FEIGIN & CHERRY'S
TEXTBOOK OF
PEDIATRIC INFECTIOUS DISEASES

FEIGIN & CHERRY'S
TEXTBOOK OF
PEDIATRIC INFECTIOUS DISEASES

SIXTH EDITION

VOLUME 1

Ralph D. Feigin, M.D.

J. S. Abercrombie Professor
Chairman, Department of Pediatrics
Distinguished Service Professor
Baylor College of Medicine
Physician-in-Chief
Texas Children's Hospital
Physician-in-Chief, Service of Pediatrics
Ben Taub General Hospital
Chief, Pediatric Service
The Methodist Hospital
Houston, Texas

James D. Cherry, M.D., M.Sc.

Professor of Pediatrics
David Geffen School of Medicine at UCLA
Member, Division of Infectious Diseases
Mattel Children's Hospital UCLA
Los Angeles, California

Gail J. Demmler-Harrison, M.D.

Professor of Pediatrics
Baylor College of Medicine
Attending Physician, Infectious Diseases Service
Director, Diagnostic Virology Laboratory
Texas Children's Hospital
Houston, Texas

Sheldon L. Kaplan, M.D.

Professor and Vice-Chairman of Clinical Affairs
Head, Section of Pediatric Infectious Diseases
Department of Pediatrics
Baylor College of Medicine
Chief, Infectious Diseases Service
Texas Children's Hospital
Houston, Texas

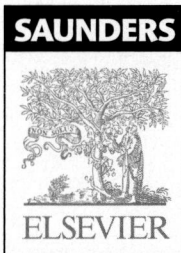

SAUNDERS

ELSEVIER

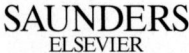

SAUNDERS
ELSEVIER

1600 John F. Kennedy Boulevard
Suite 1800
Philadelphia, PA 19103-2899

Volume 1: Part no. 9996036847
Volume 2: Part no. 9996036901

FEIGIN & CHERRY'S TEXTBOOK OF PEDIATRIC   Two-volume set ISBN: 978-1-4160-4044-6
INFECTIOUS DISEASES

Notice

Knowledge and best practice in this field are constantly changing. As new research and experience broaden our knowledge, changes in practice, treatment, and drug therapy may become necessary or appropriate. Readers are advised to check the most current information provided (i) on procedures featured or (ii) by the manufacturer of each product to be administered to verify the recommended dose or formula, the method and duration of administration, and contraindications. It is the responsibility of practitioners, relying on their own experience and knowledge of their patients, to make diagnoses and the best treatment for each individual patient, and to take all appropriate safety precautions. To the fullest extent of the law, neither the Publisher nor the Editors assume any liability for any injury and/or damage to persons or property arising out of or related to any use of the material contained in this book.

The Publisher

Library of Congress Cataloging-in-Publication Data

Feigin & Cherry's textbook of pediatric infectious diseases / [edited by] Ralph D. Feigin . . . [et al.].
—6th ed.
   p. ; cm.
   Rev. ed. of: Textbook of pediatric infectious diseases / [edited by] Ralph D. Feigin . . . [et al.]. 5th ed.
c2004
   Includes bibliographical references and index.
   ISBN 978-1-4160-4044-6
   1. Communicable diseases in children. I. Feigin, Ralph D. II. Textbook of pediatric infectious diseases. III. Title: Textbook of pediatric infectious diseases.
   [DNLM: 1. Communicable Diseases. 2. Child. 3. Pediatrics—methods. WC 100 F297 2009]
RJ401.T49 2009
618.92'98—dc22   2008015063

Acquisitions Editor: Judy Fletcher
Developmental Editor: Melissa Dudlick
Publishing Services Manager: Frank Polizzano
Project Manager: Lee Ann Draud
Design Direction: Ellen Zanolle

Printed in the United States of America

Last digit is the print number: 9 8 7 6 5 4 3 2 1

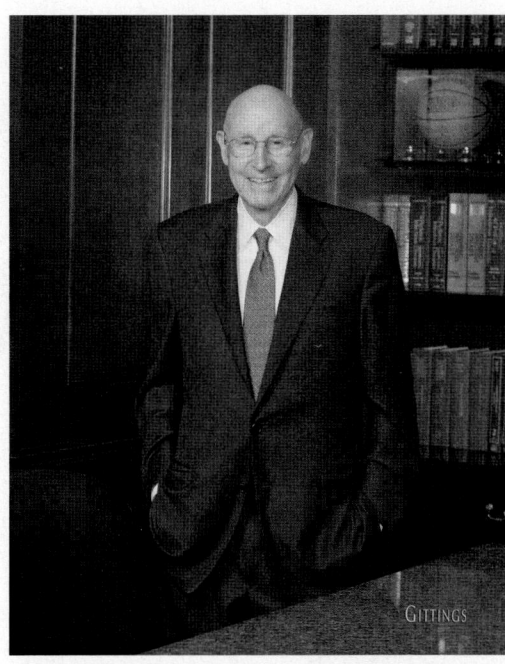

Ralph D. Feigin, M.D.
April 3, 1938–August 14, 2008

With great sadness, we dedicate this sixth edition of the *Textbook of Pediatric Infectious Diseases* to Ralph D. Feigin. As everyone in pediatrics and, in particular, pediatric infectious diseases, knows, Ralph was an extraordinary individual, and his untimely death leaves a void that will never be filled.

Ralph Feigin was born in New York City on April 3, 1938. He graduated from Columbia College in New York City in 1958 and received his M.D. from Boston University School of Medicine in 1962. He married Judith S. Zobel, a childhood friend, in 1960 while in medical school. Ralph completed his first two years of pediatric residency at Boston City Hospital and his third year at the Massachusetts General Hospital. He then fulfilled his military service requirement at the United States Army Research Institute of Infectious Diseases, Ft. Detrick, Frederick, Maryland. While at the United States Army Research Institute, he participated in significant studies relating to circadian periodicity and susceptibility to infections, as well as other studies that resulted in eight publications for which he was the first author. After completing his service commitment, he was Chief Resident at Massachusetts General Hospital during the 1967-68 academic year.

Ralph was recruited to Washington University in St. Louis by Phil Dodge in 1968, and soon thereafter he and one of us (JDC), who was then at St. Louis University, got together and forged an academic and personal friendship that continued until the time of his death. Almost 40 years ago, the two investigators recognized the need for a comprehensive book on pediatric infectious diseases, but because of their busy schedules the plan was put on hold, and in 1973 Jim moved to California. In 1976, the pediatric research meetings were held in St. Louis, and at this time Jim and Ralph met with W. B. Saunders representatives, and the book was conceived. The first edition of the textbook was published 5 years later in the fall of 1981. In comparison with this 6th edition, it was a modest effort, with 44 chapters and 124 contributors.

At Washington University and St. Louis Children's Hospital, Ralph developed one of the finest infectious diseases divisions in the country. His "Feigin Rounds" were an unparalleled learning experience and were legendary among medical students and residents. In 1977, Ralph moved to Houston, Texas, to accept the challenge of being the Chair of Pediatrics for Baylor College of Medicine and the Physician-in-Chief at Texas Children's Hospital. During the ensuing 30 years, the Department grew from 43 faculty members to almost 500. One of us (SLK) came under Ralph's spell in St. Louis and moved to Houston with him. The other one of us (GJD-H), an intern in Houston in 1977, was waiting for Dr. Feigin when he arrived.

In Houston, Ralph served as the Chair of Pediatrics for Baylor College of Medicine and the Physician-in-Chief at Texas Children's Hospital for 31 years. For 7 years of his tenure, he also served as President and CEO of Baylor College of Medicine. In addition to his commitments in Houston, Ralph served in leadership roles on more than 100 local, regional, and national committees and professional societies. His efforts in persuading government officials of all ranks helped children in Texas, the United States, and in all parts of the world. Many consider him to be the foremost pediatrician in the world.

As will be noted in the table of contents of this 6th edition of Feigin and Cherry, Ralph made his usual contributions to the text. In spite of his illness, he contributed to the book and made decisions relating to it until right before his death. Not only was Dr. Feigin a powerhouse of energy, speed, and unsurpassed accomplishments, but he also was a gentleman, full of compassion, warmth, and kindness, and a man who kept people and patients first in his heart and mind. He was a loving husband to his wife, Judy, and a proud father to his three children, Susan, Debra, and Michael; doting grandfather to his six grandchildren, Rebecca, Matthew, Sarah, Rachel, Jacob, and Eli; and a mentor to so many of us in the field of pediatrics and pediatric infectious diseases. Ralph Feigin is missed by everyone who knew him, particularly by Judy Feigin and the family as well as by the three of us.

JDC
SLK
GJD-H

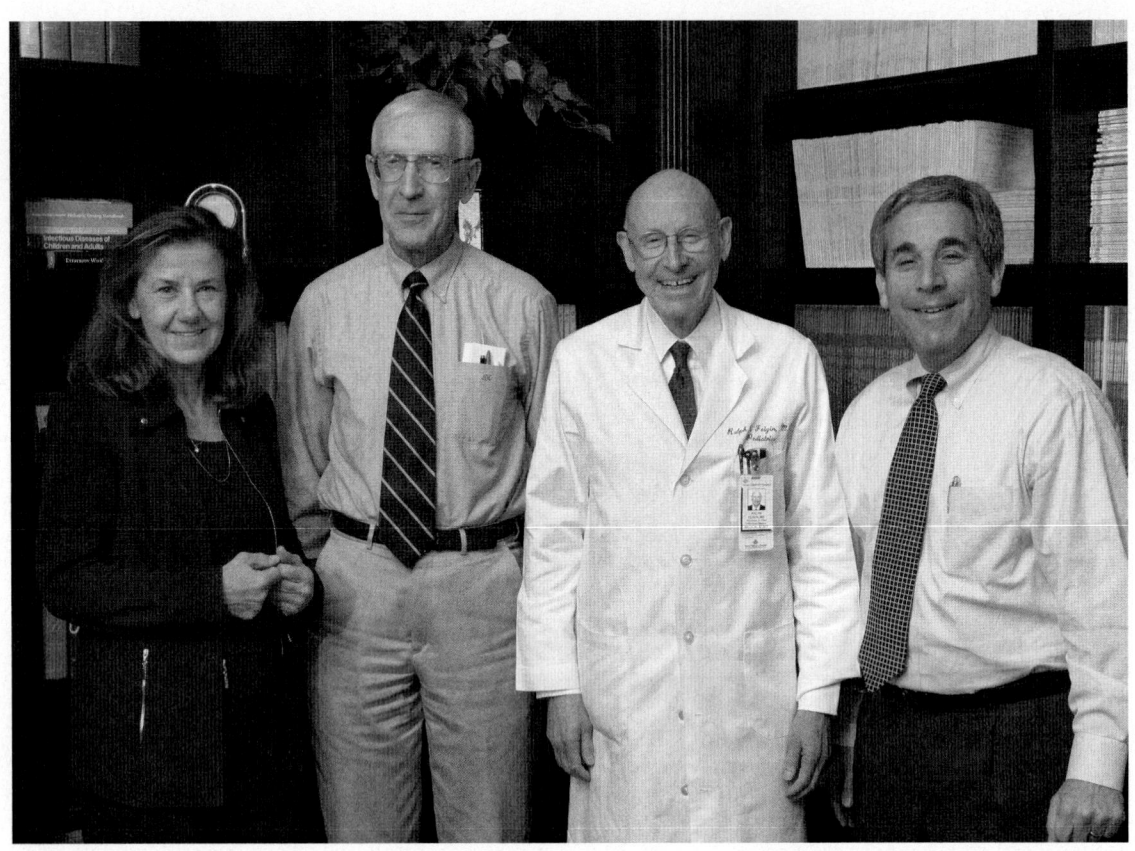

To our spouses—
Judith Feigin, Jeanne Cherry, Neil Harrison, and Marsha Kaplan

our children—
Susan Feigin Harris and Jonathan Harris, Michael and Barbara Feigin,
Debra Feigin Sukin and Steven Sukin;
James Cherry, Jeffrey Cherry and
Kass Hogan, Susan Cherry, Kenneth and Jennifer Cherry;
Emily Demmler Wolfe and Joshua Wolfe, Matthew Demmler, Amy Demmler, Anna Rose Demmler,
Kelly Harrison, and Haley Harrison;
and Lauren Kaplan, Mindy Kaplan Langland and Lance Langland

and our grandchildren—
Rebecca and Sarah Harris, Matthew and Rachel Feigin, Jacob and Eli Sukin; Ferguson,
Dennis, and Siena Rose Cherry; and Reece Langland

John G. Aaskov, Ph.D.
School of Life Sciences, Queensland University of Technology, Brisbane, Queensland, Australia
Alphaviruses: Ross River Virus Arthritis; Flaviviruses: Murray Valley Encephalitis

Susan M. Abdel-Rahman, Pharm.D.
Associate Professor of Pediatrics, University of Missouri at Kansas City School of Medicine; Director, Pharmacokinetic and Pharmacodynamic Care Laboratory, Children's Mercy Hospital and Clinics, Kansas City, Missouri
The Pharmacokinetic-Pharmacodynamic Interface: Determinants of Anti-infective Drug Action and Efficacy in Pediatrics

Christoph Aebi, M.D.
Head, Pediatric Infectious Diseases Unit, Department of Pediatrics and Institute for Infectious Diseases, University of Bern, Bern, Switzerland
Flaviviruses: Tick-Borne Encephalitis

Marvin E. Ament, M.D.
Professor of Pediatrics, David Geffen School of Medicine at UCLA; Chief, Division of Gastroenterology, Mattel Children's Hospital UCLA, Los Angeles, California
Esophagitis

Marsha S. Anderson, M.D.
Assistant Professor of Pediatrics, University of Colorado Denver School of Medicine; Attending Physician, Children's Hospital, Aurora, Colorado
Meningococcal Infections

Stephen S. Arnon, M.D.
Founder and Chief, Infant Botulism Treatment and Prevention Program, California Department of Health Services, Richmond, California
Infant Botulism

Ann M. Arvin, M.D.
Vice Provost and Dean of Research, Stanford University; Professor of Microbiology and Immunology and Lucile Salter Packard Professor of Pediatrics, Stanford University School of Medicine, Stanford; Attending Physician, Lucile Packard Children's Hospital, Palo Alto, California
Herpes Simplex Viruses 1 and 2

Jane T. Atkins, M.D.
Consultant, Pediatric Infectious Diseases, and Hospital Epidemiologist, Methodist Children's Hospital of South Texas, San Antonio, Texas
Cyclosporiasis, Isosporiasis, and Microsporidiosis

Robert L. Atmar, M.D.
Professor, Departments of Medicine and Molecular Virology and Microbiology, Baylor College of Medicine; Chief, Infectious Diseases Service, Department of Medicine, Ben Taub General Hospital, Houston, Texas
Rhinoviruses

Carol J. Baker, M.D.
Professor of Pediatrics and Molecular Virology and Microbiology, Baylor College of Medicine; Attending Physician, Infectious Diseases Service, Texas Children's Hospital, Houston, Texas
Cervical Lymphadenitis; Group B Streptococcal Infections

Robert S. Baltimore, M.D.
Professor of Pediatrics, Epidemiology, and Public Health, Yale University School of Medicine; Attending Physician in Pediatrics and Associate Hospital Epidemiologist, Yale–New Haven Children's Hospital, New Haven, Connecticut
Epidemiology of Infectious Diseases

Stephen J. Barenkamp, M.D.
Professor of Pediatrics and Molecular Biology, St. Louis University School of Medicine; Director, Division of Pediatric Infectious Diseases, Cardinal Glennon Children's Medical Center, St. Louis, Missouri
Haemophilus influenzae; Other Haemophilus Species (aphrophilus, ducreyi, haemolyticus, influenzae Biogroup Aegyptius, parahaemolyticus, and parainfluenzae)

Elizabeth D. Barnett, M.D.
Associate Professor of Pediatrics, Boston University School of Medicine; Section of Pediatric Infectious Diseases, Boston Medical Center, Boston, Massachusetts
Malaria

Robert D. Basow, M.D.
Community Preceptor Attending, Department of Community Pediatrics, University of Massachusetts Medical Center, Worcester, Massachusetts
Streptobacillus moniliformis (Rat-Bite Fever); Spirillum minus (Rat-Bite Fever)

William R. Beisel, M.D.
Adjunct Professor (retired), W. Harry Feinstone Department of Molecular Microbiology and Immunology, Johns Hopkins School of Hygiene and Public Health, Baltimore, Maryland
Metabolic Response of the Host to Infections

Beth P. Bell, M.D., M.P.H.
Associate Director for Epidemiologic Science, National Center for Immunization and Respiratory Diseases, Centers for Disease Control and Prevention, Atlanta, Georgia
Hepatitis A Virus

Gil Benard, M.D., Ph.D.
Medical Researcher, Faculty of Medicine, University of São Paulo, São Paulo, Brazil
Paracoccidioidomycosis

David I. Bernstein, M.D., M.A.
Professor, Department of Pediatrics, University of Cincinnati College of Medicine; Director, Division of Infectious Diseases, Cincinnati Children's Hospital Medical Center, Cincinnati, Ohio
Rotaviruses

Kathrin M. Bernt, M.D.
Pediatrician, Boston, Massachusetts
Interaction of Infection and Nutrition

Andrea A. Berry, M.D.
Fellow, Department of Pediatrics, Division of Infectious Diseases and Tropical Pediatrics, University of Maryland School of Medicine, Baltimore, Maryland
Diarrhea-Causing and Dysentery-Causing Escherichia coli

Charles D. Bluestone, M.D.
Eberly Professor of Pediatric Otolaryngology, Department of Otolaryngology, University of Pittsburgh School of Medicine; Director, Department of Pediatric Otolaryngology, Children's Hospital of Pittsburgh, Pittsburgh, Pennsylvania
Otitis Media

Jeffrey L. Blumer, M.D., Ph.D.
Professor of Pediatrics and Pharmacology, Case Western Reserve University; Director, Rainbow Regional Network Development, Rainbow Babies and Children's Hospital, Cleveland, Ohio
Antibiotic Resistance

Robert Bortolussi, M.D., F.R.C.P.C.
Professor of Pediatrics and Microbiology and Immunology, Dalhousie University Faculty of Medicine; Staff Consultant, IWK Health Centre, Halifax, Nova Scotia, Canada
Listeriosis

Bobby L. Boyanton, Jr., M.D.
Medical Director, Clinical Microbiology, William Beaumont Hospital, Royal Oak, Michigan
Bacterial Laboratory Diagnosis

Kenneth M. Boyer, M.D.
Woman's Board Professor of Pediatrics, Rush Medical College; Chairman, Department of Pediatrics, Rush Children's Hospital of Rush University Medical Center, Chicago, Illinois
Nonbacterial Pneumonia; Congenital Toxoplasmosis; Borrelia (Relapsing Fever); Toxoplasmosis

John S. Bradley, M.D.
Director, Division of Infectious Diseases, Rady Children's Hospital–San Diego, San Diego, California
Peritonitis and Intra-abdominal Abscess; Retroperitoneal Infections; Outpatient Intravenous Antimicrobial Therapy for Serious Infections

Michael T. Brady, M.D.
Chair and Professor, Department of Pediatrics, College of Medicine, The Ohio State University; Physician-in-Chief, Nationwide Children's Hospital, Columbus, Ohio
Pseudomonas and Related Genera

William J. Britt, M.D.
Professor of Pediatrics and Microbiology, The University of Alabama at Birmingham School of Medicine; Attending Physician, Children's Hospital of Alabama, Birmingham, Alabama
Transmissible Spongiform Encephalopathies (Creutzfeldt-Jakob Disease, Gerstmann-Sträussler-Scheinker Disease, Kuru, Fatal Familial Insomnia, New Variant Creutzfeldt-Jakob Disease, Sporadic Fatal Insomnia)

Annemarie Broderick, M.D.
Consultant/Clinician-Scientist, Our Lady's Hospital for Sick Children, Dublin, Ireland
Hepatitis B and D Viruses

David E. Bronstein, M.D., M.S.
Department of Pediatrics, Southern California Permanente Medical Group, Palmdale, California
Aseptic Meningitis and Viral Meningitis; Encephalitis and Meningoencephalitis

David A. Bruckner, Sc.D.
Department of Pathology and Laboratory Medicine, David Geffen School of Medicine at UCLA, Los Angeles, California
Nomenclature for Aerobic and Anaerobic Bacteria; Classification of Fungi; Fungal Laboratory Analysis: Specimen Collection, Direct Detection, and Culture; Parasitic Laboratory Diagnosis

Steven C. Buckingham, M.D.
Associate Professor, Department of Pediatrics, Division of Pediatric Infectious Diseases, University of Tennessee Health Science Center; Attending Physician, Le Bonheur Children's Medical Center, Memphis, Tennessee
Other Anaerobic Infections

Ana Burgos, M.D.
Pediatric Hematology/Oncology, Duke University Medical Center, Durham, North Carolina
Aspergillus and Aspergillosis

Carrie L. Byington, M.D.
Professor of Pediatrics and Associate Chair for Clinical Research, University of Utah School of Medicine, Salt Lake City, Utah
Streptobacillus moniliformis (Rat-Bite Fever); *Spirillum minus* (Rat-Bite Fever)

Judith R. Campbell, M.D.
Associate Professor of Pediatrics, Section of Pediatric Infectious Diseases, Baylor College of Medicine; Attending Physician, Pediatric Infectious Diseases Service, Texas Children's Hospital, Houston, Texas
Parotitis; Peritonitis and Intra-abdominal Abscess

Samson Cantu, M.D.
Fellow, Pediatric Gastroenterology, Hepatology, and Nutrition, Baylor College of Medicine, Houston, Texas
Helicobacter pylori

Mariam R. Chacko, M.D.
Professor of Pediatrics, Section of Adolescent Medicine and Sports Medicine, Baylor College of Medicine; Attending Physician, Texas Children's Hospital; Medical Director, Baylor Teen Health Clinics, Houston, Texas
Genital Infections; *Calymmatobacterium granulomatis*; *Trichomonas* Infections

Louisa E. Chapman, M.D., M.S.P.H.
Captain, U.S. Public Health Service, and Medical Epidemiologist, National Center for Zoonotics, Vector-Borne and Enteric Diseases, Centers for Disease Control and Prevention, Atlanta, Georgia
Hantaviruses

Rémi N. Charrel, M.D., Ph.D.
Associate Professor of Virology, Unité des Virus Emergents, Faculté de Médecine, Université de la Méditerranée, Marseille, France
Lymphocytic Choriomeningitis Virus Infection; Arenaviral Hemorrhagic Fevers; Toscana Virus

Tempe K. Chen, M.D.
Pediatric Family Center, Long Beach, California
Adenoviruses

James D. Cherry, M.D., M.Sc.
Professor of Pediatrics, David Geffen School of Medicine at UCLA; Member, Division of Infectious Diseases, Mattel Children's Hospital UCLA, Los Angeles, California
The Common Cold; Pharyngitis (Pharyngitis, Tonsillitis, Tonsillopharyngitis, and Nasopharyngitis); Herpangina; Pharyngoconjunctival Fever; Sinusitis; Mastoiditis; Epiglottitis; Croup (Laryngitis, Laryngotracheitis, Spasmodic Croup, Laryngotracheobronchitis, Bacterial Tracheitis, and Laryngotracheobroncho-pneumonitis); Acute Bronchitis; Aseptic Meningitis and Viral Meningitis; Encephalitis and Meningoencephalitis; Cutaneous Manifestations of Systemic Infections; Roseola Infantum (Exanthem Subitum); *Mycoplasma* and *Ureaplasma* Infections of the Neonate; Pertussis and Other *Bordetella* Infections; Tetanus; Human Parvovirus B19; Human Bocaviruses; Adenoviruses; Smallpox (Variola Virus); Monkeypox and Other Poxviruses; Enteroviruses and Parechoviruses; Reoviruses; Rubella Virus; Measles Virus; Mumps Virus; Human Metapneumovirus; *Mycoplasma* and *Ureaplasma* Infections

P. Joan Chesney, M.D.
Professor of Pediatrics, Division of Infectious Diseases, University of Tennessee, Memphis, College of Medicine; Active Staff, Department of Pediatrics, Le Bonheur Children's Medical Center; Director, Office of Academic Programs, St. Jude Children's Research Hospital, Memphis, Tennessee
Toxic Shock Syndrome

Madhuri C. Chilakapati, M.D.
Staff Physician, Kelsey Seybold Clinic, Houston, Texas
Ocular Infectious Diseases

Javier Chinen, M.D., Ph.D.
Assistant Professor, Department of Pediatrics, Baylor College of Medicine; Attending Physician, Allergy and Immunology Service, Texas Children's Hospital, Houston, Texas
Primary Immunodeficiencies

Natascha Ching, M.D.
Assistant Clinical Professor of Pediatrics, David Geffen School of Medicine at UCLA; Attending Physician, Division of Pediatric Infectious Diseases, Mattel Children's Hospital UCLA, Los Angeles, California
Arcanobacterium haemolyticum

H. Fred Clark, D.V.M., Ph.D.
Research Professor, Department of Pediatrics, University of Pennsylvania School of Medicine; Adjunct Professor, Wistar Institute, Philadelphia, Pennsylvania
Rabies Virus

Thomas G. Cleary, M.D.
Professor of Pediatrics, Division of Pediatric Infectious Diseases, University of Texas–Houston Medical School; Professor of Pediatrics, Department of Pediatric Infectious Diseases, Memorial Hermann Children's Hospital, Houston, Texas
Bacillus cereus; *Shigella*; *Salmonella*

David K. Coats, M.D.
Professor of Ophthalmology and Pediatrics, Department of Ophthalmology, Baylor College of Medicine; Chief, Ophthalmology Service, Texas Children's Hospital, Houston, Texas
Ocular Infectious Diseases

Armando G. Correa, M.D.
Assistant Professor of Pediatrics, Baylor College of Medicine; Attending Physician, Infectious Diseases Service, Texas Children's Hospital, Houston, Texas
Acinetobacter

J. Thomas Cross, Jr., M.D., M.P.H.
Vice President for Education, MedStudy Corporation, Colorado Springs, Colorado
Fungal Meningitis; Other Mycobacteria

William B. Cutrer, M.D.
Fellow, Pediatric Critical Care, Baylor College of Medicine; Attending Physician, Texas Children's Hospital, Houston, Texas
Bacterial Meningitis beyond the Neonatal Period

Ronald Dagan, M.D.
Professor of Pediatrics and Infectious Diseases, Faculty of Health Sciences, Ben-Gurion University of the Negev; Director, Pediatric Infectious Disease Unit, Soroka University Medical Center, Beer-Sheva, Israel
Pneumococcal Infections

David E. Dassey, M.D., M.P.H.
Acute Communicable Disease Control Program, Los Angeles, California
Public Health Aspects of Infectious Disease Control

Jeffrey P. Davis, M.D.
Adjunct Professor, Departments of Pediatrics and Preventative Medicine, University of Wisconsin Medical School; Chief Medical Officer and State Epidemiologist for Communicable Diseases, Bureau of Public Health, Wisconsin Division of Health, Madison, Wisconsin
Toxic Shock Syndrome

Gail J. Demmler-Harrison, M.D.
Professor of Pediatrics, Baylor College of Medicine; Attending Physician, Infectious Diseases Service, and Director, Diagnostic Virology Laboratory, Texas Children's Hospital, Houston, Texas
Hepatitis; Viral Infections of the Fetus and Neonate; Yeast and Fungal Infections of the Fetus and Neonate; Opportunistic Infections in Kidney Transplantation; Human Papillomaviruses; Cytomegalovirus; Antiviral Agents

Penelope H. Dennehy, M.D.
Professor of Pediatrics and Vice Chair for Academic Affairs for Pediatrics, The Warren Alpert Medical School of Brown University; Director, Division of Pediatric Infectious Diseases, Hasbro Children's Hospital, Providence, Rhode Island
Active Immunizing Agents

Minh L. Doan, M.D.
Assistant Professor of Pediatrics, Uniformed Services University of the Health Sciences F. Edward Hébert School of Medicine, Bethesda, Maryland; Pediatric Pulmonologist, Tripler Army Medical Center, Honolulu, Hawaii
Children's Interstitial Lung Disease and Hypersensitivity Pneumonitis

Simon R. Dobson, M.D., F.R.C.P.C.
Clinical Associate Professor, University of British Columbia Faculty of Medicine; Division of Infectious and Immunological Diseases, British Columbia Children's Hospital, Vancouver, British Columbia, Canada
Syphilis

Jan E. Drutz, M.D.
Professor of Pediatrics and Director, Pediatric Continuity Training Program, Baylor College of Medicine, Houston, Texas
Arthropods

Paul H. Edelstein, M.D.
Professor of Pathology and Laboratory Medicine, University of Pennsylvania School of Medicine; Director, Clinical Microbiology Laboratory, Hospital of the University of Pennsylvania, Philadelphia, Pennsylvania
Legionnaires' Disease, Pontiac Fever, and Related Illnesses

Kathryn M. Edwards, M.D.
Professor of Pediatrics, Vanderbilt University School of Medicine; Attending Physician, Monroe Carell Jr. Children's Hospital at Vanderbilt, Nashville, Tennessee
Bartonella (Cat-Scratch Disease)

Morven S. Edwards, M.D.
Professor of Pediatrics, Baylor College of Medicine; Attending Physician, Infectious Diseases Service, Texas Children's Hospital, Houston, Texas
Mediastinitis; Anthrax; Rickettsial and Ehrlichial Diseases; Animal Bites

B. Keith English, M.D.
Professor of Pediatrics, University of Tennessee Health Science Center; Chief, Division of Infectious Diseases, Le Bonheur Children's Medical Center, Memphis, Tennessee
Enterococcal and *Viridans* Streptococcal Infections

Dora Estripeaut, M.D.
Professor of Pediatrics and Infectious Diseases, University of Panama School of Medicine; Attending Physician in Pediatric Infectious Diseases, Hospital del Niño, Panama City, Panama
Perinatal Bacterial Diseases

Leland L. Fan, M.D.
Professor of Pediatrics, Baylor College of Medicine; Attending Physician, Pulmonary Service, Texas Children's Hospital, Houston, Texas
Children's Interstitial Lung Disease and Hypersensitivity Pneumonitis

Ralph D. Feigin, M.D.
Formerly J. S. Abercrombie Professor and Chairman, Department of Pediatrics, and Distinguished Service Professor, Baylor College of Medicine; Physician-in-Chief, Texas Children's Hospital; Physician-in-Chief, Service of Pediatrics, Ben Taub General Hospital; Chief, Pediatric Service, The Methodist Hospital, Houston, Texas
Metabolic Response of the Host to Infections; Interaction of Infection and Nutrition; Bacterial Meningitis beyond the Neonatal Period; Fever without Source and Fever of Unknown Origin; Diphtheria; *Aeromonas;* Tularemia; Leptospirosis; Rickettsial and Ehrlichial Diseases

George D. Ferry, M.D.
Professor of Pediatrics, Baylor College of Medicine; Chief, Inflammatory Bowel Disease Center, Texas Children's Hospital, Houston, Texas
Antibiotic-Associated Colitis

Anthony E. Fiore, M.D.
Deputy Branch Chief, Epidemiology and Prevention Branch, Influenza Division, National Center for Immunization and Respiratory Diseases, Centers for Disease Control and Prevention, Atlanta, Georgia
Hepatitis A Virus

Philip R. Fischer, M.D.
Professor of Pediatrics, Mayo Clinic; Medical Director, Mayo Eugenio Litta Children's Hospital, Rochester, Minnesota
Cestodes; Trematodes; Schistosomiasis

Randall G. Fisher, M.D.
Associate Professor of Pediatrics, Eastern Virginia Medical School; Medical Director, Division of Infectious Diseases, and Attending Physician, Children's Hospital of The King's Daughters, Norfolk, Virginia
Miscellaneous Gram-Positive Cocci; *Erysipelothrix rhusiopathiae;* Miscellaneous Gram-Positive Bacilli; *Citrobacter; Enterobacter; Klebsiella; Morganella morganii; Proteus; Providencia; Serratia;* Miscellaneous Enterobacteria; *Vibrio vulnificus;* Miscellaneous Non-Enterobacteriaceae Fermentative Bacilli; *Achromobacter (Alcaligenes); Eikenella corrodens; Elizabethkingia* and *Chryseobacterium* Species

Patricia M. Flynn, M.D., M.S.
Professor, Departments of Pediatrics and Preventive Medicine, University of Tennessee Health Science Center; Member, Department of Infectious Diseases, St. Jude Children's Research Hospital, Memphis, Tennessee
Candidiasis

Thomas R. Flynn, D.M.D.
Associate Professor of Oral and Maxillofacial Surgery, Harvard School of Dental Medicine; Associate Visiting Surgeon, Department of Oral and Maxillofacial Surgery, Massachusetts General Hospital; Boston, Massachusetts
Infections of the Oral Cavity

Lisa M. Frenkel, M.D.
Professor of Pediatrics, Division of Infectious Diseases, and Professor of Laboratory Medicine, Division of Virology, University of Washington School of Medicine; Co-Director, Virology Clinic, and Associate and Attending Physician, Division of Pediatric Infectious Diseases, Seattle Children's Hospital, Seattle, Washington
Dientamoeba fragilis Infections

Ellen M. Friedman, M.D.
Professor of Otolaryngology and Pediatrics and Bobby Alford Chair of Pediatric Otolaryngology, Baylor College of Medicine; Chief, Otolaryngology, Speech, Language and Learning, and Auditory Services, Texas Children's Hospital, Houston, Texas
Otitis Externa

Richard A. Friedman, M.D., M.B.A.
Professor of Pediatrics, Baylor College of Medicine; Chief, Arrhythmia and Pacing Services, and Chief, Cardiology Clinic, Texas Children's Hospital, Houston, Texas
Infectious Pericarditis

Lynne S. Garcia, M.S., M.T.
Director, LSG & Associates, Santa Monica, California
Classification and Nomenclature of Human Parasites; Leishmaniasis; Trypanosomiasis

Patrick J. Gavin, M.D.
Department of Pathology and Laboratory Medicine, Evanston Northwestern Healthcare, Evanston, Illinois
Naegleria, Acanthamoeba, and *Balamuthia*

Michael A. Gerber, M.D.
Professor of Pediatrics, University of Cincinnati College of Medicine; Division of Infectious Diseases, Cincinnati Children's Hospital Medical Center, Cincinnati, Ohio
Group A, Group C, and Group G Beta-Hemolytic Streptococcal Infections

Anne A. Gershon, M.D.
Professor of Pediatrics, Columbia University College of Physicians and Surgeons; Attending Physician, Morgan Stanley Children's Hospital, New York, New York
Varicella-Zoster Virus

Mark A. Gilger, M.D.
Professor of Pediatrics, Baylor College of Medicine; Chief of Service, Gastroenterology, Hepatology, and Nutrition, Texas Children's Hospital, Houston, Texas
Whipple Disease; *Helicobacter pylori*

Susan L. Gillespie, M.D., Ph.D.
Assistant Professor, Department of Pediatrics, Baylor College of Medicine; Baylor International Pediatric AIDS Initiative, Houston, Texas
Human Retroviruses: Oncoviruses (Human T-Cell Lymphotropic Viruses) and Lentiviruses (Human Immunodeficiency Virus Type 2)

Daniel G. Glaze, M.D.
Professor of Pediatrics and Neurology, Baylor College of Medicine; Director of Sleep Clinic and Sleep Laboratory, Texas Children's Hospital, Houston, Texas
Parainfectious and Postinfectious Disorders of the Nervous System

W. Paul Glezen, M.D.
Professor, Departments of Molecular Virology and Microbiology and Pediatrics, Baylor College of Medicine; Courtesy Staff, Infectious Diseases Service, Texas Children's Hospital, Houston, Texas
Influenza Viruses

Mary P. Glodé, M.D.
Professor of Pediatrics, University of Colorado Denver School of Medicine; Professor of Pediatric Infectious Diseases, Children's Hospital, Aurora, Colorado
Meningococcal Infections

Donald A. Goldmann, M.D.
Professor of Pediatrics, Harvard Medical School; Senior Associate in Infectious Diseases, Children's Hospital Boston, Boston, Massachusetts
Health Care–Associated Infections; Programs to Prevent and Control Health Care–Associated Infections

Ellie J. C. Goldstein, M.D.
Clinical Professor of Medicine, David Geffen School of Medicine at UCLA, Los Angeles; Director, R. M. Alden Research Laboratory, Culver City, California
Human Bites

Nira A. Goldstein, M.D.
Assistant Professor, Division of Pediatric Otolaryngology, State University of New York Downstate Medical Center College of Medicine; Attending Physician, Division of Pediatric Otolaryngology, University Hospital of Brooklyn, Long Island College Hospital, and Kings County Hospital Center, Brooklyn, New York
Peritonsillar, Retropharyngeal, and Parapharyngeal Abscesses

Edmond T. Gonzales, Jr., M.D.
Professor of Urology, Scott Department of Urology, Baylor College of Medicine; Head, Department of Surgery, and Chief, Pediatric Urology Service, Texas Children's Hospital, Houston, Texas
Renal Abscess; Prostatitis

Mark P. Gorman, M.D.
Instructor, Harvard Medical School; Assistant in Neurology, Children's Hospital Boston, Boston, Massachusetts
Parainfectious and Postinfectious Disorders of the Nervous System

Michael D. Green, M.D., M.P.H.
Professor of Pediatrics and Surgery, University of Pittsburgh School of Medicine; Attending Physician, Division of Infectious Diseases, and Director, Infectious Diseases Research Laboratories, Children's Hospital of Pittsburgh, Pittsburgh, Pennsylvania
Opportunistic Infections in Liver and Intestinal Transplantation

David Greenberg, M.D.
Lecturer, Faculty of Health Sciences, Ben-Gurion University of the Negev; Senior Physician, Specialist in Pediatrics and Infectious Diseases, Soroka University Medical Center, Beer-Sheva, Israel
Pneumococcal Infections

Andreas H. Groll, M.D.
Infectious Disease Research Program, Department of Pediatric Hematology/Oncology, Children's University Hospital, Münster, Germany
Antifungal Agents

Charles Grose, M.D.
Professor, Department of Pediatrics, University of Iowa Carver College of Medicine; Director of Infectious Diseases, Children's Hospital, Iowa City, Iowa
Bacterial Myositis and Pyomyositis; Human Herpesviruses 6, 7, and 8

Duane J. Gubler, M.D.
Professor and Chair, Department of Tropical Medicine and Medical Microbiology, John A. Burns School of Medicine, University of Hawaii at Manoa, Honolulu, Hawaii
Flaviviruses: Yellow Fever

Roberto A. Guerrero, M.D.
Pediatric Gastroenterologist, Loxahatchee, Florida
Whipple Disease

Javier Nieto Guevara, M.D.
Department of Pediatrics, Hospital del Niño, Panama City, Panama
Parameningeal Infections

Kathleen M. Gutierrez, M.D.
Assistant Professor, Stanford University School of Medicine, Stanford; Assistant Professor of Pediatrics, Lucile Packard Children's Hospital, Palo Alto, California
Herpes Simplex Viruses 1 and 2

Caroline Breese Hall, M.D.
Professor of Pediatrics and Medicine, University of Rochester School of Medicine and Dentistry, Rochester, New York
Parainfluenza Viruses; Respiratory Syncytial Virus

Scott B. Halstead, M.D.
Director, Supportive Research and Development, Pediatric Dengue Vaccine Initiative, International Vaccine Institute, Seoul, Korea
Alphaviruses: Chikungunya; Flaviviruses: Dengue and Dengue Hemorrhagic Fever

Shinjiro Hamano, M.D., Ph.D.
Department of Parasitology, Faculty of Medical Sciences, Kyushu University, Fukuoka, Japan
Amebiasis

Richard J. Hamill, M.D.
Professor, Departments of Medicine and Molecular Virology and Microbiology, Baylor College of Medicine; Staff Physician, Infectious Diseases Section, Michael E. DeBakey Veterans Affairs Medical Center, Houston, Texas
Cryptococcosis

Margaret R. Hammerschlag, M.D.
Professor of Pediatrics and Medicine, State University of New York Downstate Medical Center College of Medicine; Director, Division of Pediatric Infectious Diseases, State University of New York Downstate Medical Center, Kings County Hospital Center, Brooklyn, New York
Peritonsillar, Retropharyngeal, and Parapharyngeal Abscesses; *Chlamydia trachomatis* Infections in the Neonate; *Chlamydia* Infections

I. Celine Hanson, M.D.
Professor of Pediatrics, Section of Allergy and Immunology, Baylor College of Medicine; Chief, Allergy and Immunology Clinic, Texas Children's Hospital, Houston, Texas
Chronic Bronchitis; Human Retroviruses: Impact of Human Immunodeficiency Virus and Acquired Immunodeficiency Syndrome

Nada Harik, M.D.
Assistant Professor, Department of Pediatrics and Department of Microbiology and Immunology, Division of Pediatric Infectious Diseases, University of Arkansas for Medical Sciences, Little Rock, Arkansas
Nocardia

Rick E. Harrison, M.D.
Professor of Pediatrics, David Geffen School of Medicine at UCLA; Medical Director, Mattel Children's Hospital UCLA, Los Angeles, California
Tetanus

C. Mary Healy, M.D.
Assistant Professor, Department of Pediatrics, Section of Infectious Diseases, Baylor College of Medicine; Attending Physician, Infections Diseases Service, Texas Children's Hospital, Houston, Texas
Cervical Lymphadenitis

Ulrich Heininger, M.D.
Professor of Pediatrics, University of Basel Medical School; Chair, Division of Pediatric Infectious Diseases and Vaccines, University Children's Hospital, Basel, Switzerland
Pertussis and Other *Bordetella* Infections

Gloria P. Heresi, M.D.
Professor of Pediatrics, Section of Pediatric Infectious Diseases, University of Texas Health Science Center at Houston; Attending Physician, Memorial Hermann Hospital and Lyndon Baines Johnson General Hospital, Houston, Texas
Campylobacter jejuni

Peter W. Hiatt, M.D.
Associate Professor of Pediatrics, Baylor College of Medicine; Attending Physician and Medical Director, Infant Pulmonary Diagnostic Laboratory, Texas Children's Hospital, Houston, Texas
Cystic Fibrosis; Acute Respiratory Distress Syndrome in Children

Harry R. Hill, M.D.
Professor of Pathology and Pediatrics, Department of Pathology, University of Utah School of Medicine, Salt Lake City, Utah
Immunomodulating Agents

David C. Hilmers, M.D., M.P.H.
Assistant Professor of Pediatrics and Internal Medicine, Baylor College of Medicine; Attending Physician, Texas Children's Hospital, Houston, Texas
Nonvenereal Treponematoses

Jill A. Hoffman, M.D.
Associate Professor of Pediatrics, Keck School of Medicine of the University of Southern California; Division of Infectious Diseases, Children's Hospital Los Angeles, Los Angeles, California
Infections in Pediatric Lung Transplantation

Ellis K. L. Hon, M.B.B.S.
Assistant Professor, Department of Paediatrics, Chinese University of Hong Kong; Honorary Medical Officer, Prince of Wales Hospital, Shatin, Hong Kong, China
Coronaviruses and Toroviruses, Including Severe Acute Respiratory Virus Syndrome

Margaret K. Hostetter, M.D.
Jean McLean Wallace Professor and Chair, Yale School of Medicine, New Haven, Connecticut
Infectious Disease Considerations in International Adoptees and Refugees

Peter J. Hotez, M.D., Ph.D.
Distinguished Research Professor and Walter G. Ross Professor and Chair, Department of Microbiology, Immunology, and Tropical Medicine, George Washington University School of Medicine and Health Sciences; President, Sabine Vaccine Institute, Washington, D.C.
Blastocystis hominis Infection; *Entamoeba coli* Infection; *Balantidium coli* Infection; Parasitic Nematode Infections; Drugs for Parasitic Infections

Walter T. Hughes, M.D.
Lecturer, Department of Pediatrics, Johns Hopkins University School of Medicine, Baltimore, Maryland; Emeritus Chairman, Department of Infectious Diseases, St. Jude Children's Research Hospital, Memphis, Tennessee
Pneumocystis Pneumonia

Kristina G. Hulten, Ph.D.
Assistant Professor of Pediatrics, Baylor College of Medicine; Attending Physician, Texas Children's Hospital, Houston, Texas
Staphylococcus aureus Infections (Coagulase-Positive Staphylococci)

David A. Hunstad, M.D.
Assistant Professor of Pediatrics and Molecular Microbiology, Washington University in St. Louis School of Medicine, St. Louis, Missouri
Molecular Determinants of Microbial Pathogenesis

Eugene S. Hurwitz, M.D.
Clinical Assistant Professor, Department of Pediatrics, Emory University School of Medicine; Respiratory Disease Management Associates, LLC, Atlanta, Georgia
Reye Syndrome

W. Charles Huskins, M.D., M.Sc.
Assistant Professor of Pediatrics, Mayo Medical School; Consultant, Pediatric Infectious Diseases, and Hospital Epidemiologist, Mayo Eugenio Litta Children's Hospital, Mayo Clinic, Rochester, Minnesota
Health Care–Associated Infections; Programs to Prevent and Control Health Care–Associated Infections

David Y. Hyun, M.D.
Assistant Professor of Pediatrics, Division of Infectious Diseases, Children's National Medical Center, Washington, D.C.
Coagulase-Negative Staphylococcal Infections; *Vibrio parahaemolyticus*

Mary Anne Jackson, M.D.
Professor of Pediatrics, University of Missouri–Kansas City School of Medicine; Section Chief, Pediatric Infectious Diseases, Children's Mercy Hospital, Kansas City, Missouri
Bacterial Skin Infections

Michael R. Jacobs, M.B. B.Ch., Ph.D.
Professor of Pathology, Case Western Reserve University; Director of Clinical Microbiology, University Hospitals of Cleveland, Cleveland, Ohio
Pneumococcal Infections

Richard F. Jacobs, M.D., F.A.A.P.
Horace C. Cabe Professor of Pediatrics and Professor and Chairman, Department of Pediatrics, University of Arkansas for Medical Sciences; President, Arkansas Children's Hospital Research Institute; Attending Physician, Pediatric Infectious Diseases, Arkansas Children's Hospital, Little Rock, Arkansas
Pleural Effusions and Empyema; Lung Abscess; Fungal Meningitis; Other Mycobacteria; *Nocardia; Actinobacillus actinomycetemcomitans;* Actinomycosis

Jenifer L. Jaeger, M.D.
Epidemic Intelligence Service Officer, Bureau of Communicable Disease Control, Centers for Disease Control and Prevention, Albany, New York
Active Immunizing Agents

Ravi R. Jhaveri, M.D.
Assistant Professor of Pediatrics, Molecular Genetics, and Microbiology, Division of Pediatric Infectious Diseases, Duke University School of Medicine, Durham, North Carolina
Hepatitis E Virus

Samantha Johnston, M.D.
Physician, Doctors without Borders, New York, New York
Smallpox; Monkeypox and Other Poxviruses

Maureen M. Jonas, M.D.
Associate Professor of Pediatrics, Harvard Medical School; Senior Associate Physician in Medicine, Division of Gastroenterology, Children's Hospital Boston, Boston, Massachusetts
Hepatitis B and D Viruses; Hepatitis C Virus

Meena R. Julapalli, M.D.
Physician-in-Training, Department of Dermatology, Baylor College of Medicine and Texas Children's Hospital, Houston, Texas
Viral and Fungal Skin Infections

Edward L. Kaplan, M.D.
Professor of Pediatrics, Department of Pediatrics, University of Minnesota Medical School; Attending Physician, Department of Pediatrics, Fairview University Medical Center, Minneapolis, Minnesota
Group A, Group C, and Group G Beta-Hemolytic Streptococcal Infections

Sheldon L. Kaplan, M.D.
Professor and Vice-Chairman of Clinical Affairs and Head, Section of Pediatric Infections Diseases, Department of Pediatrics, Baylor College of Medicine; Chief, Infectious Diseases Service, Texas Children's Hospital, Houston, Texas
Infectious Pericarditis; Renal Abscess; Prostatitis; Pyogenic Liver Abscess; Bacteremia and Septic Shock; Infections in Pediatric Heart Transplantation; *Staphylococcus aureus* Infections (Coagulase-Positive Staphylococci); Coagulase-Negative Staphylococcal Infections

Saul J. Karpen, M.D., Ph.D
Associate Professor of Pediatrics and Molecular and Cellular Biology, and Faculty, Translational Biology and Molecular Medicine, Baylor College of Medicine; Director, Texas Children's Liver Center, Texas Children's Hospital, Houston, Texas
Cholangitis and Cholecystitis

Gregory L. Kearns, Pharm.D., Ph.D.
Professor of Pediatrics, University of Missouri–Kansas City School of Medicine; Professor of Pharmacology, University of Missouri–Kansas City School of Pharmacy; Marion Merrell Dow/Missouri Chair of Medical Research and Chairman, Department of Medical Research, Children's Mercy Hospitals and Clinics, Kansas City, Missouri
The Pharmacokinetic-Pharmacodynamic Interface: Determinants of Anti-infective Drug Action and Efficacy in Pediatrics

Margaret A. Keller, M.D.
Professor of Pediatrics, David Geffen School of Medicine at UCLA, Los Angeles; Chief, Pediatric Infectious Diseases, Harbor-UCLA Medical Center, Torrance, California
Passive Immunization

Chaouki K. Khoury, M.D., M.S.
*Assistant Professor and Assistant Residency Program Director,
Department of Neurology, University of Oklahoma Health Sciences
Center, Oklahoma City, Oklahoma*
Cyclosporiasis, Isosporiasis, and Microsporidiosis

Martin B. Kleiman, M.D.
*Professor, Department of Pediatric Infectious Diseases, Indiana
University School of Medicine; Director, Pediatric Infectious Diseases,
Riley Hospital for Children, Indianapolis, Indiana*
Histoplasmosis

Jerome O. Klein, M.D.
*Professor of Pediatrics, Boston University School of Medicine;
Division of Pediatric Infectious Diseases, Maxwell Finland
Laboratory for Infectious Diseases, Boston, Massachusetts*
Otitis Media; Bacterial Pneumonias

Mark W. Kline, M.D.
*Professor and Head, Retrovirology Section, Department of Pediatrics,
Baylor College of Medicine; President, Baylor International Pediatric
AIDS Initiative, Texas Children's Hospital, Houston, Texas*
Primary Immunodeficiencies

Katherine M. Knapp, M.D.
*Assistant Professor, Department of Pediatrics, University of
Tennessee Health Science Center; Assistant Member, Department of
Infectious Diseases, St. Jude Children's Research Hospital, Memphis,
Tennessee*
Candidiasis

Heidi M. Kokkinos, M.T.(ASCP), B.S.
*Core Technologist, Mycology Laboratory, University of California,
Los Angeles; Clinical Laboratory Scientist, Department of Pathology
and Laboratory Medicine, UCLA Medical Center, Los Angeles,
California*
Classification of Fungi

Peter J. Krause, M.D.
*Associate Research Scientist, Department of Epidemiology and Public
Health, Yale School of Medicine, New Haven; Division of Pediatric
Infectious Diseases, Connecticut Children's Medical Center, Hartford,
Connecticut*
Babesiosis

Leonard R. Krilov, M.D.
*Professor of Pediatrics, State University of New York Stony Brook
School of Medicine, Stony Brook; Chief, Pediatric Infectious Disease,
and Vice-Chairman, Department of Pediatrics, Children's Medical
Center, Winthrop University Hospital, Mineola, New York*
Chronic Fatigue Syndrome

Paul Krogstad, M.D., M.S.
*Professor of Pediatrics and Molecular and Medical Pharmacology,
Department of Pediatrics, David Geffen School of Medicine at
UCLA; Attending Physician, Mattel Children's Hospital UCLA,
Los Angeles, California*
Esophagitis; Osteomyelitis; Septic Arthritis; Enteroviruses and Parechoviruses

Thomas L. Kuhls, M.D.
*Consultant, Pediatric Infectious Diseases, Norman Regional Hospital,
Norman; Consultant, Pediatric Infectious Diseases, Baptist Medical
Center, Oklahoma City, Oklahoma*
Appendicitis and Pelvic Abscess; Pancreatitis; *Kingella* Species

Xavier de Lamballerie, M.D., Ph.D.
*Professor of Virology, Unité des Virus Emergents, Faculté de
Médecine, Université de la Méditerranée, Marseille, France*
Lymphocytic Choriomeningitis Virus Infection; Arenaviral Hemorrhagic Fevers;
    Toscana Virus

Timothy R. La Pine, M.D.
*Adjunct Professor of Pathology and Pediatrics, Department of
Pathology, University of Utah School of Medicine, Salt Lake City,
Utah*
Immunomodulating Agents

Matthew B. Laurens, M.D., M.P.H.
*Research Associate, Pediatric Infectious Diseases and Tropical
Pediatrics, University of Maryland School of Medicine, Baltimore,
Maryland*
Cholera

Charles T. Leach, M.D.
*Professor of Pediatrics, University of Texas Health Science Center
at San Antonio; Attending Physician, CHRISTUS Santa Rosa
Children's Hospital and University Hospital, San Antonio, Texas*
Epstein-Barr Virus

Robert J. Leggiadro, M.D.
*Professor of Clinical Pediatrics, Weill Medical College of Cornell
University; Chairman, Department of Pediatrics, Lincoln Medical
and Mental Health Center, Bronx, New York*
Other *Campylobacter* Species; Bioterrorism

Diana R. Lennon, M.B.Ch.B., F.R.A.C.P.
*Professor of Population Health of Children and Youth, University of
Auckland; Pediatrician in Infectious Diseases, Starship Children's
Hospital, Auckland, New Zealand*
Acute Rheumatic Fever

Carolyn Lentzsch-Parcells, M.D.
Pediatrician, Pearland, Texas
Fever: Pathogenesis and Treatment

Eric Leroy
*Institut de Recherche pour le Developpement, Université de la
Méditerranée, Marseille, France; Centre International de Recherches
Medicales de Franceville, Franceville, Gabon*
Filoviral Hemorrhagic Fever: Marburg and Ebola Virus Fevers

Chi Wai Leung, M.B.B.S.
Honorary Clinical Associate Professor, Department of Paediatrics and Adolescent Medicine, University of Hong Kong; Consultant Paediatrician and Head of Paediatric Infectious Diseases, Department of Paediatrics and Adolescent Medicine, Princess Margaret Hospital, Hong Kong, China
Coronaviruses and Toroviruses, Including Severe Acute Respiratory Syndrome

Moise L. Levy, M.D.
Chief, Pediatric Dermatology, Dell Children's Medical Center, Austin, Texas
Viral and Fungal Skin Infections

Karen Lewis, M.D.
Medical Director, Bureau of Epidemiology and Disease Control, and State Tuberculosis Control Officer, Arizona Department of Health Services, Phoenix, Arizona
Mastoiditis

Phyllis T. Losikoff, M.D., M.P.H.
Clinical Assistant Professor of Pediatrics, The Warren Alpert Medical School of Brown University, Providence; Medical Director, Rhode Island Training School, Cranston, Rhode Island
Active Immunizing Agents

Timothy Edward Lotze, M.D.
Assistant Professor of Pediatrics and Neurology, Baylor College of Medicine; Attending Physician, Neurology Service, Texas Children's Hospital, Houston, Texas
Parainfectious and Postinfectious Disorders of the Nervous System

Adam W. Lowry, M.D.
Instructor, Department of Pediatrics, Baylor College of Medicine; Air Transport Physician, Critical Care Service, Texas Children's Hospital, Houston, Texas
Leptospirosis

Timothy Mailman, M.D.
Associate Professor, Department of Pediatrics, Dalhousie University Faculty of Medicine; Staff Consultant, IWK Health Centre, Halifax, Nova Scotia, Canada
Listeriosis

Susan A. Maloney, M.D.
Chief Epidemiologist and Special Studies, Division of Global Migration and Quarantine, Centers for Disease Control and Prevention, Atlanta, Georgia
International Travel Issues for Children

Laurene Mascola, M.D., M.P.H.
Chief, Acute Communicable Disease Control, Los Angeles County Department of Health Services, Los Angeles, California
Public Health Aspects of Infectious Disease Control

Edward O. Mason, Ph.D.
Professor, Department of Pediatrics and Department of Molecular Virology and Microbiology, Baylor College of Medicine; Director, Infectious Disease Laboratory, Texas Children's Hospital, Houston, Texas
Staphylococcus aureus Infections (Coagulase-Positive Staphylococci)

David O. Matson, M.D., Ph.D.
Director, Graduate Program in Public Health, and Professor of Health Professions and Pediatrics, Eastern Virginia Medical School and Old Dominion University, Norfolk, Virginia
Caliciviruses

Alan N. Mayer, M.D., Ph.D.
Instructor, Department of Pediatrics, Harvard Medical School; Assistant, Division of Gastroenterology, Children's Hospital Boston, Boston, Massachusetts
Hepatitis C Virus

Marc A. Mazade, M.D.
Pediatric Infectious Diseases Consultant, Cook Children's, Fort Worth, Texas
Infections Related to Craniofacial Surgical Procedures

James B. McAuley, M.D., M.P.H.
Associate Professor of Pediatrics and Internal Medicine, Rush Medical College; Director, Section of Pediatric Infectious Diseases, Rush Children's Hospital of Rush University Medical Center, Chicago, Illinois
Congenital Toxoplasmosis; Toxoplasmosis

George H. McCracken, Jr., M.D.
Glaxosmithkline Distinguished Professorship of Pediatric Infectious Diseases, Sarah M. and Charles E. Sey Chair in Pediatric Infectious Diseases, and Professor, Department of Pediatrics, University of Texas Southwestern Medical School; Attending Physician, Children's Medical Center of Dallas, Dallas, Texas
Antibacterial Therapeutic Agents

Kenneth McIntosh, M.D.
Professor of Pediatrics, Harvard Medical School; Emeritus Chief, Division of Infectious Diseases, Children's Hospital Boston, Boston, Massachusetts
Coronaviruses and Toroviruses, Including Severe Acute Respiratory Syndrome

James E. McJunkin, M.D.
Professor of Pediatrics, West Virginia University Health Sciences Center–Charleston Division; Professor of Pediatrics, Women and Children's Hospital, Charleston Area Medical Center, Charleston, West Virginia
La Crosse Encephalitis and Other California Serogroup Viruses

Kelly T. McKee, Jr., M.D.
Vice President, Public Health and Government Services, Quintiles Transnational Corporation, Durham, North Carolina
Hantaviruses

Rima L. McLeod, M.D.
Jules and Doris Stein RPB Professor, Department of Visual Sciences, Pathology, Committees of Molecular Medicine, Genetics, and Immunology, University of Chicago Pritzker School of Medicine; Attending Physician, Department of Medicine, University of Chicago Hospitals; Attending Physician, Department of Ophthalmology, Medical Reese Hospital and Medical Center, Chicago, Illinois
Toxoplasmosis

Valérie A. McLin, M.D.
Assistant Professor of Pediatrics, Baylor College of Medicine; Texas Children's Liver Center, Texas Children's Hospital, Houston, Texas
Cholangitis and Cholecystitis

Maria José Soares Mendes-Giannini, M.D.
Professor, School of Pharmaceutical Sciences, Araraquara, São Paulo State University, São Paulo, Brazil
Paracoccidioidomycosis

Wayne M. Meyers, M.D., Ph.D., D.Sc. (Hon)
Visiting Scientist, Department of Environmental and Infectious Disease Sciences, Armed Forces Institute of Pathology; Registrar for Leprosy, American Registry of Pathology, Washington, D.C.
Leprosy and Buruli Ulcer: The Major Cutaneous Mycobacterioses

Marian G. Michaels, M.D., M.P.H.
Professor of Pediatrics and Surgery, University of Pittsburgh School of Medicine; Director, Pediatric HIV Center; Co-Director, Infectious Diseases Clinical Research Unit; and Attending Physician, Division of Infectious Diseases, Children's Hospital of Pittsburgh, Pittsburgh, Pennsylvania
Opportunistic Infections in Liver and Intestinal Transplantation

Ian C. Michelow, M.D.
Pediatrician, Massachusetts General Hospital, Boston, Massachusetts
Antibacterial Therapeutic Agents

Vladana Milisavljevic, M.D., M.S.
Assistant Clinical Professor, Department of Pediatrics, David Geffen School of Medicine at UCLA; Attending Physician, Mattel Children's Hospital UCLA, Los Angeles, California
Mycoplasma and *Ureaplasma* Infections of the Neonate

Aaron M. Miller, M.D.
Staff Physician, Houston Eye Associates, Tomball, Texas
Ocular Infectious Diseases

James N. Miller, Ph.D.
Professor Emeritus on Recall, Department of Microbiology, Immunology, and Molecular Genetics, David Geffen School of Medicine at UCLA, Los Angeles, California
Nonvenereal Treponematoses

Marjorie J. Miller, Ph.D.
Senior Specialist, Virology, Department of Pathology and Laboratory Medicine, UCLA Medical Center, Los Angeles, California
Classification and Nomenclature of Viruses; Viral Laboratory Diagnosis

James N. Mills, Ph.D.
Chief, Medical Ecology Unit, Special Pathogens Branch, Division of Viral and Rickettsial Diseases, National Center for Zoonosis, Vector-Borne, and Enteric Diseases, Centers for Disease Control and Prevention, Atlanta, Georgia
Hantaviruses

Linda L. Minnich, M.S.
Adjunct Assistant Professor, Robert C. Byrd Health Sciences Center, Charleston Division; Virologist, Charleston Area Medical Center, Charleston, West Virginia
La Crosse Encephalitis and Other California Serogroup Viruses

Ann Moran, M.D.
Assistant Professor, Department of Medicine, Baylor College of Medicine; Staff Physician, Infectious Diseases Section, Michael E. DeBakey Veterans Affairs Medical Center, Houston, Texas
Cryptococcosis

James R. Murphy, Ph.D.
Professor, Department of Pediatrics, Section of Pediatric Infectious Diseases, University of Texas Health Science Center, Houston, Texas
Campylobacter jejuni

Pratip K. Nag, M.D., Ph.D.
Assistant Professor of Pediatrics, Pediatric Emergency Medicine Section, Baylor College of Medicine; Attending Physician, Texas Children's Hospital, Houston, Texas
Diphtheria; Tularemia

Joseph J. Nania, M.D.
Department of Pediatrics, Division of Infectious Diseases, Vanderbilt University School of Medicine, Nashville, Tennessee
Bartonella (Cat-Scratch Disease)

James P. Nataro, M.D., Ph.D., M.B.A.
Professor of Pediatrics, Medicine, Microbiology and Immunology, and Biochemistry and Molecular Biology, Center for Vaccine Development, University of Maryland School of Medicine; Vice Chair, Department of Pediatrics, University of Maryland Hospital for Children, Baltimore, Maryland
Diarrhea-Causing and Dysentery-Causing *Escherichia coli;* Cholera

Roger K. Nicome, M.D.
Assistant Professor of Pediatrics, Pediatric Emergency Medicine Section, Baylor College of Medicine; Attending Physician, Emergency Medicine Department, Texas Children's Hospital, Houston, Texas
Aeromonas

Karin Nielsen-Saines, M.D., M.P.H.
Assistant Professor of Pediatrics, David Geffen School of Medicine at UCLA; Member, Division of Infectious Diseases, Mattel Children's Hospital UCLA, Los Angeles, California
Leishmaniasis

Delma J. Nieves, M.D.
Assistant Professor of Pediatrics, David Geffen School of Medicine at UCLA; Member, Division of Infectious Diseases, Mattel Children's Hospital UCLA, Los Angeles, California
The Common Cold

Richard A. Oberhelman, M.D.
Professor of Tropical Medicine and Pediatrics, Tulane School of Public Health and Tropical Medicine, New Orleans, Louisiana
Bacillus cereus

Theresa J. Ochoa, M.D.
Assistant Professor of Pediatrics, Universidad Peruana Cayetano Heredia, Lima, Peru; Assistant Professor of Epidemiology, University of Texas School of Public Health, Houston, Texas
Shigella; Salmonella; Cryptosporidiosis

Christopher M. Oermann, M.D.
Associate Professor, Department of Pediatrics, Baylor College of Medicine; Attending Physician, Pulmonary Medicine Service, Texas Children's Hospital, Houston, Texas
Acute Respiratory Distress Syndrome in Children

Alina Olteanu, M.D., Ph.D.
Assistant Professor of Pediatrics, Tulane University School of Medicine, New Orleans, Louisiana
Metabolic Response of the Host to Infections

Gary D. Overturf, M.D.
Professor of Pediatrics and Pathology, University of New Mexico School of Medicine; Medical Director, Infectious Diseases, TriCore Reference Laboratories, Albuquerque, New Mexico
Plague (Yersinia pestis); Clostridial Intoxication and Infection; Antimicrobial Prophylaxis

Debra L. Palazzi, M.D.
Assistant Professor of Pediatrics, Pediatric Infectious Diseases Section, Baylor College of Medicine; Attending Physician, Texas Children's Hospital, Houston, Texas
Fever without Source and Fever of Unknown Origin

Pia S. Pannaraj, M.D.
Assistant Professor of Pediatrics, Keck School of Medicine of the University of Southern California; Attending Physician, Children's Hospital Los Angeles, Los Angeles, California
Group B Streptococcal Infections

Janak A. Patel, M.D.
Professor of Pediatrics and Director, Division of Pediatric Infectious Diseases and Immunology, Children's Hospital, University of Texas Medical Branch; Consultant, Shriners Burn Hospital for Children, Galveston, Texas
Infections in Burn Patients

Christian C. Patrick, M.D., Ph.D.
Chief Medical Officer and Senior Vice President for Medical and Academic Affairs, Miami Children's Hospital, Miami, Florida
Opportunistic Infections in Hematopoietic Stem Cell Transplantation; Coagulase-Negative Staphylococcal Infections

Evelyn A. Paysse, M.D.
Associate Professor of Ophthalmology and Pediatrics, Department of Ophthalmology, Baylor College of Medicine; Clinical Physician, Department of Pediatric Ophthalmology and Strabismus, Texas Children's Hospital, Houston, Texas
Ocular Infectious Diseases

Norma Pérez, D.O.
Assistant Professor, Baylor College of Medicine; Staff Scientist, University of Texas Health Science Center, Houston, Texas
Campylobacter jejuni

C. J. Peters, M.D.
Professor of Microbiology, Immunology, and Pathology, University of Texas Medical Branch–Galveston, Galveston, Texas
Hantaviruses; Other Bunyaviridae: Rift Valley Fever

William A. Petri, Jr., M.D., Ph.D.
Professor of Medicine, Microbiology, and Pathology; Chief, Division of Infectious Diseases and International Health; Wade Hampton Frost Professor of Epidemiology, University of Virginia School of Medicine; Attending Physician, University of Virginia Hospitals, Charlottesville, Virginia
Amebiasis

Brandon Lane Phillips, M.D.
Instructor in Pediatrics, Mayo College of Medicine, and Fellow, Division of Pediatric Cardiology, Mayo Clinic, Rochester, Minnesota
Pneumococcal Infections

Larry K. Pickering, M.D.
Senior Adviser to the Director, National Center for Immunization and Respiratory Diseases, Centers for Disease Control and Prevention, Atlanta, Georgia
Approach to Patients with Gastrointestinal Tract Infections and Food Poisoning

Joseph F. Piecuch, D.M.D., M.D.
Clinical Professor, Department of Oral and Maxillofacial Surgery, University of Connecticut School of Dental Medicine, Farmington; Director, Oral and Maxillofacial Surgery Section, Hartford Hospital, Hartford, Connecticut
Infections of the Oral Cavity

Francisco P. Pinheiro, M.D.
Department of Arbovirus, Instituto Evandro Chagas, Belém, Brazil
Other Bunyaviridae: Oropouche Fever

Stanley A. Plotkin, M.D.
Emeritus Professor of Pediatrics, University of Pennsylvania School of Medicine and Wistar Institute; Former Chief, Division of Infectious Diseases, Children's Hospital of Philadelphia, Philadelphia, Pennsylvania; Adjunct Professor of International Health, Johns Hopkins University, Baltimore, Maryland; Former Medical and Scientific Director, Aventis Pasteur; and Executive Advisor to the CEO, Sanofi Pasteur, Swiftwater, Pennsylvania
Rabies Virus

Scott L. Pomeroy, M.D., Ph.D.
Bronson Crothers Professor of Neurology, Harvard Medical School; Neurologist-in-Chief, Children's Hospital Boston, Boston, Massachusetts
Parainfectious and Postinfectious Disorders of the Nervous System

Alice Pong, M.D.
Attending Physician, Division of Pediatric Infectious Diseases, Rady Children's Hospital–San Deigo, San Diego, California
Retroperitoneal Infections

David L. Pugatch, M.D.
Clinical Professor of Pediatrics, University of California, San Francisco, School of Medicine, San Francisco; Medical Director, Pediatric Infectious Diseases, Children's Hospital of Central California, Madera, California
Active Immunizing Agents

Joan S. Purcell, M.D.
Chair, Department of Pediatrics, The Woodlands Memorial Hospital; Vice President, Step Pediatrics, The Woodlands, Texas
Trichomonas Infections

Ramya Ramraj, M.D.
Pediatrician, Sugarland, Texas
Mimiviruses

Jack S. Remington, M.D.
Professor Emeritus, Department of Medicine, Stanford University School of Medicine; Palo Alto Medical Foundation, Palo Alto, California
Toxoplasmosis

Carina A. Rodriguez, M.D.
Postdoctoral Fellow, University of Tennessee, Memphis, College of Medicine, and Department of Infectious Diseases, St. Jude Children's Research Hospital, Memphis, Tennessee
Coagulase-Negative Staphylococcal Infections

José R. Romero, M.D.
Horace C. Cabe Professor of Pediatrics and Chief, Pediatric Infectious Diseases, Arkansas Children's Hospital/University of Arkansas for Medical Sciences; Director, Clinical Trials Research, Arkansas Children's Hospital Research Unit, Little Rock, Arkansas
Flaviviruses: West Nile Virus

Benjamin A. Ross, M.D.
Pediatric Neurologist, Denver, Colorado
Parainfectious and Postinfectious Disorders of the Nervous System

Lawrence A. Ross, M.D.
Professor of Clinical Pediatrics, Keck School of Medicine of the University of Southern California; Attending Physician, Division of Infectious Diseases, Children's Hospital Los Angeles, Los Angeles, California
Trypanosomiasis

Judith L. Rowen, M.D.
Associate Professor of Pediatrics and Assistant Dean for Educational Affairs, University of Texas Medical Branch–Galveston, Galveston, Texas
Miscellaneous Mycoses

Charles E. Rupprecht, V.M.D., Ph.D.
Chief, Rabies Program, Division of Viral and Rickettsial Diseases, Centers for Disease Control and Prevention, Atlanta, Georgia
Rabies Virus

Xavier Sáez-Llorens, M.D.
Professor of Pediatrics and Infectious Diseases, University of Panama School of Medicine; Vice-Chairman and Head of Infectious Diseases, Hospital del Niño, Panama City, Panama
Parameningeal Infections; Perinatal Bacterial Diseases

Lisa Saiman, M.D., M.P.H.
Associate Professor of Clinical Pediatrics, Department of Pediatrics, Columbia University College of Physicians and Surgeons; Associate Attending Pediatrician, Department of Pediatrics, and Hospital Epidemiologist, Department of Pediatrics and Epidemiology, Children's Hospital of New York, New York, New York
Cystic Fibrosis

Joseph W. St. Geme III, M.D.
Professor of Pediatrics and Molecular Genetics and Microbiology and Chair, Department of Pediatrics, Duke University School of Medicine; Chief Medical Officer, Duke University Hospital, Durham, North Carolina
Molecular Determinants of Microbial Pathogenesis

Pablo J. Sánchez, M.D.
Professor, Department of Pediatrics, Division of Neonatal-Perinatal Medicine and Pediatric Infectious Diseases, University of Texas Southwestern Medical School; Division of Neonatal-Perinatal Medicine and Pediatric Infectious Diseases, Parkland Health and Hospital Systems and Children's Medical Center of Dallas, Dallas, Texas
Viral Infections of the Fetus and Neonate; Syphilis

Laura A. Sass, M.D.
Assistant Professor of Pediatrics, Eastern Virginia Medical School; Attending Physician, Division of Pediatric Infectious Diseases, Children's Hospital of The King's Daughters, Norfolk, Virginia
Enterobacter

Carlos A. Sattler, M.D.
Senior Director, Medical Affairs and Policy, Merck Vaccines and Infectious Diseases, West Point, Pennsylvania
Stenotrophomonas (Xanthomonas) maltophilia

Danica J. Schulte, M.D.
Clinical Instructor, Department of Pediatrics, David Geffen School of Medicine at UCLA; Attending Physician, Division of Pediatric Infectious Diseases, Immunology, and Allergy, Cedars-Sinai Medical Center, Los Angeles, California
Human Parvovirus B19

Gordon E. Schutze, M.D.
Professor of Pediatrics, Section of Retrovirology, Baylor College of Medicine; Vice President, Baylor International Pediatric AIDS Initiative, Texas Children's Hospital, Houston, Texas
Human Retroviruses: Oncoviruses (Human T-Cell Lymphotropic Viruses) and Lentiviruses (Human Immunodeficiency Virus Type 2); Blastomycosis

Filiz O. Seeborg, M.D.
Assistant Professor of Pediatrics, Section of Pediatric Allergy and Immunology, Baylor College of Medicine; Attending Physician, Allergy and Immunology Service, Texas Children's Hospital, Houston, Texas
Human Retroviruses: Impact of Human Immunodeficiency Virus and Acquired Immunodeficiency Syndrome

Eugene D. Shapiro, M.D.
Professor of Pediatrics, Epidemiology, and Public Health and Investigative Medicine, Yale School of Medicine; Associate Chairperson, Yale–New Haven Children's Hospital, New Haven, Connecticut
Epidemiology of Infectious Diseases; Epidemiology and Biostatistics

Nina L. Shapiro, M.D.
Associate Professor, Division of Head and Neck Surgery, David Geffen School of Medicine at UCLA; Attending Physician, Division of Head and Neck Surgery, UCLA Medical Center, Los Angeles, California
Sinusitis; Mastoiditis

William T. Shearer, M.D., Ph.D.
Professor, Departments of Pediatrics and Immunology, and Head, Section of Pediatric Allergy and Immunology, Baylor College of Medicine; Chief, Allergy and Immunology Service, Texas Children's Hospital, Houston, Texas
Chronic Bronchitis; Primary Immunodeficiencies; Human Retroviruses: Impact of Human Immunodeficiency Virus and Acquired Immunodeficiency Syndrome

Ziad M. Shehab, M.D.
Professor of Clinical Pediatrics and Pathology, University of Arizona Health Sciences Center, Tucson, Arizona
Coccidioidomycosis

Jerry L. Shenep, M.D.
Professor of Pediatrics, University of Tennessee Health Science Center; Member, Department of Infectious Diseases, St. Jude Children's Research Hospital, Memphis, Tennessee
Enterococcal and Viridans Streptococcal Infections; Cryptococcosis

W. Donald Shields, M.D.
Professor of Neurology and Pediatrics, David Geffen School of Medicine at UCLA; Member, Division of Neurology, Mattel Children's Hospital UCLA, Los Angeles, California
Encephalitis and Meningoencephalitis

Robyn Shimizu-Cohen
University of California, Los Angeles, School of Medicine; Clinical Laboratory Scientist, University of California, Los Angeles, Healthcare, Los Angeles, California
Parasitic Laboratory Diagnosis

Stanford T. Shulman, M.D.
Virginia H. Rogers Professor of Pediatric Infectious Diseases, Feinberg School of Medicine, Northwestern University; Chief, Division of Infectious Diseases, Children's Memorial Hospital, Chicago, Illinois
Kawasaki Disease

Constantine Simos, D.M.D.
Attending Physician, Oral and Maxillofacial Surgery, Robert Wood Johnson University Hospital and Saint Peter's University Hospital, New Brunswick, New Jersey
Infections of the Oral Cavity

Arnold L. Smith, M.D.
Professor, Department of Pathobiology, University of Washington School of Public Health; Member, Department of Bacterial Pathogens, Seattle Biomedical Research Institute, Seattle, Washington
Meningococcal Infections

Jason S. Soden, M.D.
Assistant Professor of Pediatrics, University of Colorado Denver School of Medicine; Attending Physician, Pediatric Gastroenterology, The Children's Hospital, Denver, Colorado
Cholangitis and Cholecystitis

Mary Allen Staat, M.D., M.P.H.
Associate Professor, Department of Pediatrics, University of Cincinnati College of Medicine; Director, International Adoption Center, Cincinnati Children's Hospital Medical Center, Cincinnati, Ohio
Genital Infections; Rotaviruses

Jeffrey R. Starke, M.D.
Professor and Vice-Chairman of Pediatrics, Baylor College of Medicine; Chief of Pediatrics, Ben Taub General Hospital; Infection Control Officer, Texas Children's Hospital, Houston, Texas
Infective Endocarditis; Tuberculosis

Barbara W. Stechenberg, M.D.
Professor of Pediatrics, Tufts University School of Medicine, Boston; Vice-Chair, Department of Pediatrics, and Director, Pediatric Infectious Diseases, Baystate Children's Hospital, Springfield, Massachusetts
Eosinophilic Meningitis; Moraxella catarrhalis; Diphtheria; Pasteurella multocida; Bartonellosis; Borrelia (Lyme Disease)

William J. Steinbach, M.D.
Assistant Professor of Pediatrics, Duke University School of Medicine; Division of Pediatric Infectious Diseases, Duke University Medical Center, Durham, North Carolina
Aspergillus and Aspergillosis; Zygomycosis

Paul G. Steinkuller, M.D.
Associate Professor of Ophthalmology and Pediatrics, Baylor College of Medicine; Clinical Staff, Ophthalmology Service, Texas Children's Hospital, Houston, Texas
Ocular Infectious Diseases

E. Richard Stiehm, M.D.
Professor of Pediatrics, David Geffen School of Medicine at UCLA; Attending Pediatrician, Mattel Children's Hospital UCLA, Los Angeles, California
Passive Immunization

Stephanie H. Stovall, M.D.
Assistant Professor of Pediatrics, University of Arkansas for Medical Sciences; Medical Director, Clinical Microbiology and Virology Laboratory, and Co-Director, Antimicrobial Stewardship, Arkansas Children's Hospital, Little Rock, Arkansas
Blastomycosis

Jeffrey Suen, M.D.
Assistant Professor, Department of Pediatrics, David Geffen School of Medicine at UCLA; Member, Division of Infectious Diseases, Mattel Children's Hospital UCLA, Los Angeles, California
Toxic Shock Syndrome

Ciro V. Sumaya, M.D.
Dean, School of Rural Public Health, and Professor and Cox Endowed Chair in Medicine, Department of Pediatrics, Texas A & M Health Science Center, College Station; Attending Physician, Scott and White Hospital and Clinic, Temple, Texas
Epstein-Barr Virus

Andrea P. Summer, M.D.
Associate Professor of Pediatrics, Medical University of South Carolina, Charleston, South Carolina
Cestodes; Trematodes; Schistosomiasis

Douglas S. Swanson, M.D.
Associate Professor of Pediatrics, University of Missouri–Kansas City School of Medicine; Children's Mercy Hospital, Kansas City, Missouri
Indigenous Flora

Tina Q. Tan, M.D.
Associate Professor of Pediatrics, Feinberg School of Medicine, Northwestern University; Attending Physician, Infectious Diseases; Co-Director, Pediatric Travel Medicine Clinic; and Director, International Adoptee Clinic, Children's Memorial Hospital, Chicago, Illinois
Infections Related to Prosthetic or Artificial Devices; Giardiasis; *Naegleria, Acanthamoeba,* and *Balamuthia*

Herbert B. Tanowitz, M.D.
Professor of Pathology and Medicine, Department of Pathology, Albert Einstein College of Medicine of Yeshiva University; Attending Physician, Department of Medicine, Weiler Hospital–Montefiore Medical Center; Attending Physician, Departments of Medicine and Pathology, Jacobs Medical Center, Bronx, New York
Trypanosomiasis

Robert B. Tesh, M.D., M.S.
Professor, Departments of Pathology and Microbiology and Immunology, University of Texas Medical Branch–Galveston, Galveston, Texas
Other Bunyaviridae: Crimean-Congo Hemorrhagic Fever; Other Bunyaviridae: Phlebotomus Fever (Sandfly Fever)

Philip Toltzis, M.D.
Associate Professor of Pediatrics, Case Western Reserve University School of Medicine; Medical Director, Pediatric Intensive Care Unit, Rainbow Babies and Children's Hospital, Cleveland, Ohio
Antibiotic Resistance

Richard G. Topazian, D.D.S.
Professor Emeritus, Department of Oral and Maxillofacial Surgery, University of Connecticut School of Dental Medicine, Farmington, Connecticut
Infections of the Oral Cavity

Michael F. Tosi, M.D.
Director, Pediatric Infectious Diseases, Maimonides Medical Center, Brooklyn, New York
Normal and Impaired Immunologic Responses to Infection

Amelia P. A. Travassos da Rosa, B.Sc.
Visiting Scientist, Department of Pathology, University of Texas Medical Branch–Galveston, Galveston, Texas
Other Bunyaviridae: Oropouche Fever

Theodore F. Tsai, M.D., M.P.H.
Senior Vice President for Scientific Affairs, Novartis Vaccines, Cambridge, Massachusetts
Orbiviruses, Coltiviruses, and Seadornaviruses; Alphaviruses: Eastern Equine Encephalitis; Alphaviruses: Western Equine Encephalitis; Alphaviruses: Venezuelan Equine Encephalitis; Alphaviruses: Other Alphaviral Infections; Flaviviruses: St. Louis Encephalitis; Flaviviruses: Japanese Encephalitis; Flaviviruses: Tick-Borne Encephalitis; Flaviviruses: Other Flaviviral Infections

Tulio A. Valdez, M.D.
Otolaryngologist, Houston, Texas
Otitis Externa

Jesus G. Vallejo, M.D.
Associate Professor of Pediatrics, Baylor College of Medicine; Attending Physician, Infectious Diseases Service, Texas Children's Hospital, Houston, Texas
Myocarditis; Bacteremia and Septic Shock

John A. Vanchiere, M.D., Ph.D.
Assistant Professor of Pediatrics, Louisiana State University Health Sciences Center–Shreveport; Chief, Pediatric Infectious Diseases, Children's Hospital of LSUHSC Shreveport, Shreveport, Louisiana
Human Polyomaviruses

Pedro Fernando da C. Vasconcelos, M.D., Ph.D.
Chief, Department of Arbovirus, Instituto Evandro Chagas, Belém, Brazil
Other Bunyaviridae: Oropouche Fever

Jorge J. Velarde, M.D., Ph.D.
Resident, Department of Pediatrics, Cincinnati Children's Hospital Medical Center, Cincinnati, Ohio
Diarrhea-Causing and Dysentery-Causing *Escherichia coli*

James Versalovic, M.D., Ph.D.
Associate Professor of Pathology and Pediatrics, Baylor College of Medicine; Director, Microbiology Laboratories, Texas Children's Hospital, Houston, Texas
Antibiotic-Associated Colitis; Bacterial Laboratory Diagnosis

Ellen R. Wald, M.D.
Professor of Pediatrics, University of Wisconsin School of Medicine and Public Health; Chair of Pediatrics and Alfred Dorrance Daniels Professor of Diseases of Children, American Family Children's Hospital, Madison, Wisconsin
Uvulitis; Urethritis; Cystitis and Pyelonephritis; Infections in Daycare Environments

Douglas S. Walsh, M.D., M.S.
Adjunct Associate Professor of Dermatology, Uniformed Services University of the Health Sciences F. Edward Hébert School of Medicine, Bethesda, Maryland; Director, KEMRI/Walter Reed Project, Kisumu, Kenya
Leprosy and Buruli Ulcer: The Major Cutaneous Mycobacterioses

Edward E. Walsh, M.D.
Professor of Pediatrics, University of Rochester School of Medicine and Dentistry, Rochester, New York
Respiratory Syncytial Virus

Thomas J. Walsh, M.D.
Senior Investigator and Chief, Immunocompromised Host Section, Pediatric Oncology Branch, National Cancer Institute, Bethesda, Maryland
Antifungal Agents

Mark A. Ward, M.D.
Assistant Professor of Pediatrics and Director of Pediatric Housestaff Training, Baylor College of Medicine; Attending Physician, Texas Children's Hospital, Houston, Texas
Fever: Pathogenesis and Treatment

Richard L. Ward, Ph.D.
Research Professor, Department of Infectious Diseases, Cincinnati Children's Hospital Medical Center, Cincinnati, Ohio
Rotaviruses

Michelle Weinberg, M.D., M.P.H.
Division of Global Migration and Quarantine, Centers for Disease Control and Prevention, Atlanta, Georgia
International Travel Issues for Children

Robert C. Welliver, M.D.
Professor of Pediatrics, State University of New York at Buffalo School of Medicine; Co-Director, Division of Infectious Diseases, Women & Children's Hospital of Buffalo, Buffalo, New York
Bronchiolitis and Infectious Asthma

J. Gary Wheeler, M.D., M.P.S.
Professor, Department of Pediatrics, University of Arkansas for Medical Sciences; Attending Physician, Pediatric Infectious Diseases, Arkansas Children's Hospital, Little Rock, Arkansas
Pleural Effusions and Empyema; Lung Abscess

A. Clinton White, Jr., M.D.
Paul R. Stalnaker, M.D., Distinguished Professor of Internal Medicine and Director, Infectious Disease Division, Department of Internal Medicine, University of Texas Medical Branch–Galveston, Galveston, Texas
Cryptosporidiosis; Cestodes; Trematodes; Schistosomiasis

Suzanne Whitworth, M.D.
Senior Consultant, Cook Children's Healthcare System, Fort Worth, Texas
Actinobacillus actinomycetemcomitans; Actinomycosis

Bernhard L. Wiedermann, M.D., M.A.
Professor of Pediatrics, George Washington University School of Medicine and Health Sciences; Attending Physician, Infectious Diseases, Children's National Medical Center, Washington, D.C.
Sporotrichosis

Natalie Williams-Bouyer, M.D.
Director, Clinical Microbiology Laboratory, Shriners Burn Hospital for Children, Galveston, Texas
Infections in Burn Patients

Murray Wittner, M.D.
Professor of Pathology and Parasitology, Department of Pathology, Albert Einstein College of Medicine of Yeshiva University; Attending Physician, Departments of Medicine and Pathology, Montefiore Medical Center, Bronx, New York
Trypanosomiasis

Charles R. Woods, Jr., M.D., M.S.
Vice Chair for Faculty Development and Professor of Pediatrics, University of Louisville School of Medicine, Louisville, Kentucky
Genital Infections; Gonococcal Infections; Other *Yersinia* Species

Kimberly G. Yen, M.D.

Assistant Professor of Ophthalmology and Pediatrics, Baylor College of Medicine; Attending Physician, Ophthalmology Service, Texas Children's Hospital, Houston, Texas

Ocular Infectious Diseases

Ram Yogev, M.D.

Susan B. DePree Founders' Board Professor in Pediatrics, Feinberg School of Medicine, Northwestern University; Director, Section of Pediatric, Adolescent, and Maternal HIV Infection; Deputy Director for Research, Clinical Sciences; and Director, Clinical and Translational Research Program, Children's Memorial Hospital and Children's Memorial Research Center, Chicago, Illinois

Infections Related to Prosthetic or Artificial Devices

Edward J. Young, M.D., M.S.

Professor of Medicine and Molecular Virology and Microbiology, Baylor College of Medicine; Chief, Infection Control, Michael E. DeBakey Veterans Affairs Medical Center, Houston, Texas

Brucellosis

Theoklis E. Zaoutis, M.D.

Assistant Professor of Pediatrics and Epidemiology, University of Pennsylvania School of Medicine; Associate Chief, Division of Infectious Diseases, Children's Hospital of Philadelphia, Philadelphia, Pennsylvania

Zygomycosis

Preface

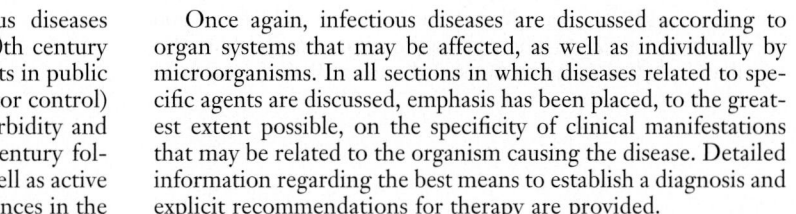

Morbidity and mortality rates related to infectious diseases decreased dramatically during the first half of the 20th century in the developed world because of major improvements in public health (e.g., clean water, adequate sanitation, and vector control) and personal health. Further major reduction in morbidity and mortality rates occurred in the second half of that century following the introduction of antimicrobial therapy, as well as active and passive immunization efforts. Despite theses advances in the 20th century, infectious diseases in the developed world remain the leading cause of morbidity in infants and children in the early 21st century. Children continue to experience three to nine respiratory infections and one to three gastrointestinal illnesses annually, requiring visits to physicians that outnumber the visits made for the purpose of well-child care. Infectious diseases also are the most common cause of school absenteeism. In more recent years, the emergence of resistance to multiple antibiotics by a large number of bacterial microorganisms (i.e., community-associated methicillin-resistant *Staphylococcus aureus*) has contributed to the morbidity and mortality related to infectious diseases processes, as have new infectious agents (i.e., bocavirus, SARS coronavirus). The developing world is confronted with the same present-day problems seen in the developed world (antimicrobial resistance and new infectious agents), and these challenges are compounded by malnutrition and lack of adequate public health services and antimicrobial agents.

The first edition of our text was written because we and many of our colleagues were concerned that no single reference text existed that comprehensively covered infectious diseases in children and adolescents. With each subsequent edition, including this one, our goal has been to provide comprehensive coverage of all subjects pertinent to the study of infectious diseases in these populations. Any attempt to summarize our present understanding of infectious diseases for serious students of the subject is a formidable task. In many areas, new information continues to accrue so rapidly that material becomes dated before it can appear in a text of this magnitude. Nonetheless, we have endeavored with the help of many of our colleagues to provide the most comprehensive and up-to-date discussion of this field. The new edition will be available online as well as in print. Purchasers can access the online version by registering their PIN number (found on the inside front cover of the book) at www.expertconsult.com. Online access includes not only fully searchable text, photos, illustrations, and tables but references linked to Pub Med access.

To provide a text as comprehensive and authoritative as possible, we have enlisted contributions from a large number of individuals whose collective expertise is responsible for whatever success we may have had in meeting our objective. We offer our most profound appreciation to the 284 fellow contributors from 108 universities or institutions in 15 countries for their professional expertise and devoted scholarship. Their cooperation and willingness to work with us leave us deeply in their debt.

Once again, infectious diseases are discussed according to organ systems that may be affected, as well as individually by microorganisms. In all sections in which diseases related to specific agents are discussed, emphasis has been placed, to the greatest extent possible, on the specificity of clinical manifestations that may be related to the organism causing the disease. Detailed information regarding the best means to establish a diagnosis and explicit recommendations for therapy are provided.

The entire text has been revised extensively. This edition continues the format that was initiated in the fourth edition in that infections with specific microorganisms have been organized to provide appropriate emphasis on the common features that may relate specific microorganisms to one another. Thus, all gram-positive coccal organisms are presented sequentially and are followed by gram-negative cocci, gram-positive bacilli, enterobacteria, gram-negative coccobacilli, Treponemataceae, anaerobic bacteria, and so forth. In addition, special sections of the text have been devoted to discussions of each of the following: molecular determinants of microbial pathogenesis; immunologic and phagocytic responses to infection; metabolic response of the host to infections; interaction of infection and nutrition; pathogenesis and treatment of fever; indigenous flora; epidemiology of infectious diseases; infections of the compromised host; Kawasaki disease; chronic fatigue syndrome; international travel issues for children; infectious disease problems of international adoptees and refugees; nosocomial infections; prevention and control of infections in hospitalized children; pharmacology and pharmacokinetics of antibacterial, antiviral, antifungal, and antiparasitic agents; immunomodulating agents; active and passive immunizing agents; public health considerations; infections in daycare environments; and use of the bacteriology, mycology, parasitology, virology, and serology laboratories. The section on infections in the compromised host has been divided into nine chapters including opportunistic infections in children with bone marrow transplantation, infections in pediatric heart transplant recipients and lung transplant recipients, opportunistic infections in children with liver and intestinal transplantation, opportunistic infections in children with kidney transplantation, infections related to prosthetics or artificial devices, infections related to craniofacial surgical procedures, and infections related to burns. This reorganization has been necessitated by the large number of individuals, particularly post-transplantation recipients, who now serve as the source of many infectious disease problems and constitute a large part of the consulting practice of many pediatric infectious disease physicians.

With some sadness, we have retained a section on bioterrorism, which is necessitated by the current state of world affairs. The section on immunomodulating agents and their potential use in the treatment of infectious diseases has been expanded because information on this subject has become more extensive since the publication of the last edition. Specific sections also have been

devoted to human and animal bites. The subject of biostatistics as applicable to the subspecialty of infectious diseases also has been included. New chapters on human bocavirus and mimiviruses have been added, and the chapters on human metapneumovirus, coronaviruses, and monkeypox have been expanded.

This project could not have been brought to fruition without the help and assistance of many people whose names do not appear in the text. No words are sufficient to adequately convey our gratitude appropriately; we hope that they know they have our heartfelt thanks.

We would like to single out certain individuals for specific mention. We cannot adequately convey our appreciation for the thousands of hours devoted by Dr. B. Lee Ligon, who edited and also proofread every word of the text that was submitted, as well as the page proofs. We are equally indebted to Mary Campbell, who spent an equivalent amount of time and who was specifically responsible for the coordination of the editorial effort, correspondence with our contributors and with the publishers, and coordination of the manuscript preparation process. She also typed and retyped many sections of the text. We also extremely

appreciate the efforts of Laura Wennstrom Sheehan, who oversaw and coordinated all events in Los Angeles. In particular, the work of Tiki Valentino and the students in the UCLA office (Lilit Gevorgyan, Judy Diep, Wendy Monteon, Robin Nguyen, Narges Moaddel, Margarita Santiago, Kelley Shin, and Karla Ortiz) deserves much praise.

We also appreciate the assistance provided to Mary Campbell and to the editors by Carrel Briley in Dr. Feigin's office.

Also appreciated were the help and support of Judith Fletcher, Melissa Dudlick, and Lee Ann Draud at Elsevier.

Finally, we thank the Baylor College of Medicine and Texas Children's Hospital in Houston, Texas, and the David Geffen School of Medicine at UCLA and the Mattel Children's Hospital UCLA in Los Angeles, California, for providing an environment that is supportive of intellectual pursuits.

Ralph D. Feigin, M.D.
James D. Cherry, M.D.
Sheldon L. Kaplan, M.D.
Gail J. Demmler-Harrison, M.D.

Contents

SECTION **XV**

UNCLASSIFIED INFECTIOUS DISEASES

PART **III**

INFECTIONS WITH SPECIFIC MICROORGANISMS   1183

SECTION **XVI**

BACTERIAL INFECTIONS

SUBSECTION **1**
Gram-Positive Cocci

SUBSECTION **2**
Gram-Negative Cocci

SUBSECTION **3**
Gram-Positive Bacilli

VOLUME 2

PART I

HOST-PARASITE RELATIONSHIPS AND THE PATHOGENESIS OF INFECTIOUS DISEASES

MOLECULAR DETERMINANTS OF MICROBIAL PATHOGENESIS

David A. Hunstad ✪ Joseph W. St. Geme III

Despite the availability of antibiotics and expansion of vaccination programs, infectious diseases remain a leading cause of morbidity and mortality worldwide. Numerous factors, including an increase in the prevalence of antimicrobial resistance, an increase in global travel, and an increase in the number of individuals with altered immunity, contribute to the continuing importance of infectious agents. In recent years, several microorganisms have been implicated in diseases previously considered noninfectious, and a variety of new and emerging pathogens have been recognized.

Pathogens are defined as microorganisms that are capable of causing disease. Not all pathogens are equal, however, with respect to their pathogenic potential (i.e., their virulence). Many pathogens are commensal organisms and live in harmony with their host under most conditions, causing disease only when normal immune mechanisms are disrupted or absent. Other pathogens produce disease even in the setting of intact immunity and almost always cause symptoms.

For a given pathogen, pathogenic potential is determined by the specific array of virulence-associated genes. Some species of bacteria are capable of natural transformation and readily acquire fragments of DNA from other organisms, expanding or altering their genetic composition, occasionally with consequences related to virulence. Many microorganisms carry virulence-associated genes on mobile genetic elements, including plasmids, transposons, and bacteriophages. These elements may equip the organism with genetic information that facilitates rapid adaptation to an unfavorable or changing environment. Comparison of genomes from pathogenic and nonpathogenic members of a single genus or species has led to the identification of *pathogenicity islands*—large blocks of chromosomal DNA that are present in pathogens and absent from related nonpathogens. These blocks are flanked by insertion sequences or repeat elements and differ in nucleotide composition relative to the surrounding genome, suggesting acquisition by horizontal exchange. Pathogenicity islands contain clusters of virulence-associated genes that encode a variety of factors, including protein secretion systems, secreted effector molecules, adhesins, and regulatory proteins.

To be successful, a pathogen must enter the host, find an appropriate niche, and multiply. Often the pathogen induces damage to the host and then spreads to other tissues, either nearby the initial site of infection or more distant. Ideally, the pathogen stops short of causing death to the host and produces symptoms, such as cough or diarrhea, that facilitate spread to another host.

This chapter addresses several key steps in the pathogenic process. In each case, we present examples that highlight pathogens and paradigms of relevance to infectious diseases in children. As a reflection of our personal bias, we focus primarily on bacterial pathogens.

COLONIZATION

Most infectious diseases begin with microbial colonization of a host surface—typically the skin, the respiratory tract, the gastrointestinal tract, or the genitourinary tract. Although colonization is insufficient for an organism to produce disease, it is a necessary prerequisite. The process of colonization requires specialized microbial factors, called *adhesins*, which promote adherence to host structures and enable the organism to overcome local defenses, such as mucociliary function, peristalsis, and urinary flow. The cognate receptors for these interactions generally are either carbohydrate or protein structures—in some cases expressed on host cells, and in others present in mucosal secretions or in submucosal tissue.

PILUS ADHESINS

Perhaps most common among bacterial adhesins are hairlike fibers called *pili* (also called *fimbriae*). Pili are polymeric structures containing a major structural subunit that usually ranges in size from 15 to 25 kd. Because of their size and morphology, most pili can be seen by negative-stain transmission electron microscopy.

The prototype example among adhesive pili is the P (or Pap) pilus, which is expressed by uropathogenic *Escherichia coli* (UPEC) and has been strongly associated with pyelonephritis. P pili recognize globoseries glycolipids, host molecules that are characterized by a core structure consisting of Gal-α1,4-Gal. The globoseries glycolipids are especially abundant in renal epithelium,[20] accounting for the predilection of P-piliated *E. coli* to adhere to kidney tissue and cause pyelonephritis. As shown in Figure 1–1, P pili are composite structures and consist of two subassemblies, including a thick rod that emanates from the bacterial surface and a thin tip fibrillum that extends distally.[141,226] The pilus rod is a right-handed helical cylinder and comprises repeating PapA subunits, whereas the tip fibrillum has an open helical configuration and contains mostly repeating PapE subunits. The two subassemblies are joined to each other by the PapK adapter protein. PapG contains the adhesive moiety and is located at the distal end of the tip fibrillum, joined to PapE by the PapF adapter.[123]

P pili are assembled in a process that involves a periplasmic chaperone, called *PapD*, and an outer membrane usher, called *PapC* (see Fig. 1–1).[50,142] The crystal structures of PapD alone and PapD interacting with the PapK pilin subunit have been solved, revealing significant insights into PapD interaction with Pap subunits and the mechanism of P pilus assembly.[225] PapD consists of two immunoglobulin-like folds oriented in an L shape with an intervening cleft. The PapK subunit consists of a single immunoglobulin-like fold but lacks the seventh, C-terminal β-strand (strand G1). The absence of this strand leaves a deep groove along the surface of PapK and exposes its hydrophobic core, predisposing the subunit to aggregation and degradation.

In the PapD-PapK complex, the G1 strand of PapD occupies the groove in PapK and completes the immunoglobulin-like fold, a phenomenon termed *donor strand complementation* (Fig. 1–2A). This interaction shields the hydrophobic core of the subunit and stabilizes the protein. Within the groove, the G1 strand of PapD interacts on one side with the C-terminal, F strand of PapK.[225] Ultimately, PapD delivers PapK and other Pap subunits to the PapC usher, which forms a dimer with twin pores in the outer membrane.[148] As the pilus is assembled on the bacterial surface, the N-terminal strand of a neighboring subunit (the one most

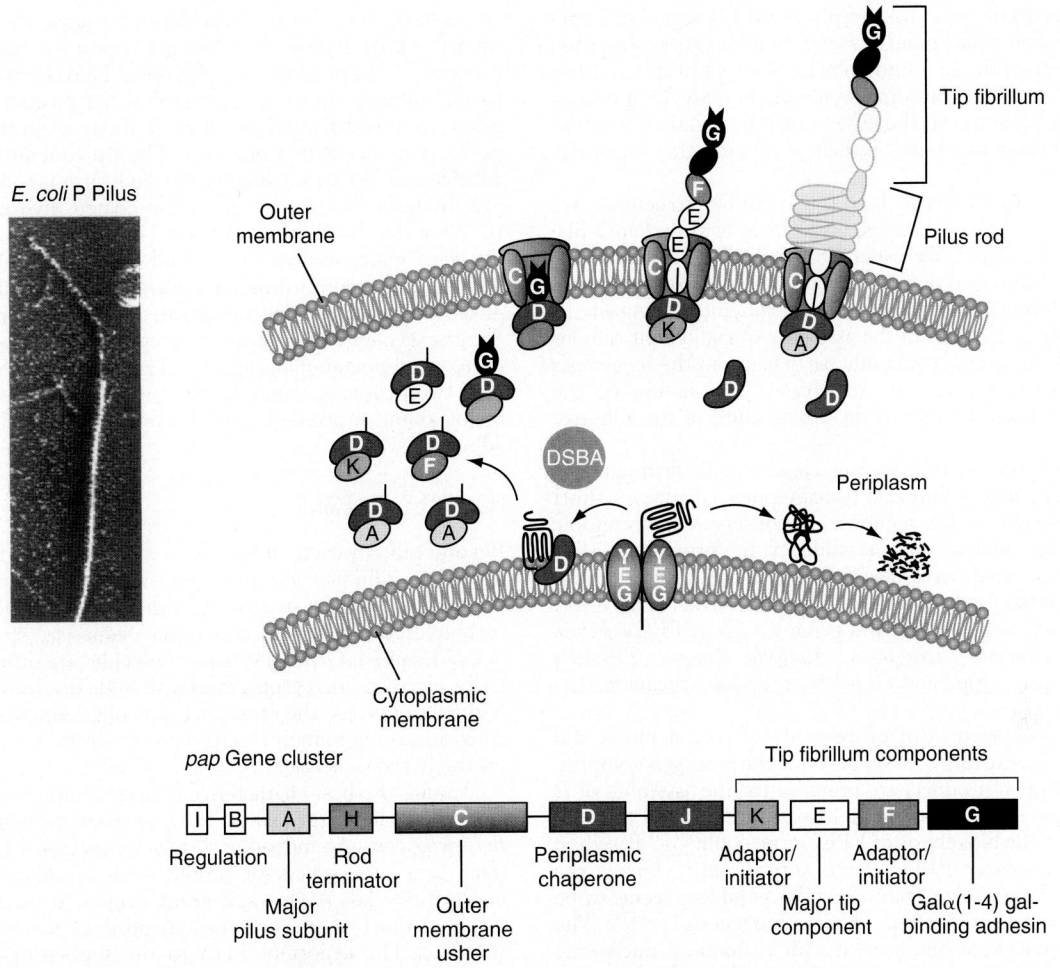

Figure 1–1 Biogenesis and structure of *Escherichia coli* P pili. The *pap* gene cluster and the function of each of the gene products are indicated in the lower portion of the figure. Nascent pilin subunits are complexed with the PapD chaperone and added to the base of the developing pilus via the PapC usher. The mature pilus rod is composed of repeating units of PapA; the tip fibrillum contains the adhesin PapG. The ultrastructure of the pilus is shown in the electron micrograph at the left side of the figure. DSBA, disulfide oxidoreductase that resides in the periplasm; YEG, sec machinery that facilitates protein export from the cytoplasm to the periplasm. *(Courtesy of S. J. Hultgren and F. J. Sauer.)*

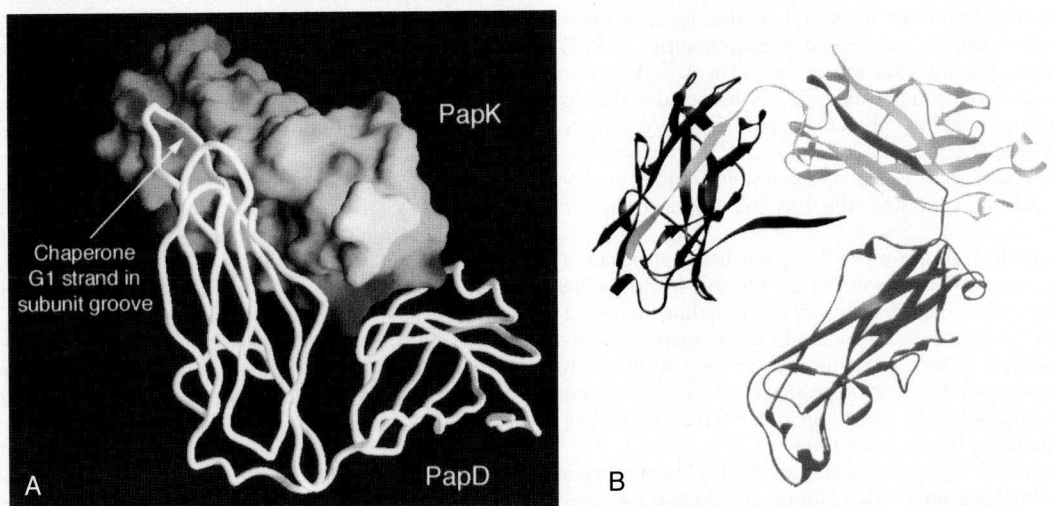

Figure 1–2 A, The G1 strand of the PapD chaperone completes the immunoglobulin-like fold of the PapK pilin subunit (donor strand complementation). **B,** The mature P pilus rod comprises a helix (3.28 subunits per turn) of repeating PapA subunits; each subunit is completed by a strand donated by its neighbor. *(Courtesy of S. J. Hultgren and F. J. Sauer.)*

recently added to the pilus base) replaces the G1 strand of PapD in a process called *donor strand exchange*. In the mature pilus, each subunit completes the immunoglobulin-like fold of its neighbor (see Fig. 1–2B).[117] The PapA major subunit employs an intramolecular "hinge" first to exit the usher vertically and then to adopt its final conformation within the helical cylinder that forms the pilus fiber.[176]

More than 30 different bacterial adhesive structures are assembled via the chaperone-usher pathway with a PapD-like chaperone and a PapC-like usher. These PapD-like chaperones can be divided into two distinct subfamilies based on conserved structural differences that occur near the subunit binding site.[118] One subfamily is involved in the assembly of rodlike pili similar to P pili, and the second subfamily participates in the biogenesis of more atypical filamentous structures. The nature of the chaperone is linked directly to the architecture of the adhesive appendage.[239]

Type 4 pili represent a second class of pili, distinguished by a methylated first amino acid (usually phenylalanine), a short positively charged leader sequence, a conserved hydrophobic amino terminal domain, and a tendency to form bundle-like structures. Type 4 pili have been identified in numerous gram-negative bacterial pathogens, including *Neisseria gonorrhoeae*, *Neisseria meningitidis*, enteropathogenic *E. coli* (EPEC), *Vibrio cholerae*, *Pseudomonas aeruginosa*, *Kingella kingae*, *Eikenella corrodens*, *Moraxella* spp., and *Dichelobacter nodosus* (formerly *Bacteroides nodosus*).*

Although the mechanism of assembly of type 4 pili is still being elucidated, existing data suggest that the process is complex. Twenty to 40 gene products are required for the assembly of *P. aeruginosa* type 4 pili, and at least 15 plasmid-encoded proteins are involved in the biogenesis of EPEC type 4 pili.[107,247] Based on studies of *P. aeruginosa*, EPEC, *Neisseria* spp., and *V. cholerae*, the presence of an inner membrane pre-pilin peptidase seems to be a general prerequisite for type 4 pilus biogenesis.[132,144,186] The involvement of at least one protein with a canonical nucleotide binding domain is another common feature. Many of the other proteins required for type 4 pilus assembly resemble proteins from filamentous phage biogenesis systems and DNA uptake and transfer systems, suggesting that similar transport and assembly mechanisms are used.[108,221] More recent evidence indicates that type 4 pili often are glycosylated, with carbohydrate decoration affecting function in at least some cases and perhaps serving to obscure antigenic epitopes.[26,157,234,268]

Despite marked differences in the assembly pathways for type 4 pili and P pili, examination by electron microscopy suggests that, in some cases, significant structural similarities may exist. Gonococcal type 4 pili are composed predominantly of PilE structural subunits polymerized into a helical rod.[195] A minor phase-variable adhesive protein called PilC is displayed at the tip of the pilus and is essential for pilus-mediated binding to epithelial cells.[127,220] These observations suggest that *N. gonorrhoeae* pili may be composite structures with a tip-associated adhesin, analogous to P pili and other pili assembled by the chaperone-usher pathway.

Although adhesive pili are more prevalent in gram-negative bacteria, they also are found in some gram-positive species. One example is *Streptococcus parasanguis*, an oral pathogen and a member of the sanguis streptococcal family. This organism binds to calcium phosphate (the primary mineral component of tooth enamel) and to other oral bacteria, epithelial cells, platelets, and fibronectin. Several adhesins, including pili referred to as *long fimbriae*, mediate these binding functions.

Based on studies of *S. parasanguis* strain FW213, long fimbriae are fashioned primarily from Fap1, a 200-kd protein that includes

an unusually long (50 amino acids) signal sequence and a cell wall sorting signal typical of other gram-positive bacterial surface proteins.[283,284] Specific glycosylation of Fap1 seems to be critical to the adhesive function of this fimbrial protein.[246] Similar to gram-negative bacterial pili, long fimbriae seem to have a composite structure with a pilus tip. The tip contains an additional adhesin called FimA, which in purified form is capable of blocking bacterial adherence to saliva-coated hydroxyapatite.[61,191] In work by Burnette-Curley and coworkers,[23] disruption of the *fimA* gene resulted in a 7-fold to 20-fold reduction in the incidence of endocarditis after intravenous inoculation of rats. A second gram-positive organism capable of expressing pili is *Streptococcus agalactiae* (group B streptococcus), a common cause of neonatal pneumonia, sepsis, and meningitis. In *S. agalactiae*, at least two genomic islands encode pilus components, including a major pilin, a pilus-associated anchor, and a pilus-associated adhesin.[55,219]

NON-PILUS ADHESINS

Beyond pili, a variety of non-pilus adhesins exist. In most cases, non-pilus adhesins are proteinaceous and are monomeric or oligomeric surface structures, although isolated examples of carbohydrate and lipid-containing adhesive structures have been identified. Generally, these molecules are difficult to visualize by electron microscopy, even with high-resolution techniques. Similar to pili, for the most part non-pilus adhesins can be classified according to their mechanism of secretion and presentation on the bacterial surface.

Among the best characterized bacterial non-pilus adhesins is filamentous hemagglutinin (FHA), a surface protein expressed by *Bordetella pertussis* and other *Bordetella* species. FHA is synthesized as a large precursor protein with a calculated molecular mass of 367 kd. A cleavage event occurs to eliminate the C-terminal third of the protein and produce the mature 220-kd species.[52] The export of FHA to the surface of the organism occurs via the so-called two-partner secretion pathway, a conserved strategy in which a secreted (TpsA) protein interacts, via specific determinants within its N-terminus, with a cognate outer membrane transporter (TpsB).[109] In *B. pertussis*, the TpsA-type protein FHA is transported by a TpsB-type outer membrane protein called *FhaC*, which has β-barrel pore-forming properties and facilitates translocation of FHA across the outer membrane.[279] Homologous TpsB proteins in other species include those that export the hemolysins of *Serratia marcescens*, *Proteus mirabilis*, and *Haemophilus ducreyi*; the *Haemophilus influenzae* heme:hemopexin binding protein (HxuA); and the *H. influenzae* HMW1 and HMW2 adhesins, among others.[7,36,194,207,264] Although crystallographic data are lacking, the C-terminal portion of FhaC is predicted to form a β-barrel pore in the outer membrane, whereas the FhaC N-terminus may participate in specific recognition of FHA on the periplasmic side.[167]

Examination of purified FHA by transmission electron microscopy and circular dichroism spectroscopy showed that the FHA molecule is 50 nm in length and adopts the shape of a horseshoe nail. It has a globular head, a 37 nm long shaft that averages 4 nm in width but tapers slightly from the head end, and a small flexible tail (Fig. 1–3).[130,156] In the crystal structure of the N-terminus of FHA (the so-called two-partner secretion domain that interacts with FhaC), a series of 19-residue repeat motifs forms a β-helix that is central to the overall structure of full-length FHA (see Fig. 1–3).[30]

Consistent with its large size, FHA contains at least four separate binding domains, three of which have been localized. The region involved in adherence to sulfated saccharides has been mapped to the N-terminus of the FHA molecule.[170] Sulfated saccharides, such as heparin and heparan sulfate, are major components of mucus and extracellular matrix in the respiratory tract

---

*See references 59, 78, 160, 172, 208, 214, 228, 249, 260, 272.

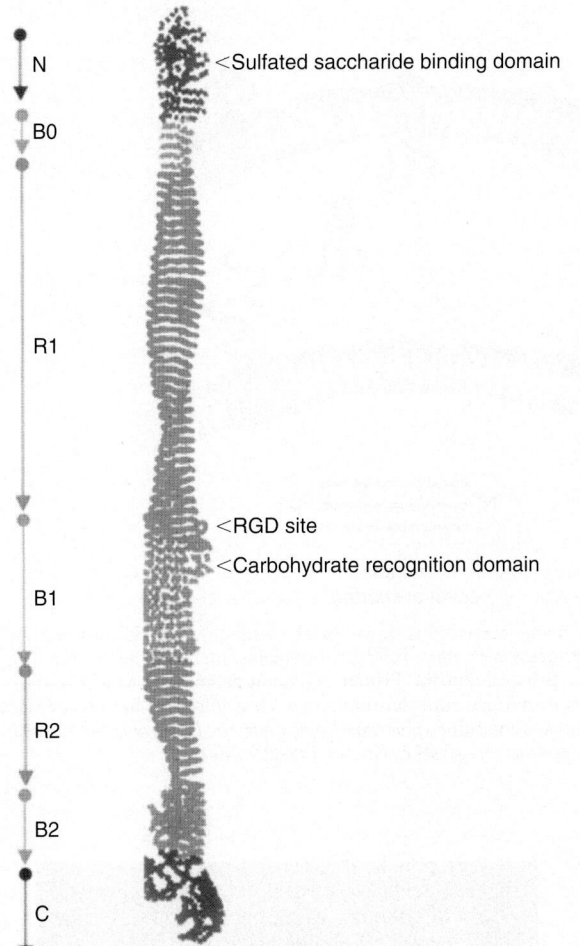

Figure 1–3 Ribbon representation model structure of filamentous hemagglutinin from *Bordetella pertussis*. There are five regions that are assigned β-helical coils, designated B0, R1, B1, R2, and B2. The N-terminus of the protein is designated with "N," and the C-terminus of the protein is designated with "C." The locations of the sulfated saccharide binding domain, the carbohydrate recognition domain, and the arginine-glycine-aspartic acid (RGD) tripeptide are noted. (See companion Expert Consult web site for color version.) *(From Kajava, A. V., Cheng, N., Cleaver, R., et al.: Beta-helix model for the filamentous haemagglutinin adhesin of* Bordetella pertussis *and related bacterial secretory proteins. Mol. Microbiol. 42:279-292, 2001.)*

and are found on the surface of epithelial cells.[162,287] The region that recognizes lactosylceramides and promotes adherence to ciliated respiratory epithelial cells and macrophages has been localized to amino acids 1141 to 1279 (the carbohydrate recognition domain).[209] An arginine-glycine-aspartic acid (RGD) tripeptide is located at amino acids 1097 to 1099 and interacts with leukocyte response integrin, a leukocyte integrin that stimulates up-regulation of complement receptor type 3 (CR3).[122] Finally, FHA recognizes CR3 (CD11b/CD18), allowing organisms to be ingested by macrophages without stimulating an oxidative burst.[215,282] The location of the CR3-binding domain is unknown.

A growing number of non-pilus adhesins belong to the so-called autotransporter family. These proteins are synthesized as precursor proteins with three functional domains: an N-terminal canonical signal sequence, an internal passenger domain, and a C-terminal outer membrane domain. The signal sequence directs the protein to the Sec machinery and is cleaved after it facilitates transport of the polypeptide from the cytoplasm to the periplasm.

The C-terminal domain inserts into the outer membrane and forms a β-barrel with a central hydrophilic channel. Ultimately, the passenger domain is presented on the surface of the organism and influences interaction with host molecules.[100]

More recent studies have established that autotransporter proteins can be separated into two distinct groups, designated *conventional autotransporters* and *trimeric autotransporters* (Fig. 1–4).[42] In conventional autotransporters, the C-terminal outer membrane domain contains roughly 300 amino acids and is a monomeric β-barrel with a single N-terminal α-helix spanning the pore (Fig. 1–5A).[192,252] In trimeric autotransporters, the C-terminal outer membrane domain contains approximately 70 amino acids and forms heat-resistant, detergent-resistant trimers in the outer membrane. Each trimer forms a β-barrel with four strands from each of the three subunits and with three N-terminal α-helices spanning the pore (see Fig. 1–5B).[168]

An example of a conventional autotransporter adhesin is the *H. influenzae* Hap protein, which was discovered based on its ability to promote adherence and low-level invasion in assays with cultured epithelial cells.[240] Hap also promotes bacterial binding to extracellular matrix proteins and bacterial microcolony formation.[63,101] Examination of chimeric proteins and studies with purified protein have shown that the adhesive activity responsible for Hap-mediated adherence, invasion, binding to extracellular matrix proteins, and microcolony formation localizes to the passenger domain, referred to as Hap$_S$.[63,101] More detailed characterization of Hap$_S$ has established that the region responsible for interaction with host epithelial cells and microcolony formation resides in the C-terminal 311 amino acids and may have utility as a vaccine antigen.[44,62,151] A prototype member of the trimeric autotransporter subfamily is the *H. influenzae* Hia adhesin. This protein is expressed in a subset of nontypeable *H. influenzae* strains and contains two homologous high-affinity trimeric binding domains, creating the potential for stable multivalent interaction with respiratory epithelial cells.[143,288]

Another group of non-pilus adhesins is typified by intimin, a protein expressed by EPEC, enterohemorrhagic *E. coli*, and the murine pathogen *Citrobacter rodentium*. Intimin contains a flexible N-terminus, a central β-barrel domain that integrates into the outer membrane, and a C-terminal binding domain that interacts with the translocated intimin receptor (Tir).[261] Tir is synthesized by the bacterium, translocated into the host cell cytoplasm via the EPEC type III secretion system,[134,281] and inserted into the host cell membrane, a process that has been modeled in vitro.[212]

The interaction between intimin and Tir triggers a series of host cell events, resulting in receptor clustering, dramatic rearrangement of the actin cytoskeleton, and formation of a distinctive pedestal referred to as an attaching and effacing (A/E) lesion (Fig. 1–6).[134,218] All of the genes essential for formation of A/E lesions are present within a 35-kb region of the EPEC chromosome termed the *locus of enterocyte effacement*, an example of a pathogenicity island.[53,163] This locus is highly conserved in content and organization across all A/E pathogens and contains the genes that encode intimin, Tir, and the EPEC type III secretion system, with a total of 41 open reading frames overall.

In recent years, investigators have identified a large family of non-pilus adhesins involved in adherence to host extracellular matrix proteins, including fibronectin, laminin, vitronectin, collagen, fibrinogen, and a variety of proteoglycans. These adhesins have been classified as *microbial surface components recognizing adhesive matrix molecules* (MSCRAMMs) and are especially prevalent among gram-positive bacteria.[199] In gram-positive organisms, these adhesins are covalently anchored to the cell wall peptidoglycan and have a characteristic primary amino acid sequence. In particular, the carboxy-terminus contains a segment rich in proline and glycine residues, an LPXTG motif (involved in sorting the protein to the cell wall), a hydrophobic

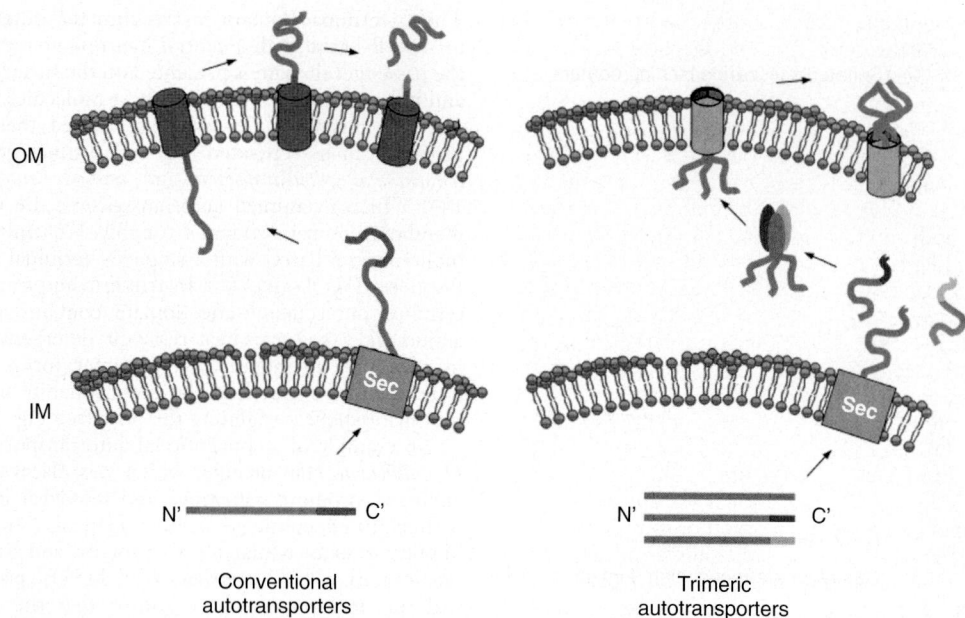

OM

IM

Sec

N'   C'

Conventional
autotransporters

Sec

N'   C'

Trimeric
autotransporters

Figure 1–4 Autotransporter protein secretion pathway. Conventional autotransporter secretion is shown on the left, and trimeric autotransporter secretion is shown on the right. Autotransporter proteins are synthesized as preproteins with three functional domains, including an N-terminal signal sequence, an internal passenger domain, and a C-terminal outer membrane β-barrel domain. Protein secretion begins with export of the protein from the cytoplasm via the inner membrane Sec machinery (Sec). Most conventional autotransporters are cleaved on the bacterial surface. IM, inner membrane; OM, outer membrane. (See companion Expert Consult web site for color version.) *(From Cotter, S. E., Surana, N. K., and St. Geme, J. W., III: Trimeric autotransporters: A distinct subfamily of autotransporter proteins. Trends Microbiol. 13:199-205, 2005.)*

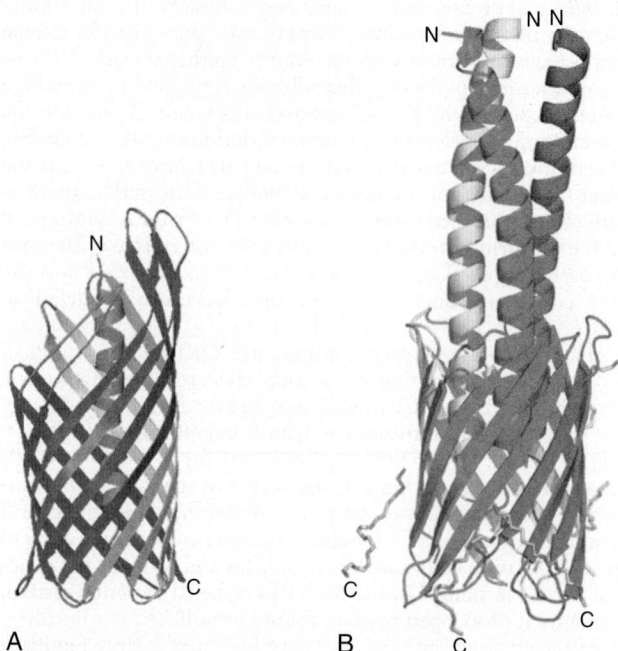

Figure 1–5 Crystal structures of the C-terminal outer membrane β-barrel of autotransporter proteins. **A,** Crystal structure of NalP, a conventional autotransporter. **B,** Crystal structure of Hia, a trimeric autotransporter. (See companion Expert Consult web site for color version.) *(A from Surana, N. K., Cotter, S. E., Yeo, H. J., et al.: Structural determinants of Haemophilus influenzae adherence to host epithelium: Variations on type V secretion. In Waksman, G., Caparon M., and Hultgren, S. [eds]: Structural Basis of Bacterial Pathogenesis. Washington, D.C., American Society for Microbiology, 2005, pp. 129-148. B from Meng, G., Surana, N. K., St. Geme, J. W., III, et al.: Structure of the outer membrane translocator domain of the Haemophilus influenzae Hia trimeric autotransporter. EMBO J. 25:2297-2304, 2006.)*

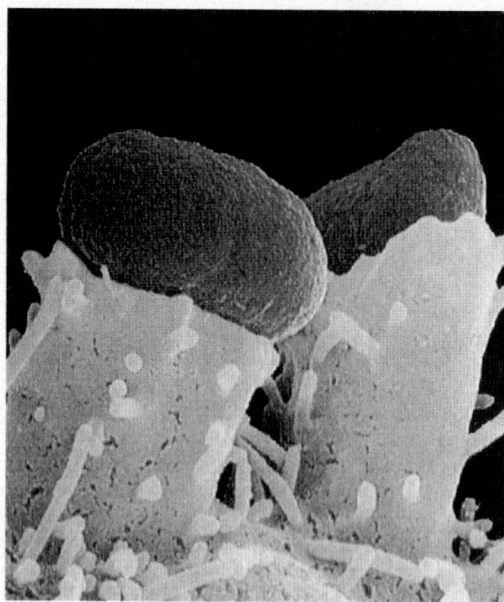

Figure 1–6 Enteropathogenic *E. coli* are perched on pedestals in the attaching and effacing lesion. *(Courtesy of B. B. Finlay; from Rosenshine, I., Ruschkowski, S., Stein, M., et al.: A pathogenic bacterium triggers epithelial signals to form a functional bacterial receptor that mediates actin pseudopod formation. EMBO J. 15:2613-2624, 1996.)*

membrane-spanning domain, and a short, positively charged segment that resides in the cytoplasm and serves as a cell wall retention signal. Adhesive functions typically are located near the N-terminus.[65]

Staphylococcus aureus is a common gram-positive pathogen in children and is capable of producing a variety of MSCRAMMs, including collagen-binding protein (Cna), fibronectin-binding protein A (FnBPA), and clumping factor (ClfA). Strains recovered from patients with septic arthritis commonly express Cna, which mediates binding to cartilage in vitro and seems to play a key role in the pathogenesis of septic arthritis in experimental mice.[198,200,253] The current model of Cna binding suggests that the two major domains (N1 and N2) and an intervening linker polypeptide together form a spherical "hole" through which the bound collagen fiber passes.[294] FnBPA shares homology with *Streptococcus pyogenes* protein F and mediates binding to fibronectin and the gamma chain of fibrinogen.[271] This protein likely is important in *S. aureus* infections of implanted biomaterials, which become coated with fibrinogen and fibrin soon after implantation. ClfA was named based on the observation that it mediates bacterial clumping in the presence of soluble fibrinogen.[164] Similar to FnBPA, ClfA mediates binding to fibrinogen-coated surfaces in vitro and probably contributes to infections of artificial surfaces. The active domain of ClfA is designated region A and contains two amino acid residues (E526 and V527) shown more recently to mediate binding to soluble fibrinogen.[95] The crystal structure of region A shows an immunoglobulin-like fold common to other *S. aureus* MSCRAMMs.[49] Vaccination with ClfA was shown to protect against subsequent development of septic arthritis and death in a mouse model of intravenous *S. aureus* infection.[128]

OTHER MECHANISMS OF ADHERENCE

Candida albicans is a common inhabitant of mucosal surfaces and an important cause of systemic disease, especially in patients with compromised immunity. *Candida* blastospores are capable of efficient adhesion to epithelial cells, leading to budding and division. In addition, germ tube formation occurs, facilitating penetration through the epithelial barrier and dissemination to distant sites.[114] In recent years, several candidate *C. albicans* adhesins have been identified.[8,113,149,290] Of particular interest is a protein called INT1, which shares functional homology with the vertebrate integrin family.

Integrins normally are expressed by cells of the human immune system (neutrophils, monocytes, macrophages) and mediate cellular binding and shape-changing functions. Each integrin is a heterodimer of an alpha chain and a beta chain. Many different alpha and beta chains have been identified, and each combination displays a unique binding specificity. INT1 is an α-integrin–like protein that recognizes the RGD sequence of the C3 fragment iC3b on epithelial cells. In in vitro assays, short peptides encompassing the RGD sequence are capable of inhibiting *C. albicans* adherence by 50 percent, confirming that INT1 plays a significant role as an adhesin and suggesting that other adhesins also exist.[114] Beyond promoting adherence to epithelium, INT1 disguises organisms as leukocytes, allowing evasion of phagocytosis. Introduction of INT1 into *Saccharomyces cerevisiae* confers a capacity for adherence and results in germ tube formation, indicating the importance of this protein in morphogenesis.[73,74]

The adhesive properties of *C. albicans* are tied closely to its morphologic state. Adherence to buccal epithelial cells is greater by organisms bearing germ tubes than by yeast forms.[138] With this information in mind, Staab and coworkers[243] searched a germ tube cDNA library and identified a putative adhesin called *hyphal wall protein 1* (Hwp1), encoded by the *hwp1* gene. Examination of the predicted amino acid sequence of Hwp1 revealed similarity to proteins that are substrates for mammalian transglutaminase enzymes. These enzymes form a cornified envelope on squamous epithelial cells (including buccal epithelial cells) by cross-linking relevant substrates.[244] The interactions of germ tubes with buccal epithelial cells resist stresses (e.g., heating or treatment with sodium dodecylsulfate [SDS]) capable of dissociating most typical microbe-host adhesive pairs, and elimination of expression of Hwp1 results in a marked reduction in adhesion to buccal epithelial cells.[18,242] Hwp1 represents a unique adhesive strategy, employing host transglutaminase enzymes to cross-link Hwp1 (via a glycosyl phosphatidylinositol remnant anchor) directly to surface proteins on buccal epithelial cells.[241]

TISSUE TROPISM

Most microorganisms show restriction in the range of hosts, tissues, and cell types that they colonize. This restriction is referred to as *tropism* and generally reflects the specificity of the interaction between a given microbial adhesin and its cognate receptor. Tropism is determined by the distribution of the relevant host receptor.

P pili of uropathogenic *E. coli* serve as the platform for presentation of one of three different PapG variants, referred to as class I, class II, and class III PapG. All three variants recognize globoseries glycolipids, but each binds with a distinct specificity to the globoseries glycolipid isotypes. Class I PapG preferentially recognizes globotriosylceramide (GbO3, Gal-α1,4-Gal-β1,3-Glc-ceramide); class II PapG preferentially recognizes globoside (GbO4, GalNAc-β1,3-Gal-α1,4-Gal-β1,3-Glc-ceramide); and class III PapG preferentially interacts with Forssman antigen (GbO5, GalNAc-α1,3-GalNAc-β1,3-Gal-α1,4-Gal-β1,3-Glc-ceramide).[250] Globoside is the dominant globoseries glycolipid expressed in human kidney, and most human isolates of *E. coli* associated with pyelonephritis express class II PapG. In contrast, Forssman antigen is the most abundant globoseries glycolipid in dog kidney, and more than 50 percent of canine urinary isolates of *E. coli* express class III PapG.[286] *E. coli* expressing P pili with class II PapG are not found as a cause of urinary tract infection in dogs. The specificity of the PapG variant at the tip of the P pilus influences host range, favoring infection of either human or dog.

The crystal structure of class II PapG bound to Gal-α1,4-Gal was solved by Dodson and coworkers,[51] uncovering the structural basis of PapG binding specificity. The PapG receptor binding site is located on the side of the molecule and must be oriented with its N-terminal to C-terminal axis parallel to the host cell membrane to allow docking to the receptor. This orientation may be facilitated by the flexibility inherent in the tip fibrillum. The PapG binding site consists of two regions. The first forms a β-barrel, and the second is composed of a central antiparallel β-sheet that is flanked on one side by two 2-stranded β-sheets and on the other side by an α-helix. When class II PapG interacts with GbO4, the arginine residue at position 170 in PapG makes contact with the GbO4 side chain. In class I PapG, a histidine residue occupies position 170, interfering with potential contact with the GbO4 side chain. Similarly, class II PapG and class III PapG differ in amino acids required for interaction with the GbO5 side chain.[51]

Group A streptococcus (*S. pyogenes*) is a common cause of infections of skin and soft tissue, including impetigo, cellulitis, and necrotizing fasciitis. Adherence to host cells by *S. pyogenes* is influenced by non-pilus adhesins called *M protein* and *protein F*. M protein forms a fiber and consists of a C-terminal region that anchors the protein in the cell wall, a coiled-coil rod region extending approximately 50 nm from the cell wall, and a short non-helical domain extending more distally.[64] Protein F is a 120-

kd protein that is notable for a tandem repeat element consisting of six repeats of 32 to 44 amino acids adjacent to the C-terminus.[93,193] Based on experiments with a series of isogenic strains that differ in expression of M protein or protein F or both, M protein clearly promotes adherence to human keratinocytes via interaction with the CD46 molecule (also called *membrane cofactor protein*), whereas protein F mediates adherence to epidermal Langerhans cells, which are located in the basal layer of the epidermis.[189,190] M protein and protein F contribute to group A streptococcal adherence to the skin, but each protein directs interaction with a different population of epidermal cells.

Early studies showed that human immunodeficiency virus type 1 (HIV-1) infects CD4+ cells and interacts with the CD4 molecule, but that CD4 alone is insufficient to permit infection. More recent observations have established that numerous host cell chemokine receptors, especially CCR5 and CXCR4, serve as co-receptors for HIV-1 and are required for viral entry into CD4+ target cells. These co-receptors seem to influence the cellular tropism displayed by different HIV-1 variants.[48] All HIV variants are able to replicate in primary T cells, but only some also can replicate in primary macrophages or in immortalized T-cell lines. Asymptomatic HIV-infected individuals carry strains that generally use CCR5 as a co-receptor (termed M5 strains) and are non–syncytium-inducing in vitro. Such strains traditionally have been described as macrophage tropic (M-tropic), but more recent experiments have shown that these M5 strains also can infect CD4+ T cells and peripheral blood mononuclear cells.[205] Rapid viral mutation caused by the error-prone HIV polymerase and HIV reverse transcriptase leads to the production within the host of syncytium-inducing, T cell–tropic (T-tropic) HIV-1 strains, which predominate in the circulation of patients with acquired immunodeficiency syndrome.[48] These variants generally are restricted to CXCR4 (expressed on T cells) as a co-receptor, although some primary syncytium-inducing variants can use CCR5 and CXCR4.[54,60,233] T-tropic, syncytium-inducing strains are characterized by positively charged residues at fixed positions of the V3 loop and changes in charge and length of the V2 region of the viral envelope glycoprotein gp120, which binds to CD4 and co-receptors before viral entry into host cells occurs.[66,67,86] Cellular tropism is closely aligned, but not synonymous, with HIV co-receptor usage.

New HIV-1 infection is selectively established by M-tropic HIV-1 strains, even if the transmitting host harbors more pathogenic non–M-tropic strains as well.[265,292] CCR5 also is expressed on the surface of rectal and vaginal epithelial cells, which may be sites of initial encounter between HIV-1 and the human host.[291] The importance of CCR5 in HIV-1 binding to CD4+ cells is underscored by the observation that individuals homozygous for a 32-bp deletion in CCR5 (the Δ32 allele) are resistant to infection with HIV-1.[116,152] The Δ32 heterozygous state does not protect against acquisition of HIV-1, although HIV disease in heterozygous patients may follow an attenuated course.

This allele is found frequently (10 to 14 percent) in white populations, leading to speculation that it provided a survival advantage during one or more historical epidemics of infectious diseases.[185] More recent data suggest, however, that the Δ32 allele may confer immunodeficiency in the face of challenge with certain viral pathogens, such as West Nile virus.[79,80] CCR5 may have a role in controlling the development of malignancy, including lymphoma, raising some concern about developing anti-HIV pharmacologic agents that target CCR5 function.[146] Finally, co-evolution of viral determinants and host cell receptors may determine the spectrum of tissue and organ involvement within the host. The chemokine receptor CCR8 may facilitate the entry of neurotropic HIV-1 strains into brain cells,[126] and envelopes derived from brain isolates of HIV are adapted to infect cells with low-level CD4/CCR5 expression, such as neuroglia and brain macrophages.[204]

BIOFILMS

After attachment to a particular surface, many pathogens are capable of forming *biofilms*—structured communities of microbial cells enclosed in a self-produced exopolysaccharide matrix.[210] Although most studies of biofilms have involved a single species, it is likely that biofilms relevant to human infection often involve multiple species sharing the advantages of biofilm existence. Human infections associated with biofilms include dental caries, lower airway infection with *P. aeruginosa* in patients with cystic fibrosis, and foreign body infection in patients with prostheses and implanted devices. In addition, formation of biofilms likely occurs during osteomyelitis and endocarditis.[39]

P. aeruginosa is a model organism for the study of biofilms; it forms pillars of stationary (sessile) bacteria held together by an extracellular polysaccharide called *alginate*. Interposed among these pillars are channels that facilitate the flow of nutrients and provide pathways for motile (planktonic) organisms to move about (Fig. 1–7A). In experiments directed at defining the early steps of *P. aeruginosa* biofilm formation, O'Toole and Kolter[187] established that flagella are required for initial bacterial attachment, presumably because these appendages promote movement toward the relevant surface (see Fig. 1–7A). After attachment occurs, type 4 pili and pilus-mediated twitching motility promote formation of microcolonies. In the context of microcolonies, transcription of *algC*, *algD*, and *algU* is activated, resulting in synthesis of alginate.[46] The alternative sigma factor σ22 positively regulates the *alg* genes and negatively regulates expression of flagella. Consistent with this observation, pulmonary isolates from patients with cystic fibrosis often are highly mucoid (reflecting expression of alginate) and lack flagella.[71,76]

Development of the complex community present within a biofilm requires intercellular communication. In the case of *P. aeruginosa*, this communication occurs via the LasR-LasI *quorum sensing* system, which involves the acyl-homoserine lactone called *N*-(3-oxododecanoyl)-L-homoserine lactone (3OC12-HSL).[47,196] 3OC12-HSL is synthesized in a reaction catalyzed by LasI and accumulates with increases in population density. Ultimately, 3OC12-HSL reaches a critical concentration and then interacts with LasR, serving to activate transcription of numerous genes. Host inflammatory pathways also are induced directly by accumulated 3OC12-HSL.[238] Organisms with a mutation in *lasI* are capable of attachment and microcolony formation, but the resulting microcolonies remain thin, undifferentiated, and sensitive to dispersion by detergents. Addition of the missing lactone signal to the *lasI* mutant restores development into structured, thick, biocide-resistant biofilms, analogous to biofilms observed with wild-type organisms.[47] Mutation in *lasI* impedes establishment of pulmonary infection in mice.[202,285]

Biofilms constitute a protected mode of growth that allows survival in a hostile environment, such as in the presence of host immune mechanisms or antimicrobial agents.[39] Based on studies of *P. aeruginosa*, sessile bacteria release antigens and stimulate production of antibodies, but these antibodies are ineffective in killing organisms within biofilms.[31] Similarly, sessile *P. aeruginosa* stimulate a diminished oxidative burst and are refractory to phagocytic uptake. In addition, organisms within biofilms are resistant to the effects of many antibiotics—in part because antibiotic agents are unable to diffuse through the biofilm, in part because these bacteria may exist in a slow-growing state, and possibly because these organisms adopt a distinct and protected phenotype.[39] Progress in understanding the mechanisms by which biofilms develop, such as the solution of the

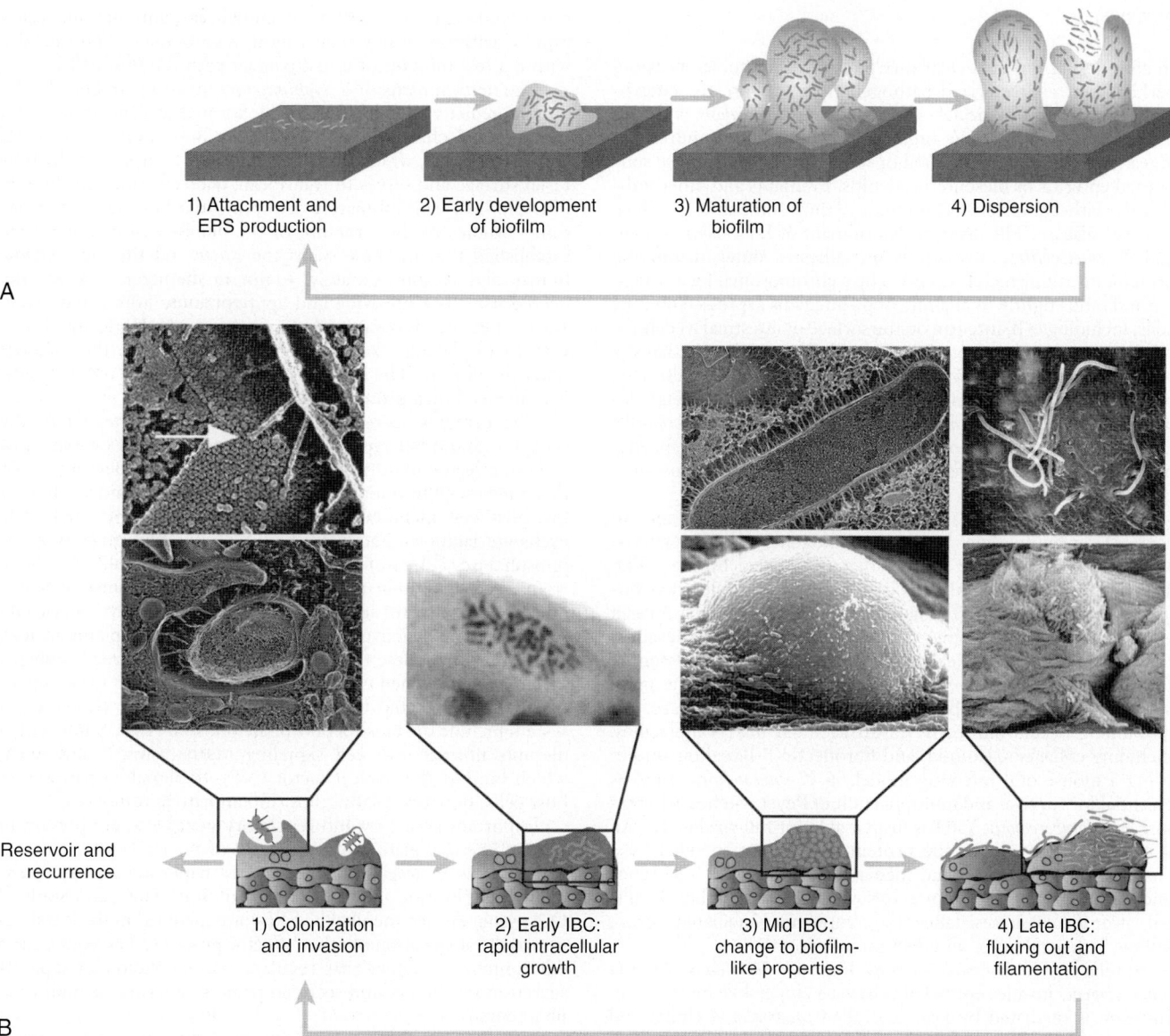

Figure 1–7 In vitro *Pseudomonas* biofilm formation and parallel stages of formation of uropathogenic *Eschericha coli* intracellular bacterial communities [IBCs]. **A,** Dynamics of *Pseudomonas aeruginosa* biofilm formation on an inert surface. Keys to the formation of the biofilm include flagella-mediated attachment, type 4 pilus-based twitching motility, and a quorum sensing system. **B,** Composite representation of the stages of IBC formation and maturation. EPS, exopolysaccharide. (See companion Expert Consult web site for color version.) (*A adapted from Kau, A. L., Hunstad, D. A., and Hultgren, S. J.: Interaction of uropathogenic* Escherichia coli *with host uroepithelium. Curr. Opin. Microbiol. 8:54-59, 2005. B from Costerton, J. W., Stewart, P. S., and Greenberg, E. P.: Bacterial biofilms: A common cause of persistent infections. Science 284:1318-1322, 1999. Copyright 1999 American Association for the Advancement of Science.*)

LasI crystal structure,[84] are likely to yield novel approaches to antimicrobial therapy, aimed at disrupting biofilm formation or persistence.

INVASION, INTRACELLULAR SURVIVAL, AND CELL-TO-CELL SPREAD

After adherence to a host surface occurs, many pathogenic organisms are able to invade and survive inside epithelial cells and other non-professional phagocytes (e.g., M cells in intestinal Peyer patches). In addition, some pathogens are able to survive inside professional phagocytes (macrophages and neutrophils). Invasion may represent a mechanism to breach host mucosal barriers and gain access to deeper or more distant tissues. Alternatively,

invasion may provide the organism with a special niche, protected from the host's immune mechanisms. Generally, the process of invasion involves a class of molecules called *invasins*, which mediate microbial adherence and entry. Invasion is an active event that relies on underlying host cell functions and is associated with rearrangement of the host cell cytoskeleton. When inside the host cell, the invading or ingested organism usually is localized within a membrane-bound vacuole that contains lysosomal enzymes. In some cases, the pathogen escapes from this vacuole and enters the cytoplasm, a more permissive environment. In others, the pathogen remains in the vacuole and neutralizes lysosomal enzymatic activity. The processes of invasion into cells, survival within cells, cell-to-cell spread, and entry into the circulation define the extent of infection and dissemination.

INVASION

In considering the molecular mechanisms of microbial invasion, perhaps best characterized pathogenic bacteria are the entero-pathogenic *Yersinia* species—*Yersinia pseudotuberculosis* and *Yersinia enterocolitica*. These organisms usually are acquired by ingestion of contaminated food or water and typically cause self-limited enteritis or mesenteric adenitis. In infants and other individuals with compromised immunity, they sometimes produce systemic disease. The primary determinant of *Y. pseudotuberculosis* and *Y. enterocolitica* invasion is an adhesive outer membrane protein, invasin, which is encoded by a chromosomal locus called *inv* and binds tightly to a family of β$_1$-integrins expressed on host cells, including α$_3$β$_1$ integrin on the surface of intestinal M cells.[121] The interaction between invasin and β$_1$-integrins initiates a cascade of signaling steps in the host cell, resulting in actin rearrangement and formation of large complexes of cytoskeletal elements (e.g., talin, vinculin, α-actinin) called *focal adhesions*.[120] Bacterial entry into the host cell occurs via a "zipper-like" mechanism, with the plasma membrane zippering around the invading organism.

Beyond invasin, two additional proteins called YadA and Ail also influence invasion by enteropathogenic *Yersinia* species. YadA is a 45-kd surface protein that is encoded by the 70-kb *Yersinia* virulence plasmid. It is highly expressed under environmental conditions (e.g., temperature of 37° C) in which invasin is repressed.[57] YadA reaches the bacterial surface via the auto-transporter pathway and exists in a trimeric form that is essential for its adhesive activity.[41] Similar to invasin, YadA promotes invasion through binding to β$_1$-integrins on the host cell surface, but its binding occurs indirectly via extracellular matrix molecules, including collagens, laminin, and fibronectin.[58] Based on studies using a mouse oral infection model, in *Y. enterocolitica*, YadA is essential for survival and multiplication in Peyer patches, whereas in *Y. pseudotuberculosis*, YadA is dispensable for full virulence.[17] Ail is a 17-kd outer membrane protein that also is encoded by a chromosomal locus (*ail*) and mediates high levels of adherence and low levels of invasion in assays with cultured epithelial cells. Ail also mediates resistance to complement-mediated serum killing, independent of an effect on invasion.[14]

Similar to *Y. enterocolitica* and *Y. pseudotuberculosis*, *Listeria monocytogenes* invades epithelial cells via a zipper-like mechanism. Invasion is mediated by proteins called *internalin A* (InlA) and *internalin B* (InlB), which are required for virulence in animal models. InlA interacts with E-cadherin, a host cell transmembrane protein with an intracellular domain that interacts with the cytoskeleton.[169] InlB interacts with C1q on host cells and promotes invasion by activating the PI-3 kinase pathway.[19] Uropathogenic strains of *E. coli* also invade epithelial cells via a zipper-like mechanism, mediated by the FimH adhesin expressed on the tip of type 1 pili. In experiments with cultured bladder epithelial cells, FimH is necessary and sufficient for entry, as shown by examination of a *fimH*$^-$ mutant and of latex beads coated with purified FimH.[161] In vitro experiments suggest further that FimH-mediated bacterial binding to a mannose-coated surface is strengthened by shear forces, such as fluid flow over the surface.[257,258] After FimH-dependent invasion into superficial epithelial cells of the murine bladder occurs, uropathogenic *E. coli* multiply rapidly to form intracellular bacterial communities, which display some features of biofilms (see Fig. 1–7B).[5,129,131] Bacteria derived from this intracellular niche ultimately form a quiescent bacterial reservoir within the epithelium, possibly serving as a seed for recurrent infections.[179]

Salmonella enterica serovar Typhimurium (*S. typhimurium*) is an example of a pathogen that invades cells by a mechanism distinct from zippering. On contact with the epithelial cell surface, *S. typhimurium* triggers a dramatic host cell response characterized by actin rearrangement, calcium and inositol phosphate fluxes, and membrane ruffling. Bacterial entry into the cell occurs rapidly, with organisms appearing in membrane-bound vacuoles within a few minutes of initial contact with the host cell.

The determinants of *S. typhimurium* invasion are encoded by a pathogenicity island called SPI-1, located at centisome 63 on the bacterial chromosome.[72] Especially important is a type III secretion system, which forms a needle-like complex on the bacterial surface and serves to translocate bacterial proteins directly into the host cell, ultimately disrupting the host cell cytoskeleton.[33] Studies of the structure of the needle-like complex have established that the base spans the inner and the outer membranes and is approximately 40 nm in diameter, whereas the needle itself is 8 nm wide and approximately 80 nm long (Fig. 1–8).[35] The base is composed of proteins PrgH, PrgK, and InvG, with InvG playing a key role in pore formation in the bacterial outer membrane. The needle is composed of PrgI, and its length is influenced by a protein called InvJ.[139,140]

The proteins secreted through the *S. typhimurium* needle complex (and other type III secretion systems) and into the host cell are referred to as *effector proteins*. SopE is an effector protein that mediates the initial rearrangement of actin and ruffling of the host cell membrane. It functions as a guanyl-nucleotide exchange factor and activates two host cell Rho guanosine triphosphatase (GTPase) proteins called Rac and Cdc42.[28,92,94] SptP is an effector protein that functions as an antagonist of SopE, mediating reversal of actin rearrangement by converting Rac and Cdc42 to the inactive forms (guanosine diphosphate forms). Consistent with these functions, SopE and SptP directly antagonize each other when co-injected into Ref52 cells.[70] Other effector proteins secreted by the *S. typhimurium* type III secretion system include the inositol phosphate phosphorylase SopB, which disrupts normal host cell signaling mechanisms,[184] and AvrA, which inhibits the nuclear factor (NF)-κB signaling pathway in host cells, down-regulating host inflammatory responses.[34]

Important accessory and regulatory genes also are present in SPI-1. The *sicA* gene is just upstream of the *sipB* and *sipC* genes and encodes an accessory protein with chaperone activity essential for stabilization and translocation of SipB, SipC, and SopE.[263] Other chaperones encoded by SPI-1 are involved in the stabilization and translocation of other effector proteins. The genetic and environmental factors that regulate the expression of type III secretion machinery and secreted proteins also are beginning to be understood.[4]

INTRACELLULAR SURVIVAL

When an organism invades a non-professional phagocyte or is ingested by a professional phagocyte, there are several potential outcomes. Often, the organism is killed. Some pathogens have developed strategies to survive and replicate inside host cells, however, in some cases within a vacuole and in others by escaping from the vacuole.

General agreement is that *S. typhimurium* resides within a membrane-bound vacuole in professional and non-professional phagocytes. The vacuole lacks several lysosomal markers typical of the main endocytic pathway (the mannose-6-phosphate receptor pathway), however, and seems to be distinct from this pathway. Insight into the molecular determinants of intravacuolar survival came in 1996, when two independent groups reported the discovery of a second *Salmonella* pathogenicity island, now called *SPI-2*.[102,188] This island maps to centisome 31 and encodes another type III secretion system, including structural proteins (*ssa* locus),[102] effector proteins (*sse* locus), and accessory proteins (*ssc* locus). In addition, this region encodes a two-component regulatory system consisting of proteins SsrA (formerly SpiR) and SsrB. SsrA is a membrane-located sensor kinase, and SsrB is a transcriptional regulator.[188] Mutations in SPI-2 result in reduced

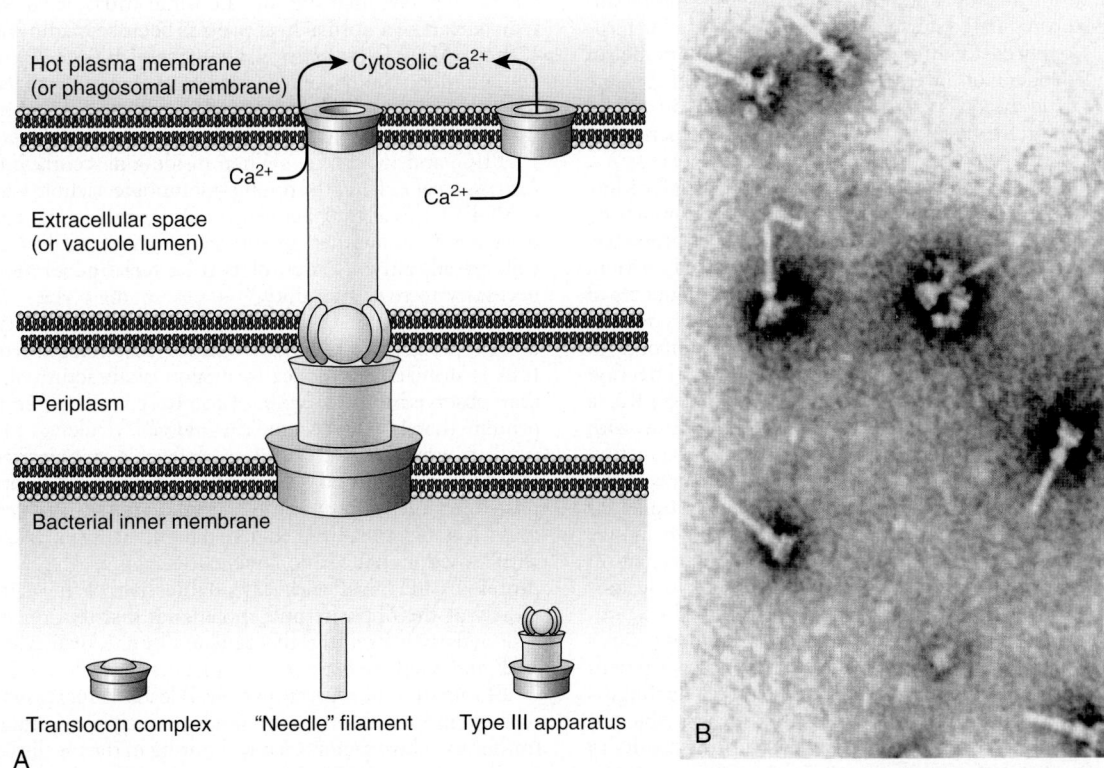

Figure 1–8 A, General structure of the gram-negative type III secretion system, represented schematically. **B,** Appearance on electron micrograph of isolated needle complexes from the *Salmonella* type III secretion system. (*A from Coombes, B. K., and Finlay, B. B.: Insertion of the bacterial type III translocon: Not your average needle stick. Trends Microbiol. 13:92-95, 2005. B courtesy of J. E. Galan; from Kubori, T., Matsushima, Y., Nakamura, D., et al.: Supramolecular structure of the* Salmonella typhimurium *type III protein secretion system. Science 280:602-605, 1998. Copyright 1998 American Association for the Advancement of Science.*)

survival inside macrophages, with no effect on adherence and invasion in assays with intestinal epithelial cells.[188]

Salmonella SPI-2 mutants show reduced virulence in experimental mice (10^4-fold reduction in 50 percent lethal dose), suggesting that survival inside macrophages is a key factor in the pathogenesis of disease.[229] Expression of SPI-2 genes within the macrophage vacuole depends at least partly on the acidic intravacuolar environment. Inhibition of macrophage vacuolar acidification using bafilomycin A1 (an inhibitor of the vacuolar proton adenosine triphosphatase [ATPase]) results in a sharp attenuation in transcription of SPI-2 genes. This effect is not reproduced by low pH alone outside the vacuole, suggesting that other environmental effects within the vacuole play a role.[29] More recent work indicates that *Salmonella* SPI-2 transcription is activated before invasion occurs, apparently preparing the pathogen for the hostile intracellular environment.[21] As a group, the SPI-2 genes seem to modulate host endocytic and exocytic transport mechanisms.[1]

A third *Salmonella* pathogenicity island called *SPI-3* also influences survival inside macrophages. This island is located at centisome 82 and was discovered by examining the *Salmonella selC* locus, a tRNA gene in which pathogenicity islands reside in some strains of *E. coli*.[10,12] SPI-3 contains the *mgtBC* operon, which permits *S. typhimurium* to grow in environments with low concentrations of Mg^{2+}, including macrophages. In particular, mutation of the *mgtBC* operon abolishes the ability of *S. typhimurium* to replicate in low Mg^{2+} liquid media and in macrophages, and addition of Mg^{2+} to the medium after phagocytosis restores the ability to survive intracellularly. Homologous *mgtBC* genes have been found in other organisms with intracellular lifestyles, such as *Brucella melitensis* and *Yersinia pestis*.[11] In *Salmonella*, the *mgtBC* genes are expressed after internalization into host cells occurs

under control of the PhoP-PhoQ two-component regulatory system, a complex that directs expression of many virulence determinants.[158]

The ability to survive within phagocytic cells may provide *Salmonella* with a means to exploit an intrinsic host pathway and disseminate to distant sites. In particular, certain phagocytes express the β_2-integrin CD18, which mediates leukocyte migration in response to various stimuli. During *S. typhimurium* infection, CD18-expressing phagocytes transfer organisms from the intestine to the spleen. Bacterial loads in the liver and spleen are reduced after oral inoculation in CD18-deficient mice, compared with infection in wild-type mice.[266] On the one hand, this function of CD18 facilitates initiation of a systemic immune response and benefits the host. On the other hand, it provides bacteria with a mechanism of transit from the gut to organs of the reticuloendothelial system and elsewhere.

Mycobacterium tuberculosis, another intracellular pathogen, uses an array of mechanisms to ensure intracellular survival. The *M. tuberculosis* vacuole lacks the usual amounts of the vesicular proton ATPase responsible for mediating acidification and fails to acidify to normal levels.[251] In addition, *M. tuberculosis* blocks fusion of the vacuole with acidic lysosomes, further preventing acidification.[222] Similar to intracellular gram-negative bacterial pathogens, *M. tuberculosis* contains an *mgtC* gene, and mutation of this gene results in impaired virulence in cultured human macrophages and in mouse spleen and lung. Low Mg^{2+} concentration and mildly acidic pH inhibit the growth of the *mgtC* mutant, suggesting that the gene is important for survival in the phagosome, where such conditions may exist.[22]

Another factor that influences *M. tuberculosis* survival within macrophages is isocitrate lyase, an enzyme of the glycolytic shunt that is essential for metabolism of fatty acids. Expression of iso-citrate lyase is up-regulated during infection of activated macrophages and is required for full virulence in a murine model of infection, independent of an effect on bacterial growth.[165] The structure of *M. tuberculosis* isocitrate lyase has been solved and may provide a target for new drug therapies against persistent infection because this enzyme is absent from vertebrates.[227,235]

During interaction with macrophages, *M. tuberculosis* (at a low to moderate multiplicity of infection) is capable of stimulating caspase-1 and inducing macrophage apoptosis. This process may be beneficial to the host, preventing systemic spread of infection; less virulent strains of *M. tuberculosis* are more potent inducers of apoptosis.[133] At the same time, *M. tuberculosis* possesses at least two anti-apoptotic mechanisms that influence the outcome of macrophage encounters further. First, *M. tuberculosis* infection enhances host macrophage production of soluble TNFR2, a protein that binds to tumor necrosis factor–α and interferes with apoptosis.[6] Second, *M. tuberculosis* infection activates production of NF-κB, a transcriptional regulator that activates anti-apoptotic pathways within the host cell.[75] Higher multiplicities of infection with virulent strains of *M. tuberculosis* can induce caspase-independent cell death in macrophages, a mechanism proposed to contribute to the formation of necrotic lesions during tuberculosis disease.[147]

Listeria monocytogenes is an example of an organism that escapes from the phagocytic vacuole in macrophages and epithelial cells and moves into the cytoplasm. This organism causes meningitis and focal brain abscesses in humans and has a predilection for the fetoplacental unit. In pregnant women, listeriosis results in fetal loss in 30 percent of cases. Escape from the vacuole is mediated primarily by listeriolysin O, a hemolysin encoded by the *hly* gene. Listeriolysin O interacts with cholesterol in host cell membranes and forms pores, leading to lysis of the phagosome.[69] Mutants defective in *hly* fail to survive intracellularly and are avirulent in mice,[267] although vacuolar escape of *hly* mutants within human cells may be complemented by other bacterial enzymes. Additional factors that contribute to escape from the phagosome include two phospholipase C molecules, one with broad-range specificity (PC-PLC) and another with phosphatidylinositol specificity (PI-PLC). In human epithelial cells, the contributions of PC-PLC and a metalloproteinase called Mpl are most important for vacuolar escape in the absence of listeriolysin O.[87,159,236]

CELL-TO-CELL SPREAD

Movement from one cell to another may help an organism gain a stronger foothold in host tissues. *L. monocytogenes* is one example of a pathogen capable of cell-to-cell spread. When this organism is free in the cytoplasm, actin begins to polymerize on the bacterial surface. Eventually, the condensed actin forms a polar tail or comet, which propels the organism through the cytoplasm and into adjacent cells. The rate of bacterial movement within a cell correlates with actin tail length.[255] Actin accumulation and condensation is mediated by the *L. monocytogenes* ActA protein, which is tightly anchored to the bacterial surface and is expressed asymmetrically over the length of the organism.[237,254] ActA is the sole *Listeria* factor required for actin polymerization because actin tails form in *Xenopus* cytoplasmic extracts containing ActA-coated beads. In these experiments, motility occurs, however, only when ActA is distributed asymmetrically on the beads.[24] ActA seems to interact directly with actin and with a variety of other host cytoskeletal proteins.[69,256] Cytochalasin D is an inhibitor of actin polymerization and inhibits the cell-to-cell spread of *L. monocytogenes* in epithelial monolayers.[45,174]

On reaching the plasma membrane, bacteria protrude from the cell in filipodium-like structures (called listeriopods),

which are engulfed by neighboring cells. This engulfment may be part of a normal host process because madin darby canine kidney (MDCK) cells show low-level endocytosis of adjacent cell membrane fragments even in the absence of bacteria.[217] The formation of listeriopods and the engulfment of these structures by neighboring cells are independent of listeriolysin O, PI-PLC, and PC-PLC.[77] When inside a nascently infected cell, *Listeria* escapes from the double-membrane vacuole via the action of PI-PLC, PC-PLC, and Mpl.[69] On arrival in the cytosol, bacteria can enter another cycle of actin-based motility and cell-to-cell spread, although one or two bacterial generations may be necessary to regain motility.[217]

A second pathogen capable of actin-based motility and cell-to-cell spread is *Shigella flexneri*. In *Shigella*, a single protein called IcsA is sufficient to induce formation of an actin tail, similar to that observed in *L. monocytogenes*. IcsA is an outer membrane protein that is encoded on the *Shigella* virulence plasmid and is distributed on the bacterial surface in a polarized fashion, possibly as a result of specialized machinery for autotransporter protein secretion near the poles of some gram-negative bacteria.[125] Initially, IcsA is distributed over the whole bacterial surface, with a predominance at one pole. Over time, a secreted bacterial protease called IcsP cleaves roughly half of the surface IcsA, mostly at the opposite pole, polarizing distribution further.[56,245] IcsP activity is itself tightly regulated by the virulence regulators VirF and VirB.[280]

Elimination of expression of IcsP leads to increased quantities of IcsA and increased actin-based motility, suggesting that IcsA (rather than host factors) is rate-limiting in the motility process.[232] Similar to ActA, IcsA is necessary and sufficient to induce polymerization of the actin tail, and the tail forms at the end where IcsA concentration is highest.[81] Despite the functional similarities between IcsA and ActA, no significant amino acid sequence homology exists between the two proteins. In contrast to ActA, no direct interaction between IcsA and actin has been shown, and IcsA is found throughout the actin tail, not only at the bacterial pole-actin tail junction.

Rickettsia spp. also are capable of actin-based motility and cell-to-cell spread. Based on examination of *Rickettsia rickettsiae*, *Rickettsia* move through the cytoplasm of infected cells 2.5 to 3 times more slowly than do *L. monocytogenes* and *S. flexneri*. In *Rickettsia conorii*, the actin tails seem to be anchored to the bacterial body in a parallel manner, differing from the actin tails in *Listeria* and *Shigella*, which are composed of much shorter actin filaments organized in a random branching network.[83] Details of the bacterial determinants of *Rickettsia* movement remain poorly defined.

DAMAGE TO THE HOST

Damage to host cells and host tissues represents a fundamental mechanism by which a pathogen is able to survive at a given site and then spread within a host. Generally, damage is induced by microbial toxins. Most toxins are released extracellularly and are capable of inducing damage at very low concentrations (exotoxins). Microbial attachment and invasion facilitate toxin delivery to target cells and target tissues and serve to enhance toxicity.

Historically, microbial toxins have been classified according to a variety of criteria, including cellular target of action (e.g., enterotoxins, leukotoxins, neurotoxins), mechanism of action (e.g., adenosine diphosphate [ADP]–ribosylating toxins, adenylate cyclase toxins, pore-forming toxins, proteolytic toxins), and major biologic effect (e.g., hemolytic toxins, edema-producing toxins). In recent years, the term *toxin* has been applied more broadly to include enzymes that mediate damaging effects via phospholipase or hyaluronidase activity.

WHOOPING COUGH AND *BORDETELLA PERTUSSIS* TOXINS

Whooping cough (*B. pertussis* infection) is a classic example of a toxin-mediated disease and involves an interplay of multiple toxins.[135] The pathogenesis of whooping cough begins with *B. pertussis* colonization of the trachea, which is facilitated by a molecule called *tracheal cytotoxin* (TCT). TCT is a naturally occurring disaccharide-tetrapeptide fragment of peptidoglycan and belongs to the family of muramyl peptides.[82] Many gram-negative organisms produce an analogous fragment during normal turnover of cell wall components, but significant extracellular release apparently occurs only in *Bordetella* spp. and gonococci. In most species, an inner membrane protein called AmpG recycles this fragment back into the bacterial cell.[40] More recent crystal structures of TCT in complex with *Drosophila* pathogen pattern recognition receptors offer insight into the specific recognition of TCT via its unique diaminopimelic acid moiety, in contrast to other muramyl peptides.[27,150] TCT is toxic to tracheal epithelial cells in vitro, stimulating nitric oxide synthase and local production of interleukin-1 and causing inhibition of ciliary motility, inhibition of DNA synthesis, and cell death.[97-99,104] During natural infection, TCT likely paralyzes the mucociliary escalator and interferes with clearance of *B. pertussis* and respiratory mucus.

Beyond TCT, *B. pertussis* elaborates a toxin called *adenylate cyclase toxin* (CyaA), which has pore-forming activity and inhibits adenylate cyclase, resulting in accumulation of cyclic adenosine monophosphate (cAMP). In phagocytic cells, the elevated levels of cAMP inhibit oxidative activity and induce apoptosis, disabling this arm of the immune system.[136,137,203] In respiratory epithelial cells, the elevated levels of cAMP may result in increased fluid and mucus secretion, impairing mucociliary function further. Adenylate cyclase toxin has homology to many other bacterial calcium-dependent, pore-forming toxins known as *RTX toxins* (named because of a repeat found in each toxin), with the prototype being the *E. coli* HlyA hemolysin.[40] These toxins create pores in the host cell plasma membrane, ultimately leading to host cell lysis. Among the family of RTX toxins, the general mechanism of pore formation and the predicted amino acid sequences are conserved, but target cell specificities differ.

Pertussis toxin is thought to be a key determinant of the clinical manifestations of whooping cough. This toxin belongs to a family of bacterial ADP-ribosyltransferase enzymes. The target of pertussis toxin is host cell G proteins, resulting in disruption of normal signaling processes. Many biological effects have been ascribed to pertussis toxin and include induction of lymphocytosis, stimulation of insulin release, sensitization to histamine, and disruption of phagocytic cell function; however, the specific relationship between the effects of pertussis toxin and the symptoms of whooping cough remains unclear.[105] *Bordetella parapertussis* is closely related to *B. pertussis* and produces a similar cough illness but fails to produce pertussis toxin because of mutations in the *ptx* promoter region.[180]

HEMOLYTIC-UREMIC SYNDROME AND SHIGA TOXINS

Numerous intestinal pathogens produce Shiga toxins, including *Shigella dysenteriae*, enterohemorrhagic *E. coli* (including *E. coli* O157:H7), and *Citrobacter freundii*, among others. Shiga toxins are classic A-B toxins, consisting of an A subunit that has toxic activity and five B subunits arranged in a pentameric ringlike structure that promotes binding to host cells and delivery of the A subunit. The B subunits interact with host cell globoseries glycolipids, especially the Pk trisaccharide moiety of globotriaosylceramide (GbO3). The A subunit is endocytosed by the host cell and traverses the cytoplasm in membrane-bound vesicles. Some of these vesicles fuse with lysosomes, resulting in degrada-

tion of toxin. Others travel in a retrograde fashion to the Golgi apparatus and the endoplasmic reticulum.[224] Within the endoplasmic reticulum, toxin binds to host 28S ribosomal RNA and cleaves a single adenine residue via N-glycosidase activity. Ultimately, this depurination event results in inhibition of protein elongation and cell death.[223]

In humans, *E. coli* O157:H7 is an important cause of hemorrhagic colitis and sometimes produces hemolytic-uremic syndrome. Infection begins with adherence to epithelial cells via intimin and other proteins encoded by the locus of enterocyte effacement, resulting in formation of attaching and effacing lesions analogous to the lesions observed in EPEC infection.[163] After adherence occurs, the organism releases Shiga toxin, which traverses the intestinal epithelial cell and enters the bloodstream.[2] Toxin circulates to distant organs and mediates damage via toxicity to endothelium. Diarrhea likely results from damage to endothelium in small mesenteric vessels, leading to ischemia and sloughing of the intestinal mucosa. The renal effects observed in human hemolytic-uremic syndrome arise from microvascular and glomerular damage with luminal occlusion by fibrin and platelets.[293] Hemolysis and thrombocytopenia likely develop as a consequence of microangiopathy.

Shiga toxins can be divided into two antigenically distinct groups, Stx1 and Stx2, which share 50 to 60 percent homology. Most isolates of *E. coli* O157:H7 recovered from patients with hemolytic-uremic syndrome express Stx2, and some express Stx1 as well.[145] Wadolkowski and colleagues[269] pretreated mice with antibodies against Stx1, Stx2, or both, and challenged these animals with an *E. coli* strain expressing Stx1 and Stx2. Consistent with the importance of Stx2, mice pretreated with antibodies against Stx2 (with or without antibodies against Stx1) were protected from severe disease, whereas 90 percent of mice pretreated with anti-Stx1 alone or anti-cholera toxin died. Pathologic examination of the kidneys showed acute renal tubular necrosis and not glomerular injury, however, suggesting that this model has deficiencies in mimicking human disease.

Understanding the interaction between Shiga toxins and human glycolipid receptors may lead to important therapeutic interventions to prevent hemolytic-uremic syndrome in children with enterohemorrhagic *E. coli* colitis.[96] One initial effort along these lines was a synthetic GbO3 analogue attached to silica particles (Synsorb Pk). Oral administration of this toxin binder did not reduce the severity of hemolytic-uremic syndrome in clinical trials.[262] A more recent strategy has been to express heterologously in nonpathogenic *E. coli* a modified lipopolysaccharide (LPS) containing a sugar moiety that is a mimic for GbO3.[197,206] Oral administration of such bacteria protects mice from subsequent infection with Shiga toxin–producing *E. coli*. Monoclonal antibodies to Shiga toxins have been designed for systemic administration, offering potential activity against toxin already absorbed from the gut; these agents show promising results in animal models of hemolytic-uremic syndrome.[177,230,231] All of these therapeutic strategies would depend on timely recognition of Shiga toxin–producing *E. coli* diarrhea; consequently, additional efforts are being directed at methods to establish this diagnosis early in the course of diarrheal illness.[155]

TISSUE-DEGRADING TOXINS

Numerous toxins have enzymatic activity and are capable of degrading tissue components. One example is hyaluronidase, which degrades hyaluronic acid, a repeating disaccharide glycosaminoglycan involved in cell motility, adhesion, and proliferation in normal hosts. Hyaluronic acid contains alternating *N*-acetylglucosamine and glucuronic acid moieties, connected by β linkages. It is prominent in extracellular matrix when cell turnover and tissue repair are prominent, such as in embryogenesis, wound healing, and carcinogenesis.[43] The primary host receptor for hyaluronic acid is CD44, which undergoes post-translational modification that varies according to host cell type. Interactions between hyaluronic acid and CD44 are crucial to T-cell and B-cell stimulation, growth of certain lymphoid malignancies, and propagation of certain inflammatory responses.[171]

In *S. pyogenes*, hyaluronidase is a 96-kd protein that is encoded by the *hylA* gene and is released extracellularly. It is proposed to promote invasion through cell layers and tissue planes and is considered one of several *S. pyogenes* spreading factors.[119] *S. pyogenes* also produces a thick "capsule" of hyaluronic acid that can interact with other host cellular and extracellular matrix proteins to contribute to tissue invasion by the organism. Other pathogens that produce a hyaluronidase include *S. agalactiae* (group B streptococcus), *Treponema pallidum*, *Candida*, *Entamoeba histolytica*, and *Ancylostoma braziliense*.[43]

EVASION OF IMMUNITY

To survive and replicate within the host, a pathogen must evade the host immune system. Initially, the organism must circumvent innate immune mechanisms, including mechanical forces, resident phagocytes, and complement activity. Over time, the organism also must overcome adaptive immunity, including the presence of specific antibodies.

ANTIPHAGOCYTIC FACTORS

As described earlier in this chapter, invasin-mediated entry into M cells plays an important role in the early stages of *Yersinia* infection. At the same time, evasion of phagocytosis is crucial to the pathogenesis of *Yersinia* disease. The ability to avoid phagocytosis depends on the *Yersinia* virulence plasmid, which encodes numerous proteins called Yops.[38,248] YopE and YopH interfere with ingestion by macrophages and neutrophils via slightly different mechanisms. YopE shares sequence homology with the *S. typhimurium* SptP protein and down-regulates all three of the Rho GTPases (Rho, Cdc42, and Rac), inhibiting actin rearrangement and blocking formation of membrane ruffles (lamellipodia) and spikes (filopodia).[13] YopH is a protein tyrosine phosphorylase that seems to act on a host cell cytosolic protein called Cas, interfering with recruitment of Rho, Cdc42, and Rac, and preventing formation of actin stress fibers, focal complexes, and focal adhesions.[9,13] YopJ is an acetyltransferase that covalently modifies and inactivates intermediate kinases in the mitogen-activated protein kinase and NF-κB signaling pathways, leading to host cell apoptosis.[178,289] Further elucidation of Yop mechanisms may lead to development of Yop inhibitors that abolish the antiphagocytic properties of this pathogen.

Shigella employs another strategy to induce apoptosis in phagocytic cells. This pathogen produces hemorrhagic enterocolitis and is an important etiology of bloody diarrhea in children. Infection begins with ingestion of organisms, which attach to intestinal M cells and cross the intestinal epithelium.[297] On entry into the subepithelial space, organisms are engulfed by resident macrophages and contained in membrane-bound vacuoles. They quickly escape from macrophage vacuoles, however, and move to the cytosol of the cell, where they induce apoptosis.[296] The mechanism of apoptosis involves a protein called IpaB, which is encoded by the *Shigella* virulence plasmid and is injected into host cell membranes via the *Shigella* type III secretion system.[15] Work by Hilbi and coworkers[106] has established that IpaB binds to cytosolic interleukin-1β converting enzyme (caspase-1), a cysteine protease that cleaves interleukin-1β to its active form. Caspase-1 is homologous to many other enzymes involved in cell death pathways, including ced-3 of *Caenorhabditis*

elegans. The *S. typhimurium* SipB protein shares homology with IpaB and induces apoptosis by interacting with caspase-1.[103] Insertion of IpaB into host membranes also may facilitate cell-to-cell spread.

EVASION OF COMPLEMENT ACTIVITY

S. pyogenes expresses at least three factors that interfere with host complement activity. Perhaps best known is M protein, which inhibits activation of the alternative complement pathway. This effect is mediated at least in part by the ability of M protein to bind complement factor H, a regulatory protein that inhibits assembly and accelerates decay of C3bBb. More recent studies indicate that serotype M1 and M57 strains express an extracellular protein called Sic (streptococcal inhibitor of complement-mediated lysis), which associates with human plasma proteins called *clusterin* and *histidine-rich glycoprotein* (HRG) and apparently blocks formation of the membrane attack complex (C5b-C9).[3] Studies of epidemic waves of M1 infection show that Sic undergoes significant variation over time, perhaps in response to the selective pressure associated with specific antibodies.[110,111,166] Nonpolar inactivation of *sic* results in reduced mucosal colonization of mice.[153] In addition, *S. pyogenes* produces a serine protease called *C5a peptidase*, which cleaves and inactivates C5a.[278] C5a is a cleavage product of C5 and serves as a powerful chemoattractant for neutrophils. C5a peptidase serves to attenuate the neutrophil response to streptococcal infection.

N. gonorrhoeae is a common cause of cervicitis, urethritis, and pelvic inflammatory disease and is capable of producing disseminated disease. Fresh clinical isolates of *N. gonorrhoeae* typically are resistant to complement-mediated killing, and resistance to complement likely is important in the pathogenesis of disease. Resistance is due in part to sialylation of lipo-oligosaccharide, which involves addition of host-derived cytidine monophospho-*N*-acetylneuraminic acid (CMP-NANA) by a bacterial sialyltransferase. Given the requirement for CMP-NANA, subcultivation in the absence of human serum or human neutrophils is associated with loss of sialylation and loss of resistance. Sialylated lipo-oligosaccharide binds factor H, resulting in down-regulation of activity of the alternative pathway C3 convertase. In addition, sialylated lipo-oligosaccharide interferes with neutrophil phagocytosis and with the normal oxidative burst in neutrophils.[216,277]

A second determinant of resistance to complement-mediated killing is Por1, an outer membrane porin protein that binds factor H and C4b binding protein (C4b BP).[213] C4b BP binds C4b and serves to inhibit assembly and accelerate decay of C4b2a, the classical pathway C3 convertase. Gonococci express a third factor that influences resistance to complement: an outer membrane protein called AniA (for anaerobically induced protein A), which has been shown to be a copper-containing nitrite reductase.[16,25]

EVASION OF HUMORAL IMMUNITY

Numerous pathogens have evolved mechanisms to vary surface-exposed immunogenic molecules, facilitating evasion of a specific antibody response. *Antigenic variation* represents one such mechanism and is characterized by the emergence of modified molecules with novel antigenic properties. *Phase variation* is a second mechanism and is typified by the reversible loss or gain of a given molecule or structure.

N. gonorrhoeae is capable of producing recurrent infection, reflecting the fact that the antibody response to infection fails to provide lasting immunity. In this context, *N. gonorrhoeae* pili are an important target of serum antibody and undergo frequent antigenic variation. Gonococcal pilin expression is controlled by the *pilE* locus (the expression locus), which contains an intact pilin gene along with promoter sequences. In addition to *pilE*, the gonococcal chromosome contains numerous copies of variant *pil* sequences, called *pilS* loci.[90] These loci are transcriptionally inactive because they lack a promoter and 5′ coding sequence. They can be introduced into the expression locus by RecA-dependent recombination, however, resulting in an altered structural subunit and antigenically variant pili.[115] Because *N. gonorrhoeae* is naturally transformable, horizontal exchange of species-related DNA possibly also contributes to the generation of new *pil* sequences.

The African trypanosomes (including *Trypanosoma brucei*) cause sleeping sickness in sub-Saharan Africa and account for more than 50,000 deaths per year. These organisms avoid humoral immunity by antigenic variation of a large family of proteins called *variable surface glycoproteins* (VSGs), which coat the entire surface of the trypanosome. VSGs are highly immunogenic and stimulate antibodies that lead to efficient and rapid clearing of parasites from the bloodstream. At any given point in time, the organism is able to express a new VSG, however, allowing some organisms to escape the antibody response against the previous VSG.

Each parasite can express more than 100 different VSGs, with variation in expression occurring spontaneously at a rate of 10^{-2} per cell per generation. Overall, the genome of *T. brucei* contains more than 1000 *vsg* genes, including so-called expression sites located near telomeres on mini-chromosomes and silent loci in non-telomeric sites on large chromosomes.[201,259] Generally, VSG antigenic variation occurs by two different mechanisms. The first is termed *in situ activation* and involves the simultaneous activation of a new expression site and inactivation of the old expression site, occurring independent of DNA rearrangement. The second involves DNA recombination, either between the expressed *vsg* and another telomeric expression site (reciprocal recombination) or between the expressed *vsg* and a silent *vsg* locus (gene conversion).[259]

In the case of *H. influenzae*, LPS likely is a key factor in facilitating colonization and is a major target of the antibody response to infection. *H. influenzae* LPS undergoes phase variation. LPS biosynthesis involves multiple enzymatic steps and numerous genes. Among these genes, *lic1A*, *lic2A*, *lic3A*, *lex-2*, *lgtC*, and an *oafA*-like gene contain long stretches of tandem 4-bp repeats within their 5′ coding region. In studies of the *lic* loci, Weiser and coworkers[273] observed that the number of repeats varies spontaneously, generating translational frame shifts with different ATG start codons falling in or out of frame. Such frame shifts result in synthesis of a protein with a different N-terminus or eliminate protein production altogether (when no in-frame start codon exists).

The mechanism of variation in repeat number is presumed to be slipped-strand mispairing, which occurs during DNA replication and involves a single repeat looping out on either the template or the replicating strand. Changes in *lic2A* and *lic3A* influence glycotransferase activity and alter reactivity with monoclonal antibodies directed against specific LPS oligosaccharide epitopes.[88] The *lic2A* gene product is responsible for the addition of a Gal-α1,4-Galβ moiety, which resembles the globoseries glycolipids and protects *H. influenzae* from antibody-mediated killing, possibly by molecular mimicry.[274] *lgtC* may be involved in formation of a Gal-β1,4-Glu moiety.[112] Variation in the *lic1A* gene affects production of a choline kinase responsible for addition of phosphorylcholine (ChoP) to the LPS molecule, a physical change that enhances binding of C-reactive protein and results in susceptibility to serum bactericidal activity.[154,275,276] Expression of *lex2* results in addition of a tetrasaccharide (Gal-α1,4-Gal-β1,4-Glc-β1,4-Glc) to the proximal heptose in LPS and increases resistance to complement-mediated serum killing.[85] Similarly, expression of the *oafA*-like gene results in LPS O-acetylation, which facilitates resistance to serum killing.[68]

ENCAPSULATION

Expression of an extracellular capsule is a common strategy to evade phagocytosis, complement activity, and humoral immunity among pathogenic bacteria, fungi, and parasites. One example is *H. influenzae*, a common cause of childhood bacteremia and meningitis in underdeveloped countries. Among isolates of *H. influenzae*, six structurally and antigenically distinct capsular types are recognized, designated serotypes a to f. Historically, serotype b isolates have accounted for greater than 95 percent of all *H. influenzae* invasive disease, reflecting the distinct virulence properties of the type b capsule, which is a polymer of ribose and ribitol-5-phosphate (PRP) and is encoded by the *cap*b locus.[175] In animal studies comparing derivatives of *H. influenzae* strain Rd expressing type a, b, c, d, e, or f capsule, the strain expressing the type b capsule was associated with the highest incidence of bacteremia after intranasal inoculation of infant rats. Similarly, this strain was associated with the highest magnitude of bacteremia and incidence of meningitis after intraperitoneal inoculation of experimental rats.[295]

In considering the mechanism by which the type b capsule promotes intravascular survival and invasive disease, in vitro studies using mouse peritoneal macrophages and human peripheral blood monocytes provide some insights. Based on work by Noel and colleagues,[183] the type b capsule has been shown to inhibit bacterial binding to macrophages in the absence of complement and a source of C3. In addition, the type b capsule interferes with ingestion by macrophages when anti-PRP antibody is lacking.[182,183] The type b capsule blocks complement deposition on the bacterial surface and resultant complement-mediated bacteriolysis. In almost all isolates of *H. influenzae* type b, the *cap*b locus is a tandem repeat of 18-kb *cap*b gene sequences.[181] As a consequence of this arrangement, the *cap*b locus serves as a template for further amplification of capsule gene sequences in vivo, resulting in increased capsule production. In a study by Corn and associates,[37] 23 of 66 minimally passaged invasive isolates had three to five copies of the 18-kb repeat. Further analysis showed that amplification of the repeat results in augmented resistance to phagocytosis and complement-mediated bacterial killing.[181]

Given the importance of the type b capsule in the pathogenesis of disease, efforts to develop a vaccine effective against *H. influenzae* type b focused on the type b polysaccharide, initially as a plain polysaccharide vaccine and eventually as a conjugate vaccine with the polysaccharide linked to an immunogenic carrier protein. Since routine immunization with conjugate vaccines has been implemented in developed countries, the incidence of invasive *H. influenzae* type b disease in these countries has plummeted.

VIRAL LATENCY

Among viral pathogens, latency represents an important mechanism for viral persistence in the face of host immunity, especially in the case of viruses belonging to the herpes family. Herpes simplex virus is one example, commonly establishing latency after gingivostomatitis and genital tract infection. After infection of a host cell occurs, herpes simplex virus replication commences. Eventually cell death occurs, resulting in cell lysis and release of viral particles, which can infect adjacent cells. This so-called lytic replication is under control of a few *immediate early* (IE) genes, which must be transcribed in moderate amounts to allow expression of the remainder of the viral genome.

IE gene expression is activated by VP16, a viral protein that binds to a sequence common to IE gene promoters.[211] After lysis of the host cell, new virions enter local nerve termini and travel up the long axon to sensory ganglia, where latency is established within days. In the latent state, viral DNA can be detected in the neuron, but infectious virions cannot be isolated. During latency, IE genes are repressed, and only one small fragment of viral DNA is actively transcribed, yielding the latency-associated transcript (LAT). No protein product has been attributed to the LAT; instead, more recent work has shown the production of a micro-RNA, transcribed from exon 1 of LAT, which maintains latency by directly inhibiting transforming growth factor–β signaling and promoting survival of infected cells.[89] LAT-deficient mutants are still able to establish initial latency, however, suggesting that IE gene expression may be under multiple controls.[270] The mechanism by which herpes simplex virus is reactivated seems to involve the viral thymidine kinase (TK) gene because TK⁻ mutants are defective in lytic replication and ordinarily do not reactivate.[32,124] Although a detailed understanding of reactivation is lacking, other viral genes suspected to support reactivation are being studied.[91,173]

CONCLUSION

With the explosion in the development of molecular techniques in recent years, understanding of the specific microbial and host factors involved in the pathogenesis of a variety of infectious diseases has expanded remarkably. As a consequence of this understanding, numerous new vaccines have been developed, including the *H. influenzae* type b and acellular pertussis vaccines. In the coming years, we likely will benefit from novel approaches for treating and preventing human infections. Possible examples might include inhibitors of type III protein secretion systems, antagonists of periplasmic chaperones, and analogues of important host cell receptors. Given the impressive adaptability of pathogenic organisms, however, as new therapeutic agents become available, we must remain vigilant for new microbial strategies allowing evasion of our interventions.

REFERENCES

1. Abrahams, G. L., and Hensel, M.: Manipulating cellular transport and immune responses: Dynamic interactions between intracellular *Salmonella enterica* and its host cells. Cell. Microbiol. *8*:728-737, 2006.
2. Acheson, D. W., Moore, R., De Breucker, S., et al.: Translocation of Shiga toxin across polarized intestinal cells in tissue culture. Infect. Immun. *64*:3294-3300, 1996.
3. Akesson, P., Sjoholm, A. G., and Bjorck, L.: Protein SIC, a novel extracellular protein of *Streptococcus pyogenes* interfering with complement function. J. Biol. Chem. *271*:1081-1088, 1996.
4. Altier, C.: Genetic and environmental control of *Salmonella* invasion. J. Microbiol. *43*(Spec. No.):85-92, 2005.
5. Anderson, G. G., Palermo, J. J., Schilling, J. D., et al.: Intracellular bacterial biofilm-like pods in urinary tract infections. Science *301*:105-107, 2003.
6. Balcewicz-Sablinska, M. K., Keane, J., Kornfeld, H., et al.: Pathogenic *Mycobacterium tuberculosis* evades apoptosis of host macrophages by release of TNF-R2, resulting in inactivation of TNF-α. J. Immunol. *161*:2636-2641, 1998.
7. Barenkamp, S. J., and St. Geme, J. W., III: Genes encoding high-molecular-weight adhesion proteins of nontypeable *Haemophilus influenzae* are part of gene clusters. Infect. Immun. *62*:3320-3328, 1994.
8. Barki, M., Koltin, Y., Yanko, M., et al.: Isolation of a *Candida albicans* DNA sequence conferring adhesion and aggregation on *Saccharomyces cerevisiae*. J. Bacteriol. *175*:5683-5689, 1993.
9. Black, D. S., and Bliska, J. B.: Identification of p130Cas as a substrate of *Yersinia* YopH (Yop51), a bacterial protein tyrosine phosphatase that translocates into mammalian cells and targets focal adhesions. EMBO J. *16*:2730-2744, 1997.
10. Blanc-Potard, A. B., and Groisman, E. A.: The *Salmonella selC* locus contains a pathogenicity island mediating intramacrophage survival. EMBO J. *16*:5376-5385, 1997.
11. Blanc-Potard, A. B., and Lafay, B.: MgtC as a horizontally-acquired virulence factor of intracellular bacterial pathogens: Evidence from molecular phylogeny and comparative genomics. J. Mol. Evol. *57*:479-486, 2003.
12. Blanc-Potard, A. B., Solomon, F., Kayser, J., et al.: The SPI-3 pathogenicity island of *Salmonella enterica*. J. Bacteriol. *181*:998-1004, 1999.
13. Bliska, J. B.: Yop effectors of *Yersinia* spp. and actin rearrangements. Trends Microbiol. *8*:205-208, 2000.
14. Bliska, J. B., and Falkow, S.: Bacterial resistance to complement killing mediated by the Ail protein of *Yersinia enterocolitica*. Proc. Natl. Acad. Sci. U. S. A. *89*:3561-3565, 1992.
15. Blocker, A., Gounon, P., Larquet, E., et al.: The tripartite type III secreton of *Shigella flexneri* inserts IpaB and IpaC into host membranes. J. Cell. Biol. *147*:683-693, 1999.
16. Boulanger, M. J., and Murphy, M. E.: Crystal structure of the soluble domain of the major anaerobically induced outer membrane protein (AniA) from pathogenic *Neisseria*: A new class of copper-containing nitrite reductases. J. Mol. Biol. *315*:1111-1127, 2002.
17. Boyd, A. P., and Cornelis, G. R.: *Yersinia. In* Groisman, E. A. (ed): Principles of Bacterial Pathogenesis. San Diego, Academic Press, 2001, pp. 227-264.
18. Bradway, S. D., and Levine, M. J.: Do proline-rich proteins modulate a transglutaminase catalyzed mechanism of candidal adhesion? Crit. Rev. Oral Biol. Med. *4*:293-299, 1993.
19. Braun, L., Nato, F., Payrastre, B., et al.: The 213-amino-acid leucine-rich repeat region of the *Listeria monocytogenes* InlB protein is sufficient for entry into mammalian cells, stimulation of PI 3-kinase and membrane ruffling. Mol. Microbiol. *34*:10-23, 1999.
20. Breimer, M. E., and Karlsson, K. A.: Chemical and immunological identification of glycolipid-based blood group ABH and Lewis antigens in human kidney. Biochim. Biophys. Acta *755*:170-177, 1983.
21. Brown, N. F., Vallance, B. A., Coombes, B. K., et al.: *Salmonella* pathogenicity island 2 is expressed prior to penetrating the intestine. PLoS Pathog. *1*:e32, 2005.
22. Buchmeier, N., Blanc-Potard, A., Ehrt, S., et al.: A parallel intraphagosomal survival strategy shared by *Mycobacterium tuberculosis* and *Salmonella enterica*. Mol. Microbiol. *35*:1375-1382, 2000.
23. Burnette-Curley, D., Wells, V., Viscount, H., et al.: FimA, a major virulence factor associated with *Streptococcus parasanguis* endocarditis. Infect. Immun. *63*:4669-4674, 1995.
24. Cameron, L. A., Footer, M. J., van Oudenaarden, A., et al.: Motility of ActA protein-coated microspheres driven by actin polymerization. Proc. Natl. Acad. Sci. U. S. A. *96*:4908-4913, 1999.
25. Cardinale, J. A., and Clark, V. L.: Expression of AniA, the major anaerobically induced outer membrane protein of *Neisseria gonorrhoeae*, provides protection against killing by normal human sera. Infect. Immun. *68*:4368-4369, 2000.
26. Castric, P., Cassels, F. J., and Carlson, R. W.: Structural characterization of the *Pseudomonas aeruginosa* 1244 pilin glycan. J. Biol. Chem. *276*:26479-26485, 2001.
27. Chang, C. I., Chelliah, Y., Borek, D., et al.: Structure of tracheal cytotoxin in complex with a heterodimeric pattern-recognition receptor. Science *311*:1761-1764, 2006.
28. Chen, L. M., Hobbie, S., and Galan, J. E.: Requirement of CDC42 for *Salmonella*-induced cytoskeletal and nuclear responses. Science *274*:2115-2118, 1996.
29. Cirillo, D. M., Valdivia, R. H., Monack, D. M., et al.: Macrophage-dependent induction of the *Salmonella* pathogenicity island 2 type III secretion system and its role in intracellular survival. Mol. Microbiol. *30*:175-188, 1998.
30. Clantin, B., Hodak, H., Willery, E., et al.: The crystal structure of filamentous hemagglutinin secretion domain and its implications for the two-partner secretion pathway. Proc. Natl. Acad. Sci. U. S. A. *101*:6194-6199, 2004.
31. Cochrane, D. M., Brown, M. R., Anwar, H., et al.: Antibody response to *Pseudomonas aeruginosa* surface protein antigens in a rat model of chronic lung infection. J. Med. Microbiol. *27*:255-261, 1988.
32. Coen, D. M., Kosz-Vnenchak, M., Jacobson, J. G., et al.: Thymidine kinase-negative herpes simplex virus mutants establish latency in mouse trigeminal ganglia but do not reactivate. Proc. Natl. Acad. Sci. U. S. A. *86*:4736-4740, 1989.
33. Collazo, C. M., and Galan, J. E.: The invasion-associated type III system of *Salmonella typhimurium* directs the translocation of Sip proteins into the host cell. Mol. Microbiol. *24*:747-756, 1997.
34. Collier-Hyams, L. S., Zeng, H., Sun, J., et al.: Cutting edge: *Salmonella* AvrA effector inhibits the key proinflammatory, anti-apoptotic NF-κB pathway. J. Immunol. *169*:2846-2850, 2002.
35. Coombes, B. K., and Finlay, B. B.: Insertion of the bacterial type III translocon: Not your average needle stick. Trends Microbiol. *13*:92-95, 2005.
36. Cope, L. D., Yogev, R., Muller-Eberhard, U., et al.: A gene cluster involved in the utilization of both free heme and heme:hemopexin by *Haemophilus influenzae* type b. J. Bacteriol. *177*:2644-2653, 1995.
37. Corn, P. G., Anders, J., Takala, A. K., et al.: Genes involved in *Haemophilus influenzae* type b capsule expression are frequently amplified. J. Infect. Dis. *167*:356-364, 1993.
38. Cornelis, G. R., Biot, T., Lambert de Rouvroit, C., et al.: The *Yersinia* yop regulon. Mol. Microbiol. *3*:1455-1459, 1989.
39. Costerton, J. W., Stewart, P. S., and Greenberg, E. P.: Bacterial biofilms: A common cause of persistent infections. Science *284*:1318-1322, 1999.
40. Cotter, P. A., and Miller, J. F.: *Bordetella. In* Groisman, E. A. (ed): Principles of Bacterial Pathogenesis. San Diego, Academic Press, 2001, pp. 619-674.
41. Cotter, S. E., Surana, N. K., Grass, S., et al.: Trimeric autotransporters require trimerization of the passenger domain for stability and adhesive activity. J. Bacteriol. *188*:5400-5407, 2006.
42. Cotter, S. E., Surana, N. K., and St. Geme, J. W., III: Trimeric autotransporters: A distinct subfamily of autotransporter proteins. Trends Microbiol. *13*:199-205, 2005.

43. Csoka, T. B., Frost, G. I., and Stern, R.: Hyaluronidases in tissue invasion. Invasion Metastasis *17*:297-311, 1997.

44. Cutter, D., Mason, K. W., Howell, A. P., et al.: Immunization with *Haemophilus influenzae* Hap adhesin protects against nasopharyngeal colonization in experimental mice. J. Infect. Dis. *186*:1115-1121, 2002.

45. Dabiri, G. A., Sanger, J. M., Portnoy, D. A., et al.: *Listeria monocytogenes* moves rapidly through the host-cell cytoplasm by inducing directional actin assembly. Proc. Natl. Acad. Sci. U. S. A. *87*:6068-6072, 1990.

46. Davies, D. G., and Geesey, G. G.: Regulation of the alginate biosynthesis gene *algC* in *Pseudomonas aeruginosa* during biofilm development in continuous culture. Appl. Environ. Microbiol. *61*:860-867, 1995.

47. Davies, D. G., Parsek, M. R., Pearson, J. P., et al.: The involvement of cell-to-cell signals in the development of a bacterial biofilm. Science *280*:295-298, 1998.

48. de Roda Husman, A. M., and Schuitemaker, H.: Chemokine receptors and the clinical course of HIV-1 infection. Trends Microbiol. *6*:244-249, 1998.

49. Deivanayagam, C. C., Wann, E. R., Chen, W., et al.: A novel variant of the immunoglobulin fold in surface adhesins of *Staphylococcus aureus*: Crystal structure of the fibrinogen-binding MSCRAMM, clumping factor A. EMBO J. *21*:6660-6672, 2002.

50. Dodson, K. W., Jacob-Dubuisson, F., Striker, R. T., et al.: Outer-membrane PapC molecular usher discriminately recognizes periplasmic chaperone-pilus subunit complexes. Proc. Natl. Acad. Sci. U. S. A. *90*:3670-3674, 1993.

51. Dodson, K. W., Pinkner, J. S., Rose, T., et al.: Structural basis of the interaction of the pyelonephritic *E. coli* adhesin to its human kidney receptor. Cell *105*:733-743, 2001.

52. Domenighini, M., Relman, D., Capiau, C., et al.: Genetic characterization of *Bordetella pertussis* filamentous haemagglutinin: A protein processed from an unusually large precursor. Mol. Microbiol. *4*:787-800, 1990.

53. Donnenberg, M. S., Kaper, J. B., and Finlay, B. B.: Interactions between enteropathogenic *Escherichia coli* and host epithelial cells. Trends Microbiol. *5*:109-114, 1997.

54. Doranz, B. J., Rucker, J., Yi, Y., et al.: A dual-tropic primary HIV-1 isolate that uses fusin and the beta-chemokine receptors CKR-5, CKR-3, and CKR-2b as fusion cofactors. Cell *85*:1149-1158, 1996.

55. Dramsi, S., Caliot, E., Bonne, I., et al.: Assembly and role of pili in group B streptococci. Mol. Microbiol. *60*:1401-1413, 2006.

56. Egile, C., d'Hauteville, H., Parsot, C., et al.: SopA, the outer membrane protease responsible for polar localization of IcsA in *Shigella flexneri*. Mol. Microbiol. *23*:1063-1073, 1997.

57. Eitel, J., and Dersch, P.: The YadA protein of *Yersinia pseudotuberculosis* mediates high-efficiency uptake into human cells under environmental conditions in which invasin is repressed. Infect. Immun. *70*:4880-4891, 2002.

58. El Tahir, Y., and Skurnik, M.: YadA, the multifaceted *Yersinia* adhesin. Int. J. Med. Microbiol. *291*:209-218, 2001.

59. Elleman, T. C., and Hoyne, P. A.: Nucleotide sequence of the gene encoding pilin of *Bacteroides nodosus*, the causal organism of ovine footrot. J. Bacteriol. *160*:1184-1187, 1984.

60. Feng, Y., Broder, C. C., Kennedy, P. E., et al.: HIV-1 entry cofactor: Functional cDNA cloning of a seven-transmembrane, G protein-coupled receptor. Science *272*:872-877, 1996.

61. Fenno, J. C., Shaikh, A., Spatafora, G., et al.: The *fimA* locus of *Streptococcus parasanguis* encodes an ATP-binding membrane transport system. Mol. Microbiol. *15*:849-863, 1995.

62. Fink, D. L., Buscher, A. Z., Green, B., et al.: The *Haemophilus influenzae* Hap autotransporter mediates microcolony formation and adherence to epithelial cells and extracellular matrix via binding regions in the C-terminal end of the passenger domain. Cell. Microbiol. *5*:175-186, 2003.

63. Fink, D. L., Green, B. A., and St. Geme, J. W., III: The *Haemophilus influenzae* Hap autotransporter binds to fibronectin, laminin, and collagen IV. Infect. Immun. *70*:4902-4907, 2002.

64. Fischetti, V. A.: Streptococcal M protein: Molecular design and biological behavior. Clin. Microbiol. Rev. *2*:285-314, 1989.

65. Foster, T. J., and Höök, M.: Surface protein adhesins of *Staphylococcus aureus*. Trends Microbiol. *6*:484-488, 1998.

66. Fouchier, R. A., Broersen, S. M., Brouwer, M., et al.: Temporal relationship between elongation of the HIV type 1 glycoprotein 120 V2 domain and the conversion toward a syncytium-inducing phenotype. AIDS Res. Hum. Retroviruses *11*:1473-1478, 1995.

67. Fouchier, R. A., Groenink, M., Kootstra, N. A., et al.: Phenotype-associated sequence variation in the third variable domain of the human immunodeficiency virus type 1 gp120 molecule. J. Virol. *66*:3183-3187, 1992.

68. Fox, K. L., Yildirim, H. H., Deadman, M. E., et al.: Novel lipopolysaccharide biosynthetic genes containing tetranucleotide repeats in *Haemophilus influenzae*, identification of a gene for adding O-acetyl groups. Mol. Microbiol. *58*:207-216, 2005.

69. Fsihi, H., Steffen, P., and Cossart, P.: *Listeria monocytogenes*. *In* Groisman, E. A. (ed): Principles of Bacterial Pathogenesis. San Diego, Academic Press, 2001, pp. 751-803.

70. Fu, Y., and Galan, J. E.: A *Salmonella* protein antagonizes Rac-1 and Cdc42 to mediate host-cell recovery after bacterial invasion. Nature *401*:293-297, 1999.

71. Gacesa, P.: Bacterial alginate biosynthesis—recent progress and future prospects. Microbiology *144*:1133-1143, 1998.

72. Galan, J. E.: Molecular genetic bases of *Salmonella* entry into host cells. Mol. Microbiol. *20*:263-271, 1996.

73. Gale, C., Finkel, D., Tao, N., et al.: Cloning and expression of a gene encoding an integrin-like protein in *Candida albicans*. Proc. Natl. Acad. Sci. U. S. A. *93*:357-361, 1996.

74. Gale, C. A., Bendel, C. M., McClellan, M., et al.: Linkage of adhesion, filamentous growth, and virulence in *Candida albicans* to a single gene, INT1. Science *279*:1355-1358, 1998.

75. Gao, L., and Abu Kwaik, Y.: Hijacking of apoptotic pathways by bacterial pathogens. Microbes Infect. *2*:1705-1719, 2000.

76. Garrett, E. S., Perlegas, D., and Wozniak, D. J.: Negative control of flagellum synthesis in *Pseudomonas aeruginosa* is modulated by the alternative sigma factor AlgT (AlgU). J. Bacteriol. *181*:7401-7404, 1999.

77. Gedde, M. M., Higgins, D. E., Tilney, L. G., et al.: Role of listeriolysin O in cell-to-cell spread of *Listeria monocytogenes*. Infect. Immun. *68*:999-1003, 2000.

78. Giron, J. A., Ho, A. S., and Schoolnik, G. K.: An inducible bundle-forming pilus of enteropathogenic *Escherichia coli*. Science *254*:710-713, 1991.

79. Glass, W. G., Lim, J. K., Cholera, R., et al.: Chemokine receptor CCR5 promotes leukocyte trafficking to the brain and survival in West Nile virus infection. J. Exp. Med. *202*:1087-1098, 2005.

80. Glass, W. G., McDermott, D. H., Lim, J. K., et al.: CCR5 deficiency increases risk of symptomatic West Nile virus infection. J. Exp. Med. *203*:35-40, 2006.

81. Goldberg, M. B., Barzu, O., Parsot, C., et al.: Unipolar localization and ATPase activity of IcsA, a *Shigella flexneri* protein involved in intracellular movement. Infect. Agents Dis. *2*:210-211, 1993.

82. Goldman, W. E., Klapper, D. G., and Baseman, J. B.: Detection, isolation, and analysis of a released *Bordetella pertussis* product toxic to cultured tracheal cells. Infect. Immun. *36*:782-794, 1982.

83. Gouin, E., Gantelet, H., Egile, C., et al.: A comparative study of the actin-based motilities of the pathogenic bacteria *Listeria monocytogenes*, *Shigella flexneri* and *Rickettsia conorii*. J. Cell. Sci. *112*:1697-1708, 1999.

84. Gould, T. A., Schweizer, H. P., and Churchill, M. E.: Structure of the *Pseudomonas aeruginosa* acyl-homoserine lactone synthase LasI. Mol. Microbiol. *53*:1135-1146, 2004.

85. Griffin, R., Cox, A. D., Makepeace, K., et al.: Elucidation of the monoclonal antibody 5G8-reactive, virulence-associated lipopolysaccharide epitope of *Haemophilus influenzae* and its role in bacterial resistance to complement-mediated killing. Infect. Immun. *73*:2213-2221, 2005.

86. Groenink, M., Fouchier, R. A., Broersen, S., et al.: Relation of phenotype evolution of HIV-1 to envelope V2 configuration. Science *260*:1513-1516, 1993.

87. Grundling, A., Gonzalez, M. D., and Higgins, D. E.: Requirement of the *Listeria monocytogenes* broad-range phospholipase PC-PLC during infection of human epithelial cells. J. Bacteriol. *185*:6295-6307, 2003.

88. Gulig, P. A., Patrick, C. C., Hermanstorfer, L., et al.: Conservation of epitopes in the oligosaccharide portion of the lipooligosaccharide of *Haemophilus influenzae* type b. Infect. Immun. *55*:513-520, 1987.

89. Gupta, A., Gartner, J. J., Sethupathy, P., et al.: Anti-apoptotic function of a microRNA encoded by the HSV-1 latency-associated transcript. Nature *442*:82-85, 2006.

90. Hagblom, P., Segal, E., Billyard, E., et al.: Intragenic recombination leads to pilus antigenic variation in *Neisseria gonorrhoeae*. Nature *315*:156-158, 1985.

91. Halford, W. P., and Schaffer, P. A.: ICP0 is required for efficient reactivation of herpes simplex virus type 1 from neuronal latency. J. Virol. *75*:3240-3249, 2001.

92. Hall, A.: Rho GTPases and the actin cytoskeleton. Science *279*:509-514, 1998.

93. Hanski, E., and Caparon, M.: Protein F, a fibronectin-binding protein, is an adhesin of the group A streptococcus *Streptococcus pyogenes*. Proc. Natl. Acad. Sci. U. S. A. *89*:6172-6176, 1992.

94. Hardt, W. D., Chen, L. M., Schuebel, K. E., et al.: *S. typhimurium* encodes an activator of Rho GTPases that induces membrane ruffling and nuclear responses in host cells. Cell *93*:815-826, 1998.

95. Hartford, O. M., Wann, E. R., Höök, M., et al.: Identification of residues in the *Staphylococcus aureus* fibrinogen-binding MSCRAMM clumping factor A (ClfA) that are important for ligand binding. J. Biol. Chem. *276*:2466-2473, 2001.

96. Haslam, D. B.: Molecular decoys: Novel approaches to the prevention of hemolytic uremic syndrome. Pediatr. Res. *48*:267-268, 2000.

97. Heiss, L. N., Flak, T. A., Lancaster, J. R., Jr., et al.: Nitric oxide mediates *Bordetella pertussis* tracheal cytotoxin damage to the respiratory epithelium. Infect. Agents Dis. *2*:173-177, 1993.

98. Heiss, L. N., Lancaster, J. R., Jr., Corbett, J. A., et al.: Epithelial autotoxicity of nitric oxide: Role in the respiratory cytopathology of pertussis. Proc. Natl. Acad. Sci. U. S. A. *91*:267-270, 1994.

99. Heiss, L. N., Moser, S. A., Unanue, E. R., et al.: Interleukin-1 is linked to the respiratory epithelial cytopathology of pertussis. Infect. Immun. *61*:3123-3128, 1993.

100. Henderson, I. R., and Nataro, J. P.: Virulence functions of autotransporter proteins. Infect. Immun. *69*:1231-1243, 2001.

101. Hendrixson, D. R., and St. Geme, J. W., III: The *Haemophilus influenzae* Hap serine protease promotes adherence and microcolony formation, potentiated by a soluble host protein. Mol. Cell *2*:841-850, 1998.

102. Hensel, M., Shea, J. E., Raupach, B., et al.: Functional analysis of *ssaJ* and the *ssaK/U* operon, 13 genes encoding components of the type III secretion apparatus of *Salmonella* pathogenicity island 2. Mol. Microbiol. *24*:155-167, 1997.
103. Hersh, D., Monack, D. M., Smith, M. R., et al.: The *Salmonella* invasin SipB induces macrophage apoptosis by binding to caspase-1. Proc. Natl. Acad. Sci. U. S. A. *96*:2396-2401, 1999.
104. Hewlett, E. L.: Pertussis: Current concepts of pathogenesis and prevention. Pediatr. Infect. Dis. J. *16*:S78-S84, 1997.
105. Hewlett, E. L.: A commentary on the pathogenesis of pertussis. Clin. Infect. Dis. *28*:S94-S98, 1999.
106. Hilbi, H., Moss, J. E., Hersh, D., et al.: *Shigella*-induced apoptosis is dependent on caspase-1 which binds to IpaB. J. Biol. Chem. *273*:32895-32900, 1998.
107. Hobbs, M., Collie, E. S., Free, P. D., et al.: PilS and PilR, a two-component transcriptional regulatory system controlling expression of type 4 fimbriae in *Pseudomonas aeruginosa*. Mol. Microbiol. 7:669-682, 1993.
108. Hobbs, M., and Mattick, J. S.: Common components in the assembly of type 4 fimbriae, DNA transfer systems, filamentous phage and protein-secretion apparatus: A general system for the formation of surface-associated protein complexes. Mol. Microbiol. *10*:233-243, 1993.
109. Hodak, H., Clantin, B., Willery, E., et al.: Secretion signal of the filamentous haemagglutinin, a model two-partner secretion substrate. Mol. Microbiol. *61*:368-382, 2006.
110. Hoe, N. P., Kordari, P., Cole, R., et al.: Human immune response to streptococcal inhibitor of complement, a serotype M1 group A streptococcus extracellular protein involved in epidemics. J. Infect. Dis. *182*:1425-1436, 2000.
111. Hoe, N. P., Nakashima, K., Lukomski, S., et al.: Rapid selection of complement-inhibiting protein variants in group A streptococcus epidemic waves. Nat. Med. *5*:924-929, 1999.
112. Hood, D. W., Deadman, M. E., Allen, T., et al.: Use of the complete genome sequence information of *Haemophilus influenzae* strain Rd to investigate lipopolysaccharide biosynthesis. Mol. Microbiol. *22*:951-965, 1996.
113. Hostetter, M. K.: Adhesins and ligands involved in the interaction of *Candida* spp. with epithelial and endothelial surfaces. Clin. Microbiol. Rev. 7:29-42, 1994.
114. Hostetter, M. K.: Linkage of adhesion, morphogenesis, and virulence in *Candida albicans*. J. Lab. Clin. Med. *132*:258-263, 1998.
115. Howell-Adams, B., and Seifert, H. S.: Molecular models accounting for the gene conversion reactions mediating gonococcal pilin antigenic variation. Mol. Microbiol. *37*:1146-1158, 2000.
116. Huang, Y., Paxton, W. A., Wolinsky, S. M., et al.: The role of a mutant CCR5 allele in HIV-1 transmission and disease progression. Nat. Med. *2*:1240-1243, 1996.
117. Hung, D. L., and Hultgren, S. J.: Pilus biogenesis via the chaperone/usher pathway: An integration of structure and function. J. Struct. Biol. *124*:201-220, 1998.
118. Hung, D. L., Knight, S. D., Woods, R. M., et al.: Molecular basis of two subfamilies of immunoglobulin-like chaperones. EMBO J. *15*:3792-3805, 1996.
119. Hynes, W. L., Dixon, A. R., Walton, S. L., et al.: The extracellular hyaluronidase gene (hylA) of *Streptococcus pyogenes*. FEMS Microbiol. Lett. *184*:109-112, 2000.
120. Isberg, R. R.: Uptake of enteropathogenic *Yersinia* by mammalian cells. Curr. Top. Microbiol. Immunol. *209*:1-24, 1996.
121. Isberg, R. R., and Leong, J. M.: Multiple beta 1 chain integrins are receptors for invasin, a protein that promotes bacterial penetration into mammalian cells. Cell *60*:861-871, 1990.
122. Ishibashi, Y., Claus, S., and Relman, D. A.: *Bordetella pertussis* filamentous hemagglutinin interacts with a leukocyte signal transduction complex and stimulates bacterial adherence to monocyte CR3 (CD11b/CD18). J. Exp. Med. *180*:1225-1233, 1994.
123. Jacob-Dubuisson, F., Heuser, J., Dodson, K., et al.: Initiation of assembly and association of the structural elements of a bacterial pilus depend on two specialized tip proteins. EMBO J. *12*:837-847, 1993.
124. Jacobson, J. G., Ruffner, K. L., Kosz-Vnenchak, M., et al.: Herpes simplex virus thymidine kinase and specific stages of latency in murine trigeminal ganglia. J. Virol. *67*:6903-6908, 1993.
125. Jain, S., van Ulsen, P., Benz, I., et al.: Polar localization of the autotransporter family of large bacterial virulence proteins. J. Bacteriol. *188*:4841-4850, 2006.
126. Jinno, A., Shimizu, N., Soda, Y., et al.: Identification of the chemokine receptor TER1/CCR8 expressed in brain-derived cells and T cells as a new coreceptor for HIV-1 infection. Biochem. Biophys. Res. Commun. *243*:497-502, 1998.
127. Jonsson, A. B., Nyberg, G., and Normark, S.: Phase variation of gonococcal pili by frameshift mutation in *pilC*, a novel gene for pilus assembly. EMBO J. *10*:477-488, 1991.
128. Josefsson, E., Hartford, O., O'Brien, L., et al.: Protection against experimental *Staphylococcus aureus* arthritis by vaccination with clumping factor A, a novel virulence determinant. J. Infect. Dis. *184*:1572-1580, 2001.
129. Justice, S. S., Hung, C., Theriot, J. A., et al.: Differentiation and developmental pathways of uropathogenic *Escherichia coli* in urinary tract pathogenesis. Proc. Natl. Acad. Sci. U. S. A. *101*:1333-1338, 2004.
130. Kajava, A. V., Cheng, N., Cleaver, R., et al.: Beta-helix model for the filamentous haemagglutinin adhesin of *Bordetella pertussis* and related bacterial secretory proteins. Mol. Microbiol. *42*:279-292, 2001.
131. Kau, A. L., Hunstad, D. A., and Hultgren, S. J.: Interaction of uropathogenic *Escherichia coli* with host uroepithelium. Curr. Opin. Microbiol. *8*:54-59, 2005.
132. Kaufman, M. R., Seyer, J. M., and Taylor, R. K.: Processing of TCP pilin by TcpJ typifies a common step intrinsic to a newly recognized pathway of extracellular protein secretion by gram-negative bacteria. Genes Dev. *5*:1834-1846, 1991.
133. Keane, J., Balcewicz-Sablinska, M. K., Remold, H. G., et al.: Infection by *Mycobacterium tuberculosis* promotes human alveolar macrophage apoptosis. Infect. Immun. *65*:298-304, 1997.
134. Kenny, B., DeVinney, R., Stein, M., et al.: Enteropathogenic *E. coli* (EPEC) transfers its receptor for intimate adherence into mammalian cells. Cell *91*:511-520, 1997.
135. Kerr, J. R., and Matthews, R. C.: *Bordetella pertussis* infection: Pathogenesis, diagnosis, management, and the role of protective immunity. Eur. J. Clin. Microbiol. Infect. Dis. *19*:77-88, 2000.
136. Khelef, N., and Guiso, N.: Induction of macrophage apoptosis by *Bordetella pertussis* adenylate cyclase-hemolysin. FEMS Microbiol. Lett. *134*:27-32, 1995.
137. Khelef, N., Zychlinsky, A., and Guiso, N.: *Bordetella pertussis* induces apoptosis in macrophages: Role of adenylate cyclase-hemolysin. Infect. Immun. *61*:4064-4071, 1993.
138. Kimura, L. H., and Pearsall, N. N.: Relationship between germination of *Candida albicans* and increased adherence to human buccal epithelial cells. Infect. Immun. *28*:464-468, 1980.
139. Kubori, T., Matsushima, Y., Nakamura, D., et al.: Supramolecular structure of the *Salmonella typhimurium* type III protein secretion system. Science *280*:602-605, 1998.
140. Kubori, T., Sukhan, A., Aizawa, S. I., et al.: Molecular characterization and assembly of the needle complex of the *Salmonella typhimurium* type III protein secretion system. Proc. Natl. Acad. Sci. U. S. A. *97*:10225-10230, 2000.
141. Kuehn, M. J., Heuser, J., Normark, S., et al.: P pili in uropathogenic *E. coli* are composite fibres with distinct fibrillar adhesive tips. Nature *356*:252-255, 1992.
142. Kuehn, M. J., Normark, S., and Hultgren, S. J.: Immunoglobulin-like PapD chaperone caps and uncaps interactive surfaces of nascently translocated pilus subunits. Proc. Natl. Acad. Sci. U. S. A. *88*:10586-10590, 1991.
143. Laarmann, S., Cutter, D., Juehne, T., et al.: The *Haemophilus influenzae* Hia autotransporter harbours two adhesive pockets that reside in the passenger domain and recognize the same host cell receptor. Mol. Microbiol. *46*:731-743, 2002.
144. Lauer, P., Albertson, N. H., and Koomey, M.: Conservation of genes encoding components of a type IV pilus assembly/two-step protein export pathway in *Neisseria gonorrhoeae*. Mol. Microbiol. *8*:357-368, 1993.
145. Law, D.: Virulence factors of *Escherichia coli* O157 and other Shiga toxin-producing *E. coli*. J. Appl. Microbiol. *88*:729-745, 2000.
146. Lederman, M. M., Penn-Nicholson, A., Cho, M., et al.: Biology of CCR5 and its role in HIV infection and treatment. J. A. M. A. *296*:815-826, 2006.
147. Lee, J., Remold, H. G., Ieong, M. H., et al.: Macrophage apoptosis in response to high intracellular burden of *Mycobacterium tuberculosis* is mediated by a novel caspase-independent pathway. J. Immunol. *176*:4267-4274, 2006.
148. Li, H., Qian, L., Chen, Z., et al.: The outer membrane usher forms a twin-pore secretion complex. J. Mol. Biol. *344*:1397-1407, 2004.
149. Li, R. K., and Cutler, J. E.: Chemical definition of an epitope/adhesin molecule on *Candida albicans*. J. Biol. Chem. *268*:18293-18299, 1993.
150. Lim, J. H., Kim, M. S., Kim, H. E., et al.: Structural basis for preferential recognition of diaminopimelic acid-type peptidoglycan by a subset of peptidoglycan recognition proteins. J. Biol. Chem. *281*:8286-8295, 2006.
151. Liu, D. F., Mason, K. W., Mastri, M., et al.: The C-terminal fragment of the internal 110-kilodalton passenger domain of the Hap protein of nontypeable *Haemophilus influenzae* is a potential vaccine candidate. Infect. Immun. *72*:6961-6968, 2004.
152. Liu, R., Paxton, W. A., Choe, S., et al.: Homozygous defect in HIV-1 coreceptor accounts for resistance of some multiply-exposed individuals to HIV-1 infection. Cell *86*:367-377, 1996.
153. Lukomski, S., Hoe, N. P., Abdi, I., et al.: Nonpolar inactivation of the hypervariable streptococcal inhibitor of complement gene (*sic*) in serotype M1 *Streptococcus pyogenes* significantly decreases mouse mucosal colonization. Infect. Immun. *68*:535-542, 2000.
154. Lysenko, E., Richards, J. C., Cox, A. D., et al.: The position of phosphorylcholine on the lipopolysaccharide of *Haemophilus influenzae* affects binding and sensitivity to C-reactive protein-mediated killing. Mol. Microbiol. *35*:234-245, 2000.
155. MacConnachie, A. A., and Todd, W. T.: Potential therapeutic agents for the prevention and treatment of haemolytic uraemic syndrome in shiga toxin producing *Escherichia coli* infection. Curr. Opin. Infect. Dis. *17*:479-482, 2004.
156. Makhov, A. M., Hannah, J. H., Brennan, M. J., et al.: Filamentous hemagglutinin of *Bordetella pertussis*: A bacterial adhesin formed as a 50-nm monomeric rigid rod based on a 19-residue repeat motif rich in beta strands and turns. J. Mol. Biol. *241*:110-124, 1994.
157. Marceau, M., and Nassif, X.: Role of glycosylation at Ser63 in production of soluble pilin in pathogenic *Neisseria*. J. Bacteriol. *181*:656-661, 1999.
158. Marcus, S. L., Brumell, J. H., Pfeifer, C. G., et al.: *Salmonella* pathogenicity islands: Big virulence in small packages. Microbes Infect. *2*:145-156, 2000.

159. Marquis, H., Doshi, V., and Portnoy, D. A.: The broad-range phospholipase C and a metalloprotease mediate listeriolysin O-independent escape of *Listeria monocytogenes* from a primary vacuole in human epithelial cells. Infect. Immun. *63*:4531-4534, 1995.

160. Marrs, C. F., Schoolnik, G., Koomey, J. M., et al.: Cloning and sequencing of a *Moraxella bovis* pilin gene. J. Bacteriol. *163*:132-139, 1985.

161. Martinez, J. J., Mulvey, M. A., Schilling, J. D., et al.: Type 1 pilus-mediated bacterial invasion of bladder epithelial cells. EMBO J. *19*:2803-2812, 2000.

162. Mawhinney, T. P., Adelstein, E., Morris, D. A., et al.: Structure determination of five sulfated oligosaccharides derived from tracheobronchial mucus glycoproteins. J. Biol. Chem. *262*:2994-3001, 1987.

163. McDaniel, T. K., Jarvis, K. G., Donnenberg, M. S., et al.: A genetic locus of enterocyte effacement conserved among diverse enterobacterial pathogens. Proc. Natl. Acad. Sci. U. S. A. *92*:1664-1668, 1995.

164. McDevitt, D., Francois, P., Vaudaux, P., et al.: Molecular characterization of the clumping factor (fibrinogen receptor) of *Staphylococcus aureus*. Mol. Microbiol. *11*:237-248, 1994.

165. McKinney, J. D., Höner zu Bentrup, K., Munoz-Elias, E. J., et al.: Persistence of *Mycobacterium tuberculosis* in macrophages and mice requires the glyoxylate shunt enzyme isocitrate lyase. Nature *406*:735-738, 2000.

166. Mejia, L. M., Stockbauer, K. E., Pan, X., et al.: Characterization of group A streptococcus strains recovered from Mexican children with pharyngitis by automated DNA sequencing of virulence-related genes: Unexpectedly large variation in the gene (*sic*) encoding a complement-inhibiting protein. J. Clin. Microbiol. *35*:3220-3224, 1997.

167. Meli, A. C., Hodak, H., Clantin, B., et al.: Channel properties of TpsB transporter FhaC point to two functional domains with a C-terminal protein-conducting pore. J. Biol. Chem. *281*:158-166, 2006.

168. Meng, G., Surana, N. K., St. Geme, J. W., III, et al.: Structure of the outer membrane translocator domain of the *Haemophilus influenzae* Hia trimeric autotransporter. EMBO J. *25*:2297-2304, 2006.

169. Mengaud, J., Ohayon, H., Gounon, P., et al.: E-cadherin is the receptor for internalin, a surface protein required for entry of *L. monocytogenes* into epithelial cells. Cell *84*:923-932, 1996.

170. Menozzi, F. D., Mutombo, R., Renauld, G., et al.: Heparin-inhibitable lectin activity of the filamentous hemagglutinin adhesin of *Bordetella pertussis*. Infect. Immun. *62*:769-778, 1994.

171. Menzel, E. J., and Farr, C.: Hyaluronidase and its substrate hyaluronan: biochemistry, biological activities and therapeutic uses. Cancer Lett. *131*:3-11, 1998.

172. Meyer, T. F., Billyard, E., Haas, R., et al.: Pilus genes of *Neisseria gonorrhoeae*: Chromosomal organization and DNA sequence. Proc. Natl. Acad. Sci. U. S. A. *81*:6110-6114, 1984.

173. Miller, C. S., Danaher, R. J., and Jacob, R. J.: ICP0 is not required for efficient stress-induced reactivation of herpes simplex virus type 1 from cultured quiescently infected neuronal cells. J. Virol. *80*:3360-3368, 2006.

174. Mounier, J., Ryter, A., Coquis-Rondon, M., et al.: Intracellular and cell-to-cell spread of *Listeria monocytogenes* involves interaction with F-actin in the enterocyte-like cell line Caco-2. Infect. Immun. *58*:1048-1058, 1990.

175. Moxon, E. R., and Kroll, J. S.: The role of bacterial polysaccharide capsules as virulence factors. Curr. Top. Microbiol. Immunol. *150*:65-85, 1990.

176. Mu, X. Q., and Bullitt, E.: Structure and assembly of P-pili: A protruding hinge region used for assembly of a bacterial adhesion filament. Proc. Natl. Acad. Sci. U. S. A. *103*:9861-9866, 2006.

177. Mukherjee, J., Chios, K., Fishwild, D., et al.: Human Stx2-specific monoclonal antibodies prevent systemic complications of *Escherichia coli* O157:H7 infection. Infect. Immun. *70*:612-619, 2002.

178. Mukherjee, S., Keitany, G., Li, Y., et al.: *Yersinia* YopJ acetylates and inhibits kinase activation by blocking phosphorylation. Science *312*:1211-1214, 2006.

179. Mulvey, M. A., Schilling, J. D., and Hultgren, S. J.: Establishment of a persistent *Escherichia coli* reservoir during the acute phase of a bladder infection. Infect. Immun. *69*:4572-4579, 2001.

180. Nicosia, A., and Rappuoli, R.: Promoter of the pertussis toxin operon and production of pertussis toxin. J. Bacteriol. *169*:2843-2846, 1987.

181. Noel, G. J., Brittingham, A., Granato, A. A., et al.: Effect of amplification of the *capb* locus on complement-mediated bacteriolysis and opsonization of type b *Haemophilus influenzae*. Infect. Immun. *64*:4769-4775, 1996.

182. Noel, G. J., Hoiseth, S. K., and Edelson, P. J.: Type b capsule inhibits ingestion of *Haemophilus influenzae* by murine macrophages: Studies with isogenic encapsulated and unencapsulated strains. J. Infect. Dis. *166*:178-182, 1992.

183. Noel, G. J., Mosser, D. M., and Edelson, P. J.: Role of complement in mouse macrophage binding of *Haemophilus influenzae* type b. J. Clin. Invest. *85*:208-218, 1990.

184. Norris, F. A., Wilson, M. P., Wallis, T. S., et al.: SopB, a protein required for virulence of *Salmonella dublin*, is an inositol phosphate phosphatase. Proc. Natl. Acad. Sci. U. S. A. *95*:14057-14059, 1998.

185. Novembre, J., Galvani, A. P., and Slatkin, M.: The geographic spread of the CCR5 Δ32 HIV-resistance allele. PLoS Biol. *3*:e339, 2005.

186. Nunn, D. N., and Lory, S.: Product of the *Pseudomonas aeruginosa* gene *pilD* is a prepilin leader peptidase. Proc. Natl. Acad. Sci. U. S. A. *88*:3281-3285, 1991.

187. O'Toole, G. A., and Kolter, R.: Flagellar and twitching motility are necessary for *Pseudomonas aeruginosa* biofilm development. Mol. Microbiol. *30*:295-304, 1998.

188. Ochman, H., Soncini, F. C., Solomon, F., et al.: Identification of a pathogenicity island required for *Salmonella* survival in host cells. Proc. Natl. Acad. Sci. U. S. A. *93*:7800-7804, 1996.

189. Okada, N., Liszewski, M. K., Atkinson, J. P., et al.: Membrane cofactor protein (CD46) is a keratinocyte receptor for the M protein of the group A streptococcus. Proc. Natl. Acad. Sci. U. S. A. *92*:2489-2493, 1995.

190. Okada, N., Pentland, A. P., Falk, P., et al.: M protein and protein F act as important determinants of cell-specific tropism of *Streptococcus pyogenes* in skin tissue. J. Clin. Invest. *94*:965-977, 1994.

191. Oligino, L., and Fives-Taylor, P.: Overexpression and purification of a fimbria-associated adhesin of *Streptococcus parasanguis*. Infect. Immun. *61*:1016-1022, 1993.

192. Oomen, C. J., van Ulsen, P., van Gelder, P., et al.: Structure of the translocator domain of a bacterial autotransporter. EMBO J. *23*:1257-1266, 2004.

193. Ozeri, V., Tovi, A., Burstein, I., et al.: A two-domain mechanism for group A streptococcal adherence through protein F to the extracellular matrix. EMBO J. *15*:989-998, 1996.

194. Palmer, K. L., and Munson, R. S., Jr.: Cloning and characterization of the genes encoding the hemolysin of *Haemophilus ducreyi*. Mol. Microbiol. *18*:821-830, 1995.

195. Parge, H. E., Forest, K. T., Hickey, M. J., et al.: Structure of the fibre-forming protein pilin at 2.6 Å resolution. Nature *378*:32-38, 1995.

196. Parsek, M. R., and Greenberg, E. P.: Acyl-homoserine lactone quorum sensing in gram-negative bacteria: A signaling mechanism involved in associations with higher organisms. Proc. Natl. Acad. Sci. U. S. A. *97*:8789-8793, 2000.

197. Paton, A. W., Morona, R., and Paton, J. C.: A new biological agent for treatment of Shiga toxigenic *Escherichia coli* infections and dysentery in humans. Nat. Med. *6*:265-270, 2000.

198. Patti, J. M., Bremell, T., Krajewska-Pietrasik, D., et al.: The *Staphylococcus aureus* collagen adhesin is a virulence determinant in experimental septic arthritis. Infect. Immun. *62*:152-161, 1994.

199. Patti, J. M., and Höök, M.: Microbial adhesins recognizing extracellular matrix macromolecules. Curr. Opin. Cell. Biol. *6*:752-758, 1994.

200. Patti, J. M., Jonsson, H., Guss, B., et al.: Molecular characterization and expression of a gene encoding a *Staphylococcus aureus* collagen adhesin. J. Biol. Chem. *267*:4766-4772, 1992.

201. Pays, E., and Nolan, D. P.: Expression and function of surface proteins in *Trypanosoma brucei*. Mol. Biochem. Parasitol. *91*:3-36, 1998.

202. Pearson, J. P., Feldman, M., Iglewski, B. H., et al.: *Pseudomonas aeruginosa* cell-to-cell signaling is required for virulence in a model of acute pulmonary infection. Infect. Immun. *68*:4331-4334, 2000.

203. Pearson, R. D., Symes, P., Conboy, M., et al.: Inhibition of monocyte oxidative responses by *Bordetella pertussis* adenylate cyclase toxin. J. Immunol. *139*:2749-2754, 1987.

204. Peters, P. J., Bhattacharya, J., Hibbitts, S., et al.: Biological analysis of human immunodeficiency virus type 1 R5 envelopes amplified from brain and lymph node tissues of AIDS patients with neuropathology reveals two distinct tropism phenotypes and identifies envelopes in the brain that confer an enhanced tropism and fusigenicity for macrophages. J. Virol. *78*:6915-6926, 2004.

205. Peters, P. J., Sullivan, W. M., Duenas-Decamp, M. J., et al.: Non-macrophage-tropic human immunodeficiency virus type 1 R5 envelopes predominate in blood, lymph nodes, and semen: Implications for transmission and pathogenesis. J. Virol. *80*:6324-6332, 2006.

206. Pinyon, R. A., Paton, J. C., Paton, A. W., et al.: Refinement of a therapeutic Shiga toxin-binding probiotic for human trials. J. Infect. Dis. *189*:1547-1555, 2004.

207. Poole, K., Schiebel, E., and Braun, V.: Molecular characterization of the hemolysin determinant of *Serratia marcescens*. J. Bacteriol. *170*:3177-3188, 1988.

208. Potts, W. J., and Saunders, J. R.: Nucleotide sequence of the structural gene for class I pilin from *Neisseria meningitidis*: Homologies with the *pilE* locus of *Neisseria gonorrhoeae*. Mol. Microbiol. *2*:647-653, 1988.

209. Prasad, S. M., Yin, Y., Rodzinski, E., et al.: Identification of a carbohydrate recognition domain in filamentous hemagglutinin from *Bordetella pertussis*. Infect. Immun. *61*:2780-2785, 1993.

210. Pratt, L. A., and Kolter, R.: Genetic analyses of bacterial biofilm formation. Curr. Opin. Microbiol. *2*:598-603, 1999.

211. Preston, C. M.: Repression of viral transcription during herpes simplex virus latency. J. Gen. Virol. *81*:1-19, 2000.

212. Race, P. R., Lakey, J. H., and Banfield, M. J.: Insertion of the enteropathogenic *Escherichia coli* Tir virulence protein into membranes in vitro. J. Biol. Chem. *281*:7842-7849, 2006.

213. Ram, S., Mackinnon, F. G., Gulati, S., et al.: The contrasting mechanisms of serum resistance of *Neisseria gonorrhoeae* and group B *Neisseria meningitidis*. Mol. Immunol. *36*:915-928, 1999.

214. Rao, V. K., and Progulske-Fox, A.: Cloning and sequencing of two type 4 (N-methylphenylalanine) pilin genes from *Eikenella corrodens*. J. Gen. Microbiol. *139*:651-660, 1993.

215. Relman, D., Tuomanen, E., Falkow, S., et al.: Recognition of a bacterial adhesion by an integrin: macrophage CR3 (alpha M beta 2, CD11b/CD18) binds filamentous hemagglutinin of *Bordetella pertussis*. Cell *61*:1375-1382, 1990.

216. Rest, R. F., and Frangipane, J. V.: Growth of *Neisseria gonorrhoeae* in CMP-N-acetylneuraminic acid inhibits nonopsonic (opacity-associated outer membrane protein-mediated) interactions with human neutrophils. Infect. Immun. *60*:989-997, 1992.

217. Robbins, J. R., Barth, A. I., Marquis, H., et al.: *Listeria monocytogenes* exploits normal host cell processes to spread from cell to cell. J. Cell. Biol. *146*:1333-1350, 1999.

218. Rosenshine, I., Ruschkowski, S., Stein, M., et al.: A pathogenic bacterium triggers epithelial signals to form a functional bacterial receptor that mediates actin pseudopod formation. EMBO J. *15*:2613-2624, 1996.

219. Rosini, R., Rinaudo, C. D., Soriani, M., et al.: Identification of novel genomic islands coding for antigenic pilus-like structures in *Streptococcus agalactiae*. Mol. Microbiol. *61*:126-141, 2006.

220. Rudel, T., Scheurerpflug, I., and Meyer, T. F.: *Neisseria* PilC protein identified as type-4 pilus tip-located adhesin. Nature *373*:357-359, 1995.

221. Russel, M.: Phage assembly: A paradigm for bacterial virulence factor export? Science *265*:612-614, 1994.

222. Russell, D. G.: What does "inhibition of phagosome-lysosome fusion" really mean? Trends Microbiol. *6*:212-214, 1998.

223. Sandvig, K., and van Deurs, B.: Endocytosis, intracellular transport, and cytotoxic action of Shiga toxin and ricin. Physiol. Rev. *76*:949-966, 1996.

224. Sandvig, K., and van Deurs, B.: Entry of ricin and Shiga toxin into cells: Molecular mechanisms and medical perspectives. EMBO J. *19*:5943-5950, 2000.

225. Sauer, F. G., Futterer, K., Pinkner, J. S., et al.: Structural basis of chaperone function and pilus biogenesis. Science *285*:1058-1061, 1999.

226. Sauer, F. G., Knight, S. D., Waksman, G., et al.: PapD-like chaperones and pilus biogenesis. Semin. Cell. Dev. Biol. *11*:27-34, 2000.

227. Sharma, V., Sharma, S., Höner zu Bentrup, K., et al.: Structure of isocitrate lyase, a persistence factor of *Mycobacterium tuberculosis*. Nat. Struct. Biol. *7*:663-668, 2000.

228. Shaw, C. E., and Taylor, R. K.: *Vibrio cholerae* O395 *tcpA* pilin gene sequence and comparison of predicted protein structural features to those of type 4 pilins. Infect. Immun. *58*:3042-3049, 1990.

229. Shea, J. E., Hensel, M., Gleeson, C., et al.: Identification of a virulence locus encoding a second type III secretion system in *Salmonella typhimurium*. Proc. Natl. Acad. Sci. U. S. A. *93*:2593-2597, 1996.

230. Sheoran, A. S., Chapman-Bonofiglio, S., Harvey, B. R., et al.: Human antibody against shiga toxin 2 administered to piglets after the onset of diarrhea due to *Escherichia coli* O157:H7 prevents fatal systemic complications. Infect. Immun. *73*:4607-4613, 2005.

231. Sheoran, A. S., Chapman, S., Singh, P., et al.: Stx2-specific human monoclonal antibodies protect mice against lethal infection with *Escherichia coli* expressing Stx2 variants. Infect. Immun. *71*:3125-3130, 2003.

232. Shere, K. D., Sallustio, S., Manessis, A., et al.: Disruption of IcsP, the major *Shigella* protease that cleaves IcsA, accelerates actin-based motility. Mol. Microbiol. *25*:451-462, 1997.

233. Simmons, G., Wilkinson, D., Reeves, J. D., et al.: Primary, syncytium-inducing human immunodeficiency virus type 1 isolates are dual-tropic and most can use either Lestr or CCR5 as coreceptors for virus entry. J. Virol. *70*:8355-8360, 1996.

234. Smedley, J. G., III, Jewell, E., Roguskie, J., et al.: Influence of pilin glycosylation on *Pseudomonas aeruginosa* 1244 pilus function. Infect. Immun. *73*:7922-7931, 2005.

235. Smith, C. V., Sharma, V., and Sacchettini, J. C.: TB drug discovery: Addressing issues of persistence and resistance. Tuberculosis (Edinburgh) *84*:45-55, 2004.

236. Smith, G. A., Marquis, H., Jones, S., et al.: The two distinct phospholipases C of *Listeria monocytogenes* have overlapping roles in escape from a vacuole and cell-to-cell spread. Infect. Immun. *63*:4231-4237, 1995.

237. Smith, G. A., and Portnoy, D. A.: How the *Listeria monocytogenes* ActA protein converts actin polymerization into a motile force. Trends Microbiol. *5*:272-276, 1997.

238. Smith, R. S., Harris, S. G., Phipps, R., et al.: The *Pseudomonas aeruginosa* quorum-sensing molecule N-(3-oxododecanoyl)homoserine lactone contributes to virulence and induces inflammation in vivo. J. Bacteriol. *184*:1132-1139, 2002.

239. St. Geme, J. W., III: Bacterial adhesins: Determinants of microbial colonization and pathogenicity. Adv. Pediatr. *44*:43-72, 1997.

240. St. Geme, J. W., III, de la Morena, M. L., and Falkow, S.: A *Haemophilus influenzae* IgA protease-like protein promotes intimate interaction with human epithelial cells. Mol. Microbiol. *14*:217-233, 1994.

241. Staab, J. F., Bahn, Y. S., Tai, C. H., et al.: Expression of transglutaminase substrate activity on *Candida albicans* germ tubes through a coiled, disulfide-bonded N-terminal domain of Hwp1 requires C-terminal glycosylphosphatidylinositol modification. J. Biol. Chem. *279*:40737-40747, 2004.

242. Staab, J. F., Bradway, S. D., Fidel, P. L., et al.: Adhesive and mammalian transglutaminase substrate properties of *Candida albicans* Hwp1. Science *283*:1535-1538, 1999.

243. Staab, J. F., Ferrer, C. A., and Sundstrom, P.: Developmental expression of a tandemly repeated, proline-and glutamine-rich amino acid motif on hyphal surfaces on *Candida albicans*. J. Biol. Chem. *271*:6298-6305, 1996.

244. Steinert, P. M., Candi, E., Kartasova, T., et al.: Small proline-rich proteins are cross-bridging proteins in the cornified cell envelopes of stratified squamous epithelia. J. Struct. Biol. *122*:76-85, 1998.

245. Steinhauer, J., Agha, R., Pham, T., et al.: The unipolar *Shigella* surface protein IcsA is targeted directly to the bacterial old pole: IcsP cleavage of IcsA occurs over the entire bacterial surface. Mol. Microbiol. *32*:367-377, 1999.

246. Stephenson, A. E., Wu, H., Novak, J., et al.: The Fap1 fimbrial adhesin is a glycoprotein: Antibodies specific for the glycan moiety block the adhesion of *Streptococcus parasanguis* in an in vitro tooth model. Mol. Microbiol. *43*:147-157, 2002.

247. Stone, K. D., Zhang, H. Z., Carlson, L. K., et al.: A cluster of fourteen genes from enteropathogenic *Escherichia coli* is sufficient for the biogenesis of a type IV pilus. Mol. Microbiol. *20*:325-337, 1996.

248. Straley, S. C., Skrzypek, E., Plano, G. V., et al.: Yops of *Yersinia* spp. pathogenic for humans. Infect. Immun. *61*:3105-3110, 1993.

249. Strom, M. S., and Lory, S.: Cloning and expression of the pilin gene of *Pseudomonas aeruginosa* PAK in *Escherichia coli*. J. Bacteriol. *165*:367-372, 1986.

250. Stromberg, N., Marklund, B. I., Lund, B., et al.: Host-specificity of uropathogenic *Escherichia coli* depends on binding specificity to Gal-α1,4-Gal-containing isoreceptors. EMBO J. *9*:2001-2010, 1990.

251. Sturgill-Koszycki, S., Schlesinger, P. H., Chakraborty, P., et al.: Lack of acidification in *Mycobacterium* phagosomes produced by exclusion of the vesicular proton-ATPase. Science *263*:678-681, 1994.

252. Surana, N. K., Cotter, S. E., Yeo, H. J., et al.: Structural determinants of *Haemophilus influenzae* adherence to host epithelium: Variations on type V secretion. *In* Waksman, G., Caparon, M., and Hultgren, S. (eds): Structural Basis of Bacterial Pathogenesis. Washington, D.C., American Society for Microbiology, 2005, pp. 129-148.

253. Switalski, L. M., Patti, J. M., Butcher, W., et al.: A collagen receptor on *Staphylococcus aureus* strains isolated from patients with septic arthritis mediates adhesion to cartilage. Mol. Microbiol. *7*:99-107, 1993.

254. Theriot, J. A.: The cell biology of infection by intracellular bacterial pathogens. Annu. Rev. Cell. Dev. Biol. *11*:213-239, 1995.

255. Theriot, J. A., Mitchison, T. J., Tilney, L. G., et al.: The rate of actin-based motility of intracellular *Listeria monocytogenes* equals the rate of actin polymerization. Nature *357*:257-260, 1992.

256. Theriot, J. A., Rosenblatt, J., Portnoy, D. A., et al.: Involvement of profilin in the actin-based motility of *L. monocytogenes* in cells and in cell-free extracts. Cell *76*:505-517, 1994.

257. Thomas, W. E., Nilsson, L. M., Forero, M., et al.: Shear-dependent "stick-and-roll" adhesion of type 1 fimbriated *Escherichia coli*. Mol. Microbiol. *53*:1545-1557, 2004.

258. Thomas, W. E., Trintchina, E., Forero, M., et al.: Bacterial adhesion to target cells enhanced by shear force. Cell *109*:913-923, 2002.

259. Tomlinson, S., and Raper, J.: The lysis of *Trypanosoma brucei brucei* by human serum. Nat. Biotechnol. *14*:717-721, 1996.

260. Tonjum, T., Marrs, C. F., Rozsa, F., et al.: The type 4 pilin of *Moraxella nonliquefaciens* exhibits unique similarities with the pilins of *Neisseria gonorrhoeae* and *Dichelobacter* (*Bacteroides*) *nodosus*. J. Gen. Microbiol. *137*:2483-2490, 1991.

261. Touze, T., Hayward, R. D., Eswaran, J., et al.: Self-association of EPEC intimin mediated by the beta-barrel-containing anchor domain: A role in clustering of the Tir receptor. Mol. Microbiol. *51*:73-87, 2004.

262. Trachtman, H., Cnaan, A., Christen, E., et al.: Effect of an oral Shiga toxin-binding agent on diarrhea-associated hemolytic uremic syndrome in children: a randomized controlled trial. J. A. M. A. *290*:1337-1344, 2003.

263. Tucker, S. C., and Galan, J. E.: Complex function for SicA, a *Salmonella enterica* serovar typhimurium type III secretion-associated chaperone. J. Bacteriol. *182*:2262-2268, 2000.

264. Uphoff, T. S., and Welch, R. A.: Nucleotide sequencing of the *Proteus mirabilis* calcium-independent hemolysin genes (*hpmA* and *hpmB*) reveals sequence similarity with the *Serratia marcescens* hemolysin genes (*shlA* and *shlB*). J. Bacteriol. *172*:1206-1216, 1990.

265. van't Wout, A. B., Kootstra, N. A., Mulder-Kampinga, G. A., et al.: Macrophage-tropic variants initiate human immunodeficiency virus type 1 infection after sexual, parenteral, and vertical transmission. J. Clin. Invest. *94*:2060-2067, 1994.

266. Vazquez-Torres, A., Jones-Carson, J., Baumler, A. J., et al.: Extraintestinal dissemination of *Salmonella* by CD18-expressing phagocytes. Nature *401*:804-808, 1999.

267. Vicente, M. F., Mengaud, J., Chenevert, J., et al.: Reacquisition of virulence of haemolysin-negative *Listeria monocytogenes* mutants by complementation with a plasmid carrying the *hlyA* gene. Acta Microbiol. Hung. *36*:199-203, 1989.

268. Virji, M., Stimson, E., Makepeace, K., et al.: Posttranslational modifications of meningococcal pili: Identification of a common trisaccharide substitution on variant pilins of strain C311. Ann. N. Y. Acad. Sci. *797*:53-64, 1996.

269. Wadolkowski, E. A., Sung, L. M., Burris, J. A., et al.: Acute renal tubular necrosis and death of mice orally infected with *Escherichia coli* strains that produce Shiga-like toxin type II. Infect. Immun. *58*:3959-3965, 1990.

270. Wagner, E. K., and Bloom, D. C.: Experimental investigation of herpes simplex virus latency. Clin. Microbiol. Rev. *10*:419-443, 1997.

271. Wann, E. R., Gurusiddappa, S., and Hook, M.: The fibronectin-binding MSCRAMM FnbpA of *Staphylococcus aureus* is a bifunctional protein that also binds to fibrinogen. J. Biol. Chem. *275*:13863-13871, 2000.

272. Weir, S., and Marrs, C. F.: Identification of type 4 pili in *Kingella denitrificans*. Infect. Immun. *60*:3437-3441, 1992.

273. Weiser, J. N., Maskell, D. J., Butler, P. D., et al.: Characterization of repetitive sequences controlling phase variation of *Haemophilus influenzae* lipopolysaccharide. J. Bacteriol. *172*:3304-3309, 1990.

274. Weiser, J. N., and Pan, N.: Adaptation of *Haemophilus influenzae* to acquired and innate humoral immunity based on phase variation of lipopolysaccharide. Mol. Microbiol. *30*:767-775, 1998.

275. Weiser, J. N., Pan, N., McGowan, K. L., et al.: Phosphorylcholine on the lipopolysaccharide of *Haemophilus influenzae* contributes to persistence in the respiratory tract and sensitivity to serum killing mediated by C-reactive protein. J. Exp. Med. *187*:631-640, 1998.

276. Weiser, J. N., Shchepetov, M., and Chong, S. T.: Decoration of lipopolysaccharide with phosphorylcholine: A phase-variable characteristic of *Haemophilus influenzae*. Infect. Immun. *65*:943-950, 1997.

277. Wetzler, L. M., Barry, K., Blake, M. S., et al.: Gonococcal lipooligosaccharide sialylation prevents complement-dependent killing by immune sera. Infect. Immun. *60*:39-43, 1992.

278. Wexler, D. E., Chenoweth, D. E., and Cleary, P. P.: Mechanism of action of the group A streptococcal C5a inactivator. Proc. Natl. Acad. Sci. U. S. A. *82*:8144-8148, 1985.

279. Willems, R. J., Geuijen, C., van der Heide, H. G., et al.: Mutational analysis of the *Bordetella pertussis fim/fha* gene cluster: Identification of a gene with sequence similarities to haemolysin accessory genes involved in export of FHA. Mol. Microbiol. *11*:337-347, 1994.

280. Wing, H. J., Yan, A. W., Goldman, S. R., et al.: Regulation of IcsP, the outer membrane protease of the *Shigella* actin tail assembly protein IcsA, by virulence plasmid regulators VirF and VirB. J. Bacteriol. *186*:699-705, 2004.

281. Wolff, C., Nisan, I., Hanski, E., et al.: Protein translocation into host epithelial cells by infecting enteropathogenic *Escherichia coli*. Mol. Microbiol. *28*:143-155, 1998.

282. Wright, S. D., and Silverstein, S. C.: Receptors for C3b and C3bi promote phagocytosis but not the release of toxic oxygen from human phagocytes. J. Exp. Med. *158*:2016-2023, 1983.

283. Wu, H., and Fives-Taylor, P. M.: Identification of dipeptide repeats and a cell wall sorting signal in the fimbriae-associated adhesin, Fap1, of *Streptococcus parasanguis*. Mol. Microbiol. *34*:1070-1081, 1999.

284. Wu, H., Mintz, K. P., Ladha, M., et al.: Isolation and characterization of Fap1, a fimbriae-associated adhesin of *Streptococcus parasanguis* FW213. Mol. Microbiol. *28*:487-500, 1998.

285. Wu, H., Song, Z., Givskov, M., et al.: *Pseudomonas aeruginosa* mutations in *lasI* and *rhlI* quorum sensing systems result in milder chronic lung infection. Microbiology *147*:1105-1113, 2001.

286. Xu, H., Storch, T., Yu, M., et al.: Characterization of the human Forssman synthetase gene: An evolving association between glycolipid synthesis and host-microbial interactions. J. Biol. Chem. *274*:29390-29398, 1999.

287. Yanagishita, M., and Hascall, V. C.: Cell surface heparan sulfate proteoglycans. J. Biol. Chem. *267*:9451-9454, 1992.

288. Yeo, H. J., Cotter, S. E., Laarmann, S., et al.: Structural basis for host recognition by the *Haemophilus influenzae* Hia autotransporter. EMBO J. *23*:1245-1256, 2004.

289. Yoon, S., Liu, Z., Eyobo, Y., et al.: *Yersinia* effector YopJ inhibits yeast MAPK signaling pathways by an evolutionarily conserved mechanism. J. Biol. Chem. *278*:2131-2135, 2003.

290. Yu, L., Lee, K. K., Sheth, H. B., et al.: Fimbria-mediated adherence of *Candida albicans* to glycosphingolipid receptors on human buccal epithelial cells. Infect. Immun. *62*:2843-2848, 1994.

291. Zhang, L., He, T., Talal, A., et al.: In vivo distribution of the human immunodeficiency virus/simian immunodeficiency virus coreceptors: CXCR4, CCR3, and CCR5. J. Virol. *72*:5035-5045, 1998.

292. Zhu, T., Mo, H., Wang, N., et al.: Genotypic and phenotypic characterization of HIV-1 patients with primary infection. Science *261*:1179-1181, 1993.

293. Zoja, A., and Remuzzi, G.: The pivotal role of the endothelial cell in the pathogenesis of HUS. *In* Kaplan, B. S., Trompeter, R. S., and Moake, J. I. (eds): Hemolytic Uremic Syndrome and Thrombotic Thrombocytopenic Purpura. New York, Marcel Dekker, 1992, pp. 389-404.

294. Zong, Y., Xu, Y., Liang, X., et al.: A "collagen hug" model for *Staphylococcus aureus* CNA binding to collagen. EMBO J. *24*:4224-4236, 2005.

295. Zwahlen, A., Kroll, J. S., Rubin, L. G., et al.: The molecular basis of pathogenicity in *Haemophilus influenzae*: Comparative virulence of genetically-related capsular transformants and correlation with changes at the capsulation locus *cap*. Microb. Pathog. 7:225-235, 1989.

296. Zychlinsky, A., Prevost, M. C., and Sansonetti, P. J.: *Shigella flexneri* induces apoptosis in infected macrophages. Nature *358*:167-169, 1992.

297. Zychlinsky, A., and Sansonetti, P. J.: Apoptosis as a proinflammatory event: What can we learn from bacteria-induced cell death? Trends Microbiol. 5:201-204, 1997.

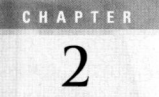

CHAPTER 2

NORMAL AND IMPAIRED IMMUNOLOGIC RESPONSES TO INFECTION

Michael F. Tosi

This chapter provides an overview of immunologic responses to infection and considers host interactions with different classes of pathogens, normal innate and adaptive immune mechanisms, the developing host responses of neonates, specific primary and secondary immunodeficiencies, and approaches to the evaluation of pediatric patients suspected to have impaired immunity. Human immunodeficiency virus (HIV) and acquired immunodeficiency syndrome (AIDS) are not considered here because they are addressed fully in Chapter 204A. This chapter is intended to supply sufficient information for the development of a basic understanding of mechanisms involved in normal host responses to infection, an appreciation of the underlying basis and clinical presentation of important immunodeficiencies, and a familiarity with general principles of evaluations and management of patients with suspected or documented disorders of immunity. For greater depth and detail regarding specific topics, readers are referred to many excellent reviews.

HOST-PARASITE INTERACTIONS

GENERAL FEATURES OF HOST-PARASITE INTERACTIONS

Humans constantly are exposed to a daunting number and diversity of microorganisms that can cause infection. Many organisms that usually coexist harmoniously with the human host on the skin or on mucous membranes of the oral cavity, upper airways, or lower gastrointestinal tract may invade and become pathogens if the balance of the commensal relationship is disrupted. Other organisms are more virulent, and they overtly attack the host's normal surface barriers and internal defense mechanisms. The human host has evolved a complex array of protective mechanisms designed to defend itself against these continuous microbial challenges.[626] To understand the pathogenesis, pathology, and natural history of infectious diseases, one must be familiar with the features of infectious agents that confer virulence, which are addressed elsewhere in this book. It is equally important to understand the elements of the host's response that contribute to containment, elimination, and protection against subsequent infection with these agents. It is important further to recognize that host responses to infections also may contribute to the pathophysiology of infectious diseases and may injure the host in other ways.

The characteristic features of specific infectious diseases are determined by the interactions of structural components and released products of microbial pathogens with host tissue, cells, and their products. Virulence tactics commonly employed by organisms include adherence to host cell surfaces, internalization within or invasion of host cells, production of toxins, elaboration of surface barriers such as bacterial polysaccharide capsules, usurpation of host synthetic mechanisms, and direct inhibition of specific defense mechanisms within host cells. The successful evolution of host strategies to protect against microbial attack has resulted in defenses designed to interfere with or to counteract many of these modes of microbial virulence.[626] In recent years, some of humanity's oldest microbial adversaries (e.g., smallpox, poliomyelitis, measles) systematically have been, or are being, eradicated. In the meantime, previously unrecognized human pathogens, such as HIV-1 and Ebola virus, have emerged as new challenges. Many of our oldest nemeses (e.g., tuberculosis, malaria) continue to elude our efforts to bring them under control, and they remain serious problems world-wide. Continued research at the interface between microbial pathogenesis and immunologic mechanisms is essential for the development of innovative approaches that can support and augment human immune responses to old and new microbial challenges.

MAIN FEATURES OF HOST RESPONSES TO SPECIFIC CLASSES OF INFECTIOUS AGENTS

Viruses

Viruses are obligate intracellular parasites that consist of genetic material in the form of either DNA or RNA that usually is surrounded by a protein coat and may or may not be bound by a lipid envelope.[395] Diseases caused by viruses are remarkably diverse, ranging from mild and merely inconvenient to rapidly fatal and from acute or brief to chronic or lifelong. Certain features are common to the pathogenesis of most viral infections, however. First, viruses must enter host cells to replicate. Viral entry ordinarily is initiated by attachment of a viral surface protein to a specific receptor molecule on the host cell. The specific viral ligands or their corresponding host cell receptors have been identified for numerous viruses. Rhinovirus has evolved a capsid protein that binds to human intercellular adhesion molecule-1 (ICAM-1) on respiratory epithelium[255]; the envelope glycoproteins of HIV-1 interact with CD4 on T lymphocytes and distinct chemokine receptors on lymphocytes or macrophages[163,327,623]; and internalization of adenoviruses depends on interaction between a specific peptide sequence in the penton base complex of the viral capsid and α_V integrins on host cell surfaces.[618]

After the virus has entered the host cell, the cellular synthetic machinery is redirected to the synthesis of viral components. As with many native proteins made by the host cell, a portion of viral protein is processed into peptides and presented on the infected cell surface by major histocompatibility complex (MHC) class I molecules (see later). The host mechanisms most important in defense against most viral pathogens include the production of specific neutralizing antibodies against viral surface proteins, the development of specific CD8+ cytotoxic T-cell responses that eliminate infected cells, and the production of interferons (IFNs) that disrupt viral replication.[367,369,504]

Other host defenses also may exhibit antiviral activity, although the importance of some of these mechanisms in protection against viral infection in humans has not been established as firmly. It is possible that natural killer (NK) cells mediate the destruction of infected host cells[126,542] and that antibody-dependent cellular cytotoxicity (ADCC) may ensue after IgG antibodies bind to viral antigens on the infected cell, permitting subsequent attachment of NK cells or cytotoxic T cells via IgG Fc receptors.[209] IFNs and other cytokines may enhance NK and ADCC activity, and cytokines such as tumor necrosis factor-α (TNF-α) may exert cytotoxic actions on cells infected with certain viruses.[369] Additionally, opsonic complement components bound to viral surfaces can interfere with cell attachment, and the complement-derived membrane attack complex (MAC) can lyse enveloped viruses.[63]

Bacteria

The human host is colonized with a large variety of bacteria at skin and mucous membrane surfaces.[113,482] The integrity of these mechanical barriers ordinarily prevents systemic invasion of local commensal bacteria.[93] The epithelial cells that constitute these barriers, on recognition of an organism as a pathogen, also can release defensins and other microbicidal molecules.[235] In healthy hosts, circulating polymorphonuclear leukocytes (PMNs) help keep the resident flora in check by leaving the bloodstream at the mucosal sites containing the highest bacterial burdens, such as the oral cavity and the lower intestine.[29] This phenomenon helps account for the increased risk of developing local and systemic infection caused by oral and intestinal organisms in patients with severe neutropenia, including patients who receive prolonged chemotherapy for malignancies, and in patients with phagocytic migratory function disorders, such as leukocyte adhesion deficiency syndromes.[29] Important host defenses against most bacteria that invade the human host systemically include the complement system, specific antibodies that promote the opsonic and the bacteriolytic functions of complement, and phagocytes.[2,29,63,279,310]

Fungi

Host mechanisms crucial for defense against fungi are less well understood than are the defense mechanisms directed at bacteria and viruses, but phagocytes and cell-mediated immunity seem to be most important.[197,223] The relative importance of these factors seems to depend on the specific organisms involved, as is shown by clinical observations in patients with isolated defects of one or the other. Severe mucosal infections caused by *Candida* spp. are common occurrences in patients with acquired or primary cell-mediated immune deficits, such as HIV infection, thymic aplasia (see later), chronic mucocutaneous candidiasis, and some forms of severe combined immunodeficiency (SCID), and in patients with disorders of leukocyte migration.[29,197] Disseminated candidiasis more often is attributed to iatrogenic factors, such as prolonged antimicrobial therapy and indwelling vascular catheters. Patients with malignancies, complicated postsurgical courses, and burns also seem to be at increased risk. Although neutrophils from patients with myeloperoxidase (MPO) deficiency kill *Candida* organisms more slowly than do neutrophils from healthy individuals, these patients usually do not develop *Candida* infections, suggesting that this aspect of neutrophil function is not crucial.[29,197]

In contrast to *Candida*, *Aspergillus* infections are not as great a problem for patients with cell-mediated immune defects as they are for patients with defects in phagocytic host defenses, such as chemotherapy-induced neutropenia, or genetic defects in phagocyte killing, such as chronic granulomatous disease (CGD).[61,622] Fungi such as *Histoplasma* and *Cryptococcus*, similar to *Candida*, tend to cause severe infections in patients with defects in cell-mediated immunity, although phagocytes are required for optimal clearance of these organisms.[305,616] The main role of antibodies and complement in protection from fungi probably is to provide opsonic activity to enhance phagocyte function.[181]

Parasites

Parasites, such as protozoa and helminths, comprise such a widely varying group of pathogenic organisms that generalizing about mechanisms of immunity to these organisms as a group is difficult. The importance of specific host mechanisms in defense against certain parasites may be appreciated, however, by considering the characteristic host responses mobilized by parasitic infection or infestations and examples of special susceptibilities to certain parasites among patients with impairments of different components of immunity. Many helminths induce production by host cells of chemokines that recruit eosinophils and stimulate their production, suggesting a likely role for these cells in antiparasitic defenses; eosinophils have been shown to be important in protection against helminths such as *Strongyloides* and other parasites in this group that can invade tissues. Among the immunoglobulins, IgE seems to play a special role, often in concert with eosinophils, in antihelminthic defenses. IgG also may be important, based on the susceptibility of individuals with hypogammaglobulinemia to hyperinfection with *Strongyloides*. Patients with hypogammaglobulinema or IgA deficiency also are at risk for developing chronic or severe infestations with the flagellate intestinal parasite, *Giardia lamblia*, suggesting a role for some degree of antibody-mediated protection in normal hosts. Patients with primary or acquired disorders of cell-mediated immunity are prone to development of serious central nervous system and ocular manifestations of infection with the protozoan *Toxoplasma gondii*, an obligate intracellular parasite, and hyperinfection with *Strongyloides*.[318,407,454]

FEATURES OF NORMAL IMMUNE FUNCTION

The organization of the immune system often has been viewed as consisting of several separate arms or compartments, such as complement, phagocytes, cell-mediated immunity, and humoral immunity. A more current approach often considers two broader categories—innate immunity and adaptive immunity. The former encompasses the more rapid and phylogenetically primitive, nonspecific responses to infection, such as surface defenses, cytokine elaboration, complement activation, and phagocytic responses, and the latter involves more slowly developing, persistent, and highly evolved antigen-specific responses, such as cell-mediated immunity and antibody production, which exhibit extraordinarily diverse ranges of specificities. Although the individual components of innate and adaptive immunity are addressed separately, the various arms of the immune system engage in a wide range of interactions that may enhance or regulate functions of other components of immunity and add to the already remarkable complexity of the human immune response, and numerous examples of such interactions are provided.

INNATE IMMUNE RESPONSES

Epithelia, Defensins, and Other Antimicrobial Peptides

The epithelium of skin and mucosal tissue functions as a mechanical barrier to the invasion of microbial pathogens. In the last 2 decades, it has become clear that epithelial cells also are a major source of antimicrobial peptides that play important roles in local host defense.[50,233-235,445] Studies of their structure, sources, expression, and actions also have revealed an unexpected range of immunologic activities for these molecules, the functions of which previously were considered mainly antimicrobial in nature.[3,35]

Epithelial cells of mucous membranes of the airways and intestines and keratinocytes express the human β-defensins, HBD-1, HBD-2, HBD-3, and HBD-4. These small cationic peptides are similar to the α-defensins stored in the azurophilic granules of neutrophils, and they display antimicrobial activity against a broad range of bacteria, fungi, chlamydiae, and enveloped viruses.[50,233,235,445] Their production by epithelial cells may be constitutive, as for HBD-1, or inducible, as for HBD-2, HBD-3, and HBD-4. More recent evidence indicates that epithelial

cells of the airway or intestine can produce HBD-2 in response to activation by bacterial products via the Toll-like receptors (TLRs), TLR2 or TLR4 (see later), on the epithelial cells.[275,602,608] Stimulation of epithelium by cytokines, including interleukin-1 (IL-1) or TNF-α, also can induce production of defensins.[50,235]

Defensins have been reported to exert their antimicrobial action either by the creation of membrane pores or by membrane disruption resulting from electrostatic interaction with the polar head groups of membrane lipids, with more evidence now favoring the latter mechanism.[50,288] Some microorganisms have evolved mechanisms for evading the action of defensins. Bacterial polysaccharide capsules may limit access of microbial peptides to the cell membrane,[118] and an exoprotein of *Staphylococcus aureus*, staphylokinase, neutralizes the microbicidal action of neutrophil α-defensins.[304]

Several immunoregulatory properties of defensins and related peptides, distinct from their antimicrobial actions, have been documented.[233] Several of these peptides have been shown to facilitate post-translational processing of IL-1β.[464] Some of the β-defensins have been shown to function as chemoattractants for neutrophils, memory T cells, and immature dendritic cells by binding to the chemokine receptor CCR-6.[287,427,445] Separately, HBD-2 has been shown to activate immature dendritic cells via a mechanism that requires TLR4.[72,625] The activation of immature dendritic cells by these mechanisms also promotes their maturation. The β-defensins also act as a chemoattractant for mast cells by an undefined mechanism, and they can induce mast cell degranulation.[426] HBD-2 and several other antimicrobial peptides can interfere with binding between bacterial lipopolysaccharide (LPS) and LPS-binding protein.[522]

Additional antimicrobial peptides of epithelial cells include lysozyme and cathelicidin. Lysozyme, an antimicrobial peptide also found in neutrophil granules, attacks the peptidoglycan cell walls of bacteria and may be released from cells by mechanisms that involve activation of TLR.[456] Cathelicidin, or LL37, similar to lysozyme, is released from neutrophils and epithelial cells. It exhibits broad antimicrobial activity and can inhibit lentiviral replication.[287,556] Cathelicidin also exhibits chemotactic activity for neutrophils, monocytes, and T lymphocytes. This activity is mediated by a formyl peptide receptor-like molecule, FPRL1, rather than the chemokine receptor CCR6 bound by β-defensins.[624]

The release of defensins in response to activation of TLRs and the many actions of these peptides, including their direct antimicrobial activities, their chemoattractant actions for a wide range of immune cells, and their activation of dendritic cell maturation, already suggest a highly complex and regulatory role in the development of host defense and immunity. More recent genomic evidence for the possible existence of 25 additional human defensins that have not yet been characterized suggests that current knowledge describes only a small sample of the overall contribution of these peptides to immune responses.[50,519]

Toll-Like Receptors

Mononuclear phagocytes, including circulating monocytes and tissue macrophages, other phagocytic cells, and many epithelial cells, express a family of receptors that is highly homologous to the *Drosophila* receptor called *Toll*.[99,275,393,602,608] These receptors mediate a phylogenetically primitive, non-clonal mechanism of pathogen recognition based on binding, not to specific antigens, but to structurally conserved pathogen-associated molecular patterns.[9,442,443,629] At least 10 human TLRs bind a range of microbial ligands, such as gram-negative bacterial LPS, bacterial lipoproteins, lipoteichoic acids of gram-positive bacteria, bacterial cell wall peptidoglycans, cell wall components of yeast and mycobacteria, unmethylated CpG dinucleotide motifs in bacterial DNA, and viral RNA.[9,442,443,629]

Gram-positive cell wall components bind mainly to TLR2, and TLR2 also can bind components of herpes simplex virus.[345,568] Gram-negative LPS activates TLR4 indirectly by first binding to LPS-binding protein, which binds to CD14 at the cell surface. The bound CD14 has no transmembrane domain, but it associates directly with an extracellular domain of TLR4.[443,568] TLR5 has been identified as the receptor for bacterial flagellin, TLR9 recognizes CpG motifs of bacterial DNA, and TLR3 has been shown to bind synthetic and viral double-stranded RNA.[59,265,341,345]

Signaling via TLRs occurs via a well-described pathway in which receptor binding generates a signal via an adapter molecule, MyD88, which leads to intracellular association with IL-1 receptor–associated kinase. This association leads to activation of TNF receptor–associated factor-6, which results in nuclear translocation of nuclear factor-κB.[140] NF-κB is an important transcription factor that activates the promoters of the genes for a broad range of cytokines and other proinflammatory products, such as TNF-α, IL-1, IL-6, and IL-8. This signaling pathway, based on studies with TLR4, is similar to, but not identical to, the signaling pathways activated by other TLRs.[140] The activation of cytokine production by TLRs plays an important role in recruiting other components of innate host defense against bacterial pathogens. With large-scale release of cytokines, the deleterious effects of sepsis or other forms of the systemic inflammatory response syndrome show, however, that these pathways have beneficial and potentially harmful effects for the host.[140] Genetic polymorphisms in TLRs may play a role in determining the balance of these effects in certain individuals responding to the challenge of systemic infection.[140,373,374]

In addition to their "first responder" roles in generating an inflammatory response to invading pathogens, TLRs may network with other components of innate and adaptive immunity. TLR4 function is suppressed by activation of cells via the chemokine receptor CXCR4.[326] Activation of some TLRs also can induce expression of the co-stimulatory molecule B7 on antigen-presenting cells (APCs), which is required for activation of naive T cells.[393]

Cytokines

A heterogeneous group of soluble small polypeptide or glycoprotein mediators, often collectively called *cytokines*, form part of a complex network that helps regulate the immune and inflammatory responses. Included in this group of mediators, molecular weights of which range from approximately 8 kd to approximately 45 kd, are the interleukins (ILs), IFNs, growth factors, and chemokines (see separately subsequently). Most cells of the immune system and many other host cell types release cytokines, respond to cytokines via specific cytokine receptors, or both.

New cytokines are being discovered and characterized regularly, and the range of sources and effects of cytokines and their actions and interrelationships are of such complexity that they cannot be addressed here in detail. A list of cytokines and related molecules that play a role in immune function, with selected characteristics, is provided in Table 2–1.[344,445,468] Excellent general reviews are available.[344,369,446,468] Numerous cytokines are considered in subsequent sections because they play important roles in the functions of various immune cells. Two cytokines, IL-1 and TNF-α, are of such fundamental importance in acute host responses to infection that they warrant specific attention here.

IL-1 and TNF-α are small polypeptides, each with a molecular weight of approximately 17 kd, which exhibit a broad range of effects on immunologic responses, inflammation, metabolism, and hematopoiesis.[69,446] IL-1 originally was described as "endogenous pyrogen," referring to its ability to produce fever in experimental animals, and TNF-α, which produces some of the same effects produced by IL-1, originally was named *cachectin* after the wasting syndrome it produced when injected chronically in mice.[69,446] Many of the physiologic changes associated with gram-negative sepsis can be reproduced by injecting experimental animals with these cytokines in the absence of microorganisms. Depending on the doses injected, these effects may include fever, hypotension, and either neutrophilia or leukopenia.[69,446]

In the production of endotoxic shock secondary to gram-negative sepsis, IL-1 and TNF-α are produced by mononuclear phagocytes in response to activation of TLRs by bacterial LPS. They activate the production of other cytokines and chemokines, lipid mediators such as platelet-activating factor and prostaglandins, and reactive oxygen species. They also induce expression of adhesion molecules of endothelial cells and leukocytes, stimulating recruitment of leukocytes by inducing release of the chemokine IL-8 and activating neutrophils for phagocytosis, degranulation, and oxidative burst activity.[69,140]

These all are important, usually beneficial, host responses to infection. At high levels of activation, pathophysiologic effects of this proinflammatory cascade, including vascular instability, decreased myocardial contractility, capillary leak, tissue hypoperfusion, coagulopathy, and multiple organ failure, may occur.[140] For some systemic actions, notably the production of hemodynamic shock, IL-1 and TNF-α are synergistic. IL-1 and TNF-α also induce production of IL-6, a less potent cytokine that exhibits some of the actions of IL-1 and TNF-α.[446] The human host produces several soluble antagonists of IL-1 and TNF-α, including IL-1 receptor antagonist, soluble TNF-α receptor, and anti-inflammatory cytokines, especially IL-10,[140] that can modulate their effects.

The importance of effects mediated by IL-1 and TNF-α in the pathophysiology of septic shock has prompted much active research aimed at blocking their effects to reduce morbidity and mortality. Monoclonal antibodies against TNF-α and other inhibitors of TNF-α or IL-1 have shown early promise in vitro and in animal models of septic shock.[30,45,140,222,446] They have been far more effective at preventing the effects of cytokines than reversing them, however. More recent attempts to address the issue of the timing of intervention have been directed at the intracellular signaling mechanisms activated through the TNF-α receptor or at mediators that appear later than TNF-α. Lipophilic inhibitors of protein tyrosine kinases, enzymes that propagate the cellular signals via TNF-α receptors, have been found to enhance survival in experimental animals, even when administered 2 hours after systemic injection with endotoxin.[594]

Additionally, monoclonal antibodies against a cytokine-like, non-histone nucleoprotein product of macrophages, high mobility group B1 (which appears much later than TNF-α or IL-1 after LPS stimulation) were found to rescue mice from endotoxin shock, when given 2 hours after an otherwise lethal dose of LPS was administered.[606] More recently, clinical trials with activated protein C, a regulatory protein in the coagulation cascade, have shown beneficial effects in selected patients with septic shock by mechanisms that may involve inhibition of activation of NF-κB.[100,482] To date, despite progress, clinical strategies to interfere with the cytokine-induced cascade that leads to endotoxin shock have continued, overall, to meet with limited success.

Chemokines

A specialized group of small cytokine-like polypeptides, chemokines, all of which share the feature of being ligands for G protein–coupled, seven transmembrane–segment receptors, plays an increasingly appreciated and complex role in the immune response as cellular activators that induce directed cell migration, mainly of immune and inflammatory cells.[46,300,324,386,419,500] The chemokines and their receptors have been classified into four families, based on the motif displayed by the first two cysteine

TABLE 2-1   Features of Selected Human Cytokines and Growth Factors

	Main Cellular Sources	Biologic Effects
IL-1	Mo, TL, BL, NK, PMN, others	Broad range of cellular activation in inflammatory and immune responses
IL-2	TL, BL, NK	TL, BL proliferation and activation; enhances TL and NK cytotoxicity
IL-3	TL	General stimulation of hematopoiesis
IL-4	TL, BL, Mast, Mo	TL, BL proliferation; BL isotype switching; stimulates IgE synthesis; enhances MHC class II expression
IL-5	TL	Stimulation of Eo production
IL-6	TL, BL, Mo	Broad inflammatory activity; stimulates BL differentiation and megakaryocyte production
IL-7	Marrow and thymus stromal cells	TL, BL growth and differentiation
IL-8	Mac, Mo, Endo, Epi, PMN, Eo	Activation and chemotaxis of PMN, Eo
IL-9	TL	Mast growth and differentiation; growth of activated TL
IL-10	TL, BL, Mast, Mac	Broad anti-inflammatory actions; inhibits synthesis of several other cytokines (TNF, IL-2, IL-3, IFN-γ)
IL-11	Marrow stromal cells	General stimulation of hematopoiesis; BL growth and differentiation
IL-12	BL, Mo	Stimulation of TL growth; induction of IFN-γ production; enhancement of TL and NK cytotoxicity
IL-13	TL	BL proliferation and isotype switching; enhances MHC class II expression; inhibits production of cytokines by Mac
IL-14	TL, malignant BL	Induces BL growth
IL-15	Epi, Endo, Mo, Mac, marrow stromal cells	Enhances NK growth, development, function; enhances TL growth/migration
IL-17	TL	Enhances TL growth; induces Mac cytokine release
IL-18	Kupffer cells, Epi, spleen, Mac	Promotes TL, BL, NK cytokine release; promotes TL, BL cytotoxicity
IL-21	TL	Promotes BL, TL proliferation; NK cytoxicity
IL-23	Dendritic cells, Mac	Similar to IL-12
IL-25	TL (T_H2), Mast	TL, Mac T_H2 cytokine secretion
IL-27	Dendritic cells, Mac	TL responsiveness to IL-12
IFN-α	Mo, TL	Interference with viral replication; increases MHC class I expression
IFN-β	Epi, Fibro	Similar to IFN-α
IFN-γ	TL, NK	Similar to IFN-α, IFN-β; stimulates Mac inflammatory functions
TNF-α	Mo, Mac, TL, NK	Broad inflammatory effects; fever; cachexia; stimulates catabolism; activation of leukocytes and Endo
GM-CSF	TL, BL, Mo, PMN, Eo, Fibro, Mast, Endo	Growth of PMN, Eo, Mo, and Mac precursors; enhances leukocyte function
G-CSF	Mo, Epi, Fibro	Enhances production and function of granulocytes
M-CSF	Mo, TL, BL, Endo, Fibro	Promotes Mo production; stimulates Mo and Mac function

BL, B lymphocyte; Endo, endothelial cell; Eo, eosinophil; Epi, epithelial cell; Fibro, fibroblast; GM-CSF, granulocyte-macrophage colony-stimulating factor; IFN, interferon; IL, interleukin; Mac, macrophage; Mast, mast cell; MHC, major histocompatibility complex; Mo, monocyte; NK, natural killer cell; PMN, polymorphonuclear leukocyte; TL, T lymphocyte; TNF, tumor necrosis factor.

residues of the respective chemokine peptide sequence. Each of at least 16 CXC chemokines binds to one or more of the CXCRs, CXCR1 through CXCR6. Examples of CXC chemokines include IL-8 and Gro-α. Similarly, at least 28 CC chemokines, such as MIP-1α, RANTES, and eotaxin-1, eotaxin-2, and eotaxin-3, bind to one or more of the CCRs, CCR1 through CCR10. The sole CX3C chemokine, fractalkine, or neurotaxin, binds to CX3CR1, currently the only receptor in its family. The two XC chemokines, including lymphotaxin, bind to the sole receptor in this family, XCR1.

A new nomenclature has been proposed to designate each of the chemokines as a numbered ligand for its respective receptor family. In this system, Gro-α is CXC ligand (L)-1 (or CXCL-1), and IL-8 now becomes CXCL-8. Similarly, RANTES becomes CCL-5, fractalkine is CX3CL-1, and lymphotactin is XCL-1.[300,500] An update of this nomenclature system has been published, tabulating the members of each family with their respective ligands and receptors and the traditional names in human and murine systems.[300]

Virtually every cell type of the immune system expresses receptors for one or more of the chemokines. The cells of virtually any inflamed tissue can release a variety of chemokines, and tissues infected with different bacteria or viruses release chemokines that recruit characteristic sets of immune cells.[244,324] Rhinoviruses induce the release of chemokines that result mainly in recruitment of neutrophils (early in the course of infection), whereas Epstein-Barr virus induces a set of chemokines that result in recruitment of B cells, NK cells, and CD4$^+$ and CD8$^+$ T cells.[244] Almost mutually exclusive sets of chemokines are induced by cytokines associated with T_H1 (IL-12, IFN-γ) versus T_H2 (IL-4, IL-13) immune responses, indicating a tight interplay between cytokines and chemokines in determining the type of immune response to specific infectious challenges generated under different conditions.[75] The specificity of such cellular responses is influenced strongly by the type of chemokines released by specific tissues, the vascular adhesion molecules expressed in those tissues, the chemokine receptors expressed by different populations of leukocytes, and the specific adhesion molecules expressed by leukocytes.[75,244,324]

Modulation of chemokine function may occur by several mechanisms. Chemokines themselves may be potentiated or inactivated by tissue proteases, including tissue peptidases and matrix metalloproteinases.[392,444] Heparan sulfate–related proteoglycans on endothelial cell surfaces tether chemokines locally, where they can activate circulating leukocytes for adhesion most efficiently (see later). Similar proteoglycans free in the extracellular environment may act to bind and sequester chemokines, however, preventing them from interacting with their cellular receptors.[145,346] Finally, in addition to the well-described use of chemokine receptors as co-receptors for viral entry by HIV-1, other viruses, especially members of the herpesvirus family, encode soluble decoy receptors that compete with native host receptors for chemokine binding, disrupting normal host responses.[145,497]

Natural Killer Cells

NK cells are an important cellular feature of innate immunity. They are lymphoid cells that do not express clonally distributed receptors, such as TCRs or surface immunoglobulin, for specific antigens.[411,412,542] They respond in an antigen-independent manner to help contain viral infections before the development of adaptive immune responses, and they aid in the control of malignant tumors.[542,543] NK cells are found in the peripheral circulation and in the spleen and bone marrow. Similar to many other leukocytes, they can be recruited to sites of inflammation by chemokines and other chemoattractants. They seem to be important for the control of tumors in vivo and serve a crucial function in host defense against viral infections, especially infections caused by members of the herpesvirus family.[126,542] Activated NK cells also are an important source of IFN-γ, which limits tumor angiogenesis and promotes the development of specific protective immune responses.[411,412,542,543]

Regulation of NK cell activity involves a balance between activating and inhibitory signals. Several cytokines can activate NK cell proliferation, cytotoxicity, or IFN-γ production, including IL-12, IL-15, IL-18, IL-21, and IFN-αβ.[542] Activating signals via other receptors on NK cells, such as NKG2D, may lead to cytotoxicity or cytokine production, or both, depending on the receptor's association with distinct intracellular adapter proteins that signal via different kinases.[542,598] Other molecules on NK cells may act as co-stimulatory or adhesion receptors, including CD27, CD28, CD154 (CD40 ligand), and LFA-1 (CD11a/CD18).[53,543] Additionally, FcγRIII (CD16), can contribute to NK cell cytotoxic activity by mechanisms that include ADCC.[209,412]

NK cells are able to distinguish normal cells of self origin via receptors that recognize specific MHC class I molecules. Activation of such receptors provides an inhibitory signal that protects healthy host cells from NK cell–mediated lysis. Virus-infected cells and malignant cells may express MHC class I molecules at reduced levels and may be less able to generate inhibitory NK cell signals, rendering them more susceptible to attack by NK cells.[126,542] NK cell inhibitory receptors, which are not well characterized, seem to contain intracytoplasmic tyrosine-based inhibition motifs and to antagonize NK cell activation pathways via protein tyrosine phosphatases.[480,542] The regulation of the phosphorylation state of specific tyrosine residues by activating kinases and inhibitory phosphatases seems to be a pivotal determinant of NK cell activation.

NK cells kill infected or malignant cells by the release of perforin and granzymes from granular storage compartments and by binding of the death receptors Fas and TRAIL-R on target cells via their respective NK cell ligands.[513,542,543] The mechanisms by which perforin and granzymes mediate target cell death are not fully understood. The best available evidence suggests that perforin and one or more of five human granzymes, released along with perforin from cytotoxic granules of NK cells, associate with the cell membranes of target cells, either by binding via the mannose 6-phosphate receptor or by another mechanism that remains to be defined. One or more of the granzymes seems to activate intracellular pathways leading to target apoptosis via pathways that involve the mitochondria or caspases or both.[319,584] Separately, binding of the death receptors also activates caspases, causing target cell apoptosis.[542] Although some tumor cells do not express Fas, NK cells can induce Fas expression on these targets by releasing IFN-γ, then proceed to kill them by binding to the newly expressed Fas.[523]

NK cells engage in several kinds of interactions with other cells of the immune system, including dendritic cells and other APCs. Dendritic cells can influence the proliferation and activation of NK cells by release of cytokines, including IL-12, and by cell surface interactions, including CD40/CD40 ligand (CD40L),

LFA-1/ICAM-1, and CD27/CD70.[173] In return, NK cells can provide signals that result in either dendritic cell maturation or apoptosis.[126,542]

Complement System

The complement system consists of more than 30 different free and membrane-bound activation and regulatory proteins. It has multiple key roles in the clearance of invading microbes, including opsonization, recruitment of inflammatory cells, and lytic destruction of pathogens.[62,178,196,198,217,305,308,309,416] Complement and antibody often act synergistically in host defense against infection. Traditionally, they have been known as the heat-labile (complement) and heat-stable (antibody) factors, which contribute to serum opsonic and bactericidal activity. Activation of the complement response to the initial encounter with an organism usually occurs earlier than that of antibody because some components of complement activation are independent of antibodies and can be initiated before specific antibody can be produced. When specific antibody is available, it serves to activate complement more efficiently and to direct complement binding to locations on the microbial surface that support the optimal execution of its effector functions, such as opsonization and killing.

Approximately 90 percent of complement proteins are synthesized in the liver, but some components can be produced locally at sites of infection by tissue mononuclear phagocytes and fibroblasts.[143,463] In healthy individuals, most complement is found in the circulation; less than 10 percent is in mucosal secretions, and little is detectable in cerebrospinal fluid. Circulating complement levels vary over time, particularly in the presence of inflammation. The inflammatory response may lead to increases in levels of complement components such as C3 that are acute-phase reactants or to decreases in individual components and total complement activity as a result of consumption.

The importance of normal complement component levels and activity in host defense has been well established and is based primarily on the increased susceptibility of patients with specific complement component deficiencies to recurrent and severe infections.[176,178,196,305,308] Although the complement response to infection usually is beneficial to the host, it also may be associated with adverse clinical manifestations, such as septic shock and acute respiratory distress syndrome.[212,610]

COMPLEMENT ACTIVATION

Complement proteins are activated in a specific sequence or "cascade" via one of at least three pathways—the classical pathway, the alternative pathway, and the more recently described mannan-binding lectin (MBL) pathway (Fig. 2–1). These pathways converge at C3, and the complement cascade downstream from C3 proceeds identically, regardless of the pathway by which activation occurs. The C3 convertases, C4b2a for the classical and MBL pathways, and C3bBb for the alternative pathway, cleave the C3 molecule at exactly the same location, producing C3b, which binds to the target surface, and C3a, which is released into the fluid phase. Cleavage and activation of C3 lead to a conformational change in C3b that transiently renders its reactive thioester group capable of forming covalent ester or amide bonds with acceptor molecules on the target surface.[291,353]

If the acceptor molecules are situated on the surface of a microorganism, the bound C3b can act as an opsonin to promote phagocytosis, or it can bind with the classical and alternative pathway C3 convertases to form the C5 convertases, C4b2a3b and C3bBb3b. C5 convertases bind and then cleave C5, with release of the C5a fragment into the fluid phase. The bound C5b fragment can initiate formation of the MAC by the sequential incorporation of the remaining terminal components, C6, C7, C8, and multiple molecules of C9. The MAC can insert into the

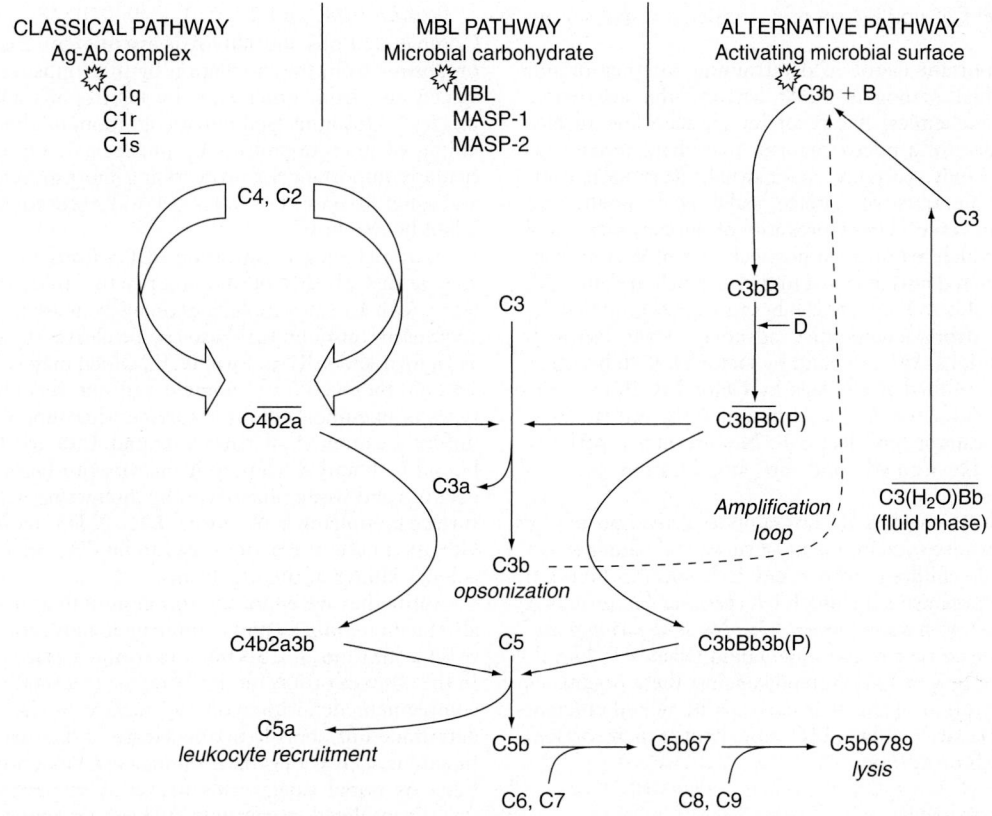

CLASSICAL PATHWAY
Ag-Ab complex

MBL PATHWAY
Microbial carbohydrate

ALTERNATIVE PATHWAY
Activating microbial surface

Figure 2–1 The complement cascade. The initial binding events of the classical, mannan-binding lectin (MBL), and alternative pathways are indicated by a *starburst*. These pathways intersect at the conversion of C3 to C3b. This is followed by activation of the terminal components, beginning with the binding and cleavage of C5, releasing C5a and leaving bound C5b to initiate assembly of the remaining components to form the membrane attack complex (C5b, 6, 7, 8, 9). Enzymatically active proteases, or convertases, of the classical and alternative pathways that cleave and activate subsequent components are shown by convention with an *overbar*. The alternative pathway C3 and C5 convertases are shown associated with properdin (P), which increases their stability.

outer membrane of target cells, such as erythrocytes or gram-negative bacteria, and cause cell lysis and death.[309]

Classical Pathway
Ordinarily, the classical pathway is activated by IgM or IgG bound to microbial antigenic targets or by other kinds of antigen-antibody complexes.[178] IgM activates complement more efficiently than does IgG because only one molecule of polymeric IgM is required compared with at least two molecules of IgG.[151] Activation is initiated when C1q binds directly to an immuno-globulin molecule on the surface of an organism or, less often, to a surface molecule of the organism itself. C1r and C1s are activated and bound to C1q sequentially, forming C1qrs. The enzymatic activity of this complex, which resides in the C1s molecule, can cleave multiple molecules of C4 and C2 into two fragments each. The C4a and C2b fragments are released into the environment, whereas C4b and C2a remain bound to each other on the surface of the target to form the classical pathway C3 convertase, C4b2a. C4bC2a can cleave and activate C3 and localize C3b binding to nearby sites on the target surface. As noted previously, some C3b binds with C4b2a to form the classical pathway C5 convertase, C4b2a3b. Activation of the classical pathway ordinarily is not initiated by complexes of antigens with IgG4, IgA, IgD, or IgE.

Alternative Pathway
The classical pathway requires specific antibody and contributes to host defense in immune individuals, whereas the alternative pathway is more important in protection of non-immune

hosts, such as premature infants who have low levels of transplacentally acquired antibody and older infants and young children whose maternal antibody has waned, but who have not yet produced their own specific antibodies. The alternative pathway can be initiated by microbial surface macromolecules (e.g., polysaccharide, LPS, teichoic acid), although, as noted earlier, in some circumstances, specific antibody increases alternative pathway efficiency and may direct the location of C3b binding.[309]

A spontaneous low level of hydrolysis of the thioester of C3 in the fluid phase results in an activated form of C3, C3(H2O). This activated form of C3 can bind factor B, and the latter then is cleaved by factor D to form the fluid-phase C3 convertase C3(H2O)Bb. The constitutive presence of small amounts of this convertase in the fluid phase ensures that a small amount of C3b always is available to bind to microbial surfaces and initiate the alternative pathway.[457] The alternative pathway protein factor B has structural and functional similarities to C2, including the ability to bind to surface-bound C3b. When bound to C3b, factor B undergoes proteolytic cleavage by factor D to release a small soluble fragment, Ba, leaving the larger fragment, Bb, associated with C3b. C3bBb, the alternative pathway C3 convertase, is analogous to the classical pathway C3 convertase, C4b2a. Properdin stabilizes the C3 convertase C3bBb, permitting more efficient activation of C3 to form more C3b, creating the C3 amplification loop (see Fig. 2–1).[211,214] Alternative pathway activation of C3 by this mechanism is several times less efficient than activation via the classical pathway, but it is vital to host defense because it is the principal means by which a non-immune host can activate C3 until a specific antibody response can be mounted.[175,214]

The most important factor in determining whether or not a specific microbial pathogen would activate the alternative pathway is the biochemical nature of its surface. The surface biochemical features of a microorganism that characterize it as an activator are only partially understood. Microorganisms that bear large amounts of surface sialic acid usually are non-activators, however. The expression of surface sialic acid is one means by which mammalian host cells are protected from complement-mediated lysis in vivo. On surfaces rich in sialic acid, bound C3b is less able to bind factor B because another molecule, factor H, has a strong competitive advantage over factor B under these conditions. When bound by factor H, C3b becomes highly susceptible to further cleavage by factor I (C3b inactivator), resulting in C3bi (or iC3b). Although C3bi can function as an opsonin, it cannot bind factor B. No alternative pathway convertases can be formed, and no amplification loop is established.[62,416]

Organisms whose surfaces do not support activation of the alternative pathway are some of the most successful pathogens in infants and young children, who often lack specific humoral immunity. These organisms include K1 *Escherichia coli*, groups A and B streptococci, *Streptococcus pneumoniae*, *Neisseria meningitidis*, *Haemophilus influenzae* type b, and some salmonellae.[121,309] Development of specific IgG or IgM antibody against these organisms permits some activation of the alternative pathway and efficient activation of the classical pathway of complement at their surfaces and correlates with protection.

Mannan-Binding Lectin Pathway

A third complement activation pathway, the MBL pathway, has been described more recently. It is similar to the classical pathway, but it does not involve antibodies. MBL is a serum protein of the collectin family that has structural and functional similarities to those of C1q. It does not require antigen-antibody complexes to initiate its complement-activating function, however. MBL binds to mannose-containing carbohydrates on microbial surfaces, leading to its association at the microbial surface with activated MBL-associated serine proteases (MASP-1 and MASP-2). These latter proteases seem to have structural and functional similarities to those of C1r and C1s and result in activation of C4, with sequential binding of C4b and C2a and formation of C4b2a, the C3 convertase of the classical pathway. C3 is activated, and the cascade proceeds as described. A more detailed characterization of the MBL pathway and its role in immune responses to infection may be found in an excellent review.[465]

EFFECTOR FUNCTIONS OF COMPLEMENT IN HOST DEFENSE

All complement effector functions in host defense against infection require activation of the complement cascade through at least C3. The cascade needs to be activated through only C3 for effective opsonization, stimulation of leukocytosis, and immune regulation. Activation through C5 is required to produce a normal inflammatory response, including recruitment of phagocytes to sites of inflammation, and activation through C8 is needed for formation of the MAC. Complement may be activated and bound to cell surfaces but may not be able to carry out its effector functions if it is bound at a disadvantageous location.[97,250,290] C3b bound to a pneumococcal cell wall underneath a thick polysaccharide capsule is not accessible to CR1 on phagocytes and does not promote effective opsonophagocytosis. Similarly, complement-mediated killing of some strains of *Salmonella* is prevented when the MAC is bound to long LPS molecules distant from the organism's cell membrane.[309]

Opsonic Activity

Complement opsonic activity is essential for effective removal of organisms from the circulation by macrophages in the liver and spleen and from other sites by neutrophils and tissue macrophages.[82] Opsonins facilitate recognition, binding, ingestion, and killing of microorganisms by phagocytes. Opsonization is particularly important for protection against gram-positive bacteria and fungi because their thick cell walls prevent them from being killed by the MAC.

As noted earlier, activation of C3 leads to a conformational change in C3b that permits its reactive thioester to bind covalently with acceptor molecules on microbial surfaces, where it can serve as an opsonin. C3b also can be cleaved by inactivators such as factor I and CR1 to form iC3b, which may be a more efficient opsonin than C3b.[250,291] Some organisms, including certain serotypes of pneumococci, have surfaces that support degradation of differing amounts of surface-bound C3b to iC3b.[290] Surface-bound C3b and iC3b permit microbes to be recognized by circulating and tissue phagocytes by interacting with the phagocyte surface complement receptors, CR1 (CD35) and CR3 (CD11b/CD18). These interactions lead to binding, ingestion, and intracellular killing of the organisms.[250,291,353]

Antibodies are important opsonins in their own right, but they also facilitate more rapid complement activation and more effective localization of C3b binding to the surface of the organism. In the absence of specific antibody to direct complement binding, complement deposition on the surface of the target would be determined principally by the nature of the surface, and effector functions such as opsonization may not be performed as successfully. As noted earlier, this matter is of particular importance for encapsulated organisms, such as pneumococci, because in the absence of specific anticapsular antibody, C3b would be deposited at the cell wall, where it is inaccessible to phagocyte receptors.[97,290,311]

Inflammation

The cleavage products of several complement proteins contribute to the development of an inflammatory response. C3a stimulates an increase in the number of circulating granulocytes, and C5a serves as a potent stimulus for migration of monocytes, neutrophils, and eosinophils toward the source of C5a gradients being produced at infected tissue sites. C5a also up-regulates phagocytes' expression of CR1 and CR3 and stimulates them to release stored enzymes and other granular contents that also are important mediators of inflammation, aggregation, and production of microbicidal oxidants. C5a-induced neutrophil aggregation and stasis in the pulmonary circulation can be an important feature of the respiratory distress syndrome associated with sepsis.[610]

The anaphylotoxins, C4a, C3a, and especially C5a, induce release of histamine from mast cells and basophils, causing increased vascular dilation and permeability, which permit local influx of other inflammatory mediators.[294] In this way, they help produce the hallmark clinical manifestations of inflammation, swelling, and erythema. When large quantities of anaphylotoxins are released rapidly, they can contribute to septic shock.[212] Carboxypeptidase treatment of C4a, C3a, and C5a destroys their anaphylatoxin activity, but the C5a cleavage product $C5a_{des\ arg}$ maintains some chemoattractant-activating and phagocyte-activating activity.[323]

Microbicidal Activity

Complement can act directly on certain bacteria to kill them. As noted earlier, C5b and the terminal complement proteins C6, C7, C8, and C9 form the MAC, which can kill and lyse target cells such as gram-negative bacteria by penetrating their outer membranes.[309] The C5b-C8 complex serves as a polymerization site for several molecules of C9.[71] Although C9 is not essential to membrane penetration, its presence as poly-C9 allows it to proceed more efficiently.[569] Electron microscopy of the MAC shows that it is composed of a ringlike structure at the outer surface of the target cell membrane and a perpendicular cylindrical component that penetrates the cell membrane. As has been noted, the MAC cannot penetrate the thick cell walls of gram-positive bacteria and fungi and cannot kill these organisms directly.

The MAC can lyse some virus-infected host cells and some enveloped viruses themselves.[152] Additionally, C1 and C4 can enhance neutralization of virus by antibody.

Immune Regulation

Complement components and fragments can modulate several features of the immune response—directly by binding to CR1, CR2, and CR3 on the surfaces of T cells, B cells, and other cells involved in antigen recognition and indirectly by stimulating the synthesis and release of cytokines.[204] The C3b cleavage product, C3dg, when covalently bound to antigen, brings the antigen close to B cells by binding to B-cell CR2 (CD21).[73,88,119,178,439] Complement decreases the amount of antigen required to induce an immune response and increases the efficiency of the process by facilitating presentation and localization of antigen. C3 influences antigenic localization within germinal centers, and it is involved in anamnestic responses and isotype switching. The importance of complement in the immune response has been shown by the finding that C1-deficient, C2-deficient, C4-deficient, and C3-deficient animals have decreased antibody responses that can be restored by providing the missing protein.[73,88,119,178,439] Deficiency of early complement components, such as C2, in humans also has been associated with antibody deficiencies.[17,119]

Phagocytes

The first recognized cellular mechanism of host defense was the accumulation of phagocytic host cells around a foreign body in starfish observed by Metchnikoff.[397] PMNs, the most abundant circulating phagocytes in the human host, serve as a model here for discussing phagocyte functions. These cells constitute a major line of defense against invading bacteria and fungi. The proliferation of myeloid marrow progenitors and their differentiation into mature progeny are regulated by specific growth factors and cytokines.[47,367,576] The normal half-life of circulating PMNs is approximately 8 to 12 hours.[604] In the absence of active infection, most PMNs leave the circulation via the gingival crevices and the lower gastrointestinal tract, where the resident flora stimulate ongoing local extravasation of PMNs, a process that helps maintain the integrity of these tissues.[30] In response to invasive bacterial infection, circulating PMNs engage in three major functions: (1) migration to the site of infection, (2) recognition and ingestion of invading microorganisms, and (3) killing and digestion of these organisms.

PHAGOCYTE RECRUITMENT TO INFECTED SITES

Activation of endothelial cells that line the microvessels of acutely infected tissue occurs via locally produced cytokines, eicosanoid compounds, and microbial products.[115,534] As a result, the endothelial cells rapidly up-regulate their surface expression of P-selectin and then E-selectin.[70,537] These selectins engage in lectin-like interactions with the fucosylated tetrasaccharide moiety sialyl Lewis X, which is presented on constitutively expressed glycoproteins on PMNs, including L-selectin and P-selectin glycoprotein ligand-1.[350,366,631] These early interactions slow the PMNs in this first adhesive phase of leukocyte recruitment, sometimes described as "slow rolling."[70,115,534]

Within several hours, newly synthesized ICAM-1 is expressed at the endothelial surface.[115,534,556] The slowly rolling PMNs are activated by transient selectin-mediated interactions and locally produced mediators, especially endothelium-derived chemokines, such as IL-8.[365] These chemokines are most effective in activating the PMNs when they are bound by complex proteoglycans at the endothelial cell surface.[346] The activated PMNs produce a conformational activation of their surface β_2 integrins LFA-1 and Mac-1[179,595] and translocate an additional large quantity of Mac-1 from intracellular storage pools to the cell surface.[63,84] The newly translocated Mac-1 also may undergo this activation as the PMN is exposed to increasing concentrations of activating mediators.[179,282]

These activated β_2 integrins interact with the endothelial cell ICAM-1 in this second, firm adhesion phase mediated by integrin-ICAM interactions, which ultimately is necessary for transendothelial migration of the PMNs.[63,115,179,365,525,534,536] Other chemoattractants, such as C5a, N-formyl bacterial oligopeptides, and leukotrienes (e.g., leukotriene B4), which diffuse from the site of infection, activate PMNs further and provide a chemotactic gradient for migration of PMNs into tissue.[241,419] The receptors for these chemoattractants, similar to the chemokine receptors, are G protein–coupled and have a seven transmembrane–domain structure.[241,419] They constitute important sensory mechanisms of the PMNs for activating adhesion, directional orientation, and the contractile protein-dependent lateral movement of adhesion sites in the PMN membrane necessary for migration.[26,241,419,561]

A scheme for recruitment of PMNs from the microcirculation into infected tissue is presented in Figure 2–2, and a more detailed diagram depicting the surface molecules that mediate PMN-endothelial adhesion is provided in Figure 2–3. Although the specific stimuli and adhesion molecules may vary, this general scheme applies to the local recruitment of virtually all circulating cells of the immune system.[75,244,324]

PHAGOCYTOSIS

After PMNs reach the site of infection, they must recognize and ingest, or phagocytose, the invading bacteria. Opsonization, especially with IgG and fragments of C3, greatly enhances phagocytosis.[290,310] Although non-opsonic phagocytosis may occur, only opsonin-mediated phagocytosis is discussed here. CR1 and CR3, respectively, are the main phagocytic receptors for opsonic C3b and iC3b.[63,213] When PMNs are activated by chemoattractants or other stimuli, CR1 and CR3 are translocated rapidly to the cell surface from intracellular storage compartments, increasing surface expression 10-fold.[63,213] CR3 is identical to the adhesion-mediating integrin Mac-1.[36,63] CR1 and CR3 act synergistically with receptors for the Fc portion of antibodies, especially IgG.[36,310]

Phagocytic cells may express three different types of IgG Fc receptors, or FcγRs, all of which can mediate phagocytosis.[209,587] FcγRI (CD64) is a high-affinity receptor that is expressed mainly on mononuclear phagocytes.[587] The two FcγRs ordinarily expressed on circulating PMNs are FcγRII (CD32) and FcγRIII (CD16).[576,587] FcγRII is conventionally anchored in the cell membrane, exhibits polymorphisms that determine preferences for binding of certain IgG subclasses, and can activate PMN oxidative burst activity directly.[576,587,588] FcγRIII is expressed on PMNs as a glycolipid-anchored protein, although it is anchored conventionally on NK cells and macrophages.[587] Most phagocytes also express IgA receptors. The best-characterized FcαR, CD89, binds monomeric IgA and promotes phagocytosis and killing of IgA-opsonized bacteria.[292,409]

The engagement of phagocyte receptors with microbial opsonins on microbes locally activates cytoskeletal contractile elements, leading to invagination of the phagocyte membrane at

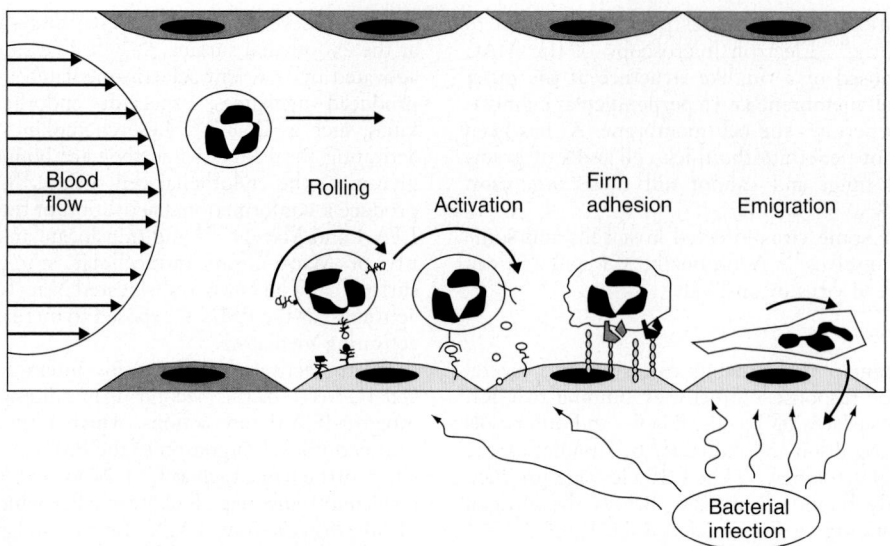

Figure 2–2 Events during polymorphonuclear leukocyte (PMN) recruitment to infected sites. Interactions between microorganisms in infected tissue and host cells and proteins result in elaboration of mediators that diffuse to the local microcirculation and stimulate the endothelial cells. This stimulation induces new surface expression of P-selectin and E-selectin, release of interleukin-8 and other chemokines, and new surface intercellular adhesion molecule 1 (ICAM-1). The endothelial selectins bind to constitutively expressed carbohydrate ligands on circulating PMNs and slow the passage of the PMNs through the microvessels. As the PMNs slow further, they become activated by interaction with chemokines bound to complex glycopeptides on the endothelial surface. This activation of PMNs increases their expression and binding activity of the β_2 (CD11/CD18) integrins, Mac-1 and lymphocyte function-associated antigen 1 (LFA-1). Interactions between these integrins and ICAM-1 (and ICAM-2 in the case of LFA-1) lead to tight adhesion and spreading on the endothelial surface. These latter adhesive interactions also are used for migration between endothelial cells and through the subjacent extracellular matrix in response to the gradient of chemoattractants, such as C5a and bacterial peptides, released at the infected site. Homophilic interactions between platelet–endothelial cell adhesion molecule-1 (PECAM-1) on the PMNs and endothelial cells also seem to contribute to transendothelial migration. *(Drawing courtesy of Dr. Scott Seo.)*

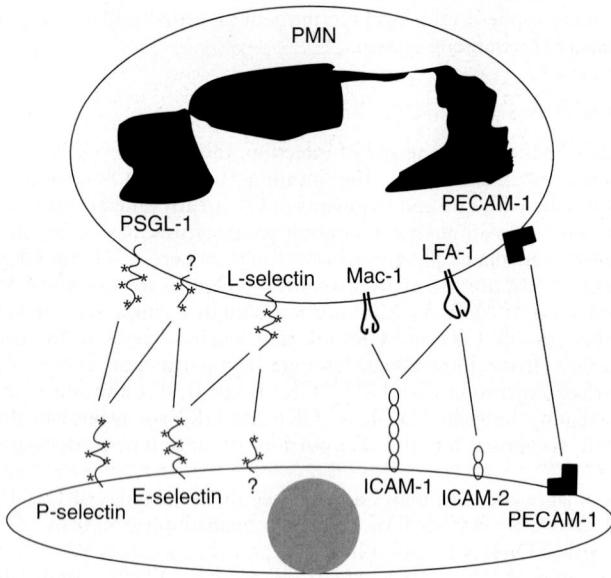

Figure 2–3 Molecular interactions that mediate polymorphonuclear leukocyte (PMN)–endothelial adhesion. The selectins, P-selectin and E-selectin on endothelium and L-selectin on leukocytes, bind to oligosaccharide moieties, including sialyl Lewis X (sLeX), which decorate the selectins and other glycoproteins on the opposite cell, including P-selectin glycoprotein ligand-1 (PSGL-1) on leukocytes. These interactions mediate the early adhesive phase of leukocyte recruitment. The β_2 integrins macrophage antigen 1 (Mac-1) (CD11b/ CD18) and lymphocyte function-associated antigen 1 (LFA-1) (CD11a/ CD18) on PMNs bind intercellular adhesion molecule 1 (ICAM-1) on endothelial cells. LFA-1 also can bind ICAM-2, which is expressed constitutively on endothelium. Platelet–endothelial cell adhesion molecule-1 (PECAM-1) molecules interact with each other and are expressed on PMNs and endothelial cells.

the site of initial engagement and the extension of pseudopods around the microbe. The ligation of additional opsonin-receptor pairs leads to engulfment of the microbe within a sealed phagosome,[560] as depicted in Figure 2–4. This engulfment is followed by fusion of the phagosome with lysosomal compartments containing the phagocyte's array of microbicidal products.

PHAGOCYTE MICROBICIDAL MECHANISMS

The microbicidal mechanisms of PMNs usually are categorized as either oxygen-dependent or oxygen-independent,[492] and intracellular killing usually occurs after the phagosome fuses with one or more types of lysosomal granules that contain many of the cell's microbicidal weapons. The contents of the three major populations of intracellular granules of PMNs, which contain many of the PMN's microbicidal molecules, either free within the granules or anchored in the granule membrane, are shown in Table 2–2.[84,85,235] Oxygen-dependent microbicidal mechanisms of phagocytes depend on a complex enzyme, nicotinamide adenine dinucleotide phosphate (NADPH) oxidase, which converts molecular oxygen (O_2) into superoxide anion (O_2^-).[42,135] This enzyme is assembled at the activated cell membrane from six or more components that include a cytochrome (*a* and *b* subunits, designated gp91*phox* and p22*phox* ["phox" refers to phagocyte oxidase]), a flavoprotein, and a quinone, all of which are associated with the cell membrane, and at least two cytoplasmic proteins, p47*phox* and p67*phox*, which assemble with the membrane-associated components to form the active enzyme complex.[42,84,135] Each of the main oxidant products derived from these reactions exhibits microbicidal activity, including the earliest products, O_2^- and hydrogen peroxide (H_2O_2), which are less potent than the downstream products hypochlorite (OCl^-) and chloramines (NH_3Cl, RNH_2Cl), chloramines being the most stable.[492] Figure 2–5 shows the sequence of the main oxidative reactions of PMN after the formation of superoxide anion.

TABLE 2–2 Stored Contents of Neutrophil Granules and Vesicles

Primary (Azurophilic) Granules	Secondary (Specific) Granules[a]	Tertiary Granules[b]	Secretory Vesicles[c]
Elastase	Lactoferrin	Gelatinase	Alkaline phosphatase
Cathepsin G	Vitamin B_{12}–binding protein		
Myeloperoxidase	Lysozyme		
Defensins	Gelatinase		
Bactericidal/permeability-increasing protein			
"p15s"			
Cathelicidin (LL37)			
Lysozyme			

Selected membrane-bound proteins in intracellular granules and vesicles:
f-met-leu-phe receptor[a,b,c]
type 1 complement receptor (CR1)[c]
CD11b/CD18 (CR3, Mac-1)[a,b,c]
cytochrome b_{558}[a,b,c]
type III Fcγ receptor (CD16)[c]

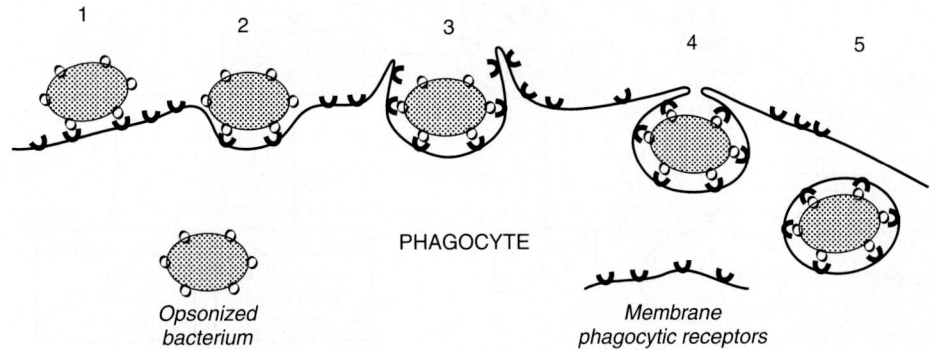

PHAGOCYTE

Opsonized bacterium

Membrane phagocytic receptors

Figure 2–4 Opsonin-receptor-mediated phagocytosis. Phagocytes such as polymorphonuclear leukocytes (PMNs) that reach the site of bacterial infection are activated for enhanced recognition, attachment, and ingestion of bacteria that have been coated with opsonic C3 fragments, IgG, or both via specific receptors on the PMN surface. Binding of opsonized bacteria to opsonin receptors (1) activates contractile elements of the cytoskeleton to produce an invagination at the initial site of attachment (2), with subsequent extension of membrane pseudopods around the organism (3). This process allows engagement of additional opsonin-receptor pairs, as the organism becomes engulfed (4). Finally, the plasma membrane fuses completely around the bacteria to create the phagosome (5), which soon fuses with lysosomal granules, exposing the bacterium to the microbicidal components of the phagocyte.

1. $2O_2 + NADPH \xrightarrow{\text{NADPH oxidase}} 2O_2^- + NADP^+ + H^+$

2. $2O_2^- + 2H^+ \xrightarrow{\substack{\text{Spontaneous or}\\\text{catalyzed by dismutase}}} H_2O_2 + O_2$

3. $H_2O_2 + H^+ + Cl^- \xrightarrow{\text{Myeloperoxidase}} H^+ + OCl^- + H_2O$

4. $H^+ + OCl^- + RNH_2 \longrightarrow RNHCl + H_2O$

Figure 2–5 Major reactions in the evolution of oxygen-dependent polymorphonuclear leukocyte microbicidal activity. The conversion of molecular oxygen to superoxide anion (O_2^-) by nicotinamide adenine dinucleotide phosphate (NADPH) oxidase is the initial event in the sequence of production of antimicrobial oxidants. Shown in order are the subsequent reactions for production of hydrogen peroxide (H_2O_2), hypochlorite (OCl^-), and chloramines (RNH_2Cl).

Oxygen-independent microbicidal activity of PMNs resides mainly in a group of proteins and peptides stored within primary (azurophilic) granules. Lysozyme is contained in the primary and the secondary (specific) granules of PMN.[551] It cleaves important linkages in the peptidoglycan of bacterial cell walls and is most effective when it can act in concert with the complement MAC.[310] The primary granules contain several cationic proteins with important microbicidal activity. A 59-kd protein, bactericidal/permeability-increasing protein, is active against only gram-negative bacteria.[612] Smaller arginine-rich and cysteine-rich peptides, the α-defensins, similar to the β-defensins of epithelial cells, are active against a range of bacteria, fungi, chlamydiae, and enveloped viruses, and other related molecules include cathelicidin and a group of peptides called p15s.[230,234,235,363] The mechanisms of action of these peptides are not fully understood, although they are addressed in the earlier section on antimicrobial peptides of epithelial cells. Some of these PMN proteins and peptides may interact with each other synergistically to enhance overall antimicrobial activity.[362]

Important Interactions among Innate Immune Mechanisms

A schematic overview of many of the main features of innate immunity discussed previously, along with some of their important interactions, is diagrammed in Figure 2–6. Several levels of interactions are depicted, from initial host-pathogen contact, through a variety of activating signals, to the attack by host effector mechanisms on pathogenic targets.

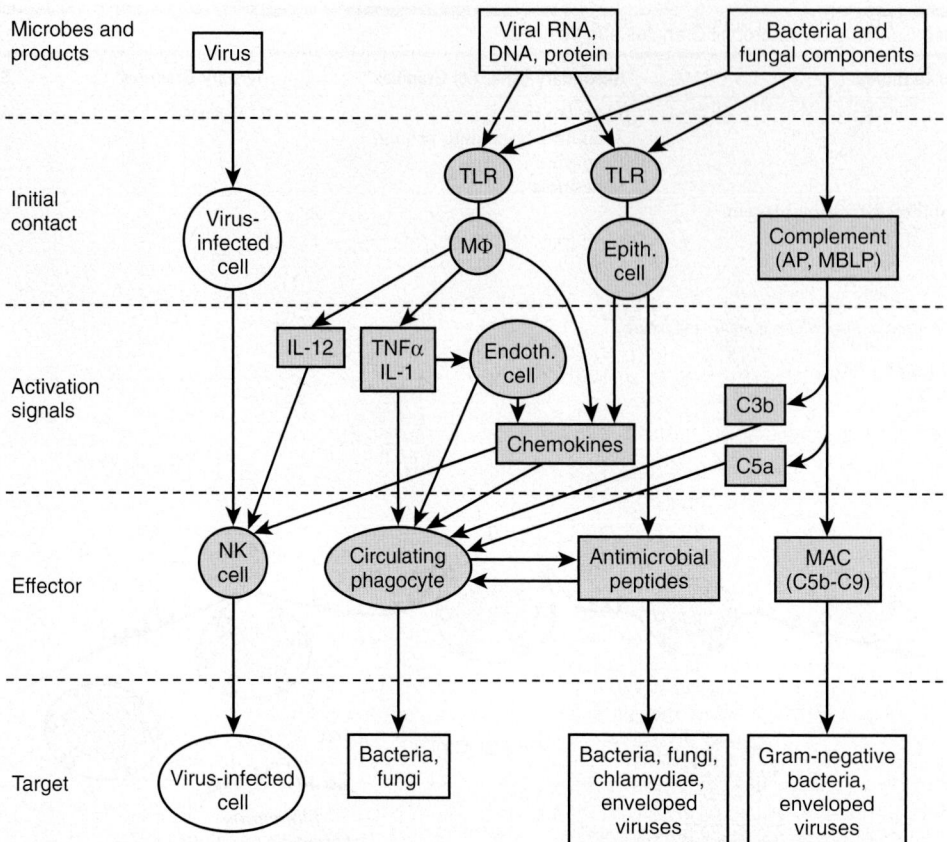

Figure 2–6 Innate immunity: first contact, intermediate signals, and effector mechanisms. Diagrammed are important host responses to infection that are independent of specific cell-mediated immunity or antibodies. Initial contact between the host and microbes or their products may result in viral infection of cells, activation of Toll-like receptors (TLRs) on macrophages (MΦ) and epithelial cells, and activation of the alternative pathway (AP) or mannose-binding lectin pathway (MLBP) of complement. The resulting activation signals, including cytokines (e.g., interleukin-12 [IL-12], tumor necrosis factor–α [TNF-α], IL-1), chemokines, and products of the complement cascade, mobilize cellular (natural killer [NK] cells, phagocytes) and humoral (antimicrobial peptides, membrane attack complex [MAC]) effectors, which attack their respective microbial targets. *(From Tosi, M. F.: Innate immune responses to infection. J. Allergy Clin. Immunol. 116:241-249, 2005.)*

ADAPTIVE IMMUNE RESPONSES

Adaptive immunity involves the host's antigen-specific responses to infectious challenges that, once modified, can help clear some infections and can provide specific protection against subsequent challenges. The major steps in the development of adaptive immunity include processing and presentation of specific antigens by APCs, activation of T lymphocytes for specific cytotoxic T-cell activity, T-cell cytokine production, and T-cell help in activating and maturing of antigen-specific B cells for the production of specific antibodies. Innate immune responses often occur in minutes to hours and may activate early cellular responses that are essential for the development of adaptive immunity. The full development of most adaptive immune responses requires days to weeks. When developed, however, adaptive immune responses often can provide durable protection. Figure 2–7 depicts the major events in the adaptive immune response to infection.

Antigen Presentation and Specific Cell-Mediated Immunity

Specific cell-mediated immunity provides T-cell help for production of antibodies by B cells, cytokine production for the stimulation and regulation of a range of immune responses, and cytotoxic T-cell activity against host cells infected with viruses.[184,414,461] The development of cell-mediated immunity requires complex inter-

actions to occur between T cells and APCs via several types of surface molecules on the respective cell surfaces. These interactions include binding of an antigen-specific T-cell receptor (TCR) on the T lymphocyte to a peptide antigen presented on the class I or class II MHC by the APC, with concurrent binding of the class I or class II MHC by CD8 or CD4,[574] as shown in Figure 2–8. Other respective pairs of accessory cell/surface molecules that enhance interactions between T cells and APCs include CD40L/CD40, LFA-1/ICAM-1, and CD28/B7. An additional molecule, cytotoxic T lymphocyte antigen-4, expressed on activated T cells, also can bind to B7 molecules on APCs to generate a suppressive signal that may terminate T-cell activation.[574] The sustained physical interface between T cells and APCs at which these molecular interactions take place has been characterized as the *immunologic synapse*.[96,252]

CLASS I MAJOR HISTOCOMPATIBILITY COMPLEX

Virtually all human cells except neurons express class I MHC.[161] The class I MHC molecule presents antigenic peptides to CD8+ cytotoxic T lymphocytes.[431,565] It consists of a heavy chain that contains the peptide-binding domain and a transmembrane domain and a smaller extracellular subunit, β2-microglobulin.[77] The three major types of class I MHC heavy chains in humans— HLA-A, HLA-B, and HLA-C—have at least 22, 31, and 12 different alleles, respectively.[630] This polymorphism permits a great diversity in the peptide-binding repertoire in individuals and

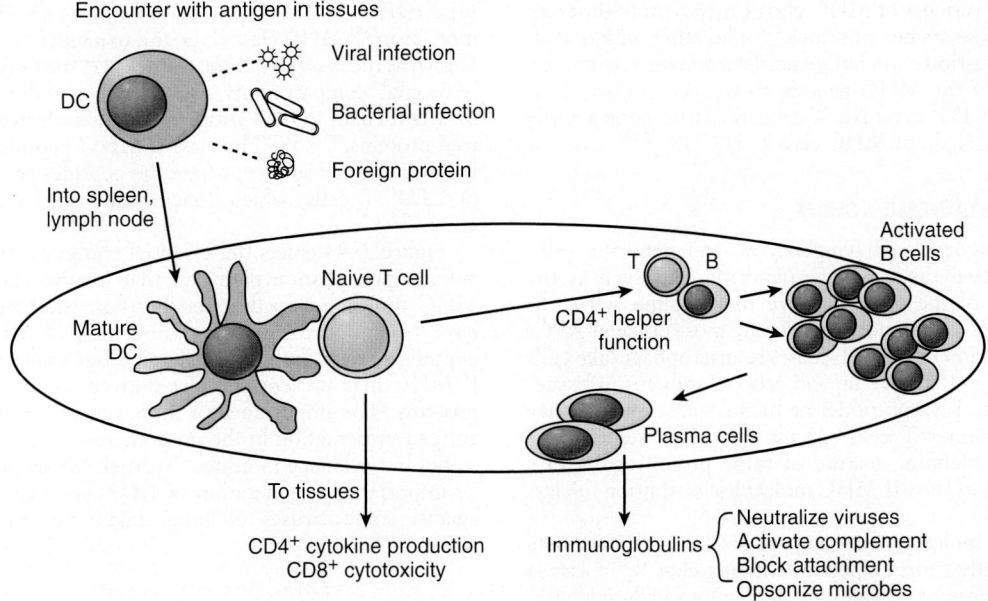

Figure 2–7 A simplified scheme of major events in the development of adaptive immune responses. When antigen-presenting cells, such as dendritic cells (DC), encounter and internalize microbes or their protein antigens in peripheral tissues, they process the microbial proteins and present the resulting antigenic peptides on either class I or class II major histocompatibility complex (MHC) molecules. The activated antigen-presenting cells migrate to lymphoid tissue, where they undergo maturation. When mature DC encounter naive CD4+ or CD8+ T cells expressing T-cell receptors (TCRs) specific for the peptides presented in the appropriate MHC context (CD4/MHC-II; CD8/MHC-I), binding between the cells occurs via TCR/peptide, MHC/CD4+ or MHC/CD8+, and other pairs of accessory molecules, all necessary for stimulating the T cells to become effector cells. Cytotoxic effector CD8+ T cells migrate into the periphery and kill virus-infected cells that present viral peptides via MHC class I. Effector CD4+ cells produce cytokines or provide help for proliferation of antigen-specific B cells in the lymphoid germinal centers and eventual production by plasma cells of specific antibodies that can neutralize viruses, prevent microbial attachment, opsonize microorganisms, or activate complement.

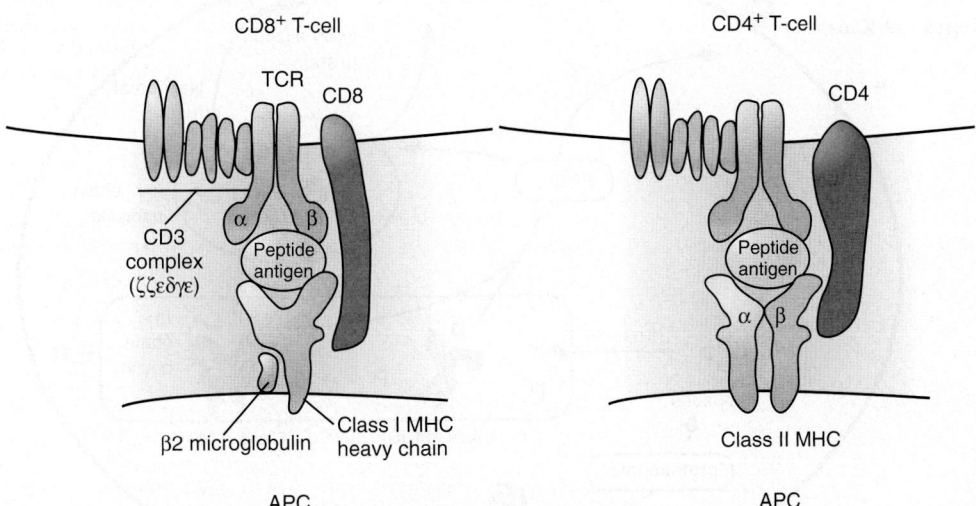

Figure 2–8 Principal cell surface interactions between CD8+ and CD4+ T lymphocytes and peptide antigens complexed with major histocompatibility complex (MHC) class I and class II molecules, respectively. CD3 (composed of six subunits, ζ, ζ, ε, δ, γ, ε) is associated closely with the T-cell receptor (TCR), which recognizes a specific peptide presented on MHC molecules. Class I and class II MHC determinants are recognized by CD8+ and CD4+. Additional or accessory interactions are discussed in the text. APC, antigen-presenting cell. *(Adapted from Lewis, D. B., and Wilson, C. B.: Developmental immunology and role of host defenses in neonatal susceptibility to infection. In Remington, J. S., and Klein, J. O. [eds.]: Infectious Diseases of the Fetus and Newborn Infant. 6th ed. Philadelphia, W. B. Saunders, 2006, p. 92.)*

within populations. A restricted degree of MHC genetic polymorphism has been invoked as a possible explanation for the predisposition of certain populations to develop infections.[78]

Class I MHC molecules within the cell ordinarily bind peptides derived from recently synthesized proteins, either of self origin or of infecting viruses.[207,208] A portion of newly synthesized

proteins is processed into peptides at a cytoplasmic site termed the *proteasome*.[245] These peptides actively are transported into the endoplasmic reticulum, where they are bound in the peptide-binding cleft of MHC class I. Suitable peptides usually are restricted to 8 to 10 amino acids in length, and they must contain certain amino acids at specific "anchor" positions on the peptide to bind.[295] Allelic variants of MHC class I may require different amino acids at these anchor positions.[227] The other amino acids of the peptide constitute the antigenic determinant recognized, after trafficking of the MHC-peptide to the cell surface, by a specific TCR on CD8+ cytotoxic T cells, the latter concurrently binding the heavy chain of MHC class I via CD8.[227,295]

CLASS II MAJOR HISTOCOMPATIBILITY COMPLEX

Mononuclear phagocytes, B lymphocytes, and dendritic cells, including specialized tissue-specific dendritic cells such as the Langerhans cells of the skin, all serve the immune system as "professional" APCs.[597] Dendritic cells, the most efficient APCs for primary activation of naive T cells, are macrophage-like cells of a distinct lineage that take up and process antigens in tissues and migrate to local lymph nodes or to the spleen, where they are likely to encounter T cells specific for the presented antigens.[191,263,489,565] A defining feature of these professional APCs is their expression of class II MHC molecules in addition to class I MHC.[161]

Class II MHC molecules are composed of an alpha and a beta chain, which together form a peptide-binding cleft.[98,503] Class II MHC molecules present peptides, 13 to 17 amino acids in length, derived from proteins that are internalized by endocytosis or during phagocytosis of microorganisms.[261,296,503] There are three major types of class II MHC alpha and beta chains—HLA-DR, HLA-DP, and HLA-DQ—each exhibiting a high degree of polymorphism.[383] MHC class II, bound to a separate smaller molecule known as the *invariant chain*, trafficks via the Golgi to endosomal/lysosomal compartments, where it must dissociate from the invariant chain to bind antigenic peptides derived from internalized proteins.[487,572,573] The class II MHC-peptide complexes then move to the cell surface, where the peptides are bound by TCRs of CD4+ T cells, which concurrently bind class II MHC via CD4.[192,372]

Figure 2–9 depicts the essential features of the conventional antigen presentation pathways that involve class I and class II MHC molecules, as described earlier. Alternative mechanisms have been documented by which class I MHC can present peptides derived from internalized exogenous proteins, and class II MHC may present peptides derived from newly synthesized proteins. The importance of these unconventional pathways of antigen presentation in the immune response is not fully understood, but evidence indicates that such "cross-presentation" may be important for generation of CD8+ cytotoxic T-cell response against some viruses or fungi taken up via endocytosis by APCs.[38,313]

CD1 FAMILY OF ANTIGEN-PRESENTING MOLECULES

The CD1 family comprises proteins with significant homology and structural similarity to the MHC class I heavy chain, but

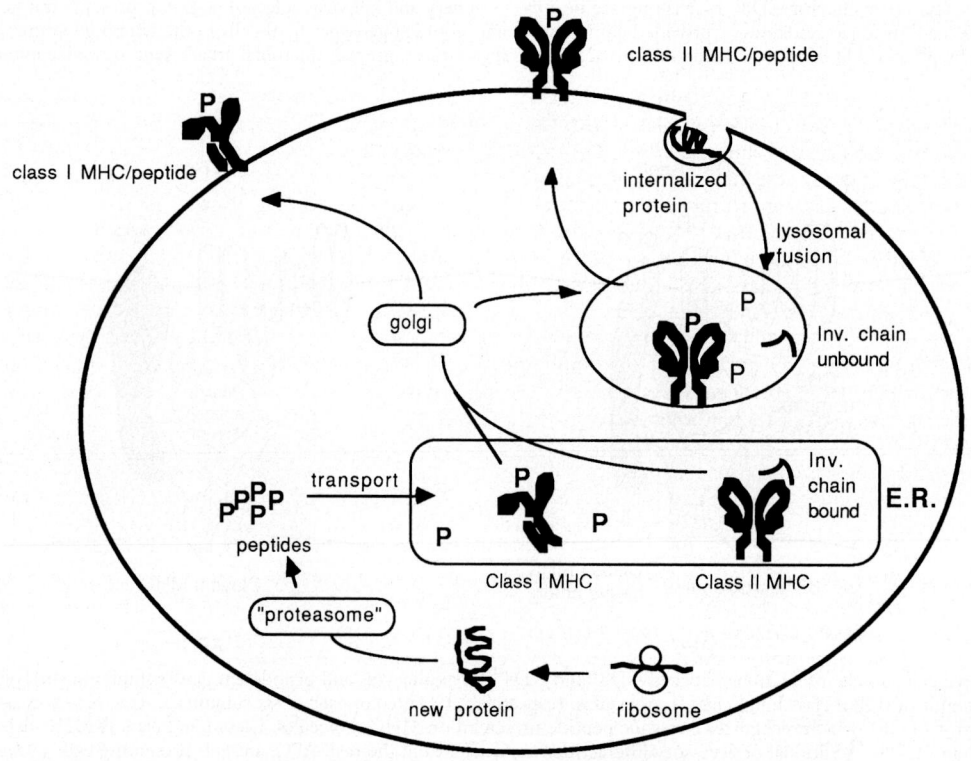

Antigen-Presenting Cell

Figure 2–9 Conventional pathways for peptide antigen presentation by class I and class II major histocompatibility complex (MHC) molecules. In the antigen-presenting cell, a proportion of newly synthesized proteins undergoes proteolysis into peptides by enzymes that constitute the "proteasome." The peptides actively are transported into the endoplasmic reticulum (E.R.), where peptides with the appropriate length and sequence bind to MHC class I molecules. MHC class II cannot bind peptides in the E.R. because of interference by the associated "invariant chain." The class I MHC/peptide complex is transported via the Golgi to the cell surface, where it may be recognized by CD8+ lymphocytes. Class II MHC molecules pass via the Golgi to a lysosomal compartment, where conditions favor the release of the invariant chain. This release permits class II MHC to bind peptides derived from internalized proteins that have entered the lysosomal compartment via fusion of endosomes or phagosomes with the lysosome. The lysosome translocates to the cell surface, where the class II MHC/peptide complex may be recognized by CD4+ lymphocytes.

which present lipid and glycolipid antigens. All mammalian species express one or more members of the CD1 family, principally on professional APCs. Four human CD1 proteins—CD1a, CD1b, CD1c, and CD1d—have been identified, each tightly associated with a β_2-microglobulin subunit. Mycolic acid, lipoarabinomannans, and other related components of mycobacteria are the best-documented foreign antigens presented by CD1 molecules, and internalized antigens and antigens synthesized within the APCs by ingested mycobacteria may be presented via distinct trafficking patterns of the CD1-antigen complexes.

Researchers have hypothesized that other antigens, such as the lipoteichoic acids of gram-positive bacteria, the complex capsular polysaccharides of *H. influenzae* and *N. meningitidis*, and the glycosylphosphatidylinositol components of glycosylphosphatidylinositol-linked proteins of malarial parasites and trypanosomes, also could be presented by CD1 molecules. Antigens presented on APC by CD1 molecules are recognized by a specialized subset of CD1-restricted T cells that usually lack CD4 and CD8, known as NK/T cells. These cells share characteristics of NK cells and T cells, exhibiting a limited range of TCR specificity. They represent a sizeable fraction of the T cell compartment, although their function in the immune response is incompletely understood. Greater detail regarding the structure, function, phylogeny, trafficking, expression, and T cell interactions for members of the CD1 family may be found in an extensive review.[470]

T Lymphocytes

The development of T lymphocytes, or T cells, begins when prothymocytes leave the marrow and enter the subcapsular region of the thymus.[190] By mechanisms that are poorly understood, the thymic environment induces the rearrangement of TCR V (variable), D (diversity), and J (joining) gene segments with the eventual expression of mature alpha-beta TCRs complexed with CD3. The T cells, now co-expressing CD4 and CD8, migrate to the thymic cortex, where they undergo screening for TCR specificity to optimize the repertoire for distinguishing self from non-self and to eliminate TCR rearrangements that result in undesirably high self-reactivity. The mechanism by which this screening occurs is the subject of intense investigation and theoretical controversy, and several reviews of the subject are cited here.[249,317,387,396] Thymocytes that do not pass this dual screening procedure receive signals that induce programmed cell death (apoptosis).[396,417,600] Only approximately 5 percent of the original thymocytes pass this screening, after which they express either CD4 or CD8, but not both.[396,417,600]

Mature thymocytes are released into the periphery, where the CD4+ cells serve as the main source of IL-2 and provide help for B-cell antibody production, and the CD8+ cells engage in specific cytotoxic activity. This discussion of T cells and TCRs specifically relates to T cells that express TCRs composed of alpha and beta chains, or alpha-beta T cells. T cells of a distinct type, gamma-delta T cells, are far less numerous in most tissues (intestinal epithelium is a notable exception); exhibit much less TCR diversity than do alpha-beta T cells; may not require an intact thymus for development; and play a role in host responses to certain intracellular bacterial pathogens, including *Listeria* and mycobacteria.[110,264]

Antigen specificity of alpha-beta T cells resides in their TCRs, which are integral membrane proteins that exhibit structural homology with immunoglobulins. TCR diversity results from a rearrangement of V, D, and J segments. There are 100 different V segments, 1 D segment, and 100 different J segments in the complete germline configuration of the TCR genes. Rearrangement of these gene segments into a mature VDJ sequence occurs by the action of a recombinase enzyme complex formed by two proteins, RAG-1 and RAG-2.[440,516] TCR diversity is generated by several factors, including the range of possible combinations of

V, D, and J segments; the imprecise action of the recombinase complex; the variability in the number of nucleotides deleted during rearrangement; and the action of another enzyme, *terminal deoxytransferase*, which seems to add nucleotides at random to extend segments during rearrangement.[215,533] The actions of Artemis and DNA ligase IV, two enzymes crucial for the processing and joining of DNA ends, introduce additional sources of variability.[103,200,376] Researchers have estimated that 10^{15} different TCR specificities theoretically could result from the several mechanisms involved in TCR segment rearrangement.[168]

Stimulation of naive CD4+ or CD8+ T cells occurs as they circulate through peripheral lymphoid tissue and encounter dendritic cells and other professional APCs. Localized T-cell migration is highly regulated by specific chemokines and adhesive interactions with local endothelium and involves mechanisms similar to the mechanisms discussed earlier for circulating phagocytes.[194,342] When T cells engage APCs presenting specific peptide antigens on the appropriate MHC molecules, they are activated via their TCR and several costimulatory molecules, especially CD28, to produce IL-2 and to proliferate and differentiate into effector T cells.[134,299] Effector CD4+ T cells may be of the T_H1 or T_H2 type, and this type is influenced by several factors, including the specific cytokines elicited by a particular microbial pathogen. Naive T cells activated in the presence of IL-12 and IFN-γ are likely to develop into T_H1 cells, whereas IL-4 and IL-6 tend to drive development in the direction of T_H2 cells.[413,421] Preferential development of T_H1 effector cells leads mainly to macrophage activation and cell-mediated immunity, whereas T_H2 effector cells, which provide more effective B-cell help, drive the development of humoral immunity.[418]

Activation of naive CD8+ T cells by antigen binding, co-stimulation by accessory binding molecules on APCs, and exposure to cytokines, including IL-2, leads to clonal proliferation of specific CD8+ cells and their differentiation into cytotoxic effector cells. Effector CD4+ T cells bound in common to an APC may play a role in activating naive CD8+ T cells, either by releasing IL-2 or by activating the APC to provide greater co-stimulation to the CD8+ T cell to make its own IL-2.[33] Antigenically experienced effector CD8+ T cells respond to specific antigen and co-stimulatory molecules on infected host cells by activating cytotoxic mechanisms similar to those described earlier for NK cells, including the release of perforin and granzymes and generation of receptor-mediated signals for target cell apoptosis.[367,504,583]

T-CELL MEMORY

Some proportion of activated CD4+ and CD8+ T cells become endowed with the capacity for long-term antigenic memory and rapidly can become effectors on re-exposure to specific antigen. Whether these cells develop directly from naive T cells or previously have been effector cells, or both, is uncertain, and the mechanisms by which they become memory T cells is poorly understood. Among the features of memory T cells are high levels of expression of CD45RO, the ability to suppress activation of naive T cells of the same specificity, and a homeostatic level of ongoing proliferation in bone marrow and peripheral lymphoid organs.[314,378,509]

T-CELL ACTIVATION BY SUPERANTIGENS

The term *superantigen* describes a class of protein antigens, mainly microbial exotoxins, including most staphylococcal enterotoxins, staphylococcal toxic shock syndrome toxin-1 (TSST-1), and related streptococcal TSST-1-like toxins. These bacterial toxins are potent pyrogens, can induce a potentially lethal toxic shock syndrome, and share binding domains for TCR V regions and MHC class II molecules. Superantigens bypass normal antigen processing and presentation pathways by binding directly to class II MCH molecules on APCs and to specific variable regions on the beta chain of the T-cell antigen receptor. Through these interactions, superantigens induce a polyclonal activation of T cells at orders of magnitude above levels induced by antigen-specific activation, resulting in massive release of cytokines from T cells and APCs, including TNF-α, TNF-β, IL-1, IL-2, and IFN-γ, which are thought to be responsible for the most severe features of toxic shock syndromes.[16,476]

REGULATORY T CELLS

The existence of T suppressor cells was long a subject of debate among immunologists. Only since the 1990s has solid evidence been developed to support the existence of suppressor T cells, now referred to as *regulatory T cells*. These cells were discovered when thymectomized mice were noted to develop autoimmune disease. Transfer of T cells that expressed CD25, the alpha chain of the IL-2 receptor, from normal adult mice to thymectomized mice prevented autoimmune disease. This population of CD4+CD25+ regulatory T cells can suppress the activity of other immune cells and has been shown to prevent graft-versus-host disease and allograft rejection. The mechanism of suppression by regulatory T cells is uncertain but may involve direct contact with other cells or secretion of inhibitory cytokines, including IL-10. These inhibitory cytokines can interfere with T-cell proliferation and inhibit the ability of antigen-presenting dendritic cells to promote T-cell activation. The role of regulatory T cells in immunity to infection is only beginning to be studied; some current evidence suggests that the action of regulatory T cells with specificity for microbial antigens may suppress protective immune responses to some infections but also may suppress excessive or injurious host responses.[475]

B Lymphocytes and Immunoglobulins

B LYMPHOCYTES

B lymphocytes (B cells) are the source of humoral immunity in the form of specific immunoglobulin. The earliest recognizable marrow precursors of B cells are pro-B cells, surfaces of which bear the pan-B marker CD19. Further differentiation produces pre-B cells and then mature B cells, the latter expressing cell-surface immunoglobulin by which they recognize and bind antigen. B lymphocytes constitute approximately 20 percent of the lymphocytes in the circulation and peripheral lymphoid tissues, including the lymph nodes, spleen, bone marrow, tonsils, and intestines, and they are identified by the presence of surface immunoglobulin and the pan-B differentiation markers CD19 and CD20.[114,394]

B-cell activation is initiated by recognition and binding of specific antigens to B-cell surface immunoglobulins. Early activation leads to increased expression of receptors that either bind cytokines (e.g., IL-2, IL-4, IL-6) or interact with T cells,[349,459] leading to clonal proliferation and differentiation into memory B cells and plasma cells in the germinal centers of peripheral lymphoid tissue.[321] Some data suggest that B-cell differentiation into memory B cells is favored by exposure to the CD40L on dendritic cells in lymphoid organs, whereas differentiation into plasma cells is favored by exposure to CD23, IL-1a, IL-6, and IL-10.[321,571] The plasma cells, later found in bone marrow and liver and peripheral lymphoid tissue, are responsible for most free production of immunoglobulin.[571]

The B-cell response to protein antigens depends on T-cell help. B cells can process and present antigen to CD4+ T cells they encounter in the lymph nodes and spleen.[320,321,571] B-cell surface immunoglobulin binds to a protein antigen, which is internalized, processed, and presented to the T cell via class II

MHC molecules. B cell-mediated activation of T cells during antigen presentation is much more effective for memory T cells, whereas naive T cells are more likely to be turned off or rendered tolerant.[206,229] T-cell help is provided for B-cell proliferation and production of antibody against the specific protein antigen. It is mediated by signaling via CD40L interactions with CD40 on the B cell and by the release of cytokines, which also can induce isotype switching.[429,555] Most B-lymphocyte responses to polysaccharide antigens proceed largely without formal T-cell help, although antibody responses to some such antigens may be enhanced in the presence of T cells.[408]

IMMUNOGLOBULIN

Immunoglobulin molecules may be bound at the surface of B cells or free in the circulation, mucosal secretions, or tissues. Free immunoglobulins function in host defense against infection by binding to microbial surfaces to prevent microbial attachment, activating complement via the classical pathway, neutralizing viruses and toxins, and participating in the formation of immune complexes.[134]

Immunoglobulin molecules are composed of two identical heavy and two identical light chains, as diagrammed in Figure 2–10.[195] The carboxyl terminus of the immunoglobulin molecule is the heavy chain constant, or Fc, region. The amino acid sequence of this region determines the immunoglobulin isotype. The heavy chain is encoded by V, D, J, and constant (C) regions on chromosome 14.[66,605] Each immunoglobulin molecule has a pair of either kappa or lambda light chains, defined by distinct C regions. The variable region of the immunoglobulin molecule contains the antigen binding site. Similar to the TCR, the Fab region consists of two identical heavy and light chain pairs; similarly, broadly diverse antigen specificity results from the variable nature of recombinase-mediated DNA rearrangements of the three hypervariable, or complementarity-determining, regions

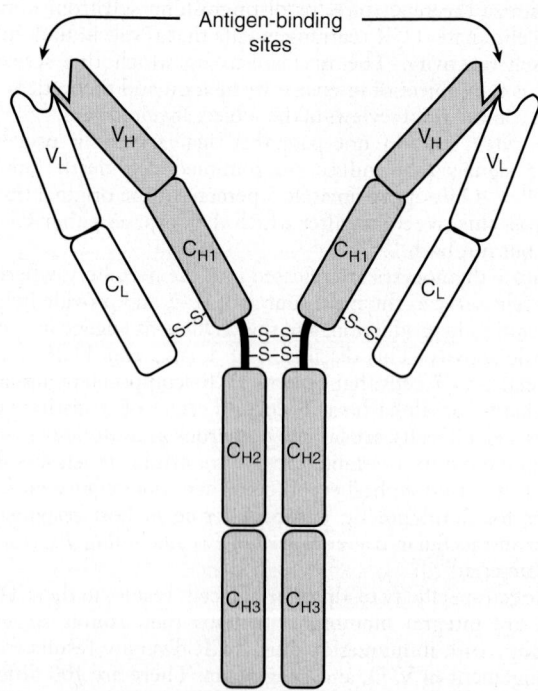

Figure 2–10 Structure of an immunoglobulin molecule. The schematic structure of IgG is shown, depicting the variable (V) and constant (C) regions of the heavy (H) and light (L) chains, the disulfide bonds that link the two heavy chains at the hinge region and the CL region with CH1, and the antigen-binding sites formed by the complementarity-determining regions of VH and VL.

(CDR1, CDR2, and CDR3) and the four framework regions during development of B cells.[210,381]

The imprecision inherent in this rearrangement, involving mechanisms similar to those described for the TCR, leads to the generation of more than 10^{12} potential antigenic specificities. Somatic hypermutation of variable regions after gene rearrangement occurs adds to the repertoire, and further diversity results from differences in approximation of the three complementarity-determining regions in relation to each other, affecting the three-dimensional structure of the antigen recognition site.[406,458] In contrast to most TCRs, which recognize specific peptide sequences, immunoglobulin molecules can recognize the three-dimensional structures of antigens.[165]

All immunoglobulin is derived from B cells expressing surface IgM. B cells may change immunoglobulin isotype when they differentiate into plasma cells, which produce only one class or subclass of immunoglobulin each. Isotypes other than IgM are the result of isotype switching by replacing a part of the constant region of the immunoglobulin heavy chain with another isotype-specific segment.[555] As already noted, isotype switching primarily depends on specific B-cell interactions with cytokines and T cells. The variable region remains unchanged during isotype switching; no change occurs in antigen specificity. Important features of immunoglobulins, including half-life, localization in tissues, and interactions with cellular IgG receptors, are directly determined by isotype, however.[166]

IMMUNOGLOBULIN ISOTYPES

IgG accounts for approximately 80 percent of circulating immunoglobulin and includes the subclasses IgG1, IgG2, IgG3, and IgG4. The half-life of IgG ordinarily is approximately 21 days (7 days for IgG3).[303] Initial exposure to most microbial protein antigens first induces IgM and then an IgG response consisting of IgG1 and IgG3. IgG2 and IgG4 usually are produced during the secondary immune response. IgG1 usually is made in response to protein antigens.[303] In adults, the main antibody response to polysaccharides is IgG2, whereas in infants, IgG1 predominates.[19] The functions of IgG in host defense include blocking microbial attachment, opsonization, complement activation, toxin and virus neutralization, and promotion of ADCC. IgG1, IgG2, and IgG3, but not IgG4, can trigger complement activation via the classical pathway by binding to C1q.[95]

Free IgM usually exists as an immunoglobulin pentamer that has a molecular weight of approximately 950,000 and is stabilized by a single J chain.[195,336,398,458] Present mainly in the circulation, its half-life is approximately 8 to 10 days. The IgM response is the earliest of the isotype responses, appearing within the first few days of infection, but it is transient. The formation of an IgM response in the absence of an IgG response to infection is not associated with the formation of memory B cells. The main function of IgM in host defense is the activation of complement to promote opsonization and lysis of microorganisms.[166,398]

IgA exists in monomeric circulating and polymeric secretory forms and has a half-life of approximately 7 days.[303] Both forms are produced mainly by plasma cells that have migrated to mucosal sites. Secretory IgA is composed of two or three IgA molecules joined by a stabilizing J segment that is secreted by plasma cells and a secretory component produced by mucosal epithelial cells.[322,336] The secretory component permits delivery of IgA to mucosal surfaces.[430] There are two subclasses, IgA1 and IgA2, which differ in the composition of their heavy chains. Most IgA in the circulation is IgA1, whereas most IgA in secretions is IgA2. IgA1, but not IgA2, may be cleaved at mucosal sites by bacterial proteases.[335] IgA neutralizes viruses at mucosal sites, may block bacterial adhesion, and can act directly as an opsonin to promote phagocytosis and killing of microbes via Fcα receptors.[292,322]

The IgE molecule has a molecular weight of 200,000 and a half-life of only 2.3 days.[303] Most IgE is produced by plasma cells in lymphoid tissue near gastrointestinal and respiratory mucosal surfaces and released into the circulation.[301,564] IgE acts via Fcε receptors to trigger activation of mast cells and basophils, leading to immediate hypersensitivity reactions.[564] Individuals with intestinal metazoan parasites often have elevated serum levels of IgE, and IgE may have a role in protecting against parasitic disease by stimulating mediator release from mast cells, causing intestinal smooth muscle contraction and expulsion of parasites.[564]

IgD has a molecular weight of approximately 180,000 and a half-life of 3 days.[303] It is expressed along with IgM on surfaces of naive B cells but is present in normal adult serum and secretions in very low concentrations. Some antigenic specificity for IgD has been shown, and, although its function in host defense is unclear, it may serve as a secondary antigen receptor on B cells, where it may regulate the development of B-cell antibody responses.[80]

CLINICAL CONDITIONS ASSOCIATED WITH DEFICIENT HOST RESPONSES TO INFECTION

IMMATURE HOST RESPONSES OF THE NEWBORN

A mild febrile respiratory illness in a 10-month-old infant might prompt little more than gentle reassurance over the telephone from the child's pediatrician. If the patient is an infant in the first few weeks of life, however, the physician's response is likely to include an evaluation for systemic bacterial infection and administration of parenteral antibiotics in the hospital until a serious infection can be ruled out. Similarly, in an older infant, the appearance of a few cutaneous perioral vesicles characteristic of herpes simplex virus usually evokes little concern and no specific treatment. The same condition in the first 3 weeks of life is likely to lead to a prolonged hospitalization for antiviral therapy because of the risk of developing serious central nervous system or disseminated infection.[617] It is a well-recognized fact that newborns are much more susceptible to serious disease from many types of organisms than are older children and adults. This predisposition to infection is even more profound in infants born prematurely.[364] The basis for this special vulnerability of neonates is complex and encompasses all arms of the immune system. This vulnerability is of such importance that the clinical approach to possible infections in infants during the first month of life usually is far more aggressive than that in older children.

Cell-Mediated Immunity

Antigen presentation per se, via the mechanisms discussed earlier, seems to be intact in the newborn. Expression of class I and class II MHC molecules has been documented in a broad range of fetal tissues by 12 weeks' gestation,[284,441] and levels of expression are sufficient to mediate normal MHC class II–restricted antigen presentation by neonatal monocytes to maternal or paternal CD4+ T cells and to induce vigorous rejection of allogeneic fetal tissue by CD8+ cytotoxic T cells.[269,283]

By about 20 weeks' gestation, the fetal repertoire of diversity of TCRs has developed fully.[593] At the time of birth, although most basic functions of cell-mediated immunity are present, a high proportion of immature T cells are present in the peripheral circulation and can be identified by their co-expression of CD4 and CD8.[364] This phenotype typifies type II thymocytes, which usually are not found in the periphery in older individuals.

Neonatal T cells seem to be deficient in most of their major functions, including CD8+ T cell–mediated cytotoxicity, delayed hypersensitivity, and T-cell help for B-cell differentiation.

Diminished production of cytokine by neonatal T cells likely accounts for much of this deficiency. The naive status of most neonatal T cells may account for reduced production of cytokine because memory T cells are much more efficient in all of these functions.[364]

B Cells and Antibody

B CELLS

Pre-B cells are found in the fetal liver and omentum by 8 weeks' gestation and in the fetal bone marrow by 13 weeks' gestation.[237,364,545] Pre-B cells with surface IgM have been detected by 10 weeks' gestation. After 30 weeks' gestation and delivery, pre-B cells are seen only in the bone marrow. Mature B cells are present in the circulation by the 11th week of gestation, and have reached adult levels in the bone marrow, blood, and spleen by the 22nd week of gestation.[170,237,545]

Fetal B cells express only IgM, whereas most adult B cells express IgM and IgD. Neonatal B cells may express three immunoglobulin isotypes (e.g., different combinations of IgG, IgA, IgM, and IgD) on their surfaces.[237,260] Data from experiments in mice suggest that exposing B cells with surface IgM, but not IgD, to antigens leads to anergy, or B-cell inactivation. The absence of surface IgD on fetal B cells has been speculated to contribute to the induction of tolerance to self- and, possibly, maternal antigens in utero. In addition, the fetus has a higher proportion of the functionally immature CD5[+], or B1, cells than adults do. These cells produce autoantibodies and may play a role in the development of tolerance to self-antigens, maternal antigens, or both.

Although germinal centers are not present in lymphoid tissue at birth, they begin to develop in the first few months of life concomitant with the infant's exposure to antigens.[575] Despite conflicting in vitro data, neonatal T-cell help for B cells probably is comparable to that of adult T cells, as is reflected by the

excellent T cell–dependent antibody response of the newborn to immunization with protein antigens such as tetanus toxoid.[174] Neonatal T-cell help is associated with secretion of IgM alone, however, not other isotypes, possibly because neonatal T cells have diminished production of cytokines crucial for promoting isotype switching. Addition of cytokines such as IL-2, IL-4, and IL-6 helps overcome neonatal B-cell dysfunction in vitro.[364] In contrast to adult B cells, neonatal B cells cannot respond to polysaccharides without help from T cells.

ANTIBODY

Maternal IgG accounts for most of the newborn's circulating immunoglobulin because almost none is made by the healthy fetus, and IgG is the only isotype of maternal immunoglobulin that crosses the placenta.[333,384] Maternal transport of IgG can be detected by 8 weeks' gestation, and the newborn's IgG level is directly proportional to gestational age, reaching 100 mg/dL by 17 to 20 weeks' gestation and 50 percent of the maternal level by 30 weeks' gestation (Fig. 2–11).[49,305] By term, the infant has 5 to 10 percent more IgG than the mother does because maternal antibody is transported not only passively but also actively via trophoblast Fc receptors. Trophoblast Fc receptors have higher affinity for IgG1 and IgG3 than for IgG2 and IgG4, and so more of those subclasses are transported from the mother.[199,358] Newborns may have higher proportions of IgG1 and IgG3 than IgG2 and IgG4 compared with adults, and term newborns' IgG1 levels may exceed maternal levels.

By approximately 2 months of chronologic age, the term infant has quantitative IgG that is of approximately half maternal and half infant origin. The physiologic nadir of IgG in all infants is approximately 3 to 4 months of age and ranges from less than 100 mg/dL in very-low-birth-weight preterm infants to about 400 mg/dL in term infants (Table 2–3; see Fig. 2–11).[49,559] Maternal IgG essentially is gone by the time the infant is approximately 12 months old, at which time infant levels are approximately 60

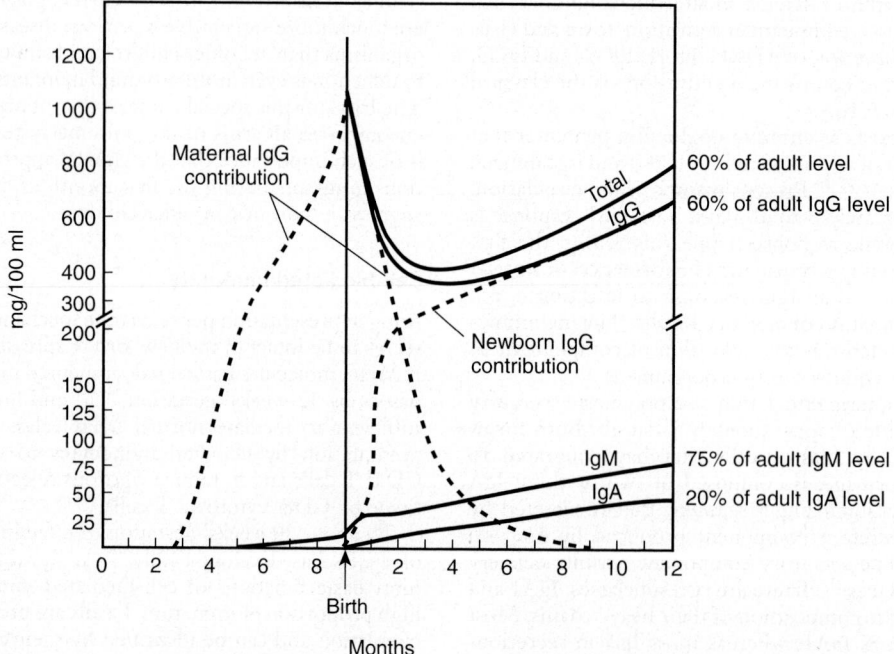

Figure 2–11 Immunoglobulin (IgG, IgM, and IgA) levels in the fetus and infant in the first year of life. The IgG of the fetus and newborn is solely of maternal origin. The maternal IgG disappears by the time the infant is 9 months of age, by which time endogenous synthesis of IgG by the infant is well established. The IgM and IgA of the neonate are synthesized entirely endogenously because maternal IgM and IgA do not cross the placenta. *(After Braun, J., and Stiehm, E. R.: The B-lymphocyte system. In Stiehm, E. R. [ed.]: Immunologic Disorders in Infants and Children. 4th ed. Philadelphia, W. B. Saunders, 1996, p. 67.)*

TABLE 2–3   Levels of Immunoglobulins in Sera of Normal Subjects, by Age

Age (mo)	IgG (mg/dL)	IgG (mg/dL)	IgG (mg/dL)	Total Immunoglobulin (mg/dL)
Newborn	1031 ± 200*	11 ± 5	2 ± 3	1044 ± 201
1-3	430 ± 119	30 ± 11	21 ± 13	481 ± 127
4-6	427 ± 186	43 ± 17	28 ± 18	498 ± 204
7-12	661 ± 219	54 ± 23	37 ± 18	752 ± 242
13-14	762 ± 209	58 ± 23	50 ± 24	870 ± 258
25-36	892 ± 183	61 ± 19	71 ± 37	1024 ± 205

Values were derived from measurements made in 296 children and 30 adults. Levels were determined by the radial diffusion plate method using specific rabbit antisera to human immunoglobulins. Values are ± 1 SD.
Modified from Stiehm, E. R., and Fudenberg, H. H.: Serum levels of immune globulins in health and disease: A survey. Pediatrics 37:715-727, 1966. Copyright American Academy of Pediatrics, 1966.

percent of adult levels. Production of IgG1 and IgG3 matures more rapidly than that of IgG2 and IgG4, reaching adult levels by the time the child is approximately 8 years old versus 10 and 12 years of age for IgG2 and IgG4.[437]

The fetus normally produces little IgM, IgA, IgE, or IgD, and none is transported from the mother.[285] The presence of IgM levels greater than 20 mg/dL at birth suggests an intrauterine infection. Serum IgA levels at birth in preterm and term infants usually are less than 5 mg/dL and consist of IgA1 and IgA2. Secretory IgA is not detectable until after birth, but it usually is present within the first few weeks of life. IgM and IgA reach approximately 60 percent and 20 percent of adult levels by the time the infant reaches 1 year of age (see Fig. 2–11). Secretory IgA reaches adult levels by the time the child is 6 to 8 years old.[364]

The IgG transferred from the mother to the fetus has been shown to protect the newborn from many infectious agents, including viruses such as varicella, polio, measles, mumps, and rubella, and bacteria such as tetanus, diphtheria, H. influenzae type b, and group B streptococcus.[146,147] The infant is not protected by the mother, however, if she does not have specific IgG antibody, even if she is immune to a given organism. The mother may have low or absent levels of circulating IgG antibody but good memory B cells capable of mounting a booster response. In this case, the mother is protected, but she cannot transfer protection to her infant. Similarly, because no IgM is transferred to the fetus, the mother cannot protect her newborn effectively against many gram-negative enteric organisms, even if she is immune.[148,403]

The concept of passive transfer of protective IgG is being used to develop vaccines for maternal immunization before or during pregnancy so that passive transfer of vaccine-induced antibody would result in protection during the neonatal period. Examples of organisms for which such strategies have been investigated include group B streptococcus, H. influenzae type b, meningococcus, pneumococcus, rotavirus, and respiratory syncytial virus.[48,203,297]

Researchers have documented that the fetus can respond to antigenic stimulation in the form of maternal immunization with tetanus toxoid vaccine and be primed for a secondary antibody response to repeat immunization after birth.[242,243] Some fetuses near term also can make IgM and IgA antibody to organisms such as toxoplasmosis, rubella, cytomegalovirus, or herpes.[201,422] The amount of fetal antibody produced in response to intrauterine antigenic stimulation is proportional to gestational age.[171,557]

Maternal antibody inhibits the infant's ability to respond to vaccines against certain organisms, such as measles, but it does not prevent the infant from mounting protective immune responses to most normal childhood vaccine antigens, such as tetanus, diphtheria, polio, hepatitis B, and protein-conjugated polysaccharide vaccines.[14] Generally, neonates have protective responses to T cell–dependent antigens, although they may

produce less antibody to some antigens than do older infants and adults.[13,164,174,218,540,541]

The newborn's response to T cell–independent type 1 (TI-1) antigens is slightly decreased and to TI-2 antigens is poor.[246] The antibody response to most TI-2 antigens, including the polysaccharide capsules of group B streptococcus, pneumococcus, and H. influenzae type b, is not mature until the infant is 18 to 24 months old, although infants 3 months of age can respond to group A meningococcal polysaccharide.[538] In contrast, in the first few weeks of life, infants mount excellent antibody responses to T cell–independent polysaccharide antigens that have been rendered T cell–dependent by covalent conjugation of the polysaccharide to a protein carrier.[7]

A proposal is that immunologic tolerance may be induced in infants by early exposure to some antigens. The subject is controversial, but some data suggest that immunization to pertussis in the newborn period results in lower levels of antibody to subsequent doses of vaccine than does initially immunizing the infant at 1 month of age.[47,52] No evidence indicates, however, that tolerance is induced by administration of tetanus, diphtheria, or oral polio vaccines in the newborn period.[174,518]

The response of premature infants to most routine childhood vaccines, including diphtheria, tetanus, pertussis, and oral and inactivated polio, is comparable to that of 2-month-old term infants.[8,68,122,541] That premature infants do not respond as well to hepatitis B vaccine is well documented; the reasons are unclear.[201,352]

The data are conflicting, but small-for-gestational-age infants may have lower total levels of IgG at birth than those of normal-weight newborns,[199,531,627] possibly because of placental insufficiency. Their response to most routine vaccines is good, but it may be slightly decreased to inactivated polio vaccine.[128]

Complement

Complement proteins do not cross the placenta, but studies of mothers with congenital complement component deficiencies, studies of mother-infant pairs discordant for variants of individual components, and studies of fetal tissues have provided evidence for fetal synthesis of complement beginning as early as 5½ weeks' gestation. Most complement proteins are present by 10 weeks' gestation.[144,333] Levels of complement activity and of individual complement components vary significantly among infants, but generally classical pathway hemolytic activity of term neonates ranges from 50 to 80 percent of maternal values (Table 2–4). Because serum complement levels are elevated during pregnancy, term neonates' levels are approximately 60 to 90 percent of normal adult values.[197,307,628] Alternative pathway hemolytic activity is decreased more consistently than classical pathway activity, and ranges from approximately 50 to 70 percent of normal adult values at term (see Table 2–4).[6,193,434,531] Complement activity usually is lower in premature infants than

TABLE 2–4   Summary of Published Complement Levels in Neonates

	Mean Percentage of Adult Levels	
Complement Component	Term Neonate	Preterm Neonate
CH$_{50}$	56-90 (4)*	45-71 (3)
AP$_{50}$	49-65 (3)	40-51 (2)
C1q	65-90 (3)	27-58 (2)
C4	60-100 (4)	42-91 (3)
C2	76-100 (2)	96 (1)
C3	60-100 (5)	39-78 (4)
C5	75 (1)	—
C6	47 (1)	—
C7	67 (1)	—
C8	20 (1)	—
C9	<20 (2)	—
B	35-59 (8)	36-50 (3)
P	33-71 (5)	13-65 (2)
H	61 (1)	—
C3bi	55 (1)	—

*Number of studies.
Data from Lewis, D. B., and Wilson, C. B.: Developmental immunology and role of host defenses in neonatal susceptibility to infection. In Remington, J. S., and Klein, J. O. (eds.): Infectious Diseases of the Fetus and Newborn Infant. 4th ed. Philadelphia, Pa, W. B. Saunders, 1995, p. 65.

in term infants, with hemolytic activity of both pathways and serum levels of most complement proteins usually corresponding directly with gestational age.[193] Small-for-gestational-age infants have complement levels comparable to levels of infants of the same gestational age who are not small for gestational age.[434,531]

Hemolytic activity of the classical and the alternative pathways increases rapidly and reaches adult levels by the time the infant is 3 to 6 months old (classical pathway) and approximately 6 to 18 months old (alternative pathway). In addition to hemolytic activity, complement-mediated opsonic and bactericidal activity is decreased in newborn sera and generally correlates with C3 and factor B levels.[197] Studies of opsonic and bactericidal activity of newborn sera have been reviewed in detail elsewhere.[197,307,308] Levels of individual complement proteins do not correlate always with their functional activity.[238,291] Zach and Hostetter[628] reported not only that total C3 levels were decreased as measured by enzyme-linked immunosorbent assay, but also that C3 thioester reactivity was decreased, and that it correlated with gestational age. Because the opsonic function of C3 is mediated by its thioester, such a defect may contribute to the newborn's deficiency in functional complement activity. Although complement levels and activity are decreased significantly in most newborns, these abnormalities are mild compared with the abnormalities seen in hereditary complement deficiencies, in which levels of an individual component often are nil. Despite studies in vitro that suggest increased risk of development of infection, the extent to which lower neonatal complement levels predispose the infant to infection in vivo is uncertain.

Phagocytes

The newborn exhibits quantitative and qualitative deficits in phagocytic defenses. Although the number of circulating PMNs usually does not differ greatly from those in older children and adults, under conditions of stress, including systemic infection, the availability of marrow reserves of PMNs is impaired markedly.[131] The ratio of marrow neutrophil reserves to circulating cells in older individuals is nearly 15:1, whereas this ratio in newborns is 2:1 to 3:1.[131,380] Neutropenia is more likely to develop during severe systemic infections in newborns than in older children and adults.[131] The resulting deficiency in PMNs available for delivery to infected sites under conditions of stress

is a serious disadvantage for the neonate in containing bacterial and fungal infections. Distinct from this quantitative deficiency in marrow reserves of PMNs are functional impairments of PMNs, which also are important in understanding neonatal phagocytic defenses.

The most important and best-documented functional impairments of neonatal PMNs are related to defective adherence and chemotaxis.[4,5,25-28,339,390,400] Numerous specific structural, functional, and biochemical abnormalities have been documented, any or all of which may contribute to the overall impairment in adhesion and migration of these cells.[280] Impaired adhesion of neonatal PMNs to endothelial cells and other biologic substrates has been linked with deficiencies in the expression or function of the β_2 integrins Mac-1 (CD11b/CD18) and LFA-1 (CD11a/CD18).[4,28,99,312,390] Perhaps the best-documented of these deficiencies is the diminished level of surface expression of Mac-1 on activated neonatal PMNs, although expression on resting PMNs is similar to that of adults.[99,312] The deficiency in stimulated Mac-1 surface expression can be explained sufficiently by the observation that the total cell content of Mac-1 in PMNs from term neonates is only approximately 60 percent of that in adult PMNs.[4] The total PMN content of Mac-1 at the time of birth is related directly to gestational age, and PMNs from very early premature infants (<30 weeks' gestation) may contain less than 20 percent of the Mac-1 content of adult PMNs.[390] The PMN content of LFA-1, which is normal at term, seems to be reduced in infants born before 35 weeks' gestation.[390] In addition to reduced expression of these integrins, reduced adhesive function of the β_2 integrin molecules themselves at the surface of activated PMNs has been documented.[28]

Several other defects of neonatal PMNs that are likely to influence chemotaxis have been documented. They include defective redistribution of surface adhesion sites,[26] impaired uropod formation during stimulated shape change,[27] reduced cell deformability,[310] impaired microtubule assembly,[27] deficient F-actin polymerization,[262,506] reduced lactoferrin content and release,[25] reduced ability to effect membrane depolarization and intracellular calcium ion transients,[507] and impaired uptake of glucose during stimulation by chemoattractants.[5] The importance of each of these individual impairments to the overall deficiency in chemotaxis by neonatal PMNs has not been determined.

Evidence suggests that the number and binding efficiencies of receptors for chemoattractants, including C5a and synthetic bacterial peptides such as the formyl peptide N-f-met-leu-phe, are normal.[26,507,562] Phagocytosis and microbicidal activity of neonatal PMNs have been found in several studies to be similar to that of adult PMNs.[399,400] In some studies in which the assay conditions are designed to expose a potential defect in these functions (e.g., limiting concentrations of opsonins and high bacterial inocula), defects in phagocytosis and killing have been documented, however.[399,400] Whether these potential deficiencies play a role in impaired neonatal phagocyte defenses in vivo is unclear.

PRIMARY OR HERITABLE IMMUNOLOGIC DEFICIENCIES

Physicians who care for children often are faced with the problem of a child who has a predilection for recurrent infections. Most of these children are normal infants or toddlers who have been exposed to a succession of common respiratory infections when they entered daycare or a similar setting for the first time.[117] For most of these children, repeated exposure elicits relative immunity to many or most of the infectious agents. It is an important challenge for the physician to identify infants and children who do not fit into the normal pattern, but who are unusually susceptible to development of infection with respect to frequency, severity, type of causative agent, and response to appropriate treatment. This challenge usually falls to the pediatrician or family physician because, with few exceptions, the primary immunodeficiencies manifest during infancy and early childhood.[149]

As suggested earlier, an infant or toddler who experiences six to eight presumed viral upper respiratory infections during the course of a winter season, without other complications, ordinarily would not be considered likely to have an immunodeficiency. In contrast, a child who has experienced five episodes of acute otitis media in the previous 4 months, several episodes accompanied by sinusitis or pneumonia, has displayed reasonable cause to suspect a humoral immunodeficiency.[149] For certain organisms, infection in the healthy host is so rare that even a single episode should prompt a high suspicion of impaired host defenses. *Pneumocystis jiroveci* pneumonia strongly suggests a severe defect of T-cell number or function.[149] Similarly, lymphadenitis or osteomyelitis caused by gram-negative enteric bacilli suggests a defect of phagocytic killing, such as CGD.[306,474] The following discussion of specific immunologic defects, their genetic basis, if known, and their infectious consequences focuses on well-characterized prototypic disorders within each class of defects, but addresses other related disorders.

Antibody Deficiencies

Humoral immunity is provided by antibody and plays an important role in host defense against most pathogens, as illustrated by the finding that patients with significant antibody deficiencies develop recurrent and sometimes life-threatening infections.[148,156,439] These patients particularly are prone to otitis media, sinusitis, bronchitis, pneumonia, sepsis, and meningitis. Antibodies participate in complement-dependent and complement-independent opsonization, bactericidal activity, virus and toxin neutralization, and the formation of immune complexes that can be cleared by the reticuloendothelial system.[134,270] The role of immunoglobulins globally and of distinct isotypes and subclasses in humoral immunity is elucidated by the nature of infections found in patients with the specific deficiencies addressed subsequently.

X-LINKED AGAMMAGLOBULINEMIA

X-linked agammaglobulinemia (XLA), first described by Bruton, is a primary immunodeficiency disorder of the B-cell lineage and is the most serious disorder of humoral immunity.[102,357,439,494] XLA is characterized by absent or severely decreased numbers of circulating B lymphocytes and absent or extremely low levels of all classes of circulating immunoglobulins. It is caused by several different mutations in the gene encoding for a B cell–specific tyrosine kinase, *Btk*, which maps to the long arm of the X chromosome at Xq22.[585,596] This abnormality in kinase activity results in an arrest in the development of B cells, usually at the pre-B cell stage, and few B cells or their progeny (e.g., plasma cells) are in the circulation or lymphoid tissues.[248]

Most individuals with XLA develop chronic or recurrent pyogenic bacterial sinopulmonary or gastrointestinal infections, and they may have recurrent skin infections.[102,357,439] Systemic disease, such as sepsis, and serious focal infections resulting from bacteremia, such as meningitis, osteomyelitis, and septic arthritis, do not occur as frequently as do respiratory and gastrointestinal infections, but they occur more commonly and are more severe than in normal hosts. The causative agents of most of these infections are *S. pneumoniae* and *H. influenzae*, but *S. aureus* and *Pseudomonas aeruginosa* and other gram-negative organisms may be implicated. The most troublesome gastrointestinal infections in XLA are caused by *Salmonella*, *Campylobacter*, and chronic infestation with *Giardia lamblia*. Although they have no increased susceptibility to most viruses, these patients have been found to have unusually severe or chronic enterovirus infections, which can be

manifested by chronic meningoencephalitis, dermatomyositis, hepatitis, or a combination thereof, and several patients with XLA have developed vaccine-related paralytic poliomyelitis after receiving the live oral polio vaccine.[357]

The only abnormality on physical examination that is not related directly to infections is a paucity of normal B cell–containing lymphoid tissues, such as tonsils, adenoids, and peripheral lymph nodes.[439] Patients who are diagnosed and treated early in life have normal physical examination, growth, and development.

Older individuals with XLA have very low serum levels of IgG, IgM, IgA, and IgE. The diagnosis can be confirmed by studying lymphocyte markers.[439] These patients have a lack of circulating cells that stain for surface immunoglobulin or of B cell–specific monoclonal antibodies against CD19, CD20, or both. The number and function of T lymphocytes are normal in XLA. Establishing the diagnosis in the newborn period may be difficult because maternally derived immunoglobulin bestows normal IgG levels. If there are other reasons to suspect this diagnosis, such as a newborn boy with a documented family history, the diagnosis can be established by documenting a paucity of circulating B cells.

Advances in genetic techniques have enabled maternal carrier detection.[148] In contrast to carriers of some other X-linked genetic diseases, X chromosome inactivation is not random in carriers of XLA. Instead of the two populations of B cells in normal individuals, B lymphocytes of XLA carriers express only one population of B cells—those with the normal allele on the X chromosome—suggesting that B cells with the mutant allele are at a selective disadvantage and do not develop. Prenatal diagnosis is made by genetic studies of amniotic fluid cells or quantitation of fetal circulating B cells.

The prognosis for patients with XLA has improved markedly with earlier diagnosis, high-dose intravenous immunoglobulin (IVIG) therapy, and aggressive use of antibiotics.[439] Before the availability of IVIG, most patients who survived to the third decade of life had chronic lung disease from pulmonary infections and hearing loss from recurrent otitis media.[357]

IgG SUBCLASS DEFICIENCY

Individuals with IgG subclass deficiencies have levels of one or more IgG subclasses that are more than two standard deviations below normal for age, normal to slightly decreased total IgG, normal levels of other immunoglobulin isotypes, and, often, a poor antibody response to certain antigens.* Patients with IgG subclass deficiency who also have IgM and IgA deficiency may have another immunodeficiency disorder, such as common variable immunodeficiency (CVID).

Patients with individual or combined deficiencies of IgG1, IgG2, and IgG3 may be at increased risk for development of infection, particularly if the deficiency is associated with an abnormal antibody response to antigenic stimulation. The most common kinds of infections in patients with IgG subclass deficiency involve the upper respiratory tract. Ordinarily, these patients do not have life-threatening systemic infections.

Because this subclass accounts for approximately 60 percent of total IgG, deficiency of IgG1 is most likely to be associated with subnormal levels of total IgG, and it usually is associated with other subclass deficiencies.[18,19,521,527-529] IgG1-deficient individuals may have recurrent pulmonary infections that can lead to chronic lung disease. IgG2 deficiency usually is associated with normal total serum IgG levels and is more likely to be clinically significant if accompanied by IgG4 or IgA deficiency. Patients with IgG2 deficiency have poor antibody responses to polysac-

---

*See references 272-274, 410, 437, 450, 451, 520, 521, 526-530.

charide antigens but normal responses to protein antigens. Their infections are localized primarily to the respiratory tract, but some patients have had recurrent meningococcal meningitis or disseminated pneumococcal disease. IgG3 deficiency has been associated with low total levels of serum IgG and recurrent respiratory infections, which also may lead to chronic pulmonary disease.[437] IgG4 deficiency is difficult to diagnose because many normal individuals have low serum levels of IgG4, and most normal infants have no detectable IgG4.[437] IgG4 deficiency seems to be of clinical significance if it is associated with IgG2 and IgA deficiency.

The treatment for children with IgG subclass deficiency usually is individualized according to the frequency and severity of symptoms. Noninvasive infections usually can be treated successfully with appropriate antibiotics. Patients with more severe presentations may benefit from IVIG therapy, but patients who also are IgA-deficient should be followed closely for the formation of anti-IgA antibodies and treated only with IgA-depleted IVIG preparations.

HYPER-IgM SYNDROME

Immunoglobulin deficiency with increased IgM is characterized by low levels of IgG, IgA, and IgE but normal to increased levels of IgM in the circulation and normal numbers of circulating B cells.[433,437] The disorder is caused by an intrinsic T-cell abnormality that alters switching from IgM to other isotypes. The basis for the various genetic forms of this defect is in one of several possible defects that involve interactions between CD40 on B cells and CD40L on T cells. In normal individuals, CD40 on the surface of B cells interacts with CD40L on activated T cells to cause B-cell differentiation into memory B cells and switching from IgM to other isotypes. B cells from patients with hyper-IgM syndrome make only IgM antibody, and their B cells express only surface IgM and IgD. The originally described and most common form of the defect is X-linked recessive and results from a mutation in the gene encoding CD40L, a protein expressed transiently on activated T cells.[14,39] More recently described autosomal recessive forms of this disorder involve mutations either in CD40 itself[216] or in a CD40-activated RNA editing enzyme, activation-induced cytidine deaminase.[481] Other cells have surface CD40, and immunologic abnormalities such as the neutropenia and the increased incidence of infections caused by *Pneumocystis* and of malignancies in patients with the hyper-IgM syndrome also may be the result of impaired cell interactions via CD40.

Clinically, hyper-IgM syndrome is manifested by recurrent bacterial infections, especially of the respiratory tract, beginning after maternal immunoglobulin levels subside during the first few months of life.[433,437] Such individuals are susceptible to the same kinds of recurrent pyogenic infections that are associated with other immunoglobulin deficiencies and to infections with organisms more commonly encountered in patients with T-cell defects (e.g., *P. jiroveci*).[51] Some patients with this syndrome have recurrent diarrhea caused by *G. lamblia* and *Cryptosporidium* that is severe enough to require parenteral nutrition. Life-threatening peritonsillar and peritracheal soft tissue infections also have been observed. Approximately half of patients also have persistent or recurrent neutropenia. Patients with autoantibodies may have thrombocytopenia, hemolytic anemia, nephritis, hypothyroidism, or arthritis, as noted earlier.

Physical examination usually is normal except for the sequelae of infections and lymphoid hyperplasia, which probably is caused by constant antigenic stimulation. Arthritis and arthralgia may be the result of chronic infection or the production of autoantibodies. The diagnosis of X-linked hyper-IgM syndrome may be established by using immunofluoresence to document absent expression of CD40L on activated T cells or absent CD40 expression on B cells, or by showing a mutation in one of the genes

encoding CD40, CD40L, or the enzyme activation-induced cytidine deaminase.

IVIG treatment of patients with hyper-IgM syndrome usually results in marked clinical improvement.[51] Patients who have neutropenia with granulocyte colony-stimulating factor (G-CSF) and patients with arthritis or other autoimmune symptoms may need to be treated with steroids. Patients with hyper-IgM syndrome usually do not do as well as patients with XLA because, in addition to their immunoglobulin deficiency, they have an increased incidence of neutropenia, autoimmune disease, and malignancy.

IgA DEFICIENCY

IgA deficiency is the most common immunodeficiency, occurring with a frequency of 1 : 400. Most of the functions of serum IgA can be performed by IgG and IgM.[156,437] Although deficiencies of secretory IgA may lead to recurrent respiratory or gastrointestinal tract infections, deficiency of serum IgA usually is not associated with increased susceptibility to systemic infections.[24] IgA deficiency has been associated with many other conditions, including recurrent infections, IgG2 deficiency, a family history of immunodeficiency (e.g., relatives with CVID), autoimmune disorders, and malignancy.[23] Recurrent infections are most likely to occur in the subset of IgA-deficient patients who also have IgG2 deficiency.[156,450]

Infections usually are mild and involve the upper respiratory and gastrointestinal tracts. Chronic gastrointestinal disease can be caused by *G. lamblia* infections, nodular lymphoid hyperplasia, lactose intolerance, malabsorption, ulcerative colitis, regional enteritis, or autoimmune disorders (e.g., chronic hepatitis, cirrhosis, pernicious anemia). Approximately 20 percent of IgA-deficient patients have allergies, and many have elevated levels of IgE.[156] Food allergy is a common finding and may be the result of abnormal processing of antigen at mucosal surfaces. Other autoimmune diseases that are associated with IgA deficiency include rheumatoid arthritis, systemic lupus erythematosus, thyroiditis, transfusion reactions, pulmonary hemosiderosis, myasthenia gravis, and vitiligo.[156] IgA deficiency seems to occur sporadically, but familial cases have been described.[24,156]

Serum IgA levels less than 5 mg/dL can be clinically significant because patients with levels this low who receive transfusions may make antibody against donor IgA and have severe reactions when transfused again.[517] Reactions to IVIG also may occur because IVIG preparations contain varying amounts of IgA. IgA-depleted preparations are available and usually are well tolerated.

IgE DEFICIENCY

The clinical significance of selective IgE deficiency is unclear because it has been described in healthy individuals. Some patients with profound antibody and cellular immunodeficiencies lack serum IgE, but several partial cellular immunodeficiency syndromes are characterized by elevated levels of IgE (e.g., DiGeorge syndrome, Wiskott-Aldrich syndrome, Hodgkin disease).[437] The absence of IgE does not correlate with an enhanced susceptibility to infection in developed countries, but it has not been investigated in the developing world, where its role in immunity to parasites may be more important.

TRANSIENT HYPOGAMMAGLOBULINEMIA OF INFANCY

Hypogammaglobulinemia is a normal physiologic phenomenon occurring in all infants beginning about 3 to 4 months of age, when maternal antibody wanes and infant synthesis of immunoglobulin has not compensated yet.[437] The syndrome of transient hypogammaglobulinemia of infancy can be differentiated from physiologic hypogammaglobulinemia by the fact that immunoglobulin levels of normal infants begin to increase by the time they are approximately 6 months old, whereas the immunoglobulin levels of infants with transient hypogammaglobulinemia of infancy do not begin to increase until they are 18 to 36 months old.[437] Infants suspected to have this syndrome should be evaluated for XLA and CVID (see later) and followed closely until their immunoglobulin levels normalize for age.

ANTIBODY DEFICIENCY WITH NORMAL OR ELEVATED LEVELS OF IMMUNOGLOBULINS

Some individuals with normal levels of all circulating immunoglobulin isotypes are at increased risk of acquiring infection.[18,20,437] The cause of this disorder remains poorly defined, but it may be related to an inability to respond to specific antigens or the induction of tolerance by exposure to certain antigens very early in development. The most common infections in these patients are recurrent sinopulmonary infections, although a few patients have developed pneumococcal sepsis.[20]

Such individuals can be identified by their inability to make antibody in response to stimulation with specific antigens. They do not have abnormal total serum immunoglobulin classes or subclasses or B-cell or T-cell quantity or function. They can respond to some, but not all, antigenic stimulation. It is important to test these individuals with a variety of stimuli. A good way to test for this syndrome is to immunize with protein antigens, such as tetanus and diphtheria toxoids, and with polysaccharide antigens, such as pneumococcal and *H. influenzae* type b capsular polysaccharide vaccines. Patients who can respond to protein but not to polysaccharide antigens usually respond to protein-polysaccharide conjugates. Treatment with IVIG may help prevent recurrent infections in these patients, although their normal overall levels of immunoglobulin could pose difficulties in determining the appropriate doses of IVIG and intervals between infusions.

Defects of Cell-Mediated Immunity: DiGeorge Syndrome

The prototypic pure T-cell defect, DiGeorge syndrome, is characterized clinically by congenital heart disease (usually involving the aortic arch), hypocalcemic tetany, unusual facial features, and recurrent infections.[182] In the classic or complete form of this disorder, there is absence or hypoplasia of the thymus and parathyroid glands, cardiac or aortic arch deformities, and a stereotypic constellation of abnormal facial features.[182,340,567] Although the condition usually is considered to be associated with immunodeficiency because of the thymic hypoplasia, only approximately 25 percent of patients actually exhibit an immunologic defect.[58] Although currently out of favor, the term *partial DiGeorge syndrome* has been used to describe patients with the typical anatomic findings, but without immunodeficiency, or with mild immunologic impairment.[286]

Some sources designate this disorder as an "anomaly" or "sequence," rather than a syndrome, because of confusion about its relationship to 22q11 deletion syndrome (del22q11) or to the more recently defined microdeletion, del22p11.2, a deletion also associated with velocardiofacial syndrome. Robin and Shprintzen[486] hold that the findings that comprise the DiGeorge "sequence," although often associated with del22q11.2, are etiologically heterogeneous and have been associated with other chromosomal deletions, such as del10p and del17p, or del10q13. Numerous individuals with del22p11.2 exhibit abnormalities distinct from those of the DiGeorge sequence.[253,254,286,348,462,486] This genetic and phenotypic heterogeneity should be considered when evaluating patients with the classic facial and cardiac findings that so often have been associated with a serious T-cell defect.

DiGeorge syndrome usually is recognized in the newborn period by the presence of unusual but characteristic facial features, hypocalcemic tetany in the first 2 days of life, or the presence of serious cardiovascular manifestations, most commonly associated with an interrupted aortic arch or truncus arteriosus.[286,371] Because of the serious nature of the cardiovascular defect, many patients with DiGeorge syndrome have not survived long enough for the immune defect to become a clinical problem.[286] However, with improvements in aggressive surgical treatment of the heart defects, more of these infants are surviving long enough to display manifestations of the immunodeficiency that results in an increased frequency and severity of viral and fungal infections and *Pneumocystis* pneumonia. In such patients, management often has included prophylaxis against *Pneumocystis*, periodic immunoglobulin infusions, and avoidance of live virus vaccines.[286] Transplantation of fetal or postnatal thymic tissue has corrected the immunologic problem for the long-term in approximately a third of such attempts.[247,286] More recently, HLA-matched bone marrow transplantation has been successful in some cases.[87,247,286]

Combined Defects of Cellular and Humoral Immunity

SEVERE COMBINED IMMUNODEFICIENCY DISEASE

SCID describes a heterogeneous group of heritable immunodeficiencies that involve serious impairments of cellular and humoral immunity with recurrent severe infections by a wide range of viral, bacterial, and fungal organisms. SCID has many different forms, which have been reviewed in greater detail elsewhere.[104,107,501] At this writing, there are at least 10 genes, abnormalities of which are known to result in SCID. X-linked SCID, the most common form of SCID, is caused by a mutation in the common gamma chain of the receptor for IL-2 and several other cytokines (γ_c).[104,361] The other known forms of SCID are either known or presumed to be autosomal recessive. They include a deficiency of adenosine deaminase (a purine salvage pathway enzyme), a deficiency in Janus kinase 3 (a cytokine receptor signaling molecule), and a defect in the alpha chain of the IL-7 receptor.[104,315] Mutation of one of at least six different genes whose products play a role in TCR or immunoglobulin gene recombination or TCR signaling, including RAG1, RAG2, Artemis, DNA ligase IV, CD3-delta, and CD3-epsilon, also results in SCID.[104,200,315,377] Additionally, SCID is caused by a mutation in CD45, a phosphatase that regulates signaling thresholds in immune cells.[315]

Long-term management of patients with SCID involves modalities employed in T-cell and B-cell disorders, including prophylaxis against pneumocystis pneumonia, avoidance of live viral vaccines, and immunoglobulin replacement therapy.[104] Bone marrow transplantation from HLA-matched siblings has corrected the defect in many cases and is considered the current treatment of choice.[106] Considerable effort has been expended toward development of gene therapy to treat SCID.[361] Adenosine deaminase deficiency is of historical interest in that it is the first heritable disorder for which gene therapy was attempted, although early success was limited.[79,106] More recent advances in retroviral gene therapy for X-linked SCID initially appeared to be successful. However, at least three patients have developed lymphoproliferative disorders similar to lymphocytic leukemia, with malignant cells showing insertion of the vector into the promoter or first intron of a proto-oncogene, LMO2.[83,107,124,220,472]

COMMON VARIABLE IMMUNODEFICIENCY

CVID is a heterogeneous group of combined immunodeficiencies that differ from most other primary immunodeficiencies in that they usually manifest in the second or third decade of life, although they may manifest at any age.[155,157] Some sources indicate that CVID may be the most common symptomatic primary immunodeficiency. Patients with CVID have normal or only slightly decreased numbers of circulating B cells; low, but not absent, levels of IgG, IgM, and IgA; poor responsiveness to antigens; and abnormal T-lymphocyte function.[159]

Although T-cell and B-cell abnormalities often can be shown, the clinical presentation usually is comparable to that in patients with humoral or B-cell defects (i.e., recurrent bacterial otitis media and sinopulmonary infections).[155,271,494] Occasionally, in addition to having the organisms causing infections in patients with XLA, these patients also have infections with organisms found more commonly in individuals with T-lymphocyte abnormalities, such as *P. jiroveci*, *Mycoplasma pneumoniae*, recurrent herpes simplex virus, and herpes zoster virus infections. Chronic gastrointestinal problems may be caused by *G. lamblia* or other intestinal pathogens. Patients with CVID are prone to development of nodular lymphoid hyperplasia, autoimmune diseases, and malignancies. CVID occasionally has been reported to be familial, and it has been described in families with IgA deficiency. Several gene mutations that have been found more recently in patients with CVID include the genes encoding for CD19, TACI (transmembrane activator and CAML interactor), BAFF-R (receptor for B-cell activating factor of the TNF receptor family), and ICOS (inducible co-stimulatory molecule).[120,514,592]

Patients with CVID usually can benefit from therapy with IVIG, which reduces the incidence of acute infections. Most patients with CVID, even some who undergo long-term treatment with IVIG, develop chronic sinopulmonary disease.[157,449]

Defects of the Interferon-γ and Interleukin-12 Pathways

Macrophages infected by intracellular pathogens, especially mycobacteria or salmonellae, are stimulated via a TLR4-dependent mechanism to release IL-12, along with IL-18, IL-23, and IL-27. These cytokines stimulate T cells and NK cells to produce IFN-γ, via interactions with cellular receptors for the aforementioned cytokines. The released IFN stimulates the macrophage further to release more IL-12 and to activate killing. The mechanism by which this intracellular killing occurs is unknown. This cycle of mutual activation is essential for normal defense against mycobacterial pathogens, and numerous genetic defects of these cytokines, their cellular receptors, or related molecules crucial for receptor-mediated signaling have been associated with increased susceptibility to mycobacterial infections. Deficiencies in this system have resulted from mutations in either of the two receptors for IFN-γ, IFN-γR1 and IFN-γR2, and mutations in STAT1, a molecule crucial for transducing signals from both IFN-γ receptors. Mutations also have been described in the 40-kd subunit of IL-12, IL-12p40, and in the IL-12 receptor, IL-12Rb1. These disorders are uncommon, all involving fewer than 100 known patients.[498]

Mutation of either of the IFN-γ receptors is associated with increased risk of developing mycobacterial infections. Deficiencies of IFN-γR1 may be autosomal recessive or dominant and complete or partial. Most recessive defects are complete and result in absent IFN-γ responsiveness. Dominant IFN-γR1 deficiency is associated with mutations that result in heterozygous truncations of the cytoplasmic domain of the receptor with excessive accumulation of nonfunctional receptor at the cell surface, leading to reduced, but not absent, responsiveness to IFN-γ. Patients with the recessive complete form of this deficiency have a much more severe clinical phenotype than that of patients with the dominant partial form, although the latter have a fivefold greater frequency of nontuberculous mycobacterial osteomyeli-

tis. Defects in IFN-γR2, much less common, also may be recessive or dominant in inheritance and complete or partial. Rare deficiencies in the receptor signaling molecule STAT1 have led to an increased number of mycobacterial infections in a partial deficiency or, in two patients with a recessive complete form, to post-vaccination disseminated bacille Calmette-Guérin disease followed later by death from severe viral infections. The latter probably relates to the additional role of STAT1 in development of IFN-α/β-mediated antiviral activity.[498]

Deficiencies of IL-12p40 or its receptor IL-12Rβ1 are associated with disseminated nontuberculous mycobacterial infections, tuberculosis, and *Salmonella* infections. The receptor deficiency results in unresponsiveness to IL-12. This defect apparently is autosomal recessive with variable clinical penetrance. Deficiency of IL-12p40 also varies in its clinical phenotype and has resulted in deaths caused by severe mycobacterial infections.[452,498,554]

Diagnosis of defects of the IFN-γ pathway usually first involves immunofluorescence flow cytometry to examine cells for deficient or abnormally excessive expression of IFN-γR1. If these studies are normal, studies of STAT1 phosphorylation in response to IFN-γ stimulation may reveal a defect in IFN-γR2 function or expression. For evaluation of the IL-12 pathway, IL-12p40 can be measured in cell supernatants with an enzyme immunoassay, and IL-12Rb1 expression function can be assessed with flow cytometry and, if necessary, by measuring STAT4 phosphorylation after stimulation with IL-12. These studies ordinarily should be done only in a highly specialized reference laboratory.[498]

Complement Deficiencies

Approximately 0.03 percent of the general population have complement deficiencies resulting from acquired or congenital abnormalities of single or multiple complement components or regulatory proteins. Excellent reviews of complement deficiencies are available elsewhere.[175,176,178,185,277,308,499,614]

The most common complement deficiencies are acquired and are transient. They include the relative complement deficiencies in infants (see earlier) and complement deficiencies that result from complement consumption in various inflammatory states, such as connective tissue disorders and acute or chronic infections.[175,176,178,308] Acquired complement deficiencies usually are associated with low levels of more than one complement component.[176] These deficiencies generally are incomplete and are of doubtful clinical significance in host defense against infection.

In contrast, congenital or hereditary deficiencies more often are manifested by abnormality or complete absence of a single complement protein. Deficiencies of individual components may have profound clinical implications because they have been well documented to predispose to acquiring life-threatening infections. Most primary complement abnormalities (C1q dysfunction and C1rs, C4, C2, C3, C5, C6, C7, C8, and C9 deficiencies) are inherited as autosomal co-dominant traits.[176]

Patients with homozygous or heterozygous deficiency of the early classical pathway proteins—C1, C2, and C4—are more prone to develop collagen vascular disease than infections, for reasons that are not fully understood. Approximately 20 percent of patients with homozygous deficiency of early components have problems, however, with recurrent or severe infections that are similar to those seen in C3 deficiency.[176,217,499] Ordinarily, these patients do not have as serious or as frequent problems with infections as do patients with alternative pathway deficiencies because they always can protect themselves via the alternative pathway whether or not they have specific antibody to the infecting organism. Their predilection to development of collagen vascular disease probably is due partly to abnormal solubilization and removal of immune complexes. Although cases of deficiency of one of the isotypes of C4 (C4B) have been reported to be associated with increased susceptibility to infection caused by encapsulated organisms, subsequent studies have not confirmed this finding.[74,121] C2 deficiency has been associated with antibody deficiencies in individuals with recurrent infections.[17,119]

Deficiencies of alternative pathway proteins predispose to development of serious, often fatal, infections because of the lack of ability to respond promptly to organisms not previously encountered.[176] Although the classical pathway is intact, patients with alternative pathway deficiencies often die before they have the opportunity to make the specific antibody required for its activation. No homozygous factor B–deficient patients have been reported. Properdin deficiency, the only X-linked complement deficiency, has been associated with fulminant, usually fatal, meningococcal infection.[177] Factor D deficiency is rare and seems to predispose to recurrent neisserial infection.[330]

More recently, mutations or variants in the gene for MBL, the initiator of the MBL pathway (see earlier), have been associated with an increased risk of having recurrent infections.[185,277,563] In particular, homozygosity for such mutations or variants was found to be associated with an increased risk for developing systemic meningococcal disease.[223]

Because all three complement activation pathways converge at the activation of C3, patients who are deficient in C3 are unable to mobilize any of the three main effector functions of complement in host defense—opsonization, phagocyte recruitment, or bacteriolysis. One is not surprised that the most serious complement deficiency state is the total absence of C3.[176] Congenital C3 deficiency is rare and results from decreased production of C3.[217,499] Patients with deficiencies of factors H and I have low, but detectable, levels of C3 because absence of either of these regulatory factors allows continuous activation of the alternative pathway and uncontrolled C3 consumption. Patients with C3 deficiency caused by any of these mechanisms have increased susceptibility to infections caused by encapsulated bacteria, such as pneumococci, meningococci, and *H. influenzae* type b. Many of these infections involve the respiratory tract (otitis, sinusitis, bronchitis, and pneumonia), but C3-deficient patients also are predisposed to development of sepsis and meningitis.[176,217,499] In addition, some C3-deficient patients develop one of several different autoimmune diseases.[176,217,499]

Deficiencies of terminal complement proteins C5, C6, C7, and C8 greatly increase the risk of developing systemic infections caused by *N. meningitidis* or *Neisseria gonorrhoeae*.[76] Because C9 is not absolutely required for bacteriolysis—although it renders this process more efficient—C9 deficiency increases the risk of infection to a lesser degree than deficiencies of other terminal components. C9 deficiency was found to be present in approximately 0.1 percent of the population in Japan, and the risk of acquiring meningococcal disease was increased 5000-fold in C7-deficient patients and 700-fold in C9-deficient patients.[420]

The risk of developing infection is higher in patients with C5 deficiency than in patients with deficiencies of other terminal proteins because, in addition to the role of C5 in initiating assembly of the MAC, the free C5 fragment, C5a, is an important chemoattractant and is crucial for leukocyte recruitment to sites of microbial invasion and for bactericidal activity.[175] Although a rare patient with C5 deficiency had recurrent subcutaneous skin infections, as might characterize a disorder of chemotaxis, most patients with this disorder are at increased risk for acquiring meningococcal and disseminated gonococcal infections.

At least one episode of meningococcal disease occurs in approximately 60 percent of individuals who have been identified as having C5, C6, C7, C8, or properdin deficiency, and 75 to 85 percent of documented bacterial infections in complement-deficient patients are meningococcal.[176,217,499] Conversely, approximately 14 percent of patients presenting with sporadic meningococcal diseases may be expected to have a defect in one of the late complement components, and this percentage increases

to approximately one third among individuals with two or more meningococcal infections.

Differences in the features of meningococcal disease between individuals with complement component deficiencies and normal hosts have been noted. First, meningococcal disease occurs in older individuals (mean age 17 years versus 3 years), and a higher proportion of disease is caused by groups Y, W135, and X in complement-deficient individuals than in normal individuals.[176] Additionally, the mortality rate in meningococcal infection is much lower than in normal individuals, probably because many patients with one of these deficiencies have developed antibodies to meningococci that can activate the classical pathway leading to normal opsonization and phagocyte activation, functions upstream in the cascade from the MAC. In contrast, individuals with normal complement levels who develop meningococcal infection usually do so because they do not have specific antibodies with which to activate the classical pathway, and meningococci are poor activators of the alternative pathway.

Currently, no specific treatment exists for patients with hereditary complement deficiencies. Replacement of missing complement proteins has been attempted with fresh-frozen plasma, but it is not practical because of the short half-life of most of the components.[55,351,502] Immunization of complement-deficient patients and their close household contacts against encapsulated organisms may reduce the risk of acquiring infections caused by these organisms.

Disorders of Phagocyte Function

GENERAL FEATURES OF PHAGOCYTE DISORDERS

The most frequent reminder of the importance of having an adequate supply of well-functioning phagocytes comes from patients who develop neutropenia after undergoing chemotherapy for malignancies. The high risk of developing bacterial and fungal infections in these patients mainly is the result of a lack of circulating neutrophils available for delivery to infected tissue.[467] The qualitative disorders of phagocyte function discussed in this section result in similar susceptibilities to these infections, either because the circulating cells are unable to migrate to an infected site or because, even having migrated to the infected tissue, they are unable to effect normal microbicidal activity. Some overlap exists among the types of infectious complications associated with disorders of migration versus killing. As a rule, defects of neutrophil migration tend to be associated with infections at skin and mucous membrane sites. In contrast, killing defects are more likely to result in infections of soft tissues and internal organs, although skin infections are common findings.

INTRINSIC DISORDERS OF CELL MIGRATION

Type 1 Leukocyte Adhesion Deficiency

In the late 1970s and the first half of the 1980s, several reports described patients with recurrent bacterial infections, diminished neutrophil motility, and delayed separation of the umbilical cord.[2,29-31,37,89,154,221,268] The neutrophils of these patients were discovered to be markedly deficient in adherence to natural and artificial surfaces, in response to complement-opsonized particles, and in expression of surface glycoproteins in the molecular weight range of 150 to 180 kd. The deficient glycoproteins were found to be members of a family of heterodimeric glycoproteins, LFA-1, Mac-1, and p150,95, each defined by its own unique alpha subunit, CD11a, CD11b, and CD11c, respectively, but sharing a common 95-kd beta subunit designated CD18.[30,31,36,37,552] A fourth alpha subunit, CD11d, the importance of which remains poorly understood, has been described more recently.

These proteins, also called the β_2 leukocyte integrins, were identified as crucial determinants of adhesion-dependent functions on neutrophils and other phagocytic cells, and their absence seemed to be directly responsible for the striking adherence-dependent defects that characterized the function of leukocytes from patients with this disorder.[29-31,36,37,552] Variously called Mac-1 deficiency, MO1 deficiency, LFA-1 deficiency, CD11/CD18 deficiency, or CR3 deficiency, this disorder, now usually termed *type 1 leukocyte adhesion deficiency* (LAD-1), is an autosomal recessive disorder with one of numerous mutations in the β_2 integrin subunit, CD18, localized to chromosome 21.[31,36,552,553] It has been identified in more than 150 individuals worldwide and has a broad ethnic diversity.[31,36] Patients may exhibit a moderate or severe phenotype, depending on the extent of the defect in protein expression.[30,31] The documented mutations of CD18 that result in LAD-1 have been diverse, leading to abnormalities ranging from complete absence of the protein to extensions of the molecule, truncations of the extracellular portion or of the cytoplasmic domain of the molecule, small deletions, and point mutations.[33,36,282]

Patients with LAD-1 develop recurrent necrotic skin and soft tissue infections with poor or absent formation of pus, and they exhibit poor wound healing.[30,31] They develop a severe generalized form of gingivitis or periodontitis, often losing most or all of their primary and secondary dentition along with some of their alveolar bone.[30,31] They also may develop enterocolitis similar to that seen in neutropenic patients.[30,31] Delayed separation of the umbilical cord, presumably caused by an impaired inflammatory response, is a common feature of the more severe phenotype of this disorder,[30,31] but this finding alone in infants without infectious complications or other characteristic features is of doubtful significance.[619] Pronounced leukocytosis is a common feature of LAD-1, even in the absence of active infection.[30,31] The reason for this feature is not completely understood. The fact that LAD-1 neutrophils are incapable of normal egress from the circulation via the oral cavity or lower intestinal tract was long thought to provide the principal explanation for the high circulating neutrophil counts. More recent studies in CD18-null LAD-1 mice reveal abnormally high circulating G-CSF levels, however, and suggest that a more likely explanation involves the absence of a negative feedback mechanism on production of G-CSF that occurs during normal transendothelial migration of leukocytes and involves IL-17. Absent ongoing transendothelial migration results in failure of this putative feedback mechanism, resulting in elevated G-CSF levels and higher circulating granulocyte counts.[225]

Functional studies of neutrophils from patients with LAD-1 reveal a marked impairment of adherence-dependent functions that require the β_2 integrins, including attachment to various surfaces, orientation in a chemotactic gradient, chemotaxis through nitrocellulose filters or under agarose gels, aggregation, phagocytosis of iC3b-opsonized particles, degranulation or activation of the oxidative metabolic burst in response to such particles, and recruitment of PMNs in vivo to Rebuck skin windows or dermal suction blisters.[29-31,111,232] In contrast, neutrophil functions that are independent of CD11/CD18-mediated interactions, including degranulation or oxidative burst activation in response to soluble stimuli or polarized shape change in suspension in response to chemoattractants, are normal.[29-31] PMNs and NK cells from patients with LAD-1 exhibit impaired ADCC for virus-infected target cells, suggesting that CD11/CD18-mediated cell-cell adhesion is essential for normal killing of virus-infected cells by this mechanism[331] and that the increased severity of viral infections in a few of the most severely affected patients could be related to defective ADCC. Currently, the specific diagnosis of LAD usually is made by showing absent or markedly deficient expression of the CD11/CD18 family of glycoproteins on circulating leukocytes by immunofluorescence flow cytometry, although various other methods have been used.[29-31,37]

Careful attention given to skin and oral hygiene, aggressive management of infections, and meticulous local care of wound sites are important in the care of patients with LAD-1 or any serious disorder of neutrophil migration. Prophylactic antibiotics, usually trimethoprim-sulfamethoxazole, have been used in many of these patients, but their efficacy has not been well established. Granulocyte transfusions have been used with some success to treat severe infections in a few patients with LAD-1.[31,89] Bone marrow transplantation with HLA-matched allogeneic marrow has led to missed results, ranging from complete correction of the phagocytic defect to death from graft-versus-host disease 9 months after transplantation.[31,221] The human CD18 gene has been cloned and sequenced, and human LAD-1 cells have been corrected successfully in vitro with the normal CD18 complementary DNA carried by retrovirus vectors, hinting at the future promise of gene therapy for patients with LAD-1.[31,32] The development of genetic knockout mice deficient in CD18 may provide a useful model for studying gene therapy in vivo and for helping to elucidate features of the underlying deficiency itself.[31,338]

Type 2 Leukocyte Adhesion Deficiency

In 1992, two unrelated patients were reported, both products of consanguineous matings, who exhibited clinical characteristics virtually identical to those described for LAD-1.[228] Expression of the β_2 (CD18) integrins on leukocytes was normal, however. In addition to defects in neutrophil motility, these children exhibited short stature, psychomotor retardation, and the Bombay (hh) erythrocyte phenotype (homozygous for absence of the H antigen). Phagocytosis by PMNs was normal.

This defect has been documented to be caused by one or more mutations of a specific guanosine diphosphate–fucose transporter,[375] resulting in the absence of fucosyl residues on sialyl Lewis X, the tetrasaccharide moiety that serves as an important ligand for members of the selectin family of adhesion molecules.[228,350,600] In vivo and in vitro studies comparing the adhesive functions of PMNs from LAD-1 and this new disorder, now called LAD-2, have provided elegant validation of the distinct roles of selectins and integrins in the recruitment of leukocytes in vivo, with the initial selectin-mediated "rolling" stage (deficient in LAD-2) required first for the second integrin-mediated "firm adhesion and extravasation" stage (deficient in LAD-1) to occur.[600] A deficiency in either mechanism results in defective delivery of PMNs to infected sites and is manifested clinically as a form of LAD. The other somatic and neurologic features of LAD-2 may be related to more widespread consequences of the generalized defect in fucosylation of glycoproteins.[375] Because of the generalized nature of this deficiency, a proposal has been made to designate this disorder *type IIc congenital disorder of glycosylation*.[375]

Type 3 Leukocyte Adhesion Deficiency (Integrin Activation Defect)

In recent years, at least four patients have been reported who have clinical phenotypes that include features of type 1 LAD and Glanzmann thrombasthenia, a bleeding disorder associated with mutations in the αIIbβ3 integrin on platelets. Laboratory studies of these patients revealed markedly deficient integrin-mediated adhesive functions of leukocytes and platelets despite normal surface expression of leukocyte and platelet integrins. Further studies led to the conclusion that this defect in integrin function was the result of defective "inside-out" signaling pathways that normally lead to integrin activation.[205,325,389] Although the precise molecular defect in this disorder remains uncharacterized, cells from one patient with this disorder have been reported to exhibit deficient activation of a small guanosine triphosphatase, Rap1, an important regulator of inside-out integrin activation.[325] A growing consensus is that this defect of integrin activation be termed *type 3 leukocyte adhesion deficiency* (LAD-3), although this nomenclature does not include reference to the defect in platelet function.[205,325]

Specific Granule Deficiency

Rare patients with hereditary specific granule deficiency have been reported, beginning with the original description by Spitznagel and colleagues in 1972.[90,231,550] These patients exhibited recurrent and severe infections, primarily of the skin and mucous membranes, sometimes involving the lung and, in one patient, the mastoid. Normal human neutrophils contain azurophilic (primary) granules and specific (secondary) granules, the contents of which have been summarized previously. Neutrophils from patients with this disorder exhibit bilobed nuclei and absent specific granules on Wright-stained blood smears. Lactoferrin released from specific granules reduces the negative surface charge of the plasma membrane, contributing to nonspecific adhesiveness of the cell.[231]

The specific granule membrane also contains some of the intracellular store of the important adhesion molecule Mac-1 (CD11b/CD18) that is mobilized to the plasma membrane on stimulation by chemoattractants or other stimuli that induce granule secretion.[63,85] Specific granule deficiency results in marked impairment of adhesion and migration of neutrophils, probably on the basis of diminished intracellular pools of adhesive proteins and the inability to effect the change in surface charge caused by lactoferrin. This impairment leads to the recurrent skin and mucous membrane infections caused by *S. aureus*, gram-negative bacilli, and *Candida* that characterize the natural history of patients with this disorder.[90,231,550] Neutrophils in this disorder also exhibit diminished microbicidal activity, presumably because of diminished amounts of the cytochrome b_{558} component of NADPH oxidase that are stored in the membrane of specific granules.

Although the disorder is probably too rare to make such generalizations, specific granule deficiency likely is autosomal recessive in its mode of inheritance because males and females are represented equally. The documentation of a specific granule deficiency phenotype in mice rendered genetically null for an important myeloid cell transcription factor known as *CCAAT/enhancer binding protein epsilon* (C/EBPε) has led to studies in a few patients with specific granule deficiency that confirmed a deletion in the C/EBPε gene, with absent expression of this transcription factor, although not all patients with this disorder have a mutation of this gene.[183,360] Specific granule deficiency may be diagnosed in a patient with recurrent skin and mucous membrane infections whose neutrophils exhibit the characteristic absence of specific granules on Wright stain and a marked impairment of chemotaxis in vivo and in vitro.

Chédiak-Higashi Syndrome

Chédiak-Higashi syndrome is a complex, rare autosomal recessive disorder characterized by partial oculocutaneous albinism, recurrent pyogenic infections, peripheral neuropathy, and neutropenia.[81] The illness also may involve an accelerated lymphoproliferative phase.[81] Granular cells, including neutrophils, contain giant lysosomal granules that are the apparent result of spontaneous intracellular fusion of azurophilic granules and, to a lesser extent, specific granules.[81] Corresponding disorders of intracellular pigment granules and vesicle trafficking in axons account for the albinism and other manifestations of this disease.[81] Similar disorders have been described in Aleutian mink, beige mice, albino Hereford cattle, and albino whales.[81] The genetic basis of the defect now is known to involve either a nonsense or a frameshift mutation in the gene encoding a large protein called the *lysosomal trafficking regulator*, homologous to the "beige" gene in mice, with all mutations studied so far resulting in a truncated protein.[54,125]

Patients with Chédiak-Higashi syndrome develop recurrent skin and mucosal infections, most often caused by *S. aureus*, which are characteristic of those observed in defects of phagocyte migration.[31,81] They have a consistent defect in cell migration that seems to be related to abnormal regulation of microtubule polymerization on stimulation by chemoattractant agents.[81] The possible role of intracellular levels of cyclic adenosine monophosphate (cAMP) and guanylic acid in this microtubule abnormality has been suggested,[93] but the relationship between cyclic nucleotides and the microtubule dysfunction in Chédiak-Higashi syndrome has not been established. Ascorbic acid has been shown in at least one study to normalize the elevated levels of cAMP and the number of microtubules present within the cell.[93] Studies of two brothers with Chédiak-Higashi syndrome showed abnormally increased tyrosinylation of the alpha subunit of tubulin.[81,423] Phagocytosis is normal, but killing of ingested bacteria is defective or delayed. The reason for this deficient or delayed killing is uncertain but may involve defective phagolysosomal fusion or abnormalities in levels of microbicidal defensins, which also are stored in primary granules.[235]

The diagnosis of Chédiak-Higashi syndrome usually is suspected clinically on the basis of partial oculocutaneous albinism and recurrent pyogenic infections. A Wright stain showing giant lysosomal granules and laboratory studies showing defective cell migration are confirmatory.

Neutrophil Actin Dysfunction

Filamentous actin constitutes the main contractile mechanism of neutrophils for migration and phagocytosis.[560] An extremely rare and apparently heterogeneous disorder, neutrophil actin dysfunction, has been characterized by recurrent skin infections caused by *S. aureus* and *Candida albicans*. Biopsy samples of infected skin lesions in one child showed necrotic tissue with a notable absence of neutrophils. In vivo and in vitro studies revealed severely impaired neutrophil chemotaxis and phagocytosis.[91] The capacity for polymerization of actin from cell extracts also was diminished markedly. PMNs from family members of this patient also were found to be variably deficient in the CD11/CD18 family of glycoproteins that are the basis of LAD-1.[547,548] The nature and significance of this association is uncertain.

Another infant reported to have recurrent skin and mucosal infections and defective neutrophil chemotaxis was found to have abnormally high levels of a 47-kd protein, now identified as *lymphocyte-specific protein–1*, which exhibits actin-binding activity.[138] More recently, a 12-year-old patient with recurrent infections, mental retardation, and abnormal neutrophil chemotaxis was reported to be heterozygous for a substitution of lysine for glutamic acid-364 in non-muscle β-actin.[435] This substitution lies in a region important for binding to profilin and other actin-regulatory molecules. This patient's neutrophils also exhibited reduced production of superoxide, suggesting a possible role for normal actin function in the assembly of the NADPH oxidase complex.

Glycogen Storage Disease Type 1B

Beaudet and colleagues[60] first reported the association of recurrent infection, neutropenia, and impaired neutrophil migration with glycogen storage disease (GSD) type 1B, a metabolic disorder characterized by defective microsomal transport of glucose-6-phosphate. In 1985, Ambruso and coworkers[21] reviewed the features of 21 patients with GSD type 1B, 15 of whom had frequent infections, especially of the skin and subcutaneous tissues. Osteomyelitis, pneumonitis, sinusitis, and septicemia also were reported. Seventeen of these 21 patients were found to have serum inhibitors of myeloid stem cell proliferation, which were presumed to account for their chronic neutropenia. Impaired neutrophil motility was found in 8 of 11 patients in whom this condition was evaluated. Assays of neutrophil microbicidal capacity generally were normal. A specific relationship between the underlying metabolic defect in GSD type 1B and the mechanism of impaired cell motility has not been established. However, exogenous glucose is an important energy source for chemotaxis,[611] and the uptake of glucose by PMNs in response to chemoattractant stimulation is impaired in patients with GSD type 1B and in neonates, both examples of patients with impaired PMN migration.[5,56]

EXTRINSIC OR SECONDARY DEFECTS OF POLYMORPHONUCLEAR LEUKOCYTE MIGRATION

Defective Neutrophil Chemotaxis Associated with Serum Inhibitors of Cell Function

Many investigators have reported the presence of inhibitors of PMN chemotaxis in the serum of patients with recurrent infection.[337,415,535,546,590,609] In most cases, the pathophysiologic mechanisms of these inhibitors are unknown. In many of the patients described, other associated immunologic disorders could account for at least part of the increased susceptibility to infection. In each case, the patient's neutrophils exhibited diminished chemotaxis in the presence of autologous serum or plasma, whereas identical assays in the presence of control serum or plasma resulted in a normal chemotactic response. Most such inhibitors seem to be immunoglobulins or immunoglobulin-like molecules.

Hyper-IgE Syndrome

In 1966, Davis and colleagues[169] described two young girls with coarse facial features, reddish hair, fair skin, severe eczema, dystrophic nails, staphylococcal skin abscesses, and recurrent sinopulmonary infections. The absence of classic signs of inflammation accompanying the staphylococcal abscesses led to their being characterized as cold abscesses. The term *Job syndrome* was suggested, referring to the similar biblical affliction. Additional patients, including a patient who exhibited a defect in neutrophil chemotaxis reported in 1973 by Clark and associates,[137] were described with a similar disorder, first associated by Buckley and colleagues[109] with very high serum IgE levels.

Subsequent reports of similar patients have shown that certain features are common to all patients with the disease, now called *hyper-IgE syndrome*. These consistent features include a history of staphylococcal infections of the skin and sinopulmonary tract beginning in infancy or early childhood and serum levels of IgE that are greater that 2000 IU/mL.[105,109,188] Other characteristic, but variable, features of this disorder include coarse facies, cold abscesses of the skin and subcutaneous tissues, a chronic eczematoid rash, eosinophilia, and mucocutaneous candidiasis.[105,188] Comprehensive reviews have provided detailed characterizations of the abnormalities of patients with this poorly understood disorder.[105,188] Consistent abnormalities of cell-mediated immune functions in patients with hyper-IgE syndrome suggest that the pathogenic basis involves a defect of T-cell regulation.[239] Documented abnormalities include diminished reactivity to *Candida* and tetanus toxoid in delayed hypersensitivity skin testing, decreased in vitro lymphocyte proliferative responses to these antigens, and reduced numbers of T cells with the CD45RO memory T-cell phenotype.[108,132,188]

A more recent extensive study of 30 patients with hyper-IgE syndrome and 70 of their relatives concluded that this disorder is inherited as a single-locus autosomal dominant trait with variable expressivity.[256] Although the specific gene defect or defects responsible for this disorder remain unknown, a study of 19 kindreds has revealed a genetic locus for hyper-IgE syndrome on chromosome 4, in the proximal 4q region.[257,258] More recently, a novel autosomal recessive form of hyper-IgE syndrome has been described that includes some patients who have developed severe viral infections or a form of autoimmune vasculitis involving the central nervous system.[83,257]

Although hyper-IgE syndrome more properly may belong in discussions of defective T-cell regulation, some patients with hyper-IgE syndrome may have a defect in neutrophil chemotaxis.[188] The defect, if observed at all, usually is intermittent. In several cases, the presence of a serum inhibitor of chemotaxis has been recognized.[188] Donabedian and Gallin[187] showed an inhibitor of granulocyte chemotaxis in supernatants from cultured peripheral blood monocytes from patients with hyper-IgE syndrome. The persistence of infectious complications in this disorder, at times when chemotaxis has been found to be normal and the presence of large purulent collections within cold abscesses, raises questions about the significance of a chemotactic disorder in explaining the markedly increased susceptibility of these patients to recurrent infections.

Impaired Generation of Serum-Derived Chemotaxins

A deficiency in the host's ability to produce chemotaxins derived from serum components may have profound consequences for the recruitment of PMNs to an infected site. The most important serum-derived chemotaxin is the fragment of the fifth component of complement, C5a, and its des-arg form. Several kindreds have been described with either absent or defective C5.[495] The chemoattractant activity measured in activated normal serum virtually is absent in C5-deficient serum.[496] The risk of developing systemic *Neisseria* infections owing to deficient activation of the lytic terminal complement sequence seems far more significant than any phagocytic recruitment defect caused by impaired production of chemotaxins.[62,217] Patients with C3 deficiency also have impaired chemotaxigenesis because C5 cannot be activated. Host impairment usually is more severe because of the importance of C3 in opsonization and its role in the activation of the remainder of the complement cascade.[499]

OTHER SECONDARY OR POORLY DEFINED DISORDERS OF POLYMORPHONUCLEAR LEUKOCYTE MIGRATION

Patients with protein-calorie malnutrition have defective PMN chemotaxis that seems to be based on systemic pre-activation of circulating cells owing to chronic low-level endotoxemia that results from impaired intestinal mucosal integrity.[128,512] Shwachman-Diamond syndrome, is associated with defective PMN migration in addition to pancreatic insufficiency, neutropenia, and growth retardation.[11] Two kindreds with congenital ichthyosis and an associated defect of PMN migration have been described.[402] Patients with severe thermal injuries develop an acquired form of specific granule deficiency with impaired PMN migration beginning approximately 14 days after injury.[231] Children with juvenile periodontitis of various types may exhibit reduced PMN chemotaxis.[437] In some of these patients, this condition has been associated with gingival infections caused by *Capnocytophaga*, an anaerobic gram-negative organism that can elaborate factors that markedly impair PMN migration in vitro.[532] In one such patient, the ultimate diagnosis was LAD-1, a finding that raises some uncertainty about the role of *Capnocytophaga* in such disorders.[282] Several reports have been published of a poorly defined disorder of neutrophil migration termed *lazy leukocyte syndrome*,[10,401] which is characterized by recurrent staphylococcal skin infections, rhinitis, gingivitis, stomatitis, neutropenia despite adequate marrow precursors, and diminished in vivo and in vitro migration of neutrophils.

DEFECTS IN PHAGOCYTE MICROBICIDAL ACTIVITY

As described earlier, the broad array of available phagocyte microbicidal mechanisms may be divided into oxygen-dependent and oxygen-independent mechanisms. To date, no isolated deficiency of a specific oxygen-independent microbicidal mechanism has been described. This section is concerned mainly with the known deficiencies of oxygen-dependent microbicidal mechanisms of phagocytes, especially CGD, the prototypic defect in this group. PMN migration usually is normal in these killing defects. Monocytes and the fixed phagocytes of the reticuloendothelial system generally share in the deficient microbicidal activity.

Chronic Granulomatous Disease

CGD was one of the earliest syndromes of phagocyte dysfunction to be characterized[474] and probably is the most extensively studied among individual phagocyte defects. It is recognized now to be a family of biochemically and genetically heterogeneous disorders of distinct components of the phagocyte NADPH oxidase complex.[87,128,183] CGD results in the inability of phagocytes to generate superoxide anion and other reactive oxygen species.[183] Organisms that produce catalase pose a special problem for patients with CGD[183,189,306,355] and encompass a broad range of pathogens that includes staphylococci, gram-negative enteric bacteria, *Pseudomonas* spp., yeast, fungi, *Nocardia* spp., and numerous other pathogenic species.[189,306,355,622]

Most microorganisms produce H_2O_2, which might be used, even by the CGD phagocyte, as an effective microbicidal weapon because it feeds into the sequence of oxidant reactions downstream from the defective oxidase enzyme (see Fig. 2–5).[492] Organisms that produce catalase are able to survive within these deficient cells because catalase is an enzyme that degrades H_2O_2 to oxygen and water.[306,492] Infections with catalase-negative bacteria, such as *S. pneumoniae*, *H. influenzae*, and *N. meningitidis*, do not occur with increased frequency in patients with CGD,[622] and these organisms are killed normally in vitro by CGD phagocytes. Phagocyte functions not related directly to oxidative mechanisms of intracellular killing, including adherence, chemotaxis, phagocytosis, and degranulation, usually are normal in patients with CGD.[44,405,474,544]

The genetic defect in CGD may be inherited by X-linked recessive or autosomal recessive mechanisms.[87,160] In the female obligate carriers of X-linked CGD, the proportion of cells that express the defect usually is 35 to 65 percent, depending on the proportion of cells in which random inactivation of the normal versus the affected X chromosome occurs.[376,622] In most of the autosomal recessive forms of CGD, the quantity of the cytochrome in cells is normal, but there is a deficiency in one of two cytosolic proteins, $p47^{phox}$ and $p67^{phox}$, each of which is a crucial component of the fully assembled NADPH oxidase complex.[42,87,136] In the report of a recently created registry of 368 patients with CGD in the United States,[622] greater than two thirds of the patients had the X-linked recessive form with absent $gp91^{phox}$, the larger subunit of the cytochrome b_{558}; approximately 12 percent had an autosomal recessive form with absent $p47^{phox}$; and fewer than 5 percent each had autosomal recessive disease with absence of the $p67^{phox}$ or absence of $p22^{phox}$, the smaller subunit of the cytochrome b_{558}. Approximately 12 percent had an unknown genetic form of the disease.

A more recent review[276] indicates that approximately 5 percent of patients with CGD have normal levels of an abnormal protein that is inactive and that at least 410 different mutations have been reported to result in CGD. These genetically diverse defects all result in defective function of the oxidase and the characteristic CGD phenotype. Included in the above-mentioned registry were two rare adult women whose sons had X-linked disease and who exhibited clinical signs of the CGD phenotype because of dramatically skewed X-chromosome inactivation with 5 percent or less of their phagocytes showing oxidase activity. Overall, patients with X-linked disease have more severe courses and experience higher yearly death rates than do patients with autosomal recessive forms of the disease.[622]

Patients with CGD experience recurrent serious bacterial and fungal infections, usually beginning in the first few months of life. *S. aureus* and gram-negative bacilli, especially *Serratia* and *Burkholderia cepacia*, are the most common causes of infection in patients with CGD, but fungi, especially *Aspergillus* spp., also are prominent etiologic agents.[355,479,622] Infections caused by *Aspergillus* are the most common cause of death in patients with CGD.[622] Lymphadenopathy associated with lymphadenitis and chronic suppuration with poor healing is a common presenting feature of CGD. Granuloma formation at infected sites is a histologic hallmark of this disorder.[306,479] Pulmonary infections and their complications have been the reported cause of death in 50 percent of patients with CGD in some series, and *Aspergillus* predominates.[622]

These infections often are protracted and respond slowly to appropriate antibiotic therapy.[306,479] Progression to lung abscess, empyema, or both occurs in approximately 20 percent of patients with CGD and pneumonia.[306] Liver abscesses occur in approximately half of patients with CGD and may be recurrent.[62,133] The hepatosplenomegaly common in patients with CGD may result from these infections but probably is more likely to result from chronic infections at various sites with systemic lymphoid hyperplasia.[47,306] Osteomyelitis occurs in approximately one third of patients with CGD.[306,479,622] In contrast to normal children, in whom this infection usually involves the metaphyseal area of long bones, patients with CGD more often develop infections of the small bones of the hands and feet. In normal children, *S. aureus* is the most common etiologic agent, and this agent does cause a significant proportion of cases in CGD. However, gram-negative bacilli and *Aspergillus* seem to be the predominant etiologies, and other agents, including *Nocardia*, also may be important etiologic agents in CGD.[462,566,622] Skin infections in patients with CGD may include pyoderma, purulent dermatitis, and cutaneous or subcutaneous abscesses and often are preceded by a chronic eczematoid skin rash[479] but are less of a problem than in patients with leukocyte migration defects.

Although localized infections are the rule in patients with CGD, these patients also may develop septicemia.[306,479,622] The most common cause of septicemia in most series has been *Salmonella*, but other gram-negative enteric bacilli also have been prominent.[306,355] *S. aureus*, the most common etiologic agent of localized infections in CGD, is a proportionally less common cause of septicemia in these patients.[479,622] Other infections sometimes seen in patients with CGD include recurrent urinary tract infections in approximately 6 to 8 percent of patients; ocular infections with conjunctivitis, blepharitis, or both in approximately 20 percent of patients; and, rarely, chorioretinitis.[385,479]

Granuloma formation adjacent to hollow viscera in patients with CGD has been found to produce clinically significant obstruction. Reported examples of this problem include obstruction of the gastric outlet, esophagus, small intestine, and ureters.[22,129,189] This complication usually responds to treatment with corticosteroids.[129]

CGD should be suspected in patients with a history of recurrent indolent infections caused by catalase-positive organisms such as those described earlier, especially if granulomas are found in biopsy specimens of lymph nodes or other tissues. Confirmation of the diagnosis usually rests on the demonstration of an absent or nearly absent oxidative metabolic burst in the patient's phagocytes. This burst can be detected by the slide nitroblue tetrazolium test (Fig. 2–12) or by other measurements of oxidative burst activity, such as cytochrome reduction, lucigenin-enhanced or luminol-enhanced chemiluminescence, oxygen consumption, H_2O_2 production, and flow cytometry of cells loaded with oxidant-sensitive fluorescent dyes.[15,42,57,391,491,579] Prenatal diagnosis has been achieved by the use of the slide nitroblue tetrazolium test with blood from placental vessels obtained at fetoscopy.[425]

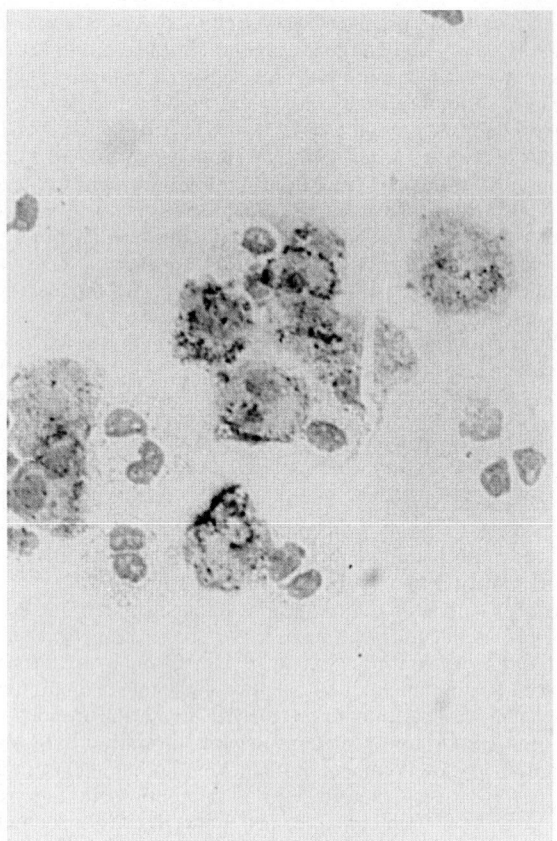

Figure 2–12 Photomicrograph of a slide nitroblue tetrazolium (NBT) test of polymorphonuclear leukocytes (PMNs) isolated from the blood of a maternal carrier of X-linked recessive chronic granulomatous disease. Because of random inactivation of either the normal or the affected X chromosome in maternal carriers of this disorder, approximately half of the PMNs exhibit the granular blue-black staining characteristic of the oxidative reduction of NBT by normal PMNs. In contrast, the remaining PMNs, which express the reduced nicotinamide adenine dinucleotide phosphate (NADPH) oxidase defect of chronic granulomatous disease, are visible only by their nuclear counterstain.

The management of patients with CGD traditionally has relied on antibiotic prophylaxis, usually with trimethoprim-sulfamethoxazole or an oral antistaphylococcal penicillin, and an aggressive approach to the specific diagnosis and treatment of acute infections.[479] The use of antifungal prophylaxis with itraconazole or newer azole derivatives that also have activity against *Apergillus* has become standard in most centers. Granulocyte transfusions have been reported to be at least partially beneficial in a few cases.[112,142] Bone marrow transplantation met with limited success in the late 1970s and early 1980s, with only one successful long-term engraftment reported among four separate attempts in different patients.[251,316,477,615] Allogeneic peripheral blood stem cell transplantation from HLA-identical sibling donors, with prior myeloablative conditioning, has been considerably more promising, as suggested by the European experience from 1985 to 2000—22 of 23 patients "cured," with median follow-up of 12 years.[524] Longer term follow-up is necessary, however, to confirm the promise of this approach to treatment.

One of the most important developments in the treatment of patients with CGD is the administration of IFN-γ. A multicenter study initially showed that daily subcutaneous injections of this agent reduced the requirement for hospitalization of patients with CGD for serious infections by approximately two thirds.[298] IFN-γ does not increase oxidase activity in neutrophils, and the

mechanism by which IFN-γ exerts its beneficial effect in CGD has not been determined. Long-term follow-up of patients being treated with IFN-γ has indicated that it continues to reduce the rate of serious infections over the course of many years and generally is well tolerated.[382] This treatment carries some mild systemic side effects, such as fever, fatigue, and myalgia,[298] but it has become part of the standard regimen for managing most patients with CGD.

The definition of the molecular basis for CGD and the cloning of the genes responsible for the various forms of this defect have led to correction of some forms of the defect in cultured cells and the development of animal models of CGD in mice,[183,301,469,599] both of which are crucial steps in developing gene therapy for patients with this disorder in the future. Preclinical studies of gene therapy in mice with CGD have shown promise when bone marrow cells are transduced using retroviral vectors ex vivo and transplanted into irradiated syngeneic recipients.[183] Fifty to eighty percent of circulating neutrophils were oxidase-positive 12 to 14 weeks post-transplantation, and protection from respiratory challenge with *Aspergillus* was achieved.[183] Early human phase I trials with autosomal recessive (p47*phox*) and X-linked CGD, using autologous peripheral blood stem cells retrovirally transduced ex vivo and then re-infused without prior marrow conditioning, have yielded a maximum of 0.2 percent oxidase-corrected neutrophils in the circulation.[379] This accomplishment is still far short of what probably must be achieved to produce a clinically meaningful correction.[183]

Deficiencies of Glucose-6-Phosphate Dehydrogenase and Glutathione Peroxidase

The normal activity of the NADPH oxidase enzyme complex depends on the continued availability of NADPH to reduce molecular oxygen to form superoxide anion.[40,135,491] The primary source of NADPH for this enzyme is the hexose monophosphate shunt. It is provided with the hexose substrate, 6-phosphoglucose, by the enzyme glucose-6-phosphate dehydrogenase, which also generates NADPH in a coupled reaction.[492] The reactions of the hexose monophosphate shunt itself are coupled to two other enzymes, glutathione reductase and glutathione peroxidase, which recycle oxidized and reduced glutathione.[492]

The absence of any of these three enzymes results in a lack of available NADPH to drive the NADPH oxidase. Deficiencies in any of these other three enzymes may result in a phagocyte killing defect similar to that of CGD. Patients with deficiencies of glucose-6-phosphate dehydrogenase or glutathione peroxidase have been described with functional oxidative metabolic defects and presentations that are clinically indistinguishable from CGD caused by defects in the NADPH oxidase itself.[43,505] Glucose-6-phosphate dehydrogenase deficiency usually involves erythrocytes and is associated with hemolytic anemia, especially in conjunction with the administration of sulfonamides.[150] Only when the defect also involves myeloid cells and is severe or complete (<5 percent of normal enzyme levels) is the CGD-like disorder manifested.[43,505] A partial deficiency of glutathione reductase has been reported, with hemolytic anemia and early cataracts, but no increased incidence of infection was noted.[490]

Glutathione Synthetase Deficiency

Glutathione, along with glutathione peroxidase and glutathione reductase, the two enzymes involved in its recycling between oxidized and reduced forms, constitutes a protective mechanism in PMNs against membrane damage mediated by reactive oxygen intermediates formed during PMN activation.[490] The synthesis of an adequate supply of glutathione is crucial to these cells. Two brothers with glutathione synthetase deficiency who presented with neutropenia, hemolytic anemia, acidosis, 5-oxoprolinuria, and recurrent infection were reported by Spielberg and colleagues.[92,549] The PMNs from these patients exhibited elevated cytosolic H_2O_2 levels, diminished oxidative microbicidal activity, and impaired microtubule assembly. Antioxidant therapy with vitamin E normalized the in vitro abnormalities of the patients' PMNs, and these patients had no further difficulty with recurrent infections.[92] This result suggested that vitamin E protected the cell membranes by scavenging excess H_2O_2 produced during PMN activation and prevented or minimized oxidant-induced membrane damage.

Myeloperoxidase Deficiency

Congenital deficiency of neutrophil MPO, previously thought to be a rare disorder, has come to be recognized as the most common heritable disorder of neutrophil function. Its clinical significance remains in doubt, however. Population surveys made possible with the advent of automated flow cytochemical techniques have indicated an incidence of MPO deficiency of approximately 1 in 2000 individuals.[424,460] Approximately half of these patients have complete absence of this neutrophil enzyme, and the remainder have a partial deficiency. The precise mode of inheritance of this defect has not been established, but MPO is known to be a product of a single gene on chromosome 17.[591] The reaction of MPO with H_2O_2 and chloride, causing the formation of hypochlorite, is one of the most effective microbicidal mechanisms of neutrophils, and cells from some patients with MPO deficiency have been found to exhibit delayed killing of *C. albicans* and *S. aureus*. MPO deficiency rarely has been associated with unusual infectious complications, however.

IMPORTANT EXAMPLES OF SECONDARY IMMUNODEFICIENCY (NOT INCLUDING HUMAN IMMUNODEFICIENCY VIRUS INFECTION)

Asplenia

Fulminant infections can occur in patients who have anatomic or functional asplenia.[512] The mortality rate from these infections in asplenic patients ranges from 40 to 80 percent.[621] The most common pathogens are encapsulated bacteria, including *S. pneumoniae* (50 to 70%), *H. influenzae*, and *N. meningitidis*.[621] Other streptococci, *S. aureus*, *Salmonella*, and other gram-negative bacilli are important but less common pathogens. All can cause fulminant, often fatal, disease characterized by rapid onset of shock. Malaria and babesiosis also are more severe in asplenic individuals. Infections can occur at any time but are most common within the first 2 years after patients undergo splenectomy.

The liver and the spleen are important in phagocytic clearance of bacteria from the circulation, and the spleen is an important site for antibody production. The spleen is more important than the liver in processing antigen in the naive host. The younger the individual is when splenic function is lost, the higher is the risk for developing serious infection. Young children who become asplenic are much more susceptible to fulminant infection than are adults because adults are more likely than are children to have encountered antigens before undergoing splenectomy. Individuals whose indication for splenectomy is thalassemia or Hodgkin disease are at higher risk of dying of overwhelming infection than are individuals who have functional asplenia from sickle-cell disease. Patients who undergo removal of their spleens for spherocytosis or idiopathic thrombocytopenia have a lower risk of developing infection. The lowest risk group consists of adults whose spleens are removed surgically after trauma, who are at little or no increased risk of developing infection.[147]

Congenital asplenia usually is associated with complex congenital cardiac disease and occasionally with structural abnormalities of the gastrointestinal or genitourinary tracts. Asplenia should be suspected in any patient with congenital heart disease and sepsis caused by encapsulated organisms. Anatomic or functional asplenia also should be suspected in patients with erythrocytes that contain Howell-Jolly bodies because these bodies are normally removed from the circulation by the normally functioning spleen. A radionuclide liver spleen scan or other modes of abdominal imaging usually can confirm asplenia or significant hyposplenia.[512]

Elective splenectomy for conditions such as hereditary spherocytosis should be delayed as long as possible, and splenic repair or subtotal splenectomy should be performed whenever possible after trauma. Asplenic patients are managed using prophylactic antibiotics, usually penicillin V or amoxicillin until at least 5 years of age.[147] They also should be immunized against encapsulated organisms at the appropriate ages (e.g., *H. influenzae* type b and pneumococcal conjugate vaccines beginning at 2 months and meningococcal polysaccharide vaccines at 2 years).[147] Patients should be warned about their increased risk of acquiring serious infections caused by malaria and babesiosis.

Sickle-Cell Disease

Immunodeficiency in patients with sickle-cell disease is due largely to their functional asplenia.[512] Part of the risk of developing infection stems from local infarction and tissue necrosis caused by sickling, which causes sludging and resultant tissue hypoxia. The reticuloendothelial system also may be obstructed by having to deal with chronic hemolysis. Patients with sickle-cell disease are protected partially from *Plasmodium falciparum* malaria but have a high incidence of fulminant sepsis and meningitis caused by encapsulated organisms (e.g., *S. pneumoniae*, *H. influenzae* type b, *N. meningitidis*) and *Salmonella*.[224] The relative risk of pneumococcal meningitis developing in children with sickle-cell disease is approximately 500 times that of normal children. *Salmonella* infections often are associated with osteomyelitis or meningitis.[202]

Patients with sickle-cell disease seem to have normal antibody response to most antigens, including age-appropriate responses to vaccines. A deficiency in heat-labile opsonic activity has been reported and may be due to a defect in the alternative pathway of complement. Rare cases of patients with sickle-cell disease who have deficiencies of factor B have been reported, but patients with sickle-cell disease have normal CH_{50} and normal levels of properdin, C3, and factor I.[308] Patients with sickle-cell disease should be managed with prophylactic antibiotics until they are at least 5 years old and should be immunized against *H. influenzae* type b, pneumococci, and meningococci at the appropriate ages.[147]

Cystic Fibrosis

Cystic fibrosis (CF) is an autosomal recessive disorder caused by mutations in both alleles of the gene encoding the protein called *cystic fibrosis transmembrane conductance regulator* (CFTR), a cAMP-regulated chloride channel expressed at the luminal surface of airway epithelial cells.[613] Most patients with CF develop chronic endobronchial infection with *P. aeruginosa* of the mucoid phenotype. This infection is accompanied by an intense chronic airway inflammation with an exuberant influx of neutrophils that leads to bronchiectasis and destruction and fibrosis of lung and airway tissue and early death.[130,334] No systemic disorder of immunity has been documented in CF, but local factors in the airway inflammatory milieu, including neutrophil-derived proteases such as elastase, contribute to secondary impairments in opsonic and phagocytic host defenses by cleaving opsonic antibody and complement fragments and important phagocytic receptors for these opsonins.[581]

Mucociliary clearance of bacteria from the CF airway is impaired because of viscous, dehydrated epithelial lining fluid, although the early pathogenesis of the unique chronic endobronchial infection in CF and its relationship to the underlying genetic defect have remained obscure. Several possible explanations have been offered. Researchers have suggested that CFTR on airway epithelial cells may function as a receptor for *Pseudomonas* that the cells normally use to internalize the organisms before being sloughed and cleared by mucociliary action and that this internalization may be deficient in CF epithelial cells.[466] Other evidence suggests that microbicidal peptides of or related to the defensin family, released from airway epithelial cells as a local defense mechanism, may be inactivated by abnormal salt concentrations at the airway epithelial surface, thwarting an important first line of local antibacterial defense.[539]

None of the aforementioned explanations has proved satisfactory. A reduction in cell surface sialic acid on CF epithelial cells unmasks the glycoprotein asialo-GM-1, which seems to function as an epithelial receptor for adhesion by *P. aeruginosa* and may promote early airway colonization.[508] More recently, investigators have proposed that reduced expression of inducible nitric oxide synthase by CF airway epithelial cells may impair airway host defenses against early small inocula of bacteria, but the unresolved question of the relationship between the CF genetic defect and *Pseudomonas* chronic lung infection continues to stimulate active research.[130]

EVALUATION FOR IMMUNODEFICIENCY IN A CHILD WITH RECURRENT OR SEVERE INFECTIONS

Most immunodeficiency disorders can be diagnosed readily by employing a methodical process that begins with careful analysis of the child's presenting history and physical examination.[149,156,178,285,439,512,515] This information serves as the foundation for a rational laboratory evaluation. It is important to bear in mind that it is normal for children to have several infections every year. Normal children who are exposed to other children, particularly older school-aged siblings or classmates, develop approximately one infection per month. Most infections in immunocompetent children are characterized by being mild and localized to the gastrointestinal or upper respiratory tracts, and they either are self-limited or respond rapidly to conventional therapy. Immunocompromised hosts tend to have more frequent, severe, and unusual infections that may not respond readily to appropriate therapy.

HISTORY

A detailed history alone is sufficient to determine whether or not an immunologic evaluation should be pursued in many children who have recurrent or severe infections. If tests for immunity are indicated, the history also serves as a guide to the types of studies that should be performed initially. Table 2–5 provides a list of historical information that is valuable in assessing the likelihood the patient has an immunodeficiency. Whenever possible, the child's complete medical records (including growth charts) should be obtained, particularly if several physicians have provided care, because the history often is complicated, and incomplete or inaccurate information may be misleading.

The age of onset of suspicious infections usually helps define the underlying problem. Children with isolated immunoglobulin deficiencies tend to do well during the first few months of life because they are protected by maternal antibody. They usually start developing serious infections later in the first year of life. Children with cell-mediated or phagocytic disorders may begin developing infections in the newborn period (see earlier). In contrast, healthy children who have been cared for at home by

TABLE 2–5   History in the Evaluation of a Child with Recurrent or Severe Infections

Age at onset of infections
Number, frequency, and periodicity of infections
Nature of infections
  Location on body
  Organism(s)
  Severity
  Duration
Nature and duration of therapy
Response to therapy
Hospitalizations
Surgery
Growth pattern
Periodontal disease
Allergies
Immunizations
Exposure history
  Contagious diseases in family, school, or community
  Number and ages of siblings
  Parents' occupations
  Babysitting or daycare arrangements
  Foreign travel
  Parental smoking
  Wood furnaces
Family history (especially in males)
  Immunodeficiency
  Recurrent, severe, or unusual infections
  Cause of early deaths
  Autoimmune disease
  Allergy
  Consanguinity
Days of school missed (and why)

their mothers and who have no siblings often have few infections in the first few years of life but may present for immunologic evaluation when they develop recurrent respiratory infections beginning the first few weeks after entering daycare, preschool, or kindergarten, owing to new exposure to various respiratory viral pathogens.

The number, nature, and severity of infections help in determining how aggressively to pursue an immunologic evaluation. Certain clinical presentations of disease and causative organisms are associated with a high likelihood of an immunodeficiency. Antibody or complement deficiencies, or functional asplenia, should be suspected in children with recurrent or life-threatening infections, such as sepsis and meningitis caused by encapsulated organisms (e.g., *S. pneumoniae*, *H. influenzae* type b).[102,178,308,357,439,493] Complement deficiencies should be considered in individuals with recurrent or severe neisserial disease.[175] CGD should be suspected in the presence of recurrent or unusual deep tissue infections, such as liver abscess, lymphadenopathy, pneumonia, or osteomyelitis, especially when caused by unusual gram-negative bacteria, such as *Serratia marcescens*, or by *Aspergillus* spp.[622] Pneumonia caused by *Pneumocystis* suggests a T-cell deficiency, either hereditary or due to HIV infection.

Recurrent or even severe infections with group A streptococci have not been associated with immunodeficiency. Recurrent urinary tract infections usually are associated with anatomic abnormalities of the urinary tract and not immunodeficiency.

An essential part of the history is documentation of the child's growth pattern. Children who are thriving, particularly those older than 2 years of age, are much less likely to have serious immune disorders than children with failure to thrive.

The immunization history should be documented carefully because it may prove to be useful in evaluating the child's ability to mount an antibody response to specific vaccine antigens. The history of recent live viral immunization should be obtained in children who have clinical presentations compatible with polio or measles because infection caused by vaccine strains of these viruses is the first indication of immunodeficiency in some children.

Exposures to contagious diseases may lead to recurrent and occasionally even severe infections in individuals with normal host defenses. Children who never leave the house may have recurrent infections from organisms brought home by older siblings, other relatives, or neighbors. One must assume that children who attend daycare facilities or schools constantly are being exposed to common infections. Familiarity with community patterns of disease, such as prevalent clinical manifestations of enterovirus infection or the beginning of croup, respiratory syncytial virus, influenza, or rotavirus seasons, can be used to reassure families of normal children with frequent mild infections. Environmental pollutants, such as cigarette smoke and wood-burning stoves, also have been associated with an increased risk of acute lower respiratory illnesses developing in children.[485]

Because many immunodeficiencies are hereditary, a detailed family history should be obtained that includes questions about the presence of immunodeficiency, recurrent or severe infections, contributing factors to any early deaths, the gender of affected individuals, and consanguinity. A history of recurrent or severe infections in more than one male relative is highly suspicious of a familial immunodeficiency disorder. Autoimmune diseases may suggest a familial disorder of complement or cell-mediated immunity.[175]

A thorough history of school absenteeism and the reasons the child stays home may be helpful in differentiating medical from psychosocial problems in older children who present for evaluation for recurrent infections, particularly when symptoms are unusual or inconsistent with physical findings. Prolonged absences for vague problems with no physical findings, particularly in the presence of normal growth, are less likely to be caused by infections than are those characterized by well-defined physical or laboratory findings and poor growth. Generally, recurrent severe infections beginning before the child reaches age 1 year, failure to thrive, invasive disease caused by encapsulated or unusual organisms, or family histories of such infections should prompt consideration of an immunologic evaluation.

PHYSICAL EXAMINATION

Physical examination may provide valuable clues as to the nature of the immune disorder. In certain cases, such as some patients with hyper-IgE syndrome[105,281] and DiGeorge syndrome[182] who exhibit the characteristic facies, it may be diagnostic. As noted earlier, one of the most obvious signs that a child may have a serious underlying medical problem is failure to thrive. Every immunologic evaluation *must* include documentation of current growth parameters and a comparison with past growth.

Many immunodeficiency disorders have dermatologic manifestations. Eczematoid rashes are seen in patients with the hyper-IgE syndrome and CGD.[105,281] CGD also is characterized by slow wound healing and the development of hypertrophic scars.[622] Patients with Chédiak-Higashi syndrome have partial albinism.[81] Severe gingival disease and early loss of teeth are prominent clinical features in disorders of neutrophil migration, such as LAD.[30,31]

The chest should be evaluated for physical signs of active disease, such as rales and rhonchi, and evidence of chronic infection, such as an increased anterior-posterior diameter. Pneumonia, bronchitis, bronchiectasis, and scarring can occur with most immunodeficiencies but are associated most frequently with immunoglobulin deficiencies.[102,271,439] Cardiac abnormalities may be associated with primary asplenia or immunodeficiency disor-

ders such as DiGeorge syndrome,[182] and situs inversus should alert the clinician to the possibility of ciliary dyskinesia.[149] Although hepatosplenomegaly may be found in many types of primary immunodeficiency disease, it occurs more frequently in patients with disorders of phagocyte function, especially CGD.[622]

LABORATORY STUDIES

The laboratory evaluation should be guided by the history and physical findings. Simple, inexpensive screening tests often can help narrow the differential diagnosis and streamline the evaluation. One of the first tests that should be performed is a complete blood count with differential and evaluation of the blood smear. This simple test can detect several immunologic abnormalities, including neutropenia, lymphopenia associated with HIV-1 or forms of SCID, the abnormal neutrophil granules associated with the Chédiak-Higashi syndrome, Howell-Jolly bodies found with asplenia, and some malignancies. Chest radiographs should be examined for thymic tissue, mediastinal lymphadenopathy, pneumonia, bronchiectasis, and other evidence of pulmonary infections. Consideration also should be given to evaluating patients with chronic pulmonary disease for CF with a sweat chloride test.

Quantitative immunoglobulin levels provide a useful screening test for evaluating patients with suspected humoral immunodeficiency. IgG2 deficiency often is not reflected in the IgG level, however, because it makes up such a relatively small proportion of total IgG. Patients with suspected humoral immunodeficiency usually should be tested for IgG subclasses and quantitative IgG, IgA, and IgM. Enumeration of B cells and marker studies by immunofluorescence flow cytometry should be considered if more severe forms of humoral deficiency, such as XLA or some forms of CVID, are suspected. Very high IgE levels may be helpful in establishing the diagnosis of hyper-IgE syndrome, although an elevated IgE level is much more common in patients with allergies than immunologic abnormalities. Immunoglobulin levels may be extremely elevated in children with HIV-1 infection.

Children who have normal quantitative immunoglobulin and IgG subclass levels but who continue to have frequent sinopulmonary infections that do not respond well to appropriate medical and surgical management (e.g., ventilation tubes) also can be evaluated by measuring antibody responses to specific antigens, such as tetanus and diphtheria toxoids and *H. influenzae* type b and meningococcal and pneumococcal capsular polysaccharides. Antibody levels can be measured before immunization and approximately 1 to 2 months after immunization is administered to evaluate the child's ability to respond to different kinds of antigens, including T cell–dependent antigens such as diphtheria and tetanus toxoid or T cell–independent antigens such as unconjugated pneumococcal capsular polysaccharide vaccine.

The complement system should be evaluated in individuals with recurrent or life-threatening neisserial disease, including systemic gonococcal infections and sporadic meningococcal disease. The best screening test for hemolytic complement is the CH_{50}. A normal CH_{50} reflects a normal quantity and function of classical pathway proteins (C1, C4, C2), C3, and terminal components through C8, as noted earlier.[143] The alternative pathway proteins can be measured in a similar assay employing rabbit erythrocytes instead of antibody-coated sheep cells. Alternative pathway deficiencies are extremely rare; demonstration of a normal CH_{50} generally is a sufficient indicator of normal complement activity. An abnormal CH_{50} should be repeated immediately, taking care that the specimen is handled correctly. Complement abnormalities may be quantitative or qualitative. If a very low CH_{50} is confirmed, determining the serum levels of individual complement proteins and their functional activity in consultation with a reference laboratory is important.

Delayed hypersensitivity skin testing with antigens such as *Candida* or mumps antigens may be useful to assess cell-mediated immunity, but results are not always reliable. T-lymphocyte subset quantitation may be helpful in diagnosing such conditions as SCID and HIV, but more sophisticated testing of lymphocyte function, such as mitogen and antigen stimulation, should be done in patients with recurrent or severe fungal infection. These studies ideally should be directed by a clinical immunologist.

Similarly, suspected phagocyte function disorders should be evaluated in consultation with experts in phagocyte function because lack of proper standardization and expertise often leads to misleading results from commercial laboratories. Phagocyte function studies should be directed toward adherence and migration in patients with recurrent skin and mucosal infections, poor or absent formation of pus, and persistent leukocytosis suggestive of a leukocyte adhesion defect. Tests of oxidative metabolic activity and killing should be performed in patients with recurrent staphylococcal or unusual gram-negative or fungal tissue infections suggestive of CGD.

Whenever clinical suspicion of an inherited immunodeficiency is confirmed by appropriate functional laboratory studies, arranging for specific genetic testing to determine the precise nature of a patient's genetic mutation or variation, when such testing is available, may be desirable. This testing may assist greatly in subsequent genetic counseling and would add important information to the clinical database on patients with the specific disorder.

MANAGEMENT OF IMMUNODEFICIENCY DISORDERS

Proper management of immunodeficiency disorders (as described earlier) can enhance markedly the quality of life and life expectancy. Although some children with immunodeficiency disorders have serious problems with autoimmune disease, malignancy, or both, most morbidity and mortalities result from infections. This discussion is limited to the general principles of managing infectious complications of immunodeficiency.

EDUCATION

After the immunologic abnormality has been thoroughly characterized, the first step in management is to educate the family and, when he or she is old enough, the patient regarding environmental risks, how to take medications, and precisely when and where to seek medical care. Families of patients with inherited disorders should receive genetic counseling and be offered the option of prenatal screening if it is available for the disease in question.

EVALUATION FOR INFECTION

Patients with known immunodeficiency disorders should be evaluated promptly and thoroughly for unexplained fevers or any other indication of infection. Immunodeficient individuals are susceptible to a wide variety of pathogens, their responses to appropriate therapy may be slow, and they often require prolonged treatment. Every effort should be made to identify the infecting organism so that treatment can be specific. Unless the pathogen is known, extended courses of empiric broad-spectrum coverage may be required, which may lead to superinfection caused by multidrug-resistant pathogens.

TREATMENT OF INFECTIONS

Many aspects of disease-specific therapy already have been discussed. Generally, patients with immunodeficiency who are susceptible to bacterial infections should be treated empirically and aggressively with antibiotics at the first indication of infection. Antifungal therapy should be added empirically in patients with increased risk of developing fungal infection (e.g., patients with cell-mediated immune and neutrophil disorders) if a prompt response to antibacterial therapy does not occur. When a definitive etiology has been established, treatment should be tailored to the pathogen. The duration of therapy must be individualized, but generally patients with abnormal immune systems should be treated longer than normal hosts who have similar infections.

PREVENTION OF INFECTION

Patients and household members should be immunized with appropriate vaccines as soon as possible after a diagnosis of immunodeficiency has been established.[147] Although many immunodeficient patients, such as those with XLA, cannot respond to immunizations, immunization of household members and other close contacts with vaccines may reduce the patients' likelihood of developing infection. Patients with complement deficiencies, asplenia, and sickle-cell disease should be immunized with vaccines directed against encapsulated organisms, such as meningococci, pneumococci, and *H. influenzae* type b. These patients may not have normal responses to immunization, however, and, if possible, their antibody responses to these vaccines should be measured; if they are low, these patients should receive extra doses of the vaccines. Live viral vaccines should not be administered to patients with primary defects in cell-mediated immunity.

Patients with disorders characterized by recurrent or severe bacterial or fungal infections may require prophylactic antibacterial or antifungal therapy. The benefits of long-term antimicrobial therapy must be weighed carefully against the risks of rapid emergence of multidrug-resistant organisms.

PROSPECTS FOR CORRECTION OF SERIOUS PRIMARY IMMUNODEFICIENCIES

Bone marrow or stem cell transplants have been successful in a few patients with specific immunologic disorders, including SCID,[104,124] Wiskott-Aldrich syndrome,[453] LAD, and CGD.[31,221,615] Gene therapy has raised new possibilities for correcting certain immunologic defects, having shown early promise for some forms of SCID and early success in animal models of CGD.[183,472] The development of malignancies associated with retroviral gene therapy in some cases raises serious concerns about the ultimate feasibility of this approach,[107,472] but the means of overcoming these and other potential obstacles to gene therapy will continue to be sought.

REFERENCES

1. Abraham, E., Wunderink, R., Silverman, H., et al.: Efficacy and safety of monoclonal antibody to human tumor necrosis factor-α in patients with sepsis syndrome. J. A. M. A. *273*:934-941, 1995.
2. Abramson, J. S., Mills, E. L., Sayer, M. K., et al.: Recurrent infections and delayed separation of the umbilical cord in an infant with abnormal phagocytic cell locomotion and oxidative response during opsonized particle phagocytosis. J. Pediatr. *99*:887-894, 1981.
3. Abramson, J. S., Wheeler, J. G., and Quie, P. G.: The polymorphonuclear leukocyte system. *In* Stiehm, E. R. (ed.): Immunologic Disorders in Infants and Children. 4th ed. Philadelphia, W. B. Saunders, 1996, pp. 94-112.

4. Abughali, N., Berger, M., and Tosi, M. F.: Deficient total cell content of CR3 (CD11b) in neonatal neutrophils. Blood *83*:1086-1092, 1994.

5. Abughali, N., Dubyak, G., and Tosi, M. F.: Impairment of chemoattractant-stimulated hexose uptake in neonatal neutrophils. Blood *82*:2182-2187, 1993.

6. Adamkin, D., Stitzel, A., Urmson, J., et al.: Activity of the alternative pathway of complement in the newborn infant. J. Pediatr. *93*:604-608, 1978.

7. Adderson, E. E., Schackelford, P. G., Quinn, A., et al.: Restricted Ig H chain V gene usage in the human antibody response to *Haemophilus influenzae* type b capsular polysaccharide. J. Immunol. *147*:1667-1674, 1991.

8. Adenyi-Jones, S. C. A., Faden, H., Ferdon, M. B., et al.: Systemic and local immune responses to enhanced-potency inactivated poliovirus vaccine in premature and term infants. J. Pediatr. *120*:686-689, 1992.

9. Aderem, A., and Ulevitch, R. J.: Toll-like receptors in the induction of the innate immune response. Nature *406*:782-787, 2000.

10. Aggarwal, J., Khan, A. J., Diamond, S., et al.: Lazy leukocyte syndrome in a black infant. J. Natl. Med. Assoc. 77:928-931, 1985.

11. Aggett, P. J., Harries, J. T., Harvey, B. A. M., et al.: An inherited defect of neutrophil mobility in Shwachman syndrome. J. Pediatr. *94*:391-394, 1979.

12. Albelda, S. M., Muller, W. A., Buck, C. A., et al.: Molecular and cellular properties of PECAM-1 (endoCAM/CD31): A novel vascular cell-cell adhesion molecule. J. Cell. Biol. *114*:1059-1068, 1991.

13. Alford, C. A., Stagno, S., and Reynold, D. W.: Diagnosis of chronic perinatal infections. Am. J. Dis. Child. *129*:455-463, 1975.

14. Allen, R. C., Armitage, R. J., Conley, M. E., et al.: CD40 ligand gene defects responsible for X-linked hyper-IgM syndrome. Science *259*:990-993, 1993.

15. Allen, R. C., and Loose, L. D.: Phagocytic activation of a luminol-dependent chemiluminescence in rabbit alveolar and peritoneal macrophages. Biochem. Biophys. Res. *69*:245-252, 1976.

16. Alouf, J. E., and Muller-Alouf, H.: Staphylococcal and streptococcal superantigens: Molecular, biological and clinical aspects. Int. J. Med. Microbiol. *292*:429-440, 2003.

17. Alper, C. A., Xu, J., Cosmopoulos, K., et al.: Immunoglobulin deficiencies and susceptibility to infection among homozygotes and heterozygotes for C2 deficiency. J. Clin. Immunol. *23*:297-305, 2003.

18. Ambrosino, D. M., Siber, G. R., Chilmonczyk, B. A., et al.: An immunodeficiency characterized by impaired antibody responses to polysaccharides. N. Engl. J. Med. *316*:790-793, 1987.

19. Ambrosino, D. M., Sood, S. K., Lee, M. C., et al.: IgG1, IgG2, and IgM responses to two *Haemophilus influenzae* type b conjugate vaccines in young infants. Pediatr. Infect. Dis. J. *11*:855-859, 1992.

20. Ambrosino, D. M., Umetsu, D. T., Siber, G. R., et al.: Selective defect in the antibody response to *Haemophilus influenzae* type b in children with recurrent infections and normal serum IgG subclass levels. J. Allergy Clin. Immunol. *81*:1175-1179, 1988.

21. Ambruso, D. R., Edward, R. B., McCabe, M. D., et al.: Infectious and bleeding complications in patients with glycogenosis 1b: Relationship to neutrophil and platelet function. Am. J. Dis. Child. *139*:691-697, 1985.

22. Ament, M. E., Ochs, H. D., and Davis, S. D.: Structure and function of the gastrointestinal tract in primary immunodeficiency syndromes: A study of 39 patients. Medicine *52*:227-248, 1973.

23. Ammann, A. J., and Hong, R.: Selective IgA deficiency and autoimmunity. Clin. Exp. Immunol. 7:833-838, 1970.

24. Ammann, A. J., and Hong, R.: Selective IgA deficiency: Presentation of 30 cases and a review of the literature. Medicine *60*:223-236, 1971.

25. Anderson, D. C., Freeman, K. B., Hughes, B. J., et al.: Secretory determinants of impaired adherence and mobility of neonatal PMNs. Pediatr. Res. *19*:257A, 1985.

26. Anderson, D. C., Hughes, B. J., and Smith, C. W.: Abnormal mobility of neonatal polymorphonuclear leukocytes: Relationship to impaired redistribution of surface adhesion sites by chemotactic factor or colchicine. J. Clin. Invest. *68*:863-874, 1981.

27. Anderson, D. C., Hughes, B. J., Wible, L. J., et al.: Impaired motility of neonatal PMN leukocytes: Relationship to abnormalities of cell orientation and assembly of microtubules in chemotactic gradients. J. Leukoc. Biol. *36*:1-15, 1984.

28. Anderson, D. C., Rothlein, R., Martin, S. D., et al.: Impaired transendothelial migration of neonatal neutrophils: Abnormalities of MAC-I (CD11/CD18) dependent adherence reactions. Blood 76:2613-2621, 1990.

29. Anderson, D. C., Schmalstieg, F. C., Arnaout, M. A., et al.: Abnormalities of polymorphonuclear leukocyte function associated with a heritable deficiency of high molecular weight surface glycoproteins (gp 138): Common relationship to diminished cell adherence. J. Clin. Invest. *74*:546-557, 1984.

30. Anderson, D. C., Schmalstieg, F., Finegold, M. J., et al.: The severe and moderate phenotypes of heritable MAC-1, LFA-1, P150,95 deficiency: Their quantitative definition and relation to leukocyte dysfunction and clinical features. J. Infect. Dis. *152*:668-689, 1985.

31. Anderson, D. C., and Smith, C. W.: Leukocyte adhesion deficiencies and other disorders of leukocyte motility. *In* Scriver, C. R., Beaudet, A. L., Sly, W. S., et al. (eds): The Metabolic Basis of Inherited Disease. 8th ed. New York, McGraw-Hill, 2001, pp. 4829-4856.

32. Anderson, D. C., Wibble, L. J., Hughes, B. J., et al.: Cytoplasmic microtubules in polymorphonuclear leukocytes: Effects of chemotactic stimulation and colchicine. Cell *31*:719-729, 1982.

33. Andreasen, S. O., Christensen, J. E., Marker, O., and Thomsen, A. R.: Role of CD40 ligand and CD28 in induction and maintenance of antiviral CD8+ effector T cell responses. J. Immunol. *164*:3689-3697, 2000.

34. Appleman, L. J., Berezovskaya, A., Grass, I., and Boussiotis, V. A.: CD28 costimulation mediates T cell expansion via IL-2-independent and IL-2-dependent regulation of cell cycle progression. J. Immunol. *164*:144-151, 2000.

35. Arai, K.-I., Lee, F., Miyajima, A., et al.: Cytokines: Coordinators of immune and inflammatory responses. Annu. Rev. Biochem. *59*:783-836, 1990.

36. Arnaout, M. A.: Structure and function of the leukocyte adhesion molecules CD11/CD18. Blood 75:1037-1050, 1990.

37. Arnaout, M. A., Pitt, J., Cohen, H. J., et al.: Deficiency of a granulocyte membrane glycoprotein (gp 150) in a boy with recurrent bacterial infections. N. Engl. J. Med. *306*:693-699, 1982.

38. Arrode, F., Boccaccio, C., Abastado, J. P., and Davrinche, C.: Cross-presentation of human cytomegalovirus pp565 (UL83) to CD8+ T cells is regulated by virus-induced soluble-mediator-dependent maturation of dendritic cells. J. Virol. 76:142-150, 2002.

39. Aruffo, A., Farrington, M., Hollenbaugh, D., et al.: The CD40 ligand, gp39, is defective in activated T cells from patients with X-linked hyper-IgM syndrome. Cell *72*:291-300, 1993.

40. Babior, B. M.: The nature of the NADPH oxidase. *In* Gallin, J. I., and Fauci, A. S. (eds.): Advances in Host Defense Mechanisms. New York, Raven Press, 1983, pp. 91-119.

41. Babior, B. M., Kipnes, R. S., and Curnutte, J. T.: Biological defense mechanisms: The production by leukocytes of superoxide, a potential bactericidal agent. J. Clin. Invest. *52*:741-744, 1973.

42. Babior, B. M., Rosin, R. E., McMurrich, B. J., et al.: Arrangement of the respiratory burst oxidase in the plasma membrane of the neutrophil. J. Clin. Invest. *67*:1724-1730, 1981.

43. Baehner, R. L., Johnston, R. B., and Nathan, D. G.: Comparative study of the metabolic and bactericidal characteristics of severely glucose-6-phosphate dehydrogenase–deficient polymorphonuclear leukocytes and leukocytes from children with chronic granulomatous disease. J. Reticul. Soc. *12*:150-160, 1972.

44. Baehner, R. L., Karnovsky, M. J., and Karnovsky, M. L.: Degranulation of leukocytes in chronic granulomatous disease. J. Clin. Invest. *48*:187-192, 1969.

45. Bagby, G. J., Plessala, K. J., Wilson, L. A., et al.: Divergent efficacy of antibody to tumor necrosis factor-α in intravascular and peritonitis models of sepsis. J. Infect. Dis. *163*:83-88, 1991.

46. Baggiolini, M.: Chemokines in pathology and medicine. J. Intern. Med. *250*:91-104, 2001.

47. Bainton, D. F.: Developmental biology of neutrophils and eosinophils. *In* Gallin, J. I., Goldstein, I. M., and Snyderman, R. (eds.): Inflammation: Basic Principles and Clinical Correlates. 2nd ed. New York, Raven Press, 1992, pp. 303-324.

48. Baker, C. J., and Edwards, M. S.: Group B streptococcal infections. *In* Remington, J. S., and Klein, J. O. (eds.): Infectious Diseases of the Fetus and Newborn Infant. 4th ed. Philadelphia, W. B. Saunders, 1995, pp. 980-1054.

49. Ballow, M., Cates, K. L., Rowe, J. C., et al.: Development of the immune system in very low birth weight (less than 1500 g) premature infants: Concentrations of plasma immunoglobulins and patterns of infections. Pediatr. Res. *20*:899-904, 1986.

50. Bals, R.: Epithelial antimicrobial peptides in host defense against infection. Respir. Res. *1*:141-150, 2000.

51. Banatvala, N., Davies, J., Kanariou, M., et al.: Hypogammaglobulinaemia associated with normal or increased IgM (the hyper IgM syndrome): A case series review. Arch. Dis. Child. 71:150-152, 1994.

52. Baraff, L. J., Leake, R. D., Burstyn, D. G., et al.: Immunologic response to early and routine DTP immunization in infants. Pediatrics 73:37-42, 1984.

53. Barber, D. F., Faure, M., and Long, E. O.: LFA-1 contributes an early signal for NK cell cytotoxicity. J. Immunol. *173*:3653-3659, 2004.

54. Barbosa, M. D., Nguyen, Q. A., Tchernev, V. T., et al.: Identification of the homologous beige and Chediak-Higashi syndrome genes. Nature *382*:262-265, 1996.

55. Barrett, D. J., and Boyle, M. D. P.: Restoration of complement function in vivo by plasma infusion in factor I (C3b inactivator) deficiency. J. Pediatr. *104*:76-81, 1984.

56. Bashan, N., Potashnik, R., Hagay, Y., et al.: Impaired glucose transport in polymorphonuclear leukocytes in glycogen storage disease 1b. Inherit. Metab. Dis. *10*:234-239, 1987.

57. Bass, D. A., Parce, J. W., Dechatelet, L. R., et al.: Flow cytometric studies of oxidative product formation by neutrophils: A graded response to membrane stimulation. J. Immunol. *130*:1910-1917, 1983.

58. Bastian, J., Law, S., Vogler, L., et al.: Prediction of persistent immunodeficiency in the DiGeorge anomaly. J. Pediatr. *115*:391-396, 1989.

59. Bauer, S., Kirschning, C. J., Hacker, H., et al.: Human TLR9 confers responsiveness to bacterial DNA via species-specific CpG motif recognition. Proc. Natl. Acad. Sci. U. S. A. *98*:9237-9242, 2001.

60. Beaudet, A. L., Anderson, D. C., Michels, V. V., et al.: Neutropenia and impaired neutrophil migration in type 1B glycogen storage disease. J. Pediatr. *97*:906-910, 1980.

61. Bennett, J. E.: *Aspergillus* species. *In* Mandell, G. L., Bennett, J. E., and Dolin, R. (eds.): Principles and Practice of Infectious Diseases. 4th ed. New York, Churchill Livingstone, 1995, pp. 2306-2311.

62. Berger, M., and Frank, M. M.: The serum complement system. *In* Stiehm, E. R. (ed.): Immunologic Disorders in Infants and Children. 4th ed. Philadelphia, W. B. Saunders, 1996, pp. 133-158.

63. Berger, M., O'Shea, J., Cross, A. S., et al.: Human neutrophils increase expression of C3bi as well as C3b receptors upon activation. J. Clin. Invest. 74:1566-1571, 1984.

64. Berger, M., Wetzler, E., August, J. T., et al.: Internalization of Type 1 complement receptors and de novo multivesicular body formation during chemoattractant-induced endocytosis in human neutrophils. J. Clin. Invest. 94:1113-1125, 1994.

65. Berger, M., Wetzler, E. M., Wallis, R. S.: Tumor necrosis factor is the major monocyte product that increases complement receptor expression on mature human neutrophils. Blood 71:151-158, 1988.

66. Berman, J. E., Mellis, S. J., Pollock, R., et al.: Content and organization of the human Ig V_H locus: Definition of three new V_H families and linkage to the Ig C_H locus. E. M. B. O. J. 7:727-738, 1988.

67. Berman, S., Lee, B., Nuss, R., et al.: Immunoglobulin G, total and subclass, in children with or without recurrent otitis media. J. Pediatr. 121:249-251, 1992.

68. Bernbaum, J. C., Daft, A., Anolik, R., et al.: Response of preterm infants to diphtheria-tetanus-pertussis immunizations. J. Pediatr. 107:184-188, 1985.

69. Beutler, B., and Cerami, A.: The biology of cachectin/TNF-α primary mediator of the host response. Annu. Rev. Immunol. 7:625-655, 1989.

70. Bevilacqua, M. P., and Nelson, R. M.: Selectins. J. Clin. Invest. 91:379-387, 1993.

71. Bhakdi, S., and Tranum-Jensen, J.: Complement lysis: A hole is a hole. Immunol. Today 12:318-320, 1991.

72. Biragyn, A., Ruffini, P. A., Leifer, C. A., et al.: Toll-like receptor 4-dependent activation of dendritic cells by beta-defensin 2. Science 298:1025-1029, 2002.

73. Bird, P., and Lachmann, P. J.: The regulation of IgG subclass production in man: Low serum IgG4 in inherited deficiencies of the classical pathway of C3 activation. J. Immunol. 18:1217-1222, 1988.

74. Bishof, N. A., Welch, T. R., and Beischel, L. S.: C4B deficiency: A risk factor for bacteremia with encapsulated organisms. J. Infect. Dis. 162:248-250, 1990.

75. Bisset, L. R., and Schmid-Grendelmeier, P.: Chemokines and their receptors in the pathogenesis of allergic asthma: progress and perspective. Curr. Opin. Pulm. Med. 11:35-42, 2005.

76. Bjorkman, P. J., Saper, M. A., Samraoui, B., et al.: The foreign antigen binding site and T cell recognition regions of class I histocompatibility antigens. Nature 329:512-518, 1987.

77. Bjorkman, P. J., Saper, M. A., Samraoui, B., et al.: Structure of the human class I histocompatibility antigen, HLA-A2. Nature 329:506-512, 1987.

78. Black, F. L.: Why did they die? Science 258:1739-1740, 1992.

79. Blaese, R. M.: Development of gene therapy for immunodeficiency: Adenosine deaminase deficiency. Pediatr. Res. 33:S49-S55, 1993.

80. Blattner, F. R., and Tucker, P. W.: The molecular biology of immunoglobulin D. Nature 307:417-422, 1984.

81. Blume, R. S., and Wolff, S. M.: The Chediak-Higashi syndrome: Studies in four patients and a review of the literature. Medicine 51:247-280, 1972.

82. Bohnsack, J. F., and Brown, E. J.: The role of the spleen in resistance to infection. Annu. Rev. Med. 37:49-59, 1986.

83. Bonilla, F. A., and Geha, R. S.: Update on primary immunodeficiency diseases. J. Allergy Clin. Immunol. 117:S435-S441, 2006.

84. Borregaard, N., Heiple, J. M., Simons, E. R., et al.: Subcellular localization of the b-cytochrome component of the human neutrophil microbicidal oxidase: Translocation during activation. J. Cell Biol. 97:52-61, 1983.

85. Borregaard, N., Kjeldsen, L., Lollike, K., et al.: Granules and vesicles of human neutrophils: The role of endomembranes as source of plasma membrane proteins. Eur. J. Haematol. 51:318-322, 1993.

86. Borregaard, N., Kjeldsen, L., Sengelov, H., et al.: Changes in subcellular localization and surface expression of L-selectin, alkaline phosphatase, and Mac-1 in human neutrophils during stimulation with inflammatory mediators. J. Leukoc. Biol. 56:80-87, 1994.

87. Borzy, M. S., Ridgway, D., Noya, F. J., et al.: Successful bone marrow transplantation with split lymphoid chimerism in DiGeorge syndrome. J. Clin. Immunol. 9:386-392, 1989.

88. Bottger, E. C., and Bitter-Suermann, D.: Complement and the regulation of humoral immune responses. Immunol. Today 8:261-264, 1987.

89. Bowens, T. S., Ochs, H. D., Altman, L. C., et al.: Severe recurrent bacterial infections associated with defective adherence and chemotaxis in two patients with neutrophils deficient in cell-associated glycoproteins. J. Pediatr. 101:932-940, 1982.

90. Boxer, L. A., Coates, T. D., Haak, R. A., et al.: Lactoferrin deficiency associated with altered granulocyte function. N. Engl. J. Med. 307:404-410, 1982.

91. Boxer, L. A., Hedley-Whyte, E. T., and Stossel, T. P.: Neutrophil actin dysfunction and abnormal neutrophil behavior. N. Engl. J. Med. 29:1093-1099, 1974.

92. Boxer, L. A., Oliver, J. M., Spielberg, S. P., et al.: Protection of granulocytes by vitamin E in glutathione synthetase deficiency. N. Engl. J. Med. 301:901-905, 1979.

93. Boxer, L. A., Wantanbe, A. M., Rister, M., et al.: Correction of leukocyte function in Chediak-Higashi syndrome by ascorbate. N. Engl. J. Med. 295:1041-1045, 1976.

94. Braun, J., and Stiehm, E. R.: The B-lymphocyte system. *In* Stiehm, E. R. (ed.): Immunologic Disorders in Infants and Children. 4th ed. Philadelphia, W. B. Saunders, 1996, pp. 35-74.

95. Bredius, R. G., Van de Winkel, J. G., Weening, R. S., and Out, T. A.: Effector functions of IgG subclass antibodies. Immunodeficiency 4:51-53, 1993.

96. Bromley, S. K., Burack, W. R., Johnson, K. G., et al.: The immunological synapse. Annu. Rev. Immunol. 19:375-396, 2001.

97. Brown, E. J.: Interaction of gram-positive microorganisms with complement. Curr. Top. Microbiol. Immunol. 121:159-197, 1985.

98. Brown, J. H., Jardetzky, T., Saper, M. A., et al.: A hypothetical model of the foreign antigen binding site of class II histocompatibility molecules. Nature 353:845-850, 1988.

99. Bruce, M. C., Baley, J. E., Medvik, K. A., et al.: Impaired surface membrane expression of C3bi but not C3b receptors on neonatal neutrophils. Pediatr. Res. 21:306-311, 1987.

100. Brueckmann, M., Hoffmann, U., Dvortsak, E., et al.: Drotrecogin alfa (activated) inhibits NF-kappa B activation and MIP-1-alpha release from isolated mononuclear cells of patients with severe sepsis. Inflamm. Res. 53:528-533, 2004.

101. Brunet, A., Gabau, E., Perich, R. M., et al.: Microdeletion and microduplication 22q11.2 screening in 295 patients with features of DiGeorge/velocardiofacial syndrome. Am. J. Med. Genet. 140:2426-2432, 2006.

102. Bruton, O. C.: Agammaglobulinemia. Pediatrics 9:722-728, 1952.

103. Buck, D., Moshous, D., de Chasseval, R., et al.: Severe combined immunodeficiency and microcephaly in siblings with hypomorphic mutations in DNA ligase IV. Eur J. Immunol. 36:224-235, 2006.

104. Buckley, R., Schiff, R. I., Schiff, S. E., et al.: Human severe combined immunodeficiency: Genetic, phenotypic, and functional diversity in one hundred eight infants. J. Pediatr. 130:378-387, 1997.

105. Buckley, R. H.: Disorders of the IgE system. *In* Stiehm, E. R. (ed.): Immunologic Disorders in Infants and Children. 4th ed. Philadelphia, W. B. Saunders, 1996, pp. 409-422.

106. Buckley, R. H.: Molecular defects in human severe combined immunodeficiency and approaches to immune reconstitution. Annnu. Rev. Immunol. 22:625-655, 2004.

107. Buckley, R. H.: The multiple causes of human SCID. J. Clin. Invest. 114:1409-1411, 2004.

108. Buckley, R. H., Schiff, S. E., and Hayward, A. R.: Reduced frequency of CD45RO+ T lymphocytes in blood of hyper IgE syndrome patients. J. Allergy Clin. Immunol. 87:313-321, 1991.

109. Buckley, R. H., Wray, B. B., and Belmaker, E. Z.: Extreme hyperimmunoglobulinemia E and undue susceptibility to infection. Pediatrics 49:59-70, 1972.

110. Bucy, R. P., Chan, C.-L., and Cooper, M. D.: Tissue localization and CD8 accessory molecule expression of T$\gamma\delta$ cells in humans. J. Immunol. 142:3045-3049, 1989.

111. Buescher, E. S., Gaither, T., Nath, J., et al.: Abnormal adherence-related function of neutrophils, monocytes, and EB virus-transformed B cells in a patient with C3bi receptor deficiency. Blood 65:1382-1390, 1985.

112. Buescher, E. S., and Gallin, J. I.: Leukocyte transfusions in chronic granulomatous disease. N. Engl. J. Med. 307:800-803, 1982.

113. Burnett, G. W., and Scherp, H. W.: Oral Microbiology and Infectious Disease. Baltimore, Williams & Wilkins, 1968.

114. Burrows, P. D., and Cooper, M. D.: B cell development and differentiation. Curr. Opin. Immunol. 9:239-244, 1997.

115. Butcher, E. C.: Leukocyte-endothelial cell recognition: Three (or more) steps to specificity and diversity. Cell 67:1033-1036, 1991.

116. Cabau, N., Levy, F. M., Zivy, D., et al.: Evolution of titre of serum IgG in newborn. Med. Microbiol. Immunol. 162:251-258, 1974.

117. Campbell, A. D., Long, M. W., and Wicha, M. S.: Haemonectin, a bone marrow adhesion protein specific for cells of granulocyte lineage. Nature 329:744, 1987.

118. Campos, M. A., Vargas, M. A., Regueiro, V., et al.: Capsule polysaccharide mediates bacterial resistance to antimicrobial peptides. Infect. Immun. 72:7107-7114, 2004.

119. Carroll, M. C.: The complement system in B cell regulation. Mol. Immunol. 41:141-146, 2004.

120. Castigli, E., Wilson, S. A., Garibyan, L., et al.: TACI is mutant in common variable immunodeficiency and IgA deficiency. Nat. Genet. 37:829-834, 2005.

121. Cates, K. L., Densen, P., Lockman, J. D., et al.: C4B deficiency is not associated with meningitis or bacteremia with encapsulated bacteria. J. Infect. Dis. 165:942-944, 1992.

122. Cates, K. L., Goetz, C., Rosenberg, N., et al.: Longitudinal development of specific and functional antibody in very low birth weight premature infants. Pediatr. Res. 23:14-22, 1988.

123. Cates, K. L., and Levine, R. P.: C3 binding to bacterial surfaces. *In* Cabello, F., and Pruzzo, C. (eds.): Bacteria, Complement, and the Phagocytic Cell. NATO ASI Series. New York, Springer-Verlag, 1988, pp. 109-128.

124. Cavazzana-Calvo, M., Lagresie, C., Hacein-Bey-Abina, S., and Fischer, A.: Gene therapy for severe combined immunodeficiency. Annu. Rev. Med. 56:585-602, 2005.

125. Certain, S., Barrat, F., Pastural, E., et al.: Protein truncation test of LYST reveals heterogeneous mutations in patients with Chediak Higashi syndrome. Blood 95:979-983, 2000.

126. Cerwenka, A., and Lanier, L. L.: Natural killer cells, viruses and cancer. Nat. Rev. Immunol. *1*:41-49, 2001.

127. Chan, K., and Puck, J.: Development of population-based newborn screening for severe combined immunodeficiency. J. Allergy Clin. Immunol. *115*:391-398, 2005.

128. Chandra, R. K.: Fetal malnutrition and postnatal immunocompetence. Am. J. Dis. Child. *29*:450-454, 1975.

129. Chin, T. W., Stiehm, E. R., Faloon, J., and Gallin, J. I.: Corticosteroids in treatment of obstructive lesions of chronic granulomatous disease. J. Pediatr. *111*:349-352, 1987.

130. Chmiel, J., and Davis, P.: State of the art: Why do the lungs of patients with cystic fibrosis become infected and why can't they clear the infection? Resp. Res. *4*:8-19, 2003.

131. Christensen, R. D.: Hematopoiesis in the fetus and neonate. Pediatr. Res. *26*:531-535, 1989.

132. Church, J. A., Frenkel, L. D., and Wright, D. G.: T lymphocyte dysfunction, hyperimmunoglobulinemia E, recurrent bacterial infections, and defective neutrophil chemotaxis in a negro child. J. Pediatr. *88*:982-984, 1976.

133. Chusid, M. J.: Pyogenic hepatic abscess in infancy and childhood. Pediatrics *62*:554-559, 1978.

134. Clark, M. R.: IgG effector mechanisms. Chem. Immunol. *65*:88-110, 1997.

135. Clark, R. A., Leidal, K. G., Pearson, D. W., and Nauseef, W. M.: NADPH oxidase of human neutrophils: Subcellular localization and characterization of an arachidonate-activatable superoxide-generating system. J. Biol. Chem. *262*:4065-4074, 1987.

136. Clark, R. A., Malech, H. L., Gallin, J. I., et al.: Genetic variants of chronic granulomatous disease: Prevalence of deficiencies of two cytosolic components of the NADPH oxidase system. N. Engl. J. Med. *321*:647-652, 1989.

137. Clark, R. A., Root, R. K., Kimball, H. R., et al.: Defective neutrophil chemotaxis and cellular immunity in a child with recurrent infection. Ann. Intern. Med. *78*:515-519, 1973.

138. Coates, T. D., Torkildson, J. C., Torres, M., et al.: An inherited defect of neutrophil motility and microfilamentous cytoskeleton associated with abnormalities in 47-Kd and 89-Kd proteins. Blood *78*:1338-1346, 1991.

139. No reference cited.

140. Cohen, J.: The immunopathogenesis of sepsis. Nature *420*:885-891, 2002.

141. Cohn, M.: The a priori principles which govern immune responsiveness. *In* Cellular Basis of Immune Modulation. New York, Liss, 1989, pp. 11-44.

142. Cohen, M. S., Isturiz, R. E., and Malech, H. L.: Fungal infection in chronic granulomatous disease: The importance of the phagocyte in defense against fungi. Am. J. Med. *71*:59-66, 1981.

143. Colten, H. R.: Complement biogynthesis. Clin. Immunol. Allergy *5*:287-300, 1985.

144. Colten, H. R., and Goldberger, G.: Ontogeny of serum complement proteins. Pediatrics *64*(Suppl.):775-780, 1979.

145. Comerford, I., and Nibbs, R. J.: Post-translational control of chemokines: A role for decoy receptors? Immunol. Lett. *96*:163-174, 2005.

146. Committee on Infectious Diseases: Update on timing of hepatitis B vaccination for premature infants and for children with lapsed immunization. Pediatrics *94*:403-404, 1994.

147. Committee on Infectious Diseases: 2006 Red Book: Report of the Committee on Infectious Diseases. 27th ed. Elk Grove Village, IL, American Academy of Pediatrics, 2006.

148. Conley, M. E., and Puck, J. M.: Carrier detection in typical and atypical X-linked agammaglobulinemia. J. Pediatr. *112*:688-694, 1988.

149. Conley, M. E., and Stiehm, E. R.: Immunodeficiency disorders: General considerations. *In* Stiehm, E. R. (ed.): Immunologic Disorders in Infants and Children. 4th ed. Philadelphia, W. B. Saunders, 1996, pp. 201-252.

150. Cooper, M. R., DeChatelet, L. R., and McCall, C. E.: Complete deficiency of leukocyte glucose-6-phosphate dehydrogenase with defective bactericidal activity. J. Clin. Invest. *51*:769-778, 1972.

151. Cooper, N. R.: The classical complement pathway: Activation and regulation of the first complement component. Adv. Immunol. *37*:151-216, 1985.

152. Cooper, N. R., and Nemerow, G. R.: Complement-dependent mechanisms of virus neutralization. *In* Ross, G. D. (ed.): Immunobiology of the Complement System. Orlando, Academic Press, 1986, pp. 139-162.

153. Croft, M., Duncan, D. D., and Swain, S. L.: Response of naive antigen-specific CD4+ T cells in vitro: Characteristics and antigen-presenting cell requirements. J. Exp. Med. *176*:1431-1437, 1992.

154. Crowley, C. A., Curnutte, J. T., Roskin, R. E., et al.: An inherited abnormality of neutrophil adhesion: Its genetic transmission and its association with a missing protein. N. Engl. J. Med. *302*:1163-1168, 1980.

155. Cunningham-Rundles, C.: Clinical and immunologic analyses of 103 patients with common variable immunodeficiency. J. Clin. Immunol. *9*:22-33, 1989.

156. Cunningham-Rundles, C.: Disorders of the IgA system. *In* Stiehm, E. R. (ed.): Immunologic Disorders in Infants and Children. 4th ed. Philadelphia, W. B. Saunders, 1996, pp. 423-442.

157. Cunningham-Rundles, C.: Common variable immunodeficiency. Curr. Allergy Asthma Rep. *1*:421-429, 2001.

158. Cunningham-Rundles, C., Zhou, Z., Mankarious, S., et al.: Long-term use of IgA depleted intravenous immunoglobulin in immunodeficient subjects with anti-IgA antibodies. J. Clin. Immunol. *13*:272-278, 1993.

159. Cunningham-Rundles, S., Cunningham-Rundles, C., Ma, D. I., et al.: Impaired proliferative response to B lymphocyte activators in common variable immunodeficiency. J. Clin. Immunol. *1*:65-72, 1981.

160. Curnutte, J. T.: Classification of chronic granulomatous disease. Hematol. Oncol. Clin. N. Am. *2*:241-252, 1988.

161. Daar, A. S., Fuggle, S. V., Fabre, J. W., et al.: The detailed distribution of MHC class II antigens in normal human organs. Transplantation *38*:293-298, 1984.

162. Daar, A. S., Fuggle, S. V., Fabre, J. W., et al.: The detailed distribution of HLA-A, B, C antigens in normal human organs. Transplantation *38*:287-292, 1984.

163. Dalgleish, A., Beverly, P., Clapham, P., et al.: The CD4 (T4) antigen is an essential component of the receptor for the AIDS retrovirus. Nature *312*:763-767, 1984.

164. Dancis, J., Osburn, J. J., and Kunz, H. W.: Studies of immunology of the newborn infant, IV: Antibody formation in the premature infant. Pediatrics *12*:151-156, 1953.

165. Davies, D. R., and Cohen, G. H.: Interactions of protein antigens with antibodies. Proc. Natl. Acad. Sci. U. S. A. *93*:7-12, 1996.

166. Davies, D. R., and Metzger, H.: Structural basis of antibody function. Annu. Rev. Immunol. *1*:87-117, 1983.

167. Davis, A. E., III: C1 inhibitor and hereditary angioneurotic edema. Annu. Rev. Immunol. *6*:595-628, 1988.

168. Davis, M. D., and Bjorkman, P. J.: T-cell antigen receptor genes and T-cell recognition. Nature *334*:395-402, 1988.

169. Davis, S. D., Schaller, J., and Wedgewood, R. J.: Job's syndrome: Recurrent "cold" staphylococcal abscesses. Lancet *1*:1013-1015, 1966.

170. DeBiagi, M., Andreani, M., and Centis, F.: Immune characterization of human fetal tissues with monoclonal antibodies. Prog. Clin. Biol. Res. *193*:89-94, 1985.

171. Decoster, A., Darcy, F., Caron, A., et al.: Anti-P30 IgA antibodies as prenatal markers of congenital toxoplasma infection. Clin. Exp. Immunol. *87*:310-315, 1992.

172. Defrance, T., Vanbervliet, F., Briere, F., et al.: Interleukin 10 and transforming growth factor β cooperate to induce anti-CD40-activated naive human B cells to secrete immunoglobulin A. J. Exp. Med. *175*:671-682, 1992.

173. Degli-Esposti, M. A., and Smyth, M. J.: Close encounters of different kinds: Dendritic cells and NK cells take centre stage. Nat. Rev. Immunol. *5*:112-124, 2005.

174. Dengrove, J., Lee, E. J., Heiner, D. C., et al.: IgG and IgG subclass specific antibody responses to diphtheria and tetanus toxoids in newborns and infants given DTP immunization. Pediatr. Res. *20*:735-739, 1986.

175. Densen, P.: Human complement deficiency states and infection. *In* Whaley, K., Loos, M., and Weiler, J. M. (eds.): Complement in Health and Disease. Dordrecht, The Netherlands, Kluwer Academic Publishers, 1993, pp. 173-197.

176. Densen, P.: Complement. *In* Mandell, G. L., Bennett, J. E., and Dolin, R. (eds.): Principles and Practice of Infectious Diseases. 4th ed. New York, Churchill Livingstone, 1995, pp. 58-78.

177. Densen, P., McRill, C., and Ross, S. C.: The contribution of the alternative and classical complement pathways to gonococcal killing and C3 fixation. *In* Poolman, J. T., Zanen, H. C., Meyer, T. F., et al.: (eds.): Gonococci and Meningococci. Dordrecht, The Netherlands, Kluwer Academic Publishers, 1988, pp. 693-697.

178. Densen, P., Weiler, J. M., Griffiss, J. M., et al.: Familial properdin deficiency and fatal meningococcemia: Correction of the bactericidal defect by vaccination. N. Engl. J. Med. *316*:922-926, 1987.

179. Diamond, M. S., and Springer, T. A.: A subpopulation of Mac-1 (CD11b/CD18) molecules mediates neutrophil adhesion to ICAM-1 and fibrinogen. J. Cell. Biol. *120*:545-556, 1993.

180. Diamond, R. D.: *Cryptococcus neoformans. In* Mandell, G. L., Bennett, J. E., and Dolin, R. (eds.): Principles and Practice of Infectious Diseases. 4th ed. New York, Churchill Livingstone, 1995, pp. 2331-2340.

181. Diamond, R. D., Root, R. K., and Bennett, J. E.: Factors influencing killing of *Cryptococcus neoformans* by human leukocytes in vitro. J. Infect. Dis. *163*:1108-1113, 1972.

182. DiGeorge, A. M.: A new concept of the cellular basis of immunity (discussion). J. Pediatr. *67*:907-908, 1965.

183. Dinauer, M. C., Lekstrom-Himes, J. A., and Dale, D. C.: Inherited neutrophil disorders: Molecular basis and new therapies. Hematology (Am. Soc. Hematol. Educ. Program) 303-318, 2000.

184. Doherty, P. C., Allan, W., and Eichelberger, M.: Roles of αβγδ T cell subsets in viral immunity. Annu. Rev. Immunol. *10*:123-151, 1992.

185. Dommett, R. M., Klein, N., and Turner, M. W.: Mannose-binding lectin in innate immunity: Past, present and future. Tissue Antigens *68*:193-209, 2006.

186. Donabedian, H., and Gallin, J. I.: Deactivation of human neutrophil chemotaxis by chemoattractants: Effect on receptors for the chemotactic factor f-met-leu-phe. J. Immunol. *127*:839-844, 1981.

187. Donabedian, H., and Gallin, J. I.: Mononuclear cells from patients with the hyperimmunoglobulin E-recurrent infection syndrome produce an inhibitor of leukocyte chemotaxis. J. Clin. Invest. *69*:115-124, 1982.

188. Donabedian, H., and Gallin, J. I.: The hyperimmunoglobulin E recurrent infection (Job's) syndrome: A review of the NIH experience and the literature. Medicine *62*:195-207, 1983.

189. Donowitz, G. R., and Mandell, G. L.: Clinical presentation and unusual infections in chronic granulomatous disease. *In* Gallin, J. I., and Fauci, A. S.

(eds.): Advances in Host Defense Mechanisms. New York, Raven Press, 1983, pp. 55-75.

190. Donskoy, E., and Goldschneider, I.: Thymocytopoiesis is maintained by blood-borne precursors throughout postnatal life: A study of parabiotic mice. J. Immunol. *148*:1604-1612, 1992.

191. Douglas, S. D., and Yoder, M. C.: The mononuclear phagocyte and dendritic cell systems. *In* Stiehm, E. R. (ed.): Immunologic Disorders in Infants and Children. 4th ed. Philadelphia, W. B. Saunders, 1996, pp. 113-132.

192. Doyle, C., and Stominger, J. L.: Interaction between CD4 and class II MHC molecules mediates cell adhesion. Nature *330*:256-259, 1987.

193. Drew, J. H., and Arroyave, C. M.: The complement system of the newborn infant. Biol. Neonate *37*:209-217, 1980.

194. Ebnet, K., Kaldjian, E. P., Anderson, A. O., and Shaw, S.: Orchestrated information transfer underlying leukocyte endothelial interactions. Annu. Rev. Immunol. *14*:155-177, 1996.

195. Edelman, G. M.: Antibody structure and molecular immunology. Scand. J. Immunol. *34*:1-22, 1991.

196. Edwards, J. E.: *Candida* species. *In* Mandell, G. L., Bennett, J. E., and Dolin, R. (eds.): Principles and Practice of Infectious Diseases. 4th ed. New York, Churchill Livingstone, 1995, pp. 2289-2306.

197. Edwards, M. S.: Complement in neonatal infections: An overview. Pediatr. Infect. Dis. *5*:S168-S170, 1986.

198. Eichenfield, L. F., and Johnston, R. B., Jr.: Secondary disorders of the complement system. Am. J. Dis. Child. *143*:595-602, 1989.

199. Einhorn, M. S., Granoff, D. M., Nahm, M. H., et al.: Concentrations of antibodies in paired maternal and infant sera: Relationship to IgG subclass. J. Pediatr. *111*:783-788, 1987.

200. Enders, A., Fisch, P., Schwartz, K., et al.: A severe form of human combined immunodeficiency due to mutations in DNA ligase IV. J. Immunol. *176*:5060-5068, 2006.

201. Enders, G.: Serologic test combinations for safe detection of rubella infections. Rev. Infect. Dis. *7*:S113-S122, 1985.

202. Engh, C. A., Hughes, J. L., Abrams, R. C., et al.: Osteomyelitis in the patient with sickle-cell disease. J. Bone Joint Surg. *53*:1-15, 1971.

203. Englund, J. A., Glezen, W. P., Turner C., et al.: Transplacental antibody transfer following maternal immunization with polysaccharide and conjugate *Haemophilus influenzae* type b vaccines. J. Infect. Dis. *171*:99-105, 1995.

204. Erdei, A., Fust, G., and Gergely, J.: The role of C3 in the immune response. Immunol. Today *12*:332-337, 1991.

205. Etzione, A., and Alon, R.: Leukocyte adhesion deficiency, III: A group of integrin activation defects in hematopoietic lineage cells. Curr. Opin. Allergy Clin. Immunol. *4*:485-490, 2004.

206. Eynon, E. E., and Parker, D. C.: Small B cells as antigen-presenting cells in the induction of tolerance to soluble protein antigens. J. Exp. Med. *175*:131-138, 1992.

207. Falk, K., Rotzschke, O., Deres, K., et al.: Identification of naturally processed viral nonapeptides allows their quantification in infected cells and suggests an allele-specific T cell epitope forecast. J. Exp. Med. *174*:425-434, 1991.

208. Falk, K., Rotzschke, O., Stevanovic, S., et al.: Allele-specific motifs revealed by sequencing of self-peptides eluted from MHC molecules. Nature *351*:290-296, 1991.

209. Fanger, M., Shen, L., Graziano, R., and Guyre, P.: Cytotoxicity mediated by human Fc receptors for IgG. Immunol. Today *10*:92-99, 1989.

210. Fanning, L. J., Connor, A. M., and Wu, G. E.: Development of the immunoglobulin repertoire. Clin. Immunol. Immunopathol. *79*:1-14, 1996.

211. Fearon, D. T., and Austen, K. F.: Properdin: Binding to C3b and stabilization of the C3b-dependent C3 convertase. J. Exp. Med. *142*:856-863, 1975.

212. Fearon, D. T., and Austen, K. F.: The alternative pathway of complement: A system for host resistance to microbial infection. N. Engl. J. Med. *303*:259-263, 1980.

213. Fearon, D. T., and Collins, L. A.: Increased expression of C3b receptors on polymorphonuclear leukocytes induced by chemotactic factors and by purification procedures. J. Immunol. *130*:370-375, 1983.

214. Fearon, D. T., Ruddy, S., Schur, P. H., et al.: Activation of the properdin pathway of complement in patients with gram-negative bacteremia. N. Engl. J. Med. *292*:937-940, 1975.

215. Ferguson, S. E., and Thompson, C. B. A.: A new break in V(D)J recombination. Curr. Biol. *3*:51-53, 1993.

216. Ferrari, S., Giliani, S., Insalaco, A., et al.: Mutations of CD40 gene cause an autosomal recessive form of immunodeficiency with hyper-IgM. Proc. Natl. Acad. Sci. U. S. A. *98*:12614-12619, 2001.

217. Figueroa, J. E., and Densen, P.: Infectious diseases associated with complement deficiencies. Clin. Microbiol. Rev. *4*:359-395, 1991.

218. Fink, C. W., Miller, W. E., Dorward, B., et al.: The formation of macroglobulin antibodies, II: Studies on neonatal infants and older children. J. Clin. Invest. *41*:1422-1428, 1962.

219. Fischer, A., de Saint Basile, G., and Le Deist, F.: CD3 deficiencies. Curr. Opin. Allergy Immunol. *5*:491-495, 2005.

220. Fischer, A., Hacein-Bey, S., Le Deist, F., et al.: Gene therapy of severe combined immunodeficiencies. Immunol. Rev. *178*:13-20, 2000.

221. Fisher, A., Trung, P. H., Descamps-Latsdra, B., et al.: Bone marrow-transplantation for inborn error of phagocytic cells associated with defective adherence, chemotaxis, and oxidative response during opsonized particle phagocytosis. Lancet *2*:473-475, 1983.

222. Fisher, C. J., Jr., Dhainaut, J. F., Opal, S. M., et al.: Recombinant human interleukin 1 receptor antagonist in the treatment of patients with sepsis syndrome. J. A. M. A. *271*:1836-1843, 1994.

223. Fleishmann, J., and Lehrer, R. I.: Phagocytic mechanism in host response. *In* Howard, D. H. (ed.): Fungi Pathogenic for Humans and Animals, Part B2. New York, Marcel Dekker, 1985, pp. 123-149.

224. Fleming, A. F., Storey, J., Molineaux, L., et al.: Abnormal haemoglobins in the Sudan savanna of Nigeria, I. Prevalence of haemoglobins and relationships between sickle cell trait, malaria, and survival. Ann. Trop. Med. Parasitol. *73*:161-172, 1979.

225. Forlow, S. B., Schurr, J. R., Kolls, J. K., et al.: Increased granulopoiesis through interleukin-17 and granulocyte colony-stimulating factor in leukocyte adhesion deficient mice. Blood *98*:3309-3314, 2001.

226. Freeman, A. F., Kleiner, D. E., Nadiminti, H., et al.: Causes of death in hyper-IgE syndrome. J. Allergy Clin. Immunol. *119*:1234-1240, 2007.

227. Fremont, D. H., Matsumura, M., Stura, E. A., et al.: Crystal structures of two viral peptides in complex with murine MHC class I H-2K^b. Science *257*:919-927, 1992.

228. Frydman, M., Etzioni, A., Eidlitz-Markus, T., et al.: Rambam-Hasharon syndrome of psychomotor retardation, short stature, defective neutrophil motility, and Bombay phenotype. Am. J. Med. Genet. *44*:297-302, 1992.

229. Fuchs, E. J., and Matzinger, P. B.: B cells turn off virgin but not memory T cells. Science *258*:1156-1159, 1992.

230. Gabbay, J. E., and Almeida, R. P.: Antibiotic peptides and serine protease homologs in human polymorphonuclear leukocytes: Defensins and azurocidin. Curr. Opin. Immunol. *5*:97-102, 1993.

231. Gallin, J. I.: Neutrophil specific granule deficiency. Annu. Rev. Med. *36*:263-274, 1985.

232. Garibyan, L., Lobito, A. A., Siegel, R. M., et al.: Dominant negative effect of the heterozygous C104R TACI mutation in common variable immunodeficiency (CVID). J. Clin. Invest. *117*:1550-1557, 2007.

233. Ganz, T.: Defensins: Antimicrobial peptides of innate immunity. Nat. Rev. Immunol. *3*:710-720, 2003.

234. Ganz, T., and Lehrer, R. I.: Antimicrobial peptides of vertebrates. Curr. Opin. Imunol. *10*:41-44, 1998.

235. Ganz, T., and Weiss J.: Antimicrobial peptides of phagocytes and epithelia. Semin. Hematol. *34*:343-354, 1997.

236. Garcia, K. C., Teyton, L., Wilson, I. A.: Structural basis of T cell recognition. Annu. Rev. Immunol. *17*:369-397, 1999.

237. Gathings, W. E., Lawton, A. R., and Cooper, M. D.: Immunofluorescent studies of the development of pre-B cells, B lymphocytes and immunoglobulin isotype diversity in humans. Eur. J. Immunol. *7*:804-810, 1977.

238. Geelan, S. P. M., Bazemer, A., Gerards, L. J., et al.: Deficiencies in opsonic defense to pneumococci in the human newborn despite adequate levels of complement and specific IgG antibodies. Pediatr. Res. *27*:514-518, 1990.

239. Geha, R. S., Reinherz, E., Leung, D., et al.: Deficiency of suppressor T cells in the hyperimmunoglobulin E syndrome. J. Clin. Invest. *68*:783-791, 1981.

240. Gelfand, E. W., and Finkel, T. H.: The T-lymphocyte system. *In* Stiehm, E. R. (ed.): Immunologic Disorders in Infants and Children. 4th ed. Philadelphia, W. B. Saunders, 1996, pp. 14-34.

241. Gerard, C., and Gerard, N.: C5a anaphylatoxin and its seven transmembrane-segment receptor. Annu. Rev. Immunol. *12*:775-808, 1994.

242. Gill, T. J., Repetti, C. F., Metlay, L. A., et al.: Transplacental immunization of the human fetus to tetanus by immunization of the mother. J. Clin. Invest. *72*:987-996, 1983.

243. Gill, T. J., III, Karasic, R. B., Antoncic, J., and Rabbin, B. S.: Long-term follow-up of children born to women immunized with tetanus toxoid during pregnancy. Am. J. Reprod. Immunol. *25*:69-71, 1991.

244. Glass, W. G., Rosenberg, H. F., and Murphy, P. M.: Chemokine regulation of inflammation during acute viral infection. Curr. Opin. Allergy Clin. Immunol. *3*:467-473, 2003.

245. Goldberg, A. L., and Rock, K. L.: Proteolysis, proteasomes and antigen presentation. Nature *357*:375-379, 1992.

246. Golding, B., Muchmore, A. V., and Blaese, R. M.: Newborn and Wiskott-Aldrich patient B cells can be activated by TNP-*Brucella abortus*: Evidence that TNP-*Brucella abortus* behaves as a T-independent type 1 antigen in humans. J. Immunol. *133*:2966-2971, 1984.

247. Goldsobel, A. B., Haas, A., and Stiehm, E. R.: Bone marrow transplantation in DiGeorge syndrome. J. Pediatr. *111*:40-44, 1987.

248. Good, R. A.: Studies on agammaglobulinemia, II: Failure of plasma cell formation in the bone marrow and lymph nodes of patients with agammaglobulinemia. J. Lab. Clin. Med. *46*:167-181, 1955.

249. Goodnow, C. C.: Balancing immunity, autoimmunity, and self-tolerance. Ann. N. Y. Acad. Sci. *815*:55-66, 1997.

250. Gordon, D. L., and Hostetter, M. K.: Complement and host defense against microorganisms. Pathology *18*:365-375, 1986.

251. Goudemand, J., Anssens, R., Delmas-Marsalet, Y., et al.: Essai de traitement d'un cas de granulomatose familiale chronique par greffe de moelle osseuse allogenique. Arch. Fr. Pediatr. *33*:121-129, 1976.

252. Grakoui, A., Bromley, S. K., Sumen, C., et al.: The immunological synapse: A molecular machine controlling T cell activation. Science *285*:221-227.

253. Greenberg, F., Crowder, W. E., Paschall, V., et al.: Familial DiGeorge syndrome and associated partial monosomy of chromosome 22. Hum. Genet. *65*:317-319, 1984.

254. Greenberg, F., Elder, F. F. B., Haffner, P., et al.: Cytogenic findings in a prospective series of patients with DiGeorge anomaly. Am. J. Hum. Genet. 43:605-611, 1988.

255. Greve, J. M., Davis, G., Meyer, A. M., et al.: The major human rhinovirus receptor is ICAM-1. Cell 56:839-847, 1989.

256. Grimbacher, B., Holland, S. M., Gallin, J. I., et al.: Hyper-IgE syndrome with recurrent infections—an autosomal dominant multisystem disorder. N. Engl. J. Med. 340:692-702, 1999.

257. Grimbacher, B., Holland, S. M., and Puck, J. M.: Hyper-IgE syndromes. Immunol. Rev. 203:244-250, 2005.

258. Grimbacher, B., Schaffer, A. A., Holland, S. M., et al.: Genetic linkage of hyper-IgE syndrome to chromosome 4. Am. J. Hum. Genet. 65:735-744, 1999.

259. Grisham, M. B., Jefferson, M. M., Melton, D. F., and Thomas, E. L.: Chlorination of endogenous amines by isolated neutrophils: Ammonia-dependent bactericidal, cytotoxic, and cytolytic activities of the chloramines. J. Biol. Chem. 259:10404-10413, 1984.

260. Gupta, S., Rahwa, R., O'Reilly, R., et al.: Ontogeny of lymphocyte subpopulations in human fetal liver. Proc. Natl. Acad. Sci. U. S. A. 73:919-922, 1976.

261. Harding, C. V., Collins, D. S., Slot, J. W., et al.: Liposome-encapsulated antigens are processed in lysosomes, recycled, and presented to T cells. Cell 64:393-401, 1991.

262. Harris, B. H., Shalit, M., and Southwick, F. S.: Diminished actin polymerization by neutrophils from newborn infants. Pediatr. Res. 33:27-31, 1992.

263. Hart, D. N. J.: Dendritic cells: Unique leukocyte populations which control the primary immune response. Blood 90:3245-3287, 1997.

264. Havran, W. L., and Boismenu, R.: Activation and function of gamma delta T cells. Curr. Opin. Immunol. 6:442-446, 1994.

265. Hayashi, F., Smith, K. D., Ozinsky, A., et al.: The innate immune response to bacterial flagellin is mediated by Toll-like receptor 5. Nature 410:1099-1103, 2001.

266. Hayashi, S.-I., Kundisada, T., Ogawa, M., et al.: Stepwise progress of B lineage differentiation supported by interleukin 7 and other stromal cell molecules. J. Exp. Med. 171:1683-1695, 1990.

267. Hayward, A. R.: Development of lymphocyte responses and interactions in the human fetus and newborn. Immunol. Rev. 57:39-60, 1981.

268. Hayward, A. R., Leonard, J., Wood, C. B. S., et al.: Delayed separation of the umbilical cord, widespread infections and defective neutrophil mobility. Lancet 1:1099-1101, 1979.

269. Heath, W. R., Kane, K. P., Mescher, M. F., et al.: Alloreactive T cells discriminate among a diverse set of endogenous peptides. Proc. Natl. Acad. Sci. U. S. A. 88:5101-5105, 1991.

270. Heinzel, F.: Antibodies. In Mandell, G. L., Bennett, J. E., and Dolin, R. (eds.): Principles and Practice of Infectious Diseases. 4th ed. New York, Churchill Livingstone, 1995, pp. 36-57.

271. Hermaszewski, R. A., and Webster, A. D. B.: Primary hypogammaglobulinaemia: A survey of clinical manifestations and complications. Q. J. M. 86:31-42, 1993.

272. Herrod, H. G.: Management of the patient with IgG subclass deficiency and/or selective antibody deficiency. Ann. Allergy 70:3-11, 1993.

273. Herrod, H. G.: Clinical significance of IgG subclasses. Curr. Opin. Pediatr. 5:696-699, 1993.

274. Herrod, H. G., Gross, S., and Insel, R.: Selective antibody deficiency to Haemophilus influenzae type b capsular polysaccharide vaccination in children with recurrent respiratory tract infection. J. Clin. Immunol. 9:429-434, 1989.

275. Hertz, C. J., Wu, Q., Porter, E. M., et al.: Activation of Toll-like receptor 2 on human tracheobronchial epithelial cells induces the antimicrobial peptide human beta defensin-2. J. Immunol. 171:6820-6826, 2003.

276. Heyworth, P. G., Cross, A. R., and Curnutte, J. T.: Chronic granulomatous disease. Curr. Opin. Clin. Immunol. 15:578-584, 2003.

277. Hibberd, M. L., Sumiya, M., Summerfield, J. A., et al.: Association of variants of the gene for mannose-binding lectin with susceptibility to meningococcal disease. Lancet 353:1049-1053, 1999.

278. Hibbs, M. L., Wardlaw, A. J., Stacker, S. A., et al.: Transfection of cells from patients with leukocyte adhesion deficiency with an intergrin B subunit (CD18) restores lymphocyte function-associated antigen-1 expression and function. J. Clin. Invest. 85:674-681, 1990.

279. Hill, H. R.: Clinical disorders of leukocyte functions. In Snyderman, R. (ed.): Current Topics in Immunology. New York, Plenum Press, 1984, pp. 345-393.

280. Hill, H. R.: Biochemical, structural, and functional abnormalities of polymorphonuclear leukocytes in the neonate. Pediatr. Res. 22:375-382, 1987.

281. Hill, H. R., and Quie, P. G.: Raised serum IgE levels and defective neutrophil chemotaxis in three children with eczema and recurrent bacterial infections. Lancet 1:183-187, 1974.

282. Hixson, P., Smith, C. W., Shurin, S. B., and Tosi, M. F.: Unique CD18 mutations involving a deletion in the extracellular stalk region and a major truncation of the cytoplasmic domain in a patient with leukocyte adhesion deficiency type I. Blood 103:1105-1113, 2004.

283. Hoffman, A. A., Hayward, A. R., Kurnick, J. T., et al.: Presentation of antigen by human newborn monocytes to maternal tetanus toxoid-specific T-cell blasts. J. Clin. Immunol. 1:217-221, 1981.

284. Hofman, F. M., Danilovs, J. A., and Taylor, C. R.: HLA-DR (Ia)-positive dendritic-like cells in human fetal nonlymphoid tissues. Transplantation 27:590-594, 1984.

285. Holland, S. M., and Gallin, J. I.: Evaluation of the patient with suspected immunodeficiency. In Mandell, G. L., Bennett, J. E., and Dolin, R. (eds.): Principles and Practice of Infectious Diseases. 4th. ed. New York, Churchill Livingstone, 1995, pp. 149-158.

286. Hong, R.: Disorders of the T-cell system. In Stiehm, E. R. (ed.): Immunologic Disorders in Infants and Children. 4th ed. Philadelphia, W. B. Saunders, 1996, pp. 339-408.

287. Hoover, D. M., Boulegue, C., Yang, D., et al.: The structure of human macrophage inflammatory protein-3alpha CCL20: Linking antimicrobial and CC chemokine receptor-6-binding activities with human beta-defensins. J. Biol. Chem. 277:37647-37654, 2002.

288. Hoover, D. M., Rajashankar, K. R., Blumenthal, R., et al.: The structure of human beta-defensin-2 shows evidence of higher order oligomerization. J. Biol. Chem. 275:32911-32918, 2000.

289. Horwitz, M. A.: Interactions between Legionella pneumophilia and human mononuclear phagocytes. In Thornsberry, C., Balows, A., Feeley, J. C., et al.: (eds.): Legionella. Proceedings of the 2nd International Symposium. Washington, D. C., American Society for Microbiology, 1984, pp. 159-166.

290. Hostetter, M. K.: Serotypic variations among virulent pneumococci in deposition and degradation of covalently bound C3b: Implications for phagocytosis and antibody production. J. Infect. Dis. 153:682-693, 1986.

291. Hostetter, M. K., Kreuger, R. A., and Schmeling, D. J.: The biochemistry of opsonization: Central role of the reactive thiolester of the third component of complement. J. Infect. Dis. 150:653-661, 1984.

292. Hostoffer, R. W., Krukovets, I., and Berger, M.: Enhancement by tumor necrosis factor-α of Fcα receptor expression and IgA-mediated superoxide generation and killing of Pseudomonas aeruginosa by polymorphonuclear leukocytes. J. Infect. Dis. 170:82-87, 1994.

293. Hudson, A. W., and Ploegh, H. L.: The cell biology of antigen presentation. Exp. Cell Res. 272:1-7, 2002.

294. Hugli, T. E.: Structure and function of the anaphylatoxins. Springer Semin. Immunopathol. 7:193-220, 1984.

295. Hunt, D. F., Henderson, R. A., Shababowitz, J., et al.: Characterization of peptides bound to the class I MHC molecule HLA-A2.1 by mass spectrometry. Science 255:1261-1263, 1992.

296. Hunt, D. F., Michel, H., Dickinson, T. A., et al.: Peptides presented to the immune system by the murine class II major histocompatibility complex molecule I-A^d. Science 256:1817-1820, 1992.

297. Insel, R. A., Amstey, M., Woodin, K., et al.: Maternal immunization to prevent infectious diseases in the neonate or infant. Int. J. Technol. Assess. Health Care 10:143-153, 1994.

298. International Chronic Granulomatous Disease Cooperative Study Group: A controlled trial of interferon gamma to prevent infection in chronic granulomatous diseases. N. Engl. J. Med. 324:509-516, 1991.

299. Itano, A. A., and Jenkins, M. K.: Antigen presentation to naive CD4 T cells in the lymph node. Nat. Immunol. 4:733-739, 2003.

300. IUIS/WHO Subcommittee on Chemokine Nomenclature: Chemokine/chemokine receptor nomenclature. Cytokine 21:48-49, 2003.

301. Jackson, S. H., Gallin, J. I., and Holland, S. M.: The p47$_{phox}$ mouse knockout model of chronic granulomatous disease. J. Exp. Med. 182:751-758, 1995.

302. Janeway, C. A., and Medzhitov, R.: Innate immune recognition. Annu. Rev. Immunol 20:197-216, 2002.

303. Janeway, C. A., Jr., Travers, P., Walport, M., and Schlomchik, M. J.: The generation of lymphocyte antigen receptors. In Immunobiology: The Immune System in Health and Disease. 6th ed. New York, Garland Science, 2005, pp. 135-168.

304. Jin, T., Bokarewa, M., Foster, T., et al.: Staphylococcus aureus resists human defensins by production of staphylokinase, a novel bacterial evasion mechanism. J. Immunol. 172:1169-1176, 2004.

305. Johnston, R. B., and Baehner, R. L.: Chronic granulomatous disease: Correlation between pathogenesis and clinical findings. Pediatrics 48:730-737, 1971.

306. Johnston, R. B., and Newman, S. L.: Chronic granulomatous disease. Pediatr. Clin. North Am. 24:365-376, 1977.

307. Johnston, R. B., Jr.: The complement system in host defense and inflammation: The cutting edges of a double edged sword. Pediatr. Infect. Dis. J. 12:933-941, 1993.

308. Johnston, R. B., Jr.: Disorders of the complement system. In Stiehm, E. R. (ed.): Immunologic Disorders in Infants and Children. 4th ed. Philadelphia, W. B. Saunders, 1996, pp. 133-158.

309. Joiner, K. A.: Complement evasion by bacteria and parasites. Ann. Rev. Microbiol. 42:201-230, 1988.

310. Joiner, K. A., Brown, E. J., and Frank, M. M.: Complement and bacteria: Chemistry and biology in host defense. Ann. Rev. Immunol. 2:461-491, 1984.

311. Joiner, K. A., Fries, L. F., and Frank, M. M.: Studies of antibody and complement function in host defense against bacterial infection. Immunol. Lett. 14:197-202, 1987.

312. Jones, D. H., Schmalsteig, F. C., Dempsey, K., et al.: Subcellular distribution and mobilization of Mac-1 (CD11b/CD18) in neonatal neutrophils. Blood 75:488-498, 1990.

313. Lin, J. S., Yang, C. W., Wang, D. W., and Wu-Hsieh, B. A.: Dendritic cells cross-present exogenous fungal antigens to stimulate a protective CD8 T cell response to infection by Histoplasama capsulatum. J. Immunol. 174:6282-6291, 2005.

314. Kaech, S. M., Hemby, S., Kersh, E., and Ahmed, R.: Molecular and functional profiling of memory CD8 T cell differentiation. Cell *111*:837-851, 2002.

315. Kalman, L., Lindergren, M. L., Koibrynski, L., et al.: Mutations in genes required for T-cell development: IL7R, CD45, IL2RG, JAK3, RAG1, RAG2, ARTEMIS, and ADA and severe combined immunodeficiency: HuGE review. Genet. Med. *6*:16-26, 2004.

316. Kamani, N., August, C. S., Douglas, S. D., et al.: Transplantation in chronic granulomatous disease. J. Pediatr. *105*:42-46, 1984.

317. Kappler, J. W., Roehm, N., and Marrack, P.: T cell tolerance by clonal elimination in the thymus. Cell *49*:273-280, 1987.

318. Keiser, P. B., and Nutman, T. B.: *Strongyloides stercoralis* in the immunocompromised population. Clin. Microbiol. Rev. *17*:208-217, 2004.

319. Kelly, J. M., Waterhouse, N. J., Cretney, E., et al.: Granzyme M mediates a novel form of perforin-dependent cell death. J. Biol. Chem. *279*:22236-22242, 2004.

320. Kelsoe, G.: The germinal center: A crucible for lymphocyte selection. Semin. Immunol. *8*:179-184, 1996.

321. Kelsoe, G. F., and Zheng, B.: Sites of B cell activation in vivo. Curr. Opin. Immunol. *5*:418-422, 1993.

322. Kerr, M. A.: The structure and function of human IgA. Biochem. J. *271*:285-296, 1990.

323. Kew, R. R., and Wester, R. O.: Gelglobulin (vitamin D-binding protein) enhances the neutrophil chemotactic activity of C5a and C5a des arg. J. Clin. Invest. *82*:364-369, 1988.

324. Kim, C. H.: Chemokine-chemokine receptor network in immune cell trafficking. Curr. Drug Targets Immune Endocr. Metabol. Disord. *4*:343-361, 2004.

325. Kinashi, T., Aker, M., Sokolovsky-Eisenberg, M., et al.: LAD-III, a leukocyte adhesion deficiency syndrome associated with defective Rap1 activation and impaired stabilization of integrin bonds. Blood *103*:1033-1036, 2004.

326. Kishore, S. P., Bungum, M. K., Platt, J. L., and Brunn, G. J.: Selective suppression of Toll-like receptor 4 activation by chemokine receptor 4. FEBS Lett. *579*:699-704, 2005.

327. Klatzman, D., Champagne, E., Chamaret, S., et al.: T-lymphocyte T4 molecule behaves as a receptor for human retrovirus LAV. Nature *312*:767-770, 1984.

328. Klein, J. O., and Marcy, S. M.: Bacterial sepsis and meningitis. *In* Remington, J. S., and Klein, J. O. (eds.): Infectious Diseases of the Fetus and Newborn Infant. 4th ed. Philadelphia, W. B. Saunders, 1995, pp. 835-890.

329. Klein, R. B., Fisher, T. J., Gard, S. E., et al.: Decreased mononuclear and polymorphonuclear chemotaxis in human newborn infants and young children. Pediatrics *60*:467-472, 1977.

330. Kluin-Nelemans, H. C., van Velzen-Blad, H., van Helden, H. P. T., et al.: Functional deficiency of complement factor D in a monozygous twin. Clin. Exp. Immunol. *58*:724-730, 1984.

331. Kohl, S., Springer, T. A., Shmalsteig, F. C., et al.: Defective natural killer cytotoxicity and polymorphonuclear leukocyte antibody-dependent cellular cytotoxicity in patients with LFA-1/OKM-1 deficiency. J. Immunol. *133*:2972-2981, 1984.

332. Kohler, P. F.: Maturation of the human complement system, I: Onset of the time and site of fetal C1q, C4, C3 and C5 synthesis. J. Clin. Invest. *52*:671-677, 1973.

333. Kohler, P. F., and Farr, R. S.: Elevation of cord over maternal IgG immunoglobulin—evidence for an active placental IgG transport. Nature *210*:1070-1071, 1966.

334. Konstan, M., and Berger, M.: Infection and inflammation in the lung in cystic fibrosis. *In* Davis, P. (ed.): Cystic Fibrosis. New York, Marcel Dekker, 1993, pp. 221-276.

335. Kornfeld, S. J., and Plaut, A. G.: Secretory immunity and the bacterial IgA proteases. Rev. Infect. Dis. *3*:521-534, 1981.

336. Koshland, M. E.: The coming of age of the immunoglobulin J chain. Annu. Rev. Immunol. *3*:425-453, 1985.

337. Kramer, N., Perez, H. D., and Goldstein, I. M.: An immunoglobulin (IgG) inhibitor of polymorphonuclear leukocyte motility in a patient with recurrent infection. N. Engl. J. Med. *303*:1253-1258, 1980.

338. Kraus, J. C., Mayo-Bond, L., Rogers, C. E., et al.: An in vivo animal model of gene therapy for leukocyte adhesion deficiency. J. Clin. Invest. *88*:1412-1417, 1991.

339. Krause, P. J., Maderazo, E. G., and Scroggs, M.: Abnormalities of neutrophil adherence in newborns. Pediatrics *69*:184-187, 1982.

340. Kretschmer, R., Say, B., Brown, D., et al.: Congenital aplasia of the thymus gland (DiGeorge's syndrome). N. Engl. J. Med. *279*:1295-1301, 1968.

341. Kulka, M., Alexopoulou, L., Flavell, R. A., and Metcalfe, D. D.: Activation of mast cells by double-stranded RNA: Evidence for activation through Toll-like receptor 3. J. Allergy Clin. Immunol. *114*:174-182, 2004.

342. Kunkel, E. J., and Butcher, E. C.: Chemokines and the tissue-specific migration of lymphocytes. Immunity *16*:1-4, 2002.

343. Kunkel, S., Standiford, T., Chensue, S. W., et al.: Cellular and molecular mechanisms of cytokine networking. Agents Actions Suppl. *32*:205-218, 1991.

344. Kunkel, S. L., and Strieter, R. M.: Cytokine networking in lung inflammation. Hosp. Pract. *25*:63-76, 1990.

345. Kurt-Jones, E. A., Belko, J., Yu, C., et al.: The role of toll-like receptors in herpes simplex infection in neonates. J. Infect. Dis. *191*:746-748, 2005.

346. Kuschert, G. S., Coulin, F., Power, C. A., et al.: Glycosaminoglycans interact selectively with chemokines and modulate receptor binding and cellular responses. Biochemistry *38*:12959-12968, 1999.

347. Lachmann, P. J.: The control of homologous lysis. Immunol. Today *12*:312-315, 1991.

348. Lammer, E. J., and Opitz, J. M.: The DiGeorge anomaly as a developmental field defect. Am. J. Med. Genet. *2*(Suppl.):113-127, 1986.

349. Lane, P., Traunecker, A., Hubele, S., et al.: Activated human T cells express a ligand for the human B cell-associated antigen CD40 which participates in T cell-dependent activation of B lymphocytes. Eur. J. Immunol. *22*:2573-2578, 1992.

350. Lasky, L. A.: Selectins: Interpreters of cell-specific carbohydrate information during inflammation. Science *258*:964-969, 1992.

351. Lassiter, H. A., Wilson, J. L., Feldhoff, R. C., et al.: Supplemental complement component C9 enhances the capacity of neonatal serum to kill multiple isolates of pathogenic *Escherichia coli*. Pediatr. Res. *35*:389-396, 1994.

352. Lau, Y.-L., Tam, A. Y. C., and Ng, K. W.: Clinical laboratory observations: Response of preterm infants to hepatitis B vaccine. J. Pediatr. *121*:962-965, 1992.

353. Law, S. K., Lichtenberg, N. A., and Levine, R. P.: Covalent binding and hemolytic activity of complement proteins. Proc. Natl. Acad. Sci. U. S. A. *77*:7194-7198, 1980.

354. Lawton, A. R., and Cooper, M. D.: Development and function of the immune system. *In* Stiehm, E. R. (ed.): Immunologic Disorders in Infants and Children. 4th ed. Philadelphia, W. B. Saunders, 1996, pp. 1-13.

355. Lazarus, G. M., and Neu, H. C.: Agents responsible for infection in chronic granulomatous disease of childhood. J. Pediatr. *86*:415-417, 1975.

356. Lebecque, S. G., and Gearhart, P. J.: Boundaries of somatic mutation in rearranged immunoglobulin genes: 5′ boundary is near the promoter, and 3′ boundary is >1 kb from V(D)J gene. J. Exp. Med. *172*:1717-1727, 1990.

357. Lederman, H. M., and Winkelstein, J. A.: X-linked agammaglobulinemia: An analysis of 96 patients. Medicine *64*:145-156, 1985.

358. Lee, S. I., Heiner, D. C., and Wara, D.: Development of serum IgG subclass levels in children. Monogr. Allergy *19*:108-121, 1986.

359. Lehrer, R. I., and Ganz, T.: Antimicrobial polypeptides of human neutrophils. Blood *76*:2169-2181, 1990.

360. Lekstrom-Himes, J. A., Dorman, S. E., Kopar, P., et al.: Neutrophil specific granule deficiency results from a novel mutation with loss of function of the transcription factor CCAAT/enhancer binding protein epsilon. J. Exp. Med. *189*:1847-1852, 1999.

361. Leonard, W. J.: X-linked severe combined immunodeficiency: From molecular cause to gene therapy within seven years. Mol. Med. Today *6*:403-407, 2000.

362. Levy, O., Ooi, C. E., Weiss, J., et al.: Individual and synergistic effects of rabbit granulocyte proteins on *Escherichia coli*. J. Clin. Invest. *94*:672-682, 1994.

363. Levy, O., Weiss, J., Zarember, K., et al.: Antibacterial 15-kDa protein isoforms (p15s) are members of a novel family of leukocyte proteins. J. Biol. Chem. *268*:6058-6063, 1993.

364. Lewis, D. B., and Wilson, C. B.: Developmental immunology and role of host defenses in fetal and neonatal susceptibility to infection. *In* Remington, J. S., and Klein, J. O. (eds.): Infectious Diseases of the Fetus and Newborn Infant. 5th ed. Philadelphia, W. B. Saunders, 2001, pp. 25-138.

365. Ley, K.: Integration of inflammatory signals by rolling neutrophils. Immunol. Rev. *186*:8-18, 2002.

366. Ley, K.: The role of selectins in inflammation and disease. Trends Mol. Med. *9*:263-268, 2003.

367. Lieberman, J.: The ABCs of granule-mediated cytotoxicity: New weapons in the arsenal. Nat. Rev. Immunol. *3*:361-370, 2003.

368. Lieschke, G. J., and Burgess, A. W.: Granulocyte colony-stimulating factor and granulocyte-macrophage colony-stimulating factor, parts I and II. N. Engl. J. Med. *327*:28-35, 99-106, 1992.

369. Liles, W. C., and Van Voorhis, W. C.: Review: Nomenclature and biologic significance of cytokines involved in inflammation and the host immune response. J. Infect. Dis. *172*:1573-1580, 1995.

370. Liu, Y.-J., Cairns, J. A., Holder, M. J., et al.: Recombinant 25-kDa CD23 and interleukin 1α promote the survival of terminal center B cells: Evidence for bifurcation in the development of centrocytes rescued from apoptosis. Eur. J. Immunol. *21*:1107-1114, 1991.

371. Lodewyk, H. S., Van Mierop, M. D., and Kutsche, L. M.: Cardiovascular anomalies in DiGeorge syndrome and importance of neural crest as a possible pathogenic factor. Am. J. Cardiol. *58*:133-137, 1986.

372. Long, E. O.: Antigen processing for presentation to CD4+ T cells. New Biol. *4*:274-282, 1992.

373. Lorenz, E., Mira, J. P., Cornish, K. L., et al.: A novel polymorphism in the toll-like receptor 2 gene and its potential association with staphylococcal infection. Infect. Immun. *68*:6398-6401, 2000.

374. Lorenz, E., Mira, J. P., Frees, K. L., and Schwartz, D. A.: Relevance of mutations in the TLR4 receptor in patients with gram-negative septic shock. Arch. Intern. Med. *162*:1028-1032, 2002.

375. Lubke, T., Marquardt, T., Etzioni, A., et al.: Complementation cloning identifies CDG-IIc, a new type of congenital disorders of glycosylation, as a GDP-fucose transporter deficiency. Nat. Genet. *28*:73-76, 2001.

376. Lyon, M. F.: Some milestones in the history of X-chromosome inactivation. Annu. Rev. Genet. *26*:17-28, 1992.

377. Ma, Y., Pannicke, U., Schwartz, K., and Lieber, M. R.: Hairpin opening and overhang processing by an Artemis/DNA-dependent protein kinase complex in nonhomologous end joining and V(D)J recombination. Cell 108:781-794, 2002.

378. Macallan, D. C., Wallace, D., Zhang, Y., et al.: Rapid turnover of effector-memory CD4(+) T cells in healthy humans. J. Exp. Med. 200:255-260, 2004.

379. Malech, H., Horwitz, M., Linton, G., et al.: Prolonged production of NADPH oxidase-corrected granulocytes after gene therapy of chronic granulomatous disease. Proc. Natl. Acad. Sci. U. S. A. 94:12133-12138, 1997.

380. Manroe, B., Weinberg, A. G., Rosenfeld, C. R., et al.: The neonatal blood count in health and disease, I: Reference values for neutrophilic cells. J. Pediatr. 64:60-64, 1979.

381. Marchalonis, J. J., Jensen, I., and Schluter, S. F.: Structural, antigenic and evolutionary analyses of immunoglobulins and T cell receptors. J. Mol. Recognit. 15:260-271, 2002.

382. Marciano, B. E., Wesley, R., De Carlo, E. S., et al.: Long-term interferon-γ therapy for patients with chronic granulomatous disease. Clin. Infect. Dis. 39:692-699, 2004.

383. Marsh, S. G. E., and Bodmer, J. G.: HLA class II nucleotide sequences. Hum. Immunol. 31:207-227, 1991.

384. Martensson, L., and Fudenberg, H. H.: Gm genes and gamma G-globulin synthesis in the human fetus. J. Immunol. 94:514-520, 1965.

385. Martyn, L. J., Lischner, H. W., and Pileggi, A. J.: Chorioretinal lesions in familial chronic granulomatous disease of childhood. Trans. Am. Ophthalmol. Soc. 69:84-112, 1971.

386. Matsukawa, A., Hogaboam, C. M., Lukacs, N. W., and Kunkel, S. L.: Chemokines and innate immunity. Rev. Immunogenet. 2:339-358, 2000.

387. Matzinger, P.: Tolerance, danger and the extended family. Annu. Rev. Immunol. 12:991-1045, 1994.

388. Mauer, A. M., Athens, J. W., Ashenbrucker, H., et al.: Leukokinetic studies, II: A method for labeling granulocytes in vitro with radioactive di-isopropyl-fluorophosphate (DFP32). J. Clin. Invest. 39:1482-1489, 1960.

389. McDowall, A., Inwald, D., Leitinger, B., et al.: A novel form of integrin dysfunction involving β1, β2, and β3 integrins. J. Clin. Invest. 111:51-60, 2003.

390. McEvoy, L. T., Zakem-Cloud, H., and Tosi, M. F.: Total cell content of CR3 (CD11b/CD18) and LFA-1 (CD11a/CD18) in neonatal neutrophils: Relationship to gestational age. Blood 87:392-3933, 1996.

391. McPhail, L. C., DeChatelet, L. R., and Shirley, P. S.: Deficiency of NADPH oxidase activity in chronic granulomatous disease. J. Pediatr. 90:213-217, 1977.

392. McQuibban, G. A., Butler, G. S., Gong, J. H., et al.: Matrix metalloproteinase activity inactivates the CXC chemokine stromal cell-derived factor-1. J. Biol. Chem. 276:43503-43508, 2001.

393. Medzhitov, R., Preston-Hurlburt, P., and Janeway, C. A., Jr.: A human homologue of the Drosophila Toll protein signals activation of adaptive immunity. Nature 388:394-397, 1997.

394. Melchers, F., ten Boekel, E., Seidl, T., et al.: Repertoire selection by pre-B-cell receptors and B-cell receptors, and genetic control of B-cell development from immature to mature B cells. Immunol. Rev. 175:33-46, 2000.

395. Melnick, J. L.: Nomenclature and classification of viruses. In Feigin, R. D., and Cherry, J. D. (eds.): Textbook of Pediatric Infectious Diseases. 3rd ed. Philadelphia, W. B. Saunders, 1992, pp. 1374-1389.

396. Merkenschlager, M., Graf, D., Lovatt, M., et al.: How many thymocytes audition for selection? J. Exp. Med. 186:1149-1158, 1997.

397. Metchnikoff, E.: Immunity in Infectious Diseases. (F. G. Binnie.) London, Cambridge University Press, 1905.

398. Metzger, H.: Structure and function of gamma M macroglobulins. Adv. Immunol. 12:57-116, 1970.

399. Miller, M. E.: Phagocytosis in the newborn infant: Humoral and cellular factors. J. Pediatr. 74:255-259, 1969.

400. Miller, M. E.: Chemotactic function in the human neonate: Humoral and cellular aspects. Pediatr. Res. 5:487-492, 1971.

401. Miller, M. E.: Developmental maturation of human neutrophil motility and its relationship to membrane deformity. In Bellanti, J. A., and Dayton, D. H. (eds.): Phagocytic Cell in Host Resistance. New York, Raven Press, 1975, pp. 295-314.

402. Miller, M. E.: Phagocytic function in the neonate: Selected aspects. Pediatrics 64:S709-S712, 1979.

403. Miller, M. E., Norman, M. E., Koblenzer, P. J., et al.: A new familial defect of neutrophil movement. J. Lab. Clin. Med. 82:1-8, 1973.

404. Miller, M. E., Oski, F. A., and Harris, M. B.: Lazy leukocyte syndrome: A new disorder of neutrophil function. Lancet 1:665-669, 1971.

405. Mills, E. L., and Quie, P. G.: Congenital disorders of the functions of polymorphonuclear neutrophils. Rev. Infect. Dis. 2:505-517, 1980.

406. Milstein, C.: From antibody structure to immunological diversification of immune response. Science 231:1261-1268, 1986.

407. Mir, A., Benahmed, D., Igual, R., et al.: Eosinophil-selective mediators in human strongyloidiasis. Parasite Immunol. 28:397-400, 2006.

408. Mond, J. J., Vos, Q., Lees, A., and Snapper, C. M.: T cell independent antigens. Curr. Opin. Immunol. 7:349-354, 1995.

409. Monteiro, R. C., Cooper, M. D., and Kubagawa, H.: Molecular heterogeneity of Fcα receptors detected by receptor-specific monoclonal antibodies. J. Immunol. 148:1764-1771, 1992.

410. Morell, A., Skvaril, F., and Hitzig, W. H.: IgG subclass: Development of the serum concentrations in "normal" infants and children. J. Pediatr. 80:960-964, 1972.

411. Moretta, A., Bottino, C., Mingari, M. C., et al.: What is natural killer cell? Nat. Immunol. 3:6-8, 2002.

412. Moretta, L., Bottino, C., Pende, D., et al.: Human natural killer cells: Their origin, receptors and function. Eur. J. Immunol. 32:1205-1211, 2002.

413. Moser, M., and Murphy, K. M.: Dendritic cell regulation of T_H1-T_H2 development. Nat. Immunol. 1:199-205, 2000.

414. Mosmann, T. R., Li, L., Hengartner, H., et al.: Differentiation and functions of T cell subsets. Ciba Found. Symp. 204:148-154, 1997.

415. Moy, J. N., Nelson, R. D., Richards, K. L., and Hostetter, M. K.: Identification of an IgA inhibitor of neutrophil chemotaxis and its membrane target for the metabolic burst. Immunology 69:257-262, 1990.

416. Muller-Eberhard, H. J.: Complement: Chemistry and pathways. In Gallin, J. I., and Snyderman, R. (eds.): Inflammation: Basic Principles and Clinical Correlates. 2nd ed. New York, Raven Press, 1992, pp. 33-61.

417. Murphy, K. M., Heimberger, A. B., and Loh, D. Y.: Induction by antigen of intrathymic apoptosis of CD4+ CD8+ TCRlo thymocytes in vivo. Science 250:1720-1723, 1990.

418. Murphy, K. M., and Reiner, S. L.: The lineage decisions of helper T cells. Nat. Rev. Immunol. 2:933-944, 2002.

419. Murphy, P. M.: The molecular biology of leukocyte chemoattractant receptors. Annu. Rev. Immunol. 12:593-633, 1994.

420. Nagata, M., Hara, T., Aoki, T., et al.: Inherited deficiency of ninth component of complement: An increased risk of meningococcal meningitis. J. Pediatr. 114:260-264, 1989.

421. Nakamura, T., Kamogawa, Y., Bottomly, K., and Flavell, R. A.: Polarization of IL-4- and IFN-gamma-producing CD4+ T cells following activation of naive CD4+ T cells. J. Immunol. 158:1085-1094, 1997.

422. Naot, Y. D., Desmonts, G., and Remington, J. S.: IgM enzyme-linked immunosorbent assay test for the diagnosis of congenital Toxoplasma infection. J. Pediatr. 98:32-36, 1981.

423. Nath, J., Flavin, M., and Gallin, J. I.: Tubulin tyrosinolation in human polymorphonuclear leukocytes: Studies in normal subjects and in patients with Chédiak-Higashi syndrome. J. Cell. Biol. 95:519-526, 1982.

424. Nauseef, W. M., Root, R. K., and Malech, H. L.: Biochemical and immunologic analysis of hereditary myeloperoxidase deficiency. J. Clin. Invest. 71:1307-1307, 1983.

425. Newburger, P. E., Cohen, H. J., Rothchild, S. B., et al.: Prenatal diagnosis of chronic granulomatous disease. N. Engl. J. Med. 300:178-181, 1979.

426. Niyonsaba, F., Iwabuchi, K., Matsuda, H., et al.: Epithelial cell-derived human beta-defensin-2 acts as a chemotaxin for mast cells through a pertussis toxin-sensitive and phospholipase C-dependent pathway. Int. Immunol. 14:421-426, 2002.

427. Niyonsaba, F., Ogawa, H., and Nagaoka, I.: Human beta-defensin-2 functions as a chemotactic agent for tumour necrosis factor-alpha-treated human neutrophils. Immunology 111:273-281, 2004.

428. Noble, W. C.: Skin microbiology: Coming of age. J. Med. Microbiol. 17:1-12, 1984.

429. Noelle, R. J., Ledbetter, J. A., and Aruffo, A.: CD40 and its ligand, an essential ligand-receptor pair for thymus-dependent B-cell activation. Immunol. Today 13:431-433, 1992.

430. Norderhaug, I. N., Johansen, F. E., Schjerven, H., and Brandtzaeg, P.: Regulation of the formation and external transport of secretory immunoglobulins. Crit. Rev. Immunol. 19:481-508, 1999.

431. Norment, A. M., Salter, R. D., Parham, P., et al.: Cell-cell adhesion mediated by CD8 and MHC class I molecules. Nature 336:79-81, 1988.

432. Nossal, G. J. V.: The molecular and cellular basis of affinity maturation in the antibody response. Cell 68:1-2, 1992.

433. Notarangelo, L. D., Chirico, G., Chiara, A., et al.: Activity of classical and alternative pathways of complement in preterm and small for gestational age infants. Pediatr. Res. 18:281-285, 1984.

434. Notarangelo, L. D., Duse, M., and Ugazio, A. G.: Immunodeficiency with hyper-IgM (HIM). Immunodefic. Rev. 3:101-122, 1992.

435. Nunoi, H., Yamazaki, T., Tsuchiya, H., et al.: A heterozygous mutation of β-actin associated with neutrophil dysfunction and recurrent infection. Proc. Natl. Acad. Sci. U. S. A. 96:8693-8698, 1999.

436. Ochs, H. D., Nonoyama, S., Zhu, Q., et al.: Regulation of antibody responses: The role of complement and adhesion molecules. Clin. Immunol. Immunopathol. 67:S33-S40, 1993.

437. Ochs, H. D., and Wedgwood, R. J.: IgG subclass deficiencies. Annu. Rev. Med. 38:325-340, 1987.

438. Ochs, H. D., Wedgwood, R. J., Heller, S. R., et al.: Complement, membrane glycoproteins and complement receptors: Their role in regulation of the immune response. Clin. Immunol. Immunopathol. 40:94-104, 1986.

439. Ochs, H. D., and Winkelstein, J.: Disorders of the B-cell system. In Stiehm, E. R. (ed.): Immunologic Disorders in Infants and Children. 4th ed. Philadelphia, W. B. Saunders, 1996, pp. 296-338.

440. Oettinger, M. A., Schatz, D. G., Gorka, C., et al.: RAG-1 and RAG-2, adjacent genes that synergistically activate V(D)J recombination. Science 248:1517-1523, 1990.

441. Oliver, A. M., Sewell, H. F., Abramovich, D. R., et al.: The distribution and differential expression of MHC class II antigens (HLA-DR, DP, and DQ) in

human fetal adrenal, pancreas, thyroid and gut. Transplant. Proc. *21*:651-652, 1989.

442. O'Neill, L. A., and Greene, C.: Signal transduction pathways activated by the IL-1 receptor family: Ancient signaling machinery in mammals, insects, and plants. J. Leukoc. Biol. *63*:650-657, 1998.

443. O'Neill, L. A. J.: TLRs: Professor Mechnikov, sit on your hat. Trends Immunol. *25*:687-693, 2004.

444. Opdenakker, G., Van den Steen, P. E., Dubois, B., et al.: Gelatinase B functions as regulator and effector in leukocyte biology. J. Leukoc. Biol. *69*:851-859, 2001.

445. Oppenheim, J. J., Biragyn, A., Kwak, L. W., and Yang, D.: Roles of antimicrobial peptides such as defensins in innate and adaptive immunity. Ann. Rheum. Dis. *62*(Suppl. 2):17-21, 2003.

446. Oppenheim, J. J., and Feldman, M.: Introduction to the role of cytokines in innate host defense and adaptive immunity. *In* Oppenheim, J. J., Feldman, M., Durum, S. K., et al.: (eds): Cytokine Reference. San Diego, Academic Press, 2001, pp. 3-20.

447. Ott, M. G., Schmidt, M., Schwartzwaelder, K., et al.: Correction of X-linked chronic granulomatous disease by gene therapy, augmented by insertional activation of MDS1-EVI1, PRDM16, or SETBP1. Nat. Med. *12*:401-409, 2006.

448. Otternhoff, T. H., De Boer, T., van Dissel, J. T., and Verreck, F. A. Human deficiencies in type 1 cytokine receptors reveal the essential role of type 1 cytokines in immunity to intracellular bacteria. Adv. Exp. Med. Biol. *531*:279-294, 2003.

449. Ouinti, I., Soresinsa, A., Spadaro, G., et al.: Long-term follow-up and outcome of a large cohort of patients with common variable immunodeficiency. J. Clin. Immunol. *27*:308-316, 2007.

450. Oxelius, V.-A.: IgG subclass levels in infancy and childhood. Acta Paediatr. Scand. *68*:23-27, 1979.

451. Oxelius, V.-A., Laurell, A. B., Linquist, B., et al.: IgG subclasses in selective IgA deficiency. N. Engl. J. Med. *304*:1476-1477, 1981.

452. Ozen, M., Mehmet, C., Ozden, S., et al.: Recurrent *Salmonella* bacteremia in interleukin-12 receptor β1 deficiency. J. Trop. Pediatr. *52*:296-298, 2006.

453. Ozsahin, H., Le Deist, F., Benkerrou, M., et al.: Bone marrow transplantation in 26 patients with Wiskott-Aldrich syndrome from a single center. J. Pediatr. *129*:238-244, 1996.

454. Padigel, U. M., Lee, J. J., Nolan, T. J., et al.: Eosinophils can function as antigen-presenting cells to induce primary and secondary immune responses to *Strongyloides stercoralis*. Infect. Immun. *74*:3232-3238, 2006.

455. Padlan, E. A.: Anatomy of the antibody molecule. Mol. Immunol. *31*:169-217, 1994.

456. Palaniyar, N., Nadesalingam, J., and Reid, K. B.: Pulmonary innate immune proteins and receptors that interact with gram-positive bacterial ligands. Immunobiology *205*:575-594, 2002.

457. Pangburn, M. K.: The alternative pathway. *In* Ross, G. D. (ed.): Immunobiology of the Complement System. Orlando, Academic Press, 1986, pp. 45-62.

458. Papavasiliou, F. N., and Schatz, D. G.: Somatic hypermutation of immunoglobulin genes: Merging mechanisms for genetic diversity. Cell *109*(Suppl.): S35-S44, 2002.

459. Parker, D. C.: T cell-dependent B-cell activation. Annu. Rev. Immunol. *11*:331-340, 1993.

460. Parry, M. F., Root, R. K., Metcalf, J. A., et al.: Myeloperoxidase deficiency: Prevalence and clinical significance. Ann. Intern. Med. *95*:293-301, 1981.

461. Paul, W. E.: Pleiotropy and redundancy: T cell-derived lymphokines in the immune response. Cell *57*:521-524, 1989.

462. Perez, E., and Sullivan, K. E.: Chromosome 22q11.2 deletion syndrome (DiGeorge and velocardiofacial syndromes). Curr. Opin. Pediatr. *14*:678-683, 2002.

463. Perlmuter, D. H., and Colten, H. R.: Molecular immunobiology of complement biosynthesis: A model of single-cell control of effector-inhibitor balance. Annu. Rev. Immunol. *4*:231-251, 1986.

464. Perregaux, D. G., Bhavsar, K., Contillo, L., et al.: Antimicrobial peptides initiate IL-1 beta posttranslational processing: A novel role beyond innate immunity. J. Immunol. *168*:3024-3032, 2002.

465. Peterson, S. V., Thiel, S., and Jensenius, J. C.: The mannan-binding lectin pathway of complement activation: biology and disease association. Mol. Immunol. *38*:133-149, 2001.

466. Pier, G. B., Grout, M., Zaidi, T. S., et al.: Role of mutant CFTR in hypersusceptibility of cystic fibrosis patients to lung infections. Science *271*:64-67, 1996.

467. Pizzo, P. A., Robechaud, K. J., Gill, F. A., et al.: Empiric antibiotic and antifungal therapy for cancer patients with prolonged fever and granulocytopenia. Am. J. Med. *72*:101-111, 1982.

468. Plaeger, S. F.: Principal human cytokines. *In* Stiehm, E. R. (ed.): Immunologic Disorders in Infants and Children. 4th ed. Philadelphia, W. B. Saunders, 1996, pp. 1063-1065.

469. Pollack, J. D., Williams, D. A., Gifford, M. A., et al.: Mouse model of X-linked chronic granulomatous disease, an inherited defect in phagocyte superoxide production. Nat. Genet. *9*:202-209, 1995.

470. Porcelli, S. A., and Modlin, R. L.: The CD1 system: Antigen-presenting molecules for T cell recognition of lipids and glycolipids. Annu. Rev. Immunol. *17*:297-329, 1999.

471. Provenzano, R. W., Wetterlow, L. H., and Sullivan, C. L.: Immunization and antibody response in the newborn infant. N. Engl. J. Med. *273*:959-965, 1965.

472. Puck, J. M., and Malech, H. L.: Gene therapy for immune disorders: Good news tempered by bad news. J. Allergy Clin. Immunol. *117*:865-869, 2006.

473. Purkerson, J., and Isakson, P.: A two-signal model for regulation of immunoglobulin isotype switching. F. A. S. E. B. J. *6*:3245-3252, 1992.

474. Quie, P. G., White, J. G., Holmes, B., et al.: In vitro bactericidal capacity of human polymorphonuclear leukocytes: Diminished activity in chronic granulomatous disease of childhood. J. Clin. Invest. *46*:668-679, 1967.

475. Raghavan, S., and Holmgren, J.: CD4+CD25+ suppressor T cells regulate pathogen induced inflammation and disease. F. E. M. S. Immunol. Med. Microbiol. *44*:121-127, 2004.

476. Rago, J. V., and Schlievert, P. M.: Mechanisms of pathogenesis of staphylococcal superantigens. Curr. Top. Microbiol. Immunol. *225*:81-97, 1998.

477. Rappeport, J. M., Newburger, P. E., Goldblum, R. M., et al.: Allogeneic bone marrow transplantation for chronic granulomatous disease. J. Pediatr. *101*:952-955, 1982.

478. Rawal, N., and Pangburn, M. K.: Structure/function of C5 convertases of complement. Int. Immunopharmacol. *1*:415-422, 2001.

479. Regelmann, W., Hays, N., and Quie, P. G.: Chronic granulomatous disease: Historical perspective and clinical experience at the University of Minnesota Hospitals. *In* Gallin, J. I., and Fauci, A. S. (eds.): Advances in Host Defense Mechanisms. Vol. 3. New York, Raven Press, 1983, pp. 3-23.

480. Regunathan, J., Chen, Y., Wang, D., and Malarkannan, S.: NKG2D receptor-mediated NK cell function is regulated by inhibitory Ly49 receptors. Blood *105*:233-240, 2005.

481. Revy, P., Muto, T., Levy, Y., et al.: Activation-induced cytidine deaminase (AID) deficiency causes the autosomal recessive form of the hyper-IgM syndrome (HIGM2). Cell *102*:565-575, 2000.

482. Rice, T. W., and Bernard, G. R.: Therapeutic intervention and targets for sepsis. Annu. Rev. Med. *56*:225-248, 2005.

483. Rieux-Laucat, F., Hivroz, C., Lim, A., et al.: Inherited and somatic CD3zeta mutations in a patient with T-cell deficiency. N. Engl. J. Med. *354*:1913-1921, 2006.

484. Robey, E. A., Fowlkes, B. J., Gordon, J. W., et al.: Thymic selection in CD8 transgenic mice supports an instructive model for commitment to a CD4 or CD8 lineage. Cell *64*:99-107, 1991.

485. Robin, L. F., Lees, P. S. J., Winget, M., et al.: Wood-burning stoves and lower respiratory illnesses in Navajo children. Pediatr. Infect. Dis. J. *15*:859-865, 1996.

486. Robin, N. H., and Shprintzen, R. J.: Defining the clinical spectrum of deletion 22q11.2. J. Pediatr. *147*:90-96, 2005.

487. Roche, P. A., and Cresswell, P.: Invariant chain association with HLA-DR molecules inhibits immunogenic peptide binding. Nature *345*:615-618, 1990.

488. Rock, K. L., Gamble, S., Rothstein, L., et al.: Dissociation of β2-microglobulin leads to the accumulation of a substantial pool of inactive class I MHC heavy chains on the cell surface. Cell *85*:611-620, 1991.

489. Romani, N., Koide, S., Crowley, M., et al.: Presentation of exogenous protein antigens by dendritic cells to T cell clones: Intact protein is presented best by immature, epidermal Langerhans cells. J. Exp. Med. *169*:1169-1178, 1989.

490. Roos, D., Weening, R. S., Voteman, A. A., et al.: Protection of phagocytic leukocytes by endogenous glutathione: Studies in a family with glutathione reductase deficiency. Blood *53*:851-857, 1979.

491. Root, R. K., and Cohen, M. S.: The microbicidal mechanisms of human neutrophils and eosinophils. Rev. Infect. Dis. *3*:565-598, 1981.

492. Root, R. K., Metcalf, J., Oshino, N., et al.: H2O2 release from human granulocytes during phagocytosis, I. Documentation, quantitation, and some regulating factors. J. Clin. Invest. *55*:945-955, 1975.

493. Rosen, F. S., Cooper, M. D., and Wedgwood, R. J.: The primary immunodeficiencies. N. Engl. J. Med. *311*:235-242, 1984.

494. Rosen, F. S., and Janeway, C. A.: The gamma globulins, III: The antibody deficiency syndromes. N. Engl. J. Med. *275*:769-775, 1966.

495. Rosenfield, S. I., Baum, J., Steigbigel, R. T., et al.: Hereditary deficiency of the fifth component of complement in man, II: Biological properties of C5-deficient human serum. J. Clin. Invest. *57*:1635-1643, 1976.

496. Rosenfield, S. I., Kelly, M. E., and Leddy, J. P.: Hereditary deficiency of the fifth component of complement in man, I: Clinical, immunochemical, and family studies. J. Clin. Invest. *57*:1626-1634, 1976.

497. Rosenkilde, M. M.: Virus-encoded chemokine receptors—putative novel antiviral drug targets. Neuropharmacology *48*:1-13, 2005.

498. Rosenzweig, S. D., and Holland, S. M.: Defects in the interferon-γ and interleukin-12 pathways. Immmunol. Rev. *203*:38-47, 2005.

499. Ross, S. C., and Densen, P.: Complement deficiency states and infection: Epidemiology, pathogenesis, and consequences of neisserial and other infections in an immune deficiency. Medicine *63*:243-273, 1984.

500. Rossi, D., and Zlotnik, A.: The biology of chemokines and their receptors. Annu. Rev. Immunol. *18*:217-242, 2000.

501. Rudd, C. E.: Disabled receptor signaling and new primary immunodeficiency disorders. N. Engl. J. Med. *354*:1874-1877, 2006.

502. Ruddy, S., Carpenter, C. B., Chin, K. W., et al.: Human complement metabolism: An analysis of 144 studies. Medicine *54*:165-178, 1975.

503. Rudensky, A. Y., Preston-Hurlburt, P., Hong, S. C., et al.: Sequence analysis of peptides bound to MHC class II molecules. Nature *353*:622-627, 1991.

504. Russel, J. H., and Ley, T. J.: Lymphocyte-mediated cytotoxicity. Annu. Rev. Immunol. *20*:323-370, 2002.

505. Rutenberg, W. D., Yang, M. C., Doberstyn, B., et al.: Multiple leukocyte abnormalities in chronic granulomatous disease: A familial study. Pediatr. Res. 11:158-163, 1977.

506. Sacchi, F., Augustine, N. H., and Hill, H. R.: Abnormality in actin polymerization associated with defective chemotaxis in neutrophils from neonates. Int. Arch. Allergy Appl. Immunol. 84:32-39, 1987.

507. Sacchi, F., and Hill, H. R.: Defective membrane potential changes in neutrophils from human neonates. J. Exp. Med. 160:1247-1252, 1984.

508. Saiman, L., and Prince, A.: *Pseudomonas aeruginosa* pili bind to asialoGM1 which is increased on the surface of cystic fibrosis epithelial cells. J. Clin. Invest. 92:1875-1880, 1993.

509. Sallusto, F., Lenig, D., Forster, R., et al.: Two subsets of memory T lymphocytes with distinct homing potentials and effector functions. Nature 401:708-712, 1999.

510. Salmon, J. E., Edberg, J. C., and Kimberly, R. P.: Fcγ receptor III on human neutrophils: Allelic variants have functionally distinct capacities. J. Clin. Invest. 85:1287-1295, 1990.

511. Salmon, J. E., Kapur, S., and Kimberly, R. P.: Opsonin-independent ligation of Fcγ receptors; the 3G8-bearing receptors on neutrophils mediate the phagocytosis of concanavalin A-treated erythrocytes and non-opsonized *E. coli*. J. Exp. Med. 166:1798-1813, 1987.

512. Sandberg, E. T., Kline, M. W., and Shearer, W. T.: The secondary immunodeficiencies. *In* Stiehm, E. R. (ed.): Immunologic Disorders in Infants and Children. 4th ed. Philadelphia, W. B. Saunders, 1996, pp. 553-601.

513. Sato, K., Hida, S., Takayanagi, H., et al.: Antiviral response by natural killer cells through TRAIL gene induction by IFN-alpha/beta. Eur. J. Immunol. 31:3138-3146, 2001.

514. Schaffer, A. A., Salzer, U., Hammmarstrom, L., and Grimbacher, B.: Deconstructing common variable immunodeficiency by genetic analysis. Curr. Opin. Genet. Dev. 17:201-212, 2007.

515. Schaffer, F. M., and Ballow, M.: Immunodeficiency: The office work-up. J. Respir. Dis. 16:523-546, 1995.

516. Schatz, D. G., Oettinger, M. A., and Schlissel, M. S.: V (D) J recombination: Molecular biology and regulation. Annu. Rev. Immunol. 10:359-384, 1992.

517. Schmidt, A. P., Taswell, H. F., and Gleich, G. J.: Anaphylactic transfusion reaction associated with anti-IgA antibody. N. Engl. J. Med. 280:188-193, 1969.

518. Schoub, B. D., Johnson, S., McAnerney, J., et al.: Monovalent neonatal polio immunization—a strategy for the developing world. J. Infect. Dis. 147:836-839, 1988.

519. Schur, P. H.: IgG subclasses: A historical perspective. Monogr. Allergy 23:1-11, 1988.

520. Schur, P. H., Rosen, F., and Norman, M. E.: Immunoglobulin subclasses in normal children. Pediatr. Res. 13:181-183, 1979.

521. Schutte, B. C., Mitros, J. P., Bartlett, J. A., et al.: Discovery of five conserved beta-defensin gene clusters using a computational search strategy. Proc. Natl. Acad. Sci. U. S. A. 99:2129-2133, 2002.

522. Scott, M. G., Vreugdenhil, A. C., Buurman, W. A., et al.: Cutting edge: Cationic antimicrobial peptides block the binding of lipopolysaccharide (LPS) to LPS binding protein. J. Immunol. 164:549-553, 2000.

523. Screpanti, V., Wallin, R. P., Ljunggren, H. G., and Grandien, A.: A central role for death receptor-mediated apoptosis in the rejection of tumors by NK cells. J. Immunol. 167:2068-2073, 2001.

524. Seger, R. A., Gungor, T., Belohradsky, B. H., et al.: Treatment of chronic granulomatous disease with myeloablative conditioning and an unmodified hemopoietic allograft: A survey of the European exerience. Blood 100:4344-4350, 2002.

525. Seo, S. M., McIntire, L. V., and Smith, C. W.: Effects of IL-8, Gro-alpha, and LTB(4) on the adhesive kinetics of LFA-1 and Mac-1 on human neutrophils. Am. J. Physiol. Cell. Physiol. 281:C1568-C1578, 2001.

526. Shackelford, P. G.: IgG subclasses: Importance in pediatric practice. Pediatr. Rev. 14:291-296, 1993.

527. Shackelford, P. G., and Granoff, D. M.: IgG subclass composition of the antibody response of healthy adults, and normal or IgG2-deficient children and to immunization with *H. influenzae* type b polysaccharide vaccine or Hib PS-protein conjugate vaccines. Monogr. Allergy 23:269-281, 1988.

528. Shackelford, P. G., Granoff, D. M., Madassery, J. V., et al.: Clinical and immunologic characteristics of healthy children with subnormal serum concentrations of IgG2. Pediatr. Res. 27:16-21, 1990.

529. Shackelford, P. G., Granoff, D. M., Polmar, S. H., et al.: Subnormal serum concentrations of IgG2 in children with frequent infections associated with varied patterns of immunologic dysfunction. J. Pediatr. 116:529-538, 1990.

530. Shackelford, P. G., Polmar, S. H., Mayus, J. L., et al.: Spectrum of IgG2 subclass deficiency in children with recurrent infections: Prospective study. J. Pediatr. 108:647-653, 1986.

531. Shapiro, R., Beatty, D. W., Woods, L. I., et al.: Serum complement and immunoglobulin values in small-for-gestational-age infants. J. Pediatr. 99:139-141, 1981.

532. Shurin, S. B., Socransky, S. S., Sweeney, E., and Stossel, T. P.: A neutrophil disorder induced by *Capnocytophaga*, a dental micro-organism. N. Engl. J. Med. 301:849-854, 1979.

533. Siu, G., Kronenberg, M., Strauss, E., et al.: The structure, rearrangement and expression of D$_\beta$ gene segments of the murine T-cell antigen receptor. Nature 311:344-350, 1984.

534. Smith, C. W.: Molecular determinants of neutrophil adhesion. Am. J. Respir. Cell. Mol. Biol. 2:487-489, 1990.

535. Smith, C. W., Hollers, J. C., Dupree, E., et al.: A serum inhibitor of leukotaxis in a child with recurrent infections. J. Lab. Clin. Med. 79:878-883, 1972.

536. Smith, C. W., Marlin, S. D., Rothlein, R., et al.: Cooperative interaction of LFA-1 and Mac-1 with intercellular adhesion molecule-1 in facilitating adherence and transendothelial migration of human neutrophils in vitro. J. Clin. Invest. 83:2008-2017, 1989.

537. Smith, C. W., Rothlein, R., Hughes, B. J., et al.: Recognition of an endothelial determinant for CD18-dependent human neutrophil adherence and transendothelial migration. J. Clin. Invest. 82:1746-1756, 1988.

538. Smith, D. H., Peter, G., Ingram, D. L., et al.: Responses of children immunized with the capsular polysaccharide of *Haemophilus influenzae*. Pediatrics 52:637-644, 1973.

539. Smith, J. J., Travis, S. M., Greenberg, E. P., and Welsh, M. J.: Cystic fibrosis airway epithelia fail to kill bacteria because of abnormal airway surface fluid. Cell 86:1-20, 1996.

540. Smith, R. T., Eitzman, D. V., Catlin, M. E., et al.: The development of the immune response. Pediatrics 33:163-183, 1964.

541. Smolen, P., Bland, R., Heiligenstein, E., et al.: Antibody response to oral polio vaccine in premature infants. J. Pediatr. 103:917-920, 1983.

542. Smyth, M. J., Cretney, E., Kelly, J. M., et al.: Activation of NK cell cytotoxicity. Mol. Immunol. 42:501-510, 2005.

543. Smyth, M. J., Hayakawa, Y., Takeda, K., and Yagita, H.: New aspects of natural-killer-cell surveillance and therapy of cancer. Nat. Rev. Cancer 2:850-861, 2002.

544. Snyderman, R., Pike, M. C., and Altman, L. C.: Abnormalities of leukocyte chemotaxis in human disease. Ann. N. Y. Acad. Sci. 256:386-388, 1975.

545. Solvason, N., and Kearney, J. F.: The human fetal omentum: A site of B cell generation. J. Exp. Med. 175:397-404, 1992.

546. Soriano, R. B., South, M. A., Goldman, A. S., and Smith, C. W.: Defect of neutrophil motility in a child with recurrent bacterial infections and disseminated cytomegalovirus infection. J. Pediatr. 83:951-955, 1973.

547. Southwick, F. S., Holbrook, T., Howard, T., et al.: Neutrophil actin dysfunction is associated with a deficiency of Mol. Clin. Res. 34:533A, 1986.

548. Southwick, F. S., Howard, T. H., Holbrook, T., et al.: The relationship between CR3 deficiency and neutrophil actin assembly. Blood 73:1973-1979, 1989.

549. Spielberg, S. P., Boxer, L. A., Oliver, J. M., et al.: Oxidative damage to neutrophils in glutathione synthetase deficiency. Br. J. Haematol. 42:215-223, 1979.

550. Spitznagel, J. K., Cooper, M. R., McCall, A. E., et al.: Selective deficiency of granules associated with lysozyme and lactoferrin in human polymorphs with reduced microbicidal capacity. J. Clin. Invest. 51:93A, 1972.

551. Spitznagel, J. K., Dalldorf, F. G., Leffell, M. S., et al.: Character of azurophil and specific granules purified from human polymorphonuclear leukocytes. Lab. Invest. 30:774-785, 1974.

552. Springer, T. A., and Anderson, D. C.: The importance of adherence, chemotaxis, and migration into inflammatory sites: Insights from an experiment of nature. *In* Evered, D., Nugent, J., and O'Connor, M. (eds.): Biochemistry of Macrophages. Ciba Foundation Symposium. London, Pittman, 1986, pp. 102-126.

553. Springer, T. A., Thompson, W. S., Miller, J., et al.: Inherited deficiency of the Mac-1, LFA-1, P150,95 glycoprotein family and its molecular basis. J. Exp. Med. 160:1901-1918, 1984.

554. Staretz-Haram, O., Melamed, R., and Lifshitz, M.: Interleukin-12 receptor β1 deficiency presenting as recurrent *Salmonella* infection. Clin. Infect. Dis. 37:137-140, 2003.

555. Stavnezer, J.: Immunoglobulin class switching. Curr. Opin. Immunol. 8:199-205, 1996.

556. Steinstraesser, L., Tippler, B., Mertens, J., et al.: Inhibition of early steps in the lentiviral replication cycle by cathelicidin host defense peptides. Retrovirology 2:2-13, 2005.

557. Stepick-Biek, P., Thulliez, P., Araujo, F. G., et al.: IgA antibodies for diagnosis of acute congenital and acquired toxoplasmosis. J. Infect. Dis. 162:270-273, 1990.

558. Stevens, R., Dichek, D., Keld, B., et al.: IgG$_1$ is the predominant subclass of in vivo- and in vitro-produced anti-tetanus toxoid antibodies and also serves as the membrane IgG molecule for delivering inhibitory signals to anti-tetanus toxoid antibody-producing B cells. J. Clin. Immunol. 3:65-69, 1983.

559. Stiehm, E. R., and Fudenberg, H. H.: Serum levels of immune globulins in health and disease: A survey. Pediatrics 37:715-727, 1966.

560. Stossel, T. P.: Phagocytosis: Recognition and ingestion. Semin. Hematol. 12:83, 1975.

561. Stossel, T. P.: The mechanical responses of white blood cells. *In* Gallin, J. I., Goldstein, I. M., and Snyderman, R. (eds.): Basic Principles and Clinical Correlates. New York, Raven Press, 1992, pp. 459-475.

562. Strauss, R. G., and Snyder, E. L.: Chemotactic peptide binding by intact neutrophils from human neonates. Pediatr. Res. 18:63-66, 1984.

563. Summerfield, J. A., Sumiya, M., Levin, M., and Turner, M. W.: Association of mutations in mannose binding protein gene with childhood in consecutive hospital series. B. M. J. 314:1229-1232, 1997.

564. Sutton, B. J., and Gould, H. J.: The human IgE network. Nature 366:421-428, 1993.

565. Swain, S.: T cell subsets and the recognition of MHC class. Immunol. Rev. 74:129-142, 1983.

566. Tack, K. J., Rham, F. S., Brown, B., et al.: *Aspergillus* osteomyelitis: Report of four cases and review of the literature. Am. J. Med. 73:295-300, 1982.
567. Taitz, L. S., Zarate-Salvador, C., and Schwartz, E.: Congenital absence of the parathyroid and thymus glands in an infant (III and IV pharyngeal pouch syndrome). Pediatrics 38:412-418, 1966.
568. Takeuchi, O., Hoshino, K., Kawai, T., et al.: Differential roles of TLR2 and TLR4 in recognition of gram-negative and gram positive bacterial cell wall components. Immunity 11:443-451, 1999.
569. Taylor, P. W.: Bactericidal and bacteriolytic activity of serum against gram-negative bacteria. Microbiol. Rev. 47:46-83, 1983.
570. Tenen, D. G., Hromas, R., Licht, J. D., and Zhang, D. E.: Transcription factors, normal myeloid development, and leukemia. Blood 90:489-519, 1997.
571. Tew, J. G., DiLosa, R. M., Burton, G. F., et al.: Germinal centers and antibody production in bone marrow. Immunol. Rev. 126:99-112, 1992.
572. Teyton, L., O'Sullivan, D., Dickson, P. W., et al.: Invariant chain distinguishes between the exogenous and endogenous antigen presentation pathways. Nature 348:39-44, 1990.
573. Teyton, L., and Peterson, P. A.: Assembly and transport of MHC class II molecules. New Biol. 4:441-447, 1992.
574. Thery, C., and Amigorena, S.: The cell biology of antigen presentation in dendritic cells. Curr. Opin. Immunol. 13:45-51, 2001.
575. Timens, W., Boes, A., Rozeboom-Uiterwijk, T., and Poppema, S.: Immaturity of the human splenic marginal zone in infancy: Possible contribution to the deficiency infant immune response. J. Immunol. 143:3200-3206, 1989.
576. Tosi, M., and Berger, M.: Functional differences between the 40 kDa and 50 to 70 IgG Fc receptors on human neutrophils revealed by elastase treatment and antireceptor antibodies. J. Immunol. 141:2097-2103, 1988.
577. Tosi, M. F.: Innate immune responses to infection. J. Allergy Clin. Immunol. 116:241-249, 2005.
578. Tosi, M. F., Anderson, D. C., Barrish, J., et al.: Effect of piliation on interactions of *Haemophilus influenzae* type b with human polymorphonuclear leukocytes. Infect. Immun. 47:780-785, 1985.
579. Tosi, M. F., and Hamedani, A.: A rapid, specific assay for superoxide release from phagocytes in small volumes of whole blood. Am. J. Clin. Pathol. 97:566-573, 1992.
580. Tosi, M. F., and Zakem, H.: Surface expression of Fcγ receptor III (CD16) on chemoattractant-stimulated neutrophils is determined by both surface shedding and translocation from intracellular storage compartments. J. Clin. Invest. 90:462-470, 1990.
581. Tosi, M. F., Zakem, H., and Berger, M.: Neutrophil elastase cleaves C3bi on opsonized *Pseudomonas* as well as CR1 on neutrophils to create a functionally important opsonin-receptor mismatch. J. Clin. Invest. 86:300-308, 1990.
582. Townsend, A., and Bodmer, H.: Antigen recognition by class I-restricted T lymphocytes. Annu. Rev. Immunol. 7:601-624, 1989.
583. Trambas, C. M., and Griffiths, G. M.: Delivering the kiss of death. Nat. Immunol. 4:399-403, 2003.
584. Trapani, J. A., and Smyth, M. J.: Functional significance of the perforin/granzyme cell death pathway. Nat. Rev. Immunol. 2:735-747, 2002.
585. Tsukada, S., Saffran, D. C., Rawlings, D. J., et al.: Deficient expression of a B cell cytoplasmic tyrosine kinase in human X-linked agammaglobulinemia. Cell 72:279-290, 1993.
586. Uckun, F. M., Dibirdik, I., Smith R., et al.: Interleukin 7 receptor ligation stimulates tyrosine phosphorylation, inositol phospholipid turnover, and clonal proliferation of human B-cell precursors. Proc. Natl. Acad. Sci. U. S. A. 88:3589-3593, 1991.
587. Unkeless, J. C., Shen, Z., Lin, C. W., and DeBeus, E.: Function of human Fc gamma RIIA and Fc gamma RIIIB. Semin. Immunol. 7:37-44, 1995.
588. van der Pol, W.-L., and van de Winkel, J. G. J.: IgG receptor polymorphisms: Risk factors for disease. Immunogenetics 48:222-232, 1998.
589. Van Dyke, T. E., Horoszewicz, H. U., and Genco, R. J.: The polymorphonuclear leukocyte (PMNL) locomotor defect in juvenile periodontitis: Study of random migration, chemokinesis and chemotaxis. J. Peridontol. 53:682-687, 1982.
590. Van Epps, D., Palmer, D. L., and Williams, R. C.: Characterization of serum inhibitors of neutrophil chemotaxis is associated with anergy. J. Immunol. 113:189-200, 1974.
591. van Tuinen, P., Johnson, K. R., Ledbetter, S., et al.: Localization of myeloperoxidase to the long arm of human chromosome 17: Relationship to the 15:17 translocation of acute promyelocytic leukemia. Oncogene 1:319-326, 1987.
592. van Zelm, M. C., Reisli, I., vander Burg, M., et al.: An antibody deficiency syndrome due to mutations in the CD19 gene. N. Engl. J. Med. 354:1901-1912, 2006.
593. Vanderkerckhove, B. A. E., Baccala, R., Jones, D., et al.: Thymic selection of the human T-cell receptor Vβ repertoire in SCID-hu mice. J. Exp. Med. 176:1619-1624, 1992.
594. Vanichkin, A., Patya, M., Gazit, A., et al.: Late administration of lipophilic tyrosine kinase inhibitor prevents lipopolysaccharide and *Escherichia coli*-induced lethal toxicity. J. Infect. Dis. 173:927-933, 1996.
595. Vedder, N. B., and Harlan, J. M.: Increased surface expression of CD11b/CD18 (Mac-1) is not required for stimulated neutrophil adherence to cultured endothelium. J. Clin. Invest. 81:676-682, 1988.
596. Vetrie, D., Vorechovsky, I., Sideras, F., et al.: The gene involved in X-linked agammaglobulinemia is a member of the *src* family of protein-tyrosine kinases. Nature 361:226-233, 1993.
597. Villadangos, J. A.: Presentation of antigens by MHC class II molecules: Getting the most out of them. Mol. Immunol. 38:329-346, 2001.
598. Vivier, E., Nunes, J. A., and Vely, F.: Natural killer cell signaling pathways. Science 306:1517-1519, 2004.
599. Volpp, B. D., Nauseef, W. M., Donelson, J. E., et al.: Cloning of the cDNA and functional expression of the 47 kilodalton cytosolic component of the human neutrophil respiratory burst oxidase. Proc. Natl. Acad. Sci. U. S. A. 86:7195-7199, 1989.
600. von Andrian, U. H., Berger, E. M., Ramezani, L., et al.: In vivo behavior of neutrophils from two patients with distinct inherited leukocyte adhesion deficiency syndromes. J. Clin. Invest. 91:2893-2897, 1993.
601. von Boehmer, H., Teh, H. S., and Kisielow, P.: The thymus selects the useful, neglects the useless and destroys the harmful. Immunol. Today 10:57-61, 1989.
602. Vora, P., Youdim, A., Thomas, L. S., et al.: Beta-defensin-2 expression is regulated by TLR signaling in intestinal epithelial cells. J. Immunol. 173:5398-5405, 2004.
603. Waage, A., Halstensen, A., and Espevik, T.: Association between tumor necrosis factor in serum and fatal outcome in patients with meningococcal disease. Lancet 1:355-357, 1987.
604. Walker, R. I., and Willemze, R.: Neutrophil kinetics and the regulation of granulopoiesis. Rev. Infect. Dis. 2:282-292, 1980.
605. Walter, M. A., Surti, U., Hofker, M. H., et al.: The physical organization of the human immunoglobulin heavy chain gene complex. E. M. B. O. J. 9:3303-3313, 1990.
606. Wang, H., Bloom, O., Zhang, M., et al.: HMG-1 as a late mediator of endotoxin lethality in mice. Science 285:248-251, 1999.
607. Wang, L., Fuster, M., Sriramarao, P., and Esko, J. D.: Endothelial heparan sulfate deficiency impairs L-selectin- and chemokine-mediated neutrophil trafficking during inflammatory resonses. Nat. Immunol. 6:902-910, 2005.
608. Wang, X., Zhang, Z., Louboutin, J. P., et al.: Airway epithelia regulate expression of human beta-defensin 2 through Toll-like receptor 2. F. A. S. E. B. J. 17:1727-1729, 2003.
609. Ward, P. A., and Schlegel, R. J.: Impaired leukotactic responsiveness in a child with recurrent infection. Lancet 2:344-347, 1969.
610. Weaver, L. J., Craddock, P. R., and Jacob, H. S.: Association of complement activation and elevated plasma-C5a with adult respiratory distress syndrome: Patholophysiological relevance and possible prognostic value. Lancet 1:947-949, 1980.
611. Weisdorf, D. J., Craddock, P. R., and Jacob, H. S.: Granulocytes utilize different energy sources for movement and phagocytosis. Inflammation 6:245-251, 1982.
612. Weiss, J., Victor, M., and Elsbach, P.: Role of charge and hydrophobic interactions in the action of the bactericidal/permeability-increasing protein of neutrophils on gram-negative bacteria. J. Clin. Invest. 71:540-549, 1983.
613. Welsh, M. J., and Smith, A. E.: Molecular mechanisms of CFTR chloride channel dysfunction in cystic fibrosis. Cell 73:1251-1254, 1993.
614. Wen, L., Atkinson, J. P., and Giclas, P. C.: Clinical and laboratory evaluation of complement deficiency. J. Allergy Clin. Immunol. 113:585-593, 2004.
615. Westminster Hospitals Bone-Marrow Transplant Team: Bone marrow transplant from an unrelated donor for chronic granulomatous disease. Lancet 1:210-213, 1977.
616. Wheat, L. J., Connolly-Stringfield, P. A., and Baker, R. L.: Disseminated histoplasmosis in the acquired immune deficiency syndrome: Clinical findings, diagnosis and treatment, and review of the literature. Medicine 69:361-374, 1990.
617. Whitley, R. J., and Arvin, A. M.: Herpes simplex virus infections. *In* Remington, J. S., Klein, J. O. (eds.): Infectious Diseases of the Fetus and Newborn Infant. 4th ed. Philadelphia, W. B. Saunders, 1995, pp. 354-376.
618. Wickham, T. J., Mathias, P., Cheresh, D. A., and Nemerow, G. R.: Integrins αvβ3 and αvβ5 promote adenovirus internalization but not virus attachment. Cell 73:309-319, 1993.
619. Wilson, C. B., Ochs, H. D., Almquiest, J., et al.: When is umbilical cord separation delayed? J. Pediatr. 107:292-293, 1985.
620. Wilson, R. K., Lai, E., Concannon, P., et al.: Structure, organization and polymorphism of murine and human T-cell receptors αβ chain gene families. Immunol. Rev. 101:149-172, 1988.
621. Winkelstein, J. A., Lambert, G. H., and Swift, A.: Pneumococcal serum opsonizing activity in splenectomized children. J. Pediatr. 87:430-433, 1975.
622. Winkelstein, J. A., Marino, M. C., Johnston, R. B., et al.: Chronic granulomatous disease: Report on a national registry of 368 patients. Medicine 79:155-169, 2000.
623. Wu, L., Gerard, N. P., Wyatt, R., et al.: CD4-induced interaction of primary HIV-1 gp120 glycoproteins with the chemokine receptor CCR-5. Nature 384:179-183, 1996.
624. Yang, D., Chen, Q., Schmidt, A. P., et al.: LL-37, the neutrophil granule- and epithelial cell-derived cathelicidin, utilizes formyl peptide receptor-like 1 (FPRL1) as a receptor to chemoattract human peripheral blood neutrophils, monocytes, and T cells. J. Exp. Med. 192:1069-1074, 2000.
625. Yang, D., Chertov, O., Bykovskaia, S. N., et al.: Beta-defensins: Linking innate and adaptive immunity through dendritic and T cell CCR6. Science 286:525-528, 1999.
626. Yang, K. D., and Hill, H. R.: Immune responses to infectious diseases: An evolutionary perspective. Pediatr. Infect. Dis. J. 15:355-364, 1996.

627. Yeung, C. Y., and Hobbs, J. R.: Serum-gamma G-globulin levels in normal, premature, post-mature and "small-for-dates" newborn babies. Lancet 1:1167-1170, 1968.
628. Zach, T. L., and Hostetter, M. K.: Biochemical abnormalities of the third component of complement in neonates. Pediatr. Res. 26:116-120, 1989.
629. Zarember, K. A., and Godowski, P. J.: Tissue expression of human toll-like receptors and differential regulation of toll-like receptor mRNAs in leukocytes

in response to microbes, their products, and cytokines. J. Immunol. 168:554-561, 2002.
630. Zemmour, J., and Parham, P.: HLA class I nucleotide sequences. Hum. Immunol. 31:195-206, 1991.
631. Zimmerman, G. A.: Two by two: The pairings of P-selectin and P-selectin glycoprotein ligand-1. Proc. Natl. Acad. Sci. U. S. A. 98:10023-10024, 2001.

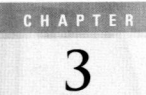

METABOLIC RESPONSE OF THE HOST TO INFECTIONS

Alina Olteanu ◦ Ralph D. Feigin ◦ William R. Beisel

Although infectious microorganisms constitute a continuing threat at all ages of life, they are particularly dangerous in neonates, infants, and young children. Despite the availability of modern sanitation, public health measures, vaccines, and antibiotics, most children have many discrete episodes of acute infection before reaching adulthood. Depending on their severity and duration, infectious illnesses can interrupt normal growth patterns. More importantly, if closely spaced in time, a series of infections can initiate a downhill health spiral, leading to malnutrition, chronic debilitation, immune system dysfunction, and death.[12,14,86,87,129] This possibility is of greatest concern in newborns and weaning children, especially in Third World areas.

The human host normally protects itself against invading microorganisms by maintaining a broad array of general defensive mechanisms and immunologic responses. This array includes the initiation of acute-phase reactions triggered by the release of proinflammatory cytokines from macrophages, monocytes, and other cells.[7,12,14,42] The resulting nonspecific defensive measures typically include fever and anorexia, slow-wave sleep, accelerated production of phagocytic cells, hormonal responses, and participation of many biochemical pathways and molecular mechanisms within body cells.[7,8,10-12,14,170] The acute-phase reaction produces stereotyped patterns of transient metabolic sequelae (diagrammed in Fig. 3–1), which accompany and follow most acute, generalized infectious illnesses and some localized ones.[60] A pediatrician should anticipate these metabolic changes so as to recognize dangerous complications, such as hypoglycemia and electrolyte imbalance, that may occur during an acute infection.

The array of metabolic changes depicted in Figure 3–1 typically is shared as a group of common responses during all generalized acute infectious diseases.[6-9,12,13,141] Similar changes are seen during other types of disease or trauma when they are accompanied by fever or inflammatory reactions.[75] These common acute-phase responses are composed of a hypermetabolic admixture of anabolic and catabolic components. Each 1° C of fever causes basal cellular oxygen consumption to increase approximately 13 percent.[8] The resultant increase in cellular energy expenditure comes at a time when food intake and intestinal absorption are diminished by anorexia and sometimes by vomiting and diarrhea. In the absence of an adequate intake of nutrients, body energy needs are met mostly by the oxidation of metabolic substrates that are derived from nutrient stores already contained within body tissues. The hypermetabolic effects of acute fever are fueled primarily by carbohydrates (some of which are derived from the metabolism of amino acids),[8] but if infectious illnesses become subacute or chronic, body fats become the important sustaining fuel.

Generalized acute-phase metabolic responses may be modified by numerous factors, such as the severity of an infectious process, its duration, and its possible progression to a subacute or chronic disease.[7-12,14] The age and sex of the patient, the presence of genetic resistance (or susceptibility) factors or partial immunity, the adequacy of nonspecific defensive mechanisms and de novo immune responsiveness, the preexisting nutritional status, and the presence or absence of other diseases all combine to modify host metabolic responses through their diverse influences on the infectious process per se.

Superimposed on this general array of common host metabolic responses are additional metabolic changes that occur when an infectious process becomes localized within certain anatomic sites or organ systems. Diarrhea that develops during gastrointestinal infections can lead to depletion of fluids and electrolytes, hepatic infections can lead to derangements of carbohydrate and amino acid metabolism, and infections of the central nervous system that cause neuronal destruction are accompanied by muscle paralysis and atrophy. Other infections localized within the cranial vault often produce an inappropriate secretion of antidiuretic hormone, leading to development of dangerous overhydration in children.[14] The development of shock syndromes during infectious diseases imposes additional metabolic derangements because of progressive stagnant hypoxia.[10,135]

In recent years, the role of genetic variations in host genes important in the immune response to infections has been studied. Wide variations in individual response to several microorganisms, such as *Chlamydia trachomatis*[38] and *Candida albicans*, have been documented.[148]

The total number of discrete metabolic responses known to occur during acute and chronic infectious illnesses continues to expand.[10] The most widely recognized of these multiple responses are grouped for discussion into major categories, including changes in nitrogen, amino acid, carbohydrate, lipid, electrolyte, vitamin, and trace element metabolism. Another important mechanism involved in the host response to infection is oxidative stress, which plays a major role in the systemic inflammatory response in bacterial[153] and viral infections.[147] The important initiating and control mechanisms provided by cytokines, antioxidants, and the endocrine system also are discussed.

Importantly, each of the many individual metabolic changes that occur during the course of an infection must be interpreted in a manner that reflects its longitudinal development and progression over time and its relationship to the evolving phases of the infectious process.[7] Some metabolic changes may be detected during the incubation period, many other responses occur at the onset of fever, and still other phenomena develop during the recovery phase of illness or later during convalescence.

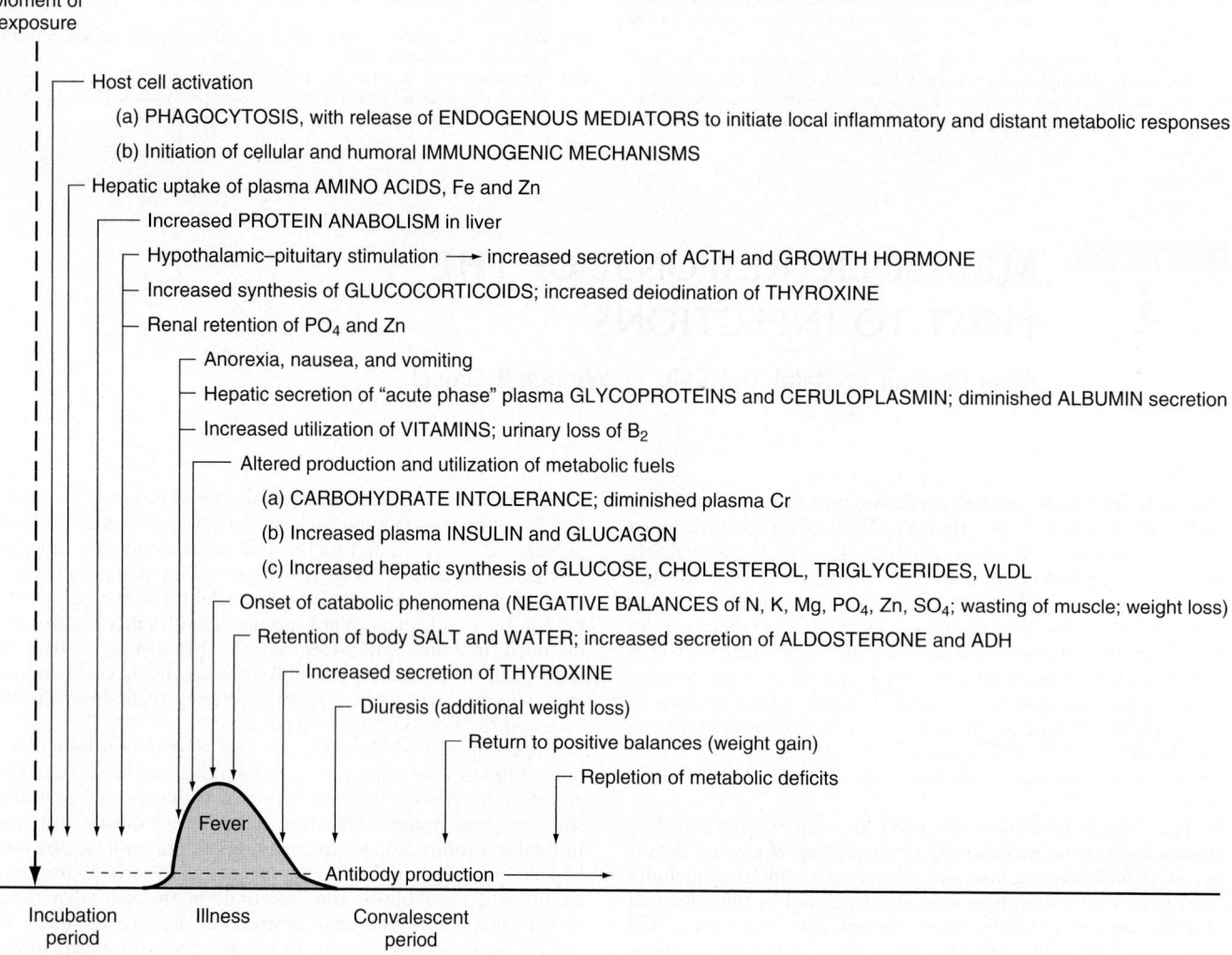

Figure 3–1 Onset time of various host metabolic responses in relation to the sequential phases of a "model" acute, self-limited, generalized infectious illness. *(From McKigney, J. I., and Munro, H. N. [eds.]: Nutrient Requirements in Adolescence. Cambridge, MA, MIT Press, 1976, p. 250.)*

NITROGEN METABOLISM

Fever and its accompanying hypermetabolic state, as induced by acute-phase responses during infectious illnesses, trigger a complex assortment of changes in protein, amino acid, and nitrogen metabolism.[9] Although the catabolic destruction of skeletal muscle protein is most obvious clinically, important anabolic events occur simultaneously. These events involve the synthesis of new proteins and cells that are important in host defense mechanisms. Increases in whole-body protein turnover involve catabolic and anabolic events in chronic infections also, as shown by leucine kinetic studies in patients with human immunodeficiency virus (HIV) infections.[82] Using amino acids isotope tracing techniques to measure muscle protein synthesis, researchers also showed that high plasma HIV RNA interferes with muscle amino acid synthesis and muscle proteolysis.[174]

NITROGEN BALANCE STUDIES

Because the ability of body cells to synthesize new proteins is a fundamental necessity for maintaining all known host defensive mechanisms, including the immunologic ones, understanding the changes that occur in the nitrogen metabolism of an infected individual is important.[110] When the availability of free amino acids within body pools is restricted by diet or disease, the catabolism of certain existing body proteins (chiefly the contractile proteins of skeletal muscle) generates the free amino acids required to synthesize new body proteins with higher priorities in terms of the many new proteins needed for defensive purposes. Information about these metabolic responses has been gained through quantitative analyses of proteins and other nitrogen-containing compounds in tissues, body fluids, and excretions, and through kinetic studies with tagged molecules.[82,99,107,122,158]

One useful approach has been the measurement of nitrogen balance throughout the sequential course of an infectious process.[9,10,110] Daily measurements of nitrogen intake and all nitrogen losses that occur via different routes are obtained to determine whether the body is losing or retaining nitrogen. Other investigative techniques are needed to provide specific information about the molecular mechanisms involved in producing any observed changes in nitrogen balance. Nonetheless, the use of balance techniques has provided information concerning the typical losses of body nitrogen and muscle mass during acute generalized infections (Fig. 3–2). Quantitation of these catabolic losses provides an important framework of reference for more detailed studies of changes in nitrogen metabolism.

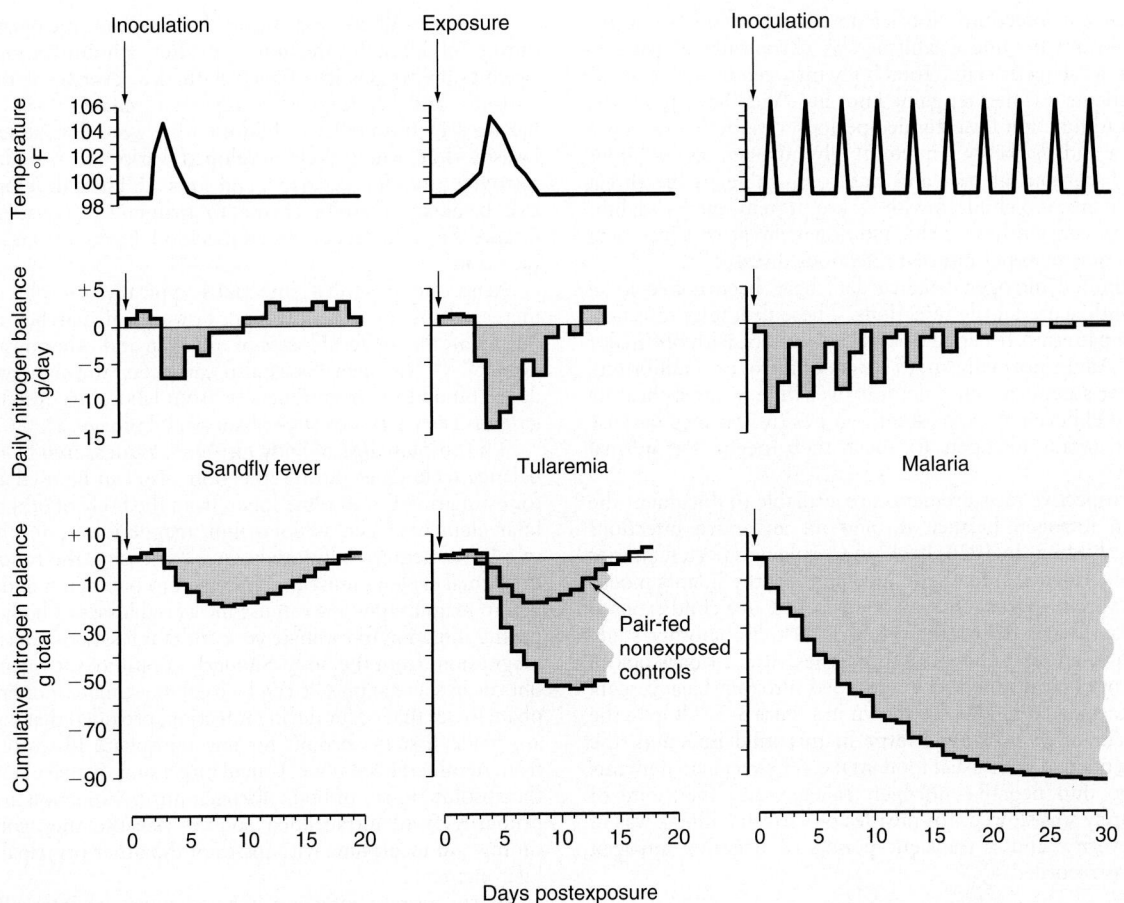

Figure 3–2 Comparisons between the occurrence of fever (top) and changes in daily nitrogen balance (middle) and cumulative nitrogen (bottom) in patients with viral, bacterial, and generalized parasitic infections. Cumulative balance values for pair-fed healthy control subjects show the amounts of body nitrogen loss that can be ascribed to diminished food intake during infection. *(From McKigney, J. I., and Munro, H. N. [eds.]: Nutrient Requirements in Adolescence. Cambridge, MA, MIT Press, 1976, p. 261.)*

A comprehensive series of nitrogen balance studies was obtained in young adult male volunteers subjected to different kinds of experimentally induced infections during the course of studies to test vaccine efficacy.[9] Extensive normal baseline data were obtained on each volunteer before the time of his or her inoculation with or exposure to infectious bacteria, viruses, or rickettsiae. Longitudinal serial measurements made throughout the course of the infectious process allowed for a comprehensive, prospective evaluation of metabolic balance changes in nitrogen and other elements to be obtained.[9]

Nitrogen balances did not change from baseline values during the incubation periods of the infectious diseases studied (see Fig. 3–2). The body began to lose nitrogen only after symptoms and fever had begun. These losses persisted for a period encompassing the acute illness. In convalescence, the subjects began to retain nitrogen so that gradually, over the course of several weeks, body nitrogen losses were regained. Similar nitrogen balance studies were conducted in healthy control volunteers who were not infected.[9,13,15] Instead, these controls were subjected to (1) partial food deprivation to mimic the anorexia-induced reduction in dietary intake measured in the patients with infection, (2) a 24-hour exposure to artificially induced high environmental temperatures to produce an increase in body temperature comparable to that seen in patients with infection, (3) treatment with antibiotic therapy in courses identical to those given to patients with infections, or (4) treatment with oral hydrocortisone using sequentially changing daily doses to mimic the measured adrenal responses of infected subjects.

These balance studies showed that the major losses in body nitrogen resulted from the combined effects of a reduced intake of food plus a continued (or increased) loss of nitrogen via the urine.[9] In contrast, simple starvation produced a prompt decrease in the daily losses of nitrogen via the urine. A patient with an acute infectious illness differed markedly from someone subjected to only simple dietary deprivation. Urinary nitrogen losses did not decline appreciably, or they increased in the presence of fever, whether the fever was caused by an active infection or an artificial increase in environmental temperatures.[15] The control studies also showed that the negative nitrogen balances that occurred during infection were not caused by adrenal glucocorticoid hormones or the antibiotics used in therapy.[7,13] Rather, by terminating infection quickly, antibiotics helped to reverse the loss of body nitrogen, allowing a more rapid restoration of nitrogen stores.

Because the loss of sizable quantities of nitrogen has important nutritional consequences, the same balance data were used to determine patterns of cumulative loss of body nitrogen.[7,9,10] As shown in Figure 3–2, total losses of body nitrogen grew progressively larger as the acute febrile phase of illness continued; the cumulative total loss of body nitrogen persisted throughout early convalescence. When nitrogen balances finally became positive, nitrogen was recovered over the course of weeks as body stores were accumulated slowly.

Studies performed in adult patients with infections such as tuberculosis and malaria suggested that the depletion of body stores of protein nitrogen did not continue unabated during subacute or chronic infection.[67] Rather, a new state of relative nitrogen equilibrium became established as chronically ill patients lapsed into a cachectic state. Total body nitrogen in such chronically ill patients was neither gained nor lost. Vital body processes continued to function for extended periods, despite the presence of cachexia and markedly depleted body nitrogen stores.[8] This state was hazardous at best and was comparable to the threat faced by infants and children with severe protein-energy malnutrition, who constantly face the additional threat of developing dangerous new or superimposed infectious diseases.[86,87,104,129]

Only limited nitrogen balance data have been collected in children with acute febrile infections. These data tend to reflect closely the patterns of change described in adults, with one major exception. Adults normally are in a state of nitrogen equilibrium, with neither a net gain nor a net loss over time, whereas healthy infants and children are consistently in positive balance because they must retain nitrogen to meet their needs for normal growth.

Few prospective measurements are available to document the changes in nitrogen balance throughout an entire infectious process in children. In 1926, Beck[6] in Germany reported a series of metabolic balance studies conducted in healthy infants inoculated with vaccinia virus. One study was begun in a child exposed to varicella 15 days before the onset of pustules; another study was begun in an infant exposed to measles virus 14 days before the onset of clinical illness. The grouped nitrogen balance data from the vaccinated infants are shown in Figure 3–3. Despite the development of a short-lived fever in this mild infection, the infants maintained their usual food intake. The vaccinated infants did not go into negative nitrogen balance, and their rate of growth barely was slowed.[6] In measles or varicella, illness was of greater severity, and a transient period of negative nitrogen balance was recorded.

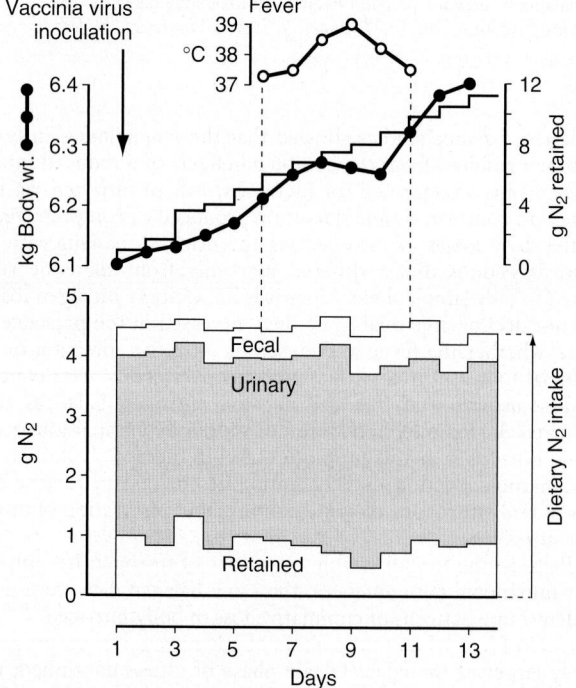

Figure 3–3 Sequential measurements of body weight and cumulative nitrogen balance (top) and daily nitrogen balance (bottom) in a group of five healthy infants inoculated with vaccinia virus. Nitrogen intake values (plotted upward from baseline) and fecal and urinary losses (plotted downward from intake) reveal that the growing infants continued to retain nitrogen despite having brief periods of fever. *(Drawn from numerical data published by Beck.[6])*

Similarly, Viteri and Behar[156] measured nitrogen balance during childhood infections or after administration of live vaccines. Nitrogen loss varied with the severity of the illness. Wilson and colleagues[172] reported changes in nitrogen balances in hospitalized children who were convalescing from kwashiorkor when they developed varicella. A reduction in nitrogen retention occurred, and some children developed negative balances. Despite efforts to maintain a constant dietary intake, the children consumed less food during the course of the infection.

Acute nondiarrheal infections typically do not cause an increased loss of fecal nitrogen; however, if diarrhea is present during an illness, fecal losses of nitrogen and other nutrients can occur.[104,126] Nitrogen losses also can occur through sweat, exudates, blood loss (from illness or from laboratory tests), sputum, gaseous exchanges, or sites of surgical drainage.[9,15]

The absolute loss of body nitrogen, as measured by metabolic balance techniques during infection, also can be used as a guide for estimating the absolute losses from the body of other intracellular elements, such as potassium, magnesium, phosphate, and, to a lesser degree, sulfur and zinc.[9,10] By using the ratios present in normal skeletal muscle of nitrogen to potassium and of nitrogen to magnesium, one can use measured losses of body nitrogen during infection to estimate concomitant losses of potassium and magnesium from the body. Similarly, a ratio of nitrogen to phosphorus in skeletal muscle can be used to estimate inorganic phosphate losses that occur during infection, provided that corrections are made first to account for any phosphate losses originating from demineralized bone. Calculations such as these suggest that the absolute losses of body nitrogen during infection are derived primarily from intracellular sources because they correlate in timing and magnitude with losses of the other principal intracellular elements.[9]

In contrast to infection-induced losses of intracellular elements, the losses of extracellular ions, sodium and chloride, follow an independent course during infection. Calcium losses are minimal in acute infection in the absence of long-term bed rest or paralysis with body immobilization.[9,168]

A newer method to measure total protein metabolism involves the use of a single oral dose of [15N] glycine. This method was used to study children with septic shock as a result of meningococcemia and showed that the protein metabolism of these patients is increased significantly compared with healthy children.[41] A similar method was used previously in children with malaria, HIV, and measles.[41]

URINARY EXCRETION OF NITROGEN-CONTAINING COMPOUNDS

The onset of fever typically is accompanied by an increased urinary loss of creatinine. This loss usually is followed within 1 day by increased losses of urea and ammonia.[9] Although alpha-amino nitrogen losses may increase transiently at the onset of fever in some infections, this excretion tends to be lower than baseline measurements during the remainder of the illness and throughout convalescence. When measured prospectively, excretion of urinary alpha-amino nitrogen or most individual free amino acids did not change appreciably during sandfly fever, a mild virus infection.[159] In contrast, urinary losses of 3-methylhistidine and phenylalanine increased. The increased loss of phenylalanine seemed to reflect its increased concentrations in plasma.[160] Studies using radioactive compounds in rats suggested that most of the excess urea excreted during an acute infection was generated by the deamination of endogenous amino acids derived principally from skeletal muscle.[10]

Increased excretion of one of the amino acids, 3-methylhistidine, serves to indicate the extent of skeletal muscle catabolism.

This amino acid cannot be reused after its release from contractile proteins.[80,178]

Uric acid excretion may increase during febrile periods, but the greatest changes have been reported during infectious mononucleosis.[102] Uric acid losses are ascribed to an accelerated turnover of nucleic acids and enhanced purine degradation.

An increased excretion of urinary diazo reactants commonly occurs during most acute infectious illnesses, especially typhoid fever. These reactants include metabolites, such as kynurenine, 3-hydroxykynurenine, o-aminohippuric acid, xanthurenic acid, and anthranilic acid, which are created during the accelerated hepatic metabolism of tryptophan via the kynurenine pathway.[118]

A sudden, dramatic increase in urinary nitrate excretion occurs during acute infections. This increase is a reflection of the cytokine-stimulated production of nitric oxide as a host defensive measure.[44,139,144,157]

METABOLISM OF FREE AMINO ACIDS

The distribution, use, and metabolism of free amino acids undergo profound alterations during the course of acute infectious illness. Measurements in patients show patterns of change that can be explained by studies performed in experimental laboratory animals.[46,110,113,161] As some proteins are produced, others are degraded, and many of the released amino acids are redistributed throughout the body before they are reused.

A diminution in the concentration of most free individual amino acids in plasma may begin before the onset of symptoms. Hypoaminoacidemia generally persists throughout the febrile period of an illness, the largest decreases occurring in the branched-chain amino acids, leucine, isoleucine, and valine.[99] The decline in branched-chain amino acids is caused primarily by an accelerated uptake of free amino acids by the liver. This increased flux from plasma to liver has been shown to occur in several species of animals during a variety of infections.[99] The amino acids that enter the liver are used for a variety of purposes. Amino acids may be metabolized to other compounds, oxidized, or reused for the synthesis of new proteins. Interleukin-6 (IL-6) seems to trigger many of the alterations in hepatic protein and amino acid metabolism that occur during an acute infection.[12,133]

Amino acids become important sources of energy during the hypermetabolic phase of acute infections. Some amino acids are oxidized directly in muscle, whereas others are transformed progressively into glucose and glucagon. Gluconeogenic amino acids, such as alanine, are deaminated; their carbon skeletons are used as the principal substrate for producing glucose; and their nitrogen is used to create urea for excretion.

Serum and the total body pool of certain amino acids are depleted in various infections, presumably to diminish the substrate that some microorganism may use to replicate. Interferon-γ secretion causes a depletion of the body pool of tryptophan to retard the progression of *Chlamydia* infection.[116] A complete spectrum of amino acids is required for the synthesis of new body proteins generated during infection, including hepatic enzymes,[119] such as tryptophan oxygenase and tyrosine transaminase, and the lipoproteins and glycoproteins released into the plasma.[10,110,111] This group of glycoproteins constitutes the "acute-phase reactants," which include alpha₁-antitrypsin, amyloid, alpha₁-acid glycoprotein, haptoglobin, C-reactive protein, fibrinogen (the third component of complement), and ceruloplasmin.

These acute-phase reactant proteins are produced in excess during infections, even in protein-deficient children who exhibit acute kwashiorkor.[108] Some of the potentially beneficial functions attributed to acute-phase reactants include an amplification of humoral and cell-mediated immunity, antiproteinase effects that could limit or contain harmful enzymes liberated during inflammatory reactions, oxidase activities, and the detoxification of free hemoglobin.[110]

In addition to the accelerated synthesis of proteins within the liver, infection increases the production of phagocytic and lymphoid cells. A need to produce increased quantities of such diverse proteins as the cytokines, complement and kinin components, fibronectin, and the several classes of immunoglobulins also exists. All of these requirements involve the need for free amino acids.

Proinflammatory cytokines and interferon-γ stimulate the production of nitric oxide from arginine, its sole precursor.[44,157] Among the many important biologic effects of nitric oxide are the effects resulting from its being a highly potent microbicidal, parasiticidal, and tumoricidal agent,[139] and from having major immunomodulatory functions.[84] Research also has shown that nitric oxide may act as an antiviral agent against adenoviruses and other similar viruses.[25]

The importance of nitric oxide in these roles may rival those of free oxygen radicals in potency and effectiveness.[144] This newly recognized host defense agent is generated when cytokine-induced nitric oxide synthase initiates the oxygenation of one of arginine's guanido nitrogen groups to produce citrulline and nitric oxide.[139] During sepsis, arginine balance becomes negative, as consumption of arginine exceeds the rate of synthesis. Because arginine is the sole source of nitric oxide, it becomes an essential amino acid in critically ill children.[4] Arginine also plays an important role in wound healing. In patients with infected chronic wounds, total plasma arginine is decreased, and wound healing is impaired secondary to defective usage of arginine.[36]

AMINO ACID AVAILABILITY

In the presence of anorexia and a diminished intake of food nutrients, the body in large measure must use endogenous sources to supply its increased amino acid needs. The principal sources of potentially available endogenous amino acids are the proteins of somatic tissues, including skeletal muscle and skin. The free amino acid pool contains the equivalent of approximately 12.5 g of protein in a normal man, an amount that represents only 0.1 percent of total body protein.[158] Because the normal turnover of protein in a healthy adult is approximately 200 to 250 g each day, the free amino acid pool must be resupplied continually from endogenous and exogenous sources. During infections, the absorption of individual amino acids from the intestine may be depressed and delayed[93] or increased,[33] depending on the infection.

Protein synthesis is not stopped entirely within body somatic tissues during an infection, but it is slowed markedly. At the same time, the rates of degradation of somatic proteins are accelerated so that a net loss of muscle, skin, and other somatic proteins occurs through catabolic wasting. Catabolic degradation of skeletal muscle protein can be initiated by IL-1,[5,8,31,42] which triggers muscular proteases via the intracellular production of prostaglandin E₂. The body apparently sacrifices contractile proteins of skeletal muscle to obtain the free amino acids needed for higher priority requirements.

Some of the amino acids liberated during muscle protein catabolism are lost directly to the plasma. Others, such as the branched-chain group, are used in situ as sources of energy for muscle fibers; after oxidation, their amino groups are used to manufacture new glutamine and alanine, which can be used elsewhere for gluconeogenesis.[80] Because the branched-chain amino acids can be oxidized within skeletal muscle, their rate of release from muscle is decreased, which exaggerates the decline in their concentrations in plasma.[10,99,158] Branched-chain amino acids also play a major role in protein synthesis for lymphocytes and in immunity.[23] Some of the free amino acids liberated within muscle are retained within contractile cells and reused for the slowed but continuing process of muscle protein anabolism.

This catabolic breakdown of somatic protein to supply amino acids for use in other parts of the body is a highly visible clinical phenomenon. In this regard, the proteins of skin, skeletal muscle, and other somatic structures seem to constitute the principal body pool of "labile" nitrogen, which is called on to maintain protein homeostasis and the physiologic functions of visceral tissues during periods of infectious illness or other stresses. Because infants and small children have very little muscle protein (and a very small "bank" of readily available amino acids), the infection-induced need for free amino acids puts them at a special disadvantage.

To study the complex interrelationships involved in amino acid metabolism, workers have used isotopes to measure the simultaneous rates of anabolism and catabolism in the protein of skeletal muscle and other tissues of experimental animals during the course of infection.[122] In addition, clinically useful estimates of skeletal muscle degradation can be obtained in patients through the quantitative daily measurements of 3-methylhistidine excretion into urine. More than 90 percent of the total body content of 3-methylhistidine is associated with the peptide chains of actin in all muscle and of myosin in white muscle fibers.[178] This unique amino acid is formed in situ through the transmethylation of histidine, but only after the histidine first has been incorporated into the amino acid structure of myofibrillar proteins. When released, 3-methylhistidine cannot be reused by the body and instead is lost via the urine.

The increase in excretion of 3-methylhistidine during acute infections is in keeping with other estimates of skeletal muscle wasting. The extent to which proteolysis occurs during periods of severe surgical sepsis also has been quantified by measuring the differences among concentrations of glucose, lactate, free fatty acids, ketones, and alanine in femoral arterial and venous blood.[106] Neither free fatty acid nor ketone use was increased during occurrences of acute fevers, but an increased oxidation of glucose and of amino acids derived from protein was used to fuel cellular hypermetabolism. Although infection stimulates a sizable increase in the rates of body protein synthesis, the acceleration of protein catabolism is increased even further, and the body experiences a net loss of somatic proteins and even some visceral ones.[158]

Phenylalanine is one of the amino acids released by the accelerated catabolism of somatic proteins. Only limited amounts of phenylalanine can be used, however, for the synthesis of new proteins or for its conversion into tyrosine.[158,160] Phenylalanine concentrations in the circulating free amino acid pool tend to increase rather than decrease during periods of fever. These increases occur coincidentally with the typical declines in plasma values for tyrosine and most other free amino acids. The exaggerated phenylalanine-to-tyrosine ratio can be useful for evaluating these opposing changes during febrile illnesses. An increase in this ratio is a useful clinical index of the severity of infection-induced alterations in amino acid metabolism.[158] During occurrences of infections of great severity and infections with hepatocellular dysfunction, hypoaminoacidemia may be replaced by an excessive accumulation of many other free amino acids in plasma.[10,135,170]

Free tryptophan, also liberated from degrading protein, undergoes an accelerated metabolism via several different metabolic pathways in the liver.[10,96,97,112] In response to the increased hepatic availability of tryptophan or the increased synthesis of tryptophan oxygenase, or both, excess tryptophan enters the kynurenine pathways, where it is converted into different diazo-reactant compounds and pyrimidine nucleotides.[112] At the same time, tryptophan enters other pathways, leading possibly to increased synthesis of serotonin or indoleacetic acid.[118]

CARBOHYDRATE METABOLISM

During the febrile phase of infectious illnesses, carbohydrate metabolism provides much of the additional energy needed by body cells. An increased demand for metabolizable energy is met by a resetting of the endocrine control mechanisms to permit a marked acceleration of the synthesis and release of glucose from the liver.[35,54,171] Although some glucose is derived from hepatocellular glycogen, most additional requirements for glucose during acute infections are met by accelerated hepatic gluconeogenic mechanisms. Recycled lactate and amino acids, especially amino acids with gluconeogenic potential, such as alanine, are the principal substrates used by the liver to increase its output of newly synthesized glucose; glycerol (derived from the metabolism of triglyceride lipids) and pyruvate also are used.[80]

Early in acute infectious illnesses, basal blood glucose concentrations tend to become elevated. Diabetic patients who require insulin often develop glycosuria at the onset of febrile infections, and more insulin must be given to maintain their control. The tendency for acute infections to be accompanied by an early modest hyperglycemia also is seen in laboratory animals. Modest hyperglycemia often is noted in animals after they have been injected with bacterial endotoxin.[21,89]

Although an early hyperglycemic response seems to be the initial change in carbohydrate metabolism, the ability of the body to sustain an accelerated production of glucose may be lost. Hypoglycemia may emerge as an important clinical problem. Hypoglycemia generally results from one of two major pathogenic mechanisms: a diminished availability of substrate molecules required for gluconeogenesis or a failure of the metabolic mechanisms needed to produce hepatic glucose. Carbohydrate pathway defects at the molecular level have not been found in overwhelming bacterial infections in laboratory animals.[61,103] Carbohydrate depletion during overwhelming or terminal infections can be ascribed to nonavailability of substrate. If hepatic cells are injured during an infectious disease, such as viral hepatitis, hypoglycemia can result from a failure of gluconeogenic processes.[10,47,126]

The depletion of substrate for adequate gluconeogenesis occurs primarily as a dangerous clinical complication of neonatal sepsis. Infants are born with only minimal amounts of skeletal muscle protein. Because muscle contains the principal "labile nitrogen" pool for supplying amino acids that can be converted into glucose, neonatal infants lack a sufficient quantity of potential substrate molecules for sustaining long-term gluconeogenesis. Newborns especially are prone to develop severe hypoglycemia whenever a septic process becomes established.[176] Hypoglycemia that results from a breakdown of hepatic gluconeogenic mechanisms occurs primarily when liver cells are damaged by an infectious or toxemic process. Hypoglycemia can become an important complicating factor in severe viral hepatitis, yellow fever, or endotoxemia during gram-negative sepsis.[47,89] These conditions can cause hepatocellular damage and a breakdown of enzyme-synthesizing mechanisms within the liver.[89]

A change in glucose tolerance can be detected within hours after the onset of a febrile infection.[121,132] Baseline blood glucose values may be elevated, and disappearance of glucose is slowed moderately as a component aspect of a febrile illness. Under these circumstances, the pancreatic islets produce insulin in excess quantities. Despite an increase in plasma insulin concentrations, glucose disappearance rates are slowed; these combined metabolic changes resemble the changes caused by mild insulin resistance. In low-birth-weight neonates, hyperglycemia could be an ominous sign and suggests the presence of systemic fungal infections.[85]

Bacterial and viral infections also cause increased secretion of pancreatic glucagon,[121,124] which, together with release of catecholamines accompanying infection,[58,60,171] provides hormonal stimuli for accelerating gluconeogenesis within the liver. These hormonal stimuli initiate their hepatic effects during infection by activating adenylate cyclase.[35] The unusual simultaneous increase in basal concentrations of insulin and glucagon in plasma results from direct cytokine stimulation of pancreatic islet cells.[8,53,175] Because of these hormonal changes and high plasma glucocorticoid values in patients with severe bacterial sepsis, infusions of glucose may fail to suppress hepatic gluconeogenesis.[80,81] The resultant increase in glucose pool size helps to explain the apparent slowing of glucose disappearance and the hyperinsulinemia that occur during infections.

Certain viral infections in children seem prone to initiate acute juvenile-type, insulin-requiring diabetes mellitus. Although the evidence for a viral cause of diabetes has not been established fully in humans, epidemiologic findings indicate that juvenile diabetes may develop several months after onset of certain viral illnesses, especially mumps, coxsackievirus B (type 4) infection, rubella, or cytomegalovirus infection.[101] Additional epidemiologic evidence is based on a tendency for new cases of juvenile-type diabetes to appear in clusters.

Susceptibility to juvenile diabetes also may be influenced by genetic make-up. A high incidence of human leukocyte antigen types B8 and Bw15 has been detected in juvenile diabetics.[127] Studies in laboratory animals suggest that genetically susceptible species may have virus receptor sites on their insulin-producing beta cells. These receptors in species with high-risk haplotypes allow viruses to be absorbed by the pancreatic beta cells, with subsequent destruction of insulin-producing cells.

The cytokine granulocyte colony-stimulating factor influences the uptake of glucose by phagocytic cells and their mobilization during inflammatory reactions.[77] Availability of glucose contributes directly to the respiratory burst that accompanies phagocytosis and to the production of the myeloperoxidase enzymes needed to kill engulfed organisms.

LIPID METABOLISM

As Table 3–1 shows, numerous changes in lipid metabolism have been documented during infection. In contrast to the stereotyped patterns of change in nitrogen and amino acid metabolism and in the accelerated production of glucose, responses involving body lipids vary more from infection to infection. Plasma lipid changes also may be biphasic during the course of a single infection. This complexity results partly from the multiple factors that control the metabolism of lipids during infectious illnesses,[10,135] including the need for hepatic synthesis of serum lipoproteins, variations in the production and use of free fatty acids and ketones as sources of cellular energy, and variable changes in rates of uptake or release of lipids from body fat depots.[10,135]

Lipids have another function that is crucial during acute-phase reactions. This function involves the cytokine-stimulated use of polyunsaturated fatty acids localized within cell walls to serve as precursor molecules for various families of eicosanoids (prostaglandins, prostacyclins, thromboxanes, and lipoxins). These eicosanoid lipids trigger many of the diverse cellular responses seen during infection, inflammation, and immune responses.[73,123]

PLASMA LIPIDS AND LIPOPROTEINS

Because the concentrations of individual lipid moieties in plasma depend on the algebraic summation of input and removal rates, the mechanisms that control the release or uptake of individual lipids must be studied throughout the course of various kinds of infectious illnesses. Concentrations of cholesterol have been reported to increase, to decrease, or to remain unchanged.[10] In

TABLE 3–1 Basic Mechanisms Leading to Observed Effects of Infection on Lipid Metabolism of the Host

Effects Associated with the Presence of Invading Microorganisms
1. Direct effects
   a. Microorganism use of host lipids for replication
   b. Disruption of host cell metabolism by intracellular microorganisms
   c. Localized destruction of fat cells by infectious process
2. Indirect effects
   a. Alterations in host metabolism caused by bacterial exotoxins, endotoxins, or bacterial enzymes
   b. Activation of lipases and other lipid-affecting enzymes within host phagocytes

Effects Secondary to Development of Generalized Illness Due to Infection
1. Decreased dietary fat intake
2. Interference with intestinal digestion and absorption of lipids
3. Alterations in lipid transport
   a. Changing concentrations of lipid transport proteins
   b. Decreased lipoprotein lipase activity (caused by tumor necrosis factor), which allows triglycerides to accumulate in plasma
4. Altered lipid metabolism within host cells caused by proinflammatory cytokines
   a. Activation of cell wall phospholipases by proinflammatory cytokines
   b. Creation, from cell wall polyunsaturated fatty acids, of intracellular arachidonic or eicosapentanoic acids or both
   c. Transformation of arachidonic and eicosapentanoic acids into various eicosanoids (prostaglandins, prostacyclin, thromboxanes, and lipoxins)
5. Other alterations of lipid metabolism within host cells
   a. Altered rates of hormone-mediated lipolysis within fat depots
   b. Accelerated fatty acid synthesis within the liver
   c. Depressed hepatic ketogenesis
   d. Altered rates of lipid uptake and use by peripheral tissues
6. Participation of newly formed eicosanoids in inflammatory and immunologic responses, and coagulation mechanisms
7. Effects related to prior nutritional status of the patient
8. Terminal pathologic hyperlipidemic effects associated with gram-negative sepsis and hypotensive shock

severe meningococcal sepsis, high-density lipoprotein and low-density lipoprotein levels are low, and the severity of total hypocholesterolemia correlates with the severity of disease.[152] Other studies have shown that hypocholesterolemia in sepsis may have prognostic value. Decrease of cholesterol parallels increase of C-reactive protein, fibrinogen, and white blood cells in septic patients.[28]

Mild viral infections often are associated with a transient decline in serum cholesterol values. When longitudinal studies were conducted during the course of experimentally induced sandfly fever in young adult male volunteers, plasma values for total and esterified cholesterol, phospholipids, and free fatty acids all declined in conjunction with, or immediately before, the onset of fever.[78] This decline in concentration included the cholesterol and the protein components of the low-density beta-lipoproteins. In contrast, the plasma triglyceride values showed a biphasic pattern of change: An initial decline was followed by an increase above baseline control concentrations during the early convalescent period. Depressions of total serum cholesterol values also have been reported to occur during pneumococcal pneumonia, cholera, tuberculosis, and malaria.

When studied in rhesus monkeys experimentally infected with *Streptococcus pneumoniae* or *Salmonella typhimurium*, rates of [³H] mevalonic acid incorporation into free cholesterol were accelerated,[48] and no evidence of an inhibition of squalene synthesis or its conversion to cholesterol was found. In contrast, the synthesis of cholesterol was blocked partially when monkeys with diet-induced hypercholesterolemia were subjected to a pneumococcal infection.[48]

Marked increases in the concentrations of total serum lipids and triglycerides are found consistently in patients with infections caused by gram-negative bacilli,[10,69,135] but this response is minimized or fails to occur in patients with viral or gram-positive coccal infections. A similar difference has been noted in monkeys with either *S. pneumoniae* or *S. typhimurium* infection.[70] Tumor necrosis factor, a proinflammatory cytokine with a unique additional function that inhibits the enzyme lipoprotein lipase, seems to be of central importance in accounting for these differences.[69]

Although a release of tumor necrosis factor from activated macrophages may occur in many infections, its release is stimulated markedly by bacterial endotoxins released during gram-negative infections.[10,92] Hypertriglyceridemia occurring during periods of *S. typhimurium* infection in monkeys was generated by tumor necrosis factor–induced mechanisms that reduced the clearance of lipids from plasma and the activity of heparin-sensitive plasma lipoprotein lipase. Hypertriglyceridemia that accompanied pneumococcal infections was far less severe than that observed with gram-negative infections. After endotoxin was administered,[69] hypertriglyceridemia developed chiefly as the result of an impaired lipid disposal mechanism, secondary to release of tumor necrosis factor from macrophages.[8] An acceleration in the rate of hepatic production of triglycerides from free fatty acid precursors also occurred.

LIPIDS AND ENERGY METABOLISM DURING INFECTION

Requirements for cellular energy during periods of chronic infections in laboratory animals seem to be met largely through the catabolism of stored body fat.[82] In contrast, fat wasting does not seem to be as prominent during rapidly lethal bacterial infections. Ketogenesis also seems to be blunted during periods of acute infections.[103] Concentrations of free fatty acid in plasma normally are increased by the actions of catecholamines, growth hormone, and glucagon, which are increased during the course of infection.[10] Concomitantly high concentrations of plasma insulin apparently serve to inhibit lipolysis and ketogenesis.[10,103] The contribution of free fatty acids to energy production during an infection is influenced by the interplay of these hormones, the availability of glucose, and the functional capacity of the liver to take up fatty acids and convert them to triglycerides.[48,49,53,54]

Finally, brown fat is thought to contribute importantly to heat production in newborns via sympathetic nerve activation of this tissue. Because numerous viruses are known to proliferate in brown fat,[136] fever that occurs with neonatal viral infections may involve brown fat thermogenesis.

Acute infectious illnesses produce few effects on the intestinal absorption of fat, although it may be reduced with intestinal infections and parasitemic or enterotoxemic illnesses.[109,126] Lipid precursors needed for the replication of microorganisms within host tissues must be supplied from metabolic pools within the host. Malarial parasites obtain their structural lipids from red blood cell precursors; lipid-containing viruses apparently obtain the lipid components needed for their assembly from lipid-rich membranes already present within host cells.

LIPID METABOLISM AND HOST DEFENSIVE MEASURES

Rapid metabolic responses by cell wall lipids play a major role in initiating a panoply of intracellular events during acute-phase reactions. The attachment of proinflammatory cytokines to cell wall receptors triggers the conversion of polyunsaturated fatty acid in cell wall membranes to a variety of biologically active eicosanoids. Lipids of various eicosanoid families become the messenger molecules that are responsible for many of the acute-phase metabolic and cellular responses[8,42] that occur with infection. These short-lived eicosanoids are biopotent at nanomolar to picomolar concentrations.

In addition to their importance within lymphocytes of the immune system, eicosanoid lipids transmit stimulatory or inhibitory signals between other cells and tissues in health and disease.[73,123] Although they do not initiate disease processes, various eicosanoid lipids (i.e., prostaglandins, leukotrienes, prostacyclin, lipoxins, and thromboxanes) are important components of the pathogenic progression of infectious diseases.[73,123]

Eicosanoids also have important effects on other white blood cells and platelets and on such diverse organs as the brain, lungs, stomach, and kidneys. These eicosanoids seem to be components of complex, often overlapping, regulatory mechanisms that interconnect the immune system, the central nervous system, the endocrine glands, and the functions of many other organs and tissues. These homeostatic (and at times pathogenic) mechanisms are characterized by numerous duplications, amplifications, checks and balances, and feedback control loops.

Biochemical details now are well established concerning the intracellular synthesis of individual eicosanoids from *n*-3 and *n*-6 polyunsaturated fatty acid precursors.[73,123] After cytokines interact with cell wall receptors, they activate cell membrane phospholipase enzymes. These enzymes initiate the release (into the cell interior) of arachidonic acid from cell wall (*n*-6) polyunsaturated fatty acid or eicosapentanoic acid from (*n*-3) polyunsaturated fatty acid. These first steps of eicosanoid synthesis can be blocked by adrenocorticoid hormones. In target cells having cyclooxygenase enzymes, arachidonic acid is oxygenated into 4-series leukotrienes, 2-series prostaglandins, or thromboxanes and prostacyclin. If a cell possesses lipooxygenase enzymes, arachidonic acid is oxygenated into the sometimes less potent 5-series leukotrienes, 3-series prostaglandins, or lipoxins.[123] The highly active eicosanoid molecules are degraded rapidly. Importantly, synthesis of prostaglandins of the 2-series and the 4-series can be blocked by certain nonsteroidal anti-inflammatory drugs, such as aspirin, indomethacin, and ibuprofen.[73,123]

Other fatty acids may participate in defense mechanisms of the host and occasionally even may be involved in pathogenic events of a harmful nature. An increase in the fat content of vital organs is a common occurrence in patients dying of severe bacterial infections; fatty metamorphosis especially is prominent in the liver, kidney, and heart.[66] Hyperlipemia in gram-negative septicemia may be accompanied by fat embolization to the lungs. Other deleterious actions of body lipids involve the liberation of phospholipids from platelets and their subsequent participation in the activation of the blood-clotting cascade leading to disseminated intravascular coagulation. Chronic *Chlamydia* pneumonia infection leads to oxidation of low-density lipoprotein, which promotes atherogenesis.[43]

ELECTROLYTE AND ACID-BASE METABOLISM

Many life-threatening medical emergencies faced by infants and children with acute infectious diseases involve problems in the areas of salt and water or acid-base balance. Some infections cause severe overhydration, and others produce dehydration with hypovolemic shock. Pathogenic mechanisms that come into play during various infections can lead to metabolic alkalosis or acidosis, to respiratory alkalosis or acidosis, or to complex admixtures of these pathophysiologic perturbations.[8,18]

The onset of fever typically is accompanied by tachypnea and accelerated respiratory gas exchange, which leads to an exaggerated loss of dissolved carbon dioxide from blood and a state of uncompensated respiratory alkalosis.[10] Alkalosis may persist as long as febrile tachypnea lasts, and gas exchange within the alveoli remains unimpeded.

Conversely, infections that produce extensive pulmonary consolidation can impair carbon dioxide exchange and cause respiratory acidosis. Respiratory acidosis also is a complication in patients whose pulmonary musculature no longer can function effectively, such as patients with poliomyelitis, tetanus, botulism, or respiratory distress syndrome.

Metabolic acidosis generally develops whenever an infectious disease process becomes severe. With the hypotension, vascular stasis, and cellular anoxia seen during gram-negative sepsis, the generation of excessive lactic acid and other acidic metabolic products exceeds the capacity of the body's buffering systems.[10,135]

Diarrheal diseases can be accompanied by two other forms of metabolic acid-base derangement.[18,126,163] Toxigenic diarrhea characterized by high-volume stool loss, such as that seen in Asiatic cholera or *Escherichia coli* enterotoxemia, causes an excessive loss of fecal bicarbonate and an alkaline stool, with a resultant decline in blood pH. Bicarbonate is secreted actively in the lower ileum and cannot be reabsorbed completely by the colonic mucosa if high-volume losses of watery stool occur.[18]

In contrast, diarrhea accompanied by only low-volume stool losses, as in rotavirus infections,[126] tends to be associated with an acid stool associated with an exaggerated loss of fecal potassium rather than bicarbonate. If fecal potassium losses persist chronically for a long time or occur rapidly as part of the massive fluid loss of acute secretory diarrhea, such as in pediatric cholera, body potassium can be depleted severely. The loss of cellular potassium can produce metabolic alkalosis, cardiac arrhythmia, paralytic ileus, and weakness in children and the occurrence of hypokalemic vacuolization in cells of the myocardium and renal tubular epithelium. Even if the balance of fluid is restored promptly in these patients, a prolonged state of metabolic alkalosis can persist until body potassium stores are replenished.

The importance of diarrheal diseases in infants and small children is great, with an estimated 2 to 3 million deaths occurring worldwide each year.[104] Life-threatening dehydration can result from the loss of body water and electrolytes during an episode of high-volume diarrhea. Because massive diarrhea produces an iso-osmotic loss of body water and electrolytes, the fluid losses come from the extracellular rather than the intracellular space.[163] The circulating blood becomes thick and viscous because of a relative increase in hematocrit values and a progressive concentration of serum proteins, which can increase to more than twice their normal values. Despite serious dehydration, concentrations of plasma sodium remain normal, when expressed in terms of plasma water.[163] This type of acute, massive diarrhea can lead to the rapid onset of hypovolemic shock, renal failure, and death.

Dehydration usually does not become a problem in infectious diseases that lack protracted vomiting, diarrhea, or prominent sweat loss. Instead, severe generalized infections in children may be accompanied by some retention of body water and salt. Soon after the onset of a febrile illness, the adrenal secretion of aldosterone increases,[9,17] and this mineralocorticoid stimulates the renal retention of sodium and chloride. These electrolytes virtually may disappear from the urine during a severe febrile illness. Retention of salt tends to be accompanied by a retention of body water throughout the illness.[10] Generalized edema is an infection-induced manifestation of kwashiorkor and can be seen during severe infections in well-nourished children. Accumulations of excess water and salt typically are excreted after the acute phase of illness by a transient period of diuresis during the early convalescent period.

Some infections, particularly infections that become localized within the central nervous system, also are complicated by an inappropriate secretion of antidiuretic hormone from the posterior pituitary.[45,169] The ensuing retention of body water may dilute the sodium and chloride in plasma. Redistribution of sodium also may contribute to the development of hyponatremia during infections. Sodium may begin to accumulate within body cells, apparently because the sodium-pumping mechanisms in extracellular membranes may fail to maintain internal electrolyte homeostasis.[10] This form of sodium sequestration is evidence of severe illness. It is not reversed easily and may be a major complication in patients with severe infections, such as meningococcemia or Rocky Mountain spotted fever.

VITAMIN METABOLISM

Although few measurement data are available concerning infection-induced changes in vitamin metabolism, the consensus is that the use or metabolism of most vitamins is accelerated.[16,155] Scattered reports suggest that infectious diseases in humans may be followed by classic scurvy, beriberi, pellagra, or xerophthalmia.[129]

More recent attention has focused on vitamin A, which previously was termed the anti-infection vitamin. Declining concentrations of plasma vitamin A during episodes of childhood infections are accompanied or perhaps caused by a marked urinary loss of this vitamin.[1,142] Not only does the heightened vitamin A deficiency induced by infection contribute to the subsequent development of ocular and conjunctival pathologies, but also subclinical deficiencies of vitamin A and their associated immunologic dysfunctions can heighten the mortality associated with childhood infections,[130] as shown most dramatically in measles.[138] Depressed plasma concentrations of several other vitamins have been reported.[10] In addition to the urinary losses of vitamin A,[1,142] increased excretion of urinary riboflavin and vitamin C may occur in conjunction with negative nitrogen balance.[16]

Vitamins are known to participate in metabolic processes activated during host defensive mechanisms.[8] The rapid synthesis of steroid hormones by the adrenal cortex is accompanied by a decline in the adrenal content of vitamin C. The B group vitamins, vitamin C, and folate all participate in the metabolism of activated phagocytic cells.

Controversy continues to exist over whether massive daily doses of vitamin C can suppress or prevent the common cold and other viral respiratory infections. More than 2 decades ago, the American Academy of Pediatrics Committee on Drugs[2] failed to find sufficient scientific evidence to support Pauling's claim, but new data subsequently were introduced.[63] Concentrations of vitamin C in neutrophils decline during infectious diseases. Vitamin C is recognized for its importance in the locomotive activity of phagocytic cells and its contributions to the immune system.[3]

Intestinal parasites, such as tapeworms, may take up sufficient vitamin B_{12} from the succus entericus to diminish vitamin B_{12} absorption and lead to the development of megaloblastic anemia. The intestinal absorption of fat-soluble vitamins and folate also may be impaired for a time in children with enteric infections or parasitic diseases.[83]

The antioxidant role of several vitamins (A, C, and E) has been recognized more recently. Antioxidants act to reduce oxidative stress within the body by serving as scavengers of singlet oxygen radicals. The antioxidant functions of several other provitamin-A carotenoids are of still greater importance. They include beta carotene, lycopene (the red pigment found in tomatoes and other brightly colored fruits), lutein (from spinach), and zeaxanthin (from kale and other dark green collard greens). Lycopene is more abundant in plasma than is beta carotene and twice as powerful in quenching free oxygen radicals. Lutein and zeaxanthin are retinal pigments, with lutein being found throughout the retina and zeoxanthin being concentrated in the macula. Antioxidants are thought to protect cell membranes, DNA, and arteries to augment the immune system and the function of natural killer cells and to help prevent heart attacks, macular degeneration, and various cancers, especially prostate cancer. Little is known about the probable role of antioxidants during episodes of infectious diseases of children.

More recent studies on a small sample of adults have suggested that vitamin D is decreased in patients with HIV infection, and that vitamin D levels correlate directly with the CD4 count and inversely with mortality in HIV-infected patients.[154] Vitamin C seems to be decreased in patients with HIV infection, whereas vitamin E concentrations are similar to those in healthy subjects.[143] Oxidative damage is known to play an important role in inflammation, but the exact mechanism by which vitamin C is involved in the antioxidant host defense is unclear. One study that looked at *Klebsiella pneumoniae* infection showed that vitamin C does not prevent lipid and protein oxidation. Another study suggests that vitamin C is protective against oxidative stress, at least partly by decreasing lipid peroxidation.[72] Vitamin C seems to protect against infections in mouse models.[52]

TRACE ELEMENT METABOLISM

As Table 3–2 shows, infectious illnesses often are accompanied by changes in the concentration of several of the trace elements in plasma. The most consistent responses include a decrease in the concentrations of plasma iron and zinc and an increase in plasma copper.[10] This triad of trace-element changes has been reported in bacterial, viral, rickettsial, and parasitic infections. In acute viral hepatitis, serum iron values tend to increase, however, in the second and third weeks of illness. Hepatitis also is associated with an unusual change in the binding of zinc to various ligands.[65] Soon after the acute onset of jaundice, plasma zinc is found to be bound almost entirely as microligands to small molecules, such as the amino acids. This phenomenon contrasts with the normal propensity for approximately 95 percent of plasma zinc to bind predominantly as a macroligand with either albumin or alpha$_2$-macroglobulin. In any event, plasma zinc is sequestered

rapidly in the liver, where it becomes tightly bound during acute infections to newly synthesized metallothioneins.[137]

CHANGES IN IRON METABOLISM

An abrupt depression in serum iron concentrations has been observed in virtually all infections in which iron values have been measured except acute viral hepatitis, with pyogenic infections causing the greatest effects. This hypoferremia has been ascribed primarily to an accelerated flux of iron from plasma into the liver, where it becomes localized in reticuloendothelial cells and hepatocytes. There the iron becomes sequestered as intracellular hemosiderin molecules or as a complex with ferritin.[8] Tumor necrosis factor and IL-1 seem to trigger this sequestration of iron by inducing the formation of ferritin,[24] some of which may be found in plasma. Plasma ferritin values provide a valuable clue concerning the quantities of body iron available in storage depots. When iron has become sequestered, it is not released readily until the infection is terminated.

Hepcidin is a peptide involved in major iron metabolic pathways. Hepcidin's secretion in the liver is induced during infections, likely by cytokines such as IL-6. Increased production of hepcidin leads to decreased plasma iron, which can be detrimental to the host but nonetheless acts as a host defense mechanism by reducing the iron available to different microorganisms.[51] Despite a low pool of plasma iron, some microorganisms, such as mycobacteria, have developed survival mechanisms by using the iron stored intracellularly in macrophages.[128]

During acute and chronic infections, the normal mechanisms that allow for the continuing release from tissue stores of the iron needed for use in erythropoiesis seem to be inhibited. If an infection persists for a prolonged period, anemia may develop. Although the "anemia of infection" resembles iron-deficiency anemia in its peripheral manifestations, it develops in the presence of adequate quantities of iron in storage sites and cannot be reversed by the therapeutic administration of iron.[8]

Other factors that influence iron metabolism during episodes of infection include an accelerated destruction of red blood cells and their direct loss in diseases in which hemolysis or bleeding

TABLE 3–2   Infection-Related Changes in Trace Elements

Trace Element	Observed Change during Infection	Suggested Pathophysiologic Mechanisms
Iron	Hyposideremia (common)	Flux of iron into liver and reticuloendothelial system cells
		Increased synthesis of ferritin
		Sequestration of iron in tissue stores
		Diminished iron absorption
	Anemia	Accelerated red blood cell destruction
		Direct blood loss
		Inhibition of erythropoiesis
	Reduced serum iron-binding capacity	Reduced synthesis of transferrin
	Hypersideremia (selective)	Hepatocyte damage during hepatitis
Zinc	Hypozincemia	Accelerated flux of zinc into liver
		Hepatic synthesis of additional metallothioneins
		Negative body balance of zinc
	Hyperzincuria	Hepatitis-induced inhibition of zinc binding to plasma proteins
Copper	Hypercupremia	Accelerated hepatic synthesis and release of ceruloplasmin
Chromium	Hypochromia	Unknown
Manganese	Hypermanganemia	Hepatocyte damage during hepatitis
Cobalt	Hypercobaltemia	Hepatocyte damage during hepatitis
	Macrocytic anemia	Intestinal parasitic competition for available vitamin B$_{12}$
Gallium	Hypergallemia	Hepatocyte damage during hepatitis
	Accumulation in sites of localized infection	Unknown
Iodine	Accelerated deiodination of thyroid hormones	Increased cellular metabolic rates
		Increased iodine availability for cellular bactericidal functions

is a factor. Excessive laboratory testing of blood samples can occur. In malaria, serum iron values tend to decline, despite the unusually large amounts of hemoglobin released from parasitized red blood cells. The released hemoglobin rapidly complexes with haptoglobin and is taken up by reticuloendothelial cells.[42] As in other forms of hemolytic anemia, a depression of serum haptoglobin values in malaria can serve as an index of the severity of red blood cell destruction.

An inhibition of iron absorption in the intestinal tract also can contribute to an infection-induced depression of serum iron values.[166] Studies using radioactive iron showed that a febrile illness or the febrile response of infants or young children to immunization could depress intestinal iron absorption for several days.[20]

The abrupt decrease in serum iron concentration, which can reach virtually undetectable values, occurs without any appreciable change in total serum iron-binding capacity. Although concentrations of serum transferrin decline along with concentrations of albumin during states of severe protein deficiency, they decline only slowly, if at all, during occurrences of acute infections. The combination of a normal iron-binding capacity and a markedly depressed concentration of serum iron in previously well-nourished children results in an increase in the concentration of serum unsaturated transferrin.[8] Unsaturated transferrin may play an important host defensive role by competing with siderophores of bacteria, which need to acquire iron for their growth and replication.[165] Because of its high affinity constant for iron, unsaturated transferrin is an important potential mechanism for inhibiting bacterial replication.

Increased concentrations of serum iron have been reported during bacillary dysentery, typhoidal infections, and, most commonly, acute viral hepatitis. The increase in concentrations of serum iron is delayed in hepatitis until several weeks after the initial appearance of jaundice; this increase may be large enough virtually to saturate the iron-binding capacity of serum. An impairment of mechanisms accounting for the normal daily hepatic removal of iron from serum has been thought to explain the hyperferremia noted during infections associated with liver cell dysfunction. An alternative hypothesis suggests that hepatitis-induced hyperferremia is caused by an escape of iron from the damaged hepatocytes. The latter explanation also is used to explain the reported increase in concentrations of serum manganese, gallium, and cobalt during acute hepatitis.[10]

CHANGES IN ZINC METABOLISM

Concentrations of zinc decline during episodes of various infectious diseases, as they do with a large variety of other diseases characterized by the presence of an inflammatory process.[10,111] Zinc values rarely decrease, however, as much as iron values do. This difference apparently is because of the large amount of plasma zinc that is bound tightly to alpha$_2$-macroglobulin. This plasma protein remains constant during periods of infection.[10]

Similar to iron, zinc seems to move into the liver at an accelerated rate during episodes of acute infections. This increased flux of zinc from serum to liver apparently is triggered by the action of proinflammatory cytokines released from activated monocytes and macrophages.[8,10] The hepatic uptake and sequestration of zinc are associated with an increased synthesis of zinc-binding metallothioneins within the hepatic cells.[137] The reason for this flux of zinc from serum to liver has not been explained in terms of host defense.

Body balances of zinc are thought to become negative during episodes of infectious diseases because of a combination of factors, including a reduction in dietary zinc intake, a diminished absorption from the intestinal tract, and a concomitant continuation (or increase) of zinc losses via the urine and possibly via the feces and

sweat. During periods of acute infectious hepatitis, a marked increase in the urinary loss of zinc occurs. This loss is caused by enhanced glomerular filtration and excretion of zinc microligands.[65] The increased formation of zinc microligands with amino acids, such as histidine and cysteine, permits plasma zinc to be excreted from the body via the urine. Whether an increased binding of zinc to amino acid microligands occurs with infections other than acute hepatitis is unknown; this phenomenon was not detected with sandfly fever. Zinc deficiency is important particularly in developing countries, where zinc deficiency is widespread and plays a significant role in diarrhea, pneumonia, tuberculosis, and malaria.[34]

CHANGES IN COPPER METABOLISM

Concentrations of plasma copper increase in virtually all infections. This increase apparently accompanies the accelerated synthesis and release from the liver of ceruloplasmin, the copper-binding protein of plasma. The increase in plasma ceruloplasmin resembles that of other acute-phase reactant proteins produced by the liver during inflammatory states when triggered by IL-6 and other proinflammatory cytokines.[8] Increases in ceruloplasmin and copper occur later than do the abrupt depressions in serum iron and zinc. The increase in copper values tends to persist longer than the changes in zinc and iron do, apparently as a result of the long in vivo half-disappearance time of ceruloplasmin from plasma. Body balances of copper have not been studied during an episode of an infectious illness.

PROINFLAMMATORY CYTOKINES

The generalized metabolic and physiologic responses to febrile infections are initiated and sustained by a unique control mechanism. This mechanism involves the secretion by various body cells of hormone-like cytokines (mainly monokines and lymphokines).[42] The cytokines include ILs, interferons, colony-stimulating factors, and tumor necrosis factor. Cytokines also function during localized infections.[117]

Complex interactions of cytokines that occur during illness only now are being unraveled.[8,42] Cytokines are not classified as hormones because they are produced by a variety of different cells located throughout the body, rather than by anatomically distinct glands; because cytokines are effective at far lower concentrations than are hormones; and because their interacting array of checks and balances is far more complex than that of hormones. Although cytokines are not components of either the central nervous or the endocrine systems, they interact with and trigger responses by both of these major regulatory control systems.[8,111]

Proinflammatory cytokines (which include IL-1, IL-6, and IL-8, and tumor necrosis factor) initiate and orchestrate the highly complex but stereotyped admixture of concomitant anabolic and catabolic events that make up the generalized host response to febrile infections. Individual components of this generalized response form distinct patterns. Some metabolic responses begin during the incubation period; some, at the onset of fever; some, late in the course of fever; and some, during convalescence.[8,10-12,14,21] No matter which type of microorganism causes an acute, generalized, febrile infection, the onset of most metabolic, biochemical, or physiologic responses seems to occur at consistent, predictable times. These many responses can be categorized temporally by their relationships to the time of onset of clinical symptoms and fever.[8] Virtually every metabolic or biochemical process is influenced in some manner by the body's response to an acute infection. The duration and magnitude of individual components of the generalized response show some variability from infection to infection. More must be learned about how the cytokines influence this variability in host metabolic responses.

In today's terminology, this overall response is termed an *acute-phase response*, an *acute-phase reaction*, or the *systemic inflammatory response syndrome*. This acute-phase response may accompany other severe medical and surgical problems, in addition to infection.[75] This complex response, which also activates complement and stimulates the immune system, seems to help defend the body.[8,75] On the negative side, acute-phase responses generate important nutritional costs,[8,10,125] costs that can produce severe, life-threatening malnutrition. In addition, acute-phase responses that become excessive or overly prolonged can lead to hypotensive shock, multiorgan dysfunction, and death.[42,79,106,125]

Acute-phase responses are initiated and controlled by the proinflammatory cytokines.[42,62,64,71,79,134,140,167] The cytokine interferon-α also can contribute to the wasting syndrome of acute infections.[32] The acute-phase reaction may be modified by bacterial endotoxins, which uniquely stimulate an exaggerated release of tumor necrosis factor, a cytokine that inhibits lipoprotein lipase enzymes, to account for the high concentrations of plasma triglycerides that develop during gram-negative sepsis.[8,69]

The primary control mechanisms that initiate acute-phase responses normally exist in a standby mode but can be turned on whenever necessary by the activation of macrophages, blood monocytes, or other body cells, and by the subsequent rapid release of proinflammatory cytokines.[8,42,92] The many diverse types of stimuli that can activate these cells include the phagocytosis of microorganisms, tissue debris, or other particulate matter; the effects of polynucleotides, certain drugs and chemicals, antigen-antibody complexes, and bacterial toxins; and the actions of other cytokines. During infectious illnesses, proinflammatory cytokines can be detected in body fluids, body secretions, urine, and stools.[55,88,117,120]

After their release from producing cells, proinflammatory cytokines circulate via the plasma or diffuse through tissue fluids to stimulate cell populations in many locations throughout the body. These cytokines have multiple, often overlapping, actions, and they stimulate the release of companion cytokines. IL-1 previously was termed *endogenous pyrogen, leukocytic endogenous mediator*, and *lymphocyte-activating factor*,[42] and tumor necrosis factor previously was termed *cachectin*. Proinflammatory cytokines stimulate the hypothalamic temperature-regulating center to initiate fever,[8,42] endocrine glands to secrete hormones, the liver to take up amino acids and trace elements and to synthesize many different proteins,[8,111,134] the pancreatic islets to release insulin and glucagon,[53,175] and the muscle cells to catabolize contractile proteins.[5,31] These cytokines also stimulate the bone marrow to produce and release neutrophils[111] and synovial cells and fibroblasts to activate collagenase.[42] Proinflammatory cytokines also may affect growth during certain viral infections by exerting a direct effect on bone remodeling.[141] Marrow stimulation involves the effect of IL-1 on progenitor cells[98] and its ability to trigger the release of various colony-stimulating cytokines.[8,59,98] In this regard, IL-1 has been found to be identical with hematopoietin.[98] The proinflammatory cytokines also activate the immune system and cause certain subsets of T lymphocytes to secrete IL-2, IL-3, IL-4, and IL-5.[8,42]

Proinflammatory cytokines are thought to function, after attachment to their specific cell wall receptors, by activating phospholipase A_2 within the cell walls, leading to the intracellular release of arachidonic acid or eicosapentanoic acid, or both, from cell wall polyunsaturated fatty acid phospholipids.[42] Subsequent responses by the cytokine-stimulated cell are determined by the intracellular enzymes that can metabolize these acids to one of many possible eicosanoids.

CONTROL MECHANISMS FOR PROINFLAMMATORY CYTOKINE ACTIONS

Similar to the action of hormones, proinflammatory cytokine actions are regulated by numerous checks and balances. To act on a cell, a cytokine first must attach itself to a protein receptor on an exterior cell wall. Cells produce other similar receptor proteins, however, which are released to float free in plasma.[76,107] Freely circulating receptors can intercept and inactivate their matching cytokine.[50,56] Other unique plasma protein molecules, receptor antagonists, also are produced.[149] They can attach to and block the cellular receptors for specific cytokines.[76,107] Cytokine inhibitor proteins have been identified.[27,150] Other cytokines, such as IL-4 and IL-10, can suppress the cellular production of proinflammatory cytokines.[39,57,76,115,145] Cytokine stimulation of release of cortisol has complex feedback effects because cortisol can block the intracellular formation of eicosanoids stimulated by the cytokines. Cortisol and epinephrine also can stimulate the production of cytokines.[79]

CYTOKINE DETECTION IN BIOLOGIC FLUIDS

Individual components of this complex cytokine system of checks and balances now can be measured in body fluids, and their relationships can be studied throughout the course of an acute-phase reaction.[22,26,42,71,76,140,150] These cytokines and their free receptors can be found in mucosal fluids and in plasma.[105,114,120] Cytokine measurements may have diagnostic and prognostic value.[26,134] Identification of IL-8 in amniotic cord sera was reported to be a specific marker for preterm chorioamnionitis.[134] Raqib and colleagues[120] described longitudinal measurements of cytokines and receptor antagonists in the plasma and stools of patients with acute shigellosis. Concentrations of tumor necrosis factor-α; IL-1β, IL-6, and IL-8; and IL-1 receptor antagonist in stools were quite high when patients with shigellosis first were seen and gradually returned to normal values during the next 2 weeks.[134] IL-6 and IL-8 can be used as markers for neonatal sepsis with coagulase-negative staphylococci and to differentiate between bacterial and enteroviral infections.[151] Proinflammatory cytokines also are responsible for the cachexia associated with acute or chronic inflammatory diseases.[37] The pathogenic or physiologic effects of these interacting molecules in either systemic or localized diseases still are not fully understood.

HORMONAL RESPONSES

Infectious illnesses are accompanied by a variety of endocrine responses, which especially include increased secretion of the hormones that regulate carbohydrate and energy metabolism and the hormones that influence salt and water retention. These hormonal responses are secondary to and often are initiated by the primary release of proinflammatory cytokines from activated cells.

In addition to their participation in physiologic responses, endocrine functions also may be affected by pathologic complications of an infectious process that results in the direct destruction or dysfunction of hormone-producing cells. The adrenal glands may be destroyed if tubercle bacilli localize in these glands or if hemorrhagic necrosis becomes a complication of such infections as acute meningococcemia. Pancreatic islet cells may be destroyed during episodes of viral infections of experimental animals, and the same pathogenic possibility may initiate insulin-requiring diabetes in children. Thyroid function may be impaired after occurrence of a viral infection that triggers an autoimmune thyroiditis, and gonadal tissues may be the site of localization and destruction by the mumps virus.

PITUITARY GLAND FUNCTIONS

Secretion of certain of the trophic hormones produced by the anterior pituitary is increased during infection. An increase in adrenocorticotropic hormone production (stimulated by proinflammatory cytokines) triggers an increased secretion of several adrenocorticoids. Concentrations of plasma growth hormone generally are increased in acute infections in which this hormone has been measured,[19,121] but the increases do not seem to correlate directly in timing or magnitude with the presence or severity of fever.[7,10] This increase in plasma growth hormone may be due partly to its production by mononuclear leukocytes.[164] Concentrations of plasma growth hormone increase rapidly in a paradoxical manner if an intravenous infusion of glucose is given to a patient or a laboratory animal with an acute infection.[121] Thyroid-stimulating hormone does not respond during the early phases of an acute febrile illness but may increase during the convalescent period. No increases in the gonadotropic hormones have been documented during an episode of an infection. A release of several anterior pituitary hormones can be stimulated by fever-producing doses of bacterial endotoxin. Such responses have been used in the clinical testing of anterior pituitary function.[74,95]

As described in the earlier discussion of salt and water imbalances, inappropriate secretion of antidiuretic hormone may occur in patients with severe infectious diseases.[45] This phenomenon also seems to be a characteristic response in patients whose infectious process becomes localized within the cranial vault.

ADRENAL FUNCTIONS

Although the adrenocortical hormones are known to influence the ability of a patient to respond to stressful situations, few data define the duration and magnitude of the adrenal response or characterize the spectrum of specific steroid hormones produced in excess.[17,94] Available data suggest that acute generalized infections typically are accompanied by a transient increase in the adrenal output of glucocorticoid hormones that is of short duration. Although these responses generally are limited in magnitude, they serve to maintain a constant concentration of cortisol in plasma throughout the early periods of fever.[17]

The usual diurnal decline in plasma 17-hydroxycorticosteroid values fails to occur during the afternoon and evening hours if fever is present. Cortisol-binding proteins have not been observed to change in plasma during periods of acute infection.[10] The plasma concentrations of unbound, physiologically active cortisol are maintained at or higher than the normal peak early morning values throughout the initial period of a febrile illness.[10,17] The total increase in glucocorticoid secretion rates during early illness ranges from two to five times normal values in infections that have been studied. Lesser degrees of increase have been noted in the adrenocortical output of pregnanetriol and the weak ketosteroid androgens.[17] If an infectious illness becomes chronic, adrenal output generally returns to or even falls below baseline values, and diminished adrenal responsiveness to adrenocorticotropic hormone may occur.

Extremely high concentrations of plasma 17-hydroxycorticosteroids may develop during gram-negative septicemia or before death in patients with other severe acute infections.[91,94] These high terminal values may be ascribed to failures in the hepatic clearance of cortisol from plasma and the metabolic pathways for converting cortisol to water-soluble metabolites; high plasma values are not the result of an extraordinary increase in adrenal secretion rates.[91] In a detailed study of adrenal function in children with meningitis, Migeon and coworkers[94] reported a maximum average increase in cortisol secretion rate of approximately threefold during uncomplicated aseptic or bacterial meningitis. This increase was accompanied by a threefold increase in the excretion of urinary 17-hydroxycorticosteroids during the first few days of illness. On admission to the hospital, these children had concentrations of plasma cortisol that ranged from high normal to twice normal values. Severely ill patients who were dying of adrenal hemorrhage generally had values that were depressed or absent.

Mechanisms by which small increases in adrenal glucocorticoid secretion might protect the host have not been defined. The ability of the liver to produce some of its proteins during periods of infection is known, however, to depend on the permissive presence of glucocorticoid hormones.[17]

The increase in production of aldosterone seems to lag behind the increase in production of cortisol during periods of acute infections and then persists longer. Increases in aldosterone stimulate the intense retention of sodium and chloride by the kidney during episodes of acute infections.[13]

The adrenomedullary secretion of catecholamines may increase in severe infectious diseases.[60,171] High plasma epinephrine and norepinephrine values develop in patients with gram-negative sepsis and bacterial meningitis. The catecholamine response contributes significantly to the acceleration of gluconeogenesis during periods of infection.

CARBOHYDRATE-REGULATING HORMONES

Hormones that serve in the normal regulation of carbohydrate metabolism also participate in the host response to infection. In addition to the heightened secretion of the glucocorticoids, catecholamines, and growth hormone, the major pancreatic hormones insulin and glucagon circulate in increased concentrations in the plasma of patients with acute infectious diseases.[171] The combined effect of these hormonal actions is to accelerate the production of glucose within the liver and to stimulate the release of glucose from stored glycogen. These actions cause the glucose pool size to increase twofold or threefold to provide an important source of metabolizable energy during the early febrile periods of acute infections.

Intravenous glucose tolerance tests performed early in the course of febrile infections in young adult subjects[121,132] led to an exaggerated increase of concentrations of plasma insulin in magnitude and duration, to an appropriate decline in elevated fasting concentrations of plasma glucagon, and to a paradoxical stimulation of release of growth hormone. Extreme hyperinsulinism also was observed after glucose infusions were given to dogs with endotoxic shock.[21]

The modest increase in concentrations of fasting plasma insulin that occurs during periods of infection seems to account for an inhibition of ketogenesis and fat depot lipolysis, two responses that would be expected to occur because of concomitant starvation or semistarvation. The simultaneous combination of high fasting plasma glucagon and insulin values and their effects on the liver and peripheral fat depots and somatic tissues helps to explain the observed differences between the anorexia-induced semistarvation associated with infectious illnesses and the starvation caused by food deprivation.

THYROID HORMONES

Thyroid hormones do not seem to initiate or sustain the hypermetabolic response to fever. Nonetheless, thyroxine (T_4) and triiodothyronine (T_3) are deiodinated at accelerated rates within the body tissues, especially in the liver, during the early phases of infections studied in humans and experimental animals.[40,162,173] This acceleration in the metabolism of peripheral thyroid hormones accounts for an early decline in serum protein-bound iodine values.[131] Only after an infectious illness has progressed for several days does the thyroid gland hormone output seem to increase. This increase in thyroid secretion persists into early convalescence so that for a time the production of thyroid hormones exceeds apparent body requirements. As a result, protein-bound iodine values in serum are increased in the convalescent period. This sequence of events produces a biphasic response pattern with an initial decrease and a late increase in concentrations of thyroid hormones. Serum concentrations of "reverse T_3" increase during febrile illnesses.[29] Because reverse T_3 has an apparent role in regulating the peripheral cellular actions of T_4 and T_3, its function during acute infectious illness remains to be elucidated.

In studies of patients with falciparum malaria infection, serum T_3 values declined abruptly, whereas serum T_4 values were stable or increased slightly.[162] The decline in serum T_3 concentrations was accompanied by reciprocal increases in reverse T_3. The slowing of T_4 turnover during periods of malaria may be caused by an impaired ability of hepatocytes to metabolize or deiodinate T_4. Hypothalamic suppression in early stages of malaria seems to result in a decreased release of thyroid-stimulating hormone from the anterior pituitary and a secondary decrease in T_4 and T_3 secretion from the thyroid gland. In patients with sepsis and septic shock, thyroid hormones (total and free T_3, T_4, and thyroid-stimulating hormone) are decreased and are associated with poor prognosis.[177]

PROCALCITONIN

Procalcitonin, discovered in the early 1960s, is a prohormone, the precursor of the hormone calcitonin. Multiple studies have shown that procalcitonin is involved in the pathogenesis of infections, and that it can be a useful diagnostic marker for infections such as bacterial pneumonia,[68] bacterial sepsis and septic shock, meningitis, infectious endocarditis, pancreatitis, and urinary tract infections.[30,100,146]

The role of calcitonin is unclear; most likely, it had an evolutionary role, and it currently is nonessential in humans.[30] Serum concentrations of procalcitonin and other precursors of mature calcitonin are elevated significantly during episodes of sepsis and other infectious and noninfectious causes of inflammation. Serum concentration of procalcitonin also is elevated in patients with malaria. The serum concentration of procalcitonin usually correlates with the severity of infection and with mortality.[30]

Secretion of procalcitonin is stimulated by IL-1β and tumor necrosis factor–α in patients with bacterial infections and by interferon-γ in patients with viral infections. The target tissues are lung, liver, kidney, adipose tissue, and muscle.

Several studies have suggested procalcitonin could be used as a marker for bacterial sepsis and could be used to differentiate infectious from noninfectious causes of inflammation. Although procalcitonin has been shown possibly to have greater specificity and sensitivity compared with C-reactive protein as a marker for bacterial infections, it should not be used without evaluation of other clinical and laboratory data in making therapeutic decisions because serum procalcitonin concentration may be normal in patients with sepsis or increased in some individuals with no clinical symptoms.[30]

REFERENCES

1. Alvarez, J. O., Salazar-Lindo, E., Kohatsu, J., et al.: Urinary excretion of retinol in children with acute diarrhea. Am. J. Clin. Nutr. 61:1273-1276, 1995.
2. American Academy of Pediatrics Committee on Drugs: Vitamin C and the common cold. Nutr. Rev. (Suppl):39-40, 1974.
3. Anderson, R., Smit, M. J., Joone, G. K., and Van Staden, A. M.: Vitamin C and cellular immune functions: Protection against hypochlorous acid-mediated inactivation of glyceraldehyde-3-phosphate dehydrogenase and ATP generation in human leukocytes as a possible mechanism of ascorbate-mediated immunostimulation. Ann. N. Y. Acad. Sci. 587:34-48, 1990.
4. Argaman, Z., Young, V. R., Noviski, N., et al.: Arginine and nitric oxide metabolism in critically ill septic pediatric patients. Crit. Care Med. 31:591-597, 2003.
5. Baracos, V., Rodemann, H. P., Dinarello, C. A., and Goldberg, A. L.: Stimulation of muscle protein degradation and prostaglandin E2 release by leukocytic pyrogen (interleukin-1): A mechanism for the increased degradation of muscle proteins during fever. N. Engl. J. Med. 308:553-558, 1983.
6. Beck, O.: Weitere untersuchungen zub fieberstoffwechsel des sauglings: Die qualitativen Veranderungen des Stickstoffwechsel im Fiber. Jahrb. Kinderh. 112:184-216, 1926.
7. Beisel, W.: The influence of infection or injury on nutritional requirements during adolescence. In McKingey, J. I., and Munro, H. N. (eds.): Nutrient Requirements in Adolescents. Cambridge, MA, MIT Press, 1976.
8. Beisel, W.: Nutrition and infection. In Linder, M. C. (ed.): Nutrional Biochemistry and Metabolism. 2nd ed. New York, Elsevier Science, 1991, pp. 508-542.
9. Beisel, W., Sawyer, W. D., Ryell, E. D., et al.: Metabolic effects of intracellular infections in man. Ann. Intern. Med. 67:755-779, 1967.
10. Beisel, W. R.: Metabolic effects of infection. Progr. Food Nutr. Sci. 8:43-75, 1984.
11. Beisel, W. R.: Nutrition, infection, specific immune response, and nonspecific host defenses: A complex interaction. In Watson, R. (ed.): Nutrition, Disease Resistance and Immune Function. New York, Marcel Dekker, 1984, pp. 3-34.
12. Beisel, W. R.: Herman Award Lecture, 1995: Infection-induced malnutrition—from cholera to cytokines. Am. J. Clin. Nutr. 62:813-819, 1995.
13. Beisel, W. R., Bruton, J., Anderson, K. D., et al.: Adrenocortical responses during tularemia in human subjects. J. Clin. Endocrinol. Metab. 27:61-69, 1967.
14. Beisel, W. R., Feigin, R. D., et al.: Proceedings of a workshop: Impact of infection on nutritional status of the host. Am. J. Clin. Nutr. 30:1203-1371, 1439-1566, 1977.
15. Beisel, W. R., Goldman, R. F., and Joy, R. J. T.: Metabolic balance studies during induced hyperthermia in man. J. Appl. Physiol. 24:1-10, 1968.
16. Beisel ,W. R., Herman, Y. F., Sauberlich, H. E., et al.: Experimentally induced sandfly fever and vitamin metabolism in man. Am. J. Clin. Nutr. 25:1165-1173, 1972.
17. Beisel, W. R., and Rapoport, M. I.: Inter-relation between adrenocortical functions and infectious illness. N. Engl. J. Med. 280:569-604, 1969.
18. Beisel, W. R., Watten, R. H., Blackewell, Q., et al.: The role of bicarbonate pathophysiology and therapy in Asiatic cholera. Am. J. Med. 35:58-66, 1963.
19. Beisel, W. R., Woeber, K. A., Bartelloni. P. J., et al.: Growth hormone response during sandfly fever. J. Clin. Endocrinol. Metab. 28:1220-1223, 1968.
20. Beresford, C. H., Neale, R. J., and Brooks, O. G.: Iron absorption and pyrexia. Lancet 1:568-575, 1971.
21. Blackard, W. G., Anderson, J. H., Jr., and Spitzer, J. J.: Hyperinsulinism in endotoxin shock dogs. Metabolism 25:675-684, 1976.
22. Brown, C. C., Poli, G., Lubaki, N., et al.: Elevated levels of tumor necrosis factor-α in Zairian neonate plasmas: Implications for perinatal infection with the human immunodeficiency virus. J. Infect. Dis. 169:975-980, 1994.
23. Calder, P. C.: Branched-chain amino acids and immunity. J. Nutr. 136:288S-293S, 2006.
24. Campbell, C. H., Solgonick, R. M., Linder, M. C.: Translational regulation of ferritin synthesis in rat spleen: Effects of iron and inflammation. Biochem. Biophys. Res. Commun. 160:453-459, 1989.
25. Cao, W., Baniecki, M. L., McGrath, W. J., et al.: Nitric oxide inhibits the adenovirus proteinase in vitro and viral infectivity in vivo. Faseb. J. 17:2345-2346, 2003.
26. Casey, L. C., Balk, R. A., and Bone, R. C.: Plasma cytokine and endotoxin levels correlate with survival in patients with sepsis syndrome. Ann. Intern. Med. 119:771-778, 1993.
27. Chang, D. M., and Shaio, M. F.: Production of interleukin-1 (IL-1) and IL-1 inhibitor by human monocytes exposed to dengue virus. J. Infect. Dis. 170:811-817, 1994.
28. Chiarla, C., Giovannini, I., Siegel, J. H.: The relationship between plasma cholesterol, amino acids and acute phase proteins in sepsis. Amino Acids 27:97-100, 2004.
29. Chopra, I. J., Chopra, U., Smith, S. R., et al.: Reciprocal changes in serum concentrations of 3,3N5N-triiodothyronine (reverse T3) and 3,3N5-triiodothyronine (T3) in systemic illness. J. Clin. Endocrinol. Metab. 41:1043-1049, 1975.
30. Christ-Crain, M., and Muller, B.: Procalcitonin in bacterial infections—hype, hope, more or less? Swiss. Med. Wkly. 135:451-460, 2005.
31. Clowes, G. H., Jr., George, B. C., Villee, C. A., Jr., and Saravis, C. A.: Muscle proteolysis induced by a circulating peptide in patients with sepsis or trauma. 1983. Nutrition (Burbank, Los Angeles County, Calif) 11:775; discussion 774, 776-777, 1995.

32. Constans, J., Pellegrin, I., Pellegrin, J. L., et al.: Plama alpha-interpheron and the wasting syndrome in patients with human deficiency virus. Clin. Infect. Dis. *20*:1069-1070, 1995.

33. Cook, G. C.: Increased glycine absorption rate associated with acute bacterial infections in man. Br. J. Nutr. *29*:377-386, 1973.

34. Cuevas, L. E., and Koyanagi, A.: Zinc and infection: A review. Ann. Trop. Paediatr. *25*:149-160, 2005.

35. Curnow, R. T., Rayfield, E. J., George, D. T., et al.: Altered hepatic glycogen metabolism and glucoregulatory hormones during sepsis. Am. J. Physiol. *230*:1296-1301, 1973.

36. Debats, I. B., Booi, D., Deutz, N. E., et al.: Infected chronic wounds show different local and systemic arginine conversion compared with acute wounds. J. Surg. Res. *134*:205-214, 2006.

37. Delano, M. J., and Moldawer, L. L.: The origins of cachexia in acute and chronic inflammatory diseases. Nutr. Clin. Pract. *21*:68-81, 2006.

38. den Hartog, J. E., Ouburg, S., Land, J. A., et al.: Do host genetic traits in the bacterial sensing system play a role in the development of *Chlamydia trachomatis*-associated tubal pathology in subfertile women? B.M.C. Infect. Dis. *6*:122, 2006.

39. Derkx, B., Marchant, A., Goldman, M., et al.: High levels of interleukin-10 during the initial phase of fulminant meningococcal septic shock. J. Infect. Dis. *171*:229-232, 1995.

40. DeRubertis, F. R., and Woeber, K. A.: Accelerated cellular uptake and metabolism of L-thyroxine during acute *Salmonella typhimurium* sepsis. J. Clin. Invest. *52*:78-87, 1973.

41. van Waardenburg, D. A., Deutz, N. E., Hoos, M. B., et al.: Assessment of whole body protein metabolism in critically ill children: Can we use the [15N]glycine single oral dose method? Clin. Nutr. *23*:153-160, 2004.

42. Dinarello, C. A.: The proinflammatory cytokines interleukin-1 and tumor necrosis factor and treatment of the septic shock syndrome. J. Infect. Dis. *163*:1177-1184, 1991.

43. Dittrich, R., Dragonas, C., Mueller, A., et al.: Endothelial *Chlamydia pneumoniae* infection promotes oxidation of LDL. Biochem. Biophys. Res. Commun. *319*:501-505, 2004.

44. Drapier, J. C., Wietzerbim, J., and Hibbs, J. B., Jr.: Interferon-gamma and tumor necrosis factor induct the L-arginine-dependent cytotoxic effector mechanism in murin macrophages. J. Immunol. *18*:1587-1592, 1988.

45. Feigin, R. D., and Kaplan, S.: Inappropriate secretion of antidiuretic hormone (ADH) in children with bacterial meningitis. Am. J. Clin. Nutr. *30*:1482-1484, 1977.

46. Feigin, R. D., Middelkamp, J. N., and Reed, C. A.: Murine myocarditis due to coxsackie B 3 virus: Blood amino acid, virologic, and histopathologic correlates. J. Infect. Dis. *126*:574-584, 1972.

47. Felig, P., Brown, W., Levine, R. A., et al.: Glucose homeostasis in viral hepatitis. N. Engl. J. Med. *283*:1436-1440, 1970.

48. Fiser, R. H., Denniston, J. C., and Beisel, W. R.: Infection with *Diplococcus pneumoniae* and *Salmonella typhimurium* in monkeys: Changes in plasma lipids and lipoproteins. J. Infect. Dis. *125*:54-60, 1972.

49. Fiser, R. H., Denniston, J. C., Kastello, M. D., et al.: Cholesterolgenesis during acute infection in chronically hypercholesterolemic rhesus monkeys. Proc. Soc. Exp. Biol. Med. *140*:314-318, 1972.

50. Frieling, J. T. M., van Deuren, M., Wijdens, J., et al.: Circulating interleukin-6 receptor in patients with sepsis syndrome. J. Infect. Dis. *171*:469-472, 1995.

51. Ganz, T.: Hepcidin—a peptide hormone at the interface of innate immunity and iron metabolism. Curr. Topics Microbiol. Immunol *306*:183-198, 2006.

52. Gaut, J. P., Belaaouaj, A., Byun, J., et al.: Vitamin C fails to protect amino acids and lipids from oxidation during acute inflammation. Free Rad. Biol. Med. *40*:1494-1501, 2006.

53. George, D. T., Abels, F. B., Mapes, C. A., et al.: Effect of leukocytic endogenous mediators on endocrine pancreas secretory responses. Am. J. Physiol. *233*:E240-E245, 1977.

54. George, D. T., Rayfield, E. J., and Wannemacher, R. W., Jr.: Altered glucoregulatory hormones during acute pneumococcal sepsis in the rhesus monkey. Diabetes *23*:544-549, 1974.

55. Girardin, E., Grau, G. E., Dayer, J. M., et al.: Tumor necrosis factor and interleukin-1 in the serum of children with severe infectious purpura. N. Engl. J. Med. *319*:397-400, 1988.

56. Godfried, M. H., van der Poll, T., Weverling, G. J., et al.: Soluble receptors for tumor necrosis factor as predictors of progression to AIDS in asymptomatic human deficiency virus type 1 infection. J. Infect. Dis. *169*:739-745, 1994.

57. Gomez-Jimenez, J., Martin, M. C., Sauri, R., et al.: Interleukin-10 and the monocyte/macrophage-induced inflammatory response in septic shock. J. Infect. Dis. *171*:472-475, 1995.

58. Griffiths, J., Groves, A. C., and Leung, F. Y.: Hypertriglyceridemia and hypoglycemia in gram-negative sepsis in the dog. Surg. Gynecol. Obstet. *136*:897-903, 1973.

59. Groofman, J. E., Molina, J. M., and Scadden, D. T.: Hematopoietic growth factors. N. Engl. J. Med. *321*:1449-1459, 1989.

60. Groves, A. C., Griffiths, J., Leung, F., et al.: Plasma catecholamines in patients with serious postoperative infection. Ann. Surg. *178*:102-107, 1973.

61. Guckian, J. C.: Role of metabolism in pathogenesis of bacteremia due to *Diplococcus pneumoniae* in rabbits. Infect. Dis. *127*:1-8, 1973.

62. Halstensen, A., Ceska, M., Brandtzaeg, P., et al.: Interleukin-8 in serum and cerebrospinal fluid from patients with meningococcal disease. J. Infect. Dis. *167*:471-475, 1993.

63. Hemila, H., Herman, Z. S.: Vitamin C and the common cold: A retrospective analysis of Chalmers' review. J. Am. Coll. Nutr. *14*:116-123, 1995.

64. Heney, D., Lewis, I. J., Evans, S. W., et al.: Interleukin-6 and its relationship to C-reactive protein and fever in children with febrile neutropenia. J. Infect. Dis. *165*:886-890, 1992.

65. Henkin, R. I., and Smith, F. R.: Zinc and copper metabolism in acute viral hepatitis. Am. J. Med. Sci. *264*:401-409, 1972.

66. Hirsch, R. L., McKay, D. G., Travers, R. I., et al.: Hyperlipidemia, fatty liver, and bromsulfophthalein retention in rabbits injected intravenously with bacterial endotoxins. J. Lipid Res. *5*:563-568, 1964.

67. Howard, J. E., Bighan, R. S., Jr., and Mason, R. E.: Studies on convalescence, V: Observations on the altered protein metabolism during induced malarial infections. Trans. Assoc. Am. Physicians *59*:242-247, 1946.

68. Jereb, M., and Kotar, T.: Usefulness of procalcitonin to differentiate typical from atypical community-acquired pneumonia. Wien. Klin. Wochenschr. *118*:170-174, 2006.

69. Kauffmann, R. L., Matson, C. F., and Beisel, W. R.: Hypertriglyceridemia produced by endotoxin: Role of impaired triglyceride disposal mechanism. J. Infect. Dis. *133*:548-555, 1976.

70. Kauffmann, R. L., Matson, C. F., Rowberg, A. H., et al.: Defective lipid disposal mechanisms during bacterial infection in rhesus monkeys. Metabolism *25*:615-624, 1976.

71. Keuter, M., Dharmana, E., Gasem, M. H., et al.: Patterns of proinflammatory cytokines and inhibitors during typhoid fever. J. Infect. Dis. *169*:1306-1311, 1994.

72. Kim, J. Y., and Lee, S. M.: Vitamins C and E protect hepatic cytochrome P450 dysfunction induced by polymicrobial sepsis. Eur. J. Pharm. *534*:202-209, 2006.

73. Kinsella, J. E., Lokesh, B., Broughton, S., and Whelan, J.: Dietary polyunsaturated fatty acids and eicosanoids: Potential effects on the modulation of inflammatory and immune cells: An overview. Nutrition (Burbank, Los Angeles County, Calif) *6*:24-44; discussion 59-62, 1990.

74. Kohler, P. O., O'Malley, B. W., Rayford, P. L., et al.: Effect of pyrogen on blood levels of pituitary trophic hormones: Observations of the usefulness of the growth hormone response in the detection of pituitary disease. J. Clin. Endocrinol. Metab. *27*:219-226, 1967.

75. Koj, A.: The role of interleukin-6 as the hepatocyte stimulating factor in the network of inflammatory cytokines. Ann. N. Y. Acad. Sci. *557*:1-8, 1989.

76. Kuhns, D. B., Alvord, W. G., and Gallin, J. I.: Increased circulating cytokines, cytokine antagonists, and E-selectin after intravenous administration of endotoxin in humans. J. Infect. Dis. *171*:145-152, 1995.

77. Lang, C. H., Bagby, G. J., and Dobrescu, C.: Effect of granulocyte colony-stimulating factor on sepsis-induced changes in neutrophil accumulation and organ glucose uptake. J. Infect. Dis. *166*:336-342, 1992.

78. Lees, R. S., Fiser, R. H., Beisel, W. R., Jr., et al.: Effects of an experimental viral infection on plasma lipid and lipoprotein metabolism. Metabolism *21*:825-833, 1972.

79. Liao, J., Keiser, J. A., Scales, W. E., et al.: Role of epinephrine in TNF and IL-6 production from isolated perfused rat liver. Am. J. Physiol. *268*:R896-R901, 1995.

80. Long, C. L., Haverber, L. N., Young, V. R., et al.: Metabolism of 3-methylhistidine in man. Metabolism *24*:929-935, 1974.

81. Long, C. L., Kinney, J. M., and Geiger, J. W.: Nonsuppressibility of gluconeogenesis by glucose in septic patients. Metabolism *25*:193-201, 1976.

82. Macallan, D. C., McNurlan, M. A., Milne, E., et al.: Whole-body protein turnover from leucine kinetics and the response to nutrition in human immunodeficiency virus infection. Am. J. Clin. Nutr. *61*:818-826, 1995.

83. Mahalanabis, D., Jalan, K. N., Maitra, T. K., and Agarwal, S. K.: Vitamin A absorption in ascariasis. Am. J. Clin. Nutr. *29*:1372-1375, 1976.

84. Mannick, J. B.: Immunoregulatory and antimicrobial effects of nitrogen oxides. Proc. Am. Thor. Soc. *3*:161-165, 2006.

85. Manzoni, P., Castagnola, E., Mostert, M., et al.: Hyperglycaemia as a possible marker of invasive fungal infection in preterm neonates. Acta Paediatr. *95*:486-493, 2006.

86. Mata, L.: Malnutrion-infection interaction in the tropics. Am. J. Trop. Med. Hyg. *24*:564-574, 1975.

87. Mata, L. J., Kronmal, R. A., Urrutia, J. J., et al.: Antenatal events and postnatal growth and survival of children: Prospective observation in a rural Guatemalan village. *In* White, P. L. (ed.): Proceedings of the Western Hemisphere Nutrition Congress IV. Acton, MA, Publishing Sciences Group, 1975.

88. Maury, C. P. J., Salo, E., and Pelekonen, P.: Circulating interleukin-1b in patients with Kawasaki disease. N. Engl. J. Med. *319*:1670-1671, 1988.

89. McCallum, R. E., Seale, T. W., and Stith, R. D.: Influence of endotoxin treatment on dexamethasone induction of hepatic phosphoenolpyruvate carboxykinase. Infect. Immun. *39*:213-219, 1983.

90. McKigney, J. I., and Munro, H. N. (eds.): Nutrient Requirements in Adolescence. Cambridge, MA, MIT Press, 1976.

91. Melby, J. C., and Spink, W. W.: Comparative studies on adrenal cortical function and cortisol metabolism in healthy adults and in patients with shock due to infection. J. Clin. Invest. *37*:1791-1798, 1958.

92. Michie, H. R., Manogue, K. R., Sprigs, D. R., et al.: Detection of circulating tumor necrosis factor after endotoxinc administration. N. Engl. J. Med. *318*:1481-1486, 1988.

93. Migasena, P., and Maegraith, B. G.: Intestinal absorption in malaria, I: The absorption of an amino acid (AIB-i-14C) across the gut membrane in normal and in *Plasmodium knowlesi*-infected monkeys. Ann. Trop. Med. Parasitol. *63*:439-448, 1969.

94. Migeon, C. J., Kenny, F. M., Hung, W., et al.: Study of adrenal function in children with meningitis. Pediatrics *40*:163-183, 1967.

95. Moberg, G. P.: Site of action endotoxins on hypothalamic-pituitary-adrenal axis. Am. J. Physiol. *220*:397-400, 1971.

96. Moon, R. J., Tremblay, E. S., and Morris, K. M.: Distribution and metabolism of 14C-tryptophan in normal and endotoxic-poisoned mice. Infect. Immun. *8*:604-611, 1973.

97. Morris, K. M., and Moon, R. J.: Quantitative analysis of serotonin biosynthesis in endotoxemia. Infect. Immun. *10*:340-346, 1974.

98. Morrissey, P. J., and Mochizuki, D. Y.: Interleukin-1 is identical to hematopoietin, 1: Studies on its therapeutic effects of myelopoiesis and lymphopoiesis. Biotherapy *1*:281-291, 1989.

99. Moyer, E. D.: Amino acid metabolism during infectious illness. *In* Powanda, M. (ed.): Infection: The Physiologic and Metabolic Responses of the Host. Amsterdam, Elsevier/North Holland, 1981.

100. Muller, B., and Becker, K. L.: Procalcitonin: How hormone became a marker and mediator of sepsis. Swiss Med. Wkly. *131*:595-602, 2001.

101. Nelson, P. G., Pyke, D. A., and Gamble, D. R.: Viruses and the aetiology of diabetes: A study in identical twins. B. M. J. *4*:249-251, 1975.

102. Nessan, V. J., Geerken, R. C., and Ulvilla, J.: Uric acid excretion in infectious mononucleosis: A function of increased purine turnover. J. Clin. Endocrinol. Metab. *38*:652-654, 1974.

103. Neufeld, H. A., Pace, J. A., Kaminski, M. Y., et al.: A probable endocrine basis for the depression of ketone bodies during infections or inflammatory state in rats. Endocrinology *107*:596-601, 1980.

104. Nichols, B. L., and Soriano, H. A.: A critique of oral therapy of dehydration due to diarrheal syndromes. Am. J. Clin. Nutr. *30*:1457, 1977.

105. Noah, T. L., Henderson, F. W., Wortman, I. A., et al.: Nasal cytokine production in viral acute upper respiratory infection of childhood. J. Infect. Dis. *171*:584-592, 1995.

106. O'Donnel, T. F., Clowes, G. H., Jr., Blackburn, G. L., et al.: Proteolysis associated with a deficit of peripheral energy fuel substrates in septic man. Surgery *80*:192-200, 1976.

107. Paris, M. M., Friedland, I. R., Ehrett, S., et al.: Effect of interleukin-1 receptor antagonist and soluble tumor necrosis factor receptor in animal models of infection. J. Infect. Dis. *171*:161-169, 1995.

108. Patwardhan, V. N., Maghrabi, R. H., Mousa, W., et al.: Serum glycoproteins in protein-calorie deficiency disease. Am. J. Clin. Nutr. *24*:906-912, 1971.

109. Pawlowski, Z. S.: Implications of parasite-nutrition interactions from a world perspective. Fed. Proc. *43*:256-260, 1984.

110. Powanda, M.: Change in body balance of nitrogen and other key nutrients: Description and underlying mechanism. Am. J. Clin. Nutr. *30*:1254-1268, 1977.

111. Powanda, M. C., and Beisel, W. R.: Hypothesis: Leukocyte endogenous mediator/endogenous pyrogen/lymphocyte-activating factor modulates the development of nonspecific immunity and affects nutritional status. Am. J. Clin. Nutr. *35*:762-768, 1982.

112. Powanda, M. C., Dinterman, R., Wannemacher, R. W., Jr., et al.: Tryptophan metabolism in relation to amino acid alterations during typhoid fever. Acta Vitaminol. Enzymol. *29*:164-168, 1975.

113. Powanda, M. C., Wannemacher, R. W., Jr., and Cockerell, G. L.: Nitrogen metabolism and protein synthesis during pneumococcal sepsis in rats. Infect. Immun. *6*:266-271, 1972.

114. Proud, D., Gwaltney, J. M., Jr., Hendley, J. O., et al.: Increased levels of interleukin-1 are detected in nasal secretions of volunteers during experimental rhinovirus colds. J. Infect. Dis. *169*:1007-1013, 1994.

115. Puccetti, P., Mencacci, A., Cenci, E., et al.: Cure of murine candidiasis by recombinant soluble interleukin-4 receptor. J. Infect. Dis. *169*:1325-1331, 1994.

116. Rahman, M. A., Azuma, Y., Fukunaga, H., et al.: Serotonin and melatonin, neurohormones for homeostasis, as novel inhibitors of infections by the intracellular parasite chlamydia. J. Antimicrob. Chemother. *56*:861-868, 2005.

117. Ramsey, K. H., Schneider, H., Cross, A. S., et al.: Inflammatory cytokines produced in response to experimental human gonorrhea. J. Infect. Dis. *172*:186-191, 1995.

118. Rapoport, M. I., and Beisel, W. R.: Studies of tryptophan metabolism in experimental animals and man during infectious ilness. Am. J. Clin. Nutr. *24*:807-814, 1971.

119. Rapoport, M. I., Lust, G., and Beisel, W. R.: Host enzyme induction of bacterial infection. Arch. Intern. Med. *121*:11-16, 1968.

120. Raqib, R., Wretlind, B., Anderson, J., et al.: Cytokine secretion in acute shigellosis is correlated to disease activity and directed more to stool than to plasma. J. Infect. Dis. *171*:376-384, 1995.

121. Rayfield, E. J., Curnow, R. T., George, D. T., et al.: Impaired carbohydrate metabolism during a mild viral illness. N. Engl. J. Med. *289*:618-621, 1973.

122. Reiss, E.: Protein metabolism in infection: Change in certain visceral proteins studies with glycin-N[15]. Metabolism *8*:151-159, 1959.

123. Robinson, D. R.: Lipid mediators of inflammation. Rheum. Dis. Clin. North Am. *13*:385-405, 1987.

124. Rocha, D. M., Santeusanio, F., Faloona, G. R., et al.: Abnormal pancreatic alpha-cell function in bacterial infections. N. Engl. J. Med. *288*:700-703, 1973.

125. Roubenoff, R., Roubenoff, R. A., Cannon, J. G., et al.: Rheumatoid cachexia: Cytokine-driven hypermetabolism accompanying reduced body cell mass in chronic inflammation. J. Clin. Invest. *93*:2379-2386, 1994.

126. Sack, D., Rohads, M., Molla, A., et al.: Carbohydrate malabsorption in infants with rotavirus diarrhea. Am. J. Clin. Nutr. *36*:1112-1118, 1982.

127. Sasazuki, T., McDevitt, H. O., and Grumet, F. C.: The association between genes in the major histocompatibility complex and disease susceptibility. J. Clin. Nutr. *36*:1982, 1977.

128. Schaible, U. E., and Kaufmann, S. H.: Iron and microbial infection. Nat. Rev. *2*:946-953, 2004.

129. Scrimshaw, N. S., and Gordon, J. E.: Interaction of Nutrition and Infection. Geneva, World Health Organization, 1968.

130. Semba, R. D.: Vitamin A, immunity, and infection. Clin. Infect. Dis. *19*:489-499, 1994.

131. Shambaugh, G. E., III, and Beisel, W. R.: Early alterations in thyroid hormone physiology during acute infections in man. J. Clin. Endocrinol. Metab. *27*:1667-1673, 1967.

132. Shambaugh, G. E., III, and Beisel, W. R.: Insulin response during tularemia in man. Diabetes *16*:369-376, 1967.

133. Shaw, A. R.: Molecular biology of cytokines: An introduction. *In* Thompson, A. W. (ed.): The Cytokine Handbook. New York, Academic Press, 1991, pp. 19-42.

134. Shimoya, K., Matsuzaki, N., Taniguchi, T., et al.: Interleukin-8 in cord sera: A sensitive and specific marker for the detection of preterm chorioamnionitis. J. Infect. Dis. *165*:957-960, 1992.

135. Siegel, J. H., Cerra, F. B., Coleman, B., et al.: Physiological and metabolic correlations in human sepsis: Invited commentary. Surgery *86*:163-193, 1979.

136. Smith, R. E., and Horwitz, B. A.: Brown fat and thermogenesis. Physiol. Rev. *49*:330-425, 1969.

137. Sobocinski, P. Z., Canterbury, W. J., Jr., Mapes, C. A., and Dinterman, R. E.: Involvement of hepatic metallothioneins in hypozincemia associated with bacterial infection. Am. J. Physiol. *234*:E399-E406, 1978.

138. Sommer, A.: Vitamin A, infectious disease, and childhood mortality: A 2c solution? J. Infect. Dis. *167*:1003-1007, 1993.

139. Stamler, J. S., Singel, D. J., and Loscalzo, J.: Biochemistry of nitric oxide and its redox-activated forms. Science *258*:1891-1902, 1992.

140. Steinmetz, C. B., Alvarez, J. O., Kohatsu, J., et al.: Vitamin A is excreted in the urine during acute infection. Am. J. Clin. Nutr. *60*:388-392, 1994.

141. Stephensen, C. B.: Burden of infection on growth failure. J. Nutr. *129*:534S-538S, 1999.

142. Stephensen, C. B., Alvarez, J. O., Kohatsu, J., et al.: Vitamin A is excreted in the urine during acute infection. Am. J. Clin. Nutr. *60*:388-392, 1994.

143. Stephensen, C. B., Marquis, G. S., Jacob, R. A., et al.: Vitamins C and E in adolescents and young adults with HIV infection. Am. J. Clin. Nutr. *83*:870-879, 2006.

144. Stuehr, D. J., and Nathan, C. F.: Nitric oxide: A macrophage product responsible for cytostasis and respiratory inhibition of tumor target cells. J. Exp. Med. *169*:1543-1555, 1989.

145. te Vede, M., Huijbens, R. J. F., Heije, K., et al.: Interleukin-4 (IL-4) inhibits secretion of IL-1 beta, tumor necrosis factor alpha, and IL-6 by human monocytes. Blood *76*:1392-1397, 1990.

146. Uzzan, B., Cohen, R., Nicolas, P., et al.: Procalcitonin as a diagnostic test for sepsis in critically ill adults and after surgery or trauma: A systematic review and meta-analysis. Crit. Care Med. *34*:1996-2003, 2006.

147. Valyi-Nagy, T., and Dermody, T. S.: Role of oxidative damage in the pathogenesis of viral infections of the nervous system. Histol. Histopathol. *20*:957-967, 2005.

148. Van der Graaf, C. A., Netea, M. G., Morre, S. A., et al.: Toll-like receptor 4 Asp299Gly/Thr399Ile polymorphisms are a risk factor for *Candida* bloodstream infection. Eur. Cytokine Network *17*:29-34, 2006.

149. van der Pool, T., van Deventer, S. J. H., ten Cate, H., et al.: Tumor necrosis factor is involved in the appearance of interleukin-1 receptor antagonist in endotoxemia. J. Infect. Dis. *169*:665-667, 1994.

150. van Deuren, M., van der Ven-Jongekrijg, J., and Demacker, P. M. N.: Differential expression of proinflammatory cytokines and their inhibitors during the course of meningococcal infections. J. Infect. Dis. *169*:157-161, 1993.

151. Verboon-Maciolek, M. A., Thijsen, S. F., Hemels, M. A., et al.: Inflammatory mediators for the diagnosis and treatment of sepsis in early infancy. Pediatr. Res. *59*:457-461, 2006.

152. Vermont, C. L., den Brinker, M., Kakeci, N., et al.: Serum lipids and disease severity in children with severe meningococcal sepsis. Crit. Care Med. *33*:1610-1615, 2005.

153. Victor, V. M., Rocha, M., Esplugues, J. V., and De la Fuente, M.: Role of free radicals in sepsis: Antioxidant therapy. Curr. Pharmaceut. Design *11*:3141-3158, 2005.

154. Villamor, E.: A potential role for vitamin D on HIV infection? Nutr. Rev. *64*:226-233, 2006.

155. Vitale, J. J.: The impact of infection on vitamin metabolism: An unexplored area. Am. J. Clin. Nutr. *30*:1473-1477, 1977.

156. Viteri, F. E., and Behar, M.: Efectos de diversas infecctiones sobre la nutricion del preschtolar especialmente el sarampi. Bole. Ofic. Sani. Panam. 78:226-240, 1975.
157. Wagner, D. A., and Tannenbaum, S. R.: Enhancement of nitrate biosynthesis by *Escherichia coli* lipopolysaccharides. *In* McGee, P. N. (ed.): Nitrosamines and Human Cancer. Cold Spring Harbor, NY, Cold Spring Harbor Laboratories, 1982, pp. 437-441.
158. Wannemacher, R. W., Jr.: Key role of individual amino acids in host response to infection. Am. J. Clin. Nutr. 30:1269-1280, 1977.
159. Wannemacher, R. W., Jr., Dinterman, R. E., Pekarek, R. S., et al.: Urinary amino acid excretion during experimentally induced sandly fever in man. Am. J. Clin. Nutr. 28:110-118, 1975.
160. Wannemacher, R. W., Jr., Klainer, A. S., Dinterman, R. E., et al.: The significance and mechanism of an increased serum phenylalanine-tyrosine ratio during infection. Am. J. Clin. Nutr. 29:997-1006, 1976.
161. Wannemacher, R. W., Jr., Powanda, M. C., and Dinterman, R. E.: Amino acid flux and protein synthesis after exposure of rats to either *Diplococcus pneumoniae* or *Salmonella typhimurium*. Infect. Immun. 10:60-65, 1974.
162. Wartofsky, L., Burman, K. D., Dimond, R. C., et al.: Studies on the nature of thyroidal suppression during acute falciparum malaria: Integrity of pituitary response to TRH and alterations in serum T₃ and reverse T₃. J. Clin. Endocrinol. Metab. 14:85-90, 1977.
163. Watten, R. H., Morgan, F. M., Songkhla, Y. N., et al.: Water and electrolyte studies in cholera. J. Clin. Invest. 38:1879-1889, 1959.
164. Weigent, D. A., Baxter, J. B., Wear, W. E., et al.: Production of immunoreactive growth hormone by mononuclear leukocytes. FASEB. J. 2:2812-2818, 1988.
165. Weinberg, E. D.: Iron and susceptibility to infectious disease. Science 184:952-956, 1974.
166. West, H. D., Jackson, A. H., Elliott, R. R., et al.: The utilization of ingested iron in disease. South. Med. J. 45:629-633, 1952.
167. Westerdorp, R. G. J., Langermans, J. A. M., de Bel, C. E., et al.: Release of tumor necrosis factor: An innate host characteristic that may contribute to the outcome of meningococcal disease. J. Infect. Dis. 171:1057-1060, 1995.
168. Whedon, G. D., and Shorr, E.: Metabolic studies in paralytic acute anterior polyomyelitis, II: Alterations in calcium and phosphorus metabolism. J. Clin. Invest. 36:966-981, 1957.
169. White, M. G., Carter, N. W., Rector, F. C., et al.: Pathophysiology of epidemic St. Louis encephalitis. Ann. Intern. Med. 71:691-702, 1969.
170. Wiles, J. B., Cerra, F. B., Siegel, J. H., and Border, J. R.: The systemic septic response: Does the organism matter? Crit. Care Med. 8:55-60, 1980.
171. Wilmore, D. W., Long, J. M., Mason, A. D., Jr., et al.: Catecholamines: Mediator of the hypermetabolic response to thermal injury. Ann. Surg. 180:653-669, 1974.
172. Wilson, D., Bressani, R., and Scrimshaw, N. S.: Infection and nutritional status, I: The effect of chicken pox on nitrogen metabolism in children. Am. J. Clin. Nutr. 9:154-158, 1961.
173. Woeber, K. A.: Alterations in thyroid hormone economy during acute infection with *Diplococcus pneumoniae* in the rhesis monkey. J. Clin. Invest. 50:378-387, 1971.
174. Yarasheski, K. E., Smith, S. R., and Powderly, W. G.: Reducing plasma HIV RNA improves muscle amino acid metabolism. Am. J. Physiol. 288:E278-E284, 2005.
175. Yelish, C. Y., and Filkins, J. P.: Mechanism of hyperinsulinism in endotoxicosis. Am. J. Physiol. 239:E156-E161, 1980.
176. Yeung, C. Y.: Hypoglycemia in neonatal sepsis. J. Pediatr. 77:812-817, 1970.
177. Yildizdas, D., Onenli-Mungan, N., et al.: Thyroid hormone levels and their relationship to survival in children with bacterial sepsis and septic shock. J. Pediatr. Endocrinol. Metab. 17:1435-1442, 2004.
178. Young, V. R., Alexis, S. D., Maliga, B. S., et al.: Metabolism of administered 3-methylhistidine: Lack of muscle transfer ribonucleic acid charging and quantitative excretion as 3-methylhistidine and its *N*-acetyl derivative. J. Biol. Chem. 247:3592-3600, 1972.

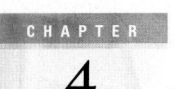

INTERACTION OF INFECTION AND NUTRITION

4

Ralph D. Feigin ◉ Kathrin M. Bernt

The introduction to the World Health Organization (WHO) report on nutrition and infection, published in 1965, stated the following[343]:

> The concept that malnutrition could make man more susceptible to infectious disease and also alter the course and outcome of the resulting illness has long been current in the history of medicine and public health. Circumstantial evidence is plentiful, principally based on clinical experience. Well controlled observations have been few, and hence clear proof in support of the concept has been slow to accumulate. It has been much easier to demonstrate that infection is often directly responsible for lowering the state of nutrition.

The 2005 WHO report estimated that 1 million children would die before reaching 5 years of age. Infections, including acute respiratory infections (19%), diarrheal diseases (17%), neonatal infections (including neonatal tetanus) (14%), malaria (8%), measles (4%), and human immunodeficiency virus (HIV) (3%),[347] account for most of these deaths. More than half of these deaths are associated with malnutrition.[46] This problem has been called "silent genocide" by WHO officials and is one of the most underreported health problems facing humans.

The association of malnutrition with infection has been documented repeatedly. The devastating effects of long-term semistarvation in infants and small children were described by physicians trapped in the Jewish ghetto of Warsaw by the prolonged Nazi siege.[41,341] They observed gross and microscopic evidence of lymphoid tissue atrophy and the disappearance of delayed hypersensitivity reactions and acute inflammation, as well as the disappearance of clinical allergies, blood eosinophils, and gastric acid in severely malnourished children. More recent data also support the concept that malnutrition renders individuals more susceptible to acquisition of infection. Metabolic, biochemical, and clinical evidence has accumulated that strongly supports the concept that nutrition affects profoundly the progress of infection within the host. The normal host response to infection is described in detail in Chapter 3. Virtually every normal metabolic or endocrine function is altered in some manner by the presence of an infectious illness.

Traditionally, clinical inquiries into the interaction of nutrition and infection have focused on patients with protein-calorie malnutrition. Nutrition is a crucial determinant of immunocompetence and risk for development of illness. Young children with protein-calorie malnutrition exhibit increased morbidity and mortality rates largely secondary to infectious diseases.[59] These children often have isolated deficiencies of single nutrients, and single-nutrient deficiencies and protein-calorie malnutrition are associated with impaired immune responses.

In light of the well-recognized biologic synergism that exists between malnutrition and infection, it is noteworthy that malnutrition has not received comparable attention in child health and survival strategies. This oversight may occur partly because data on mortality gathered from health facilities in developing countries report only the proximate cause of death (usually infectious diseases), such that only the severe cases of nutritional deficiency are recorded as nutritional causes of death.[237]

PROTEIN-CALORIE MALNUTRITION

Protein-calorie malnutrition describes a wide range of clinical conditions resulting from mild to severe undernutrition. The

WHO estimated in 1996[345] that 174 million children younger than 5 years of age in the developing world were malnourished, as indicated by low weight for age, and that 230 million were stunted. Mild protein-calorie malnutrition may be detected primarily by poor growth because when energy consumption is low, amino acids from dietary protein are used for energy, rather than for protein synthesis and growth.

The conditions of kwashiorkor and marasmus represent manifestations of severe protein-calorie malnutrition. Both conditions result from consumption of a diet deficient in protein and calories, but infections also play an important role. Frequently, an acute infection is incriminated as the event precipitating kwashiorkor.[13,117,134,306] Marasmus is characterized by severe wasting, whereas kwashiorkor is manifested by the presence of edema. In marasmus, the prognosis on refeeding is good, whereas treatment of kwashiorkor is more difficult, and the prognosis often is poor.[122] African studies have estimated the mortality rate in kwashiorkor to be 25 to 31 percent.[112,188] In these children, infection was second only to electrolyte abnormalities as a leading cause of death. Inadequate diet, including insufficient intake of energy, protein, and micronutrients (e.g., iron, vitamins, and minerals), leads to weight loss, retarded growth rate, diminished immunity, and mucosal damage. These factors exacerbate the incidence, severity, and duration of infectious diseases, which lead to the loss of nutrients, malabsorption, altered metabolism, and loss of appetite that lead to further inadequate dietary intake.[35]

That various infectious diseases interfere with or influence the responses of host defense is well known. Metabolic responses of the host to infection include increased use of proteins, carbohydrates, lipids, minerals, electrolytes, trace elements, vitamins, and hormones. The normal host responds to infection by initiating an immediate and marked stimulus for protein anabolism. The chemical changes in protein-calorie malnutrition include low serum albumin, low concentrations of essential amino acids in serum, generalized aminoaciduria, lower glycosylated hemoglobin levels, and decreased activity of many enzymes. Reduction in the activity of diphosphopyridine nucleotide, cytochrome *c* reductase, plasma esterase, and leukocyte pyruvate kinase has been documented.

A patient with kwashiorkor, depleted of amino acids and protein, cannot initiate the necessary anabolic response when challenged by infection, which seems to alter the capacity of the host to resist the debilitating effects of infection. Decreased activity of the various enzymes that help to resist infection and the inability to synthesize new enzymes necessary for energy-producing reactions in the body impose an additional burden on an individual with protein-calorie malnutrition. If the diet does not replace calories and protein sufficiently, the individual becomes progressively depleted with each episode of infection. Repeated episodes of infection may be a major factor in precipitating frank kwashiorkor in children on a borderline diet with regard to protein and calories. In many instances, whether the malnutrition or the infection was the event that initiated the ultimate deterioration of the patient cannot be determined.

Postmortem studies have confirmed that acute bacterial infections are the major cause of death in patients with severe protein-calorie malnutrition. Septicemia is the most dreaded infectious complication of protein-calorie malnutrition and has been reported in 31 percent of hospitalized patients. Gram-negative enteric bacilli are the most common cause; less frequent agents include *Haemophilus influenzae*, *Shigella flexneri*, *Pseudomonas aeruginosa*, *Corynebacterium diphtheriae*, *Streptococcus* spp., *Staphylococcus aureus*, and *Neisseria* spp. Tuberculosis occurs more frequently, is more virulent, spreads faster, and reinfects more readily individuals with protein-calorie malnutrition. The rate of urinary tract infections in malnourished children is increased significantly, with gram-negative enteric bacilli encountered most frequently. Diarrhea is a common occurrence in malnourished children, the most common infectious cause being enteric pathogens, such as *Salmonella enteritidis*, enteropathogenic *Escherichia coli*, and nontyphi *Salmonella* spp.[286] The occurrence of *Pneumocystis carinii* infection in malnourished individuals also has been highlighted.[134] Additionally, viral diseases, such as measles, varicella, hepatitis, and herpes simplex, are prevalent in patients with protein-calorie malnutrition.[13,117,306]

Almost all cases of severe protein-calorie malnutrition exhibit biochemical or clinical evidence of micronutrient deficiencies, such as vitamin A deficiency or iron-deficiency anemia. Little evidence exists, however, that any one micronutrient deficiency is the main cause of protein-calorie malnutrition or by itself is responsible for the edema of kwashiorkor.

Although protein is an essential and important nutrient, protein-calorie malnutrition is associated more often with deficient food intake than with protein intake. When commonly consumed cereal-based diets meet caloric needs, they *usually* meet protein needs, especially if the diet also provides modest amounts of legumes and vegetables. Control and prevention of protein-calorie malnutrition should focus on improvements in the quantity and quality of food consumed, immunization, provision of oral rehydration therapy for diarrhea, early treatment of common diseases, regular deworming, and attention given to the underlying causes of protein-calorie malnutrition, such as poverty and inequity.[173]

IN UTERO EFFECTS OF MALNUTRITION

The medical literature reports widespread occurrence of infant low birth weight throughout the nations of the world in which malnutrition is prevalent. Hytten,[137] discussing the relationship of maternal diet to the size of the infant's body, called attention to the fact that dietary status in pregnancy is only part of the broad environmental picture. He emphasized that the mother's nutrition throughout life may be as important as nutrition during pregnancy in ensuring the birth of an infant of normal size. A well-fed mother deprived of food during pregnancy may have been able to lay down a sufficient energy reserve to protect the fetus during intrauterine life despite deficiencies in day-to-day intake. Short maternal stature, which is influenced by biosocial factors, large family size, malnutrition, and chronic disease, frequently becomes intergenerational. Women who were growth retarded as newborns tend to give birth to infants who also are growth retarded, which may be a reflection of poor maternal nutritional status during childhood and adolescence.[183]

Severe nutritional deprivation during pregnancy may affect the size and vitality of the fetus. Abrams and Laros[1] showed that underweight women and women with poor weight gain during pregnancy had an increased risk for delivering an infant weighing less than 2500 g.

Maternal malnutrition results in impaired placental function and chronic vascular insufficiency, which leads to symmetric growth retardation. As nutritional deprivation becomes more severe, first weight, then length, and finally brain mass are affected. Acute placental insufficiency results in asymmetric growth retardation. When the nutritional insult occurs late in pregnancy, when length velocity is declining and weight velocity is increasing, the amount of muscle, fat, and hepatic glycogen is affected adversely. This type of growth retardation is seen in postmature infants; in these infants, placental function no longer is adequate to meet fetal needs, and the fetus must mobilize its own fat and carbohydrate stores.[183]

Maternal malnutrition before or during pregnancy and maternal infection during pregnancy may act alone or in concert to influence the size, gestational age at birth, and vitality of the fetus. Infection during pregnancy occurs commonly in the areas of the world where malnutrition is prevalent. In a prospective study in four Guatemalan villages, 12 percent of village women who were tested serologically throughout pregnancy for cytomegalovirus, herpes simplex, rubella, syphilis, and *Toxoplasma* spp. infection showed seroconversion during pregnancy to one of these agents.[144] The aforementioned infections, varicella, HIV, malaria, and trypanosomiasis are associated with intrauterine growth retardation.[32]

Infant size at birth correlates to a great extent with neonatal survival. Village infants who are small for gestational age at birth have a greater risk for developing subsequent malnutrition and infection than do term infants with an adequate birth weight. Infants with low birth weight (predominantly small for gestational age) have higher rates of infection with *Shigella* spp., *Entamoeba histolytica*, and *Giardia* spp. in the first month of life and exhibit higher occurrences of diarrhea and oral candidiasis in the first 6 months than do term infants.

A case-control study in rural Africa suggests this susceptibility to infectious disease extends far beyond the first 6 months of life.[212] As late as adolescence, increased infectious mortality rates were seen in individuals who had been born during the "hungry season" compared with those born during the "harvest season." These findings suggest that nutritionally mediated growth retardation may impair development of immune function permanently. Animal models highlight these long-term effects of intrauterine malnutrition by showing impaired T-cell–dependent immune responses in the first-generation and second-generation offspring of animals subjected to prenatal nutritional deprivation.[54]

Even if caloric requirements are met during pregnancy, micronutrient deficiencies have been linked to adverse pregnancy outcomes, and the worldwide prevalence of these deficiencies varies greatly.[280] In particular, iodine and folic acid are two micronutrients with proven roles in embryonic/fetal development. Deficiencies are endemic in certain parts of the world and may have devastating consequences for affected infants. More recently, zinc deficiency during pregnancy has been implicated in postnatal immune dysfunction and increased risk for development of infections.[338]

Even in industrialized countries, the consequences of low birth weight can be extensive. Providing enteral nourishment to very-low-birth-weight infants can be difficult because of systemic illnesses, such as respiratory distress syndrome and gastrointestinal tract immaturity. Many of these infants ultimately develop clinical and biochemical signs of malnutrition during the early postnatal period. This malnutrition may compromise an already inadequate immune system and alter host susceptibility to infection. Reductions in spleen, thymus, and body weights were noted in rats after experiencing intrauterine protein-calorie deprivation. After nutritional restoration was achieved in these animals, thymic tissue remained depleted of lymphocytes and significantly reduced in weight.

Newborn infants may develop similar long-term immunologic defects after in utero or early postnatal malnutrition. Low-birth-weight infants born to malnourished mothers have decreased thymus and spleen size and diminished cell-mediated immune responses, reduced transfer of maternal-fetal IgG, and decreased number of T lymphocytes. Infants with fetal growth retardation have shown diminished neutrophil chemotaxis, abnormal nitroblue tetrazolium oxidative reduction, and deficient microbicidal activity.[55,121] After birth, nutritional deprivation may create the environment for frequent episodes of infection. Mechanisms responsible for the increased number and severity of infections in the malnourished host are detailed subsequently.

BREAST-FEEDING

The nutritional, immunologic, psychosocial, and child-spacing benefits of breast-feeding are recognized universally. According to numerous reports, breast-fed infants seem to be less susceptible than are bottle-fed infants to certain infections. The protective effect is most evident for upper respiratory infections, otitis media, and gastroenteritis and has been studied most extensively in developing countries; the impact of breast-feeding on other infections and in more developed countries also is under investigation. Many studies are investigating the specific agents present in human milk that may be important in imparting protection to the infant. In addition to its anti-infective properties, breast milk has been shown to exhibit other advantages over infant formula; however, despite its many benefits, in certain situations, breast-feeding is contraindicated.

The antimicrobial system in human milk constitutes a complex group of biochemical agents that differ widely in structure but have a common effect at the mucosa. These agents include lysozyme, lactoperoxidase, lactoferrin, interferon, complement components, immunoglobulins, leukocytes, lipids, and retinol. These anti-infective factors transmitted by breast milk protect primarily by noninflammatory mechanisms and act to reduce the risk for development of mucosal infection in the gut. Proteins present in breast milk are thought to escape digestion in young infants as a result of low acid, reduced protease activity in gastric and pancreatic secretions, and the presence of protease inhibitors in breast milk.

The component most important to the newborn may be secretory IgA, which is found in high concentrations in colostrum and early milk. Secretory IgA constitutes more than 90 percent of the immunoglobulins in human milk and is formed by intricate processes that may be regulated by cytokines and hormones produced late in pregnancy or during lactation. During this process, B cells producing IgA against respiratory and gastrointestinal infectious agents migrate to the mammary gland in a higher proportion than their percentage of the total IgA-secreting B-cell pool. IgA possesses virus-neutralizing and antibacterial properties and is capable of activating the alternate complement pathway, providing local protection in the gastrointestinal tract.

Lactoferrin is an iron-binding glycoprotein that competes with siderophilic bacteria for ferric iron and interferes with the multiplication of organisms. Lactoferrin also may have a positive influence on cell growth and a negative effect on inflammation. Lysozyme is found in high concentrations in external secretions, including human milk, and lysis-susceptible bacteria by hydrolyzing β-1,4 linkages between *N*-acetylmuramic acid and 2-acetylamino-2-deoxy-D-glucose residues in cell walls. Lysozyme is resistant to digestion by trypsin and denaturation caused by acid. Fibronectin is a high-molecular-weight protein found in breast milk that facilitates the uptake of particulates by phagocytic cells.

Human milk also is rich in carbohydrate moieties that act as receptor homologues and inhibit attachment of pathogenic bacteria, such as *Vibrio cholerae*, *Streptococcus pneumoniae*, *H. influenzae*, and *E. coli*, onto epithelial cells.[72] Certain oligosaccharides in human milk promote the growth of *Bifidobacterium* spp. and lactobacilli in the lower intestinal tract, which produce acetic acid and inhibit the multiplication of bacterial pathogens such as *E. coli* and *Salmonella* and *Shigella* spp. Additionally, lactadherin, a component of human milk, has been found to bind specifically to rotavirus and inhibit its replication in vitro.[222] A study of rotavirus infection in Nicaraguan children supports this finding by showing an association between a longer duration of breast-feeding and decreased symptoms with rotavirus infection.[92]

A plethora of cytokines have been isolated from human milk, many in concentrations exceeding maternal serum, which suggests an active transport mechanism. Viable leukocytes are found in human milk and have been proposed to play a role in protection against infections and immune modulation.[33]

Epidemiologic studies of the association between infections and breast-feeding have come under great scrutiny. Strong evidence has shown that in developing countries, infant morbidity is reduced by breast-feeding. A pooled analysis[348] of studies performed in the Philippines, Brazil, and Pakistan indicates that breast-feeding offers protection against the risks of diarrhea and of mortality from acute respiratory infection. The greatest protection is offered early in infancy and then steadily declines. Multiple small studies from Mexico,[181,330] India,[335] Belarus (diarrhea only; no protective effect against respiratory infections),[163] Haiti,[157] and Nicaragua[92] confirm these results. In a study from Nicaragua, protection against *Giardia* infections depended on the maternal antibody status: breast-fed infants of nonimmune mothers had a higher risk of developing giardiasis and experienced more severe symptoms compared with breast-fed infants of immune mothers.[310]

Many researchers consider that infants in more developed countries have similar benefits.[56,69,233,333,349] In a longitudinal analysis of infants in the United States, the risk for developing otitis media or diarrhea increased as the amount of breast milk received decreased.[265] The effect against otitis media may be the result of transmission of humoral or cellular immune components to the infant or the result of positioning during bottle feeding, which may predispose the infant to otitis media. Data showing general protection against infection are supplemented by studies that investigate the effects of breast milk on specific pathologic organisms. Formula-fed infants are more likely than are breast-fed infants to have colonization[130] or invasive disease[287] caused by *H. influenzae* and a higher risk for acquiring invasive pneumococcal disease.[176] Other studies have shown decreased risk for developing respiratory illnesses,[38,223] meningococcal disease,[210] urinary tract infections,[189] salmonellosis,[255] and human herpesvirus-7[172] infection with breast-feeding.

Despite studies such as these, the evidence in highly developed countries remains controversial. Bauchner and associates[21] presented a meta-analysis of the association between breast-feeding and infections in industrialized countries. Of 20 studies in the meta-analysis, only 6 met strict methodologic standards. These investigators concluded that the evidence supports only a minimally protective effect of breast-feeding. In 1990, a group from Denmark reported their results after following 500 infants prospectively for the first year of life.[258] They were unable to document a protective effect of breast-feeding against infectious illness. A case-control study of 13,224 mother-infant pairs, the largest study published to date, found no measurable association between breast-feeding and risk of neonatal respiratory infections in boys and only a small protective effect in girls.[290] These differences highlight the importance of environmental factors, such as socioeconomic status, parental education, exposure in daycare centers, and parental smoking, to the incidence of infectious disease in infants. Nonetheless, a report of the Department of Health and Human Services Office on Women's Health[83] recommends exclusive breast-feeding except in special situations in which contraindications to breast-feeding exist.

Breast-feeding has distinct advantages over bottle feeding in situations in which infection is not an important factor. Numerous studies in various parts of the world have investigated the possible prevention of atopic or allergic diseases by breast-feeding. Three more recent meta-analyses concluded that there was a lower incidence of asthma[111] and allergic rhinitis[205] in breast-fed infants and a lower incidence of eczema in breast-fed versus formula-fed infants with a family history of atopy.[110] A study analyzing cytokine profiles in formula-fed or breast-fed infants with respiratory syncytial virus (RSV) bronchiolitis suggested that the protective effect of breast milk against infections together with its potential immune-modulatory properties act together to protect infants from more severe RSV disease.[252]

The effect of breast-feeding on the prevention of atopic diseases has not been unchallenged—a cohort study from Brazil found an increased risk for development of asthma associated with being breast-fed for 9 months or longer.[71] The data currently available point toward a protective effect of breast-feeding, however, during the first 6 months of life on allergic or atopic diseases. Although evidence is inconclusive, some studies have implied that breast-feeding provides protection against sudden infant death syndrome, obesity, type 1 and type 2 diabetes, hypercholesterolemia, arteriosclerosis, celiac disease, and other metabolic disorders, and enhances neurodevelopment.[8,149]

Colostrum and early milk contain hormones and growth factors, such as epidermal growth factor, prostaglandins, insulin, and thyroid hormones, that may benefit children whose gut integrity has been compromised by malnutrition and gastrointestinal disease.[242] Whether these components are present in amounts sufficient to have any physiologic effect after the first few months of lactation is unclear, however. Breast milk also contains the digestive enzymes amylase, bile salt–stimulated lipase, and bile salt–stimulated esterase in measurable quantities after 6 months of lactation. Children whose digestive functions are compromised by malnutrition or small bowel overgrowth may benefit from the addition of breast milk enzymes. The combined effects of protection against infections, immune modulation, and maintenance of the integrity and promotion of growth of the intestinal mucosa may work together to explain a much decreased incidence of sepsis and necrotizing enterocolitis in a cohort study of Norwegian extremely-low-birth-weight infants in whom early enteral feeding with human milk was established.[253]

In certain circumstances, breast-feeding is contraindicated. The most common of these situations is maternal infection with HIV, a topic that has been the focus of much recent research. More recent studies estimate that one third to one half of mother-to-child transmissions of HIV occur through breast milk.[164,314] A randomized clinical trial of 401 mother-infant pairs in Kenya[218] showed that the risk for transmission in breast milk was 16.2 percent and that the use of formula feeding prevented 44 percent of infant infections. Risk for transmission is approximately 14 percent in chronic maternal HIV infection and increases to 29 percent in acute infection.

Other factors that may increase transmission of HIV through breast milk include longer duration of breast-feeding, mastitis in the mother, lower maternal CD4 counts, and mixed feedings (i.e., infants fed breast milk and formula).[314] The mechanism by which mixed feedings increase transmission is currently under debate. Some researchers theorize that a subclinical mastitis caused by milk stasis is responsible, whereas others hypothesize that an inflammatory or immunologic response in the infant gut may play a role. Currently, breast-feeding by HIV-infected women is contraindicated in areas where safe alternative sources of infant nutrition exist. Some researchers argue that in areas where environmental contamination precludes the safe use of other infant feeding regimens, exclusive breast-feeding should be promoted. A more recent study conducted in Kenya showed, however, that with access to clean water, formula feeding can decrease HIV transmission rates significantly without substantially increasing morbidity and mortality rates from diarrhea and pneumonia even in resource-poor settings.[194]

Breast-feeding also is contraindicated in mothers who are sputum-positive for *Mycobacterium tuberculosis* or who are carriers of hepatitis B virus. Breast milk has been implicated in the transmission of rubella, cholera, Q fever, human T-cell lymphotropic virus 1, and cytomegalovirus in selected individuals. Human milk also can transmit environmental toxins, such as polychlorinated biphenyl compounds and dichlorodiphenyltrichloroethane. Toxic side effects can occur in nursing infants secondary to passive excretion of medicines taken by the mother.[88,149] On balance, breast milk is preferable except in unusual circumstances and helps diminish the role of infection during infancy.

IMMUNE SYSTEM AND MALNOURISHED HOST

MUCOSAL IMMUNITY

The first barrier to potential pathogens is the physical integrity of the skin and mucous membranes. This barrier involves single or multiple layers of cells, mechanical clearance mechanisms such as the cilia of the respiratory epithelium, complex carbohydrate structures in the intestinal epithelium, lubricants such as sebum or mucus, and soluble factors such as antibodies and lysozyme.

A "mucosal immune system" has been described in the gut, where tissue resident cells of the monocyte/macrophage lineage and specialized enterocytes act as antigen-presenting cells to lymphocytes. Primed lymphocytes migrate to the Peyer patches, where they proliferate and differentiate. A subset also enters the circulation to reach central immune organs, such as the spleen, bone marrow, and possibly thymus, where the lymphocytes undergo further clonal expansion. Eventually, they become IgA-producing cells that re-enter the circulation and by a selective homing process migrate to the mucosa of the gut and to salivary, lacrimal, bronchial, and lactating mammary glands.[243]

The physical integrity of the cell layers of skin or mucous membranes is affected in numerous nutritional deficiencies. Examples include the metaplastic hyperkeratosis caused by avitaminosis A; the dermatitis, cheilitis, and angular stomatitis from iron, riboflavin, and pyridoxine deficiencies; the mucosal atrophy and dermatosis of pellagra; the acrodermatitis enteropathica associated with zinc deficiency; the spongy gums and subcutaneous hemorrhages of scurvy; and the atrophy of skin and gastrointestinal mucosa of severe protein deficiency.

The carbohydrate composition of intestinal epithelium has been shown to vary according to dietary influences, and a decreased risk for gastrointestinal infections in breast-fed infants is thought to be due partly to decreased carbohydrate receptor sites for intestinal pathogens. Severe protein malnutrition and xerophthalmia have been shown to suppress significantly the secretion of lysozyme in the tears of children.[344] Diminished secretory IgA has been noted in malnutrition, which may increase host susceptibility to infection by permitting increased penetration of infectious agents into the circulation.[292,301] Malnutrition also affects other parts of the "mucosal immune system": Malnourished children have a reduced number of lymphocytes and plasma cells in the interstitial space, and the migration of lymphoblasts from the mesentery is decreased.[63]

HUMORAL IMMUNITY

Numerous studies of B-cell function have been done in patients with protein-calorie malnutrition, albeit with conflicting results. The total number of circulating B cells has been reported to be normal or increased,[312] or diminished.[217,248] Serum immunoglobulin concentrations may be normal or elevated.[293] Cohen and Hansen[65] showed that children with protein-calorie malnutrition and infection synthesized gamma-globulin at three times the rate of uninfected malnourished individuals, documenting the fact that synthesis of gamma-globulin was not rate-limited in malnutrition at the expense of other protein synthesis, such as that of albumin. In protein-calorie malnutrition, antibody affinity is decreased, which may explain the higher frequency of antigen-antibody complexes found in malnourished patients.

In protein-calorie malnutrition, the most dramatic change in humoral immunity concerns IgE. Serum IgE concentrations in healthy, well-nourished children are extremely low. Significant elevations of serum IgE in malnourished children have been reported in the absence of allergy or parasitic infections, possibly caused by an imbalance in T-lymphocyte regulation of IgE-producing B-cell function. The defect in cell-mediated immunity in patients with protein-calorie malnutrition could initiate an exaggerated IgE response during infections with respiratory pathogens, such as RSV or parainfluenza virus, and increase the risk for developing severe bronchiolitis.[153]

Antibody production after immunization with antigen is the best functional measure of humoral immunity. Much of the data on specific serum antibody responses in human malnutrition are conflicting. The serum antibody response to many protein antigens, such as tetanus or diphtheria toxoid, is well preserved. The responses to immunization with viral antigens vary. Responses to yellow fever vaccine, hepatitis, and killed influenza A have been reported to be impaired in protein-calorie malnutrition. Chronic malnutrition also is associated with a poor response to measles vaccine.[331] A diminished antibody response to polysaccharide antigens, such as killed typhoid vaccine (polysaccharide typhoid O antigen), is seen in severe protein-calorie malnutrition. The degree of malnutrition may play a role; mild protein-calorie malnutrition had no impact on the response to a meningococcal group C polysaccharide vaccine.[120]

A diminished antibody response to polysaccharide antigens may be caused by a selective impact on the IgG subclasses that contain antibody to polysaccharide antigens, IgG2 and IgG4.[153] Studies in rats deficient in vitamin A support this hypothesis[156]; however, total serum levels and IgG subclasses in 109 malnourished children from Ghana were found to be normal.[248] Further studies investigating the relationship between IgG subclasses and protein-calorie malnutrition are needed.

CELLULAR IMMUNITY

In patients with malnutrition, the cellular immune system (T-cell system) seems to be the component of the immune system affected most significantly. Impairments have been shown at nearly all levels of T-cell development and function. Histological studies of lymphoid tissues show severe depletion of T-cell areas in malnourished hosts.[197] The total number of circulating T cells, particularly the helper CD4 subset, is decreased.[217] Little change occurs in the number of suppressor T cells; the helper-to-suppressor ratio is decreased significantly.[62,234] The levels of circulating immature (CD1a$^+$, or CD4$^-$CD8$^-$ "null cell") T cells have been found to be increased in several studies, pointing toward a defect in maturation.[234] Indirect evidence, such as decreased deoxynucleotide transferase activity and increased adenosine deaminase in the serum of malnourished children, also suggests a defect in T-cell maturation.[206]

T-cell function in malnourished hosts seems to be impaired as well. Several studies have shown decreased responses to mitogenic stimuli and decreased production of cytokine, particularly type 1 cytokines (interleukin-2 [IL-2], interferon-γ).[89,251,266] Finally, the level of circulating memory T cells (CD45RO$^+$) has been found to be decreased in malnourished children.[216]

The observed abnormalities in T-cell numbers and function are clinically reflected in decreased responses to skin testing for antigens that normally induce delayed hypersensitivity responses. Chandra[60] reported that malnourished children had a decreased ability to respond to tuberculin antigen after receiving bacille Calmette-Guérin (BCG) immunization, and, in most cases, they could not be sensitized to dinitrochlorobenzene. Smythe and associates[293] reported similar findings in malnourished children and noted lymphocyte depletion in the thymus glands of 118 children with kwashiorkor or marasmus at necropsy. Bhaskaram and coworkers[36] showed that malnutrition did not influence the ability of BCG-vaccinated children to localize tuberculosis infection; however, malnourished children who did not receive the vaccine had a significantly greater incidence of systemic tuberculosis infection than did BCG-vaccinated malnourished children. Another study of 69 children with protein-calorie malnutrition and 20 healthy controls showed an association between all levels of protein-calorie malnutrition and decreased absolute lymphocyte count, but a decreased response to tuberculin antigen was found only in children with moderate or severe malnutrition.[206]

A few contradicting studies regarding the influence of malnutrition on cellular immunity have been published. McFarlane[195] reported that skin transplants in malnourished rats were rejected, suggesting that all aspects of cell-mediated immunity may not be impaired simultaneously or to the same extent. Good and colleagues[115] have evaluated many aspects of the effect of nutritional status (including chronic protein deficiency) on cellular immune functions, including tumor immunity in animal models. Their results suggest an enhancement of cell-mediated immunity in chronic protein deficiency in the absence of infection. The mechanism for this enhancement and the implications of these findings in humans are unclear.

Most significant is the clinical and epidemiologic evidence for impaired cellular immunity in malnutrition. Numerous studies show that malnourished children are much more susceptible to tuberculosis, measles, disseminated herpes simplex, hepatitis, *P. carinii*, and many other diseases for which prevention requires optimal function of the cellular immune system.

THYMUS

Dourov[85] reviewed the morphologic response of the thymus in malnutrition. In 1845, Simon recognized that the thymus was an "early critical barometer of nutrition." In protein-calorie malnutrition, the severe nutritional defect leads to thymic atrophy and fibrotic changes, with the cortex affected sooner than is the medulla. In contrast to atrophy of liver, kidney, or cardiac muscle, thymic atrophy is characterized more by a loss of cells than by a decrease in cell size. Histologically, corticomedullary differentiation is lost, and fewer lymphoid cells are present. Hassall bodies are enlarged, degenerated, and occasionally calcified. These changes are noted after 5 days of starvation and can be reversed after 6 days of refeeding. In contrast to other organs, thymic tissue does not regain normal size after refeeding. Histopathologic studies on the thymuses of 19 malnourished children at necropsy showed that the degree of lymphocyte depletion correlates with an increase in the extracellular matrix.[186]

In addition to substrate deficiency, stress-related factors may play a role in thymic atrophy. Generally, stress-induced immunosuppression seems to be adrenal-mediated. The stress of malnutrition has been associated with an increase of serum glucocorticoids, a lower binding capacity for steroids, and an increase in their metabolically active forms. Schlesinger and associates[267] found elevated levels of norepinephrine in the thymuses of rats with protein-calorie malnutrition that correlated with decreased immune response.

Functional changes resulting from thymic atrophy also are under investigation. Thymic factors, such as thymosin and thymopoietin, have been incubated with isolated T cells from malnourished children, resulting in a normalization of the maturational characteristics of the lymphocytes.[138,227,234] These observations were confirmed when the results were controlled for infection and zinc content.[140]

The nutritional influence on early thymic development may have lifelong consequences. In rural Gambia, being born during the "hungry" season (July through December) predicts increased infection-related adult mortality. Serial sonographic measurements of thymic indices in children born during the "hungry" season were lower than the measurements in children born during the harvest season, and measurements in all children regardless of birth month were lower when assessed during "hungry" versus "harvest" months. This difference persisted even when adjusted for current weight and infectious markers, pointing toward severe long-term effects of starvation on thymic development and function.[67]

MEDIATORS (CYTOKINES, CHEMOKINES, AND COMPLEMENT SYSTEM)

Data are conflicting with regard to circulating cytokine levels and malnutrition. Normal, decreased, and increased tumor necrosis factor–α (TNF-α) production all have been reported in malnourished children.[17,89] In several studies, a T-helper cell type 1 (T$_H$1) to T$_H$2 type shift in cytokine profiles has been reported, with increased levels of IL-4 and IL-10 and decreased levels of IL-2 and interferon-γ.[89,251] These results suggest a diminished ability of malnourished children to mount a T$_H$1 response important for the elimination of pathogens. The observed skewing of the serum cytokine profile and the reported increased IgE production and increased severity of RSV bronchiolitis in malnourished children also point toward inappropriately hyperactive T$_H$2 responses and, consequently, more severe tissue damage than in children with intact nutritional status. The available data on cytokine profiles in malnourished children should be interpreted with caution because many confounders, such as chronic infections and living in extremely stressful environments, are likely to coexist in this population and have been shown to influence cytokine profiles.

The proteins of the complement system seem to be sensitive to nutritional stress.[62] Seth and Chandra[278] noted low serum complement in patients with protein-calorie malnutrition. Sirisinha and associates[291] also reported low serum concentrations of all complement components except C4 in malnourished children. Children with kwashiorkor had levels lower than those of children with marasmus. These data are consistent with more recent animal studies that show significantly decreased levels of C1, C2, C3, and C4 in malnourished rats compared with controls.[260]

The cause of the hypocomplementemia is unclear. Electrophoretically distinct C3 breakdown products have been detected in one study, as have increased titers of immunocoagglutinin, an antibody directed to the C423b complex of activated complement. Alternatively, activation of the complement pathway may be a consequence of infection. Complement serum concentrations also may decrease in the malnourished individual as a result of a consumption complementopathy, or a decreased ability to synthesize complement de novo. Complement-derived chemotactic factors and opsonic factors also are depressed. These functional deficits may contribute to an enhanced susceptibility to infection.

Despite these changes, complement may be less susceptible to nutritional stress than other aspects of the immune system. Complement activity seems to be preserved better in patients with severe protein-calorie malnutrition than cell-mediated immunity and it recovers more rapidly after refeeding.[259,261]

PHAGOCYTOSIS

Phagocyte function can be divided into three main phases: (1) adherence and chemotaxis; (2) recognition, opsonization, and engulfment; and (3) postphagocytic events, which include formation of phagocytic vacuoles or phagosomes followed by fusion of lysosomes with phagosomes and degranulation of lysosomal enzymes, microbicidal activity, and associated metabolic changes.[122] Phagocytosis and intracellular microbicidal activity of neutrophils and macrophages depend on various components of the complement system, antibodies against surface microbial antigens, and possibly acute-phase reactants, such as C-reactive protein. Appropriate phagocytic function also requires adequate pool sizes of neutrophils and mononuclear phagocytes at inflammatory sites and adequate capacity of the bone marrow to produce and mobilize these cells. More recent research suggests that an association exists between low neutrophil count and decreased weight-for-height measurements in children.[321] Protein deprivation in mice results in a marked decrease in phagocyte precursor cell pool sizes as measured colony-forming units in the spleen.[122]

In malnourished individuals, defects in phagocytosis and killing have been identified, but these deficits are subtle. Research has shown that neutrophils from malnourished children have enhanced baseline adhesion; however, after being stimulated with chemotactic factors, the adherence response is decreased, and neutrophil chemotaxis is diminished. These abnormalities reverse with nutritional recovery.[10,122] Schopfer and Douglas[269] investigated the neutrophil function of 46 children with kwashiorkor. Chemotactic response was reduced at early intervals (30, 60, and 120 minutes) and reached values achieved by controls only after 180 minutes, which suggests an early migration defect.

Studies of opsonization and phagocytosis of cells in malnourished animals and humans indicate that neutrophil membrane receptors for Fc-IgG and complement (C3b) are intact. Serum from malnourished patients is deficient in opsonic activity, however, and kinetic studies in malnourished children suggest that the defect in opsonization is related to complement deficiencies.[121] An indirect measure of opsonic activity is fibronectin, and reduced levels of fibronectin have been reported in starvation in rats and in protein-calorie malnutrition in infants. The levels of fibronectin increase to greater than normal values after nutritional rehabilitation.[121]

No evidence has been found for any abnormalities in lysosomal fusion or degranulation in leukocytes of malnourished hosts. Nonetheless, intracellular killing seems to be impaired in malnourished states. Schopfer and Douglas[269] noted that neutrophils from children with kwashiorkor did not kill *Candida albicans* intracellularly as well as did control cells. Seth and Chandra[278] reported impaired intracellular bactericidal killing in patients with kwashiorkor. De la Fuente and Munoz[77] showed a decrease in nitroblue tetrazolium reduction in stimulated and nonstimulated macrophages from mice with protein-calorie malnutrition. Because the nitroblue tetrazolium dye reduction test in nonstimulated phagocytes indirectly measures intracellular hexose monophosphate shunt activity, protein-calorie malnutrition may interfere with this metabolic pathway. Studies from children with kwashiorkor show diminished neutrophil iodination during phagocytosis,[121] suggesting an abnormality in the myeloperoxidase-halide–mediated system.

SINGLE NUTRIENTS

Many barriers exist to analyzing the clinical significance of single nutrients in maintaining normal immune function. First, nourishment is a combination event, and nutrient-nutrient interaction can be of major consequence. Competition for transport may affect absorption or excretion in intracellular and extracellular environments. Second, a hierarchy exists for some nutrient requirements. If an element subserves several functions, as does iron, the prerequisite amount may vary with the function. Third, experimental animal models do not always allow for extrapolation to human medicine. Most species, with the notable exception of the guinea pig, make indigenous vitamin C, and no animal model exists for studying cobalamin deficiency. Finally, infection can affect body stores of essential nutrients. Chandra[58] suggested a framework for evaluation of micronutrients. Alterations in immune responses occur early in the course of reduced intake,

and these alterations may predict the risk for developing infection and mortality.[324] In the case of many nutrients, excessive intake also is associated with immune abnormalities.

IRON

Iron deficiency is the most common nutritional deficiency in the world and results in systemic disease involving all cell systems. The role of iron in chronic and acute infection is complex. Experimental and clinical studies have been published that support an impaired immune function in iron deficiency on one hand and a protective role of low iron states against certain infections on the other.[228]

Experimental data suggesting impaired immune function in iron deficiency exist for almost any part of the immune system. Severely iron-deficient rats have an increased number of phagocytes in whole blood, but granulocytic activity as measured by nitroblue tetrazolium dye reduction is decreased significantly.[284] The rate at which granulocytes killed staphylococci was decreased in 819 iron-deficient patients studied by Joynson and coworkers.[147] Retention of iron in the reticuloendothelial system may enable macrophages to detoxify bacterial toxins. Iron in monocytes may enhance antibacterial activity of these cells.[144] Iron also may activate lysosomal hydrolases.[141] Cellular development of lymphoid tissues has been shown to be diminished in iron deficiency; lymphoid tissue from iron-deficient rats shows reduced cellularity, decreased lymphopoiesis, and deranged histology.[284]

In humans with iron deficiency, reduced numbers of circulating T cells and decreased in vitro lymphocyte response to mitogens have been reported.[81] The bactericidal capacity of leukocytes also is reduced, which may be caused by deficient function of iron-dependent myeloperoxidase and cytochrome enzymes.[60] Natural killer cell activity is impaired significantly in moderate and severe iron deficiency compared with controls. In iron-deficient patients studied by Macdougall and coworkers,[184] impaired leukocyte responsiveness, decreased bactericidal capacity, increased IgA, and increased C3 concentrations were observed. Restoration of normal bactericidal function occured before any increase in hemoglobin concentrations was noted, suggesting that tissue iron depletion rather than anemia was an etiologic factor in depressing bactericidal function. Clinically, impairment of delayed cutaneous hypersensitivity responses are found in humans with iron deficiency.[81]

Humoral immunity also may be affected by iron deficiency. In studies in iron-deficient rats, baseline plasma IgG levels were normal, and IgM was low only in severe iron deficiency, but rates of de novo synthesis of IgM and IgG after stimulation were found to be decreased significantly. Although circulating plasma immunoglobulin may be normal in iron-deficiency anemia, iron deficiency may result in diminished antibody production. Cytokine and chemokine production is impaired in individuals with iron deficiency, as has been shown for IL-1 and migration inhibitory factor.[147,269]

Taken together, these studies imply that appropriate iron stores and availability of iron within cells, particularly in selected tissue, is beneficial to the host. Numerous studies suggest, however, that free iron may be detrimental to the host during bacterial infection. Iron may stimulate the growth of the pathogen with which the host is infected, may inhibit bactericidal proteins, and may enhance bacterial metabolism.[337] The percentage of saturation of transferrin with iron in plasma correlates directly with the ability of the sera to support the growth of various microorganisms. Iron in fluids such as plasma, milk, nasal secretions, and saliva is to a greater or lesser extent unavailable to many bacteria and fungi because of the presence of the iron-binding proteins transferrin and lactoferrin.[174,191] Microorganisms produce iron chelators termed *siderophores*. If the supply of iron in the host is so high that the physiologic processes to with-hold it are exceeded, the invading microbes can obtain iron for growth.[284]

The administration of iron to animals by the intravenous, intramuscular, or intraperitoneal route reduces the LD_{50} for *P. aeruginosa*, *Salmonella typhosa*, streptococci, *Klebsiella pneumoniae*, *Salmonella typhimurium*, and *Listeria monocytogenes*.[337] Similarly, the administration of iron intramuscularly to children with kwashiorkor has resulted in overwhelming infection and death. Clinicians in these cases concluded that iron therapy should be deferred until transferrin synthesis was restored by protein nutrition. No evidence exists, however, that gradual oral replenishment of iron predisposes children to more severe infection.

Secondary bacterial infection occurs commonly in patients with bartonellosis and malaria,[175] and bacterial infection, particularly that caused by *S. pneumoniae* and *Salmonella* spp., occurs more frequently in individuals with sickle cell anemia.[19,175] This evidence has been cited by some investigators to support the concept that iron is detrimental to the host during infection. This theory is not justified because patients with these diseases are known to have other deficits that intrinsically increase propensity for infection. The increased incidence of bacterial infection in these individuals cannot be attributed specifically to an increase in free iron.

Malaria frequently is cited as a situation in which iron-deficient states are protective to the host. Field researchers in malaria-endemic countries noted that treatment of iron deficiency, especially with parenteral iron, often was associated with an increase in the incidence of smear-positive malaria. Other studies have manipulated iron availability by using desferrioxamine, which is an iron chelator. In vitro and in vivo, desferrioxamine inhibits the growth of malaria parasites. The effect of desferrioxamine seems to be directly on parasitized erythrocytes, which behave as if they contain a chelation-labile iron pool.[152] In a study of Indian children, no statistical difference was found, however, in the incidence or prevalence of malaria or in the severity of *Plasmodium falciparum* parasitemia at different hemoglobin or nutritional levels.[98]

Several studies[9,185] of iron supplementation have reported fewer episodes of respiratory and gastrointestinal illnesses in iron-supplemented infants, but because of difficulties defining and statistically evaluating infectious episodes, the significance of these findings is not compelling. In a study in Colombia[11] in which iron deficiency was severe, nutritional supplementation and medical care had no impact on the mortality caused by infectious diseases, but supplemented groups experienced an impressive reduction in enteric infections. The relative contributions of iron and other supplements in decreasing morbidity could not be ascertained. Significantly improved iron status and reduced morbidity from upper respiratory tract infections were found in a placebo-controlled trial of iron supplementation in a study on 363 low-income children from Sri Lanka.[78]

Taken together, the depletion of tissue levels of iron as noted in iron deficiency are likely to be detrimental to optimal performance of the inflammatory and immune systems. To date, no studies have identified the point at which iron deprivation interferes with immunologic states. The diverse role of iron in multiple enzyme systems, mammalian and bacterial, may be understood best in a hierarchy of functions in which optimal activity of the different systems may be at different elemental concentrations. The suggestion that iron deficiency protects humans against infection cannot be supported, although caution against rapid parenteral iron repletion in states of acute infection may be advised. Recognizing the importance of maintaining appropriate iron stores, the WHO recommended iron and folic acid supplementation of flour in developing countries as a strategy for breaking the vicious cycle of malnutrition and infection.[327]

SELENIUM

Selenium has three major functions in the tissues and cells of the immune system: reduction of organic and inorganic peroxides, metabolism of hydroperoxides, and modulation of the respiratory burst. Glutathione peroxidase and phospholipid hydroperoxide glutathione peroxidase are selenium-containing enzymes that catalyze the reduction of peroxides formed from general metabolism, drugs, and other initiators of free radical chain reactions. Both of these enzymes also are involved in steps in the synthesis of thromboxane A_2, prostaglandins, leukotrienes, and lipoxins.

Research has shown reduction of eicosanoid biosynthesis in the absence of selenium and glutathione peroxidase. Selenium and the glutathione peroxidases also modulate the production of the oxidizing products of the respiratory burst: O^+_2, H_2O_2, CLO^+, and chloramines, which are used in the phagolysosome to lyse and destroy phagocytized cells. As predicted from these roles, selenium supplementation prevents oxidative stress–induced damage to immune cells. Selenium deficiency in experimental animals is associated with decreased glutathione peroxidase activity in phagocytic cells, release of increased amounts of H_2O_2 by macrophages and peritoneal granulocytes, and increased superoxide formation in macrophages.[58,196,297]

Selenium also apparently boosts cellular immunity by up-regulating the expression of the T-cell high-affinity IL-2 receptor, enhancing T-cell response. Splenic leukocytes from selenium-deficient rats proliferated less after mitogenic stimulation than did leukocytes from control rats.[241] Controversy still surrounds the role of selenium in the prevention of infections in humans. Deficiency has been associated with generalized immunosuppression affecting neutrophil function, antibody production, and lymphocyte proliferation. A more recent study investigating selenium levels in 134 patients in intensive care units (ICUs) found that the mean plasma selenium concentration of these patients was 2 standard deviations below that of the general population.[106] This study also showed an inverse correlation between plasma selenium and severity of sepsis in these patients. The treatment of patients in ICUs with supplemental selenium has not been investigated.

In Keshan, China, selenium deficiency has been implicated in the pathogenesis of a dilated cardiomyopathy known as Keshan disease. The seasonal and annual incidences of Keshan disease were characteristic of an infectious disease, and screening of tissues from patients revealed the presence of numerous viruses, including coxsackieviruses. These findings are significant in light of Beck and Levander's[26] studies showing increased virulence of certain coxsackieviruses in selenium-deficient animals.

ZINC

Zinc is a cofactor for more than 300 cellular enzymes, with functions ranging from signal transduction to transcription to replication. Zinc deficiency in humans has been associated with poor growth and development, impaired wound healing, and impaired sensory perception. The low levels of zinc in acrodermatitis enteropathica may be related to the thymic atrophy and high frequency of serious bacterial, viral, and fungal infections seen in these patients because pharmacologic zinc supplementation can reverse all of these symptoms.[219]

Multiple animal models show the association of zinc deficiency with altered nonspecific and specific immune responses.[271,338] Lower zinc levels have been found in serum and hair of otherwise well-nourished children with pneumonia compared with healthy controls in Bangladesh.[281] Patients maintained on parenteral nutrition lacking in zinc showed reduced T-lymphocyte proliferation in response to mitogenic stimulation, which markedly increased after repletion of zinc.[285] A trial in Indian children showed increased CD3 and CD4 cell counts and an increased CD4/CD8 ratio in children given zinc supplementation compared with controls.[264] Deficiencies in zinc also are associated with reduction in thymulin activity and slower neutrophil chemotaxis; these changes are reversed with the zinc supplementation.[58] Zinc deficiency impairs the function of antigen-presenting cells.[270] Conversely, excessive supplementation with zinc has been shown to cause reduced chemotactic and phagocytic activities and a suppressive effect on lymphocyte proliferation.[70] The inhibition of T-cell proliferation seems to be caused by inhibition of an IL-1 receptor–associated protein kinase by zinc ions at higher concentrations.[339]

Several randomized, double-blind, placebo-controlled trials of zinc supplementation have been done with children in developing countries, most of whom exhibit some manifestations of malnutrition.[231,256,257,263,322] These studies showed the association of zinc supplementation with decreased incidence of and morbidity from respiratory infections and reduced morbidity from diarrhea. Micronutrient deficiencies may be of particular clinical significance in malnourished children with chronic diarrhea or intestinal parasitic infections. Treatment of the infection has been shown to increase serum zinc levels without nutritional intervention, suggesting a vicious cycle comprising malabsorption, immune dysfunction, and inability to clear the infection.[226]

The immunologic consequences of zinc deficiency during pregnancy have received increased attention more recently. Animal studies have shown reduced thymic and spleen size and decreased active and passive immunity in the offspring, which was not fully reversible by postnatal zinc supplementation and partially persisted into the next generation.[338]

OTHER TRACE ELEMENTS

Copper facilitates absorption of iron from the gastrointestinal tract and is essential for the production of red blood cells. It also is crucial for several oxidative enzyme systems. Copper deficiency has been shown to cause anemia of varying degrees and gross ataxia in neonates of many species and defects in formation of connective tissue. Neutropenia has been documented in children with a copper-deficient diet. Copper deficiency is associated with depressed function of the reticuloendothelial system, reduced microbicidal activity of granulocytes, decreased response of splenic lymphocytes to T-cell and B-cell mitogens, and impaired natural killer cell cytotoxicity in animal models. The reduced microbicidal activity of granulocytes is attributed to the role of copper in superoxide dismutase and cytochrome-*c* oxidase enzyme systems.[285] Copper-deficient patients are more susceptible to contracting bronchopneumonia and bacterial sepsis, especially with *E. coli*. Copper-deficient animals show increased mortality rates when exposed to *S. typhimurium*, *L. monocytogenes*, and coxsackievirus B.

The role of chromium in disease control is undefined. Excess amounts adversely affect macrophage and lymphocyte cultures.[109,332] Chromium acts as a cofactor for the potentiation of insulin at the cellular level, and deficiency is characterized by impaired glucose use.[198,236] The role of chromium in impaired glucose homeostasis in kwashiorkor has been documented.[51]

Manganese is another essential trace element necessary for optimal growth. It affects the primary sites of chondroitin sulfate synthesis. In humans, manganese deficiency is characterized by weight loss, transient dermatitis, occasional nausea and vomiting, changes in hair color, hypocholesterolemia, and teratogenicity.

Lymphocyte and neutrophil functions in iodine deficiency are diminished. Iodide interacts with neutrophil peroxidases to form the halide-superoxide system, which is modulated by the amount of thyroid hormone, which supplies the iodide molecule. In hypothyroid patients, the bactericidal activity is decreased and restored after treatment with thyroid hormone.[58]

VITAMIN A

Three of the fat-soluble vitamins—A, D, and E—have recognized effects on immune system function. Before the discovery of antibiotics, researchers noted that urinary tract infections in children responded to vitamin A therapy. In the modern era, vitamin A deficiency is well documented to be a major risk factor for infections in Third World countries. Vitamin A levels in the serum have been used as markers of malnutrition; the independent effects of vitamin A deficiency are significant. Researchers have suggested that improving the vitamin A status of all children who are deficient would prevent approximately 1 to 3 million deaths each year, curtailing the incidence and severity of infectious episodes, especially respiratory and diarrheal infections.[135]

Vitamin A plays an important role in maintaining the integrity of epithelial surfaces. In animals and humans, vitamin A deficiency is associated with keratinizing metaplasia of mucus-secreting epithelial surfaces, particularly of the respiratory, gastrointestinal, and genitourinary tracts, and corneal tissues. This histopathologic alteration is conducive to an overgrowth of bacteria and secondary infections of loculated areas obstructed by keratinized debris. A classic example of this type of alteration is a Bitot spot, a triangular patch of xerotic conjunctiva characteristic of xerophthalmia, which is composed largely of keratin debris and a heavy growth of *Xerosis bacillus*, a saprophytic diphtheroid.

Immune changes in patients with vitamin A deficiency are characterized by disruption of the skin and epithelial barriers, increased bacterial binding to epithelial cells, reduced thymic weight, decreased lymphocyte proliferation, reduced immunoglobulin production, decreased T-helper cell activity, and decreased cytokine production. Vitamin A deficiency also is characterized by reduced phagocytosis, diminished nitroblue tetrazolium dye reduction by neutrophils, and reduced macrophage function.[60,113,275] Lysozyme is a vitamin A–dependent glycoprotein; the activity of this protein is decreased markedly in vitamin A deficiency.[340]

Vitamin A deficiency in children seems to increase their susceptibility to various types of infections. In a malnutrition ward in Bangladesh, 78 percent of children with xerophthalmia had bacteriuria determined by urine culture obtained by bladder tap compared with 17 percent of malnourished peers without xerophthalmia.[44] Studies from South Africa[86] and Israel[66] showed a strong association between poor vitamin A status and increased incidence and severity of acute respiratory infections.

Vitamin A supplementation may reverse some of these susceptibilities. A double-blind, placebo-controlled trial in a malaria-endemic area of Papua New Guinea showed that children supplemented with vitamin A had fewer febrile episodes and decreased parasite counts compared with unsupplemented controls.[282] In contrast, a study from Nigeria failed to establish a relationship between the use of red palm oil, a local oil rich in vitamin A, and decreased disease severity from malaria, whereas such a relationship existed for the overall nutritional status.[68] Finally, a meta-analysis of randomized trials of vitamin A supplementation in developing countries indicated a significant decrease in rates of respiratory and diarrheal disease mortality with vitamin A supplementation compared with placebo in children with no overt deficiency.[113] Vitamin A supplementation may be of particular importance in states of baseline increased susceptibility to infections, such as in children with HIV.[87,100]

Children in Third World countries frequently are caught in a vicious cycle in which infection leads to vitamin A deficiency, which increases the risk for subsequent development of infection. The impact that vitamin A supplementation would have on childhood morbidity and mortality depends on several factors, including the prevalence and severity of deficiency, aggravating conditions (e.g., protein-calorie malnutrition), associated nutrient defects, virulence of the infectious agents to which they are exposed, and adequacy of supplementation.[296]

The effects of retinoids on the maintenance of the integrity and differentiation of epithelial surfaces on one hand, and their various immunologic effects on the other, raise the interesting question whether retinoid supplementation might help to prevent human papillomavirus–associated cervical dysplasia. In a more recent study, *trans*-leukopene and *cis*-leukopene (but not retinol, tocopherols, vitamin B12, and folic acid) levels correlated with higher rates of clearing of an established infection with oncogenic strains of human papillomavirus.[273]

VITAMIN D

Vitamin D serves as an immunoregulatory hormone and as a lymphocyte-differentiating hormone in addition to its classic role of mineral homeostasis. 1,25-Dihydroxyvitamin D_3 functions in the manner of a steroid hormone in many different cell types. Receptors for 1,25-dihydroxyvitamin D_3 have been identified on the surface of T lymphocytes, monocytes, and macrophages,[326] and an extensive number of RNA polymerase II–transcribed genes that govern lymphokine expression are regulated by this vitamin-hormone.[27] Although vitamin D must be present at a certain concentration for proper immune function, high-dose supplementation also may have detrimental effects. One study has shown suppression of the delayed hypersensitivity response in patients with vitamin D deficiency and in individuals receiving high doses of vitamin D.[145] Activated vitamin D may inhibit T-lymphocyte proliferation and natural killer cell cytotoxicity and decrease concentrations of interferon-γ, IL-2, and IL-12.[180] Additionally, the differentiation of immature dendritic cells into antigen-presenting cells is inhibited in culture by activated vitamin D.[239]

A more recent case-control study from India found subclinical vitamin D deficiency to be a risk factor for pneumonia in children younger than 5 years old.[335] A case-control study from Jordan reported longer hospital stays in children with rickets and pneumonia compared with the nonrachitic controls.[215]

VITAMIN E

Vitamin E enhances immune responses and phagocytosis by acting as an antioxidant to prevent lipid peroxidation of cell membranes. Rapidly proliferating cells of the specific immune and phagocytic systems are prone to peroxidative damage by free radicals, peroxides, and superoxides. In vitro studies of rat alveolar macrophages show that high levels of vitamin E suppress the release of reactive oxygen species after stimulation.[235] These findings suggest that vitamin E may reduce self-inflicted damage to macrophages and surrounding tissue during infection. The antioxidant effect of vitamin E also modulates the biosynthesis and activity of prostaglandins, thromboxane, and leukotrienes.[311]

Several studies have shown that vitamin E deficiency impairs cell-mediated and humoral immunity in different animal models. Some studies suggest that vitamin E deficiency may contribute to the decreased immune function of neonates, especially premature infants.[199] In humans, vitamin E deficiency impairs T-cell–mediated function, which is reversible by vitamin E supplementation. Supplementation in an amount 2 to 10 times greater than the present recommended dose significantly increased humoral and cell-mediated immune responses and

phagocytic functions in laboratory animals and humans.[311] Vitamin E seems to interact with other micronutrients in immune modulation. The heightened humoral response noted with vitamin E is synergistic with selenium[124] and copper.[311] In addition, zinc deficiency, even when marginal, can decrease markedly vitamin E serum concentrations.[249]

WATER-SOLUBLE VITAMINS

Among the water-soluble vitamins, B_1, B_6, B_{12}, and C have been implicated in immune function. Vitamin B_6 deficiency impairs immunity by slowing the rate of production of one-carbon units necessary for nucleic acid synthesis in these rapidly proliferating cells. Animal models deficient in vitamin B_6 exhibit impaired antibody production, a delay in IgM-to-IgG class switching, and altered cell-mediated immunity with reduced delayed-type hypersensitivity responses.[315] Humans consuming a diet low in vitamin B_6 or being treated with deoxypyridoxine (vitamin B_6 antagonist) have a decreased number of circulating lymphocytes and reduced antibody production and a mild decrease in the percentage of helper T cells.[200] The thymus is smaller, and thymic hormone activity is decreased in patients with vitamin B_6 deficiency.

Vitamin B_{12} also seems to affect immunity. Patients with vitamin B_{12} deficiency were found to have decreased numbers of lymphocytes, decreased CD8 cells, an altered CD8/CD4 ratio, and suppressed natural killer cell cytotoxicity.[308] All of these parameters improved with supplementation of vitamin B_{12}. Osawa[230] first suggested that thiamine deficiency may predispose to the occurrence of tropical pyomyositis, a hematogenous pyogenic infection characterized by abscess formation in various muscle tissues. Muscle tissue generally is resistant to infection, but lack of thiamine may change the biochemical milieu of the muscle, rendering it more susceptible to infection.

Physiologic quantities of ascorbic acid are necessary for normal metabolism of lipids and iron. One of the major functions of vitamin C is as an antioxidant that protects the alpha$_1$ proteinase inhibitor from inactivation by free radical products of the respiratory burst. Alpha$_1$ proteinase inhibitor is present in plasma, where it reacts with elastase, protecting the extracellular space from escaped proteases from damaged cells. The concentration of intracellular vitamin C is approximately 50 times that found in plasma, which suggests that vitamin C may protect intracellular regions from oxidants that leak into the cytoplasm.

Host susceptibility to infection is increased in scurvy. Vitamin C deficiency is associated with impaired phagocytic activity. Microtubule organization is responsible for phagocytosis and locomotion and depends on the redox state of the cell; vitamin C may modulate it by an antioxidant effect on tubulin tyrosinolation.[126] Macrophages from mice supplemented with vitamin C, vitamin E, or both showed increased random migration, chemotaxis, ingestion, and superoxide anion production compared with controls.[80] Because vitamin C is associated with chemotactic activation of phagocytes, its use has been suggested in patients with disorders of phagocyte function, such as Chédiak-Higashi syndrome.[268]

The possibility that vitamin C may be important in preventing upper respiratory infections has received widespread publicity in the medical and lay presses. Chalmers[53] reported, however, after reviewing 14 clinical trials of ascorbic acid in the prevention and treatment of the common cold, that differences between supplemented and nonsupplemented subjects were minor and insignificant. Nonetheless, in most studies, the severity of symptoms was worse in patients who received placebo. Miller and colleagues[201] performed a double-blind, co-twin controlled study on 44 monozygotic twins of school age. During the 5-month study period, no statistically significant difference in the number or severity of illness episodes was noted between the recipients of vitamin C and a placebo control group. Several studies have shown a consistent decrease in the duration of the common cold episodes; although most of the results are not statistically significant, all of them point consistently in the same direction.[126] Administration of ascorbic acid is not a panacea for upper respiratory infections. Also, although lack of vitamin C is detrimental, excess intake is of no proven value.

Vitamin deficiencies interfere with host defenses. Infections also may cause or exacerbate certain vitamin deficiencies. Concentrations of vitamins A, B$_6$, and C have been reported to be lower than normal during acute bacterial and viral infections, and reduced concentrations of folic acid in blood and serum have been found in infants with diarrhea or acute bacterial infection[193] and in adults with tuberculosis or malaria.[250] Severe xerophthalmia in Indian children often is preceded by diarrhea, measles, or a respiratory infection and may have been precipitated by a decline in serum vitamin A and retinol-binding protein concentrations during the course of the infection. A study in children with shigellosis showed increased urinary excretion of vitamin A during infection, which was attributed to impaired renal tubular absorption of low-molecular-weight proteins, such as retinol-binding protein bound to retinol.[207] Infections may alter plasma retinol levels because activation of the acute-phase response may decrease the synthesis of the circulating proteins that transport retinol.[313]

Altered concentrations of circulating vitamins during infection also may be caused by several other mechanisms, including impaired absorption from the gastrointestinal tract, liver cell damage, and altered rates of vitamin excretion. Transient malabsorption of folic acid and vitamin B$_{12}$ has been noted during and after recovery from acute intestinal infections, including cholera and salmonellosis.[178] The urinary excretion of the group B vitamins and vitamin C also has been observed to change during hepatitis and tuberculosis.[125,146]

Taken together, in vitro studies show alterations in immune cell function; animal models and clinical studies show an enhanced susceptibility to infection with deficiencies of macronutrients and micronutrients. More studies are needed, however, to assess particularly mild micronutrient deficiencies, possible synergistic effects, and optimal substitution regimens.

CONSIDERATIONS OF NUTRITION AND INFECTION IN SPECIAL POPULATIONS

Overall, the prevalence of malnutrition in industrialized nations is considerably less than that in developing countries; however, in industrialized nations, certain populations are at increased risk for developing malnutrition. Malnutrition is a common complication in HIV-positive individuals, regardless of their geographic location or economic situation. Critically ill patients have an increased risk for development of malnutrition and infection. Finally, burn patients, premature neonates, cancer patients, and children with cystic fibrosis have special nutritional requirements and metabolic changes that highlight the interactions of infection and nutrition.

HUMAN IMMUNODEFICIENCY VIRUS AND NUTRITION

Acquired immunodeficiency syndrome (AIDS) has become one of the most pressing public health problems, with more than 40 million HIV-infected individuals worldwide (WHO estimate 2005[346]) and more than 1 million in the United States. Infection with HIV has a devastating effect on nutritional status. Malnutrition was one of the earliest recognized complications of AIDS, and unexplained weight loss remains one of the most common

initial AIDS-defining diagnoses reported to public health authorities. Patients may lose 30 to 50 percent of their body mass before dying of AIDS. The onset of depletion of body cell mass occurs early in HIV infection and may predate any significant immunodeficiency, suggesting that the virus itself may be responsible.[161]

Most commonly, the malnutrition associated with HIV is multifactorial. Decreased caloric intake, malabsorption of nutrients, and elevated energy expenditure, especially during systemic opportunistic infections, all contribute to malnutrition in these patients. Protein-calorie malnutrition is encountered frequently, as are individual or combined micronutrient deficiencies. All contribute to the growth failure seen in children with HIV, emphasizing the need for early and intensive nutritional intervention and treatment in these patients.

Two major paradigms of weight loss that contribute in patients with HIV infection are starvation and cachexia.[18] Starvation refers to a voluntary or involuntary deprivation of food that leads to increased losses of body fat and extracellular water, with relative sparing of lean body mass. In contrast, cachexia is characterized by a disproportionate loss of lean body mass resulting from specific alterations in metabolism. These alterations during cachexia are caused by shifts in cytokine levels and may include changes in protein metabolism or energy expenditure, appetite changes, or derangement of the sleep-wake cycle.

Investigation of energy metabolism in HIV-infected individuals has produced conflicting results. Some studies report increased resting energy expenditure, and others report that energy expenditure was decreased. A study of 36 HIV-infected children between infancy and 10 years of age showed that cardiac muscle mass and heart rate were correlated inversely with weight and skeletal muscle mass.[204] This finding is inconsistent with the decreased energy expenditure of hypometabolic compensation that occurs in starvation; instead, it suggests that these children have cachexia and intrinsic metabolic changes.

Animal and human studies have found correlations between cytokine levels and anorexia, cachexia, and altered lipid metabolism. Serum levels of interferon-α are increased in some patients with AIDS and are correlated significantly with elevated serum triglyceride levels. Adult patients with AIDS and with wasting were found to have higher plasma concentrations of TNF-α and cholecystokinin octapeptide sulfate, an appetite neuropeptide, and lower levels of β-endorphins compared with well-nourished patients with AIDS and healthy controls.[12] These changes may inhibit appetite pathologically and contribute to weight loss.

Very different metabolic changes have been observed more recently in patients with HIV who are receiving antiretroviral therapy. Lipodystrophy, or fat redistribution syndrome, seems to be associated more strongly with the administration of protease inhibitors than are other antiretroviral agents. Patients with this condition develop a dorsocervical fat pad; abdominal adiposity; and facial, extremity, and buttocks wasting. Increased breast size also is seen in female patients. Other changes include hyperlipidemia with increased levels of total cholesterol and low-density lipoprotein and decreased levels of high-density lipoprotein. These patients also may develop insulin resistance. The mechanism of this syndrome and its long-term consequences are unclear. A study examining the effect of protease inhibitors on growth of children found that despite the protease inhibitor–induced metabolic abnormalities, protease inhibitor therapy had a positive effect on growth parameters, including height, weight, and muscle mass, likely through reducing viral load and improving disease control.[203]

Involvement of the gastrointestinal tract in patients with HIV infections also undoubtedly plays a role in weight loss. Chronic weight loss often is related to gastrointestinal disease and malabsorption. The pathogenesis of malabsorption involves a combination of factors, including primary enterocyte injury with partial villous atrophy and crypt hyperplasia, ileal dysfunction with bile salt wasting and fat malabsorption, and exudative enteropathy.[162] Small intestine pathology or pancreatic insufficiency may lead to malabsorption of fat, weight loss, and depletion of fat-soluble vitamins.[171] Hypochlorhydria has been found in almost 75 percent of patients with AIDS and can allow for enteric infections and reduced absorption of micronutrients, such as folate and iron. Malabsorption of lactose is a common finding and is more severe in symptomatic than asymptomatic HIV-infected children.[353] Subclinical malabsorption may play a role in early HIV disease, whereas overt malabsorption is found more frequently in advanced HIV infection.

Along with the direct effects of HIV, immunosuppression leads to an increased frequency of gastrointestinal infections, which exacerbate weight loss caused by diarrhea and malabsorption. Protozoal infections can disrupt mucosal architecture in the small intestine, resulting in severe malnutrition. Studies indicate that HIV-infected patients with diarrhea caused by enteric infections experience greater weight loss than do HIV-infected patients with diarrhea for which no pathogen can be identified.[50]

Protein-calorie malnutrition is a common occurrence in patients with AIDS and is considered a predominant cause of morbidity in AIDS. In the United States, 30 to 50 percent of children followed in HIV programs have evidence of protein-calorie malnutrition.[202] The immune effects of protein-calorie malnutrition and HIV infection are similar: Decreased CD4 cells, reversal of the helper-to-suppressor T-cell ratio, impairment of delayed hypersensitivity reactions, and abnormal humoral responses occur in both conditions. A child with protein-calorie malnutrition and HIV infection is likely to have an outcome worse than that of a child with either condition alone.

Low levels of vitamins A, E, B_6, B_{12}, and C and of carotenoids, selenium, and zinc are common findings in many HIV-infected populations. These deficiencies may be caused by decreased dietary intake, diarrhea, malabsorption, impaired storage, or altered metabolism of micronutrients.[277] Some researchers attribute the low levels of zinc in HIV-infected patients to direct use of zinc by the virus for gene expression, multimerization, and integration into the host genome.[23]

More recently, the prognostic significance of the status of selenium has received much attention. Several studies[22,24,49] have shown that selenium deficiency is associated more strongly than other micronutrient deficiencies with mortality in HIV-infected patients. Selenium-deficient, HIV-infected patients had a 10-fold to 20-fold increase in mortality rates compared with HIV-infected patients with adequate selenium levels. Among HIV-infected children who died, children with low selenium levels died at a younger age (mean age at death of 4.3 years versus 8 years), suggesting a more rapid progression of disease in patients with selenium deficiency.[49] The relationship between selenium deficiency and early death in HIV may be associated with the role of selenium in preventing oxidative stress, which may be involved in maintaining viral latency in an infected cell. An in vitro study of HIV-infected monocytes and T lymphocytes emphasized this role by showing that selenium supplementation partially suppresses the TNF-α–mediated replication of the virus.[131]

Controversy currently surrounds the role of maternal micronutrient status, particularly vitamin A, in the perinatal transmission of HIV. Several studies[119,275] show an increased risk for perinatal HIV transmission with maternal vitamin A deficiency; one study[275] showed that the risk for perinatal transmission was correlated inversely with concentration of maternal serum retinol. Other studies showed no association, however, between maternal vitamin A level and risk for transmission of HIV to the infant.[47,48,98,99,303] Further research is required before any conclusions can be drawn. In contrast, administration of vitamin A

supplementation in children starting at 6 months of age has been shown to be beneficial in reducing mortality rates and morbidity among HIV-infected children.[100]

In children with HIV, the combination of diarrhea, malabsorption, protein-calorie malnutrition, and micronutrient deficiencies can have devastating effects on growth. HIV-infected infants may exhibit growth failure, failure to thrive, developmental delay, or frank malnutrition by 4 months of age.[101] A retrospective, cross-sectional analysis of 54 children with perinatally acquired HIV showed an early decline in the rate of linear growth (growth failure) with relative preservation of weight for age.[240] A prospective study of HIV-infected infants in Uganda[30] showed an association between mortality and the severity of growth failure. The exact nature of the relationship between growth failure and mortality in HIV infection is unclear. Poor nutritional parameters may represent frequent opportunistic infections and debilitation in infants with already advanced disease; conversely, poor nutritional status may accelerate the progression from asymptomatic HIV infection to symptomatic AIDS.

Nutritional intervention is important for all HIV-infected patients, but it is particularly crucial in the management of infants and children. In 2000, the American Dietetic Association and Dieticians of Canada recommended that children should be referred for a full nutrition evaluation as soon as possible after receiving the diagnosis of HIV infection.[101] Nutrition intervention should begin early in the course of HIV infection in the hopes of stabilizing weight loss and preventing growth failure. Evaluation should address stages of growth and development, anthropometrics, dietary intake assessment, medical data, and any psychosocial or economic issues that may be barriers to establishing adequate nutrition.

Specific dietary interventions include maximizing intake of high-calorie, nutrient-dense foods and vitamin and mineral supplements, especially vitamins A, B_6, B_{12}, E, and C, and riboflavin, zinc, and selenium. In addition, dietary counseling should emphasize the importance of daily ingestion of a full complement of amino acids. If adequate nutritional status cannot be maintained orally, enteral supplementation should be used. To maximize absorption and minimize diarrhea, formulas that have low residue or low lactose and that contain peptides and medium-chain triglycerides should be used. If the patient has intractable diarrhea or impaired function of the gastrointestinal tract, or if nutrient needs are not met by enteral nutrition, home total parenteral nutrition (TPN) may be considered for long-term use; however, TPN therapy may be complicated by metabolic abnormalities (hypertriglyceridemia, hyperglycemia, fluid and electrolyte imbalance) and problems related to catheters, such as infection, hemorrhage, and pneumothorax. Standard nutritional recommendations for patients with AIDS have not been established because of the heterogeneous nature of the complications of this disease.

ROUTE AND COMPOSITION OF NUTRITION IN CRITICALLY ILL PATIENTS

The effects of quality and quantity of nutrients on the immune system have been shown, but the route of administration of nutrition also has been shown to affect host susceptibility to infection. The first experimental evidence that the route of nutrition plays a role in host defense came from Kudsk and associates[166] in the early 1980s. Well-nourished rats were fed the same solution through either gastrostomy or central catheter for 12 days, after which hemoglobin–*E. coli* peritonitis was induced. The 48-hour survival was 60 percent in the enterally fed group compared with 20 percent in the parenterally fed group. Improved survival also was observed in malnourished rats under similar experimental conditions.[165]

Analyses of infection rates in hospitalized patients seem to confirm an association between TPN and susceptibility to infection. In a meta-analysis of data from eight prospective, randomized trials of early enteral versus parenteral feeding of high-risk surgical patients, Moore and colleagues[211] found a 35 percent risk for development of septic complications in patients receiving TPN compared with an 18 percent risk in patients fed enterally. Similar increases in infection rates have been observed in children. Several prospective cohort studies of patients in neonatal and pediatric ICUs have shown that TPN is the most significant risk factor for acquiring a nosocomial infection.[42,114,289]

Numerous hypotheses have been proposed to explain the increased risk for development of infection in parenterally fed patients. Intravenous nutrition may induce immunosuppression directly. In vitro studies of whole blood from infants receiving long-term TPN showed impaired phagocytosis and intracellular killing in response to challenge with coagulase-negative staphylococci, a model for bacteremia.[224,225] The intracellular killing was correlated negatively with duration, but not amount, of parenteral feeding and was found to normalize after the addition of small enteral feeding.[225] Correction of this immune defect with enteral feeding implies the involvement of the gastrointestinal tract in the increased infection risk with parenteral feeding.

Enteral feeding helps to maintain barrier function of the gut through increased gastric acidity, mucus production, and intact peristalsis.[7] Gastrointestinal tract "starvation" in animal models produces mucosal atrophy, bacterial overgrowth, decreased secretory IgA, increased intestinal permeability and translocation of bacteria or toxins, and atrophy of gut-associated lymphoid tissue.[155,177,225] The preliminary evidence suggests that enteral feeding may maintain immunologic integrity in the gut and result in increased resistance to infection.

The composition of enteral diets has been another area of more recent investigation. Certain key nutrients are being recognized for their ability to modulate a variety of inflammatory, metabolic, and immune processes when ingested in increased amounts. Nutritional components such as dietary nucleotides, omega-3 fatty acids, glutamine, and arginine are being called "immune-enhancing agents" because of their potential roles in bolstering and maintaining host defenses against infection.

Nucleotides are thought to have immune-modulating properties because of their role as structural units for DNA, RNA, adenosine triphosphate, and cyclic adenosine monophosphate. The unaltered human gastrointestinal tract contains bacteria, the continuous turnover of which provides an adequate supply of nucleotides, but this flora may be altered in critically ill patients.[20] Periods of rapid growth or certain disease states also may create increased demands for nucleotides. Under these conditions, supplemental dietary nucleotides may spare the energy of de novo synthesis and optimize the function of rapidly proliferating cells of the immune system.[52] Numerous studies have shown the immune-modulating effects of nucleotides in vitro and in animal models.[148,167] More recent studies in children also show these effects. Studies in infants showed that infants receiving nucleotide-supplemented formula had increased natural killer cell cytotoxicity, increased IL-2 production by stimulated mononuclear cells, and higher serum concentrations of IgM and IgA compared with infants fed standard formulas, and they were less likely to experience diarrhea.[52,190,350]

Omega-3 fatty acids may regulate immune function by modulating formation of prostaglandins and regional blood flow. Some inflammatory mediators of shock and sepsis, including prostaglandins, leukotrienes, and platelet-activating factor, are metabolites of omega-6 fatty acids, the primary fat source in many nutritional formulations. Substitution of omega-3 fatty acids for omega-6 fatty acids has been shown to have anti-inflammatory effects.[20] Parenterally fed rats receiving supplemental omega-3 fatty acids had increased splanchnic blood flow in response to

endotoxin challenge compared with parenterally fed rats without supplementation.[245] They also had decreased viable bacteria in mesenteric lymph nodes and liver, which may represent decreased bacterial translocation from the gastrointestinal tract or improved bactericidal activity.

Glutamine is the most abundant amino acid in human muscle and plasma and is used as a fuel source for lymphocytes, macrophages, and enterocytes. It also is a precursor of glutathione and nucleotide synthesis. Glutamine is a nonessential amino acid; however, during catabolic illness, glutamine uptake by small intestinal and immune cells may exceed synthesis and release from skeletal muscle, rendering it conditionally essential.[20] Studies of glutamine supplementation to enteral feeding solutions in adult trauma patients have shown significantly less pneumonia, bacteremia, and sepsis in supplemented groups compared with controls.[132] Small individual trials have suggested a beneficial effect of glutamine supplementation in preterm infants.[220] A Cochrane review examining the effect of enteral and parenteral glutamine supplementation on mortality, sepsis, necrotizing enterocolitis, duration of hospitalization, and neurodevelopmental outcome found no clinically significant benefit, however.[317]

Arginine, a nonessential amino acid, has received considerable attention for its immune-enhancing properties. Arginine is a precursor for nitric oxide in vascular endothelial cells, macrophages, and neutrophils, and infusion of arginine stimulates release of growth hormone, glucagon, somatostatin, prolactin, and insulin.[20] A meta-analysis of 15 randomized, controlled trials comparing standard enteral nutrition with commercially available immune-enhancing enteral formulations containing arginine, with or without glutamine, nucleotides, and omega-3 fatty acids, found no effect on mortality, but patients receiving the immune-enhancing formulations showed a decreased risk for developing infection and had shorter hospital stays.[25]

Finally, probiotics such as lactobacillus have received increasing attention as potentially promising supplements for critically ill patients, given their beneficial effects on the gastrointestinal flora in patients with infectious diarrhea or inflammatory bowel disease.[29] Most clinical trials available to date that investigated lactobacillus supplementation in critically ill neonates and adults established safety but were unable to measure any clinical benefit.[74,139]

NUTRITION IN PRETERM INFANTS

Critically ill preterm infants represent a particular nutritional challenge. In addition to all the immunologic abnormalities seen in patients in the ICU, the preterm infant's immune system is immature. Immaturity of the gastrointestinal system renders enteral nutrition particularly difficult and is associated with potentially lethal conditions such as necrotizing enterocolitis, which is not seen in adults. The nutritional requirements of preterm infants exceed the requirements of older patients several-fold in terms of total calories and specific nutrients, calcium, phosphorus, iron, and vitamins. Nutritional management of the critically ill preterm infant is particularly difficult and, at the same time, of utmost importance.

Specialized preterm formulas or human milk fortifiers try to meet the preterm infant's nutritional needs. These formulas are optimized in their caloric content, composition of carbohydrates, type of protein, type of fat, electrolyte and mineral composition, iron content, vitamins, and trace elements. Introduction of enteral feeding often is delayed, however, because of intolerance, immaturity, or an intercurrent episode of infection, hemodynamic decompensation, or necrotizing enterocolitis. Most very-low-birth-weight infants at some point during hospitalization have nutritional deficiencies of vitamin A, vitamin E, or iron, from decreased bone mineralization and growth retardation.

An important strategy in the nutrition of preterm infants is the concept of "trophic feeds." Very small amounts of enteral nutrition, which contribute only minimally to the overall caloric intake, have been shown to avoid many of the devastating consequences of TPN, such as gut atrophy and short gut syndrome. The role of the gut-associated immune system in the overall acquisition of immunocompetence is likely of great importance, and (even trophic) enteral feeds are thought to enhance the development and improve the function of this important part of the immune system. Studies suggest beneficial immunologic effects of early enteral feeds manifesting in decreased incidence of sepsis.[103,250,304] Despite a plethora of studies, the minimal amount at which a clinically significant effect of trophic feeds can be expected is controversial.

BURNS, INFECTION, AND NUTRITION

In the United States, approximately 2.5 million people seek medical care for burns each year. More than 100,000 individuals are hospitalized with burns each year, and 12,000 die. During the past 50 years, great strides have been made in the treatment and management of patients who have sustained thermal injuries. A marked decrease in burn mortality rates, particularly in patients younger than age 35 years, has occurred.[214]

Infection always has been the predominant determinant of wound healing and outcome of burn patients. The incidence of infectious complications in burn patients increases in proportion to the fraction of the body surface injured. The direct effects of heat on skin and underlying tissue render the burn wound particularly susceptible to infection; the denatured protein in burn-injured tissue serves as a rich medium for microbial growth. The thermal thrombosis that renders the eschar avascular precludes delivery of the cellular components of the host defense system and limits delivery of blood-borne antibiotics to the infected wound site. Further microbial proliferation occurs at the interface between viable tissue and the eschar, termed the *subeschar space*. If host defenses are adequate, the eschar is sloughed; however, microbial invasion of the viable tissue occurs if host defenses are deficient.

Pneumonia is the most frequent infection occurring in burn patients. Other infectious complications, such as suppurative thrombophlebitis and septicemia, have been decreasing in incidence as a result of improvements in patient management, wound care, and infection control.[244]

A larger role in the development of sepsis has been attributed more recently to the gastrointestinal tract. The gastrointestinal barrier normally is highly effective in containing its flora. Critically ill patients often experience a breakdown of the barrier, followed by translocation of inert particles and microorganisms across the intestinal wall. This event may play a role in the colonization of burn wounds by gram-negative organisms. Alteration of the indigenous microbial flora, which may be caused by the stress of injury, antibiotics, or composition of enteral feedings, has been shown to influence translocation markedly.

Translocation of bacteria and their toxins from ischemic bowel causes a massive release of cytokines and inflammatory mediators.[79] This "cytokine storm" is associated with depressed cytotoxic activity of T cells, decreased ratio of helper-to-suppressor T lymphocytes, depressed phagocytic activity, reduced intracellular killing, increased superoxide formation, decreased serum concentrations of immunoglobulins, and activation of complement with release of anaphylatoxins.[123]

Major thermal injury is associated with extreme hypermetabolism and catabolism, which occur shortly after successful resuscitation from the shock phase of the burn injury. This hypermetabolic state is characterized by elevated cardiac output, increased energy expenditure, erosion of lean body mass, negative nitrogen balance, and disturbances in glucose metabolism.[316]

The role of nutrition in maintaining immunocompetence and modulating hypermetabolism in burned patients has become increasingly important. The use of early enteral nutrition combined with early excision of nonviable tissue has resulted in reduced energy requirements in burned children.[127] Providing proper nutrition by the enteral route when possible may satisfy caloric needs, regulate microflora, and maintain the integrity of the mucosa of the gut, but it also may blunt the hypermetabolic response after thermal injury.[143]

CANCER AND NUTRITION

Cancer predisposes patients to malnutrition through several mechanisms. Often, patients with cancer have experienced a period of weight loss before being diagnosed with a malignancy. This loss varies for different forms of cancer. Acute lymphoblastic leukemia typically is of rapid onset, and only 6 percent of children have lost a substantial amount of weight at diagnosis. In contrast, 50 percent of patients with stage IV neuroblastoma present with at least some degree of malnutrition.[6]

Malnutrition in patients with cancer originates from a combination of anorexia (i.e., decreased intake) and cachexia (i.e., increased metabolic demand). The latter is particularly evident in children with a very high tumor burden.[238] Anorexia in patients with cancer is due to the malignancy itself and is a common side effect of various cancer treatments. Chemotherapy and radiation often induce substantial nausea, altered smell or taste, vomiting, mucositis, gastric ulcers, or colitis. Certain chemotherapeutic agents, such as vinca alkaloids, can cause severe constipation, as do narcotics, which often are needed to control pain. Pain, malaise, and infections decrease oral intake and are frequent occurrences as a manifestation of the malignancy (bone marrow infiltration leading to immune dysfunction) and as a side effect of therapy. Antibiotics and antifungal agents can cause gastric irritation and diarrhea. Some agents, such as amphotericin B, also may lead to a tubulopathy with urinary losses of electrolytes, amino acids, and trace elements.

Supporting enteral nutrition with nasogastric or gastrostomy tube feeds in patients with cancer is complex. Mucositis and nausea decrease the tolerance for, and compliance with, nasogastric feeds, whereas poor healing and infectious complications affect gastrostomy feedings. Despite these drawbacks, enteral nutrition is much preferred over TPN for its beneficial effect on the gastrointestinal flora and on the structural and functional integrity of the gastrointestinal tract, which helps to prevent translocation of bacteria from the gut into the bloodstream with the associated risk of gram-negative septicemia. In contrast, TPN is associated with a high complication rate, such as central line infections and sepsis, and TPN cholestasis. Nonetheless, both types of nutritional support are used currently in children with cancer.

A variety of clinical studies have highlighted the importance of maintaining adequate nutrition in children with cancer. Malnourished children undergoing cancer chemotherapy have more infectious complications and experience more therapy-related toxicity than do children undergoing therapy with normal nutritional status.[82,151,169,307] In addition to the risks for adverse outcomes from the complications themselves, infections and delayed recovery between cycles of chemotherapy may lead to delays and dose reductions in subsequent cycles. In Brazil, malnutrition has been linked to an increased risk for relapse after treatment for acute lymphoblastic leukemia.[328] Particularly mild nutritional deficits have not been linked conclusively to a decreased rate of overall or event-free survival, however.[232,323] Currently, no national or international standards have been established regarding the nutritional management of children with cancer, and nutritional support practices vary widely even among centers of the Children's Oncology Group. An urgent need exists for more conclusive studies to be performed on the impact of nutrition on toxicity, infectious complications, and, particularly, survival and on the different types of nutritional support for children undergoing cancer treatment.[168]

CYSTIC FIBROSIS

Malnutrition and growth failure are two common presenting signs of cystic fibrosis with pancreatic insufficiency. The failure to thrive seen in these patients is mostly a consequence of malabsorption; however, chronic infections with repeated exacerbations likely also play a role. Particularly crucial is the absorption of fat-soluble vitamins. The importance of vitamins A, D, and E for the development of the immune system and host defenses against infections has been reviewed earlier in this chapter. Later in life, many children with cystic fibrosis also develop insulin-dependent diabetes mellitus, which decreases further their ability to fight off infections.

Based on the multiple levels of interplay among growth, nutrition, development of the immune system, maintenance of immunologic functions, infections, and pulmonary damage, newborn screening for cystic fibrosis has been proposed. Nutritional deficits have been identified through screening in asymptomatic infants 2 months of age.[247] Early recognition and nutritional intervention not only may prevent failure to thrive but also strengthen host defenses and decrease or delay the severity of pulmonary colonization and infections, and ultimately improve overall survival.

Many studies have addressed this hypothesis and have found conflicting results. Data from the Cystic Fibrosis Foundation Registry suggest that early diagnosis is associated with a survival advantage.[170] Almost all studies confirm that early nutritional optimization through early diagnosis helps to avoid malnutrition and stunting, with benefits measurable in adolescence. Although some studies suggest fewer infectious complications, decreased colonization rate with *P. aeruginosa*, and improved pulmonary function tests in 20-year-old patients who were diagnosed through newborn screens,[2,288,302] other studies have been unable to confirm improved pulmonary function or improved survival through early intervention.[96,288] Malnourished *CFTR* knockout mice showed similar levels of cytokine production, inflammatory cells in bronchoalveolar lavage, and survival after challenge with *P. aeruginosa* as wild-type and nonmalnourished *CFTR* knockout mice.[324]

One also must bear in mind that early intervention is likely to lead to not only early and more targeted nutritional intervention, but also to more aggressive monitoring of pulmonary function tests and colonization with pathogens, with earlier and more aggressive antibiotic intervention. Although most data on newborn screening for cystic fibrosis point toward a beneficial effect of early diagnosis, the exact role of nutritional optimization in preventing colonization and infections needs to be studied in more detail.

OBESITY AND INFECTIONS

In industrialized countries, the burden of morbidity and mortality continues to shift toward chronic diseases. Research has focused on the effects of surfeit nutrition, especially obesity.

Numerous animal studies suggest that obesity increases the susceptibility for, and interferes with the ability to respond appropriately to, infection. When dogs were fed a high-calorie diet, a greater susceptibility to distemper virus and a shorter survival time were noted than in control animals fed a normal diet.[221] Chickens on a high-protein diet experienced greater mortality and morbidity from Newcastle disease agent than did controls that were fed normally.[40] Swiss mice made obese by high-fat diets were less resistant to infection by *S. typhimurium* and *K. pneumoniae* compared with mice fed a standard laboratory diet.[300] High-fat diets result in consistently depressed host resistance to tuberculosis and malaria in rats and to pneumococcal infections in chickens.[187] Erickson and associates[90,91] discovered that high levels of dietary fat, particularly polyunsaturated fat, suppressed the response of lymphocytes to T-cell mitogens. Animal models also have shown the adverse effects of excess cholesterol. Fiser and coworkers[102] found that hypercholesterolemic monkeys developed altered humoral and cellular immune function. Hypercholesterolemia also has been found to increase mortality rates in mice infected with group B coxsackieviruses.[182]

Epidemiologic and clinical data in patients support the concept of obesity-related disturbances in immune function. A cross-sectional study of 1129 preadolescent children suggests that obesity in children may be a predisposing factor to acute respiratory disease.[142] The study showed that children with a body mass index greater than or equal to 20 had twice as high a risk for acquiring acute respiratory infections compared with children with a lower body mass index. Chandra[57] examined the immunocompetence of obese children, adolescents, and adults. Approximately one third of the obese group showed a variable impairment of cell-mediated immune responses and a reduction of intracellular bacterial killing by neutrophils. The obese group had moderately low concentrations of serum zinc and iron, and therapy with these micronutrients for 4 weeks resulted in improvement in immunologic responses.

Obese adolescents and adults experience a greater risk for developing sepsis and wound infections after surgery than do lean control subjects.[97,300] Obese individuals exhibit a slight impairment of delayed cutaneous hypersensitivity responses, reduced helper T-cell populations, decreased lymphocyte response to mitogens, and reduced bactericidal capacity of neutrophils. Humoral immunity also may be affected by obesity. A randomized clinical trial of immunogenicity of hepatitis B vaccine found obesity to be a risk factor for nonresponse to the vaccine.[16] Obese subjects were 2.1 times more likely to be nonresponders than were lean subjects.

Obesity also is implicated in altering cytokine responses. Animal studies have shown that elevated levels of TNF are associated with insulin resistance; Boeck and associates[39] reported that obese patients with significant insulin resistance had little or no detectable plasma TNF compared with control subjects. Genetically obese rodents have attenuated production of TNF and IL-6 in response to lipopolysaccharide compared with their lean littermates.[179] These findings may reflect a refractive state in obesity in which production of TNF is down-regulated. Kolterman and colleagues[158] reported reduced release of migration inhibitory factor by stimulated lymphocytes from moderately obese, non-hyperglycemic subjects to 36 percent of the level of normal-weight controls.

A variety of cell-mediated immune responses have been evaluated in genetically obese animals. Reduced numbers of T lymphocytes in peripheral blood, spleen, and thymus were described in obese rats compared with nonobese littermates. The proliferative response of splenocytes to mitogens and natural killer cell activity also was significantly lower in the obese rats.[309] When obese mice were immunized with lymphoma cells, the cytotoxic response of spleen cells was markedly lower than that of lean controls.[60] When lymphocytes from obese and lean mice were sensitized in vitro rather than in vivo, however, they performed similarly. This observation suggests that the microenvironment of obese animals, which includes hyperlipidemia, hyperglycemia, and altered levels of insulin, glucagon, cortisol, and adrenocorticotropic hormone, may be responsible for impaired cellular responses.

Studies indicate that leptin, a protein known to regulate appetite and energy expenditure, may play a role in the altered immune responses associated with obesity. The molecular structure of leptin is similar to that of IL-6, whereas its receptor is a member of the class I cytokine receptor superfamily. Studies of rodents with genetic abnormalities of leptin or leptin receptor revealed deficits in cell-mediated and humoral specific immunity[192] and in macrophage proliferation and phagocytosis.[108,179]

In humans, genetic leptin deficiency is associated with increased susceptibility to infections. Administration of recombinant leptin to two children with congenital leptin deficiency restored mitogenic responses and cytokine responses of T lymphocytes. This result raises the question as to whether, and if so to what extent, low leptin levels contribute to the immune dysfunction seen in malnutrition. Animal data suggest that malnutrition-induced immunosuppression is reversed, at least partially, through administration of leptin. Weight gain in malnourished children has been shown to lead to an increase in leptin serum concentrations and cytokine production and proliferative responses in T cells. A study conducted in mildly undernourished children in Gambia found that, although leptin serum concentrations were low and correlated well with nutritional status, an association between low leptin levels and depressed immune function as measured by vaccine and delayed hypersensitivity responses could not be established in this population.[213]

The role of leptin in the clinically observed increased susceptibility to infections in obese patients is even less clear. Some researchers have hypothesized that increased serum concentrations of leptin in obesity lead to down-regulation of the leptin receptor and leptin resistance in the target cell. The net effect on a cellular level may be that of decreased leptin signaling in obesity and starvation.[192] Characterizing intracellular signaling pathways through leptin in malnutrition and obesity may help to understand better the influence of different nutritional states on leptin's effect on immune responses. It is hoped that animal and clinical studies will help to define the interrelationship among leptin, infections, and obesity or malnutrition and may aid the discovery of new targets for therapeutic interventions.

EFFECT OF NUTRITION ON RESISTANCE TO SPECIFIC INFECTIONS

When malnutrition diminishes resistance to infection or when infection aggravates malnutrition, the relationship between the two can be described as synergistic. In other situations, malnutrition impedes the multiplication of the agent more than it diminishes resistance of the host. In this case, the interaction between infection and malnutrition can be considered antagonistic. Vitamin A deficient patients have been reported to have a higher incidence of tuberculosis, bronchitis, otitis media, urinary tract infections, and bronchopneumonia. Protein deficiency leaves patients more susceptible to typhus, hepatitis, amebic dysentery, diarrheal disease, and tuberculosis. A reasonable assumption is that most deficiency states decrease host resistance to infection.

EXPERIMENTAL VIRAL INFECTION

The effects of malnutrition on experimental viral infection have been studied, but results have not been uniform. Most studies published before 1965 suggested that starved, fasted, or underfed animals are more resistant to viral infections than are normal animals and that the severity of viral infection is decreased.[28,76,246,298,299,336] Despite some contradicting reports, the concept that healthy animals are more susceptible than are their malnourished counterparts to experimental viral infection gained broad acceptance.[272] This antagonistic effect of malnutri-

tion on viral infection was attributed by some investigators to starvation of the virus at the cellular level, with restriction of viral replication.[34,107]

The first studies to cast doubt on this prevailing concept were done by Woodruff and Kilbourne.[342] Their studies convincingly showed an increased severity of infection with coxsackievirus B3 in male albino mice that were subjected to sustained postweaning undernutrition. Severity of infection was proportional to the magnitude of malnutrition. Virus persisted in the heart, spleen, pancreas, and liver of severely malnourished animals, and mortality rates were highest in these groups. If a quantitatively optimal diet was fed to previously malnourished mice at the time of infection, they were protected from further viremia and death.

Further studies of coxsackievirus B in mice with specific nutrient deficiencies were done by Beck and Levander.[26] In these studies, a normally benign strain of coxsackievirus B behaved more virulently and induced cardiomyopathy in selenium-deficient and vitamin E–deficient mice. The increased virulence was caused by genotypic changes in the virus so that the sequence of the normally benign virus now resembles that of more virulent strains. These viral genotypic changes may be secondary to a decreased immune response in the host, leading to increased viral replication and risk for mutation. Alternatively, the increased oxidative stress in a selenium-deficient or vitamin E–deficient host may result in an increase in free radicals that could damage viral RNA directly and result in mutations. This study is the first example of a host diet having a direct effect on the genetic composition of a pathogen.

Overall, the broad consensus is that malnutrition leads to increased susceptibility, morbidity, and mortality from almost all viral infections. Dengue fever seems to constitute an exception, however: Malnourished children apparently have a lower risk of contracting dengue fever than do children with normal nutritional status.[150] The mechanism underlying this observation is unclear.

MEASLES

Measles may be the most extreme example of a childhood disease that is benign in industrialized populations but associated with high mortality rates in developing nations. This difference can be attributed to many factors, including vaccination patterns, concurrent disease, and available medical care. One of the most important causes of this differential mortality is varying nutritional status. Measles influences the nutritional and immune status by several mechanisms. Similar to any other febrile illness, measles contributes to severe reduction in food intake, vomiting, and increased metabolic losses. Measles also can produce a viral enteritis that results in a protein-losing enteropathy. Measles induces prolonged immunosuppression characterized by a decrease in the number of circulating T cells and impaired proliferation of T lymphocytes that has been shown to last for nearly 6 months.

A study in India revealed a close association between protein-calorie malnutrition and measles, with nearly 25 percent of children hospitalized for severe protein-calorie malnutrition reporting an episode of measles in the preceding 3 to 6 months.[36] In a prospective study done in the urban slums of Hyderabad, measles was associated with a weight loss of 2 to 12 percent of initial body weight. These children also were shown to have retarded growth 6 months after the initial infection, and 4 percent developed clinical signs of kwashiorkor or marasmus. All children with severe protein-calorie malnutrition in the post-measles period were undernourished before contracting the infection, which highlights the importance of nutritional status as a major determinant of the severity of nutritional deficiencies and growth failure that occur in the post-measles period.[36]

In the malnourished host, the epithelial surfaces are affected severely by measles, with eye and mouth involvement, laryngitis, bronchopneumonia, and gastroenteritis. These children carry and transmit the virus three times longer than do children with normal nutritional status, and they are more susceptible to viral and bacterial superinfection. A study in Nigeria found a mortality rate of 26 percent, with respiratory complications accounting for more than 90 percent of deaths.[94]

Vitamin A deficiency may cause some of the severe manifestations of measles that occur in malnourished hosts. As mentioned previously, vitamin A is essential for maintenance of epithelial surfaces and for the synthesis of the ground substance of the corneal stroma. The striking occurrence of post-measles blindness in approximately 1 percent of all children with measles in developing countries demonstrates the crucial role of vitamin A metabolism in the malnourished host. Vitamin A supplementation in patients with measles in developing countries is associated with significantly decreased morbidity and mortality rates.[113,136] Patients given vitamin A supplementation showed increased serum concentrations of IgG and faster resolution of virus-induced lymphopenia compared with controls, suggesting an increased immunoresponsiveness to the disease. Hyporetinemia is associated with increased severity of measles,[113] but the relationship between cause and effect is unclear. In the case of malnutrition, exhaustion of hepatic stores accounts for decreased retinol and may predispose the patient to severe measles. Alternatively, hepatic stores of retinol may be mobilized inadequately during severe measles.

Vaccination is an extremely important tool in preventing measles and its associated infections. Often, tuberculosis and malnutrition are considered contraindications for administering measles vaccination. In contrast to the natural measles infection, the attenuated virus has no immunosuppressive effect and is unlikely to activate latent tuberculosis.[36] Several studies in undernourished children have shown high rates of seroconversion to the measles vaccine except in cases of severe protein-calorie malnutrition, indicating the efficacy of immunization against measles in undernourished children.[37,75]

BACTERIAL INFECTION

Bacteremia, the most dreaded infective complication of severe malnutrition, varies in incidence among different studies from 2 to 31 percent. Most commonly, bacteremia is caused by gram-negative enteric bacilli, especially *Salmonella* spp. and *E. coli*, and the common organisms that infect normal hosts. Malnourished patients with bacteremia have an increased risk for organ failure and mortality compared with patients with adequate nutrition. Malnutrition also may modify the response of the immune system to bacterial infections and increase the risk for development of long-term sequelae. In a study of Bangladeshi children with antecedent group A beta-hemolytic streptococcal throat infections, poor nutritional status was associated with an increased risk for developing rheumatic fever.[351] This finding is consistent with the steady decline of the incidence of rheumatic fever in the industrialized countries in the first half of the 20th century, before the advent of penicillin, which was due largely to better socioeconomic conditions and consequently better nutrition of large parts of the population.

More recent research has examined the association between nutrition and *Helicobacter pylori* infection. *H. pylori* infection often is acquired in early childhood. The prevalence of *H. pylori* infection has been reported to be higher in breast-fed compared with formula-fed children, and infection rates seemed to correlate with the duration of breast-feeding.[254] A study in Colombian children found an increased incidence of *H. pylori* infection in children with lower consumption of fruits and vegetables, vitamin C, and beta carotene.[116] Because *H. pylori* is associated with depressed gastric acid secretion and loss of the gastric acid barrier,

it predisposes hosts to enteric infections and may exacerbate malnutrition. A study in Gambian children reported decreased weight for age in infants with sustained *H. pylori* infections compared with uninfected controls.[73] In contrast, an association between *H. pylori* and decreased adult height could not be shown conclusively in an industrialized setting and may not exist without established baseline malnutrition.[208]

Urinary tract infections usually are caused by bacteria that are physiologically present in the stool. Researchers hypothesized that certain foods, by means of altering the composition of the gastrointestinal flora, may affect the incidence of urinary tract infections. In addition, certain foods may alter the urinary pH and render the bladder milieu more or less conducive to bacterial growth. Based on these theories, dietary modifications have been proposed as preventive and therapeutic interventions. Consumption of berry juices or food items containing probiotic bacteria seems to decrease the incidence of urinary tract infections. Some studies showed a therapeutic effect of cranberries or blueberry products on established urinary tract infections, but a therapeutic effect of probiotic bacteria could not be established.[159] Breast-feeding has been shown to decrease the incidence of urinary tract infections in neonates.[189] Whether this effect is due to transferred immunity, alteration of the infant's immune system, local effects on the bladder milieu, or the bacterial composition of the stool is unclear.

PARASITIC INFECTION

Parasitic disease in humans has been estimated to affect more than 1 billion people, particularly children who are living in developing countries in Africa, Asia, and Latin America, where protein-calorie malnutrition is endemic. The same conditions of poverty, overcrowding, and inadequate sanitation that are associated with parasitic infections also are associated with individuals who are at the highest risk for having malnutrition. A particularly vulnerable time for children seems to be from the time they are 4 months old until they are approximately 5 years old. During this period, the transition from breast-feeding to a home diet occurs, and the exposure to disease in the environment increases. Parasitic diseases may reduce intake, interfere with absorption from the intestine, or cause increased losses of nutrients through gastrointestinal, urinary, or blood loss. Evidence suggests that parasitic infections in humans may reduce voluntary food intake by immunologic mechanisms that cause anorexia. Zwingenberger and associates[354] found elevated levels of TNF and cachectin in humans infected with *Schistosoma mansoni*, which normalized after treatment.

Schistosoma haematobium causes urinary schistosomiasis and is endemic in 52 African and eastern Mediterranean countries. *S. mansoni* and *Schistosoma japonicum* cause intestinal schistosomiasis. *S. mansoni* is endemic in Africa, the Middle East, and a few countries in South America and the Caribbean. Schistosomiasis has been implicated as a major contributor to the two most important forms of malnutrition in the Third World—protein-calorie malnutrition and iron-deficiency anemia. The larval and the adult stages of the infection can alter nutritional status by reducing food and nutrient intake, increasing nutrient excretion (mainly through blood loss, vomiting, and diarrhea), or altering nutrient metabolism within the body.[354]

S. haematobium infection is characterized by hematuria and proteinuria. Infected subjects had mean hemoglobin levels 0.9 to 1.3 g/dL lower than the levels of uninfected controls from their areas. The daily urinary protein losses in urinary schistosomiasis are an average of 1 g/day. *S. haematobium* infection may cause splenomegaly and hepatomegaly. Splenomegaly may be related to increased destruction of erythrocytes and can predispose to anemia, whereas hepatomegaly may alter nutrient metabolism.

Hepatomegaly and splenomegaly are reversible with adequate treatment.[354]

S. mansoni infection is associated with blood loss in the stool. Farid and associates[95] estimated the daily fecal blood loss in seven chronically infected Egyptian patients to be equivalent to 3.3 mg/day of iron. These iron losses are sufficient to produce anemia if persistent and if the daily intake of iron is inadequate. Severe infection with *S. mansoni* has been reported to result in significantly lower height for age and skin-fold thickness than milder or no infection. In particular, hepatosplenic involvement has been associated with lower insulin-like growth factor–I, lower insulin-like growth factor binding protein 3, and lower body mass index in affected children.[229] Increasing evidence indicates that mild and moderate infections also have deleterious effects on childhood nutrition. A double-blind, placebo-controlled trial in Brazilian schoolchildren showed that treatment of mild to moderate intensity *S. mansoni* infections was associated with improvement in height, weight, and body mass index in boys.[15]

The effects of *S. japonicum* are similar to those of *S. mansoni*; however, they tend to be more severe because *S. japonicum* produces 10 times as many eggs per worm pair as does *S. mansoni*. Studies from China report that the presence and intensity of *S. japonicum* infection are related directly to reduced arm circumference, skin-fold thickness, height, weight, and weight-for-height ratios.[352]

Hookworms and *Trichuris* spp. are associated with significant intestinal blood losses. Foo[105] showed that children with hookworm infection were on average 1 kg lighter and 2.4 cm shorter and had hemoglobin levels 1.1 g/dL lower. *Ascaris lumbricoides* infection has been shown to interfere with the absorption of fat and is associated with reduced weight and height and reduced serum concentrations of albumin and vitamin A and C.[128] In addition to reducing fat absorption, *Giardia intestinalis* and *A. lumbricoides* reduce intestinal lactase activity, resulting in lactose intolerance. *Strongyloides stercoralis* infection is associated with a protein-losing enteropathy resulting in significant hypoalbuminemia. To a lesser degree, *Giardia lamblia* has been associated with a protein-losing enteropathy without hypoalbuminemia.[305] Several more recent studies[64,209] have shown an association between infection with *Cryptosporidium parvum* and poor linear growth in children, with more marked and lasting effects seen with younger age at infection.

Malnutrition also may affect reinfection rates after successful eradication of enteral parasites. Follow-up of 585 Brazilian children from a poor neighborhood of São Paulo showed higher reinfection rates in malnourished children; the results maintained borderline statistical significance when corrected for confounding variables, such as income or literacy.[262]

Many parasitic infections are caused by crowded living conditions and poor sanitation. At the same time, parasitic infections place an enormous economical and social burden on societies in which they are widespread. In this context, two more recent studies reported parasitic infections as an independent risk factor for poor cognitive function, even when controlled for socioeconomic or nutritional status.[31,93]

DIARRHEAL DISEASE

Disease of the intestinal tract is the most obvious link between the mutually aggravating conditions of infection and malnutrition.[43] Historically, diarrhea has been a primary cause of childhood morbidity and mortality in developing countries. Poor nutrition increases susceptibility to diarrhea, and diarrhea contributes to deteriorating nutrition. Overcrowding and poor sanitation, conditions that coexist with poverty, also act synergistically with malnutrition to enhance the risk for and morbidity of diarrhea. Steps to improve nutrition and to provide oral rehydration

therapy in acute situations can contribute to decreasing diarrheal disease and its effects.

The risk for developing diarrheal disease seems to increase proportionally with the degree of malnutrition. A study of children in the Sudan[160] showed that mild to moderate wasting was associated with a 9 percent increased risk for developing diarrhea, severe wasting was associated with a 34 percent increased risk, and very severe wasting was associated with a 50 percent increased risk compared with normally nourished controls. Gracey[118] has suggested that protein-calorie malnutrition predisposes an individual to having chronic diarrhea by causing changes in the intestinal mucosa. The changes include thinning of the gut wall, flattening of the intestinal villi, inflammatory infiltration of the lamina propria, and alteration of the enterocytes from columnar to cuboidal or squamous.

The gastric mucosa also is abnormal in malnourished states. Chronic gastritis has been noted in Indonesian children in association with a reduction of secretion of gastric acid. This condition may lead to heavy bacterial infestation of the upper gut. The changes seen in the gastrointestinal tracts of children with malnutrition may account for their altered susceptibility to various pathogenic organisms. A cohort study of children in Bangladesh revealed that shigellosis and cholera were common causes of diarrhea in severely malnourished children, whereas rotavirus was seen more often in well-nourished children with diarrhea.[84] Exposure to different pathogens depending on the socioeconomic status also is likely to play a role in this epidemiology.

The mechanisms of nutrient loss in diarrhea that lead to malnutrition include maldigestion resulting in insufficient breakdown of substrates, malabsorption characterized by inefficient uptake, and excessive wastage of nutrients from the body. Bile salt pool depletion and impaired micelle formation in malnutrition cause steatorrhea. Carbohydrate intolerance and malabsorption occur partly because of enterocyte damage and loss of brush border enzymes and partly because of bacterial overgrowth. All of these mechanisms act synergistically with the enteric pathogen to exacerbate the ill effects of malnutrition on the individual.[129,295]

In addition, nonenteral infections commonly coexist and worsen the prognosis. Nutritional restitution is vital and a key factor in survival. It may be initiated through oral feedings or by a modified parenteral route in children who are unable to tolerate oral feedings. Ahmed and coworkers[5] tested a protocol for treating severely malnourished patients with diarrhea that emphasized oral rehydration, immediate refeeding, routine micronutrient supplementation, and broad-spectrum antibiotics. A 47 percent reduction in mortality rates was observed compared with treatment with the conventional protocol, which focused on immediate parenteral rehydration and delayed feeding without routine micronutrient supplementation. Specialized formulas, such as lactose-free formulas or probiotics, may assist further in the treatment of diarrhea, malabsorption, and dehydration, although this approach may be difficult to implement in situations where meeting the most basic needs, such as clean water, is a challenge.[14,294]

Several studies have suggested that breast-feeding and immunization against major pathogens (e.g., measles, rotavirus, cholera) play a protective role in reducing the incidence of morbidity and mortality from diarrhea.[45,133,329] Steps such as improving water quality and availability, ensuring proper food and personal hygiene, controlling zoonotic reservoirs, and improving waste disposal and sanitation would minimize transmission of pathogens to individuals at risk.[129]

RESPIRATORY INFECTION

In the underdeveloped world, acute respiratory infections rank with diarrheal disease as a leading cause of morbidity and mortality. In developing countries, acute respiratory infections account for approximately 28 percent of childhood deaths and are even more frequent than diarrheal episodes. The annual incidence of pneumonia for children younger than 5 years of age in industrialized countries is 3 to 4 percent compared with 10 to 20 percent in most developing countries. This increased incidence of lower respiratory infection likely relates to the increased incidence of malnutrition in these areas.[283]

Malnourished infants are 10 to 20 times as likely to contract pneumonia as are children of normal weight for age.[66] Severe complications, such as empyema and bronchiectasis, also are more likely to occur in the face of nutritional deficiencies. A community-based study in the Philippines showed that malnutrition was the most important determinant of mortality associated with respiratory disease.[320] Such evidence supports WHO recommendations that in areas of prevalent malnutrition the use of antibiotic therapy be determined on the basis of clinical signs that can be recognized by minimally trained health care workers.[344] The presentation of a child with cough, chest indrawing, inability to drink, or a respiratory rate of more than 50 breaths per minute meets the requirement for antimicrobial therapy.

The World Bank Health Sector Review on Acute Respiratory Infections suggested that the most cost-effective interventions to reduce mortality from respiratory infections are case management, promotion of breast-feeding, vaccination against childhood communicable diseases, reduction of malnutrition, and pneumococcal vaccination. Pneumococcal vaccines such as PCV-7 may not be as efficient in preventing severe infections in Third World countries because the spectrum of the most prevalent strains differs in different parts of the world, and antigens of regionally common strains may not be present in vaccines that are directed toward marketing in industrialized countries. Reduction in malnutrition probably is the most important preventive intervention because mortality correlates directly with nutritional status. Other studies also have stressed the importance of vitamin A supplementation in malnourished children, improved access to health care services, adequate housing, and proper waste management in reducing the transmission and development of acute respiratory diseases in children.[133,318,319,325]

PROPHYLAXIS AND IMMUNIZATION

The link between malnutrition and infection must be considered from biologic and social viewpoints. Strategies for improving the control of disease in the developing world have been reviewed by Keusch and Scrimshaw.[154] Immediate interventions include immunizations, oral rehydration programs, promotion of breast-feeding, adequate weaning foods with increased protein, continued feeding during infection, nutrient fortification, and growth monitoring. Complex measures, such as improved sanitation and general education, are important long-term goals.

The effect of malnutrition on the ability of a child to establish immunity after vaccination varies for different types of vaccines and for different degrees and types of malnutrition. Several investigators have concluded that the immune response to immunization remains unimpaired in balanced mild to moderate malnutrition; however, severe forms of protein-calorie malnutrition, especially when maintained for long periods, may affect negatively the ability to seroconvert after immunization.[3,4,75,276] Response rates to tetanus and diphtheria toxoid are well preserved even in children with severe malnutrition. In contrast, impaired responses to measles, yellow fever vaccine, hepatitis, killed influenza A, and killed typhoid vaccine all have been described in moderate to severe protein-calorie malnutrition. Cell-mediated immune responses after BCG immunization in Indian schoolchildren correlated positively with adequate nutri-

tion and waned more rapidly in malnourished than in normal individuals.[279]

Despite these concerns, most data on vaccine campaigns indicate that virtually every immunization program among populations with malnourished children has been at least partially successful.[312] Adequate studies to define the extent of immunization failure in malnourished populations have not been done. The route of vaccination also may play a role. Flo and associates[104] showed that malnourished rats, after receiving oral immunization with cholera toxin, had diminished levels of total IgA in intestinal fluid and an impaired ability to neutralize cholera toxin in vitro compared with well-nourished controls. This finding suggests that oral immunizations have a diminished capacity to evoke an immune response compared with systemic immunizations in severe malnutrition.

Further research may help to improve the immune response after vaccinations in children with severe protein-calorie malnutrition. Of greater importance, no data are available to answer important questions regarding the possible harmful effects of live viral vaccines in malnourished children.

CONCLUSION

Attempts to reduce the mortality and morbidity referable to infection in a malnourished individual must be predicated on a more comprehensive understanding of this process than that presently available; the need for further research is clear. In the interim, every effort must be expended to control infection and improve nutrition and living conditions throughout the world. Meeting these goals requires education, improvement in sanitation, improvement in prenatal care to reduce the incidence of prematurity, and either greater access to appropriate food supplies or education directed toward improving the use of food of appropriate nutritional quality when it already is available.

Mounting evidence indicates that fine-tuning nutritional interventions in premature neonates, critically ill patients, and children with chronic diseases helps to prevent or decrease the development of infectious complications of these various conditions. It is hoped that further reductions in morbidity and mortality rates can be achieved in these patients as more is learned about the various levels of interplay between nutrition and immune function.

The possible link between cardiovascular disease and the immunologic consequences of obesity, such as increased susceptibility to infections and a chronic inflammatory state, constitutes an interesting platform for new therapeutic intervention in the fight against the number one killer in industrialized countries. It also underscores the importance of fighting obesity early in life. Pediatricians will be asked to play an ever more important role in educating their patients to prevent overweight; helping obese children to stabilize or lose weight; advocating for healthier school lunches and sports; and treating the increasingly more prevalent consequences of obesity, such as hypertension, type 2 diabetes, and obstructive sleep apnea, which were previously rare findings in pediatric patients.

REFERENCES

1. Abrams, B. F., and Laros, R. K., Jr.: Prepregnancy weight, weight gain, and birth weight. Am. J. Obstet. Gynecol. *154*:503-509, 1986.
2. Accurso, F. J., Sontag, M. K., and Wagener, J. S.: Complications associated with symptomatic diagnosis in infants with cystic fibrosis. J. Pediatr. *147*(Suppl.):S37-S41, 2005.
3. Adeiga, A., Akinosho, R. O., and Onyewuche, J.: Evaluation of immune response in infants with different nutritional status: Vaccinated against tuberculosis, measles, and poliomyelitis. J. Trop. Pediatr. *40*:345-350, 1994.

4. Ahmed, F., Jones, D. B., and Jackson, A.: Effect of under-nutrition on the immune response to rotavirus infection in mice. Ann. Nutr. Metab. *34*:21-31, 1990.

5. Ahmed, T., Ali, M., Ullah, M. M., et al.: Mortality in severely malnourished children with diarrhoea and use of a standardised management protocol. Lancet *353*:1919-1922, 1999.

6. Alexander, H. R., Rickard, K. A., and Godshall, B.: Nutritional supportive care. *In* Pizzo, P. A., and Poplack, D. G. (eds.): Principles and Practices of Pediatric Oncology. 3rd ed. Philadelphia, Lippincott-Raven Publishers, 1997, pp. 1167-1182.

7. Alverdy, J., Chi, H. S., and Sheldon, G. F.: The effect of parenteral nutrition on gastrointestinal immunity: The importance of enteral stimulation. Ann. Surg. *202*:681-684, 1985.

8. American Academy of Pediatrics Policy Statement: Breastfeeding and the use of human milk. Pediatrics *115*:496-506, 2005.

9. Andelman, M. B., and Sered, B. R.: Utilization of dietary iron by term infants: A study of 1048 infants from a low socioeconomic population. Am. J. Dis. Child. *111*:45-55, 1966.

10. Anderson, D. C., Krishna, G. S., Hughes, J. B., et al.: Impaired polymorphonuclear leukocyte motility in malnourished infants: Relationship to functional abnormalities of cell adherence. J. Lab. Clin. Med. *101*:881-895, 1983.

11. Arbeter, A., Echeverri, L., Franco, D., et al.: Nutrition and infection. Fed. Proc. *30*:1421-1428, 1971.

12. Arnalich, F., Martinez, P., Hernanz, A., et al.: Altered concentrations of appetite regulators may contribute to the development and maintenance of HIV-associated wasting. AIDS *11*:1129-1134, 1997.

13. Ascoli, W., Guzman, M. A., Scrimshaw, N. S., et al.: Nutrition and infection: Field study in Guatemalan villages, 1959-1964, IV. Death of infants and preschool children. Arch. Environ. Health *15*:439-449, 1967.

14. Ashraf, H., Ahmed, S., Fuchs, G. J., et al.: Persistent diarrhoea: Associated infections and response to a low lactose diet. J. Trop. Pediatr. *48*:142-148, 2002.

15. Assis, A. M., Barreto, M. L., Prado, M. S., et al.: *Schistosoma mansoni* infection and nutritional status in schoolchildren: A randomized, double-blind trial in northeastern Brazil. Am. J. Clin. Nutr. *68*:1247-1253, 1998.

16. Averhoff, F., Mahoney, F., Coleman, P., et al.: Immunogenicity of hepatitis B vaccines: Implications for persons at occupational risk of hepatitis B virus infection. Am. J. Prev. Med. *15*:1-8, 1998.

17. Azevedo, Z. M., Luz, R. A., Victal, S. H., et al.: Increased production of tumor necrosis factor-alpha in whole blood cultures from children with primary malnutrition. Braz. J. Med. Biol. Res. *38*:171-183, 2005.

18. Babameto, G., and Kotler, D. P.: Malnutrition in HIV infection. Gastroenterol. Clin. North Am. *26*:393-415, 1997.

19. Barrett-Connor, E.: Bacterial infection and sickle cell anemia: An analysis of 250 infections in 166 patients and a review of the literature. Medicine (Baltimore) *50*:97-112, 1971.

20. Barton, R. G.: Immune-enhancing enteral formulas: Are they beneficial in critically ill patients? Nutr. Clin. Pract. *12*:51-62, 1997.

21. Bauchner, H., Leventhal, J. M., and Shapiro, E. D.: Studies of breast-feeding and infections. J.A.M.A. *256*:887-892, 1986.

22. Baum, M. K., and Shor-Posner, G.: Micronutrient status in relationship to mortality in HIV-1 disease. Nutr. Rev. *56*:S135-S139, 1998.

23. Baum, M. K., Shor-Posner, G., and Campa, A.: Zinc status in human immunodeficiency virus infection. J. Nutr. *130*(Suppl. 5):1421S-1423S, 2000.

24. Baum, M. K., Shor-Posner, G., Lai, S., et al.: High risk of HIV-related mortality is associated with selenium deficiency. J. Acquir. Immune Defic. Syndr. Hum. Retrovirol. *15*:370-374, 1997.

25. Beale, R. J., Bryg, D. J., and Bihari, D. J.: Immunonutrition in the critically ill: A systematic review of clinical outcome. Crit. Care Med. *27*:2799-2805, 1999.

26. Beck, M. A., and Levander, O. A.: Host nutritional status and its effect on a viral pathogen. J. Infect. Dis. *182*(Suppl. 1):S93-S96, 2000.

27. Beisel, W. R.: Vitamins and the immune system. Ann. N. Y. Acad. Sci. *585*:5-8, 1990.

28. Bendinelli, M., Ruschi, A., and Santopadre, G.: Replicazione virale e produzione di interferone intopi a dieta carente infettai con virus mengo. Riv. Ital. Ig. *25*:191-204, 1965.

29. Bengman, S., Garcia de Lorenzo, A., and Culebras, J. M.: Use of pro-, pre- and synbiotics in the ICU—future options. Nutr. Hosp. *16*:239-256, 2001.

30. Berhane, R., Bagenda, D., Marum, L., et al.: Growth failure as a prognostic indicator of mortality in pediatric HIV infection. Pediatrics *100*:E7, 1997.

31. Berkman, D. S., Lescano, A. G., Gilman, R. H., et al.: Effects of stunting, diarrhoeal disease, and parasitic infection during infancy on cognition in late childhood: A follow-up study. Lancet *359*:564-571, 2002.

32. Bernstein, P. S., and Divon, M. Y.: Etiologies of fetal growth restriction. Clin. Obstet. Gynecol. *40*:723-729, 1997.

33. Bernt, K. M., and Walker, W. A.: Human milk and the response of intestinal epithelium to infection. *In* Newburg D. S. (ed.): Bioactive Components in Human Milk, 1st ed. New York, Kluwer Academic/Plenum Publishers, 2001, pp. 11-30.

34. Beveridge, W. I. B.: Immunity to viruses. *In* Betts, A. O., and York, C. J. (eds.): Viral and Rickettsial Infections of Animals. Vol. 1. New York, Academic Press, 1967.

35. Bhaskaram, P.: The vicious cycle of malnutrition-infection with special reference to diarrhea, measles, and tuberculosis. Natl. Inst. Nutr. Indian Council Med. Res. *29*:805-813, 1992.

36. Bhaskaram, P., Hemalatha, P., and Rao, K. V.: BCG vaccination in malnourished child population. Indian Pediatr. *29*:39-44, 1992.

37. Bhaskaram, P., Madhusudan, J., Radhakrishna, K. V., et al.: Immunological response to measles vaccination in poor communities. Hum. Nutr. Clin. Nutr. *40C*:295-300, 1986.

38. Blaymore-Bier, J. A., Oliver, T., Ferguson, A., et al.: Human milk reduces outpatient upper respiratory symptoms in premature infants during their first year of life. J. Perinatol. *22*:354-359, 2002.

39. Boeck, M. A., Chin, C., and Cunningham-Rundles, S.: Altered immune function in a morbidly obese pediatric population. Ann. N. Y. Acad. Sci. *587*:253-256, 1990.

40. Boyd, F. M., and Edwards, H. M., Jr.: The effect of dietary protein on the course of various infections in the chick. J. Infect. Dis. *112*:53-56, 1963.

41. Braude-Heller, A., Ratbalsam, I., and Elbinger, R.: Clinical aspects of hunger disease in children. *In* Winick, M. (ed.): Hunger Disease. New York, John Wiley & Sons, 1959, pp. 45-68.

42. Brodie, S. B., Sands, K. E., Gray, J. E., et al.: Occurrence of nosocomial bloodstream infections in six neonatal intensive care units. Pediatr. Infect. Dis. J. *19*:56-65, 2000.

43. Brown, K. H.: Diarrhea and malnutrition. J. Nutr. *133*:S328-S332, 2003.

44. Brown, K. H., Gaffar, A., and Alamgir, S. M.: Xerophthalmia, protein-calorie malnutrition, and infections in children. J. Pediatr. *95*:651-656, 1979.

45. Brown, K. R., Black, G., Lopez, R., et al.: Infant feeding practices and their relationship with diarrheal and other diseases in Huascar (Lima), Peru. Pediatrics *83*:31-40, 1989.

46. Brundtland, G. H.: Nutrition and infection: Malnutrition and mortality in public health. Nutr. Rev. *58*:S1-S4, 2000.

47. Burger, H., Kovacs, A., Weiser, B., et al.: Maternal serum vitamin A levels are not associated with mother-to-child transmission of HIV-1 in the United States. J. Acquir. Immune Defic. Syndr. Hum. Retrovirol. *14*:321-326, 1997.

48. Burns, D. N., FitzGerald, G., Semba, R., et al.: Vitamin A deficiency and other nutritional indices during pregnancy in human immunodeficiency virus infection: Prevalence, clinical correlates, and outcome. Women and Infants Transmission Study Group. Clin. Infect. Dis. *29*:328-334, 1999.

49. Campa, A., Shor-Posner, G., Indacochea, F., et al.: Mortality risk in selenium-deficient HIV-positive children. J. Acquir. Immune Defic. Syndr. Hum. Retrovirol. *20*:508-513, 1999.

50. Carbonnel, F., Beaugerie, L., Abou Rached, A., et al.: Macronutrient intake and malabsorption in HIV infection: A comparison with other malabsorptive states. Gut *41*:805-810, 1997.

51. Carter, J. P., Kattab, A., Abd-el-hadi, K., et al.: Chromium (3) in hypoglycemia and in impaired glucose utilization in kwashiorkor. Am. J. Clin. Nutr. *21*:195-202, 1968.

52. Carver, J. D., Pimentel, B., Cox, W. I., et al.: Dietary nucleotide effects upon immune function in infants. Pediatrics *88*:359-363, 1991.

53. Chalmers, T. C.: Effects of ascorbic acid on the common cold. Am. J. Med. *58*:532-536, 1975.

54. Chandra, R. K.: Antibody formation in first and second generation offspring of nutritionally deprived rats. Science *190*:289-290, 1975.

55. Chandra, R. K.: Fetal malnutrition and postnatal immunocompetence. Am. J. Dis. Child. *129*:450-454, 1975.

56. Chandra, R. K.: Prospective studies of the effect of breastfeeding on incidence of infection and allergy. Acta Paediatr. Scand. *68*:691-694, 1979.

57. Chandra, R. K.: Immune response in overnutrition. Cancer Res. *41*:3795-3796, 1981.

58. Chandra, R. K.: Micronutrients and immune functions. Ann. N. Y. Acad. Sci. *587*:9-16, 1990.

59. Chandra, R. K.: Immunocompetence is a sensitive and functional barometer of nutritional status. Acta Paediatr. Scand. *374*(Suppl.): S129-S132, 1991.

60. Chandra, R. K.: Nutrition and immunity: Lessons from the past and new insights into the future. Am. J. Clin. Nutr. *53*:1087-1101, 1991.

61. Chandra, R. K.: Nutrition and immunoregulation: Significance for host resistance to tumors and infectious diseases in humans and rodents. J. Nutr. *122*(Suppl. 3):754-757, 1992.

62. Chandra, R. K., Gupta S., and Singh, H.: Induce and suppressor T cells subsets in protein-energy malnutrition: Analysis by monoclonal antibodies. Nutr. Res. *2*:21-26, 1982.

63. Chandra, R. K., and Wadhwa, M.: Nutritional modulation of intestinal mucosal immunity. Immunol. Invest. *18*:119-126, 1989.

64. Checkley, W., Epstein, L. D., Gilman, R. H., et al.: Effects of *Cryptosporidium parvum* infection in Peruvian children: Growth faltering and subsequent catch-up growth. Am. J. Epidemiol. *148*:497-506, 1998.

65. Cohen, S., and Hansen, J. D. L.: Metabolism of albumin and γ-globulin in kwashiorkor. Clin. Sci. *23*:351-359, 1962.

66. Coles, C. L., Fraser, D., Givon-Lavi, N., et al.: Nutritional status and diarrheal illness as independent risk factors for alveolar pneumonia. Am. J. Epidemiol. *162*:999-1007, 2005.

67. Collinson, A. C., Moore, S .E., and Cole, T. J.: Birth season and environmental influences on patterns of thymic growth in rural Gambian infants. Acta Paediatr. *92*:994-996, 2003.

68. Cooper, K. A., Adelekan, D. A., Esimai, A. O., et al.: Lack of influence of red palm oil on severity of malaria infection in pre-school Nigerian children. Trans. R. Soc. Trop. Med. Hyg. 96:216-223, 2002.

69. Cunningham, A. S.: Morbidity in breast fed and artificially fed infants. J. Pediatr. 95:685-689, 1979.

70. Cunningham-Rundels, S., Bockman R. S., Lin, A., et al.: Physiological and pharmacological effects of zinc on immune response. Ann. N. Y. Acad. Sci. 587:113-122, 1990.

71. da Costa Lima, R., Victora, C. G., Menezes, A. M., et al.: Do risk factors for childhood infections and malnutrition protect against asthma? A study of Brazilian male adolescents. Am. J. Public Health 93:1858-1864, 2003.

72. Dai, D., and Walker, W. A.: Protective nutrients and bacterial colonization in the immature human gut. Adv. Pediatr. 46:353-382, 1999.

73. Dale, A., Thomas, J. E., Darboe, M. K., et al.: *Helicobacter pylori* infection, gastric acid secretion, and infant growth. J. Pediatr. Gastroenterol. Nutr. 26:393-397, 1998.

74. Dani, C., Biadaioli, R., Bertini, G., et al.: Probiotics feeding in prevention of urinary tract infection, bacterial sepsis and necrotizing enterocolitis in preterm infants: A prospective double-blind study. Biol. Neonate 82:103-108, 2002.

75. Dao, H., Delisle, H., and Fournier, P.: Anthropometric status, serum preal-bumin level, and immune response to measles vaccination in Mali children. J. Trop. Pediatr. 38:179-184, 1992.

76. Davies, W. L., Smith, S. C., Pond, W. L., et al.: Effect of dietary restriction on susceptibility of mice to infection with Theiler's GDVII virus. Proc. Soc. Exp. Med. 72:528-531, 1949.

77. De la Fuente, M., and Munoz, M. L.: Impairment of phagocytic process in macrophages from young and old mice by protein malnutrition. Ann. Nutr. Metab. 36:41-47, 1992.

78. de Silva, A., Atukorala, S., Weerasinghe, I., et al.: Iron supplementation improves iron status and reduces morbidity in children with or without upper respiratory tract infections: A randomized controlled study in Colombo, Sri Lanka. Am. J. Clin. Nutr. 77:234-241, 2003.

79. Deitch, E. A.: The management of burns. N. Engl. J. Med. 323:1249-1253, 1990.

80. Del Rio, M., Ruedas, G., Medina, S., et al.: Improvement by several antioxi-dants of macrophage function in vitro. Life Sci. 63:871-881, 1998.

81. Delafuente, J. C.: Nutrients and immune response. Rheum. Dis. Clin. North Am. 17:203-211, 1991.

82. den Broeder, E., Lippens, R. J., van't Hof, M. A., et al.: Association between the change in nutritional status in response to tube feeding and the occurrence of infections in children with a solid tumor. Pediatr. Hematol. Oncol. 17:567-575, 2000.

83. Department of Health and Human Services Office on Women's Health: Benefits of breastfeeding. Nutr. Clin. Care 6:125-131, 2003.

84. Dewan, N., Faruque, A. S., and Fuchs, G. J.: Nutritional status and diarrhoeal pathogen in hospitalized children in Bangladesh. Acta Paediatr. 87:627-630, 1998.

85. Dourov, N.: Thymic atrophy and immune deficiency in malnutrition. Curr. Top. Pathol. 75:127-150, 1986.

86. Dudley, L., Hussey, G., Huskissen, J., et al.: Vitamin A status, other risk factors and acute respiratory infection morbidity in children. S. Afr. Med. J. 87:65-70, 1997.

87. Duggan, C., and Fawzi, W.: Micronutrients and child health: Studies in inter-national nutrition and HIV infection. Nutr. Rev. 59:358-369, 2001.

88. Edelman, R.: Infant nutrition and immunity. Ann. N. Y. Acad. Sci. 587:232-235, 1990.

89. Enwonwu, C. O., Phillips, R. S., and Savage, K. O.: Inflammatory cytokine profile and circulating cortisol levels in malnourished children with necrotiz-ing ulcerative gingivitis. Eur. Cytokine Netw. 16:240-248. 2005.

90. Erickson, K. L.: Dietary fat modulation of immune response. Int. J. Immunopharmacol. 8:529-543, 1986.

91. Erickson, K. L., Adams, D. A., and Scibienski, R. J.: Dietary fatty acid modula-tion of murine B-cell responsiveness. J. Nutr. 116:1830-1840, 1986.

92. Espinoza, F., Paniagua, M., Hallander, H., et al.: Rotavirus infections in young Nicaraguan children. Pediatr. Infect. Dis. J. 16:564-571, 1997.

93. Ezeamama, A. E., Friedman, J. F., Acosta, L. P., et al.: Helminth infection and cognitive impairment among Filipino children. Am. J. Trop. Med. Hyg. 72:540-548, 2005.

94. Fagbule, D., and Orifunmishe, F.: Measles and childhood mortality in semi-urban Nigeria. Afr. J. Med. Sci. 17:181-185, 1988.

95. Farid, Z., Bassily, S., Schulert, A. R., et al.: Blood loss in chronic S. *mansoni* infection in Egyptian farmers. Trans. R. Soc. Trop. Med. Hyg. 61:289-314, 1967.

96. Farrell, P. M., Lai, H. J., Li, Z., et al.: Evidence on improved outcomes with early diagnosis of cystic fibrosis through neonatal screening: Enough is enough! J. Pediatr. 147(Suppl.):S30-S36, 2005.

97. Fasol, R., Schindler, M., Schumacher, B., et al.: The influence of obesity on perioperative morbidity: Retrospective study of 502 aortocoronary bypass operations. Thorac. Cardiovasc. Surg. 40:126-129, 1992.

98. Fawzi, W. W., Msamanga, G., Hunter, D., et al.: Influence of nutritional and haemoglobin status on malaria infection in children. Indian J. Pediatr. 62:321-326, 1995.

99. Fawzi, W. W., Msamanga, G., Hunter, D., et al.: Randomized trial of vita-min supplements in relation to vertical transmission of HIV-1 in Tanzania. J. Acquir. Immune Defic. Syndr. 23:246-254, 2000.

100. Fawzi, W., Msamanga, G., Spiegelman, D., et al.: Studies of vitamins and minerals and HIV transmission and disease progression. J. Nutr. 135:938-944, 2005.

101. Fields-Gardner, C., and Ayoob, K. T.: Position of the American Dietetic Association and Dietitians of Canada: Nutrition intervention in the care of persons with human immunodeficiency virus infection. J. Am. Diet. Assoc. 100:708-717, 2000.

102. Fiser, R. H., Jr., Denniston, J. C., McGann, V. G., et al.: Altered immune functions in hypercholesterolemic monkeys. Infect. Immunol. 8:105-109, 1973.

103. Flidel-Rimon, O., Friedman, S., Lev, E., et al.: Early enteral feeding and nosocomial sepsis in very low birthweight infants. Arch. Dis. Child. Fetal Neonatal Ed. 89:F289-F292, 2004.

104. Flo, J., Roux, M., and Massouh, E.: Deficient induction of the immune response to oral immunization with cholera toxin in malnourished rats during suckling. Infect. Immun. 62:4948-4954, 1994.

105. Foo, L.: Hookworm infection and protein-energy malnutrition: Transverse evidence from two Malaysian ecological groups. Trop. Geogr. Med. 42:8-12, 1990.

106. Forceville, X., Vitoux, D., Gauzit, R., et al.: Selenium, systemic immune response syndrome, sepsis, and outcome in critically ill patients. Crit. Care Med. 26:1536-1544, 1998.

107. Foster, C., Jones, J. H., Henle, W., et al.: Comparative effects of vitamin B₁ deficiency and restriction of food intake on the response of mice to the Lansing strain of poliomyelitis virus, as determined by the paired feeding technique. J. Exp. Med. 80:257-264, 1944.

108. Gainsford, T., Willson, T. A., Metcalf, D., et al.: Leptin can induce prolifera-tion, differentiation, and functional activation of hemopoietic cells. Proc. Natl. Acad. Sci. U. S. A. 93:14564-14568, 1996.

109. Gallagher, K., Matarazzo, W., and Gray, I.: Trace metal modification of lym-phocyte transformation in vitro. Fed. Proc. 37:377, 1978.

110. Gdalevich M., Mimouni D., David M., et al.: Breast-feeding and the onset of atopic dermatitis in childhood: A systematic review and meta-analysis of prospective studies. J. Am. Acad. Dermatol. 45:520-527, 2001.

111. Gdalevich M., Mimouni D., and Mimouni M.: Breast-feeding and the risk of bronchial asthma in childhood: A systematic review and meta-analysis of prospective studies. J. Pediatr. 139:261-266, 2001.

112. Gernaat, H. B., Dechering, W. H., and Voorhoeve, H. W.: Mortality in severe protein-energy malnutrition at Nchelenge, Zambia. J. Trop. Pediatr. 44:211-217, 1998.

113. Gerster, H.: Vitamin A: Functions, dietary requirements and safety in humans. Int. J. Vitam. Nutr. Res. 67:71-90, 1997.

114. Gilio, A. E., Stape, A., Pereira, C. R., et al.: Risk factors for nosocomial infec-tions in a critically ill pediatric population: A 25-month prospective cohort study. Infect. Control Hosp. Epidemiol. 21:340-342, 2000.

115. Good, R. A., Fernandes, E. J., Yunis, W. C., et al.: Nutritional deficiency, immunologic function and disease. Am. J. Pathol. 84:599-614, 1976.

116. Goodman, K. J., Correa, P., Tengana Aux, H. J., et al.: Nutritional factors and *Helicobacter pylori* infection in Colombian children. J. Pediatr. Gastroenterol. Nutr. 25:507-515, 1997.

117. Gordon, J. E., Ascoli, W., Mata, L. J., et al.: Nutrition and infection: Field study in Guatemalan villages, 1959-1964. Arch. Environ. Health 16:424-437, 1968.

118. Gracey, M.: Chronic diarrhoea in protein-energy malnutrition. Paediatr. Indones. 21:235-239, 1981.

119. Greenberg, B. L., Semba, R. D., Vink, P. E., et al.: Vitamin A deficiency and maternal-infant transmissions of HIV in two metropolitan areas in the United States. AIDS 11:325-332, 1997.

120. Greenwood, B. M., Bradley, A. K., Blakebrough, I. S., et al.: The immune response to a meningococcal polysaccharide vaccine in an African village. Trans. R. Soc. Trop. Med Hyg. 74:340-346, 1980.

121. Harris, M. C., and Douglas, S. D.: Nutritional influence on neonatal infections in animal models and man. Ann. N. Y. Acad. Sci. 587:246-255, 1990.

122. Harris, M. C., and Douglas, S. D.: Nutritional modulation of phagocyte func-tion with special emphasis on the newborn. Indian J. Pediatr. 57:147-158, 1990.

123. Heideman, M., and Bengtsson, A.: The immunologic response to thermal injury. World J. Surg. 16:53-56, 1992.

124. Heinzerling, R. H., Nockels, C. F., Quarles, C. L., et al.: Protection of chicks against E. *coli* infections by dietary supplementation with vitamin E. Proc. Soc. Exp. Biol. Med. 146:279-283, 1974.

125. Heise, F. H., and Martin, G. J.: Ascorbic acid metabolism in tuberculosis. Proc. Soc. Exp. Biol. Med. 34:642-644, 1936.

126. Hemila, H.: Vitamin C and the common cold. Br. J. Nutr. 67:3-16, 1992.

127. Hildreth, M. A., Herndon, D. N., Desai, M. H., et al.: Current treatment reduces calories required to maintain weight in pediatric patients with burns. J. Burn Care Rehabil. 11:405-409, 1990.

128. Hlaing, T.: Ascariasis and childhood malnutrition. Parasitology 107:S125-S136, 1993.

129. Hodges, M.: Diarrhoeal disease in early childhood: Experiences from Sierra Leone. Parasitology 107:S37-S51, 1993.

130. Hokama, T., Yara, A., Hirayama, K., et al.: Isolation of respiratory bacte-rial pathogens from the throats of healthy infants fed by different methods. J. Trop. Pediatr. 45:173-176, 1999.

131. Hori, K., Hatfield, D., Maldarelli, F., et al.: Selenium supplementation suppresses tumor necrosis factor alpha-induced human immunodeficiency virus type 1 replication in vitro. AIDS Res. Hum. Retroviruses 13:1325-1332, 1997.

132. Houdijk, A. P., Rijnsburger, E. R., Jansen, J., et al.: Randomised trial of glutamine-enriched enteral nutrition on infectious morbidity in patients with multiple trauma. Lancet 352:772-776, 1998.

133. Huffman, S. L., and Martin, L.: Child nutrition, birth spacing, and child mortality. Ann. N. Y. Acad. Sci. 585:236-247, 1990.

134. Hughes, W. T., Price, R. A., Sisko, F., et al.: Protein-calorie malnutrition. Am. J. Dis. Child. 128:44-52, 1974.

135. Humphrey, J. H., West, K. P., Jr., and Sommer, A.: Vitamin A deficiency and attributable mortality among under-5-year-olds. Bull. W. H. O. 70:225-232, 1992.

136. Hussey, G. D., and Klein, M.: A randomized, controlled trial of vitamin A in children with severe measles. N. Engl. J. Med. 323:160-164, 1990.

137. Hytten, S. E.: Nutritional aspects of foetal growth. In: Nutrition and Early Growth, Sixth International Congress of Nutrition. Edinburgh, Churchill Livingstone, 1964.

138. Jackson, T. M., and Zaman, S. N.: The in vitro effect of the thymic thymopoietin on a subpopulation of lymphocytes from severely malnourished children. Clin. Exp. Immunol. 39:717-721, 1980.

139. Jain, P. K., McNaught, C. E., Anderson, A. D., et al.: Influence of synbiotics containing Lactobacillus acidophilus La5, Bifidobacterium lactis Bb 12, Streptococcus thermophilus, Lactobacillus bulgaricus and oligofructose on gut barrier function and sepsis in critically ill patients: A randomised controlled trial. Clin. Nutr. 223:467-475, 2004.

140. Jambon, B., Ziegler, O., Maire, B., et al.: Thymulin (facteur thymique serique) and zinc contents of the thymus glands of malnourished children. Am. J. Clin. Nutr. 48:335-342, 1988.

141. Janoff, A.: The role of iron in macrophages. J. Theoret. Biol. 7:168-170, 1964.

142. Jedrychowski, W., Maugeri, U., Flak, E., et al.: Predisposition to acute respiratory infections among overweight preadolescent children: An epidemiologic study in Poland. Public Health 112:189-195, 1998.

143. Jenkins, M. E., Gottschlich, M. M., and Warden, G. D.: Enteral feeding during operative procedures in thermal injuries. J. Burn Care Rehabil. 15:199-205, 1994.

144. Jiang, X., and Balwin, C. L.: Iron augments macrophage mediated killing of Brucella abortus alone and in conjunction with interferon-gamma. Cell. Immunol. 148:397-407, 1993.

145. Jones, G., Strugnell, S. A., and DeLuca, H. F.: Current understanding of the molecular actions of vitamin D. Physiol. Rev. 78:1193-1231, 1998.

146. Jones, P. N., Mills, E. H., and Capps, R. B.: The effect of liver disease on serum vitamin B_{12} concentrations. J. Lab. Clin. Med. 49:910-922, 1957.

147. Joynson, D. H., Walker, D. M., Jacobs, A., et al.: Defect of cell-mediated immunity in patients with iron-deficiency anaemia. Lancet 2:1058-1059, 1972.

148. Jyonouchi, H.: Nucleotide actions on humoral immune responses. J. Nutr. 124(Suppl. 1):138S-143S, 1994.

149. Kacew, S.: Adverse effects of drugs and chemicals in breast milk on the nursing infant. J. Clin. Pharmacol. 33:213-221, 1993.

150. Kalayanarooj, S., and Nimmannitya, S.: Is dengue severity related to nutritional status? Southeast Asian J. Trop. Med. Public Health 36:378-384, 2005.

151. Kennedy, D. D., Tucker, K. L., Ladas, E. D., et al.: Low antioxidant vitamin intakes are associated with increases in adverse effects of chemotherapy in children with acute lymphoblastic leukemia. Am. J. Clin. Nutr. 79:1029-1036, 2004.

152. Keusch, G. T.: Micronutrients and susceptibility to infection. Ann. N. Y. Acad. Sci. 587:181-187, 1990.

153. Keusch, G. T.: Nutritional effects of response of children in developing countries to respiratory tract pathogens: Implications for vaccine development. Rev. Infect. Dis. 13(Suppl. 6):S486-S491, 1991.

154. Keusch, G. T., and Scrimshaw, N. S.: Selective primary health care: Strategies for control of disease in the developing world, XXIII: Control of infection to reduce the prevalence of infantile and childhood malnutrition. Rev. Infect. Dis. 8:273-287, 1986.

155. King, B. K., and Kudsk, K. A.: Can an enteral diet decrease sepsis after trauma? Adv. Surg. 31:53-78, 1997.

156. Kinoshita, M., and Ross, A. C.: Vitamin A status and immunoglobulin G subclasses in rats immunized with tetanus toxoid. Faseb. J. 7:1277-1282, 1993.

157. Kirkpatrick, B. D., Daniels, M. M., Jean, S. S., et al.: Cryptosporidiosis stimulates an inflammatory intestinal response in malnourished Haitian children. J. Infect. Dis. 186:94-101, 2002.

158. Kolterman, O. G., Olefsky, J. M., Kurahara, C., et al.: A defect in cell-mediated immune function in insulin-resistant diabetic and obese subjects. J. Lab. Clin. Med. 96:535-543, 1980.

159. Kontiokari, T., Nuutinen, M., and Uhari, M.: Dietary factors affecting the susceptibility to urinary tract infections. Pediatr. Nephrol. 19:378-383, 2004.

160. Kossmann, J., Nestel, P., Herrera, M. G., et al.: Undernutrition in relation to childhood infections: A prospective study in the Sudan. Eur. J. Clin. Nutr. 54:463-472, 2000.

161. Kotler, D. P.: Management of nutritional alterations and issues concerning quality of life. J. Acquir. Immune Defic. Syndr. Hum. Retrovirol. 16(Suppl. 1):S30-S35, 1997.

162. Kotler, D. P.: Human immunodeficiency virus-related wasting: Malabsorption syndromes. Semin. Oncol. 25(Suppl. 6):70-75, 1998.

163. Kramer, M. S., Guo, T., Platt, R. W., et al.: Infant growth and health outcomes associated with 3 compared with 6 mo of exclusive breastfeeding. Am. J. Clin. Nutr. 78:291-295, 2003.

164. Kreiss, J.: Breastfeeding and vertical transmission of HIV-1. Acta. Paediatr. Suppl. 421:113-117, 1997.

165. Kudsk, K. A., Carpenter, G., Petersen, S., et al.: Effect of enteral and parenteral feeding in malnourished rats with E. coli-hemoglobin adjuvant peritonitis. J. Surg. Res. 31:105-110, 1981.

166. Kudsk, K. A., Stone, J. M., Carpenter, G., et al.: Enteral and parenteral feeding influences mortality after hemoglobin-E. coli peritonitis in normal rats. J. Trauma 23:605-609, 1983.

167. Kulkarni, A. D., Rudolph, F. B., and Van Buren, C. T.: The role of dietary sources of nucleotides in immune function: A review. J. Nutr. 124(Suppl. 8):1442S-1446S, 1994.

168. Ladas, E. J., Sacks, N., Brophy, P., et al.: Standards of nutritional care in pediatric oncology: Results from a nationwide survey on the standards of practice in pediatric oncology. A Children's Oncology Group study. Pediatr. Blood Cancer 46:339-344, 2006.

169. Ladas, E. J., Sacks, N., Meacham, L., et al.: A multidisciplinary review of nutrition considerations in the pediatric oncology population: A perspective from children's oncology group. Nutr. Clin. Pract. 20:377-393, 2005.

170. Lai, H. J., Cheng, Y., and Farrell, P. M.: The survival advantage of patients with cystic fibrosis diagnosed through neonatal screening: Evidence from the United States Cystic Fibrosis Foundation registry data. J. Pediatr. 147(Suppl): S57-S63, 2005.

171. Lake-Bakaar, G., Quadros, E., Beidas, S., et al.: Gastric secretory failure in patients with acquired immunodeficiency syndrome (AIDS). Ann. Intern. Med. 109:502-504, 1988.

172. Lanphear, B. P., Hall, C. B., Black, J., et al.: Risk factors for the early acquisition of human herpesvirus 6 and human herpesvirus 7 infections in children. Pediatr. Infect. Dis. J. 17:792-795, 1998.

173. Latham, M. C.: Protein-energy malnutrition: Its epidemiology and control. J. Environ. Pathol. Toxicol. Oncol. 10:168-169, 1990.

174. Laurell, C. B.: Metal-binding plasma proteins and cation transport. In Putnam, F. W. (ed.): The Plasma Proteins, I. New York, Academic Press, 1960, pp. 229-264.

175. Lehmann, H., Huntsman, R. G., and Ager, J. A. M.: The hemoglobinopathies and thalassemia. In Stanbury, J. B., Wyngaarden, J. B., and Fredrickson, D. S. (eds.): The Metabolic Basis of Inherited Disease. 2nd ed. New York, McGraw-Hill, 1966, pp. 1100-1136.

176. Levine, O. S., Farley, M., Harrison, L. H., et al.: Risk factors for invasive pneumococcal disease in children: A population-based case-control study in North America. Pediatrics 103:E28, 1999.

177. Li, J., Kudsk, K. A., Gocinski, B., et al.: Effects of parenteral and enteral nutrition on gut-associated lymphoid tissue. J. Trauma 39:44-51, 1995.

178. Lindenbaum, J.: Malabsorption during and after recovery from acute intestinal infection. B. M. J. 2:326-329, 1965.

179. Loffreda, S., Yang, S. Q., Lin, H. Z., et al.: Leptin regulates proinflammatory immune responses. Faseb. J. 12:57-65, 1998.

180. Long, K. Z., and Santos, J. I.: Vitamins and the regulation of the immune response. Pediatr. Infect. Dis. J. 18:283-290, 1999.

181. Lopez-Alarcon, M., Villalpando, S., and Fajardo, A.: Breast-feeding lowers the frequency and duration of acute respiratory infection and diarrhea in infants under six months of age. J. Nutr. 127:436-443, 1997.

182. Loria, R. M., Kibrick, S., and Madge, G. E.: Infection of hypercholesterolemic mice with coxsackievirus B. J. Infect. Dis. 133:655-662, 1976.

183. Luke, B.: Nutritional influences on fetal growth. Clin. Obstet. Gynecol. 37:538-549, 1994.

184. Macdougall, L. G., Anderson, R., McNab, G. M., et al.: The immune response in iron-deficient children: Impaired cellular defense mechanisms with altered humoral components. J. Pediatr. 86:833-843, 1975.

185. MacKay, H. M.: Anaemia in infancy: Its prevalence and prevention. Arch. Dis. Child. 3:117-144, 1928.

186. Madi, K., Maeda, C. T., and Savino, W.: Thymic extracellular matrix in human malnutrition. J. Pathol. 171:231-236, 1993.

187. Maki, P. A., and Newberne, P. M.: Dietary lipids and immune function. J. Nutr. 122(Suppl. 3):610-614, 1992.

188. Manary, M. J., and Brewster, D. R.: Intensive nursing care of kwashiorkor in Malawi. Acta Paediatr. 89:203-207, 2000.

189. Marild S., Hansson S., Jodal U., et al.: Protective effect of breast feeding against urinary tract infection. Acta Paediatr. 93:164-166, 2004.

190. Martinez-Augustin, O., Boza, J. J., Navarro, J., et al.: Dietary nucleotides may influence the humoral immunity in immunocompromised children. Nutrition 13:465-469, 1997.

191. Masson, P. L., and Heremans, J. F.: Studies on lactoferrin, the iron-binding protein of secretions. In Peeters, H. (ed.): Protides of the Biological Fluids. Vol. 14. Amsterdam, Elsevier, 1967, pp. 115-124.

192. Matarese, G., Moschos, S., and Mantzoros, C. S.: Leptin in immunology. J. Immunol. 174:3137-13142, 2005.

193. Matoth, Y., Zamir, R., and Bar-shani, S.: Studies on folic acid in infancy, II: Folic and folinic acid blood levels in infants with diarrhea, malnutrition and infection. Pediatrics 33:694-699, 1964.

194. Mbori-Ngacha, D., Nduati, R., John, G., et al.: Morbidity and mortality in breastfed and formula-fed infants of HIV-1 infected women: A randomized clinical trial. JAMA 286:2413-2420, 2001.

195. McFarlane, H.: Cell-mediated immunity in protein-calorie malnutrition. Lancet 2:1146-1147, 1971.

196. McKenzie, R. C., Rafferty, T. S., and Beckett, G. J.: Selenium: An essential element for immune function. Immunol. Today 19:342-345, 1998.

197. McMurray, D. N.: Cell-mediated immunity in nutritional deficiency. Prog. Food Nutr. Sci. 8:193-228, 1984.

198. Mertz, W.: Chromium occurrence and function in biological systems. Physiol. Rev. 49:163-239, 1969.

199. Meydani, S. N., and Beharka, A. A.: Recent developments in vitamin E and immune response. Nutr. Rev. 56:S49-S58, 1998.

200. Meydani, S. N., Hayek, M., and Coleman, L.: Influence of vitamins E and B_6 on immune response. Ann. N. Y. Acad. Sci. 585:125-137, 1990.

201. Miller, J. Z., Nance, W. E., Norton, J. A., et al.: Therapeutic effect of vitamin C: A co-twin control study. J. A. M. A. 237:248S-251S, 1977.

202. Miller, T. L.: Nutrition in paediatric human immunodeficiency virus infection. Proc. Nutr. Soc. 59:155-162, 2000.

203. Miller, T. L., Mawn, B. E., Orav, E. J., et al.: The effect of protease inhibitor therapy on growth and body composition in human immunodeficiency virus type-1 infected children. Pediatrics 107:e77, 2001.

204. Miller, T. L., Orav, E. J., Colan, S. D., et al.: Nutritional status and cardiac mass and function in children infected with the human immunodeficiency virus. Am. J. Clin. Nutr. 66:660-664, 1997.

205. Mimouni-Bloch, A., Mimouni, D., Mimouni, M., et al.: Does breastfeeding protect against allergic rhinitis during childhood? A meta-analysis of prospective studies. Acta Paediatr. 91:275-279, 2002.

206. Mishra, O. P., Agrawal, S., Ali, Z., et al.: Adenosine deaminase activity in protein-energy malnutrition. Acta Paediatr 87:1116-1119, 1998.

207. Mitra, A. K., Alvarez, J. O., Guay-Woodford, L., et al.: Urinary retinol excretion and kidney function in children with shigellosis. Am. J. Clin. Nutr. 68:1095-1103, 1998.

208. Moayyedi, P., Forman, D., Duffett, S., et al.: Association between *Helicobacter pylori* infection and adult height. Eur. J. Epidemiol. 20:455-465, 2005.

209. Molbak, K., Andersen, M., Aaby, P., et al.: *Cryptosporidium* infection in infancy as a cause of malnutrition: A community study from Guinea-Bissau, West Africa. Am. J. Clin. Nutr. 65:149-152, 1997.

210. Moodley, J. R., Coetzee, N., and Hussey, G.: Risk factors for meningococcal disease in Cape Town. S. Afr. Med. J. 89:56-59, 1999.

211. Moore, F. A., Feliciano, D. V., Andrassy, R. J., et al.: Early enteral feeding, compared with parenteral, reduces postoperative septic complications: The results of a meta-analysis. Ann. Surg. 216:172-183, 1992.

212. Moore, S. E., Cole, T. J., Collinson, A. C., et al.: Prenatal or early postnatal events predict infectious deaths in young adulthood in rural Africa. Int. J. Epidemiol. 28:1088-1095, 1999.

213. Moore, S. E., Morgan, G., Collinson, A. C., et al.: Leptin, malnutrition and immune response in rural Gambian children. Arch. Dis. Child 87:192-197, 2002.

214. Muller, M. J., and Herndon, D. N.: The challenge of burns. Lancet 343:216-220, 1994.

215. Najada, A. S., Habashneh, M. S., and Khader, M.: The frequency of nutritional rickets among hospitalized infants and its relation to respiratory disease. J. Trop. Pediatr. 50:364-368, 2004.

216. Nájera, O., González, C., Toledo, G., et al.: CD45RA and CD45RO isoforms in infected malnourished and infected well-nourished children. Clin. Exp. Immunol. 126:461-465, 2001.

217. Nájera, O., González, C., Toledo, G., et al.: Flow cytometry study of lymphocyte subsets in malnourished and well-nourished children with bacterial infections. Clin. Diagn. Lab. Immunol. 11:577-580, 2004.

218. Nduati, R., John, G., Mbori-Ngacha, D., et al.: Effect of breastfeeding and formula feeding on transmission of HIV-1: A randomized clinical trial. J. A. M. A. 283:1167-1174, 2000.

219. Neldner, K. H., and Hambidge, K. M.: Zinc therapy of acrodermatitis enteropathica. N. Engl. J. Med. 292:879-882, 1975.

220. Neu, J., Roig, J. C., Meetze, W. H., et al.: Enteral glutamine supplementation for very low birth weight infants decreases morbidity. J. Pediatr. 131:691-699, 1997.

221. Newberne, P. M.: Overnutrition on resistance of dogs to distemper virus. Fed. Proc. 25:1701-1710, 1966.

222. Newburg, D. S., Peterson, J. A., Ruiz-Palacios, G. M., et al.: Role of human-milk lactadherin in protection against symptomatic rotavirus infection. Lancet 351:1160-1164, 1998.

223. Oddy, W. H., Sly, P. D., de Klerk, N. H., et al.: Breast feeding and respiratory morbidity in infancy: A birth cohort study. Arch. Dis. Child. 88:224-228, 2003.

224. Okada, Y., Klein, N. J., van Saene, H. K., et al.: Bactericidal activity against coagulase-negative staphylococci is impaired in infants receiving long-term parenteral nutrition. Ann. Surg. 231:276-281, 2000.

225. Okada, Y., Klein, N., van Saene, H. K., et al.: Small volumes of enteral feedings normalise immune function in infants receiving parenteral nutrition. J. Pediatr. Surg. 33:16-19, 1998.

226. Olivares, J. L., Fernandez, R., Fleta, J., et al.: Serum mineral levels in children with intestinal parasitic infection. Dig. Dis. 21:258-261, 2003.

227. Olusi, S. O., Thurman, G. B., and Goldstein, A. L.: Effect of thymosin on T-lymphocyte rosette formation in children with kwashiorkor. Clin. Exp. Immunopathol. 15:687-691, 1980.

228. Oppenheimer, S. R.: Iron and its relation to immunity and infectious disease. J. Nutr. 131:S616-S633, 2001.

229. Orsini, M., Rocha, R. S., Disch, J., et al.: The role of nutritional status and insulin-like growth factor in reduced physical growth in hepatosplenic *Schistosoma mansoni* infection. Trans. R. Soc. Trop. Med. Hyg. 95:453-456, 2001.

230. Osawa, Y.: Ueber die Entstenung der Polymositis acuta purulenta in Japan. Beitr. Klin. Chirg. 146:621-653, 1929.

231. Osendarp, S. J., Santosham, M., Black, R. E., et al.: Effect of zinc supplementation between 1 and 6 mo of life on growth and morbidity of Bangladeshi infants in urban slums. Am. J. Clin. Nutr. 76:1401-1408, 2002.

232. Ovesen, L., Allingstrup, L., Hannibal, J., et al.: Effect of dietary counseling on food intake, body weight, response rate, survival, and quality of life in cancer patients undergoing chemotherapy: A prospective, randomized study. J. Clin. Oncol. 11:2043-2039, 1993.

233. Paine, R., and Coble, R. J.: Breast-feeding and infant health in a rural US community. Am. J. Dis. Child. 136:36-38, 1980.

234. Parent, G., Chevalier, P., Zalles, L., et al.: In vitro lymphocyte-differentiating effects of thymulin (Zn-FTS) on lymphocyte subpopulations of severely malnourished children. Am. J. Clin. Nutr. 60:274-278, 1994.

235. Pathania, V., Syal, N., Pathak, C. M., et al.: Vitamin E suppresses the induction of reactive oxygen species release by lipopolysaccharide, interleukin-1beta and tumor necrosis factor-alpha in rat alveolar macrophages. J. Nutr. Sci. Vitaminol. (Tokyo) 45:675-686, 1999.

236. Pekarek, R. S., Hauer, E. C., Rayfield, E. J., et al.: Relationship between serum chromium concentrations and glucose utilization in normal and infected subjects. Diabetes 24:350-353, 1975.

237. Pelletier, D. L., Frongillo, E. A., Jr., Schroeder, D. G., et al.: A methodology for estimating the contribution of malnutrition to child mortality in developing countries. J. Nutr. 124(Suppl. 10):2106S-2122S, 1994.

238. Pencharz, P. B.: Aggressive oral, enteral or parenteral nutrition: prescriptive decisions in children with cancer. Int. J. Cancer Suppl. 11:73-75, 1998.

239. Penna, G., and Adorini, L.: 1 Alpha,25-dihydroxyvitamin D3 inhibits differentiation, maturation, activation, and survival of dendritic cells leading to impaired alloreactive T cell activation. J. Immunol. 164:2405-2411, 2000.

240. Peters, V. B., Rosh, J. R., Mugrdtichian, L., et al.: Growth failure as the first expression of malnutrition in children with human immunodeficiency virus infection. Mt. Sinai J. Med. 65:1-4, 1998.

241. Pighetti, G. M., Eskew, M. L., Reddy, C. C., et al.: Selenium and vitamin E deficiency impair transferrin receptor internalization but not IL-2, IL-2 receptor, or transferrin receptor expression. J. Leukoc. Biol. 63:131-137, 1998.

242. Prentice, A.: Breast-feeding and the older infant. Acta Paediatr. Scand. Suppl. 374:78-88, 1991.

243. Prindull, G., and Ahmad, M.: The ontogeny of the gut mucosal immune system and the susceptibility to infections in infants of developing countries. Eur. J. Pediatr. 152:786-792, 1993.

244. Pruit, B. A., and MacManus, A. T.: The changing of epidemiology of infection in burn patients. World J. Surg. 16:57-66, 1992.

245. Pscheidl, E., Schywalsky, M., Tschaikowsky, K., et al.: Fish oil-supplemented parenteral diets normalize splanchnic blood flow and improve killing of translocated bacteria in a low-dose endotoxin rat model. Crit. Care Med. 28:1489-1496, 2000.

246. Rasmussen, A. F., Jr., Waisman, H. A., Elvehjem, C. A., et al.: Influence of the level of thiamine intake on the susceptibility of mice to poliomyelitis virus. J. Infect. Dis. 74:41-47, 1944.

247. Reardon, M. C., Hammond, K. B., Accurso, F. J., et al.: Nutritional deficits exist before 2 months of age in some infants with cystic fibrosis identified by screening tests. J. Pediatr. 105:271-274, 1984.

248. Rikimaru, T., Taniguchi, K., Yartey, J. E., et al.: Humoral and cell-mediated immunity in malnourished children in Ghana. Eur. J. Clin. Nutr. 52:344-350, 1998.

249. Rivlin, R. S.: The clinical significance of micro-nutrients in relation to immune functions. Ann. N. Y. Acad. Sci. 585:55-57, 1990.

250. Roberts, P. D., Hoffbrand, A. V., and Mullin, D. L.: Iron and folate metabolism in tuberculosis. B. M. J. 2:198-202, 1966.

251. Rodriguez, L., Gonzalez, C., and Flores, L.: Assessment by flow cytometry of cytokine production in malnourished children. Clin. Diagn. Lab. Immunol. 12:502-507, 2005.

252. Roine, I., Fernandez, J. A., Vasquez, A., et al.: Breastfeeding reduces immune activation in primary respiratory syncytial virus infection. Eur. Cytokine Netw. 16:206-210, 2005.

253. Ronnestad, A., Abrahamsen, T. G., Medbo, S., et al.: Late-onset septicemia in a Norwegian national cohort of extremely premature infants receiving very early human milk feeding. Pediatrics 115:e269-e276, 2005.

254. Rothenbacher, D., Bode, G., and Brenner, H.: History of breast feeding and *Helicobacter pylori* infection in pre-school children: Results of a population based study from Germany. Int. J. Epidemiol. 31:632-637, 2002.

255. Rowe, S. Y., Rocourt, J. R., Shiferaw, B., et al.: Breast-feeding decreases the risk of sporadic salmonellosis among infants in FoodNet sites. Clin. Infect. Dis. 38:S262-S270, 2004.

256. Roy, S. K., Tomkins, A. M., Akramuzzaman, S. M., et al.: Randomised controlled trial of zinc supplementation in malnourished Bangladeshi children with acute diarrhoea. Arch. Dis. Child. 77:196-200, 1997.
257. Roy, S. K., Tomkins, A. M., Haider, R., et al.: Impact of zinc supplementation on subsequent growth and morbidity in Bangladeshi children with acute diarrhoea. Eur. J. Clin. Nutr. 53:529-534, 1999.
258. Rubin, D. H., Leventhal, J. M., Krasilnikoff, P. A., et al.: Relationship between infant feeding and infectious illness: A prospective study of infants during the first year of life. Pediatrics 85:464-471, 1990.
259. Sakamoto, M., and Nishioka, K.: Complement system in nutritional deficiency. World Rev. Nutr. Diet 67:114-139, 1992.
260. Sakamoto, M., Fujisawa, Y., and Nishioka, K.: Physiologic role of the complement system in host defense, disease, and malnutrition. Nutrition 14:391-398, 1998.
261. Sakamoto, M.: The sequence of recovery of the complement systems and phytohemagglutinin skin reactivity in malnutrition. Nutr. Res. 2:137-145, 1982.
262. Saldiva, S. R., Carvalho, H. B., Castilho, V. P., et al.: Malnutrition and susceptibility to enteroparasites: Reinfection rates after mass chemotherapy. Paediatr. Perinat. Epidemiol. 16:166-171, 2002.
263. Sazawal, S., Black, R. E., Jalla, S., et al.: Zinc supplementation reduces the incidence of acute lower respiratory infections in infants and preschool children: A double-blind, controlled trial. Pediatrics 102:1-5, 1998.
264. Sazawal, S., Jalla, S., Mazumder, S., et al.: Effect of zinc supplementation on cell-mediated immunity and lymphocyte subsets in preschool children. Indian Pediatr. 34:589-597, 1997.
265. Scariati, P. D., Grummer-Strawn, L. M., and Fein, S. B.: A longitudinal analysis of infant morbidity and the extent of breastfeeding in the United States. Pediatrics 99:E5, 1997.
266. Schlesinger, L. A., Olbaum, L., Grez, L., et al.: Cell mediated immune studies in marasmic children from Chile: Delayed hypersensitivity, lymphocyte transformation and interferon production. In Suskind, R. M. (ed.): Malnutrition and the Immune Response. New York, Raven Press, 1977, pp. 91-98.
267. Schlesinger, L., Munoz, C., Arevalo, M., et al.: Depressed immune response in malnourished rats correlates with increased thymic noradrenaline level. Int. J. Neurosci. 77:229-236, 1994.
268. Schmidt, K.: Interaction of antioxidative micronutrients with host defense mechanisms: A critical review. Int. J. Vitam. Nutr. Res. 67:307-311, 1997.
269. Schopfer, K., and Douglas, S. D.: Neutrophil function in children with kwashiorkor. J. Lab. Clin. Med. 88:450-461, 1976.
270. Scott, M. E., and Koski, K. G.: Zinc deficiency impairs immune responses against parasitic nematode infections at intestinal and systemic sites. J. Nutr. 130(Suppl. 5):1412S-1420S, 2000.
271. Scrimshaw, N. S., and SanGiovanni, J. P.: Synergism of nutrition, infection, and immunity: An overview. Am. J. Clin. Nutr. 66:464S-477S, 1997.
272. Scrimshaw, N. S.: Nutrition and infection. Prog. Food Nutr. Sci. 1:393-420, 1975.
273. Sedjo, R. L., Papenfuss, M. R., Craft, N. E., et al.: Effect of plasma micronutrients on clearance of oncogenic human papillomavirus (HPV) infection. Cancer Causes Control. 14:319-326, 2003.
274. Semba, R. D.: The role of vitamin A and related retinoids in immune function. Nutr. Rev. 56:S38-S48, 1998.
275. Semba, R. D., Miotti, P. G., Chiphangwi, J. D., et al.: Maternal vitamin A deficiency and mother-to-child transmission of HIV-1. Lancet 343:1593-1597, 1994.
276. Semba, R. D., Muhilal, Scott, A., et al.: Depressed immune response to tetanus in children with vitamin A deficiency. J. Nutr. 121:101-107, 1992.
277. Semba, R. D., and Tang, A. M.: Micronutrients and the pathogenesis of human immunodeficiency virus infection. Br. J. Nutr. 81:181-189, 1999.
278. Seth, V., and Chandra, R. K.: Opsonic activity, phagocytosis, and bactericidal capacity of polymorphs in undernutrition. Arch. Dis. Child. 47:282-284, 1972.
279. Seth, V., Kukreja, R. K., Saundaram, K. R., et al.: Waning of cell mediated immune response in preschool children given BCG at birth. Indian J. Med. Res. 76:710-715, 1982.
280. Shah, D., and Sachdev, H. P.: Maternal micronutrients and fetal outcome. Indian J. Pediatr. 71:985-990, 2004.
281. Shakur, M. S., Malek, M. A., Bano, N., et al.: Zinc status in well nourished Bangladeshi children suffering from acute lower respiratory infection. Indian Pediatr. 41:478-481, 2004.
282. Shankar, A. H., Genton, B., Semba, R. D., et al.: Effect of vitamin A supplementation on morbidity due to Plasmodium falciparum in young children in Papua New Guinea: A randomised trial. Lancet 354:203-209, 1999.
283. Shell-Duncan, B., and Wood, J. W.: The evaluation of delayed-type hypersensitivity responsiveness and nutritional status as predictors of gastro-intestinal and acute respiratory infection: A prospective field study among traditional nomadic Kenyan children. J. Trop. Pediatr. 43:25-32, 1997.
284. Sherman, A. R.: Influence of iron on immunity and disease resistance. Ann. N. Y. Acad. Sci. 587:140-146, 1990.
285. Sherman, A. R.: Zinc, copper, and iron nutriture and immunity. J. Nutr. 122(Suppl. 3):604-609, 1992.
286. Shimeles, D., and Lulseged, S.: Clinical profile and pattern of infection in Ethiopian children with severe parasite-energy malnutrition. East Afr. Med. J. 71:264-267, 1994.

287. Silfverdal, S. A., Bodin, L., Hugosson, S., et al.: Protective effect of breastfeeding on invasive Haemophilus influenzae infection: A case-control study in Swedish preschool children. Int. J. Epidemiol. 26:443-450, 1997.
288. Sims, E. J., McCormick, J., Mehta, G., et al.: Neonatal screening for cystic fibrosis is beneficial even in the context of modern treatment. J. Pediatr. 147(Suppl.):S42-S46, 2005.
289. Singh-Naz, N., Sprague, B. M., Patel, K. M., et al.: Risk assessment and standardized nosocomial infection rate in critically ill children. Crit. Care Med. 28:2069-2075, 2000.
290. Sinha A., Madden J., Ross-Degnan D., et al.: Reduced risk of neonatal respiratory infections among breastfed girls but not boys. Pediatrics 112:e303, 2003.
291. Sirisinha, S., Edelman, R., Suskind, R., et al.: Complement and C3-proactivator levels in children with protein-calorie malnutrition and effect of dietary treatment. Lancet 1:1016-1020, 1973.
292. Sirisinha, S., Suskind, R., Edelman, R., et al.: Secretory and serum IgA in children with protein calorie malnutrition. Pediatrics 55:166-170, 1975.
293. Smythe, P. M., Brereton-Stiles, G. G., Grace, H. J., et al.: Thymolymphatic deficiency and depression of cell-mediated immunity in protein-calorie malnutrition. Lancet 2:939-943, 1971.
294. Solis, B., Samartin, S., Gomez, S., et al.: Probiotics as a help in children suffering from malnutrition and diarrhoea. Eur. J. Clin. Nutr. 56:S57-S59, 2002.
295. Solomons, N. W.: Pathways to the impairment of human nutritional status by gastrointestinal pathogens. Parasitology 107:S19-S35, 1993.
296. Sommer, A: Vitamin A status, resistance to infection and childhood mortality. Ann. N. Y. Acad. Sci. 585:17-23, 1990.
297. Spallholz, J. E., Boylan, L. M., and Larsen, H. S.: Advances in understanding selenium's role in the immune system. Ann. N. Y. Acad. Sci. 587:123-139, 1990.
298. Sprunt, D. H.: Effect of undernourishment on the susceptibility of rabbit to infection with vaccinia. J. Exp. Med. 75:297-304, 1942.
299. Squibb, R. L., and Grun, J.: Effect of nutritional status on resistance to infection in the avian species. Fed. Proc. 25:1695-1700, 1966.
300. Stallone, D. D.: The influence of obesity and its treatment on the immune system. Nutr. Rev. 52:37-50, 1994.
301. Steihm, E. D.: Humoral immunity in malnutrition. Fed. Proc. 39:3093-3097, 1980.
302. Steinkamp, G., and Wiedemann B.: Relationship between nutritional status and lung function in cystic fibrosis: Cross sectional and longitudinal analyses from the German CF quality assurance (CFQA) project. Thorax 57:596-601, 2002.
303. Stephensen, C. B.: Vitamin A, beta-carotene, and mother-to-child transmission of HIV. Nutr. Rev. 61:280-284, 2003.
304. Strodtbeck, F.: The role of early enteral nutrition in protecting premature infants from sepsis. Crit. Care Nurs. Clin. North Am. 15:79-87, 2003.
305. Sullivan, P. B., Marsh, M. N., Phillips, M. B., et al.: Prevalence and treatment of giardiasis in chronic diarrhoea and malnutrition. Arch. Dis. Child. 65:304-306, 1990.
306. Suskind, R. M., Olson, L. C., and Olson, R. E.: Protein calorie malnutrition and infection with hepatitis-associated antigen. Pediatrics 51:525-530, 1973.
307. Taj, M. M., Pearson, A. D., Mumford, D. B., et al.: Effect of nutritional status on the incidence of infections in childhood cancer. Pediatr. Hematol. Oncol. 10:283-287, 1993.
308. Tamura, J., Kubota, K., Murakami, H., et al.: Immunomodulation by vitamin B12: Augmentation of CD8+ T lymphocytes and natural killer (NK) cell activity in vitamin B12-deficient patients by methyl-B12 treatment. Clin. Exp. Immunol. 116:28-32, 1999.
309. Tanaka, S. I., Isoda, F., Yamakawa, T., et al.: T lymphopenia in genetically obese rats. Clin. Immunol. Immunopathol. 86:219-225, 1998.
310. Tellez, A., Winiecka-Rusnell, J., Paniagua, M., et al.: Antibodies in mother's milk protect children against giardiasis. Scand. J. Infect. Dis. 35:322-325, 2003.
311. Tengerdy, R. P.: The role of vitamin E in immune response and disease resistance. Ann. N. Y. Acad. Sci. 585:24-33, 1990.
312. The National Health Research Council, National Academy of Science: Immune response in the malnourished child. Subcommittee on Interactions of Nutrition and Infection. Committee on International Nutrition Programs, May 1976.
313. Thurnham, D. I., and Northrop-Clewes, C. A.: Optimal nutrition: Vitamin A and the carotenoids. Proc. Nutr. Soc. 58:449-457, 1999.
314. Tomkins, A.: Malnutrition, morbidity and mortality in children and their mothers. Proc. Nutr. Soc. 59:135-146, 2000.
315. Trakatellis, A., Dimitriadou, A., and Trakatelli, M.: Pyridoxine deficiency: New approaches in immunosuppression and chemotherapy. Postgrad. Med. J. 73:617-622, 1997.
316. Tredget, E. E., and Yu, Y. M.: The metabolic effects of thermal injury. World J. Surg. 16:68-79, 1992.
317. Tubman, T. R., Thompson, S. W., and McGuire, W.: Glutamin supplementation to prevent morbidity and mortality in preterm infants. Cochrane Database Syst. Rev. CD001457, 2005.
318. Tupasi, T. E., deLeon, L. E., Lupsia, S., et al.: Community based studies of acute respiratory tract infections in young children. Rev. Infect. Dis. 12:S940-S949, 1990.
319. Tupasi, T. E., Lucerno, M. G., Magdangal, D. M., et al.: Etiology of acute lower respiratory tract infection in children from Alabang. Metro. Manila 12:S929-S939, 1990.

320. Tupasi, T. E., Velmonte, M. E., Sanvictores, M. E., et al.: Determinants of morbidity and mortality due to acute respiratory infections: Implications for intervention. J. Infect. Dis. 157:615-623, 1988.
321. Ulijaszek, S. J.: Immunology and growth faltering of Anga children, Papua New Guinea: Preliminary work. Am. J. Phys. Anthropol. 106:515-520, 1998.
322. Umeta, M., West, C. E., Haidar, J., et al.: Zinc supplementation and stunted infants in Ethiopia: A randomised controlled trial. Lancet 355:2021-2026, 2000.
323. Van Eys J.: Benefits of nutritional intervention on nutritional status, quality of life and survival. Int. J. Cancer Suppl. 11:66-68, 1998.
324. van Heeckeren, A. M., Schluchter, M., Xue, L., et al.: Nutritional effects on host response to lung infections with mucoid Pseudomonas aeruginosa in mice. Infect. Immun. 72:1479-1486, 2004.
325. Vathanophas, K., Sangchai, R., Raktham, S., et al.: A community-based study of acute respiratory tract infection in Thai children. Rev. Infect. Dis. 12:S957-S965, 1990.
326. Veldman, C. M., Cantorna, M. T., and DeLuca, H. F.: Expression of 1, 25-dihydroxyvitamin D(3) receptor in the immune system. Arch. Biochem. Biophys. 374:334-338, 2000.
327. Verster, A.: Food fortification: Good to have or need to have? East. Mediterr. Health J. 10:771-777, 2004.
328. Viana, M. B., Murao, M., Ramos, G., et al.: Malnutrition as prognostic factor in lymphoblastic leukemia: A multivariant analysis. Arch. Dis. Child. 71:304-310, 1994.
329. Victora, C. G., Vaughan, J. P., Lombardi, C., et al.: Evidence for protection by breast-feeding against infant deaths from infectious diseases in Brazil. Lancet 2:319-322, 1987.
330. Villalpando, S., and Lopez-Alarcon, M.: Growth faltering is prevented by breast-feeding in underprivileged infants from Mexico City. J. Nutr. 130:546-552, 2000.
331. Waibale, P., Bowlin, S. J., Mortimer, E. A., Jr., et al.: The effect of human immunodeficiency virus-1 infection and stunting on measles immunoglobulin-G levels in children vaccinated against measles in Uganda. Int. J. Epidemiol. 28:341-346, 1999.
332. Waters, M. D., Gardner, D. E., Arany, C., et al.: Metal toxicity for rabbit alveolar macrophages in vitro. Environ. Res. 9:32-47, 1975.
333. Watkins-Leeder, S. R., and Corkhill, R. T.: The relationship between breast and bottle-feeding and respiratory illness in the first year of life. J. Epidemiol. Community Health 33:180-182, 1979.
334. Watson, R. R.: Nutrition, disease resistance and age. Food Nutr. News 51:1-6, 1979.
335. Wayse, V., Yousafzai, A., Mogale, K., et al.: Association of subclinical vitamin D deficiency with severe acute lower respiratory infection in Indian children under 5 y. Eur. J. Clin. Nutr. 58:563-567, 2004.
336. Weaver, H. M.: Resistance of cotton rats to virus of poliomyelitis as affected by intake of vitamin A, partial inanition and sex. J. Pediatr. 28:14-23, 1946.
337. Weinberg, E. D.: Roles of iron in host-parasite infections. J. Infect. Dis. 124:401-410, 1971.
338. Wellinghausen, N.: Immunobiology of gestational zinc deficiency. Br. J. Nutr. 85:S81-S86, 2001.
339. Wellinghausen, N., Martin, M., and Rink, L.: Zinc inhibits interleukin-1-dependent T cell stimulation. Eur. J. Immunol. 27:2529-2535, 1997.
340. West, C. E., Rombout, J. H., van der Zijpp, A. J., Sijtsma, S. R.: Vitamin A and immune function. Proc. Nutr. Soc. 50:251-262, 1991.
341. Winick, M. (ed.): Hunger Disease: Studies by the Jewish Physicians in the Warsaw Ghetto. New York, John Wiley & Sons, 1959.
342. Woodruff, J. F., and Kilbourne, E. D.: The influence of quantitated post-weaning undernutrition on coxsackievirus B3 infection of adult mice, I: Viral persistence and increased severity of lesions. J. Infect. Dis. 121:137-163, 1970.
343. World Health Organization (WHO): Nutrition and infection: Report of a WHO Expert Committee. W. H. O. Tech. Rep. Ser. 314:5-30, 1965.
344. World Health Organization (WHO): Technical Advisory Group on Acute Respiratory Infections: A programme for controlling acute respiratory infections in children: A memorandum from a WHO meeting. Bull. W. H. O. 62:47-58, 1984.
345. World Health Organization (WHO): Childhood Malnutrition. World Health Organization Fact Sheet No. 119, reviewed November 1996. Available at: http://www.who.ch.
346. World Health Organization (WHO): AIDS Epidemic Update: December 2005. Available at: http://www.who.int/hiv/pub/epidemiology/epiupdate2005/en/index.html.
347. World Health Organization (WHO): The WHO World Health Report 2005. Available at: http://www.who.int/whr/2005/whr2005_en.pdf.
348. World Health Organization (WHO) Collaborative Study Team on the Role of Breastfeeding on the Prevention of Infant Mortality: Effect of breastfeeding on infant and child mortality due to infectious diseases in less developed countries: A pooled analysis. Lancet 355:451-455, 2000.
349. Wright, A. L., Bauer, M., Naylor, A., et al.: Increasing breastfeeding rates to reduce infant illness at the community level. Pediatrics 101:837-844, 1998.
350. Yau, K. I., Huang, C. B., Chen, W., et al.: Effect of nucleotides on diarrhea and immune responses in healthy term infants in Taiwan. J. Pediatr. Gastroenterol. Nutr. 36:37-43, 2003.
351. Zaman, M. M., Yoshiike, N., Chowdhury, A. H., et al.: Nutritional factors associated with rheumatic fever. J. Trop. Pediatr. 44:142-147, 1998.
352. Zhou, H., Ohtsuka, R., He, Y., et al.: Impact of parasitic infections and dietary intake on child growth in the schistosomiasis-endemic Dongting Lake Region, China. Am. J. Trop. Med. Hyg. 72:534-539, 2005.
353. Zuin, G., Fontana, M., Monti, S., et al.: Malabsorption of different lactose loads in children with human immunodeficiency virus infection. J. Pediatr. Gastroenterol. Nutr. 15:408-412, 1992.
354. Zwingenberger, K., Irschick, E., Vergetti, S., et al.: Tumor necrosis factor in hepatosplenic schistosomiasis. Scand. J. Immunol. 31:205-211, 1990.

CHAPTER 5

FEVER: PATHOGENESIS AND TREATMENT

Mark A. Ward ☉ Carolyn Lentzsch Parcells

Fever is defined as a thermoregulated increase in body temperature above normal as the result of a coordinated response to a pathologic insult. Fever has two essential features: abnormal elevation in body temperature and being the end-product of a coordinated physiologic response. The first feature differentiates fever from normal regulated elevations in body temperature (e.g., elevations associated with the circadian rhythm), whereas the latter distinguishes it from conditions in which the regulatory mechanisms are overwhelmed or dysfunctional (e.g., heat stroke). In children, the pathologic insult most likely to result in fever is infection. A variety of other conditions, including malignancies and autoimmune diseases, also may result in this phenomenon, however.

NORMAL BODY TEMPERATURE

Although the general public and physicians alike often refer to "*the*" body temperature, the implication that a single number can

represent the thermal state of the entire body is inaccurate. Depending on the site of measurement, body temperature may vary by 1° C or more.[34] These regional variations in temperature do not have a fixed relationship to each other. Although axillary temperatures are consistently lower than rectal temperatures, the absolute difference between the two varies greatly.[4] In addition, even in the healthy state, body temperature is not constant; it varies depending on numerous factors, such as time of day, level of activity, and phase of the menstrual cycle. Generally, clinicians have been most interested in the core body temperature, defined as the temperature of the internal organs of the trunk and head. Under normal circumstances, core temperature is higher than the temperature of more superficial tissues such as skin. Even within these two anatomic regions, temperature gradients exist, however.

The most widely accepted definition of normal body temperature is 37° C (98.6° F).[45] This number is derived from studies performed in the 19th century by Wunderlich.[82] He reportedly arrived at this figure based on the result of several million measurements conducted in approximately 25,000 individuals. Other, more recent studies have found slightly lower mean temperatures in healthy individuals, despite the fact that these more recent studies are based on oral or rectal temperatures, whereas Wunderlich's studies relied on axillary temperatures.[28] Mackowiak and colleagues[46] determined the mean oral temperature in adults to be 36.8° C (98.2° F), with the upper limit of normal ranging from 37.2° C (98.9° F) at 6:00 A.M. to 37.7° C (99.9° F) at 4:00 P.M. Given the limitations imposed by the technology available at the time, however, perhaps the most surprising aspect of the value reported by Wunderlich is how closely it approximates these more recent determinations.

As noted previously, body temperature fluctuates depending on numerous normal physiologic factors. Core temperature shows a diurnal variation of 1° C, the nadir occurring in the early morning hours and the peak in the late afternoon.[36,46] After exercise and in the postprandial state, body temperature increases.[51,65] In addition, variations in the normal body temperature of women associated with the menstrual cycle are well described, with increases in baseline temperature occurring after ovulation.[15]

THERMOREGULATION

Humans, similar to other mammals, are homeothermic, indicating that they regulate body temperature within a narrow range despite wide variations in the ambient temperature. Regulation of temperature is mediated by a variety of physiologic (e.g., vasoconstriction, sweating) and behavioral (e.g., moving to a warmer environment, putting on additional clothing) responses.

The principal thermoregulatory area is located within the brain in the preoptic area and anterior hypothalamus. Although it frequently is conceptualized as a single center, no single neuronal structure seems to control all aspects of temperature regulation.[10] Rather, a complex interplay occurs among a variety of neural pathways, with the final result being the maintenance of the body's temperature within a narrow range. Regardless of the precise nature of central regulation, body temperature ultimately is a function of the balance between heat gain and heat loss.

Heat energy is a by-product of the inefficiency of the body's normal metabolic processes. It is this "waste" heat that renders the homeothermic state possible. During exercise, the increased metabolic activity in muscle tissue results in increased production of heat, leading to an increase in the body's temperature.[63] Shivering, an involuntary form of muscle activity, is the primary means by which the body generates additional heat under conditions of cold stress. Heat also may be generated by a process known as *non-shivering thermogenesis*. Originally described in rats, non-shivering thermogenesis has been found to occur in a variety of mammals, including humans. It seems to be of greater importance in newborns than in adults. Although this process has been shown to occur in a variety of tissues, brown adipose tissue seems to be the most important site for this phenomenon. Under the control of the adrenergic system, production of free fatty acid is increased, resulting in an uncoupling of oxidative phosphorylation and the production of large amounts of heat.[9,27]

Four mechanisms are responsible for heat transfer: radiation, conduction, convection, and evaporation. Heat loss owing to radiation occurs when heat is transferred directly between two objects not in direct contact. Conduction involves the transfer of heat energy between two objects in contact with each other. Convection is the result of the movement of a fluid or gas across the surface of the body (e.g., as the result of fanning). Evaporative heat loss occurs in association with the energy required to convert liquid to gas form.

Under normal conditions, radiation accounts for most of the body's heat loss. By contrast, conductive losses are smaller under normal circumstances. Conductive losses may become substan-

tial, however, under conditions in which a substantial portion of the individual's body surface is in direct contact with a cooler object (e.g., an unclothed infant in an unheated bassinet). Convective losses are proportional to the amount of air moving over the body surface; these losses are greatest in windy conditions. Conductive and convective heat losses are particularly important in infants and children because of their relatively greater body surface area compared with that of adults. Evaporative losses occur when fluids such as sweat evaporate from the skin's surface. In addition, substantial evaporative losses are associated with respiration.

PATHOGENESIS OF FEVER

In the classic model of fever pathogenesis, exogenous pyrogens stimulate the release of circulating endogenous pyrogens, which act via prostaglandins to increase the set-point of the hypothalamic thermoregulatory center.[17] In this model, exogenous pyrogens are substances extrinsic to the body, primarily various bacterial microorganisms or the products of those microorganisms. Conversely, endogenous pyrogens are a varied group of proteins produced within the human body that share the intrinsic ability to induce fever. The first endogenous pyrogen was described originally more than 60 years ago and was derived from leukocytes, primarily granulocytes, and now is known as interleukin-1.[18] Numerous other cytokines that qualify as endogenous pyrogens, including tumor necrosis factor, interferon-α, interferon-γ, and interleukin-6, have been identified.[44,83]

A variety of alternative and complementary theories of fever pathogenesis have been proposed.[52] The actual mechanisms involved likely are more varied and complex than just described. A variety of intrinsically produced substances (e.g., antigen-antibody complexes) may act as "exogenous" pyrogens.[61] The classic model provides a reasonable framework, however, for understanding most of the observed phenomena associated with the febrile response.

Regardless of the precise pathogenesis, the height of fever seems to be a limit. Retrospective studies of hyperpyrexia in children have found that it is unusual for the body temperature to rise above 41.1° C (106° F), and it rarely rises above 41.7° C (107° F).[56,75] Children with temperatures exceeding this range almost always have an element of heat illness.

EFFECTS OF FEVER

Attempts to treat fever often are predicated on the assumption that fever has harmful effects and that reduction in temperature would abrogate such harm. The evidence with regard to these premises is mixed, however.

ADVERSE EFFECTS

Some animal studies have found that high fever may impair certain immunologic responses, including phagocytosis of staphylococci by polymorphonuclear leukocytes[5,21,22] and lymphocyte transformation in response to mitogens.[60] Whether these isolated in vitro phenomena observed in animal models are relevant to human infection is unknown.

Fever may cause seizures, a phenomenon observed most frequently in young children. The onset generally occurs in infants 6 to 30 months of age. Recurrence is common, occurring in approximately one third of children experiencing an initial febrile seizure. The primary adverse consequences of febrile seizures are the emotional distress experienced by patients and their families and the need for medical evaluation, which may involve invasive testing and substantial expense. Febrile seizures do not cause brain injury and are not associated with subsequent intellectual or neurologic deficits.[20,77]

BENEFICIAL EFFECTS

Fever may be beneficial—by enhancing the host response to infection and by directly inhibiting the infecting agent. Several studies have illustrated that the immune system responds to mildly elevated body temperature by increasing migration of leukocytes, production of interferon, and lymphocyte transformation and phagocytosis.[2,7,60,62] Studies of bacterial infection in reptiles and fish have shown an increased survival rate in groups maintained at approximately 4° C (reptiles) and 2.5° C (fish) above baseline.[14,37] Kluger and Vaughn[39] showed that rabbits infected with *Pasteurella multocida* had improved survival rates at body temperatures of approximately 4.5° C above normal. Although these data are impressive, their clinical significance with regard to humans has yet to be determined.

Fever also may inhibit the growth and survival of some infectious agents. One potential mechanism for this inhibition is the decrease in serum iron and increase in ferritin that are associated with fever, coupled with the increased iron requirement of many bacteria at higher temperatures.[5,38] Fever therapy was used historically to treat neurosyphilis and gonococcal urethritis, correlating with more recent studies that show that certain gonococci and *Treponema* are eradicated at temperatures of 40° C (104° F) and greater.[12,35] Finally, growth of some pneumococci and viruses seems to be impaired at higher temperatures.[26,71,79]

Several studies have found that the treatment of fever with antipyretics is associated with adverse consequences, providing indirect evidence of a beneficial effect of fever. Ahmady and Samadi[2] reported that the use of aspirin in children with measles prolonged the duration of the illness and was associated with an increase in prevalence of respiratory complications and diarrhea. Other investigators have reported that the length of time to total scabbing in varicella was significantly longer in children treated with acetaminophen compared with children treated with placebo.[19] Several studies in animal models and in humans have found prolongation of viral shedding, depressed neutralizing antibody response, and increased nasal symptoms in association with the use of antipyretics.[24,31,74] Although these studies establish that an association exists between reduction of fever and adverse outcomes, they do not prove a causal relationship. The adverse effects possibly are mediated by some direct physiologic effects of antipyretics, rather than indirectly by their impact on fever.

CLINICAL THERMOMETRY

TYPES OF THERMOMETERS

For many years, glass thermometers containing mercury were the most common type of thermometer used to measure body temperature. This type of thermometer is reasonably accurate for most clinical purposes. Although they are still available, use of mercury-containing thermometers has diminished greatly because of environmental concerns about mercury exposure from broken or discarded thermometers. These thermometers have been replaced largely by digital thermometers or glass thermometers containing liquids other than mercury.

Electronic thermometers (often referred to as *digital thermometers*) previously were used primarily in the hospital and office setting. As their cost has decreased, they are used more frequently in the home as well. Electronic thermometers have the advantage over mercury thermometers of requiring a significantly shorter dwell time, that is, the time they must remain in situ to obtain an accurate reading. Hospital-grade electronic thermometers typically have two modes: monitor and predictive. In the monitor mode, these thermometers function similarly to mercury thermometers in that they must remain in place until equilibration occurs, a process that may require several minutes. In the predictive mode, a complex algorithm is used to estimate the final temperature based on measurements made during the first few seconds. Because the predictive mode produces a temperature reading within seconds, it is the mode used most often in clinical settings. Determinations of temperatures using these two modes have been found to correlate well.[22,53]

Infrared thermometers are a more recent addition to the clinician's armamentarium. Devices that determine the temperature by detecting infrared radiation emitted from the ear drum are used most frequently. Tympanic temperature should provide an accurate estimation of the core temperature because its blood supply is derived from the carotid artery. Additional advantages of this type of thermometer are its speed, acceptance by patients, and decreased risk of cross-contamination compared with oral or rectal thermometers. Studies of the accuracy of tympanic thermometers have yielded mixed results, with numerous studies finding tympanic thermometers inaccurate compared with mercury in glass or electronic thermometers.[13,49] Discrepancies seem to be particularly common in infants who are in the first few months of life.[68] Tympanic thermometers should not be used in young infants because of the importance of fever in making management decisions in these patients.[16]

Even more recently, the temporal artery (TA) thermometer has been introduced. TA thermometers use an infrared sensor to determine skin temperature as the device is passed across the forehead and temporal area. The site of highest measured temperature is assumed to represent that of the temporal artery. An algorithm is applied to the measured temperature to estimate the core temperature. Studies to date suggest that TA thermometer temperatures correlate significantly better with rectal and core temperatures than with temperatures determined by tympanic thermometers. The initial data also suggest that TA thermometers are more sensitive at detecting fever in children than in adults. TA thermometers do not seem to correlate well enough with rectal or core temperature measurements, however, to replace rectal thermometry in clinical situations in which accurate measurement of fever is crucial for making decisions about management. The accuracy of TA thermometer readings is adversely affected by sweating and may be affected by vascular constriction or dilation. In addition, data comparing TA and axillary thermometry are lacking.[25,73]

Several other types of thermometers have been developed. Among them are electronic pacifier thermometers, used for obtaining an oral temperature in infants. Although they are appealing in theory, this type of thermometer has the disadvantage of requiring a prolonged dwell time and has not been found to be sufficiently accurate to recommend its use.[57] Another approach to measuring temperature is the use of liquid crystal thermometers that are applied to the skin of the forehead. Results generally have been disappointing when these thermometers have been compared with more standard techniques.[40,66]

MEASUREMENT SITE

The most common locations for measuring body temperature are the mouth, rectum, axilla, and tympanic membrane. Because of the previously noted regional variations in body temperature, each of these sites has its own range of normal temperatures. The oral cavity historically has been the preferred site for measuring temperature in older children and adults. When taking a temperature orally, one should place the thermometer in the sublingual space because the blood supply for structures in this region is derived from branches of the carotid arteries and should reflect the core temperature accurately. Younger children usually are unable to cooperate adequately to permit the use of oral thermometers. In addition, the oral temperature may be affected by recent ingestion of hot or cold liquids, and it may be altered by tachypnea.

Rectal temperatures are used frequently in younger children. The rectal temperature correlates well with the core body temperature. The rectal temperature may exceed the core temperature (using the pulmonary artery temperature as the reference standard), however, possibly because of the effects of bacterial activity in the rectum. The use of rectal thermometry has the disadvantage of causing the patient discomfort and is contraindicated in patients with neutropenia because of the risks of causing invasive infection via trauma to the rectal mucosa.

Axillary temperatures are appealing because of the ready accessibility of the axillae. Considerable variability occurs in the readings obtained, however, particularly in younger children. One should not rely on axillary temperatures, particularly in neonates and young children.

TREATMENT

As noted previously, fever may have numerous beneficial effects, convincing evidence of harm owing to fever is lacking, and treatment of fever may be associated with undesirable effects. Routine intervention to reduce fever is not warranted. Rather, physicians should individualize the decision to treat fever and the specific method chosen to do so.

INDICATIONS

Antipyretic therapy often is considered for children who have an increased risk of having febrile seizures, either because of age or because of a history of febrile seizures. Although treatment seems rational in this situation, studies of antipyretic therapy to prevent febrile seizures have failed to show its efficacy.[11,65,76] Even this indication should be considered relative rather than absolute.

Antipyretic therapy also should be considered for children with poorly compensated underlying cardiac or pulmonary disease, significant neurologic impairment, or sepsis, and for children with significant alterations of fluid and electrolyte balance. Definitive controlled trials to support these indications are lacking. Rather, the recommendations are based on the metabolic consequences of fever and their potential adverse impact on the underlying disease.

Perhaps the most frequent indication for the use of antipyretics is to improve the patient's comfort. Despite the absence of definitive studies to support this practice and the potential adverse consequences of using antipyresis, such an approach is reasonable in the absence of definitive evidence to the contrary. In some circumstances, improving the patient's comfort may enhance the ability to assess the seriousness of the patient's illness accurately.[6]

ANTIPYRETICS

A wide variety of antipyretic agents is available. In the United States, the drugs used most frequently for treatment of fever in children are acetaminophen and ibuprofen. Previously, aspirin was the antipyretic used most frequently. Aspirin has fallen into disuse for the management of fever in children, however, primarily because of its association with Reye syndrome, particularly when used in managing children with varicella or influenza.[30] In addition, aspirin has a variety of other adverse effects, including inhibition of platelet function, gastritis and gastrointestinal

bleeding, and provocation of asthma exacerbations, although this third complication occurs more frequently in adults.[32,59,67] Aspirin has greater toxicity in situations of overdose than do acetaminophen and ibuprofen.

Each of these agents acts to restore normal body temperature by reducing the set-point of the temperature regulatory center in the hypothalamus. The specific mechanism of action seems to be interference with prostaglandin synthesis in the PAOH. When selecting among the available antipyretic agents, one should consider efficacy and potential toxicity.

Similar to aspirin, ibuprofen inhibits prostaglandin synthesis in a variety of tissues outside the central nervous system. It shares many of the toxicities associated with aspirin. One exception is that ibuprofen lacks the association with Reye syndrome.[58] Ibuprofen inhibits platelet function because of its effect on prostaglandin synthesis, but this effect is reversible with discontinuation of the drug, and platelet dysfunction is short-lived compared with the effect of aspirin.[54] Because prostaglandins are important to the integrity of the gastrointestinal mucosa, inhibition by ibuprofen may result in gastrointestinal upset and bleeding. Although ibuprofen has been associated with exacerbations of asthma in some children, the risk seems to be small and may not be greater than that associated with the use of acetaminophen.[41,42]

Acetaminophen has a lengthy track record of safety. When used in the usual therapeutic doses, it has few adverse effects. Acetaminophen inhibits prostaglandin synthase activity, but this action is inhibited by peroxide. Because peroxide is generated at sites of inflammation, acetaminophen has little anti-inflammatory activity. It also lacks the adverse gastrointestinal and platelet effects of aspirin and ibuprofen.

Recommended dosing of ibuprofen is 5 to 10 mg/kg every 6 hours as needed. Acetaminophen is administered at a dose of 10 to 15 mg/kg every 4 hours, but no more frequently than five times per day. An important note for individuals administering these agents is that a variety of over-the-counter combination medications contain one or the other of these agents. Co-administration may result in inadvertent overdosing.

In addition, recognizing that ibuprofen and acetaminophen come in a variety of formulations is important. Acetaminophen is available as infant drops (concentration 10 mg/mL) and children's liquid (concentration 32 mg/mL). Substitution of children's liquid for infant drops without adjusting the volume administered to reflect the difference in concentration may result in serious toxicity. Acetaminophen also is available in suppository form. Absorption varies, however, and is delayed compared with oral administration. In addition, the medication is not distributed uniformly throughout the suppository, resulting in potential dosing errors if the suppositories are divided before use.[8] The use of acetaminophen in suppository form should be discouraged.

The antipyretic efficacy of acetaminophen and ibuprofen has been the subject of numerous clinical trials.[33,78,80,81] These trials have shown uniformly that both are effective antipyretic agents. Ibuprofen seems to result in a greater decrease in temperature than does acetaminophen, however. In addition, the antipyretic effect of ibuprofen is more prolonged, not surprising in light of ibuprofen's longer half-life compared with acetaminophen. These observations were confirmed in a meta-analysis of trials comparing ibuprofen and acetaminophen.[55]

Acetaminophen and ibuprofen frequently are used in combination.[43] Use of alternating doses often is advocated by practicing physicians.[48] The pathways for metabolism of these drugs are distinct, and, theoretically, metabolism of one should not affect the metabolism of the other. Controlled trials documenting safety and efficacy of combination or alternating use are sparse, however. In the only such study to date, using alternate doses of acetaminophen (12.5 mg per dose) and ibuprofen (5 mg/kg per dose) every 4 hours was found to be associated with a more rapid reduction in fever, lower mean temperature, and fewer caregiver days absent from work and infant days absent from daycare compared with use of either agent alone.[64] The groups assigned to a single agent received dosing that was either on the low end or infrequent, however, compared with usual practice in the United States.

Another approach to antipyretic treatment frequently employed is the use of a second antipyretic when the initial agent is judged to have resulted in an inadequate response. Theoretically, some individuals may have a better antipyretic response to one agent than another. Although the premise is reasonable, sequential use of acetaminophen and ibuprofen remains unproven in terms of efficacy and safety.

Acetaminophen and ibuprofen have been proven to be remarkably safe when used in the recommended doses. Although ibuprofen may be slightly more efficacious in producing and sustaining fever reduction, acetaminophen remains the antipyretic of choice because of its longer track record and more favorable side-effects profile. Because acetaminophen lacks significant anti-inflammatory activity, ibuprofen or another nonsteroidal anti-inflammatory drug may be preferred in febrile conditions for which anti-inflammatory activity is desired (e.g., juvenile arthritis). Limited data suggest that use of acetaminophen and ibuprofen in combination may be safe and more efficacious than is either agent alone. Prudence suggests, however, that combined therapy seldom is warranted for this generally benign condition. Perhaps most important, patients and their parents should be educated to the benign nature of fever and the lack of evidence to indicate that routine treatment, particularly complete suppression, is either necessary or beneficial.

EXTERNAL COOLING

The use of external cooling in the management of fever has a long history. Compared with standard antipyretics, sponging with tepid water is inferior in fever reduction at 2 to 3 hours, although sponging was found to reduce the temperature more quickly than did antipyretics in one trial.[1,3] External cooling without concomitant administration of antipyretics makes little sense from a physiologic standpoint, however. In a febrile patient whose temperature regulatory center set-point has not been reset by administration of an antipyretic agent, external cooling inevitably results in an increase in the body's heat-production mechanisms.

When used in conjunction with an antipyretic agent, the usual goal of external cooling is to reduce the body's temperature more rapidly or to a greater degree. Several studies have compared the use of external cooling combined with antipyretics with antipyretics alone. Results have been mixed; some studies showed no difference in efficacy of the two approaches, whereas others found combination therapy to be superior.[23,29,47,69,72] Even in the studies in which a difference was found, the superiority of combination therapy was shown primarily in the very early phase of treatment. In addition, the use of external cooling usually is uncomfortable for the patient. When external cooling is to be used, sponging with tepid water is preferred. Alcohol and solutions containing alcohol should not be used for this purpose. Absorption of alcohol vapors via the lungs may occur in sufficient quantities to produce toxicity and even death.[50]

REFERENCES

1. Agbolosu, N. B., Cuevas, L. E., Milligan, P., et al.: Efficacy of tepid sponging versus paracetamol in reducing temperature in febrile children. Ann. Trop. Paediatr. 17:283-288, 1997.
2. Ahmady, A. S., and Samadi, A. R.: The adverse effects of antipyretics in measles. Indian Pediatr. 18:49-52, 1981.
3. Aksoylar, S., Aksit, S., Caglayan S., et al.: Evaluation of sponging and antipyretic medication to reduce body temperature in febrile children. Acta Paediatr. Jpn. 39:215-217, 1997.
4. Anagnostakis, D., Matsaniotis, N., Grafakos, S., et al.: Rectal-axillary temperature difference in febrile and afebrile infants and children. Clin. Pediatr. 32:268-272, 1993.
5. Austin, T. W., and Truant, G.: Hyperthermia, antipyretics and function of polymorphonuclear leukocytes. Can. Med. Assoc. J. 118:493-495, 1978.
6. Baker, R. C., Tiller, T., Bellet, P. S., et al.: Severity of disease correlated with fever reduction in febrile infants. Pediatrics 83:1016-1019, 1989.
7. Bernheim, H. A., Bodel, P. T., Askenase, P. W., et al.: Effects of fever on host defense mechanisms after infection in the lizard, Dipsosaurus dorsalis. Br. J. Exp. Pathol. 59:76-84, 1978.
8. Birmingham, P. K., Tobin, M. J., Henthorn, T. K., et al.: Twenty-four-hour pharmacokinetics of rectal acetaminophen in children: An old drug with new recommendations. Anesthesiology 87:244-252, 1997.
9. Boulant, J. A.: Thermoregulation. In Mackowiak, P. A. (ed.): Fever—Basic Mechanisms and Management. 2nd ed. Philadelphia, Lippincott-Raven Publishers, 1997, pp. 38-58.
10. Boulant, J. A.: Role of the preoptic-anterior hypothalamus in thermoregulation and fever. Clin. Infect. Dis. 31:S157-S161, 2000.
11. Camfield, P. R., Camfield, C. S., Shapiro, S. H., et al.: The first febrile seizure: Antipyretic instruction plus either phenobarbital or placebo to prevent recurrence. J. Pediatr. 97:16-21, 1980.
12. Carmichael, L. E., Barnes, F. D., and Percy, D. H.: Temperature as a factor in resistance of young puppies to canine herpesvirus. J. Infect. Dis. 120:669-678, 1969.
13. Chamberlain, J. M., Grandner, J., Rubinoff, J. L., et al.: Comparison of a tympanic thermometer to rectal and oral thermometers in a pediatric emergency department. Clin. Pediatr. 30:24-29, 1991.
14. Covert, J. B., and Reynolds, W. W.: Survival value of fever in fish. Nature 267:43-45, 1977.
15. Coyne, M. D., Kesick, C. M., and Doherty, T. J.: Circadian rhythm in core temperature over the menstrual cycle: Method for noninvasive monitoring. Am. J. Physiol. Regul. Integr. Comp. Physiol. 279:1316-1320, 2000.
16. Craig, J. V., Lancaster, G. A., Taylor, S., et al.: Infrared ear thermometry compared with rectal thermometry in children: A systematic review. Lancet 360:603-609, 2002.
17. Dinarello, C. A.: Thermoregulation and the pathogenesis of fever. Infect. Dis. Clin. North Am. 10:433-449, 1996.
18. Dinarello, C. A.: Cytokines as endogenous pyrogens. In Mackowiak, P. A. (ed.): Fever—Basic Mechanisms and Management. 2nd ed. Philadelphia, Lippincott-Raven Publishers, 1997, pp. 87-116.
19. Doran T. F., De Angelis C., Baumgardner R. A., et al.: Acetaminophen: More harm than good for chickenpox? J. Pediatr. 114:1045-1048, 1989.
20. Ellenberg, J. H., and Nelson, K. B.: Febrile seizures and later intellectual performance. Arch. Neurol. 35:17-21, 1978.
21. Ellingson, H. V., and Clark, P. F.: The influence of artificial fever on mechanisms of resistance. J. Immunol. 43:65-83, 1942.
22. Fallis, W. M., and Christiani, P.: Neonatal axillary temperature measurements: A comparison of electronic thermometer predictive and monitor modes. Obstet. Gynecol. Neonatal. Nurs. 28:389-394, 1999.
23. Friedman, A. D., Barton, L. L., and the Sponging Study Group: Efficacy of sponging vs. acetaminophen for reduction of fever. Pediatr. Emerg. Care. 6:6-7, 1990.
24. Graham, N. M., Burrell, C. J., Douglas, R. M., et al.: Adverse effects of aspirin, acetaminophen, and ibuprofen on immune function, viral shedding, and clinical status in rhinovirus-infected volunteers. J. Infect. Dis. 162:1277-1282, 1990.
25. Greenes, D. S., and Fleisher, G. R.: Accuracy of a noninvasive temporal artery thermometer for use in infants. Arch. Pediatr. Adolesc. Med. 155:376-381, 2001.
26. Grieger, T. A., and Kluger, M. J.: Fever and survival: The role of serum iron. J. Physiol. 279:187-196, 1978.
27. Himms-Hagen, J.: Nonshivering thermogenesis. Brain Res. Bull. 12:151-160, 1984.
28. Horvath, S. M., Menduke, H., and Perso, G. M.: Oral and rectal temperatures of man. J. A. M. A. 144:1562-1565, 1950.
29. Hunter, J.: Study of antipyretic therapy in current use. Arch. Dis. Child. 48:313-315, 1973.
30. Hurwitz, E. S., Barrett, M. J., Bregman, D., et al.: Public health service study of Reye's syndrome and medications: Report of the Main study. J. A. M. A. 257:1905, 1987.
31. Husseini, R. H., Sweet, C., Collie, M. H., and Smith, H.: Elevation of nasal viral levels by suppression of fever in ferrets infected with influenza viruses of differing virulence. J. Infect. Dis. 145:520-524, 1982.
32. Jenkins, C., Costello, J., and Hodge, L.: Systematic review of prevalence of aspirin induced asthma and its implications for clinical practice. B. M. J. 328:434, 2004.
33. Kauffman, R. E., Sawyer, L. A., and Scheinbaum, M. L.: Antipyretic efficacy of ibuprofen vs acetaminophen. Am. J. Dis. Child. 146:622-625, 1992.
34. Kelly, G.: Body temperature variability (Part 1): A review of the history of body temperature and its variability due to site selection, biological rhythms, fitness, and aging. Altern. Med. Rev. 11:278-293, 2006.
35. Kendell, H. W.: Fever Therapy. Springfield, IL, Charles C Thomas, 1935, pp. 67-83.

36. Kleitman, N., Titelbaum, S., and Hoffmann, H.: The establishment of the diurnal temperature cycle. Am. J. Physiol. *119*:48-54, 1937.
37. Kluger, M. J., Ringler, D. H., and Anver, M. R.: Fever and survival. Science *188*:166-168, 1975.
38. Kluger, M. J., and Rothenberg, B. A.: Fever and reduced iron: Their interaction as a host defense response to bacterial infection. Science *203*:374-376, 1979.
39. Kluger, M. J., and Vaughn, L. K.: Fever and survival in rabbits infected with *Pasteurella multocida*. J. Physiol. *282*:243-251, 1978.
40. Kongpanichkul, A., and Bunjongpak, S.: A comparative study on accuracy of liquid crystal forehead, digital electronic axillary, infrared tympanic with glass-mercury rectal thermometer in infants and young children. J. Med. Assoc. Thai. *83*:1068-1076, 2000.
41. Lesko, S. M., and Mitchell, A. A.: An assessment of the safety of pediatric ibuprofen: A practitioner-based randomized clinical trial. J. A. M. A. *273*:929-933, 1995.
42. Lesko, S. M., and Mitchell, A. A.: The safety of acetaminophen and ibuprofen among children younger than two years old. Pediatrics *104*:e39, 1999.
43. Li, S. F., Lacher, B., and Crain, E. F.: Acetaminophen and ibuprofen dosing by parents. Pediatr. Emerg. Care. *16*:394-397, 2000.
44. Luheshi, F., and Rothwell, N.: Cytokines and fever. Int. Arch. Allergy. Immunol. *109*:301-307, 1996.
45. Mackowiak, P. A., and Wasserman, S. S.: Physicians' perceptions regarding body temperature in health and disease. South. Med. J. *88*:934-938, 1995.
46. Mackowiak, P. A., Wasserman, S. S., and Levine, M. M.: A critical appraisal of 37° C (98.6° F), the upper limit of the normal body temperature, and other legacies of Carl Reinhold August Wunderlich. J. A. M. A. *268*:1578-1580, 1992.
47. Mahar, A. F. T., Allen, S. J., Milligan, P., et al.: Tepid sponging to reduce temperature in febrile children in a tropical climate. Clin. Pediatr. *33*:227-231, 1994.
48. Mayoral, C. E., Marino, R. V., Rosenfeld, W., et al.: Alternating antipyretics: Is this an alternative? J. Pediatr. *105*:1009-1012, 2000.
49. Modell, J. G., Katholi, C. R., Kumaramangalam, S. M., et al.: Unreliability of the infrared tympanic thermometer in clinical practice: A comparative study with oral mercury and oral electronic thermometers. South. Med. J. *91*:649-654, 1998.
50. Moss, M. H.: Alcohol-induced hypoglycemia and coma caused by alcohol sponging. Pediatrics *46*:445-447, 1970.
51. Narumi Nagaia, N., Sakanec, N., Hamadaa, T., et al.: The effect of a high-carbohydrate meal on postprandial thermogenesis and sympathetic nervous system activity in boys with recent onset of obesity. Metabolism *54*:430-438, 2005.
52. Netea, M. G., Kullberg, F. J., and Vander Meer, J. W. M.: Circulating cytokines as mediators of fever. Clin. Infect. Dis. *31*:S178-S184, 2000.
53. Nuckton, T. J., Godlreich, D., Wendt, F. C., et al.: A comparison of 2 methods of measuring rectal temperatures with digital thermometers. Am. J. Crit. Care *10*:146-150, 2001.
54. Parks, W. M., Hoak, J. C., and Czervionke, R. L.: Comparative effect of ibuprofen on endothelial and platelet prostaglandin synthesis. J. Pharmacol. Exp. Ther. *219*:415-419, 1981.
55. Perrott, D. A., Piira, T., Goodenough, B., and Champion, D.: Efficacy and safety of acetaminophen vs ibuprofen for treating children's pain or fever. Arch. Pediatr. Adolesc. Med. *158*:521-526, 2004.
56. Press, S.: Association of hyperpyrexia with serious disease in children. Clin. Pediatr. *33*:19-25, 1994.
57. Press, S., and Quinn, B. J.: The pacifier thermometer: Comparison of supralingual with rectal temperatures in infants and young children. Arch. Pediatr. Adolesc. Med. *151*:551-554, 1997.
58. Prior, M. J., Nelson, E. B., Temple, A. R.: Pediatric ibuprofen use increases while incidence of Reye's syndrome continues to decline. Clin. Pediatr. *39*:245-247, 2000.
59. Rachelefsky, G. S., Coulson, A., Siegel, S. C., et al.: Aspirin intolerance in chronic childhood asthma: Detected by oral challenge. Pediatrics *56*:443-448, 1975.
60. Roberts, N. J., and Steigbigel, R. T.: Hyperthermia and human leukocyte function: Effects on response of lymphocytes to mitogens and antigen and bactericidal capacity of monocytes and neutrophils. Infect. Immunol. *18*:673-679, 1977.

61. Root, R. K., and Wolff, S. M.: Pathogenetic mechanisms in experimental immune fever. J. Exp. Med. *128*:309-323, 1968.
62. Ruiz-Gomez, J., and Isaacs, A.: Interferon production by different viruses. Virology *19*:8-12, 1963.
63. Saltin, B., and Hermansen, L.: Esophageal, rectal, and muscle temperature during exercise. J. Appl. Physiol. *21*:1757-1762, 1966.
64. Sarrell, M. E., Wielunsky, E. W., and Cohen, H. A.: Antipyretic treatment in young children with fever: Acetaminophen, ibuprofen, or both alternating in a randomized, double-blind study. Arch. Pediatr. Adolesc. Med. *160*:197-202, 2006.
65. Schnaiderman, D., Lahat, E., Sheefer, T., et al.: Antipyretic effectiveness of acetaminophen in febrile seizures: Ongoing prophylaxis versus sporadic use. Eur. J. Pediatr. *152*:747-749, 1993.
66. Scholefield, J. M., Gerber, M. A., and Dwyer, P.: Liquid crystal forehead temperature strips: A clinical appraisal. Am. J. Dis. Child. *136*:198-201, 1982.
67. Schuhl, J. F., and Pereyra, J. G.: Oral acetylsalicylic acid (aspirin) challenge in asthmatic children. Clin. Allergy *9*:83-88, 1979.
68. Selfridge, J., and Shea, S. S.: The accuracy of the tympanic membrane thermometer in detecting fever in infants aged 3 months and younger in the emergency department setting. J. Emerg. Nurs. *19*:127-130, 1993.
69. Sharber, J.: The efficacy of tepid sponge bathing to reduce fever in young children. Am. J. Emerg. Med. *15*:188-192, 1997.
70. Sinha, Y., and Cranswick, N. E.: Prescribing safely for children. J. Paediatr. Child Health *43*:112-116, 2007.
71. Small, P. M., Tauber, M. G., Hackbarth, C. J., et al.: Influence of body temperature on bacterial growth rates in experimental pneumococcal meningitis in rabbits. Infect. Immunol. *52*:484-487, 1986.
72. Steele, R. W., Tanaka, P. T., Lara, R. P., and Bass, J. W.: Evaluation of sponging and of oral antipyretic therapy to reduce fever. J. Pediatr. *77*:824-829, 1970.
73. Suleman, M. I., Doufas, A. G., Akca, O., et al.: Insufficiency in a new temporal-artery thermometer for adult and pediatric patients. Anesth. Analg. *95*:67-71, 2002.
74. Toms, G. L., Davies, J. A., Woodward, C. G., et al.: The relation of pyrexia and nasal inflammatory response to virus levels in nasal washings of ferrets infected with influenza viruses of differing virulence. Br. J. Exp. Pathol. *58*:444-458, 1977.
75. Trautner, B. W., Caviness, A. C., Gerlacher, G. R., et al.: Prospective evaluation of the risk of serious bacterial infection in children who present to the emergency department with hyperpyrexia (temperature of 106° F or higher). Pediatrics *118*:34-40, 2006.
76. Uhari, M., Rantala, H., Vainionpaa, L., et al.: Effect of acetaminophen and of low intermittent doses of diazepam on prevention of recurrences of febrile seizures. J. Pediatr. *126*:991-995, 1995.
77. Verity, C. M., Greenwood, R., and Golding, J.: Long-term intellectual and behavioral outcomes of children with febrile convulsions. N. Engl. J. Med. *338*:1723-1728, 1998.
78. Walson, P. D., Galletta, G., Chomilo, F., et al.: Comparison of multidose ibuprofen and acetaminophen therapy in febrile children. Am. J. Dis. Child. *146*:626-632, 1992.
79. Walter, D. L., and Boring, W. D.: Factors influencing host-virus interactions, III: Further studies on the alteration of Coxsackie virus infection in adult mice by environmental temperature. J. Immunol. *80*:39-44, 1958.
80. Wilson, J. T., Brown, R. D., Kearns, G. L., et al.: Single-dose, placebo-controlled comparative study of ibuprofen and acetaminophen antipyresis in children. J. Pediatr. *119*:803-811, 1991.
81. Wong, A., Sibbald, A., Ferrero, F., et al.: Antipyretic effects of dipyrone versus ibuprofen versus acetaminophen in children. Clin. Pediatr. *40*:313-324, 2001.
82. Wunderlich, C., and Seguin, E.: Medical Thermometry, and Human Temperature. New York, W. Wood & Co., 1871.
83. Zetterstrom, M., Lundkvist, J., Malinowsky, D., et al.: Interleukin-1 mediated febrile responses in mice and interleukin-1β activation of NFκB in mouse primary astrocytes, involves the interleukin-1 receptor accessory protein. Eur. Cytokine Netw. *9*:131-138, 1998.

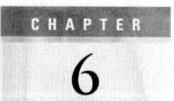

CHAPTER 6

INDIGENOUS FLORA

Douglas S. Swanson

The terms *indigenous flora* and *normal flora* describe the microorganisms that colonize the internal and external surfaces of healthy individuals.[113] Colonization is the presence of replicating microorganisms on or within a host, without evidence of the development of disease. The microbial agents that compose the normal flora are called *commensal, colonizing,* or *endogenous* organisms. They usually do not cause injury to the host and can be divided into categories of resident or transient flora.[29,159] Resident flora are organisms that are present routinely in a specified anatomic location. *Staphylococcus epidermidis* is a resident organism of the skin, and *Escherichia coli* is a resident organism of the gastrointestinal tract. Transient flora are organisms that are present only temporarily in a certain anatomic location, such as *Staphylococcus aureus* on the skin or *Pseudomonas aeruginosa* in the gastrointestinal tract. Blood, cerebrospinal fluid, urine, bile, and synovial fluid are considered sterile fluids and have no normal flora.

Environmental factors, host characteristics, and microbial properties all can influence the composition of the indigenous flora. Disruption of the balance among these various factors can have a profound impact on the normal flora and their subsequent potential for pathogenicity. Pathogens are microorganisms that are able to cause disease in the host. Strict pathogens, such as *Neisseria gonorrhoeae* and the rabies virus, always are associated with disease and are not considered part of the normal flora. Organisms such as *P. aeruginosa*, *S. epidermidis*, and *Serratia marcescens* are opportunistic pathogens and do not cause disease except in immunocompromised hosts or in special circumstances that support their dissemination. Central venous catheters can become contaminated with *S. epidermidis*, resulting in a bloodstream infection. Similarly, after a dental procedure, transient bacteremia can cause viridans streptococcal endocarditis in a patient with an abnormal heart valve.

Facultative pathogens fall somewhere between strict and opportunistic pathogens. They have the capacity to cause disease in healthy individuals and compose much of the indigenous flora found in the body (e.g., *Streptococcus pneumoniae*, *E. coli*, and *S. aureus*).[149,159]

It is useful for clinicians to have a general understanding of the normal human microbial flora. First, familiarity with the organisms that compose the normal flora may help with the interpretation of culture reports, such as the isolation of diphtheroids from a peripheral blood culture. Second, when an infectious disease is present, knowledge of the indigenous flora can assist in determining the likely causative agents and provide a basis for determining the initial antimicrobial therapy. This knowledge is especially important because of the increasing number of immunocompromised individuals who are vulnerable to endogenous infections. Third, an understanding of the normal flora may assist in making the decision to withhold antimicrobial therapy when a culture report identifies an organism that is considered to be a pathogen but is not for that patient's particular clinical presentation. The isolation of *S. pneumoniae* from a throat culture of a patient with pharyngitis can be disregarded if one recognizes that this organism is a normal part of the nasopharyngeal microbial environment and an unlikely cause of pharyngitis. Finally, clinicians may prescribe broad-spectrum antimicrobial agents more judiciously if they have an appreciation for the role that indigenous flora play as part of the host's defense system.[138]

ACQUISITION OF INDIGENOUS FLORA BY THE NEWBORN

The fetus normally is in a sterile environment in the uterus. The newborn begins to acquire indigenous microbial flora during delivery. Maternal flora provide the initial source of colonizing organisms. Exposure to organisms from other people and environmental sources contributes to the formation of the neonate's eventual normal flora.[139]

The gestational age, mode of delivery, and type of feeding all can affect the formation of a newborn's indigenous flora. Premature infants requiring prolonged hospitalization have a delay in bacterial colonization and more frequently are colonized with hospital flora, especially *Klebsiella*, *Enterobacter*, and *Citrobacter* spp., compared with healthy term newborns.[49,56,63] Infant-to-infant transmission by the hands of health care workers is an important factor contributing to gram-negative colonization of premature neonates.[56] Infants born by cesarean delivery have delayed intestinal colonization with anaerobic bacteria, and gut colonization can remain altered for 6 months after birth.[21,68,106,144] The intestinal flora also are influenced by the newborn's diet. *Bifidobacterium* spp. and a few other anaerobic bacteria dominate the intestinal flora of breast-fed newborns, whereas infants fed formula have a more complex intestinal microbial flora.[6,13,41,109,156,183] As the infant gets older, the composition of the indigenous flora begins to resemble more closely that of an adult.

MECHANISMS OF COLONIZATION

The normal flora differ substantially among the various anatomic sites because of local barriers to colonization. Environmental conditions, such as moisture, pH, oxygen tension, and nutritional supply, influence the ability of microorganisms to establish residence.[55,113] In certain anatomic regions, mucociliary clearance, epithelial cell turnover, and the flow of secretions restrict colonization to specific species of microbes.[113] Additional barriers include specific and nonspecific immune factors, the production of lysozyme, local attachment-blocking proteins, and microbial competition.[37]

The primary mechanisms of bacterial colonization are adherence to epithelial cells, colonization of mucus, and attachment to other colonizing organisms.[37] Adherence of bacteria to epithelial cells occurs primarily by specific binding between microbial surface antigens (adhesins) and epithelial receptor molecules.[12,72,95] Oral bacteria colonize specific sites within the mouth. *Streptococcus salivarius* binds to the epithelial cells of the tongue and buccal mucosa, whereas *Streptococcus mutans* and *Streptococcus sanguis* bind to tooth enamel.[138,180] Normal flora also can be established by the colonization of the mucous layer without bacterial attachment to host cells, as shown in the intestinal tract.[37] Finally, microbes can attach to colonizing organisms through adhesin-receptor binding. This means is established most clearly in the formation of dental plaque.[180]

EXOGENOUS INFLUENCES ON THE NORMAL FLORA

An individual's normal flora tends to remain stable and consistent but can be affected by a variety of exogenous factors. Antibacterial soaps, topical antiseptics, and deodorants can temporarily suppress the skin flora.[14,74,93] Similarly, brushing teeth with fluoride toothpaste reduces dental microflora. Eating fresh fruits and vegetables may provide a source of transient intestinal colonization with *P. aeruginosa*.[96,134] Cigarette smoke has been found to alter the normal flora and increase the number of potential pathogens in the nasopharynx.[26,27] Viral infections can disrupt the normal flora and predispose the patient to development of bacterial superinfections.[32,50,52,61,70,71,107,132,161] Influenza virus infection increases susceptibility to bacterial pneumonia, otitis media, and bacteremia partly by facilitating the adherence of pathogenic bacteria to respiratory epithelial cells.[61,146,184]

Medications can influence the composition of the normal flora. Acid reduction therapy may permit bacterial overgrowth within the stomach and small intestine, resulting in deconjugation of bile salts and malabsorption.[42,67,92,141,164,166,181] Gastric acid suppression also may reduce the number of ingested pathogens needed to cause enteric disease.[181] Antimicrobial agents can alter significantly the indigenous flora and promote colonization with potential pathogens by eliminating susceptible commensals.[10,40,60,76,82,117,122,123] Such changes can lead to superinfections with overgrowing organisms.[5,23,108,185] Antibiotics can reduce the barrier effect of the normal intestinal flora, permitting *Clostridium difficile* to propagate and produce toxins, resulting in pseudomembranous colitis.[9] Antimicrobial effects on the indigenous flora depend on the type of antibiotic, route, dose, and duration of administration.

Severe or chronic illnesses alone can cause changes in an individual's indigenous flora.[79,89,90,103] Hospitalized patients with severe illness are much more likely to develop pharyngeal colonization with gram-negative bacilli than are hospitalized patients who are physiologically normal.[89,90] Medical devices may alter the host's normal flora. Thomas and colleagues[165] showed that patients requiring placement of nasogastric tubes had significantly greater nasopharyngeal colonization with aerobic gram-negative bacilli compared with patients in a control group.

BACTERIAL COMPOSITION AT SPECIFIC LOCATIONS

SKIN

Because of the presence of moisture and sebum, most skin flora are associated with sweat glands (Table 6–1). Bacterial concentrations are highest on the face, on the neck, in the finger and toe webs, and in the axillae and groin.[115,116] The organisms occupy the most superficial layers of the epidermis and are found primarily around the hair follicles, although some are located deeper within follicles.[11,115,121] Although soaps and other skin cleansers

TABLE 6–1   Common Indigenous Flora at Various Anatomic Sites

Body Site and Type of Pathogen	Resident Flora	Transient Flora
Skin		
Opportunistic pathogens	*Corynebacterium, Staphylococcus epidermidis, Micrococcus, Peptococcus, Brevibacterium, Acinetobacter, Demodex folliculorum*	Viridans streptococci, *Enterococcus, Malassezia*
Facultative pathogens	*Propionibacterium acnes, Pityrosporum*	*Staphylococcus aureus, Enterobacter, Escherichia coli, Klebsiella, Proteus,* group A streptococci, *Candida, Trichophyton*
Eye		
Opportunistic pathogens	Coagulase-negative staphylococci, *Corynebacterium, Micrococcus*	*Bacillus,* viridans streptococci, *Propionibacterium*
Facultative pathogens	*Haemophilus*	*S. aureus, Streptococcus pneumoniae*
Mouth and Oropharynx		
Opportunistic pathogens	Viridans streptococci, coagulase-negative staphylococci, *Haemophilus,* non–group A beta-hemolytic streptococci, *Treponema, Veillonella, Porphyromonas, Prevotella, Lactobacillus, Peptostreptococcus, Bacteroides,* nonmeningococcal *Neisseria, Corynebacterium, Gemella, Granulicatella*	*Eikenella corrodens*
Facultative pathogens	*Fusobacterium, Streptococcus mutans,* * *Actinomyces**	Group A streptococci, *Lactobacillus,* * *Neisseria meningitidis, Kingella, S. pneumoniae, Moraxella, Candida,* cytomegalovirus, herpes simplex virus
Nose and Nasopharynx		
Opportunistic pathogens	Coagulase-negative staphylococci, viridans streptococci, *Corynebacterium*	Nonmeningococcal *Neisseria*
Facultative pathogens	—	*S. aureus, N. meningitidis, S. pneumoniae, Moraxella*
Stomach		
Opportunistic pathogens	—	*Streptococcus, Lactobacillus*
Facultative pathogens	—	*Helicobacter pylori*
Small Intestine		
Opportunistic pathogens	*Lactobacillus, Streptococcus, Veillonella, Prevotella, Porphyromonas, Bifidobacterium*	*Candida, Entamoeba coli, Endolimax nana, Iodamoeba bütschlii, Trichomonas hominis, Chilomastix mesnili*
Facultative pathogens	*Bacteroides,* Enterobacteriaceae, *Clostridium*	*Blastocystis hominis*
Large Intestine		
Opportunistic pathogens	*Bifidobacterium, Peptostreptococcus, Lactobacillus, Veillonella, Eubacterium, Fusobacterium, Prevotella, Porphyromonas, Enterococcus, Peptococcus, Ruminococcus*	*Candida, Corynebacterium, Pseudomonas, Mycobacterium avium* complex, *E. coli, E. nana, I. bütschlii, T. hominis, C. mesnili*
Facultative pathogens	*Bacteroides, Clostridium,* Enterobacteriaceae	*Aeromonas, B. hominis,* enterovirus
Anterior Urethra		
Opportunistic pathogens	*Corynebacterium,* coagulase-negative staphylococci, viridans streptococci, *Lactobacillus* (women)	*Mycobacterium smegmatis, Bacteroides, Fusobacterium*
Facultative pathogens	—	Enterobacteriaceae, *Enterococcus, Ureaplasma, Mycoplasma*
Vagina		
Opportunistic pathogens	*Lactobacillus, Streptococcus,* coagulase-negative staphylococci	*Enterococcus*
Facultative pathogens	*Gardnerella vaginalis, Mobiluncus, Prevotella, Actinomyces*	Group B streptococci, *Candida, Trichomonas vaginalis*

*Contribute to dental caries.

substantially reduce the number of most surface bacteria, organisms within hair follicles and sweat glands quickly re-establish the normal flora.[74,93]

The normal skin flora are primarily of coagulase-negative *Staphylococcus* spp. (especially *S. epidermidis*), *Propionibacterium acnes*, *Corynebacterium* spp. (diphtheroids), and *Micrococcus* spp. *P. acnes* emerges at the onset of puberty, occupies hair follicles and sebaceous glands, and is a major contributing cause of acne. *S. aureus* and group A streptococci are not usual residents of the skin but may cause transient colonization.[152] *Acinetobacter* spp. are a common resident of the toe webs. Other gram-negative organisms, such as *Klebsiella*, *Proteus*, and *Enterobacter* spp. and *E. coli*, are uncommon findings and transient residents of the skin. The fungus *Pityrosporum* (*ovale* and *orbiculare*) normally inhabits the skin,[135,136] but *Candida* spp. do not.[34] Many other microorganisms come in contact with the skin, but because of the skin's dryness and presence of organic fatty acids, they are present only briefly and do not propagate.

Newborns

Within hours, a normal full-term infant's skin becomes colonized with microbes. In addition to typical normal skin flora, potential pathogens (group B streptococci, *E. coli*, *Klebsiella* spp.) frequently are recovered from cultures of the external ear canal.[110,125] Obtaining routine surveillance cultures in an attempt to identify infants at risk for acquiring invasive disease is not recommended, however, because their predictive value is limited.[87,110,125]

CONJUNCTIVAE

The mechanical actions of the eyelids and the washing effect of tears containing antimicrobial substances inhibit microbial colonization of the eye; however, normal flora do exist. The conjunctival flora probably originate from the eyelids and the nasolacrimal ducts. The organisms most commonly isolated are coagulase-negative staphylococci, *Corynebacterium*, *Micrococcus*, and *Propionibacterium* spp. Other isolates include *S. aureus*, *Haemophilus* spp., viridans streptococci, *S. pneumoniae*, and *Bacillus* spp.[102,129,138,177]

RESPIRATORY TRACT

The mouth and oropharynx contain several unique microbial habitats. Viridans (alpha-hemolytic and nonhemolytic) streptococci are the most prominent commensals and include *S. mutans*, *S. sanguis*, *S. salivarius*, *Streptococcus milleri*, and *Streptococcus mitis*.[97,138,159] The flora of the gingival crevice include a diverse collection of facultative and anaerobic organisms. More common isolates include *S. mitis*, *S. mutans*, *Actinomyces*, *Fusobacterium*, *Treponema*, *Veillonella*, and *Peptostreptococcus*. *Bacteroides* spp., *S. sanguis*, and *S. mitis* are the initial colonizers of the tooth surface. Dental plaque forms when *S. mutans* and *Actinomyces*, *Fusobacterium*, *Treponema*, and *Veillonella* spp., along with other organisms, attach to the initial bacterial cell layer and each other.[127,180] The buccal mucosa, tongue, and saliva are colonized most heavily by *S. salivarius*, *S. mitis*, and *Veillonella*, *Gemella*, *Granulicatella*, and *Lactobacillus* spp.[1] Asymptomatic pharyngeal carrier rates of group A streptococci in children range from 3 to 50 percent, with the highest prevalence rates associated with school outbreaks of pharyngitis.[35,45,53,78,130,154,157,178,182]

Compared with flora of the mouth and oropharynx, the microbial flora of the nose and nasopharynx are less diverse. Coagulase-negative staphylococci, viridans streptococci, *Corynebacterium* spp., and *S. aureus* are the most prevalent strains isolated. Nasal carriage rates of *S. aureus* average 20 to 35

percent, and the prevalence of methicillin-resistant *S. aureus* nasal colonization has been increasing, with estimates ranging from 0.2 to 22 percent, depending on demographic characteristics.[2,3,31,77,85,98,150,158,170] Colonization of children with *Neisseria*, *Haemophilus*, *Moraxella* spp., and *S. pneumoniae* is a common occurrence.

Pneumococcal colonization of the nasopharynx generally is transient, averaging in duration from 1 to 4 months.[51,66] Increased colonization is seen with younger age, overcrowding, attendance at a daycare center, winter season, and exposure to tobacco smoke. Nasopharyngeal carriage rates of *S. pneumoniae* average 40 to 50 percent in children and 20 to 30 percent in adults.[59] Nasopharyngeal colonization occurs even with the implementation of pneumococcal protein conjugate vaccine; several studies indicate a change in serotype distribution with an increased presence of drug-resistant strains.[54,83,86] Despite the presence of potential pathogens in the nasopharynx, no convincing evidence supports the use of nasopharyngeal cultures to predict the etiology of acute otitis media, pneumonia, or sinusitis.[58,173]

The sinuses and lower respiratory tract generally are assumed to be sterile. In actuality, bacteria from the mouth and nose probably reach these regions daily but are cleared promptly by local defense mechanisms.[138]

During the first week of life, the newborn's oropharynx usually is colonized by maternal vaginal flora, primarily *Lactobacillus* spp. and *Streptococcus viridans*.[28,119] These bacteria gradually are replaced by mouth flora from the mother and caretakers. *S. salivarius* and *S. mitis* predominate. Anaerobes, *S. mutans*, and *S. sanguis* are uncommon findings until teeth erupt.[97] *Ureaplasma* spp. and *Mycoplasma* spp. from the maternal vagina readily colonize the newborn's respiratory tract.[160] They are a suspected, yet still undetermined, cause of chronic lung disease in premature infants.[75,124,176] Enteric bacilli can be recovered from the throats of more than half of normal infants older than 2 months of age.[7]

GASTROINTESTINAL TRACT

The gastrointestinal tract consists of the esophagus, stomach, small intestine, and colon. The esophagus usually is sterile, and the stomach generally harbors only a few bacteria. The digestive enzymes and acid in the stomach destroy most swallowed organisms, or they pass promptly into the small intestine. Among the microflora of the stomach are acid-tolerant organisms, such as lactobacilli and streptococci,[147] and *Helicobacter pylori*, which survives within the mucous layer overlaying the gastric mucosal epithelium.[22,57,91] The worldwide prevalence of *H. pylori* colonization in children ranges from 10 to 90 percent.[162] Factors associated with colonization include lower socioeconomic status, household crowding, ethnicity, and household contact with carriers.[65,128,168] When the gastric pH is increased, nasopharyngeal and fecal-type flora may colonize the stomach.[181]

Low concentrations of *Streptococcus*, *Lactobacillus*, *Veillonella*, and rare *Bacteroides* spp. can be found in the upper small intestine.[17,30,44] Higher concentrations of the same bacteria plus *Bifidobacterium*, *Clostridium*, and Enterobacteriaceae are present in the lower small intestine.[18,114] Small bowel bacterial overgrowth can occur under conditions of gastric achlorhydria, a blind loop, or dysmotility. This syndrome may result in malabsorption and diarrhea.[94]

The colon contains a large and diverse population of microorganisms.[64,151] More microbes occur in this location than anywhere else in the body. For many years, because of inadequate techniques available for culturing strict anaerobic bacteria, *E. coli* was thought to be the principal resident of the large intestine. It has become apparent that the strict anaerobes outnumber the facultative microbes by 1000 to 1, with hundreds of different anaerobic species being isolated from the colon.[147] Molecular analysis of fecal flora has expanded understanding of the microbial diversity found in the gastrointestinal tract.[48,175] *Bacteroides* and *Bifidobacterium* spp. comprise the largest percentage of fecal flora. Other major organisms in the colon include *Peptostreptococcus*, *Peptococcus*, *Ruminococcus*, *Enterococcus*, Enterobacteriaceae, *Prevotella*, *Porphyromonas*, *Fusobacterium*, *Clostridium*, *Lactobacillus*, and *Eubacterium* spp.

Newborns

The newborn's intestinal flora usually are derived from organisms within the mother's birth canal and from the newborn's environment. Diet can influence the composition of the infant's intestinal flora.[37,41,106,111] Full-term, breast-fed infants are colonized predominantly with *Bifidobacterium* spp. Formula-fed infants have a more complex intestinal flora in which *Bifidobacterium*, *Bacteroides*, *Enterobacter*, *Clostridia*, and *Enterococcus* spp. are prevalent.[6,13,41,109,156,183] Infants delivered by cesarean section have 6 months' delay in colonization with anaerobic organisms.[21,68,106] At 12 months of age, after the introduction of solid foods, all infants have intestinal flora that more closely resemble those of an adult.[41]

Intestinal colonization of very-low-birth-weight infants is delayed, and the development of anaerobic flora is diminished. Anaerobes, especially *Bifidobacterium* and *Lactobacillus* spp., are thought to protect the host against invasion by pathogens. Paucity of these organisms permits bacterial overgrowth with potential pathogens, especially *E. coli*, *Klebsiella*, *Enterobacter*, and *Citrobacter* spp. Researchers suspect that this aberrant intestinal colonization of premature infants contributes to the pathogenesis of necrotizing enterocolitis.[33,43,101,126]

GENITOURINARY TRACT

The endogenous flora of the genitourinary tract normally are confined to the distal portion of the urethra and the vaginal mucosa. The anterior urethra in men and women commonly is colonized with skin flora (coagulase-negative staphylococci, *Corynebacterium* spp., and streptococci) and may contain *Mycobacterium smegmatis* and *Bacteroides*, *Fusobacterium*, *Enterococcus*, and Enterobacteriaceae. The female anterior urethra also contains *Lactobacillus* spp. Asymptomatic colonization with *Ureaplasma urealyticum*, and to a lesser extent with *Mycoplasma hominis*, is a common event in sexually active individuals.[120,163]

The microbial flora of the vagina is influenced profoundly by hormonal factors.[99,100] During the first few weeks of life, estrogen from the maternal circulation creates in the newborn girl a vaginal environment conducive for the growth of *Lactobacillus* spp. This event is followed by development of a scant vaginal flora, containing mostly coagulase-negative staphylococci, *Corynebacterium*, and occasionally Enterobacteriaceae and *Streptococcus* spp. With the onset of puberty, lactobacilli again become the predominant organisms isolated. Coagulase-negative staphylococci and *Corynebacterium* spp. and various anaerobic streptococci also are common findings.[8,73,133] *Enterococcus*, Enterobacteriaceae, and *Candida* spp. are found less frequently.[8] *U. urealyticum* is present in approximately half of premenopausal women, and *M. hominis* is found in fewer numbers.[120,163] The vaginal colonization rate of group B streptococci in pregnant women is 5 to 35 percent.[4] Heavy colonization with *Gardnerella vaginalis*, *Trichomonas vaginalis*, and *Mobiluncus* and *Prevotella* spp. is associated with bacterial vaginosis.[153]

BENEFICIAL EFFECTS OF INDIGENOUS FLORA

It is generally recognized that pathogens first need to colonize the host before causing disease. The indigenous flora help to protect the host against infections through colonization resistance, also called *bacterial interference*.* Colonization resistance is accomplished by several mechanisms, including competition for nutrients, competition for epithelial cell receptors, production of toxins and bacteriocins, and stimulation of the immune response.[19,24,25,169,179] Suppression of the normal flora with antimicrobial therapy correlates with an increased susceptibility to candidiasis,[148] *C. difficile* colitis,[9] and *Salmonella* infection.[81] Use of probiotic agents, live microbial food supplements (e.g., *Lactobacillus*, *Bifidobacterium* spp.), helps restore the normal intestinal microflora during antibiotic therapy and inhibits the growth of potential pathogens.[36,69,143]

The endogenous intestinal flora seem to stimulate the cellular and humoral mucosal immune system.[16,131,167,174] This relationship influences the development of the newborn's immune system. Germ-free animals have underdeveloped, poorly differentiated lymphoidal tissues and low serum immunoglobulin concentrations. These animals have increased susceptibility to experimental challenges with pathogenic microbes.[47] The intestinal microflora also may affect the development of atopic disease and allergy.[20]

The normal flora provide some nutritional supplement for the host. The intestinal microflora ferment undigested carbohydrates into short-chain fatty acids. The short-chain fatty acids affect colonic epithelial cell transport and serve as an energy source for colonic epithelial cells, the liver, and muscle.[39,137,140,142] The intestinal flora also participate in the enterohepatic recirculation of biliary metabolites and the degradation of toxins and carcinogens.[62,114] In addition, normal flora microbes produce essential vitamins, such as vitamins K and B_{12}. Whether humans use these vitamins in any substantial manner is uncertain.[46]

ADVERSE EFFECTS OF THE INDIGENOUS FLORA

The indigenous flora can have unpleasant or even harmful effects on the host and are the source of intestinal gas and body odor. Oral flora are associated with dental caries and periodontal disease. In special circumstances, bacterial overgrowth of normal flora in the small intestine can result in malabsorption, diarrhea, and weight loss.[84,94] Other clinical conditions can create the potential for bacterial translocation, the invasion of indigenous bowel flora across the intestinal mucosa.[15,104] Intestinal toxins from endogenous bacteria may contribute to the encephalopathy, renal failure, and coagulopathy seen in hepatic failure.[37] Injury to the host from endotoxic shock may be caused to some extent by a hypersensitivity response induced by endotoxin from intestinal flora because germ-free animals are highly resistant to the effects of injected endotoxin.[159] Intestinal flora are speculated to cause cancer by metabolically activating carcinogens or by making carcinogenic products.[112] Finally, the intestinal normal flora may have a causative role in failure to thrive, arthritis, and autoimmune disorders.[37]

SUMMARY

The indigenous flora of humans are unique to specific anatomic locations. They are influenced by intrinsic microbial properties, host characteristics, and exogenous factors. Indigenous flora provide clear benefits to the host and potential adverse affects. Familiarity with the normal flora should help clinicians provide improved care for their patients.

---

*See references 25, 38, 80, 88, 105, 118, 145, 155, 171, 172.

REFERENCES

1. Aas, J. A., Paster, B. J., Stokes. L, N., et al.: Defining the normal bacterial flora of the oral cavity. J. Clin. Microbiol. *43*:5721-5732, 2005.

2. Abudu, L., Blair, I., Fraise, A., et al.: Methicillin-resistant *Staphylococcus aureus* (MRSA): A community-based prevalence survey. Epidemiol. Infect. *126*:351-356, 2001.

3. Alfaro, C., Mascher-Denen, M., Fergie, J., and Purcell, K.: Prevalence of methicillin-resistant *Staphylococcus aureus* nasal carriage in patients admitted to Driscoll Children's Hospital. Pediatr. Infect. Dis. J. *25*:459-461, 2006.

4. American Academy of Pediatrics: Group B streptococcal infections. *In* Pickering, L. K. (ed.): 2000 Red Book: Report of the Committee on Infectious Diseases. 25th ed. Elk Grove Village, IL, American Academy of Pediatrics, 2000, pp. 537-544.

5. Asay, L. D., and Koch, R.: *Pseudomonas* infections in infants and children. N. Engl. J. Med. *262*:1062-1066, 1960.

6. Balmer, S. E., and Wharton, B. A.: Diet and faecal flora in the newborn: Breast milk and infant formula. Arch. Dis. Child. *64*:1672-1677.

7. Baltimore, R. S., Duncan, R. L., Shapiro, E. D., et al.: Epidemiology of pharyngeal colonization of infants with aerobic gram-negative rod bacteria. J. Clin. Microbiol. *27*:91-95, 1989.

8. Bartlett, J. G., and Polk, B. F.: Bacterial flora of the vagina: Quantitative study. Rev. Infect. Dis. *6*(Suppl. 1):S67-S72, 1984.

9. Bartlett, J. G., Chang, T. W., Gurwith, M., et al.: Antibiotic-associated pseudomembranous colitis due to toxin-producing clostridia. N. Engl. J. Med. *298*:531-534, 1978.

10. Barza, M., Giuliano, M., Jacobus, N. V., et al.: Effect of broad-spectrum parenteral antibiotics on "colonization resistance" of intestinal microflora of humans. Antimicrob. Agents Chemother. *31*:723-727, 1987.

11. Baxby, D., and Woodroffe, R. C. S.: The location of bacteria in the skin. J. Appl. Bacteriol. *28*:316-321, 1965.

12. Beachey, E. H.: Bacterial adherences: Adhesion-receptor interactions mediating the attachment of bacteria to mucosal surfaces. J. Infect. Dis. *143*:325-345, 1981.

13. Benno, Y., Sawada, K., and Mitsuoka, T.: The intestinal microflora of infants: Composition of fecal flora in breast-fed infants and bottle-fed infants. Microbiol. Immunol. *28*:975-986, 1984.

14. Benohanian, A.: Antiperspirants and deodorants. Clin. Dermatol. *19*:398-405, 2001.

15. Berg, R. D., and Savage, D. C.: Immune responses of specific pathogen-free and gnotobiotic mice to antigens of indigenous and nonindigenous microorganisms. Infect. Immun. *11*:320-329, 1975.

16. Berg, R. D.: Bacterial translocation from the gastrointestinal tract. Trends Microbiol. *3*:149-154, 1995.

17. Bernhardt, H., and Knoke, M.: Recent studies on the microbial ecology of the upper gastrointestinal tract. Infection *17*:259-263, 1989.

18. Bhat, P., Albert, M. J., Rajan, D., et al.: Bacterial flora of the jejunum: A comparison of luminal aspirate and mucosal biopsy. J. Med. Microbiol. *13*:247-256, 1980.

19. Bibel, D. J., Aly, R., Bayles, C., et al.: Competitive adherence as a mechanism of bacterial interference. Can. J. Microbiol. *29*:700-703, 1983.

20. Bjorksten, B., Sepp, E., Julge, K., et al.: Allergy development and the intestinal microflora during the first year of life. J. Allergy Clin. Immunol. *108*:516-520, 2001.

21. Blakey, J. L., Lubitz, L., Barnes, G. L., et al.: Development of gut colonisation in pre-term neonates. J. Med. Microbiol. *15*:519-529, 1982.

22. Blaser, M. J.: Hypothesis: The changing relationships of *Helicobacter pylori* and humans: Implications for health and disease. J. Infect. Dis. *179*:1523-1530, 1999.

23. Bonhogg, M., Drake, B. L., and Miller, C. P.: Effect of streptomycin on susceptibility of intestinal tracts to experimental *Salmonella* infection. Proc. Soc. Exp. Biol. Med. *86*:132-137, 1954.

24. Borriello, S. P.: The influence of the normal flora on *Clostridium difficile* colonisation of the gut. Ann. Med. *22*:61-67, 1990.

25. Brook, I.: Bacterial interference. Crit. Rev. Microbiol. *25*:155-172, 1999.

26. Brook, I., and Gober, A. E.: Recovery of potential pathogens and interfering bacteria in the nasopharynx of smokers and nonsmokers. Chest. *127*:2072-2075, 2005.

27. Brook, I., and Gober, A. E.: Effect of smoking cessation on the microbial flora. Arch. Otolaryngol. Head Neck Surg. *133*:135-138, 2007.

28. Carlsson, J., Grahnen, H., Jonsson, G., et al.: Early establishment of *Streptococcus salivarius* in the mouths of infants. J. Dent. Res. *49*:415-418, 1970.

29. Casadevall, A., and Pirofski, L. A.: Host-pathogen interactions: Basic concepts of microbial commensalism, colonization, infection, and disease. Infect. Immun. *68*:6511-6518, 2000.

30. Challacombe, D. N., Richardson, J. M., and Anderson, C. M.: Bacterial microflora of the upper gastrointestinal tract in infants without diarrhea. Arch. Dis. Child. *49*:264-269, 1974.

31. Charlebois, E. D., Bangsberg, D. R., Moss, N. J., et al.: Population-based community prevalence of methicillin-resistant *Staphylococcus aureus* in the urban poor of San Francisco. Clin. Infect. Dis. *34*:425-433, 2002.

32. Chonmaitree, T., and Heikkinen, T.: Viruses and acute otitis media. Pediatr. Infect. Dis. J. *19*:1005-1007, 2000.

33. Claud, E. C., and Walker, W. A.: Hypothesis: Inappropriate colonization of the premature intestine can cause neonatal necrotizing enterocolitis. Faseb. J. *15*:1398-1403, 2001.

34. Clayton, Y. M., and Noble, W. C.: Observations on the epidemiology of *Candida albicans*. J. Clin. Pathol. *19*:76-78, 1966.

35. Cockerill, F. R., MacDonald, K. L., Thompson, R. L., et al.: An outbreak of invasive group A streptococcal disease associated with high carriage rates of the invasive clone among school-aged children. J. A. M. A. *277*:38-43, 1997.

36. Collins, M. D., and Gibson, G. R.: Probiotics, prebiotics, and synbiotics: Approaches for modulating the microbial ecology of the gut. Am. J. Clin. Nutr. *69*:1052S-1057S, 1999.

37. Cooperstock, M. S.: Indigenous flora in host economy and pathogenesis. *In* Feigin, R. D., and Cherry, J. D. (eds.): Textbook of Pediatric Infectious Diseases. 3rd ed. Philadelphia, W. B. Saunders, 1992, pp. 91-119.

38. Crowe, C. C., Sanders, W. E., Jr., and Longley, S.: Bacterial interference, II: Role of the normal throat flora in prevention of colonization by group A *Streptococcus*. J. Infect. Dis. *128*:527-532, 1973.

39. Cummings, J. H., and Macfarlane, G. T.: Role of intestinal bacteria in nutrient metabolism. J. Parenter. Enteral Nutr. *21*:357-365, 1997.

40. Dagan, R., Leibovitz, E., Cheletz, G., et al.: Antibiotic treatment in acute otitis media promotes superinfection with resistant *Streptococcus pneumoniae* carried before initiation of treatment. J. Infect. Dis. *183*:880-886, 2001.

41. Dai, D., and Walker, W. A.: Protective nutrients and bacterial colonization in the immature human gut. Adv. Pediatr. *46*:353-382, 1999.

42. Deane, S., Youngs, D., Poxon, V., et al.: Cimetidine and the gastric microflora. Br. J. Surg. *67*:371, 1980.

43. Deitch, E. A.: Role of bacterial translocation in necrotizing enterocolitis. Acta Paediatr. Suppl. *396*:33-36, 1994.

44. Dickman, M. D., Chappelka, A. R., and Schaedler, R. W.: The microbial ecology of the upper small bowel. Am. J. Gastroenterol. *65*:57-62, 1976.

45. Dierksen, K. P., Inglis, M., and Tagg, J. R.: High pharyngeal carriage rates of *Streptococcus pyogenes* in Dunedin school children with a low incidence of rheumatic fever. N. Z. Med. J. *113*:496-499, 2000.

46. Donaldson, R. M., Jr.: Normal bacterial populations of the intestine and their relation to intestinal function. N. Engl. J. Med. *270*:938-946, 994-1000, 1050-1056, 1964.

47. Dubos, R. J., and Schaedler, R. W.: The effect of the intestinal flora on the growth rate of mice, and on their susceptibility to experimental infections. J. Exp. Med. *111*:407-417, 1960.

48. Eckburg, P. B., Bik, E. M., Bernstein, C. N., et al.: Diversity of the human intestinal microbial flora. Science *308*:1635-1638, 2005.

49. Ehrenkranz, N. J.: Bacterial colonization of newborn infants and subsequent acquisition of hospital bacteria. J. Pediatr. *76*:839-847, 1970.

50. Eichenwald, H. F., Kotsevalov, O., and Fasso, L. A.: Some effects of viral infection on aerial dissemination of staphylococci and on susceptibility to bacterial colonization. Bacteriol. Rev. *25*:274-281, 1961.

51. Ekdahl, K., Ahlinder, I., Hansson, H. B., et al.: Duration of NP carriage of PRP: Experiences from the South Swedish Pneumococcal Intervention Project. Clin. Infect. Dis. *25*:1113-1117, 1997.

52. Elahmer, O. R., Raza, M. W., Ogilvie, M. M., et al.: The effect of respiratory virus infection on expression of cell surface antigens associated with binding of potentially pathogenic bacteria. Adv. Exp. Med. Biol. *408*:169-177, 1996.

53. Engelgau, M. M., Woernle, C. H., Schwartz, B., et al.: Invasive group A streptococcus carriage in a child care centre after a fatal case. Arch. Dis. Child. *71*:318-322, 1994.

54. Farrell, D. J., Klugman, K. P., and Pichichero, M.: Increased antimicrobial resistance among nonvaccine serotypes of *Streptococcus pneumoniae* in the pediatric population after the introduction of 7-valent pneumococcal vaccine in the United States. Pediatr. Infect. Dis. J. *26*:123-128, 2007.

55. Freter, R.: Interactions between mechanisms controlling the intestinal microflora. Am. J. Clin. Nutr. *27*:1409-1416, 1974.

56. Fryklund, B., Tullus, K., Berglund, B., et al.: Importance of the environment and the faecal flora of infants, nursing staff, and parents as sources of gram-negative bacteria colonizing newborns in three neonatal wards. Infection *20*:253-257, 1992.

57. Ganga-Zandzou, P. S., Michaud, L., Vincent, P., et al.: Natural outcome of *Helicobacter pylori* infection in asymptomatic children: A two-year follow-up study. Pediatrics *104*:216-221, 1999.

58. Gehanno, P., Lenoir, G., Barry, B., et al.: Evaluation of nasopharyngeal cultures for bacteriologic assessment of acute otitis media in children. Pediatr. Infect. Dis. J. *15*:329-332, 1996.

59. Ghaffar, F., Friedland, I. R., and McCracken, G. H.: Dynamics of nasopharyngeal colonization by *Streptococcus pneumoniae*. Pediatr. Infect. Dis. J. *18*:638-646, 1999.

60. Giuliano, M., Barza, M., Jacobus, N. V., et al.: Effect of broad-spectrum parenteral antibiotics on composition of intestinal microflora of humans. Antimicrob. Agents Chemother. *31*:202-206, 1987.

61. Glezen, W. P.: Prevention of acute otitis media by prophylaxis and treatment of influenza virus infections. Vaccine *19*(Suppl. 1):S56-S58, 2000.

62. Goldin, B. R.: Intestinal microflora: Metabolism of drugs and carcinogens. Ann. Med. *22*:43-48, 1990.

63. Goldmann, D. A., Leclair, J., and Macone, A.: Bacterial colonization of neonates admitted to an intensive care environment. J. Pediatr. *93*:288-293, 1978.

64. Gorbach, S. L.: Intestinal microflora. Gastroenterology *60*:1110-1129, 1971.

65. Graham, D. Y., Malaty, H. M., Evans, D. J., et al.: Epidemiology of *Helicobacter pylori* in an asymptomatic population in the United States: Effect of age, race, and socioeconomic status. Gastroenterology *100*:1495-1501, 1991.

66. Gray, B. M., Converse, G. M., III, and Dillon, H. C., Jr.: Epidemiologic studies of *Streptococcus pneumoniae* in infants: Acquisition, carriage, and infection during the first 24 months of life. J. Infect. Dis. *142*:923-933, 1980.

67. Gray, J. D., and Shiner, M.: Influence of gastric pH on gastric and jejunal flora. Gut *8*:574-581, 1967.

68. Gronlund, M. M., Lehtonen, O. P., Eerola, E., et al.: Fecal microflora in healthy infants born by different methods of delivery: Permanent changes in intestinal flora after cesarean delivery. J. Pediatr. Gastroenterol. Nutr. *28*:19-25, 1999.

69. Guarner, F., and Malagelada, J. R. Gut flora in health and disease. Lancet *361*:512-519, 2003.

70. Gwaltney, J. M., Jr., Sande, M. A., Austrian, R., et al.: Spread of *Streptococcus pneumoniae* in families, II: Relation of transfer of *S. pneumoniae* to incidence of colds and serum antibody. J. Infect. Dis. *132*:62-68, 1975.

71. Hakansson, A., Kidd, A., Wadell, G., et al.: Adenovirus infection enhances in vitro adherence of *Streptococcus pneumoniae*. Infect. Immun. *62*:2707-2714, 1994.

72. Hamada, S., Amano, A., Kimura, S., et al.: The importance of fimbriae in the virulence and ecology of some oral bacteria. Oral Microbiol. Immunol. *13*:129-138, 1998.

73. Hammerschlag, M. R., Alpert, S., Onderdonk, A., et al.: Anaerobic microflora of the vagina in children. Am. J. Obstet. Gynecol. *131*:853-856, 1978.

74. Hartmann, A. A.: Daily bath and its effect on the normal human skin flora: Quantitative and qualitative investigations of the aerobic skin flora. Arch. Dermatol. Res. *265*:153-164, 1979.

75. Heggie, A. D., Bar-Shain, D., Boxerbaum, B., et al.: Identification and quantification of ureaplasma colonizing the respiratory tract and assessment of their role in the development of chronic lung disease in preterm infants. Pediatr. Infect. Dis. J. *20*:854-859, 2001.

76. Heikkinen, T., Saeed, K. A., McCormick, D. P., et al.: A single intramuscular dose of ceftriaxone changes nasopharyngeal bacterial flora in children with acute otitis media. Acta Paediatr. *89*:1316-1321, 2000.

77. Herold, B. C., Immergluck, L. C., Maranan, M. C., et al.: Community-acquired methicillin-resistant *Staphylococcus aureus* in children with no identified predisposing risk. J. A. M. A. *279*:593-598, 1998.

78. Hoffmann, S.: The throat carrier rate of group A and other beta hemolytic streptococci among patients in general practice. Acta Pathol. Microbiol. Immunol. Scand. *93*:347-351, 1985.

79. Holdeman, L. V., Good, I. J., and Moore, W. E. C.: Human fecal flora: Variation in bacterial composition within individuals and a possible effect of emotional stress. Appl. Environ. Microbiol. *31*:359-375, 1976.

80. Holm, S. E., and Grahn, E.: Bacterial interference in streptococcal tonsillitis. Scand. J. Infect. Dis. Suppl. *39*:73-78, 1983.

81. Holmberg, S. D., Osterholm, M. T., Senger, K. A., et al.: Drug-resistant *Salmonella* from animals fed antimicrobials. N. Engl. J. Med. *311*:617-622.

82. Hooker, K. D., and Di Piro, J. T.: Effect of antimicrobial therapy on bowel flora. Clin. Pharm. *7*:878-888, 1988.

83. Huang, S. S., Platt, R., Rifas-Shiman, S. L., et al.: Post-PCV7 changes in colonizing pneumococcal serotypes in 16 Massachusetts communities, 2001 and 2004. Pediatrics. *116*:e408-e413, 2005.

84. Husebye, E.: Gastrointestinal motility disorders and bacterial overgrowth. J. Intern. Med. *237*:419-427, 1995.

85. Hussain, F. M., Boyle-Vavra, S., and Daum, R. S.: Community-acquired methicillin-resistant *Staphylococcus aureus* colonization in healthy children attending an outpatient pediatric clinic. Pediatr. Infect. Dis. J. *20*:763-767, 2001.

86. Jacobs, M. R., Good, C. E., Sellner, T., et al.: Nasopharyngeal carriage of respiratory pathogens in children undergoing pressure equalization tube placement in the era of pneumococcal protein conjugate vaccine use. Laryngoscope *117*:295-298, 2007.

87. Jarvis, W. R.: The epidemiology of colonization. Infect. Control Hosp. Epidemiol. *17*:47-52, 1996.

88. Johanson, W. G., Jr., Blackstock, R., Pierce, A. K., et al.: The role of bacterial antagonism in pneumococcal colonization of the human pharynx. J. Lab. Clin. Med. *75*:946-952, 1970.

89. Johanson, W. G., Jr., Pierce, A. K., Sanford, J. P., et al.: Nosocomial respiratory infections with gram-negative bacilli: The significance of colonization of the respiratory tract. Ann. Intern. Med. *77*:701-706, 1972.

90. Johanson, W. G., Pierce, A. K., and Sanford, J. P.: Changing pharyngeal bacterial flora of hospitalized patients: Emergence of gram-negative bacilli. N. Engl. J. Med. *281*:1137-1140, 1969.

91. Karlsson, K. A.: The human gastric colonizer *Helicobacter pylori*: A challenge for host-parasite glycobiology. Glycobiology *10*:761-771, 2000.

92. Karmeli, Y., Stalnikowitz, R., Eliakim, R., et al.: Conventional dose of omeprazole alters gastric flora. Dig. Dis. Sci. *40*:2070-2073, 1995.

93. Keswick, B. H., Berge, C. A., Bartolo, R. G., et al.: Antimicrobial soaps: Their role in personal hygiene. *In* Aly, R., Beutner, K. R., and Maibach, H. (eds.): Cutaneous Infection and Therapy. New York, Marcel Dekker, 1997, pp. 49-82.

94. Kirsch, M.: Bacterial overgrowth. Am. J. Gastroenterol. *85*:231-237, 1990.

95. Klemm, P., and Schembri, M. A.: Bacterial adhesins: Function and structure. Int. J. Med. Microbiol. *290*:27-35, 2000.

96. Kominos, S. D., Copeland, C. E., Grosiak, B., et al.: Introduction of *Pseudomonas aeruginosa* into a hospital via vegetables. Appl. Microbiol. *24*:567-570, 1972.

97. Kononen, E.: Development of oral bacterial flora in young children. Ann. Med. *32*:107-112, 2000.

98. Kuehnert, M. J., Kruszon-Moran, D., Hill, H. A., et al.: Prevalence of *Staphylococcus aureus* nasal colonization in the United States, 2001-2002. J. Infect. Dis. *193*:172-179, 2006.

99. Larsen, B., and Galask, R. P.: Vaginal microbiol flora: Composition and influences of host physiology. Ann. Intern. Med. *96*:926-930, 1982.

100. Larsen, B., and Monif, G. R.: Understanding the bacterial flora of the female genital tract. Clin. Infect. Dis. *32*:69-77, 2001.

101. Lawrence, G., Bates, J., and Gaul, A.: Pathogenesis of neonatal necrotizing enterocolitis. Lancet *1*:137-139, 1982.

102. Levine, J., and Snyder, R. W.: Practical ophthalmic microbiology. J. Ophthalmic Nurs. Technol. *18*:50-59, 1999.

103. Li, L., Wu, Z., Ma, W., et al.: Changes in intestinal microflora in patients with chronic severe hepatitis. Chin. Med. J. *114*:869-872, 2001.

104. Lichtman, S. M.: Bacterial translocation in humans. J. Pediatr. Gastroenterol. Nutr. *33*:1-10, 2001.

105. Liljemark, W. F., and Gibbons, R. J.: Suppression of *Candida albicans* by human oral streptococci in gnotobiotic mice. Infect. Immun. *8*:846-849, 1973.

106. Long, S. S., and Swenson, R. M.: Development of anaerobic fecal flora in healthy newborn infants. J. Pediatr. *91*:298-301, 1977.

107. Loukides, S., Panagou, P., Kolokouris, D., et al.: Bacterial pneumonia as a suprainfection in young adults with measles. Eur. Respir. J. *13*:356-360, 1999.

108. Louria, D. B., and Kaminski, T.: The effects of four antimicrobial drug regimens on sputum superinfection in hospitalized patients. Am. Rev. Respir. Dis. *85*:649-665, 1962.

109. Lundquist, B., Nord, C. E., and Winberg, J.: The composition of the faecal microflora in breast fed and bottle fed infants from birth to eight weeks. Acta Paediatr. Scand. *74*:45-51, 1985.

110. MacGregor, R. R., and Tunnessen, W. W.: The incidence of pathogenic organisms in the normal flora of the neonate's external ear and nasopharynx. Clin. Pediatr. *12*:697-700, 1973.

111. Mackie, R. I., Sghir, A., and Gaskins, H. R.: Developmental microbial ecology of the neonatal gastrointestinal tract. Am. J. Clin. Nutr. *69*(Suppl.):1035S-1045S, 1999.

112. Mackowiak, P. A.: Microbial oncogenesis. Am. J. Med. *82*:79-97, 1987.

113. Mackowiak, P. A.: The normal microbial flora. N. Engl. J. Med. *307*:83-93, 1982.

114. Mallory, A., Kern, F., Smith, J., et al.: Patterns of bile acids and microflora in the human small intestine, I: Bile acids. Gastroenterology *64*:26-33, 1973.

115. Marples, M. J.: The normal flora of the human skin. Br. J. Dermatol. *81*(Suppl. 1):2-13, 1969.

116. Marples, R.: The normal flora of different sites in the young adult. Curr. Med. Res. Opin. 7(Suppl. 2): 67-70, 1982.

117. Marples, R. R., and Kligman, A. M.: Ecological effects of oral antibiotics on the microflora of human skin. Arch. Dermatol. *103*:148-153, 1971.

118. Martin, R. R., and White, A.: The reacquisition of staphylococci by treated carriers: A demonstration of bacterial interference. J. Lab. Clin. Med. *71*:791-797, 1968.

119. McCarthy, C., Snyder, M. L., and Parker, R. B.: The indigenous oral flora of man, I: The newborn to one year old infant. Arch. Oral. Biol. *10*:61-70, 1965.

120. McCormak, W. M., Rosner, B., Alpert, S., et al.: Vaginal colonization with *Mycoplasma hominis* and *Ureaplasma urealyticum*. Sex. Transm. Dis. *13*:67-70, 1986.

121. Montes, L. F., and Wilborn, W. H.: Location of bacterial skin flora. Br. J. Dermatol. *81*(Suppl. I):23-26, 1969.

122. Nord, C. E., Heimdahl, A., and Kager, L.: Antimicrobial induced alterations of the human oropharyngeal and intestinal microflora. Scand. J. Infect. Dis. Suppl. *49*:64-72, 1986.

123. Norrby, S. R.: Ecological consequences of broad spectrum versus narrow spectrum antibacterial therapy. Scand. J. Infect. Dis. Suppl. *49*:189-195, 1986.

124. Ollikainen, J., Heiskanen-Kosma, T., Korppi, M., et al.: Clinical relevance of *Ureasplasma urealyticum* colonization in preterm infants. Acta Paediatr. *87*:1075-1078, 1998.

125. Ostfeld, E., Segal, J., Segal, A., et al.: Bacterial colonization of the nose and external ear canal in newborn infants. Isr. J. Med. Sci. *19*:1046-1049, 1983.

126. Panigrahi P: Necrotizing enterocolitis: A practical guide to its prevention and management. Pediatr. Drugs *8*:151-165, 2006.

127. Paster, B. J., Boches, S., Galvin, J. L., et al.: Bacterial diversity in human subgingival plaque. J. Bacteriol. *183*:3770-3783, 2001.

128. Peek, R. M.: The biological impact of *Helicobacter pylori* colonization. Semin. Gastrointest. Dis. *12*:151-166, 2001.

129. Perkins, R. E., Kundsin, R. B., Pratt, M. V., et al.: Bacteriology of normal and infected conjunctiva. J. Clin. Microbiol. *1*:147-149, 1975.

130. Pichichero, M. E., Marsocci, S. M., Murphy, M. L., et al.: Incidence of streptococcal carriers in private pediatric practice. Arch. Pediatr. Adolesc. Med. 153:624-628, 1999.

131. Pickard, K. M., Bremner, A. R., Gordon, J. N., and MacDonald, T. T.: Microbial-gut interactions in health and disease: Immune responses. Best Pract Res Clin Gastroenterol. 18:271-285, 2004.

132. Ramirez-Ronda, C. H., Fuxench-Lopez, Z., and Nevarez, M.: Increased pharyngeal bacterial colonization during viral illness. Arch. Intern. Med. 141:1599-1603, 1981.

133. Redondo-Lopez, V., Cook, R. L., and Sobel, J. D.: Emerging role of lactobacilli in the control and maintenance of the vaginal bacterial microflora. Rev. Infect. Dis. 12:856-872, 1990.

134. Remington, J. S., and Schimpff, S. C.: Occasional notes: Please don't eat the salads. N. Engl. J. Med. 304:433-435, 1981.

135. Roberts, S. O.: *Pityrosporum orbiculare*: Incidence and distribution on clinically normal skin. Br. J. Dermatol. 81:264-269, 1969.

136. Roberts, S. O.: The mycology of the clinically normal scalp. Br. J. Dermatol. 81:626-628, 1969.

137. Roediger, W. E.: Role of anaerobic bacteria in the metabolic welfare of the colonic mucosa in man. Gut 21:793-798, 1980.

138. Roscoe, D. L., and Chow, A. W.: Normal flora and mucosal immunity of the head and neck. Infect. Dis. Clin. N. Am. 2:1-19, 1988.

139. Rotimi, V. O., and Duerden, B. I.: The development of the bacterial flora in normal neonates. J. Med. Microbiol. 14:51-62, 1981.

140. Royall, D. R., Wolever, T. M., and Jeejeebhoy, K. N.: Clinical significance of colonic fermentation. Am. J. Gastroenterol. 80:1307-1312, 1990.

141. Ruddell, W. S., Axon, A. T., Findlay, J. M., et al.: Effect of cimetidine on the gastric bacterial flora. Lancet 1:672-674, 1980.

142. Ruppin, H., Bar-Meir, S., Soergel, K. H., et al.: Absorption of short chain fatty acids by the colon. Gastroenterology 78:1500-1507, 1980.

143. Saavedra, J. M.: Clinical applications of probiotic agents. Am. J. Clin. Nutr. 73:1147S-1151S, 2001.

144. Sakata, H., Yoshioka, H., and Fujita, K.: Development of the intestinal flora in very low birth weight infants compared to normal full-term infants. Eur. J. Pediatr. 144:186-190, 1985.

145. Sanders, E.: Bacterial interference, I: Its occurrence among the respiratory tract flora and characterization of inhibition of group A streptococci by viridans streptococci. J. Infect. Dis. 120:698-707, 1969.

146. Sanford, B. A., Shelokov, A., and Ramsay, M. A.: Bacterial adherence to virus-infected cells: A cell culture model of bacterial superinfection. J. Infect. Dis. 137:176-181, 1978.

147. Savage, D. S.: Microbial ecology of the gastrointestinal tract. Annu. Rev. Microbiol. 31:107-133, 1977.

148. Seelig, M. S.: The role of antibiotics in the pathogenesis of *Candida* infections. Am. J. Med. 40:887-917, 1966.

149. Sharp, S. E.: Commensal and pathogenic microorganisms of humans. In Murray, P. A., Baron, E. J., Pfaller, M. A., et al. (eds.): Manual of Clinical Microbiology. 7th ed. Washington, D.C., ASM Press, 1999, pp. 23-32.

150. Shopsin, B., Mathema, B., Martinez, J., et al.: Prevalence of methicillin-resistant and methicillin-susceptible *Staphylococcus aureus* in the community. J. Infect. Dis. 182:359-362, 2000.

151. Simon, G. L., and Gorbach, S. L.: Intestinal flora in health and disease. Gastroenterology 86:174-193, 1984.

152. Somerville, D. A.: The normal flora of the skin in different age groups. Br. J. Dermatol. 81:248-258, 1969.

153. Spiegel, C. A.: Bacterial vaginosis. Clin. Microbiol. Rev. 4:485-502, 1991.

154. Spitzer, J., Hennessy, E., and Neville, L.: High group A streptococcal carriage in the Orthodox Jewish community of North Hackney. Br. J. Gen. Pract. 51:101-105, 2001.

155. Sprunt, K., and Redman, W.: Evidence suggesting importance of role in interbacterial inhibition in maintaining balance of normal flora. Ann. Intern. Med. 68:579-590, 1968.

156. Stark, P. L., and Lee, A.: The microbial ecology of the large bowel of breast-fed and formula-fed infants during the first year of life. J. Med. Microbiol. 15:189-203, 1982.

157. Stromberg, A., Schwan, A., and Cars, O.: Throat carrier rates of beta-hemolytic streptococci among healthy adults and children. Scand. J. Infect. Dis. 20:411-417, 1988.

158. Suggs, A. H., Maranan, M. C., Boyle-Vavra, S., et al.: Methicillin-resistant and borderline methicillin-resistant asymptomatic *Staphylococcus aureus* colonization in children without identifiable risk factors. Pediatr. Infect. Dis. J. 18:410-414, 1999.

159. Swartz, M. N., Gibbons, R., and Socransky, S.: Indigenous bacteria: Oral microbiology. In Davis, B. D., Dulbecco, R., Eisen, H. N., et al. (eds.): Microbiology. 4th ed. Philadelphia, J. B. Lippincott, 1990, pp. 727-736.

160. Syringiannopoulos, G. A., Kapatais-Zoumbos, K., Decavalas, G. O., et al.: *Ureaplasma urealyticum* colonization of full term infants: Perinatal acquisition and persistence during early infancy. Pediatr. Infect. Dis. J. 9:236-240, 1990.

161. Takase, H., Nitanai, H., Yamamura, E., et al.: Facilitated expansion of pneumococcal colonization from the nose to the lower respiratory tract in mice preinfected with influenza virus. Microbiol. Immunol. 43:905-907, 1999.

162. Taylor, D. N., and Blaser, M. J.: The epidemiology of *Helicobacter pylori* infection. Epidemiol. Rev. 13:42-59, 1991.

163. Taylor-Robinson, D., and McCormack, W. M.: The genital mycoplasmas. N. Engl. J. Med. 302:1003-1010, 1063-1067, 1980.

164. Theisen, J., Nehra, D., Citron, D., et al.: Suppression of gastric acid secretion in patients with gastroesophageal reflux disease results in gastric bacterial overgrowth and deconjugation of bile acids. J. Gastrointest. Surg. 4:50-54, 2000.

165. Thomas, S., Raman, R., Idikula, J., et al.: Alterations in oropharyngeal flora in patients with a nasogastric tube: A cohort study. Crit. Care. Med. 20:1677-1680, 1992.

166. Thorens, J., Froehlich, F., Schwizer, W., et al.: Bacterial overgrowth during treatment with omeprazole compared with cimetidine: A prospective randomised double blind study. Gut 39:54-59, 1996.

167. Tlaskalova-Hogenova, H., Sterzl, J., Stepankova, R., et al.: Development of immunological capacity under germfree and conventional conditions. Ann. N. Y. Acad. Sci. 409:96-113.

168. Torres, J., Perez-Perez, G., Goodman, K. J., et al.: A comprehensive review of the natural history of *Helicobacter pylori* infection in children. Arch. Med. Res. 31:431-469, 2000.

169. Tramont, E. C., and Hoover, D. L.: Innate (general or nonspecific) host defense mechanisms. In Mandell, G. L., Bennett, J. E., and Dolin, R. (eds.): Principles and Practice of Infectious Diseases. 5th ed. Philadelphia, Churchill Livingstone, 2000, pp. 31-38.

170. Vanden Bergh, M. F., Yzerman, E. P., van Belkum, A., et al.: Follow-up of *Staphylococcus aureus* nasal carriage after 8 years: Redefining the persistent carrier state. J. Clin. Microbiol. 37:3133-3140, 1999.

171. van der Waaij, D., Berghuis-de Vries, J. M., and Lekkerkerk van der Wees, J. E. C.: Colonization resistance of the digestive tract in conventional and antibiotic-treated mice. J. Hyg. 69:405-411, 1971.

172. Vollaard, E. J., and Clasener, H. A.: Colonization resistance. Antimicrob. Agents Chemother. 38:409-414, 1994.

173. Wald, E. R., Milmoe, G. J., Bowen, A., et al.: Acute maxillary sinusitis in children. N. Engl. J. Med. 304:749-754, 1981.

174. Walker, W. A.: Role of nutrients and bacterial colonization in the development of intestinal host defense. J. Pediatr. Gastroenterol. Nutr. 30(Suppl. 2):S2-7, 2000.

175. Wang, M., Ahrne, S., Antonsson, M., and Molin, G.: T-RFLP combined with principal component analysis and 16S rRNA gene sequencing: an effective strategy for comparison of fecal microbiota in infants of different ages. J. Microbiol. Methods 59:53-69 2004.

176. Wang, E. E., Ohlsson, A., and Kellner, J. D.: Association of *Ureaplasma urealyticum* colonization with chronic lung disease of prematurity: Results of a metaanalysis. J. Pediatr. 127:40-644, 1995.

177. Weiss, A., Brinser, J. H., and Nazar-Stewart, V.: Acute conjunctivitis in childhood. J. Pediatr. 122:10-14, 1993.

178. Weiss, K., Laverdiere, M., Lovgren, M., et al.: Group A *Streptococcus* carriage among close contacts of patients with invasive infections. Am. J. Epidemiol. 149:863-868, 1999.

179. Wells, C. L., Maddaus, M. A., Jechorek, R. P., et al.: Role of intestinal anaerobic flora in colonization resistance. Eur. J. Clin. Microbiol. Infect. Dis. 7:107, 1988.

180. Whittaker, C. J., Klier, C. M., and Kolenbrander, P. E.: Mechanisms of adhesion by oral bacteria. Annu. Rev. Microbiol. 50:513-552, 1996.

181. Williams, C.: Occurrence and significance of gastric colonization during acid-inhibitory therapy. Best Pract. Res. Clin. Gastroenterol. 15:511-521, 2001.

182. Yagupsky, P., Landau, D., Beck, A., et al.: Carriage of *Streptococcus pyogenes* among infants and toddlers attending day-care facilities in closed communities in southern Israel. Eur. J. Clin. Microbiol. Infect. Dis. 14:54-58, 1995.

183. Yoshioka, H., Iseki, K., and Fujita, K.: Development and differences of intestinal flora in the neonatal period in breast-fed and bottle-fed infants. Pediatrics 72:317-321, 1983.

184. Young, L. S., LaForce, F. M., Head, J. J., et al.: A simultaneous outbreak of meningococcal and influenza infections. N. Engl. J. Med. 287:5-9, 1972.

185. Yow, M.: Development of *Proteus* and *Pseudomonas* infection during antimicrobial therapy. J. A. M. A. 149:1184-1188, 1952.

CHAPTER 7

EPIDEMIOLOGY OF INFECTIOUS DISEASES

Robert S. Baltimore ✪ Eugene D. Shapiro

Epidemiology is concerned primarily with describing and explaining the occurrence of disease in populations. This chapter is a general review of epidemiology as it relates to infectious diseases important in pediatrics. Readers concerned with the epidemiology of a particular disease should consult the appropriate chapter for the relevant information. The principles and methods of epidemiology must be meshed with biostatistics (presented in detail in Chapter 266) and with information from other fields, including, but not limited to, clinical medicine, microbiology, pathophysiology, immunology, demography, and sociology.

The three types of epidemiology are descriptive, analytic or causative, and experimental. All three types are important in infectious diseases.

Descriptive epidemiology provides accounts of the health experiences of populations, including morbidity and mortality. It may or may not be used to support a hypothesis. The data are of two types—incidence and prevalence. *Incidence* is used to denote the numbers of new cases of or deaths from a given disorder that occurs in a defined population during a specified period. Sequential temporal comparisons often are used for assessing trends, and incidence data frequently are useful for setting public health priorities.

Prevalence is used to denote the number of cases of a disorder in the population (or sample) at a single moment in time. Prevalence data are applicable largely to chronic disorders, such as diabetes mellitus, tuberculosis, or human immunodeficiency virus (HIV) infection, and have no utility when applied to acute disorders, such as measles or infection with respiratory syncytial virus. In addition, in studies of infectious diseases, the prevalence of serologic markers may be used to estimate the immune status of a population or the proportion of a group that has had previous exposure to an infectious agent. Examples that have been useful for vaccine development include meningococcal infections[13] and *Haemophilus influenzae* infections.[2] For certain infections such as tuberculosis and diphtheria, skin testing may serve as a substitute for serologic testing to estimate previous exposure to the agent (or to a vaccine).

Analytic, or *causative,* epidemiology searches for clues to the cause of disease. It is based on the principle that disease does not occur at random in the population and classically considers time, person, and place. In other words, differences exist between individuals who acquire a given disorder and individuals who do not. Identification of these differences may lead to ascertainment of causation, inferences about pathogenic mechanisms, or means of control. These differences may be inherent in the individuals themselves and include biologic characteristics (e.g., hereditary, such as race; acquired, such as immunity) and lifestyle. They may be external and consist largely of environmental risk factors for disease, including various factors that influence the likelihood of exposure to an agent, such as geography, weather, contact with vectors (including other humans), and social and economic conditions. In studies of infectious diseases, considerable overlap exists between descriptive and analytic epidemiology because differences in the distribution of disease by person, place, and time often are obvious in descriptive data and provide clues for further study. Analysis of data may lead to the development of useful hypotheses for studies that then generate new data.

Analytic epidemiologic studies of infectious diseases and studies related to other types of conditions generally fall into three categories. The least frequently used, but nonetheless

useful, category is the cross-sectional study. Such studies can be conducted in one of two ways. One might examine apparently comparable populations with differing prevalence rates of a given infection for characteristics that might explain these different rates. Alternatively, if a disorder is sufficiently common, one can determine rates of disease in individuals with and individuals without a suspected risk factor. A classic example is the relationship of sickle-cell trait to resistance to *Plasmodium falciparum* malaria, which was examined in both ways.[1] In studies of variations in the prevalence of the sickle-cell gene in Africa, researchers noted that the trait seemed to be more prevalent in areas with a high incidence of malaria. Based on this observation, other studies were conducted and showed that in hyperendemic areas, individuals with the sickle-cell trait might have some resistance to malaria, permitting selective survival in these areas. This observation led to additional studies of the mechanism of this phenomenon, including examinations of the roles of blood groups and other characteristics of erythrocytes that influence the risk of acquiring malaria.

Another type of causative or analytic epidemiologic study is the *longitudinal cohort study*. In this type of study, incidence of infection and routes of transmission may be determined by examining groups of individuals with differences in exposure, which may include timing, duration, intimacy of contact, or disparate sources or mechanisms of potential transmission. The classic studies of the transmission of group A streptococcal infection in military recruits are excellent examples. One particular finding was that transmission of infection from individuals with streptococcal pharyngitis to others in military barracks occurred at rates inversely related to distances between bunks, which established that transmission occurred largely by intimate respiratory contact with droplets containing hundreds or thousands of organisms, rather than by airborne droplet nuclei.[34] Other studies showed that fomites, naturally contaminated with streptococci, did not contribute significantly to the transmission of infection.[26] Studies by Goldschneider and colleagues,[13] by following a cohort of Army recruits at a training camp, showed that recruits without bactericidal antibody against the prevalent strain of meningococcus were susceptible to infection.

Studies of the transmission of staphylococci to newborns are another example of prospective epidemiologic observation. In the 1950s, outbreaks of staphylococcal disease, sometimes severe, occurred in newborn nurseries. In an effort to determine how these organisms were transmitted to infants by personnel or other infants, researchers investigated nurseries with persistently high rates of colonization of infants.[23] Two types of prospective cohort studies were conducted. One consisted of instituting measures that prevented transmission by all but one or two routes, permitting assessment of the importance of those routes in transmission. The other method was the reverse: Some suspected routes of transmission were blocked, and subsequent colonization of infants was monitored. These studies showed that transmission of organisms from personnel who were carriers or from previously colonized infants occurred primarily via the hands of personnel.

Another type of analytic epidemiologic study useful in infectious disease is the *case-control study*. In cohort studies, the investigator compares individuals who are exposed or not exposed to a given agent. The outcome measure of the study is infection or no infection. In contrast, in a case-control study, the samples being studied comprise individuals who have the infection compared with similar individuals who do not have the infection. From individuals in both groups, historical data about previous exposure are obtained. In a case-control study, the investigator starts with diseased individuals and searches for exposure; in a cohort study, the investigator starts with exposure and follows subjects forward in time for development of the outcome. Case-control studies can be used to show a vaccine's effectiveness in actual field conditions after it has been licensed. Rather than having to show efficacy by following many thousands of volunteers, Shapiro and colleagues[31] showed the efficacy of pneumococcal vaccine by comparing 1054 people with invasive pneumococcal infections with 1054 matched controls, looking at the rate of vaccination in each group. Of the case patients, 13 percent had received pneumococcal vaccine, whereas 20 percent of the controls had received the vaccine (effectiveness was 47 percent for all patients and 56 percent for serotypes represented in the vaccine).

Case-control studies are of particular utility when the disease is rare because a cohort study might require an unwieldy number of subjects. A disadvantage of retrospective studies is that they do not provide an estimate of the risk or rate of disease occurring after exposure (i.e., the proportion of exposed or of unexposed individuals in whom the disorder in question actually did develop).

A third type of epidemiologic study useful in infectious diseases is an *experimental* study—*the clinical trial*. Clinical trials are actually a special kind of cohort study in which the investigator determines which subjects are exposed to an intervention. Clinical trials generally are used to determine the efficacy of preventive or therapeutic measures. As such, they often require previous information from analytic epidemiologic studies and from other basic and clinical studies. Sometimes, studies that are, in effect, clinical trials may provide useful information regarding the cause or routes of transmission of an infection. If a vaccine composed of a single purified antigen is associated with elimination of the disease, this information provides strong evidence that antibody directed against that antigen is protective.

To assess the efficacy of either therapeutic or preventive measures, experimental epidemiologic studies require comparison groups of individuals who do not receive the measure in question. Generally, these individuals are given an older agent, an alternative agent, a placebo, or an agent that would have no effect on the infection in question. Having contemporaneous controls is especially important for diseases that have significant year-to-year variation in incidence, to ensure that a decrease in incidence after introducing an intervention was not just a natural event.

An important component of a controlled clinical trial is that treatment and control groups be as similar as possible in characteristics that may affect the outcome. Clinical trials designed to assess the efficacy of either therapeutic or preventive measures must take into consideration many such factors, which usually include age, sex, socioeconomic status, co-morbid diseases, and likelihood of exposure. In any trial, an effort should be made to balance treated and untreated subjects in terms of recognized factors. Not all variables that may lead to bias in the results are recognized in advance, however. To try to ensure as far as possible that these characteristics are distributed approximately equally between the two groups, the process of randomization almost always is necessary. In addition, true randomization must occur; methods involving odd-versus-even record numbers or birth dates, alternate days of the week, and the like are inappropriate. An optimal method is a system of random numbers, as published in most textbooks of biostatistics or available as computer programs. Randomization avoids selection bias, best defined as underlying differences between the treatment and control groups, whether internal (inherent) or external (e.g., the likelihood of exposure). Randomization ensures only lack of bias because one has no assurance in a small clinical trial that

unrecognized confounders are distributed equally among groups being compared. If the size of the sample is large, however, unequal distribution, although not impossible, becomes unlikely. Chapter 266 provides a more extensive discussion of types of bias.

Although the principles discussed here and in Chapter 266 apply to all epidemiologic studies, in studies of infectious diseases, three additional factors contribute uniquely to who is and who is not affected: (1) The cause is a specific external agent (the infecting organism); (2) transmission of the organism to the host is required; and (3) certain host factors, such as immunity to infection or disease, may affect the outcome. Recognition of these factors (the infecting agent, transmission, and immunity) evolved gradually over many years.

HISTORICAL PERSPECTIVES

Epidemiology evolved from the study of great epidemic diseases such as plague, cholera, and smallpox. The periodic waves of these diseases, which were associated with high mortality rates, stimulated the first serious efforts to explain the occurrence of disease on the basis of factors other than supernatural or divine forces.

Fundamental to such explanations was the concept of contagion. This factor long had been implicit in attitudes toward victims of leprosy, as exemplified by such early Christian practices as conducting antemortem funerals for lepers, who then were given a bell and cup and forbidden further human contact or, more drastically, were buried alive or burned at the stake.[28] The English physician Thomas Sydenham (1624-1689) introduced laudanum (derived from opium) as a painkiller; recognized the efficacy of Peruvian bark (quinine) in malaria; and revived the Hippocratic idea of "epidemic constitutions" (of atmospheric nature), which by grafting onto existing illness, gave all concurrent illnesses the character reflecting the then prevailing "constitution." These views persisted in colonial America, where they were expounded by such eminent individuals as Noah Webster (of dictionary fame) and Dr. Benjamin Rush of Philadelphia.[37]

Nonetheless, by the mid-18th century, the theory of contagion had gained acceptance for particular diseases, including measles, syphilis, and smallpox. The theory is alleged to have been exploited in an early act of biologic warfare: Massachusetts colonists reportedly presented the blankets of smallpox victims as gifts to the Indians, who then suffered a decimating epidemic.[9a]

The true origin of the concept of immunity is uncertain, but it was applied first in relation to smallpox. Variolation (inoculation of young people with lesion material expected to induce modified, but immunizing, disease) was practiced in China in the 11th or 12th century and in England and the American colonies in the early 18th century. Also popular in rural England at this time was the theory that cowpox, the minor disease acquired from afflicted cattle, induced immunity to smallpox. This theory was verified by Edward Jenner (reported in 1798) and resulted years later in general acceptance of cowpox vaccine (vaccinia) to protect against smallpox.

The germ theory of disease was stated explicitly in 1855 by John Snow, an English anesthesiologist who took up cholera epidemiology as an avocation. Snow argued that the causative agent of cholera was a living cell that multiplied with great rapidity but was too small to be seen under the microscopes then in use.[32] Louis Pasteur (1822-1895) formally validated the germ theory by showing that the microorganisms responsible for fermentation were not generated spontaneously but came from the air.[25] On this basis, Joseph Lord Lister revolutionized surgery by using carbolic acid to combat atmospheric germs and minimize "putrification" in surgical procedures.[30]

In Pasteur's wake, bacteria were cultured with great frequency from ill individuals and often were identified erroneously as causal agents. Robert Koch (1843-1910), who first isolated the bacterial causes of tuberculosis and cholera, also was the first to introduce scientific rigor into the proof of primary causation. His famed "postulates," to be satisfied before a causal relationship between a bacterium and a disease could be accepted, required that (1) the presence of the agent be shown in every case by its recovery in pure culture; (2) the agent not be found in cases of other disease; (3) the agent, when isolated, be capable of reproducing the disease in experimental animals; and (4) the agent be recovered in pure culture from such experimental disease.[12]

Koch's postulates since have been modified, largely to meet problems posed by viruses. As obligate intracellular parasites, viruses cannot be "cultivated in pure culture." In addition, they often are host-specific and do not produce disease in an animal model. Other considerations that were invoked as elements of proof included the significance of recovery of the agent from diseased tissues, the demonstration of an increase in titer of specific antibody in temporal relation to the disease, and, most conclusive, the specific preventive effect of vaccines containing the viral antigen.[16] One further situation not recognized by Koch is that infections with true pathogens do not always cause disease. We now recognize pathogenicity (defined as the proportion of infections that result in disease) as an important characteristic of infectious disease agents.

CAUSE OF DISEASE

GENERAL CONCEPTS

Causation of infectious diseases is defined in terms of the *primary cause* and *contributing factors* (or secondary causes). The former is the specific microorganism (the agent of disease) without which the particular disease cannot occur. Contributing factors affect the likelihood that infection will occur and help determine that disease will result, given infection. Identification of the causative agent may lead to the development of effective means for providing specific protective immunization (e.g., diphtheria and tetanus toxoids, vaccines against polio and measles). Finding the cause of a disease also may lead to other means of control. An example is the discovery of *Legionella pneumophila* as the cause of legionnaires' disease. The discovery of the organism led to the understanding of how the disease is transmitted—via aerosols from cooling towers, which serve as reservoirs for the bacteria.[8,22] Disinfection of these towers has helped to control legionnaires' disease.

Infection and disease are not synonymous, although infection is necessary for disease to occur. *Infection* denotes colonization, multiplication, and completion of the entire pathogenetic process of the organism in the host, usually including induction of an immune response, but without necessarily producing recognizable pathologic and clinical manifestations. *Disease* is present when pathologic and clinical changes occur with infection. There are many examples of infections that may be either asymptomatic or the cause of serious disease in the host, such as poliomyelitis and mumps. When disease occurs, it may vary in severity among infected individuals. Some infections produce full-blown disease in all infected susceptible individuals; measles is an example. Simple *colonization*, in contrast to infection and disease, is a state in which the organism parasitizes the host at an appropriate site, replicates, and may persist, but it fails to proceed further with the processes of infection and disease, including induction of immunity. The *carrier state*, in which the organism persists over time and can be infective for others, may occur after colonization, infection, or disease. Examples of organisms that behave in this way include group A streptococcus and *Neisseria meningitidis*.

Many contributing factors, largely related to the host and to the conditions of exposure, determine whether colonization occurs and whether the subsequent processes of infection and disease occur. These contributing or risk factors are many and varied, and from the standpoint of the host may include, but are not limited to, age, sex, race, immune status, genetic constitution, and general state of health, including underlying diseases. Similarly, contributing factors unrelated to the host may include climate, the presence of vectors, quality of sanitation, intimacy of exposure, and socioeconomic conditions. These contributing factors vary among infectious diseases and are discussed in chapters about specific infectious agents.

AGENT FACTORS

What characteristics of living parasites are significant epidemiologically? Properties directly important to the occurrence of disease are properties that relate to perpetuation of the agent as a species, properties that govern the type of contact required to infect humans, and properties that determine the production of disease. Also important are characteristics useful in classification and specific identification of agents. Some important characteristics are *intrinsic*, in that they can be described after appropriate direct examination of the agent. Others can be described only on the basis of the behavior of the agents in the host; they are *host related*.

Intrinsic Properties

Precise classification and identification of agents are basic to the specific recognition of infections and related disease. Both depend on intrinsic properties, including morphology (which alone provides the basis for identifying most higher parasites), chemical composition (the type of nucleic acid being important in viral classification), and antigenic character. The last is central to specific identification of agent isolates and antibodies induced by infection. Requirements for growth or replication provide keys to the identification of some bacteria (e.g., sugar fermentation) and many viruses that replicate optimally or only in cultures of certain types of cells incubated at specified temperatures. Rhinoviruses replicate best in human diploid cells incubated at 33° C.

In recent years, rapid development of species detection and classification by genome identification has occurred. The use of whole-genome analysis, molecular analysis of gene fragments, and various methods of polymerase chain reaction has resulted in reclassification of some microorganisms and of rapid identification of pathogens, including microorganisms that cannot be cultivated by conventional means. Developments in this field are expected to shift the clinical microbiology laboratory from morphologic and biochemical tests to molecular tests in the coming years.

Several intrinsic properties relate to transmission and long-term survival of infectious agents. Persistence in the free state outside the host depends on requirements for replication (viruses replicate only within the cells of their host, whereas the nutrient requirements of bacteria often exist in food or milk) and on viability under natural conditions of temperature, moisture, and radiation. The ability of agents to persist determines whether transmission requires direct contact, as with influenza viruses, or can involve indirect mechanisms operating over longer periods. Examples include polioviruses, typhoid bacilli, and the bacterial cause of legionnaires' disease.

The spectrum of animals and arthropods that an agent can parasitize (the host range) helps determine the possibilities for successful links in the transmission and reservoir mechanisms. The broader the range, the greater the possibilities. Agents that use arthropod vectors include St. Louis encephalitis virus and

Borrelia burgdorferi, the cause of Lyme disease. The former can infect many avian and mammalian species and a wide range of mosquitoes, whereas the latter is restricted to a few tick species. Among agents requiring no vector, many infect only humans (diphtheria bacillus, the meningococcus, and measles virus), whereas others have multiple natural hosts (rabies virus, most of the *Salmonella* group of bacteria).

Elaboration of exotoxins is an intrinsic attribute of many bacteria and contributes in varying degrees to disease pathogenesis and indirectly to immunity in many infections. Another attribute, which can operate in two opposing ways, is susceptibility to chemotherapeutic agents or antibiotics. Successful treatment may shorten the period of communicability, as in group A streptococcal and *Bordetella pertussis* infections, but it may lead to relaxed precautions against infection; syphilis and gonorrhea are notable examples.

The instability of some intrinsic characteristics as a result of the emergence of genetically different populations because of mutations, selective pressure, gene or plasmid transfer between bacteria, or genetic recombination can be important. One example is the resistance to chemotherapeutic or antibiotic agents that may result from selective pressure (the probable explanation for the rapid acquisition of multiple antibiotic resistance by gonococci and in HIV or plasmid transfer of resistance to antibiotics among enteric bacteria). Antibiotic resistance is of increasing importance, as exemplified by the appearance of multidrug-resistant *Mycobacterium tuberculosis*, penicillin-resistant pneumococci, and methicillin-resistant staphylococci.

Change in antigenic character can diminish the effectiveness of immunity and complicate specific recognition of infection. Influenza A virus is the classic example, with periodic major changes (shift) occurring in either or both crucial surface antigens, hemagglutinin and neuraminidase, associated with pandemic disease and progressive minor changes in hemagglutinin in the interpandemic period. Finally, the emergence of new diseases, such as St. Louis encephalitis, which first affected humans in Paris, Illinois, in 1932, or the appearance of a known disease in a new reservoir, possibly exemplified by the emergence of West Nile virus in North America, can be the result of adaptation of the agent to a new host.[3,4]

Host-Related Properties

Some epidemiologically important properties of infectious agents can be defined only with reference to specific hosts. Such properties include infectivity, pathogenicity, virulence, and immunogenicity.

INFECTIVITY

Infectivity (ability to invade and multiply in a host) is measured conceptually in terms of the minimal number of infective particles required to establish an infection. This number, which can vary from one host to another and within the same host, depending on the portal of entry, host age, and, in some cases, medications, can be determined only experimentally. Except for benign agents such as rhinoviruses or vaccine strains of polioviruses with which challenge of human volunteers is permissible, the infectivity of agents for humans must be inferred from the facility with which they spread in populations or, more directly, from the frequency with which infection develops in exposed susceptible individuals within a reasonable incubation period (*secondary attack rate*). Some researchers have used prisoners to study infectivity of *Salmonella* and *Shigella*, but the ethics of such studies has been questioned. Measles, varicella, and polioviruses are highly infective because they require few infective particles to cause infection; rubella, mumps, and rhinoviruses have intermediate infectivity; and typhoid and tubercle bacilli have low infectivity. Infectivity

and pathogenicity may vary among strains of the same organism. The infectivity of group A streptococci is related directly to the amount of M protein in the cell wall, and strains of *Staphylococcus aureus* that appear identical in the laboratory may differ strikingly in infectivity and virulence. Additionally, some evidence indicates that strains of influenza A may vary in infectivity and virulence independent of preexisting immunity in the host. Contemporary studies show that variation in certain genes that are not ordinarily expressed in the clinical diagnostic laboratory are responsible for these variations in infectivity.

PATHOGENICITY

Pathogenicity (ability to induce disease) is measured in terms of the proportion of infections that result in disease. It ordinarily can be determined readily by studies of the incidence and outcome of naturally occurring infections in humans. This proportion may be affected by the size of the infecting dose and numerous host factors, including age. Highly pathogenic agents include typhoid bacilli, rabies, measles, varicella, and rhinoviruses. Agents of intermediate pathogenicity include rubella, mumps, and adenoviruses; polioviruses and the tubercle bacillus have low pathogenicity.

VIRULENCE

Virulence, offered as a synonym for *pathogenicity* in medical dictionaries, is defined more usefully as a measure of the severity of the disease that does occur. Various criteria may be used: days confined to bed, serious sequelae such as persisting paralysis, and death. The measure of virulence is the number of severe cases over the total number of cases, which when death is the criterion becomes the familiar *case-fatality rate*. With this as our measure, the viral agents previously mentioned fall into a different gradient from that based on pathogenicity. Rabies virus (with a case-fatality rate of nearly 100 percent) qualifies as highly virulent, and poliovirus (with a case-fatality rate of 7 to 10 percent for paralytic disease) can be classed as moderately virulent. Measles, with an occasional death from encephalitis or pneumonia, is far down the scale but is still ahead of mumps, varicella, non-fetal rubella, and rhinoviruses, for which the case-fatality rates are very low. Outcomes of severity short of death can be used in a similar fashion.

IMMUNOGENICITY

Immunogenicity (ability to induce specific immunity) is measured best in terms of the degree and duration of resistance conferred by infection. Although agents may differ with respect to the immunogenicity of their intrinsic "protective antigens," more important factors are the sites of primary infection and disease, and the amount of antigen formed during infection to stimulate a host response. Superficial sites, such as the respiratory mucosa, are guarded chiefly by secretory antibody, which is poorly persistent; agents such as rhinoviruses, which replicate only at such sites, are ineffective stimulants of the systemic immune response. The amounts of the respective toxins released during clinical tetanus and diphtheria usually do not induce satisfactory immunity. In contrast, systemic viral infections, as with measles and yellow fever viruses, induce solid and long-lasting immunity.

Agent-Host Relationship

The infected host provides a shelter in which the agent can multiply and from which it may spread. Key questions involve how long the agent can persist in the host and over what period and by what avenues it can escape. The time relationships and descrip-

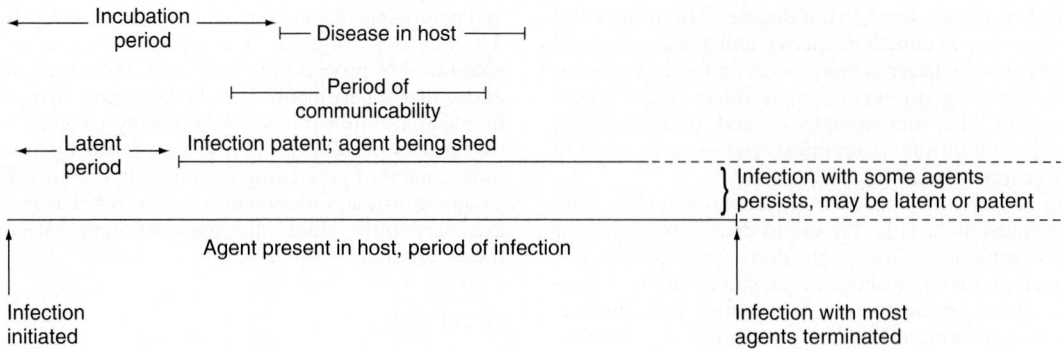

Figure 7–1 Important phases of infection in vertebrate hosts.

tive terms of different phases of infection are suggested schematically in Figure 7–1.

When the agent is not readily recoverable but perhaps is hidden within host cells or at some other site, infection is termed *latent*. Conversely, when the agent is being shed, as in feces or respiratory secretions, or can be recovered from blood or tissues, infection is said to be *patent*. Infections are necessarily latent at first (the *latent period*) and become patent when the agent has multiplied sufficiently for shedding to begin. The *period of communicability* commonly starts soon after initial shedding begins and continues as long as the level of shedding is sufficient for transmission. The rapidity with which disease is spread is related to the length of the latent period, which almost always is shorter (sometimes much shorter) than the better known *incubation period* (time until disease develops). The period of communicability has no consistent relationship to either the occurrence or the duration of disease.

Persistence in the host is important to the agent for as long as escape remains possible. The period of persistence (see Fig. 7–1) varies widely among agents. Infection terminates completely within 2 to 3 weeks with many agents, such as most respiratory viruses, and after a few months with some agents, such as polioviruses or adenoviruses. Truly persistent lifelong infections may become permanently latent as with some herpesvirus group (Epstein-Barr virus, cytomegalovirus) infections. Infection may remain permanently patent (approximately 3 percent of typhoid cases, numerous hepatitis B virus infections), may be intermittently patent (herpes simplex virus infections [HSV]), or after years of latency may recrudesce with patency and associated disease (tuberculosis, Brill disease caused by *Rickettsia prowazekii*, varicella-zoster virus [herpes zoster]).

RESERVOIRS OF INFECTIOUS AGENTS

Reservoir is defined here as the total mechanism responsible for perpetuation of an infectious agent. The reservoir is a continuing chain of transmission from one host to another (including vertebrate and invertebrate species). Chains with long links requiring infrequent transmission are especially favorable to survival of agent species.

Among agents for which humans are the only natural vertebrate host, many contrasting patterns exist. The most common is exemplified by infections with most respiratory viruses, which are characterized by short latent periods (1 to several days) and short periods of communicability (rarely >1 week). The links are short, and frequent transmission is necessary. At the other extreme are long-persisting infections associated with continuous (typhoid carriers, hepatitis B virus, HIV) or intermittent (HSV) patency or shedding. The links in this case may be as long as the

post-infection life of the host and render generation-to-generation transmission possible. Such transmission also may occur via congenital infection, as in mice infected with lymphocytic choriomeningitis virus. Examples in humans include cytomegalovirus and hepatitis B virus infections. Long links also occur in persistent infections that after many years of latency recrudesce to cause disease and renewed shedding (varicella-zoster virus and *R. prowazekii*).

When infection of invertebrate hosts (vectors) is a link in the chain of transmission, a wide range of reservoir patterns is possible. The simplest involves agents for which humans are the only natural vertebrate hosts (malarial parasites, *R. prowazekii*, dengue virus), with the chain consisting of alternating links of human and vector infection. More commonly, the basic reservoir is a similar alternating chain primarily involving lower vertebrate hosts, with humans being an opportunistic and usually blind-end host. Examples include murine typhus rickettsiae and plague bacillus (both cycling primarily in rats and rat fleas), Lyme disease, and various arboviruses (yellow fever, St. Louis encephalitis). In the case of the latter, the broad vertebrate (numerous avian and mammalian species) and invertebrate (various mosquito species) host range results in very complex patterns that in a given area are defined by the prevalent susceptible host species. The links in these chains are defined temporally by the persistence of patent infection in the vertebrate host and the short life span of the invertebrate host.

Several aspects of infection of the invertebrate (vector) host are important. Typically, infection is acquired in a blood meal and endures for (and does not influence) the life span of the arthropod. Hibernating arthropods may be the long link in the chain by which the agent survives the winter. In at least two instances, infection kills the vector: *R. prowazekii* in the body louse and plague bacilli in the rat flea. As with malaria, infection of the arthropod also may permit completion of an essential stage in the developmental cycle of the agent. Finally, transmission of infection from arthropod to arthropod may be alternate or necessary links in the chain. Transovarial transmission of *Rickettsia tsutsugamushi* (scrub typhus) in mites is essential because the individual mite feeds only once, during the larval stage, on vertebrate hosts. Transovarial transmission also occurs in ticks infected with *Rickettsia rickettsii* (Rocky Mountain spotted fever) and in *Aedes triseriatus* mosquitoes infected with La Crosse virus (California encephalitis), in both cases affording an overwintering mechanism. Venereal transmission of La Crosse virus between mosquitoes also has been shown.[33]

Finally, the inanimate environment can play a role in the reservoir mechanism. Examples are bacteria that can multiply in the free state (salmonellae and staphylococci in food) and agents endowed with unusual survival capacity (tetanus bacillus and *Histoplasma capsulatum*, both of which form highly resistant spores).

It also occurs when a brief sojourn under proper environmental conditions is required for a necessary stage in the life cycle (e.g., hookworm eggs from human feces must hatch into larvae to become infectious).

MECHANISMS OF TRANSMISSION

Transmission, in this context, is defined as the transport of an agent from one vertebrate host to another. It involves escape from the source host and conveyance to and entry into the recipient host. The basic interdependence of these sequential steps is illustrated in Table 7–1, which also presents specific examples of diseases. Although humans are the usual or only source for most agents of human disease, lower vertebrates serve as the major or only (rabies virus) source for some pathogens.

Fomites are intimate personal articles, such as handkerchiefs, playthings, and eating utensils. *Direct contact* includes not only physical contact (shaking hands, kissing, sexual intercourse) but also, in practice, short-range (within 3 ft), airborne transmission by large droplets (>5 μm) containing hundreds or thousands of organisms that descend rapidly to the ground or floor. These heavy droplets are the primary route of transmission of group A streptococcal pharyngitis,[34] pertussis, and influenza virus.

Indirect transmission for respiratory and some other infections includes the acquisition of organisms from dust (e.g., tubercle bacilli), from fomites (inanimate objects in the environment such as bedding), and from airborne droplet nuclei (<5 μm) containing only one or a few organisms that promptly dry, float in the air for long periods, and may be wafted for moderately long distances, such as between rooms or floors in a hospital. Transmission by airborne droplet nuclei is limited to highly infectious agents such as varicella virus. Because respiratory colonization with group A streptococci requires a large inoculum, airborne droplet nuclei play no role in their transmission. Other forms of indirect transmission include inanimate vectors such as food, milk, and water, which are frequent vehicles for spread, particularly of intestinal infections. Another source of indirect transmission is animate vectors, which either may function as a vehicle for transport (as with flies that carry organisms from feces to food) or may be infected. In the latter case, multiplication and transformation in the vector are required for transmission, as with African trypanosomiasis and the tsetse fly.

Conveyance ends when the agent reaches a portal of entry, which to be effective must provide ready access to a tissue in which the pathogen can lodge and multiply. For a given agent, a particular portal (nasal or genital mucosa, oral) often is obligatory or usual, but alternative portals may be possible. Rhinoviruses replicate only in nasal mucosa, whereas typhus rickettsiae typically enter through skin broken by a louse bite but also can infect via ocular or respiratory mucous membranes.

HOST FACTORS

Many biologic and behavioral characteristics of the human host influence the occurrence of infection and subsequent disease. Although the host characteristics to be considered are of widely differing nature, they operate by influencing one or more of the following: degree of exposure, innate susceptibility to infection, and the likelihood of specific immunity. Although much of the following discussion focuses on the individual human host, factors that influence individuals also affect whole human populations.

Infection of the Host

A key principle to be emphasized is the usual existence of a gradient of response to exposure to an infectious agent. Because of this gradient, the occurrence of characteristic overt disease is a notably unreliable measure of the extent of activity of a disease agent. Given a particular exposure, infection may not occur, disease may not result, or the consequences may range from trivial to the fully developed syndrome "characteristic" of the agent. Accumulating data indicate that specific host genes may be responsible for differences in host susceptibility.

An inadequate challenge dose, an unsuitable portal of entry, or specific host immunity also may explain failure of infection to develop. Whether infection causes disease and the extent, nature, and outcome of the resulting disease are determined partly by host-related properties of the agent (pathogenicity and virulence) and partly by host defense mechanisms, a variety of which confront an infectious agent that has reached a site of primary infection. Bacteria and other extracellular parasites stimulate an inflammatory response at the site in an effort to localize the invaders by a retaining fibrin network, and the invaders are destroyed by congregating numerous phagocytic cells. Invader organisms meet sinusoidal passages lined by phagocytic cells in regional (lymph nodes) and bloodstream (bone marrow, spleen, and liver) filters. In addition, clinicians are beginning to understand the importance of so-called innate immunity. This complex network of receptors and responders prevents invader microorganisms from gaining access to tissues. In addition to physical barriers already mentioned, the innate immune system includes a family of receptors known as the Toll-like receptors. These recognition molecules signal the host to activate numerous protective mechanisms. They are discussed in other chapters in this textbook.

Several aspects of the outcome of infection are important, the first being survival of the host. Death is an unsatisfactory outcome not only for the host but also for the many agents for which survival as a species depends on the host. The remaining aspects relate to the surviving host. Was recovery from disease complete,

TABLE 7–1   Typical Modes of Transmission from Host, Conveyance, and Portal of Entry

Agent Shed via	How Conveyed	Portal of Entry	Disease Example
Respiratory secretions	Airborne droplets, fomites, or direct contact	Respiratory	Common cold, influenza, respiratory syncytial virus
Feces	Food, fomites, water, flies	Oral	Poliomyelitis, typhoid, rotavirus
Blood	Arthropod vector, transfusion, needle-stick	Skin—via insect bite, intravenous device	Typhus, dengue, malaria, human immunodeficiency virus, hepatitis B and C
Lesion exudate	Direct contact, sexual intercourse, fomites, flies	Skin, genital or ocular mucous membrane	Syphilis, trachoma, staphylococcal abscess
Aerosols	Droplet nuclei, direct inhalation	Respiratory	Tuberculosis, varicella

or were permanent sequelae present? If the latter, were they stationary (as in paralysis resulting from polioviruses) or potentially progressive (rheumatic heart disease resulting from streptococcal infection, pulmonary tuberculosis)? Another aspect, persistence of the agent, was discussed previously under agent-host relationships. The final aspect is the state of post-infection resistance. If it is incomplete, the recovered host may experience reinfection, with or without disease, and again become a source of infection for others.

Biologic Factors

Biologic factors include characteristics such as age, sex, and race (ethnic group), which are so important and easily ascertained that determining their relationship to occurrence of disease is a usual first step in an epidemiologic description. Biologic factors also include genetic make-up, general health status, and specific immunity.

AGE

The influence of age is illustrated best by patterns of common diseases such as varicella, measles, and mumps before the advent of vaccines. All three diseases occur predominantly in young children, who are affected because of their usual lack of immunity and their high risk of exposure to other children, among whom most infections occur. Older individuals are likely to be immune and, unless they are parents of young children, are unlikely to be exposed to infected individuals. Vaccines that provide only temporary immunity could cause a shift to an older age of presentation in the population.

Age also often is related to the outcome of infections in nonimmune individuals. Demonstration of the influence of age requires that all infections be recognized and classified according to the severity of the resulting disease (if any). When many or most infections are subclinical (as with polioviruses and other enteroviruses), the increase in the case-fatality rate with age is apparent immediately, but special studies to document asymptomatic or mild infections are required to show that the proportion of infections that resulted in clinical disease also increased with age. In contrast, the case-fatality rate for pertussis is highest in young infants. With measles and varicella-zoster virus, initial infection at any age usually results in characteristic disease, but the frequency of serious disease increases with age.

SEX AND RACE OR ETHNIC GROUP

That sex may be a factor is illustrated by the fact that most infectious diseases typically occur more frequently in males than females. The question, with respect to any particular disease, is whether these differences between sexes reflect innate differences in susceptibility to disease or can be attributed to sex-associated differences in behavior, occupation, or stress.

The incidence of many diseases varies greatly between groups defined by race or ethnic group. This variation may be explained by differences in behavior or environment for which socioeconomic status is a marker. Ethnic groups share many genetically determined traits, however, which may include either heightened susceptibility or increased resistance to specific infectious agents. Selective evolutionary pressure may be invoked to explain the greater resistance of whites to tuberculosis and the heightened resistance of blacks to malaria. Differences in host susceptibility based on race, familial clustering, and ethnicity is beginning to be investigated at the genomic level now that the code for the whole human genome has been elucidated. Future investigations likely will be directed at discovering polymorphisms of genes that involve the immune response.

GENERAL HEALTH STATUS

General health status includes the physiologic state, nutritional status, presence of intercurrent disease, and stress. The importance of such factors is commonly accepted in many cases but rarely documented by well-controlled studies. Infancy, during which immune mechanisms are immature, is a period of special vulnerability to many infectious diseases. HSV, enteroviruses, and group B streptococci manifest as disseminated infections in neonates, in marked contrast to their presentation in older individuals. Puberty, associated with rapid growth and change in endocrine balance, is a period of vulnerability to acne and tuberculosis. Pregnancy predisposes to tuberculosis and paralytic poliomyelitis, and varicella is more severe.

Gross protein malnutrition causes definite impairment in the cell-mediated immune response,[17a] a correspondingly increased susceptibility to bacterial and parasitic infections, and increased morbidity and mortality in many viral infections. Viral infections may depress cell-mediated immunity (and increase susceptibility further) to other concurrent infections. In the developing world, where malnutrition may be epidemic, the consequences of diarrhea, measles, and other respiratory virus infections are many times more devastating. Diarrheal diseases also may be the cause and the consequence of malnutrition. Diabetics are especially vulnerable to bacterial infections; measles and pertussis may reactivate quiescent tuberculosis; and, perhaps of greatest importance, otherwise benign respiratory viral infections, notably influenza, may pave the way for development of serious bacterial pneumonia. HIV infection enhances the susceptibility to and severity of tuberculosis, toxoplasmosis, and many other infections.

Finally, stress induced by widely divergent stimuli (including strong emotions, physical exertion, trauma, or excessive heat or cold), according to Selye,[29] may operate through a pituitary-adrenocortical hormonal path to decrease resistance to infections. Widely accepted examples include physical exertion, child-bearing, and rearing of children as factors predisposing to paralytic poliomyelitis and pregnancy and rapid growth during puberty as causes of reactivation of quiescent tuberculosis.

IMMUNITY AND IMMUNE RESPONSE

Immunity and immune response to viruses warrant special attention. Although important in recovery from bacterial infection, antibody response is of questionable significance in viral infections because viruses within cells are inaccessible to antibody, and by the time antibody appears, many or most susceptible cells have been infected already. Nonetheless, the importance of antibody in viral infections is suggested by the great vulnerability of immunodeficient children to vaccine strains of poliovirus, other enteroviruses, and varicella and by the sometimes beneficial effect of passive immunotherapy in progressive vaccinia. The benefits of previous experience with viruses can be seen with the decreased severity of rotavirus infections following the first bout of rotavirus and the protection afforded by varicella-zoster immunoglobulin in highly vulnerable children.

At its maximum (exemplified by post-infection immunity to measles), protection against infection is virtually absolute. At the other extreme (exemplified by many respiratory viral infections), susceptibility to infection persists or wanes as with pertussis, although the severity of related disease may be reduced. In most instances, protection seems to be mediated by antibody, but cell-mediated immunity also may be important. Children with defects in cell-mediated immunity are at particular risk for acquiring infection with varicella, *Pneumocystis carinii*, and otherwise noninvasive fungi.

To the extent that immunity protects the individual against infection or acts to minimize shedding of the agent when infection occurs, an immune host can play little or no part in the spread of an infectious agent in the population. If a sufficient proportion of a population is immune, an agent transmitted via contact cannot spread, and non-immune members of the population would be spared exposure. The concept of herd immunity assumes that a non-immune individual is protected from a communicable infection by being surrounded by immune individuals. What proportion must be immune to achieve effective *herd immunity* usually is unknown.[10] This concept is valid only in homogeneous, randomly mixing populations in which all possible pairs of individuals have the same probability of making effective contact. Although measles vaccine has been used extensively in the United States, outbreaks of measles continue to occur in segments of the population that failed to accept vaccine, often defined by beliefs, race, economic status, and social behavior.

Human Behavior

Governed largely by habits of the individual and the customs and culture of groups, human behavior greatly influences exposure to and modes of transmission of infectious agents. Cultural factors also underlie attitudes toward preventive and curative practices.

Water is a potential vehicle for many agents. When commonly imbibed without boiling, as in the United States, community water systems constitute potential channels for transmission that usually are well-guarded. Occasional operational failures occur, as exemplified by failure of a water quality–monitoring device in a filtration plant that resulted in an outbreak of *Cryptosporidium* diarrhea affecting an estimated 403,000 individuals in Milwaukee in 1993.[20] Foods and milk, especially items that are consumed raw or after minimal cooking, likewise are excellent vehicles for transmission of disease. Well-known examples include trichinosis from undercooked pork; bacterial enteritis from unpasteurized milk; fish tapeworm from raw fish; and various forms of food poisoning caused by bacterial contamination during handling, poor refrigeration, and inadequate cooking. In recent years, outbreaks of hemorrhagic diarrhea caused by *Escherichia coli* O157:H7, sometimes associated with hemolytic-uremic syndrome, have occurred as a result of improperly prepared products of bovine origin, particularly ground beef.[14]

Closely related to water and foods is the disposal of human excreta. Casual defecation near habitations or in or near running water leads to dissemination of enteric pathogens by filth flies and by water. The use of human feces (night soil) to fertilize crops commonly eaten raw, such as strawberries and lettuce, has an obvious similar potential.

Many more individual types of behavior also are important. Infrequent bathing and laundering of clothes favor infestation with body lice. Inadequate clothing increases exposure to arthropod vectors and, as in young children lightly clad for summer weather, facilitates the exchange of feces. Going barefoot provides exposure to hookworm larvae. Handwashing minimizes the role of hands in indirect transmission of enteric (fecal) and respiratory (nasal secretion) pathogens. Rhinovirus infections result from inserting contaminated fingers into the nose and eyes.[15] Intimate personal contact such as hand shaking, kissing, and play among young children fosters the spread of a wide variety of agents. Even recreation, such as travel, picnics, and camping, may lead to unusual exposure to infectious agents. Sexual behavior is associated with the transmission of numerous infections, including HIV, syphilis, gonorrhea, group B streptococci, and hepatitis B.

ENVIRONMENTAL FACTORS

The environment in concept embraces all that is external to the individual human host. There are three broad environmental areas: *physical*, which includes geologic and climatologic or mete-orologic features; *biologic*, which consists of all flora and fauna and all living microbial pathogens; and *socioeconomic*, which encompasses the interrelationships of humans. Environmental factors often act through indirect paths, and some have the potential to affect the agent, the host, and the agent-host relationship. Solar radiation is lethal for many pathogens in the free state, helps humans synthesize vitamin D, and can provoke recrudescence of a latent HSV infection and result in recurrent fever blisters. The capacity of humans to modify adverse environmental conditions beneficially is another important factor.

Geographic and Geologic Factors

Spread of infectious agents on a global scale requires their transport, which is influenced by distance alone and by geographic features—mountain ranges, oceans, rivers—that assist or impede travel. The importance of these factors declines as the extent and speed of travel increase, but it remains substantial, especially in developing countries. The minimal effect of geographic barriers in containing highly infective agents is overcome by modern travel, and rapid spread by airline travel is exemplified by epidemics of severe acute respiratory syndrome, which spread from China throughout the world in a matter of weeks.

The natural paths of travel (including waterways), natural harbors, and the location of mineral deposits help determine where populations concentrate. Water supply, dependent in part on geologic formations, is a factor limiting population size and, together with fossil fuels and mineral deposits, influences the type, extent, and location of industrial development. Soil types vary greatly in their ability to hold and purify water and in their capacity to support vegetation, which influences the type and abundance of animal life. Soil is a determinant of the type and importance of agriculture and a major factor influencing the biologic environment.

Climate

The term *climate* describes the typical annual pattern, along with its seasonal variation, of climatologic conditions in a specified region. Such conditions (climatologic factors) include solar radiation, temperature, humidity, barometric pressure, winds, precipitation (and drought), and lightning. These factors can affect infectious disease agents directly. Many microbial agents in the free state are vulnerable to excessive heat and radiation and uncontrolled drying. The life cycles and reservoir mechanisms of many pathogens, including higher parasites, depend on appropriate temperature and humidity. Maturation and hatching of hookworm larvae from ova deposited in the soil require warmth and reasonable humidity, and the multiplication of malarial parasites and arboviruses in their mosquito vectors and the abundance of the vectors are favored by warm temperatures.

The usual seasonal variation in the incidence of specific infectious diseases suggests important influences of climatologic factors, but how they operate may be hard to determine. Overall, respiratory infections occur more frequently in colder months, but within this period (roughly October through mid-May in the Northern Hemisphere), the prevalence of the many respiratory pathogens varies greatly. Rhinoviruses peak in the early fall and spring, and influenza viruses are most active in midwinter. Parainfluenza virus type 1 and 2 infections usually peak in the fall. Increased congregation of people indoors facilitates transmission, and fluctuations in temperature and humidity not only affect the viability of agents in airborne droplet nuclei or on fingers or fomites but also may affect host susceptibility to infection.

Enterically transmitted infections occur most frequently in the warmer months, presumably largely because of season-related changes in host behavior. The outdoor play of scantily clad children facilitates the spread of skin infection and fecally shed agents such as enteroviruses. Rotavirus infections are an exception in that they occur most frequently in colder months. More completely understood are the seasonal patterns of infections spread by arthropod vectors; these patterns reflect seasonal variations in the abundance and activity of the vectors and the various lower vertebrate host species, which together constitute the reservoir mechanisms of the specific infectious agents. Climate overall, as a major determinant of the biologic environment, helps determine the abundance and the particular species of flora and fauna in a given area.

Longer term changes in climate have been associated with changes in patterns of infection. The hantavirus outbreak in the southwestern United States in 1993 has been attributed to unusually heavy precipitation in the spring of 1993 after 6 years of drought. This precipitation resulted in marked proliferation of the deer mouse population, the reservoir of the virus.[35]

Socioeconomic Environment

Socioeconomic factors depend on the density and distribution of populations; the available natural resources; the level of social, political, cultural, and scientific development; and, most importantly, the interrelationships of people. These factors typically affect health by indirect means, and, because they often are interrelated closely, evaluating the impact of individual factors is very difficult.

The relationship of population distribution and density to the occurrence of infectious diseases is substantial. Increasing density favors the spread of infectious agents to humans from human and nonhuman sources and the occurrence of related disease and development of immunity. In large and dense populations, agents such as measles virus typically infect in early childhood and persist because a sufficient number of new susceptible individuals are added continuously by birth. In smaller populations, the agents are unable to persist and are reintroduced at unpredictable intervals; as a result, manifestations of "childhood" diseases may be delayed for long periods. Populations of urban and rural areas differ not only in relative density, but also in other important ways. Exposure to zoonotic agents, especially agents prevalent in wildlife and livestock, is greater in rural areas, although rats and stray dogs may abound in city slums. Environmental sanitation (protection of water and milk supplies, safe disposal of sewage) often is a personal problem for rural residents but is handled by cooperative effort in urban populations. In addition, the importance of schools and school buses in facilitating exchange of infectious agents is greater in rural areas, where isolation of farm residents otherwise restricts contact between young children.

The basic population unit is *the household*, membership in which has similar implications for health in rural and urban areas. Family members are similar genetically; share a common diet and economic status; are subject to the same cultural, religious, and educational influences; and are exposed to a common local physical and biologic environment. Most important for contact-transmitted diseases, intrafamilial contact is prolonged and increases in intimacy with household crowding. In the wintertime, many homes are insulated, and the windows are closed so that air exchange is poor and exposure to airborne organisms is great. Prolonged contact is especially important for persisting infections such as HSV and tuberculosis. Family size, regardless of the degree of crowding, is particularly important for acute infections because it determines the number of potential introducers who bring home infections acquired elsewhere. The likelihood of exposure in early childhood increases with family size. Except for early infancy, a period of special vulnerability to some agents (e.g., respiratory syncytial virus, pertussis), early exposure is beneficial because most resulting infections are less apt to have serious consequences.

A population with a highly developed *social and political structure*, through its capacity for cooperative action, enjoys many advantages that directly or indirectly benefit health, including provision of preventive and curative health services, effective environmental sanitation, and well-developed educational facilities. Education closely relates to personal health practices that are based on understanding what individuals should do to minimize disease hazards. Schools, where the educational process begins, have been identified already as important factors in the exchange of infectious agents among children, especially agents spread by contact and airborne droplet nuclei. This matter is offset partly by the benefits derived from school-based immunization programs.

Economic status affects the occurrence of diseases indirectly through its relationship to adequacy of housing, nutrition, level of education, and availability and use of health services. It also is related closely to occupation, which may be associated with exposure to specific infections, such as Rocky Mountain spotted fever (forest workers and hikers in the south Atlantic coast states) and ornithosis (workers in poultry-processing plants).

DISEASE OCCURRENCE IN POPULATIONS

Patterns of occurrence of disease that are not random, but instead reflect the influence of underlying causes (risk factors), not only help predict future occurrence of disease but also provide important clues to understanding causation. Describing the pattern of occurrence of disease begins with definition and classification of disease in the individual so that cases can be identified and counted reliably. The occurrence of disease in defined populations can be expressed quantitatively.

INFECTION AND DISEASE IN THE INDIVIDUAL

Epidemiologic interest focuses on the specific etiologic identification of *infection* and *disease*, terms that are not synonyms. Technically, any deviation from normal function or state constitutes *disease*. Because virtually all infections cause at least some deviation from the normal state (e.g., a change in the white cell pattern in blood and mobilization of such cells at the site of infection), they cause disease. In practice, many infections result in no clinical evidence of disease and are important to the individual only for the reason that they induce immunity. Because subclinical infections help define the overall pattern of occurrence of infection and often play a significant role in its spread, their recognition is important epidemiologically. Subclinical infections go unrecognized except when healthy individuals are observed for infection in longitudinal or case-control studies.

Only infections resulting in disease usually come to the attention of the medical community. To the extent that they are recognized etiologically, they provide the earliest and most available indicator of the pattern of infection in the population.

With few exceptions, such as measles and chickenpox, typical clinical syndromes are not pathognomonic and require the clinician to develop a differential diagnosis. Basically, clinical manifestations depend more on the site or sites of disease than on the infecting agent. Because the number of possible disease targets in the body is small and the number of potential agents is large, reasonably distinct clinical entities may be caused by any of several agents. Notable examples include "common colds," approximately 40 percent of which are caused by rhinoviruses and 60 percent by any of many other viruses, and aseptic meningitis, which may be caused by such agents as mumps virus, many enteroviruses, or *B. burgdorferi*.

Infection with a specific agent may have several possible clinical outcomes. Infection with polioviruses usually is (perhaps

80%) subclinical, but can result in brief febrile illness (approximately 15%), aseptic meningitis (4-5%), or classic paralytic disease (<1 percent). The response to agents with multiple potential targets varies even more widely. Group B coxsackieviruses can cause such disparate entities as acute upper respiratory disease, aseptic meningitis, polio-like paralytic disease, myocarditis, and epidemic pleurodynia (Bornholm disease).

Knowledge of the agents active in the community when a given illness occurs helps narrow the differential diagnosis, but confirming etiologic diagnosis requires laboratory assistance: by culturing the agent, direct visualization in specimens, antigen detection, genome identification using molecular techniques, or demonstration of a specific antibody response in tests of "acute" and "convalescent" serum pairs. The diagnosis is most secure when both approaches suggest infection with the same agent. Although demonstration of the agent in relation to the disease site carries special weight (e.g., in a pharyngeal swab specimen from a respiratory illness), its presence could be the result of preexisting persisting infection unrelated to the current illness. Antibody response indicates a newly acquired infection.

DESCRIBING INFECTION AND DISEASE IN POPULATIONS

Sources of Information

Many sources provide data regarding the incidence of infectious diseases, including U.S. Vital Statistics, which tabulates only fatal cases; the Centers for Disease Control and Prevention (CDC), which receives reports of specific notifiable diseases from state health departments and summarizes them in the *Morbidity and Mortality Weekly Report*; and state and local health departments. In the absence of a focused surveillance project, these data vary in their completeness by source and by disease because of underreporting, subjects who are not seen, and errors in diagnosis.

Among the different states, reporting requirements vary, and adherence to these requirements by providers also varies. Reporting is most complete for uncommon but characteristic disorders of unusual interest, particularly if they are severe or fatal and require hospitalization, such as rabies, anthrax, trichinosis, plague, and diphtheria. Reporting is enhanced by outbreaks, as with measles, mumps, and classic pertussis in recent years. Some notifiable infections, such as leptospirosis and atypical pertussis in partially immune individuals, often are unrecognized and are under-reported. Reporting requirements may change from year to year based on CDC or state interests (neonatal sepsis and West Nile infection) or concerns about bioterrorism. Another source of data, often useful in certain areas, is state health department laboratories, which perform specific microbiologic or serologic tests for providers.

Infectious diseases that are not notifiable by law pose a difficult problem. Although necessarily limited in scale, longitudinal studies of defined populations of families have yielded valuable information. Finally, researchers now can use well-designed serosurveys to make reliable estimates of rates of previous infection with agents that induce long-persisting antibody.

International data on the incidence of infectious diseases are less precise except in well-developed countries. For the developing world, the World Health Organization (WHO) and the United Nations International Children's Emergency Fund provide estimates of the incidence of morbidity and mortality from various infectious diseases in different nations based on local reports, which are not always collected systematically. Continuing collection of such data is important for monitoring the effects of the Expanded Program of Immunization, which is directed at controlling the major vaccine-preventable diseases of childhood. More difficult to develop are definitive data about the

incidence and causation of the respiratory and diarrheal diseases, which are estimated to kill 6 million children annually in the developing world (approximately 5% of the yearly birth cohort).

For developing these kinds of statistics, it is important to have a definition of disease that is as useful as possible, which means that the sensitivity and specificity of the definition should be so balanced that as many cases of the disease as possible are identified, while avoiding the confusion that occurs when other disorders with overlapping manifestations meet criteria that are too nonspecific. A well-known example of a useful definition of disease is the Jones criteria for the diagnosis of rheumatic fever, established in 1944 at the request of the National Research Council in an effort to bring order out of chaos at a time when the disease was a major problem in the civilian and military populations.[17] These criteria subsequently have been modified to enhance their specificity by making evidence of a previous group A streptococcal infection a sine qua non for the reason that too many cases of polyarthritis of other causes met the original criteria.[9] Similarly, the criteria for the diagnosis of Kawasaki disease were revised more recently to avoid missing some episodes in infants and missing the opportunity to prevent coronary artery aneurysms by using intravenous immunoglobulin.[24]

Recognizing the importance of standardized diagnostic criteria for surveillance of infectious diseases of public health importance, the CDC published in 1990 case definitions for reportable infections.[36] Optimal use of these criteria and reporting of confirmed and probable cases to the proper authorities are of particular importance currently, when for a variety of reasons, some formerly well-controlled contagious diseases are becoming recrudescent (e.g., mumps, pertussis). All states mandate reporting contagious diseases of major public health importance, particularly diseases affecting children.

Definitions of Terms and Rates

Two commonly used (and often misused) terms, *incidence* and *prevalence*, have significantly distinct meanings. *Incidence* refers to new occurrences of infection or disease, in a population of individuals uninfected or without disease at baseline, during a specified period, commonly a year, whereas *prevalence* refers to the state (infected, ill, immune) of individuals in a population at a specified point in time (point prevalence).

To describe variations in occurrence over limited periods within a single population, such as a city or a state, a simple *numerical incidence* (number of cases or infections) often is used—daily or weekly (during an epidemic), monthly (to reflect seasonal patterns), or annually (to compare successive years). Comparisons among different populations or subgroups within a population or at widely separated times in the same population require use of the *incidence rate*, or *attack rate*, which is defined as follows:

$$\frac{\text{No. new occurrences (cases, infections) within a specified period}}{\text{Population at risk at midperiod}} \times 100, 1000, 10,000$$

If 10,000 cases of influenza occurred in a city of 200,000 people in a year, the incidence (or attack) rate would be expressed as 5 per 100 per year. In contrast to *incidence*, which is useful for determining acute and chronic conditions, *prevalence* is applied usefully only in describing conditions of long duration (months or years), such as immunity, persisting infection, and chronic disease. In relation to an acute disease such as influenza, we speak of the incidence of disease and the prevalence of immunity (reflected by antibody). Because most interest is in comparisons of different populations or subgroups, prevalence is expressed customarily as the *prevalence rate*, which is defined as follows:

$$\frac{\text{No. persons (infected, ill or immune)}}{\text{Population at that time}} \times 100, 1000, 10,000$$

For infections transmitted by contact, the frequency with which infection or disease occurs among exposed susceptible individuals provides a measure of the infectivity of the agent. This frequency, called the *secondary attack rate*, is defined as follows:

$$\frac{\text{No. contacts becoming infected or ill}}{\text{Total number of "susceptibles" exposed}} \times 100$$

The secondary attack rate is applied usefully only to closed groups, households, or classrooms, where exposure safely can be presumed for all members. The first, or primary, case is the presumed source of exposure; other cases that occur within the minimal incubation period are called *co-primary cases*. In calculating the secondary attack rate, primary and co-primary cases are excluded from the numerator and the denominator. Cases that occur subsequently within the maximal incubation period constitute the secondary cases. Cases that develop later are excluded as being derived from outside sources or from tertiary spread. The exclusion of immune individuals from the denominator is feasible only for diseases sufficiently characteristic clinically that the history serves to identify them (e.g., measles, chickenpox). Although immune individuals are not readily identifiable in the case of common respiratory diseases, the secondary attack rate based on all exposed members of the group still remains a useful tool. Its value decreases, however, when the period of communicability of the primary case (as with *Mycoplasma pneumoniae*) is longer than the incubation period because distinguishing between secondary and tertiary cases becomes difficult. Finally, the occurrence of death caused by a specific disease is expressed in two different ways. One, the *cause-specific mortality rate*, is defined as follows:

$$\frac{\text{No. deaths from the disease in a given year in a population}}{\text{Total population at midyear}} \times 100,000$$

It is a measure of the effect of the disease on the population. The potential significance of the disease to the affected individual is suggested by the *case-fatality rate*, which is defined as follows:

$$\frac{\text{No. deaths from the disease within a specified period}}{\text{No. cases in the same period}} \times 100$$

RELATING INFECTION AND DISEASE TO PERSONAL CHARACTERISTICS

Multiple characteristics may serve to distinguish one individual from another. Some factors are determined at conception—age, sex, ethnicity, genetic make-up, and birth order. Others, far more numerous, are acquired subsequently. They may be biologic (specific immunity, nutritional state), behavioral (smoking, dietary, recreational habits), or socioeconomic (occupation, educational level, marital status). Many of these characteristics relate to exposure to infectious agents or to susceptibility or resistance to the

effects of such agents and to the occurrence and severity of disease.

Relative Usefulness and Importance of Characteristics

Although almost any potentially relevant characteristic of an individual patient can be identified, it is not useful for purposes of description unless we can estimate how many people in the population also possess the characteristic. From census data or other accessible records, numbers of people in groups defined by age, sex, race, occupation, or marital status can be estimated easily. Special surveys would need to be conducted to estimate the prevalence of specific immunity or possibly significant exposure, such as to household pets.

The importance of personal characteristics to the description of a disease varies in two ways. One is in the degree of association that exists between a characteristic and a specific disease. Age is associated strongly with disease caused by prevalent contagious agents, whereas sex usually is not. The second way is in the independence or relative interdependence of characteristics as variables. Inherent characteristics, such as age, sex, and ethnic origin, are independent of one another, whereas acquired characteristics rarely are. The nature of interpersonal contacts, degree of personal hygiene, and usual forms of recreation are associated closely with age or sex or both. The common interdependence of characteristics means that before making an inference from a particular association, one should explore association with other, possibly correlated, characteristics.

Age Patterns

The occurrence of infection and disease generally is related so strongly to age that until possible differences in age distribution are taken into account, differences in occurrence among population subgroups defined by other characteristics cannot be interpreted meaningfully. Age as a characteristic is ascertained easily and reliably for affected individuals and the total membership of the relevant population. Description of the age pattern involves computing a series of *age-specific rates* for sequential age groups, usually defined in intervals of 5 years or multiples thereof (e.g., 0 to 4, 5 to 9, 10 to 19). For conditions of pediatric concern, the use of single-year intervals (<1, 1, 2, 3, and 4 years) to cover early childhood may be more informative. In some cases, especially in the first 2 years of life, a breakdown by months of age would be informative.

Affected individuals in an age group form the numerator, and all individuals in the population in that age group serve as the denominator. Rates so computed describe the age profile of immunity at a specified point in time (age-specific antibody prevalence rates), the age profile of new infections or disease (age-specific incidence rates), or the age profile of deaths caused by a disease (disease-specific and age-specific mortality rates). Age-specific incidence rates for acute infectious diseases indicate the risk of disease occurring in each age group and, depending on the disease agent, more or less accurately reflect the underlying age-specific infection rates.

Age Adjustment of Rates

The need to take age distribution into account when comparing disease in different populations is indicated when (1) the rates vary with age and (2) the distribution of the populations by age differs substantially. From published U.S. mortality data for 1983 and 1984, one can compare pneumonia and influenza mortality rates for Alaska and Florida. During those years, 89 deaths were recorded among 986,000 Alaskans at risk, for an annual mortality rate of 9/100,000. In contrast, in Florida, 4703 deaths occurred from pneumonia and influenza among the 21,792,000 residents at risk for those 2 years, for a rate of 21.6/100,000, nearly 2.5 times that of Alaska. These rates are called *crude mortality rates.* In this instance, these rates are misleading for the reasons that the likelihood of death occurring from pneumonia and influenza increases with age and the age distributions of the populations of these two states differ markedly. National death rates from these infections are nearly 10-fold greater in people 65 to 74 years of age than in people 55 to 64 years of age. For those years, 17.5 percent and 3 percent of the Florida and Alaska populations were 65 years or older.

To make a valid comparison of the pneumonia and influenza mortality rates for these two states, one must perform an age adjustment; this is a simple process that is not detailed here because the method can be found in available texts of biostatistics and epidemiology. Briefly, one determines mortality rates for specific age groups (usually 5 or 10 years) for the two populations and calculates the deaths that would be expected in a common (or standard) population for the same age groupings by using the age-specific rates of the populations being compared, in this instance those of Alaska and Florida. Summation of these expected deaths permits calculation of the rates that would have occurred in the standard population if the age-specific rates of Alaska applied and if the age-specific rates of Florida applied. In this example, the age-adjusted mortality rate for pneumonia and influenza for Alaska is 35.2/100,000, and that for Florida is 21.8/100,000, nearly the reverse of the crude rates. (The combined population of the two states was used as the standard.)

These age-adjusted rates are not true rates; they are used for comparison. Although often applicable to infectious diseases, age-adjusted rates almost always are required for comparisons of morbidity and mortality from chronic diseases.

Sex Patterns

Because sex is a readily ascertained characteristic of the membership of populations, the occurrence of infections and disease in relation to sex is described easily. Its simplest form is the *sex ratio*, or the ratio of cases in males to cases in females. This ratio is meaningful only when, as in childhood, the population is divided approximately equally by sex. Although males exceed females at birth (106:100), the death rate for males exceeds that for females at all ages (average 1.5:1). From approximately age 20 years on, females outnumber males, the difference increasing with age, which means that when comparing sex-specific rates, age adjustment must be made, or, better yet, the age profiles for the sexes should be compared directly so that important differences in the contour can be seen.

Ethnic or Racial Patterns

A third characteristic by which members of the population can be grouped in describing occurrence of disease is race or ethnic origin, the usefulness of which has decreased with the increasing frequency of mixed marriages. The U.S. census classification is based on information collected regarding race and native origin. Individuals of mixed racial parentage are classified by the race of the nonwhite parent or, if both are nonwhite, by that of the father. People of foreign birth are classified by country. Native-born children of foreign-born parents are identified as "foreign stock" and grouped according to parental origin. Census data provide estimates of population subgroups belonging to several "races" (white, black, Native American, Chinese, Japanese) or "foreign stocks" (including foreign born and first generation).

Although controversial currently, this method yields differences in the occurrence of many infections and other diseases among such population subgroups. Knowledge of such differences is useful in case finding and organizing the application of specific preventive measures. Subgroups defined by ethnicity possess some similarity in genetic constitution that may determine susceptibility or resistance to specific agents. They also may be affected distinctively by environmental factors because of voluntary or involuntary differences in behavior and patterns of living.

Disease Patterns in Kinships

Genetically determined susceptibility and resistance to specific infectious agents have not yet been associated clearly with recognized genetic markers that could serve as a basis for defining population subgroups. Most efforts to look for genetic influences have been studies of occurrence of diseases in individuals of differing degrees of relationship within kinships or in the total memberships of different kinships. With rapid advancement in the database of the human genome, considerable interest has been generated in polymorphisms at loci that may define susceptibility to infectious diseases on a genetic basis. Populations with a high prevalence of certain alleles and known to have an increased risk of certain infections could be studied to determine whether the risk is due to abnormal function of the specified gene.

Family Episodes of Infection and Disease

With respect to contact-transmitted infectious diseases, the family is more important as the basic epidemiologic subgroup of a population than for its shared genes. Observation of family units for episodes of infection and related illnesses has contributed significantly to knowledge of the epidemiology of widely prevalent infectious agents. The situation in all family studies begins with one member's infection, acquired from outside the house. That member then exposes the other family members. The introductory infection and any infections in family members who are exposed constitute a family episode, which is described basically in terms of the times of onset of the related infections and the identities (age, sex, position in the family) of the introducer and the infected and uninfected contacts.

Analysis of cumulated episodes of common respiratory illness, observed in the early studies, identified children as the most frequent introducers (important in community spread). Analysis also yielded estimates of the risk of cross-infection occurring within the family, expressed in terms of secondary attack rates among specified members (e.g., younger children) exposed to specified introducers (e.g., a schoolchild or a parent). Generally, the risk in contacts was related inversely to age overall, as a result of the influence of immunity, and to intimacy of within-family contact (ready exchange between spouses and between children nearest in age). Finally, the relationship of time between the onset of illness in the introducer and onset in family members exposed serves to define the range of incubation periods.

Analysis of the episodes can yield additional information concerning such crucial aspects as mode and duration of the agent's shedding; the spectrum of clinical response to infection, including the proportion that is subclinical; and the significance of previous immunity in the face of close exposure, as measured by the frequency and clinical consequences of the reinfections that result. The results of the analysis of adenovirus episodes in the Virus Watch program are illustrative.[11] Virus appears regularly in the feces and less often (approximately 50%) in the pharynx, and shedding may be abortive (a few days only) or continue intermittently for many months. Overall, 50 percent of infections are subclinical, and illness, typically febrile and respiratory, occurs more commonly with pharyngeal excretion (65%) than with only fecal shedding (31%). Immunity is 85 percent protective against infection; re-infections that do occur usually are subclinical. Young children and especially infants younger than 2 years of age are the usual introducers, and within-family spread depends more on duration than on the mode of virus excretion by the introducer.

Socioeconomic Patterns

Socioeconomic status covers a complex of characteristics, including levels of education and income and, less tangibly, "social standing." The problem is to discover a useful single indicator. One possibility is area of residence as classified by median income or measures that reflect housing standards, such as type of plumbing and average number of individuals per room. Relevant data are available for census tracts, which have proved useful when the tracts are homogeneous.

Occupation of the head of a household seems to be the one attribute most closely reflecting socioeconomic status. On this basis, the British have defined five broad social classes that directly apply to employed adults and can be extended to cover their dependents. These classes, in descending order, are professional, intermediate, skilled, partly skilled, and unskilled occupations. For use in the United States, based on census-recorded occupations, these terms have been translated as follows:

- Professional workers
- Non-farm technical, administrative, and managerial workers
- Clerical, sales, and skilled workers
- Semiskilled workers
- Non-farm laborers
- Farm workers of whatever level are included in a sixth group as agricultural workers

RELATING INFECTION AND DISEASE TO PLACE

Place is of interest, epidemiologically, when occupied by humans and, unless indicated as relating to work, recreation, or travel, refers here to residence. Place usually is classified geographically (hemisphere, continent, nation) but also can be classified usefully by environmental characteristics such as climate, altitude, stage of economic development, population density, and urban or rural nature. Variations in occurrence of disease with place reflect parallel variations in the operation of causative factors and raise the question of whether these factors are to be found in the characteristics of the physical and biologic environment inherent to the place or in the characteristics of the inhabitants. The former is suggested when the age-adjusted risk of disease increases for immigrants and decreases for emigrants, when risk does not vary among the ethnic groups present, and when similar ethnic groups in other places enjoy a lower risk. One also must consider possible differences in reliability and completeness of recognition and reporting of disease.

Global Variation

On the global scale, the WHO collects and publishes information concerning the occurrences of diseases derived from statistics compiled routinely within nations for morbidity from notifiable infectious diseases and for causes of death. The great variations among nations in the quality and availability of medical care and other health services result in corresponding variations in the reliability and completeness of the data collected by the WHO. Generally, basic demographic data and the quality and availability of health services are equally good in well-developed countries, so specific disease rates can be compared. In less-developed countries, demographic data may be inaccurate and medical services may be inconsistent in quality and concentrated in urban populations, within which their availability varies with economic status. Many illnesses and deaths are unattended medically, especially in rural areas, and births commonly are attended by midwives.

Because infant deaths are reported more completely than births are, infant mortality rates may be unreliable.

With respect to infectious and parasitic diseases, knowledge of the frequency of disease is less important than is qualitative knowledge of the distribution and spread of disease. Such knowledge guides the application and enforcement of international control measures and is the basis for advice given by physicians to prospective foreign travelers. Important diseases, such as yellow fever, plague, and cholera, because of their high case-fatality rate and characteristic clinical picture, are almost certain to come to attention when substantial numbers of cases occur. Such knowledge may not be publicized, however, or may not be promptly available. Some countries, in the hope that a new outbreak (perhaps of cholera) will be controlled soon, may withhold information to avoid discouraging economically important tourists.

Two additional considerations are relevant to evaluating the disease hazards of foreign travel. One is the fact that recognized occurrence of disease in the indigenous population may be an inaccurate index of risk to a newcomer. Particular agents, such as polioviruses in the past and hepatitis A virus and Epstein-Barr virus at present, may be so prevalent that infections in natives occur so early in life that they usually are subclinical. The second consideration is the nature of the proposed travel. The usual tourist or business traveler visits chiefly larger population centers and popular tourist attractions, where the most important hazards are pathogens transmitted by food or water. Travelers whose activities bring them into more intimate contact with the people and the biologic environment (Peace Corps workers, military personnel) may encounter additional hazards, such as rabies and the locally prevalent arthropod-transmitted pathogens.

As suggested in considering geographic influences on occurrence of disease, the distribution of many diseases is influenced by relevant environmental factors, rather than political boundaries. In depicting (or predicting) the global distribution of a particular disease, identifying regions defined by the presence of factors thought to be important to disease occurrence is useful.

For most agents pathogenic for humans, the chief environmental requisite is a susceptible human population, and most such agents already exist wherever the size and density of the population are sufficient for them to persist. Concern about global spread is limited to a few important pathogens, such as the cholera vibrio and influenza virus. Cholera is a special case in that its spread also depends on poor sanitation. Neither persistence nor even limited spread should occur after its introduction into highly developed areas. Influenza A virus continues to be a major, and so far unstoppable, threat by virtue of its ability to emerge at irregular intervals in a new antigenic coat, which largely negates the pre-existing widespread immunity.

Local Patterns of Infection and Disease

"Local" units of population for which demographic data are readily available in the United States include "large" units, such as counties, metropolitan areas, and large cities, which contain smaller units (smaller cities and towns [within counties] and census tracts [within metropolitan areas and large cities]). The smaller units, including unincorporated areas within counties, often can be characterized by variables (urban or rural nature, population density, socioeconomic status, racial or ethnic group) that may help explain observed differences in the occurrence of specific infections and related diseases.

Particularly in relation to outbreaks of acute infectious diseases, spot maps commonly are used to show the local distribution of individual cases. Placing new pins (a different color each week) to mark the residences of newly reported cases serves to visualize the outbreak's geographic progression. The final distribution of the pins may help identify a major source of infection.

A classic example is the 1854 outbreak of cholera in the Golden Square district of London, in which the clustering of residences of fatal cases helped Snow incriminate the Broad Street pump as the source.[32] Sometimes, place of work is a better guide to the source of infection than place of residence. In another classic study, that of endemic typhus in Montgomery, Alabama, in the early 1920s, the residences of cases (Fig. 7–2) were scattered widely, whereas the workplaces (Fig. 7–3) were concentrated in relation to feed stores and food-handling businesses, all heavily

rat-infested. This finding led Maxcy[21] to perform studies showing the basic role of rats and rat fleas in this disease.

TEMPORAL PATTERNS OF INFECTION AND DISEASE

Definitions

The unit of time used can vary from hours to decades to centuries. In describing acute outbreaks, the units are short—hours for

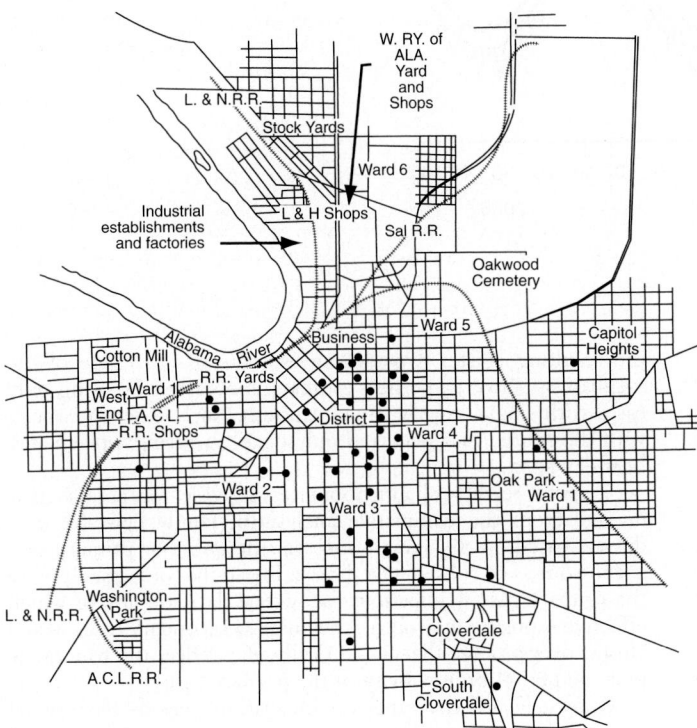

Figure 7–2 Cases of mild typhus (Brill disease) in Montgomery, Alabama, 1922 to 1925, spotted according to residence. *(From Maxcy, K. F.: An epidemiological study of endemic typhus [Brill disease] in the southeastern United States. Public Health Rep. 41:2967-2995, 1926.)*

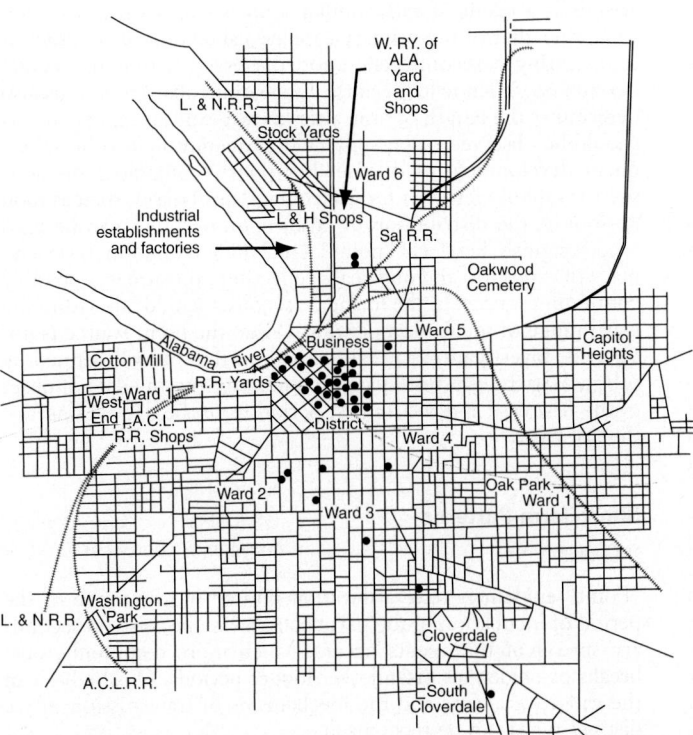

Figure 7–3 Cases of mild typhus (Brill disease) in Montgomery, Alabama, 1922 to 1925, spotted according to place of employment or, if unemployed, according to place of residence. *(From Maxcy, K. F.: An epidemiological study of endemic typhus [Brill disease] in the southeastern United States. Public Health Rep. 41:2967-2995, 1926.)*

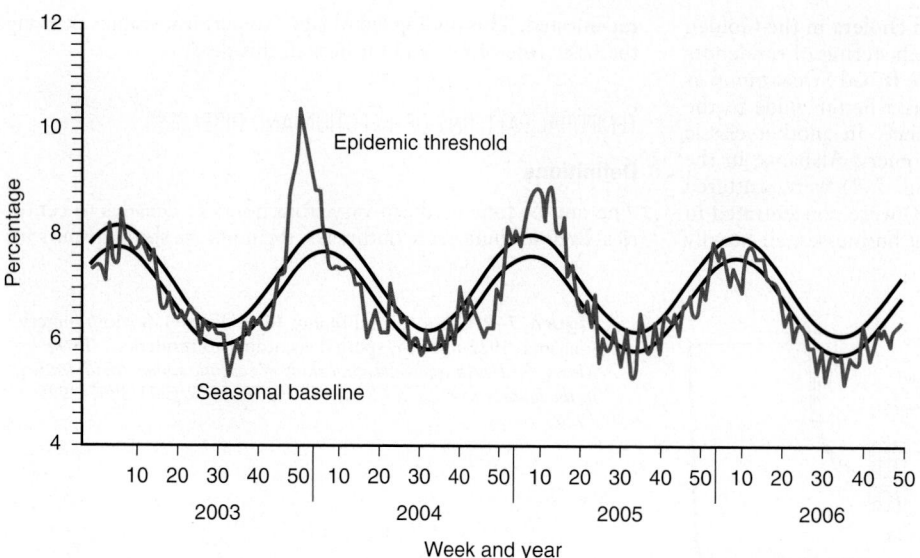

Figure 7–4 Percentage of all deaths attributed to pneumonia and influenza reported by the 122 Cities Mortality Reporting System, by week and year—United States, week ending December 9, 2006. *(From M. M. W. R. Morb. Mortal. Wkly. Rep. 55:1345-1375, 2006.)*

food poisoning, days or weeks for most infectious diseases—whereas long-term time trends are described in longer units of years or decades. Comparisons extending over 1 or more decades may be complicated by changes in diagnostic standards and reporting.

Finally, the meanings of two words commonly used to describe the occurrence of disease over time in a given area should be defined clearly. *Endemic* refers to diseases regularly present. The usual frequency, including expected seasonal variations, is called the *endemic level*. The term *epidemic* applies to any number of cases, small or large, that is a significant increase over the usual, or endemic, level (although just what constitutes a "significant increase" is not clearly defined).

This principle underlies the monitoring of many infectious diseases, deaths, and pneumonia caused by influenza by the CDC. Such monitoring is illustrated in Figure 7–4, in which the weekly ratios of deaths caused by pneumonia and influenza to the total deaths observed from 2003 to 2006 are compared with the ratios expected from use of the time series method[7] and "epidemic threshold," which depicts the upper 95 percent confidence limit. When the observed value exceeds the expected one for 2 successive weeks, an influenza epidemic is indicated. On this basis, epidemics began in week 48 of 2003 and week 9 of 2005.

In practice, especially at the local level, health authorities use the term *outbreak*, rather than *epidemic* (unless the number of cases is very large), to minimize public alarm. The term *pandemic* is used to describe excess disease occurring in many countries, as influenza did in 1957 and 1968.

Time Clusters

Time clusters relate to the recognition and interpretation of events (infections and disease) that occur with some increased frequency within a limited period or clustering in time. An important determinant of clustering of infections is the incubation period. Infection resulting from a known exposure is manifested within a predictable range of time by the initiation of shedding of the agent and the onset of disease (if it occurs). Although the average incubation period of a given disease is remarkably constant, the usual range broadens as the incubation period increases. This range can be estimated by accumulating cases for which the time of exposure is known precisely or approximately and, with this point as day 0 on the time axis, plotting the day of onset of each subsequent case. The width of

the resulting cluster provides an estimate of the range of the incubation period. The best estimate is obtained by using only cases with single, clearly timed exposure, such as when contact with the source case occurred only once, as during a playmate's birthday party.

A more readily obtained but less precise estimate is that derived from the cumulative analysis of family episodes of a disease based on the assumption that the initial or primary case is the source of subsequent disease in family contacts. Because the primary case is infectious for several days, on any of which effective exposure may occur, the onset of secondary cases would cluster over a range that theoretically may reflect the true range plus the period of infectivity of the primary case.

Knowledge of the range of incubation periods has several practical implications. For contagious diseases, it can be used to distinguish true secondary cases that occur in families from others arising as a result of extrafamilial sources (cases with onset too soon after that of the primary case are called *co-primary cases*) or representing a second generation of spread within the family (*tertiary cases*). Knowledge of the range of incubation periods also determines the length of time after known exposure that contacts should be observed or possibly held in quarantine for the subsequent development of disease. For poorly contagious diseases, such as typhoid fever, or for noncontagious diseases, such as food poisoning, the distribution of onset in an outbreak can be used to distinguish between "point" epidemics (common time and place of exposure) and outbreaks reflecting exposure to a possibly continuing source. In the former case, onset would fall within the usual range of incubation periods. When the point source is not obvious, investigation can be focused on the interval defined by subtracting the shortest incubation period from the date of onset of the first case and the longest period from the date of onset of the last case.

Short-Term Patterns

EPIDEMICS

"Point" epidemics have a duration limited by the range of the period of incubation of the particular disease because no secondary spread of the agents occurs. Much more commonly, outbreaks or epidemics extend over longer periods. On the basis of the causative agents and the mechanisms of transmission, three distinct types can be recognized.

The first type typically consists of outbreaks of poorly contagious or noncontagious diseases; such outbreaks reflect the new but persisting activity of a source that must be identified and terminated quickly. One example of such a "continuing source" type of outbreak was a community-wide outbreak of salmonellosis in Madeira, California, in 1965, which was traced quickly to the water supply.[27] Unrecognized typhoid carriers working as food handlers and shellfish harvested from sewage-polluted waters contaminated with hepatitis A virus are other examples of outbreaks requiring prompt epidemiologic investigation to identify the source. One of the major causes of point epidemics is food contaminated with *E. coli* O157:H7. More recent outbreaks, such as the contamination of spinach at the growing source, have been reported by the CDC.[6] Often the CDC posts interim reports of investigations on the CDC website (www.cdc.gov) before publication in *Morbidity and Mortality Weekly Reports.*

The element of contagion distinguishes the second type of epidemic, in which disease spreads from person to person. Such epidemics generally are self-limited, and the curve describing them often resembles the bell-shaped curve of a normal distribution. Modification of this curve, as in an abrupt decline from the peak, is the expected result of successful efforts to control the epidemic. Epidemics of contagious diseases occur when the population in which the agent persists or is newly introduced contains a sufficient number of susceptible individuals with contact with one another that is adequate to permit transfer of infection from each new case to, on average, more than one susceptible individual. When this average falls below 1, the curve declines, and when the probability of successful transfer of infection approaches zero, the epidemic stops (typically well before the supply of susceptible individuals has been exhausted).

Reasons that underlie this decline and termination of transmission include seasonal changes in environmental factors that affect viability of the agent, such as temperature and humidity; changes in the behavior of hosts that affect the intimacy of contact, such as indoor school versus outdoor play; and the progressive conversion of individuals from susceptible to immune. Institution of appropriate hygienic precautions likely was an important facet of control and termination of the worldwide outbreak of severe acute respiratory syndrome in 2003.[5] If one assumes constant units on the time axis, the slope of the ascending limb of the epidemic curve is determined by the incubation period (interval between successive cases) and by factors that influence transmission (infectivity of the agent, frequency of adequate contact between susceptible individuals). In the absence of effective control measures, the duration of epidemics of a particular disease depends on the size of the susceptible population and the persistence of favorable environmental factors.

Epidemics of "diseases in nature" constitute the third type. Because susceptible individuals usually are abundant in the human population, these epidemics typically reflect increases in the number of sources of infection in nature. With zoonoses such as arbovirus encephalitis, the initiation, slope of the curve, and duration of the epidemic are determined by the number of susceptible lower vertebrate hosts, the seasonally determined abundance of the vector mosquitoes, and the length of the extrinsic incubation period in the vector. The occurrence of West Nile virus in the United States, which began in August 1999 and has continued with outbreaks in the late summer of each succeeding year in mosquitoes and humans is an example.[3,4]

SEASONAL AND CYCLIC VARIATIONS

Predictable periodic variations in disease take two forms, seasonal and cyclic, neither of which is understood completely in the case of agents infecting only humans. *Seasonal* variations presumably reflect the influence of changes in temperature, precipitation, and length of daylight on the activity of the agent. This variation is readily apparent with respect to diseases, such as Lyme disease (the peak incidence of which typically occurs in the summer months), which depend on lower vertebrate hosts and arthropod vectors, the abundance and activity of which are determined seasonally. Similarly, the increased occurrence of enteric bacterial infections (spread by indirect means) in the warmer months is explainable largely by more rapid bacterial growth in unrefrigerated milk and food, the increase in abundance of flies, and the lack of sanitary precautions associated with summer recreational activities.

The mode of transmission is only a partial determinant of the seasonal pattern. Although the enteroviruses (including polio), the rotaviruses that cause acute gastroenteritis, and hepatitis A virus all are spread chiefly by fecal-oral mechanisms (direct and indirect), the seasonal patterns are distinctly different (late summer and fall for enteroviruses and late winter for rotaviruses and hepatitis A virus). Similarly, although infections with agents present in respiratory secretions and spread by either airborne mechanisms or contaminated fomites occur infrequently in the summer, their seasonal peaks occur at significantly different times. The season of respiratory diseases coincides roughly with the school year. Infections with rhinoviruses occur most frequently in the early fall and late spring, and infections with parainfluenza virus types 1 and 2 occur most frequently in the fall. The annual peaks of RSV vary among fall, winter, and spring. Mumps peaks in late fall, influenza in late winter or early spring, and measles typically in the spring.

Plotting variation over a series of years reveals a roughly regular cyclic variation for some diseases. In larger metropolitan areas, the usual biennial measles epidemic appears as an enlarged annual wave. Before 1950, deaths caused by meningococcal meningitis occurred on a nationwide basis in cycles of 7 to 9 years, a phenomenon presumably terminated by the advent of prophylactic antibiotics. Pandemic influenza A, which provides the most dramatic example of cycling, is explainable by a major change in the antigenic character of the agent.

Long-Term Trends

Except for poliomyelitis during the first half of the 20th century, clearly defined long-term trends in the occurrence of infectious diseases in the United States usually have been downward, and in no case has description or understanding of the mechanisms posed a major difficulty. In the case of poliomyelitis, the increase in the rate of paralytic disease that began about 1880 is attributable to numerous factors, including improved sanitation, which resulted in an expanding proportion of infection occurring among older children and young adults without previous exposure to the viruses. In young infants, most poliovirus infections are benign but produce long-lasting immunity; the older an individual is when infected, the more likely that individual will have paralysis. The frequency of paralytic poliomyelitis is related inversely to the level of sanitation. In the United States, the increase in paralytic disease with epidemics of polio continued unabated (with an apparent sharp increase around 1940 because of changes in reporting criteria) until the widespread use of polio vaccines.

The post-1955 decline in poliomyelitis; the much earlier decline in pertussis and diphtheria; the disappearance of smallpox; and the more recent marked decline in measles, rubella, *H. influenzae* type b, and varicella all are attributable chiefly to widespread use of effective specific vaccines. Similarly, the disappearance of indigenous malaria and the decline of rabies to a negligible level in humans in certain areas reflect the application of a variety of effective control measures.

Emerging Infections

Although in the 1980s one might have said that most infectious disorders had been explored thoroughly epidemiologically and that little was left to do, this conclusion no longer is the case. Infectious disease epidemiology has become increasingly challenging, and in many ways the problems are more complex and necessitate greater cooperation with additional disciplines, such as microbiology and molecular biology.

In part, this increased complexity is due to so-called *emerging infections*, a term that has come into vogue in recent years and refers to two different groups of disorders. The first is associated with the appearance of previously unrecognized or possibly heretofore nonexistent infections in humans. Well-known examples are legionellosis, hantavirus pulmonary disease, acquired immunodeficiency syndrome (AIDS), Lyme disease, hemorrhagic colitis caused by *E. coli* O157:H7, and Ebola virus infection. The other group includes previously recognized human infections that exhibit changes in epidemiologic behavior or biologic characteristics that enhance their transmission or virulence. These changes usually can be attributed to external influences, such as altered demographics including increasing population and rural-urban migration, international travel, new technology or technologic failure, changes in land use, adaptation of infecting organisms to various influences, and inadequate or underused public health measures.[18] To this list should be added changes in host factors such as immune defenses.

No clear dividing line exists between new infections and old ones that exhibit new behavior. Examples of some with new behavior include multidrug-resistant tuberculosis, penicillin-resistant pneumococcal infections, invasive group A streptococcal (popularly known as flesh-eating bacteria) infections, staphylococcal toxic shock syndrome, community-acquired methicillin-resistant staphylococcal infections, H5N1 influenza ("bird flu"), cryptosporidiosis, and numerous infections that are fostered by immunosuppression or various therapeutic measures such as antibiotics and catheters.

These emerging infections are not minor threats. Although in some instances small populations have been affected to date, the potential for widespread disease of epidemic or even of pandemic proportions exists. This potential can be expected to increase because the demographic and other conditions that have predisposed to the emergence of these infections continue to grow and intensify. Maximal efforts must be expended to reverse this process. To achieve this goal requires worldwide collaborative effort among various disciplines, including epidemiology, microbiology, entomology, immunology, clinical medicine, demography, nutrition, sanitation, and even political science.

The responsibilities of epidemiologists regarding emerging infections may be described in three categories. The first category is surveillance, including recognition of the appearance of a previously unrecognized infection or a new variant of an existing disease. Optimal surveillance requires systematic observations and specific diagnostic criteria to ensure precision. An important part of surveillance is to determine who, when, and where: who is affected (e.g., age and other personal characteristics, contact with others who are ill), when the disorder occurs (e.g., year-to-year variations, season, temporal course of the outbreak), and where it occurs (e.g., geographic locations, urban or rural, local ecology). Second, an important task is to use surveillance and other data to develop an understanding of the epidemiology of the infection, which often provides clues to its etiology and pathogenesis and to approaches to controlling the disease. The third role of epidemiologists is that of monitoring the effects of various control measures, including assessment of the safety and efficacy of new vaccines, such as those for H5N1 influenza, malaria, and AIDS. Chapter 266 contains a description of how the efficacy of vaccines is determined.

The increasing magnitude and speed of international travel enhance the likelihood of global spread of disease and complicate approaches to prevent or contain epidemic infections. Many of the emerging infections are not limited geographically by their

ecologic requirements. The nations of the world increasingly depend on each other for surveillance, a task that is not accomplished easily given the logistics; costs (in the face of other needs and priorities, particularly of many developing countries); and the required standardization, collaboration, communication, coordination, and centralized resource for assembly and analysis of surveillance. Although the WHO, the Pan American Health Organization, the U.S. Military and Public Health Service, and various other organizations maintain surveillance systems and laboratories in various parts of the world, these efforts at present are considered to be inadequate except for some infections and in some areas. The development of comprehensive national and worldwide surveillance systems has been urgently recommended.[18]

REFERENCES

1. Allison, A. C.: Protection afforded by sickle-cell trait against subtertian malarial infection. B. M. J. *1*:290-294, 1953.
2. Anderson P., Johnston R. B., and Smith, D. H.: Human serum activities against *Hemophilus influenzae*, type b. J. Clin. Invest. *51*:31-38, 1972.
3. Asnis, D. S., Conetta, R., Teixeira, A. A., et al.: The West Nile virus Outbreak of 1999 in New York: The Flushing Hospital Experience. Clin. Infect. Dis. *30*:413-418, 2000.
4. Centers for Disease Control and Prevention: West Nile virus activity—United States, 2001. M. M. W. R. Morb. Mortal. Wkly. Rep. *51*:497-501, 2002.
5. Centers for Disease Control and Prevention: Public Health guidance for community-level preparedness and response to severe acute respiratory syndrome (SARS). Supplement D: Community containment measures, including nonhospital isolation and quarantine. January 8, 2004. Available at http://www.cdc.gov/ncidod/sars/guidance/D/pdf/d.pdf. Accessed January 1, 2007.
6. Centers for Disease Control and Prevention: Ongoing multistate outbreak of *Escherichia coli* type O157:H7 infections associated with consumption of fresh spinach—United States. M. M. W. R. Morb. Mortal. Wkly. Rep. *55*:1045-1046, 2006.
7. Choi, K., and Thacker, S. B.: An evaluation of influenza mortality surveillance, 1962-1979, I: Time series forecasts of expected pneumonia and influenza deaths, and II: Percentage of pneumonia and influenza as an indicator of influenza activity. Am. J. Epidemiol. *113*:216-226 and 227-235, 1981.
8. Donsero, T. J., Rendtorff, R. C., Mallison, G. F., et al.: An outbreak of Legionnaires' disease associated with a contaminated air-conditioning cooling tower. N. Engl. J. Med. *302*:365-370, 1980.
9. Ferrieri, P., for the Jones Criteria Working Group: AHA Scientific Statement. Proceedings of the Jones criteria workshop. Circulation *106*:2521, 2002.
9a. Fothergill, L. C.: Biological warfare and its defense. Public Health Rep. *72*:865-871, 1957.
10. Fox, J. P., and Elveback, L. R.: Herd immunity: Changing concepts. *In* Notkins, A. L. (ed.): Viral Immunology and Immunopathology. New York, Academic Press, 1975, pp. 273-290.
11. Fox, J. P., Hall, C. E., and Cooney, M. K.: The Seattle Virus Watch. VII: Observations of adenovirus infections. Am. J. Epidemiol. *105*:362-386, 1977.
12. Frobisher, M.: Fundamentals of Microbiology. 7th ed. Philadelphia, W. B. Saunders, 1962, p. 354.
13. Goldschneider, I., Gotschlich, E. C., and Artenstein, M. S.: Human immunity to the meningococcus, I: The role of humoral antibodies. J. Exp. Med. *129*:1307-1326, 1969.
14. Griffin, P. M., and Tauxe, R. V.: The epidemiology of infections caused by *Escherichia coli* O157:H7, other enterohemorrhagic *E. coli* and the associated hemolytic-uremic syndrome. Epidemiol. Rev. *13*:60-98, 1991.
15. Gwaltney, J. M., Jr., and Hendley, J. O.: Rhinovirus transmission: One if by air, two if by hand. Am. J. Epidemiol. *107*:357-361, 1978.
16. Huebner, R. J.: The virologist's dilemma. Ann. N. Y. Acad. Sci. *67*:430-438, 1957.
17. Jones, T. D.: Diagnosis of rheumatic fever. J. A. M. A. *126*:481-484, 1944.
17a. Katz, M., and Stiehm, E. R.: Host defenses in malnutrition. Pediatrics *59*:490-495, 1977.
18. Lederberg, J., Shope, R. E., and Oaks, S. C., Jr., (eds.): Emerging Infections: Microbial Threats to Health in the United States. Washington, D. C., National Academy Press, 1992.
19. Levine, M. M., DuPont, H. L., Formal, S. B., et al.: Pathogenesis of *Shigella dysenteriae* 1 (Shiga) dysentery. J. Infect. Dis. *127*:261-270, 1973.
20. MacKenzie, W. R., Hoxie, N. J., Proctor, M. E., et al.: A massive outbreak in Milwaukee of *Cryptosporidium* infection transmitted through the public water supply. N. Engl. J. Med. *331*:161-167, 1994.
21. Maxcy, K. F.: An epidemiological study of endemic typhus (Brill's disease) in the southeastern United States. Public Health Rep. *41*:2967-2995, 1926.
22. McDade, J. E., Shepard, C. C., Fraser, D. W., et al.: Legionnaires' disease: Isolation of a bacterium and demonstration of its role in other respiratory disease. N. Engl. J. Med *297*:1197-1203, 1977.

23. Mortimer, E. A., Jr.: Hospital staphylococcal infections: Interruption of transmission as a means of control. Med. Clin. North Am. *47*:1247-1256, 1963.

24. Newburger, J. W., Takahashi, M., Gerber, M. A., et al.: Diagnosis, treatment, and long-term management of Kawasaki disease: A statement for health professionals from the Committee on Rheumatic Fever, Endocarditis and Kawasaki Disease, Council on Cardiovascular Disease in the Young, American Heart Association. Circulation *110*:2747-2771, 2004.

25. Pasteur, L.: The physiological theory of fermentation. *In* Eliot, C. (ed.): Scientific Papers. New York, P. F. Collier & Sons, 1910, pp. 289-381.

26. Perry, W. D., Siegel, A. C., Rammelkamp, C. H., Jr., et al.: Transmission of group A streptococci, I: The role of contaminated bedding. Am. J. Hyg. *66*:85-101, 1957.

27. Renteln, H. A., and Hinman, A. R.: A waterborne epidemic of gastroenteritis in Madeira, California. Am. J. Epidemiol. *86*:1-10, 1967.

28. Rosen, G.: A History of Public Health. New York, M.D. Publications, 1958, pp. 62-64.

29. Selye, H.: The Physiology and Pathology of Exposure to Stress. Montreal, Acta, 1950.

30. Sigerist, H. E.: The Great Doctors. New York, W. W. Norton, 1933, pp. 100-108, 375-379.

31. Shapiro, E. D., Berg, A. T., Austrian, R., et al.: The protective efficacy of polyvalent pneumococcal polysaccharide vaccine. N. Engl. J. Med *325*:1453-1460, 1991.

32. Snow on Cholera, being a reprint of two papers by John Snow, M. D., together with a biographical memoir by B. W. Richardson and an introduction by Wade Hampton Frost. New York, Commonwealth Fund, 1936.

33. Thompson, W. H., and Beaty, B. J.: Venereal transmission of La Crosse (California encephalitis) arbovirus in *Aedes triseriatus* mosquitoes. Science *196*:530-531, 1977.

34. Wannamaker, L. W.: The epidemiology of streptococcal infections. *In* McCarty, M. (ed.): Streptococcal Infections. New York, Columbia University Press, 1954, p. 157.

35. Wenzel, R. P.: A new hantavirus infection in North America. N. Engl. J. Med. *330*:1004-1005, 1994.

36. Wharton, M., Chorba, T. L., Vogt, R. L., et al.: Case definitions for public health surveillance. M. M. W. R. Recomm. Rep. *39*(RR-13):1-43, 1990.

37. Winslow, C. E. A.: The Colonial era and the first years of the Republic (1606-1799): The pestilence that walketh in darkness, No. 1. *In* Top, F. H. (ed.): The History of American Epidemiology. St. Louis, C. V. Mosby, 1954, pp. 31-44.

PART II

INFECTION OF SPECIFIC
ORGAN SYSTEMS

UPPER RESPIRATORY TRACT INFECTIONS

CHAPTER
8

THE COMMON COLD

James D. Cherry ⊛ Delma J. Nieves

The common cold is an acute, communicable, viral disease characterized by nasal stuffiness, sneezing, coryza, throat irritation, and no or minimal fever. Although the terms *upper respiratory infection* and *nasopharyngitis* are used frequently as synonyms for the common cold by physicians and other health care workers, the practice should be discouraged; the term *upper respiratory infection* is too broad, and pharyngitis is not present in most colds. To add to the confusion regarding terminology, "a cold" frequently has an even more inclusive connotation to the layperson.

HISTORY

Although the common cold undoubtedly has had an impact on the events of history, the specific symptom complex in ancient times was overshadowed by more severe contagious problems (influenza, plague, smallpox) and by septic diseases (otitis, mastoiditis, pneumonia) that were complications of upper respiratory viral infections. The name *common cold* most certainly arose from the fact that the onset of symptoms included the feeling of chilliness on exposure to cold. This association was perceived as a cause-and-effect relationship. More than 200 years ago, Benjamin Franklin pointed out that colds were caught from other people rather than by exposure to cold.[140]

In 1914, Kruse[114] showed that colds could be transmitted by the nasal instillation in healthy adults of Berkefeld-filtered nasal washings from ill individuals and that the causative agent was smaller than common bacteria. These findings were confirmed clearly in 1930 by Dochez and associates.[51] The way was paved for more extensive study of respiratory viral infections in 1933 when Smith and colleagues[158] reported the isolation and cultivation of an influenza A virus from a human.

The greatest contribution to the present understanding of the common cold has been the use of human volunteers under carefully controlled conditions. The Common Cold Research Unit at Salisbury, England, was established in 1946,[5,179] and volunteer studies at this institution and studies done in the United States* are responsible for the present understanding of colds in adults.

Although studies of respiratory illness in children also have been extensive, controlled virus challenge trials have not been done. Pediatric studies have been most useful in delineating the spectrum of clinical manifestations by age group and seasonal prevalence rates of the different respiratory viruses.

ETIOLOGIC AGENTS

Initial investigations into the etiology of the common cold were based on the hypothesis that only one etiologic agent needed to

be discovered. Subsequent studies revealed that many different groups of viruses were involved etiologically and that many types frequently existed within each group. Table 8–1 lists the agents associated with colds. Each of these agents is covered more fully in other chapters; this chapter presents only an overview. As a group, rhinoviruses are the most common cause of colds in children and adults. Also of major importance in the etiology of colds are reinfections with parainfluenza viruses and respiratory syncytial virus (RSV). Although the quantitative contribution of coronaviruses to colds in children is unknown, they probably are significant contributors. More recent studies also indicate that human metapneumovirus causes colds and lower respiratory infections in children.[38,146,185,186]

Enteroviruses and adenoviruses have been implicated frequently in upper respiratory illnesses, but in most instances, the illnesses do not conform to strictly defined colds. Reoviruses cause colds, but their contribution to the overall incidence is unknown. *Mycoplasma pneumoniae*, *Chlamydia pneumoniae*, *Streptococcus pneumoniae*, and *Haemophilus influenzae* infections were identified serologically in one study involving young adults with colds, but in most instances, concomitant viral infections also were noted.[121] The more recently identified human bocavirus also causes coldlike illnesses in some children.[8] Other agents, such as *Coccidioides immitis*, *Histoplasma capsulatum*, *Bordetella pertussis*, *Bordetella parapertussis*, *Bordetella bronchiseptica*, *Chlamydia psittaci*, and *Coxiella burnetii*, also have been associated with illnesses with initial coldlike symptoms.

TABLE 8–1 Infectious Agents Associated with the Common Cold

Category	Agents
Common viruses that usually cause the common cold	Rhinoviruses Parainfluenza viruses Respiratory syncytial virus Coronaviruses Human metapneumovirus
Common infectious agents that occasionally cause illness with common cold symptoms	Adenoviruses Enteroviruses Influenza viruses Reoviruses Human bocavirus
Illnesses with initial symptoms suggestive of the common cold	*Coccidioides immitis* *Histoplasma capsulatum* *Bordetella pertussis, Bordetella parapertussis, Bordetella bronchiseptica* *Chlamydia psittaci* *Coxiella burnetii*

*See references 1, 25, 41, 44, 46-49, 79-82, 85-88, 101, 102, 108, 124, 128, 172, 173, 175, 177, 178.

TABLE 8–2   Comparative Incidence of Upper Respiratory Infection by Age: London, 1952-1953; Seattle, 1965-1969; and Cleveland, 1948-1950

London		Seattle		Cleveland	
Age (yr)	**Illnesses/Person/Yr**	**Age (Yr)**	**Illnesses/Person/Yr**	**Age (yr)**	**Illnesses/Person/Yr**
0-4	5	<1	3.5	<1	6.9
5-9	3.6	1	3.8	1	8.3
10-16	4.1	2-5	3.7	2-5	8.3
Adult	2.9	6-9	2.7	6-9	6.1
		10-19	1.6	10->11	5.5
		Adult	2.9	Adult	4.8

Data modified from Brimblecombe et al.,[22] Fox et al.,[69] and Badger et al.[10]

EPIDEMIOLOGY

The common cold is an exceedingly frequent illness in childhood. For rhinoviruses alone, more than 100 serologically different viral types can cause this illness. Nonetheless, a general predictability of incidence and seasonal occurrence exists for the common cold. Numerous epidemiologic studies have been conducted on the occurrence of respiratory illnesses, but calculating a precise incidence of the common cold from these studies is difficult because criteria of disease classification have been different. The findings in three carefully performed studies are presented in Table 8–2. Two of these studies were done more than 50 years ago, and the other was done more than 35 years ago. These studies involved a wide range of family life settings, and the average number of colds per year in children varied from three to eight.[10-13,22,69] Adults had on the average approximately one half the number of colds as their children.

In more recent times and in the era of the common use of daycare facilities, studies of the scope and magnitude of those presented in Table 8–2 have not been done. In one study published in the 1980s, the incidence of acute respiratory infections in daycare attendees peaked at 10 per child-year during the second 6 months of life.[46] A study by Wald and associates[181] found that children in home care had 4.7 illnesses per year, whereas the illness rate was 7.1 per year in children in daycare. Of the illnesses, 89 percent in daycare attendees were respiratory infections.

In a study in Arizona, researchers found that 52 percent of 2-year-old children who attended large daycare centers had six to nine colds per year.[15] The conventional spread of colds has its initial focus in the school.[10,13,22] School-age children become infected and introduce secondary infections into the home. Under these conditions, the secondary attack rate was highest in other school-age children and preschool-age children. Generally, the secondary attack rate in adult family members was approximately one half that of the children. The introduction of infection into the family by adults is unusual. In crowded settings, such as a university, infection is common and can be associated with substantial morbidity. In a cohort study of more than 3000 college students, colds and influenza-like illness were common findings and were associated with missed classes, poor performance on class assignments, missed extracurricular activities, and increases in use of medical care.[132]

As noted previously, the present trend toward the use of daycare centers and preschool programs has increased the number of primary infections in younger children and has made them the source from which secondary family infections frequently occur.[130] In a study that involved 606 children who received care at home or in a daycare program during the first 3 years of life, researchers found that children who attended a large daycare facility (six or more unrelated children) had more frequent colds at year 2 and less frequent colds at years 6 through 11 than did the children with home care only.[15]

Close personal contact between children is necessary for the transmission of viruses that cause colds. In the typical pediatric practice office setting, no increased risk for the acquisition of respiratory illnesses by well infants has been shown.[119] Among children, boys tend to have more colds than girls do.[10,22] In the conventional family setting, mothers tend to have at least one more cold a year than their spouses have.[10,22,69,70] The usual incubation period of colds is 1 to 5 days.

In all nonisolated populations, colds occur more frequently during the winter months than during the summer.[50,71,121,179] This seasonal discrepancy in incidence is as apparent in areas of high wintertime mean temperatures as it is in locations with extremely low temperatures. In the tropics, colds are more prevalent during the rainy season. Colds occur throughout the world. In isolated populations in which the number of people is few (e.g., members of Antarctic exploration teams and isolated island communities), colds do not occur unless introduced by a visiting person.[95]

Although colds can be produced regularly in volunteers, the method of transmission of viruses, which results in colds under natural circumstances, is unclear.* In individuals infected with respiratory viruses that cause colds, the greatest concentration of virus is in the nasal secretions. Children tend to have greater concentrations of virus than do adults, and they tend to shed virus for longer periods. Neither secretions related to coughing nor saliva contains appreciable amounts of virus, and both are unlikely sources of contagion. During the process of talking, little virus is disseminated into the air. The greatest amount of virus from an infected individual is contributed to the surrounding environment by sneezing, nose blowing, and the general contamination of external surfaces (including the sufferer's hands) with nasal secretions.

The route of acquisition of virus is by the nose and possibly the conjunctiva. With these facts in mind, one can easily see that a susceptible individual can become infected by the inhalation of virus in droplet nuclei (small particles) resulting from a sneeze, by the direct nasal hit of virus containing large droplets from a sneeze, by nose blowing, or by the inoculation of virus (usually by the fingers of the recipient) from nasal secretions from disseminators that have been transmitted directly or indirectly. In children, most likely the spread either involves close contact with large droplets of nasal secretions containing virus that are applied to the nose from the hands of the future host or occurs by close-range airborne acquisition.

Considerable folklore is related to the catching of a cold. All available evidence to date indicates, however, that cold weather

---

*See references 23, 26, 41, 44, 45, 49, 79, 81, 85, 93, 101, 106, 124, 150, 168, 179.

per se, chilling, wet feet, and drafts neither cause nor increase the susceptibility of individuals to colds.[52,101] A study of 180 subjects showed that acute cooling of the feet was associated with the onset of common cold symptoms.[107] On day 4, after the cooling of the feet or the control procedure, significantly more subjects in the chilled group thought they were suffering from a cold (14.4%) compared with the control group (5.6%). The subjects who thought they were suffering from a cold had a history of more colds each year compared with subjects who did not develop cold symptoms. In this study, no virologic studies were done, so no evidence exists that the cold symptoms observed were caused by viral infections.

In contrast, in controlled studies in which virologic studies were performed, no increased susceptibility to colds after exposure to chilling conditions was found.[5,52,62] In adults, risk factors for increased susceptibility to colds include stress, smoking, high basal levels of catecholamines, infrequent exercise, low intake of vitamin C, low sleep efficiencies, and lack of diverse social networks.[40,163] Physical stress, as opposed to mental stress, does not seem to be associated with increased susceptibility to colds. In a study of nine healthy men who were competitive cyclists who underwent intensive internal training, the men experienced enhanced performance but had no change in white blood cells, cytokine levels, or the frequency of upper respiratory infections.[56]

PATHOPHYSIOLOGY

The pathophysiology of human infections with viruses that cause colds is presented in the sections of this book covering the individual infectious agents. A general overview is presented here. Few studies on the pathophysiology of respiratory infections have been done in children; the material presented in this section has been derived mainly from studies in adults.* The clinical syndrome of the common cold can occur in association with more than 100 different viral types and in many instances can occur with either a primary infection or a reinfection with a particular viral type.

Although the primary site of virus inoculation in some colds may be on the conjunctival surface, most result from inhalation or self-inoculation of virus onto the nasal mucosa. After acquisition of a virus has occurred, infection of the cells of the local respiratory epithelium develops. This infection varies in the degree of cytopathology on the basis of the viral agent. The infection spreads locally, resulting in an increase in nasal secretions with an increased protein content. Symptoms (nasal stuffiness and throat irritation followed by sneezing) begin on the second or third day and are caused by cellular damage and irritation. Virus shedding is at its maximum in 2 to 7 days, although some shedding may continue for another 2 weeks.

Hilding[94] examined biopsy specimens, scrapings, and smears of nasal secretions and noted that submucosal edema occurred initially, followed by shedding of the ciliated epithelial cells. By the fifth day, the epithelial damage had reached its maximum, with regeneration occurring during the next 10 days. Winther and associates[189] performed similar studies and noted the sloughing of epithelial cells, but they found that the epithelial lining remained continuous with normal cell borders. On the second day of disease, an increase in the number of neutrophils in the epithelium and in the lamina propria occurred. Epithelial mast cells were not involved in the inflammation. The nasal discharge during the second to the seventh day is mucopurulent, owing to its content of desquamated epithelial cells and polymorphonuclear leukocytes.

In experimental rhinovirus colds in adults, little or no discernible damage to the nasal epithelium has been shown.[80,168,188,190] Arruda and associates[9] noted in adults infected with rhinovirus types 14 and 39 that virus replicates in ciliated and nonciliated cells in the nasopharynx and that only a very small proportion of the cells were infected.

Because damage to the nasal epithelium is not noted in rhinovirus colds, apparently cell death is not the cause of symptoms. Naclerio and colleagues[129] and Proud and associates[147] have found that kinins are generated locally and that their concentrations correlate with the severity of symptoms. The cause-and-effect relationship between kinins and symptoms is questionable, however, because treatment with a bradykinin antagonist failed to lessen symptoms.[176] In addition, steroid therapy was found to reduce the concentration of kinins in nasal wash fluid, but it did not affect clinical symptoms.

More recently, researchers have noted that interleukin-1 (IL-1) may contribute to the pathogenesis of rhinovirus infections.[148] Ongoing molecular and biochemical research has provided information about methods by which rhinoviruses interfere with the host response, induce epithelial expression of IL-6 and IL-8, and mediate infection via activation of kinases and receptor binding activity.[58,111,126,139] Similarly, research into the other viruses of the common cold has helped in the understanding of their similarities and differences, such as the cell-mediated immune response to human metapneumovirus and RSV.[55]

In studies in children with acute upper respiratory infections, IL-1β, IL-8, IL-6, and tumor necrosis factor-α were found to be elevated markedly in nasal lavage fluid.[133] Pacifico and associates[136] found that IL-8 concentrations and white blood cell and neutrophil counts were significantly greater in children with rhinovirus colds than in well children. In an adult volunteer study, Turner and colleagues[178] noted a significant rank correlation between nasal obstruction severity, rhinorrhea severity, and nasal-wash albumin concentrations and the increase in IL-8 concentration from baseline on days 2 to 4 after virus challenge. In a study of 285 children with a parental history of asthma or other respiratory allergy or both, blood specimens were obtained at birth and at 1 year of age.[73] The cytokine responses of mononuclear cells when incubated with phytohemagglutinin, RSV, and a rhinovirus were analyzed. Vigorous IL-13 and interferon-γ responses to phytohemagglutinin and a marked secretion of interferon-γ in response to the viruses were associated with a reduced risk of developing wheezing with viral infections in the first year of life.

Pedersen and colleagues[138] studied nasal mucociliary transport in naturally acquired colds and noted that transport was reduced markedly during the acute illness and that slight impairment remained for approximately 1 month. They point out that because some children have four to six colds during a winter season, these children may have constantly impaired mucociliary transport.

Although viremia has been noted during infections with some of the viruses that cause colds, viremia is not known to occur during the typical common cold. The infection is restricted to the epithelial surfaces of the upper respiratory air passages, including the sinuses and the eustachian tubes. With infection, local interferon is produced and presumably has a major role in controlling the infection.[35] Serum antibody and secretory antibody regularly result from infection. The roles of cell-mediated factors in immunity and disease pathogenesis of colds are unknown.

Levandowski and associates[117] noted in rhinovirus-challenged volunteers that total T cells, and particularly helper T cells, were depressed. The magnitude of this finding correlated with progression of infection and symptoms. In a study in which volunteers received rhinovirus type 39, Skoner and associates[155] found a slight increase in helper (CD4+) and suppressor (CD8+) T cells

---

*See references 9, 36, 53, 109, 133, 136, 148, 155, 168, 178, 179, 188, 193.

during illness. Noting that asthma exacerbations and rhinovirus infections are associated with decreased pH and ammonium levels in exhaled breath condensates, Carraro and colleagues[29] studied whether a direct rhinovirus infection or the host immune response to the infection or both decreased the airway epithelial cell surface pH in vitro. They found that airway epithelial cell pH is affected partly by T-helper type 1 cytokines. This decrease in pH can provide an innate host defense, inhibiting viral replication in the lower airways. By mechanisms not well understood, within already infected cells, low pH is thought to trigger uncoating of rhinoviral RNA from within the endosome, enabling viral replication.[21]

The role of antibody (serum and secretory) in the protection against reinfection and clinical colds is complicated. High levels of secretory and serum antibodies seem to be protective against reinfections.* Clinically abortive colds probably are reinfection colds with early antibody recall. Fleet and colleagues[67] have demonstrated a short-lived heterologous resistance to rhinovirus colds, which probably is not caused by interferon or antibody.

Unexplained constitutional factors also seem to control the clinical manifestations of colds.[152] Although studies have shown genetic disease susceptibility patterns related to tissue types, no studies relating to common respiratory infections have been done.[37] In experimental coronavirus infections in adults, clinical severity correlated with detectable IgE in nasal secretions.[27] This finding suggests that atopy may be related to symptoms in colds caused by coronaviruses. Although clinical symptoms and virologic data suggest that colds are upper respiratory diseases, some studies of pulmonary function also have indicated occult lower respiratory tract involvement.[6,33,142]

CLINICAL PRESENTATION

Because the common cold is caused by more than 100 different viral types, considerable variation in the clinical manifestations occurs. As indicated in the beginning of this chapter, the limits of illness to be considered under the diagnosis of the common cold have been set arbitrarily but rigidly. A disappointing note is that although many comprehensive studies of respiratory viral illnesses of children have been done, little attention has been given to the details of upper respiratory infections.

Illness in children must be considered under two categories—infants and older children. The latter is similar to illness in adults. In studies involving 100 young adults, Jackson and colleagues[99] noted that virtually all patients complained of nasal discharge, nasal obstruction, and sore throat; approximately 80 percent had malaise, postnasal discharge, headache, and cough; slightly fewer than 50 percent reported a feverish feeling and chilliness; and approximately 25 percent noted burning eyes and nasal membranes and muscle aching. In older children, the onset of illness is heralded by dryness and irritation in the nose and a scratchy feeling in the throat.[131] The initial symptoms are followed within a few hours by sneezing and watery nasal discharge; chilly feelings and occasionally muscular aches also are noted. Other complaints include headache, general malaise, anorexia, and low-grade fever.

After a variable period of 1 to 3 days, the illness changes; the nasal secretions become thicker and frequently develop a purulent appearance. Persistent nasal discharge, associated with the trauma of repeated blowing of the nose, leads to excoriation around the nose. Nasal obstruction leads to mouth breathing, which causes drying of the throat, increasing the discomfort in

the throat. The usual duration of illness is approximately 7 days, but lingering cough and nasal discharge may persist for 2 weeks or more.[54]

In infants, the manifestations of illness may be more varied. The onset of illness in infants is associated more often with fever (38° C to 39° C [100.4° F to 102.2° F]) than it is in older children. Nasal manifestations in infants are similar to manifestations in older children, but the only other manifestations are irritability and restlessness. Occasionally, coryza is the only symptom. Nasal obstruction may interfere significantly with feeding and sleeping. Vomiting and diarrhea also may occur.

DIFFERENTIAL DIAGNOSIS

Because the clinical entity of the common cold is an arbitrary grouping of signs and symptoms limited to anatomic boundaries and is caused by many different viral types, the approach to the differential diagnosis must consider clinical and etiologic criteria. Many upper respiratory illnesses are caused by numerous infectious agents that should not be confused with colds. A diagnosis of the common cold should not be considered if objective pharyngitis, other enanthema, or evidence of obstructive airway disease is present. Because the common cold is an acute, self-limited disease, the diagnosis should not be considered in a child who has persistent nasal signs or symptoms. Subacute or chronic illness should suggest the possibility of adenoiditis or sinusitis.

The most important differential diagnostic considerations are clinical entities of noninfectious etiology. Allergic rhinitis is a particularly important possibility in a child with "recurrent colds." Careful attention to family history, a search for allergies, the presence or absence of nasal eosinophilia, and the serum IgE value help confirm or exclude this consideration.

Although not reported particularly in pediatric patients, mental stress can lead to vasomotor responses and rhinitis in some susceptible patients. Chemical irritants can cause coldlike symptoms; the clinical response varies greatly among different individuals. Early symptoms of many illnesses, such as pertussis, epiglottitis, measles, and diphtheria, are those of a cold, but in a short time, the more serious nature of the actual illness becomes apparent.

SPECIFIC DIAGNOSIS

The epidemiologic history is the most important aspect of specific diagnosis. In children, if exposure history is requested, a contact usually is uncovered. If strict attention to clinical criteria of the common cold has been adopted, routine laboratory study is unnecessary. Frequently, the physician has an urge to take a throat culture to rule out the possibility of group A streptococcal infection. Usually, one is unnecessary because nasal symptoms are not characteristic of acute streptococcal illness except in infancy, and pharyngitis is not within the limits of the diagnosis of the common cold. The white blood cell count also is of little use.

A specific diagnosis can be made by the isolation of virus from the nasal secretions. It is performed best by using either a nasal-wash technique[84] or a nasopharyngeal swab or aspirate. With laboratory techniques of diagnostic virologic facilities such as those in many university hospitals, parainfluenza viruses, RSV, and most rhinoviruses and influenza viruses are recovered. Direct antigen-detection techniques can be used to identify infections caused by RSV, parainfluenza viruses, adenoviruses, and influenza viruses. Coronaviruses and some rhinoviruses and influenza strains can be recovered only by special laboratory techniques.

---

*See references 32, 34, 67, 99, 100, 102, 103, 116, 156, 167.

TREATMENT

Although literally hundreds of cold remedies are available, few offer any benefit to the pediatric patient, and many may be harmful.* No clinically available antiviral agents have been shown to be effective in the treatment of colds.

In the approach to a child with a cold, the best assumption is that no therapy is indicated in most cases. Specific symptomatic care can be added in the individual case when it is needed. Many children and adults feel miserable when they have a cold, and therapy with an analgesic often is used. Because aspirin is a risk factor for Reye syndrome in children, the use of acetaminophen rather than aspirin is prudent. The dose per single administration of acetaminophen by year of age is the following: younger than 1 year, 60 mg; 1 to 3 years, 60 to 120 mg; 3 to 6 years, 120 mg; 6 to 12 years, 150 to 300 mg; older than 12 years, 325 to 650 mg. Administration may be repeated three to four times daily in young children and every 4 hours in older children. Acetaminophen rarely should be given to infants younger than 6 months of age.

In adult volunteers with rhinovirus infections, acetaminophen was found to be associated with suppression of the serum neutralizing antibody response, and an increase in nasal symptoms was noted compared with subjects who received a placebo.[77] In another adult volunteer study, administration of naproxen resulted in a reduction in headache, malaise, myalgia, and cough compared with placebo.[161]

Relief of nasal obstruction is the most important therapeutic consideration in young children. Locally applied or orally administered, systemically active decongestants are used frequently, but neither their true efficacy nor their adverse effects have been evaluated carefully. Excessive use of sprays and drops with vasoconstrictive drugs can lead to rebound obstruction, which prolongs the illness. The associated drying effect of vasoconstrictive drugs administered orally can be expected to be deleterious to normal mechanisms of clearance. In young infants, sympathomimetic-antihistamine mixtures in oral drop dosage forms particularly are dangerous because respiratory depression may occur.[75] In addition, in a controlled trial, brompheniramine maleate–phenylpropanolamine hydrochloride was found to be no better than a placebo in relieving cold symptoms in children 6 months to 5 years of age.[39] If vasoactive drugs are used, their use should be restricted to times when maximum benefit would occur (i.e., bedtime), and they should be discontinued within 3 days.

The use of isotonic saline drops and gentle aspiration can be very effective in the temporary relief of nasal obstruction in an infant. Also useful is the general humidification of room air because this moisture tends to dilute tenacious nasal mucus so that its elimination is facilitated.

Antibiotics have no place in the routine therapy of common colds.[76,97,105,112,115,118,135,151,159] Occasionally in children, persistent cough is a problem of such magnitude that it disturbs sleep. For cough, codeine and dextromethorphan often are used.[3] No well-controlled studies support either the efficacy or the safety of codeine or dextromethorphan as an antitussive in children, however. Eccles[61] suggested that the apparent efficacy of liquid cough syrups may be due to the sweetness of the products rather than their active ingredients. The proposed mechanism is that a sweet taste may effect cough at the level of the nucleus tractus solitarius by stimulating the production of endogenous opioids.

In the past, antihistamines often have been given to children with colds, but efficacy had not been shown.[184] In more recent years, first-generation antihistamines, but not second-generation

products, have been shown to lessen rhinorrhea in adults with colds.[127,128,168,169,176] Doxylamine succinate, clemastine fumarate, chlorpheniramine maleate, and brompheniramine all have been shown to offer benefit in controlled trials. The effect of these antihistamines is due to their anticholinergic properties. To date, no studies in children have been reported.

A major controversy relates to the efficacy of vitamin C in the common cold prophylactically and therapeutically. In two carefully controlled volunteer studies, the administration of 3 g of ascorbic acid per day did not prevent or alter the symptoms of experimental colds.[153,183] In addition, several large controlled trials in which vitamin C and placebo preparations have been used to prevent and to treat colds have been conducted.[4,28,42,43,63,108,143] In some of these studies, some benefit was reported, whereas in others, no efficacy was noted. Most probably, the reported benefits are a result of statistical artifacts and placebo effect owing to poor study design, rather than specific pharmacologic drug effects. The antihistaminic action of vitamin C[180,194] probably afforded relief to some patients with allergic rhinitis, who thought that their illnesses were colds. Because of the many toxic effects of ascorbic acid,[16] and because its use in treating respiratory illnesses is questionable at best, giving children vitamin C in excess of normal daily requirements seems unwarranted.

For many years, efforts have been made to develop effective rhinovirus chemotherapy, but showing convincing efficacy in natural infection has been a challenge.[137] Interferon alfa-2b administered intranasally has been shown to have some efficacy in the prevention of rhinovirus colds in controlled clinical trials.[160] The effect is variable, however, and adverse effects of the medication are frequent occurrences.[164] Intranasal interferon alfa-2b was ineffective in the treatment of naturally occurring colds but showed some benefit in experimental coronavirus colds.[89,173] Studies in adults using an antiviral anti-inflammatory combination for the treatment of the common cold showed some benefit compared with either agent used alone.[83] However, the irritation caused by intranasal interferon alfa-2b and the drowsiness associated with first-generation antihistamines render these drug combinations suboptimal.

Zinc lozenges have been used to treat the common cold, and the internet and lay literature are full of claims of efficacy. In well-done controlled studies, efficacy has not been shown, however.[59,60,65,104,120,144,172,181] The use of intranasal zinc preparations also is not well validated and raises some concern because of the possible development of the zinc-induced anosmia syndrome.[2,19] In a double-blind, placebo-controlled trial, the use of intranasal corticosteroid (fluticasone propionate) offered no clinical benefit in young adults with colds and induced prolonged shedding of rhinovirus.[149]

In a controlled trial in adults, a soluble intercellular adhesion molecule-1 product (tremacamra) reduced the severity of rhinovirus colds.[177] The antiviral pleconaril induced an early reduction in severity of symptoms in adults with colds caused by rhinovirus.[90] Pleconaril is an antipicornavirus drug that interacts directly with viral capsid proteins. It blocks attachment of virus to cells through intercellular adhesion molecule-1 and subsequent uncoating and release of viral RNA.

In another randomized, double-blind, placebo-controlled trial, the symptomatic efficacy of pleconaril was linked to its in vivo antiviral effects and to the drug susceptibility of the infecting virus.[140] In March 2002, the Antiviral Drugs Advisory Committee of the U.S. Food and Drug Administration voted against recommending pleconaril for approval of its use in the treatment of the common cold in adults. This decision was based on drug interactions, poor risk-to-benefit ratio, and concerns of development of resistant virus.[137]

Clarithromycin, a macrolide antibiotic, enhances mucosal immunity in mice by increasing levels of IL-12, IgA, and IgG.[110]

*See references 2, 7, 14, 18-20, 24, 30, 31, 47, 57, 59, 60, 72, 74, 75, 83, 92, 96, 98, 113, 122, 123, 134, 137, 141, 145, 157, 162, 165, 170, 181, 192.

In a controlled trial, clarithromycin had no effect on the severity of cold symptoms, however. The intranasal administration of nedocromil sodium has been observed to have a beneficial effect on rhinoviral infections in adult volunteers.[17] Mucolytics have emerged as potential therapeutics for modulating the function of airway epithelial cells and altering the course of viral infections.[8,192] Leukoprotease inhibitors and pulmonary surfactant have been shown to be up-regulated by ambroxol—a mucolytic and antioxidant agent.[7,134]

In one study, adults who took sauna baths once or twice a week were found to have fewer colds than did members of a non–sauna-bathing control group.[64] In another study, volunteers with colds did not benefit from inhaling heated vapor.[68]

The list of available and proposed complementary and alternative medicines thought to be useful for the common cold is long.[20,24,57,191] Blinding subjects in placebo-controlled trials can be difficult, and the placebo effect seems to play a significant role in the popularity of all complementary and alternative medicines.[18,20,31,47,92,170] Fluid extracts of *Echinacea* spp. are popular for the prevention and the treatment of colds.[78,168,175] Because several species of *Echinacea* have been used in prevention and treatment studies, criticism of the negative results in some studies has been expressed by *Echinacea* advocates.[20,30,74,113,154,162,165,170]

In a controlled trial, Taylor and associates[166] evaluated *Echinacea* for the treatment of upper respiratory tract infections in children aged 2 to 11 years old. No benefit was noted, and the *Echinacea*-treated children had an increased occurrence of rash. Preparations of North American ginseng have been reported to decrease the frequency of colds in adults.[14,123,145] No controlled studies have been done in children.

PROGNOSIS

The prognosis of common colds in children is excellent. Secondary complications do occur, however, and frequently they require careful and prolonged therapy. The most common complications are otitis media, sinusitis, bacterial adenoiditis, bacterial pharyngitis, and lower respiratory bacterial infections. The primary viral pathogens identified in hospitalized children with lower respiratory tract infections include RSV, influenza A and B viruses, human matapneumovirus, parainfluenza viruses, adenoviruses, rhinoviruses, and enteroviruses.[112] Infections with multiple agents also occur.

PREVENTION

Studies in isolated populations have shown that when a particular respiratory viral infection has run through the entire group, no further respiratory viral illnesses can occur until a new infected individual enters the population. This type of evidence indicates that quarantine or isolation-type practices could prevent colds. The average urban society of today is so complex, however, that prevention through isolation procedures is impractical. Efforts to control the spread of respiratory virus should be minimal and practical. For children with undue susceptibility to complications, contact with crowds or with infected children and adults should be avoided.

The use of virucidal nasal tissues has been shown to reduce markedly the spread of rhinovirus colds in human volunteers and to reduce modestly colds in the family setting, but as yet no commercial products are available.[48,66] Heikkinen and associates[91] found that the intranasal administration of an immunoglobin preparation by nasal sprays twice a day significantly reduced the occurrence of rhinitis in children attending daycare centers. If confirmed, this form of prophylaxis might be useful for selected children. A study showed that organic acids commonly used in over-the-counter skin care and cosmetic products had substantial virucidal activity against rhinoviruses. The amount of acid applied to the hands correlated directly with the prevention of infection in the deliberate infection model.[171,174]

REFERENCES

1. Abisheganaden, J. A., Avila, P. C., Kishiyama, J. L., et al.: Effect of clarithromycin on experimental rhinovirus-16 colds: A randomized, double-blind, controlled trial. Am. J. Med. *108*:453-459, 2000.
2. Alexander, T. H., and Davidson, T. M.: Intranasal zinc and anosmia: The zinc-induced anosmia syndrome. Laryngoscope *116*:217-220, 2006.
3. American Academy of Pediatrics Committee on Drugs: Use of codeine- and dextromethorphan-containing cough remedies in children. Pediatrics *99*:918-920, 1997.
4. Anderson, T. W., Beaton, G. H., Corey, P. N., et al.: Winter illness and vitamin C: The effect of relatively low doses. Can. Med. Assoc. J. *112*:823-826, 1975.
5. Andrewes, C. H.: The natural history of the common cold. Lancet *1*:71-75, 1949.
6. Aquilina, A. T., Hall, W. J., Douglas, R. G., Jr., et al.: Airway reactivity in subjects with viral upper respiratory tract infections: The effects of exercise and cold air. Am. Rev. Respir. Dis. *122*:3-10, 1980.
7. Arnold, J. C., Singh, K. K., Spector, S. A., et al.: Human Bocavirus: Prevalence and clinical spectrum at a Children's Hospital. Clin. Infect. Dis. *43*:283-288, 2006.
8. Arroll, B.: Non-antibiotic treatments for upper-respiratory tract infections (common cold). Respir. Med. *99*:1477-1484, 2005.
9. Arruda, E., Boyle T. R., Winther, B., et al.: Localization of human rhinovirus replication in the upper respiratory tract by in situ hybridization. J. Infect. Dis. *171*:1329-1333, 1995.
10. Badger, G. F., Dingle, J. H., Feller, A. E., et al.: A study of illness in a group of Cleveland families, II: Incidence of the common respiratory diseases. Am. J. Hyg. *58*:31-40, 1953.
11. Badger, G. F., Dingle, J. H., Feller, A. E., et al.: A study of illness in a group of Cleveland families, III: Introduction of respiratory infections into families. Am. J. Hyg. *58*:41-46, 1953.
12. Badger, G. F., Dingle, J. H., Feller, A. E., et al.: A study of illness in a group of Cleveland families, IV: The spread of respiratory infections within the home. Am. J. Hyg. *58*:174-178, 1953.
13. Badger, G. F., Dingle, J. H., Feller, A. E., et al.: A study of illness in a group of Cleveland families, V: Introductions and secondary attack rates as indices of exposure to common respiratory diseases in the community. Am. J. Hyg. *58*:179-182, 1953.
14. Bakalar, N.: Ginseng may reduce number and severity of colds. The New York Times. November 1, 2005.
15. Ball, T. M., Holberg, C. J., Aldous, M. B., et al.: Influence of attendance at day care on the common cold from birth through 13 years of age. Arch. Pediatr. Adolesc. Med. *156*:121-126, 2002.
16. Barness, L. A.: Safety considerations with high ascorbic acid dosage. Ann. N. Y. Acad. Sci. *258*:523-528, 1975.
17. Barrow, G. I., Higgins, P. G., Al-Nakib, W., et al.: The effect of intranasal nedocromil sodium on viral upper respiratory tract infections in human volunteers. Clin. Exp. Allergy *20*:45-51, 1989.
18. Barton, R.: Efficacy of Echinacea for the common cold. Correspondence. Clin. Infect. Dis. *41*:761-762, 2005.
19. Belongia, E. A., Berg, R., and Liu, K.: A randomized trial of zinc nasal spray for the treatment of upper respiratory illness in adults. Am. J. Med. *111*:103-108, 2001.
20. Berman, J. D., and Straus, S. E.: Complementary and alternative medicines for infectious diseases. *In* Mandell, G. L., Bennett, J. E., and Dolin, R. (eds.): Principles and Practice of Infectious Diseases. 6th ed. Philadelphia, W. B. Saunders, 2005, pp. 603-611.
21. Blacklow, S. C.: Catching the common cold. Nat. Struct. Molec. Biol. *11*:388-390, 2004.
22. Brimblecombe, F. S. W., Cruickshank, R., Masters, P. L., et al.: Family studies of respiratory infections. B. M. J. *1*:119-128, 1958.
23. Buckland, F. E., and Tyrrell, D. A. J.: Experiments on the spread of colds, I: Laboratory studies on the dispersal of nasal secretion. J. Hyg. Camb. *62*:365-377, 1964.
24. Buechi, S., Vogelin, R., Mennet-von Eiff, M., et al.: Open trial to assess aspects of safety and efficacy of a combined herbal cough syrup with ivy and thyme. Forsch. Komplementarmed. Klass. Naturheilkd. *12*:328-332, 2005.
25. Bush, R. K., Busse, W., Flaherty, D., et al.: Effects of experimental rhinovirus 16 infection on airways and leukocyte function in normal subjects. J. Allergy Clin. Immunol. *61*:80-87, 1978.
26. Bynoe, M. L.: The common cold. Practitioner *197*:739-746, 1966.
27. Callow, K. A., Tyrrell, D. A. J., Shaw, R. J., et al.: Influence of atopy on the clinical manifestations of coronavirus infection in adult volunteers. Clin. Allergy *18*:119-129, 1988.
28. Carr, A. B., Einstein, R., Lai, L. Y. C., et al.: Vitamin C and the common cold: Using identical twins as controls. Med. J. Aust. *2*:411-412, 1981.

29. Carraro, S., Doherty, J., Zaman, K., et al.: S-nitrosothiols regulate cell-surface pH buffering by airway epithelial cells during the human immune response to rhinovirus. Am. J. Physiol. Lung Cell Mol. Physiol. *290*:L827-L832, 2006.

30. Caruso, T. J., and Gwaltney, J. M., Jr.: Treatment of the common cold with Echinacea: A structured review. Clin. Infect. Dis. *40*:807-810, 2005.

31. Caruso, T. J., and Gwaltney, J. M., Jr.: Reply to Barton and Hemila. Correspondence. Clin. Infect. Dis. *41*:763-764, 2005.

32. Cate, T. R., Couch, R. B., and Johnson, K. M.: Studies with rhinoviruses in volunteers: Production of illness, effect of naturally acquired antibody, and demonstration of a protective effect not associated with serum antibody. J. Clin. Invest. *43*:56-67, 1964.

33. Cate, T. R., Douglas, R. G., Jr., and Couch, R. B.: Interferon and resistance to upper respiratory virus illness. Proc. Soc. Exp. Biol. Med. *131*:631-636, 1969.

34. Cate, T. R., Roberts, J. S., Russ, M. A., et al.: Effects of common colds on pulmonary function. Am. Rev. Respir. Dis. *108*:858-865, 1973.

35. Cate, T. R., Rossen, R. D., Douglas, R. G., Jr., et al.: The role of nasal secretion and serum antibody in the rhinovirus common cold. Am. J. Epidemiol. *84*:352-363, 1966.

36. Cherry, J. D.: Newer respiratory viruses: Their role in respiratory illnesses of children. Adv. Pediatr. *20*:225-289, 1973.

37. Cherry, J. D.: Comments. Pediatr. Res. *11*:250-251, 1977.

38. Ciancio, B.: Understanding the socioeconomic burden of human metapneumovirus in childhood: Italian study recommends further research. Eurosurveillance *v10*, Feb 10, 2005.

39. Clemens, C. J., Taylor, J. A., Almquist, J. R., et al.: Is an antihistamine-decongestant combination effective in temporarily relieving symptoms of the common cold in preschool children? J. Pediatr. *130*:463-466, 1997.

40. Cohen, S., Doyle, W. J., Skoner, D. P., et al.: Social ties and susceptibility to the common cold. J. A. M. A. *277*:1940-1944, 1997.

41. Couch, R. B., Cate, T. R., Douglas, R. G., Jr., et al.: Effect of route of inoculation on experimental respiratory viral disease in volunteers and evidence for airborne transmission. Bacteriol. Rev. *30*:517-529, 1966.

42. Coulehan, J. L.: Ascorbic acid and the common cold: Reviewing the evidence. Postgrad. Med. *66*:153-160, 1979.

43. Coulehan, J. L., Eberhard, S., Kapner, L., et al.: Vitamin C and acute illness in Navajo schoolchildren. N. Engl. J. Med. *18*:973-977, 1976.

44. D'Alessio, D. J., Meschievitz, C. K., Peterson, J. A., et al.: Short-duration exposure and the transmission of rhinoviral colds. J. Infect. Dis. *150*:189-194, 1984.

45. D'Alessio, D. J., Peterson, J. A., Dick, C. R., et al.: Transmission of experimental rhinovirus colds in volunteer married couples. J. Infect. Dis. *133*:28-36, 1976.

46. Denny, F. W., Collier, A. M., and Henderson, F. W.: Acute respiratory infections in day care. Rev. Infect. Dis. *8*:527-532, 1986.

47. Desbiens, N. A.: Lessons learned from attempts to establish the blind in placebo-controlled trials of zinc for the common cold. Editorial. Ann. Intern. Med. *133*:302-303, 2000.

48. Dick, E. C., Hossain, S. U., Mink, K. A., et al.: Interruption of transmission of rhinovirus colds among human volunteers using virucidal paper handkerchiefs. J. Infect. Dis. *153*:352-356, 1986.

49. Dick, E. C., Jennings, L. C., Mink, K. A., et al.: Aerosol transmission of rhinovirus colds. J. Infect. Dis. *156*:442-448, 1987.

50. Dingle, J. H., Badger, G. F., Feller, A. E., et al.: A study of illness in a group of Cleveland families, I: Plan of study and certain general observations. Am. J. Hyg. *58*:16-30, 1953.

51. Dochez, A. R., Shibley, G. S., and Mills, K. C.: Studies in the common cold, IV: Experimental transmission of the common cold to anthropoid apes and human beings by means of a filtrable agent. J. Exp. Med. *52*:701-716, 1930.

52. Douglas, R. G., Jr.: Pathogenesis of rhinovirus common colds in human volunteers. Ann. Otol. Rhinol. Laryngol. *79*:563-571, 1970.

53. Douglas, R. G., Jr., Lindgren, K. M., and Couch, R. B.: Exposure to cold environment and rhinovirus common cold: Failure to demonstrate effect. N. Engl. J. Med. *279*:742-747, 1968.

54. Doust, J., and Del Mar, C.: Diagnosing coughs and colds. Editorials. Br. J. Gen. Pract. *Jan.*:5-6, 2004.

55. Douville, R. N., Bastien, N., Li, Y., et al.: Human metapneumovirus elicits weak IFN-γ memory response compared with respiratory syncytial virus. J. Immunol. *176*:5848-5855, 2006.

56. Dressendorfer, R. H., Petersen, S. R., Moss Lovshin, S. E., et al.: Performance enhancement with maintenance of resting immune status after intensified cycle training. Clin. J. Sport Med. *12*:301-307, 2002.

57. Duenwald, M.: Keeping colds at bay: Or maybe not. The consumer. The *New York Times*, February 1, 2005.

58. Dumitru, C. A., Dreschers, S., and Gulbins, E.: Rhinoviral infections activate p38MAP-kinases via membrane rafts and rhoA. Cell Physiol. Biochem. *17*:159-166, 2006.

59. Eby, G. A.: Elimination of efficacy by additives in zinc acetate lozenges for common colds. Correspondence. Clin. Infect. Dis. *32*:1520, 2001.

60. Eby, G. A., and Halcomb, W. W.: Ineffectivenes of zinc gluconate nasal spray and zinc orotate lozenges in common-cold treatment: A double-blind, placebo-controlled clinical trial. Altern. Ther. Health Med. *12*:34-38, 2006.

61. Eccles, R.: Mechanisms of the placebo effect of sweet cough syrups. Respir. Physiol. Neurobiol. *152*:340-348, 2006. Epub 2005.

62. Dowling, H. F., Jackson, G. G., Spiesman, I. G., et al.: Transmission of the common cold to volunteers under controlled conditions, II: The effect of chilling of the subject upon susceptibility. Am J. Hyg. *66*:59-65, 1958.

63. Elwood, P. C., Hughes, S. J., and St. Leger, A. S.: A randomized controlled trial of the therapeutic effect of vitamin C in the common cold. Practitioner *218*:133-137, 1977.

64. Ernst, E., Pecho, E., Wirz, P., and Saradeth, T.: Regular sauna bathing and the incidence of common colds. Ann. Med. *22*:225-227, 1990.

65. Farr, B. M., Conner, E. M., Betts, R. F., et al.: Two randomized controlled trials of zinc gluconate lozenge therapy of experimentally induced rhinovirus colds. Antimicrob. Agents Chemother. *31*:1183-1187, 1987.

66. Farr, B. M., Hendley, J. O., Kaiser, D. L., et al.: Two randomized controlled trials of virucidal nasal tissues in the prevention of natural upper respiratory infections. Am. J. Epidemiol. *128*:1162-1172, 1988.

67. Fleet, W. F., Couch, R. B., Cate, T. R., et al.: Homologous and heterologous resistance to rhinovirus common cold. Am. J. Epidemiol. *82*:185-196, 1965.

68. Forstall, G. J., Macknin, M. L., Yen-Lieberman, B. R., and Medendorp, S. V.: Effect of inhaling heated vapor on symptoms of the common cold. J. A. M. A. *271*:1109-1111, 1994.

69. Fox, J. P., Hall, C. E., Cooney, M. K., et al.: The Seattle virus watch, II: Objectives, study population and its observation, data processing and summary of illnesses. Am. J. Epidemiol. *96*:270-285, 1972.

70. Foy, H. M., Cooney, M. K., Hall, C., et al.: Case-to-case intervals of rhinovirus and influenza virus infections in households. J. Infect. Dis. *157*:180-182, 1988.

71. Frost, W. H., and Gover, M.: The incidence and time distribution of common colds in several groups kept under continuous observation. *In* Maxcy, K. F. (ed.): Papers of Wade Hampton Frost. New York, Commonwealth Fund, 1941, pp. 359-392.

72. Gadomski, A., and Horton, L.: The need for rational therapeutics in the use of cough and cold medicine in infants. Pediatrics *89*:774-776, 1992.

73. Gern, J. E., Brooks, G. D., Meyer, P., et al.: Bidirectional interactions between viral respiratory illnesses and cytokine responses in the first year of life. J. Allergy Clin. Immunol. *117*:72-78, 2006.

74. Goel, V., Lovlin, R., Chang, C., et al.: A proprietary extract from the Echinacea plant (*Echinacea pupurea*) enhances systemic immune response during the common cold. Phytother. Res. *19*:689-694, 2005.

75. Goldbloom, R. B.: Nasopharyngitis (the common cold). *In* Gellis, S. S., and Kagan, B. M. (eds.): Current Pediatric Therapy. 11th ed. Philadelphia, W. B. Saunders, 1984, p. 93.

76. Gordon, M., Lovell, S., and Dugdale, A. E.: The value of antibiotics in minor respiratory illness in children: A controlled trial. Med. J. Aust. *1*:304-306, 1974.

77. Graham, N. M. H., Burrell, C. J., Douglas, R. M., et al.: Adverse effects of aspirin, acetaminophen, and ibuprofen on immune function, viral shedding, and clinical status in rhinovirus-infected volunteers. J. Infect. Dis. *162*:1277-1282, 1990.

78. Grimm, W., and Müller, H.: A randomized controlled trial of the effect of fluid extract of *Echinacea purpurea* on the incidence and severity of colds and respiratory infections. Am. J. Med. *106*:138-143, 1999.

79. Gwaltney, J. M., Jr., and Hendley, J. O.: Transmission of experimental rhinovirus infection by contaminated surfaces. Am. J. Epidemiol. *116*:828-833, 1982.

80. Gwaltney, J. M., Jr., Hendley, J. O., Simon, G., et al.: Rhinovirus infections in an industrial population, I: The occurrence of illness. N. Engl. J. Med. *275*:1261-1268, 1966.

81. Gwaltney, J. M., Jr., Moskalski, P. B., and Hendley, J. O.: Hand-to-hand transmission of rhinovirus colds. Ann. Intern. Med. *88*:463-467, 1978.

82. Gwaltney, J. M., Jr., Moskalski, P. B., and Hendley, J. O.: Interruption of experimental rhinovirus transmission. J. Infect. Dis. *142*:811-815, 1980.

83. Gwaltney, J. M., Jr., Winther, B., Patrie, J. T., et al.: Combined antiviral-antimediator treatment for the common cold. J. Infect. Dis. *186*:147-154, 2002.

84. Hall, C. B., and Douglas, R. G., Jr.: Clinically useful method for the isolation of respiratory syncytial virus. J. Infect. Dis. *131*:1-5, 1975.

85. Hall, C. B., Douglas, R. G., Jr., Schnabel, K. C., et al.: Infectivity of respiratory syncytial virus by various routes of inoculation. Infect. Immunol. *33*:779-783, 1981.

86. Harris, J. M., II, and Gwaltney, J. M., Jr.: Incubation periods of experimental rhinovirus infection and illness. Clin. Infect. Dis. *23*:1287-1290, 1996.

87. Hayden, F. G., and Gwaltney, J. M., Jr.: Intranasal interferon α2 for prevention of rhinovirus infection and illness. J. Infect. Dis. *148*:543-550, 1983.

88. Hayden, F. G., and Gwaltney, J. M., Jr.: Intranasal interferon α2 treatment of experimental rhinoviral colds. J. Infect. Dis. *150*:174-180, 1984.

89. Hayden, F. G., Kaiser, D. L., and Albrecht, J. K.: Intranasal recombinant alfa-2b interferon treatment of naturally occurring common colds. Antimicrob. Agents Chemother. *32*:224-230, 1988.

90. Hayden, F. G., Kim, K., Hudson, S. A., et al.: Pleconaril treatment provides early reduction of symptom severity in viral respiratory infection due to picornaviruses. Abstract 414. *In* Program and Abstracts 39th Annual Meeting of the Infectious Diseases Society of America, San Francisco, October 25-28, 2001.

91. Heikkinen, T., Ruohola, A., Ruuskanen, O., et al.: Intranasally administered immunoglobulin for the prevention of rhinitis in children. Pedriatr. Infect. Dis. *17*:367-372, 1998.

92. Hemila, H.: Echinacea, vitamin C, the common cold and blinding. Correspondence. Clin. Infect. Dis. *41*:762-763, 2005.

93. Hendley, J. O., Wenzel, R. P., and Gwaltney, J. M., Jr.: Transmission of rhinovirus colds by self-inoculation. N. Engl. J. Med. *288*:1361-1364, 1973.

94. Hilding, A.: The common cold. Arch. Otolaryngol. *12*:133-150, 1930.

95. Holmes, M. J., and Allen, T. R.: Viral respiratory diseases in isolated communities: A review. Br. Antarct. Surv. Bull. *35*:23-31, 1973.

96. Hrastinger, A., Dietz, B., Bauer, R., et al.: Is there clinical evidence supporting the use of botanical dietary supplements in children? J. Pediatr. *146*:311-317, 2005.

97. Huang, N., Morlock, L., Lee, C., et al.: Antibiotic prescribing for children with nasopharyngitis (common colds), upper respiratory infections, and bronchitis who have health-professional parents. Pediatrics *116*:826-832, 2005.

98. Hutton, N., Wilson, M. H., Mellits, E. D., et al.: Effectiveness of an antihistamine-decongestant combination for young children with the common cold: A randomized, controlled clinical trial. J. Pediatr. *118*:125-130, 1991.

99. Jackson, G. G.: Understanding of viral respiratory illnesses provided by experiments in volunteers. Bacteriol. Rev. *28*:423-430, 1964.

100. Jackson, G. G., Dowling, H. F., Akers, L. W., et al.: Immunity to the common cold from protective serum antibody: Time of appearance, persistence and relation to reinfection. N. Engl. J. Med. *266*:791-796, 1962.

101. Jackson, G. G., Dowling, H. F., and Anderson, T. O.: Neutralization of common cold agents in volunteers by pooled human globulin. Science *128*:27-28, 1958.

102. Jackson, G. G., Dowling, H. F., Anderson, T. O., et al.: Susceptibility and immunity to common upper respiratory viral infections: The common cold. Ann. Intern. Med. *53*:719-738, 1960.

103. Jackson, G. G., Dowling, H. F., and Muldoon, R. L.: Present concepts of the common cold. Am. J. Public Health *52*:940-945, 1962.

104. Jackson, J. L., Peterson, C., and Lesho, E.: A meta-analysis of zinc salts lozenges and the common cold. Arch. Intern. Med. *157*:2373-2376, 1997.

105. Jacobs, R. F.: Judicious use of antibiotics for common pediatric respiratory infections. Pediatr. Infect. Dis. J. *19*:938-943, 2000.

106. Jennings, L. C., Dick, E. C., Mink, K. A., et al.: Near disappearance of rhinovirus along a fomite transmission chain. J. Infect. Dis. *158*:888-892, 1988.

107. Johnson, C., and Eccles, R.: Acute cooling of the feet and the onset of common cold symptoms. Fam. Pract. 22:608-613, 2005.

108. Karlowski, T. R., Chalmers, T. C., Frenkel, L. D., et al.: Ascorbic acid for the common cold: A prophylactic and therapeutic trial. J. A. M. A. *231*:1038-1042, 1975.

109. Kaul, P., Singh, I., and Turner, R. B.: Effect of nitric oxide on rhinovirus replication and virus-induced interleukin-8 elaboration. Am. J. Respir. Crit. Care Med. *159*:1193-1198, 1999.

110. Kido, H., Okumura, Y., Yamada, H., et al.: Secretory leukoprotease inhibitor and pulmonary surfactant serve as principal defenses against influenza A virus infection in the airway and chemical agents up-regulating their levels may have therapeutic potential. Biol. Chem. *385*:1029-1034, 2004.

111. Kim, J., Sanders, S. P., Siekerski, E. S., et al.: Role of NF-κB in cytokine production induced from human airway epithelial cells by rhinovirus infection. J. Immunol. *165*:3384-3392, 2000.

112. Klig, J. E.: Office pediatrics: Current perspectives on the outpatient evaluation and management of lower respiratory infections in children. Curr. Opin. Pediatr. *18*:71-76, 2006.

113. Knight, V.: Echinacea treatment for the common cold. Editorial commentary. Clin. Infect. Dis. *40*:811-812, 2005.

114. Kruse, W.: Die erreger von husten und schnupfen. München Med. Wochenschr. 61:1547, 1914.

115. Kuyvenhoven, M., Van Essen, G., Schellevis, F., et al.: Management of upper respiratory tract infections in Dutch general practice: Antibiotic prescribing rates and incidence in 1987 and 2001. Fam. Pract. *23*:175-179, 2006.

116. Lefkowitz, L. B., Jr., Jackson, G. G., and Dowling, H. F.: The role of immunity in the common cold and related viral infections. Med. Clin. North Am. *47*:1171-1184, 1963.

117. Levandowski, R. A., Ou, D. W., and Jackson, G. G.: Acute-phase decrease of T lymphocyte subsets in rhinovirus infection. J. Infect. Dis. *153*:743-748, 1986.

118. Lexomboon, U., Duangmani, C., Kusalasai, V., et al.: Evaluation of orally administered antibiotics for treatment of upper respiratory infections in Thai children. J. Pediatr. *78*:771-778, 1971.

119. Lobovitz, A. M., Freeman, J., Goldmann, D. A., et al.: Risk of illness after exposure to a pediatric office. N. Engl. J. Med. *313*:425-428, 1985.

120. Mackin, M. L., Piedmonte, M., Calendine, C., et al.: Zinc gluconate lozenges for treating the common cold in children: A randomized controlled trial. J. A. M. A. *279*:1962-1967, 1998.

121. Mäkelä, M. J., Puhakka, T., Ruuskanen, O., et al.: Viruses and bacteria in the etiology of the common cold. J. Clin. Microbiol. *36*:539-542, 1998.

122. Marinetti, L., Lehman, L., Casto, B., et al.: Over-the-counter cold medications—postmortem findings in infants and the relationship to cause of death. J. Analyt. Toxicol. *29*:738-743, 2005.

123. McElhaney, J. E., Goel, V., Toane, B., et al.: Efficacy of COLD-fX in the prevention of respiratory symptoms in community dwelling adults: A randomized, double-blinded, placebo controlled trial. J. Altern. Complem. Med. *12*:153-157, 2006.

124. Meschievitz, C. K., Schultz, S. B., and Dick, E. C.: A model for obtaining predictable natural transmission of rhinoviruses in human volunteers. J. Infect. Dis. *150*:195-201, 1984.

125. Monto, A. S., Cavallaro, J. J., and Keller, J. B.: Seasonal patterns of acute infection in Tecumseh, Mich. Arch. Environ. Health *21*:408-417, 1970.

126. Moser, R., Snyers, L., Wruss, J., et al.: Neutralization of a common cold virus by concatemers of the third ligand binding module of the VLDL-receptor strongly depends on the number of modules. Virology *338*:259-269, 2005.

127. Mossad, S. B.: Treatment of the common cold. B. M. J. *317*:33-36, 1998.

128. Muether, P. S., and Gwaltney, J. M., Jr.: Variant effect of first- and second-generation antihistamines as clues to their mechanism of action on the sneeze reflex in the common cold. Clin. Infect. Dis. *33*:1483-1488, 2001.

129. Naclerio, R. M., Proud, D., Lichtenstein, L. M., et al.: Kinins are generated during experimental rhinovirus colds. J. Infect. Dis. *157*:133-142, 1988.

130. Nafstad, P., Hagen, J. A., Øie, L., et al.: Day care centers and respiratory health. Pediatrics *103*:753-758, 1999.

131. Nelson, W. E.: Infections of the upper respiratory tract. *In* Nelson, W. E. (ed.): Textbook of Pediatrics. 6th ed. Philadelphia, W. B. Saunders, 1954, pp. 770-786.

132. Nichol, K. L., D'Heilly, S., and Ehlinger, E.: Colds and influenza-like illness in university students: Impact on health, academic and work performance, and health care use. Clin. Infect. Dis. *40*:1263-1270, 2005.

133. Noah, T. L., Henderson, F. W., Wortman, I. A., et al.: Nasal cytokine production in viral acute upper respiratory infection of childhood. J. Infect. Dis. *171*:584-592, 1995.

134. Nobata, K., Fujimara, M., Ishiura, Y., et al.: Ambroxol for the prevention of acute respiratory disease. Clin. Exp. Med. 6:79-83, 2006.

135. Nyquist, A., Gonzales, R., Steiner, J., et al.: Antibiotic prescribing for children with colds, upper respiratory tract infections, and bronchitis. J. A. M. A. *279*:875-877, 1998.

136. Pacifico, L., Iacobini, M., Viola, F., et al.: Chemokine concentrations in nasal washings of infants with rhinovirus illness. Clin. Infect. Dis. *31*:834-838, 2000.

137. Patrick, A. K.: Rhinovirus chemotherapy. Antivir. Res. *71*:391-396, 2006.

138. Pedersen, M., Sakakura, Y., Winther, B., et al.: Nasal mucociliary transport, number of ciliated cells, and beating pattern in naturally acquired common colds. Eur. J. Respir. Dis. *64*(Suppl.):355-364, 1983.

139. Peng, T., Kotla, S., Bumgarner, R. E., et al.: Human rhinovirus attenuates the type 1 interferon response by disrupting activation of interferon regulatory factor 3. J. Virol. *80*:5021-5031, 2006.

140. Pepper, W.: The Medical Side of Benjamin Franklin. Philadelphia, W. J. Campbell, 1911, pp. 50-51, 60-65, 72-73.

141. Pevear, D. C., Hayden, F. G., Demenczuk, T., et al.: Relationship of pleconaril susceptibility and clinical outcomes in treatment of common colds caused by rhinoviruses. Antimicrob. Agents Chemother. 49:4492-4499, 2005.

142. Picken, J. J., Niewoehner, D. E., and Chester, E. H.: Prolonged effects of viral infections of the upper respiratory tract upon small airways. Am. J. Med. 52:738-746, 1972.

143. Pitt, H. A., and Costrini, A. M.: Vitamin C prophylaxis in marine recruits. J. A. M. A. *241*:908-911, 1979.

144. Prasad, A. S., Fitzgerald, J. T., Bao, B., et al.: Duration of symptoms of plasma cytokine levels in patients with the common cold treated with zinc acetate. Ann. Intern. Med. *133*:245-252, 2000.

145. Predy, G. N., Goel, V., Lovlin, R., et al.: Efficacy of an extract of North American ginseng containing poly-furanosyl-saccharides for preventing upper respiratory tract infections: A randomized controlled trial. Can. Med. Assoc. J. *173*:1043-1048, 2005.

146. Principi, N., Bosis, S., and Esposito, S.: Human metapneumovirus in paediatric patients. Review. Clin. Microbiol. Infect. *12*:301-308, 2006.

147. Proud, D., Gwaltney, J. M., Hendley, J. O., et al.: Increased levels of interleukin-1 are detected in nasal secretions of volunteers during experimental rhinovirus colds. J. Infect. Dis. *169*:1007-1013, 1994.

148. Proud, D., Naclerio, R. M., Gwaltney, J. M., et al.: Kinins are generated in nasal secretions during natural rhinovirus colds. J. Infect. Dis. *161*:120-123, 1990.

149. Puhakka, T., Mäkelä, M. J., Malmström, K., et al.: The common cold: Effects of intranasal fluticasone proportionate treatment. J. Allergy Clin. Immunol. *101*:726-731, 1998.

150. Reed, S. E.: An investigation of the possible transmission of rhinovirus colds through indirect contact. J. Hyg. Camb. *75*:249-258, 1975.

151. Rosenstein, N., Phillips, W. R., Gerber, M., et al.: The common cold—principles of judicious use of antimicrobial agents. Pediatrics *101*:181-184, 1998.

152. Sargent, F., Lombard, O. M., and Sargent, V. W.: Further studies on stability of resistance to the common cold: The importance of constitution. Am. J. Hyg. *45*:29-32, 1947.

153. Schwartz, A. R., Togo, Y., Hornick, R. B., et al.: Evaluation of the efficacy of ascorbic acid in prophylaxis of induced rhinovirus 44 infection in man. J. Infect. Dis. *128*:500-505, 1973.

154. Sharma, M., Arnason, J. T., and Hudson, J. B.: Echinacea extracts modulate the pattern of chemokine and cytokine secretion in rhinovirus-infected and uninfected epithelial cells. Phytother. Res. *20*:147-152, 2006.

155. Skoner, D. P., Whiteside, T. L., Wilson, J. W., et al.: Effect of rhinovirus 39 infection on cellular immune parameters in allergic and nonallergic subjects. J. Allergy Clin. Immunol. *92*:732-743, 1993.

156. Smith, C. B., Purcell, R. H., Bellanti, J. A., et al.: Protective effect of antibody to parainfluenza type I virus. N. Engl. J. Med. *275*:1145-1152, 1966.

157. Smith, M. B. H., and Feldman, W.: Over-the-counter cold medications: A critical review of clinical trials between 1950 and 1991. J. A. M. A. *269*:2258-2263, 1993.

158. Smith, W., Andrewes, C. H., and Laidlaw, P. P.: A virus obtained from influenza patients. Lancet *2*:66-68, 1933.

159. Soyka, L. F., Robinson, D. S., Lachant, N., et al.: The misuse of antibiotics for treatment of upper respiratory tract infections in children. Pediatrics *55*:552-556, 1975.

160. Sperber, S. J., and Hayden, F. G.: Chemotherapy of rhinovirus colds. Antimicrob. Agents Chemother. *32*:409-419, 1988.

161. Sperber, S. J., Hendley, J. O., Hayden, F. G., et al.: Effects of naproxen on experimental rhinovirus colds: A randomized, double-blind, controlled trial. Ann. Intern. Med. *117*:37-41, 1992.

162. Sperber, S. J., Shah, L. P., Gilbert, R. D., et al.: Echinacea purpurea for prevention of experimental rhinovirus colds. Clin. Infect. Dis. *38*:1367-1371, 2004.

163. Takkouche, B., Regueira, C., and Gestal-Otero, J.: A cohort study of stress and the common cold. Epidemiology *11*:345-349, 2001.

164. Tannock, G. A., Gillett, S. M., Gillett, R. S., et al.: A study of intranasally administered interferon A (rIFN-alpha 2A) for the seasonal prophylaxis of natural viral infections of the upper respiratory tract in healthy volunteers. Epidemiol. Infect. *101*:611-621, 1988.

165. Taylor, J. A., Weber, W., and Calabrese, C.: Echinacea for treating colds in children. Letters. J. A. M. A. *291*:1323-1324, 2004.

166. Taylor, J. A., Weber, W., Standish, L., et al.: Efficacy and safety of Echinacea in treating upper respiratory tract infections in children. J. A. M. A. *290*:2824-2830, 2003.

167. Tremonti, L. P., Lin, J. S. L., and Jackson, G. G.: Neutralizing activity in nasal secretions and serum in resistance of volunteers to parainfluenza virus type 2. J. Immunol. *101*:572-577, 1968.

168. Turner, R. B.: The common cold. Pediatr. Ann. *27*:790-795, 1998.

169. Turner, R. B.: The treatment of rhinovirus infections: Progress and potential. Antiviral Res. *49*:1-14, 2001.

170. Turner, R. B.: Studies of "natural" remedies for the common cold: Pitfalls and pratfalls. Commentary. Can. Med. Assoc. J. *173*:1051-1052, 2005.

171. Turner, R. B., Biedermann, K. A., Morgan, J. M., et al.: Efficacy of organic acids in hand cleaners for prevention of rhinovirus infections. Antimicrob. Agents Chemother. *48*:2595-2598, 2004.

172. Turner, R. B., and Cetnarowski, W. E.: Effect of treatment with zinc gluconate or zinc acetate on experimental and natural colds. Clin. Infect. Dis. *31*:1202-1208, 2000.

173. Turner, R. B., Felton, A., Kosak, K., et al.: Prevention of experimental coronavirus colds with intranasal alpha-2b interferon. J. Infect. Dis. *154*:443-447, 1986.

174. Turner, R. B., and Hendley, O.: Virucidal hand treatments for prevention of rhinovirus infection. J. Antimicrob. Chemother. 56:805-807, 2005.

175. Turner, R. B., Riker, D. K., and Gangemi, J. D.: Ineffectiveness of Echinacea for prevention of experimental rhinovirus colds. Antimicrob. Agents Chemother. *44*:1708-1709, 2000.

176. Turner, R. B., Sperber, S. J., Sorrentino, J. V., et al.: Effectiveness of clemastine fumarate for treatment of rhinorrhea and sneezing associated with the common cold. Clin. Infect. Dis. *25*:824-830, 1997.

177. Turner, R. B., Wecker, M. T., Pohl, G., et al.: Efficacy of tremacamra, a soluble intercellular adhesion molecule 1, for experimental rhinovirus infection: A randomized clinical trial. J. A. M. A. *281*:1797-1804, 1999.

178. Turner, R. B., Weingand, K. W., Yeh, C., et al.: Association between interleukin-8 concentration in nasal secretions and severity of symptoms of experimental rhinovirus colds. Clin. Infect. Dis. *26*:840-846, 1998.

179. Tyrrell, D. A. J.: Common Colds and Related Diseases. Baltimore, Williams & Wilkins, 1965.

180. Valic, F., and Zuskin, E.: Pharmacological prevention of acute ventilatory capacity reduction in flax dust exposure. Br. J. Indian Med. *30*:381-384, 1973.

181. Wald, E. R., Dashefsky, B., Byers, C., et al.: Frequency and severity of infections in day care. J. Pediatr. *112*:540-546, 1988.

182. Walker, C. F., and Black, R. E.: Zinc and the risk of infectious disease. Annu. Rev. Nutr. *24*:255-275, 2004.

183. Walker, G. H., Bynoe, M. L., and Tyrrell, D. A. J.: Trial of ascorbic acid in prevention of colds. B. M. J. *1*:603-606, 1967.

184. West, S., Brandon, B., Stolley, P., et al.: A review of antihistamines and the common cold. Pediatrics *56*:100-107, 1975.

185. Wilkesmann, A., Schildgen, O., Eis-Hubinger, A. M., et al.: Human metapneumovirus infections cause similar symptoms and clinical severity as respiratory syncytial virus infections. Eur. J. Pediatr. *165*:467-475, 2006.

186. Wilkesmann, A., Schildgen, O., Eis-Hubinger, A. M., et al.: Human metapneumovirus in hospitalized children—a review. Kin. Padiatr. *219*:58-65, 2007. Epub 2006.

187. Williams, J. V., Wang, C. K., Yang, C., et al.: The role of human metapneumovirus in upper respiratory tract infections in children: A 20 year experience. J. Infect. Dis. *193*:387-395, 2006.

188. Winther, B., Brofeldt, S., Christensen, B., et al.: Light and scanning electron microscopy of nasal biopsy material from patients with naturally acquired common colds. Acta Otolaryngol. (Stockh.) *97*:309-318, 1984.

189. Winther, B., Farr, B., Turner, R. B., et al.: Histopathologic examination and enumeration of polymorphonuclear leukocytes in the nasal mucosa during experimental rhinovirus colds. Acta Otolaryngol. (Stockh.) *413*(Suppl.):19-24, 1984.

190. Winther, B.: Effects on the nasal mucosa of upper respiratory viruses (common cold). Danish Med. *41*:193-204, 1994.

191. Xie, Y., Cao, S., Jiang, X., et al.: Preparation of bupleurum nasal spray and evaluation on its safety and efficacy. Chem. Pharm. Bull. *54*:48-53, 2006.

192. Yasuda, H., Yamaya, M., Sasaki, T., et al.: Carbocisteine reduces frequency of common colds and exacerbations in patients with chronic obstructive pulmonary disease. Letters. J. Am. Geriatr. Soc. *54*:378-380, 2006.

193. Zhu, Z., Tang, W., Gwaltney, J. M., Jr., et al.: Rhinovirus stimulation of interleukin-8 in vivo and in vitro: Role of NF-κB. Am. J. Physiol. *273*:L814-L824, 1997.

194. Zuskin, E., Lewis, A. J., and Bouhuys, A.: Inhibition of histamine-induced airway constriction by ascorbic acid. J. Allergy Clin. Immunol. *51*:218-226, 1973.

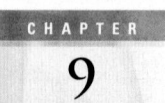

INFECTIONS OF THE ORAL CAVITY

Constantine Simos ❂ Thomas R. Flynn ❂ Joseph F. Piecuch ❂ Richard G. Topazian

Although most infections of the oral cavity in children are odontogenic and may be treated simply with local measures, the occasional spread of these infections to adjacent or distant fascial spaces or to the maxilla and mandible may result in life-threatening complications. Consequently, careful attention, including liberal use of the dental consultation, should be given to such infections.[16,53]

MICROBIOLOGIC CONSIDERATIONS IN DENTAL INFECTIONS

NORMAL FLORA

That the oral cavity provides an environment favorable to the growth of microorganisms is substantiated by reports of bacterial counts of 10^8 to 10^{11} organisms/mL of saliva.[3,6] More than 30 species of bacteria normally can be identified in saliva in varying proportions, depending on a dynamic interaction of different microbial ecosystems, including the tongue, the gingival crevice, and the presence of plaque.[50,57] Age, anatomic relationships, eruption of teeth, presence of decayed teeth, diet, oral hygiene, antibiotic therapy, systemic disease, cancer chemotherapy,[51] and hospitalization can modify the microbial population. In the older literature, emphasis was placed on the role of *Streptococcus* and *Staphylococcus* spp. in producing odontogenic infections, to the exclusion of most anaerobic bacteria. This emphasis probably was the result of failure to culture satisfactorily for anaerobic organisms, and it is now well known that the ratio of anaerobic to aerobic organisms ranges from 3:1 to 10:1.[3,7]

The nomenclature of the oral flora is changing rapidly owing to the improved understanding of the genetic make-up of these bacteria provided by molecular biology techniques. Table 9–1 summarizes changes in nomenclature among selected members

TABLE 9–1   Terminology Changes for Selected Oral Pathogens

Older Terminology	Current Terminology
Streptococcus viridans	Streptococcus anginosus
	Streptococcus intermedius
	Streptococcus constellatus
	Streptococcus mutans
	Streptococcus sanguis
	Streptococcus mitis
	Streptococcus salivarius
	Streptococcus vestibularis
Streptococcus milleri	Streptococcus anginosus
	Streptococcus intermedius
	Streptococcus constellatus
Bacteroides melaninogenicus	Prevotella melaninogenica
	Prevotella intermedia
	Prevotella oralis
	Prevotella buccae
	Prevotella denticola
	Prevotella nigrescens
	Porphyromonas asaccharolytica
	Porphyromonas gingivalis
	Porphyromonas endodontalis
	Porphyromonas salivosa
	Porphyromonas circumdentaria
Streptococcus faecalis	Enterococcus faecalis
Streptococcus faecium	Enterococcus faecium
Peptococcus species	Peptostreptococcus species (main oral pathogen is P. micros)

TABLE 9–2   Most Frequent Pathogens Isolated from Orofacial Infections in Two Studies

Microorganism	Percentage of Cases	
	Lewis et al.*	Sakamoto et al.†
Streptococcus milleri	50	65
Peptostreptococcus species	64	65
Other anaerobic streptococci	8	9
Bacteroides (Prevotella) oralis	40	74
Bacteroides (Prevotella) gingivalis	28	‡
Bacteroides (Porphyromonas) melaninogenicus	24	17
Fusobacterium species	14	52

*Data from Lewis, M. A. O., MacFarlane, T. W., and McGowan, D. A.: Quantitative bacteriology of acute dentoalveolar abscesses. J. Med. Microbiol. 21:101-104, 1986.
†Data from Sakamoto, H., Kato, H., Sato, T., and Sasaki, J.: Semiquantitative bacteriology of closed odontogenic abscesses. Bull. Tokyo Dent. Coll. 39:103-107, 1998.
‡This organism was not reported in this study.

of the oral flora.[8,61,62] Molecular methods based on the polymerase chain reaction allow direct identification of bacterial species to be made from the oral flora and odontogenic infections by isolation of their DNA or RNA or both. These methods have led to appreciation of the true oral flora, for which 60 percent of species are unculturable. In recent years, many new species and phylotypes have been identified in the normal and pathologic oral flora.

The flora of children is similar to that of adults, with several exceptions. At birth, the oral cavity is sterile, but colonization with *Streptococcus salivarius* occurs rapidly. This organism has been found in 80 percent of cultures taken from 1-day-old infants.[63] The percentage of *Streptococcus* spp. decreases from 98 percent at day 1 to 70 percent at 4 months[48] as other organisms become established. *Staphylococcus* spp., *Neisseria*, *Veillonella*, *Actinomyces*, *Nocardia*, *Fusobacterium*, *Bacteroides*, *Corynebacterium*, *Candida*, and a variety of coliforms gradually become established by the time the child reaches 1 year of age. As the deciduous dentition erupts, anaerobic organisms become well established in the gingival crevice, yet the spirochetes, *Bacteroides* and *Prevotella* spp., and related oral anaerobes, which commonly are associated with the gingival crevice in adults, seem to be present in fewer numbers in patients younger than 13 to 16 years.[6,63] Eruption of deciduous teeth also is associated with the establishment of *Streptococcus mutans* and *Streptococcus sanguis*, which adhere to the enamel surface.

PATHOGENIC ORGANISMS

Not all residents of the oral flora are pathogens. In the odontogenic infections caries and periodontal disease, a progression from initiating infections caused by oral streptococci toward a predominance of oral anaerobes in the more severe and longstanding infections apparently occurs. Caries is initiated primarily by *S. mutans*, a member of the alpha-hemolytic *Streptococcus viridans* group. As tooth decay progresses toward the dental pulp,

Lactobacillus and *Actinomyces* spp. join the carious milieu. Severe pulpal infections generally are caused by a combination of these same oral facultative streptococci plus obligate anaerobes, such as *Porphyromonas endodontalis*, formerly classified as *Bacteroides melaninogenicus*.[66]

Periodontal infections also are polymicrobial; gram-positive aerobes, primarily streptococci, predominate in gingivitis, and the gram-negative anaerobic rods predominate in bone-destroying periodontitis. Juvenile periodontitis (formerly called *periodontosis*), a particularly aggressive periodontal infection in children and adolescents, shows a predominance of *Actinobacillus actinomycetemcomitans* in its cultivable flora.

Orofacial odontogenic infections that spread beyond the teeth and alveolar processes are polymicrobial, yielding on average four to six isolates per case.[5,34,46] With the use of molecular methods, even greater numbers of species can be identified in these infections, ranging from 5 to 18 species per case.[14] Severe orofacial infections have been associated statistically with *Fusobacterium nucleatum*.[24] The concept of the progression from aerobic streptococci to anaerobic gram-negative rods in orofacial infections is supported further by studies that have found a predominance of streptococci in early infections (in the first 3 days of symptoms) and a predominance of anaerobes in late infections.[34] Table 9–2 lists the frequency with which the major pathogens in orofacial infections were isolated in two studies.[26,36,59]

Infections originating from nonodontogenic causes (facial trauma, surgical manipulation, tonsillitis) are included in most studies of soft tissue and fascial space infections, and contamination from the skin or oropharynx might allow aerobic organisms, such as *Staphylococcus aureus* and aerobic *Streptococcus* spp., to become established.[6] In contrast, infections originating solely from the dental periapical tissues are much more likely to be predominantly anaerobic.

A pitfall in the identification of organisms as described in the older literature was the failure to culture satisfactorily for anaerobic organisms. The more current literature recognizes this fact.[37,49] The preponderance of anaerobic organisms in odontogenic infections mandates the use of anaerobic and aerobic culturing techniques in situations in which cultures are indicated.

ANATOMIC CONSIDERATIONS

Most severe orofacial infections develop consequent to dental infection—periapical, periodontal, or pericoronal. Spread occurs along anatomic pathways of least resistance.[3,7,27,35,65] Periodontal and pericoronal infections rarely have major sequelae because

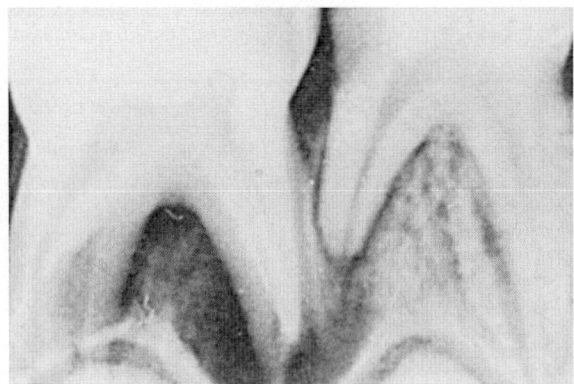

Figure 9–1 Radiolucency representing a chronic periapical abscess involving the mesial root of the deciduous second molar and the distal root of the deciduous first molar. The developing mandibular bicuspids are seen inferior to the deciduous roots. The cause of the abscess is the deep carious lesions in both teeth, which appear to have penetrated the pulp chambers.

they generally drain from the gingival sulcus along the surface of the tooth into the oral cavity. Infections associated with the root apices generally are confined within the bony alveolar process (Fig. 9–1). Should spontaneous intraoral drainage occur through either the periodontium or the pulp chamber, further spread through the marrow spaces is unlikely to occur. If such drainage does not occur, spread through bone (osteomyelitis) or perforation of the cortical plate of the affected jaw may occur. Infections associated with root apices close to the buccal cortical plate generally spread buccally, whereas infections close to the lingual or palatal cortical plate or to the maxillary sinus spread in those directions (Fig. 9–2). When penetration of the cortical plate occurs, infection involves the adjacent soft tissues and may manifest as cellulitis or a soft tissue abscess, which eventually may perforate mucous membrane or skin as a sinus tract (Fig. 9–3).

Perforation of periapical infections through bone follows a typical pattern that results from the position of the root apices in relation to the bony cortex and to muscle attachments (Fig. 9–4). Infections involving maxillary anterior teeth and buccal roots of maxillary posterior teeth generally perforate labially or buccally, whereas infections involving palatal roots of posterior teeth perforate palatally or rarely into the maxillary sinus. The presence of the buccinator muscle attachment superior to the root apices usually confines these infections and fistulas to the oral cavity. In children, maxillary root apices often are superior to the buccinator, however, and infections may spread to the buccal or infraorbital space or to the periorbital tissues. They eventually may drain through the skin.

Infections of the mandibular incisor or canine tooth may spread either labially or lingually because the alveolar process is thin in this area. Labial perforation, which occurs more commonly, may be confined intraorally if the root apices are superior to the origin of the mentalis muscle but may spread extraorally if the apices are inferior to the mentalis attachment (Fig. 9–5). Infections of the mandibular premolar and first molar often perforate buccally, whereas the second and third molars perforate lingually.

When spread of mandibular infections occurs medially, the relationship of the tooth apices to the mylohyoid muscle origin is significant (Fig. 9–6). From the first molar forward, the dental root apices are superior to the mylohyoid, and these infections localize intraorally in the floor of the mouth (sublingual space). The apices of the second and third molars generally are inferior to the mylohyoid, and so the submandibular space is involved, with an extraoral presentation. As in maxillary infections, the

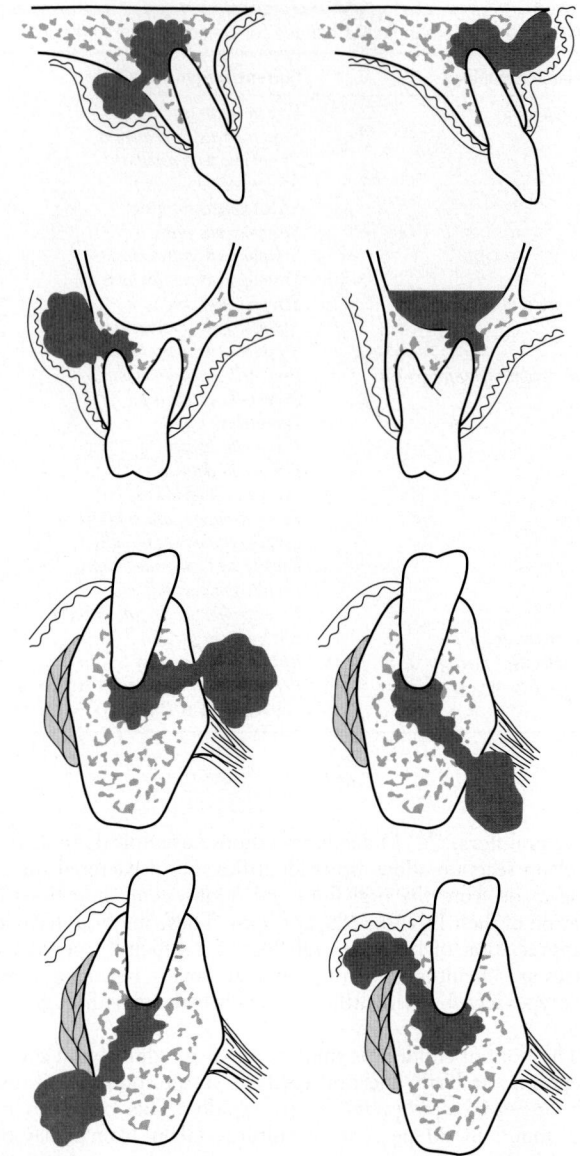

Figure 9–2 Possible pathways of spread of periapical infection. *(From Shafer, W. G., Hine, M. K., and Levy, B. M.: Textbook of Oral Pathology. 2nd ed. Philadelphia, W. B. Saunders, 1963.)*

relationship of the buccinator muscle to the root apices determines whether the infection spreads intraorally or extraorally.

Two fascial spaces commonly associated with odontogenic infections are the submandibular and masticator spaces.[19,20,35] The submandibular space is formed within the superficial layer of deep cervical fascia inferior to the mylohyoid muscle and inferomedial to the mandible. Anteriorly and posteriorly, it is limited by the bellies of the digastric muscle. Within this space lies the submandibular gland and portions of the facial artery and anterior facial vein. This space is closely approximated to the sublingual and masticator spaces. Infections of the submandibular space may originate in these adjacent spaces and in mandibular posterior teeth.

The masticator space also is formed within the superficial layer of deep cervical fascia. Its name is appropriate because its contents include the masseter, internal and external pterygoid, and temporalis muscles, as well as the mandibular ramus and the inferior alveolar neurovascular bundle. The submandibular, lateral pharyngeal, and retropharyngeal spaces are adjacent.

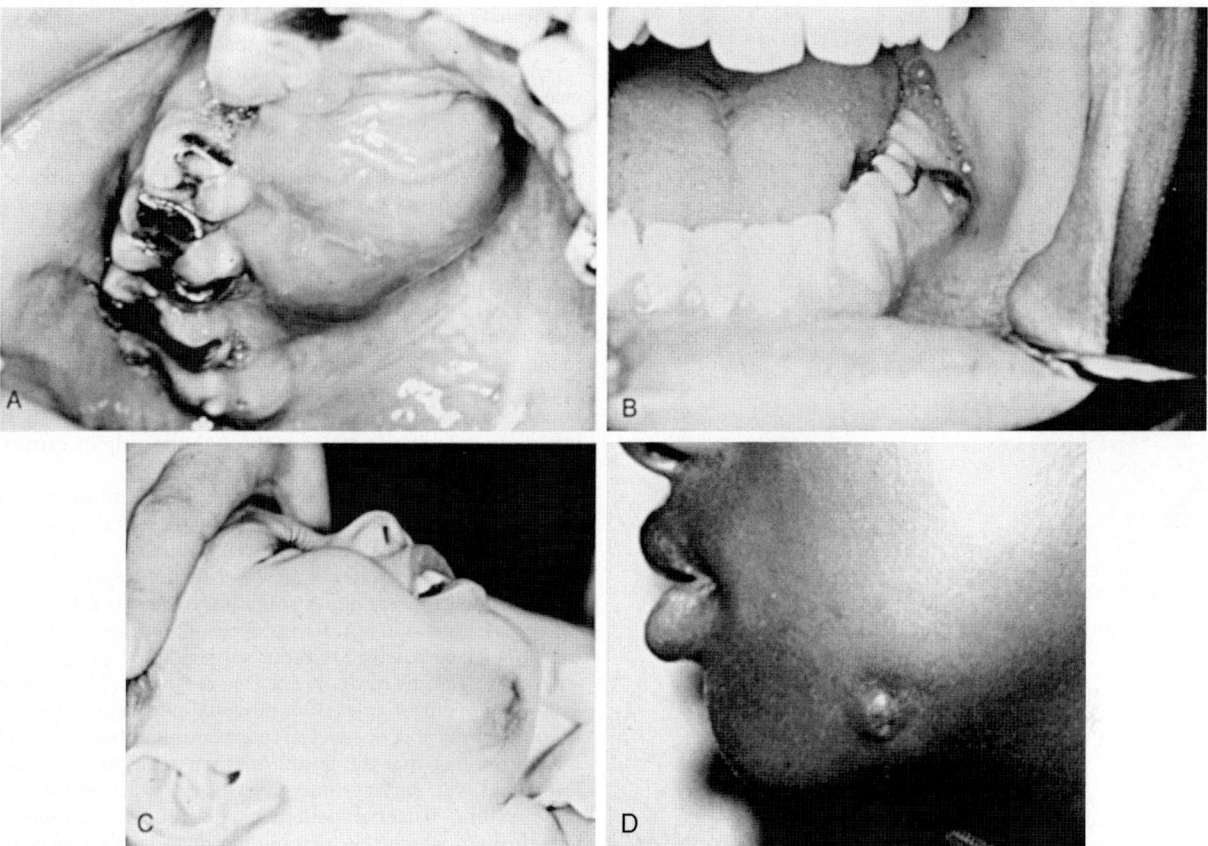

Figure 9-3 Spread of odontogenic infection. **A,** Palatal abscess resulting from infected first premolar. **B,** Intraoral mucosal fistula from periapical abscess of mandibular left first molar. **C,** Soft tissue infection secondary to periapical abscess. **D,** Draining cutaneous sinus tract from a chronically infected lower molar in an adolescent girl. *(A from Piecuch, J.: Odontogenic infections. Dent. Clin. North Am. 26:129-145, 1982. D from Flynn, T. R., and Topazian, R. G.: Infections of the oral cavity. In Waite, D. E. [ed.]: Textbook of Practical Oral and Maxillofacial Surgery. Philadelphia, Lea & Febiger, 1987.)*

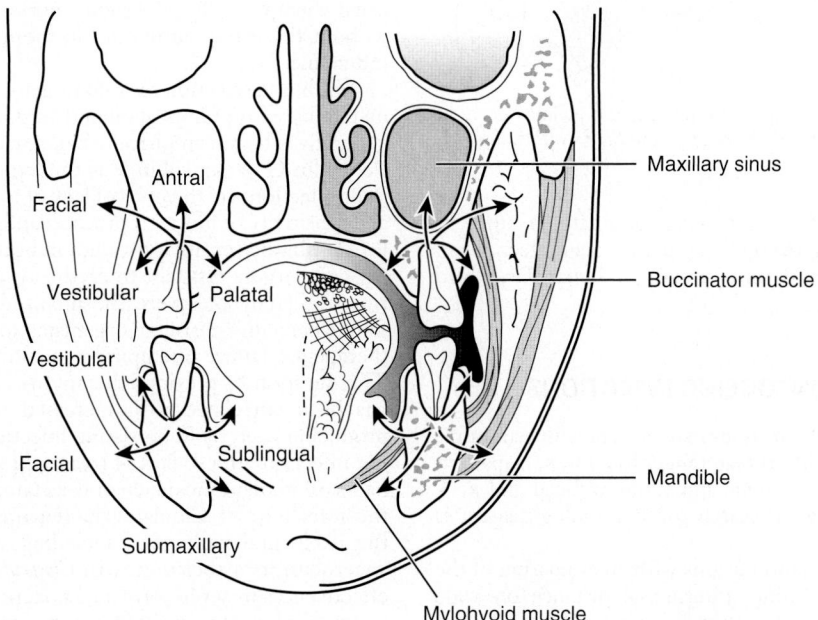

Figure 9-4 Common pathways of spread of periapical infection. *(From Kruger, G.: Textbook of Oral Surgery. 4th ed. St. Louis, C. V. Mosby, 1980.)*

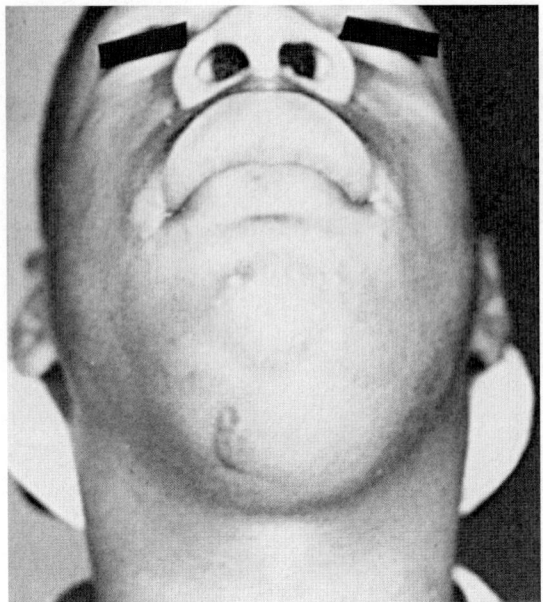

Figure 9–5   Submental space abscess.

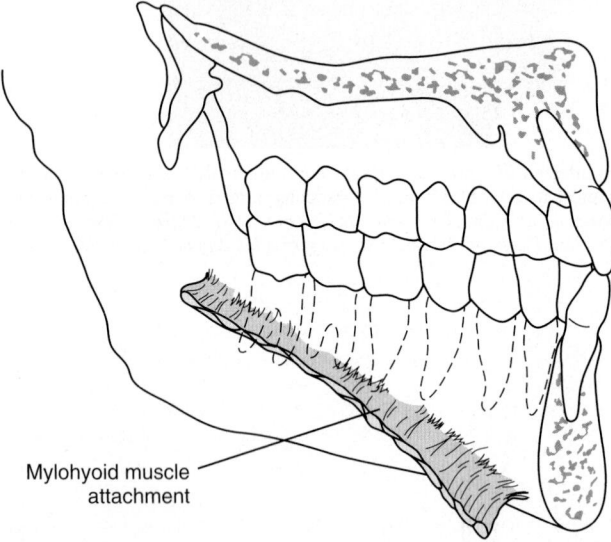

Mylohyoid muscle
attachment

Figure 9–6   Relation of tooth apices to the origin of mylohyoid muscle. *(From Waite, D.: Textbook of Practical Oral Surgery. Philadelphia, Lea & Febiger, 1978.)*

Infections of the masticator space may originate in adjacent spaces or spread to it from periapical or pericoronal infections of the mandibular second and third molars and maxillary third molar.

TREATMENT OF ODONTOGENIC INFECTIONS

Patients with odontogenic infections may present with symptoms ranging from minor to life-threatening. Too often, a patient may be given a thorough systemic and extraoral head and neck evaluation while the intraoral search for the etiologic agent is overlooked.

A thorough oral examination begins with an evaluation of the degree of mandibular opening. Interincisal distance on wide opening extends 40 mm or more, even in young children. Painful limitation of the oral opening, or trismus, is associated with

inflammation of the muscles of mastication and indicates spread of the infection to the masticator space. In association with a high fever, it can represent a serious turn of events. Teeth are inspected visually for caries by percussion for tenderness and by electric sensitivity or hot and cold stimulation for the pulpal pain response. Gingival tissues are probed for periodontal defects, and salivary glands are palpated for tenderness and milked to observe for purulent discharge from the duct orifices.

GENERAL THERAPEUTIC PRINCIPLES

As with infections elsewhere in the body, the principles of treatment of oral infections involve surgical drainage and antibiotics. Surgical drainage may comprise standard incision and drainage of an orofacial swelling or, in the case of localized periapical infection, endodontic drainage through the pulp or extraction of the offending tooth.

Surgical treatment of odontogenic infections is primary. Dodson and colleagues,[10] in a review of head and neck infections requiring hospitalization of children, found that facial infections of the regions at or above the level of the upper lip and teeth most frequently were upper respiratory or sinus related and that lower face infections primarily were odontogenic. Infections of the upper face resolved without surgery in 65 percent of cases, whereas infections of the lower face resolved without surgery in only 25 percent of cases. Odontogenic infections almost always required some sort of surgical intervention. This finding may be due to the fact that the portal of entry in respiratory infections is through the surface mucosa, whereas the tooth roots carry the invading bacterial pathogens deep into the bone of the jaw, through which the surrounding deep fascial spaces become infected.

Respiratory pathogens frequently are viral, and odontogenic infections almost uniformly are bacterial, which may explain the propensity of odontogenic infections to form abscesses that need to be drained. Odontogenic infections treated with antibiotics only almost always recur in worse form than did their previous manifestation. The indications for treating with antibiotics in addition to appropriate dental surgical therapy are fever, trismus, lymphadenopathy, osteomyelitis, and compromise of the immune system. Minor infections localized to the alveolar processes can be treated by tooth extraction, gingival curettage, or root canal therapy, with or without intraoral incision and drainage, without the use of antibiotics in the non-immunocompromised individual.

Antibiotic selection for odontogenic infections, although ultimately based on Gram stain and aerobic and anaerobic cultures, generally is begun empirically before culture results are available. Penicillin G or penicillin V is the logical first choice for outpatient infections on the basis of lack of toxicity, bactericidal nature, and sensitivity of most streptococci and oral anaerobes to penicillin. Antibiotic sensitivity studies indicate that the oral anaerobes now are largely resistant to erythromycin and most cephalosporins.[52] A study of severe (hospitalized) odontogenic infections found penicillin-resistant organisms in 54 percent of cases and therapeutic failure of empiric penicillin in 21 percent of cases.[13] The duration of previous therapy with β-lactam antibiotics also has been correlated with increased numbers of β-lactamase–producing bacteria in persisting infections. Patients with persisting infection after 3 days of treatment with a β-lactam antibiotic had a 50 percent incidence of β-lactamase–producing bacteria in the infection.[23,31] Clindamycin remains highly effective against the likely oral pathogens, including streptococci and the oral anaerobes; its association with *Clostridium difficile* colitis and its effectiveness in severe orofacial infections indicate that it should be reserved, in this era of increasing microbial resistance to antibiotics, for the most severe cases.

TABLE 9–3 Empiric Antibiotics of Choice for Odontogenic Infections*

Type of Infection	Antibiotic of Choice
Outpatient infections	Penicillin
	Clindamycin
	Azithromycin
Penicillin allergy	Clindamycin
	Azithromycin
Inpatient infections	Clindamycin
	Ampicillin + metronidazole
	Ampicillin + sulbactam
Penicillin allergy	Clindamycin
	Third-generation cephalosporin IV (if the penicillin allergy was not the anaphylactoid type—use caution)

Empiric antibiotic therapy is used before culture and sensitivity reports are available. Cultures should be taken in severe infections that threaten vital structures.

The aforementioned considerations suggest that the empiric antibiotics of choice are penicillin in mild odontogenic infections and clindamycin for severe cases or in a patient with penicillin allergy. Table 9–3 lists our recommendations for empiric antibiotic therapy in odontogenic infections.

Second-line antibiotics in odontogenic infections are the cephalosporins, to which effectiveness against the oral anaerobes has been waning, and metronidazole, which is effective against obligate anaerobes only. The safety and effectiveness of metronidazole in children have been established only for treatment of amebiasis.

Other considerations that may be important in the selection of antibiotics for individual cases are as follows: (1) *Eikenella corrodens*, an occasional pathogen in odontogenic infections, is uniformly resistant to clindamycin, which may explain the lack of effectiveness of clindamycin in some cases. (2) Some cephalosporins do not cross the blood-brain barrier in high concentrations, which may be a factor in selection of an antibiotic for an odontogenic infection that is approaching the cranial cavity. Ceftazidime and ceftriaxone cross the blood-brain barrier well. Penicillin is able to cross the blood-brain barrier when the meninges are inflamed. Metronidazole crosses the blood-brain barrier, and its use may be justified in severe odontogenic infections approaching the brain in children. (3) Tetracycline is incorporated permanently into newly formed dentin, causing permanent disfiguring discoloration of the dentition. It should not be used in children until they are at least 9 years old, when all but the third molar teeth would have full crown formation. (4) β-Lactamase inhibitors used in combination with β-lactam antibiotics may improve their effectiveness against resistant anaerobes. A clear clinical advantage of amoxicillin-clavulanate over amoxicillin alone has not been established in adult studies of odontogenic infections, however.[36] (5) Staphylococci are uncommon pathogens in odontogenic infections, and coverage for staphylococci is not indicated in empiric therapy for these infections, although their role in upper respiratory and sinus infections is well known.

NURSING BOTTLE CARIES

Nursing bottle caries is a pattern of tooth decay affecting mainly the primary upper incisors and frequently the upper and lower primary molars in children of bottle-feeding age. It is caused by a practice of putting the child to bed with a nursing bottle filled with a sugar-containing drink, such as milk, fruit juice, or a soft drink. The child sucks on the bottle intermittently during sleep, when salivary secretion is low, and the sugar-containing liquid

stays in the mouth for extended periods. This situation provides an excellent environment for the growth of caries-producing organisms, such as *S. mutans*. Nursing-bottle caries can destroy virtually the entire primary dentition of a child as it erupts. Pediatric physicians and dentists should instruct parents to avoid putting their children to bed with nursing bottles or, if they must do so, to use water only in the bedtime drink.

PERIAPICAL ABSCESS

Extension of microorganisms through the root apex leads to the formation of an abscess. Early in this process, the acute abscess is indistinguishable clinically and radiographically from an acute pulpitis, particularly because radiographic evidence of bone destruction may take 7 to 14 days or more to develop. Sensitivity to heat stimulus (relieved by cold), exquisite sensitivity to percussion, and tenderness to finger pressure on the alveolar process are indications that the tooth has become abscessed. Electric pulp testing may be diagnostic if the tooth shows no response to the electric stimulus, but a positive pain response may be equivocal in multirooted teeth. Chronic abscesses are diagnosed more easily by looseness of the tooth, suppuration from draining sinuses or from the gingival crevice (see Fig. 9–3), and radiolucency on the radiographs (see Fig. 9–1). Depending on the path of least resistance, fluctuant areas may be noted in the buccal or lingual mucosa. Spread through the tissues, or cellulitis, may lead to the classic presentation of swollen face, pain, elevated temperature, and malaise.

In 1951, Krogh[31] showed a 3 percent complication rate when 2626 infected teeth were removed at the time of initial presentation. In 1975, Martis and Karakasis[45] published a similar study in which they treated 1376 acute dentoalveolar abscesses by immediate extraction. A 3 percent complication rate was found in this study as well. A complication was defined as further extension of the infection, requiring additional treatment. Hall and associates[22] published a report in 1968 in which 350 patients with odontogenic cellulitis were divided randomly into two groups. The first group had extractions performed on the day of initial presentation, whereas the second group waited (with antibiotics) until the fourth day for surgical treatment to be performed after "localization" had occurred. The investigators' observations showed that extraction did not spread the cellulitis in either group. Patients with earlier extractions recovered more rapidly, whereas patients with delayed treatment had a greater need for incision and drainage, which was twice as likely to be extraoral than intraoral. In 1978, Martis and colleagues[44] showed in a series of more than 2000 patients that extraction without antibiotics in the presence of periapical infection led to the same complication rate as did extraction of noninfected teeth.

Considering the prospect of early relief of symptoms and a 97 percent chance that extraction (or occasionally root canal treatment) will cure the infection, early surgical intervention is mandatory. The use of antibiotics must be determined on an individual basis according to principles outlined previously (Table 9–4).

PERIODONTAL INFECTIONS

Surrounding the teeth is a distinctive, pink keratinized mucosa, the gingiva (Fig. 9–7A). Normal gingiva is attached firmly to the alveolar bone and extends between the teeth as the interdental papilla. A thin cuff of free (nonattached) gingiva surrounds each tooth, and the resulting crevice between the free gingiva and the tooth normally is 1 to 3 mm in depth. It is represented by a thin roll of tissue along each tooth in Figure 9–7A.

Accumulation of food deposits and bacteria in the gingival crevice may result in gingivitis, a localized inflammation of the free gingiva that manifests as an erythematous, nonpainful swelling of the interdental papillae. In severe cases (see Fig. 9–7B), the gingival architecture may become distorted, and accumulations of plaque are evident. Although gingivitis is prevalent at all ages, affecting more than 50 percent of children[47] and almost all adults to some degree, it often is most severe in compromised hosts, including patients with diabetes and immunosuppressed patients. Poor oral hygiene is the usual precipitating factor for development of gingivitis, and this condition generally responds to dental scaling and improved oral hygiene.

In adolescents and in adults, gingivitis may progress to periodontitis, a progressively severe infection that is characterized by hypertrophied gingivae, tooth mobility caused by irreversible resorption of alveolar bone, and a purulent exudate. This insidious condition usually is painless and may progress for years

TABLE 9–4 Indications for Antibiotic Therapy in Odontogenic Infections

Antibiotic therapy is necessary
Acute-onset facial or oral swelling
Swelling inferior to the mandible
Trismus
Dysphagia
Lymphadenopathy
Fever >38.3°C (>101°F)
Pericoronitis
Osteomyelitis

Antibiotic therapy is *not* necessary*
Asymptomatic periapical abscess
Parulis (draining sinus tract)
Dry socket (alveolar osteitis)
Periodontal disease
Dental extractions
Root canal therapy

With coexisting immune system compromise, antibiotic therapy may be indicated in some of these conditions.

before being recognized. Localized periodontal treatment and meticulous oral hygiene may arrest the condition.

A rare variant, juvenile periodontitis,[34] usually is localized to the molar and incisor regions of younger, otherwise healthy children. Deep gingival pocketing and severe bone resorption are characteristic of this process and may result in loss of the dentition in these areas. The etiology is thought to involve a gram-negative anaerobe, *A. actinomycetemcomitans*, and localized bacterial inhibition of leukocyte function. Tetracycline in older patients has been useful in combination with periodontal surgery and meticulous home care.

Acute necrotizing ulcerative gingivitis (see Fig. 9–7C) is a specific infection caused by fusiform bacilli and spirochetes. Synonyms include trench mouth and Vincent infection. Erythema at the tips of the interdental papillae soon is supplanted by frank ulceration and foci of spontaneous bleeding. A pseudomembranous necrotic exudate forms along the marginal gingivae and the interdental papillae. The papillae later become blunted. Acute necrotizing ulcerative gingivitis is characterized by pain, foul breath and taste, thick ropy saliva, malaise, and occasionally fever. Theories suggest a concomitant viral etiology. Treatment consists initially of penicillin therapy followed within a few days by localized gingival curettage and oral rinses with 0.5 percent hydrogen peroxide or 0.12 percent chlorhexidine.[40] The safety and effectiveness of chlorhexidine in children have not been established.

PERICORONITIS

Impaction of microorganisms and debris under the soft tissue overlying the crown of a tooth, often a mandibular third molar, or any erupting permanent tooth leads to the development of inflammation. Drainage usually occurs spontaneously from under the flap, localizing the problem. Blockage of natural drainage may lead to spread of infection to adjacent soft tissues and fascial spaces (Fig. 9–8).

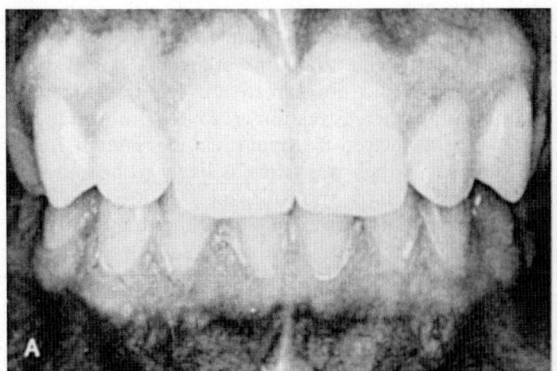
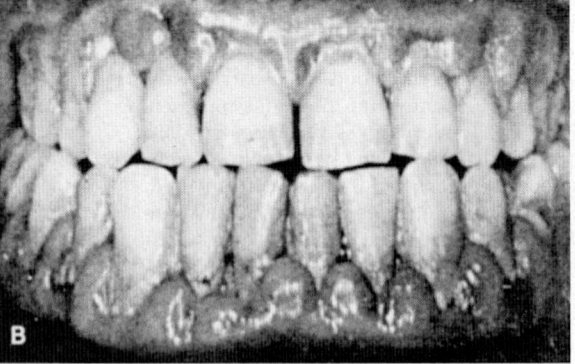
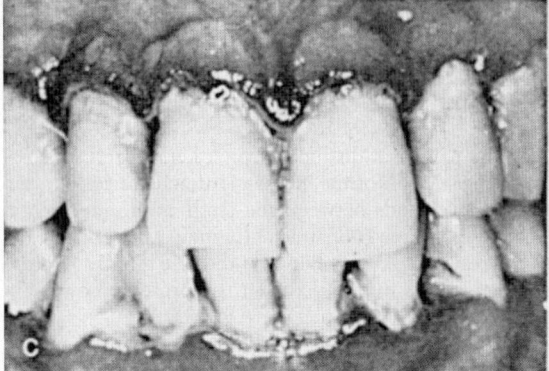

Figure 9–7 A, Normal gingivae. **B,** Severe gingivitis. The maxillary gingivae exhibit mild inflammation; the mandibular interdental papillae are distorted grossly in form. Accumulations of plaque are prominent adjacent to the mandibular incisors. **C,** Acute necrotizing ulcerative gingivitis.

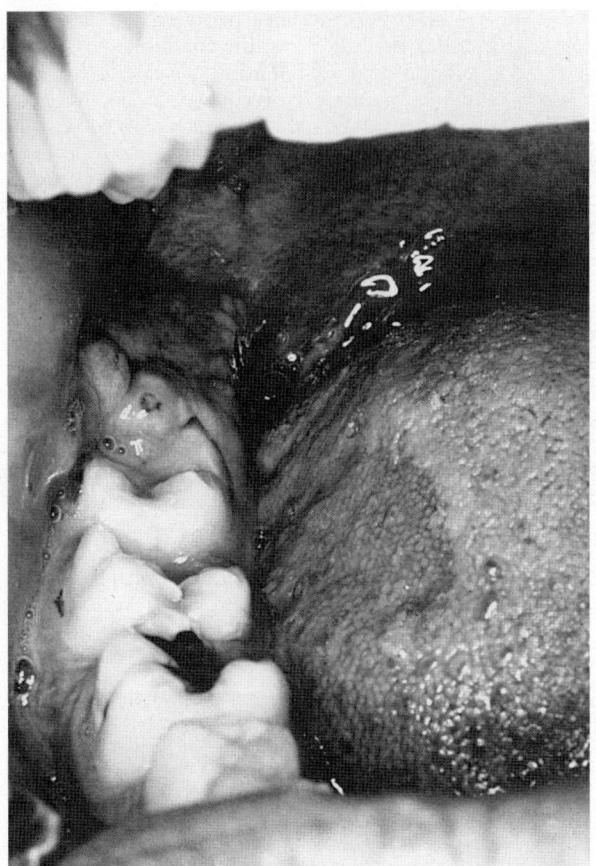

Figure 9–8 Pericoronitis.

Pericoronitis is a polymicrobial infection; the periodontal pathogens *Prevotella* and *Porphyromonas* spp. and oral spirochetes, such as *Treponema denticola*, usually are the causative organisms. The *Streptococcus milleri* group bacteria also have been found to have a significant role in acute pericoronitis.[26] These organisms usually are sensitive to penicillin or penicillin combined with metronidazole. Pericoronitis most frequently occurs around the posterior portion of the crown of the lower third molar because it erupts during adolescence. In most cases, partial eruption of the third molar is caused by insufficient length of the horizontal ramus of the mandible to house all of the teeth. Part of the third molar is trapped under the oral mucosa covering the buccinator muscle and the superior pharyngeal constrictor because they form the most anterior portion of the oropharynx. In cases in which room is insufficient for the eruption of the third molar, the pericoronitis becomes recurrent or chronic, and the impacted third molar should be removed.

Lower third molars lie in proximity to the pterygomandibular space, a portion of the masticator space. When these infections spread to involve this space, trismus results, which obscures the infection to clinical examination. The presence of trismus with a history of pain in the third molar region is an ominous sign of infection involving the masticator space, which, although not manifested by external facial swelling, may begin to involve the deeper parapharyngeal spaces. These infections may become life-threatening. The lower third molar is the most frequent offending tooth in severe odontogenic infections requiring hospitalization, and these infections occur most frequently in adolescents and young adults.[24]

Various treatment modalities, including local incision and drainage and extraction of the tooth, are applicable to pericoronitis.[44,58] Antibiotic therapy is used if fever, trismus, or lymphade-

nopathy is present (see Table 9–4). Resolution of symptoms should occur in less than 1 week.

ORAL MANIFESTATIONS OF HUMAN IMMUNODEFICIENCY VIRUS INFECTION IN CHILDREN

The most common oral lesions found in children with human immunodeficiency virus (HIV) disease are oral candidiasis, herpes simplex virus infections, linear gingival erythema, parotid salivary gland enlargement, and recurrent aphthous ulcerations. In contradistinction to adult HIV infection, HIV-associated periodontitis and gingivitis are much less common. Neoplastic oral manifestations of HIV infection, such as Kaposi sarcoma, non-Hodgkin lymphoma, and hairy leukoplakia, continue to be rare findings. In contrast to adults, children infected with HIV have a greater susceptibility to bacterial infections, especially with encapsulated organisms, such as *Streptococcus pneumoniae* and *Haemophilus influenzae*. Septicemia from an oral focus of infection can become a life-threatening problem in an HIV-infected child, and optimal oral health must be established and vigorously maintained in these children.[33] Routine use of chlorhexidine gluconate 0.12 percent mouth rinse may be helpful in minimizing gingivitis, candidiasis, and bacterial superinfections of the oral cavity, although its safety and effectiveness have not been shown in children.

Oral candidiasis usually is of the pseudomembranous type, which is seen in the oral cavity as a creamy white plaque that is rubbed off easily, leaving a reddened surface mucosa exposed. Because oral candidiasis is rare in normal children older than 6 months, persistence of oral candidiasis for 2 months or more in a child older than 6 months who has not received antibiotic therapy in the past 2 weeks is suggestive of HIV infection. Persistent oral candidiasis indicates acquired immunodeficiency category P-2D3 (symptomatic infection with secondary infectious diseases) in the Centers for Disease Control and Prevention classification of HIV infection in children younger than 12 years.[30]

Oral candidiasis was associated with a decreased survival time in a study of 99 children with perinatally acquired HIV infection. The median time from birth to the manifestation of the first lesion of oral candidiasis was 2.4 years, and the median time from the appearance of lesions to death was 3.4 years, with a relative hazard rate of 14.2.[29]

Treating oral candidiasis lesions is difficult because of frequent recurrence of oral fungal infection with resistant biotypes of *Candida albicans* or colonization by related but more resistant species, such as *Candida krusei*, *Candida parapsilosis*, and *Candida guilliermondii*. Treatment regimens may progress from nystatin to clotrimazole, fluconazole, and amphotericin B, depending on the extent of disease, clinical response, and culture and sensitivity results.[43] Sudden onset of rampant dental caries has been associated with prolonged oral use of sucrose-containing antifungal antibiotic preparations.[69]

Linear gingival erythema, formerly referred to as HIV gingivitis, is the most common form of periodontal disease seen in children with HIV infection. It is described as a fiery red, 2- to 3-mm-wide linear band of inflammation of the gingiva. Pain is not associated with the lesion, but the gingivae are likely to bleed during tooth brushing or even spontaneously. The microbiology of this lesion is unclear, but *Candida* spp. may be a possible cause.

Parotid salivary gland enlargement, which may be painful and become secondarily infected, has been reported in 14 to 30 percent of HIV-infected children. The enlargement apparently is caused by infiltration of the glands by T8 lymphocytes and has been associated with increased survival time. The median time was 4.6 years from birth to development of parotid enlargement and 5.4 years from development of lesions to death, with a relative hazard rate of 0.38.[29]

Herpes simplex virus infections, although common occurrences in normal children, seem to be particularly severe and recur more often in HIV-infected children. The lesions appear first as multiple clustered vesicles on the lips or keratinized oral mucosa, which soon rupture to leave painful irregular oral ulcers or crusted labial ulcers. Fever and dysphagia may warrant hospital admission for hydration, nutrition, and therapy with parenteral acyclovir. Less severe cases may be treated with oral acyclovir.

Dental caries is increased in pediatric HIV cohorts. The cause of this finding is unclear. It may be due to xerostomia secondary to parotid enlargement in some cases, prolonged use of sucrose-containing antifungal agents in others, and nursing-bottle caries in still others. The association of nursing bottle caries with pediatric HIV infection may be due to their common increased prevalence in urban dwellers with limited economic resources, although nursing-bottle caries also is found frequently in children with other chronic diseases.[69]

COMPLICATIONS OF ODONTOGENIC INFECTIONS

FASCIAL SPACE INFECTIONS

Spread of infection to the fascial spaces may result in dramatic facial swelling and high fever and, if untreated, respiratory embarrassment. The characteristics of the more common fascial space infections related to odontogenic infection are described here.

Infraorbital space infections generally are related to maxillary anterior teeth and are well localized to the infraorbital fossa by the levator labii superioris and levator anguli oris muscles. Facial swelling lateral to the nose is prominent, as is decreased mobility of the upper lip caused by inflammation of these muscles. If the area is fluctuant, intraoral incision and drainage with placement of a small Penrose drain for 1 to 2 days generally are sufficient treatment. Antibiotics are indicated for all infections of the fascial spaces.

Trismus is the hallmark of infection of the masticator space. Trismus is caused by spasm in the muscles of mastication, which define this large potential space. The resulting inability to open the mouth hinders access to the airway for endotracheal intubation. In addition, abscesses of the masticator space may rupture into the oropharynx, causing aspiration of pus, or they may pass easily around the medial pterygoid muscle to involve the lateral pharyngeal and retropharyngeal spaces. Figure 9–9 shows a 6-year-old boy whose lower primary molar abscesses spread to involve the buccal, pterygomandibular, and lateral pharyngeal spaces. Extraoral and intraoral drainage, prolonged intubation, and extraction of the offending teeth were required.

Infections of the submandibular space (Fig. 9–10) may be localized unilaterally or may involve bilateral structures. Treatment of submandibular space infection is via extraoral incision and drainage.

First described in 1836, Ludwig angina consists of infection of the sublingual and submandibular spaces bilaterally and is characterized by hard, brawny swelling and a minimum of suppuration. The tongue often is edematous and raised to the roof of the mouth, with little mobility (Fig. 9–11). Airway obstruction should be considered imminent; the greatest cause of death in Ludwig angina is blockage of the airway by soft tissue swelling, pus, or blood, which occurred in more than 50 percent of its victims in the pre-antibiotic era.[21] In 1940, Williams[72] published a series of 37 cases of Ludwig angina, which reported a 54 percent mortality rate. The airway management policy at that time was emergency tracheotomy if necessary. Three years later, Williams and Guralnick[73] published a series of 20 cases of Ludwig angina

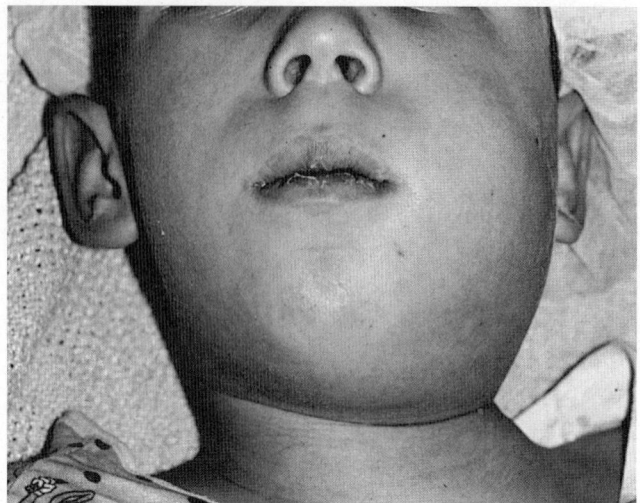

Figure 9–9 Lateral pharyngeal space abscess in a 6-year-old boy. Note the swelling above the hyoid bone and anterior to the sternocleidomastoid muscle. Swelling also occurs in the buccal and submandibular spaces.

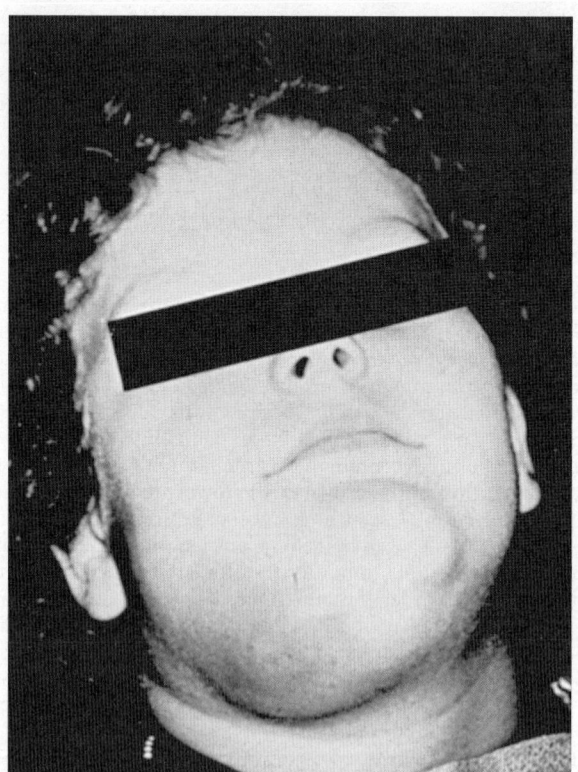

Figure 9–10 Submandibular space abscess.

treated with a new policy of immediate establishment of airway security by intubation or tracheotomy and aggressive incision and drainage of all anatomic spaces affected by the infection. By these measures, they were able to reduce the mortality rate of this dreaded infection to 20 percent only 3 years later. Antibiotics were unavailable during the course of these two studies. These studies underscore the importance of airway security and aggressive surgical management in the treatment of severe odontogenic infections.

Today, death rarely occurs from severe odontogenic infections, although the need for tracheotomy or prolonged endotracheal intubation is common. The cause of this infection often is odontogenic infection but may include laceration of the floor of the mouth and mandibular fracture. Usually a disease of middle-aged adults, it is a rare occurrence in children but may occur in greater frequency in immunologically compromised children.[18] Surgical drainage of all four spaces, accompanied by vigorous antibiotic therapy, is indicated.

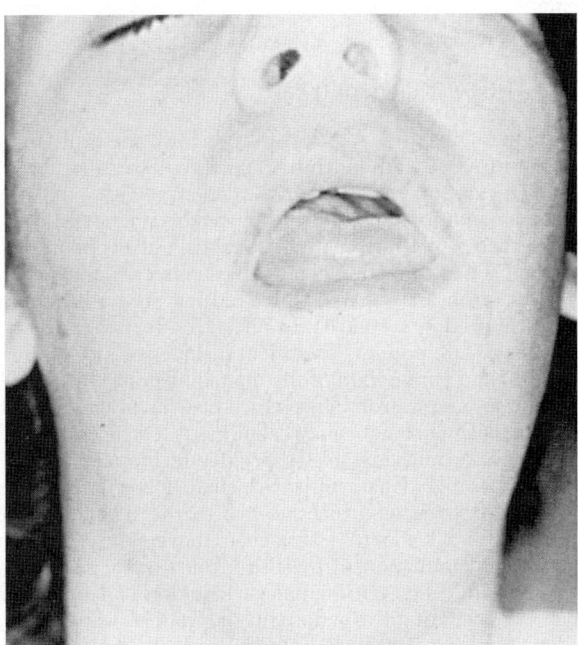

Figure 9–11 Ludwig angina.

NECROTIZING FASCIITIS

Necrotizing fasciitis, which causes a frightening loss of skin and underlying tissues, has received considerable notoriety in the press. Cervicofacial necrotizing fasciitis often is odontogenic and typically causes a superficial spreading of cellulitis that follows the platysma muscle from the cheek down the entire neck to the anterior chest wall (Fig. 9–12A). Figure 9–12B illustrates such a swelling in an 8-year-old boy. The presumptive cause was odontogenic infection of the primary molars, which caused a high fever and a rapidly progressive cellulitis extending from the cheek to the chest. The cause of these infections often is group A streptococci, but a wide variety of microorganisms may be involved.

Wide-spectrum antibiotic therapy is indicated empirically, along with hydration, transfusions if necessary, and support of electrolyte balance, especially with calcium, which may be sequestered by necrotic fat molecules.[1] Timely surgery is important in the management of necrotizing fasciitis. Incision and drainage of the involved spaces, débridement of necrotic tissue, and fasciotomy often are performed as soon as possible after the patient's admission.[71] Hyperbaric oxygen therapy has been advocated as an adjunct in the treatment of necrotizing fasciitis. A significant reduction in the mortality rate and length of hospitalization associated with necrotizing fasciitis has been shown in adults.[71] Necrotizing fasciitis is cited as an indication for hyperbaric oxygen therapy in infants and children and should be considered if available.[70]

ODONTOGENIC SINUSITIS

A significant percentage of cases of sinusitis are odontogenic, especially in adults, because the maxillary sinus follows the erupting permanent tooth roots into the alveolar process. This pneumatization of the alveolar process progresses throughout life and is accelerated by loss of the upper posterior teeth. Dental infections of the periapical upper posterior teeth occasionally rupture through the maxillary sinus floor to involve the paranasal sinuses.

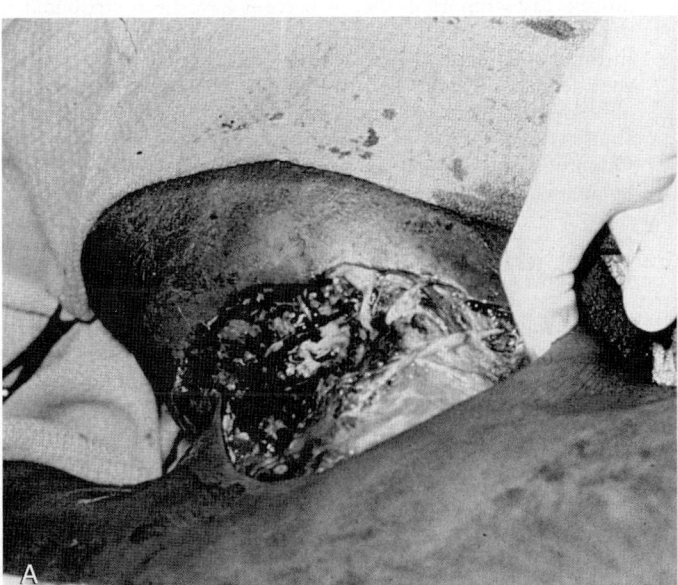

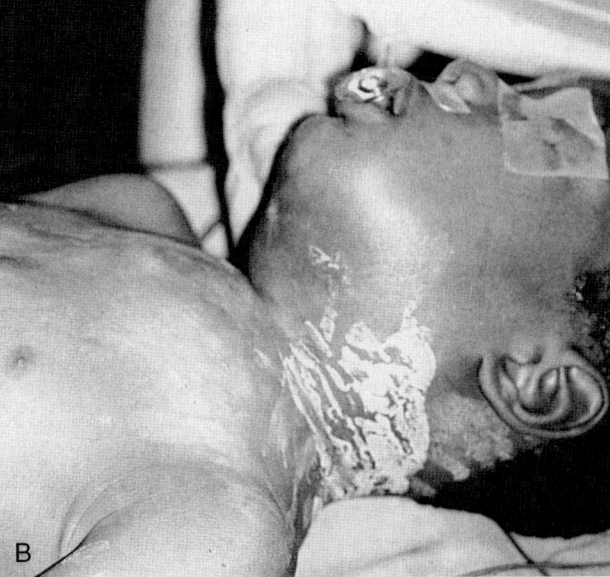

Figure 9–12 A, Surgical débridement of necrotic skin and platysma muscle of the left neck of a diabetic female patient with necrotizing fasciitis. Note how easily blunt finger dissection can undermine the skin in the plane of the necrotic platysma muscle. **B,** Necrotizing fasciitis in an 8-year-old boy. Note the swelling extending from the buccal space down the neck and onto the anterior chest wall, following the extent of the platysma muscle. The chalky material on the posterior neck is calamine lotion placed by the patient's mother for vesicles that resembled poison ivy.

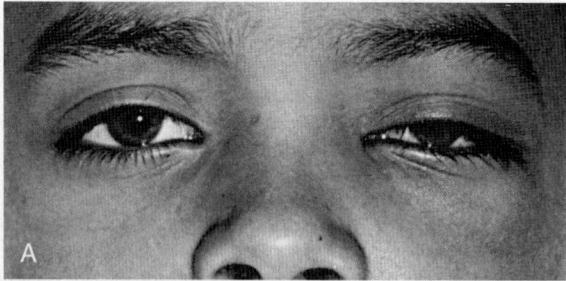
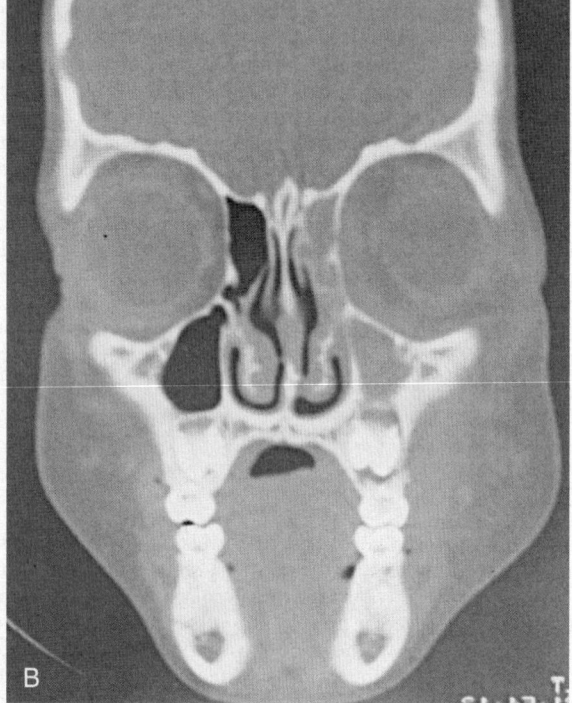

Figure 9–13 A, A 9-year-old boy with a left pansinusitis and an abscess of the upper left first primary molar. Note the left periorbital discoloration and swelling, with partial ptosis and displacement of the globe laterally. **B,** Computed tomography scan of the same patient. Note the left maxillary sinus opacification close to the infected tooth, opacification of the ethmoid sinuses, elevation of the periosteum away from the medial orbital wall, and displacement of the globe laterally within the orbit.

Dental infection should be eliminated in the complete treatment of severe recurrent sinusitis in children.

Figure 9–13 illustrates a case in a 9-year-old boy of left pansinusitis, including ethmoiditis and a subperiosteal orbital abscess associated with infected upper primary molars. His treatment involved a team approach of the dental and otolaryngology services for tooth extraction, incision and drainage of the buccal and infraorbital spaces, endoscopic sinus surgery, and external drainage of the orbital abscess.

BUCCAL AND PERIORBITAL CELLULITIS

A child occasionally presents with an acute buccal or periorbital space swelling and cellulitis with no clinically apparent odontogenic cause. These infections tend to occur in young children, usually younger than 36 months. They usually have a history of recent upper respiratory infection or sinusitis. *H. influenzae* type b and *S. pneumoniae* have been implicated as pathogens in these

conditions, although the widespread use of conjugated vaccines has reduced drastically the incidence of invasive disease from *H. influenzae.*[17] A possible mechanism for the inoculation of the soft tissues is migration of organisms through emissary veins piercing the thin cortical bone overlying the lateral surface of the maxillary sinus, in cases with existing sinusitis. Unless the infection is severe, incision and drainage usually are unnecessary, and treatment with antibiotics is successful. Blood cultures frequently are positive in more severe cases. The role of lumbar puncture remains controversial in the overall management of infants and young children. The incidence of this infection has declined significantly as a result of the widespread use of *H. influenzae* vaccine.

ORBITAL AND INTRACRANIAL COMPLICATIONS

Odontogenic infections that spread to involve the orbit and the brain are rare. Orbital and intracranial abscesses may have an odontogenic origin, however, and the dental condition of patients with these conditions should be evaluated by a dentist. Probably no more than 5 to 10 percent of orbital cellulitis is odontogenic in origin.[28,74] This infection generally is unilateral and is characterized by proptosis, chemosis, lid edema, and restriction of extraocular motion secondary to edema.[54] No nerve palsies or visual changes are present. Treatment includes surgical drainage, antibiotics, and elimination of the dental infection.

Cavernous sinus thrombosis, which may be difficult to differentiate clinically from orbital cellulitis, is considerably more serious because microorganisms proliferate intracranially. The risk of death is high. Characteristics include bilateral involvement with rapid progression from one eye to the other, proptosis, chemosis, and lid edema. Extraocular movements are limited because of inflammation of the third, fourth, and sixth cranial nerves. Systemic signs of meningeal irritation and ophthalmoscopic evidence of obstruction of the retinal veins also are present.[7,54,65] Treatment includes high doses of parenteral antibiotics, elimination of the causative dental pathosis, and incision and drainage of infected fascial spaces.

Brain abscess and subdural empyema are rare findings today compared with several decades ago. Of the large series of brain abscess cases reported, 0 to 4 percent have been attributed to dental causes.[41,68] All of the studies in which the individual case histories are described disclose a pansinusitis intervening between the dental infection and the brain.[42,60] Odontogenic brain abscesses seem to occur by direct extension through the paranasal sinuses, usually to the frontal lobe through the frontal sinuses. Odontogenic cavernous sinus thrombosis seems to be propagated by an ascending thrombophlebitis.

OSTEOMYELITIS OF THE JAWS IN CHILDREN

Osteomyelitis of the jaws in children usually results from periodontal or, more commonly, periapical infection. Open fracture of the jaws with delayed treatment also is a significant cause of osteomyelitis. Extension from contiguous infections, such as otitis, parotitis, and mastoiditis, occurs much less often.

Osteomyelitis of the jaws occurring in children must be viewed with great concern because it may result in the following problems: (1) loss of primary and permanent teeth; (2) sequestration of segments of the jaws; (3) growth defects, such as mandibular hypoplasia, asymmetry, and ankylosis[12]; (4) disfiguring facial scars and cutaneous fistulas; and (5) lesions suggestive of malignancy, which require open biopsy. For these reasons, osteomyelitis of the jaws in children should be diagnosed rapidly and treated aggressively. Table 9–5 presents a useful classification of this disease.[67]

TABLE 9-5 Osteomyelitis of the Jaws

Suppurative	Nonsuppurative
Acute suppurative	Chronic sclerosing
Chronic suppurative	Facial sclerosing
Primary	Diffuse sclerosing
Secondary	Garré sclerosing
Infantile	Actinomycotic
	Radiation osteomyelitis and necrosis

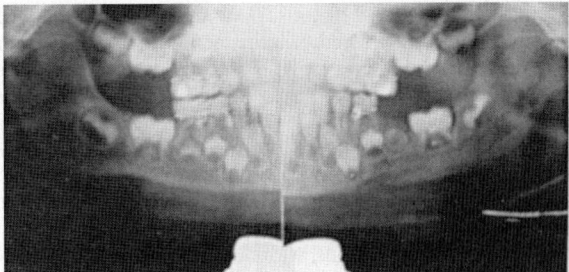

Figure 9–14 Radiograph of the jaws of a 4-year-old girl with suppurative osteomyelitis of the left mandible. The film shows marked destruction of the body and ramus of the mandible.

PREDISPOSING FACTORS

Preexisting systemic disease with accompanying alteration of host resistance plays a major role in the initiation of osteomyelitis of the jaws. It includes such conditions as uncontrolled diabetes, agranulocytosis, leukemia, sickle-cell disease, and febrile illnesses. Conditions that alter the vascularity of bone and the ability to combat infections, including bone tumors, fibrous dysplasia, Paget disease, and radiation to the jaws, also are important predisposing conditions. Major maxillofacial injuries resulting in open fractures of the jaws, especially fractures that are not treated immediately, are an important cause of osteomyelitis.

MICROBIOLOGY

Because the etiology of osteomyelitis of the jaws includes causes other than purely odontogenic infections, the bacterial spectrum is broad. Most instances of osteomyelitis of the jaws are caused by aerobic streptococci (alpha-hemolytic streptococci, *Streptococcus* viridans group), anaerobic streptococci, and other anaerobes, particularly peptostreptococci, fusobacteria, and *Bacteroides* and related genera.[52] Only occasional cases are caused by *S. aureus*, with entry through the skin being the probable route. Other bacteria involved include oral anaerobes, aerobic and microaerophilic cocci, and gram-negative organisms. Specific forms of osteomyelitis are caused by *Actinomyces israelii*, *Treponema pallidum*, and *Mycobacterium tuberculosis*. *Salmonella* organisms have been associated with osteomyelitis of the jaws in patients with sickle-cell anemia.[9]

CLINICAL FINDINGS

Osteomyelitis involves the mandible far more frequently than the maxilla because the poor blood supply to the mandible comes primarily from one major vessel and the periosteal blood supply. Four major forms of the disease, which may be distinguished clinically, are (1) acute suppurative; (2) secondary chronic, which begins as an acute osteomyelitis and becomes chronic; (3) primary chronic, which has no acute phase and always has seemed to be a low-grade infection; and (4) nonsuppurative osteomyelitis. The forms most often seen in children are the acute suppurative, the secondary chronic, and one nonsuppurative form, Garré sclerosing osteomyelitis. These conditions are described in some detail.

SUPPURATIVE OSTEOMYELITIS

Suppurative osteomyelitis usually begins with deep and intense pain in the jaws, high intermittent fever, and an obvious cause, most often a deeply carious or discolored tooth. In the early stages, mental nerve paresthesia occasionally is present. During the course of several days, facial swelling develops, and in 10 to 14 days, teeth begin to loosen, pus exudes around the gingival

sulcus, and multiple mucosal or cutaneous sinus tracts form. In addition to the draining sinuses, a firm cellulitis is present in the soft tissues accompanied by trismus and cervical lymphadenopathy. A leukocytosis, ranging typically from 8000 to 15,000 cells/mm^3, is present, although it does not ordinarily reach the levels that are seen in acute osteomyelitis of the long bones. After 10 days to 2 weeks, radiographs may show scattered areas of bone destruction suggestive of a moth-eaten appearance (Fig. 9–14), and periosteal reaction characterized by the laying down of new bone commonly is seen. Smears of specimens and cultures, including cultures of bone sequestra, should be taken whenever possible. Interpretation of cultures must be made with caution because of the possibility of skin and oral contaminants in the specimen.

Initially, antibiotic doses adjusted for age may be given empirically, but the selection of the antibiotic is determined by culture and sensitivity testing of specimens taken directly from the infected site.[15] The antibiotics of choice in mandibular osteomyelitis include amoxicillin-clavulanate, clindamycin, and fluoroquinolones. Fluoroquinolones are excellent choices because of their complete absorption from the gastrointestinal tract and high penetration of bone, but these drugs generally should be avoided in children because they are chondrotoxic during growth. As results from smears and culture are obtained, antibiotics may be changed, unless the infection is responding favorably, in which case no change is made. The involved tooth is removed as early as possible to allow drainage and to provide material for culture.

Antibiotic therapy is continued for at least 2 to 4 weeks after all symptoms subside. If the infection persists, repeated cultures are obtained, and the antibiotic is changed if necessary. The greater vascularity of the jaws may explain their more rapid response to antibiotic therapy and surgery compared with long bones. The duration of intravenous antibiotic therapy in osteomyelitis of the jaws may not need to be as prolonged as in that of the long bones. Consideration should be given to sequestrectomy, saucerization, or the placement of closed-wound irrigation and suction. Saucerization involves the removal of teeth in the immediate area and removal of the overlying buccal plate of bone, allowing access to the medullary portion and sequestra that may be present. Placement of catheters through an extraoral approach occasionally is necessary for closed irrigation and suction. It permits instillation of antibiotics, allowing direct contact with the bone. Hyperbaric oxygen treatment may be considered in chronic cases refractory to antibiotic treatment.[47]

INFANTILE OSTEOMYELITIS

Osteomyelitis of the jaws in a newborn is an uncommon occurrence but warrants special mention because of its serious sequelae. It occurs most often a few weeks after birth and usually involves the maxilla. It is not odontogenic in origin, but is thought to arise from neonatal trauma to oral tissues, hematogenous spread (from skin, middle ear, mastoid, or tonsils), or an infected nipple.[56] The patient presents with a facial cellulitis centered around the orbit (Fig. 9–15). Irritability and malaise precede development of cellulitis and are followed by marked elevation in temperature, anorexia, and dehydration. Extraorally, inner canthal swelling, palpebral edema with closure of the eye, conjunctivitis, and proptosis may be seen together with a purulent discharge from the nose or from the inner canthus. Oral examination shows swelling of the maxilla on the affected side extending to the buccal and the palatal regions, with fluctuation often present with multiple sinus tracts. *S. aureus* is the organism usually found.

Aggressive, prompt treatment must be undertaken to prevent permanent optic damage, neurologic complications, loss of tooth buds and bone, and extension to the dural sinuses. Intravenous penicillin and a penicillinase-resistant penicillin are given simultaneously with surgical drainage of all fluctuant areas, repeated Gram smears, and culture and sensitivity testing. Antibiotics are continued orally for 2 to 4 weeks after all signs of the infection have disappeared. If sequestra form, they should be removed conservatively. Tooth buds may be lost, and surviving teeth may be deformed or discolored after eruption.

GARRÉ SCLEROSING OSTEOMYELITIS

Garré sclerosing osteomyelitis, also known as chronic nonsuppurative sclerosing osteomyelitis and proliferative osteomyelitis of Garré,[4] is notable because of the similarity of some of its characteristics to those of other neoperiostoses. It is characterized by a localized, hard, nontender swelling of the mandible (Fig. 9–16). Lymphadenopathy, hyperpyrexia, and leukocytosis are not present. Garré osteomyelitis is associated commonly with a carious tooth, usually the lower first molar (Fig. 9–17), and a

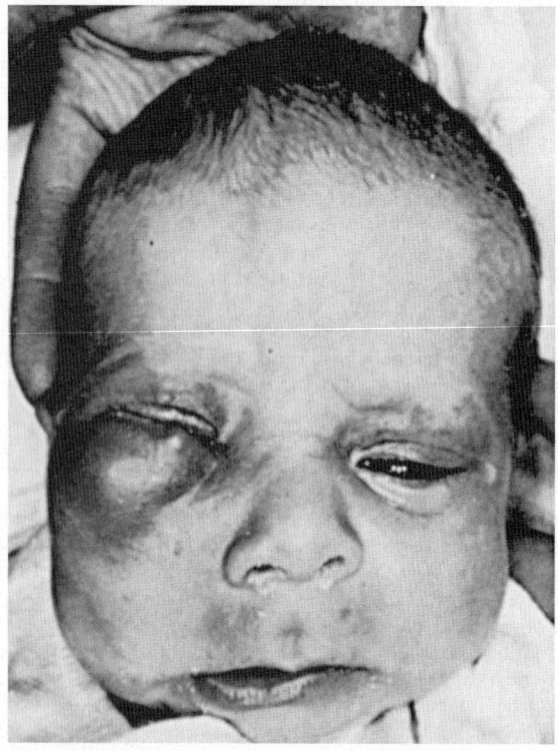

Figure 9–15 Characteristic clinical picture of a 3-week-old child with infantile osteomyelitis. *(Courtesy of Dr. M. Michael Cohen, Sr.)*

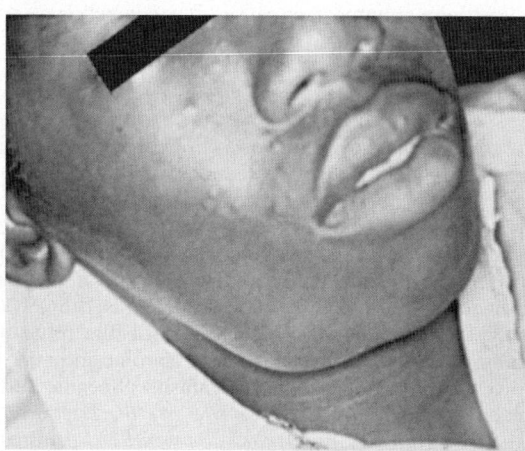

Figure 9–16 Enlargement of the right side of the mandible in a 12-year-old patient with Garré sclerosing osteomyelitis. The swelling is hard and nontender.

Figure 9–17 Radiograph of a deeply carious lower first molar tooth with periapical spread of infection. It is the usual cause of Garré osteomyelitis.

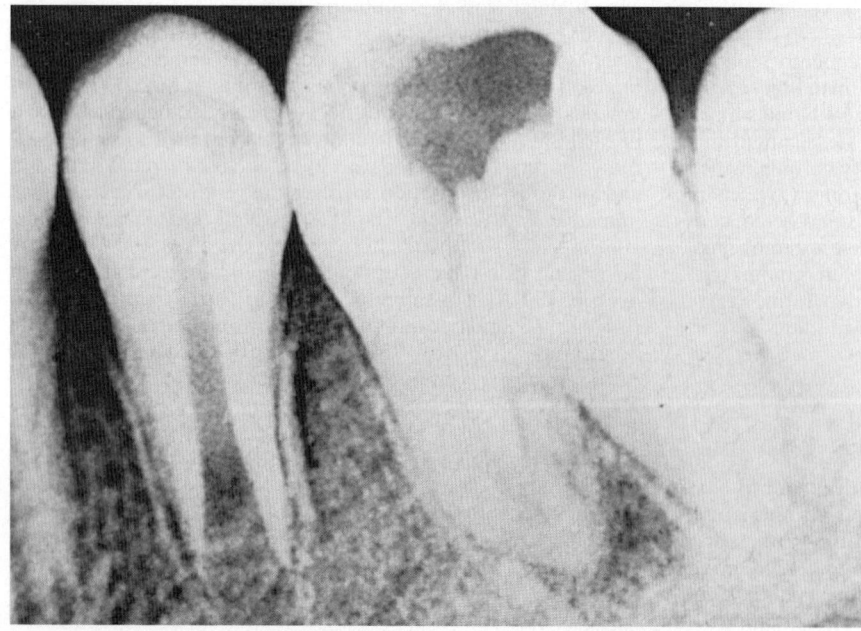

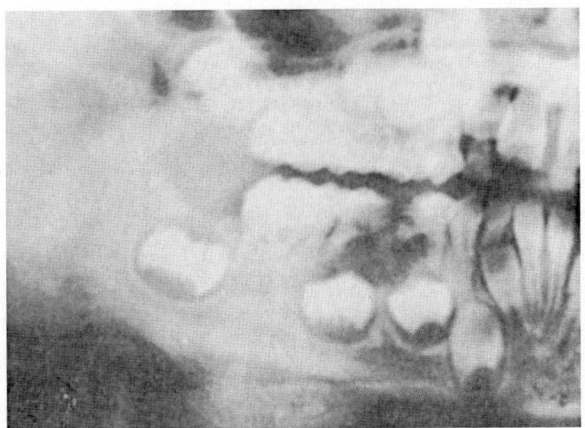

Figure 9–18 Characteristic radiograph of Garré osteomyelitis showing the laminated or onion-peel appearance of the mass. *(Courtesy of Dr. Larry J. Peterson.)*

history of a past toothache. It also may be associated with a recent dental extraction or an infected flap of tissue over an erupting tooth.[39] Radiographs are impressive, showing a focal area of well-calcified bone proliferation that is smooth and that often has a laminated or onion-peel appearance (Fig. 9–18).

Garré osteomyelitis is thought to be a response to a low-grade stimulus, such as a dental infection, which influences the potentially active periosteum of young individuals. Its appearance resembles that of infantile cortical hyperostosis (Caffey disease), osteosarcoma, and Ewing sarcoma, and it must be distinguished from these conditions.[11] Treatment consists of extraction or endodontic treatment of the involved tooth, with continued clinical and radiographic follow-up of the patient to ensure that the new bone formation does not progress. Ordinarily, remodeling occurs over the course of time, but biopsy should be done to rule out neoplasm if the lesion does not regress. No antibiotic therapy is necessary.

HERPES SIMPLEX VIRUS INFECTIONS

Herpes simplex virus type 1 infections[64] commonly are manifested as herpetic gingivostomatitis. Five stages of infection have been identified: (1) primary mucocutaneous infection, (2) acute infection of ganglia, (3) establishment of latency, (4) reactivation, and (5) recurrent infection.

Primary infection is established by direct contact either with individuals who have draining lesions or with an asymptomatic carrier who may continue to shed the virus despite the lack of symptoms. The highest incidence of primary infection seems to be in children 2 to 4 years old. Infants are protected by maternal antibodies, which may explain why this infection is not found in infants younger than 6 months. It appears to have no seasonal variation or male-female difference in incidence.

The incubation period is thought to be approximately 6 days, followed by the development of small vesicles that may coalesce to form larger lesions or ulcers. In severe cases, the lips, gingivae, oral mucosa, and pharynx may be involved. Many patients with primary herpes labialis may be asymptomatic, however, and symptoms may not develop. Healing occurs in 1 to 2 weeks, with gradual crusting of the lesions followed by re-epithelialization.

Latency is thought to continue throughout life, with reactivation occurring at various times, possibly triggered by actinic radiation and emotional or physical stress. Recurrent disease is manifested by vesicles at the mucocutaneous border, which are painful for about 2 days, followed by crusting and complete healing in 7 to 8 days.

Fifty percent of the adult population in industrialized countries and a higher percentage in less-developed countries may have recurrent herpes labialis. Many, if not most, adults who have recurrent "cold sores" are not aware that they can transmit the disease and should be counseled in this regard. Likewise, medical, dental, and nursing personnel should be advised that occurrence of cutaneous lesions (the herpetic whitlow) is possible after direct contact of the practitioner's fingers with lesions during the physical examination.

In treating recurrent herpes labialis in non-immunocompromised adults, acyclovir has been shown to decrease the duration of symptoms by 12 to 24 hours, at a cost of approximately $75.00 per day. Frequent use of acyclovir also may promote the spread of resistant viral strains. The use of acyclovir for treatment of recurrent herpes labialis in non-immunocompromised individuals seems to offer little benefit at significant expense and risk.[55]

REFERENCES

1. Balcerak, R. J., Sisto, J. M., and Bosack, R. C.: Cervicofacial necrotizing fasciitis: Report of three cases and literature review. J. Oral Maxillofac. Surg. 46:450-459, 1988.
2. Barkin, R., Bonis, S., Elzhammer, R., et al.: Ludwig's angina in children. J. Pediatr. 87:563-565, 1975.
3. Bartlett, J. G., and Gorbach, S. L.: Anaerobic infections of the head and neck. Otolaryngol. Clin. North Am. 9:655-678, 1976.
4. Benca, P. G., Mostofi, R., and Kuo, P.: Proliferative periostitis (Garré's osteomyelitis). Oral Surg. 63:258-260, 1987.
5. Brook, I., Frazier, E. H., and Gher, M. E.: Aerobic and anaerobic microbiology of periapical abscess. Oral Microbiol. Immunol. 6:123-125, 1991.
6. Busch, D. E.: Anaerobes in infections of the head and neck and ear, nose, and throat. Rev. Infect. Dis. 6:S115-S122, 1984.
7. Chow, A. W., Roser, S. M., and Brady, F. A.: Orofacial odontogenic infections. Ann. Intern. Med. 88:392-402, 1978.
8. Coykendall, A. L.: Classification and identification of the viridans streptococci. Clin. Microbiol. Rev. 2:315-328, 1989.
9. Daramola, J. O.: Massive osteomyelitis of the mandible complicating sickle cell disease: Report of case. J. Oral Surg. 39:144-146, 1981.
10. Dodson, T. B., Perrott, D. H., and Kaban, L. B.: Pediatric maxillofacial infections: A retrospective study of 113 patients. J. Oral Maxillofac. Surg. 47:327-330, 1989.
11. Eversole, L. R., Lieder, A. S., Gorwin, J. O., et al.: Proliferative periostitis of Garré: Its differentiation from other neoperiostoses. J. Oral Surg. 37:725-731, 1979.
12. Fisher, A. D.: Osteomyelitis of the mandible in a child. J. Oral Surg. 353:60-63, 1977.
13. Flynn, T. R., Shanti, R. M., Levy, M., et al.: Severe odontogenic infections, part one: Prospective report. J. Oral Maxillofac. Surg. 64:1093-1103, 2006.
14. Flynn, T. R., Stokes, L. N., Lee, A. M., et al.: Molecular microbiology of orofacial infections [abstract]. J. Oral Maxillofac. Surg. 60(Suppl. 1):72, 2002.
15. Gilbert, D. N., Moellering, R. C., Jr., Eliopoulos, G. M., and Sande, M. A.: The Sanford Guide to Antimicrobial Therapy. 36th ed. Sperryville, VA, Antimicrobial Therapy, Inc., 2006, p. 5.
16. Gilmore, W. C., Jacobus, N. V., Gorbach, S. L., et al.: A prospective double-blind evaluation of penicillin versus clindamycin in the treatment of odontogenic infections. J. Oral Maxillofac. Surg. 46:1065-1070, 1988.
17. Givner, L. B., Mason, E. O., Barson, W. J., et al.: Pneumococcal facial cellulitis in children. Pediatrics 106:E61, 2000.
18. Goldberg, M. H., and Topazian, R. G.: Odontogenic infection and deep fascial space infection of dental origin. In Topazian, R. G., and Goldberg, M. H. (eds.): Oral and Maxillofacial Infections. 3rd ed. Philadelphia, W. B. Saunders, 1994, pp. 198-250.
19. Granite, E. L.: Anatomic considerations in infections of the face and neck. J. Oral Surg. 34:34-44, 1976.
20. Grodinsky, M., and Holyoke, E.: The fascia and fascial spaces of the head and neck and adjacent regions. Am. J. Anat. 63:367-407, 1938.
21. Gross, S., and Nieburg, P.: Ludwig's angina in childhood. Am. J. Dis. Child. 131:291-292, 1977.
22. Hall, H. D., Gunter, J. W., Jr., Jamison, H. C., et al.: Effect of time of extraction on resolution of odontogenic cellulitis. J. Am. Dent. Assoc. 77:626-631, 1968.
23. Handal, T., and Olsen, I.: Antimicrobial resistance with focus on oral beta-lactamases. Eur. J. Oral Sci. 108:163-174, 2000.
24. Haug, R. H., Hoffman, M. J., and Indresano, A. T.: An epidemiologic and anatomic survey of odontogenic infections. J. Oral Maxillofac. Surg. 49:976-980, 1991.
25. Heidrun, P. L., Reichart, E., Schmitt, W., et al.: Investigation of infectious organisms causing pericoronitis of the mandibular third molar. J. Oral Maxillofac. Surg. 58:611-616, 2000.

26. Heimdahl, A., Von Konow, L., Satoh, T., et al.: Clinical appearance of orofacial infections of odontogenic origin in relation to microbiological findings. J. Clin. Microbiol. 22:299-302, 1985.

27. Howe, G.: Orofacial infections and their management. In Howe, G. (ed.): Minor Oral Surgery. Bristol, John Wright & Sons, 1966.

28. Kaban, L., and McGill, T.: Orbital cellulitis of dental origin: Differential diagnosis and the use of computed tomography as a diagnostic aid. J. Oral Surg. 38:682-685, 1980.

29. Katz, M. H., Mastrucci, M. T., Leggott, P. J., et al.: Prognostic significance of oral lesions in children with perinatally acquired human immunodeficiency virus infection. Am. J. Dis. Child. 147:45-48, 1993.

30. Ketchem, L., Berkowitz, R. J., McIlveen, L., et al.: Oral findings in HIV-seropositive children. Pediatr. Dent. 12:143-146, 1990.

31. Krogh, H. W.: Extraction of teeth in the presence of acute infections. J. Oral Surg. 9:136-151, 1951.

32. Kuriyama, T., Nakagawa, K., Karasawa, T., et al.: Past administration of beta-lactam antibiotics and increase in the emergence of beta-lactamase-producing bacteria in patients with orofacial odontogenic infections. Oral Surg. Oral Med. Oral Pathol. Oral Radiol. Endod. 89:186-192, 2000.

33. Leggott, P. J.: Oral manifestations of HIV infection in children. Oral Surg. 73:187-192, 1992.

34. Lesco, B., and Brownstein, M. P.: Recognition of periodontal disease in children. Pediatr. Clin. North Am. 29:457-474, 1982.

35. Levitt, G. W.: Cervical fascia and deep neck infections. Otolaryngol. Clin. North Am. 9:703-716, 1976.

36. Lewis, M. A., Carmichael, F., MacFarlane, T. W., and Milligan, S. G.: A randomised trial of co-amoxiclav (Augmentin) versus penicillin V in the treatment of acute dentoalveolar abscess. Br. Dent. J. 17:5169-5174, 1993.

37. Lewis, M. A. O., MacFarlane, T. W., and McGowan, D. A.: Quantitative bacteriology of acute dentoalveolar abscesses. J. Med. Microbiol. 21:101-104, 1986.

38. Lewis, M. A. O., MacFarlane, T. W., McGowan, D. A., et al.: Assessment of the pathogenicity of bacterial species plated from acute dentoalveolar abscesses. J. Med. Microbiol. 27:109-116, 1988.

39. Lichty, G., Langlais, R. P., and Aufdemorte, T.: Garré's osteomyelitis: Literature review and case report. Oral Surg. 50:309-313, 1980.

40. Magnusson, B. O., Matsson, L., and Modeen, T.: Gingivitis and periodontal disease in children. In Magnusson, B. O., Koch, B., and Poulsen, S. (eds.): Pedodontics: A Systematic Approach. Copenhagen, Munksgaard, 1981.

41. Mampalam, T. J., and Rosenblum, M. L.: Trends in the management of bacterial brain abscesses: A review of 102 cases over 17 years. Neurosurgery 23:451-458, 1988.

42. Maniglia, A. J., Goodwin, W. J., Arnold, J. E., et al.: Intracranial abscesses secondary to nasal, sinus, and orbital infections in adults and children. Arch. Otolaryngol. Head Neck Surg. 115:1424-1429, 1989.

43. Marchisio, P., and Principi, N.: Treatment of oropharyngeal candidiasis in HIV-infected children with oral fluconazole. Eur. J. Clin. Microbiol. Infect. Dis. 13:338, 1994.

44. Martis, C. S., Karabouta, I., and Lazaridis, N.: Extraction of impacted mandibular wisdom teeth in the presence of acute infection. Int. J. Oral Surg. 7:541-548, 1978.

45. Martis, C. S., and Karakasis, D. T.: Extractions in the presence of acute infections. J. Dent. Res. 54:59-61, 1975.

46. Marx, R., Johnson, R., and Kline, S.: Prevention of osteoradionecrosis: A randomized prospective clinical trial of hyperbaric oxygen vs. penicillin. J. Am. Dent. Assoc. 111:49-54, 1985.

47. Massler, M.: Epidemiology of gingivitis in children. J. Am. Dent. Assoc. 45:319, 1952.

48. McCarthy, C., Snyder, M. G., and Parker, R. B.: The indigenous oral flora of man, I: The newborn to one-year-old infant. Arch. Oral Biol. 10:61-70, 1975.

49. Moenning, J., Nelson, C., and Kohler, R.: The microbiology and chemotherapy of odontogenic infections. J. Oral Maxillofac. Surg. 43:976-985, 1989.

50. Morhert, R. E., and Fitzgerald, R. J.: Nutritional determinants of the ecology of the oral flora. Dent. Clin. North Am. 42:473-489, 1976.

51. O'Sullivan, E. A., Duggal, M. S., Bailey, C. C., et al.: Changes in the oral microflora during cytotoxic chemotherapy in children being treated for acute leukemia. Oral Surg. 76:161-168, 1993.

52. Peterson, L. J.: Microbiology of head and neck infections. Oral Maxillofac. Clin. N. Am. 3:247, 1991.

53. Piecuch, J. F.: Odontogenic infections. Dent. Clin. North Am. 26:129-145, 1982.

54. Price, C. D., Hameroff, S. B., and Richards, R. D.: Cavernous sinus thrombosis and orbital cellulitis. South. Med. J. 64:1243-1247, 1971.

55. Raborn, G. W., McGaw, W. T., Grace, M., et al.: Oral acyclovir and herpes labialis: A randomized, double-blind, placebo-controlled study. J. Am. Dent. Assoc. 115:38-42, 1987.

56. Raymon, Y., Oberman, M., Horowitz, I., et al.: Osteomyelitis of the maxilla in the newborn. Int. J. Oral Surg. 6:90-94, 1977.

57. Rogers, A. H.: The oral cavity as a source of potential pathogens in focal infection. Dent. Clin. North Am. 42:245-248, 1976.

58. Rud, J.: Removal of impacted lower third molars with acute pericoronitis and necrotizing gingivitis. Br. J. Oral Surg. 7:153-160, 1970.

59. Sakamoto, H., Kato, H., Sato, T., and Sasaki, J.: Semiquantitative bacteriology of closed odontogenic abscesses. Bull. Tokyo Dent. Coll. 39:103-107, 1998.

60. Schwaber, M. K., Pensak, M. L., and Bartels, L. J.: The early signs and symptoms of neurotologic complications of chronic suppurative otitis media. Laryngoscope 99:373-375, 1989.

61. Shah, H. N., and Collins, D. M.: Proposal for reclassification of Bacteroides asaccharolyticus, Bacteroides gingivalis, and Bacteroides endodontalis in a new genus, Porphyromonas. Int. J. Syst. Bacteriol. 38:128, 1988.

62. Shah, H. N., and Collins, D. M.: Prevotella, a new genus to include Bacteroides melaninogenicus and related species formerly classified in the genus Bacteroides. Int. J. Syst. Bacteriol. 40:205-208, 1990.

63. Socransky, S., and Manganiello, S.: The oral microbiota of man from birth to senility. J. Periodontol. 42:485-496, 1971.

64. Straus, S. E. (moderator): Herpes simplex virus infection: Biology, treatment, prevention. NIH Conference. Ann. Intern. Med. 103:404, 1985.

65. Summers, G. W.: The diagnosis and management of dental infections. Otolaryngol. Clin. North Am. 9:717-728, 1976.

66. Sundqvist, G.: Taxonomy, ecology, and pathogenicity of the root canal flora. Oral Surg. 78:522-530, 1994.

67. Topazian, R. G.: Uncommon infections of the oral and maxillofacial regions. In Topazian, R. G., and Goldberg, M. H. (eds.): Oral and Maxillofacial Infections. 3rd ed. Philadelphia, W. B. Saunders, 1994, pp. 407-429.

68. Traub, W. H.: Brain abscess and acute purulent meningitis: Recent developments in clinical microbiology. In Schiefer, W., Klinger, M., and Brock, M. (eds.): Brain Abscess and Meningitis: Subarachnoid Hemorrhage: Timing Problems. New York, Springer-Verlag, 1981.

69. Valdez, I. H., Pizzo, P. A., and Atkinson, J. C.: Oral health of pediatric AIDS patients: A hospital-based study. J. Dent. Child. 61:114-148, 1994.

70. Waisman, D., Shupak, A., Weisz, G., and Melamed, Y.: Hyperbaric oxygen therapy in the pediatric patient: The experience of the Israel Naval Medical Institute. Pediatrics 102:53-61, 1998.

71. Whitesides, L., Cotto-Cumba, C., and Myers, R. A. M.: Cervical necrotizing fasciitis of odontogenic origin: A case report and review of 12 cases. J. Oral Maxillofac. Surg. 58:144-151, 2000.

72. Williams, A. C.: Ludwig's angina. Surg. Gynecol. Obstet. 70:140, 1940.

73. Williams, A. C., and Guralnick, W. C.: The diagnosis and treatment of Ludwig's angina: A report of twenty cases. N. Engl. J. Med. 228:443, 1943.

74. Woods, R.: Pyogenic dental infections: A ten-year review. Aust. Dent. J. 23:107-111, 1978.

CHAPTER

10

PHARYNGITIS (PHARYNGITIS, TONSILLITIS, TONSILLOPHARYNGITIS, AND NASOPHARYNGITIS)

James D. Cherry

Pharyngitis is an inflammatory illness of the mucous membranes and underlying structures of the throat. The clinical diagnostic category includes tonsillitis, tonsillopharyngitis, and nasopharyngitis; inflammation also frequently involves the nasopharynx, uvula, and soft palate. Illness usually is acute but also may be subacute or chronic. Establishing the diagnosis of pharyngitis requires objective evidence of inflammation (erythema, exudate,

or ulceration). The symptom of sore throat invariably accompanies pharyngitis, but it should not be used as the sole criterion; sore throat is a common complaint of children with colds in whom no objective evidence of pharyngeal inflammation is present.

Although the clinical finding of pharyngitis suggests an almost exclusive group A streptococcal etiology to many physicians, etiologic considerations should include a multitude of viruses, bacteria, and other infectious and noninfectious agents. Etiologically, pharyngitis is subdivided into two categories: illness with nasal symptoms (nasopharyngitis) and illness without nasal involvement (pharyngitis or tonsillopharyngitis). In acute illness, nasopharyngitis nearly always is of viral origin, whereas pharyngitis without nasal signs has diverse etiologic possibilities, including bacteria, viruses, fungi, and other infectious agents. In this chapter, nasopharyngitis and pharyngitis without nasal involvement are considered separately.

HISTORY

Although throat inflammation undoubtedly has been a physical finding of disease throughout human existence, only in more recent years has attention been given to pharyngitis as a primary complaint. The throat findings of diphtheria were mentioned in the 3rd century AD,[164] and Vincent angina was noted in the military before the Christian era,[47] but group A streptococcal infection and pharyngitis were not clearly associated until World War II.[30,141] Although Glover and Griffith[62] mentioned streptococcal tonsillitis in 1931, the major reference to streptococci in the preantibiotic era was in association with scarlet fever, erysipelas, and suppurative processes.[23]

NASOPHARYNGITIS

ETIOLOGIC AGENTS

Etiologic agents of nasopharyngitis, categorized by type of lesion, frequency, season of occurrence, and duration of illness, are listed in Table 10–1. The relative importance of nasal and pharyngeal manifestations also is presented. Although Table 10–1 shows three bacterial agents and one rickettsia, most occurrences of nasopharyngitis are caused by viral infections. The specific infectious agents are discussed fully in their respective sections of this book; only an overview is presented here.

Adenoviruses are the most common cause of nasopharyngitis; types 1, 2, 3, 4, 5, 6, 7, 7a, 9, 14, and 15 account for most illnesses.* Nasopharyngitis also commonly occurs with influenza and parainfluenza viral infections.† Although rhinoviral, respiratory syncytial viral, human metapneumovirus, and human bocavirus infections are common occurrences in children and all always have nasal manifestations (coryza), the occurrence of objective pharyngeal manifestations is less common.[20,51,74,77-80,87,111,130,151] Respiratory symptoms with cough, nasal discharge, and pharyngitis frequently occur in children with rotaviral gastroenteritis.[69,100,143]

EPIDEMIOLOGY

Nasopharyngitis is a common illness of childhood. It tends to be most prevalent in young children, in association with primary infections with respiratory viruses. Nasal symptoms with enteroviruses occur less frequently in school-aged children than in preschool-aged children. In contrast, older children rarely have pharyngitis with respiratory syncytial viral, parainfluenza viral, and rhinoviral infections. Nasopharyngitis caused by adenoviral infection is a particularly frequent occurrence in adolescents and young adults in military training.[33,153,170]

Nasopharyngitis occurs more commonly during the cold weather months (see Table 10–1). No apparent sex predilection

---

*See references 11, 21, 33, 35, 87, 116, 133, 153, 157, 170.
†See references 7, 71, 79, 80, 87, 88, 122, 130-132, 139, 140, 147, 160.

has been found. The method of transmission is similar to that of other respiratory viral infections (see Chapter 8).

PATHOPHYSIOLOGY

The pathophysiology of nasopharyngitis is discussed in Chapter 8, in the pharyngitis section of this chapter, and in the chapters discussing the individual viral agents. In nasopharyngitis associated with *Haemophilus influenzae* and *Neisseria meningitidis*, the nasal symptoms may result from a concomitant respiratory viral infection.[23]

CLINICAL PRESENTATION

Because nasopharyngitis is caused by many different etiologic agents, a reasonable expectation is varied clinical manifestations. These differences are highlighted in Table 10–1. Fever occurs in nearly all cases of nasopharyngitis. With adenoviral and influenza viral disease, the pharyngeal findings are most prominent; with the other respiratory viruses, coryza is more notable than are pharyngeal complaints. In adenoviral infections, follicular pharyngitis is the rule, and exudate is a common manifestation. In contrast, patients with the other respiratory viral infections usually present with pharyngeal erythema only. Nasopharyngitis of a viral etiology most often is an acute, self-limited disease lasting 4 to 10 days. Generally, adenoviral illnesses tend to be more prolonged than are illnesses resulting from the other respiratory viruses. Other symptoms in nasopharyngitis are related to the causative virus. Parainfluenza and respiratory syncytial viral infections also might have lower respiratory tract findings (laryngotracheitis, pneumonia, or bronchiolitis), and influenza might be associated with more severe, generalized complaints.

Although respiratory symptoms in association with rotaviral gastroenteritis have been noted frequently, little careful clinical study of the respiratory manifestations has been performed. Lewis and associates,[100] in a careful study, observed a statistically significant occurrence of nasal discharge, cough, and red throat in children with rotaviral diarrhea compared with children with diarrhea caused by other agents.

Nasopharyngitis with *H. influenzae* or *N. meningitidis* infections has been noted mainly in patients with septicemia and meningitis. The nasal symptoms (coryza) usually preceded the pharyngitis and severe systemic disease by a few to several days. In Q fever, the predominant finding is pneumonia. With diphtheria, the exudative pharyngitis and constitutional symptoms are most prominent.

PHARYNGITIS, TONSILLITIS, AND TONSILLOPHARYNGITIS

ETIOLOGIC AGENTS

Etiologic agents of pharyngitis categorized by type of lesion, frequency of occurrence, and duration of illness are presented in Table 10–2. Numerous diverse possibilities exist for the differential diagnosis of pharyngitis. The specific agents or factors are presented in their respective sections of this book, and only an overview is given here.

As with all infectious diseases, etiologic prevalence depends on multiple factors (status of the host, age, season, environment, exposure, and type of lesion) that must be considered in each individual case. In otherwise healthy children, the following infectious agents account for more than 90 percent of acute infections with pharyngeal involvement: *Streptococcus pyogenes*; adenoviruses; influenza viruses A and B; parainfluenza viruses

TABLE 10-1   Etiologic Agents of Nasopharyngitis

Etiologic Agent	Type of Pharyngeal Lesion*			Relative Importance of Nasal and Pharyngeal Symptoms†		Frequency of Pharyngitis‡	Main Season	Duration of Pharyngitis
	Erythematous	Follicular	Exudative	Nasal	Pharyngeal			
Bacteria								
Corynebacterium diphtheriae[181]	+++		++++	+	+++	+	Fall, winter, spring	Acute, subacute
Haemophilus influenzae[174]	++			++	++	+	Fall, winter, spring	Acute, subacute
Neisseria meningitidis[154]	++			+	+++	+	Fall, winter, spring	Acute, subacute
Viruses								
Adenoviruses[11,21,33,35,40,116,133,153,157,170]	++++	++++	++	+	+++	++++	All seasons	Acute
Enteroviruses (polio, coxsackieviruses A and B, echovirus)[24,32,90,91,116,149,150,175]	+++		+	+	+++	+++	Summer, fall	Acute
Influenza A and B[90,131,139,147,160]	+++			+	+++	++	Fall, winter	Acute
Parainfluenza[1-4,7,71,79,80,88,122,140,146,150,152,160]	++		+	+++	+	++	Fall, winter, spring	Acute
Respiratory syncytial[20,77,80,111,130]	++			+++	+	+	Fall, winter, spring	Acute
Rhinoviruses[74,90]	+			+++	+	+	Fall, winter, spring	Acute
Human metapneumovirus[151]	++			+++	+	+	Fall, winter, spring	Acute
Human bocavirus[51]	++			+++	+	+	Fall, winter, spring	Acute
Rotaviruses[70,100,111,143]	++			++	++	++	Fall, winter, spring	Acute
Rickettsia								
Coxiella burnetii[86]	++			++	++	+	All seasons	Acute

*Plus signs indicate the relative degree and severity of the lesion (++++, most marked; +, minimal).
†Each +, 25%.
‡++++, 76 to 100 percent; +++, 51 to 75 percent; ++, 26 to 50 percent; +, 1 to 25 percent.

1, 2, and 3; Epstein-Barr virus; enteroviruses; and *Mycoplasma pneumoniae*.*

Although group A streptococci are suggested frequently[25] as the only worthy bacterial consideration in the etiology of pharyngitis, the data in Table 10–2 indicate broader possibilities. When streptococci with beta-hemolysis recovered from children and adolescents with pharyngitis are typed, group B, C, and G strains occasionally are found.[5,26,28,58,75,166,167] Turner and associates[166] found that of the group C streptococci, only *Streptococcus equisimilis* caused pharyngitis; *Streptococcus anginosus* (*Streptococcus milleri*) was part of the normal oropharyngeal flora.

Laboratory accidents have provided evidence that *H. influenzae* can cause pharyngitis,[129,173] and children with systemic illnesses caused by *H. influenzae* and *N. meningitidis* frequently have an associated marked pharyngitis.[152,174,178] *Arcanobacterium haemolyticum* and *Corynebacterium ulcerans* occasionally cause an illness mimicking diphtheria.[15,68,89,93,107,134] *A. haemolyticum* also causes an illness that has been confused with streptococcal scarlet fever.[46,89,104,107]

Because anaerobic microorganisms are universal constituents of the normal throat flora, assigning etiologic significance to these agents in throat infections frequently is difficult. Vincent stomatitis and angina seem to result from mixed infections with anaerobes.[48,65,106,169] Brook and Gober[14] noted a significant

association between encapsulated organisms of the *Bacteroides melaninogenicus* group (*Prevotella melaninogenica*) and acute tonsillitis in children. My impression is that acute and subacute infections with anaerobes account for numerous pharyngeal infections in adolescents in which cultures do not reveal group A streptococci and infectious mononucleosis test results are negative. Gonococcal and treponemal infections should be considered in sexually active or known exposed teenagers and other children.[17,31,49,84,177]

Adenoviral types 1, 2, 3, 4, 5, 6, 7, 7a, 9, 11, 14, 15, and 16 are the most common causes of pharyngitis in young children, and they are prominent etiologic agents in older children and adolescents.* Pharyngeal involvement frequently is overshadowed by other respiratory symptoms (e.g., cough, coryza) in parainfluenza viral infections and by systemic complaints (e.g., fever, exanthem, meningitis) in enteroviral infections.† An enteroviral etiology should be suspected when small ulcerative lesions are noted that involve the soft palate and uvula and the posterior pharyngeal wall (see Chapter 11). Infection with Epstein-Barr virus causes infectious mononucleosis with pharyngeal involvement similar to that resulting from group A streptococcal infection.[76,171] The clinical manifestations of Epstein-Barr virus are age-related; young children rarely have marked pharyngeal involvement.

---

*See references 1, 7, 11, 12, 24, 25, 32, 33, 37, 43, 61, 66, 71, 76, 79, 80, 88, 90, 91, 115-117, 122, 130-133, 139, 140, 146-150, 153, 155, 157, 158, 170, 171, 175.

*See references 11, 18, 33, 36, 116, 119, 133, 153, 157, 170.
†See references 1, 7, 24, 32, 71, 79, 80, 88, 91, 116, 122, 130, 132, 140, 146, 149, 150, 155, 160, 175.

TABLE 10–2 Etiologic Agents of Pharyngitis

Etiologic Agent or Factor	Type of Lesion*					Frequency of Occurrence†	Duration of Pharyngitis
	Erythematous	Follicular	Exudative	Ulcerative	Petechial		
Bacteria							
Streptococcus pyogenes[12,37,45,61,115,117,148,158]	++++	++	+++		+++	++++	Acute
Other streptococci (groups B, C, and G)[2,26-28,53,75,102,166,167]	+++	+	++			++	Acute
Corynebacterium diphtheriae[112,148,181]	+++		++++			+	Acute
Corynebacterium pyogenes[172]	++++		++++			+	Acute
Corynebacterium ulcerans[104,134,163]	++++		+++			+	Acute
Arcanobacterium haemolyticum[4,15,46,63,89,93,107]	++++	++	+++			+	Acute
Mixed anaerobes (Prevotella spp., Peptostreptococcus, Fusobacterium spp.)[13,14,16,43,63,106,169]	++++		+	++++		++	Subacute
Actinomyces spp.[48]	+			+		+	Chronic
Francisella tularensis[85,168,179]	++++		+++			+	Acute
Haemophilus influenzae[129,159,173,174,178]	++					++	Acute, subacute
Legionella pneumophila[120]	++++					+	Acute
Neisseria meningitidis[152]	++		+			++	Acute
Neisseria gonorrhoeae[84,177]	++		+			+	Acute, subacute, chronic
Leptospira spp.[81,135]	++++					+	Acute
Treponema pallidum[17,31,49,70]	+	+		+		+	Subacute
Borrelia spp.[97]	++++					+	Acute
Streptobacillus moniliformis[138]	+					+	Acute
Yersinia enterocolitica[142,161]	++++		++			+	Acute
Yersinia pseudotuberculosis[145]	+					+	Acute
Streptococcus pneumoniae[109]	+			+		+	Acute
Salmonella typhi[3,121]	+					+	Acute
Rothia dentocariosa[124]	+		+			+	Acute
Mycobacterium tuberculosis[29]				+		+	Chronic
Chlamydia							
Chlamydia pneumoniae[42,67]	++++					++	Acute
Chlamydia trachomatis[123]	++	+	+			+	Acute, recurrent
Viruses							
Adenoviruses[11,35,116,119,133,153,170]	++++	++++	++			++++	Acute
Influenza A and B[131,139,147,160]	+++					+++	Acute
Parainfluenza[1-4,7,71,79,80,122,130,132,140,146,160]	++					+++	Acute
Respiratory syncytial[20,77-80,111,130]	++					+	Acute
Enteroviruses (polio, coxsackieviruses A and B, echovirus)[1,24,82,91,149,150,155,175,176]	+++		+	++		+++	Acute
Epstein-Barr[76,171]	+++	+	++++		++	+++	Acute, subacute
Reoviruses[99,180]	++					+	Acute
Cytomegalovirus[10,95]	+					+	Acute
Herpes simplex[19,23,43,116,176]	++		++	++++		++	Acute
Measles[22]	+++				+	++	Acute
Rubella[22,50]					++	+	Acute
Rhinoviruses[74]	+					+	Acute
HIV[6]	++						Acute
Mycoplasma							
Mycoplasma pneumoniae[25,42,61,66,80]	++	+	+			++	Acute
Mycoplasma hominis[118]	+		+			+	Acute
Rickettsia							
Coxiella burnetii[41,86,126]	++					+	Acute
Fungi							
Candida spp.[98,154]	+		++++			+++	Acute, subacute, chronic
Parasites							
Toxoplasma gondii[96]	+					+	Acute

Continued

TABLE 10–2   Etiologic Agents of Pharyngitis—cont'd

Etiologic Agent or Factor	Type of Lesion*					Frequency of Occurrence†	Duration of Pharyngitis
	Erythematous	Follicular	Exudative	Ulcerative	Petechial		
Recognized Illnesses of Uncertain Etiology							
Aphthous stomatitis[64,144]	+			++++		++	Acute, recurrent
PFAPA[45,53,82,85,105,110,125,162]	++		++	++		+	Acute, recurrent
Behçet syndrome[108]	+			++++		+	Chronic, recurrent
Kawasaki disease[73,114]	++	+				+	Acute
Stevens-Johnson syndrome[22]	+		+	++++		+	Acute
Illness in which Host Factors or Therapeutic Agents are Primary Causes							
Neutropenia, other immunodeficiencies, cancer, chemotherapeutic agents, generalized neoplastic disease[22]	+			++++		++	Chronic

*Plus signs indicate the relative degree and severity of the lesion (++++, most marked; +, minimal).
†++++, 76 to 100 percent; +++, 51 to 75 percent; ++, 26 to 50 percent; +, 1 to 25 percent.
HIV, human immunodeficiency virus; PFAPA, periodic fever, aphthous stomatitis, pharyngitis, and adenitis (syndrome).

Acquired cytomegalovirus infection causes an infectious mononucleosis–like syndrome, but pharyngitis occurs less commonly than it does in Epstein-Barr virus mononucleosis.[95] Primary and recurrent herpes simplex virus infections occasionally have pharyngeal manifestations.[19,23,43,116] Many illnesses that are ascribed clinically to herpes simplex virus actually are misidentified instances of aphthous stomatitis, however. Virtually all instances of herpes simplex virus infections with pharyngitis also reveal lesions in the anterior mouth and externally around the mouth. Although Koplik spots are known universally as the enanthem of measles, many physicians are unaware of the diffuse nature of the associated measles pharyngitis.[22] Primary infection with human immunodeficiency virus may cause the acute retroviral syndrome with fever, nonexudative pharyngitis, lymphadenopathy, exanthem, arthralgia, myalgia, and lethargy.[6]

The role of *Chlamydia* spp. in the cause of pharyngitis is unclear. Grayston and associates[65,67] noted the occurrence of pharyngitis in adolescents and young adults infected with *Chlamydia pneumoniae*. In a study in children, IgM antibody to *Chlamydia trachomatis* was found in children with pharyngitis.[72] Because cross-reactivity between *C. trachomatis* and *C. pneumoniae* exists, the illnesses studied were likely to be caused by *C. pneumoniae*, rather than by *C. trachomatis*. Ogawa and colleagues[123] noted prolonged and recurrent tonsillitis in association with sexually transmitted *C. trachomatis*.

Mild pharyngitis occurs in young children with *M. pneumoniae* infections; in older children, pharyngeal involvement is more pronounced.[25,61,66,80] In young adult volunteers, *Mycoplasma hominis* was noted to cause pharyngitis.[103] Although lower respiratory tract findings and systemic complaints are most marked in Q fever, moderate subjective and mild objective evidence of pharyngitis also is noted.[41,86,126] Exudative pharyngeal involvement with *Candida* spp. commonly occurs.[98,154] *Candida* infection most commonly occurs in children whose normal throat flora has been disrupted and in children who have a compromised immunologic response.

Recurrent aphthous stomatitis usually involves the anterior oral cavity, but occasionally is noted with extensive pharyngeal and soft palate lesions.[64,144] Although L-forms (spheroplasts) of *Streptococcus sanguinis* can be recovered consistently from the lesions of this disease,[64] their role in the etiology is unclear. In 1987, Marshall and colleagues[110] described a new syndrome, periodic fever, aphthous stomatitis, pharyngitis, and adenitis (PFAPA), and it subsequently has been observed by others.[45,53,82,85,105,125,162]

In 1999, Thomas and associates[162] presented an analysis of data in their PFAPA registry of 94 cases. The male-to-female ratio was 1.8:1, and the mean age of PFAPA onset was 2.8 years (95% confidence interval 2.4 to 3.3). The children had an average 11.5 febrile episodes per year, and the average symptom-free interval between episodes was 28.2 days (99% confidence interval 26 to 30.4 days). The average duration of an episode was 4.8 days, with the temperature being greater than 38.3° C for 3.8 days. The average maximum temperature per episode was 40.5° C (95% confidence interval 40.4 to 40.6° C). Along with the periodic fevers, the children also experienced aphthous stomatitis (67%), pharyngitis (65%), cervical lymphadenopathy (77%), chills (80%), headache (65%), abdominal pain (45%), nausea (52%), diarrhea (30%), cough (20%), coryza (18%), and rash (15%). In addition to fever, 97 percent had one or more of the following: aphthous stomatitis, pharyngitis, or adenopathy. The mean leukocyte count was 13,000 with 62 percent polymorphonuclear leukocytes, and the mean erythrocyte sedimentation rate was 41 mm/hr.

In PFAPA, the episodes persist for several years with unchanged findings and periodicity. In the Nashville data, 41 percent of the children had stopped having episodes after a mean of 4.5 years. Before remission, the episodes decreased in frequency over an extended period.[162] Treatment modalities that have offered relief include ibuprofen (85%) and prednisone (90%). Thomas and associates[162] recommend prednisone or prednisolone treatment (1 mg/kg at the beginning of an attack and the same dose on the next morning and 0.5 mg/kg on days 3 and 4). Tonsillectomy, adenoidectomy, and prophylactic cimetidine administration have been associated with remission in some children.

In Behçet syndrome, the ulcerative lesions are subacute or chronic and usually are not associated with surrounding pharyngeal inflammation.[108] In Kawasaki disease, the pharyngeal mucosa is deeply erythematous.[114]

Pharyngeal involvement is a common occurrence in noninfectious illnesses in which host resistance has been altered. The lesions usually are ulcerative, but secondary bacterial or fungal overgrowth can lead to marked erythematous and exudative findings.

EPIDEMIOLOGY

Pharyngitis is a common occurrence in children and, as noted in Table 10–2, is the result of many different infectious agents. Generally, bacterial pharyngitis occurs more commonly in the cold weather seasons; an enteroviral etiology is most common in the summer and fall. In younger children, viral pharyngitis tends to occur more frequently than does bacterial disease.[36] It has no apparent sex predilection.

Most diseases associated with pharyngitis require close person-to-person contact for spread. Pathogens are transmitted directly by close-range airborne dissemination or indirectly by the hands of the future host. Several food-borne outbreaks of streptococcal pharyngitis have been reported.[44,52] Prechewing of food by adults also may be a cause of streptococcal pharyngitis in infants.[156]

PATHOPHYSIOLOGY

The pathology and pathophysiology of diseases in which pharyngitis is prominent are presented in the chapters of this book on specific infectious agents (in particular, see Chapters 93, 168, and 178).

CLINICAL PRESENTATION

The clinical findings in pharyngitis are highlighted in Table 10–2. Manifestations related to individual pathogens are detailed in the chapters of this book dealing with the specific agents. The onset of pharyngitis usually is sudden and accompanied by fever and the complaint of sore throat. Frequently, parents observe that the child's breath is not normal, and that the throat and particularly the tonsils are red. Other initial complaints include headache, nausea, vomiting, and sometimes abdominal pain. Anorexia is the rule, as is some degree of lessened activity. Parents also report frequently that the child's cervical lymph nodes are enlarged and tender.

Physical examination usually substantiates the parents' observations—the child is febrile with moderate to severe pharyngeal erythema and some degree of cervical adenitis. As noted in Table 10–2, the pharyngeal response varies. With acute common infections, the basic lesion is erythema. Associated with erythema can be follicular, ulcerative, and petechial lesions and generalized or circumscribed exudative areas. Follicular lesions are most characteristic of adenoviral infections, whereas exudative lesions occur most commonly in group A streptococcal infections and in infectious mononucleosis. Meland and associates[113] noted that the absence of cough and the presence of swollen lymph nodes had the highest specificity in predicting a streptococcal cause of pharyngitis. Ulcerative lesions are observed most frequently in enteroviral infections (see Chapter 178). Petechiae on the soft palate frequently are seen in group A streptococcal infections, but also commonly occur in infectious mononucleosis, measles, and rubella.

Occurrences of pharyngitis in children almost always are acute, self-limited diseases. Pharyngitis of viral origin lasts 4 to 10 days, and pharyngitis caused by group A streptococci, if untreated, lasts slightly longer. Subacute and chronic pharyngeal disease is an uncommon occurrence in children, but the etiologic possibilities are numerous (see Table 10–2).

DIFFERENTIAL DIAGNOSIS

As noted in Table 10–2, the differential diagnoses in pharyngitis are numerous, as in nasopharyngitis (see Table 10–1). Although considerable overlap exists in the spectrum of illness in pharyngeal infections, many clues help in ruling in or out certain diagnostic possibilities. The diagnosis of pharyngitis requires carefully eliciting epidemiologic and other historical data (i.e., exposure, season, incubation period, age of patient, associated clinical findings), in addition to observing pharyngeal physical findings.

Most acute instances of nasopharyngitis are of viral origin (see Table 10–1), with adenoviruses accounting for the greatest number of cases. Nasopharyngitis also occurs during epidemic influenza A and B and parainfluenza 1 and 2 infections, and with sporadic parainfluenza 3 infections. In all cases, proper epidemiologic and historical data should be elicited so that early diphtheria and other unusual but treatable illnesses are not diagnosed incorrectly. Retrospective study has indicated that nasopharyngitis occasionally occurs in severe infections from *H. influenzae* and meningococci, so the possible presence of these infections should be considered when the epidemiology suggests it.

Although most cases of pharyngitis without nasal symptoms are caused by viral infections, numerous other etiologic possibilities exist. The approach taken frequently by many physicians is to consider all pharyngitis as being of bacterial origin and to treat it with antibiotics. The initial consideration in a child with pharyngitis should be the duration of illness. Subacute, chronic, and recurrent illnesses (see Table 10–2) generally suggest more unusual problems and require a more deliberate approach. In all instances of acute pharyngitis, ruling out streptococcal disease is mandatory.

SPECIFIC DIAGNOSIS

The epidemiologic history and careful clinical categorization are the most important aspects of specific diagnosis. The most pressing diagnostic need in upper respiratory infections in everyday pediatric practice is distinguishing bacterial from viral disease—who and who not to treat with antibiotics. An approach to the problem is presented in Table 10–3.

A child with the common cold, herpangina, or pharyngoconjunctival fever has a viral disease and does not need therapy with antibiotics. In most instances, when these clinical diagnoses are apparent, performing throat cultures for bacterial pathogens is unnecessary. A child with severe acute pharyngitis with exudate and fever and cervical lymphadenitis also is treated easily because most of these children have disease resulting from group A streptococci.

Only a few children have illnesses at the extremes of those shown in Table 10–3. Most illnesses seen routinely by the physi-

TABLE 10–3 Treatment Considerations in Upper Respiratory Tract Infections

Clinical Entity	Etiology
Common cold, herpangina, pharyngoconjunctival fever	Viral, 100%
↓ Never-Never Land ↓	
Marked pharyngitis with exudate and fever and cervical lymphadenitis	Bacterial, 70%

Modified from Cherry, J. D.: Newer respiratory viruses: Their role in respiratory illness of children. In Schulman, I., et al. (eds.): Advances in Pediatrics. Vol. 20. Chicago, Year Book Medical Publishers, Inc., © 1973. Used by permission.

cian treating children fall into the large middle area—"never-never land." On clinical grounds, no certain way to make an etiologic diagnosis and specifically to rule out infection caused by *S. pyogenes* exists. Until more recently, the usually recommended approach to management of pharyngitis and nasopharyngitis was to obtain a throat culture to determine whether group A streptococci were present. Because several rapid tests (rapid antigen detection tests [RADT]) for the detection of group A streptococci are available, establishing the immediate diagnosis and providing treatment of streptococcal pharyngitis are possible in the practice setting.* Generally, these rapid tests have high specificity, but sensitivity is suboptimal. If early treatment is desirable today, a reasonable approach to establishing the diagnosis of streptococcal pharyngitis is to do a rapid test. If the test result is positive, specific therapy is instituted. In the case of a negative rapid test result, a routine throat culture is done, and therapy is withheld pending the culture results.[9,39,137]

A question exists regarding whether early treatment of streptococcal pharyngitis is desirable.[40,55,57,136,137] In the public clinic, where following up children with positive throat cultures often is difficult, providing immediate diagnosis and treatment is important. As Pichichero and associates[136,137] and El-Daher and colleagues[40] have shown, early treatment may result in a decreased desirable antibody response, allowing reinfection with type-specific organisms to occur. In settings in which the communication between physicians and parents is satisfactory, an advisable approach in many instances is to withhold the institution of treatment for 1 or 2 days. Gerber and associates[55,57] argue against this approach because providing immediate therapy can reduce the risk of transmission of infection, and they challenge the interpretation of the findings of Pichichero and associates[136,137] and El-Daher and colleagues.[40]

Cultures for other pathogens should be reserved for unusual situations, such as persistent symptoms, indicative epidemiology, or other pertinent historical data. Because *H. influenzae* and *Streptococcus pneumoniae* frequently are part of the normal flora, their isolation is not always etiologically significant. If cultures reveal predominant growths of either *H. influenzae* or *S. pneumoniae*, however, they are likely contributing to the disease process, and antibiotic therapy directed at the specific pathogen would benefit the patient.[23,109,178] When the possibility of disease because of anaerobic agents exists, a Gram-stained smear from an exudative area may be rewarding. When the pharyngeal findings are unique, or when many cases of a similar illness are observed, a viral culture from the throat is indicated.

TREATMENT

The specific treatments of diseases with nasopharyngitis and pharyngitis are discussed in chapters of this book that deal with the individual pathogens. That antimicrobial agents are prescribed inappropriately in children with sore throat and pharyngitis is common knowledge. Based on the etiologic agents noted in Tables 10–1 and 10–2, it is apparent that many infectious agents are associated with nasopharyngitis and pharyngitis, which can be treated effectively with antimicrobial agents. Except in rare specific circumstances, the only common pathogens that require treatment are group A streptococci. The treatment of streptococcal pharyngitis is discussed in detail in Chapter 93. A study noted that physicians prescribed antibiotics to 53 percent of children with sore throat, which is far greater than the 15 to 36 percent likelihood of a group A streptococcal infection.[103] This study also noted that this rate of antimicrobial

usage is an improvement from 1995, when the prescribing rate was 66 percent.

Although a multitude of proprietary remedies are available for respiratory infections, and sore throat specifically, none has a place in the care of pediatric patients. Particularly to be condemned are throat lozenges that contain numerous useless ingredients, many potentially harmful. Antibiotic-containing lozenges particularly are to be condemned because they may allow streptococcal disease to go unrecognized. Antiseptic mouthwashes have no value, and decongestants and antihistamines have no proven efficacy and frequently lead to troublesome side effects.

Because children with pharyngitis frequently feel ill, therapy with an analgesic is reasonable. Formerly, aspirin was the analgesic usually recommended. However, because aspirin is an etiologic factor in influenza-associated Reye syndrome and because differentiating influenza viral infections from other respiratory viral infections is difficult clinically, using acetaminophen rather than aspirin is prudent. The dose per single administration of acetaminophen by year of age is as follows: younger than 1 year, 60 mg; 1 to 3 years, 60 to 120 mg; 3 to 6 years, 120 mg; 6 to 12 years, 150 to 300 mg; older than 12 years, 325 to 650 mg. Administration may be repeated three or four times daily in young children and every 4 hours in older children. Acetaminophen rarely should be given to infants younger than 6 months old. In young children, careful attention to adequate hydration is particularly necessary.

PROGNOSIS

Almost all occurrences of nasopharyngitis and pharyngitis are self-limited, and the overall prognosis is excellent. Keeping a constant vigil for streptococcal and other more serious diseases is necessary, however. Failure to diagnose and to treat group A streptococcal infections, syphilis, and other more unusual infections can lead to serious short-term and long-term difficulties.

PREVENTION

Because pharyngitis and nasopharyngitis are caused by infections with many different respiratory pathogens, no practical specific approach to prevention exists. Occasionally, streptococcal disease can be prevented by the judicious use of prophylactic penicillin. For young children or others with undue susceptibility to serious disease with common respiratory pathogens, reducing contact situations (e.g., daycare centers) is prudent. In the 1980s, Paradise and colleagues[127] studied the effect of tonsillectomy on the rate of recurrent throat infections in severely affected children. In this controlled study, children needed to have a history of seven or more episodes of tonsillitis in the preceding year, or five or more episodes in each of 2 preceding years, or three or more episodes in the 3 preceding years. The findings in this study indicated that children in the surgical group had significantly fewer throat infections than occurred in the nonsurgical control group during the ensuing 2 years of follow-up. In a more recent but similar study with less stringent criterion for surgery, Paradise and colleagues[128] found that tonsillectomy or adenotonsillectomy conferred a modest benefit. They concluded, however, that the modest benefit of tonsillectomy or adenotonsillectomy in children with recurrent throat infections does not justify the risks, morbidity, and cost of the operations.

REFERENCES

1. Ager, E. A., Felsenstein, W. C., Alexander, E. R., et al.: An epidemic of illness due to coxsackievirus group B, type 2. J. A. M. A. *187*:251-256, 1964.

---

*See references 6, 8, 9, 34, 38, 39, 54, 56, 59, 60, 78, 94, 101, 136, 165.

2. Arditi, M., Shulman, S. T., Davis, A. T., et al.: Group C β-hemolytic strepto-coccal infections in children: Nine pediatric cases and review. Rev. Infect. Dis. 2:34-45, 1989.
3. Ash, I., McKendrick, G. D. W., Robertson, M. H., et al.: Outbreak of typhoid fever connected with corned beef. B. M. J. 1:1474-1478, 1964.
4. Banck, G., and Nyman, M.: Tonsillitis and rash associated with *Corynebacterium haemolyticum*. J. Infect. Dis. 154:1037-1039, 1986.
5. Benjamin, J. T., and Perriello, V. A., Jr.: Pharyngitis due to group C hemolytic streptococci in children. J. Pediatr. 89:254-256, 1976.
6. Bisno, A. L.: Acute pharyngitis. N. Engl. J. Med. 344:205-211, 2001.
7. Bisno, A. L., Barratt, N. P., Swanston, W. H., et al.: An outbreak of acute respiratory disease in Trinidad associated with para-influenza viruses. Am. J. Epidemiol. 91:68-77, 1970.
8. Bisno, A. L., Gerber, M. A., Gwaltney, J. M., et al.: Diagnosis and manage-ment of group A streptococci pharyngitis: A practice guideline. Clin. Infect. Dis. 25:574-583, 1997.
9. Bisno, A. L., Gerber, M. A., Gwaltney, J. M., et al.: Practice guidelines for the diagnosis and management of group A streptococcal pharyngitis. Clin. Infect. Dis. 35:113-125, 2005.
10. Bonkowsky, H. L., Lee, R. V., and Klatskin, G.: Acute granulomatous hepati-tis: Occurrence in cytomegalovirus mononucleosis. J. A. M. A. 233:1284-1288, 1975.
11. Brandt, C. D., Kim, H. W., Vargosko, A. J., et al.: Infections in 18,000 infants and children in a controlled study of respiratory tract disease, I: Adenovirus pathogenicity in relation to serologic type and illness syndrome. Am. J. Epidemiol. 90:484-500, 1969.
12. Breese, B. B.: Streptococcal pharyngitis and scarlet fever. Am. J. Dis. Child. 132:612-616, 1978.
13. Brook, I.: The role of anaerobic bacteria in tonsillitis. Int. J. Pediatr. Otorhinolaryngol. 69:9-19, 2005.
14. Brook, I., and Gober, A. E.: *Bacteroides melaninogenicus*: Its recovery from ton-sils of children with acute tonsillitis. Arch. Otolaryngol. 109:818-819, 1983.
15. Carlson, P., Kontianinen, S., Renkonen, O. V., et al.: *Arcanobacterium haemo-lyticum* and streptococcal pharyngitis in Army conscripts. Scand. J. Infect. Dis. 27:17-18, 1995.
16. Carrie, S., and Fenton, P. A.: Necrobacillosis: An unusual case of pharyngo-tonsillitis. J. Laryngol. Otol. 108:1097-1098, 1994.
17. Catalano, P. M., and Schragger, A. H.: Early and latent syphilis. Arch. Dermatol. 92:433-435, 1965.
18. Centers for Disease Control: Adenovirus type 16-Long Island, New York. M. M. W. R. Morb. Mortal. Wkly. Rep. 28:530-532, 1979.
19. Cesario, T. C., Poland, J. D., Wulff, H., et al.: Six years' experience with her-pes simplex virus in a children's home. Am. J. Epidemiol. 90:416-422, 1969.
20. Chanock, R. M., Parrott, R. H., Vargosko, A. J., et al.: Respiratory syncytial virus. Am. J. Public Health 52:918-925, 1962.
21. Chen, H. L., Chiou, S. S., Hsiao, H. P., et al.: Respiratory adenoviral infec-tions in children: A study of hospitalized cases in southern Taiwan in 2001-2002. J. Trop. Pediatr. 50:279-284, 2004.
22. Cherry, J. D.: Personal observations, 1964, 1971.
23. Cherry, J. D.: Newer respiratory viruses: Their role in respiratory illness of children. Adv. Pediatr. 20:225-290, 1973.
24. Cherry, J. D., and Jahn, C. L.: Herpangina: The etiologic spectrum. Pediatrics 36:632-634, 1965.
25. Cherry, J. D., and Welliver, R. C.: *Mycoplasma pneumoniae* infections of adults and children. West. J. Med. 125:47-55, 1976.
26. Chretien, J. H., McGinniss, C. G., Thompson, J., et al.: Group B beta-hemolytic streptococci causing pharyngitis. J. Clin. Microbiol. 10:263-266, 1979.
27. Cimolai, N., Elford, R. W., Bryan, L., et al.: Do the β-hemolytic non-group A streptococci cause pharyngitis? Rev. Infect. Dis. 10:587-601, 1988.
28. Cimolai, N., Morrison, B. J., MacCulloch, L., et al.: Beta-haemolytic non-group A streptococci and pharyngitis: A case-control study. Eur. J. Paediatr. 150:776-779, 1991.
29. Cinar, U., Seven, H. S., Vural, C., et al.: Tuberculosis tonsillitis. Otalaryngol. Head Neck Surg. 126:448-449, 2002.
30. Commission on Acute Respiratory Diseases: Endemic exudative pharyngitis and tonsillitis: Etiology and clinical characteristics. J. A. M. A. 125:1163-1169, 1944.
31. Conant, M. A., and Lane, B.: Secondary syphilis misdiagnosed as infectious mononucleosis. Calif. Med. 109:462-464, 1968.
32. Cramblett, H. G., Moffet, H. L., Black, J. P., et al.: Coxsackievirus infections: Clinical and laboratory studies. J. Pediatr. 64:406-414, 1964.
33. Dascomb, H. E., and Hilleman, M. R.: Clinical and laboratory studies in patients with respiratory disease caused by adenoviruses (RI-APC-ARD agents). Am. J. Med. Aug.:161-174, 1956.
34. Denny, F. W.: Current problems in managing streptococcal pharyngitis. J. Pediatr. 111:797-806, 1987.
35. Dominguez, O., Rojo, P., De Las Heras, S., et al.: Clinical presentation and characteristics of pharyngeal adenovirus infections. Pediatr. Infect. Dis. J. 24:733-734, 2005.
36. Douglas, R. M., Miles, H., Hansman, D., et al.: Acute tonsillitis in children: Microbial pathogens in relation to age. Pathology 16:79-82, 1984.
37. Dyment, P. G., Klink, L. B., and Jackson, D. W.: Hoarseness and palatal petechiae as clues in identifying streptococcal throat infections. Pediatrics 41:822-823, 1968.
38. Ebell, M. H., Smith, M. A., Barry, H. C., et al.: Does this patient have strep throat? J. A. M. A. 284:2912-2918, 2000.
39. Edmonson, M. B., and Farwell, K. R.: Relationship between the clinical likelihood of group A streptococcal pharyngitis and the sensitivity of a rapid antigen-detection test in a pediatric practice. Pediatrics 115:280-285, 2005.
40. El-Daher, N. T., Hijazi, S. S., Rawashedeh, N. M., et al.: Immediate vs. delayed treatment of group A beta-hemolytic streptococcal pharyngitis with penicillin V. Pediatr. Infect. Dis. J. 10:126-130, 1991.
41. Eshchar, J., Waron, M., and Alkan, W. J.: Syndromes of Q fever. J. A. M. A. 195:146-149, 1966.
42. Esposito, S., Bosis, S., Begliatti, E., et al.: Acute tonsillopharyngitis associated with atypical bacterial infection in children: Natural history and impact of macrolide therapy. Clin. Infect. Dis. 43:206-209, 2006.
43. Evans, A. S., and Dick, E. C.: Acute pharyngitis and tonsillitis in University of Wisconsin students. J. A. M. A. 190:699-708, 1964.
44. Farley, T. A., Wilson, S. A., Mahoney, F., et al.: Direct inoculation of food as the cause of an outbreak of group A streptococcal pharyngitis. J. Infect. Dis. 167:1232-1235, 1993.
45. Feder, H. M., Jr.: Periodic fever, aphthous stomatitis, pharyngitis, adenitis: A clinical review of a new syndrome. Curr. Opin. Pediatr. 12:253-256, 2000.
46. Fell, H. W. K., Nagington, J., Naylor, G. R. E., et al.: *Corynebacterium haemo-lyticum* infections in Cambridgeshire. J. Hyg. Camb. 79:269-275, 1977.
47. Finegold, S. M., Bartlett, J. G., Chow, A. W., et al.: Management of anaerobic infections. Ann. Intern. Med. 83:375-389, 1975.
48. Finegold, S. M., and Rosenblatt, J. E.: Practical aspects of anaerobic sepsis. Medicine (Baltimore) 52:311-322, 1973.
49. Fiumara, N. J., and Berg, M.: Primary syphilis in the oral cavity. Br. J. Vener. Dis. 50:463-464, 1974.
50. Forchheimer, F.: The enanthem of German measles. Phila. Med. J. II:15-17, 1898.
51. Foulongne, V., Olejnik, Y., Perez, V., et al.: Human bocavirus in French children. Emerg. Infect. Dis. 12:1251-1253, 2006.
52. Fries, S. M.: Diagnosis of group A streptococcal pharyngitis in a private clinic: Comparative evaluation of an optical immunoassay method and culture. J. Pediatr. 126:933-936, 1995.
53. Galanakis, E., Papadakis, C. E., Giannoussi, E., et al.: PFAPA syndrome in children evaluated for tonsillectomy. Arch. Dis. Child. 86:434-435, 2002.
54. Gallo, G., Berzero, R., Cattai, N., et al.: An outbreak of group A food-borne streptococcal pharyngitis. Eur. J. Epidemiol. 8:292-297, 1992.
55. Gerber, M. A.: Effect of early antibiotic therapy on recurrence rates of strep-tococcal pharyngitis. Pediatr. Infect. Dis. J. 10:S56-S60, 1991.
56. Gerber, M. A.: Comparison of throat cultures and rapid strep tests for diagno-sis of streptococcal pharyngitis. Pediatr. Infect. Dis. 8:820-824, 1989.
57. Gerber, M. A., Randolph, M. F., DeMeo, K. K., et al.: Lack of impact of early antibiotic therapy for streptococcal pharyngitis on recurrence rates. J. Pediatr. 117:853-858, 1990.
58. Gerber, M. A., Randolph, M. F., Martin, N. J., et al.: Community-wide out-break of group G streptococcal pharyngitis. Pediatrics 87:598-603, 1991.
59. Gerber, M. A., Spadaccini, L. J., Wright, L. L., et al.: Latex agglutination tests for rapid identification of group A streptococci directly from throat swabs. J. Pediatr. 105:702-705, 1984.
60. Gerber, M. A., Tanz, R. R., Kabat, W., et al.: Optical immunoassay test for group A β-hemolytic streptococcal pharyngitis: An office-based, multicenter investigation. J. A. M. A. 277:899-903, 1997.
61. Glezen, W. P., Clyde, W. A., Jr., Senior, R. J., et al.: Group A strepto-cocci, mycoplasmas, and viruses associated with acute pharyngitis. J. A. M. A. 202:455-460, 1967.
62. Glover, J. A., and Griffith, F.: Acute tonsillitis and some of its sequels: Epidemiological and bacteriological observations. B. M. J. Sept. 19:521-527, 1931.
63. Gorbach, S. L., and Bartlett, J. G.: Anaerobic infections (three parts). N. Engl. J. Med. 290:1177-1184, 1237-1245, 1289-1294, 1974.
64. Graykowski, E. A., Barile, M. F., Lee, W. B., et al.: Recurrent aphthous sto-matitis: Clinical, therapeutic, histopathologic, and hypersensitivity aspects. J. A. M. A. 196:637-644, 1966.
65. Grayston, J. T.: *Chlamydia pneumoniae* (TWAR) infections in children. Pediatr. Infect. Dis. J. 13:675-685, 1994.
66. Grayston, J. T., Alexander, E. R., Kenny, G. E., et al.: *Mycoplasma pneumoniae* infections: Clinical and epidemiologic studies. J. A. M. A. 191:369-374, 1965.
67. Grayston, J. T., Campbell, L. A., Kuo, C. C., et al.: A new respiratory tract pathogen: *Chlamydia pneumoniae* strain TWAR. J. Infect. Dis. 161:618-625, 1990.
68. Green, S. L., and LaPeter, K. S.: Pseudodiphtheritic membranous pharyngitis caused by *Corynebacterium hemolyticum*. J. A. M. A. 245:2330-2331, 1981.
69. Gurwith, M., Wenman, W., Hinde, D., et al.: A prospective study of rotavirus infection in infants and young children. J. Infect. Dis. 144:218-224, 1981.
70. Hamlyn, E., Marriott, D., and Gallagher, R. M.: Secondary syphilis presenting as tonsillitis in three patients. J. Laryngol. Otol. 120:602-604, 2006.
71. Harris, D. J., Wulff, H., Ray, C. G., et al.: Viruses and disease, II: An outbreak of parainfluenza type 2 in a children's home. Am. J. Epidemiol. 87:419-425, 1968.
72. Harrison, H. R., Magder, L. S., Boyce, W. T., et al.: Acute *Chlamydia tracho-matis* respiratory infection in childhood: Serologic evidence. Am. J. Dis. Child. 140:1068-1071, 1986.

73. Hathursinghe, H. R., Patel, S., Uppal, H. S., et al.: Acute tonsillitis: An unusual presentation of Kawasaki syndrome: A case report and review of the literature. Eur. Arch. Otorhinolaryngol. *263*:336-338, 2006.

74. Higgins, P. G., Ellis, E. M., Woolley, D. A., et al.: Viruses associated with acute respiratory infections in Royal Air Force personnel. J. Hyg. Camb. *68*:647-654, 1970.

75. Hill, H. R., Caldwell, G. G., Wilson, E., et al.: Epidemic of pharyngitis due to streptococci of Lancefield group G. Lancet *2*:371-374, 1969.

76. Hoagland, R. J.: Clinical manifestations of infectious mononucleosis: A report of two hundred cases. Am. J. Med. Sci. *240*:21-28, 1960.

77. Hoekstra, R. E., Herrmann, E. C., Jr., and O'Connell, E. J.: Virus infections in children: Clinical comparison of overlapping outbreaks of influenza A2/Hong Kong/68 and respiratory syncytial virus infections. Am. J. Dis. Child. *120*:14-16, 1970.

78. Hofer, C., Binns, H. J., and Tanz, R. R.: Strategies for managing group A streptococcal pharyngitis. Arch. Pediatr. Adolesc. Med. *151*:824-829, 1997.

79. Holzel, A., Parker, L., Patterson, W. H., et al.: Virus isolations from throats of children admitted to hospital with respiratory and other diseases, Manchester 1962-4. B. M. J. *1*:614-619, 1965.

80. Horn, M. E. C., Brain, E., Gregg, I., et al.: Respiratory viral infection in childhood: A survey in general practice, Roehampton 1967-1972. J. Hyg. Camb. *74*:157-168, 1975.

81. Humphrey, T., Sanders, S., and Stadius, M.: Leptospirosis mimicking MLNS. J. Pediatr. *91*:853-854, 1977.

82. Isaacs, D., and May, M.: Recurrent episodes of fever with tonsillitis, mouth ulcers and adenopathy. J. Paediatr. Child Health *39*:627-628, 2003.

83. Jacobs, R. F., Condrey, Y. M., and Yamauchi, T.: Tularemia in adults and children: A changing presentation. Pediatrics *76*:818-822, 1985.

84. Jamsky, R. J.: Gonococcal tonsillitis: Report of a case. Oral Surg. *44*:197-200, 1977.

85. John, C. C., and Gilsdorf, J. R.: Recurrent fever in children. Pediatr. Infect. Dis. J. *20*:1071-1080, 2002.

86. Johnson, J. E., III, and Kadull, P. J.: Laboratory-acquired Q fever: A report of fifty cases. Am. J. Med. *41*:391-403, 1966.

87. Jordan, W. S., Jr.: Acute respiratory diseases of viral etiology, I: Ecology of respiratory viruses-1961. Am. J. Public Health *52*:897-945, 1962.

88. Kapikian, A. Z., Chanock, R. M., Reichelderfer, T. E., et al.: Inoculation of human volunteers with parainfluenza virus type 3. J. A. M. A. *178*:537-546, 1961.

89. Karpathios, T., Drakonaki, S., Zervoudaki, A., et al.: *Arcanobacterium haemolyticum* in children with presumed streptococcal pharyngotonsillitis or scarlet fever. J. Pediatr. *121*:735-737, 1992.

90. Kellner, G., Popow-Kraupp, T., Kundi, M., et al.: Contribution of rhinoviruses to respiratory viral infections in childhood: A prospective study in a mainly hospitalized infant population. J. Med. Virol. *25*:455-469, 1988.

91. Kibrick, S.: Current status of Coxsackie and ECHO viruses in human disease. Prog. Med. Virol. *6*:27-70, 1964.

92. Komaroff, A. L., Aronson, M. D., Pass, T. M., et al.: Serologic evidence of chlamydial and mycoplasmal pharyngitis in adults. Science *222*:927-928, 1983.

93. Kovatch, A. L., Schuit, K. E., and Michaels, R. H.: *Corynebacterium hemolyticum* peritonsillar abscess mimicking diphtheria. J. A. M. A. *249*:1757-1758, 1983.

94. Kurtz, B., Kurtz, M., Roe, M., et al.: Importance of inoculum size and sampling effect in rapid antigen detection for diagnosis of *Streptococcus pyogenes* pharyngitis. J. Clin. Microbiol. *38*:279-281, 2000.

95. Lajo, A., Borque, C., Del Castillo, F., et al.: Mononucleosis caused by Epstein-Barr virus and cytomegalovirus in children: A comparative study of 124 cases. Pediatr. Infect. Dis. J. *13*:56-60, 1994.

96. Lascari, A. D., and Bapat, V. R.: Syndromes of infectious mononucleosis. Clin. Pediatr. *9*:300-305, 1970.

97. Le, C. T.: Tick-borne relapsing fever in children. Pediatrics *66*:963-966, 1980.

98. Lehner, T.: Oral thrush, or acute pseudomembranous candidiasis: A clinicopathologic study of forty-four cases. Oral Surg. *18*:27-37, 1964.

99. Lerner, A. M., Cherry, J. D., Klein, J. O., et al.: Infections with reoviruses. N. Engl. J. Med. *267*:947-952, 1962.

100. Lewis, H. M., Parry, J. V., Davies, H. A., et al.: A year's experience of the rotavirus syndrome and its association with respiratory illness. Arch. Dis. Child. *54*:339-346, 1979.

101. Lieu, T. A., Fleisher, G. R., and Schwartz, J. S.: Cost-effectiveness of rapid latex agglutination testing and throat culture for streptococcal pharyngitis. Pediatrics *85*:246-256, 1990.

102. Lindbaek, M., Høiby, E. A., Lermark, G., et al.: Clinical symptoms and signs in sore throat patients with large colony variant β-haemolytic streptococci groups C or G versus group A. Br. J. Gen. Pract. *55*:615-619, 2005.

103. Linder, J. A., Bates, D. W., Lee, G. M., et al.: Antibiotic treatment of children with sore throat. J. A. M. A. *294*:2315-2322, 2005.

104. Lipsky, B. A., Goldberger, A. C., Tompkins, L. S., et al.: Infections caused by nondiphtheria corynebacteria. Rev. Infect. Dis. *4*:1220-1235, 1982.

105. Long, S.: Syndrome of periodic fever, aphthous stomatitis, pharyngitis, and adenitis (PFAPA)—what it isn't. What is it? J. Pediatr. *135*:1-5, 1999.

106. Macdonald, J. B., Socransky, S. S., and Gibbons, R. J.: Aspects of the pathogenesis of mixed anaerobic infections of mucous membranes. J. Dent. Res. *42*(Suppl.):529-544, 1963.

107. Mackenzie, A., Fuite, L. A., Chan, F. T. H., et al.: Incidence and pathogenicity of *Arcanobacterium haemolyticum* during a 2-year study in Ottawa. Clin. Infect. Dis. *21*:177-181, 1995.

108. Mamo, J. G., and Baghdassarian, A.: Behçet's disease: A report of 28 cases. Arch. Ophthalmol. *71*:4-14, 1964.

109. Markowitz, M.: Cultures of the respiratory tract in pediatric practice. Am. J. Dis. Child. *105*:12-18, 1963.

110. Marshall, G. S., Edwards, K. M., Butler, J., et al.: Syndrome of periodic fever, pharyngitis, and aphthous stomatitis. J. Pediatr. *110*:43-46, 1987.

111. Maynard, J. E., Fletz, E. T., Wulff, H., et al.: Surveillance of respiratory virus infections among Alaskan Eskimo children. J. A. M. A. *200*:927-931, 1967.

112. McCloskey, R. V., Eller, J. J., Green, M., et al.: The 1970 epidemic of diphtheria in San Antonio. Ann. Intern. Med. *75*:495-503, 1971.

113. Meland, E., Digranes, A., and Skjaerven, R.: Assessment of clinical features predicting streptococcal pharyngitis. Scand. J. Infect. Dis. *25*:177-183, 1993.

114. Melish, M. E., Hicks, R. M., and Larson, E. J.: Mucocutaneous lymph node syndrome in the United States. Am. J. Dis. Child. *130*:599-607, 1976.

115. Moffet, H. L., Cramblett, H. G., and Smith, A.: Group A streptococcal infections in a children's home, II: Clinical and epidemiologic patterns of illness. Pediatrics *33*:11-17, 1964.

116. Moffet, H. L., Siegel, A. C., and Doyle, H. K.: Nonstreptococcal pharyngitis. J. Pediatr. *73*:51-60, 1968.

117. Mortimer, E. A., Jr., and Boxerbaum, B.: Diagnosis and treatment: Group A streptococcal infections. Pediatrics *36*:930-932, 1965.

118. Mufson, M. A.: *Mycoplasma hominis 1* in respiratory tract infections. Ann. N. Y. Acad. Sci. *174*:798-808, 1970.

119. Nakayama, M., Miyazaki, C., Ueda, K., et al.: Pharyngoconjunctival fever caused by adenovirus type 11. Pediatr. Infect. Dis. J. *11*:6-9, 1992.

120. Nigro, G., Pastoris, M. D., Fantasia, M. M., et al.: Acute cerebellar ataxia in pediatric legionellosis. Pediatrics *72*:847-849, 1983.

121. Nourmand, A., and Ziai, M.: Typhoid and paratyphoid fever in children: Review of symptoms and therapy in 165 cases. Clin. Pediatr. *8*:235-238, 1969.

122. Numazaki, Y., Yano, N., Shigeta, S., et al.: Studies on parainfluenza virus infections among infants and children in Sendai, II: Serologic and epidemiologic investigation. Jpn. J. Microbiol. *12*:343-351, 1968.

123. Ogawa, H., Hashiguchi, K., and Kazuyama, Y.: Prolonged and recurrent tonsillitis associated with sexually transmitted *Chlamydia trachomatis*. J. Laryngol. Otol. *107*:27-29, 1993.

124. Ohashi, M., Yoshikawa, T., Akimoto, S., et al.: Severe acute tonsillitis caused by *Rothia dentocariosa* in a healthy child. Pediatr. Infect. Dis. J. *24*:466-467, 2005.

125. Padeh, S., Brezniak, N., Zemer, D., et al.: Periodic fever, aphthous stomatitis, pharyngitis, and adenopathy syndrome: Clinical characteristics and outcome. J. Pediatr. *135*:98-101, 1999.

126. Pappas, G., Giannoutsos, C., Christou, L., et al.: *Coxiella burnetii*: An unusual ENT pathogen. Am. J. Otolaryngol. *25*:263-265, 2004.

127. Paradise, J. L., Bluestone, C. D., Bachman, R. Z., et al.: Efficacy of tonsillectomy for recurrent throat infection in severely affected children. N. Engl. J. Med. *310*:674-683, 1984.

128. Paradise, J. L., Bluestone, C. D., Colborn, D. K., et al.: Tonsillectomy and adenotonsillectomy for recurrent throat infection in moderately affected children. Pediatrics *110*:7-15, 2002.

129. Park, W. H., and Cooper, G. V.: Accidental inoculation of influenza bacilli on the mucous membranes of healthy persons with development of infection in at least one: Persistence of type characteristics of the bacilli. J. Immunol. *6*:81-85, 1921.

130. Parrott, R. H.: Viral respiratory tract illnesses in children. Bull. N. Y. Acad. Med. *39*:629-648, 1963.

131. Parrott, R. H., Kim, H. W., Vargosko, A. J., et al.: Serious respiratory tract illness as a result of Asian influenza and influenza B infections in children. J. Pediatr. *61*:205-213, 1962.

132. Parrott, R. H., Vargosko, A., Luckey, A., et al.: Clinical features of infection with hemadsorption viruses. N. Engl. J. Med. *260*:731-738, 1959.

133. Pereira, M. S.: Adenovirus infections. Postgrad. Med. J. *49*:798-801, 1973.

134. Pers, C.: Infection due to *Corynebacterium ulcerans* producing diphtheria toxin: A case report from Denmark. Acta Pathol. Microbiol. Immunol. Scand. *95*:361-362, 1987.

135. Peter, G.: Leptospirosis: A zoonosis of protean manifestations. Pediatr. Infect. Dis. *1*:282-288, 1982.

136. Pichichero, M. E., Disney, F. A., Talpey, W. B., et al.: Adverse and beneficial effects of immediate treatment of group A beta-hemolytic streptococcal pharyngitis with penicillin. Pediatr. Infect. Dis. *6*:635-643, 1987.

137. Pichichero, M. E., Disney, F. A., Green, J. L., et al.: Comparative reliability of clinical, culture, and antigen detection methods for the diagnosis of group A beta-hemolytic streptococcal tonsillopharyngitis. Pediatr. Ann. *21*:798-805, 1992.

138. Place, E. H., and Sutton, L. E.: Erythema arthriticum epidemicum (Haverhill fever). Arch. Intern. Med. *54*:659-684, 1934.

139. Podosin, R. L., and Felton, W. L., II: The clinical picture of Far East influenza occurring at the Fourth National Boy Scout Jamboree: Report of 616 cases. N. Engl. J. Med. *258*:778-782, 1958.

140. Poland, J. D., Wulff, H., Welton, E. R., et al.: Viruses and disease: Studies in a children's home. Am. J. Epidemiol. *84*:92-102, 1966.

141. Rantz, L. A., Boisvert, P. J., and Spink, W. W.: Hemolytic streptococci and nonstreptococcic diseases of the respiratory tract: A comparative clinical study. Arch. Intern. Med. 78:369-386, 1946.

142. Rodriguez, W. J., Controni, G., Cohen, G. J., et al.: *Yersinia enterocolitica* enteritis in children. J. A. M. A. 242:1978-1980, 1979.

143. Rodriguez, W. J., Kim, H. W., Arrobio, J. O., et al.: Clinical features of acute gastroenteritis associated with human reovirus-like agent in infants and young children. J. Pediatr. 91:188-193, 1977.

144. Rogers, R. S., III: Recurrent aphthous stomatitis: Clinical characteristics and evidence for an immunopathogenesis. J. Invest. Dermatol. 69:499-509, 1977.

145. Saari, T. N., and Triplett, D. A.: *Yersinia pseudotuberculosis* mesenteric adenitis. J. Pediatr. 85:656-659, 1974.

146. Saliba, G. S., Glezen, W. P., and Chin, T. D. Y.: Etiologic studies of acute respiratory illness among children attending public schools. Am. Rev. Respir. Dis. 95:592-602, 1967.

147. Schmidt, J. P., Metcalf, T. G., and Miltenberger, F. W.: An epidemic of Asian influenza in children at Ladd Air Force Base, Alaska, 1960. J. Pediatr. 61:214-220, 1962.

148. Schmidt, W. C., and Rammelkamp, C. H., Jr.: Bacterial infections of the nasopharynx, with particular reference to the prevention of rheumatic fever and glomerulonephritis. Pediatr. Clin. Feb.:139-154, 1957.

149. Scott, T. F.: Clinical syndromes associated with entero virus and REO virus infections. Adv. Virus Res. 8:165-197, 1961.

150. Siegel, W., Spencer, F. J., Smith, D. J., et al.: Two new variants of infection with coxsackievirus group B, type 5, in young children: A syndrome of lymph-adenopathy, pharyngitis and hepatomegaly or splenomegaly, or both, and one of pneumonia. N. Engl. J. Med. 268:1210-1216, 1963.

151. Sloots, T. P., Mackay, I. M., Bialasiewicz, S., et al.: Human metapneumovirus, Australia, 2001-2004. Emerg. Infect. Dis. 12:1263-1266, 2006.

152. Smith, H. W., Thomas, L., Dingle, J. H., et al.: Meningococcic infections: Report of 43 cases of meningococcic meningitis and 8 cases of meningococcemia. Ann. Intern. Med. 20:12-32, 1944.

153. Sohier, R., Chardonnet, Y., and Prunieras, M.: Adenoviruses: Status of current knowledge. Prog. Med. Virol. 7:253-325, 1965.

154. Solomon, P.: Oral moniliasis complicating combined broad-spectrum-antibiotic and antifungal therapy. N. Engl. J. Med. 265:847-848, 1961.

155. Steigman, A. J., Lipton, M. M., and Braspennickx, H.: Acute lymphonodular pharyngitis: A newly described condition due to coxsackie A virus. J. Pediatr. 61:331-336, 1962.

156. Steinkuller, J. S., Chan, K., and Rinehouse, S. E.: Prechewing of food by adults and streptococcal pharyngitis in infants. J. Pediatr. 120:563-564, 1992.

157. Sterner, G.: Adenovirus infection in childhood: An epidemiological and clinical survey among Swedish children. Acta Paediatr. 142:5-30, 1962.

158. Stillerman, M., and Bernstein, S. H.: Streptococcal pharyngitis: Evaluation of clinical syndromes in diagnosis. Am. J. Dis. Child. 101:476-489, 1961.

159. Stollerman, G. H.: Sore throat: A diagnostic and therapeutic dilemma. J. A. M. A. 189:145-146, 1964.

160. Sutton, R. N. P.: Respiratory viruses in a residential nursery. J. Hyg. Camb. 60:51-67, 1962.

161. Tacket, C. O., Davis, B. R., Carter, G. P., et al.: *Yersinia enterocolitica* pharyngitis. Ann. Intern. Med. 99:40-42, 1983.

162. Thomas, K. T., Feder, H. M., Jr., Lawton, A. R., et al.: Periodic fever syndrome in children. J. Pediatr. 135:15-21, 1999.

163. Tomlinson, A. J. H.: Human pathogenic coryneform bacteria: Their differentiation and significance in public health today. J. Appl. Bacteriol. 29:131-137, 1966.

164. Top, F. H., Sr.: Diphtheria. *In* Top, F. H., Sr., and Wehrle, P. F. (eds.): Communicable and Infectious Diseases. St. Louis, C. V. Mosby, 1972, pp. 190-207.

165. Tsevat, J., and Kotagal, U. R.: Management of sore throats in children. Arch. Pediatr. Adolesc. Med. 153:681-688, 1999.

166. Turner, J. C., Fox, A., Fox, K., et al.: Role of group C beta-hemolytic streptococci in pharyngitis: Epidemiologic study of clinical features associated with isolation of group C streptococci. J. Clin. Microbiol. 31:808-811, 1993.

167. Turner, J. C., Hayden, G. F., Kiselica, D., et al.: Association of group C beta-hemolytic streptococci with endemic pharyngitis among college students. J. A. M. A. 264:2644-2647, 1990.

168. Tyson, H. K.: Tularemia: An unappreciated cause of exudative pharyngitis. Pediatrics 58:864-866, 1976.

169. Uohara, G. I., and Knapp, M. J.: Oral fusospirochetosis and associated lesions. Oral Surg. 24:113-123, 1967.

170. Van Der Veen, J.: The role of adenoviruses in respiratory disease. Am. Rev. Respir. Dis. 88:167-180, 1963.

171. Veltri, R. W., Sprinkle, P. M., and McClung, J. E.: Epstein-Barr virus associated with episodes of recurrent tonsillitis. Arch. Otolaryngol. 101:552-556, 1975.

172. Von Graevenitz, A.: Which bacterial species should be isolated from throat cultures? Eur. J. Clin. Microbiol. 2:1-3, 1983.

173. Walker, J. E.: Infection of laboratory worker with bacillus influenzae. J. Infect. Dis. 43:300-305, 1928.

174. Walker, S. H.: The respiratory manifestations of systemic *Hemophilus influenzae* infection. J. Pediatr. 62:386-392, 1963.

175. Ward, R.: Poliomyelitis. Pediatr. Clin. North Am. 7:947-963, 1960.

176. Wat, P. J., Strickler, J. G., Myers, J. L., et al.: Herpes simplex infection causing acute necrotizing tonsillitis. Mayo Clin. Proc. 69:269-271, 1994.

177. Wiesner, P. J., Tronca, E., Bonin, P., et al.: Clinical spectrum of pharyngeal gonococcal infection. N. Engl. J. Med. 288:181-185, 1973.

178. Willard, C. Y., and Hansen, A. E.: Bacterial flora of the nasopharynx in children: Influence of respiratory infections and previous antimicrobial therapy. Am. J. Dis. Child. 97:318-325, 1959.

179. Wills, P. I., Gedosh, E. A., and Nichols, D. R.: Head and neck manifestations of tularemia. Laryngoscope 92:770-773, 1982.

180. Zalan, E., Leers, W. D., and Labzoffsky, N. A.: Occurrence of reovirus infection in Ontario. Can. Med. Assoc. J. 87:714-715, 1962.

181. Zalma, V. M., Older, J. J., and Brooks, G. F.: The Austin, Texas, diphtheria outbreak: Clinical and epidemiological aspects. J. A. M. A. 211:2125-2129, 1970.

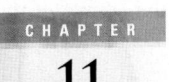

HERPANGINA

James D. Cherry

Herpangina, a fairly frequent, acute febrile illness that occurs in the summer and fall in temperate climates, is characterized by papular, vesicular, and ulcerative lesions on the anterior tonsillar pillars, soft palate, tonsils, pharynx, and posterior buccal mucosa. It is caused by many different enteroviruses.

HISTORY

Zahorsky[48,49] generally is credited with the identification and characterization of the disease spectrum of herpangina. In his first publication in 1920 entitled "Herpetic Sore Throat," he presented the findings in 82 cases. In 1924, he introduced the term *herpangina* so that the clinical entity would not be confused with other diseases of the mouth and throat. In both articles, Zahorsky noted that Moro previously had referred to a similar illness in 1906. Johnsson and Lindahl[19] also reported that similar syndromes had been observed by Trousseau in 1906 and Marfan in

1924 and Moro in 1906. In 1939, Levine and associates[26] described epidemic herpangina in three summer camps, and in 1941, Breese[4] reported 28 cases that he observed during the summers of 1938 and 1940. In 1951, Huebner and associates[18] and Parrott and colleagues[35] established the etiologic relationship of group A coxsackieviruses to herpangina. In 1965, Cherry and Jahn[10] noted from the literature and from their own observations that herpangina resulted from infection with many echoviruses and group B coxsackieviruses as well as group A coxsackieviruses.

ETIOLOGIC AGENTS

Virologic studies in the early 1950s that used suckling mice inoculation indicated that several group A coxsackieviruses were the cause of epidemic herpangina.[18,20,22,35,39,45] In subsequent years, tissue culture techniques became widely used in diagnostic virology, and many studies revealed additional enteroviral types asso-

TABLE 11-1   Etiologic Agents Found in Association with Sporadic or Epidemic Herpangina Occurrence

Virus	Occurrence		Reference
	Epidemic	*Sporadic*	
Coxsackievirus A			
1	+		20, 44, 45
2	+		20, 39, 44, 45
3	+		20, 39, 44, 45
4	+		20, 39, 44, 45
5	+		9, 20, 44, 45, 47
6	+		20, 39, 44, 45, 47
7		+	20, 37
8	+		20, 39, 44, 45
9		+	10, 20, 25, 37
10	+		20, 39, 44, 45
12		+	47
16		+	7, 10, 20
22	+		20, 44, 45
Coxsackievirus B			
1	+	+	10, 14, 30, 37, 44, 45
2		+	1, 14, 20, 28, 37, 44, 45
3		+	13-15, 20, 24, 33, 37, 44-46
4		+	2, 3, 10, 11, 14, 20, 36, 37, 44, 45
5		+	2, 14, 20, 37, 42, 44, 45
Echovirus			
6		+	20
9		+	10, 20, 23, 37, 42
11		+	31, 43
16	+	+	20, 34
17		+	10
25	+		32
Parechovirus 1		+	31
Enterovirus 71	+		5-8, 16, 17, 21, 27, 40
Herpes simplex		+	12, 29

ciated with herpangina.[10] Except for the initial interest in herpangina in 1950, careful study of the etiology of epidemic disease has not been done. Most herpangina virus-illness associations that have been made during the last 50 years have resulted from secondary findings in other investigations.* Table 11-1 lists viral agents associated with herpangina. In recent years, group B coxsackieviruses and enterovirus 71 have been implicated most frequently. Diagnostic studies using suckling mice inoculation have been performed only rarely during the last 40 years, however. As noted in Table 11-1, herpes simplex virus also can cause a clinical picture suggestive of herpangina.[12,29] Zahorsky[49] suggested that the cause of poliomyelitis also could be etiologic in herpangina because a similar enanthem had been observed in sporadic and epidemic poliomyelitis.

EPIDEMIOLOGY

For a discussion of epidemiology, see sections on coxsackieviruses and echoviruses in Chapter 178.

PATHOPHYSIOLOGY

The pathophysiology of coxsackievirus and the pathophysiology of echovirus infections are discussed in their respective sections in Chapter 178. Simkova and Petrovicova[41] presented specific

---

*See references 1-3, 5-8, 10-17, 21, 23-25, 27-32, 34, 36-38.

experimental data related to herpangina. In rhesus monkeys, these investigators found that oropharyngeal lesions typical of herpangina developed 2 to 7 days after oral, intravenous, or subcutaneous administration of coxsackievirus A4. This study indicated that the oropharyngeal lesions were the result of multiplication of virus at the secondary infection site after viremia, rather than a primary manifestation of initial cellular involvement.

CLINICAL MANIFESTATIONS

Although Zahorsky[48,49] and others[18,35] have considered herpangina a specific febrile disease, perhaps a more appropriate approach is to restrict the term *herpangina* to the characteristic oropharyngeal lesions. Herpangina is one of the protean manifestations of enteroviral infections, and it can occur in association with exanthem, aseptic meningitis, encephalitis, acute flaccid paralysis, and other clinical constellations.

The onset of herpangina is typical of most enteroviral infections and is characterized by the sudden awareness of fever.[4,35,48,49] No characteristic prodrome usually is present, but young children may be irritable and occasionally listless and anorexic for a few hours before the febrile state is recognized. The initial temperature can vary, with a range from normal to 41° C (106° F). Generally, the temperature tends to be higher in younger patients. Breese[4] noted that the most common temperature in young children was 39.5° C to 40° C (103° F to 104° F). Older children frequently complain of headache and backache. Vomiting occurs in approximately 25 percent of children younger than 5 years. In one outbreak of illness caused by coxsackievirus A4,[12] initial symptoms were anorexia and drooling (100%); sore throat (50%); coryza (45%); headache (18%); and vomiting, diarrhea, or both (36%).

In most instances of herpangina, the oropharyngeal lesions are present on the first examination at the time of fever or shortly after fever is noted. In the coxsackievirus A4 outbreak described by Forman and Cherry,[12] the enanthem was not observed until 24 to 48 hours after the onset of initial nonspecific symptoms. The characteristic lesions in herpangina are small (1 to 2 mm) vesicles and ulcers. These lesions apparently start as papules, become vesicular, and ulcerate in a short but variable period. In my experience, the lesions most commonly observed are ulcers. Breese[4] noted in many children seen early in the course of the illness that a petechial appearance preceded the appearance of typical vesicular-ulcerative enanthem.

The lesions usually are discrete, with an average of five per patient; some patients have only 1 or 2 lesions, whereas others may have 14 or more. When seen early, the vesicular lesions are observed to enlarge from 1 to 2 mm to 3 to 4 mm during a 2- to 3-day period.[35] Each vesicular and ulcerative lesion is surrounded by an erythematous ring that varies in size up to 10 mm in diameter. The most common site of the lesions is the anterior tonsillar pillars. Lesions also occur on the soft palate, uvula, tonsils, and pharyngeal wall and occasionally on the posterior buccal surfaces. In some cases, additional lesions have been noted on the dorsum or tip of the tongue. By definition, cases in which the primary involvement is on the tongue or anterior mouth and in which the lesions are of a general size greater than 5 mm are not considered to be herpangina.

Aside from the specific lesions, the remainder of the throat appears normal, minimally injected, or mildly erythematous. The usual duration of signs and symptoms is 3 to 6 days. Most cases of herpangina are mild and without complications, but aseptic meningitis and other severe enteroviral manifestations also occur occasionally. More recently, severe neurologic manifestations have been observed in children with herpangina caused by enterovirus 71.[5,6,8,16,17,21,27,40] During epidemic disease in Taiwan in 1998, children with herpangina and aseptic meningitis, acute flaccid paralysis, and rhombencephalitis were described.[16,17,40] In one study, a biphasic course was described, with herpangina occurring first and neurologic manifestations appearing 2 to 5 days later.[17]

Routine laboratory studies are of little value in herpangina. The total white blood cell count may be normal or slightly elevated; the differential count most often is normal.

DIFFERENTIAL DIAGNOSIS

The classic appearance of the oropharynx in herpangina renders establishing the diagnosis easy. Herpangina can be differentiated clearly from bacterial pharyngitis on clinical grounds, so obtaining bacterial cultures seldom is necessary. The follicular lesions of adenoviral infections can be confused with herpangina, but they frequently are exudative, not ulcerative, and associated with a more marked, generalized, erythematous pharyngitis than is seen in herpangina. Additional differential considerations are discussed elsewhere (see Chapters 10 and 178).

SPECIFIC DIAGNOSIS

In most instances, a clinical diagnosis is all that is necessary. Because herpangina is a good indicator of enteroviral disease in a community, however, submission of throat or rectal specimens to a viral diagnostic center can be rewarding.

TREATMENT, PROGNOSIS, AND PREVENTION

No treatment is necessary other than attention to hydration and observation for signs of more severe enteroviral illness. Except in rare instances (associated myocarditis, encephalitis), the prognosis is excellent. No general preventive measures are necessary, but a wise policy is not to expose young children unnecessarily to individuals known to be afflicted.

REFERENCES

1. Ager, E. A., Felsenstein, W. C., Alexander, E. R., et al.: An epidemic of illness due to Coxsackie virus group B, type 2. J. A. M. A. 187:251-256, 1964.
2. Artenstein, M. S., Cadigan, F. C., Jr., and Buescher, E. L.: Epidemic Coxsackie virus infection with mixed clinical manifestations. Ann. Intern. Med. 60:196-203, 1964.
3. Artenstein, M. S., Cadigan, F. C., Jr., and Buescher, E. L.: Clinical and epidemiological features of Coxsackie group B virus infections. Ann. Intern. Med. 63:597-603, 1965.
4. Breese, B. B., Jr.: Aphthous pharyngitis. Am. J. Dis. Child. 61:669-674, 1941.
5. Chang, L. Y., Hsia, S. H., Wu, C. T., et al.: Outcome of enterovirus 71 infections with or without stage-based management: 1998 to 2002. Pediatr. Infect. Dis. J. 23:327-331, 2004.
6. Chang, L. Y., King, C. C., Hsu, K. H., et al.: Risk factors of enterovirus 71 infection and associated hand, foot, and mouth disease/herpangina in children during an epidemic in Taiwan. Pediatrics 109:e88, 2002.
7. Chang, L. Y., Lin, T. Y., Huang, Y. C., et al.: Comparison of enterovirus 71 and coxsackie-virus A16 clinical illnesses during the Taiwan enterovirus epidemic, 1998. Pediatr. Infect. Dis. J. 12:1092-1096, 1999.
8. Chang, L. Y., Lin, T. Y., Hsu, K. H., et al.: Clinical features and risk factors of pulmonary oedema after enterovirus-71-related hand, foot, and mouth disease. Lancet 354:1682-1686, 1999.
9. Chawareewong, S., Kiangsiri, S., Lokaphadhana, K., et al.: Neonatal herpangina caused by Coxsackie A-5 virus. J. Pediatr. 93:492-494, 1978.
10. Cherry, J. D., and Jahn, C. L.: Herpangina: The etiologic spectrum. Pediatrics 36:632-634, 1965.
11. Felici, A., and Gregorig, B.: Contribution to the study of diseases in Italy caused by the Coxsackie B group of viruses, II: Epidemiological, clinical and virological data obtained in the course of a summer outbreak caused by Coxsackie B4 virus. Arch. Ges. Virusforsch. 9:317-328, 1959.
12. Forman, M. L., and Cherry, J. D.: Enanthems associated with uncommon viral syndromes. Pediatrics 41:873-882, 1968.
13. Glick, S. M., and Stroud, R.: An unusual case of Coxsackie B infection. Arch. Intern. Med. 109:97-101, 1962.
14. Hable, K. A., O'Connell, E. J., and Herrmann, E. C., Jr.: Group B coxsackieviruses as respiratory viruses. Mayo Clin. Proc. 45:170-176, 1970.
15. Hierholzer, J. C., Mostow, S. R., and Dowdle, W. R.: Prospective study of a mixed coxsackie virus B3 and B4 outbreak of upper respiratory illness in a children's home. Pediatrics 49:744-752, 1972.
16. Ho, M., Chen, E. R., Hsu, K. H., et al.: An epidemic of enterovirus 71 infection in Taiwan. N. Engl. J. Med. 341:929-935, 1999.
17. Huang, C. C., Liu, C. C., Chang, Y. C., et al.: Neurologic complications in children with enterovirus 71 infection. N. Engl. J. Med. 341:936-942, 1999.
18. Huebner, R. J., Cole, R. M., Beeman, E. A., et al.: Herpangina: Etiological studies of a specific infectious disease. J. A. M. A. 145:628-633, 1951.
19. Johnsson, T., and Lindahl, J.: Herpangina: A clinical and virological study. Arch. Ges. Virusforsch. 2:96-109, 1953.
20. Kibrick, S.: Current status of Coxsackie and ECHO viruses in human disease. Prog. Med. Virol. 6:27-70, 1964.
21. Komatsu, H., Shimizu, Y., Takeuchi, Y., et al.: Outbreak of severe neurologic involvement associated with enterovirus 71 infection. Pediatr. Neurol. 20:17-23, 1999.
22. Kravis, L. P., Hummeler, K., Sigel, M. M., et al.: Herpangina: Clinical and laboratory aspects of an outbreak caused by group A Coxsackie viruses. Pediatrics 11:113-119, 1953.
23. Lepow, M. L., Carver, D. H., and Robbins, F. C.: Clinical and epidemiologic observations on enterovirus infection in a circumscribed community during an epidemic of ECHO 9 infection. Pediatrics 26:12-26, 1960.
24. Lerner, A. M., Klein, J. O., and Finland, M.: Infection with Coxsackie virus group B, type 3, with vesicular eruption: Report of two cases. N. Engl. J. Med. 263:1305, 1960.
25. Lerner, A. M., Klein, J. O., Levin, H. S., et al.: Infections due to Coxsackie virus group A, type 9, in Boston, 1959, with special reference to exanthems and pneumonia. N. Engl. J. Med. 263:1265-1272, 1960.
26. Levine, H. B., Hoerr, S. O., and Allanson, J. C.: Vesicular pharyngitis and stomatitis: An unusual epidemic of possible herpetic origin. J. A. M. A. 112:2020-2022, 1939.
27. Liu, C. C., Tseng, H. W., Wang, S. M., et al.: An outbreak of enterovirus 71 infection in Taiwan, 1998: Epidemiologic and clinical manifestations. J. Clin. Virol. 17:23-30, 2000.
28. Marchessault, V., Pavilanis, V., Podoski, M. O., et al.: An epidemic of aseptic meningitis caused by Coxsackie B type 2 virus. Can. Med. Assoc. J. 85:123-126, 1961.
29. Marks, M. I.: Herpangina and pleurodynia associated with herpes simplex virus. Pediatrics 48:305-307, 1971.
30. McLean, D. M., Coleman, M. A., Larke, R. P. B., et al.: Viral infections of Toronto children during 1965, I: Enteroviral disease. Can. Med. Assoc. J. 94:839-843, 1966.
31. Moore, M.: Enteroviral disease in the United States, 1970-1979. J. Infect. Dis. 146:103-108, 1982.
32. Moritsugu, Y., Sawada, K., Hinohara, M., et al.: An outbreak of type 25 echovirus infections with exanthem in an infant home near Tokyo. Am. J. Epidemiol. 87:599-608, 1968.
33. Nakayama, T., Urano, T., Osano, M., et al.: Outbreak of herpangina associated with coxsackievirus B3 infection. Pediatr. Infect. Dis. 8:495-498, 1989.
34. Neva, F. A., Feemster, R. F., and Gorbach, I. J.: Clinical and epidemiological features of an unusual epidemic exanthem. J. A. M. A. 155:544-548, 1954.
35. Parrott, R. H., Ross, S., Burke, F. G., et al.: Herpangina: Clinical studies of a specific infectious disease. N. Engl. J. Med. 245:275-280, 1951.
36. Ray, C. G., Plexico, K. L., Wenner, H. A., et al.: Acute respiratory illness associated with Coxsackie B4 virus in children. Pediatrics 39:220-226, 1967.
37. Reinhard, K. R.: Ecology of enteroviruses in the western Arctic. J. A. M. A. 183:410-418, 1963.
38. Sabin, A. B.: Role of ECHO viruses in human disease. In Rose, H. M. (ed.): Viral Infections of Infancy and Childhood. Symposium No. 19, Section on Microbiology, New York Academy of Medicine. New York, Hoeber-Harper, 1960, pp. 78-100.
39. Scott, T. F. M.: Clinical syndromes associated with enterovirus and reovirus infection. Adv. Virus Res. 8:165-197, 1962.
40. Shen, W. C., Tsai, C., Chiu, H., et al.: MRI of enterovirus 71 myelitis with monoplegia. Neuroradiology 42:124-127, 2000.
41. Simkova, A., and Petrovicova, A.: Experimental infection of rhesus monkeys with Coxsackie A 4 virus. Acta Virol. 16:250-257, 1972.
42. St. Geme, J. W., Jr., and Prince, J. T.: Vesicular pharyngitis associated with Coxsackie virus group B, type 5. N. Engl. J. Med. 265:1255-1256, 1961.
43. Suzuki, N., Ishikawa, K., Horiuchi, T., et al.: Age-related symptomatology of ECHO 11 virus infection in children. Pediatrics 65:284-286, 1980.
44. Wenner, H. A.: The enteroviruses. Am. J. Clin. Pathol. 57:751-761, 1972.
45. Wenner, H. A.: Virus diseases associated with cutaneous eruptions. Prog. Med. Virol. 16:269-336, 1973.
46. Winsser, J., and Altieri, R. H.: A three-year study of Coxsackie virus, group B, infection in Nassau County, part I: Fecal studies of patients. Am. J. Med. Sci. 247:269-273, 1964.
47. Yamashita, T., Ito, M., Taniguchi, A., and Sakae, K.: Prevalence of coxsackievirus A5, A6, and A10 in patients with herpangina in Aichi prefecture, 2005. Jpn. J. Infect. Dis. 58:390-391, 2005.
48. Zahorsky, J.: Herpetic sore throat. South. Med. J. 13:871-872, 1920.
49. Zahorsky, J.: Herpangina: A specific infectious disease. Arch. Pediatr. 41:181-184, 1924.

CHAPTER
12
PHARYNGOCONJUNCTIVAL FEVER
James D. Cherry

Pharyngoconjunctival fever is an acute, communicable disease syndrome characterized by fever, pharyngitis, and conjunctivitis. It is caused by several serologic types of adenovirus. Illness is epidemic and sporadic.

HISTORY

Shortly after the first isolation of adenoviruses in tissue culture by Rowe and associates[54] in 1953, the clear association of infection with certain adenoviral types and the syndrome of fever, pharyngitis, and conjunctivitis were established.[52] For an approximate 5-year period after the discovery of the adenoviral etiology of pharyngoconjunctival fever, the literature contained numerous confirmatory reports from throughout the world.* In almost all reports, the association between swimming and the contraction of the syndrome was noted. A quick perusal of the reports would suggest that the syndrome and the etiologic agents were new discoveries. Epidemics of pharyngoconjunctival fever–like illness have been noted throughout the 20th century, however. In 1907, Béal[4] in France was perhaps the first to note the syndrome. In the 1920s, epidemics of febrile disease with conjunctivitis associated with swimming in public pools and lakes were noted in Germany[51] and the United States.[2] It is likely that "swimming bath conjunctivitis," as described by Derrick[16] in 1943, was caused by adenoviral infection. An epidemic of conjunctivitis studied by Cockburn and associates[12] in Greeley, Colorado, in 1951 later was proved to have been caused by adenovirus type 3.

In more recent years, reports of pharyngoconjunctival fever have been relatively few.** My experience suggests that this paucity is not because of a decrease in prevalence of the syndrome but because of a general disinterest in the differential diagnosis of viral respiratory disease.

ETIOLOGIC AGENTS

In epidemic pharyngoconjunctival fever, the most likely etiologic agent is adenovirus type 3.† The next most prevalent adenovirus associated with epidemic disease is type 7.[9,17,22,73] One or more epidemics also have been noted with adenoviruses 2, 4, 7a, 11, and 14.[1,7,15,18,19,48,66,67,76] Sporadic occurrences of pharyngoconjunctival fever have been observed in association with infections with adenoviruses 1, 2, 3, 4, 5, 6, 7, 7a, 8, 14, 19, and 13/30 (an intermediate type).‡

EPIDEMIOLOGY

Pharyngoconjunctival fever occurs in large community-wide epidemics, in focal outbreaks, and as sporadic cases. Most major community epidemics have occurred in the summer and have

been centered around public swimming facilities. Two community outbreaks involving primarily swimmers have occurred in the winter.[9,23] In swimming-associated outbreaks, infection probably occurs by conjunctival inoculation of adenoviruses from contaminated water. To date, however, the virus has been recovered from the incriminated water in only two outbreaks.[15,46] In one outbreak, adenovirus type 4 was recovered from water samples on two occasions 14 days apart.[15] More recently, adenovirus type 3 was recovered from a pool in which 681 campers had symptoms.[46] In this outbreak, the frequency of swimming and the history of towel sharing increased the risk of acquiring illness. Adenovirus type 3 also was recovered from a sewage outlet area in a lake that was close to a swimming beach.[42]

The incubation period of swimming-associated infections is approximately 5 to 7 days.[6,23,36,67] Secondary cases regularly occur in contacts (most often family members) of swimming-acquired cases. In these instances, the incubation period frequently is slightly longer (9 days).[3,23] This longer period of incubation may be due to a delay in the time of spread of the virus to the contact, rather than an actual prolongation of incubation. Secondary cases probably result from large-droplet respiratory spread to the conjunctiva, the upper respiratory tract, or both. An alternative method would be the contamination of the recipient's hands with eye discharge followed by autoinoculation of the conjunctiva.

In non–swimming-associated outbreaks of adenoviral respiratory illness with appropriate serotypes, conjunctivitis occurs only rarely.[8,21,30,35,41,63] This fact, in conjunction with the finding that pharyngoconjunctival fever occurred after conjunctival administration of virus, but not after nasopharyngeal application in volunteers,[7,58,71] suggests that the conjunctiva must be inoculated directly for the syndrome to occur. After conjunctival inoculation, pharyngeal spread and systemic illness occur. After direct respiratory inoculation, the conjunctiva does not become involved, unless respiratory secretions containing virus are applied to the conjunctiva, presumably by autoinoculation. Hospital outbreaks of pharyngoconjunctival fever–like illnesses have been reported.[20,43] Most instances have occurred in intensive care units. An outbreak of pharyngoconjunctival fever also has been noted in a daycare center.[11]

Although some early epidemic investigations suggested that boys were more susceptible to disease than were girls,[22,66] the incidence of pharyngoconjunctival fever in children does not differ by sex.[6,60] In some cultures, boys had more exposure to swimming and accounted for more cases of illness. In an outbreak that occurred in children hospitalized in Japan for long-term treatment of bronchial asthma, the attack rate was 68.2 percent in boys and only 6.3 percent in girls. This sex difference was attributed to the fact that the boys and girls took separate daily communal baths. Secondary cases in adult family members occur more commonly in mothers than in fathers, presumably because of greater contact with the children.[7,23]

PATHOPHYSIOLOGY

The route of infection with adenoviruses that are capable of causing pharyngoconjunctival fever determines the pathologic manifestations. Conjunctival biopsy specimens in volunteer studies revealed an inflammatory response with lymphocytic infiltration of the submucosal layer.[5,7] Biopsy material from pala-

---

*See references 1, 3, 5, 7, 8, 12, 17, 19, 21, 22, 25-28, 32-37, 39-42, 47-50, 57, 59-61, 63, 65-67, 69, 71.
**See references 9, 10, 13, 15, 18, 23, 24, 28, 31, 32, 45, 46, 48, 53, 54, 56, 58, 64, 68, 70, 72, 73, 76.
†See references 3, 6, 7, 8, 12, 23, 25, 26, 33, 36-38, 42, 45, 46, 49, 52, 59, 66, 72, 76.
‡See references 5, 7, 10, 24, 26, 30-32, 35, 39-41, 47, 55, 56, 60-65, 68, 70.

TABLE 12-1 Frequency of Symptoms in Epidemic Pharyngoconjunctival Fever

Symptoms	Frequency*
Throat Complaints	++++
Soreness	++++
Cough	++
Foreign body sensation	++
Dry feeling	+
Eye Complaints	+++
Aching or soreness	+++
Burning sensation	++
Lacrimation	+
Photophobia	+
Nasal Complaints	+++
Coryza	++
Stuffiness or blockage or both	++
Sneezing	+
Epistaxis	+
Other Complaints	++++
Headache	++++
Anorexia	+++
Malaise	++
Generalized aches and pains	++
Nausea	++
Vomiting	+
Diarrhea	+
Abdominal pain	+

*++++, 76 to 100 percent; +++, 51 to 75 percent; ++, 26 to 50 percent; +, 1 to 25 percent.
Data from references 5, 9, 22, 25, 36, 39, 40, 45, 52, 57, 58, 66.

TABLE 12-2 Frequency of Signs in Epidemic Pharyngoconjunctival Fever

Signs	Frequency*
Throat Findings	++++
Erythema and infection	++++
Hypertrophied lymphatic tissue	++++
Particulate exudate	++
Eye Findings	++++
Erythema and infection of palpebral and bulbar conjunctiva	++++
Edema	+++
Granular and follicular involvement	++
Eyes unequally affected	++
Superficial punctate keratitis	+
Lymph Node Enlargement	++++
Cervical	++++
Preauricular	+
Generalized	+
Fever	++++
≥39° C (≥102.2° F)	+++
Other	
Flushed face	+++
Enlarged liver or spleen or both	+

*++++, 76 to 100 percent; +++, 51 to 75 percent; ++, 26 to 50 percent; +, 1 to 25 percent.
Data from references 5, 9, 22, 25, 29, 40, 52, 57, 58, 66.

tine tonsils of infected volunteers revealed hypertrophy and hyperplasia of the lymphoid tissue, with congestion and edema of the surrounding connective tissue.

CLINICAL PRESENTATION

By definition, pharyngoconjunctival fever is a syndrome characterized by fever, pharyngitis, and conjunctivitis. During epidemics, not all children and adults who have the same infection have the complete syndrome triad. Some patients have only pharyngitis, and some have only conjunctivitis. For purposes of this discussion, all descriptions of frequency of signs and symptoms are calculated from the starting point of 100 percent fever, pharyngitis, and conjunctivitis.

Tables 12–1 and 12–2 summarize the frequencies of specific symptoms and signs.* Although some patients have noted mild prodromal symptoms of headache and malaise, the usual onset of illness is abrupt, with sore throat, generalized aches and pains, eye irritation or pain, and fever. Throat complaints vary from mild to severe. In some patients, only a dry, scratchy feeling is reported; others have noted the feeling of a foreign body. On examination, the tonsils and pharyngeal lymphoid tissue are hypertrophied. The degree of pharyngeal redness and infection varies considerably from patient to patient. Approximately one third of affected patients have follicular exudative lesions that cannot be differentiated from streptococcal disease on clinical grounds. Follicular lesions also have been noted on the soft palate, and the papillae of the tongue may be hypertrophied.

Hypertrophy of the adenoids occurs, which results in nasal blockage. Coryza is a common occurrence. Posterior nasal discharge is a common occurrence and leads to cough in many instances. In some investigations, epistaxis has occurred in 20 percent of the cases.[57,66]

Generally, complaints related to conjunctivitis are fewer than might be suggested by the usual physical appearance. Most patients note some aching or soreness; photophobia and lacrimation are unusual occurrences. The appearance of the palpebral conjunctiva usually is granular. The lesions may be almost microscopic or 2 to 3 mm in diameter. Hemorrhages occasionally are noted on the bulbar surface. Frequently, involvement starts in one eye and does not involve the other eye until 2 or 3 days later. Occasionally, the involvement is restricted to one eye.

Some degree of anterior and posterior cervical lymphadenopathy occurs in most patients. Preauricular involvement occurs surprisingly infrequently when the degree of eye involvement is taken into consideration. Generalized lymphadenopathy is observed in 10 to 20 percent of affected patients, and liver and spleen enlargement occurs frequently.

Most patients complain of generalized symptoms, but the degree varies considerably among affected patients. Temperatures greater than 39° C (102.2° F) occur in more than 50 percent of the patients, and headache is the rule. General malaise and anorexia are common occurrences; gastrointestinal symptoms occur in approximately 25 percent of cases. Vomiting and diarrhea occur most commonly in younger age groups.

Compared with other respiratory viral infections, the duration of illness with pharyngoconjunctival fever is long. In most patients, the fever is sustained or remittent for 3 to 4 days, then temperature gradually returns to normal within 24 to 48 hours. Approximately 10 percent of patients have fever that lasts longer than 7 days. Throat and eye findings usually are improved considerably by the seventh day of illness, but these findings and nasal complaints, fatigue, and headache may persist for 14 days.

Early in the illness, the total white blood cell count is within normal limits or slightly elevated, with a normal differential count or one with a slight increase in polymorphonuclear leukocytes. During convalescence, many patients have a moderate leukopenia with an equal number of lymphocytes and polymorphonuclear cells. Smears from affected conjunctivae usually do not reveal abnormalities on cytologic examination.

DIFFERENTIAL DIAGNOSIS

Because the symptom triad of fever, pharyngitis, and conjunctivitis is virtually unique to pharyngoconjunctival fever, establishing the diagnosis should be easy. The only difficulty on clinical grounds is in trying to assign a specific type of adenovirus. Generally, major epidemic disease is most likely to be caused by type 3 or 7; sporadic cases can occur with types 1 to 8, 14, 19, and 13/30. Manifestations by different adenoviral types have no known differences.

Of some concern in the differential diagnosis is picornavirus epidemic conjunctivitis (acute hemorrhagic conjunctivitis).[44,74,75] Two enteroviruses (coxsackievirus A24 and enterovirus 70) have been implicated etiologically in several extensive outbreaks of disease. Affected patients have had severe conjunctivitis with preauricular lymphadenitis, but fever and pharyngitis have not been prominent associated signs. In one outbreak, 23 percent of patients studied had upper respiratory tract symptoms.[44]

Generalized diseases that occasionally might be confused with pharyngoconjunctival fever include leptospirosis, psittacosis, *Mycoplasma pneumoniae* infection, Q fever, Newcastle disease virus infection, and prodromal measles. Of these illnesses, all but Newcastle disease virus infection have generalized symptoms that are disproportionately more important than the symptoms of either conjunctivitis or pharyngitis. Human infection with Newcastle disease virus could be confused easily on clinical grounds with pharyngoconjunctival fever. A history of exposure to chickens or other fowl should aid in establishing the diagnosis.

Of more difficulty in making a differential diagnosis are illnesses usually characterized by either pharyngitis or conjunctivitis. Occasionally, infections with influenza viruses, parainfluenza viruses, enteroviruses (other than coxsackievirus A24 and enterovirus 70), and Epstein-Barr virus are confusing. Although eye complaints do occur in these illnesses, severe conjunctivitis usually does not occur.

The differential diagnosis of conjunctivitis includes bacterial infections caused by *Haemophilus influenzae*, *Streptococcus pneumoniae*, *Streptococcus pyogenes*, and *Neisseria gonorrhoeae*. In all of these infections, purulent discharge is greater than that usually observed in pharyngoconjunctival fever. *Chlamydia trachomatis* infections are perhaps the most troublesome in the differential diagnosis. In the past, many cases of swimming pool conjunctivitis were attributed to chlamydial infections. Many such reported cases in reality probably were adenoviral infections. *C. trachomatis* infections can be diagnosed by showing characteristic inclusions in Giemsa-stained scrapings from the palpebral conjunctivae, by direct immunofluorescence, by enzyme immunoassay, or by culture. Epidemic adenoviral keratoconjunctivitis is another differential diagnostic consideration. Other differential diagnostic possibilities that should cause no difficulty include cat-scratch fever, tularemia, *Acanthamoeba* keratitis, and allergic conjunctivitis.

SPECIFIC DIAGNOSIS

In most instances, a clinical diagnosis is all that is necessary. Specific viral diagnosis can be accomplished with ease in any routinely equipped diagnostic virology laboratory. Diagnosis can be made by isolation of virus in tissue culture or by direct antigen detection by indirect immunofluorescence, enzyme-linked immunosorbent assay, or polymerase chain reaction analysis.[11,14,53,68] Cultures from the conjunctivae generally are more diagnostically specific than are cultures from the throat. The recovery of an adenovirus (particularly type 2) from the throat in an isolated case does not indicate an etiologic role for the recovered virus. An adenoviral etiology also can be verified by studying paired serum samples for a titer increase to the adenoviral group antigen.

TREATMENT

Generally, no treatment is necessary or effective in pharyngoconjunctival fever. If conjunctivitis persists and becomes purulent, an investigation for bacterial pathogens and appropriate topical antimicrobial therapy are indicated. Use of steroid-containing ophthalmic ointments should be avoided.

PROGNOSIS

The prognosis generally is excellent. Although superficial keratitis occasionally occurs, permanent scarring is not a problem. Sinusitis, otitis media, and bacterial conjunctivitis are rare secondary complications that, if untreated, can result in long-term difficulties.

PREVENTION

Volunteer studies have clearly indicated that infection and presumable resultant antibody are protective against future disease. Protection theoretically could be achieved through immunization, but priority given to study and to implement an immunization program is low. Because the major cause of pharyngoconjunctival fever caused by adenoviruses is swimming in contaminated water, discretion in bathing locations is advised. Swimming pool water should be chlorinated adequately, and pool filtration systems should be inspected daily. Ill individuals should be excluded from swimming pools during their illness and for at least 2 weeks after recovery.

REFERENCES

1. Albano, A., Salvaggio, L., and Morrone, G.: Episodio epidemico de febbre faringocongiuntivale da adenovirus di tipo 2. Boll. Ist. Sieroter. Milan *40*:580-584, 1961.
2. Bahn, C. A.: Swimming bath conjunctivitis. New Orleans Med. Surg. J. *79*:586-590, 1927.
3. Barr, J., Kjellén L., and Svedmyr, A.: Hospital outbreak of adenovirus type 3 infections: A clinical and virologic study on 38 patients partly involved in a nosocomial outbreak. Acta Pediatr. *47*:365-382, 1958.
4. Béal, R.: Sur une forme particulière de conjonctivité aigue avec follicules. Ann. D'Oculistique *Jan.*:1-33, 1907.
5. Bell, J. A.: Clinical manifestations of pharyngoconjunctival fever. Am. J. Ophthalmol. *43*:11-14, 1957.
6. Bell, J. A., Rowe, W. P., Engler, J. I., et al.: Pharyngoconjunctival fever: Epidemiological studies of a recently recognized disease entity. J. A. M. A. *157*:1083-1092, 1955.
7. Bell, J. A., Ward, T. G., Huebner, R. J., et al.: Studies of adenoviruses (APC) in volunteers. Am. J. Public Health *46*:1130-1146, 1956.
8. Bell, T. M., Turner, G., MacDonald, A., et al.: Type-3 adenovirus infection. Lancet *2*:1327-1329, 1960.
9. Caldwell, G. G., Lindsey, N. J., Wulff, H., et al.: Epidemic of adenovirus type 7 acute conjunctivitis in swimmers. Am. J. Epidemiol. *99*:230-234, 1974.
10. Chen, H. L., Chiou, S. S., Hsiao, H. P., et al.: Respiratory adenoviral infections in children—a study of hospitalized cases in southern Taiwan in 2001-2002. J. Trop. Pediatr. *50*:279-284, 2004.
11. Chomel, J. J., Szymczyszyn, P., Honneger, D., et al.: An epidemic of adenovirus type 1 conjunctivitis. Pediatr. Infect. Dis. J. *8*:885-886, 1989.
12. Cockburn, T. A., Rowe, W. P., and Huebner, R. J.: Relationship of the 1951 Greeley, Colorado, outbreak of conjunctivitis and pharyngitis to type 3 APC virus infection. Am. J. Hyg. *63*:250-253, 1956.
13. Cooper, R. J., Hallett, R., Tullo, A. B., and Klapper, P. E.: The epidemiology of adenovirus infections in Greater Manchester, UK, 1982-96. Epidemiol. Infect. *125*:333-345, 2000.
14. Cooper, R. J., Yeo, A. C., Bailey, A. S., and Tullo, A. B.: Adenovirus polymerase chain reaction assay for rapid diagnosis of conjunctivitis. Invest. Ophthalmol. Vis. Sci. *40*:90-95, 1999.

15. D'Angelo, L. J., Hierholzer, J. C., Keenlyside, R. A., et al.: Pharyngoconjunctival fever caused by adenovirus type 4: Report of a swimming pool-related outbreak with recovery of virus from pool water. J. Infect. Dis. *140*:42-47, 1979.
16. Derrick, E. H.: Swimming-bath conjunctivitis, with a report of 3 probable cases and a note on its epidemiology. Med. J. Aust. *2*:334-336, 1943.
17. Duxbury, A. E., McCutchan, R., White, J., et al.: Epidemic adenovirus infection in a Victorian migrant centre presenting as pharyngoconjunctival fever. Med. J. Aust. *2*:413-417, 1960.
18. Ellis, A. W., McKinnon, G. T., Lewis, F. A., et al.: Adenovirus type 4 in Melbourne, 1969-1971. Med. J. Aust. *1*:209-211, 1974.
19. Epshtein, F. G., Agarkova, L. G., Dreizin, E. Y., et al.: Acute respiratory diseases in children caused by adenovirus of 7a type. Sov. Med. *2*:81-85, 1962.
20. Faden, H., Gallagher, M., Ogra, P., et al.: Nosocomial outbreak of pharyngoconjunctival fever due to adenovirus type 4: New York. M. M. W. R. Morb. Mortal. Wkly. Rep. *27*:49, 1978.
21. Forssell, P., Halonen, H., Stenstrom, R., et al.: An adenovirus epidemic due to types 1 and 2. Ann. Pediatr. Fenn. *8*:35-44, 1962.
22. Forssell, P., Lapinleimu, K., Strandström, H., et al.: Febrile pharyngitis and conjunctivitis: An epidemic associated with APC virus infection. Ann. Med. Exp. Biol. Fenn. *34*:287-292, 1956.
23. Foy, H. M., Cooney, M. K., and Hatlen, J. B.: Adenovirus type 3 epidemic associated with intermittent chlorination of a swimming pool. Arch. Environ. Health *17*:795-802, 1968.
24. Foy, H. M., and Grayston, J. T.: Adenoviruses. In Evans, A. S. (ed.): Viral Infections of Humans: Epidemiology and Control. New York, Plenum, 1976.
25. Fukumi, H., Nishikawa, F., Mizutani, H., et al.: An epidemic of adenovirus type 3 infections among school children in an elementary school in Tokyo. Jpn. J. Med. Sci. Biol. *11*:129-140, 1958.
26. Fukumi, H., Nishikawa, F., Nakamura, K., et al.: Studies on the adenovirus as an etiological agent of pharyngoconjunctival fever. Jpn. J. Med. Sci. Biol. *10*:79-85, 1957.
27. Fukumi, H., Nishikawa, F., Nakamura, K., et al.: Further studies of the cases associated with adenoviruses. Jpn. J. Med. Sci. Biol. *10*:407-418, 1957.
28. Fukumi, H., Nishikawa, F., Takemura, M., et al.: Isolation of adenovirus possessing both the antigens of types 3 and 7. Jpn. J. Med. Sci. Biol. *14*:173-181, 1961.
29. Harley, D., Harrower, B., Lyon, M., and Dick, A.: A primary school outbreak of pharyngoconjunctival fever caused by adenovirus type 3. Commun. Dis. Intell. *25*:9-12, 2001.
30. Harris, D. J., Wulff, H., Ray, C. G., et al.: Viruses and disease, III: An outbreak of adenovirus type 7a in a children's home. Am. J. Epidemiol. *93*:399-402, 1971.
31. Herrmann, E. C., Jr.: Experiences in laboratory diagnosis of adenovirus infections in routine medical practice. Mayo Clin. Proc. *43*:635-644, 1968.
32. Huebner, R. J., Rowe, W. P., and Chanock, R. M.: Newly recognized respiratory tract viruses. Annu. Rev. Microbiol. *12*:49-76, 1958.
33. Jansson, E., Wager, O., Forssel, P., et al.: Epidemic occurrence of adenovirus type 7 infection in Helsinki. Ann. Paediatr. Fenn. *8*:24-34, 1962.
34. Jones, B. R.: Sporadic ocular disease associated with adenovirus infection in London. Proc. R. Soc. Med. *50*:758-760, 1957.
35. Jordan, W. S., Jr., Badger, G. F., Curtiss, C., et al.: A study of illness in a group of Cleveland families, X: The occurrence of adenovirus infections. Am. J. Hyg. *64*:336-348, 1956.
36. Kaji, M., Kamiya, S., Tatewaki, E., et al.: An epidemic of pharyngoconjunctival fever in Moji, Kyushu. Kyushu J. Med. Sci. *12*:241-249, 1961.
37. Kaji, M., Kimura, M., Kamiya, S., et al.: An epidemic of pharyngoconjunctival fever among school children in an elementary school in Fukuoka prefecture. Kyushu J. Med. Sci. *12*:1-8, 1960.
38. Kawana, R., Kaneko, M., Matsumoto, I., et al.: An outbreak of pharyngoconjunctival fever due to adenovirus type 3. Jpn. J. Microbiol. *10*:149-157, 1966.
39. Kendall, E. J. C., Riddle, R. W., Tuck, H. A., et al.: Pharyngoconjunctival fever: School outbreaks in England during the summer of 1955 associated with adenovirus types 3, 7, and 14. B. M. J. *2*:131-136, 1957.
40. Kimura, S. J., Hanna, L., Nicholas, A., et al.: Sporadic cases of pharyngoconjunctival fever in Northern California, 1955-1956. Am. J. Ophthalmol. *43*:14-16, 1957.
41. Kjellén, L., Sterner, G., and Svedmyr, A.: On the occurrence of adenoviruses in Sweden. Acta Paediatr. *46*:164-176, 1957.
42. Kjellén, L., Zetterberg, B., and Svedmyr, A.: An epidemic among Swedish children caused by adenovirus type 3. Acta Paediatr. *46*:561-568, 1957.
43. Larsen, R. A., Jacobson, J. T., Jacobson, J. A., et al.: Hospital-associated epidemic of pharyngitis and conjunctivitis caused by adenovirus (21/H21 + 35). J. Infect. Dis. *154*:706-709, 1986.
44. Lim, K. H., and Yin-Murphy, M.: An epidemic of conjunctivitis in Singapore in 1970. Singapore Med. J. *12*:247-249, 1971.
45. Martone, W. J., Hierholzer, J. C., Keenlyside, R. A., et al.: An outbreak of adenovirus type 3 disease at a private recreation center swimming pool. Am. J. Epidemiol. *111*:229-237, 1980.
46. McMillan, N. S., Martin, S. A., Sobsey, M. D., et al.: Outbreak of pharyngoconjunctival fever at a summer camp: North Carolina, 1991. M. M. W. R. Morb. Mortal. Wkly. Rep. *41*:342-343, 1992.
47. Merchant, R. K., Rowe, W. P., Kasel, J. A., et al.: Pharyngoconjunctival fever due to type 1 adenovirus: Report of three cases. N. Engl. J. Med. *258*:131-133, 1958.
48. Nakayama, M., Miyazaki, C., Ueda, K., et al.: Pharyngoconjunctival fever caused by adenovirus type 11. Pediatr. Infect. Dis. J. *11*:6-9, 1992.
49. Oker-Blom, N., Wager, W., Strandström, H., et al.: Adenoviruses associated with pharyngoconjunctival fever: Isolation of adenovirus type 7 and serological studies suggesting its etiological role in an epidemic in Helsinki. Ann. Med. Exp. Biol. Fenn. *35*:342-351, 1957.
50. Ormsby, H. L., and Aitchison, W. S.: The role of the swimming pool in the transmission of pharyngeal-conjunctival fever. Can. Med. Assoc. J. *73*:864-866, 1975.
51. Paderstein, R.: Was ist Schwimmbad-Konjunktivitis? Klin. Monat. Augenh. *74*:634-642, 1925.
52. Parrott, T. H., Rowe, W. P., Huebner, R. J., et al.: Outbreak of febrile pharyngitis and conjunctivitis associated with type 3 adenoidal-pharyngeal-conjunctival virus infections. N. Engl. J. Med. *251*:1087-1090, 1954.
53. Player, V., and Westmoreland, D.: Rapid diagnosis of adenovirus pharyngoconjunctival fever: Use of a monoclonal antibody-based ELISA test during an outbreak. J. Virol. Methods *24*:307-312, 1989.
54. Rowe, W. P., Huebner, R. J., Gilmore, L. K., et al.: Isolation of a cytopathogenic agent from human adenoids undergoing spontaneous degeneration in tissue culture. Proc. Soc. Exp. Biol. Med. *84*:570-573, 1953.
55. Schaap, G. J. P., DeJong, J. C., Van Bijsterveld, O. P., et al.: A new intermediate adenovirus type causing conjunctivitis. Arch. Ophthalmol. *97*:2336-2338, 1979.
56. Schwartz, H. S., Vastine, D. W., Yamashiroya, H., et al.: Immunofluorescent detection of adenovirus antigen in epidemic keratoconjunctivitis. Invest. Ophthalmol. *15*:199-207, 1976.
57. Sobel, G., Aronson, B., Aronson, S., et al.: Pharyngoconjunctival fever. Am. J. Dis. Child. *92*:596-612, 1956.
58. Sohier, R., Chardonnet, Y., and Prunieras, M.: Adenoviruses: Status of current knowledge. Prog. Med. Virol. *7*:253-325, 1965.
59. Sterner, G.: Infections with adenovirus type 7 in children and their relationship to acute respiratory disease. Acta Paediatr. *48*:287-298, 1959.
60. Sterner, G.: Adenovirus infection in childhood: An epidemiological and clinical survey among Swedish children. Acta Paediatr. *51*:1-30, 1962.
61. Sterner, G., Gerzen, P., Ohlson, M., et al.: Acute respiratory illness and gastroenteritis in association with adenovirus type 7 infections. Acta Paediatr. *50*:457-468, 1961.
62. Sutton, R. N. P., Pullen, H. J. M., Blackledge, P., et al.: Adenovirus type 7; 1971-74. Lancet *2*:987-991, 1976.
63. Tyrrell, D. A. J., Balducci, D., and Zaiman, T. E.: Acute infections of the respiratory tract and the adenoviruses. Lancet *2*:1326-1330, 1956.
64. Van Bijsterveld, O. P., DeJong, J. C., Muzerie, C. J., et al.: Pharyngoconjunctival fever caused by adenovirus type 19. Ophthalmologica *177*:134-139, 1978.
65. Van Der Veen, J.: The role of adenoviruses in respiratory disease. Am. Rev. Respir. Dis. *88*:167-180, 1963.
66. Van Der Veen, J., and Van Der Ploeg, G.: An outbreak of pharyngoconjunctival fever caused by types 3 and 4 adenovirus at Waalwijk, the Netherlands. Am. J. Hyg. *68*:95-105, 1958.
67. Van Horne, R. G., Saslaw, S., Anderson, G. R., et al.: An intrafamilial epidemic of pharyngoconjunctival fever. Arch. Intern. Med. *99*:70-73, 1957.
68. Vastine, D. W., Schwartz, H. S., Yamashiroya, H. M., et al.: Cytologic diagnosis of adenoviral epidemic keratoconjunctivitis by direct immunofluorescence. Invest. Ophthalmol. *16*:195-200, 1977.
69. Wallis, A. L.: An unusual epidemic. Lancet *2*:290-291, 1955.
70. Ward, T. G.: Viruses of the respiratory tract. Prog. Med. Virol. *15*:126-158, 1973.
71. Ward, T. G., Huebner, R. J., Rowe, W. P., et al.: Production of pharyngoconjunctival fever in human volunteers inoculated with APC viruses. Science *122*:1086-1087, 1955.
72. Yamadera, S., Yamashita, K., Akatsuka, M., et al.: Adenovirus surveillance, 1982-1993. A report of the National Epidemiological Surveillance of Infectious Agents in Japan. Jpn. J. Med. Sci. Biol. *48*:199-210, 1995.
73. Yamadera, S., Yamashita, K., Akatsuka, M., et al.: Trend of adenovirus type 7 infection, an emerging disease in Japan. A report of the National Epidemiological Surveillance of Infectious Agents in Japan. Jpn. J. Med. Sci. Biol. *51*:43-51, 1998.
74. Yin-Murphy, M.: Simple tests for the diagnosis of picornavirus epidemic conjunctivitis (acute haemorrhagic conjunctivitis). Bull. World Health Organ. *54*:675-679, 1976.
75. Yin-Murphy, M., and Lim, K. H.: Picornavirus epidemic conjunctivitis in Singapore. Lancet *1*:857-858, 1972.
76. Yodfat, Y., and Nishmi, M.: Successive overlapping outbreaks of febrile pharyngitis and pharyngoconjunctival fever associated with adenovirus types 2 and 7, in a kibbutz. Isr. J. Med. Sci. *10*:1505-1509, 1974.

13

UVULITIS

Ellen R. Wald

Infections of the uvula have been reported infrequently in the medical literature. When the uvula is the most inflamed structure in the posterior pharynx of a febrile child, acute infection should be suspected. Other causes of uvulitis include trauma (from instrumentation), inhalant irritation (from cannabis use), vasculitis, and allergy.[3,5,11]

ETIOLOGY

The main bacterial agents that cause uvulitis in children include *Haemophilus influenzae* type b (Hib) and *Streptococcus pyogenes*.[6] Uvulitis caused by *H. influenzae* may occur concurrently with epiglottitis or as an isolated infection.[8,14] Uvulitis caused by *S. pyogenes* seems always to occur in concert with pharyngitis. Brook[2] reported two cases of uvulitis caused by anaerobic bacteria, *Fusobacterium nucleatum* and *Prevotella intermedia*. No search for viral agents has been conducted. Several cases of uvulitis caused by *Candida albicans* have been described in immunocompetent toddlers.[7] In adults, *Streptococcus pneumoniae* and *H. influenzae* have been reported to cause uvulitis.[4,13] In many patients, an associated epiglottitis has been present.[10,13]

EPIDEMIOLOGY

The epidemiology of uvulitis is the epidemiology of its two etiologic agents, *S. pyogenes* and Hib. It occurs in school-age children 5 to 15 years old (the so-called streptococcal age group) in association with pharyngitis. Similarly, it can be seen in the *H. influenzae* age group (3 months to 5 years) if a child has not received the now routine and universally recommended conjugate vaccine to prevent infections caused by Hib. Cases of uvulitis in association with epiglottitis have been reported in the United States and in England.[2,6,12] Infections caused by *S. pyogenes* and *H. influenzae* occur primarily in the winter and spring, but both types can occur throughout the year.

PATHOGENESIS

Uvulitis is an acute cellulitis characterized by dramatic swelling and erythema. Infection of the uvula probably arises from direct invasion by *S. pyogenes* or Hib; both are recognized as normal nasopharyngeal flora. In the latter case, epiglottitis also may arise by direct extension, and the bacteremia may result secondarily from either the uvula or the epiglottis as a primary site of infection.

Uvulitis that is noninfectious may result from injury, chemical irritation, or allergic inflammation. A child ultimately diagnosed to have Kawasaki disease presented with uvulitis.[5]

CLINICAL MANIFESTATIONS

In a review of five patients with streptococcal uvulitis, all had associated pharyngitis.[6] The patients presented with low-grade fever and sore throat. Three of the five patients experienced a choking or gagging sensation in the pharynx that induced coughing and spitting; one of these patients also presented with drool-

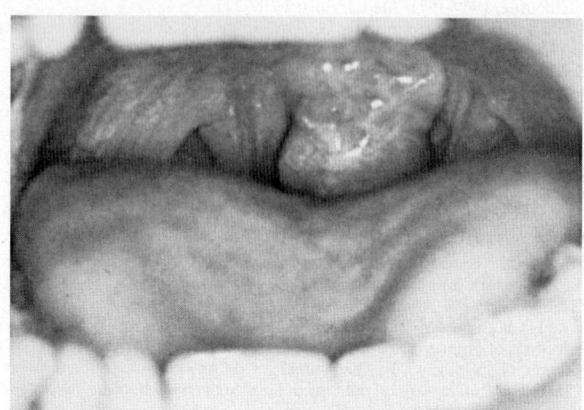

Figure 13–1 Swollen (two to three times normal size) and erythematous uvula in a patient without epiglottitis or pharyngitis.

ing. Although pharyngitis was noted on physical examination, the swelling and erythema of the uvula were most dramatic (Fig. 13–1). None of the patients had evidence of respiratory distress.

In most children with uvulitis and epiglottitis, the presentation usually is typical for epiglottitis, with sudden onset of high fever, dysphagia, and increasing respiratory distress. Rapkin[12] reported a case of uvulitis and epiglottitis, however, in which the epiglottitis initially was unsuspected. The same observation has been made in some adults with uvulitis and epiglottitis.[4,10] Lateral neck radiography (performed in one case to evaluate the possibility of a retropharyngeal abscess) belatedly alerted the clinicians to the correct diagnosis.

In patients with uvulitis and no epiglottitis, the presentation may be similar to that of epiglottitis (acute onset of fever, odynophagia, and drooling) or less specific, with fever and irritability or decreased appetite.[8,14] The diagnosis in these cases is provided by physical examination of the oropharynx, which shows a swollen and erythematous uvula (see Fig. 13–1).

DIAGNOSIS

The diagnosis of streptococcal uvulitis is suspected when a school-age child presents with low-grade fever, pharyngitis, and uvulitis. The diagnosis is confirmed by the recovery of *S. pyogenes* from a surface culture of the throat or uvula or both.

The diagnosis of uvulitis caused by *H. influenzae* is suspected in a highly febrile infant or preschool-age child who has uvular inflammation on physical examination. Lateral neck radiography must be performed to evaluate the possibility of epiglottitis, unless obvious signs of upper respiratory obstruction are present, in which case immediate endoscopy is warranted. If epiglottitis is discovered, the airway must be secured, and appropriate parenteral antimicrobials must be initiated after blood and surface culture specimens are obtained. Any surface culture specimen obtained to search for *H. influenzae* must be plated onto chocolate agar. After appropriate culture specimens are obtained, parenteral antimicrobials should be initiated, as in other infections associated with bacteremia caused by *H. influenzae*.

DIFFERENTIAL DIAGNOSIS

The differential diagnosis of a patient with acute onset of fever, dysphagia, and drooling includes herpes simplex gingivostomatitis, uvulitis, epiglottitis, severe pharyngitis, and peritonsillar or retropharyngeal abscess. Although being extremely cautious in examining the pharynx of any patient with suspected epiglottitis is appropriate, some children tolerate attempted visualization of the oral cavity without becoming unduly upset. Instrumentation with a tongue blade should be avoided. If the examination does not show gingivostomatitis or peritonsillar abscess, lateral neck radiography should be performed. If epiglottitis or retropharyngeal abscess is confirmed, management of the airway and administration of antimicrobials are indicated for epiglottitis, and incision and drainage and antimicrobials are indicated for retropharyngeal abscess. If the lateral neck is normal and the uvula is inflamed, uvulitis with or without pharyngitis is confirmed.

TREATMENT

Management of uvulitis is guided primarily by the associated pharyngitis or epiglottitis, if either is present. In the case of streptococcal pharyngitis, penicillin therapy for 10 days is most appropriate. These patients usually can be treated orally with penicillin V, 25 to 50 mg/kg/day, administered in two divided doses.

In the case of uvulitis and epiglottitis, management of the airway is most important and can be accomplished by performing nasotracheal intubation or tracheotomy. Appropriate parenteral antibiotic therapy usually is initiated.

In the case of uvulitis without epiglottitis in an infant or preschool-age child, antimicrobial therapy should be planned for possible Hib bacteremia. Generally, approximately 50 percent of respiratory isolates of *H. influenzae* are β-lactamase producing. Administration of an advanced-generation cephalosporin, such as cefotaxime at 200 mg/kg/day in four divided doses or ceftriaxone at 100 mg/kg/day in one dose or two divided doses, is appropriate. In a patient with serious penicillin hypersensitivity, aztreonam at 100 mg/kg/day in three divided doses also is a satisfactory

regimen. After the patient has defervesced and has improved clinically, an oral antimicrobial agent can be substituted. The results of blood and surface cultures now can guide therapy. For an ampicillin-sensitive *H. influenzae* infection, amoxicillin at 45 mg/kg/day in two divided doses should be prescribed to complete a 7- to 10-day course of treatment. For β-lactamase-producing *H. influenzae*, a variety of oral agents, including cefixime at 10 mg/kg in a single daily dose, cefuroxime at 30 mg/kg/day in two divided doses, or amoxicillin-potassium clavulanate at 45 mg/kg/day of amoxicillin in two divided doses, can be prescribed.

Resolution was prompt in the two cases of uvulitis allegedly caused by *C. albicans*. One child was treated with topical nystatin, and the other had spontaneous improvement.[7]

REFERENCES

1. Boyce, S. H., and Quigley, M. A.: Uvulitis and partial upper airway obstruction following cannabis inhalation. Emerg. Med. *14*:106-108, 2002.
2. Brook, I.: Uvulitis caused by anaerobic bacteria. Pediatr. Emerg. Care *13*:221, 1997.
3. Butterton, J. R., and Clawson-Simons, J.: Hymenoptera uvulitis. N. Engl. J. Med. *317*:1291, 1987.
4. Jerrard, D. A., and Olshaker, J.: Simultaneous uvulitis and epiglottitis without fever or leukocytosis. Am. J. Emerg. Med. *14*:551-552, 1996.
5. Kazi, A., Gauthier, M., Lebel, M. H., et al.: Uvulitis and supraglottitis: Early manifestations of Kawasaki disease. J. Pediatr. *120*:564-567, 1992.
6. Kotloff, K. L., and Wald, E. R.: Uvulitis in children. Pediatr. Infect. Dis. *2*:392-393, 1983.
7. Krober, M. S., and Weir, M. R.: Acute uvulitis apparently caused by *Candida albicans*. Pediatr. Infect. Dis. J. *10*:73, 1991.
8. Li, K. I., Kiernan, S., and Wald, E. R.: Isolated uvulitis due to *Hemophilus influenzae* type b. Pediatrics *74*:1054-1057, 1984.
9. McNamara, R.: Clinical characteristics of acute uvulitis. Am. J. Emerg. Med. *12*:51-52, 1994.
10. McNamara, R., and Koobatian, T.: Simultaneous uvulitis and epiglottitis in adults. Am. J. Emerg. Med. *15*:161-163, 1997.
11. Peghini, P. L., Salcedo, J. A., and Al-Kavas, F. H.: Traumatic uvulitis: A rare complication of upper GI endoscopy. Gastrointest. Endosc. *53*:818-820, 2001.
12. Rapkin, R. H.: Simultaneous uvulitis and epiglottitis. J. A. M. A. *43*:1843, 1980.
13. Westerman, E. L., and Hutton, J. P.: Acute uvulitis associated with epiglottitis. Arch. Otolaryngol. Head Neck Surg. *112*:448-449, 1986.
14. Wynder, S. G., Lampe, R. M., and Shoemaker, M. E.: Uvulitis and *Hemophilus influenzae* bacteremia. Pediatr. Emerg. Care *2*:23-25, 1986.

CHAPTER 14

PERITONSILLAR, RETROPHARYNGEAL, AND PARAPHARYNGEAL ABSCESSES

Nira A. Goldstein • Margaret R. Hammerschlag

A deep neck abscess is a collection of pus in a potential space bounded by fascia.[6] These potential spaces are areas of least resistance to the spread of infection. An infection may begin with a minimal area of cellulitis and progress to a deep neck abscess, which may extend to invade adjacent potential spaces; these spaces frequently encompass vital structures in the neck. Destruction and dysfunction of these structures represent the major complications of deep neck infections.[44]

EPIDEMIOLOGY OF HEAD AND NECK SPACE INFECTIONS IN CHILDREN

Data concerning the frequency of head and neck space infections in children are limited. A survey conducted by the American

Academy of Otolaryngology found the incidence of peritonsillar abscesses to be approximately 30 per 100,000 person-years, or approximately 45,000 cases annually in the United States and Puerto Rico.[32] A retrospective study from the Children's Hospital of Pittsburgh identified 117 children with head and neck space infections seen between 1986 and 1992.[72] The patients ranged in age from 1 month to 18 years (mean age 7.8 years).[72] Peritonsillar space infections (cellulitis and abscesses) occurred most frequently, accounting for 61 (49%) cases, followed by retropharyngeal space infections, accounting for 27 (22%) cases. Only three (2%) parapharyngeal space infections were seen during the period of the study. Broughton[14] reported seeing 14 pediatric patients, 15 months to 17 years of age, with retropharyngeal and parapharyngeal space infections during a 9-year period at the University of Kentucky Medical Center. Craig and Schunk[18] described 64 cases of retropharyngeal abscesses in children at the Primary Children's Medical Center in Salt Lake City, Utah, from 1993 to 1998, a higher number of cases than previously reported. Kirse and Roberson[40] reported 73 cases of retropharyngeal space infection from 1989 to 1998, with a twofold to fivefold increase in the number of patients treated in the last 4 years of the study compared with the first 6 years.

Peritonsillar abscesses rarely occur in young children. They occur most frequently in patients in their late teens and early 20s. The mean age of the children with peritonsillar infection in Pittsburgh was 11 years, whereas the mean age of the patients with retropharyngeal space infections was 4 years, similar to the mean age of 4.5 years reported by Thompson and associates[71] in their 36-year review of 65 children with retropharyngeal abscesses treated at the Children's Hospital of Los Angeles. Retropharyngeal abscesses have been reported to occur more frequently in young children. In the Salt Lake City series, the median age was 3 years, and 75 percent of the children were younger than 5 years.[18]

All of the peritonsillar infections were associated with tonsillitis, and 15 percent had antecedent infectious mononucleosis shown by positive monospot test results.[72] Results of a meta-analysis of 15 previously reported series of patients with peritonsillar abscess reported by Herzon[32] found prior tonsillar infection rates ranging from 11 to 56 percent, with an overall rate of 36 percent. The high incidence of peritonsillar abscess reported in the American Academy of Otolaryngology study raised the possibility that the decreasing rate of tonsillectomy might increase the risk for development of peritonsillar abscess.[32]

PERITONSILLAR ABSCESS (QUINSY)

A peritonsillar abscess (quinsy) is circumscribed medially by the fibrous wall of the tonsil capsule and laterally by the superior constrictor muscle. Pus may be localized in the superior pole, midpoint, or inferior pole or rarely may be dispersed, with multiple loculations in the peritonsillar space. The superior pole is the most common location, with a frequency range of 41.2 to 70 percent; the remaining inferior locations account for the balance.[7,10,46]

The etiology of peritonsillar abscesses is not constant. They may occur after any "virulent" tonsillitis, with extension through the fibrous tonsil capsule.

CLINICAL MANIFESTATIONS

The recent history may include a sore throat with occasional unilateral ear pain, malaise, low-grade pyrexia, chills, diaphoresis, dysphagia, reduced oral intake, trismus, and a muffled "hot potato voice." Trismus results from irritation and reflex spasm of the internal pterygoid muscle. Sixty-three percent of the children with peritonsillar infection from the Pittsburgh series had trismus.[72] Impaired palatal motion from edema contributes to the muffled voice.

Physical examination reveals minimal to moderate toxicity, dehydration, and drooling. Inspection of the oropharynx may be compromised by trismus. The soft palate is displaced toward the unaffected side, swollen and red, and frequently palpably fluctuant. The edematous uvula is pushed across the midline (Fig. 14–1). The displaced tonsil and its crypts rarely are coated with exudate. The breath is fetid, and ipsilateral, tender, cervical adenopathy is present. The white blood cell count is elevated, with a predominance of polymorphonuclear leukocytes.

Brodsky and associates[11] attempted to identify the clinical signs that might distinguish peritonsillar abscess from peritonsillar cellulitis in a group of 21 children admitted to the Children's Hospital of Buffalo from 1985 through 1987. No significant difference in age, duration of sore throat, fever, or white blood cell count was noted, although a greater degree of pharyngotonsillar bulge and muffled voice was found in the patients with abscess. Patients with peritonsillar cellulitis improved after receiving 24 hours of intravenous antibiotics, whereas patients with peritonsillar abscess had no change or worsening of symptoms. Blotter and colleagues[8] confirmed these findings in 102 patients admitted to Children's Hospital of Columbus, Ohio, between 1995 and 1998.

In uncomplicated cases, computed tomography (CT) scan has not been as useful as clinical assessment and follow-up evaluation in the management of peritonsillar abscess. CT scans are useful in young children with suspected peritonsillar abscess who are

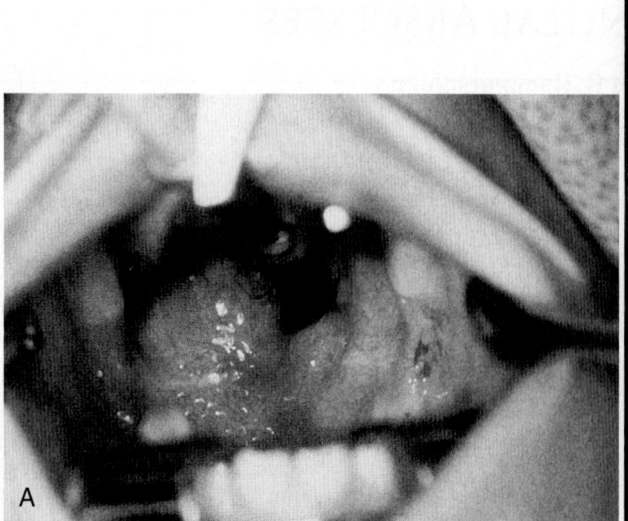
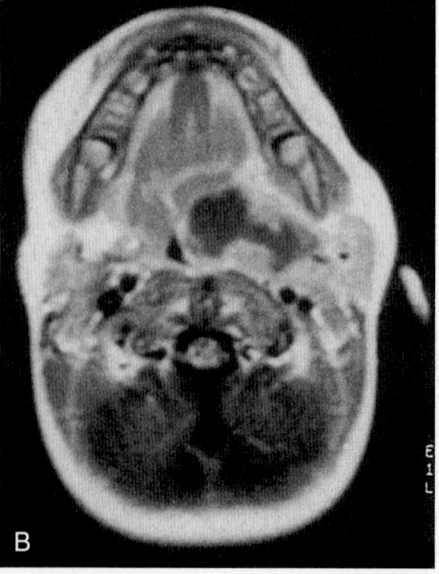

Figure 14–1 Left peritonsillar abscess in an 18-month-old child. *(From Wiatrak, B. J., and Woolley, A. L.: Pharyngitis and adenotonsillar disease. In Cummings, C. W., Flint, P. W., Harker, L. A., et al. [eds.]: Otolaryngology: Head and Neck Surgery. 4th ed. Philadelphia, Elsevier, 2005, p. 4144.)*

not cooperative with examination or children with other suspected deep neck infections.[27]

TREATMENT

Traditionally, management of peritonsillar abscess in children involved hospital admission for intravenous hydration, antibiotic therapy and analgesia, and either intraoral incision and drainage of the abscess or "acute quinsy tonsillectomy" with removal of the medial wall of the abscess. Although older children may tolerate incision and drainage under local anesthetic, the procedure is not well tolerated in young children and carries the risk of potential injury to adjacent vascular structures. The administration of a general anesthetic is required for tonsillectomy in all age groups and often is required for incision and drainage in young children. Acute tonsillectomy often was done to prevent future recurrence of the peritonsillar abscess.

Although it is a commonly accepted clinical observation, a high recurrence rate of peritonsillar abscess has not been well documented. A meta-analysis reported by Herzon[32] of 19 studies from the United States, Europe, and Israel involving 1399 patients found recurrence rates of 10 to 15 percent for peritonsillar abscess. The rates of recurrence seem to be lower in the United States (0 to 17%) than in the series reported from Europe and Israel (3 to 22%). A retrospective analysis of 290 patients treated for peritonsillar abscess found that patients who had a history of recurrent tonsillitis before development of the abscess had a fourfold greater rate of recurrence than patients with no history (40 versus 9.6%).[41] The authors recommended that patients with a history of recurrent tonsillitis before admission be treated with tonsillectomy.[41]

The risks of acute tonsillectomy are not greater than the risks associated with delayed tonsillectomy.[45,51,77] In addition, the morbidity caused by two hospitalizations involving two procedures is reduced by acute tonsillectomy.[4,9,10] An additional benefit of acute tonsillectomy is the ability to evacuate inferior pole abscesses that technically are difficult to drain by needle aspiration or incision and drainage.[46]

Studies have suggested that many peritonsillar abscesses can be managed by simple needle aspiration combined with antibiotic therapy on an outpatient basis.[11,32,58,60,61,66,72,74] An extensive meta-analysis of 10 studies conducted from 1961 through 1994 involving 496 patients with peritonsillar abscesses found that needle aspiration had an overall success rate of 94 percent (range 85 to 100%).[32] This success rate compares favorably with that reported for incision and drainage. Weinberg and associates[74] successfully performed needle aspiration in 41 of 43 children 7 to 18 years old (mean age 13.9 years). All were admitted for intravenous antibiotic therapy, two (5%) required repeated aspiration for resolution, and five (12%) did not respond and required acute tonsillectomy. A pooled analysis of three prospective studies comparing needle aspiration versus incision and drainage showed no significant difference in resolution rates (93.7% for incision and drainage and 91.6% for needle aspiration), but the power was low because of the small sample size.[36] Other studies, which have included adults and children with peritonsillar abscesses, have reported that 0 to 48 percent of patients require hospitalization.[32,51,58,66]

Younger children often require admission to correct dehydration.[27] Younger children also are more likely than are older children to respond to intravenous antibiotics alone and to have negative findings at surgical drainage.[8] The use of conscious sedation has been reported to be a safe and effective approach for the drainage of peritonsillar abscesses in children.[48,67]

In a 10-year retrospective review of 83 children with peritonsillar abscesses by Schraff and colleagues,[61] 65 percent were treated by incision and drainage (51% knife versus 14% needle

aspiration), 31 percent had quinsy tonsillectomy, and 4 percent were admitted and treated by intravenous antibiotics alone. Of patients treated surgically, 51 percent of the procedures were done in the emergency department, and 49 percent were done in the operating room. Forty-eight percent of the children required admission, and the average length of stay was 0.9 days (standard deviation 1.37).

A suggested approach to the management of children with peritonsillar abscess is as follows.[33] Cooperative children should undergo needle aspiration of the abscess and treatment with antibiotics. Children who can tolerate liquids orally may be managed as outpatients, and the remainder should be admitted for hydration and administration of intravenous antibiotics. Approximately 4 percent of children require a repeated aspiration for resolution.[32] Children who remain symptomatic after undergoing needle aspiration require incision and drainage or acute quinsy tonsillectomy, depending on the prior history of recurrent tonsillitis. Children who cannot tolerate needle aspiration on initial presentation are admitted for administration of intravenous antibiotics. If no response occurs within 24 hours, incision and drainage or acute tonsillectomy is done, depending on the prior history of recurrent tonsillitis. Delayed tonsillectomy is reserved for children who recover from the peritonsillar abscess without general anesthesia but have a history of recurrent tonsillitis or prior peritonsillar abscess.

Untreated peritonsillar abscess may point, with spontaneous rupture, or extend to the pterygomaxillary space, with potentially fatal complications. Upper airway obstruction, septicemia, and vascular catastrophe may occur. Necrotizing fasciitis also has been reported in adults with peritonsillar abscess.[28,75]

RETROPHARYNGEAL ABSCESS (POSTERIOR VISCERAL SPACE, RETROVISCERAL SPACE, AND RETROESOPHAGEAL SPACE ABSCESSES)

The anterior wall of the retropharyngeal space is the middle layer of the deep cervical fascia, which abuts the posterior esophageal wall (the superior pharyngeal constrictor muscle). The deep layer of the deep cervical fascia circumscribes the posterior wall of this potential space. Inferiorly, these two fasciae fuse to limit the depth of this pocket at a level between the first and second thoracic vertebrae. A retropharyngeal abscess can erode inferiorly through the junction of these fasciae to extend posteriorly into the prevertebral space (Fig. 14–2). Subsequently, pus in the prevertebral space can descend inferiorly below the diaphragm to the psoas muscles.

The retropharyngeal space contains two paramedial chains of lymph nodes that receive drainage from the nasopharynx, adenoids, posterior paranasal sinuses, middle ear, and eustachian tube. These structures are prominent in early childhood and atrophy at puberty.[29] Retropharyngeal abscesses are common occurrences in young children and are thought to be secondary to suppurative adenitis of these retropharyngeal nodes.[3] Other sources of infection are penetrating foreign bodies, endoscopy, trauma, pharyngitis, vertebral body osteomyelitis, petrositis, dental procedures,[72] and branchial cleft anomalies.[35] In one series of 17 cases of retropharyngeal abscesses at the Children's Hospital, Denver, Colorado, 7 children (41%), including 2 neonates (most likely associated with attempts at intubation), had perforations of the hypopharynx or esophagus.[53] In the Pittsburgh series, 63 percent of the children with retropharyngeal abscess had antecedent tonsillitis, pharyngitis, or viral upper respiratory tract infection.[72] Two children had previous trauma; however, no details on the type of trauma were given.

In adults, tuberculosis and syphilis were common causes of retropharyngeal abscesses in the pre-antibiotic era.[56] Four of

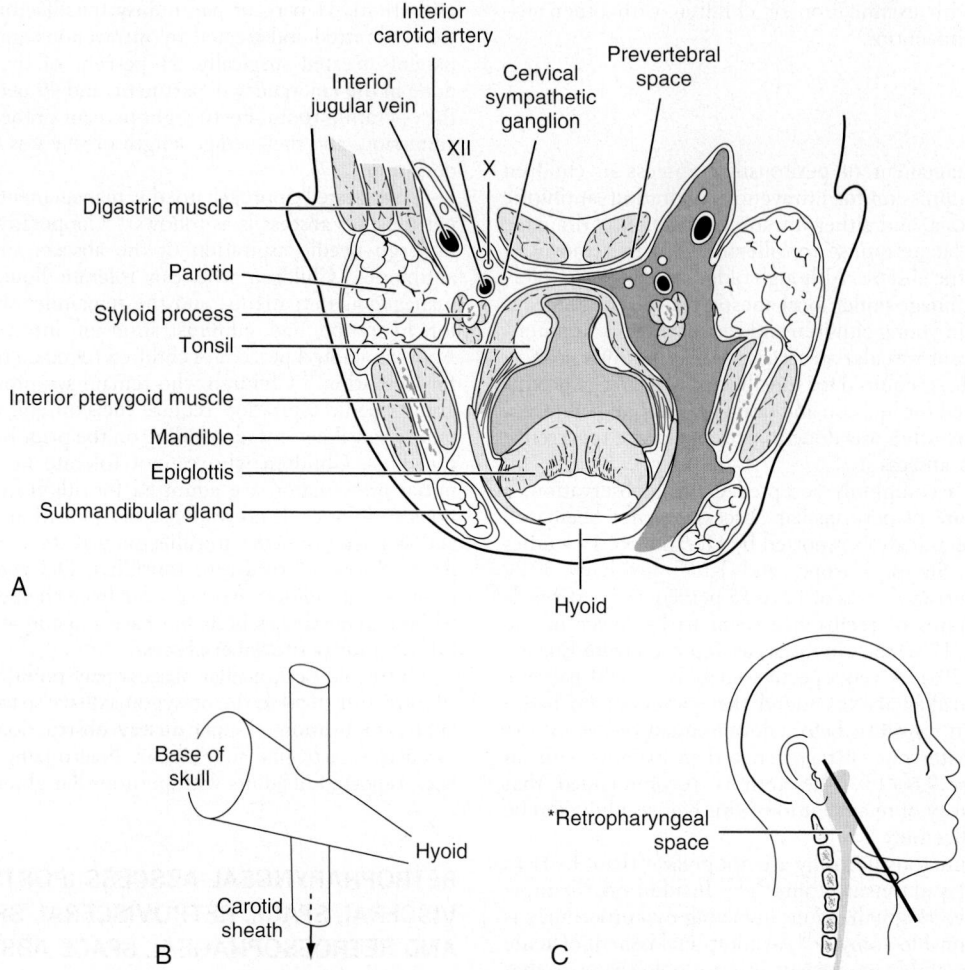

Figure 14–2 A, Oblique transverse section of the oropharynx posterosuperiorly and the hypopharynx anteroinferiorly. Depicted are a peritonsillar abscess on the right and a pterygomaxillary space abscess on the left. The *asterisk* in **C** indicates the location of the retropharyngeal space. **B,** The "cone" of the potential pterygomaxillary space with its carotid sheath. **C,** The vertical dimensions of the retropharyngeal space. The black oblique line represents the level of the drawing in **A.**

seven patients treated for retropharyngeal abscess at Columbia-Presbyterian Medical Center in New York during a 6-year period had serologic evidence of acute primary Epstein-Barr viral infection.[69]

CLINICAL MANIFESTATIONS

The symptoms of retropharyngeal abscess frequently begin insidiously after mild antecedent infection. Signs and symptoms include sore throat, fever, limitation of neck motion, torticollis, neck pain, neck mass, drooling, odynophagia, poor oral intake, and lethargy. Airway stridor or respiratory distress from edema, cellulitis, or an obstructing mass occasionally occurs.[17,18,20,73] Thirty-three percent of the 27 children with retropharyngeal abscess in the Pittsburgh series had torticollis or limitation of neck motion,[72] compared with 53 of the 94 children (83%) in the Las Vegas series.[18] In adults, the symptoms may be milder. Complaints of chest pain by an adult may reflect mediastinal extension.

Early in the course, midline or unilateral swelling of the posterior pharynx occurs. Later, gentle palpation may show a large fluctuant mass in the posterior pharynx. Vigorous palpation should be avoided because it may cause the abscess to rupture into the upper airway. As with other abscesses, the

white blood cell count is increased, with a predominance of granulocytes.

Plain films of the neck often are the initial radiologic study, but they must be obtained with the patient in a true lateral position, with the neck in extension, and on inspiration, or the child's retropharyngeal soft tissues may appear abnormally thickened. Widening of the prevertebral soft tissues exceeding the antero-posterior diameter of the contiguous vertebral bodies, or thickening of the retropharyngeal space greater than 7 mm at C2 in children and adults, or 14 mm at C6 in children or 22 mm at C6 in adults suggests retropharyngeal inflammation. Rarely, a prevertebral soft tissue mass, air-fluid level, or gas may be seen. The normal cervical lordosis may be lost or reversed secondary to muscle spasm or local inflammation (Fig. 14–3).

CT scan has rendered the diagnosis and management of deep neck space infections more precise.[12,23,40,43,70,73,76] In contrast to conventional radiologic studies, CT scan distinguishes cellulitis of the neck, which usually does not require surgical treatment, from a deep neck abscess, which does require surgical drainage. With its ability to define differences in tissue density, CT scanning permits an accurate determination of the extent of the abscess and its extension and involvement of adjacent spaces to be made. An abscess is distinguished from cellulitis by a low-attenuation homogeneous area surrounded by a ring enhancement of contrast material (see Fig. 14–3). Kirse and Roberson[40]

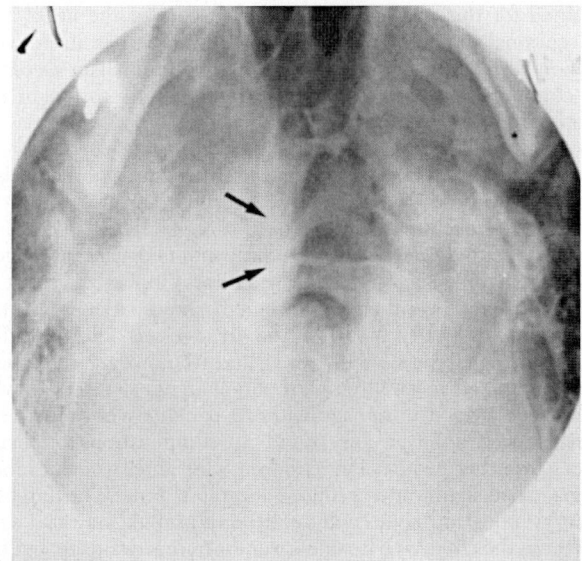

Figure 14–3 Lateral neck radiograph showing a retropharyngeal abscess.

reported scalloping of the abscess wall to be a more useful predictor of the presence of pus than ring enhancement. When more than one space is involved, accurate assessment of these spaces may ensure sufficient surgical drainage. Vascular structures can be identified, as can potential complications such as venous thrombosis. Gas also may be detected by CT.

A 10-year retrospective study from the Massachusetts Eye and Ear Infirmary compared preoperative CT scans with intraoperative findings in 38 patients who underwent surgical exploration of the parapharyngeal or retropharyngeal space within 48 hours after the scans were performed. Overall, the intraoperative findings confirmed the CT scan interpretation in 76.3 percent of the patients.[43] Of the 38 patients, 5 (13.2%) had CT scans indicative of abscesses that were not confirmed at surgery. Exploration of the parapharyngeal or retropharyngeal space revealed cellulitis. The false-negative rate was 10.5 percent. The sensitivity of CT scanning for detection of parapharyngeal or retropharyngeal space abscess was 87.9 percent. Similar findings were reported in the Pittsburgh series; the sensitivity of CT scanning for differentiating an abscess from cellulitis was 91 percent.[72] In three cases, the radiologist's blinded CT scan interpretation did not correlate with the operative findings. Two patients with false-positive interpretations had retropharyngeal infections and underwent needle aspiration. The positive predictive value of CT scans in detection of abscess versus cellulitis was 83 percent. Additional studies have reported that the accuracy of CT in predicting surgical findings was 63 percent, 73 percent, 76 percent, and 92 percent.[23,65,73,76]

TREATMENT

The treatment of choice is administration of intravenous antibiotics and incision and drainage. If the mass is small, a peroral incision with the patient in the Rose position (supine with the neck hyperextended) may provide some drainage, but a slight risk of aspiration exists. If the mass is large and extends lateral to the great vessels, or if fever persists after peroral drainage is performed, an external incision is preferred. A tracheotomy may be required if risk of compromising the airway exists.

Posterior mediastinitis can result from the spread of infection from the retropharyngeal area into the prevertebral space. Other complications may be seen when the abscess extends to the parapharyngeal space and involves the great vessels and cranial nerves.

Reports have documented that patients with small retropharyngeal abscesses may respond to treatment with intravenous antibiotics alone. Broughton[14] described the experience at the University of Kentucky Medical Center, where 8 of 14 patients with deep neck infections seen during a 9-year period were treated successfully by antibiotics alone. All were reported to have small abscesses on CT scan. Possibly some had only cellulitis, however. In the Pittsburgh study, 15 of the children with parapharyngeal or retropharyngeal space infections underwent surgical intervention; 11 (73%) underwent incision and drainage, and 4 (27%) underwent needle aspiration.[72] All had successful outcomes. Twelve (44%) of the children with retropharyngeal infections were treated with intravenous antibiotics alone, and all did well. Ten (37%) of 27 patients in the Las Vegas series with well-defined abscess on CT scan were treated with intravenous antibiotics alone, and no treatment failures occurred.[18]

McClay and colleagues[50] used intravenous antibiotics alone to treat 11 children with deep neck abscesses (retropharyngeal in 8, both retropharyngeal and parapharyngeal in 2) without severe symptoms or airway compromise. Ten children responded and showed clinical improvement within 48 hours, whereas one child required surgical drainage. Close clinical follow-up is mandatory for children treated with intravenous antibiotics alone. Children who do not improve within 24 to 48 hours require surgical drainage.

PARAPHARYNGEAL ABSCESS (PTERYGOMAXILLARY, PHARYNGOMAXILLARY, LATERAL, AND PHARYNGEAL SPACE ABSCESSES)

The potential parapharyngeal or pterygomaxillary space is an inverted conical cavity (see Fig. 14–2B) lying along an oblique axis roughly parallel to the ramus of the mandible (see Fig. 14–2C). The base of the skull at the jugular foramen forms the base of the "cone," and its apex is at the hyoid bone (see Fig. 14–2B). The buccopharyngeal fascia, lateral to the superior pharyngeal constrictor, delineates the medial boundary, and the parotid gland and its partially dehiscent deep layer of the superficial cervical fascia form the lateral wall of this cone. The internal pterygoid muscle and mandible demarcate the cone on its anterolateral aspect. The parapharyngeal space is contiguous with the peritonsillar, submandibular, and retropharyngeal spaces, all of which are potential avenues of egress for an extending parapharyngeal space abscess (see Fig. 14–2A).

The posterior portion of the cone contains the contents of the carotid sheath (carotid artery and internal jugular vein), cranial nerves IX through XII, and the cervical sympathetic chain. The internal pterygoid muscle and fatty connective tissue are anterior.

Involvement of these structures determines the clinical manifestations and complications of the parapharyngeal space abscess. An abscess in the posterior compartment may show medial displacement of the lateral pharyngeal wall and parotid space induration and swelling, with variable overlying facial nerve weakness, carotid artery erosion and hemorrhage,[42] internal jugular vein thrombosis, decreased gag reflex and dysphagia, ipsilateral vocal cord paralysis, weakness of the ipsilateral trapezius muscle, ipsilateral lingual deviation, and Horner syndrome from cervical sympathetic chain involvement.[16]

Extension of the abscess into the anterior compartment causes trismus from irritation of the internal pterygoid muscle. Induration at the angle of the jaw and medial displacement of the tonsil and pharyngeal wall also occur with an anterior compartment abscess.

By the time a patient with an abscess seeks medical attention, the source of the parapharyngeal space infection may be unclear. Reports indicate variable causes, including incompletely or inadequately treated bacterial pharyngitis, tonsillitis,[3] peritonsillar abscess, dental infections, bacterial parotitis, otitis, mastoiditis (Bezold abscess from a mastoid tip infection traveling along the digastric muscles), petrositis, cervical adenitis with suppuration, cervical vertebral tubercular adenitis in the adult,[5,54] foreign bodies,[16,19] trauma, intravenous drug abuse,[31] branchial cleft anomalies,[68] and cat-scratch disease.[78] Parapharyngeal abscesses seem to be less common than are peritonsillar and retropharyngeal abscesses in children. Only three cases of parapharyngeal abscess and cellulitis were reported in the Pittsburgh series,[72] and only three cases were reported in a 15-year review of pediatric neck abscesses from Rainbow Babies and Children's Hospital in Cleveland, Ohio.[22] Amar and Manoukian[1] reported on 25 children with parapharyngeal abscesses during an 11-year period at Montreal Children's Hospital. Parapharyngeal abscesses occur throughout childhood, with an average age at presentation of 4 to 6 years.[1,63]

CLINICAL MANIFESTATIONS

In addition to the symptoms noted in the preceding description, tender cervical swelling, induration and erythema of the side of the neck, torticollis, sore throat, dysphagia, trismus, hoarseness, malaise, chills, and diaphoresis may occur. Variable low-grade pyrexia with occasional temperature spikes occurs. Examination discloses variable toxicity, respiratory tract distress, laryngeal edema, medial displacement of the lateral pharyngeal wall and inferior tonsil pole, trismus, and, infrequently, drooling. Palpation of the neck reveals a tender, high cervical mass, initially diffuse and later fluctuant. Pharyngeal blood clots may presage erosion of the carotid artery. The complications of parapharyngeal abscesses are related to the structures involved: Involvement of the carotid artery can produce hemiplegia from emboli; internal jugular vein thrombosis with cephalad extension may lead to a cavernous sinus thrombosis, whereas inferior extension leads to internal jugular vein thrombosis. Internal jugular vein thrombosis is characterized by spiking temperature, toxicity with intense diaphoresis, headaches, and increased intracranial pressure. Septic pulmonary emboli occasionally are present.

Extension into the retropharyngeal region by a parapharyngeal abscess may lead to a posterior mediastinitis. Airway obstruction occurring secondary to laryngeal edema and aspiration pneumonia from suppuration of the abscess into the pharynx have been reported. Initially, the parapharyngeal abscess may be difficult to differentiate from a peritonsillar abscess, but the latter usually is less toxic and has a distinct, soft palatal fluctuation.

As described for the diagnosis of retropharyngeal abscess, CT is an extremely useful tool for distinguishing parapharyngeal abscess from cellulitis and for localizing the abscess for surgical planning. In a review of 47 children who presented with deep neck infections to the Children's Hospital of Buffalo during a 5.5-year period, CT scan showed that 34 (77%) of 44 patients who underwent CT scan had involvement of the parapharyngeal and retropharyngeal spaces.[55] The involvement of both spaces had implications for the approach to surgical drainage.

TREATMENT

Intravenous antibiotic therapy with incision and drainage is the primary treatment. An otolaryngologic consultation should be

obtained for this potentially complex surgery of the neck. The conventional method of approaching this abscess is an external incision with sufficient exposure to provide immediate access to the common carotid artery for ligation, should erosion of the carotid artery be present.[47]

An intraoral drainage procedure traditionally has been condemned because rapid access to the vital structures of the neck is impossible with this approach. Nagy and associates[55] used an intraoral approach, however, to treat successfully 21 of 22 children with either parapharyngeal or combined parapharyngeal and retropharyngeal abscesses. The authors emphasized that CT with intravenous contrast enhancement showed that all of the abscesses were located medial to the great vessels and were adjacent to the pharyngeal wall. Amar and Manoukian[1] retrospectively compared 15 children with parapharyngeal abscesses who underwent intraoral drainage with 10 patients who underwent external neck drainage and found no complications or recurrences in either group. The children who underwent intraoral drainage had significantly reduced anesthesia time. The duration of intravenous antibiotics and duration of hospital stay also were shorter in the children who underwent intraoral drainage, but the differences between groups were not statistically significant. Cable and coworkers[15] described 12 children presenting to three centers with superior parapharyngeal space abscesses medial to the great vessels who were treated successfully by intraoral drainage using CT-guided systems to assist with localization of the abscess cavity.

The use of CT has made it possible for some patients with parapharyngeal abscesses to be managed with intravenous antibiotics. The number of reported cases is small, however, and usually analyzed with cases of retropharyngeal abscess.[14,55] Nagy and associates[55] used intravenous antibiotics alone to treat 3 (13%) of 24 children with small parapharyngeal abscesses. Sichel and associates[63] used intravenous antibiotics alone to treat successfully 12 children prospectively with infection limited to the parapharyngeal space abscess. Close clinical follow-up is necessary for children with parapharyngeal cellulitis or small parapharyngeal abscesses that are treated conservatively with intravenous antibiotics. Surgical drainage should be performed in children who do not improve within 24 to 48 hours.

In another report, Sichel and colleagues[62] reviewed the CT scans of 29 patients with infections of the parapharyngeal space and divided the patients into two groups: 22 patient with posterior parapharyngeal space infections and 7 patients with anterior parapharyngeal space infections. The patients with posterior infections generally were children who responded well to intravenous antibiotics and did not develop complications. The patients with anterior infections of the parapharyngeal space more commonly were adults who required external drainage in addition to intravenous antibiotics and developed complications including septic shock, respiratory distress, mediastinitis, pericarditis, and lung empyema. The authors suggested that the location of the infection in the fat of the anterior parapharyngeal space resulted in liquefaction of the fat, with formation of pus and rapid spread of the infection to other anatomic spaces.

MICROBIOLOGY OF DEEP NECK ABSCESSES

Group A streptococci (*Streptococcus pyogenes*) and *Staphylococcus aureus* have been considered to be the organisms most frequently associated with pharyngeal space infections. Studies have shown the presence of oral anaerobes in these infections, however; these organisms may be responsible for the gas seen on lateral neck radiographs. This finding is not surprising because the main portals of entry for pharyngeal space infections are the nasopharynx, oropharynx, paranasal sinuses, mastoid, and lower molars, all areas that are colonized with anaerobes.

The most complete microbiologic data available are from studies of peritonsillar abscesses. Flödstrom and Hallander[26] in 1976 reported the results of bacterial cultures on aspirates of pus from 37 patients with peritonsillar abscesses. The ages of the patients were not given. Group A streptococci were isolated from 17 of these patients, whereas 15 had an increase in their anti-streptolysin O or anti-DNAase titers. Anaerobes were found in 28 of the cultures, including those of eight patients that also disclosed the presence of streptococci. The most common anaerobic species isolated were fusobacteria (13), peptostreptococci (16), and *Bacteroides* spp. (18). Among the aerobic organisms, *S. aureus* was isolated four times, and *Haemophilus influenzae* was isolated twice. No isolates of aerobic gram-negative enteric organisms were present.

Jokipii and colleagues[37] performed semiquantitative cultures of aspirated pus from 42 peritonsillar abscesses and found similar results. Group A streptococci, the aerobic bacteria isolated most frequently, were isolated in pure culture 4 of 10 times. Anaerobes were more abundant than were aerobes; the most important species, in frequency and quantitatively, were *Bacteroides*, *Peptostreptococcus*, and *Fusobacterium*. Most of the infections were polymicrobial, with two to seven bacteria in 83 percent of the specimens. Subsequent studies from the United States and Finland have reported similar findings.[13,38,60,64]

Kieff and associates[39] found that streptococci were the most frequent isolates; group A streptococci and other non–group A beta-hemolytic streptococci were present in more than 30 percent of patients, and alpha-hemolytic streptococci accounted for another 27.2 percent. The pathogenic role of anaerobic bacteria in peritonsillar abscesses has been reinforced by reports of complications caused by fusobacterial infection in children.[57,59] *Fusobacterium* and *Bacteroides* spp. have been associated with septic thrombophlebitis and pulmonary emboli from the jugular veins.

Data on the microbiology of retropharyngeal and parapharyngeal abscesses in children are more limited. The organisms isolated are similar to those found in peritonsillar abscesses, but with a higher number of anaerobic species. Brook[12] examined aspirated pus from 14 children, 1 to 6 years old (median age 3 years, 2 months), with retropharyngeal abscesses. Anaerobes were isolated from all patients; they were the only organisms isolated in two patients (14%) and were mixed with aerobes in the remainder (86%). The predominant anaerobic species were *Bacteroides*, *Peptostreptococcus*, and *Fusobacterium*. The predominant aerobic species were alpha-hemolytic and gamma-hemolytic streptococci, *S. aureus*, *Haemophilus* spp., and group A beta-hemolytic streptococci. Seventy-one percent of the isolates were β-lactamase–positive and included all isolates of the *S. aureus* group, 6 of 18 of the *Bacteroides melaninogenicus* group (33%), and 2 of 3 of the *Bacteroides oralis* group.

Dodds and Maniglia[22] reported the results of cultures from nine retropharyngeal and three parapharyngeal abscesses from children and adolescents. The organisms isolated were similar to those reported by Brook,[12,13] but the microbiology was not as complete because the study was retrospective and not all specimens may have been processed for anaerobic culture. Streptococcal species were the isolates that occurred most frequently, followed by *S. aureus* and *H. influenzae*. One isolate each of *Fusobacterium necrophorum*, *Escherichia coli*, and *Klebsiella pneumoniae* was found. Asmar[2] performed cultures on material from 17 children with retropharyngeal abscesses; viridans streptococci were isolated from 11 of the abscesses, *S. aureus* from 8, and group A streptococci from 6. The most frequently identified anaerobes were *Peptostreptococcus* spp. Overall, 45 aerobic and 18 anaerobic species were identified.

Rarely, retropharyngeal abscess may result from anterior extension from cervical osteomyelitis. This condition has been described with tuberculosis[56] and atypical mycobacteria causing a retropharyngeal abscess in a similar clinical setting. Barratt and

colleagues[3] reported one case of retropharyngeal abscess caused by *Coccidioides immitis* in a 24-year-old woman with Hodgkin disease. The infection also was secondary to cervical vertebral osteomyelitis. Other rare and unusual causes of deep neck abscesses include cat-scratch disease (*Bartonella*),[78] *Streptococcus pneumoniae*,[52] and Kawasaki disease.[34]

Because a large variety of organisms can be found in pharyngeal space infections, obtaining adequate culture specimens is crucial. The optimal material for culture is an aspirate of the pus obtained at operation. Throat swabs or swabs of the abscess obtained after drainage usually are inadequate because of contamination with normal oropharyngeal flora. The pus, when obtained, can be transported in a capped syringe if anaerobic transport media are unavailable. Most pathogenic obligate anaerobes can survive in a purulent exudate, despite extended periods of exposure to air.[25] A Gram stain of the exudate would provide important clues to the bacterial etiology. A Gram stain showing a mixture of organisms suggests a mixed aerobic-anaerobic infection.

Although use of a β-lactamase-resistant antibiotic may be necessary in the treatment of deep neck abscesses because of the presence of β-lactamase-producing bacteria, including *S. aureus* and *Bacteroides* spp.,[12,13,72] results of two studies suggest that penicillin alone was equivalent to broad-spectrum antibiotics for treatment of peritonsillar abscesses.[39,79] Yilmaz and colleagues[79] compared procaine penicillin with intramuscular administration of ampicillin-sulbactam in outpatient treatment of 40 patients with peritonsillar abscesses that were drained perorally. No statistical difference in duration of symptoms and clinical recovery was found between the two groups. Kieff and associates[39] retrospectively evaluated 103 patients with peritonsillar abscesses who were treated with incision and drainage. Fifty-eight patients were treated with broad-spectrum antibiotics including ampicillin-sulbactam, clindamycin, cephalosporins, and metronidazole, alone and in combination; 45 patients were treated with penicillin alone. All patients were hospitalized after drainage, and the clinical outcomes, including duration of hospitalization and fever, did not differ significantly between the two groups. No significant difference in the organisms isolated was found, and failure and complication rates did not differ.

No comparative treatment studies for retropharyngeal or parapharyngeal abscesses have been reported. Treatment in these cases should be based on the results of cultures, as stated before. Drugs that may be effective include penicillin-lactamase inhibitor combinations such as ampicillin-sulbactam, ticarcillin-clavulanic acid, and piperacillin-tazobactam; expanded-spectrum cephalosporins such as ceftriaxone; or penicillinase-resistant penicillins including oxacillin or nafcillin. Cephalosporins, oxacillin, or nafcillin should be used in combination with clindamycin or metronidazole for adequate anaerobic coverage. Erythromycin and other macrolides (azithromycin, clarithromycin) are less satisfactory because of increasing macrolide resistance in group A streptococci and less activity against *Bacteroides fragilis* and *Fusobacterium*.

A study by Hanna and colleagues[30] reported macrolide resistance in 26 percent of group A streptococcal isolates obtained from peritonsillar abscesses seen between August 2001 and July 2002. The routine use of aminoglycoside antibiotics is not indicated because aerobic gram-negative enteric rods rarely are found in these infections. Antibiotic therapy is effective only in conjunction with adequate surgical drainage.

REFERENCES

1. Amar, Y. G., and Manoukian, J. J.: Intraoral drainage: Recommended as the initial approach for the treatment of parapharyngeal abscesses. Otolaryngol. Head Neck Surg. *130*:676-680, 2004.

2. Asmar, B. I.: Bacteriology of retropharyngeal abscess in children. Pediatr. Infect. Dis. J. 9:595-596, 1990.
3. Barratt, G. E., Koopmann, C. F., and Coulthard, S. W.: Retropharyngeal abscess: A ten-year experience. Laryngoscope 94:455-463, 1984.
4. Bateman, G. H., and Kodicek, J.: Primary quinsy tonsillectomy. Ann. Otol. Rhinol. Laryngol. 68:315-321, 1959.
5. Beck, A. L.: Deep neck infection. Ann. Otol. Rhinol. Laryngol. 56:722-765, 1947.
6. Beck, A. L.: Deep neck infection. Ann. Otol. Rhinol. Laryngol. 56:439-481, 1947.
7. Beeden, A. G., and Evans, J. N. G.: Quinsy tonsillectomy: A further report. J. Laryngol. Otol. 84:443-448, 1970.
8. Blotter, J. W., Yin, L., Glynn, M., and Wiet, G. J.: Otolaryngology consultation for peritonsillar abscess in the pediatric population. Laryngoscope 110:1698-1701, 2000.
9. Bonding, P.: Tonsillectomy à chaud. J. Laryngol. Otol. 81:1171-1182, 1973.
10. Brandon, E. C., Jr.: Immediate tonsillectomy for peritonsillar abscess. Trans. Am. Acad. Ophthalmol. Otolaryngol. 77:412-416, 1973.
11. Brodsky, L., Sobie, S. R., Korwin, D., et al.: A clinical prospective study of peritonsillar abscess in children. Laryngology 98:780-783, 1988.
12. Brook, I.: Microbiology of retropharyngeal abscesses in children. Am. J. Dis. Child. 141:202-204, 1987.
13. Brook, I.: Microbiology and management of peritonsillar, retropharyngeal, and parapharyngeal abscesses. J. Oral. Maxillofac. Surg. 62:1545-1550, 2004.
14. Broughton, R. A.: Nonsurgical management of deep neck infections in children. Pediatr. Infect. Dis. J. 11:14-18, 1992.
15. Cable, B. E., Brenner, P., Bauman, N. B., and Mair, E. A.: Image-guided surgical drainage of medial parapharyngeal abscesses in children: A novel adjuvant to a difficult approach. Ann. Otol. Rhinol. Laryngol. 113:115-120, 2004.
16. Chassaignae, E.: Traite Pratique de la Suppuration et du Drainage Chirurgal. Vol. II. Paris, Masson, 1859.
17. Coticchia, J. M., Getnick, G. S., Yun, R. D., and Arnold, J. E.: Age-, site-, and time-specific differences in pediatric deep neck abscesses. Arch. Otolaryngol. Head Neck Surg. 130:201-207, 2004.
18. Craig, F. W., and Schunk, J. E.: Retropharyngeal abscess in children: Clinical presentation, utility of imaging, and current management. Pediatrics 111:1394-1398, 2003.
19. Danforth, H. B., and Brown, A. K., Jr.: A foreign body etiology of pterygomaxillary space abscess. Laryngoscope 73:1485, 1963.
20. Daya, H., Lo, S., Papsin, B. C., et al.: Retropharyngeal and parapharyngeal infections in children: The Toronto experience. Int. J. Pediatr. Otorhinolaryngol. 69:81-86, 2005.
21. de Marie, S., Tham, R., van der Mey, A. G. L., et al.: Clinical infections and nonsurgical treatment of parapharyngeal space infections complicating throat infection. Rev. Infect. Dis. 11:975-982, 1989.
22. Dodds, B., and Maniglia, A. J.: Peritonsillar and neck abscesses in the pediatric age group. Laryngoscope 98:956-959, 1988.
23. Elden, L. M., Grundfast, K. M., and Vezina, G.: Accuracy and usefulness of radiographic assessment of cervical neck infections in children. J. Otolaryngol. 30:82-89, 2001.
24. Endicott, J. N., Nelson, R. J., and Saraceno, C. A.: Diagnosis and management decisions in infections of the deep fascial spaces of the head and neck utilizing computerized tomography. Laryngoscope 92:630-633, 1982.
25. Finegold, S. M.: Anaerobic Bacteria in Human Disease. New York, Academic Press, 1977, pp. 129-141.
26. Flödstrom, A., and Hallander, H. O.: Microbiological aspects of peritonsillar abscesses. Scand. J. Infect. Dis. 8:157-160, 1976.
27. Friedman, N. R., Mitchell, R. B., Pereira, K. D., et al.: Peritonsillar abscess in early childhood: Presentation and management. Arch. Otolaryngol. Head Neck Surg. 123:630-632, 1997.
28. Greinwald, J. H., Wilson, J. F., and Haggerty, P. G.: Peritonsillar abscess: An unlikely cause of necrotizing fasciitis. Ann. Otol. Rhinol. Laryngol. 104:133-137, 1995.
29. Grodinsky, M.: Retropharyngeal and lateral pharyngeal abscesses: An anatomic and clinical study. Ann. Surg. 110:177-199, 1939.
30. Hanna, B. C., Mc Mullan, R., Gallagher, G., and Hedderwick, S.: The epidemiology of peritonsillar abscess disease in Northern Ireland. J. Infect. 52:247-253, 2006.
31. Har-El, G., Aroesty, J. H., Shaha, A., and Lucente, F. E.: Changing trends in deep neck abscess: A retrospective study of 110 patients. Oral Surg. Oral Med. Oral Pathol. 77:446-450, 1994.
32. Herzon, F. S.: Peritonsillar abscess: Incidence, current management practices, and a proposal for treatment guidelines. Laryngoscope 105:1-17, 1995.
33. Herzon, F. S., and Nicklaus, P.: Pediatric peritonsillar abscess: Management guidelines. Curr. Probl. Pediatr. 26:270-278, 1996.
34. Homicz, M. R., Carvalho, D., Kearns, D. B., et al.: An atypical presentation of Kawasaki disease resembling a retropharyngeal abscess. Int. J. Pediatr. Otolaryngol. 54:45-49, 2000.
35. Huang, R. Y., Damrose, E. J., Alavi, S., et al.: Third branchial cleft anomaly presenting as a retropharyngeal abscess. Int. J. Pediatr. Otolaryngol. 54:167-172, 2000.
36. Johnson, R. F., Stewart, M. G., and Wright, C. C.: An evidence-based review of the treatment of peritonsillar abscess. Otolaryngol. Head Neck Surg. 128:332-343, 2003.
37. Jokipii, A. M. M., Jokipii, L., Sipila, P., et al.: Semiquantitative culture results and pathogenic significance of obligate anaerobes in peritonsillar abscesses. J. Clin. Microbiol. 26:957-961, 1988.
38. Jousimies-Somer, H., Savolainen, S., Makitie, A., et al.: Bacteriologic findings in peritonsillar abscesses in young adults. Clin. Infect. Dis. 16:S292-S298, 1993.
39. Kieff, D. A., Bhattacharyya, N., Siegel, N. S., and Salman, S. D.: Selection of antibiotics after incision and drainage of peritonsillar abscesses. Otolaryngol. Head Neck Surg. 120:57-61, 1999.
40. Kirse, D. J., and Roberson, D. W.: Surgical management of retropharyngeal space infections in children. Laryngoscope 111:1413-1422, 2001.
41. Kronenberg, J., Wolf, M., and Leventon, G.: Peritonsillar abscess: Recurrence rate and the indication for tonsillectomy. Am. J. Otolaryngol. 8:82-84, 1987.
42. Langenbrunner, D. J., and Dajani, S.: Pharyngomaxillary space abscess with carotid artery erosion. Arch. Otolaryngol. 94:447-457, 1971.
43. Lazor, J. B., Cunningham, J., Eavey, R. D., et al.: Comparison of computed tomography and surgical findings in deep neck infections. Otolaryngol. Head Neck Surg. 111:746-750, 1994.
44. Leavitt, G. W.: Cervical fascia and deep neck infections. Otolaryngol. Clin. North Am. 9:703-716, 1976.
45. Lee, K. J., Traxler, J. H., Smith, A. W., et al.: Tonsillectomy: Treatment of peritonsillar abscess. Trans. Am. Acad. Ophthalmol. Otolaryngol. 77:417-421, 1973.
46. Licameli, G. R., and Grillone, G. A.: Inferior pole peritonsillar abscess. Otolaryngol. Head Neck Surg. 118:95-99, 1998.
47. Liston, R. L.: On a variety of false aneurysm. Br. Foreign Med. Rev. 15:155-161, 1843.
48. Luhmann, J. D., Kennedy, R. M., McAllister, J. D., and Jaffe, D. M.: Sedation for peritonsillar abscess drainage in the pediatric emergency department. Pediatr. Emerg. Care 18:1-3, 2002.
49. Mattucci, K., and Samet, C.: Pterygomaxillary space abscess. N. Y. State J. Med. 74:1409-1412, 1974.
50. McClay, J. E., Murray, A. D., and Booth, T.: Intravenous antibiotic therapy for deep neck abscesses defined by computed tomography. Arch. Otolaryngol. Head Neck Surg. 129:1207-1212, 2003.
51. McCurdy, J. A., Jr.: Peritonsillar abscess. Arch. Otol. 103:414-415, 1977.
52. Medina, M., Goldfarb, J., Traquina, D., et al.: Cervical adenitis and deep neck infection caused by Streptococcus pneumoniae. Pediatr. Infect. Dis. J. 16:823-824, 1997.
53. Morrison, J. E., Jr., and Pashley, N. R.: Retropharyngeal abscess in children: A 10-year review. Pediatr. Emerg. Care 4:9-11, 1988.
54. Mosher, H. P.: The submaxillary fossa approach to deep pus in the neck. Trans. Am. Acad. Ophthalmol. Otolaryngol. 34:19-36, 1926.
55. Nagy, M., Pizzuto, M., Backstrom, J., and Brodsky, L.: Deep neck infections in children: A new approach to diagnosis and treatment. Laryngoscope 107:1627-1634, 1997.
56. Neumann, J. L., and Schlueter, D. P.: Retropharyngeal abscess as the presenting feature of tuberculosis of the cervical spine. Am. Rev. Respir. Dis. 110:508-511, 1974.
57. Oleske, J. M., Starr, S. E., and Nahmias, A. J.: Complications of peritonsillar abscess due to Fusobacterium necrophorum. Pediatrics 57:570-571, 1976.
58. Ophir, D., Bawnik, J., Porat, M., et al.: Peritonsillar abscess: A prospective evaluation of outpatient management by needle aspiration. Arch. Otolaryngol. 114:661-663, 1988.
59. Rubinstein, E., Onderdonk, A. B., and Rahal, J. J.: Peritonsillar infection and bacteremia caused by Fusobacterium gonidiaformans. J. Pediatr. 85:673, 1974.
60. Savolainen, S., Jousimies-Somer, H. R., Makitie, A. A., et al.: Peritonsillar abscess. Arch. Otolaryngol. Head Neck Surg. 119:521-524, 1993.
61. Schraff, S., McGinn, J. D., and Derkay, C. S.: Peritonsillar abscess in children: A 10-year review of diagnosis and management. Int. J. Pediatr. Otorhinolaryngol. 57:213-218, 2001.
62. Sichel, J.-Y., Attal, P., Hocwald, E., and Eliashar, R.: Redefining parapharyngeal space infections. Ann. Otol. Rhinol. Laryngol. 115:117-123, 2006.
63. Sichel, J.-Y., Dano, I., Hocwald, E., et al.: Nonsurgical management of parapharyngeal space infections: A prospective study. Laryngoscope 112:906-910, 2002.
64. Sprinkle, P. M., Veltri, R. W., and Kantor, C. M.: Abscesses of the head and neck. Laryngoscope 84:1142-1148, 1974.
65. Stone, M. E., Walner, D. L., Koch, B. L., et al.: Correlation between computed tomography and surgical findings in retropharyngeal inflammatory processes in children. Int. J. Pediatr. Otorhinolaryngol. 49:121-125, 1999.
66. Stringer, S. P., Schaefer, S. D., and Close, L. G.: A randomized trial for outpatient management of peritonsillar abscess. Arch. Otolaryngol. 114:278-298, 1988.
67. Suskind, D. L., Park, J., Piccirillo, J. F., et al.: Conscious sedation: A new approach for peritonsillar abscess drainage in the pediatric population. Arch. Otolaryngol. Head Neck Surg. 125:1197-1200, 1999.
68. Takimoto, T., and Itoh, M.: Parapharyngeal abscess associated with the second pharyngeal pouch. J. Laryngol. Otol. 107:456-457, 1993.
69. Takoudes, T. G., and Haddad, J.: Retropharyngeal abscess and Epstein-Barr virus infection in children. Ann. Otol. Rhinol. Laryngol. 107:1072-1075, 1998.
70. Thawley, S. E., Godo, M., and Fuller, T. R.: Computerized tomography in the evaluation of head and neck lesions. Laryngoscope 88:451-459, 1978.

71. Thompson, J. W., Cohen, S. R., and Reddix, P.: Retropharyngeal abscess in children: A retrospective and historical analysis. Laryngoscope *98*:589-592, 1988.
72. Ungkanont, K., Yellon, R. F., Weissman, J. L., et al.: Head and neck space infections in infants and children. Otolaryngol. Head Neck Surg. *112*:375-382, 1995.
73. Vural, C., Gungor, A., and Comerci, S.: Accuracy of computerized tomography in deep neck infections in the pediatric population. Am. J. Otolaryngol. *24*:143-148, 2003.
74. Weinberg, E., Brodsky, L., Stanievich, J., et al.: Needle aspiration of peritonsillar abscess in children. Arch. Otolaryngol. Head Neck Surg. *119*:169-172, 1993.
75. Wenig, B. L., Shikowitz, M. J., and Abramson, A. L.: Necrotizing fasciitis as a lethal complication of peritonsillar abscess. Laryngoscope *94*:1576-1579, 1984.
76. Wetmore, R. F., Mahboubi, S., and Soyupak, S. K.: Computed tomography in the evaluation of pediatric neck infections. Otolaryngol. Head Neck Surg. *119*:624-627, 1998.
77. Windfuhr, J. P., and Chen, Y.-S.: Immediate abscess tonsillectomy—a safe procedure? Auris Nasus Larynx *28*:323-327, 2001.
78. Yeh, S. H., Zangwill, K. M., Hall, B., et al.: Parapharyngeal abscess due to cat-scratch disease. Clin. Infect. Dis. *30*:599-601, 2000.
79. Yilmaz, T., Ünal, Ö. F., Figen, G., et al.: A comparison of procaine penicillin with sulbactam-ampicillin in the treatment of peritonsillar abscesses. Eur. Arch. Otolaryngol. *255*:163-165, 1998.

CERVICAL LYMPHADENITIS

C. Mary Healy ✪ Carol J. Baker

Cervical lymphadenopathy is enlargement of the lymph nodes in the neck. *Cervical lymphadenitis* implies that there is inflammation of one or more nodes. The inflammatory response by the host is triggered by some form of injury or invasion proximal to the involved lymph node or nodes. The nodes become affected secondarily by drainage through connecting afferent lymphatic channels. The injury may be acute or chronic, infectious or non-infectious. Proper anatomic definition of the inflamed node or nodes,[78] combined with knowledge of the structures of the head and neck drained by them, may allow a portal of entry for infectious agents, the most common cause of cervical lymphadenitis in infants and children, to be identified.

Figure 15–1 illustrates the regional lymph nodes commonly affected in infants and children with cervical lymphadenitis. The superficial cervical lymph nodes lie on top of the sternocleidomastoid muscle along the course of the external jugular vein. They receive afferents from the superficial tissues of the neck, mastoid, superficial parotid (preauricular) nodes, and submaxillary glands. Their efferents terminate in the upper deep cervical lymph nodes. The mastoid lymph nodes overlie the mastoid process of the temporal bone and receive drainage from the parietal scalp and inner surface of the pinna. The occipital lymph nodes lie on the upper part of the trapezius and receive afferents from the occipital scalp and superficial portions of the upper posterior neck. Their efferents terminate in the deep cervical glands, as do the efferents from the mastoid nodes.

The deep cervical lymph nodes lie deep to the sternomastoid muscle along the whole length of the internal jugular vein and are divided into upper and lower groups. The jugulodigastric gland, a member of the upper group, lies at the angle of the jaw below the posterior belly of the digastric muscle. The lymphoid tissue of the palatine tonsil is drained into this gland; it frequently becomes enlarged in patients with "tonsillitis" or with tuberculous infection originating from the tonsils. The larynx, trachea, thyroid gland, and esophagus drain into the lower deep cervical glands. The submental lymph nodes, which lie between the digastric muscles below the myohyoid, receive superficial and deep drainage from the anterior tongue, lower lip, and chin, from both sides of the midline. They send efferents to the submandibular and upper deep cervical glands. The submandibular lymph nodes lie adjacent to the submandibular salivary gland and receive wide, superficial drainage from the lateral aspect of the lower lip, the vestibule of the nose, the cheeks, the medial parts of the eyelids, and the forehead. Deep drainage to these nodes arises from the posterior part of the mouth, gums, teeth, and tongue and from superficial and submental lymph nodes.

Because most of the lymphatic drainage of the head and neck goes to the submaxillary and deep cervical nodes, these glands are involved in more than 80 percent of cases of cervical adenitis in young children. Submental and superficial cervical lymphadenitis is observed less frequently.

EPIDEMIOLOGY

The epidemiology of infectious cervical adenitis is that of its infectious agents. Although cervical lymphadenitis can be a manifestation of focal viral infections of the oropharynx or respiratory tract, often it is part of a more generalized reticuloendothelial response to systemic infection. Viruses commonly associated

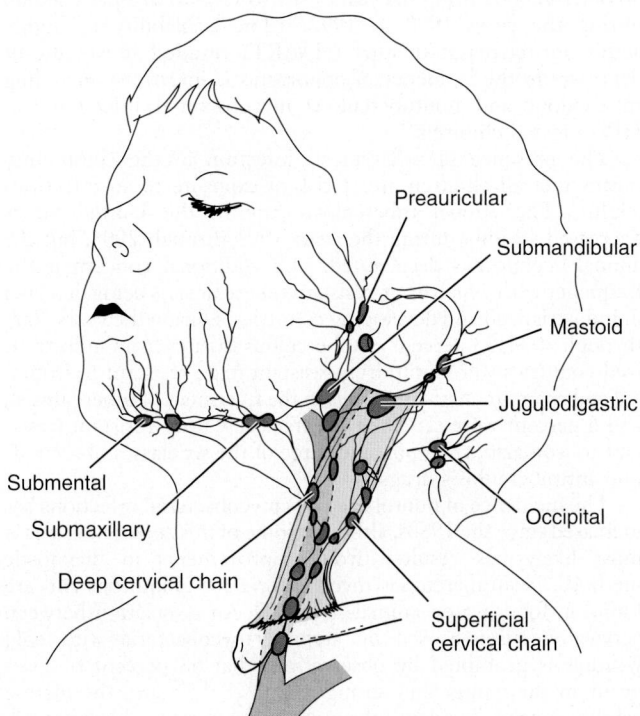

Figure 15–1 The lymphatic drainage and lymph nodes involved in infants and children with cervical lymphadenitis.

with prominent cervical adenitis include Epstein-Barr virus, cytomegalovirus, and human immunodeficiency virus (HIV). In HIV-infected children, cervical adenopathy either may herald or may be a part of the more generalized lymphadenopathy associated with this infection. Although human herpesvirus-6 (HHV-6), the cause of roseola in infants (exanthem subitum), is associated with the development of a mononucleosis syndrome and cervical adenopathy in adults,[3] lymphadenitis is not a prominent feature in children with primary infection.[55] Adenoviral and enteroviral infections are causes of generalized lymphadenopathy rather than of cervical adenitis alone. The epidemiology of cervical adenitis varies with age, geographic location, and socioeconomic status. Generally, lower socioeconomic status is associated with a higher incidence of infection in younger children.

When bacterial in origin, with the exception of group A streptococci and *Mycobacterium tuberculosis*, the agents isolated from these glands are the normal inhabitants of the nose, mouth, pharynx, and skin—*Staphylococcus aureus*, anaerobes, nontuberculous mycobacteria, *Actinomyces* spp.—and person-to-person transmission does not occur. In contrast, group A streptococci and *M. tuberculosis* infection of cervical lymph nodes results from contact with human infection by way of airborne droplets. Except in neonates, for whom male dominance has been reported in cases caused by group B streptococci,[11] infectious lymphadenitis has no gender or seasonal predilection.[13,35]

Any age group may be affected. In neonates, *S. aureus* and group B streptococci are the most common pathogens. Suppurative cervical lymphadenitis caused by *Staphylococcus epidermidis* in an otherwise healthy infant has been reported.[125] Nonetheless, despite the high frequency of nasal colonization by this organism, it remains a rare etiologic agent. There are rare reports of *Streptococcus pneumoniae* causing suppurative adenitis[94] in older children. Some studies[35,141,159] indicate that *S. aureus* has the leading role in infants, whereas in children, either group A streptococci or *S. aureus* is equally likely to be pathogenic. Other reports have varied regarding the relationship between age and probable etiologic agent.[13,24]

Overall, *S. aureus* and *Streptococcus pyogenes* accounted for 65 to 89 percent of consecutive cases in prospectively evaluated series.[13,35,159] Methicillin-resistant *S. aureus* (MRSA) must be strongly considered as a possible etiology because of the increased incidence of nosocomial MRSA and community-associated methicillin-resistant *S. aureus* (CA-MRSA) infections in the United States and elsewhere,[21,42,49,59,61,63,99] and recognition that the highest rates of CA-MRSA colonization and disease are found in children.[42,99] Many studies have shown that CA-MRSA strains predominantly cause skin and soft tissue infections, but a wide spectrum of illness is reported, and invasive CA-MRSA has been associated with a variety of clinical manifestations, including severe illness and death.[59,61,63,101] The impact of the CA-MRSA "epidemic" on pediatric cervical adenitis is less easy to define; however, retrospective and more recent prospective case series report that 6 to 10 percent of CA-MRSA infections manifest as adenitis.[61,63,99] One single-center study found that MRSA was the infectious etiology of no head and neck abscesses from July 1999 through December 2001 but accounted for 34 percent of cases from January 2002 through June 2004.[108]

The epidemiology of bacterial lymphadenitis varies by geographic location. Resurgence of infection with *Yersinia pestis* in the southwestern United States means that, in areas where it is endemic, it also must be considered in the differential diagnosis. Epidemic diphtheria, reported in the Russian Federation in 1990, subsequently spread to several newly independent states in the European region, with the number of reported cases (50,425) peaking in 1995. Although the number of diphtheria cases declined after the implementation of diphtheria control measures, 176 cases from the European region were reported to the World Health Organization (WHO) in 2004, 88 percent from

TABLE 15-1   Differentiation of *Mycobacterium tuberculosis* and Nontuberculous Mycobacterial Cervical Adenitis

	NTM MCA	*M. tuberculosis*
Age	1-6 yr	All ages
Ethnicity	White	Black, Asian, Hispanic
Exposure to tuberculosis	Absent	Present
Abnormal chest radiographs	Rare	Often
Residence	Suburban	Urban
TST >15 mm	Uncommon	Often
Bilateral involvement	Rare	Not uncommon

NTM, nontuberculous mycobacteria; TST, tuberculin skin test.

newly independent states. Diphtheria must be added to the list of possible causes of cervical lymphadenitis in that region of the world.[156]

The distinctive epidemiologic features of mycobacterial infection are summarized in Table 15-1. Scrofula caused by *M. tuberculosis* is a rare disease. When it does occur, it usually affects adults and older children. In contrast, children with atypical mycobacterial infection almost always are 1 to 6 years old, live in suburban or rural communities, and have no history of contact with *M. tuberculosis*.* Although *M. tuberculosis* is an infection acquired primarily by inhalation, the gastrointestinal tract or the respiratory tract may serve as the primary portal of entry for nontuberculous mycobacteria.[47,104,114,119] There seems to be an ethnic predilection for nontuberculous mycobacterial infection to occur in whites and for tuberculous infections to occur in blacks, Hispanics, Asians, and the Australian Aboriginal population.[103,139]

The advent of the HIV pandemic had a major impact on the nature and frequency of mycobacterial infections. A marked increase in the incidence of tuberculous infection occurred in HIV-infected adults and children, with annualized case rates for tuberculosis in HIV-infected children increasing from 58 per 100,000 during the years 1981 to 1985 to 478 per 100,000 during the years 1990 to 1992.[51] The availability of highly active antiretroviral therapy (HAART) resulted in significant decreases in the incidence of opportunistic infections, including tuberculous and nontuberculous mycobacterial infections, in HIV-infected children.[48]

The presence of tuberculosis infection in the community means that all children are at risk of exposure to an infectious adult.[20] The annual tuberculosis rate in the United States decreased steadily during the years 1993 through 2005, but the annual decline has decelerated.[31] Of additional concern is the frequency with which drug-resistant tuberculosis is being detected in industrialized and developing countries. During the years 2000 through 2004, 33 percent of tuberculous isolates from industrialized countries were multidrug-resistant (e.g., resistant to isoniazid and rifampin, first-line drugs in the treatment of tuberculosis), and 6 percent were classified as extensively drug-resistant (resistant to isoniazid, rifampin, and three of the six classes of second-line antituberculosis drugs).[32]

The incidence of nontuberculous mycobacterial infections has increased since the 1980s, although some of this apparent increase most likely has resulted from improvements in diagnostic methods. Nontuberculous mycobacteria are ubiquitous and are found in food, water, animals, and soil. An association between cervical adenitis caused by atypical mycobacteria with cold weather is prompted by observations that 68 percent of cases occur in the winter and spring months,[83,112,155] and the disease exhibits a steady incidence throughout the year in cold climates.[47]

---

*See references 19, 33, 36, 41, 47, 69, 80, 84, 112, 120, 134, 149, 155.

A 10-year Canadian retrospective study reported that 70 percent of cases occurred in girls; however, most reports suggest no gender difference.[112]

Until the 1970s, *Mycobacterium scrofulaceum* was the usual etiologic agent isolated from children, followed by *Mycobacterium avium–intracellulare*.[155] This trend has reversed, with *M. avium–intracellulare* now accounting for 50 to 98 percent of culture-proven cases.[43,58,79,83,102,103,142,155] Previously uncommon species, such as *Mycobacterium kansasii*, *Mycobacterium malmoense*, *Mycobacterium fortuitum*, *Mycobacterium haemophilum*, and *Mycobacterium bohemicum*, also are being detected more frequently.* Some of these uncommon species probably are responsible for many cases of culture-negative mycobacterial lymphadenitis because of their fastidious growth requirements. New diagnostic methods have led to case reports of cervical adenitis secondary to slow-growing species, such as *Mycobacterium lentiflavum* and *Mycobacterium interjectum*.[37,53,57,116,136] Cervical lymphadenitis caused by *Mycobacterium chelonae* is rare, usually involves the submandibular glands, and typically occurs in patients with an antecedent history of dental pathology.[5]

Cervical lymphadenopathy may be the direct result of infection with HIV per se. The development of acute tender adenitis in an HIV-infected child should provoke a search for another etiology, however. Although the typical childhood pathogens remain the most common pathogens in this setting, as in other immunocompromised children, opportunists also should be sought.[51] Patients with HIV infection beginning therapy with potent antiretroviral agents may develop new-onset mycobacterial lymphadenitis (tuberculous and nontuberculous mycobacteria). When this lymphadenitis occurs, it is more localized, is associated with more sinus formation, and is more often caused by nontuberculous mycobacteria (*M. avium–intracellulare*) than by *M. tuberculosis*.[115]

Cat-scratch disease is a common cause of lymphadenitis in children and young adults.[23] In 1988, English and associates[40] first isolated a pleomorphic gram-negative bacillus, later identified as *Afipia felis*, from lymph nodes of patients with cat-scratch disease. *Bartonella henselae* (formerly called *Rochalimaea henselae*), a morphologically similar but genetically distinct pleomorphic gram-negative bacillus, now is recognized as the cause of most cat-scratch disease.[1]

The cervical nodes are the second most common site of cat-scratch disease involvement. Although unusual and severe manifestations of this infection have been described, it remains mostly a mild, self-limited infection in children and adolescents, with no ethnic predilection. Seasonal variation with an increased incidence in fall, winter, and early spring does occur in temperate zones. A history of animal contact with cats usually can be elicited.[26] The importance of bites and scratches by kittens in transmitting this disease has been well defined.[91] However, the absence of a history of traumatic contact with cats in a substantial number of cases has raised the possibility that other modes of transmission exist. Zangwill and associates[161] suggested that fleas might serve as vectors of transmission. Their hypothesis is strengthened by the detection of *Bartonella* DNA by polymerase chain reaction in collections of fleas from cats owned by two infected patients.[161]

PATHOPHYSIOLOGY

Although cervical lymphadenitis is a common entity in pediatric clinical practice, little information exists regarding its pathogenesis. Viral cervical adenitis may be part of either a local response to viruses invading the oropharynx or respiratory tract (e.g.,

adenoviruses, coxsackieviruses) or a more generalized reticuloendothelial response to systemic viral infection (e.g., Epstein-Barr virus, cytomegalovirus, HHV-6, HIV). Infection attributed to group A streptococci and *S. aureus* is presumed to enter the cervical lymphatics from the oropharynx (group A streptococci) and anterior nares (*S. aureus*). In a patient with group A streptococcal pharyngitis or tonsillitis, whether infection remains localized at the pharyngotonsillar tissues or spreads to cervical lymph nodes and results in suppuration primarily is a function of host response. Although peak attack rates for group A streptococcal pharyngitis are observed among school-age children, suppurative cervical adenitis is an uncommon occurrence. In contrast, infants and children younger than 3 years old rarely have group A streptococci isolated from throat cultures, but this age group more commonly has suppurative cervical lymphadenitis.[118]

In infections attributed to *S. aureus*, colonization of the anterior nares is thought to be a prerequisite for cervical lymphadenitis. Brook and Winter[22,23] arrived at this conclusion because organisms of identical phage types were isolated from the anterior nares and the cervical abscesses of their patients. An investigation of children in St. Louis found no such correlation between isolates from nasal and cervical node cultures.[13] The role of *S. aureus* as a primary pathogen has been the subject of some debate. In most series, 30 percent of aspirates yield mixed cultures of *S. aureus* and group A streptococci, and frequently significant elevations of antistreptolysin O titer are found in the sera of patients whose lymph nodes yielded a pure culture of *S. aureus*.

In a California study, 65 percent of patients had node aspirates yielding a pure culture of *S. aureus*, and 41 percent exhibited an immune response to one or more of the extracellular antigens of group A streptococci.[159] Similarly, the finding that many children improve with penicillin or ampicillin treatment, despite the high prevalence of penicillin resistance among *S. aureus*, suggests that, although streptococci and staphylococci may coexist in these nodes, staphylococci may play a subsidiary role as secondary invaders. Most children with isolates of *S. aureus* from suppurative lymph nodes show no evidence of coexistent streptococcal infection or viral upper respiratory infection. In this more common circumstance, *S. aureus* apparently has the capacity to be a primary invader.

Recovery of anaerobic bacteria from cervical nodes suggests invasion of the lymphatics by mouth flora, often as a result of local tissue destruction by periodontal disease.[24] The delineation of the pathophysiology of cervical lymphadenitis of diverse bacterial etiology requires an understanding of the interaction between a given microorganism (e.g., inoculum size, elaboration of extracellular enzymes, ability to adhere to epithelium) and the host (e.g., humoral and surface immune capacity, degree of trauma).

Tuberculous cervical lymphadenopathy occurs within months of the initial exposure, through pulmonary infection and involvement of the regional and then more distant lymph nodes. It is a rapid process; chest radiographic evidence of active pulmonary disease often is seen. Nontuberculous mycobacteria are ubiquitous in the environment. Oropharyngeal acquisition and local infection lead to lymph node involvement. Most children with nontuberculous mycobacterial cervical lymphadenitis are immunocompetent, although a more recent study suggests that children who develop necrotic nodes may have deficient production of interferon-γ.[102] Despite *M. avium* skin test positivity being linked with pet birds, no clear relationship with lymphadenitis has been shown.[75] The observation that discontinuation of childhood bacille Calmette-Guérin vaccination has been associated with an increase in atypical mycobacterial infection in many countries suggests that this vaccine may have a protective effect.[150] Progressive cervical adenitis developing after bacille Calmette-Guérin vaccination also has been reported.[105]

---

*See references 10, 43, 58, 79, 83, 102, 103, 111, 112, 142, 155.

CLINICAL PRESENTATION

The clinical manifestations of cervical lymphadenitis vary considerably but are consistent with the diverse etiologies associated with cervical node enlargement in infants and children. To categorize the mode of presentation as either acute or subacute and chronic is useful because, although the boundaries are ill-defined and much overlap exists, common etiologies tend to fall consistently within one or another category. Cervical lymphadenitis of acute onset may be categorized further as either bilateral or unilateral. In most situations, acute, bilateral cervical adenitis is either part of a generalized reticuloendothelial response to a systemic infection or a localized reaction to acute pharyngitis. The presence or absence of associated features (e.g., pharyngitis, enanthems or exanthems, generalized adenopathy, hepatosplenomegaly) aids in making the differentiation.

Acute unilateral cervical lymphadenitis is caused by streptococcal or staphylococcal infection in 53 to 89 percent of cases.[13,35,62,159] In newborns, *S. aureus* is the most common cause, and clinical features are similar to those seen in older children. Group B streptococci have been described as causative in a "cellulitis-adenitis" syndrome in infancy.[11] These infants differ from infants with staphylococcal adenitis in that they are younger; more often are male; and have a greater incidence of systemic symptoms, irritability, and anorexia; 94 percent have associated bacteremia. The typical patient presents with fever, facial or submandibular cellulitis, and ipsilateral otitis media.[11] Isolated cervical adenitis caused by group B streptococci also has been described.[44]

Patients with disease attributed to *S. aureus* or group A streptococci typically are 1 to 4 years old (70-80% of cases), and the male-to-female ratio is equal. Clinically, there is little that helps to differentiate streptococcal from staphylococcal infections. Cervical adenitis can occur as part of the "streptococcosis" syndrome of infancy, with an onset heralded by coryza, an irregular low-grade fever, nasal discharge with excoriation and crusting around the nares, vomiting, and loss of appetite. Lymph node enlargement occurs within a few days of onset and resolves, as do other symptoms, without treatment within 6 to 8 weeks.[118] Suppuration of cervical glands may occur at any time during this interval but seldom does so if antimicrobial therapy is given early in the illness. Group A streptococci also should be suspected as a cause of cervical adenitis in a patient with typical vesiculopustular or crusted lesions of impetigo involving the face or scalp.

Systemic symptoms in children with staphylococcal or streptococcal cervical adenitis usually are minimal or absent unless associated with cellulitis, metastatic foci of infection, or bacteremia. The primary site of lymph node involvement by frequency is submandibular (50-60%), upper cervical (25-30%), submental (5-8%), occipital (3-5%), and lower cervical (2-5%).[13,35,157] Involved nodes generally vary in size from 2 to 6 cm in diameter, and one fourth to one third suppurate. Patients with lymphadenitis caused by *S. aureus* are more likely to have suppuration and a longer duration of symptoms and signs before diagnosis than are patients with disease caused by other bacterial agents (Fig. 15-2).[13,141] Among patients who develop suppurative adenitis, 86 percent do so within 2 weeks of onset.[157]

Approximately one third of patients in one study had concomitant lymphadenopathy at other anatomic sites.[13] A history of recent upper respiratory tract symptoms, including sore throat (40%), earache or coryza (16%), and impetigo (32%), is a frequent finding, as are signs of pharyngitis, tonsillitis, or otitis media.[13,35] These factors do not help to delineate the etiology, however. Hepatomegaly or splenomegaly is a rare occurrence and, if present, should suggest bacteremia or generalized disease processes (e.g., infectious mononucleosis, reticuloendotheliosis, tuberculosis, HIV infection).

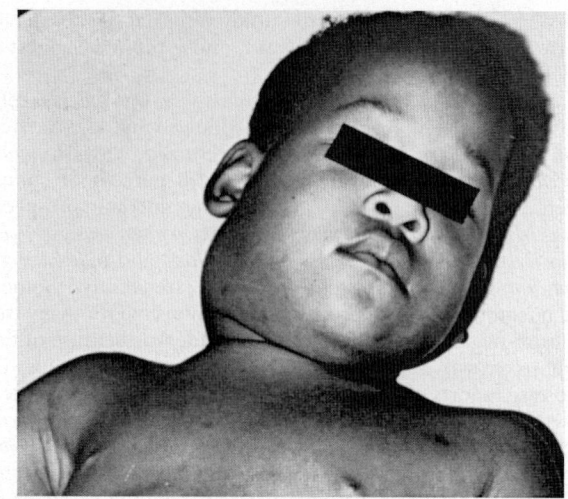

Figure 15-2 A 2-year-old boy with fever and unilateral inflammation of the cervical lymph nodes of 2 days' duration. Needle aspirate culture of this nonfluctuant node grew *Staphylococcus aureus*. Antistaphylococcal therapy resulted in complete resolution of adenitis without surgical drainage.

Kawasaki disease may manifest as a febrile illness associated with bilateral or unilateral cervical lymphadenopathy and may be confused with more common acute pyogenic infections.[152] Other features (e.g., conjunctivitis, oral manifestations, changes in the peripheral extremities, polymorphic erythematous rash) are required criteria for the diagnosis.[95] Although originally termed *mucocutaneous lymph node syndrome*, unilateral lymph node enlargement of at least 1.5 cm is the most inconsistent feature.[15,95] Lymphadenopathy usually subsides when the fever subsides, although in some cases it may follow a more chronic course.

The rapid development of painful lymphadenitis, quickly succeeding the sudden onset of fever, chills, weakness, and headache, is a classic presentation of infection caused by *Y. pestis* (bubonic plague). The groin is the site most often involved. Other locations, including the cervical area, may be affected, however. Establishing the diagnosis and providing treatment quickly are crucial because infection can be fulminant.

In cases of diphtheria, cervical adenopathy develops secondary to infection of the posterior structures of the mouth and proximal pharynx. A whitish gray membrane covers the mucosal surfaces. In severe cases, the cervical adenopathy, which typically is bilateral, can result in a "bull neck" appearance.

Careful physical examination of the head and neck, particularly areas drained by affected lymph nodes, may yield important clues about etiology. The presence of periodontal disease is associated with a higher incidence of anaerobic organisms causing adenitis[24]; the history or presence of tick bites suggests the possibility of tularemia[135]; and the presence of papular or pustular lesions, suggesting an inoculation site, raises the possibility of rarer causes of infection, including *Nocardia*, actinomycosis, sporotrichosis, plague, cutaneous diphtheria, and cat-scratch disease.

Mycobacterial infections, cat-scratch disease, and toxoplasmosis are more common entities presenting as subacute or chronic lymphadenitis. The epidemiologic and clinical features that aid in the differentiation of typical and nontuberculous mycobacterial infections are summarized in Table 15-1. The clinical manifestations virtually are identical (Fig. 15-3).[19,30,97] Typically, a child presents with a history of painless, (so-called cold) cervical node swelling. The submandibular cervical nodes

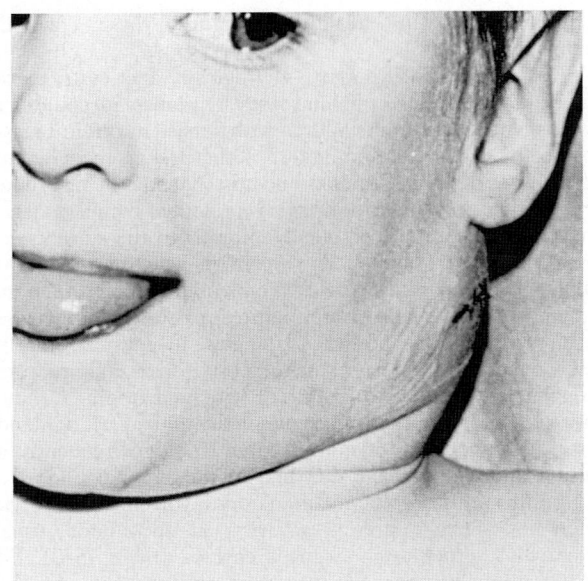

Figure 15–3 A 4-year-old boy who had bilateral nontender enlargement of lymph nodes of 6 weeks' duration without other symptoms. Placement of a TST resulted in 18-mm induration, excisional biopsy acid-fast stain was positive, and cultures grew *Mycobacterium tuberculosis.*

usually are involved in nontuberculous mycobacterial infection,* whereas other cervical nodes are involved more frequently with *M. tuberculosis.*[4,19,65,90,127] As the infection progresses, the skin overlying the node may develop a pinkish or violaceous discoloration caused by increased vascularity, although the skin temperature is not increased. This finding may be followed by adherence of the skin to the underlying mass. If left untreated, fluctuance and spontaneously draining sinus tracts may develop.

A patient with *M. tuberculosis* is more likely than one with atypical mycobacterial disease to be older than 4 years of age and to have generalized lymphadenopathy (10-20% of cases), bilateral node enlargement (10% of cases), a history of exposure to tuberculosis (93% of cases), and an urban residence.[19,90,107] No differences have been noted, however, with regard to duration of adenopathy, fever, and presence or absence of constitutional symptoms. An abnormal chest radiograph has been noted in 28 to 71 percent of cases caused by *M. tuberculosis,*[127,128,138,149] in contrast to the 98 to 100 percent of normal chest radiographs found in patients with nontuberculous mycobacterial adenitis.[47,126,127,142,148]

In a summary of 447 reported childhood cases of nontuberculous mycobacterial infections from 15 countries, Lincoln and Gilbert[74] detected only 6 cases of bilateral cervical node involvement, 4 with abnormal chest radiographs, and none with nodal enlargement other than cervical. Similar findings have been reported by other investigators.[126,148] Intradermal tuberculin skin testing with purified protein derivative uncommonly produces more than 15 mm of induration at 48 hours in a child with nontuberculous mycobacterial infection, but reactions between 5 and 15 mm are common.[76,86] Reactions of 10 to 20 mm can occur with *Mycobacterium marinum* and *M. fortuitum* infection.[114] Tuberculin skin test positivity may persist, even when children are retested many years after infection.[155]

Cat-scratch disease may manifest days to weeks after the initial inoculation. Characteristically, a history of contact with a cat or kitten or a scratch is present. Later, when the primary lesion may

have healed, tender regional adenopathy appears. Although axillary nodes most frequently are affected, 25 percent of children have isolated cervical node involvement. Middle cervical and parotid nodes are involved more often than are submandibular ones.[122] Constitutional symptoms, present early in the course of the illness, usually are mild and may have resolved by the time the adenitis appears. Fever is observed in one fourth of patients and, if present, has a mean duration of 5 to 7 days.[85] Nodes suppurate in one tenth to one third of patients.[28,29] Rare manifestations include Parinaud syndrome,[26] encephalopathy,[82] exanthems[28] (usually of the erythema nodosum type), and osteolytic lesions.[27]

Acquired toxoplasmosis may manifest as regional lymphadenopathy, frequently with posterior cervical node involvement.[93,121,146] Most children exhibit few, if any, constitutional symptoms. If present, fatigue and generalized myalgia are prominent. The characteristic location combined with a history of exposure to cats or of eating undercooked meats should raise this diagnostic possibility, and the diagnosis may be confirmed by appropriate serologic testing. It is an uncommon etiology for cervical adenopathy in children living in the United States.

Chronic, recurrent cervical adenitis forms part of the periodic fever, aphthous ulcers, pharyngitis, cervical adenitis (PFAPA) syndrome, a chronic syndrome first described in 1987.[92] It is characterized by periodic episodes of high fever greater than 39° C lasting 3 to 6 days and recurring every 3 to 8 weeks in association with aphthous ulcers, pharyngitis, and cervical adenitis, although symptoms such as abdominal pain, nausea, diarrhea, and headache also are described in 20 to 73 percent of children.[147] In most children, the onset of disease occurs before they reach 5 years of age, the syndrome is self-limited, and recovery without long-term sequelae is the rule. Oral corticosteroids are effective in aborting an attack.[72,109,147]

Kikuchi-Fujimoto disease, also called *subacute necrotizing lymphadenitis,* is an uncommon disorder of uncertain etiology that also may manifest as cervical adenopathy, with or without fever. This disorder was described first in 1972 and seems to have a predilection for Asian women 25 to 30 years old, who generally have a benign course with spontaneous resolution over 3 to 4 months.[46,151] Kikuchi-Fujimoto disease also has been reported in children, typically adolescents, although cases in children 2 years old are documented.[34,71,73,153]

In contrast to the 4:1 female predominance documented in adult series, pediatric Kikuchi-Fujimoto disease occurs more commonly in boys (male-to-female ratio ranges from 1.2:1 to 1.9:1). The most common presentation is unilateral or bilateral lymphadenopathy of multiple nodes. In most cases, posterior cervical chain nodes are involved, and affected nodes may be painful and tender. Fever is an inconsistent symptom. Extranodal manifestations include malaise, nightsweats, weight loss, maculopapular skin rashes, gastrointestinal symptoms, hepatosplenomegaly, arthritis, and aseptic meningitis. Associated laboratory findings include leukopenia (33-100% of cases with prolonged fever), elevated erythrocyte sedimentation rate, mild anemia, elevated C-reactive protein, and elevated liver enzymes.

Diagnosis is established by biopsy of the lymph nodes and not by fine-needle aspiration cytology, showing lymphadenitis with focal proliferation of reticular cells accompanied by histiocytes and extensive nuclear debris. Lymph node biopsy also has been associated with prompt resolution of fever.[34] Treatment generally is supportive, although steroids are reported to provide more rapid resolution of symptoms. The prognosis is favorable; most cases of Kikuchi-Fujimoto disease resolve within 6 months, although a recurrence rate of 3 to 4 percent is recorded. Some children subsequently develop autoimmune disorders, most commonly systemic lupus erythematosus, and regular clinical follow-up looking for signs of evolving autoimmune disorder is

---

*See references 4, 19, 43, 58, 79, 83, 84, 90, 126, 127, 142, 148, 155.

required.[100,132,153] Whether Kikuchi-Fujimoto disease is infectious or genetic in nature, perhaps the result of infection with a single novel agent or a nonspecific host response to any of a variety of agents, remains to be determined.

Another rare but important cause of cervical lymphadenitis in association with generalized lymphadenopathy or hepatosplenomegaly is hemophagocytic syndrome. This diagnosis should be considered if the aforementioned features occur with prolonged fever, cytopenia in at least two cell lines, low fibrinogen, and high ferritin and triglyceride serum levels.[110] Other features include rash, respiratory distress, hypotension, and coagulopathy. The diagnosis is confirmed by showing hemophagocytosis in bone marrow or lymph node biopsy specimens. Finally, when presented with a history of subacute or chronic lymphadenitis, careful physical examination should be undertaken to exclude obvious local causes (e.g., seborrhea, head lice, tinea capitis, chronic otitis media) before an extensive diagnostic work-up is initiated.

DIFFERENTIAL DIAGNOSIS

Cervical swellings are encountered frequently in pediatric practice, and most of them represent lymph nodes. When considering the diagnostic possibilities in patients with cervical lymphadenitis, one first must ascertain whether or not the pathologic process involves a lymph node, then whether or not its cause is infectious, and, if infectious, the likely etiologic agent. The duration of the cervical swelling aids in the differential diagnosis because most tumors or developmental anomalies have been noted for weeks. Rapid enlargement may occur in the latter, but usually it occurs as a result of secondary infection. Location is a helpful clue because midline masses rarely represent lymph nodes and the most common neck masses of congenital origin (thyroglossal duct cyst, branchial cleft cyst, and cystic hygromas) all have characteristic anatomic locations.

Of the midline masses, thyroglossal duct cysts are the most common.[66,117] These cysts may occur anywhere from the foramen cecum to the thyroid, are midline, and move on protrusion of the tongue. They may have an associated sinus tract, midline or just lateral to it, from which cloudy mucus sometimes can be expressed. They may become infected secondarily, but, in the noninfected state, these cysts are nontender, smooth, and round with well-defined margins. Thyroglossal duct cysts must be differentiated from other midline masses, including epidermoid cysts, lipomas, thyroid tumors, and the rare midline lymph node.

The second most common benign congenital neck mass is the branchial cleft cyst. It usually arises from the second branchial cleft and lies at the anterior border of the sternocleidomastoid muscle. Although such cysts usually manifest as skin dimples, they may become infected secondarily and manifest as inflammatory swellings or draining sinus tracts. A careful examination should detect a sinus tract. Branchial cleft cysts can occur in individuals of any age, but usually occur in school-age children.

Cystic hygromas, considerably less common than thyroglossal duct or branchial cleft cysts, are the third most frequent cause of congenital neck masses. These arise from lymphatics derived from either the jugular vein or the mesenchymal tissue. They may occur elsewhere but usually are found posterior to the sternocleidomastoid muscle in the supraclavicular fossa. Most cystic hygromas appear in the first 2 years of life, many being noted at birth or soon thereafter. They are soft, compressible tumors that transilluminate well, and, although benign in themselves, they may cause symptoms through pressure exerted on surrounding structures. Confusion may arise when cystic hygromas increase in size in association with an upper respiratory tract infection. The latter causes increased lymph flow so that the hygroma persists while other lymph nodes decrease in size after resolution of the infection. In most circumstances, palpation

and transillumination readily distinguish these congenital malformations.

These four cervical masses—thyroglossal duct cysts, thyroid tumors, branchial cleft cysts, and cystic hygromas—accounted for 63.7 percent of lesions in children with persistent cervical masses reported by Moussatos and Baffes.[97] Other lesions included neurogenic tumors, parotid tumors, and miscellaneous benign tumors (12.3%). The remainder of masses represented lymph nodes. As a rule, masses located completely anterior to the sternocleidomastoid muscle are benign. The exception is the thyroid tumor.[97] Malignancies that mimic cervical lymph nodes usually are located in the posterior triangle or are multiple masses extending across the anterior and the posterior triangles. In contrast, approximately 50 percent of masses in the posterior triangle represent malignancies, most of which are of lymphoid origin. Although most cysts and tumors manifest as solitary, unilateral, nontender masses, lymph nodes of noninfectious etiology frequently are multiple and bilateral, and they may be mildly tender.

Noninfectious chronic inflammatory involvement of cervical lymph nodes may represent a variety of uncommon, usually benign, but sometimes malignant entities (Table 15–2). Fifty percent of malignant neck masses in children are caused by Hodgkin and non-Hodgkin lymphomas. Neuroblastoma is the second most common malignancy, accounting for 15 percent. The likelihood of a given diagnosis is age-dependent, with neuroblastoma being more common than Hodgkin disease in younger age groups.[62] Thyroid tumors are the third most frequent neck

TABLE 15–2   Noninfectious Etiology of Cervical Adenitis

	Isolated Cervical	Cervical Associated with Generalized Adenopathy
Malignancy		
Hodgkin disease	+	+
Non-Hodgkin lymphomas	+	+
Rhabdomyosarcoma	+	–
Neuroblastoma	+	+
Leukemia	+	+
Metastatic carcinoma	+	–
Thyroid tumors	+	–
Drugs		
Isoniazid	–	+
Phenytoin (Dilantin)	–	+
Serum Sickness	–	+
Collagen Vascular Disease		
Juvenile rheumatoid arthritis	–	+
Systemic lupus erythematosus	–	+
Miscellaneous		
Sarcoidosis	–	+
Reticuloendotheliosis	–	+
Sinus histiocytosis with massive lymphadenopathy	+	+
Histiocytosis X	–	+
Postvaccinial	+	–
Storage disorders	–	+
Kawasaki disease	+	+
Hemophagocytic syndrome	–	+
PFAPA syndrome	+	–
Kikuchi-Fujimoto disease	+	+
Masses Simulating Adenopathy		
Cystic hygroma	+	–
Branchial cleft cyst	+	–
Thyroglossal duct cyst	+	–
Epidermoid cyst	+	–
Sternocleidomastoid tumor	+	–

PFAPA, periodic fever, aphthous ulcers, pharyngitis, cervical adenitis.

TABLE 15–3   Infectious Etiology of Cervical Adenitis

	Isolated Cervical	Cervical Associated with Generalized Adenopathy
Bacterial		
Staphylococcus aureus	+	–
Group A streptococci	+	+
Mycobacterium tuberculosis	+	+
Nontuberculous mycobacteria	+	–
Bartonella henselae	+	–
Gram-negative enterics	+	–
Anaerobes	+	–
Haemophilus influenzae	+	–
Yersinia pestis	–	+
Actinomyces israelii	+	–
Diphtheria	+	–
Tularemia	+	–
Brucellosis	–	+
Syphilis	+	+
Viral		
Measles	+	+
Rubella	+	+
Epstein-Barr virus	+	+
Herpes simplex	+	–
Human herpesvirus 6	+	+
Cytomegalovirus	+	+
Mumps	+	–
Varicella	+	+
HIV	+	+
Fungal		
Histoplasmosis	+	+
Cryptococcus	+	–
Aspergillosis	+	–
Candida	+	–
Sporotrichosis	+	–
Parasitic		
Toxoplasma gondii	+	+

HIV, human immunodeficiency virus.

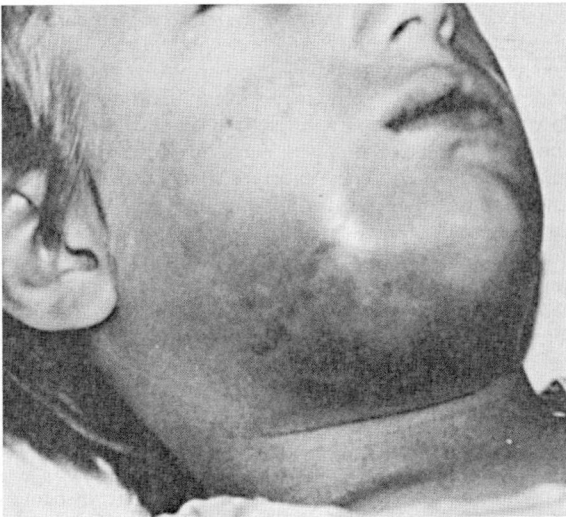

Figure 15–4 A 9-year-old boy who developed high fever and markedly tender submental lymph node inflammation after a tooth extraction. Cultures from this fluctuant mass grew three anaerobes and viridans streptococci.

malignancies. Other entities to be included in the differential diagnosis include leukemia,[25] metastatic carcinoma,[97] phenytoin-induced pseudolymphoma,[25] serum sickness,[25] storage disorders (Gaucher disease, Niemann-Pick disease), collagen vascular disease,[25] sarcoidosis,[64] sinus histiocytosis with massive lymphadenopathy,[12,124] and reticuloendotheliosis or histiocytosis X. Except for malignancies, these disease entities almost always are associated with lymphadenopathy that is not limited to the cervical region and have a variety of clinical and laboratory findings that allow the correct diagnosis to be made.

Numerous infectious agents have been reported in association with cervical adenitis in infants and children (Table 15–3). Among patients evaluated prospectively with needle aspirate cultures of affected lymph nodes, *S. aureus* or group A streptococci are the organisms most frequently isolated.[13,24,35,141,159] No significant difference has been reported that distinguishes between patients with adenitis caused by streptococci or staphylococci with respect to gender, ethnicity, dental problems, symptoms, presence of fever, or site or size of lymph nodes. In patients from whom *S. aureus* is isolated, a longer duration of disease before diagnosis is established, a larger percentage of fluctuant lymph nodes,[13,141] and a tendency toward slower resolution are found.[34] Most patients with bacterial cervical lymphadenitis, including patients with mycobacterial infection, are 1 to 6 years old. Older children are more likely to have negative lymph node aspirate cultures.[13,134,141]

In early studies, anaerobes rarely were associated with cervical adenitis.[13,35] Proper bacteriologic techniques for the isolation of these fastidious organisms allowed Brook[24] to report anaerobes alone in 18 percent and mixed anaerobic and aerobic bacteria in 20 percent of patients, suggesting that anaerobic organisms may play a more significant role in the etiology of cervical lymphadenitis than recognized previously. An older child with "negative" cultures, especially a child with poor dental hygiene or periodontal disease, may have anaerobic infection, as did the 9-year-old boy in Figure 15–4. Needle aspiration of this cervical mass yielded *Peptococcus, Peptostreptococcus, Bacteroides fragilis,* and viridans streptococci. Resolution of the lymphadenitis occurred promptly after incision and drainage and penicillin therapy.

Dental disease or manipulation also should suggest the possibility of cervicofacial actinomycosis (lumpy jaw). These patients have a chronic submandibular mass and frequently a fistula from the skin to the oral cavity.[16] Less frequently occurring bacteria,[70] viruses, fungi, and parasites can cause cervical lymphadenitis in children, but these patients usually have less evidence of acute inflammation, with or without adenopathy at additional sites, and historical and physical findings that suggest unusual causes of cervical lymph gland enlargement.

SPECIFIC DIAGNOSIS

A detailed history to ascertain preceding dental problems, presence of skin lesions, animal exposure (including exposure to fleas and ticks), duration of illness, presence of associated symptoms, contact with tuberculosis, presence of risk factors for HIV infection, drug usage (especially phenytoin) or other unusual ingestions (undercooked meat, unpasteurized dairy products), recent travel outside the geographic region of residence, and sites of occult infection drained by the affected node may yield important diagnostic clues in a patient with cervical lymphadenitis. Physical examination should include careful inspection for the presence of dental disease, noncervical lymphadenopathy, hepatosplenomegaly, and oropharyngeal or skin lesions.

Radiologic evaluation of adenitis is unnecessary in most mild to moderate cases. Ultrasonography often is performed when the presenting neck mass is very large, is increasing in size, or has not responded to initial antibiotic therapy. It is useful in diagnosing suppuration and expediting incision and drainage. High-resolution and color Doppler ultrasonography (with or without contrast enhancement) defining longitudinal-to-transverse nodal ratio and vascularity patterns has had some success in differentiating benign and malignant lymph nodes in adults.[2,96,98,158,160]

In children in whom most adenopathy is infectious or reactive in etiology, ultrasonography is less discriminating. In one study of 35 children, ultrasonography showed significant differences in lymph nodes in 22 children with a diagnosis of Kawasaki disease compared with 8 children with bacterial lymphadenitis, but findings were similar to those of children with lymphadenitis secondary to Epstein-Barr virus infection.[144]

In another study of 146 children, unilateral lymph nodes and cystic necrosis were found only in lymphadenitis caused by cat-scratch disease or bacterial or tuberculous infection.[113] Individual sonographic findings were nonspecific for diagnosis, although these findings combined with clinical signs were helpful. No patients with nontuberculous mycobacterial adenitis were evaluated in this study. Nodal calcifications and spread of nodal masses into the subcutaneous tissues by ultrasonography and characteristic low-density, ring-enhancing lesions with minimal or absent inflammatory stranding of subcutaneous fat seen on computed tomography and magnetic resonance imaging have been reported with nontuberculous mycobacterial adenitis in children.[54,58,77,123] These findings may be helpful in differentiating this etiology from other bacterial causes when the diagnosis is not suspected clinically or early in the course. Differences in clinical presentation between the two entities should obviate the need for such imaging, however, in all but the most complicated of cases.

In the acute stage of cervical lymphadenitis, needle aspiration of the affected node is a valuable diagnostic tool. Sixty to eighty-eight percent of patients with acute cervical lymphadenitis subjected to needle aspiration of the affected node for bacterial and mycobacterial culture have an etiologic agent recovered.[13,24,65,159] Only inflamed nodes should be aspirated, but they need not be fluctuant. No serious complications of this procedure have been recorded.

The largest or most fluctuant node should be selected, and the skin should be cleansed and anesthetized. Skin anesthesia can be induced effectively using a topical anesthetic cream (e.g., lidocaine-prilocaine [EMLA]) placed on the selected aspiration site under an occlusive dressing 30 to 45 minutes before the procedure. An 18- or 20-gauge needle attached to a 20-mL syringe is used. If no material is aspirated, 1 to 2 mL of sterile *nonbacteriostatic* saline is injected into the node, and it is reaspirated. The aspirate should be inoculated directly from the syringe onto aerobic (including chocolate agar) and anaerobic media, onto Sabouraud agar (fungi), and into a broth medium suitable for the early detection of mycobacteria, such as the Bactec radiometric assay. In the last-mentioned system, the release of labeled carbon dioxide in an automated ion chamber system can detect mycobacteria 12 to 17 days after inoculation of the broth.[133] Gram and acid-fast stains are mandatory, and their reading serves as a guide to initial antimicrobial therapy.

Polymerase chain reaction assays used to identify tuberculous and nontuberculous mycobacteria have successfully confirmed their presence in gastric aspirates and in specimens obtained from lymph nodes by aspiration or biopsy.[39,45,52,53,131,136] This technique shows great promise in rapidly providing a specific diagnosis, but it is not yet routinely available.

Thioglycolate broth and anaerobically incubated blood agar plates are incapable of providing optimal conditions for the isolation of many anaerobic bacteria.[13] Optimal methods for cultivation of fastidious anaerobes should be employed because anaerobic organisms may be recovered in 20 percent of cases.[24] Cultures of infected skin lesions and exudates on tonsils also should be done, but not to the exclusion of needle aspiration.

Isolation of group A streptococci from the throat or skin cultures of a patient with lymphadenitis does *not* confirm the etiology of the lymph node inflammation. Patients have been noted to have isolation of group A streptococci from throat and of

S. aureus from lymph node aspirate cultures.[13,118] Tuberculin skin tests should be performed. Induration of 15 mm or greater suggests infection with *M. tuberculosis*, whereas reactions of 5 to 14 mm may be caused by either a tuberculous or a nontuberculous mycobacterial infection.[86]

In an attempt to develop a rational approach to the use and interpretation of differential skin testing, Huebner and associates,[60] using tuberculin skin tests and nontuberculous mycobacterial antigens, studied 144 children with chronic cervical adenopathy, of whom 123 had mycobacterial culture results available. The low incidence of tuberculosis within the study population (four cases) precluded making an interpretation regarding the utility of these antigens in distinguishing disease caused by *M. tuberculosis* from that caused by other mycobacteria. Children with culture-confirmed mycobacterial lymphadenopathy had significantly larger reactions to nontuberculous mycobacterial antigens than did children with microscopy-negative and culture-negative results. The study was terminated prematurely because of an unacceptably high incidence of a blistering skin reaction to nontuberculous mycobacterial antigens.

Intradermal skin testing, using a crude extract from affected nodes, historically has been used to establish the diagnosis of cat-scratch disease.[28] A diagnosis usually is reached, however, based on the presence of regional adenopathy, a history of cat exposure (particularly if the patient has a history of a scratch or a primary skin lesion), and negative laboratory studies for other causes of lymphadenopathy. *B. henselae*, the more common etiologic agent of this disease, can be isolated from blood if lysis-centrifugation blood cultures or the Bactec blood culture system is used. Isolates may be identified using a commercially available system (Microscan Rapid Anaerobe Panel; Baxter, Sacramento, CA).[1] Serologic methods for the detection of IgG antibodies to *B. henselae* are available[1,161] and should be considered the gold standard diagnostic method. In few cases, a lymph node biopsy should be undertaken to exclude other, more serious, pathologies.

If, after the aforementioned evaluation, the etiology of adenitis remains uncertain, or lymphadenopathy has persisted with no detectable response to antimicrobial therapy, a more intense diagnostic evaluation is indicated. Studies may include a complete blood count; serology for Epstein-Barr virus, cytomegalovirus, HHV-6, HIV, histoplasmosis, coccidioidomycosis, toxoplasmosis, tularemia, *B. henselae*, and *Brucella*; and a radiograph of the chest. If the diagnosis remains in doubt, and the node persists, enlarges, is hard, or is fixed to the adjacent structures, biopsy *should* be performed. Biopsy material should be submitted for the studies outlined earlier for lymph node aspirate cultures and for routine histology; Giemsa, periodic acid–Schiff, and methenamine silver stains; and, in select cases only, viral cultures. If the histology reveals noncaseating granulomas and the child has a history of cat exposure, the most likely diagnosis is cat-scratch disease,[85,87] and serologic testing is indicated. Sarcoidosis involving lymph nodes would have a similar histology but is rare in children and a condition in which isolated cervical node involvement has not been observed.[64,130]

Older children are more likely to have negative cultures of lymph node aspirates[13,141] and to be more frequent candidates for excisional lymph node biopsy. They also are more likely to have lymphomas. It is important that appropriate tissue be excised, especially from adolescents, so that precise diagnostic interpretation can be done. This interpretation can be facilitated by the proper selection of a lymph node to be biopsied; intact removal of the node chosen; and proper fixation, cutting, and staining of the specimen. If only one node or one anatomic group of nodes is enlarged, the largest node should be excised. If several groups of lymph nodes are involved, the site for biopsy should be selected according to the likelihood of diagnostic yield. Biopsy specimens from the lower neck and supraclavicular area have the highest yields.[67] Other areas, including the upper cervical, submandibular, axillary, and parotid lymph nodes, are much more likely to be affected by reactive hyperplasia, which may or may not be related to the underlying disease process. If lymphoma is suspected, needle biopsies or frozen sections are contraindicated.[18,25]

Even under optimal conditions, many reactive processes, including rheumatoid arthritis, toxoplasmosis, phenytoin-induced adenopathy, dermatopathic adenitis, and infectious mononucleosis, have been noted to simulate lymphoma.[25] Obtaining a thorough history and performing appropriate serologic studies should provide sufficient information for the physician to exclude reactive processes known to simulate lymphoma.

TREATMENT

Optimal management of a child with cervical lymphadenitis depends on an accurate assessment of the underlying etiology. Because almost all cases are associated with infectious agents, every effort should be made to ascertain the etiologic agent so that specific therapy can be initiated. Aspiration of the affected lymph node for Gram and acid-fast stains serves as a guide for initial therapy, and culture and antimicrobial susceptibility form the basis for prescribing specific treatment in patients with bacterial lymphadenitis.[13,35] When the patient presents with typical findings of acute bacterial lymphadenitis, however, empiric therapy may be undertaken without prior needle aspiration. In this situation, close follow-up is essential because failure to show some clinical response after 48 hours of therapy is an indication for this diagnostic procedure to be done.

Acute suppurative cervical lymphadenitis most frequently is caused by infection with S. aureus or group A streptococci.[13,22,35,129,141,159] In nodes that progress to abscess formation, S. aureus is the most frequent agent isolated,[13,35,129] and drainage is mandatory. Because of the frequency of infection caused by S. aureus or group A streptococci, empiric antimicrobial therapy should be directed against these two agents. Penicillinase-resistant penicillins should be used. If the patient requires parenteral therapy and CA-MRSA is not common in the area, oxacillin, nafcillin (150 mg/kg/day), or cefazolin (75 to 100 mg/kg/day) may be used.

When oral therapy is deemed to be adequate, cloxacillin (50 mg/kg/day), dicloxacillin (25 mg/kg/day), or cephalexin (25 to 50 mg/kg/day) is recommended. Augmentin, the fixed combination of amoxicillin and clavulanic acid, provides good activity against methicillin-susceptible staphylococci and streptococci and has an expanded spectrum of activity against the oral anaerobic organisms. These features, combined with its palatability, render it an attractive alternative to the traditional penicillinase-resistant penicillins. Clavulanate-associated diarrhea can be problematic in some children, however. In penicillin-allergic patients, cephalosporins may be used. Once-daily ceftriaxone (50 to 100 mg/kg/day) is an attractive and effective alternative to the parenteral antibiotics that require more frequent administration.

In areas where CA-MRSA is prevalent, clindamycin (30 mg/kg/day) for parenteral or oral use is appropriate for empiric or alternative therapy. In addition to its good activity against anaerobes and methicillin-susceptible S. aureus, clindamycin is effective against most CA-MRSA isolates. Because of reports that clindamycin resistance is increasing among CA-MRSA isolates, however, close clinical follow-up to ensure a therapeutic response has been achieved is mandatory when clindamycin therapy is chosen.[42,59,61,63,99] In a severely ill child needing hospitalization or with signs of airway compromise, vancomycin (45 mg/kg/day) is appropriate in combination with another agent until culture results are obtained. Trimethoprim-sulfamethoxazole (10 mg/kg/day of the trimethoprim component) is an alternative choice for oral therapy of CA-MRSA infections[42,59,61,99] but should

not be used initially because it is not active against group A streptococci.

Antibiotic therapy may need to be modified if an obvious primary focus of infection suggests a different etiologic agent. In a patient with periodontal or dental disease, adequate anaerobic activity is mandatory, and therapy with penicillin V (50 mg/kg/day), augmentin (40 mg/kg/day), or clindamycin (30 mg/kg/day) should be initiated, pending results of cultures.

Patients with marked lymph node enlargement, moderate to severe systemic symptoms, or concomitant cellulitis frequently require parenteral therapy for the first few days. This therapy allows for a high concentration of the antimicrobial agent within the inflamed tissue and may promote more rapid localization, especially in patients with staphylococcal adenitis. Although the use of parenteral drugs has to be individualized, most infants and children with staphylococcal or streptococcal lymphadenitis respond to orally administered antimicrobials.

Adenitis caused by group A streptococci should be treated with penicillin G (100,000 IU/kg/day) or penicillin V (50 mg/kg/day) for a total of 10 days. In a child with penicillin allergy, erythromycin ethyl succinate (40 mg/kg/day) or cephalexin (25 to 50 mg/kg/day) may be used. Both drugs have been shown to be effective in the treatment of cervical lymphadenitis.[13,22] Treatment should be continued for at least 10 days or approximately 5 days after signs of local inflammation and systemic toxicity have disappeared, whichever is longer. If required, analgesics should be given and not overlooked in infants and children too young to verbalize their discomfort. The average duration of antibiotic therapy is 10 days, unless abscess formation occurs late in the first or early in the second week of treatment.[13] In this situation, incision and drainage are indicated,[13,23,35] and therapy should be continued until resolution of the acute process occurs, usually within another 5 to 7 days.

Some clinical improvement is to be expected within 48 hours after initiation of therapy and is manifested by a decrease in inflammation and tenderness of the lymph node and a decrease in the maximum daily temperature. The size of the lymph node may not show evidence of regression at this stage, and total resolution of fever should not be expected. It is important to record accurate measurements of the node at the time of presentation because a subjective evaluation is an unreliable indicator of lymph node evolution during therapy. If no clinical improvement is noted by 48 hours, needle aspiration is recommended. The history and physical examination should be reassessed, and a more detailed laboratory evaluation should be initiated.

In a study of 284 children admitted to the hospital with acute cervical adenitis, age younger than 1 year and node involvement for more than 48 hours before admission predicted the need for node aspiration.[81] Regression of the size of a lymph node is slow, usually requiring 4 to 6 weeks or more. Persistence of significant enlargement beyond 6 to 8 weeks, even in the face of good initial response to antimicrobial therapy, demands that an underlying disorder be excluded. When signs of acute inflammation have resolved, prolonged antimicrobial therapy is of little value because penetration of antimicrobials through the fibrous capsule of the node is poor.[22] Spontaneous regression occurs in most patients, although it may require several weeks. Uncommonly, reactivation of inflammation may occur, and a meticulous search for an untreated primary source of bacterial infection, such as secondarily infected dermatitis, infestation, foreign body, or dental abscess, should be undertaken. Re-treatment should include specific measures to eliminate the predisposing condition.

If Gram stain of the lymph node aspirate suggests a microorganism other than S. aureus or group A streptococci, initial antimicrobial therapy should be directed at the most likely agent until culture results are known. Because attempts to perform careful Gram stains and careful anaerobic cultures of lymph node aspirates in most reported series have been limited, the large number of infants and children with sterile aspirates may be attributed partly to a failure to isolate fastidious anaerobes indigenous to the mouth. These microorganisms should respond to penicillin G therapy. For penicillin-resistant organisms, clindamycin is a useful alternative drug.

For infants in the first 2 months of life, group B streptococci and *S. aureus* are important pathogens to consider in selecting initial therapy. Penicillinase-resistant penicillins are active against both agents, unless the occurrence of CA-MRSA is frequent, in which case clindamycin or vancomycin should be considered for initial therapy. If group B streptococci are isolated, penicillin G can be substituted. Final bacteriologic identification and antimicrobial susceptibility tests should be the ultimate guide to selecting specific antimicrobial therapy in all patients. Treatment of cervical lymph node infections associated with rarely encountered bacteria, fungi, and parasites listed in Table 15-3 is discussed under those specific disease entities.

Although controversy exists as to whether cervical adenitis associated with *M. tuberculosis* in a child is truly a localized process, only rarely do patients have disseminated infection.[36,51,106] When infection is not localized, pulmonary or hilar lymph node involvement is a common finding.[36,65,107,159] A 2-month regimen of isoniazid (10 mg/kg/day), rifampin (15 to 20 mg/kg/day), pyrazinamide (30 mg/kg/day), and ethambutol (15 mg/kg/day) is recommended for the treatment of uncomplicated pulmonary tuberculosis or isolated cervical lymphadenitis in children. Triple therapy is given daily for the first 2 months of therapy, after which isoniazid and rifampin are administered, either daily or on a twice-weekly basis, for the ensuing 4 months. Directly observed therapy is preferred.[6]

In areas where multiple-drug resistance in *M. tuberculosis* is prevalent, streptomycin (20 to 40 mg/kg/day) or another aminoglycoside (kanamycin, amikacin, or capreomycin) is added for initial treatment until drug susceptibilities are known.[6] The addition of a fifth drug should occur after consultation with an expert in the field because these drugs may have toxic effects, and careful assessment of the risks and benefits is warranted. Detailed discussion of the treatment of tuberculosis in children is provided in Chapter 107. Response to antituberculous therapy is usual, with rapid resolution of symptoms and marked regression of lymph nodes within 3 months. Nodes remain palpable for months, however, because scarring and fibrosis are regular accompaniments to resolution of disease. Draining sinuses, a common complication of lymph node aspiration or incision, and drainage before the advent of effective antituberculous chemotherapy no longer develop.[107]

Cervical lymphadenitis attributed to nontuberculous mycobacteria is much more common in a young child than that caused by *M. tuberculosis*. These microorganisms exhibit in vitro resistance to commonly employed antituberculous drugs. Resistance particularly is common among *M. scrofulaceum* and *M. intracellulare*. Surgical excision is the treatment of choice for nontuberculous mycobacterial lymphadenitis,* and total removal of all the visibly affected nodes is recommended.[4,8,30,56,112,114,120,126,155] Early (within 1 month of onset) removal of affected nodes was associated significantly with better esthetic results in one series.[83] Thorough curettage has been found to be effective,[84,106] but results in higher relapse rates.[43]

Antimicrobial therapy alone is less effective.[90] The new macrolides clarithromycin and azithromycin, rifampin and its analogue rifabutin, ethambutol, amikacin, and cefoxitin show activity against nontuberculous mycobacteria.[38,143] Clarithromycin monotherapy and combination therapy with clarithromycin and ethambutol or rifampin have had some success in the treatment of nontuberculous lymphadenitis.[17,50,58,79,80,84,145] In the

largest retrospective case series, 22 children received clarithromycin either alone or in combination with other antimycobacterial agents without surgery, and only one recurrence was documented.[80]

In another study, 10 children (7 of whom had initial incision and drainage or aspiration) were treated for 1 to 14 months with a regimen of clarithromycin (20 to 30 mg/kg/day) in combination with ethambutol (12.5 to 19 mg/kg/day) or rifampin (6 to 20 mg/kg/day). Five children were cured; the remainder needed further surgical procedures.[58] Six of seven patients treated for 6 months in another series had not relapsed after a mean follow-up of 3 years.[79] Rifabutin was used in all children in this study, resulting in side effects in four (neutropenia, yellow skin pigmentation), which disappeared after dose reduction. In HIV-infected children receiving protease inhibitors, rifabutin generally is contraindicated, but it can be given at a much reduced dosage (indinavir or nelfinavir is the preferred protease inhibitor) if deemed necessary.[8]

Despite the lack of prospective studies, macrolide-containing regimens are promising options for the treatment of nontuberculous mycobacterial adenitis for which complete excision of the affected node would endanger the facial nerve or its branches, or if a reduction in size of the swelling would facilitate a complete and esthetic excision at a later stage. The optimal duration of therapy is unknown, but regimens of 4 to 6 months or longer are usual. Expert opinion should be sought, especially as new mycobacterial species are described. Currently, macrolide (clarithromycin or azithromycin) monotherapy or combination therapy should be viewed as a valuable adjunct when surgery is not feasible or is refused.

Cat-scratch disease usually is a benign, self-limited disorder requiring no specific therapy. The use of antimicrobials is controversial, but rifampin, trimethoprim-sulfamethoxazole, azithromycin, ciprofloxacin, and parenteral gentamicin may be useful in promoting fever defervescence and in clinical resolution of systemic cat-scratch disease.[7,9,14,89] If the lymph node progresses to fluctuance, needle aspiration may hasten resolution and relieve discomfort. Surgical excision may be required in a few patients who have persistent problems despite having needle aspiration, or who develop draining sinuses.

PROGNOSIS

With effective antimicrobial therapy, complete resolution of cervical lymphadenitis caused by *S. aureus*, group A streptococci, and *M. tuberculosis* is the rule. Delay in establishing the diagnosis or initiating therapy may prolong the clinical course and may result in complications or sequelae, such as sinus tracts (mycobacteria),[19,33,107] abscess formation,[23] cellulitis or bacteremia (*S. aureus* and *S. pyogenes*),[13] acute glomerulonephritis (group A streptococci),[35] disseminated disease (*M. tuberculosis*),[65] or mycotic carotid artery aneurysm.[154] Except for abscess formation, these complications are rare events. Although lymph node infection caused by *S. aureus* is more likely to result in abscess formation, at least one study has noted a significantly greater duration of infection before treatment in patients in whom *S. aureus* was isolated from the abscess cavity cultures.[13] The extracellular products of this organism (e.g., coagulase, fibrinolysin, hyaluronidase) partly explain its propensity for abscess formation, which may occur in 50 to 70 percent of patients.[23,35,157]

Even in patients whose course is complicated by suppuration, appropriate drainage in conjunction with specific antimicrobial therapy results in prompt resolution of signs and symptoms, and relapse occurs only rarely. Today, surgical excision of affected nodes seldom is recommended except when the disease is caused by nontuberculous mycobacteria, in which case surgical excision remains the treatment of choice. Antimicrobial therapy has been

---

*See references 8, 38, 43, 83, 88, 112, 114, 120, 137, 142.

responsible for the disappearance of the events commonly associated with cervical adenitis historically, including thrombosis of the internal jugular vein, rupture of the carotid artery, generalized septic embolic phenomena, mediastinal abscess, purulent pericarditis, and even death.[68,140,157]

With the advent of effective antituberculous agents, the prognosis for tuberculous cervical or adenitis also is excellent. When surgical excision is performed early in the course of lymphadenitis caused by nontuberculous mycobacterial infection, resolution can be anticipated.[43,83,112,120,126,137] Persistent and recurrent disease is the most frequent complication encountered.[155] Macrolide monotherapy and combination therapy are useful in ameliorating these complications or in cases for which surgery is not feasible.[114,137] Cat-scratch disease usually is a benign, self-limited disorder only rarely requiring therapeutic intervention, such as needle aspiration, to relieve pain.

PREVENTION

Providing appropriate medical and, occasionally, surgical therapy of predisposing conditions (e.g., dental caries, abscess, group A streptococcal pharyngitis or nasopharyngitis, purulent otitis media, impetigo, other infections involving the face and scalp) and minimizing the exposure of infants and children to adults with active tuberculosis should reduce the incidence of cervical lymphadenitis. Some authors suggest that decreased exposure to animals may result in fewer infections,[13] especially for adenitis attributed to toxoplasmosis or *Bartonella*.[29,121]

REFERENCES

1. Adal, K. A., Cockerell, C. J., and Petri, W. A., Jr.: Cat scratch disease, bacillary angiomatosis, and other infections due to *Rochalimaea*. N. Engl. J. Med. *330*:1509-1515, 1994.
2. Ahuja, A. T., Ying, M., Ho, S. S., and Metreweli, C.: Distribution of intranodal vessels in differentiating benign from metastatic neck nodes. Clin. Radiol. *56*:197-201, 2001.
3. Akashi, K., Eizuru, Y., Sumiyoshi, Y., et al. Brief report: Severe infectious mononucleosis-like syndrome and primary human herpes 6 infection in an adult. N. Engl. J. Med. *329*:168-171, 1993.
4. Altman, R. P., and Margileth, A. M.: Cervical lymphadenopathy from atypical mycobacteria: Diagnosis and surgical treatment. J. Pediatr. Surg. *10*:419-422, 1975.
5. Alvi, A., and Myssiorek, D.: *Mycobacterium chelonae* causing recurrent neck abscess. Pediatr. Infect. Dis. J. *12*:617-618, 1993.
6. American Academy of Pediatrics: Tuberculosis. *In* Pickering, L. K., Baker, C. J., Long, S. S., and McMillan, J. A. (eds.): Red Book: 2006 Report of the Committee on Infectious Diseases. 27th ed. Elk Grove Village, IL: American Academy of Pediatrics, 2006, pp. 678-698.
7. American Academy of Pediatrics: Cat-scratch disease. *In* Pickering, L. K., Baker, C. J., Long, S. S., and McMillan, J. A. (eds.): Red Book: 2006 Report of the Committee on Infectious Diseases. 27th ed. Elk Grove Village, IL: American Academy of Pediatrics, 2006, pp. 246-248.
8. American Academy of Pediatrics: Diseases caused by nontuberculous mycobacteria. *In* Pickering, L. K., Baker, C. J., Long, S. S., and McMillan, J. A. (eds.): Red Book: 2006 Report of the Committee on Infectious Diseases. 27th ed. Elk Grove Village, IL: American Academy of Pediatrics, 2006, pp. 698-704.
9. Arisoy, E. S., Correa, A. G., Wagner, M. L., et al.: Hepatosplenic cat-scratch disease in children: Selected clinical features and treatment. Clin. Infect. Dis. *28*:778-784, 1999.
10. Armstrong, K. L., James, R. W., and Dawson, D. J., et al.: *Mycobacterium haemophilum* causing perihilar or cervical lymphadenitis in healthy children. J. Pediatr. *121*:202-205, 1992.
11. Baker, C. J.: Group B streptococcal cellulitis-adenitis in infants. Am. J. Dis. Child. *136*:631-633, 1982.
12. Bankaci, M., Morris, R. F., Stool, S. E., et al.: Sinus histiocytosis with massive lymphadenopathy: Report of its occurrence in two siblings with retropharyngeal involvement in both. Ann. Otol. Rhinol. Laryngol. *87*:327-331, 1978.
13. Barton, L. L., and Feigin, R. D.: Childhood cervical lymphadenitis: A reappraisal. J. Pediatr. *84*:846-852, 1974.
14. Bass, J. W., Freitas, B. C., Freitas, A. D., et al.: Prospective randomized double blind placebo-controlled evaluation of azithromycin for treatment of cat-scratch disease. Pediatr. Infect. Dis. J. *17*:447-452, 1998.
15. Bell, D. M., Morens, D. M., Holman, R. C., et al.: Kawasaki syndrome in the United States. Am. J. Dis. Child. *137*:211-214, 1983.
16. Bennhoff, D. F.: Actinomycosis: Diagnostic and therapeutic considerations and a review of 32 cases. Laryngoscope *94*:1198-1217, 1984.
17. Berger, C., Pfyffer, G. E., and Nadal, D.: Treatment of nontuberculous mycobacterial lymphadenitis with clarithromycin plus rifabutin. J. Pediatr. *128*:383-386, 1996.
18. Betsill, W. L., Jr., and Hajdu, S. I.: Percutaneous aspiration biopsy of lymph nodes. Am. J. Clin. Pathol. *73*:471-479, 1980.
19. Black, B. G., and Chapman, J. S.: Cervical adenitis in children due to human and unclassified mycobacteria. Pediatrics *33*:887-893, 1984.
20. Braun, M. M., and Cauthen, G.: Relationship of the human immunodeficiency virus epidemic to pediatric tuberculosis and bacillus Calmette-Guérin immunization. Pediatr. Infect. Dis. J. *11*:220-227, 1992.
21. Bronzwaer, S. L., Buchholz, U., Kool, J. L., et al.: EARSS activities and results: Update. Eur. Surveill. *6*:2-5, 2001.
22. Brook, A. H., and Winter, G. B.: Cervico-facial suppurative lymphadenitis due to staphylococcal infection in childhood. Br. J. Oral Surg. *8*:257-263, 1971.
23. Brook, A. H., and Winter, G. B.: Staphylococcal cervico-facial lymphadenitis in children. Lancet *2*:660-661, 1972.
24. Brook, I.: Aerobic and anaerobic bacteriology of cervical adenitis in children. Clin. Pediatr. *19*:693-696, 1980.
25. Butler, J. J.: Non-neoplastic lesions of lymph nodes of man to be differentiated from lymphomas. Natl. Cancer Inst. Monogr. *32*:233-249, 1969.
26. Carithers, H. A.: Oculoglandular disease of Parinaud: A manifestation of cat-scratch disease. Am. J. Dis. Child. *132*:1195-1200, 1978.
27. Carithers, H. A.: Cat-scratch disease associated with an osteolytic lesion. Am. J. Dis. Child. *137*:968-970, 1983.
28. Carithers, H. A.: Cat-scratch disease: An overview based on a study of 1200 patients. Am. J. Dis. Child. *139*:1124-1133, 1985.
29. Carithers, H. A., Carithers, C. M., and Edwards, R. O., Jr.: Cat-scratch disease: Its natural history. J. A. M. A. *207*:312-316, 1969.
30. Castro, D. J., Hoover, L., Castro, D. J., et al.: Cervical mycobacterial lymphadenitis. Arch. Otolaryngol. *111*:816-819, 1985.
31. Centers for Disease Control and Prevention: Trends in tuberculosis—United States, 2005. M. M. W. R. Morb. Mortal. Wkly. Rep. *55*:305-308, 2006.
32. Centers for Disease Control and Prevention: Emergence of *Mycobacterium tuberculosis* with extensive resistance to second-line drugs—worldwide, 2000-2004. M. M. W. R. Morb. Mortal. Wkly. Rep. *55*:301-305, 2006.
33. Chapman, J. S., and Guy, L. R.: Scrofula caused by atypical mycobacteria. Pediatrics *23*:323-331, 1959.
34. Chuang, C. H., Yan, D. C., Chiu, C. H., et al.: Clinical and laboratory manifestations of Kikuchi's disease in children and differences between patients with and without prolonged fever. Pediatr. Infect. Dis. J. *24*:551-554, 2005.
35. Dajani, A. S., Garcia, R. E., and Wolinsky, E.: Etiology of cervical lymphadenitis in children. N. Engl. J. Med. *268*:1329-1333, 1963.
36. Davis, S. D., and Comstock, G. W.: Mycobacterial cervical adenitis in children. J. Pediatr. *58*:771-778, 1961.
37. De Baere, T., Moerman, M., Rigouts, L., et al.: *Mycobacterium interjectum* as causative agent of cervical lymphadenitis. J. Clin. Microbiol. *39*:725-727, 2001.
38. Diagnosis and treatment of disease caused by nontuberculous mycobacteria. This official statement of the American Thoracic Society was approved by the Board of Directors, March 1997. Medical Section of the American Lung Association. Am. J. Respir. Crit. Care Med. *156*:S1-25, 1997.
39. El Amin, N. M., Hanson, H. S., Petterson, B., et al.: Identification of nontuberculous mycobacteria: 16S rRNA gene sequence analysis vs. conventional methods. Scand. J. Infect. Dis. *32*:47-50, 2000.
40. English, C. K., Wear, D. J., Margileth, A. M., et al.: Cat-scratch disease: Isolation and culture of the bacterial agent. J. A. M. A. *259*:1347-1352, 1988.
41. Evans, A. K., and Cunningham, M. J.: Atypical mycobacterial cervicofacial lymphadenitis in children: A disease as old as mankind, yet a persistent challenge. Am. J. Otolaryngol. *26*:337-343, 2005.
42. Fergie, J. E., and Purcell, K.: Community-acquired methicillin-resistant *Staphylococcus aureus* infections in South Texas children. Pediatr. Infect. Dis. J. *20*:860-863, 2001
43. Flint, D., Mahadevan, M., Barber, C., et al.: Cervical lymphadenitis due to non-tuberculous mycobacteria: Surgical treatment and review. Int. J. Pediatr. Otorhinolaryngol. *53*:187-194, 2000.
44. Fluegge, K., Greiner, P., and Berner, R.: Late onset group B streptococcal disease manifested by isolated cervical lymphadenitis. Arch. Dis. Child. *88*:1019-1020, 2003.
45. Frevel, T., Schafer, K. L., Totsch, M., et al.: PCR based detection of mycobacteria in paraffin wax embedded material routinely processed for morphologic examination. J. Clin. Pathol. *52*:283-288, 1999.
46. Fujimori, T., Shioda, K., and Sussman, E. B.: Subacute necrotising lymphadenitis: A clinicopathologic study. Acta Pathol. Jpn. *31*:791-797, 1981.
47. Gill, M. J., Fanning, E. A., and Chomyc, S.: Childhood lymphadenitis in a harsh northern climate due to atypical mycobacteria. Scand. J. Infect. Dis. *19*:77-83, 1987.
48. Gona, P., Van Dyle, R. B., Williams, P. L., et al.: Incidence of opportunistic and other infections in HIV-infected children in the HAART era. J. A. M. A. *296*:292-300, 2006.

49. Gorak, E. J., Yamada, S. M., and Brown, J. D.: Community-acquired methicillin-resistant *Staphylococcus aureus* in hospitalized adults and children without known risk factors. Clin. Infect. Dis. 29:797-800, 1999.

50. Green, P. A., von Reyn, C. F., and Smith, R. P., Jr.: *Mycobacterium avium* complex parotid lymphadenitis: Successful therapy with clarithromycin and ethambutol. Pediatr. Infect. Dis. J. 12:615-617, 1993.

51. Gutman, L. T., Moye, J., Zimmer, B., et al.: Tuberculosis in human immunodeficiency virus-exposed or -infected United States children. Pediatr. Infect. Dis. J. 13:963-968, 1994.

52. Haas, W. H., Amthor, B., Engelmann, G., et al.: Preoperative diagnosis of *Mycobacterium avium* lymphadenitis in two immunocompetent children by polymerase chain reaction of gastric aspirates. Pediatr. Infect. Dis. J. 17:1016-1020, 1998.

53. Haase, G., Kentrup, H., Skopnik, H., et al.: *Mycobacterium lentiflavum*: An etiologic agent of cervical lymphadenitis. Clin. Infect. Dis. 25:1245-1246, 1997.

54. Haber, H. P., Warmann, S. W., and Fuchs, J.: Cervical atypical mycobacterial lymphadenitis in childhood: Findings on sonography. Ultraschall. Med. 27:462-466, 2006.

55. Hall, C. B., Long, C. E., Schnabel, K. C., et al.: Human herpesvirus-6 infection in children. N. Engl. J. Med. 331:432-438, 1994.

56. Harris, B. H., Webb, W., Wilkinson, A. H., et al.: Mycobacterial lymphadenitis. J. Pediatr. Surg. 17:589-590, 1982.

57. Hazra, R., Floyd, M. M., Sloutsky, A., et al.: Novel mycobacterium related to *Mycobacterium triplex* as a cause of cervical lymphadenitis. J. Clin. Microbiol. 39:1227-1230, 2001.

58. Hazra, R., Robson, C. D., Perez-Atayde, A. R., et al.: Lymphadenitis due to nontuberculous mycobacteria in children: Presentation and response to therapy. Clin. Infect. Dis. 28:123-129, 1999.

59. Herold, B. C., Immergluck, L. C., Maranan, M. C., et al.: Community-acquired methicillin-resistant *Staphylococcus aureus* in children with no identified predisposing risk. J. A. M. A. 279:593-598, 1998.

60. Huebner, R. E., Schein, M. F., Cauthen, G. M., et al.: Usefulness of skin testing with mycobacterial antigens in children with cervical lymphadenopathy. Pediatr. Infect. Dis. J. 11:450-456, 1992.

61. Hulten, K. G., Kaplan, S. L., Gonzalez, B. E., et al.: Three-year surveillance of community onset health care-associated *Staphylococcus aureus* infections in children. Pediatr. Infect. Dis. J. 25:349-353, 2006.

62. Jaffe, B. F.: Pediatric head and neck tumors: A study of 178 cases. Laryngoscope 83:1644-1651, 1973.

63. Kaplan, S. L., Hulten, K. G., Gonzalez, B. E., et al.: Three-year surveillance of community-acquired *Staphylococcus aureus* infections in children. Clin. Infect. Dis. 40:1785-1791, 2005.

64. Kendig, E. L. Jr.: The clinical picture of sarcoidosis in children. Pediatrics 54:289-292, 1974.

65. Kent, D. C: Tuberculous lymphadenitis: Not a localized disease process. Am. J. Med. Sci. 254:866-873, 1967.

66. Knight, P. J., Hamoudi, A. B., and Vassy, L. E.: The diagnosis and treatment of midline neck masses in children. Surgery 93:603-611, 1983.

67. Knight, P. J., Mulne, A. F., and Vassy, L. E.: When is lymph node biopsy indicated in children with enlarged peripheral nodes? Pediatrics 69:391-396, 1982.

68. Kratz, R. C., Stine, F. A., Grover, J. W., et al.: Suppurations of the neck. Arch. Otolaryngol. 70:692-695, 1959.

69. Lai, K. K., Stottmeier, K. D., Sherman, I. H., et al.: Mycobacterial cervical lymphadenopathy: Relation of etiologic agents to age. J. A. M. A. 251:1286-1288, 1984.

70. Lampe, R. M., Baker, C. J., Septimus, E. J., et al.: Cervicofacial nocardiosis in children. J. Pediatr. 99:593-595, 1981.

71. Lee, K. Y., Yeon, Y. H., and Lee, B. C.: Kikuchi-Fujimoto disease with prolonged fever in children. Pediatrics 114:e752-e756, 2004.

72. Leong, S. C. L., Karkos, P. D., and Apostolidou, M. T.: Is there a role for the otolaryngologist in PFAPA syndrome? A systematic review. Int. J. Pediatr. Otorhinolaryngol. 70:1841-1845, 2006.

73. Lin, H. C., Su, C. Y., and Huang, S. C.: Kikuchi's disease in Asian children. Pediatrics 115:e92-e96, 2005.

74. Lincoln, E. M., Gilbert, L. A.: Disease in children due to mycobacteria other than *Mycobacterium tuberculosis*. Am. Rev. Respir. Dis. 105:683-714, 1972.

75. Lind, A., Larsson, L. O., Bentzon, M. W., et al.: Sensitivity to sensitins and tuberculin in Swedish children, I: A study of school-children in an urban area. Tubercle 72:29-36, 1991.

76. Lindeboom, J. A., Kuijper, E. J., Prins, J. M., et al.: Tuberculin skin testing is useful in the screening for nontuberculous mycobacterial cervicofacial lymphadenitis in children. Clin. Infect. Dis. 43:1547-1551, 2006.

77. Lindeboom, J. A., Smets, A. M., Kuijper, E. J., et al.: The sonographic characteristics of nontuberculous mycobacterial cervicofacial lymphadenitis in children. Pediatr. Radiol. 36:1063-1067, 2006.

78. Lockhart, R. D., Hamilton, G. F., and Fyfe, F. W.: Anatomy of the Human Body. Philadelphia, J. B. Lippincott, 1959, pp. 662-664.

79. Losurdo, G., Castagnola, E., Cristino, E., et al.: Cervical lymphadenitis caused by nontuberculous mycobacteria in immunocompetent children: Clinical and therapeutic experience. Head Neck 20:245-249, 1998.

80. Luong, A., McClay, J. E., Hasan, S. J., et al.: Antibiotic therapy for nontuberculous mycobacterial cervicofacial lymphadenitis. Laryngoscope 115:1746-1751, 2005.

81. Luu, T. M., Chevalier, I., Gauthier, M., et al.: Acute adenitis in children: Clinical course and factors predictive of surgical drainage. J. Paediatr. Child. Health 41:273-277, 2005.

82. Lyon, L. W.: Neurologic manifestations of cat-scratch disease: Report of a case and review of the literature. Arch. Neurol. 25:23-27, 1971.

83. Maltezou, H. C., Spyridis, P., and Kafetzis, D: Nontuberculous mycobacterial lymphadenitis in children. Pediatr. Infect. Dis. J. 18:968-970, 1999.

84. Mandell, D. L., Wald, E. R., Michaels, M. G., et al.: Management of nontuberculous mycobacterial cervical lymphadenitis. Arch. Otolaryngol. Head Neck Surg. 129:341-344, 2003.

85. Margileth, A. M.: Cat scratch disease: Nonbacterial regional lymphadenitis: The study of 145 patients and a review of the literature. Pediatrics 42:803-818, 1968.

86. Margileth, A. M.: The use of purified protein derivative mycobacterial skin test antigens in children and adolescents: Purified protein derivative skin test results correlated with mycobacterial isolates. Pediatr. Infect. Dis. J. 2:225-231, 1983.

87. Margileth, A. M.: Cat-scratch disease update. Am. J. Dis. Child. 138:711-713, 1984.

88. Margileth, A. M.: Management of nontuberculous (atypical) mycobacterial infections in children and adolescents. Pediatr. Infect. Dis. J. 4:119-121, 1985.

89. Margileth, A. M.: Antibiotic therapy for cat-scratch disease: Clinical study of therapeutic outcome in 268 patients and a review of the literature. Pediatr. Infect. Dis. J. 11:474-478, 1992.

90. Margileth, A. M., Chandra, R., and Altman, R. P.: Chronic lymphadenopathy due to mycobacterial infection: Clinical features, diagnosis, histopathology, and management. Am. J. Dis. Child. 138:917-921, 1984.

91. Margileth, A. M., Wear, D. J., Hadfield, T. L., et al.: Cat-scratch disease: Bacteria in skin at the primary inoculation site. J. A. M. A. 252:928-931, 1984.

92. Marshall, G. S., Edwards, K. M., Butler, J., et al.: Syndrome of periodic fever, pharyngitis, and aphthous stomatitis. J. Pediatr. 110:43-46, 1987.

93. McCabe, R. E., Brooks, R. G., Dorfman, R. F., et al.: Clinical spectrum in 107 cases of toxoplasmic lymphadenopathy. Rev. Infect. Dis. 9:754-774, 1987.

94. Medina, M., Goldfarb, J., Traquinna, D., et al.: Cervical adenitis and deep neck infection caused by *Streptococcus pneumoniae*. Pediatr. Infect. Dis. J. 16:823-824, 1997.

95. Melish, M. E., Hicks, R. V., and Reddy, R.: Kawasaki syndrome: An update. Hosp. Pract. 17:99-105, 1982.

96. Moritz, J. D., Ludwig, A., and Oestmann, J. W.: Contrast-enhanced color Doppler sonography for evaluation of enlarged cervical lymph nodes in head and neck tumors. A. J. R. Am. J. Roentgenol. 174:1279-1284, 2000.

97. Moussatos, G. H., and Baffes, T. G.: Cervical masses in infants and children. Pediatrics 32:251-256, 1963.

98. Na, D. G., Lim, H. K., Byun, H. S., et al.: Differential diagnosis of cervical lymphadenopathy: Usefulness of color Doppler sonography. A. J. R. Am. J. Roentgenol. 168:1311-1316, 1997.

99. Naimi, T. S., LeDell, K. H., Boxrud, D. J., et al.: Epidemiology and clonality of community-acquired methicillin-resistant *Staphylococcus aureus* in Minnesota, 1996-1998. Clin. Infect. Dis. 33:990-996, 2001.

100. Nambiar, S., Chandra, R. S., Schwartz, R. H., et al.: Seven-year-old Indian girl with fever and cervical lymphadenitis: Kikuchi-Fujimoto disease. Pediatr. Infect. Dis. J. 20:464-465, 2001.

101. Naidu, S. I., Donepudi, S. K., Stocks, R. M. S., et al.: Methicillin-resistant *Staphylococcus aureus* as a pathogen in deep neck abscesses: A pediatric case series. Int. J. Pediatr. Otorhinolaryngol. 69:1367-1371, 2005.

102. Nylen, O., Berg-Kelly, K., and Andersson, B.: Cervical lymph node infections with non-tuberculous mycobacteria in preschool children: Interferon gamma deficiency as a possible cause of clinical infection. Acta Paediatr. 89:1322-1325, 2000.

103. O'Brien, D. P., Currie, B. J., and Krause, V. L.: Nontuberculous mycobacterial disease in Northern Australia: A case series and review of the literature. Clin. Infect. Dis. 31:958-968, 2000.

104. O'Brien, R. J., Geiter, L. J., and Snider, D. E., Jr.: The epidemiology of nontuberculous mycobacterial diseases in the United States. Am. Rev. Respir. Dis. 135:1007-1014, 1987.

105. Oguz, F., Mujgan, S., Alper, G., et al.: Treatment of bacillus Calmette Guérin associated lymphadenitis. Pediatr. Infect. Dis. J. 11:87, 1992.

106. Olson, N. R.: Nontuberculous mycobacterial infections of the face and neck: Practical considerations. Laryngoscope 91:1714-1726, 1981.

107. Ord, R. J., and Matz, G. J.: Tuberculous cervical lymphadenitis. Arch. Otolaryngol. 99:327-329, 1974.

108. Ossowski, K., Chun, R. H., Suskind, D., et al.: Increased isolation of methicillin-resistant *Staphylococcus aureus* in pediatric head and neck abscesses. Arch. Otolaryngol. Head Neck Surg. 132:1176-1181, 2006.

109. Padeh, S., Brezniak, N., Zemer, D., et al.: Periodic fever, aphthous stomatitis, pharyngitis, and adenopathy syndrome: Clinical characteristics and outcome. J. Pediatr. 135:98-101, 1999.

110. Palazzi, D. L., McClain, K. L., and Kaplan, S. L.: Hemophagocytic syndrome in children: An important diagnostic consideration in fever of unknown origin. Clin. Infect. Dis. 36:306-312, 2003.

111. Palca, A., Aebi, C., Weimann, R., et al.: *Mycobacterium bohemicum* cervical lymphadenitis. Pediatr. Infect. Dis. J. 21:982-984, 2002.

112. Panesar, J., Higgins, K., Daya, H., et al.: Nontuberculous mycobacterial cervical adenitis: A ten-year retrospective review. Laryngoscope *113*:149-154, 2003.
113. Papakonstantinou, O., Bakantaki, A., Paspalaki, P., et al.: High-resolution and color Doppler ultrasonography of cervical lymphadenopathy in children. Acta Radiol. *42*:470-476, 2001.
114. Perlman, D. C., D'Amico, R., and Salomon, N.: Mycobacterial infections of the head and neck. Curr. Infect. Dis. Rep. *3*:233-241, 2001.
115. Phillips, P., Kwiatkowski, M. B., Copland, M., et al.: Mycobacterial lymphadenitis associated with the initiation of combination antiretroviral therapy. J. AIDS *20*:122-128, 1999.
116. Piersimoni, C., Goteri, G., Nista, D., et al.: *Mycobacterium lentiflavum* as an emerging causative agent of cervical lymphadenitis. J. Clin. Microbiol. *42*:3894-3897, 2004.
117. Pounds, L. A.: Neck masses of congenital origin. Pediatr. Clin. North Am. *28*:841-844, 1981.
118. Powers, G. F., and Boisvert, P. L.: Age as a factor in streptococcosis. J. Pediatr. *25*:481-504, 1944.
119. Prince, D. S., Peterson, D. D., Steiner, R. M., et al.: Infection with *Mycobacterium avium* complex in patients without predisposing conditions. N. Engl. J. Med. *321*:863-868, 1989.
120. Pumberger, W., Hallwirth, U., Pawlowsky, J., et al.: Cervicofacial lymphadenitis due to atypical mycobacteria: A surgical disease. Pediatr. Dermatol. *21*:24-29, 2004.
121. Rafaty, F. M.: Cervical adenopathy secondary to toxoplasmosis. Arch. Otolaryngol. *103*:547-549, 1977.
122. Ridder, G. J., Richter, B., Disko, U., et al.: Gray-scale sonographic evaluation of cervical lymphadenopathy in cat-scratch disease. J. Clin. Ultrasound *29*:140-145, 2001.
123. Robson, C. D., Hazra, R., Barnes, P. D., et al.: Nontuberculous mycobacterial infection of the head and neck in immunocompetent children: CT and MR findings. A. J. N. R. Am. J. Neuroradiol. *20*:1829-1835, 1999.
124. Rosai, J., and Dorfman, R. F.: Sinus histiocytosis with massive lymphadenopathy: A newly recognized benign clinicopathological entity. Arch. Pathol. *87*:63-70, 1969.
125. Ryan-Poirier, K., and Patrick, C. C.: Cervical adenitis caused by *Staphylococcus epidermidis*. J. Clin. Microbiol. *31*:426-427, 1993.
126. Schaad, U. B., Votteler, T. P., McCracken, G. H., et al.: Management of atypical mycobacterial lymphadenitis in childhood: A review based on 380 cases. J. Pediatr. *95*:356-360, 1979.
127. Schroder, K. E., Elverland, H. H., Mair, I. W. S., et al.: Granulomatous cervical lymphadenitis. J. Otolaryngol. *8*:127-131, 1979.
128. Schuit, K. E., and Powell, D. A.: Mycobacterial lymphadenitis in childhood. Am. J. Dis. Child. *132*:675-677, 1978.
129. Scobie, W. G.: Acute suppurative adenitis in children: Review of 964 cases. Scott. Med. J. *14*:352-354, 1969.
130. Siltzbach, L. E., and Greenberg, G. M.: Childhood sarcoidosis: A study of 18 patients. N. Engl. J. Med. *279*:1239-1244, 1968.
131. Singh, K., Muralidar, M., Kumar, A., et al.: Comparison of in house polymerase chain reaction techniques for the detection of *Mycobacterium tuberculosis* DNA in granulomatous lymphadenopathy. J. Clin. Pathol. *53*:355-361, 2000.
132. Smith, H. L., II: Necrotizing lymphadenitis (Kikuchi's disease). Pediatrics *91*:152, 1993.
133. Sommers, H. M., and Good, R. C.: Mycobacterium. *In* Lennette, E. H., Balows, A., Hausler, W. J., Jr., et al. (eds.): Manual of Clinical Microbiology. 4th ed. American Society for Microbiology, Washington, D. C. 1985, pp. 216-240.
134. Spark, R. P., Fried, M. L., Bean, C. K., et al.: Nontuberculous mycobacterial adenitis of childhood. Am. J. Dis. Child. *142*:106-108, 1988.
135. Speert, D. P., Britt, W. J., and Kaplan, E. L.: Tick-borne tularemia presenting as ulcerative lymphadenitis. Clin. Pediatr. *18*:239-241, 1979.
136. Springer, B., Kirschner, P., Rost-Meyer, G., et al.: *Mycobacterium interjectum*, a new species isolated from a patient with chronic lymphadenitis. J. Clin. Microbiol. *31*:3083-3089, 1993.
137. Starke, J. R.: Management of nontuberculous mycobacterial cervical adenitis. Pediatr. Infect. Dis. J. *19*:674-675, 2000.
138. Starke, J. R., and Taylor-Watts, K. T.: Tuberculosis in the pediatric population of Houston, Texas. Pediatrics *84*:28-35, 1989.
139. Stout, J. E., Saharia, K. K., Nageswaran, S., et al.: Racial and ethnic disparities in pediatric tuberculosis in North Carolina. Arch. Pediatr. Adolesc. Med. *160*:631-637, 2006.
140. Stuteville, O. H.: Otorhinolaryngologic surgery: The spread of infections in the head and neck. J. Int. Coll. Surg. *29*:750-754, 1958.
141. Sundaresh, H. P., Kumar, A., Hokanson, J. T., et al.: Etiology of cervical lymphadenitis in children. Am. Fam. Physician *24*:147-151, 1981.
142. Suskind, D. L., Handler, S. D., Tom, L. W. C., et al.: Nontuberculous mycobacterial cervical adenitis. Clin. Pediatr. (Phila.) *36*:403-409, 1997.
143. Tartaglione, T.: Treatment of nontuberculous mycobacterial infections: Role of clarithromycin and azithromycin. Clin. Ther. *19*:626-638, 1997.
144. Tashiro, N., Matsurba, T., Uchida, M., et al.: Ultrasonographic evaluation of cervical lymph nodes in Kawasaki disease. Pediatrics *109*:E77, 2002.
145. Tessier, M.-H., Amoric, J. C., Mechinaud, F., et al.: Clarithromycin for atypical mycobacterial lymphadenitis in nonimmunocompromised children. Lancet *344*:1778, 1994.
146. Thomaidis, T., Anastassea-Vlachou, K., Mandalenaki-Lambrou, C., et al.: Chronic lymphoglandular enlargement and toxoplasmosis in children. Arch. Dis. Child. *52*:403-407, 1977.
147. Thomas, K. T., Feder, H. M., Jr., Lawton, A. R., et al.: Periodic fever syndrome in children. J. Pediatr. *135*:15-21, 1999.
148. Thompson, J. N., Watanabe, M. J., Greene, G. R., et al.: Atypical mycobacterial cervical adenitis: Clinical presentation. Laryngoscope *90*:287-294, 1980.
149. Tomblin, J. L., and Roberts, F. J.: Tuberculous cervical lymphadenitis. Can. Med. Assoc. J. *121*:324-330, 1979.
150. Trinka, L., Dankova, D., and Svandova, E.: Six years experience with the discontinuation of the BCG vaccination, IV: Protective effect of BCG vaccination against *Mycobacterium avium intra-cellulare* complex. Tubercle Lung Dis. *75*:348-352, 1994.
151. Turner, R. R., Martin, J., and Dorfman, R. F.: Necrotizing lymphadenitis: A study of 30 cases. Am. J. Surg. Pathol. *7*:115-123, 1983.
152. Waggoner-Fountain, L. A., Hayden, G. F., and Hendley, J. O.: Kawasaki syndrome masquerading as bacterial lymphadenitis. Clin. Pediatr. *34*:185-189, 1995.
153. Wang, T. J., Yang, Y. H., Lin, Y. T., et al.: Kikuchi-Fujimoto disease in children: Clinical features and disease course. J. Microbiol. Immunol. Infect. *37*:219-224, 2004.
154. Wells, R. G., and Sty, J. R.: Cervical lymphadenitis complicated by mycotic carotid artery aneurysm. Pediatr. Radiol. *21*:402-403, 1991.
155. Wolinsky, E.: Mycobacterial lymphadenitis in children: A prospective study of 105 nontuberculous cases with long-term follow-up. Clin. Infect. Dis. *20*:954-963, 1995.
156. World Health Organization: Vaccine-Preventable Diseases and Immunization: Diphtheria Control. Available at: http://www.euro.who.int/vaccine/20030724_3.
157. Wright, N. L.: Cervical infections. Am. J. Surg. *113*:379-386, 1967.
158. Wu, C. H., Lee, M. M., Huang, K. C., et al.: A probability prediction rule for malignant cervical lymphadenopathy using sonography. Head Neck *22*:223-228, 2000.
159. Yamauchi, T., Ferrieri, P., and Anthony, B. F.: The aetiology of acute cervical adenitis in children: Serological and bacteriological studies. J. Med. Microbiol. *13*:37-43, 1980.
160. Ying, M., Ahuja, A., and Brook, F.: Accuracy of sonographic vascular features in differentiating different causes of cervical lymphadenopathy. Ultrasound Med. Biol. *30*:441-447, 2004.
161. Zangwill, K. M., Hamilton, D. H., Perkins, B. A., et al.: Cat scratch disease in Connecticut: Epidemiology. Risk factors, and evaluation of a new diagnostic test. N. Engl. J. Med. *329*:8-13, 1993.

PAROTITIS

CHAPTER 16

Judith R. Campbell

Parotitis, inflammation of the parotid gland, is caused by a variety of infectious agents and noninfectious systemic illnesses. Several terms are used to describe the clinical presentations and etiologic processes that lead to parotid gland swelling and inflammation. *Suppurative parotitis*, first described in the 1800s, is a serious bacterial infection in neonates and postsurgical patients.[49] *Epidemic parotitis*, particularly prevalent in the pre-vaccine era, was caused primarily by mumps virus infection.[56] In the postvaccine era, this form of parotitis also is caused by other viral pathogens and is referred to as *viral parotitis*. Rarely, a more indolent, slowly progressive, granulomatous infection may occur that is referred to as *granulomatous parotitis*. *Recurrent parotitis of childhood* is a unique illness that is characterized by multiple episodes of acute and subacute parotid gland swelling. The histologic findings in

TABLE 16–1   Predisposing Factors for Parotitis

Drug-Induced Xerostomia
Anticholinergics
Antihistamines
Antidepressants
Phenothiazines
Beta blockers
Diuretics
General anesthesia

Disease-Related Xerostomia
Sjögren syndrome
Diabetes mellitus
Chronic liver disease
Cystic fibrosis

Obstruction
Dental appliances
Oral tumors
Radiation therapy
Trauma

TABLE 16–2   Reported Infectious Etiologies of Parotitis

Aerobic Bacteria
Staphylococcus aureus
Streptococcus pneumoniae
Streptococcus pyogenes
Viridans streptococci
Francisella tularensis
Haemophilus spp.
Moraxella catarrhalis
Pseudomonas aeruginosa
Escherichia coli
Proteus spp.
Salmonella spp.
Klebsiella spp.
Brucella spp.

Anaerobic Bacteria
Peptostreptococcus spp.
Prevotella spp.
Fusobacterium spp.
Actinomyces spp.

Mycobacteria
Mycobacterium tuberculosis
Mycobacterium avium–intracellulare
Other mycobacteria

Viruses
Mumps
Coxsackieviruses A and B
Echoviruses
Epstein-Barr virus
Influenza A
Parainfluenza viruses 1 and 3
Cytomegalovirus
Herpes simplex virus type 1
Human herpesvirus 6
Lymphocytic choriomeningitis virus
Human immunodeficiency virus

this disease include architectural changes in the ducts and chronic inflammation. Many noninfectious systemic illnesses cause persistent or recurrent parotid gland swelling and inflammation, which is referred to as *chronic parotitis*. Bilateral parotid enlargement is a frequent presentation of human immunodeficiency virus (HIV) infection as part of *diffuse infiltrative lymphocytosis syndrome*.

PATHOPHYSIOLOGY

Despite the various agents that cause parotitis, involvement of the gland occurs mainly by three mechanisms. The most common mechanism is a localized infection limited to the gland and surrounding structures. Parotitis may be a manifestation of a systemic infection, as in mumps, or rarely may develop secondary to hematogenous seeding during periods of transient bacteremia. Several common contributing factors and pathophysiologic mechanisms lead to swelling of the gland. The parotid is well encapsulated and consists of superficial and deep lobes that are separated by the facial nerve. The parotid duct (Stensen duct) traverses the buccal soft tissue anteriorly and exits opposite the second upper molar. Thin, watery secretions from the parotid gland cleanse the ductal system and have some bacteriostatic properties, preventing accumulation of bacteria and debris.[36] Factors that predispose individuals to the development of parotitis include side effects of certain drugs and diseases that lead to dehydration, xerostomia, or ductal obstruction (Table 16–1).[36,49] Decreased salivary flow allows retrograde migration of bacteria. Stasis in the ductal system, caused by ductal ectasia, inflammation, calculi, or strictures, allows proliferation of bacteria and inflammation within the gland.

ETIOLOGY

Infectious parotitis may be caused by aerobes, anaerobes, mycobacteria, and viruses (Table 16–2). In all age groups, *Staphylococcus aureus* is the organism most commonly associated with suppurative parotitis.[47,49] Gram-negative pathogens (e.g., *Escherichia coli* and *Klebsiella* and *Pseudomonas* spp.) also may cause suppurative parotitis, particularly in neonates and debilitated or hospitalized patients.[11,31,48,49] The role of anaerobic organisms in this infection has become apparent, especially when poor oral hygiene and oral pathology are associated features.[4,5,39] In cases of recurrent parotitis of childhood, *Streptococcus* spp. are the bacteria most commonly isolated.[21,42,46] Granulomatous parotitis most often is caused by *Mycobacterium tuberculosis* and may occur in the absence of systemic or disseminated tuberculous disease.[36,44,52] Other causes of granulomatous parotitis include *Mycobacterium avium–intracellulare*, *Actinomyces* spp., and gram-negative intracellular organisms (*Francisella tularensis* and *Brucella* spp.).[25,36,59]

In the postvaccine era, the most common viral cause of parotitis still is the paramyxovirus mumps virus. Coxsackieviruses, Epstein-Barr virus, influenza A virus, parainfluenza viruses, adenovirus, human herpes virus–6, herpes simplex virus, cytomegalovirus, and lymphocytic choriomeningitis virus all have been implicated in cases of parotitis.[1,2,16,28,30,32,35,36]

CLINICAL PRESENTATION AND DIAGNOSIS

A detailed history and physical examination are crucial in assisting the clinician in determining the most likely etiology of parotid gland swelling. One should determine the onset and duration of symptoms, their periodicity, and the character of salivary secretions. In addition, the presence of a systemic disease must be excluded. Examination of the parotid gland is achieved best by simultaneous palpation of the intraoral and extraoral salivary structures. Gentle external pressure should be applied to the gland, and the parotid duct should be examined for evidence of purulent secretions or surrounding erythema.

Suppurative parotitis occurs most commonly in neonates or patients with dehydration, poor oral hygiene, malnutrition, immunosuppression, oral trauma, sepsis, or any medication or disease that decreases salivary secretions.[18] Most often, the disease is unilateral; however, bilateral suppurative parotitis may occur in 17 percent of cases.[42] The disease is characterized by acute onset of pain, swelling, warmth, and induration of the involved gland and purulent discharge from the Stensen duct. Associated physical findings include fever, trismus, malaise, and cervical adenitis. In suppurative parotitis, Gram stain and culture (aerobic and anaerobic) of purulent material from the duct can provide a specific microbiologic diagnosis. In addition, elevation of the white blood cell count with a neutrophil predominance may help differentiate this form of parotitis from viral parotitis and parotid disease of a noninfectious etiology.

Mumps is the most common form of viral parotitis and is characterized by a prodrome of fever, malaise, anorexia, and headache. Usually, the following day, unilateral or bilateral earache and parotid tenderness develop. The gland or glands enlarge during the subsequent 2 to 3 days, and the orifice of the Stensen duct is erythematous and swollen, yet secretions from the duct are clear. At the point of maximal swelling, the angle of the jaw is obliterated, and the earlobe is lifted upward and out. The other salivary glands are involved in 10 percent of cases.[42] Rare systemic manifestations of mumps infection include epididymo-orchitis, meningitis, meningoencephalitis, and oophoritis. More recent outbreaks of confirmed and probable mumps emphasize that this infection may occur in highly immunized populations.[6] In 2006, more than 5000 cases of probable mumps were reported to the Centers for Disease Control and Prevention. Of these, 54 percent were laboratory confirmed or linked epidemiologically to a confirmed case. Although the median age was 22 years, patients ranged in age from 1 month to 96 years. Most cases were from the Midwest (Iowa, Kansas, Wisconsin, Illinois, Nebraska, and South Dakota), and many of the patients had received two doses of measles-mumps-rubella (MMR) vaccine.[6]

Other viral agents may produce similar clinical manifestations and can be differentiated from mumps only by culture and hemagglutination inhibition, complement fixation, or enzyme-linked immunosorbent assay serology.[16] In viral parotitis, the white blood cell count may be normal, slightly elevated, or depressed, with a lymphocytic predominance.

Granulomatous parotitis typically manifests as a painless, slowly enlarging mass without surrounding inflammation. It may be misdiagnosed as a slow-growing tumor until the correct diagnosis often is made by biopsy and culture. *M. tuberculosis* and *M. avium–intracellulare* may cause infection in the parenchyma of the gland or in intraglandular or periglandular lymph nodes.[43,59] Clinical evidence of systemic tuberculous disease usually is absent. Parotitis has been observed as an extension of nontuberculous cervical adenitis.[59] Actinomycosis of the parotid gland causes a slowly enlarging, nodular, nontender gland; associated oral or cervicofacial infection usually is present. Fistulas draining yellow or white material with sulfur granules are common findings.[25]

Recurrent parotitis of childhood is rare, with onset that typically occurs before the child reaches 10 years of age and a peak incidence at approximately 6 years of age.[17,42] Some authors hypothesize that an underlying congenital abnormality, such as sialectasis, is a common predisposing feature.[33,43] Others suggest that selective IgA deficiency may be a contributing variable.[19] Clinically, these children experience repeated episodes of fever, pain, and unilateral swelling of the parotid gland. Purulent material often can be expressed from the Stensen duct and, when cultured, often yields streptococcal organisms. Sialography and ultrasound reveal multiple areas of sialectasis throughout the parotid glands bilaterally, even if only one side is symptomatic. The frequency of attacks varies, and each episode of parotitis may last 2 weeks, when it resolves spontaneously.[10] Several authors have noted that recurrences become less frequent with increasing age and that the disease tends to cease at the onset of puberty or early adulthood.[17,42]

HUMAN IMMUNODEFICIENCY VIRUS AND PAROTID ENLARGEMENT

Salivary gland enlargement has been recognized as a common finding in children infected with HIV since before the era of highly active antiretroviral therapy. The prevalence of this manifestation in HIV-infected individuals is 0 to 58 percent.[46] More recently, in a retrospective report of oral lesions in a cohort of HIV-infected children from Brazil, Miziara and colleagues[40] noted the prevalence of parotid gland enlargement to be 7.6 percent. Although parotid enlargement occurred more commonly in children older than 5 years of age, the prevalence did not differ between children who were receiving antiretroviral therapy without protease inhibitors and children who were receiving highly active antiretroviral therapy.

The exact pathophysiology is unknown, but proposed mechanisms include lymphoepithelial cysts, lymph node enlargement within the gland, cytomegalovirus or Epstein-Barr virus infection, and diffuse infiltrative lymphocytosis syndrome of the gland.[46] This entity in HIV-positive children possibly is associated with the HLA-DR5 and HLA-DR11 phenotype, but the significance of this finding is unclear.[27,46,55] Bilateral parotid enlargement frequently is seen as part of diffuse infiltrative lymphocytosis syndrome, which is characterized by proliferation of CD8+ lymphocytes within the circulation and is of unclear etiology. Growth of the parotid is secondary to infiltration of CD8 lymphocytes into the gland, follicular hyperplasia of intraparotid lymphoid tissue (as occurs in lymph nodes throughout the body in HIV infection), and development of diffuse intraparotid, lymphoepithelial cysts.[8,37] Epstein-Barr virus has been proposed as an impetus for CD8 lymphoproliferation because the virus has been isolated from parotid tissue of some affected patients.[9] The absence of positive serology for the virus renders it an unlikely causative agent, however. HIV, which may be the inciting agent, has been detected in dendritic cells, macrophages, and lymphocytes isolated from the parotid glands of affected patients.[9]

Parotid enlargement may be present in 20 to 50 percent of children with HIV infection and acquired immunodeficiency syndrome (AIDS).[29,33,54,57] The median time from birth to development of parotid enlargement is 4.6 years, and often it is the first manifestation of HIV infection acquired during the perinatal period in an otherwise healthy older child.[27,29] HIV-positive children with enlarged parotid glands tend to have a slower progression to death than do HIV-positive children with oral herpes or candidiasis.[29] Usually, both parotid glands are involved, and an affected patient presents with enlarged, tender parotid glands, xerostomia, and increased serum amylase level.[7] Severity of pain and size of the gland tend to fluctuate without apparent cause. This manifestation of HIV infection and AIDS is still commonly seen in developing countries where access to antiretroviral therapy is limited.

The differential diagnoses for parotid enlargement in an HIV-positive patient include viral and bacterial parotitis. Some patients have preexisting xerostomia that may increase their susceptibility to parotitis. In addition, the immunocompromised state of patients with AIDS may predispose them to development of infection of the parotid gland with other agents, such as cytomegalovirus, Epstein-Barr virus, bacteria, mycobacteria, and fungi.[23,51,58,61] Noninfectious etiologies, such as non-Hodgkin lymphoma or Kaposi sarcoma, also should be included in the differential diagnosis of parotid gland enlargement in an HIV-infected patient, although these manifestations usually are observed in adults.

DIFFERENTIAL DIAGNOSIS

Parotitis most often is diagnosed based on clinical presentation, microbiology, serology, and response to empiric therapy. Ultrasound may be useful as a screening tool to prompt more sensitive modalities if the ultrasound scan is abnormal.[41] Computed tomography is most useful in the presence of anatomic defects, radiolucent calculi, or abscess formation in the parotid gland.[50] X-ray sialography is the gold standard in examining the parotid gland ducts; however, sialography is contraindicated in the setting of acute infection. Magnetic resonance sialography is a promising alternative and has several advantages. In contrast to x-ray sialography, magnetic resonance sialography is not contraindicated during acute parotitis and does not require injection of contrast material or involve manipulation of the Stensen duct.[20] Nonetheless, experience with magnetic resonance sialography is limited, and this mode alone may not be sufficiently sensitive to detect tertiary salivary ductules or calculus disease.[20,61]

Noninfectious causes of parotid swelling and inflammation include collagen vascular diseases (Sjögren syndrome and systemic lupus erythematosus), metabolic disorders (hepatic disease, hyperlipoproteinemia, hyperuricemia), endocrine disorders (diabetes mellitus, hypothyroidism), tumors, leukemic infiltration, drugs (antineoplastic chemotherapy), and poisons (iodine).[36,42,47] Sjögren syndrome, the most common cause of noninfectious parotitis, is caused by lymphocyte-mediated destruction of the exocrine glands.[24,47] Patients with this disease have diminished or absent glandular secretions and mucosal dryness; xerostomia and keratoconjunctivitis sicca are prominent clinical features. In addition, the parotid glands are enlarged bilaterally, are firm, and have an irregular contour. Sialography reveals sialectasia, and saliva from these patients has unique biochemical characteristics. Antibodies to nuclear antigens SS-A and SS-B can be detected in the sera of patients with Sjögren syndrome.[47] Patients with chronic noninfectious parotitis have changes in the ductular architecture or strictures that can predispose them to episodes of infectious parotitis.

TREATMENT

Treatment of parotitis includes rehydration, parotid massage, discontinuation of any medications that diminish salivary flow, and sialalogues (e.g., lemon drops, hard candy, chewing gum), which increase salivary flow.[3,36,47,49] In cases of suspected suppurative parotitis, a broad-spectrum antibiotic regimen that is effective against *S. aureus*, *Streptococcus* spp., gram-negative organisms, and anaerobes should be administered empirically, pending specific culture results. Antibiotic regimens frequently employed include penicillinase-resistant penicillins, first-generation cephalosporins, and clindamycin in combination with an aminoglycoside.[3] Vancomycin should be used if MRSA is the likely pathogen. If the patient has been hospitalized for a prolonged period, or if the predominant organisms on Gram stain of the purulent discharge are gram-negative, ceftazidime should be considered as initial empiric therapy.[47,49]

Surgical incision and drainage of purulent fluid are indicated if there is slow or no response to medical therapy or fluctuant increases.[53] The treatment of viral parotitis consists of antipyretics, analgesia, and hydration. In cases of mycobacterial infection, excision of the gland may be required, in addition to administration of specific antimycobacterial therapy.[44,52] Reports have described successful treatment with clarithromycin and azithromycin of parotitis caused by atypical mycobacteria.[22] In contrast, actinomycosis of the parotid gland is managed medically with penicillin G.[25] Children with recurrent parotitis should be treated with antibiotics during acute episodes, but chronic suppressive antimicrobial therapy is not recommended.

Tympanic neurectomy involves severing the parasympathetic secretomotor fibers of the tympanic plexus to the parotid. This procedure attenuates secretion from the gland and relieves sialectasis and further episodes of parotitis in more than 70 percent of patients.[15,45] Only 10 to 20 percent of these patients require parotidectomy for persistence of symptoms beyond puberty.[13] Although it is the optimal treatment for complete resolution of recurrent parotitis, parotidectomy carries a risk for facial nerve injury. More recently, Nahlieli and colleagues[43] described the use of endoscopy to diagnose and endoscopic irrigation to treat children with recurrent parotitis.

COMPLICATIONS

With improved fluid management of postsurgical patients and the use of broad-spectrum antimicrobial agents, complications secondary to infectious parotitis now are rare events. In neonates or immunocompromised patients, sepsis may be a severe complication of this infection. Abscess formation may result from delayed or ineffective therapy. Compromise of the facial nerve may occur and can resolve with successful treatment of the infected gland.[38] The most serious and rare complication is extension to other structures of the head and neck and along fascial planes to the face, external auditory canal, jugular vein, mandible, and mediastinum.

PREVENTION

Suppurative parotitis can be prevented in postsurgical patients by maintaining adequate hydration and good oral hygiene. The most common form of viral parotitis, mumps, can be prevented by appropriate vaccination. Between 1968 and 1993, a 99 percent reduction in the incidence of new cases of mumps occurred.[60] In the mid-1980s and more recently in 2006, a resurgence of the incidence of mumps in previously vaccinated populations was noted.[6,12,26] The most recent outbreaks occurred among college students and young adults in several states, raising concern of waning immunity in this highly vaccinated population.[6] The current recommendation is to provide two doses of live mumps vaccine for school-age children (i.e., grades kindergarten through 12) with MMR vaccine and to ensure that students in college or other post–high school educational institutions also have received two doses of MMR vaccine.[6,14]

REFERENCES

1. Arditi, M., Langman, C. B., Christensen, M., et al.: Probable herpes simplex virus type 1-related acute parotitis, nephritis and erythema multiforme. Pediatr. Infect. Dis. J. 7:427-429, 1988.
2. Brill, S. J., and Gilfillan, R.: Acute parotitis associated with influenza type A: A report of twelve cases. N. Engl. J. Med. 296:1391-1392, 1977.
3. Brook, I.: Diagnosis and management of parotitis. Arch. Otolaryngol. Head Neck Surg. 118:469-471, 1992.
4. Brook, I., and Finegold, S. M.: Acute suppurative parotitis caused by anaerobic bacteria: Report of two cases. Pediatrics 62:1019-1020, 1978.
5. Brook, I., Frazier, E. H., and Thompson, D. H.: Aerobic and anaerobic microbiology of acute suppurative parotitis. Laryngoscope 101:170-172, 1991.
6. CDC: Update: Mumps activity—United States, January 1-October 7, 2006. M. M. W. R. Morb. Mortal. Wkly. Rep. 55:1152-1153, 2006.
7. Chanock, S. J., and McIntosh, K.: Pediatric infection with the human immunodeficiency virus: Issues for the otorhinolaryngologist. Otolaryngol. Clin. North Am. 22:637-660, 1989.
8. Chapnik, J. S., Noyek, A. M., Berris, B., et al.: Parotid gland enlargement in HIV infection: Clinical/imaging findings. J. Otolaryngol. 19:189-194, 1990.
9. Chetty, R., Vaithilingum, M., and Thejpal, R.: Epstein-Barr virus status and the histopathological changes of parotid gland lymphoid infiltrates in HIV-positive children. Pathology 31:413-417, 1999.
10. Chitre, V. V., and Premchandra, D. J.: Recurrent parotitis. Arch. Dis. Child. 77:359-363, 1997.

11. Chiu, C., and Lin, T.: Clinical and microbiological analysis of six children with acute suppurative parotitis. Acta Paediatr. *85*:106-108, 1996.

12. Cochi, S. L., Preblud, S. R., and Orenstein, W. A.: Perspectives on the relative resurgence of mumps in the United States. Am. J. Dis. Child. *142*:499-507, 1988.

13. Cohen, H. A., Gross, S., Nussinovitch, M., et al.: Recurrent parotitis. Arch. Dis. Child. *67*:1036-1037, 1992.

14. Committee on the Control of Infectious Diseases, American Academy of Pediatrics: 1994 Red Book: Report of the Committee on the Control of Infectious Diseases. 23rd ed. Evanston, IL, American Academy of Pediatrics, 1994.

15. Daud, A. S., and Pahor, A. L.: Tympanic neurectomy in the management of parotid sialectasis. J. Laryngol. Otol. *109*:1155-1158, 1995.

16. Davidkin, I., Jokinen, S., Leinikki, P., and Peltola, H.: Etiology of mumps-like illnesses in children and adolescents vaccinated for measles, mumps and rubella. J. Infect. Dis. *191*:719-723, 2005.

17. Ericson, S., Zetterlund, B., and Ohman, J.: Recurrent parotitis and sialectasis in childhood: Clinical, radiologic, immunologic, bacteriologic, and histologic study. Ann. Otol. Rhinol. Laryngol. *100*:527-535, 1991.

18. Fathalla, B., Collins, D., and Ezhuthachan, S.: Acute suppurative parotitis: Uncommon presentation in a premature infant. J. Perinatol. *1*:57-59, 2000.

19. Fazekas, T., Wiesbauer P., Schroth, B., et al.: Selective IgA deficiency in children with recurrent parotitis of childhood. Pediatr. Infect. Dis. J. *24*:461-462, 2005.

20. Fischbach, R., Kugel, H., Ernst, S., et al.: MR sialography: Initial experience using a T2-weighted fast SE sequence. J. Comput. Assist. Tomogr. *21*:826-830, 1997.

21. Giglio, M. S., Landaeta, M., and Pinto, M. E.: Microbiology of recurrent parotitis. Pediatr. Infect. Dis. J. *16*:386-390, 1997.

22. Green, P. A., von Reyn, C. F., and Smith, R. P. Jr.: *Mycobacterium avium* complex parotid lymphadenitis: Successful therapy with clarithromycin and ethambutol. Pediatr. Infect. Dis. J. *12*:615-617, 1993.

23. Hanekom, W. A., Chadwick, E. G., and Yogev, R.: Pneumococcal parotitis in a human immunodeficiency virus-infected child. Pediatr. Infect. Dis. J. *14*:1113-1114, 1995.

24. Hearth-Holmes, M., Baethge, B. A., Abreo, F., et al.: Autoimmune exocrinopathy presenting as recurrent parotitis of childhood. Arch. Otolaryngol. Head Neck Surg. *119*:347-349, 1993.

25. Hensher, R., and Bowerman, J.: Actinomycosis of the parotid gland. Br. J. Oral Maxillofac. Surg. *23*:128-134, 1995.

26. Hersh, B. S., Fine, P. E. M., Kent, W. K., et al.: Mumps outbreak in a highly vaccinated population. J. Pediatr. *119*:187-193, 1991.

27. Itescu, S.: Diffuse infiltrative lymphocytosis syndrome in children and adults infected with HIV-1: A model of rheumatic illness caused by acquired viral infection. Am. J. Reprod. Immunol. *28*:247-250, 1992.

28. Jantausch, B. A., Wiedermann, B. L., and Jeffries, B.: Parainfluenza virus type 2 meningitis and parotitis in an 11-year-old child. South. Med. J. *88*:230-231, 1995.

29. Katz, M. H., Mastrucci, M. T., Leggot, P. J., et al.: Prognostic significance of oral lesions in children with perinatally acquired human immunodeficiency virus infection. Am. J. Dis. Child. *147*:45-48, 1993.

30. Krilov, L. R., and Swenson, P.: Acute parotitis associated with influenza A infection. J. Infect. Dis. *152*:853, 1985.

31. Leake, D., and Leake, R.: Neonatal suppurative parotitis. Pediatrics *46*:203-207, 1970.

32. Lee, A. C. W., Lim, W. L., and So, K. T.: Epstein-Barr virus associated parotitis. J. Paediatr. Child Health *33*:177-178, 1997.

33. Leerdam, C. M., Martin, H. C. O., and Isaacs, D.: Recurrent parotitis of childhood. J. Paediatr. Child Health *41*:631-634, 2005.

34. Lepage, P., Van de Perre, P., Van Vliet, G., et al.: Clinical and endocrinologic manifestations in perinatally human immunodeficiency virus type 1-infected children aged 5 years or older. Am. J. Dis. Child. *145*:1248-1251, 1991.

35. Lewis, J. M., and Utz, J. P.: Orchitis, parotitis and meningoencephalitis due to lymphocytic-choriomeningitis virus. N. Engl. J. Med. *265*:776-780, 1961.

36. Loughran, D. H., and Smith, L. G.: Review: Infectious disorders of the parotid gland. N. J. Med. *85*:311-314, 1988.

37. Mandel, L., Kim, D., and Uy, C.: Parotid gland swelling in HIV diffuse infiltrate CD8 lymphocytosis syndrome. Oral Surg. Oral Med. Oral Pathol. Oral Radiol. Endod. *85*:565-568, 1998.

38. Mathur, N. B., Goyal, R. K., and Khalil, A.: Neonatal suppurative parotitis with facial palsy. Indian Pediatr. *25*:806-807, 1988.

39. Matlow, A., Korentager, R., Keystone, E., et al.: Parotitis due to anaerobic bacteria. Rev. Infect. Dis. *10*:420-423, 1988.

40. Miziara, I. D., Araujo Filho, B. C., Weber, R.: Oral lesions in Brazilian HIV-infected children undergoing HAART. Int. J. Pediatr. Otorhinolaryngol. *70*:1089-1096, 2006.

41. Murray, M. E., Buckenham, T. M., and Joseph, A. E. A.: The role of ultrasound in screening patients referred for sialography: A possible protocol. Clin. Otolaryngol. *21*:21-23, 1996.

42. Myer, C., and Cotton, R. T.: Salivary gland disease in children: A review, Part 1: Acquired non-neoplastic disease. Clin. Pediatr. *25*:314-322, 1986.

43. Nahlieli, O., Shacham, R., Shlesinger, M., and Eliav, E.: Juvenile recurrent parotitis: A new method of diagnosis and treatment. Pediatrics *114*:9-12, 2004.

44. O'Connell, J. E., George, M. K., Speculand, B., et al.: Mycobacterial infection of the parotid gland: An unusual case of parotid swelling. J. Laryngol. Otol. *107*:561-564, 1993.

45. Perera, A. M., Kumar, B. N., and Pahor, A. L.: Long-term results of tympanic neurectomy for chronic parotid sialectasis. Rev. Laryngol. Otol. Rhinol. *121*:95-98, 2000.

46. Pinto, A., and DeRossi, S. S.: Salivary gland disease in pediatric HIV patients: An update. J. Dent. Child. *71*:33-37, 2004.

47. Pou, A. M., Johnson, J. T., and Weissman, J.: Management decisions in parotitis. Compr. Ther. *21*:85-92, 1995.

48. Pruett, T. L., and Simmons, R. L.: Nosocomial gram-negative bacillary parotitis. J. A. M. A. *251*:252-253, 1984.

49. Raad, I. I., Sabbagh, M. F., and Caranasos, G. J.: Acute bacterial sialadenitis: A study of 29 cases and review. Rev. Infect. Dis. *12*:591-601, 1990.

50. Rabinov, J. D.: Imaging of salivary gland pathology. Radiol. Clin. North Am. *38*:1047-1057, 2000.

51. Redleaf, M. I., Bauer, C. A., and Robinson, R. A.: Fine-needle detection of cytomegalovirus parotitis in a patient with acquired immunodeficiency syndrome. Arch. Otolaryngol. Head Neck Surg. *120*:414-416, 1994.

52. Rowe-Jones, J. M., Vowles, R., Leighton, S. E. J., et al.: Diffuse tuberculous parotitis. J. Laryngol. Otol. *106*:1094-1095, 1992.

53. Sabatino, G., Verrotti, A., de Martino, M., et al.: Neonatal suppurative parotitis: A study of five cases. Eur. J. Pediatr. *158*:312-314, 1999.

54. Schuval, S. J., Bonagura, V. R., and Ilowite, N. T.: Rheumatologic manifestations of pediatric human immunodeficiency virus infection. J. Rheumatol. *20*:1578-1582, 1993.

55. Schuval, S. J., O'Reilly, M. E., and Bonagura, V. R.: Increased frequency of HLA-DR11 in pediatric human immunodeficiency virus-associated parotid gland enlargement. Clin. Diagn. Lab. Immunol. *4*:258-260, 1997.

56. Simpson, R. E. H.: Infectiousness of communicable diseases in the household (measles, chickenpox, and mumps). Lancet *2*:549-554, 1952.

57. Sperling, N. M., and Lin, P.: Parotid disease associated with human immunodeficiency virus infection. Ear Nose Throat J. *69*:475-477, 1990.

58. Stellbrink, H., Albrecht, H., and Greten, H.: Pneumococcal parotitis and cervical lymph node abscesses in an HIV-infected patient. Clin. Invest. *72*:1037-1040, 1994.

59. Tunkel, D. E.: Atypical mycobacterial adenitis presenting as a parotid abscess. Am. J. Otolaryngol. *16*:428-432, 1995.

60. van Loon, F. P., Holmes, S. J., Sirotkin, B. I., et al.: Mumps surveillance—United States, 1988-1993. M. M. W. R. Morb. Mortal. Wkly. Rep. *44*:1-14, 1995.

61. Vargas, P.A., Mauad, T., Bohm, G. M., and Saldiva, P. H. N.: Parotid gland involvement in advanced AIDS. Oral Dis. *9*:55-61, 2003.

62. Varghese, J. C., Thornton, F., Lucey, B. C., et al.: A prospective comparative study of MR sialography and conventional sialography of salivary disease. A. J. R. Am. J. Roentgenol. *173*:1497-1503, 1999.

CHAPTER 17

SINUSITIS

James D. Cherry ◉ Nina L. Shapiro

Sinusitis is an inflammation of the mucosal lining of one or more of the paranasal sinuses. Although this inflammation of sinus mucosa most probably occurs to some degree with every upper respiratory tract infection that produces rhinitis, most of these episodes apparently have a spontaneous resolution.[94] Studies during the last 2 decades estimate that 5 to 10 percent of upper respiratory infections are complicated by acute sinusitis.[2,167,184] This rate range represents a significant increase from earlier reports,[36] possibly because of a greater awareness of the illness and improved imaging techniques. The growing number of children in daycare has led to an actual increase in the incidence of upper respiratory tract infections.[182,184] In addition, recognition that sinus infection can have a negative effect on the health of children with chronic pulmonary disease has increased the interest in this disease.[108]

When considering a diagnosis of sinusitis in a child, the major problem is to distinguish simple upper respiratory tract infection or allergic inflammation from secondary bacterial infection of the sinuses. Unless complications such as periorbital cellulitis or cavernous sinus thrombosis render the diagnosis obvious, the clinician has no reliable way to establish a diagnosis of acute sinusitis in the office setting. Sometimes, symptoms and signs of sinusitis occur simultaneously with rhinitis, but most often, they occur after an episode of rhinitis. Infection in the sinuses usually persists after the preceding rhinitis has resolved. Sinusitis is classified by the duration of clinical symptoms: acute (≤3 weeks), subacute (3 to 10 weeks), and chronic (>10 weeks). Available data comparing acute and subacute sinusitis are sparse; both entities may have a similar etiology, diagnosis, and prognosis; the distinction seems to be arbitrary and to have no clinical significance.

HISTORY

Purulent sinusitis and its relationship to orbital inflammation have been known for more than 2000 years.[71] Highmore, a 17th-century English physician and anatomist, is given credit for the separation of dental and antral disease.[130] Hunter indicated the importance of surgical drainage in purulent sinusitis and suggested perforating the partition between the maxillary antrum and the nose.[130] During the first half of the 20th century, sinusitis was responsible for considerable morbidity and mortality, and surgical care of sinusitis frequently was lifesaving. Since the advent of antibiotics, sinusitis has had a lower medical profile. Interest in this topic has increased, however. Some factors involved in this increased interest include the advent of the newer surgical techniques of functional endoscopic sinus surgery that yield comparable results to sinus puncture and aspiration,[163] which now have been applied to children; improved diagnostic imaging studies; and the greater social importance of upper respiratory tract infections for parents who must be absent from work to seek treatment for their children.[108]

ANATOMY

All the paranasal sinuses develop as outpouchings of the nasal cavity. Three shelflike structures—the inferior, middle, and superior turbinates—are on the lateral nasal wall. The superior turbinate is not well developed in the first year of life.[194] Beneath each turbinate is the corresponding meatus into which the sinuses open; that is, the frontal, maxillary, and anterior ethmoid sinuses open into the middle meatus. The sphenoid and posterior ethmoid cells open high in the nasal vault into the superior meatus.[175]

The maxillary sinuses develop early in the second trimester of fetal life as lateral outpouchings in the posterior aspect of the middle meatus. They are present at birth,[6,115,146,194] with floors being barely below the attachment of the inferior turbinates.[175] They expand rapidly by the time the child is 4 years of age.[194] Ultimately, at full size, the lateral borders of the maxillary sinuses reach the lateral orbital rims. The position of the floors of the sinuses is determined by the eruption of the dentition.[175] The ostia of the maxillary sinuses are located high on the medial walls of the sinuses, which impedes gravitational drainage of secretions; ciliary activity is required to move secretions from the body of the maxillary sinuses through the ostia into the nose.[175]

The ethmoid sinuses develop in the fourth month of gestation[175] and are present at birth.[115,146,194] They are not a single large cavity but a grouping of cells, 3 to 15 in number, each with its own opening or ostium. They have a honeycombed radiographic appearance and are small anteriorly and large posteriorly. The walls of the ethmoid labyrinth, especially the lateral walls bordering on the orbits, are thin; they are referred to as the *lamina papyracea*.[175]

Development of the frontal sinuses is variable. In adults, 80 percent have bilateral frontal sinuses, 1 to 4 percent have agenesis of the frontal sinuses, and the remainder have unilateral hypoplasia. The position of the frontal sinuses is supraorbital after the child reaches 4 years of age, but they are not distinguished radiographically from the ethmoid sinuses until the child is 6 to 8 years old. The frontal sinuses do not reach adult size for another 8 to 10 years.[175]

The onset of development of the sphenoid sinuses occurs during the child's first 2 years of life, but they remain rudimentary until the child is approximately 6 years of age. They have reached their permanent size, although not their permanent shape, by the time the child is 12 years old.[194]

Although the full development of the sinuses may take 20 years, by the time the child is 12 years old, the nasal cavity and the paranasal sinuses nearly have completed their development and have reached adult proportions.[194] Sinus disease in postpubertal adolescents is similar to that in adults.

The mucosal lining of all the paranasal sinuses is composed of ciliated columnar epithelium and goblet cells.[149] It is continuous and similar to the lining of the nasal cavity except that the mucosa in the nose is thicker and contains more glands. The epithelium of all the paranasal sinuses and nasal cavity is covered in part by a mucus blanket.

PATHOPHYSIOLOGY

The pathogenesis of sinus infection undoubtedly is similar to that of otitis media. The middle ear, with its extension, the eustachian tube, and the paranasal sinuses normally are sterile, but their contiguous areas (nasopharynx and nose) have a dynamic microbial flora. Under normal conditions, ciliary function with mucus flow can be expected to keep the sinuses clear of pathogens. The cilia within the sinuses propel the mucus toward their respective ostia, and from there, nasal ciliary action moves the mucus blanket posteriorly toward the pharynx. Insults that damage the ciliary epithelium and affect the morphology, number, and function of cilia and insults that alter the production or viscosity of the mucus blanket lead to obstruction of the flow of mucus, however, which allows the inoculation of numerous microorganisms into the sinuses that can lead to infection. In a study in adults in whom sneezing, coughing, and nose blowing were stimulated or initiated voluntarily, intranasal pressures were measured, and the deposition of contrast medium (which before the initiation of the event had been inoculated into the nasopharynx) was determined by computed tomography (CT) scan.[66] Results of this study showed that nose blowing introduced viscous fluid into the maxillary sinuses, whereas coughing or sneezing did not generate enough pressure to propel fluid into the sinuses. When instituted, sinus infection is complicated further by inflammatory obstruction of the ostium leading to the nose.

Recurrent chronic sinusitis implies a problem with local mucociliary defense, a defect in systemic immunity, or a fixed anatomic sinus obstruction. Often, the predisposing factors work in tandem, as in a child with a septal deformity and a viral illness.[108] In chronic sinusitis, the mucosa is thickened, and marked edema, vessel dilation, and infiltration of inflammatory cells are present.[166] Goblet cells are decreased in density, and seromucous glands are increased in density compared with their presence in normal sinuses. The most important factor leading to purulent sinus infection in children and in adults is upper respiratory viral infection.[20,44,108,184]

Wald and colleagues[184] in a large prospective study involving children younger than 3 years of age showed a doubling of the rate of sinusitis (defined as upper respiratory symptoms persisting >15 days) among children in a daycare setting compared with children not in daycare. The differences presumably were due to increased exposure to viral respiratory illnesses. Radiographic studies in children with acute colds regularly indicate abnormalities of the maxillary sinuses, suggesting that the infection involves these areas.[111] These asymptomatic sinus opacifications may persist for 2 weeks after the symptoms of the upper respiratory illness have resolved.[41,92,175] Viral infection that involves the sinuses rarely is differentiated from its primary manifestations, such as the common cold, nasopharyngitis, and influenza, and recovery is the rule. If the effect of the viral infection on the mucosal surface is severe, and is associated with the inoculation of one or more pathogenic bacterial agents and obstruction of an ostium, disease occurs.

The mechanisms by which upper respiratory viral infections set the stage for secondary bacterial infection in the sinuses are complex. Using in situ hybridization, rhinovirus RNA was shown inside epithelial cells of maxillary sinus in 50 percent of a small number of adults with acute sinusitis.[128] This finding is remarkable because in experimental rhinovirus infections, only a small percentage of nasal epithelial cells were noted to contain rhinovirus RNA.[7] These differences may reflect only differences in inoculum between experimental and natural infection, but they may indicate heavier infection in the sinuses than in the nose. Symptoms in upper respiratory viral infections are not caused by extensive damage to ciliated nasal epithelium, but rather to aspects of the host response (see Chapter 8).[7,67,120,122,126,131,132,193]

Other irritants can set the stage for sinus infection. Swimming in ocean, lake, or chlorinated pool water can lead to sinus involvement. Drying of the nasal mucosa, which occurs commonly during the winter in cold climates, may be a precipitating factor. Children with respiratory allergies are prone to sinusitis,[53,101,135-137] and allergy probably is the second most prevalent predisposing factor in childhood sinusitis, acting through mucosa congestion and perhaps depressing local and systemic immune responses.[108,151] The treatment of respiratory allergies may contribute to sinusitis because ciliary damage occurring after the administration of nasal decongestants has been shown in organ culture and animal studies.[41,42,116] Richards and colleagues[141] reported a diagnosis of atopy in 62 percent of a selected cohort of pediatric patients who had documented recurrent sinusitis and were referred to allergy clinics in Los Angeles. Dental infections or extractions also can lead to maxillary sinusitis if the tooth root is adjacent to the maxillary sinus floor.[32]

Sudden change in pressure, as with diving or during descent in an airplane, physically can overcome local mucociliary defense mechanisms and lead to the sudden onset of acute sinusitis.[119] Defects of ciliary function, such as those occurring in the immotile cilia syndrome and Kartagener syndrome, predispose a child to chronic sinusitis.[47,78,89,137,146,155] Refractory sinusitis also occurs commonly in children with primary and acquired immunodeficiency diseases.[28,108,117,147,152,168,179] A growing population of immunocompromised children undergoing treatment for malignancies and organ transplantations and young patients with maternally transmitted and blood-transmitted acquired immunodeficiency syndrome constitute another growing population with a potential for developing sinusitis that is difficult to manage. Finally, anatomic obstruction caused by septal deformities, craniofacial anomalies, foreign bodies, adenoidal hypertrophy, or nasal masses or polyps predisposes children to sinusitis. Nasal polyps in young children usually are not caused by allergies and should be an indication for evaluation for cystic fibrosis.[108]

Immunologic mechanisms are important in the pathogenesis of sinus infections, as indicated by the high prevalence of chronic sinus infections in children with immunodeficiencies.[28,108,117,147,152,168] Sinus and nasal mucus contains IgA, IgG, and IgM and lysozymes.[25,145] Secretory IgA, which is produced locally, is the predominant immunoglobulin in nasal mucus.[69] IgG antibodies in nasal mucus result from passive leakage from plasma cells in the epithelium and submucosa and from the serum.[16] Generally, with the patient's increasing age and as a result of previous exposures, these immunoglobulins develop species-specific and type-specific antibodies that block epithelial colonization by specific microorganisms.

Shapiro and associates[152] studied 61 children with refractory sinusitis and found that 34 had abnormal immunologic studies. Abnormal findings included poor response to pneumococcal type 7 antigen after immunization, IgG3 subclass deficiency, low serum IgA or IgG values, and elevated serum IgE values.

ETIOLOGY

Although most studies on the etiology of sinusitis have involved adults, adequate pediatric data are available. The findings in studies of adults can be applied appropriately to adolescents.

Examining the results of anterior nasal cultures from normal subjects and from subjects with respiratory illnesses is important to clear up confusion regarding the make-up of normal flora. During early investigations of the common cold, Shibley and associates[153] noted that in a group of 13 subjects followed for 4 to 9 months, neither *Haemophilus influenzae* nor hemolytic streptococci were obtained from nasal culture when the subjects were well. When the study subjects were ill with colds, *H. influenzae* was recovered from 9 percent of the cultures, and hemolytic streptococci were recovered from 6 percent. In a study of 500 consecutive medical patients, Jacobson and Dick[83] noted in all but two instances that the recovery of pneumococci and hemolytic streptococci from the nose correlated with nasal or sinus disease. Studies in children have disclosed more varied results. Dunlap and Harvey[44,70] recovered *H. influenzae*, pneumococci, and hemolytic streptococci from the noses of normal children with some consistency. These investigators were interested in carriage and spread of organisms, however, and the state of well-being of their subjects was not delineated clearly.

Orobello and colleagues[123] found that cultures of ipsilateral middle meatus correlated well with maxillary (83%) and ethmoid (80%) sinus cultures. Nasopharyngeal cultures correlated less well, however, with only 45 percent and 40 percent of maxillary and ethmoid sinus cultures being similar.

Yang[195] studied children in a day nursery and noted that neither pneumococci nor *H. influenzae* could be recovered from the noses of well children. Hays and Mullard[73] only rarely could find *Streptococcus pneumoniae*, beta-hemolytic streptococci, or *H. influenzae* in nose cultures from normal children. In an extensive study, Box and associates[15] noted pneumococci in nasal specimens of 38 percent of children without respiratory illness, but in only 3 percent was the growth of great magnitude (>100 colonies per plate). In the same study, *Haemophilus* spp. and beta-hemolytic streptococci were recovered from 14 percent and 1 percent of the cultured specimens from noses. In comparison, in the same study, pneumococci and *Haemophilus* spp. were recovered from 57 percent and 25 percent of the cultures of patients with respiratory illness.

In a more recent study involving 49 children with sinusitis, Ilki and associates[81] found a strong correlation with throat cultures positive for *H. influenzae*, *S. pneumoniae*, or *Moraxella catarrhalis*. Similar organisms were recovered from sinus aspirates.

TABLE 17–1 Etiologic Agents in Sinusitis Analyzed by Patient Age and Type of Illness

	Frequency				Age Group (yr)		
	Overall	Acute	Subacute	Chronic	≤5	6-12	>12
Aerobic Bacteria							
Haemophilus influenzae	++++	++++	++++	++++	++++	++++	++++
Streptococcus pneumoniae	++++	++++	++++	++++	++++	++++	++++
Moraxella catarrhalis	+++	+++	++	+	+++	+	++
Staphylococcus aureus	++	+	+	++	++	++	++
Streptococcus pyogenes	++	++	++	++	+	++	++
Alpha-hemolytic and nonhemolytic streptococci	+		+	+			++
Staphylococcus epidermidis	+		+	+		+	++
Alcaligenes spp.	+		+	+			++
Escherichia coli	+			+			++
Klebsiella pneumoniae	+			+			++
Pseudomonas aeruginosa	+			+			++
Other*	+			+			++
Anaerobic Bacteria							
Peptostreptococcus spp.	++	+	+	+++		+	++
Prevotella and *Porphyromonas* spp.	++			++		+	++
Fusobacterium spp.	++			++			
Propionibacterium spp.	++			++			
Bifidobacterium spp.	+			+			
Bacteroides fragilis	+	+	+	+			+
Veillonella spp.	+	+	+	+			
Fungi							
Aspergillus spp.	+	+		+	+	++	++
Alternaria spp.	+	+		+	+	+	+
Penicillium spp.	+			+	+	+	+
Curvularia spp.	+		+	+	+	+	+
Drechslera spp.	+			+	+	+	+
Bipolaris spp.	+			+	+	+	+
Mucor spp. and other Zygomycetes	+	+			+	+	+
Mycoplasma and ***Chlamydia***							
Mycoplasma pneumoniae	+	+					+
Chlamydia pneumoniae				+	+	+	+
Other							
L-forms	+			+			++
Mixed aerobes and anaerobes	++	+	+	++			++
Mixed *H. influenzae* with other organisms	++	+	+	++		+	++
Rhinovirus, adenovirus	+	+		+		+	+

Serratia spp., diphtheroids, *Enterococcus* spp., *Neisseria* spp., *Haemophilus* spp., *Proteus* spp., *Acinetobacter* spp., *Citrobacter* spp., *Eikenella corrodens*, *Arcanobacterium haemolyticum*.
Data from references *8, 14, 18-20, 23, 28, 31, 43, 45, 50, 51, 60, 86, 87, 90, 93, 103, 107, 125, 137, 172-174, 181, 185, 186.*

In a study performed in the Finnish military, nasal cultures from 183 healthy recruits revealed the following frequencies of specific organisms: *H. influenzae,* 4 percent; *S. pneumoniae,* 1 percent; *M. catarrhalis,* 3 percent; and *Streptococcus pyogenes,* 0 percent.[87] In contrast, in 185 recruits with acute maxillary sinusitis, the percentages of nasal isolates for the same organisms were 61 percent, 25 percent, 7 percent, and 6 percent, respectively. In 91 percent of cases in which a sinus aspirate culture yielded an isolate, the same organism was found in a nasal sample. Similar results have been obtained in other studies done in adults with acute sinusitis, in which nontypeable *H. influenzae* and *S. pneumoniae* account for approximately 74 percent of all bacterial strains recovered in sinus aspirates.[68] In all studies, *Staphylococcus aureus* clearly is part of the normal nasal flora. *S. aureus* is present in well or sick children approximately 50 percent of the time.

Pneumococci, *H. influenzae,* *M. catarrhalis,* and *S. pyogenes* seldom are found in the nose of a healthy child and should suggest a nasal or paranasal infectious illness. The recovery of *S. aureus* cannot be correlated with disease, however.

A review of many reports of children indicates that *S. pneumoniae,* *H. influenzae,* and *M. catarrhalis* are the etiologic agents that occur most commonly in acute and subacute ethmoid and maxillary sinusitis.* In one of the studies[186] of sinus aspirates from 50 children, *S. aureus* was not isolated from the maxillary sinus. Several studies of pediatric patients with chronic sinusitis suggest an increased importance of anaerobes and staphylococcal species.[19,21,39,179] In other studies in children with chronic sinusitis who have undergone surgery, a predominance of coagulase-negative staphylococci, viridans streptococci, and *S. aureus* was noted.[118,123] Several studies[55,71,190] documenting that *S. pneumoniae,* *H. influenzae,* and *M. catarrhalis* were the most common etiologic agents were concerned primarily with orbital involvement; 50 to 85 percent of cases of orbital cellulitis had radiographic evidence of sinusitis. Orbital complications of ethmoiditis primarily affect children. *Staphylococcus* spp., *S. pneumoniae,* and other streptococci have been found in children with orbital involvement from ethmoiditis[3] or frontal sinusitis.[54]

Table 17–1 lists etiologic agents of sinusitis by age of patient and type of illness. In all age groups and in acute, subacute, and chronic disease, *H. influenzae* and *S. pneumoniae* are the principal pathogens in most cases. Also, a large number of different

*See references 55, 71, 73, 77, 78, 107, 115, 172-174, 181, 186, 190.

bacterial species have been recovered from the sinuses of affected patients. In young children, more than 90 percent of all cases of sinusitis are caused by five organisms: *H. influenzae*, *S. pneumoniae*, *M. catarrhalis*, *S. aureus*, and *S. pyogenes*. In adolescents, the same organisms, plus largely penicillin-sensitive anaerobes, account for most cases. As noted in Table 17–1, a variety of gram-negative enteric and other bacilli have been recovered from patients with sinusitis, in most instances from patients who have had various forms of antibiotic therapy before culture. Organisms previously considered to be nonpathogens, such as *Staphylococcus epidermidis*, have been implicated etiologically.

Although clinically recognized sinusitis has occurred rarely in patients with *Mycoplasma pneumoniae* infection, Griffin and Klein[61] noted radiographic evidence of sinusitis in approximately two thirds of a group of Navy recruits with *M. pneumoniae* pneumonia. In adults with chronic suppurative maxillary sinusitis, mycoplasmas have been sought but not recovered.[14,60,161] Bhattacharyya and colleagues[14] noted L-forms in 21 percent of all sinuses in patients with chronic disease.

In a study of 25 adults with chronic rhinosinusitis, *Chlamydia pneumoniae* was recovered from nasopharyngeal samples in 2 patients, but not from any of 10 healthy controls.[45] In addition, the patients were more likely than control subjects (20 percent) to have serum IgG antibody titers to *C. pneumoniae* of 1:64 or greater (72%). IgA antibody titers to *C. pneumoniae* of 1:32 or greater also were more prevalent in the patients (48%) than in the controls (10%). In a study involving 20 children with chronic sinusitis, Cultrara and colleagues[31] cultured material from 13 bilateral endoscopic ethmoidectomies with maxillary antrostomies, 10 adenoidectomies, and 3 bilateral maxillary sinus lavages. They isolated *C. pneumoniae* from a nasopharyngeal swab and adenoid tissue from a 6-year-old child.

Fungal diseases of the sinuses have been well described in adults.[188] Acute fulminate fungal sinusitis is seen in immunosuppressed individuals and is associated with high morbidity and mortality rates.[33,158] *Aspergillus* spp. are the most common fungal causes of sinusitis. Many cases of chronic sinusitis from which a microorganism is not recovered have been thought to be caused by *Aspergillus* spp. infections.[88] The presence of eosinophils, Charcot-Leyden crystals, and hyphae found retrospectively, and not noted on the original examination, in mucus recovered from sinuses suggests that some cases of chronic sinusitis may represent *Aspergillus* hypersensitivity. This allergic aspergillosis in the sinuses is similar to allergic bronchopulmonary aspergillosis. In a series of six patients who were 8 to 16 years of age and had allergic aspergillosis sinusitis, all presented with nasal polyposis and facial deformity, indicating advanced disease.[110] Mucormycosis, an infection caused by Zygomycetes (formerly Phycomycetes), is seen in immunocompromised children and adults.[85] *Drechslera* spp., *Bipolaris* spp., and *Curvalaria lunata* have been added to the list of fungi that can cause sinusitis in children.[13,23,51,157]

Although sinusitis has been reported as a complication of Epstein-Barr virus infection, the sinus infections seem to be a complication of steroid treatment and not specifically the viral infection.[57] *Nocardia* spp. have been reported as a cause of acute sinusitis in an adult transplant recipient[142] and of chronic sinusitis in immunocompetent and immunocompromised individuals.[170]

EPIDEMIOLOGY

Although sinus involvement occurs commonly with respiratory viral infection, sinusitis seldom is identified as a specific illness in previously healthy children. In a survey of all office visits, totaling 2613, Breese and colleagues[17] noted only 6 children (0.23%) in whom the initial diagnosis was sinusitis. The true incidence of sinusitis in childhood is unknown. In 1989, Wald and colleagues[181]

estimated that 0.5 to 5 percent of upper respiratory tract infections are complicated by acute sinusitis. More recent estimates by the same authors have been 10 percent.[184] The most recent estimates of greater incidence could be related to a heightened awareness and concern for lost work days by working parents, a possible correlation between pulmonary problems in an increasing number of children with chronic lung disease, better imaging techniques, increased interest in endoscopic sinus surgery,[163] more disease because of more exposure as a result of more children being in daycare,[108] and an increased recognition or perhaps incidence of allergy-related illness.[140,141] Seasonal prevalence has not been studied, but a reasonable assumption is that disease would increase during the cold weather months because it is the time of greatest respiratory viral activity. Cases in older children also can be expected to occur more frequently in association with swimming.

Although it is not well documented, sinusitis seems to be more of a problem in geographic areas where marked temperature changes occur. In children, sinusitis seems to occur more commonly in boys than in girls.[72,115] Ueda and Yoto[167] found abnormal findings in the maxillary sinuses in 135 (6.7%) of 2013 children who presented to an outpatient department with upper respiratory symptoms; of this group, 65 percent were boys, and 35 percent were girls. Manning and associates[109] found similar distribution in a group of 60 children diagnosed by CT or magnetic resonance imaging (MRI). Host factors are important in sinusitis because the illness occurs more commonly in allergic children; in children with chronic ear infections; and in patients with cystic fibrosis, primary humoral immunodeficiencies, and Kartagener syndrome.[22,78,121,146] Although an association between sinus disease and asthma seems to exist, controversy continues regarding whether sinusitis and other upper airway stimuli can induce asthma.[52,141,150,196] A review of hospital admissions of patients with status asthmaticus at the Children's Hospital of Los Angeles showed a marked increase in admissions, and sinusitis was diagnosed in 23 percent.[140] Children with various immunologic defects frequently have sinusitis.

Sinusitis is noncontagious from person to person, but point-source outbreaks are possible from swimming in heavily contaminated water. A cluster of seven cases of invasive nosocomial fungal sinusitis in severely neutropenic patients has been described. It was caused by the release of airborne fungal spores from soil reservoirs that were distributed during hospital construction during a 2-year period.[104]

CLINICAL PRESENTATION

The clinical symptoms of sinusitis vary by age. Older children and adolescents have localized complaints similar to those of adults, whereas in young children, the findings are related less clearly to the sinuses.[176] Table 17–2 presents the overall frequencies of symptoms, signs, and laboratory findings for acute, subacute, and chronic disease.

In young children, disease involves only the ethmoid and maxillary sinuses. In these children, illness frequently has its onset after they have had an upper respiratory viral infection. A period of general improvement may occur, however, between the acute respiratory illness and the onset of symptoms related to sinus infection. The most prominent symptom in all children, and particularly in children younger than 10 years of age, is persistent rhinorrhea. The discharge frequently is purulent, but it occasionally can be serous or watery. Associated with rhinorrhea is cough, which becomes more prominent with increasing duration of disease. The cough particularly is troublesome at night because it is caused by the stimulation of the sinus drainage as it traverses the pharyngeal wall. The posterior drainage also occasionally causes vomiting. Fever is of variable occurrence in

TABLE 17–2 Clinical Findings in Acute, Subacute, and Chronic Sinusitis of Children

	Occurrence (%)	
	Acute and Subacute Sinusitis	Chronic Sinusitis
Symptoms		
Fever	50	20
Rhinorrhea	80	80
Cough (persistent and evening)	50	90
Pain/headache	30	30
Sore throat	20	20
Periorbital swelling	30	0
Vomiting	20	10
Allergic history	20	40
Malodorous breath	20	20
Signs		
Rhinorrhea	80	80
Temperature ≥38.3°C (≥101°F)	20	0
Sinus tenderness	20	10
Otitis media	40	60
Posterior pharyngeal pus	0	10
Transillumination positive	30	10
Periorbital swelling	30	0
Malodorous breath	20	20
Laboratory		
Abnormal radiographs	100	100
Maxillary	90	90
Ethmoid	40	40
Frontal and sphenoid	10	10
Unilateral	70	10
Bilateral	30	90
Erythrocyte sedimentation rate elevation	50	10
White blood cell count elevation with an increased percentage of band form neutrophils	40	10

Data from references 3, 10, 72, 75, 84, 89, 91, 115, 121, 141, 146, 159, 178, 187.

sinusitis and generally is related inversely to age and duration of illness. Malodorous breath often is reported by parents. The first evidence of illness in some children is fever and periorbital swelling. In most instances, periorbital cellulitis is a manifestation of ethmoid sinusitis.

Although facial pain and headache are frequent complaints of sinus disease in adults, they have been noted in only approximately one third of the cases in children and are unusual occurrences in young children. The main symptom in older children and adolescents is rhinorrhea. In older patients with more chronic disease, the nasal symptoms may be minimal or absent. Troublesome postnasal drip is a frequent complaint.

Acute isolated sphenoid sinusitis in children is rare but often misdiagnosed because the symptoms are vague and there are no specific physical findings.[112] Findings include fever, headache, and neurologic symptoms. Swimming and diving are possible predisposing factors.

Physical signs in sinusitis also differ by age. Nasal discharge is the most frequent finding in all age groups. Young children are more likely to have a serous or watery discharge, however, than are adolescents. Elevation of temperature occurs more commonly in acute disease and in association with orbital cellulitis. Sinus tenderness, a common finding in older patients, is noted only rarely in children. Particularly significant is tenderness with percussion of the upper molars. Examination of the throat frequently reveals free exudate. Occasionally, the breath is malodorous.

The ears are abnormal in almost half of all patients with sinusitis. In acute disease in young children, it can be acute otitis media, but usually the findings are more suggestive of serous disease. Acute sinusitis frequently is unilateral, whereas chronic disease more often is bilateral.

Children with chronic sinusitis frequently have only minimal complaints. The parent notes that the child does not feel well and frequently reports that the child has had a persistent respiratory infection for months. In a series of children with chronic (>3 months) upper respiratory complaints who were referred to allergy clinics, 60 percent had sinusitis.[121] In this study, the combination of moderate to severe rhinorrhea and cough with minimal sneezing was reported to have a specificity of 95 percent and a sensitivity of 38 percent in predicting the presence of chronic sinusitis. In the referred children in this study, sinusitis was found in 63 percent of atopic children and in 75 percent of non-atopic children.

Laboratory studies other than cultures and radiography are not useful in the evaluation of a child with sinusitis. Herz and Gfeller[75] noted that in their study, erythrocyte sedimentation rates were elevated in only approximately half of the patients, and leukocytosis occurred in only one third. Generally, younger children with orbital cellulitis and ethmoid sinusitis are more likely to have elevated sedimentation rates and white blood cell counts. The American Academy of Pediatrics (AAP) Subcommittee of Sinusitis and Committee on Quality Improvement has recommended that the diagnosis of acute bacterial sinusitis be based on clinical criteria in children who present with upper respiratory symptoms that are either persistent (nasal or postnasal discharge of any quality with or without daytime cough for >10 to 14 days) or severe (temperature >39° C and purulent nasal discharge present concurrently for at least 3 or 4 consecutive days in a child who appears ill).[4]

COMPLICATIONS

Serious complications, including meningitis, osteomyelitis, cavernous sinus thrombosis, and epidural, subdural, brain, and orbital abscesses, occur in untreated sinusitis.* Signs and symptoms of neurologic involvement in sinusitis frequently call for aggressive surgical management of the sinusitis and the intracranial and paracranial lesions. Osteomyelitis of the frontal bone may be a complication of frontal sinusitis[9] and may manifest as Pott puffy tumor if a subperiosteal abscess also is present.

DIFFERENTIAL DIAGNOSIS

Differential considerations in sinusitis are few and are more concerned with whether sinus involvement in a particular child is the primary event or a secondary problem related to a more general host defect. Children with recurrent and chronic sinusitis should be evaluated for respiratory allergy, cystic fibrosis, immunologic deficiency, and Kartagener and other immotile-cilia syndromes.

Foreign bodies in the nose can be mistaken for sinusitis, as can cysts in the maxillary antra. Nasal structural defects (congenital and acquired), such as palatal clefts, unilateral choanal atresia, nasal polyps, and septal deviation, can be confused with sinusitis, but more commonly these problems are predisposing factors in sinus infections.

Dental infections frequently are mistaken for maxillary sinus disease. Dental infections can lead by direct extension to sinus involvement. Primary infections in the region of the eye also

---

*See references 1, 46, 56, 57, 96, 113, 124, 133, 148, 189, 192.

occur without sinus disease. In young children, a chronic infection of the adenoids can be confused clinically with sinusitis. Infections with *Bordetella pertussis* can be confused with subacute sinusitis.

SPECIFIC DIAGNOSIS

Although persistent nasal symptoms and the presence of other clinical findings as listed in Table 17–2 indicate a diagnosis of sinusitis, the only certain way to make the diagnosis is by obtaining radiographs and cultures reflecting sinus flora. Although some physicians have suggested that maxillary sinus radiographs frequently are abnormal for normal children,[111,154] other data indicate that normal children older than 1 year of age seldom have abnormal radiographs.[92] During infancy, the maxillary sinuses are so small that minimal mucosal edema may "opacify" a sinus on a radiograph. In young children, radiographic examination should consist of two views: lateral and Waters. In older children, Caldwell and basal projections also should be performed. Radiographs in acute upper respiratory viral infections as a rule are abnormal; these radiographs are not false-positive ones, but are the result of viral infections. From a therapeutic point of view, sinus radiographs usually should not be obtained unless nasal symptoms in an upper respiratory illness have not shown signs of improvement after 5 to 7 days.

Plain-film radiographic examination has been supplanted mainly by CT and MRI for the diagnosis of sinusitis. Many endoscopic sinus surgeons consider CT to be a mandatory part of the preoperative evaluation. MRI is useful in cases that may be complicated by orbital or intracranial extension. The high prevalence of incidental sinus opacification in asymptomatic infants and children noted radiographically has been confirmed by CT studies.[35,58,76] Since the advent of MRI, researchers have realized that many incidental sinus abnormalities also occur in adults. These findings in children and adults may be from subclinical or resolving respiratory infections or may be due to unrecognized allergies.[34]

CT has been recognized widely as the standard for the diagnosis of paranasal sinus disease.[12] In particular, coronal thin-section images offer excellent delineation of lesions in the osteomeatal complex.[197] Obtaining axial images is useful for evaluating periorbital and intraorbital complications.[49] In some institutions, a so-called screening CT of the sinuses is performed with a limited number of slices.[64] It can be offered at a cost and radiation exposure that are similar to those associated with plain-film studies, but with much greater accuracy. Some young children and infants require sedation for CT, which limits its suitability.

The AAP Subcommittee of Sinusitis and Committee on Quality Improvement has recommended that imaging studies are not necessary to confirm a diagnosis of clinical sinusitis in children 6 years of age or younger.[4] The need for radiographic evidence as a confirmatory test in children older than 6 years with severe symptoms is controversial. The American College of Radiology considers that the diagnosis of acute uncomplicated sinusitis should be made only on clinical grounds.[114] CT scans of the sinuses should be reserved for patients in whom surgery is being considered as a management strategy.[4] In a meta-analysis of acute uncomplicated sinusitis in children,[82] poor concordance was observed among clinical criteria, plain radiographs, CT scans, ultrasonography, and fluid aspiration. More studies are necessary to determine the optimal set of clinical criteria and other laboratory or radiologic studies for diagnosis of this condition.

Which radiographic technique (plain radiography, CT, or MRI) is selected for evaluation of a child with presumed sinusitis should be determined by availability of techniques and the expertise of the radiologist and by clinical symptoms. Radiographs, in most instances, should not be obtained early in the illness of children with uncomplicated upper respiratory complaints because of the high incidence of transient abnormalities.[5] Radiography is indicated for children with continuing symptoms of sinusitis after extensive medical therapy or for children with possible complications of sinusitis. CT is optimal.[5] A limited CT scan with axial cuts may be obtained. It allows for excellent visualization of sinus anatomy and pathology while limiting the radiation exposure to the child. A limited sinus CT scan has radiation similar to that of a sinus plain-film series. In the absence of low-cost screening CT, plain radiography should be the initial imaging study in most children who have symptoms of sinus disease.[34] Children who have periorbital swelling or proptosis should undergo immediate contrast-enhanced CT studies in axial and coronal planes. If symptoms or CT findings suggest intracranial extension, MRI should be performed.[5,34]

Although ultrasonography would seem to offer an alternative to sinus radiography, some question remains about its dependability unless one normal air-filled maxillary sinus or one opacified maxillary sinus is present for comparison.[174,185] The hallmark of specific diagnosis in sinusitis is similar to that of other infectious diseases: the culture of infected material. Many physicians erroneously considered it an impossible task because of the inability of obtaining material directly from the sinuses of children. As discussed in the section on etiology, nasal cultures that are properly performed reveal the causative organism in most instances. Nasal culture should be taken from the region of the maxillary ostium in the middle meatus. Culture specimens should be obtained from this area and not from the nasopharynx. Wald and associates[185] found no correlation between bacteria isolated directly from the maxillary sinuses and nasopharyngeal and throat culture isolates. Best results are obtained when a vasoconstrictor, such as 0.25 percent phenylephrine hydrochloride, is administered first and the culture specimen is obtained with a wire-cotton swab under direct vision. With this technique, material frequently can be obtained as it comes from the sinus ostium. Bilateral cultures always should be obtained. In serious cases, such as in children with neurologic complications or in treatment failures, performing antral puncture for culture can be lifesaving. Anaerobic and aerobic cultures should be performed on any material recovered by antral puncture.

TREATMENT

ACUTE AND SUBACUTE SINUSITIS

The successful treatment of acute and subacute sinusitis in children depends primarily on the administration of an appropriate antibiotic in adequate dosage for a sufficient period.[4,180] In most instances, therapy should be instituted before obtaining the results of cultures. Antibiotic selection in this situation is not a great problem in children because the etiologic agent is *H. influenzae*, *S. pneumoniae*, *M. catarrhalis*, *S. aureus*, or *S. pyogenes* in more than 90 percent of acute cases.

Initial selection of an antibiotic should be based on the severity of the clinical illness and must take into consideration the antibiotic resistance patterns of the common causative organisms and the cost and ease of administration of the treatment regimen. Today, approximately 50 percent of nontypeable *H. influenzae* and 100 percent of *M. catarrhalis* strains produce β-lactamases and are resistant to amoxicillin.[37,38] In addition, 15 to 38 percent of *S. pneumoniae* strains have either intermediate (7-19%) or complete (7-19%) penicillin resistance.[11,26,40]

The AAP Subcommittee of Sinusitis and Committee on Quality Improvement, in their "Clinical Practice Guideline: Management of Sinusitis," recommended amoxicillin as first-line therapy for children younger than 2 years of age suspected of having acute bacterial sinusitis of mild to moderate severity, who do not attend daycare, and who have not been treated recently with an antimicrobial agent.[4] They recommend an amoxicillin dose of either 45 mg/kg/day in two divided doses or 90 mg/kg/day in two divided doses. They recommend cefdinir (14 mg/kg/day in one or two doses), cefuroxime (30 mg/kg/day in two divided doses), or cefpodoxime (10 mg/kg/day once daily) for the child who is "allergic" to amoxicillin if the past allergic reaction was not a type 1 hypersensitivity reaction. If the past allergic reaction was of a type 1 nature, they recommend clarithromycin (15 mg/kg/day in two divided doses) or azithromycin (10 mg/kg/day on day 1 followed by 5 mg/kg/day as a single dose for 4 days). They suggest clindamycin (30 to 40 mg/kg/day in three divided doses) as an alternative therapy for the penicillin-allergic patient who is known to be infected with a penicillin-resistant pneumococcal strain. Their recommendation is based on the safety, tolerability, low cost, and narrow spectrum of amoxicillin, and a calculated success rate based on data regarding treatment of acute otitis media.

The AAP committees further recommended that children who did not improve while receiving the lower amoxicillin dose, children with more severe illness, and children who attend daycare should be treated with high-dose amoxicillin-clavulanate (80 to 90 mg/kg/day of amoxicillin component in two divided doses). For children with vomiting, a single dose of ceftriaxone (50 mg/kg/day) given either intravenously or intramuscularly is suggested. After this regimen, the child's therapy is switched to an oral regimen.

The committees' suggestions presented above applied only to children younger than 2 years of age; however, because the spectrum of etiologic agents is similar to that for older children, it should also apply for those older than 2 years of age.

In contrast to the AAP committees' recommendations, we consider that a more appropriate approach is to use only high-dose amoxicillin or amoxicillin-clavulanate (90 mg/kg/day in two divided doses). The duration of treatment in the outpatient setting has not been studied adequately. Wald[178] suggests that therapy should be continued for 7 days after the child becomes symptom-free.

A seriously ill child should be hospitalized, and therapy for β-lactamase–producing staphylococci and highly resistant pneumococci should be implemented, in addition to coverage for amoxicillin-resistant *H. influenzae* and *M. catarrhalis*. This coverage is achieved with vancomycin (40 mg/kg per 24 hours every 6 hours) and cefotaxime (100 to 200 mg/kg per 24 hours every 6 hours) or ceftriaxone (100 mg/kg per 24 hours every 12 hours). Therapy should be adjusted on the basis of clinical response and culture results. The dosage and duration of antimicrobial therapy in sinusitis are crucial considerations. Penicillins penetrate the sinuses poorly.[9,48,65,85,105] The duration of therapy should be a minimum of 10 days.

The relief of obstruction at the sinus ostia and the establishment of drainage are time-honored principles of therapy. To achieve these goals, locally applied and systemically active vasoconstrictive drugs are used. To date, no evidence supports their therapeutic effectiveness, however. The beneficial effects of oral, systemically active, vasoconstrictive drugs are hampered by the fact that their drying effect may be deleterious to the mucus blanket. Topical vasoconstrictor drugs (e.g., phenylephrine hydrochloride and oxymetazoline) are plagued by rebound vasodilation. We consider that these drugs should be used rarely in acute disease; their main use is to relieve pain caused by obstruction, and they should be used only for 2 to 3 days.

CHRONIC AND RECURRENT SINUSITIS

Allergic disorders are common in chronic and recurrent sinusitis.[108,177] Children should be evaluated for allergy, and, when identified, specific treatment should be employed. Specific allergens and irritants should be avoided (e.g., through air filtering, removal of pets, avoidance of tobacco smoke), and pharmacologic management should be implemented.

Nasal saline washes (twice daily in each nostril) are useful because they liquefy secretions and enhance mucociliary transport, which improves sinus drainage and ventilation. Antihistamines may be useful if allergic rhinitis is a contributing factor to the chronic sinus infection. Anti-inflammatory agents also may be useful. In selected cases, use of either topically applied corticosteroids or cromolyn sodium may be beneficial. Corticosteroids should be used carefully because their use occasionally can lead to superinfection in the sinuses with *Pseudomonas* spp., other highly resistant gram-negative bacilli, or fungi. For effective corticosteroid use, Wald[177] suggests using a topical decongestant first so that the steroid preparation can reach the affected areas better.

In chronic or recurrent disease, antimicrobial treatment should be based on culture and sensitivity data. Specific antimicrobial agents are the same as the agents used in acute and subacute disease, but treatment should be prolonged for 3 weeks or more and for 7 days after the resolution of symptoms. *Aspergillus* and *Bipolaris* spp. and other fungal infections require prolonged therapy with an antifungal agent to which the specific agent is susceptible. Itraconazole, ketoconazole, and fluconazole all have been effective in selected cases. Allergic fungal sinusitis can be treated with endoscopic sinus débridement of all fungal and polypoid disease, followed by topical and systemic corticosteroids and close follow-up, including frequent endoscopic cleaning.[30,96,97,134] Allergic aspergillosis of the sinuses can be managed with topical steroids without specific antifungal therapy (see Chapter 28).

In the past, surgical therapy for sinusitis in children was of questionable benefit. Surgical therapy included diagnostic and therapeutic irrigation; permanent drainage procedures in children with complications of sinusitis and in children who had immune defects; and such procedures as adenoidectomy,[99,169] septoplasty, and turbinectomy to relieve anatomic obstructions to improve nasal and sinus ventilation. In one uncontrolled study of children with otitis media with effusion and sinusitis, the sinusitis was improved 6 months after adenoidectomy in 56 percent of children, whereas only 24 percent of similar children who did not undergo surgery had similar improvement.[162]

Historically, creating nasoantral windows was the most common major surgical procedure for treating chronic sinusitis in children.[62,118] Long-term success with this procedure was poor, however, because of the high rate of closure of the windows. A new interest in sinus surgery has resulted from the introduction of endoscopic techniques. Several studies have found endoscopic surgery to be safe and effective.[63,98,106,129,144] Pediatric endoscopic sinus surgery now is recognized as a viable option for children with chronic recurrent sinusitis refractory to medical therapy.[27,102,138] A meta-analysis of 832 children who underwent endoscopic sinus surgery from 1986 to 1996 revealed an overall 88.4 percent positive outcome after surgery.[74]

The goal of functional endoscopic sinus surgery is to remove obstruction at the osteomeatal complex where the mucociliary flow from the frontal, maxillary, and ethmoid sinuses converges.[98,144] This removal results in improved drainage and restoration of normal physiologic function of the frontal, maxillary, and ethmoid sinuses. Surgery involves an anterior ethmoidectomy and enlargement of the natural ostium of the maxillary sinus. Follow-up surgery performed 2 to 3 weeks after the initial surgery sometimes is necessary to remove crusts, blood clots, any stenting material, granulative tissue, and adhesions.[187]

In a study of 210 children with a history of chronic sinusitis for 3 months or longer, functional endoscopic sinus surgery resulted in successful outcomes in 165 (79%).[98] The follow-up period was 3 to 36 months (mean 18 months), and all of the infections in these children had failed to respond to prior extensive medical management. In this series, no major complications occurred.

Functional endoscopic sinus surgery should be considered for children with chronic or recurrent sinusitis that has failed extensive, prolonged, and adequate medical management.[102] Many pediatric otolaryngologists have resumed performing adenoidectomy as a surgical intervention before proceeding with functional endoscopic sinus surgery.[156] This management includes specific antimicrobial therapy for specific organisms identified by culture; the diagnosis and treatment of allergic and other contributing conditions, such as cystic fibrosis, asthma, or immunologic disorders; and a trial of prophylactic antimicrobial agents.

Orbital and intracranial abscesses and cavernous sinus thrombosis secondary to sinus infection require emergency surgery, which often is lifesaving.[143,148,189,192] Cellulitis, osteomyelitis, and meningitis also frequently require surgery if they do not respond to antimicrobial therapy.[143] Surgery in these cases involves drainage of the sinuses and abscesses. Endoscopic techniques may allow for intranasal drainage and avoidance of development of facial scars.[6] If an intracranial complication involves an intracranial abscess, concomitant craniotomy along with functional endoscopic sinus surgery may be required.[59] Surgical procedures also may be indicated for a child with acute or chronic disease resulting from an identified underlying problem, such as an immunologic deficiency.[191]

PROGNOSIS

The prognosis of identified and adequately treated sinusitis in otherwise normal children is excellent. Frequently, children have subnormal health because sinusitis goes unrecognized; it may be treated only partially because of other clinical impressions, which contributes to the chronicity of the problem. Sinusitis is likely to be recurrent in children with a history of previous chronic disease and in children with repeated adverse exposure, such as swimming in contaminated or irritating water. Children with allergic respiratory disease also are likely to have frequent recurrences. Sinusitis in an immunocompromised child frequently is resistant to cure; long-term continuous therapy can be beneficial in such patients. Signs and symptoms of neurologic involvement in sinusitis frequently call for aggressive surgical management of the sinusitis and the intracranial and paracranial lesions.

Paranasal sinusitis also has been noted occasionally to be associated with bronchial asthma.[127,136] Its successful treatment has resulted in clearing of the asthma.[80,150]

PREVENTION

Sinusitis, as such, is not preventable in most instances. In some individuals, change of lifestyle can do much to improve the situation, however. Sinusitis in some children is related to their swimming habits and can be controlled by elimination of swimming or perhaps by the use of nose plugs. Good allergic management, including intranasal corticosteroid or cromolyn therapy, prevents sinus disease in certain atopic children. Relief of nasal airway obstruction caused by allergic rhinitis, enlarged adenoids, or other anatomic problems also should help to prevent sinusitis. Early attention given to persistent nasal discharge also can be expected to lessen the damage associated with sinus infection.

REFERENCES

1. Adame, N., Hedlund, G., and Byington, C. L.: Sinogenic intracranial empyema in children. Pediatrics 116:461-467, 2005.
2. Aitken, M., and Taylor, J. A.: Prevalence of clinical sinusitis in young children followed by primary care pediatricians. Arch. Pediatr. Adolesc. Med. 152:244-248, 1998.
3. Alfaro, V. R.: Nasal sinus disease in children. Pediatr. Clin. North Am. 9:1061-1072, 1962.
4. American Academy of Pediatrics Subcommittee on Management of Sinusitis and Committee on Quality Improvement: Clinical practice guideline: Management of sinusitis. Pediatrics 108:798-808, 2001.
5. April, M. M., Zinreich, J., Baroody, F. M., et al.: Coronal CT scan abnormalities in children with chronic sinusitis. Laryngoscope 103:985-990, 1993.
6. Arjmand, E. M., Lusk, R. P., and Muntz, H. R.: Pediatric sinusitis and subperiosteal orbital abscess formation: Diagnosis and treatment. Otolaryngol. Head Neck Surg. 109:886-894, 1993.
7. Arruda, E., Boyle, T. R., Winther, B., et al.: Localization of human rhinovirus replication in the upper respiratory tract by in situ hybridization. J. Infect. Dis. 171:1329-1333, 1995.
8. Axelsson, A., and Brorson, J. E.: The correlation between bacteriological findings in the nose and maxillary sinus in acute maxillary sinusitis. Laryngoscope 88:2003-2011, 1973.
9. Axelsson, A., Grebelius, N., Jensen, C., et al.: Treatment of acute maxillary sinusitis, IV: Ampicillin, cephradine and erythromycin estolate with and without irrigation. Acta Otol. 79:466-472, 1975.
10. Axelsson, A., and Runze, U.: Symptoms and signs of acute maxillary sinusitis. Otol. Rhinol. Laryngol. 38:298-308, 1976.
11. Baquero, F., and Loza, E.: Antibiotic resistance of microorganisms involved in ear, nose and throat infections. Pediatr. Infect. Dis. J. 13:S9-S14, 1994.
12. Berry, A. J., Kerkering, T. M., Giordano, A. M., et al.: Phaeohyphomycotic sinusitis. Pediatr. Infect. Dis. 3:150-152, 1984.
13. Bhattacharyya, N., Jones, D. T., Hill, M., et al.: The diagnostic accuracy of computed tomography in pediatric chronic rhinosinusitis. Arch. Otolaryngol. Head Neck Surg. 130:1029-1032, 2004.
14. Bhattacharyya, T. K., Mehra, Y. N., and Agarwal, S. C.: Incidence of bacterial, L-form and mycoplasma in chronic sinusitis. Acta Otol. 74:293-296, 1972.
15. Box, Q. T., Cleveland, R. T., and Willard, C. Y.: Bacterial flora of the upper respiratory tract, I: Comparative evaluation by anterior nasal, oropharyngeal, and nasopharyngeal swabs. Am. J. Dis. Child. 102:293-301, 1961.
16. Brandtzaeg, P.: Mucosal immunology: With special reference to specific immune defense of the upper respiratory tract. Otorhinolaryngology 50:225-235, 1988.
17. Breese, B. B., Disney, F. A., and Talpey, W.: The nature of a small pediatric group practice: Part I. Pediatrics 38:264-277, 1966.
18. Brook, I.: Beta-lactamase-producing bacteria in head and neck infection. Laryngoscope 98:428-431, 1988.
19. Brook, I.: Bacteriologic features of chronic sinusitis in children. J. A. M. A. 246:967-969, 1981.
20. Brook, I.: The role of anaerobic bacteria in sinusitis. Anaerobe 12:5-12, 2006.
21. Brook, I., Yocum, P., and Shah, K.: Aerobic and anaerobic bacteriology of concurrent chronic otitis media with effusion and chronic sinusitis in children. Arch. Otolarynol. Head Neck Surg. 126:174-176, 2000.
22. Buering, I., Friedrich, B., Schaaf, J., et al.: Chronic sinusitis refractory to standard management in patients with humoral deficiencies. Clin. Exp. Immunol. 109:468-472, 1997.
23. Campbell, J. M., Graham, M., Gray, H. C., et al.: Allergic fungal sinusitis in children. Ann. Allergy Asthma Immun. 96:286-290, 2006.
24. Carenfelt, C., and Lundberg, C.: Purulent and nonpurulent maxillary sinus secretions with respect to pO2, pCO2, and pH. Acta Otol. 84:138-144, 1977.
25. Carenfelt, C., Lundberg, C., and Karlen, K.: Immunoglobulins in maxillary sinus secretion. Acta Otol. 82:123-130, 1976.
26. Centers for Disease Control and Prevention: Geographic variation in penicillin resistance in Streptococcus pneumoniae-selected sites, United States, 1997. M. M. W. R. Morb. Mortal. Wkly. Rep. 48:656-661, 1999.
27. Chan, K. H., Winslow, C. P., Levin, M. J., et al.: Clinical practice guidelines for the management of chronic sinusitis in children. Otolaryngol. Head Neck Surg. 120:328-334, 1999.
28. Cherry, J. D.: Infection in the compromised host. In Stiehm, E. R. (ed.): Immunologic Disorders in Infants and Children. 4th ed. Philadelphia, W. B. Saunders, 1996, pp. 975-1013.
29. Colman, B. H.: Sinusitis. Practitioner 215:725-731, 1975.
30. Corey, J. P., Delsupene, K. G., and Ferguson, B. J.: Allergic fungal sinusitis: Allergic, infectious, or both? Otolaryngol. Head Neck Surg. 113:110-119, 1995.
31. Cultrara, A., Goldstein, N. A., Ovchinsky, A., et al.: The role of Chlamydia pneumoniae infection in children with chronic sinusitis. Arch. Otolaryngol. Head Neck Surg. 129:1094-1097, 2003.
32. Dawes, J. D. K.: Diagnosis and treatment of sinusitis. B. M. J. 1:843-845, 1966.
33. de Shazo, R. D., O'Brien, M., Chapin, K., et al.: A new classification and diagnostic criteria for invasive fungal sinusitis. Arch. Otolaryngol Head Neck Surg. 127:1181-1188, 1997.

34. Diament, M. J.: The diagnosis of sinusitis in infants and children: X-ray, computed tomography, and magnetic resonance imaging: Diagnostic imaging of pediatric sinusitis. J. Allergy Clin. Immunol. 90:442-444, 1990.

35. Diament, M. J., Senac, M. O., Jr., Gilsanz, V., et al.: Prevalence of incidental paranasal sinuses opacification in pediatric patients: A CT study. J. Comput. Assisted Tomogr. 11:426-431, 1987.

36. Dingle, J. H., Badjer, D. F., and Jordan, W. S., Jr.: Patterns of Illness: Illness in the Home. Cleveland, Western Reserve University, 1964, p. 347.

37. Doern, G. V., Brueggemann, A. B., Pierce, G., et al.: Antibiotic resistance among clinical isolates of *Haemophilus influenzae* in the United States in 1994 and 1995 and detection of beta-lactamase-positive strains resistant to amoxicillin-clavulanate: Results of a national multicenter surveillance study. Antimicrob. Agents Chemother. 41:292-297, 1997.

38. Doern, G. V., Jones, R. N., Pfaller, M. A., et al.: *Haemophilus influenzae* and *Moraxella catarrhalis* from patients with community-acquired respiratory tract infections: Antimicrobial susceptibility patterns from the SENTRY Antimicrobial Surveillance Program (United States and Canada, 1997). Antimicrob. Agents Chemother. 43:385-389, 1999.

39. Don, D. M., Yellon, R. F., Casselbrant, M. L., et al.: Efficacy of a stepwise protocol that includes intravenous antibiotic therapy for the management of chronic sinusitis in children and adolescents. Arch. Otolaryngol. Head Neck Surg. 127:1093-1098, 2001.

40. Dowell, S. F., Butler, J. C., Giebink, G. S., et al.: Acute otitis media: Management and surveillance in an era of pneumococcal resistance—a report from the Drug-Resistant *Streptococcus pneumoniae* Therapeutic Working Group. Pediatr. Infect. Dis. J. 18:1-9, 1999.

41. Dudley, J. P., and Cherry, J. D.: The effect of mucolytic agents and topical decongestants on the ciliary activity of chicken tracheal organ cultures. Pediatr. Res. 11:904-906, 1977.

42. Dudley, J. P., and Cherry, J. D.: Effects of topical nasal decongestants on the cilia of a chicken embryo tracheal organ culture system. Laryngoscope 88:110-116, 1978.

43. Dudley, J. P., Goldstein, E. J. C., George, W. L., et al.: Sinus infection due to *Eikenella corrodens*. Arch. Otol. 104:462-463, 1978.

44. Dunlap, M. B., and Harvey, H. S.: Host influence on upper respiratory flora. N. Engl. J. Med. 255:640-646, 1956.

45. Edvinsson, M., Asplund, M. S., Hjelm, E., et al.: *Chlamydophila pneumoniae* in chronic rhinosinusitis. Acta Oto-Laryngol. 126:952-957, 2006.

46. El-Hakim, H., Malik, A. C., Aronyk, K., et al.: The prevalence of intracranial complications in pediatric frontal sinusitis. Int. J. Pediatr. Otorhinolaryngol. 70:1383-1387, 2006.

47. Eliasson, R., Mossberg, B., Camner, P., et al.: The immotile cilia syndrome: A congenital ciliary abnormality as an etiologic factor in chronic airway infections and male sterility. N. Engl. J. Med. 297:1-6, 1977.

48. Eneroth, C. M., Lundberg, C., and Wretlind, B.: Antibiotic concentrations in maxillary sinus secretions and in the sinus mucosa. Chemotherapy 21(Suppl. 1):1-7, 1975.

49. Fernbach, S. K., and Naidich, T. P.: CT diagnosis of orbital inflammation in children. Neuroradiology 22:7-13, 1981.

50. Frederick, J., and Braude, A. I.: Anaerobic infection of the paranasal sinuses. N. Engl. J. Med. 290:135-137, 1974.

51. Frenkel, L. M., Kuhls, T. L., Nitta, K., et al.: Recurrent bipolaris sinusitis following surgical and antifungal therapy. Pediatr. Infect. Dis. 6:1130-1132, 1987.

52. Friday, G. A., and Fireman, P.: Sinusitis and asthma: Clinical pathogenic relationships. Clin. Chest Med. 9:557-565, 1988.

53. Friedman, R., Ackerman, M., Wald, E., et al.: Asthma and bacterial sinusitis in children. J. Allergy Clin. Immunol. 74:185-189, 1984.

54. Garcia, C. E., Cunningham, M. J., Randall, A. C., et al.: The etiologic role of frontal sinusitis in pediatric orbital abscesses. Am. J. Otolaryngol. 14:449-452, 1993.

55. Gellady, A. M., Shulman, S. T., and Ayoub, E. M.: Periorbital and orbital cellulitis in children. Pediatrics 61:272-277, 1978.

56. Germiller, J. A., Monin, D. L., Sparano, A. M., et al.: Intracranial complications of sinusitis in children and adolescents and their outcomes. Arch. Otolaryngol. Head Neck Surg. 132:969-976, 2006.

57. Givner, L. B., McGehee, D., Taber, L. H., et al.: Sinusitis, orbital cellulitis and polymicrobial bacteremia in a patient with primary Epstein-Barr virus infection. Pediatr. Infect. Dis. 3:254-256, 1984.

58. Glasier, C. M., Archer, D. P., and Williams, K. D.: Incidental paranasal sinus abnormalities on CT of children: Clinical correlation. A. J. N. R. Am. J. Neuroradiol. 7:861-864, 1986.

59. Glickstein, J. S., Chandra, R. K., and Thompson, J. W.: Intracranial complications of pediatric sinusitis. Otolaryngol. Head Neck Surg. 134:733-736, 2006.

60. Gnarpe, H., and Lundberg, C.: L-phase organisms in maxillary sinus secretions. Scand. J. Infect. Dis. 3:257-259, 1971.

61. Griffin, J. P., and Klein, E. W.: Role of sinusitis in primary atypical pneumonia. Clin. Med. 78:23-27, 1971.

62. Gross, C. W.: Surgical management: An otolaryngologist's perspective. Pediatr. Infect. Dis. 4:567, 1985.

63. Gross, C. W., Gurucharri, M. J., Lazar, R. H., et al.: Functional endonasal sinus surgery (FESS) in the pediatric age group. Laryngoscope 99:272-275, 1989.

64. Gross, C. W., McGeady, S. J., Kerut, T., et al.: Limited-slide CT in the evaluation of paranasal sinus disease in children. A. J. R. Am. J. Roentgenol. 156:367-369, 1991.

65. Gullers, K., Lundberg, C., and Malmborg, A. S.: Penicillin in paranasal sinus secretions. Chemotherapy 14:303-307, 1969.

66. Gwaltney, M. J., Jr., Hendley, J. O., Phillips, C. D., et al.: Nose blowing propels nasal fluid into the paranasal sinuses. Clin. Infect. Dis. 30:387-391, 2000.

67. Gwaltney, M. J., Jr., Hendley, J. O., Simon, G., et al.: Rhinovirus infections in an industrial population, I: The occurrence of illness. N. Engl. J. Med. 275:1261-1268, 1966.

68. Hamory, B. H., Sande, M. A., Sydnor, A., Jr., et al.: Etiology and antimicrobial therapy of acute maxillary sinusitis. J. Infect. Dis. 139:197-202, 1979.

69. Hansson, L. A., Ahlstedt, S., Andersson, B., et al.: Mucosal immunity. Ann. N. Y. Acad. Sci. 409:1-21, 1983.

70. Harvey, H. S., and Dunlap, M. B.: Seasonal prevalence of upper respiratory pathogens. N. Engl. J. Med. 264:684-686, 1961.

71. Hawkins, D. B., and Clark, R. W.: Orbital involvement in acute sinusitis: Lessons from 24 childhood patients. Clin. Pediatr. 16:464-471, 1977.

72. Haynes, R. E., and Cramblett, H. G.: Acute ethmoiditis: Its relationship to orbital cellulitis. Am. J. Dis. Child. 114:261-267, 1967.

73. Hays, G. C., and Mullard, J. E.: Can nasal bacterial flora be predicted from clinical findings? Pediatrics 49:596-599, 1972.

74. Hebert, R. L., and Bent, J. P.: Meta-analysis of pediatric functional endoscopic sinus surgery. Laryngoscope 108:796-799, 1998.

75. Herz, G., and Gfeller, J.: Sinusitis in paediatrics. Chemotherapy 23:50-57, 1977.

76. Hill, M., Bhattacharyya, N., Hall, T. R., et al.: Incidental paranasal sinus imaging abnormalities and the normal Lund score in children. Otolaryngol. Head Neck Surg. 130:171-175, 2004.

77. Holdaway, M. D., and Turk, D. C.: Capsulated *Haemophilus influenzae* and respiratory tract disease. Lancet 1:358-360, 1967.

78. Hoshaw, T. C., and Nickman, N. J.: Sinusitis and otitis in children. Arch. Otol. 100:194-195, 1974.

79. Huijssoon, E., Woerdeman, P. A., van Diemen-Steenvoorde, R. A. A. M., et al.: An 8-year-old boy with a Pott's puffy tumor. Int. J. Pediatr. Otorhinolaryngol. 67:1023-1026, 2003.

80. Ikeda, K., Tanno, N., Tamura, G., et al.: Endoscopic sinus surgery improves pulmonary function in patients with asthma associated with chronic sinusitis. Ann. Otol. Rhinol. Laryngol. 108:355-359, 1999.

81. Ilki, A., Ulger, N., Inanli, S., et al.: Microbiology of sinusitis and the predictive value of throat culture for the aetiology of sinusitis. Clin. Microbiol. Infect. 11:407-410, 2005.

82. Ioannidis, J. P., and Lau, J.: Technical report: Evidence for the diagnosis and treatment of acute uncomplicated sinusitis in children: A systematic overview. Pediatrics 108:E57, 2001.

83. Jacobson, L. O., and Dick, G. F.: Normal and abnormal bacterial flora of the nose. J. A. M. A. 117:2222-2225, 1941.

84. Jaffe, B. F.: Chronic sinusitis in children: Comments on pathogenesis and management. Clin. Pediatr. 13:944-948, 1974.

85. Jeppesen, F., and Illum, P.: Concentration of ampicillin in antral mucosa following administration of ampicillin sodium and privampicillin. Acta Otol. 73:428-432, 1972.

86. Jousimies-Somer, H. R., Savolainen, S., and Ylikoski, J. S.: Bacteriological findings of acute maxillary sinusitis in young adults. J. Clin. Microbiol. 26:1919-1925, 1988.

87. Jousimies-Somer, H. R., Savolainen, S., and Ylikoski, J. S.: Comparison of the nasal bacterial floras in two groups of healthy subjects and in patients with acute maxillary sinusitis. J. Clin. Microbiol. 27:2736-2743, 1989.

88. Katzenstein, A. L., Sale, S. R., and Greenberger, P. A.: Pathologic findings in allergic aspergillus sinusitis. Am. J. Surg. Pathol. 7:439-443, 1983.

89. Kern, E. B.: Sinusitis. J. Allergy Clin. Immunol. 73:25-31, 1984.

90. Kim, H. J., Lee, K., Yoo, J. B., et al.: Bacteriological findings and antimicrobial susceptibility in chronic sinusitis with nasal polyp. Acta Oto-Laryngol. 126:489-497, 2006.

91. Kogutt, M. S., and Swischuk, L. E.: Diagnosis of sinusitis in infants and children. Pediatrics 52:152-156, 1973.

92. Kovatch, A. L., Wald, E. R., Ledesma-Medina, J., et al.: Maxillary sinus radiographs in children with nonrespiratory complaints. Pediatrics 73:306-308, 1984.

93. Krajina, Z., Koskovic, F., and Babic, I.: The bacteriology of the respiratory tract in various pathological conditions. Acta Otol. 67:453-459, 1969.

94. Kristo, A., Uhari, M., Luotonen, J., et al.: Paranasal sinus findings in children during respiratory infection evaluated with magnetic resonance imaging. Pediatrics 111:586-589, 2003.

95. Kuczkowski, J., Naronzny, W., Mikaszewski, B., et al.: Suppurative complications of frontal sinusitis in children. Clin. Pediatr. 44:675-682, 2005.

96. Kupferberg, S. B., and Bent, J. P.: Allergic fungal sinusitis in the pediatric population. Arch. Otolaryngol. Head Neck Surg. 122:1381-1384, 1996.

97. Kupferberg, S. B., Bent J. P., and Kuhn, F. A.: Prognosis for allergic fungal sinusitis. Otolaryngol. Head Neck Surg. 117:35-41, 1997.

98. Lazar, R. H., Ramzi, R. Y., and Gross, C. W.: Pediatric functional endonasal sinus surgery: A review of 210 cases. Head Neck 14:92-98, 1992.

99. Lee, D., and Rosenfeld, R. M.: Adenoid bacteriology and sinonasal symptoms in children. Otolaryngol. Head Neck Surg. 116:301-307, 1997.

100. Lehrer, R. I., Howard, D. H., Sypherd, P. S., et al.: Mucormycosis. Ann. Intern. Med. 93:93-108, 1980.
101. Lehtinen, P., Jartti, T., Virkki, R., et al.: Bacterial coinfections in children with viral wheezing. Eur. J. Clin. Microbiol. Infect. Dis. 25:463-469, 2006.
102. Lieser, J. D., and Derkay, C. S.: Pediatric sinusitis: When do we operate? Curr. Opin. Otolaryngol. Head Neck Surg. 13:60-66, 2005.
103. Limjoco-Antonio, A. D., Janda, W. M., and Schreckenberger, P. C.: *Arcanobacterium haemolyticum* sinusitis and orbital cellulitis. Pediatr. Infect. Dis. J. 22:465-467, 2003.
104. Lueg, E. A., Ballagh, R. H., and Forte, V.: Analysis of the recent cluster of invasive fungal sinusitis at the Toronto Hospital for Sick Children. J. Otolaryngol. 25:366-370, 1996.
105. Lundberg, C., and Malmburg, A. S.: Studies of antibiotics in sinus secretions. Rhinology 9:166-168, 1971.
106. Lusk, R. P., and Muntz, H. R.: Endoscopic sinus surgery in children with chronic sinusitis: A pilot study. Laryngoscope 100:654-658, 1990.
107. Lystad, A., Berdal, P., and Lund-Iversen, L.: The bacterial flora of sinusitis with an in vitro study of the bacterial resistance to antibiotics. Acta Otol. 188(Suppl.):390-399, 1963.
108. Manning, S. C.: Pediatric sinusitis. Otolaryngol. Clin. North Am. 26:623-638, 1993.
109. Manning, S. C., Biavati, M. J., and Phillips, D. L.: Correlation of clinical sinusitis signs and symptoms to imaging findings in pediatric patients. Int. J. Pediatr. Otorhinolaryngol. 37:65-74, 1996.
110. Manning, S. C., Vuitch, F., Weinberg, A. G., et al.: Allergic aspergillosis: A newly recognized form of sinusitis in the pediatric population. Laryngoscope 99:681-685, 1989.
111. Maresh, M. M., and Washburn, A. H.: Paranasal sinuses from birth to late adolescence, II: Clinical and roentgenographic evidence of infection. Am. J. Dis. Child. 60:841-861, 1940.
112. Marseglia, G. L., Pagella, F., Licari, A., et al.: Acute isolated sphenoid sinusitis in children. Int. J. Pediatr. Otorhinolaryngol. 70:2027-2031, 2006.
113. May, M. L. A.: Severe consequences of sinusitis. J. Paediatr. Child Health 40:311-314, 2004.
114. McAllister, W. H., Parker, B. R., Kushner, D. C., et al.: Sinusitis in the pediatric population. In ACR Appropriateness Criteria. Reston, VA, American College of Radiology, 2000. Available at: http://www.acr.org/cgi-bin/ fr?tmpl: appcrit,pdf:0811-818 sinusitis-ac.pdf.
115. McLean, D. C.: Sinusitis in children: Lessons from 25 patients. Clin. Pediatr. 9:342-345, 1970.
116. Min, Y. G., Kim, H. S., Suh, S. H., et al.: Paranasal sinusitis after long-term use of topical nasal decongestants. Acta Otolaryngol. 116:465-471, 1996.
117. Mofenson, L. M., Korelitz, J., Pelton, S., et al.: Sinusitis in children infected with human immunodeficiency virus: Clinical characteristics, risk factors, and prophylaxis. Clin. Infect. Dis. 21:1175-1181, 1995.
118. Muntz, H. R., and Lusk, R. P.: Nasal antral windows in children: A retrospective study. Laryngoscope 100:643-646, 1990.
119. Muntz, H. R., and Lusk, R. P.: Bacteriology of the ethmoid bullae in children with chronic sinusitis. Arch. Otolaryngol. Head Neck Surg. 117:179-181, 1991.
120. Naclerio, R. M., Proud, D., Lichtenstein, L. M., et al.: Kinins are generated during experimental rhinovirus colds. J. Infect. Dis. 157:133-142, 1988.
121. Nguyen, K. L., Corbett, M. L., Garcia, D. P., et al.: Chronic sinusitis among pediatric patients with chronic respiratory complaints. J. Allergy Clin. Immunol. 92:824-830, 1993.
122. Noah, T. L., Henderson, F. W., Wortman, I. A., et al.: Nasal cytokine production in viral acute upper respiratory infection of childhood. J. Infect. Dis. 171:584-592, 1995.
123. Orobello, P. W., Park, R. I., Belcher, L. J., et al.: Microbiology of chronic sinusitis in children. Arch. Otolaryngol. Head Neck Surg. 117:980-983, 1991.
124. Oxford, L. E., and McClay, J.: Complications of acute sinusitis in children. Otolaryngol. Head Neck Surg. 133:32-37, 2005.
125. Palva, T., Grumlaut-Onroos, J. A., and Palva, A.: Bacteriology and pathology of chronic maxillary sinusitis. Acta Otol. 54:159-175, 1962.
126. Pedersen, M., Sakakura, Y., Winther, B., et al.: Nasal mucociliary transport, number of ciliated cells, and beating pattern in naturally acquired common colds. Eur. J. Respir. Dis. 128(Suppl.):355-364, 1983.
127. Phipatanakul, C. S., and Slavin, R. G.: Bronchial asthma produced by paranasal sinusitis. Arch. Otol. 100:109-112, 1974.
128. Pitkaranta, A., Starck, M., Savolainen, S., et al.: Rhinovirus RNA in the maxillary sinus epithelium of adult patients with acute sinusitis. Clin. Infect. Dis. 33:909-911, 2001.
129. Poole, M. D.: Pediatric sinusitis is not a surgical disease. Ear Nose Throat J. 71:622-623, 1992.
130. Proctor, D. F.: The historical background of modern otolaryngology. In Ravitch, M. M. (ed.): The Nose, Paranasal Sinuses and Ears in Childhood. Springfield, IL, Charles C Thomas, 1963, pp. 3-19.
131. Proud, D., Gwaltney, J. M., Hendley, J. O., et al.: Increased levels of interleukin-1 are detected in nasal secretions of volunteers during experimental rhinovirus colds. J. Infect. Dis. 169:1007-1013, 1994.
132. Proud, D., Naclerio, R. M., Gwaltney, J. M., et al.: Kinins are generated in nasal secretions during natural rhinovirus colds. J. Infect. Dis. 161:120-123, 1990.
133. Quraishi, H., and Zevallos, J. P.: Subdural empyema as a complication of sinusitis in the pediatric population. Int. J. Pediatr. Otorhinolaryngol. 70:1581-1586, 2006.
134. Quraishi, H. A., and Ramadan, H. H.: Endoscopic treatment of allergic fungal sinusitis. Otolaryngol. Head Neck Surg. 117:29-34, 1997.
135. Rachelefsky, G. S., Katz, R. M., and Siegel, S. C.: Chronic sinusitis in children with respiratory allergy: The role of antimicrobials. J. Allergy Clin. Immunol. 69:382-387, 1982.
136. Rachelefsky, G. S., Katz, R. M., and Siegel, S. C.: Chronic sinus disease with associated reactive airway disease in children. Pediatrics 73:526-529, 1984.
137. Rachelefsky, G. S., Katz, R. M., and Siegel, S. C.: Chronic sinusitis in the allergic child. Pediatr. Clin. North Am. 35:1091-1101, 1988.
138. Ramadan, H. H.: Surgical management of chronic sinusitis in children. Laryngoscope 114:2103-2109, 2004.
139. Rantanen, T., and Arvilommi, H.: Double-blind trial of doxycycline in acute maxillary sinusitis: A clinical and bacteriological study. Acta Otol. 76:58-62, 1973.
140. Richards, W.: Hospitalization of children with status asthmaticus: A review. Pediatrics 84:111-118, 1989.
141. Richards, W., Roth, R., and Church, F.: Underdiagnosis and undertreatment of chronic sinusitis in children. Clin. Pediatr. 30:88-92, 1991.
142. Roberts, S. A., Bartley, J., Braatvedt, G., et al.: *Nocardia asteroides* as a cause of sphenoidal sinusitis: Case report. Clin. Infect. Dis. 21:1041-1042, 2001.
143. Rosenfeld, R. A., and Rowley, A. H.: Infectious intracranial complications of sinusitis, other than meningitis, in children: 12-year review. Clin. Infect. Dis. 18:750-754, 1994.
144. Rosenfeld, R. M.: Pilot study of outcomes in pediatric rhinosinusitis. Arch. Otol. Head Neck Surg. 121:729-736, 1995.
145. Rossen, R. D., Butler, W. T., Cate, T. R., et al.: Protein composition of nasal secretion during respiratory virus infection. Proc. Soc. Exp. Biol. Med. 119:1169-1176, 1965.
146. Rulon, J. T.: Sinusitis in children. Postgrad. Med. 48:107-112, 1970.
147. Rynnel-Dagoo, B., Forsgren, J., Freijd, A., et al.: Rationale for antibiotic therapy in pediatric ear, nose and throat infections: Immunologic issues. Pediatr. Infect. Dis. J. 13:15-20, 1994.
148. Sable, N. S., Hengerer, A., and Powell, K. R.: Acute frontal sinusitis with intracranial complications. Pediatr. Infect. Dis. 3:58-61, 1984.
149. Schenck, N. L., and Rauchbach, E.: Frontal sinus disease, IV: Cellular response to experimentally induced infection. Laryngoscope 86:1726-1733, 1976.
150. Senior, B. A., Kennedy, D. W., Tanabodee, J., et al.: Long-term impact of functional endoscopic sinus surgery on asthma. Otolaryngol. Head Neck Surg. 121:66-68, 1999.
151. Shapiro, G. G.: The role of nasal airway obstruction in sinus disease and facial development. J. Allergy Clin. Immunol. 82:935-940, 1988.
152. Shapiro, G. G., Virant, F. S., Furukawa, C. T., et al.: Immunologic defects in patients with refractory sinusitis. Pediatrics 87:311-316, 1991.
153. Shibley, G. S., Hanger, F. M., and Dochez, A. R.: Studies in the common cold, I: Observations of the normal bacterial flora of nose and throat with variations occurring during colds. J. Exp. Med. 43:415-431, 1926.
154. Shopfner, C. E., and Rossi, J. O.: Roentgenogram evaluation of the paranasal sinuses in children. A. J. R. Am. J. Roentgenol. 118:176-186, 1973.
155. Shurin, P. A.: Etiology and antimicrobial therapy of paranasal sinusitis in children. Ann. Otol. Rhinol. Laryngol. 90(Suppl.):72-74, 1981.
156. Sobol, S. E., Samadi, D. S., Kazahaya, K., et al.: Trends in the management of pediatric chronic sinusitis: Survey of the American Society of Pediatric Otolaryngology. Laryngoscope 115:78-80, 2005.
157. Sobol, S. M., Love, R. G., Stutman, H. R., et al.: Phaeohyphomycosis of the maxilloethmoid sinus caused by *Drechslera spicifera*: A new fungal pathogen. Laryngoscope 94:620-627, 1984.
158. Sohail, M. A., Al Khabori, M., Hyder, J., et al.: Acute fulminant fungal sinusitis: Clinical presentation, radiological findings and treatment. Acta Trop. 80:177-185, 2001.
159. Sparrevohn, U. R., and Buch, A.: The bacteriology of maxillary sinusitis, I: Technique. Acta Otol. 34:425-436, 1946.
160. Spector, S. L., English, G. M., McIntosh, K., et al.: Adenovirus in the sinuses of an asthmatic patient with apparent selective antibody deficiencies. Am. J. Med. 55:227-231, 1973.
161. Sprinkle, P.: Current status of mycoplasmatales and bacterial variants in chronic otolaryngic disease. Laryngoscope 82:737-747, 1972.
162. Takahashi, H., Fujita, A., and Hanjo, I.: Effect of adenoidectomy on otitis media with effusion, tubal function, and sinusitis. Am. J. Otol. 10:208-213, 1989.
163. Talbot, G. H., Kennedy, D. W., Scheld, W. M., et al.: Rigid nasal endoscopy versus sinus puncture and aspiration for microbiologic documentation of acute bacterial maxillary sinusitis. Clin. Infect. Dis. 33:1668-1675, 2001.
164. Taxy, J. B.: Paranasal fungal sinusitis: Contributions of histopathology to diagnosis. Am. J. Surg. Pathol. 30:713-720, 2006.
165. Tinkelman, D. G., and Silk, H. J.: Clinical and bacteriologic features of chronic sinusitis in children. Am. J. Dis. Child. 143:938-941, 1989.
166. Tos, M., and Mogensen, C.: Mucus production in chronic maxillary sinusitis. Acta Otol. 97:151-159, 1984.
167. Ueda, D., and Yoto, Y.: The ten-day mark as a practical diagnostic approach for acute paranasal sinusitis in children. Pediatr. Infect. Dis. 15:576-579, 1996.

168. Umetsu, D. J., Ambrosino, D. M., Quinti, I., et al.: Recurrent sinopulmonary infection and impaired antibody response to bacterial capsular polysaccharide antigen in children with selective IgG subclass deficiency. N. Engl. J. Med. *313*:1247-1251, 1985.
169. Ungkanont, K., and Damrongsak, S.: Effect of adenoidectomy in children with complex problems of rhinosinusitis and associated diseases. Int. J. Pediatr. Otorhinolaryngol. *68*:447-451, 2004.
170. Unzaga, M. J., Crovetto, M. A., Santamaria, J. M., et al.: Maxillary sinusitis caused by *Nocardia nova*. Clin. Infect. Dis. *23*:184-185, 1996.
171. Urdal, K., and Berdal, P.: The microbial flora in 81 cases of maxillary sinusitis. Acta Otol. *37*:20-25, 1949.
172. Van Cauwenberge, P., Verschraegen, G., and Van Renterghem, L.: Bacteriological findings in sinusitis (1963-1975). Scand. J. Infect. Dis. *9*:72-77, 1976.
173. Wald, E. R.: Epidemiology, pathophysiology and etiology of sinusitis. Pediatr. Infect. Dis. *4*:S51-S81, 1985.
174. Wald, E. R.: Sinusitis in children. Pediatr. Infect. Dis. 7:S150-S153, 1988.
175. Wald, E. R.: Rhinitis and acute and chronic sinusitis. *In* Bluestone, C. D., Stool, S. E., and Scheetz, M. D. (eds.): Pediatric Otorhinolaryngology. 2nd ed. Philadelphia, W. B. Saunders, 1990, pp. 729-944.
176. Wald, E. R.: Sinusitis in infants and children. Ann. Otol. Rhinol. Laryngol. Suppl. *155*:37-41, 1992.
177. Wald, E. R.: Chronic sinusitis in children. J. Pediatr. *127*:339-347, 1995.
178. Wald, E. R.: Sinusitis. Pediatr. Ann. 27:811-818, 1998.
179. Wald, E. R.: Microbiology of acute and chronic sinusitis in children and adults. Am. J. Med. Sci. *316*:13-20, 1998.
180. Wald, E. R.: Beginning antibiotics for acute rhinosinusitis and choosing the right treatment. Clin. Rev. Allerg. Immun. *30*:143-151, 2006.
181. Wald, E. R., Byers, C., Guerra, N., et al.: Subacute sinusitis in children. J. Pediatr. *115*:28-32, 1989.
182. Wald, E. R., Dashefky, B., Byers, C., et al.: Frequency and severity of infections in day care. J. Pediatr. *112*:540-546, 1988.
183. Wald, E. R., Chiponis, D., and Ledesma-Medina, J.: Comparative effectiveness of amoxicillin and amoxicillin-clavulanate potassium in acute paranasal sinus infections in children: A double-blind, placebo-controlled trial. Pediatrics 77:795-800, 1986.
184. Wald, E. R., Guerra, N., and Byers, C.: Upper respiratory tract infection in young children: Duration and frequency of complications. Pediatrics *87*:129-133, 1991.
185. Wald, E. R., Milmoe, G. J., Bowen, A. D., et al.: Acute maxillary sinusitis in children. N. Engl. J. Med. *304*:749-754, 1981.
186. Wald, E. R., Reilly, J. S., Casselbrant, M., et al.: Treatment of acute maxillary sinusitis in childhood: A comparative study of amoxicillin and cefaclor. J. Pediatr. *104*:297-302, 1984.
187. Walner, D. L., Falaglia, M., Willging, J. P., et al.: The role of second-look nasal endoscopy after pediatric functional endoscopic sinus surgery. Arch. Otolaryngol. Head Neck Surg. *124*:425-428, 1998.
188. Washburn, R. G., Kennedy, D. W., Begley, M. G., et al.: Chronic fungal sinusitis in apparently normal hosts. Medicine 67:231-247, 1988.
189. Wassermann, D.: Acute paranasal sinusitis and cavernous sinus thrombosis. Arch. Otol. *86*:99-103, 1967.
190. Watters, E. C., Wallar, P. H., Hiles, D. A., et al.: Acute orbital cellulitis. Arch. Ophthalmol. *94*:785-788, 1976.
191. Whiatick, B. J., Willging, P., Myer, C. M., et al.: Functional endoscopic sinus surgery in the immunocompromised child. Otolaryngol. Head Neck Surg. *105*:818-825, 1991.
192. Whitaker, C. W.: Intracranial complications of ear, nose, and throat infections. Laryngoscope *81*:1375-1380, 1971.
193. Winther, B.: Effects on the nasal mucosa of upper respiratory viruses (common cold). Danish Med. Bull. *41*:193-204, 1994.
194. Wold, G., Anderhuber, W., and Kuhn, F.: Development of the paranasal sinuses in children: Implications for paranasal sinus surgery. Ann. Otol. Rhinol. Laryngol. *102*:705-711, 1993.
195. Yang, H. S.: Nasal flora of the children in a day nursery. Am. J. Dis. Child. *61*:262-272, 1941.
196. Zimmerman, B., Stringer, D., Feanning, S., et al.: Prevalence of abnormalities found by sinus x-ray in childhood asthma: Lack of relation to severity of asthma. J. Allergy Clin. Immunol. *80*:268-273, 1987.
197. Zinreich, S. J., Kennedy, D. W., Rosenbaum, A. E., et al.: Paranasal sinuses: CT imaging requirements for endoscopic surgery. Radiology *163*:769-775, 1987.

OTITIS EXTERNA

Ellen M. Friedman ⊙ Tulio A. Valdez

Otitis externa constitutes one of the most common otolaryngologic encounters in the emergency department. This condition is addressed commonly as *swimmer's ear* or *tropical ear* because it often occurs after a history of repeated water exposure and it occurs more commonly in warm and humid environments. This condition became of significant interest to the medical field during World War II because of its high incidence among the troops in the South Pacific. During World War II, otitis externa accounted for 50 to 70 percent of the caseload for otolaryngologists in the South Pacific.[22]

Today, otitis externa accounts for 7.5 million annual ototopical prescriptions in the United States and is a significant cause of discomfort because of the associated pain and conductive hearing loss.[36] This chapter discusses knowledge of the basic anatomy of the external canal, different etiologies of otitis externa, and treatment and prevention that are needed by the pediatric practitioner managing this condition.

NORMAL ANATOMY

The external ear is composed of the auricle and external auditory canal (EAC). The auricle of the ear is a skin-covered cartilaginous structure on the temporal region of the head and is an extension of the EAC. The EAC is divided into two regions—a lateral cartilaginous portion and a medial bony portion that ends at the tympanic membrane.

The cartilaginous portion of the canal makes up approximately 40 percent of its 2.5 cm total length and typically is directed slightly upward and backward. This shape and the presence of cerumen help to prevent water and foreign objects from entering the canal.[24] In the anterior portion of the cartilaginous canal are the fissures of Santorini, which provide a route for the spread of infection from the canal into the adjacent parotid and surrounding tissues. The bony canal makes up the remainder of the canal length and is directed slightly downward and anterior. The isthmus, which is the narrowest portion of the canal, corresponds to the bony-cartilaginous junction.

The sensory innervation of the EAC is complex and includes contributions from the fifth, seventh, ninth, and tenth cranial nerves. This sensory innervation is responsible for the exquisite pain associated with otitis externa.[24] The skin of the entire EAC consists of keratinizing stratified squamous epithelium. It is the only keratinizing epithelium that lacks eccrine sweat glands.

Differences exist in the canal skin of the cartilaginous canal and the bony canal. The cartilaginous canal skin is thicker and contains rete pegs, dermis, dermal papillae, hair follicles, and sebaceous and cerumen glands, which are absent in the bony canal. The thinner skin of the bony canal lacks dermal papillae and rete pegs. The lack of subcutaneous tissue in the bony canal allows the tight attachment of the skin to the underlying periosteum, rendering the bony canal wall more vulnerable to trauma.

PROTECTIVE MECHANISMS OF THE EXTERNAL EAR

Three major defense mechanisms protect the EAC and lateral surface of the tympanic membrane: the tragus and antitragus, the skin with its cerumen coat, and the isthmus of the canal. The tragus and antitragus provide a partial barrier to the entrance of the foreign bodies into the EAC.

The skin of the cartilaginous canal contains many hair cells and sebaceous and apocrine glands, such as cerumen glands. Together, these three adnexal structures are termed the *pilosebaceous unit* and provide a protective function in the EAC. Migration of the skin of the EAC also helps to keep the canal free of debris. The pattern of migration is from the tympanic membrane laterally and radially away from the umbo.[1,24] Glandular secretions combine with sloughed squamous epithelium to form an acidic coat of cerumen, one of the primary barriers to infection of the canal. Cerumen is composed of lipids that are hydrophobic, and its major function is to waterproof the canal. Racial and gender differences that exist in the characteristics of cerumen do not seem to have any major clinical significance. Whites and African-Americans produce cerumen with higher levels of lipids compared with Asians, who produce cerumen with higher levels of proteins. Cerumen in males also has been shown to be higher pH than that in females.[18] The acidic nature of cerumen has been shown to inhibit bacterial and fungal growth.[11,18,23]

The canal normally is a self-protecting and self-cleansing structure. The cerumen coat gradually works its way to the lateral part of the canal and sloughs externally. Instrumentation and excessive cleansing of the canal can alter this primary protective barrier and may lead to infection (Table 18–1).

NORMAL BACTERIAL FLORA

The normal bacterial flora of the EAC is a combination of aerobic (80%) and anaerobic (20%) organisms.[9] Aerobic bacteria include *Staphylococcus epidermidis*, alpha-hemolytic streptococci, diphtheroids, and *Pseudomonas aeruginosa*.

In a study by Stroman and colleagues[42] of 291 bacteria isolated from cerumen, 99 percent were gram-positive, whereas of 302 bacteria isolated from the canal, 96 percent were gram-positive. Staphylococci accounted for 63 percent of the cerumen bacteria and the canal bacteria. *Staphylococcus auricularis* is the isolate found most frequently (23% in cerumen and 21% in canal), and *S. epidermidis* is the second most commonly isolated bacteria from cerumen and canal (14% and 17%, respectively). After staphylococci, the coryneform bacteria (diphtheroids) are the organisms most frequently isolated. The third most frequently recovered bacteria belong to the streptococci and enterococci groups. *Alloiococcus otitidis* was isolated with the greatest frequency (>95%) in the cerumen and the canal.[42]

In addition, seven species of *Bacillus* were isolated in the canal and cerumen. From the Micrococcaceae family, *Micrococcus luteus* was isolated most frequently from the canal and cerumen. *Turicella otitidis* was the primary coryneform recovered: 58 percent

---

TABLE 18–1 Predisposing Factors for Otitis Externa

Hot and humid environment
Water exposure
Instrumentation of ear canal
Previous radiation therapy
Eczema
Draining ear
Contact dermatitis

---

from cerumen and 65 percent from the canal. *Corynebacterium auris* was the second most frequently isolated coryneform: 12.5 percent from the canal and 12.3 percent from cerumen. Twenty-one other species of coryneforms (including 10 previously undefined species of *Corynebacterium* and 4 of *Microbacterium*) were isolated as well. Coryneforms represented 22 percent of the bacteria in cerumen and 19 percent in the canal. *Propionibacterium acnes* and a variety of *Peptococcus* spp. make up the anaerobic flora.[42]

ACUTE OTITIS EXTERNA

Acute otitis externa is an infection of the EAC that often is the end result of a combination of factors. Bacterial and fungal infections of the EAC occur when the natural defenses break down, resulting in a significant reduction in the amount of cerumen, an injury to the skin of the canal, or a shift of the normal canal flora. Humidity, heat, and maceration all produce itching, which often leads to manipulation and instrumentation of the canal, which in turn leads to additional trauma. Otitis externa may be caused by insults that result in the removal of the protective lipid film from the canal, allowing the entrance of organism to the apopilosebaceous unit. Rapid proliferation of bacteria occurs as a result of the warm, dark, and moist canal environment.

Inflammation and infection can cause canal edema or complete obstruction of the canal in severe cases, with purulent discharge. If the infectious process goes untreated, it leads to cellulitis of the auricle and surrounding area.

Symptoms of otitis externa, in addition to pruritus and drainage, include pain and tenderness on palpation or manipulation of the external ear. Pain arises as the soft tissues and skin of the canal distract the periosteal lining of the bony canal. Pain is severe enough to interfere with daily activities and is the major reason for medical consultation.

HISTORY AND PHYSICAL EXAMINATION

Otitis externa is a clinical diagnosis. Interrogation often reveals a history of exposure to water, previous auricular instrumentation, or trauma. The physician should inquire about predisposing factors, such as diabetes, immunosuppression, history of eczema, or previous radiation therapy, all of which may predict a more complicated course.

On physical examination, the pinna may appear swollen or erythematous or may be protruding. Primary care practitioners and emergency department personnel frequently establish the diagnosis of mastoiditis based on auricular protrusion. On manipulation of the auricle, the patient often experiences severe pain. Tragal tenderness is another key feature of this disease. A hand-held otoscope often suffices to establish the diagnosis, but the microscope is recommended for full cleaning of the ear canal. The pinna may appear erythematous with edema and eczematization (Fig. 18–1). The canal appears swollen with various grades of patency, depending on the severity of the infection. Purulent discharge combined with keratin debris usually fills the canal. It is important to attempt to visualize the tympanic membrane if the canal is not completely obstructed. Absence of drainage from the middle ear confirms the diagnosis of otitis externa.

PATHOGENS IN ACUTE OTITIS EXTERNA

Common bacterial pathogens that cause otitis externa include *P. aeruginosa*, *Staphylococcus aureus*, *Escherichia coli*, and *Proteus* spp. (Table 18–2). *Pseudomonas* have been found to be the

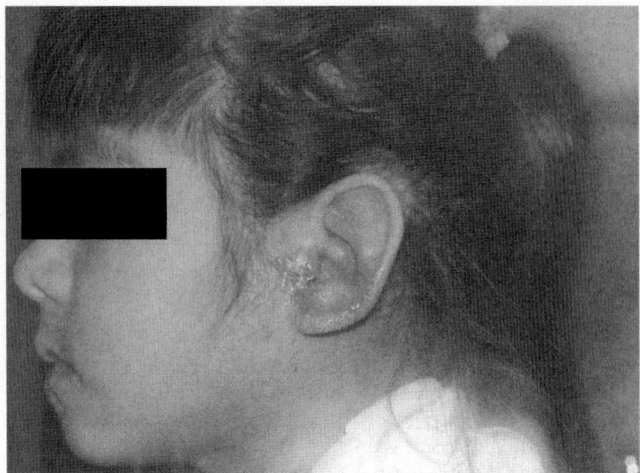

Figure 18–1 Patient with acute otitis externa, with purulent drainage from the ear canal with mild edema and erythema of the pinna. (See companion Expert Consult web site for color version.)

TABLE 18–2   Common Pathogens in Otitis Externa

Gram-Negative Organisms
Pseudomonas aeruginosa
Pseudomonas spp. Nov. "otitidis"
Proteus mirabilis
Serratia marcescens

Gram-Positive Organisms
Staphylococcus aureus
Staphylococcus epidermidis
Corynebacterium auris
Enterococcus faecalis

Fungi and Yeasts
Aspergillus fumigatus
Candida albicans
Candida parapsilosis

predominant organism in various studies.[4,7,35,38] Historically, *Pseudomonas* have accounted for 50 to 80 percent of bacteria isolated from cases of chronic otitis externa.[4,29,31,35,38] In a study by Roland and Stroman,[35] gram-negative bacteria accounted for 53 percent of recovered organisms; 45.3 percent were gram-positive. In this same study, *P. aeruginosa* accounted for 37.7 percent of the total number of isolates, whereas a newly identified species, *Pseudomonas otitidis*, accounted for 2.3 percent of recovered organisms.[35]

Staphylococci are the most common gram-positive organism recovered in cases of otitis externa, accounting for 25 percent of the cases. *S. epidermidis* is the most common staphylococcal species recovered, followed by *S. aureus*. Coryneforms are the second largest group of gram-positive bacteria isolated from cases of otitis externa.[35]

Other organisms that have been identified as pathogens include *Enterobacter*, *Klebsiella*, *Serratia*, *Proteus*, and *E. coli*. Although *Microbacterium* spp. previously were considered normal flora, more recently they have been identified at a 10 times higher rate in infected ears compared with normal controls. *Microbacterium* also have been the single recovered isolate in treatment failures and re-infections.[35]

MANAGEMENT OF ACUTE OTITIS EXTERNA

No consensus exists about the most effective treatment for otitis externa. Treatment usually includes thorough cleaning and suctioning of the purulent debris and application of topical agents. Topical treatment has been shown to be effective and is the mainstay of treatment. A wick usually is placed in the canal to provide adequate delivery of the topical solution. Without the wick and adequate cleaning of the canal, the topical drops may not achieve adequate penetration and are ineffective. When topical therapy is prescribed, various options, including multiple antibiotics, antiseptics, steroids, and combination agents, are available.[9,10,18,34,36] Topical antimicrobial therapy increased absolute clinical cure rates of acute otitis externa by 46 percent and bacteriologic cure rates by 61 percent compared with placebo.[36] Freedman[20] compared topical neomycin/colistin/hydrocortisone with topical placebo and found less severe edema and itching by day 3 and less severe edema, itching, redness, scaling, and weeping by day 7.[36] Without treatment, approximately 15 percent of patients with acute otitis externa have clinical cure within 10 days; however, the cure rate increases to 65 to 85 percent when topical antimicrobial therapy is administered.[20,36]

Rosenfeld and colleagues[36] performed a meta-analysis to assess topical antiseptics and antibiotics and found comparable clinical cures at 7 to 14 days. The most common antiseptics used in the treatment of otitis externa include acetic acid, boric acid/ethyl alcohol and aluminum acetate, and *N*-chlorotaurine.

Topical antibiotic preparations usually are divided into two groups: quinolones and non-quinolone antibiotics. Non-quinolone antibiotics, such as polymyxin, neomycin, gentamicin, tobramycin, and oxytetracycline, have been the mainstay of treatment for otitis externa for several decades. Most of these agents have some degree of ototoxicity, however, which renders them undesirable in the case of a tympanic membrane perforation or a patent pressure equalizing tube.[26,32] The introduction of quinolones in the late 1980s for management of otitis externa and malignant external otitis provided a non-ototoxic alternative treatment. Topical antibiotic therapy allows for the administration of high concentrations of antibiotics, which can overcome organisms with high minimal inhibitory concentrations. Rosenfeld and colleagues[36] reported comparable clinical cure rates for topical quinolone antibiotics compared with non-quinolones at 3 to 4 days, 7 to 10 days, and 14 to 28 days. This same study found no differences in adverse effects between the two antibiotic groups.

More recent studies have reported pseudomonal resistance to fluoroquinolones. Berenholz and colleagues[6] reported 33 percent ciprofloxacin resistance in cases of necrotizing otitis externa.[6] Other studies have shown strains of *S. aureus* and *S. epidermidis* that have developed quinolone resistance.[34] One of the most common mistakes in the treatment of otitis externa is not identifying a tympanic membrane perforation and draining middle ear as the source of the infection, which may have treatment implications because of the ototoxicity of some compounds.

CHRONIC OTITIS EXTERNA

Chronic otitis externa is an inflammatory condition of the ear canal skin. This condition generally is caused by the loss of the protective coating of cerumen and oils secondary to constant mechanical débridement, such as with cotton applicators or with repeated water exposure. Associated pruritus leading to self-cleaning perpetuates the vicious cycle. The ear canal with chronic otitis externa often is more vulnerable to bacterial superinfection.[33] *S. aureus* and *P. aeruginosa* have been shown to secrete proteases that may continue to establish pathologic skin conditions in the EAC in cases of chronic otitis externa.[27] Treatment of chronic otitis externa involves débridement and application of topical anti-inflammatory agents, such as corticosteroids. Cessation of habitual canal manipulation is necessary for achieving a positive response. For recalcitrant cases, surgical removal of the canal skin and replacement with skin grafts may be required.

OTOMYCOSIS

Otomycosis is a fungal infection of the skin of the external canal. Otomycosis often is the result of superinfection of chronic bacterial infection of the external canal or middle ear. All fungi have three basic growth requirements—moisture, warmth, and darkness—all of which commonly are present in the EAC. The most common fungus is *Aspergillus* spp., although *Candida* spp., *Actinomyces* spp., and Phycomycetes also have been reported.[7] Pruritus is the primary clinical manifestation. Patients also complain of feeling moisture in their ears. Physical examination commonly shows a white, black, or dotted gray membrane in the EAC. Diagnosis often is confirmed with a fungal culture.

Thorough cleaning with removal of the matted fungal debris and topical application of an acidifying solution, such as aluminum sulfate–calcium acetate (Domeboro), or of a drying powder, such as boric acid, often is adequate treatment. Antifungals such as clotrimazole cream or solution (Lotrimin) also may be used. It is important to assess for perforation of the tympanic membrane because antifungals can be ototoxic.[16,26] Gentian violet usually is well tolerated in patients with mastoid cavities, but it permanently stains skin and clothing. Many patients with refractory otomycotic infections have had previous canal wall mastoid surgery and require a hearing aid with a closed mold. Because the patient relies on the hearing aid virtually all day, trauma associated with placing and removing the hearing aid throughout the day can cause a significant problem. Ointments are not recommended for patients with closed hearing aids because they may promote fungal growth secondary to the accumulation of moisture.

NECROTIZING OTITIS EXTERNA

Necrotizing otitis externa is an infection of the EAC that spreads to the surrounding subcutaneous tissues and can lead to osteomyelitis of the skull base.[15] This condition was described first by Chandler[12,14] and was referred to as *malignant otitis externa* because of the aggressive extension of the disease and the poor outcome. Survival rates have improved during the past 2 decades as a result of increased awareness, allowing for earlier diagnosis and treatment.[15,16] Patients often are diabetic, immunocompromised, or undergoing post-radiation therapy.[5,37,39] The infection often begins as any other acute otitis externa involving the bony-cartilaginous junction and often extends through the fissures of Santorini to involve the parotid region. Facial paralysis can occur as a complication of this disease and does so more commonly in children than in adults in cases of necrotizing otitis externa.[30] Facial nerve paralysis in necrotizing otitis externa often is permanent.[13]

P. aeruginosa is the most common pathogen in necrotizing otitis externa. *Proteus mirabilis* also has been reported as a causal agent in some cases.[15,16] Necrotizing otitis externa should be suspected in the presence of a pseudomonal infection that does not resolve and may be associated with facial nerve paralysis. The presence of granulation in the external canal at the bony-cartilaginous junction also should raise suspicion of necrotizing otitis externa.

Diagnostic imaging, including computed tomography or magnetic resonance imaging, of the temporal region often is required.[21] The most common finding of extension beyond the ear canal is retrocondylar fat infiltration.[25] A gallium 67 scan often is diagnostic in the early course of the disease and provides a good way to monitor the efficacy of treatment. A positive technetium 99m scan is diagnostic for acute osteolytic osteomyelitis because it measures osteoclastic activity, but it may remain positive long after the infection has subsided. For this reason, a technetium 99m scan is not ideal for monitoring treatment response.[41]

Treatment of necrotizing otitis externa often involves multiple surgical débridements combined with topical and intravenous antibiotics. Hyperbaric oxygen also has been tried in patients, with some success.[17] In diabetic patients or immunocompromised patients, coadjuvant treatment to control the primary condition is crucial and should be initiated immediately.

DIFFERENTIAL DIAGNOSIS

Not every condition that manifests with pain and purulent discharge from the EAC is otitis externa. Multiple other entities that may manifest with one or more similar symptoms include relapsing polychondritis, suppurative otitis media, and herpetic infections.

Relapsing polychondritis is a progressive inflammatory disorder affecting cartilage. When it involves the ear, it usually involves the pinna and the cartilaginous portion of the EAC, manifesting as swelling and erythema.[3] This condition can affect any cartilaginous structure, including the trachea, the nasal septum, and the larynx. Destruction of the cartilage by inflammatory infiltrates is followed by granulation, fibrosis, and calcifications. It often is accompanied by arthralgias involving one or more joints and rarely affects only one ear.

Herpes simplex and herpes zoster also can affect the EAC. Both conditions manifest with painful vesicles along the EAC (Fig. 18–2) and can be accompanied by facial nerve paralysis (Ramsay Hunt syndrome or herpes zoster oticus).[2,43] Treatment is with antivirals, such as acyclovir or famciclovir.

Dermatologic conditions also can give the appearance of otitis externa. Allergic and contact dermatitis can manifest with erythema, weeping areas, and itching. Allergic dermatitis is a delayed hypersensitivity reaction resulting from substances such as poison

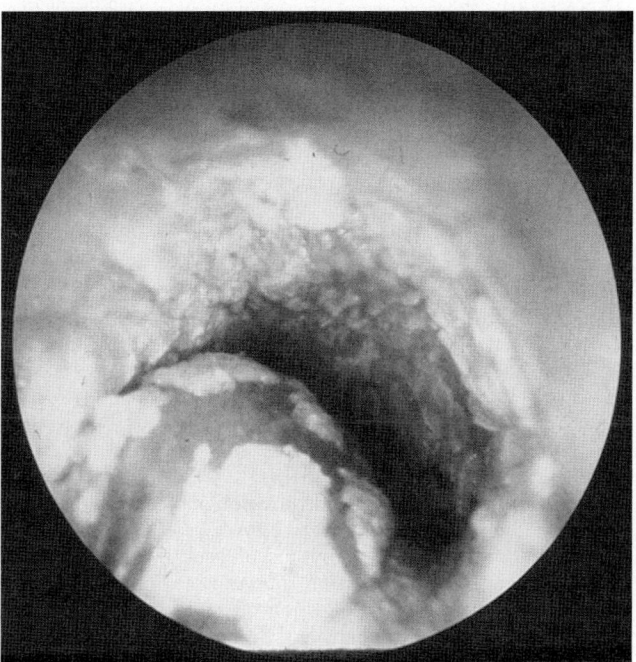

Figure 18–2 Ear canal with multiple vesicles from herpes zoster oticus. (See companion Expert Consult web site for color version.)

ivy, rubber, and nickel compounds.[28,40] Treatment is with administration of topical steroids and removal of the causative agent.

CONCLUSION

Understanding the external ear anatomy and its physiology allows clinicians to comprehend better the natural history of the diseases that affect this region. Despite improvements in diagnostic imaging techniques, no substitute exists for a good history and physical examination to differentiate among various conditions with a similar presentation. Treatment of otitis externa should focus on achieving relief of the acute condition; at the same time, clinicians should try to help prevent recurrences in patients with higher risk factors.

REFERENCES

1. Alberti, P. W.: Epithelial migration on the tympanic membrane. J. Laryngol. Otol. 78:808-830, 1964.
2. Aleksic, S N., Budzilovich, G. N., and Lieberman, A. N.: Herpes zoster oticus and facial paralysis (Ramsay Hunt syndrome): Clinico-pathologic study and review of literature. J. Neurol. Sci. 20:149-159, 1973.
3. Bachor, E., Blevins, N. H., Karmody, C., and Kuhnel, T.: Otologic manifestations of relapsing polychondritis: Review of literature and report of nine cases. Auris Nasus Larynx 33:135-141, 2006.
4. Beers, S. L., and Abramo, T. J.: Otitis externa review. Pediatr. Emerg. Care 20:250-256, 2004.
5. Benuck, I., and Traisman, H. S.: Malignant external otitis in a diabetic adolescent. J. Adolesc. Health Care 7:57-59, 1986.
6. Berenholz, L., Katzenell, U., and Harell, M.: Evolving resistant pseudomonas to ciprofloxacin in malignant otitis externa. Laryngoscope 112:1619-1622, 2002.
7. Bojrab, D. I., Bruderly, T., and Abdulrazzak, Y.: Otitis externa. Otolaryngol. Clin. North Am. 29:761-782, 1996.
8. Brook, I.: Microbiological studies of the bacterial flora of the external auditory canal in children. Acta Otolaryngol. 91:285-287, 1981.
9. Brook, I.: Treatment of otitis externa in children. Paediatr. Drugs 1:283-289, 1999.
10. Buchalter, G. M.: Near synchronous methicillin-resistant *Staphylococcus aureus* external auditory canal abscesses in 2 pediatric siblings. Otolaryngol. Head Neck Surg. 127:238-240, 2002.
11. Chai, T. J., and Chai, T. C.: Bactericidal activity of cerumen. Antimicrob. Agents Chemother. 18:638-641, 1980.
12. Chandler, J. R.: Malignant external otitis. Laryngoscope 78:1257-1294, 1968.
13. Chandler, J. R.: Malignant external otitis and facial paralysis. Otolaryngol. Clin. North Am. 7:375-383, 1974.
14. Chandler, J. R.: Malignant external otitis: Further considerations. Ann. Otol. Rhinol. Laryngol. 86:417-428, 1977.
15. Chandler, J. R.: Malignant external otitis and osteomyelitis of the base of the skull. Am. J. Otol. 10:108-110, 1989.
16. Chandler, J. R., Grobman, L., Quencer, R., and Serafini, A.: Osteomyelitis of the base of the skull. Laryngoscope 96:245-251, 1986.
17. Davis, J. C., Gates, G. A., Lerner, C., et al.: Adjuvant hyperbaric oxygen in malignant external otitis. Arch. Otolaryngol. Head Neck Surg. 118:89-93, 1992.
18. Fabricant, N. D., and Kolb, L. W.: External auditory canal and lobule temperature. Arch. Otolaryngol. 74:340-341, 1961.
19. Fairbanks, D. N.: Otic topical agents. Ear Nose Throat J. 60:239-242, 1981.
20. Freedman, R.: Versus placebo in treatment of acute otitis externa. Ear Nose Throat J. 57:198-204, 1978.
21. Gherini, S. G., Brackmann, D. E., and Bradley, W. G.: Magnetic resonance imaging and computerized tomography in malignant external otitis. Laryngoscope 96:542-548, 1986.
22. Gordon, A.: Otitis externa. Bull. U. S. Army Med. Dept. 8:245-246, 1948.
23. Hyslop, N. E., Jr.: Ear wax and host defense. N. Engl. J. Med. 284:1099-1100, 1971.
24. Kelly, K. E., and Mohs, D. C.: The external auditory canal: Anatomy and physiology. Otolaryngol. Clin. North Am. 29:725-739, 1996.
25. Kwon, B. J., Han, M. H., Oh, S. H., et al.: MRI findings and spreading patterns of necrotizing external otitis: Is a poor outcome predictable? Clin. Radiol. 61:495-504, 2006.
26. Marsh, R. R., and Tom, L. W.: Ototoxicity of antimycotics. Otolaryngol. Head Neck Surg. 100:134-136, 2002.
27. Miedzobrodzki, J., Kaszycki, P., Bialecka, A., and Kasprowicz, A.: Proteolytic activity of *Staphylococcus aureus* strains isolated from the colonized skin of patients with acute-phase atopic dermatitis. Eur. J. Clin. Microbiol. Infect. Dis. 21:269-276, 2002.
28. Nakada, T., Iijima, M., Nakayama, H., and Maibach, H. I.: Role of ear piercing in metal allergic contact dermatitis. Contact Dermat. 36:233-236, 1997.
29. Nichols, A. C., and Perry, E. T.: Studies on the growth of bacteria in the human ear canal. J. Invest. Dermatol. 27:165-170, 1956.
30. Nir, D., Nir, T., Danino, J., and Joachims, H. Z.: Malignant external otitis in an infant. J. Laryngol. Otol. 104:488-490, 1990.
31. Perry, E. T.: A practical approach to external otitis. J. A. M. A. 163:161-164, 1957.
32. Roland, P. S.: Clinical ototoxicity of topical antibiotic drops. Otolaryngol. Head Neck Surg. 110:598-602, 1994.
33. Roland, P. S.: Chronic external otitis. Ear Nose Throat J. 80(Suppl. 6):12-16, 2001.
34. Roland, P. S., and Stroman, D. W.: Microbiology of acute otitis externa. Laryngoscope 112:1166-1177, 2002.
35. Roland, P. S., Pien, F. D., Schultz, C. C., et al.: Efficacy and safety of topical ciprofloxacin/dexamethasone versus neomycin/polymyxin B/hydrocortisone for otitis externa. Curr. Med. Res. Opin. 20:1175-1183, 2004.
36. Rosenfeld, R. M., Singer, M., Wasserman, J. M., and Stinnett, S. S.: Systematic review of topical antimicrobial therapy for acute otitis externa. Otolaryngol. Head Neck Surg. 134(Suppl. 4):S24-S48, 2006.
37. Rubin, J., Yu, V. L., and Stool, S. E.: Malignant external otitis in children. J. Pediatr. 113:965-970, 1988.
38. Senturia, B. H.: Diffuse external otitis: Pathogenesis and treatment, II. Laryngoscope 65:313-321, 1955.
39. Sobie, S., Brodsky, L., and Stanievich, J. F.: Necrotizing external otitis in children: Report of two cases and review of the literature. Laryngoscope 97:598-601, 1987.
40. Stevenson, O. E., and Finch, T. M.: Allergic contact dermatitis from rectified camphor oil in Earex ear drops. Contact Dermat. 49:51, 2003.
41. Stokkel, M. P., Takes, R. P., van Eck-Smit, B. L., and Baatenburg de Jong, R. J.: The value of quantitative gallium-67 single-photon emission tomography in the clinical management of malignant external otitis. Eur. J. Nucl. Med. 24:1429-1432, 1997.
42. Stroman, D. W., Roland, P. S., Dohar, J., and Burt, W.: Microbiology of normal external auditory canal. Laryngoscope 111:2054-2059, 2001.
43. Vest, C., Munneke, J. A., and Smith, R.: Herpes zoster oticus: Uncommon but recognizable cause of facial paralysis. Postgrad. Med. 65:143-150, 1979.

CHAPTER
19 OTITIS MEDIA

Jerome O. Klein ☉ Charles D. Bluestone

The term *otitis media* denotes inflammation of the mucoperiosteal lining of the middle ear. *Acute otitis media (AOM)* is the rapid onset of signs and symptoms of acute infection within the middle ear. *Otitis media with effusion* is an inflammation of the middle ear in which a collection of liquid is present in the middle ear space, and no signs or symptoms of acute infection are present. *Middle ear effusion* denotes liquid in the middle ear. The effusion may be serous, a thin, watery liquid; mucoid, a thick, viscid, mucus-like liquid; purulent; or a combination of these forms. Fluctuating or persisting loss of hearing is present in most patients who have middle ear effusion; hearing impairment is the most frequent complication of AOM or otitis media with effusion. Suppurative complications of otitis media occur when inflammation and infection extend beyond the mucoperiosteal lining of the middle ear (e.g., mastoiditis, epidural abscess). An extended review of otitis media in infants and children was written by the authors and published in 2007.[25]

INCIDENCE AND EPIDEMIOLOGY OF ACUTE OTITIS MEDIA

AOM is one of the most common infectious diseases of childhood. A survey of diagnoses made in office practices in the United States in 1990 identified 24.5 million visits for which the principal diagnosis was otitis media; the number of diagnoses of otitis media had increased from 9.91 million visits recorded in 1975.[171] In Boston, Teele and associates[187] found that about 33 percent of pediatric office visits for illness of any kind were attributable to AOM or otitis media with effusion. The same group of investigators reported that 62 percent of children had had at least one episode of AOM by the time they reached 1 year of age, and 17 percent had experienced three or more episodes.[188] By 3 years of age, more than 80 percent of children had experienced at least one episode of AOM, and 46 percent had had three or more episodes. A similar preponderance of cases of AOM during the first or second year of life with a decline in incidence rate thereafter has been reported by investigators from locations as diverse geographically as Finland[152,175]; Sweden[88]; Cleveland, Ohio[118]; Huntsville, Alabama[86]; and Galveston, Texas.[17] The results of these studies suggest that by the time children reach 3 years of age, they may be categorized into three groups of about equal size relative to acute infections of the middle ear: one group is free of ear infections; a second group may have occasional episodes of otitis media, usually associated with infections of the respiratory tract; and a third group is otitis-prone, subject to repeated (three or more) episodes of acute infection.

A prospective study beginning in 1991 of more than 2000 children in Pittsburgh, Pennsylvania, surveyed during the first 2 years of life provided insight into the prevalence of otitis media, the amount of antibiotic used, and the proportion of children who required surgery for severe and recurrent disease.[142] Middle ear effusion was present 20.4 percent and 16.6 percent of the time during the first and second years of life, respectively; mean number of days of antimicrobial therapy for otitis media was 41.9 and 48.6 in the first and second years of life, respectively (>90% of all antibiotic treatment in the first 2 years of life was for otitis media); and 1.8 percent and 4.2 percent of the children had myringotomy and insertion of tympanostomy tubes in the first and second years of life, respectively.

Three factors are likely to alter the incidence and epidemiology of AOM in the United States in the next few years: (1) the introduction of the seven-valent pneumococcal conjugate vaccine (PCV7) in 2000; (2) the publication of management guidelines by the American Academy of Pediatrics (AAP) and the American Academy of Family Physicians (AAFP) in 2004, which included minimal criteria for establishing the diagnosis of AOM and an option of "watchful waiting," rather than immediate use of antimicrobial drugs; and (3) the educational campaign of the Centers for Disease Control and Prevention (CDC) and other professional groups to influence parents and physicians to avoid inappropriate uses of antimicrobial agents for trivial, usually viral, respiratory tract infections because of concern for development of multidrug resistance. Any one or all of these factors may play a role in decreasing the number of diagnoses of AOM, altering the microbiology of AOM, decreasing the number of surgical procedures for severe and recurrent otitis media, and reducing the volume of antimicrobial agents used in infants and children.

HOST RISK FACTORS

Table 19–1 lists the risk factors for developing severe and recurrent AOM. The peak age-specific attack rate occurs between 6 and 18 months of age. The frequent occurrence of otitis media in otherwise healthy infants is partly a reflection of the fact that the eustachian tube of the young child is shorter, floppier,

TABLE 19–1   Risk Factors for Severe and Recurrent Acute Otitis Media

Male gender
Familial aggregation—disease in siblings and parents
Very low birth weight (<1500 g) and gestational age <33 wk
Early onset of disease
Race—Native American, Alaskan Eskimo, Australian Aborigine
Poverty—crowded living conditions, poor sanitation, lack of access to medical care
Prone sleeping position
Use of pacifier
Not breast-fed
Group daycare
Exposure to smoke and environmental antigens
Congenital or acquired immunodeficiency

straighter, and more horizontal than the eustachian tube of the older child. Organisms from the nasopharynx reach the middle ear more readily than they do in older children. By 3 years of age, the incidence of AOM decreases because of changes in the child's anatomy and physiology and maturing immune mechanisms. Children who have had little or no experience with otitis media by the time they reach age 3 years are unlikely to develop problems with middle ear infections, unless some predisposing factor, such as tumor or fracture of the base of the skull or a facial bone or acquired immunodeficiency, occurs.

AOM, similar to most bacterial infections in children, seems to occur more commonly in boys than in girls.[188] A genetic predisposition to AOM has been shown by a study in twins.[37] Histories of severe and recurrent ear infections in siblings and parents are found frequently in families with an otitis-prone child.[61,188] Although prematurity has not been associated previously with predisposition to middle ear infection, a study from the Netherlands suggests that a gestational age of younger than 33 weeks and very low birth weight (<1500 g) are risk factors for developing recurrent otitis media.[51] Age at first episode of AOM is associated significantly with recurrent episodes.[188]

Race and ethnicity as predisposing factors may be difficult to separate from poor social and economic conditions. Particularly high rates of the disease have been observed among Eskimos,[94,153,163] Native Americans,[141] and Australian Aboriginal children.[126] Factors of poverty predisposing children to development of respiratory infections and otitis media include crowded living conditions, poor sanitation, and limited access to medical care.[121]

Although most children with recurrent and severe otitis media have no obvious predisposing factor, a few have altered host defenses, including anatomic changes (e.g., cleft palate or uvula, submucous cleft), alterations of normal physiologic defenses (e.g., patulous eustachian tube, barotrauma), and congenital or acquired immunologic deficiencies (e.g., immunoglobulin deficiency, chronic granulomatous disease, malignancy). Active middle ear disease is a constant event in children with cleft palate.[134,136] Children with acquired immunodeficiency syndrome have a higher age-specific incidence of otitis media beginning at 6 months of age compared with uninfected children.[8] Nasotracheal intubation has been identified as a factor in the development of AOM and otitis media with effusion in neonates and older children.[15,48,145]

ENVIRONMENTAL RISK FACTORS

An increased incidence of respiratory infections, including otitis media, among children in group daycare compared with children receiving home care has been documented in the United States,[78,128,165] Sweden,[80] and Finland.[3,174] A survey of children in Memphis, Tennessee, found that children in daycare experienced more episodes of otitis media and were more likely to have placement of ventilation tubes.[9] By the second year of life, 21 percent of children in Pittsburgh observed from birth who were in group daycare (7 children or more) had surgical procedures for middle ear disease (almost all were myringotomy and placement of tubes) compared with only 3 percent of children in home care.[198] The increase in incidence of otitis media from 9.91 million office visits in 1975 to 24.5 million office visits in 1990 is associated with increased usage of group daycare for young infants.[171]

Placing infants in daycare usually is necessitated by the professional needs of one or both parents. Paid maternal leave, as is fostered in some European countries, results in an increased proportion of mothers who are breast-feeding and delayed entry of infants into out-of-home daycare. In the Czech Republic, paid maternal leave is available to all women for 9 months after giving birth and is optional to the child's third birthday. Paid parental leave now is reaching a stage of discussion and experimental programs in the United States. The Federal Family and Leave Act guarantees 6 weeks of unpaid leave, but more generous programs are available in Massachusetts, Vermont, Maryland, and Washington.

Infants who are breast-fed have fewer incidents of ear disease than infants who are bottle-fed. In a Boston, Massachusetts, study,[188] breast-feeding for 3 months or more was associated with decreased risk of developing AOM in the first year of life. Although bottle-fed infants are placed in a reclining or horizontal position and breast-fed infants are held in a vertical position, the data suggest that a constituent of breast milk is the important factor and not position during feeding. Of children with cleft palate who were provided breast milk or formula in a similar container, children who received breast milk had fewer cases of middle ear effusion.[139]

Sleep position and use of a pacifier have been identified as risk factors for recurrent episodes of AOM. More episodes of AOM were identified in infants who slept prone (compared with infants who slept supine) in an investigation of 14,000 infants in Bristol, England.[62] Use of a pacifier increased the risk for development of recurrent AOM in Finnish children attending daycare centers.[129] More than three episodes of AOM occurred in 29.5 percent of children younger than 2 years of age using pacifiers compared with 20.6 percent of children not using pacifiers; in children 2 to 3 years old, the incidences of recurrent AOM were 30.6 percent and 13.2 percent, respectively.

Allergy to environmental antigens plays a role in congestion of the mucosa of the eustachian tube. Exposure to smoke can result in goblet cell hyperplasia, mucus hypersecretion, ciliostasis, and decreased mucociliary transport.[192] The availability of a biochemical marker, cotinine, in saliva, serum, or urine has rendered documentation of passive exposure to tobacco smoke more reliable than that provided by history alone. High concentrations of serum cotinine were associated by Etzel and colleagues[53] with increased incidence of AOM and increased duration of middle ear effusion. Kim and colleagues[98] in Houston, Texas, documented the association of invasive pneumococcal infections in children and adults with increased environmental exposures to sulfur dioxide (a marker for air pollution) and higher counts of ragweed pollen.

Studies in the United Kingdom and the United States show seasonal variation in the occurrence of AOM. The pattern within a period of 1 year is sinusoidal, with the peak incidence in December through March and lowest incidence in July through September.[87,123] These findings do not correlate with general climatic conditions because the U.S. studies were performed in Texas and Washington, D.C., and the United Kingdom study was done in northern England. The incidence coincides, however, with the peak incidence of respiratory infections in both countries.

COST ANALYSES

Analyses of cost of management of otitis media have provided additional insights into the epidemiology of otitis media. Direct costs of an episode of otitis media include health care visits, cost of drugs, consultations, surgical procedures, audiometry and remedial speech and language visits, and hospitalizations related to severe AOM or its complications. Indirect costs include transportation, babysitters, and lost time from work. The average total cost of treating an episode of otitis media was estimated to be $116[93] to $131 in 1997 and 2000.[32] In 1996, the combined cost of AOM and its sequelae was estimated to be more than $5 billion every year. Mean costs of surgical procedures for severe and recurrent AOM in a managed care population in northern California for 1997 included myringotomy and placement of tympanostomy tube at $1400, mastoidectomy at $5062, and adenoidectomy at $1500.[32]

ETIOLOGIC AGENTS

The microbiology of otitis media has been documented by cultures of middle ear effusions obtained by needle aspiration (Table 19–2). In 1906, German investigators studied the bacteriology of AOM by aspiration of middle ear fluids. Many microbiologic studies were done, most in European otolaryngologic centers, before the introduction of antimicrobial agents. In the 1960s, investigative studies of the bacteriology of AOM were done in pediatric clinics and offices. Group A streptococcus was the dominant pathogen throughout the early studies but diminished in importance as more cases of mild and moderate disease were studied in pediatric programs, in contrast to the more severe disease referred to otolaryngologic centers. *Streptococcus pneumoniae*, which had been second to group A streptococci in frequency in the studies before 1960, now became the pathogen most frequently identified, followed by *Haemophilus influenzae* and *Moraxella catarrhalis*. More recent studies suggest the extensive use of the conjugate pneumococcal vaccine may have resulted in a decrease in the number of episodes of AOM caused by *S. pneumoniae* and a proportional increase in the incidence of disease caused by *H. influenzae* and *M. catarrhalis*.[21,34]

Bacteria may be isolated from middle ear fluid in approximately two thirds of patients with AOM. The finding that approximately one third of patients have sterile cultures may reflect limitations of bacterial culture methods because antigen detection tests often indicate the presence of pneumococcal capsular polysaccharide in sterile middle ear fluids.[107,113] In addition,

TABLE 19–2 Bacterial Pathogens Isolated from Middle Ear Aspirates in Infants and Children with Acute Otitis Media (Percentage of Children with Pathogen, 1985-1992)*

Pathogen	Mean	Range
Streptococcus pneumoniae	38	27-52
Haemophilus influenzae	27	16-52
Moraxella catarrhalis	10	2-15
Group A *Streptococcus*	3	0-11
Staphylococcus aureus	2	0-16
Miscellaneous bacteria	8	0-24
None or nonpathogens	28	12-35

*Percentage >100 because of more than one pathogen per middle ear effusion.
From Bluestone, C. D., and Klein, J. O.: Otitis Media in Infants and Children. 4th ed. Hamilton, Ontario, B. C. Decker, 2007.

polymerase chain reaction for bacterial genome sequences has identified DNA of *S. pneumoniae*, *H. influenzae*, and *M. catarrhalis* in patients with otitis media with effusion whose cultures were negative for these bacterial species.[149] Concomitant isolation of two or more organisms in the same effusion occurs in 7 percent of cases. Disparate results of cultures in children with bilateral AOM occur in approximately 20 percent of cases.[144] The detection of bacterial biofilms in the middle ear mucosa of children with chronic otitis media raises the possibility of metabolically active bacteria in culture-negative middle ear effusions.[71,149]

Several clinical situations warrant special consideration: (1) The occurrence of purulent conjunctivitis in association with AOM (conjunctivitis-otitis syndrome) usually is attributable to nontypeable *H. influenzae*[27,28]; (2) AOM occurs commonly among children hospitalized in intensive care units, and the bacteriology may be reflective of the hospital environment[48]; (3) renewed signs of AOM within 14 days usually represent relapse, whereas signs occurring 21 or more days after a prior infection are likely to indicate a new infection or recurrence[33]; and (4) children with tympanostomy tubes may develop AOM caused by organisms associated with otitis externa and AOM (e.g., *Staphylococcus aureus, Pseudomonas aeruginosa, Staphylococcus epidermidis, S. pneumoniae*, and *H. influenzae*).[164]

The bacteriology of otitis media with effusion mimics that of AOM.[64,65,124,155,170,181] In contrast, the etiologic agents of chronic suppurative otitis media with persistent perforation include *P. aeruginosa, S. aureus*, anaerobic bacteria, and enteric gram-negative bacilli.[29,96,133] *Mycobacterium tuberculosis* is a rare but important cause of chronic suppurative otitis media with persistent perforation.[200]

Bacteria found in middle ear aspirates usually are present in the nasopharynx of children with AOM, but multiple pathogens may be present in the nasopharynx that are not present in the middle ear.[54] Although not useful for specific microbiologic diagnosis of AOM, nasopharyngeal cultures are valuable for monitoring antibiotic susceptibility patterns of bacterial pathogens associated with AOM. Several investigators have noted quantitative differences in the nasopharyngeal flora of patients with and without otitis media, and these differences may play a role in the pathogenesis of middle ear disease. Long and colleagues[111] described a significant association between the recovery of abundant *H. influenzae* (at least 50% total colony count) from the nasopharynx and bacteriologically confirmed otitis media. An additional finding was that a semiquantitative nasopharyngeal culture was sensitive and specific in predicting the middle ear pathogen. Similar nasopharyngeal colonization rates for *S. pneumoniae* occur in ill and healthy children.[79,110,111] Gray and coworkers[70] have correlated the occurrence of AOM with nasopharyngeal acquisition of new serotypes of *S. pneumoniae*.

S. pneumoniae is the most frequent cause of severe AOM and suppurative complications. Of the 90 antigenically distinct pneumococcal serotypes, only few serotypes are responsible for most cases of otitis media. In more recent surveys, the most common types responsible for AOM in order of decreasing frequency were types 19F, 23, 14, 6B, and 3 (Table 19–3). All of these types except serotype 3 are included in the conjugate vaccine, PCV7. The serotypes responsible for sequential episodes of AOM were described by Austrian and colleagues.[5] Of interest is the constancy of the four most frequently isolated types in recurrent episodes. Other features of interest in the study are (1)

TABLE 19–3 Distribution of Pneumococcal Serotypes in Children with Acute Otitis Media (%)

Year of Study	1948-1951		1985-1989				2000-2002
City	Turku	1970-1977	Birmingham	1994-2000	1995-1999	1996-1999	Czech Republic
Country	Finland	U.S.	U.S.	Multinational	Finland	U.S.	and Slovakia
No. Strains	239	958	228	5520	414	500	189
Serotype							
1	10*	2.7	1.8	1.6	—	—	—
3	33.9	6.3	6.1	4	3.1	9.6	9
4	1.7	3.5	0.9	0.7	1	0.4	1.6
5	3.3	0.2	—	1	—	0.4	—
6	5.9	—	14				
6A	—	4.9	—	7.3	10.9	9.6	5.8
6B	—	7.3	—	10.1	13.5	10.8	12.7
7	3.8	2.2	0.4	0.8	—	0.4	—
8	2.9	1.9	—	—	—	—	—
9	—	—	4.4	—	—	—	—
9N	—	0.8	—	—	1.9	—	2.1
9V	—	7.1	—	4.6	—	5.2	—
10	—	1.2	—	—	—	—	—
11	1.3	1.2	3.1	1.3	5.8	—	—
14	1.7	10.2	10.9	13.1	6.3	15.8	11.6
15	1.3	4	—	2.1	5.6	—	—
18	3.8	5.3	2.2	—	0.2	1.4	3.7
19	10	—	33.2				
19A		5.5		6.6		5.4	1.6
19F		15.7		16.1	14	23.8	22.8
23	5	12.5	14	—		0.4	1.1
23A		0.1	—		1	0.4	1.1
23F	—	11.4	—	14.9	19.8	10	9.5
27	3.3	0.1	—	—			—
35	—	0.1	—		2.4		—
Author	Lahikainen, 1953[106]	Austrian et al., 1977[5]	Orange and Gray, 1993[132]	Hausdorff et al., 2002[76]	Eskola et al., 2001[52]	Joloba et al., 2001[89]	Prymula et al., 2006[151]

Four most frequent serotypes are shaded.

simultaneous infection of the middle ear fluid by two pneumococcal types, (2) isolation of the same type in consecutive episodes, and (3) isolation of the same type after an intercurrent episode caused by another type. At present, monitoring of pneumococcal serotypes responsible for AOM and invasive pneumococcal diseases is important in determining the durability of efficacy of the conjugate pneumococcal vaccine.

Otitis media caused by *H. influenzae* almost always is associated with nontypeable strains.[84,85,178] The clinical presentation of AOM caused by nontypeable *H. influenzae* usually is less severe than acute infection caused by *S. pneumoniae*, as measured by temperature elevation, ear pain, suppurative complications, and perforation of the tympanic membrane. Before the introduction of the conjugate *H. influenzae* type b vaccine, approximately 10 percent of children with *Haemophilus* spp. otitis had disease caused by type b, and approximately one fourth of these children had concurrent or subsequent bacteremia or meningitis.[74] *H. influenzae* causes AOM in all age groups, including older children and adolescents.[166,168] Of *H. influenzae* strains isolated from middle ear fluids, 30 to 60 percent produce β-lactamase.[105,173,195]

Although *S. pneumoniae* and *H. influenzae* are responsible for most cases of bacterial otitis media, *M. catarrhalis* and group A streptococci are responsible for some cases and should be considered in choosing appropriate antimicrobial agents. The incidence of AOM caused by *M. catarrhalis* in most studies is less than 10 percent but was noted to be 22 percent and 27 percent in 1983 reports from Pittsburgh[105] and Cleveland,[173] respectively, and 18.4 percent in a study of Finnish children observed between 1995 and 1997.[97] Most strains of *M. catarrhalis* isolated from middle ear fluids produce β-lactamase, and some patients fail to improve if they are treated with a β-lactamase-susceptible drug.

During the pre-antibiotic era, otitis media caused by group A streptococci frequently was associated with scarlet fever and often was of a severe and destructive form. In recent years, group A streptococci have been isolated frequently in some studies from Scandinavia but have been found infrequently in most studies from the United States. A survey of Israeli children identified group A streptococci in 350 of 11,311 episodes (3.1%) of AOM during 1999 to 2003. The incidence of mastoiditis was higher for patients with streptococcal AOM than for patients with other pathogens.[169]

Tuberculous otitis was an occasional cause of severe middle ear disease at the turn of the 20th century in the United States and western Europe and still occurs in developing countries. Otitis caused by *M. tuberculosis* is characterized by a painless, watery otorrhea through single or multiple perforations of the tympanic membrane.[176] Other bacteria, including *S. aureus* (which occurs infrequently in the United States but is the etiologic agent in 10% of cases in Japan[6]), gram-negative enteric bacilli (responsible for approximately 20% of otitis media cases in neonates, but a rare finding in older infants), anaerobic bacteria, *Clostridium tetani*, and *Corynebacterium diphtheriae*, are responsible for occasional cases of AOM.

Chlamydia trachomatis[190] has been identified in infants 6 months of age and younger, often associated with pneumonia. The role of *Chlamydia pneumoniae* in AOM is uncertain.[131,183]

The clinical history suggests that viral infection serves as a frequent initiating event of AOM by producing congestion of the mucosa of the upper respiratory tract. Epidemiologic data support an association between viral respiratory infection and the occurrence of AOM.[77] Upper respiratory tract infection with respiratory syncytial virus, influenza viruses, and adenoviruses was associated with a greater risk for developing otitis media than was infection with other viruses. Early studies identified a low viral isolation rate from middle ear fluid in patients with otitis media. A virus was isolated from only 29 of 663 (4.4%) specimens obtained by tympanocentesis and reviewed by Klein and Teele

in 1976.[104] A higher virus identification rate in middle ear fluid using culture and antigen detection has been reported.[41,99,162]

Pitkaranta and colleagues[148] used reverse transcriptase polymerase chain reaction to identify viruses in middle ear fluids of children with AOM and otitis media with effusion; evidence of rhinovirus was found in 22 percent and 19 percent, respectively, and respiratory syncytial virus was found in 18 percent and 8 percent, respectively. Ruuskanen and colleagues[159] summarized eight studies published between 1982 and 1990 using immunoassay or isolation; virus was identified in middle ear fluids in 17 percent of the samples—as a single agent in 6 percent and in combination with a bacterial pathogen in 11 percent. Viruses identified in middle ear fluids have included respiratory syncytial virus, influenza viruses, adenoviruses, parainfluenza viruses, enteroviruses, and rhinoviruses.

Concomitant isolation of viral and bacterial pathogens from middle ear fluid seems to be a common finding.[41,162] A survey of the microbiology of new-onset otorrhea in 79 children with tympanostomy tubes identified bacteria in 92 percent, viruses in 70 percent, and bacteria and viruses in 66 percent.[158] In an accompanying commentary, Chonmaitree[40] noted that AOM no longer should be considered a pure bacterial disease and that antibacterial treatment may not result in optimal outcome in some cases because of viral co-infection.

ETIOLOGY IN NEONATES

Clinical investigators have performed needle tympanocentesis to isolate bacterial pathogens causing otitis media in the first 6 weeks of life. Four studies included 169 infants.[14,20,172,189] Bacteria were isolated from middle ear fluid in 68 percent of cases. As in older children, *S. pneumoniae* and *H. influenzae* were the organisms most frequently isolated. Other than the more frequent occurrence of disease caused by gram-negative enteric organisms (approximately 20% cases) and the occasional isolation of other neonatal pathogens (e.g., group B streptococci), the bacteriology of otitis media in this age group was similar to that in older children.

PATHOGENESIS

The pathogenesis of otitis media is likely to follow a similar sequence of events in most children. The patient has an antecedent event (usually caused by an upper respiratory viral infection) that results in congestion of the respiratory mucosa throughout the respiratory tract, including the nose, nasopharynx, eustachian tube, and middle ear; congestion of the mucosa in the eustachian tube results in obstruction of the narrowest portion of the tube, the isthmus. The obstruction results in negative pressure in the middle ear and then development of middle ear effusion. The secretions of the mucosa of the middle ear, which usually drain through the eustachian tube, now have no egress and accumulate in the middle ear. The effusion may be asymptomatic (i.e., lacking the signs and symptoms of acute infection) and is termed *otitis media with effusion*. If pathogenic bacteria or viruses that colonize the nasopharynx are present in the middle ear after obstruction of the eustachian tube has occurred, the organisms multiply, resulting in an acute suppurative infection, with an abscess, and characterized by signs and symptoms of acute infection such as fever and otalgia.[24,25,66,161] For children with recurrent episodes of AOM or otitis media with effusion, anatomic or physiologic abnormalities of the eustachian tube seem to be predisposing factors.

It also is possible that subtle changes in immune response occur that predispose a child to frequent episodes of otitis media. Experimental studies provide evidence that virus-induced

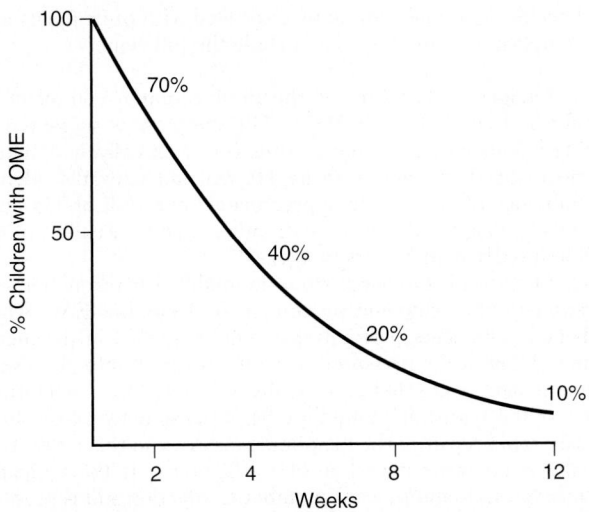

Figure 19–1 Persistence of middle ear effusion after onset of acute otitis media. OME, otitis media with effusions. *(Modified from Teele, D. W., Klein, J. O., and Rosner, B. A.: Epidemiology of otitis media in children. Ann. Otol. Rhinol. Laryngol. 89:5-6, 1980; in Bluestone, C. D., and Klein, J. O.: Otitis Media in Infants and Children. 4th ed. Hamilton, Ontario, B. C. Decker, 2007, p. 80.)*

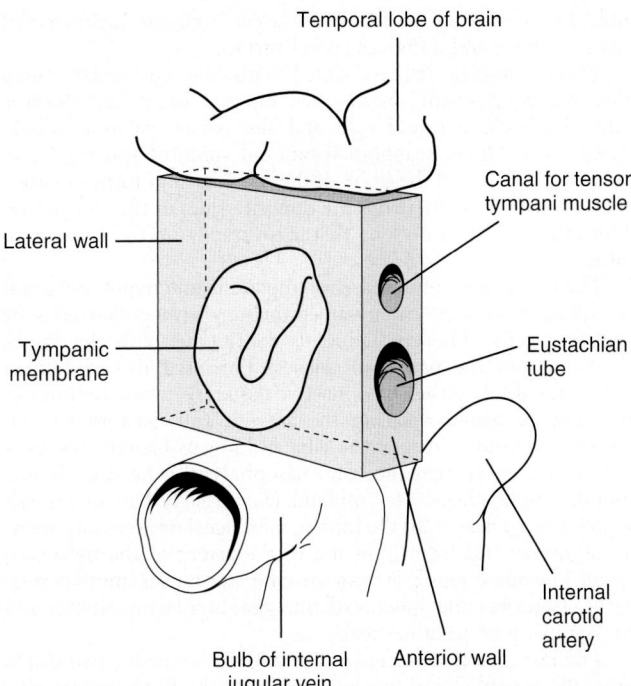

Figure 19–2 The middle ear. *(From Klein, J. O., and Daum, R. S.: The Diagnosis and Management of the Patient with Otitis Media. Copyright Biomedical Information Corporation, New York, 1985.)*

impairments in neutrophil migration and bacterial killing also may be important in the pathogenesis of AOM.[2]

With growth of the skull and change in the position, length, and width of the eustachian tube over the course of time, the predilection to otitis media in accompanying acute infections of the upper respiratory tract in the first 3 years of life diminishes, and the patient has fewer episodes of AOM. Children younger than 3 years of age with similar respiratory infections are predisposed to the complication of acute infection of the middle ear, whereas older children challenged by the same microorganism have signs of upper respiratory infection but need not have a complicating ear infection.

The pathogenesis of persistent middle ear effusion or otitis media with effusion is uncertain. An effective antimicrobial agent sterilizes the acute bacterial infection of AOM. The middle ear effusion, now sterile, may persist for weeks to months. The median duration of middle ear effusion after AOM is approximately 23 days (Fig. 19-1). The type of antibacterial drug used does not seem to alter the duration of fluid in the middle ear after acute infection occurs.

PATHOPHYSIOLOGY

TYMPANIC MEMBRANE

In the presence of otitis media, changes in the tympanic membrane occur rapidly. The presence of congested blood vessels, edema (which obscures normal landmarks), and bulging or sagging of Shrapnell membrane indicate not only a myringitis (inflammation of the tympanic membrane) but also the presence of fluid in the middle ear space. Blebs that appear on the surface epithelium are a consequence of AOM or edema or hydropic degeneration of the membrane.

Inflammation may occur on outer epithelial or inner mucosal sides of the fibrous layer (middle layer) of the drum. In severe cases, infection may involve the fibrous layer itself. The membrane thickens as a result of edema and infiltration of polymorphonuclear leukocytes. All three layers of the drum may undergo dissolution, owing to pressure necrosis resulting from the expanding middle ear abscess or thrombophlebitis of tympanic veins,

with resulting perforation. With evacuation of the contents of the middle ear abscess, healing may be rapid, and the perforation usually seals within a few days. In the process of healing, metaplasia of the epithelium, hyaline degeneration, calcium deposition, and scar formation may occur.

Occasionally, when a perforation is close to the margin of the annulus or occurs in Shrapnell membrane, the skin of the external auditory canal (EAC) and the surface squamous epithelium of the tympanic membrane may grow through the aperture and invade the middle ear. This event may lead to formation of a cholesteatoma (epidermal inclusion cyst). Even if the perforation heals, a differential in gas pressure across the tympanic membrane caused by malfunction of the eustachian tube may result in resorption of gas in the middle ear cavity and negative pressure in the middle ear, which causes retraction of Shrapnell membrane or an atrophic scar into the middle ear or mastoid attic.

EUSTACHIAN TUBE

The eustachian tube is approximately 3.8 cm long in an adult. It opens in the fossa of Rosenmüller and extends upward, backward, and laterally to open in the upper anterior wall of the tympanic cavity (protympanum). In a child, the tube is shorter and floppier. The eustachian tube is composed of two portions: the cartilaginous portion extending into the nasopharynx and the bony portion originating in the middle ear. The upper third of the tube is bony; the middle ear opening is the widest; and the medial end (the part joining the cartilaginous eustachian tube), or isthmus, is the narrowest. Pneumatic peritubal air cells arising from the middle ear cavity surround it and can extend to the petrous apex. The internal carotid artery lies anteromedial to this region (Fig. 19-2).

The lower two thirds of the eustachian tube is a narrow, slit-like, fibrocartilaginous passage. It makes a 160-degree angle with the bony portion at its junction. The cross section of the tube looks like a shepherd's crook, with a cartilaginous superior and medial surface and a fibrous lateral surface.

Three muscles are associated with the eustachian tube. The tensor tympani muscle lies on top of it; the levator palatini muscle lies under it; and the tensor palatini muscle arises on the tube, scaphoid fossa, and spine of sphenoid and then courses around the hook of the hamulus and forms an aponeurosis with its mate (from the opposite side) in the soft palate. This muscle is the only one that acts directly on the eustachian tube.

The eustachian tube area, protympanum, and hypotympanum are lined by ciliated columnar epithelium with goblet cells or secretory cells. The epithelium is continuous with the upper airway system and paranasal sinuses. This area also contains a well-defined subepithelial connective tissue layer, which thins out and may be absent nearing the antrum and mastoid air cell system. The movement of the cilia and mucus blanket always is toward the eustachian tube and nasopharynx. The tube is surrounded by a plexus of lymphoid channels. It has an arterial supply from a branch of the middle meningeal or accessory meningeal artery and from branches of the artery of the pterygoid canal. The nerve supply is from the tympanic plexus (ninth cranial nerve) (sensory) and sphenopalatine ganglion (sympathetics and parasympathetic palatine fiber).

The bony portion is rigid and patulous; the medial two thirds normally is held closed by elastic recoil of the fibrocartilaginous tissue. Contraction of the tensor palatini muscle that inserts in the anterolateral wall opens the tube on swallowing. On average, an adult swallows once per minute while awake and once every 5 minutes while asleep. Suckling infants usually swallow five times per minute.

Mucus and ciliary action flow from the middle ear to the eustachian tube. The eustachian tube acts as a unidirectional valve that favors outflow from the middle ear to the pharynx. Reverse flow can be induced by an increase in pressure in the nasopharynx (Valsalva, barotrauma). During occlusion of the eustachian tube, oxygen and carbon dioxide (and other gases) are absorbed from the middle ear by diffusion into the rich vasculature, and a negative pressure is created. A patent eustachian tube is a crucial prerequisite for subsidence of middle ear disease.

DIAGNOSIS

To establish uniformity of diagnosis, the clinical practice guideline published by the AAP and the AAFP proposed criteria for diagnosis of AOM.[4] The diagnosis required (1) a history of acute onset of signs and symptoms, (2) the presence of middle ear effusion, and (3) signs and symptoms of middle ear inflammation. The presence of middle ear effusion was identified by any of the following: (1) bulging of the tympanic membrane, (2) limited or absent mobility of the tympanic membrane, (3) air-fluid level behind the tympanic membrane, or (4) otorrhea. Signs or symptoms of middle ear inflammation were identified by either erythema of the tympanic membrane or otalgia that results in interference with or precludes normal activity or sleep. The following sections expand these definitions.

CLINICAL PRESENTATION

Children with AOM may have nonspecific signs and symptoms, including fever, irritability, headache, apathy, anorexia, vomiting, and diarrhea. Signs of respiratory viral infection, including cough and coryza, usually are present before the specific signs of ear infection occur. Fever occurs in approximately one third[167] to two thirds[127] of children with otitis media.

Specific signs and symptoms associated with otitis media and its complications and sequelae include the following:

1. Otalgia, or ear pain, is the most common complaint of infants and children with AOM. The symptom is suggested in young infants who are pulling at the ear or excessively irritable. Some infants do not have earache; Hayden and Schwartz[77] identified absence of ear pain in approximately one fifth of 335 consecutively diagnosed episodes of otitis media, usually among children older than 2 years of age.

2. Otorrhea is discharge from the middle ear through a perforation in the tympanic membrane or from the EAC when inflamed. The acute perforation usually is central in the membrane. Relief of the pressure on the tympanic membrane results in immediate pain relief and usually a decrease in temperature. Because the tympanic membrane has a dense network of blood vessels, rapid repair of the membrane occurs, and the perforation usually is unapparent within 24 to 72 hours. If the tympanic membrane seals and mucous membrane infection still is present, fluid may reaccumulate with renewed acute signs of otitis media.

3. Hearing loss occurs whenever fluid fills the middle ear space, whether the fluid is associated with acute infection or with otitis media with effusion. When fluid fills the middle ear space, the median hearing loss is 25 dB (the equivalent of having plugs in the ear canals).[59]

4. Vertigo occurs but is not a common complaint of children with otitis media. Vertigo occurs more commonly in unilateral than bilateral disease and may be caused by labyrinthitis. Older children describe a feeling of spinning, whereas younger children may not be able to verbalize these symptoms but manifest disequilibrium by falling or stumbling.

5. Tinnitus is an uncommon complaint in children, but when it does occur, the symptom often is caused by otitis media and eustachian tube dysfunction.

6. Swelling around the ear, especially in the postauricular area, may be a sign of mastoiditis.

7. Facial paralysis in children occurs as a complication of AOM or chronic otitis media with perforation of the tympanic membrane or as a result of an enlarging cholesteatoma.

8. Conjunctivitis has been associated with AOM caused by nontypeable strains of H. influenzae. The conjunctivae are injected, with tearing or purulent discharge.[28]

9. Craniofacial anomalies, such as cleft palate, mandibulofacial dysostosis, and Down syndrome, may predispose to frequent ear disease. Hypernasal speech suggests velopharyngeal insufficiency.

EXAMINATION OF THE EAR

OTOSCOPY

Examination of the ear should begin with observation of the auricle and the external auditory meatus. Palpation of the periauricular areas should be done to indicate presence of periostitis or diffuse external otitis. The ear canal should be examined for inflammation or cerumen that obstructs vision of the tympanic membrane.

For proper assessment of the tympanic membrane and its mobility, a pneumatic otoscope in which the diagnostic head has a secure seal should be used. The speculum should have the largest lumen that can fit comfortably into the child's cartilaginous external auditory meatus. The important landmarks of the tympanic membrane that can be visualized with the otoscope are indicated in Figure 19–3. The otoscopic examination should include observation of the following conditions of the tympanic membrane:

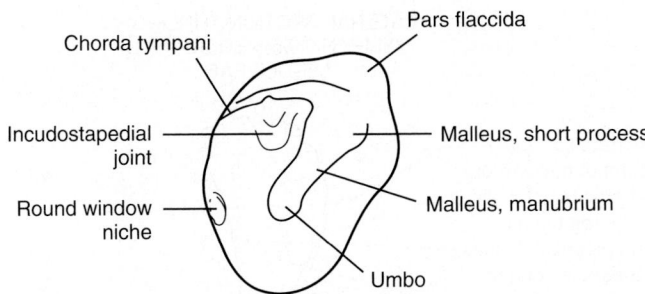

Figure 19–3 Important landmarks of the tympanic membrane that usually can be visualized with the otoscope. *(From Bluestone, C. D., and Klein, J. O.: Otitis Media in Infants and Children. 4th ed. Hamilton, Ontario, B. C. Decker, 2007, p. 156.)*

- *Position*: Normal is slightly convex; bulging indicates increased pressure from positive air pressure or fluid; a retracted drum indicates negative pressure with or without effusion; fullness of the tympanic membrane is apparent initially in the posterosuperior portion of the pars tensa and the pars flaccida because these two areas are the most highly compliant parts of the membrane.
- *Appearance and color*: The normal color is pearly gray and translucent; any congestion of the mucous membrane of the middle ear would be reflected in congestion of the vessels of the tympanic membrane and appear pink; a blue discoloration suggests blood in the middle ear associated sometimes with basal skull fracture; the inflamed middle ear mucosa usually is reflected in a bright red tympanic membrane.
- *Integrity of the membrane*: All four quadrants of the tympanic membrane should be inspected for presence or absence of perforation, retraction pockets, or cholesteatoma.
- *Mobility*: Application of positive and negative pressures by the pneumatic otoscope enables the viewer to determine the presence of an air-filled space (rapid excursion of the membrane on positive and negative pressures) or a fluid-filled space (limited or no excursion of the membrane); a middle ear with negative pressure does not respond to otoscopic negative pressure, and a middle ear with high positive pressure does not respond to otoscopic positive pressure (Fig. 19–4).

TYMPANOMETRY

Tympanometry measures the compliance of the tympanic membrane (Fig. 19–5).[30,45,120,150,154,191] Under normal circumstances, the pressure in the middle ear virtually is the same as the external ambient pressure; the eustachian tube functions to equate middle ear pressure to atmospheric pressure. If for any reason a pressure differential occurs across the tympanic membrane, stress is applied to the drum. Middle ear compliance varies as a function of the pressure differential across the tympanic membrane. When blockage of the eustachian tube with no fluid in the middle ear occurs, the tympanometry curve has a shape similar to that observed on a normal tympanogram, but the point of maximal compliance is shifted to the negative pressure side because maximal compliance is reached when the tympanic membrane reaches a peak of compliance (i.e., when EAC pressure is reduced to the same level as in the middle ear).

If ossicular discontinuity or a flaccid or atrophic tympanic membrane is present, the drum is highly compliant, and a highly peaked tympanogram is obtained. Abnormal tympanograms obtained in the presence of fluid in the middle ear are characterized by the following:

1. Reduced height of the curve (i.e., the middle ear has reduced compliance)

2. Shift to negative pressure sides of the curve and point of maximal compliance (i.e., eustachian tube blockage)

3. A flat curve without definite peak, the most characteristic feature

Although tympanometry with the electroacoustic impedance bridge has proved to be a satisfactory method for detecting the presence of fluid in the middle ear cavity, technical difficulties exist in obtaining accurate readings in infants and children, including the requirement for a secure seal of the probe in the ear canal, the need for a period of quiet to obtain an accurate reading, and decreased accuracy in infants younger than 7 months of age (because of the highly compliant EAC in infants <7 months).[143] In addition, only a few of many instruments currently on the market in the United States have data about sensitivity and specificity based on tympanometric patterns of otoscopic results before myringotomy.[57,130] Less persuasive data are available from studies correlating tympanometry and otoscopy findings.[30,120,150]

ACOUSTIC REFLECTOMETRY

The acoustic otoscope, or reflectometer (Ear Check Pro; Innova Medical, Lenexa, KS), is a handheld instrument that uses a microphone in the probe tip placed in the opening of the child's external ear canal. A professional and a consumer model were developed. The tip measures the level of transmitted and reflected sound from a less than 90 dB sound source that varies from 1800 to 4400 Hz in a 750-msec period. Acoustic energy is reflected back toward the probe tip from the ear canal and eardrum. The operating principle is based on the fact that a sound wave in a closed tube would be reflected when it strikes the end of the tube. Sound reflectivity is measured in units that indicate the status of a fluid-filled or air-filled middle ear.[44] Babonis and associates[7] found that tympanometry and reflectometry had comparable accuracy in predicting middle ear effusion documented by myringotomy. Acoustic reflectometry has some technical advantages compared with tympanometry: Accurate readings can be obtained in crying children, and a secure seal of the probe tip in the ear canal is not required.

AUDIOMETRIC TESTS

Audiometric testing may be employed to measure auditory acuity and evaluate conductive hearing losses, but assessment of hearing is an inaccurate method for identifying middle ear effusion. Hearing loss is the most prevalent complication of otitis media and is present uniformly whenever fluid fills the middle ear. The audiogram usually reveals a mild to moderate conductive hearing loss (median 25 dB).[59] Obstruction of the eustachian tube early in the clinical course of otitis media results in absorption of gases from the middle ear and drum retraction. The reduced compliance of the drum results in increased stiffness in the ossicular chain system. The audiogram reveals a low-frequency conductive hearing loss. As serous effusion appears and the middle ear fills with serum and pus, the ossicular system has an increased mass applied to it, and the audiogram flattens out, resulting in a high-frequency conductive hearing loss.

TYMPANOCENTESIS AND MYRINGOTOMY

Tympanocentesis, a needle aspiration of the middle ear effusion, is used primarily for establishing the presence or absence of an effusion and for microbiologic study. Because cultures of the

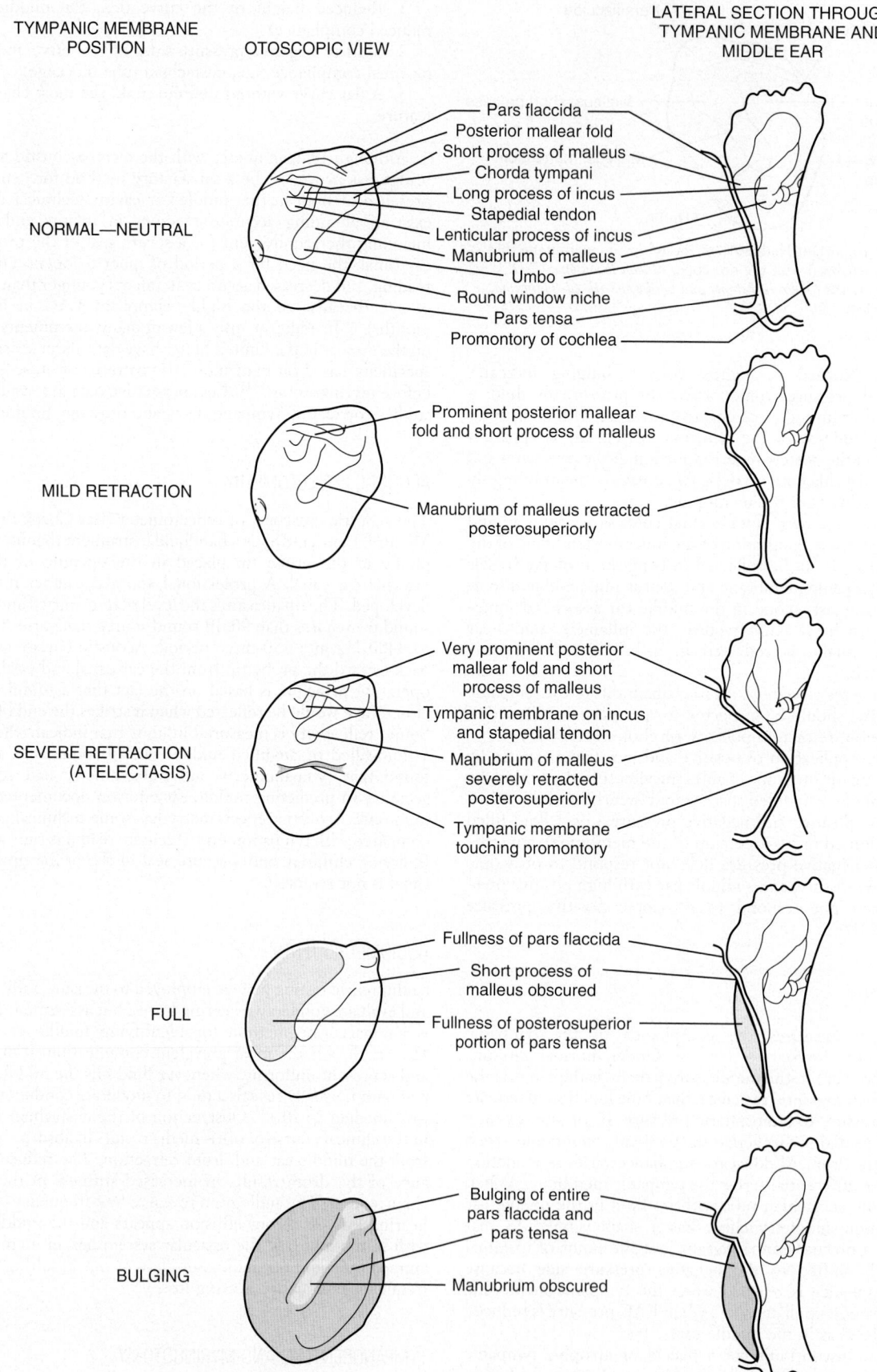

TYMPANIC MEMBRANE
POSITION

OTOSCOPIC VIEW

LATERAL SECTION THROUGH
TYMPANIC MEMBRANE AND
MIDDLE EAR

NORMAL—NEUTRAL

- Pars flaccida
- Posterior mallear fold
- Short process of malleus
- Chorda tympani
- Long process of incus
- Stapedial tendon
- Lenticular process of incus
- Manubrium of malleus
- Umbo
- Round window niche
- Pars tensa
- Promontory of cochlea

MILD RETRACTION

Prominent posterior mallear
fold and short process of malleus

Manubrium of malleus retracted
posterosuperiorly

SEVERE RETRACTION
(ATELECTASIS)

Very prominent posterior
mallear fold and short
process of malleus

Tympanic membrane on incus
and stapedial tendon

Manubrium of malleus
severely retracted
posterosuperiorly

Tympanic membrane
touching promontory

FULL

Fullness of pars flaccida

Short process of
malleus obscured

Fullness of posterosuperior
portion of pars tensa

BULGING

Bulging of entire
pars flaccida and
pars tensa

Manubrium obscured

Figure 19–4 Otoscopic views and corresponding lateral sections through the tympanic membranes and middle ear show the various positions of the drum with their respective anatomic landmarks. *(From Bluestone, C. D., and Klein, J. O.: Otitis Media in Infants and Children. 4th ed. Hamilton, Ontario, B. C. Decker, 2007, p. 153.)*

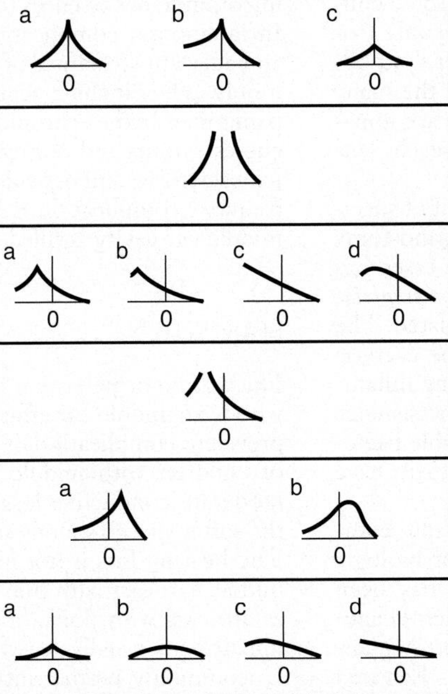

TYMPANOGRAM TYPES	COMMON VARIANTS	PRESUMPTIVE DIAGNOSIS OF TYMPANIC MEMBRANE MIDDLE EAR CONDITION
1. Normal		Normal
2. High compliance (normal pressure)		Flaccid tympanic membrane or ossicular discontinuity
3. Negative pressure (normal compliance)		High negative pressure with or without middle ear effusion
4. High negative pressure and high compliance		Flaccid tympanic membrane and high negative pressure (or ossicular discontinuity and high negative pressure)
5. High positive pressure		High positive pressure with or without middle ear effusion
6. Low compliance		Middle ear effusion and/or thickened tympanic membrane and/or ossicular fixation and/or adhesive otitis media

Figure 19–5 Tympanogram types related to presumptive conditions of the middle ear. *(From Bluestone, C. D., and Klein, J. O.: Otitis Media in Infants and Children. 4th ed. Hamilton, Ontario, B. C. Decker, 2007, p. 171.)*

upper respiratory tract are of limited value in providing specific microbiologic diagnosis of otitis media, only materials obtained by aspiration of the middle ear abscess can be considered a true reflection of the etiology of AOM. Myringotomy is an incision in the anterior lower quadrant of the tympanic membrane for therapeutic drainage. Tympanocentesis or myringotomy should be considered in patients who at onset appear toxic or are seriously ill, in patients who are toxic after initiation of antimicrobial therapy, in the presence of suppurative complications (including mastoiditis and meningitis), and in immunologically deficient patients in whom an unusual organism may be present.

RADIOGRAPHY

Radiographic evaluation of the temporal bone is indicated when complications or sequelae of otitis media are suspected or present. Plain radiographs are of limited value in the diagnosis of osteitis of the mastoid or cholesteatoma; computed tomography and magnetic resonance imaging are more precise and should be obtained if a suppurative intratemporal or intracranial complication is suspected.

DIFFERENTIAL DIAGNOSIS

Inflammation or foreign body in the external ear canal may produce ear pain simulating that of AOM. When external otitis or furunculosis of the EAC is present, the patient often has severe itching in the ear canal and pain elicited by manipulation of the pinna. The canal may be narrowed and so tender that performing an otoscopic examination is impossible.

An erythematous tympanic membrane may be caused by an upper respiratory tract infection with congestion of the mucosa lining the entire respiratory tract, including the middle ear. A

"red drum" also may be produced by trauma or aggressive examination of the EAC and may appear suddenly in a crying child.

Otalgia may be associated with infections of the tonsils, adenoids, teeth, nasopharynx, hypopharynx, or larynx. Tumors in those regions can refer pain to the ipsilateral ear along the tenth cranial nerve. Lymphomas, leukemias, and rhabdomyosarcomas involving the palate, nasopharynx, or base of the skull eventually occlude one or both eustachian tubes, producing serous effusions and otalgia.

AOM must be differentiated from an acute exacerbation of an unrelated disease in a patient with persistent middle ear effusion. Because fluid persists for weeks to months after each episode of AOM, an intercurrent infection, not associated with middle ear disease, may be misdiagnosed as AOM because of the presence of acute systemic signs of an infectious illness plus a middle ear effusion. This event may be one of the reasons for overdiagnosis of AOM. At present, no technique, other than tympanocentesis, is readily available to distinguish a relapse of AOM from a new and recurrent episode of AOM or from an intercurrent and unrelated infection associated with persistent middle ear effusion.

OTITIS MEDIA WITH EFFUSION

The presence of an asymptomatic middle ear effusion has many synonyms, such as secretory, nonsuppurative, and serous otitis media, but the most acceptable term is *otitis media with effusion*. After every episode of AOM, fluid persists in the middle ear for weeks to months (see Fig. 19–1).[186] In a study of children with AOM in Boston, 70 percent of the patients still had effusion at 2 weeks, 40 percent had effusion at 1 month, 20 percent had effusion at 2 months, and 10 percent had effusion at 3 months. Similar results of persistent middle ear effusion after an episode of AOM have been noted in all other clinical studies of AOM. The incidence or prevalence of otitis media with effusion that is unrecognized by parents and not brought to medical attention has been studied extensively.[35,56,147] The prevalence of effusion varied with age and the time of year. Incidence of otitis media with effusion peaked during the second year of life and was more prevalent in winter than in summer months.[56,147,182] In some children, the duration of otitis media with effusion may be only 1 or several days.[18] Because hearing loss is present whenever fluid fills the middle ear space, physicians are concerned about the many children with prolonged time spent with effusion; the accompanying hearing loss; and possible adverse effects on speech, language, and cognitive development.

Bacteria can be recovered from one third to one half of specimens obtained at the time of myringotomy or tympanostomy tube insertion.[64,65,124,155,170] The bacteriology in such cases has mimicked closely the bacteriology of AOM, with *S. pneumoniae* and *H. influenzae* being the predominant organisms isolated. The significance of this finding at present is unknown. The bacteria merely may colonize middle ear fluid without producing inflammation, or they may play a role in the production or persistence of middle ear fluid. In addition to live bacteria, nonviable bacteria, pneumococcal capsular polysaccharide, and endotoxin have been found in chronic middle ear effusions.[47,64,107]

Much attention has been given to the nature and composition of the middle ear effusion. The presence of biologic mediators of inflammation in the middle ear fluid has been shown[16,108,177]; they include chemotactic factors, macrophage-inhibiting factors, activated complement, histamine, prostaglandins, leukotrienes,[90,91,125] and immune complexes.[197] Elevated levels of IgA, IgE, IgM, and IgG also have been noted in serous effusions.

Clinical evaluation depends on otologic examination and audiologic and tympanometric testing. Symptoms of this disease include conductive deafness, which usually is fluctuant and may be position-dependent. The patient may have a dull ear ache or a sensation of fullness in the ear. The eardrum usually is dull with a poor light reflex and may be retracted. Color may be pale pink or have a ground-glass appearance.

COMPLICATIONS AND SEQUELAE

Intracranial suppurative complications of otitis media, including meningitis, brain abscess, and lateral sinus thrombosis, are uncommon occurrences today in developed countries (Fig. 19–6). Intratemporal complications that occur within the aural cavity and adjacent structures of the temporal bone are seen more commonly. They include acute and chronic perforation of the tympanic membrane, chronic suppurative otitis media, mastoiditis, cholesteatoma and retraction pocket, adhesive otitis media, tympanosclerosis, and ossicular discontinuity and fixation. The most frequent complication is hearing loss that occurs whenever the middle ear cavity is filled with fluid.

HEARING LOSS

Fluctuating or persisting hearing loss is present in most children who have middle ear effusion; impairment of hearing is the most prevalent complication of otitis media with effusion. Audiograms of children with middle ear effusion usually reveal a mild to moderate conductive loss of 15 to 40 dB.[59] With such deficits, the softer speech sounds and voiceless consonants may be missed. The hearing loss is not influenced by the quality of fluid in the middle ear; ears with thin fluids are impaired to the same degree as are ears with fluids of gluelike consistency.[31,199] The hearing impairment usually is reversed with resolution of the effusion. Uncommonly, permanent conductive hearing loss occurs because of irreversible changes from the inflammatory reaction, resulting in adhesive otitis media or ossicular discontinuity. High negative pressure in the middle ear or atelectasis in the absence of effusion also may cause conductive loss.

Sensorineural hearing loss after a case of AOM may occur as a result of increased tension and stiffness of the round-window membrane and is reversible. A permanent sensorineural loss may occur as a result of spread of infection or products of inflammation through the round-window membrane.[112]

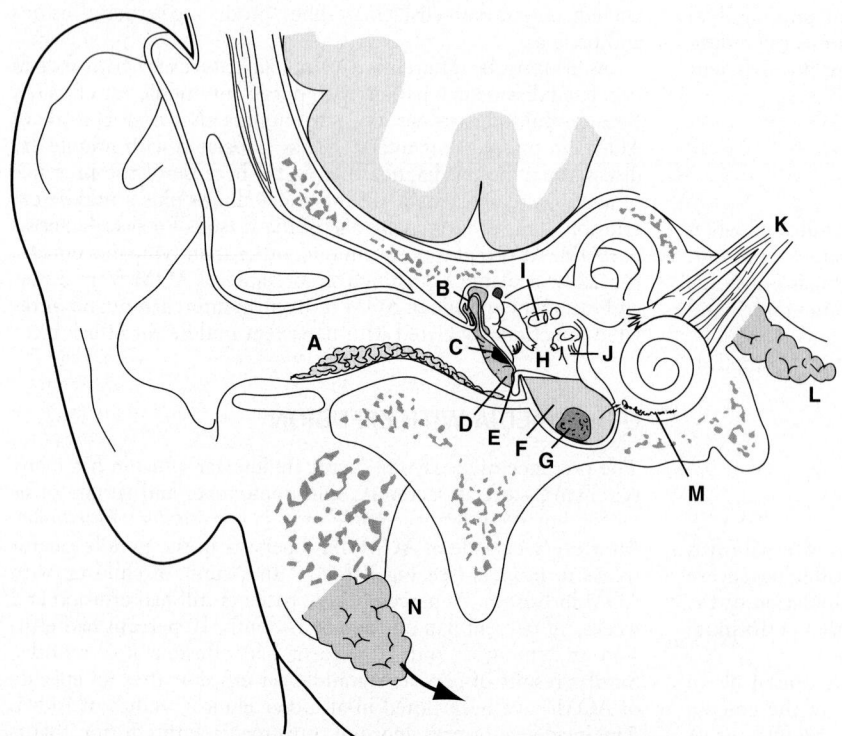

Figure 19–6 Intratemporal complications and sequelae of otitis media include the following: A, Infectious eczematoid dermatitis. B, Cholesteatoma. C, Retraction pocket of tympanic membrane. D, Tympanosclerosis. E, Perforation of tympanic membrane. F, Chronic suppurative otitis media. G, Cholesterol granuloma. H, Ossicular discontinuity. I, Facial paralysis. J, Adhesive otitis media with fixation of the ossicles. K, Hearing loss. L, Petrositis. M, Labyrinthitis. N, Mastoiditis with extension into the neck (Bezold abscess). *(From Bluestone, C. D., and Klein, J. O.: Otitis Media in Infants and Children. 4th ed. Hamilton, Ontario, B. C. Decker, 2007, p. 329.)*

EFFECTS OF OTITIS MEDIA ON DEVELOPMENT OF THE CHILD

Children with severe or recurrent otitis media have prolonged time spent with middle ear effusion. Hearing impairment accompanies the effusion in most children. If the hearing impairment occurs at a time of rapid intellectual growth, the result may be impaired development of speech, language, and cognitive abilities (Fig. 19–7). Because language acquisition is dynamic during infancy, any problems in receiving or interpreting sound signals might have a significant effect on development of speech and language. Softer speech sounds and voiceless consonants, in particular, may be missed or confused when effusion is present in the middle ear.

Although many studies have been done and are reviewed in a clinical practice guideline (*Otitis Media with Effusion in Young Children*) published by the Agency for Health Care Policy and Research of the U.S. Department of Health and Human Services,[182] the limitations of design of many of the studies and inconsistencies of the results limit the ability to make conclusions about the effect of otitis media on development. The interested reader should consult the guideline for a valuable review and extensive bibliography. A study by Paradise and colleagues[140] indicates that early placement of ventilating tubes in children with prolonged time spent with middle ear fluid did not measurably improve developmental outcomes at age 3 years. Nonetheless, some infants and young children with recurrent otitis media and prolonged time spent with middle ear effusion possibly have substantive loss in potential for development of speech, language, and cognitive abilities. Selected references about long-term outcomes of otitis media include studies by Gravel and Wallace,[69] Teele and colleagues,[185] and Friel-Patti and associates[60] and reviews by Berman[13] and Klein.[103]

CHILD BEHAVIOR AND QUALITY-OF-LIFE OUTCOMES

Disturbances in the child's behavior associated with otitis media have been reported to include restlessness, frequent disobedience, impaired task orientation in the classroom, short attention span and distractibility, attention deficits, and restricted social interaction. Only selected children may be most affected. Paradise and colleagues[141] found that stress in the parent-child relationship and behavior problems were highest among children from the most socioeconomically disadvantaged homes.

A working parent who has spent a sleepless night attending to a child who is fretful because of ear pain may have work-related

and home-related stress. Chase[39] described the response of parents of 1-year-old children to structured interaction tasks; parents of a child who had one or more episodes of otitis media were less effective in gaining the child's attention, less able to respond effectively when the child was distracted from the task, and less able to help the child understand and perform the task.

PERFORATION OF THE TYMPANIC MEMBRANE

Acute perforation (not caused by trauma) usually is secondary to AOM but also may occur during the course of otitis media with effusion. The perforation occurs because of pressure of the expanding middle ear contents on the membrane, resulting in local ischemia and tissue damage, usually in the central portion of the membrane. With rupture, the middle ear contents are discharged into the external ear canal, with instant relief of pain and defervescence in acute infection occurring. Because the membrane is highly vascular, the perforation may seal quickly and not be evident within hours to days. If the mucous membrane of the middle ear remains inflamed, fluid may reaccumulate behind the resealed tympanic membrane.

Chronic perforation may occur after an acute episode, spontaneous extrusion, or removal of a tympanostomy tube. If squamous epithelium grows at the edges of the perforation, healing may be prevented, and the perforation persists. The term *chronic suppurative otitis media* is limited to a stage of ear disease in which chronic inflammation of the middle ear and mastoid occurs and in which a nonintact tympanic membrane (caused by perforation or tympanostomy tube) and otorrhea are present. Mastoiditis usually is present, and a cholesteatoma may have formed.

CHOLESTEATOMA

A cholesteatoma usually is a cystic structure lined by squamous epithelium resting on a fibrous strand. The contents of the cyst are the products of desquamation, keratinization, and pus formulation. A cholesteatoma may invade, causing local bone erosion and destruction of the ossicular chain. Aural cholesteatomas can be classified as congenital or acquired.

A congenital cholesteatoma is a congenital rest of epithelial tissue and appears as a white cystlike structure within the middle ear or temporal bone. Acquired cholesteatoma may be secondary to implantation of epithelial tissue or may be a sequela of otitis media or a retraction pocket, or both. Implantation cholesteatoma may develop either from epithelium that has migrated through a perforation of the tympanic membrane or from intraaural epithelium remaining after middle ear or mastoid surgery. Infection caused by such organisms as *S. aureus, P. aeruginosa, Proteus* spp., nonhemolytic streptococci, and *Aspergillus* spp. may be present. The process of alternating infection and healing causes the advancement of squamous epithelium into the middle ear and antrum.[55,109,160] The persistent infection also stimulates proliferation of the mucoperiosteum of the attic region, creating an accelerated tissue growth (increased production of collagenase) and a destructive and expansive process. It is characterized by a foul smell, pus, squames, and bone destruction.

Management of cholesteatoma is surgical removal of the entire cyst. Antimicrobial therapy may be necessary if secondary infection is present.

ADHESIVE OTITIS MEDIA

Adhesive otitis media is a result of healing after chronic inflammation of the middle ear and mastoid. Fibrous tissue proliferates in the muscosal lining and may impair movement of the ossicles

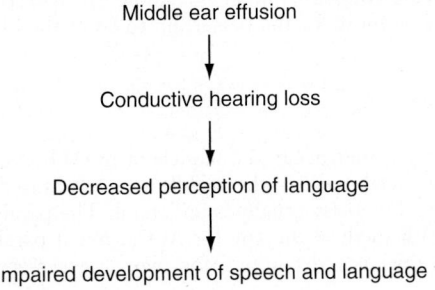

Middle ear effusion

↓

Conductive hearing loss

↓

Decreased perception of language

↓

Impaired development of speech and language

↓

Lower scores on tests of cognitive abilities

↓

Poor performance in school

Figure 19–7 Long-term sequelae of middle ear effusion. *(From Bluestone, C. D., and Klein, J. O.: Otitis Media in Infants and Children. 4th ed. Hamilton, Ontario, B. C. Decker, 2007, p. 333.)*

and result in conductive hearing loss. Adhesive changes may bind the eardrum to the ossicles and surrounding middle ear structures and cause resorption of the ossicles.

TYMPANOSCLEROSIS

Tympanosclerosis, or scarring of the tympanic membrane, may be a sequela of chronic middle ear inflammation or trauma. White plaques are present in the tympanic membrane, with nodular deposits in the submucosal layers. The histopathology is marked by hyaline degeneration resulting from a healing reaction characterized by fibroblastic invasion of the submucosa followed by thickening and fusion of the fibers.

OSSICULAR DISCONTINUITY AND FIXATION

Ossicular chain abnormalities, including osteitis, may be secondary to chronic inflammation in the middle ear or the presence of a retraction pocket or cholesteatoma. The long process of the incus most commonly is involved. Erosion of the blood supply, cholesteatoma, or adhesive otitis media may be the cause of the bone erosion and disarticulation. Conductive hearing loss is present to a varying degree. Diagnosis may be assisted by computed tomography or magnetic resonance imaging.

MASTOIDITIS

Reports from Denmark,[146] Italy,[114] and the United States[95] indicate that mastoiditis continues to be an important complication of AOM in developed countries, although at a low rate. In developing countries, untreated otitis media may lead to persistent perforation of the tympanic membrane, dysarticulation of ossicles, and mastoiditis. Berman[12] estimated that mastoiditis occurred as a complication of otitis media in developing countries in 0.74 percent of cases of otitis, based on community and school surveys, and in 1.7 to 18 percent, based on hospital clinical record reviews. In a survey of eight children's hospitals in the United States between 1993 and 1998 for pneumococcal diseases, Kaplan and colleagues[95] identified 34 children with pneumococcal mastoiditis; serogroup 19 accounted for 57 percent of the isolates. The cases occurred primarily in children younger than 2 years of age.

At birth, the mastoid consists of a single cell, the antrum, connected to the middle ear by a small channel, the aditus ad antrum. Pneumatization of the mastoid bone occurs soon after birth and usually is extensive by the time the child reaches 2 years of age. Likely, whenever AOM occurs, some degree of mastoiditis is present. With healing of the middle ear infection, healing of the mastoid also occurs. In a few cases, mastoid disease progresses with hyperemia and edema of the mucosal lining of the pneumatized cells, accumulation of serous and then purulent exudates in the cells, demineralization of the cellular walls and necrosis of bone, and formation of abscess cavities caused by coalescence of adjacent cells after destruction of the cell walls. Pus may escape into contiguous areas, including the posterior cranial fossa, middle cranial fossa, sigmoid and lateral sinuses, canal of the facial nerve, semicircular canals, and petrous tip of the temporal bone.

Signs of acute mastoiditis with periostitis include fever, otalgia, postauricular erythema, tenderness, and slight swelling. The pinna may be displaced inferiorly and anteriorly.

Initial management of acute mastoiditis includes administration of parenteral antibiotics and myringotomy to provide drainage of the middle ear and mastoid contents. Surgical drainage of the mastoid should be performed if the symptoms of the acute

infection, including fever and otalgia, persist. If the infection progresses, causing destruction of the bony trabeculae, a mastoid empyema, mastoidectomy should be performed to prevent spread of the infection to adjacent structures.

PETROSITIS

Petrositis occurs when suppurative infection extends from the middle ear and mastoid into the petrous portion of the temporal bone. Signs of petrositis include pain behind the eye, deep ear pain, persistent ear discharge, and sixth nerve palsy. The triad of pain behind the eye, aural discharge, and sixth nerve palsy is termed *Gradenigo syndrome*. Management is similar to that described earlier for mastoiditis.

LABYRINTHITIS

Spread of AOM into the cochlear and vestibular apparatus through the round (less commonly, the oval) window results in inflammation of the labyrinth. The signs of labyrinthitis include sudden, progressive, or fluctuating sensorineural hearing loss or vertigo in association with otitis media or mastoiditis. Signs of suppurative labyrinthitis (in the absence of meningitis) warrant performing aggressive otologic surgery and administering parenteral antimicrobial therapy.

MENINGITIS

Meningitis may be associated with middle ear infections in three circumstances:

1. *Direct invasion*: A suppurative focus in the middle ear or mastoid spreads through the dura, extends to the pia-arachnoid, and causes generalized meningitis.
2. *Inflammation in an adjacent area*: The meninges may become inflamed if there is suppuration in an adjacent area, such as the mastoid air cells.
3. *Concurrent infection*: Otitis media arises by spread of bacteria from the upper respiratory tract, and meningitis concurrently invades the blood from the upper respiratory focus.

Children with cochlear implants are at risk for development of meningitis. Although the implant has been implicated in the subsequent development of meningitis, some children likely had an underlying congenital inner or middle ear malformation that provided a pathway for the bacterium to enter the brain.[23]

FACIAL PARALYSIS

Facial paralysis may occur as a sequela of AOM because of exposure of the facial nerve in the middle ear cleft caused by a bony dehiscence. The palsy usually is unilateral. The paralysis usually resolves with medical therapy for AOM, but if paralysis of the facial nerve persists, decompression may be necessary.

OTHER SUPPURATIVE COMPLICATIONS

The middle ear and mastoid air cells are adjacent to the dura of the posterior and middle cranial fossa, the sigmoid venous sinus of the brain, and the inner ear (Fig. 19–8). Suppuration in the middle ear or mastoid may spread to these structures, producing suppurative complications, such as meningitis, extradural abscess, subdural empyema, focal encephalitis, brain abscess, and lateral

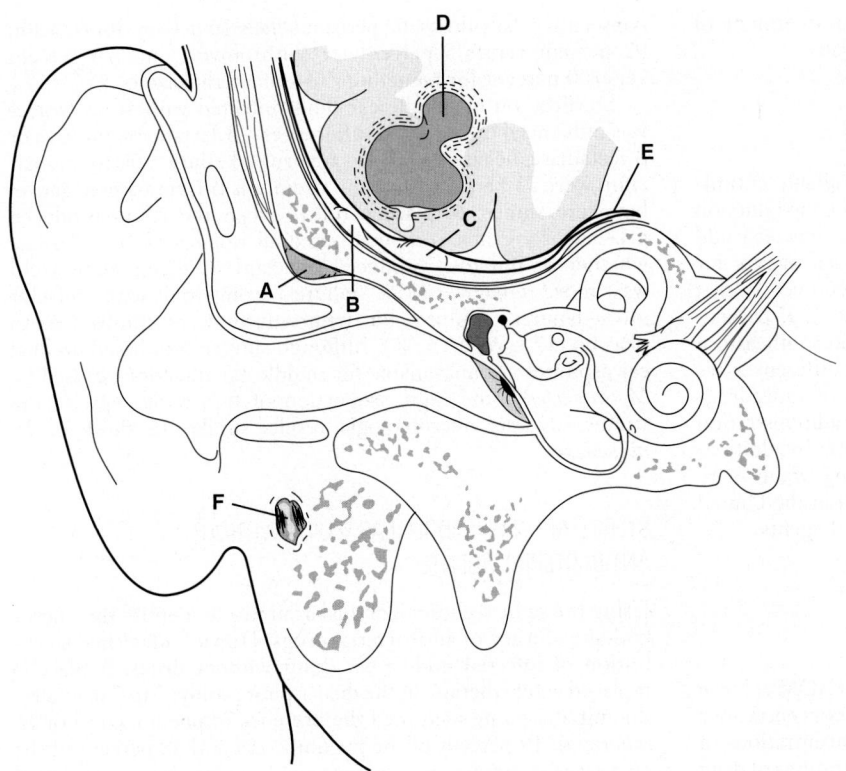

Figure 19–8 Suppurative complications of otitis media and mastoiditis. A, Subperiosteal abscess. B, Extradural abscess. C, Subdural empyema. D, Brain abscess. E, Meningitis. F, Lateral sinus thrombosis. *(From Bluestone, C. D., and Klein, J. O.: Otitis Media in Infants and Children. 4th ed. Hamilton, Ontario, B. C. Decker, 2007, p. 434.)*

sinus thrombosis. Intracranial complications should be suspected when a child with acute or chronic otitis media develops persistent and severe headache, severe otalgia, and change in affect or level of responsiveness. Conversely, children with diagnosed intracranial infection, such as meningitis, should have middle ear or mastoid disease assessed as the origin of the central nervous system disease.

Intracranial extension of infection from the middle ear into the intracranial area may occur because of any of the following:

1. Progressive thrombophlebitis, permitting infection to spread through the intact bone
2. Erosion of the bony walls of the middle ear or mastoid
3. Extension along preformed pathways, such as the round window, dehiscent sutures, skull fractures, and congenital or surgically acquired bony dehiscences.

The microbiology, pathogenesis, diagnosis, and management of intracranial complications of otitis media and mastoiditis are discussed extensively elsewhere (see Chapters 20, 37, 38, and 42).

MANAGEMENT OF ACUTE OTITIS MEDIA

Management of AOM focuses on the choice of an appropriate antimicrobial agent or an option to observe initially rather than treat. Decongestants and antihistamines may provide some comfort for a patient who has congestion of the upper respiratory tract, but they provide no benefit in terms of earlier resolution of the middle ear infection. The antimicrobial agent should have a spectrum of activity that includes *S. pneumoniae* and *H. influenzae* and have documented clinical and microbiologic efficacy, limited side effects, availability in a convenient dosage schedule, palatability when provided in suspension, and reasonable cost. When treated with appropriate antimicrobial therapy, a patient should have substantial resolution of signs and symptoms within

TABLE 19–4   Daily Dosage Schedule for Antimicrobial Agents Useful in Acute Otitis Media

Agent	24-Hr Dosage
Amoxicillin	40-80 mg/kg in 2-3 doses
Amoxicillin-clavulanate	40-80 mg/kg in 2 doses (90 mg/kg in 2 doses for Augmentin ES-600)
Cefprozil	30 mg/kg in 2 doses
Cefpodoxime	10 mg/kg in 2 doses
Cefaclor	40 mg/kg in 2-3 doses
Cefixime	8 mg/kg in 1 dose
Cefuroxime axetil	30 mg/kg in 2 doses
Loracarbef	30 mg/kg in 2 doses
Ceftriaxone	50 mg/kg in 1 dose* (1-3 days)
Ceftibuten	9 mg/kg in 1 dose
Cefdinir	14 mg/kg in 1-2 doses
Erythromycin-sulfisoxazole	50 mg/kg erythromycin, 150 mg/kg sulfisoxazole in 4 doses
Clarithromycin	15 mg in 2 doses
Azithromycin	30 mg/kg in 1 dose (1 day)
	10 mg/kg in 1 dose (3 days)
	10 mg/kg in 1 dose (day 1); 5 mg/kg in 1 dose (days 2-5)
Trimethoprim-sulfamethoxazole	8 mg trimethoprim, 40 mg sulfamethoxazole in 2 doses

Intramuscular route.

72 hours and absence of signs of relapse, recurrence, or suppurative sequelae.

Table 19–4 lists the daily dosage schedules of 15 oral or parenteral antimicrobial agents approved for the indication of therapy of AOM. In addition, ofloxacin otic and ciprofloxacin (combined with dexamethasone) otic have been approved by the

U.S. Food and Drug Administration (FDA) for treatment of AOM in children with tympanostomy tubes in place.

CLINICAL IMPLICATIONS OF ANTIBIOTIC RESISTANCE

Increased resistance of bacterial pathogens to available antimicrobial agents has been a constant concern since the introduction of antimicrobial agents. Multidrug-resistant pneumococci add complexity to the choice of optimal antimicrobial agents for AOM. At present, the incidence of strains of pneumococci that are nonsusceptible to penicillin averages approximately 25 percent in the United States but is more than twice that in southeastern and southwestern states. Reasons for the regional differences are unknown. The major risk factors for presence of multidrug-resistant pneumococci are recent (within 30 days) administration of an antimicrobial agent and attendance in daycare. In addition, the increasing proportion of β-lactamase–producing strains of *H. influenzae* and *M. catarrhalis*, now 30 to 75 percent in the United States, warrants consideration in choice of optimal agents.

DIFFUSION OF ANTIMICROBIAL AGENTS INTO MIDDLE EAR FLUIDS

Most antimicrobial agents of value for treatment of AOM achieve significant concentrations in middle ear fluid. The concentrations are generally parallel to, although lower than, concentrations of drug in serum. Purulent fluids have higher concentrations of drug than do mucoid or serous fluids. Penicillins and cephalosporins achieve concentrations in middle ear fluids that are approximately one fifth to one third the levels present in serum. Sulfonamides and erythromycin achieved middle ear concentrations that were approximately 50 percent of serum concentrations. An extensive review of concentrations achieved in middle ear fluids is provided in the textbook *Pediatric Otolaryngology*, edited by Bluestone, Stool, and Kenna.[26]

STERILIZATION OF MIDDLE EAR FLUIDS BY ANTIMICROBIAL AGENTS

To define the ability of antimicrobial agents to eradicate bacterial pathogens from middle ear fluids of children with AOM, investigators have used serial aspirates of the infected fluids.[46,82,83,119,122] The initial aspirate identifies the bacterial pathogen of the acute middle ear infection; the second aspirate, obtained days after initiation of therapy, defines the ability of the drug to eradicate the infection. The results of these tests generally are consistent with data available from in vitro assays of the drugs against the major bacterial pathogens and the concentrations of drug achieved in the middle ear fluids.[100] Penicillin-susceptible pneumococcal infections were sterilized by most penicillins, cephalosporins, and macrolides; failure rates of 10 percent or more were identified only in infections treated with cefaclor, cefixime, and cefpodoxime; sulfonamides alone were ineffective, but trimethoprim-sulfamethoxazole was effective.

Dagan[46] reviewed sterilization of middle ear fluids by antimicrobial agents for pneumococci that were penicillin-susceptible and penicillin-nonsusceptible. The sterilization of middle ear fluids infected with susceptible strains was consistent with prior data. Nonsusceptible strains were less readily eradicated from the middle ear fluid, and the failure rates were twofold or more than those for penicillin-susceptible strains. The failure rates for penicillin-nonsusceptible versus penicillin-susceptible strains were 20 percent versus 10 percent for amoxicillin, 53 percent versus 0 percent for ceftriaxone administered as one dose, 9 percent versus 0 percent for ceftriaxone administered as three

consecutive daily doses, 62 percent versus 10 percent for cefaclor, 92 percent versus 5 percent for azithromycin, and 79 percent versus 0 percent for trimethoprim-sulfamethoxazole.

Sterilization of middle ear fluids infected with *H. influenzae* was influenced by the strain differences—β-lactamase–positive or β-lactamase–negative for β-lactam drugs. Failure rates for amoxicillin were 21 percent when the strain was β-lactamase–negative, but were similar to placebo (60%) when the strain produced β-lactamase. Ceftriaxone eradicated all isolates of *H. influenzae* whether or not they produced β-lactamase. Cefuroxime axetil was more effective (15% failures) compared with cefaclor (40% failures). Failures for azithromycin were comparable to placebo (57% versus 52%). Although similar data based on dual ear aspirates are unavailable for middle ear infections caused by *M. catarrhalis*, the high proportion of β-lactamase–producing strains suggests microbiologic results similar to those of *H. influenzae*.

STERILIZATION OF MIDDLE EAR FLUIDS WITHOUT ANTIBACTERIAL AGENTS

Using the same technique of dual aspirates to identify the microbiologic efficacy of antibacterial drugs, Howie[81] identified sterilization of infected middle ear fluids without drugs. A placebo replaced active therapy in the dual aspirate study: 2 to 7 days after the initial aspirate identified the presence of pneumococci or *H. influenzae*, 19 percent of the pneumococci and 48 percent of the *Haemophilus* strains no longer were present. The differential clearing of the bacteria with persistence of most pneumococci but resolution of one half of the infections caused by nontypeable *H. influenzae* likely is associated with some immune or bacteriostatic factor in the middle ear inflammatory exudate that acts to inhibit growth of these organisms. These data of spontaneous resolution need to be considered in evaluating the efficacy of new and old antibacterial drugs.

INITIAL OBSERVATION RATHER THAN ANTIMICROBIAL AGENT THERAPY

Before the introduction of sulfonamides in 1936, management of AOM included watchful waiting or, when the suppurative process produced severe clinical signs, use of myringotomy to drain the middle ear abscess. Spread of infection to the mastoid, meninges, or other intracranial foci was a feared complication of otitis media. Early therapeutic trials identified the value of using antimicrobial agents for resolution of clinical signs and decreased incidence of suppurative complications. Most children with AOM respond clinically without use of antimicrobial agents. Children who improve without antimicrobial drugs include one third with AOM who have a bacteriologically sterile effusion and are presumed to have a viral infection and children who have bacterial infections that clear without antimicrobial agents (19% of pneumococcal infections, 48% of infections caused by nontypeable strains of *H. influenzae*, and approximately 75% of AOM caused by *M. catarrhalis*).[100] Because of the increased incidence of bacterial pathogens resistant to available antimicrobial agents, and the data associating extensive use of the drugs with development of resistant strains, limiting the use of antimicrobial agents for children with AOM has been suggested. The option of observation and symptomatic treatment rather than initial antibiotic treatment has been advocated in Western Europe based on studies by van Buchem and colleagues.[193,194] In the United States, interest in this management increased with concerns for multidrug resistance resulting from the extensive use of antimicrobial agents, but the recommendations of the CDC and the AAP in 1998 focused on increasing the accuracy of diagnosis, avoiding use of antimicrobial agents for otitis media with effusion, and continuing use of these drugs for treatment of AOM.[50]

The AAP and the AAFP in 2004 altered their positions and for the first time provided a guideline for an observation option for selected patients.[4] The guideline recommended that observation without use of antimicrobial agents could be considered in a child older than 24 months of age with uncomplicated AOM with nonsevere signs (mild otalgia, temperature <39° C orally in the past 24 hours) when follow-up was ensured, and antibacterial agents could be started if symptoms persisted or worsened. Table 19–5 lists the options considered in the guidelines.

CHOICE OF ANTIMICROBIAL AGENTS

Oral amoxicillin remains the first-line antimicrobial agent for treating AOM because of the expected low failure rates. The drug-resistant *S. pneumoniae* Therapeutic Working Group of the CDC[49] and the 2004 guidelines of the AAP and the AAFP[4] suggested that an increase in dosage used of amoxicillin for empiric treatment from 40 to 45 mg/kg/day to 80 to 90 mg/kg/day would be effective for more nonsusceptible strains of *S. pneumoniae*. The 2004 guidelines for initial treatment and treatment failures are listed in Table 19–6.

The guideline differentiates treatment choice of drug by severity of signs. Children with nonsevere disease may be treated initially with high-dose amoxicillin, but children with severe signs should be treated with amoxicillin-clavulanate. The use of high-dose amoxicillin-clavulanate responds to concern about failure of amoxicillin in cases of AOM caused by β-lactamase–producing

H. influenzae. If failure occurred because of a high-level resistant strain of *S. pneumoniae*, however, the same dosage of amoxicillin in the combination would not be advantageous. Cefuroxime axetil, cefpodoxime, and cefdinir have equivalent profiles in vitro against *S. pneumoniae* and *H. influenzae*. Because of bitter taste, cefuroxime and cefpodoxime are not well accepted by young patients, and the better taste of cefdinir increased acceptability and compliance. Intramuscular ceftriaxone was most effective in eradicating nonsusceptible pneumococci when provided in three daily doses, but an alternative regimen is to provide a single dose and, if signs do not resolve at 48 hours, to proceed to a second or third dose.[102]

DOSAGE SCHEDULES

Dosage schedules of the antimicrobial agents of value for therapy of AOM have been determined on the basis of studies of the pharmacokinetics and results of clinical trials (see Table 19–4).

DURATION OF THERAPY

Duration of therapy is based on clinical trials and tradition. Most clinical trials and standard pediatric practice include a 10-day course of an antimicrobial agent. The FDA approved a 5-day schedule of once-a-day azithromycin administered orally based on studies comparing the clinical efficacy of 5-day azithromycin with 10-day amoxicillin-clavulanate courses. These data suggest that short courses of therapy may be appropriate for many children with AOM, although some children (likely children with severe and recurrent disease) would require more prolonged schedules.

CLINICAL COURSE AFTER INITIATION OF THERAPY

The clinical course of a child who receives appropriate antimicrobial therapy includes significant resolution of acute signs within 48 to 72 hours. Instructions to the parent should indicate the need to contact the physician if the signs or symptoms worsen at any time or are unimproved at 72 hours. Persistent ear pain or systemic signs, such as fever, signal the need for re-evaluation to examine for other foci of infections, to determine the need for another antimicrobial agent, or to perform tympanocentesis or myringotomy to incise and drain the middle ear abscess and culture the fluid to identify the pathogen. If a new antibiotic is

TABLE 19–5 Guidelines for Management of Acute Otitis Media from the American Academy of Pediatrics and American Academy of Family Physicians[4]

Age (mo)	Certain Diagnosis*	Uncertain Diagnosis
<6	Antibiotics	Antibiotics
6-24	Antibiotics	Antibiotics if severe; observe if not severe†
>24	Antibiotics if severe; observe if not severe†	Observe

*Certain diagnosis = middle ear effusion, rapid onset, symptoms of middle ear inflammation.
†Not severe = mild otalgia; temperature <39°C orally or <39.5°C rectally in past 24 hr.

TABLE 19–6 Recommended Antibacterial Agents for Patients Who Are Being Treated Initially with Antibacterial Agents or Who Have Failed Initial Management with Antibacterial Agents

	At Diagnosis for Patients Being Treated Initially with Antibacterial Agents*		Clinically Defined Treatment Failure at 48-72 Hr after Initial Management with Antibacterial Agents	
Temperature ≥39° C and/or Severe Otalgia	Recommended	Alternative for Penicillin Allergy	Recommended	Alternative for Penicillin Allergy
No	Amoxicillin 80-90 mg/kg/day	Non–type I: cefdinir, cefuroxime, cefpodoxime Type I: azithromycin, clarithromycin	Amoxicillin-clavulanate (90 mg/kg/day of amoxicillin component, with 6.4 mg/kg/day of clavulanate)	Non–type I: ceftriaxone—3 days Type I: clindamycin
Yes	Amoxicillin-clavulanate (90 mg/kg/day of amoxicillin with 6.4 mg/kg/day of clavulanate)	Ceftriaxone—1 or 3 days	Ceftriaxone—3 days	Tympanocentesis, clindamycin

*Choices are the same for patients who were initially managed with observation but require therapy at 48-72 hours.
From American Academy of Pediatrics.[4]

needed, one with β-lactamase stability and activity against penicillin-resistant pneumococci (if such information is available from local surveillance studies) should be chosen.

Follow-up visits should be made to determine that the child has recovered from the acute infection and to diagnose persistent middle ear effusion if it is present. The utility of the traditional 10- to 14-day visit was reassessed by Hathaway and coworkers[75] and Mandel and colleagues[116]; these investigators concluded that the follow-up visit can be extended to 4 to 6 weeks after onset of treatment in children whose parents thought the disease had resolved at 10 to 14 days. For children who still had signs or symptoms of disease (other than persistent middle ear effusion), the 10- to 14-day visit was recommended. Visits at 4 to 6 weeks and repeated at 1-month intervals if effusion is present are valuable in determining the duration of middle ear effusion after the acute episode and identifying children who may be candidates for placement of tympanostomy tubes.

SYMPTOMATIC THERAPY

Administration of antipyretics and analgesics and application of local heat usually are helpful in treating a child with an acute painful and febrile episode. Acetaminophen or ibuprofen is recommended for children with mild to moderate pain. Topical agents such as benzocaine may provide brief benefit in patients older than 5 years of age. Narcotic analgesia with codeine or analogues should be reserved for patients with moderate or severe pain. An oral decongestant, such as pseudoephedrine hydrochloride, may relieve nasal congestion, and antihistamines may help patients with known or suspected nasal allergy. The efficacy of antihistamines and decongestants for resolution of middle ear effusion is unproven.

MANAGEMENT OF ACUTE OTITIS MEDIA IN A CHILD WITH TYMPANOSTOMY TUBES

Children with tympanostomy tubes also experience AOM. Because the tube permits drainage of the middle ear fluid and an abscess does not develop, the major pathology is inflammation of the mucous lining of the middle ear, and the dominant clinical sign is otorrhea. The bacterial pathogens include those responsible for AOM (*S. pneumoniae, H. influenzae,* and *M. catarrhalis*) and bacteria that may invade the middle ear from the EAC (*S. aureus* and *P. aeruginosa*). Although amoxicillin or amoxicillin-clavulanate is the usual choice for treatment of AOM in a child with tympanostomy tubes, ofloxacin otic and ciprofloxacin-dexamethasone otic were effective for children who presented with acute otorrhea. The efficacy of the otic suspensions for AOM in children with tympanostomy tubes indicates that high concentrations of drug reach the middle ear mucosa and result in eradication of bacterial pathogens. Additional advantages of otic versus systemic antimicrobial administration include lesser systemic adverse events (e.g., diarrhea) and absence of effect on the upper respiratory flora, and absence of selection of resistant bacteria.[67,157]

MANAGEMENT OF OTITIS MEDIA WITH EFFUSION

The following options have been investigated for management of a child with prolonged middle ear fluid or with otitis media with effusion:

1. Another 10-day course of a broad-spectrum antimicrobial agent that has activity against β-lactamase–producing organisms has been recommended because bacterial pathogens are found in approximately one fourth of patients with otitis media with effusion; a meta-analysis of blinded studies identified resolution of effusion in 14 percent of cases.[182]

2. Myringotomy or myringotomy and tympanostomy tubes drain the middle ear fluid, aerate the middle ear space, and permit the middle ear mucosa to return to normal.[117]

3. Adenoidectomy with or without tonsillectomy for children who have recurrences after an initial placement of tympanostomy tubes is controversial.[63] A Finnish study concluded that adenoidectomy did not reduce the incidence of AOM in otitis-prone children younger than 4 years of age who received tympanostomy tubes.[72]

4. Steroid therapy alone or with an antibiotic has been shown to be effective in some children with otitis media with effusion. Berman[11] recommended a regimen of prednisone, 1 mg/kg/day (given orally in two doses) for 7 days, with an antibiotic for 14 to 21 days. Children without a history of varicella infection who have been exposed to the virus in the month before receiving treatment should not be given prednisone because of the risk for developing disseminated disease. The guidelines published by the Agency for Health Care Policy and Research concluded that the data were insufficient in sample size or duration of observation to recommend use of steroids for otitis media with effusion.[182]

Topical or systemic nasal decongestants, antihistamines, and anti-inflammatory agents,[1,196] alone or in combination, have been found to be of limited or no value in the management of otitis media with effusion.

We favor an initial course of a broad-spectrum antibiotic for children with otitis media with effusion for 3 or more months. If the effusion does not resolve, use of tympanostomy tubes is the most efficient method for managing prolonged middle ear effusion. The use of tympanostomy tubes first was suggested more than 100 years ago by Politzer, but the procedure did not become readily available until it was reintroduced by Armstrong in 1954. Myringotomy and placement of ventilating tubes result in the following immediate benefits to the patient with otitis media with effusion:

- The effusion is drained, and the fluid-filled space is aerated.
- The middle ear secretions, which constantly are being formed by the secretory cells of the mucosa, are drained.
- The chronically diseased mucosa (characterized by hypertrophic secretory cells) returns to normal.
- The hearing impairment caused by the middle ear fluid disappears.
- Concern for effects of hearing loss on development of speech and cognitive abilities is diminished.
- The child who was not responsive or attentive (a condition often unrecognized as hearing impairment by the parent) becomes more social and more involved with siblings, parents, and playmates.

The procedure may be disadvantageous for the following reasons:

- General anesthesia is required.
- The cost is significant.
- Although uncommon, sequelae, such as persistent otorrhea, permanent perforation, scarring of the membrane, and cholesteatoma, may occur.

In addition, developmental outcomes may not be improved after early rather than delayed insertion of tympanostomy tubes.[138]

Current recommendations for pediatric otitis media with effusion include follow-up visits for 1 to 2 months after the acute episode. When the effusion persists for 3 or more months, the child should receive medical treatment with a course of antibiotics (2 to 3 weeks) or in conjunction with a 7-day regimen of prednisone. If the effusion fails to resolve with medical management, the child should be referred to an otolaryngologist for consideration of placement of tympanostomy tubes with or without adenoidectomy.[117,137]

PREVENTION

ADVISING PARENTS

Parents of children who have severe and recurrent otitis media or risk factors for developing middle ear infections should be advised of measures that may reduce the incidence of infection, such as breast-feeding; enrolling children in small, rather than large, group daycare centers; and reducing exposure to tobacco smoke. In addition, data about the risks for developing recurrent otitis media associated with the prone sleeping position and use of a pacifier, although requiring corroboration, may be added to the discussion with the parent. Physicians also may advise parents that the seasonal incidence of otitis media suggests that their child's condition is expected to improve in late spring and summer and that aggressive measures of management, including chemoprophylaxis and surgery, may be postponed until the course of disease has been determined in the next respiratory season.

PNEUMOCOCCAL VACCINES

A pneumococcal polysaccharide vaccine was introduced in the United States in the 1970s, but it had limited efficacy in infants 2 years of age and younger and only a modest effect in prevention of AOM. In February 2000, the FDA approved a safe and effective seven-valent conjugate pneumococcal vaccine (PCV7) that was immunogenic in infants 2 months of age. By December 2005, more than 80 million doses had been distributed in the United States (Peter Paradiso, personal communication). PCV7 has been effective in decreasing the incidence of invasive disease and, to a lesser extent, the incidence of AOM. The results of two large PCV7 clinical trials have been published: (1) an evaluation of the efficacy of the vaccine for prevention of invasive bacterial disease, pneumonia, and otitis media in approximately 38,000 Northern California infants[19,58] and (2) a clinical and microbiologic study of the efficacy of PCV7 for prevention of AOM in 1662 Finnish infants.[52] A clinical trial of an 11-valent polysaccharide vaccine conjugated with an outer membrane protein of nontypeable *H. influenzae* was found to be effective in infants in the Czech Republic and Slovakia against AOM caused by *S. pneumoniae* and *H. influenzae*.[151] A 13-valent vaccine is currently being studied for safety and immunogenicity. Table 19–7 lists the serotypes included in the various pneumococcal vaccines.

In the Northern California study, the efficacy of PCV7 for prevention of episodes of AOM was based on clinical criteria. The vaccine was 7.8 percent effective in preventing episodes of AOM, antibiotic prescriptions decreased by 5.8 percent, and 24.9 percent fewer surgical procedures (most were placement of ventilating tubes) were performed in children immunized with PCV7 compared with children who received the control vaccine (conjugate polysaccharide meningococcal group C).

The Finnish trial provided microbiologic data based on aspirates of middle ear fluids in children who had AOM. Children who received PCV7 had 6 percent fewer episodes of AOM; culture-confirmed pneumococcal episodes were reduced by 34 percent. Children who received PCV7 experienced a 57 percent reduction in episodes caused by pneumococcal serotypes included

TABLE 19–7 Serotypes in Pneumococcal Vaccines—2008

Serotype	Polysaccharide 23 Type (Merck)	Polysaccharide Conjugates		
		7 Type (Wyeth)	13 Type* (Wyeth)	11 Type* (GSK)
1	+		+	+
2	+			
3	+		+	+
4	+	+	+	+
5	+		+	+
6A	−		+	
6B	+	+	+	+
7F	+			+
7V	−		+	
8	+			
9N	+			
9V	+	+	+	+
10A	+			
11A	+			
12F	+			
14	+	+	+	+
15B	+			
17F	+			
18C	+	+	+	+
19A	+		+	
19F	+	+	+	+
20	+			
22F	+			
23F	+	+	+	+
33F	+			

Not approved by the FDA as of May 2008.

TABLE 19–8 Efficacy of PCV7 in Finnish Children with Acute Otitis Media (AOM)

End-Point	AOM Episodes		Vaccine Efficacy Point Estimate
	PCV7 (N = 831)	Control (N = 831)*	
Any AOM	1251	1345	6
Pneumococcal AOM	271	414	34
Vaccine serotypes	107	250	57
Cross-reactive serotypes	41	84	51
Nonvaccine serotypes	125	95	−33
Haemophilus influenzae AOM	315	287	−11
Moraxella catarrhalis AOM	379	381	−1

Hepatitis B vaccine.
Adapted from data published in Eskola, J., Kilpi, T., Palmu, A., et al.: Efficacy of a pneumococcal conjugate vaccine against acute otitis media. N. Engl. J. Med. 344:403-409, 2001.

in the vaccine and a 51 percent reduction in episodes caused by cross-reactive pneumococcal serotypes. A 33 percent increase in episodes of AOM caused by nonvaccine pneumococcal serotypes and an 11 percent increase in episodes caused by *H. influenzae* occurred (Table 19–8).

An 11-valent pneumococcal polysaccharide vaccine conjugated with an outer membrane protein of nontypeable *H. influenzae* was found to be effective against AOM caused by *S. pneumoniae* and *H. influenzae* (GlaxoSmithKline Biologics), but it has not been approved (as of May 2008) for immunization of infants in the United States or elsewhere.[151] The vaccine prevented 52 percent of episodes of AOM caused by pneumococcal vaccine serotypes and 35.3 percent of episodes caused by nontypeable *H. influenzae*.

The 23-type polysaccharide vaccine currently available produces an independent antibody response in children 2 years of age or older and in adults. Studies of polysaccharide vaccines in Finland and the United States have indicated that the vaccines were effective in preventing type-specific pneumococcal otitis media if an adequate immune response occurred, but the number of types producing an adequate response in children younger than 2 years was limited.[115,179,184] Administration of the polysaccharide vaccine in older children may provide protection against types not included in PCV7 and has been recommended by the AAP and the Advisory Committee on Immunization Practices of the Surgeon General for high-risk children ages 2 years and older who have received PCV7. For children 2 years old and older who continue to have severe and recurrent AOM, use of the polysaccharide vaccine after administration of PCV7 may be valuable for protection against additional pneumococcal serotypes.

INFLUENZA VIRUS VACCINES

Influenza virus vaccine resulted in a reduction in cases of influenza A and a 36 percent decline in otitis media in children attending a daycare center.[42] A similar reduction (30%) in episodes of febrile otitis media also was reported in children after administration of a live, attenuated cold-adapted intranasal vaccine.[10] Annual administration of influenza virus vaccines should be part of the strategy for reducing the incidence of AOM for children with recurrent and severe disease.

CHEMOPROPHYLAXIS

Use of chemoprophylaxis has succeeded in reducing the number of new symptomatic episodes of AOM in children who have a history of recurrent infections. Children at risk for developing severe and recurrent disease should be considered for chemoprophylaxis despite the concern for development of resistant strains of bacterial pathogens after use of the regimen of a modified dosage of an antimicrobial agent. Results of controlled clinical trials of modified courses of antimicrobial agents compared with trials in which placebo or historical controls were used have been reviewed.[101] Most of these studies used a sulfonamide or a broad-spectrum penicillin. Most reports indicated benefit to the enrollees in reduction of new episodes when they were compared with controls: Amoxicillin efficacy was 44 to 67 percent, and sulfonamide efficacy was 40 to 88 percent (although the efficacy of sulfonamides was reported as only 8% in one study).

We recommend the following protocol based on the results of these studies. Criteria for enrollment should include three documented episodes of AOM in 6 months or four episodes in 12 months. Because children who have episodes of acute infection early in life or have siblings with severe and recurrent ear infections are prone to develop otitis media, prophylaxis also should be considered for children who have one episode in the first 6 months of life plus a family history of ear infections or who have two episodes in the first year of life.

A sulfonamide or amoxicillin is the agent used most often and provides the advantages of demonstrated efficacy, safety, and low cost. The drug is administered at half the therapeutic dose (administered once a day). Amoxicillin is given at a dose of 40 mg/kg, and sulfisoxazole is given at a dose of 50 mg/kg. Chemoprophylaxis should be provided during the fall, winter, and early spring months (when respiratory tract infections are most frequent) for 6 months.

Children, when free of signs of acute infection, should be examined at approximately 2-month intervals to determine whether middle ear effusion is present. Management of prolonged middle ear effusion should be considered separately from prevention of recurrences of acute infection.

Acute infections are expected to occur, although at a lower rate, during the course of prophylaxis. The infection should be treated with an alternative regimen. Amoxicillin-clavulanate or intramuscular ceftriaxone would be a suitable alternative, regardless of the prophylactic agent used.

SURGICAL OPTIONS

When nonsurgical methods of prevention fail to prevent recurrent otitis media, surgery is a reasonable option. Among the options that have been shown to be effective is insertion of tympanostomy tubes, with or without adenoidectomy. Casselbrant and colleagues[36] randomly assigned children into treatment groups receiving amoxicillin, tympanostomy tube placement, or placebo and found that amoxicillin and insertion of the tympanostomy tube were effective. With the current concern about the association of low-dose, long-term antimicrobial prophylaxis and emergence of resistant otitis pathogens,[49] myringotomy and placement of tympanostomy tubes may be more desirable than antimicrobial prophylaxis. When tympanostomy tubes extrude and the child continues to have recurrent episodes of otitis media, replacement of the tympanostomy tubes in conjunction with adenoidectomy has been shown to be effective.[137] As shown by Paradise and coworkers,[135] neither adenoidectomy nor adenotonsillectomy is effective in children not treated previously with tympanostomy tubes, when prevention of otitis media is the only indication.

REFERENCES

1. Abramovich, S., O'Grady, J., Fuller, A., et al.: Naproxen in otitis media with effusion. J. Laryngol. Otol. 100:263-266, 1986.
2. Abramson, J. S., Giebink, G. S., Mills, E. L., et al.: Polymorphonuclear leukocyte dysfunction during influenza virus infection in chinchillas. J. Infect. Dis. 143:836-845, 1981.
3. Alho, O. P., Koivu, M., Sorri, M., et al.: Risk factors for recurrent acute otitis media and respiratory infection in infancy. Int. J. Pediatr. Otorhinolaryngol. 19:151-161, 1990.
4. American Academy of Pediatrics and American Academy of Family Physicians: Clinical Practice Guidelines—Subcommittee on Management of Acute Otitis Media: Diagnosis and management of acute otitis media. Pediatrics 113:1451-1465, 2004.
5. Austrian, R., Howie, V. M., and Ploussard, J. H.: The bacteriology of pneumococcal otitis media. Johns Hopkins Med. J. 141:104-111, 1977.
6. Baba, S.: Recent aspects of clinical bacteriology in otitis media. Presented at Presymposium on Management of Otitis Media. Kyoto, January 12, 1985.
7. Babonis, T. R., Weir, M. R., and Kelly, P. C.: Impedance tympanometry and acoustic reflectometry at myringotomy. Pediatrics 87:475-480, 1991.
8. Barnett, E. D., Klein, J. O., Pelton, S. I., et al.: Otitis media in children born to human immunodeficiency virus-infected mothers. Pediatr. Infect. Dis. J. 11:360-364, 1992.
9. Bell, D. W., Gleiber, D. W., Mercer, A. A., et al.: Illness associated with child day care: A study of incidence and cost. Am. J. Public Health 79:479-484, 1989.
10. Belshe, R. B., Mendelman, P. M., Treanor, J., et al.: The efficacy of live attenuated, cold-adapted trivalent, intranasal influenza virus vaccine in children. N. Engl. J. Med. 338:1459-1461, 1998.
11. Berman, S.: Otitis media in children. N. Engl. J. Med. 332:1560-1565, 1995.
12. Berman, S.: Otitis media in developing countries. Pediatrics 96:126-131, 1995.
13. Berman, S.: Management of otitis media and functional outcomes related to language, behavior, and attention: Is it time to change our approach? Pediatrics 107:1175-1177, 2001.
14. Berman, S. A., Balkany, T. J., and Simmons, M. A.: Otitis media in infants less than 12 weeks of age: Differing bacteriology among in-patients and out-patients. J. Pediatr. 93:453-454, 1978.
15. Berman, S. A., Balkany, T. J., and Simmons, M. A.: Otitis media in the neonatal intensive care unit. Pediatrics 62:168, 1978.
16. Bernstein, J. M.: Biologic mediators of inflammation in middle ear effusion. Ann. Otol. Rhinol. Laryngol. 85(Suppl. 25):90-96, 1976.
17. Biles, R. E., Bufler, P. A., and O'Donnell, A. A.: Epidemiology of otitis media: A community study. Am. J. Public Health 70:593-598, 1980.

18. Birch, L., and Elbrond, O.: Daily impedance audiometric screening of children in a day-care institution: Changes through one month. Scand. Audiol. *14*:5-8, 1985.

19. Black, S., Shinefield, H., Fireman, B., et al.: Efficacy, safety and immunogenicity of heptavalent pneumococcal conjugate vaccine in children. Northern California Kaiser Permanente Vaccine Study Center Group. Pediatr. Infect. Dis. J. *19*:187-195, 2000.

20. Bland, R. D.: Otitis media in the first six weeks of life: Diagnosis, bacteriology and management. Pediatrics *49*:187-197, 1972.

21. Block, S. L., Hedrick, J., Harrison, C. J., et al.: Community-wide vaccination with the heptavalent pneumococcal conjugate vaccine significantly alters the microbiology of acute otitis media. Pediatr. Infect. Dis. J. *23*:829-833, 2004.

22. Bluestone, C. D.: Management of otitis media in infants and children: Current role of old and new antimicrobial agents. Pediatr. Infect. Dis. *7*:S129-S136, 1988.

23. Bluestone, C. D.: Prevention of meningitis: Cochlear implants and inner-ear abnormalities. Arch. Otolaryngol. Head Neck Surg. *129*:279-281, 2003.

24. Bluestone, C. D.: Eustacian Tube: Structure, Function, and Role in Otitis Media. Humilton, Ontario, B. C. Decker, 2005.

25. Bluestone, C. D., Klein, J. O.: Otitis Media in Infants and Children, 4th ed. Hamilton, Ontario, B. C. Decker, 2007.

26. Bluestone, C. D., Stool, S. E., Kenna, M. A. (eds.): Pediatric Otolaryngology. 3rd ed., Vol. 1. Philadelphia, W. B. Saunders, 2003, pp. 603-604.

27. Bodor, F. F.: Systemic antibiotics for treatment of the conjunctivitis-otitis media syndrome. Pediatr. Infect. Dis. *8*:287-290, 1989.

28. Bodor, F. F., Marchant, C. D., Shurin, P. A., et al.: Bacterial etiology of conjunctivitis-otitis media syndrome. Pediatrics *76*:26-28, 1985.

29. Brook, I.: Prevalence of beta-lactamase-producing bacteria in chronic suppurative otitis media. Am. J. Dis. Child. *139*:280-283, 1985.

30. Brooks, D. N.: Hearing screening: A comparative study of an impedance method and pure tone testing. Scand. Audiol. *2*:67-72, 1973.

31. Brown, D. T., Marsh, R. R., and Potsic, W. P.: Hearing loss induced by viscous fluids in the middle ear. Int. J. Pediatr. Otorhinolaryngol. *5*:39-46, 1983.

32. Capra, A. M., Lieu, T. A., Black, S. B., et al.: The costs of otitis media in a managed care population. Pediatr. Infect. Dis. J. *19*:354-355, 2000.

33. Carlin, S. A., Marchant, C. D., Shurin, P. A., et al.: Early recurrences of otitis media: Reinfection or relapse? J. Pediatr. *110*:20-25, 1987.

34. Casey, J. R., and Pichichero, M. E.: Changes in frequency and pathogens causing acute otitis media in 1995-2003. Pediatr. Infect. Dis. *23*:824-828, 2004.

35. Casselbrant, M. D., Brostoff, L. M., Cantekin, E. I., et al.: Otitis media with effusion in preschool children. Laryngoscope *95*:428-436, 1985.

36. Casselbrant, M. L., Kaleida, P. H., Rockette, H. E., et al.: Efficacy of antimicrobial prophylaxis and tympanostomy tube insertion for prevention of recurrent acute otitis media: Results of randomized clinical trial. Pediatr. Infect. Dis. J. *11*:278-286, 1992.

37. Casselbrant, M. L., Mandel, E. M., Fall, P. A., et al.: The heritability of otitis media: A twin and triplet study. J. A. M. A. *202*:2125-2130, 1999.

38. Chang, M. J., Rodriguez, W. J., and Mohla, C.: *Chlamydia trachomatis* in otitis media in children. Pediatr. Infect. Dis. *1*:95-97, 1982.

39. Chase, C.: Hearing loss and development: A neuropsychologic perspective. *In* Eavey, R. D., and Klein, J. O. (eds.): Hearing Loss in Childhood: A Primer. Report of the 102nd Ross Conference on Pediatric Research. Columbus, OH, Ross Laboratories, 1992, pp. 88-94.

40. Chonmaitree, T.: Acute otitis media is not a pure bacterial disease. Clin. Infect. Dis. *43*:1423-1425, 2006.

41. Chonmaitree, T., Howie, V. M., and Truant, A. L.: Presence of respiratory viruses in middle ear fluids and nasal wash specimens from children with acute otitis media. Pediatrics *77*:698-702, 1986.

42. Clements, D. A., Langdon, L., Bland, C., and Walter, E.: Influenza A vaccine decreased the incidence of otitis media in 6- to 30-month old children in day care. Arch. Pediatr. Adolesc. Med. *149*:1113-1117, 1997.

43. Coffey, J. D., Jr., Martin, A. D., and Booth, H. N.: *Neisseria catarrhalis* in exudative otitis media. Arch. Otolaryngol. *86*:403-406, 1967.

44. Combs, J. T.: Two useful tools for exploring the middle ear. Contemp. Pediatr. *10*:60-75, 1993.

45. Cooper, J. E., Jr., Gates, G. A., Owen, J. H., et al.: An abbreviated impedance bridge technique for school screening. J. Speech Hear. Disord. *40*:260-269, 1975.

46. Dagan, R.: Treatment of acute otitis media: Challenges in the era of antibiotic resistance. Vaccine *19*:S9-S16, 2001.

47. DeMaria, T. F., Prior, R. B., Briggs, B. R., et al.: Endotoxin in middle ear effusions from patients with chronic otitis media with effusion. *In* Lim, D. J., Bluestone, C. D., Klein, J. O., et al. (eds.): Recent Advances in Otitis Media with Effusion. Philadelphia, B. C. Decker, 1984, pp. 123-125.

48. Derkay, C. S., Bluestone, C. D., Thompson, A. E., et al.: Otitis media in the pediatric intensive care unit: A prospective study. Otolaryngol. Head Neck Surg. *100*:292-299, 1989.

49. Dowell, S. F., Butler, J. C., Giebink, G. S., et al.: Acute otitis media management and surveillance in an era of pneumococcal resistance: A report from the Drug-Resistant *Streptococcus pneumoniae* Therapeutic Working Group. Pediatr. Infect. Dis. J. *18*:1-9, 1999.

50. Dowell, S. F., Marcy, S. M., Phillips, W. R., et al.: Principles of judicious use of antimicrobial agents for pediatric upper respiratory tract infections. Pediatrics *101*(Suppl.):163-165, 1998.

51. Engel, J. A. M., Anteunis, L. J. C., Hendriks, J. J. T., et al.: Epidemiological aspects of otitis media with effusion in infancy. *In* Abstracts of the Sixth International Symposium on Recent Advances in Otitis Media. Fort Lauderdale, June 4-8, 1995, p. 15.

52. Eskola, J., Kilpi, T., Palmu, A., et al.: Efficacy of a pneumococcal conjugate vaccine against acute otitis media. N. Engl. J. Med. *344*:403-409, 2001.

53. Etzel, R. A., Pattishall, E. N., Haley, N. J., et al.: Passive smoking and middle ear effusion among children in day care. Pediatrics *90*:228-232, 1992.

54. Faden, H., Stanievich, J., Brodsky, L., et al.: Changes in nasopharyngeal flora during otitis media of childhood. Pediatr. Infect. Dis. J. *9*:623, 1990.

55. Fernandez, C., Lindsay, J. R., Moskowitz, M.: Some observations on the pathogenesis of middle ear cholesteatoma. Arch. Otolaryngol. *69*:537-546, 1959.

56. Fiellau-Nikolajsen, M.: Tympanometry in three-year-old children, II: Seasonal influence on tympanometric results in nonselected groups of three-year-old children. Scand. Audiol. *8*:181-185, 1979.

57. Finitzo, T., Friel-Patti, S., Chinn, K., et al.: Tympanometry and otoscopy prior to myringotomy: Issues in diagnosis of otitis media. Int. J. Pediatr. Otorhinolaryngol. *24*:101-110, 1992.

58. Fireman, B., Black, S. B., Shinefield, H. R., et al.: Impact of the pneumococcal conjugate vaccine on otitis media. Pediatr. Infect. Dis. J. *22*:10-16, 2003.

59. Fria, T. J., Cantekin, E. I., and Eichler, J. A.: Hearing acuity of children with otitis media with effusion. Arch. Otolaryngol. Head Neck Surg. *111*:10-16, 1985.

60. Friel-Patti, S., Finitzo-Hieber, T., Conti, G., et al.: Language delay in infants associated with middle ear disease and mild fluctuating hearing impairment. Pediatr. Infect. Dis. *1*:104-109, 1982.

61. Fry, J., Dillane, J. B., Jones, R. F. M., et al.: The outcome of acute otitis media. Br. J. Prev. Soc. Med. *23*:205-209, 1969.

62. Gannon, M. M., Haggard, M. P., Golding, J., et al.: Sleeping position: A new environmental risk factor for otitis media? *In* Abstracts of the Sixth International Symposium on Recent Advances in Otitis Media. Fort Lauderdale, June 4-8, 1995, p. 24.

63. Gates, G. A., Avery, C. A., Prihoda, T. A., et al.: Effectiveness of adenoidectomy and tympanostomy tubes in the treatment of chronic otitis media with effusion. N. Engl. J. Med. *317*:1444-1451, 1987.

64. Giebink, G. S., Juhn, S. K., Weber, M. L., et al.: The bacteriology and cytology of chronic otitis media with effusion. Pediatr. Infect. Dis. *1*:98-103, 1982.

65. Giebink, G. S., Mills, E. L., Huff, J. S., et al.: The microbiology of serous and mucoid otitis media. Pediatrics *63*:915-919, 1979.

66. Giebink, G. S., and Quie, P. G.: Otitis media: The spectrum of middle ear inflammation. Annu. Rev. Med. *29*:285-306, 1978.

67. Goldblatt, E. L., Dohar, J., Nozza, R. J., et al.: Topical ofloxacin versus systemic amoxicillin/clavulanate in purulent otorrhea in children with tympanostomy tubes. Int. J. Pediatr. Otorhinolaryngol. *46*:91-101, 1998.

68. Goo, Y. A., Hori, M. K., Voorhres, J. H., Jr., et al.: Failure to detect *Chlamydia pneumoniae* in ear fluids from children with otitis media. Pediatr. Infect. Dis. J. *14*:1000-1001, 1995.

69. Gravel, J. S., and Wallace, I. F.: Listening and language at 4 years of age: Effects of early otitis media. J. Speech Hear. Res. *35*:588-595, 1992.

70. Gray, B. M., Converse, G. M., III, and Dillon, H. C., Jr.: Serotypes of *Streptococcus pneumoniae* causing disease. J. Infect. Dis. *140*:979-983, 1979.

71. Hall-Stoodley, L., Hu, F. Z., Gieseke, A., et al.: Direct detection of bacterial biofilms on the middle-ear mucosa of children with chronic otitis media. J. A. M. A. *296*:202-211, 2006.

72. Hammaren-Malmi, S., Saxen, H., Tarkkanen, J., and Mattila, P. S.: Adenoidectomy does not significantly reduce the incidence of otitis media in conjunction with the insertion of tympanostomy tubes in children who are younger than 4 years: A randomized trial. Pediatrics *116*:185-189, 2005.

73. Hammerschlag, M. R., Hammerschlag, P. E., and Alexander, E. R.: The role of *Chlamydia trachomatis* in middle ear effusions in children. Pediatrics *66*:615-617, 1980.

74. Harding, A. L., Anderson, P., Howie. V. M., et al.: *Hemophilus influenzae* isolated from children with otitis media. *In* Sell, S. H., and Karzon, D. T. (eds.): *Hemophilus influenzae*. Nashville, Vanderbilt University Press, 1973.

75. Hathaway, T. J., Katz, H. P., Dershewitz, R. A., et al.: Acute otitis media: Who needs post-treatment follow-up? Pediatrics *94*:143, 1994.

76. Hausdorff, W. P., Yothers, G., Dagan, R., et al.: Multinational study of pneumococcal serotypes causing acute otitis media in children. Pediatr. Infect. Dis. J. *21*:1008-1016, 2002.

77. Hayden, G. F., and Schwartz, R. H.: Characteristics of earache among children with acute otitis media. Am. J. Dis. Child. *139*:721-723, 1985.

78. Henderson, F. W., Collier, A. M., Sanyal, M. A., et al.: A longitudinal study of respiratory viruses and bacteria in the etiology of acute otitis media with effusion. N. Engl. J. Med. *306*:1377-1383, 1982.

79. Hendley, J. O., Sande, M. A., Stewart, P. M., et al.: Spread of *Streptococcus pneumoniae* in families: Carriage rates and distribution of types. J. Infect. Dis. *132*:55-68, 1975.

80. Hesselvik, L.: Respiratory infections among children in day nurseries. Acta. Paediatr. Scand. *74*(Suppl.):33-103, 1949.

81. Howie, V. M.: Eradication of bacterial pathogens from middle ear infections. Clin. Infect. Dis. *14*(Suppl. 2):209-210, 1992.

82. Howie, V. M.: Otitis media. Pediatr. Rev. *18*:320-323, 1993.

83. Howie, V. M., and Ploussard, J. H.: The "in vivo" sensitivity test: Bacteriology of middle ear exudate during antimicrobial therapy in otitis media. Pediatrics *44*:940-944, 1969.

84. Howie, V. M., and Ploussard, J. H.: Bacterial etiology and antimicrobial treatment of exudative otitis media: Relation of antibiotic therapy to relapses. South. Med. J. *64*:233-239, 1971.

85. Howie, V. M., Ploussard, J. H., and Lester, R. L., Jr.: Otitis media: A clinical and bacteriological correlation. Pediatrics *45*:29-35, 1970.

86. Howie, V. M., Ploussard, J. H., and Sloyer, J.: The "otitis-prone" condition. Am. J. Dis. Child. *129*:676-678, 1975.

87. Howie, V. M., and Schwartz, R. H.: Acute otitis media: One year in general pediatric practice. Am. J. Dis. Child. *137*:155-158, 1983.

88. Ingvarsson, L., Lundgren, A., and Oloffson, B.: Epidemiology of acute otitis media in children: A cohort study in an urban population. *In* Lim, D. J., Bluestone, C. D., Klein, J. O., et al. (eds.): Recent Advances in Otitis Media with Effusion. Philadelphia, B. C. Decker, 1984, pp. 19-22.

89. Joloba, M. L., Windau, A., Bajaksouzian, S., et al.: Pneumococcal conjugate vaccine serotypes of *Streptococcus pneumoniae* isolates and the antimicrobial susceptibility of such isolates in children with otitis media. Clin. Infect. Dis. *33*:1489-1494, 2001.

90. Jung, T. T. K., Juhn, S. K., and Michael, A. F.: Localization of prostaglandin-forming cyclooxygenase in middle ear and external canal tissue. Otolaryngol. Head Neck Surg. *91*:187-192, 1983.

91. Jung, T. T. K., Smith, D. M., Juhn, S. K., et al.: Prostaglandins and otitis media: Studies in the chinchilla. Otolaryngol. Head Neck Surg. *88*:316-323, 1980.

92. Kamme, C., Ageberg, M., and Lundgren, K.: Distribution of *Diplococcus pneumoniae* types in acute otitis media in children and influence of the types on the clinical course in penicillin V therapy. Scand. J. Infect. Dis. *2*:183-190, 1970.

93. Kaplan, B., Wandstrat, T. L., and Cunningham, J. R.: Overall cost in the treatment of otitis media. Pediatr. Infect. Dis. J. *16*:S9-S11, 1997.

94. Kaplan, G. J., Fleshman, J. K., Bender, T. R., et al.: Long-term effects of otitis media: A 10-year cohort study of Alaskan Eskimo children. Pediatrics *52*:577-585, 1973.

95. Kaplan, S. L., Mason, E. O., Wald, E. R., et al.: Pneumococcal mastoiditis in children. Pediatrics *106*:695-699, 2000.

96. Kenna, M. A.: Intravenous antibiotics for otorrhea. *In* Alper, C. M., Bluestone, C. D., Casselbrant, M. L., et al. (eds.): Advanced Therapy of Otitis Media. Hamilton, Ontario, B. C. Decker, 2004.

97. Kilpi, T., Herva, E., Kaijalainen, T., et al.: Bacteriology of acute otitis media in a cohort of Finnish children followed for the first two years of life. Pediatr. Infect. Dis. J. *20*:654-662, 2001.

98. Kim, P. E., Musher, D. M., Glezen, W. P., et al.: Association of invasive pneumococcal disease with season, atmosphere conditions, air pollution and the isolation of respiratory viruses. Clin. Infect. Dis. *22*:100-106, 1996.

99. Klein, B. S., Dollete, F. R., and Yolken, R. H.: The role of respiratory syncytial virus and other viral pathogens in acute otitis media. J. Pediatr. *101*:16-20, 1982.

100. Klein, J. O.: Microbiologic efficacy of antibacterial drugs for acute otitis media. Pediatr. Infect. Dis. *12*:973-975, 1993.

101. Klein, J. O.: Preventing recurrent otitis: What role for antibiotics? Contemp. Pediatr. *11*:44-60, 1994.

102. Klein, J. O.: Review of consensus reports on management of acute otitis media. Pediatr. Infect. Dis. J. *18*:1150-1153, 1999.

103. Klein, J. O.: The burden of otitis media. Vaccine *19*:S2-S8, 2001.

104. Klein, J. O., and Teele, D. W.: Isolation of viruses and mycoplasmas from middle ear effusions: A review. Ann. Otol. Rhinol. Laryngol. *85*(Suppl. 25):140-144, 1976.

105. Kovatch, A. L., Wald, E. R., and Michaels, R. H.: β-Lactamase-producing *Branhamella catarrhalis* causing otitis media in children. J. Pediatr. *102*:261-263, 1983.

106. Lahikainen, E. A.: Clinico-bacteriologic studies on acute otitis media: Aspiration of tympanum as diagnostic and therapeutic method. Acta Otolaryngol. (Stockh.) (Suppl.) *107*:7-82, 1953.

107. Leinonen, M. K.: Detection of pneumococcal capsular polysaccharide antigens by latex agglutination, counterimmunoelectrophoresis, and radioimmunoassay in middle ear exudates in acute otitis media. J. Clin. Microbiol. *11*:135-140, 1980.

108. Lim, D. J., Bluestone, C. D., Saunders, W. H., et al.: Report of research committee on middle ear effusions. Ann. Otol. Rhinol. Laryngol. *85*(Suppl. 25):1-295, 1976.

109. Lim, D. J., and Saunders, W. H.: Acquired cholesteatoma: Light and electron microscopic observations. Ann. Otol. Rhinol. Laryngol. *81*:1-11, 1972.

110. Loda, F. A., Collier, A. M., Glezen, W. P., et al.: Occurrence of *Diplococcus pneumoniae* in the upper respiratory tract of children. J. Pediatr. *87*:1087-1093, 1975.

111. Long, S. S., Heuretig, F. M., Teter, M. J., et al.: Nasopharyngeal flora and acute otitis media. Infect. Immunol. *41*:987-991, 1983.

112. Lundman, L., Juhn, S. K., Bagger-Sjoback, D., et al.: Permeability of the normal round window membrane to *Haemophilus influenzae* type b endotoxin. Acta. Otolaryngol. *112*:524-529, 1992.

113. Luotonen, J., Herva, E., Karma, P., et al.: The bacteriology of acute otitis media in children with special reference to *Streptococcus pneumoniae* as studied by bacteriological and antigen detection methods. Scand. J. Infect. Dis. *113*:177-183, 1981.

114. Magliulo, G., Vingola, G. M., Petti, R., et al.: Acute mastoiditis in pediatric age group. Int. J. Otorhinolaryngol. *31*:147-151, 1995.

115. Makela, P. H., Leinonen, M., Pukander, J., et al.: A study of the pneumococcal vaccine in prevention of clinically acute attacks of recurrent otitis media. Rev. Infect. Dis. *3*(Suppl.):124-133, 1981.

116. Mandel, E. M., Casselbrant, M. L., Rockette, H. E., et al.: Efficacy of 20- vs. 10-day antimicrobial treatment for acute otitis media. Pediatrics *96*:5-13, 1995.

117. Mandel, E. M., Rockette, H. E., Bluestone, C. D., et al.: Myringotomy with and without tympanostomy tubes for chronic otitis media with effusion. Arch. Otolaryngol. Head Neck Surg. *115*:1217-1224, 1989.

118. Marchant, C. D., Shurin, P. A., Turczyk, V. A., et al.: Course and outcome of otitis media in early infancy: A prospective study. J. Pediatr. *104*:826-831, 1984.

119. Marchant, C. D., Shurin, P. A., Turcyzk, V. A., et al.: A randomized controlled trial of cefaclor compared with trimethoprim-sulfamethoxazole for treatment of acute otitis media. J. Pediatr. *105*:633-638, 1984.

120. McCandless, G. A., and Thomas, G. K.: Impedance audiometry as a screening procedure for middle ear disease. Trans. Am. Acad. Ophthalmol. Otolaryngol. *78*:98-102, 1974.

121. McEldowney, D., and Kessner, D. M.: Review of the literature: Epidemiology of otitis media. *In* Gloric, A., and Gerwin, K. S. (eds.): Otitis Media. Springfield, IL, Charles C Thomas, 1972.

122. McLinn, S. E.: Cefaclor in treatment of otitis media and pharyngitis in children. Am. J. Dis. Child. *134*:560-563, 1980.

123. Medical Research Council Working Party Report: Acute otitis media in general practice. Lancet *2*:510-514, 1957.

124. Meyerhoff, W. L., and Giebink, G. S.: Pathology and microbiology of otitis media. Laryngoscope *92*:273-277, 1982.

125. Mogi, G.: Secretory IgA and antibody activities in middle ear effusions. Ann Otol Rhinol Laryngol *85*(Suppl. 25):97-102, 1976.

126. Morris, P. S.: A systematic review of otitis media in Australian Aboriginal children. *In* Abstracts of the Sixth International Symposium on Recent Advances in Otitis Media. Fort Lauderdale, June 4-8, 1995, p. 11.

127. Mortimer, E. A., Jr., and Watterson, R. L., Jr.: A bacteriologic investigation of otitis media in infancy. Pediatrics *17*:359-366, 1956.

128. Murwitz, E. S., Gunn, W. J., Pinsky, P. F., et al.: Risk of respiratory illness associated with day-care attendance: A nationwide study. Pediatrics *87*:62-69, 1991.

129. Niemela, M., Uhari, M., and Mottonen, M.: A pacifier increases the risk of recurrent acute otitis media in children in day care centers. Pediatrics *96*:884-888, 1995.

130. Nozza, R. J., Bluestone, C. D., Kardatzke, D., et al.: Towards the validation of aural acoustic immittance measures for the diagnosis of middle ear effusion in children. Ear Hearing *13*:442-453, 1992.

131. Ogawa, H., Fujisawa, T., and Kazuyama, Y.: Isolation of *Chlamydia pneumoniae* from middle ear aspirates of otitis media with effusion: A case report. J. Infect. Dis. *162*:1000-1001, 1990.

132. Orange, M., and Gray, B. M.: Pneumococcal serotypes causing disease in children in Alabama. Pediatr. Infect. Dis. J. *12*:244-246, 1993.

133. Papastavros, T., Giamarellou, H., and Varlejides, S.: Role of aerobic and anaerobic microorganisms in chronic suppurative otitis media. Laryngoscope *96*:438-442, 1986.

134. Paradise, J. L., and Bluestone, C. D.: Early treatment of the universal otitis media of infants with cleft palate. Pediatrics *53*:48-54, 1974.

135. Paradise, J. L., Bluestone, C. D., Colburn, D. K., et al.: Adenoidectomy and tonsillectomy for recurrent acute otitis media: Parallel randomized and non-randomized trials. J. A. M. A. *263*:2066-2073, 1990.

136. Paradise, J. L., Bluestone, C. D., and Felder, H.: The universality of otitis media in 50 infants with cleft palate. Pediatrics *44*:35-42, 1969.

137. Paradise, J. L., Bluestone, C. D., Rogers, K. D., et al.: Efficacy of adenoidectomy for recurrent otitis media in children previously treated with tympanostomy tube placement: Results of parallel randomized and nonrandomized trials. J. A. M. A. *263*:2066-2073, 1990.

138. Paradise, J. L., Campbell, T. F., Dollaghan, C. A., et al.: Developmental outcomes after early or delayed insertion of tympanostomy tubes. N. Engl. J. Med. *353*:576-586, 2005.

139. Paradise, J. L., Elster, B. A., and Tan, L.: Evidence in infants with cleft palate that breast milk protects against otitis media. Pediatrics *94*:853, 1994.

140. Paradise, J. L., Feldman, H. M., Campbell, T. F., et al.: Effect of early or delayed insertion of tympanostomy tubes for persistent otitis media on developmental outcomes at the age of three years. N. Engl. J. Med. *334*:1179-1187, 2001.

141. Paradise, J. L., Feldman, H. M., Colborn, D. K., et al.: Parental stress and parent-rated child behavior in relation to otitis media in the first three years of life. Pediatrics *104*:1264-1273, 1999.

142. Paradise, J. L., Rockette, H. E., Colburn, D. K., et al.: Otitis media in 2253 Pittsburgh-area infants: Prevalence and risk factors during the first two years of life. Pediatrics *99*:318-333, 1997.

143. Paradise, J. L., Smith, C. G., and Bluestone, C. D.: Tympanometric detection of middle ear effusion in infants and young children. Pediatrics 56:198-210, 1976.
144. Pelton, S. I., Teele, D. W., Shurin, P. A., et al.: Disparate cultures of middle ear fluids in bacterial otitis media. Am. J. Dis. Child. 134:951-953, 1980.
145. Persico, M., Barker, G. A., and Mitchell, D. P.: Purulent otitis media: A "silent" source of sepsis in the pediatric intensive care unit. Otolaryngol. Head Neck Surg. 93:330, 1985.
146. Petersen, C. G., Oveson, T., and Petersen, C. B.: Acute mastoidectomy in a Danish county from 1977 to 1996 with focus on the bacteriology. Int. J. Pediatr. Otorhinolaryngol. 45:21-29, 1998.
147. Pitkaranta, A., Jero, J., Aruda, E., et al.: Polymerase chain reaction-based detection of rhinovirus, respiratory syncytial virus and coronavirus in otitis media with effusion. J. Pediatr. 133:390-394, 1998.
148. Pitkaranta, A., Virolainen, A., Jero, J., et al.: Detection of rhinovirus, respiratory syncytial virus and coronavirus infections in acute otitis media by reverse transcriptase polymerase chain reaction. Pediatrics 102:291-299, 1998.
149. Post, J. C., Preston, R. A., Aul, J. J., et al.: Molecular analysis of bacterial pathogens in otitis media with effusion. J. A. M. A. 273:1598-1604, 1995.
150. Poulsen, G., and Tos, M.: Screening tympanometry in newborn infants and during the first six months of life. Scand. Audiol. 7:159-166, 1978.
151. Prymula, R., Peeters, P., Chrobok, V., et al.: Pneumococcal capsular polysaccharides conjugated to protein D for prevention of acute otitis media caused by both Streptococcus pneumoniae and non-typable Haemophilus influenzae: A randomized double-blind efficacy study. Lancet 367:740-748, 2006.
152. Pukander, J., Luotonen, J., Sipila, M., et al.: Incidence of acute otitis media. Acta Otolaryngol. 93:447-453, 1982.
153. Reed, D., and Brody, J.: Otitis media in urban Alaska. Alaska Med. 8:64-67, 1966.
154. Renvall, U., and Holmquist, J.: Tympanometry revealing middle ear pathology. Ann. Otol. Rhinol. Laryngol. 85(Suppl. 25):209-215, 1976.
155. Riding, K. H., Bluestone, C. D., Michaels, R. H., et al.: Microbiology of recurrent and chronic otitis media with effusion. J. Pediatr. 93:739-743, 1978.
156. Rifkind, D. R., Chanock, R., Kranetz, H., et al.: Ear involvement (myringitis) and primary atypical pneumonia following inoculation of volunteers with Eaton agent. Am. Rev. Respir. Dis. 85:479-489, 1962.
157. Roland, P. S., Kreisler, L. S., Reese, B., et al.: Topical ciprofloxacin/dexamethasone otic suspension is superior to ofloxacin otic solution in the treatment of children with otorrhea through tympanostomy tubes. Pediatrics 114:127(e40), 2004.
158. Ruohola, A., Meurman, O., Nikkari, S., et al.: Microbiology of acute otitis media in children with tympanostomy tubes: Prevalence of bacteria and viruses. Clin. Infect. Dis. 43:1417-1422, 2006.
159. Ruuskanen, O., Arola, M., Heikkinen, T., et al.: Viruses in acute otitis media: Increasing evidence for clinical significance. Pediatr. Infect. Dis. J. 10:425, 1991.
160. Ruedi, L.: Cholesteatoma formation in the middle ear in animal experiments. Acta. Otolaryngol. 50:233-242, 1959.
161. Sanyal, M. A., Henderson, F. W., Stempel, E. C., et al.: Effect of upper respiratory tract infection on eustachian tube ventilatory function in the preschool child. J. Pediatr. 97:11-15, 1980.
162. Sarkkinen, H., Ruuskanen, I., Meurman, O., et al.: Identification of respiratory virus antigens in middle ear fluids of children with acute otitis media. J. Infect. Dis. 151:444-448, 1985.
163. Schaefer, O.: Otitis media and bottle feeding: An epidemiological study of infant feeding habits and incidence of recurrent and chronic middle ear disease in Canadian Eskimos. Can. J. Public Health 62:478-489, 1971.
164. Schneider, M. L.: Bacteriology of otorrhea from tympanostomy tubes. Arch. Otolaryngol. Head Neck Surg. 115:1225-1226, 1989.
165. Schwartz, B., Giebink, G. S., Henderson, F. W., et al.: Respiratory infections in day care. Pediatrics 84:1018-1020, 1994.
166. Schwartz, R. H., and Rodriguez, W. J.: Acute otitis media in children eight years old and older: A reappraisal of the role of Hemophilus influenzae. Am. J. Otolaryngol. 2:19-21, 1981.
167. Schwartz, R. H., Rodriguez, W. J., Brook, I., et al.: The febrile response in acute otitis media. J. A. M. A. 245:2057-2058, 1981.
168. Schwartz, R. H., Rodriguez, W. J., Khan, W. N., et al.: Acute purulent otitis media in children older than 5 years: Incidence of Hemophilus as a causative organism. J. A. M. A. 238:1032-1033, 1977.
169. Segal, N., Givon-Lavi, N., Leibovitz, E., et al.: Acute otitis media caused by Streptococcus pyogenes in children. Clin. Infect. Dis. 41:35-41, 2005.
170. Senturia, B. H.: Classification of middle ear effusion. Ann. Otol. Rhinol. Laryngol. 79:358-370, 1970.
171. Schappert, S. M.: Office visits for otitis media: United States, 1975-90. From Vital and Health Statistics of the Centers for Disease Control/National Center for Health Statistics 214:1-18, 1992.
172. Shurin, P. A., Howie, V. M., Pelton, S. I., et al.: Bacterial etiology of otitis media during the first 6 weeks of life. J. Pediatr. 92:893-896, 1978.
173. Shurin, P. A., Marchant, C. D., Kim, C. H., et al.: Emergence of beta-lactamase-producing strains of Branhamella catarrhalis as important agents of acute otitis media. Pediatr. Infect. Dis. 2:34-38, 1983.
174. Sipila, M., Karma, P., Pukander, J., et al.: The Bayesian approach to the evaluation of risk factors in acute and recurrent acute otitis media. Acta. Otolaryngol. 106:94-101, 1988.
175. Sipila, M., Pukander, J., and Karma, P.: Incidence of acute otitis media up to the age of 1½ years in urban infants. Acta Otolaryngol. 104:138-145, 1987.
176. Skolnik, P. R., Nadol, J. B., Jr., and Baker, A. S.: Tuberculosis of the middle ear: Review of the literature with an instructive case report. Rev. Infect. Dis. 8:403, 1986.
177. Skoner, D. P., Stillwagon, P. K., Casselbrandt, M. L., et al.: Inflammatory mediators in chronic otitis media with effusion. Arch. Otolaryngol. Head Neck Surg. 114:1131-1133, 1988.
178. Sloyer, J. L., Jr., Cate, C. C., Howie, V. M., et al.: Immune response to acute otitis media in children, II: Serum and middle ear fluid antibody in otitis media due to H. influenzae. J. Infect. Dis. 132:685-688, 1975.
179. Sloyer, J. L., Jr., Ploussard, J. H., and Howie, V. M.: Efficacy of pneumococcal polysaccharide vaccine in preventing acute otitis media in infants in Huntsville, Alabama. Rev. Infect. Dis. 3(Suppl.):119-123, 1981.
180. Spivey, G. H., and Hirschhorn, N.: A migrant study of adopted Apache children. Johns Hopkins Med. J. 140:43-46, 1977.
181. Sriwardhana, K. B., Howard, A. J., and Dunkin, K. T.: Bacteriology of otitis media with effusion. J. Laryngol. Otol. 103:253-256, 1989.
182. Stool, S. E., Berg, A. O., Berman, S., et al.: Otitis Media with Effusion in Young Children: Clinical Practice Guideline. Number 12. AHCPR Publication No. 94-0622. Rockville, MD, Agency for Health Care Policy and Research, Public Health Service, U.S. Department of Health and Human Services, July 1994.
183. Storgaard, M., Storgaoard, L., Jensen, J. S., et al.: Chlamydia pneumoniae in children with otitis media. Clin. Infect. Dis. 25:1090-1093, 1997.
184. Teele, D. W., Klein, J. O., Bratton, L., et al.; for the Greater Boston Collaborative Otitis Media Study Group: Use of pneumococcal vaccine for prevention of recurrent acute otitis media in infants in Boston. Rev. Infect. Dis. 3(Suppl.):113-118, 1981.
185. Teele, D. W., Klein, J. O., Chase, C., et al.: Otitis media in infancy and intellectual ability, school achievement, speech, and language at age 7 years. J. Infect. Dis. 162:685-694, 1990.
186. Teele, D. W., Klein, J. O., and Rosner, B. A.: Epidemiology of otitis media in children. Ann. Otol. Rhinol. Laryngol. 89(Suppl. 68):5-6, 1980.
187. Teele, D. W., Klein, J. O., Rosner, B., et al.: Middle ear disease and the practice of pediatrics. J. A. M. A. 249:1026-1029, 1983.
188. Teele, D. W., Klein, J. O., Rosner, B., et al.: Epidemiology of otitis media during the first seven years of life in children in greater Boston: A prospective cohort study. J. Infect. Dis. 160:83-94, 1989.
189. Tetzlaff, T. R., Ashworth, C., and Nelson, J. D.: Otitis media in children less than 12 weeks of age. Pediatrics 59:827-832, 1977.
190. Tipple, M. A., Beem, M. O., and Saxon, E. M.: Clinical characteristics of the afebrile pneumonia associated with Chlamydia trachomatis infection in infants less than 6 months of age. Pediatrics 63:192-197, 1979.
191. Tos, M., Poulson, G., and Hancke, A. B.: Screening tympanometry during the first year of life. Acta. Otolaryngol. 88:388-394, 1979.
192. U.S. Department of Health and Human Services: The health consequences of smoking: A report from the Surgeon General. Department of Health. Human Services Publication (DHS)84-50205. Rockville, MD, Office on Smoking and Health, 1984, p. 292.
193. van Buchem, F. L., Dunk, J. H. M., and van't Hof, M. A.: Therapy of acute otitis media: Myringotomy, antibiotics or neither? A double-blind study in children. Lancet 2:883-887, 1981.
194. van Buchem, F. L., Peeters, M. F., and van't Hof, M. A.: Acute otitis media: A new treatment strategy. B. M. J. 290:1033-1037, 1985.
195. Van Hare, G. F., Shurin, P. A., Marchant, C. D., et al.: Acute otitis media caused by Branhamella catarrhalis: Biology and therapy. Rev. Infect. Dis. 9:16-27, 1987.
196. Varsano, I. B., Volovitz, B. M., and Grossman, J. E.: Effect of naproxen, a prostaglandin inhibitor, on acute otitis media and persistence of middle ear effusion in children. Ann. Otol. Rhinol. Laryngol. 98:389-392, 1989.
197. Veltri, R. W., and Sprinkle, P. M.: Secretory otitis media: An immune complex disease. Ann. Otol. Rhinol. Laryngol. 85(Suppl. 25):135-319, 1976.
198. Wald, E. R., Dashefsky, B., Byers, C., et al.: Frequency and severity of infections in day care. J. Pediatr. 112:540-564, 1988.
199. Weiderhold, M. L., Zajtchuk, J. T., Vap, J. G., et al.: Hearing loss in relation to physical properties of middle ear effusions. Ann. Otol. Rhinol. Laryngol. 85:185-189, 1980.
200. Yaniv, E.: Tuberculous otitis: An underdiagnosed disease. Am. J. Otolaryngol. 8:356-360, 1987.

CHAPTER
20   MASTOIDITIS

Karen Lewis ◎ Nina L. Shapiro ◎ James D. Cherry

Mastoiditis, a suppurative infection of the mastoid air cells, is a potential complication of all cases of otitis media caused by the continuity of the mucoperiosteal lining of the mastoid with that of the middle ear.[20] The spectrum of disease in mastoiditis ranges from asymptomatic cases with apparent spontaneous resolution to progressive disease with life-threatening complications.[7] Since the advent of antibiotic therapy, mastoiditis is seen much less frequently, but the complications remain similar.[17,19,21,81] With mastoiditis occurring less commonly, physicians are less apt to consider the diagnosis, especially when the clinical picture has been masked by antibiotic therapy or when the process is chronic and of low grade. Appropriate antibiotic therapy, often accompanied by surgical drainage, can halt and prevent serious complications if mastoiditis is diagnosed early.

HISTORY

Before the advent of antibiotics, mastoiditis was a frequent complication of otitis media that could be treated only by expectant waiting or surgery.[32,36] When surgery was used, many patients with mastoiditis were cured by simple mastoid drainage alone, with a mortality rate quoted at 2 percent.[36] Intracranial complications of mastoiditis carried a very grave prognosis, however. In the pre-antibiotic era, between 1928 and 1933, 25 of every 1000 deaths at Los Angeles County Hospital in California were caused by intracranial complications of otitis media, such as meningitis, venous sinus thrombosis, and brain abscess. In contrast, between 1949 and 1954, only 2.5 per 1000 deaths at the same hospital were caused by complications of otitis or mastoiditis. The use of antibiotics in treating mastoiditis initially led to a marked decrease in the surgical approach to treatment of this illness.[7,81] The realization that infection can persist and that complications of mastoiditis can occur even while the patient is receiving antibiotic therapy has resulted in the present-day approach of combined antibiotics and surgery.*

BACTERIOLOGY

The bacteriology of acute mastoiditis differs from that of acute otitis media (AOM) (Table 20–1). For decades, the predominate bacterial cause of AOM was *Streptococcus pneumoniae*, with *Haemophilus influenzae* being the second most common isolate. Since the introduction of pneumococcal conjugate vaccine, nontypeable *H. influenzae* is the most frequent pathogen isolated (57%) in AOM, with *S. pneumoniae* being the second most common (31%), *Moraxella catarrhalis* the third most common (7-10%), and group A beta-hemolytic streptococcus the fourth most common (3-10%).[59] Studies on acute mastoiditis (defined as symptoms of <1 month's duration) show that *S. pneumoniae* is the most common isolate, with *Streptococcus pyogenes* and *Staphylococcus aureus* as the second and third most common isolates, respectively.[17,19,25,28,49,54,80]

H. influenzae has been isolated from the middle ear of patients with mastoiditis, but less often than one would expect, given its frequent recovery in AOM without mastoiditis. Gram-negative bacteria, enterococci, anaerobes, and *Mycobacterium tuberculosis*

also have been isolated occasionally in patients with acute mastoiditis. An increased incidence of penicillin-resistant *S. pneumoniae* infections has occurred, leading to a higher likelihood of mastoiditis being a complication of otitis media.[53,80] The percentage of pneumococcal mastoiditis caused by penicillin-resistant strains increased from 25 to 44 percent between 1994 and 1998, without an increase in the total number of cases of pneumococcal mastoiditis.[30] Although *M. catarrhalis* is a common cause of otitis media, it rarely is noted in association with mastoiditis.[35]

The bacteriologic spectrum of chronic mastoiditis differs from that of acute mastoiditis. Aerobic cultures of chronic mastoiditis and chronic otitis media show predominantly *S. aureus* and gram-negative bacilli, especially *Pseudomonas aeruginosa*.[4,13,61] In addition, a wide variety of anaerobic organisms can be isolated from an infected mastoid and middle ear.[4,13] Brook[4] studied the aerobic and anaerobic bacteriology of chronic otitis media (of ≥3 months' duration) in 24 children. Anaerobic isolates alone were found in 17 percent, aerobic organisms alone were found in 4 percent, and mixed aerobic and anaerobic infections were found in 79 percent. All cases had from two to seven different bacterial isolates. *Peptococcus* spp., *Actinomyces* spp., and *Bacteroides melaninogenicus* (*Prevotella melaninogenica*) were the most commonly isolated anaerobic organisms. Seventeen patients were infected with β-lactamase–producing organisms (i.e., *S. aureus* or *P. melaninogenica*, *Bacteroides fragilis*, or other *Bacteroides* spp. that were resistant to ampicillin).

M. tuberculosis currently is an uncommon cause of mastoiditis in the United States but continues to be a cause of chronically draining ears in lower socioeconomic groups and immigrants from endemic areas.[5,45,47] Case reports of mastoiditis implicate such organisms as nontuberculous mycobacteria,[52] *Aspergillus fumigatus*,[23] *Paragonimus*-like trematodes,[55] *Nocardia asteroides*,[43] *Actinomyces* spp.,[67] *Blastomyces dermatitidis*,[30] and *Histoplasma capsulatum*.[43] *Pneumocystis carinii* otitis media and mastoiditis have occurred as the first manifestation of acquired immunodeficiency syndrome.[18]

ANATOMY AND PATHOPHYSIOLOGY

The mastoid process comprises the posterior part of the temporal bone and, as such, is adjacent to many important structures. Within the mastoid is an interconnecting system of air cells divided by bony septa that drain superiorly into the middle ear via a narrow aditus.[7,20] Only the superior portion of the mastoid airspace, the antrum, is present at birth; pneumatization of the mastoid starts soon after birth and usually is completed by the time the child is 2 years of age.[2,36] Structures lying anteromedial to the mastoid process include the middle ear and ossicles, the facial nerve, the posterior bony wall of the external auditory canal, the jugular vein, and the internal carotid artery. Posteromedially, the mastoid borders the posterior cranial fossa and the sigmoid sinus. Superiorly, the mastoid borders the middle cranial fossa. Medially, the mastoid cortex encases the cochlea and semicircular canals. The soft tissues and muscles of the lateral neck are located inferiorly. Any or all of these adjacent structures can be affected by extension of a suppurative process in the mastoid.

A certain amount of mastoid inflammation accompanies all cases of otitis media because the mastoid airspaces are continuous with the middle ear cavity and both are lined by a continuous mucoperiosteum.[2,20] The first stage of an ear and mastoid

---

*See references 21, 22, 25, 39, 44, 49, 54, 68, 79.

TABLE 20–1 Summary of Bacterial Isolates from the Middle Ear, Subperiosteal Abscess, or Mastoid of Children with Mastoiditis in Seven Studies

Isolates	Acute Mastoiditis						Chronic Mastoiditis
	Ginsburg et al., 1955-1979[19]	Hoppe et al., 1975-1992[28]	Ogle and Lauer, 1973-1984[54]	Nadal et al., 1971-1988[49]	Ghaffar et al., 1983-1999[17]	Zapalac et al., 1993-2000[80]	Brook, 1976-1980[4]
Streptococcus pneumoniae	14	13	5	9	20*	15†	1
Streptococcus pyogenes	8	4	3	4	4	10	2
Staphylococcus aureus	8	2	1	4	5	3	8
Staphylococcus epidermidis	1	2	2	6	7	12	—
Other aerobic gram-positive cocci	3	—	1	2	2	—	4
Haemophilus influenzae	1	—	2	1	—	1	—
Pseudomonas aeruginosa	2	—	—	3	5	—	7
Other aerobic gram-negative rods	1‡	1	1	—	4§	—	7**
Anaerobic cocci	1	—	—	1	—	—	23
Anaerobic gram-positive bacilli	—	—	—	1	—	—	14
Anaerobic gram-negative bacilli	1	—	1	—	—	—	24
Other	1¶	—	4	—	—	10¶¶	—
Total patients with cultures	49	28	30	54	49	64	24

*Four of 12 tested isolates were penicillin resistant.
†Nine of 15 isolates were penicillin resistant.
‡Citrobacter spp.
§Escherichia coli, Klebsiella oxytoca, Proteus mirabilis, Serratia marcescens.
¶Mycobacterium tuberculosis.
¶¶Pseudomonas, Prevotella, and Bacillus spp.
**Polymicrobial—unspecified.
**E. coli (5), Klebsiella pneumoniae (2).

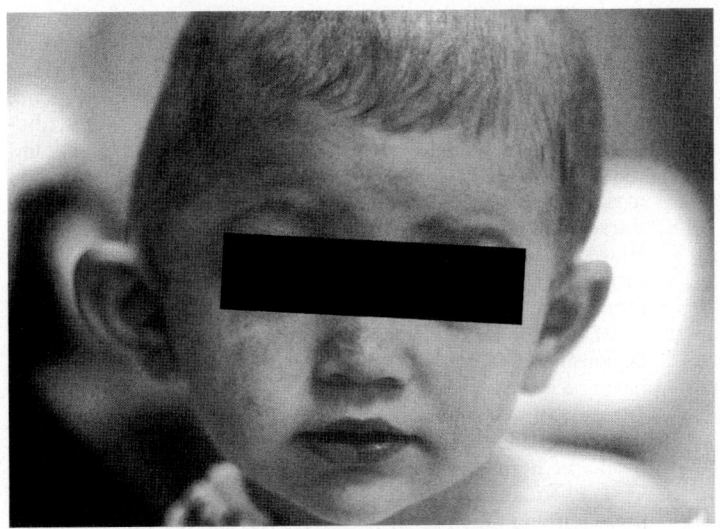

Figure 20–1 An 18-month-old child with right-sided mastoiditis and proptotic right auricle.

infection is associated with hyperemia of the middle ear and the mastoid air cell mucosa. If the infection persists, an exudative stage develops, with serum, fibrin, polymorphonuclear cells, and red blood cells accumulating in the middle ear and mastoid. The accumulation of purulent exudate increases the middle ear pressure, eventually resulting in perforation of the tympanic membrane, followed by drainage of mucopurulent matter from the middle ear and mastoid air cells. Some children also have such marked mucoperiosteal swelling that the drainage of pus from the mastoid is blocked. The pus under pressure creates an environment of local acidosis, hypoxia, and ischemia, causing decalcification and resorption of the bony septa. The term *coalescent mastoiditis* is applied to this process because, with the destruction of the bony septa, the mastoid air cells coalesce into large cavities. Osteomyelitis of the adjacent bone may develop, with subsequent bony erosion and eventual extension of the infection into surrounding structures.[2,20]

Congenital cholesteatomas usually manifest as a "squamous pearl" in the anterosuperior quadrant of the middle ear, abutting the tympanic membrane. They may be associated with recurrent otitis media.[42] Acquired cholesteatomas often are a result of chronic infections and tympanic membrane perforation. The perforation allows for squamous material from the external auditory canal to enter the middle ear space.[57] This tissue contains osteolytic enzymes, leading to bony erosion or mastoid air cell obstruction.[50] Cholesteatomas also may cause slow, insidious erosion of underlying bone, predisposing the patient to extramastoid spread of infection months or years later.[20,61]

CLINICAL PRESENTATION

The classic presentation of acute mastoiditis is a febrile child with ear pain, postauricular swelling, and postauricular tenderness developing days to weeks after the beginning of development of AOM (Fig. 20–1).[17,19,49,54,80] If antibiotics were used to treat AOM, the child may have seemed to improve, only to become ill again while still receiving therapy or after the antibiotics were stopped;

conversely, the child may not have responded to the antibiotics at all. Examination of the tympanic membrane in acute mastoiditis usually shows that it is abnormal.[19,25,49] Early in the course of illness, periosteal inflammation produces swelling and tenderness and sometimes redness over the mastoid process.[2,19] Palpable postauricular fluctuance occurs later, when pus from the mastoid air cells breaks through the underlying bony cortex and forms a subperiosteal abscess.[24] In children older than 1 year of age, the most common area where fluctuance is felt lies behind the ear, where it pushes the earlobe up and out; however, in children younger than 1 year, the fluctuance often may occur above the ear, pushing the pinna down and out.[19]

Chronic mastoiditis is a much more indolent disease process than is acute mastoiditis. It develops when long-standing middle ear disease, usually having a duration of months to years, has been present.[61] Fever and postauricular swelling may or may not be present. Persistent or intermittent drainage of mucopurulent matter from a previously perforated eardrum suggests chronic mastoiditis. Hearing loss and ear pain also may accompany chronic mastoiditis.[61] All these symptoms can be mild enough to be ignored until serious intracranial suppuration occurs. Persistent ear drainage, persistent ear pain, or an otitis media nonresponsive to antibiotics should prompt a search for mastoiditis.

COMPLICATIONS

Complications of mastoiditis include subperiosteal abscess,[24] Bezold abscess,[15,63] facial nerve paralysis,[71] meningitis,[7,19] brain abscess,[7,19] cerebellar abscess,[2] epidural abscess,[2] subdural empyema,[3] labyrinthitis,[20] venous sinus thrombophlebitis,[12,33,56,73] bacteremia,[7,44] benign intracranial hypertension,[3] osteomyelitis of the temporal bone with occasional extension to adjacent bones,[2,20] hearing loss,[58] septic pulmonary emboli,[29] and cerebrospinal fluid otorrhea.[20] Subperiosteal abscesses appear as a postauricular fluctuant mass that obscures the postauricular sulcus. They occur when pus in the mastoid breaks through the bony cortex or extends along vascular channels and dissects under the overlying periosteum.[24]

A Bezold abscess develops when a mastoid infection erodes through the bony cortex of the inferior aspect of the mastoid tip and dissects down the tissue planes to form a deep neck abscess. Fluctuance over the mastoid is not felt. Rather, swelling and tenderness are present below the mastoid process and under the sternocleidomastoid muscle.[15]

The facial nerve runs close to the mastoid and the middle ear, rendering it vulnerable to injury when extension of mastoid or middle ear infection occurs.[20] Pressure on and inflammation of the facial nerve from symptomatic or asymptomatic mastoiditis can lead to transient or permanent facial nerve paralysis that usually is unilateral, although bilateral facial palsy from mastoiditis can occur.[2,71]

Because the temporal bone that houses the mastoid air cells constitutes the floor of the middle and posterior cranial fossae, bony erosion from osteomyelitis, preexisting bony defects, or spread of infection along vascular channels can allow for intracranial spread of mastoid infections into the middle and posterior cranial fossae. The infection may remain confined to the extradural space as an extradural abscess, or it may penetrate the dura and produce a subdural empyema, a brain abscess, a cerebellar abscess, or meningitis.[2,20]

Invasion of infection into the bony labyrinth through the oval or round window triggers a labyrinthitis. Initial tinnitus, hearing loss, nausea, and dizziness progress to severe vertigo, ear pain, vomiting, nystagmus, and difficulties with balance.[20]

Intracranial venous sinus thrombophlebitis is a rare but potentially fatal complication of mastoiditis.[2,20,33,56,69,73] The lateral aspect of the sigmoid sinus is formed by the temporal bone. Venous sinus thrombophlebitis results when an underlying mastoiditis extends through the temporal bone in close proximity to the lateral or sigmoid venous sinus. A perisinus abscess initially is formed, followed by formation of a mural thrombus in the sinus wall. The thrombus eventually may occlude the entire sinus, or it may suppurate and spread along the sinus, resulting in septicemia, increased intracranial pressure, septic emboli, and extension of infection to other intracranial structures.[12,16] The classic findings of a septic thrombosis of the lateral sinus are spiking fevers, shaking chills, and tenderness along the jugular vein associated with acute or chronic otitis. A palpable "cord" at the jugular vein (indicating a jugular vein thrombus) also may be present. When only a perisinus abscess is present, or if the patient is being treated partially with antibiotics, the only symptoms may be a low-grade fever and headache.[22,69]

Benign intracranial hypertension can be seen in association with lateral sinus obstruction secondary to mastoiditis and is termed *otitic hydrocephalus*. Rarely, otitic hydrocephalus can be seen with mastoiditis in the absence of lateral sinus thrombosis. The decreased venous drainage caused by the venous sinus obstruction results in increased intracranial pressure, headache, papilledema, and sixth nerve palsy without enlarged ventricles or a space-occupying lesion.[20,22]

Permanent conductive hearing loss occurs when the middle ear mastoid infection is severe enough to damage or destroy the ossicles. Tuberculous mastoiditis classically manifests with marked conductive hearing loss that often is irreversible.[40]

Osteomyelitis secondary to mastoiditis can spread to adjacent bones. Involvement of the petrous portion of the temporal bone produces a syndrome, described by Gradenigo in 1907, with a triad of abducens paralysis or paresis, severe pain in the distribution of the trigeminal nerve, and suppurative otitis media; additional cranial nerve deficits also may occur.[6,39] Antibiotics may mask the classic signs of petrositis and allow progression to severe intracranial complications, such as meningitis and epidural abscess. Petrositis may be suspected only when antibiotic and surgical management for mastoiditis fails to control chronic ear drainage.[20]

M. tuberculosis mastoiditis is an uncommon finding but should be considered in children who have chronic ear discharge despite having received antibiotic therapy.[40,45] Children can go for months or years with chronic draining ears before the diagnosis of tuberculous mastoiditis is considered.[5,47] Children from lower socioeconomic homes, immigrants from endemic areas, and children with tuberculosis contacts in the family are at risk. The classic presentation in the pre-antibiotic era was an afebrile young child with painless persistent watery ear drainage, an enlarged preauricular lymph node, a history of tuberculosis contact, and often facial nerve paralysis.[64,72]

Tuberculous mastoiditis not always is painless.[76] Sometimes, the diagnosis initially is suspected only when a mastoidectomy wound does not heal.[38,61] Early in the course of the disease, physical examination may reveal small yellow spots (caseating granulomas) on a thickened and hyperemic tympanic membrane. These spots coalesce early and produce tympanic membrane perforations.[38] The discharge through these perforations initially is watery, but later it becomes purulent.[37] Pale, avascular granulation tissue is abundant throughout the middle ear and mastoid and often is seen in the external auditory canal and around the tympanic membrane perforation.[5,64,76] Preauricular and postauricular nontender, enlarged lymph nodes may be present,[37,43] and early and severe hearing loss is characteristic.[76] Often, there is evidence of tuberculosis elsewhere in the body.[76] A 5–tuberculin unit purified protein derivative skin test usually, but not always, is positive.[47]

DIFFERENTIAL DIAGNOSIS

Postauricular swelling, a chronically draining ear, or radiographic evidence of mastoid abnormalities also can appear in other disease entities. Postauricular lymphadenopathy can occur secondary to a scalp infection, causing postauricular swelling. The swelling would be discrete, would not displace the pinna, and would not obliterate the postauricular sulcus.[19] Severe otitis externa may lead to periauricular cellulitis, with postauricular swelling, erythema, and tenderness.[27] Mumps can cause parotid swelling, pushing the earlobe up and out, but the swelling is over the parotid gland, rather than located postauricularly. Histiocytosis,[41] acute lymphocytic leukemia,[48] acute myelogenous leukemia,[70] Burkitt lymphoma,[74] aneurysmal bone cysts,[10] and other benign and malignant tumors of the mastoid bone[8] also can manifest with symptoms clinically suggestive of mastoiditis. Kawasaki disease may mimic acute mastoiditis with postauricular lymph node swelling and ear pain.[62] Children with severe and recurrent ear infections may have an underlying congenital or acquired immunodeficiency.

SPECIFIC DIAGNOSIS

The diagnosis of mastoiditis can be made on clinical grounds alone when a child has an acute episode of fever, otitis media, and posterior auricular tenderness and fluctuance. Temporal bone computed tomography (CT) always is recommended to confirm the diagnosis. Mastoiditis is much less likely when swelling and tenderness over the mastoid process are absent, such as when an infection has been masked by antibiotic treatment or when it has extended to an area other than over the mastoid process. Mastoiditis needs to be considered in all cases of otitis media not responding to antibiotics and in all intracranial suppurative diseases that do not have an apparent focus.

Obtaining an aspirate from the middle ear is an important part of properly diagnosing and managing mastoiditis. Gram stains of aspirates from the middle ear are quite accurate and, as such, can help in the initial selection of antibiotic therapy for chronic mastoiditis. Brook[4] found that in 24 children with tympanocentesis, half of the Gram stains showed a complete correlation with subsequent culture results and the other half showed a partial correlation (one bacterial species was not seen). Leukocytes were seen on all the Gram stains. In addition, cultures from the middle ear accurately reflect mastoid disease.[19,44]

Ginsburg and associates[19] compared the results of cultures of middle ear aspirates and mastoid cultures in 16 patients with acute mastoiditis and found that the same bacterial species was isolated from both sites. A sterile aspiration through an intact tympanic membrane gives the most accurate culture information. If the tympanic membrane is perforated, the purulent drainage may be contaminated by colonizing ear canal flora. An aspirate for culture generally should be obtained from the ear drainage, preferably from as close to the perforation as possible. Aspiration of postauricular fluctuance also is useful in identifying the responsible organisms.[24,54] In addition, specimens should be obtained directly from the mastoid at surgery. All of them should be sent for aerobic and anaerobic cultures with proper anaerobic transport technique. If the child has had a chronic ear infection, or if the child is in a high-risk population for acquiring tuberculosis, mycobacterial stains and cultures also should be obtained and a purified protein derivative should be placed.

A lumbar puncture should be performed if the clinical presentation suggests meningeal irritation. A CT scan should be obtained before performing the lumbar puncture if papilledema or a suggestion of focal intracranial extension is present. Lymphocytosis of the cerebrospinal fluid suggests a parameningeal

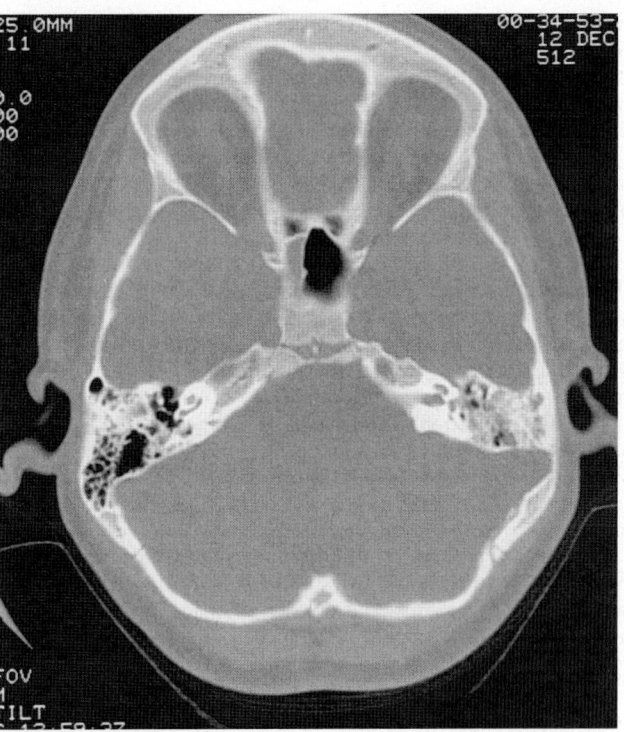

Figure 20–2 Computed tomography scan of the head of a 12-year-old boy with left lateral sinus thrombosis and increased intracranial pressure complicating left mastoiditis. The left mastoid air cells are opacified with marked loss of the fine bony septa, in contrast to the right mastoid air cells.

focus of infection. An immunologic evaluation should be considered if a child has had recurrent episodes of otitis media leading to mastoiditis.

Peripheral white blood cell counts in mastoiditis may be normal or elevated, often with an increase in band-form neutrophils.[25,49] The erythrocyte sedimentation rate often is elevated in acute mastoiditis, but it usually is normal in chronic mastoiditis.[58]

Mastoiditis often can be diagnosed on clinical findings alone. When a patient is not improving on medical therapy, radiologic imaging of the temporal bone is needed. Changes in the temporal bone are seen best by CT scan.[66] Early in the course of mastoiditis, nonspecific clouding of the middle ear and mastoid is seen. With time, necrosis and coalescence of the bony septa occur. Other CT findings in mastoiditis include hypoaeration of the mastoid and adjacent bony destruction. Figure 20–2 shows a CT scan of a child with unilateral mastoiditis complicated by lateral sinus thrombosis and elevated intracranial pressure. Magnetic resonance imaging is valuable to search for suppurative intracranial complications of mastoiditis.[65,66] In addition, sometimes magnetic resonance angiography or venography (or both) is indicated to diagnose sigmoid sinus thrombosis.[8]

TREATMENT

The pediatrician and the otolaryngologist should work together in the management of a child with suspected or proven mastoiditis because all children with mastoid infections are potential surgical candidates. Some kind of drainage for the middle ear should be provided early in the course of therapy for therapeutic and diagnostic purposes. The drainage could consist of tympanocentesis with subsequent tympanostomy tubes or a myringotomy.[19,25,49,54,80] A specific etiologic diagnosis is more important today than in the past because of the increasing incidence of infections caused by penicillin-resistant pneumococci and methicillin-resistant, coagulase-positive staphylococci.[1,14,26,31,51,60,75]

If the patient has an acute onset of posterior auricular swelling and tenderness with minimal or no posterior auricular fluctuance and no signs of intracranial complications, he or she is likely to respond to antibiotic therapy alone.[25,49,54,79]

Indications for surgical intervention include postauricular fluctuance; a history of chronic ear drainage with postauricular swelling or bony changes on radiographs; facial nerve palsy; nausea, vomiting, and vertigo suggestive of labyrinthitis; meningitis; brain abscess; venous sinus thrombosis with or without intracranial hypertension; epidural or subdural empyema; and petrositis. In addition, if the patient initially is treated medically, a mastoidectomy is indicated if progression of postauricular swelling or fluctuance or persistence of fever, ear pain, or purulent ear drainage occurs while the child is receiving parenteral antibiotics.[17,20,25,49,54,68]

All surgical treatment should include culture of the middle ear or mastoid, either by tympanocentesis or during surgery. If a notable middle ear effusion is present, drainage of the middle ear and equalization of pressure should be done by placement of a tympanostomy tube or a wide circumferential myringotomy.

If postauricular subperiosteal abscess or a Bezold abscess is present, incision and drainage need to be performed. Incision and drainage should be combined with myringotomy and tube placement. In addition, consideration should be given to performing a simple mastoidectomy to remove any diseased mastoid cells or inflammatory mucosa. When a mastoidectomy is done, a biopsy specimen of the inflammatory tissue should be sent to the laboratory for examination to exclude lesions such as eosinophilic granuloma or rhabdomyosarcoma.

For intracranial complications (e.g., subdural or cerebral abscess), a mastoidectomy needs to be performed. Draining the mastoid at the same time as draining the intracranial abscess has been done safely in the same operative setting.[34]

If a patient is found to have a cholesteatoma, a modified radical mastoidectomy, with complete removal of the cholesteatoma, should be performed. A child with a cholesteatoma is likely to need a second-look operation at a later date to monitor for recurrent disease.

Ototopical drops should be included in the postoperative care. Ciprofloxacin ear drops seem to be less toxic than aminoglycoside drops.[11,77,78] All children with mastoiditis should have audiograms performed to help distinguish a purely conductive loss (indicative of middle ear involvement) from a sensorineural loss (a sign of inner ear involvement).

The initial choice of antibiotics for mastoiditis must be made empirically, based on the knowledge of the most likely organisms. Because acute mastoiditis most often is caused by S. pneumoniae or S. pyogenes and less often by S. aureus and H. influenzae, oxacillin (150 mg/kg/day divided every 6 hours) and cefotaxime (200 mg/kg/day divided every 6 hours) can be recommended. In cases of severe illness or when possible central nervous system involvement is present, initial administration of vancomycin (60 mg/kg/day intravenously every 6 hours) instead of oxacillin often is desirable because of the possibility that resistant pneumococci or staphylococci are present.

In cases of chronic mastoiditis in which symptoms have been present for longer than 1 month, S. aureus, gram-negative bacilli (especially P. aeruginosa), and anaerobes are seen more frequently. A broad-spectrum combination of intravenous antibiotics is recommended: an aminoglycoside, such as gentamicin (7.5 mg/kg/day divided every 8 hours), for gram-negative bacillary coverage and a semisynthetic penicillin, such as ticarcillin-clavulanate or piperacillin-tazobactam (200 to 300 mg/kg/day divided every 6

hours). These semisynthetic penicillins are synergistic with gentamicin against P. aeruginosa, and they are effective against anaerobes and methicillin-sensitive S. aureus. The antibiotics can be adjusted based on the identification and sensitivities of the organisms isolated from the pretherapy cultures. For an intracranial extension of infection caused by P. aeruginosa, better penetration of cerebrospinal fluid can be obtained with an antipseudomonal cephalosporin such as cefepime (150 mg/kg/day divided every 8 hours) rather than ticarcillin-clavulanate or piperacillin-tazobactam.

The approach to antibiotic therapy for acute and chronic bacterial mastoiditis should conform to the principles of therapy for osteomyelitis. Treatment is begun with intravenous antibiotics. Intracranial extension of infection or mastoiditis with an organism for which no effective oral antibiotic (e.g., P. aeruginosa) exists requires long-term intravenous antibiotic therapy. Otherwise, after the patient has responded well clinically, high-dose oral antibiotic therapy can be considered (e.g., two or three times the normal dose of an oral cephalosporin).[46] Total duration of therapy should be for a minimum of 3 weeks and possibly longer, depending on the severity of illness, the causative organism, and the clinical response. Optimally, the causative organisms and their sensitivities should be known, and an oral agent to which the organisms are sensitive is needed. An oral regimen should not be attempted if vomiting or diarrhea is present because either one would prevent adequate oral absorption. Following the sedimentation rate may be helpful in monitoring treatment. The oral antibiotic should be given strictly every 6 hours rather than four times a day to ensure around-the-clock therapeutic drug levels.

No study has examined the optimal antituberculous chemotherapy for mastoiditis. If M. tuberculosis mastoiditis is probable or diagnosed, antituberculous chemotherapy should be started as recommended for tuberculosis of the bone (see Chapter 107).

If fever, purulent ear drainage, or ear pain persists despite antibiotic therapy and surgery, further evaluation is needed to search for either resistant organisms or a persistent site of infection that requires additional surgical drainage. In addition, a slow response to therapy should raise the possibility of an underlying immunodeficiency.

PROGNOSIS

The prognosis of mastoiditis depends on the extent of the infection and the causative organism. Mastoiditis that is treated adequately early in the course of illness before the onset of intracranial extension has a very good prognosis. Facial nerve paralysis is reversible early on,[64,71] and benign intracranial hypertension resolves with treatment of the mastoiditis.[20] Permanent neurologic deficits and death may occur if mastoiditis extends to cause meningitis, brain abscesses, epidural abscess, subdural empyema, or venous sinus thrombophlebitis. Symptoms of mastoiditis may recur if antibiotic therapy is of insufficient duration or if surgical débridement of an infected bone or of an infected cholesteatoma is inadequate. Sensorineural and conductive hearing deficits are reversible early on in mastoiditis; however, chronic infection may produce irreversible hearing loss.

PREVENTION

Early adequate antibiotic treatment of otitis media reduces significantly a child's risk for developing mastoiditis. In addition, rapid treatment of known mastoiditis along with early investigation of persistent ear drainage, persistent ear pain, or an otitis media that is not responding to antibiotic management decreases the risk for developing suppurative complications associated with mastoiditis.

REFERENCES

1. Antonelli, P. J., Dhanani, N., Giannoni, C. M., et al.: Impact of resistant pneumococcus on rates of acute mastoiditis. Otolaryngol. Head Neck Surg. *121*:190-194, 1999.
2. Bluestone, C. D., and Klein, J. O.: Otitis Media in Infants and Children. Philadelphia, W. B. Saunders, 1988, pp. 233-244.
3. Bluestone, C. D., and Klein, J. O.: Intracranial suppurative complications of otitis media and mastoiditis. *In* Bluestone, C. D., Stool, S. E., and Kenna, M. A. (eds.): Pediatric Otolaryngology. 3rd ed. Philadelphia, W. B. Saunders, 1996, pp. 636-648.
4. Brook, I.: Aerobic and anaerobic bacteriology of chronic mastoiditis in children. Am. J. Dis. Child. *135*:478-479, 1981.
5. Buchanan, G., and Rainer, E. H.: Tuberculous mastoiditis. J. Laryngol. Otol. *102*:440-446, 1988.
6. Burson, B. J., Pretorius, P. M., and Ramsden, J. D.: Gradenigo's syndrome: Successful conservative treatment in adult and paediatric patients. J. Laryngol. Otol. *119*:325-329, 2005.
7. Davison, F. W.: Otitis media: Then and now. Laryngoscope *65*:142-151, 1955.
8. Davison, S. P., Facer, G. W., McGough, P. F., et al.: Use of magnetic resonance imaging and magnetic resonance angiography in diagnosis of sigmoid sinus thrombosis. Ear Nose Throat J. 76:436-441, 1997.
9. De, S. K., and Dey, D. D.: Tumours of the mastoid temporal bone. J. Laryngol. Otol. *102*:582-587, 1988.
10. deVries, E. J., Kamerer, D. B., and Rafalko, D.: Aneurysmal bone cyst masquerading as acute mastoiditis. Otolaryngol. Head Neck Surg. *100*:613-616, 1989.
11. Dohar, J. E., Alper, C. M., Rose, E. A. M., et al.: Treatment of chronic suppurative otitis media with topical ciprofloxacin. Ann. Otol. Rhinol. Laryngol. *107*:865-871, 1998.
12. Doyle, K. J., and Jackler, R. K.: Otogenic cavernous sinus thrombosis. Otolaryngol. Head Neck Surg. *104*:873-877, 1991.
13. Finegold, S. M.: Anaerobic infections in otolaryngology. Ann. Otol. Rhinol. Laryngol. *90*(Suppl. 84):13-16, 1981.
14. Fridkin, S. K., Hageman, J. C., Morrison, M., et al.: Methicillin-resistant *Staphylococcus aureus* in disease in three communities. N. Engl. J. Med. *352*:1436-1444, 2005.
15. Gaffney, R. J., O'Dwyer, T. P., and Maguire, A. J.: Bezold's abscess. J. Laryngol. Otol. *105*:765-766, 1991.
16. Garcia, R. D. J., Baker, A. S., Cunningham, M. J., et al.: Lateral sinus thrombosis associated with otitis media and mastoiditis in children. Pediatr. Infect. Dis. J. *14*:617-623, 1995.
17. Ghaffar, F. A., Wordemann, M., and McCracken, G. H. Jr.: Acute mastoiditis in children: A seventeen-year experience in Dallas, Texas. Pediatr. Infect. Dis. J. *20*:376-380, 2001.
18. Gherman, C. R., Ward, R. R., and Bassis, M. L.: *Pneumocystis carinii* otitis media and mastoiditis as the initial manifestation of the acquired immunodeficiency syndrome. Am. J. Med. *85*:250-252, 1988.
19. Ginsburg, C. M., Rudoy, R., and Nelson, J. D.: Acute mastoiditis in infants and children. Clin. Pediatr. *19*:549-553, 1980.
20. Glasscock, M. E., and Shambaugh, G. E., Jr. (eds.): Surgery of the Ear. Philadelphia, W. B. Saunders, 1990.
21. Goldstein N. A., Casselbrant, M. L., Bluestone, C. D., et al.: Intratemporal complications of acute otitis media in infants and children. Otolaryngol. Head Neck Surg. *119*:444-454, 1998.
22. Goycoolea, M. V., and Jung, T. T. K.: Complications of suppurative otitis media. *In* Paparella, M. M., Shumrick, D. A., Gluckman, J. L., and Meyerhoff, W. L. (eds): Otolaryngology. 3rd ed. Philadelphia, W. B. Saunders, 1991, pp. 1381-1404.
23. Hall, P. J.: *Aspergillus* mastoiditis. Otolaryngol. Head Neck Surg. *108*:167-170, 1993.
24. Hawkins, D. B., and Dru, D.: Mastoid subperiosteal abscess. Arch. Otolaryngol. *109*:369-371, 1983.
25. Hawkins, D. B., Dru, D., House, J. W., et al.: Acute mastoiditis in children: A review of 54 cases. Laryngoscope 93:568-572, 1983.
26. Hofmann, J., Cetron, M. S., Farley, M. M., et al.: The prevalence of drug-resistant *Streptococcus pneumoniae* in Atlanta. N. Engl. J. Med. *333*:481-486, 1995.
27. Hopkin, R. J., Bergeson, P. S., Pinckard, K. C., et al.: Otitis externa posing as mastoiditis. Arch. Pediatr. Adolesc. Med. *148*:1346-1349, 1994.
28. Hoppe, J. E., Koster, S., Bootz, F., et al.: Acute mastoiditis: Relevant once again. Infection 22:178-182, 1994.
29. Hughes, C. E., Spear, R. K., Shinabarger, C. E., et al.: Septic pulmonary emboli complicating mastoiditis: Lemierre's syndrome revisited. Clin. Infect. Dis. *18*:633-635, 1994.
30. Istorico, L. J., Sanders, M., Jacobs, R. F., et al.: Otitis media due to blastomycosis: Report of two cases. Clin. Infect. Dis. *14*:355-358, 1992.
31. Kaplan, S. L., Mason, E. O., Wald, E. R., et al.: Pneumococcal mastoiditis in children. Pediatrics *106*:695-699, 2000.
32. Keeler, J. C.: Modern Otology. Philadelphia, F. A. Davis, 1930, pp. 417-481.
33. Koitschiev, A., Simon, C., Lowenheim, H., et al.: Delayed otogenic hydrocephalus after acute otitis media in pediatric patients: The changing presentation of a serious otologic complication. Acta Oto-Laryngol. *125*:1230-1235, 2005.
34. Kurien, M., Job, A., Mathew, J., et al.: Otogenic intracranial abscess: Concurrent craniotomy and mastoidectomy—changing trends in a developing country. Arch. Otolaryngol. Head Neck Surg. *124*:1352-1356, 1998.
35. Leskinene, K., and Jero, J.: Acute mastoiditis caused by *Moraxella catarrhalis*. Int. J. Pediatr. Otorhinol. *67*:31-33, 2003.
36. Levine, M.: Practical Otology. Philadelphia, Lea & Febiger, 1938.
37. Lincoln, E. M., and Sewell, E. M.: Tuberculosis in Children. New York, McGraw-Hill, 1963.
38. Lucente, F. E., Tobias, G. W., Parisier, S. C., et al.: Tuberculous otitis media. Laryngoscope *88*:1107-1116, 1978.
39. Lutter, S. A., Kerschner, J. E., and Chusid, M. J.: Gradenigo syndrome, a rare but serious complication of otitis media. Pediatr. Emerg. Care *21*:384-386, 2005.
40. MacAdam, A., and Rubio, T.: Tuberculosis otomastoiditis. Am. J. Dis. Child. *131*:152-156, 1977.
41. McCaffrey, T. V., and McDonald, T. J.: Histiocytosis X of the ear and temporal bone: Review of 22 cases. Laryngoscope *89*:1735-1742, 1979.
42. McGill, T. J., Merchant, S., Healy, G. B., et al.: Congenital cholesteatoma of the middle ear in children: A clinical and histopathological report. Laryngoscope *101*:606-613, 1991.
43. Meyerhoff, W. L.: Granulomas and other specific diseases of the ear and temporal bone. *In* Paparella, M. M., and Shumrick, D. A. (eds.): Otolaryngology. 2nd ed. Philadelphia, W. B. Saunders, 1980, pp. 1548- 1575.
44. Moloy, P. J.: Anaerobic mastoiditis: A report of two cases with complications. Laryngoscope *92*:1311-1315, 1982.
45. Mongkolrattanothai, K., Oran, R., Redleaf, M., et al.: Tuberculous otitis media with mastoiditis and central nervous system involvement. Pediatr. Infect. Dis. J. *22*:453-456, 2003.
46. Moore, J. A., Wei, J. L., Smith, H. J., et al.: Treatment of pediatric suppurative mastoiditis: Is peripherally inserted central catheter (PICC) antibiotic therapy necessary? Otolaryngol. Head Neck Surg. *135*:106-110, 2006.
47. Mumtaz, M. A., Schwartz, R. H., Grundfast, K. M., et al.: Tuberculosis of the middle ear and mastoid. Pediatr. Infect. Dis. *2*:234-236, 1983.
48. Nabors, M. W., Narayan, R. K., and Poplack, D. G.: Intracranial and otological presentation of acute lymphocytic leukemia. Neurosurgery *17*:309-312, 1985.
49. Nadal, D., Herrmann, P., Baumann, A., et al.: Acute mastoiditis: Clinical, microbiological, and therapeutic aspects. Eur. J. Pediatr. *149*:560-564, 1990.
50. Nadol, J. B.: Chronic otitis media. *In* Nadol, J. B., and Schuknecht, H. F. (eds.): Surgery of the Ear and Temporal Bone. New York, Raven Press, 1993, pp. 155-170.
51. Nelson, C. T., Mason, E. O., Jr., and Kaplan, S. L.: Activity of oral antibiotics in middle ear and sinus infections caused by penicillin-resistant *Streptococcus pneumoniae*: Implications for treatment. Pediatr. Infect. Dis. J. *13*:585-589, 1994.
52. Nylen, O., Alestig, K., Fasth, A., et al.: Infections of the ear with nontuberculous mycobacteria in three children. Pediatr. Infect. Dis. J. *13*:653-656, 1994.
53. Oestreicher-Kedem, Y., Raveh, E., Kornreich, L., et al.: Complications of mastoiditis in children at the onset of a new millennium. Ann. Otol. Rhinol. Laryngol. *114*:147-152, 2005.
54. Ogle, J. W., and Lauer, B. A.: Acute mastoiditis. Am. J. Dis. Child. *140*:1178-1182, 1986.
55. Oyediran, A. B. O. O., Fajemisin, A. A., Abioye, A. A., et al.: Infection of the mastoid bone with a *Paragonimus*-like trematode. Am. J. Trop. Med. Hyg. *24*:268-273, 1975.
56. Ozdemir, D., Cakmakci, H., Ikiz, A. O., et al.: Sigmoid sinus thrombosis following mastoiditis, early diagnosis enhances good prognosis. Pediatr. Emerg. Care *21*:606-609, 2005.
57. Palva, A., Karma, P., and Karja, J.: Cholesteatoma in children. Arch. Otolaryngol. Head Neck Surg. *103*:74-77, 1977.
58. Palva, T., and Pulkkinen, K.: Mastoiditis. J. Laryngol. Otol. *72*:573-588, 1959.
59. Pichichero, M. E.: Pathogen shifts and changing cure rates for otitis media and tonsillopharyngitis. Clin. Pediatr. *45*:493-502, 2006.
60. Pikis, A., Akram, S., Donkersloot, J. A., et al.: Penicillin-resistant pneumococci from pediatric patients in the Washington, D.C., area. Arch. Pediatr. Adolesc. Med. *149*:30-35, 1995.
61. Procter, B.: Chronic otitis media and mastoiditis. *In* Paparella, M. M., and Shumrick, D. A. (eds.): Otolaryngology. 2nd ed. Philadelphia, W. B. Saunders, 1980, pp. 1455-1489.
62. Puczynski, M. S., Stankiewicz, J. A., and Ow, P. E.: Mucocutaneous lymph node syndrome mimicking acute coalescent mastoiditis. Am. J. Otol. 7:71-73, 1986.
63. Schondorf, H. J., Roth, B., and Streppel, M.: Bezold's abscess following chronic mastoiditis in a newborn. Ann. Otol. Rhinol. Laryngol. *113*:843-845, 2004.
64. Singh, B.: Role of surgery in tuberculous mastoiditis. J. Laryngol. Otol. *105*:907-915, 1991.
65. Swartz, J. D.: Temporal bone inflammatory disease. *In* Som, P. M., and Curtin, H. D. (eds.): Head and Neck Imaging. 3rd ed. St. Louis, Mosby, 1996, pp. 1391-1431.
66. Swartz, J. D., and Harnsberger, H. R.: Imaging of the Temporal Bone. 2nd ed. New York, Thieme Medical Publishers, 1992, pp. 105-153.
67. Tarabichi, M., and Schloss, M.: Actinomycosis otomastoiditis. Arch. Otolaryngol. Head Neck Surg. *119*:561-562, 1993.
68. Taylor, M. F., and Berkowitz, R. G.: Indications for mastoidectomy in acute mastoiditis in children. Ann. Otol. Rhinol. Laryngol. *113*:69-72, 2004.
69. Teichgraeber, J. F., Per-Lee, J. H., and Turner, J. S.: Lateral sinus thrombosis: A modern perspective. Laryngoscope *92*:744-751, 1982.
70. Todd, N. W., and Bowman, C. A.: Acute myelogenous leukemia presenting as atypical mastoiditis with facial paralysis. Int. J. Pediatr. Otorhinolaryngol. 7:173-177, 1984.

71. Tovi, F., and Leiberman, A.: Silent mastoiditis and bilateral simultaneous facial palsy. Int. J. Pediatr. Otorhinolaryngol. 5:303-307, 1983.
72. Turner, A. L.: Tuberculosis of the middle ear cleft in children. J. Laryngol. Rhinol. Otol. 30:209-247, 1915.
73. Van den Bosch, M. A. A. J., Vos, J. A., De Letter, M. A. C. J., et al.: MRI findings in a child with sigmoid sinus thrombosis following mastoiditis. Pediatr. Radiol. 33:877-879, 2003.
74. Welling, D. B., and McCabe, B. F.: American Burkitt's lymphoma of the mastoid. Laryngoscope 97:1038-1042, 1987.
75. Whitney, C. G., Farley, M. M., Hadler, J., et al.: Increasing prevalence of multidrug-resistant *Streptococcus pneumoniae* in the United States. N. Engl. J. Med. 343:1917-1924, 2000.
76. Windle-Taylor, P. C., and Bailey, C. M.: Tuberculous otitis media: A series of 22 patients. Laryngoscope 90:1039-1044, 1980.
77. Wintermeyer, S. M., Hart, M. C., and Nahata, M.C.: Efficacy of ototopical ciprofloxacin in pediatric patients with otorrhea. Otolaryngol. Head Neck Surg. 116:450-453, 1997.
78. Wong, D. L. H., and Rutka, J. A.: Do aminoglycoside otic preparations cause ototoxicity in the presence of tympanic membrane perforations? Otolaryngol. Head Neck Surg. 116:404-410, 1997.
79. Zanetti, D., and Nassif, N.: Indications for surgery in acute mastoiditis and their complications in children. Int. J. Pediatr. Otorhinol. 70:1175-1182, 2006.
80. Zapalac, J. S., Billings, K. R., Schwade, N. D., et al.: Suppurative complications of acute otitis media in the era of antibiotic resistance. Otolaryngol. Head Neck Surg. 128:660-663, 2006.
81. Zoller, H.: Acute mastoiditis and its complications: A changing trend. South. Med. J. 65:477-480, 1972.

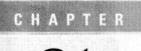

CHAPTER 21

EPIGLOTTITIS (SUPRAGLOTTITIS)

James D. Cherry

Epiglottitis (supraglottitis) is an illness characterized by inflammation and edema of the epiglottis and frequently also of the arytenoepiglottic folds and ventricular bands at the base of the epiglottis.[43] This disorder usually is caused by *Haemophilus influenzae* type b (Hib), and it mainly is a disease of children. The illness is characterized by rapid onset and progression, and without treatment, death caused by obstruction of the airway occurs. Epiglottitis in children is a pediatric otolaryngologic emergency.

HISTORY

The early history of epiglottitis is obscure, probably because of the importance of diphtheritic croup.[44] In 1887, Baron[9] described in detail a 30-year-old woman with epiglottitis who recovered after treatment with hot poultices and steam with tincture of benzoin. In 1900, Theisen[200] described three cases in the United States. Not until the early 1940s did acute epiglottitis become recognized as a definite clinical entity caused by Hib.[3,18,183] In 1948, Rabe,[155] in a study of 347 children with "infectious croup," presented evidence for the division of the clinical illness into three etiologic categories: diphtheritic croup, viral croup, and Hib croup (acute epiglottitis). Since the early 1990s, a dramatic decrease in the number of cases of epiglottitis has occurred in developed countries because of the widespread use of Hib conjugate vaccines.[4,34,64,70,78,80,126,136,138,152,209,215,227]

EPIDEMIOLOGY

In the pre-vaccine era, the epidemiology of invasive Hib disease varied markedly among different population groups.[215,216] Epiglottitis also differed by population group, but this variation was not related necessarily to the rate of overall Hib invasive disease in the population. For example, among Alaskan Eskimos and Navajo Native Americans, whose risk for acquiring invasive Hib disease was 4 to 10 times that of most other American populations, epiglottitis was not recognized among 295 patients with invasive Hib illness.[49,216]

Of Hib invasive disease, the percentage of cases of epiglottitis varied markedly among different localities. For example, in Israel, only 0.3 percent of invasive Hib infections were epiglottitis, whereas in Ireland, Wales, northeast England, Sydney (Australia), and Denmark, the percentage of epiglottitis cases varied

between 16 and 32 percent.[50,68,91,109,135,154] In Minnesota and Dallas County, Texas, only 6 and 3 percent, respectively, of invasive Hib infections were epiglottitis.[142] In contrast with these findings in the United States, Europe, and Australia, the most common manifestation of invasive Hib infection in Sweden was epiglottitis.[46,206] In Sweden, the incidence of epiglottitis in children 14 years of age or younger in 1981 to 1983 was 10 per 100,000 per year. The annual incidence in Minnesota and Dallas County, Texas, in children 5 years of age or younger in 1982 to 1984 was 5.4 and 4.4 cases, respectively, per 100,000 per year.[143]

In children in the United States in the pre-vaccine era, the peak occurrence of epiglottitis was during the third year of life, and 72 percent of all cases occurred in children 1 to 5 years of age.[13,16,20,47,65,97] The disease occurred more commonly in boys than in girls; in 8 studies with 611 cases, 58 percent of cases were in boys.[13,16-18,20,47,65,97,141]

In specific geographic areas, marked differences in the yearly percentage of cases of epiglottitis occurred, but no intercity, national, or international cycles of illness were demonstrated.[13,16,47,65,97,141] Seasonal prevalence varied by locality but was not marked. The greatest number of cases in three studies occurred in the winter and spring,[20,97,141] whereas Baxter[16] observed more cases during the summer and in November, and Cohen and Chai[47] found no seasonal pattern.

Epiglottitis is a disease that occurs most commonly in temperate climates.[67,100] In several U.S. military hospitals, a wide geographic variation in incidence was noted; no cases were found among 4625 admissions at Gorgas Hospital in Panama, whereas 1 of 600 admissions to Elmendorf Hospital in Alaska was for epiglottitis.[13] In the past, acute epiglottis had not been reported in either Taiwan or Hong Kong.[96]

Epiglottitis also occurs in adults but less commonly than in children.[71,133,195,207] Annual rates in Rhode Island, Denmark, Finland, and northern California were 1.0, 0.9, 0.2, and 1.8 per 100,000, respectively. In both Ireland and Israel, rates of reported epiglottitis in adults appear to be increasing.[19,84] Whether these increases are true increases or are the result of increased awareness is not apparent.

In the present Hib conjugate vaccine era, the incidence of epiglottitis has fallen dramatically in all countries employing routine immunization, as has the incidence of all invasive disease caused by *H. influenzae*.[4,34,64,73,80,126,136,138,152,209,215,227] In northern Finland, the incidence in children 4 years of age or younger fell from 7.6 per 100,000 before 1988 to 0 per 100,000 after 1988.[4] In Sweden, in the 10-year period from 1986 to 1996, the rate of epiglottitis in children younger than 14 years fell from 8.2 per 100,000 to less than 1 per 100,000.[74] At the Children's Hospital of Philadelphia, the average annual incidence of epiglottitis declined from 10.9 per 10,000 admissions before 1990 to 1.8 per 10,000 admissions from 1990 through 1992.[80] In this study, investigators also noted that the median age of patients increased from 35.5 months before 1990 to 80.5 months in the post-1989 period.

In recent years, an increase in incidence of invasive Hib disease, including acute epiglottitis, has been reported in England.[136] Many of the cases have occurred in children who had received Hib conjugate vaccine at 2, 3, and 4 months of age but not a booster dose in the second year of life.

ETIOLOGY

Acute supraglottitis in children in the pre-vaccine era almost always was caused by Hib. Lemierre and colleagues[120] and Sinclair[183] first called attention to "Hib laryngitis." This variant of laryngitis was characterized by marked swelling of the epiglottis and arytenoid regions, high fever, and shock. All 10 children described by Sinclair[183] had Hib bacteremia. Rabe[155] recognized a form of "croup" associated with epiglottitis and Hib bacteremia; 25 of 28 blood cultures (89%) yielded this organism. Table 21–1 summarizes 34 pediatric series from the pre-vaccine era with reported blood culture data. In children, 1570 of 2279 (69%) had blood cultures performed; Hib was isolated from 1191 of 1570 (76%).

As the clinical entity gained recognition, the frequency with which blood cultures were obtained and the yield of Hib increased. During 17 years of experience with epiglottitis in Denver, Colorado,[141] researchers found that 40 percent of all blood cultures yielded Hib; however, 70 percent yielded this organism during the last 5 years of the study.

Supraglottitis with bacteremia caused by other organisms in children rarely occurs, but cases have been noted more frequently during the last decade. The following pathogens have been impli-

TABLE 21–1　Etiology of Epiglottitis in Children

Author and Year of Study	Number of Patients	Number of Patients Having Blood Cultures (%)		Patients with Blood Cultures Yielding *Haemophilus influenzae* Type b (%)		Other Bacteria Isolated from Blood (%)*
Sinclair,[183] 1941	10	10	(100)	10	(100)	None
Rabe,[155] 1948	28	28	(100)	25	(89)	None
Berenberg and Kevy,[19] 1958	42	16	(38)	11	(69)	*Streptococcus pneumoniae*
Vetto,[213] 1960	37	2	(5)	2	(100)	None
Margolis et al.,[131] 1972	15	15	(100)	13	(87)	None
Johnson et al.,[97] 1974	55	33	(60)	20	(61)	None
Bass et al.,[13] 1974	97	6	(6)	1	(17)	*Staphylococcus aureus*
Milko et al.,[139] 1974	41	33	(80)	33	(100)	None
Branefors-Helander and Jeppsson,[30] 1975	15	14	(93)	13	(93)	None
Margolis et al.,[130] 1975	32	32	(100)	30	(94)	None
Battaglia and Lockhart,[14] 1975	40	40	(100)	13	(33)	None
Rapkin,[157] 1975	4	4	(100)	4	(100)	None
Smith and Ingram,[189] 1975	8	8	(100)	8	(100)	None
Benjamin and O'Reilly,[18] 1976	61	51	(84)	36	(71)	None
Molteni,[141] 1976	72	29	(40)	10	(34)	None
Breivik and Klaastad,[31] 1978	27	9	(33)	5	(56)	*S. aureus*
Cohen and Chai,[47] 1978	147	49	(33)	28	(57)	*H. influenzae*, not type b
Faden,[65] 1979	48	48	(100)	48	(100)	*S. pneumoniae*[†]
Bottenfield et al.,[28] 1980	24	22	(92)	18	(82)	None
Briggs and Altenau,[32] 1980	53	44	(83)	30	(68)	*H. influenzae* type a *H. influenzae*, nontypable *Haemophilus parainfluenzae*
Baugh and Baker,[15] 1982	24	22	(92)	18	(82)	None
Broughton and Warren,[35] 1984	24	19	(80)	19	(100)	None
Drake-Lee et al.,[60] 1984	25	19	(76)	19	(100)	None
Sly et al.,[188] 1984	171	89	(52)	71	(80)	None
Claesson et al.,[46] 1984	211	85	(40)	74	(81)	*H. parainfluenzae*
McGregor et al.,[134] 1985	31	31	(100)	19	(61)	None
Vernon and Sarnaik,[212] 1986	60	56	(93)	54	(96)	None
Gerber and Pfenninger,[75] 1986	137	126	(92)	83	(66)	None
Hodge and Ganzel,[90] 1987	25	24	(96)	14	(58)	None
Blackstock et al.,[24] 1987	14	12	(86)	10	(83)	None
Butt et al.,[38] 1988	349	234	(67)	187	(80)	None
Brilli et al.,[33] 1989	41	41	(100)	39	(95)	None
Losek et al.,[127] 1990	169	169	(100)[§]	131	(78)	*Bacillus* species *S. pneumoniae* *S. aureus*[‡]
Gorelick and Baker,[80] 1994	142	142	(100)	95	(67)	None
Totals	2,279	1,570	(69)	1,191	(76)	12 (1)

*Each organism represents one patient.
[†]One patient had S. pneumoniae and H. influenzae type b bacteremia.
[‡]One patient had S. aureus and H. influenzae type b bacteremia.
[§]Only patients with blood cultured and no prior antibiotic treatment reported.

cated in this regard: *Streptococcus pneumoniae*[20,65,127]; *Staphylococcus aureus* (including one case in a 5-day-old baby)[11,31,61,127]; *Haemophilus parainfluenzae*[32,204]; group A,[17,112,186,222] group B,[125,228] group C,[8,176] and group G[92] streptococci; *Pseudomonas aeruginosa*[113] (in a patient with severe combined immunodeficiency syndrome); untypeable and *H. influenzae* type a[32]; and *Bacillus* spp.[127] *Candida tropicalis* was isolated from the blood of a 3½-year-old girl with supraglottitis who had been the recent recipient of an autologous bone marrow transplant.[214]

Candida albicans was noted in a case in a newborn whose mother had vaginal candidiasis and in a 6-year-old boy with chronic mucocutaneous candidiasis.[2] *Candida* spp. epiglottitis was noted in two children infected with human immunodeficiency virus (HIV),[145,181] and *C. albicans* epiglottitis was observed recently in a 2-year-old girl who was immunocompromised as a result of receiving chemotherapy for a primitive neuroectodermal tumor.[132]

The possibility that supraglottitis could be caused by a virus has been noted: a 16-month-old child with type 1 herpes simplex virus stomatitis complicated by stridor and respiratory distress had an epiglottis and arytenoepiglottic folds that were edematous and covered with vesicular lesions resembling those in the oral mucosa.[26] An 18-year-old girl had supraglottitis that also was caused by herpes simplex virus.[138] In addition, parainfluenza type 3 and influenza type B viruses were isolated from the nasopharynx of two children with supraglottic inflammation.[83] *Haemophilus paraphrophilus*[101] was recovered from the epiglottic surface of a single patient, as was *Moraxella catarrhalis* in another patient.[211]

In adults, Hib also has been the major cause of epiglottitis, but other organisms occur more commonly in adults than in children.[9,29,30,43,45,51,66,71,72,76,77,86,88,94,95,99,106,108,133,146,147,162,175,182,186,193,195,205,206] In 1992, Daum and Smith[54] reviewed 474 published cases of epiglottitis in adults, 293 of whom had blood cultures performed; 79 of those cultures (27%) yielded *H. influenzae*. Of these positive cultures, 43 were Hib; 35 isolates were not typed, and one isolate was not Hib. Trollfors and associates[206] in Sweden found that blood cultures were obtained from 185 of 356 (52%) adult patients, and *H. influenzae* was isolated from 53 percent of them. Of these, 53 were Hib, and the type of the remaining 45 was not known.

S. pneumoniae was reported to be isolated from the blood of 18 adults with supraglottitis, 10 of whom were receiving immunosuppressive therapy or were infected with HIV-1,[23,30,93,104,106,118,155,163,164,179] and *H. parainfluenzae* was isolated from the blood of 5 patients.[45,69,128,172,218] In Denmark between 1995 and 2002, *H. influenzae* type f was recovered from 13 cases of epiglottitis in adults.[36] Numerous other infectious agents have been implicated in case reports of adults with supraglottitis.[27,29,56,72,76,77,94,95,98,103,124,129,137,144,146,147,159,160,165,175,185,192,230] These agents include *Pasteurella multocida*, *Kingella kingae*, *Klebsiella pneumoniae*, group A and B streptococci, *Bacteroides* spp., *Fusobacterium necrophorum*, *Vibrio vulnificus*, *Serratia marcescens*, *S. aureus*, *Neisseria meningitidis*, *Aspergillus flavus*, and herpes simplex virus. Epiglottitis has been reported as a complication of infectious mononucleosis caused by Epstein-Barr virus infection.[39]

Epiglottitis also can result from noninfectious causes. Hot foods and water can cause thermal epiglottitis, as can poisoning with corrosive agents including cocaine alkaloid.[16,105,110,115] Hereditary angioedema may manifest with findings typical of epiglottitis.[149]

ANATOMY

The thin, elastic, leaflike epiglottic cartilage is attached to the anterior surface of the thyroid cartilage by the thyroepiglottic ligament (Fig. 21–1). The hyoepiglottic ligament also provides support and anchors the epiglottis to the hyoid bone. The superior aspect of the epiglottis arches slightly posteriorly. Stratified squamous epithelium covers the anterior surface of the epiglottis and the superior third of the posterior portion; respiratory epithelium covers the remaining posterior surface. The stratified squamous epithelium is loosely adherent and creates a large potential space for the accumulation of inflammatory cells and edema fluid.

The arytenoepiglottic folds arise from the epiglottis and terminate posteriorly near the paired arytenoid cartilages. These structures commonly are involved in the supraglottic infection and occasionally are the site of serious disease without epiglottitis per se.[16] Immediately anterior to the epiglottis are the valleculae epiglotticae, where saliva pools before deglutition.

PATHOPHYSIOLOGY

Supraglottic cellulitis with marked edema involving the epiglottis, arytenoepiglottic folds, ventricular bands, and arytenoids is the hallmark of this illness. As the edema increases, the epiglottis curls posteriorly and inferiorly. Inspiration tends to draw the inflamed supraglottic ring into the laryngeal inlet, whereas expiration is unopposed.[177] This "ball-valve" mechanism is thought to produce slight hypoxia without hypercapnia.[167] Diffuse infiltration with polymorphonuclear leukocytes, hemorrhage, edema, and fibrin deposition can be seen microscopically; this infiltration can progress to microabscesses, with Hib occasionally seen in the tissue.[100,162] Frank abscess formation has been documented in adults.[19,124,129,160,165,192,219,225] Infection of the supraglottic larynx

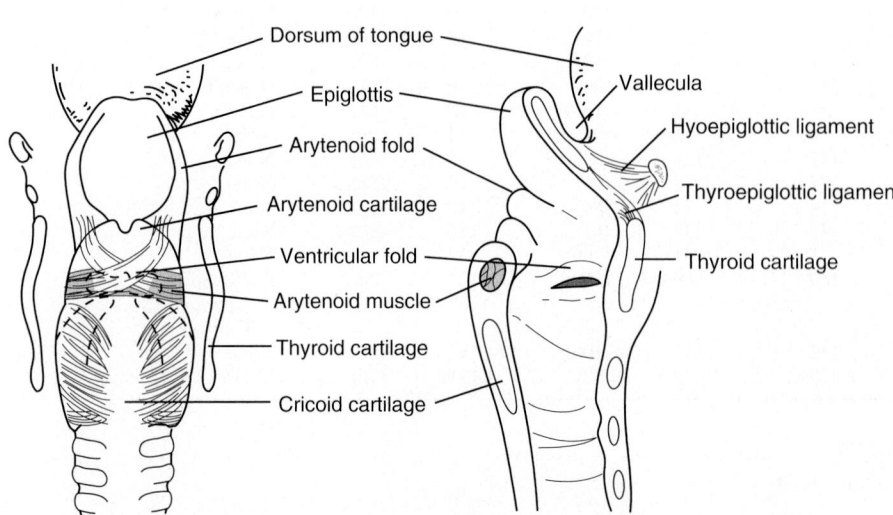

Figure 21–1 Anatomic relationships of the supraglottic larynx. Posterior view (*left*) and sagittal view (*right*).

Dorsum of tongue
Epiglottis
Arytenoid fold
Arytenoid cartilage
Ventricular fold
Arytenoid muscle
Thyroid cartilage
Cricoid cartilage
Vallecula
Hyoepiglottic ligament
Thyroepiglottic ligament
Thyroid cartilage

may spread inferiorly to involve the paraglottic space,[87] but as a rule, neither upward extension into the laryngeal lymphatics nor downward extension into the subglottic region occurs.[18,100]

Infection of the supraglottic structures probably arises from direct invasion by Hib with subsequent development of bacteremia. The bacteremia appears to be relatively short in duration and of low concentration, as suggested by several observations: (1) the serum concentration of the capsular polysaccharide is directly proportional to the concentration and duration of bacteremia,[168] (2) children with epiglottitis have less Hib capsular polysaccharide in their sera than do patients with meningitis,[217] and (3) the density of Hib in blood is significantly lower in patients with epiglottitis than in patients with meningitis.[117,166,194] In 23 patients with epiglottitis, the geometric mean number of organisms was 123 colony-forming units (CFU)/mL, whereas the geometric mean number in 43 patients with meningitis was 2203 CFU/mL ($p < .001$).[117]

What predisposes the epiglottitis to infection is unknown. Possibly, mild trauma to the epiglottis occurs during food intake. This trauma could result in damage to the mucosal surface, which, in turn, could allow the invasion of organisms that already were present in the upper respiratory tract. Also possible is that a viral infection damages the mucosal surface and thus predisposes the patient to secondary bacterial infection.

Acute-phase sera in most children with epiglottitis lack specific bactericidal and hemagglutinating antibody. Seroconversion regularly occurs after infection.[30,130]

Conflicting evidence exists relating to a possible genetic difference between patients with Hib epiglottitis and other individuals.[5,82,198,225] Whisnant and associates[225] surveyed human leukocyte antigens (HLA) and erythrocytic antigens among 30 children with epiglottitis and 20 patients with meningitis. HLA-A11 was found in 17 and 3 percent of the patients with meningitis and epiglottitis, respectively ($p < .01$). HLA-B5 occurred in 13 and 3 percent of patients with epiglottitis and meningitis, respectively ($p < .05$), whereas HLA-B40 occurred more often (23% versus 10%) in patients with meningitis than in those with epiglottitis ($p < .05$). Moreover, the frequency of HLA-A28 and HLA-B17 was higher among the patients with epiglottitis than in uninfected control subjects.[225] However, the results of another study did not confirm these observations.[82]

The distribution and frequency of MNS erythrocyte antigens in patients with epiglottitis may differ from those observed in others. For example, the NNSS genotype occurred in 6.4 percent of patients with epiglottitis and in 0.5 percent of healthy control subjects ($p < .0002$),[225] but this difference was not confirmed.[82] However, the results of two studies suggest that the MNS genotype occurs less often in patients with Hib meningitis than in patients with epiglottitis.[82,225] In one study, white children with Hib meningitis lacked G2m(n), an allotype antigen of IgG2 subclass heavy chains, more frequently than did control subjects.[5] In another study in a white population in Finland, however, this difference was not noted.[197] The frequency of the Km(1) immunoglobulin allotype in children with epiglottitis did not differ significantly from the prevalence of that marker in blacks or whites. However, in blacks with Hib meningitis, the Km(1) marker occurred less frequently in patients than in control subjects.[82] The identification of one outer-membrane protein subtype of Hib that was associated relatively infrequently with epiglottitis suggests that isotype-specific differences in the propensity of Hib to cause epiglottitis may exist.[196]

CLINICAL MANIFESTATIONS

The classic onset of epiglottitis in children is abrupt, and progression of disease is rapid; careful history on occasion reveals the

occurrence of a trivial antecedent upper respiratory tract infection.* The total duration of illness before hospitalization usually is less than 24 hours and occasionally is as short as 2 hours. In one study in which 142 medical records of children with epiglottitis were reviewed, the duration of illness before tracheotomy was performed was found to be 12 hours or less in 73 percent and more than 24 hours in only four patients.[47]

The most common presentation of acute epiglottitis in children includes the sudden onset of fever, severe sore throat, dysphagia, and drooling. Airway obstruction always occurs and is rapidly progressive. It is manifested by distress on inspiration, a choking sensation, irritability, restlessness, and anxiety. The speech is muffled or thick sounding, but hoarseness usually does not occur. The child usually insists on sitting up in a characteristic posture with the arms back, the trunk leaning forward, the neck hyperextended, and the chin pushed forward. This posture increases the diameter of the obstructed airway.

In contrast to acute laryngotracheitis, in which marked inspiratory stridor occurs, the degree of observed stridor in epiglottitis often is not severe. This apparent lack of respiratory distress often leads the unwary physician to underestimate the severity of the child's illness. With progression, the air exchange becomes progressively worse, and hypoxia, hypercapnia, and acidosis develop. These developments cause increased irritability, restlessness, and disorientation, and if an artificial airway is not established, the child will experience sudden cardiorespiratory arrest.

Fever occurs in virtually all children; most temperatures are between 38.8° C and 40.0° C (101.8° F and 104° F). Blood leukocyte counts almost always are elevated; the mean total count was approximately 20,000 cells/mm³ in five studies.[4,20,47,97,221] The differential cell count reveals an increased percentage of neutrophils and band forms; most patients have absolute band counts that are more than 500 cells/mm³.

The clinical picture of epiglottitis in adults is more indolent than that in children.[19,86,191,231] Berger and associates[20] reviewed 118 cases of acute epiglottitis seen between 1986 and 2000. Of these patients, 33 percent were admitted to the hospital within 1 day of the onset of symptoms, and 77 percent were admitted within 3 days of onset. Symptoms on admission were as follows: sore throat, 85 percent; odynophagia, 83 percent; temperature elevation, 38 percent; respiratory difficulties, 34 percent; muffled voice, 25 percent; and drooling, 7 percent. In two other studies, an average of 1 to 3 days elapsed before medical aid was sought. The mean temperature was 38.2° C (100.7° F), and some patients were afebrile; the temperature range was 36.6° C to 40.0° C (97.8° F to 104° F). Blood leukocyte counts averaged 17,000/mm³ (range, 8000 to 32,000/mm³).[86,191] Sore throat and dysphagia were universal occurrences. Zwahlen and Regamy[231] reviewed the clinical features of 100 reported adult cases of epiglottitis. Of these patients, 78 percent had dyspnea, 49 percent had dysphonia, 41 percent had cyanosis, and 38 percent had stridor. Forty-six percent had edema of the neck. A precordial purring or fluttering sensation was described by one adult patient.[169] In three cases in adults, Ehara[63] noted on physical examination that all had tenderness of the anterior neck over the hyoid bone.

DIFFERENTIAL DIAGNOSIS

The hallmarks of the successful management of acute epiglottitis are an awareness of the condition and an understanding of the rapidity of its progression. A correct early diagnosis frequently is lifesaving. Acute epiglottitis must be differentiated from seven other conditions with symptoms of acute upper airway obstruction. Aspects of the differential diagnosis are presented in the text in Chapter 22 and in Table 22–4.

---

*See references 13, 14, 18, 20, 30, 33, 47, 65, 86, 97, 99, 122, 127, 130, 131, 141, 150, 155, 184, 213, 224.

In epiglottitis, the important differential points are as follows: the lack of a croupy cough; the presence of a swollen, cherry-red epiglottis; the sitting posture of the child with the chin pushed forward, as well as a reluctance or refusal to lie down; and the relatively greater apprehension and anxiety of the child than the degree of chest retraction suggests. In contrast, the child with acute laryngotracheitis has a normal epiglottis on examination, always has a typical barking cough, is comfortable in a supine position, and frequently appears to have only minimal apprehension in spite of retractions in which the sternum appears to be indenting 2 inches or more.

Acute angioneurotic edema that involves the epiglottis can mimic acute epiglottitis. However, in this condition, the temperature usually is normal, and the patient appears less toxic. This condition usually is brought on by a specific allergic reaction after the ingestion of a food or medication.

Supraglottitis should be considered in children with uvulitis because the clinical features of these disorders may overlap, and both infections may be present. Concomitant uvulitis and epiglottitis were described in association with Hib bacteremia in children[107,158] and with *S. pneumoniae* bacteremia in an adult.[223] Isolated uvulitis has been associated with Hib bacteremia and group A beta-hemolytic streptococcal pharyngitis.[107,123] Uvulitis in the absence of epiglottitis was described in a child with odynophagia, drooling, and Hib bacteremia.[123]

A foreign body lodged in a vallecula or the larynx or in penetrating posterior pharyngeal tissues may cause signs and symptoms that mimic those of acute supraglottitis.[220] A paravertebral collection of pus, from cervical osteomyelitis or parapharyngeal abscess, rarely can spread anteriorly and can produce acute "croup." Congenital anomalies and laryngeal papillomas can be excluded by their chronic course. *C. albicans* has caused neonatal laryngeal obstruction without radiologic epiglottitis.[153]

Infection of supraglottic structures by *Mycobacterium tuberculosis* occurs less commonly than does glottic involvement; tuberculous laryngitis is an exceedingly rare occurrence in children and always is associated with pulmonary lesions.[62] The onset is considerably more insidious than is that of Hib supraglottitis. Nasopharyngeal diphtheria may mimic acute epiglottitis and may be associated with a serosanguineous nasal discharge.

Chronic epiglottic enlargement with edema was observed in two children with cancer who had received radiation therapy to the neck. These clinical features were not confused with those of acute supraglottitis, although one patient had dysphagia and snored.[229] Severe, chronic inflammatory epiglottitis with associated granulomatous lymphangitis was found on histologic examination of tissue obtained from a 19-month-old black child who had epiglottic enlargement without erythema for 3 months.[220] "Tuberculoid" granulomatous lesions were seen at histologic examination of an epiglottic biopsy specimen obtained from a 22-year-old man, HIV status unknown, who presented with weight loss, sore throat, and dysphonia of 1 month's duration.[140] The epiglottitis and arytenoepiglottic folds of this patient were erythematous and edematous.

Lymphangiectasis of the epiglottis produced airway obstruction with stridor and intermittent cyanosis in a 4-month-old white boy. On histologic examination, the epiglottis consisted of multiple dilated lymphatic vessels lined by a single layer of epithelial cells with no discernible wall. The stroma contained scattered lymphocytes and a few neutrophils. This lesion spontaneously regressed, and the child's condition was normal at 1 year of age.[208]

SPECIFIC DIAGNOSIS

The clinical picture of sore throat, dysphagia, drooling, anxiety, and inspiratory distress without significant stridor and the char-

acteristic sitting position should suggest the presumptive diagnosis in most cases. The definitive anatomic diagnosis is made by the visualization of the epiglottis, and the etiologic diagnosis is confirmed by culture of an organism from the blood or the surface of the epiglottis. An Hib origin also can be established by the demonstration of antigenemia or antigenuria.[189,217]

In the typical case, the epiglottis is fiery red and greatly swollen. In children, the epiglottis can be seen by simple depression of the tongue with a tongue blade. In older children and adults, indirect or direct laryngoscopy usually is necessary to confirm the diagnosis. On occasion, the obstruction is caused by swelling of the ventricular bands and the arytenoepiglottic folds so that the epiglottis may appear relatively normal.

Major controversy exists concerning the safety of using a tongue depressor to examine a child with suspected epiglottitis because sudden cardiorespiratory arrest has been noted to occur. However, most instances of cardiorespiratory arrest that I am aware of occurred after the child was forced into a supine position rather than because of the examination itself.[42] In many instances, patients with presumptive epiglottitis can be examined, while they are in an upright position, by using tongue blade or indirect laryngoscopy.

Case management should be individualized. In the child with moderate or advanced disease, the clinical diagnosis should be apparent without having to do an intraoral examination. In this situation, intraoral examination should not be performed, but the child should be prepared for the establishment of an airway. This preparation should be rapid but controlled so that intubation can be performed in an operating room.

The diagnosis of epiglottitis can be established by the classic appearance on a lateral neck radiograph (Fig. 21–2).[156,221]

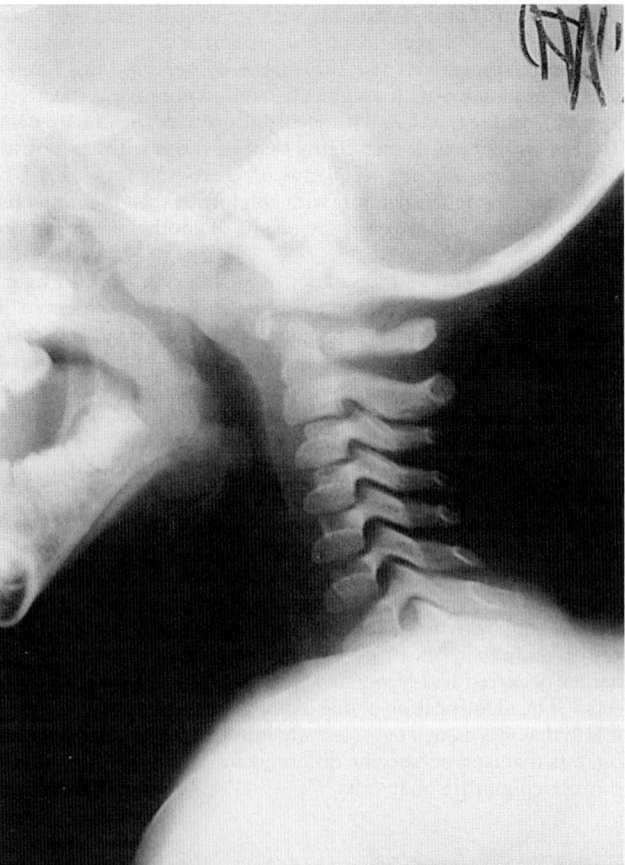

Figure 21–2 Acute epiglottitis. A lateral neck radiograph from a child with acute epiglottitis showing the swollen epiglottis (thumb sign) encroaching on the airway. (*Courtesy of Dr. Ines Bouchat.*)

However, my opinion is that this radiographic procedure rarely is necessary; all too often, it leads to a delay in providing the necessary definitive therapy.[47,100,139] The use of the lateral neck radiograph should be reserved for subacute cases in which the specific diagnosis after completion of a clinical examination is not clear.

The lateral film of the neck, delineating the soft tissues, taken with the patient upright, gives the best view of the upper airway anatomy (see Fig. 21–2). The hypopharynx is dilated; normal cervical lordosis may be replaced by a straight or kyphotic contour. The valleculae are narrowed and may be obliterated. A thickened mass of tissue stretching from the valleculae to the arytenoids emphasizes the appropriateness of the term *supraglottitis*. In adults with epiglottitis, the widths of the epiglottis and arytenoepiglottic folds uniformly exceed 8 and 7 mm, respectively.[174]

When performed, radiography of the neck in the anteroposterior projection usually reveals that tracheal narrowing is absent. However, some children with acute supraglottitis have localized subglottic narrowing indistinguishable from that found in acute laryngotracheitis.[178,187]

All patients with suspected epiglottitis should have a blood culture, and a culture specimen should be obtained from the surface of the epiglottis when an artificial airway is established. Today, cultures are of increasing importance because of the change in epidemiology of Hib infection and the resulting increased likelihood that an organism other than Hib may be causing the illness. A white blood cell count with a differential also may provide useful information. In children who have received antimicrobial treatment before cultures were obtained, performing a direct antigen test for Hib on the blood and urine is worthwhile.

TREATMENT

The treatment of acute epiglottitis should be relatively simple in that it involves only two main aspects of therapy: an airway must be established, and an appropriate antimicrobial agent needs to be administered. However, in the past, the mortality rate from epiglottitis varied from 0 to 32 percent,[47,86] a finding suggesting major differences in the implementation of treatment.

Most deaths occur in transit to the hospital or within the first few hours after arrival. Once the diagnosis is suspected, the patient should be attended constantly by individuals skilled in resuscitation with appropriate equipment for airway stabilization and ventilatory support. Delays of 2 or 3 hours have proved fatal; every effort should be made to reduce the time needed to secure a patient's airway and to initiate antibiotic therapy, before which unnecessary stress should be avoided. In most cases, radiographic confirmation should be omitted. Blood tests, extensive history taking, and delay in transport should be eliminated.

Medical centers and pediatric services that have planned protocols for the diagnostic investigation and treatment of patients with suspected acute epiglottitis generally have better morbidity and mortality statistics than do services that do not have such protocols in place. Pediatricians, radiologists, otolaryngologists, and anesthetists may contribute to the assessment and management of a case; defining roles and responsibilities of each service in advance minimizes confusion and renders the institution of care easier.

SECURING THE AIRWAY

In general, the cornerstone of all management plans is the establishment of an airway in all children in whom the diagnosis of epiglottitis is made.[44] In 1938, Sinclair[183] recognized that trache-

ostomy was lifesaving. Berenberg and Kevy[19] advocated hospitalization for all patients with epiglottitis but tracheostomy only "if necessary." However, Bass and associates[13] presented a compelling argument for performing routine tracheostomy. Among 83 patients with documented epiglottitis, 11 of whom were adults, these authors noted that 16 (19%) had life-threatening obstruction when they were first seen. An additional 14 (17%) progressed to this point within 6 hours of admission; 9 of the 83 (11%) required emergency tracheostomy while they were hospitalized. Of these 9, 2 died, and 1 suffered anoxic brain damage. All 9 were being monitored carefully, with bedside tracheostomy equipment available and trained personnel nearby. Six of the adults required tracheostomy for survival.[13] Margolis and colleagues[131] noted that elective tracheostomy, performed at the time of diagnosis, eliminated fatalities in 15 consecutive patients. This observation was in contrast to 4 deaths in 20 patients observed until tracheostomy "was required."

A large body of literature attests to the safety and efficacy of nasotracheal intubation as a replacement for tracheostomy,* which has a complication rate of 50 percent.[199,224] Biologically inert tubes, with their decreased risk of complicating subglottic stenosis,[180] and the recollection that endotracheal tube insertion was a universal approach before tracheostomy[139] was an accepted procedure led to the routine use of nasotracheal intubation in this disease. Nasotracheal intubation requires a shorter duration of airway maintenance: 32 patients with epiglottitis managed with tracheostomy had a mean duration of intubation of 7.5 days and a mean hospitalization of 8.8 days. In contrast, a nasotracheal tube was used for a mean of 38 hours with a 6.5-day hospitalization in 5 patients.[139] Diaz and Lockhart[57] managed 104 patients with nasotracheal intubation. The mean intubation time was 53 ± 14.9 hours; 7 patients (6.8%) extubated themselves, and 2 required reintubation. Laryngeal edema occurred in 3 patients (2.9%) who had been intubated. In 2 patients, subglottic granulations required excision.

My position, as well as that of Daum and Smith,[54] is that the argument for performing elective tracheostomy or, preferably, intubation in all children with supraglottitis is compelling, and the procedure should be performed immediately after the diagnosis is established. Whether this "stimulus-response" approach is necessary for adults with epiglottitis is controversial.[12,70,86,151,177,182,191,226] Mayo Smith and associates[133] compared selected clinical features in adults with epiglottitis at the time of diagnosis who died or who received an artificial airway with those of adults who recovered without airway intervention. Few differences emerged. Patients who died or who were managed with airway intervention had respiratory distress and bacteremia more often than did those who recovered without airway intervention. Obviously, the presence of bacteremia was not known on presentation. Moreover, the mortality rate among all adults managed expectantly was 4.6 percent, a figure comparable to the mortality rate (6.1%) of children in a series reported before recommendations were made for routine securing of the airway at diagnosis.[40,133] The preponderance of evidence until very recently has suggested that securing the airway in all adults with supraglottitis by nasotracheal intubation should reduce mortality rates.[7,10,12,13,21,22,51,106,133] However, Frantz and associates[71] reported an analysis of 129 cases of acute epiglottitis in adults in which no deaths occurred in the cohort, and 85 percent of these patients were managed without airway intervention.

In the large series reported by Berger and colleagues[20] involving 118 cases, 19 had airways established on admission (16 endotracheal intubation, 2 tracheotomy, 1 cricothyrotomy), and 6 other patients subsequently required either endotracheal intubation or tracheotomy. The remaining 93 patients were managed successfully without the need for airway intervention. Fifty-eight

---

*See references 14, 48, 89, 114, 131, 150, 157, 171, 173, 180, 199, 201.

TABLE 21-2   Size of Nasotracheal Tubes Recommended for Children with Acute Supraglottitis

Age	Size (mm)
Birth-6 mo	3.0
6 mo-3 yr	3.5
3-5 yr	4.0
>5 yr	4.5

Data from Rabe, E. F.: Infectious croup: III. Haemophilus influenzae type b croup. Pediatrics 2:559-566, 1948.

of the patients were treated with intravenous corticosteroids in addition to antibiotics, and these patients tended to have more prolonged hospital stays than those who did not receive steroids (5.7 ± 4.1 days versus 4.7 ± 4.3 days; $p = .2$).

To aid in intubation and to reduce long-term sequelae, most investigators have advocated use of a nasotracheal tube 0.5 to 1.0 mm smaller than that predicted by the patient's age.[89,139,171] Recommendations for tube size are shown in Table 21-2. Published criteria for extubation (summarized in reference 14) include those based on duration of therapy and those based on daily examination of the epiglottis and supraglottic structures by direct laryngoscopy[55] or fiberoptic bronchoscopy.[148,210]

Long-term complications of nasotracheal intubation are rare. Thirty-three children with epiglottitis who were managed with nasotracheal intubation (mean duration of intubation, 55 hours) were evaluated 1 to 8 years later. By history and measurement of peak expiratory flow rates, no complications were found.[171] Although additional long-term data are necessary to ensure absence of residua, elective nasotracheal intubation appears to be the procedure of choice.

Several reports documented the recognition of idiopathic pulmonary edema before[119] or, more commonly, after[25,55,59,73,102,190,202] insertion of an endotracheal tube to relieve laryngeal obstruction caused by epiglottitis. One hypothesis to explain this phenomenon is that airway obstruction produces markedly negative intrapleural pressure with increased venous return to the right side of the heart, with decreased left ventricular output and increased pulmonary blood volume.[116] These changes increase the pulmonary microvascular pressure and produce pulmonary hyperemia and edema. Endotoxemia may play a role in altering vascular permeability, but it is not necessary for recognition of this complication of airway obstruction because abrupt onset of pulmonary edema was described when airway obstruction caused by croup, foreign body, and malignant neoplasm was relieved acutely.[37] The frequency of pulmonary edema as a complication of intubation in supraglottitis was approximately 9 percent,[187] and it has occurred in an adult.[161] Continuous positive airway pressure in all intubated patients with epiglottitis probably will provide prophylaxis against this complication,[57,73] but controlled data are lacking.

ANTIBIOTICS

The mainstay of antibiotic therapy for acute epiglottitis in the recent past has been ceftriaxone (50 to 100 mg/kg/day given every 12 hours intravenously) or cefotaxime (100 to 200 mg/kg/day given every 6 hours intravenously) because virtually all cases in both children and adults were caused by Hib. However, in the present conjugate vaccine era, the incidence of all invasive Hib disease has decreased dramatically. Therefore, in children previously vaccinated, the cause is likely to be another organism. Culture results today have added significance because one possible cause that would require a change in therapy is *S. aureus*.

No controlled data exist about the duration of antimicrobial administration, but a course of 7 days seems appropriate. In the event that group A streptococci are isolated from the airway, penicillin is the drug of choice. A first-generation semisynthetic penicillinase-resistant penicillin or vancomycin (if methicillin-resistant *S. aureus* is suspected) should be used for *S. aureus*, whereas erythromycin is indicated for *Corynebacterium diphtheriae*.

OTHER SUPPORTIVE MEASURES

Some authors have advocated corticosteroid therapy on the basis of anecdotal experience in patients with epiglottitis, but no controlled data exist to support its use, and such therapy may be hazardous: among 91 patients with epiglottitis who received corticosteroid therapy, 4 (4%) had evidence of bleeding from the gastrointestinal tract that was sufficient in 2 patients to require transfusion,[58] a phenomenon observed by other investigators.[111] Therapy with racemic epinephrine is without benefit.

Expert respiratory nursing care is essential. Inadvertent extubation must be avoided, particularly in the first 24 hours. Judicious use of sedatives that do not appreciably depress respiration may be appropriate.

COMPLICATIONS

Extraepiglottic complications are not common occurrences in children with acute epiglottitis. In a study involving 72 children with epiglottitis, investigators noted that 25 percent had pneumonia, 25 percent had cervical adenitis, 8 percent had tonsillitis, and 5 percent had otitis media.[141] The other common invasive manifestations of Hib infections (meningitis, arthritis, and cellulitis) rarely are found in conjunction with epiglottitis.[141,170]

PREVENTION

PROPHYLAXIS OF HOUSEHOLD CONTACTS

In the pre–conjugate vaccine era, household contacts of patients with Hib infection were at increased risk for acquiring Hib infection.[81] Whether an increased risk occurred in daycare contacts was unresolved.[53] Although contacts of patients with Hib epiglottitis younger than 5 years are colonized less frequently than are contacts of patients with other Hib invasive infections,[52] secondary disease was described in household contacts when an index patient had epiglottitis.[1,78,79,203] Secondary Hib epiglottitis was described in a child[1] and two adults who were household contacts of a patient with Hib meningitis.[78,79] Hib epiglottitis occurred in two siblings who presented with the condition within 1 day.[85]

Rifampin prophylaxis, 20 mg/kg/day (600 mg/dose maximum) for 4 days, is recommended for all unvaccinated members of a patient's contact group when the index patient has Hib epiglottitis and at least one contact in the group is 4 years of age or younger.[6,41]

The recognition that adults occasionally may acquire secondary infection, particularly epiglottitis, on exposure to children with invasive Hib infection prompted some experts to extend prophylaxis to all of a patient's contact groups, regardless of the presence of one or more contacts who are 4 years of age or younger. All experts, however, recommended that adults and older children be made aware of the signs and symptoms of Hib disease, particularly when the patient's contact group would not receive prophylaxis under current guidelines.

REFERENCES

1. Addy, M. G., Ellis, P. D. M., and Turk, D. C.: *Haemophilus* epiglottitis: Nine recent cases in Oxford. Br. Med. J. *1*:40-41, 1972.
2. Alba, D., Perna, C., Torres, E., et al.: Isolated candidal epiglottitis: Report of a fatal case. Clin. Infect. Dis. *22*:732-733, 1996.
3. Alexander, H. E., Ellis, C., and Leidy, C.: Treatment of type-specific *H. influenzae* infections in infancy and childhood. J. Pediatr. *20*:673-698, 1942.
4. Alho, O.-P., Jokinen, K., Pirila, T., et al.: Acute epiglottitis and infant conjugate *Haemophilus influenzae* type b vaccination in northern Finland. Arch. Otolaryngol. Head Neck Surg. *121*:898-902, 1995.
5. Ambrosino, D. M., Schiffman, G., Gottschlich, E. C., et al.: Correlation between G2m(n) immunoglobulin allotype and human antibody response and susceptibility to polysaccharide encapsulated bacteria. J. Clin. Invest. *75*:1935-1942, 1985.
6. American Academy of Pediatrics: *Haemophilus influenzae* infections. *In* Pickering, L. K. (ed.): 2000 Red Book: Report of the Committee on Infectious Diseases. 25th ed. Elk Grove Village, IL, American Academy of Pediatrics, 2000, pp. 203-217.
7. Andreassen, U. K., Husum, B., Tos, M., et al.: Acute epiglottitis in adults: A management based on a 17-year material. Acta Anaesthesiol. Scand. *28*:155-157, 1984.
8. Barnham, M., Kerby, J., Chandler, R. S., et al.: Group C streptococci in human infection: A study of 308 isolates with clinical correlations. Epidemiol. Infect. *102*:379-390, 1989.
9. Baron, B. J.: Comments on a case of extremely acute edematous laryngitis. Br. Med. J. *2*:1328, 1887.
10. Bass, J. W.: Routine tracheotomy for epiglottitis: What are the odds? J. Pediatr. *83*:510-511, 1973.
11. Bass, J. W.: Personal communication, 1977.
12. Bass, J. W.: Response to CPC. N. Engl. J. Med. *298*:342-343, 1978.
13. Bass, J. W., Steele, R. W., and Wiebe, R. A.: Acute epiglottitis: A surgical emergency. JAMA. *229*:671-675, 1974.
14. Battaglia, J. D., and Lockhart, C. H.: Management of acute epiglottitis by nasotracheal intubation. Am. J. Dis. Child. *129*:334-336, 1975.
15. Baugh, R., and Baker, S. R.: Epiglottitis in children: Review of 24 cases. Otolaryngol. Head Neck Surg. *90*:157-162, 1982.
16. Baxter, J. D.: Acute epiglottitis in children. Laryngoscope *77*:1358-1367, 1967.
17. Belfer, R. A.: Group A beta-hemolytic streptococcal epiglottitis as a complication of varicella infection. Pediatr. Emerg. Care *12*:203-204, 1996.
18. Benjamin, B., and O'Reilly, B.: Acute epiglottitis in infants and children. Ann. Otol. *85*:565-572, 1976.
19. Berenberg, W., and Kevy, S.: Acute epiglottitis in childhood: A serious emergency, readily recognized at the bedside. N. Engl. J. Med. *258*:870-874, 1958.
20. Berger, G. B., Landau, T., Berger, S., et al.: The rising incidence of adult acute epiglottis and epiglottic abscess. Am. J. Otolaryngol. *24*:374-383, 2003.
21. Bishop, M. L.: Epiglottitis in the adult. Anesthesiology *55*:701-702, 1981.
22. Bishop, M. J., and Weymuller, E. A.: Adult epiglottitis revisited. Anesthesiology *57*:545-546, 1982.
23. Black, M. J., Harbour, J., Remsen, K. A., et al.: Acute epiglottitis in adults. J. Otolaryngol. *10*:23-27, 1981.
24. Blackstock, D., Adderley, R. J., and Steward, D. J.: Epiglottitis in young infants. Anesthesiology *69*:97-100, 1987.
25. Blankson, V. N.: Pulmonary edema complicating epiglottitis. J. Med. Soc. N. J. *80*:939-941, 1983.
26. Bogger-Goren, S.: Acute epiglottitis caused by herpes simplex virus. Pediatr. Infect. Dis. *6*:1133, 1987.
27. Bolivar, R., Gomez, L. G., Luna, M., et al.: *Aspergillus* epiglottitis. Cancer *51*:367-370, 1983.
28. Bottenfield, G. W., Arcinue, E. L., Sarnaik, A., et al.: Diagnosis and management of acute epiglottitis: Report of 90 consecutive cases. Laryngoscope *90*:822-825, 1980.
29. Bower, C. M., and Suen, J. Y.: Adult acute epiglottitis caused by *Serratia marcescens*. Otolaryngol. Head Neck Surg. *115*:156-159, 1996.
30. Branefors-Helander, P., and Jeppsson, P. H.: Acute epiglottitis: A clinical, bacteriological and serological study. Scand. J. Infect. Dis. *7*:103-111, 1975.
31. Breivik, H., and Klaastad, O.: Acute epiglottitis in children. Br. J. Anaesth. *50*:505-509, 1978.
32. Briggs, W. H., and Altenau, M. M.: Acute epiglottitis in children. Otolaryngol. Head Neck Surg. *88*:665-669, 1980.
33. Brilli, R. J., Benzing, G., and Cotcamp, D. H.: Epiglottitis in infants less than two years of age. Pediatr. Emerg. Care *5*:16-21, 1989.
34. Broadhurst, L. E., Erickson, R. L., and Kelley, P. W.: Decreases in invasive *Haemophilus influenzae* diseases in US Army children, 1984 through 1991. JAMA. *269*:227-231, 1993.
35. Broughton, S. J., and Warren, R. E.: A review of *Haemophilus influenzae* infections in Cambridge 1975-1981. J. Infect. *9*:30-42, 1984.
36. Bruun, B., Gahrn-Hansen, B., Westh, H., et al.: Clonal relationship of recent invasive *Haemophilus influenzae* serotype f isolates from Denmark and the United States. J. Med. Microbiol. *53*:1161-1165, 2004.
37. Burtner, D. D., and Goodman, M.: Anesthetic and operative management of potential upper airway obstruction. Arch. Otolaryngol. *104*:657-661, 1978.
38. Butt, W., Shann, F., Walker, C., et al.: Acute epiglottitis: A different approach to management. Crit. Care Med. *16*:43-47, 1988.
39. Caballero, M., Sabater, F., Traserra, J., et al.: Epiglottitis and necrotizing fasciitis: A life-threatening complication of infectious mononucleosis. Acta Otolaryngol. *125*:1130-1133, 2005.
40. Cantrell, R. W., Bell, R. A., and Morioka, W. T.: Acute epiglottitis: Intubation versus tracheostomy. Laryngoscope *88*:994-1005, 1978.
41. Centers for Disease Control and Prevention: Immunization Practices Advisory Committee: *Haemophilus* b conjugate vaccine for prevention of *Haemophilus influenzae* type b disease among infants and children 2 months of age and older. M. M. W. R. Morb. Mortal. Wkly Rep. *40*:1-7, 1991.
42. Cherry, J. D.: Unpublished data, 1973.
43. Cherry, J. D.: Acute epiglottitis, laryngitis, and croup. *In* Remington, J. S., and Swartz, M. N. (eds.): Current Clinical Topics in Infectious Diseases. New York, McGraw-Hill, 1981, pp. 1-30.
44. Cherry, J. D.: Croup. *In* Kiple, K. F. (ed.): The Cambridge World History of Human Disease. Cambridge, Cambridge University Press, 1993, pp. 654-657.
45. Chow, A. W., Bushkell, L. L., Yoshikawa, T. T., et al.: *Haemophilus parainfluenzae* epiglottitis with meningitis and bacteremia in an adult. Am. J. Med. Sci. *267*:365-368, 1974.
46. Claesson, B., Trollfors, B., Ekström-Jodal, B., et al.: Incidence and prognosis of acute epiglottitis in children in a Swedish region. Pediatr. Infect. Dis. *3*:534-538, 1984.
47. Cohen, S. R., and Chai, J.: Epiglottitis: Twenty-year study with tracheotomy. Ann. Otol. *87*:461-467, 1978.
48. Coker, S. B., and Scherz, R. G.: Safe alternative to tracheostomy in acute epiglottitis. Am. J. Dis. Child. *129*:136, 1975.
49. Coulehan, J. L., Michaels, R. H., Hallowell C., et al.: Epidemiology of *Haemophilus influenzae* type b disease among Navajo Indians. Public Health Rep. *99*:404-409, 1984.
50. Dagan, R., and the Israeli Pediatric Bacteremia and Meningitis Group: A two-year prospective, nationwide study to determine the epidemiology and impact of invasive childhood *Haemophilus influenzae* type b infection in Israel. Clin. Infect. Dis. *15*:720-725, 1992.
51. Darnell, J. C.: Acute epiglottitis in adults: Report of a case and review of the literature. J. Indiana State Med. Assoc. *69*:21-23, 1976.
52. Daum, R. S., Glode, M. P., Goldmann, D. A., et al.: Rifampin chemoprophylaxis for household contacts of patients with invasive infections due to *Haemophilus influenzae* type b. J. Pediatr. *98*:485-491, 1981.
53. Daum, R. S., Granoff, D. M., Gilsdorf, J., et al.: *H. influenzae* type b infections in day care attendees: Implications for management. Rev. Infect. Dis. *8*:46-55, 1986.
54. Daum, R. S., and Smith, A. L.: Epiglottitis (supraglottitis). *In* Feigin, R. D., and Cherry, J. D. (eds.): Textbook of Pediatric Infectious Diseases. 3rd ed. Philadelphia, W. B. Saunders, 1992, pp. 197-209.
55. Davis, H. W., Gartiner, J. C., Galvis, A. G., et al.: Acute upper airway obstruction: Croup and epiglottitis. Pediatr. Clin. North Am. *28*:859-880, 1981.
56. Devita, M. A., and Wagner, I. J.: Acute epiglottitis in the adult. Crit. Care Med. *14*:1082-1083, 1986.
57. Diaz, J. H., and Lockhart, C. H.: Early diagnosis and airway management of acute epiglottitis in children. South. Med. J. *75*:399-403, 1982.
58. DiTirro, F. R., Silver, M. H., and Hengerer, A. S.: Acute epiglottitis: Evolution of management in the community hospital. Int. J. Pediatr. Otorhinolaryngol. *7*:145-152, 1984.
59. Donnelly, J., Overtun, J. H., and Mellis, C. M.: Pulmonary oedema following relief of epiglottitis. Anaesth. Intensive Care *9*:290-291, 1981.
60. Drake-Lee, A. B., Broughton, S. J., and Grace, A.: Children with epiglottitis. Br. J. Clin. Pract. *38*:218-220, 1984.
61. Dudley, J. P.: Supraglottitis and *Haemophilus parainfluenzae*: Pathogenic potential of the organism. Ann. Otol. Rhinol. Laryngol. *96*:400-402, 1987.
62. Dworetzky, J. P., and Risch, O. C.: Laryngeal tuberculosis: A study of 500 cases of pulmonary tuberculosis with a resume based on twenty-eight years of experience. Ann. Otol. Rhinol. Laryngol. *50*:745-761, 1941.
63. Ehara, H.: Tenderness over the hyoid bone can indicate epiglottitis in adults. J. Am. Board Fam. Med. *19*:517-520, 2006.
64. Faden, H.: The dramatic change in the epidemiology of pediatric epiglottis. Pediatr. Emerg. Care *22*:443-444, 2006.
65. Faden, H. S.: Treatment of *Haemophilus influenzae* type b epiglottitis. Pediatrics *63*:402-407, 1979.
66. Farley, M. M., Stephens, D. S., Brachman, P. S., Jr., et al.: Invasive *Haemophilus influenzae* disease in adults: A prospective, population-based surveillance. Ann. Intern. Med. *116*:806-812, 1992.
67. Fearon, B. W., and Bell, R. D.: Acute epiglottitis: A potential killer. Can. Med. Assoc. J. *112*:760-766, 1975.
68. Fogarty, J., Moloney, A. C., and Newell, J. B.: The epidemiology of *Haemophilus influenzae* type b disease in the Republic of Ireland. Epidemiol. Infect. *114*:451-463, 1995.
69. Fontanarosa, P. B., Polsky, S. S., and Goldman, G. E.: Adult epiglottitis. J. Emerg. Med. *7*:223-231, 1989.
70. Frantz, T. D., and Rasgon, B. M.: Acute epiglottitis: Changing epidemiologic patterns. Otolaryngol. Head Neck Surg. *109*:457-460, 1993.
71. Frantz, T. D., Rasgon, B. M., and Quesenberry, C. P., Jr.: Acute epiglottitis in adults: Analysis of 129 cases. J. A. M. A. *272*:1358-1360, 1994.

72. Freeman, L., and Wolford, R.: Acute epiglottitis caused by methicillin-resistant *Staphylococcus aureus* in adults. Clin. Infect. Dis. *26*:1240-1241, 1998.

73. Galvis, A. G., Stool, S. E., and Bluestone, C. D.: Pulmonary edema following relief of acute upper airway obstruction. Ann. Otol. *89*:124-128, 1980.

74. Garpenholt, O., Hugosson, S., Fredlund, H., et al.: Epiglottitis in Sweden before and after introduction of vaccination against *Haemophilus influenzae* type b. Pediatr. Infect. Dis. J. *18*:490-493, 1998.

75. Gerber, A. C., and Pfenninger, J.: Acute epiglottitis: Management by short duration of intubation and hospitalisation. Intensive Care Med. *12*:407-411, 1986.

76. Giani, G., Quirino, F., Sacrini, A., et al.: Supraglottitis due to herpes simplex virus type 1 in an adult. Clin. Infect. Dis. *22*:382-383, 1996.

77. Glickman, M., and Klein, R. S.: Acute epiglottitis due to *Pasteurella multocida* in an adult without animal exposure. Emerg. Infect. Dis. *3*:408-409, 1997.

78. Glode, M. P.: Post exposure prophylaxis for bacterial meningitis. *In* Sande, M. A., Smith, A. L., and Root, R. K. (eds.): Bacterial Meningitis. New York, Churchill Livingstone, 1985.

79. Glode, M. P., Halsey, N. A., Murray, M., et al.: Epiglottitis in adults: Association with *Haemophilus influenzae* type b colonization and disease in children. Pediatr. Infect. Dis. *3*:548-551, 1984.

80. Gorelick, M. H., and Baker, M. D.: Epiglottitis in children, 1979 through 1992: Effects of *Haemophilus influenzae* type b immunization. Arch. Pediatr. Adolesc. Med. *148*:47-50, 1994.

81. Granoff, D. M., and Daum, R. S.: Spread of *Haemophilus influenzae* type b: Recent epidemiologic and therapeutic considerations. J. Pediatr. *97*:854-860, 1980.

82. Granoff, D. M., Pandey, J. P., Boies, E., et al.: Response to immunization with *Haemophilus influenzae* type b polysaccharide–pertussis vaccine and risk of *Haemophilus* meningitis in children with the Km(1) immunoglobulin allotype. J. Clin. Invest. *74*:1708-1714, 1984.

83. Grattan-Smith, T., Forer, M., Kilham, H., et al.: Viral supraglottitis. J. Pediatr. *110*:434-435, 1987.

84. Hafidh, M. A., Sheahan, P., Keogh, I., et al.: Acute epiglottitis in adults: A recent experience with 10 cases. J. Laryngol. Otol. *120*:310-313, 2005.

85. Handler, S. D., Plotkin, S. A., Potsic, W. P., et al.: *Haemophilus influenzae* epiglottitis occurring concurrently in two siblings. Clin. Pediatr. *21*:634-635, 1982.

86. Hawkins, D. B., Miller, A. H., Sachs, G. B., et al.: Acute epiglottitis in adults. Laryngoscope *83*:1211-1220, 1973.

87. Healy, G. B., Hyams, V. J., and Tucker, G. F.: Paraglottic laryngitis in association with epiglottitis. Ann. Otol. Rhinol. Laryngol. *94*:618-621, 1985.

88. Hébert, P. C., Ducic, Y., Boisvert, D., et al.: Adult epiglottitis in a Canadian setting. Laryngoscope *108*:64-69, 1998.

89. Heldtander, P., and Lee, G.: Treatment of acute epiglottitis in children by long-term intubation. Acta Otolaryngol. *75*:379-381, 1973.

90. Hodge, K. M., and Ganzel, T. M.: Diagnostic and therapeutic efficiency in croup and epiglottitis. Laryngoscope *97*:621-625, 1987.

91. Howard, A. J., Dunkin, K. T., Musser, M., et al.: Epidemiology of *Haemophilus influenzae* type b invasive disease in Wales. BMJ. *303*:441-445, 1991.

92. Isaacson, G., and Isaacson, D. M.: Pediatric epiglottitis caused by group G beta-hemolytic *streptococcus*. Pediatr. Infect. Dis. J. *22*:846-847, 2003.

93. Isenberg, D. A., Lipkin, D. P., Mowbray, J. F., et al.: Fatal pneumococcal epiglottitis in lupus overlap syndrome. Clin. Rheumatol. *3*:529-532, 1984.

94. Jenkins, W. A.: *Pasteurella multocida* as a cause of acute adult epiglottitis. Am. J. Emerg. Med. *15*:323, 1997.

95. Jerrard, D. A., and Olshaker, J.: Simultaneous uvulitis and epiglottitis without fever or leukocytosis. Am. J. Emerg. Med. *14*:551-552, 1996.

96. Jiang, J., Chiu, N., Lin, Y., et al.: Acute epiglottitis caused by *Haemophilus influenzae* type b: A case report. J. Microbiol. Immunol. Infect. *36*:69-71, 2003.

97. Johnson, G. K., Sullivan, J. L., and Bishop, L. A.: Acute epiglottitis: Review of 55 cases and suggested protocol. Arch. Otolaryngol. *100*:333-337, 1974.

98. Johnson, R. H., and Rumans, L. W.: Unusual infections caused by *Pasteurella multocida*. JAMA. *237*:146-147, 1977.

99. Johnstone, J. M., and Lawy, H. S.: Acute epiglottitis in adults due to infection with *Haemophilus influenzae* type b. Lancet *2*:134-136, 1967.

100. Jones, H. M.: Acute epiglottitis: A personal study over twenty years. Proc. R. Soc. Med. *63*:706-712, 1970.

101. Jones, R. N., Slepack, J., and Bigelow, J.: Ampicillin-resistant *Haemophilus paraphrophilus* laryngoepiglottitis. J. Clin. Microbiol. *4*:405-407, 1976.

102. Kanter, R. K., and Watchko, J. F.: Pulmonary edema associated with upper airway obstruction. Am. J. Dis. Child. *138*:356-358, 1984.

103. Kennedy, C. A., and Rosen, H.: *Kingella kingae* bacteremia and adult epiglottitis in a granulocytopenic host. Am. J. Med. *85*:701-702, 1988.

104. Kessler, H. A., Schade, R., and Trenhome, G. M.: Acute pneumococcal epiglottitis in immunocompromised adults. Scand. J. Infect. Dis. *12*:207-210, 1980.

105. Kharasch, S., Vinci, R., and Reece, R.: Esophagitis, epiglottitis, and cocaine alkaloid ("crack"): "Accidental" poisoning or child abuse? Pediatrics *86*:117-119, 1990.

106. Khilanani, U., and Khatib, R.: Acute epiglottitis in adults. Am. J. Med. Sci. *287*:65-70, 1984.

107. Kotloff, K. L., and Wald, E. R.: Uvulitis in children. Pediatr. Infect. Dis. *2*:392-393, 1983.

108. Kristensen, K.: *Haemophilus influenzae* type b infections in adults. Scand. J. Infect. Dis. *21*:651-653, 1989.

109. Kristensen, K., Kaaber, K., Ronne, T., et al.: Epidemiology of *Haemophilus influenzae* type b infections among children in Denmark in 1985 and 1986. Acta Paediatr. Scand. *79*:587-592, 1990.

110. Kulick, R. M., Selbst, S. M., Baker, M.D., et al.: Thermal epiglottitis after swallowing hot beverages. Pediatrics *81*:441-444, 1988.

111. Kyrcz, R. W., and Indyk, D.: Atypical acute epiglottitis with gastrointestinal bleeding. J. Fam. Pract. *27*:102-103, 1988.

112. Lacroix, J., Ahronheim, G., Arcand, P., et al.: Group A streptococcal supraglottitis. J. Pediatr. *109*:20-24, 1986.

113. Lacroix, J., Ahronheim, G., and Girouard, G.: *Pseudomonas aeruginosa* supraglottitis in a six-month-old child with severe combined immunodeficiency syndrome. Pediatr. Infect. Dis. J. *7*:739-741, 1988.

114. Lacroix, J., Blanc, V. F., Weber, M., et al.: Étude de 100 cas consécutifs d'epiglottite aiguë. Union Med. Can. *11*:774-779, 1982.

115. Lai, S. H., Wong, K. S., Liao, S. L., et al.: Noninfectious epiglottitis in children: Two case reports. Int. J. Pediatr. Otorhinolaryngol. *55*:57-60, 2000.

116. Lang, S. A., Duncan, P. G., Shephard, D. A. E., et al.: Pulmonary edema associated with airway obstruction. Can. J. Anaesth. *37*:210-218, 1990.

117. La Scolea, L. J., Rosales, S. V., Welliver, R. C., et al.: Mechanisms underlying the development of meningitis or epiglottitis in children after *Haemophilus influenzae* type b bacteremia. J. Infect. Dis. *151*:1162-1165, 1985.

118. Lederman, M. M., Lowder, J., and Lerner, P. I.: Bacteremic pneumococcal epiglottitis in adults with malignancy. Am. Rev. Respir. Dis. *125*:117-118, 1982.

119. Lee, S. C., Meislin, H., and Iserson, K. V.: Epiglottitis presenting as acute pulmonary edema. Ann. Emerg. Med. *14*:60-63, 1985.

120. Lemierre, A., Meyer, A., and Laplane, R.: Maladies infectieuses: Les septicemies à bacille de Pfeiffer. Ann. Med. *39*:97-119, 1936.

121. Levison, H., Tabachnik, E., and Newth, C. J. L.: Wheezing in infancy, croup and epiglottitis. Curr. Probl. Pediatr. *12*:1-65, 1982.

122. Lewis, J. K., Gartner, J. C., and Galvis, A. G.: A protocol for management of acute epiglottitis. Clin. Pediatr. *17*:494-496, 1978.

123. Li, K. I., Kiernan, S., Wald, E. R., et al.: Isolated uvulitis due to *Haemophilus influenzae* type b. Pediatrics *74*:1054-1057, 1984.

124. Lindquist, J. R., Franzen, R. E., and Ossoff, R. H.: Acute infectious supraglottitis in adults. Ann. Emerg. Med. *9*:256-259, 1980.

125. Lipson, A., Kronick, J. B., Tewfik, L., et al.: Group B streptococcal supraglottitis in a 3-month-old infant. Am. J. Dis. Child. *140*:411-412, 1986.

126. Liptak, G. S., McConnochie, K. M., Roghmann, K. J., et al.: Decline of pediatric admissions with *Haemophilus influenzae* type b in New York State, 1982 through 1993: Relation to immunizations. J. Pediatr. *130*:923-930, 1997.

127. Losek, J. D., Dewitz-Zink, B. A., Melzer-Lange, M., et al.: Epiglottitis: Comparison of signs and symptoms in children less than 2 years old and older. Ann. Emerg. Med. *19*:55-58, 1990.

128. Mace, S. E.: Acute epiglottitis in adults. Am. J. Emerg. Med. *3*:543-550, 1985.

129. Macneil, A., Campbell, A. M., and Clark, L. J.: Adult acute epiglottitis in association with infection of an epiglottic cyst. Anaesth. Intensive Care *17*:211-212, 1989.

130. Margolis, C. Z., Colletti, R. B., and Grundy, G.: *Haemophilus influenzae* type b: The etiologic agent in epiglottitis. J. Pediatr. *87*:322-323, 1975.

131. Margolis, C. Z., Ingram, D. L., and Meyer, J. H.: Routine tracheotomy in *Haemophilus influenzae* type b epiglottitis. J. Pediatr. *81*:1150-1153, 1972.

132. Mathur, K. K., and Mortelliti, A. J.: *Candida* epiglottitis. Ear Nose Throat J. *83*:13, 2004.

133. Mayo Smith, M. F., Hirsch, P. J., Wodzinski, S. F., et al.: Acute epiglottitis in adults. N. Engl. J. Med. *314*:1133-1139, 1986.

134. McGregor, A. R., Dawson, K. P., and Abbott, G. D.: Acute epiglottitis in childhood, Christchurch 1970-84. N. Z. Med. J. *98*:1011-1013, 1985.

135. McIntyre, P. B., Leeder, S. R., and Irwig, L. M.: Invasive *Haemophilus influenzae* type b disease in Sydney children 1985-1987: A population-based study. Med. J. Aust. *154*:832-837, 1991.

136. McVernon, J., Slack, M. P. E., and Ramsay, M. E.: Changes in the epidemiology of epiglottitis following introduction of *Haemophilus influenzae* type b (Hib) conjugate vaccines in England: a comparison of two data sources. Epidemiol. Infect. *134*:570-572, 2006.

137. Mehtar, S., Bangham, L., Kalmanovitch, D., Wren, M.: Adult epiglottitis due to *Vibrio vulnificus*. Br. Med. J. (Clin. Res. Ed.) *296*:827-828, 1988.

138. Midwinter, K. I., Hodgson, D., and Yardley, M.: Paediatric epiglottitis: The influence of the *Haemophilus influenzae* b vaccine, a ten-year review in the Sheffield region. Clin. Otolaryngol. *24*:447-448, 1999.

139. Milko, D. A., Marshak, G., and Striker, T. W.: Nasotracheal intubation in the treatment of acute epiglottitis. Pediatrics *53*:674-677, 1974.

140. Mitchell, D. B., and Drake-Lee, A. B.: Chronic nonspecific granulomatous epiglottitis. J. Laryngol. Otol. *99*:1305-1308, 1985.

141. Molteni, R. A.: Epiglottitis: Incidence of extraepiglottis infection: Report of 72 cases and review of the literature. Pediatrics *58*:526-531, 1976.

142. Murphy, T. V., Granoff, D. M., Pierson, L. M., et al.: Invasive *Haemophilus influenzae* type b disease in children <5 years of age in Minnesota and in Dallas County, Texas, 1983-1984. J. Infect. Dis. *165*(Suppl. 1):S7-S10, 1992.

143. Murphy, T. V., Osterholm, M. T., Pierson, L. M., et al.: Prospective surveillance of *Haemophilus influenzae* disease in Dallas County, Texas, and in Minnesota. Pediatrics *79*:173-180, 1987.

144. Musharrafieh, U. M., Araj, G. F., and Fuleihan, N. S.: Viral supraglottitis in an adult: A case presentation and literature update. J. Infect. 39:157-160, 1999.
145. Myer, C. M., 3rd.: *Candida* epiglottitis: Clinical implications. Am. J. Otolaryngol. 18:428-430, 1997.
146. Nelson, K., Watanakunakorn, C., and Watkins, D. A.: Acute epiglottitis due to serogroup Y *Neisseria meningitidis* in an adult. Clin. Infect. Dis. 23:1192-1193, 1996.
147. Nguyen, R., and Leclerc, J.: Cervical necrotizing fasciitis as a complication of acute epiglottitis. J. Otolaryngol. 26:129-131, 1997.
148. Nussbaum, E.: Fiberoptic laryngoscopy as a guide to tracheal extubation in acute epiglottitis. J. Pediatr. 102:269-270, 1983.
149. O'Bier, A., Muniz, A. E., and Foster, R. L.: Hereditary angioedema presenting as epiglottitis. Ped. Emerg. Care 21:27-30, 2005.
150. Oh, T. H., and Motoyama, E. K.: Comparison of nasotracheal intubation and tracheostomy in management of acute epiglottitis. Anaesthesiology 46:214-216, 1977.
151. Park, K. W., Darvish, A., and Lowenstein, E.: Airway management for adult patients with acute epiglottitis: A 12-year experience at an academic medical center (1984-1995). Anesthesiology 88:254-261, 1998.
152. Peltola, H.: *Haemophilus influenzae* type b disease and vaccination in Europe: Lessons learned. Pediatr. Infect. Dis. J. 17:S126-S132, 1998.
153. Perrone, J. A.: Laryngeal obstruction due to *Monilia albicans* in a newborn. Laryngoscope 80:288-291, 1970.
154. Quigley, C., Kaczmarski, E. B., Jones, D. M., et al.: *Haemophilus influenzae* type b disease in north-west England. J. Infect. 26:215-220, 1993.
155. Rabe, E. F.: Infectious croup: III. *Haemophilus influenzae* type b croup. Pediatrics 2:559-566, 1948.
156. Rapkin, R. H.: The diagnosis of epiglottitis: Simplicity and reliability of radiographs of the neck in the differential diagnosis of the croup syndrome. J. Pediatr. 80:96-98, 1972.
157. Rapkin, R. H.: Nasotracheal intubation in epiglottitis. Pediatrics 56:110-112, 1975.
158. Rapkin, R. H.: Simultaneous uvulitis and epiglottitis. JAMA. 243:1843, 1980.
159. Richens, J., and Montgomery, J.: Acute epiglottitis (supraglottitis) in the puerperium caused by infection with group A *Streptococcus*. Papua New Guinea Med. J. 31:293-294, 1988.
160. Ridgeway, N. A., Verghese, A., Perlman, P. E., et al.: Epiglottic abscess due to group B *Streptococcus* communication. Ann. Otol. Rhinol. Laryngol. 93:277-278, 1984.
161. Rivera, M., Hadlock, F. P., and O'Meara, M. I.: Pulmonary edema secondary to acute epiglottitis. A. J. R. Am. J. Roentgenol. 132:991-992, 1979.
162. Robbins, J. P., and Fitz-Hugh, G. S.: Epiglottitis in the adult. Laryngoscope 81:700-706, 1971.
163. Rose, F. E., Garman, R. F., Falkenberg, K. J., et al.: Adult epiglottitis, cellulitis and *Streptococcus pneumoniae* bacteremia. Scand. J. Infect. Dis. 14:301-302, 1982.
164. Rothstein, S. G., Persky, M. S., Edelman, B. A., et al.: Epiglottitis in AIDS patients. Laryngoscope 99:389-392, 1989.
165. Russell, G. A., Gresham, G. A., and Wight, D. G. D.: Acute epiglottitis in adults not due to *Haemophilus*. J. Laryngol. Otol. 99:1035-1038, 1985.
166. Santosham, M., and Moxon, E. R.: Detection and quantitation of bacteremia in childhood. J. Pediatr. 91:719-721, 1977.
167. Scheidemandel, H. H. E., and Page, R. S.: Special considerations in epiglottitis in children. Laryngoscope 85:1738-1745, 1975.
168. Scheifele, D. W., Daum, R. S., Syriopoulou, V., et al.: Comparison of two antigen detection techniques in a primate model of H. influenzae type b infection. Infect. Immun. 26:827-831, 1979.
169. Schiffman, F. J., and Lichtman, H. C.: Paroxysmal precordial purring sign in epiglottitis. Lancet 335:609, 1990.
170. Schuh, S., Huang, A., and Fallis, J. C.: Atypical epiglottitis. Ann. Emerg. Med. 17:168-170, 1988.
171. Schuller, D. E., and Birch, H. G.: The safety of intubation in croup and epiglottitis: An eight-year follow-up. Laryngoscope 85:33-46, 1975.
172. Schultes, A., and Agia, G. A.: Acute *Haemophilus parainfluenzae* epiglottitis in an adult. Postgrad. Med. 75:207-211, 1984.
173. Schultz, R. L., and Morrison, W. V.: Short term intubation in children with acute epiglottitis. South. Med. J. 75:158-160, 1982.
174. Schumaker, H. M., Doris, P. E., and Birnbaum, G.: Radiographic parameters in adult epiglottitis. Ann. Emerg. Med. 13:588-590, 1984.
175. Schwam, E., and Cox, J.: Fulminant meningococcal supraglottitis: An emerging infectious syndrome? Emerg. Infect. Dis. 5:464-467, 1999.
176. Schwartz, R. H., Knerr, R. J., Hermansen, K., et al.: Acute epiglottitis caused by β-hemolytic group C streptococci. Am. J. Dis. Child. 136:558-559, 1982.
177. Scully, R. E., Galdabini, J. J., and McNeely, B. U.: Presentation of case. N. Engl. J. Med. 297:878-883, 1977.
178. Shackelford, G. D., Siegel, M. J., and McAlister, W. H.: Subglottic edema in acute epiglottitis in children. A. J. R. Am. J. Roentgenol. 131:603-605, 1978.
179. Shalit, M., Gross, D. J., and Levo, Y.: Pneumococcal epiglottitis in systemic lupus erythematosus on high-dosage corticosteroids. Ann. Rheum. Dis. 41:615-616, 1982.
180. Shann, F. A., Phelan, P. D., Stocks, J. G., et al.: Prolonged nasotracheal intubation of tracheostomy in acute laryngotracheobronchitis and epiglottitis? Aust. Paediatr. J. 11:212-217, 1975.

181. Sharma, N., Berman, D. M., Scott, G. B., et al.: *Candida* epiglottitis in an adolescent with acquired immunodeficiency syndrome. Pediatr. Infect. Dis. J. 24:91-92, 2005.
182. Shih, L., Hawkins, D. B., and Stanley, R. B., Jr.: Acute epiglottitis in adults: A review of 48 cases. Ann. Otol. Rhinol. Laryngol. 97:527-529, 1988.
183. Sinclair, S. E.: *Haemophilus influenzae* type b in acute laryngitis with bacteremia. JAMA. 117:170-173, 1941.
184. Singer, J. I., and McCabe, J. B.: Epiglottitis at the extremes of age. Am. J. Emerg. Med. 6:228-231, 1988.
185. Sivalingam, P., and Tully, A. M.: Acute meningococcal epiglottitis and septicaemia in a 65-y-old man. Scand. J. Infect. Dis. 30:196-198, 1998.
186. Slack, C. L., Allen, G. C., Morrison, J. E., et al.: Post-varicella epiglottitis and necrotizing fasciitis. Pediatrics 105:e13, 2000.
187. Slovis, T. L., and Arcinue, E.: Subglottic edema in acute epiglottitis in children. Letter. A. J. R. Am. J. Roentgenol. 132:500, 1979.
188. Sly, P. D., Landau, L. I., and Wagener, J. S.: Acute epiglottitis in childhood: Report of an increased incidence in Victoria. Aust. N. Z. J. Med. 14:131-134, 1984.
189. Smith, E. W. P., and Ingram, D. L.: Counterimmunoelectrophoresis in *Haemophilus influenzae* type b epiglottitis and pericarditis. J. Pediatr. 85:571-573, 1975.
190. Soliman, M. G., and Richer, P.: Epiglottitis and pulmonary edema in children. Can. Anaesth. Soc. J. 25:270-276, 1978.
191. Solomon, P., Weisbrod, M., Irish, J. C., et al.: Adult epiglottitis: The Toronto Hospital experience. J. Otolaryngol. 27:332-336, 1998.
192. Stanley, R. E., and Liange, T. S.: Acute epiglottitis in adults (the Singapore experience). J. Otolaryngol. 102:1017-1021, 1988.
193. Stuart, M. J., and Hodgetts, T. J.: Adult epiglottitis: Prompt diagnosis saves lives. BMJ. 308:329-330, 1994.
194. Sullivan, T. D., La Scotea, L. J., and Neter, E.: Relationship between the magnitude of bacteremia and the clinical disease. Pediatrics 69:669-702, 1982.
195. Takala, A., Eskola, J., and Alphen, L.: Spectrum of invasive *Haemophilus influenzae* type b disease in adults. Arch. Intern. Med. 150:2573-2576, 1990.
196. Takala, A., Eskola, J., Bol, P., et al.: *Haemophilus influenzae* type b strains of outer membrane subtypes 1 and 1c cause different types of invasive disease. Lancet 2:647-649, 1987.
197. Takala, A. K., Sarvas, H., Kela, E., et al.: Susceptibility to invasive *Haemophilus influenzae* type b disease and the immunoglobulin G2m(n) allotype. J. Infect. Dis. 163:637-639, 1991.
198. Tejani, A., Mahadevan, R., Dobias, B., et al.: Occurrence of HLA types in H. influenzae type b disease. Tissue Antigens 17:205-211, 1981.
199. Templer, J. W.: Trauma to the larynx and cervical trachea. *In* English, G. M. (ed.): Otolaryngology. Hagerstown, MD, Harper & Row, 1976.
200. Theisen, D. F.: Angina epiglottidea anterior: Report of three cases. Albany Med. Ann. 21:395-405, 1900.
201. Tos, M.: Nasotracheal intubation instead of tracheotomy in acute epiglottitis in children. Acta Otolaryngol. 75:382-383, 1973.
202. Travis, K. W., Todres, I. D., and Shannon, D. C.: Pulmonary edema associated with croup and epiglottitis. Pediatrics 59:695-698, 1977.
203. Trollfors, B.: Invasive *Haemophilus influenzae* infections in household contacts of patients with *Haemophilus influenzae* meningitis and epiglottitis. Acta Paediatr. Scand. 80:795-797, 1991.
204. Trollfors, B., Brorson, J. E., Clarsson, B., et al.: Invasive infections caused by *Haemophilus* species other than *Haemophilus influenzae* infection. Infection 13:12-14, 1985.
205. Trollfors, B., Nylen, O., Carenfelt, C., et al.: Aetiology of acute epiglottitis in adults. Scand. J. Infect. Dis. 30:49-51, 1998.
206. Trollfors, B., Nylen, O., and Strangert, K.: Acute epiglottitis in children and adults in Sweden 1981-1983. Arch. Dis. Child. 65:491-494, 1990.
207. Tveteras, K., and Kristensen, S.: Acute epiglottitis in adults: Bacteriology and therapeutic principles. Clin. Otolaryngol. 12:337-343, 1987.
208. Tyler, D. C., and Haas, J. E.: Airway obstruction due to epiglottic lymphangiectasis: A case report. Int. J. Pediatr. Otorhinol. 6:285-289, 1983.
209. Valdepena, H. G., Wald, E. R., Rose, E., et al.: Epiglottitis and *Haemophilus influenzae* immunization: The Pittsburgh experience. A five-year review. Pediatrics 96:424-427, 1995.
210. Vauthy, P. A., and Reddy, R.: Acute upper airway obstruction in infants and children: Evaluation by the fiberoptic bronchoscope. Ann. Otol. Rhinol. Laryngol. 89:417-418, 1980.
211. Vernham, G. A., and Crowther, J. A.: Acute myeloid leukaemia presenting with acute *Branhamella catarrhalis* epiglottitis. J. Infect. 26:93-95, 1993.
212. Vernon, D. D., and Sarnaik, A. P.: Acute epiglottitis in children: A conservative approach to diagnosis and management. Crit. Care Med. 14:23-25, 1986.
213. Vetto, R. R.: Epiglottitis: A report of thirty-seven cases. JAMA. 173:990-994, 1960.
214. Walsh, T. J., and Gray, W. C.: *Candida* epiglottitis in immunocompromised patients. Chest 91:482-485, 1987.
215. Ward, J.: *Haemophilus influenzae*. *In* Feigin, R. D., and Cherry, J. D. (eds.): Textbook of Pediatric Infectious Diseases. 4th ed. Philadelphia, W. B. Saunders, 1998.
216. Ward, J. I., Lum, M. K. W., Margolis, H. S., et al.: *Haemophilus influenzae* disease in Alaskan Eskimos: Characteristics of a population with an unusual incidence of invasive disease. Lancet 1:1281-1285, 1981.

217. Ward, J. I., Siber, G. R., Scheifele, D. W., et al.: Rapid diagnosis of *Haemophilus influenzae* type b infections by latex particle agglutination and counterimmunoelectrophoresis. J. Pediatr. *93*:37-42, 1978.
218. Warner, J. A., and Finlay, W. E. I.: Fulminating epiglottitis in adults: Report of three cases and review of the literature. Anaesthesia *40*:348-352, 1985.
219. Warshawski, J., Havas, T. E., McShane, D. P., et al.: Adult epiglottitis. J. Otolaryngol. *15*:362-364, 1986.
220. Watts, F. B., Jr., and Slovis, T. L.: The enlarged epiglottis. Pediatr. Radiol. *5*:133-136, 1977.
221. Weber, M. L., Desjardins, R., Perreault, G., et al.: Acute epiglottitis in children: Treatment with nasotracheal intubation: Report of 14 consecutive cases. Pediatrics *57*:152-155, 1976.
222. Wenger, J. K.: Supraglottitis and group A *Streptococcus*. Pediatr. Infect. Dis. J. *16*:1005-1007, 1997.
223. Westerman, E. L., and Hutton, J. P.: Acute uvulitis associated with epiglottitis. Arch. Otolaryngol. Head Neck Surg. *112*:448-449, 1986.
224. Wetmore, R. F., and Handler, S. D.: Epiglottitis: Evolution in management during the last decade. Ann. Otol. *88*:822-826, 1979.

225. Whisnant, J. K., Rogentine, G. N., Gralnick, M. A., et al.: Host factors and antibody response in *Haemophilus influenzae* type b meningitis and epiglottitis. J. Infect. Dis. *133*:448-455, 1976.
226. Wolf, M., Strauss, B., Kronenberg, J., et al.: Conservative management of adult epiglottitis. Laryngoscope *100*:183-185, 1990.
227. Wood, N., Menzies, R., and McIntyre, P.: Epiglottitis in Sydney before and after the introduction of vaccination against *Haemophilus influenzae* type b disease. Intern. Med. J. *35*:530-535, 2005.
228. Young, N., Finn, A., and Powell, C.: Group B streptococcal epiglottitis. Pediatr. Infect. Dis. J. *15*:95-96, 1996.
229. Yousefzadeh, D. K., Tewfik, H. H., and Franken, E. A.: Epiglottic enlargement following radiation treatment and head and neck tumors. Pediatr. Radiol. *10*:165-168, 1981.
230. Yousuf, K., Lui, B., Lemckert, R., et al.: Recurrent adult epiglottitis: Contiguous spread from group A streptococcus lingual tonsillitis. J. Otol. *35*:65-67, 2006.
231. Zwahlen, A., and Regamy, C.: Les épiglottites aiguës de l'adulte. Schweiz. Med. Wochenschr. *108*:447-482, 1978.

CHAPTER 22

CROUP (LARYNGITIS, LARYNGOTRACHEITIS, SPASMODIC CROUP, LARYNGOTRACHEOBRONCHITIS, BACTERIAL TRACHEITIS, AND LARYNGOTRACHEOBRONCHOPNEUMONITIS)

James D. Cherry

The term *croup* is used to identify several different respiratory illnesses characterized by varying degrees of inspiratory stridor, cough, and hoarseness resulting from obstruction in the region of the larynx. The etiology of croup syndromes is diverse, and the consideration of noninfectious possibilities in the differential diagnosis is of major importance. Table 22–1 classifies etiologic considerations in supraglottic, laryngeal, and infraglottic acute obstructions.

Epiglottitis (see Chapter 21) and diphtheria (see Chapter 101) are mentioned here only for historical perspective and as a consideration in differential diagnosis. Croup is discussed under the subheadings of laryngitis, laryngotracheitis, spasmodic croup, laryngotracheobronchitis, bacterial tracheitis, and laryngotracheobronchopneumonitis.

TABLE 22–1 Clinical Considerations in Acute Supraglottic, Laryngeal, and Infraglottic Obstructions

Infectious
Acute epiglottitis
Laryngitis
Laryngeal diphtheria
Laryngotracheitis
Laryngotracheobronchitis
Laryngotracheobronchopneumonitis
Bacterial tracheitis
Spasmodic croup

Mechanical
Foreign body
Secondary to trauma resulting from intubation
Extrinsic or intrinsic mass

Allergic
Acute angioneurotic edema

Data from references 33, 34, 42, 69, 73, 74, 162, 179, 239.

HISTORICAL ASPECTS

The word *croup* is derived from the Anglo-Saxon word *kropan*, "to cry aloud."[55] Until the 20th century, most crouplike illnesses were thought to be diphtheria. Diphtheritic croup is an ancient disease that has been traced to the time of Homer. The historical trail of diphtheria disappeared in the 5th century and did not reappear until 1100 years later. In the 16th century, epidemics were noted in Europe. Top[217] credits Bretonneau for differentiating diphtheritic croup from spasmodic croup in 1826. In the middle third of the 20th century, the history of croup was marked by three important events: (1) the rapid decline in incidence of diphtheria associated with the use of toxoid; (2) the introduction and widespread use of antibiotics; and (3) the advent of tissue culture techniques, resulting in the establishment of viruses as etiologic agents. After these three events occurred, a prevalent academic view was that all croup was of viral etiology, and bacteria generally were dismissed as causative agents.[36,42,64,180] A careful review of many publications from the first half of the 20th century indicates, however, a causative role for several bacteria, in addition to *Corynebacterium diphtheriae*, in croup.* Bacterial croup (bacterial tracheitis) was rediscovered in 1979.†

In the 1940s, Davison[48] separated spasmodic croup from other, more severe forms of croup. The clinical and pathologic aspects of this entity were poorly defined, and today it often is not separated clinically from more severe forms of croup.

---

*See references 9, 19, 20, 48, 49, 68, 81, 102, 110, 150, 161, 167, 184, 185.
†See references 33, 34, 39, 53, 58, 59, 63, 65, 67, 85, 89, 91, 98, 111, 116, 136, 137, 148, 153, 160, 162, 201, 208, 209, 213, 227, 236.

TABLE 22–2 Classification and Definition of Infectious Illnesses Involving the Larynx and Infraglottic Region

Category	Other Terms	Definitions
Laryngitis		Inflammation of larynx resulting in hoarseness; usually occurs in older children and adults in association with common upper respiratory viral infection
Laryngeal diphtheria	Membranous croup, true croup, diphtheritic croup	Infection involving larynx and other areas of upper and lower airway due to *Corynebacterium diphtheriae*, resulting in gradually progressive obstruction of airway and associated inspiratory stridor
Laryngotracheitis	False croup, virus croup, acute obstructive subglottic laryngitis	Inflammation of larynx and trachea usually caused by infection with parainfluenza and influenza viruses
Laryngotracheobronchitis and laryngotracheobronchopneumonitis	Membranous laryngotracheobronchitis, pseudomembranous croup	Inflammation of larynx, trachea, and bronchi or lung or both; usually similar in onset to laryngotracheitis, but more severe illness; bacterial infection frequently has causative role
Bacterial croup	Bacterial tracheitis, membranous croup, membranous tracheitis, membranous laryngotracheobronchitis, pseudomembranous croup	Severe form of laryngotracheitis, laryngotracheobronchitis, or laryngotracheobronchopneumonitis due to bacterial infection
Spasmodic croup	Spasmodic laryngitis, catarrhal spasm of the larynx, subglottic allergic edema	Illness characterized by sudden onset at night of inspiratory stridor; associated with mild upper respiratory infection without inflammation or fever but with edema in subglottic region

Data from references 33, 50, 69, 162.
Modified from Cherry, J. D.: Acute epiglottitis, laryngitis, and croup. In Remington, J. S., and Swartz, M. N. (eds.): Current Clinical Topics in Infectious Diseases. Vol. 2. New York, McGraw-Hill, 1981. Reproduced with permission of The McGraw-Hill Companies.

TERMINOLOGY

The terminology and classification of infectious illnesses involving the larynx and infraglottic region have evolved over time. Classifications often have mixed etiologic systems with anatomic systems and have led to confusion. Croup often has been presented in articles under the heading of *laryngotracheobronchitis* when the authors actually were discussing laryngotracheitis and spasmodic croup.[112,138,149,176,188,196,214] The term *membranous croup* has been used as the title for articles dealing with bacterial croup.[53,89] This use is confusing because membranous croup historically was diphtheria. Many articles dealing with bacterial croup also have been titled *bacterial tracheitis*.* This term seems inappropriate because most cases of bacterial croup seen today have lower respiratory tract involvement in addition to tracheal findings. Table 22–2 lists the classifications and definitions used in this chapter. In the present era, the physician's knowledge of the clinical symptoms of croup and of the relationship of history and physical findings to the needs of therapy and general prognosis basically has declined.

ETIOLOGY

The etiologic agents in laryngitis, laryngotracheitis, spasmodic croup, laryngotracheobronchitis, and laryngotracheobronchopneumonitis are presented by frequency and severity of illness in Table 22–3. Laryngitis is a common manifestation of infection with many respiratory viruses in older children, adolescents, and adults. Outbreaks of laryngitis in closed population groups (e.g., boarding schools and military training camps) most frequently are caused by adenovirus types 4 and 7, and community outbreaks most often are noted in association with epidemic influenza. Sporadic instances of laryngitis most often are caused by adenoviral infections. Laryngitis also has been reported in association

with group A streptococcal infections; the incidence of this association has varied from 2 to 40 percent.[17,155,222]

Generally accepted today is that acute laryngotracheitis and spasmodic croup, which rarely are differentiated clinically, are caused by infection with many different viruses. Although numerous studies of respiratory viral infection exist, almost no attempt has been made to delineate the differences in etiologic spectrum by severity of illness.

Parainfluenza virus type 1 is the most common cause of acute laryngotracheitis and is responsible for frequent and clearly delineated fall and winter epidemics. Croup with parainfluenza type 2 virus seldom is severe but occasionally is related to small outbreaks. Parainfluenza virus type 3 is a frequent cause of sporadic but severe illness.

The most severe laryngotracheitis has been noted in association with influenza A viral infections. Respiratory syncytial virus and several different adenoviruses frequently are isolated in croup. Generally, these illnesses are not severe, but lower respiratory involvement occasionally is a problem. Laryngeal, tracheal, and bronchial involvement commonly occurs in measles.[36] Although rhinoviruses, *Mycoplasma pneumoniae*, enteroviruses, herpes simplex virus, and reoviruses have been associated with croup, they generally cause only minimal distress. More recently, croup has been noted in association with infection with the novel coronavirus NL63, human bocavirus,[8a] and human metapneumovirus.[5a,38,224] Recurrent croup may be due to infection with a human papillomavirus.[239]

Bacteria, other than *Haemophilus influenzae* in epiglottitis and *C. diphtheriae* in membranous croup, generally were dismissed as causative agents in croup until more recently.[42,64,180] Many publications on laryngotracheobronchitis from the first half of the 20th century indicate a role for several common bacterial pathogens.* In 1979, bacterial croup was rediscovered,[111] and numerous reports of this illness have been published since then.†

*See references 39, 58, 59, 63, 65, 67, 98, 111, 116, 136, 137, 160, 201, 227, 236.

*See references 9, 19, 20, 39, 47, 48, 58, 65, 68, 81, 85, 102, 110, 150, 161, 167, 184, 185, 208, 213, 227.
†See references 11, 53, 59, 63, 67, 89, 91, 98, 116, 136, 137, 148, 153, 160, 162, 201, 209, 236.

TABLE 22-3 Etiologic Agents in Laryngitis, Spasmodic Croup, Laryngotracheitis, Laryngotracheobronchitis, and Laryngotracheobronchopneumonitis Presented by Frequency and Severity of Illness

Category	Etiologic Agents	Frequency*	Associated with Outbreaks	Severity†	References
Laryngitis	Adenoviruses				
	Types 4 and 7	++++	Yes	+ to +++	46, 97, 222, 306
	Types 2, 3, 5, 8, 11, 14, and 21	+++	No	+ to +++	
	Influenza viruses	++++	Yes	+ to ++++	6, 97, 169, 222
	Parainfluenza viruses				
	Type 1	++	Yes	+ to +++	97, 222
	Types 2 and 3	+	Yes	+ to ++	
	Coronavirus	++	Yes	++	8
	Rhinoviruses and respiratory syncytial virus	++	No	+ to ++	84, 155, 163, 198
	Enteroviruses	+	No	+	97, 222
	Streptococcus pyogenes	+ to +++	Yes	+ to ++	17, 155
Laryngotracheitis and spasmodic croup	Parainfluenza viruses	++++		+ to +++	12, 28-30, 32, 54, 56, 78, 79, 82, 92, 96, 99, 128, 133, 139, 140, 143, 158, 169, 173, 174, 177, 225
	Type 1	++++	Yes		
	Type 2	++	Yes		
	Type 3	++	No		
	Influenza viruses	++			22, 28, 29, 32, 54, 56, 66, 72, 78, 82, 99, 100, 139, 143, 158, 169, 173, 174, 177, 225
	Type A	+++	Yes	+ to ++++	
	Type B	+	Yes	+ to ++	
	Respiratory syncytial virus	++	No	+ to ++	27-30, 32, 54, 56, 77, 78, 82, 99, 128, 140, 154, 173, 174, 176, 218, 226, 232, 237
	Human metapneumovirus	++	Yes	+	5a
	Coronavirus	++	Yes	++	38, 224
	Human bocavirus	+	No	+	8a
	Measles virus	++	Yes	+ to +++	36
	Adenoviruses	++	No	+ to ++	16, 28-30, 32, 54, 82, 96, 99, 128, 133, 139, 140, 158, 173, 174, 176, 204, 218, 225, 226
	Unspecified types and types 1, 2, 3, 5, 6, and 7				
	Rhinoviruses	+	No	+	32, 78, 112, 139, 158
	Mycoplasma pneumoniae	+	No	+	28, 30, 32, 54-56, 82, 99, 140
	Enteroviruses	+	No	+	29, 36, 43, 77, 78, 82, 99, 107, 139, 154, 205, 218, 232
	Coxsackievirus type A9	+	No	+	
	Coxsackievirus types B4 and B5	+	No	+	
	Echoviruses types 4, 11, and 21	+	No	+	
	Herpes simplex viruses	+	No	+	99, 104, 129, 158, 205
	Reoviruses	+	No	+	237
	Human papillomavirus	+	No	+ to +++	239
Laryngotracheobronchitis and laryngotracheobronchopneumonitis	Parainfluenza viruses types 1, 2, and 3	+	No	+++	19, 77, 83, 96, 140, 150, 171, 173
	Influenza viruses types A and B	+	No	++++	66, 72, 100, 174
	Staphylococcus aureus, *S. pyogenes*, *Streptococcus pneumoniae*, *Haemophilus influenzae*, and *Moraxella catarrhalis*	++	No	++++	9, 11, 19, 20, 47, 48, 53, 59, 63, 67, 68, 81, 89, 91, 98, 102, 110, 111, 116, 136, 137, 148, 149, 161, 162, 167, 184, 185, 201, 236
	Other bacteria	±	No	++++	67, 89, 94, 116, 136, 153, 236
	Cryptosporidium	−	No	++	90

*++++, most frequent; +++, frequent; ++, occasional; +, rare; −, questionable.
†++++, most severe; +++, severe; ++, not severe; +, minimal distress.

In the reports from the preantibiotic era, *Streptococcus pyogenes* was the pathogen implicated most frequently. Since 1979, *Staphylococcus aureus* has been the agent implicated most commonly. Other important bacteria are *Streptococcus pneumoniae* and *H. influenzae*. More recently, *Moraxella catarrhalis* has been found to be the causative agent in several cases.[11,67,116,236] In most instances, bacterial croup is likely to be the result of bacterial superinfection in viral disease.* *Cryptosporidium* also has been recovered from the trachea of an infant with a subacute illness.[90]

EPIDEMIOLOGY

Croup accounts for approximately 15 percent of lower respiratory tract disease seen in pediatric practice. In a large 11-year study in a pediatric practice in Chapel Hill, North Carolina, Denny and associates[56] noted the incidence of croup by age and sex. The highest attack rate occurred in children 7 to 36 months of age. Few cases occurred after the sixth birthday. Hoekelman[94] studied the occurrence of illness prospectively in 246 full-term, first-born, well infants during their first year of life. Three infants (1.2%) had croup during the study year. The analysis of a pediatric practice with approximately 3000 active records and approximately 10,000 yearly visits of children younger than 5 years old disclosed five cases of croup in a group of 50 consecutive hospitalized patients.[18]

Although croup occurs occasionally in older children, most cases occur within the first 3 years of life. A review of 211 children hospitalized for croup during a 2-year period at Cardinal Glennon Memorial Hospital for Children in St. Louis showed that 26 percent of the cases were in infants younger than 1 year old, and 73 percent were in children younger than 3 years.[75] Similar data on age have been reported by others.[56,64,69,188,195]

Croup occurs more commonly in boys than in girls.[56] In our studies, two of every three hospitalized children were boys.[75] Berg,[10] Kravitz,[130] and Rosales and Davenport[188] noted similar sex-related illness ratios. Figure 22–1 shows the 3-year seasonal pattern of croup as manifested by emergency department visits at Cardinal Glennon Memorial Hospital for Children. In each of the years, late fall–early winter peaks occurred. In the Chapel Hill studies, an increase was noted in the number of croup cases beginning in September, with a peak in October and November and then a decrease during the next 7-month period.[56] In a 2-year emergency department study in Toronto involving 1700 cases, the peak month of visits and hospital admissions was found to be October.[195] Marx and associates[144] reviewed the National Hospital Discharge Survey data for hospitalizations for croup between 1979 and 1993. They also examined Centers for Disease Control and Prevention laboratory-based surveillance data and published reports with virus isolation studies. Major peaks in hospitalizations for croup occurred in October of odd-number years at the time of peak parainfluenza virus type 1 activity. Minor peaks in hospitalizations for croup occurred each year in February when influenza A, influenza B, and respiratory syncytial viral infections were common occurrences. Epidemic peaks of acute laryngotracheitis reflect community-wide activity with parainfluenza 1 and 2 viruses or influenza A or B outbreaks.[56,83,144]

In the Toronto study, the time of the visit to the emergency department was analyzed.[195] The peak number of visits occurred between 10 P.M. and 4 A.M. During this period, approximately 17 percent of the children seen were admitted to the hospital. In contrast, of children seen between noon and 6 P.M., approximately 50 percent were admitted to the hospital. A study of croup hospitalizations in Ontario over 14 years from

*See references 23, 39, 63, 89, 110, 137, 148, 159, 160, 162, 166.

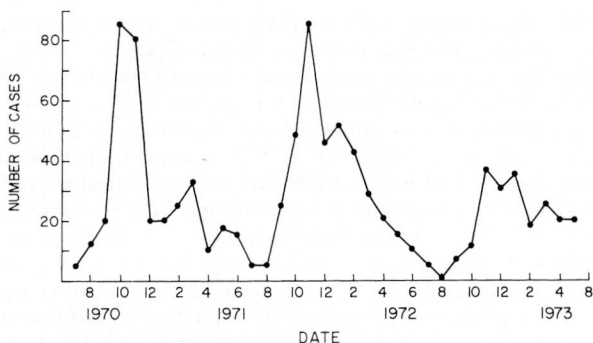

Figure 22–1 Seasonal occurrence of croup, Cardinal Glennon Memorial Hospital for Children emergency department, July 1970 to June 1973.

1988 to 2002 noted a biennial midautumn peak and an annual summer trough throughout the entire study period.[194] A striking finding in this study was a marked decrease in hospitalizations for croup after the winter of 1993-1994. This decrease continued in linear fashion for the remainder of the study duration. The authors suggest that the decreasing trend in croup hospitalizations was likely due to the increasing use of corticosteroid treatment in patients who presented to emergency departments with croup.

Because croup is caused by the same viruses that cause other respiratory illnesses, the method of spread probably is similar for all (see discussion of the common cold in Chapter 8). In children, most spread involves close person-to-person contact, with large droplets of virus-containing nasal secretions being applied to the nose from the hands of the future host or by close-range airborne acquisition. Parainfluenza viruses are common causes of colds in adults, so older individuals with trivial illnesses may be the source of more severe childhood croup.

PATHOLOGY

Laryngoscopic studies in acute laryngotracheitis reveal redness and swelling of the lateral walls of the trachea, just below the vocal cords.[48,49,211] Because the subglottic trachea is surrounded by a firm cartilaginous ring, the inflammatory swelling can occur only by encroaching on the patency of the airway; the subglottic space often is reduced to a slit 1 to 2 mm wide. As the disease progresses, the tracheal lumen becomes obstructed further by a fibrinous exudate, and its surface is covered by pseudomembranes composed of the exudative material. The vocal cords frequently are swollen, and their mobility is impaired.

Histologic study of postmortem material from the larynx and trachea reveals marked edema and cellular infiltration in the lamina propria, submucosa, and adventitia. The cellular infiltrate includes histiocytes, lymphocytes, plasma cells, and polymorphonuclear leukocytes.[19,20,157,167,185] The cotton rat model of laryngotracheitis caused by human parainfluenza virus type 3 reveals pathologic findings similar to those noted in human postmortem studies.[168] This model also indicates the time course of events. Early in the course of an infection (first 2 to 4 days), moderate mucosal and submucosal inflammatory infiltrates were noted in the subglottic and proximal tracheal regions. The infiltrates initially contained lymphocytes and neutrophils, and subsequently a mononuclear infiltrate with lymphocytes and macrophages in the submucosa was noted. Cell injury was most marked on days 6 to 8 after infection. The ciliated epithelial cells were blunted, with loss of cilia in large patches. By 12 days after infection, the region reverted to a nearly normal appearance.

The older literature indicates that classic laryngotracheobronchitis and the same disease with pneumonia represent the extension of disease from the trachea to the bronchi and alveoli. The progressive obstructive disease with exudate and pseudomembrane obstruction at the bronchial and bronchiolar levels usually is the result of secondary bacterial involvement. In bacterial croup, the tracheal wall is infiltrated with inflammatory cells, and ulceration, pseudomembranes, and microabscess formation occur.* In addition to the findings in laryngotracheitis of viral origin, thick pus is present within the lumen of the trachea and lower air passages.[91,116,136,148] Spasmodic croup is an enigma because it occurs in association with respiratory viral infections similar to those that cause more severe laryngotracheitis. Using direct laryngoscopy, Davison[49] noted that the subglottic tissues in spasmodic croup showed noninflammatory edema.

PATHOGENESIS

Although the eventual site of clinically important pathologic change in laryngotracheitis is within the larynx and trachea, the initial acquisition of infection is similar to that of other respiratory viral infections and occurs within the upper air passages, including the nasal and pharyngeal epithelial surfaces. After acquisition of virus, infection of the cells of the local respiratory epithelium develops and spreads locally to involve the larynx and trachea. The initial symptoms of nasal stuffiness and throat irritation reflect the primary sites of involvement. Studies in organ culture systems and in the cotton rat model have shown that several respiratory viruses inhibit tracheal ciliary function and eventually lead to marked destruction of the epithelium and evidence of viral infection in the lamina propria.[126,168,182] In uncomplicated croup, failure of gas exchange within the lung, in addition to hypoxia resulting from subglottic tracheal obstruction, may occur.[163,214]

Parainfluenza viruses types 1, 2, and 3 all are significant causes of respiratory infections in children (see Chapter 191). Infection with parainfluenza virus type 3 occurs in most infants, whereas infections with types 1 and 2 generally occur more frequently in older children. Only a third of children have antibodies against these two viral types by the time they reach age 4 years.

Because parainfluenza viral infections are common occurrences in young children, and because only a few get croup, host factors probably are important factors in the pathogenesis. In contrast with the numerous studies of the pathogenesis of bronchiolitis and respiratory syncytial virus infection, few similar studies relating to parainfluenza viruses and croup have been reported.[37]

The above-presented pathologic data suggest that the findings in laryngotracheitis are directly virus-related (parainfluenza viruses types 1, 2 and 3 and influenza virus types A and B) owing to the direct cytopathic effect of a virus or related to the concomitant host response or perhaps both.[37] In the cotton rat model, the use of topical steroid therapy led to a significant reduction in the degree of inflammatory infiltrates and cell injury, which suggests that the host response contributes to the pathologic findings.[168] The pathogenesis of laryngotracheobronchitis and laryngotracheobronchopneumonitis is similar to that described previously, but with the extension of infection to the lower respiratory tract and, usually, the occurrence of secondary bacterial infection.

Many studies suggest that allergic factors play a role in recurrent croup.[24,93,165,223,229,230,231,238,235] Welliver and associates[230] found that children with croup caused by parainfluenza viral infections

had titers of IgE-specific antibody in their nasopharyngeal secretions that were 3.6-fold higher than titers of similarly infected children with only upper respiratory infections. The children with croup had a cell-mediated immune response to parainfluenza virus that was 1.6-fold greater than that of the children with only upper respiratory infections.

In a subsequent review, investigators noted that an atopic disposition might be associated with the development of croup.[229] Children with croup caused by a parainfluenza virus had specific IgE antibodies and released histamine into the airway more frequently than did control patients with parainfluenzal viral upper respiratory infections. They also noted that children with recurrent croup had several atopic features, such as positive skin tests to environmental allergens, and were more likely to develop asthma when they grew older. Also, some children with a history of recurrent croup develop stridor with histamine challenge.

The above-mentioned studies by Welliver and associates[229,230] and other reports make it easy to accept a role of atopy in recurrent croup. What is difficult to explain, however, is why many apparent primary infections result in only spasmodic croup. As I have suggested previously, initial sensitization may be parainfluenza virus group–specific and not type-specific.[37] This proposal suggests that early infection (primary infection) with parainfluenza virus type 3 would set the stage for spasmodic croup with parainfluenza viral types 1 and 2. The primary infection itself could have been mild owing to transplacentally acquired antibody.

CLINICAL PRESENTATION

ACUTE LARYNGITIS

Table 22–4 summarizes clinical characteristics of laryngitis. Laryngitis is mainly a disease of older children, adolescents, and adults that is disturbing but self-limited. The specific clinical manifestation is hoarseness. Other symptoms depend on the causative infectious agent. Adenoviruses and influenza viruses cause the most severe instances of laryngitis. With these viruses, fever usually occurs, and sore throat, headache, muscle aches and pains, and prostration are common symptoms. In contrast, patients with laryngitis resulting from rhinoviral, parainfluenza viral, or respiratory syncytial viral infections have minimal or no fever and few systemic complaints. They usually have pronounced nasal symptoms (coryza and stuffiness), however. Occasionally, hoarseness may persist, which may be a result of secondary bacterial infection of the upper respiratory tract.

ACUTE LARYNGOTRACHEITIS

Although the clinical spectrum of acute laryngotracheitis varies considerably, its manifestations usually are significantly different from the manifestations of the other acute diseases with obstruction in the region of the larynx (see Table 22–4). Onset of illness usually is not alarming and suggests the onset of a cold. Initial symptoms are nasal complaints and include dryness, irritation, and coryza. Ordinary cough and the complaint of sore throat occur frequently. Fever is a usual occurrence within the first 24 hours, which is not true of the common cold. After a period as short as a few hours, but usually after 12 to 48 hours, upper airway obstructive signs and symptoms are seen. The cough first becomes "croupy" (sounding like a barking seal), and then evidence of respiratory stridor (difficulty associated with inspiration) gradually increases. Examination at this time reveals a child with a hoarse voice, coryza, a normal or minimally inflamed pharynx, and a slightly increased respiratory rate with a prolonged inspiratory phase. Temperature nearly always is between 37.8° C and 40.5° C (100° F and 105° F).

---

*See references 2, 31, 33-35, 39, 53, 58, 59, 63, 67, 85, 91, 98, 111, 116, 136-138, 162, 166, 201, 209.

TABLE 22-4 Differential Diagnosis of Acute Obstruction in the Region of the Larynx

Category	Acute Epiglottitis	Laryngeal Diphtheria	Laryngitis	Acute Laryngotracheitis	Laryngotracheobronchitis and Laryngotracheobronchopneumonitis (Including Bacterial Tracheitis)	Spasmodic Croup	Foreign Body	Acute Angioneurotic Edema
Common age of occurrence	1-8 yr	All ages	Older children and adults	3 mo to 3 yr	3 mo to 3 yr	3 mo to 3 yr	All ages	All ages
Past and family history	Not contributory	No or inadequate immunization	Not contributory	Family history of croup	May be family history of croup	Family history of croup; perhaps previous attack	Occasional history of ingestion	Allergic history; perhaps previous attack
Prodrome	Occasionally coryza	Usually pharyngitis	Usually stuffy nose or coryza	Usually coryza	Usually coryza	Minimal coryza	None	Occasionally cutaneous allergic manifestations
Onset (time to full-blown disease)	Rapid; 4-12 hr	Slowly for 2- to 3-day period	Variable; 12 hr to 4 days	Moderate but variable; 12-48 hr	Usually gradually progressive; 12 hr to 7 days	Sudden; always at night	Usually sudden	Rapid
Symptoms on presentation Fever	Yes; usually 39.5° C (103° F)	Yes; usually 37.8° C to 38.5° C (100° F to 101° F)	Yes; 37.8° C to 39.4° C (100° F to 103° F) with adenoviral and influenza viral infections; usually minimal with other viruses	Yes; variable, 37.8° C to 40.5° C (100° F to 105° F)	Yes; variable, 37.8° C to 40.5° C (100° F to 105° F)	No	No, unless secondary infection	No
Hoarseness and barking cough	No	Yes	Yes	Yes	Yes	Yes	Usually no	No
Dysphagia	Yes; usually severe	Usually yes	No	No	No	No	Frequently yes	Yes
Inspiratory stridor	Yes; moderate to severe	Yes; minimal to severe	No	Yes; minimal to severe	Yes; usually severe	Yes; moderate	Variable	Yes

TABLE 22-4   Differential Diagnosis of Acute Obstruction in the Region of the Larynx—cont'd

Category	Acute Epiglottitis	Laryngeal Diphtheria	Laryngitis	Acute Laryngotracheitis	Laryngotracheobronchitis and Laryngotracheobronchopneumonitis (Including Bacterial Tracheitis)	Spasmodic Croup	Foreign Body	Acute Angioneurotic Edema
Toxic appearance	Severe	Usually no	No	Usually minimal	Usually moderate; may be severe	No	No	No
Signs on presentation								
Oral cavity	Pharyngitis and excessive salivation	Membranous pharyngitis	Normal or mild to moderate pharyngitis	Usually minimal pharyngitis	Usually minimal pharyngitis	Normal	Normal	Pale appearance
Epiglottis	Cherry-red and swollen	Usually normal; may contain membrane	Normal	Normal	Normal	Normal	Normal	Swollen and pale
Radiographs	Swollen epiglottis on lateral film	Not useful	Not useful	Subglottic narrowing on PA film	Subglottic narrowing on PA film; irregular soft tissue densities within trachea on lateral film	Not useful	May reveal foreign body	Swollen epiglottis on lateral film
Laboratory								
Leukocyte count	Usually markedly elevated with increased percentage of band forms	Usually elevated with increased percentage of band forms	Usually normal	Mildly elevated with >70% polymorphonuclear cells	Variable; usually mildly elevated with 70% polymorphonuclear cells; may be increased band count	Normal	Normal, unless secondary infection	Normal; sometimes eosinophilia
Bacteriology	Throat and blood cultures yield *Haemophilus influenzae* type b	Smear and culture from membrane reveal organism	Usually normal flora in throat; occasionally *Streptococcus pyogenes* in throat	Only important if secondary infection suspected	Normal throat flora; tracheal culture often yields *S. pyogenes*, *Staphylococcus aureus*, *Streptococcus pneumoniae*, or *H. influenzae*	Normal flora	Only important if secondary infection suspected	Normal flora
Clinical course	Rapidly progressive; cardiorespiratory arrest occurs within hours if not treated	Slowly progressive obstruction of airway	Hoarseness persists at a constant degree about 4-7 days; occasionally persists 2-3 wk	Variable speed of progression of obstruction; usually does not require surgical intervention	Degree of obstruction usually severe; persists 7-14 days; frequently requires surgical intervention	Symptoms of short duration with treatment; repeated attacks common	Variable depending on size and substance of foreign body	Variable; sometimes leads to rapid asphyxia without therapy

Data from references 48, 49, 53, 63, 70, 76, 89, 91, 111, 136, 137, 152, 215.

The speed of progression and final degree of upper airway obstruction vary. Some children have hoarseness and barking cough but no other evidence of obstruction; in these cases, the symptoms last approximately 3 to 7 days, with a gradual return to normal. In other cases, the obstruction is progressive and leads to severe respiratory distress with supraclavicular and infraclavicular and sternal retractions, cyanosis of varying degrees, and apprehension. With hypoxia, the cardiac rate increases, and the child becomes restless. Without intervention, asphyxial death occurs rapidly in some children. In others, the problem of hypoxia is more prolonged, and respiratory fatigue may lead to the patient's demise. The duration of illness in a severely affected child, regardless of therapy, is rarely less than 7 days and frequently is 14 days.

Laboratory study in acute laryngotracheitis is of only minimal value. The white blood cell count frequently is greater than 10,000 cells/mm³, and polymorphonuclear cells predominate.[32,164] Very high white blood cell counts (>20,000/mm³) with numerous band-form neutrophils should suggest bacterial superinfection or the possibility of acute epiglottitis. The posteroanterior chest radiograph reveals the subglottic narrowing (steeple sign), and a lateral neck radiograph indicates the size of the epiglottis.

ACUTE LARYNGOTRACHEOBRONCHITIS AND LARYNGOTRACHEOBRONCHOPNEUMONITIS (BACTERIAL TRACHEITIS)

Laryngotracheobronchitis and laryngotracheobronchopneumonitis are far less common occurrences than are laryngotracheitis and spasmodic croup; however, these illnesses occur more commonly than generally realized.[*] These entities may be considered an extension of acute laryngotracheitis, as numerous descriptions in the literature suggest.[†] The severity of the illness is due to secondary bacterial infection. Initial symptoms and signs are similar to those of laryngotracheitis (see Table 22-4). An afflicted child usually has mild to moderately severe illness for 2 to 7 days and then suddenly becomes markedly worse. Occasionally, upper and lower airway obstructions seem to occur simultaneously. In many children, the distress from tracheal obstruction is of such magnitude that the symptoms and signs of lower respiratory involvement go unnoticed. Symptoms and signs associated with extension of disease to the bronchi, bronchioles, and lung substance include rales, air trapping, wheezing, and a further increase in the respiratory rate. Obstruction in these illnesses usually is of such a degree that either intubation or tracheostomy is necessary.

Several instances of laryngotracheobronchopneumonitis with toxic shock syndrome have been observed.[21,31,166,202,209] Generally, children with these staphylococcal infections initially have the onset of croup, then the more severe manifestations of bacterial tracheitis develop, and finally the exanthem and other manifestations of toxic shock syndrome develop. An infant with tracheitis and supraglottitis caused by *M. catarrhalis* has been described.[2] Other findings in laryngotracheobronchitis and laryngotracheobronchopneumonitis are presented in Table 22-4.

SPASMODIC CROUP

In recent years, the clinical entity of spasmodic croup has been incorporated by many physicians into the overall diagnosis of croup. Although distinguishing mild cases of laryngotracheitis

from spasmodic croup is difficult at the onset in some instances, the delineation of the two entities is important from prognostic and therapeutic perspectives (see Table 22-4).

Spasmodic croup occurs in children 3 months to 3 years old. The onset always is at night, and the characteristic presentation occurs in a child who previously was thought to be well or to have had a mild cold with coryza as the only symptom. The child awakens at night with sudden dyspnea, croupy cough, and inspiratory stridor. There is no fever. The symptoms apparently are the result of sudden subglottic edema; relief is achieved easily by general reassurance and administration of moist air. The occurrence of spasmodic croup tends to run in families, with repeated attacks occurring in some children. After one attack, the child is likely to have another attack the same evening and on three or four successive evenings. These attacks can be prevented by employing mild sedation at bedtime and ensuring that the bedroom air is adequately humidified.

DIFFERENTIAL DIAGNOSIS

The therapeutic approaches to the various acute obstructions in the region of the larynx vary markedly. Establishing a correct diagnosis is essential and frequently lifesaving. Table 22-4 lists the differential points of eight conditions with symptoms and signs of acute upper airway obstruction.

The most frequent serious differential diagnostic problem is the recognition of acute epiglottitis and its separation from the less fulminant laryngotracheitis. In epiglottitis (a rare disease in children today because of universal immunization with *H. influenzae* type B conjugate vaccines), the important differential points are lack of a croupy cough; the presence of a swollen, cherry-red epiglottis; the sitting posture of the child with the chin pushed forward and a reluctance or refusal to lie down; and the relatively greater apprehension and anxiety of the patient than the degree of chest retraction suggests. In contrast, a child with acute laryngotracheitis has a normal epiglottis on examination, always has a typical barking cough, is comfortable in a supine position, and frequently appears to have only minimal apprehension, despite retractions in which the sternum appears to be indenting 2 inches or more.

Early in the course of epiglottitis, the diagnosis can be confirmed only by the observation of the epiglottis, which can be done without difficulty.[127] Later in the disease, the posture of the child and the history of rapidly progressing disease render the differential from laryngotracheitis readily apparent, so examination of the epiglottis directly (a dangerous procedure if the child is forced to lie down) or indirectly by a lateral neck radiograph rarely is indicated and usually is contraindicated.

Laryngotracheobronchitis and laryngotracheobronchopneumonitis can be recognized by signs of lower respiratory involvement (rales, air trapping, wheezing, and pulmonary infiltrates on the radiograph). Bacterial disease should be suspected in laryngotracheobronchitis and laryngotracheobronchopneumonitis and when symptoms and signs become worse in laryngotracheitis. A lateral radiograph can be useful in the evaluation because it may reveal soft tissue densities within the trachea. Lateral neck and chest radiographs are regarded by many physicians as definitive tests to determine whether to rule out epiglottitis and laryngotracheitis. In a careful study by Stankiewicz and Bowes,[203] the sensitivity and specificity of both radiographs were low, however.

Although a rare occurrence today, laryngeal diphtheria always should be considered and ruled out in croup. Important in this regard are the history of immunization, the pharyngeal evidence of diphtheria, the relative slowness of the disease to progress, and a greater degree of hoarseness caused by direct laryngeal membrane formation.

---

*See references 11, 34, 39, 53, 58, 59, 63, 67, 85, 89, 91, 98, 111, 116, 136, 137, 148, 153, 160, 209, 236.
†See references 9, 19, 20, 47, 48, 68, 81, 102, 116, 150, 167, 180, 181, 184, 185.

Spasmodic croup rarely should be confused with acute laryngotracheitis, but a perusal of the literature indicates that the two entities most commonly are considered laryngotracheitis, which is unfortunate because prognostic considerations for the two entities are different. Spasmodic croup always is of sudden onset at night, occurs without fever, and is relieved by simple therapeutic modalities.

The possibility of a foreign body and angioneurotic edema always must be considered in upper airway obstructive disease. Differential points are presented in Table 22–4. Rarely, acute upper airway obstruction occurs in adolescents as a result of psychogenic and emotional factors.[80,120,192]

SPECIFIC DIAGNOSIS

The epidemiologic history frequently is an important factor in establishing a specific diagnosis. Obtaining bacterial culture specimens from the throat, laryngeal region, and blood is helpful in diagnosing epiglottitis and important in identifying laryngotracheitis, laryngotracheobronchitis, and laryngotracheobronchopneumonitis when secondary infection is suspected. The white blood cell count should be obtained because it can be helpful when secondary bacterial infection is considered.

A specific etiologic diagnosis can be made by the isolation of virus or its identification by a direct antigen test from a nasopharyngeal specimen. The diagnostic virologic facilities of many medical centers enable rapid identification of parainfluenza viruses, respiratory syncytial viruses, adenoviruses, most rhinoviruses, and influenza viruses to be established.

TREATMENT

During the last 65 years, the treatment of croup has created considerable controversy: tracheostomy versus no tracheostomy, intubation versus tracheostomy, warm versus cold humidification, antibiotics versus no antibiotics, corticosteroids versus no corticosteroids, sedation versus no sedation, and racemic epinephrine therapy versus mist therapy alone. Few of these controversies have been resolved scientifically, but the passage of time has lessened the importance of some of the discrepant opinions.

Of most importance in the evaluation of therapeutic modalities and the specific approach to therapy in croup is making an accurate differential diagnosis. A look at the most important controversy (the use of steroids) indicates that in most instances, cases of spasmodic croup, in which a favorable outcome invariably can be expected, were not separated clinically from cases of laryngotracheitis, in which the outcome is less predictable.

ACUTE LARYNGOTRACHEITIS AND SPASMODIC CROUP

In managing acute laryngotracheitis and spasmodic croup, each case must be treated individually; one child may need minimal therapy, whereas another may require consideration of all modalities. In all children with acute laryngotracheitis, attention should be given to the anxiety and apprehension of the patient and parents. The parents should be reassured immediately, and it is important that the child is not separated from them. Physical examination should be done rapidly by one physician, and all but absolutely necessary procedures should be deferred.

In the past, mist therapy was the cornerstone of management of croup. In more recent years, the value of this therapy has been questioned.[15,135,156,193] It had been my opinion, as expressed in previous editions of this book, that mist therapy in croup was useful. The results of a large randomized controlled trial[193] and the extensive review by Moore and Little[156] indicate, however, that mist treatment offers no benefit in treatment.

Oxygen should be administered to a child who is hypoxemic from respiratory distress. The studies of Newth and associates[163] and Taussig and colleagues[214] indicate that mild hypoxemia occurs more commonly than is realized clinically. The drying effect of oxygen is counterproductive to the removal of tracheal exudate, so it should not be used routinely.

Since 1952, numerous communications in the English medical literature have described the use of corticosteroids in croup. Nine double-blind, controlled studies were conducted before 1989.[61,62,107,127,132,134,199,207,210] In 1964, Eden and Larkin[62] noted no difference between control and methylprednisolone therapy in a study of 50 children with acute croup. In 1967, Eden and colleagues[61] studied another 50 patients and could find no benefit from dexamethasone compared with a control preparation. Sussman and colleagues[210] also could not show any benefit from dexamethasone therapy.

In contrast to these three studies, Skowron and coworkers[199] noted a slight benefit regarding duration of stridor, retractions, fever, and days in the hospital in a group receiving dexamethasone. They suggested, however, that steroids not be used routinely for laryngotracheitis because the overall benefits were minimal, and a potential risk exists in administration of steroids. In 1969, James[107] noted that dexamethasone-treated patients recovered from obstructive symptoms more quickly than did the control group. In another study involving 30 children, Leipzig and associates[134] concluded that dexamethasone in an adequate dose (0.3 mg/kg initially and repeated in 2 hours) given intramuscularly hastens the recovery from uncomplicated croup. This study and its predecessors have major inadequacies in design.[33,220] In a study with 72 children, Koren and colleagues[127] noted that dexamethasone did not offer any benefit to patients with laryngotracheitis but did decrease significantly the respiratory rate in children with spasmodic croup compared with placebo-treated control subjects. Although these findings were statistically significant, the benefits were not clinically significant.

Two additional modest studies of the use of dexamethasone in croup were published in 1988 and 1989, as was a meta-analysis of the evidence from the various randomized trials and a set of related editorials and a review.[4,115,132,198,200,207] Kuusela and Vesikari[132] concluded that dexamethasone was beneficial in acute spasmodic croup, and Super and associates[207] concluded that dexamethasone is beneficial in reducing the overall severity of moderate to severe acute laryngotracheitis during the first day of treatment.

The 1989 meta-analysis suggested that the use of steroids in children hospitalized with croup resulted in a significantly increased number with clinical improvement 12 hours and 24 hours after treatment and a reduced incidence of endotracheal intubation than occurred in the control subjects.[115] In this analysis, improvement at 12 hours was noted to be greater in the children who received higher initial doses of steroid (≥125 mg of cortisone) than in children who received lower doses.

In the early 1990s, nebulized steroids were evaluated in the treatment of croup, which led to another round of testimonials, controlled studies, and treatment articles supporting the efficacy of steroids.* Since the 1989 meta-analysis, more than 15 additional, controlled, steroid treatment trials have been performed, and another meta-analysis was published in 1999.[5] Finally, a large

---

*See references 5, 45, 84, 86, 101, 106, 108, 114, 122-125, 186, 187, 198, 229.

controlled trial of oral dexamethasone for mild croup was published in 2004, and a comprehensive meta-analysis was published in 2005.[13,190] Also published more recently are many articles comparing doses, types, and methods of administration of steroids and a further round of commentaries.*On the basis of the three meta-analyses and the specific studies analyzed, most reviews on the management of croup recommend the routine use of steroids (administered orally, intramuscularly, or by nebulization) in the treatment of croup.†

In the past, when I reviewed the data on the use of steroids in croup, what concerned me was that the specific clinical entity that was being treated was poorly defined and that no evidence indicated that steroids worked in any illness other than spasmodic croup.[33] Of most concern to me today is that the risks of steroid use have not been evaluated and that, because of small sample sizes in all but two of the available studies, they cannot be evaluated by meta-analysis.

I have seen lower respiratory tract complications develop in three children receiving steroid treatment for croup. In one case, an adenoviral pneumonia worsened, and in the other cases, bacterial tracheitis with pneumonia occurred. In these three cases, they all received corticosteroid treatment over the course of several days and not single-dose treatment. In the study of Super and colleagues,[207] two steroid-treated patients developed pneumonia during therapy; none of the control subjects developed pneumonia. In a more recent trial in which 28 children received nebulized dexamethasone, two children with neutropenia developed bacterial tracheitis.[108] Burton and associates[23] reported the occurrence of *Candida* laryngotracheitis as a complication of corticosteroid and antibiotic treatment in a child with croup, and Myers and colleagues[159] reported an infant who developed multiple pulmonary abscesses caused by *Legionella pneumophila* after receiving prolonged corticosteroid treatment of severe croup.

Today, the standard of care for the initial treatment of laryngotracheitis and spasmodic croup is the use of corticosteroids administered orally, intramuscularly, or by nebulization.[3,14,70] Recommended therapy is a single dose of intramuscular or oral dexamethasone. The limited use of nebulized budesonide also is effective. In the most definitive study, the treatment dose was dexamethasone (0.6 mg/kg) given orally once.[13] In a subsequent review, Bjornson and Johnson[14] noted that the standard dose of dexamethasone is 0.6 mg/kg (oral or intramuscular); they suggested that oral is preferable because absorption is excellent, and peak serum concentrations are achieved as rapidly as with intramuscular administration.

As noted earlier, I and others have observed bacterial and fungal infections as complications in children who have received multiple doses of steroids in croup. It is disturbing to me to note that in pediatric practice many children are receiving 3- to 5-day treatment courses rather than the recommended single-dose schedule. The data from the cotton rat model of human parainfluenza virus type 3 laryngotracheitis provides strong evidence supporting the limited use of steroids in croup.[168] In this model, topical steroid therapy significantly reduced the degree of inflammatory infiltrates and cell damage. The steroid therapy increased the virus load but did not prolong virus shedding.

I believe the most dramatic evidence supporting the use of steroid therapy in laryngotracheitis and spasmodic croup is the marked decrease in the number of hospitalizations for croup in Ontario, which coincided with the 1992 recommendation by the Canadian Pediatrics Society to use dexamethasone for treat-

ment.[103,194] Steroids should not be used in laryngotracheobronchitis, laryngotracheobronchopneumonitis, or epiglottitis.

Because laryngotracheitis is a disease of viral etiology, what seems apparent is that antibiotic therapy would not be indicated and consequently not employed. In our analysis of more than 200 hospitalized children with laryngotracheitis, we noted that antibiotics had been administered to 85 percent.[75] A review of the records in many instances revealed that the physician had given antibiotic therapy because the possibility of epiglottitis had not been ruled out adequately. In several instances, the epiglottis had been observed and thought to be reddened or questionably enlarged.

A second consideration with regard to antibiotic therapy in croup is that the most dramatic reduction in mortality rates coincides with the introduction and widespread use of antibiotics. In my opinion, many of the deaths attributed to croup in the preantibiotic era were caused by secondary bacterial infections. Although use of antibiotics contributed to the reduction in the number of deaths caused by croup, other factors may be important. At about the same time that antibiotics were introduced, disease caused by *S. pyogenes* decreased in incidence and severity. Reasons for the decreased frequency of streptococcal disease were not clear.

Most patients with laryngotracheitis today do not need antibiotic therapy. In severe cases in which bacterial sepsis cannot be ruled out, however, antibiotic therapy should be employed. The pathogens to consider include pneumococci, group A streptococci, *S. aureus*, and *H. influenzae*. In patients with laryngotracheitis in whom fever persists or signs change, secondary infection should be considered. In these instances, appropriate culture specimens should be obtained before therapy is initiated (see the section on laryngotracheobronchitis for specific antibiotic therapy).

The use of nebulized racemic epinephrine, which was introduced by Jordan[112] in 1966 and popularized by Jordan and other members of the Utah group,[1,113] has been adopted widely throughout the United States and elsewhere.[118,131,138,152,189,196] The usual method of nebulization of racemic epinephrine is by intermittent positive-pressure breathing. This form of therapy was associated with a marked reduction in tracheostomies in several series.

In 1973, Gardner and associates[76] performed the first double-blind, controlled study in which racemic epinephrine was nebulized by a compressor without intermittent positive-pressure breathing. They found that saline-treated patients responded as well to therapy as did the racemic epinephrine recipients. In retrospect, this study can be criticized because the investigators failed to differentiate spasmodic croup from laryngotracheitis. In 1975, Taussig and associates[214] reported a small but carefully conducted study with intermittent positive-pressure breathing and racemic epinephrine in which they noted acute improvement in all cases, recurrence of symptoms in 2 hours, and no change in partial pressure of oxygen with clinical improvement; 24 to 36 hours after therapy, treated and untreated children were clinically similar. In another significant study that involved children hospitalized with severe croup without improvement after admission to a high-humidity mist room, Westley and colleagues[233] showed that racemic epinephrine therapy caused definite short-term improvement in children compared with saline treatment. This study is particularly important because a parainfluenza viral etiology was documented in more than 65 percent of the study's subjects, and all cases were clearly laryngotracheitis and not spasmodic croup.

The following points can be made about the use of racemic epinephrine in the treatment of croup: (1) Many children with croup respond to moist air alone; (2) significant rebound occurs after racemic epinephrine therapy, so it frequently needs to be repeated many times; (3) in a hospitalized child with severe acute

*See references 14, 26, 37, 57, 70, 71, 79, 121, 142, 186, 216.
†See references 3, 13, 14, 44, 51, 52, 70, 71, 84, 86, 103, 106, 107, 121-123, 125, 186, 187, 216.

laryngotracheitis, racemic epinephrine should be used. Tracheotomy or endotracheal intubation can be prevented in some cases. The most important issue today regarding the use of racemic epinephrine is whether it can be used safely for outpatient therapy.[40,117,178] In the past, most experts advised against the use of racemic epinephrine in the outpatient setting because of the known rebound that occurs. Some data suggest that with careful observation for a sufficient period (at least 2 hours) after administration, patients can be managed safely, and the number of hospitalizations can be decreased.[40,117,178] In a small study, investigators found that the administration of a helium-oxygen mixture (heliox) resulted in improvement in children with croup similar to that with racemic epinephrine treatment.[228]

The establishment of a mechanical airway seldom is necessary today in patients with laryngotracheitis. The planned procedure has a better outcome than does the procedure performed under emergency conditions. Traditionally, tracheostomy was the preferred method when a mechanical airway was needed.[7,74,240] When careful attention is given to tube size and other aspects of placement and maintenance, however, nasotracheal intubation compares favorably with tracheostomy.[7,240] The management of a child with a mechanical airway requires trained pediatric intensive care physicians and the facilities of an adequately staffed intensive care unit.

Five antiviral drugs have activity against viruses that cause laryngotracheitis.[88,105,146,212,234] Amantadine and rimantadine are approved for use in treating influenza A viral infections, and ribavirin is active against parainfluenza viruses, influenza A and B viruses, and respiratory syncytial virus (see Chapters 251 and 190). The neuraminidase inhibitors, zanamivir and oseltamivir, are active against influenza A and B types.[25,41] At present, consideration of therapy for severe croup that occurs during documented epidemics caused by influenza A or B viruses would seem reasonable. Because of high levels of resistance of influenza A strains to amantadine and rimantadine, treatment with the neuraminidase inhibitors is recommended.[25]

LARYNGOTRACHEOBRONCHITIS AND LARYNGOTRACHEOBRONCHOPNEUMONITIS (BACTERIAL TRACHEITIS)

Generally, all the treatment considerations discussed for laryngotracheitis except corticosteroids and racemic epinephrine by aerosol apply to laryngotracheobronchitis and laryngotracheobronchopneumonitis. Most important, however, because most patients have bacterial disease, antibiotics should be administered to all patients after appropriate culture specimens are obtained. Empiric therapy should be directed against *S. aureus*, *S. pyogenes*, *S. pneumoniae*, and *H. influenzae*. At present, initial treatment with vancomycin (40 mg/kg/day intravenously every 6 hours) and a third-generation cephalosporin, such as cefotaxime (150 mg/kg/day every 6 hours intravenously), is reasonable. If methacillinsensitive *S. aureus* is isolated, treatment should be changed to oxacillin (150 mg/kg/day every 6 hours intravenously) or a similar agent.

Most children with advanced laryngotracheobronchitis or laryngotracheobronchopneumonitis need the placement of a mechanical airway. Whenever possible, this procedure should be done electively rather than as an emergency.

LARYNGITIS

Patients with laryngitis should rest their voices as much as possible. Increased fluid intake and perhaps the use of a vaporizer may help liquefy secretions and might provide symptomatic relief. Because group A streptococcal infection is a cause of lar-

yngitis, culture should be performed. If it is positive, penicillin or a suitable alternative antimicrobial agent should be administered. In children and adolescents with prolonged hoarseness, sinusitis should be considered. Radiographs of the sinuses and a quantitative culture from the nose should be performed in search of a predominant abnormal bacterial flora. If either is positive, therapy with appropriate antibiotics is indicated. If laryngeal symptoms are persistent, the child should undergo laryngoscopic examination and other appropriate studies to exclude tumor, foreign body, and other chronic diseases.

PROGNOSIS

The prognosis of acute laryngotracheitis has improved markedly during the last 50 years. Today, a child with croup only rarely requires a mechanical airway, and virtually all deaths should be preventable. The child should be observed for the following complications: hypoxemia and cardiorespiratory failure, pulmonary edema, pneumothorax and pneumomediastinum, mechanical problems caused by tracheotomies and nasotracheal tubes, and secondary bacterial infections. Children with a history of croup have a higher prevalence of increased bronchial reactivity than children without such history.[87,141,229]

PREVENTION

At present, acute laryngotracheitis is not preventable. The widespread use of influenza vaccines could reduce the incidence of croup caused by influenza A and B viruses.

REFERENCES

1. Adair, J. C., Ring, W. H., Jordan, W. S., et al.: Ten-year experience with IPPB in the treatment of acute laryngotracheobronchitis. Anesth. Analg. *50*:649-655, 1971.
2. Alligood, G. A., and Kenny, J. F.: Tracheitis and supraglottitis associated with *Branhamella catarrhalis* and respiratory syncytial virus. Pediatr. Infect. Dis. *8*:190, 1989.
3. American Academy of Pediatrics: Parainfluenza viral infections. *In* Pickering, L. K., Baker, C. J., Long, S. S., McMillan, J. A (eds.): Red Book: 2006 Report of the Committee on Infectious Diseases. 27th ed. Elk Grove Village, IL, American Academy of Pediatrics, 2006, pp. 479-481.
4. Anonymous: Steroids and croup. Lancet *2*:1134-1136, 1989.
5. Ausejo, M., Saenz, A., Pham, B., et al.: The effectiveness of glucocorticoids in treating croup: Meta-analysis. B. M. J. *319*:595-600, 1999.
5a. Baer, G., Schaad, U. B., and Heininger, U.: Clinical findings and unusual epidemiologic characteristics of human metapneumovirus infections in children in the region of Basel, Switzerland. Eur. J. Pediatr. *167*:63-69, 2008.
6. Banatvala, J. E., Reiss, B. B., Anderson, T. B., et al.: Asian influenza in 1963 in two general practices in Cambridge, England. Can. Med. Assoc. J. *93*:593-597, 1965.
7. Barker, G. A.: Current management of croup and epiglottitis. Pediatr. Clin. North Am. *26*:565-579, 1979.
8. Bastien, N., Anderson, K., Hart, L., et al.: Human coronavirus NL63 infection in Canada. J. Infect. Dis. *191*:503-506, 2005.
8a. Bastien, N., Chui, N., Robinson, J. L., et al.: Detection of human bocavirus in Canadian children in a 1-year study. J. Clin. Microbiol. *45*:610-613, 2007.
9. Baum, H. L.: Acute laryngotracheobronchitis. J. A. M. A. *91*:1097-1102, 1928.
10. Berg, R. B.: Weight and sex of children hospitalized with infectious croup: An analysis of 850 cases. Pediatrics *31*:18-21, 1963.
11. Bernstein, T., Brilli, R., and Jacobs, B.: Is bacterial tracheitis changing? A 14-month experience in a pediatric intensive care unit. Clin. Infect. Dis. *27*:458-462, 1998.
12. Bisno, A. L., Barratt, N. P., Swanston, W. H., et al.: An outbreak of acute respiratory disease in Trinidad associated with para-influenza viruses. Am. J. Epidemiol. *91*:68-77, 1970.
13. Bjornson, C. L., Klassen, T. P., Williamson, J., et al.: A randomized trial of a single dose of oral desamethasone for mild croup. N. Engl. J. Med. *351*:1306-1313, 2004.

14. Bjornson, C. L., and Johnson, D. W.: Croup—treatment update. Pediatr. Emerg. Care 21:863-873, 2005.

15. Bourchier, D., Dawson, K. P., and Ferguson, D. M.: Humidification in viral croup: A controlled trial. Aust. Paediatr. J. 20:289-291, 1984.

16. Brandt, C. D., Kim, H. W., Vargosko, A. J., et al.: Infections in 18,000 infants and children in a controlled study of respiratory tract disease, I: Adenovirus pathogenicity in relation to serologic type and illness syndrome. Am. J. Epidemiol. 90:484-500, 1969.

17. Breese, B. B.: Diagnosis of streptococcal pharyngitis. In Breese, B. B., and Hall, C. B. (eds.): Beta Hemolytic Streptococcal Diseases. Boston, Houghton Mifflin, 1978, pp. 79-96.

18. Breese, B. B., Disney, F. A., and Talpey, W.: The nature of a small pediatric group practice, Part I. Pediatrics 38:264-277, 1966.

19. Brennemann, J., Clifton, W. M., Frank, A., et al.: Acute laryngotracheobronchitis. Am. J. Dis. Child. 55:667-695, 1938.

20. Brighton, G. R.: Laryngotracheobronchitis. Ann. Otol. Rhinol. Laryngol. 49:1070-1082, 1940.

21. Britto, J., Habibi, P., Walters, S., et al.: Systematic complications associated with bacterial tracheitis. Arch. Dis. Child. 74:249-250, 1996.

22. Brocklebank, J. T., Court, S. D. M., McQuillin, J., et al.: Influenza-A infection in children. Lancet 2:497-500, 1972.

23. Burton, D. M., Seid, A. B., Kearns, D. B., et al.: Candida laryngotracheitis: A complication of combined steroid and antibiotic usage in croup. Int. J. Pediatr. Otorhinol. 23:171-175, 1992.

24. Castro-Rodriguez, J. A., Holberg, C. J., Morgan, W. J., et al.: Relation of two different subtypes of croup before age three to wheezing, atopy, and pulmonary function during childhood: a prospective study. Pediatrics 170:512-518, 2001.

25. Centers for Disease Control and Prevention: Prevention and control of influenza. M. M. W. R. Morb. Mortal. Wkly. Rep. 55(No. RR-10):1-42, 2006.

26. Cetinkaya, F., Tufekci, B. S., and Kutluk, G.: A comparison of nebulized budesonide, and intramuscular, and oral dexamethasone for treatment of croup. Int. J. Pediatr. Otorhinol. 68:453-456, 2004.

27. Chanock, R. M., Parrott, R. H., Johnson, K. M., et al.: Myxoviruses: Parainfluenza. Am. Rev. Respir. Dis. 88(Pt. 2):152-166, 1962.

28. Chanock, R., Chambon, L., Chang, W., et al.: WHO respiratory disease survey in children: A serological study. Bull. World Health Organ. 37:363-369, 1967.

29. Chanock, R. M., and Parrott, R. H.: Acute respiratory disease in infancy and childhood: Present understanding and prospects for prevention: E. Mead Johnson Address, October 1964. Pediatrics 36:21-39, 1965.

30. Chapman, R. S., Henderson, F. W., Clyde, W. A., Jr., et al.: The epidemiology of tracheobronchitis in pediatric practice. Am. J. Epidemiol. 114:786-797, 1981.

31. Chenaud, M., Leclerc, F., and Martinot, A.: Bacterial croup and toxic shock syndrome. Eur. J. Pediatr. 145:306-307, 1986.

32. Cherry, J. D.: Newer respiratory viruses: Their role in respiratory illnesses of children. In Schulman, I. (ed.): Advances in Pediatrics. Vol. 20. Chicago, Year Book Medical Publishers 1973, pp. 225-289.

33. Cherry, J. D.: The treatment of croup: Continued controversy due to failure of recognition of historic, ecologic, etiologic and clinical perspectives. J. Pediatr. 94:352-354, 1979.

34. Cherry, J. D.: Acute epiglottitis, laryngitis and croup. In Remington, J. S., and Swartz, M. N. (eds.): Current Clinical Topics in Infectious Diseases. New York, McGraw-Hill, 1981, pp. 1-30.

35. Cherry, J. D.: Croup. In Kiple, K. F. (ed.): The Cambridge World History of Human Disease. Cambridge, Cambridge University Press, 1993, pp. 654-657.

36. Cherry, J. D.: Measles. In Feigin, R. D., and Cherry, J. D. (eds.): Textbook of Pediatric Infectious Diseases. 4th ed. Philadelphia, W. B. Saunders, 1998.

37. Cherry, J. D.: State of the evidence for standard-of-care treatments for croup: Are we where we need to be? Pediatr. Infect. Dis. J. 24:S198-S202, 2005.

38. Chiu, S. S., Chan, K. H., Chu, K. W., et al.: Human coronavirus NL63 infection and other coronavirus infections in children hospitalized with acute respiratory disease in Hong Kong, China. Clin. Infect. Dis. 40:1721-1729, 2005.

39. Conley, S. F., Beste, D. J., and Hoffmann, R. G.: Measles-associated bacterial tracheitis. Pediatr. Infect. Dis. J. 12:414-415, 1993.

40. Cornell, H. M., and Bolte, R. G.: Outpatient use of racemic epinephrine in croup. Am. Fam. Phys. 46:683-684, 1992.

41. Couch, R.B.: Prevention and treatment of influenza. N. Engl. J. Med. 343:1778-1787, 2000.

42. Cramblett, H. G.: Croup: Present day concept. Pediatrics 25:1071-1076, 1960.

43. Cramblett, H. G., Moffett, H. L., Black, J. P., et al.: Coxsackie virus infections: Clinical and laboratory studies. J. Pediatr. 64:406-414, 1964.

44. Cressman, W. R., and Myer, C. M., III: Diagnosis and management of croup and epiglottitis. Pediatr. Clin. North Am. 41:265-276, 1994.

45. Cruz, M. N., Stewart, G., and Rosenberg, N.: Use of dexamethasone in the outpatient management of acute laryngotracheitis. Pediatrics 96:220-223, 1995.

46. Dascomb, H. E., and Hilleman, M. R.: Clinical and laboratory studies in patients with respiratory disease caused by adenoviruses (R1-APC-ARD agents). Am. J. Med. 21:161, 1956.

47. Davison, F. W.: Acute laryngotracheobronchitis: Further studies on treatment. Arch. Otolaryngol. 47:455-464, 1948.

48. Davison, F. W.: Acute obstructive laryngitis in children. Penn. Med. J. 53:250-254, 1950.

49. Davison, F. W.: Acute laryngeal obstruction in children. J. A. M. A. 171:1301-1305, 1959.

50. Davison, F. W.: Inflammatory diseases of the larynx of infants and small children. Ann. Otol. Rhinol. Laryngol. 76:753, 1967.

51. Dawson, K., Cooper, D., Cooper, P., et al.: The management of acute laryngo-tracheo-bronchitis (croup): A consensus view. J. Paediatr. Child Health 28:223-224, 1992.

52. DeBoeck, K.: Croup: A review. Eur. J. Pediatr. 154:432-436, 1995.

53. Denneny, J. C., and Handler, S. D.: Membranous laryngotracheobronchitis. Pediatrics 70:705-707, 1982.

54. Denny, F. W., and Clyde, W. A., Jr.: Acute lower respiratory tract infections in nonhospitalized children. J. Pediatr. 108:635-646, 1986.

55. Denny, F. W., Clyde, W. A., Jr., and Glezen, W. P.: Mycoplasma pneumoniae disease: Clinical spectrum, pathophysiology, epidemiology, and control. J. Infect. Dis. 123:74-92, 1971.

56. Denny, F. W., Murphy, T. F., Clyde, W. A., Jr., et al.: Croup: An 11-year study in a pediatric practice. Pediatrics 71:871-876, 1983.

57. Donaldson, D., Poleski, D., Knipple, E., et al.: Intramuscular versus oral dexamethasone for the treatment of moderate-to-severe croup: A randomized, double-blind trial. Acad. Emerg. Med. 10:16-21, 2003.

58. Donnelly, B. W., McMillan, J. A., and Weiner, L. B.: Bacterial tracheitis: Report of eight new cases and review. Rev. Infect. Dis. 12:729-735, 1990.

59. Dudin, A. A., Thalji, A., and Rambaud-Cousson, A.: Bacterial tracheitis among children hospitalized for severe obstructive dyspnea. Pediatr. Infect. Dis. 9:293-295, 1990.

60. Dulfano, M. J., Adler, K., and Wooten, O.: Physical properties of sputum, IV: Effects of 100 percent humidity and water mist. Am. Rev. Respir. Dis. 107:130-132, 1972.

61. Eden, A. N., Kaufman, A., and Yu, R.: Corticosteroids and croup: Controlled double-blind study. J. A. M. A. 200:403-404, 1967.

62. Eden, A. N., and Larkin, V. D. P.: Corticosteroid treatment of croup. Pediatrics 33:768-769, 1964.

63. Edwards, K. M., Dundon, M. C., and Altemeier, W. A.: Bacterial tracheitis as a complication of viral croup. Pediatr. Infect. Dis. 2:390-391, 1983.

64. Eichenwald, H. F.: Respiratory infections in children. Hosp. Pract. 11:81-90, 1976.

65. Eid, N. S., and Jones, V. F.: Bacterial tracheitis as a complication of tonsillectomy and adenoidectomy. J. Pediatr. 125:401-402, 1994.

66. Eller, J. J., Fulginiti, V. A., Plunket, D. C., et al.: Attack rates for hospitalized croup in children in a military population: Importance of A2 influenza infection. Pediatr. Res. 6:386, 1972.

67. Ernst, T. N., and Philp, M.: Bacterial tracheitis caused by Branhamella catarrhalis. Pediatr. Infect. Dis. 6:574, 1987.

68. Everett, A. R.: Acute laryngotracheobronchitis: An analysis of 1,175 cases with 98 tracheotomies. Laryngoscope 61:113-123, 1951.

69. Fearon, B.: Acute obstructive laryngitis in infants and children. Hosp. Med. 4:51-67, 1968.

70. Fitzgerald, D. A.: The assessment and management of croup. Paediatr. Resp. Rev. 7:73-81, 2006.

71. Fitzgerald, D., and Kilham, H. A.: Croup: assessment and evidence-based management. Med. J. Aust. 179:372-377, 2003.

72. Forbes, J. A.: Severe effects of influenza viral infection. Med. J. Aust. 44:75-79, 1958.

73. Foskey, G., Jr., and Singer, J.: Artificial nail aspiration masquerading as refractory croup. Pediatr. Emerg. Care 21:523-526, 2005.

74. Fried, M. P.: Controversies in the management of supraglottitis and croup. Pediatr. Clin. North Am. 26:931-942, 1979.

75. Gardner, H. G., Powell, K. R., and Cherry, J. D.: Unpublished data, 1973.

76. Gardner, H. G., Powell, K. R., Roden, V. J., et al.: The evaluation of racemic epinephrine in the treatment of infectious croup. Pediatrics 52:68-71, 1973.

77. Gardner, P. S.: Virus infections and respiratory disease of childhood. Arch. Dis. Child. 43:629-645, 1968.

78. Gardner, P. S., McQuillin, J., McGuckin, R., et al.: Observations on clinical and immunofluorescent diagnosis of parainfluenza virus infections. Br. Med. J. 2:7-12, 1971.

79. Geelhoed, G. C.: Budesonide offers no advantage when added to oral dexamethasone in treatment of croup. Pediatr. Emerg. Care 21:359-362, 2005.

80. Geist, R., and Tallett, S. E.: Diagnosis and management of psychogenic stridor caused by a conversion disorder. Pediatrics 86:315-317, 1990.

81. Gittens, T. R.: XXXIII: Laryngitis and tracheobronchitis in children: Special reference to nondiphtheritic infections. Ann. Otol. Rhinol. Laryngol. 41:422-438, 1932.

82. Glezen, W. P., Loda, F. A., Clyde, W. A., Jr., et al.: Epidemiologic patterns of acute lower respiratory disease of children in a pediatric group practice. J. Pediatr. 78:397-406, 1971.

83. Glezen, W. P., Loda, F. A., and Denny, F. W.: The parainfluenza viruses. In Evans, A. S. (ed.): Viral Infections of Humans: Epidemiology and Control. New York, Plenum, 1976, pp. 337-349.

84. Godden, C. W., Campbell, M. J., Hussey, M., et al.: Double blind placebo controlled trial of nebulised budesonide for croup. Arch. Dis. Child. 76:155-158, 1997.

85. Gold, S. M., Shott, S. R., and Myer, C. M., III: Radiological case of the month. Arch. Pediatr. Adolesc. Med. *150*:97-98, 1996.
86. Griffin, S., Ellis, S., Fitzgerald-Barron, A., et al.: Nebulised steroid in the treatment of croup: A systematic review of randomized controlled trials. Br. J. Gen. Pract. *50*:135-141, 2000.
87. Gurwitz, D., Corey, M., and Levison, H.: Pulmonary function and bronchial reactivity in children after croup. Am. Rev. Respir. Dis. *122*:95-99, 1980.
88. Hall, C. B., McBride, J. T., Walsh, E. E., et al.: Aerosolized ribavirin treatment of infants with respiratory syncytial viral infection: A randomized double-blind study. N. Engl. J. Med. *308*:1443-1447, 1983.
89. Han, B. K., Dunbar, J. S., and Striker, T. W.: Membranous laryngotracheobronchitis (membranous croup). A. J. R. Am. J. Roentgenol. *133*:53-58, 1979.
90. Harari, M. D., West, B., and Dwyer, B.: *Cryptosporidium* as cause of laryngotracheitis in an infant. Lancet *1*:1207, 1986.
91. Henry, R. L., Mellis, C. M., and Benjamin, B.: Pseudomembranous croup. Arch. Dis. Child. *58*:180-183, 1983.
92. Herrmann, E. C., Jr., and Hable, K. A.: Experiences in laboratory diagnosis of parainfluenza viruses in routine medical practice. Mayo Clin. Proc. *45*:177-188, 1970.
93. Hide, D. W., and Guyer, B. M.: Recurrent croup. Arch. Dis. Child. *60*:585-586, 1985.
94. Hoekelman, R. A.: Infectious illness during the first year of life. Pediatrics *59*:119-121, 1977.
95. Holdaway, M. D.: Croup and epiglottitis: Diagnosis and action. Drugs *13*:452-457, 1977.
96. Holzel, A., Parker, L., Patterson, W. H., et al.: Virus isolations from throats of children admitted to hospital with respiratory and other diseases, Manchester 1962-4. Br. Med. J. *1*:614-619, 1965.
97. Hope-Simpson, R. E., and Higgins, P. G.: A respiratory virus study in Great Britain: Review and evaluation. Prog. Med. Virol. *11*:354-407, 1969.
98. Hopkins, A., Lahiri, T., Salerno, R., et al.: Changing epidemiology of life-threatening upper airway infections: The reemergence of bacterial tracheitis. Pediatrics *118*:1418-1421, 2006.
99. Horn, M. E. C., Brain, E., Gregg, I., et al.: Respiratory viral infection in childhood: A survey in general practice, Roehampton 1967-1972. J. Hyg. Camb. *74*:157-168, 1975.
100. Howard, J. B., McCracken, G. H., Jr., and Luby, J. P.: Influenza A₂ virus as a cause of croup requiring tracheotomy. J. Pediatr. *81*:1148-1150, 1972.
101. Husby, S., Agertoft, L., Mortensen, S., et al.: Treatment of croup with nebulised steroid (budesonide): A double-blind, placebo-controlled study. Arch. Dis. Child. *68*:352-355, 1993.
102. Hyde, C. I., and Ruchman, J.: Acute infectious edematous laryngitis in which recovery followed tracheotomy. Arch. Pediatr. *48*:124-129, 1931.
103. Infectious Diseases and Immunization Committee, Canadian Paediatric Society: Steroid therapy for croup in children admitted to hospital. Can. Med. Assoc. J. *147*:429-430, 1992.
104. Inglis, A. F., Jr.: Herpes simplex virus infection: A rare cause of prolonged croup. Arch. Otolaryngol. Head Neck Surg. *119*:551-552, 1993.
105. Jackson, G. G., and Stanley, E. D.: Prevention and control of influenza by chemoprophylaxis and chemotherapy: Prospects from examination of recent experience. J. A. M. A. *235*:2739-2742, 1976.
106. Jaffe, D.M.: The treatment of croup with glucocorticoids. N. Engl. J. Med. *339*:553-555, 1998.
107. James, J. A.: Dexamethasone in croup: A controlled study. Am. J. Dis. Child. *117*:511-516, 1969.
108. Johnson, D. W., Schuh, S., Koren, G., et al.: Outpatient treatment of croup with nebulized dexamethasone. Arch. Pediatr. Adolesc. Med. *150*:349-355, 1996.
109. Johnson, D. W., Jacobson, S., Edney, P. C., et al.: A comparison of nebulized budesonide, intramuscular dexamethasone, and placebo for moderately severe croup. N. Engl. J. Med. *339*:498-503, 1998.
110. Johnson, M. C.: Acute laryngotracheobronchitis in infants: Report of three cases. Arch. Otolaryngol. *17*:230-234, 1933.
111. Jones, R., Santos, J. I., and Overall, J. C., Jr.: Bacterial tracheitis. J. A. M. A. *242*:721-726, 1979.
112. Jordan, W. S.: Laryngotracheobronchitis: Evaluation of new therapeutic approaches. Rocky Mt. Med. J. *63*:69, 1966.
113. Jordan, W. S., Graves, C. L., and Elwyn, R. A.: New therapy for postintubation laryngeal edema and tracheitis in children. J. A. M. A. *212*:585-588, 1970.
114. Kaditis, A. G., and Wald, E. R.: Viral croup: A current diagnosis and treatment. Pediatr. Infect. Dis. J. *17*:827-834, 1998.
115. Kairys, S. W., Olmstead, E. N., and O'Connor, G. T.: Steroid treatment of laryngotracheitis: A meta-analysis of the evidence from randomized trials. Pediatrics *83*:683-693, 1989.
116. Kasian, G. F., Bingham, W. T., Steinberg, J., et al.: Bacterial tracheitis in children. Can. Med. Assoc. J. *140*:46-50, 1989.
117. Kelley, P. B., and Simon, J. E.: Racemic epinephrine use in croup and disposition. Am. J. Emerg. Med. *10*:181-183, 1992.
118. Kepes, E. R., Martinez, L. R., Andrews, I. C., et al.: Racemic epinephrine in postintubation laryngeal edema. N. Y. State J. Med. *72*:583-584, 1972.
119. Kibrick, S.: Current status of coxsackie and ECHO viruses in human disease. Prog. Med. Virol. *6*:27-70, 1964.
120. Kissoon, N., Kronick, J. B., and Frewen, T. C.: Psychogenic upper airway obstruction. Pediatrics *81*:714-717, 1988.
121. Klass, P.: Croup—the bark is worse than the bite. N. Engl. J. Med. *351*:1283-1284, 2004.
122. Klassen T.P.: Croup: A current perspective. Emerg. Med. *46*:1167-1178, 1999.
123. Klassen, T. P., Craig, W. R., Moher, D., et al.: Nebulized budesonide and oral dexamethasone for treatment of croup: A randomized controlled trial. J. A. M. A. *279*:1629-1632, 1998.
124. Klassen, T. P., Feldman, M. E., Watters, L. K., et al.: Nebulized budesonide for children with mild to moderate croup. N. Engl. J. Med. *331*:285-289, 1994.
125. Klassen, T. P., Watters, L. K., Feldman, M. E., et al.: The efficacy of nebulized budesonide in dexamethasone-treated outpatients with croup. Pediatrics *97*:463-466, 1996.
126. Klein, J. D., and Collier, A. M.: Pathogenesis of human parainfluenza type 3 virus infection in hamster tracheal organ culture. Infect. Immunol. *10*:883-888, 1974.
127. Koren, G., Frand, M., Barzilay, Z., et al.: Corticosteroid treatment of laryngotracheitis vs spasmodic croup in children. Am. J. Dis. Child. *137*:941-944, 1983.
128. Korppi, M., Halonen, P., Kleemola, M., et al.: The role of parainfluenza viruses in inspiratory difficulties in children. Acta Paediatr. Scand. *77*:105-111, 1988.
129. Krause, I., Schonfeld, T., Ben Ari, J., et al.: Prolonged croup due to herpes simplex virus infection. Eur. J. Pediatr. *157*:567-569, 1998.
130. Kravitz, H.: Sex distribution of hospitalized children with acute respiratory diseases, gastroenteritis and meningitis. Clin. Pediatr. *4*:484-491, 1965.
131. Kristjansson, S., Berg-Kelly, K., and Winso, E.: Inhalation of racemic adrenaline in the treatment of mild and moderately severe croup: Clinical symptom score and oxygen saturation measurements for evaluation of treatment effects. Acta Paediatr. *83*:1156-1160, 1994.
132. Kuusela, A. L., and Vesikari, T.: A randomized double-blind, placebo-controlled trial of dexamethasone and racemic epinephrine in the treatment of croup. Acta Paediatr. Scand. *77*:99-104, 1988.
133. Laxdal, O. E., Robertson, H. E., Braaten, V., et al.: Acute respiratory infections in children, I: An intensive study of etiology in an open community. Can. Med. Assoc. J. *88*:1049-1054, 1963.
134. Leipzig, B., Oski, F. A., Cummings, C. W., et al.: A prospective randomized study to determine the efficacy of steroids in treatment of croup. J. Pediatr. *94*:194-196, 1979.
135. Lenney, W., and Milner, A. D.: Treatment of acute viral croup. Arch. Dis. Child. *53*:704-706, 1978.
136. Liston, S. L., Gehrz, R. C., and Jarvis, C. W.: Bacterial tracheitis. Arch. Otolaryngol. *107*:561-564, 1981.
137. Liston, S. L., Gehrz, R. C., Siegel, L. G., et al.: Bacterial tracheitis. Am. J. Dis. Child. *137*:764-767, 1983.
138. Lockhart, C. H., and Battaglia, J. D.: Croup (laryngotracheal bronchitis) and epiglottitis. Pediatr. Ann. *6*:262-269, 1977.
139. Loda, F. A., Clyde, W. A., Jr., Glezen, W. P., et al.: Studies on the role of viruses, bacteria, and *M. pneumoniae* as causes of lower respiratory tract infections in children. J. Pediatr. *72*:161-176, 1968.
140. Loda, F. A., Glezen, W. P., and Clyde, W. A., Jr.: Respiratory disease in group day care. Pediatrics *49*:428-437, 1972.
141. Loughlin, G. M., and Taussig, L. M.: Pulmonary function in children with a history of laryngotracheobronchitis. J. Pediatr. *94*:365-369, 1979.
142. Luria, J. W., Gonzalez-del-Rey, J. A., DiGiulio, G. A., et al.: Effectiveness of oral or nebulized dexamethasone for children with mild croup. Arch. Pediatr. Adolesc. Med. *155*:1340-1345, 2001.
143. Macasaet, F. F., Kidd, P. A., Bolano, C. R., et al.: The etiology of acute respiratory infections, III: The role of viruses and bacteria. J. Pediatr. *72*:829-839, 1968.
144. Marx, A., Török, T. J., Holman, R. C., et al.: Pediatric hospitalizations for croup (laryngotracheobronchitis): Biennial increases associated with human parainfluenza virus 1 epidemics. J. Infect. Dis. *176*:1423-1427, 1997.
145. Mauro, R. D., Poole, S. R., and Lockhart, C. H.: Differentiation of epiglottitis from laryngotracheitis in the child with stridor. Am. J. Dis. Child. *142*:679-682, 1988.
146. McClung, H. W., Knight, V., Gilbert, B. E., et al.: Ribavirin aerosol treatment of influenza B virus infection. J. A. M. A. *249*:2671-2674, 1983.
147. McDonogh, A. J.: The use of steroids and nebulised adrenaline in the treatment of viral croup over a seven-year period at a district hospital. Anaesth. Intensive Care *22*:175-178, 1994.
148. McKenzie, M., Norman, M. G., Anderson, J. D., et al.: Upper respiratory tract infection in a 3-year-old girl. J. Pediatr. *105*:129-133, 1984.
149. McLean, D. M., Roy, T. E., O'Brien, M. J., et al.: Parainfluenza viruses in association with acute laryngotracheobronchitis, Toronto, 1960-61.Can. Med. Assoc. J. *85*:290-294, 1961.
150. McNab, J. C. G.: Acute streptococcal infection of the trachea in an infant, aged fifteen months. J. Laryngol. *30*:337-338, 1915.
151. Meade, R. H., III: Laryngeal obstruction in children. Pediatr. Clin. North Am. *9*:233-262, 1962.
152. Melnick, A., Berger, R., and Green, G.: Spasmodic croup in children: Personal experiences with intermittent positive pressure breathing in therapy. Clin. *11*:615-617, 1972.
153. Miller, B. R., Arthur, J. D., Parry, W. H., et al.: Atypical croup and *Chlamydia trachomatis*. Lancet *1*:1022, 1982.

154. Miller, D. G., Gabrielson, M. O., and Horstmann, D. M.: Clinical virology and viral surveillance in a pediatric group practice: The use of double-seeded tissue culture tubes for primary virus isolation. Am. J. Epidemiol. 88:245-256, 1968.

155. Mogabgab, W. J.: Beta-hemolytic streptococcal and concurrent infections in adults and children with respiratory disease, 1958 to 1969. Am. Rev. Respir. Dis. 102:23-34, 1970.

156. Moore, M., and Little, P.: Humidified air inhalation for treating croup. Cochrane Database Syst. Rev. 3:1-16, 2006.

157. Morgan, E. A., and Wishart, D. E. S.: Laryngo-tracheobronchitis: A statistical review of 549 cases. Can. Med. Assoc. J. 56:8-15, 1947.

158. Mufson, M. A., Krause, H. E., Mocega, H. E., et al.: Viruses, *Mycoplasma pneumoniae* and bacteria associated with lower respiratory tract disease among infants. Am. J. Epidemiol. 91:192-202, 1970.

159. Myers, C., Corbelli, R., Schrenzel, J., et al.: Multiple pulmonary abscesses caused by *Legionella pneumophila* infection in an infant with croup. Pediatr. Infect. Dis. J. 25:753-754, 2006.

160. Naqvi, S. H., and Dunkle, L. M.: Bacterial tracheitis and viral croup. Pediatr. Infect. Dis. 3:282-283, 1984.

161. Neffson, A. H.: Acute laryngotracheobronchitis: A 25-year review. Am. J. Med. Sci. 208:524-547, 1944.

162. Nelson, W. E.: Bacterial croup: A historical perspective. J. Pediatr. 105:52-55, 1984.

163. Newth, C. J. L., Levison, H., and Bryan, A. C.: The respiratory status of children with croup. J. Pediatr. 81:1068-1073, 1972.

164. Nichol, K. P., and Cherry, J. D.: Bacterial-viral interrelations in respiratory infections of children. N. Engl. J. Med. 277:667-672, 1967.

165. Nicolai, T., and Mutius, E.: Risk of asthma in children with a history of croup. Acta Paediatr. 85:1295-1299, 1996.

166. Nijssen-Jordan, C., Donaldson, J. D., and Halperin, S. A.: Bacterial tracheitis associated with respiratory syncytial virus infection and toxic shock syndrome. Can. Med. Assoc. J. 142:233-234, 1990.

167. Orton, H. B., Smith, E. L., Bell, H. O., et al.: Acute laryngotracheobronchitis: Analysis of sixty-two cases with report of autopsies in eight cases. Arch. Otolaryngol. 33:926-960, 1941.

168. Ottolini, M. G., Porter, D. D., Blanco, J. C. G., et al.: A cotton rat model of human parainfluenza 3 laryngotracheitis: Virus growth, pathology, and therapy. J. Infect. Dis. 186:1713-1717, 2002.

169. Paisley, J. W., Bruhn, F. W., Lauer, B. A., et al.: Type A2 influenza viral infections in children. Am. J. Dis. Child. 132:34-36, 1978.

170. Parks, C. R.: Mist therapy: Rationale and practice. J. Pediatr. 76:305-313, 1970.

171. Parrott, R. H.: Viral respiratory tract illnesses in children. Bull. N. Y. Acad. Med. 39:629-648, 1963.

172. Parrott, R. H., Kim, H. W., Vargosko, A. J., et al.: Serious respiratory tract illness as a result of Asian influenza and influenza B infections in children. J. Pediatr. 61:205-213, 1962.

173. Parrott, R. H., Vargosko, A. J., Kim, H. W., et al.: Acute respiratory diseases of viral etiology, III: Myxoviruses: Para influenza. Am. J. Public Health 52:907-917, 1962.

174. Parrott, R. H., Vargosko, A. J., Kim, H. W., et al.: Clinical syndromes among children. Am. Rev. Respir. Dis. 88:73-76, 1962.

175. Person, D. A., and Herrmann, E. C., Jr.: Experiences in laboratory diagnosis of rhinovirus infections in routine medical practice. Mayo Clin. Proc. 45:517, 1970.

176. Plachtova-Pecenkova, I., Brockova, M., Fecova, D., et al.: Note on the aetiology of acute laryngotracheobronchitis in children: Findings in the autumn of 1965 and the spring of 1966. J. Hyg. Epidemiol. Microbiol. Immunol. 12:227-237, 1968.

177. Poland, J. D., Welton, E. R., and Chin, T. D. Y.: Influenza virus B as a cause of acute croup syndrome. Am. J. Dis. Child. 107:54, 1964.

178. Prendergast, M., Jones, J. S., and Hartman, D.: Racemic epinephrine in the treatment of laryngotracheitis: Can we identify children for outpatient therapy? Am. J. Emerg. Med. 12:613-616, 1994.

179. Rabe, E. F.: Infectious croup, I. Etiology. Pediatrics 2:255-265, 1948.

180. Rabe, E. F.: Infectious croup, II. "Virus" croup. Pediatrics 2:415-427, 1948.

181. Rabe, E. F.: Acute inflammatory disorders of the larynx and laryngotracheal area. Pediatr. Clin. North Am. 4:169-182, 1957.

182. Reed, S. E., and Boyde, A.: Organ cultures of respiratory epithelium infected with rhinovirus or parainfluenza virus studied in a scanning electron microscope. Infect. Immunol. 6:68-76, 1972.

183. Reilly, C. M., Hoch, S. M., Stokes, J., Jr., et al.: Clinical and laboratory findings in cases of respiratory illness caused by coryzaviruses. Ann. Intern. Med. 57:515-525, 1962.

184. Richards, L.: Fulminating laryngo-tracheo-bronchitis. Ann. Otol. Rhinol. Laryngol. 42:1014-1040, 1933.

185. Richards, L.: A further study of the pathology of acute laryngo-tracheo-bronchitis in children. Ann. Otol. Rhinol. Laryngol. 47:326-341, 1938.

186. Rittichier, K. K., and Ledwith, C. A.: Outpatient treatment of moderate croup with dexamethasone: Intramuscular versus oral dosing. Pediatrics 106:1344-1348, 2000.

187. Roberts, G. W., Master, V. V., Staugas, R. E., et al.: Repeated dose inhaled budesonide versus placebo in the treatment of croup. J. Paediatr. Child Health 35:170-174, 1999.

188. Rosales, J. K., and Davenport, H. T.: Acute laryngotracheobronchitis and epiglottitis. Can. Anaesth. Soc. J. 9:467-478, 1962.

189. Rull, J., and Hargitai, R.: Laryngitis subglottica kezelese mikronephrin tulnyomasos belelegeztetesevel. Orvosi Hetilap 115:2727-2731, 1974.

190. Russel, K., Wiebe, N., Saenz, A., et al.: Glucocorticoids for croup. Cochrane Database Syst. Rev. 4:1-67, 2003.

191. Sasaki, C. T., and Suzuki, M.: The respiratory mechanism of aerosol inhalation in the treatment of partial airway obstruction. Pediatrics 59:689-694, 1977.

192. Schalen, L., and Andersson, K.: Differential diagnosis and treatment of psychogenic voice disorder. Clin. Otolaryngol. 17:225-230, 1992.

193. Scolnik, D., Coates, A. L., Stephens, D., et al.: Controlled delivery of high vs. low humidity vs. mist therapy for croup in emergency departments. J. A. M. A. 295:1274-1280, 2006.

194. Segal, A. O., Crighton, E. J., Moineddin, R., et al.: Croup hospitalizations in Ontario: A 14-year time-series analysis. Pediatrics 116:51-55, 2005.

195. Sendi, K., Crysdale, S., and Yoo, J.: Tracheitis: Outcome of 1,700 cases presenting to the emergency department during two years. J. Otolaryngol. 21:20-24, 1992.

196. Singer, O. P., and Wilson, W. J.: Laryngotracheobronchitis: 2 years' experience with racemic epinephrine. Can. Med. Assoc. J. 115:132-134, 1976.

197. Skolnik, N.: Croup. J. Fam. Pract. 37:165-170, 1993.

198. Skolnik, N. S.: Treatment of croup: A critical review. Am. J. Dis. Child. 143:1045-1049, 1989.

199. Skowron, P. N., Turner, J. A. P., and McNaughton, G. A.: The use of corticosteroid (dexamethasone) in the treatment of acute laryngotracheitis. Can. Med. Assoc. J. 94:528-531, 1966.

200. Smith, D. S.: Corticosteroids in croup: A chink in the ivory tower? J. Pediatr. 115:256-257, 1989.

201. Sofer, S., and Chernick, V.: Increased need for tracheal intubation for croup in relation to bacterial tracheitis. Can. Med. Assoc. J. 128:160-161, 1983.

202. Solomon, R., Truman, T., and Murray, D. L.: Toxic shock syndrome as a complication of bacterial tracheitis. Pediatrics 4:298-299, 1985.

203. Stankiewicz, J. A., and Bowes, A. K.: Croup and epiglottitis: A radiologic study. Laryngoscope 95:1159-1160, 1985.

204. Sterner, G., Gerzen, P., Ohlson, M., et al.: Acute respiratory illness and gastroenteritis in association with adenovirus type 7 infections. Acta Paediatr. 50:457-468, 1961.

205. Stott, E. J., Bell, E. J., Eadie, M. B., et al.: A comparative virological study of children in hospital with respiratory and diarrhoeal illnesses. J. Hyg. Camb. 65:9-23, 1967.

206. Stuart-Harris, C. H.: The adenoviruses and respiratory disease in man. Lectures on the Scientific Basis of Medicine 8:148-164, 1958-59.

207. Super, D. M., Cartelli, N. A., Brooks, L. J., et al.: A prospective randomized double-blind study to evaluate the effect of dexamethasone in acute laryngotracheitis. J. Pediatr. 115:323-329, 1989.

208. Suresh, G. K., Dhawan, A., and Kohli, V.: Tracheal diphtheria mimicking bacterial tracheitis. Pediatr. Infect. Dis. J. 11:502, 1992.

209. Surh, L., and Read, S. E.: Staphylococcal tracheitis and toxic shock syndrome in a young child. J. Pediatr. 104:585-587, 1984.

210. Sussman, S., Grossman, M., Magoffin, R., et al.: Dexamethasone (16 alpha-methyl, 9 alpha-fluoroprednisolone) in obstructive respiratory tract infections in children: A controlled study. Pediatrics 34:851-855, 1964.

211. Szpunar, J., Glowacki, J., Laskowski, A., et al.: Fibrinous laryngotracheobronchitis in children. Arch. Otolaryngol. 93:173-178, 1971.

212. Taber, L. H., Knight, V., Gilbert, B. E., et al.: Ribavirin aerosol treatment of bronchiolitis associated with respiratory syncytial virus infection in infants. Pediatrics 72:613-618, 1983.

213. Tan, A. K. W., and Manoukian, J. J.: Hospitalized croup (bacterial and viral): The role of rigid endoscopy. J. Otolaryngol. 21:48-53, 1992.

214. Taussig, L. M., Castro, O., Beaudry, P. H., et al.: Treatment of laryngotracheobronchitis (croup): Use of intermittent positive-pressure breathing and racemic epinephrine. Am. J. Dis. Child. 129:790-793, 1975.

215. Temple, A. R.: Recent advances in diagnosis and management of croup. J. Fam. Pract. 2:85-89, 1975.

216. Tenenbein, M.: The steroid odyssey in croup. Pediatrics 116:230-231, 2005.

217. Top, F. H., Sr.: Diphtheria. In Top, F. H., Sr., and Wehrle, P. F. (eds.): Communicable and Infectious Diseases. St. Louis, C. V. Mosby, 1972, pp. 190-207.

218. Toth, M., and Major, V.: Virological investigation of hospitalized cases of pseudocroup and acute laryngotracheobronchitis. Acta Microbiol. 12:189-200, 1965.

219. Travis, K. W., Todres, I. D., and Shannon, D. C.: Pulmonary edema associated with croup and epiglottitis. Pediatrics 59:695-698, 1977.

220. Tunnessen, W. W., Jr., and Feinstein, A. R.: The steroid-croup controversy: An analytic review of methodologic problems. J. Pediatr. 96:751-756, 1980.

221. Tyeryar, F. J., Jr., Richardson, L. S., and Belshe, R. B.: Report of a workshop on respiratory syncytial virus and parainfluenza viruses. J. Infect. Dis. 137:835-846, 1978.

222. Tyrrell, D. A. J.: Common Colds and Related Diseases. Baltimore, Williams & Wilkins, 1965.

223. Van Bever, H. P., Wieringa, M. H., Weyler, J. J., et al.: Croup and recurrent croup: Their association with asthma and allergy. Pneumology 158:253-257, 1999.

224. Van der Hoek, L., Sure, K., Ihorst, G., et al.: Croup is associated with the novel coronavirus NL63. Plos Med. 2:764-770, 2005.

225. Vargosko, A. J., Chanock, R. M., Huebner, R. J., et al.: Association of type 2 hemadsorption (parainfluenza 1) virus and Asian influenza A virus with infectious croup. N. Engl. J. Med. 261:1-9, 1959.

226. Vihma, L.: Surveillance of acute viral respiratory diseases in children. Acta Paediatr. Scand. 192(Suppl.):8-53, 1969.

227. Walker, P., and Crysdale, W. S.: Croup, epiglottitis, retropharyngeal abscess, and bacterial tracheitis: Evolving patterns of occurrence and care. Int. Anesth. Clin. 30:57-70, 1992.

228. Weber, J. E., Chudnofsky, C. R., Younger, J. G., et al.: A randomized comparison of helium-oxygen mixture (Heliox) and racemic epinephrine for the treatment of moderate to severe croup. Pediatrics 107:E96, 2001.

229. Welliver, R.C.: Croup: Continuing controversy. Semin. Pediatr. Infect. Dis. 6:90-95, 1995.

230. Welliver, R. C., Sun, M., and Rinaldo, D.: Defective regulation of immune response in croup due to parainfluenza virus. Pediatr. Res. 19:716-720, 1985.

231. Welliver, R. C., Wong, D. T., Middleton, E., Jr., et al.: Role of parainfluenza virus-specific IgE in pathogenesis of croup and wheezing subsequent to infection. J. Pediatr. 101:889-896, 1982.

232. Wenner, H. A., Christodoulopoulou, G., Weston, J., et al.: The etiology of respiratory illnesses occurring in infancy and childhood. Pediatrics 31:4-17, 1963.

233. Westley, C. R., Cotton, E. K., and Brooks, J. G.: Nebulized racemic epinephrine by IPPB for the treatment of croup: A double-blind study. Am. J. Dis. Child. 132:484-487, 1978.

234. Wilson, S. Z., Gilbert, B. E., Quarles, J. M., et al.: Treatment of influenza A (H1N1) virus infection with ribavirin aerosol. Antimicrob. Agents Chemother. 26:200-203, 1984.

235. Wolf, I. J.: Allergic factors in the etiology of spasmodic croup and laryngotracheitis. Ann. Allergy 24:79-82, 1966.

236. Wong, V. K., and Mason, W. H.: *Branhamella catarrhalis* as a cause of bacterial tracheitis. Pediatr. Infect. Dis. 6:945-946, 1987.

237. Wulff, H., Kidd, P., and Wenner, H. A.: Etiology of respiratory infections: Further studies during infancy and childhood. Pediatrics 33:30-44, 1964.

238. Zach, M. S.: Airway reactivity in recurrent croup. Eur. J. Respir. Dis. 128(Suppl.):81-88, 1983.

239. Zacharisen, M. C., and Conley, S. F.: Recurrent respiratory papillomatosis in children: Masquerader of common respiratory diseases. Pediatrics 118:1925-1931, 2006.

240. Zulliger, J. J., Schuller, D. W., Beach, T. P., et al.: Assessment of intubation in croup and epiglottitis. Ann. Otol. Rhinol. Laryngol. 91:403-406, 1982.

LOWER RESPIRATORY TRACT INFECTIONS

23 ACUTE BRONCHITIS
James D. Cherry

Bronchitis is a common diagnosis in pediatric practice, although little unanimity exists among physicians regarding its exact clinical constellation, and in the true pathologic sense, it probably never occurs as an isolated entity. Acute bronchitis is a febrile illness with cough, rhonchi, and referred breath sounds.[15] Asthmatic bronchitis (infectious asthma), similar to acute bronchitis, but with associated wheezing and expiratory distress, is discussed in Chapter 25. On pathologic examination, the clinical illness of acute bronchitis reflects acute inflammatory disease of the larger air passages, including the trachea and the large and medium-sized bronchi.[25]

ETIOLOGY

Table 23–1 lists various infectious agents associated with acute bronchitis. Infections with adenoviruses, influenza viruses, parainfluenza viruses, respiratory syncytial virus, and *Mycoplasma pneumoniae* account for most cases of acute bronchitis in children. These agents, plus many rhinoviruses, a few enteroviruses, and perhaps human metapneumovirus, human bocavirus, and the newer human coronaviruses, account for virtually all cases in the United States today.

Of the adenoviruses, type 7 has been associated most commonly with acute bronchitis in children. In military recruits, including adolescents, adenovirus types 4 and 7 cause epidemic acute respiratory disease, in which bronchitis is a usual occurrence.[22,64]

Influenza A virus infection is a common cause of severe acute bronchitis, particularly at the time of antigenic shift of influenza A virus subtype and pandemic disease. Acute bronchitis caused by influenza A virus also is a regular occurrence between pandemics in new susceptible individuals (young children) in the population. Influenza B virus also is an important cause of bronchitis, and it was a more common causative agent than was influenza A virus in one large longitudinal study.[13]

All cases of measles involve the bronchi, but measles has been an uncommon occurrence since the advent of widespread use of vaccines. Of the parainfluenza viruses, type 3 is associated most commonly with acute bronchitis. Respiratory syncytial virus is a common cause of acute bronchitis, particularly in very young children. The more recently identified human metapneumovirus is another cause of acute bronchitis.[57]

Of the bacterial agents listed in Table 23–1, only *Haemophilus influenzae* clearly can be incriminated. *Bordetella pertussis* infection involves the trachea and bronchi, but fever is an uncommon event, and the illness is outside the definition of acute bronchitis. When sought, *M. pneumoniae* is a common cause of bronchitis. *Chlamydia pneumoniae* has been found to be the cause of bronchitis in adolescents and young adults.[32]

EPIDEMIOLOGY

The epidemiology of the common viruses that are associated with bronchitis is presented in Section XVII. Chapman and associates[13] published the results of a study of acute bronchitis in a single private group pediatric practice in Chapel Hill, North Carolina. The study occurred during a 104-month period, during which 5489 episodes of lower respiratory illness occurred. Of these illnesses, 40.1 percent were acute bronchitis. The bronchitis attack rate was highest in children in the second year of life (6.71%), and then it decreased gradually to approximately 2 percent in teenagers. In contrast to the age-specific attack rates, the ratio of bronchitis cases to all lower respiratory illness cases increased with age. In the first year of life, the ratio was 0.29; in children 12 years old or older, it was 0.69.

During the first 6 years of life, respiratory syncytial virus and parainfluenza virus type 3 were the most common etiologic agents noted in the Chapel Hill study. During the first 2 years of life, adenoviruses also commonly were associated with bronchitis. In patients older than 6 years, *M. pneumoniae* and influenza A and B viruses were the most common etiologic agents. In a study of cough illnesses of 6 days' duration or longer in university students, investigators found that 15 of 31 students with laboratory evidence of *Bordetella* spp. infection were considered by their primary care providers to have bronchitis.[46]

The incidence of acute bronchitis peaks in the winter months, declines to midsummer, and increases again through the fall. Attack rates generally are higher in boys than in girls.[13,39,65] A sex difference is most pronounced during the first 6 years of life.

PATHOPHYSIOLOGY AND PATHOLOGY

Because acute bronchitis is an illness characterized by clinical features and one not usually associated with death, knowledge of its pathophysiology and pathology is meager. The general pathophysiology of human infections with viruses and *M. pneumoniae* that cause acute bronchitis is presented more completely in the sections of this book related to the individual infectious agents.

In virtually all cases of acute bronchitis, evidence of upper respiratory viral infection (pharyngitis, rhinitis) also is present. Tracheal and bronchial infection apparently is the result of distal spread. In bronchitis, the clinical features result from damage to the ciliated epithelium of the lower trachea and the large and medium-sized bronchi.[25] Although the cytopathologies of the various infectious agents is different,[71] the resulting obstruction of the air passages leads to similar symptoms. The duration of symptoms depends to some extent on the specific initial infectious agent and, in cases of prolonged illness, on secondary bacterial infection.

TABLE 23-1 Infectious Agents Associated with Acute Bronchitis

Agent	Importance in Causation*	References
Viruses		
Adenovirus types 1-7, 12	+++	1, 2, 5, 10-12, 14, 23, 27, 28, 35, 36, 42, 54, 59, 62, 65, 66, 70
Enterovirus	+	30, 35, 36, 59
Coxsackieviruses B	+	12
Echoviruses 8, 12, 14	+	63
Polioviruses	+	27, 63
Herpes simplex	+	27, 59, 63
Influenza virus	+++	1, 6, 8, 10-13, 14, 23, 28, 30, 61, 63
A	++	6, 10, 12, 13, 30, 35, 36, 61, 63
B	++	10, 12, 13, 30, 35
C	+	1
Measles	+	14, 25, 52
Mumps	+	63
Parainfluenza	+++	1, 6, 10-13, 14, 27-30, 33, 35, 42, 59, 61, 63, 66
1	++	10-13, 23, 30, 33
2	++	6, 10-12, 30, 33
3	+++	1, 2, 6, 10-13, 23, 30, 33, 36, 61
4	+	29
Respiratory syncytial virus	+++	1-3, 8, 10-13, 14, 23, 27, 28, 30, 34-36, 38, 45, 55, 59, 60, 62, 63, 66
Human metapneumovirus	+	57
Human bocavirus	+	37
Human coronavirus	+	4, 17, 26
Rhinovirus	++	12, 14, 27, 28, 30, 35, 36, 51, 58, 59
Bacteria		
Bordetella pertussis	+	25, 46
Bordetella parapertussis	–	
Haemophilus influenzae	–	42, 67
Moraxella catarrhalis	–	21, 31
Streptococcus pneumoniae	–	42
Streptococcus pyogenes	–	42, 50, 59
Other		
Chlamydia psittaci	+	10
Chlamydia pneumoniae	+	32
Mycoplasma pneumoniae	+++	10-13, 14, 23, 30, 35, 41, 53, 68

*+++, *very common*; ++, *common*; +, *rare*; –, *of questionable etiologic significance.*

In acute bronchitis, the larynx and subglottic trachea are not involved prominently. Conversely, today, bronchial involvement is seen only occasionally in croup.

CLINICAL PRESENTATION

Initial manifestations of acute bronchitis are upper respiratory in nature and, depending on the etiologic agent, are predominantly nasal, as in the common cold, or show additional objective evidence of pharyngitis, as in nasopharyngitis. Fever usually is present, and temperatures vary from 37.8° C to 39° C (100° F to 103° F) on most occasions. Cough always is present, and its onset can be insidious or abrupt. Initially, the cough is dry and harsh and often brassy in younger children. As the illness progresses, the cough becomes looser. In older children, purulent sputum is raised and expectorated. In younger children, the swallowing of often tenacious sputum frequently leads to gagging and vomiting. Older children may complain of chest pain resulting from coughing.

On initial physical examination, a variable degree of rhinitis usually is present; many patients have diffuse pharyngeal erythema. As the disease progresses, these upper respiratory signs generally decrease. Examination of the chest reveals rhonchi and referred breath sounds. Coarse, changing rales are noted frequently.

In the usual case of acute bronchitis, the illness can be separated into three phases: (1) a 1- to 2-day prodromal period when fever and upper respiratory symptoms predominate, (2) a 4- to 6-day period of marked tracheobronchial symptoms with some fever and general discomfort, and (3) a recovery period that may last 1 or 2 weeks and is characterized by cough and expectoration. Occasionally, the recovery period is particularly distressing and is associated with a low-grade fever, suggesting secondary bacterial infection. Bronchitis caused by *C. pneumoniae* often is insidious in onset and frequently associated with or preceded by pharyngitis.[32,40] Illness persists for several weeks but responds to appropriate antibiotic therapy.

Laboratory study in acute bronchitis is of limited use. Children in whom throat cultures reveal pathogenic bacteria in predominant growth tend to have more severe illness than do children with only viral infections.[16,47] The white blood cell count usually is greater than 10,000 cells/mm³, and approximately one third of the cases have a predominance of neutrophils.[47] The chest radiograph is normal unless associated pulmonary involvement is present.

DIFFERENTIAL DIAGNOSIS AND SPECIFIC DIAGNOSIS

Because acute bronchitis is a clinical entity caused by multiple etiologic agents, the most difficult differential aspect of diagnosis is the selection of the specific infectious cause. Also important is the separation of acute, self-limited bronchitis from chronic, more serious problems, such as cystic fibrosis, allergic respiratory disease, and sinusitis.

An epidemiologic history frequently can help in assigning a particular virus, *M. pneumoniae*, *C. pneumoniae*, or *B. pertussis*, as the presumptive etiologic agent. If epidemic bronchiolitis is occurring in the community, respiratory syncytial virus would be a likely cause. Similarly, predictions of causation by influenza virus, parainfluenza virus, adenoviruses, *M. pneumoniae*, *C. pneumoniae*, or *B. pertussis* can be made through clinical epidemiologic observations. Specific etiologic diagnosis can be established through the isolation of an organism or its identification by a direct antigen test from the nasopharyngeal secretions. Serologic study on paired sera may be useful for the diagnosis of *M. pneumoniae*, *C. pneumoniae*, and *B. pertussis*.

Children with protracted illnesses or febrile exacerbations should be examined by culture, radiograph, and perhaps further imaging studies for secondary bacterial infection of the tracheobronchial tree or the lungs or both. Children with chronic recurrent illnesses should be tested for cystic fibrosis, allergic conditions, and anatomic problems, such as gastroesophageal reflux and tracheoesophageal fistula.

TREATMENT

Treatment of acute bronchitis is distinguished more by what *not* to do than by specific modalities. In most mild cases, no specific therapy is indicated.

For children who feel miserable during the initial phases of acute bronchitis, analgesic therapy may be useful. Formerly, aspirin was the recommended analgesic. Because aspirin is an etiologic factor in influenza-associated Reye syndrome and because differentiating influenza viral infections from other respiratory viral infections is difficult, it is prudent to use acetaminophen rather than aspirin. The dose per single administration of acetaminophen by year of age is as follows: younger than 1 year, 60 mg; 1 to 3 years, 60 to 120 mg; 3 to 6 years, 120 mg; 6 to 12 years, 150 to 300 mg; older than 12 years, 325 to 650 mg. Administration may be repeated three or four times daily in young children and every 4 hours in older children. Acetaminophen rarely should be given to infants younger than 6 months of age.

As a result of widespread advertising, a common practice of individuals with acute bronchitis is to use an array of cold remedies, which contain various combinations of antihistamines, decongestants, and antitussives. None has been shown to be useful in acute bronchitis, and in certain stages of illness, they may aggravate the recovery process. Repeated bouts of coughing occasionally result in emesis, exhaustion, or insomnia, and the careful use of antitussive agents (codeine or dextromethorphan) can be helpful.[19] Cough suppressants should be used with caution when a cough is productive.

Intake of fluids should be encouraged to prevent overall dehydration and to decrease the viscosity of new secretions. Use of mist therapy also may help in thinning the exudate-containing respiratory secretions.[24,49]

In severe cases of acute bronchitis, treatment with specific antiviral agents should be considered. When influenza A virus is the likely etiologic agent, amantadine, rimantadine, zanamivir, or oseltamivir therapy may be beneficial.[9]

As noted in Table 23–1, most cases of acute bronchitis are caused by viruses, so antibiotic therapy would not be indicated.[48,69] In cases in which fever returns or no trend toward recovery is seen by the seventh day of illness, the possibility of a secondary bacterial infection should be considered. The association of sinusitis or a throat culture with a predominant growth of a respiratory pathogen (*Streptococcus pneumoniae*, *Streptococcus pyogenes*, *Moraxella catarrhalis*, *H. influenzae*) is an indication for

therapy. Infection with *M. pneumoniae* also should be treated, but in contrast to treatment of pneumonia, the therapy usually does not show an impressive response. Bronchitis caused by *C. pneumoniae* should be treated with erythromycin (50 mg/kg/day divided every 6 hours) for 10 to 14 days.[32]

PROGNOSIS

The prognosis in acute bronchitis usually is excellent. Although the duration of cough can be disturbing to the parent and the child, full recovery is the rule. Several studies suggest that lower respiratory illness in the first few years of life may be associated with persistent respiratory symptoms and with abnormalities in lung function in later life.[7,18,43,44] Although none of these studies has followed children with acute bronchitis specifically, the findings in other illnesses (bronchiolitis and croup) indicate a need to observe children with episodes of acute bronchitis carefully as well.

PREVENTION

At present, no practical method of prevention of acute bronchitis in children exists. Because most cases result from infections with common respiratory viruses, the development of vaccines could be expected to be helpful.

REFERENCES

1. Aitken, C. J. D., Moffat, M. A. J., and Sutherland, J. A. W.: Respiratory illness and viral infection in an Edinburgh nursery. J. Hyg. Camb. *65*:25-36, 1967.
2. Avila, M. M., Carballal, G., Rovaletti, H., et al.: Viral etiology in acute lower respiratory infections in children from a closed community. Am. Rev. Respir. Dis. *140*:634-637, 1989.
3. Berglund, B., and Strahlmann, C. H.: Respiratory syncytial virus infections in hospitalized children: Evaluation of the virus isolation and complement-fixation techniques in the virological diagnosis: Clinical and epidemiological characteristics. Acta Paediatr. Scand. *56*:1-10, 1967.
4. Boivin, G., Baz, M., Cote, S., et al.: Infections by human coronavirus-NL in hospitalized children. Pediatr. Infect. Dis. J. *24*:1045-1048, 2005.
5. Brandt, C. D., Kim, H. W., Vargosko, A. J., et al.: Infections in 18,000 infants and children in a controlled study of respiratory tract disease, I: Adenovirus pathogenicity in relation to serologic type and illness syndrome. Am. J. Epidemiol. *90*:484-500, 1969.
6. Brocklebank, J. T., Court, S. D. M., McQuillin, J., et al.: Influenza A infection in children. Lancet *1*:497-500, 1972.
7. Burrows, B., Knudson, R. J., and Lebowitz, M. D.: The relationship of childhood respiratory illness to adult obstructive airway disease. Am. Rev. Respir. Dis. *115*:751-760, 1977.
8. Caul, E. O., Waller, D. K., Clarke, S. K. R., et al.: A comparison of influenza and respiratory syncytial virus infections among infants admitted to hospital with acute respiratory infections. J. Hyg. Camb. *77*:383-392, 1976.
9. Centers for Disease Control and Prevention: Prevention and control of influenza. M. M. W. R. Morb. Mortal. Wkly. Rep. *55*(No. RR-10):1-31, 2006.
10. Chanock, R., Chambon, L., Chang, W., et al.: WHO respiratory disease survey in children: A serological study. Bull. World Health Organ. *37*:363-369, 1967.
11. Chanock, R. M., Mufson, M. A., and Johnson, K. M.: Comparative biology and ecology of human virus and mycoplasma respiratory pathogens. Prog. Med. Virol. *7*:208-252, 1965.
12. Chanock, R. M., and Parrott, R. H.: Acute respiratory disease in infancy and childhood: Present understanding and prospects for prevention. E. Mead Johnson Address, October 1964. Pediatrics *36*:21-39, 1965.
13. Chapman, R. S., Henderson, F. W., Clyde, W. A., Jr., et al.: The epidemiology of tracheobronchitis in pediatric practice. Am. J. Epidemiol. *114*:786-797, 1981.
14. Cherry, J. D.: Personal observations over 45 years.
15. Cherry, J. D.: Newer respiratory viruses: Their role in respiratory illnesses of children. *In* Schulman, I. (ed.): Advances in Pediatrics. Vol. 20. Chicago, Year Book Medical Publishers, 1973, pp. 225-290.
16. Cherry, J. D., Diddams, J. A., and Dick, E. C.: Rhinovirus infections in hospitalized children: Provocative bacterial interrelationships. Arch. Environ. Health *14*:390-396, 1967.
17. Chiu, S. S., Chan, K. H., Chu, K. W., et al.: Human coronavirus NL63 infection and other coronavirus infections in children hospitalized with acute respiratory disease in Hong Kong, China. Clin. Infect. Dis. *40*:1721-1729, 2005.

18. Colley, J. R. T., Douglas, J. W. B., and Reid, D. D.: Respiratory disease in young adults: Influence of early childhood lower respiratory tract illness, social class, air pollution, and smoking. B. M. J. 8:195-198, 1973.

19. Committee on Drugs: Use of codeine- and dextromethorphan-containing cough syrups in pediatrics. Pediatrics 62:118-122, 1978.

20. Couch, R. B.: Prevention and treatment of influenza. N. Engl. J. Med. 343:1778-1787, 2000.

21. Darelid, J., Lofgren, S., and Malmvall, B. E.: Erythromycin treatment is beneficial for longstanding *Moraxella catarrhalis* associated cough in children. Scand. J. Infect. Dis. 25:323-329, 1993.

22. Dascomb, H. E., and Hilleman, M. R.: Clinical and laboratory studies in patients with respiratory disease caused by adenoviruses (RI-APC-ARD agents). Am. J. Med. 21:161-174, 1956.

23. Denny, F. W., and Clyde, W. A., Jr.: Acute lower respiratory tract infections in nonhospitalized children. J. Pediatr. 108:635-646, 1986.

24. Dulfano, M. J., Adler, K., and Wooten, O.: Physical properties of sputum, IV: Effects of 100 percent humidity and water mist. Am. Rev. Respir. Dis. 107:130-132, 1973.

25. Edwards, G.: Acute bronchitis: Aetiology, diagnosis, and management. B. M. J. 1:963-966, 1966.

26. Esper, F., Weibel, C., Ferguson, D., et al.: Evidence of a novel human coronavirus that is associated with respiratory tract disease in infants and young children. J. Infect. Dis. 191:492-498, 2005.

27. Gardner, P. S.: Virus infections and respiratory disease of childhood. Arch. Dis. Child. 43:629-645, 1968.

28. Gardner, P. S.: How etiologic, pathologic, and clinical diagnoses can be made in a correlated fashion. Pediatr. Res. 11:254-261, 1977.

29. Gardner, S. D.: The isolation of parainfluenza 4 subtypes A and B in England and serological studies of their prevalence. J. Hyg. Camb. 67:545-550, 1969.

30. Glezen, W. P., Loda, F. A., Clyde, W. A., Jr., et al.: Epidemiologic patterns of acute lower respiratory disease of children in a pediatric group practice. J. Pediatr. 78:397-406, 1971.

31. Gottfard, P., and Brauner, A.: Children with persistent cough: Outcome with treatment and role of *Moraxella catarrhalis*? Scand. J. Infect. Dis. 26:545-551, 1994.

32. Grayston, J. T., Campbell, L. A., Kuo, C. C., et al.: A new respiratory tract pathogen: *Chlamydia pneumoniae* strain TWAR. J. Infect. Dis. 161:618-625, 1990.

33. Herrmann, E. C., Jr., and Hable, K. A.: Experiences in laboratory diagnosis of parainfluenza viruses in routine medical practice. Mayo Clin. Proc. 45:177-188, 1970.

34. Hilleman, M. R.: Respiratory syncytial virus. Am. Rev. Respir. Dis. 88(Suppl.):181-189, 1963.

35. Horn, M. E. C., Brain, E., Gregg, I., et al.: Respiratory viral infection in childhood: A survey in general practice, Roehampton 1967-1972. J. Hyg. Camb. 74:157-168, 1975.

36. Kellner, G., Popow-Kraupp, T., Kundi, M., et al.: Contribution of rhinoviruses to respiratory viral infections in childhood: A prospective study in a mainly hospitalized infant population. J. Med. Virol. 25:455-469, 1988.

37. Kesebir, D., Vazquez, M., Weibel, C., et al.: Human bocavirus infection in young children in the United States: Molecular epidemiological profile and clinical characteristics of a newly emerging respiratory virus. J. Infect. Dis. 194:1276-1282, 2006.

38. Kim, H. W., Arrobio, J. O., Brandt, C. D., et al.: Epidemiology of respiratory syncytial virus infection in Washington, D.C., I: Importance of the virus in different respiratory tract disease syndromes and temporal distribution of infection. Am. J. Epidemiol. 98:216-225, 1973.

39. Kravitz, H.: Sex distribution of hospitalized children with acute respiratory diseases, gastroenteritis and meningitis. Clin. Pediatr. 4:484-491, 1965.

40. Kuo, C. C., Jackson, L. A., Campbell, L. A., et al.: *Chlamydia pneumoniae* (TWAR). Clin. Microbiol. Rev. 8:451-461, 1995.

41. Kuroki, H., Morozumi, M., Chiba, N., et al.: Characterization of children with *Mycoplasma pneumoniae* infection detected by rapid polymerase chain reaction technique. J. Infect. Chemother. 10:65-67, 2004.

42. Laxdal, O. E., Robertson, H. E., Braaten, V., et al.: Acute respiratory infections in children, I: An intensive study of etiology in an open community. Can. Med. Assoc. J. 88:1049-1054, 1963.

43. Lebowitz, M. D., and Burrows, B.: The relationship of acute respiratory illness history to the prevalence and incidence of obstructive lung disorders. Am. J. Epidemiol. 105:544-554, 1977.

44. Leeder, S. R., Woolcock, A. J., and Blackburn, C. R. B.: Prevalence and natural history of lung disease in New South Wales schoolchildren. Int. J. Epidemiol. 3:15-23, 1974.

45. McClelland, L., Hilleman, M. R., Hamparian, V. V., et al.: Studies of acute respiratory illnesses caused by respiratory syncytial virus, 2: Epidemiology and assessment of importance. N. Engl. J. Med. 264:1169-1175, 1961.

46. Mink, C. A. M., Cherry, J. D., Christenson, P., et al.: A search for *Bordetella pertussis* infection in university students. Clin. Infect. Dis. 14:464-471, 1992.

47. Nichol, K. P., and Cherry, J. D.: Bacterial-viral interrelations in respiratory infections of children. N. Engl. J. Med. 277:667-672, 1967.

48. O'Brien, K. L., Dowell, S. F., Schwartz, B., et al.: Cough illness/bronchitis—principles of judicious use of antimicrobial agents. Pediatrics 101:178-181, 1998.

49. Parks, C. R.: Mist therapy: Rationale and practice. J. Pediatr. 76:305-313, 1970.

50. Pereira, M. S.: Adenovirus infections. Postgrad. Med. J. 49:798-801, 1973.

51. Person, D. A., and Herrmann, E. C., Jr.: Experiences in laboratory diagnosis of rhinovirus infections in routine medical practice. Mayo Clin. Proc. 45:517-526, 1970.

52. Robbins, F. C.: Measles: Clinical features. Am. J. Dis. Child. 103:266-273, 1962.

53. Saliba, G. S., Glezen, W. P., and Chin, T. D. Y.: *Mycoplasma pneumoniae* infection in a resident boys' home. Am. J. Epidemiol. 86:408-418, 1967.

54. Similä, S., Jouppila, R., Salmi, A., et al.: Encephalomeningitis in children associated with an adenovirus type 7 epidemic. Acta Paediatr. Scand. 59:310-316, 1970.

55. Spence, L., and Barratt, N.: Respiratory syncytial virus associated with acute respiratory infections in Trinidadian patients. Am. J. Epidemiol. 88:257-266, 1968.

56. Sterner, G., Gerzen, P., Ohlson, M., et al.: Acute respiratory illness and gastroenteritis in association with adenovirus type 7 infections. Acta Paediatr. 50:457-468, 1961.

57. Stockton, J., Stephenson, I., Fleming, D., and Zambon, M.: Human *Metapneumovirus* as a cause of community-acquired respiratory illness. Emerg. Infect. Dis. 8:897-901, 2002.

58. Stott, E. J., Eadie, M. B., and Grist, N. R.: Rhinovirus infections of children in hospital: Isolation of three possibly new rhinovirus serotypes. Am. J. Epidemiol. 90:45-52, 1969.

59. Stuart-Harris, C. H.: The present status of the respiratory viruses and acute respiratory disease in man. Israel J. Med. Sci. 2:255-268, 1966.

60. Suto, T., Yano, N., Ikeda, M., et al.: Respiratory syncytial virus infection and its serologic epidemiology. Am. J. Epidemiol. 82:211-224, 1965.

61. Sutton, R. N. P.: Respiratory viruses in a residential nursery. J. Hyg. Camb. 60:51-67, 1962.

62. Toth, M., Barna, M., and Voltay, B.: Aetiology of acute respiratory diseases in infants and children. Acta Paediatr. Hung. 6:367-374, 1965.

63. Urquhart, G. E. D., Moffat, M. A. J., Calder, M. A., et al.: An aetiological study of respiratory infection in children, Edinburgh City Hospital, 1961-1963. J. Hyg. Camb. 63:187-199, 1965.

64. van der Veen, J.: The role of adenoviruses in respiratory disease. Am. Rev. Respir. Dis. 88:167-180, 1963.

65. van Lierde, S., Corbeel, L., and Eggermont, E.: Clinical and laboratory findings in children with adenovirus infections. Eur. J. Pediatr. 148:423-525, 1989.

66. Vihma, L.: Surveillance of acute viral respiratory diseases in children. Acta Paediatr. Scand. 192(Suppl.):7-53, 1969.

67. Walker, S. H.: The respiratory manifestations of systemic *Haemophilus influenzae* infection. J. Pediatr. 62:386-392, 1963.

68. Waites, K. B., and Talkington, D. F.: *Mycoplasma pneumoniae* and its role as a human pathogen. Clin. Microbiol. Rev. 17:697-728, 2004.

69. Watson, R. L., Dowell, S. F., Jayaraman, M., et al.: Antimicrobial use for pediatric upper respiratory infections: Reported practice, actual practice, and parent beliefs. Pediatrics 104:1251-1257, 1999.

70. Yodfat, Y., and Nishmi, M.: Successive overlapping outbreaks of febrile pharyngitis and pharyngoconjunctival fever associated with adenovirus types 2 and 7, in a Kibbutz. Israel J. Med. Sci. 10:1505-1509, 1974.

71. Zinserling, A.: Peculiarities of lesions in viral and mycoplasmal infections of the respiratory tract. Virchows Arch. A 356:259-273, 1972.

CHAPTER 24

CHRONIC BRONCHITIS

I. Celine Hanson ✧ William T. Shearer

Chronic bronchitis is a serious and costly health problem in adults.[17] In a U.S. review of the epidemiology of chronic bronchitis, affected adult morbidity estimates were greater than 900,000 hospitalizations and 10 to 14 million physician visits each year.[24] The World Health Organization estimates 23.6 million

adults have chronic obstructive pulmonary disease, representing more than 15 percent of the adult population, and many of these cases meet the definition for chronic bronchitis.[5] In the adult literature, the accepted definition of chronic bronchitis includes daily excessive production of sputum with manifestation of cough present on most days for 3 months in a year for not less than 2 successive years.[46]

For most pediatricians, the clinical entity of chronic bronchitis is ill-defined. Chronic cough complex can be associated with other, more common respiratory or cardiac diseases that must be excluded before a diagnosis of chronic bronchitis is considered.[11] Chronic bronchitis usually is described in the literature as chronic productive cough and is synonymous with asthmatic bronchitis.[8,43] The lack of uniform or standardized definitions of pediatric chronic bronchitis leads to wide discrepancies in reported childhood prevalence (Table 24–1). In affected patients, causal relationships and acute exacerbations have been linked to exposure to a noxious inhaled agent (e.g., environmental/industrial pollution, cigarette smoke), specific host factors (e.g., genetic predisposition), and infectious respiratory pathogens. The pathology of the disease entity is unclear. Bronchoscopy of pediatric patients with chronic bronchitis has revealed findings similar to those noted in children with asthma, which reflects the inclusion of asthma in the spectrum of the chronic bronchitis complex.[27]

Pediatric bronchoscopic evaluation yields heterogeneous histologic findings (granulocyte and mononuclear cell predominance at lavage and biopsy) that are distinct from findings in adults with chronic bronchitis.[43]

DIFFERENTIAL DIAGNOSIS

Because chronic bronchitis is accepted by most physicians as being a complex of symptoms characterized by persistent cough with or without wheezing, it is imperative that the physician evaluate the patient for diseases that include chronic bronchitis within their spectrum of signs and symptoms. Figure 24–1 includes disorders that have clinical manifestations of chronic cough for longer than 3 months and provides guidelines for diagnostic evaluation of children with chronic cough.[26]

Heading the differential list is asthma,[10] defined as reversible obstructive airways disease with a significant inflammatory component leading to increased edema and production of mucus.

TABLE 24–1   Prevalence of Childhood Bronchitis

Author	Year	Study Subjects	Prevalence (%)	Acute/Chronic Bronchitis
Bland et al.	1974	Kent schoolchildren	5.5	Acute/chronic
Burrows and Lebowitz	1975	Arizona children	7.1	Chronic
Burrows et al.	1977	Arizona retrospective	46.4	Chronic
Kubo et al.	1978	Japanese children	1.4	Chronic
Peat et al.	1980	Sydney schoolchildren	20	Acute/chronic

Modified from Morgan, W. T., and Taussig, L. M.: The chronic bronchitis complex in childhood. Pediatr. Clin. North Am. 31:851-864, 1984.)

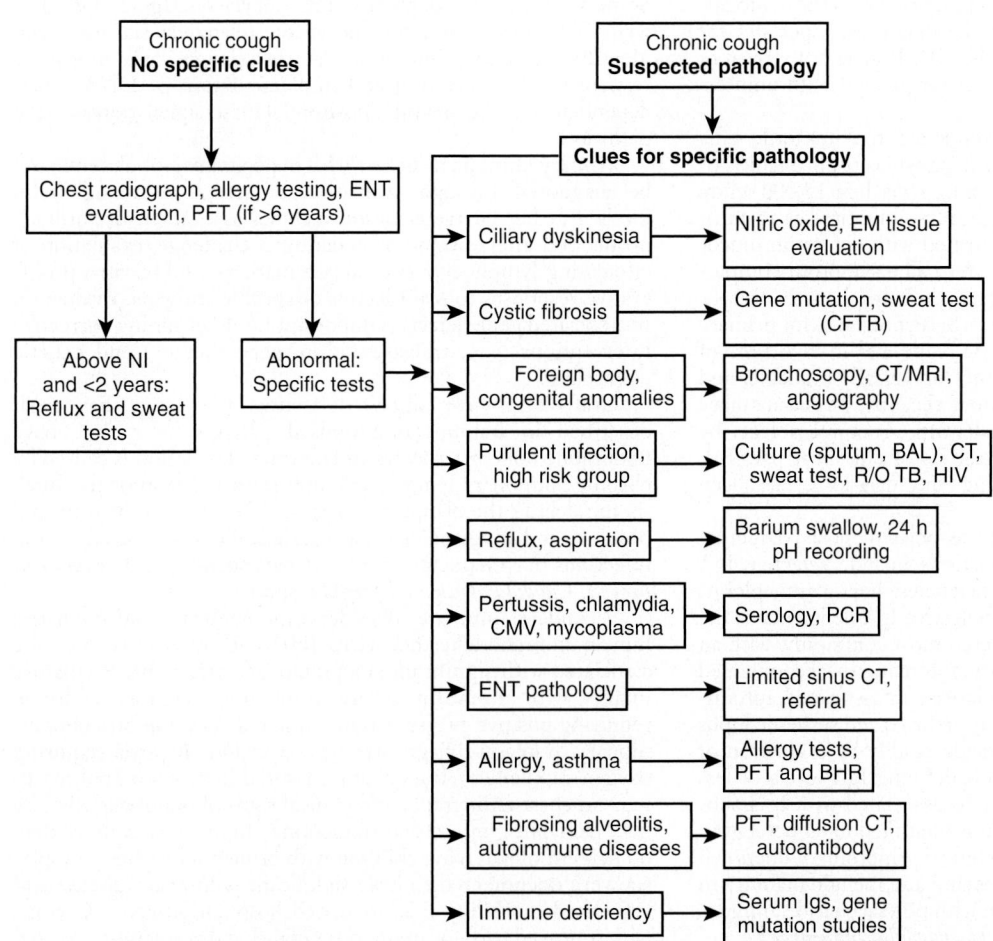

Figure 24–1 Diagnostic evaluation of children with chronic cough. BAL, bronchoalveolar lavage; BHR, bronchial hyperreactivity; CFTR, cystic fibrosis transmembrane conductance regulator; CMV, cytomegalovirus; CT, computed tomography; EM, electron microscopy; ENT, ear, nose, throat; HIV, human immunodeficiency virus; MRI, magnetic resonance imaging; NI, no information; PCR, polymerase chain reaction; PFT, pulmonary function test; TB, tuberculosis. (*Modified from Morice, A. J., Fontana, G. A., Sovijarvi, A. R., et al.: Diagnoses and management of chronic cough. Eur. Respir. J. 24:487, 2004.*)

Asthma is a common pediatric lower respiratory disease, affecting more than 6.3 million children younger than 18 years old in the United States.[1] Asthma can be distinguished from chronic bronchitis by pulmonary function evaluation documenting reversal of airway obstruction after delivery of pulmonary bronchodilators. Recurrent episodes of acute bronchitis often can be interpreted as chronic bronchitis, although the intermittent nature of these episodes and absence of a persistent cough usually distinguish this group of patients clinically.[4]

Specific viral infections (e.g., rhinovirus, parainfluenza virus) in children with or without allergic rhinitis may provoke airway hyperreactivity and late asthmatic reactions, which may be confused symptomatically with chronic bronchitis.[6,20] Persistent lower respiratory tract infections (i.e., *Chlamydia* spp., pertussis, *Mycoplasma* spp., and *Mycobacterium* spp.) frequently manifest with the complex of symptoms described and are evaluated best with chest radiographs in a search for enlarged hilar nodes or interstitial lung infiltrates. Respiratory tract secretions for appropriate bacterial and viral culture and serum for determinations of antibacterial antibodies should be obtained. In the case of tuberculosis, a delayed hypersensitivity skin test for *Mycobacterium tuberculosis* antigen should be applied.

Cystic fibrosis is a recessively inherited illness occurring in approximately 1 in 3700 live births, with clinical manifestations of failure to thrive, steatorrhea, nasal polyps, and recurrent lower respiratory tract symptoms. The disorder is associated with mutation of the cystic fibrosis transmembrane conductance regulator (CFTR) gene.[38] Cystic fibrosis can be diagnosed by newborn screening methodologies including identifying typical CFTR gene mutation patterns in DNA extracted from dot blots or other collected blood specimens at or after birth or by detecting abnormally elevated chloride levels (>60 mEq/L) as measured by the sweat iontophoresis test.[40] In clinical practice, one or both modalities may be used for establishing the diagnosis, especially for patients with genetic variations of the CFTR gene not typical of the classic cystic fibrosis phenotype or for patients with uninterpretable sweat test outcomes.

Primary ciliary dyskinesia encompasses the immotile cilia disorders and Kartagener syndrome (rhinosinusitis, bronchitis or bronchiectasis, and situs inversus) and affects 1 in 15,000 white births. Primary ciliary dyskinesia typically is inherited as an autosomal recessive disorder and is associated with defects in mucociliary transport in the respiratory tree. The symptom complex also has been associated with polycystic kidneys, hepatic disease, and central nervous system symptoms. Screening tests for primary ciliary dyskinesia include nasal nitric oxide and in vivo tests of ciliary motility, but these tests are not universally available, and standardization is problematic.[31] More recently, physicians have used tissue biopsy specimens to identify structural defects by electron microscopy, high-speed analysis of cilia beat patterns, and cell culture when establishing the diagnosis has been difficult.[29]

The primary immune disorders associated most frequently with recurrent sinopulmonary infections include selective IgA deficiency, functional antibody deficiencies, hypogammaglobulinemia, and ataxia telangiectasia.[3] Selective IgA deficiency is the primary immune disorder encountered most commonly, with an incidence of 1 in 500. It may be asymptomatic or accompanied by a propensity for atopy and an increase in associated autoimmune disease (most often rheumatoid arthritis and systemic lupus erythematosus). The diagnosis is made readily by evaluation of quantitative serum immunoglobulins defining IgA levels of less than 10 mg/dL. IgA deficiency may be associated with IgG subclass deficiencies (IgG2 deficiency was identified in 85 percent in a series of >150) with or without clinical symptoms. Functional antibody deficiencies have been detected and include inability to respond serologically to vaccination with polysaccharide antigens such as *Streptococcus pneumoniae* or *Haemophilus influenzae*.[13]

Patients with hypogammaglobulinemia represent a diverse group having primary immune disorders that include X-linked agammaglobulinemia, common variable immune deficiency (CVID), and hyper-IgM syndrome. X-linked agammaglobulinemia typically affects boys, with recurrent sinopulmonary infections with onset occurring postnatally as maternal antibody wanes. X-linked agammaglobulinemia is associated with deficiency of a B-cell maturation enzyme, Bruton tyrosine kinase, and is characterized by the absence of circulating mature B lymphocytes. CVID is a disorder of young adults, with immune findings of agammaglobulinemia and variable T-cell defects. Clinical presentation includes lower respiratory and sinus disease. Inherited CVID disorders have been described and include defects in inducible T-cell costimulator gene and transmembrane activator and calcium-modulator and cyclophilin ligand interactor (TACI).[3] Patients with TACI defect and CVID may lack circulating mature B lymphocytes. More often, patients with CVID normally express B-cell markers on circulating lymphocytes. Hyper-IgM syndrome is a rare disorder associated with elevated IgM and low IgG and IgA and recurrent infections including sinopulmonary and hepatic infections. Different gene defects have been identified in patients with hyper-IgM syndrome; patients with defects in nucleotide-modifying enzymes located only in B cells have no associated T-cell defect.

Patients with ataxia telangiectasia have depressed serum IgA concentrations and marked dysfunction of the swallowing mechanism, leading to recurrent lower respiratory tract infections probably secondary to recurrent aspiration. These patients are identified by telangiectasias of the skin and conjunctivae in association with aberrant and progressively deteriorating neurologic symptoms and immunodeficiency (depressed IgA and IgE and aberrant T-cell–mediated immunity). Some patients have depressed IgG subclasses (IgG2, IgG4) as well. The gene mutation in ataxia telangiectasia has been identified as disruption of the ataxia telangiectasia molecules responsible for detection and implementation of DNA repair dependent on phosphatidylinositol-3-kinase signal transduction pathways.

Primary immune disorders with hypogammaglobulinemia can be diagnosed through evaluation of serum immunoglobulin levels. Further characterization includes assessment of antibody production after vaccine or neoantigen challenge, evaluation of circulating lymphocyte cell surface markers, and in vitro proliferative responses to plant lectins or specific antigens. Evaluation of associated gene defects is important for determining corrective interventions (e.g., transplantation, gene therapy) and genetic counseling.

Graft-versus-host disease affecting the lungs has been described in immunocompromised patients after they have undergone bone marrow transplantation. The lesion is caused by chronic pulmonary lymphocytic infiltrates and pulmonary fibrosis mimicking the symptom complex of chronic bronchitis and often is indistinguishable radiographically or clinically from infections that characteristically are pathogenic (i.e., *Pneumocystis jiroveci*, *Candida albicans*, *Aspergillus* spp.).

Secondary immune disorders (prematurity and pediatric human immunodeficiency virus [HIV] infection) also may be associated with significant sinopulmonary infections. Premature infants with attendant severe respiratory distress syndrome requiring positive-pressure ventilation may develop bronchopulmonary dysplasia. Diagnostic criteria include hypoxia requiring oxygen supplementation, characteristic diffuse interstitial markings on chest radiograph, and clinical signs of pulmonary disease (i.e., tachypnea, intercostal retractions). In one series, more than 60 percent of surviving children with bronchopulmonary dysplasia were documented to have significant pulmonary disease and associated morbidity (i.e., increased hospitalizations).[33] Continued improved care for premature infants and resultant decreased incidence of mortality may increase the population of infants with bronchopulmonary dysplasia.

Pediatric HIV infection is estimated to affect approximately 1.5 percent of infants born to HIV-infected mothers in the United States.[28] This reduced infection rate can be attributed to (1) availability and use of highly active antiretroviral therapy (HAART) to pregnant women and their newborn infants, (2) U.S. practices that minimize exposure to breast milk, and (3) obstetric practices that minimize exposure to infected blood products (cesarean delivery and practices that decrease time from membrane rupture to delivery). For infants in the United States who continue to be infected, with noncompliance to treatment or lack of treatment, HIV is associated with serious lower respiratory tract illness.

In previous years, lymphoid interstitial pneumonitis/hyperplasia, reported in 25 percent of all children with acquired immunodeficiency syndrome, was associated with chronic cough, but this HIV-associated outcome rarely is reported with the advent of improved antiviral medications to suppress replication of HIV. Despite restoration of immunocompetence with HAART, lower respiratory tract infections (viral, bacterial, fungal) are still common occurrences in children infected with HIV.[23] In the face of improved survival for HIV-infected children, the incidence of chronic radiographic lung changes (parenchymal consolidations and nodular disease for >3 months) has been described in 33 percent of children by the time they are 4 years of age.[30] An unexpected consequence of HAART therapy in HIV-infected children may lead to increased risk of developing asthma through an immune reconstitution mechanism.[14] The diagnosis of HIV infection is established by viral diagnostic assays (polymerase chain reaction, p24 antigen) for perinatally exposed infants younger than 18 months of age and by serology (enzyme-linked immunosorbent assay and confirmational assays [Western blot analysis, indirect fluorescent antibody assay]) for perinatally exposed infants 18 months or older.[35]

Anatomic lesions that lead to pulmonary obstructive airway disease can simulate the complex of chronic bronchitis. An infant with chronic cough, poor feeding habits, and failure to thrive should undergo evaluation for gastroesophageal reflux and tracheoesophageal fistula, which are identified most easily by barium swallow or pH probe monitoring. Mediastinal tumors can produce extrinsic obstruction, leading to recurrent cough and wheezing. Congenital heart disease should be considered in this patient group and can be evaluated with chest radiography, electrocardiography, and echocardiography.

Respiratory tract irritants have been implicated as a cause of chronic cough, as documented in adult populations of industrial European nations.[44] An assessment of the public health impact of pollution in Austria, France, and Switzerland concluded that air pollution caused 6 percent of all mortality, or 40,000 attributable cases per year.[19] Nonindustrial, rural communities, such as the forest zone of Nigeria, report virtually no chronic bronchitis, whereas metropolitan New York reports an increased risk for development of upper and lower respiratory tract infections in adults and children who reside in parts of the city with the highest ambient air levels of sulfur dioxide and particulate air pollution.[22] After exposure to urban air particulate matter, animal models with induced chronic bronchitis (exposure to 200 ppm of sulfur dioxide for 6 weeks) have shown pathologic changes consistent with exacerbation of chronic bronchitis—changes in ventilatory capacity and marked pulmonary inflammation.[9]

A correlation between tobacco smoking and reduced ventilatory capacity in adults has been reported by many investigators. Peat and associates[34] described teenagers in Sydney, Australia, with recurrent episodes of bronchitis with worsened lung function when coupled with tobacco smoking. A meta-analysis of 21 relevant publications on relationships between exposure to environmental tobacco smoke and lower respiratory tract infection in infancy and early childhood concluded that exposure to environmental smoke resulted in adverse childhood respiratory outcomes.[21] The outcomes included an increased number of lower respiratory tract infections and an increased number of hospitalizations for these infections. These data suggest that it is imperative for physicians to obtain a smoking history not only for the patient but also for other household members.

Other noxious agents associated with outdoor pollution have been associated with poor control of chronic cough complex diseases such as asthma. In Los Angeles, adults with asthma were more poorly controlled if they resided near areas of heavy traffic.[25] Similar findings of poorly controlled lung disease associated with traffic pollution have been documented in adult and pediatric patients in Lima, Peru.[7] Occupational exposures long have been cited for exacerbating pulmonary diseases. Blanc and colleagues[2] evaluated the risk for developing chronic lung disease from occupational exposure and identified the population attributable risk at 15 percent for chronic bronchitis and chronic obstructive pulmonary disease. Classic examples of occupational exposure to dust leading to increased risk of developing chronic cough are described in coal miners in Great Britain, foundry workers in the Rhine-Ruhr area of Germany, potters in West Virginia, and farmers in Croatia.[47] After the disaster of September 11, 2001, in New York City, firefighters with existing sarcoidosis (reported at higher frequency in firefighters before the disaster) reported increased incidence of bronchial hyperreactivity measured by pulmonary challenge testing.[16]

EPIDEMIOLOGY AND ETIOLOGY

Differentiating the impact of clinical, social, and environmental factors on lower respiratory tract disease, including chronic bronchitis, has been problematic and has led to conflicting outcomes in epidemiologic assessments.[12,42] In addition, the lack of a standardized definition of chronic bronchitis in the pediatric literature leads to confusing interpretation of data when attempting to appreciate the prevalence or etiology of the disease complex.[43] In Table 24–1, the data from Kubo and associates[18] separate acute recurrent bronchitis, asthmatic bronchitis, and chronic bronchitis, leading to a decrease in the prevalence from a proposed 46.4 percent (in the Arizona questionnaire) to 1.4 percent.[27]

Considerable overlap also exists in evaluating etiologic agents for chronic bronchitis. The same viral agents proposed as the exacerbating factors of asthmatic bronchitis (see Chapter 25) are implicated in exacerbations of chronic bronchitis,[1,15] including rhinoviruses, parainfluenza viruses, respiratory syncytial virus, influenza A and B viruses, adenoviruses, and enteroviruses. Persistent adenovirus infection has been implicated as a cause of childhood chronic bronchitis. In a study of 11 children with chronic bronchitis, transbronchial biopsy specimens revealed no evidence of persistent adenovirus infection (culture or polymerase chain reaction),[36] suggesting that viral infections may precipitate cough, but their roles in the pathologic findings associated with chronic bronchitis should be questioned.

Table 24–2 lists predominant bacterial pathogens isolated from washed sputum for a group of 40 pediatric patients with chronic bronchitis and exacerbations of cough and fever; these pathogens include *H. influenzae*, *S. pneumoniae*, and *Staphylococcus aureus*.[18] These bacteria also are implicated as etiologic agents in the triggering of asthmatic bronchitis. Neither *Mycoplasma* nor human metapneumovirus was included in this listing, but this simply may reflect the time-frame (late 1970s) when the Kubo study was conducted.[32,45] Treatment of exacerbations of chronic bronchitis with antibiotic therapy usually is effective in reducing the volume of sputum and purulence during the acute infection but shows no parallel elimination of the cultured microorganisms.

TABLE 24-2 Predominant Pathogens in Washed Sputum of Chronic Bronchitis (40 Cases)

Pathogen	No. Cases
Haemophilus influenzae and *Streptococcus pneumoniae*	21 (52.5%)
H. influenzae	17 (42.5%)
Staphylococcus aureus	2 (5%)
Superinfection with gram-negative rods	
Pseudomonas aeruginosa	4
Klebsiella pneumoniae	2
Escherichia coli	1
Enterobacter cloacae	1

From Kubo, S., Funabashi, S., Uehara, S., et al.: Clinical aspects of "asthmatic bronchitis" and chronic bronchitis in infants and children. J. Asthma Res. 15:99-132, 1978.

TREATMENT

When a specific diagnosis is found in association with chronic cough or wheezing, therapy is directed toward the primary disease entity and the clinical presentation of cough. Bronchodilators (beta-adrenergic agents, cromolyn sodium, corticosteroids) and anticholinergic agents are used, when appropriate, for the treatment of chronic cough associated with asthma or acute exacerbations of chronic obstructive pulmonary disease.[41] Appropriate positioning techniques (prone 30 degrees), feeding schedules, and medications (e.g., prokinetics or cholinergics) are indicated in the approach to infants with gastroesophageal reflux. Patients with hypogammaglobulinemia can be helped with supplemental intravenous immunoglobulin preparations currently available commercially (400 to 600 mg/kg per dose every 3 to 4 weeks) in an attempt to decrease the incidence of infections.

It is imperative that patients with chronic pulmonary diseases such as cystic fibrosis, asthma, or ciliary dyskinesias understand the pulmonary irritant effect of tobacco smoking, dust exposure, and air pollution. A change of occupation may be essential for their well-being. It also is imperative to stress the irritant effect of parental smoking on the already compromised pulmonary function of the child.

Antibiotic therapy for chronic bronchitis usually is reserved for patients with severe illness in whom the likelihood of developing a secondary bacterial infection is great. In these instances, antibiotic therapy can be considered and usually consists of amoxicillin (45 to 90 mg/kg per 24 hours), erythromycin (40 mg/kg per 24 hours), or, in adolescents and adults, tetracycline (25 to 50 mg/kg per 24 hours) or quinolones for 5 to 10 days. There do not seem to be significant differences in short-term effectiveness in adults with these outlined treatment regimens.[39] Methylxanthine therapy is used less frequently in chronic bronchitis care. When it is used, certain antibiotics, such as erythromycin, lead to elevated serum concentrations of theophylline, which renders toxicity more likely to occur. Treatment with mucolytic agents in chronic pulmonary disease has not proven to have a significant impact except in adults with already advanced disease with multiple hospitalizations, and no evidence suggests that they are beneficial in children.[37]

As with patients with obstructive lung disease, attention must be aimed at careful and sequential monitoring of pulmonary function. The prognosis for chronic bronchitis varies and is dependent on the specific etiology of this syndrome.

REFERENCES

1. Asthma in children fact sheet. American Lung Association, 2004.
2. Blanc, P. D., and Toren, K.: Int. J. Tuberc. Lung Dis. 11:251-257, 2007.
3. Bonilla, F. A., and Geha, R. S.: Update on primary immunodeficiency diseases. J. Allergy Clin. Immunol. 117:S435-S441, 2006.
4. Boule, M., Gaultier, C., Tournier, G., et al.: Lung function in children with recurrent bronchitis. Respiration 38:127-134, 1979.
5. Braman, S. S.: Chronic cough due to chronic bronchitis. ACCP evidence-based clinical practice guidelines. Chest 129:104S-115S, 2006.
6. Busse, W. W.: Respiratory infections: Their role in airway responsiveness and the pathogenesis of asthma. J. Allergy Clin. Immunol. 85:671-684, 1990.
7. Carbajal-Arroyo, L., Barraza-Villarreal, A., Durand-Pardo, R., et al.: Impact of traffic flow on the asthma prevalence among school children in Lima, Peru. J. Asthma 44:197-202, 2007.
8. Carter, E. R., Debley, J. S., and Redding, G. R.: Chronic productive cough in school children: Prevalence and associations with asthma and environmental tobacco smoke exposure. Cough 2:11, 2006.
9. Clarke, R. W., Catalano, P. J., Koutrakis, P., et al.: Urban air particulate inhalation alters pulmonary function and induces pulmonary inflammation in a rodent model of chronic bronchitis. Inhal. Toxicol. 11:637-656, 1999.
10. Cloutier, M. M., and Laughlin, G. M.: Chronic cough in children: A manifestation of airway hyperreactivity. Pediatrics 67:6-12, 1981.
11. DeJongste, J. C., and Shields, M. D.: Cough, 2: Chronic cough in children. Thorax 58:998-1003, 2003.
12. Dodge, R., Burrows, B., Lebowitz, M. D., et al.: Antecedent features of children in whom asthma develops during the second decade of life. J. Allergy Clin. Immunol. 92:744-749, 1993.
13. Edwards, E., Razvi, S., and Cunningham-Rundles, C.: IgA deficiency: Clinical correlates and responses to pneumococcal vaccine. Clin. Immunol. 111:93-77, 2004.
14. Foster, S. B., Paul, M. E., Kozinetz, C. A., et al.: Prevalence of asthma in children and young adults with HIV infection. J. Allergy Clin. Immunol. 119:750-752, 2007.
15. Horn, M. E. C., and Gregg, I.: Role of viral infection and host factors in acute episodes of asthma and chronic bronchitis. Chest 63:44-85, 1973.
16. Izbicki, G., Chavko, R., Banauch, G. I., et al.: World Trade Center 'sarcoid-like' granulomatous pulmonary disease in New York City Fire Department rescue workers. Chest 131:1414-1423, 2007.
17. Kim, N., and Leeper, K. V., Jr.: Epidemiology of chronic bronchitis and acute infective exacerbations of chronic bronchitis. Semin. Respir. Crit. Care Med. 21:73-78, 2000.
18. Kubo, S., Funabashi, S., Uehara, S., et al.: Clinical aspects of "asthmatic bronchitis" and chronic bronchitis in infants and children. J. Asthma Res. 15:99-132, 1978.
19. Kunzli, N., Kaiser, R., Medina, S., et al.: Public-health impact of outdoor and traffic-related air pollution: A European assessment. Lancet 356:795-801, 2000.
20. Lemanske, R. F., Dick, E. C., Swenson, C. A., et al.: Rhinovirus upper respiratory tract infection increases airway hyperreactivity and late asthmatic reactions. J. Clin. Invest. 83:1-10, 1989.
21. Li, J. S., Peat, J. K., Zuan, W., et al.: Meta-analysis on the association between environmental tobacco smoke (ETS) exposure and the prevalence of lower respiratory tract infection in early childhood. Pediatr. Pulmonol. 27:5-13, 1999.
22. Love, G. T., Lan, S. P., Shy, C. M., et al.: The incidence and severity of acute respiratory illness in families exposed to different levels of air pollution, New York metropolitan area 1971-1972. Arch. Environ. Health 36:66-74, 1981.
23. Mato, S. P., and Van Dyke, R. B.: Pulmonary infections in children with HIV infection. Semin. Respir. Infect. 17:33-46, 2002.
24. McGuire, A., Irwin, D. E., Fenn, P., et al.: The excess cost of acute exacerbations of chronic bronchitis in patients aged 45 and older in England and Wales. Value Health 4:370-375, 2001.
25. Meng, Y. Y., Wilhelm, M., Rull, R. P., et al.: Traffic and outdoor air pollution levels near residences and poorly controlled asthma in adults. Ann. Allergy Asthma Immunol. 98:455-463, 2007.
26. Morice, A. J., Fontana, G. A, Sovijarvi, A. R., et al.: Diagnoses and management of chronic cough. Eur. Respir. J. 24:487, 2004.
27. Morgan, W. T., and Taussig, L. M.: The chronic bronchitis complex in childhood. Pediatr. Clin. North Am. 31:851-864, 1984.
28. Newel, M. L., Huang, S., Fiore, S., et al.: Characteristics and management of HIV-1-infected pregnant women enrolled in a randomized trial: differences between Europe and the USA. B. M. C. Infect. Dis. 7:60, 2007.
29. Noone, P., Leigh, M. S., Sannuti, A., et al.: Primary ciliary dyskinesia: Diagnostic and phenotypic features. Am. J. Respir. Crit. Care Med. 169:459-467, 2004.
30. Norton, K. I., Kattan, M., Rao, J. S., et al.: Chronic radiographic lung changes in children with vertically transmitted HIV-1 infection. A. J. R. Am. J. Roentgenol. 176:1553-1558, 2001.
31. O'Callaghan, C., Chilvers, M., Hogg, C., et al: Diagnosing primary ciliary dyskinesia. Thorax 62:656-657, 2007.
32. Park, Y.: Asthma and *Mycoplasma* pneumonia infection. J. Allergy Clin. Immunol. 119:S24, 2007.
33. Payne, N. R., LaCorte, M., Karna, P., et al.: Reduction of bronchopulmonary dysplasia after participating in the Breathsavers group of the Vermont Oxford Network Neonatal Intensive Care quality improvement collaboration. Pediatrics 118:S73-S77, 2006.

34. Peat, J. K., Woolcock, A. J., Leider, S. R., et al.: Asthma and bronchitis in Sydney school children, I: Prevalence during a six-year study. Am. J. Epidemiol. *111*:721-727, 1980.
35. Perinatal HIV Guidelines Working Group: Public Health Service Task Force recommendations for use of antiretroviral drugs in pregnant HIV-1 infected women for maternal health and interventions to reduce perinatal HIV-1 transmission in the United States. October 12, 2006 1-65. Available at: http://aidsinfo.nih.gov/ContentFiles/PerinatalGL.pdf. Accessed August 20, 2007.
36. Pichler, M., Herrmann, G., Schmidt, H., et al.: Persistent adenoviral infection and chronic obstructive bronchitis in children: Is there a link? Pediatr. Pulmonol. *32*:367-371, 2001.
37. Poole, P. J., and Black, P. N.: Mucolytic agents for chronic bronchitis and chronic obstructive pulmonary disease. Cochrane Database Syst. Rev. *19*: CD001287, 2006.
38. Rich, D. P., Anderson, M. P., Gregory, R. J., et al.: Expression of cystic fibrosis transmembrane regulator corrects defective chloride channel regulations in cystic fibrosis airway epithelial cells. Nature *347*:358-363, 1990.
39. Siempos, I. I., Dimopoulos, G., Korbila, I. P., et al.: Macrolides, quinolones and amoxicillin/clavulanate for chronic bronchitis: A meta-analysis. Eur. Respir. J. *29*:1127-1137, 2007.
40. Southern, K. W., and Peckham, D.: Establishing a diagnosis of cystic fibrosis. Chron. Respir. Dis. *1*:205-210, 2004.
41. Stoller, J. K.: Acute exacerbations of chronic obstructive pulmonary disease. N. Engl. J. Med. *346*:988-994, 2002.
42. Strachan, D. P., Seagrott, V., and Cook, D. G.: Chest illness in infancy and chronic respiratory disease in later life: An analysis by month of birth. Int. J. Epidemiol. *23*:1060-1068, 1994.
43. Taussig, L. M., Smith, S. M., and Blumenfeld, R.: Chronic bronchitis in childhood: What is it? Pediatrics *67*:1-5, 1981.
44. Wanner, H. U.: Effects of atmospheric pollution on human health. Experientia *49*:754-758, 1993.
45. Williams, J. V., Harris, P. A., Tollefson, S. J., et al.: Human metapneumovirus and lower respiratory tract disease in otherwise healthy infants and children. N. Engl. J. Med. *350*:443-450, 2004.
46. Wilson, R., Tillotson, G., and Ball, P.: Clinical studies in chronic bronchitis: A need for better definition and classification of severity. J. Antimicrob. Chemother. *37*:205-208, 1996.
47. Zock, J. P., Sunyer, J., Kogevinas, M., et al.: Occupation, chronic bronchitis, and lung function in young adults: An international study. Am. J. Respir. Crit. Care Med. *163*:1572-1577, 2001.

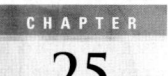

BRONCHIOLITIS AND INFECTIOUS ASTHMA

25

Robert C. Welliver

Bronchiolitis and infectious asthma, which also is called *asthmatic bronchitis*, *wheezy bronchitis*, or *virus-induced asthma*, are common illnesses of children, characterized by symptoms of upper respiratory tract infection and signs of obstructive airway disease, particularly wheezing. Bronchiolitis and infectious asthma often are considered to be distinct entities, and not all infants who develop bronchiolitis have infectious asthma in later life. Although the two illnesses are similar in terms of clinical presentation and have some mediators in common, the pathologic findings may contrast in some cases. Differences in terms of etiologic agents that precipitate episodes of illness or in terms of response to therapy are more a function of the patient's age (particularly older or younger than 3 years) than of any underlying disease process. *Infectious asthma* is considered as a term defining the occurrence of repeated episodes of bronchiolitis, and the two conditions are discussed together.

DEFINITIONS

Bronchiolitis is an acute communicable disease predominantly manifesting in infancy and characterized by cough, coryza, fever, grunting, tachypnea, retractions, inspiratory crackles, expiratory wheezing, and air trapping. The first (and the most severe) episodes occur most frequently in infants aged 2 to 6 months. *Infectious asthma* is a term that generally refers to infection-induced wheezing occurring beyond infancy. Nonetheless, a patient may experience bronchiolitis during the first months of life and a recurrent episode caused by the same virus in the second year, suggesting an identical underlying nature of the two illnesses. Certain viruses (e.g., respiratory syncytial virus [RSV] and influenza viruses) seem capable of causing bronchiolitis in all children; in contrast, other agents (rhinovirus in particular) seem to induce wheezing only in atopic children.

HISTORY

Although all practicing pediatricians today are familiar with the term *bronchiolitis* and associate it with an acute clinical illness with the signs and symptoms of obstructive emphysema, it has been recognized in the medical literature for only a relatively brief period. In the early years of the 20th century, the term *capillary bronchitis* was used to describe an inflammatory illness of the smallest alveoli.[56] The condition could not be distinguished clinically from pneumonia, however, and whether the pathologic entity (i.e., bronchiolitis) ever occurred separately from pneumonia was doubted. In the 11th edition of *Holt's Diseases of Infancy and Childhood*,[73] published in 1940, capillary bronchitis is discussed only briefly and is considered under pneumococcal pneumonia. Acute bronchiolitis finally was listed as a heading in the sixth edition of the *Textbook of Pediatrics*,[118] published in 1954; even at that time, bronchiolitis was associated with interstitial pneumonitis.

In contrast to the delayed textbook recognition of bronchiolitis, good clinical descriptions were presented in journals. In 1941, Hubble and Osborn[76] published "Acute Bronchiolitis in Children," in which they described an epidemic of bronchiolitis involving 50 hospitalized children. Pratt[131] in 1944 and Nelson and Smith[119] in 1945 published excellent clinical articles. Studies in the late 1950s and early 1960s established the etiologic association of RSV and other viruses with acute bronchiolitis.[6,21,22,24,25,145]

ETIOLOGIC AGENTS

RSV is the major cause of bronchiolitis in infancy and virtually the only important etiologic consideration when major epidemics are occurring. Other agents cause smaller annual outbreaks. Table 25–1 presents the frequency of infectious agents in the overall cause of bronchiolitis. These data were compiled from 12 reports in which respiratory illness in children was observed over an extended period, and in most instances, numerous clinical illness categories were being studied. During major epidemics in the colder months in temperate climates, virologic and serologic studies indicate RSV as the cause in 80 percent or more of the cases, especially in the more severe ones. In nonepidemic situations, more than 50 percent of the isolates or instances of serologic evidence of infection are infectious agents other than RSV.

Sporadic disease rarely is associated with more than a 50 percent association of infectious agent and illness, despite the fact that infections undoubtedly are the cause of sporadic and epidemic bronchiolitis.[107]

Children surviving infantile bronchiolitis often have recurrent episodes of wheezing that, on clinical grounds, seem to be precipitated by upper respiratory infections. Studies designed to determine the infectious agents responsible for these repeated wheezing episodes have yielded variable results, presumably because they involve patients of different ages followed during different seasons of the year.[8,55,98,108-111]

A comprehensive study based on more than a decade of observation of children from birth through 15 years of age[68] revealed that viruses and *Mycoplasma pneumoniae* are the most common etiologic agents (Table 25-2). RSV is the most common cause of recurrent, wheezing-associated respiratory illness occurring in young children, including children who previously experienced bronchiolitis, which strongly suggests the identical nature of infection-related wheezing episodes occurring in children of different ages. With increasing patient age, rhinoviruses and *M. pneumoniae* account for most infection-induced wheezing episodes. The parainfluenza viruses and influenza viruses are important causes of such wheezing episodes throughout childhood, whereas coronaviruses and adenoviruses are less common causes in infancy. Human metapneumovirus and bocaviruses are more recently identified causes of bronchiolitis, and their relative importance as etiologic agents is being determined. RSV remains an important cause of wheezing in adolescents[68] and can cause airway obstruction in middle-aged and elderly individuals.[175]

The role of bacteria as primary agents, synergistically active participants, or secondary invaders in bronchiolitis

has interested investigators for many years. No evidence has been found of a primary role for bacteria in bronchiolitis of infants.[6,94] The data on synergistic viral-bacterial infections also are unconvincing. Wood and colleagues[189] in 1954 and Sell[149] in 1960 reported results of studies in which bacteriologic and serologic evidence tended to associate *Haemophilus influenzae* infections with bronchiolitis. Some of the children from these studies later were shown serologically to have had RSV infection.[26] Later studies showed evidence of mixed viral-bacterial infections in bronchiolitis[99,121] and other lower respiratory illnesses.[121]

These serologically defined mixed infections were found no more commonly among patients with bronchiolitis than among patients with mild upper respiratory tract disease, whereas RSV was recovered 10 times as often from patients with lower respiratory tract disease as from patients with upper respiratory tract disease alone.[99] A significant role for mixed viral-bacterial infection in bronchiolitis of infancy is unlikely to exist. Bacterial superinfection is an uncommon occurrence in bronchiolitis (at least in developed countries), as is discussed later in the section on complications and prognosis.

The association of asthma and infectious illnesses was appreciated throughout the 20th century. Initial reports tended to relate bacterial agents to wheezing; in 1909, Carmalt-Jones[19] reported improvement of patients with asthma in association with injections of a bacterial vaccine. Throughout the first half of the 20th century, "bacterial allergy" was the main consideration in infection-related wheezing, and controversy raged about the therapeutic merits of bacterial vaccines. Despite widespread use of bacterial vaccines in the treatment of infectious asthma, no evidence exists that bacterial organisms of the normal flora precipitate asthmatic attacks.[64,74,112,113,173] More recent, large retrospective reviews have shown the rarity with which bacterial infection complicates bronchiolitis, even in severe cases.[133,134] Generally, after a diagnosis of RSV or parainfluenza virus infection has been established, antibiotic courses started empirically can be safely stopped.

TABLE 25-1 Infectious Agents Associated with Acute Bronchiolitis

Infectious Agent	Relative Frequency (%)
Respiratory syncytial virus	50
Parainfluenza viruses	25
Type 1	8
Type 2	2
Type 3	15
Adenoviruses	5
Mycoplasma pneumoniae	5
Rhinoviruses	5
Influenza viruses	5
Type A	3
Type B	2
Metapneumovirus	5-10
Enteroviruses	2
Herpes simplex virus	2
Mumps virus	<1

EPIDEMIOLOGY

Bronchiolitis predominantly is a disease of infancy, although an identical disease occurring in older children arbitrarily may be referred to as another diagnostic entity. In a study involving 1148 children, the peak age of incidence was 2 to 6 months, with more than 80 percent of the cases occurring during the first year of life.[126] In a study of families in or near Houston, Texas, rates of RSV infection were 68.8 per 100 children in the first year of life and 82.6 per 100 children in the second year, including many reinfections. Lower respiratory illness was caused by RSV in 22.4 of 100 children in the first year of life. Of all RSV infections

TABLE 25-2 Principal Agents Recovered from Children of Different Ages with Wheezing Precipitated by Infection

Agent*	Frequency of Isolation of Each Age Group[†]			
	0-2 years	2-5 years	5-9 years	9-15 years
Respiratory syncytial virus	++++	+++	++	++
Adenovirus	++	++	+	0
Parainfluenza viruses	++	++	++	++
Rhinoviruses	+	++ to +++	++ to +++	+++
Metapneumovirus	++	+	+	0
Mycoplasma pneumoniae	+	++	+++	++++

Other agents that more rarely precipitate wheezing include enteroviruses, herpes simplex virus, cytomegalovirus, coronaviruses, influenza viruses, mumps virus, varicella-zoster virus, Bordetella pertussis, and Coxiella burnetii.
[†]*++++, very common; +++, common; ++, occasional; +, uncommon; 0, unknown.*
Data from references 7, 40, 45, 51, 68, 74, 94, 99, 107, 109, 115, 149.

TABLE 25–3 Attack Rates of Respiratory Syncytial Virus

Age in months [per Welliver] (n)	Infections per 100 Child-Years	LRI per 100 Child-Years	LRI per 100 Infections
0-12 (125)	68.8	22.4	32.6
13-24 (92)	82.6	13	15.8
25-36 (65)	46.2	10.8	23.3
37-48 (39)	33.3	7.7	23.1

LRI, lower respiratory tract infections.
From Glezen, W. P., Taber, L.H., Frank, A. L., et al.: Risk of primary infection and reinfection with respiratory syncytial virus. Am. J. Dis. Child. 140:543-546, 1986.

occurring in children younger than 12 months of age, one third were accompanied by lower respiratory illness. Although the attack rate of RSV decreased with age, the frequency with which lower respiratory disease occurred among individuals infected remained constant (Table 25–3), at least until they reached 4 years of age.[53] In Tucson, Arizona, a study of 1179 children enrolled in a health maintenance organization found that the rate of lower respiratory illness in the first year of life was 32.9 episodes per 100 children; 60 percent of these episodes were diagnosed as bronchiolitis.[192]

Studies in the Washington, D.C., area[84] and in North Carolina[68] estimated the risk of hospitalization for bronchiolitis among infants 0 to 12 months old to be 10 per 1000. A combined study involving 10 centers in Great Britain[28] concluded that the frequency of hospitalization for lower respiratory tract disease (predominantly wheezing) caused by RSV was 1 per 114 infants younger than 1 year of age and 1 per 476 children younger than 5 years. Peak rates of hospitalization were observed for children 1 to 3 months old (1 in 56).

More recent studies suggest that the rate of hospitalization for bronchiolitis may be higher currently than in the above-mentioned older studies. A study of the Tennessee Medicaid population found that the frequency of hospitalization for bronchiolitis was 4.4 and 1.5 per 100 child-years of observation for infants infected in the first and second 6 months of life, respectively.[10] Approximately 123,000 infants younger than 1 year of age are hospitalized annually with bronchiolitis, with RSV infection accounting for 51,000 to 82,000 of these hospitalizations. Including cases diagnosed as pneumonia, RSV infection results in 70,000 to 120,000 hospitalizations.[150]

Between 1979 and 1997, an average of 95 bronchiolitis-associated deaths occurred annually, with 77 percent occurring during the RSV epidemic season. Including fatal cases of bronchiolitis or pneumonia, RSV infection might have resulted in 171 to 510 deaths annually.[151] The yearly incidence of hospitalization for bronchiolitis increased from 12.9 per 1000 infants in 1980 to 31.2 per 1000 in 1996, suggesting an increased severity of illness developing during this interval.[150]

Epidemic bronchiolitis caused by RSV is markedly seasonal in temperate climates, with peak activity occurring from January to April and virtually no activity seen from August to October.[84] Sporadic bronchiolitis cases caused by other agents are seen throughout the year. In their study of 1179 cases, Kim and associates[84] found that 77 percent of the cases of RSV infection occurred between December and June. The lowest incidence occurred in August (2%). Regional differences can be striking. In Miami, RSV activity is year-round, with the maximum number of cases occurring in September and October. Epidemics usually begin in October in other southern states, although still earlier than in the Northeast. Further north (Winnipeg, Canada, and Alaska), the duration of the RSV season again becomes longer, and cases occur essentially year-round. Near the equator, temperature and humidity are positively associated with the number of bronchi-

olitis cases. In contrast, further from the equator (in either direction), temperature and humidity are inversely associated with bronchiolitis cases. Ultraviolet radiation is negatively associated with bronchiolitis in several regions.[194]

Bronchiolitis occurs more frequently in boys; the male-to-female ratio is approximately 1.5:1.[45] In older children, wheezing attributable to viral and mycoplasmal infections also occurs more frequently in boys (male-to-female ratio 1.35:1) until they reach 9 years of age, when the incidence becomes equal for the sexes.[68] Crowding may be a major determinant of hospitalization rates for lower respiratory illness caused by RSV, with the incidence of hospitalization for infants 1 to 3 months old residing in rural, urban, and heavily industrialized areas of Great Britain being 1 in 80, 1 in 60, and 1 in 40, respectively. The figures for all children younger than 5 years of age were 1 in 714, 1 in 588, and 1 in 227, respectively.[28] Studies from Tucson, Arizona, indicate that many socioeconomic factors, including absence of breast-feeding, low level of maternal education, and exposure to cigarette smoke, are associated with an increased risk of developing lower respiratory infection at the time of infection with RSV. The greatest risk was conferred by sharing sleeping quarters with two or more individuals.[192]

CLINICAL PRESENTATION

Acute bronchiolitis occurs most commonly in infants 1 to 12 months of age. In most instances, the patient's history reveals exposure to an adult or older child with a common cold or other trivial respiratory infection. Occasionally, as in the daycare setting, the child is exposed to other children with more marked respiratory illness. After exposure, the incubation period is approximately 5 to 7 days. The initial signs include copious nasal discharge (often serous in the early stage), cough, irritability, poor feeding, and vomiting in some cases. Slightly more than 50 percent of infants have fever, with rectal temperatures ranging from normal to 40.6° C (105.4° F) (mean, 39° C [102° F]).[137] Nasal congestion with tenacious secretions and progressive cough and dyspnea dominate the clinical picture.

Symptoms of upper respiratory infection persist for several days, and the onset of lower respiratory infection usually is precipitous, with the time of the onset of wheezing often being recognizable from the caretaker's description of the illness. The maximum severity of illness generally is attained within 24 to 36 hours of the first signs of lower respiratory illness. Apnea may occur and may be sufficiently severe to require mechanical ventilation.[12]

At the time of hospital admission, all patients have cough and evidence of respiratory distress. The pulse is rapid, and the respiratory rate usually is 40 to 80 breaths/min. The breathing is labored, with flaring of the alae nasae; grunting; abdominal breathing; and supraclavicular, subcostal, and intercostal retractions. The degree of retraction of the lower chest wall may be an accurate indicator of the severity of the illness. Wheezing often is audible without the use of a stethoscope, and the chest is full. Hyperresonance may be detected on percussion, and auscultation generally reveals harsh rhonchi, high-pitched or low-pitched expiratory wheezes, or fine inspiratory rales. Occasionally, wheezing is not audible despite other evidence of airway obstruction. A prolonged expiratory phase of breathing may occur, suggesting the presence of a more severe degree of illness. Cyanosis also occurs in severe cases.

Other findings include a mild conjunctivitis in one third of cases, pharyngitis of varied severity in approximately half of affected infants, and otitis media in 5 to 15 percent of cases. The abdomen frequently appears distended, and the liver and spleen usually are palpable; the organs are not enlarged but are pushed down because of emphysema and the flattened diaphragm.

The duration of the hospital course of bronchiolitis varies. Significant improvement occurred in half of the cases within 2 days in one large study.[1] In the same study, approximately one third of the cases had a gradual course without evidence of clear-cut improvement at any one time; 71 percent of the patients were afebrile by the third hospital day. In another study done more than 25 years later,[54] the average duration of hospitalization was 3.4 days. Longer stays were required for infants with initial oxygen saturations of less than 90 percent and infants younger than 6 weeks at the onset of illness. Reasonable criteria for admission in otherwise healthy infants seem to include hypoxia (i.e., oxygen saturation of <90-92%), age younger than 6 weeks, and a degree of respiratory distress sufficient to reduce fluid intake to inadequate levels. Other criteria include apnea, immunodeficiency, premature birth, and the presence of significant underlying heart or lung disease. Most patients can be discharged from the hospital within 2 to 3 days after admission, although mild wheezing still may be present.

In 121 hospitalized patients, the total white blood cell count was less than 12,500/mm^3 in 74 percent, and in 15 determinations had more than 60 percent neutrophils.[1] In another study, a mean leukocyte count of 16,000/mm^3 was determined for children with lower respiratory tract disease, including bronchiolitis, as was an increased percentage of band form neutrophils compared with that of a control group.[137] As in most infections, eosinophil counts in peripheral blood are reduced at the time of acute RSV infection.[48] Nonetheless, some patients maintain detectable eosinophilia in peripheral blood; these infants may be more likely to develop childhood asthma.[37]

Abnormalities of oxygenation frequently are present. Cyanosis may not be evident, even in the presence of markedly reduced oxygenation.[31,152] The respiratory rate is related inversely to the degree of oxygenation except when respiratory failure is imminent. In mild to moderate cases, carbon dioxide retention does not occur because the alveoli that are functioning can compensate for alveoli that are not ventilated. In severe disease, the blood pH is low, and the Paco$_2$ is elevated.[31,152] The technique of pulse oximetry has obviated the need for arterial blood gas sampling except perhaps in severe cases in which hypercarbia is a concern.

In certain patients, clinical findings (e.g., degree of chest wall retractions, wheezing) often are out of proportion to the degree of hypoxia as measured by pulse oximetry.[116,178] Infants with marked dyspnea must be evaluated carefully because respiratory failure may occur precipitously, despite their reassuring oximetry readings. A more meaningful scoring system to assess severity of illness has been developed.[57]

The radiographic appearance of the chest in bronchiolitis varies considerably.[88] Anteroposterior x-rays may be normal in mild cases. In moderate to severe illness, radiographs often appear exceptionally clear because of hyperinflation. The diaphragms often are flattened or depressed. The costophrenic angle is less acute, and the hilar vascular shadows are stretched. Frequently, areas of atelectasis give the appearance of pneumonitis, although true consolidation is a rare occurrence. The heart usually appears small. On the lateral radiograph, the diaphragm is depressed markedly, and reversal of the normal convexity frequently may be seen. The anteroposterior diameter of the chest is increased.

With recurrent wheezing episodes, the prodrome may be considerably shorter in duration with little or no fever and minimal coryza. In these children, differentiation of infection-induced wheezing from more conventional asthma becomes essentially impossible clinically.[186]

PATHOPHYSIOLOGY

The pathophysiology of bronchiolitis deservedly has been the focus of numerous investigations. Several original theories can be discounted reliably, whereas others warrant further study. Pathologic examinations of the lung in bronchiolitis or human airways in organ culture[70] reveal necrosis of the respiratory epithelium with destruction of the ciliated layer; mononuclear cell invasion of the peribronchial tissues; edema of the submucosa and adventitia; and obstruction of small airways with dense plugs consisting of dying epithelial cells, fibrin, and inflammatory cells. In contrast to asthma, mucin (periodic acid-Schiff positive material) usually is absent in fatal bronchiolitis.[184] An associated interstitial pneumonitis often is present, and patchy areas of atelectasis frequently are noted.[188]

The predominant cell types present in the lung of fatal cases are macrophages and neutrophils. Lymphocytes bearing CD4 (helper cells), CD8 (cytotoxic cells), and CD56 (natural killer cells) antigens are almost absent.[184] Even in surviving infants, CD8 lymphocyte counts are less than 1 percent of the total cells in bronchoalveolar lavage fluids,[41] and cytokines characteristically released by CD4 and CD8 cells (interleukin-2 [IL-2], IL-4, IL-5, IL-13, and interferon-γ) are present in low concentrations in nasopharyngeal and tracheal secretions.[184] Adaptive immune responses seem to be poorly developed in infants with severe forms of bronchiolitis. In contrast, staining for markers of apoptosis (caspase 3 and Fas) is positive in infected epithelial cells,[184] suggesting that recovery from primary infection depends on the antiviral activity of phagocytic cells, induction of apoptosis, and perhaps the activity of other innate immune mechanisms.

Recovery from bronchiolitis apparently is complete histologically,[117,187] although plugging of the airway still was prominent in an infant 5 weeks after having an acute episode of bronchiolitis. This infant had experienced an apparent full clinical recovery before eventually dying of acute pneumococcal pneumonia.[117]

Infants may be particularly prone to the development of severe illness as a result of infection of the small airways for many reasons, including the small diameters of their airways. The infant lung is deficient in collateral alveolar ventilation through the pores of Kohn, which develop only in later life.[100] Atelectatic areas cannot be re-expanded readily. Other studies have shown that the small airways in children younger than age 5 years contribute fivefold to sevenfold more to total airway resistance than do small airways of adults.[72] Viral infections involving small airways in young children are more likely to manifest as serious clinical illnesses than are similar infections in adults. Nonetheless, these abnormalities exist in all infants. In contrast, most infants infected with RSV do not develop lower respiratory illness, which suggests that host or environmental factors may be involved in determining the pathogenesis of RSV infection. Table 25-4 lists environmental factors, and potentially important host factors are described later.

TABLE 25-4   Factors Associated with an Increased Risk and Severity of Bronchiolitis and of Postbronchiolitic Morbidity

Factor	Increase in Frequency	Increase in Severity	Increase in Later Morbidity
Crowding	+++	+++	?
Passive smoking	+++	+++	++
Male gender	+	++	++
Absence of breast-feeding	+	+	?
Family history of asthma	±	±	±
Personal atopy	−	−	+++
Congenitally small airways	++	?	−
Airway hyperreactivity	−	+	++
RSV-specific IgE responses	++	++	++

+++, *implies strong relationship; ++, implies moderate relationship; +, implies weak relationship; ±, implies controversial relationship; −, implies no relationship; ?, implies unknown relationship.*
RSV, respiratory syncytial virus.
Data from references 16, 28, 52, 60, 68, 89, 97, 102-104, 154, 163, 179, 180, 183, 185, 191-193, 195.

One factor that may predispose to the development of lower respiratory illness on RSV infection is the infecting dose of virus. Infants with greater quantities of RSV in their nasopharyngeal secretions are more likely to exhibit severe illness.[15] In fatal cases, abundant virus is evident in epithelial cells plugging the airway lumen by immunohistochemical staining.[184] The fact that crowding is associated with greater risk of developing lower respiratory infection also suggests the importance of the initial inoculum.[187]

Another risk factor for the development of lower respiratory infection may be the relative diameter (or degree of intrinsic constriction) of the airway. When pulmonary function testing is completed on healthy infants before lower respiratory infection occurs, certain infants have lower air flows in smaller airways (and presumably more narrow airways) than do other infants. When followed prospectively, these infants are more likely to develop wheezing early in life than are infants with better air flow.[102] These abnormalities of lung function no longer are associated with an increased risk of wheezing after the child reaches 3 years of age. Instead, evidence of atopy becomes the principal risk factor for recurrent wheezing.[104]

Studies of adolescents reveal reversibility of their airway narrowing after receiving bronchodilator treatment, indicating the airways were constricted, but not stenotic, in early life.[160] Several studies have shown that the airways of infants are intrinsically more reactive to bronchospastic stimuli than are airways of older children,[92,169] particularly children from families with asthma.[193] How long this increased reactivity persists is unknown, and no study has shown that infants with greater degrees of hereditary airway hyperreactivity are more likely to develop bronchiolitis or recurrent virus-induced wheezing. In later childhood, repeated occurrences of viral infections are necessary to sustain this increased reactivity.[177]

In addition to the hereditary airway hyperreactivity, viruses themselves may induce increases in reactivity. Viral infections that clinically appear to be restricted to the upper respiratory tract in adults and children nonetheless result in transient, increased constrictive responses of the airway to a variety of stimuli, including histamine, irritants, and other agents, and small airway dysfunction.[2,3,9,30,39,93] Whether these minor changes contribute to the airway obstruction observed in bronchiolitis is doubtful, in that they are of much lesser magnitude than is the markedly increased reactivity that is observed in asthmatic individuals after exposure to allergens. These virus-induced changes were observed in all infected individuals, including subjects who did not experience wheezing at the time of the virus infection. If airways already are hyperreactive in infants, on a hereditary basis or as a result of a preceding viral infection, the subsequent stimulus of RSV infection may be sufficient to cause airway obstruction.

Immunologic deficits may be expected to lead to more severe forms of virus-induced respiratory illness. Studies of the antibody response to RSV infection in serum and in respiratory secretions show, however, that the nature of responses generally is similar among patients with bronchiolitis or simple upper respiratory illness alone caused by this agent.[82,181] Antibody-directed cellular cytotoxicity expressed against tissue culture cells infected with RSV also is similar in patients with all forms of illness caused by this agent.[80,147] Although investigators have shown that cells infected with RSV can activate complement through classic and alternative pathways,[159] studies suggest that in vivo activation of the complement cascade occurs with equal frequency among patients with all forms of illness caused by the virus.[81]

The concept that serum IgG antibody to RSV, acquired by vaccination or transplacentally, might sensitize the host has been dispelled by results of studies showing that severe bronchiolitis may occur in the absence of circulating antibody[126] and that titers of maternal antibody correlate with protection against infection caused by the virus.[52,123]

Lymphocyte hypersensitivity has been suggested to play a role in the development of severe bronchiolitis. Original field trials showed that a formalin-inactivated RSV (FI-RSV) vaccine induced humoral and cell-mediated immune responses to the virus. Nonetheless, vaccinated subjects manifested more severe forms of illness than did unvaccinated controls when subjects in each group subsequently were infected naturally.[85] Cell-mediated immune responses to viral antigen were greater among recipients of this FI-RSV vaccine compared with control subjects who previously had experienced natural infection.[86] The resulting disease in vaccine recipients was similar in form to bronchiolitis, and the idea that natural RSV bronchiolitis is a consequence of lymphocyte hypersensitivity to the virus has persisted.

Nonetheless, reasons to doubt that the illness that followed FI-RSV vaccination is the same as that following natural bronchiolitis exist. The two FI-RSV vaccine recipients who died after having subsequent natural infection had numerous lymphocytes and eosinophils present in the lung, which is not the case after natural RSV infection.[85,184] Infants surviving RSV infection after receiving the FI-RSV vaccine had high eosinophil counts in peripheral blood, which also is unusual in natural RSV infection.[48] In addition, cytotoxic T-lymphocyte activity is not detected easily in infants after they have had bronchiolitis,[4] and more recent autopsy studies have shown the virtual absence of CD4 and CD8 antigen-positive cells in the lung.[184] Although the development of cell-mediated cytotoxic antiviral responses may be protecting individuals with milder disease, little reason exists to contend that lymphocyte hyperresponsiveness contributes to severe bronchiolitis.

Immediate hypersensitivity to viral antigens has received much consideration as a potential contributing factor in bronchiolitis. The association of a family history of asthma with the development of bronchiolitis in infancy remains controversial.[89,154,161,195] Production of virus-specific IgE and subsequent release of mediators of bronchoconstriction have been documented, however, in infants hospitalized with bronchiolitis caused by RSV and the parainfluenza viruses.[16,179,182,183] In bronchiolitis caused by RSV, the quantities of virus-specific IgE produced and histamine present in respiratory secretions correlate with the severity of illness, as measured by degree of arterial oxygen tension.[183] Leukotriene C_4 is a product of mast cells and eosinophils primarily, but also epithelial cells and macrophages, and is a potent stimulant of airway smooth muscle constriction and mucus secretion. This mediator is released into the airway in acute bronchiolitis,[176] as is histamine,[183] and histamine is found in increased concentrations in plasma of patients with bronchiolitis.[156] In addition, prostaglandins and metabolites can be detected in secretions and blood after bronchiolitis.[156]

A possible role for eosinophils in the pathogenesis of bronchiolitis is supported by the finding of increased concentrations of eosinophil cationic protein in secretions of infants with bronchiolitis and (among high responders) an overall correlation of concentrations of this protein with the degree of hypoxia.[48,49] Peripheral blood eosinophil counts are depressed during the acute phase of most infectious diseases, including RSV infection. Nonetheless, eosinophil counts in peripheral blood are higher in infants with bronchiolitis than in infants with upper respiratory illness only, particularly in boys.[48] This finding is notable because boys generally have more severe forms of bronchiolitis. A contrasting viewpoint is that eosinophils contribute to the clearance of viruses after infection. This view is supported by the fact that eosinophils contain enzymes with ribonuclease activity, which inactivates RSV.[34,35] IgE-dependent and eosinophil-dependent mechanisms may be important in recovery from viral infections, much as they are in parasitic infections.

The airways of asthmatic individuals are infiltrated by T lymphocytes (predominantly T-helper lymphocytes) and eosinophils. T-helper cells can be classified as type 1 (T_H1), which produce primarily interferon-γ and IL-2, or type 2 (T_H2), which produce IL-4, IL-5, IL-13, and others. This finding is important because IL-4, IL-5, and IL-13 are important factors in promoting IgE synthesis and eosinophil migration. Asthma is thought by some researchers to be a result of a T_H2 bias in the airway. An attractive hypothesis is that RSV infection induces airway obstruction and wheezing by inciting the same type of T_H2 responses as observed in asthma. Interferon-γ and IL-4 are found in respiratory secretions of infants with RSV bronchiolitis, but IL-5 and IL-13 rarely are detectable in serum or secretions,[50,174] suggesting that bronchiolitis is not characterized by a T_H2 lymphocyte bias.

Chemokines are proteins released by airway epithelial cells, inflammatory cells, fibroblasts, and other cell types that are chemotactic for leukocytes. Certain chemokines (e.g., IL-8) are active on a broad variety of leukocytes. Others, such as macrophage inflammatory protein 1-alpha (MIP-1α); monocyte chemotactic protein, types 1 through 4; eotaxin; and regulated on activation, normal T-cell expressed and secreted (RANTES), are more selective for eosinophils, basophils, mast cells, and T lymphocytes. These chemokines represent an alternative to T_H2 lymphocytes in terms of initiating the inflammatory response in asthma and bronchiolitis. Studies suggest that MIP-1α, eotaxin, and monocyte chemotactic protein may be particularly important in the pathogenesis of bronchiolitis because they correlate with the degree of hypoxia observed during acute illness.[50] Abnormalities of chemokine responses, rather than T-helper cell responses, may underlie the pathogenesis of bronchiolitis and represent therapeutic targets.

DIAGNOSIS

DIFFERENTIAL DIAGNOSIS

A tendency exists to attribute all infantile respiratory distress occurring after the immediate newborn period to bronchiolitis. The list of causes of infantile dyspnea consists of conditions that are associated with upper and lower airway obstruction, however. Recognition of upper airway obstructive disease should cause little difficulty because the problem is one of distress with inspiration, rather than air trapping. Illnesses that cause lower airway obstructive disease and diseases that suggest this problem are listed in Table 25–5.

The differential diagnosis of allergic disease causes the most difficulty. Generally, the first episode of allergic respiratory disease, when associated with infection, cannot be separated from bronchiolitis by any objective measures. Anatomic defects such as vascular rings can cause obstruction of the airway at many locations; inspiratory or expiratory distress, or a combination, can occur. Frequently, a child with an anatomic defect does not have any detectable difficulty until a trivial respiratory infection occurs, which complicates the diagnostic picture.

Foreign bodies should be considered even in very young infants. Gastroesophageal reflux disease has become recognized as a frequent cause of wheezing in young infants. Because of its obvious therapeutic implications, bacterial pneumonia is the most important differential consideration, although wheezing occurs rarely in association with bacterial pneumonia.[98,99]

SPECIFIC DIAGNOSIS

Because bronchiolitis and infectious asthma are clinical diseases with arbitrary boundaries and multiple etiologic agents, outlining a method for establishing specific diagnosis is difficult. When

TABLE 25–5 Differential Diagnostic Considerations in Acute Bronchiolitis and Infectious Asthma

Allergy
Asthma
Allergic pneumonias (e.g., allergic aspergillosis)
Anatomic cause
Vascular ring, lung cysts, lobar emphysema
Pneumothorax, hydrothorax, chylothorax
Foreign body
Circulatory failure
Congenital and acquired heart disease
Anemia
Nephritis
Infections
Viral, chlamydial, rickettsial, mycoplasmal, bacterial, and fungal
  pneumonias
Migrating parasites
Irritants
Inhalation of toxic substances (e.g., chlorine gas)
Aspiration pneumonia
Gastroesophageal reflux
Metabolic cause
Poisons (e.g., salicylate)
Acidosis

illness is epidemic, RSV usually is the cause. In nonepidemic situations, a careful history and appropriate laboratory studies and radiographs should be considered to exclude the other differential diagnostic possibilities that are listed in Table 25–5.

A specific etiologic diagnosis can be made by the isolation of virus from the nasopharynx. The diagnostic virologic facilities of many medical centers enable the isolation in tissue culture of RSV, parainfluenza viruses, influenza viruses, adenoviruses, rhinoviruses, enteroviruses, and herpesviruses. The use of the shell vial technique has been applied to RSV infection with success.[158] The polymerase chain reaction technique also shows promise in amplification of small quantities of RSV RNA from clinical specimens, although its having superiority to other methods for testing of infants does not seem likely.[128] Rapid detection of viral antigen of RSV directly in nasopharyngeal secretions by commercially available (e.g., enzyme-linked immunosorbent assay) or fluorescent antibody techniques is the method of choice in most laboratories for several reasons.

The accuracy of these techniques often is superior to that of standard cell culture (at least in infants) because antigens remain stable under transport conditions that inactivate live virus. Results also are available several days earlier than by cell culture. Infections with influenza viruses, parainfluenza viruses, and adenoviruses also can be identified by rapid detection techniques, and reliable commercial kits permitting simultaneous testing for each of these agents are the standard in most laboratories.

TREATMENT

The cornerstone of therapy for bronchiolitis is the administration of oxygen because sicker patients usually are hypoxemic.[36,152] Oxygen saturation should be maintained at 92 percent or higher. Usually, an oxygen concentration of 30 percent or 40 percent can achieve this goal, and the patient's respiratory status can be monitored by pulse oximetry; however, blood gas determinations should be obtained when indicated by clinical findings (e.g., cyanosis, agitation). A common practice is to place children with bronchiolitis in tents and administer mist vigorously. Although oxygen should be humidified, the use of mists and aerosols except to deliver specific antiviral therapy is discouraged; mist can act as an irritant, causing reflex bronchoconstriction, and the water usually does not reach the lower airways.[5]

Although dehydration is a potential problem in children with bronchiolitis because of vomiting and lack of intake, care must be taken not to overhydrate such patients. Because edema is an important part of the pathology of bronchiolitis, excess water may contribute to obstruction of the airway.

Beta-adrenergic bronchodilators have been used frequently in bronchiolitis. Slight improvements in air flow, in oxygenation, and in clinical illness scores have been reported,[63,87,91,143,144] but these effects are not likely to be meaningful clinically; hospitalization is not prevented, and hospital stays are not shortened.[33,43] Improvements observed after the administration of the first dose of these compounds usually are not observed after administration of subsequent doses. In one study, oral and aerosolized beta-adrenergic agents were compared with inactive substances given by the corresponding route. The degree of improvement was the same in all four groups.[47] Combinations of salbutamol and dexamethasone also have no objective effect.[167]

In the past, epinephrine often was administered subcutaneously to older infants in an attempt to differentiate allergic disease from true bronchiolitis. This approach rarely was successful in differentiating one illness from the other or in improving the condition of the patient. Studies have suggested, however, that use of aerosolized, racemic epinephrine produced greater improvement than the use of beta-adrenergic aerosols alone.[144] Other studies of alpha-adrenergic agents have resulted in the same conclusion. Generally, the minor improvements in pulmonary function obtained using alpha-adrenergic agents or racemic epinephrine are not clinically meaningful; the mortality rate is not improved, and the duration of stay in the intensive care unit or in the hospital is not reduced.

Aerosolized sympathomimetic drugs are used frequently in older children with wheezing presumed to be caused by viral infections, with better results than those in infants.[77,91,129,143] Nonetheless, no evidence exists that this form of therapy reduces the need for hospitalization of these patients. Aerosols of ipratropium also have been administered in bronchiolitis without observable benefit.[148] Possible explanations for poor responses to bronchodilators include a paucity of beta-adrenergic receptors in infancy[139]; decreased amounts of smooth muscle capable of responding to bronchodilators surrounding the terminal airways[136]; the nature of the airway obstruction itself (intense plugging with cellular debris)[184,188]; and, presumably, persistence of virus in the airway, stimulating continued inflammation or release of bronchoconstrictive mediators, or both.

Trials of alpha-adrenergic or beta-adrenergic aerosols may be attempted in seriously ill patients,[13,36] although persistence with either of these approaches in the absence of an initial response may prove harmful.[77,124] Most infants hospitalized with bronchiolitis recover quickly with no other intervention than supplemental oxygen and fluid replacement as necessary. A child treated for croup with multiple doses of racemic epinephrine developed ventricular tachycardia and a small myocardial infarction,[18] emphasizing the need to avoid the careless use of these compounds in viral respiratory infections.

Corticosteroids have been employed repeatedly in treating bronchiolitis. Controlled studies have failed to reveal any benefit in terms of prevention of hospitalization, reduced duration of hospitalization, reduced need for intubation, or reduced frequency of recurrent wheezing episodes after bronchiolitis.[8,14,31,32,44,90,138] In a child with nonrespiratory indications for the administration of corticosteroids, these drugs need not be withheld because of fear of complications, although the duration of viral shedding may be extended in individuals treated with steroids.

Early experience with the antiviral substance ribavirin in bronchiolitis suggested that mild subjective benefits and improvement in oxygenation occurred after near-continuous aerosol administration of this compound.[60,61,141,165] The degree of improvement in patients treated with ribavirin was not marked. No study has shown whether the administration of ribavirin could prevent deaths, avoid the need for mechanical ventilation, or shorten the duration of hospital stays.[105,112,157] A meta-analysis of studies using ribavirin showed slight benefits in morbidity and mortality rates that were not statistically significant.[135]

Ribavirin is quite expensive and is difficult to use because of the need for prolonged aerosol administration. Although the drug may precipitate in ventilatory circuits of mechanical ventilators, it can be administered safely if filters are used to prevent plugging of the circuits.[124,125] Because ribavirin is teratogenic in rodents, concern has arisen regarding the safety of health care workers exposed to aerosols of the drug.[65,140] Although absorption may occur in hospital workers, the amount absorbed is negligible.

Other approaches to therapy of RSV infection include the use of interferon-α,[27] vitamin A,[120] DNase,[106] and nitric oxide.[127] The results of these studies were negative. Surfactant[83,171] and leukotriene receptor antagonists[155] have been used in very small studies of bronchiolitis or virus-induced wheezing, with positive effects that require confirmation. Preparations containing a very high titer of neutralizing antibody against RSV have been tested in the prevention and treatment of RSV infection in high-risk populations.[57,66,170] The results of the prophylaxis studies were positive, as discussed later. A significant therapeutic effect of these compounds could not be identified after RSV infection was established, however.[101]

Because bronchiolitis is a viral disease, antibiotics are not useful or necessary. In many instances, the radiographic picture suggests pneumonia, and the blood leukocyte count is elevated; the physician feels compelled to administer antibiotics. Most authorities do not use antibiotics in bronchiolitis or discontinue their use after RSV infection is confirmed because bacterial infection of the lung is rare in bronchiolitis even when infiltrates are identified on chest radiographs. In one large study, secondary bacterial infection occurred in no more than 7 (1.2%) of 565 children with RSV infection.[62] Institution of antibiotics should be considered during the course of therapy when a change in illness suggests the possibility of secondary bacterial infection.

A child with bronchiolitis generally is more comfortable in the supine position with the head end of the crib slightly elevated. Infant seats are used frequently, but are not optimal because the child's head tends to fall to the side or forward, which constricts the upper airway. The sitting position also causes a possibly deleterious upward pressure on the diaphragm. If respiratory failure occurs (virtually absent inspiratory breath sounds, severe inspiratory retractions, inability to maintain an oxygen saturation of >90% in 40% ambient oxygen, cyanosis in 40% oxygen, decreased or absent response to painful stimuli, and a $Paco_2$ of ≥65 mm Hg), ventilatory assistance, such as nasotracheal intubation, neuromuscular blockade, and positive-pressure ventilation,[36,124] is indicated.

PREVENTION

The development of a method to prevent RSV infection is a high priority. The initial adverse experience with formalin-inactivated vaccine (described earlier) has nearly prevented further investigation of inactivated vaccines.[85,172] Later, a live, temperature-sensitive vaccine was developed by adapting RSV to grow at low temperatures in cell culture. This attenuated vaccine was designed to grow at the lower temperatures of the upper respiratory tract but be inactive at the higher temperatures in the lung. In initial field trials, the vaccine strain caused febrile respiratory illnesses in seronegative vaccinees but did not replicate adequately in seropositive subjects.[23] Further trials of temperature-sensitive mutant RSV strains as vaccines showed improved immunogenicity and some protection, at least against rechallenge with the vaccine strain. Nasal congestion that could cause apnea was common in recipients, however.[78] Numerous other vaccine candidates, including RSV nucleic acid vaccines, bovine RSV strains, parainfluenza virus strains bearing RSV antigens, and human RSV strains with gene deletions or given with immunologically active adjuvants, have been developed. Many of them are in early clinical trials, but development of a successful vaccine is not imminent.

In contrast to the largely negative experience with vaccine development, protection against serious illness caused by RSV infection was achieved using a pooled preparation of human serum obtained from donors with very high titers of neutralizing antibody against RSV.[57] This compound, when administered during the RSV season on a monthly basis to infants and young children with a history of birth at less than 32 weeks' gestation or with bronchopulmonary dysplasia, caused a marked reduction in the severity of illness and rate of hospitalization after RSV infection.

These trials have been repeated successfully using a mouse monoclonal antibody against the RSV fusion protein.[170] The antibody is reconstructed so that it has more than 95 percent of the protein structure of a human antibody. This compound is approximately 50 percent effective in preventing RSV-related hospitalization when administered to high-risk infants, and it has received approval for use in infants born prematurely with or without lung disease of premature birth. Separate trials in infants with hemodynamically significant congenital heart disease have shown a similar reduction in the rate of hospitalization for RSV-related illness, and the compound is now approved for use in these infants as well.[42]

COMPLICATIONS AND PROGNOSIS

Virtually all cases of bronchiolitis in healthy children resolve without acute complications. Secondary bacterial infection in bronchiolitis now is a rare occurrence, at least in developed countries. Scott and colleagues[146] identified minor electrocardiographic abnormalities in 2 percent of 188 children with bronchiolitis. Involvement of other organs apparently does not occur.

The overall mortality rate in bronchiolitis is low. Before the modern era of improved ventilatory support, mortality rates ranged from 2 to 5.5 percent.[36,67,71] A multicenter study in Great Britain published in 1978[28] estimated the mortality rate owing to RSV infection in infancy at 0.5 percent. Deaths should occur rarely except among infants with severe underlying cardiac or pulmonary disease; even in these cases, mortality rate should not exceed 1 percent of cases.[42] Between 1979 and 1997, an average of 95 bronchiolitis-associated deaths occurred annually in the United States, with 20 percent occurring in infants with underlying heart disease, lung disease, or premature birth.[151]

The association of bronchiolitis with the subsequent development of asthma has long been controversial. Fifty percent of patients with bronchiolitis have recurrent episodes of wheezing, although this figure decreases to approximately 10 percent by adolescence and may not be above that of the general population by this time.[96,97,160] Whether this recurrent wheezing is caused by RSV infection or, alternatively, suggests that RSV infection in early life is an indicator of a tendency toward airway obstruction is still being investigated. Recurrent wheezing after having a case of bronchiolitis could reflect an inherited asthmatic trait. Some studies find a strong correlation between atopic family history and postbronchiolitic wheezing,[38,46,142,186,195] whereas others, particularly studies from Great Britain,[132,153,154] do not. Titers of total

serum IgE[130,161] and peripheral blood eosinophil counts[37,103,195] have some predictive value for the development of recurrent wheezing after having bronchiolitis. Two studies showed that peripheral blood eosinophilia during viral infections, particularly RSV bronchiolitis, predicts the development of recurrent wheezing in school-aged children.[37,103] Atopy seems to explain a great deal of the recurrent wheezing that occurs after bronchiolitis.

RSV infection in early infancy could damage the developing airway, rendering the airway more prone to obstruction in later life. Pulmonary function tests performed in former patients with bronchiolitis 12 years after an episode of bronchiolitis reveal an increased frequency of airway hyperreactivity in response to challenge with exercise or chemical agents, increased ratios of residual volume to total lung capacity, and reduced expiratory air flow at low lung volumes.[58,79,132,153,162,163,169,190] Although these abnormalities are observed commonly in individuals with asthma, they could not be explained in several of the previous studies simply by the presence of a personal or family history of atopy.[59,132,154] Some of these retrospective studies showed, however, that a single episode of RSV bronchiolitis was not associated with long-term lung dysfunction; abnormal lung function was observed only if at least two episodes of lower respiratory illness had occurred before the patient had reached age 2 years.[69,177]

Prospective studies show that recurrent wheezing in children through age 3 years after bronchiolitis (but not beyond) is related to abnormalities of lung function that existed before RSV infection occurred.[102] Wheezing persisting beyond age 3 years was related, at least partially, to the atopic status of the host.[103,104] No study has shown a relationship between the severity of the initial bronchiolitis episode and the degree of abnormality of long-term lung function.[58,59,132,153] Personal atopy is responsible for many of the long-term manifestations proposed to be sequelae of bronchiolitis. Some factor other than atopy may determine in part the apparent lung abnormalities seen after a case of bronchiolitis,[96,179,191,192] but no direct evidence indicates that this other factor is the initial episode of RSV infection itself.

RSV infection could induce persistent airway hyperreactivity. Retrospective studies have shown that airway reactivity is greater in individuals 1 decade after having an episode of infantile bronchiolitis than in control populations without a history of bronchiolitis.[58,132] Airway reactivity in all children (even children never experiencing bronchiolitis) is greater than that in adults, however, and it is greatest in children of atopic families and in children exposed to cigarette smoke.[193] Airway hyperreactivity occurring after bronchiolitis is not a reflection of the RSV infection itself. One prospective study found no relationship between RSV bronchiolitis and the degree of airway reactivity at age 2 years.[2]

RSV infection possibly can promote sensitization to allergens. In animal models, critically timed RSV infection can enhance temporarily the degree of airway reactivity induced after sensitization to an allergen. Whether this phenomenon occurs in humans is unknown. The absence of T_H2-like cytokine responses at the time of having RSV bronchiolitis[50] suggests, however, that RSV infection in infancy likely does not promote a persistent atopic state in the host.

RSV infection more likely results in the release of mediators of airway obstruction, such as histamine and leukotrienes, through a mechanism other than T_H2 cytokine responses. Chemokines such as MIP-1α, which cause mast cell and basophil degranulation, are possible candidates. Release of these mediators at the time of having RSV infection may result in wheezing in susceptible individuals. These same individuals may develop wheezing again at the time of having allergen exposure in childhood (particularly if they are atopic), but the relationship of bronchiolitis in infancy and such subsequent childhood wheezing would not be causal, but rather would be based on the underlying susceptibility of the airway to obstruction.

The overall outlook for infantile bronchiolitis generally is excellent. In a follow-up study conducted at the author's institution,[179] severe lung disease was not observed in former bronchiolitis patients. All oxygen saturation levels were greater than 95 percent, and at least some of the air flow obstruction present in patients aged 7 to 9 years was reversible with a single bronchodilator treatment, as was confirmed later.[160] Single episodes of infantile bronchiolitis (in the absence of passive smoke exposure and without recurrent wheezing episodes) have not been associated with abnormalities of lung function or airway hyperreactivity in later childhood.[79,163,177]

The natural history of postbronchiolitic wheezing in childhood is for episodes of wheezing to become progressively milder,[58,97,132,153] and the frequency of postbronchiolitic wheezing eventually decreases to essentially the same rate as that of children who did not experience bronchiolitis in infancy.[69,97,160] Nonetheless, the overall prognosis is not entirely benign, and exposure to noxious environmental elements may result in an accelerated deterioration of lung function in later life.[27,186,190] The combination of respiratory tract illness in early life and subsequent cigarette smoking especially may be harmful.[166] Individuals who develop bronchiolitis in infancy should avoid smoking in later life and occupations that are associated with exposure to respiratory irritants.

REFERENCES

1. Ackerman, B. D.: Acute bronchitis: A study of 207 cases. Clin. Pediatr. 1:75-81, 1962.
2. Adler, A., Ngo, L., and Tager, I. B.: Association of tobacco smoke exposure and respiratory syncytial virus infection with airways reactivity in early childhood. Pediatr. Pulmonol. 32:418-427, 2001.
3. Aquilina, A. T., Hall, W. J., Douglas, G., et al.: Airway reactivity in subjects with viral upper respiratory tract infections: The effects of exercise and cold air. Am. Rev. Respir. Dis. 122:3-10, 1980.
4. Bangham, R. M., Cannon, M. J., Karzon, D. T., et al.: Cytotoxic T-cell response to respiratory syncytial virus in mice. J. Virol. 56:55-59, 1985.
5. Bau, S. K., Aspin, N., Wood, D. E., et al.: The measurement of fluid deposition in humans following mist tent therapy. Pediatrics 48:605-612, 1971.
6. Beem, M., Wright, F. H., Fasan, D. M., et al.: Observations on the etiology of acute bronchiolitis in infants. J. Pediatr. 61:864-869, 1962.
7. Beem, M., Wright, F. H., Hamre, D., et al.: Association of the chimpanzee coryza agent with acute respiratory disease in children. N. Engl. J. Med. 263:523-530, 1960.
8. Berger, I., Argaman, Z., Schwartz, S. B., et al.: Efficacy of corticosteroids in acute bronchiolitis: Short-term and long-term follow-up. Pediatr. Pulmonol. 26:162-166, 1998.
9. Boushey, H. A., Holtzman, M. J., Sheller, J. R., et al.: Bronchial hyperreactivity. Am. Rev. Respir. Dis. 121:389-413, 1980.
10. Boyce, T. G., Mellen, B. G., Mitchel, E. F., Jr., et al.: Rates of hospitalization for respiratory syncytial virus infection among children in Medicaid. J. Pediatr. 137:865-870, 2000.
11. Brandt, C. D., Kim, H. W., Arrobio, J. O., et al.: Epidemiology of respiratory syncytial virus infection in Washington, D.C., III: Composite analysis of eleven consecutive yearly epidemics. Am. J. Epidemiol. 98:355-364, 1973.
12. Bruhn, F. W., Mokrohisky, S. T., and McIntosh, K.: Apnea associated with respiratory syncytial virus infection in young infants. J. Pediatr. 90:382-386, 1977.
13. Brooks, L. J., and Cropp, G. J. A.: Theophylline therapy in bronchiolitis: A retrospective study. Am. J. Dis. Child. 135:934-936, 1981.
14. Brunette, M. G., Lands, L., and Thibodeau, L.: Childhood asthma: Prevention of attacks with short-term corticosteroid treatment of upper respiratory tract infection. Pediatrics 81:624-629, 1988.
15. Buckingham, S. C., Bush, A. J., and Devincenzo, J. P.: Nasal quantity of respiratory syncytial virus correlates with disease severity in hospitalized infants. Pediatr. Infect. Dis. J. 19:113-117, 2000.
16. Bui, R. H. D., Molinaro, G. A., Kettering, J. D., et al.: Virus-specific IgE and IgG4 antibodies in serum of children infected with respiratory syncytial virus. J. Pediatr. 110:87-90, 1987.
17. Burrows, B., Knudson, R. J., and Lebowitz, M. D.: The relationship of childhood respiratory illness to adult obstructive airway disease. Am. Rev. Respir. Dis. 115:751-760, 1977.
18. Butte, M. J., Nguyen, B. X., Hutchison, T. J., et al.: Pediatric myocardial infarction after racemic epinephrine administration. Pediatrics 104:103-104, 1999.
19. Carmalt-Jones, D. W.: The treatment of bronchial asthma by a vaccine. B. M. J. 2:1049-1050, 1909.
20. Chanock, R., Chambon, L., Chang, W., et al.: WHO Respiratory Disease Survey in Children: A serologic study. Bull. World Health Org. 37:363-369, 1967.
21. Chanock, R. M., Kim, H. W., Vargosko, A. J., et al.: Respiratory syncytial virus, I: Virus recovery and other observations during a 1960 outbreak of bronchiolitis, pneumonia, and minor respiratory diseases in children. J. A. M. A. 176:647-653, 1961.
22. Chanock, R. M., Mufson, M. A., and Johnson, K. M.: Comparative biology and ecology of human virus and mycoplasma respiratory pathogens. Prog. Med. Virol. 7:208-252, 1965.
23. Chanock, R. M., and Murphy, B. R.: Use of temperature-sensitive and cold-adapted mutant viruses in immunoprophylaxis of acute respiratory tract disease. Rev. Infect. Dis. 2:421-431, 1980.
24. Chanock, R. M., and Parrott, R. H.: Acute respiratory disease in infancy and childhood: Present understanding and prospects for prevention. Pediatrics 36:21-39, 1965.
25. Chanock, R. M., Parrott, R. H., Vargosko, A. J., et al.: IV: Respiratory syncytial virus. Am. J. Public Health 52:918-925, 1962.
26. Cherry, J. D.: Newer respiratory viruses: Their role in respiratory illness of children. Adv. Pediatr. 20:225-290, 1973.
27. Chipps, B. E., Sullivan, W. F., and Portnoy, J. M.: Alpha-2a-interferon for treatment of bronchiolitis caused by respiratory syncytial virus. Pediatr. Infect. Dis. J. 12:653-658, 1993.
28. Clarke, S. K. R., Gardner, P. S., Poole, P. M., et al.: Respiratory syncytial virus infection: Admissions to hospital in industrial, urban, and rural areas. B. M. J. 2:796-798, 1978.
29. Colley, J. R. T., Douglas, J. W. B., and Reid, D. D.: Respiratory disease in young adults: Influence of early childhood lower respiratory tract illness, social class, air pollution, and smoking. B. M. J. 3:195-198, 1973.
30. Collier, A. M., Pimmel, R. L., Hasselblad, V., et al.: Spirometric changes in normal children with upper respiratory infections. Am. Rev. Respir. Dis. 117:47-53, 1978.
31. Connolly, J. H., Field, C. M. B., Glasgow, J. F. T., et al.: A double blind trial of prednisolone in epidemic bronchiolitis due to respiratory syncytial virus. Acta Paediatr. Scand. 58:116-120, 1969.
32. Dabbous, I. A., Tkachyk, J. S., and Stamm, S. J.: A double blind study on the effects of corticosteroids in the treatment of bronchiolitis. Pediatrics 37:477-484, 1966.
33. Dobson, J. V., Stephens-Grof, S. M., McMahon, S. R., et al.: The use of albuterol in hospitalized infants with bronchiolitis. Pediatrics 101:361-368, 1998.
34. Domachowske, J. B., Bonville, C. A., Dyer, K. D., et al.: Evolution of antiviral activity in the ribonuclease A gene superfamily: Evidence for a specific interaction between eosinophil-derived neurotoxin (EDN/RNase 2) and respiratory syncytial virus. Nucleic Acids Res. 26:5327-5332, 1998.
35. Domachowske, J. B., Dyer, K. D., Bonville, C. A., et al.: Recombinant human eosinophil-derived neurotoxin/RNase 2 functions as an effective antiviral agent against respiratory syncytial virus. J. Infect. Dis. 177:1458-1464, 1998.
36. Downes, J. J., Wood, D. W., Striker, T. W., et al.: Acute respiratory failure in infants with bronchiolitis. Anesthesiology 29:426-434, 1968.
37. Ehlenfield, D. R., Cameron, K., and Welliver, R. C.: Eosinophilia at the time of bronchiolitis predicts childhood reactive airway disease. Pediatrics 105:79-83, 2000.
38. Eisen, A. H., and Bacal, H. L.: The relationship of acute bronchiolitis to bronchial asthma: A 4 to 14 year follow-up. Pediatrics 31:859-861, 1963.
39. Empey, D. W., Laitinen, L. A., Jacobs, L., et al.: Mechanisms of bronchial hyperreactivity in normal subjects after upper respiratory tract infection. Am. Rev. Respir. Dis. 113:131-139, 1976.
40. Esper, F., Martinello, R. A., Boucher, D., et al.: A 1-year experience with human metapneumovirus in children aged <5 years. J. Infect. Dis. 189:1388-1396, 2004.
41. Everard, M. L., Swarbrick, A., Wrightham, M., et al.: Analysis of cells obtained by bronchial lavage of infants with respiratory syncytial virus infection. Arch. Dis. Child. 71:428-432, 1994.
42. Feltes, T. F., Cabalka, A. K., Meissner, H. C., et al.: Palivizumab prophylaxis reduces hospitalization due to respiratory syncytial virus in young children with hemodynamically significant congenital heart disease. J. Pediatr. 143:532-540, 2003.
43. Flores, G., and Horwitz, R.: Efficacy of β_2-agonists in bronchiolitis: A reappraisal and meta-analysis. Pediatrics 100:233-239, 1997.
44. Fox, G. F., Everard, M. E., Marsh, M. J., and Milner, A. D.: Randomized controlled trial of budesonide for the prevention of post-bronchiolitis wheezing. Arch. Dis. Child. 80:343-347, 1999.
45. Foy, H. M., Cooney, M. K., Maletzky, A. J., et al.: Incidence and etiology of pneumonia, croup and bronchiolitis in preschool children belonging to a pre-paid medical care group over a four-year period. Am. J. Epidemiol. 97:80-92, 1973.
46. Freeman, G. L., and Todd, R. H.: The role of allergy in viral respiratory tract infections. Am. J. Dis. Child. 104:330-334, 1962.
47. Gadomski, A. M., Aref, G. H., Badr El Din, O., et al.: Oral versus nebulized albuterol in the management of bronchiolitis in Egypt. J. Pediatr. 124:131-138, 1994.
48. Garofalo, R., Dorris, A., Ahlstedt, S., et al.: Peripheral blood eosinophil counts and eosinophil cationic protein content of respiratory secretions in bronchio-

litis: Relationship to severity of disease. Pediatr. Allergy Immunol. *5*:111-117, 1994.

49. Garofalo, R., Kimpen, J. L. L., Welliver, R. C., et al.: Eosinophil degranulation in naturally acquired respiratory syncytial virus infection. J. Pediatr. *120*:28-32, 1992.

50. Garofalo, R. P., Patti, J., Hintz, K. E., et al.: Macrophage inflammatory protein-1α (not T-helper type 2 cytokines) is associated with severe forms of respiratory syncytial virus bronchiolitis. J. Infect. Dis. *184*:383-389, 2001.

51. Glezen, W. P., Loda, F. A., Clyde, W. A., Jr., et al.: Epidemiologic patterns of acute lower respiratory disease of children in a pediatric group practice. J. Pediatr. *78*:397-406, 1971.

52. Glezen, W. P., Paredes, A., Allison, J. E., et al.: Risk of respiratory syncytial virus infection for infants from low-income families in relationship to age, sex, ethnic group, and maternal antibody level. J. Pediatr. *98*:708-715, 1981.

53. Glezen, W. P., Taber, L. H., Frank, A. L., et al.: Risk of primary infection and reinfection with respiratory syncytial virus. Am. J. Dis. Child. *140*:543-546, 1986.

54. Green, M., Brayer, A. F., Schenkman, K. A., et al.: Duration of hospitalization in previously well infants with respiratory syncytial virus infection. Pediatr. Infect. Dis. J. *8*:601-605, 1989.

55. Gregg, I.: The role of viral infection in asthma and bronchitis. *In* Proudfoot, A. T. (ed.): Symposium on Viral Diseases. Edinburgh, T. A. Constable, 1975, pp. 82-98.

56. Griffith, J. P. C., and Mitchell, A. G.: The Diseases of Infants and Children. Vol. II. Philadelphia, W. B. Saunders, 1927, pp. 274-355.

57. Groothuis, J. R., Simoes, E. A. F., Levin, M. J., et al.: Prophylactic administration of a respiratory syncytial virus immune globulin to high-risk infants and young children. N. Engl. J. Med. *329*:1524-1530, 1993.

58. Gurwitz, D., Mindorf, C., and Levison, H.: Increased incidence of bronchial reactivity in children with a history of bronchiolitis. J. Pediatr. *98*:551-555, 1981.

59. Hall, C. B., Hall, W. J., Gala, C. L., et al.: Long-term prospective study in children after respiratory syncytial virus infection. J. Pediatr. *105*:358-364, 1984.

60. Hall, C. B., McBride, J. T., Gala, C. L., et al.: Ribavirin treatment of respiratory syncytial virus infection in infants with underlying cardiopulmonary disease. J. A. M. A. *254*:3047-3051, 1985.

61. Hall, C. B., McBride, J. T., Walsh, E. E., et al.: Aerosolized ribavirin treatment of infants with respiratory syncytial viral infection. N. Engl. J. Med. *308*:1443-1447, 1983.

62. Hall, C. B., Powell, K. R., Schnabel, K. C., et al.: Risk of secondary bacterial infection in infants hospitalized with respiratory syncytial viral infection. J. Pediatr. *113*:266-271, 1988.

63. Hammer, J., Numa, A., and Newth, C. J. L.: Albuterol responsiveness in infants with respiratory failure caused by respiratory syncytial virus infection. J. Pediatr. *127*:485-490, 1995.

64. Hampton, S. F., Johnson, M. C., and Galakatos, E.: Studies of bacterial hypersensitivity in asthma, I: The preparation of antigen of *Neisseria catarrhalis*, the induction of asthma by aerosols, the performance of skin and passive transfer tests. J. Allergy *34*:63-95, 1963.

65. Harrison, R., Bellows, J., Rempel, D., et al.: Assessing exposures of health-care personnel to aerosols of ribavirin: California. M. M. W. R. Morb. Mortal. Wkly. Rep. *37*:560-563, 1988.

66. Hemming, V. G., and Prince, G. A.: Immunoprophylaxis of infections with respiratory syncytial virus: Observations and hypothesis. Rev. Infect. Dis. *12*:S470-S475, 1990.

67. Henderson, A. T., and Rosenzweig, S.: Bronchiolitis in infancy: Clinical study with special emphasis on the cardiac complications. U. S. Armed Forces Med. J. *2*:943-952, 1951.

68. Henderson, F. W., Clyde, W. A., Jr., Collier, A. M., et al.: The etiologic and epidemiological spectrum of bronchiolitis in pediatric practice. J. Pediatr. *95*:183-190, 1979.

69. Henderson, F. W., Stewart, P. W., Burchinal, M. R., et al.: Respiratory allergy and the relationship between early childhood lower respiratory illness and subsequent lung function. Am. Rev. Respir. Dis. *145*:283-290, 1992.

70. Henderson, J. W., Hu, S. C., and Collier, A. M.: Pathogenesis of respiratory syncytial virus infection in ferret and fetal human tracheas in organ culture. Am. Rev. Respir. Dis. *118*:29-37, 1978.

71. Heycock, J. B., and Noble, T. C.: 1,230 Cases of acute bronchiolitis in infancy. B. M. J. *5309*:879-881, 1962.

72. Hogg, J. C., Williams, J., Richardson, J. B., et al.: Age as a factor in the distribution of lower-airway conductance and in the pathologic anatomy of obstructive lung disease. N. Engl. J. Med. *282*:1283-1287, 1970.

73. Holt, L. E., and Howland, J.: Diseases of the lungs: Peculiarities of the thorax in children. *In* Holt, L. E., and McIntosh, R. (eds.): Holt's Diseases of Infancy and Childhood. 11th ed New York, D. Appleton-Century, 1940, pp. 498-513.

74. Horn, M. E. C., Brain, E., Gregg, I., et al.: Respiratory viral infection in childhood: A survey in general practice, Roehampton 1967-1972. J. Hyg. (Camb.) *74*:157-168, 1975.

75. Horn, M. E. C., Brain, E., Gregg, I., et al.: Respiratory viral infection and wheezy bronchitis in childhood. Thorax *34*:23-28, 1979.

76. Hubble, D., and Osborn, G. R.: Acute bronchitis in children. B. M. J. *1*:107-110, 1941.

77. Hughes, D. M., Lesouef, P. N., and Landau, L. I.: Effect of salbutamol on respiratory mechanics in bronchiolitis. Pediatr. Res. *22*:83-86, 1987.

78. Karron, R. A., Wright, P. F., Belshe, R. B., et al.: Identification of a recombinant live attenuated respiratory syncytial virus vaccine candidate that is highly attenuated in infants. J. Infect. Dis. *191*:1093-1104.

79. Kattan, M., Keens, T. G., Lapierre, J. G., et al.: Pulmonary function abnormalities in symptom-free children after bronchiolitis. Pediatrics *59*:683-688, 1977.

80. Kaul, T. N., Welliver, R. C., and Ogra, P. L.: Development of antibody dependent cell-mediated cytotoxicity in the respiratory tract after natural infection with respiratory syncytial virus. Infect. Immun. *37*:492-498, 1982.

81. Kaul, T. N., Welliver, R. C., and Ogra, P. L.: Appearance of complement components and immunoglobulins on nasopharyngeal epithelial cells following naturally acquired infection with respiratory syncytial virus. J. Med. Virol. *9*:149-158, 1982.

82. Kaul, T. N., Welliver, R. C., Wong, D. T., et al.: Secretory antibody response to respiratory syncytial virus infection. Am. J. Dis. Child. *135*:1013-1016, 1981.

83. Kerr, M. H., and Paton, J. Y.: Surfactant protein levels in severe respiratory syncytial virus infection. Am. J. Respir. Crit. Care Med. *159*:1115-1118, 1999.

84. Kim, H. W., Arrobio, J. O., Brandt, C. D., et al.: Epidemiology of respiratory syncytial virus infection in Washington, D.C., I: Importance of the virus in different respiratory tract disease syndromes and temporal distribution of infection. Am. J. Epidemiol. *98*:216-225, 1973.

85. Kim, H. W., Canchola, J., Brandt, C. D., et al.: Respiratory syncytial virus disease in infants despite prior administration of antigenic inactivated vaccine. Am. J. Epidemiol. *89*:422-434, 1969.

86. Kim, H. W., Leikin, S. L., Arrobio, J., et al.: Cell-mediated immunity to respiratory syncytial virus induced by inactivated vaccine or by infection. Pediatr. Res. *10*:75-78, 1976.

87. Klassen, T. P., Rowe, P. C., Sutcliffe, T., et al.: Randomized trial of salbutamol in acute bronchiolitis. J. Pediatr. *118*:807-811, 1991.

88. Koch, D. A.: Roentgenologic considerations of capillary bronchiolitis. Am. J. Roentgenol. Radiat. Ther. Nucl. Med. *82*:433-436, 1959.

89. Laing, I., Riedel, F., Yap, P. L., et al.: Atopy predisposing to acute bronchiolitis during an epidemic of respiratory syncytial virus. B. M. J. *284*:1070-1072, 1982.

90. Leer, J. A., Jr., Green, J. L., Heimlich, E. M., et al.: Corticosteroid treatment in bronchiolitis: A controlled, collaborative study in 297 infants and children. Am. J. Dis. Child. *117*:495-502, 1969.

91. Lenney, W., and Milner, A. D.: Alpha and beta adrenergic stimulants in bronchiolitis and wheezy bronchitis in children under 18 months of age. Arch. Dis. Child. *53*:707-709, 1978.

92. Lesouef, P. N., Geelhoed, G. C., Turner, D. J., et al.: Response of normal infants to inhaled histamine. Am. Rev. Respir. Dis. *139*:62-66, 1989.

93. Little, J. W., Hall, W. J., Douglas, R. G., et al.: Airway hyperreactivity and peripheral airway dysfunction in influenza A infection. Am. Rev. Respir. Dis. *118*:295-303, 1978.

94. Loda, F. A., Clyde, W. A., Jr., Glezen, W. P., et al.: Studies on the role of viruses, bacteria, and *M. pneumoniae* as causes of lower respiratory tract infections in children. J. Pediatr. *72*:161-176, 1968.

95. Loda, F. A., Glezen, W. P., and Clyde, W. A., Jr.: Respiratory disease in group day care. Pediatrics *49*:428-437, 1972.

96. McConnochie, K. M., and Roghmann, K. J.: Bronchiolitis as a possible cause of wheezing in childhood: New evidence. Pediatrics *74*:1-10, 1984.

97. McConnochie, K. M., and Roghmann, K. J.: Wheezing at age 8 and 13 years: Changing importance of bronchiolitis and passive smoking. Pediatr. Pulmonol. *6*:138-146, 1989.

98. McGeorge, M.: Severe obstructive bronchiolitis in infancy: Treatment with hydrocortisone. Clin. Pediatr. *3*:11-18, 1964.

99. Macasaet, F. F., Kidd, P. A., Bolano, C. R., et al.: The etiology of acute respiratory infections, III: The role of viruses and bacteria. J. Pediatr. *72*:829-839, 1968.

100. Macklin, C. C.: Alveolar pores and their significance in the human lung. Arch. Pathol. *21*:202, 1936.

101. Malley, R., DeVincenzo, J., Ramilo, O., et al.: Reduction of respiratory syncytial virus in tracheal aspirates in intubated infants by use of humanized monoclonal antibody to RSV F protein. J. Infect. Dis. *178*:1555-1561, 1998.

102. Martinez, F. D., Morgan, W. J., Wright, A. L., et al.: Diminished lung function as a predisposing factor for wheezing respiratory illness in infants. N. Engl. J. Med. *319*:1112-1117, 1988.

103. Martinez, F. D., Stern, D. A., Wright, A. L., and Taussig, L. M.: Differential immune responses to acute lower respiratory illnesses in early life and subsequent development of persistent wheezing and asthma. J. Allergy Clin. Immunol. *102*:915-920, 1998.

104. Martinez, F. D., Wright, A. L., Taussig, L. M., et al.: Asthma and wheezing in the first six years of life. N. Engl. J. Med. *332*:133-138, 1995.

105. Meert, K. L., Sarnaik, A. P., Gelmini, M. J., et al.: Aerosolized ribavirin in mechanically ventilated children with respiratory syncytial virus lower respiratory tract disease: A prospective, double-blind, randomized trial. Crit. Care Med. *22*:566-572, 1994.

106. Merkus, P. J., de Hoog, M., van Gent, R., et al.: DNase treatment for atelectasis in infants with severe respiratory syncytial virus bronchiolitis. Eur. Respir. J. *18*:734-737, 2001.

107. Miller, D. G., Gabrielson, M. O., and Horstmann, D. M.: Clinical virology and viral surveillance in a pediatric group practice: The use of double-seeded tissue culture tubes for primary virus isolation. Am. J. Epidemiol. 88:245-256, 1968.

108. Minor, T. E., Baker, J. W., Dick, F. C., et al.: Greater frequency of viral respiratory infections in asthmatic children as compared with their nonasthmatic siblings. J. Pediatr. 85:472-477, 1974.

109. Minor, T. E., Dick, E. C., De Meo, A. N., et al.: Viruses as precipitants of asthmatic attacks in children. J. A. M. A. 227:292-298, 1974.

110. Minor, T. E., Dick, E. C., Baker, J. W., et al.: Rhinovirus and influenza type A infections as precipitants of asthma. Am. Rev. Respir. Dis. 113:149-153, 1976.

111. Mitchell, I., Inglis, J. M., and Simpson, H.: Viral infection as a precipitant of wheeze in children: Combined home and hospital study. Arch. Dis. Child. 53:106-111, 1978.

112. Moler, F. W., Bandy, K. P., and Custer, J. R.: Ribavirin therapy for acute bronchiolitis: Need for appropriate controls. J. Pediatr. 119:509, 1991.

113. Mueller, H. L.: The dual role of infection in asthma of childhood. Postgrad. Med. 50:225-229, 1971.

114. Mueller, H. L., and Lanz, M.: Hyposensitization with bacterial vaccine in infectious asthma: A double-blind study and a longitudinal study. J. A. M. A. 208:1379-1383, 1969.

115. Mufson, M. A., Krause, H. E., Mocega, H. E., et al.: Viruses, *Mycoplasma pneumoniae* and bacteria associated with lower respiratory tract disease among infants. J. Epidemiol. 91:192-202, 1970.

116. Mulholland, E. K., Olinsky, A., and Shann, F.: Clinical findings and severity of acute bronchiolitis. Lancet 335:1259-1261, 1990.

117. Neilson, K. A., and Yunis, E. J.: Demonstration of respiratory syncytial virus in an autopsy series. Pediatr. Pathol. 10:491-502, 1990.

118. Nelson, W. E.: Viral or probable viral infections. *In* Nelson, W. E. (ed.): Pediatrics. 6th ed. Philadelphia, W. B. Saunders, 1954, pp. 823-828, 1438-1446.

119. Nelson, W. E., and Smith, L. W.: Generalized obstructive emphysema in infants. J. Pediatr. 26:36-55, 1945.

120. Neuzil, K. M., Gruber, W. C., Chytil, F., et al.: Safety and pharmacokinetics of vitamin A therapy for infants with respiratory syncytial virus infections. Antimicrob. Agents Chemother. 39:1191-1193, 1995.

121. Nichol, K. P., and Cherry, J. D.: Bacterial-viral interrelations in respiratory infections of children. N. Engl. J. Med. 277:667-672, 1967.

122. O'Callaghan, C., Milner, A. D., and Swarbrick, A.: Paradoxical deterioration in lung function after nebulised salbutamol in wheezy infants. Lancet 2:1424-1425, 1986.

123. Ogilvie, M. M., Vathenen, S., Radford, M., et al.: Maternal antibody and respiratory syncytial virus infection in infancy. J. Med. Virol. 7:263-271, 1981.

124. Outwater, K. M., and Crone, R. K.: Management of respiratory failure in infants with acute viral bronchiolitis. Am. J. Dis. Child. 138:1071-1075, 1984.

125. Outwater, K. M., Meissner, C., and Peterson, M. B.: Ribavirin administration to infants receiving mechanical ventilation. Am. J. Dis. Child. 142:512-515, 1988.

126. Parrott, R. H., Kim, H. W., Arrobio, J. O., et al.: Epidemiology of respiratory syncytial virus infection in Washington, D.C., II: Infection and disease with respect to age, immunologic status, race and sex. Am. J. Epidemiol. 98:289-300, 1973.

127. Patel, N. R., Hammer, J., Nichani, S., et al.: Effect of nitric oxide on respiratory mechanics in ventilated infants with RSV bronchiolitis. Intensive Care Med. 25:81-87, 1999.

128. Paton, A. W., Paton, J. C., Lawrence, A. J., et al.: Rapid detection of respiratory syncytial virus in nasopharyngeal aspirates by reverse transcription and polymerase chain reaction amplification. J. Clin. Microbiol. 30:901-904, 1992.

129. Phelan, P. D., and Williams, H. E.: Sympathomimetic drugs in acute viral bronchiolitis: Their effect on pulmonary resistance. Pediatrics 44:493-497, 1969.

130. Polmar, S. H., Robinson, L. D., Jr., and Minnefor, A. B.: Immunoglobulin E in bronchiolitis. Pediatrics 50:279-284, 1972.

131. Pratt, E. L.: Acute bronchiolitis in infants. Med. Clin. North Am. 28:1098-1107, 1944.

132. Pullan, C. R., and Hey, E. N.: Wheezing, asthma, and pulmonary dysfunction 10 years after infection with respiratory syncytial virus in infancy. B. M. J. 284:1665-1669, 1982.

133. Purcell, K., and Fergie, J.: Concurrent serious bacterial infections in 912 infants and children hospitalized for treatment of respiratory syncytial virus lower respiratory tract infection. Pediatr. Infect. Dis. J. 23:267-269, 2004.

134. Randolph, A. G., Reder, L., Englund, J. A.: Risk of bacterial infection in previously healthy respiratory syncytial virus-infected young children admitted to the intensive care unit. Pediatr. Infect. Dis. J. 23:990-994, 2004.

135. Randolph, A. G., and Wang, E. E. L.: Ribavirin for respiratory syncytial virus infection: A systematic overview. Arch. Pediatr. Adolesc. Med. 150:942-947, 1996.

136. Reid, L.: Influence of the pattern of structural growth of lung on susceptibility to specific infectious diseases in infants and children. Pediatr. Res. 11:210-215, 1977.

137. Reilly, C. M., Stokes, J., Jr., McClelland, L., et al.: Studies of acute respiratory illnesses caused by respiratory syncytial virus, 3: Clinical and laboratory findings. N. Engl. J. Med. 264:1176-1182, 1961.

138. Richter, H., and Seddon, P.: Early nebulized budesonide in the treatment of bronchiolitis and the prevention of postbronchiolitis wheezing. J. Pediatr. 132:849-853, 1998.

139. Roan, Y., and Galant, S. P.: Decreased neutrophil beta adrenergic receptors in the neonate. Pediatr. Res. 16:591-593, 1982.

140. Rodriguez, W. J., Bui, R. H. D., Connor, J. D., et al.: Environmental exposure of primary care personnel to ribavirin aerosol when supervising treatment of infants with respiratory syncytial virus infections. Antimicrob. Agents Chemother. 31:1143-1146, 1987.

141. Rodriguez, W. J., Kim, H. W., Brandt, C. D., et al.: Aerosolized ribavirin in the treatment of patients with respiratory syncytial virus disease. Pediatr. Infect. Dis. J. 6:159-163, 1987.

142. Rooney, J. C., and Williams, H. E.: The relationship between proved viral bronchiolitis and subsequent wheezing. J. Pediatr. 79:744-747, 1971.

143. Rutter, N., Milner, A. D., and Hiller, E. J.: Effect of bronchodilators on respiratory resistance in infants and young children with bronchiolitis and wheezy bronchitis. Arch. Dis. Child. 50:719-722, 1975.

144. Sanchez, I., De Koster, J., Powell, R., et al.: Effect of racemic epinephrine and salbutamol on clinical score and pulmonary mechanics in infants with bronchiolitis. J. Pediatr. 122:145-151, 1993.

145. Sandiford, B. R., and Spencer, B.: Respiratory syncytial virus in epidemic bronchiolitis of infants. B. M. J. 5309:881-882, 1962.

146. Scott, L. P., III, Gutelius, M. F., and Parrott, R. H.: Children with acute respiratory tract infections: An electrocardiographic survey. Am. J. Dis. Child. 119:111-113, 1970.

147. Scott, R., DeLandazuri, M. O., Gardner, P. S., et al.: Human antibody-dependent cell-mediated cytotoxicity against target cells infected with respiratory syncytial virus. Clin. Exp. Immunol. 28:19-26, 1977.

148. Seidenberg, J., Masters, I. B., Hudson, I., et al.: Effect of ipratropium bromide on respiratory mechanics in infants with acute bronchiolitis. Aust. Paediatr. J. 23:169-172, 1987.

149. Sell, S. H. W.: Some observations on acute bronchiolitis in infants. Am. J. Dis. Child. 100:31-39, 1960.

150. Shay, D. K., Holman, R. C., Roosevelt, G. E., et al.: Bronchiolitis-associated mortality and estimates of respiratory syncytial virus-associated deaths among US children, 1979-1997. J. Infect. Dis. 183:16-22, 2001.

151. Shay, D. K., Holman, R. C., Newman, R. D., et al.: Bronchiolitis-associated hospitalizations among US children, 1980-1996. J. A. M. A. 282:1440-1446, 2001.

152. Simpson, H., Matthew, D. J., Inglis, J. M., et al.: Virological findings and blood gas tensions in acute lower respiratory tract infections in children. B. M. J. 2:629-632, 1974.

153. Sims, D. G., Downham, M. A. P. S., Gardner, P. S., et al.: Study of 8-year-old children with a history of respiratory syncytial virus bronchiolitis in infancy. B. M. J. 1:11-14, 1978.

154. Sims, D. G., Gardner, P. S., Weightman, D., et al.: Atopy does not predispose to RSV bronchiolitis or postbronchiolitic wheezing. B. M. J. 282:2086-2088, 1981.

155. Skoner, D.: Montelukast in 2- to 5-year-old children with asthma. Pediatr. Pulmonol. 21:46-48, 2001.

156. Skoner, D. P., Fireman, P., Caligiuri, L., et al.: Plasma elevations of histamine and a prostaglandin metabolite in acute bronchiolitis. Am. Rev. Respir. Dis. 142:359-364, 1990.

157. Smith, D. W., Frankel, L. R., Mathers, L. H., et al.: A controlled trial of aerosolized ribavirin in infants receiving mechanical ventilation for severe respiratory syncytial virus infection. N. Engl. J. Med. 325:24-29, 1991.

158. Smith, M. C., Creutz, C., and Huang, Y. T.: Detection of respiratory syncytial virus in nasopharyngeal secretions by shell vial technique. J. Clin. Microbiol. 29:463-465, 1991.

159. Smith, T. F., McIntosh, K., Fishaut, M., et al.: Activation of complement by cells infected with respiratory syncytial virus. Infect. Immun. 33:43-48, 1981.

160. Stein, R. T., Sherrill, D., Morgan, W. J., et al.: Respiratory syncytial virus in early life and risk of wheeze and allergy by age 13 years. Lancet 354:541-545, 1999.

161. Stempel, D. A., Clyde, W. A., Jr., Henderson, F. W., et al.: Serum IgE levels and the clinical expression of respiratory illnesses. J. Pediatr. 97:185-190, 1980.

162. Stokes, G. M., Milner, A. D., Hodges, I. G. C., et al.: Lung function abnormalities after acute bronchiolitis. J. Pediatr. 98:871-874, 1981.

163. Strope, G. L., Stewart, P. W., Henderson, F. W., et al.: Lung function in school-age children who had mild lower respiratory illnesses in early childhood. Am. Rev. Respir. Dis. 144:665-662, 1991.

164. Sturdy, P. M., McQuillin, J., and Gardner, P. S.: A comparative study of methods for the diagnosis of respiratory virus infections in childhood. J. Hyg. (Camb.) 67:659-670, 1969.

165. Taber, L. H., Knight, V., Gilbert, B. E., et al.: Ribavirin aerosol treatment of bronchiolitis associated with respiratory syncytial virus infection in infants. Pediatrics 72:613-618, 1983.

166. Tager, I. B., Weiss, S. T., Munoz, A., et al.: Longitudinal study of the effects of maternal smoking on pulmonary function in children. N. Engl. J. Med. 309:699-703, 1983.

167. Tal, A., Bavilski, C., Yohai, D., et al.: Dexamethasone and salbutamol in the treatment of acute wheezing in infants. Pediatrics 71:13-18, 1983.

168. Taussig, L. M.: Clinical and physiologic evidence of the persistence of pulmonary abnormalities after respiratory illnesses in infancy and childhood. Pediatr. Res. 11:216-218, 1977.

169. Tepper, R. S., Rosenberg, D., and Eigen, H.: Airway responsiveness in infants following bronchiolitis. Pediatr. Pulmonol. 13:6-10, 1992.

170. The Impact RSV study group: Palivizumab, a humanized respiratory syncytial virus monoclonal antibody, reduces hospitalization from respiratory syncytial virus infection in high-risk infants. Pediatrics 102:531-537, 1998.

171. Tibby, S. M., Hatherill, M., Wright, S., et al.: Exogenous surfactant supplementation in infants with respiratory syncytial virus bronchiolitis. Am. J. Respir. Crit. Care Med. 162:1251-1256, 2000.

172. Tristram, D. A., Welliver, R. C., Mohar, C. K., et al.: Immunogenicity and safety of respiratory syncytial virus subunit vaccine in seropositive children 18-36 months old. J. Infect. Dis. 167:191-195, 1993.

173. Twarog, F. J., and Colten, H. R.: Rational management of allergic disease: The role of immunotherapy. Pediatrics 60:320-323, 1977.

174. van Schaik, S. M., Tristram, D. A., Nagpal, I. S., et al.: Increased production of interferon-γ and cysteinyl leukotrienes in virus-induced wheezing. J. Allergy Clin. Immunol. 103:630-636, 1999.

175. Vikerfors, T., Grandien, M., and Olcen, P.: Respiratory syncytial virus infections in adults. Am. Rev. Respir. Dis. 136:561-564, 1987.

176. Volovitz, B., Welliver, R. C., DeCastro, G., et al.: The release of leukotrienes in the respiratory tract during infection with respiratory syncytial virus: Role in obstructive airway disease. Pediatr. Res. 24:504-507, 1988.

177. Voter, K. Z., Henry, M. M., Stewart, P. W., et al.: Lower respiratory illness in early childhood and lung function and bronchial reactivity in adolescent males. Am. Rev. Respir. Dis. 137:302-307, 1988.

178. Wang, E. E. L., Milner, R. A., Navas, L., et al.: Observer agreement for respiratory signs and oximetry in infants hospitalized with lower respiratory infections. Am. Rev. Respir. Dis. 145:106-109, 1992.

179. Welliver, R. C., and Duffy, L.: The relationship of RSV-specific immunoglobulin E antibody responses in infancy, recurrent wheezing, and pulmonary function at age 7-8 years. Pediatr. Pulmonol. 15:19-27, 1993.

180. Welliver, R. C., Kaul, T. N., and Ogra, P. L.: The appearance of cell-bound IgE in respiratory-tract epithelium after respiratory-syncytial-virus infection. N. Engl. J. Med. 303:1198-1202, 1980.

181. Welliver, R. C., Kaul, T. N., Putnam, T. I., et al.: The antibody response to primary and secondary infection with respiratory syncytial virus: Kinetics of class-specific responses. J. Pediatr. 96:808-813, 1980.

182. Welliver, R. C., Wong, D. T., Middleton, E., Jr., et al.: Role of parainfluenza virus-specific IgE in pathogenesis of croup and wheezing subsequent to infection. J. Pediatr. 101:889-896, 1982.

183. Welliver, R. C., Wong, D. T., Sun, M., et al.: The development of respiratory syncytial virus-specific IgE and the release of histamine in nasopharyngeal secretions after infection. N. Engl. J. Med. 305:841-846, 1981.

184. Welliver, T. P., Garofalo, R. P., Hintz, K. H., et al.: Severe human lower respiratory tract illness caused by respiratory syncytial virus and influenza virus is characterized by the absence of pulmonary cytotoxic lymphocyte responses. J. Infect. Dis. 195:1126-1136, 2007.

185. Williams, H., and McNicol, K. N.: Prevalence, natural history, and relationship of wheezy bronchitis and asthma in children: An epidemiological study. B. M. J. 4:321-325, 1969.

186. Wittig, H. J., Cranford, N. J., and Glasner, J.: The relationship between bronchiolitis and childhood asthma: A follow-up study of 100 cases of bronchiolitis in infancy. J. Allergy 30:19-23, 1959.

187. Wohl, M. E. B., and Chernick, V.: Bronchiolitis. Am. Rev. Respir. Dis. 118:759-781, 1978.

188. Wohl, M. E. B., Stigol, L. C., and Mead, J.: Resistance of the total respiratory system in healthy infants and infants with bronchiolitis. Pediatrics 43:495-509, 1969.

189. Wood, S. H., Buddingh, G. J., and Abberger, B. F., Jr.: An inquiry into the etiology of acute bronchiolitis of infants. Pediatrics 13:363-372, 1954.

190. Woolcock, A. J., Leeder, S. R., Peat, J. K., et al.: The influence of lower respiratory illness in infancy and childhood and subsequent cigarette smoking on lung function in Sydney schoolchildren. Am. Rev. Respir. Dis. 120:5-14, 1979.

191. Wright, A. L., Holberg, C., Martinez, F. D., et al.: Relationship of parental smoking to wheezing and nonwheezing lower respiratory tract illnesses in infancy. J. Pediatr. 118:207-214, 1991.

192. Wright, A. L., Taussig, L. M., Ray, C. G., et al.: The Tucson children's respiratory study, II: Lower respiratory illness in the first year of life. Am. J. Epidemiol. 129:1232-1246, 1989.

193. Young, S., Le Souf, P., Geelhoed, G., et al.: The influence of a family history of asthma and parental smoking on airway responsiveness in early infancy. N. Engl. J. Med. 324:1168-1174, 1991.

194. Yusuf, S., Piedimonte, G., Auais, A., et al.: The relationship of meteorological conditions to the epidemic activity of respiratory syncytial virus. Epidemiol. Infect. 135:1077-1090, 2007.

195. Zweiman, B., Schoenwetter, W. F., Pappano, J. E., Jr., et al.: Patterns of allergic respiratory disease in children with a past history of bronchiolitis. J. Allergy Clin. Immunol. 48:283-289, 1971.

NONBACTERIAL PNEUMONIA

CHAPTER 26

Kenneth M. Boyer

Nonbacterial pneumonias remain the most frequent pulmonary infections encountered in pediatrics. In recent years, conjugate vaccines against invasive *Haemophilus influenzae* type b (Hib) and *Streptococcus pneumoniae* infections have decreased significantly the importance of these bacterial pathogens.[33,34] Relatively less progress has been made in creating effective vaccines against the most common nonbacterial pathogens that cause pneumonia. Work is progressing on several attenuated viral vaccines,[128] however, and the recommendations for annual influenza vaccination of children have been broadened considerably.[208]

Numerous terms, based on causes, clinical manifestations, or histologic features, are used for these pulmonary infections. Although the connotations differ, viral pneumonia, viral lower respiratory tract infection, atypical pneumonia, infant pneumonitis, and interstitial pneumonia are encountered frequently. The varied causes, excluding bacteria and fungi, cover a broad taxonomic spectrum. With improvements in microbiologic techniques, the number of known causative agents continues to increase. Defining the origin of these infections once was the province of the epidemiologist and virologist, but a sufficient body of knowledge has accumulated to permit informed diagnostic judgment to be made by practicing physicians and rapid

specific diagnosis to be confirmed by clinical microbiology laboratories. Although most nonbacterial pneumonias have a good prognosis, occasionally they are life-threatening. Therapy directed against the causative agent may shorten the duration of the course of illness or may avert serious complications. At times, it is lifesaving. This chapter provides an overview of pneumonia syndromes caused by viruses, mycoplasmas, and chlamydiae, as well as by *Coxiella burnetii* (a rickettsia) and *Pneumocystis jiroveci* (an apicomplexan parasite).

HISTORICAL ASPECTS

The development of systematic bacteriology in the late 19th century led to the widespread consensus that pneumonias were bacterial infections with differences in manifestations (bronchial, lobular, lobar) that primarily were the result of differences in anatomic localization. During the 1918 influenza pandemic, most postmortem examinations of patients with pneumonia revealed numerous bacteria in the lungs. Various different species were identified, not exclusively *H. influenzae*, the organism at that time regarded as the cause of influenza. However, in a few cases in which no bacteria were found, Goodpasture[89] and Winternitz and colleagues[253] found distinctive histopathologic lesions in the lung that they concluded were induced by a nonbacterial agent. Isolation of influenza A virus by Smith and associates[234] in 1933 confirmed their observations, altered the prevailing bacteriologic and anatomic concepts of pneumonia, and ushered in a new era of etiologic diagnosis of respiratory syndromes.

The first isolation of influenza virus and subsequent isolation of *Chlamydia psittaci* (psittacosis) and *C. burnetii* (Q fever) involved transmission of infection to experimental animals such as ferrets and chick embryos. The development of tissue culture techniques in the 1950s enabled researchers to identify numerous other common respiratory viruses: adenoviruses, parainfluenza viruses, respiratory syncytial virus (RSV), enteroviruses, and rhinoviruses. The major etiologic agent of primary atypical pneumonia had been passed to experimental animals in the 1940s, but it was not identified as a mycoplasma definitively until 1962.[42]

In the 1960s and 1970s, the most valuable studies of nonbacterial respiratory infection in pediatrics were comprehensive longitudinal investigations in which epidemiologic and clinical patterns of illness were defined. These studies established that most lower respiratory tract infections in infants and young children are caused by nonbacterial agents, principally respiratory viruses and *Mycoplasma pneumoniae*.

The attention of current investigators is being directed increasingly at developing methods for rapid diagnosis, chemotherapy, and prevention. However, more refined tissue culture and nucleic acid amplification techniques have enabled researchers to identify numerous new agents, including Sin Nombre hantavirus,[111,245] human metapneumovirus,[247] human bocavirus (HBoV),[3] and several strains of coronavirus, including the virus that caused the global epidemic of severe acute respiratory syndrome (SARS).[56,139,247,256]

ETIOLOGY

Three *Mycoplasma* spp., a single *Rickettsia* sp., 3 *Chlamydia* spp., 1 protozoan parasite, and at least 16 different virus groups have been associated with pneumonia syndromes in children. The overall importance of these agents is not measured simply by their incidence. Some agents, although quite common, generally give rise to mild illness; others, less frequently encountered, characteristically cause serious disease. In Table 26–1, the major agents in various age groups are presented by their overall frequency, their typical degree of severity, and their mode of access to the lung. Although the incidence data are representative of numerous major epidemiologic studies,* one should recall that the proportion of pneumonias of unproven cause in most such studies has been approximately 50 percent. Possible explanations for the high percentage of such cases include the following: a bacterial origin[175]; partial treatment with antimicrobial agents[127]; late collection of viral cultures and sera[71]; suboptimal storage, transport, or cultivation of specimens[83,218]; and as yet unidentified agents. The use of antigen tests for bacterial pathogens and of immunoassays and polymerase chain reaction (PCR) assays for viruses accounts for the higher rates of diagnosis in some studies.[110,127,258]

RSV generally is accepted as the agent found most frequently in pediatric pneumonias, particularly those associated with bronchiolitis.† Although infection with this virus is quite common in all age groups, lower respiratory tract involvement is especially prominent in infancy.

The three parainfluenza viruses (types 1, 2, and 3) are second only to RSV as causes of lower respiratory tract disease in infants and younger children. Parainfluenza virus type 3 is the agent most frequently found in pneumonia[85,86,117,198]; infection with parainfluenza virus types 1 and 2 generally produces laryngotracheitis.

Human metapneumovirus, described in children with upper and lower respiratory tract infection in the Netherlands,[246] is thought to account for 10 percent of otherwise unexplained respiratory infections. The clinical symptoms in infected children resemble those caused by RSV.[188,246]

Influenza A and B viruses are not as prevalent overall as are RSV and parainfluenza viruses, but during periods of epidemic spread, they may become predominant isolates in hospitalized children with lower respiratory tract disease.[15,26,81,134,193,197,226] The threat of a pandemic of influenza A, secondary to a recombination event resulting in a "humanized" avian virus, keeps influenza in the forefront of concern for global public health agencies.[81,204]

Adenoviruses commonly are isolated in children with pneumonia* and pertussis syndrome.[25,48,186,190] The overall impact of these viruses in the origin of nonbacterial pneumonia in children probably is somewhat less than that of the aforementioned agents; however, many fatal illnesses have been reported. Their common asymptomatic carriage and potential for endogenous activation by unrelated illnesses can render causation difficult to prove.[68,186] Of the 51 known adenoviruses, types 1, 2, 3, 4, 5, 7, 14, 21, and 35 clearly have been associated with pneumonia.[25,135] In certain aboriginal populations such as the Maori, Native Americans, and Inuit, adenoviruses commonly produce severe infection.[114,140] In military recruits, adenoviruses are second to *M. pneumoniae* as a cause of atypical pneumonia.[54]

Rhinoviruses[15,79,199,215,240] have been associated less frequently with pneumonia, although upper respiratory infection with the multiple serotypes of these organisms is common. Some degree of lower respiratory involvement by rhinoviruses also is indicated by the documented role of these viruses in exacerbations of asthma[176] and bronchitis.[171] Among the enteroviruses, primary viral pneumonia has been documented best with coxsackieviruses A9[146] and B1,[58] although coxsackieviruses A16, B4, and B5 and echoviruses 9, 11, 19, 20, and 22 also have been reported.[42,97,230]

Coronaviruses HCo-OC43 and HCo-229E have been implicated as causes of pneumonia since the 1960s, but until recently, this family of viruses was considered a rare cause of human disease.[132,168] The worldwide epidemic of SARS that occurred in 2002 to 2004 focused new interest on these pathogens and led to a new appreciation of their reservoirs in domestic animals and their potential to cause severe pneumonia and respiratory failure.[56,139] Fortunately, the SARS-CoV, no longer circulating, appears to be unique in its pathogenic potential. Two other strains of coronavirus, HCo-NL63[247] and HCo-HKU1,[256] have been discovered more recently. They appear to be among the less common causes of lower respiratory infections, but their clinical manifestations are similar to those caused by the other common respiratory viruses.[61,212]

The respiratory virus most recently described that can cause pneumonia is HBoV.[3] It is a parvovirus closely related to bovine parvovirus and canine parvovirus. (The "bo" in "bocavirus" derives from "bovine," the "ca" from canine.) It was identified using a novel technique based on amplification of nonspecific viral nucleotide sequences, a method that holds promise for identification of other previously uncultivated human viral pathogens. Because only a few population-based studies have been per-

---

*See references 37, 38, 42, 47, 52, 53, 69, 70, 71, 83, 87, 88, 118, 122, 129, 145, 149, 152, 155, 158, 180, 183, 187, 194, 196, and 244 (major epidemiologic studies).
†See references 18, 20, 24, 27, 112, 123, 133, 165, 179, 235, and 242 (RSV).

---

*See references 7, 9,19, 25, 28, 39, 83, 113, 115, 116, 126, 185, 202, 234, and 257 (adenoviruses).

TABLE 26-1   Etiologic Agents in Nonbacterial Pneumonia

Etiologic Agents	Frequency*			Usual Degree of Severity†			Mode of Access to Lung
	0-3 mo	4 mo-5 yr	6-16 yr	0-3 mo	4 mo-5 yr	6-16 yr	
Virus							
Respiratory syncytial virus	+++	++++	+	++	++	++	Respiratory
Human metapneumovirus	+	++	?	++	++	?	Respiratory
Parainfluenza viruses							
Type 1	+	++	+	++	++	+	Respiratory
Type 2	+	+	+	++	++	+	Respiratory
Type 3	++	+++	++	++	++	+	Respiratory
Influenza viruses							
Type A	++	+++	+++	++	++	++	Respiratory
Type B	++	++	+	++	++	+	Respiratory
Adenoviruses‡	+	++	++	+++	++	+	Respiratory
Rhinoviruses§	+	±	+	–	++	+	Respiratory
Enteroviruses¶	+	+	+	++	++	+	Respiratory (hematogenous)
Coronaviruses							
Human¶	+	+	+	–	+	+	Respiratory
Severe acute respiratory syndrome	–	+	+	–	++	+++	Respiratory
Human bocavirus	?	±	+	?	?	?	Respiratory
Measles virus	+	++	++	+++	++	++	Respiratory (hematogenous)
Rubella virus	+	–	–	++	–	–	Hematogenous
Human immunodeficiency virus	+	++	+	++	++	++	Hematogenous
Varicella-zoster virus	+	+	+	+++	+++	+++	Hematogenous (respiratory)
Cytomegalovirus	+++	+	+	++	+++	+++	Hematogenous (respiratory)
Epstein-Barr virus	–	+	++	–	++	+	Hematogenous (respiratory)
Herpes simplex virus	++	+	+	++++	+++	+++	Hematogenous (respiratory)
Mycoplasmas							
Mycoplasma pneumoniae	–	+	++++	–	++	+	Respiratory
Mycoplasma hominis	?	–	–	?	–	–	Respiratory
Ureaplasma urealyticum	?	–	–	?	–	–	Respiratory
Chlamydiae							
Chlamydia pneumoniae	–	+	+++	–	+	+	Respiratory
Chlamydia psittaci	+	+	+	–	++	++	Respiratory
Chlamydia trachomatis	++++	–	–	++	–	–	Respiratory
Rickettsiae							
Coxiella burnetii	–	+	+	–	++	++	Respiratory (hematogenous)
Protozoa							
Pneumocystis jiroveci	+	++	+	+++	+++	+++	Respiratory

*++++, most frequent; +++, frequent; ++, infrequent; +, rare; –, no reported cases; ?, uncertain.
†++++, often fatal; +++, severe; ++, usually hospitalized; +, home management; –, no reported cases; ?, uncertain.
‡Types 1, 2, 3, 4, 5, 7, 14, and 21.
§Ninety or more types known.
¶Coxsackieviruses A9, A16, B1, B4, and B5; echoviruses 9, 11, 19, 30, and 22.
¶Human coronaviruses.
Data from references 5, 7, 17, 23, 26, 35, 76, 106, 108, 119, 174, 191, 225, and 240.

formed, the contribution of HBoV to the overall epidemiology of pediatric pneumonia remains uncertain. It has been identified in serum and feces, as well as in respiratory specimens[73] and was found to be a relatively common (19%) finding in a Finnish study of children with asthma exacerbations.[2]

Pneumonia is the most frequent serious complication of measles. Kohn and Koiransky[137] demonstrated, by careful radiographic study, that 55 percent of patients with routine measles cases had pulmonary infiltrates early in the illness, a finding suggesting a viral rather than a bacterial cause. Secondary bacterial pneumonia in measles is caused by common respiratory pathogens: *S. pneumoniae*, *H. influenzae*, *Streptococcus pyogenes*, and *Staphylococcus aureus*. Progressive, fatal, primary measles pneumonia (Hecht giant-cell pneumonia) occurs in immunocompromised patients, particularly those with hematologic malignancy or infection with human immunodeficiency virus type 1 (HIV-1).[138,159,228,229] The typical measles rash often is absent. In some persons immunized with killed measles virus vaccine during the 1960s, unusual nodular pneumonia, along with vasculitis of the distal extremities, developed after infection with wild measles virus. Although no longer seen, atypical measles remains important because its pathogenetic mechanism has implications for the development of new vaccines.[74]

Viruses that may attack the lungs by hematogenous spread include varicella-zoster virus (VZV), Epstein-Barr virus (EBV), rubella virus, cytomegalovirus (CMV), herpes simplex virus (HSV), and HIV. Rubella virus, CMV, and HSV may cause interstitial pneumonia in congenitally or perinatally infected infants.[10,106,255,261] CMV and VZV are causes of life-threatening pneumonia in immunocompromised hosts[120,203,252] Pneumonia has been noted in association with primary EBV infections.[8,62] Pulmonary infiltration also is a component of the fatal X-linked lymphoproliferative syndrome caused by EBV.[211] One of the characteristic features of HIV infection in children is lymphocytic interstitial pneumonitis, an indolent but progressive process that occurs in approximately one fourth of children in whom acquired immunodeficiency syndrome (AIDS) develops.[221] Both HIV RNA and EBV DNA have been demonstrated in the lung tissue of affected children.[6] The relative contributions of the two agents to the pathogenesis of lymphocytic interstitial pneumonitis are not understood clearly, although EBV is suspected to be the trigger.[131]

Of the 15 known *Mycoplasma* spp. that infect humans, only *M. pneumoniae* is a well-established cause of pneumonia. In children younger than 2 years of age, infection is a common occurrence, but pneumonia is unusual. In children older than 5 years of age, *M. pneumoniae* is the most common cause of nonbacterial pneumonia.[44,71] Studies have associated genital mycoplasmas, in particular *Ureaplasma urealyticum* and *Mycoplasma hominis*, with congenitally and perinatally acquired pneumonia.[32,107]

Three *Chlamydia* spp. have been associated with pneumonia. *C. psittaci* is the well-recognized cause of psittacosis (ornithosis). *Chlamydia trachomatis*, the established agent of inclusion blennorrhea in neonates, causes a characteristic afebrile pneumonitis syndrome in infants aged 4 to 14 weeks.[17] In urban areas in the United States where the condition first was studied carefully (Chicago, Seattle, San Francisco, and Birmingham, Alabama), it was the most frequent cause of pneumonia in that age group.[57,109] With widespread screening and treatment of pregnant women for *Chlamydia*, the incidence of this condition appears to be decreasing. *Chlamydia pneumoniae* was isolated first in 1965 and was recognized as a cause of pneumonia in 1986.[91] It now is considered to be the second most frequent cause of pneumonia in older children and young adults.[92,223]

Of the rickettsiae, only *C. burnetii* is associated with pneumonia, in the form of Q fever. This infection may be severe, but because of its restricted zoonotic niche in domestic farm animals, it is a rare occurrence in children.

P. jiroveci, a protozoan parasite, is an important cause of pneumonia in compromised hosts,[120,203,252] although its incidence in children receiving chemotherapeutic regimens for malignancy has been reduced dramatically with the use of trimethoprim-sulfamethoxazole (TMP-SMX) prophylaxis.[119] *P. jiroveci* is an established cause of pneumonia in premature and debilitated infants,[77] and, with *C. trachomatis*, CMV, and genital mycoplasmas, it has been associated with the afebrile pneumonitis syndrome of infancy.[57,201,237,238] *P. jiroveci* is the most frequent cause of death in infants with HIV infection, although the incidence is reduced markedly in U.S. populations as a result of early diagnosis and treatment of perinatal HIV infection and by the institution of chemoprophylaxis with TMP-SMX.[216,231]

EPIDEMIOLOGY

The major contributors to the overall epidemiology of nonbacterial pneumonia in children are RSV, parainfluenza viruses, *M. pneumoniae*, and, to a lesser extent, influenza viruses A and B.[53] Because of their brief incubation periods and high degree of communicability, these agents often spread through communities in well-defined waves[83,85] (Fig. 26–1). During intervals between epidemics, RSV, parainfluenza viruses types 1 and 2, and influenza viruses A and B rarely are isolated. Between peaks, *M. pneumoniae* and parainfluenza virus type 3 tend to persist endemically. During seasons of respiratory disease in the colder months, an interference phenomenon has been noted whereby peaks of infection by particular agents seldom occur simultaneously[83] (Fig. 26–2).

Annual incidence rates of childhood pneumonia show a rough inverse correlation with age. These rates range from

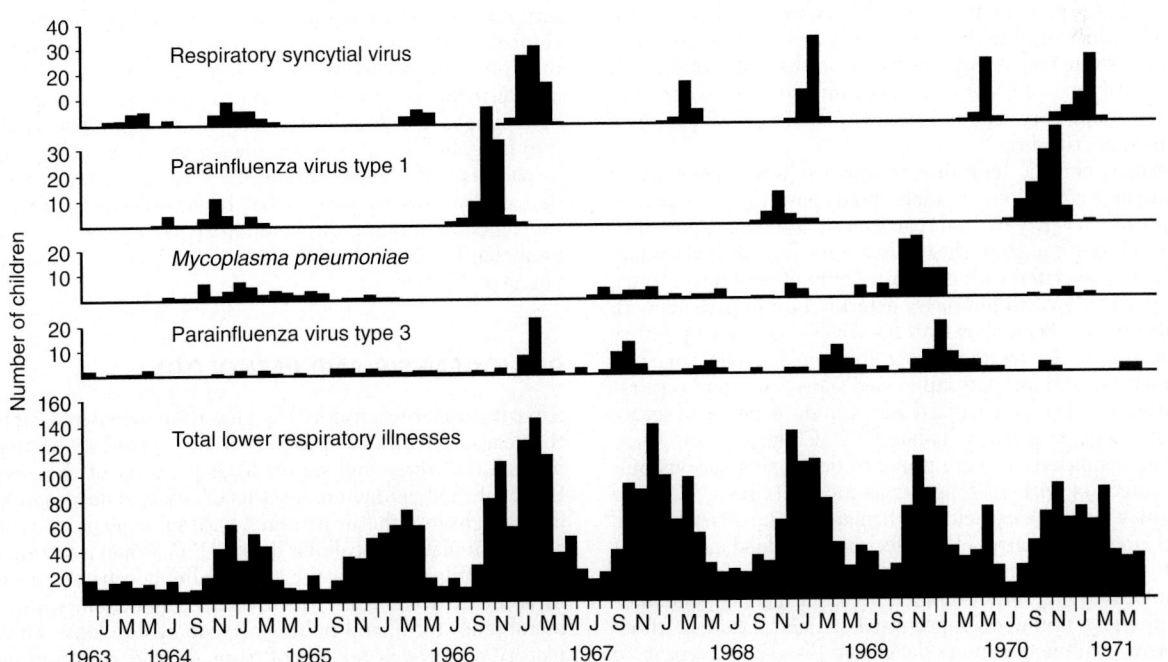

Figure 26-1 Number of isolations, according to month, of four major respiratory pathogens from children with lower respiratory illnesses in Chapel Hill, North Carolina. (*From Glezen, W. P., and Denny, F. W.: Epidemiology of acute lower respiratory disease in children. N. Engl. J. Med. 288:500, 1973. Reprinted with permission from the New England Journal of Medicine.*)

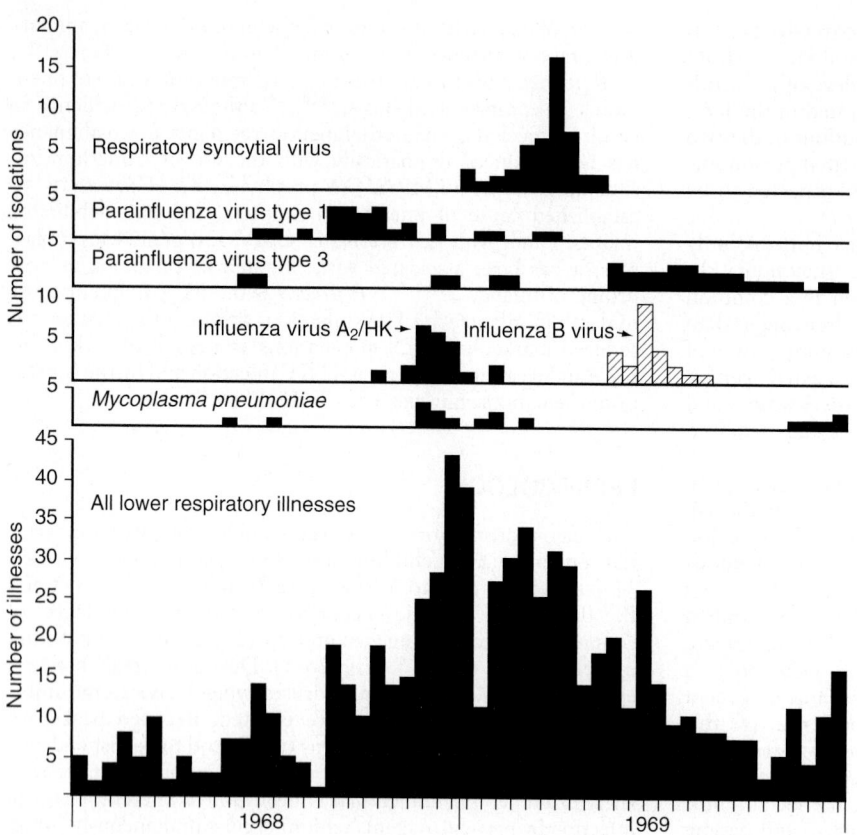

Figure 26-2 Weekly isolations, in 1968 and 1969, of respiratory pathogens from children with lower respiratory illnesses in Chapel Hill, North Carolina. *(From Glezen, W. P., and Denny, F. W.: Epidemiology of acute lower respiratory disease in children. N. Engl. J. Med. 288:500, 1973. Reprinted with permission from the New England Journal of Medicine.)*

40 per 1000 in children younger than 5 years of age to 7 per 1000 in adolescents aged 12 to 15 years.[71,183] RSV is the most common etiologic agent in children younger than 5 years of age; in those older than 5 years, *M. pneumoniae* is the most common.[71] Most studies have shown a male preponderance in pediatric lower respiratory infections on the order of 1.25 : 1. The increased rates of lower respiratory infection in lower socioeconomic groups correlate best with family size, a reflection of environmental crowding.[83]

Pregnancy, chronic lung disease, valvular heart disease, and neuromuscular conditions in adults predispose them to experiencing greater severity of viral, particularly influenzal, pneumonia.[154] In children, congenital heart disease and bronchopulmonary dysplasia are associated with greater severity of viral pneumonia, especially with RSV.[156] Pulmonary deterioration in patients with cystic fibrosis has been shown to be accelerated by respiratory viral infection.[249] In treated hematologic malignancy, marrow transplantation, and immunosuppressed states, common respiratory viruses have been recognized increasingly as causes of severe pneumonia and respiratory failure.[104,108] Children with these underlying conditions also are prone to developing serious pulmonary infection with such agents as measles virus, VZV, and CMV, which have the capacity for hematogenous dissemination and viral latency. Pediatric HIV infection has added a new category of immunocompromised children susceptible to these pathogens, as well as to the common bacterial agents of pneumonia. Profoundly immunocompromised patients, such as those with severe combined immunodeficiency disease, are prone to acquiring progressive and prolonged pulmonary disease caused by common respiratory viruses.[125]

Transmission of the more common agents of lower respiratory tract disease most often occurs by means of droplet spread from relatively close contact with a source case. Direct inoculation at the alveolar level probably does not occur in most cases because of the extremely small size of aerosolized particles necessary for such transmission to be accomplished. Studies of nosocomially transmitted RSV infection have shown the importance of adults with relatively trivial upper respiratory tract infection as intermediates in transmission to susceptible young infants.[100] School-aged children often introduce respiratory viral agents into households and thus are the source of secondary infections in parents and younger siblings.[83] The increasing use of group daycare by working parents has been associated with enhanced transmission of numerous respiratory pathogens,[151,210] and it certainly has extended the definition of "school age" to increasingly younger children.

PATHOGENESIS AND PATHOLOGY

After the upper respiratory tract has been inoculated, viral agents that cause pneumonia proliferate and spread by contiguity to involve the lower and more distal portions of the respiratory tract. Infected epithelium loses its ciliary appendages, rounds up, and sloughs into the air passages, with subsequent stasis of mucus and accumulation of cellular debris.[1,31,262] When infection extends to the terminal airways, the alveolar lining cells lose their structural integrity. As a result, surfactant production is lost, hyaline membranes form, and pulmonary edema develops. The inflammatory response at the site of tissue damage results in mononuclear infiltration of submucosal and interstitial structures, which further contributes to narrowing of air passages and alveolocapillary block of gas exchange. Relative expiratory obstruction gives rise to hyperinflation and air trapping. Complete obstruction or stop-valve mechanisms result in atelectasis. Ventilation-perfusion mismatch further exacerbates the hypoxia.

The relative rarity of fatal outcomes in patients with the common causes of nonbacterial pneumonia has resulted in a narrow view of the characteristic pathologic features, limited largely to autopsy studies of overwhelming illness in infants and military recruits. The pathology associated with infection by RSV, adenoviruses, and influenza virus A has been studied most extensively in humans. Studies of the pathology of RSV, parainfluenza virus, and *Mycoplasma* infection have been aided by animal model systems such as mice,[90] the Syrian hamster,[84] and the cotton rat.[95]

Five major pathologic findings have been described in fatal human infections, any or all of which may be present in a given case: acute bronchiolitis, necrotizing bronchiolitis, interstitial pneumonia, alveolar pneumonia, and diffuse alveolar damage. Acute bronchiolitis is characterized by relatively superficial and reversible destruction of ciliated respiratory epithelium, along with accompanying mononuclear infiltration. Necrotizing bronchiolitis extends to the deeper submucosal layers lining the respiratory tract and may not be as readily reversible. It is associated particularly with adenoviral pneumonia.[16] Interstitial pneumonia is a diffuse process in which the inflammatory mononuclear response predominantly involves the peribronchial alveolar septa. In alveolar pneumonia, the alveoli are filled with degenerating lining cells and mononuclear or polymorphonuclear inflammatory cells with or without hyaline membranes. Hyaline membranes consist of fibrin deposits triggered by local release of tissue factor–factor VII complexes, as well as inhibitors of fibrinolysis.[21] When hyaline membranes are present, the process is described as *diffuse alveolar damage*. It is the histopathologic hallmark of the acute phase of the adult respiratory distress syndrome.[219,220] Acute bronchiolitis and interstitial pneumonia are observed in most cases of fatal nonbacterial pneumonia, regardless of cause.[1] Alveolar pneumonia may reflect bacterial superinfection, adult respiratory distress syndrome, or agonal changes associated with intensive ventilator support and oxygen toxicity.

Three important factors that influence the pathologic expression of nonbacterial pneumonia in children are anatomy, preexisting pulmonary disease, and immunity. In young infants, the small caliber of the terminal airways and the absence of interconnections between alveolar spaces (pores of Kohn) contribute to the development of wheezing and lobular atelectasis.[182,254] Preexisting pulmonary disease (e.g., bronchopulmonary dysplasia) is characterized by emphysema, squamous metaplasia of the tracheobronchial tree, hypertrophied goblet cells, and enhanced airway smooth muscle reactivity. An inability to clear the excessive secretions triggered by infection in patients with bronchopulmonary dysplasia often leads to bronchospasm, atelectasis, and respiratory failure.

Immunopathologic mechanisms have been invoked to explain the disparity between infants and older children in the clinical expression of infection by RSV and *M. pneumoniae*.[36,169] Investigators have widely accepted that both viral replication and inappropriately enhanced immune responses contribute to the severity of RSV disease in infants. In a recent study, however, quantities of lymphocyte-derived cytokines were unexpectedly minimal in respiratory secretions, and CD8-positive lymphocytes and natural killer cells were nearly absent in autopsy lung tissue. Thus, it now appears that the severity of RSV in infants relates to inadequate (rather than excessive) adaptive immune responses to robust viral replication and apoptosis of respiratory epithelium.[250] In contrast, cumulative immunity that develops after repeated natural infections with *M. pneumoniae* may account for the more impressive clinical expression of illness in older children and adults.[66] Specific cell-mediated immunity, detectable at low levels in young children but increased in adults, probably contributes to the pathogenesis.

Opportunistic nonbacterial pathogens generally take advantage of the defects in cell-mediated immunity induced by immunosuppressive therapy or HIV infection. Various unique pathologic manifestations of viral pneumonia, including giant-cell pneumonia (leukemia or HIV infection with superimposed measles),[159,228,229] lymphoid interstitial pneumonitis or pulmonary lymphoid hyperplasia (HIV with associated EBV infection),[6,221] and graft-versus-host disease (bone marrow allograft with associated CMV infection), may ensue in these circumstances.[60,241,252]

CLINICAL MANIFESTATIONS

Acute nonbacterial pneumonia in infants and young children generally occurs after 1 or 2 days of coryza, decreased appetite, and low-grade fever. The onset usually is gradual, with increasing fretfulness, respiratory congestion, vomiting, cough, and fever. In very young infants, fever may be minimal, and apneic spells may be the most prominent (and frightening) initial complaint.[29] The most reliable physical findings are those of respiratory distress: tachypnea (respiratory rate =50/min[41]), tachycardia, nasal flaring, and retractions, but without the stridor characteristic of upper airway obstruction. In patients with atelectasis or air trapping, grunting may be present. Cyanosis generally accompanies the apneic spells or coughing attacks, but it may be present at rest in patients with advanced disease or in those with underlying chronic cardiopulmonary conditions.

Other physical findings are quite variable and, in fact, may be normal. Wheezing occurs in infants with associated bronchiolitis or bronchospasm. Hyperresonance may be noted if air trapping is present. Diminished local percussion or breath sounds may indicate lobar consolidation or atelectasis. In interstitial pneumonia, fine crackling rales may be present diffusely or locally. Also important in initial assessment is an evaluation of the young child's state of hydration because increased insensible loss from fever and hyperventilation, coupled with anorexia, can result in significant deficits in fluid.

The afebrile pneumonitis syndrome of young infants, in contrast to the usual acute viral pneumonias affecting this age group, is subacute to chronic in its development and is nonseasonal. Characteristic features include the absence of fever, a "staccato" cough pattern (individual coughs separated by inspirations), and diffuse rales on auscultation.[17] Radiographic findings usually consist of interstitial infiltrates with subsegmental atelectasis. Hypergammaglobulinemia and mild eosinophilia are abnormalities frequently detected in the laboratory.

Most infants with HIV/AIDS and *P. jiroveci* pneumonia have a progressive febrile course leading to respiratory failure over the course of 1 to 3 weeks. Typical upper respiratory symptoms may be absent, and these infants fail to respond to conventional antibiotic therapy. When pneumonia actually is detected by chest radiography, the severity of involvement may not be appreciated because abnormalities often are subtle early in the course. However, even with mild radiographic abnormalities, hypoxia may be obvious and severe. Frequently, the discovery of HIV seropositivity first raises this diagnostic possibility. An important observation is that *P. jiroveci* pneumonia may develop in infants with HIV/AIDS who have CD4 lymphocyte counts in the "normal" range.[231]

Nonbacterial pneumonia in older children and adolescents clinically is more nearly like the pattern seen in adults. Premonitory complaints generally include such systemic symptoms as malaise, myalgia, and anorexia, in addition to upper respiratory symptoms. "Chilliness" may occur, but rigors generally are absent. Cough usually is irritative and nonproductive. A temperature higher than 39° C (102.2° F) is unusual. Although tachypnea, flaring, and retractions typically are present, they may be less apparent than in an infant or young child. Findings on examination of the chest are more reliable than in infancy and may include local percussion dullness or diminished breath sounds and local or diffuse fine rales. Because apnea rarely occurs in older patients, cyanosis is an ominous sign of advanced disease and respiratory failure. Progression to acute respiratory failure occurred in a disturbingly high proportion of patients with SARS.[143,207] Although mild dehydration often is present, generally it is not evident on examination. Nonspecific rash suggests a viral or mycoplasmal cause.[43]

Radiologic findings in nonbacterial pneumonia are variable and depend on the child's age and the infecting agent.[49,50,160,163,192,217,232] In infants and young children, bilateral air trapping and perihilar infiltrates are the most frequent findings. Patchy areas of consolidation may represent lobular atelectasis or alveolar pneumonia. In older children and adolescents, lobar involvement more frequently is definable, but typically the affected areas are not consolidated completely. Although lobar consolidation may occur in nonbacterial pneumonia, this finding should be distinguished from atelectasis and is more consistent with a bacterial origin. Similarly, although small pleural effusions may be detected on decubitus films in patients with nonbacterial pneumonia,[67] effusions are much more suggestive of a bacterial cause.

Peripheral leukocyte counts are quite variable in nonbacterial pneumonia.[71,187,206] Leukocytosis occurs most frequently in children with influenza and parainfluenza pneumonia,[71] but high counts are more consistent with a bacterial origin.[71,164] Gram staining of sputum or tracheal secretions from patients with nonbacterial pneumonia tends to show epithelial cells as the predominant cell type, with a mixed bacterial population representing the patient's pharyngeal flora. A predominance of neutrophils may be seen, but this finding generally reflects bacterial superinfection or preexisting chronic pulmonary disease.

DIFFERENTIAL DIAGNOSIS

In the differential diagnosis of nonbacterial pneumonia, the following factors need to be considered: status of the host, whether normal or compromised; the environment, whether animate (human and other animal exposure) or inanimate; the age of the patient; and, finally, the season. In certain epidemiologic settings, the diagnosis of nonbacterial pneumonia may be made with relative certainty. Often, however, this category of pulmonary infection is a diagnosis of exclusion. The major conditions to be differentiated include the following: noninfectious pulmonary disease; bacterial pneumonia amenable to conventional antibiotics; and the more unusual bacterial, fungal, or parasitic infections that may require specialized forms of therapy.

Noninfectious conditions that may simulate nonbacterial pneumonia are summarized in Table 26–2. These conditions are particularly relevant to consider in a child with persistent or recurrent pulmonary disease. The line of demarcation between infectious and noninfectious conditions may be blurred. In a child with sickle-cell anemia, for example, pulmonary vascular occlusive crisis is manifested as fever, leukocytosis, and patchy pulmonary infiltrates (the acute chest syndrome).[13,205] Differentiating it from pneumococcal, *Haemophilus*, or mycoplasmal pneumonia, to which a child with sickle-cell anemia has increased susceptibility, may be difficult or impossible. Early recognition of noninfectious conditions either mimicking or underlying pneumonia may prevent recurrence or improve the prognosis. Aspiration resulting from gastroesophageal reflux, for example, is a relatively common correctable cause of recurrent diffuse pneumonia.[45] Early recognition of and initiation of treatment for cystic fibrosis as an underlying condition have clear beneficial effects in reducing irreversible pulmonary damage.[191]

Pneumonias caused by pyogenic bacteria are classically lobar in distribution and exhibit consolidation on radiographs. Atelectasis, conversely, is a common event in viral pneumonia and must be distinguished from true consolidation. Pleural effusions, circular infiltrates, consolidations with convex margins, and pneumatoceles all favor a bacterial cause. In a young child, high fever with significant leukocytosis also suggests a bacterial origin.[166] In contrast to patients with lower counts, children with pneumonia who had leukocyte counts greater than 15,000/mm^3 were found to have a high probability of rapid defervescence with antimicrobial therapy in one emergency department study, presumably on the basis of a bacterial origin.[164]

Other laboratory investigations, such as erythrocyte sedimentation rate, C-reactive protein, and reduction of nitroblue tetrazolium by leukocytes, frequently are positive in children with bacterial respiratory infection.[63,162,189] However, these tests add little to careful initial clinical examination, roentgenographic findings, a differential white count, and, if accessible, Gram stain and culture of tracheal secretions in excluding a bacterial cause.[164] Specific detection techniques for bacterial antigens, used with urine or respiratory secretions, occasionally are helpful. However,

---

TABLE 26–2   Noninfectious Conditions That May Simulate Nonbacterial Pneumonia in Children

Technical	Damage by Physical Agents	Collagen Disease (SLE, JRA)
Poor inspiratory film	Lipoid pneumonia	Sarcoidosis
Underpenetrated film	Kerosene pneumonia	Neoplasm
Physiologic	Near drowning	Histiocytosis X
Prominent thymus	Smoke inhalation	Bronchogenic cyst
Breast shadows	Iatrogenic pulmonary damage	Vascular ring
Chronic pulmonary disease	Drugs (bleomycin, nitrofurantoin)	Pulmonary sequestration
Asthma	Radiation pneumonitis	Cystic adenomatoid malformation
Bronchiectasis	Graft-versus-host disease	Congenital lobar emphysema
Bronchopulmonary dysplasia	Atelectasis	Alpha$_1$-antitrypsin deficiency
Pulmonary fibrosis	Mucus plug	Allergic alveolitis
Cystic fibrosis	Foreign body	Dust (farmer's lung)
Recurrent aspiration	Congestive heart failure	Mold (allergic aspergillosis)
Gastroesophageal reflux	Pulmonary infarction	Excreta (pigeon breeder's lung)
Tracheoesophageal fistula	Sickle vaso-occlusive crisis	Pulmonary hemosiderosis
Cleft palate	Fat embolism	Desquamative interstitial pneumonitis
Neuromuscular disorders	Pleural effusion	Adult respiratory distress syndrome
Familial dysautonomia	Pleural reaction	

JRA, juvenile rheumatoid arthritis; SLE, systemic lupus erythematosus.

false-negative results occur frequently. Because a bacterial cause cannot be excluded with certainty, these tests seldom are used in clinical laboratories.[122,222]

Positive cultures of blood, pleural fluid, or lung aspirates provide definite evidence of the origin of bacterial pneumonia. Because of the common asymptomatic carriage of potential pulmonary pathogens in children, however, the diagnostic value of upper respiratory tract and tracheal bacterial cultures is debated.[14,86,150] In a child with a suspected nonbacterial pneumonia, the finding of "normal flora" in endotracheal secretions generally is reassuring but may reflect aspiration. In a child who is not doing well, a predominant pathogen in such cultures can be helpful in selecting or altering antimicrobial therapy.[22,42]

Among the less common causes of pneumonia, tuberculosis should never be forgotten. Tuberculin testing should be considered in the initial evaluation and is especially important in children residing in urban areas, in recent immigrants, and in Native Americans. Fungal pneumonia, particularly coccidioidomycosis, histoplasmosis, and blastomycosis, should be considered in children residing in or visiting endemic areas. Often a suggestive history, such as exposure to excavations (backyard swimming pools, geologic or archaeologic "digs"), clean-up chores in old sheds and barns, and exposure to dust storms, may be elicited. Erythema nodosum and eosinophilia are common clinical clues to these entities. Immunodiffusion serologic testing, urine antigen detection, biopsy of skin lesions, and bronchoscopy often are required for establishing the diagnosis. Other fungal pneumonias, such as aspergillosis and cryptococcosis, occur in the setting of immunosuppression. These conditions, coupled with the possibility of *Pneumocystis*, fungal, resistant bacterial, and CMV pneumonia, warrant the use of bronchoalveolar lavage or open lung biopsy as a definitive approach to diagnosis in compromised hosts.[72,255] In an appropriate epidemiologic setting, progressive or recurrent pneumonia should prompt obtaining serologic testing for HIV. At present, pulmonary disease is the most common defining condition in pediatric AIDS.[221] Pulmonary paragonimiasis caused by the lung fluke *Paragonimus westermani* has been recognized as a cause of chronic pneumonia in Indochinese immigrants in the United States.[30]

SPECIFIC DIAGNOSIS

Isolation of virus can be performed in most major medical centers and public health laboratories. With the possible exception of HSV and adenoviruses, respiratory viruses rarely are carried asymptomatically. Thus, identification of an agent in upper respiratory secretions is strong evidence for its causative role in pneumonia. Conventional virologic techniques provide the most sensitive and specific means of identification (see Chapter 264). However, most of the common respiratory viral pathogens, as well as chlamydiae and mycoplasmas, now are identified readily by "rapid" techniques. The available methods and reagents are expanding rapidly and include fluorescent antibody techniques, enzyme-linked immunosorbent assay, direct DNA probes, and PCR.[40,59,78,148,177] Clinical specimens may be tested directly or after pre-incubation in tissue culture systems. In an individual case, serologic diagnosis of acute respiratory viral infection is, in general, less satisfactory than is virologic diagnosis. The difficulty with serology relates to timing of specimens, choice of antigens to test, and variation in the quality and specificity of available reagents.

In contrast, laboratory facilities for the actual isolation of chlamydiae, mycoplasmas, and rickettsiae are less readily available to the clinician. Thus, serologic techniques are important means for establishing a specific diagnosis. Acute-phase reactants (e.g., cold agglutinins in *M. pneumoniae* infection) are of greatest diagnostic help during acute illness but are not invariably present.

Serologic tests also can be helpful in diagnosing chlamydial pneumonitis in infants; high levels of immunoglobulin G–specific antibodies are found uniformly at initial evaluation.[17] *Pneumocystis* infection usually is diagnosed by visualizing organisms in specimens obtained by bronchoalveolar lavage during bronchoscopy or by open lung biopsy. Silver impregnation and direct immunofluorescence staining techniques have the greatest sensitivity. Noninvasive diagnosis by serologic and molecular biologic techniques has not proven to be effective.[147,200,238]

Because of the epidemiologic behavior of nonbacterial respiratory infections, a reasonable guess regarding the specific cause often can be based on such factors as age, season, and associated clinical features. If the presence of a particular nonbacterial agent in a community can be established by isolation or serologic means, however, the probability that other patients with similar manifestations will have illness caused by that agent is increased greatly. Regional viral surveillance programs, such as those performed in Rochester, New York,[99] and Houston,[82] can be particularly helpful to practicing pediatricians in this regard.

TREATMENT

Therapy for nonbacterial pneumonia primarily is expectant and supportive. However, specific therapies are available for some of these conditions. Rapid etiologic diagnosis permits appropriate use of these therapies, particularly for hospitalized patients and compromised hosts. Although these treatments shorten the course of illness, they frequently have a less dramatic therapeutic effect than do specific antibiotic therapies for bacterial infections.

The course of uncomplicated viral pneumonia is not influenced by the administration of antibiotics. However, in most cases in which pulmonary involvement is uncovered, antibiotic therapy is administered because bacterial disease cannot be ruled out with certainty, and combined viral-bacterial infection is a common occurrence.[127] In all but the most mild cases, this approach is both reasonable and practical. Of importance, however, is that antibiotic therapy in routine cases be appropriate for the most common bacterial pathogens (*S. pneumoniae* and *H. influenzae*). The increasing prevalence of penicillin-resistant pneumococci now renders treatment with ceftriaxone or cefotaxime a reasonable choice. Concomitant treatment with a macrolide drug such as erythromycin or azithromycin should be considered in children younger than 3 months and older than 6 years because of the high prevalence of chlamydial and mycoplasmal causes.[124,167] In immunocompromised hosts or when secondary infection is a possibility, *S. aureus* (including methicillin-resistant strains) and other hospital-associated and opportunistic pathogens must be considered.[154]

In fulminant viral pneumonia caused by VZV in a compromised host, specific antiviral chemotherapy with acyclovir may be lifesaving, but as many as 50 percent of patients with this condition have complicating bacterial sepsis that requires antibiotic therapy as well.[64] Treatment with zanamivir or oseltamivir should be considered in children with viral pneumonia in the context of a community epidemic of influenza. Treatment of lymphocytic interstitial pneumonia in pediatric patients with AIDS includes antiretroviral therapy with prednisone pulses for increasing hypoxia.[170] Progressive CMV interstitial pneumonia in bone marrow or solid organ transplant recipients is treated best with ganciclovir and intravenous immunoglobulin, ideally with high-titer antibody activity.[60]

TMP-SMX and pentamidine are equally effective for treating *P. jiroveci* pneumonitis, but the former combination is the drug regimen of choice because of its lower toxicity. TMP-SMX may be given orally (20 mg/kg/day of the TMP component divided every 6 hours) or intravenously (15 mg/kg/day divided every 8 hours). Pentamidine should be reserved for patients who are intolerant of TMP-SMX. Atovaquone is a third therapeutic option, pending more complete information on its pharmacokinetic profile in pediatrics. Completion of a course of therapy with any agent should be followed by direct transition to long-term chemoprophylaxis.

Inhalational administration of the antiviral compound ribavirin has been used successfully to treat viral pneumonia caused by RSV and influenza.[80,103,136] Anecdotal experience and in vitro activity suggest that it also may be beneficial in parainfluenza and measles virus infection.[11] Early studies indicated that ribavirin was of particular value for the treatment of RSV infection in nonventilated infants with underlying cardiopulmonary disease,[102] as well as in previously normal infants with RSV pneumonia and respiratory failure.[233] However, several multicenter re-evaluations of the use of ribavirin therapy for RSV-infected infants with and without respiratory failure yielded equivocal results.[142,172,178,251] These observations, coupled with the high cost of the drug,[65] concerns about its possible teratogenicity in medical personnel,[5] and the complexity of its administration during mechanical ventilation,[51] led to reassessment of its use and a change in American Academy of Pediatrics recommendations from "should be used"[5] to "may be considered."[213]

Bronchospasm is present in a substantial proportion of nonbacterial pneumonias. Airway reactivity may be preexisting, or it may arise as part of the pathogenesis of the pneumonia itself. In most hospitals, intervention with inhaled bronchodilators has become part of the routine management of any patient with wheezing, regardless of age or mechanism. Rigorous pulmonary function studies have shown that only approximately 50 percent of previously normal infants with RSV-associated respiratory failure respond to inhaled albuterol.[105] However, in several double-blind controlled trials, inhaled albuterol and racemic epinephrine both showed a statistically significant overall benefit.[173,214,224,227] Other studies of the use of albuterol and ipratropium in mildly ill infants were less convincing.[75,248] None of the available studies of ribavirin therapy for RSV bronchiolitis and pneumonia controlled for the effects of concomitant inhaled bronchodilator therapy.

The use of systemic corticosteroids in nonbacterial pneumonia should be approached with caution. In patients with preexisting asthma or bronchopulmonary dysplasia and acute deterioration triggered by pneumonia, steroids are a noncontroversial element of treatment. In adult patients with AIDS and rapidly progressive *P. jiroveci* pneumonia, short-course steroid therapy clearly is beneficial.[23,76] Comparable data do not exist for pediatric patients with HIV/AIDS. In infants and children without preexisting lung disease, steroid therapy for viral bronchiolitis with or without concomitant pneumonia has shown neither consistent benefit nor harm.[144,236] The value of steroids probably strikes a balance between their anti-inflammatory effects in short-term use and their immunosuppressive effects with more prolonged administration.

Other key elements of supportive therapy include the following: maintenance of adequate hydration, high humidity, and oxygenation and ventilation; mobilization of lower respiratory secretions; and, particularly in young infants, continuous monitoring of respiration. Because of increased insensible loss caused by fever, hyperventilation, and anorexia, mild dehydration frequently is observed initially, and continuing fluid loss is expected during the acute phase of illness. Thus, restoration of deficits and adequate maintenance of fluid intake are desirable. Maintaining nutrition often is difficult when respiratory distress is present; oral feeding is limited or contraindicated. Parenteral nutrition through peripheral veins is adequate during acute self-limited pneumonia. Situations involving more prolonged hospitalization or mechanical ventilation should lead to early consideration of central alimentation.

Mist tents have fallen into disuse because they hinder observation and because mist has little direct therapeutic benefit.[195] However, high humidity is required to prevent the drying effects of supplemental oxygen therapy; slowing evaporation probably also serves to reduce the viscosity of mucous secretions and the magnitude of insensible fluid loss. Mobilization of respiratory secretions by means of vibration and postural drainage is indicated in nonbacterial pneumonias complicated by atelectasis,[153] but it is not helpful in the absence of excessive secretions or mucus plugging.[184] Progression of infiltrates and hypoxia occasionally occurs secondary to pulmonary edema. If it is recognized, diuretic therapy may be beneficial.

Because of the presence of ventilation-perfusion abnormalities and alveolocapillary block, most children with nonbacterial pneumonia have some degree of hypoxemia. In a child with respiratory distress, provision of supplemental oxygen reduces anxiety and ventilation rates. Increases in inspired oxygen to approximately 30 percent are provided easily by nasal cannulas, which are the most convenient means of administration. More severe respiratory distress or cyanosis requires documentation of respiratory status by means of arterial blood gas determination and more exact regulation of inspired oxygen administered by mask or hood. Noninvasive monitoring by means of oximetry can reduce the need for frequent blood gas sampling and arterial lines.[101] Consistent oxygen saturations of 95 percent or more should be the target. In respiratory failure, mechanical ventilation may be required to maintain oxygenation and to control retention of carbon dioxide.[55,161,243] In this instance, management in an intensive care unit setting, with invasive monitoring of gas exchange, is mandated.

Apnea and bradycardia occur commonly in young infants with RSV, parainfluenza, and influenza viral pneumonia.[29,46] These complications are particularly frequent in infants with a history of premature birth. Although the mechanism for these episodes is uncertain, continuous cardiorespiratory monitoring of any young infant with viral pneumonia is prudent.

Acetaminophen or ibuprofen should be used to control high fever and will benefit the patient in terms of comfort as well as reduction in oxygen and nutritional requirements. Expectorants, antihistamines, and cough suppressants, although widely prescribed for upper respiratory tract infections in children and adults, probably have no place in the management of acute nonbacterial pneumonia. In convalescence, persistent irritative coughing that interferes with sleep may be alleviated by the judicious use of antihistamines or dextromethorphan.[4]

PROGNOSIS

In the pre-antibiotic era, pneumonia (of which most cases were "bronchopneumonia") was the most frequent cause of death in children. At present, a fatal outcome rarely occurs but always is a possibility. It is most likely to occur in young infants or compromised hosts.

The incidence of long-term complications of nonbacterial pneumonia is unknown. However, these conditions probably play a role in the development of some cases of bronchiectasis, chronic pulmonary fibrosis, desquamative interstitial pneumonitis, bronchiolitis obliterans, and unilateral hyperlucent lung (Swyer-James syndrome). These complications are well-documented sequelae of measles and adenoviral and influenza viral pneumonia.[130,140,141,157] They occur most frequently today in children who have survived complex and prolonged hospitalization involving aggressive ventilator management of respiratory failure.[219,220]

At a minimum, children with pneumonia should be re-evaluated clinically 2 to 3 weeks after being diagnosed. Provided the child is asymptomatic, has returned to normal activities, and has a benign physical examination, a follow-up radiograph is not required.[94] Repeated chest radiographs are necessary for children with complicated clinical courses, underlying pulmonary disease, or previous episodes of pneumonia, or if signs or symptoms of respiratory difficulty persist at the time of follow-up. Approximately 20 percent of patients with even uncomplicated pneumonias will show persistent radiographic abnormalities 3 to 4 weeks after the diagnosis has been established, but a selective approach to follow-up films permits early recognition of atelectasis, unresolved infiltrates, or progressive disease.

PREVENTION

Nosocomial spread of respiratory viruses occurs readily in pediatric wards and involves intermediate carriage by medical personnel who have acquired mild upper respiratory tract infections.[98] A reasonable approach to interdicting nosocomial transmission is to group patients with pneumonia and to exclude from ward duties personnel with symptomatic respiratory illness. With the exception of measles, varicella, and SARS, mask or gown isolation has no effect on transmission. Contact precautions, washing hands, and wearing glasses or goggles will minimize the incidence of respiratory infections among personnel and secondary spread. Blood and secretion precautions (universal precautions) are recommended for all hospitalized patients.

Of the common viral causes of pneumonia, vaccines at present are available for only influenza A and B viruses. Annual influenza vaccination with "split-product" vaccines is now recommended for all children aged 6 to 59 months and for children of any age with chronic respiratory, cardiovascular, renal, hepatic, hematologic, or metabolic disorders; with HIV infection; or receiving long-term aspirin therapy. Immunization also is recommended for health care personnel and the household contacts and caregivers of children with predisposing medical conditions.[208] Adenoviral vaccines have been used widely in the military, but their manufacture was discontinued recently. Attenuated, inactivated, and subunit vaccines against RSV, parainfluenza virus type 3, and *M. pneumoniae* have received considerable investigative effort but have not yet proved to be effective.[121,128,181] They present problems in vaccine development because of the possibility of triggering immunopathologic phenomena that could potentiate rather than prevent illness.[169,250]

In compromised hosts, intramuscular passive immunization with pooled immunoglobulin or varicella-zoster immunoglobulin is an established postexposure measure to prevent the acquisition of measles and varicella pneumonia, respectively.[35] Palivizumab is a "humanized" mouse monoclonal antibody specific for the fusion protein of RSV and is administered intramuscularly.[259] It has replaced RSV-specific intravenous immunoglobulin as a means of preventing RSV lower respiratory tract infection in infants with prematurity or other high-risk conditions.[93,209] Other products, such as specific Fab immunoglobulin fragments produced by recombinant DNA technology, are being studied.[12]

P. jiroveci pneumonia can be prevented in pediatric patients with hematologic malignancy or HIV/AIDS by prophylactic administration of TMP-SMX. This medication has become a part of the routine management of these conditions and has reduced the incidence of *P. jiroveci* infection dramatically.[96,119,216] Unless HIV infection can be excluded reasonably by serial PCR studies, seropositive HIV-exposed infants should receive chemoprophylaxis from 4 to 6 weeks of age up to 12 months of age, regardless of their immune status. Infected children aged 1 to 5 years should continue to receive prophylaxis if their CD4 counts are less than 500 cells/μL or the CD4 percentage is less than 15. The criterion for prophylaxis in older children and adults is a

CD4 count less than 200 cells/μL or a percentage less than 15. The recommended dosage of TMP-SMX is 150 mg/m^2/day of TMP divided into two doses given on 3 successive days each week.[216]

Opportunistic CMV pneumonia, a major hazard in seronegative high-risk premature infants and recipients of allogeneic bone marrow transplants, can be prevented effectively by the exclusive use of CMV-free blood products.[260,261] In bone marrow transplant recipients who are seropositive and thus are at risk for reactivation of disease, prophylactic acyclovir, ganciclovir, and intravenous immunoglobulin have been shown to reduce rates of infection and interstitial pneumonia.[174,225,241]

REFERENCES

1. Aherne, W., Bird, T., Court, S. D. M., et al.: Pathological changes in virus infection of the lower respiratory tract in children. J. Clin. Pathol. 23:7-18, 1970.
2. Allander, T., Jartti, T., Gupta S., et al.: Human bocavirus and acute wheezing in children. Clin. Infect. Dis. 44:904-910, 2007.
3. Allander, T., Tammi, M. T., Eriksson, M., et al.: Cloning of a human parvovirus by molecular screening of respiratory tract samples. Proc. Natl. Acad. Sci. U. S. A. 102:12891-12896, 2005.
4. American Academy of Pediatrics Committee on Drugs: Use of codeine- and dextromethorphan-containing cough syrups in pediatrics. Pediatrics 62:118-122, 1978.
5. American Academy of Pediatrics Committee on Infectious Diseases: Use of ribavirin in the treatment of respiratory syncytial virus infection. Pediatrics 92:501-504, 1993.
6. Andiman, W. A., Eastman, R., Martin, K., et al.: Opportunistic lymphoproliferations associated with Epstein-Barr viral DNA in infants and children with AIDS. Lancet 2:1390-1393, 1985.
7. Andiman, W. A., Jacobson, R. I., and Tucker, G.: Leukocyte-associated viremia with adenovirus type 2 in an infant with lower-respiratory-tract disease. N. Engl. J. Med. 297:100-101, 1977.
8. Andiman, W. A., McCarthy, P., Markowitz, R. I., et al.: Clinical, virologic, and serologic evidence of Epstein-Barr virus infection in association with childhood pneumonia. J. Pediatr. 99:880-886, 1981.
9. Angella, J. J., and Connor, J. D.: Neonatal infection caused by adenovirus type 7. J. Pediatr. 72:474-478, 1968.
10. Ballard, R. A., Drew, W. L., Hufnagle, K. G., et al.: Acquired cytomegalovirus infection in preterm infants. Am. J. Dis. Child. 133:482-485, 1979.
11. Banks, G., and Fernandez, H.: Clinical use of ribavirin in measles: A summarized review. *In* Smith, R. A., Knight, V., and Smith, J. A. D. (eds.): Clinical Applications of Ribavirin. New York, Academic Press, 1984, pp. 203-209.
12. Barbas, C. F., Crowe, J. E., Cababa, D., et al.: Human monoclonal Fab fragments derived from a combinatorial library bind to respiratory syncytial virus F glycoprotein and neutralize infectivity. Proc. Natl. Acad. Sci. U. S. A. 89:10164-10168, 1992.
13. Barrett-Connor, E.: Acute pulmonary disease and sickle cell anemia. Am. Rev. Respir. Dis. 104:159, 1971.
14. Barrett-Connor, E.: The nonvalue of sputum culture in the diagnosis of pneumococcal pneumonia. Am. Rev. Respir. Dis. 103:845-848, 1971.
15. Bauer, C. R., Elie, K., Spene, L., et al.: Hong Kong influenza in a neonatal unit. J. Am. Med. Assoc. 223:1233-1235, 1973.
16. Becroft, D. M. O.: Histopathology of fatal adenovirus infection of the respiratory tract in young children. J. Clin. Pathol. 20:561-569, 1967.
17. Beem, M., and Saxon, E.: Respiratory-tract colonization and a distinctive pneumonia syndrome in infants infected with *Chlamydia trachomatis*. N. Engl. J. Med. 296:306-310, 1977.
18. Beem, M., Wright, F. H., Hamre, D., et al.: Association of the chimpanzee coryza agent with acute respiratory disease in children. N. Engl. J. Med. 263:523-530, 1960.
19. Benyesh-Melnick, M., and Rosenberg, H. S.: The isolation of adenovirus type 7 from a fetal case of pneumonia and disseminated disease. J. Pediatr. 64:83-87, 1964.
20. Berkovich, S., and Taranko, L.: Acute respiratory illness in the premature nursery associated with respiratory syncytial virus infections. Pediatrics 34:735-760, 1964.
21. Bertozzi, P., Astedt, B., Zenzius, L., et al.: Depressed bronchoalveolar urokinase activity in patients with adult respiratory distress syndrome. N. Engl. J. Med. 322:890-897, 1990.
22. Boyer, K. M., and Cherry, J. D.: Pneumonias in children. Curr. Top. Pediatr. 1:169-182, 1979.
23. Bozzette, S. A., Sattler, F. R., Chin, J., et al.: A controlled trial of early adjunctive treatment with corticosteroids for *Pneumocystis carinii* pneumonia in the acquired immunodeficiency syndrome. N. Engl. J. Med. 323:1451-1457, 1990.

24. Brandt, C. D., Kim, H. W., Arrobio, J. O., et al.: Epidemiology of respiratory syncytial virus infection in Washington, DC. III. Composite analysis of eleven consecutive yearly epidemics. Am. J. Epidemiol. *98*:355-364, 1973.
25. Brandt, C. D., Kim, H. W., Vargosko, A. J., et al.: Infections in 18,000 infants and children in a controlled study of respiratory tract disease. I. Adenovirus pathogenicity in relation to serologic type and illness syndrome. Am. J. Epidemiol. *90*:484-500, 1969.
26. Brocklebank, J. T., Court, S. D. M., McQuillin, J., et al.: Influenza-A infection in children. Lancet *2*:497-500, 1972.
27. Brodie, H. R., and Spencer, L. P.: Respiratory syncytial virus infections in children in Montreal: A retrospective study. Can. Med. Assoc. J. *109*:1199-1201, 1973.
28. Brown, R. S., Nogrady, M. B., Spence, L., et al.: An outbreak of adenovirus type 7 infection in children in Montreal. Can. Med. Assoc. J. *108*:434-439, 1973.
29. Bruhn, F. W., Mokrohisky, S. T., and McIntosh, K.: Apnea associated with respiratory syncytial virus infection in young infants. J. Pediatr. *40*:382-386, 1977.
30. Burton, K., Yogev, R., London, N., et al.: Pulmonary paragonimiasis in Laotian refugee children. Pediatrics *70*:246-248, 1982.
31. Carson, J. L., Collier, A. M., and Hu, S. S.: Acquired ciliary defects in nasal epithelium of children with acute viral upper respiratory infections. N. Engl. J. Med. *312*:463-468, 1985.
32. Cassell, G. H., Waites, K. B., Crouse, D. T., et al.: Association of *Ureaplasma urealyticum* infection of the lower respiratory tract with chronic lung disease and death in very-low-birthweight infants. Lancet *2*:240-245, 1988.
33. Centers for Disease Control and Prevention: Progress toward elimination of *Haemophilus influenzae* type b invasive disease among infants and children: United States, 1998-2000. M. M. W. R. Morb. Mortal. Wkly. Rep. *51*:234-236, 2002.
34. Centers for Disease Control and Prevention: Direct and indirect effects of routine vaccination of children with 7-valent pneumococcal conjugate vaccine on incidence of invasive pneumococcal disease: United States, 1998-2003. M. M. W. R. Morb. Mortal. Wkly. Rep. *54*:893-897, 2005.
35. Centers for Disease Control and Prevention: Prevention of varicella: Recommendations of the Advisory Committee on Immunization Practices (ACIP.) M. M. W. R. Morb. Mortal. Wkly. Rep. *56*:P-48, 2007.
36. Chanock, R. M., Kapikian, A. Z., Mills, J., et al.: Influence of immunological factors in respiratory syncytial virus disease. Arch. Environ. Health *21*:347-356, 1970.
37. Chanock, R. M., Mufson, M. A., and Johnson, K. M.: Comparative biology and ecology of human virus and mycoplasma respiratory pathogens. Prog. Med. Virol. 7:208-252, 1965.
38. Chanock, R. M., and Parrott, R. H.: Acute respiratory disease in infancy and childhood: Present understanding and prospects for prevention. Pediatrics *36*:21-39, 1965.
39. Chany, C., Lepine, P., Lelong, M., et al.: Severe and fatal pneumonia in infants and young children associated with adenovirus infections. Am. J. Hyg. *67*:367-378, 1958.
40. Chao, R. K., Fishaut, M., Schwartzman, J. D., et al.: Detection of respiratory syncytial virus in nasal secretions from infants by enzyme-linked immunosorbent assay. J. Infect. Dis. *139*:483-486, 1979.
41. Cherian, T., John, T. J., Simoes, E., et al.: Evaluation of simple clinical signs for the diagnosis of acute lower respiratory tract infection. Lancet *2*:125-128, 1988.
42. Cherry, J. D.: Newer respiratory viruses: Their role in respiratory illnesses of children. Adv. Pediatr. *20*:225-290, 1973.
43. Cherry, J. D., Hurwitz, E. S., and Welliver, R. C.: *Mycoplasma pneumoniae* infections and exanthems. J. Pediatr. *87*:369-373, 1975.
44. Cherry, J. D., and Welliver, R. C.: *Mycoplasma pneumoniae* infections of adults and children. West. J. Med. *125*:47-55, 1976.
45. Christie, D. L., O'Grady, L. R., and Mack, D. V.: Incompetent lower esophageal sphincter and gastroesophageal reflux in recurrent acute pulmonary disease of infancy and childhood. J. Pediatr. *93*:23-27, 1978.
46. Church, N. R., Anas, N. G., Hall, C. B., et al.: Respiratory syncytial virus-related apnea in infants: Demographics and outcome. Am. J. Dis. Child. *138*:247-250, 1984.
47. Claesson, B. A., Trollfors, B., Brolin, I., et al.: Etiology of community-acquired pneumonia in children based on antibody responses to bacterial and viral antigens. Pediatr. Infect. Dis. J. *8*:856-862, 1989.
48. Connor, J. D.: Evidence for an etiologic role of adenoviral infection in pertussis syndrome. N. Engl. J. Med. *283*:390-394, 1970.
49. Conte, P., Heitzman, E. R., and Marakarian, B.: Viral pneumonia: Roentgen pathological correlations. Radiology *95*:267-272, 1970.
50. Courtnoy, I., Lande, A. E., and Turner, R. B.: Accuracy of radiographic differentiation of bacterial from nonbacterial pneumonia. Clin. Pediatr. (Phila) *28*:261-264, 1989.
51. Demers, R. R., Parker, J., Frankel, L. R., et al.: Administration of ribavirin to neonatal and pediatric patients during mechanical ventilation. Respir. Care *31*:1188-1196, 1986.
52. Dennehy, P. H., and McIntosh, K.: Viral pneumonia in childhood. *In* Weinstein, L., and Fields, B. N. (eds.): Seminars in Infectious Disease. Vol. 5. Pneumonias. New York, Thieme-Stratton, 1983.
53. Denny, F. W.: The replete pediatrician and the etiology of lower respiratory tract infections. Pediatr. Res. *3*:463-470, 1969.
54. Dingle, J., and Langmuir, A. D.: Epidemiology of acute respiratory disease in military recruits. Am. Rev. Respir. Dis. *97*:1-65, 1968.
55. Downes, J. J., Wood, D. W., Striker, T. W., et al.: Acute respiratory failure in infants with bronchiolitis. Anesthesiology *29*:426-434, 1968.
56. Drosten, C., Günther, S., Preiser, W., et al.: Identification of a novel coronavirus in patients with severe acute respiratory syndrome. N. Engl. J. Med. *348*:1967-1976, 2003.
57. Dworsky, M., and Stagno, S.: Newer agents causing pneumonitis in early infancy. Pediatr. Infect. Dis. J. *1*:188-195, 1982.
58. Eckert, H. L., Portnoy, B., Salvatore, M. A., et al.: Group B Coxsackie virus infection in infants with acute lower respiratory disease. Pediatrics *39*:526-531, 1967.
59. Eisenstein, B. J.: The polymerase chain reaction: A new method of using molecular genetics for medical diagnosis. N. Engl. J. Med. *322*:178-183, 1990.
60. Emanuel, D., Cunningham, I., Jules-Elysee, K., et al.: Cytomegalovirus pneumonia after bone marrow transplantation successfully treated with the combination of ganciclovir and high-dose intravenous immune globulin. Ann. Intern. Med. *109*:777-782, 1988.
61. Esper, F., Weibel, C., Ferguson, D., et al.: Coronavirus HKU1 in the United States. Emerg. Infect. Dis. *12*:775-779, 2006.
62. Evans, A. S.: Infectious mononucleosis in University of Wisconsin students: Report of a five-year investigation. Am. J. Hyg. *71*:342-362, 1960.
63. Feigin, R. D., Shackelford, P. G., Choi, S. C., et al.: Nitroblue tetrazolium dye test as an aid in the differential diagnosis of febrile disorders. J. Pediatr. *78*:230-237, 1971.
64. Feldman, S., Hughes, W. T., and Daniel, C. B.: Varicella in children with cancer: Seventy-seven cases. Pediatrics *56*:388-397, 1975.
65. Feldstein, T. J., Swegarden, J. L., Atwood, G. F., et al.: Ribavirin therapy: Implementation of hospital guidelines and effect on usage and cost of therapy. Pediatrics *46*:14-17, 1995.
66. Fernald, G. W., and Clyde, W. A.: Pulmonary immune mechanisms in *Mycoplasma pneumoniae* disease. *In* Kirkpatrick, C. H., and Reynolds, H. Y. (eds.): Immunologic and Infectious Reactions in the Lung. New York, Marcel Dekker, 1976, pp. 101-130.
67. Fine, N. L., Smith, L. R., and Sheedy, P. F.: Frequency of pleural effusions in mycoplasmal and viral pneumonias. N. Engl. J. Med. *283*:790-793, 1970.
68. Fox, J. P., Brandt, C. D., Wasserman, F. E., et al.: The Virus Watch Program: A continuing surveillance of viral infections in metropolitan New York families. VI. Observations of adenovirus infections, virus excretion patterns, antibody response, efficiency of surveillance, patterns of infection, and relation to illness. Am. J. Epidemiol. *89*:25-50, 1969.
69. Fox, J. P., and Hall, C. E.: Viruses in Families: Surveillance of Families as a Key to Epidemiology of Virus Infections. Littleton, MA, PSG Publishing, 1980.
70. Foy, H. M., Cooney, M. K., Maletzky, A. J., et al.: Incidence and etiology of pneumonia, croup and bronchiolitis in preschool children belonging to a pre-paid medical care group over a four-year period. Am. J. Epidemiol. *97*:80-92, 1973.
71. Foy, H. M., Cooney, M. K., McMahon, R., et al.: Viral and mycoplasmal pneumonia in a prepaid medical care group during an eight-year period. Am. J. Epidemiol. *97*:93-102, 1973.
72. Frankel, L. R., Smith, D. W., and Lewiston, N. J.: Bronchoalveolar lavage for diagnosis of pneumonia in the immunocompromised child. Pediatrics *81*:785-788, 1988.
73. Fry, A. M., Lu, X., Chittaganpitch, M.: Human bocavirus: A novel parvovirus epidemiologically associated with pneumonia requiring hospitalization in Thailand. J. Infect. Dis. *195*:1038-1045, 2007.
74. Fulginiti, V. A., Eller, J. J., Downie, A. W., et al.: Altered reactivity to measles virus: Atypical measles in children previously immunized with inactivated measles virus vaccines. J. Am. Med. Assoc. *202*:1075-1080, 1967.
75. Gadomski, A. M., Lichtenstein, R., Horton, L., et al.: Efficacy of albuterol in the management of bronchiolitis. Pediatrics *43*:907-912, 1994.
76. Gagnon, S., Boota, A. M., Fischl, M. A., et al.: Corticosteroids as adjunctive therapy for severe *Pneumocystis carinii* pneumonia in the acquired immunodeficiency syndrome: A double-blind, placebo-controlled trial. N. Engl. J. Med. *323*:1444-1450, 1990.
77. Gajdusek, D. C.: *Pneumocystis carinii [jerovici]:* Etiologic agent of interstitial plasma cell pneumonia of premature and young infants. Pediatrics *19*:543-565, 1957.
78. Gardner, P. S.: How etiologic, pathologic, and clinical diagnoses can be made in a correlated fashion. Pediatr. Res. *11*:254-261, 1977.
79. George, R. B., and Mogabgab, W. J.: Atypical pneumonia in young men with rhinovirus infections. Ann. Intern. Med. *71*:1073-1078, 1969.
80. Gilbert, B. E., Wilson, S. Z., Knight, V., et al.: Ribavirin small-particle aerosol treatment of infections caused by influenza virus strains A/Victoria/7/83 (H1N1) and B/Texas/1/84. Antimicrob. Agents Chemother. *27*:309-313, 1985.
81. Gilllin-Ross, L., Subbarao, K.: Emerging respiratory viruses: Challenges and vaccine strategies. Clin. Microbiol. Rev. *19*:614-636, 2006.
82. Glezen, W. P.: Acute Respiratory Disease Update. Houston, Baylor College of Medicine, 1985.
83. Glezen, W. P., and Denny, F. W.: Epidemiology of acute lower respiratory disease in children. N. Engl. J. Med. *288*:498-505, 1973.

84. Glezen, W. P., and Denny, F. W.: Effect of passive antibody on parainfluenza virus type 3 pneumonia in hamsters. Infect. Immun. *14*:212-216, 1976.

85. Glezen, W. P., and Denny, F. W.: The parainfluenza viruses. *In* Evans, A. S. (ed.): Viral Infections of Humans: Epidemiology and Control. 4th ed. New York, Plenum, 1997, pp. 551-567.

86. Glezen, W. P., Frank, A. L., Taber, L. H., et al.: Parainfluenza virus type 3: Seasonality and risk of infection and reinfection in young children. J. Infect. Dis. *150*:851-857, 1984.

87. Glezen, W. P., Loda, F. A., Clyde, W. A., et al.: Epidemiologic patterns of acute lower respiratory disease of children in a pediatric group practice. J. Pediatr. *78*:397-406, 1971.

88. Glezen, W. P., Paredes, A., and Taber, L. H.: Influenza in children: Relationship to other respiratory agents. J. A. M. A. *243*:1345-1349, 1980.

89. Goodpasture, E. W.: The significance of certain pulmonary lesions in relation to the etiology of influenza. Am. J. Med. Sci. *158*:863-870, 1919.

90. Graham, B., Davis, T., Tang, Y., et al.: Immunoprophylaxis and immunotherapy of respiratory syncytial virus–infected mice with respiratory syncytial virus–specific immune serum. Pediatr. Res. *34*:167-172, 1993.

91. Grayston, J. T., Campbell, L. A., Kuo, C.-C., et al.: A new respiratory tract pathogen: *Chlamydia pneumoniae* strain TWAR. J. Infect. Dis. *161*:618-625, 1990.

92. Grayston, J. T., Kuo, C.-C., Wang, S. P., et al.: A new *Chlamydia psittaci* strain, TWAR, isolated in acute respiratory tract infection. N. Engl. J. Med. *315*:161-168, 1986.

93. Groothius, J. R., Simoes, E. A., Levin, M. J., et al.: Prophylactic administration of respiratory syncytial virus immune globulin to high-risk infants and young children. N. Engl. J. Med. *329*:1524-1530, 1993.

94. Grossman, L. K., Wald, E. R., Nair, P., et al.: Roentgenographic follow-up of acute pneumonia in children. Pediatrics *63*:30-31, 1979.

95. Gruber, W., Wilson, S., Throop, P., et al.: Immunoglobulin administration and ribovirus infection of the cotton rat. Pediatr. Res. *21*:270-274, 1987.

96. Guidelines for prophylaxis against *Pneumocystis carinii [jerovici]* pneumonia for children infected with human immunodeficiency virus. M. M. W. R. Recomm. Rep. *40*:1-13, 1991.

97. Hable, K. A., O'Connell, E. J., and Herrmann, E. C., Jr.: Group B Coxsackieviruses as respiratory viruses. Mayo Clin. Proc. *45*:170-176, 1970.

98. Hall, C. B.: The shedding and spreading of respiratory syncytial virus. Pediatr. Res. *11*:236-239, 1977.

99. Hall, C. B.: Infectious Disease Newsletter. Rochester, NY, University of Rochester School of Medicine, 1985.

100. Hall, C. B., Douglas, R. G., Geiman, J. M., et al.: Nosocomial respiratory syncytial virus infections. N. Engl. J. Med. *293*:1343-1346, 1975.

101. Hall, C. B., Hall, W. J., and Speers, D. M.: Clinical and physiological manifestations of bronchiolitis and pneumonia: Outcome of respiratory syncytial virus. Am. J. Dis. Child. *133*:798-802, 1979.

102. Hall, C. B., McBride, J. T., Gala, L. L., et al.: Ribavirin treatment of respiratory syncytial viral infection in infants with underlying cardiopulmonary disease. JAMA *254*:3047-3051, 1985.

103. Hall, C. B., McBride, J. T., Walsh, E. E., et al.: Aerosolized ribavirin treatment of infants with respiratory syncytial virus infection: A randomized double-blind study. N. Engl. J. Med. *308*:1443-1447, 1983.

104. Hall, C. B., Powell, K. R., MacDonald, N. E., et al.: Respiratory syncytial viral infection in children with compromised immune function. N. Engl. J. Med. *315*:77-81, 1986.

105. Hammer, J., Numa, A., and Neroth, C. J.: Albuterol responsiveness in infants with respiratory failure caused by respiratory syncytial virus infection. J. Pediatr. *127*:485-490, 1995.

106. Hanshaw, J. B., and Dudgeon, J. A.: Viral Diseases of the Fetus and Newborn. Philadelphia, W. B. Saunders, 1978.

107. Hardy, R. D., and Ranilo, O: Mycoplasmal infections. *In* Remington, D. S., Klein, J. O., Baker, C. J., and Wilson, C. B. (eds.): Infectious Diseases of the Fetus and Newborn Infant. 6th ed. Philadelphia, Saunders Elsevier, 2006, pp. 499-512.

108. Harrington, R. D., Hooton, T. M., Hackman, R. C., et al.: An outbreak of respiratory syncytial virus in a bone marrow transplant center. J. Infect. Dis. *165*:987-993, 1992.

109. Harrison, H. R., English, M. G., Lee, C. K., et al.: *Chlamydia trachomatis* infant pneumonitis: Comparison with matched controls and other infant pneumonitis. N. Engl. J. Med. *298*:702-708, 1978.

110. Heiskanen-Kosma, T., Korppi, M., Jokimen, C., et al.: Etiology of childhood pneumonia: Serologic results of a prospective, population-based study. Pediatr. Infect. Dis. J. *17*:986-991, 1998.

111. Heiskanen-Kosma, T., Korppi, M., Laurila, A., et al.: *Chlamydia pneumoniae* is an important cause of community-acquired pneumonia in school-aged children: Serologic results of a prospective, population-based study. Scand. J. Infect. Dis. *31*:255-259, 1999.

112. Henderson, F. W., Clyde, W. A., Collier, A. M., et al.: The etiologic and epidemiologic spectrum of bronchiolitis in pediatric practice. J. Pediatr. *95*:183-190, 1979.

113. Henson, D., and Mufson, M. A.: Myocarditis and pneumonitis with type 21 adenovirus infection: Association with fatal myocarditis and pneumonitis. Am. J. Dis. Child. *121*:334-336, 1971.

114. Herbert, F. A., Mahon, W. A., Wilkinson, D., et al.: Pneumonia in Indian and Eskimo infants and children. I. A clinical study. Can. Med. Assoc. J. *96*:257-265, 1967.

115. Herbert, F. A., Wilkinson, D., Burchak, E., et al.: Adenovirus type 3 pneumonia causing lung damage in childhood. Can. Med. Assoc. J. *116*:274-276, 1977.

116. Herrmann, E. C., Jr.: Experiences in laboratory diagnosis of adenovirus infections in routine medical practice. Mayo Clin. Proc. *43*:635-644, 1968.

117. Herrmann, E. C., Jr., and Hable, K. A.: Experiences in laboratory diagnosis of parainfluenza viruses in routine medical practice. Mayo Clin. Proc. *45*:177-188, 1970.

118. Horn, M. E. C., Brain, E., Gregg, I., et al.: Respiratory viral infection in childhood: A survey in general practice, Roehamptom, 1967-1972. J. Hyg. (Camb.) *74*:157-168, 1975.

119. Hughes, W. T.: Five-year absence of *Pneumocystis carinii [jerovici]* pneumonitis in a pediatric oncology unit. J. Infect. Dis. *150*:305-306, 1984.

120. Hughes, W. T., Feldman, S., and Cox, F.: Infectious diseases in children with cancer. Pediatr. Clin. North Am. *21*:583-615, 1974.

121. Institute of Medicine, National Academy of Sciences: New Vaccine Development: Establishing Priorities. Diseases of Importance in the United States. Washington, D. C., National Academy Press, 1985.

122. Isaacs, D.: Problems in determining the etiology of community-acquired childhood pneumonia. Pediatr. Infect. Dis. J. *8*:143-148, 1989.

123. Jacobs, J. W., Peacock, D. B., Corner, B. D., et al.: Respiratory syncytial and other viruses associated with respiratory disease in infants. Lancet *1*:871-876, 1971.

124. Jadavji, T., Law, B., Lebel, M. H., et al.: A practical guide for the diagnosis and treatment of pediatric pneumonia. C. M. A. J. *156*(Suppl.):703-711, 1997.

125. Jarvis, W. R., Middleton, P. J.: and Gelfand, E. W.: Significance of viral infections in severe combined immunodeficiency disease. Pediatr. Infect. Dis. J. *2*:187-192, 1983.

126. Jasson, E., Wager, O., Forssell, P., et al.: Epidemic occurrence of adenovirus type 7 infection in Helsinki. Ann. Paediatr. Fenn. *8*:24-34, 1962.

127. Juven, T., Mertsola, J., Waris, M., et al.: Etiology of community-acquired pneumonia in 254 hospitalized children. Pediatr. Infect. Dis. J. *19*:293-298, 2000.

128. Karron, R. A., Wright, P. F., Belshe, R. B., et al.: Identification of a recombinant live attenuated respiratory syncytial virus vaccine candidate that is highly attenuated in infants. J. Infect. Dis. *191*:1043-1104, 2005.

129. Kaslow, R. A., and Evans A. S.: Epidemiologic concepts and methods. *In* Evans, A. S. (ed.): Viral Infections of Humans. Epidemiology and Control. 4th ed. New York, Plenum, 1997, pp. 3-58.

130. Kattan, M., Keens, T. G., LaPierre, J. G., et al.: Pulmonary function abnormalities in symptom-free children after bronchiolitis. Pediatrics *59*:683-688, 1977.

131. Katz, B. Z., Berkman, A. B., and Shapiro, E. D.: Serologic evidence of active Epstein-Barr virus infection in Epstein-Barr virus–associated lymphoproliferative disorders of children with acquired immunodeficiency syndrome. J. Pediatr. *120*:228-232, 1992.

132. Kaye, H. S., Marsh, H. B., and Dowdle, W. R.: Seroepidemiologic survey of coronavirus (strain OC 43) related infections in a children's population. Am. J. Epidemiol. *94*:43-49, 1971.

133. Kim, H. W., Arrobio, J. O., Brandt, C. D., et al.: Epidemiology of respiratory syncytial virus infection in Washington, D.C. I. Importance of the virus in different respiratory tract disease syndromes and temporal distribution of infection. Am. J. Epidemiol. *98*:216-225, 1973.

134. Kim, H. W., Brandt, C. D., Arrobio, J. O., et al.: Influenza A and B virus infection in infants and young children during the years 1957-1976. Am. J. Epidemiol. *109*:464-479, 1979.

135. Kim, K. S., and Gohd, R. S.: Fatal pneumonia caused by adenovirus type 35. Am. J. Dis. Child. *135*:473-475, 1981.

136. Knight, V., Wilson, S. Z., Quarles, J. M., et al.: Ribavirin small-particle aerosol treatment of influenza. Lancet *2*:945-950, 1981.

137. Kohn, J. L., and Koiransky, H.: Successive roentgenograms of the chest of children during measles. Am. J. Dis. Child. *38*:258-270, 1929.

138. Krasinski, K., and Borkowsky, W.: Measles and measles immunity in children infected with human immunodeficiency virus. JAMA *261*:2512-2516, 1989.

139. Ksiazek, T. G., Erdman, D., Goldsmith, C. S., et al.: A novel coronavirus associated with severe acute respiratory syndrome. N. Engl. J. Med. *348*:1953-1966, 2003.

140. Lang, W. R., Howden, C. W., Laws, J., et al.: Bronchopneumonia with serious sequelae in children with evidence of adenovirus type 21 infection. Br. Med. J. *1*:73-79, 1969.

141. Laraya-Cuasay, L. R., Deforest, A., Huff, D., et al.: Chronic pulmonary complications of early influenza virus infection in children. Am. Rev. Respir. Dis. *116*:617-625, 1977.

142. Law, B. J., Wang, E. E., and Stephens, D.: Ribavirin does not reduce hospital stay in patients with respiratory syncytial virus lower respiratory tract infection. Abstract. Pediatr. Res. *37*:110, 1995.

143. Lee, N., Hui, D. H., Wu, A., et al.: A major outbreak of severe acute respiratory syndrome in Hong Kong. N. Engl. J. Med. *348*:1986-1994, 2003.

144. Leer, J. A., Bloomfield, N. J., Green, J. L., et al.: Corticosteroid treatment in bronchiolitis: A controlled collaborative study in 297 infants and children. Am. J. Dis. Child. *117*:495-503, 1969.
145. Lepow, M. L., Balassanian, N., Emmerich, J., et al.: Interrelationships of viral, mycoplasmal, and bacterial agents in uncomplicated pneumonia. Am. Rev. Respir. Dis. *97*:533-545, 1968.
146. Lerner, A. M., Klein, J. O., Levin, H. S., et al.: Infections due to Coxsackie virus group A, type 9, in Boston, 1959, with special reference to exanthems and pneumonia. N. Engl. J. Med. *263*:1265-1272, 1960.
147. Liebovitz, E., Pollack, H., Moore, T., et al.: Comparison of PCR and standard cytological staining for detection of *Pneumocystis carinii [jerovici]* from respiratory specimens from patients with or at high risk for infection by human immunodeficiency virus. J. Clin. Microbiol. *33*:3004-3007, 1995.
148. Liu, C.: Diagnosis of influenzal infection by means of fluorescent antibody. Am. Rev. Respir. Dis. *83*(Suppl.):130-138, 1960.
149. Loda, F. A., Clyde, W. A., Jr., Glezen, W. P., et al.: Studies on the role of viruses, bacteria, and *M. pneumoniae* as causes of lower respiratory tract infections in children. J. Pediatr. *72*:161-176, 1968.
150. Loda, F. A., Collier, A. M., Glezen, W. P., et al.: Occurrence of *Diplococcus pneumoniae* in the upper respiratory tract of children. J. Pediatr. *87*:1087-1093, 1975.
151. Loda, F. A., Glezen, W. P., and Clyde, W. A., Jr.: Respiratory disease in group daycare. Pediatrics *49*:428-437, 1972.
152. Long, S. S.: Treatment of acute pneumonia in infants and children. Pediatr. Clin. North Am. *30*:297-321, 1983.
153. Lough, M. D., Doershuk, C. F., and Stern, R. C.: Pediatric Respiratory Therapy. 3rd ed. Chicago, Year Book, 1985.
154. Louria, D. B., Blumenfield, H. L., Ellis, J. T., et al.: Studies on influenza in the pandemic of 1958-59. II. Pulmonary complications of influenza. J. Clin. Invest. *38*:213-265, 1959.
155. Macasaet, F. F., Kidd, P. A., Bolanco, C. R., et al.: The etiology of acute respiratory infections. III. The role of viruses and bacteria. J. Pediatr. *72*:829-839, 1968.
156. MacDonald, N. E., Hall, C. B., Suffin, S. D., et al.: Respiratory syncytial viral infection in infants with congenital heart disease. N. Engl. J. Med. *307*:397-400, 1982.
157. MacPherson, R. I., Cumming, G., and Chernick, V.: Unilateral hyperlucent lung in childhood: A complication of viral pneumonia. J. Can. Assoc. Radiol. *20*:225-231, 1969.
158. Maletzky, A. J., Cooney, M. K., Luce, R., et al.: Epidemiology of viral and mycoplasmal agents associated with childhood lower respiratory illness in a civilian population. J. Pediatr. *78*:407-414, 1971.
159. Markowitz, L. E., Chandler, F. W., Boldan, E. O., et al.: Fatal measles pneumonia without rash in a child with AIDS. J. Infect. Dis. *158*:480-483, 1988.
160. Markowitz, R. I., and Ruchelli, E.: Pneumonia in infants and children: Radiological-pathological correlation. Semin. Roentgenol. *33*:151-162, 1998.
161. Martin, L. D., Bratton, S. L., and Walker, L. K., et al.: Principles of respiratory support and mechanical ventilation. *In* Rogers, M. C. (ed.): Textbook of Pediatric Intensive Care. 3rd ed. Baltimore, Williams & Wilkins, 1996, pp. 265-330.
162. McCarthy, P. L., Frank, A. L., Ablow, R. C., et al.: Value of the C-reactive protein test in the differentiation of bacterial and viral pneumonia. J. Pediatr. *92*:454-456, 1978.
163. McCarthy, P. L., Spiesel, S. Z., Stashwick, C. A., et al.: Radiographic findings and etiologic diagnosis in ambulatory childhood pneumonias. Clin. Pediatr. (Phila.) *20*:686-691, 1981.
164. McCarthy, P. L., Tomasso, L., and Dolan, T. F.: Predicting fever responses of children with pneumonia treated with antibiotics. Clin. Pediatr. (Phila.) *19*:753-760, 1980.
165. McClelland, L., Hilleman, M. R., Hamparian, V. V., et al.: Studies of acute respiratory illnesses caused by respiratory syncytial virus. II. Epidemiology and assessment of importance. N. Engl. J. Med. *264*:1169-1175, 1961.
166. McGowan, J. E., Bratton, L., Klein, J. D., et al.: Bacteremia in febrile children seen in a "walk-in" pediatric clinic. N. Engl. J. Med. *288*:1309-1312, 1973.
167. McIntosh, K.: Community-acquired pneumonia in children. N. Engl. J. Med. *346*:429-437, 2002.
168. McIntosh, K., Chao, R. K., Krause, H. E., et al.: Coronavirus infection in acute lower respiratory tract disease of infants. J. Infect. Dis. *130*:502-507, 1974.
169. McIntosh, K., and Fishaut, J. M.: Immunopathologic mechanisms in lower respiratory tract disease in infants due to respiratory syncytial virus. Prog. Med. Virol. *26*:94-118, 1980.
170. McKinney, R. E., Maha, M. A., Connor, E. M., et al.: A multicenter trial of oral zidovudine in children with advanced human immunodeficiency virus disease. N. Engl. J. Med. *324*:1018-1025, 1991.
171. McNamara, M. J., Phillips, I. A., and Williams, O. B.: Viral and *Mycoplasma pneumoniae* infections in exacerbations of chronic lung disease. Am. Rev. Respir. Dis. *100*:19-24, 1969.
172. Meert, K. L., Sarnaik, A. P., Gelmino, M. J., et al.: Aerosolized ribavirin in mechanically ventilated children with respiratory syncytial virus lower respiratory tract disease: A prospective, double-blind, randomized trial. Crit. Care Med. *22*:566-572, 1994.
173. Menon, K., Sutcliffe, T., and Klassen, T. P.: A randomized trial comparing the efficacy of epinephrine with salbutamol in the treatment of acute bronchiolitis. J. Pediatr. *126*:1004-1007, 1995.
174. Meyers, J. D., Reed, E. C., Shepp, D. H., et al.: Acyclovir for prevention of cytomegalovirus infection and disease after allogeneic marrow transplantation. N. Engl. J. Med. *318*:70-75, 1988.
175. Mimica, L., Donoso, E., Howard, J. E., et al.: Lung puncture in the etiological diagnosis of pneumonia. Am. J. Dis. Child. *122*:278-282, 1971.
176. Minor, T. E., Dick, E. C., DeMeo, A. N., et al.: Viruses as precipitants of asthmatic attacks in children. J. Am. Med. Assoc. *227*:292-298, 1974.
177. Mintz, L., Ballard, R. A., Sniderman, S. H., et al.: Nosocomial respiratory syncytial virus infections in an intensive care nursery: Rapid diagnosis by direct immunofluorescence. Pediatrics *64*:149-153, 1979.
178. Moler, F. W., Steinhart, C. M., Ohmit, S. E., et al.: Effectiveness of ribavirin in otherwise well infants with respiratory syncytial virus- associated respiratory failure. J. Pediatr. *128*:422-428, 1996.
179. Morrell, R. E., Marks, M. I., Champlin, R., et al.: An outbreak of severe pneumonia due to respiratory syncytial virus in isolated Arctic populations. Am. J. Epidemiol. *101*:231-237, 1975.
180. Mufson, M. A., Krause, H. E., Mocega, H. E., et al.: Viruses, *Mycoplasma pneumoniae*, and bacteria associated with lower respiratory tract disease among infants. Am. J. Epidemiol. *91*:912-202, 1970.
181. Murphy, B. R., Hall, S. L., Kulkarni, A. B., et al.: An update on approaches to the development of respiratory syncytial virus and parainfluenza virus type 3 vaccines. Virus Res. *32*:13-36, 1994.
182. Murphy, S., and Florman, A. L.: Lung diseases against infection: A clinical correlation. Pediatrics *72*:1-15, 1983.
183. Murphy, T. F., Henderson, F. W., Clyde, W. A., Jr., et al.: Pneumonia: An eleven-year study in a pediatric practice. Am. J. Epidemiol. *113*:12-21, 1981.
184. Murray, J. F.: The ketchup-bottle method. N. Engl. J. Med. *300*:1155-1157, 1979.
185. Nahmias, A. J., Griffith, D., and Snitzer, J.: Fatal pneumonia associated with adenovirus type 7. Am. J. Dis. Child. *114*:36-41, 1967.
186. Nelson, K. E., Gavitt, F., Batt, M. D., et al.: The role of adenoviruses in the pertussis syndrome. J. Pediatr. *86*:335-341, 1975.
187. Nichol, K. P., and Cherry, J. D.: Bacterial-viral interrelationships in respiratory infections of children. N. Engl. J. Med. *277*:667-672, 1967.
188. Nissen, M. D., Siebert, D. J., Mackay, I. M., et al.: Evidence of human metapneumovirus in Australian children. Med. J. Aust. *176*:188, 2002.
189. Nohynek, H., Valkeila, E., Leinonen, M., et al.: Erythrocyte sedimentation rate, white blood cell count and serum C-reactive protein in assessing etiologic diagnosis of acute lower respiratory infection in children. Pediatr. Infect. Dis. J. *14*:484-490, 1995.
190. Olson, L. C., Miller, G., and Hanshaw, J. B.: Acute infectious lymphocytosis presenting as a pertussis-like illness: Its association with adenovirus type 12. Lancet *1*:200-201, 1964.
191. Orenstein, D. M., Boat, T. F., Stern, R. C., et al.: The effect of early diagnosis and treatment in cystic fibrosis. Am. J. Dis. Child. *131*:973-975, 1977.
192. Osborne, D.: Radiologic appearance of viral disease of the lower respiratory tract in children. A. J. R. Am. J. Roentgenol. *130*:29-33, 1978.
193. Paisley, J. W., Bruhn, F. W., Lauer, B. A., et al.: Type A$_2$ influenza viral infections in children. Am. J. Dis. Child. *132*:34-36, 1978.
194. Paisley, J. W., Lauer, B. A., McIntosh, K., et al.: Pathogens associated with acute lower respiratory tract infection in young children. Pediatr. Infect. Dis. *3*:14-19, 1984.
195. Parks, C. R.: Mist therapy: Rationale and practice. J. Pediatr. *76*:305-313, 1970.
196. Parrott, R. H.: Viral respiratory tract illness in children. Bull. N. Y. Acad. Med. *39*:629-648, 1963.
197. Parrott, R. H., Kim, H. W., Vargosko, A. J., et al.: Serious respiratory tract illness as a result of Asian influenza and influenza B infections in children. J. Pediatr. *61*:205-213, 1962.
198. Parrott, R. H., Vargosko, A., Luckey, A., et al.: Clinical features of infection with hemadsorption viruses. N. Engl. J. Med. *260*:731-738, 1959.
199. Person, D. A., and Herrmann, E. C., Jr.: Experiences in laboratory diagnosis of rhinovirus infections in routine medical practice. Mayo Clin. Proc. *45*:517-526, 1970.
200. Pifer, L. L.: *Pneumocystis carinii [jerovici]:* A diagnostic dilemma. Pediatr. Infect. Dis. *2*:177-183, 1983.
201. Pifer, L. L., Hughes, W. J., Stagno, S., et al.: *Pneumocystis carinii [jerovici]* infection: Evidence for high prevalence in normal and immunosuppressed children. Pediatrics *61*:35-41, 1978.
202. Pinkerton, H., and Carroll, S.: Fatal adenovirus pneumonia in infants: Correlation of histologic and electron microscopic observations. Am. J. Pathol. *65*:543-548, 1971.
203. Pizzo, P. A.: Fever in immunocompromised patients. N. Engl. J. Med. *341*:893-900, 1999.
204. Poland, G. A.: Vaccines against avian influenza: A race against time. N. Engl. J. Med. *354*:1411-1413, 2006.
205. Poncz, M., Kane, E., and Gill, F. M.: Acute chest syndrome in sickle cell disease: Etiology and clinical correlates. J. Pediatr. *107*:861-866, 1985.
206. Portnoy, B., Hanes, B., Salvatore, M. A., et al.: The peripheral white blood count in respirovirus infection. J. Pediatr. *68*:181-188, 1966.

207. Poutanen, S. M., Low, D. E., Henry, B., et al.: Identification of severe acute respiratory syndrome in Canada. N. Engl. J. Med. *348*:1995-2005, 2003.

208. Prevention and control of influenza: Recommendations of the Advisory Committee on Immunization Practices (ACIP). M. M. W. R. Morb. Mortal. Wkly. Rep. *56*:1-54, 2007.

209. Prevention of respiratory syncytial virus infections: Indications for the use of palivizumab and update on the use of RSV-IGIV. American Academy of Pediatrics Committee on Infectious Diseases and Committee on Fetus and Newborn. Pediatrics *102*:1211-1216, 1998.

210. Public health considerations of infectious diseases in child day care centers: The Child Day Care Infectious Disease Study Group. J. Pediatr. *105*:683-701, 1984.

211. Purtilo, D. T., Sakamoto, K., Barnabei, V., et al.: Epstein-Barr virus induced diseases in boys with X-linked lymphoproliferative syndrome. Am. J. Med. *73*:49-56, 1982.

212. Pyrc, K., Berkhout, B., Van der Hoek, L.: The novel human coronaviruses NL63 and HKU1. J. Virol. *81*:3051-3057, 2007.

213. Reassessment of the indications for ribavirin therapy in respiratory syncytial virus infection: American Academy of Pediatrics Committee on Infectious Diseases. Pediatrics *97*:137-140, 1996.

214. Reijowen, T., Korppi, M., Pitkakangas, S., et al.: The clinical efficacy of nebulized racemic epinephrine and albuterol in acute bronchiolitis. Arch. Pediatr. Adolesc. Med. *149*:686-692, 1995.

215. Reilly, C. M., Hoch, S. M., Stokes, J., Jr., et al.: Clinical and laboratory findings in cases of respiratory illness caused by coryzaviruses. Ann. Intern. Med. *57*:515-525, 1962.

216. 1995 Revised Guidelines for Prophylaxis against *Pneumocystis carinii [jerovici]* Pneumonia for Children Infected with or Perinatally Exposed to Human Immunodeficiency Virus. National Pediatric and Family HIV Resource Center and National Center for Infectious Diseases, Centers for Disease Control and Prevention. Atlanta, Centers for Disease Control and Prevention, 1995.

217. Rice, R. P., and Loda, F. A.: A roentgenographic analysis of respiratory syncytial virus pneumonia in infants. Radiology *87*:1021-1027, 1966.

218. Ross, C. A., Stott, E. J., McMichael, S., et al.: Problems of laboratory diagnosis of respiratory syncytial virus infection in childhood. Arch. Virusforsch. *14*:553-562, 1964.

219. Royall, J. A., and Levin, D. L.: Adult respiratory distress syndrome in pediatric patients. I. Clinical aspects, pathophysiology, pathology, and mechanisms of lung injury. J. Pediatr. *112*:169-180, 1988.

220. Royall, J. A., and Levin, D. L.: Adult respiratory distress syndrome in pediatric patients. II. Management. J. Pediatr. *112*:335-347, 1988.

221. Rubinstein, A., Morecki, R., Silverman, B., et al.: Pulmonary disease in children with acquired immune deficiency syndrome and AIDS-related complex. J. Pediatr. *108*:498-503, 1986.

222. Rusconi, F., Rancilio, L., Assael, B. M., et al.: Counter immunoelectrophoresis and latex particle agglutination in the etiologic diagnosis of presumed bacterial pneumonia in pediatric patients. Pediatr. Infect. Dis. J. *7*:781-785, 1988.

223. Saikku, P., Ruutu, P., Leinonen, M., et al.: Acute lower-respiratory-tract infection associated with chlamydial TWAR antibody in Filipino children. J. Infect. Dis. *158*:1095-1097, 1988.

224. Sanchez, I., DeKoster, J., Powell, R. E., et al.: Effect of racemic epinephrine and salbutamol on clinical score and pulmonary mechanics in infants with bronchiolitis. J. Pediatr. *122*:145-151, 1993.

225. Schmidt, G. M., Horak, D. A., Niland, J. C., et al.: A randomized, controlled trial of prophylactic ganciclovir for cytomegalovirus pulmonary infections in recipients of allogeneic bone marrow transplants. N. Engl. J. Med. *324*:1005-1011, 1991.

226. Schmidt, J. P., Metcalf, T. G., and Miltenberger, F. W.: An epidemic of Asian influenza in children at Ladd Air Force Base, Alaska, 1960. J. Pediatr. *61*:214-220, 1962.

227. Schuh, S., Canny, G., Reisman, J. J., et al.: Nebulized albuterol in acute bronchiolitis. J. Pediatr. *117*:633-637, 1990.

228. Siegel, M. M., Walter, T. K., and Ablin, A. R.: Measles pneumonia in childhood leukemia. Pediatrics *60*:38-40, 1977.

229. Siegel, S., Johnston, S., and Adair, S.: Isolation of measles virus in primary rhesus monkey cells from a child with acute interstitial pneumonia who cytologically had giant-cell pneumonia without a rash. Am. J. Clin. Pathol. *94*:464-469, 1990.

230. Siegel, W., Spencer, F. J., Smith, D. J., et al.: Two new variants of infection with Coxsackie virus group B, type 5, in young children: A syndrome of lymphadenopathy, pharyngitis and hepatomegaly or splenomegaly, or both, and one of pneumonia. N. Engl. J. Med. *268*:1210-1216, 1963.

231. Simonds, R. J., Lindegren, M. L., Thomas, P., et al.: Prophylaxis against *Pneumocystis carinii* pneumonia among children with perinatally acquired human immunodeficiency virus infection in the United States. N. Engl. J. Med. *332*:786-790, 1995.

232. Simpson, W., Hacking, P. M., Court, S. D. M., et al.: The radiological findings in respiratory syncytial virus infection in children. II. The correlation of radiological categories with clinical and virological findings. Pediatr. Radiol. *2*:155-160, 1974.

233. Smith, D. W., Frankel, L. R., Mathers, L. H., et al.: A controlled trial of aerosolized ribavirin in infants receiving mechanical ventilation for severe respiratory syncytial virus infection. N. Engl. J. Med. *325*:24-29, 1991.

234. Smith, W., Andrewes, C. H., and Laidlaw, P. P.: A virus isolated from influenza patients. Lancet *2*:66-68, 1933.

235. Spence, L., and Barratt, N.: Respiratory syncytial virus associated with acute respiratory infections in Trinidadian patients. Am. J. Epidemiol. *88*:257-266, 1968.

236. Springer, C., Bar-Yishay, E., Uwayyad, K., et al.: Corticosteroids do not affect the clinical or physiological status of infants with bronchiolitis. Pediatr. Pulmonol. *9*:181-185, 1990.

237. Stagno, S., Brasfield, D. M., Brown, M. B., et al.: Infant pneumonitis associated with cytomegalovirus, *Chlamydia*, *Pneumocystis* and *Ureaplasma*: A prospective study. Pediatrics *68*:322-329, 1981.

238. Stagno, S., Pifer, L. L., Hughes, W. T., et al.: *Pneumocystis carinii* pneumonitis in young immunocompetent infants. Pediatrics *66*:56-62, 1980.

239. Steen-Johnsen, J., Orstavik, I., and Attramadal, A.: Severe illnesses due to adenovirus type 7 in children. Acta Paediatr. Scand. *58*:157-163, 1969.

240. Stott, E. J., Eadie, M. B., and Grist, N. R.: Rhinovirus infections of children in hospital: Isolation of three, possibly new rhinovirus serotypes. Am. J. Epidemiol. *90*:45-52, 1969.

241. Sullivan, K. M., Kopecky, K. J., and Jocom, J.: Immunomodulatory and antimicrobial efficacy of intravenous immunoglobulin in bone marrow transplantation. N. Engl. J. Med. *323*:705-712, 1990.

242. Suto, T., Yano, N., Ikeda, M., et al.: Respiratory syncytial virus infection and its serologic epidemiology. Am. J. Epidemiol. *82*:211-224, 1965.

243. Toro-Figueroa, L. O., Barton, R. P., Luckett, P. M., and Perkin, R. M.: Mechanical ventilation and oxygen support systems. *In* Levin, D. L., and Morris, F. C. (eds.): Essentials of Pediatric Intensive Care. 2nd ed. New York, Churchill Livingstone, 1997, pp. 1416-1452.

244. Turner, R. B., Lande, A. E., Chase, P., et al.: Pneumonia in pediatric outpatients: Cause and clinical manifestations. J. Pediatr. *111*:194-200, 1987.

245. Update: Hantavirus pulmonary syndrome—United States, 1999. M. M. W. R. Morb. Mortal. Wkly. Rep. *48*:521-525, 1999.

246. van den Hoogen, B. G., de Jong, J. C., Groen, J., et al.: A newly discovered human pneumovirus isolated from young children with respiratory disease. Nat. Med. *7*:719-724, 2001.

247. van der Hoek, L., Pyrc, K., Jebbink, M. F., et al.: Identification of a new human coronavirus. Nat. Med. *10*:368-373, 2004.

248. Wang, E. E., Milner, R., Allen, U., et al.: Bronchodilators for treatment of mild bronchiolitis: A factorial randomized trial. Arch. Dis. Child. *67*:289-293, 1992.

249. Wang, E. E. L., Prober, C. G., Manson, B., et al.: Association of respiratory viral infections with pulmonary deterioration in patients with cystic fibrosis. N. Engl. J. Med. *311*:1653-1658, 1984.

250. Welliver, T. P., Garofalo, R. P., Hosakote, Y., et al.: Severe human lower respiratory tract illness caused by respiratory syncytial virus and influenza virus is characterized by the absence of pulmonary cytotoxic lymphocyte responses. J. Infect. Dis. *195*:1126-1136, 2007.

251. Wheeler, J. G., Wofford, J., and Turner, R. B.: Historical cohort evaluation of ribavirin efficacy in respiratory syncytial virus infection. Pediatr. Infect. Dis. J. *12*:209-213, 1993.

252. Winston, D. J., Gale, R. P., Meyer, D. V., et al.: Infectious complications of human bone marrow transplantation. Medicine (Baltimore) *58*:1-31, 1979.

253. Winternitz, M. C., Wason, I. M., and McNamara, F. P.: The Pathology of Influenza. New Haven, CT, Yale University Press, 1920.

254. Wohl, M. E. B.: Developmental physiology of the respiratory system. *In* Chernick, V., Boat, T. F., Wilmott, R. W., Bush, A. (eds.): Kendig's Disorders of the Respiratory Tract in Children. 7th ed. Philadelphia, Saunders Elsevier 2006, pp. 23-28.

255. Wolff, L. J., Bartlett, M. S., Baehner, R. L., et al.: The causes of interstitial pneumonitis in immunocompromised children: An aggressive systematic approach to diagnosis. Pediatrics *60*:41-45, 1977.

256. Woo, P. C., Lan, S. K., Chu, C. M., et al.: Characterization and complete genome sequence of a novel coronavirus, Coronavirus HKU1, from patients with pneumonia. J. Virol. *79*:884-895, 2005.

257. Wright, H. T., Jr., Beckwith, J. B., and Gwinn, J. L.: A fatal case of inclusion body pneumonia in an infant infected with adenovirus type 3. J. Pediatr. *64*:528-533, 1964.

258. Wubbel, L., Muniz, L., Ahmed, A., et al.: Etiology and treatment of community-acquired pneumonia in ambulatory children. Pediatr. Infect. Dis. J. *18*:98-104, 1999.

259. Wyde, P. R., Moore, D. K., Hepburn, T., et al.: Evaluation of the protective efficacy of reshaped human monoclonal antibody RSHZ19 against respiratory syncytial virus in cotton rats. Pediatr. Res. *38*:543-550, 1995.

260. Yeager, A. S.: Transfusion-acquired cytomegalovirus infection in newborn infants. Am. J. Dis. Child. *128*:478-483, 1974.

261. Yeager, A. S., Grumet, F. C., Hafleigh, E. G., et al.: Prevention of transfusion-acquired cytomegalovirus infections in newborn infants. J. Pediatr. *98*:281-287, 1981.

262. Zinserling, A.: Peculiarities of lesions in viral and *Mycoplasma* infections of the respiratory tract. Virchows Arch. Pathol. Anat. *356*:259-273, 1972.

BACTERIAL PNEUMONIAS
JEROME O. KLEIN

Bacterial pneumonia is an inflammation of the lung caused by a bacterial pathogen. Pneumonias may be classified in anatomic terms, such as lobar pneumonia, bronchopneumonia, and interstitial pneumonia. The disease usually is categorized by the etiologic agent, however, as in pneumococcal or staphylococcal pneumonia.

HISTORY

Pneumonia has been a frequent and serious human illness throughout recorded history. Histologic examination of Egyptian mummies (1250 to 1000 BCE) revealed hepatization of the lungs compatible with acute pneumococcal pneumonia. The disease was well known to the Greeks and Romans, and the symptoms and management (including a drainage procedure for empyema) were described by Hippocrates. Laennec described the pathologic changes and physical signs of pneumonia and pleurisy in 1819, and Rokitansky distinguished lobar pneumonia from bronchopneumonia in 1842. The early history of pneumonias was reviewed by white.[113a]

In 1881, Pasteur in France and Sternberg in the United States independently isolated, cultured, and described the pneumococcus. Each researcher used inoculation of rabbits with human saliva. Pasteur used saliva from a child who had died of clinical rabies, whereas Sternberg used material from a normal subject. A fatal septicemia resulted in the rabbits, and the organisms were isolated from their blood. In 1882, Friedländer described the pneumococcus in pathologic sections of lung and pleura and in fluid obtained by lung puncture from living patients with pneumonia. In the same laboratory, Gram exposed the sections to a sequence of dyes: aniline-gentian violet, a weak solution of iodine, ethanol, and Bismarck brown. Pairs of elongated cocci retained the dark aniline-gentian violet dye. The organism was referred to as *pneumococcus* by Fraenkel in 1886 because of its role as a cause of pulmonary infection.

Early methods of treating pneumonia included bloodletting; leeching; inhalation of chloroform; subcutaneous injection of gold, silver, and platinum solutions; and oral administration of mercury, quinine, and digitalis. The investigations of the pneumococcus in the late 19th century led to the use in 1891 of small subcutaneous doses of rabbit serum for treatment of patients with pneumonia. These treatments usually failed, but after the many antigenically separable types of the pneumococcus were recognized, specific antisera were prepared. These type-specific sera provided prompt and striking symptomatic improvement and a marked reduction in the fatality rate for pneumococcal pneumonia. Problems arose because of hypersensitivity reactions to the animal sera and the difficulty of making type-specific diagnoses. Responses to these problems included partial elimination of some of the animal protein and adaptation of the Neufeld technique for typing of pneumococci in sputum and body fluids. Use of rabbit antisera resulted in a significant increase in survival rates of patients with pneumonia caused by *Haemophilus influenzae*, and antistreptococcal horse serum or human serum obtained from patients convalescing from scarlet fever was used with success in patients with group A streptococcal pneumonia. Serotherapy was discarded after the introduction of the sulfonamides and penicillin.

Soon after the introduction of the sulfonamides for clinical use in 1935, sulfapyridine was identified as the most potent of the compounds for treatment of pneumococcal disease. By 1943, sulfonamide-resistant strains were reported, however.[101] Abraham and colleagues in 1941[3] and Keefer and colleagues in 1943[56] reported the efficacy of penicillin in treatment of life-threatening infections caused by gram-positive cocci, including *Streptococcus pneumoniae*. Penicillin-resistant pneumococci were identified in epidemic form in South Africa in the 1970s and since have been identified throughout the world.

The approval of a heptavalent conjugate polysaccharide vaccine (Prevnar; Wyeth Lederle Vaccines, Pearl River, NY) by the U.S. Food and Drug Administration (FDA) in February 2000 was the culmination of more than a century of efforts to provide protection for infants, the age group with the highest attack rates for pneumococcal diseases. Whole-cell vaccines had been investigated at the turn of the 20th century and were administered to more than 1 million individuals without serious adverse events, but with uncertain benefit. The importance of capsular polysaccharides to provide serotype-specific antigens was described in the 1930s, and a quadrivalent capsular polysaccharide pneumococcal vaccine was successful in reducing the incidence of serotype-specific pneumonia in military recruits.[63] The results of the military trial led to licensure of a hexavalent capsular polysaccharide vaccine for general use after World War II. The introduction of penicillin and other potent antimicrobials focused physicians' attention on treatment rather than prevention, however, and use of the vaccine lagged. As a result of limited use, the first polysaccharide vaccines were withdrawn in the 1950s.

A 14-valent pneumococcal polysaccharide vaccine was introduced in the United States in 1977, and a 23-valent vaccine was introduced in 1983. Most of the polysaccharides were poor immunogens for children younger than 2 years of age, and the vaccines were used only in children who were 2 years old or older and at risk for contracting invasive pneumococcal infections (e.g., children with sickle-cell disease, functional asplenia, or nephrosis). In October 1990, a conjugate polysaccharide vaccine for *H. influenzae* type b was approved by the FDA. Use of the vaccine has led to a significant decrease in the incidence of invasive disease, including pneumonia caused by *H. influenzae* type b. Similar technology was used to produce a pneumococcal conjugate vaccine. Approval of the pneumococcal conjugate vaccine by the FDA in 2000 resulted in recommendations for universal immunization in infants and selected children aged 2 to 5 years old. By spring 2008, more than 180 million doses of the pneumococcal conjugate vaccine had been distributed worldwide.

Further information about early studies of the pneumococcus and bacterial pneumonias is provided in two reference works of great value that were reprinted in 1979 by the Harvard University Press: *The Biology of the Pneumococcus* by Benjamin White and *Pneumonia* by Roderick Heffron. These works were published first in 1938 (White) and 1939 (Heffron) by the Commonwealth Fund, New York.

Watson and colleagues[112] wrote a brief history of the pneumococcus, highlighting landmarks in infectious disease discovery, including the development of Gram stain, the role of the capsule in resistance to phagocytosis, use of polysaccharides as vaccines, and evidence that DNA encodes genetic information. Podolsky[84] wrote an extensive and insightful review of the therapy of pneumonia before the advent of antimicrobial agents, including a description of early views of treatment of pneumonia by physiologic support and development of specific pneumococcal serum therapy, concluding with the introduction of the sulfonamides. Of interest are the description of U.S. Public Health Service policy in the 1930s that defined health care as a right and the recognition by states and the federal government that pneumococcal pneumonia was a public health responsibility.[84] Hager[45] wrote a description of the quest for antimicrobials by Domagk and colleagues at the German chemical manufacturer, I. G. Farben, leading to discovery of the sulfonamides, the first successful antimicrobial drug for therapy of bacterial pneumonias. Symposia proceedings have focused on the pneumococcus,[87] polysaccharide pneumococcal vaccines,[55] *H. influenzae*,[30] and lower respiratory tract infections in children in developing countries.[9,35]

MICROBIOLOGY

Because of the difficulty of documenting the microbiology of pneumonia in infants and young children, accurate data concerning the incidence and specific agents of bacterial pneumonia in children are lacking. Austrian[7] estimated that bacteria are responsible for one tenth to one third of all cases of acute pneumonias. Of 540 children with community-acquired pneumonia without empyema diagnosed between 1993 and 1999, only 6.5 percent had a positive blood culture, but 42 percent of children with empyema had a positive blood or pleural fluid culture.[21] A presumptive diagnosis of bacterial or mixed bacterial and viral infection based on antigen detection and antibody assays was made in 45 percent of Finnish children who were hospitalized for lower respiratory tract infections.[75] A reduction of 23 percent of pneumonias in children who received the pneumococcal conjugate vaccine suggests that *S. pneumoniae* is responsible for more than one quarter of pneumonias in infants and children.[64] Bacteriologic findings based on results of lung punctures from 1069 children in developing countries identified *S. pneumoniae*, *H. influenzae*, and *Staphylococcus aureus* as the leading pathogens.[92]

Now, as in the past, *S. pneumoniae* is the leading bacterial cause of pneumonia in all age groups except newborns. *H. influenzae* type b was an important cause of pneumonia in young infants in the United States until the introduction of the heptavalent conjugate polysaccharide vaccine in October 1990. In areas with high rates of immunization, pneumonia and invasive disease caused by *H. influenzae* now are uncommon occurrences. Other species of bacteria are important in special groups: Group B streptococci, *S. aureus*, and some gram-negative enteric bacilli are responsible for pneumonia in newborns; group A streptococci may cause pneumonia in children with viral infections, particularly measles, chickenpox, and influenza; and *S. aureus* and gram-negative enteric bacilli causing pneumonia are a concern in children with malignancy or children who have altered host defense mechanisms. Anaerobic bacteria play significant roles in aspiration pneumonia and lung abscess. Only a few cases of pneumonia caused by *Legionella pneumophila* have been reported in children. Other bacteria responsible for occasional cases of pneumonia include *Neisseria meningitidis*, *Bordetella pertussis*, *Bartonella henselae*,[1] *Bacillus anthracis*, *Salmonella typhi*, *Francisella tularensis*, and *Leptospira* causing leptospirosis (associated with pulmonary hemorrhage).[115]

STREPTOCOCCUS PNEUMONIAE

Although approximately 90 immunologically distinct types of *S. pneumoniae* have been identified on the basis of capsular polysaccharide antigens, relatively few types are responsible for most disease in children. Types 1, 3, 6, 7, 14, 18, 19, and 23 are the types most frequently implicated in pneumonia in children; all types but 1 and 3 are included in the heptavalent pneumococcal conjugate polysaccharide vaccine.

The spectrum of lower respiratory tract illness caused by *S. pneumoniae* ranges from a mild to moderate disease that can be managed without hospitalization to a severe, life-threatening disease that may be complicated by empyema or extrapulmonary manifestations, including meningitis and septic shock. The usual case has a sudden onset, lobar involvement, abrupt termination after appropriate chemotherapy is instituted, and rapid restoration of the involved area of the lung to normal. Although the classic pattern of pneumococcal pneumonia has a lobar distribution, bronchopneumonia and interstitial pneumonia are frequent occurrences.

Multidrug-resistant strains of pneumococci were reported from South Africa[5] in 1977. Some of the strains were highly resistant to penicillin G, requiring more than 4 µg/mL for inhibition, and were resistant to other drugs. The increase in resistance to penicillin has been accompanied by increased resistance to other antimicrobial agents, including other β-lactam drugs, tetracyclines, chloramphenicol, macrolides, clindamycin, trimethoprim-sulfamethoxazole, and other sulfonamides. Resistance of pneumococci to fluoroquinolones is uncommon, and no vancomycin-resistant strains of pneumococci have been reported.[40] The rate of multidrug resistant pneumococci varies in different countries. Incidence is highest in the Far East, with Korea, Taiwan, and Thailand reporting resistance rates of greater than 80 percent. Spain and France have the highest rates of pneumococcal resistance in Europe (30-40%), whereas the Netherlands and Germany have resistance rates of less than 5 percent.

Resistance of *S. pneumoniae* to penicillin is caused by alterations of penicillin-binding proteins. Penicillin resistance is defined by the minimal inhibitory concentrations (MIC) of pneumococci, as follows: less than 0.1 µg/mL = susceptibility; 0.1 µg/mL or higher = nonsusceptibility; among nonsusceptible strains, 0.1 to 1 µg/mL = intermediate status; and 2 µg/mL or greater = high-level resistance. No clinical features distinguish infection caused by a resistant pneumococcal strain, and virulence of infection does not seem to be increased in resistant strains.

Prevalence of multidrug resistance varies by region, with rates highest occurring in the Southeast United States and lowest in the Northeast and Pacific regions. These regional differences are unexplained. Results of surveys of antimicrobial resistance of pneumococcal strains are published frequently; a source of current information is available on the Centers for Disease Control and Prevention (CDC) website (www.cdc.gov). A report[32] of antimicrobial resistance among clinical isolates of *S. pneumoniae* in the United States during 1999 to 2000 revealed 34 percent were nonsusceptible to penicillin, including 21.5 percent with high-level resistance; MICs to all β-lactam antimicrobials increased as penicillin MICs increased. Resistance rates among non–β-lactam agents were 25 percent for macrolides, 9 percent for clindamycin, and 30 percent for trimethoprim-sulfamethoxazole. Resistance to vancomycin was not detected. A trend analysis from the same group extending the surveillance to 2002 to 2003 indicated that the rates of resistance to multiple drugs either have plateaued or have begun to decrease.[33]

The clinical implications of in vitro antibiotic resistance are variable. Daneman and colleagues[29] found high rates of clinical failure among patients with bacteremic pneumococcal disease treated with a macrolide antibiotic to which the organism was resistant; clinical failures were significantly more common among cases of pneumococcal bacteria with isolates having an erythromycin MIC of 1 µg/mL or greater than among isolates exhibiting MICs of less than 0.25 µg/mL. Less certain is the association of penicillin resistance with clinical failure in hospitalized patients treated with a penicillin; results of a study of adults with bacteremic pneumonia caused by penicillin-resistant pneumococci suggested that patients with highly resistant strains (MICs 4-8 µg/mL) failed to respond to a penicillin, whereas patients with strains with lower MICs did respond.[80] A meta-analysis of 3430 adult patients identified a mortality rate of 19.4 percent in the penicillin-nonsusceptible cases of *S. pneumoniae* pneumonia, in contrast to a 15.7 percent mortality rate in the penicillin-susceptible *S. pneumoniae* group.[102]

HAEMOPHILUS INFLUENZAE

H. influenzae type b accounts for most cases of pneumonia caused by *Haemophilus* spp. Pneumonia caused by *H. influenzae* types a, c, or d is reported rarely, but in a study of serotypes isolated from children with pneumonia in developing countries, types a, c, d, e, or f were responsible for 10 percent of cases.[93] Nontypeable strains are responsible for an uncertain proportion of cases of pneumonia and bronchitis, bronchiectasis, and acute exacerbations of pulmonary disease in patients with cystic fibrosis.

In developing countries, nontypeable strains of *H. influenzae* are important causes of pneumonia. The nontypeable strains gain access to the lung through spread from the upper respiratory tract but are less likely than are type b strains to invade the bloodstream. The diagnosis of nontypeable *H. influenzae* pneumonia in a living child is made only by lung aspiration or blood culture.[93] Of 32 isolates of *H. influenzae* obtained from blood or lung puncture of children with pneumonia in Papua New Guinea, 18 were nontypeable, 8 were types other than b, and 6 were type b; all 6 patients with type b obtained from culture of the lung aspirate also were bacteremic. Only 4 of 18 patients with nontypeable *H. influenzae* in the lung puncture were bacteremic.[94] Of 105 isolates of *Haemophilus* spp. from cultures of blood from children with lower respiratory tract infection in Pakistan, 10 were *Haemophilus parainfluenzae*, 61 were *H. influenzae* type b, and 34 were nontypeable.[113] Similar data were reported in patients with lobar pneumonia in the Gambia.[108]

Nontypeable *H. influenzae* is unlikely to be diagnosed as the cause of pneumonia if microbiologic diagnosis relies on cultures of blood alone. These data also suggest that pneumonia caused by nontypeable *H. influenzae* probably is underdiagnosed in developed and developing countries.

The clinical presentation of pneumonia caused by *H. influenzae* is indistinguishable from that caused by *S. pneumoniae* and includes mild, moderate, and severe disease. In a series of cases in children seen at the Boston City Hospital, 17 children with pneumonia and bacteremia caused by *H. influenzae* type b were identified in a 5-year period; only 4 of the children were judged to be sufficiently ill for admission to a hospital.[68] All 13 children with mild to moderate pneumonia and bacteremia were treated successfully as outpatients. The mild course of pneumonia in these patients contrasts with findings of other investigators who based their reports on the records of children admitted to the hospital.[6,19,53,85] A report of 65 children with *H. influenzae* pneumonia hospitalized at Parkland Memorial Hospital in Dallas during the 14-year period beginning July 1964 included 24 children with pleural effusion, 7 with pneumothorax, and 1 who developed pneumatoceles; 10 children had associated meningitis, and 3 had purulent pericarditis.[42] *H. influenzae* type b was the pathogen cultured most frequently from empyema fluids in children receiving care in Bethesda during the period 1974 to 1987.[19]

Beginning in the 1970s, β-lactamase–producing strains of nontypeable and type b *H. influenzae* were reported throughout the United States.[109] The enzyme cleaves the β-lactam ring of susceptible penicillins, rendering the antibiotic inactive against the enzyme-producing strain. In the United States, 33.5 percent and 41.6 percent of strains of *H. influenzae* in two 1997 surveys were β-lactamase–positive.[52,100] Strains of *H. influenzae* that were β-lactamase–negative but resistant to amoxicillin and amoxicillin-clavulanate also have been identified. A survey in the

United States in 1994 and 1995[31] identified 38.9 percent of *H. influenzae* resistant to amoxicillin, including 4.5 percent of strains resistant to amoxicillin-clavulanate (presumably resistant on the basis of a mechanism other than production of β-lactamase).

STAPHYLOCOCCUS AUREUS

Pneumonia and other serious infections caused by *S. aureus* are of particular concern in newborns, patients with altered host defenses, and patients with prior viral respiratory infection (e.g., influenza). In the United States and western Europe, the most severe problem with staphylococcal disease in newborns occurred in the 1950s and ended around 1965. The cyclic appearance and disappearance of virulent strains of *S. aureus* has no satisfactory explanation. The phage type 80/81, which was so devastating in the 1950s, no longer is a major problem in the United States or Europe. Nonetheless, cases of fatal and rapidly progressive staphylococcal pneumonia still occur[78] and are likely to become more frequent occurrences with the widespread increased incidence of community-acquired methicillin-resistant *S. aureus* (CA-MRSA).

The mechanism of β-lactam drug resistance of CA-MRSA is based on the MEC A gene, which confers resistance by encoding a penicillin-binding protein with decreased affinity for β-lactam antibiotics. Although the β-lactam antibiotics act by inhibiting bacterial cell wall synthesis in susceptible organisms, the penicillin-binding protein of CA-MRSA permits cell wall synthesis despite the presence of β-lactam antibiotics. Hospital-acquired MRSA usually is multidrug resistant but susceptible to vancomyin and linezolid. CA-MRSA strains are resistant to β-lactam drugs and macrolides, but they usually are susceptible to clindamycin, trimethoprim-sulfamethoxazole, and some tetracyclines (minocycline and doxycycline). Strains of CA-MRSA (but not hospital-acquired MRSA) carry a gene for a cytolytic toxin, Panton-Valentine leukocidin, which is associated with enhanced inflammatory response and increased necrosis and tissue damage. Although most CA-MRSA infections cause disease of the skin and soft tissues, CA-MRSA was the most frequent cause of pleural empyemas in children in Houston based on a retrospective chart review for the period 1993 to 2002.[91]

In older children, staphylococcal pneumonia may not be differentiated clinically or radiologically from other bacterial pneumonias. In young infants, the course usually is severe; the onset is abrupt, with tachypnea, significant dyspnea, and restlessness. Progression of the disease is rapid, and empyema, abscesses, and pneumatoceles are common findings. Although pneumatoceles are associated with staphylococcal pneumonia, they also may be seen in children with pneumonia caused by *S. pneumoniae*, group A streptococci, and *H. influenzae*. Pneumatoceles may persist for many months but are not a significant cause of morbidity, and they usually require no specific therapy.

GROUP A STREPTOCOCCI

Pneumonia caused by group A streptococci is an uncommon occurrence. Surveys of children hospitalized with pneumonia in Dallas[103] during a 9-year period and in Denver[72] and Chicago[53] during a 5-year period identified only five (Dallas), three (Denver), and two (Chicago) cases caused by group A streptococci. A rare outbreak of group A streptococcal pneumonia occurred among 34 U.S. Marines at a military facility in California.[25] Pneumonia caused by group A streptococci may develop after viral infection, such as influenza, measles, and chickenpox, but it also occurs in children without previous illness. The disease is characterized by necrosis of respiratory tract mucosa and lung tissue with edema and localized hemorrhage. Clinical signs include chills, high and prolonged fever, dyspnea, and pleuritic chest pain. Patients remain febrile for a mean of 10 days,[103] but patients often remain febrile for 2 to 3 weeks after initiation of therapy with appropriate antibacterial drugs. Bacteremia and pleural effusion are frequent occurrences, and pneumatoceles may occur. The typical pleural effusion begins as a serous fluid, progresses to be serosanguineous, and may become fibrinopurulent.

GROUP B STREPTOCOCCI

Early-onset disease in newborns caused by group B streptococci manifests as a multisystem illness during the first week of life and frequently is characterized by pneumonia, the clinical and radiologic pattern of which simulates respiratory distress syndrome.[2] The pattern of group B streptococci on chest radiograph includes diffuse pulmonary granularity and air bronchograms, similar to the pattern seen in infants with respiratory distress syndrome. Apnea and shock are frequent developments, but pneumonias caused by group B streptococci require lower respiratory pressures on mechanical ventilation than does respiratory distress syndrome. At autopsy, hyaline membranes similar to those seen in infants with respiratory distress syndrome have been observed in the lungs of infants who died of pneumonia caused by group B streptococci, and gram-positive cocci were identified within the hyaline membranes.

ANAEROBIC BACTERIA

Improvements in techniques for isolation and identification of the various genera and species of anaerobic bacteria have provided a better understanding of the anaerobic flora of humans and the roles of these organisms in disease. Anaerobes are present on the skin, in the mouth, in the intestines, and in the genital tract. Anaerobic bacteria may be responsible for pneumonia and lung abscesses in a host who is subject to aspiration. Anaerobic bacteria most commonly responsible for pulmonary infection include *Fusobacterium* spp., *Bacteroides melaninogenicus*, *Bacteroides fragilis*, *Peptococcus*, and *Peptostreptococcus*. The initial lesion of anaerobic infection of the lower respiratory tract is a pneumonitis with a slowly progressive clinical course. Lung abscess and necrotizing pneumonia may be a late consequence of the anaerobic pneumonitis.[12,20]

LEGIONELLA PNEUMOPHILA

In August 1976, 221 cases of respiratory illness caused by an unknown agent occurred among 4500 participants at an American Legion convention in Philadelphia. The disease was marked by high fever, recurrent chills, prominent myalgia, abnormal liver function, and a toxic encephalopathy in addition to respiratory signs. Patients had nonproductive coughs, and their radiologic patterns showed patchy bronchopneumonia, which in some cases progressed to lobar consolidation. Some patients responded promptly to therapy with erythromycin.

Investigators at the CDC isolated small pleomorphic rods from lung tissues taken at autopsy. The rods were stained with silver-impregnation methods and were visualized by direct immunofluorescence; however, they were seen poorly or not at all with Gram stain. The organism was designated *Legionella pneumophila*.

The genus *Legionella* includes aerobic, fastidious, gram-negative rods that require cysteine and some form of iron for growth. Eighteen separable species have been identified. The natural habitat of *L. pneumophila* is aquatic reservoirs, including rivers, lakes, air-conditioning cooling towers, and water distribu-

tion systems. Almost all cases of respiratory infection in children have been associated with *L. pneumophila* except for one case caused by *Legionella micdadei* (the Pittsburgh pneumonia agent).[60] Diagnosis is made by culture on buffered yeast extract agar, direct fluorescent antibody staining of respiratory tract secretions, demonstration of antibody by indirect immunofluorescence, and polymerase chain reaction (PCR).

Seroepidemiologic studies suggest that subclinical or minor infections occur in children.[73,88] Prospective studies of children with lower respiratory disease identified few cases caused by *L. pneumophila*, however.[4,79] The development of legionellosis in children with leukemia in relapse,[60] with chronic granulomatous disease,[82] receiving immunosuppressive therapy,[110] or with corticosteroid-induced immunosuppression (a patient with multiple pulmonary abscesses)[74] indicates that the organism should be added to the list of agents that cause pneumonia in immunocompromised children.

NEISSERIA MENINGITIDIS

N. meningitidis usually is associated with asymptomatic carriage in the upper respiratory tract, and pneumonia seldom develops. When pneumonia caused by *N. meningitidis* does occur, it usually is caused by group Y and is accompanied in some cases by bacteremia[51,114] and, rarely, empyema.[43] No distinctive clinical pattern occurs in children, and the diagnosis usually is made by culture of blood.[10,44]

GRAM-NEGATIVE ENTERIC BACILLI

Pneumonia caused by gram-negative enteric bacilli occurs in newborns and children with altered host defense mechanisms but is seen rarely in normal infants and children. Pneumonia caused by *Pseudomonas aeruginosa* and, to a lesser extent, by *Burkholderia cepacia* is a particular problem in children with cystic fibrosis and may occur as a severe, progressive disease leading to a fatal, necrotizing bronchopneumonia. Pneumonia caused by *Klebsiella pneumoniae* is severe, with fever, chills, and a pattern of necrosis and destruction of lung tissue. *Salmonella typhimurium* was cultured by lung aspirate from a specimen of lung in a Malawian child with human immunodeficiency virus (HIV) and lobar pneumonia.[66]

EPIDEMIOLOGY

The respiratory pathogens *S. pneumoniae*, *H. influenzae*, group A streptococci, and *S. aureus* are common inhabitants of the upper respiratory tract. These organisms may be isolated from many healthy children, and it is important to differentiate the many children who are colonized (i.e., multiplication of microorganisms without signs or symptoms of disease and without immune response), children who have asymptomatic or inapparent infection (i.e., multiplication of organisms without signs or symptoms of disease but with immune response), and children with disease (i.e., clinical signs or symptoms that result from multiplication of microorganisms). Colonization may persist for several months. The reason for colonization in some individuals and inapparent infection or disease in others is unknown.

Humans are the only known source for the common bacterial pathogens responsible for respiratory disease. Transmission occurs in most cases by droplet spread—the brief passage of the infectious agent through the air when the source and the patient are near each other (usually within several feet). Spread also occurs during talking or sneezing. The incidence of airborne spread in some cases of staphylococcal infection in children diminished after introduction of the conjugate pneumococcal vaccine in 2000.[39,98]

Bacterial pneumonia occurs uncommonly in epidemic form in the community, although the incidence of disease increases during periods of epidemic viral infection, as occurs with influenza outbreaks. Legionnaires' disease usually occurs in clusters of cases; most outbreaks have been related to airborne spread from contaminated air-conditioning cooling towers. Hospital-acquired infection may be epidemic (e.g., infections in newborn nurseries during the period of prevalence of virulent strains of *S. aureus*). Common-source outbreaks of pneumonia caused by gram-negative enteric bacilli may result from contaminated aqueous solutions used in humidification equipment.

Pneumonia is of particular concern in developing countries. In 1995, pneumonia caused 2.1 million deaths in children younger than 5 years of age; more children died because of pneumonia than because of acquired immunodeficiency disease (AIDS), malaria, and measles combined.[110] Half of the pneumonias were caused by *S. pneumoniae*.[95] In African countries, rates of pneumonia and invasive pneumococcal disease rates are 10-fold higher than in developed countries.[27] Severe and recurrent pneumonias were associated with development of bronchiectasis in indigenous children living in central Australia.[106]

PATHOGENESIS

The most important factors in development of bacterial pneumonias are the virulence of the pathogen, the absence of specific humoral immunity, and the presence of viral respiratory tract infection. Most bacterial pneumonias are a result of colonization of the nasopharynx, followed by aspiration or inhalation of organisms. The lung is protected from bacterial infection by a variety of mechanisms, including filtration of particles in the nares, prevention of aspiration of infected secretions by the epiglottal reflex, expulsion of aspirated materials by the cough reflex, entrapment and expulsion of organisms by mucus-secreting and ciliated cells, ingestion and killing of bacteria by alveolar macrophages, neutralization of bacteria by local and systemic nonspecific and specific immune substances (i.e., complement, opsonins, and antibodies), and transport of particles from the lung by lymphatic drainage. Pulmonary infection may occur when one or more of these barriers are altered, inhibited, or destroyed. Hematogenous spread to the lung by means of infected emboli arising from a suppurative focus, such as an abscess of the skin or soft tissue caused by *S. aureus*, is an infrequent occurrence.

Animal models suggest that the inflammatory responses in the lung are caused by cell wall components of gram-positive organisms or endotoxins of gram-negative bacteria.[26,104] An increase in cell wall components and endotoxin may occur after antibiotic-caused cell death, with resulting increase in inflammation. The first stage in the healing produced by appropriate antimicrobial drugs may be accompanied by clinical deterioration caused by an early increase in inflammation in the lung.

Pneumonia caused by *S. pneumoniae* begins with acute inflammation and hyperemia of the lower respiratory mucosa, exudation of edema fluid, deposition of fibrin, and infiltration of alveoli by polymorphonuclear leukocytes (i.e., "red hepatization"), followed by predominance of fibrin deposition and macrophage activity (i.e., "white hepatization"). Exudate in the alveoli is digested enzymatically and absorbed or removed by coughing. Resolution then occurs, with return of lung morphology and physiology to normal. In contrast, when the pneumonia is caused by *S. aureus* or *K. pneumoniae*, destruction of tissue and formation of multiple small abscesses frequently occur.

Clinicians have observed that symptoms and signs of minor respiratory infection caused by viruses frequently precede development of bacterial pneumonia. The respiratory virus may act by destruction of respiratory epithelium or up-regulation of bacterial adhesion molecules. Studies in animal models of infection with influenza and reoviruses[58] show a limited period of vulnerability of the lung to bacterial challenge after viral infection. The effects of the viral infection seem to be mediated by alterations in the activity of the alveolar macrophage. A brief period of impaired function of these phagocytic cells results from the viral infection. Staphylococcal[38,69] or pneumococcal pneumonias[36,37] may occur during or shortly after infection caused by influenza virus. Severe pneumococcal pneumonia has been associated with outbreaks of influenza,[77] and increased mortality rates from pneumonia in children occur during epidemics of influenza.[34]

Infections with other respiratory viruses were thought to be uncommon antecedents to bacterial pneumonias.[69] Hall and colleagues[46] found that the risk of secondary bacterial infection developing in infants hospitalized with respiratory syncytial viral infection was low (1.2% of 565 children studied over 9 years). In contrast, the conjugate pneumococcal vaccine was effective in reducing chest x-ray–defined alveolar consolidation associated with respiratory syncytial virus by 12 percent, with parainfluenza types 1 to 3 by 44 percent, and with human metapneumovirus by 40 percent, suggesting that concurrent pneumococcal infection was frequent in virus-associated pneumonias.[64,65] By documenting the decrease of pneumonias in immunized patients, the conjugate pneumococcal vaccine has been valuable in identifying the proportion of pneumonias caused by *S. pneumoniae* and identifying the roles of viral and pneumococcal co-infections.

Anatomic, physiologic, or immune defects predispose patients to single episodes and recurrent lower respiratory tract infection.[83] These defects include congenital anomalies (i.e., cleft palate, tracheoesophageal fistula, or sequestration of lung), congenital or acquired defects in immune function, aspiration (e.g., in children with familial dysautonomia, in a comatose patient, in a child who has a nasogastric feeding tube in place, after seizure, during anesthesia),[67] and alterations in the quality of mucus secretions (e.g., in patients with cystic fibrosis) or impairments in cough or swallowing or mucociliary clearance mechanisms.

Various types of pulmonary infections may develop in children who are being treated with cytotoxic and immunosuppressive drugs for malignancy or for collagen vascular disease or who are recipients of organ transplants. Patients with immune deficits may develop pneumonia caused by aerobic and anaerobic gram-negative bacilli, staphylococci, *Legionella* spp., *Nocardia*, various fungi (including *Aspergillus* and *Candida* spp. and *Pneumocystis carinii*), and viruses such as cytomegalovirus. Some infections in patients with depressed immune response represent reactivation of a latent infection. Newborns can acquire pneumonia by several routes, including transplacental infection, aspiration of organisms present in the birth canal during delivery, and postnatal infection in the nursery or at home from human sources or contaminated equipment or materials.

CLINICAL MANIFESTATIONS

The signs and symptoms of bacterial pneumonia vary with the bacterial pathogen, the age of the patient, and the severity of the disease. Some organisms are associated with a specific pattern of disease, such as the lobar pneumonia of *S. pneumoniae* and the empyema, abscess, and pneumatocele formation caused by *S. aureus*; however, any of these manifestations may result from infection caused by any of the bacterial pathogens. In young infants, signs may be nonspecific, and findings may be sparse on physical examination. Radiologic evidence of pneumonia may be found in infants who appear to have minimal disease or whose signs are more likely to be associated with upper respiratory tract infection. In older children, most cases are mild, and undoubtedly many cases occur and remain unrecognized because signs of disease do not warrant radiography of the chest. A child with pneumonia who requires hospitalization represents a small but unknown fraction of all children with pneumonia.

Symptoms and signs of pneumonia in children may be classified for convenience into five categories: (1) nonspecific manifestations of infection and toxicity, (2) general signs of lower respiratory tract disease, (3) signs of pneumonia, (4) signs of pleural fluid, and (5) signs of extrapulmonary disease. Nonspecific manifestations of infection and toxicity include fever, headache, malaise, gastrointestinal complaints, restlessness, and apprehension. Rigors may occur and vary from symptoms of chilliness to a sign of teeth-chattering chills.

General signs of lower respiratory tract disease include tachypnea; dyspnea, including shallow or grunting respirations; cough; expectoration of sputum; and flaring of the alae nasae. Because of the importance of tachypnea as a sign of lower respiratory tract disease, reference values for normal patients should be known.[89] Respiratory rates are correlated inversely with age during the first 3 years of life and vary from a median of 47 breaths/min in the first months of life to 38 breaths/min at the end of the first year to 28 breaths/min by 3 years of age. In older children, rates are 15 to 25 breaths/min. Subjects who are asleep have lower respiratory rates than do awake subjects. On the basis of these data, definitions of tachypnea for the purpose of diagnosing lower respiratory tract infection are 50 breaths/min in infants 1 to 11 months old, 40 breaths/min in children 1 to 4 years old, and 30 breaths/min in children 5 years old or older.[59]

Other general signs of pneumonia include a protective position and abdominal findings. The patient may lie on the affected side of the lung with legs drawn up because of chest pain. Abdominal distention may result from gastric dilation because of swallowed air or paralytic ileus. The liver may be displaced downward by the right diaphragm or may be enlarged if congestive heart failure complicates the pneumonia.

Signs of pneumonia may be subtle in young infants. Percussion usually is not valuable in an infant or older child if distribution of the pneumonia is patchy. Dullness to percussion is associated more often in young children with the presence of pleural fluid than with the involvement of the parenchyma of the lung. Auscultatory findings may include rales, but findings are less consistent than in older children. Abnormal findings in older children include dullness to percussion, decreased tactile and vocal fremitus on palpation, and decreased breath sounds and rales over involved areas on auscultation. Intercostal retraction indicates recruitment of accessory muscles, which becomes necessary to assist respiration when significant involvement of the lung is present.

Irritation of the pleura is accompanied by chest pain that may be severe and may limit chest movement. A friction rub may be detected over the involved area of pleura. As the effusion enlarges, dyspnea may increase, but pleuritic pain may diminish and become a dull ache. The pain of pleural irritation may be present at the site of inflammation. If the involved area includes the diaphragm, the pain may be referred to the posterior and lateral neck. Abdominal pain may be so severe as to suggest acute appendicitis. Pleural irritation over the right upper lobe may elicit meningismus, a sign of meningeal irritation without evidence of inflammation. Empyema may extend to involve the mediastinum or pericardium, or it may penetrate the chest wall to manifest as a soft tissue abscess (i.e., empyema necessitatis). Signs of extension of empyema should be sought in a patient who does not respond appropriately to chemotherapy and surgical drainage.

Extrapulmonary infection, including abscesses of the skin and soft tissues, otitis media, sinusitis, and meningitis, may occur concomitantly with bacterial pneumonia. Pericarditis and epiglottitis are particularly likely to be associated with pneumonia caused by *H. influenzae* type b.

DIAGNOSIS

MICROBIOLOGIC DIAGNOSIS

Effective chemotherapy is available to treat all forms of bacterial pneumonia in children. Optimal treatment requires definition of the etiologic agent, however. The physician must differentiate viral or mycoplasmal from bacterial pneumonia; if the agent is bacterial, the probable species must be considered. An effort should be made to obtain adequate materials, including sputum, secretions from the posterior nasopharynx, and blood, for bacteriologic diagnosis. The physician also should consider tracheal aspiration in young children unable to produce sputum, thoracentesis when pleural fluid is present, percutaneous lung aspiration in children who are critically ill, and lung biopsy when tissue diagnosis is important.

Methods for Obtaining Material for Examination and Culture

Sputum usually is not available from children until they are 5 years old; younger children usually swallow their secretions. A Gram-stained smear of sputum is valuable in providing immediate information about the bacterial pathogen; the presence of a significant number of organisms associated with or ingested by polymorphonuclear leukocytes suggests the likely pathogen, whereas the presence of epithelial cells indicates that the material is from the mouth and that further attempts should be made to obtain sputum. The adequacy of the specimen for microbiologic evaluation may be defined by the presence of 10 or more polymorphonuclear cells per low-power field and less than 25 squamous epithelial cells per low-power field.

Secretions from the nasopharynx include organisms that may be responsible for pneumonia, but results of culture of the nasopharynx may be unrevealing or misleading because of the high rate of carriage of bacterial pathogens. Tracheal aspiration through a catheter may be of diagnostic assistance when it is performed with direct laryngoscopy, but it is less valuable when the catheter is passed through the nose or mouth because of contamination with organisms present in the upper respiratory tract. Use of a double-lumen catheter ensures that the specimen remains free of contaminants.

Culture of blood provides specific bacteriologic diagnosis. Bennett and Beeson[14] suggested that most patients with pneumococcal pneumonia have bacteremia at some time during their illness. Reports of pneumococcal pneumonia in adults indicate an incidence of bacteremia of approximately 25 percent.[8,50] Data on the occurrence of bacteremia in children are less well documented. In a study of children in Boston,[99] bacteremia occurred in 8 of 100 consecutive febrile children younger than 2 years of age with radiologic evidence of pneumonia who were seen in a "walk-in" clinic. This and other studies of febrile children seen in clinics for ambulatory children reveal many cases of unsuspected bacteremia in children with pneumonia caused by *S. pneumoniae*,[17] *H. influenzae*,[68] and *N. meningitidis*.[10] The proportion of children with pneumonia who are bacteremic is uncertain, but some data are available from studies of concurrent cultures of blood and lung aspirate. Of 43 Gambian children younger than 10 years of age with pneumonia who had concurrent cultures of blood and lung aspirate, bacterial pathogens were cultured from lung aspirates in 19 children, from blood in 4, and from blood and lung in 10.[108]

The availability of flexible bronchoscopy and bronchoalveolar lavage has added another approach to obtain optimal specimens for microbiologic diagnosis of pneumonia.[13] The technique provides a direct view of bronchial and lung pathology, may provide evidence of endobronchial obstructions, and may identify and remove mucus or mucopurulent plugs. These techniques have been of particular value in the diagnosis of pulmonary disease in children with AIDS.[15]

Thoracentesis should be considered whenever fluid is present in the pleural space and microbiologic diagnosis is unrevealed by cultures of sputum, blood, or tracheal aspirate. Pleural biopsy should be performed at the time of thoracentesis if tuberculosis or tumor is in the differential diagnosis. The area to be aspirated is defined by physical examination (i.e., the point of maximal dullness), chest radiography, and ultrasonography. Gram or acid-fast stain of the fluid may provide immediate information about the pathogen. Fluid should be sent for culture; cytology; and determination of glucose, protein, and pH.

Aspiration of pulmonary exudate (i.e., lung puncture) can provide direct, specific, and immediate information about the causative agent of pneumonia. The procedure is performed similar to a thoracentesis. Lung puncture should be considered for a child who is critically ill and for whom a specific diagnosis is of immediate importance in guiding antimicrobial therapy, a child whose condition deteriorates after receiving initial therapy and for whom an etiologic agent has not been identified, and a child who has an underlying disease complicating the pneumonia or who is receiving drugs limiting normal host defense mechanisms.[57] A reappraisal of lung puncture in children indicated that a bacteriologic cause was identified in approximately 50 percent of cases and that adverse events were few.[107] Performing open or closed lung biopsy is necessary if tissue diagnosis is important.

Transtracheal aspiration is a safe and useful method of obtaining secretions from the lower respiratory tract of adults with pneumonia who are unable to produce adequate sputum. This method bypasses the mouth flora and permits the investigator to obtain direct culture of tracheal secretions. Transtracheal aspiration has not been used in young children with pneumonia because pediatricians lack experience with the technique and are concerned about the safety of the procedure. Only one report is available; Brook and Finegold[20] used transtracheal aspiration without apparent morbidity to determine the bacteriology of lung abscesses in 10 institutionalized children aged 23 months to 14 years.

Special Methods of Isolation and Identification

Clinical microbiology laboratories have facilities for isolation and identification of aerobic bacterial pathogens associated with pneumonia, but anaerobic bacteria require special techniques. Because many anaerobic bacteria are exquisitely sensitive to oxygen, anaerobic transport media must be provided and special methods must be used to handle materials on arrival in the laboratory.

Identification of bacterial antigens from secretions and body fluids is possible with the use of precipitin reaction, counterimmunoelectrophoresis, latex agglutination, and enzyme-linked immunosorbent assay. Identification of antigen is particularly helpful when prior administration of antimicrobial agents prevents successful isolation of bacteria.

Counterimmunoelectrophoresis of nasopharyngeal secretions may distinguish patients with pneumococcal pneumonia from patients who are carriers of this organism.[24] Detection in urine of polysaccharide antigens of *S. pneumoniae* and *H. influenzae* type b has been used for establishing rapid diagnosis of pneumonia.[18,105] Questions about sensitivity and specificity of the technique need to be answered. Preliminary studies suggest value for PCR for detection of *S. pneumoniae* in whole blood and serum in patients with pneumonia.[90,116] Michelow and colleagues[71] reviewed the diagnosis of lower respiratory infections caused by *S. pneumoniae* by culture, PCR (i.e., whole blood, buffy coat, or plasma), serology, and urinary antigen. A similar study was done by Le Monnier and associates of the microbiologic diagnosis of

empyema in children by evaluation of culture, PCR, and pneumococcal antigen detection in pleural fluids.[61]

Laboratory Tests

Elevated white blood cell counts (>15,000 cells/mm³) frequently, but not invariably, occur in patients with bacterial pneumonia. A white blood cell count less than 5000 cells/mm³ usually is associated with severe and overwhelming disease. Determinations of erythrocyte sedimentation rate and measurement of C-reactive protein did not distinguish virus from bacterial pneumonia in Finnish children.[78]

The presence of an immune response to infection may be used to document bacterial pneumonia in retrospect. Serologic tests for bacterial pathogens of importance in pneumonia are available only from investigative laboratories.

Chest Radiography

Although the diagnosis of pneumonia may be suggested by clinical signs, pneumonia is defined by chest radiography. In addition to plain radiography, tomography and computed tomography may be used to provide special detail about cavitation, calcification, and patency of central airways.

Radiographic findings may not correlate with clinical signs in young infants. Significant pneumonia may be found by radiography in the absence of clinical signs. Pleural effusion may be identified only with the use of a radiograph taken in the lateral decubitus position. The radiologic pattern may lag behind clinical improvement for weeks to months.

A chest radiograph should be obtained at the conclusion of the illness to determine that the pneumonia has cleared and that no underlying process, such as foreign body, congenital malformation, or residual atelectasis, is present. The precise timing for performing such a study is uncertain, but it should be done when resolution is expected, approximately 4 to 6 weeks after initial signs appear.

To establish uniformity of radiologic diagnosis of pneumonia, the World Health Organization (WHO) created in 2001 the Pneumonia Vaccine Trial Investigator's Group to develop criteria for evaluating chest radiographs. The WHO criteria were used to reinterpret radiographs obtained during the clinical trial of PCV7 in Northern California.[47] The WHO working group established the following criteria:

- *Category 1.* Consolidation/pleural effusion—alveolar consolidation, a dense or fluffy opacity that occupies a portion or whole of a lobe or entire lung and that may or may not contain air bronchograms; or pleural effusion—fluid in the lateral space and not just in the minor or oblique tissue; spatially associated with a pulmonary parenchymal infiltrate or obliterated enough of the hemithorax to obscure an opacity.
- *Category 2.* Interstitial pattern/infiltrate—the presence of linear patchy densities in a lacy pattern involving both lungs and featuring peribronchial thickening and multiple areas of atelectasis.
- *Category 3.* Absence of consolidation/infiltrate/effusion.
- *Category 4.* Radiograph quality insufficient for reading.

Of particular interest in the clinical trial of the heptavalent conjugate pneumococcal vaccine conducted in Northern California (see section on prevention) was the insight obtained in the proportion of radiologically identifiable pneumonias that were caused by the pneumococcus.[16] Children immunized with the conjugate pneumococcal vaccine had approximately one third fewer episodes of radiographically confirmed pneumonia than children who received the control vaccine. Because approximately 80 percent of the pneumococcal types thought to be responsible for pneumonia in infants were in the vaccine, these data suggest that the pneumococcus was responsible for roughly 40 percent of pneumonias identified by abnormal radiographs. Because lobar pneumonia frequently is caused by the pneumococcus, the 63 percent decrease in radiographically confirmed lobar consolidation in infants who had received the pneumococcal conjugate vaccine was less surprising.

DIFFERENTIAL DIAGNOSIS

The differential diagnosis of bacterial pneumonia includes non-bacterial pneumonias and noninfectious causes of pulmonary disease. During each period of life, certain nonbacterial agents are prominent causes of pneumonia. Pneumonia in neonates may result from congenital infection or infection acquired at the time of delivery because of rubella, toxoplasmosis, herpes simplex infection, cytomegalovirus infection, or syphilis. In infants 2 weeks to 6 months old, *Chlamydia trachomatis* is an important cause of a syndrome of afebrile pneumonia. Throughout childhood, most pneumonias are caused by respiratory viruses, including adenoviruses, influenza viruses, parainfluenza viruses, respiratory syncytial virus, echoviruses, and coxsackieviruses A and B. *Mycoplasma pneumoniae* is an uncommon cause of pneumonia in preschool-aged children, but is an important cause of pneumonia in school-aged children, adolescents, and young adults. Nonbacterial pneumonias that are susceptible to available antimicrobial agents include disease caused by fungi (e.g., histoplasmosis, blastomycosis), *Rickettsia* (i.e., Q fever), and *Chlamydia* (i.e., TWAR agent and psittacosis).

An important consideration is tuberculosis in children with persistent pulmonary disease who do not respond to penicillin or alternatives to penicillin. All children living in areas that have a high risk for tuberculosis should have a tuberculin skin test if admitted to the hospital with a lower respiratory tract infection.

Noninfectious causes of pulmonary lesions include aspiration of gastric contents, aspiration of foreign body, drug reactions, sequestration of lobe, congestive heart failure, atelectasis, sarcoidosis, malignancy or tumor, alveolar proteinosis, pulmonary hemosiderosis, and desquamating interstitial pneumonia.

Bacterial causes of acute empyema include *S. aureus*, *S. pneumoniae*, *H. influenzae*, gram-negative bacilli, and anaerobic bacteria.[19] Bloody exudates (when thoracentesis occurs without trauma) suggest malignancy, infarct of the lung, connective tissue disorder, pancreaticopleural fistula, or tuberculosis.

CLINICAL GUIDELINES IN DEVELOPING COUNTRIES

Acute infections of the lower respiratory tract are the most important cause of death in children younger than 5 years of age in developing countries.[97] The authors of the Programme for the Control of Respiratory Infections of the WHO developed clinical guidelines for case diagnosis of pneumonia for use in developing countries. In these areas, diagnosis and management are provided for children by health care personnel who work in facilities where laboratory and radiologic tests are limited or do not exist.[86] The goals of the program are to simplify diagnosis to the smallest number of readily identifiable signs, to provide a system for classification of the illness, and to define the basis for use of antibacterial agents. The guidelines include assessment of fever, nutrition, lethargy, and color (i.e., presence or absence of cyanosis); measurement of the respiratory rate; observations of chest wall movement to detect retractions; and auscultation for stridor and wheezes.

The guidelines distinguish levels of disease for purposes of management. *Very severe pneumonia* includes central cyanosis and an inability to drink. *Severe pneumonia* includes chest indrawing, without cyanosis, and the ability to drink. *Pneumonia* includes no chest indrawing, but sustained tachypnea (>60 breaths/min for infants <2 months old, >50 breaths/min for children 2 to 12 months old, or >40 breaths/min for children 12 months to 5 years old). *No pneumonia* includes cough in the absence of chest indrawing and tachypnea. Suggested management includes hospitalization and administration of parenteral antibiotics for children with very severe and severe pneumonia, home care and administration of oral antibiotics for children with pneumonia, and no antibiotics but assessment and treatment of other problems for children with cough but without signs of severe respiratory illness.

Simoes and McGrath[96] evaluated the ability of nurses and nursing assistants in Swaziland to recognize pneumonia using the WHO's protocols. Signs of severe disease, including stridor and abnormal sleepiness, often were overlooked, as was audible wheeze, but tachypnea and chest wall retractions were well recognized. In a study of Chinese children, tachypnea (50 cycles/min for infants 2 to 11 months old and 40 cycles/min for children 1 to 5 years old) was a good predictor of radiologically defined pneumonia and was recommended for use by village health care workers in diagnosing pneumonia. Nasal flaring, retractions, stridor, and cyanosis of the tongue had high predictive values but were observed infrequently.[28] A respiratory rate of more than 50 cycles/min or retractions was predictive of pneumonia in children with cough evaluated in Papua New Guinea.[48]

MANAGEMENT

Therapy should be initiated promptly after bacterial pneumonia is diagnosed or strongly suspected. Initial therapy is guided by knowledge of the likely bacterial pathogens in the child's age group because examination of the sputum or tracheal aspirate usually is unavailable in patients younger than school age. The physician must decide whether hospitalization is required for optimal management of the child. Most children with mild to moderate disease can be treated at home. Hospitalization is required for children with severe disease who require hydration, oxygen, or observation; children who are toxic and have a significant degree of pulmonary dysfunction; and children whose families lack the ability to provide therapy and supportive care. Special concern is warranted for infants in the first year of life, when signs of respiratory disease are subtle and disease may progress rapidly.

INITIAL CHOICE OF ANTIMICROBIAL AGENTS BY AGE GROUP

Neonatal Pneumonia

The treatment of neonatal pneumonia is similar to treatment of other severe neonatal infections. Initial therapy must include coverage for gram-positive cocci, particularly group B streptococci, and gram-negative bacilli.

A penicillin is the drug of choice for gram-positive organisms. Penicillin G or ampicillin is used. The latter drug may provide a theoretical advantage because of greater in vitro activity against some enterococci and some gram-negative bacilli, particularly *Escherichia coli* and *Proteus mirabilis*, when used alone or in combination with an aminoglycoside. If the physician has reason to suspect staphylococcal infection, a penicillinase-resistant penicillin is chosen. Infants with pulmonary signs suggestive of severe staphylococcal pneumonia (e.g., abscesses, pneumatoceles, and/or empyema) should be treated with drugs having known efficacy for multidrug-resistant staphylococci, such as vancomycin or linezolid.

Choice of therapy for suspected gram-negative bacillary infection depends on the antibiotic susceptibility pattern for recent isolates obtained from newborns. An aminoglycoside such as gentamicin has an effective range of in vitro activity. Amikacin and tobramycin have similar activity but may be effective for strains of gram-negative enteric bacilli that are resistant to gentamicin.

Initial therapy is reevaluated when the results of cultures are available. Duration of therapy depends on the causative agent. Pneumonia caused by group B streptococci or gram-negative enteric bacilli is treated for 7 to 10 days; disease caused by *S. aureus* requires 3 to 6 weeks of antimicrobial therapy, according to the severity of the disease.

Pneumonias in Children 1 Month to 10 Years of Age

Most cases of bronchopneumonias in children aged 1 month to 10 years are caused by respiratory viruses. If the initial clinical and radiologic findings are consistent with viral infection, and the child can be observed closely, antimicrobial agents may be withheld pending the results of cultures. *S. pneumoniae* and *H. influenzae* (nontypeable and type b) are the major bacterial agents responsible for bacterial pneumonia in this age group. The rate of disease caused by *H. influenzae* type b is low in children who were immunized previously with the conjugate vaccine. Although multidrug-resistant organisms among pneumococci vary, the concentrations of parenteral ampicillin are sufficient to achieve concentrations in the blood and lung that can inhibit and kill all but the most resistant strains.

If the child is critically ill, vancomycin should be substituted for ampicillin because pneumococci are not resistant to it. Strains of β-lactamase–producing *H. influenzae* resistant to amoxicillin and other susceptible penicillins have been isolated throughout the United States. Nonetheless, amoxicillin still is appropriate initial therapy for a young child with mild disease. If the child is moderately or seriously ill, drugs with efficacy against *S. pneumoniae* and β-lactamase–producing *H. influenzae*, including ampicillin-sulbactam or cephalosporins (i.e., cefuroxime, ceftriaxone, cefotaxime, or ceftazidime), should be administered by parenteral routes.

S. aureus now is an uncommon cause of pneumonia in this age group. If clinical signs compatible with staphylococcal disease are present, however, initial therapy should include a parenteral penicillinase-resistant penicillin. If the disease is severe, drugs of known efficacy for MRSA, such as vancomycin or linezolid, should be used.

Because *M. pneumoniae* and *Chlamydia pneumoniae* are common causes of pneumonia in school-aged children and adolescents, presumptive therapy should include coverage for *S. pneumoniae*, *M. pneumoniae*, and *C. pneumoniae* in children older than 5 years. Erythromycin, azithromycin, and clarithromycin are appropriate drugs for coverage of both pathogens.

Pneumonia in Children 10 Years of Age or Older

S. pneumoniae, *M. pneumoniae*, and *C. pneumoniae* are the major treatable causes of pneumonia in children 10 years of age or older. *H. influenzae* occurs infrequently, and initial therapy need not include coverage for this organism. Therapy outlined earlier for school-aged children is appropriate for children 10 years or older.

CHEMOTHERAPY FOR SPECIFIC PATHOGENS

Pneumococcal Pneumonia

Penicillin G is the drug of choice for children with pneumonia caused by *S. pneumoniae*. For most children with mild to moderately severe disease, an oral penicillin is suitable. Phenoxymethylpenicillin (penicillin V) administered orally provides significant antibacterial activity and approximately twice the peak serum level provided by an equivalent dose of buffered oral penicillin

G. Children who appear to be toxic, who have underlying disease, or who have complications (e.g., abscesses, empyema) require the higher serum and tissue antibacterial activity that is provided by aqueous penicillin G administered intravenously or intramuscularly.

Strains of nonsusceptible *S. pneumoniae* have become prevalent in most communities in the United States. Clinical failures have occurred in some patients with meningitis caused by penicillin-resistant pneumococci, but few failures have been identified in cases of sepsis or pneumonia treated with a penicillin or cephalosporin in an adequate dosage schedule. Susceptibility tests should be done on all isolates of *S. pneumoniae* from sputum and body fluids (i.e., blood, cerebrospinal fluid, and pleural fluid). Presumptive therapy for mild to moderate pneumonias need not be altered because of concern for resistant pneumococci, but severe pneumonias should be treated with high-dose parenteral therapy providing high serum and tissue concentrations and stability to β-lactamases, such as intravenous ceftriaxone and cefotaxime. The most appropriate regimen is chosen when results of culture and susceptibility tests are available. Vancomycin is effective uniformly against all pneumococci, including highly resistant strains, and should be considered if susceptibility tests indicate the strain is multidrug-resistant and uniquely susceptible to vancomycin.

The dosage schedule for mild to moderate disease and severe disease is provided in Chapter 235. The duration of therapy depends on the clinical response, but therapy should be continued for at least 3 days after defervescence and significant resolution of radiologic and clinical signs; usually 5 to 7 days is sufficient.

Pneumonia Caused by *Haemophilus influenzae*

Nontypeable and type b strains of *H. influenzae* are susceptible to various antimicrobial agents, including ampicillin or amoxicillin (non–β-lactamase producers), oral or parenteral cephalosporins, sulfonamides, and aminoglycosides. All of these agents have been used with success in systemic infections (including pneumonia) caused by this agent. Amoxicillin is considered the drug of choice for treating young children with mild to moderate pulmonary disease. Because of the concern for β-lactamase–producing strains of *H. influenzae*, a parenteral second-generation (cefuroxime) or third-generation (ceftriaxone, cefotaxime, or ceftazidime) cephalosporin should be used as initial therapy in patients with severe disease when this microorganism is known or strongly suspected to be the pathogen.

A child with mild to moderate disease should be treated for a minimum of 7 days, including a period without fever of at least 3 days. A child with severe disease should be treated for 2 to 3 weeks.

Staphylococcal Pneumonia

The high incidence of staphylococci resistant to penicillin G, in the hospital and in the community, requires the use of a penicillinase-resistant penicillin whenever staphylococcal pneumonia is diagnosed or suspected. Subsequently, if the culture and sensitivity data indicate that the organism is susceptible to penicillin G, the drug should be used because of its greater efficacy and lower cost. Clinical trials indicate that all penicillinase-resistant penicillins are equally effective in treating staphylococcal pneumonia. The increased incidence of CA-MRSA suggests that initial therapy of patients with pulmonary signs suggestive of staphylococcal infection (e.g., abscesses, pneumatoceles, and emypema) should include parenteral drugs of known efficacy, such as vancomycin or linezolid.

The rapid development of empyema, pneumatoceles, and abscesses demands close observation and meticulous nursing care. The antibiotic should be administered parenterally using a high-dose schedule for 2 to 3 weeks; an oral preparation then may be given for 1 to 3 weeks. The total duration of antibiotic therapy depends on the initial response, the presence of pulmonary and extrapulmonary complications, and the rapidity of resolution of the pneumonia.

Pneumonia Caused by Anaerobic Bacteria

Most anaerobic bacteria that cause pneumonia, including strains of B. fragilis, are highly susceptible to penicillin G. Some strains of B. fragilis may be resistant to penicillin G and susceptible to chloramphenicol, clindamycin, or cefoxitin. The duration of therapy depends on the extent of the disease; pneumonia without complications clears rapidly with appropriate therapy; 7 days of therapy usually is sufficient.

Pneumonia Caused by Gram-Negative Bacilli

The initial choice of therapy is guided by the following factors: the source of the infection, the disease process present (e.g., burn, cystic fibrosis), the host susceptibility to infection (e.g., deficient immune mechanisms), and the antimicrobial susceptibility pattern for these organisms in the community or hospital. The basis for choice of antibiotic is similar to that outlined for neonatal pneumonia suspected to be caused by gram-negative bacilli. The duration of therapy must be tailored to the clinical course and the response to therapy. Cases of pneumonia with minimal pulmonary lesions and limited symptoms should be treated for at least 3 days after defervescence. Severe cases of pneumonia should be treated for 2 to 3 weeks.

Therapy for Penicillin-Allergic Children

A child who has a significant history of allergic reaction to any of the penicillins must be considered allergic to all of them, and alternative antimicrobial agents must be considered for therapy. If the patient has a history consistent with IgE-mediated reaction to penicillin, cephalosporins also should be avoided. If the patient has a history of a penicillin reaction that was not IgE-mediated and not serious, administration of a cephalosporin usually is safe.[83] Cephalothin, cefazolin, ceftriaxone, and cefotaxime have been used with success in the treatment of pneumococcal pneumonia. Erythromycin, the new macrolides clarithromycin and azithromycin, and clindamycin are active in vitro against gram-positive cocci, but use for pneumococcal and staphylococcal pneumonias should be determined on the basis of susceptibility tests. Because there are no vancomycin-resistant pneumococci and only rare cases of staphylococci that are resistant, vancomycin is the drug of choice for presumptive therapy of a patient who is allergic to penicillin and who has severe pneumonia likely caused by staphylococcal or pneumococcal infections.

Adjuncts to Chemotherapy

Administration of antimicrobial agents is only part of the management of a child with pneumonia. Close observation, nursing care (including suction of excess secretions), and the following supportive measures are crucial:

1. Maintenance of fluid and electrolyte balance
2. Humidification provided by cool mist
3. Oxygen for severe dyspnea
4. Cleansing of the mouth
5. Sparing use of antipyretics because the temperature course provides a guideline for the therapeutic response

More extensive procedures may be required in special circumstances, as follows:

1. Bronchoscopy is important in documenting the presence of a foreign body, tumor, or congenital anomaly.
2. Intubation of the trachea or tracheotomy may be considered when the patient has difficulty clearing secretions and more efficient suction of the lower respiratory tree is required.
3. Drainage of pleural effusions may be necessary when an accumulation of fluid compromises respiration. Thick, tenacious empyema may require intercostal tube drainage or closed-tube thoracostomy. Empyema caused by S. aureus may require placement of a tube, whereas the less viscid effusion associated with S. pneumoniae and Streptococcus pyogenes rarely requires more than frequent thoracentesis. Empyema caused by H. influenzae may be thick and viscid, requiring placement of a chest tube, or less viscid, requiring only thoracentesis. Single or multiple thoracenteses are adequate when the volume of fluid is small and the quality of the fluid allows ready drainage, as usually is the case with empyema caused by S. pneumoniae or group A streptococci. When large amounts of fluid are present or the fluid is thick and viscid, a closed drainage system with intercostal chest tube under negative pressure is placed; this placement frequently is necessary for empyema caused by S. aureus. The tube should be removed as soon as its drainage function is completed because delay might result in local tissue injury, secondary infection, or sinus formation. The use of video-assisted thoracoscopy early in the course of empyema (within 48 hours after admission to hospital) has significantly decreased the duration of fever and the length of hospitalization for patients with pleural empyemas.[91]
4. Intrapleural instillation of antibiotics or fibrinolytics should be considered in cases of empyema when the fluid is loculated because of fibrous adhesions. If a chest tube is in place, antibiotics can be instilled after irrigation through the tube. In susceptible infections, aqueous penicillin G (10,000 to 50,000 U), ampicillin (10 to 50 mg), or a penicillinase-resistant penicillin or cephalosporin (10 to 50 mg) may be inoculated in 10 mL of diluent (i.e., sterile water or normal saline) after the tube is clamped. The clamp is maintained for 1 hour and then released for drainage. The instillations should be repeated three to four times each day that the tube remains in place. Hawkins and colleagues[49] reported successful resolution of 54 of 58 children with empyema who underwent intrapleural placement of catheters and administration of fibrinolytics consisting of tissue plasminogen activator.

PROGNOSIS

In uncomplicated cases of pneumococcal pneumonia in children in the United States, the mortality rate is very low (<1%). A review of mortality from pneumonia in children in the United States, 1939 through 1996, identified reductions in mortality rates that were thought to reflect expanded access to medical care for poor children.[34] In developing countries, pneumonia is a major cause of mortality, accounting for more than one fourth of deaths in children younger than 5 year old. Half of the pneumonia-related mortality occurs in children younger than 1 year old. The WHO estimates that approximately 4 million childhood deaths are caused each year by pneumonia.

Lung morphology and physiology usually return to normal after completion of appropriate antimicrobial therapy. Fibrothorax is a rare occurrence; almost all children resolve thickened pleurae with no effect on lung growth and function. Even after having extensive disease associated with empyema caused by S. aureus or H. influenzae, children have normal growth and development and normal pulmonary function after recovery.[70] Deaths still result from bacterial pneumonias; however, most deaths of children result from abrupt, overwhelming disease. Asmar and colleagues[6] reported two deaths in 43 children with pneumonia caused by H. influenzae; both deaths occurred before antibiotics could be administered.

PREVENTION

PNEUMOCOCCAL VACCINES

The approval of a conjugate polysaccharide pneumococcal vaccine by the FDA in February 2000, followed by the recommendations of various authoritative groups (e.g., American Academy of Pediatrics, American Academy of Family Physicians, and Advisory Committee on Immunization Practices of the Surgeon General) for universal immunization of infants and selective immunization of children at risk who are 2 to 5 years of age, added the most effective mode of prevention of pneumococcal diseases yet available. The available vaccine (Prevnar; Wyeth Lederle Vaccines, Pearl River, NY) is a heptavalent vaccine in which the individual polysaccharides have been purified and directly conjugated to the protein carrier CRM 197, a nontoxic variant of diphtheria toxin. The conjugate vaccine induces type-specific antibodies in infants 2 months of age. The vaccine currently is distributed in 73 countries, and more than 180 million doses have been distributed worldwide (Paradiso P, personal communication May 2008).

The safety and efficacy of the vaccine for prevention of pneumonia were studied in a trial of approximately 38,000 children in Northern California by Black and colleagues at the Kaiser Permanente Vaccine Study Center.[16] Children were randomly assigned to receive the conjugate pneumococcal vaccine or a conjugate polysaccharide meningococcal group C vaccine. Pneumonia was defined clinically and radiologically. Infants and children who had received the pneumococcal vaccine had a 4.3 percent reduction in clinical episodes of pneumonia and a 20 percent decrease in radiographically confirmed pneumonia. Similar results have been reported from developing countries; a nine-valent pneumococcal conjugate vaccine was found to be effective compared with placebo in prevention of 7 percent of clinical pneumonias and 37 percent of first episodes of radiologically diagnosed pneumonias.[27]

The 23-type pneumococcal polysaccharide vaccine produces a satisfactory independent antibody response, but only in children older than 2 years. The polysaccharide vaccine is recommended for children 2 years of age and older who are at risk for developing invasive disease (e.g., sickle-cell disease, HIV infection or other immunodeficiencies, malignancy, nephrosis) after they have received the appropriate number of doses of the conjugate vaccine.

HAEMOPHILUS INFLUENZAE VACCINES

A polysaccharide vaccine for prevention of H. influenzae type b disease was introduced in the United States in April 1985. As was true of other polysaccharide vaccines, infants younger than 18 months of age had an inadequate immune response to the capsular polysaccharide. The development of a conjugate vaccine by coupling the capsular saccharide of H. influenzae type b and a protein resulted in protective antibodies in infants 2 months of age. The conjugate H. influenzae type b vaccine was approved by the FDA in fall 1990 and has resulted in virtual elimination of disease caused by H. influenzae type b in infants and children. The conjugate vaccine has had varying efficacy in different regions. The incidence of pneumonia associated with alveolar consolidation or pleural effusion was reduced by 22 percent in Chilean infants, whereas the vaccine had limited efficacy in prevention of clinical or radiologically confirmed pneumonias in Indonesian children.

Because nontypeable strains of H. influenzae are important causes of otitis media, sinusitis, and pneumonia, investigators have sought vaccine candidates, including outer membrane proteins, bacterial adherence proteins, and lipo-oligosaccharides.

Questions of strain heterogeneity and choice of the number of antigens needed for optimal protection remain unanswered, and no products have moved beyond preclinical testing.[11]

INFLUENZAVIRUS VACCINE

Secondary bacterial pneumonia may complicate primary influenza virus infections. Extensive use of conjugate pneumococcal vaccines in children (and widespread use of influenza vaccines) should limit the incidence and morbidity of the combined infections. Brundage[21] reviewed the epidemiologically and clinically important interactions between influenza and secondary bacterial respiratory pathogens during the 1918 and subsequent influenza pandemics.

CHEMOPROPHYLAXIS

Chemoprophylaxis for prevention of bacterial pneumonias is limited to patients with immunodeficiency. Children who have sickle-cell anemia or who have functional or anatomic asplenia are at risk for developing overwhelming disease caused by S. pneumoniae. Daily antimicrobial prophylaxis is recommended for these children, regardless of their immunization status. The chemoprophylactic regimen used most commonly is daily administration of oral penicillin V (125 mg twice daily for children <5 years; 250 mg twice daily for children >5 years). Children with HIV should receive a regimen of trimethoprim-sulfamethoxazole for prophylaxis against infection caused by P. carinii.

PREVENTION OF HEALTH CARE–ASSOCIATED PNEUMONIA

Because a hospitalized child is exposed to a variety of pathogens, including bacteria capable of causing pneumonia, and may undergo procedures that compromise the airway, health care providers should be familiar with techniques for limiting exposures. The CDC periodically has provided guidelines for prevention of health care–associated pneumonia, most recently in 2004.[22,23]

REFERENCES

1. Abbasi, S., and Chesney, P. J.: Pulmonary manifestations of cat-scratch disease: A case report and review of the literature. Pediatr. Infect. Dis. J. 14:547-548, 1995.
2. Ablow, R. C., Driscoll, S. G., Effmann, E. L., et al.: A comparison of early-onset group B streptococcal neonatal infection and the respiratory distress syndrome of the newborn. N. Engl. J. Med. 294:65-70, 1976.
3. Abraham, E. P., Gardner, A. D., Chain, E., et al.: Further observations on penicillin. Lancet 2:177-189, 1941.
4. Anderson, R. D., Lauer, B. A., Fraser, D. W., et al.: Infections with Legionella pneumophila in children. J. Infect. Dis. 13:386-390, 1981.
5. Applebaum, P. C., Bhamjee, A., Scragg, J. N., et al.: Streptococcus pneumoniae resistant to penicillin and chloramphenicol. Lancet 2:995, 1977.
6. Asmar, B. I., Slovis, T. L., Reed, J. O., et al.: Haemophilus influenzae type b pneumonia in 43 children. J. Pediatr. 93:389-393, 1978.
7. Austrian, R.: Treatment of pneumonia. Mod. Treat. 1:909-923, 1964.
8. Austrian, R., and Gold, J.: Pneumococcal bacteremia with especial reference to bacteremic pneumococcal pneumonia. Ann. Intern. Med. 60:759-776, 1964.
9. Bale, J. R.: Creation of a research program to determine the etiology and epidemiology of acute respiratory tract infection in children in developing countries. Rev. Infect. Dis. 12(Suppl. 8):S861-S866, 1990.
10. Baltimore, R. S., and Hammerschlag, M.: Meningococcal bacteremia: Clinical and serologic studies of infants with mild illness. Am. J. Dis. Child. 131:1001-1004, 1977.
11. Barenkamp, S. J.: Rationale and prospects for a nontypable Haemophilus influenzae vaccine. Pediatr. Infect. Dis. J. 23:461-462, 2004.
12. Bartlett, J. G.: Anaerobic bacterial pneumonitis. Am. Rev. Respir. Dis. 119:19-23, 1979.
13. Baselski, V. S., and Wunderink, R. G.: Bronchoscopic diagnosis of pneumonia. Clin. Microbiol. Rev. 7:533-558, 1994.

14. Bennett, I. L., Jr., and Beeson, P. B.: Bacteremia: A consideration of some experimental and clinical aspects. Yale J. Biol. Med. 26:241-262, 1954.
15. Birriel, J. A., Jr., Adams, J. A., Saldana, M. A., et al.: Role of flexible bronchoscopy and bronchoalveolar lavage in the diagnosis of pediatric acquired immunodeficiency syndrome-related pulmonary disease. Pediatrics 87:897-899, 1991.
16. Black, S., Shinefield, H., Ling, S., et al.: Efficacy of heptavalent pneumococcal conjugate vaccine in children younger than five years of age for prevention of pneumonia. Pediatr. Infect. Dis. J. 21:810-815, 2002.
17. Bratton, L., Teele, D. W., and Klein, J. O.: Outcome of unsuspected pneumococcemia in children not initially admitted to the hospital. J. Pediatr. 90:703-706, 1977.
18. Bromberg, K., Tannis, G., and Rodgers, A.: Pneumococcal C and type polysaccharide detection in the concentrated urine of patients with bacteremia. Med. Microbiol. Immunol. 179:335-338, 1990.
19. Brook, I.: Microbiology of empyema in children and adolescents. Pediatrics 85:722-726, 1990.
20. Brook, I., and Finegold, S. M.: Bacteriology and therapy of lung abscess in children. J. Pediatr. 94:10-12, 1979.
21. Brundage, J. F.: Interactions between influenza and bacterial respiratory pathogens: Implications for pandemic preparedness. Lancet Infect. Dis. 6:303-312, 2006.
22. Byington, C. L., Spencer, L. Y., Johnson, T. A., et al.: An epidemiological investigation of a sustained high rate of pediatric parapneumonic empyema: Risk factors and microbiological associations. Clin. Infect. Dis. J. 34:434-440, 2002.
23. Centers for Disease Control and Prevention: Guidelines for preventing health-care-associated pneumonia, 2003: Recommendations of CDC and the Healthcare Infection Control Practices Advisory Committee. M. M. W. R. Morb. Mortal. Wkly. Rep. 53(No. RR-3):1-36, 2003.
24. Congeni, B. L., and Nankervis, G. A.: Diagnosis of pneumonia by counterimmunoelectrophoresis of respiratory secretions. Am. J. Dis. Child. 1132:684-688, 1978.
25. Crum, N. F., Russell, K. L., Kaplan, E. L., et al.: Pneumonia outbreak associated with group A Streptococcus species at a military training facility. Clin. Infect. Dis. 49:511-518, 2005.
26. Cundell, D., Masure, H. R., and Tuomanen, E. I.: The molecular basis of pneumococcal infection: A hypothesis. Clin. Infect. Dis. 21(Suppl. 3):S204-S212, 1995.
27. Cutts, F. T., Zaman, S. M. A., Enwere, G., et al.: Efficacy of nine-valent pneumococcal conjugate vaccine against pneumonia and invasive pneumococcal disease in The Gambia: Randomized, double-blind, placebo-controlled trial. Lancet 365:1139-1146, 2005.
28. Dai, Y., Foy, H. M., Zonghan, Z., et al.: Respiratory rate and signs in roentgenographically confirmed pneumonia among children in China. Pediatr. Infect. Dis. J. 14:48-50, 1995.
29. Daneman, N., McGeer, A., Green, K., et al.: Macrolide resistance in bacteremic pneumococcal disease: Implications for patient management. Clin. Infect. Dis. 43:432-438, 2006.
30. Daum, R. S., Granoff, D. M., Mäkelä, P. H., et al. (guest eds.): Epidemiology, pathogenesis, and prevention of Haemophilus influenzae disease. J. Infect. Dis. 165(Suppl. 1):S1-S206, 1992.
31. Doern, G. V., Brueggemann, A. B., Pierce, G., et al.: Antibiotic resistance among clinical isolates of Haemophilus influenzae in the United States in 1994-1995 and detection of β-lactamase-positive strains resistant to amoxicillin-clavulanate: Results of a national multicenter surveillance study. Antimicrob. Agents Chemother. 41:292-297, 1997.
32. Doern, G. V., Heilman, K. P., Huynh, H. K., et al.: Antimicrobial resistance among clinical isolates of Streptococcus pneumoniae in the United States during 1999-2000 including a comparison of resistance rates since 1994-1995. Antimicrob. Agents Chemother. 45:1721-1729, 2001.
33. Doern, G. V., Richter, S. S., Miller, A., et al.: Antimicrobial resistance among Streptococcus pneumoniae in the United States: Have we begun to turn the corner on resistance to certain antimicrobial classes? Clin. Infect. Dis. 41:1139-1148, 2005.
34. Dowell, S. F., Kupronis, B. A., Zell, E. R., and Shay, D. K.: Mortality from pneumonia in children in the United States, 1939 through 1996. N. Engl. J. Med. 342:1399-1407, 2000.
35. Edelstein, P. H.: Antimicrobial chemotherapy for legionnaires' disease: A review. Clin. Infect. Dis. 21(Suppl. 3):S265-S276, 1995.
36. Finland, M., Barnes, M. W., and Samper, B. A.: Influenza virus isolations and serological studies made in Boston during the winter of 1943-1944. J. Clin. Invest. 24:192-208, 1945.
37. Finland, M., Ory, E. M., Meads, M., et al.: Influenza and pneumonia: Serological studies during and after an outbreak of influenza. Br. J. Lab. Clin. Med. 33:32-46, 1948.
38. Finland, M., Peterson, O. L., and Strauss, E.: Staphylococcic pneumonia occurring during an epidemic of influenza. Arch. Intern. Med. 70:183-205, 1942.
39. Flannery, B., Schrag, S., Bennett, N. M., et al.: Impact of childhood vaccination on racial disparities in invasive Streptococcus pneumoniae infections. J. A. M. A. 291:2197-2203, 2004.
40. Friedland, E. R., and McCracken, G. H., Jr.: Management of infections caused by antibiotic-resistant Streptococcus pneumoniae. N. Engl. J. Med. 331:377-382, 1994.

41. Gessner, B. D., Sutanto, A., Linehan, M., et al.: Incidence of vaccine-preventable Haemophilus influenzae type b pneumonia and meningitis in Indonesian children: Hamlet-randomised vaccine-probe trial. Lancet 365:43-52, 2005.
42. Ginsburg, C. M., Howard, J. B., and Nelson, J. D.: Report of 65 cases of Haemophilus influenzae b pneumonia. Pediatrics 64:283-286, 1979.
43. Glikman, D., Matushek, S. M., Kahana, M. D., and Daum, R. S.: Pneumonia and empyema caused by penicillin-resistant Neisseria meningitidis: A case report and literature review. Pediatrics 117:e1061-e1066, 2006.
44. Goldwater, P. N., and Rice, M. S.: Primary meningococcal pneumonia in a nineteen-month-old child. Pediatr. Infect. Dis. J. 14:155-156, 1995.
45. Hager, T.: The Demon Under the Microscope: From Battlefield Hospitals to Nazi Labs, One Doctor's Heroic Search for the World's First Miracle Drug. New York, Harmony Books, 2006.
46. Hall, C. B., Powell, K. R., Schnabel, K. C., et al.: Risk of secondary bacterial infection in infants hospitalized with respiratory syncytial viral infection. J. Pediatr. 113:266-271, 1988.
47. Hansen, J., Black, S., Shinefield, H., et al.: Effectiveness of heptavalent pneumococcal conjugate vaccine in children younger than 5 years of age for prevention of pneumonia: Updated analysis using World Health Organization standardized interpretation of chest radiographs. Pediatr. Infect. Dis. J. 25:779-781, 2006.
48. Harari, M., Shann, F., Spooner, V., et al.: Clinical signs of pneumonia in children. Lancet 338:928-930, 1991.
49. Hawkins, J. A., Scaife, E. S., Hillman, N. D., and Feola, G. P.: Current treatment of pediatric empyema. Semin. Thorac. Cardiovasc. Surg. 16:193-200, 2004.
50. Heffron, R.: Pneumonia with Special Reference to Pneumococcus Lobar Pneumonia. New York, Commonwealth Fund, 1939, pp. 308, 312, 549; reissued by Harvard University Press, Boston, 1979.
51. Hersh, J. H., Gold, R., and Lepow, M. L.: Meningococcal group Y pneumonia in an adolescent female. J. Pediatr. 64:222-224, 1979.
52. Jacobs, M. R., Bajaksouzian, S., Zilles, A., et al.: Susceptibilities of Streptococcus pneumoniae and Haemophilus influenzae to 10 oral antimicrobial agents based on pharmacodynamic parameters: 1997 US surveillance study. Antimicrob. Agents Chemother. 43:1901-1908, 1999.
53. Jacobs, N. M., and Harris, V. J.: Acute Haemophilus pneumonia in childhood. Am. J. Dis. Child. 133:603-605, 1979.
54. Jacobs, R. F.: Nosocomial pneumonia in children. Infection 19:64-72, 1991.
55. Kass, E. H. (ed.): Assessment of the pneumococcal polysaccharide vaccine. Rev. Infect. Dis. 3(Suppl.):S1-S197, 1981.
56. Keefer, C. S., Blake, F. G., Marshall, E. K., Jr., et al.: Penicillin in the treatment of infections: A report of 500 cases. J. A. M. A. 122:1217-1224, 1943.
57. Klein, J. O., and Gellis, S. S.: Diagnostic needle aspiration in pediatric practice. Pediatr. Clin. North Am. 18:219-231, 1971.
58. Klein, J. O., Green, G. M., Tilles, J. G., et al.: Effect of intranasal reovirus infection on antibacterial activity of mouse lung. J. Infect. Dis. 119:43-50, 1969.
59. Korppi, M.: Physical signs in childhood pneumonia. Pediatr. Infect. Dis. J. 14:405-406, 1995.
60. Kovatch, A. L., Jardine, D. S., Dowling, J. N., et al.: Legionellosis in children with leukemia in relapse. Pediatrics 73:811-815, 1984.
61. Le Monnier, A., Carbonnelle, E., Zahar, J.-R., et al.: Microbiological diagnosis of empyema in children: Comparative evaluations by culture, polymerase chain reaction, and pneumococcal antigen detection in pleural fluids. Clin. Infect. Dis. 42:1135-1140, 2006.
62. Levine, O. S., Lagos, R., Munoz, A., et al.: Defining the burden of pneumonia in children preventable by vaccination against Haemophilus influenzae type b. Pediatr. Infect. Dis. J. 18:1060-1064, 1999.
63. MacLeod, C. M., Hodges, R., Heidelberger, M., et al.: Prevention of pneumococcal pneumonia by immunization. J. Exp. Med. 82:445-465, 1945.
64. Mahdi, S. A., Klugman, K. P., and The Vaccine Trialist Group: A role for Streptococcus pneumoniae in virus-associated pneumonia. Nat. Med. 10:811-813, 2004.
65. Madhi, S. A., Ludewick, H., Kuwanda, L., et al.: Pneumococcal co-infection with human metapneumovirus. J. Infect. Dis. 193:1236-1243, 2006.
66. Mankhambo, L. A., Chiwaya, K. W., Phiri, A., and Graham, S. M.: Lobar pneumonia caused by nontyphoidal Salmonella in a Malawian child. Pediatr. Infect. Dis. J. 25:1190-1192, 2006.
67. Marik, P. E.: Aspiration pneumonitis and aspiration pneumonia. N. Engl. J. Med. 344:665-671, 2001.
68. Marshall, R., Teele, D. W., and Klein, J. O.: Unsuspected bacteremia due to Haemophilus influenzae: Outcome in children not initially admitted to hospital. J. Pediatr. 95:690-695, 1979.
69. Martin, C. M., Kunin, C. M., Gottlieb, L. S., et al.: Asian influenza A in Boston, 1957-1958, II: Severe staphylococcal pneumonia complicating influenza. Arch. Intern. Med. 103:532-542, 1959.
70. McLaughlin, F. J., Goldmann, D. A., Rosenbaum, D. M., et al.: Empyema in children: Clinical course and long-term follow-up. Pediatrics 73:587-593, 1984.
71. Michelow, I. C., Lozano, J., Olsen, K., et al.: Diagnosis of Streptococcus pneumoniae lower respiratory infection in hospitalized children by culture, polymerase chain reaction, serology and urinary antigen. Clin. Infect. Dis. [Pubmed:] 34:E1-11 34:134, 2002.
72. Molteni, R. A.: Group a beta-hemolytic streptococcal pneumonia: Clinical course and complications of management. Am. J. Dis. Child. 131:1366-1371, 1977.

73. Muldoon, R. L., Jaecker, D. L., and Kiefer, H. K.: Legionnaires' disease in children. Pediatrics 67:329-332, 1981.
74. Myers, C., Corbelli, R., Schrenzel, J., and Gervaix, A.: Multiple pulmonary abscesses caused by *Legionella pneumophila* infection in an infant with croup. Pediatr. Infect. Dis. J. 25:753-754, 2006.
75. Nohynek, H., Eskola, J., Laine, E., et al.: The causes of hospital-treated acute lower respiratory tract infection in children. Am. J. Dis. Child. 145:618-622, 1991.
76. Nohynek, H., Valkeila, E., Leinonen, M., et al.: Erythrocyte sedimentation rate, white blood cell count and serum C-reactive protein in assessing etiologic diagnosis of acute lower respiratory infections in children. Pediatr. Infect. Dis. J. 14:484-490, 1995.
77. O'Brien, K. L., Walters, M. I., Sellman, J., et al.: Severe pneumococcal pneumonia in previously healthy children: The role of preceding influenza infection. Clin. Infect. Dis. 30:784-789, 2000.
78. Olcay, L., Secmeer, G., Gogus, S., and Akcoren, Z.: Pathological case of the month: Fatal hemorrhagic staphylococcal pneumonia. Arch. Pediatr. Adolesc. Med. 149:925-926, 1995.
79. Orenstein, W. A., Overturf, G. D., Leedom, J. M., et al.: The frequency of *Legionella* infection prospectively determined in children hospitalized with pneumonia. J. Pediatr. 99:403-406, 1981.
80. Pallares, R., Linares, J., Vadillo, M., et al.: Resistance to penicillin and cephalosporin and mortality from severe pneumococcal pneumonia in Barcelona, Spain. N. Engl. J. Med. 333:474-480, 1995.
81. Panitch, H. B.: Evaluation of recurrent pneumonia. Pediatr. Infect. Dis. J. 24:265-266, 2005.
82. Peerless, A. G., Liebhaber, M., Anderson, S., et al.: *Legionella* pneumonia in chronic granulomatous disease. J. Pediatr. 106:783-785, 1985.
83. Pichichero, M.: A review of evidence supporting the American Academy of Pediatrics recommendation for prescribing cephalosporin antibiotics for penicillin-allergic patients. Pediatrics 115:1048-1057, 2005.
84. Podolsky, S. H.: Pneumonia Before Antibiotics: Therapeutic Evolution and Evaluation in Twentieth-Century America. Baltimore, Johns Hopkins University Press, 2006.
85. Potter, A. R., and Fischer, G. W.: *Haemophilus influenzae*, the predominant cause of bacterial pneumonia in Hawaii. Pediatr. Res. 11:504, 1977.
86. Programme for the Control of Acute Respiratory Infections: Acute Respiratory Infections in Children: Case Management in Small Hospitals in Developing Countries. Geneva, World Health Organization, 1990.
87. Quie, P. G., Giebink, G. S., and Winkelstein, J. A. (guest eds.): The pneumococcus. Rev. Infect. Dis. 3:183-396, 1981.
88. Renner, E. D., Helms, C. M., Hierholzer, W. J., Jr., et al.: Legionnaires' disease in pneumonia patients in Iowa: A retrospective seroepidemiologic study, 1972-1977. Ann. Intern. Med. 90:603-606, 1979.
89. Rusconi, R., Castagneto, M., Gagliardi, L., et al.: Reference values for respiratory rate in the first 3 years of life. Pediatrics 94:350-355, 1994.
90. Salo, P., Ortqvist, A., and Leinonen, M.: Diagnosis of bacteremic pneumococcal pneumonia by amplification of pneumolysin gene fragment in serum. J. Infect. Dis. 171:479-482, 1995.
91. Schultz, K. D., Fan, L., Pinsky, J., et al.: The changing face of pleural empyemas in children: Epidemiology and management. Pediatrics 113:1735-1740, 2004.
92. Shann, F.: The management of pneumonia in children in developing countries. Clin. Infect. Dis. 21(Suppl. 3):S218-S225, 1995.
93. Shann, F: *Haemophilus influenzae* pneumonia: Type b or non-type b? Lancet 354:1488-1490, 1999.
94. Shann, F., Germer, S., Hazlett, D., et al.: Aetiology of pneumonia in children in Goroka Hospital, Papua New Guinea. Lancet 2:537-541, 1984.
95. Shann, F., and Steinhoff, M. C.: Vaccines for children in rich and poor countries. Lancet 354:7-11, 1999.
96. Simoes, E. A. F., and McGrath, E. J.: Recognition of pneumonia by primary health care workers in Swaziland with a simple clinical algorithm. Lancet 340:1502-1503, 1992.
97. Steinhoff, M. C. (ed.): Belagio conference on the pathogenesis and prevention of pneumonia in children in developing regions. Rev. Infect. Dis. 13(Suppl. 6), 1991.
98. Talbot, R. R., Poehling, K. A., Hartert, T. V., et al.: Elimination of racial differences in invasive pneumococcal disease in young children after introduction of the conjugate pneumococcal vaccine. Pediatr. Infect. Dis. J. 23:726-731, 2004.
99. Teele, D. W., Pelton, S. E., Grant, J. A., et al.: Bacteremia in febrile children under 2 years of age: Results of cultures of blood of 600 consecutive febrile children seen in a "walk-in" clinic. J. Pediatr. 87:227-231, 1975.
100. Thornsberry, C., Ogilvie, P. T., Holley, H. P., Jr., and Sahm, D. F.: Survey of susceptibilities of *Streptococcus pneumoniae*, *Haemophilus influenzae* and *Moraxella catarrhalis* isolates to 26 antimicrobial agents: A prospective US study. Antimicrob. Agents Chemother. 43:2612-2623, 1999.
101. Tillett, W. S., Cambier, M. J., and Harris, W. H., Jr.: Sulfonamide-fast pneumococci: A clinical report of two cases of pneumonia together with experimental studies on the effectiveness of penicillin and tyrothricin against sulfonamide-resistant strains. J. Clin. Invest. 22:249-255, 1943.
102. Tleyjeh, I., Tlaygeh, H. M., Hejal, R., et al.: The impact of penicillin resistance on short-term mortality in hospitalized adults with pneumococcal pneumonia: A systematic review and meta-analysis. Clin. Infect. Dis. 42:778-797, 2006.
103. Trujillo, M., and McCracken, G. H., Jr.: Prolonged morbidity in children with group A beta-hemolytic streptococcal pneumonia. Pediatr. Infect. Dis. J. 13:411-412, 1994.
104. Tuomanen, E. I., Austrian, R., and Masure, H. R.: Pathogenesis of pneumococcal infection. N. Engl. J. Med. 332:1280-1284, 1995.
105. Turner, R. B., Hayden, F. G., and Hendley, J. O.: Counterimmunoelectrophoresis of urine for diagnosis of bacterial pneumonia in pediatric outpatients. Pediatrics 71:780-783, 1983.
106. Valery, P. C., Torzillo, P. J., Mulholland, K., et al.: Hospital-based case-control study of bronchiectais in indigenous children in central Australia. Pediatr. Infect. Dis. J. 23:902-908, 2004.
107. Vuori-Holopainen, E., and Peltola, H.: Reappraisal of lung tap: Review of an old method for better etiologic diagnosis of childhood pneumonia. Clin. Infect. Dis. 32:715-726, 2001.
108. Wall, R. A., Corrah, P. T., Mabey, D. C. W., et al.: The etiology of lobar pneumonia in the Gambia. Bull. World Health Organ. 64:553-558, 1986.
109. Ward, J. I., Tsai, T. F., Filice, G. A., et al.: Prevalence of ampicillin- and chloramphenicol-resistant strains of *Haemophilus influenzae* causing meningitis and bacteremia: National survey of hospital laboratories. J. Infect. Dis. 138:421-424, 1978.
110. Wardlaw, T., Salarna, P., Johansson, E. W., and Mason, E.: Pneumonia: The leading killer of children. Lancet 368:1048-1050, 2006.
111. Watson, A. M., Boyce, T. G., and Wylam, M. E.: *Legionella* pneumonia: Infection during immunosuppressive therapy for idiopathic pulmonary hemosiderosis. Pediatr. Infect. Dis. J. 23:82-84, 2004.
112. Watson, D. A., Musher, D. M., Jacobson, J. W., et al.: A brief history of the pneumococcus in biomedical research: A panoply of scientific discovery. Clin. Infect. Dis. 17:913-924, 1993.
113. Weinberg, G. A., Ghafoor, A., Ishaq, Z., et al.: Clonal analysis of *Hemophilus influenzae* isolated from children from Pakistan with lower respiratory tract infections. J. Infect. Dis. 160:634-643, 1989.
113a. White, B.: The biology of the pneumococcus. Oxford University Press, London, 1938.
114. Winstead, J. M., McKinsey, D. S., Tasker, S., et al.: Meningococcal pneumonia: Characterization and review of cases seen over the past 25 years. Clin. Infect. Dis. 30:87-94, 2000.
115. Zaki, S. R., Shieh, W.-J., and the Epidemic Working Group at Ministry of Health in Nicaragua, Pan American Health Organization, U.S. Department of Agriculture, and Centers for Disease Control and Prevention: Leptospirosis associated with outbreak of acute febrile illness and pulmonary hemorrhage, Nicaragua, 1995. Lancet 347:535-536, 1996.
116. Zhang, Y., Isaacman, D. J., Wadowsky, R. M., et al.: Detection of *Streptococcus pneumoniae* in whole blood by PCR. J. Clin. Microbiol. 33:596-601, 1995.

CHAPTER 28

CHILDREN'S INTERSTITIAL LUNG DISEASE AND HYPERSENSITIVITY PNEUMONITIS

Minh L. Doan ⊙ Leland L. Fan

Children's interstitial lung disease (ILD) encompasses a large, heterogeneous group of mostly rare, diffuse lung disorders of known and unknown etiology.[43] In many of these disorders, injury to the alveolar wall gives rise to an inflammatory response with subsequent repair that potentially can lead to pulmonary fibrosis.

Infections of the lung, either chronic or acute with postinfectious sequelae, form the largest category of children's ILD in the immunocompetent and immunocompromised host. This chapter focuses on the entities that are caused by or associated with infection and the entities that mimic community-acquired pneumonia.

CLASSIFICATION

Table 28–1 presents a general classification of children's ILD. Although a complete description of each disorder is beyond the scope of this chapter, certain conditions warrant brief mention because major differences exist between adult ILD and children's ILD in terms of types and distribution of disease. Usual interstitial pneumonitis, a progressive and fatal disorder, is the most common form of adult idiopathic ILD, but it probably does not occur in children. Also, hypersensitivity pneumonitis (HP) in adults is caused by a variety of occupational exposures but in children usually is caused by exposures to avian antigen. In addition, several entities, such as neuroendocrine cell hyperplasia of infancy and pulmonary interstitial glycogenosis, have been identified more recently and seem to be unique to infants and young children. Finally, the genetic basis for certain types of familial lung diseases has been linked to mutations in genes involved in surfactant metabolism.[97,98,131] With the exception of surfactant protein C deficiency, because of high mortality rates, these disorders have been found mostly in children.

DISORDERS ASSOCIATED WITH INFECTION

The role of infectious agents, such as adenovirus,[146] influenza,[76] *Mycoplasma*,[137] and *Chlamydia*,[56] in the development of chronic lung disease in children has been well documented. Virtually any organism that infects the lower respiratory tract is capable of producing chronic, diffuse lung disease if the injury is severe

TABLE 28–1 Classification of Pediatric Interstitial Lung Diseases

Pediatric Interstitial Lung Diseases of Known Etiology
Aspiration syndromes
Chronic infection (viral, bacterial, fungal, parasitic)
  Immunocompetent host
  Immunocompromised host
Bronchopulmonary dysplasia
Hypersensitivity pneumonitis (and other environmental exposures)
Lipid storage diseases
Pulmonary alveolar microlithiasis

Pediatric Interstitial Lung Diseases of Unknown Etiology
Primary Pulmonary Disorders
Desquamative interstitial pneumonitis
Lymphocytic interstitial pneumonitis and related disorders
Nonspecific interstitial pneumonitis
Cryptogenic organizing pneumonia
Alveolar hemorrhage syndromes
Pulmonary infiltrates with eosinophilia
Bronchiolitis obliterans
Pulmonary alveolar proteinosis
Pulmonary vascular disorders (proliferative and congenital)
Pulmonary lymphatic disorders

Systemic Disorders with Pulmonary Involvement
Connective tissue disease
Malignancies
Histiocytosis
Sarcoidosis
Neurocutaneous syndromes

Unique Forms of Interstitial Lung Disease in Infancy
Lung growth abnormalities[152]
Neuroendocrine cell hyperplasia of infancy[108]
Follicular bronchitis/bronchiolitis[63]
Cellular interstitial pneumonitis of infancy[123]/pulmonary interstitial glycogenosis[13]
Acute idiopathic pulmonary hemorrhage of infancy[36]
Chronic pneumonitis of infancy[68]/inborn errors of surfactant metabolism[97,98,131]

enough, although most infected children have acute, self-limited disease that resolves completely.

Bronchiolitis Obliterans

Probably the best example of postinfectious chronic lung disease is found in children who develop bronchiolitis obliterans after having severe adenovirus pneumonia.[146] Bronchiolitis obliterans is characterized by a fibrosing process of the small airways that results in severe, irreversible obstruction of the airways. Clinically, patients present with tachypnea, crackles, wheezing, and a productive cough that persist for more than 6 weeks after the initial illness. Chest radiographs show air trapping and atelectasis; on high-resolution computed tomography (CT) scans, mosaic perfusion, central bronchiectasis, vascular attenuation, and atelectasis are common findings.[24] Occasionally, severe involvement of one lung leads to the development of a unilateral, small, hyperlucent lung, known as Swyer-James syndrome.[146]

Patients with severe adenovirus pneumonia have been shown to have immune complexes containing adenovirus antigen in the lung and increased serum levels of interleukin-6, interleukin-8, and tumor necrosis factor-α.[92,93] These studies suggest that abnormal or excessive host immunologic and inflammatory responses may be important in the development of chronic lung disease from adenovirus in infants and young children. Although lower respiratory tract infection with respiratory syncytial virus, parainfluenza, influenza, measles, varicella,[148] *Mycoplasma*, and pertussis[18] also can result in bronchiolitis obliterans, adenovirus is the most common etiologic agent. The need for mechanical ventilation during the initial illness is a strong independent risk factor for the subsequent development of bronchiolitis obliterans.[24]

Lymphocytic Interstitial Pneumonitis

Well recognized because it is an acquired immunodeficiency syndrome (AIDS)–defining condition in children infected with human immunodeficiency virus (HIV),[15] lymphocytic interstitial pneumonitis (LIP) also occurs in association with autoimmune disorders[81,141] and other immunodeficiencies[22] and in idiopathic and familial forms.[99] LIP is not a true interstitial pneumonitis but rather is a form of pulmonary lymphoproliferative disease. It is characterized histologically by a diffuse infiltrate of mature lymphocytes, along with smaller numbers of plasma cells and histiocytes, in the pulmonary interstitium and alveolar wall.[70,71] The infiltrate also may be found along lymphatic pathways and is evident in the bronchovascular bundle and interlobular septa, but it usually spares the pleura. The lymphocytes are small noncleaved cells that may accumulate as small nodules, sometimes with germinal centers. Generally, the lymphocytes are polyclonal, with B cells and a variety of T cells being identified.[106] Although Epstein-Barr virus has been isolated from the lungs of some AIDS-infected[4,39] and non–AIDS-infected patients with LIP,[85] its role in the development of LIP is unclear. Neither fibrosis nor airspace disease is prominent in this disease.

LIP occurs in 30 percent of children infected perinatally with HIV and typically manifests between the second and third years of life with an insidious onset of cough, tachypnea, dyspnea, and hypoxemia.[65,106,117-119,125] Chest radiographs characteristically reveal a diffuse, symmetric reticulonodular or nodular pattern, occasionally with mediastinal or hilar adenopathy.[86] Among HIV-infected children, the incidence of acute lower respiratory tract infection is higher in children with LIP,[128] and these patients ultimately may develop bronchiectasis.[130]

Other Conditions

Other pediatric chronic lung diseases have been associated with various infectious agents. Perinatal infection or colonization with

Ureaplasma urealyticum has been implicated in inducing pulmonary inflammation and subsequent development of bronchopulmonary dysplasia in premature neonates.[64] A more recent meta-analysis suggested, however, that reporting bias may be partially responsible for this association.[122] Parvovirus has been linked to autoimmune disease associated with ILD and other organ involvement.[9] Finally, attempts have been made to link *Stachybotrys chartarum* and its mycotoxins to acute and recurrent pulmonary hemorrhage in infants, although a causal relationship has not been proven.

In a prospective study of immunocompetent children with chronic diffuse infiltrates, Fan and coworkers[45] found an infectious agent as the underlying cause in 10 (20%) of 51 children with ILD. Identified agents included adenovirus alone in four patients, adenovirus and cytomegalovirus in two, varicella in one, Epstein-Barr virus in one, *Chlamydia* in one, and *Toxocara* in one. Chronic infections or long-term sequelae from acute infections account for many cases of ILD of known etiology in children.

ENTITIES THAT MAY MIMIC COMMUNITY-ACQUIRED PNEUMONIA
Acute Eosinophilic Pneumonia

Acute eosinophilic pneumonia is the most severe form of the idiopathic eosinophilic pneumonias. It is characterized by very large numbers of eosinophils infiltrating the alveoli and interstitium, with resultant acute respiratory failure. Acute eosinophilic pneumonia can be idiopathic or result from inciting triggers such as drugs (minocycline, sertraline) and inhalational exposures (new-onset cigarette smoking). Patients present with acute onset of fever, cough, tachypnea, and dyspnea; pleuritic chest pain; and myalgias. On examination, crackles are present in 80 percent of patients; wheezing is a rare manifestation. Hypoxemia is uniformly present, and patients can progress rapidly to respiratory failure. In contrast to patients with other eosinophilic lung diseases, patients with acute eosinophilic pneumonia generally do not have significant peripheral eosinophilia (>350 cells/mm³) on presentation as a diagnostic clue. Chest radiographs and CT scans show reticular markings with Kerley B lines and alveolar infiltrates and pleural effusions in 50 percent of cases. Bronchoalveolar lavage (BAL) fluid shows marked eosinophilia (>20%) in most patients. Pleural fluid also has increased eosinophils and a high pH, caused by the basic eosinophil granule contents. Treatment with corticosteroids (methylprednisolone, 2 to 4 mg/kg/day) usually results in a rapid and complete resolution.[3,113]

Pulmonary Vasculitis

In children, the spectrum of pulmonary vasculitides includes Wegener granulomatosis, Churg-Strauss syndrome, microscopic polyangiitis, and pulmonary capillaritis. These disorders can manifest as diffuse alveolar hemorrhage, with fever, dyspnea, hemoptysis (not present in one third of patients), anemia, and patchy alveolar infiltrates on chest radiographs. Other patients may have fever and cavitary or nodular lesions on imaging.[60] Diffuse alveolar hemorrhage can be diagnosed with BAL, when sequentially recovered aliquots of fluid show persistently bloody return. Renal involvement may be present sometimes, with microscopic hematuria and red blood cell casts seen on urinalysis. A positive serum antineutrophil cytoplasmic antibody (ANCA) may be seen with Wegener granulomatosis (especially cytoplasmic ANCA), Churg-Strauss syndrome, and microscopic polyangiitis, and the presence of peripheral and pulmonary eosinophilia would support the diagnosis of Churg-Strauss syndrome.[11] Pulmonary capillaritis is associated with a variety of conditions and requires an open lung biopsy for diagnosis because it may

manifest as an ANCA-negative, hematuria-negative diffuse alveolar hemorrhage syndrome.[52] Therapeutic options for pulmonary vasculitis include systemic corticosteroids, cyclophosphamide, and intravenous immunoglobulin; aggressive treatment is required in severe cases.

Connective Tissue Disorders

Pulmonary manifestations can precede other systemic findings in children with systemic lupus erythematosus[23] and juvenile rheumatoid arthritis,[114] and these patients may present with acute respiratory symptoms associated with fever. In acute lupus pneumonitis, signs and symptoms include high fevers, dyspnea, tachypnea, crackles, and cyanosis. Chest radiographs may show areas of consolidation and pleural effusions and interstitial infiltrates and elevation of the hemidiaphragms.[87] Other pulmonary manifestations of systemic lupus erythematosus include pulmonary hemorrhage, pulmonary hypertension, ILD, pneumothorax, and shrinking lung syndrome. Multisystem involvement, including renal and skin, may provide clues to the underlying diagnosis. Treatment usually requires corticosteroids.[23]

Hypersensitivity Pneumonitis

Acute and chronic HP can manifest with fever, cough, dyspnea, and pulmonary infiltrates. HP is discussed in detail later.

CLINICAL PRESENTATION

Most children with ILD have insidious symptoms that may go unrecognized for years. Some children have been misdiagnosed as having asthma and have been treated with bronchodilators.[49] Although a history of wheezing can be elicited in half of patients, it can be documented by physical examination in only approximately 20 percent of cases. Clinical suspicion for children's ILD should arise when patients meet at least three of the four following criteria: (1) presenting symptoms of dyspnea, tachypnea, retractions, cough, exercise intolerance, or respiratory failure; (2) presenting signs of crackles, failure to thrive, clubbing, or respiratory failure; (3) hypoxemia; and (4) diffuse abnormality on chest radiographs or CT not attributable to other known processes.[42]

A careful history should be taken to assess the severity of the disease and to obtain information that may contribute to establishing a diagnosis. A search for precipitating factors should include a history of feeding difficulties that may suggest aspiration; any prior acute or severe respiratory infections; and environmental exposures, especially to birds or molds. Hemoptysis may indicate a pulmonary vascular disorder or hemosiderosis. Joint disease or rash may indicate a systemic process, such as a connective tissue disease. A family history of relatives or siblings with similar respiratory conditions may be clues to genetic or familial lung diseases, such as a defect in surfactant proteins.

On physical examination, tachypnea and retractions often are observed, and crackles commonly are heard, particularly at the bases. In severe cases, cyanosis, clubbing, an accentuated pulmonic component of the second heart sound, and evidence of growth failure are seen. Oxygen saturation usually is normal under all conditions in most patients with mild disease, but desaturation may occur with exercise or during sleep as the disease progresses, and ventilation-perfusion mismatch ensues. Patients with more advanced disease are hypoxemic at rest.

DIAGNOSTIC EVALUATION

A systematic approach to children's ILD is essential to physicians confronted with such a large differential of rare conditions.

TABLE 28–2 Diagnostic Studies for Pediatric Interstitial Lung Disease

To Assess Extent and Severity of Disease
Chest films, high-resolution computed tomography scans
Pulmonary function studies—spirometry, pulse oximetry and
    arterial blood gases (resting, sleeping, and with exercise),
    diffusion, pressure-volume curve, infant studies
Electrocardiogram, echocardiogram

To Identify Primary Disorders That Predispose to Interstitial
Lung Disease
HIV
Immune studies—immunoglobulins including IgE, skin tests for
    delayed hypersensitivity, response to immunizations, T and B
    subsets, complement, others as indicated
Barium swallow, pH probe
DNA analyses for mutations in the surfactant protein B, surfactant
    protein C, and *ABCA3* genes

To Identify Primary Interstitial Lung Disease
Antinuclear antibody
Angiotensin-converting enzyme
Antineutrophil cytoplasmic antibody
Antiglomerular basement membrane antibody
Hypersensitivity screen
Infectious disease evaluation—cultures, titers, skin tests
Cardiac catheterization (in selected cases)
Bronchoalveolar lavage and transbronchial biopsy
Transthoracic biopsy

HIV, human immunodeficiency virus.
From Fan, L. L.: Pediatric interstitial lung disease. In Schwarz, M. I., and King, T. E. (eds.): Interstitial Lung Disease, 4th ed. Hamilton, Ontario, B. C. Decker, 2003, pp. 134-151.

Diagnostic studies can be divided into studies used to assess the extent and severity of disease, to identify disorders that predispose to ILD, and to identify the primary ILD (Table 28–2). In adults with ILD, Raghu[109] suggested a diagnostic process that employs a thorough history and physical examination first, noninvasive tests next, and then invasive studies, including BAL and transbronchial biopsy followed by open lung biopsy if the previous less invasive studies do not provide a specific diagnosis. Based on experience from a retrospective chart review of 48 children with ILD, Fan and colleagues[49] independently developed an algorithm remarkably similar to that of Raghu's and used it prospectively in the evaluation of 51 children presenting with ILD.[45] In that study, a specific diagnosis was established by history and physical examination alone in 1 patient; noninvasive studies alone in 8 others; and invasive studies, including lung biopsy, in another 26. Of the remaining patients, eight had a suggestive diagnosis, and eight had no specific diagnosis. This study suggests that a systematic approach to the diagnosis of children's ILD is useful and that some patients can be diagnosed with noninvasive studies, but most patients require invasive studies, including lung biopsy.

PULMONARY FUNCTION TESTS

In children who are old enough to undergo pulmonary function tests, standard spirometry typically shows a pattern of restrictive lung disease, with reduced forced vital capacity (FVC), forced expiratory volume in 1 second (FEV$_1$), and a normal or elevated FEV$_1$/FVC ratio.[49] On measurement of lung volumes, although the total lung capacity (TLC) often is low, the residual volume (RV) may be normal or elevated, resulting in an increased RV/TLC ratio that suggests air trapping and a mixed restrictive/obstructive pattern. These findings also can be documented in infants and young children with the use of infant pulmonary function testing techniques.

HIGH-RESOLUTION COMPUTED TOMOGRAPHY

In the evaluation of children's ILD, high-resolution CT is an important diagnostic modality used to provide precise detail about the extent and distribution of parenchymal disease and to select favorable sites for biopsy. To evaluate the lung parenchyma best with CT scanning, thin sections are necessary to avoid the volume averaging that occurs with 2.5- to 5-mm sections, which obscures the fine parenchymal detail and airway abnormalities. High-resolution CT samples thin sections (usually 1 mm in thickness) at wide intervals (usually 10 mm). With the development of multidetector array or multislice CT, contiguous thin section studies of the entire chest can be performed in a shorter time and with less radiation exposure than with conventional CT.[10]

Inspiratory and expiratory CT scans should be obtained whenever possible. In younger children and infants in whom cooperation is impossible and in whom rapid respiratory rates can cause motion artifact, a controlled-ventilation CT technique using mask ventilation of a sedated patient can be used.[80] Giving several assisted deep breaths to these young children results in a short period of apnea during which the lungs can be inflated to obtain inspiratory images, followed by expiratory images after passive deflation. General anesthesia produces similar results, although frequent large sigh breaths are necessary to prevent dependent atelectasis, which occurs within minutes of intubation.

High-resolution CT may increase the level of diagnostic confidence for the diagnosis of children's ILD, improve diagnostic accuracy, and provide a useful classification system. In a study of 20 children with biopsy-proven ILD, 56 percent of the confident first-choice diagnoses on high-resolution CT were correct.[82] Diseases were classified into five distinct groups based on dominant high-resolution CT features: (1) geographic hyperlucency (bronchiolitis obliterans or bronchocentric granulomatosis), (2) septal thickening (lymphangiomatosis, hemangiomatosis, microlithiasis), (3) ground-glass opacification (desquamative interstitial pneumonitis, LIP, HP), (4) lung cysts and nodules (histiocytosis), and (5) consolidation (aspiration, bronchiolitis obliterans organizing pneumonia). First-choice diagnoses based on high-resolution CT were accurate in 61 percent of cases in a similar study.[25]

BRONCHOALVEOLAR LAVAGE

BAL via flexible bronchoscopy allows for sampling of the cellular and biochemical components of alveolar lining fluid and may be helpful in the evaluation of certain cases of children's ILD. Normal indices for pediatric BAL fluid have been described, against which abnormal results can be compared.[37]

The most common indication for pediatric BAL has been to detect infection in the immunocompromised host, with a diagnostic yield of approximately 50 percent in non–AIDS-infected patients and 75 percent in patients with AIDS.[41] The use of quantitative bacterial cultures may help to differentiate whether recovered organisms represent true infection, colonization, or contamination. Examination of BAL fluid also can identify aspiration or pulmonary hemorrhage by the detection of lipid-laden or hemosiderin-laden macrophages. The presence of lipid-laden or hemosiderin-laden macrophages in BAL may be sensitive but not specific for aspiration or alveolar hemorrhage syndromes.[48] In a murine model, investigators showed that hemosiderin-laden macrophages first appear at 3 days, peak at 1 week, and persist in small numbers for 2 months after a single episode of hemorrhage.[35] BAL also has been used to diagnose pulmonary alveolar proteinosis, lysosomal storage disorders, and histiocytosis.[48]

In immunocompetent children with ILD, Fan and colleagues[48] found that BAL was diagnostic of a primary disorder in only 5 of 29 patients—aspiration was detected in 3, and infection in 2. The differential diagnosis was narrowed in 15 patients by the presence of lymphocytosis, neutrophilia, or eosinophilia. A secondary disorder was uncovered in eight patients. This study suggests that BAL provides some useful information in children with ILD, but that its ability to determine the primary cause is limited.

LUNG BIOPSY

As in adult ILD, lung biopsy is the gold standard for establishing the diagnosis of children's ILD because most diseases are classified in terms of previously defined histopathologic patterns. Although transbronchial or percutaneous needle biopsy may be helpful in certain conditions, a transthoracic approach by either conventional open lung biopsy or video-assisted thoracoscopic surgery (VATS) remains the gold standard for obtaining tissue adequate for diagnosis.

The use of VATS is rapidly becoming the method of choice for lung biopsy in children. Technical modifications have allowed its use even in infants.[116] In a prospective study in a small group of immunocompetent children with ILD, Fan and coworkers[46] found that the diagnostic yield for open lung biopsy (57%) and VATS (54%) was comparable, but the morbidity from VATS was lower in terms of duration of surgery, chest tube insertion, and hospitalization.[46] Although multiple lobe biopsies directed by high-resolution CT have been advocated for the diagnosis of adult and children's ILD, this study did not show a difference in diagnostic yield for single-lobe versus multiple-lobe biopsies. Depending on the handling of the specimen and the expertise of the reviewing pathologist, the diagnostic yield from transthoracic lung biopsy (open lung biopsy and VATS) can be quite high, especially in light of the more recent advances in the understanding of children's ILD.

Lung biopsy material must be handled in a consistent manner to ensure optimal interpretation, and a protocol for such handling was published based on the recommendations of the chILD Pathology Group.[75] A general scheme for division of the biopsy specimen is as follows: (1) microbiology cultures, 35 percent; (2) snap-frozen for polymerase chain reaction or other molecular studies, 10 percent; (3) snap-frozen in cryomatrix for immuno-fluorescent, laser capture, or other studies requiring frozen sections, 10 percent; (4) fixed in glutaraldehyde for electron microscopy, less than 5 percent; (5) imprints for cytologic examination or rapid identification of organisms, 0 percent; and (6) expanded and fixed in formalin (methods previously described[47]) for light microscopy, 40 percent. It is crucial that the biopsy material be interpreted by a pathologist with considerable expertise in pediatric lung disease because the normal lung of an infant differs greatly from that of an older child or adolescent, and any pathologic finding needs to be interpreted in light of the normal age-dependent variations of lung architecture.

TREATMENT

Supportive care includes providing adequate nutrition, annual influenza vaccination, and aggressive treatment of intercurrent infections; engaging the patient in a carefully supervised fitness and exercise program; having the patient avoid inhalant hazards such as tobacco smoke; and providing selective use of bronchodilators and oxygen for chronic hypoxemia. Patients with underlying systemic disorders need primary treatment for that disorder, such as intravenous gamma globulin for hypogammaglobulinemia. Specific therapy for primary ILD, such as anti-infective therapy for chronic infections, interferon-α for pulmonary hem-

angiomatosis,[146] and lung lavage for pulmonary alveolar proteinosis, should be used when possible.[84] When environmental agents such as bird antigens are causative, avoiding contact with them is crucial (see the section on HP).

Generally, corticosteroids remain the treatment of choice for most patients with ILD on the presumption that suppression of inflammation may reduce the risk of developing fibrosis.[47] Although controlled clinical studies are lacking, corticosteroids have been used to treat such diverse types of diffuse lung diseases as desquamative interstitial pneumonitis, LIP, and HP.[41] In a retrospective study of pediatric ILD by Fan and coworkers,[49] corticosteroids were judged to be effective in 40 percent (12 of 30) of treated children in terms of improved clinical status, decreased oxygen requirements, and improved pulmonary function. A trial of prednisone or equivalent corticosteroid (1 to 2 mg/kg/day) for at least 6 to 8 weeks probably is warranted.

Alternative but unproven therapy includes pulse steroid therapy, hydroxychloroquine, azathioprine, cyclophosphamide, methotrexate, cyclosporine, and intravenous gamma globulin. Of these, hydroxychloroquine probably has been used most frequently.[5,49,128,133] The precise mechanism of action is unknown, but chloroquine and hydroxychloroquine have shown immunosuppressive effects with the ability to inhibit the functional capabilities of monocytes and the generation of antibody-forming cells. Hydroxychloroquine is preferred over chloroquine because the former has less retinal toxicity. The recommended dose in children for the treatment of ILD is 10 mg/kg/day. A more recent case report described the successful use of infliximab, an anti–tumor necrosis factor-α monoclonal antibody, in reversing bronchiolitis obliterans in a hematopoietic stem cell transplant recipient.[51]

The fact that many alternative pharmacologic approaches are considered for children and adults with ILD implies that conventional therapy often is ineffective. New strategies are being developed based on animal models of pulmonary fibrosis and more recent advances in the cellular and molecular biology of inflammatory reactions. Such therapies would be directed against the action of certain cytokines, oxidants, and growth factors that may be involved in the fibrotic process. The potential to deliver specific inflammatory inhibitors or inhibitors of collagen biosynthesis directly to the lung via aerosolization suggests that disease processes in the lung may be more amenable to novel therapies than are disease processes in other internal organs.

More children are receiving lung transplantation for end-stage ILD. According to the 2006 Registry of the International Society for Heart and Lung Transplantation, between 1991 and 2005, there were 30 reported pediatric lung transplantations worldwide for "idiopathic pulmonary fibrosis," 20 for "interstitial pneumonitis," 14 for "pulmonary fibrosis, other," 8 for "surfactant protein B deficiency," and 7 for "bronchopulmonary dysplasia," together constituting 9 percent of all pediatric lung transplantations.[144] Although the overall 5-year survival after transplantation is still disappointing at approximately 50 percent,[144] outcomes for infants undergoing transplantation for surfactant protein B deficiency seem to be at least similar to the outcomes of infants transplanted for other reasons.[104] A case of recurrent pulmonary alveolar proteinosis in the lung allografts of a child who underwent heart-lung transplantation for lysinuric protein intolerance has been reported.[121]

OUTCOME

The prognosis of children with ILD varies. Infants with neuroendocrine cell hyperplasia of infancy generally do well, although they may be symptomatic and require oxygen for years.[108] At the other end of the spectrum, children with growth failure, pulmonary hypertension, and severe fibrosis do poorly.

The overall mortality rates for children's ILD remain high. In a series of 25 children with fibrosing alveolitis or desquamative interstitial pneumonitis, Sharief and associates[129] reported a poor response to treatment in nine patients, with four deaths. In a review of 28 patients with desquamative interstitial pneumonitis, Stillwell and colleagues[136] reported that only 17 patients survived. In another series of children with a variety of more recently described ILD, Nicholson and coworkers[95] reported four deaths in 17 patients with available follow-up data.

Fan and Kozinetz[44] reviewed the outcome of 99 children with chronic ILD seen in Denver, Colorado, over 15 years (1980 to 1994). As expected, a wide variety of disorders were encountered, and 15 recorded deaths occurred, with a probability that a patient would survive to 24 months, 48 months, and 60 months after onset of symptoms of 83 percent, 72 percent, and 64 percent, respectively. Of the clinical features present at the time of initial evaluation, weight less than fifth percentile, crackles, clubbing, family history of ILD, and symptom duration were not associated with decreased survival rates. A severity of illness score, based on increasing levels of hypoxemia and the presence or absence of pulmonary hypertension, was related significantly to survival, with an increasing score associated with a higher probability of decreased survival rates. A simple scoring system seems to be a useful measure of outcome in children with ILD.

HYPERSENSITIVITY PNEUMONITIS

HP, also known as *extrinsic allergic alveolitis*, is a form of immune-mediated ILD that develops in response to repeated inhalation of finely dispersed organic antigens.[27] HP should be considered in the differential diagnosis of a child who presents with acute or chronic respiratory symptoms associated with fever, and obtaining an environmental exposure history is essential to arrive at the proper diagnosis. A wide variety of organic particles, including mammalian and avian proteins, fungi, thermophilic bacteria, and certain low-molecular-weight volatile and nonvolatile chemical compounds, are known to induce HP in susceptible individuals.[54] Certain systemic medications, such as ciprofloxacin,[134] dapsone,[140] and methotrexate,[28] also have been reported as triggers.

Acute and chronic forms of HP have been described, and repeated exposure can lead to irreversible lung damage. Although exposure to antigens capable of provoking HP occurs commonly in the home and work environment, the overall incidence of the condition in the general population is low. An estimated 5 to 15 percent of individuals exposed to high levels of a specific organic antigen develop clinical disease.

PATHOLOGY AND PATHOGENESIS

Pathologically, HP is characterized by a diffuse, predominantly mononuclear cell inflammation of the small airways and pulmonary parenchyma, often associated with poorly formed, nonnecrotizing granulomas.[126] Foamy macrophages are seen commonly in the airspaces. With advanced disease, interstitial and intra-alveolar fibrosis develops that is indistinguishable from other causes of pulmonary fibrosis.

The mechanisms by which organic dusts induce these characteristic pathologic features of the disease are poorly understood. Evidence supports a type III and a type IV hypersensitivity reaction, as defined by Gell and Coombs.[52b,77] A type III reaction is suggested by the presence of precipitating antibody to the offending antigen, immune complex deposition, and activation of complement. A type IV reaction is suggested by an increased percentage of T lymphocytes in BAL fluid, with a strong predominance of CD8⁺ subsets and a low CD4/CD8 ratio, and the

presence of granulomas on lung biopsy specimen. Considering the small proportion of exposed individuals who develop clinical symptoms, complex interactions among the nature of the antigen, the intensity and duration of the exposure, and the host response in susceptible individuals most likely are involved.

ETIOLOGY

As shown in Table 28–3, HP in adults is caused by a wide variety of occupational and environmental exposures.[126] In contrast, in children, HP is caused mainly by exposure to an array of domestic birds (71%) and fungi (28%), based on a review of 133 reported pediatric cases.* HP also has been reported in a child receiving methotrexate.[28] Familial cases have been identified, with one report describing a mother (who died from the disease) and all of her five children who developed HP from exposure to wild city pigeons.[32]

CLINICAL PRESENTATION

Although a wide variety of antigens can induce HP, the immunologic response and clinical presentation are similar. In the reported pediatric cases referenced previously, the mean age (± standard deviation) was 9.6 (± 3.9) years. The youngest reported patient with HP developed symptoms at 10 weeks of age.[139]

In the acute form, symptoms mimic a flulike illness, with high fevers, chills, dry cough, dyspnea, myalgias, and malaise. These symptoms begin several hours after exposure and diminish during the next 12 to 24 hours, provided that no additional exposure occurs. Physical examination reveals a dyspneic, ill-appearing child, often with bibasilar crackles. Transient hypoxemia and nodular pulmonary infiltrates often are present.

In the subacute form, children have insidious and progressive symptoms. In the reported pediatric cases in which the following specific symptoms were recorded, exercise intolerance was present in 97 percent (93 of 96), cough was present in 96 percent (101 of 105), weight loss was present in 87 percent (46 of 53), and fever was present in 70 percent (51 of 73). On physical examination, crackles were present in 72 percent (66 of 91), and clubbing was present in 35 percent (16 of 46) of cases. The chronic form of HP is an extension of the subacute form resulting from continued antigen exposure, with development of irreversible pulmonary fibrosis.

DIAGNOSIS

A careful and thorough environmental history is a critical component in detecting potential antigens. The presence of the following six predictors can help to establish a clinical diagnosis of HP in adults: (1) exposure to a known offending antigen, (2) positive precipitating antibodies to the offending antigen, (3) recurrent episodes of symptoms, (4) inspiratory crackles on physical examination, (5) symptoms occurring 4 to 8 hours after exposure, and (6) weight loss.[74] Compatible findings on chest radiographs (Fig. 28–1), pulmonary function testing, BAL, and open lung biopsy also aid in establishing the diagnosis.

Detecting precipitating IgG antibodies to the offending antigen can be useful in confirming the diagnosis in a patient with documented exposure and typical clinical features (Fig. 28–2). Fifty percent of individuals who are exposed to a particular antigen develop precipitating antibodies, however, and only a

---

*See references 1, 2, 6, 7, 12, 14, 16, 17, 20, 21, 29, 32-34, 38, 54, 55, 58, 59, 61, 62, 66, 67, 69, 72, 73, 78, 79, 88, 91, 94, 100, 102, 103, 105, 107, 112, 115, 120, 127, 135, 138, 139, 141, 143, 147, 149-151.

TABLE 28–3   Etiologic Agents of Hypersensitivity Pneumonitis

Disease	Antigen	Source
Fungal and Bacterial		
Farmer's lung	*Faeni rectivirgula*	Moldy hay, grain, silage
Ventilation pneumonitis; humidifier lung; air conditioner lung	*Thermoactinomyces vulgaris, Thermoactinomyces sacchari, Thermoactinomyces candidus, Klebsiella oxytoca*	Contaminated forced air systems, water reservoirs
Bagassosis	*T. vulgaris*	Moldy sugarcane (i.e., bagasse)
Mushroom worker's lung	*T. sacchari*	Moldy mushroom compost
Suberosis	*Thermoactinomyces viridis, Penicillium glabrum*	Moldy cork
Detergent lung; washing powder lung	*Bacillus subtilis* enzymes	Detergents (during processing or use)
Malt worker's lung	*Aspergillus fumigatus, Aspergillus clavatus*	Moldy barley
Sequoiosis	*Graphium, Pullularia,* and *Trichoderma* spp.; *Aureobasidium pullulans*	Moldy wood dust
Maple bark stripper's lung	*Cryptostroma corticale*	Moldy maple bark
Cheese washer's lung	*Penicillium casei, A. clavatus*	Moldy cheese
Woodworker's lung	*Alternaria* spp., wood dust	Oak, cedar, and mahogany dust; pine and spruce pulp
Paprika slicer's lung	*Mucor stolonifer*	Moldy paprika pods
Sauna taker's lung	*Aureobasidium* spp., other sources	Contaminated sauna water
Familial HP	*B. subtilis*	Contaminated wood dust in walls
Wood trimmer's lung	*Rhizopus* spp., *Mucor* spp.	Contaminated wood trimmings
Composter's lung	*T. vulgaris, Aspergillus* spp.	Compost
Basement shower HP	*Epicoccum nigrum*	Mold on unventilated shower
Hot-tub lung	*Cladosporium* spp.	Hot-tub mists, mold on ceiling
Wine maker's lung	*Botrytis cinerea*	Mold on grapes
Woodsman's disease	*Penicillium* spp.	Oak and maple trees
Thatched-roof lung	*Saccharomonospora viridis*	Dead grasses and leaves
Tobacco grower's lung	*Aspergillus* spp.	Tobacco plants
Potato riddler's lung	*Thermophilic actinomycetes, F. rectivirgula, T. vulgaris, Aspergillus* spp.	Moldy hay around potatoes
Summer-type pneumonia	*Trichosporon cutaneum*	Contaminated old houses
Dry rot lung	*Merulius lacrymans*	Rotten wood
Stipatosis	*A. fumigatus, T. actinomycetes*	Esparto dust
Machine operator's lung	*Pseudomonas fluorescens*	Aerosolized metal-working fluid
Amebae		
Humidifier lung	*Naegleria grubeni, Acanthamoeba polyphaga, Acanthamoeba castellani*	Contaminated water
Animal Proteins		
Pigeon breeder's or pigeon fancier's disease	Avian droppings, feathers, serum	Parakeets, budgerigars, pigeons, chickens, turkeys
Pituitary snuff taker's lung	Pituitary snuff	Bovine and porcine pituitary proteins
Fish meal worker's lung	Fish meal	Fish meal dust
Bat lung	Bat serum protein	Bat droppings
Furrier's lung	Animal fur dust	Animal pelts
Animal handler's lung; laboratory worker's lung	Rats, gerbils	Urine, serum, pelts, proteins
Insect Proteins		
Miller's lung	*Sitophilus granarius*	Dust-contaminated grain (i.e., wheat weevil)
Lycoperdonosis	Puffball spores	Lycoperdon puffballs
Chemical		
Pauli's reagent alveolitis	Sodium diazobenzene sulfate	Laboratory reagent
Chemical worker's lung	Isocyanates, trimellitic anhydride	Polyurethane foams, spray paints, elastomers, special glues
Vineyard sprayer's lung	Copper sulfate	Bordeaux mixture
Pyrethrum HP	Pyrethrum	Pesticide
Epoxy resin lung	Phthalic anhydride	Heated epoxy resin
Dental technician's lung	Methyl methacrylate	Dental prosthesis
Unknown		
Bible printer's lung		Moldy typesetting water
Coptic lung (mummy handler's lung)		Cloth wrappings of mummies
Grain measurer's lung		Cereal grain
Coffee worker's lung		Coffee bean dust
Tap water lung		Contaminated tap water
Tea grower's lung		Tea plants
Mollusk-shell HP		Sea-snail shell
Swimming pool worker's lung		Aerosolized endotoxin from pool water, sprays, and fountains

HP, hypersensitivity pneumonitis.
From Selman, M.: Hypersensitivity pneumonitis. In Schwarz, M. I., and King, T. E. (eds.): Interstitial Lung Disease, 4th ed. Hamilton, Ontario, B. C. Decker, 2003, pp. 452-484.

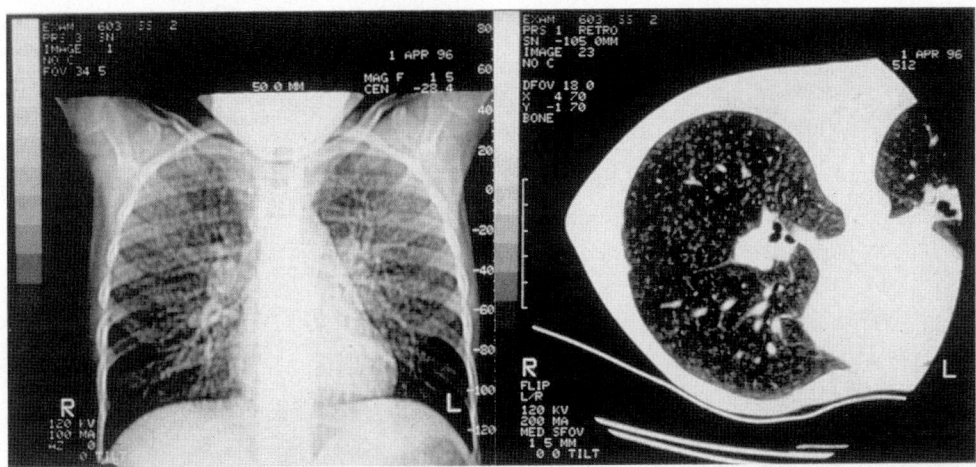

Figure 28–1 Hypersensitivity pneumonitis from cockatiel antigens in an adolescent. Chest radiograph shows bilateral reticulonodular infiltrates. High-resolution computed tomography scan shows diffuse, multiple fine nodules. *(Courtesy of Robin Deterding, M.D., University of Colorado, Denver, CO. From Fan, L. L. Pediatric interstitial lung disease. In Schwarz, M. I., and King, T. E. [eds.]: Interstitial Lung Disease, 4th ed. Hamilton, Ontario, B. C. Decker, 2003, pp. 134–151.)*

small percentage of these develop HP.[27] Long-term follow-up has shown that the simple presence of precipitins does not increase the likelihood of developing the condition.[26] Conversely, not all individuals with symptomatic HP have positive precipitins. In reported pediatric cases, positive precipitins were found in 93 percent (120 of 129) of the children tested. Because the quality of antigen material may vary in commercial laboratories, it is preferable to obtain a sample of the suspected antigen directly from the original source and test it against the patient's serum in a reputable laboratory. Researchers have reported using fluorometry to quantify serum IgG antibody against pigeon antigens, with decreasing antibody titers used as a measure of successful antigen avoidance.[89]

To document recurrence of symptoms shortly after exposure to a putative antigen, provocation challenge (inhalation of the antigen in controlled laboratory conditions) has been used in adults.[110] It has not been employed often in children, however, with only 23 of the 133 children reported in the literature having undergone such a challenge, in which 14 (61%) were positive. An in vitro measurement of antigen-induced lymphocyte proliferation compared with unstimulated lymphocyte cultures obtained from BAL or blood also has been described.[101]

Classic features of acute HP on chest radiographs and high-resolution CT scans include poorly defined centrilobular micronodules, with predominance in the upper and middle lung zones (see Fig. 28–1). On high-resolution CT, additional characteristic features are widespread ground-glass attenuation and air trapping, which is especially prominent on expiratory scans.[132] A small percentage of patients also may have lung cysts.[50] In the more chronic phase, diffuse interstitial infiltrates may predominate, with progression to fibrosis and honeycombing that are indistinguishable from usual interstitial pneumonia.[83] Instances

of negative CT examinations in patients with biopsy-proven disease have been reported.[57] In the reported pediatric cases of HP, chest radiographs were abnormal in 93 percent (113 of 132).

Pulmonary function tests typically show a restrictive defect, sometimes with an obstructive component. In reported pediatric cases, the mean (± standard deviation) FEV_1 and FVC in the children tested were 54.1 percent (± 19.8) and 52.4 percent (± 20.2) predicted. The pressure-volume curve is shifted down and to the right, consistent with decreased compliance. Low lung volumes and diminished diffusion capacity also are present.[32] Although resting room air oxygen saturation may be normal, desaturation with exercise or sleep may occur. With long-standing disease, resting oxygen desaturation can be seen. In the pediatric cases in which oxygenation was documented, 82 percent (59 of 72) had hypoxemia at rest. Pulmonary hypertension may be present with advanced disease, but in contrast to other forms of pediatric ILD, it may reverse completely with successful treatment.

BAL fluid, obtained by flexible fiberoptic bronchoscopy, typically shows a significant lymphocytosis. In adults, a low CD4/CD8 ratio frequently accompanies the lymphocytosis. The reported normal ratio (mean [± standard error of the mean]) varies from 1.9 (± 0.2) in young normal controls to 7.6 (± 1.5) in elderly controls.[90] Children with HP also have marked lymphocytosis in the BAL compared with healthy pediatric controls (80% versus 12%). Although the CD4/CD8 ratio also may be low compared with that of healthy adults, it is not significantly different from the ratio (0.6) reported in healthy children without lung disease.[111] As with positive precipitins, the presence of BAL lymphocytosis in exposed individuals who are asymptomatic does not predict the development of HP.[26] Analysis of induced sputum shows that it does not reflect accurately the lymphocytosis seen in BAL.[31]

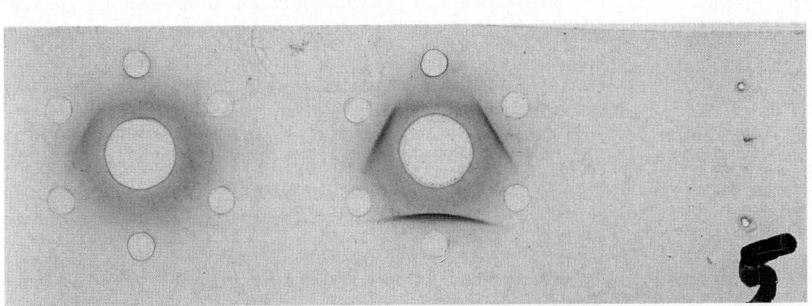

Figure 28–2 Serum-precipitating antibodies against cockatiel antigens in the patient shown in Figure 28-1. *(Courtesy of Robin Deterding, M.D., University of Colorado, Denver, CO.)*

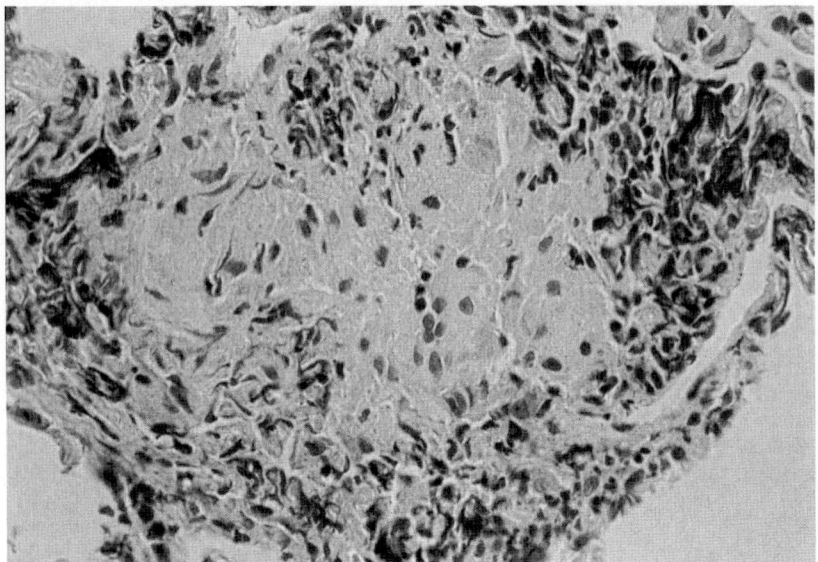

Figure 28–3 Transbronchial biopsy specimen from the patient in Figure 28–1 shows a poorly formed granuloma consistent with hypersensitivity pneumonitis. *(Courtesy of Robin Deterding, M.D., University of Colorado, Denver, CO.)*

Lung tissue obtained by transbronchial (limited to older children and adults) or transthoracic biopsy shows the characteristic histologic features described previously (Fig. 28–3). Of the 83 reported pediatric cases of HP, nine biopsy specimens were obtained, and all showed typical histologic changes.

TREATMENT AND OUTCOME

The mainstay of treatment is eliminating exposure to the offending antigen. In the literature, exposure was eliminated in 97 percent of the pediatric cases (100 of 103), with improvement achieved in all but one fatal case.

The use of corticosteroids often results in rapid improvement of symptoms and reversal of radiographic and lung function abnormalities unless irreversible changes in the lung have occurred. Corticosteroids were used in 70 percent (74 of 106) of the reported pediatric cases, with a positive response occurring in all but the one fatal case. Generally, prednisone was given at 0.5 to 2 mg/kg daily for 2 to 4 weeks, followed by a taper, although specific regimens have not been studied scientifically. Pulsed methylprednisolone also has been used.[19]

The outcome of children with HP, when properly diagnosed and treated, is excellent. In the 106 pediatric cases of HP with reported outcomes, 104 improved or became asymptomatic, 1 patient remained unchanged, and 1 patient died. In this last case, an 11-year-old girl developed classic features after several years of exposure to budgerigars and other birds.[143] Despite removal of the offending antigens and treatment with corticosteroids and penicillamine, she died of respiratory failure 13 months later. The overall prognosis for children with HP is excellent, provided that a prompt diagnosis is made and appropriate treatment consisting of antigen removal and the judicious use of corticosteroids is instituted.

REFERENCES

1. Aebischer, C. C., Frey, U., and Schoni, M. H.: Hypersensitivity pneumonitis in a five-year-old boy: An unusual antigen source. Pediatr. Pulmonol. *33*:77-78, 2002.
2. Allen, D. H., Basten, A., Williams, G. V., and Woolcock, A. J.: Familial hypersensitivity pneumonitis. Am. J. Med. *59*:505-514, 1975.
3. Allen, J.: Acute eosinophilic pneumonia. Semin. Respir. Crit. Care Med. *27*:142-147, 2006.
4. Andiman, W. A., Eastman, R., Martin, K., et al.: Opportunistic lymphoproliferations associated with Epstein-Barr viral DNA in infants and children with AIDS. Lancet *2*:1390-1393, 1985.
5. Avital, A., Godfrey, S., Maayan, C., et al.: Chloroquine treatment of interstitial lung disease in children. Pediatr. Pulmonol. *18*:356-360, 1994.
6. Balasubramaniam, S. K., O'Connell, E. J., Yunginger, J. W., et al.: Hypersensitivity pneumonitis due to dove antigens in an adolescent. Clin. Pediatr. *26*:174-176, 1987.
7. Barker, P. M., and Warner, J. O.: 'Atypical pneumonia' due to parakeet sensitivity: Bird fancier's lung in a 10-year-old girl. Br. J. Dis. Chest *78*:404-407, 1984.
8. Bokulic, R. E., and Hilman, B. C.: Interstitial lung disease in children. Pediatr. Clin. North Am. *41*:543-567, 1994.
9. Bousvaros, A., Sundel, R., Thorne, G. M., et al.: Parvovirus B19-associated interstitial lung disease, hepatitis, and myositis. Pediatr. Pulmonol. *26*:265-369, 1998.
10. Brody, A. S.: Imaging considerations: Interstitial lung disease in children. Radiol. Clin. North Am. *43*:391-403, 2005.
11. Brown, K. K.: Pulmonary vasculitis. Proc. Am. Thorac. Soc. *3*:48-57, 2006.
12. Bureau, M. A., Fecteau, C., Patriquin, H., et al.: Farmer's lung in early childhood. Am. Rev. Respir. Dis. *119*:671-675, 1979.
13. Canakis, A. M., Cutz, E., Manson, D., and O'Brodovich, H.: Pulmonary interstitial glycogenosis: A new variant of neonatal interstitial lung disease. Am. J. Respir. Crit. Care Med. *165*:1557-1565, 2002.
14. Carlsen, K. H., Leegaard, J., Lund, O. D., and Skjaervik, H.: Allergic alveolitis in a 12-year-old boy: Treatment with budesonide nebulizing solution. Pediatr. Pulmonol. *12*:257-259, 1992.
15. CDC: 1994 revised classification system for human immunodeficiency virus infection in children less than 13 years of age. M. M. W. R. Morb. Mortal. Wkly. Rep. Recomm. Rep. *43*(RR-12):1-10, 1994.
16. Ceviz, N., Kaynar, H., Olgun, H., et al.: Pigeon breeder's lung in childhood: Is family screening necessary? Pediatr. Pulmonol. *41*:279-282, 2006.
17. Chandra, S., and Jones, H. E.: Pigeon fancier's lung in children. Arch. Dis. Child. *47*:716-718, 1972.
18. Chang, A. B., Masel, J. P., and Masters, B.: Post-infectious bronchiolitis obliterans: Clinical, radiological and pulmonary function sequelae. Pediatr. Radiol. *28*:23-29, 1998.
19. Chen, C., Kleinau, I., Niggemann, B., et al.: Treatment of allergic alveolitis with methylprednisolone pulse therapy. Pediatr. Allergy Immunol. *14*:66-70, 2003.
20. Chetty, A., Bhuyan, U. N., Mitra, D. K., et al.: Cryptogenic fibrosing alveolitis in children. Ann. Allergy *58*:336-340, 1987.
21. Chiron, C., Gaultier, C., Boule, M., et al.: Lung function in children with hypersensitivity pneumonitis. Eur. J. Respir. Dis. *65*:79-91, 1984.
22. Church, J. A., Isaacs, H., Saxon, A., et al.: Lymphoid interstitial pneumonitis and hypogammaglobulinemia in children. Am. Rev. Respir. Dis. *124*:491-496, 1981.
23. Ciftci, E., Yalcinkaya, F., Ince, E., et al.: Pulmonary involvement in childhood-onset systemic lupus erythematosus: A report of five cases. Rheumatology *43*:587-591, 2004.
24. Colom, A. J., Teper, A. M., Vollmer, W. M., and Diette, G. B.: Risk factors for the development of bronchiolitis obliterans in children with bronchiolitis. Thorax *61*:503-506, 2006.

25. Copley, S. J., Coren, M., Nicholson, A. G., et al.: Diagnostic accuracy of thin-section CT and chest radiography of pediatric interstitial lung disease. A. J. R. Am. J. Roentgenol. *174*:549-554, 2000.

26. Cormier, Y., Letourneau, L., and Racine, G.: Significance of precipitins and asymptomatic lymphocytic alveolitis: A 20-yr follow-up. Eur. Respir. J. *23*:523-525, 2004.

27. Craig, T. J., and Richerson, H. B.: Update on hypersensitivity pneumonitis. Compr. Ther. *22*:559-564, 1996.

28. Cron, R. Q., Sherry, D. D., and Wallace, C. A.: Methotrexate-induced hypersensitivity pneumonitis in a child with juvenile rheumatoid arthritis. J. Pediatr. *132*:901-902, 1998.

29. Cunningham, A. S., Fink, J. N., and Schlueter, D. P.: Childhood hypersensitivity pneumonitis due to dove antigens. Pediatrics *58*:436-442, 1976.

30. Cutz, E., Wert, S., Nogee, L. M., and Moore, A. M.: Deficiency of lamellar bodies in alveolar type II cells associated with fatal respiratory disease in a full-term infant. Am. J. Respir. Crit. Care Med. *161*:608-614, 2000.

31. D'Ippolito, R., Chetta, A., Foresi, A., et al.: Induced sputum and bronchoalveolar lavage from patients with hypersensitivity pneumonitis. Respir. Med. *98*:977-983, 2004.

32. du Marchie Sarvaas, G. J., Merkus, P. J., and de Jongste, J. C.: A family with extrinsic allergic alveolitis caused by wild city pigeons: A case report. Pediatrics *105*:E62, 2000.

33. Eisenberg, J. D., Montanero, A., and Lee, R. G.: Hypersensitivity pneumonitis in an infant. Pediatr. Pulmonol. *12*:186-190, 1992.

34. El-Hefny, A., Ekladious, E. M., El-Sharkawy, S., et al.: Extrinsic allergic bronchiolo-alveolitis in children. Clin. Allergy *10*:651-658, 1980.

35. Epstein, C. E., Elidemir, O., Colasurdo, G. N., and Fan, L. L.: Time course of hemosiderin production by alveolar macrophages in a murine model. Chest *120*:2013-2020, 2001.

36. Epstein, C. E., and Fan, L. L.: Alveolar hemorrhage syndromes: Update on pulmonary hemosiderosis. J. Respir. Dis. Pediatr. *3*:49-56, 2001.

37. ERS Task Force on Bronchoalveolar Lavage in Children: Bronchoalveolar lavage in children. Eur. Respir. J. *15*:217-231, 2000.

38. Ettlin, M. S., Pache, J. C., Renevey, F., et al.: Bird breeder's disease: A rare diagnosis in young children. Eur. J. Pediatr. *165*:55-61, 2006.

39. Fackler, J. C., Nagel, J. E., Adler, W. H., et al.: Epstein-Barr virus infection in a child with acquired immunodeficiency syndrome. Am. J. Dis. Child. *139*:1001-1004, 1985.

40. Fan, L. L.: Evaluation and therapy of chronic interstitial pneumonia in children. Curr. Opin. Pediatr. *6*:248-254, 1994.

41. Fan, L. L.: Pediatric interstitial lung disease. *In* Schwarz, M. I., and King, T. E. (eds.): Interstitial Lung Disease. 4th ed. Hamilton, Ontario, B. C. Decker, 2003, pp. 134-151.

42. Fan, L. L., and Deterding, R. R.: Surfactant dysfunction mutations in children's interstitial lung disease and beyond. Am. J. Respir. Crit. Care Med. *172*:940-941, 2005.

43. Fan, L. L., Deterding, R. R., and Langston, C.: Pediatric interstitial lung disease revisited. Pediatr. Pulmonol. *38*:369-378, 2004.

44. Fan, L. L., and Kozinetz, C. A.: Factors influencing survival in children with chronic interstitial lung disease. Am. J. Respir. Crit. Care Med. *156*:939-942, 1997.

45. Fan, L. L., Kozinetz, C. A., Deterding, R. R., and Brugman, S. M.: Evaluation of a diagnostic approach to pediatric interstitial lung disease. Pediatrics *101*:82-85, 1998.

46. Fan, L. L., Kozinetz, C. A., Wojtczak, H. A., et al.: Diagnostic value of transbronchial, thoracoscopic, and open lung biopsy in immunocompetent children with chronic interstitial lung disease. J. Pediatr. *131*:565-569, 1997.

47. Fan, L. L., and Langston, C.: Chronic interstitial lung disease in children. Pediatr. Pulmonol. *16*:184-196, 1993.

48. Fan, L. L., Lung, M. C., and Wagener, J. S.: The diagnostic value of bronchoalveolar lavage in immunocompetent children with chronic diffuse pulmonary infiltrates. Pediatr. Pulmonol. *23*:8-13, 1997.

49. Fan, L. L., Mullen, A. L., Brugman, S. M., et al.: Clinical spectrum of chronic interstitial lung disease in children. J. Pediatr. *121*:867-872, 1992.

50. Franquet, T., Hansell, D. M., Senbanjo, T., et al.: Lung cysts in subacute hypersensitivity pneumonitis. J. Comput. Assist. Tomogr. *27*:475-478, 2003.

51. Fullmer, J. J., Fan, L. L., Dishop, M. K., et al.: Successful treatment of bronchiolitis obliterans in a bone marrow transplant patient with tumor necrosis factor-alpha blockade. Pediatrics *116*:767-770, 2005.

52a. Fullmer, J. J., Langston, C., Dishop, D. K., and Fan, L. L.: Pulmonary capillaritis in children: A review of eight cases with comparison to other alveolar hemorrhage syndromes. J. Pediatr. *146*:376-381, 2005.

52b. Gell, P. G. H., and Coombs, R. R. A. (eds.): Clinical Aspects of Immunology. 1st ed. Oxford, England, Blackwell, 1963.

53. Grammer, L. C.: Occupational allergic alveolitis. Ann. Allergy Asthma Immunol. *83*:602-606, 1999.

54. Grammer, L. C., Roberts, M., Lerner, C., and Patterson, R.: Clinical and serologic follow-up of four children and five adults with bird-fancier's lung. J. Allergy Clin. Immunol. *85*:655-660, 1990.

55. Grech, V., Vella, C., and Lenicker, H.: Pigeon breeder's lung in childhood: Varied clinical picture at presentation. Pediatr. Pulmonol. *30*:145-148, 2000.

56. Harrison, H. R., Taussig, L. M., and Fulginiti, V. A.: *Chlamydia trachomatis* and chronic lung disease in childhood. Pediatr. Infect. Dis. *1*:29-33, 1982.

57. Hartman, T. E.: The HRCT features of extrinsic allergic alveolitis. Semin. Respir. Crit. Care Med. *24*:419-426, 2003.

58. Heersma, J. R., Emanuel, D. A., Wenzel, F. J., and Gray, R. L.: Farmer's lung in a 10-year-old girl. J. Pediatr. *75*:704-706, 1969.

59. Highland, K. B., and Flume, P. A.: A 12-year-old girl with dyspnea and a normal chest radiographic finding: Hypersensitivity pneumonitis. Chest *120*:1372-1376, 2001.

60. Hoffman, G. S., Kerr, G. S., Leavitt, R. Y., et al.: Wegener granulomatosis: An analysis of 158 patients. Ann. Intern. Med. *116*:488-498, 1992.

61. Hogan, M. B., Patterson, R., Pore, R. S., et al.: Basement shower hypersensitivity pneumonitis secondary to *Epicoccum nigrum*. Chest *110*:854-856, 1996.

62. Hughes, W. F., Mattimore, J. M., and Arbesman, C. E.: Farmer's lung in an adolescent boy. Am. J. Dis. Child. *118*:777-780, 1969.

63. Hull, J., Chow, C. W., and Robertson, C. F.: Chronic idiopathic bronchiolitis of infancy. Arch. Dis. Child. *77*:512-515, 1997.

64. Jobe, A. H., and Bancalari, E.: Bronchopulmonary dysplasia. Am. J. Respir. Crit. Care Med. *163*:1723-1729, 2001.

65. Joshi, V. V., Oleske, J. M., Minnefor, A. B., et al.: Pathologic pulmonary findings in children with the acquired immunodeficiency syndrome: A study of ten cases. Hum. Pathol. *16*:241-246, 1985.

66. Karakurum, M., Doraswamy, B., and Bennuri, S. S.: Index of suspicion: Case 1. Hypersensitivity pneumonitis. Pediatr. Rev. *20*:53-54, 1999.

67. Katz, R. M., and Kniker, W. T.: Infantile hypersensitivity pneumonitis as a reaction to organic antigens. N. Engl. J. Med. *288*:233-237, 1973.

68. Katzenstein, A. L., Gordon, L. P., Oliphant, M., and Swender, P. T.: Chronic pneumonitis of infancy: A unique form of interstitial lung disease occurring in early childhood. Am. J. Surg. Pathol. *19*:439-447, 1995.

69. Keith, H. H., Holsclaw, D. S., and Dunsky, E. H.: Pigeon breeder's disease in children: A family study. Chest *79*:107-110, 1981.

70. Koss, M. N.: Pulmonary lymphoid disorders. Semin. Diagn. Pathol. *12*:158-171, 1995.

71. Kradin, R. L., and Mark, E. J.: Benign lymphoid disorders of the lung, with a theory regarding their development. Hum. Pathol. *14*:857-867, 1983.

72. Krasnick, J., Patterson, R., Stillwell, P. C., et al.: Potentially fatal hypersensitivity pneumonitis in a child. Clin. Pediatr. *34*:388-391, 1995.

73. Kristiansen, J. D., and Lahoz, A. X.: Riding-school lung? Allergic alveolitis in an 11-year-old girl. Acta Pediatr. Scand. *80*:386-388, 1991.

74. Lacasse, Y., Selman, M., Costabel, U., et al.: Clinical diagnosis of hypersensitivity pneumonitis. Am. J. Respir. Crit. Care Med. *168*:952-958, 2003.

75. Langston, C., Patterson, K., Dishop, M. K., et al.; chILD Pathology Group: A protocol for the handling of tissue obtained by operative lung biopsy: Recommendations of the child Pathology Co-operative Group. Pediatr. Dev. Pathol. *9*:173-180, 2006.

76. Laray-Cuasay, L. R., DeForest, A., Huff, D., et al.: Chronic pulmonary complications of early influenza virus infection in children. Am. Rev. Respir. Dis. *116*:617-625, 1977.

77. Larsen, G. L.: Hypersensitivity lung disease. Annu. Rev. Immunol. *3*:59-85, 1985.

78. Lee, S. K., Kim, S. S., Nahm, D. H., et al.: Hypersensitivity pneumonitis caused by *Fusarium napiforme* in a home environment. Allergy *55*:1190-1193, 2000.

79. Levenson, T., and Patterson, R.: Chronic cough in a child. Ann. Allergy Asthma Immunol. *76*:311-316, 1996.

80. Long, F. R., and Castile, R. G.: Technique and clinical applications of full-inflation and end-exhalation controlled-ventilation chest CT in infants and young children. Pediatr. Radiol. *31*:413-422, 2001.

81. Lovell, D., Lindsley, C., and Langston, C.: Lymphoid interstitial pneumonia in juvenile rheumatoid arthritis. J. Pediatr. *105*:947-950, 1984.

82. Lynch, D. A., Hay, T., Newell, J. D., et al.: Pediatric diffuse lung disease: Diagnosis and classification using high-resolution CT. A. J. R. Am. J. Roentgenol. *173*:713-718, 1999.

83. Lynch, D. A., Newell, J. D., Logan, P. M., et al.: Can CT distinguish hypersensitivity pneumonitis from idiopathic pulmonary fibrosis? A. J. R. Am. J. Roentgenol. *165*:807-811, 1995.

84. Mahut, B., Delacourt, C., Scheinmann, P., et al.: Pulmonary alveolar proteinosis: Experience with eight pediatric cases and a review. Pediatrics *97*:117-122, 1996.

85. Malamou-Mitsi, V., Tsai, M. M., Gal, A. A., et al.: Lymphoid interstitial pneumonia not associated with HIV infection: Role of Epstein-Barr virus. Mod. Pathol. *5*:487-491, 1992.

86. Marks, M. J., Haney, P. J., McDermott, M. P., et al.: Thoracic disease in children with AIDS. RadioGraphics *17*:1349-1362, 1996.

87. Matthay, R. A., Schwartz, M. I., Petty, T. L., et al.: Pulmonary manifestations of systemic lupus erythematosus: Review of 12 cases of acute lupus pneumonitis. Medicine (Baltimore) *54*:397-409, 1975.

88. McClellan, J. S., Albers, G. M., Noyes, B. E., et al.: B-lymphocyte aggregates in alveoli from a child with hypersensitivity pneumonitis (bird breeders lung). Ann. Allergy Asthma Immunol. *83*:357-360, 1999.

89. McSharry, C., Dye, G. M., Ismail, T., et al.: Quantifying serum antibody in bird fanciers' hypersensitivity pneumonitis. B. M. C. Pulm. Med. *6*:16, 2006.

90. Meyer, K. C., and Soergel, P.: Variation of bronchoalveolar lymphocyte phenotypes with age in the physiologically normal human lung. Thorax *54*:697-700, 1999.

91. Miller, M. M., Patterson, R., Fink, J. N., and Roberts, M.: Chronic hypersensitivity lung disease with recurrent episodes of hypersensitivity pneumonitis due to a contaminated central humidifer. Clin. Allergy *6*:451-462, 1976.

92. Mistchenko, A. S., Diez, R. A., Mariani, A. L., et al.: Cytokines in adenoviral disease in children: Association of interleukin-6, interleukin-8, and tumor necrosis factor alpha levels with clinical outcome. J. Pediatr. *124*:714-720, 1994.

93. Mistchenko, A. S., Lenzi, H. L., Thompson, F. M., et al.: Participation of immune complexes in adenovirus infection. Acta Paediatr. *81*:983-988, 1992.

94. Nacar, N., Kiper, N., Yalcin, E., et al.: Hypersensitivity pneumonitis in children: Pigeon breeder's disease. Ann. Trop. Paediatr. *24*:349-355, 2004.

95. Nicholson, A. G., Kim, H., Corrin, B., et al.: The value of classifying interstitial pneumonitis in childhood according to defined histological patterns. Histopathology *33*:203-211, 1998.

96. Nogee, L. M.: Surfactant protein-B deficiency. Chest *111*:129S-135S, 1997.

97. Nogee, L. M., deMello, D. E., Dehner, L. P., and Colten, H. R.: Deficiency of pulmonary surfactant protein B in congenital alveolar proteinosis. N. Engl. J. Med. *328*:406-410, 1993.

98. Nogee, L. M., Dunbar, A. E., Wert, S. E., et al.: A mutation in the surfactant protein C gene associated with familial interstitial lung disease. N. Engl. J. Med. *344*:573-579, 2001.

99. O'Brodovich, H. M., Moser, M. M., and Lu, L.: Familial lymphoid interstitial pneumonia: A long-term follow-up. Pediatrics *65*:523-528, 1980

100. O'Connell, E. J., Zora, J. A., Gillespie, D. N., and Rosenow, E. C.: Childhood hypersensitivity pneumonitis (farmer's lung): Four cases in siblings with long-term follow-up. J. Pediatr. *114*:995-997, 1989.

101. Ohtani, Y., Saiki, S., Sumi, Y., et al.: Clinical features of recurrent and insidious chronic bird fancier's lung. Ann. Allergy Asthma Immunol. *90*:604-610, 2003.

102. Olesen, H. V., Thelle, T., and Moller, J. C.: Childhood hypersensitivity pneumonitis probably caused by cat hair. Acta Pediatr. *87*:811-813, 1998.

103. Ostergaard, J. R.: Reversible pulmonary arterial hypertension in a 6-year-old girl with extrinsic allergic alveolitis. Acta Pediatr. Scand. *78*:145-148, 1989.

104. Palomar, L. M., Nogee, L. M., Sweet, S. C., et al.: Long-term outcomes after infant lung transplantation for surfactant protein B deficiency related to other causes of respiratory failure. J. Pediatr. *149*:548-553, 2006.

105. Park, S. M., and Tremper, L.: Hypersensitivity pneumonitis in pediatric patients. Immunol. Allergy Pract. *9*:420-423, 1987.

106. Pitt, J.: Lymphocytic interstitial pneumonia. Pediatr. Clin. North Am. *38*:89-95, 1991.

107. Purtilo, D. T., Brem, J., Ceccaci, L., et al.: A family study of pigeon breeders' disease. J. Pediatr. *86*:569-571, 1975.

108. Pye, C., Fan, L. L., and Langston, C.: Pulmonary neuroendocrine cell hyperplasia in persistent tachypnea of infancy. Mod. Pathol. *11*:4P, 1998.

109. Raghu, G.: Interstitial lung disease: A diagnostic approach: Are CT scan and lung biopsy indicated in every patient? Am. J. Respir. Crit. Care Med. *151*:909-914, 1995.

110. Ramirez-Venegas, A., Sansores, R. H., Perez-Padilla, R., et al.: Utility of a provocation test for diagnosis of chronic pigeon breeder's disease. Am. J. Respir. Crit. Care Med. *158*:862-869, 1998.

111. Ratjen, F., Costabel, U., Griese, M., and Paul, K.: Bronchoalveolar lavage fluid findings in children with hypersensitivity pneumonitis. Eur. Respir. J. *21*:144-148, 2003.

112. Reiss, J. S., Weiss, N. S., Payette, K. M., and Strimas, J.: Childhood pigeon breeder's disease. Ann. Allergy *32*:208-212, 1974.

113. Ribeiro, J. D., and Fischer, G. B.: Eosinophilic lung diseases. Paediatr. Respir. Rev. *3*:278-284, 2002.

114. Rochat, I., Sayegh, Y., Gervaix, A., et al.: Acute hypoxic respiratory failure as the first manifestation of systemic-onset juvenile rheumatoid arthritis in a child. Pediatr. Pulmonol. *38*:483-487, 2004.

115. Rosal-Sanchez, M., Alvarez, J., Torres, M. J., et al.: Pigeon fancier's lung after low exposure. Allergy *57*:649, 2002.

116. Rothenberg, S. S., Wagner, J. S., Chang, J. H., and Fan, L. L.: The safety and efficacy of thoracoscopic lung biopsy for diagnosis and treatment in infants and children. J. Pediatr. Surg. *31*:100-103, 1996.

117. Rubinstein, A., Bernstein, L. J., Charytan, M., et al.: Corticosteroid treatment for pulmonary lymphoid hyperplasia in children with the acquired immune deficiency syndrome. Pediatr. Pulmonol. *4*:13-17, 1988.

118. Rubinstein, A., Morecki, R., and Goldman, H.: Pulmonary disease in infants and children. Clin. Chest Med. *9*:507-517, 1988.

119. Rubinstein, A., Morecki, R., Silverman, B., et al.: Pulmonary disease in children with acquired immune deficiency syndrome and AIDS-related complex. J. Pediatr. *108*:498-503, 1986.

120. Saltos, N., Saunders, N. A., Bhagwandeen, S. B., and Jarvie, B.: Hypersensitivity pneumonitis in a mouldy house. Med. J. Aust. *2*:244-246, 1982.

121. Santamaria, F., Brancaccio, G., Parenti, G., et al: Recurrent fatal pulmonary alveolar proteinosis after heart-lung transplantation in a child with lysinuric protein intolerance. J Pediatr *145*:268-272, 2004.

122. Schelonka, R. L., Katz, B., Waites, K. B., and Benjamin, D. K.: Critical appraisal of the role of *Ureaplasma* in the development of bronchopulmonary dysplasia with metaanalytic techniques. Pediatr. Infect. Dis. J. *24*:1033-1039, 2005.

123. Schroeder, S. A., Shannon, D. C., and Mark, E. J.: Cellular interstitial pneumonitis in infants: A clinicopathologic study. Chest *101*:1065-1069, 1992.

124. Schuyler, M., and Cormier, Y.: The diagnosis of hypersensitivity pneumonitis. Chest *111*:534-536, 1997.

125. Scott, G. B., Hutto, C., Makuch, R. W., et al.: Survival in children with perinatally acquired human immunodeficiency virus type 1 infection. N. Engl. J. Med. *321*:1791-1796, 1989.

126. Selman, M.: Hypersensitivity pneumonitis. *In* Schwarz, M. I., and King, T. E. (eds.): Interstitial Lung Disease, 4th ed. Hamilton, Ontario, B. C. Decker, 2003, pp. 452-484.

127. Shannon, D. C., Andrews, J. L., Recavarren, S., and Kazemi, H.: Pigeon breeder's lung disease and interstitial pulmonary fibrosis. Am. J. Dis. Child. *117*:504-510, 1969.

128. Sharland, M., Gibb, D. M., and Holland, F.: Respiratory morbidity from lymphocytic interstitial pneumonitis (LIP) in vertically acquired HIV infection. Arch. Dis. Child. 76:334-336, 1997.

129. Sharief, N., Crawford, O. F., and Dinwiddie, R.: Fibrosing alveolitis and desquamative interstitial pneumonitis. Pediatr. Pulmonol. *17*:359-365, 1994.

130. Sheikh, S., Madiraju, K., Steiner, P., and Rao, M.: Bronchiectasis in pediatric AIDS. Chest *112*:1202-1207, 1997.

131. Shulenin, S., Nogee, L. M., Annilo, T., et al.: ABCA3 gene mutations in newborns with fatal surfactant deficiency. N. Engl. J. Med. *350*:1296-1303, 2004.

132. Small, J. H., Flower, C. D., Traill, Z. C., and Gleeson, F. V.: Air-trapping in extrinsic allergic alveolitis on computed tomography. Clin. Radiol. *51*:684-688, 1996.

133. Springer, C., Maayan, C., Katzir, Z., et al.: Chloroquine treatment in desquamative interstitial pneumonia. Arch. Dis. Child. *62*:76-77, 1987.

134. Steiger, D., Bubendorf, L., Oberholzer, M., et al.: Ciprofloxacin-induced acute interstitial pneumonia. Eur. Respir. J. *23*:172-174, 2004.

135. Stiehm, E. R., Reed, C. E., and Tooley, W. H.: Pigeon breeder's lung in children. Pediatrics *39*:904-915, 1967.

136. Stillwell, P. C., Norris, D. G., O'Connell, E. J., et al.: Desquamative interstitial pneumonitis in children. Chest *77*:165-171, 1980.

137. Stokes, D., Sigler, A., Khouri, N. F., and Talamo, R. C.: Unilateral hyperlucent lung (Swyer-James syndrome) after severe *Mycoplasma pneumoniae* infection. Am. Rev. Respir. Dis. *117*:145-152, 1978.

138. Swingler, G. H.: Summer-type hypersensitivity pneumonitis in southern Africa: A report of 5 cases in one family. S. Afr. Med. J. 77:104-107, 1990.

139. Thorshauge, H., Fallesen, I., and Ostergaard, P. A.: Farmer's lung in infants and small children. Allergy *44*:152-155, 1989.

140. Tobin-D'Angelo, M. J., Hoteit, M. A., Brown, K. V., et al.: Dapsone-induced hypersensitivity pneumonitis mimicking *Pneumocystis carinii* pneumonia in a patient with AIDS. Am. J. Med. Sci. *327*:163-165, 2004.

141. Tsai, E., Couture, D., and Hughes, D. M.: A pediatric case of pigeon breeder's disease in Nova Scotia. Can. Respir. J. *5*:507-510, 1998.

142. Uziel, Y., Hen, B., Cordoba, M., and Wolach, B.: Lymphocytic interstitial pneumonitis preceding polyarticular juvenile rheumatoid arthritis. Clin. Exp. Rheumatol. *16*:617-619, 1998.

143. Vergesslich, K. A., Gotz, M., and Kraft, D.: [Bird breeder's lung with conversion to fatal fibrosing alveolitis]. Dtsch. Med. Wochenschr. *108*:1238-1242, 1983.

144. Waltz, D. A., Boucek, M. M., Edwards, L. B., et al.: Registry of the International Society for Heart and Lung Transplantation: Ninth Official Pediatric Lung and Heart-Lung Transplantation Report—2006. J. Heart Lung Transplant. *25*:904-911, 2006.

145. White, C. W., Sondheimer, H. M., Crouch, E. C., et al.: Treatment of pulmonary hemangiomatosis with recombinant interferon alfa-2a. N. Engl. J. Med. *320*:1197-1200, 1989.

146. Wohl, M. E. B., and Chernic, V.: Bronchiolitis. Am. Rev. Respir. Dis. *118*:759-781, 1978.

147. Wolf, S. J., Stillerman, A., Weinberger, M., and Smith, W.: Chronic interstitial pneumonitis in a 3-year-old child with hypersensitivity to dove antigens. Pediatrics 79:1027-1029, 1987.

148. Yalcin, E., Dogru, D., Haliloglu, M., et al.: Postinfectious bronchiolitis obliterans in children: Clinical and radiological profile and prognostic factors. Respiration 70:371-375, 2003.

149. Yalcin, E., Kiper, N., Gocmen, A., et al.: Pigeon-breeder's disease in a child with selective IgA deficiency. Pediatr. Int. *45*:216-218, 2003.

150. Yee, W. F., Castile, R. G., Cooper, A., et al.: Diagnosing bird fancier's disease in children. Pediatrics 85:848-852, 1990.

151. Zacharisen, M. C., Schlueter, D. P., Kurup, V. P., and Fink, J. N.: The long-term outcome in acute, subacute, and chronic forms of pigeon breeder's disease hypersensitivity pneumonitis. Ann. Allergy Asthma Immunol. 88:175-182, 2002.

152. Zwerdling, R.: Abnormalities of lung growth and development. Clin. Chest Med. *8*:711-719, 1987.

CHAPTER
29
PLEURAL EFFUSIONS AND EMPYEMA
J. Gary Wheeler ☉ Richard F. Jacobs

Collections of fluid in the pleural space have been described in the literature as transudates, pleural effusions, exudates, purulent pleurisy, parapneumonic effusions, empyema, and complicated empyema. A great deal of inexactitude exists in the use of these terms, and comparing methods of diagnosis and management from one study to another is difficult. Standardized definitions are used in this chapter to describe pleural fluid collections.

The term *transudative pleural effusion* refers to fluid in the pleural space that is a nonpurulent effusion and typically nonpneumonic in origin. The term *purulent effusions* refers to effusions that are more cellular (exudative) and typically pneumonic in origin. The term *empyema* describes purulent effusions with chemical or microbial evidence of a severe process requiring drainage. *Complicated empyema* describes the processes associated with loculations or a fibropurulent rind requiring aggressive manipulations for cure. *Parapneumonic effusion* is a general term referring to any pleural exudative process resulting from an inflammatory process in the lung. Although these definitions are arbitrary and the literature is inconsistent in the use of these terms, a standard approach to the classification of these four types of effusions and their management has evolved.

The first description of parapneumonic infection is attributed to Hippocrates, who in the 4th century BCE advocated incision and drainage of empyema 2 weeks after the onset of symptoms. Since then, the physiology and microbiology of effusions have been described, and parapneumonic diseases and the management of fluid collections of the pleural space have been defined. In most cases, the directions of Hippocrates still are relevant: ". . . set him upon a stool, which is not wobbly; someone should hold his hands, then shake him by the shoulders and listen to see on which side a noise is heard. And right at this place—preferably on the left—make an incision, then it produces death more rarely."[58]

This description of open drainage to normal atmospheric pressures was recognized to be associated with significant mortality rates from hemodynamic instability in 1918, when the Empyema Commission of the United States Army recommended that the practice be abandoned[57]; thereafter, closed-tube drainage was introduced, and mortality rates decreased. Developments in radiology, antimicrobials, and surgery resulted in further improvements in care. Today, the major cause of mortality is related to the underlying disease because the management of parapneumonic effusions in children is largely successful and without residual morbidity. The physician must understand the risks for development of pleural effusion and empyema and indications for thoracentesis, implications of the results of pleural fluid studies, and the optimal medical and surgical management of the effusions and empyema.

EPIDEMIOLOGY

Parapneumonic effusions are known and expected complications in children with respiratory tract infections. The frequency of effusions may be 20 percent of patients with viral or mycoplasmal pneumonia[28,34,86] and 75 percent of patients with proven *Staphylococcus aureus* pneumonia.[7] Empyema has been reported to occur in 6.3 to 23 of 1000 admissions of children,[64,89] and as a complication of pneumonia in 1 percent of children in the United States.[19] One of the most extensive studies of empyema in children was from Dallas, Texas; 12 episodes per year during a 19-year period

were described.[30] A more recent report from Houston, Texas, suggested an increase in the overall number of hospitalizations per 10,000 admissions for empyema from 1993 to 1998 compared with 1999 to 2002 (8.5 versus 17.8)[89]; investigators elsewhere also have reported increases.[16,83]

In adults, empyema follows a primary pulmonary process in 55 to 60 percent of cases, surgery in 20 percent, trauma in 6 percent, spontaneous pneumothorax in 35 percent, and other causes in 2 percent.[57,84] Hoff and associates[41] found that 11 percent of cases in children had an underlying illness, including hyper-IgE syndrome, hypogammaglobulinemia, acute lymphocytic leukemia, cerebral palsy, Down syndrome, and postsurgical and congenital thrombocytopenia. The remaining cases were related to a primary pulmonary process. Freij and associates[30] found a rate of 8.3 percent with similar risk factors. The mortality rate is highest in the first 2 years of life. After reaching 2 years of age, children have better outcomes than do adults; generally, they have less intrinsic lung disease, have greater elasticity of their chest wall, and heal more quickly than older patients do.[15,35]

PATHOPHYSIOLOGY

The pleurae are mesodermally derived tissues that are approximately 30 to 40 μm thick and permeable to liquid and gas.[9,51] The parietal pleurae, which adhere to the chest wall, are fed from the intrathoracic and superior phrenic arteries and have sensory innervation. The visceral pleurae are splanchnic in origin, with blood flow from the pulmonic and pericardiophrenic arteries and no sensory innervation. The lymphatic structures of the visceral pleurae are microscopic vessels called *lacunae*. They are denser in the lower lobes to accommodate greater venous pressure. Parietal structures called *stomas* are 4- to 10-μm-diameter pores that connect the pleurae to lymphatics. These stomas have valvular function during expiration and inspiration and can filter large structures, such as red blood cells and macrophages.[51] The venous drainage of visceral pleura is into the pulmonic veins and from the parietal pleura into intercostal and bronchial veins. Lymphatic structures are woven below and around the mesothelial cells and ultimately drain into mediastinal, intercostal, and mammary nodes. The structure of the pleura is a surface of mesothelial cells and layers of lymphatic sinuses and pores, elastic fibers, and loose vascular connective tissue, with a fibroelastic layer covering the lungs and chest wall.[51]

The precise flow and distribution of pleural fluid have been debated for some time. Because of the differences in venous pressure in the intercostal and pulmonary veins, fluid is thought to flow from the parietal venous system to the visceral system by drifting from the high-pressure parietal tissues into the negative-pressure pleural space, with reabsorption on the visceral side. The latter is caused by a low venous pressure system on the parietal side and the high oncotic pressure of the pulmonic venous system compared with the pleural space.

The dynamics of this process are described in Starling's equation:

$$\text{Fluid movement} = k \cdot [\{HP_c - HP_{ip}\} - \{COP_c - COP_{ip}\}]$$

in which *k* is the filtration coefficient (a measure of the permeability of capillaries to fluid), *HP* is the hydrostatic pressure, and

TABLE 29-1   Characteristics of Pleural Effusions

	Transudative	Purulent Effusion	Empyema	Complicated Empyema
Appearance	Serous	Thin exudate	Turbid	Thick pus
Mean WBC	1000	5300	25,500	55,000
PMN (%)	50	>90	>95	>95
Protein (fluid/serum ratio)	<0.5	>0.5	>0.5	>0.5
LDH (fluid/serum ratio)	<0.6	>0.6	>0.6	>0.6
LDH (IU/L)		>200	>200	>1000
Glucose (mg/dL)	>60	<60	<60	<40
pH*	7.4-7.5	7.35-7.45	7.2-7.35	<7.2
Imaging	Fluid	Fluid	Fluid	Loculations, thick peel, scoliosis

Should be examined immediately or stored at 0° C.
LDH, lactate dehydrogenase; PMN, polymorphonuclear neutrophils; WBC, white blood cell count.

COP is the colloid osmotic pressure of capillaries (*c*) and the intrapleural compartment (*ip*).[14] The consensus is that although the impact of Starling forces on venous flow may play a role in the normal situation, parietal lymphatics absorb most of the excess fluids in pathologic situations and play an important role in normal physiology as well, removing 250 to 500 mL/day in adults.[92] They are the only mechanism for absorbing cells and other debris from the pleura.

A few studies in the past have shown that 20 mL of pleural fluid is found normally in 30 percent of resting adults, 70 percent of exercising adults,[7] and 46 to 67 percent of postpartum women.[41] Some fluid may be transported from the peritoneum to the pleura through small communications.[7] This hypothesis is supported by reports of patients with infected abdominal fluid and pleural effusions in whom the same organisms are recovered in both sites.[13]

The *raison d'être* of the pleural space is unknown. Some mammals, such as elephants, do not have a pleural space.[103] This fact has served as the rationale for using some methods of management of pleural disease that have included chemical obliteration of the pleural space. In the normal situation, pleural fluid in small amounts is a necessary requirement for optimal lubrication of the pleural space and for mechanical coupling of the lung and chest wall.[51] The accumulation of excess fluid (i.e., effusion) occurs in a limited set of circumstances, through excess production or deficient absorption. Increased production occurs when vessels are leaky (e.g., in septic shock) or active secretion of fluid with mesothelial inflammation (e.g., pleural infection) is present. Decreased absorption occurs with decreased oncotic pressure (e.g., nephrosis), increased pulmonary hydrostatic pressure (e.g., congestive heart failure), or lymphatic obstruction (e.g., malignancy).[102]

The mechanisms behind pleural effusions may vary among different infectious diseases. Effusion can be a "sympathetic" pleural response to a bacterial infection in the lung associated with inflammatory cytokines and altered venous or lymphatic drainage because of local edema. Direct or hematogenous extension of a bacterial process can occur in the pleura. *Mycoplasma* particularly is pathogenic in patients with sickle-cell disease, presumably because of pulmonary sludging, which increases pulmonic venous drainage pressures and results in accumulation of effusions. In pneumococcal disease, effusions often develop several days after the acute infection, when bacteria no longer can be recovered. These effusions may be related to immune complex disease.[14] In patients with tuberculosis, the most common cause of pleural effusions is thought to be the rupture of an old granuloma into the pleural space, with a hypersensitivity response similar to the skin test response,[15] which partly explains the low yield in cultures.

After an inflammatory process is initiated, it tends to progress through three classic stages.[3] The first, defined as a *purulent effusion*, is the acute exudative stage, with a thin pleural exudate

characterized by normal glucose, lactate dehydrogenase (LDH), and pH. The second transitional fibropurulent stage, categorized as *empyema*, is characterized by turbid fluid, decreased glucose concentration (<60 mg/dL) and pH (7.2 to 7.35), and elevated LDH (>200 U/L). The third chronic organizing stage is notable for a very low pH (<7.2) and glucose level (<40 mg/dL), LDH concentration greater than 1000 U/L, and development of loculations and peel. This fluid is found in patients with *complicated empyema*.

Often, the pleural fluid quality can be predicted without sampling the fluid based on the clinical course of the patient. A patient with anasarca caused by heart failure or nephrosis with bilateral effusions may not need to have an effusion analyzed if otherwise stable. If the same patient has fever, examination of the fluid is necessary to exclude a secondary bacterial infection. Analysis of the pleural fluid is most helpful when the underlying disease is unknown or when a primary pulmonic process is suspected. When patients have effusions caused by hydrostatic imbalance, the effusion is a transudate. Its protein and cell count do not exceed the range of normal pleural fluid (5000 cells/mm³ and <2 g of protein).[7,92] Patients who have an active inflammatory process may have an exudate (defined by excess protein and cells). In children, the most common cause of exudative pleural processes is pneumonia. In adults, most pleural effusions are related to congestive heart failure or malignancy,[56] but pneumonia is the most common cause of empyema.[71] Table 29-1 summarizes the general differences among pleural effusions.

Table 29-2 lists causes of effusions. Some of these causes, particularly iatrogenic causes, such as invasive procedures and drugs, are important to consider in the differential diagnosis of a difficult case. Others are associated with specific syndromes, such as adult respiratory distress syndrome[64] and yellow nail lymphedema syndrome.[97] Motor vehicle accidents have been identified as a common cause of serosanguineous effusions when disruption of normal mechanical lung function and hematoma occur.[81]

MICROBIOLOGY

Among children with parapneumonic effusions, no prospective study has established firmly the frequency with which effusions occur and how many are associated with particular microbes. Although respiratory viruses infrequently cause symptomatic effusions, the sheer number of cases and the presence of asymptomatic cases likely would implicate viral infection as the most common cause. Definite viral disease has been associated with cytomegalovirus, Epstein-Barr virus, measles, and adenovirus.[30,31,45,63] Other pathogens, such as *Mycoplasma* and *Chlamydia*, are difficult to diagnose but may account for a significant number of pneumonic infections in older children and adolescents that

TABLE 29-2   Causes of Pleural Effusion

Capillary leak
Sepsis syndrome
Vasculitis associated with immune complex disease
Connective tissue diseases
Inflammatory bowel disease
Malignancy (lymphoreticular, sarcoma, neuroblastoma)
Toxins (e.g., TSST-1)
Drugs (phenytoin, isoniazid, nitrofurantoin, amiodarone, methotrexate, bleomycin)
Myxedema
Trauma

Increased hydrostatic pressure
Congestive heart failure
Sickle-cell disease
Pulmonary venous hypertension
Superior vena cava syndrome
Pregnancy

Decreased oncotic pressure
Nephrosis
Cirrhosis
Protein malnutrition

Obstructed lymphatics
Congenital lymphangiectasia
Yellow nail syndrome
Radiation injury
Neoplasia (metastatic disease)
Pneumonia

Pleural inflammation
Pneumonia
Lung abscess with pleural fistula
Pleural infection (e.g., tuberculosis)
Esophageal rupture
Pancreatitis

Iatrogenic
Drugs
Central line misplacement

TSST-1, Toxic shock syndrome toxin-1.

may be associated with effusions in 20 percent of cases.[28,31,86] Viral, mycoplasmal, and chlamydial organisms rarely are isolated in patients with effusions requiring intervention.

The bacteriology of empyema is constantly evolving. Several past articles have established the role of different bacterial pathogens in childhood effusions. A study of 227 children by Freij and colleagues[30] published in 1984 found *Staphylococcus aureus* (29%), *Streptococcus pneumoniae* (22%), and *Haemophilus influenzae* (18%) as the three most frequent causes of parapneumonic effusions (Table 29-3). Subsequent studies show that the frequency of these pathogens has been affected by vaccine[1,16] and antibiotic use. Pathogens are shown in Table 29-4. *H. influenzae* and *S. pneumoniae* vaccines have led to a decreased incidence of these agents as a cause of empyema, whereas *S. aureus* has become the leading cause with antibiotic-resistant strains, accounting for most cases in community-acquired disease.[89] Among cases of *S. pneumoniae* infections, nonvaccine strains are increasing in number and may become a more severe threat.[17,24] Certain groups of children (e.g., neonates,[30] immunocompromised hosts, patients with preexisting chest tubes that become infected with nosocomial pathogens, patients with a ruptured viscus, and patients with foreign body aspiration) are at higher risk for acquiring gram-negative infections.

Administration of antibiotics before the diagnosis of empyema is made influences the recovery of organisms. In one report, the incidence of prethoracentesis antibiotics was 71 percent in culture-negative effusions and only 41 percent in culture-positive effusions.[41] Pretreatment with antibiotics may be associated with a decrease in the number of positive blood cultures and in the number of patients from whom *S. pneumoniae* are recovered.[71] Freij and associates[30] reported the frequency of parapneumonic effusions occurring in children with pneumonia caused by specific pathogens. The rates of effusion by organism were as follows: group A streptococcus, 86 to 91 percent; *S. aureus*, 72 to 76 percent; *S. pneumoniae*, 57 percent; *H. influenzae*, 49 to 75 percent; *Mycoplasma*, 21 percent; and adenoviruses, 11 to 33 percent.

TABLE 29-3   Distribution of Pathogens by Age

Pathogen	No. Cases					
	0-6 Months	7-12 Months	13-24 Months	25 Months–5 Years	6-15 Years	Total
Staphylococcus aureus	27 (41)*	11 (17)	10 (15)	6 (9)	12 (18)	66 (100)
Streptococcus pneumoniae	7 (14)	13 (27)	16 (33)	8 (16)	5 (10)	49 (100)
Haemophilus spp.	4 (10)	15 (38)	18 (45)	3 (7)	0	40 (100)
Sterile	3 (6)	9 (17)	17 (31)	11 (20)	14 (26)	54 (100)
Mixed bacteria	6 (60)	1 (10)	0	1 (10)	2 (20)	10 (100)
Streptococci	1 (20)	0	1 (20)	2 (40)	1 (20)	5 (100)
Gram-negative rods	2 (67)	0	1 (33)	0	0	3 (100)
All cases	50 (22)	49 (21)	63 (28)	31 (14)	34 (15)	227 (100)

*Numbers in parentheses = percentage of cases.
From Freij, B. J., Kusmiesz, H., Nelson, J. D., et al.: Parapneumonic effusions and empyema in hospitalized children: A retrospective review of 227 cases. Pediatr. Infect. Dis. J. 3:578-591, 1984.

TABLE 29-4   Percentage of Pathogens Recovered in Purulent Effusions from Children

Site/Years (No. Patients)	Staphylococcus aureus	Streptococcus pneumoniae	Haemophilus influenzae	Other Pathogens	Sterile	Reference
Dallas/1964-1982 (227)	29	22	18	8	24	30
Nashville/1977-1989 (61)	11	34	3	11	39	40
Washington, D.C./1973-1985 (33)	15	12	21	52	NR	13
Nigeria/1989-1991 (57)	63	NR	NR	37	NR	58
Israel/1972-1981 (37)	14	41	NR	35	11	63
Dallas/1992-1998 (135)	8	32	1	13	46	23
Houston/2001-2002 (47)	19	9	NR	4	68	89

NR, not reported.

Anaerobes were sought carefully by Brook and Frazier,[13] who found them infrequently in patients younger than 6 years of age. The anaerobes rarely were found in patients with primary pneumonia, occurring most often in patients with lung abscess and aspiration pneumonia.[13] In older patients (7-17 years old), anaerobes were recovered as isolated pathogens in 44 percent of cases.[13] Virtually every bacterial organism has been associated with pleural effusion at one time or another. *Brucella*,[47] *Francisella tularensis*,[82] and *Yersinia enterocolitica*[44] may be associated with the development of pleural effusions. The diagnosis in such cases often is suggested by a unique history in the patient.

Mycobacterial and fungal effusions are rare in children but are well described. In four published reviews, only two patients (from Nigeria) were reported to have *Mycobacterium tuberculosis*.[30,41,59,63] In a series of 303 children younger than 2 years of age with tuberculosis, 3.3 percent had an effusion.[40] In adolescents with tuberculosis, the incidence of effusion likely approximates that of adult disease. In one series of adult patients with primary tuberculous disease, pleural effusion occurred in 29 percent of cases.[20] In another adult series, primarily of reactivation disease, pleural effusion occurred in only 1 percent of the patients.[35] Whether or not co-infection with human immunodeficiency virus (HIV) is increasing the incidence of disease is controversial.[27]

Histoplasmosis has been associated with pleural effusion in 0 to 6 percent of childhood histoplasmosis cases.[73] Blastomycosis has been associated with pleural effusions in 0 to 40 percent of cases.[72,90] Effusions resulting from other fungi (e.g., *Coccidioides*, *Aspergillus*) have been described.[57] Parasitic diseases manifesting with effusions are uncommon but are found in patients with *Entamoeba histolytica* disease, most often from rupture of a hepatic abscess into the pleural space.[57] Echinococcal disease also has been reported.[29]

Pleural effusion associated with adult HIV infection has been reported in 14.6 percent of hospital admissions in one series in which 67 of 160 cases were infectious. Of those cases, 50 were associated with bacterial pneumonia, 10 with tuberculosis, and 5 with *Pneumocystis carinii* pneumonia.[2] Another report on patients infected with HIV suggested that empyema was seen primarily in patients with intravenous drug abuse.[10] We have not seen empyema frequently in our HIV-infected patients, perhaps because of the more recent use of more effective antiretroviral therapy.

Drug resistance in community-acquired pneumonia complicates the management of parapneumonic effusions. Intermediate or fully resistant *S. pneumoniae* were found in 12.8 percent and 10.1 percent of isolates in a study from multiple pediatric centers from 1993 to 2000; 7.5 percent were cephalosporin-resistant.[96] Methicillin-resistant *S. aureus* (MRSA) is a growing concern in empyema. Reports since 2000 have shown that 22 to 78 percent of isolates of *S. aureus* were methicillin-resistant, with many being community acquired.[43]

DIAGNOSIS

CLINICAL PRESENTATION

The clinical presentation of transudative effusions compared with purulent effusions ordinarily is distinctive, but a continuum of symptoms is shared by both. Many of the symptoms associated with pleural processes are caused by the underlying disease that precipitated the effusion, rendering a distinct syndrome difficult to recognize in patients. Disease caused by some pathogens (e.g., anaerobes, fungi, mycobacteria) also may follow a more insidious course, obscuring the symptoms of effusion. A history always should be obtained to identify systemic diseases, such as immunodeficiency diseases, cancer, and rheumatic diseases, or medications that may be associated with effusions.

Symptoms most specific for parapneumonic processes are dyspnea and pleuritic pain. Dyspnea occurs when the volume of the effusion mechanically interferes with breathing, or when pain prevents adequate gas exchange. Pain occurs with irritation of the parietal pleura and on inspiration (i.e., pleurisy). Fever is generated by the inflammatory response and pathogen-specific components (e.g., lipopolysaccharide, toxins). With an acute bacterial process, the fever can be high and hectic, mimicking the fever that occurs with an abscess. Patients in the chronic organizational phase generally have less fever. Cough and malaise are secondary symptoms. Hemoptysis and purulent sputum also may occur. The onset of symptoms of a purulent effusion may be delayed in time and distinct from the symptoms found at the onset of the pneumonia in older children; infants usually have no symptom-free period.[15] In the early phases of effusions, the patient may have no symptoms.

The physical examination usually is revealing. The child is tachypneic in more than 70 percent of cases, but breathing is shallow as a result of the child's attempt to minimize pain. Fever and cough usually occur in more than 90 percent of patients with purulent effusions.[59] The patient may appear toxic, with acute infection. Patients often posture toward the affected side. Classically, auscultation reveals a decrease in breath sounds and occasionally detects a pleural rub, but pleural rubs often are absent in a very young child. Rales from an associated pneumonia may be heard. Depending on the stage of the process, percussion may reveal a level of dullness associated with free-flowing effusion. As the process organizes, it may be less evident. Empyemas can erode through the chest wall into the subcutaneous tissue (i.e., empyema necessitatis) or into a bronchus (i.e., bronchopleural fistula).

IMAGING

The diagnosis most often is made by radiographic examination of the chest. Consolidation of a lobe of the lung is present, with an effusion obscuring the diaphragm (Fig. 29–1). A standard posteroanterior standing view reveals blunting of the costal diaphragmatic gutter. As fluid tracks along the lateral and posterior chest wall, a meniscus configuration is seen. Distinguishing it from pleural thickening may be difficult, and in such cases, a decubitus or cross-table view of the chest allows free-flowing fluid to layer out on the dependent chest wall. In older children and adults, a decubitus layer of fluid of more than 10 mm is considered a sufficient volume of fluid to attempt to extract by thoracentesis.[54] With large volumes of fluid (>1000 mL),[85] compression of the lung and shift of the trachea away from the effusion (Fig. 29–2) may occur. As an empyema develops and organizes, discrete pockets of fluid (i.e., loculations) may form within the pleural cavity (see Fig. 29–2). Occasionally, loculations are confused with lung abscess. Scoliosis also is well defined by the chest radiograph and occasionally is used as an indication for surgery.[41] The observation of an air-fluid level in the pleural space signifies that air has been generated in the pleural space by gas-forming organisms or has entered through a pneumothorax, perforated viscus, or bronchopleural fistula.

Ultrasonography has shown great utility in providing better guidance for thoracentesis of pleural fluid. It is noninvasive and allows empyema to be defined by showing internal echoes and septations (see Fig. 29–2).[90,105] Transudates uniformly are anechoic, although approximately one third of exudates also are anechoic.[105] Ultrasonography is not as precise as is computed tomography (CT) in differentiating a lung abscess from an empyema. CT and magnetic resonance imaging occasionally are required to distinguish parenchymal from pleural disease, identify a non-opaque foreign body, or locate a fistula.[92] CT particularly is useful in a patient whose chest radiograph shows total

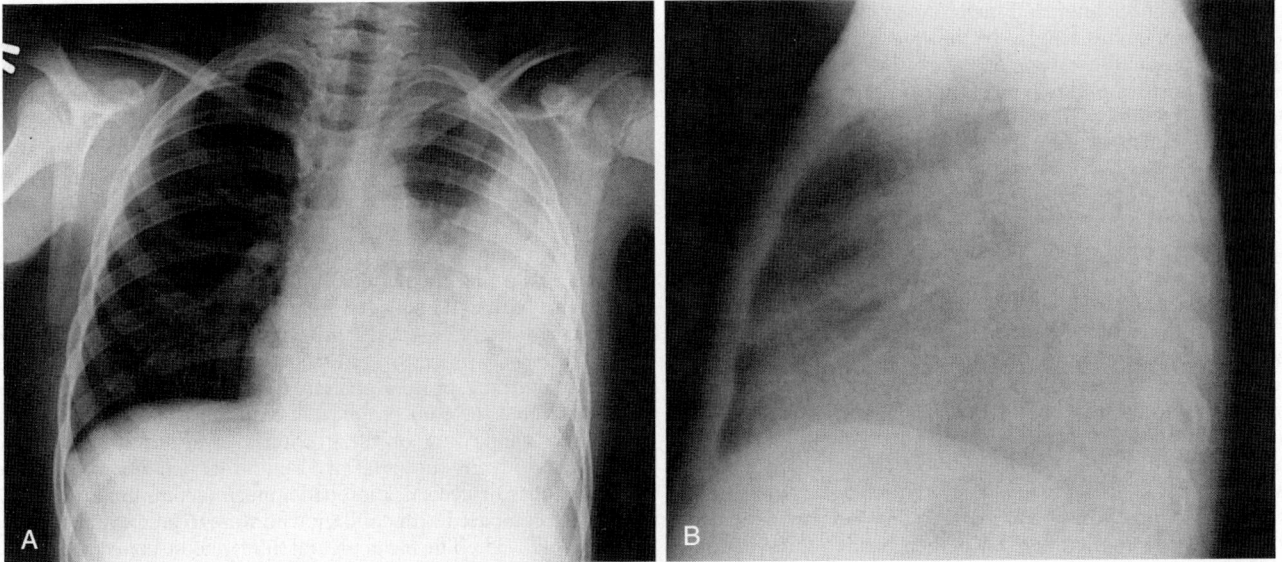

Figure 29–1 Posterior **(A)** and lateral **(B)** chest radiographs show a left pleural effusion in a 9-year-old girl who had symptoms of chest wall pain, fever, and vomiting. After 1 week, chest wall pain and shortness of breath continued, and she was admitted to the hospital and treated with cefuroxime and erythromycin for pneumonia. An ultrasound examination performed 2 days later showed a large pleural effusion that was drained, with a glucose level less than 20 mg/dL, lactate dehydrogenase level greater than 99,000 U/L, protein level 4.5 g/dL, and white blood cell count 51,000 mm³. Gram stain of the fluid showed gram-positive cocci, but the culture was negative. After failure to respond to intravenous antibiotics alone, the patient was taken to the operating room, where an empyema and several small abscesses were drained, along with decortication and repair of multiple bronchopleural fistulas. The patient was discharged 9 days later and received an additional 10 days of intravenous imipenem-cilastatin. She was well 1 month after hospital discharge.

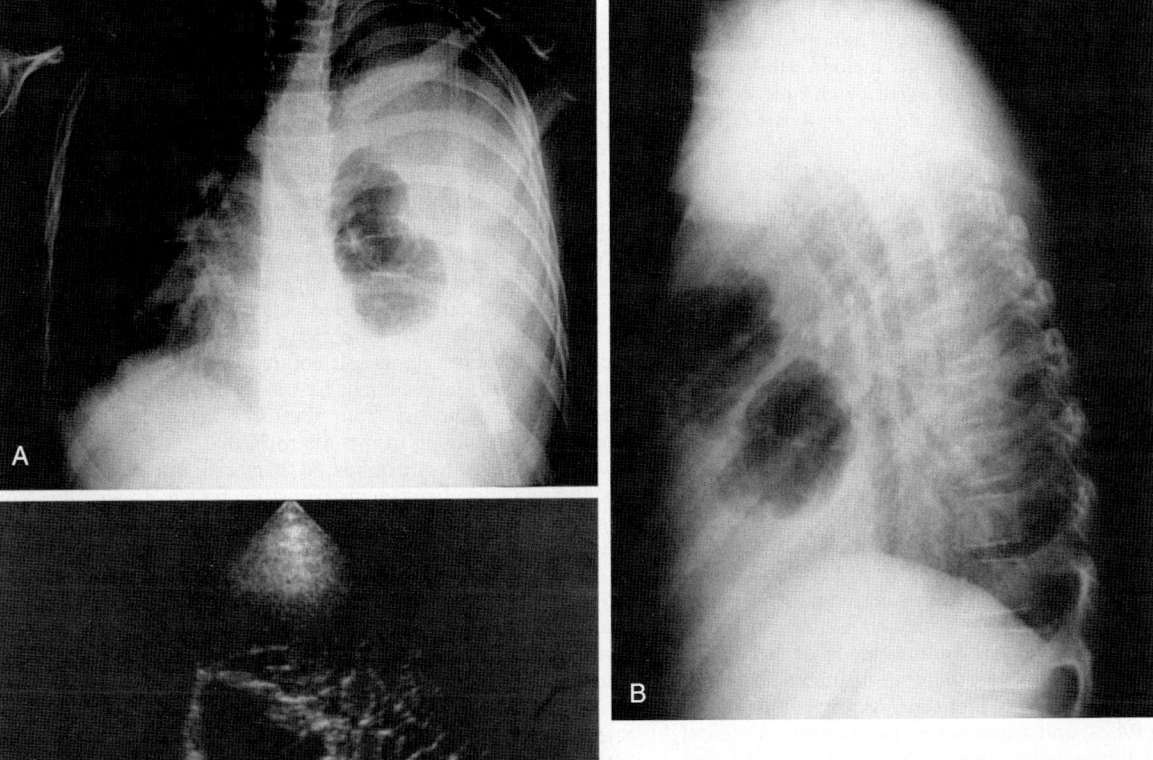

Figure 29–2 A-C, Chest radiograph and ultrasound examination images from a 7-year-old boy with a 5-day history of vomiting, diarrhea, and low-grade fever. He had a history of varicella 2 weeks earlier. The patient was hospitalized for dehydration and developed left-sided chest pain and a mild cough. Intravenous nafcillin was begun, but his condition deteriorated over the next 4 days, with an enlarging effusion and tracheal shift. Loculations were found on ultrasound **(C)**. He had a thoracotomy performed on day 6 with decortication and removal of a fibrinous rind. The patient was afebrile within 24 hours and received 1 week of intravenous antibiotics and 1 week of oral antibiotics. He was well on follow-up examination after discharge.

opacification of the lung, and such tomographic scanning is considered by some physicians to be the study of choice in this situation.[41] Ultrasound can have false-negative results, and CT can have false-positive findings on examination of pleural effusions. One study of adults showed that neither ultrasound nor CT effectively predicted the stage of the effusion or predicted the surgical outcome.[46]

THORACENTESIS

Thoracentesis plays an important role in the management of parapneumonic effusions and in 90 percent of adult cases yields useful information.[22] Some investigators would argue that primary video-assisted thoracic surgery (VATS) should be performed without thoracentesis.[23] Fluid should be obtained from the pleural cavity if fluid is adequate in volume and anatomically accessible and if a microbial diagnosis has not been made or presumed and antibiotic therapy is intended, or if pulmonary function is compromised by the effusion and imaging does not reveal evidence of organization to determine whether further intervention is necessary.

The volume and location of the fluid can be determined precisely by ultrasound examination if the physical examination does not allow localization of the fluid. When a healthy child with apparent or culture-confirmed pneumococcal pneumonia that is community acquired has a small pleural effusion, thoracentesis usually is not required. Small effusions generally can resorb, and a 10 to 50 percent chance of recovering the etiologic organism from blood cultures exists in empyema.[5,30] We suggest, however, that when the clinical presentation is atypical or a moderately sized effusion exists, thoracentesis usually is indicated to define the microbial process. Atypical situations include a history of trauma, foreign body aspiration, prolonged or chronic disease, and underlying systemic diseases (e.g., congestive heart failure, malignancy).

In a classic article published in 1972, Light and associates[56] established the methodology by which transudates could be differentiated from exudates. Such criteria are valuable in determining if antibiotic treatment is indicated, particularly in patients with underlying diseases that predispose them to sterile effusions but who may have a comorbid infectious condition. An exudate was defined by any of the following criteria: a fluid-to-serum protein ratio of greater than 0.5, a LDH fluid-to-serum ratio of greater than 0.6, a glucose concentration less than 50 mg/dL, and a pH less than 7.2. This study was based on the results from 150 adult patients, 103 of whom had exudates.[56]

The criteria of Light and associates have been accepted and are used as guidelines in the management of parapneumonic effusions in adults and children. In 1984, Peterman and Speicher,[69] using adult data, recommended a two-step process to separate transudates from exudates using only the protein and LDH serum-to-fluid ratios in the initial evaluation. If a patient had an apparent exudate, additional studies, including cultures, stains, pH, and glucose, were indicated. Another study of 297 adults compared several criteria for separating transudates and exudates and concluded that the criteria of Light and associates still yielded a high sensitivity (98%) and a specificity of 77 percent. A pleural fluid cholesterol concentration greater than 60 mg/dL also was used and had a sensitivity of 88 percent and specificity of 91 percent for exudates.[79] Although the cholesterol was not recommended for routine use, it was suggested as an extra screening test for patients with congestive heart failure in whom diuretic therapy might lead to increased concentration of pleural fluid protein.[19,38,79]

After an exudate is verified, it must be decided whether chest-tube drainage or other procedures such as VATS are needed. This decision is made by examining several aspects of the pleural

fluid. In 1980, Light and associates[55] described pleural fluid findings in adults with exudates in an attempt to determine which patients needed early chest-tube drainage of effusions. Thirty-seven adults with acute pneumonia and parapneumonic effusions were studied. Ten patients were considered to have complicated cases if they required chest tubes or had positive cultures at the time of thoracentesis. No clinical differences were found between the complicated and uncomplicated cases. Patients who required chest tubes had a pleural fluid pH of less than 7.0 and a glucose level less than 40 mg/dL. All patients with uncomplicated effusions had a pH greater than 7.2 and LDH less than 1000 mL. Patients with a pH between 7.0 and 7.2 fell into both categories. Anaerobes were recovered from 6 of 10 complicated cases, and *S. pneumoniae* was recovered from 15 of 27 uncomplicated cases. Cell count and protein analysis were not helpful in separating complicated from uncomplicated cases.

The application of these criteria to children has received limited study. In one series of 61 children, patients who required chest tubes or decortication had a mean pleural fluid pH of 7.24 or 7.10 compared with children who were treated with antibiotics only (pH 7.35). The mean pleural fluid glucose concentration was 74 g/L in the group treated with antibiotics, 10 g/L in the group treated with chest tubes, and 24 g/L in the group treated by decortication.[41] Another, more recent study confirmed that a pH less than 7.2 and low glucose were predictors of re-intervention.[65] These data suggest that the criteria of Light and associates for glucose are appropriate in children, but that the pH at which chest tubes are indicated may be higher for children than for adults. Availability of glucometers and pH meters at the site of thoracentesis is uncommon and might enhance decision-making.

Standard Gram stain and bacterial culture (aerobic and anaerobic) are indicated when thoracentesis is performed in patients in whom diagnosis of infection is considered. The Gram stain usually is positive in patients with bacterial infections; when such infections exist, Gram stain may be used to direct empiric therapy until culture results are known. In one study of children, 12 of 54 sterile effusions from patients with negative blood cultures had a positive Gram stain.[30] Some experts consider that a positive Gram stain indicates a more severe process and that such patients are more likely to require more invasive surgical procedures.[15]

When the total white blood cell count and differential are performed, supportive information may be gained. The results of a peripheral white blood cell count rarely change the clinical management of the patient. The total white blood cell count in empyema fluid can vary from 5000 to 625,000 cells/mm³, with median values ranging from 5000 to 55,000 cells/mm³.[30,41] Virtually all cells are neutrophils in bacterial infections. Marked eosinophilia may be seen in parasitic, fungal, tuberculous, or hypersensitivity disease and when blood is found in the pleural space.[15] Numerous small lymphocytes suggest malignancy, tularemia, or tuberculosis.[26,37,69,104] Other studies are required when the history suggests another underlying process. When tuberculosis is suspected by history, specific mycobacterial stains and cultures should be obtained. Identification of mycobacteria by stain and culture may be equivalent to the rate of identification of the disease process by pleural biopsy (approximately 25%).[67] Specific mycobacterial and fungal stains also should be obtained using a Ziehl-Neelsen/auramine stain and potassium hydroxide. Application of newer methods for diagnosis, such as polymerase chain reaction (PCR) and tuberculostearic acid by mass spectroscopy, may be indicated.

When malignancy or metastases are suspected, cytology is necessary.[37] Most effusions in children that prove to be malignant are of lymphoreticular origin. Amylase sometimes is measured and is elevated in cases of esophageal rupture, acute hemorrhagic peritonitis, or pulmonary infarction.[53,85] Countercurrent immunoelectrophoresis and other antigen detection systems occasionally are used for diagnosis and are useful in pretreated individuals. They are widely available only for disease caused by *S. pneumoniae* and *H. influenzae* type b and not for disease caused by *S. aureus* or anaerobes. Samples for antigen detection require special preparation before analysis because of increased levels of pleural fluid protein, which can create false-positive test results.

Molecular diagnostics is bringing promising advances to the bacteriologic diagnosis of empyema. PCR technology has been compared with routine culture and bacterial antigen and has shown increased sensitivity and good specificity for the diagnosis of *S. pneumoniae* using 16S rDNA or MRSA using the mec-300 gene probe.[24,83] Turnaround times can be quite rapid, exceeding traditional culture methods. The sensitivity of PCR for tuberculous effusions ranges from 20 to 81 percent, and specificity ranges from 78 to 100 percent.[27]

ADDITIONAL DIAGNOSTIC STUDIES

An intradermal test should be applied to any child with a parapneumonic effusion to evaluate tuberculosis as a possible cause. One third of patients with tuberculous effusions have a negative purified protein derivative skin test result.[8] Early morning gastric aspirates are recommended if tuberculosis is suspected.[98] Blood cultures also are indicated because one third of patients can have positive blood cultures and negative pleural fluid Gram stain and culture results.[30] Sputum is a less reliable source from which to determine the microbial cause of an effusion but may be helpful in a patient with purulent sputum and a single predominant organism. It can be diagnostic in older children with reactivation or cavitary tuberculosis and in cases of blastomycosis and histoplasmosis. Cold agglutinins or *Mycoplasma* serology may confirm the cause of a pleural effusion, although the nonspecificity of cold agglutinins and the delay in the increase in antibody titers render these data of marginal use in the acute management of the patient. Viral cultures are useful in only the more unusual cases and generally provide information that is not helpful in the initial management of the patient. Rapid diagnostic antigen assays, such as the rapid tests for influenza A and B, may be useful in defining the primary cause of respiratory disease but do not help exclude secondary bacterial pathogens causing pneumonia and a parapneumonic effusion. When other diseases, such as Wegener granulomatosis[6] and systemic lupus erythematosus, are suspected, disease-specific tests, such as antineutrophil cytoplasmic antibody and antinucleic acid antibody are indicated.

MANAGEMENT

If a patient has an underlying disease process associated with pleural effusion and thoracentesis has excluded bacterial infection (e.g., normal protein and LDH fluid-to-serum ratio, normal glucose level, negative cultures, and Gram stain results), no further treatment is indicated other than treatment of the underlying disease. These patients continue to be at risk for developing infection of the effusion and may require repeat examination of pleural fluid at a later time if infection is suggested clinically.

If a purulent effusion is suggested by imaging, thoracentesis, or surgical findings, empiric antibiotic therapy is indicated. Therapy always should include antimicrobials that are effective against *S. aureus*, *S. pneumoniae*, and *Streptococcus pyogenes*. Empiric therapy choices are becoming more complex as drug resistance patterns continue to change and the ability to make a rapid diagnosis improves (e.g., PCR). In the past, acceptable regimens included nafcillin, first-generation cephalosporins, cefuroxime, and clindamycin. For patients without a confirmed microbial pathogen and sensitivity profile and low incidence of resistant organisms (community-acquired MRSA and penicillin-resistant

S. pneumoniae), these past regimens based on the level of illness can be used. For mildly ill patients, one can begin with cefazolin or cefuroxime. For moderately ill patients, one can use clindamycin. We use vancomycin therapy for very ill patients and vancomycin and nafcillin for critically ill patients. For moderate to severe disease, cefotaxime or ceftriaxone is added.

In areas with high levels of antibiotic resistance (community-acquired MRSA, penicillin-resistant *S. pneumoniae*), in mild to moderate disease, clindamycin is indicated. For severely ill patients, vancomycin and a third-generation cephalosporin are appropriate. Some experts would add nafcillin, gentamicin, or both to this regimen. In patients who are vaccinated fully against *H. influenzae* (primary series and booster) and for whom the Gram stain is negative, empiric coverage against *H. influenzae* is not required. If *H. influenzae* is suspected, addition of a third-generation cephalosporin (i.e., ceftriaxone or cefotaxime) or single-drug use of cefuroxime or ampicillin-sulbactam would be effective. Ticarcillin-clavulanate, imipenem-cilastatin, meropenem, and piperacillin-tazobactam are useful if anaerobes are considered, particularly if aspiration is thought to play a role, such as in patients with abnormal swallowing. *Streptococcus milleri* has proven exceptionally difficult to manage and can be clindamycin-resistant.

In patients at risk for acquiring gram-negative disease (e.g., neonates, postsurgical patients), addition of an aminoglycoside or an advanced-generation cephalosporin (i.e., cefepime, ceftriaxone, or cefotaxime) is required. Extended-spectrum, semi-synthetic penicillins (e.g., ticarcillin-clavulanate, piperacillin-tazobactam) also are effective, as are carbapenems. Cefepime is helpful in nosocomial pneumonia/empyema because of its current efficacy for *Enterobacter* spp. In patients with renal failure or cephalosporin hypersensitivity, aztreonam is effective therapy for gram-negative infections. Ceftazidime or cefepime, broad-spectrum β-lactams with or without a β-lactamase inhibitor (i.e., ticarcillin–clavulanic acid, imipenem cilastatin, meropenem, or piperacillin-tazobactam), or aminoglycosides are indicated for *Pseudomonas* infection.

Surgical drainage is considered to be a crucial factor in resolving anaerobic infection. Clindamycin and metronidazole are effective, particularly when postsurgical infection or a ruptured gastrointestinal viscus is present. Upper respiratory tract anaerobes may be resistant to penicillins because of β-lactamase–producing oral flora (particularly *Prevotella* and *Porphyromonas* spp.).[13] In these situations, penicillin sensitivity should be documented before a penicillin is used as primary therapy.

For patients who have drug-resistant *S. pneumoniae*, most lung infections without associated central nervous system disease respond to high-dose penicillin (minimal inhibitory concentration >2 µg/mL) or cephalosporins (minimal inhibitory concentration >2 µg/mL).[52,68] In one study, the rates of effusion were similar between penicillin-susceptible and nonsusceptible *S. pneumoniae* isolates.[95] When the pneumococcus is highly resistant to penicillin and cephalosporins and the patient's disease fails to improve, therapy with vancomycin, clindamycin, or both may be required. Recovery of MRSA may require vancomycin therapy. Clindamycin sensitivity should be determined because many MRSA and methicillin-susceptible *S. aureus* isolates are resistant to clindamycin.[88] Susceptibility should be confirmed with performance of a "D" test. Intravenous clindamycin can be switched to oral clindamycin, offering a management advantage over vancomycin. New drugs such as linezolid have limited use at this time because of high cost but may have a role if vancomycin resistance becomes an issue. Daptomycin is specifically avoided in the lung because of its inactivation by surfactant.

With appropriate antibiotic therapy, the duration of fever in uncomplicated cases of purulent effusions usually is less than 48 to 72 hours.[66] When fever persists beyond 72 hours, surgical drainage may be required. The duration of antibiotic therapy is based on the response of the patient to the medical and surgical therapy provided. In one series of pediatric patients, the total duration of antibiotic therapy for patients with severe pleural infections who did or did not have surgical drainage was comparable (approximately every 12 days).[41] The duration of combined intravenous and oral therapy was 12 to 24 days in the study reported by Freij and associates,[30] with patients with *S. pneumoniae* infection receiving the shortest courses of antibiotic therapy and patients infected with *S. aureus* being treated for longer periods (Table 29–5). A prudent standard is to continue treatment for a minimum of 1 week beyond the last febrile day.

Closed-chest-tube drainage has been the standard treatment of parapneumonic effusions in four classes of patients: (1) patients in whom thick, purulent material is found at thoracentesis; (2) patients with a pleural fluid pH level less than 7.35 and glucose level less than 60 mg/dL; (3) patients for whom antibiotic therapy has not been associated with a timely clinical response (72 hours); and (4) patients in whom pulmonary function is compromised, as shown by severe hypoxemia or hypercapnia. The chest tube is left in place until minimal drainage is noted (usually <50 mL/day).[25]

When closed-chest-tube drainage is not associated with clinical improvement and defervescence of disease, or if the lung parenchyma is trapped by the fibrinopurulent peel or fever persists, decortication often is required. If the pleural involvement is limited, a small incision (minithoracotomy) can be employed.[74] Ultrasonography and CT are required to define these conditions.

Decortication has been advocated as a more expedient way to manage patients. One study reported that patients who had decortication had shorter hospital stays (11.6 days) compared with patients who had thoracentesis or tube thoracostomy (28.3 days).[32] The total number of hospital days also was reduced in another study when patients treated with decortication (16.6 days) were compared with patients treated by chest-tube drainage (21.4 days).[41] In both cases, morbidity from the operative procedure was minimal. Decortication seems to have an advantage in advanced disease in which fibrosis in the pleural cavity has resulted in a large peel. Hoff and associates[41] used an empyema scoring system to assess the need for decortication. Any two of the following are considered indicative of severe disease and need for decortication: anaerobic infection, pH less than 7.2, glucose level less than 40 mg/dL, scoliosis, and lung entrapment.[41]

Other surgical techniques to reduce operative mortality and promote earlier hospital discharge have been proposed.[48,49] VATS is the most popular technique and is gaining support in many centers. Although general anesthesia is required for thoracoscopy, only two small incisions are needed—one through the existing chest-tube tract for a telescope and the second through which operating instruments are passed. This procedure allows adhesiolysis and débridement and should be performed before a thick peel develops.

Proponents of VATS argue that a brief operative procedure and the attendant risks of anesthesia outweigh the child's suffering during thoracentesis (and chest-tube placement) and postoperatively. More importantly, a definitive procedure is done, rather than running the risk of having to perform subsequent chest-tube placements and thoracotomy. The hospital stay is shortened. Doski and colleagues[23] reported a series of 139 children who were studied from 1992 to 1998. By comparing historical cohorts, they showed a shorter length of stay (7 days versus 11 and 12 days) for children who underwent VATS than for groups of children who had thoracentesis, chest-tube drainage, or fibrinolytic therapy and rescue VATS for failure. Twelve of 98 patients who received traditional therapy required thoracotomy, whereas none in the primary VATS group did. A small, randomized study of 20 patients was conducted from 1994 to 1996 and showed that VATS was superior to chest-tube drainage with fibrinolytic therapy. Compared with chest-tube drainage with fibrinolytic therapy, VATS resulted in a higher primary success rate (91% vs 44%), fewer hospital days (8.7 days vs 12.8 days), and lower costs (about $16,000 vs $24,000).[101] Other studies have shown similar results.[33,46,62,76]

The use of radiologist-directed thoracentesis with pigtail catheters (smaller bore than standard chest tubes) for drainage with fibrinolytic therapy has been promoted as a way to reduce the number of operative procedures and achieve shorter hospital stays.[80] This therapy may have value in patients with organizing pleural inflammation and inadequate drainage caused by loculations of pleural fluid without a peel.

TABLE 29–5   Summary of Surgical Management

			No. Cases				
Procedures	*Staphylococcus aureus*	*Streptococcus pneumoniae*	*Haemophilus*	Sterile	Mixed	*Streptococcus*	GNR
DT only	5 (7.5)*	15 (31)	16 (40)	25 (46)	0	1 (20)	0
MT	5 (7.5)	5 (10)	5 (12)	2 (4)	0	0	0
D ± T	56 (85)	29 (59)	19 (48)	27 (50)	10 (100)	4 (80)	3 (100)
Thoracotomy	1 (2)	0	1 (3)	1 (2)	0	1 (20)	0
Open drainage	1 (2)	2 (4)	0	0	1 (10)	1 (20)	0
Decortication	2 (3)	0	0	3 (6)	0	0	0

			Duration of Drainage (days)[†]				
	n = 39	n = 24	n = 15	n = 22	n = 7	n = 4	n = 2
Range	1-43	2-12	3-41	1-20	4-54	3-6	3
Median	7	4.5	6	4.5	7	5.5	3
Mean	11.8	5.5	9.4	6.4	15.4	5	3
SD	11.1	3.0	9.6	4.7	18.5	1.4	0

*Numbers in parentheses = percentage of cases.
†Includes only surviving children who required closed-chest-tube drainage only and in whom the exact duration of drainage was known.
DT, diagnostic thoracentesis; D ± T, closed drainage with or without initial thoracentesis; GNR, gram-negative rods; MT, multiple thoracenteses; SD, standard deviation.
From Freij, B. J., Kusmiesz, H., Nelson, J. D., et al.: Parapneumonic effusions and empyema in hospitalized children: A retrospective review of 227 cases. Pediatr. Infect. Dis. J. 3:578-591, 1984.

The use of streptokinase in children with pleural effusion was reported in 1993.[80] The occasional side effects caused by streptokinase reported in adults have generated concern about its safety,[11,78] and its utility has been challenged in adults in a randomized study showing no benefit.[60] Urokinase is less expensive than is streptokinase and has been used in children with minimal adverse effects.[39,50,78,93] In adults and children, these different agents seem to be equivalent,[5,12] although commercial shortages of the products have occurred. Tissue-type plasminogen activator is the fibrinolytic therapy most commonly used at this time. It is less likely to promote allergic reactions.

An early report questioned the benefits of interventional radiologist-placed catheters with fibrinolytics for empyema.[77] A meta-analysis of eight evaluable reports from 2000 to 2004 of operative and nonoperative approaches to empyema suggested that the failure of primary therapy was intermediate for fibrinolytic therapy (9.4%), compared with simple chest-tube drainage (23.6% and either VATS (2.8%) or thoracotomy (3.1%).[4] The differences among these approaches are patient- and center-dependent, and some suggest that with patience even the most severe cases of pleural disease ultimately heal without sequelae.[87] The British Thoracic Society published clinical guidelines for management and concluded that fibrinolytic therapy shortened the hospital stay,[5] as seen in the meta-analysis,[4] but that failure should prompt early consideration of thoracic surgery. The physician must monitor clinical progress carefully and try at the earliest point to identify patients with more complicated disease who would benefit from surgical intervention. The American College of Chest Physicians has suggested that patients requiring surgery include adult patients with large effusions (more than half the hemithorax, loculations, pleural thickening, positive cultures or Gram stains, pH < 7.2, or frank pus).[21] Use of ultrasound also can identify patients with early organization of pleural fluid who have shorter hospitalizations if operative approaches are used.[75] Currently based on limited data, some experts prefer chest-tube and fibrinolytic therapy, whereas other experts choose VATS or minithoracotomy.

Rarely are full thoracotomy and pneumonectomy required for severe pneumonic and parapneumonic disease. An occasional complication of empyema is persistent, organized fluid or air collections in the pleural space, particularly in adults. A high rate of success has been reported using talc pleurodesis in these situations and in patients with noninfectious persistent effusions.[99,103] Long-term complications of this therapy include development of bronchogenic carcinoma and mesothelioma (asbestos-free preparations presumably are not associated with the development of these neoplastic conditions).

One frequent cause of bloody pleural effusions is motor vehicle accidents.[57,81] In one series of 100 children, 56 percent had pleural effusions associated with pulmonary contusions. They were treated with closed-chest-tube drainage; no antibiotics were used, and no infectious complications occurred.[81] Management of pleural hematoma secondary to trauma occasionally is complicated by infection because the bloody pleural fluid is an

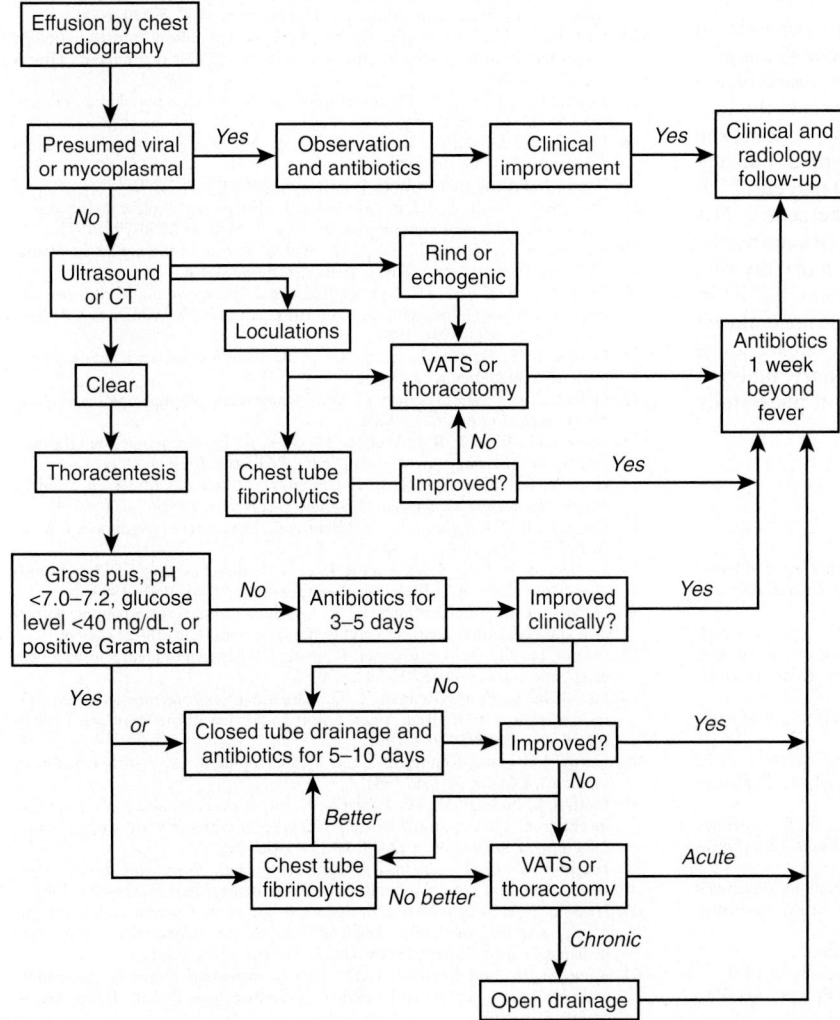

Figure 29–3 Algorithm for the management of pleural fluid collections. CT, computed tomography; VATS, video-assisted thoracic surgery.

excellent growth medium. One study suggested that empyema is less common in post-traumatic effusion with closed-chest-tube drainage than in repeated thoracentesis.[100]

Different biases exist in the management of parapneumonic effusions in children. In suspected empyema based on the clinical history and chest radiograph, we consider that a practical and effective approach is to perform an ultrasound study. If the study suggests complicated empyema (rind or loculations), primary VATS should be performed. If the study result is negative, thoracentesis should be done, and if consistent with empyema, chest-tube placement or VATS should be done. Figure 29–3 is an algorithm incorporating alternatives for the management of pleural collections. Complications from closed-chest-tube drainage include bleeding, infection of the exit wound, bronchopleural fistula, and laceration of the lung. Because of these rare complications, chest-tube placement, performed in the past by the pediatrician, now is delegated more frequently to the surgeon.

In cases of chronic empyema, other approaches are used. A closed tube can be converted into an open drainage tube. This conversion is accomplished safely a minimum of 10 to 14 days into the course of an empyema when the visceral and parietal pleurae fuse, and a pneumothorax can be avoided safely.[57] Other options include open drainage by rib resection and creation of a pleural window. The window ultimately closes with lung expansion and granulation, with disappearance of the pleural space.

PROGNOSIS AND LONG-TERM OUTCOME

The long-term outcome of patients with effusions depends on the underlying cause of the effusion. Patients with empyema who previously were well recover satisfactorily in most cases. Occasional rare complications, such as temporary paralysis of the diaphragm, have been reported.[64] In three retrospective reviews, the percentage of patients who required closed-chest-tube drainage or other surgical procedures ranged from 62 to 80 percent.[30,41,64] The rate of decortication ranged from 4[30] to 43 percent.[41] The relationship of surgical management to the pathogen causing the infection is shown in Table 29–5. The immediate mortality rate for children in recent years has been 0 to 10.8 percent.[30,41,59,64] In one of these studies, the mortality rate was highest for children younger than 1 year old.[30] Studies conducted to evaluate long-term, specific pulmonary disability using pulmonary function tests and lung volumes have shown normalization of these study results over time.[66]

REFERENCES

1. Adams, W. G., Deaver, K. A., Cochi, S. L., et al.: Decline of childhood *Haemophilus influenzae* type b (Hib) disease in the HIB vaccine era. J. A. M. A. 269:221-226, 1993.
2. Afessa, B.: Pleural effusion and pneumothorax in hospitalized patients with HIV infection—the pulmonary complications, ICU support, and prognostic factors of hospitalized patients with HIV (PIP) study. Chest 117:1031-1037, 2000.
3. Andrews, N. C., Parker, E. F., Shaw, R. R., et al.: Management of nontuberculous empyema. Am. Rev. Respir. Dis. 85:935, 1962.
4. Avansino, J. R., Goldman, B., Sawin, R. S., et al.: Primary operative versus nonoperative therapy for pediatric empyema: A meta-analysis. Pediatrics 115:1652-1659, 2005.
5. Bafour-Lynn, I. M., Abrahamson, E., Cohen, G., et al.: BTS guidelines for the management of pleural infection in children. Thorax 60(Suppl.):i1-i21, 2005.
6. Bambery, P., Sakhuja, V., Behera, D., et al.: Pleural effusions in Wegener's granulomatosis: Report of five patients and a brief review of the literature. Scand. J. Rheumatol. 20:445-447, 1991.
7. Baum, G. L.: Diseases of the pleura. Hosp. Med. 5:6-25, 1969.
8. Berger, H. W., and Mejia, E.: Tuberculous pleurisy. Chest 63:43-50, 1973.
9. Black, L. F.: The pleural space and pleural fluid. Mayo Clin. Proc. 47:494-506, 1972.

10. Borge, J. H., Michavila, I. A., Mendez, J. M., et al.: Thoracic empyema in HIV-infected patients—microbiology, management, and outcome. Chest 113:732-738, 1998.
11. Bouros, D., Schiza, S., Panagou, P., et al.: Role of streptokinase in the treatment of acute loculated parapneumonic pleural effusions and empyema. Thorax 49:852-855, 1994.
12. Bouros, D., Schiza, S., Patsourakis, G., et al.: Intrapleural streptokinase versus urokinase in the treatment of complicated parapneumonic effusions—a prospective, double-blind study. Am. J. Respir. Crit. Care Med. 115:291-295, 1997.
13. Brook, I., and Frazier, E. H.: Aerobic and anaerobic microbiology of empyema. Chest 103:1502-1507, 1993.
14. Brown, R. B., and Weinstein, L.: Pleural effusions. In Feigin, R. D., and Cherry, J. D. (eds.): Textbook of Pediatric Infectious Diseases. 3rd ed. Philadelphia, W. B. Saunders, 1992, pp. 309-315.
15. Brusch, J. L., and Weinstein, L.: Pleural empyema. In Feigin, R. D., and Cherry, J. D. (eds.): Textbook of Pediatric Infectious Diseases. 3rd ed. Philadelphia, W. B. Saunders, 1992, pp. 315-320.
16. Byington, C. L., Korgenski, K., Daly, J., et al.: Impact of the pneumococcal conjugate vaccine on pneumococcal parapneumonic empyema. Pediatr. Infect. Dis. J. 125:250-254, 2006.
17. Byington, C. L., Samore, M. L., Stoddard, G. J., et al.: Temporal trends of invasive disease due to *Streptococcus pneumoniae* among children in the intermountain west: Emergence of non-vaccine strains. Clin. Infect. Dis. 41:21-29, 2005.
18. Chartrand, S. A., and McCracken, G. H., Jr.: Staphylococcal pneumonia in infants and children. Pediatr. Infect. Dis. J. 1:19-23, 1982.
19. Chonmaitree, T., and Powell, K. R.: Parapneumonic pleural effusion and empyema in children. Clin. Pediatr. 22:414-419, 1983.
20. Choyke, P. L., Sostman, H. D., Curtis, A. M., et al.: Adult onset of pulmonary tuberculosis. Radiology 148:357, 1983.
21. Colice, G. L., Curtis, A., Deslauriers, J., et al.: Medical and surgical treatment of parapneumonic effusions: An evidence-based guideline. Chest 18:1158-1171, 2000.
22. Collins, T. R., and Dahn, S. A.: Thoracentesis: Clinical value, complications, technical problems and patient experience. Chest 91:817-822, 1987.
23. Doski, J. J., Lou, D., Hicks, B. A., et al.: Management of parapneumonic collections in infants and children. J. Pediatr. Surg. 35:265-270, 2000.
24. Eastham, K. M., Freeman, R., Kearns, A. M., et al.: Clinical features, aetiology and outcome of empyema in children in the north east of England. Thorax 59:522-525, 2004.
25. Efrati, O., and Barak, A.: Pleural effusions in the pediatric population. Pediatr. Rev. 23:417-426, 2002.
26. Epstein, D. M., Kline, L. R., Albeida, S. M., et al.: Tuberculous pleural effusions. Chest 91:106-109, 1987.
27. Ferrer, J.: Pleural tuberculosis. Eur. Respir. J. 10:42-47, 1997.
28. Fine, N. L., Smith, L. R., and Sheedy, P. E.: Frequency of pleural effusions in mycoplasma and viral pneumonias. N. Engl. J. Med. 283:790-793, 1970.
29. Fitzgerald, D., Harvey, J., Isaacs, D., et al.: The case of the persistent pleural effusions. Pediatr. Infect. Dis. J. 10:475, 479-480, 1991.
30. Freij, B. J., Kusmiesz, H., Nelson, J. D., et al.: Parapneumonic effusions and empyema in hospitalized children: A retrospective review of 227 cases. Pediatr. Infect. Dis. J. 3:578-591, 1984.
31. Gathof, B. S., Kamilli, I., Keller, C., et al.: Pleural effusions in acute mononucleosis. Bildgebung. 58:218-220, 1991.
32. Golladay, E. S., and Wagner, C. W.: Management of empyema in children. Am. J. Surg. 158:618-621, 1989.
33. Grewal, H., Jackson, R. J., Wagner, C. W., et al.: Early video-assisted thoracic surgery in the management of empyema. Pediatrics 103:1-5, 1999.
34. Grix, A., and Giammona, J. T.: Pneumonitis with pleural effusion in children due to *Mycoplasma pneumoniae*. Am. Rev. Respir. Dis. 109:665-671, 1974.
35. Groff, D. B., Randolph, J. G., and Blader, B.: Empyema in childhood. J. A. M. A. 195:572-574, 1966.
36. Hadlock, F. P., Park, S. K., Awe, R. J., et al.: Unusual findings in adult pulmonary tuberculosis. A. J. R. Am. J. Roentgenol. 134:1015-1018, 1980.
37. Hallman, J. R., and Geisinger, K. R.: Cytology of fluids from pleural, peritoneal and pericardial cavities in children. Cytol. Fluids 38:209-217, 1994.
38. Hamm, H., Brohan, U., Bohmer, R., et al.: Cholesterol in pleural effusions: A diagnostic aid. Chest 92:296-302, 1987.
39. Handman, H. P., and Reuman, P. D.: The use of urokinase for loculated thoracic empyema in children: A case report and review of the literature. Pediatr. Infect. Dis. J. 12:958-959, 1993.
40. Hardy, J. B., and Kendy, E. L., Jr.: Tuberculous pleurisy with effusion in infancy. J. Pediatr. 26:138, 1945.
41. Hoff, S. J., Neblett, W. W., Edwards, K. M., et al.: Parapneumonic empyema in children: Decortication hastens recovery in patients with severe pleural infections. Pediatr. Infect. Dis. J. 10:194-199, 1990.
42. Hughson, W. G., Friedman, P., Feigin, D. S., et al.: Postpartum pleural effusion: A common radiographic finding. Ann. Intern. Med. 97:856-858, 1982.
43. Hussain, F. M., Boyle-Vavra, S., Bethel, C. D., et al.: Current trends in community acquired methicillin resistant *Staphylococcus aureus* at a tertiary care pediatric facility. Pediatr. Infect. Dis. J. 19:1163-1166, 2000.
44. Kane, D. R., and Reuman, P. D.: *Yersinia enterocolitica* causing pneumonia and empyema in a child and a review of the literature. Pediatr. Infect. Dis. J. 11:591-593, 1992.

45. Kato, Y., Miyata, I., Sakuma, S., et al.: A case of cytomegalovirus mononucleosis associated with pleural effusion. Acta Paediatr. Jpn. *36*:280-283, 1994.

46. Kearney, S. E., Davies, C. W. H., Davies, R. J. O., et al.: Computed tomography and ultrasound in parapneumonic effusions and empyema. Clin. Radiol. *55*:542-547, 2000.

47. Kerem, E., Diav, O., Navon, P., et al.: Pleural fluid characteristics in pulmonary brucellosis. Thorax *49*:89-90, 1994.

48. Kercher, K. W., Attorri, R. J., Hoover, J. D., et al.: Thoracoscopic decortication as first-line therapy for pediatric parapneumonic empyema—a case series. Chest *118*:24-27, 2000.

49. Kern, J. A., and Rodgers, B. M.: Thoracoscopy in the management of empyema in children. J. Pediatr. Surg. *28*:1128-1132, 1993.

50. Kornecki, A., and Sivan, Y.: Treatment of loculated pleural effusion with intrapleural urokinase in children. J. Pediatr. Surg. *32*:1473-1475, 1997.

51. Lee, K. F., and Olak, J.: Anatomy and physiology of the pleural space. Chest Surg. Clin. North Am. *4*:391-403, 1994.

52. Leggiadro, R. J., Davis, Y., and Tenover, F. C.: Outpatient drug-resistant pneumococcal bacteremia. Pediatr. Infect. Dis. J. *13*:1144-1145, 1995.

53. Light, R. W.: Pleural effusions. Med. Clin. North Am. *61*:1339-1351, 1977.

54. Light, R. W.: Pleural Diseases. Philadelphia, Lea & Febiger, 1983.

55. Light, R. W., Girard, W. M., Jenkinson, S. G., et al.: Parapneumonic effusions. Am. J. Med. *69*:507-512, 1980.

56. Light, R. W., Macgregor, M. I., Luchsinger, P. C., et al.: Pleural effusions: The diagnostic separation of transudates and exudates. Ann. Intern. Med. *77*:507-513, 1972.

57. Magovern, C. J., and Rusch, V. W.: Parapneumonic and post-traumatic pleural space infections. Chest Surg. Clin. North Am. *4*:561-582, 1994.

58. Major, R. H.: Classic Descriptions of Disease. 2nd ed. Springfield, IL, Charles C Thomas, 1939, p. 620.

59. Mangete, E. D. O., Kombo, B. B., and Legg-Jack, T. E.: Thoracic empyema: A study of 56 patients. Arch. Dis. Child. *69*:587-588, 1993.

60. Maskell, N. A., Davies C. W. H., Nunn, A. J., et al.: U.K. controlled trial of intrapleural streptokinase for pleural infections. N. Engl. J. Med. *352*:865-874, 2005.

61. Mazzare, M. A., and Park, M. K.: Empyema causing paralysis of hemidiaphragm. Arch. Pediatr. Adolesc. *149*:342-343, 1995.

62. Meier, A. H., Smith, B., Raghavan, A., et al.: Rational treatment of empyema in children. Arch. Surg. *135*:907-912, 2000.

63. Meyer, K., Girgis, N., and McGravey, V.: Adenovirus associated with congenital pleural effusion. Clin. Lab. Observ. *107*:433, 1985.

64. Meyerovitch, J., Shohet, I., and Rubinstein, E.: Analysis of thirty-seven cases of pleural empyema. Eur. J. Clin. Microbiol. *4*:337-339, 1985.

65. Mitri, R. K., Brown, S. D., Zurakowski, D., et al.: Outcomes of primary image-guided drainage of parapneumonic effusions in children. Pediatrics *110*:e37, 2002.

66. Murphy, D., Lockhart, C. H., and Todd, J. K.: Pneumococcal empyema. Am. J. Dis. Child. *134*:659-662, 1980.

67. Nance, K. V., Shermer, R. W., and Askin, F. B.: Diagnostic efficacy of pleural biopsy as compared with that of pleural fluid examination. Mod. Pathol. *4*:320-324, 1991.

68. Pallares, R., Linares, J., Vadillo, M., et al.: Resistance to penicillin and cephalosporin and mortality from severe pneumococcal pneumonia in Barcelona, Spain. N. Engl. J. Med. *333*:474-480, 1995.

69. Peterman, T. A., and Speicher, C. E.: Evaluating pleural effusions: A two-stage laboratory approach. J. A. M. A. *252*:1051-1053, 1984.

70. Pettersson, T.: Similar pleural fluid findings in pleuropulmonary tularemia and tuberculous pleurisy. Chest *109*:572-575, 1996.

71. Pothula, V., and Krellenstein, D. J.: Early aggressive surgical management of parapneumonic empyemas. Chest *105*:832-836, 1994.

72. Powell, D. A., and Schult, K. E.: Acute pulmonary blastomycosis in children: Clinical course and follow-up. Pediatrics *63*:736-740, 1979.

73. Quasney, M. W., and Leggiadro, R. J.: Pleural effusion associated with histoplasmosis. Pediatr. Infect. Dis. J. *12*:415-418, 1993.

74. Raffensperger, J. G., Luck, S. R., Shkolnik, A., et al.: Mini-thoracotomy and chest tube insertion for children with empyema. J. Thorac. Cardiovasc. Surg. *84*:497-504, 1982.

75. Ranmath, R. R., Heller, R. M., Ben-Ami, T., et al.: Implications of early sonographic evaluation of parapneumonic effusions in children with pneumonia. Pediatrics *101*:68-71, 1998.

76. Rescorla, F. J., West, K. W., Gingalewski, C. A., et al.: Efficacy of primary and secondary video-assisted thoracic surgery in children. J. Pediatr. Surg. *35*:134-138, 2000.

77. Roberts, J. S., Bratton, S. L., and Brogan, T. V.: Efficacy and complications of percutaneous pigtail catheters for thoracostomy in pediatric patients. Chest *114*:1116-1121, 1998.

78. Robinson, L. A., Moulton, A. L., Fleming, W. H., et al.: Intrapleural fibrinolytic treatment of multiloculated thoracic empyemas. Ann. Thorac. Surg. *57*:803-814, 1994.

79. Romero, S., Candela, A., Martin, C., et al.: Evaluation of different criteria for the separation of pleural transudate from exudates. Chest *104*:399-404, 1993.

80. Rosen, H., Nadkarni, V., Therous, M., et al.: Intrapleural streptokinase as adjunctive treatment for persistent empyema in pediatric patients. Chest *103*:1190-1192, 1993.

81. Roux, P., and Fisher, R. M.: Chest injuries in children: An analysis of 100 cases of blunt chest trauma from motor vehicle accidents. J. Pediatr. Surg. *27*:551-555, 1992.

82. Rubin, S. A.: Radiographic spectrum of pleuropulmonary tularemia. A. J. R. Am. J. Roentgenol. *131*:277-281, 1978.

83. Saglani, S., Harris, K. A., Wallis, C., et al.: Empyema: The use of broad range 16S rDNA PCR for pathogen detection. Arch. Dis. Child. *90*:70-73, 2005.

84. Sahn, S. A.: Pleural manifestations of pulmonary disease. Hosp. Pract. *16*:73-89, 1981.

85. Sahn, S. A.: The differential diagnosis of pleural effusions. West. J. Med. *137*:99-108, 1982.

86. Sahn, S. A.: Pleural effusions in the atypical pneumonias. Semin. Respir. Infect. *3*:322-334, 1988.

87. Satish, B., Bunker, M., and Seddon, P.: Management of thoracic empyema in childhood: Does the pleural thickening matter? Arch. Dis. Child. *88*:918-921, 2003.

88. Schreckenberger, P. C., Ilendo, E., and Ristow, K. L.: Incidence of constitutive and inducible clindamycin resistance in *Staphylococcus aureus* and coagulase-negative staphylococci in a community and a tertiary care hospital. J. Clin. Microbiol. *42*:2777-2779, 2004.

89. Schultz, K. D, Fan, L. L., Pinsky, J., et al.: The changing face of pleural empyemas in children: Epidemiology and management. Pediatrics *113*:1735-1740, 2004.

90. Schutze, G. S.: Blastomycosis. Clin. Infect. Dis. *22*:496-502, 1996.

91. Sherman, M. M., Subramanian, V., and Berger, R. L.: Management of thoracic empyema. Am. J. Surg. *133*:474-479, 1977.

92. Stewart, P. B.: The rate of formation and lymphatic removal of fluid in pleural effusions. J. Clin. Invest. *42*:258-262, 1963.

93. Stringel, G., and Hartman A. R.: Intrapleural instillation of urokinase in the treatment of loculated pleural effusions in children. J. Pediatr. Surg. *29*:1539-1540, 1994.

94. Tagliabue, M., Casella, T. C., Zincone, G. E., et al.: CT and chest radiography in the evaluation of adult respiratory distress syndrome. Acta Radiol. *35*:230-234, 1994.

95. Tan, T. Q., Mason, E. O., Barson, W. J., et al.: Clinical characteristics of children with pneumonia attributable to penicillin-susceptible and penicillin-nonsusceptible *Streptococcus pneumoniae*. Pediatrics *102*:1369-1375, 1998.

96. Tan, T. Q., Mason, E. O., Wald, E. R., et al.: Clinical characteristics of children with complicated pneumococcal pneumonia caused by *Streptococcus pneumoniae*. Pediatrics *110*:1-6, 2002.

97. Tita, J. A., Wiedemann, H. P., and Weinstein, C. E.: Pleural effusions and abnormal nails. Hosp. Pract. *21*:65-68, 1986.

98. Vallejo, J. T., Ong, L. T., and Starke, J. R.: Clinical features, diagnosis and treatment of tuberculosis in infants. Pediatrics *94*:1-7, 1994.

99. Vargas, F. S., Milanez, J. R., Filomeno, L. T., et al.: Intrapleural talc for the prevention of recurrence in benign or undiagnosed pleural effusions. Chest *106*:1771-1775, 1994.

100. Varkey, B., Rose, H. D., Kutty, C. P. K., et al.: Empyema thoracis during a ten-year period: Analysis of 72 cases and comparison to a previous study (1952-1967). Arch. Intern. Med. *141*:1771-1776, 1981.

101. Wait, M. A., Sharma, S., Hohn, J., et al.: A randomized trial of empyema therapy. Chest *111*:1548-1551, 1997.

102. Weiner-Kronish, J. P., and Broaddus, V. C.: Interrelationship of pleural and pulmonary interstitial liquid. Annu. Rev. Physiol. *55*:209-226, 1993.

103. Weissberg, D., and Ben-Zeev, I.: Talc pleurodesis. J. Thorac. Cardiovasc. Surg. *106*:689-695, 1993.

104. Yam, L. T.: Diagnostic significance of lymphocytes in pleural effusions. Ann. Intern. Med. *66*:972-982, 1967.

105. Yang, P. C., Luh, K. T., Chang, D. B., et al.: Value of sonography in determining the nature of pleural effusion: Analysis of 320 cases. Am. J. Radiol. *159*:29-33, 1992.

LUNG ABSCESS

J. Gary Wheeler ❂ Richard F. Jacobs

A lung abscess is an area of necrotic material in the parenchyma of the lung initiated or complicated by infectious organisms. Although possibly originating from a pneumonia, it is distinguished by liquefaction and destruction of parenchymal tissue, organization, and cavitation. Necrotizing pneumonia, which on imaging lacks the "rim" representing the organization of the abscess, has a different clinical course and management.[18] A lung abscess may erupt and form an adjacent empyema. Empyema is defined strictly by involvement of the pleural tissues, however.

In the past, lung abscess was described as a disease of male alcoholics that was managed with surgery.[38] Lung abscess in children was recognized early on as having a different etiology and course than lung abscess in adults.[53] As is true of many infectious diseases, it continues to change as the human host and the microbial environment change. The incidence of lung abscess has declined precipitously in the modern era. Smith[46] reported lung abscesses in 0.33 percent of pediatric admissions in 1934, and Emanuel and Shulman[14] reported a rate of 0.012 percent from 1985 to 1990. In major pediatric referral centers in Chicago, Houston, Dallas, and Montreal, the incidence of lung abscesses has ranged in the last 2 decades from 1.5 to 4.7 cases per year.[4,14,28,48] Many of these cases developed in compromised hosts.

Improvements in pediatric diagnosis and care have resulted in a decrease in the numbers of cases related to underlying diseases. The morbidity and mortality rates also have decreased with use of antibiotic therapy and modern critical care. In 1920, Wessler and Schwarz[53] reported a 33 percent mortality rate, with "invalidism" and hemiplegia occurring in another 27 percent. The mortality rates in the two latest U.S. reports of lung abscess were 11 percent (1982-1993)[14] and 4 percent (1985-1990),[47] and 18.5 percent mortality was reported in Taiwan (1987-2003).[10]

Although lung abscesses occur in children of all ages, two studies have suggested that the trend is away from children younger than 5 years of age to an older population.[14,34] In other studies, the median age ranged from 7 to 9.5 years.[4,7,10,14,18,47] No consistent racial or sexual predisposition to this condition in children has been identified. In the 1950s, one series found boys to be more at risk than girls.[24] In adults, a twofold greater risk exists for men.[32,38] Table 30–1 lists specific risk factors for development of lung abscess in pediatric patients. Most factors are related to some predisposition to aspiration, hematogenous spread, or compromised immunity.

TABLE 30–1   Underlying Risks for 46 Secondary Lung Abscesses in Pediatric Patients

Risk	No.
Neuropsychiatric causes	16
Hematologic/oncologic disorders	11
Primary pulmonary disease	8
Immunodeficiency	4
Congenital heart disease	2
Solvent aspiration	1
Foreign body aspiration	1
Prematurity	1
Chromosomal disorder	1
Endocrinopathy	1

Data from references 13 and 44, and unpublished data from Little Rock, Arkansas, 1989 to 1994.

PATHOPHYSIOLOGY

Two main mechanisms explain formation of a lung abscess. The first mechanism is the introduction of pathogens directly into the airspaces, which typically results in solitary abscesses. The abscess typically follows aspiration, with a resultant neutrophilic reaction and necrosis. Aspiration is thought to be the predominant precipitating factor in adults, particularly in individuals with significant dental disease.[6] Most lung abscesses related to aspiration are polymicrobial and include anaerobes. The prevalence of fluoride and the low incidence of dental disease in children may be additional factors for the reduced incidence of lung abscess in children, although aspiration pneumonia does occur in the absence of dental disease.

The second mechanism in the formation of lung abscess is hematogenous spread. Hematogenous seeding of the lung can lead to an initial pneumonia that develops into an abscess with further organization and cavitation. Primary pneumonia rarely progresses to necrosis and abscess in modern times; this phenomenon is explained largely by the ready accessibility of antibiotics. Emboli from the venous circulation (i.e., septic thrombophlebitis) and right side of the heart (i.e., endocarditis) can cause single or multiple lung abscesses, which often are subpleural. Infection in the head and neck area also is a risk factor for vascular spread to the lung, with resultant lung abscess.[43] This complication occurred commonly in past eras. Lung abscesses complicated tonsillectomies in one third of cases in a 1920 report.[53] The abscesses were theorized to result from aspiration during the operative procedure[46] and characteristically developed 13 to 14 days after the procedure.[53] Great improvements in modern pediatric anesthesia with careful efforts made to prevent aspiration have rendered this complication uncommon today.

A lung abscess tends to have irregular margins, with occasional bullae, and it can dissect into adjacent tissues, such as the mediastinum, bronchi, and pleural space. If the abscess ruptures into a bronchus, air enters and an air-fluid level can be seen radiographically. Dissection into the pleural space creates a purulent effusion, with air noted only if an anaerobic process is present. Dissection into the mediastinum causes a widening of the mediastinum. Air is detected if communication occurs with a bronchus or in the presence of anaerobes. Multiple lung abscesses occur more frequently in hematogenous or embolic disease and are found more often with more sensitive tools, such as computed tomography (CT). Modern reviews of children have suggested that single abscesses are found more frequently than are multiple abscesses.[7,14,47]

Microscopically, a lung abscess is definable by a collection of necrotic material (i.e., highly neutrophilic inflammation); a surrounding irregular, fibrotic wall; and microvascular infarcts. Lymphocytes often are present and seem to play a regulatory role in the formation of the abscess.[44] The infrequency of lung abscesses in patients with human immunodeficiency virus (HIV) infection may be explained by this observation.

The role of preceding viral infection in undermining phagocytic host defenses is supported by the observations of preceding respiratory symptoms in patients with lung abscesses.[1] They manifest primarily in cold weather[4,14] and typically after well-defined viral illnesses, such as varicella, measles, and influenza.[24,26,52] The impact of chemotherapy on phagocytes also may explain the increased numbers of lung abscesses in patients with leukemia and other cancers.

On a macroscopic scale, lung abscesses tend to develop in all parts of the lung. If associated with aspiration, the anatomic site depends on whether the subject was supine or erect at the time of aspiration. Supine patients develop abscesses in the posterior upper and lower lobes, and erect patients develop infection in the middle and basilar lower lobes. Generally, the tendency is for aspiration-related abscesses to develop more on the right side than on the left, presumably because of the more vertical anatomy of the right stem bronchus.[14,23]

Physicians have grouped lung abscesses into primary and secondary categories, presuming that primary and secondary abscesses have different microbiologic factors, management approaches, and outcomes. The arbitrary nature of this distinction is apparent when appreciating how much the microbiology, clinical course, management, and outcome of both conditions overlap.[32] Primary abscesses occur in previously normal hosts without a history of trauma or aspiration of a foreign body. Secondary abscesses occur in the setting of underlying medical illnesses predisposing to infection, airway obstruction, embolization, or aspiration. In an earlier series, secondary abscesses were found more often in children younger than 1 year of age,[26] but this difference was not corroborated in a later study.[14] Primary abscesses were found in 64 percent of patients in Chicago,[14] 33 percent in Houston,[47] 45 percent in Little Rock (1989 to 1994) (unpublished data), 30 percent in Toronto (1956 to 1965),[26] and 30 percent in Taiwan (1987-2003).[10]

In the modern era, lung abscess should trigger a search to exclude underlying factors that may have prognostic value and lead to treatment of the underlying disease. The classic lung abscess syndrome in adults is represented by an alcoholic who aspirates during an alcoholic stupor. In children, a classic presentation would be any child with altered mental status, associated swallowing dysfunction, or both conditions. Foreign bodies can obstruct normal clearance of pathogens and precipitate the development of a lung abscess.[14,27] Obstruction also predisposes to lung abscess in adults who have carcinoma of the lung and rarely in children with metastatic disorders. Ineffective cough in patients with neurodegenerative or myopathic disorders is another risk factor for developing lung abscess, similar to that in an adult alcoholic. Patients with leukemia and patients who are receiving chemotherapy also are at increased risk. Occasionally, a bronchogenic cyst can become infected and mimic a lung abscess. Tricuspid or pulmonary valve endocarditis in children with complicated congenital heart disease places them at risk for developing lung abscesses.

Immunodeficiency is another risk factor for development of a lung abscess. Patients with chronic granulomatous disease and hyper-IgE syndrome typically are found to have lung abscesses. Patients with hypogammaglobulinemia may develop abscesses, although bronchiectasis is the more characteristic finding. The same is true for patients with immotile cilia syndromes and cystic fibrosis, although in the latter group, disease abscesses are uncommon.[10] Among pediatric patients, HIV-1 infection has not been reported as a risk factor in series from Chicago and Houston.[14,47] Additional causes are listed in Table 30-1.

MICROBIOLOGY

The microbiology of lung abscesses seems to be evolving as patients and antibiotics change.[38] In the preantibiotic era, streptococci and *Mycobacterium tuberculosis* were the most commonly reported causes of lung abscesses. After penicillin use began and tuberculosis skin testing, treatment, and control programs became widespread, staphylococci most frequently were recovered from lung abscesses.[39] Development of better culture techniques also increased the identification of anaerobes in lung abscess material; in past eras, these organisms probably were present but not

recovered. Anaerobes were suspected by the fetid odor of abscesses, the time course of postoperative aspiration infections, and Gram stains of tissue and pus, which showed fusobacteria and spirochetes.[46,53] Table 30-2 summarizes the microbiology of pediatric lung abscesses reported from 1976 to 2006.

The primary role of anaerobes in lung abscesses has been assumed in aspiration pneumonias. Anaerobes are prominent in the oral cavity and have been recovered from the abscesses of patients with dental disease.[6] In many past studies, lung abscess materials were not transported and cultured for optimal anaerobic growth, however. Successful growth was described when specimens were transported in a closed syringe, with culture inoculation beginning in less than 10 minutes.[7] Later studies, in which optimal culture methods were employed, corroborated the role of anaerobes in lung abscesses in children.[7,47] In one study of mentally retarded children with seizure disorders, poor dental care, and suspected aspiration, transtracheal polymicrobial infections with aerobes were found in 9 of 10 samples.[7] An average of 6.2 isolates were recovered per patient. *Peptostreptococcus* and *Bacteroides* spp. were the anaerobes recovered most frequently.[7] In a larger group of 45 children, 15 of whom had primary abscesses, 14 had polymicrobial infections.[47] Older children with neurologic disorders were the primary patients with anaerobes in both studies. Anaerobes, *Streptococcus pneumoniae*, nontypeable *Haemophilus influenzae*, and *Staphylococcus aureus* have been recovered from normal patients.[47]

The role of tissue lysins and toxins depends on the pathogen and is thought to be crucial for the development of lung abscesses. In mixed infections, synergy probably occurs among the pathogens as proposed by Smith in 1934.[46]

Nosocomial pathogens are becoming more frequent causes of lung abscesses as a result of the increased numbers of patients with extended hospitalizations and use of advanced-generation antibiotics. The widespread use of third-generation cephalosporins has resulted in resistant *Enterobacter* spp. and other gram-negative organisms being recovered in secondary lung abscesses.

TABLE 30-2   Microbiology of Pediatric Lung Abscess

Organism	No.
Staphylococcus aureus	22
Coagulase-negative staphylococci	2
Streptococcus pyogenes	5
Streptococcus pneumoniae	15
Alpha-hemolytic streptococcus	17
Other aerobic streptococci	7
Enterococci	2
Branhamella catarrhalis	3
Escherichia coli	10
Klebsiella	8
Pseudomonas	13
Serratia	1
Eikenella	1
Haemophilus	7
Other gram-negative organisms	2
Bacteroides	19
Peptostreptococcus	12
Other anaerobes	26
Candida	4
Aspergillus	5
Mucor	3
Mycobacterium tuberculosis	1
Total	185

These data were reported in the literature from 1976 to 2006. The isolates were recovered by direct aspiration of abscess contents, bronchoscopic aspiration, transtracheal aspiration, blood culture, or culture of surgical specimens. Data from case reports focused on procedures are included, whereas data from case reports focused on the organism recovered are not.[4,7,10,12,14,20,22,24,25,27,28,34,36,45,47,48,51]

In the report by Tan and associates,[47] fungal abscesses always were associated with debilitated, chronically hospitalized patients. Immunosuppression no doubt contributes to the recovery of other unsuspected organisms (e.g., *Legionella, Neisseria mucosa, S. pneumoniae, Citrobacter*)[13,19,40,42] and underscores the value of obtaining specimens in chronically hospitalized patients, atypical cases, and patients not responding to empiric treatment.

Among otherwise normal hosts, tuberculosis can be a cause of single and multiple abscesses. The number of tuberculosis cases manifesting as lung abscess has increased dramatically, and tuberculosis is likely to be associated more frequently with lung abscesses in the future. In patients with an international travel history, unusual pathogens such as parasites (e.g., hydatid cysts)[15] and regional bacteria (e.g., *Pseudomonas pseudomallei*) should be considered.

An important lesson for the physician is the relevance of various respiratory cultures to the microbiology of lung abscesses. Rarely is sputum useful in defining the pathogens in a lung abscess because of three factors: (1) sputum typically is contaminated with abundant mouth flora; (2) if the lung abscess is not ruptured, no direct communication of the pathogens in the abscess occurs with the airway; and (3) sputum is difficult to obtain in preadolescent children. Obtaining cough cultures, performed by gagging a young child and culturing the coughed sputum collected on a swab before it can be swallowed, frequently is unsuccessful. A skilled clinician occasionally can acquire useful information, however.

Bronchoscopy is effective in recovering relevant organisms if the abscess has ruptured and has therapeutic value because it may assist in clearing secretions from the airway. It has been performed infrequently in pediatric practice in the past because of a lack of skilled personnel and pediatric equipment. Rigid bronchoscopy rarely is used to drain the abscess but when performed, highly informative microbiologic information may be obtained. Transtracheal aspirates, likewise performed in few pediatric patients, have similar value. The upper airway frequently is colonized in debilitated patients, and microbiologic information obtained must be interpreted with care. Direct aspiration of the abscess, typically under CT or ultrasound guidance,[49] is an ideal way to provide microbiologic data and plan antimicrobial therapy. Aspiration may have therapeutic value in decompressing the abscess.

CLINICAL FEATURES

Most patients with lung abscesses have had symptoms 1 to 3 weeks before being hospitalized.[14] Fever is reported to be associated with 100 percent of primary abscesses[14,26] and 84 percent of a mixed group of primary and secondary abscesses.[47] All patients with secondary abscesses in a small series had fever.[7] Cough occurs in 53 to 67 percent of cases[26,47] and initially may be nonproductive, becoming purulent when rupture into a bronchus occurs. With necrosis, hemoptysis can occur. Ipsilateral chest or shoulder pain also has been described in some patients, particularly older children.[14,27] Weight loss may be present if the abscess is of more than a few days' duration. Other symptoms are listed in Table 30–3.[47]

Some differences in presentation by age exist. Neonates and young infants typically are febrile, without localizing symptoms. Older children also are febrile but may have more cough or tachypnea and focal pain.

The clinical features of a lung abscess vary with the causative organisms and patient risk factors. Patients with bacterial pneumonia can present with dramatic onset of fever and overwhelming respiratory failure, such as in staphylococcal pneumonia. In these cases, the patient often has a recent history of influenza or varicella infection. Staphylococcal abscesses may not be noticed

TABLE 30–3 Symptoms and Signs in Patients with Lung Abscess

Symptom	No. Cases	%
Fever	38	84
Cough	24	53
Dyspnea	17	38
Chest pain	11	24
Anorexia	9	20
Purulent sputum	8	18
Rhinorrhea	7	16
Malaise/lethargy	5	11
Hemoptysis	4	9
Diarrhea	4	9
Nausea/vomiting	3	7
Irritability	3	7
Otitis media	2	4
Convulsions	2	4
Weight loss	1	2
Sore throat	1	2
Lymphadenopathy	1	2

From Tan, T. Q., Seilheimer, D. K., and Kaplan, S. L.: Pediatric lung abscess: Clinical management and outcome. Pediatr. Infect. Dis. J. 14:51-55, 1995.

on chest radiographs until the patient already is on ventilatory support because of the time required for an abscess to organize. Similar presentations are typical of group A beta-hemolytic streptococcus and *S. pneumoniae* infections. Often, a patient has received antibiotics, and a temporary defervescence occurs before the hectic fevers of an abscess re-emerge. In the latter situation, the respiratory symptoms may be less notable but virtually always are present.[14] This biphasic presentation was described more than 70 years ago in postoperative aspiration[46] and continues to be typical of many lung abscesses.

Subacute presentations are typical in patients with tuberculosis or fungal abscesses and usually are associated with other chronic systemic symptoms, such as anorexia, weight loss, and malaise. Cough may be prominent. Aspiration pneumonia may take an indolent or acute course, depending primarily on the organisms in the abscess, the volume of aspirated material, and the status of the host.

The physical findings in lung abscess are limited. Children usually have fever,[26,47] whereas adults present with fever less frequently (19%).[38] Tachypnea is a variable finding. Typically, auscultation is unrevealing except in cases of very large abscesses, in which loss of normal breath sounds is perceived. Adults and older children seem to have more discrete physical findings, with rales and decreased breath sounds in approximately one third of adult cases,[38] but they are uncommon findings in young children.[3]

An abscess can rupture into the bronchus, the mediastinum, or the pleura. In all cases, these complications are significant. In children, all organisms seem capable of causing these complications, but polymicrobial and anaerobic infections are suspected most often. Rupture into the bronchus may not be harmful if the volume of the abscess cavity does not overwhelm the host's ability to cough and clear the material. In an immunocompromised host, rupture may lead to disseminated pneumonia and further abscesses or death. Among adult patients who died of lung abscess, 22 percent were found to have died of aspiration of the abscess contents.[16]

In an otherwise healthy individual, rupture into the bronchus can be beneficial because it decompresses the abscess and allows the affected tissues to heal more rapidly. It is associated with the sudden production of foul-smelling, abundant, and sometimes blood-stained sputum. Frank hemoptysis is uncommon. Rupture into the mediastinum can be life-threatening, can be associated with chest pain and cardiac compromise, and requires surgery to drain the resulting mediastinitis. Rupture into the pleural space results in pleuritic pain, enhancement of symptoms on inspiration, and often a more toxic presentation, and may require drainage.

Routine laboratory information is of limited help. The white blood cell count and erythrocyte sedimentation rate are elevated nonspecifically, and a left shift of the white blood cell differential count typically occurs.[14] Certain laboratory tests, such as the purified protein derivative tuberculosis skin test, HIV serology, or sweat chloride test, may be helpful in revealing an underlying cause. Except for the tuberculosis skin test, such studies should not be performed routinely and should be directed by a family history or other findings, such as chronic diarrhea or lymphadenopathy. Blood cultures are helpful but are positive in fever than 10 percent of cases.[14,47]

DIFFERENTIAL DIAGNOSIS

The major differential diagnoses in the management of a lung abscess are anatomic. A lung abscess must be differentiated from pneumonia, necrotizing pneumonia, pneumatocele, loculated empyema, and a purulent pleural effusion with a bronchopleural fistula. CT or ultrasound may confirm an abscess by documenting central cavitation and differentiating pleural from parenchymal tissues. An abscess may be confused with a congenital cyst, pseudocyst, hydatid cyst, saccular bronchiectasis, pneumatocele, or sequestration. Chest CT allows definition of these entities in many cases by identifying the associated structures, such as the vascular supply and pleural borders.

Apart from the anatomic and infectious causes of lung abscess, the other very rare cause is cancer. Unrecognized metastatic disease from Ewing sarcoma or osteosarcomas with associated central necrosis can mimic an abscess or, by obstructing a bronchus, can promote abscess formation.

DIAGNOSIS

The diagnosis of lung abscess almost always is made by imaging the lung. In most cases, the plain radiograph is adequate to define a lung abscess (Fig. 30–1), showing a thickened cavity with an air-fluid level that can be accentuated by placing the patient in the lateral decubitus or erect position. Atelectasis often occurs as an expanding abscess compressing adjacent tissues. Pleural thickening may occur if the abscess is subpleural. Hilar adenopathy occurs in subacute situations. Visualization can be obtained with bronchoscopy if the abscess ruptures into the bronchus, but it is limited by the location of the abscess and skill of the bronchoscopist. The procedure usually is not performed for anatomic diagnosis but rather to obtain microbiologic specimens or exclude a foreign body.

CT is optimal in its ability to identify smaller or multiple abscesses, document the impact of the abscess on adjacent tissues, identify cystic processes mimicking an abscess, and define an abscess for which an organized pneumonia obscures an air-fluid level on plain film.[20] CT scan of a lung abscess reveals an air-fluid level with an active rim, and the abscess is distinguished from necrotizing pneumonia, which lacks enhancement on contrast studies and lacks a distinct air-fluid level.[18] Nuclear imaging is described[11] but used rarely and adds little to the information obtained by CT.

After a presumed abscess is defined by imaging, needle aspiration of the abscess or bronchoscopic recovery of abscess fluid should allow confirmation and identification of the infectious cause of the process. Based on available pediatric studies, whether either procedure hastens recovery or reveals the microbiologic cause in pretreated individuals cannot be predicted. In a case

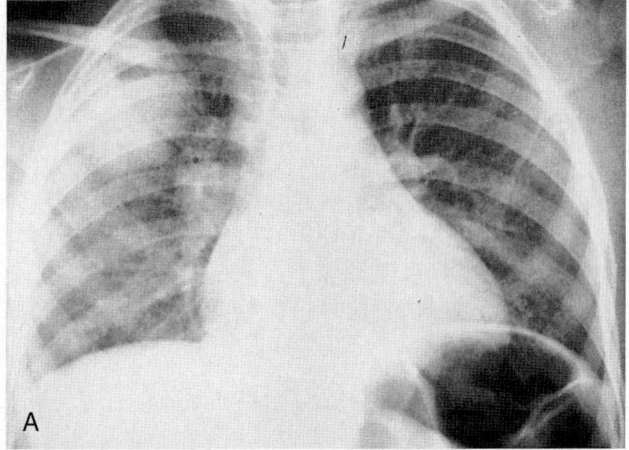

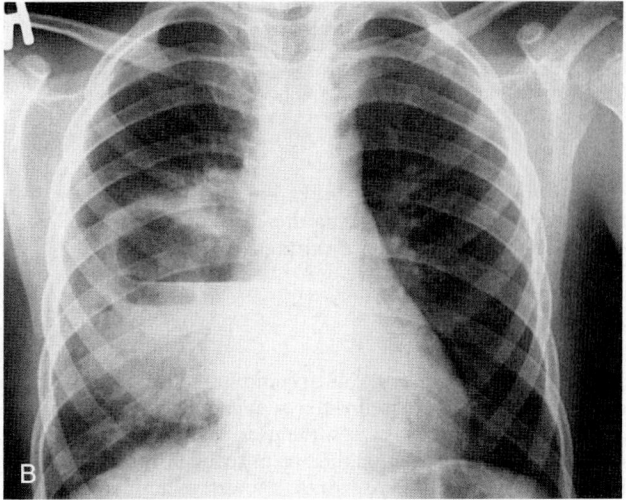

Figure 30–1 A, Plain chest film of a 4-year-old African-American boy with symptoms, including cough and fever of 104° F, for 4 days. He was treated initially with oral cefaclor and re-presented with this radiograph showing an air-fluid level in the right upper lobe. On intravenous cefuroxime, he was afebrile in 48 hours and went home on oral cefuroxime axetil after 4 days. **B,** Plain chest film of a 6-year-old African-American boy who presented after 5 days of symptoms with high fever, productive cough, dyspnea, and abdominal pain. The plain chest film reveals multiple air-fluid levels. Nafcillin and cefotaxime were begun. On day 4, an ultrasound-guided diagnostic aspiration recovered thick purulent material, but Gram stain and all cultures, including anaerobic and fungal, were negative. He was afebrile in 7 days and went home on amoxicillin-clavulanic acid at 10 days.

report in which an infant had abscesses in both lungs, the time to recovery was equal in the abscess that was drained and the other abscesses that were treated medically.[29] An adult study using thin-needle aspiration showed positive cultures in 92 percent of patients not pretreated with antibiotics and in 70 percent of patients pretreated.[37]

Directly aspirating a lung abscess may be difficult or unsuccessful if the abscess is not large or peripheral, and complications such as lung laceration and sterile pleural effusions are real risks. Two groups[18,47] have had satisfactory pediatric experience using direct aspiration under CT guidance (Fig. 30–2). Bronchoscopy particularly is valuable if foreign bodies are suspected or pus can be recovered. When material is obtained, a putrid quality is a clue that anaerobic organisms are present. Typically, the abscess contains pure neutrophils. Occasionally, counterimmune electrophoresis or other antigen detection systems may assist in the microbiologic diagnosis when cultures are negative.[16] Because of

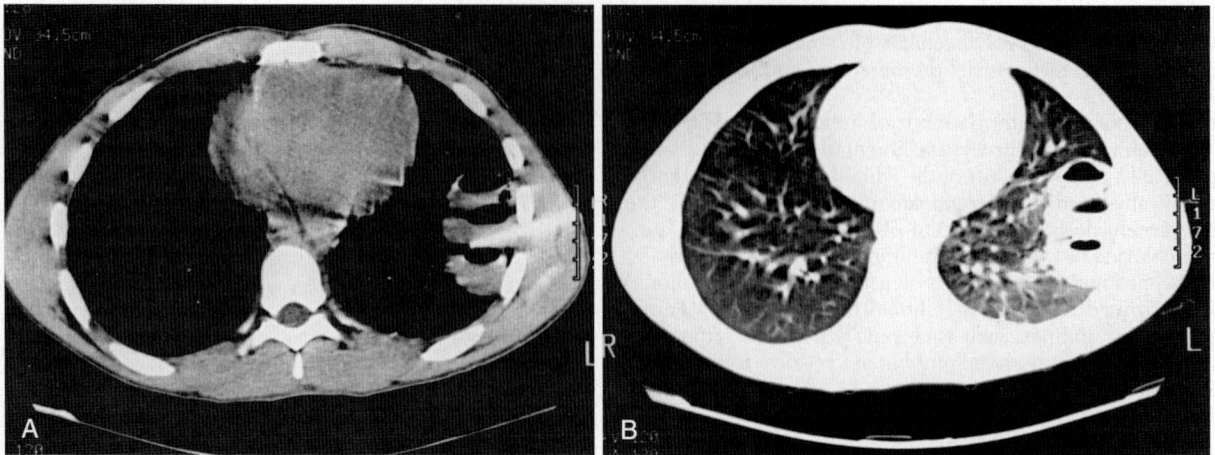

Figure 30–2 A and **B,** Computed tomography (CT) scans of a 15-year-old white boy who, 4 days before admission, reported a mild aspiration during fresh-water swimming. He awoke the next day with chest and back pain. He then developed low-grade fever. A plain chest film showed a large, thick-walled abscess in the left lower lobe. CT scans show insertion of a 20-gauge needle into the abscess on the first day of admission **(A)** and detail of the wall thickness and cavitation **(B).** *Haemophilus influenzae* grew from the aspirate. Ampicillin-sulbactam was initiated and continued for 14 days.

the special handling required, these technologies usually are employed only after standard cultures have failed.

TREATMENT

Although surgery has a role in specific situations, the treatment of lung abscess in children often is successful when antibiotics alone are used.[39] In most cases, the need for surgery is limited to instances of failed antibiotic therapy or to an abscess complicated by rupture into adjacent tissues. Newer techniques, such as hyperbaric oxygen,[8] have been proposed as adjuvant therapy.

The initial choice of antibiotics almost always is presumptive because abscess material may be unavailable. For primary lung abscesses in which no risk factors are identified and in the absence of positive blood cultures, the recommended approach is to begin therapy with a regimen that covers *S. aureus*, *S. pneumoniae*, and the anaerobic microorganisms that normally are found in the upper respiratory tract. Clindamycin, ampicillin plus sulbactam, and ticarcillin plus clavulanate frequently are used in this setting.

For patients at risk for aspiration or who are immunocompromised, gram-negative pathogens also must be considered. This spectrum of pathogens can be addressed with one of several drug regimens: clindamycin and cefotaxime (or an aminoglycoside); ticarcillin plus clavulanate or piperacillin plus tazobactam; or nafcillin (or cefazolin), gentamicin, and metronidazole. The possible emergence of more penicillin-resistant species, such as *Streptococcus milleri* and *Klebsiella*, in community-acquired disease of adults and children supports these broad-spectrum regimens in children.[21,41] Patients with cystic fibrosis are particularly vulnerable to *Pseudomonas* spp. and should receive an aminoglycoside plus an additional antipseudomonal penicillin or cephalosporin. Carbapenem therapy would be an alternative. When endocarditis is present, treatment (e.g., vancomycin plus gentamicin with or without anaerobic coverage) should be provided for staphylococci, streptococci, and enterococci while awaiting results of blood cultures.

S. pneumoniae has been isolated infrequently in lung abscesses (see Table 30–2). Most patients with resistant organisms are still clinically sensitive to achievable doses of penicillins (penicillin G, minimum inhibitory concentrations of 0.12 to 2.0).[35] Drug resistance to *S. aureus* is a much more concerning issue in lung abscess, and empiric therapy with vancomycin is required if

methicillin-resistant *S. aureus* is suspected while waiting for confirmation. For a critically ill patient with lung abscess, some experts recommend nafcillin, gentamicin, or both.

With culture information available, therapy is directed specifically at the pathogens isolated. In most patients, oral or intravenous antibiotic therapy has been administered before aspiration of a lung abscess is done, however, and may affect which organisms are recovered.[13] For this reason, coverage should be extended to include organisms that are likely to be present but are not recovered, such as anaerobes, in a setting of aspiration.

All bacterial lung abscesses should be treated with intravenous therapy until the patient is stable and no longer toxic. In approximately two thirds to four fifths of patients, this condition occurs within 3 to 7 days of instituting intravenous therapy.[14,28] After the patient has been afebrile for 48 to 72 hours, initiation of oral therapy may be considered. Certain oral drugs, such as amoxicillin plus clavulanate and clindamycin, achieve therapeutic serum levels and are effective against the spectrum of organisms in lung abscesses.

The length of total therapy for a lung abscess should be 2 to 3 weeks. Complicated infections should be treated intravenously until fever has disappeared and no evidence of continuing inflammation exists. An additional 2 to 3 weeks of oral treatment should follow. Radiographic resolution of a lung abscess that is not drained occurs over the course of weeks. Even with drainage, resolution may not occur more rapidly. Chest radiography should be repeated every 1 to 2 weeks until complete resolution is documented.

Tuberculous lung abscesses may rupture spontaneously into the pleura. Treatment is not directed at the immediate abscess or pleuritis but at preventing spread if it erupts into a bronchus. Preventing reactivation several years later is another goal of therapy.

Clinical failure is defined by persistent fever and toxicity. The length of time treatment with intravenous antibiotics should continue before declaring therapy a failure is not clearly defined. Suggestions in the literature range from 1 to 3 weeks.[2,4,39] When clinical failure occurs, several options are available, including drainage of the abscess, which permits identification of the organisms causing the disease process.

Bronchoscopy may allow direct perforation of the abscess and evacuation of its contents. A risk of fatality occurring from aspiration of abscess contents exists, however.[19]

Needle aspiration (one or more) also is possible under fluoroscopy, ultrasonography, or CT guidance.[18,24,25] Simple CT-guided needle aspiration leads to relief of symptoms in approximately two thirds of cases within 48 hours.[18] The risk of complications seems to be low.[18,25] Percutaneous transthoracic tube drainage has been used in pediatric lung abscesses.[12,27,36,50,51] The risk is lowest if the abscess is peripheral, and adhesion of the opposing pleural surfaces is a consequence of the inflammatory process. When this adhesion occurs, the needle or catheter does not traverse the pleural space. Catheter drainage may be attempted in abscesses larger than 20 cm³ or 4 cm in diameter[2,18] using 8 to 10 French pigtail catheters. Smaller abscesses are technically difficult to manage.

Chest tube thoracostomy previously was the standard therapy of lung abscesses[31,33]; it is now recommended when conservative therapy fails and may play a role in patients with large abscesses if the abscess abuts the parietal pleura and provides a direct path from the exterior surface to the abscess.[30] A 25-year review of the literature found that significant complications, such as hemothorax, pneumothorax, bronchopleural fistula, empyema, and catheter occlusion, occurred in 9.7 percent of cases, with an overall mortality rate of 4.8 percent.[50]

Surgery for lung abscess is not well described in the pediatric literature. One report that combines surgery for lung abscess and necrotizing pneumonia had no mortality in the postsurgery period and a reversible complication rate of 10 percent.[48] Indications for surgery included associated pyopneumothorax, size of the abscess, and tension pneumatocele. Another possible surgical indication is proximity of a lung abscess to the mediastinum. In the face of antibiotic failure, an open lung procedure and wedge resection may be required, depending on the location of the abscess.[5] The procedure typically is successful and often obviates the need to perform a lobectomy.[22,53] In a complicated case, such as with a gangrenous lung, lobar resection may be necessary. Managing an infant with a lung abscess has required surgery more often than in older children.[45,52]

PROGNOSIS

The outcome for pediatric patients usually is very good when lung abscesses are uncomplicated, and recovery is more rapid than in adults.[32] Most patients have complete symptomatic and radiographic resolution in 3 to 6 weeks, with normal pulmonary function tests at follow-up.[4,14] Complicated disease associated with thoracostomy tubes and empyema more likely leads to residual symptoms (e.g., pleurisy) and persistent effusions or pleural thickening on radiographs. In reports published since 1982, half of patients with lung abscess have required surgical intervention, such as thoracentesis to drain an empyema, lobectomy, or decortication, and 20 percent have required lobectomy or decortication.[4,7,14,47] If patients require lung resection, they may experience immediate surgical complications; long-term exercise tolerance may be limited, and other problems, such as scoliosis, may develop. One study found normal pulmonary functions in patients studied after undergoing lobectomy, however.[34]

Rarely, a residual cavity may develop and become superinfected. The mortality rate is 4 to 11 percent[14,47] for patients with primary and secondary lung abscesses.[14,47] Higher risk of morbidity and mortality occurs in patients with secondary abscesses who have complications caused by either a decrease in host resistance or underlying disease.[14,38,47,48]

REFERENCES

1. Abramson, J. S., and Mills, E. L.: Depression of neutrophil function induced by viruses and its role in secondary microbial infections. Rev. Infect. Dis. *10*:326-341, 1988.

2. Al-Salem, A. H., and Ali, E. A.: Computed tomography-guided percutaneous needle aspiration of lung abscesses in neonates and children. Pediatr. Surg. Int. *12*:417-419, 1997.

3. Asher, M. I., and Beaudry, P. H.: Lung abscess. *In* Chernick, V., and Kendig, E. L. (eds.): Disorders of the Respiratory Tract in Children. 5th ed. Philadelphia, W. B. Saunders, 1990, pp. 429-435.

4. Asher, M. I., Spier, S., Beland, M., et al.: Primary lung abscess in childhood: The long-term outcome of conservative management. Am. J. Dis. Child. *136*:491-494, 1982.

5. Ball, W. S., Jr., Bisset, G. S., III, and Towbin, R. B.: Percutaneous drainage of chest abscesses in children. Radiology *171*:431-434, 1989.

6. Bartlett, J. G., Gorbach, S. L., Tally, F. P., et al.: Bacteriology and treatment of primary lung abscess. Am. Rev. Respir. Dis. *109*:510-518, 1974.

7. Brook, I., and Finegold, S. M.: Bacteriology and therapy of lung abscess in children. J. Pediatr. *94*:10-12, 1979.

8. Bulynin, V. I., Koshelev, P. I., and Barsukov, V. A.: Treatment of acute lung abscess using hyperbaric oxygenation. Grudnaia Serdechno-Sosudistaia Khir. *5*:37-41, 1990.

9. Canny, G. J., Marcotte, J. E., and Levison, H.: Lung abscess in cystic fibrosis. Thorax *41*:221-222, 1986.

10. Chun, P.-C., Huang, L.-M., Wu, P.-S., et al.: Clinical management and outcome of childhood lung abscess: A 16-year experience. J. Microbiol. Immunol. Infect. *38*:183-188, 2005.

11. Cook, P. S., Datz, F. L., Disbro, M. A., et al.: Pulmonary uptake in indium-111 leukocyte imaging: Clinical significance in patients with suspected occult infections. Radiology *150*:557-561, 1984.

12. Cuestas, R. A., Kienzle, G. D., and Armstrong, J. D., II: Percutaneous drainage of lung abscesses in infants. Pediatr. Infect. Dis. J. *8*:390-392, 1989.

13. Dobranowski, J., and Stringer, D. A.: Diagnosis of *Legionella* lung abscess by percutaneous needle aspiration. Can. Assoc. Radiol. J. *40*:43-44, 1989.

14. Emanuel, B., and Shulman S. T.: Lung abscess in infants and children. Clin. Pediatr. *34*:2-6, 1995.

15. Fitzgerald, D., Harvey, J., Issacs, D., et al.: The case of the persistent pleural effusion. Pediatr. Infect. Dis. J. *10*:479-480, 1991.

16. Hanukoglu, A., Gutman, R., Fried, D., et al.: Lung abscess caused by *Streptococcus pneumoniae* type 3: The importance of counterimmunoelectrophoresis in laboratory diagnosis. Infection *12*:85-86, 1984.

17. Harber, P., and Terry, P. B.: Fatal lung abscesses: Review of 11 years experience. South. Med. J. *74*:281-283, 1981.

18. Hoffer, F. A., Bloom, D. A., Colin, A. A., et al.: Lung abscess versus necrotizing pneumonia: Implications for interventional therapy. Pediatr. Radiol. *29*:87-91, 1999.

19. Hussain, Z., Lannigan, R., and Austin, T. W.: Pulmonary cavitation due to *Neisseria mucosa* in a child with chronic neutropenia. Eur. J. Clin. Microbiol. Infect. Dis. *7*:175-176, 1988.

20. Johnson, J. F., Shiels, W. E., White, C. B., et al.: Concealed pulmonary abscess: Diagnosis by computed tomography. Pediatrics *78*:283-286, 1986.

21. Kobayashi, K.: *Streptococcus milleri* as a cause of pulmonary abscess. Acta Paediatr. *90*:233-234, 2001.

22. Kosloske, A. M., Ball, W. S., Jr., Butler, C., et al.: Drainage of pediatric lung abscess by cough, catheter, or complete resection. J. Pediatr. Surg. *21*:596-600, 1986.

23. Kuhn, C.: Bacterial infections. *In* Thurlbeck, W. M., and Churg, A. M. (eds.): Pathology of the Lung. 2nd ed. New York, Thieme Medical Publishers, 1995, p. 285.

24. Levine, M. M., Ashman, R., and Heald, F.: Anaerobic (putrid) lung abscess in adolescence. Am. J. Dis. Child. *130*:77-81, 1976.

25. Lorenzo, R. L., Bradford, B. F., Black, J., et al.: Lung abscesses in children: Diagnostic and therapeutic needle aspiration. Radiology *157*:79-80, 1985.

26. Mark, P. H., and Turner, J. A.: Lung abscess in childhood. Thorax *23*:216-220, 1968.

27. Mayer, T., Matlak, M. E., Condon, V., et al.: Computed tomographic findings of neonatal lung abscess. Am. J. Dis. Child. *136*:39-41, 1982.

28. McCracken, G. H.: Lung abscess in childhood. Hosp. Pract. *13*:35-36, 1978.

29. Melhem, R. E.: Percutaneous drainage of chest abscesses in children. Radiology *173*:575-576, 1989.

30. Mengoli, L.: Giant lung abscess treated by tube thoracostomy. J. Thorac. Cardiovasc. Surg. *90*:186-194, 1985.

31. Monaldi, V.: Endocavitary aspiration in the treatment of lung abscess. Dis. Chest *29*:193-201, 1956.

32. Neild, J. E., Eykyn, S. J., and Phillips, I.: Lung abscess and empyema. Q. J. M. *57*:875-882, 1985.

33. Neuhof, H., and Touroff, A. S. W.: Acute putrid abscess of the lung: Hyperacute variety. J. Thorac. Surg. *12*:98-106, 1936.

34. Nonoyama, A., Tanaka, K., Osako, T., et al.: Surgical treatment of pulmonary abscess in children under ten years of age. Chest *85*:358-362, 1984.

35. Pallares, R., Linares, J., Vadillo, M., et al.: Resistance to penicillin and cephalosporin and mortality from severe pneumococcal pneumonia in Barcelona, Spain. N. Engl. J. Med. *333*:474-480, 1995.

36. Parker, L. A., Melton, J. W., Delany, D. J., et al.: Percutaneous small bore catheter drainage in the management of lung abscesses. Chest *92*:213-218, 1987.

37. Pena Grinan, N., Munoz Lucena, F., Vargas Romero, J., et al.: Yield of percutaneous needle lung aspiration in lung abscess. Chest *97*:69-74, 1990.

38. Pohlson, E. C., McNamara, J. J., Char, C., et al.: Lung abscess: A changing pattern of the disease. Am. J. Surg. *150*:97-101, 1985.

39. Powell, K.: Primary pulmonary abscess. Am. J. Dis. Child. *136*:489-490, 1982.

40. Purdy, G. D., Cullen, M., Yedlin, S., et al.: An unusual neonatal case presentation: *Streptococcus pneumoniae* pneumonia with abscess and pneumatocoele formation. J. Perinatol. 7:378-381, 1987.

41. Schiza, S., Siafakas, N. M.: Clinical presentation and management of empyema, lung abscess and pleural effusion. Curr. Opin. Pulm. Med. *12*:205-211, 2006.

42. Shamir, R., Horev, G., Merlob, P., et al.: *Citrobacter diversus* lung abscess in a preterm infant. Pediatr. Infect. Dis. J. 9:221-222, 1990.

43. Shanks, G. D., and Berman, J. D.: Anaerobic pulmonary abscesses: Hematogenous spread from head and neck infections. Clin. Pediatr. *25*:520-522, 1986.

44. Shapiro, M. E., Kasper, D. L., Zaleznik, D. F., et al.: Cellular control of abscess formation: Role of T cells in the regulation of abscesses formed in response to *Bacteroides fragilis*. J. Immunol. *137*:341-346, 1986.

45. Siegel, D., and McCracken, G. H., Jr.: Neonatal lung abscess: A report of six cases. Am. J. Dis. Child. *133*:947-949, 1979.

46. Smith, D. T.: The diagnosis and treatment of pulmonary abscess in children. J. A. M. A. *103*:971-974, 1934.

47. Tan, T. Q., Seilheimer, D. K., and Kaplan, S. L.: Pediatric lung abscess: Clinical management and outcome. Pediatr. Infect. Dis. J. *14*:51-55, 1995.

48. Tseng, Y.-L., Wu, M.-H., Lin, M.-Y., et al.: Surgery for lung abscess in immunocompetent and immunocompromised children. J. Pediatr. Surg. *36*:470-473, 2001.

49. van Sonnenberg, E., D'Agostino, H. B., Casola, G., et al.: Lung abscess: CT-guided drainage. Radiology *178*:347-351, 1991.

50. Wali, S. O., Shugaeri, A., Smmaman, Y. S., et al. Percutaneous drainage of pyogenic lung abscess. Scand. J. Infect. Dis. *34*:673-679, 2002.

51. Weber, T. R., Vane, D. W., Krishna, G., et al.: Neonatal lung abscess: Resection using one-lung anesthesia. Ann. Thorac. Surg. *36*:464-467, 1983.

52. Weissberg, D.: Percutaneous drainage of lung abscess. J. Thorac. Cardiovasc. Surg. *87*:308-312, 1984.

53. Wessler, H., and Schwarz, H.: Abscess of the lung in infants and children. Am. J. Dis. Child. *19*:137-140, 1920.

CHAPTER 31

CYSTIC FIBROSIS

Lisa Saiman ○ Peter W. Hiatt

Cystic fibrosis (CF) is the most common inherited lethal disease of whites. It occurs primarily among individuals of Central and Western European origin and affects more than 30,000 Americans and 60,000 people worldwide.[365] The estimated incidence in the United States is 1:2000 to 1:2600 white,[377] 1:19,000 African-American, 1:11,500 Hispanic, and 1:25,000 Asian-American live births.[226] CF has an autosomal recessive mode of inheritance. Affected individuals are phenotypic homozygotes, and both parents usually are heterozygotes or carriers. The carrier frequency in whites in the United States is approximately 1 in 25, with full siblings of children with CF having a one in four chance of being affected.

Mutations in a single gene located on the long arm of chromosome 7 account for the defective protein in CF.[365] A range of different mutations at the DNA level account for the abnormal protein. The most common mutation (ΔF508) is the absence of three sequential nucleotides, which leads to the deletion (Δ) of phenylalanine (F) at the 508 position on the CF transmembrane conductance regulator protein (CFTR). Approximately 70 percent of individuals with CF have this mutation. To date, more than 1500 mutations in the CFTR gene have been identified,[76] but fewer than 25 occur with a frequency of more than 0.1 percent.[122] Certain populations have higher frequencies of specific mutations, such as W128X in Ashkenazi Jews[226] or G551D in French Canadians.[277]

Five classes of mutations have been proposed to account for reduced CFTR chloride channel function.[141,277,366,391] Class 1 mutations are mutations in which stop codons or frame shift mutations cause early termination of mRNA translation and minimal to no protein production. In class 2 mutations (ΔF508), protein fails to mature, resulting in little expression of CFTR at the cell membrane. Class 3 and class 4 mutations are associated with defective regulation and decreased conductance of chloride at the cell membrane. Protein production and transit to the cell surface occur, but altered chloride conductance is present, or chloride conductance is nonexistent. Class 5 mutations are splice site mutations, which affect the amount of CFTR produced.

Other mutations are associated with unstable CFTR at the cell membrane. The presence of more than 1500 mutations for CFTR has prompted investigators to evaluate the association of genotype with clinical disease. The CF phenotype genotype consortium has shown that certain mutations from classes 3 to 5 are associated with pancreatic sufficiency; however, correlation of CF genotype with the severity of pulmonary disease has been poor. The wide variation in pulmonary disease observed in CF may reflect the effects of environment, patient compliance, polymorphisms in CFTR, and modifier genes that affect the function of the CFTR.

CFTR is a glycoprotein expressed at low levels by surface epithelial cells in the lung, sweat glands, pancreas, liver, large intestine, and testes.[274] Higher levels of expression have been reported in submucosal glands. CFTR protein is a member of a group of membrane transport proteins known as the *ABC-transporter superfamily*.[158] Researchers have confirmed that CFTR functions as an apical chloride channel mediated by cyclic adenosine monophosphate containing 1480 amino acids. It is composed of two membrane-spanning domains, two nucleotide-binding domains that interact with adenosine triphosphate, and a regulatory domain.[6] Activation of the channel is regulated by protein kinase A, which serves as a target for phosphorylation. CFTR in epithelial cell membranes may influence the expression of other proteins important in regulating inflammation, ion transport, and cell signaling, altering the CF phenotype.[286] CFTR regulates the activity of separate calcium-activated chloride channels and down-regulates sodium transport, balancing the rates of chloride secretion and sodium absorption.[116,175,187]

CFTR is responsible for the proper hydration of secretions in the airway, pancreas, and other tissues. An inability to secrete chloride and excessive absorption of sodium and water contribute to altered luminal secretions in patients with CF. In the lung, this alteration leads to decreased airway surface liquid, decreased mucociliary clearance, and a predisposition to chronic bacterial infections.

CLINICAL MANIFESTATIONS

Individuals with CF have exocrine gland dysfunction, which results in progressive suppurative obstructive lung disease, pancreatic insufficiency (85 to 90 percent), elevated sweat electrolytes, male infertility (>95 percent), and female infertility. Less common manifestations include hepatobiliary disease, osteoarthropathy, diabetes mellitus, nasal polyposis, and meconium ileus (Table 31-1).[56,75]

TABLE 31-1 Clinical Features of Cystic Fibrosis at Diagnosis

0-2 years
Meconium ileus
Obstructive jaundice
Hypoproteinemia/anemia
Bleeding diathesis
Heat prostration/hyponatremia
Failure to thrive
Steatorrhea
Rectal prolapse
Bronchitis/bronchiolitis
Staphylococcal pneumonia

2-12 years
Malabsorption
Recurrent pneumonia/bronchitis
Nasal polyps
Intussusception

>13 years
Chronic pulmonary disease
Clubbing
Abnormal glucose tolerance
Diabetes mellitus
Chronic intestinal obstruction
Recurrent pancreatitis
Focal biliary cirrhosis
Portal hypertension
Gallstones
Aspermia

From Maclusky, I, and Levison, H.: Kendig's Disorders of the Respiratory Tract in Children. 5th ed. Philadelphia, W. B. Saunders, 1990, p. 701.

The potential relationship between genotype (the genetic constitution of an individual) and phenotype (the physical expression of that genotype) in CF is an area of active clinical investigation. To date, the correlation of genotype to phenotype has not led to many clear associations between severity or course of pulmonary disease and type of genetic mutations.[43,173] A family-based study of CF involving monozygotic twins, dizygotic twins, and siblings reported that a significant portion of the variability in pulmonary function was attributable to heritability, independent of CFTR genotype.[358] This finding suggests that modifier genes account for a significant amount of the variance observed in CF lung disease. Numerous candidate modifier genes have been investigated to account for the variance in CF pulmonary disease, with more recent reports identifying transforming growth factor-β1 and glutamate-cysteine ligase as candidates.[91,212] In addition to modifier genes, environmental factors, including passive smoke exposure, infection, and socioeconomic status, have been associated with reduced lung function.[68,171,235,287,300] Multiple mutations, incomplete understanding of the physiologic function of CFTR, and the role of modifier genes have delayed understanding of the genotypic influence on phenotype in CF.

A strong association between pancreatic function and genotype has been reported for individuals homozygous for ΔF508.[27] Most subjects homozygous for ΔF508 have pancreatic insufficiency.[72] Obstruction of the pancreatic duct begins in utero, resulting in fibrosis and loss of exocrine pancreatic function. Pancreatic fluid from patients with CF is low in enzyme and bicarbonate concentrations, resulting in maldigestion of fat and protein. Clinically, children commonly present with steatorrhea, protein-calorie malnutrition, muscle wasting, and progressive failure to thrive. A voracious appetite is characteristic, and stools are described as bulky, greasy, and foul-smelling. Approximately 10 to 15 percent of patients have enough preservation of pancreatic function to allow for normal digestion of food (pancreatic-sufficient).[86] At least five mutations from classes 3 to 5 described earlier are associated with pancreatic sufficiency, whereas almost all patients homozygous for ΔF508 have pancreatic insufficiency.[72]

Failure to thrive is a common complication observed at the time of diagnosis. If malnutrition is severe, hypoproteinemia and edema are observed. In addition, malabsorption can lead to vitamin deficiency, especially of fat-soluble vitamins A, D, E, and K. These problems can be reversed with pancreatic enzyme replacement therapy, oral nutritional supplements, and routine vitamin supplements.

Glucose metabolism often becomes impaired with age, as fibrosis of the pancreas occurs in patients with exocrine pancreatic insufficiency. In the 2005 CF registry, 25 percent of adults were reported to have impaired glucose tolerance or CF-related diabetes with and without fasting hyperglycemia. Decreased secretion of insulin and reductions in peripheral glucose use and hepatic insulin sensitivity are observed in patients with impaired glucose tolerance.[220] CF-related diabetes has features of type 1 and 2 diabetes. The prevalence increases with age and is associated with increased morbidity and mortality.[217]

Liver disease in CF is associated with pancreatic insufficiency.[251] Approximately 25 percent of patients with CF develop focal biliary cirrhosis, but less than 5 percent progress to multilobar biliary cirrhosis and portal hypertension. In the absence of CFTR, bile becomes inspissated and associated with periductal inflammation and fibrosis. Liver function tests frequently are abnormal, as is a small, poorly functioning gallbladder. Cholelithiasis has been reported in 12 percent of patients and may be related to loss of bile acids in the stool.[66,107,108] Meconium ileus, the thick inspissated meconium that mechanically obstructs the distal ileum, occurs in 8 to 20 percent of newborns with CF. It also is associated with pancreatic insufficiency.[172] Modifier genes are thought to play an important role in the development of meconium ileus.[24] A similar syndrome (distal intestinal obstructive syndrome) mimicking meconium ileus can occur in older children and young adults with CF.

Absence of the vas deferens with secondary aspermia renders 98 percent of men with CF infertile.[87] Sexual potency is normal, and with microsurgical techniques for sperm aspiration, affected men can become biologic fathers.[211] Men with congenital absence of the vas deferens can have abnormal CF alleles with little clinical expression of disease other than the reproductive system. Infertility in women with CF may be 20 percent related to secondary amenorrhea (malnutrition) and dehydrated cervical mucus.[329]

Pulmonary disease is the primary cause of morbidity and mortality in patients with CF.[378] Expression of CFTR has been localized to the airways and submucosal glands of the lung.[348] Clinical studies in young children with CF have found significant inflammatory changes in the airways in bacterial-positive and bacterial-negative patients.[13,78,140,215,281,347] Imaging studies using high-resolution computed tomography (CT) in infants with CF describe the presence of thickened airway walls and nonhomogeneous air trapping.[80,197,206] The lungs are morphologically normal at birth; within weeks, they begin showing evidence of small airway abnormalities and inflammation. Small and medium-sized airways become obstructed, and neutrophils are the inflammatory cells primarily recovered from bronchoalveolar lavage (BAL) fluid. An intense neutrophilic response leads to the release of proteases that cause chronic injury to the respiratory epithelium and supporting airway structure. The massive numbers of neutrophils subsequently release elastase, which overwhelms the antiproteases in the airway, contributing to enhanced destruction of tissue. Large amounts of neutrophil-derived DNA and cytosol proteins are released into the airway lumen, increasing sputum viscosity and worsening airway obstruction.[78]

Progressive bronchiectasis develops with time, leading to advanced destruction of the airways and parenchyma (Figs. 31–1 and 31–2). Bronchiectatic cysts are prominent, especially in the

Many children with CF present during infancy with recurrent wheezing or persistent bronchiolitis. Most infants are asymptomatic at birth; however, many develop tachypnea, wheezing, hypoxia, and hyperinflation after having a respiratory viral infection.[146] These findings often resolve with therapy. As mucopurulent secretions increase, chronic cough develops.[56] Digital clubbing occurs gradually and correlates with severity of lung disease. On examination, there is evidence of crackles and decreased breath sounds secondary to mucopurulent secretions. Acute exacerbations may develop, requiring intravenous antibiotic therapy and frequent hospitalization. Approximately a third of patients with CF in the 2005 U.S. CF registry[75] experienced a pulmonary exacerbation requiring intravenous antibiotics. As lung disease progresses, tolerance for exercise is reduced, dyspnea increases, and respiratory failure develops. There is marked heterogeneity in the rate of progression of pulmonary disease. Some patients live to the sixth decade of life, whereas others die as a result of respiratory failure before their tenth birthday.

In 2005, the median predicted survival for individuals with CF was 36.5 years. Survival for children born in 2000 is expected to increase, with the median age approaching the fourth decade of life. In the United States, 40 percent of people with CF are 18 years old or older, and within 10 years, half are expected to be older than 18 years. As life expectancy has increased, CF has become a disease of children and adults.

DIAGNOSIS

The diagnosis of CF remains a clinical diagnosis in the face of more recent advances in technology. A consensus panel convened by the U.S. Cystic Fibrosis panel recommended a combination of phenotypic features, family history of CF, or positive newborn screen and one or more laboratory tests to diagnose CF.[284] Laboratory tests include identification of known CF mutations, abnormal bioelectric transepithelial membrane properties, and elevated concentrations of sweat chloride. The World Health Organization adopted similar recommendations.[379] Most patients continue to be diagnosed by clinical features and an elevated sweat test. Data from the 2005 U.S. CF registry reported that newborn screening accounted for 17 percent of newly diagnosed patients.[75] In the absence of newborn screening, an in utero diagnosis, or a family history of CF, a strong clinical suspicion is required for early recognition. Most children present with a history of recurrent lower respiratory tract disease and symptoms secondary to malabsorption. Approximately 15 to 20 percent of children have meconium ileus at birth or have a family history of CF or both.

The quantitative pilocarpine iontophoresis sweat test is one acceptable test to establish a diagnosis of CF.[284] A sweat chloride concentration greater than 60 mEq/L is consistent with a diagnosis of CF. Values between 40 and 60 mEq/L are considered borderline, and values less than 40 mEq/L are normal. Some data suggest that sweat chloride concentrations greater than 40 mEq/L in infants younger than 3 months old is highly suggestive of CF. The sweat test should be repeated on two separate occasions. Identification of two CF mutations by genotype is highly specific, but less sensitive. Mutational analysis can be done by several different techniques, with commercial laboratories testing for the most common 30 to 87 mutations. These laboratories identify approximately 90 percent of CF mutations but leave more than 1000 mutations unidentified. Extensive screening for the remaining 10 percent of mutations is expensive and impractical. For rare mutations, gene sequencing is available but expensive.[283,284] The ΔF508 mutation is found in 70 percent of patients with CF in the United States and a similar number of CF patients in the United Kingdom. Because each patient has two chromosomes, however, only 50 percent of patients are homozygous for ΔF508.

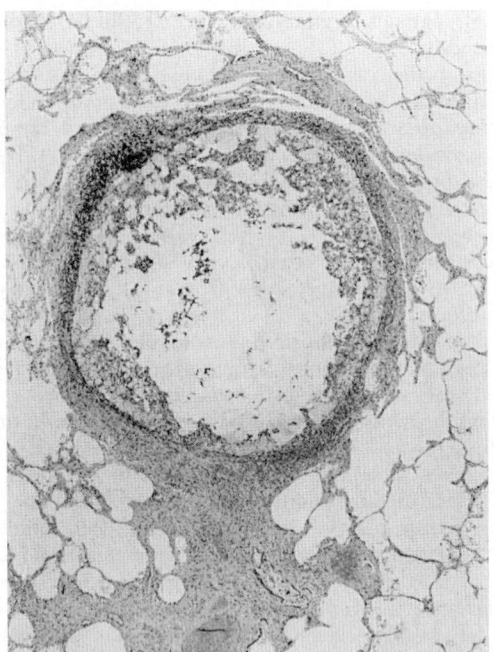

Figure 31–1 Early stages of lung disease in cystic fibrosis are shown in this lung specimen. Airway inflammation and bronchiectasis are present. The surrounding lung parenchyma is normal.

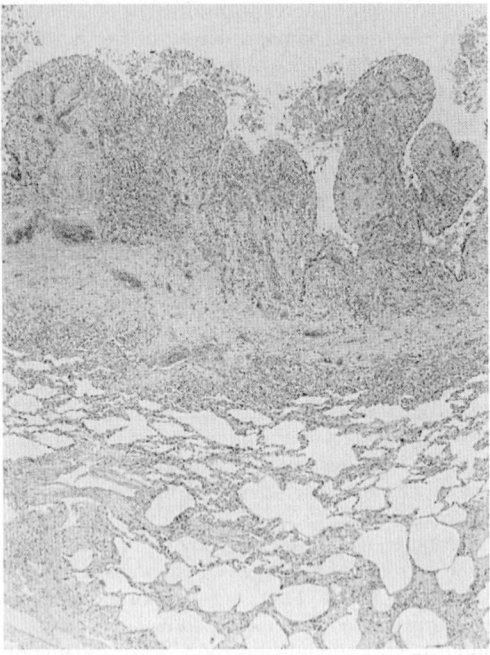

Figure 31–2 Late stages of pulmonary disease. Epithelial ulceration of the airway, loss of smooth muscle from the airway wall, inflammation, and bronchiectasis are present in the large airway at the top of the photomicrograph. Compression of the surrounding lung parenchyma occurs as bronchiectasis increases.

upper lobes. Death eventually occurs from respiratory failure. Progressive deterioration of pulmonary function occurs despite the routine use of anti-inflammatory therapy, mucolytics, airway clearance, and antimicrobial agents. Progressive destruction of the airway and increasing obstruction lead to air trapping, hyperinflation, hemoptysis, and spontaneous pneumothorax.

Nasal potential difference measurements assess the transepithelial electric potential difference that exists across nasal epithelium. Different patterns of potential difference are found in patients with CF.[284] Abnormalities in chloride transport and sodium absorption alter the transepithelial electric potential difference in CF compared with normal epithelia. The test can be useful in individuals with mild or atypical phenotypic features of CF, but it is not readily available, and it requires experienced personnel to perform.[283,284]

Newborn screening programs have been implemented in some states in the United States and the United Kingdom, Australia, and Europe. These programs identify newborns with CF using low values of trypsinogen in dried blood specimens obtained in routine screening programs for metabolic disorders. Improved nutritional status as a result of newborn screening has been reported in a controlled, randomized trial in Wisconsin.[104] Ninety percent of screened infants diagnosed with CF at birth maintained their weight greater than the 10th percentile compared with only 60 percent of unscreened controls. Children in the screened group were less likely to fall below the 10th percentile for weight and height from early childhood through 16 years of age.[44,105] In addition, cognitive function was improved significantly in the screened group.[182,183] No long-term improvements in pulmonary status were observed in the Wisconsin study; however, several observational studies have reported improved pulmonary outcomes, less colonization with *Pseudomonas aeruginosa*, decreased hospitalization for complications, and improved nutrition in children diagnosed by newborn screening.[5,106,180,188,278,282,386]

In addition to improving nutritional outcomes, newborn screening may result in improved survival rates for children. A systematic literature review of mortality in children with CF reported a survival benefit for patients diagnosed by newborn screening.[67,138] A survival effect also was shown in a study from Wales.[90] Without screening, approximately 60 percent of patients are diagnosed by the time they reach 1 year of age and almost 90 percent by the time they are 5 years. Early diagnosis through neonatal screening seems to improve nutritional outcome, with increasing evidence that these programs are associated with improved pulmonary outcomes and improved long-term survival.

The diagnosis of CF should be based on the presence of one or more clinical features (Table 31–2), a positive newborn screening test, and laboratory evidence of abnormal CFTR function. Laboratory tests include elevated sweat chloride concentration, two identifiable CF mutations, or abnormal in vivo nasal potential difference measurements made across the nasal epithelium.

PATHOGENESIS

The CFTR protein resides in the plasma membrane of epithelial cells and has several functions. In the sweat duct, it acts to absorb chloride; in the lung, it secretes chloride; and in the pancreas, it secretes chloride in exchange for bicarbonate.[342] Organs that are affected by the disease have abnormal chloride and fluid secretion, which impairs fluid movement and leads to ductular obstruction and organ damage. Five classes of CF mutations result in different amounts of CFTR expression and have been observed to produce varying clinical disease. The most common mutation, $\Delta F508$, is a class 2 mutation. The CF protein is misfolded and degraded before reaching the cell membrane.[54,273]

Other classes of mutations produce CFTR that cannot be activated, is decreased in abundance, or has altered conductance. Patients with at least one "mild" allele have some low level of CFTR expression. They retain some degree of pancreatic function, have less severe lung disease, and have sweat chloride concentrations that are borderline normal.[77,79,372] Male patients with congenital bilateral absence of the vas deferens are pancreatic sufficient, exhibit little or no lung disease, can have normal sweat chloride concentrations, and are thought to have CFTR expression that is 10 percent of normal.[9] Carriers for CFTR who are heterozygotes expressing half the expected amount of CFTR are at increased risk for developing pancreatitis, allergic bronchopulmonary aspergillosis (ABPA), and sinusitis.[49,64,93,263]

The range of severity of disease is related to the production of functioning CFTR. The amount of expression of CFTR is important in the pathogenesis of CF. Variation in the severity of disease in individuals with the same genotype indicates other factors, including the environment, genetic modifiers, and medical therapy, are important in long-term outcomes, however.

The exact mechanism by which altered salt and water transport leads to abnormal secretions in the respiratory tract, pancreas, gastrointestinal tract, sweat glands, and other exocrine glands remains under intense investigation. The isotonic, low-volume model has been proposed to account for the pathogenesis of CF.[31,32] In the lung, abnormal respiratory tract secretions leading to decreased airway surface liquid seem to decrease mucociliary clearance and impair defenses to inhaled particulate matter and various microbial pathogens. The airway surface liquid is crucial for lung defense and is composed of a gel and sol layer. The gel or mucous layer is composed of high-molecular-weight mucins with carbohydrate side chains that bind inhaled particulate matter and pathogens. The sol or periciliary liquid layer consists of low-viscosity fluid to hydrate mucins and allows ciliary movement to occur. The periciliary liquid layer is 7 μm in height, allowing cilia to beat freely.

Airway surface liquid volume is regulated by the respiratory epithelium through ion transport processes. Salt concentrations can be changed to regulate the hydration of the airway lining fluid to maintain optimal mucociliary function. The absence of CFTR in the apical cellular membrane decreases the ability of cells to secrete chloride into the periciliary fluid. CFTR inhibits the epithelial sodium channel; in its absence, excessive absorption of sodium occurs. Other channels are available for secretion of chloride (calcium-activated chloride channel) in the respiratory epithelium; however, they cannot compensate for the loss of CFTR. Chloride also can enter the cell through a chloride transporter. The net effect is increased absorption of sodium, chloride, and water, which reduces the periciliary volume, alters the composition of mucins, and decreases mucociliary clearance. The reduction in the periciliary fluid impairs ciliary movement, decreases mucus transport, markedly alters clearance, and sets the stage for airway obstruction, infection, inflammation, and progressive lung destruction.

Altered chloride channel function and fluid secretion help to explain the presence of disease in the sweat gland, intestine, pancreas, and male genital tract. The epithelial cells affected by CFTR mutations in various organs represent different channel and regulatory activities of CFTR but result in deficient secretion

---

TABLE 31–2 Diagnosis of Cystic Fibrosis

One or More Phenotypic Features
Chronic sinopulmonary disease
Gastrointestinal and nutritional abnormalities
Salt loss syndromes—acute salt depletion
Chronic metabolic alkalosis
Male urogenital abnormalities resulting in obstructive azoospermia

Plus Laboratory Evidence of CFTR Abnormality (One or More)
Elevated sweat chloride concentrations
Identification of two CFTR mutations
In vivo evidence of abnormal ion transport across nasal epithelium

CFTR, cystic fibrosis transmembrane conductance regulator.

of fluids. This deficiency causes accumulation of mucus, obstruction, and various degrees of organ damage. Plugging of pancreatic ducts leads to chronic fibrosis, pancreatic atrophy, and loss of digestive enzymes and islet cells. Similar obstruction in the biliary tract can cause inflammation and focal biliary cirrhosis. Glandular obstruction of the vas deferens causes involution of the wolffian duct and infertility in more than 95 percent of men with CF. Women with CF produce abnormally tenacious cervical mucus, with reported rates of infertility of 20 percent.

Dehydration of airway surfaces and defective mucociliary transport has been termed the *low-volume model.*[32] Obstruction of small terminal airways and of submucosal glands with thickened mucopurulent secretions are the first signs of early disease in infants with CF. Ductular dilation, neutrophil infiltration, glandular hyperplasia, and peribronchiolar inflammation are classic findings of the disease. Mucus adherent to airway surfaces serves as a site for chronic infection. Human cell culture models of normal and CF epithelia have shown the airway surface liquid is decreased in CF,[208,341] and regulation of airway surface liquid volume depends on the regulation of sodium absorption and chloride secretion. Transgenic mouse models overexpressing epithelial sodium channels to mimic CF produce airway obstruction with mucus, neutrophilic inflammation, bacterial infection, and goblet cell hyperplasia.[202]

These findings are similar to observations in humans. Mucociliary clearance is decreased in CF.[31,176,275] Submucosal glands have high expression of CFTR.[100,139] Loss of CFTR function alters the composition of mucins produced by the submucosal glands,[163,176,361] leading to ductular dilation with mucus and obstruction. Mucus is tightly adhered to the respiratory epithelium and increases airway obstruction. Failure to clear mucous plugs, continued mucin secretion, and adherent mucus to the airway surface provides the focus for infection.

The respiratory airways of patients with CF are infected with several bacterial and viral pathogens that occur in an age-dependent order. Chronic infection with *P. aeruginosa* develops in 80 percent of affected individuals by the time they reach 18 years of age.[282] *Pseudomonas* infection is associated with a more rapid decline in lung function and increased rates of mortality[99,115] and becomes the dominant organism colonizing the CF airway. Initial isolates from CF infants and toddlers are unique and suggest an environmental acquisition.[236,321,322] Evidence of person-to-person transmission from chronically colonized CF patients to younger CF children, siblings, and individuals in close contact has been documented.[11,15,53,83,184]

Multiple hypotheses have been proposed to define the mechanism of airway colonization with *P. aeruginosa.* Although several studies have assessed this problem, the exact mechanism of infection and colonization remains debated. The primary hypothesis for airway infection in CF is altered mucociliary clearance secondary to abnormal salt and water transport. As the normal function of CFTR becomes defined, additional hypotheses have been put forward to explain the mechanism of early airway infection and inflammation. They involve altered epithelial cell receptors for bacteria, abnormal mucins that enhance bacterial binding impairing airway clearance, and inactivation of epithelial-derived bactericidal activity.

Increasing evidence indicates that the low-airway-surface-liquid-volume hypothesis explains the pathogenic mechanism of lung disease in CF. Dehydration of airway surface liquid and adhesion of mucus to the airway epithelium provide an environment conducive to chronic *Pseudomonas* infection (Fig. 31–3).[380] Depletion of periciliary water decreases ciliary activity, concentrates mucins, and increases adhesion of the mucous layer to the airway surface. Secretion of mucins continues from submucosal glands and goblet cells, producing plugging and airway obstruction. These mucous plaques are poorly cleared from the airway and become the sites of initial infection. Pili extending from the

surface of the bacterium are able to bind to mucin.[308] An anaerobic gradient develops within the thickened mucous plugs. *Pseudomonas,* after binding to mucin, is able to penetrate the thickened mucus and grow in an anaerobic environment. *P. aeruginosa* is able to grow in anaerobic conditions because of the production of nitrate reductase, which allows it to cleave oxygen from nitrate.[304] When it is in the anaerobic environment, an alginate polysaccharide is formed. Biofilm-containing macrocolonies of *Pseudomonas* then are established. The established macrocolonies remain within the airway lumen. These macrocolonies are very resistant to antibiotics and host defense and allow chronic infection, inflammation, and airway destruction to occur.[151,250,380]

P. aeruginosa infection of the airway is associated with progressive respiratory impairment and death in most patients with CF. Bacterial colonization and infection of the lower respiratory tract occur early in infants with CF (Fig. 31–4), and airway inflammation often is established at the time the disease becomes clinically manifest.[14] *P. aeruginosa* infection is intermittent before chronic colonization develops.[115,136,281] Initial isolates generally are antibiotic-sensitive and nonmucoid.[37] In contrast, isolates from patients chronically colonized usually are highly antibiotic-resistant, mucoid, and increased in density.[102,324] As lung disease progresses, the phenotype changes and the bacteria adopt a mucoid biofilm mode of growth.[268] As the organism changes from a nonmucoid to mucoid state, differences in the outer membrane proteins are expressed.[143] In addition, hypermutable strains of *Pseudomonas* are isolated and show greater antibiotic resistance.[239] As *P. aeruginosa* converts from a nonmucoid to mucoid phenotype, several bacterial lipoproteins are produced that induce inflammation.[111]

Local production of cytokines and other proteins in response to bacterial infection may play an important role in modulating chronic airway inflammation.[306] Airway inflammation in CF is characterized by marked neutrophilic infiltration, with release of bioactive lipids, oxygen metabolites, myeloperoxidase, and lysozyme.[109] Proteases (e.g., elastase) derived from neutrophils and bacteria directly damage respiratory epithelium and cleave proteins important in host defense.[332,349] Chronic infection, with retention of the by-products of inflammation, ultimately leads to the severe bronchiectatic changes and derangements of gas exchange characteristic of end-stage CF.

Several in vivo studies have assessed the location of bacterial adherence within the lung of CF patients and the attachment of bacteria to CF and non-CF cells in vitro.[20,351] *P. aeruginosa* is found within the lumen of airways of patients with CF obtained from autopsy specimens.[20] These organisms are observed within the inflammatory exudates of the airway and not within epithelial cells lining the lung or in alveolar spaces. In vitro studies have shown adherence of *P. aeruginosa* in areas of epithelial cell destruction.[257,261,351] No adherence to the apical membrane of intact epithelial cells has been noted, however. In contrast, there is evidence in cell culture models that defects in CFTR enhance bacterial binding to immortalized airway epithelial cells.[290] A tetrasaccharide (asialo GM_1) is expressed more on CF than on non-CF cells and promotes *P. aeruginosa* binding to the epithelial membrane. Pseudomonal exoproducts such as neuraminidase increase the amount of asialo GM_1 available for bacterial binding and facilitate bacterial adherence to airway epithelial cells.[42,294]

Mucins also are important in binding bacteria within the airway. Sialylated and neutral forms of mucins bind *P. aeruginosa.*[264] Removal of sialylic acid from mucin by neuraminidase reduces adherence of *P. aeruginosa.* Mucus dehydration can lead to increased concentration of mucins, decreased pH, and a reduction in glutathione, which decreases mucus viscoelasticity.[287] The concentrated mucus impairs neutrophil migration, promotes an anaerobic environment, and reduces mucociliary transport. Mucin, a component of mucus, is decreased in CF, and its decreased content may promote development of infection.[288]

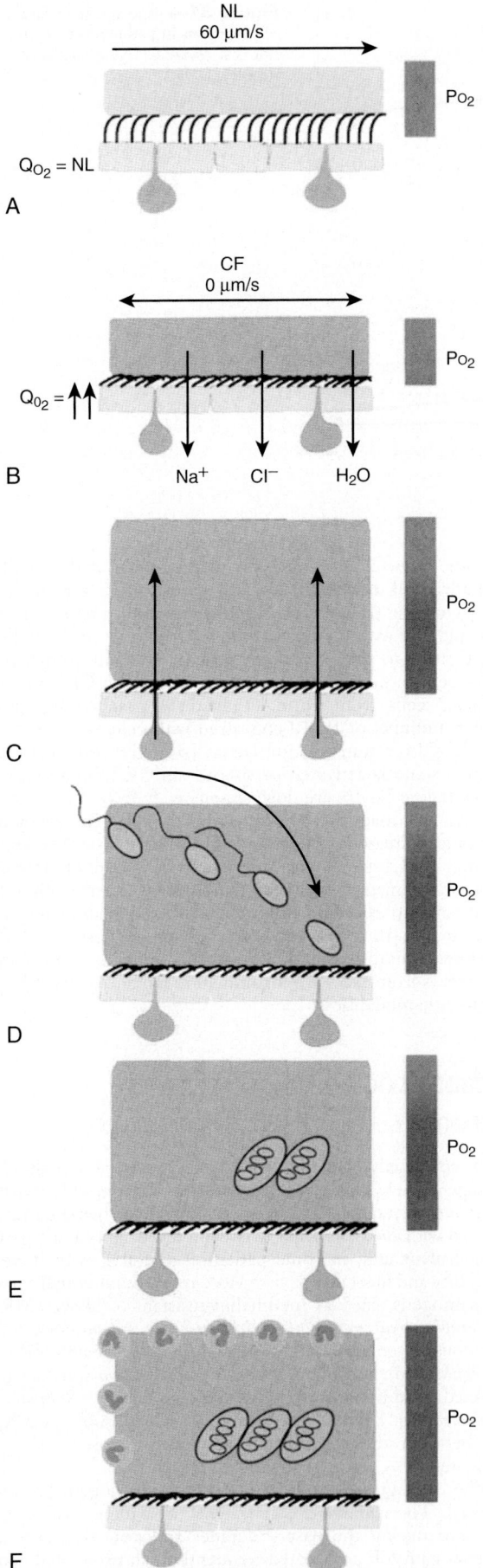

In contrast to the low-airway-surface-volume hypothesis discussed in detail earlier, the "high salt" theory proposes that CFTR maintains low concentration of salt in airway lining fluid. In the absence of CFTR, high concentrations of salt inactivate the secreted antimicrobial substances on airway surfaces.[384] Airway epithelial cells are vital in maintaining a pathogen-free environment within the airway. Smith and colleagues[311] showed that a monolayer of airway epithelial cells was able to kill bacteria when placed on their apical surface. In contrast, CF epithelia were unable to clear the bacterial load. Surface fluid washed from the normal cells showed bactericidal activity; however, fluid from the CF monolayer lacked bacterial killing properties. Goldman and colleagues[130] duplicated the results of this study using a different model. They implicated a human defensin, hBD-1, as the primary agent responsible for bacterial killing. The defensins are low-molecular-weight proteins produced by epithelial cells cytotoxic for bacteria and thought to be salt-sensitive. How deletion of CFTR affects the function of other antimicrobial substances such as lysozyme, which are produced by the respiratory epithelium, remains unclear.

Oxidant stress plays a role in tissue injury observed in CF. Reactive oxygen species are important in killing bacteria and are generated by phagocytic cells and the respiratory epithelium. Oxidants are produced from activated phagocytes, metabolic pathways, inhaled oxidants, and bacteria.[48] Increased oxidant production alters ion transport and increases secretion of mucins.[46,70,167,231,337,339] Excessive oxidant production can cause tissue injury. Increased oxidant production by CF neutrophils has been proposed as a mechanism of airway injury. Activation of reduced nicotinamide adenine dinucleotide phosphate (NADPH) within neutrophils results in production of precursors used by myeloperoxidase to generate chloramines. Chloramines are oxidants with long half-lives and, if produced in excess, potentially can damage the airway epithelium.[34]

One study has examined the activity of NADPH and myeloperoxidase with production of chloramines between CF and non-CF subjects.[374] Significant differences between groups were observed for myeloperoxidase activity and chloramine release. Myeloperoxidase activity and chloramine release were increased

Figure 31–3 Schematic model of the pathogenic events hypothesized to lead to chronic *Pseudomonas aeruginosa* infection in airways of patients with cystic fibrosis (CF). **A,** On normal airway epithelia, a thin mucous layer (*light gray*) resides atop the PCL (*clear*). The presence of the low-viscosity PCL facilitates efficient mucociliary clearance (denoted by *vector*). A normal rate of epithelial oxygen (O_2) consumption (QO_2; *left*) produces no O_2 gradients within this thin ASL. **B-F,** CF airway epithelia. **B,** Excessive CF volume depletion (denoted by *vertical arrows*) removes the PCL, mucus becomes adherent to epithelial surfaces, and mucus transport slows or stops (*bidirectional vector*). The increased O_2 consumption (*left*) associated with accelerated CF ion transport does not generate gradients in thin films of ASL. **C,** Persistent mucus hypersecretion (denoted as mucus secretory gland/goblet cell units; *dark gray*) with time increases the height of luminal mucus masses and plugs. The increased CF epithelial QO_2 generates steep hypoxic gradients in thickened mucus masses. **D,** *P. aeruginosa* bacteria deposited on mucus surfaces penetrate actively or passively or both (due to mucus turbulence) into hypoxic zones within the mucus masses. **E,** *P. aeruginosa* adapts to hypoxic niches within mucus masses with increased alginate formation and the creation of macrocolonies. **F,** Macrocolonies resist secondary defenses, including neutrophils, setting the stage for chronic infection. The presence of increased macrocolony density and, to a lesser extent, neutrophils renders the now mucopurulent mass hypoxic. (See companion Expert Consult web site for color version.) (*From Worlitzsch, D., Tarran, R., Ulrich, M., et al.: Effects of reduced mucus oxygen concentration in airway Pseudomonas infections of cystic fibrosis patients. J. Clin. Invest. 109:317-325, 2002.*)

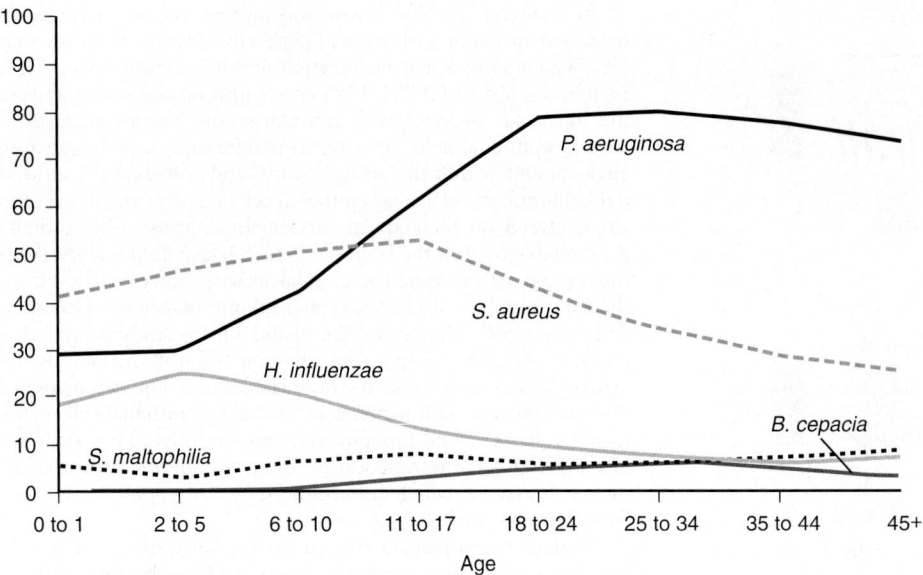

Figure 31–4 Age-specific prevalence of pathogens in patients with cystic fibrosis. *(From CF National Patient Registry, 2000.)*

in subjects with CF. Treatment of CF neutrophils with amiloride reduced oxidant generation, suggesting that altered intracellular ion concentrations or pH may regulate myeloperoxidase activity. Other investigators have suggested alternatively that the circulating neutrophils may be primed to respond to a phagocytic stimulus and that these differences in oxidant generation represent increased neutrophil activity.[135,271]

Antioxidants are produced by enzymatic and nonenzymatic pathways.[48] Mucins, reduced glutathione, alpha-tocopherol, and metal binding proteins function in the airway as antioxidants. The cysteine residues and carbohydrates of mucin account for its antioxidant properties.[71] Secretion of mucins is increased with oxidative stress. In CF, overproduction of mucus with subsequent dehydration may protect bacteria from neutrophil killing, worsening inflammation and causing more harm to the airway. In addition to affecting production of mucins, CFTR also may regulate production of glutathione.[190] Glutathione is an antioxidant found in large amounts in airway lung fluid from normal subjects[47]; however, it is reduced in patients with CF.[285] CFTR may alter glutathione transport, impairing defense to oxidant injury. Whether intracellular glutathione levels are decreased in CF, a factor that could be important in nuclear factor-κB (NF-κB) regulation, remains unclear. Increased oxidant production from neutrophils and impaired antioxidant biosynthesis can be altered by mutant CFTR, increasing the potential for oxidant injury in the CF airway.

Production of cell adherence molecules and inflammatory cytokines is intact in patients with CF.[88,174] Defects in bacterial opsonization, reduction in anti-inflammatory cytokines, and proinflammatory effects of bacterial DNA have been reported, however. Although humoral antibody responses and neutrophil phagocytosis from peripheral blood are normal, increased elastase in the CF airway can alter opsonic receptors, impairing phagocytosis. Large amounts of elastase are present in lavage fluid from airways of patients with CF, overwhelming the normal antiprotease activity. This condition can lead to local impairment in phagocytosis of bacteria within the airway lumen, contributing to bacterial persistence.

Proinflammatory mediators are elevated in BAL fluid from young patients with CF, as are macrophages expressing intracellular cytokines.[170,225,385] Increased numbers of neutrophils and interleukin (IL)-8 in BAL fluid are seen in bacterial culture–negative and bacterial culture–positive infants with CF compared with controls.[155,371] Proinflammatory mediators IL-1, IL-2, tumor

necrosis factor-α, and IL-8 are markedly elevated in children with advanced disease.[144,155,371] In contrast, some anti-inflammatory cytokines (IL-10) are found in reduced amounts in BAL from subjects with CF. These observations have prompted some investigators to assess production of IL-10 from bronchial epithelial cells in normal subjects and subjects with CF.[26] Bronchial epithelial cells from normal individuals produce significantly greater amounts of IL-10 compared with cells of subjects with CF. NF-κB is a transcription factor for several proinflammatory mediators and is activated persistently in CF. Inhibitors to NF-κB, including IL-10, are down-regulated.[85,302,360,364]

Enhanced macrophage production of proinflammatory cytokines and decreased production of IL-10 have fostered a hypothesis that the CF gene defect may result in an inability to control airway inflammation after having infections. Alternatively, CFTR could have no effect on production of anti-inflammatory cytokines, and IL-10 could be down-regulated. Although the understanding of this disease pathogenesis is incomplete, airway damage that occurs from excessive inflammation remains a target for new therapeutic modalities.

MICROBIOLOGY OF CYSTIC FIBROSIS

EPIDEMIOLOGY OF PATHOGENS IN CYSTIC FIBROSIS

Most commonly, patients with CF are infected with classic pathogens, including *Staphylococcus aureus*, nontypeable *Haemophilus influenzae*, and *P. aeruginosa*.[8,41,126,214] A few patients may be infected with *Burkholderia cepacia* complex, which can be particularly virulent and, in some patients, associated with increased morbidity and mortality.[68,132,279] More recently, potentially emerging pathogens, such as methicillin-resistant *S. aureus* (MRSA), *Stenotrophomonas maltophilia*, *Achromobacter xylosoxidans*, nontuberculous mycobacteria (NTM), and mold species (primarily *Aspergillus* spp), and, more recently, *Scedosporium* spp., are being reported. Additional potential pathogens include *Ralstonia* and *Pandoraea* spp.[62,193] As described in more detail subsequently, the link between these pathogens and lung disease is not fully elucidated.

The etiologies behind these emerging pathogens are multifactorial. The average life expectancy of patients with CF has increased during the past 4 decades and now is 36.5 years.[75] Patients with CF are treated frequently with prolonged courses of antimicrobial agents, including oral, intravenous, and aerosolized agents, placing selective pressure on their flora and leading to increased resistance.[38,75] Evidence of health care–associated acquisition of some pathogens, including B. cepacia complex, P. aeruginosa, and MRSA, is described subsequently. Finally, during the past 2 decades, detection of many potential pathogens has improved as clinical microbiology laboratories processing CF specimens use several selective media and fully speciate non–lactose-fermenting, gram-negative bacilli as described subsequently.[126,145,336,390]

AGE-SPECIFIC PREVALENCE OF PATHOGENS

The U.S. Cystic Fibrosis Foundation has maintained an annual Patient Registry since 1962.[112] The age-specific prevalence for CF pathogens in the United States as reported to this registry in 2005 is shown in Figure 31–4.[75] During the first decade of life, S. aureus is the most common pathogen and is harbored by approximately 40 percent of children and adolescents. Nontypeable H. influenzae is a less prevalent pathogen and is cultured from the respiratory tracts of 15 percent of children. Over time, P. aeruginosa becomes the most prevalent pathogen, but it can be recovered from 30 percent of infants. Approximately 80 percent of American patients with CF are infected with P. aeruginosa by the time they reach 18 years old. Overall, Burkholderia spp.[191] are recovered from 3 to 4 percent of patients and 10 percent of adults. During the late 1990s, the Cystic Fibrosis Foundation began to collect data on the prevalence of MRSA, S. maltophilia, and A. xylosoxidans. As shown in Figure 31–4, these organisms are more common than is B. cepacia complex and are harbored primarily by adult patients. As noted in patients without CF, MRSA has become increasingly common.[272]

ROLE OF THE CLINICAL MICROBIOLOGY LABORATORY

Ongoing communication between the clinical microbiology laboratory and the CF care team is crucial to ensure that appropriate methodologies are in place to provide appropriate care, to support effective infection control, and to further understanding of the epidemiology of pathogens in CF.[296] Every 5 years, the executive committee of the U.S. Cystic Fibrosis Foundation conducts site visits of accredited CF care centers and meets with the director of the clinical microbiology laboratory in efforts to ensure that standardized practices are in place.[295] In addition, a survey determined that most clinical laboratories processing CF specimens were using selective media and speciating all gram-negative bacilli,[390] which may include molecular identification strategies.

SPECIMEN PROCESSING

Respiratory tract specimens from patients with CF, including specimens obtained after lung transplantation, should be labeled "CF specimens" to ensure proper processing. Timely transport optimizes recovery of pathogens; ideally, specimens should be received by the laboratory within 3 to 4 hours of collection or stored at 4° C and processed within 24 hours. Sputum is the ideal specimen, and at least 1 mL should be collected to ensure an adequate volume is available for plating on selective media. Sputum can be Gram-stained to determine if a specimen contains bacteria and neutrophils rather than epithelial cells. Oropharyngeal cultures often are obtained in children too young to expectorate, but these cultures may not be concordant with specimens obtained from the lower airway.[280] BAL specimens generally are reserved for research protocols, lung transplant recipients, or

patients with atypical courses who cannot produce sputum. More recently, induced sputum has been promoted to assess the lower respiratory tract flora of patients with CF who cannot expectorate.[149,244]

SELECTIVE MEDIA

Selective media are needed to isolate specific pathogens, although the use of these media is costly and time-consuming. Current recommendations for selective media are shown in Table 31–3. S. aureus strains from patients with CF may be thymidine-deficient and require mannitol salt agar for growth.[295] Detection of B. cepacia complex is markedly enhanced by the use of OFBPL (oxidative fermentative bacitracin polymyxin B lactose) agar or B. cepacia selective media.[126,145] Multicenter studies conducted by the Centers for Disease Control and Prevention in the 1980s showed that the use of selective media improved the yield of Burkholderia spp. from patients with CF.[334] In addition, specimens can be plated on mycosel agar to identify Aspergillus spp., although this mold grows well on blood agar. Oropharyngeal swabs from nonexpectorating patients also should be plated on selective media.[307] If NTM are suspected, sputum should be stained for acid-fast bacilli and processed using an additional decontamination step to prevent overgrowth by P. aeruginosa.[367] This decontamination step may kill NTM present in low concentrations, however.[21] Quantitative cultures of specimens from sputum are reserved for research purposes.

ANTIMICROBIAL SUSCEPTIBILITY TESTING

The optimal methodology for antimicrobial susceptibility testing for mucoid and nonmucoid strains of P. aeruginosa has been elu-

TABLE 31–3 Recommended Media and Processing for Recovery of Cystic Fibrosis Pathogens

Organism	Recommended Media or Processing*†
Staphylococcus aureus	Mannitol salt agar Columbia/colistin–nalidixic acid agar
Haemophilus influenzae	Horse blood or chocolate agar (supplemented or not with 300 mg/L bacitracin) incubated anaerobically
Pseudomonas aeruginosa	MacConkey agar
Burkholderia cepacia complex	OFPBL agar, PC agar, BCSA
Stenotrophomonas maltophilia	MacConkey agar, VIA agar DNase agar confirmatory media or biochemical or molecular identification
Achromobacter xylosoxidans	MacConkey agar Biochemical identification assay
Mycobacterial spp.	NALC-NaOH and oxalic acid decontamination step
Yeast	Mycosel agar‡
Other gram-positive organisms	Sheep blood agar supplemented with neomycin and gentamicin (streptococcal selective agar)
Other gram-negative organisms	MacConkey agar

*Detection of some pathogens may be enhanced by prolonging incubation for 4 days to allow slow-growing colonies to become apparent.
†All media are commercially available.
‡Aspergillus spp. and other molds do not grow well on Mycosel, but do grow well (although not selectively) on many of the media used for cystic fibrosis specimens, especially OFPBL. Standard biochemical and phenotypic methods should be used for confirmation of the identification of molds.

cidated. In studies of 500 multidrug-resistant strains of *P. aeruginosa* from patients with CF, five different antimicrobial susceptibility testing methods were compared: a reference microbroth dilution assay, Kirby Bauer disks, E-tests, and the automated commercial systems Vitek and Microscan. The agar-based diffusion methods (Kirby Bauer disks and the E-test) proved most accurate compared with the reference methods.[39,289] Vitek and Microscan, the commercial systems, had unacceptably high rates of very major (i.e., false-susceptible) and major (i.e., false-resistant) errors.[40] The Clinical Laboratory Standards Institute (formerly the National Committee for Clinical Laboratory Standards) endorses the use of antibiotic-impregnated disks or reference broth microdilution assays to determine the susceptibility of multidrug-resistant strains of *P. aeruginosa* isolated from patients with CF.[229]

An intriguing concept in susceptibility testing is the potential role of susceptibility testing of bacteria grown in biofilms. As described in more detail subsequently, chronic lung infection in CF is thought to reflect a biofilm mode of growth containing bacteria in stationary phase that do not express the antibiotic targets present in log phase bacteria.[69] In vitro studies have shown that the minimal inhibitory concentration (MIC) of log phase bacteria tested in conventional susceptibility testing assays can be very different from the MIC of bacteria growing in stationary phase in biofilms.[147] Log phase–grown *P. aeruginosa* are resistant to macrolide antibiotics (MIC $\geq$ 128 μg/mL), whereas *P. aeruginosa* grown in biofilms are susceptible to these agents (MIC_{50} 2 μg/mL).[222] Studies are ongoing to compare the outcomes of pulmonary exacerbations treated using the results of conventional susceptibility testing versus the results from biofilm susceptibility testing.

SPECIFIC CYSTIC FIBROSIS PATHOGENS

VIRAL PATHOGENS

Numerous studies have evaluated the role of nonbacterial infections with pulmonary exacerbations in CF. A clear correlation between respiratory viral infection and exacerbations of lung disease has been shown in most of these reports.* Viral lower respiratory tract infections occur more often in younger children and are associated with increased pulmonary disease in 40 percent of cases in CF.[3,355] Respiratory syncytial virus (RSV) has been identified most often with CF pulmonary exacerbations; however, influenza, adenovirus, parainfluenza virus, and rhinoviruses also have been reported.[355] Respiratory viruses are isolated from patients with CF requiring hospitalization, and infection is associated with increased morbidity rates. Infants with CF infected with RSV can experience prolonged hospitalizations, mechanical ventilation, and supplemental oxygen at hospital discharge.[3] Severe viral infections in infants with CF were reported in 31 of 80 children diagnosed by newborn screening. Half of the children hospitalized had a respiratory virus identified at the time of hospitalization, and RSV infection accounted for hospitalization in 7 of the 31 children.[12]

Two studies have reported prolonged bronchiolitis-like syndromes in infants younger than 6 months of age.[119,196] These infants required intensive respiratory therapy, including bronchodilators, chest physiotherapy, and mechanical ventilation. Increased hospitalization was observed for children with CF who were infected with RSV in another study of children younger than 3 years of age.[146] Although prolonged hypoxia and respiratory failure were not observed, pulmonary function was markedly decreased after hospitalization and persisted for several months

after infection.[146] Studies in older children with CF have reported reduction in pulmonary function, clinical scores, and radiographic scores and increased hospitalization after viral infection.[65,243,315,362,373] These studies show that infection with respiratory viruses results in clinical deterioration, hospitalization, and decreases in lung function.

Mechanisms to explain the enhanced disease observed with respiratory viral infections are being investigated. Normal airway epithelia use an adenosine-regulated pathway to maintain periciliary fluid volume by regulation of sodium absorption and chloride secretion. In a CF model, this regulation can be normalized by phasic motion simulating movement of the lung. Periciliary volume is restored to normal by release of adenosine triphosphate into the periciliary liquid and activation of alternative chloride channels. Viral infections, such as RSV, up-regulate the extracellular adenosine triphosphatase activity, reducing periciliary fluid volume. Reduction in periciliary liquid volume would promote mucous stasis and plugging.[341] Other investigators have shown impaired innate defense manifested by reduced production of nitric oxide and impaired interferon-γ signaling pathway.[387,388]

The interrelationship between the acquisition of *P. aeruginosa* and viral respiratory infection is unclear. Increased colonization with *Pseudomonas* has been observed during the respiratory viral season,[166] and infection with *Pseudomonas* has been associated with hospitalization for viral respiratory illness. Antipseudomonal antibodies have been reported to increase after having RSV infection, and new infection with *Pseudomonas* has been observed during an acute respiratory illness.[65,256] Other investigators have not observed any change in bacterial infection or change in colonization associated with viral respiratory infection.[238] In cell culture models, RSV acts as a coupling agent between *P. aeruginosa* and enhances attachment to respiratory epithelial cells.[356] Petersen and colleagues[256] and Ong and associates[243] reported more severe pulmonary disease with viral infection in the presence of *P. aeruginosa* colonization, but Przyklenk and coworkers[262] found no correlation. Synergism between bacteria and respiratory virus infection was suggested by Przyklenk and coworkers[262] after an increase in the number of bacterial colony-forming units was found in sputum of subjects with CF. Hordvik and associates[153] and Efthimiou and coworkers[94] noted that patients with CF and severe pulmonary disease recovered slowly from viral infection. The underlying severity of lung disease was crucial in predicting response to viral respiratory infection.

NONTYPEABLE *HAEMOPHILUS INFLUENZAE*

H. influenzae frequently is the earliest pathogen isolated from patients with CF. The advent of the *H. influenzae* vaccine has not had an impact on the prevalence of this organism because patients with CF harbor nontypeable strains. Generally, *H. influenzae* is susceptible to a wide variety of agents and is amenable to treatment. Despite the frequent recovery of this organism from infants and children, the impact of this organism on the clinical course of CF has been difficult to assess because of the frequent occurrence of co-infection with other pathogens.

STAPHYLOCOCCUS AUREUS

Methicillin-susceptible *S. aureus* (MSSA) and MRSA are increasing in prevalence. Patients generally retain the same clone of MSSA for their lifetime.[33,301] Data from the Cystic Fibrosis Patient Registry showed that the overall prevalence of MSSA increased from 37 percent in 1995 to 51.8 percent in 2005.[75] Similarly, MRSA increased from 0.1 percent in 1995 to 17.2 percent in 2005, although the prevalence varied substantially from center to center (range per center, 0 to 24%). The causes

---

*See references 3, 94, 118, 153, 238, 243, 256, 262, 266, 327, 362, 381.

for this variability are uncertain but could reflect different laboratory practices, different clinical practices, or regional differences in community-acquired MRSA. Although MRSA generally infects older patients, it usually is persistent[272] and can be associated with deterioration in both pediatric and adult patients.[216,345] A more recent report compared the outcomes of patients with MSSA versus MRSA and showed that children (<18 years old) and adults infected with MRSA had worse lung function, more hospitalizations, and more antibiotic use.[272]

Recent hospitalization has been shown to be a risk factor for MRSA, suggesting nosocomial acquisition,[127] but the relative importance of community-acquired MRSA strains (mecA type IV and V) has not been fully elucidated. A more recent case series has suggested that community-acquired MRSA strains expressing Panton-Valentine leukocidin can be associated with increased morbidity, including focal pulmonary infiltrates with cavitary lesions and a greater decline in lung function.[96]

PSEUDOMONAS AERUGINOSA

P. aeruginosa is the most common and important pathogen in patients with CF. Initial strains are nonmucoid, antibiotic-susceptible strains that express pili, flagella, and more highly acylated lipid A component of lipopolysaccharide.[134] P. aeruginosa also produces virulence factors, including exotoxin A, exoenzyme S, leukocidin, phospholipase C, elastase, and alkaline protease, which contribute to the pathogenesis of sepsis, acute lung infections, and bacteremia.[50,318,340] These factors may be chemotactic stimuli for neutrophils, and exotoxins may increase the viscosity of secretions and impair ciliary clearance and cause small airway obstruction and ultimately lung destruction.

Over time, P. aeruginosa adapts to the CF lung and undergoes genetic and phenotypic alterations. P. aeruginosa initially attaches to solid surfaces (e.g., mucin or respiratory epithelial cells), using flagella and type IV pili.[69] Attachment activates genes that synthesize extracellular polysaccharide (alginate),[84] which confers the mucoid phenotype of P. aeruginosa unique to chronic infections in CF.[133] Strains associated with chronic infections lack pili, lack flagella, and undergo structural changes in lipopolysaccharide. These changes may render P. aeruginosa more resistant to host defenses, including defensins and the innate inflammatory response. The lasR-lasI system (quorum-sensing genes) promotes the initial formation of microcolonies, which differentiate into alginate-encased mature biofilms.[69] Bacteria in biofilms avoid ciliary clearance, evade phagocytosis, and are antibiotic-resistant.[309] Biofilms are the proposed mechanism whereby P. aeruginosa is able to infect the CF airway chronically and avoid eradication by host defenses and by antimicrobial agents. The CF lung can harbor very high concentrations of P. aeruginosa—10^8 to 10^9 organisms per gram of sputum may be present.[376]

Infection with P. aeruginosa is associated with increased morbidity and mortality rates caused by recurrent pulmonary exacerbations and a gradual deterioration in lung function.[173,247] Children who are infected with P. aeruginosa are more likely to have cough and lower chest radiograph scores than are uninfected children.[156] Investigators have shown that infants younger than 2 years infected with S. aureus and P. aeruginosa have worse pulmonary function, chest radiograph scores, and 10-year survival rates than do uninfected children.[4] The mucoid phenotype of P. aeruginosa is associated with a more rapid decline in lung function.[248]

BURKHOLDERIA CEPACIA COMPLEX

Infection with B. cepacia complex and the associated "cepacia syndrome" was reported first in 1979 among adolescent Cana-

TABLE 31–4 Members of the *Burkholderia cepacia* Complex, 2001

Species (Genomovar)	Binomial Designation	Reference
I	B. cepacia	Vandamme, 1997
II	B. multivorans	Vandamme, 1997
III	Pending	Vandamme, 1997
IV	B. stabilis	Vandamme, 1997, 2000
V	B. vietnamiensis	Vandamme, 1997; Gillis
VI	Pending	Coenye and LiPuma, 2001
VII	B. ambifaria	Coenye and Mahen, 2001
(VIII)	Pending	*
IX	B. pyrrocinia	*

*Manuscripts in preparation.

dian patients with CF.[161,335] The cepacia syndrome is characterized by a virulent course, high fevers, bacteremia, rapid deterioration in lung function, and early death. Generally, patients with CF do not have bacteremia caused by other pathogens. Different clinical courses can be associated with B. cepacia complex, however, including transient colonization, a gradual decline in lung function, or the virulent cepacia syndrome.

Through a series of genetic and phenotypic studies, researchers have discovered that B. cepacia is actually a complex of several different species, previously called genomovars, which are indistinguishable phenotypically but distinguishable genotypically.[63] The genomovars of the B. cepacia complex are shown in Table 31–4, but additional genomovars are likely to be described. Several international investigators have described the epidemiology and clinical courses associated with different genomovars, although these studies usually involved a single strain and might not be generalized to all strains of a given genomovar.[192,199,323] Most CF isolates are Burkholderia cenocepacia (genomovar III) or Burkholderia multivorans (genomovar II). The former may be associated with a more rapidly progressive clinical course,[195] whereas B. multivorans is more likely to be associated with transient colonization.[199] Patient-to-patient transmission and clinical deterioration can be associated with B. multivorans, however.[192] Most recently, an outbreak of Burkholderia dolosa (genomovar VI) occurred, and this newly described genomovar was associated with increased morbidity and mortality rates.[168]

Virulence factors for Burkholderia spp. include multidrug resistance, the ability to form biofilms, the ability to reside intracellularly, and the ability to spread from patient to patient potentially via the cable pilus[331] or the B. cepacia epidemiologic strain marker.[199] Many outbreak strains do not express these transmission factors, however. Studies are ongoing to unravel potential environmental reservoirs of Burkholderia spp.

STENOTROPHOMONAS MALTOPHILIA

S. maltophilia, an intrinsically multidrug-resistant, gram-negative bacillus, is a well-known hospital-acquired pathogen in non-CF patients and is isolated with increasing frequency from the respiratory tract of patients with CF. The overall prevalence of this organism in patients with CF is 12 percent (range 0 to 27% in individual centers).[75,82] In a multicenter, randomized, placebo-controlled study of aerosolized tobramycin conducted in 520 patients 6 years old and older with CF, the baseline prevalence of S. maltophilia determined by a core laboratory was 10.7 percent,[41] whereas the national rate among comparably aged patients reported to the Cystic Fibrosis Patient Registry was 2.9 to 3.9 percent, suggesting that many clinical laboratories were failing to identify this potential pathogen. Transient colonization also seems to be a common occurrence; Demko and colleagues[82] reported that 50 percent of patients with CF at their center had only a single positive culture for this microorganism. Increased use of antibiotics has been shown to be a potential risk factor for acquisition of *S. maltophilia*.[205,338]

The role of this organism as a pathogen in CF is still being investigated. Case-control studies have not shown that *S. maltophilia* has a significant impact on lung function or mortality.[131,205] In contrast, Demko and colleagues[82] found that the 5-year survival of patients with *S. maltophilia* (*n* = 211) with severe lung function at initial isolation of this organism was 40 percent compared with patients without *S. maltophilia* (*n* = 471), whose 5-year survival was 72 percent.

ACHROMOBACTER XYLOSOXIDANS

The clinical significance of *A. xylosoxidans* in CF also is unclear. In 1996, the first year that this organism was reported to the Cystic Fibrosis Patient Registry, 2.7 percent of patients harbored this multidrug-resistant, gram-negative bacillus.[74] As described for *S. maltophilia*, however, the nationally reported prevalence most likely is underestimated; 8.7 percent of participants in the aerosolized tobramycin trial had positive cultures for *A. xylosoxidans*.[41] Further complicating the epidemiology of this potentially emerging pathogen are the observations that *A. xylosoxidans* may be misidentified as some other non–lactose-fermenting, gram-negative bacilli, and that *P. aeruginosa*, *B. cepacia* complex, and *S. maltophilia* may be misidentified as *A. xylosoxidans*.[291] In addition, the impact of this organism is difficult to assess fully because *A. xylosoxidans* generally is cultured from patients concomitantly infected with other CF pathogens, but an association has been found between *A. xylosoxidans* and pulmonary exacerbations.[92,103]

ASPERGILLUS SPECIES AND *SCEDOSPORIUM* SPECIES

Patients with CF frequently are colonized with *Aspergillus* spp.; 24.5 percent of participants in the inhaled tobramycin trial indicated they had positive cultures for this mold.[36] Oral and aerosolized antimicrobial agents are risk factors for colonization with *Aspergillus* spp.[22,267]

Of patients with CF, 2 to 10 percent develop APBA, which can be associated with a dramatic loss of lung function.[97,121,207,224] The diagnosis of ABPA can be difficult to establish because of variability in the application of standardized diagnostic criteria, confusion regarding these criteria, and limited recognition by physicians. This immunologically mediated syndrome is marked by a brisk IgE response, specific antibody to *Aspergillus fumigatus*, peripheral eosinophilia, and symptoms of reactive airway disease. Short-lived pulmonary infiltrates may be noted on chest radiograph. Although *Aspergillus* spp. do not normally invade the parenchyma, the airways can become impacted with mucus-containing fibrin, eosinophils, and mononuclear cells, which can cause airway obstruction and bronchiectasis.[97]

A workshop sponsored by the Cystic Fibrosis Foundation sought to further understanding of the diagnostic criteria needed for ABPA in CF.[326] This committee established minimum criteria for the diagnosis, which included (1) new clinical deterioration not attributable to another cause; (2) IgE greater than 500 IU/mL; (3) immediate skin reactivity to *Aspergillus* antigen or IgE antibody to *A. fumigatus*; and (4) precipitins or IgG against *A. fumigatus*, new chest radiograph, or new chest CT findings.

Scedosporium spp. can be isolated from the lungs of patients with CF, but the clinical significance of this microorganism is unknown. In the aerosolized tobramycin trial, 2.4 percent of patients harbored saprophytic fungi,[41] and in a single center, 8.6 percent of 128 patients followed for more than 5 years were colonized or infected with *S. apiospermum*.[58]

NONTUBERCULOUS MYCOBACTERIA

Since the early 1990s, there has been an increasing appreciation that NTM may be pathogens in patients with CF. Olivier and colleagues[241] conducted a natural history study of NTM in patients with CF in 21 CF centers from 1993 to 1997. Using standardized mycobacteriologic methods,[368] these investigators found that the overall prevalence of colonization and infection with NTM is 13 percent. *Mycobacterium avium* complex (MAC) and *Mycobacterium abscessus* were most common, representing 72 percent and 16 percent of isolates, respectively. Patients with NTM were older and had better lung function, a lower prevalence of *P. aeruginosa*, and a higher prevalence of *S. aureus* compared with patients without NTM, suggestive of a "healthy survivor effect." Risk factors for NTM may include geographic proximity to large bodies of water,[241] ABPA, and steroid therapy.[227]

In an individual patient, determining if NTM is colonizing the lung or causing disease can be difficult. Signs and symptoms of mycobacterial disease are nonspecific and may be consistent with CF pulmonary exacerbations. Radiographic signs generally are nonspecific, but small nodules in the lung periphery or progressive "tree and bud" lesions may be noted on high-resolution CT scan.[242] Patients with positive acid-fast bacillus smears and two or more positive cultures are more likely to be infected than colonized with NTM.[7] Patients harboring *M. abscessus* are more likely to fulfill the American Thoracic Society diagnostic criteria for NTM disease than are patients harboring MAC.[137,240] In a study to assess the clinical impact of NTM, 60 incident-case patients with positive NTM cultures were followed for 15 months and did not have increased morbidity compared with control subjects with negative cultures.[240] Because this was a short duration of follow-up, further studies are needed to determine if NTM causes a progressive deterioration in lung function and, if so, the optimal therapy.

TREATMENT OF PATHOGENS IN CYSTIC FIBROSIS PATIENTS

A cornerstone of CF care is the aggressive use of oral, intravenous, and aerosolized antibiotics. The increasing longevity of patients with CF has paralleled the development of effective antibiotics. Antibiotics may be used during several stages of CF lung disease: (1) to prevent acquisition of pathogens, most commonly MSSA; (2) to eradicate initial acquisition of pathogens, most commonly *P. aeruginosa*, in efforts to prevent or delay chronic infection; (3) to treat pulmonary exacerbations caused by classic CF pathogens; (4) to treat patients infected with *P. aeruginosa*, as long-term suppressive therapy; and (5) to treat emerging multidrug-resistant pathogens.

PROPHYLAXIS TO PREVENT ACQUISITION OF *STAPHYLOCOCCUS AUREUS*

Few studies have been conducted on antibiotic prophylaxis in patients with CF, and these studies have focused exclusively on *S. aureus*. The rationale for this strategy is to prevent *S. aureus* infection and to delay acquisition of *P. aeruginosa*.[312,314] From 1985 to 1992, British investigators studied 42 newly diagnosed infants randomly assigned to 12 months of flucloxacillin versus standard care.[23,363] Infants treated with flucloxacillin had fewer infections with *S. aureus* and fewer hospitalizations, but both groups had similar pulmonary function. In a placebo-controlled trial conducted in the United States, 119 patients newly diagnosed with CF (mean age, 16 months) were randomly assigned to receive cephalexin or placebo for 5 to 7 years.[328] No significant differences were found in pulmonary function, the number of pulmonary exacerbations, nutritional status, or chest radiograph scores in the two groups. In contrast, subjects treated with cephalexin had decreased incidence of infection with *S. aureus* but increased incidence of infection with *P. aeruginosa*. Similarly, an analysis of the German national database showed that patients receiving antistaphylococcal agents had increased acquisition of *P. aeruginosa* and no improvement in lung function.[269]

Antistaphylococcal prophylaxis, although practiced in the United Kingdom in infants, has not been widely endorsed in the United States because of concerns about the emergence of resistance, the increased risk of acquiring *P. aeruginosa*, and the lack of impact on lung function. The different findings in these studies may reflect the different agents studied because cephalexin is broader spectrum than is flucloxacillin or the different durations of therapy, or both. In an era of increasing prevalence of MRSA, strategies to prevent MSSA may prove to be less useful. To date, no studies have been done to assess antibiotic prophylaxis for other pathogens in CF.

EARLY ERADICATION OF *PSEUDOMONAS AERUGINOSA*

An increasingly practiced therapeutic strategy is to use antibiotics to eradicate initial acquisition of *P. aeruginosa* and prevent or delay chronic infection. This strategy was described first in Europe at the Danish Cystic Fibrosis Center.[114,164,333,352,359] The rationale for this approach is that antibiotics may be effective at eradicating initial infection and colonization with *P. aeruginosa* because the organism burden is low, organisms are largely susceptible, and a biofilm has not yet been established.

The optimal regimen for successful eradication is unknown. In some CF centers in Europe, colistin and ciprofloxacin are administered every 3 months after the initial isolation of *P. aeruginosa* has occurred.[114] Compared with historic controls, patients treated with this approach had improved lung function, improved survival rates, decreased prevalence of *P. aeruginosa*, and increased resistance to the therapeutic regimen.[333] In Australia, investigators used intravenous antibiotics followed by ciprofloxacin or aerosolized agents and found that 6 of 24 children no longer had *P. aeruginosa* isolated for 12 months or longer.[13] Compared with children treated with placebo, children treated with inhaled tobramycin within 7 to 12 weeks of initial infection and colonization with *P. aeruginosa* had shorter time to conversion from a positive to negative culture.[370] All 8 subjects treated with inhaled tobramycin compared with 1 of 13 subjects treated with placebo had successful eradication of *P. aeruginosa*.[123]

Despite the concerns about the potential emergence of antimicrobial resistance and lack of long-term studies that show the durability of eradication or an improvement in lung function, the growing consensus has been that early eradication for *P. aeruginosa* has merit. Two large, placebo-controlled studies are ongoing to assess the efficacy of different eradication regimens using different durations of inhaled tobramycin with and without oral ciprofloxacin. Neither of these trials is comparing an active regimen with placebo—evidence that early eradication has been endorsed by most of CF experts.

TREATMENT OF PULMONARY EXACERBATIONS

Pseudomonas aeruginosa

Much effort has been put into standardizing and validating the definition of a pulmonary exacerbation in CF. No currently accepted definition has been adopted universally, however, for use clinically, in quality improvement initiatives, or in clinical research. A combination of clinical signs and symptoms is used to define a pulmonary exacerbation in research trials, and similar factors are used in the clinical setting.

Mild exacerbations often are treated with oral ciprofloxacin[57,150] with or without an inhaled agent such as tobramycin or colistin. Treatment trials supporting the use of inhaled antibiotics for management of an exacerbation are lacking, however.

Several pivotal trials have led to widely accepted principles for intravenous treatment of more severe pulmonary exacerbations. During the 1970s and early 1980s, placebo-controlled trials showed that participants in the placebo group had increased morbidity and mortality rates compared with participants treated with intravenous antibiotics.[128,157,369] Hospitalized participants treated with bronchodilators and chest physiotherapy alone had less improvement in lung function and less reduction in bacterial density compared with patients treated with these interventions plus a β-lactam and an aminoglycoside agent.[270] Treatment with a β-lactam (azlocillin) and an aminoglycoside (tobramycin) agent leads to a significant reduction in bacterial density and a longer time to readmission for a new exacerbation compared with treatment with azlocillin alone.[310]

Studies also have compared various agents, singly or in combination. Most studies enrolled small numbers of patients and concluded that the comparative treatment regimens were equivalent in efficacy, but the studies were insufficiently powered to detect differences.[28,61,129,162,185,213,252,299,305] Many studies showed the emergence of resistance to study drug at the completion of therapy, which did not correlate with clinical response to treatment.[165,246] A larger multicenter trial randomly assigned patients undergoing a pulmonary exacerbation to ceftazidime and tobramycin (*n* = 52) or meropenem and tobramycin (*n* = 50).[25] Participants in the meropenem-treated group had a greater improvement in lung function than did participants in the ceftazidime-treated group (mean increase in forced expiratory volume in 1 second [FEV_1] percent predicted (38.8 percent versus 29.4 percent). Finally, examination of the safety and efficacy of single daily dosing of tobramycin versus multiple daily dosing during a pulmonary exacerbation showed that single daily dosing was associated with the same efficacy and reduced nephrotoxicity; in children, the mean percentage change in creatinine in the single daily dosing group was less than the mean change in the three-times daily dosing group (4.5% vs 3.7%).[313]

Accepted treatment of a pulmonary exacerbation caused by *P. aeruginosa* consists of two parenteral agents from different antibiotic classes to provide synergy and to delay the emergence of resistance.[122,223,265,293] Most commonly, a β-lactam agent with activity against *P. aeruginosa*, such as piperacillin or ceftazidime, is combined with an aminoglycoside agent, generally tobramycin. If a patient is co-infected with another pathogen, such as MSSA, additional agents are added. Treatment trials for pulmonary exacerbations caused by other CF pathogens are unavailable, however.

Antibiotic dosages must be higher or more frequent (or both) in patients with CF because the volume of distribution and clearance are increased in CF.[81] Treatment is administered for 14 to 21 days; treatment outcomes include improved lung function, improved well-being or improved quality of life or both, and a reduction in organism burden. Eradication of pathogens does not occur, however.[245] The Epidemiologic Study of Cystic Fibrosis analyzed the relationship between pulmonary function and treatment strategies for pulmonary exacerbations; centers with patients in the upper quartile of pulmonary function treated pulmonary exacerbations more frequently than did centers in the lower quartile.[221]

Inevitably, *P. aeruginosa* develops increasing resistance to antibiotics. Molecular studies have confirmed that resistance generally develops in the infecting strains, rather than the acquisition of more resistant strains,[237] although superinfection with multidrug-resistant *P. aeruginosa* can occur as described subsequently.[209] Much interest has been generated in optimizing the treatment of pulmonary exacerbations caused by multidrug-resistant *P. aeru-*

ginosa using in vitro synergy testing. Most commonly, checkerboard broth microdilution assays and multiple combination bactericidal testing have been studied.[189,293]

At the Cystic Fibrosis Referral Center for Susceptibility and Synergy Testing at Columbia University, the activity of clinically achievable concentrations of pairs of antimicrobial agents with different mechanisms of action (e.g., a β-lactam agent paired with an aminoglycoside) is tested.[293] To determine if a combination of agents is synergistic, a fractional inhibitory concentration is calculated; synergy is defined as a fourfold reduction in the MIC of agents alone compared with agents in combination.[204] Most multidrug-resistant strains, defined as resistance to all agents in two or more classes of antibiotics,[295] can be inhibited by one or more combinations of agents, but the efficacy of this assay has not been validated in clinical trials. In contrast, a pivotal randomized trial to study the clinical efficacy of multiple combination bactericidal testing synergy studies was performed in Canada and Australia, wherein patients undergoing a pulmonary exacerbation were randomly assigned to treatment guided by multiple combination bactericidal testing versus regimens chosen by individual treating physicians.[2] No significant differences in the time that elapsed until the next pulmonary exacerbation or improvements in lung function between the two treatment strategies were noted.

CF experts have not arrived yet at a consensus regarding the efficacy of inpatient versus outpatient management of pulmonary exacerbations. Outpatient management has advantages; it is less costly, is less disruptive to patients and their families, and involves less risk of acquiring nosocomial pathogens. Patients treated at home were shown, however, to have longer treatment courses and less improvement in lung function.[228] Patients may improve more with hospitalization, as a result of better compliance with antibiotics, bed rest, chest physiotherapy, and bronchodilator treatments.[30]

Staphylococcus aureus and Methicillin-Resistant *Staphylococcus aureus*

The clinical utility of antistaphyloccocal agents is best shown by early studies of infants with CF treated with penicillin before the nearly universal acquisition of β-lactamases by *S. aureus*.[8,214] Infants treated during the antibiotic era had markedly improved survival rates. Experts advocate the use of a first-generation cephalosporin (e.g., cephazolin) or a semisynthetic penicillin (e.g., oxacillin) for treatment of a pulmonary exacerbation associated with MSSA.[122] Treatment trials justifying this approach are lacking, however.

Vancomycin generally is advocated for treatment of MRSA when this organism is considered a pathogen. Although no treatment trials in CF patients using linezolid have been conducted, a case series showed that adults with CF required 600 mg every 8 hours to provide desired pharmacokinetics.[29,298] Linezolid-resistant MRSA did emerge in a child with CF treated for approximately 3 months.[117] Because this agent is available orally and intravenously, the potential for "abuse" exists if clinicians do not use this agent judiciously. Several investigators in Europe have published small case series of various regimens for eradication of MRSA that have included oral agents (e.g., rifampin and fusidic acid) and inhaled agents (e.g., vancomycin).[120,198,201,317] Randomized treatment trials must be performed to establish the safety and efficacy of these strategies.

Burkholderia cepacia Complex

Management of *B. cepacia* complex is more problematic because of higher levels of intrinsic antibiotic resistance and a paucity of clinical trials for this pathogen. Initial isolates may be susceptible to ciprofloxacin, β-lactam antibiotics, chloramphenicol, trimethoprim-sulfamethoxazole, meropenem, and minocycline,

but with the exception of *Burkholderia gladioli*, all *Burkholderia* spp. are resistant to aminoglycosides. Temocillin has been used in Europe to treat pulmonary exacerbation caused by *B. cepacia*.[344] Resistance can develop, however, which severely limits therapeutic options. As described for the management of *P. aeruginosa*, combinations of two or three agents are used to treat a pulmonary exacerbation. Even more prolonged courses may be required to improve lung function. Meropenem and minocycline were noted to have the most in vitro activity against 652 multidrug-resistant *Burkholderia* strains isolated from patients with CF and tested at the Cystic Fibrosis Referral Center, and inhibited 28 percent and 33 percent of strains.[197] Treatment may be guided by synergy testing of two or more drug combinations with an evident improvement in pulmonary function.[1,389]

Stenotrophomonas maltophilia and *Achromobacter xylosoxidans*

There are no published treatment trials for patients with CF who are harboring *S. maltophilia* or *A. xylosoxidans* undergoing an exacerbation. Although definitive data confirming that these organisms are pathogens in CF are unavailable, clinicians target these multidrug-resistant, gram-negative bacilli if they are consistently recovered from the respiratory tract of an individual patient. At present, the Clinical Laboratory Standards Institute recommends testing ticarcillin-clavulanate, ceftazidime, minocycline, chloramphenicol, trimethoprim-sulfamethoxazole, and levofloxacin against *S. maltophilia*,[60] but CF strains frequently are resistant to these agents.[297]

Nonetheless, similar strategies are used to treat these organisms as described for *P. aeruginosa* or *B. cepacia* complex; two or more parenteral agents are chosen based on susceptibility testing and given for 2 to 3 weeks. In a survey of 263 isolates of *S. maltophilia* from 218 patients with CF isolated from 1995 to 1998, doxycycline, ticarcillin-clavulanate, piperacillin-tazobactam, and trimethoprim-sulfamethoxazole were most active and inhibited 78 percent, 39 percent, 18 percent, and 13 percent of isolates, respectively.[297,389] A survey of 94 *A. xylosoxidans* isolates from 77 patients showed that meropenem and imipenem, or piperacillin with or without tazobactam, were most active.[291]

Nontuberculous Mycobacteria

Treatment of NTM in patients with CF is challenging and guided by the clinical presentation and the mycobacterial species. Before therapy for NTM is initiated, patients should be treated aggressively for the classic CF pathogens they harbor to determine if they clinically improve without the need for specific NTM treatment. If NTM treatment is initiated, a careful history, physical examination, and pulmonary function tests should be done to determine the baseline status of the patient in efforts to monitor response to therapy. Susceptibility testing for NTM is not done routinely for patients who do not have CF. Given the increased antibiotic exposure in CF and the potential for the emergence of resistance, NTM strains isolated from patients with CF should undergo susceptibility testing at a reference laboratory. Treatment can be guided by the initial susceptibility profile.

No treatment trials have been published for NTM in CF, and generally regimens are comparable to the regimens used in patients without CF. Treatment of MAC is straightforward and includes a macrolide agent, rifabutin, and ethambutol. Treatment of *M. abscessus* is more complex. Many experts have a lower threshold for treating *M. abscessus*, given the greater apparent virulence of this species in CF, including after lung transplant.[52] Some experts recommend oral therapy, including a macrolide and linezolid because both have excellent in vitro activity, for stable patients.[35] Some experts add vitamin B$_6$ to prevent peripheral neuropathy, but the pathogenesis of peripheral neuropathy from linezolid is unknown. For more symptomatic patients, intravenous therapy, including cefoxitin or a carbapenem, depending on susceptibilities and amikacin, is recommended. Such patients need to have hearing assessed regularly. Because of the potential for different pharmacokinetic properties in CF and the fact that oral agents may not be well absorbed by patients with CF, serum levels for antimycobacterial agents should be strongly considered.[125,255]

Patients should be followed closely and have monthly sputum testing done for acid-fast bacillus smear and culture. The response to treatment generally is good for patients infected with MAC. Although the optimal duration of treatment has not been studied, experts recommend continuing therapy for 1 year after negative sputum cultures have been obtained. Cure for *M. abscessus* is less likely to occur, and the therapeutic goal may be long-term suppression. After clinical and mycobacterial improvement (i.e., a reduction in organism burden) has been achieved, intravenous antibiotics can be stopped and prolonged oral therapy with a macrolide can be initiated.

Allergic Bronchopulmonary Aspergillosis

Treatment of ABPA also can be very challenging. Although steroids are the treatment of choice because ABPA is immunologically mediated, the response to steroids varies and may have the undesirable consequence of diabetes in this vulnerable patient population. The oral antifungal therapies voriconazole[148] and itraconazole[230] have been used with reported response and toxicity, but no controlled trials have been performed.[223] Monitoring serum levels of itraconazole is desirable because this agent may be malabsorbed if the gastric pH is non-acidic.

Long-Term Suppressive Therapy

INHALED ANTIBIOTICS

Long-term suppressive antibiotic therapy has been used increasingly to treat patients with CF and infected with *P. aeruginosa* to prolong the time between pulmonary exacerbations and to slow the progression of lung deterioration. Numerous oral agents that are not cidal for *P. aeruginosa* (e.g., amoxicillin-clavulanate, trimethoprim-sulfamethoxazole, or tetracycline agents) are used empirically, sometimes in rotation, with anecdotal support coming from patients and physicians. The use of oral antibiotics is widespread; during a 6-month period, 90 percent of patients received at least one course of oral antibiotics.[41] No clinical trials support this practice, however, and it may contribute to antibiotic resistance.

For decades, inhaled agents such as tobramycin, colistin, gentamicin, amikacin, and various β-lactam antibiotics, including carbenicillin and cephaloridine, also have been used for management of chronic infections.[45] Definitive data supporting the use of inhaled agents were derived from a multicenter phase III, double-blind, placebo-controlled, randomized treatment trial of inhaled tobramycin (TOBI) in patients with CF and chronic *P. aeruginosa* infection.[267] Patients received 300 mg of tobramycin twice daily every other month for 6 months. The rationale for administering therapy every other month was to delay the emergence of resistance, to reduce cost, to increase compliance, and potentially to exploit the post-antibiotic effect of aminoglycosides. Subjects randomly assigned to inhaled tobramycin had a 10 percent improvement in FEV$_1$ compared with subjects who received placebo, who experienced a 2 percent decline in FEV$_1$. Treated patients also had a reduction in bacterial density, fewer days of hospitalization, and fewer days of intravenous antibiotics. In subset analyses, adolescents had the greatest improvement in pulmonary function. During treatment, patients receiving tobra-

mycin had increased tinnitus that was unassociated with hearing loss. There was minimal systemic absorption of tobramycin because serum levels of tobramycin generally were less than 1 µg/mL.

Although this study confirmed the efficacy of inhaled tobramycin in CF patients with chronic *P. aeruginosa* infection, several questions remain. In routine antimicrobial susceptibility testing, the breakpoint for resistance to tobramycin is MIC of 16 µg/mL or greater. The aerosol route delivers 100-fold higher concentrations of tobramycin without toxicity, however; the median concentration of tobramycin in the phase III trial was 1200 µg/g of sputum.[267] Although the conventional breakpoint for resistance to tobramycin is irrelevant for drug delivered by inhalation, the breakpoint for inhaled tobramycin is unknown. Commercially available susceptibility tests do not measure MICs greater than 8 µg/mL. During the 6-month trial, resistance to tobramycin did occur; a trend was found toward higher MICs in the treatment group (median MIC, 2 µg/mL) compared with the placebo group (median MIC, 1 µg/mL). Only a few subjects had tobramycin MIC of 128 µg/mL or greater, however, and the impact of these higher MICs on clinical efficacy could not be determined because of the small number of such patients.

Investigators also examined the emergence of intrinsically tobramycin-resistant pathogens. Although treatment-emergent *B. cepacia*, *S. maltophilia*, and *A. xylosoxidans* did not increase in the participants randomly assigned to inhaled tobramycin, the incidence of treatment-emergent *Aspergillus* spp., but not ABPA, was increased.

Buoyed by the success of aerosolized tobramycin, other aerosolized agents have been studied. Most recently, aerosolized aztreonam has been developed for long-term suppressive therapy, with a proposed strategy of alternating with aerosolized tobramycin.[124] A phase III trial has been completed, but the results are not yet published.

MACROLIDE ANTIBIOTICS

Much interest has been generated more recently in the use of macrolide agents in CF[154] as long-term suppressive therapy. The rationale for macrolide therapy in CF stems from the successful treatment of diffuse panbronchiolitis with erythromycin, azithromycin, and clarithromycin.[177,186] Diffuse panbronchiolitis is a chronic lung disease, diagnosed primarily in Asian adults, with several clinical features similar to those found in CF, including progressive lung disease caused by mucoid and nonmucoid strains of *P. aeruginosa*.[330] Long-term administration of low-dose macrolide agents to patients with diffuse panbronchiolitis has reduced morbidity and mortality rates.

In vitro studies have provided the scientific rationale for this clinical efficacy. Although macrolides are not cidal for *P. aeruginosa*, subinhibitory concentrations of macrolide agents reduce the production of several virulence factors by *P. aeruginosa*,[218,219] including the formation of biofilm.[160,179] Macrolide antibiotics also may have an anti-inflammatory effect and decrease cytokine production by neutrophils, monocytes, and bronchial epithelial cells.[159,382]

Four azithromycin trials have been conducted in patients with CF so far.[59,101,292,375] Three trials were conducted in patients chronically infected with *P. aeruginosa*[101,292,375] and had similar results; all showed improvement in lung function using similar treatment regimens of azithromycin. Improvements in secondary outcomes, such as decreased hospitalization, decreased antibiotic use, and increased weight gain, also were noted. In the more recent study performed in 82 children and adolescents, most (63 of 82, 77%) with negative cultures for *P. aeruginosa*,[59] participants in the azithromycin-treated group had fewer pulmonary exacerbations and less oral antibiotic use. No differences in lung function or intravenous antibiotics were noted, however, in the azithromycin-treated group compared with the placebo-treated group. A Cochrane review concluded that short-term (i.e., 3 to 6 months) azithromycin seemed effective in CF, but long-term safety and efficacy remain unknown.[319] Patients treated with azithromycin should be screened for NTM before initiating therapy and annually thereafter because of concern about macrolide resistance in these microorganisms.

LUNG TRANSPLANTATION

Lung transplantation currently is considered a viable therapy for selected patients with end-stage pulmonary disease of CF.[383] Bilateral lung, heart-lung, and living donor lobar lung transplantation all have been performed in patients with CF, but most operations in recent years have used the bilateral lung transplant approach with lungs from deceased donors. By 2006, more than 3000 individuals with CF had undergone lung transplantation worldwide, with nearly 250 procedures performed annually as of 2005.[350] The survival of lung transplant recipients with CF exceeds that of any other diagnostic group for all ages, with projected survival half-life of 6.2 years.[350] Patients with CF nonetheless present special challenges for successful lung transplantation. The life-threatening manifestations of CF generally are limited to the lungs except for patients with advanced liver disease with portal hypertension. Advantages of a lung transplant recipient with CF include relative young age, giving the potential of many years of productive life ahead. In addition, patients with CF have experience with complex medical regimens.

The optimal time to refer potential candidates for evaluation for lung transplant is difficult to determine because the natural history of CF cannot be predicted precisely. In May 2005 in the United States, the United Network for Organ Sharing introduced a new system of lung distribution, which assigns a lung allocation score to each potential candidate. Key parameters used in the lung allocation score include lung function testing, the need for oxygenation, the presence of diabetes mellitus, age, body mass index, the need for ventilatory support, hospitalization in the intensive care unit, and hemodynamic data from cardiac catheterization. Waiting time no longer is considered except in individuals younger than 12 years of age. There are no microbiologic criteria.[95]

Although transplanted lungs do not develop CF, they can become infected with the pretransplant pathogens because the trachea and paranasal sinuses continue to manifest the pathophysiology of CF. Lung transplant recipients with CF are at risk for development of infection via pretransplant microbial flora or newly acquired pathogens.[169,195,316,325] Controversy has ensued about whether microbiologic criteria, specifically pretransplant infection with fungi, NTM, or multidrug-resistant pathogens, should be considered contraindications to performing lung transplantation in patients with CF. Several centers have published their experiences with infections that developed from lung transplantation pathogens; they include invasive aspergillosis; sepsis with *S. maltophilia*, *B. cepacia* complex organisms, and *B. gladioli*; and sternal wound infection.[169] Other centers have reported that morbidity and mortality caused by *P. aeruginosa* infections posttransplant are not higher in patients with CF than in patients who do not have CF.[113,234]

A more recent study indicated that lung transplant recipients with CF and with panresistant, gram-negative organisms other than *Burkholderia* spp. had significantly decreased survival rates after transplantation than a comparable group with antibiotic-sensitive organisms.[142] Patients with CF who are infected with *B. cenocepacia* have increased morbidity and mortality rates from recurrent infection or sepsis or both after lung transplantation. Although Aris and colleagues[10] did not detect patient-to-patient transmission, increased mortality rates were noted with *B. cenocepacia* but not with multidrug-resistant *P. aeruginosa*. Patients infected with genomovar III had increased mortality rates after lung transplantation compared with patients infected with other genomovars before transplantation.[10]

Infection with *M. abscessus* before undergoing transplant can be associated with severe post-transplant complications and death.[55,343] Acquisition of NTM post-transplant can be treated successfully with prolonged combination of antimicrobial therapy.[55,203] Patients with CF are at risk of developing invasive aspergillosis after transplant, but at lower rates than patients without CF.[234,249] Many of these patients with CF were colonized with *Aspergillus* spp. before undergoing transplantations. Treatment with antifungal therapy after surgery should be considered. The U.S. Cystic Fibrosis Foundation held a consensus conference on lung transplantation in 1996.[383] The conferees concluded that microbiologic contraindications to transplantation were limited to active hepatitis B and human immunodeficiency virus. The decision to transplant patients infected with *B. cepacia* complex or multidrug-resistant *P. aeruginosa*, or colonized with *Aspergillus* spp., should be made on a case-by-case basis. Potentially, an understanding of the genomovar infecting a patient may be a useful predictor of mortality.

ANTI-INFLAMMATORY THERAPY

Inflammation associated with chronic bacterial colonization plays a crucial role in CF lung disease. Nonsteroidal agents and glucocorticoids have been used as potential medications for antiinflammatory therapy. A randomized trial using oral prednisone (1 to 2 mg/kg every other day) showed a reduction in the rate of decline in pulmonary function of patients with CF but was associated with significant steroid-related side effects.[16] Three short-term trials using inhaled steroids have led to mixed results and no clear direction for long-term use.[18,232,357] A systematic review of inhaled steroids for CF was equivocal with respect to efficacy.[17] A multicenter randomized trial of withdrawal of inhaled steroids in CF did not find a difference in pulmonary exacerbations, infection with *P. aeruginosa*, or pulmonary function after inhaled steroids were discontinued.[19] High-dose ibuprofen (20 to 30 mg/kg twice per day) used over a 4-year period showed a decreased rate of decline in pulmonary function with few reported side effects.[181] Macrolide antibiotics decrease inflammation by modulation of inflammatory signaling pathways and decreased cytokine production from inflammatory cells.[98] Several anti-inflammatory agents, including antiproteases, statins, and antioxidants, have been proposed as potential therapies, but they remain under investigation and are not a part of routine clinical practice.

PREVENTION

IMMUNIZATIONS

The use of currently available routine childhood and adolescent vaccines is strongly advocated for patients with CF. Although patients with CF are not at increased risk of developing *Streptococcus pneumoniae* infections, they should receive the pneumococcal vaccine, 7-valent (Prevnar). Annual influenza vaccination is recommended for patients with CF and household members.[104,110] The RSV subunit vaccine, PFP-2 (purified fusion protein vaccine is a fusion glycoprotein that induces serum neutralizing antibodies) has been studied in children with CF for two RSV seasons.[260] Initial studies showed that the RSV subunit vaccine was safe and immunogenic and that it reduced the incidence of lower respiratory tract infections.[259] A large multicenter trial in patients with mild disease failed to show a reduction in the incidence of lower respiratory tract infection, however.[258] A placebo-controlled trial of RSV monoclonal antibody (Palivizumab) was performed in 186 children.[320] Although Palivizumab was well tolerated, two children were hospitalized (one in each group); the study was not adequately powered for efficacy.

Most recently, the results of a phase III multicenter study of a *P. aeruginosa* vaccine were published.[89] Although this bivalent, antiflagella vaccine was immunogenic and was found to reduce the incidence of *P. aeruginosa* infection and serum antibody titers, it did not prevent chronic *P. aeruginosa* infection, and it did not affect lung function.

INFECTION CONTROL PRECAUTIONS

Although the sources of most pathogens in patients with CF are unknown, it is increasingly recognized that patient-to-patient spread and acquisition from the contaminated health care environment can occur. To date, reports of transmission of bacterial pathogens occurring between individuals with and without CF are rare.[127,152,210] Direct contact, indirect contact, and spread of droplets with infectious secretions all have been implicated as modes of transmission of CF pathogens. Risk factors for transmission were described first for *B. cepacia* complex as shown in Table 31–5.[51,132,194,253,254,346]

Perhaps of most concern have been several reports of clonal spread of *P. aeruginosa* among patients with CF.[209,303,354] These examples have involved obvious phenotypes that triggered an investigation of possible patient-to-patient spread, including an increase in ceftazidime-resistant *P. aeruginosa*[53] or initial colonization of young children with mucoid strains of *P. aeruginosa*.[13,233] These reports have led CF centers in Europe to favor cohorting and segregating patients with *P. aeruginosa*, particularly patients with antibiotic-resistant strains, in hospital and clinic settings.[114,178,209] In the United States, infection control strategies have focused on containment of respiratory tract secretions as described subsequently.[296] Finally, occasional cases of patient-to-patient spread of other potential pathogens, including *S. maltophilia* and *A. xylosoxidans*, have been reported in patients with CF.[276,353]

The U.S. Cystic Fibrosis Foundation convened an expert panel to develop revised recommendations for infection control that addressed inpatient, outpatient (i.e., CF clinic and pulmonary function test laboratories), and non–health care settings, as so much CF care is delivered in the home. These recommendations have implications for treatment, transplantation, and the psychosocial well-being of patients, families, and staff. Several strategies were emphasized (Table 31–6). The guidelines emphasized that all patients with CF could harbor potentially transmissible respiratory tract pathogens, and containing respiratory tract secretions is of paramount importance.

The consensus is that patients harboring *B. cepacia* complex should be cared for apart from other patients with CF and not grouped together because of concern that some strains of *B. cepacia* complex may be more virulent and replace other strains.[200] Patients are hospitalized in single rooms and seen in outpatient settings geographically or temporally apart from other patients with CF. Similarly, patients with CF and MRSA in the respiratory tract should be placed in private rooms without access to common areas.

CONCLUSION

The microbiology of patients with CF is complex and changing. Although the pathogenesis of lung infections is still under active investigation, the current hypothesis suggests multiple etiologies. Appropriate microbiologic processing of respiratory tract specimens is crucial to ensure an accurate understanding of the epidemiology of CF lung disease and to provide appropriate treatment and infection control. Current treatment strategies are directed largely at management of deteriorations of pulmonary function, but increasingly strategies are directed at prevention and preservation of lung function.

TABLE 31–5   Risk Factors Associated with Acquisition of *Burkholderia cepacia* Complex

Risk Factors	Comment
Attendance at CF summer camp[253]	Risk of acquisition (6% incidence) increased with time spent at camp and prevalence of *B. cepacia* at the camp
Slept in same cabin	
Shared a personal item	
Danced with *B. cepacia*–infected camper	
Attendance at summer educational program[194]	3 (20%) of 15 patients acquired same ribotype
Participation in adult CF group	Disband meetings thought to represent extensive social contact
Social contact[132]	
Kissing	
Intimate contact	
Prolonged car rides	
Sibling with *B. cepacia* complex	
Handshaking	2 of 68 cultures positive, 1 from patient and 1 from investigator[254]
	3 patients' hands became contaminated after coughing[132]
Inpatient exposures	Risk of acquisition increased if hospitalized within 3 mo and if hospitalized longer
	Interviews with health care workers indicated poor adherence to contact precautions
Recent hospitalization[254]	
Use of specific shower	
Sharing hospital room with another patient infected with *B. cepacia*	
Cared for by a medical student	
Respiratory therapy equipment	Reservoirs of large-volume nebulizers grew *B. cepacia*
Sharing equipment	
Hospital nebulizers	
Spirometer[161]	
Mouthpiece filters[132]	

CF, cystic fibrosis.

TABLE 31–6   Infection Control Strategies for Cystic Fibrosis

Guideline	Setting		
	Inpatient	**Outpatient**	**Non–Health Care**
Quarterly cultures of respiratory tract		X	
Appropriate processing of CF respiratory tract cultures	X	X	
Educate patients and families about proper hand hygiene	X	X	X
Implement contact precautions for MDROs, including MRSA	X	X	
Hospitalize patients with MDROs in single-patient room	X	X	
Segregate patients with *B. cepacia* complex from other CF patients	X	X	X
Clean and disinfect respiratory therapy equipment	X	X	X
Avoid socialization among CF patients	X	X	X
Maintain at least 3 ft between CF patients to prevent droplet transmission	X	X	X

CF, cystic fibrosis; MDROs, multidrug-resistant organisms; MRSA, methicillin-resistant Staphylococcus aureus.

REFERENCES

1. Aaron, S. D., Ferris, W., Henry, D. A., et al.: Multiple combination bactericidal antibiotic testing for patients with cystic fibrosis infected with *Burkholderia cepacia*. Am. J. Respir. Crit. Care Med. *161*(4 Pt 1):1206-1212, 2000.

2. Aaron, S. D., Vandemheen, K. L., Ferris, W., et al.: Combination antibiotic susceptibility testing to treat exacerbations of cystic fibrosis associated with multiresistant bacteria: A randomised, double-blind, controlled clinical trial. Lancet *366*:463-471, 2005.

3. Abman, S. H., Ogle, J. W., Butler, S. N., et al.: Role of respiratory syncytial virus in early hospitalizations for respiratory distress of young infants with cystic fibrosis. J. Pediatr. *113*:826, 1998.

4. Abman, S. H., Ogle, J. W., Harbeck, R. J., et al.: Early bacteriologic, immunologic, and clinical courses of young infants with cystic fibrosis identified by neonatal screening. J. Pediatr. *119*:211-217, 1991.

5. Accurso, F. J., Sontag, M. S., and Wagener, J. S.: Complications associated with symptomatic diagnosis in infants with cystic fibrosis. J. Pediatr. *147*:S37-S41, 2005.

6. Amaral, M. D.: Processing of CFTR: Transversing the cellular maze—how much CFTR needs to go through to avoid cystic fibrosis? Pediatr. Pulmonol. *39*:479-491, 2005.

7. American Thoracic Society: Diagnosis and treatment of disease caused by non-tuberculous mycobacteria. Am. J. Respir. Crit. Care Med. *156*:S1-S25, 1997.

8. Anderson, D. H.: Therapy and prognosis of fibrocystic disease of the pancreas. Pediatrics 406-417, 1949.

9. Anguiana, A., Oates, R. D., Amos, J. A., et al.: Congenital bilateral absence of the vas deferens: A primarily genital form of cystic fibrosis. J. A. M. A. *267*:1704-1797, 1992.

10. Aris, R. M., Gilligan, P. H., Neuringer, I. P., et al.: The effects of panresistant bacteria in cystic fibrosis patients on lung transplant outcome. Am. J. Respir. Crit. Care Med. *155*:1699-1704, 1997.

11. Armstrong, D.: *Pseudomonas aeruginosa*: Clinical research. Prog. Respir. Res. *34*:131-137, 2006.

12. Armstrong, D., Grimwood, K., Carlin, J. B., et al.: Severe viral respiratory infections in infants with cystic fibrosis. Pediatr. Pulmonol. *26*:371-379, 1998.

13. Armstrong, D. S., Grimwood, K., Carlin, J. B., et al.: Lower airway inflammation in infants and young children with cystic fibrosis. Am. J. Respir. Crit. Care Med. *156*:1197-1204, 1997.

14. Armstrong, D. S., Grimwood, K., Carzino, R., et al.: Lower respiratory infection and inflammation in infants with newly diagnosed cystic fibrosis. B. M. J. *310*:1571, 1995.

15. Armstrong, D. S., Nixon, G. M., Carzino, R., et al.: Detection of a widespread clone of *Pseudomonas aeruginosa* in a pediatric cystic fibrosis clinic. Am. J. Respir. Crit. Care Med. *166*:983-987, 2002.

16. Auberbach, H. S., Williams, M., Kirkpatrick, J. A., and Colten, H. R.: Alternate day prednisone reduced morbity and improves pulmonary function in cystic fibrosis. Lancet *2*:686-688, 1985.

17. Balfour-Lynn, I., Walters, S., and Dezateux, C.: Inhaled corticosteroids for cystic fibrosis. Cochrane Database Syst. Rev. *1*:CD001915, 2000.

18. Balfour-Lynn, I. M., Klein, N. J., and Dinwiddie, R.: Randomized controlled trial of inhaled corticosteroids fluticasone propionate in cystic fibrosis. Arch. Dis. Child. *77*:124-130, 1997.

19. Balfour-Lynn, I. M., Lees, B., Hall, P., et al.; CF WISE (Withdrawal of Inhaled Steroids Evaluation) Investigators: Multicenter randomized controlled trial of withdrawal of inhaled corticosteroids in cystic fibrosis. Am. J. Respir. Crit. Care Med. *173*:1356-1362, 2006.

20. Baltimore, R. S., Christie, C. D., and Smith, G. J.: Immunohistopathologic localization of *Pseudomonas aeruginosa* in lungs from patients with cystic fibrosis: Implications for the pathogenesis of progressive lung deterioration. Am. Rev. Respir. Dis. *140*:1650-1661, 1989.

21. Bange, F. C., and Bottger, E. C.: Improved decontamination method for recovering mycobacteria from patients with cystic fibrosis. Eur. J. Clin. Microbiol. Infect. Dis. *21*:546-548, 2002.

22. Bargon, J., Dauletbaev, N., Kohler, B., et al.: Prophylactic antibiotic therapy is associated with an increased prevalence of *Aspergillus* colonization in adult cystic fibrosis patients. Respir. Med. *93*:835-838, 1999.

23. Beardsmore, C. S., Thompson, J. R., Williams, A., et al.: Pulmonary function in infants with cystic fibrosis: The effect of antibiotic treatment. Arch. Dis. Child. *71*:133-137, 1994.

24. Blackmon, S. M., Deering-Brose, R., McWilliams, R., et al.: Relative contribution of genetic and nongenetic modifiers to intestinal obstruction in cystic fibrosis. Gastroenterology *131*:1030-1039, 2006.

25. Blumer, J. L., Saiman, L., Konstan, M. W., and Melnick, D.: The efficacy and safety of meropenem and tobramycin vs ceftazidime and tobramycin in the treatment of acute pulmonary exacerbations in patients with cystic fibrosis. Chest *128*:2336-2346, 2005.

26. Bonfield, T. L., Konstan, M. W., Burfeind, P., et al.: Normal bronchial epithelial cells constitutively produce the anti-inflammatory cytokine interleukin-10, which is downregulated in cystic fibrosis. Am. J. Respir. Cell. Mol. Biol. *13*:257-261, 1995.

27. Borgo, G., Mastella, G., Gasparini, P., et al.: Pancreatic function and gene deletion F508 in cystic fibrosis. J. Med. Genet. *27*:665, 1990.

28. Bosso, J. A., and Black, P. G.: Controlled trial of aztreonam vs. tobramycin and azlocillin for acute pulmonary exacerbations of cystic fibrosis. Pediatr. Infect. Dis. J. *7*:171-176, 1988.

29. Bosso, J. A., Flume, P. A., and Gray, S. L.: Linezolid pharmacokinetics in adult patients with cystic fibrosis. Antimicrob. Agent Chemother. *48*:281-284, 2004.

30. Bosworth, D. G., and Nielson, D. W.: Effectiveness of home versus hospital care in the routine treatment of cystic fibrosis. Pediatr. Pulmonol. *24*:42-47, 1997.

31. Boucher, R. C.: An overview of the pathogenesis of cystic fibrosis lung disease. Adv. Drug Deliv. Rev. *54*:1359-1371, 2002.

32. Boucher, R. C.: Evidence for airway surface dehydration as the initiating event in CF airway disease. J. Intern. Med. *261*:5-16, 2007.

33. Branger, C., Gardye, C., and Lambert-Zechovsky, N.: Persistence of *Staphylococcus aureus* strains among cystic fibrosis patients over extended periods of time. J. Med. Microbiol. *45*:294-301, 1996.

34. Brown, R. K., and Kelly, F. J.: Role of free radicals in the pathogenesis of cystic fibrosis. Thorax *49*:738-742, 1994.

35. Brown-Elliott, B. A., Crist, C. J., Mann, L. B., et al.: In vitro activity of linezolid against slowly growing nontuberculous mycobacteria. Antimicrob. Agent Chemother. *47*:1736-1738, 2003.

36. Burns, J. L., Emerson, J., Stapp, J. R., et al.: Microbiology of sputum from patients at cystic fibrosis centers in the United States. Clin. Infect. Dis. *27*:158-163, 1998.

37. Burns, J. L., Gibson, R. L., McNamara, S., et al.: Longitudinal assessment of *Pseudomonas aeruginosa* in young children with cystic fibrosis. J. Infect. Dis. *183*:444-452, 2001.

38. Burns, J. L., and Saiman, L.: *Burkholderia cepacia* infections in cystic fibrosis. Pediatr. Infect. Dis. J. *18*:155-156, 1999.

39. Burns, J. L., Saiman, L., Whittier, S., et al.: Comparison of agar diffusion methodologies for antimicrobial susceptibility testing of *Pseudomonas aeruginosa* isolates from cystic fibrosis patients. J. Clin. Microbiol. *38*:1818-1822, 2000.

40. Burns, J. L., Saiman, L., Whittier, S., et al.: Comparison of two commercial systems (Vitek and MicroScan-WalkAway) for antimicrobial susceptibility testing of *Pseudomonas aeruginosa* isolates from cystic fibrosis patients. Diagn. Microbiol. Infect. Dis. *39*:257-260, 2001.

41. Burns, J. L., Van Dalfsen, J. M., Shawar, R. M., et al.: Effect of chronic intermittent administration of inhaled tobramycin on respiratory microbial flora in patients with cystic fibrosis. J. Infect. Dis. *179*:1190-1196, 1999.

42. Caclano, G., Kazys, M., Saiman, L., and Prince, A.: Production of the *Pseudomonas aeruginosa* neuraminidase is increased under hyperosmolar conditions and is regulated by genes involved in alginate expression. J. Clin. Invest. *89*:1866-1874, 1992.

43. Campbell, P. W., Phillips, J. A., Krishnamani, M. R. S., et al.: Cystic fibrosis: Relationship between clinical status and F508 deletion. J. Pediatr. *118*:239, 1991.

44. Campbell, P. W., and White, T. B.: Newborn screening for cystic fibrosis: An opportunity to improve care and outcomes. J. Pediatr. *147*:S2-S5, 2005.

45. Campbell, P. W., 3rd., and Saiman, L.: Use of aerosolized antibiotics in patients with cystic fibrosis. Chest *116*:775-788, 1999.

46. Cantin, A. M., Bilodeau, G., Ouellet, C., et al.: Oxidant stress suppresses CFTR expression. Am. J. Physiol. Cell. Physiol. *290*:C262-C270, 2006.

47. Cantin, A. M., North, S. L., Hubbard, R. C., and Crystal, R. G.: Normal alveolar epithelial lining fluid contains high levels of glutathione. J. Appl. Physiol. *63*:152-158, 1987.

48. Cantin, A. M., White, T. B., Cross, C. E., et al.: Antioxidants in cystic fibrosis: Conclusions from the CF Antioxidant Workshop, Bethesda, Maryland, November 11-12, 2003. Free Rad. Biol. Med. *42*:15-31, 2007.

49. Casals, T., De Garcia, J., Gallego, M., et al.: Bronchiectasis in adult patients: An expression of heterozygosity for CFTR gene mutations? Clin. Genet. *65*:490-495, 2004.

50. Cash, H. A., Woods, D. E., McCullough, B., et al.: A rat model of chronic respiratory infection with *Pseudomonas aeruginosa*. Am. Rev. Respir. Dis. *119*:453-459, 1979.

51. Centers for Disease Control and Prevention: *Pseudomonas cepacia* at summer camps for persons with cystic fibrosis. M. M. W. R. Morb. Mortal. Wkly. Rep. *42*:456-459, 1993.

52. Chalermskulrat, W., Sood, N., Neuringer, I. P., et al.: Nontuberculous mycobacteria in end stage cystic fibrosis: Implications for lung transplantation. Thorax *61*:507-513, 2006.

53. Cheng, K., Smyth, R. L., Govan, J. R., et al.: Spread of beta-lactam-resistant *Pseudomonas aeruginosa* in a cystic fibrosis clinic. Lancet *348*:639-642, 1996.

54. Cheng, S. H., Gregory, R. J., Marshall, J., et al.: Defective intracellular transport and processing of CFTR is the molecular basis of most cystic fibrosis. Cell *63*:827-834, 1990.

55. Chernenko, S. M., Humar, A., Hutcheon, M., et al.: *Mycobacterium abscessus* infections in lung transplant recipients: The international experience. J. Heart Lung Transplant. *25*:1447-1455, 2006.

56. Chernick, V. C., and Kendig, E. L.: Disorders of the Respiratory Tract in Children. 5th ed. Philadelphia, W. B. Saunders, 1990, pp. 692-730.

57. Church, D. A., Kanga, J. F., Kuhn, R. J., et al.: Sequential ciprofloxacin therapy in pediatric cystic fibrosis: Comparative study vs. ceftazidime/tobramycin in the treatment of acute pulmonary exacerbations. The Cystic Fibrosis Study Group. Pediatr. Infect. Dis. J. *16*:97-105; discussion 23-26, 1997.

58. Cimon, B., Carrere, J., Vinatier, J. F., et al.: Clinical significance of *Scedosporium apiospermum* in patients with cystic fibrosis. Eur. J. Clin. Microbiol. Infect. Dis. *19*:53-56, 2000.

59. Clement, A., Tamalet, A., Leroux, E., et al.: Long term effects of azithromycin in patients with cystic fibrosis: A double blind, placebo controlled trial. Thorax *61*:895-902, 2006.

60. Clinical and Laboratory Standards Institute: Performance Standards for Antimicrobial Susceptibility Testing; 17th informational supplement M100-S17. Wayne, PA, Clinical and Laboratory Standards Institute, 2007.

61. Clinical Practice Guidelines for Cystic Fibrosis. Bethesda, MD, Cystic Fibrosis Foundation, 1997.

62. Coenye, T., Spilker, T., Reik, R., et al.: Use of PCR analyses to define the distribution of *Ralstonia* species recovered from patients with cystic fibrosis. J. Clin. Microbiol. *43*:3463-3466, 2005.

63. Coenye, T., Vandamme, P., Govan, J. R. W., and LiPuma, J. J.: Taxonomy and identification of the *Burkholderia cepacia* complex. J. Clin. Microbiol. *39*:3427-3436, 2001.

64. Cohn, J. A., Friedman, K. L., Noone, P. G., et al.: Relation beween mutations of the cystic fibrosis gene and idiopathic pancreatitis. N. Engl. J. Med. *339*:653-658, 1998.

65. Collinson, J., Nicholson, K. G., Cancio, E., et al.: Effects of upper respiratory tract infections in patients with cystic fibrosis. Thorax *51*:1115-1122, 1996.

66. Colombo, C., Russo, M. C., Zazzeron, L., and Romano, G.: Liver disease in cystic fibrosis. J. Pediatr. Gastroenterol. Nutr. *43*:S49-S55, 2006.

67. Comeau, A. M., Accurso, F. J., White, T. B., et al.; Cystic Fibrosis Foundation: Guidelines for implementation of cystic fibrosis newborn screening programs: Cystic Fibrosis Foundation workshop report. Pediatrics *119*:e495-e518, 2007.

68. Corey, M., and Farewell, V.: Determinants of mortality from cystic fibrosis in Canada, 1970-1989. Am. J. Epidemiol. *143*:1007-1017, 1996.

69. Costerton, J. W., Stewart, P. S., and Greenberg, E. P.: Bacterial biofilms: A common cause of persistent infections. Science *284*:1318-1322, 1999.

70. Cowley, E. A., and Linsdell, P.: Oxidant stress stimulates anion secretion from the human airway epithelial cell line Calu-3: Implications for cystic fibrosis lung disase. J. Physiol. *543*:201-209, 2002.

71. Cross, C. E., Halliwell, B., and Allen, A.: Antioxidant protection: A function of tracheobronchial and gastrointestinal mucus. Lancet *1*:1328-1330, 1984.

72. Cutting, G. R.: Genotype defect: Its effect on cellular function and phenotypic expression. Semin. Respir. Crit. Care Med. *15*:356, 1994.

73. Cystic Fibrosis Consensus Conference: Microbiology and Infectious Disease in Cystic Fibrosis. Cystic Fibrosis Foundation, Vol. V, Section 1, May 17-18, 1994, pp. 1-26.

74. Cystic Fibrosis Foundation: Patient Registry 1996. Bethesda, MD, Cystic Fibrosis Foundation, 1997.

75. Cystic Fibrosis Foundation: Patient Registry 2005. Bethesda, MD, Cystic Fibrosis Foundation, 2006.

76. CFGA Consortium: Cystic Fibrosis Mutation Database. Available at: http://www.genet.sickkids.on.ca/cftr/.

77. Cystic Fibrosis Genotype-Phenotype Consortium: Correlation between genotype and phenotype in patients with cystic fibrosis. N. Engl. J. Med. *329*:1308-1313, 1993.

78. Dakin, C. J., Numa, A. H., Wang, H., et al.: Inflammation, infection, and pulmonary function in infants and young children with cystic fibrosis. Am. J. Respir. Crit. Care Med. *165*:904-910, 2002.

79. Davis, P. B.: Cystic fibrosis since 1938. Am. J. Respir. Crit. Care Med. *173*:475-482, 2006.

80. Davis, S. D., Fordham, L. A., Brody, A. S., et al.: Computed tomography reflects lower airway inflammation and tracks changes in early cystic fibrosis. Am. J. Respir. Crit. Care Med. *175*:943-950, 2007.

81. de Groot, R., and Smith, A. L.: Antibiotic pharmacokinetics in cystic fibrosis: Differences and clinical significance. Clin. Pharm. *13*:228-253, 1987.

82. Demko, C. A., Stern, R. C., and Doershuk, C. F.: *Stenotrophomonas maltophilia* in cystic fibrosis: Incidence and prevalence. Pediatr. Pulmonol. *25*:304-308, 1998.

83. Denton, M., Kerr, K., Mooney, L., et al.: Transmission of a colistin-resistant *Pseudomonas aeruginosa* between patients attending in a pediatric cystic fibrosis center. Pediatr. Pulmonol. *34*:257-261, 2002.

84. Deretic, V., Schurr, M. J., and Yu, H.: *Pseudomonas aeruginosa*, mucoidy and the chronic infection phenotype in cystic fibrosis. Trend Microbiol. *3*:351-356, 1995.

85. DiMango, E., Ratner, A. J., Bryan, R., et al.: Activation of NFκB by adherent *Pseudomonas aeruginosa* in normal and cystic fibrosis respiratory epithelial cells. J. Clin. Invest. *101*:2598-2605, 1998.

86. Di Sant'Agnese, P. A.: Fibrocystic disease of the pancreas with normal or partial pancreatic function. Pediatrics *15*:683, 1955.

87. Dodge, J. A.: Male fertility in cystic fibrosis. Lancet *346*:587, 1995.

88. Doring, G.: Mechanisms of airway inflammation in cystic fibrosis. Pediatr. Allergy Immunol. 7:63-66, 1996.

89. Doring, G., Meisner, C., and Stern, M.: A double-blind randomized placebo-controlled phase III study of a *Pseudomonas aeruginosa* flagella vaccine in cystic fibrosis patients. Proc. Natl. Acad. Sci. U. S. A. *104*:11020-11025, 2007.

90. Doull, I. J., Ryley, H. C., Weller, P., and Goodchild, M. C.: Cystic fibrosis-related deaths in infancy and the effect of newborn screening. Pediatr. Pulmonol. *31*:363-366, 2001.

91. Drumm, M. L., Konstand, M. W., Schluchter, M. D., et al.; Gene Modifier Study Group: Genetic modifiers of lung disease in cystic fibrosis. N. Engl. J. Med. *353*:1443-1453, 2005.

92. Dunne, W. M., Jr., and Maisch, S.: Epidemiological investigation of infections due to *Alcaligenes* species in children and patients with cystic fibrosis: Use of repetitive-element-sequence polymerase chain reaction. Clin. Infect. Dis. *20*:836-841, 1995.

93. Eaton, T. E., Weiner Millar, P., Garrett, J. E., and Cutting, G. R.: Cystic fibrosis transmembrane conductance regulator gene mutations: Do they play a role in the etiology of allergic bronchopulonary aspergillosis? Clin. Exp. Allergy *32*:756-761, 2002.

94. Efthimiou, J., Hodson, M. E., Taylor, P., et al.: Importance of viruses and *Legionella pneumophila* in respiratory exacerbations of young adults with cystic fibrosis. Thorax *39*:150, 1984.

95. Egan, T. M., Murray, S., Bustami, R. T., et al.: Development of the new lung allocation system in the United States. Am. J. Transplant. *6*:1212-1227, 2006.

96. Elizur, A., Orscheln, R. C., Ferkol, T. W., et al.: Panton-Valentine leukocidin-positive methicillin-resistant *Staphylococcus aureus* lung infection in patients with cystic fibrosis. Chest *131*:1718-1725, 2007.

97. Elliott, M. W., and Newman Taylor, A. J.: Allergic bronchopulmonary aspergillosis. Clin. Exp. Allergy 27(Suppl. 1):55-59, 1997.

98. Elston, C., and Geddes, D.: Inflammation in cystic fibrosis—when and why? Friend or foe? Semin. Respir. Crit. Care Med. *28*:286-294, 2007.

99. Emerson, J., Rosenfeld, M., McNamara, S., et al.: *Pseudomonas aeruginosa* and other predictors of mortality and morbidity in young children with cystic fibrosis. Pediatr. Pulmonol. *34*:91-100, 2002.

100. Engelhardt, J. F., Yankaskas, J. R., Ernst, S. A., et al.: Submucosal glands are the predominant site of CFTR expression in the human bronchus. Nat. Genet. *2*:240-248, 1992.

101. Equi, A., Balfour-Lynn, I. M., Bush, A., and Rosenthal, M.: Long term azithromycin in children with cystic fibrosis: A randomised, placebo-controlled crossover trial. Lancet *360*:978-984, 2002.

102. Ernst, R. K., Adams, K. N., Moskowitz, S. M., et al.: The *Pseudomonas aeruginosa* lipid A deacylase: Selection for expression and loss within the cystic fibrosis airway. J. Bacteriol. *188*:191-201, 2006.

103. Fabbri, A., Tacchella, A., Manno, G., et al.: Emerging microorganisms in cystic fibrosis. Chemioterapia *6*:32-37, 1987.

104. Farrell, P. M., Kosorok, M. R., Laxova, A., et al.; Wisconsin Cystic Fibrosis Neonatal Screening Study Group: Nutritional benefits of neonatal screening for cystic fibrosis. N. Engl. J. Med. *337*:963-969, 1997.

105. Farrell, P. M., Lai, H. C., Li, Z., et al.: Evidence on improved outcomes with early diagnosis of cystic fibrosis through neonatal screening: Enough is enough! J. Pediatr. *147*:S30-S36, 2005.

106. Farrell, P. M., Li, Z., Kosorok, M. R., et al.: Bronchopulmonary disease in children with cystic fibrosis after early or delayed diagnosis. Am. J. Respir. Crit. Care Med. *168*:1100-1108, 2003.

107. Feranchak, A. P.: Hepatobiliary complications of cystic fibrosis. Curr. Gastroenterol. Rep. *6*:231-239, 2004.

108. Feranchak, A. P., and Sokol, R. J.: Cholangiocyte biology and cystic fibrosis liver disease. Semin. Liver Dis. *21*:471-488, 2001.

109. Fick, R. B., Jr., Sonoda, F., and Hornick, D. B.: Emergence and persistence of *Pseudomonas aeruginosa* in the cystic fibrosis airway. Semin. Respir. Infect. *7*:168, 1992.

110. Fiore, A. E., Shay, D. K., Haber, P., et al.: Prevention and control of influenza: Recommendations of the Advisory Committee on Immunization Practices (ACIP), 2007. M. M. W. R. *56*:1-54, 2007.

111. Firoved, A. M., Ornatowski, W., and Derectic, V.: Microarray analysis reveals induction of lipoprotein genes in mucoid *Pseudomonas aeruginosa*: Implications for inflammation in cystic fibrosis. Infect. Immun. *72*:5012-5018, 2004.

112. Fitz-Simmons, S. C.: The changing epidemiology of cystic fibrosis. J. Pediatr. *122*:1-9, 1993.

113. Flume, P. A., Egan, T. M., Paradowski, L. J., et al.: Infectious complications of lung transplantation: The impact of cystic fibrosis. Am. J. Respir. Crit. Care Med. *149*:1601-1607, 1994.

114. Frederiksen, B., Koch, C., and Hoiby, N.: Antibiotic treatment of initial colonization with *Pseudomonas aeruginosa* postpones chronic infection and prevents deterioration of pulmonary function in cystic fibrosis. Pediatr. Pulmonol. *23*:330-335, 1997.

115. Frederiksen, B., Koch, C., and Hoiby, N.: Changing epidemiology of *Pseudomonas aeruginosa* infection in Danish Cystic Fibrosis patients (1974-1995). Pediatr. Pulmonol. *28*:159-166, 1999.

116. Gabriel, S. E., Clarke, L. L., Boucher, R. C., et al.: CFTR and outward rectifying chloride channels are distinct proteins with a regulatory relationship. Nature *363*:263, 1993.

117. Gales, A. C., Sader, H. S., Andrade, S. S., et al.: Emergence of linezolid-resistant *Staphylococcus aureus* during treatment of pulmonary infection in a patient with cystic fibrosis. Int. J. Antimicrob. Agent *27*:300-302, 2006.

118. Garcia, D. F., Hiatt, P. W., Jewell, A., et al.: Human metapneumovirus and respiratory syncytial virus infections in older children with cystic fibrosis. Pediatr. Pulmonol. *42*:66-74, 2007.

119. Garland, J. S., Chan, Y. M., Kelly, K. J., et al.: Outcome of infants with cystic fibrosis requiring mechanical ventilation for respiratory failure. Chest *96*:136, 1989.

120. Garske, L. A., Kidd, T. J., Gan, R., et al.: Rifampicin and sodium fusidate reduces the frequency of methicillin-resistant *Staphylococcus aureus* (MRSA) isolation in adults with cystic fibrosis and chronic MRSA infection. J. Hosp. Infect. *56*:208-214, 2004.

121. Geller, D. E., Kaplowitz, H., Light, M. J., and Colin, A. A.: Allergic bronchopulmonary aspergillosis in cystic fibrosis: Reported prevalence, regional distribution, and patient characteristics. Scientific Advisory Group, Investigators, and Coordinators of the Epidemiologic Study of Cystic Fibrosis. Chest *116*:639-646, 1999.

122. Gibson, R. L., Burns, J. L., and Ramsey, B. W.: Pathophysiology and management of pulmonary infections in cystic fibrosis. Am. J. Respir. Crit. Care Med. *168*:918-951, 2003.

123. Gibson, R. L., Emerson, J., McNamara, S., et al.: Significant microbiological effect of inhaled tobramycin in young children with cystic fibrosis. Am. J. Respir. Crit. Care Med. *167*:841-849, 2003.

124. Gibson, R. L., Retsch-Bogart, G. Z., Oermann, C., et al.: Microbiology, safety, and pharmacokinetics of aztreonam lysinate for inhalation in patients with cystic fibrosis. Pediatr. Pulmonol. *41*:656-665, 2006.

125. Gilliam, M., Berning, S. E., Peloquin, C. A., et al.: Therapeutic drug monitoring in patients with cystic fibrosis and mycobacterial disease. Eur. Respir. J. *14*:347-351, 1999.

126. Gilligan, P. H.: Microbiology of airway disease in patients with cystic fibrosis. Clin. Microbiol. Rev. *4*:35-51, 1991.

127. Givney, R., Vickery, A., Holliday, A., et al.: Methicillin-resistant *Staphylococcus aureus* in a cystic fibrosis unit. J. Hosp. Infect. *35*:27-36, 1997.

128. Gold, R., Carpenter, S., Heurter, H., et al.: Randomized trial of ceftazidime versus placebo in the management of acute respiratory exacerbations in patients with cystic fibrosis. J. Pediatr. *111*(6 Pt. 1):907-913, 1987.

129. Gold, R., Overmeyer, A., Knie, B., et al.: Controlled trial of ceftazidime vs. ticarcillin and tobramycin in the treatment of acute respiratory exacerbations in patients with cystic fibrosis. Pediatr. Infect. Dis. J. *4*:172-177, 1985.

130. Goldman, M. N., Anderson, G. M., Stolzenbert, E. D., et al.: Human beta-defensin-1 is a salt-sensitive antibiotic in lung that is inactivated in cystic fibrosis. Cell *88*:553-560, 1997.

131. Goss, C. H., Aitken, M. L., Otto, K., and Rubenfeld, G. D.: Acquiring *Stenotrophomonas maltophilia* does not reduce survival in patients with cystic fibrosis. Pediatr. Pulmonol. *S20*:101-102, 2000.

132. Govan, J. R., Brown, P. H., Maddison, J., et al.: Evidence for transmission of *Pseudomonas cepacia* by social contact in cystic fibrosis. Lancet *342*:15-19, 1993.

133. Govan, J. R., and Deretic, V.: Microbial pathogenesis in cystic fibrosis: Mucoid *Pseudomonas aeruginosa* and *Burkholderia cepacia*. Microbiol. Rev. *60*:539-574, 1996.

134. Govan, J. R., and Nelson, J. W.: Microbiology of lung infection in cystic fibrosis. Br. Med. Bull. *48*:912-930, 1992.

135. Graft, D. R., Mischler, E., Farrell, P. M., and Busse, W.: Granulocyte chemiluminescence in patients with cystic fibrosis. Am. Rev. Respir. Dis. *125*:540-543, 1982.

136. Griese, M., Muller, I., and Reinhardt, D.: Eradication of initial *Pseudomonas aeruginosa* colonization in patients with cystic fibrosis. Eur. J. Med. Res. *7*:79-80, 2002.

137. Griffith, D. E., Aksamit, T., Brown-Elliott, B. A., et al.: An official ATS/IDSA statement: Diagnosis, treatment, and prevention of nontuberculous mycobacterial diseases. Am. J. Respir. Crit. Care Med. *175*:367-416, 2007.

138. Grosse, S. D., Rosenfeld, M., Devine, O. J., et al.: Potential impact of newborn screening for cystic fibrosis on child survival: A systematic review and analysis. J. Pediatr. *149*:362-366, 2006.

139. Guggino, W. B.: Cystic fibrosis and the salt controversy. Cell *96*:607-610, 1999.

140. Gutierrez, J. P., Grimwood, K., Armstrong, D. S., et al.: Interlobar differences in bronchoalveolar lavage fluid from children with cystic fibrosis. Eur. Respir. J. *17*:281-286, 2001.

141. Haardt, M., Benharouga, M., Lechardeur, D., et al.: C-terminal truncations destabilize the cystic fibrosis transmembrance conductance regulator without impairing its biogenesis: A novel class of mutation. J. Biol. Chem. *274*:21873-21877, 1999.

142. Hadjiliadis, D., Steele, M. P., Chaparro, C., et al.: Survival of lung transplant patients with cystic fibrosis harboring panresistant bacteria other than *Burkholderia cepacia*, compared with patients harboring sensitive bacteria. J. Heart Lung Transplant *26*:834-838, 2007.

143. Hanna, S. L., Sherman, N. E., Kinter, M. T., and Goldberg, J. B.: Comparison of proteins expressed by *Pseudomonas aeruginosa* strains representing initial and chronic isolates from a cystic fibrosis patient: An analysis by 2-D gel electrophoresis and capillary column liquid chromatography-tandem mass spectrometry. Microbiology *146*:2495-2508, 2000.

144. Hauber, H. P., Manoukian, J. J., Nguyen, L. H., et al.: Increased expression of interleukin-9, interleukin-9 receptor, and the calcium-activated chloride channel hCLCA1 in the upper airways of patients with cystic fibrosis. Laryngoscope *113*:1037-1042, 2003.

145. Henry, D., Campbell, M., McGimpsey, C., et al.: Comparison of isolation media for recovery of *Burkholderia cepacia* complex from respiratory secretions of patients with cystic fibrosis. J. Clin. Microbiol. *37*:1004-1007, 1999.

146. Hiatt, P. W., Grace, S. C., Kozinetz, C. A., et al.: Effects of viral lower respiratory tract infection on lung function in infants with cystic fibrosis. Pediatrics *103*:619-626, 1999.

147. Hill, D., Rose, B., Pajkos, A., et al.: Antibiotic susceptabilities of *Pseudomonas aeruginosa* isolates derived from patients with cystic fibrosis under aerobic, anaerobic, and biofilm conditions. J. Clin. Microbiol. *43*:5085-5090, 2005.

148. Hilliard, T., Edwards, S., Buchdahl, R., et al.: Voriconazole therapy in children with cystic fibrosis. J. Cyst. Fibros. *4*:215-220, 2005.

149. Ho, S. A., Ball, R., Morrison, L. J., et al.: Clinical value of obtaining sputum and cough swab samples following inhaled hypertonic saline in children with cystic fibrosis. Pediatr. Pulmonol. *38*:82-87, 2004.

150. Hodson, M. E., Roberts, C. M., Butland, R. J., et al.: Oral ciprofloxacin compared with conventional intravenous treatment for *Pseudomonas aeruginosa* infection in adults with cystic fibrosis. Lancet *1*:235-237, 1987.

151. Hohn, D. C., MacKay, R. D., Halliday, B., and Hun, T. K.: Effect of O2 tension on microbicidal function of leukocytes in wounds and in vitro. Surg. Forum *27*:18-20, 1976.

152. Holmes, A., Nolan, R., Taylor, R., et al.: An epidemic of *Burkholderia cepacia* transmitted between patients with and without cystic fibrosis. J. Infect. Dis. *179*:1197-1205, 1999.

153. Hordvik, N. L., Konig, P., Hamory, B., et al.: Effects of acute viral respiratory tract infections in patients with cystic fibrosis. Pediatr. Pulmonol. *7*:217, 1989.

154. Howe, R. A., and Spencer, R. C.: Macrolides for the treatment of *Pseudomonas aeruginosa* infections? J. Antimicrob. Chemother. *40*:153-155, 1997.

155. Hubeau, C., LeNaour, R., Abely, M., et al.: Dysregulation of IL-2 and IL-8 production in circulating T lymphocytes from young cystic fibrosis patients. Clin. Exp. Immunol. *135*:538-534, 2004.

156. Hudson, V. L., Wielinski, C. L., and Regelmann, W. E.: Prognostic implications of initial oropharyngeal bacterial flora in patients with cystic fibrosis diagnosed before the age of two years. J. Pediatr. *122*:854-860, 1993.

157. Hyatt, A. C., Chipps, B. E., Kumor, K. M., et al.: A double-blind controlled trial of anti-*Pseudomonas* chemotherapy of acute respiratory exacerbations in patients with cystic fibrosis. J. Pediatr. *99*:307-314, 1981.

158. Hyde, S. C., Emsley, P., Hartshorn, M. J., et al.: Structural model of ATP-binding proteins associated with cystic fibrosis, multi-drug resistance and bacterial support. Nature *346*:362, 1990.

159. Ichikawa, Y., Ninomiya, H., Koga, H., et al.: Erythromycin reduces neutrophils and neutrophil-derived elastolytic-like activity in the lower respiratory tract of bronchiolitis patients. Am. Rev. Respir. Dis. *146*:196-203, 1992.

160. Ichimiya, T., Takeoka, K., Hiramatsu, K., et al.: The influence of azithromycin on the biofilm formation of *Pseudomonas aeruginosa* in vitro. Chemotherapy *42*:186-191, 1996.

161. Isles, A., Maclusky, I., Corey, M., et al.: *Pseudomonas cepacia* infection in cystic fibrosis: An emerging problem. J. Pediatr. *104*:206-210, 1984.

162. Jackson, M. A., Kusmiesz, H., Shelton, S., et al.: Comparison of piperacillin vs. ticarcillin plus tobramycin in the treatment of acute pulmonary exacerbations of cystic fibrosis. Pediatr. Infect. Dis. J. *5*:440-443, 1986.

163. Jayaraman, S., Joo, N. S., Reitz, B., et al.: Submucosal gland secretions in airways from cystic fibrosis patients have normal [Na(+)] and pH but elevated viscosity. Proc. Natl. Acad. Sci. U. S. A. *98*:8119-8123, 2001.

164. Jensen, T., Pedersen, S. S., Hoiby, N., et al.: Use of antibiotics in cystic fibrosis: The Danish approach. Antibiot. Chemother. *42*:237-246, 1989.

165. Jewett, C. V., Ledbetter, J., Lyrene, R. K., et al.: Comparison of cefoperazone sodium vs methicillin, ticarcillin, and tobramycin in treatment of pulmonary exacerbations in patients with cystic fibrosis. J. Pediatr. *106*:669-672, 1985.

166. Johansen, H. K., and Hoiby, N.: Seasonal onset of initial colonization with chronic infection with *Pseudonomas aeruginosa* in patients with cystic fibrosis in Denmark. Thorax *47*:109-111, 1992.

167. Jung, J. S., Lee, J. Y., Oh, S. O., et al.: Effect of t-butylhydroperoxide on chloride secretion in rat tracheal epithelia. Pharmacol. Toxicol. *82*:236-242, 1998.

168. Kalish, L. A., Waltz, D. A., Dovey, M., et al.: Impact of *Burkholderia dolosa* on lung function and survival in cystic fibrosis. Am. J. Respir. Crit. Care Med. *173*:421-425, 2006.

169. Kanj, S. S., Tapson, V., Davis, D., et al.: Infections with patients with cystic fibrosis following lung transplantation. Chest *112*:924-930, 1997.

170. Kazachkov, M. Y., Muhlebach, B. S., Livasy, C. A., and Noah, T. L.: Lipid-laden macrophage index and inflammation in bronchoalveolar lavage fluids in children. Eur. Respir. J. *18*:790-795, 2001.

171. Kerem, E., Corey, M., Gold, R., and Levison, H.: Pulmonary function and clinical course in patients with CF after pulmonary colonization with *Pseudomonas aeruginosa*. J. Pediatr. *116*:714-719, 1990.

172. Kerem, E., Corey, M., Kerem, B., et al.: Clinical and genetic comparisons of patients with cystic fibrosis with and without meconium ileus. J. Pediatr. *114*:767, 1989.

173. Kerem, E., Corey, M., Kerem, B. S., et al.: The relation between genotype and phenotype in cystic fibrosis—analysis of the most common mutation (delta F508). N. Engl. J. Med. *323*:1517-1522, 1990.

174. Khair, O. A., Davies, R. J., and Devalia, J. L.: Bacterial-induced release of inflammatory mediators by bronchial epithelial cells. Eur. Respir. J. *9*:1913-1922, 1999.

175. Knowles, M., Gatzy, J., and Boucher, R.: Relative ion permeability of normal and cystic fibrosis nasal epithelium. J. Clin. Invest. *71*:1410-1417, 1983.

176. Knowles, M. R., and Boucher, R. C.: Mucus clearance as a primary innate defense mechanism for mammalian airways. J. Clin. Invest. *109*:571-577, 2002.

177. Kobayashi, H., Takeda, H., Sakayori, S., et al.: [Study on azithromycin in treatment of diffuse panbronchiolitis]. Kansenshogaku Zasshi *69*:711-722, 1995.

178. Koch, C., Frederiksen, B., and Hoiby, N.: Patient cohorting and infection control. Semin. Respir. Crit. Care Med. *24*:703-716, 2003.

179. Kondoh, K., Hashiba, M., and Baba, S.: Inhibitory activity of clarithromycin on biofilm synthesis with *Pseudomonas aeruginosa*. Acta Otolaryngol. *525*:56-60, 1996.

180. Konstan, M. W., Butler, S. M., Wohl, M. E. B., et al.: Growth and nutritional indexes in early life predict pulmonary function in cystic fibrosis. J. Pediatr. *142*:642-630, 2003.

181. Konstan, M. W., Byard, P. J., Hoppel, C. L., and Davis, P. B.: Effect of high-dose ibuprofen in patients with cystic fibrosis. N. Engl. J. Med. *332*:848-854, 1995.

182. Koscik, R. L., Farrell, P. M., Kosorok, M. R., et al.: Cognitive function of children with cystic fibrosis: Deleterious effect of early malnutrition. Pediatrics *113*:1549-1558, 2004.

183. Koscik, R. L., Lai, H. J., Laxova, A., et al.: Preventing early, prolonged vitamin E deficiency: An opportunity for better cognitive outcomes via early diagnosis through neonatal screening. J. Pediatr. *143*:S51-S56, 2005.

184. Kosorok, M. R., Jalaluddin, M., Farrell, P. M., et al.: Comprehensive analysis of risk factors for acquisition of *Pseudomonas aeruginosa* in young children with cystic fibrosis. Pediatr. Pulmonol. *26*:81-88, 1998.

185. Krilov, L. R., Blumer, J. L., Stern, R. C., et al.: Imipenem/cilastatin in acute pulmonary exacerbations of cystic fibrosis. Rev. Infect. Dis. 7(Suppl. 3):S482-S489, 1985.

186. Kudoh, S., Azuma, A., Yamamoto, M., et al.: Improvement of survival in patients with diffuse panbronchiolitis treated with low-dose erythromycin. Am. J. Respir. Crit. Care Med. *157*(6 Pt 1):1829-1832, 1998.

187. Kunzelmann, K., Schreiber, R., Nitschke, R., et al.: Control of epithelial Na+ conductance by the cystic fibrosis transmembrane conductance regulator. Pflugers Arch. *440*:193-201, 2000.

188. Lai, H. C., Kosorok, M. R., Sondel, S. A., et al.: Growth status in children with cystic fibrosis based on the National Cystic Fibrosis Patient Registry data: Evaluation of various criteria used to identify malnutrition. J. Pediatr. *132*:478-485, 1998.

189. Lang, B. J., Aaron, S. D., Ferris, W., et al.: Multiple combination bactericidal antibiotic testing for patients with cystic fibrosis infected with multiresistant strains of *Pseudomonas aeruginosa*. Am. J. Respir. Crit. Care Med. *162*:2241-2245, 2000.

190. Linsdell, R., and Hanrahan, J. W.: Glutathione permeability of CFTR. Am. J. Physiol. Cell. Physiol. *175*:C323-C326, 1998.

191. LiPuma, J. J.: *Burkholderia cepacia* epidemiology and pathogenesis: Implications for infection control. Curr. Opin. Pulm. Med. *4*:337-341, 1998.

192. LiPuma, J. J.: *Burkholderia cepacia*: A contraindication to lung transplantation in CF? Transpl. Infect. Dis. *3*:150-162, 2001.

193. LiPuma, J. J.: *Burkholderia* and emerging pathogens in cystic fibrosis. Semin. Respir. Crit. Care Med. *24*:681-692, 2003.

194. LiPuma, J. J., Dasen, S. E., Nielson, D. W., et al.: Person-to-person transmission of *Pseudomonas cepacia* between patients with cystic fibrosis. Lancet *336*:1094-1096, 1990.

195. LiPuma, J. J., Spilker, T., Gill, L. H., et al.: Disproportionate distribution of *Burkholderia cepacia* complex species and transmissibility markers in cystic fibrosis. Am. J. Respir. Crit. Care Med. *164*:92-96, 2001.

196. Lloyd-Still, J. D., Kahw, K. T., and Shwachman, H.: Severe respiratory disease in infants with cystic fibrosis. Pediatrics *53*:678, 1974.

197. Long, F. R., Williams, R. S., Adler, B. H., and Castile, R. G.: Structural airway abnormalities in infants and young children with cystic fibrosis. J. Pediatr. *144*:154-161, 2004.

198. Macfarlane, M., Leavy, A., McCaughan, J., et al.: Successful decolonization of methicillin-resistant *Staphylococcus aureus* in paediatric patients with cystic fibrosis (CF) using a three-step protocol. J. Hosp. Infect. *65*:231-236, 2007.

199. Mahenthiralingam, E., Bischof, J., Byrne, S. K., et al.: DNA-based diagnostic approaches for identification of *Burkholderia cepacia* complex, *Burkholderia vietnamiensis*, *Burkholderia multivorans*, *Burkholderia stabilis*, and *Burkholderia cepacia* genomovars I and III. J. Clin. Microbiol. *38*:3165-3173, 2000.

200. Mahenthiralingam, E., Vandamme, P., Campbell, M. E., et al.: Infection with *Burkholderia cepacia* complex genomovars in patients with cystic fibrosis: Virulent transmissible strains of genomovar III can replace *Burkholderia multivorans*. Clin. Infect. Dis. *33*:1469-1475, 2001.

201. Maiz, L., Canton, R., Mir, N., et al.: Aerosolized vancomycin for the treatment of methicillin-resistant *Staphylococcus aureus* infection in cystic fibrosis. Pediatr. Pulmonol. *26*:287-289, 1998.

202. Mall, M., Grubb, B. R., Harkema, J. R., et al.: Increased airway epithelial Na+ absorption produces cystic fibrosis-like lung disease in mice. Nat. Med. *10*:487-493, 2004.

203. Malouf, M. A., and Glanville, A. R.: The spectrum of mycobacterial infection after lung transplantation. Am. J. Respir. Crit. Care Med. *160*:1611-1616, 1999.

204. Mandell, G., Bennett, J. E., and Dolin, R.: Principles and Practice of Infectious Diseases. 6th ed. Philadelphia, W. B. Saunders, 2005.

205. Marchac, V., Equi, A., Le Bihan-Benjamin, C., et al.: Case-control study of *Stenotrophomonas maltophilia* acquisition in cystic fibrosis patients. Eur. Respir. J. *23*:98-102, 2004.

206. Martinez, T. M., Llapur, C. J., Williams, T. H., et al.: High-resolution computed tomography imaging of airway disease in infants with cystic fibrosis. Am. J. Respir. Crit. Care Med. *172*:1133-1138, 2005.

207. Mastella, G., Rainisio, M., Harms, H. K., et al.: Allergic bronchopulmonary aspergillosis in cystic fibrosis: A European epidemiological study. Epidemiologic Registry of Cystic Fibrosis. Eur. Respir. J. *16*:464-471, 2000.

208. Matsui, H., Grubb, B. R., Tarran, R., et al.: Evidence for periciliary liquid layer depletion, not abnormal ion composition, in the pathogenesis of cystic fibrosis airways disease. Cell *95*:1005-1015, 1998.

209. McCallum, S. J., Corkill, J., Gallagher, M., et al.: Superinfection with a transmissible strain of *Pseudomonas aeruginosa* in adults with cystic fibrosis chronically colonised by *P aeruginosa*. Lancet *358*:558-560, 2001.

210. McCallum, S. J., Gallagher, M. J., Corkill, J. E., et al.: Spread of an epidemic *Pseudomonas aeruginosa* strain from a patient with cystic fibrosis (CF) to non-CF relatives. Thorax *57*:559-560, 2002.

211. McCallum, S. J., Milunsky, J. M., Cunningham, D. L., et al.: Fertility in men with cystic fibrosis: An update on current surgical practices and outcomes. Chest *118*:1059, 2000.

212. McKone, E. F., Shao, J., Frangolias, D. D., et al.: Variants in the glutamate-cysteine-ligase gene are associated with cystic fibrosis lung disease. Am. J. Respir. Crit. Care Med. *174*:415-419, 2006.

213. McLaughlin, F. J., Matthews, W. J., Jr., Strieder, D. J., et al.: Clinical and bacteriological responses to three antibiotic regimens for acute exacerbations of cystic fibrosis: Ticarcillin-tobramycin, azlocillin-tobramycin, and azlocillin-placebo. J. Infect. Dis. *147*:559-567, 1983.

214. Mearns, M. B.: Treatment and prevention of pulmonary complications of cystic fibrosis in infancy and early childhood. Arch. Dis. Child. *47*:5-11, 1972.

215. Meyer, K. C., and Sharma, A.: Regional variability of lung inflammation in cystic fibrosis. Am. J. Respir. Crit. Care Med. *156*:1536-1540, 1997.

216. Miall, L. S., McGinley, N. T., Brownlee, K. G., and Conway, S. P.: Methicillin resistant *Staphylococcus aureus* (MRSA) infection in cystic fibrosis. Arch. Dis. Child. *84*:160-162, 2001.

217. Milla, C. E., Billings, J., and Moran, A.: Diabetes is associated with dramatically decreased survival in female but not male subjects with cystic fibrosis. Diabetes Care *28*:2141-2144, 2005.

218. Mizukane, R., Hirakata, Y., Kaku, M., et al.: Comparative in vitro exoenzyme-suppressing activities of azithromycin and other macrolide antibiotics against *Pseudomonas aeruginosa*. Antimicrob. Agent Chemother. *38*:528-533, 1994.

219. Molinari, G., Guzman, C. A., Pesce, A., and Schito, G. C.: Inhibition of *Pseudomonas aeruginosa* virulence factors by subinhibitory concentrations of azithromycin and other macrolide antibiotics. J. Antimicrob. Chemother. *31*:681-688, 1993.

220. Moran, A., Pyzdrowski, K. L., Weinreb, J., et al.: Insulin sensitivity in cystic fibrosis. Diabetes *43*:1020, 2004.

221. Morgan, W. J., Butler, S. M., Johnson, C. A., et al.: Epidemiologic study of cystic fibrosis: Design and implementation of a prospective, multicenter, observational study of patients with cystic fibrosis in the U.S. and Canada. Pediatr. Pulmonol. *28*:231-241, 1999.

222. Moskowitz, S. M., Foster, J. M., Emerson, J., and Burns, J. L.: Clinically feasible biofilm susceptibility assay for isolates of *Pseudomonas aeruginosa* from patients with cystic fibrosis. J. Clin. Microbiol. *42*:1915-1922, 2004.

223. Moss, R. B.: Cystic fibrosis: Pathogenesis, pulmonary infection, and treatment. Clin. Infect. Dis. *21*:839-849, 1995.

224. Moss, R. B., and King, V. V.: Management of sinusitis in cystic fibrosis by endoscopic surgery and serial antimicrobial lavage: Reduction in recurrence requiring surgery. Arch. Otolaryngol. Head Neck Surg. *121*:566-672, 1995.

225. Muhlebach, M. S., Stewart, P. W., Leigh, M. W., and Noah, T. L.: Quantitation of inflammatory responses to bacteria in young cystic fibrosis and control patients. Am. J. Respir. Crit. Care Med. *160*:186-191, 1999.

226. Murphy, T. M., and Rosenstein, B. J.: Cystic Fibrosis Lung Disease: Approaching the 21st Century. University of Chicago, Pritzker School of Medicine. Gardiner Caldwell SynerMed, 1995.

227. Mussaffi, H., Rivlin, J., Shalit, I., et al.: Nontuberculous mycobacteria in cystic fibrosis associated with allergic bronchopulmonary aspergillosis and steroid therapy. Eur. Respir. J. *25*:324-328, 2005.

228. Nazer, D., Abdulhamid, I., Thomas, R., and Pendleton, S.: Home versus hospital intravenous antibiotic therapy for acute pulmonary exacerbations in children with cystic fibrosis. Pediatr. Pulmonol. *41*:744-749, 2006.

229. NCCLS: Performance Standards for Antimicrobial Susceptibility Testing; 11th informational supplement. Vol. 21, NCCLS document M100-S11. Wayne, PA, NCCLS, 2001.

230. Nepomuceno, I. B., Esrig, S., and Moss, R. B.: Allergic bronchopulmonary aspergillosis in cystic fibrosis: Role of atopy and response to itraconazole. Chest *115*:364-370, 1999.

231. Nguyen, T. D., and Canada, A. T.: Modulation of human colonic T84 cell secretion by hydrogen peroxide. Biochem. Pharmacol. *47*:403-410, 1994.

232. Nikolaizik, W. H., and Schöni, M. H.: Pilot study to assess the effect of inhaled corticosteroids on lung function in patients with cystic fibrosis. J. Pediatr. *128*:271-274, 1996.

233. Nixon, G. M., Armstrong, D. S., Carzino, R., et al.: Clinical outcome after early *Pseudomonas aeruginosa* infection in cystic fibrosis. J. Pediatr. *138*:699-704, 2001.

234. Nunley, D. R., Grgurich, W., Iacono, A. T., et al.: Allograft colonization and infections with *Pseudomonas* in cystic fibrosis lung transplant recipients. Chest *113*:1235-1243, 1998.

235. O'Connor, G. T., Quinton, H. B., Kneeland, T., et al.: Median household income and mortality rate in cystic fibrosis. Pediatrics *111*:e333-e339, 2003.

236. Ogle, J. W., Janda, J. M., Woods, D. E., and Vasil, M. L.: Characterizations and use of a DNA probe as an epidemiological marker for *Pseudomonas aeruginosa*. J. Infect. Dis. *155*:119-126, 1987.

237. Ogle, J. W., Reller, L. B., and Vasil, M. L.: Development of resistance in *Pseudomonas aeruginosa* to imipenem, norfloxacin, and ciprofloxacin during therapy: Proof provided by typing with a DNA probe. J. Infect. Dis. *157*:743-748, 1988.

238. Olesen, H. V., Nielsen, L. P., and Schiotz, P. O.: Viral and atypical bacterial infections in the outpatient pediatric cystic fibrosis clinic. Pediatr. Pulmonol. *41*:1197-1204, 2006.

239. Oliver, A., Canton, R., Campo, P., et al.: High frequency of hypermutable *Pseudomonas aeruginosa* in cystic fibrosis lung infection. Science *288*:1251-1254, 2000.

240. Olivier, K. N., Weber, D. J., Lee, J. H., et al.: Nontuberculous mycobacteria, II: Nested-cohort study of impact on cystic fibrosis lung disease. Am. J. Respir. Crit. Care Med. *167*:835-840, 2003.

241. Olivier, K. N., Weber, D. J., Wallace, R. J., Jr., et al.: Nontuberculous mycobacteria, I: Multicenter prevalence study in cystic fibrosis. Am. J. Respir. Crit. Care Med. *167*:828-834, 2003.

242. Olivier, K. N., Yankaskas, J. R., and Knowles, M. R.: Nontuberculous mycobacterial pulmonary disease in cystic fibrosis. Semin. Respir. Infect. *11*:272-284, 1996.

243. Ong, E. L., Ellis, M. E., Webb, A. K., et al.: Infective respiratory exacerbations in young adults with cystic fibrosis: Role of viruses and atypical microorganisms. Thorax *44*:739-742, 1989.

244. Ordonez, C. L., Kartashov, A. I., and Wohl, M. E.: Variability of markers of inflammation and infection in induced sputum in children with cystic fibrosis. J. Pediatr. *145*:689-692, 2004.

245. Orenstein, D. M., Pattishall, E. N., Nixon, P. A., et al.: Quality of well-being before and after antibiotic treatment of pulmonary exacerbation in patients with cystic fibrosis. Chest *98*:1081-1084, 1990.

246. Padoan, R., Cambisano, W., Costantini, D., et al.: Ceftazidime monotherapy vs. combined therapy in *Pseudomonas* pulmonary infections in cystic fibrosis. Pediatr. Infect. Dis. J. *6*:648-653, 1987.

247. Pamukcu, A., Bush, A., and Buchdahl, R.: Effects of *Pseudomonas aeruginosa* colonization on lung function and anthropometric variables in children with cystic fibrosis. Pediatr. Pulmonol. *19*:10-15, 1995.

248. Parad, R. B., Gerard, C. J., Zurakowski, D., et al.: Pulmonary outcome in cystic fibrosis is influenced primarily by mucoid *Pseudomonas aeruginosa* infection and immune status and only modestly by genotype. Infect. Immun. *67*:4744-4750, 1999.

249. Paradowski, L. J.: Saprophytic fungal infections and lung transplantation—revisited. J. Heart Lung Transplant *16*:524-531, 1997.

250. Park, M. D., Myers, R. A., and Marzella, L.: Oxygen tensions and infections: Modulation of microbial growth, activity of antimicrobial agents, and immunologic responses. Clin. Infect. Dis. *14*:720-740, 1992.

251. Parks, R. W., and Grand, R. J.: Gastrointestinal manifestations of cystic fibrosis: A review. Gastroenterology *81*:1143, 1981.

252. Parry, M. F., and Neu, H. C.: Tobramycin and ticarcillin therapy for exacerbations of pulmonary disease in patients with cystic fibrosis. J. Infect. Dis. *134*(Suppl.):S194-S197, 1976.

253. Pegues, D. A., Carson, L. A., Tablan, O. C., et al.: Acquisition of *Pseudomonas cepacia* at summer camps for patients with cystic fibrosis. Summer Camp Study Group. J. Pediatr. *124*(5 Pt. 1):694-702, 1994.

254. Pegues, D. A., Schidlow, D. V., Tablan, O. C., et al.: Possible nosocomial transmission of *Pseudomonas cepacia* in patients with cystic fibrosis. Arch. Pediatr. Adolesc. Med. *148*:805-812, 1994.

255. Peloquin, C. A.: Using therapeutic drug monitoring to dose the antimycobacterial drugs. Clin. Chest Med. *18*:79-87, 1997.

256. Petersen, N. T., Hoiby, N., Mordhorst, C. H., et al.: Respiratory infections in cystic fibrosis patients caused by virus, chlamydia and mycoplasma—possible synergism with *Pseudomonas aeruginosa*. Acta Paediatr. Scand. *70*:623-628, 1981.

257. Philippon, S., Streckert, H. J., and Morgenroth, K.: In vitro study of the bronchial mucosa during *Pseudomonas aeruginosa* infection. Virchows Arch. A. Pathol. Anat. *423*:39-43, 1993.

258. Piedra, P. A., Cron, S. G., Jewell, A., et al.; Purified Fusion Protein Vaccine Study Group: Immunogenicity of a new purified fusion protein vaccine to respiratory syncytial virus: A multicenter trial in children with cystic fibrosis. Vaccine *21*(19-20):2448-2460, 2003.

259. Piedra, P. A., Grace, S., Jewell, A., et al.: Purified fusion protein vaccine protects against lower respiratory tract illness during respiratory syncytial virus season in children with cystic fibrosis. Pediatr. Infect. Dis. J. *15*:23-31, 1996.

260. Piedra, P. A., Grace, S., Jewell, A., et al.: Sequential annual administration of purified fusion protein vaccine against respiratory syncytial virus in children with cystic fibrosis. Pediatr. Infect. Dis. J. *17*:217-224, 1998.

261. Plotkowski, M. C., Chevillard, M., Pierrot, D., et al.: Differential adhesion of *Pseudomonas aeruginosa* to human respiratory epithelial cells in primary culture. J. Clin. Invest. *87*:2018-2028, 1991.

262. Przyklenk, B., Bauernfeind, A., Bertele, R. M., et al.: Viral infections of the respiratory tract in patients with cystic fibrosis. Serodian Immunther. Infect. Dis. *2*:217, 1988.

263. Raman, V., Clary, R., Siegrist, K. L., et al.: Increased prevalance of mutations in the cystic fibrosis transmembrane conductance regulator in children with chronic rhinosinusitis. Pediatrics *109*:E13, 2002.

264. Ramphal, R., Houdret, N., Koo, L., et al.: Differences in adhesion of *Pseudomonas aeruginosa* to mucin glycopeptides from sputa of patients with cystic fibrosis and chronic bronchitis. Infect. Immun. *57*:3066-3071, 1989.

265. Ramsey, B. W.: Management of pulmonary disease in patients with cystic fibrosis. N. Engl. J. Med. *335*:179-188, 1996.

266. Ramsey, B. W., Gore, E. J., Smith, A. L., et al.: The effect of respiratory viral infections on patients with cystic fibrosis. Am. J. Dis. Child. *143*:662, 1989.

267. Ramsey, B. W., Pepe, M. S., Quan, J. M., et al.: Intermittent administration of inhaled tobramycin in patients with cystic fibrosis. Cystic Fibrosis Inhaled Tobramycin Study Group. N. Engl. J. Med. *340*:23-30, 1999.

268. Ramsey, D. M., and Wozniak, D. J.: Understanding the control of *Pseudomonas aeruginosa* alginate synthesis and the prospects for management of chronic infections in cystic fibrosis. Mol. Microbiol. *56*:309-322, 2005.

269. Ratjen, F., Doring, G., and Nikolaizik, W. H.: Effect of inhaled tobramycin on early *Pseudomonas aeruginosa* colonisation in patients with cystic fibrosis. Lancet *358*:983-984, 2001.

270. Regelmann, W. E., Elliott, G. R., Warwick, W. J., and Clawson, C. C.: Reduction of sputum *Pseudomonas aeruginosa* density by antibiotics improves lung function in cystic fibrosis more than do bronchodilators and chest physiotherapy alone. Am. Rev. Respir. Dis. *141*(4 Pt. 1):914-921, 1990.

271. Regelmann, W. E., Lunde, N. M., Porter, P. T., and Quie, T. G.: Increased monocyte chemiluminescence in cystic fibrosis patients and in their parents. Pediatr. Res. *20*:619-622, 1986.

272. Ren, C. L., Morgan, W. J., Konstan, M. W., et al.: Presence of methicillin resistant *Staphylococcus aureus* in respiratory cultures from cystic fibrosis patients is associated with lower lung function. Pediatr. Pulmonol. *42*:513-518, 2007.

273. Riordan, J. R.: Assembly of functional CFTR chloride channels. Annu. Rev. Physiol. *67*:701-718, 2005.

274. Riordan, J. R., Rommens, J. M., Kerem, B. S., et al.: Identification of the cystic fibrosis gene: Cloning and characterization of the complimentary DNA. Science *245*:1066, 1989.

275. Robinson, M., and Bye, P. T.: Mucociliary clearance in cystic fibrosis. Pediatr. Pulmonol. *33*:293-306, 2002.

276. Ronne Hansen, C., Pressler, T., Hoiby, N., and Gormsen, M.: Chronic infection with *Achromobacter xylosoxidans* in cystic fibrosis patients: A retrospective case control study. J. Cyst. Fibros. 5:245-251, 2006.

277. Rosen, R., Schwartz, R. H., Hilm, B. C., et al.: Cystic fibrosis mutations in North American populations of French ancestry: analysis of Quebec French-Canadian and Louisiana Acadian families. Am. J. Hum. Genet. 47:606-610, 1990.

278. Rosenfeld, M.: Overview of published evidence on outcomes with early diagnosis from US observational studies. J. Pediatr. 147:S11-S14, 2005.

279. Rosenfeld, M., Davis, R., Fitz-Simmons, S., et al.: Gender gap in cystic fibrosis mortality. Am. J. Epidemiol. 145:794-803, 1997.

280. Rosenfeld, M., Emerson, J., Accurso, F., et al.: Diagnostic accuracy of oropharyngeal cultures in infants and young children with cystic fibrosis. Pediatr. Pulmonol. 28:321-328, 1999.

281. Rosenfeld, M., Gibson, R. L., McNamara, S., et al.: Early pulmonary infection, inflammation, and clinical outcomes in infants with cystis fibrosis. Pediatr. Pulmonol. 32:356-366, 2001.

282. Rosenfeld, M., Ramsey, B. W., and Gibson, R. L.: *Pseudomonas* acquisition in young patients with cystic fibrosis: Pathophysiology, diagnosis, and management. Curr. Opin. Pulm. Med. 9:492-497, 2003.

283. Rosenstein, B. J.: Cystic fibrosis diagnosis: New dilemmas for an old disorder. Pediatr. Pulmonol. 33:83-84, 2002.

284. Rosenstein, B. J., and Cutting, G. R.; Cystic Fibrosis Foundation Consensus Panel: The diagnosis of cystic fibrosis: A consensus statement. J. Pediatr. 132:589-595, 1998.

285. Roum, J. H., Buhl, R., McElvaney, N. G., et al.: Systemic deficiency of glutathione in cystic fibrosis. J. Appl. Physiol. 75:2419-2424, 1993.

286. Rowe, S. M., Miller, S., and Sorscher, E. J.: Cystic fibrosis. N. Engl. J. Med. 352:1992-2001, 2005.

287. Rubin, B. K.: Exposure of children with cystic fibrosis to environmental tobacco smoke. N. Engl. J. Med. 323:782-788, 1990.

288. Rubin, B. K.: Mucus structure and properties in cystic fibrosis. Paediatr. Respir. Rev. 8:4-7, 2007.

289. Saiman, L., Burns, J. L., Whittier, S., et al.: Evaluation of reference dilution test methods for antimicrobial susceptibility testing of *Pseudomonas aeruginosa* strains isolated from patients with cystic fibrosis. J. Clin. Microbiol. 37:2987-2991, 1999.

290. Saiman, L., Caclano, G., Gruenert, D., and Prince, A.: Comparison of adherence of *Pseudomonas aeruginosa* to respiratory epithelial cells from cystic fibrosis patients and health subjects. Infect. Immun. 60:2808-2814, 1992.

291. Saiman, L., Chen, Y., Tabibi, S., et al.: Identification and antimicrobial susceptibility of *Alcaligenes xylosoxidans* isolated from patients with cystic fibrosis. J. Clin. Microbiol. 39:3942-3945, 2001.

292. Saiman, L., Marshall, B. C., Mayer-Hamblett, N., et al.: Azithromycin in patients with cystic fibrosis chronically infected with *Pseudomonas aeruginosa*: A randomized controlled trial. J. A. M. A. 290:1749-1756, 2003.

293. Saiman, L., Mehar, F., Niu, W. W., et al.: Antibiotic susceptibility of multiply resistant *Pseudomonas aeruginosa* isolated from patients with cystic fibrosis, including candidates for transplantation. Clin. Infect. Dis. 23:532-537, 1996.

294. Saiman, L., and Prince, A.: *Pseudomonas aeruginosa* pili bind to asialoGM1 which is increased to the surface of cystic fibrosis epithelial cells. J. Clin. Invest. 92:1875-1880, 1993.

295. Saiman, L., Schidlow, D., and Smith, A.: The diagnosis of cystic fibrosis: Consensus statement. *In* Consensus Conferences Concept in Care. Cystic Fibrosis Foundation, 1996.

296. Saiman, L., and Siegel, J.; the CF Foundation Consensus Conference on Infection Control Participants: Infection control recommendations for patients with cystic fibrosis: Microbiology, important pathogens, and infection control practices to prevent patient-to-patient transmission. Infect. Control Hosp. Epidemiol. 24(Suppl. 5):S1-S52, 2003.

297. San Gabriel, P., Zhou, J., Tabibi, S., et al.: Antimicrobial susceptibility and synergy studies of *Stenotrophomonas maltophilia* isolates from patients with cystic fibrosis. Antimicrob. Agent Chemother. 48:168-171, 2004.

298. Saralaya, D., Peckham, D. G., Hulme, B., et al.: Serum and sputum concentrations following the oral administration of linezolid in adult patients with cystic fibrosis. J. Antimicrob. Chemother. 53:325-328, 2004.

299. Schaad, U. B., Wedgwood-Krucko, J., Guenin, K., et al.: Antipseudomonal therapy in cystic fibrosis: Aztreonam and amikacin versus ceftazidime and amikacin administered intravenously followed by oral ciprofloxacin. Eur. J. Clin. Microbiol. Infect. Dis. 8:858-865, 1989.

300. Schecter, M. S., Shelton, B. J., Margolis, P. A., and Fitzsimmons, S. C.: The association of socioeconomic status with outcomes in cystic fibrosis patients in the United States. Am. J. Respir. Crit. Care Med. 163:1331-1337, 2001.

301. Schlichting, C., Branger, C., Fournier, J. M., et al.: Typing of *Staphylococcus aureus* by pulsed-field gel electrophoresis, zymotyping, capsular typing, and phage typing: Resolution of clonal relationships. J. Clin. Microbiol. 31:227-232, 1993.

302. Schottelius, A. J., Mayo, M. W., Sartor, R. B., and Baldwin, A. S., Jr.: Interleukin-10 signaling blocks inhibitor of κB kinase activity and nuclear factor κB DNA binding. J. Biol. Chem. 274:31868-31874, 1999.

303. Scott, F. W., and Pitt, T. L.: Identification and characterization of transmissible *Pseudomonas aeruginosa* strains in cystic fibrosis patients in England and Wales. J. Med. Microbiol. 53(Pt. 7):609-615, 2004.

304. Scott, F. W., and Pitt, T. L.: *Pseudomonas aeruginosa*: Basic research. Prog. Respir. Res. 34:138-144, 2006.

305. Scully, B. E., Ores, C. N., Prince, A. S., and Neu, H. C.: Treatment of lower respiratory tract infections due to *Pseudomonas aeruginosa* in patients with cystic fibrosis. Rev. Infect. Dis. 7(Suppl. 4):S669-S674, 1985.

306. Shelhamer, J. H., Levine, S. J., Wu, T., et al.: NIH conference. Airway inflammation. Ann. Intern. Med. 123:288, 1995.

307. Shreve, M. R., Butler, S., Kaplowitz, H. J., et al.: Impact of microbiology practice on cumulative prevalence of respiratory tract bacteria in patients with cystic fibrosis. J. Clin. Microbiol. 37:753-757, 1999.

308. Simpson, D. A., Ramphal, R., and Lory, S.: Genetic analysis of *Pseudomonas aeruginosa* adherence: Distinct genetic loci control attachment to epithelial cells and mucins. Infect. Immun. 60:3771-3779, 1992.

309. Singh, P. K., Schaefer, A. L., Parsek, M. R., et al.: Quorum-sensing signals indicate that cystic fibrosis lungs are infected with bacterial biofilms. Nature 407:762-764, 2000.

310. Smith, A. L., Doershuk, C., Goldmann, D., et al.: Comparison of a beta-lactam alone versus beta-lactam and an aminoglycoside for pulmonary exacerbation in cystic fibrosis. J. Pediatr. 134:413-421, 1999.

311. Smith, J. J., Travis, S. M., Greenberg, E. P., and Welsh, M. J.: Cystic fibrosis airway epithelia fail to kill bacteria because of abnormal airway surface fluid. Cell 85:229-236, 1996.

312. Smyth, A.: Prophylactic antibiotics in cystic fibrosis: A conviction without evidence? Pediatr. Pulmonol. 40:471-476, 2005.

313. Smyth, A., Tan, K. H., Hyman-Taylor, P., et al.: Once versus three-times daily regimens of tobramycin treatment for pulmonary exacerbations of cystic fibrosis—the TOPIC study: A randomised controlled trial. Lancet 365:573-578, 2005.

314. Smyth, A., and Walters, S.: Prophylactic antibiotics for cystic fibrosis. Cochrane Database Syst. Rev. 3:CD001912, 2003.

315. Smyth, A. R., Smyth, R. L., Tong, C. Y., et al.: Effect of respiratory virus infections including rhinovirus on clinical status in cystic fibrosis. Arch. Dis. Child. 73:117-120, 1995.

316. Snell, G. I., de Hoyos, A., Krajden, M., et al.: *Pseudomonas cepacia* in lung transplantation recipients with cystic fibrosis. Chest 104:466-471, 1993.

317. Solis, A., Brown, D., Hughes, J., et al.: Methicillin-resistant *Staphylococcus aureus* in children with cystic fibrosis: An eradication protocol. Pediatr. Pulmonol. 36:189-195, 2003.

318. Sorensen, R. U., Waller, R. L., and Klinger, J. D.: Cystic fibrosis: Infection and immunity to *Pseudomonas*. Clin. Rev. Allergy 9(1-2):47-74, 1991.

319. Southern, K. W., Barker, P. M., and Solis, A.: Macrolide antibiotics for cystic fibrosis. Cochrane Database Syst. Rev. 2:CD002203, 2004.

320. Speer, M. E., Fernandes, C. J., Boron, M., and Groothuis, J.: Use of palivizumab in infants with cystic fibrosis: Results from the 2000-2004 Outcomes Registry. American Thoracic Society International Conference, Orlando, Florida, 2004.

321. Speert, D. P., Campbell, M. E., Farmer, S. N., et al.: Use of a pilin gene probe to study molecular epidemiology of *Pseudomonas aeruginosa*. J. Clin. Microbiol. 27:2589-2593, 1989.

322. Speert, D. P., Campbell, M. E., Henry, D. A., et al.: Epidemiology of *Pseudomonas aeruginosa* in cystic fibrosis in British Columbia, Canada. Am. J. Respir. Crit. Care Med. 166:988-999, 2002.

323. Speert, D. P., Henry, D., Vandamme, P., et al.: Epidemiology of *Burkholderia cepacia* complex in patients with cystic fibrosis in Canada: Geographical distribution and clustering of strains. Emerg. Infect. Dis. 8:181-187, 2002.

324. Spencer, D. H., Kas, A., Smith, E. E., et al.: Whole-genome sequence variation among multiple isolates of *Pseudomonas aeruginosa*. J. Bacteriol. 185:1316-1325, 2003.

325. Steinbach, S., Sun, L., Jiang, R. Z., et al.: Transmissibility of *Pseudomonas cepacia* infection in clinic patients and lung-transplant recipients with cystic fibrosis. N. Engl. J. Med. 331:981-987, 1994.

326. Stevens, D. A., Moss, R. B., Kurup, V. P., et al.: Allergic bronchopulmonary aspergillosis in cystic fibrosis—state of the art: Cystic Fibrosis Foundation Consensus Conference. Clin. Infect. Dis. 37(Suppl. 3):S225-S264, 2003.

327. Stroobant, J.: Viral infection in cystic fibrosis. J. R. Soc. Med. 79:19, 1986.

328. Stutman, H. R., Lieberman, J. M., Nussbaum, E., and Marks, M. I.: Antibiotic prophylaxis in infants and young children with cystic fibrosis: A randomized controlled trial. J. Pediatr. 140:299-305, 2002.

329. Sueblingvong, V., and Whittaker, L. A.: Fertility and pregnancy: Common concerns of the aging cystic fibrosis population. Clin. Chest Med. 28:433-443, 2007.

330. Sugiyama, Y.: Diffuse panbronchiolitis. Clin. Chest Med. 14:765-772, 1993.

331. Sun, L., Jiang, R. Z., Steinbach, S., et al.: The emergence of a highly transmissible lineage of cbl+ *Pseudomonas* (*Burkholderia*) *cepacia* causing CF centre epidemics in North America and Britain. Nat. Med. 1:661-666, 1995.

332. Suter, S.: The role of bacterial proteases in the pathogenesis of cystic fibrosis. Am. J. Respir. Crit. Care Med. 150:S118, 1994.

333. Szaff, M., Hoiby, N., and Flensborg, E. W.: Frequent antibiotic therapy improves survival of cystic fibrosis patients with chronic *Pseudomonas aeruginosa* infection. Acta Paediatr. Scand. 72:651-657, 1983.

334. Tablan, O. C., Carson, L. A., Cusick, L. B., et al.: Laboratory proficiency test results on use of selective media for isolating *Pseudomonas cepacia* from simulated sputum specimens of patients with cystic fibrosis. J. Clin. Microbiol. 25:485-487, 1987.

335. Tablan, O. C., Chorba, T. L., Schidlow, D. V., et al.: *Pseudomonas cepacia* colonization in patients with cystic fibrosis: Risk factors and clinical outcome. J. Pediatr. 107:382-387, 1985.

336. Tablan, O. C., Martone, W. J., Doershuk, C. F., et al.: Colonization of the respiratory tract with *Pseudomonas cepacia* in cystic fibrosis: Risk factors and outcomes. Chest *91*:527-532, 1987.

337. Takeyama, K., Dabbagh, K., Jeong Shim, J., et al.: Oxidative stress causes mucin synthesis via transactivation of epidermal growth factor receptor: Role of neutrophils. J. Immunol. *164*:1546-1552, 2000.

338. Talmaciu, I., Varlotta, L., Mortensen, J., and Schidlow, D. V.: Risk factors for emergence of *Stenotrophomonas maltophilia* in cystic fibrosis. Pediatr. Pulmonol. *30*:10-15, 2000.

339. Tamai, H., Kachur, J. F., Baron, D. A., et al.: Monochloramine, a neutrophil-derived oxidant, stimulates rat colonic secretion. J. Pharmacol. Exp. Ther. *257*:887-894, 1991.

340. Tang, H., Kays, M., and Prince, A.: Role of *Pseudomonas aeruginosa* pili in acute pulmonary infection. Infect. Immun. *63*:1278-1285, 1995.

341. Tarran, R., Button, B., Picher, M., et al.: Normal and cystic fibrosis airway surface liquid homeostasis. The effects of phasic shear stress and viral infections. J. Biol. Chem. *280*:35751-35759, 2005.

342. Tarran, R., Donaldson, S., and Boucher, R. C.: Rationale for hypertonic saline therapy for cystic fibrosis lung disease. Semin. Respir. Crit. Care Med. *28*:295-302, 2007.

343. Taylor, J. L., and Palmer, S. M.: *Mycobacterium abscessus* chest wall and pulmonary infection in a cystic fibrosis lung transplant recipient. J. Heart Lung Transplant. *25*:985-988, 2006.

344. Taylor, R. F., Gaya, H., and Hodson, M. E.: Temocillin and cystic fibrosis: Outcome of intravenous administration in patients infected with *Pseudomonas cepacia*. J. Antimicrob. Chemother. *29*:341-344, 1992.

345. Thomas, S. R., Gyi, K. M., Gaya, H., and Hodson, M. E.: Methicillin-resistant *Staphylococcus aureus*: Impact at a national cystic fibrosis centre. J. Hosp. Infect. *40*:203-209, 1998.

346. Thomassen, M. J., Demko, C. A., Doershuk, C. F., et al.: *Pseudomonas cepacia*: Decrease in colonization in patients with cystic fibrosis. Am. Rev. Respir. Dis. *134*:669-671, 1986.

347. Tiddens, H. A.: Detecting early structural lung damage in cystic fibrosis. Pediatr. Pulmonol. *34*:228-231, 2002.

348. Tomashefski, J. F., Konstan, M. W., Bruce, M. C., and Abramowsky, C. R.: The pathologic characteristics of interstitial pneumonia cystic fibrosis: A retrospective autopsy study. Am. J. Clin. Pathol. *91*:522-530, 1989.

349. Tosi, M. F., Zakem, H., and Berger, M.: Neutrophil elastase cleaves C3bi on opsonized *Pseudomonas* as well as CR1 on neutrophils to create a functionally important opsonin receptor mismatch. J. Clin. Invest. *86*:300, 1990.

350. Truluck, E. P., Christie, J. D., Edwards, L. B., et al.: Registry of the International Society for Heart and Lung Transplantation: Twenty-fourth Official Adult Lung and Heart-Lung Transplantation Report 2007. J. Heart Lung Transplant. *26*:782-795, 2007.

351. Ulrich, M., Herbert, S., Berger, J., et al.: Localization of *Staphylococcus aureus* in infected airways of patients with cystic fibrosis and in a cell culture model of *S. aureus* adherence. Am. J. Respir. Cell. Mol. Biol. *19*:83-91, 1998.

352. Valerius, N. H., Koch, C., and Hoiby, N.: Prevention of chronic *Pseudomonas aeruginosa* colonisation in cystic fibrosis by early treatment. Lancet *338*:725-726, 1991.

353. Van Daele, S., Verhelst, R., Claeys, G., et al.: Shared genotypes of *Achromobacter xylosoxidans* strains isolated from patients at a cystic fibrosis rehabilitation center. J. Clin. Microbiol. *43*:2998-3002, 2005.

354. Van Daele, S. G., Franckx, H., Verhelst, R., et al.: Epidemiology of *Pseudomonas aeruginosa* in a cystic fibrosis rehabilitation centre. Eur. Respir. J. *25*:474-481, 2005.

355. van Ewijk, B. E., van der Zalm, M. M., Wolfs, T. F., and van der Ent, C. K.: Viral respiratory infections in cystic fibrosis. J. Cyst. Fibros. *4*:31-36, 2005.

356. van Ewijk, B. E., Wolfs, T. F., Aerts, P. C., et al.: RSV mediates *Pseudomonas aeruginosa* binding to cystic fibrosis and normal epithelial cells. Pediatr. Res. *61*:398-403, 2007.

357. Van Haren, E. H. J., Lammers, J.-W. J., Festen, J., et al.: The effects of inhaled corticosteroid budesonide on lung function and bronchial hyperresponsiveness in adult patients with cystic fibrosis. Respir. Med. *89*:209-214, 1995.

358. Vansoy, L. L., Blackman, S. M., Collaco, J. M., et al.: Heritability of lung disease severity in cystic fibrosis. *175*:1036-1043, 2007.

359. Vazquez, C., Municio, M., Corera, M., et al.: Early treatment of *Pseudomonas aeruginosa* colonization in cystic fibrosis. Acta Paediatr. *82*:308-309, 1993.

360. Venkatakrishnan, A., Stecenko, A., King, G., et al.: Exaggerated activation of nuclear factor-κB and altered IκB-β process in cystic fibrosis bronchial epithelial cells. Am. J. Respir. Cell. Biol. *23*:396-403, 2000.

361. Verkman, A. S., Song, Y., and Thiagarajah, J. R.: Role of airway surface liquid and submucosal glands in cystic fibrosis lung disease. Am. J. Physiol. Cell. Physiol. *284*:C2-C15, 2003.

362. Wang, E. E., Prober, C. G., Manson, B., et al.: Association of respiratory viral infections with pulmonary deterioration in patients with cystic fibrosis. N. Engl. J. Med. *311*:1653-1658, 1984.

363. Weaver, L. T., Green, M. R., Nicholson, K., et al.: Prognosis in cystic fibrosis treated with continuous flucloxacillin from the neonatal period. Arch. Dis. Child. *70*:84-89, 1994.

364. Weber, A., Soong, G., Bryan, B., et al.: Activation of NfκB in airway epithelial cells is dependent on CFTR trafficking and Cl-channel function. Am. J. Physiol. Lung Cell. Mol. Physiol. *281*:L71-L78, 2001.

365. Welsh, M. J., Ramsey, B. W., Accurso, F., and Cutting, G.: Cystic fibrosis. *In* Scriver, C. R., Beaudet, A. L., Sly, W. S., and Valle, D. (eds.): The Metabolic and Molecular Basis of Inherited Diseases. 8th ed. New York, McGraw-Hill, 2001, pp. 5121-5188.

366. Welsh, M. J., and Smith, A. E.: Molecular mechanisms of CFTR chloride channel dysfunction in cystic fibrosis. Cell *73*:1251-1254, 1993.

367. Whittier, S., Hopfer, R. L., Knowles, M. R., and Gilligan, P. H.: Improved recovery of mycobacteria from respiratory secretions of patients with cystic fibrosis. J. Clin. Microbiol. *31*:861-864, 1993.

368. Whittier, S., Olivier, K., Gilligan, P., et al.: Proficiency testing of clinical microbiology laboratories using modified decontamination procedures for detection of nontuberculous mycobacteria in sputum samples from cystic fibrosis patients. The Nontuberculous Mycobacteria in Cystic Fibrosis Study Group. J. Clin. Microbiol. *35*:2706-2708, 1997.

369. Wientzen, R., Prestidge, C. B., Kramer, R. I., et al.: Acute pulmonary exacerbations in cystic fibrosis: A double-blind trial of tobramycin and placebo therapy. Am. J. Dis. Child. *134*:1134-1138, 1980.

370. Wiesemann, H. G., Steinkamp, G., Ratjen, F., et al.: Placebo-controlled, double-blind, randomized study of aerosolized tobramycin for early treatment of *Pseudomonas aeruginosa* colonization in cystic fibrosis. Pediatr. Pulmonol. *25*:88-92, 1998.

371. Wilmott, R. W., Kassab, J. T., Kilian, P. L., et al.: Increased levels of interleukin-1 in bronchoalveolar washings from children with bacterial pulmonary infections. Am. Rev. Respir. Dis. *142*:365-368, 1990.

372. Wilschanski, M., Zielenski, J., Markiewicz, D., et al.: Correlation of sweat chloride concentration with classes of the cystic fibrosis transmembrane conductance regulator gene mutations. J. Pediatr. *127*:75-710, 1995.

373. Winnie, G. B., and Cowan, R. G.: Association of Epstein-Barr virus infection and pulmonary exacerbations in patients with cystic fibrosis. Pediatr. Infect. Dis. J. *11*:722-726, 1992.

374. Witko-Sarsat, V., Callen, R. C., Paulais, M., et al.: Disturbed myeloperoxidase-dependent activity of neutrophils in cystic fibrosis homozygotes and heterozygotes, and its correction by amiloride. J. Immunol. *157*:2728-2735, 1996.

375. Wolter, J., Seeney, S., Bell, S., et al.: Effect of long term treatment with azithromycin on disease parameters in cystic fibrosis: A randomised trial. Thorax *57*:212-216, 2002.

376. Wong, K., Roberts, M. C., Owens, L., et al.: Selective media for the quantitation of bacteria in cystic fibrosis sputum. J. Med. Microbiol. *17*:113-119, 1984.

377. Wood, R. E., Board, T. F., and Doershuk, C. F.: Cystic fibrosis. Am. Rev. Respir. Dis. *113*:841, 1976.

378. Wood, R. E., Board, T. F., and Doershuk, C. F.: State of the art: Cystic fibrosis. Am. Rev. Respir. Dis. *113*:833, 1976.

379. World Health Organization: World Health Organization Classification of Cystic Fibrosis and Related Disorders. Report No. WHO/CF/HGN/00.2. Stockholm, WHO, 2000.

380. Worlitzsch, D., Tarran, R., Ulrich, M., et al.: Effects of reduced mucus oxygen concentration in airway *Pseudomonas* infections of cystic fibrosis patients. J. Clin. Invest. *109*:317-325, 2002.

381. Wright, P. F., Khaw, K. T., Oxman, M. N., et al.: Evaluation of the safety of amantadine-HCl and the role of respiratory viral infections in children with cystic fibrosis. J. Infect. Dis. *134*:144, 1976.

382. Yanagihara, K., Tomono, K., Sawai, T., et al.: Effect of clarithromycin on lymphocytes in chronic respiratory *Pseudomonas aeruginosa* infection. Am. J. Respir. Crit. Care Med. *155*:337-342, 1997.

383. Yankaskas, J. R., and Mallory, G. B.: Lung transplantation in cystic fibrosis: Consensus conference statement. Chest *113*:217-226, 1998.

384. Zabner, J., Smith, J. J., Karp, P. H., et al.: Loss of CFTR chloride channels alters salt absorption by cystic fibrosis airway epithelia in vitro. Mol. Cell. *2*:397-403, 1998.

385. Zaidy, A. G., and Davis, P. B.: Infection versus inflammation. Prog. Respir. Res. *34*:122-130, 2006.

386. Zemel, B. S., Jawad, A. F., FitzSimmons, S., and Stallings, V. A.: Longitudinal relationship among growth, nutritional status, and pulmonary function in children with cystic fibrosis: Analysis of the Cystic Fibrosis Foundation National CF Patient Registry. J. Pediatr. *137*:374-380, 2000.

387. Zheng, S., De, B. P., Choudhary, S., et al.: Impaired innate host defense causes susceptibility to respiratory virus infections in cystic fibrosis. Immunity *18*:619-630, 2003.

388. Zheng, S., Xu, W., Bose, S., et al.: Impaired nitric oxide synthase-2 signaling pathway in cystic fibrosis airway epithelium. Am. J. Physiol. Lung Cell. Mol. Physiol. *287*:L374-L381, 2004.

389. Zhou, J., Chen, Y., Tabibi, S., et al.: Antimicrobial susceptibility and synergy studies of *Burkholderia cepacia* complex isolated from patients with cystic fibrosis. Antimicrob. Agents Chemother. *51*:1085-1088, 2007.

390. Zhou, J., Garber, E., Desai, M., and Saiman, L.: Compliance of clinical microbiology laboratories in the United States with current recommendations for processing respiratory tract specimens from patients with cystic fibrosis. J. Clin. Microbiol. *44*:1547-1549, 2006.

391. Zielenski, J., and Tsui, L. C.: Cystic fibrosis: Genotypic and phenotypic variations. Annu. Rev. Genet. *29*:777-807, 1995.

INFECTIONS OF THE HEART

CHAPTER 32

INFECTIVE ENDOCARDITIS

Jeffrey R. Starke

Infective endocarditis results when microorganisms adhere to the endocardial surface of the heart. This process usually occurs on heart valves, although septal defects and mural surfaces can be affected. Most episodes of endocarditis begin on endocardium that has been altered by congenital defects, previous disease, surgery, or trauma. The clinical manifestations depend on the degree of compromise of cardiac function and the occurrence of embolic phenomena. Although bacteria are responsible for most cases, instances of infective endocarditis caused by fungi, chlamydiae, rickettsiae, and perhaps viruses have been described. Advances in the practice of general pediatrics and cardiology during the past 3 decades have contributed to changes in the predisposing conditions and etiologic agents of "modern" infective endocarditis. Before the 1950s, rheumatic fever was the major underlying condition, but its incidence has declined greatly since then.[306] Concurrently, improvements in the medical and surgical management of children with congenital heart disease have increased survival rates. At present, approximately 80 to 90 percent of children with infective endocarditis have congenital heart disease.* Many cases occur after cardiac surgery, especially for replacement of valves and creation of shunts with prosthetic materials.[338] The reported incidence of infective endocarditis in neonates is increasing, probably because of the use of sophisticated and highly invasive techniques in neonatal intensive care nurseries.[93,159,327,397]

Historically, infective endocarditis has been classified as acute or subacute, based on the progression of untreated disease.[432] The acute form has a fulminant course, with high fever, systemic toxicity, and death from sepsis in several days to 6 weeks. The most common etiologic agents are *Staphylococcus aureus*, *Streptococcus pyogenes*, and *Streptococcus pneumoniae*. Children with the acute form often have no underlying cardiac lesion. Subacute disease usually occurs in patients with previous valvular disease or those who have undergone cardiac surgical intervention. It is characterized by a more indolent course (6 weeks to several months) and with low-grade fever, vague systemic complaints, and various embolic phenomena. Viridans streptococci are the most common etiologic agents. This classification ignores the frequent overlap in clinical manifestations caused by various organisms, especially the staphylococci and fungi, which are causes of an increasing number of subacute cases in the postcardiac surgical setting. Classification based on specific etiologic agents is preferable because it has implications for the usual clinical course, predisposing factors, and appropriate medical and surgical management.[217]

EPIDEMIOLOGY

The incidence of infective endocarditis in adults has been difficult to determine because the methods of study and criteria for diag-

nosis vary among series.[30,118] Accurate figures on the incidence of infective endocarditis in children are difficult to obtain. The most common method of reporting the incidence in pediatric series expresses the number of cases of infective endocarditis as the numerator and the total number of hospital admissions during the analyzed period as the denominator. Zakrzewski and Keith[559] reported an incidence of endocarditis of 1 in 4500 pediatric admissions at the Hospital for Sick Children in Toronto from 1952 to 1962, whereas Van Hare and colleagues[507] at Case Western Reserve in Ohio found an incidence of 1 in 1280 in the period from 1972 to 1982. In a large series from Boston Children's Hospital spanning the period between 1933 and 1972, the incidence before 1963 was 1 in 4500 pediatric admissions, whereas that for 1963 to 1972 was 1 in 1800 admissions.[230] A study from a children's hospital in Australia reported an incidence of 1 in 4500 hospital admissions between 1971 and 1983.[446] More recently, one Japanese center reported an annual incidence of 0.9 cases per 1000 children seen at the cardiology clinic.[156] Although differences in referral patterns at these centers may have introduced bias into these figures, the incidence of infective endocarditis in children appears to be rising. This rise may be explained by the increased survival rate of children with all forms of cardiovascular disease and an increase in the percentage of cases that occur after cardiac surgery and are related to intravascular catheters.[143,238,420] Early surgical correction of many types of congenital heart disease along with effective perioperative antibiotic prophylaxis regimens ultimately may lower the incidence of postoperative infective endocarditis. However, the increasing use of invasive therapeutic modalities, especially intravenous catheters and pacemakers, may lead to an increased incidence of health care–associated endocarditis.[143,312,398]

The average age of children with infective endocarditis is increasing, a phenomenon that may reflect the longer life expectancy created by improved therapy for children at risk.[477] From 1930 to 1950, the mean age for children with infective endocarditis was close to 5 years.[230] Between 1960 and the present, it increased to 8.5 and then to 13 years.[156,167,264,311,420] The number of reports of infective endocarditis in children younger than 2 years had been small but has increased significantly since the late 1980s.[39,167,327,524] The clinical course of infective endocarditis in these young children often is atypical, and some cases are diagnosed at autopsy.[230,375] Before the 1950s, this disease was a rare event in neonates, with only eight autopsy cases reported.[297] Several reports suggest a rapidly increasing rate associated with the development of intensive supportive care in neonates.[46,317,332,362,363] Symchych and colleagues[475] found a 3 percent incidence of bacterial endocarditis among all neonatal autopsies. Endocarditis in neonates frequently occurs on the tricuspid valve when associated with an indwelling central venous catheter.[493] Congenital heart defects also predispose neonates to the development of infectious endocarditis.[93]

Any form of structural cardiac disease may predispose to infective endocarditis, especially with disorders associated with

---

*See references 25, 73, 89, 260, 264, 278, 285, 350, 358, 420, 477, 489.

TABLE 32–1 Underlying Heart Disease in 266 Children with Infective Endocarditis

Underlying Heart Disease	Percentage Affected (%)
Congenital heart disease	78
Tetralogy of Fallot	24
Ventricular septal defect	16
Congenital aortic stenosis	8
Patent ductus arteriosus	7
Transposition of great vessel	4
Others	19
Rheumatic heart disease	14
No heart disease	8

From Kaplan, E. L.: Infective endocarditis in the pediatric age group: An overview. In Kaplan, E. L., and Taranta, A. V. (eds.): Infective Endocarditis: An American Heart Association Symposium. Dallas, American Heart Association, 1977, pp. 51-54.

turbulence of blood flow.[163,454] In autopsy and clinical series, children with ventricular septal defect, tetralogy of Fallot, left-sided valvular disease, and systemic-pulmonary arterial communication were at highest risk, whereas those with pulmonary stenosis, coarctation of the aorta, and secundum atrial septal defect were at low risk.[412,420] Hypertrophic obstructive cardiomyopathy rarely is associated with infective endocarditis.[76] Isolated pulmonic or tricuspid valve endocarditis can occur in "otherwise normal" children and adolescents with sepsis or focal bacterial infection,[351] but usually it is associated with congenital heart disease, intravenous catheters, or intravenous drug abuse.[67,348] A bicuspid aortic valve is recognized as an important risk factor for the development of infective endocarditis, especially in elderly men.[318] The underlying heart diseases in 266 pediatric cases of infective endocarditis are listed in Table 32–1.[238]

A cooperative study on the natural history of aortic stenosis, pulmonary stenosis, and ventricular septal defect reported data from a controlled pediatric population collected over a period of 4 to 15 years.[165] In patients not undergoing surgical correction, the risk of acquiring endocarditis by 30 years of age in those with ventricular septal defects was 9.7 percent versus 1.4 percent for aortic stenosis and 0.9 percent for pulmonic stenosis. Aortic valvotomy in children with aortic stenosis actually increases the relative risk, whereas successful repair of ventricular septal defect significantly decreases long-term susceptibility to infective endocarditis.[166] Similarly, endocarditis is an extremely rare occurrence after ligation of patent ductus arteriosus has been performed. At present, palliative systemic-to-pulmonary shunting is the surgical procedure most often complicated by infective endocarditis.[420] In a review of 115 patients with tetralogy of Fallot, Kaplan and colleagues[240] reported an 8 percent incidence of infective endocarditis after placement of a Pott shunt.

The increasing use of prosthetic valves and valved conduit repairs in children with complex heart disease may lead to a larger number of cases of infective endocarditis in the future.[239,245,483] Most medical centers report an incidence of prosthetic-valve endocarditis of 2 to 4 percent after surgery,[57,168,415,454] with the aortic and mitral valves affected most frequently.[219,299]

Older studies arbitrarily divided prosthetic-valve endocarditis into two categories—early and late—based on whether the infection occurred within 60 days of valve placement or later.[34] The rationale for categorizing by time was based on apparent differences in bacteriologic, pathogenetic, and prognostic associations. So-called early cases most often were caused by coagulase-negative staphylococci (CONS), gram-negative bacilli, and fungi, whereas oral and enterococcal streptococci, along with staphylococci, predominated in late cases.[243] These older reports suggested that early cases were acquired by contamination of an intraoperative valve or were secondary to postoperative extracardiac infections, whereas late cases were acquired by the same mechanisms as native-valve endocarditis. Nosocomial bacteremia that develops at any time after the patient has undergone valve placement is a significant risk factor for development of endocarditis.[131,502] Finally, the mortality rate was thought to be higher in early versus late infection.

However, more recent studies have blurred this arbitrary time distinction between early and late prosthetic-valve endocarditis.[57,219] The risk probably is highest in the first 6 to 12 months and decreases to its lowest point beyond 1 year after valve replacement. CONS are the dominant organisms both before and after the 60th postoperative day.[57,242] Clinical and epidemiologic data also suggest that prosthetic-valve infection caused by staphylococci within the first year after placement probably is acquired at the time of surgery.[34] Identified risk factors for the development of prosthetic-valve endocarditis in adults include native-valve endocarditis, black race, male sex, a mechanical (versus biologic) prosthesis, and prolonged cardiopulmonary bypass time[219]; no comparable information is available for children.

Mitral valve endocarditis occurs frequently on an anatomically normal valve in patients with other predisposing factors.[144] An association between mitral valve prolapse and infective endocarditis has been recognized in adults and children. This heart lesion is detected with increasing frequency in adolescent girls and may be only one component of a developmental syndrome.[438] In adults, 40 to 50 percent of cases of infective endocarditis associated with isolated insufficient mitral valves occur in patients with mitral prolapse.[88] In some series of native-valve endocarditis, mitral valve prolapse has been the most common underlying lesion.[318] The reported incidence of infective endocarditis in patients with mitral valve prolapse has varied markedly among studies, from low rates of 14 per 100,000 per year to 5 of 58 patients monitored prospectively for 9 to 22 years.[199] A retrospective epidemiologic analysis involving matched cases and controls yielded an odds ratio of 8.2, indicative of a substantially higher risk for development of endocarditis in patients with mitral valve prolapse than in normal controls.[85]

That the risk of developing infective endocarditis is not uniform for all patients with mitral valve prolapse has become apparent. The risk is increased in patients with a preexisting systolic murmur (but not for those with an isolated click and no murmur), echocardiographically demonstrated regurgitation, and valvular redundancy.[95,298,308] The signs and symptoms of endocarditis associated with mitral valve prolapse may be more subtle than those of other types of left-sided endocarditis.[144,360] However, significant complications are relatively common occurrences and sometimes require valve replacement during the acute illness or during convalescence.[19,461]

Fungal endocarditis is a rare disorder in children but should be suspected in certain clinical and epidemiologic settings. It is more likely to occur after cardiac surgery and rarely occurs on native heart valves. It occurs more commonly in neonates treated in intensive care settings than in older children.[93] Other predisposing factors include (1) the presence of an indwelling vascular catheter, (2) prolonged use of antibiotics, (3) intrinsic (immunodeficiency diseases, malignancy, malnutrition) or extrinsic (corticosteroids, cytotoxic drugs) immunosuppression, (4) bowel surgery resulting in transient fungemia, (5) intravenous drug abuse, and (6) preexisting or concomitant bacterial endocarditis.

Many conditions other than structural heart disease predispose children to the development of infective endocarditis. The most important is the presence of an indwelling central venous catheter, especially in patients who are seriously ill or immunocompromised.[159,167,284,496,523] The catheter acts as a foreign body and presumably causes microscopic damage by abrading endocardial and valve surfaces; such damage results in nonbacterial thrombotic vegetation.[25] Infection of intracardiac pacemaker wires also can lead to endocarditis.[13] Infection acquired during the placement procedure and infection of the pacemaker pouch are most common. Infective endocarditis, usually of the tricuspid valve, has developed in children with ventriculoatrial shunts placed for the treatment of hydrocephalus.[238] In patients with arteriovenous fistulas created for hemodialysis, bacterial vegetations may develop in the fistula and on heart valves.[276,401] Rarely, penetrating wounds or foreign bodies can initiate endocarditis.[202,307] Piercings of various body parts also have been associated with endocarditis.[2,394] One important group of patients with an increased risk for development of infective endocarditis is intravenous drug abusers.[314,526] In this group of patients, two thirds have no evidence of underlying heart disease. A predilection for involvement of the tricuspid valve, followed by the mitral and aortic valves, has been noted.[155] Roentgenographic evidence of septic pulmonary emboli and signs of tricuspid insufficiency dominate the clinical findings.[432] Within this group of patients, increased rates of infective endocarditis and mortality are associated with infection by human immunodeficiency virus (HIV), particularly as CD4 cell counts fall to less than $200/mm^3$.[389]

Although the incidence of infective endocarditis in children may be rising, the prognosis has improved dramatically during the past several decades. Current mortality rates usually are close to 10 percent.[341,420,437] Most survivors remain hemodynamically stable at long-term follow-up.[147,437] However, patients who experience infective endocarditis appear to be at higher risk for developing recurrent endocarditis than are those with similar cardiac abnormalities who have not had previous endocarditis.[454] The patient's functional class before treatment appears to be most predictive of long-term functional status. In one study, 22 percent of children who survived infective endocarditis required surgery related to the infection, including vegetectomy, evacuation of a hematoma, atrioventricular valve replacement, and placement or replacement of a graft or intracardiac shunt.[420]

PATHOPHYSIOLOGY

Clinical observations, autopsy studies, and work with experimental animal models have demonstrated that the occurrence of several independent events is required for the development of subacute infectious endocarditis. The endocardial surface usually is disrupted by stress or injury commonly caused by the turbulence of blood. This surface damage results in the deposition of fibrin and platelets, which form nonbacterial thrombotic vegetations. If bacteria adhere to these deposits, infective endocarditis will result. The surface of the infected vegetation becomes protected by a cover of fibrin and platelets. A tremendous proliferation of organisms (as many as 10^9 colony-forming units per gram) may ensue.[119] The protective sheath isolates the organisms from the action of host neutrophils and antibiotics. The clinical manifestations and complications of infective endocarditis are related to both the hemodynamic changes caused by local infection and the occurrence of embolization and metastatic infection.

In experimental animals, the valvular surface must be damaged, usually by an intravenous catheter, to produce infective endocarditis.[20] The first step in the pathogenesis of subacute infective endocarditis in humans is the development of hemodynamic factors that favor endocardial damage. In an autopsy study of 1024 patients with infective endocarditis, Lepeschkin[277] showed that the location of the endocardial lesions correlated with the impact of pressure; this finding makes a strong argument for the role of mechanical stress as a critical factor in the evolution of the lesions. When associated with valvular insufficiency, infective endocarditis usually occurs on the atrial surface of the mitral valve and the ventricular surface of the aortic valve. Injection of a bacterial aerosol into the air stream passing through a Venturi tube demonstrates how high pressure drives an infected fluid into a

low-pressure sink.[407] This process establishes maximal deposition of bacteria in the low-pressure sink immediately beyond the orifice. Mitral insufficiency creates a Venturi effect when blood is driven from the high-pressure left ventricle into a low-pressure atrium; maximal deposition occurs around the mitral annulus on the atrial side. Similarly, with aortic valve insufficiency, the high-pressure source is the aorta and the low-pressure sink is the left ventricle, which leads to deposition on the ventricular surface of the valve.

Lesions also are created more directly by a jet stream causing endocardial damage. For example, in a small, restrictive ventricular septal defect with a left-to-right shunt, a Venturi effect leads to the development of lesions on the right ventricular septal side of the defect, whereas secondary lesions created by the jet effect are located on the right ventricular wall opposite the defect.[518] Heart defects with a surface area sufficiently large to prevent a significant pressure gradient and those in which smaller volumes minimize the gradient do not create the jet and Venturi effects. This difference helps to explain the rarity of endocarditis in patients with atrial septal defects and the increased risk of infection complicating small, but not large, ventricular septal defects.

Once endocardial damage has occurred, collagen is exposed, and platelet and fibrin deposition ensues in a manner analogous to formation of the primary plug of normal hemostasis after vascular injury.[228,519] The sterile platelet-fibrin thrombus that is formed subsequently is referred to as a nonbacterial thrombotic vegetation. In experimental animals, many exogenous stresses, including exposure to cold, high altitude, high cardiac output states, hormonal manipulations, and passage of a sterile catheter across a heart valve, lead to formation of this lesion. Formation of the vegetation reflects two pathogenic mechanisms: hypercoagulability and endothelial damage.[432] To establish experimental infective endocarditis without initial formation of the vegetation is nearly impossible. Microscopic examination demonstrates that this lesion is the one to which microorganisms attach during the early stages of experimental endocarditis. Nonbacterial thrombotic vegetations have been found in both adults and children with malignancy, chronic wasting diseases, uremia, connective tissue diseases, and congenital heart disease and after the placement of intracardiac catheters,[291,367] and they have been associated with embolism and infarction in distant organs.[42]

Once a nonbacterial thrombotic vegetation has been established, transient bacteremia or fungemia may result in colonization of the lesion. Transient bacteremias are common occurrences, especially with traumatization of a mucosal surface. Table 32–2 lists the incidence of bacteremia in adults and children after various procedures.[130,405] The bacteremia usually is of low grade and is proportional to the amount of trauma produced by the procedure and the number of organisms inhabiting the surface. In addition, "silent" bacteremia probably occurs frequently. Many persons have circulating antibodies to their own oral flora, as well as an increase in peripheral T cells sensitized to the flora of their dental plaque.[432] Some children with congenital heart disease may be at increased risk for having gingival colonization and subsequent development of bacteremia with organisms associated with infectious endocarditis, such as the HACEK (*Haemophilus* spp., *Actinobacillus actinomycetemcomitans*, *Cardiobacterium hominis*, *Eikenella corrodens*, *Kingella kingae*) microbes.[457]

The ability of microorganisms to adhere to the platelet-fibrin thrombus is a critical factor in the development of infective endocarditis.[100,188,228] In a canine model, *S. aureus* and the viridans streptococci, which frequently cause infective endocarditis, adhere more readily to normal aortic leaflets than do organisms uncommon in endocarditis.[178] Within isolates of *S. aureus*, strains devoid of microencapsulation are less capable of inducing endocarditis in an experimental model than are encapsulated strains.[21] Specific products released by these organisms, including dextran,

TABLE 32–2 Bacteremia after Various Procedures in Adults and Children

Initiating Event	Percentage of Positive Blood Cultures (%)	Predominant Organisms
Dental extraction (children)	30-65	*Streptococcus*, diphtheroids
Chewing gum, candy, paraffin	0-51	*Streptococcus*, *Staphylococcus epidermidis*
Tooth brushing	0-26	*Streptococcus*
Tonsillectomy	28-38	*Streptococcus*, *Haemophilus*, diphtheroids
Bronchoscopy (rigid scope)	15	*Streptococcus*, *S. epidermidis*
Bronchoscopy (fiberoptic)	0	
Orotracheal intubation	0	
Nasotracheal intubation/suctioning	16	*Streptococcus*, aerobic gram-negative rods
Sigmoidoscopy/colonoscopy	0-9.5	*Enterococcus*, aerobic gram-negative rods
Upper gastrointestinal endoscopy	8-12	*Streptococcus*, *Neisseria*, *S. epidermidis*, diphtheroids, other
Percutaneous liver biopsy	3-14	Pneumococcus, aerobic gram-negative rods, *Staphylococcus aureus*, other
Urethral catheterization	8	Not stated
Manipulation of *S. aureus* suppurative foci	54	

From Everett, E. D., and Hirschmann, J. U.: Transient bacteremia and endocarditis prophylaxis: A review. Medicine (Baltimore) 56:61-77, 1977. © 1977, The Williams & Wilkins Company, Baltimore.

mannan, teichoic acid, and slime, may enhance their ability to colonize the vegetation.[228,254] The amount of dextran produced by various viridans streptococci in broth correlates with both their adherence and their ability to produce endocarditis in the rabbit model.[333,435] *Candida albicans* is readily adherent and produces infective endocarditis in rabbits more easily than does *Candida krusei*, a nonadherent yeast rarely implicated in human infective endocarditis.[433] In addition, endocarditis-producing strains of streptococci and staphylococci are more potent stimulators of platelet aggregation than are other bacteria that do not produce infective endocarditis.[84,197,333] This action may accelerate the formation of an infected vegetation or may increase the removal of organisms from the circulation. The importance of adherence by organisms has been studied by pre-incubating organisms with many classes of antibiotics. After incubation at subinhibitory concentrations, adhesion of streptococcal species to fibrin-platelet matrices and damaged canine valves is decreased.[436] Antibiotics may prevent development of infective endocarditis by both bacterial killing and inhibition of adherence to the vegetation.[172]

Host tissue factors undoubtedly play an important role in adherence of bacteria to the developing thrombus. Once bacteria become adherent to a nonbacterial thrombus, activation of the coagulation system ensues. Some organisms that produce endocarditis may be able to initiate procoagulant activity through microbial enzymes. Activation of the intrinsic coagulation pathway is triggered by exposed connective tissue components and platelet aggregation.[254] However, activation of the extrinsic coagulation pathway probably is the major stimulus for growth of vegetations. Elements of the extracellular matrix, including fibronectin, laminin, and collagen, have been shown to facilitate the adherence of bacteria on fibrin-platelet matrices.[472,495] Fibronectin may be the host receptor for organisms within the nonbacterial thrombotic vegetation.[265,293] Laminin-binding proteins have been found on the cell walls of organisms recovered from patients with endocarditis.[451]

The platelet-organism interaction is complex and not understood completely. *Streptococcus sanguis* produces two cell surface antigens that promote platelet aggregation: a class I antigen promotes adhesion of *S. sanguis* to platelets, whereas coexpression of a class II antigen promotes platelet adhesion or aggregation.[198] The induced platelet aggregation appears to be an important determinant of further development of vegetation and progression of disease in experimental endocarditis. In addition, production of streptococcal exopolysaccharide inversely correlates with platelet adhesion while inhibiting aggregation, thus indicating

that surface molecules may enhance endocarditis at only certain pathogenic steps.[469] Platelets also may be involved in host defense within the vegetation. After exposure to thrombin, platelets may release microbicidal proteins with bactericidal activity against some gram-positive cocci; resistance to these proteins may be a virulence factor for *S. aureus* in the development of endocarditis.[357,536]

As bacterial colonization of a nonbacterial thrombotic vegetation progresses, it enlarges by further bacterial proliferation and platelet-fibrin deposition (Fig. 32–1).[336] Kissane[259] described three histologic zones: (1) necrotic endocardium; (2) a broad zone of bacterial colonies, pyknotic nuclear debris, and fibrin; and (3) a thin coating on the surface of fibrin and leukocytes. The location of bacterial colonies below the surface and the minimal infiltration by phagocytic cells create an environment of impaired host resistance that results in extreme bacterial proliferation. The structure of the vegetation diminishes the penetration of antibiotics into the bacterial layer. In addition, the metabolic activity of bacteria within this lesion is slowed, thus rendering antibiotics less effective. The formation of vegetations and erosion of heart valves may cause valvular incompetence and thereby may result in cardiac failure.

Immunopathologic factors may have important roles in both the development and sequelae of infective endocarditis.[32] The susceptibility of a gram-negative bacillus to complement-mediated bactericidal activity is critical to its potential to create endocarditis; only "serum-resistant" organisms produce infective endocarditis in humans and experimental animals.[117] Gram-positive cocci are a more frequent cause of infective endocarditis than are gram-negative bacilli. Gram-positive organisms are resistant to this bactericidal activity; phagocytosis is required for killing.

The frequent presence of hypergammaglobulinemia, splenomegaly, and monocytes in the blood of patients with infective endocarditis indicates stimulation of the humoral and cellular immune systems. Macroglobulins, cryoglobulins, and agglutinating, opsonic, and complement-fixing antibodies have been associated with infective endocarditis.[204,273] Studies in animals pre-immunized with heat-killed streptococci before aortic valve trauma and infection are induced suggest that circulating antibody has a protective role.[434,503] However, antibody to *S. aureus* or *Staphylococcus epidermidis* does not prevent the development of endocarditis in immunized animals, perhaps because this antibody does not enhance opsonophagocytosis.[432] The continuous antigenic challenge created by intravascular organisms leads to increased production of specific antibody (including opsonic,

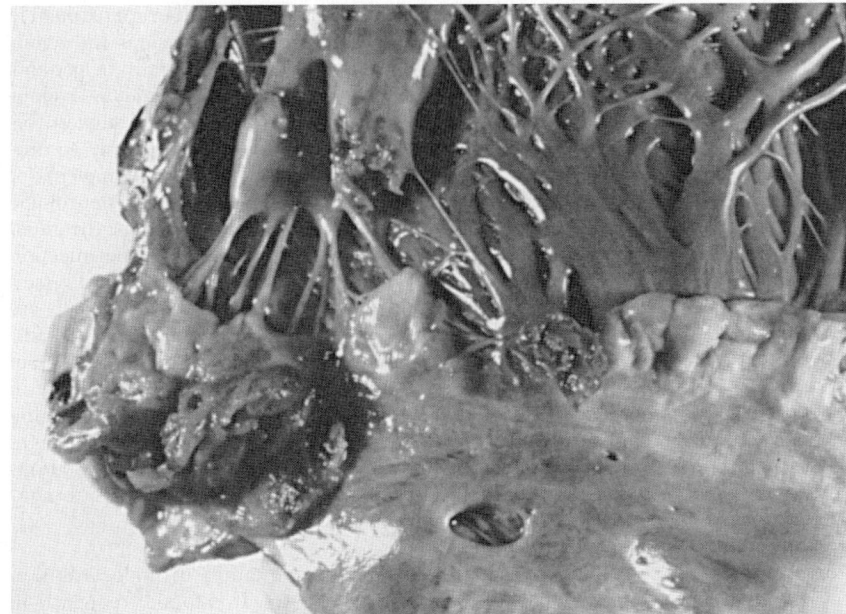

Figure 32-1 Subacute endocarditis of the mitral valve with vegetation and rupture of the papillary muscle caused by *Staphylococcus aureus*. *(Courtesy of Dr. Edith P. Hawkins, Texas Children's Hospital, Houston.)*

agglutinating, and complement-fixing antibodies), cryoglobulins, macroglobulins, and antibodies to bacterial heat shock protein,[391] as well as to the subsequent formation of circulating immune complexes. These complexes are found with increased frequency in patients with a long duration of illness, hypocomplementemia, extravalvular manifestations, and right-sided disease.[36] Quantitative levels of circulating immune complexes may be helpful in distinguishing endocarditic from non-endocarditic sepsis and in monitoring anti-infective therapy. Effective treatment usually leads to a prompt decrease in these levels,[35] whereas relapses may be characterized by rising titers.[246] The diffuse glomerulonephritis occasionally noted with infective endocarditis is caused by subepithelial deposition of immune complexes and complement.[184] Immune complexes can be demonstrated in some diffuse purpuric lesions seen with endocarditis.[292] Bacterial antigens have been found within these complexes.[216]

Further evidence of stimulation of the immune system in infective endocarditis is the development of rheumatoid factor in approximately 50 percent of adults with disease lasting longer than 6 weeks.[525] Titers of rheumatoid factor correlate with hypergammaglobulinemia and, as with immune complex levels, decrease with therapy and increase during relapse. The role of rheumatoid factor in the disease process is unknown, but it may be involved by blocking immunoglobulin G opsonic activity, stimulating phagocytosis, or accelerating microvascular damage.[432] Anti-nuclear, anti-endocardial, anti-sarcolemmal, and anti-myolemmal antibodies also have been identified in patients with infective endocarditis; their role in pathogenesis is unclear.[300]

The pathologic changes that occur in the heart in association with infective endocarditis are secondary to local extension of the infection. The vegetations vary in size from a millimeter to several centimeters; frequently they are singular, but they may be multiple. Valvular stenosis may result from large lesions. Vegetations secondary to certain organisms, especially *Candida*, *Haemophilus*, and *S. aureus* in acute cases, often are large and friable, with a propensity for embolization.[537] Ulcerative lesions may occur and may lead to perforation of the valve and subsequent congestive heart failure. Other local complications include rupture of the chordae tendineae or papillary muscle (see Fig. 32–1), valve ring abscess with subsequent fistula formation and pericardial empyema,[47,62] aneurysms of the sinus of Valsalva or ventricle,[75,160,430] myocarditis, and myocardial infarction.[135] Per-

sistent fever occurring during appropriate medical therapy for infective endocarditis may reflect a persistent vegetation, especially with right-sided disease, or extension of infection into a valve ring and adjacent structures.[113] In such cases, surgery frequently is required.

The pathologic changes in distant organs usually are secondary to embolization with subsequent infarction or metastatic infection. In many cases of infective endocarditis, the causative organism is of low pathogenicity; infections caused by septic emboli often are low-grade because of the reduced propensity of these organisms to invade tissue. However, the emboli in acute *S. aureus* endocarditis frequently cause severe metastatic infections and overwhelming sepsis. Emboli from right-sided heart lesions lodge in the lungs and cause pulmonary infarcts and abscesses, which usually are small and multiple. Left-sided lesions may embolize to any organ but most commonly affect the brain, kidney, spleen, and skin.[260,352] Cerebral emboli have been detected in 30 percent of cases in adults and children and have caused infarction, abscess, mycotic aneurysm, subarachnoid hemorrhage, meningitis, and acute hemiplegia of childhood.[59,180,191,234,313,422] Kidney abscess is a rare occurrence, but infarcts are noted in most patients at autopsy.[330] Amyloidosis involving primarily the kidneys is a rare complication of chronic infective endocarditis.[196] Splenic abscess also is a rare event but can be a fatal complication if undetected.[232] The most common manifestation of embolization to the skin is petechiae. Janeway lesions are septic emboli consisting of bacteria, neutrophils, necrosis, and subcutaneous hemorrhage. Osler nodes are areas of thrombosis and necrosis. They may be related to both immune complex deposition and septic emboli.[5]

CLINICAL MANIFESTATIONS

The signs and symptoms of infective endocarditis are determined by the extent of local cardiac disease, the continuous bacteremia, and the degree of involvement of distant organs as a result of embolization, metastatic infection, and circulating immune complexes.[24] Consequently, the clinical findings are highly variable and mimic those of many other diseases.[418] Unexplained embolic phenomena in any organ should suggest the diagnosis of endocarditis, especially in children with known heart disease.

Patients with acute bacterial endocarditis initially may be seen with florid sepsis; the endocarditis is diagnosed at autopsy. The indolent manifestations of subacute endocarditis may evolve for weeks or months before medical care is sought. Endocarditis frequently occurs in children with preexisting heart disease, so subtle changes in cardiac function may be difficult to detect early in the course. Table 32-3 lists the frequency of the major clinical manifestations of bacterial endocarditis in infants and children.

Fever is the most common symptom of infective endocarditis, but it is absent in 10 percent of cases. It usually is of low grade and has no specific pattern. Chills may accompany the fever, but they rarely are seen in children. Persistent fever during antimicrobial therapy is an uncommon occurrence. Prolonged (>2 weeks) fever is associated with certain etiologic agents (S. aureus, gram-negative bacilli, fungi), with culture-negative endocarditis, and with complications such as embolization of major vessels, intracardiac or peripheral abscess, tissue infarction, a need for cardiac surgery, and a higher mortality rate.[48,274] Nonspecific symptoms such as malaise, anorexia, weight loss, and fatigue are common findings. Arthralgia occurs in 24 percent of patients. The arthralgia frequently is multiple and most commonly affects the large joints. Although adults initially may have synovitis,[82] this finding is rare in children. Osteoarticular infection in association with infective endocarditis in adults occurs almost exclusively in intravenous drug users.[429] It is seen very rarely in children. Gastrointestinal complaints are noted in 16 percent of cases and include nausea, vomiting, and abdominal pain. Chest pain occurs in approximately 10 percent of older children and generally is mild and nonspecific. Although chest pain usually is related to diffuse myalgias, it may be secondary to pulmonary complications or cardiac lesions, especially if the tricuspid valve is involved.

Heart murmurs occur in more than 90 percent of children with infective endocarditis, but most patients have underlying heart disease with existing murmurs. The appearance of a new murmur or appreciation of a significant change in a previous one occurs in only 25 percent of cases. Significant blood flow turbulence caused by compromised valvular function must have occurred for a murmur to be detected or to change. The frequent absence of changes in the cardiac examination early in the disease contributes to the long average delay in establishing the diagnosis, especially in children with preexisting heart disease. Congestive heart failure occurs in 30 percent of children with infective endocarditis and is especially common in those in whom a new murmur of valvular insufficiency develops. Endocarditis should be suspected in any child who has rheumatic or congenital heart disease and unexplained deterioration in cardiac function. Although valvular regurgitation is the most common hemodynamic complication of endocarditis, significant obstruction of a valve or shunt requiring rapid surgery rarely occurs.[74]

Neurologic signs and symptoms are reported in approximately 20 percent of children with endocarditis. These signs and symptoms may dominate the clinical findings, especially in patients with endocarditis caused by S. aureus.[191,422] The sudden development of cerebral lesions in an infant or child should suggest this diagnosis. The manifestations are those that commonly accompany a cerebral infarct or abscess, namely, acute hemiplegia of childhood, seizures, ataxia, aphasia, sensory loss, focal neurologic deficits, and alterations in mental status.[59] They may be the initial features of endocarditis or may occur years after the infection has been eradicated.[540] Mycotic aneurysms of the cerebral vessels occur rarely in cases of pediatric endocarditis.[63] They usually are single, small, and peripheral but may lead to subarachnoid hemorrhage. Whereas computed tomographic scanning of the brain is useful for delineating central nervous system involvement in patients with infective endocarditis, magnetic resonance imaging may be more sensitive for detecting small infarctions and changes secondary to cerebral edema.[40] Other neurologic manifestations associated with endocarditis include cranial nerve palsies, neuropathy, visual changes, choreoathetosis, seizures, and toxic encephalopathy.

Splenomegaly, a common manifestation of endocarditis in children, occurs in 55 percent of cases. It is found frequently in patients with long-standing disease and other evidence of immune system activation. The spleen generally is nontender and may be associated with mild hepatomegaly. Splenic infarction and abscess are rare events but should be suspected in patients with left upper quadrant abdominal pain that radiates to the left shoulder, a pleural friction rub, or left pleural effusion.

Skin manifestations occur less commonly in children than in adults.[292] Clubbing is found in 10 to 20 percent of children with endocarditis but frequently is related to underlying heart disease. Petechiae are noted in approximately one third of patients, especially those with long-standing disease. These lesions are found most commonly on the extremities, oral mucosa, and conjunctivae. Splinter hemorrhages are linear red or brown streaks seen in the nail beds. They are present in only 5 percent of children with endocarditis and are associated with other conditions.[256] Three other types of lesions are more specific for infective endocarditis but occur in only 5 to 7 percent of patients: Osler nodes, which are small (2 to 10 mm), painful nodular lesions found in the pads of the fingers or toes[5]; Janeway lesions, which usually are painless hemorrhagic macular plaques that frequently occur on the palms and soles[133]; and Roth spots, which are small, pale retinal lesions associated with areas of hemorrhage located near the optic disk.

Other than fever and, perhaps, splenomegaly, no single sign or symptom occurs in more than 50 percent of children with endocarditis. That no classic clinical manifestation exists for this disease is obvious because the chance that even three or more signs will be present is extremely low. The appearance of any one

TABLE 32-3 Clinical Manifestations of Bacterial Endocarditis in Children

Symptom	Average (%)	Range (%)	Physical Finding	Average (%)	Range (%)
Fever	90	56-100	Splenomegaly	55	36-67
Malaise	55	40-79	Petechiae	33	10-50
Anorexia/weight loss	31	8-83	Embolic phenomena	28	14-50
Heart failure	30	9-47	New or change in heart murmur	24	9-44
Arthralgia	24	16-38	Clubbing	14	2-42
Neurologic findings	18	12-21	Osler nodes	7	7-8
Gastrointestinal findings	16	9-36	Roth spots	5	0-6
Chest pain	9	5-20	Janeway lesion	5	0-10
			Splinter hemorrhages	5	0-10

Data from references 49, 89, 91, 156, 230, 264, 311, 358, 418, 446, 453, 477, 484, and 507.

of these clinical features in a child with predisposing heart disease should raise suspicion of infective endocarditis and should lead to an appropriate diagnostic evaluation.[75]

The clinical findings of infective endocarditis in infants and neonates are less specific than are those in older children. The onset more often is acute and related to overwhelming infection.[231,321] In the pre-antibiotic era, these children often had other foci of infection, such as osteomyelitis, meningitis, and pneumonia, that dominated the clinical picture. The widespread use of antibiotics since 1941 has caused a decrease in the number of cases of infective endocarditis secondary to other suppurative infections.[321] Although early studies concluded that congenital heart disease was not an important predisposing factor to endocarditis in infants, more recent reports suggest that it is. At present, infants with heart defects undergo corrective and palliative surgery at a younger age than in the past. Infants in whom postoperative endocarditis does develop probably will have clinical findings more similar to those in older children.

Infective endocarditis is a rare occurrence in neonates and frequently is associated with indwelling vascular catheters.[159,309] It may affect the tricuspid valve and have a fairly "silent" clinical manifestation. Persistent bacteremia or fungemia should lead to a search for a cardiac focus of infection. Deterioration in pulmonary function, coagulopathies, thrombocytopenia, and low-grade murmurs often develop in neonates. Skin abscesses and hepatomegaly also are common findings. The prognosis of infective endocarditis associated with neonatal intensive care usually is favorable, perhaps because the diagnosis often is established relatively early and antibiotics are given rapidly.

Reported series of infective endocarditis in children with prosthetic valves are scarce. In early stages of disease, fever may be the only finding because the other signs of endocarditis are masked by the medical and surgical complications occurring in the immediate postoperative period. Late infections generally produce clinical findings similar to those in native-valve endocarditis. Clinical evidence of systemic embolization occurs in as many as 40 percent of patients.[77] Neurologic complications carry a particularly poor prognosis for survival.[252] A new or changing murmur often indicates valvular insufficiency caused by a paravalvular leak. Florid cardiac failure is the major manifestation if local infection or an abscess creates valve instability and acute, severe regurgitation.

The signs and symptoms of infective endocarditis in intravenous drug abusers may be similar, but these patients have several more distinctive features of their illness. Two thirds of these patients have no predisposing heart disease. The valve most commonly affected is the tricuspid, which leads to a predominance of pulmonary signs and symptoms resulting from pleural effusion, pulmonary infarction, and lung abscesses. Signs of tricuspid insufficiency (gallop rhythm, pulsatile liver, regurgitant murmur) are found in one third of cases.[432] Many patients have extracardiac sites of infection that are helpful in establishing the diagnosis.[482]

LABORATORY FINDINGS

The most important diagnostic procedure is the blood culture. Because many bacteria that usually are not pathogenic cause infective endocarditis, scrupulous aseptic technique must be used to distinguish causative agents from contaminants.[370] The yield of organisms is not increased by obtaining blood from arterial puncture or cardiac catheterization.[37] The bacteremia usually is of low grade and continuous. The first two cultures yield the organism 90 percent of the time; in two thirds of cases, all blood cultures are positive.[522] Therefore, isolated positive cultures generally are not significant. Previous outpatient antibiotic therapy may change the yield significantly.[250] In one study, culture

positivity in cases of proven endocarditis was 64 percent in patients who received antibiotics before blood was drawn for culture versus 100 percent in patients without exposure to antibiotics.[371]

When *Candida* endocarditis is suspected, several additional points should be considered. Isolation of *Candida* spp. may require incubation for 1 week or longer. All blood cultures from a patient with *Candida* endocarditis may not be positive, in contrast to the usual situation with bacterial endocarditis; several positive cultures may be interspersed among negative cultures. In patients with fungal endocarditis, *Candida* is isolated commonly from other infected sites, such as urine, sputum, synovial fluid, cerebrospinal fluid, lymph nodes, and bone marrow.[424]

Three to five samples of blood for culture should be obtained from different sites within the first 24 hours in children with suspected endocarditis. Although difficult to obtain in smaller children, 3 to 5 mL of blood per culture is desirable for optimal yield. The samples should be injected into thioglycolate and trypticase soy (or brain-heart infusion) broth and held for at least 3 weeks to detect slow-growing organisms. If gram-positive cocci grow in the broth but fail to grow on subculture, nutritionally variant streptococci should be suspected, and subculture should be performed on media with either L-cysteine or pyridoxal phosphate.[60,459] Poured plates may be used to estimate the degree of bacteremia.

Negative blood cultures are noted in 10 to 15 percent of patients with clinically diagnosed endocarditis.[498] However, when patients have not received antibiotic therapy previously and blood for culture is obtained properly, these cases account for less than 5 percent of the total. Potential reasons for negative cultures include the following: (1) right-sided endocarditis; (2) previous administration of antibiotics; (3) fungal (especially *Aspergillus*) endocarditis; (4) endocarditis caused by *Bartonella* spp., rickettsiae, chlamydiae, or viruses; (5) mural endocarditis; (6) slow growth of organisms (*Candida*, *Haemophilus*, *Brucella*, nutritionally variant streptococci); (7) anaerobic infection; and (8) nonbacterial thrombotic endocarditis or an incorrect diagnosis.[186,190,378,498] In some instances, intraleukocytic organisms may be seen in layered peripheral blood, even when cultures are negative.[386] If surgical resection of vegetations or valve replacement is performed, a cause may be demonstrated by appropriate histologic examination and stains for bacteria and fungi.[336] Organisms also may be isolated from extracardiac sites (bone marrow, urine).

Many nonspecific laboratory findings are abnormal in patients with infective endocarditis (Table 32–4). The total white blood cell count rarely is helpful, but peripheral eosinophilia may be seen with Loeffler endocarditis.[203] The erythrocyte sedimentation rate is elevated in 80 to 90 percent of cases. However, frequently it is normal or low when congestive heart failure or renal failure is present. Serum C-reactive protein levels usually are elevated initially and return to normal during the course of successful therapy.[316] An increase during therapy may result from treatment failure, but can it also be caused by drug allergy or

TABLE 32–4 Selected Laboratory Findings of Bacterial Endocarditis in Children

Laboratory Finding	Average (%)	Range (%)
Positive blood culture	87	68-98
Elevated erythrocyte sedimentation rate	80	71-96
Low hemoglobin (anemia)	44	19-79
Positive rheumatoid factor	38	25-55
Hematuria	35	28-47

Data from references 48, 89, 156, 230, 264, 311, 446, 453, 484, and 507.

intercurrent infection. Rheumatoid factor rarely has been measured in a series of pediatric patients, but when measurements have been made, they have been positive in 25 to 50 percent of children with endocarditis. A positive test may be a diagnostic aid in cases of culture-negative endocarditis when other causes are excluded. Serial measurements may provide evidence of efficacy of therapy, although a fall in the titer of rheumatoid factor may lag behind the clinical and bacteriologic response.[514] Hypocomplementemia is seen in association with glomerulonephritis. Anemia is present in approximately 40 percent of patients, especially in those with long-standing disease. Although hemolysis may occur in the areas of turbulence in the heart, more often it is anemia of chronic disease. Because many patients with cyanotic heart disease normally have a compensatory polycythemia, a serial drop in hematocrit is of more significance than is a single measurement. Leukocytosis occurs in a few patients, but leukopenia is a rare finding in the absence of acute endocarditis with overwhelming sepsis. Hematuria and proteinuria, present in 25 to 50 percent of cases, usually are secondary to microemboli in the kidneys and may be accompanied by "pyuria," casts, and bacteriuria.

Circulating immune complexes are present in most adults with subacute endocarditis, as measured by Raji cell radioimmunoassay[485] or the ^{125}I-Clq binding assay.[541] These immune complexes frequently are absent in acute endocarditis. Low levels of immune complexes have been found in 32 percent of adults with septicemia but not endocarditis, in 10 percent of normal controls, and in 40 percent of noninfected intravenous drug abusers.[36] However, levels higher than 100 µg/mL are correlated highly with the presence of endocarditis. Serial measurement of immune complex levels may aid in monitoring therapeutic efficacy.[35] Systematic investigation of immune complexes has been reported infrequently in children with endocarditis. When immune complexes have been sought, most patients, including two of three children with culture-negative endocarditis, have had significant levels.

When infective endocarditis is suspected but blood cultures remain negative, serologic testing for specific organisms may prove helpful. Several techniques measure antibody to teichoic acids, which are major components of the cell wall of *S. aureus*. These antibodies are present in more than 85 percent of adults with staphylococcal endocarditis, but the false-positive rate is as high as 10 percent.[349] False-negative results correlate with a short (<2 weeks) duration of illness. Specific information about the accuracy of this test in children is lacking, and the tests are not readily available. Serologic testing is available or under investigation for many other organisms that cause infective endocarditis, including *Bartonella, Brucella, Candida, Aspergillus, Histoplasma, Cryptococcus, Chlamydia,* and *Coxiella*.[235,257] In general, the usefulness of these tests in children with endocarditis is unproven. Some patients with non-spirochetal bacterial endocarditis who reside in locales endemic for Lyme disease have significantly elevated levels of antibodies reactive to *Borrelia burgdorferi*.[257] Diagnostic confusion may occur because the signs and symptoms of infective endocarditis and Lyme disease can be quite similar. Other techniques, such as broad-range polymerase chain reaction (PCR), have been used to identify *Bartonella* and other causative agents of endocarditis.[51,512]

Radiographic techniques have not been a great aid in establishing the diagnosis of infective endocarditis. The findings on plain chest roentgenograms are nonspecific, but evidence of complications, such as septic pulmonary emboli or congestive heart failure, may be helpful. Computed tomography may help in establishing the diagnosis of an infected shunt.[499] Immunoscintigraphy using technetium-labeled anti-granulocyte antibodies may yield useful information when the echocardiographic findings are equivocal.[334] Cineangiography is the definitive method

to determine the anatomic alterations in the heart resulting from infective endocarditis, but it rarely needs to be performed in children.

The electrocardiogram also is useful in the evaluation of patients with endocarditis because it detects arrhythmias and conduction disturbances that complicate the disease. Ventricular ectopy may be related to myocardial ischemia, myocarditis, or myocardial abscess. New conduction defects imply extension of infection beyond the valve ring into the myocardium. Any degree of atrioventricular block, a new left bundle branch block, or a new right bundle branch block with a left anterior hemiblock may represent extension of infection from the aortic valve into the ventricular septum. Junctional tachycardia, Wenckebach atrioventricular block, or complete heart block may be produced by extension of the infection from the mitral valve annulus into the atrioventricular node or proximal His bundle. In general, an unstable conduction block is more likely to develop in patients with aortic valve endocarditis than in those with mitral infection.[111]

Echocardiography has become a valuable adjunct to the diagnosis and treatment of endocarditis in children.[109,173,266,403,416,417,439] Color Doppler is a sensitive modality for detection of valvular insufficiency, and the results may influence surgical and medical treatment decisions.[145] Echocardiography can be performed by the traditional transthoracic approach or the transesophageal approach.[383] The sensitivity and specificity of transthoracic echocardiography continue to be defined, with positive results obtained in 36 to 100 percent of children in various series of pediatric patients.[52,89,109,247,278,285,420]

In general, two-dimensional echocardiography is more sensitive than is the M-mode technique, especially in cases of right-sided endocarditis,[366] and it is superior in diagnosing complications of the destructive process.[24,328] The smallest vegetation detectable is approximately 2 mm, but the acoustic impedance of the mass relative to the surrounding structures is a more important factor than is size in identifying the vegetation. Echocardiography has identified vegetations in culture-negative cases.[247] Its accuracy in prosthetic-valve endocarditis is diminished by the difficulty in resolution around the prosthetic device.[345,463] Serial evaluation of valvular vegetations generally does not assist in assessing the efficacy of antibiotic therapy because diminution or disappearance of vegetations may take place long after successful medical treatment has been completed.[258,410,511]

The use of transthoracic echocardiography to predict the clinical course and need for operative intervention in patients with endocarditis is controversial.[7,177] A synopsis of many reports that have assessed the role of transthoracic echocardiography in the diagnosis and management of infective endocarditis suggests the following: (1) because of variable sensitivity among studies for detection of vegetations, a negative study does not rule out endocarditis, especially when foreign material is present within the heart; (2) false-positive studies are quite rare (the specificity is high); (3) the reliability of transthoracic echocardiography depends on the experience of the examiner and the technical adequacy of the study; (4) transthoracic echocardiography is valuable in assessing local complications of endocarditis on native valves; and (5) in most but not all studies, patients with a vegetation identified by transthoracic echocardiography have an increased risk for the development of systemic emboli and congestive heart failure.[177,223,295,319,404,427,462]

Although some investigators contend that the presence of a vegetation should hasten early surgery, most suggest that a positive echocardiogram is adjunctive evidence that should be considered along with other clinical parameters when considering surgical intervention. One study suggested that the relative risk for having embolic events associated with echocardiographically visualized lesions is microorganism-dependent, with a significant attributable risk seen only in patients with viridans streptococcal infection.[455] The absence of a vegetation on transthoracic echocardiography may define a subset of patients at low risk for the development of embolic complications.

Transesophageal echocardiography is a newer technique that has been studied extensively in adults with infective endocarditis.[99] It uses a 5-MHz phased-array transducer with Doppler and color flow encoding capabilities mounted on the tip of a flexible endoscope.[432] Biplane transesophageal echocardiography is considered the standard technique and is superior to transthoracic echocardiography because of improved spatial resolution, lack of acoustic interference from the lungs and chest wall, and closer proximity to posterior structures, such as the mitral valve and left atrium.[98] Multiplane transesophageal echocardiography facilitates and abbreviates the examination procedure and may be more accurate in providing the dimensions of a vegetation associated with infective endocarditis.[98,226]

Transesophageal echocardiography generally is well tolerated by children, even with the use of an adult probe (when the child's weight is more than 7 kg),[439] and rarely is associated with bacteremia.[97,269,382] Transesophageal echocardiography usually is more sensitive than is transthoracic echocardiography in the detection of intracardiac vegetations and is positive in 70 to 95 percent of adults with strongly suspected endocarditis.[342,445] It is significantly more sensitive in the detection of vegetations and complications in infected prosthetic valves.[253,372,409,463,476] Transesophageal echocardiography is particularly useful for detecting an aortic root abscess or involvement of the sinus of Valsalva in adults, and it should be considered in children with aortic valve endocarditis and changing aortic root dimensions on a standard transthoracic echocardiograph.[145,319] It appears to be less helpful for detection of vegetations in right-sided endocarditis.[428] Although a negative transesophageal echocardiographic study does not exclude endocarditis,[450] the procedure should be considered for patients with suspected endocarditis and a negative transthoracic echocardiograph, when the transthoracic echocardiography windows are suboptimal, and when perivalvular extension of infection is suspected.[14,212]

To aid in establishing the diagnosis of infective endocarditis, various sets of clinical criteria have been suggested. The von Reyn criteria were described in 1982, but echocardiographic findings were not included in the case definitions.[510] In addition, isolation of a typical infective endocarditis pathogen from blood cultures was not considered. New case definitions and diagnostic criteria were proposed by investigators from Duke,[121] and they have been modified subsequently[268,283] (Tables 32–5 and 32–6). The inclusion of echocardiographic and blood culture findings in these new criteria has resulted in more flexibility, a higher proportion of "definite" cases, and a more accurate reflection of current clinical practice.[324] These criteria have been validated in large series of infective endocarditis in adults and children.[107,121,200,426] In two pediatric series of clinically defined endocarditis, no cases were rejected by the Duke criteria, whereas 25 and 19 percent were rejected by the von Reyn criteria.[107,464] In one study, three of six pathologically confirmed cases were rated as only probable or rejected by the von Reyn criteria, whereas all were definite by the Duke criteria.[107] However, a more recent study found that 12 percent of pediatric endocarditis cases were not classified as "definite" by the modified Duke criteria.[487]

MICROBIOLOGY

Many different microorganisms are capable of causing infective endocarditis in humans. Table 32–7 lists the organisms isolated from patients in major pediatric series. Gram-positive cocci are the etiologic agents in 90 percent of cases in which an organism

TABLE 32–5   Definition of Terms Used in the Modified Duke Criteria for Infective Endocarditis

Major Criteria

1. Positive blood culture
   a. Typical microorganisms for IE from ≥2 blood cultures
      (1) Viridans streptococci, *Streptococcus bovis*, HACEK group, *Staphylococcus aureus* or
      (2) Enterococci, in the absence of another primary focus, *or*
   b. Persistently positive blood cultures, with recovery of a microorganism consistent with IE from
      (1) Blood cultures drawn ≥12 hours apart *or*
      (2) All of three or a majority of four or more separate blood cultures, with first and last drawn ≥1 hour apart
2. Evidence of endocardial involvement
   a. Positive echocardiogram for IE
      (1) Oscillating intracardiac mass on valve or supporting structures, in the path of regurgitant jets, or on implanted material, in the absence of an alternative anatomic explanation, *or*
      (2) Abscess *or*
      (3) New partial dehiscence of a prosthetic valve *or*
      (4) New valvular regurgitation (increase or change in preexisting murmur is not sufficient)

Minor Criteria

1. Predisposing heart condition or intravenous drug use
2. Fever ≥38° C
3. Vascular phenomena: major arterial emboli, septic pulmonary infarcts, mycotic aneurysm, intracranial hemorrhage, conjunctival hemorrhages, Janeway lesions
4. Immunologic phenomena: glomerulonephritis, Osler nodes, Roth spots, rheumatoid factor
5. Microbiologic evidence: positive blood culture but not meeting major criteria as noted previously* or serologic evidence of active infection with organism consistent with IE

Excluding single positive cultures for coagulase-negative staphylococci and organisms that do not cause IE.

HACEK, Haemophilus species, Actinobacillus actinomycetemcomitans, Cardiobacterium hominis, Eikenella corrodens, Kingella kingae; IE, infective endocarditis.

From Li, J. S., Sexton, D. J., Mick, N., et al: Proposed modifications to the Duke criteria for the diagnosis of infective endocarditis. Clin. Infect. Dis. 30:633-638, 2000.

is isolated. Streptococci remain the bacteria isolated most frequently, although the percentage of cases caused by staphylococci and fungi has been increasing during the past 2 decades.[151,420,507,537] Polymicrobial infective endocarditis, especially in nosocomial settings, also appears to be increasing in incidence.[22] The characteristics of selected organisms and the type of disease that they produce are considered in the following subsections.

STREPTOCOCCI

Several terminologies have been used to classify streptococci. The Lancefield system defines groups (A, B, C, D, E, F, G, H) by serologic reactions. The viridans streptococci are alpha-hemolytic or nonhemolytic, may be Lancefield nontypeable (*Streptococcus milleri, Streptococcus mitior, Streptococcus salivarius,* most *Streptococcus mutans,* and *S. sanguis*) or typeable (*Streptococcus bovis* group D, some *S. sanguis* group H, some *S. milleri* group F), and display similar characteristics in vivo. They are the most frequent etiologic agents in subacute infective endocarditis and cause 40 percent of cases in children. They may cause rapidly progressive invasive disease.[205,471]

TABLE 32-6 Modified Duke Criteria for the Diagnosis of Infective Endocarditis

Definite
1. Pathologic criteria
   a. Microorganisms: demonstrated by culture or histology in a vegetation, in a vegetation that has embolized, or in an intracardiac abscess *or*
   b. Pathologic lesions: vegetation or intracardiac abscess present and confirmed by histology showing endocarditis
2. Clinical criteria (see Table 32-5)
   a. Two major criteria *or*
   b. One major and three minor criteria *or*
   c. Five minor criteria

Possible
1. One major criteria and one minor criterion, or
2. Three minor criteria

Rejected
1. Firm alternative diagnosis explaining evidence of IE *or*
2. Resolution of IE syndrome with antimicrobial therapy for ≤4 days *or*
3. No pathologic evidence of IE at surgery or autopsy with antibiotic therapy for ≤4 days

IE, infective endocarditis.
From Li, J. S., Sexton, D. J., Mick, N., et al: Proposed modifications to the Duke criteria for the diagnosis of infective endocarditis. Clin. Infect. Dis. 30:633-638, 2000.

TABLE 32-7 Etiologic Agents of Bacterial Endocarditis in Children

Organism	Average (%)	Range (%)
Streptococci		
Viridans	40.3	17-72
Enterococci	4.0	0-12
Pneumococci	3.3	0-21
Beta-hemolytic	2.7	0-8
Other	1.1	0-16
Staphylococci		
Staphylococcus aureus	23.8	5-40
Coagulase-negative	4.7	0-15
Gram-negative aerobic bacilli	4.0	0-15
Fungi	1.1	0-12
Miscellaneous bacteria	2.4	0-10
Culture-negative	12.6	2-32

Data from references 49, 58, 91, 229-231, 264, 321, 420, 453, 484, and 507.

Viridans streptococci are common pathogens in patients with underlying heart disease but are less common in postoperative patients. They are part of the indigenous flora of the human mouth and gastrointestinal tract, and procedures that disrupt mucosal integrity in these areas predispose patients to development of viridans streptococcal bacteremia. In the pediatric population, most blood and cerebrospinal fluid isolates of viridans and nonhemolytic streptococci are not from patients with infective endocarditis.[189] Most strains are exquisitely susceptible to penicillin, although previous administration of antibiotics may promote infection with resistant strains.[262,279] Nutritionally variant viridans streptococci, reclassified as *Abiotrophia defectiva* or *Granulicatella* spp., are recognized as one cause of culture-negative endocarditis in children.[72,136,286,353,393,406] These organisms grow in broth but will not grow on subculture agar-based plates. Bacteriologic failure has occurred in 40 percent of reported cases of endocarditis caused by these organisms despite susceptibility to the antibiotics used.[24,459] Most viridans streptococci have low pathogenicity; however, the *S. milleri* group has a predilection for

suppurative complications.[347] The prognosis of endocarditis caused by non-enterococcal streptococci is excellent with good medical and surgical management; the cure rate is more than 90 percent, although complications (emboli, congestive heart failure) occur in as many as 30 percent of cases.

Enterococcal endocarditis occurs much less frequently in children than in adults[322,481] and accounts for only 4 percent of pediatric cases. The organism normally inhabits the gastrointestinal and genitourinary tracts; instrumentation of these areas may cause enterococcal bacteremia. More than 40 percent of adult patients have no underlying heart disease.[402] Endocarditis should be considered in all infants and children with unexplained enterococcal bacteremia. Although the incidence of enterococcal bacteremia appears to be increasing in some neonatal intensive care units, the incidence of associated endocarditis seems to be very low. Factors that may suggest endocarditis in patients with enterococcal bacteremia include (1) preexisting heart disease, (2) community acquisition, (3) a cryptogenic source, and (4) the absence of polymicrobial bacteremia.[301] Differentiation of enterococci from other group D streptococci (*S. bovis*) is important because their respective therapeutic approaches are different.

Endocarditis caused by beta-hemolytic streptococci occurred more commonly in the pre-antibiotic era than today. Most cases are caused by Lancefield group B or G organisms,[1,16,158,517] whereas group C and A streptococci rarely cause endocarditis.[45,114,174,290,395] Group A, B, or C streptococcal infection may lead to large, bulky vegetations, easily seen by echocardiography, and to embolic complications.[17,351,423] Although group B streptococcal bacteremia is a common finding in newborn infants, endocarditis caused by this organism occurs rarely in this age group. Similarly, *S. pneumoniae* accounted for 10 to 15 percent of endocarditis cases in the pre-antibiotic era but currently causes less than 1 percent.[162,222,364] Pneumococcal endocarditis may involve either the aortic or the mitral valve.[126,171,491] In older studies, fewer than 50 percent of affected children had underlying heart disease, but in more recent series, most children have had existing heart disease.[218] The clinical course often is fulminant.[123,275,384] Concurrent meningitis or pneumonia (or both) occurs frequently. Valvular dysfunction and cardiac decompensation are common findings.[48,56,78] Early surgical intervention may be required because the mortality rate is 75 percent when medical management alone is used.[222]

STAPHYLOCOCCI

Staphylococci cause 20 to 30 percent of cases of infective endocarditis in children, but the relative incidence appears to be increasing.[151] *S. aureus* is the etiologic agent in most cases of acute endocarditis and frequently infects normal heart valves.[152,340] The course often is fulminant when the mitral or aortic valve is involved, with frequent suppurative complications occurring both in the heart (myocardial abscess, pericarditis, valve ring abscess) and in other organs.[129,236,329] *S. aureus* is responsible for more than 50 percent of cases of endocarditis in intravenous drug abusers, but the disease tends to be less severe in these patients.[70,71] The origin of the infecting organism is the addict's own nose or skin, not the injection paraphernalia.[497] Endocarditis associated with indwelling vascular catheters or prosthetic valves frequently is caused by *S. aureus*.[227] Endocarditis must be suspected in any patient with *S. aureus* bacteremia, even when a peripheral focus of infection is present. However, most patients with *S. aureus* bacteremia do not have endocarditis. The rise of methicillin-resistant *S. aureus* (MRSA) has rendered treatment more difficult but has had little impact on the rate of local complications.[210]

The incidence of endocarditis resulting from CONS is rising rapidly.[12] CONS is a common etiologic agent of endocarditis occurring after cardiac surgery,[251,287] and it is occurring more frequently on native valves.[79,80] This organism is the leading agent in prosthetic-valve endocarditis, for which it causes 25 to 67 percent of early cases and 25 to 33 percent of late cases.[168,219,242] CONS endocarditis also has been associated with mitral valve prolapse and the use of intravascular catheters in premature neonates.[23,359] Although metastatic infection rarely occurs, CONS can be locally invasive; the mortality rate of prosthetic-valve endocarditis caused by CONS approaches 75 percent when valve replacement is not performed.

GRAM-NEGATIVE ORGANISMS

Although gram-negative bacteria cause 4 to 5 percent of cases of infective endocarditis in children, the percentage of children with gram-negative enteric bacteremia in whom endocarditis develops is extremely low. Endocarditis should be suspected in patients with gram-negative infection when bacteremia persists despite administration of usually appropriate antibiotic therapy.[65] Burn patients,[214] immunosuppressed hosts, narcotic addicts, and patients with implanted endovascular devices[335] are at an increased risk for development of gram-negative endocarditis. However, in the early postoperative period after cardiac surgery, sustained gram-negative bacillary bacteremia commonly is caused by other foci of infection and does not imply the presence of endocarditis. Many species of gram-negative enteric organisms have caused infective endocarditis in children, but no clear pattern has emerged. Among the gram-negative organisms more commonly reported are *Brucella, Escherichia coli, Serratia, Klebsiella-Enterobacter, Salmonella,* and *Pseudomonas.*[108,263,294,335,473] Endocarditis caused by *Salmonella* has been reported in patients with HIV infection.[142] It most often affects previously abnormal heart valves. Endocarditis is a rare complication of tularemia.[478] Cure of left-sided endocarditis caused by the Enterobacteriaceae seldom is achieved with medical therapy alone.[432] Most information about gram-negative enteric endocarditis is limited to case reports and general medicine reviews; discussion of individual organisms is beyond the scope of this review.

Other gram-negative organisms associated with infective endocarditis are the so-called HACEK coccobacilli.[102,137,211] These organisms caused 57 percent of cases of gram-negative endocarditis seen at the Mayo Clinic in Rochester, Minnesota, from 1958 to 1979.[164] Endocarditis caused by *Haemophilus influenzae* has been reported in only four children.[96,305] Cases caused by *Haemophilus parainfluenzae* and *Haemophilus aphrophilus* occur slightly more commonly.[41,81,101,211,225,296] They generally are seen in the setting of preexisting valvular disease and run a subacute course. However, central nervous system complications and emboli to major peripheral arteries are frequent occurrences.[81] Infective endocarditis caused by other organisms of the HACEK group is an extremely rare event in children.[11,138,339,368,392,521] All the bacteria in this group are fastidious, may require 2 to 3 weeks for primary isolation, and need subculturing onto chocolate agar in an atmosphere of 5 to 10 percent carbon dioxide for optimal growth. These procedures should be performed in all cases of culture-negative endocarditis.

Neisseria gonorrhoeae was responsible for 10 percent of cases in the pre-antibiotic era, but fewer episodes have been reported since 1942.[141,220] This pathogen frequently attacks previously normal heart valves and is manifested as an acute illness.[479] Valvular destruction with a need for valve replacement occurs commonly. At present, nonpathogenic *Neisseria* spp. are isolated more frequently in endocarditis than are gonococci, but they usually attack abnormal or prosthetic valves.[53,194,206,215,381,440] Although 1 percent of cases of infective endocarditis in adults are caused by anaerobic bacteria,[139] reports of anaerobic endocarditis in children are exceedingly rare.[86,354,448,467]

GRAM-POSITIVE BACILLI

Infective endocarditis caused by *Corynebacterium* spp. is an unusual finding but may occur on normal or previously abnormal valves.[38,323] Both toxigenic[105] and nontoxigenic[182,449,486] strains of *Corynebacterium diphtheriae* cause endocarditis in children, a finding demonstrating that the toxigenic and invasive properties of the organism are independent. Infection occurs most often on native valves and may be quite aggressive and lead to major vascular complications. *Listeria monocytogenes* endocarditis rarely occurs, has a high mortality rate, and, unlike other forms of listeriosis, usually is not associated with immunocompromised hosts.[33,66] It has not been associated with listeriosis in neonates. Fewer than 40 cases of *Lactobacillus* endocarditis have been reported.[181,213,470] Endocarditis caused by *Erysipelothrix rhusiopathiae* is found predominantly in adults who are farmers or are exposed to farm animals or products.[176,192] Most cases of *Bacillus* endocarditis involve the tricuspid valve in intravenous drug users, but other patients have been affected, including those with prosthetic valves.[458] *Gemella morbillorum,* formerly known as *Streptococcus morbillorum,* is a gram-positive coccus that normally resides in the gastrointestinal tract and is a rare cause of endocarditis.[132,270]

OTHER ORGANISMS

Many different bacteria, including *Acinetobacter,*[179] *Stenotrophomonas,*[408] *Nocardia,*[516] *Actinomyces,*[267] *Streptobacillus,*[414] and *Rothia,*[468] have been associated rarely with endocarditis.[55] Mycobacterial endocarditis is an exceedingly infrequent event.[157]

Infective endocarditis caused by *Coxiella burnetii,* the causative agent of Q fever, is well documented in northern Africa, Europe, and Australia.[4,54,271,282] Most cases are chronic (occurring over a 6- to 12-month period) and involve the aortic valve.[303] Clues to establishing the diagnosis include exposure to parturient cats or rabbits, massive splenomegaly, hypergammaglobulinemia, and thrombocytopenia.[379] The diagnosis usually is confirmed by measurement of antibodies against phase I and phase II antigens, but the organism has been isolated from leukocytes in a shell vial assay and has been demonstrated by immunohistologic techniques.[54,170] At least 20 well-documented cases of infective endocarditis caused by *Chlamydia psittaci* and *Chlamydia pneumoniae* have been reported.[201,235,310,444] Most patients have had preexisting heart disease and a subacute course.[304] *Mycoplasma* endocarditis is exceedingly rare.[112] *Legionella* has been implicated in several cases of prosthetic-valve endocarditis.[492] *Bartonella quintana* and *Bartonella henselae* have been identified as the cause of endocarditis in "culture-negative" cases.[115,224,452] Most described cases have been in immunocompetent individuals.[380] The diagnosis was established by serology, PCR, or special culture techniques.[26,140,149,396,512]

Although culture of bacteria remains the primary method for establishing the microbial cause of infective endocarditis, the number of organisms causing endocarditis that cannot be cultivated by standard culture methods is growing.[148,207] More recently, universal and species-specific primers have been designed to amplify bacterial DNA directly from resected valves. Among the organisms causing endocarditis identified by these methods are *Bartonella, Tropheryma whippelii, Coxiella, Mycoplasma, Haemophilus, Abiotrophia, Gemella, Cardiobacterium,* and *Streptococcus.*[161,175,207,289,390]

FUNGI

Most cases of fungal endocarditis in children have been described as occurring after cardiovascular surgery and prolonged intravenous and antibiotic therapy.[125,326,488] More recently, cases have been reported in neonates[315] and after prosthetic-valve placement.[356] The most common causative organism is *C. albicans*, although disease has been attributed to other *Candida* spp., including *C. krusei, Candida parapsilosis, Candida stellatoidea, Candida tropicalis,* and *Candida guilliermondii.*[388,424,441] Among intravenous drug abusers, *Candida* spp. other than *C. albicans* are more common causes of endocarditis.[413] The clinical manifestation usually is indolent and not specific, with symptoms occurring weeks to months before the diagnosis is established. Signs and symptoms caused by emboli to large vessels, especially those supplying the brain, kidney, spleen, and extremities, should alert the physician to the possible presence of fungal endocarditis. Large, friable vegetations occur frequently and can be detected by echocardiography.[465] Cutaneous and ocular manifestations of systemic *Candida* infection may be present.[50] The prognosis of *Candida* endocarditis is poor and is related to the propensity for septic emboli, the tendency for invasion into the myocardium, and the poor penetration of antifungal agents into the bulky vegetation. The diagnosis frequently is delayed by the tendency for negative or intermittently positive blood cultures to occur in this disease.[233] Surgical intervention usually is required.

Aspergillus spp., including *Aspergillus flavus, Aspergillus fumigatus, Aspergillus terreus,* and *Aspergillus niger,* are the second most frequent causes of fungal endocarditis, and such infections have been reported in 16 children.[28,29] Two thirds of these patients had underlying heart disease. *Aspergillus* endocarditis has been found in immunocompromised hosts with no previous cardiac problems.[534] The most common initial manifestations are fever and embolic phenomena, especially to the central nervous system.[513] Fewer than 15 cases have been diagnosed ante mortem, three by culture of peripheral emboli. In none of the patients was the antemortem blood culture positive. Most cases occur after open heart surgery; the most likely source of the organism is airborne inoculation of the heart during the operation.[28] Surgical removal of all infected material is recommended, although only one child has been treated successfully. Other fungi that rarely cause endocarditis include *Histoplasma capsulatum, Coccidioides immitis,*[272] *Cryptococcus neoformans, Torulopsis glabrata, Trichosporon beigelii,*[249] and *Fusarium* spp.[185,208]

TREATMENT

In the pre-antibiotic era, infective endocarditis was a uniformly fatal disease. With the current improved methods of diagnosis and therapy, 80 to 90 percent of children with this disease can be expected to survive. Mortality rates are higher for acute staphylococcal infection, fungal endocarditis, and prosthetic-valve endocarditis, although the tendency toward earlier surgical intervention for these entities may improve survival rates. The cornerstone of successful therapy is selection of antibiotics with specific activity against the causative organism. Better analysis of pharmacodynamic variables, such as bactericidal activity and the post-antibiotic effects of various drugs, may assist in the selection of optimal therapeutic regimens.[90,255,529] Although persistent infection occasionally complicates treated endocarditis,[400] deterioration in cardiac function is the major cause of morbidity and mortality.

Several general principles provide the basis for the current recommendations for treatment of endocarditis. Parenteral administration of antibiotics is preferred because erratic absorption of oral antibiotics, especially in infants, can lead to therapeutic failure. Although patient selection criteria for the use of outpatient parenteral antibiotic therapy for endocarditis in adults have been suggested, no data have been published about this practice for children.[9] Prolonged treatment, usually 4 to 6 weeks or longer, is necessary to sterilize the vegetations and to prevent

relapse. Bacteriostatic antibiotics are not effective and lead to frequent relapses or failure to eradicate the infection, or both. Antibiotic combinations may produce a rapid bactericidal effect through synergistic mechanisms of action. When synergy exists, smaller doses of each drug may be used, thereby reducing toxic side effects. However, certain drug combinations (e.g., penicillin and chloramphenicol) can be antagonistic, and their use should be avoided.

Blood should be drawn for culture for several days to evaluate the effect of the antibiotics. Negative follow-up cultures do not guarantee the success of therapy, but persistent positive cultures usually require that a change or addition to the antibiotic regimen be made. Observation of the patient's clinical course is extremely important. When fever is present initially, the temperature often returns to normal within a few days after therapy is started. However, fever can persist for weeks in patients whose eventual outcome is good. Such patients must be monitored closely for cardiac arrhythmias and congestive heart failure, which may require intensive care observation and electrocardiographic monitoring. Evidence of major embolic phenomena must be sought diligently by physical examination.

Several laboratory tests may aid in monitoring therapy. In all cases of bacterial endocarditis, the minimal inhibitory concentration (MIC) and minimal bactericidal concentration (MBC) ideally is determined for the antibiotics being used because disk susceptibility testing is unreliable and is not quantitative. When combinations of antibiotics are used, tests for bactericidal synergy, such as broth dilution, "checkerboards," or time-kill curves, may give additional information. The role of monitoring the inhibitory and bactericidal activity of the patient's serum is highly controversial. The Schlichter test determines the maximal dilutions of a patient's serum that in vitro inhibit and kill an inoculum of the organism causing the endocarditis.[399] Standardization of this test is poor, with laboratories using variations in inoculum size, in composition of the broth, in timing of samples (at expected peak or trough antibiotic concentrations in serum), in methods of dilution, and in determining the bactericidal end-point. In the rabbit endocarditis model, peak serum bactericidal titers greater than 1 : 8 correlate with therapeutic success.[64] A retrospective review of 17 reports of serum bactericidal activity in patients with endocarditis failed to show any correlation between titers greater than 1 : 8 and therapeutic success.[87] A prospective study suggested adjusting antibiotic doses to achieve peak titers of 1 : 64 or greater and trough titers of 1 : 32 or greater.[520] At present, no generally accepted recommendation can be made. In general, to attempt to achieve a peak serum bactericidal titer of at least 1 : 8 or greater seems reasonable if serious drug toxicity is not encountered. However, this level may not be attainable with certain organisms such as enterococci and gram-negative bacilli. Serum bactericidal testing may be particularly useful when synergistic combinations or less well established antibiotic regimens are used or when response to therapy is suboptimal.[533]

Little information is available concerning optimal antibiotic therapy for infective endocarditis in children; most treatment regimens are adapted from studies of adults with endocarditis.[24,530] In general, these regimens have been equally successful (and generally less toxic) in children. Table 32-8 lists recommended doses of the antibiotics commonly used.

After performing the initial evaluation of a patient with suspected infective endocarditis, the physician must make a clinical judgment about when to initiate therapy. If the findings are strongly indicative of the diagnosis or the child is very ill, treatment should be started as soon as blood has been drawn for culture. Initial empiric therapy depends on the clinical setting in which the tentative diagnosis is made. If the infection is subacute, a combination of penicillin G and an aminoglycoside usually is recommended for its activity against viridans streptococci, enterococci, and most gram-negative organisms. If *S. aureus*

TABLE 32–8 Suggested Intravenous Antibiotic Doses and Schedules for Infective Endocarditis in Children

Antibiotic	Daily Dose/kg	Divided Doses Every
Aqueous crystalline penicillin G sodium	300,000 U	4-6 hr
Ampicillin sodium	300 mg	4-6 hr
Ampicillin-sulbactam	300 mg	4-6 hr
Cefazolin	100 mg	6-8 hr
Ceftriaxone	100 mg	12 hr
Ciprofloxacin	20-30 mg	12 hr
Doxycycline	2-4 mg	12 hr
Gentamicin sulfate	3 mg	8 hr or 24 hr
Imipenem/cilastatin	60-100 mg	6 hr
Linezolid	30 mg	8 hr
Nafcillin sodium	200 mg (max., 12 g)	4-6 hr
Oxacillin sodium	200 mg (max., 12 g)	4-6 hr
Rifampin	20 mg	8-12 hr
Vancomycin hydrochloride	40 mg	6-12 hr

TABLE 32–9 Suggested Regimens for Treatment of Native Valve Endocarditis Caused by Highly Penicillin-Susceptible Viridans Streptococci and *Streptococcus bovis*

Antibiotic(s)	Duration (wk)	Comments
Aqueous crystalline penicillin G sodium	4	Preferred for patients with impairment of the eighth cranial nerve or renal function
Ceftriaxone sodium	4	
Aqueous crystalline penicillin G sodium *or* Ceftriaxone *plus* Gentamicin sulfate	2 / 2	Gentamicin peak serum concentration of approximately 3 μg/mL is desirable
Vancomycin hydrochloride	4	Recommended for patients allergic to β-lactam antibiotics

From Baddour, L. M., Wilson, W. R., Bayer, A. S., et al.: Infective endocarditis: Diagnosis, antimicrobial therapy, and management of complications. Circulation 111: e394-e433, 2005.

TABLE 32–10 Suggested Therapy for Native-Valve Endocarditis Caused by Strains of Viridans Streptococci and *Streptococcus bovis* Relatively Resistant to Penicillin G (Minimum Inhibitory Concentration, 0.12 and 0.5 μg/mL)

Antibiotic(s)	Duration (wk)	Comments
Aqueous crystalline penicillin G sodium	4	Cefazolin or other first-generation cephalosporins may be substituted for penicillin in patients whose penicillin hypersensitivity is not of the immediate type
or Ceftriaxone sodium *plus* Gentamicin sulfate	4 / 2	
Vancomycin hydrochloride	4	Recommended for patients allergic to β-lactam antibiotics

From Baddour, L. M., Wilson, W. R., Bayer, A. S., et al.: Infective endocarditis: Diagnosis, antimicrobial therapy, and management of complications. Circulation 111: e394-e433, 2005.

endocarditis is a strong consideration (acute manifestation, narcotic addicts), vancomycin and a penicillinase-resistant penicillin should be added to this regimen. Patients who recently have undergone cardiac surgery, especially prosthetic-valve placement, are treated best with an aminoglycoside and vancomycin to "cover" for health care–associated infection caused by MRSA or CONS; some physicians add penicillin G to this regimen to improve activity against streptococci. When culture and susceptibility data are known, antibiotic therapy can be changed as needed.

Most strains of viridans streptococci, *S. pyogenes*, and nonenterococcal group D streptococci are exquisitely susceptible to penicillin, with an MIC of less than 0.2 μg/mL. However, 15 to 20 percent of viridans streptococci have an MIC of 0.2 μg/mL or greater and are defined arbitrarily as relatively resistant.[209] In addition, some strains (particularly *S. mutans* and *S. mitior*) demonstrate tolerance, that is, an MIC to penicillin of less than 0.1 μg/mL but an MBC that is more than 10-fold higher (1.25 to 50 μg/mL). Most strains of nutritionally dependent streptococci are tolerant to penicillin.[24] Clinical failure may occur in endocarditis caused by these tolerant organisms when penicillin alone is used for treatment.[8,209] However, except for nutritionally dependent streptococci, therapy for tolerant viridans streptococci generally should be the same as for susceptible strains.

Although most experts recommend that patients with endocarditis caused by relatively resistant streptococci be treated with high doses of penicillin combined with 2 to 4 weeks of an aminoglycoside, some authorities consider that penicillin alone usually is adequate therapy.[44,110] Synergy in vitro between penicillin or vancomycin and streptomycin, gentamicin, or kanamycin can be demonstrated against virtually all penicillin-susceptible streptococci.[515] This observation correlates with a faster rate of eradication of bacteria from cardiac vegetations in the rabbit endocarditis model when synergistic combinations of antibiotics are used.[119,122] However, streptomycin is not synergistic for strains with high-level streptomycin resistance; gentamicin is the preferred second drug for these rare isolates.[127] In pediatric patients, gentamicin usually is substituted for streptomycin because of its lower toxicity.

Several regimens have been examined in adults with penicillin-susceptible viridans streptococcal native-valve endocarditis (Table 32–9). A 2-week course of penicillin alone leads to an unacceptable relapse rate. However, a 2-week course of intramuscular procaine penicillin and streptomycin cured 99 percent of adults with penicillin-susceptible streptococcal endocarditis in one report.[531] These results are similar to those obtained with β-

lactams alone for 4 weeks[244] or with penicillin for 4 weeks combined with streptomycin for the first 2 weeks. Gentamicin may be substituted for streptomycin. The 2-week penicillin-gentamicin regimen is the least expensive and is the preferred therapy in uncomplicated cases of penicillin-susceptible streptococcal endocarditis in young adults.[432] In general, the regimen of 4 weeks of penicillin alone is preferred for patients in renal failure or at high risk for developing aminoglycoside-induced ototoxicity. Vancomycin or ceftriaxone administered for 4 weeks can be used in patients with penicillin-susceptible viridans streptococcal endocarditis who have a penicillin allergy.[153,154,442,466] The regimen of 4 weeks of penicillin plus an initial 2 weeks of gentamicin is recommended in adults with a complicated course (symptoms for >3 months)[302] or with infection caused by relatively penicillin-resistant organisms (Table 32–10). Most nutritionally deficient streptococci are tolerant to penicillin. For patients with endocarditis caused by these organisms, a course of 4 to 6 weeks of penicillin with the addition of an aminoglycoside is recommended[24,530] (Table 32–11). In patients with streptococcal

TABLE 32-11 Suggested Therapy for Endocarditis Caused by Enterococcal Strains Susceptible to Penicillin, Gentamicin, and Vancomycin and Other Selected Streptococci*

Antibiotic(s)	Duration (wk)	Comments
Aqueous crystalline penicillin G sodium	4-6	4-wk therapy recommended for patients with symptoms <3 mo in duration; 6-wk therapy recommended for patients with symptoms >3 mo in duration
plus Gentamicin sulfate	4-6	
Ampicillin sodium *plus*	4-6	
Gentamicin sulfate	4-6	
Vancomycin hydrochloride	6	Recommended for patients allergic to β-lactam antibiotics
plus Gentamicin sulfate	6	

Viridans streptococci with a minimal inhibitory concentration >0.5 µg/mL, Abiotrophia species, Granulicatella species, or Gemella species.
From Baddour, L. M., Wilson, W. R., Bayer, A. S., et al.: Infective endocarditis: Diagnosis, antimicrobial therapy, and management of complications. Circulation 111: e394-e433, 2005.

TABLE 32-12 Suggested Therapy for Endocarditis of Prosthetic Valves or Other Prosthetic Material Caused by Viridans Group Streptococci and *Streptococcus bovis*

Antibiotic(s)	Duration (wk)
Penicillin-Susceptible Strain	
Aqueous crystalline penicillin G sodium	6
or	
Ceftriaxone	6
with or without	
Gentamicin sulfate	2
Vancomycin hydrochloride	6
Penicillin Relatively or Fully Resistant	
Aqueous crystalline penicillin G sodium	6
or	
Ceftriaxone	6
plus	
Gentamicin sulfate	6
Vancomycin hydrochloride	6

From Baddour, L. M., Wilson, W. R., Bayer, A. S., et al.: Infective endocarditis: Diagnosis, antimicrobial therapy, and management of complications. Circulation 111: e394-e433, 2005.

TABLE 32-13 Suggested Therapy for Native or Prosthetic Valve Enterococcal Endocarditis Caused by Strains Resistant to Penicillin, Aminoglycoside, and Vancomycin

Antibiotic(s)	Duration (wk)
Enterococcus faecium	
Linezolid	≥8
Enterococcus faecalis	
Imipenen/cilastatin	≥8
plus	
Ampicillin sodium	≥8
or	
Ceftriaxone	≥8
plus	
Ampicillin sodium	≥8

TABLE 32-14 Suggested Therapy for Endocarditis Caused by Staphylococci in the Absence of Prosthetic Material

Antibiotic(s)	Duration	Comments
Methicillin-Susceptible Staphylococci*		
Nafcillin sodium or oxacillin sodium	6 wk	Benefit of additional aminoglycoside has not been established
optional addition of Gentamicin sulfate	3-5 days	
Cefazolin	6 wk	For patients with non–immediate-type hypersensitivity to penicillin
optional addition of Gentamicin sulfate	3-5 days	
Methicillin-Resistant Staphylococci		
Vancomycin hydrochloride	6 wk	

If Staphylococcus is penicillin-susceptible (minimal inhibitory concentration ≤0.1 µg/mL), aqueous crystalline penicillin G sodium can be used for 6 weeks instead of nafcillin or oxacillin.
From Baddour, L. M., Wilson, W. R., Bayer, A. S., et al.: Infective endocarditis: Diagnosis, antimicrobial therapy, and management of complications. Circulation 111: e394-e433, 2005.

infection of prosthetic valves or other prosthetic materials, a 6-week regimen of penicillin usually supplemented with an aminoglycoside is recommended. (Table 32–12). None of the regimens discussed has been evaluated specifically in children with endocarditis.

Most strains of enterococci have an MIC to penicillin of 0.4 µg/mL or greater and an MBC of 6.25 µg/mL or greater.[346] All β-lactam antibiotics are bacteriostatic against enterococci and cannot be used alone. However, plasmid-mediated β-lactamase production has been found in rare strains of *Enterococcus faecalis*. Ampicillin-sulbactam overcomes the enzyme production and is effective as therapy.[483] Although therapy with penicillin alone is ineffective, the combination of penicillin and an aminoglycoside

is synergistic and produces a bactericidal effect on most enterococcal strains.[323] Unfortunately, 20 to 50 percent of enterococcal strains demonstrate very high resistance (MIC >2000 µg/mL) to streptomycin, and synergy between penicillin and streptomycin does not occur.[195,431] High-level resistance to gentamicin has been found in some isolates, and the incidence is increasing in certain locales.[124,288,369] When these isolates are encountered, all aminoglycosides should be tested because the organism may be susceptible to one while resistant to others.[518] Fortunately, these strains rarely cause endocarditis.[346] Although vancomycin-resistant enterococci have emerged as important nosocomial pathogens, they rarely cause endocarditis in children. Optimal therapy for these strains has not been established, but a combination of high-dose penicillin plus vancomycin and gentamicin may be effective in some cases.[61] Vancomycin-resistant enterococcal endocarditis has been treated successfully with oral linezolid.[10,15] The usual regimens for enterococcal endocarditis are listed in Tables 32–11 and 32–13).

Most isolates of *S. aureus* are resistant to penicillin, but endocarditis caused by penicillin-susceptible (MIC <0.1 µg/mL) isolates can be treated with this agent. In general, a semisynthetic penicillinase-resistant penicillin given for 6 weeks is the drug of choice[374,456] (Table 32–14). The addition of gentamicin to nafcillin produces an enhanced bactericidal effect in vitro and in experimental staphylococcal endocarditis in rabbits.[425] However, the value of this combination in patients has not been proved, and generally it is reserved for children with overwhelming infection. In penicillin-allergic patients or in those with MRSA, vancomycin alone has been recommended, although treatment failures in children with endocarditis have been reported.[134,221,280] The addition of rifampin or the use of β-lactam drugs after desensitization is necessary in some cases.[31,340] Ciprofloxacin has been used, but treatment failures have occurred because of the emergence of resistance.[344,480] The combination of vancomycin and rifampin for at least 6 weeks, plus the addition of gentamicin for the first 2 weeks, is recommended for the treatment of endocarditis caused by MRSA, although clinical trial data are not available. Daptomycin also has been used successfully to treat endocarditis caused by MRSA.[150] Nosocomial infections with *S. epidermidis* usually are treated with vancomycin because of the high incidence of methicillin resistance among these isolates. The addition of rifampin and gentamicin to either nafcillin or vancomycin may increase bactericidal activity and is recommended in cases of prosthetic-valve endocarditis secondary to any staphylococci[24] (see Table 32–13).

Therapy for endocarditis caused by gram-negative organisms must be individualized in accordance with in vitro susceptibility and synergy studies. A regimen of 6 to 8 weeks of combination therapy with two or more drugs may be required, especially with endocarditis caused by *Klebsiella* or *Pseudomonas*.[146,373] Surgical intervention frequently is necessary, especially for infection of the mitral or aortic valves. Endocarditis caused by *Haemophilus* and other fastidious gram-negative organisms usually is responsive to ampicillin, ceftriaxone, or ciprofloxacin alone,[24] but the addition of an aminoglycoside may improve the outcome[24,81] (Table 32–15). Anaerobic bacilli generally are susceptible to penicillin, but infection caused by resistant *Bacteroides fragilis* is treated best by combinations including metronidazole, ticarcillin-clavulanate, or imipenem.

Survival rates of only 10 to 20 percent in patients with fungal endocarditis are related to the poor ability of currently available antifungal agents to sterilize the vegetations. Only rare cures with medical therapy alone have been reported.[424] Most investigators contend that early surgical intervention is mandatory in every patient who has conclusive evidence of intracardiac fungal infection.[460,500,501] Fewer than 50 cases of successful treatment of fungal prosthetic-valve endocarditis have been reported, even when surgery was performed.[169]

Although a prolonged course of antifungal therapy before surgery does not improve the outcome, chemotherapy should be given in conjunction with operative treatment. The drug of choice is amphotericin B at a dose of 0.5 to 1.0 mg/kg/day. This antibiotic may be either fungistatic or fungicidal, depending on the infecting organism. Even though the toxicity of amphotericin B appears to be less severe in children than in adults, side effects that may necessitate alterations in the usual regimen may occur and include fever, chills, phlebitis, anemia, hypocalcemia, renal tubular acidosis, nephrotoxicity, and thrombocytopenia. The optimal dosage of amphotericin B is unknown; total doses of 20 to 50 mg/kg commonly are used. 5-Fluorocytosine[320] and rifampin may act synergistically with amphotericin B against many strains of fungi, but their roles in fungal endocarditis are unproven. Fluconazole is less effective than is amphotericin B for the prophylaxis or treatment of experimental *Candida* endocarditis,[532] but it has been used successfully in a few patients.[92,508]

Treatment of culture-negative endocarditis is problematic.[27] In general, the same criteria used to choose empiric therapy for infective endocarditis can be followed. Antibiotics usually are continued for 6 weeks, and ongoing surveillance for an etiologic agent must be performed. In 52 adults with culture-negative endocarditis, survival correlated with the initial clinical response to antibiotics; most deaths were caused by systemic emboli or congestive heart failure.[378]

Surgery has become a valuable adjunct to medical therapy in the management of infective endocarditis.[30,365,377,385] Several echocardiographic findings suggest a possible need for surgical intervention[30,145] (Table 32–16). Among the generally accepted indications for surgical intervention during active endocarditis are (1) refractory congestive heart failure,[325,490,528] (2) uncontrolled infection,[304] (3) more than one serious embolic episode, (4) fungal endocarditis, (5) most cases of prosthetic-valve endocarditis,[6,104,128,419,538] and (6) local suppurative complications including perivalvular or myocardial abscess with conduction system abnormalities.[43,411,443,474,535] The usual indication for surgical intervention is congestive heart failure in left-sided lesions and persistent infection in right-sided disease.[106,509] Among children with endocarditis after cardiac surgery, repair or takedown of infected graft material commonly is the reason for surgery.[83,361] In general, operative mortality is low even if surgery is performed during the active infection.[343,355] The hemodynamic status of the patient, rather than the activity of the infection, is the critical factor in determining the timing of cardiac surgery or valve replacement.[3,241] The aortic valve is the site most often requiring surgical intervention.[337,387,494] Treatment with recombinant tissue plasminogen activator has been used successfully in some cases of endocarditis when surgery could not be performed safely.[183,281]

TABLE 32–15 Suggested Therapy for Endocarditis Caused by HACEK Organisms in Adults

Antibiotic(s)	Duration (wk)	Comments
Ceftriaxone sodium	4	Cefotaxime sodium or other third-generation cephalosporins may be substituted
Ampicillin sulbactam *or*	4	
Ciprofloxacin	4	

HACEK, *Haemophilus* species, *Actinobacillus actinomycetemcomitans*, *Cardiobacterium hominis*, *Eikenella corrodens*, *Kingella kingae*.
From Baddour, L. M., Wilson, W. R., Bayer, A. S., et al.: Infective endocarditis: Diagnosis, antimicrobial therapy, and management of complications. Circulation 111: e394-e433, 2005.

TABLE 32–16 Echocardiographic Features Suggesting a Possible Need for Surgical Intervention in Endocarditis

Vegetation
Persistent vegetation after systemic embolization
Anterior mitral valve leaflet vegetation, particularly >10 mm
Embolic event during first 2 weeks of therapy
Increase in vegetation size after 4 weeks of therapy

Valvular Dysfunction
Acute aortic or mitral insufficiency with signs of ventricular failure
Heart failure unresponsive to medical therapy
Valve perforation or rupture

Perivalvular Extension
Valvular dehiscence, rupture, or fistula
New heart block
Large abscess or extension of abscess

Data from Bayer, A.., Bolger, A., Taubert, K., et al.: Diagnosis and management of infective endocarditis and its complications. Circulation 98:2936-2948, 1998; and Ferrieri, P., Gewitz, M. H., Gerber, M. A., et al.: Unique features of infective endocarditis in children. Pediatrics 109:931-943, 2002.

PREVENTION

Accepted medical practice has been to give prophylactic antibiotics to susceptible patients in an attempt to prevent infective endocarditis.[116,248,447] The rationale for such treatment is based on studies indicating that antibiotics can reduce the incidence of bacteremia after various procedures in humans[130] and can prevent experimental endocarditis in animals.[376] However, no controlled trials have documented the efficacy of endocarditis prophylaxis in humans.[505] Prevention of bacterial infection is most likely to be successful and cost-effective when a single antibiotic is directed against a single pathogen and when the disease occurs with high frequency in the absence of prophylaxis. Prevention of endocarditis has not met these ideals because various drugs have been used against numerous organisms, and the disease rarely occurs even if prophylaxis is not given.[116] Fewer than 10 percent of all endocarditis cases can be attributed to bacteremia caused by previous medical, surgical, or dental procedures.[504] Many cases of prophylaxis failure have been reported,[120] but only 12 percent of such patients received antibiotic regimens recommended by the American Heart Association. For reasons that are not clear, mitral valve prolapse was the condition associated most frequently with failure of prophylaxis.

The most common errors in attempted prevention of endocarditis include inadequate medical histories taken by dentists and other health professionals to identify high-risk patients, initiation of prophylactic antibiotics too early, continuation of preventive therapy too long, the use of low-dose antibiotics, lack of prophylaxis for minor dental procedures, and confusion between prevention of rheumatic fever and prevention of infective endocarditis.[187,193] Several studies have shown that adult patients at risk for development of infective endocarditis often have inadequate knowledge of their cardiac lesion, endocarditis, and recommended prophylaxis.[69,261,506] One study demonstrated that the parents of children with heart defects have a low level of knowledge about the importance of good oral health in preventing endocarditis.[103] Another study cast doubt on the cost-effectiveness of endocarditis prophylaxis for urinary catheterization in children.[68]

The American Heart Association published new and radically different guidelines for the prevention of infective endocarditis in 2007.[527] These new guidelines eliminated many of the procedures for which prophylaxis previously was recommended.[94] Now, it is recommended that prophylaxis be undertaken for all dental procedures that involve manipulation of gingival tissue or the periapical region of teeth or perforation of the oral mucosa. Prophylaxis also can be considered for procedures on the respiratory tract or infected skin, skin structures, or musculoskeletal tissue. Prophylaxis no longer is recommended for gastrointestinal or genitourinary tract procedures. In addition, the number of heart lesions for which prophylaxis is recommended has been reduced to only those with the highest risk of endocarditis (Table 32–17).[527] Finally, the specific regimens for prophylaxis have been changed and simplified to encourage more judicious use (Table 32–18). Although immunization against bacteria that commonly cause endocarditis (e.g., viridans streptococci) has been proposed, this approach remains a theoretic possibility.[18]

TABLE 32–17 Heart Conditions with the Highest Risk of Adverse Outcome from Endocarditis for Which Prophylaxis with Dental Procedures Is Recommended

Prosthetic heart valve
Previous infective endocarditis
Congenital heart disease
   Unrepaired cyanotic congenital heart disease, including palliative shunts and conduits
   Completely repaired congenital heart defect with prosthetic material or device, whether placed by surgery or catheter, during the first 6 months after the procedure
   Repaired congenital heart disease with residual defects at or adjacent to the site of a prosthetic patch or device
Cardiac transplantation recipients who develop cardiac valvulopathy

From Wilson, W., Taubert, K. A., Gewitz, M., et al.: Prevention of infective endocarditis: Guidelines from the American Heart Association. Circulation 116: 1736-1754, 2007.

TABLE 32–18 Endocarditis Prophylaxis Regimens for a Dental Procedure

Situation	Agent	Regimen: Single Dose 30-60 min before Procedure	
		Adults	Children
Oral	Amoxicillin	2 g	50 mg/kg
Unable to take oral	Ampicillin	2 g IM or IV	50 mg/kg IM or IV
	or		
	Cefazolin *or* Ceftriaxone	1 g IM or IV	50 mg/kg IM or IV
Allergic to penicillins oral	Cephalexin*	2 g	50 mg/kg
	or		
	Clindamycin	600 mg	20 mg/kg
	or		
	Azithromycin or clarithromycin	500 mg	15 mg/kg
Allergic to penicillins and unable to take oral	Cefazolin	1 g IM or IV	50 mg/kg IM or IV
	or		
	Ceftriaxone*		
	or		
	Clindamycin	600 mg IM or IV	20 mg/kg IM or IV

Cephalosporins not to be used in an individual with a history of anaphylaxis, angioedema, or urticaria with penicillins.
IM, intramuscularly; IV, intravenously.
From Wilson, W., Taubert, K. A., Gewitz, M., et al.: Prevention of infective endocarditis: Guidelines from the American Heart Association. Circulation 116:1736-1754, 2007.

REFERENCES

1. Agarwala, B. N.: Group B streptococcal endocarditis in a neonate. Pediatr. Cardiol. *9*:51-53, 1988.
2. Akhondi, H., and Rahimi, A. R: *Haemophilus aphrophilus* endocarditis after tongue piercing. Emerg. Infect. Dis. *8*:850-851, 2002.
3. Aksoy, O., Sexton, D. J., Wang, A., et al.: Early surgery in patients with infective endocarditis: A propensity score analysis. Clin. Infect. Dis. *44*:364-372, 2007.
4. Al-Hajjar, S., Qadri, S. M. H., Al-Sabban E., and Jager, C.: *Coxiella burnetii* endocarditis in a child. Pediatr. Infect. Dis. J. *16*:911-912, 1997.
5. Alpert, J. S., Krous, H. F., Dalen, J. E., et al.: Pathogenesis of Osler's nodes. Ann. Intern. Med. *85*:471-476, 1976.
6. Alsip, S. G., Blackstone, E. H., Kirklin, J. W., et al.: Indications for cardiac surgery in patients with infective endocarditis. Am. J. Med. *78*:138-142, 1985.
7. Aly, A. M., Simpson, P. M., and Humes, R. A.: The role of transthoracic echocardiography in the diagnosis of infective endocarditis in children. Arch. Pediatr. Adolesc. Med. *153*:950-954, 1999.
8. Anderson, A. W., and Cruickshank, J. G.: Endocarditis due to viridans-type streptococci tolerant to beta-lactam antibiotics: Therapeutic problems. BMJ *285*:85, 1982.
9. Andrews, M. M., and von Reyn, C. F.: Patient selection criteria and management guidelines for outpatient parenteral antibiotic therapy for native valve infective endocarditis. Clin. Infect. Dis. *33*:203-209, 2001.
10. Ang, J. Y., Lua, J. L., Turner, D. R., and Asmar, B. I.: Vancomycin-resistant *Enterococcus faecium* endocarditis in a premature infant successfully treated with Linezolid. Pediatr. Infect. Dis. J. *22*:1101-1103, 2003.
11. Anolik, R., Berkowitz, R. J., Campos, J. M., et al.: *Actinobacillus* endocarditis associated with periodontal disease. Clin. Pediatr. (Phila.) *20*:633-655, 1981.
12. Arber, N., Militano, A., Ben-Yehuda, A., et al.: Native valve *Staphylococcus epidermidis* endocarditis: Report of seven cases and review of the literature. Am. J. Med. *90*:758, 1991.
13. Arber, N., Pras, E., Copperman, Y., et al.: Pacemaker endocarditis: Report of 44 cases and review of the literature. Medicine (Baltimore) *73*:299-305, 1994.
14. Ayres, N. A., Miller-Hance, W., Fyfe, D. A., et al.: Indications and guidelines for performance of transesophageal echocardiography in the patient with pediatric acquired or congenital heart disease. J. Am. Soc. Echocardiogr. *18*:91-98, 2005.
15. Babcock, H. M., Ritchie, D. J., Christiansen, E., et al.: Successful treatment of vancomycin-resistant *Enterococcus* endocarditis with oral linezolid. Clin. Infect. Dis. *32*:1373-1375, 2001.
16. Backes, R. J., Wilson, W. R., and Geraci, J. E.: Group B streptococcal infective endocarditis. Arch. Intern. Med. *145*:693-696, 1985.
17. Baddour, L. M.: Infective endocarditis caused by β-hemolytic streptococci: The Infectious Diseases Society of America's Emerging Infections Network. Clin. Infect. Dis. *26*:66-71, 1998.
18. Baddour, L. M.: Immunization for prevention of infective endocarditis. Curr. Infect. Dis. Rep. *1*:126-128, 1999.
19. Baddour, L. M., and Bisno, A. L.: Infective endocarditis complicating mitral valve prolapse: Epidemiologic, clinical and microbiological aspects. Rev. Infect. Dis. *8*:117-137, 1986.
20. Baddour, L. M., Christensen, G. D., Lowrance, J. H., et al.: Pathogenesis of experimental endocarditis. Rev. Infect. Dis. *11*:452-463, 1989.
21. Baddour, L. M., Lowrance, C., Albus, A., et al.: *Staphylococcus aureus* microcapsule expression attenuates bacterial virulence in a rat model of experimental endocarditis. J. Infect. Dis. *165*:749-753, 1992.
22. Baddour, L. M., Meyer, J., and Henry, B.: Polymicrobial infective endocarditis in the 1980's. Rev. Infect. Dis. *13*:963-970, 1991.
23. Baddour, L. M., Phillips, T. N., and Bisno, A. L.: Coagulase-negative staphylococcal endocarditis: Occurrence in patients with mitral valve prolapse. Arch. Intern. Med. *146*:119-121, 1986.
24. Baddour, L. M., Wilson, W. R., Bayer, A. S., et al.: Infective endocarditis. Diagnosis, antimicrobial therapy and management of complications. Circulation *111*:e394-e433, 2005.
25. Baltimore, R. S.: Infective endocarditis in children. Pediatr. Infect. Dis. J. *11*:907-912, 1992.
26. Baorto, E., Payne, M., Slater, L., et al.: Culture-negative endocarditis caused by *Bartonella henselae*. J. Pediatr. *132*:1051-1054, 1998.
27. Barnes, P. D., and Crook, D. W. M.: Culture negative endocarditis. J. Infect. *35*:209-213, 1997.
28. Barst, R. J., Prince, A. S., and Neu, H. C.: *Aspergillus* endocarditis: Case report and review of the literature. Pediatrics *68*:73-78, 1981.
29. Barst, R. J., Prince, A. S., and Neu, H. C.: Echocardiography in *Aspergillus* endocarditis. Pediatrics *69*:252-253, 1982.
30. Bayer, A. S., Bolger, A., Taubert, K., et al.: Diagnosis and management of infective endocarditis and its complications. Circulation *98*:2936-2948, 1998.
31. Bayer, A. S.: Infective endocarditis. Clin. Infect. Dis. *17*:313-332, 1993.
32. Bayer, A. S., and Theofilopoulos, A. N.: Immunopathogenetic aspects of infective endocarditis. Chest *97*:204-210, 1990.
33. Bayer, A. S., Chow, A. W., and Guze, L. B.: *Listeria monocytogenes* endocarditis: Report of a case and review of the literature. Am. J. Med. Sci. *273*:319-323, 1977.
34. Bayer, A. S., Nelson, R. J., and Slama, T. G.: Current concepts in prevention of prosthetic valve endocarditis. Chest *97*:1203-1207, 1990.
35. Bayer, A. S., Theofilopoulos, A. N., Dixon, F. J., et al.: Circulating immune complexes in experimental streptococcal endocarditis: A monitor of therapeutic efficacy. J. Infect. Dis. *139*:1-8, 1979.
36. Bayer, A. S., Theofilopoulos, A. N., Eisenberg, R., et al.: Circulating immune complexes in infective endocarditis. N. Engl. J. Med. *295*:1500-1505, 1976.
37. Beeson, P. B., Brannon, E. S., and Warren, J. V.: Observations on the sites of removal of bacteria from the blood in patients with bacterial endocarditis. J. Exp. Med. *81*:9-23, 1945.
38. Belmares, J., Detterline, S., Pak, J. B., and Parada, J. P.: Corynebacterium endocarditis species-specific risk factors and outcomes. B. C. M. Infect. Dis. *7*:4, 2007.
39. Berkowitz, F. E., and Dansky, R.: Infective endocarditis in black South African children: Report of 10 cases with some unusual features. Pediatr. Infect. Dis. J. *8*:787-791, 1989.
40. Bertorini, T. E., Laster, R. E., Thompson, B. F., et al.: Magnetic resonance imaging of the brain in bacterial endocarditis. Arch. Intern. Med. *149*:815-817, 1989.
41. Bieger, R. C., Brewer, N. S., and Washington, J. A.: *Haemophilus aphrophilus*: A microbiological and clinical review and report of 42 cases. Medicine (Baltimore) *57*:345-355, 1978.
42. Biller, J., Challa, V. R., Toole, J. F., et al.: Nonbacterial thrombotic endocarditis: A neurologic perspective of clinicopathologic correlations of 99 patients. Arch. Neurol. *39*:95-98, 1982.
43. Bishara, J., Leibovici, L., Gartman-Israel, D., et al.: Long-term outcome of infective endocarditis: The impact of early surgical intervention. Clin. Infect. Dis. *33*:1636-1643, 2001.
44. Bisno, A. L., Dismukes, W. E., Durack, D. T., et al.: Antimicrobial treatment of infective endocarditis due to viridans streptococci, enterococci and staphylococci. JAMA *261*:1471-1477, 1989.
45. Blair, D. C., and Martin, D. B.: Beta hemolytic streptococcal endocarditis: Predominance of non–group A organisms. Am. J. Med. Sci. *276*:269-277, 1978.
46. Blieden, L. C., Morehead, R. R., Burke, B., et al.: Bacterial endocarditis in the neonate. Am. J. Dis. Child. *124*:747-749, 1972.
47. Blumberg, E. A., Karlis, D. A., Chandrasekaran K., et al.: Endocarditis-associated paravalvular abscesses. Chest *107*:898-903, 1995.
48. Blumberg, E. A., Robbins, N., Adimora A., et al.: Persistent fever in association with infective endocarditis. Clin. Infect. Dis. *15*:983-990, 1992.
49. Blumenthal, S., Griffiths, S. P., and Morgan, B. C.: Bacterial endocarditis in children with heart disease: A review based on the literature and experience with 58 cases. Pediatrics *26*:993-1017, 1960.
50. Bodey, G. P., and Luna, M.: Skin lesions associated with disseminated candidiasis. JAMA *229*:1466-1468, 1974.
51. Bosshard, P. P., Kronenberg, A., Zbinden, R., et al.: Etiologic diagnosis of infective endocarditis by broad-range polymerase chain reaction: A 3-year experience. Clin. Infect. Dis. *37*:167-172, 2003.
52. Bricker, J., Latson, L., Huhta, J., et al.: Echocardiographic evaluation of infective endocarditis in children. Clin. Pediatr. (Phila.) *24*:312-319, 1985.
53. Brodie, E., Adler, J. L., and Daly, A. K.: Bacterial endocarditis due to an unusual species of encapsulated *Neisseria*. Am. J. Dis. Child. *122*:433-437, 1972.
54. Brouqui, P., Dumler, J. S., and Raoult, D.: Immunohistologic demonstration of *Coxiella burnetii* in the valves of patients with Q fever endocarditis. Am. J. Med. *97*:451-458, 1994.
55. Brouqui, P., and Raoult, D.: Endocarditis due to rare and fastidious bacteria. Clin. Microbiol. Rev. *14*:177-207, 2001.
56. Bruyn, G. A. W., Thompson, J., and Van Der Meer, J. W. M.: Pneumococcal endocarditis in adult patients: A report of five cases and review of the literature. Q. J. Med. *74*:33-40, 1990.
57. Calderwood, S., Swinski, L., Waternaux, C., et al.: Risk factors for the development of prosthetic valve endocarditis. Circulation *72*:31-37, 1985.
58. Caldwell, R. L., Hurwitz, R. A., and Girod, D. A.: Subacute bacterial endocarditis in children. Am. J. Dis. Child. *122*:312-315, 1971.
59. Canter, M. C., and Hart, R. G.: Neurologic complications of infective endocarditis. Neurology *41*:1015, 1991.
60. Carey, R. B., Gross, K. C., and Roberts, R. B.: Vitamin B_6–dependent *Streptococcus mitior* (*mitis*) isolated from patients with systemic infections. J. Infect. Dis. *131*:722-725, 1975.
61. Caron, F., Carbon, C., and Gutmann, L.: Triple-combination penicillin-vancomycin-gentamicin for experimental endocarditis caused by a moderately penicillin- and highly glycopeptide-resistant isolate of *Enterococcus faecium*. J. Infect. Dis. *164*:888-893, 1991.
62. Carpenter, J. L.: Perivalvular extension of infection in patients with infectious endocarditis. Rev. Infect. Dis. *13*:127-138, 1991.
63. Carr, P., Wright, M., and Handler, L. C.: Endocarditis-related cerebral aneurysms: Radiologic changes with treatment. AJNR Am. J. Neuroradiol. *16*:745, 1995.
64. Carrizosa, J., and Kaye, D.: Antibiotic concentrations in serum, serum bactericidal activity, and results of therapy of streptococcal endocarditis in rabbits. Antimicrob. Agents Chemother. *12*:479-483, 1977.
65. Carruthers, M.: Endocarditis due to enteric bacilli other than salmonellae: Case reports and literature review. Am. J. Med. Sci. *273*:203, 1977.

66. Carvajal, A., and Frederiksen, W.: Fatal endocarditis due to *Listeria monocytogenes*. Rev. Infect. Dis. *10*:616-623, 1988.

67. Cassling, R. S., Rogler, W. C., and McManus, B. M.: Isolated pulmonic valve infective endocarditis: A diagnostically elusive entity. Am. Heart J. *109*:558-567, 1985.

68. Caviness, A. C., Cantor, S. B., Allen, C. H., and Ward, M. A.: A cost-effectiveness analysis of bacterial endocarditis prophylaxis for febrile children who have cardiac lesions and undergo urinary catheterization in the emergency department. Pediatrics *113*:1291-1296, 2004.

69. Cetta, F., and Warnes, C. A.: Adults with congenital heart disease: Patient knowledge of endocarditis prophylaxis. Mayo Clin. Proc. *70*:50-54, 1995.

70. Chambers, H. F., Korzeniowski, O. M., Sande, M. A., et al.: *Staphylococcus aureus* endocarditis: Clinical manifestation in addicts and non-addicts. Medicine (Baltimore) *62*:170-174, 1983.

71. Chambers, H. F., Miller, R. T., and Newman, M. D.: Right-sided *Staphylococcus aureus* endocarditis in intravenous drug abusers: Two-week combination therapy. Ann. Intern. Med. *109*:619-624, 1988.

72. Chang, H. H., Lu, C. Y., Hsueh, P. R., et al.: Endocarditis caused by *Abiotrophia defectiva* in children. Pediatr. Infect. Dis. J. *21*:697-700, 2002.

73. Channer, K. S., Joffe, H. S., and Jordan, S. C.: Presentation of infective endocarditis in childhood and adolescence. J. R. Coll. Physicians Lond. *23*:152-155, 1989.

74. Charney, R., Keltz, T. N., Attai, L., et al.: Acute valvular obstruction from streptococcal endocarditis. Am. Heart J. *125*:544, 1993.

75. Chatzis, A. C., Saroglou, G., Giannopoulos, N. M., and Sarris, G. E.: Subtle infective endocarditis and congenital heart disease. Cardiol. Young *15*:617-620, 2005.

76. Chen, M. R.: Infective endocarditis in hypertrophic obstructive cardiomyopathy. J. Clin. Ultrasound *20*:612-614, 1992.

77. Chirouze, C., Cabell, C. H., Fowler, V. G., Jr., et al.: Prognostic factors in 61 cases of *Staphylococcus aureus* prosthetic valve infective endocarditis from the International Collaboration on Endocarditis Merged Database. Clin. Infect. Dis. *38*:1323-1327, 2004.

78. Choi, M., and Mailman, T. L.: Pneumococcal endocarditis in infants and children. Pediatr. Infect. Dis. J. *23*:166-171, 2004.

79. Chu, V. H., Cabell, C. H., Abrutyn, E., et al.: Native valve endocarditis due to coagulase-negative staphylococci: Report of 99 episodes from the International Collaboration on Endocarditis Merged Database. Clin. Infect. Dis. *39*:1527-1530, 2004.

80. Chu, V. H., Woods, C. W., Miro, J. M., et al.: Emergence of coagulase-negative staphylococci as a cause of native valve endocarditis. Clin. Infect. Dis. *46*:232-242, 2008.

81. Chunn, C. J., Jones, S. R., McCutchan, J. A., et al.: *Haemophilus parainfluenzae* infective endocarditis. Medicine (Baltimore) *56*:99-113, 1977.

82. Churchill, M. A., Geraci, J. E., and Hunder, G. G.: Musculoskeletal manifestations of bacterial endocarditis. Ann. Intern. Med. *87*:754-759, 1977.

83. Citak, M., Rees, A., and Mavroudis, C.: Surgical management of infective endocarditis in children. Ann. Thorac. Surg. *54*:755-758, 1992.

84. Clawson, C. C., Rao Gunda, H. R., and White, J. G.: Platelet interaction with bacteria. IV. Stimulation of the release reaction. Am. J. Pathol. *81*:411-417, 1975.

85. Clemens, J. O., Horwitz, R. I., Jaffee, C. C., et al.: A controlled evaluation of the risk of bacterial endocarditis in persons with mitral-valve prolapse. N. Engl. J. Med. *307*:776-781, 1982.

86. Cofsky, R. D., and Seligman, S. J.: *Peptococcus magnus* endocarditis. South. Med. J. *78*:361-362, 1985.

87. Coleman, D. L., Horwitz, R. I., and Andriole, V. T.: Association between serum inhibitory and bactericidal concentrations and therapeutic outcome in bacterial endocarditis. Am. J. Med. *73*:260-267, 1982.

88. Corrigan, D., Bolen, J., Hancock, E. W., et al.: Mitral valve prolapse and endocarditis. Am. J. Med. *63*:315-318, 1977.

89. Coward, K., Tucker, N., and Darville, T.: Infective endocarditis in Arkansan children from 1990 through 2002. Pediatr. Infect. Dis. J. *22*:1048-1052, 2003.

90. Cremieux, A. C., and Carbon, C.: Pharmacokinetics and pharmacodynamic requirements for antibiotic therapy of experimental endocarditis. Antimicrob. Agents Chemother. *36*:2069-2074, 1992.

91. Cutler, J. G., Ongley, P. A., Schwachman, H., et al.: Bacterial endocarditis in children with heart disease. Pediatrics *22*:706-714, 1958.

92. Czwerwiec, F. S., Bilsker, M. S., Kamerman, M. L., et al.: Long-term survival after fluconazole therapy of candidal prosthetic valve endocarditis. Am. J. Med. *94*:545-546, 1993.

93. Daher, A. H., and Berkowitz, F. E.: Infective endocarditis in neonates. Clin. Pediatr. (Phila.) *20*:198-206, 1995.

94. Dajani, A. S., Taubert, K. A., Wilson, W., et al.: Prevention of bacterial endocarditis: Recommendations by the American Heart Association. Clin. Infect. Dis. *75*:1448-1458, 1997.

95. Danchin, N., Voiriot, P., Briancon, S., et al.: Mitral valve prolapse as a risk factor for infective endocarditis. Lancet *1*:743-745, 1989.

96. Danford, D. A., Kugler, J. D., Cheatham, J. P., et al.: *Haemophilus influenzae* endocarditis: Successful treatment with ampicillin and early valve replacement. Neb. Med. J. *38*:88-91, 1984.

97. Daniel, W. G., Erbel, R., Kasper, W., et al.: Safety of transesophageal echocardiography: A multicenter survey of 10,419 examinations. Circulation *83*:817-821, 1991.

98. Daniel, W. G., Mugge, A., Grote, J., et al.: Evaluation of endocarditis and its complications by biplane and multiplane transesophageal echocardiography. Am. J. Card. Imaging *9*:100-105, 1995.

99. Daniel, W. G., Mugge, A., Martin, R. P., et al.: Improvement in the diagnosis of abscesses associated with endocarditis by transesophageal echocardiography. N. Engl. J. Med. *324*:795-800, 1991.

100. Dankert, J., Krijgsveld, J., van der Werff, J., et al.: Platelet microbicidal activity is an important defense factor against viridans streptococcal endocarditis. J. Infect. Dis. *184*:597-605, 2001.

101. Das, I., DeGiovanni, J. V., and Gray, J.: Endocarditis caused by *Haemophilus parainfluenzae* identified by 16 S ribosomal RNA sequencing. J. Clin. Pathol. *50*:72-74, 1997.

102. Das, M., Badley, A. D., Cockerill, F. R., et al.: Infective endocarditis caused by HACEK microorganisms. Annu. Rev. Med. *48*:25-33, 1997.

103. da Silva, D. B., Sovza, I. P., and Cunha, M. C.: Knowledge, attitudes and status of oral health in children at risk for infective endocarditis. Int. J. Pediatr. Dent. *12*:124-131, 2002.

104. David, T. E.: The surgical treatment of patients with prosthetic valve endocarditis. Semin. Thorac. Cardiovasc. Surg. *7*:47-53, 1995.

105. Davidson, S., Rotem, Y., Bogkowski, B., et al.: *Corynebacterium diphtheriae* endocarditis. Am. J. Med. Sci. *271*:351-353, 1976.

106. Delmo Walter, E. M., Musci, M., Nagdyman, N., et al.: Mitral valve repair for infective endocarditis in children. Ann. Thorac. Surg. *84*:2059-2065, 2007.

107. Del Pont, J. M., DeCicco, L. T., Vartalitis, C., et al.: Infective endocarditis in children: Clinical analyses and evaluation of two diagnostic criteria. Pediatr. Infect. Dis. J. *14*:1079-1086, 1995.

108. Delvecchio, G., Fracasetti, O., and Lorenzi N.: *Brucella* endocarditis. Int. J. Cardiol. *33*:328-329, 1991.

109. Dillon, T., Meyer, R. A., Korfhagen, J. C., et al.: Management of infective endocarditis using echocardiography. J. Pediatr. *96*:552-558, 1980.

110. DiNubile, M. J.: Treatment of endocarditis caused by relatively resistant non-enterococcal streptococci: Is penicillin enough? Rev. Infect. Dis. *12*:112-117, 1990.

111. DiNubile, M. J., Calderwood, S. B., Steinhaus, D. M., et al.: Cardiac conduction abnormalities complicating native valve active infective endocarditis. Am. J. Cardiol. *58*:1213-1217, 1986.

112. Dominguez, S. R., Littlehorn, C., and Nyquist, A. C.: *Mycoplasma hominis* endocarditis in a child with complex congenital heart disease. Pediatr. Infect. Dis. J. *25*:851-852, 2006.

113. Douglas, A., Moore-Gillon, J., and Eykyn, S.: Fever during treatment of infective endocarditis. Lancet *1*:1341-1343, 1986.

114. Downing, G. J., and Spirazza, C.: Group C beta-hemolytic streptococcal endocarditis. Pediatr. Infect. Dis. J. *5*:703-704, 1986.

115. Drancourt, M., Mainardi, J. L., Brouqui, P., et al.: *Bartonella (Rochalimaea) quintana* endocarditis in three homeless men. N. Engl. J. Med. *332*:419-423, 1995.

116. Durack, D. T.: Prevention of infective endocarditis. N. Engl. J. Med. *332*:38-44, 1995.

117. Durack, D. T., and Beeson, P. B.: Protective role of complement in experimental *Escherichia coli* endocarditis. Infect. Immun. *16*:213-214, 1977.

118. Durack, D. T., and Petersdorf, R. G.: Changes in the epidemiology of endocarditis. *In* Kaplan, E. L., Taranta, A. V. (eds.): Infective Endocarditis: An American Heart Association Symposium. Dallas, American Heart Association, 1977, p. 3.

119. Durack, D. T., Beeson, P. B., and Petersdorf, R. G.: Experimental bacterial endocarditis. III. Production and progress of the disease in rabbits. Br. J. Exp. Pathol. *54*:142-151, 1973.

120. Durack, D. T., Kaplan, E. L., and Bisno, A. L.: Apparent failure of endocarditis prophylaxis: Analysis of 52 cases submitted to a national registry. JAMA *250*:2318-2322, 1983.

121. Durack, D. T., Lukes, A. S., Bright, D. K., et al.: New criteria for diagnosis of infective endocarditis: Utilization of specific echocardiographic findings. Am. J. Med. *96*:200-209, 1994.

122. Durack, D. T., Pelletier, L. L., and Petersdorf, R. G.: Chemotherapy of experimental streptococcal endocarditis. II. Synergism between penicillin and streptomycin against penicillin-sensitive streptococci. J. Clin. Invest. *53*:829-836, 1974.

123. Edwards, K., Hruby, N., and Christy, C.: Pneumococcal endocarditis in infants and children: Report of a case and review of the literature. Pediatr. Infect. Dis. J. *9*:652-657, 1990.

124. Eliopoulos, G. M., Thauvin-Eliopoulos, C., and Moellering, R. C., Jr.: Contribution of animal models in the search for effective therapy for endocarditis due to enterococci with high-level resistance to gentamicin. Clin. Infect. Dis. *15*:58-62, 1992.

125. Ellis, M. E., Al-Abdely, H., Sandridge, A., et al.: Fungal endocarditis: Evidence in the world literature, 1965-1995. Clin. Infect. Dis. *32*:50-62, 2001.

126. Elward, K., Hruby, N., and Christy, C.: Pneumococcal endocarditis in infants and children: Report of a case and review of the literature. Pediatr. Infect. Dis. J. *9*:652-657, 1990.

127. Enzler, M. J., Rouse, M. S., Henry, N. K., et al.: In vitro and in vivo studies of streptomycin-resistant, penicillin-susceptible streptococci from patients with infective endocarditis. J. Infect. Dis. *155*:954-958, 1987.

128. Ergin, M. A.: Surgical techniques in prosthetic valve endocarditis. Semin. Thorac. Cardiovasc. Surg. *7*:54-56, 1995.

129. Esperson, F., and Frimodt-Moller, N.: *Staphylococcus aureus* endocarditis: A review of 119 cases. Arch. Intern. Med. *146*:1118-1121, 1986.

130. Everett, E. D., and Hirschmann, J. U.: Transient bacteremia and endocarditis prophylaxis: A review. Medicine (Baltimore) *56*:61-77, 1977.

131. Fang, G., Keys, T. F., Gentry, L. O., et al.: Prosthetic valve endocarditis resulting from nosocomial bacteremia. Ann. Intern. Med. *119*:560, 1993.

132. Farmaki, E., Roilides, E., Darilis, E., et al.: *Gemella morbillorum* in a child. Pediatr. Infect. Dis. J. *19*:751-753, 2000.

133. Farrior, J. B., and Silverman, M. E.: A consideration of the differences between a Janeway lesion and an Osler's node in infectious endocarditis. Chest *70*:239-243, 1976.

134. Faville, R. J., Zaska, D. E., Kaplan, E. L., et al.: *Staphylococcus aureus* endocarditis: Combined therapy with vancomycin and rifampin. JAMA *240*:1963-1965, 1978.

135. Feder, H. M., Jr., Chameides, L., and Diana, D. J.: Bacterial endocarditis complicated by myocardial infarction in a pediatric patient. JAMA *247*:1315-1316, 1982.

136. Feder, H. M., Jr., Olsen, N., McLaughlin, J. C., et al.: Bacterial endocarditis caused by vitamin B$_6$–dependent viridans group *Streptococcus*. Pediatrics *66*:309-312, 1980.

137. Feder, H. M., Jr., Roberts, J. C., Salazar, J. C., et al.: HACEK endocarditis in infants and children: Two cases and a literature review. Pediatr. Infect. Dis. J. *22*:557-562, 2003.

138. Felius, A., Fleer, A., and Mouloert, A.: *Actinobacillus actinomycetemcomitans* endocarditis in a child with a prosthetic heart valve. Infection *12*:260-261, 1984.

139. Felmer, J. M., and Dowell, V. R.: Anaerobic bacterial endocarditis. N. Engl. J. Med. *283*:1188-1192, 1970.

140. Fenollar, F., Lepidi, H., and Raoult, D.: Whipple's endocarditis: Review of the literature and comparisons with Q fever, *Bartonella* infection and blood culture-positive endocarditis. Clin. Infect. Dis. *33*:1309-1316, 2001.

141. Fernandez, G. C., Chapman, A. J., Bolli, R., et al.: Gonococcal endocarditis: A case series demonstrating modern presentation of an old disease. Am. Heart J. *108*:1326-1334, 1984.

142. Fernandez-Guerrero, M. L., Torres-Perea, R., Gomez-Rodrigo, J., et al.: Infectious endocarditis due to non–*typhi Salmonella* in patients infected with human immunodeficiency virus: Report of two cases and review. Clin. Infect. Dis. *22*:853-855, 1996.

143. Fernandez-Guerrero, M. L., Verdejo, C., Azofra, J., et al.: Hospital-acquired infectious endocarditis not associated with cardiac surgery: An emerging problem. Clin. Infect. Dis. *20*:16-23, 1995.

144. Fernicola, D. J., and Roberts, W. C.: Clinicopathologic features of active infective endocarditis isolated to the native mitral valve. Am. J. Cardiol. *71*:1186-1197, 1993.

145. Ferrieri, P., Gewitz, M. H., Gerber, M. A., et al.: Unique features of infective endocarditis in children. Pediatrics *109*:931-943, 2002.

146. Fichtenbaum, C. H., and Smith, M. J.: Treatment of endocarditis due to *Pseudomonas aeruginosa* with imipenem. Clin. Infect. Dis. *14*:353-354, 1992.

147. Fisher, R. G., Moodie, D. S., and Rice, R.: Pediatric bacterial endocarditis: Long-term follow-up. Cleve. Clin. Q. *52*:41-45, 1985.

148. Fournier, P. E., and Raoult, D.: Non-culture laboratory methods for the diagnosis of infectious endocarditis. Curr. Infect. Dis. Rep. *1*:136-141, 1999.

149. Fournier, P. E., Lelievre, H., Eykyn, S. J., et al.: Epidemiologic and clinical characteristics of *Bartonella henselae* endocarditis: A study of 48 patients. Medicine (Baltimore) *80*:245-251, 2001.

150. Fowler, V. G., Jr., Boucher, H. W., Corey, G. R., et al.: Daptomycin versus standard therapy for bacteremia and endocarditis caused by *Staphylococcus aureus*. N. Engl. J. Med. *355*:653-665, 2006.

151. Fowler, V. G., Jr., Miro, J. M., Hoen, B., et al.: *Staphylococcus aureus* endocarditis. A consequence of medical progress. JAMA *293*:3012-3021, 2005.

152. Fowler, V. G., Jr., Sanders, L. C., Kong, L. K., et al.: Infective endocarditis due to *Staphylococcus aureus*: 59 prospectively identified cases with follow-up. Clin. Infect. Dis. *28*:106-114, 1999.

153. Francioli, P., Etienne, J., Hoigue, R., et al.: Treatment of streptococcal endocarditis with a single daily dose of ceftriaxone sodium for 4 weeks: Efficacy and outpatient treatment feasibility. JAMA *267*:264-267, 1992.

154. Francioli, P., Ruch, W., Stamboulian, D., et al.: Treatment of streptococcal endocarditis with a single daily dose of ceftriaxone and netilmicin for 14 days: A prospective multicenter study. Clin. Infect. Dis. *21*:1406-1410, 1995.

155. Frontera, J. A., and Gradon, J. D.: Right-side endocarditis in injection drug users: Review of proposed mechanisms of pathogenesis. Clin. Infect. Dis. *30*:374-379, 2000.

156. Fukushige, J., Igarashi, H., and Veda, K.: Spectrum of infective endocarditis during infancy and childhood: 20-year review. Pediatr. Cardiol. *15*:127-131, 1994.

157. Galil, K., Thurer, R., Glatter, K., et al.: Disseminated *Mycobacterium chelonae* infection resulting in endocarditis. Clin. Infect. Dis. *23*:1322-1323, 1996.

158. Gallagher, P. G., and Watanakunakorn, C.: Group B streptococcal endocarditis: Report of seven cases and review of the literature. Rev. Infect. Dis. *8*:175-188, 1986.

159. Garcia-Teresa, M. A., Casado-Flores, J., Dominguez, M. A. D., et al.: Infectious complications of percutaneous central venous catheterization in pediatric patients. Intensive Care Med. *33*:466-476, 2007.

160. Garty, B., Berant, M., Weinhouse, E., et al.: False aneurysm of the right ventricle due to endocarditis in a child. Pediatr. Cardiol. *8*:275-277, 1987.

161. Gauduchon, V., Benito, Y., Celard, M., et al.: Molecular diagnosis of recurrent *Streptococcus mutans* endocarditis by PCR amplification and sequencing. Clin. Microbiol. Infect. 7:36-37, 2001.

162. Gelfand, M. S., and Threlkeld, M. G.: Subacute bacterial endocarditis secondary to *Streptococcus pneumoniae*. Am. J. Med. *93*:91, 1992.

163. Gelfman, R., and Levine, S. A.: The incidence of acute and subacute bacterial endocarditis in congenital heart disease. Am. J. Med. Sci. *204*:324-333, 1942.

164. Geraci, J. E., and Wilson, W. R.: Endocarditis due to gram-negative bacteria. Mayo Clin. Proc. *57*:145-148, 1982.

165. Gersony, W. M., and Hayes, C. J.: Bacterial endocarditis in patients with pulmonary stenosis, aortic stenosis or ventricular septal defect. Circulation *56*:84-89, 1977.

166. Gersony, W. M., Hayes, C. J., Driscoll, D. J., et al.: Bacterial endocarditis in patients with aortic stenosis, pulmonary stenosis, or ventricular septal defect. Circulation *87*(Suppl. 1):121-126, 1993.

167. Geva, T., and Frand, M.: Infective endocarditis in children with congenital heart disease: The changing spectrum, 1965-85. Eur. Heart J. *9*:1244-1249, 1988.

168. Ghann, J. W., and Dismukes, W. E.: Prosthetic valve endocarditis: An overview. Kardiovaskulare Erkrankungan *8*:320-331, 1983.

169. Gilbert, H. M., Peters, E. D., Lang, S. J., et al.: Successful treatment of fungal prosthetic valve endocarditis: Case report and review. Clin. Infect. Dis. *22*:348-354, 1996.

170. Gil-Grande, R., Aguado, J. M., Pastor, C., et al.: Conventional viral cultures and shell vial assay for diagnosis of apparently culture-negative *Coxiella burnetii* endocarditis. Eur. J. Clin. Microbiol. Infect. Dis. *14*:64-67, 1995.

171. Givner, L. B., Mason, E. O., Jr., Tan, T. Q., et al.: Pneumococcal endocarditis in children. Clin. Infect. Dis. *38*:1273-1278, 2004.

172. Glauser, M. P., Bernard, J. P., Moreillon, P., et al.: Successful single-dose amoxicillin prophylaxis against experimental streptococcal endocarditis: Evidence for two mechanisms of protection. J. Infect. Dis. *147*:568-575, 1983.

173. Goessler, M C., Riggs, T. W., DeLeon, S., et al.: Echocardiographic diagnosis of tricuspid valve endocarditis in a child with a normal heart. Pediatr. Cardiol. *2*:141-143, 1982.

174. Goldberg, P., Shulman, S. T., and Yogev, R.: Group C streptococcal endocarditis. Pediatrics *75*:114-116, 1985.

175. Goldenberg, D., Kunzli, A., Vogt, P., et al.: Molecular diagnosis of bacterial endocarditis by broad-range PCR amplification and direct sequencing. J. Clin. Microbiol. *35*:2733-2739, 1997.

176. Gorby, G. L., and Peacock, J. E.: *Erysipelothrix rhusiopathiae* endocarditis: Microbiologic, epidemiologic and clinical features of an occupational disease. Rev. Infect. Dis. *10*:317-325, 1988.

177. Gotsman, I., Meirovitz, A., Meizlish, N., et al.: Clinical and echocardiographic predictors of morbidity and mortality in infective endocarditis: The significance of vegetation size. Isr. Med. Assoc. J. *9*:365-369, 2007.

178. Gould, K., Ramirez-Ronda, C. H., Holmes, R. K., et al.: Adherence of bacteria to heart valves in vitro. J. Clin. Invest. *56*:1364-1370, 1975.

179. Gradon, J. D., Chapnick, E. K., and Lutwick, L. I.: Infective endocarditis of a native valve due to *Acinetobacter*: Case report and review. Clin. Infect. Dis. *14*:1145-1148, 1992.

180. Gransden, W. R., Eykyn, S. J., and Leach, R. M.: Neurologic presentations of native valve endocarditis. Q. J. Med. *73*:1135-1142, 1989.

181. Griffiths, J. K., Daly, J. S., and Dodge, R. A.: Two cases of endocarditis due to *Lactobacillus* species: Antimicrobial susceptibility, review and discussion of therapy. Clin. Infect. Dis. *15*:250-255, 1992.

182. Guard, R. W.: Non-toxigenic *Corynebacterium diphtheriae* causing subacute bacterial endocarditis: Case report. Pathology *11*:533-535, 1979.

183. Gunes, A. M., Bostan, O. M., Bayton, B., and Semizel, E.: Treatment of infective endocarditis with recombinant tissue plasminogen activator. Pediatr. Blood Cancer *50*:132-134, 2008.

184. Gutman, R. A., Striker, G. E., Gilliland, B. C., et al.: The immune complex glomerulonephritis of bacterial endocarditis. Medicine (Baltimore) *51*:1-5, 1972.

185. Guzman-Cottrill, J. A., Zheng, X., and Chadwick, E. G.: *Fuserium solani* endocarditis successfully treated with liposomal amphotericin B and voriconazole. Pediatr. Infect. Dis. J. *23*:1059-1061, 2004.

186. Hall, B., and Dowling, H. F.: Negative blood cultures in bacterial endocarditis: A decade's experience. Med. Clin. North Am. *50*:159-170, 1966.

187. Hall, G., Heimdahl, A., and Nord, C. E.: Bacteremia after oral surgery and antibiotic prophylaxis for endocarditis. Clin. Infect. Dis. *29*:1-10, 1999.

188. Hall, L. H., and Herndon, B. L.: Association of cell adherent glycocalyx and endocarditis production by viridans group streptococci. J. Clin. Microbiol. *28*:1698-1700, 1990.

189. Hamoudi, A. C., Hriban, M. M., Marcon, M. J., et al.: Clinical relevance of viridans and nonhemolytic streptococci isolated from blood and cerebrospinal fluid in a pediatric population. Am J. Clin. Pathol. *93*:270, 1990.

190. Hampton, J. R., and Harrison, M. J.: Sterile blood cultures in bacterial endocarditis. Q. J. Med. *36*:167-174, 1967.

191. Hart, R. G., Foster, J. W., Luther, M. F., et al.: Stroke in infective endocarditis. Stroke *21*:695-700, 1990.

192. Hayek, L. J. H. E.: *Erysipelothrix* endocarditis affecting a porcine xenograft heart valve. J. Infect. *27*:203, 1993.

193. Hayes, P. A., and Fasules, J.: Dental screening of pediatric cardiac surgical patients. A. S. D. C. J. Dent. Child. *68*:255-258, 2001.

194. Heiddal, S., Sverrisson, J. T., Ynguason, E. E., et al.: Native-valve endocarditis due to *Neisseria sicca*: Case report and review. Clin. Infect. Dis. *16*:667-670, 1993.

195. Hellinger, W. C., Rouse, M. S., Robadan, P. M., et al.: Continuous intravenous versus intermittent ampicillin therapy of experimental endocarditis caused by aminoglycoside-resistant enterococci. Antimicrob. Agents Chemother. *36*:1272-1275, 1992.

196. Herbert, M. A., Milford, D. V., Silove, E. D., et al.: Secondary amyloidosis from long-standing bacterial endocarditis. Pediatr. Nephrol. *9*:33-35, 1995.

197. Herzberg, M. C., Brintzenhote, K. C., and Clawson, C. C.: Aggregation of human platelets and adhesion of *Streptococcus sanguis*. Infect. Immun. *39*:1457-1469, 1983.

198. Herzberg, M. C., MacFarlane, G. D., Gong, K. et al.: The platelet interactivity phenotype of *Streptococcus sanguis* influences the course of experimental endocarditis. Infect. Immun. *60*:4809-4818, 1992.

199. Hickey, A. J., MacMahon, S. W., and Wilcken, D. E. L.: Mitral valve prolapse and bacterial endocarditis: When is antibiotic prophylaxis necessary? Am. Heart J. *109*:431-435, 1985.

200. Hoen, B., Selton-Suty, C., Danchin, N., et al.: Evaluation of the Duke criteria versus the Beth Israel criteria for the diagnosis of infective endocarditis. Clin. Infect. Dis. *21*:905, 1995.

201. Hoen, B., Selton-Suty, C., Lacassin, F., et al.: Infective endocarditis in patients with negative blood cultures: Analysis of 88 cases from a one-year nationwide survey in France. Clin. Infect. Dis. *20*:501-506, 1995.

202. Holland, F., II, Fernandez, L., Jacobs, J., and Bolooki, H.: Clostridial endocarditis following penetrating cardiac trauma. Clin. Infect. Dis. *24*:87-88, 1997.

203. Horenstein, M. S., Humes, R., Epstein, M. L., and Draper, D.: Loeffler's endocarditis presenting in 2 children as fever with eosinophilia. Pediatrics *110*:1014-1018, 2002.

204. Horwitz, D., Quismorio, F. P., and Friou, G. J.: Cryoglobulinemia in patients with infective endocarditis. Clin. Exp. Immunol. *19*:131-137, 1975.

205. Hosea, S. W.: Virulent *Streptococcus viridans* bacterial endocarditis. Am. Heart J. *101*:174-176, 1981.

206. Hoshimo, T., Ohkusu, K., Sudo, F., et al.: *Neisseria elongata* subsp. *nitroreducens* endocarditis in a seven year-old boy. Pediatr. Infect. Dis. J. *24*:391-392, 2005.

207. Houpikian, P., and Raoult, D.: Diagnostic methods: Current best practices and guidelines for identification of difficult-to-culture pathogens in infective endocarditis. Infect. Dis. Clin. North Am. *16*:377-392, 2002.

208. Hsu, C. M., Lee, P. I., Chen, J. M., et al.: Fatal *Fusarium* endocarditis complicated by hemolytic anemia and thrombocytopenia in an infant. Pediatr. Infect. Dis. J. *13*:1146-1148, 1994.

209. Hsu, R. B., and Lin, F. Y.: Effect of penicillin resistance on presentation and outcome of nonenterococcal streptococcal infective endocarditis. Cardiology *105*:234-239, 2006.

210. Hsu, R. B., and Lin, F. Y.: Methicillin resistance and risk factors for embolism in *Staphylococcus aureus* infective endocarditis. Infect. Control Hosp. Epidemiol. *28*:860-866, 2007.

211. Huang, S. T., Lee, H. C., Lee, N. Y., et al.: Clinical characteristics of invasive *Haemophilus aphrophilus* infections. J. Microbiol. Immunol. Infect. *38*:271-276, 2005.

212. Humpl, T., McCrindle, B. W., and Smallhorn, J. F.: The relative roles of transthoracic compared with transesophageal endocardiography in children with suspected infective endocarditis. J. Am. Coll. Cardiol. *41*:2068-2071, 2003.

213. Husni, R. N., Gordon, S. M., Washington, J. A., and Longworth, D. L.: *Lactobacillus* bacteremia and endocarditis: Review of 45 cases. Clin. Infect. Dis. *25*:1048-1055, 1997.

214. Hyams, K. C., Mader, J. T., Pollard, R. B., et al.: *Serratia* endocarditis in a pediatric burn patient. JAMA *246*:983-984, 1981.

215. Ingram, R. J. H, Cornere, B., and Ellis-Pegler, R. B.: Endocarditis due to *Neisseria mucosa*: Two case reports and review. Clin. Infect. Dis. *15*:321-324, 1992.

216. Inman, R D., Redecha, P. B., Knechtle, S. J., et al.: Identification of bacterial antigens in circulating immune complexes of infective endocarditis. J. Clin. Invest. *70*:271-280, 1982.

217. Ishiwada, N., Niwa, K., Tateno, S., et al.: Causative organism influences clinical profile and outcome of infective endocarditis in pediatric patients and adults with congenital heart disease. Circ. J. *69*:1266-1270, 2005.

218. Ishiwada, N., Niwa, K., Tateno, S., et al.: Pneumococcal endocarditis in children: A nationwide survey in Japan. Int. J. Cardiol. *123*:298-301, 2008.

219. Ivert, T. S., Dismukes, W. E., Cobbs, C. G., et al.: Prosthetic valve endocarditis. Circulation *69*:223-232, 1984.

220. Jackman, J. D., Jr., and Glamann, D. B.: Gonococcal endocarditis: Twenty-five year experience. Am. J. Med. Sci. *301*:221, 1991.

221. Jackson, M. A., and Hicks, R. A.: Vancomycin failure in staphylococcal endocarditis. Pediatr. Infect. Dis. J. *6*:750-752, 1987.

222. Jackson, M. J., and Rutledge, J.: Pneumococcal endocarditis in children. Pediatr. Infect. Dis. J. *1*:120-122, 1982.

223. Jaffe, W. M., Morgan, D. E., Pearlman, A. S., et al.: Infective endocarditis, 1983-1988: Echocardiographic findings and factors influencing morbidity and mortality. J. Am. Coll. Cardiol. *15*:1227-1233, 1990.

224. Jalava, J., Kotilainen, P., Nikkari, S., et al.: Use of the polymerase chain reaction and DNA sequencing for detection of *Bartonella quintana* in the aortic valve of a patient with culture-negative infective endocarditis. Clin. Infect. Dis. *21*:891-896, 1995.

225. Jemsek, J. G., Greenberg, S. B., Gentry, L. O., et al.: *Haemophilus parainfluenzae* endocarditis: Two cases and review of the literature in the past decade. Am. J. Med. *66*:51-57, 1979.

226. Job F. P., Franke S., Lethen H., et al.: Incremental value of biplane and multiplane transesophageal echocardiography for the assessment of active infective endocarditis. Am. J. Cardiol. 75:1033-1037, 1995.

227. John M. D., Hibberd P. L., Karchmer A. W., et al.: *Staphylococcus aureus* prosthetic valve endocarditis: Optimal management and risk factors for death. Clin. Infect. Dis. *26*:1307-1309, 1998.

228. Johnson, C. M.: Adherence events in the pathogenesis of infective endocarditis. Infect. Dis. Clin. North Am. *7*:21-36, 1993.

229. Johnson, C. M., and Rhodes, K. H.: Pediatric endocarditis. Mayo Clin. Proc. *57*:86-94, 1982.

230. Johnson, D. H., Rosenthal, A., and Nadas, A.: A forty-year review of bacterial endocarditis in infancy and childhood. Circulation *51*:581-588, 1975.

231. Johnson, D. H., Rosenthal, A., and Nadas, A.: Bacterial endocarditis in children under 2 years of age. Am. J. Dis. Child. *129*:183-186, 1975.

232. Johnson, J. D., Raff, M. J., Barnwell, P. A., et al.: Splenic abscess complicating infectious endocarditis. Arch. Intern. Med. *143*:906-912, 1983.

233. Johnson, P. G., Lee J., Domanski , M., et al.: Late recurrent *Candida* endocarditis. Chest *99*:1531-1533, 1991.

234. Jones, H. K., and Siekert, R. G.: Neurologic manifestations of infective endocarditis. Brain *112*:1295-1315, 1989.

235. Jones, R. B., Priest, J. B., and Kuo, C.: Subacute chlamydial endocarditis. JAMA *247*:655-658, 1982.

236. Julander, I.: Unfavourable prognostic factors in *Staphylococcus aureus* septicemia and endocarditis. Scand. J. Infect. Dis. *17*:179-187, 1985.

237. Kaell, A. T., Volkman, D. J., Gorevic, P. D., et al.: Positive Lyme serology in subacute bacterial endocarditis: A study of four patients. JAMA *264*:2916-2918, 1990.

238. Kaplan, E. L.: Infective endocarditis in the pediatric age group: An overview. *In* Kaplan, E. L., Taranta, A. V. (eds.): Infective Endocarditis: An American Heart Association Symposium Dallas American Heart Association 1977, pp. 51-54.

239. Kaplan, E. L., Rich, H., Gersony, W., et al.: A collaborative study of infective endocarditis in the 1970's: Emphasis on infections in patients who have undergone cardiovascular surgery. Circulation *59*:327-335, 1979.

240. Kaplan, S., Helmworth, J. A., Ahern, E. N., et al.: Results of palliative procedures for tetralogy of Fallot in infants and young children. Ann. Thorac. Surg. *5*:489-495, 1968.

241. Karalis, D. G., Blumberg, A. E., Vilaro, J. F., et al.: Prognostic significance of valvular regurgitation in patients with infective endocarditis. Am. J. Med. *90*:193-197, 1991.

242. Karchmer, A. W., Archer, G. L., and Dismukes, W. E.: *Staphylococcus epidermidis* causing prosthetic valve endocarditis: Microbiologic and clinical observations as guides to therapy. Ann. Intern. Med. *98*:447-455, 1983.

243. Karchmer, A. W., Dismukes, W. E., Buckley, M. J., et al.: Late prosthetic valve endocarditis: Clinical features influencing therapy. Am. J. Med. *64*:199-206, 1978.

244. Karchmer, A. W., Moellering, R. C., Maki, D. G., et al.: Single-antibiotic therapy for streptococcal endocarditis. JAMA *241*:1801-1806, 1979.

245. Karl, T., Wensley, D., Starke, J., et al.: Infective endocarditis in children with congenital heart disease: Comparison of selected features in patients with surgical correction or palliation and those without. Br. Heart J. *58*:57-65, 1987.

246. Kauffman, R. H., Thompson, J., Valentijn, R. M., et al.: The clinical implications and the pathogenetic significance of circulating immune complexes in infective endocarditis. Am. J. Med. *71*:17-25, 1981.

247. Kavey, R. W., Frank, D. M., Byrum ,C. J., et al.: Two-dimensional echocardiographic assessment of infective endocarditis in children. Am. J. Dis. Child. *137*:851-856, 1983.

248. Kaye, D.: Prevention of bacterial endocarditis: 1991. Ann. Intern. Med. *114*:803-804, 1991.

249. Keay, S., Denning, D. W., and Stevens, D. A.: Endocarditis due to *Trichosporon beigelii*: In vitro susceptibility of isolates and review. Rev. Infect. Dis. *13*:383-386, 1991.

250. Kennedy, M. J., Jackson, M. A., and Kearns, G. L.: Delayed diagnosis of penicillin-resistant *Streptococcus mitis* endocarditis following single-dose amoxicillin prophylaxis in a child. Clin. Pediatr. *43*:773-776, 2004.

251. Keys, T. F., and Hewitt, W. L.: Endocarditis due to micrococci and *Staphylococcus epidermidis*. Arch. Intern. Med. *132*:216-220, 1973.

252. Keyser, D. L., Biller, J., Coffman, T. T., et al.: Neurologic complications of late prosthetic valve endocarditis. Stroke *21*:472, 1990.

253. Khandheria, B. K.: Transesophageal echocardiography in the evaluation of prosthetic valves. Am. J. Card. Imaging *9*:106-114, 1995.

254. Kielhofner, M. A., and Hamill, R. J.: Role of adherence in infective endocarditis. Tex. Heart J. *16*:239-249, 1989.

255. Kihuchi, K., Enari, T., Minami, S., et al.: Postantibiotic effects and postantibiotic sub-MIC effects of benzyl penicillin on viridans streptococci isolated from patients with infective endocarditis. J. Antimicrob. Chemother. *34*:687-696, 1994.

256. Kilpatrick, Z. M., Greenberg, P. A., and Sanford, J. P.: Splinter hemorrhages: Their clinical significance. Arch. Intern. Med. *115*:730-735, 1965.

257. Kimbrough, R. C., Ormsbee, R. A., Peacock, M., et al.: Q fever endocarditis in the United States. Ann. Intern. Med. *91*:400-402, 1979.

258. King, M. E., and Weyman, A. E.: Echocardiographic findings in infective endocarditis. Cardiovasc. Clin. *13*:147-165, 1983.

259. Kissane, J. M.: Pathology of Infancy and Childhood. 2nd ed. St. Louis, C. V. Mosby, 1975, pp. 417-418.

260. Knirsch, W., Haas, N. A., Uhlemann, F., et al.: Clinical course and complications of infective endocarditis in patients growing up with congenital heart disease. Int. J. Cardiol. *101*:285-291, 2005.

261. Knirsch, W., Hassberg, D., Beyer, A., et al.: Knowledge, compliance and practice of antibiotic endocarditis prophylaxis of patients with congenital heart disease. Pediatr. Cardiol. *24*:344-349, 2003.

262. Knoll, B., Tleyjeh, I. M., Steckelberg, J. M., et al.: Infective endocarditis due to penicillin-resistant viridans group streptococci. Clin. Infect. Dis. *44*:1585-1592, 2007.

263. Komshian, S. V., Tablan, O. C., Palutke, W., et al.: Characteristics of left-sided endocarditis due to *Pseudomonas aeruginosa* in the Detroit Medical Center. Rev. Infect. Dis. *12*:693-702, 1990.

264. Kramer, H., Bourgeois, M., Liersch, R., et al.: Current clinical aspects of bacterial endocarditis in infancy, childhood and adolescence. Eur. J. Pediatr. *140*:253-259, 1983.

265. Kuypers, J. M., and Proctor, R. A.: Reduced adherence to traumatized rat heart valves by a low-fibronectin-binding mutant of *Staphylococcus aureus*. Infect. Immun. *57*:2306-2312, 1989.

266. Laird, W. P., Nelson, J. D., Weinberg, A. G., et al.: Fatal *Haemophilus influenzae* endocarditis diagnosed by echocardiography in an infant. Pediatrics *64*:292-295, 1979.

267. Lam, S., Samraj, J., Rahman, S., et al.: Primary actinomycotic endocarditis: Case report and review. Clin. Infect. Dis. *16*:481-485, 1993.

268. Lamas, C. C., and Eykyn, S. J.: Suggested modifications to the Duke criteria for the clinical diagnosis of native valve and prosthetic valve endocarditis: Analysis of 118 pathologically proven cases. Clin. Infect. Dis. *25*:713-719, 1997.

269. Lamich, R., Alonso, C., Guma, J. R., et al.: Prospective study of bacteremia during transesophageal echocardiography. Am. Heart J. *125*:1454, 1993.

270. La Scola, B., and Raoult, D.: Molecular identification of *Gemella* species from three patients with endocarditis. J. Clin. Microbiol. *36*:866-871, 1998.

271. Laufer, D., Lew, P. D., Obertianski, I., et al.: Chronic Q fever endocarditis with massive splenomegaly in childhood. J. Pediatr. *108*:535-539, 1986.

272. La Via, W. V., Koulouri, S., Ross, L. A., et al.: Right atrial mass in a child with disseminated coccidioidomycosis. Pediatr. Infect. Dis. J. *24*:470-471, 2005.

273. Laxdal, T., Messner, R. P., and Williams, R. S.: Opsonic, agglutinating and complement-fixing antibodies in patients with subacute bacterial endocarditis. J. Lab. Clin. Med. *71*:638-675, 1968.

274. Lederman, M. M., Sprague, L., Wallis, R. S., et al.: Duration of fever during treatment of infective endocarditis. Medicine (Baltimore) *71*:52, 1992.

275. Lefort, A., Mainordi, J. L., Selton-Suty, C., et al.: *Streptococcus pneumoniae* endocarditis in adults: A multi center study in France in the era of penicillin resistance (1991-1998). The Pneumococcal Endocarditis Study Group Medicine (Baltimore) *79*:327-337, 2000.

276. Leonard, A., Raij, L., and Shapiro, F. C.: Bacterial endocarditis in regularly dialyzed patients. Kidney Int. *4*:407-422, 1973.

277. Lepeschkin, E.: On the relation between the side of valvular involvement in endocarditis and the blood pressure resting on the valve. Am. J. Med. Sci. *224*:318-319, 1952.

278. Lertsapcharoen, P., Khongphatthanayothin, A., Chotirivittayatarakorn, P., et al.: Infective endocarditis in pediatric patients: An eighteen-year experience from King Chilalongkorn Hospital. J. Med. Assoc. Thai. *88*:512-516, 2005.

279. Levin, R. M., Pulliam, L., Mondry, C., et al.: Penicillin-resistant *Streptococcus constellatus* as a cause of endocarditis. Am. J. Dis. Child. *136*:42-45, 1982.

280. Levine, D. P., Fromm, B. S., and Reddy, B. R.: Slow response to vancomycin or vancomycin plus rifampin in methicillin-resistant *Staphylococcus aureus* endocarditis. Ann. Intern. Med. *115*:674-680, 1991.

281. Levitas, A., Zucker, N., Zalzstein, E., et al.: Successful treatment of infective endocarditis with recombinant tissue plasminogen activator. J. Pediatr. *143*:649-652, 2003.

282. Levy, P. Y., Drancourt, M., Etienne, J., et al.: Comparison of different antibiotic regimens for therapy of 32 cases of Q fever endocarditis. Antimicrob. Agents Chemother. *35*:533-537, 1991.

283. Li, J. S., Sexton, D. J., Mick, N., et al.: Proposed modifications to the Duke criteria for the diagnosis of infective endocarditis. Clin. Infect. Dis. *30*:633-638, 2000.

284. Liepman, M. K., Jones, P. G., and Kauffman, C. A.: Endocarditis as a complication of indwelling right atrial catheters in leukemic patients. Cancer *54*:804-807, 1984.

285. Liew, W. K., Tan, T. H., and Wong, K. Y.: Infective endocarditis in childhood: A seven-year experience. Singapore Med. J. *45*:525-529, 2004.

286. Lin, C. H., and Hsu, R. B.: Infective endocarditis caused by nutritionally variant streptococci. Am. J. Med. Sci. *334*:235-239, 2007.

287. Lina, B., Celard, M., Vandenesch, F., et al.: Infective endocarditis due to *Staphylococcus capitis*. Clin. Infect. Dis. *15*:173-174, 1992.

288. Lipman, M. L., and Silva, J.: Endocarditis due to *Streptococcus faecalis* with high-level resistance to gentamicin. Rev. Infect. Dis. *11*:325-328, 1989.

289. Lisby, G., Gutschik, E., and Durack, D. T.: Molecular methods for diagnosis of infective endocarditis. Infect. Dis. Clin. North Am. *16*:393-412, 2002.

290. Liu, V. C., Stevenson, J. G., and Smith, A. L.: Group A *Streptococcus* mural endocarditis. Pediatr. Infect. Dis. J. *11*:1060-1062, 1992.

291. Liwnicz, B. H., and Lepow, H.: Nonbacterial thrombotic endocarditis in a premature child: Clinical significance and possible relationships to subvalvular hematoma. N. Y. State J. Med. *76*:912-916, 1976.

292. Lowenstein, M. B., Urman, J. D., Abeles, M., et al.: Skin immunofluorescence in infective endocarditis. JAMA *238*:1163-1165, 1977.

293. Lowrance, J. H., Baddour, L. M., and Simpson, W. A.: The role of fibronectin binding in a rat model of experimental endocarditis caused by *Streptococcus sanguis*. J. Clin. Invest. *86*:7, 1990.

294. Lubani, M., Sharda, D., and Helin, I.: Cardiac manifestations in brucellosis. Arch. Dis. Child. *61*:569-572, 1986.

295. Lutas, E. M., Roberts, R. B., Devereux, R. B., et al.: Relation between the presence of echocardiographic vegetations and the complication rate in infective endocarditis. Am. Heart J. *112*:107-113, 1986.

296. Lynn, D. C., Kane, J. G., and Parker, R. H.: *Haemophilus parainfluenzae* endocarditis: A review of forty cases. Medicine (Baltimore) *56*:115-128, 1977.

297. Macauley, D.: Acute endocarditis in infancy and early childhood. Am. J. Dis. Child. *88*:715-721, 1954.

298. MacMahon, S. W., Hickey, A. J., Wilcken, D. E. L., et al.: Risk of infective endocarditis in mitral valve prolapse with and without precordial systolic murmurs. Am. J. Cardiol. *58*:105-108, 1986.

299. Madison, J., Wang, K., Gobel, F. L., et al.: Prosthetic aortic valve endocarditis. Circulation *51*:940-949, 1975.

300. Maisch, B., Eichstadt, H., and Kochsiek, K.: Immune reactions in infective endocarditis. I. Clinical data and diagnostic relevance of antimyocardial antibodies. Am. Heart J. *106*:329-344, 1983.

301. Maki, D. G., and Agger, W. A.: Enterococcal bacteremia: Clinical features, the risk of endocarditis and management. Medicine (Baltimore) *67*:248-269, 1988.

302. Malacoff, R. F., Frank, E., and Andriole, V. T.: Streptococcal endocarditis (non-enterococcal, non-group A): Single vs. combination therapy. JAMA *241*:1807-1810, 1979.

303. Maltezou, H. C., and Raoult, D.: Q fever in children. Lancet Infect. Dis. *2*:686-691, 2002.

304. Mansur, A. J., Grinberg, M., Lemosdaluz, P., et al.: The complications of infective endocarditis. Arch. Intern. Med. *152*:2428, 1992.

305. Marinell, P. V., Diana, D. J., and Todd, W. A.: Survival of a child after *Haemophilus influenzae* b endocarditis. Pediatr. Infect. Dis. J. *2*:46-47, 1983.

306. Markowitz, M.: The decline of rheumatic fever: Role of medical intervention. Lewis W. Wannamaker Memorial Lecture. J. Pediatr. *106*:545-550, 1985.

307. Markowitz, S. M., Szentpetery, S., Lower, R. R., et al.: Endocarditis due to accidental penetrating foreign bodies. Am. J. Med. *60*:571-576, 1976.

308. Marks, A. R., Choong, C. Y., Sanfilippo, A. J., et al.: Identification of high-risk and low-risk subgroups of patients with mitral-valve prolapse. N. Engl. J. Med. *370*:1031-1036, 1989.

309. Marks, K. A., Zucker, N., Kopelushnik, J., et al.: Infective endocarditis successfully treated in extremely low birth weight infants with recombinant tissue plasminogen activator. Pediatrics *109*:153-158, 2002.

310. Marrie, T. J., Harczy, M., Mann, O. E., et al.: Culture-negative endocarditis probably due to *Chlamydia pneumoniae*. J. Infect. Dis. *161*:127-129, 1990.

311. Martin, J. M., Neches, W. H., and Wald, E. R.: Infective endocarditis: 35 years of experience at a children's hospital. Clin. Infect. Dis. *24*:669-675, 1997.

312. Martino, P., Micozzi, A., Venditti, M., et al.: Catheter-related right-sided endocarditis in bone marrow transplant recipients. Rev. Infect. Dis. *12*:250-257, 1990.

313. Masuda, J., Yutani, C., Waki, R., et al.: Histopathologic analysis of the mechanisms of intracranial hemorrhage complicating infective endocarditis. Stroke *23*:843, 1992.

314. Mathew, J., Addai, T., Anand, A., et al.: Clinical features, site of involvement, bacteriologic findings and outcome of infective endocarditis in intravenous drug users. Arch. Intern. Med. *155*:1641-1648, 1995.

315. Mayayo, E., Moralejo, J., Camps, J., et al.: Fungal endocarditis in premature infants: Case report and review. Clin. Infect. Dis. *22*:366-368, 1996.

316. McCartney, A. C., Orange, G. U., Pringle, S. D., et al.: Serum C reactive protein in infective endocarditis. J. Clin. Pathol. *41*:44-48, 1988.

317. McGuinness, G. A., Schieken, R. M., and Maguire, G. F.: Endocarditis in the newborn. Am. J. Dis. Child. *134*:577-580, 1980.

318. McKinsey, D. S., Ratts, T. E., Bisno, A. L.: Underlying cardiac lesions in adults with infective endocarditis: The changing spectrum. Am. J. Med. *82*:681-688, 1987.

319. McMahon, C. J., Ayers, N., Pignatelli, R. H., et al.: Echocardiographic presentations of endocarditis and risk factors for rupture of a sinus of Valsalva in childhood. Cardiol. Young *13*:168-172, 2003.

320. Medoff, G., Comfort, M., and Kabayashi, G.: Synergistic action of amphotericin B and 5-fluorocytosine against yeast-like organisms. Proc. Soc. Exp. Biol. Med. *138*:571-574, 1971.

321. Mendelsohn, G., and Hutchins, G. M.: Infective endocarditis during the first decade of life. Am. J. Dis. Child. *133*:619-622, 1979.

322. Megran, D. W.: Enterococcal endocarditis. Clin. Infect. Dis. *15*:63-71, 1992.

323. Merzbach, D., Freundlich, E., Metzker, A., et al.: Endocarditis due to *Corynebacterium*. J. Pediatr. *67*:792-796, 1965.

324. Michelfelder, E. C., Ochsner, J. E., Khoury, P., and Kimball, T. R.: Does assessment of pretest probability of disease improve the utility of echocardiography in suspected endocarditis in children? J. Pediatr. *142*:263-267, 2003.

325. Middlemost, S., Wisenbaugh, T., Meyerowitz, C., et al.: A case for early surgery in native left-sided endocarditis complicated by heart failure: Results in 203 patients. J. Am. Coll. Cardiol. *18*:663-667, 1991.

326. Millar, B. C., Jugo, J., and Moore, J. E.: Fungal endocarditis in neonates and children. Pediatr. Cardiol. *26*:517-536, 2005.

327. Millard, D. D., and Shulman, S. T.: The changing spectrum of neonatal endocarditis. Clin. Perinatol. *15*:587-608, 1988.

328. Mintz, G. S., Kotler, M. N., Segal, B. L., et al.: Comparison of two-dimensional and M-mode echocardiography in the evaluation of patients with infective endocarditis. Am. J. Cardiol. *43*:738-745, 1979.

329. Miro, J. M., Anguera, I., Cabell, C. H., et al.: *Staphylococcus aureus* native valve infective endocarditis: Report of 566 episodes from the International Collaboration on Endocarditis Merged Database. Clin. Infect. Dis. *41*:507-514, 2005.

330. Mittal, B. V.: Renal lesions in infective endocarditis. J. Postgrad. Med. *33*:193-197, 1987.

331. Mohan, U. R., Walters, S., and Kroll, J. S.: Endocarditis due to group A β-hemolytic *Streptococcus* in children with potentially lethal sequelae: 2 cases and review. Clin. Infect. Dis. *30*:624-625, 2000.

332. Moodie, D. S., and Gallen, W. J.: Pneumococcal endocarditis in a 7 week old infant. Am. J. Dis. Child. *129*:980-983, 1975.

333. Moreillon, P., Que, Y. A., and Bayer, A. S.: Pathogenesis of streptococcal and staphylococcal endocarditis. Infect. Dis. Clin. North Am. *16*:297-318, 2002.

334. Morguet, A. J., Munz, D. L., Ivancevic, V., et al.: Immunoscintigraphy using technetium-99m–labeled anti-NCA-95 antigranulocyte antibodies as an adjunct to echocardiography in subacute infective endocarditis. J. Am. Coll. Cardiol. *23*:1171-1188, 1994.

335. Morpeth, S., Murdoch, D., Cabell, C. H., et al.: Non-HACEK gram-negative bacillus endocarditis. Ann. Intern. Med. *147*:829-835, 2007.

336. Morris, A. J., Drinkovic, D., Pottumarthy, S., et al.: Gram stain, culture and histopathologic examination findings from heart valves removed because of infective endocarditis. Clin. Infect. Dis. *36*:697-704, 2003.

337. Morris, A. J., Drinkovic, D., Pottumarthy, S., et al.: Bacteriological outcome after valve surgery for active infective endocarditis: Implications for duration of treatment after surgery. Clin. Infect. Dis. *41*:187-294, 2005.

338. Morris, C. D., Reller, M. D., and Menosch, V. D.: Thirty year incidence of infective endocarditis after surgery for congenital heart defect. JAMA *279*:599-603, 1998.

339. Morrison, V. A., and Wagner, K. F.: Clinical manifestations of *Kingella kingae* infections: Case report and review. Rev. Infect. Dis. *11*:776-782, 1989.

340. Mortara, L. A., and Bayer, A. S.: *Staphylococcus* bacteremia and endocarditis: New diagnostic and therapeutic concepts. Infect. Dis. Clin. North Am. 7:53-67, 1993.

341. Moy, R. J. D., George, R. H., DeGiovanni, J. V., et al.: Improving survival in bacterial endocarditis. Arch. Dis. Child. *61*:394-399, 1986.

342. Mugge, A., Daniel, W. G., Frank, G., et al.: Echocardiography in infective endocarditis: Reassessment of prognostic implications of vegetation size determined by the transthoracic and transesophageal approach. J. Am. Coll. Cardiol. *14*:631-638, 1989.

343. Mullany, C. J., Chau, Y. L., Schaff, H. V., et al.: Early and late survival after surgical treatment of culture-positive active endocarditis. Mayo Clin. Proc. *70*:517-525, 1995.

344. Munoz, P., Berenguer, J., Rodriguez-Greixems, M., et al.: Ciprofloxacin and infective endocarditis. Infect. Dis. Clin. Pract. 2:119, 1993.

345. Murphy, J. G., and Foster-Smith, K.: Management of complications of infective endocarditis with emphasis on echocardiographic findings. Infect. Dis. Clin. North Am. 7:153-165, 1993.

346. Murray, B. E.: The life and times of the *Enterococcus*. Clin. Microbiol. Rev. 3:46-65, 1990.

347. Murray, H. W., Gross, K. C., Masur, H., et al.: Serious infections caused by *Streptococcus milleri*. Am. J. Med. *64*:759-761, 1978.

348. Musewe, N. N., Hecht, B. M., Hesslein, P. S., et al.: Tricuspid valve endocarditis in two children with normal hearts: Diagnosis and therapy of an unusual clinical entity. J. Pediatr. *110*:735-738, 1987.

349. Nagel, J. G., Tuazon, C. V., Cardella, T. A., et al.: Teichoic acid serologic diagnosis of staphylococcal endocarditis. Ann. Intern. Med. *82*:13-18, 1975.

350. Nagunuma, M.: Infective endocarditis in children. Jpn. Circ. J. *49*:545-552, 1985.

351. Naidoo, D. P.: Right-sided endocarditis in the non–drug addict. Postgrad. Med. J. *69*:615-620, 1993.

352. Nakayama, D. K., O'Neill, J. A., Wagner, H., et al.: Management of vascular complications of bacterial endocarditis. J. Pediatr. Surg. *21*:636-639, 1986.

353. Narasimhan, S. L., and Weinstein, A. J.: Infective endocarditis due to a nutritionally deficient *Streptococcus*. J. Pediatr. *96*:61-62, 1980.

354. Nastro, L. J., and Finegold, S. M.: Endocarditis due to anaerobic gram-negative bacilli. Am. J. Med. *54*:482-496, 1973.

355. Nelson, R. J., Harley, D. P., French, W. J., et al.: Favorable ten-year experience with valve procedures for active infective endocarditis. J. Thorac. Cardiovasc. Surg. *87*:493-502, 1984.

356. Nguyen, M. H., Nguyen, M. L., Yu, V. L., et al.: *Candida* prosthetic valve endocarditis: Prospective study of six cases and review of the literature. Clin. Infect. Dis. *22*:262-267, 1996.

357. Nicolau, D. P., Freeman, C. D., Nightingale, C. H., et al.: Reduction of bacterial titers by low-dose aspirin in experimental aortic valve endocarditis. Infect. Immun. *61*:1593-1595, 1993.

358. Niwa, K., Nakazawa, M., Tateno, S., et al.: Infective endocarditis in congenital heart disease: Japanese national collaboration data. Heart *91*:795-800, 2005.

359. Noel, G. J., O'Loughlin, J. E., Edelson, P. J.: Neonatal *Staphylococcus epidermidis* right-sided endocarditis: Description of five catheterized infants. Pediatrics *82*:234-239, 1988.

360. Nolan, C. M., Kane, J. J., and Grunow, W. A.: Infective endocarditis and mitral prolapse: A comparison with other types of endocarditis. Arch. Intern. Med. *141*:447-450, 1981.

361. Nomura, F., Penny, D. J., and Menahem, S., et al.: Surgical intervention for infective endocarditis in infancy and childhood. Ann. Thorac. Surg. *60*:90-95, 1995.

362. O'Callaghan, C., and McDougall, P.: Infective endocarditis in neonates. Arch. Dis. Child. *63*:53-57, 1988.

363. Oelberg, D. G., Fisher, D. J., Gross, D. M., et al.: Endocarditis in high-risk neonates. Pediatrics *71*:392-397, 1983.

364. Okumura, A., Ito, K., Kondo, M., et al.: Infective endocarditis caused by highly penicillin-resistant *Streptococcus pneumoniae*: Successful treatment with cefuzonam, ampicillin and imipenem. Pediatr. Infect. Dis. J. *14*:327-329, 1995.

365. Olaison, L., and Pettersson, G.: Current best practices and guidelines: Indications for surgical intervention in infective endocarditis. Infect. Dis. Clin. North Am. *16*:453-476, 2002.

366. Panidis, I. P., Kotler, M. N., Mintz, G. S., et al.: Right heart endocarditis: Clinical and echocardiographic features. Am. Heart J. *107*:759-764, 1984.

367. Patchell, R. A., White, C. L., Clark, A. W., et al.: Nonbacterial thrombotic endocarditis in bone marrow transplant patients. Cancer *55*:631-635, 1985.

368. Patrick, W. D., Brown, W. D., Bowmer, M. I., et al.: Infective endocarditis due to *Eikenella corrodens*: Case report and review of the literature. Can. J. Infect. Dis. 1:139, 1990.

369. Patterson, J. E., and Zervos, M. J.: High-level gentamicin resistance in *Enterococcus*: Microbiology, genetic basis and epidemiology. Rev. Infect. Dis. *12*:644-652, 1990.

370. Pavlovsky, M., Press, J., Peled, N., and Yagupsky, P.: Blood culture contamination in pediatric patients: Young children and young doctors. Pediatr. Infect. Dis. J. *25*;611-614, 2006.

371. Pazin, G. J., Saul, S., and Thompson, M. E.: Blood culture positivity: Suppression by out-patient antibiotic therapy in patients with bacterial endocarditis. Arch. Intern. Med. *142*:263-269, 1982.

372. Pedersen, W. R., Walker, M., Olson, J. D., et al.: Value of transesophageal echocardiography as an adjunct to transthoracic echocardiography in evaluation of native and prosthetic valve endocarditis. Chest *100*:351-356, 1991.

373. Pefanis, A., Giamarellou, H., Karayiannakos, P., et al.: Efficacy of ceftazidime and aztreonam alone or in combination with amikacin in experimental left-sided *Pseudomonas aeruginosa* endocarditis. Antimicrob. Agents Chemother. *37*:308-313, 1993.

374. Pefanis, A., Thauvin-Eliopoulos, C., Eliopoulos, G. M., et al.: Activity of ampicillin-sulbactam and oxacillin in experimental endocarditis caused by beta-lactamase hyperproducing *Staphylococcus aureus*. Antimicrob. Agents Chemother. *37*:507-511, 1993.

375. Peled, N., Pitlik, S., Livni, G., et al.: Impact of age on clinical features and outcome of infective endocarditis. Eur. J. Clin. Microbial. Infect. Dis. 25:473-475, 2006.

376. Pelletier, L. L., Durack, D. T., and Petersdorf, R. G.: Chemotherapy of experimental streptococcal endocarditis. IV. Further observations on prophylaxis. J. Clin. Invest. *56*:319-330, 1975.

377. Perry, K. S., Tresch, D. D., Brooks, H. L., et al.: Operative approach to endocarditis. Am. Heart J. *108*:561-566, 1984.

378. Pesanti, E. L., and Smith, I. M.: Infective endocarditis with negative blood cultures: An analysis of 52 cases. Am. J. Med. *66*:43-50, 1979.

379. Peter, O., Flepp, M., Bestetti, G., et al.: Q fever endocarditis: Diagnostic approaches and monitoring of therapeutic effects. Clin. Invest. 70:932, 1992.

380. Pitchford, C. W., Creech, C. B., Peters, T. R., and Vnencak-Jones, C. L.: *Bartonella henselae* endocarditis in a child. Pediatr. Cardiol. *27*:769-771, 2006.

381. Pollack, S., Mogtader, A., Lange, M.: *Neisseria subflava* endocarditis: Case report and review of the literature. Am. J. Med. *76*:752-758, 1984.

382. Pongratz, G., Henneke, K. H., von der Grun, M., et al.: Risk of endocarditis in transesophageal echocardiography. Am. Heart J. *125*:190-193, 1993.

383. Popp, R. L.: Echocardiography. N. Engl. J. Med. *323*:165, 1990.

384. Powderly, W. G., Stanley, S. L., and Medoff, G.: Pneumococcal endocarditis: Report of a series and review of the literature. Rev. Infect. Dis. 8:786-791, 1986.

385. Powell, D. C., Bivens, B. A., Bell, R. M., et al.: Endocarditis: Increasingly a surgical disease. Am. Surg. *48*:5-10, 1982.

386. Powers, D. L., and Mandell, G. L.: Intraleukocytic bacteria in endocarditis patients. JAMA *227*:313-315, 1974.

387. Prager, R. L., Maples, M. D., Hammon, J. W., et al.: Early operative intervention in aortic bacterial endocarditis. Ann. Thorac. Surg. *32*:347-350, 1981.

388. Prinsloo, J. G., and Pretorius, P. J.: *Candida albicans* endocarditis. Am. J. Dis. Child. *111*:446-447, 1966.

389. Pulvirenti, J. J., Kerns, E., Benson, C., et al.: Infective endocarditis in injection drug users: Importance of human immunodeficiency virus serostatus and degree of immunosuppression. Clin. Infect. Dis. *22*:40-45, 1996.

390. Qin, X., and Urdahl, K. B.: PCR and sequencing of independent genetic targets for the diagnosis of culture negative bacterial endocarditis. Diagn. Microbiol. Infect. Dis. 40:145-149, 2001.
391. Qoronfleh, M. W., Weraarchakul, W., and Wilkinson, B. S.: Antibodies to a range of *Staphylococcus aureus* and *Escherichia coli* heat shock proteins in sera from patients with *S. aureus* endocarditis. Infect. Immun. 61:1567-1570, 1993.
392. Rabin, R. L., Wong, P., Noonan, J. A., et al.: *Kingella kingae* endocarditis in a child with a prosthetic aortic valve and bifurcation graft. Am. J. Dis. Child. 137:403-404, 1983.
393. Raff, G. W., Gray, B. M., Torres, A. Jr., and Hasselman, T. E.: Aortitis in a child with *Abiotrophia defectiva* endocarditis. Pediatr. Infect. Dis. J. 23:574-576, 2004.
394. Ramage, I. J., Wilson, N., and Thomson, R. B.: Fashion victim: Infective endocarditis after nasal piercing. Arch. Dis. Child. 77:187, 1997.
395. Ramirez, C. A., Naragi, S., and McCulley, D. J.: Group A beta-hemolytic streptococcus endocarditis. Am. Heart J. 108:1383-1386, 1984.
396. Raoult, D., Fournier, P. E., Dramcourt, M., et al.: Diagnosis of 22 new cases of *Bartonella* endocarditis. Ann. Intern. Med. 125:646-652, 1996.
397. Rastogi, A., Luken, J. A., Pildes, R. S., et al.: Endocarditis in the neonatal intensive care unit. Pediatr. Cardiol. 14:183-186, 1993.
398. Rech, A., Loss, J. F., Machado, A., and Brunetto, A. L.: Infective endocarditis in children receiving treatment for cancer. Pediatr Blood Cancer 43:159-163, 2004.
399. Reller, L. B.: The serum bactericidal test. Rev. Infect. Dis. 8:803-807, 1986.
400. Reymann, M. T., Holley, H. P., and Cobbs, C. G.: Persistent bacteremia in staphylococcal endocarditis. Am. J. Med. 65:729-739, 1978.
401. Ribot, S., Rothfeld, D., and Frankel, H. J.: Infectious endocarditis in maintenance hemodialysis patients. Am. J. Med. Sci. 264:183-188, 1972.
402. Rice, L. B., Calderwood, S. B., Eliopoulos, G. M., et al.: Enterococcal endocarditis: A comparison of prosthetic and native valve disease. Rev. Infect. Dis. 13:1-7, 1991.
403. Rice, M. J., McDonald, R. W., Reller, M. D., et al.: Pediatric echocardiography: Current role and a review of technical advances. J. Pediatr. 128:1-14, 1996.
404. Robbins, M. J., Frater, R. W. M., Soeiro, R., et al.: Influence of vegetation size on clinical outcome of right-sided infective endocarditis. Am. J. Med. 80:165-171, 1986.
405. Roberts, G. J., Gardner, P., and Simmons, N. A.: Optimum sampling time for detection of dental bacteremia in children. Int. J. Cardiol. 35:311-315, 1992.
406. Roberts, K. B., and Sidlak, M. J.: Satellite streptococci: A major cause of "negative" blood cultures in bacterial endocarditis? JAMA 241:2293-2294, 1979.
407. Rodbard, S.: Blood velocity and endocarditis. Circulation 27:18-28, 1963.
408. Rodero, F. G., del Mar Masia, M., Cortes, J., et al.: Endocarditis caused by *Stenotrophomonas maltophilia:* Case report and review. Clin. Infect. Dis. 23:1261-1265, 1996.
409. Rogers, J., Walker, M., Olson, J. D., et al.: Value of transesophageal echocardiography as an adjunct to transthoracic echocardiography in evaluation of native and prosthetic valve endocarditis. Chest 100:351-355, 1991.
410. Rohmann, S., Erbel, R., Darius, H., et al.: Prediction of rapid versus prolonged healing of infective endocarditis by monitoring vegetation size. J. Am. Soc. Echocardiogr. 4:465-474, 1991.
411. Rohmann, S., Seifert, T., Erbel, R., et al.: Identification of abscess formation in native-valve infective endocarditis using transesophageal echocardiography: Implications for surgical treatment. Thorac. Cardiovasc. Surg. 39:273-280, 1991.
412. Rose, A. G.: Infective endocarditis complicating congenital heart disease. S. Afr. Med. J. 53:739-743, 1978.
413. Rubinstein, E., Noreiga, E. R., Simberkoff, M. S., et al.: Fungal endocarditis: Analysis of 24 cases and review of the literature. Medicine (Baltimore) 54:331-344, 1975.
414. Rupp, M. E.: *Streptobacillus moniliformis* endocarditis: Case report and review. Clin. Infect. Dis. 14:769-772, 1992.
415. Rutledge, R., Kim, B. J., and Applebaum, R. E.: Actuarial analysis of the risk of prosthetic valve endocarditis in 1,598 patients with mechanical and bioprosthetic valves. Arch. Surg. 120:469-472, 1985.
416. Sable, C. A., Rome, J. J., Martin, G. R., et al.: Indications for echocardiography in the diagnosis of infective endocarditis in children. Am. J. Cardiol. 75:801-804, 1995.
417. Sachdev, M., Peterson, G. E., and Jollis, J. G.: Imaging techniques for diagnosis of infective endocarditis. Infect. Dis. Clin. North Am. 16:319-338, 2002.
418. Sadiq, M., Nazir, M., and Sheikh, S. A.: Infective endocarditis in children: Incidence, pattern, diagnosis and management in a developing country. Int. J. Cardiol. 78:175-182, 2001.
419. Saffle, J. R., Gardner, P., Schoenbaum, S. C., et al.: Prosthetic valve endocarditis: The case for prompt valve replacement. J. Thorac. Cardiovasc. Surg. 73:416-420, 1977.
420. Saiman, L., Prince, A., and Gersony, W. M.: Pediatric infective endocarditis in the modern era. J. Pediatr. 122:847-853, 1993.
421. Saleh, A., Dawkins, K., and Monro, J.: Surgical treatment of infective endocarditis. Acta Cardiol. 59:658-662, 2004.
422. Salgado, A. V., Furlan, A. J., Keys, T. F., et al.: Neurologic complications of endocarditis: A 12-year experience. Neurology 39:173-178, 1989.
423. Sambola, A., Miro, J. M., Tornos, M. P., et al. *Streptococcus agalactiae* infective endocarditis: Analysis of 30 cases and review of the literature, 1962-1998. Clin. Infect. Dis. 34:1576-1584, 2002.
424. Sanchez, P. J., Siegel, J. D., and Fishbein, J.: *Candida* endocarditis: Successful medical management in three preterm infants and review of the literature. Pediatr. Infect. Dis. 10:239-243, 1991.
425. Sande, M. A., and Courtney, K. B.: Nafcillin-gentamicin synergism in experimental *Staphylococcus* endocarditis. J. Lab. Clin. Med. 88:118-124, 1976.
426. Sandre, R. M., and Shatran, S. D.: Infective endocarditis: Review of 135 cases over 9 years. Clin. Infect. Dis. 22:276-286, 1996.
427. Sanfilippo, A. J., Picard, M. H., Newell, J. B., et al.: Echocardiographic assessment of patients with infectious endocarditis: Prediction of risk for complications. J. Am. Coll. Cardiol. 18:1191-1199, 1991.
428. San Roman, J. A., Vilacosta, I., Zamorano, J. L., et al.: Transesophageal echocardiography in right-sided endocarditis. J. Am. Coll. Cardiol. 21:1226-1230, 1993.
429. Sapico, F. L., Liquete, J. A., and Sarma, R. J.: Bone and joint infections in patients with infective endocarditis: Review of a 4-year experience. Clin. Infect. Dis. 22:783-787, 1996.
430. Sapsford, R. N., Fitchett, D. H., Tarin, D., et al.: Aneurysm of left ventricle secondary to bacterial endocarditis. J. Thorac. Cardiovasc. Surg. 78:79-86, 1979.
431. Scheld, W. M., and Mandell, G. L.: Enigmatic enterococcal endocarditis. Ann. Intern. Med. 100:904-905, 1984.
432. Scheld, W. M., and Sande, M. A.: Endocarditis and intravascular infections. *In* Mandell, G., Bennett, J. E., and Dolin, R. (eds.): Principles and Practices of Infectious Diseases. 4th ed. New York, Churchill Livingstone, 1995, pp. 740-782.
433. Scheld, W. M., Calderone, R. A., Alliegro, G. M., et al.: Yeast adherence in the pathogenesis of *Candida* endocarditis. Proc. Soc. Exp. Biol. Med. 168:208-217, 1981.
434. Scheld, W. M., Thomas, J. H., and Sande, M. A.: Influence of preformed antibody on experimental *Streptococcus sanguis* endocarditis. Infect. Immun. 25:781-785, 1979.
435. Scheld, W. M., Valone, J. A., and Sande, M. A.: Bacterial adherence in the pathogenesis of endocarditis: Interaction of bacterial dextran, platelets and fibrin. J. Clin. Invest. 61:1394-1398, 1978.
436. Scheld, W. M., Zak, O., Vosbeck, K., et al.: Bacterial adhesion in the pathogenesis of endocarditis: Effect of subinhibitory antibiotic concentrations on streptococcal adhesion in vitro and the development of endocarditis in rabbits. J. Clin. Invest. 68:1381, 1981.
437. Schollin, J., Bjarke, B., and Wesstrom, G.: Follow-up study on children with infective endocarditis. Acta Paediatr. 78:615-619, 1989.
438. Schulte, J. E., Gaffney, F. A., Bland, L., et al.: Distinctive anthropometric characteristics of women with mitral valve prolapse. Am. J. Med. 71:553-558, 1981.
439. Scott, P. J., Blackburn, M. E., Wharton, G. A., et al.: Transesophageal echocardiography in neonates, infants and children: Applicability and diagnostic value in everyday practice of a cardiothoracic unit. Br. Heart J. 68:488-492, 1992.
440. Scott, R. M.: Bacterial endocarditis due to *Neisseria flava.* J. Pediatr. 78:673-675, 1971.
441. Seeling, M. S., Speth, C. P., Kozinn, P. J., et al.: Patterns of *Candida* endocarditis following cardiac surgery: Importance of early diagnosis and therapy (an analysis of 91 cases). Prog. Cardiovasc. Dis. 17:125-160, 1974.
442. Sexton, D. J., Tenenbaum, M. J., Wilson, W. R., et al.: Ceftriaxone once daily for four weeks compared with ceftriaxone plus gentamicin once daily for two weeks for treatment of endocarditis due to penicillin-susceptible streptococci. Clin. Infect. Dis. 27:1470-1474, 1998.
443. Shah, F. S., Fennelly, G., Weingarten-Arams, J., et al.: Endocardial abscesses in children: Case report and review of the literature. Clin. Infect. Dis. 29:1478-1482, 1999.
444. Shapiro, D. S., Kenney, S. C., Johnson, M., et al.: *Chlamydia psittaci* endocarditis diagnosed by blood culture. N. Engl. J. Med. 326:1192-1195, 1992.
445. Shively, B. K., Gurule, F. T., Roldan, C. A., et al.: Diagnostic value of transesophageal compared with transthoracic echocardiography in infective endocarditis. J. Am. Coll. Cardiol. 18:391-397, 1991.
446. Sholler, G. F., Hawker, R. E., and Celermajer, J. M.: Infective endocarditis in childhood. Pediatr. Cardiol. 6:183-186, 1986.
447. Simmons, N. A.: Recommendations for endocarditis prophylaxis. J. Antimicrob. Chemother. 31:437-438, 1993.
448. Singhi, S. C., Singh, S., and Bidwai, P. S.: *Peptococcus* endocarditis. Indian J. Pediatr. 25:876-878, 1988.
449. Sirisanthana, V., and Sirisanthana, T.: *Corynebacterium diphtheriae* endocarditis. Pediatr. Infect. Dis. 2:470-471, 1983.
450. Sochowski, R. A., and Chan, K. L.: Implication of negative results on a monoplane transesophageal echocardiographic study in patients with suspected infective endocarditis. J. Am. Coll. Cardiol. 21:216, 1993.
451. Sommer, P., Gleyzal, C., Guerret, S., et al.: Induction of a putative laminin-binding protein of *Streptococcus gordonii* in human infective endocarditis. Infect. Immun. 60:360-365, 1992.
452. Spach, D. H., Kanter, A. S., Daniels, N. A., et al.: *Bartonella (Rochalimaea)* species as a cause of apparent "culture-negative" endocarditis. Clin. Infect. Dis. 20:1044-1047, 1995.

453. Stanton, B. F., Baltimore, R. S., and Clemens, J. D.: Changing spectrum of infective endocarditis in children. Am. J. Dis. Child. 138:720-725, 1984.

454. Steckelberg, J. M., and Wilson, W. R.: Risk factors for infective endocarditis. Infect. Dis. Clin. North Am. 7:9-19, 1993.

455. Steckelberg, J. M., Murphy, J. G., Ballard, D., et al.: Emboli in infective endocarditis: The prognostic value of echocardiography. Ann. Intern. Med. 114:635-640, 1991.

456. Steckelberg, J. M., Rouse, M. S., Tallan, B. M., et al.: Relative efficacies of broad-spectrum cephalosporins for treatment of methicillin-susceptible Staphylococcus aureus experimental infective endocarditis. Antimicrob. Agents Chemother. 37:554-558, 1993.

457. Steelman, R., Einzig, S., Balian, A., et al.: Increased susceptibility to gingival colonization by specific HACEK microbes in children with congenital heart disease. J Clin. Pediatr. Dent 25:91-94, 2000.

458. Steen, M. K., Bruno-Murtha, L. A., Chaux, G., et al.: Bacillus cereus endocarditis: Report of a case and review. Clin. Infect. Dis. 14:945-946, 1992.

459. Stein, D. S., and Nelson, K. E.: Endocarditis due to nutritionally deficient streptococci: Therapeutic dilemma. Rev. Infect. Dis. 9:908-916, 1987.

460. Steinbach, W. J., Perfect, J. R., Cabell, C. H., et al.: A meta-analysis of medical versus surgical therapy for Candida endocarditis. J. Infect. 51:230-247, 2005.

461. Sternik, L., Zehr, K. J., Orszulak, T. A., et al.: The advantage of repair of mitral valve in acute endocarditis. J Heart Valve Dis 11:91-97, 2002.

462. Stewart, J. A., Silamperi, D., Harris, P., et al.: Echocardiographic documentation of vegetative lesions in infective endocarditis: Clinical implications. Circulation 61:374-380, 1980.

463. Stewart, W. J., and Shan, K.: The diagnosis of prosthetic valve endocarditis by echocardiography. Semin. Thorac. Cardiovasc. Surg. 7:7-12, 1995.

464. Stockheim, J. A., Chadwick, E. G., Kessler, S., et al.: Are the Duke criteria superior to Beth Israel criteria for diagnosis of infective endocarditis in children? Clin. Infect. Dis. 27:1451-1456, 1998.

465. Stopfuchen, H., Benzing, F., Jungst, B., et al.: Echocardiographic diagnosis of Candida endocarditis of the tricuspid valve and of the right atrium in a young infant. Pediatr. Cardiol. 4:49-51, 1983.

466. Stramboulian, D., Bonvehi, P., Arevalo, C., et al.: Antibiotic management of outpatients with endocarditis due to penicillin-susceptible streptococci. Rev. Infect. Dis. 13(Suppl. 2):160-163, 1991.

467. Stuart, G., and Wren, C.: Endocarditis with acute mitral regurgitation caused by Fusobacterium necrophorum. Pediatr. Cardiol. 13:230-232, 1992.

468. Sudduth, E. J., Rozich, J. D., and Farrar, W. E.: Rothia dentocariosa endocarditis complicated by perivalvular abscess. Clin. Infect. Dis. 17:772-775, 1993.

469. Sullam, P. M., Costerton, J. W., Yamasaki, R., et al.: Inhibition of platelet binding and aggregation by streptococcal exopolysaccharide. J. Infect. Dis. 167:1123-1130, 1993.

470. Sussman, J. I., Baron, E. J., Goldberg, S. M., et al.: Clinical manifestations and therapy of Lactobacillus endocarditis: Report of a case and review of the literature. Rev. Infect. Dis. 8:771-776, 1986.

471. Sussman, J. I., Baron, E. J., Tenenbaum, M. J., et al.: Viridans streptococcal endocarditis: Clinical, microbiological and echocardiographic correlations. J. Infect. Dis. 154:597-603, 1986.

472. Switalski, L. M., Murchison, H., Timpl, R., et al.: Binding of laminin to oral and endocarditis strains of viridans streptococci. J. Bacteriol. 169:1095-1101, 1987.

473. Sykes, R. M.: Salmonella endocarditis in a Nigerian child. East Afr. Med. J. 61:326-327, 1984.

474. Symbas, P. N., Vlasis, S. E., Zacharupoulos, L., et al.: Immediate and long-term outlook for valve replacement in acute bacterial endocarditis. Ann. Surg. 195:721-724, 1982.

475. Symchych, P. S., Krauss, A. W., and Winchester, P.: Endocarditis following intracardiac placement of umbilical venous catheters in neonates. J. Pediatr. 90:287-289, 1977.

476. Taams, M. A., Gussenhoven, E. J., Bos, E., et al.: Enhanced morphological diagnosis in infective endocarditis by transesophageal echocardiography. Br. Heart J. 63:109-113, 1990.

477. Takeda, S., Nakanishi, T., Nakazawa, M., et al.: A 28-year trend of infective endocarditis associated with congenital heart disease: A single institute experience. Pediatr. Int. 47:392-396, 2005.

478. Tancik, C. A., and Dillaha, J. A.: Francisella tularensis endocarditis. Clin. Infect. Dis. 30:399-400, 2000.

479. Tanowitz, H. B., Alder, J. J., and Chirito, E.: Gonococcal endocarditis. N. Y. State J. Med. 42:2782-2783, 1972.

480. Tebas, P., Martinez, R., Roman, F., et al.: Early resistance to rifampin and ciprofloxacin in the treatment of right-sided Staphylococcus aureus endocarditis. J. Infect. Dis. 163:204-205, 1991.

481. Teixeira, O. H., Carpenter, B., and Vlad, P.: Enterococcal endocarditis in early infancy. Can. Med. Assoc. J. 127:612-613, 1982.

482. Thadelpall, H., and Francis, C. K.: Diagnostic clues in metastatic lesions of endocarditis in addicts. West. J. Med. 128:1-7, 1978.

483. Thal, L. A., Vazquez, J., Perri, M. B., et al.: Activity of ampicillin plus sulbactam against β-lactamase producing enterococci in experimental endocarditis. J. Antimicrob. Chemother. 31:182, 1993.

484. Thapar, M. K., Rao, P. S., Feldman, D., et al.: Infective endocarditis: A review. Paediatrician 7:65-84, 1978.

485. Theofilopoulos, A. N., Wilson, C. B., and Dixon, F. J.: The Raji cell radioimmune assay for detecting immune complexes in human sera. J. Clin. Invest. 57:169-182, 1976.

486. Tiley, S. M., Kociuba, K. R., Heron, L. G., et al.: Infective endocarditis due to nontoxigenic Corynebacterium diphtheriae: Report of seven cases and review. Clin. Infect. Dis. 16:271-275, 1993.

487. Tissieres, P., Gervaix, A., Beghetti, M., and Jaeggi, E. T.: Value and limitation of the von Reyn, Duke and modified Duke criteria for the diagnosis of infective endocarditis in children. Pediatrics 112:e467-e471, 2003.

488. Tissieres, P., Jaeggi, E. T., Beghetti, M., and Gervaix, A.: Increase in fungal endocarditis in children. Infection 33:267-272, 2005.

489. Tleyjeh, I. M., Steckelberg, J. M., Murad, H. S., et al.: Temporal trends in infective endocarditis: A population-based study in Olmstead County, Minnesota. JAMA 293:3022-3028, 2005.

490. Tolan, R. W., Jr., Kleiman, M. B., Frank, M., et al.: Operative intervention in active endocarditis in children: Report of a series of cases and review. Clin. Infect. Dis. 14:852-862, 1992.

491. Tolaymat, A., Rhatigan, R. M., and Levin, S.: Pneumococcal endocarditis in infants. South. Med. J. 72:448-451, 1979.

492. Tompkins, L. S., Roessler, B. J., Redd, S. C., et al.: Legionella prosthetic-valve endocarditis. N. Engl. J. Med. 318:530-535, 1988.

493. Tornos, M. P., Castro, A., Toran, N., et al.: Tricuspid valve endocarditis in children with normal valves. Am. Heart J. 118:624-625, 1989.

494. Tornos, M. P., Permanyer-Miralda, G., Olona, M., et al.: Long-term complications of native valve infective endocarditis in non-addicts: A 15-year follow-up study. Ann. Intern. Med. 117:567-572, 1992.

495. Toy, P. T., Lai, W., Drake, T. A., and Sande, M. A.: Effect of fibronectin on adherence of Staphylococcus aureus to fibrin thrombi in vitro. Infect. Immun. 48:83-86, 1985.

496. Tsao, M. M., and Katz, D.: Central venous catheter-induced endocarditis: Human correlate of the animal experimental model of endocarditis. Rev. Infect. Dis. 6:783-790, 1984.

497. Tuazon, C. V., and Sheagren, J. W.: Staphylococcal endocarditis in parenteral drug abusers: Source of the organism. Ann. Intern. Med. 82:788-790, 1975.

498. Tunkel, A. R., and Kaye, D.: Endocarditis with negative blood cultures. N. Engl. J. Med. 326:1215-1217, 1992.

499. Turner, S. W., Wyllie, J. P., Hamilton, J. R., and Bain, H. H.: Diagnosis of infected modified Blalock-Taussig shunt by computed tomography. Ann. Thorac. Surg. 59:1216-1217, 1995.

500. Turnier, E., Kay, J. H., Bernstein, S., et al.: Surgical treatment of Candida endocarditis. Chest 67:262-268, 1975.

501. Utley, J. R., Mills, J., and Roe, B. B.: The role of valve replacement in the treatment of fungal endocarditis. J. Thorac. Cardiovasc. Surg. 69:255-258, 1975.

502. Valente, A. M., Jain, R., Scheurer, M., et al.: Frequency of infective endocarditis among infants and children with Staphylococcus aureus bacteremia. Pediatrics 115:e15-e19, 2005.

503. van de Rijn, I.: Analysis of cross-protection between serotypes and passively transferred immune globulin in experimental nutritionally variant streptococcal endocarditis. Infect. Immun. 56:117-121, 1988.

504. van der Meer, J. T. M., Thompson, J., Valkenburg, H. A., et al.: Epidemiology of bacterial endocarditis in the Netherlands. II. Antecedent procedures and use of prophylaxis. Arch. Intern. Med. 152:1869-1873, 1992.

505. van der Meer, J. T. M., van Wijk, W., Thompson, J., et al.: Efficacy of antibiotic prophylaxis for prevention of native valve endocarditis. Lancet 339:135, 1992.

506. van der Meer, J. T. M., van Wijk, W., Thompson, J., et al.: Awareness of need and actual use of prophylaxis: Lack of patient compliance in the prevention of bacterial endocarditis. J. Antimicrob. Chemother. 29:187-194, 1992.

507. Van Hare, G. F., Ben-Shacher, G., Liebman, J., et al.: Infective endocarditis in infants and children during the past 10 years: A decade of change. Am. Heart J. 107:1235-1240, 1984.

508. Venditti, M., De Bernardis, F., Micozzi, A., et al.: Fluconazole treatment of catheter-related right-sided endocarditis caused by Candida albicans and associated with endophthalmitis and folliculitis. Clin. Infect. Dis. 14:422-426, 1992.

509. Vikram, H. R., Buenconsejo, J., Hasbun, R., and Quagliarello, V. J.: Impact of valve surgery on 6-month mortality in adults with complicated, left-sided native valve endocarditis. JAMA 290:3207-3214, 2003.

510. Von Reyn, C. F., Levy, B. S., Arbert, R. D., et al.: Infective endocarditis: An analysis based on strict case definitions. Ann. Intern. Med. 94:505-517, 1982.

511. Vuille, C., Nidor, F. M., Weyman, A., and Picard, M. H.: Natural history of vegetations during successful medical treatment of endocarditis. Am. Heart J. 128:1200-1209, 1994.

512. Walls, T., Michael, K., Trounce, J., et al.: Broad-range polymerase chain reaction for the diagnosis of Bartonella henselae endocarditis. J. Paediatr. Child Health. 42:469-471, 2006.

513. Walsh, T. J., and Hutchins, G. M.: Aspergillus mural endocarditis. Am. J. Clin. Pathol. 72:640-644, 1979.

514. Walterspiel, J. N., and Kaplan, S. L.: Incidence and clinical characteristics of "culture negative" infective endocarditis in a pediatric population. Pediatr. Infect. Dis. J. 5:328-332, 1986.

515. Watanakunakorn, C., and Glotzbecker, C.: Synergism with aminoglycosides of penicillin, ampicillin and vancomycin against nonenterococcal group D streptococci and viridans streptococci. J. Med. Microbiol. 10:133-137, 1977.

516. Watson, A., French, P., and Wilson, M.: Nocardia asteroides native valve endocarditis. Clin. Infect. Dis. 32:660-661, 2001.

517. Weinberg, A. G.: Group B streptococcal endocarditis detected by echocardiography. J. Pediatr. 92:335-336, 1978.
518. Weinstein, A. J., and Moellering, R. C.: Penicillin and gentamicin therapy for enterococcal infections. JAMA 223:1030-1032, 1973.
519. Weinstein, L., and Schlesinger, J. J.: Pathoanatomic, pathophysiologic and clinical correlations in endocarditis. N. Engl. J. Med. 291:832-837, 1122-1126, 1974.
520. Weinstein, M. P., Stratton, C. W., Ackley, A., et al.: Multicenter collaborative evaluation of a standardized bactericidal test as a prognostic indicator in infective endocarditis. Am. J. Med. 78:262-269, 1985.
521. Wells, L., Ritter, N., and Donald, F.: Kingella kingae endocarditis in a sixteen-month-old child. Pediatr. Infect. Dis. J. 20:454-455, 2001.
522. Werner, A. S., Cobbs, C. G., Kaye, D., et al.: Studies on the bacteremia of bacterial endocarditis. JAMA 202:199-203, 1967.
523. Wheeler, J. G., and Weesner, K. M.: Staphylococcus aureus endocarditis and pericarditis in an infant with a central venous catheter. Clin. Pediatr. (Phila.) 23:46-47, 1984.
524. White, P. D.: The incidence of endocarditis in earliest childhood. Am. J. Dis. Child. 32:536-549, 1926.
525. Williams, R. C., and Kunkel, H. G.: Rheumatoid factor, complement and conglutinin aberrations in patients with subacute bacterial endocarditis. J. Clin. Invest. 41:666-675, 1962.
526. Wilson, L. E., Thomas, D. L., Astemborski, J., et al.: Prospective study of infective endocarditis among injection drug users. J. Infect. Dis. 185:1761-1766, 2002.
527. Wilson, W., Taubert, K. A., Gewitz, M., et al.: Prevention of infective endocarditis: Guidelines from the American Heart Association. Circulation 116:1736-1754, 2007.
528. Wilson, W. R., Davidson, G. K., Guiliani, E., et al.: Cardiac valve replacement in congestive heart failure due to infective endocarditis. Mayo Clin. Proc. 54:223-226, 1979.
529. Wilson, W. R., Gilbert, D. N., Bisno, A. L., et al.: Evaluation of new anti-infective drugs for the treatment of infective endocarditis. Clin. Infect. Dis. 15(Suppl. 1):89-95, 1992.
530. Wilson, W. R., Karchmer, A. W., Dajani, A. S., et al.: Antibiotic treatment of adults with infective endocarditis due to streptococci, enterococci, staphylococci, and HACEK microorganisms. JAMA 274:1706-1713, 1995.
531. Wilson, W. R., Thompson, R. L., Wilkowske, C. J., et al.: Short-term therapy for streptococcal infective endocarditis. JAMA 245:360-363, 1981.
532. Witt, M. D., and Bayer, A. S.: Comparison of fluconazole and amphotericin B for prevention and treatment of experimental Candida endocarditis. Antimicrob. Agents Chemother. 35:2481-2485, 1991.
533. Wolfson, J. S., and Swartz, M. N.: Serum bactericidal activity as a monitor of antibiotic therapy. N. Engl. J. Med. 312:968-975, 1985.
534. Woods, G. L., Wood, R. P., and Shaw, B. W.: Aspergillus endocarditis in patients without prior cardiovascular surgery: Report of a case in a liver transplant recipient and review. Rev. Infect. Dis. 11:263-272, 1989.
535. Yankah, A. C., Klose, H., Petzina, R., et al.: Surgical management of acute aortic root endocarditis with viable homograft: 13 years experience. Eur. J. Cardiothorac. Surg. 21:260-267, 2002.
536. Yeaman, M. R., Norman, D. C., and Bayer, A. S.: Staphylococcus aureus susceptibility to thrombin-induced platelet microbicidal protein is independent of platelet adherence and aggregation in vitro. Infect. Immun. 60:2368-2374, 1992.
537. Yokochi, K., Sakamato, H., Mikajima, T., et al.: Infective endocarditis in children: A current diagnostic trend and the embolic complications. Jpn. Circ. J. 50:1294-1297, 1986.
538. Yu, V. L., Fang, G. D., Keys, T. F., et al.: Prosthetic valve endocarditis: Superiority of surgical valve replacement versus medical therapy alone. Ann. Thorac. Surg. 58:1073-1077, 1994.
539. Zakrzewski, T., and Keith, J. D.: Bacterial endocarditis in infants and children. J. Pediatr. 67:1179-1193, 1965.
540. Ziment, I.: Nervous system complications in bacterial endocarditis. Am. J. Med. 47:593-607, 1969.
541. Zubler, R. H., Lange, G., Lambert, P. H., et al.: Detection of immune complexes in unheated sera by a modified ^{125}I-Clq binding test. J. Immunol. 116:232-239, 1976.

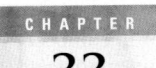

CHAPTER 33 INFECTIOUS PERICARDITIS

Sheldon L. Kaplan ❖ Richard A. Friedman

Purulent pericarditis generally refers to bacterial infection of the pericardium. Inflammation of the pericardium may result from numerous nonbacterial microorganisms, however, or may occur with a variety of noninfectious illnesses (Table 33–1). Regardless of the cause of pericarditis, the responses of the pericardium are limited to acute inflammation, effusion with or without tamponade, and fibrosis with or without constriction.[18] Because untreated purulent pericarditis is rapidly fatal, suspecting the disease early and approaching the diagnosis aggressively are important.

ANATOMY AND FUNCTION

The pericardium is composed of two loosely approximated layers: visceral and parietal. The visceral pericardium is composed of mesothelial tissue, which closely follows the contour of the heart and extends for a short distance beyond the atria and ventricles to the great vessels. The outer parietal pericardium is a more fibrous structure, composed of layers of collagen interlaced with elastic fibers. The pericardial sac is attached to the diaphragm below; to the sternum in front; and to the thoracic vertebrae, esophagus, and aorta posteriorly. It is surrounded by the lungs on either side and is related closely to the main bronchi and the mediastinal lymph nodes. The phrenic and vagus nerves supply a network of pain fibers to the parietal pericardium.

The dynamics of the pericardial fluid are poorly understood. The pericardial membrane is active in the transfer of water, electrolytes, and small molecules. Molecules of large molecular weight are absorbed poorly from the pericardial space because lymphatic channels are sparse, and drainage must occur primarily through the epicardial capillaries.[64]

Ainger[1] summarized the function of the pericardium as follows: prevention of overdistention of the heart, protection of the heart from infection and adhesions, maintenance of the heart within a fixed geometric position within the chest, and regulation of the interaction between the stroke volumes of the two ventricles.

BACTERIAL PERICARDITIS

POPULATION AND INCIDENCE

Although purulent pericarditis is not a common infection in pediatric patients, it is an important one to recognize because of its life-threatening nature. In an extensive early review of the literature on purulent pericarditis, half of 425 cases occurred in children younger than 13 years of age.[7] In a review of 162 reported children with pericarditis from 1950 to 1977, 67 percent of the children were 48 months old or younger.[27] From 1962 to 1974, 67 cases were recognized at St. Louis Children's Hospital (Table 33–2).[82] During this 12-year period, pericardial disease of all causes occurred in approximately 1 of every 850 hospital admissions.[82] Twelve (18%) of these children had purulent pericarditis.

TABLE 33–1   Causes of Pericarditis

Idiopathic
Benign
Recurrent

Infectious
Purulent
Bacterial—*Staphylococcus aureus, Haemophilus influenzae,* streptococci,
 Neisseria meningitidis, Streptococcus pneumoniae, anaerobes,
 Francisella tularensis, Salmonella, enteric bacilli, *Pseudomonas,*
 Listeria, Neisseria gonorrhoeae, Actinomyces, Nocardia
Tuberculosis
Fungal—*Histoplasma, Coccidioides, Aspergillus, Candida, Blastomyces,*
 Cryptococcus

Viral
Coxsackieviruses B
Other—influenza A and B, mumps, echoviruses, adenoviruses,
 Epstein-Barr virus, hepatitis, measles, HIV, cytomegalovirus

Other
Rickettsial—typhus, Q fever
Mycoplasmal—*Mycoplasma pneumoniae*
Parasitic—*Entamoeba histolytica, Echinococcus*
Spirochetal—syphilis, leptospirosis
Chlamydial—psittacosis
Protozoal—toxoplasmosis

Noninfectious
Postpericardiotomy syndrome
Kawasaki disease
Rheumatic fever
Connective tissue disorders—JRA, SLE, dermatomyositis,
 periarteritis nodosa
Trauma—blunt or penetrating
Metabolic—uremia, myxedema
Hypersensitivity—serum sickness, pulmonary infiltrates with
 eosinophilia, Stevens-Johnson syndrome, drugs (hydralazine,
 procainamide, chemotherapy)
Neoplasm—leukemia, metastatic
Postirradiation

HIV, human immunodeficiency virus; JRA, juvenile rheumatoid arthritis; SLE, systemic
lupus erythematosus.

TABLE 33–2   Pericarditis in Children, 1962 to 1974
(St. Louis Children's Hospital)*

Etiology	No. Patients
Unknown	28
Purulent	12
Juvenile rheumatoid arthritis	9
Acute rheumatic fever	8
Uremia	5
Viral	2
Blunt chest trauma	2
Dermatomyositis	1

Patients with postpericardiotomy pericarditis and patients with small effusions at autopsy
were excluded from consideration.
From Strauss, A. W., Santa Maria, M., and Goldring, D.: Constrictive pericarditis in
children. Am. J. Dis. Child. 129:822-826, 1975. Copyright 1975, American Medical
Association.

Most cases in younger children are infectious. Acute pericarditis was found in 20 children between 1987 and 1997 in a hospital in Iran.[72] The causes of pericarditis were bacterial in eight (40%), collagen vascular disease in six (30%), viral in four (20%), and secondary to mediastinal mass invasion in two (10%). In another series from Turkey, 18 children with purulent

pericarditis were encountered from 1990 to 2000.[11] At the Boston Children's Hospital, fewer than 10 patients seen among more than 1700 patients in consultation by the pediatric cardiologists had pericarditis during the period July 1, 2001, to June 30, 2002.[32] Although rare, purulent pericarditis also can occur in neonates.[51] In most series, a marked male predominance has been noted.

ETIOLOGY

Primary purulent pericarditis is a rare disease; it accounted for only 7 of 50 cases of pericarditis reported by Gersony and McCracken.[33] The disease is associated most often with infection from another site, with hematogenous or direct spread to the pericardium. Feldman[27] reviewed all cases of bacterial pericarditis reported in the English language literature from 1950 to 1977. Bacteria were isolated in 146 (90%) of 162 cases. No other infection was found in 10 patients. The most common concomitant site involved was the lung, especially for *Staphylococcus aureus, Haemophilus influenzae,* and *Streptococcus pneumoniae.* When septic arthritis, osteomyelitis, or skin infections were found, *S. aureus* usually was the cause of pericarditis. *Neisseria meningitidis* and *H. influenzae* most often were responsible for concomitant meningitis and pericarditis.

Before the introduction of antibiotics, pneumococcal and streptococcal organisms were the most frequent causes of purulent pericarditis in children. Most cases were associated with pulmonary infections. Nearly half of patients with streptococcal pericarditis had associated postinfluenzal pneumonia. Hemolytic streptococci were isolated most often; 10 percent were nonhemolytic streptococci, and 5 percent were viridans streptococci. Kauffman and colleagues[53] reviewed 113 cases of pneumococcal pericarditis reported since 1900. Preceding pneumonia was present in 93 percent, and empyema was present in 66 percent. Pericarditis was thought to be a late event resulting from delay in administering appropriate therapy for pneumonia.

S. aureus is the organism most commonly responsible for purulent pericarditis in children.[6,27,33,45,72] Most cases are the result of hematogenous seeding of the pericardium from staphylococcal pneumonia with empyema, acute osteomyelitis, or soft tissue abscesses. Occasionally, the pericardium is infected during the course of staphylococcal endocarditis. *S. aureus* is the most frequently recovered organism when purulent pericarditis develops within 3 months after the patient has undergone open heart surgery. The clinical course of acute staphylococcal pericarditis is dominated by severe toxemia. In addition to the necrotizing infection produced by *S. aureus,* the organism may release exotoxins, which produce shock and contribute to the high mortality.

S. aureus was isolated from 73 percent of infants who died of purulent pericarditis in the series reported by Gersony and McCracken.[33] It was responsible for 50 percent of cases in children 1 to 4 years old in the review by Feldman.[27] In seven patients younger than 1 month of age, *S. aureus* was isolated from four. This finding is corroborated in literature from other countries.[19,48,72] In one of the latest series, Thebaud and colleagues[86] reported 19 children with purulent pericarditis in a children's hospital in Paris between 1979 and 1994. The mean age of the children was 3 years (range 3 months to 10 years). The organisms isolated were *S. aureus* (three cases), *H. influenzae* (four cases), group A streptococci (three cases), *S. pneumoniae* (three cases), and *N. meningitidis* (one case). Concomitant infections included pneumonia (six cases), osteomyelitis (three cases), cellulitis (one case), and sinusitis (one case). In the series from Turkey, *S. aureus* was isolated from five patients, and *S. pneumoniae* was isolated from one patient.[11] *S. aureus* pericarditis as a complication of varicella has been reported in several children.[9]

In the prevaccine era, the second most frequently encountered organism was *H. influenzae* type b.[16] It was responsible for 22 percent (35 of 163) of the cases in Feldman's review.[27] A single site of coexisting infection, the lung, was identified in 16 of the 35 cases. Meningitis as a single other site of infection was found in 5 of 35 patients, and multiple involvement was found in 7 of 35.[27] Echeverria and colleagues[24] summarized 33 cases from the literature. Pulmonary infiltrates and empyema were seen in 64 percent of patients. Nearly 85 percent had symptoms of an upper respiratory tract infection in the preceding 5 to 12 days. Because *H. influenzae* type b conjugate vaccine has been given routinely to young infants in developed countries, this organism has been eliminated as a cause of invasive infections, including pericarditis.

Pneumococcal, streptococcal, and meningococcal pericarditis have diminished in frequency since the introduction of penicillin.[7] Go and coworkers[35] summarized the 15 reported cases of pneumococcal pericarditis from 1980 to 1998. One was a child. Only four cases did not have an underlying risk factor. In a surveillance study of invasive pneumococcal infections in eight pediatric hospitals, only three cases of pericarditis have been observed in more than 2500 cases of systemic pneumococcal infection during the 6-year period of 1993 through 1999.[52]

Pericardial involvement occurs in approximately 5 percent of young adults with meningococcemia.[21,42] The clinical course generally is milder than that observed with other types of purulent pericarditis. Pericardial involvement rarely is detected at the time of hospital admission. Pericarditis became apparent by the third day in 13 of 17 patients reported by Dixon and Sanford.[21] In some patients, it did not occur until late in the course of therapy. Whether this late-onset pericardial effusion is a part of the meningococcal infection or is related to immune complexes is unclear.[21,67,77] Primary meningococcal pericarditis that occurs without clinical evidence of meningococcemia, meningitis, or any other focal infection has been reported in 16 patients, including 6 children 18 years old or younger (range, 2 to 18 years).[3] Meningococcal serotype C was identified in 11 (79 percent) of 14 cases for which the serotype was known. Cardiac tamponade developed in 88 percent of the patients. Pericarditis also has been reported in two children with W135 meningococcal infection.[4]

Occasionally, other microorganisms cause acute purulent pericarditis. Feldman[27] reported that 11 (8%) of 146 cases of pericarditis in children were caused by *Pseudomonas aeruginosa*. *P. aeruginosa* caused pericarditis in an immunocompetent adult with cystic fibrosis.[2] Pericarditis can occur with pneumonic tularemia, salmonellosis, sepsis from enteric bacilli, listeriosis, and disseminated gonococcal disease.[7] Anaerobic bacteria should be suspected when pericarditis develops in association with lung abscess, intra-abdominal infection including ruptured appendicitis,[84] or a penetrating wound. Callanan and colleagues[12] reported the rapid development of constrictive pericarditis after purulent pericarditis caused by anaerobic streptococcal infection. The child had a history of blunt trauma to the chest with no evidence of a penetrating wound 3 weeks before cardiac tamponade developed. The incidence of anaerobic infection may be underestimated because of improper handling of specimens for culture.[27] Prolonged symptoms related to pericarditis can be associated with *Mycoplasma pneumoniae* infection.[25]

Mycobacterium tuberculosis, previously a common cause of acute pericarditis in the United States,[6] now is responsible more often for chronic pericardial disease. This infection is a complication of miliary tuberculosis and rarely a primary infection. In the series of 2500 children with tuberculosis reported by Lincoln and Savell,[59] pericarditis was diagnosed in 0.4 percent and found at necropsy in 5 percent of patients. A review of 100 cases of tuberculous pericarditis in South African blacks by Desai[20] revealed a marked male predominance (72%). The

duration of symptoms, consisting of cough and peripheral edema, in most patients was 0 to 120 days. Most patients were febrile and had congestive heart failure. Generalized lymphadenopathy occurred in nearly 30 percent of patients, pulsus paradoxus occurred in 50 percent, and a friction rub was audible in 25 percent. Of the 52 patients who had pericardiocentesis, 40 percent yielded fluid, but none was positive for acid-fast bacilli. Pericardial effusion was shown in 82 patients, 16 of whom died of tamponade, and another 16 of whom developed constricting pericarditis.

The four stages of tuberculous pericarditis have been described as dry, effusive, absorptive, and constrictive.[69] Granulomata usually are found in the dry stage and heal with no sequelae. The effusive stage occurs commonly with tuberculous lymphadenitis, and 15 to 200 mL of fluid usually accumulates in the pericardial space. The absorptive stage is characterized by thickening of the pericardium with fibrin deposition. Further fibrin deposition and calcification occur during the constrictive phase. The disease may progress through all stages or remain in one stage.

Latent infection in the mediastinal lymph nodes with spread directly into the pericardium is thought to be the mode of involvement with *M. tuberculosis*.[69] The lymph nodes at the tracheal bifurcation often are the source.

Histoplasma pericarditis generally occurs with pulmonary, rather than disseminated, disease.[71] Coccidioidomycosis[15] and, rarely, blastomycosis[41] also may cause pericardial disease. Other pathogenic fungi include *Aspergillus* and *Candida*. These fungi are more serious considerations in patients who are immunosuppressed, have serious burns, or are receiving long-term, broad-spectrum antibiotics after undergoing cardiac surgery.[74]

PATHOLOGY AND PATHOGENESIS

Pericarditis begins with fine deposits of fibrin adjacent to the great vessels; it causes the pericardial membrane to lose its smoothness and translucency. Numerous granulocytes may extend into the myocardium.[37]

Bacterial pericarditis most commonly results from direct extension of infection from involved lung and pleura. Pulmonary infections may spread to the pericardium through the bronchial circulation.[40] Pericarditis also can develop through hematogenous dissemination from infection elsewhere. Pericarditis also may be the result of an immunologically induced response to a primary infection.

As pericardial fluid accumulates, intrapericardial pressure increases. The rate of increase is a function of the speed of accumulation and the compliance of the pericardium. With slow accumulation of fluid, large volumes can be accommodated because of the gradual expansion of the parietal pericardium. As the compliance of the pericardium reaches its maximum, however, further accumulation of even small volumes of fluid results in an abrupt increase in intrapericardial pressure. If pericardial fluid accumulates at a rapid rate, marked elevation in intrapericardial pressure may occur with much smaller volumes of fluid. In a small child, 100 mL can cause severe tamponade, whereas 3 L may accumulate slowly in an older child and not result in tamponade.[1]

The most significant hemodynamic effect of pericardial effusion is restriction of ventricular filling. Ventricular end-diastolic, atrial, and venous pressures increase on the right and left sides of the heart equally. When restriction of ventricular filling becomes more pronounced, the ventricular stroke volume and cardiac output decrease. In an attempt to maintain cardiac output, tachycardia and peripheral vasoconstriction occur. Systemic arterial blood pressure and pulse pressure are reduced markedly. Tamponade occurs when these compensatory mechanisms fail to maintain adequate cardiac output.

CLINICAL MANIFESTATIONS

A diagnosis of purulent pericarditis should be suspected in any patient with septicemia who develops cardiomegaly. The classic signs and symptoms of pericarditis are precordial pain, pericardial friction rub, evidence of cardiac fluid, and muffled heart sounds.[14] Chest pain is not a common symptom, especially in small children; the reported rates vary from 15 to 80 percent.[5,7,33,45,64,68,87] Acute abdominal symptoms may be the presenting complaints of some children.[22]

The most common symptoms and signs of pericarditis are fever, tachypnea, and tachycardia. They also are presenting features of associated systemic infection. If the cardiac shadow is radiographically enlarged, with or without a friction rub, and the tachypnea and tachycardia are out of proportion to the fever, myocardial dysfunction or pericarditis should be suspected.

An evanescent or ubiquitous rub may be detected. The typical sound of a rub is that of a high-frequency murmur,[70] which may have a to-and-fro or triphasic pattern but may not have any correlation with the cardiac cycle.[28] Frequently, the rub is heard better with the patient leaning forward or kneeling.[28] A rub may be differentiated from a murmur by pressing the diaphragm of the stethoscope firmly against the chest wall; this pressure amplifies the rub, and the typical scratchy quality becomes more apparent as the examiner opposes the visceral and parietal pericardium by compression of the chest. Rubs have been known to increase with inspiration.[79] Although a rub is less likely to be heard in the presence of a large effusion, it still may exist.[28] The heart sounds usually are muffled, and the palpable ventricular impulse generally is diminished. Both findings may be present in congestive heart failure, but they may be absent with tamponade.

Cardiac tamponade may be an early complication of pericarditis associated with a systemic infection. Cardiac tamponade means that there is compression of the heart by a tense pericardial sac, usually full of fluid, resulting in a decrease in venous return to the cardiac chambers and a decrease in cardiac output. During inspiration, the intrathoracic pressure decreases, and venous return to the cavae increases. The tense pericardial sac limits the amount of blood that can enter the right atrium because of diastolic compression; a paradoxical increase in jugular venous pressure occurs during inspiration (i.e., Kussmaul sign) (Fig. 33–1).[54]

During inspiration, a small decrease in systolic blood pressure and cardiac output normally occurs and is caused by an increase in pulmonary venous capacitance. It is exaggerated with pericardial tamponade (>10 mm Hg decrease in blood pressure) because of the restricted inflow into the cardiac chambers. This clinical sign has been called *paradoxical pulse*, but it actually is an exaggeration of the normal respiratory cycle (Fig. 33–2).[36]

DIAGNOSIS

The radiographic appearance of a rapidly increasing cardiothoracic ratio without increasing pulmonary vascular markings is more suggestive of pericardial effusion than of congestive heart failure caused by myocardial dysfunction (Fig. 33–3). Fluoroscopy alone generally is of little value; myocardial dysfunction and pericarditis can impair cardiac contractility.

The size of the pericardial shadow does not indicate the severity of hemodynamic effects. It is a function of the rapidity of accumulation and the volume of pericardial fluid. When acute infection results in sudden cardiac tamponade, the heart size may be normal. A large, globular heart shadow with no evidence of increased pulmonary vasculature, particularly in a patient who has signs of right-sided heart failure, is strong evidence for pericardial disease. The lack of pulmonary overcirculation helps to distinguish this condition from myocarditis; however, determining whether pulmonary infiltrates also exist may be difficult.

A plain lateral chest radiograph may show findings consistent with a pericardial effusion.[56] Separation of more than 2 mm between the anterior mediastinal and subepithelial "fat stripes" suggests an effusion. Obliteration of the retrosternal space without evidence of thymic or right ventricular enlargement also indicates pericarditis.

The extent of electrocardiographic abnormalities may be explained by the amount of pericardial effusion and the presence of superficial myocardial injury or myocarditis. Pericardial effusion gives rise to low-voltage QRS complexes as a result of the damping effect of pericardial fluid between the chest wall and the myocardium. Accumulation of fluid and fibrin under pressure also may produce an injury pattern manifested by ST-segment deviation. More than 90 percent of patients have elevation of the ST segment, which occurs most frequently in leads I, II, V_5, and V_6. Widespread T-wave inversion indicative of epicarditis may be seen in the same leads in which ST-segment elevation occurs.

Spodick[80] described four stages of electrocardiographic changes in acute pericarditis. In stage I, ST-segment elevation is pronounced, and the PR segment may be depressed. In stage II, the ST segment begins to return to the isoelectric line, the amplitude of the T wave diminishes, and the PR segment is depressed. By stage III, the ST segment has returned to the isoelectric line, and the T-wave inversion occurs. An incompletely inverted T

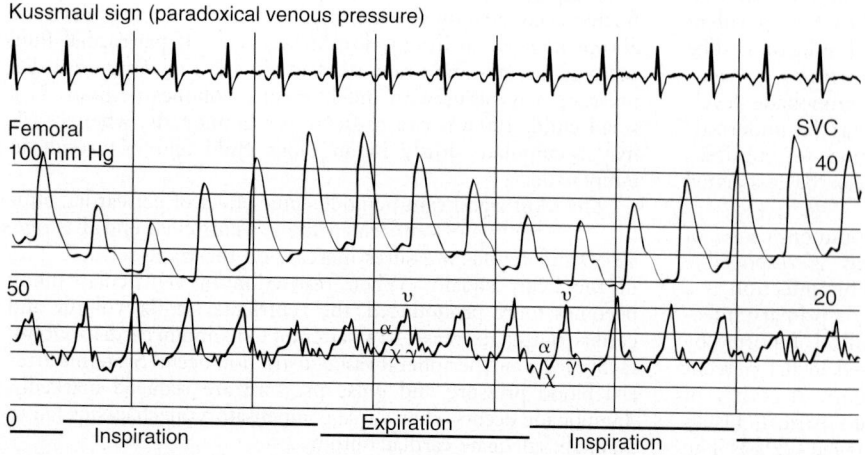

Kussmaul sign (paradoxical venous pressure)

Femoral 100 mm Hg

SVC 40

50

20

0

Inspiration — Expiration — Inspiration

Figure 33–1 Simultaneous recording of right atrial and femoral artery pressures. Notice the increased V wave and exaggerated decrease in the femoral artery pulse with inspiration.

Right Atrial and Femoral Pressures Before
Pericardiocentesis

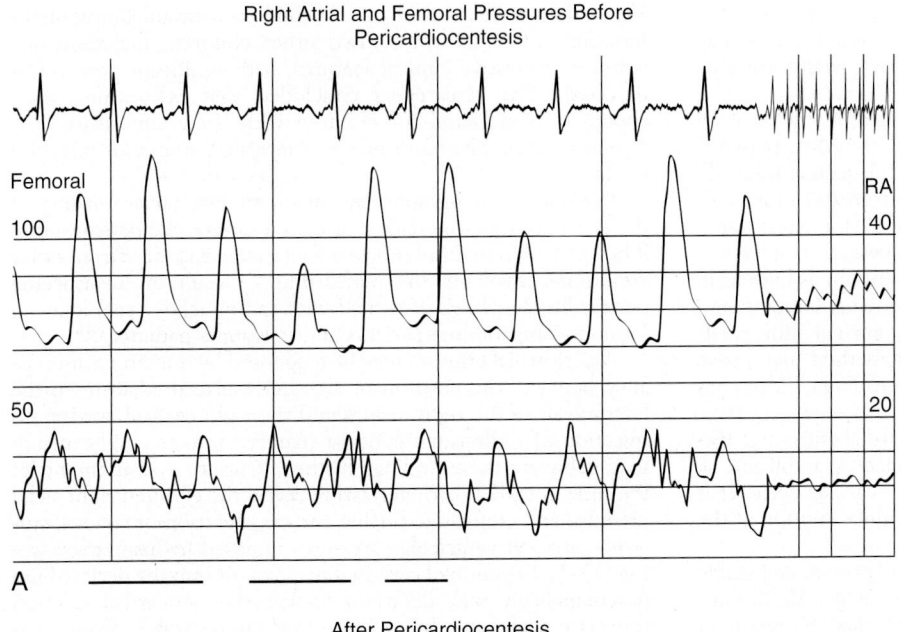

A

After Pericardiocentesis

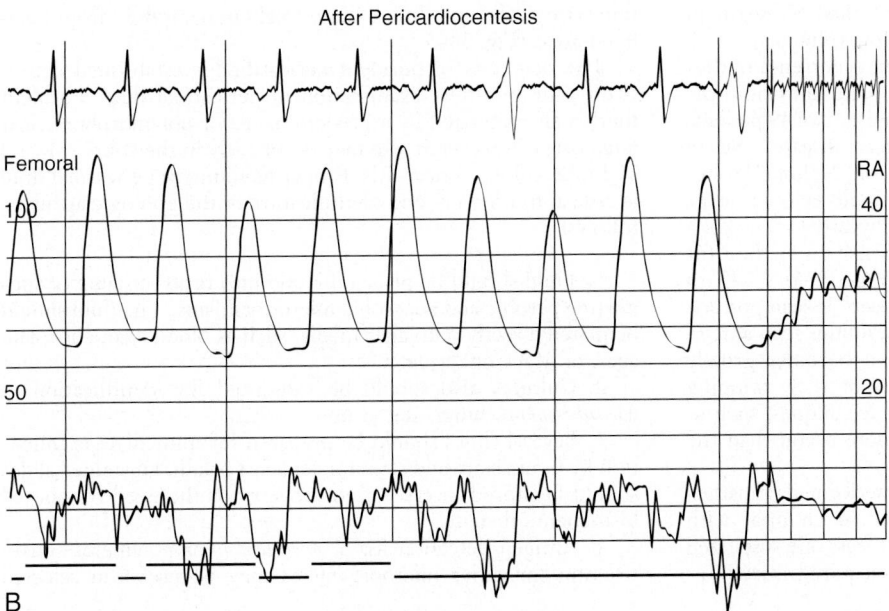

B

Figure 33–2 **A** and **B,** Recordings of femoral artery and right atrial pressures before **(A)** and after **(B)** pericardiocentesis. **A,** There is an exaggerated decrease in the fall of femoral artery pressure with inspiration and a sustained increase in right atrial pressure. **B,** The recording shows a more normal variation of femoral pressure and a lower right atrial pressure.

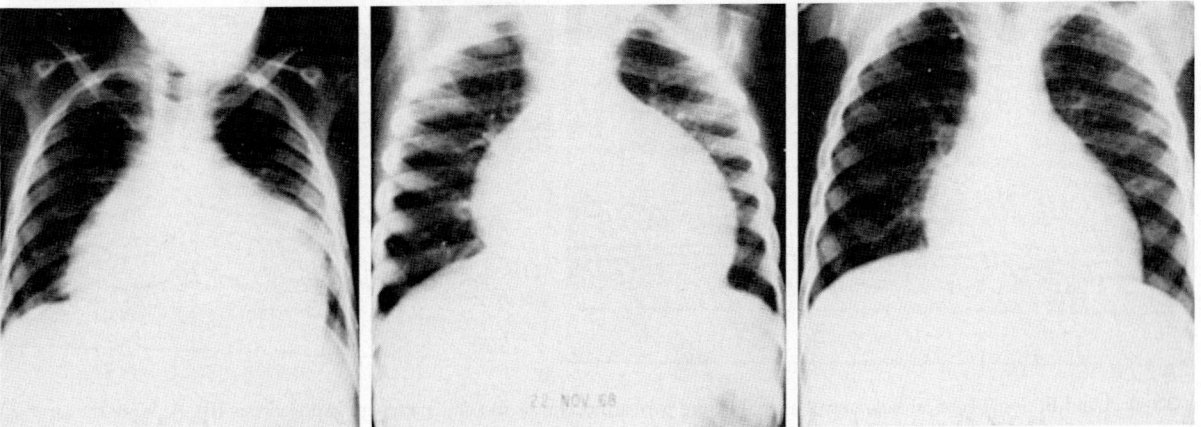

Figure 33–3 In a patient with pericarditis, the first two radiographs show an enlarged cardiac shadow without an increase in pulmonary vascular markings. The third radiograph shows a marked decrease in apparent heart size after pericardiocentesis.

wave (i.e., a diphasic wave or an upright T wave with a notched summit) sometimes is observed. In stage IV, these changes may resolve completely. T-wave abnormalities may persist for life, however, and do not indicate active disease.

Ginzton and Laks[34] compared the electrocardiograms of 19 patients with acute pericarditis with those of 20 healthy patients. By forming a ratio of the amplitude of the ST-segment and T-wave height in all patients, a value of 0.25 or greater in lead V_6 had a positive and negative predictive value of 1.0 for determining the presence of pericarditis. This finding also was true in leads I, V_4, and V_5, although the predictive values were not as high as in lead V_6. Using Spodick's criteria for their patients, Ginzton and Laks[34] were unable to distinguish healthy, normal individuals from patients with acute pericarditis. Their method may prove to be more reliable, although a large study enrolling children has not been performed.

Electrical alternans is seen in a large pericardial effusion. Electrical alternans refers to the alternation in electric amplitude of the T wave and the QRS complex with each cardiac cycle. It is thought to result from the rotational and pendular motion of the heart suspended in pericardial fluid.

Deviations from classic patterns occasionally occur, and single electrocardiographic changes are common findings. All 12 children reported by Okoroma and colleagues[68] had ST-segment elevation, whereas only 3 had concomitant low voltage.

Although many textbooks cite the frequent occurrence of dysrhythmias with pericarditis, these occurrences are unusual in the absence of coexisting heart disease. In one study, 20 of 49 patients with acute pericarditis had no underlying heart disease.[81] Seven patients had no dysrhythmias documented on 24-hour Holter monitoring, and 10 of 20 had infrequent single ectopic beats. Only three patients had supraventricular tachycardia.

M-mode echocardiography is the most sensitive method for diagnosing significant pericardial effusion (Fig. 33-4).[39,46] With a small to moderate effusion, only a "fluid space" is seen posteriorly (see Fig. 33-4B). With a larger effusion, fluid is seen anteriorly and posteriorly, and the septal motion becomes grossly abnormal. The heart may give the appearance of freely swinging (see Fig. 33-4A). Newer echocardiographic techniques, such as two-dimensional sector scanning, are not more useful than the conventional M-mode.

Friedland and colleagues[30] prospectively performed transthoracic two-dimensional echocardiography in 36 children with staphylococcal bacteremia; 89 percent had at least one suspected focus of infection, and 19 had community-acquired infections.

Vegetations were detected in four children without clinical manifestations of endocarditis. Two other children, including one without suggestive clinical features, had significant pericarditis detected. The researchers concluded that echocardiography should be considered for children with bacteremia caused by *S. aureus*, even when an obvious noncardiac source of infection exists.

Computed tomography and magnetic resonance imaging of the chest are other modalities used to examine the pericardium.[8] They may help to differentiate a bacterial pericarditis from other conditions involving the pericardium. Occult or unsuspected pericarditis has been discerned with radionuclide techniques in immunocompromised patients and in trauma patients.[38,76]

A pericardial effusion may be diagnosed by noticing a discrepancy between the position of a catheter placed adjacent to the lateral wall of the right atrium and the right cardiac border. An injection of radiopaque contrast material into the right atrium may delineate these findings further. Pressure measurements at the time of cardiac catheterization reveal the elevated right atrial pressure and emphasize further the exaggeration of venous, systemic, and left ventricular pressures imposed by inspiration (see Fig. 33-2). Injection of carbon dioxide or air into the pericardium percutaneously may delineate further the pericardial effusion fluoroscopically and differentiate freely moving fluid from loculated areas (Fig. 33-5).

The diagnosis of purulent pericarditis is established definitively only by direct examination of pericardial fluid. Purulent fluid is characterized by a predominance of polymorphonuclear leukocytes; however, it also may occur early in the course of viral and tuberculous pericarditis. Proper handling of pericardial fluid is crucial to recovery and identification of the etiologic agent, as follows:

1. Fluid should be placed directly into broth capable of supporting aerobic and anaerobic microorganisms. The fluid should be plated directly onto agar media, such as blood agar, chocolate agar, or MacConkey agar.
2. Cultures also should be submitted for identification of *M. tuberculosis*, fungi, and viruses.
3. Several slides should be prepared for immediate examination by Gram stain and stain for acid-fast bacilli. Unstained slides should be stored in case of controversy or the need for special histochemical stains.
4. Antigen detection for *S. pneumoniae* or polymerase chain reaction for other microorganisms may be useful in selected

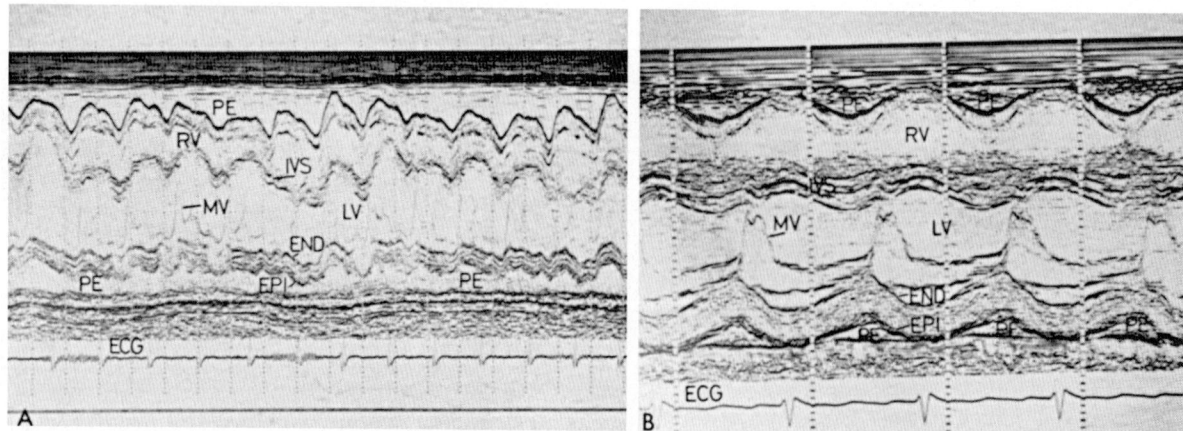

Figure 33-4 A and B, Serial echocardiograms of a child before pericardiocentesis (**A**) and after pericardiocentesis (**B**). **A**, Note the large effusion anteriorly and posteriorly with the "swinging" movement of the septum and anterior and posterior walls. **B**, The heart movement is normal, and there remains only a small effusion anteriorly and posteriorly. ECG, electrocardiogram; END, endocardium; EPI, epicardium; IVS, interventricular septum; LV, left ventricle; MV, mitral valve; PE, pericardial effusion; RV, right ventricle.

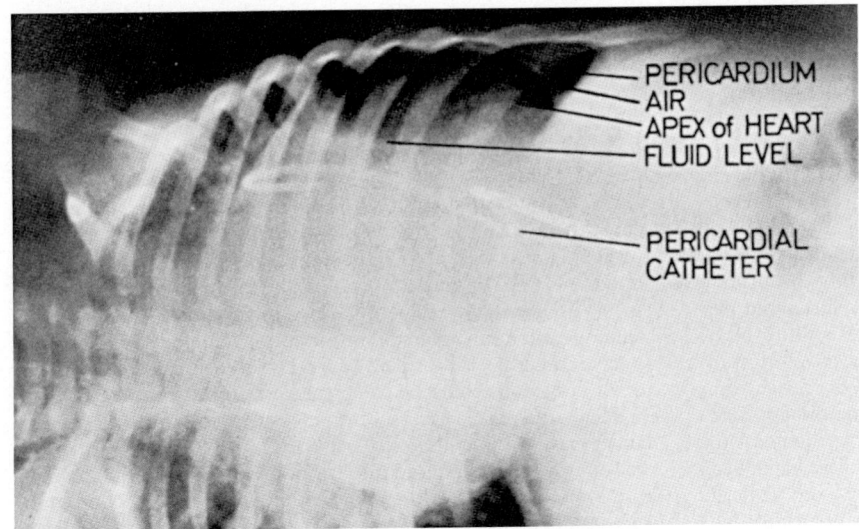

Figure 33-5 Chest radiograph of a patient lying on the right side with a catheter in the pericardium. Air has been injected through the catheter, outlining the pericardium and fluid within the sac.

cases, particularly when the patient has received prior antimicrobial therapy.[58]

The causative microorganism is isolated from blood cultures in many patients. When indicated, cerebrospinal fluid also should be cultured. Because purulent pericarditis often occurs after infections of the lung or pleural space, thoracentesis can reveal the etiologic agent in many cases. Documentation of empyema together with evidence of pericardial disease correlates highly with purulent pericarditis.

Acid-fast bacilli are seen on stained smears of pericardial fluid from 15 to 42 percent of patients with tuberculous pericarditis.[6] Examination of pericardial biopsy specimens by routine methods and with special stains such as the auramine O stain can increase the frequency of identification of *M. tuberculosis*.[66] A negative purified protein derivative skin test does not exclude the diagnosis of tuberculous pericarditis.

Grossly bloody pericardial fluid is observed frequently in patients with *Histoplasma* pericarditis, and an aspirate of the effusion reveals a predominance of mononuclear leukocytes. Growth of *Histoplasma capsulatum* from pericardial fluid rarely is successful. Showing the typical intracellular yeast forms on special stain of pericardial tissue also is helpful. Elevation of the yeast phase of the complement-fixation titer in pericardial fluid allows one to make a more rapid diagnosis.[71] Serum precipitin antibodies to *H. capsulatum* also indicate acute histoplasmosis and are helpful when present. Detecting the polysaccharide of *H. capsulatum* in urine or other body fluids is a rapid and sensitive means by which to establish the diagnosis of histoplasmosis.

DIFFERENTIAL DIAGNOSIS

Any patient with a rapidly increasing heart size in the absence of increasing pulmonary vascular markings should be suspected to have a pericardial effusion. Purulent pericarditis must be differentiated from pericardial effusion caused by collagen diseases, other infectious agents (e.g., viral, tuberculous, rickettsial, protozoan), neoplastic disorders, metabolic disorders, and congestive heart failure.[14] Glycogen storage disease, congenital heart disease, primary myocardial disease, cardiac tumors, and coronary artery aberrations (i.e., anomalous origin from the pulmonary artery, medial wall necrosis, and Kawasaki disease) may be confused with pericardial effusion.[14] Appropriate analysis of pericardial fluid usually permits differentiation of purulent pericarditis from pericarditis caused by other disorders.

TREATMENT

Purulent pericarditis is a potentially life-threatening illness that requires pericardial decompression and open drainage, appropriate antimicrobial therapy, and intense supportive therapy. Ainger[1] stated that more than half of children with purulent pericarditis require early or emergency drainage of the pericardium for relief of critical tamponade. Although bedside needle pericardiocentesis may be lifesaving or necessary for establishing a rapid diagnosis, Fowler and Manitasas[28] reported three deaths related to pericardiocentesis performed by inexperienced physicians. Complications include arrhythmias resulting from myocardial injury, laceration of the coronary arteries leading to hemopericardium and tamponade, and pneumothorax. Ledbetter[57] described a 10-year-old girl with staphylococcal pericarditis who developed an aortic aneurysm after undergoing multiple pericardiocentesis procedures for recurrent tamponade. The subxiphoid approach is recommended, and Hoffman and Stanger[44] have described the proper technique.

Decompression and drainage of the pericardium are safest in a controlled environment, such as in an operating room or under fluoroscopy in the catheterization laboratory. If the patient is awake and agitated, premedication may be required.

If pericardiocentesis does not relieve symptoms successfully, and evidence of tamponade continues, immediate surgical drainage is necessary. Multiple attempts may prove unsuccessful and can lead to serious complications. The pus surrounding the heart may be too thick to be aspirated, as has been seen especially with *H. influenzae* infection.[62] Surgical creation of a pericardial window with a drain occasionally is necessary for complete removal of fluid, which accumulates rapidly. In preparation for evacuation of the pericardial fluid during tamponade, adequate cardiac output can be maintained by stimulating the heart with pharmacologic agents that cause a chronotropic and an inotropic effect. Isoproterenol administered intravenously at a rate of 0.05 to 0.10 µg/kg/min is our drug of choice. It does not replace evacuating the fluid, but it gains time until the aspiration or drainage can be done.

Medications that tend to decrease heart rate and intravascular volume are contraindicated because they compromise the patient further. Wyler and colleagues[89] warn against the use of halothane anesthesia because of its known depressant effect on myocardial function. They described two patients who had reversible cardiac arrest when this agent was used during surgery to relieve tamponade.

Controversy exists regarding the approach and extent of surgery.[26,28,29,55,63,75] A left anterolateral thoracotomy through the fifth intercostal space or a subxiphoid approach with removal of the xiphoid process seems best. Most surgeons favor the creation of a pericardial "window"; however, some favor more extensive removal of pericardial tissue. This decision may be influenced by the severity of pericardial inflammation or the presence of bloody pericardial fluid because these conditions have greater potential for producing acute or chronic constriction. Care must be taken during the procedure not to injure the phrenic nerves.

Morgan and colleagues[62] reviewed 15 children with purulent pericarditis between 1971 and 1981. H. influenzae occurred in 7 of 15 patients. Most patients had pericardiocentesis followed by an anterior interphrenic pericardiectomy and recovered completely. In a series of nine children with H. influenzae pericarditis, all received a limited left thoracotomy with subxiphoid approach for pericardiostomy, and no deaths occurred.[16] Video-assisted thoracoscopic approaches to managing pericarditis have been described, but further experience is necessary for pediatric patients.[60] For selected patients for whom surgery cannot be performed in a timely manner, the instillation of intrapericardial streptokinase or urokinase or other thrombolytic agents has been successful in draining purulent pericarditis and preventing the need for a more extensive surgical procedure.[50]

Antimicrobial therapy alone is insufficient for the successful treatment of purulent pericarditis. The survival of patients with purulent pericarditis is improved significantly when early pericardial drainage is performed (Table 33–3). In the preantibiotic era, draining the pericardium decreased the mortality rate from nearly 100 percent to 45 percent.[7] Occasionally, patients with meningococcal pericarditis have been managed successfully without pericardial drainage.[18] Fyfe and colleagues[31] described 73 of 79 patients with H. influenzae pericarditis seen between 1928 and 1984. The mortality rate before 1960 was 64 percent (7 of 11 patients), although five of seven deaths were reported before the antibiotic era. From 1960 to 1969, the mortality rate was 36 percent, and from 1970 to 1979, it decreased to 11.5 percent. From 1980 to 1984, 25 cases with no mortality were reported.

When the etiologic agent cannot be detected rapidly, the initial antibiotic regimen should consist of two or more drugs. Because S. aureus is a major pathogen, a penicillinase-resistant penicillin, such as nafcillin or oxacillin, must be included in a dose of 200 mg/kg/24 hr (maximum 12 g). In regions where infections caused by methicillin-resistant S. aureus have occurred in the community, when strains of S. pneumoniae resistant to the extended-spectrum cephalosporins are present, or when the infection is nosocomially acquired, vancomycin should be given, 40 to 60 mg/kg/day in four divided doses (maximum 4 g). Cefotaxime (200 to 300 mg/kg/day in three or four divided doses) or ceftriaxone (100 mg/kg/day in one or two doses) should be administered to provide protection against S. pneumoniae (including penicillin-resistant strains), N. meningitidis, and H. influenzae type b for children who may be inadequately immunized.

An aminoglycoside antibiotic should be added to the above-mentioned combined drug therapy when purulent pericarditis occurs after cardiac surgery, in association with genitourinary infections, or in the immunocompromised host. For patients who are allergic to penicillin, vancomycin, clindamycin, or cefazolin is

substituted for the treatment of susceptible S. aureus; some patients who are allergic to penicillin are sensitive to cephalosporins.

The duration of therapy is empiric and is determined partly by the nature of concomitant infection. Generally, after a pathogen is isolated and the antimicrobial susceptibilities are known, the most specific antimicrobial agent is continued intravenously for 3 to 4 weeks.

Using chemotherapy to treat tuberculous pericarditis has had a major impact on mortality. Before its use, the mortality rate in the acute phase was 80 to 90 percent. The other 10 to 20 percent of patients died of constrictive pericarditis or miliary tuberculosis.[69] The use of three or four drugs, including isoniazid, pyrazinamide, rifampin, and possibly streptomycin, for 9 to 12 months is recommended. The role of corticosteroids in preventing progression to constriction or decreasing mortality is unclear.[23,61,69] In selected cases, pericardiectomy may be indicated to prevent constrictive pericarditis.

Amphotericin B, alone or with other systemic agents, is indicated for treatment of fungal pericarditis. It rarely is required for successful therapy of Histoplasma pericarditis, for which nonsteroidal anti-inflammatory drugs are recommended for 2 to 12 weeks, depending on the clinical resolution of symptoms and physical findings of pericarditis.[88] Steroids may be tried for 1 to 2 weeks. As with bacterial pericarditis, open pericardiectomy is crucial for the successful treatment of Candida pericarditis.[74]

General supportive therapy in the acute stage of infection may include the administration of oxygen, volume expansion to increase ventricular filling pressure, and isoproterenol to facilitate systolic emptying. Digitalis and diuretics should be used cautiously and only when indicated by decreased myocardial function. Serial electrocardiograms may indicate the presence of occult arrhythmias and alert the physician to the degree of myocardial involvement. The patient must be monitored carefully for signs of reaccumulation of pericardial fluid and for the development of acute constrictive pericarditis. Strauss and colleagues[82] reported this complication in 2 of 12 children with purulent pericarditis. Acute constriction may develop within weeks of the initial pericardial infection[5,10] and has been reported at 8 days.[73] Constrictive pericarditis may be suspected by increasing jugular and central venous pressure, weight gain, enlarging liver, worsening dyspnea, and decreased urinary output. The persistence of heart failure when the cardiac silhouette is becoming smaller also suggests the development of constrictive pericarditis. Complete pericardiectomy should be performed promptly when constriction is suspected.

PROGNOSIS

The current mortality rate for acute purulent pericarditis ranges from 25 to 75 percent. Accurate statistics are difficult to compute from the literature because the nature and severity of underlying disease have not been considered. Factors that contribute to mortality are delay in recognition, absence of early surgical drainage, presence of cardiac tamponade, degree of myocardial involvement, etiologic agent (particularly S. aureus), and age of the patient. Long-term follow-up of children with purulent pericarditis is recommended. They should be followed carefully for the presence of a constrictive component as a sequela to the acute infection. Most children recover fully, however, and return to normal activity.

VIRAL PERICARDITIS

In 1951, Christian[17] suggested that viral infections were responsible for cases of idiopathic or benign pericarditis. A viral cause has not been substantiated in many patients, however.

TABLE 33–3 Influence of Pericardial Drainage on Survival in Purulent Pericarditis in Children

Treatment	Survived	Died
Antibiotics alone	5	28
Antibiotics and pericardial drainage	45	10

Data from references 5, 29, 53, and 65.

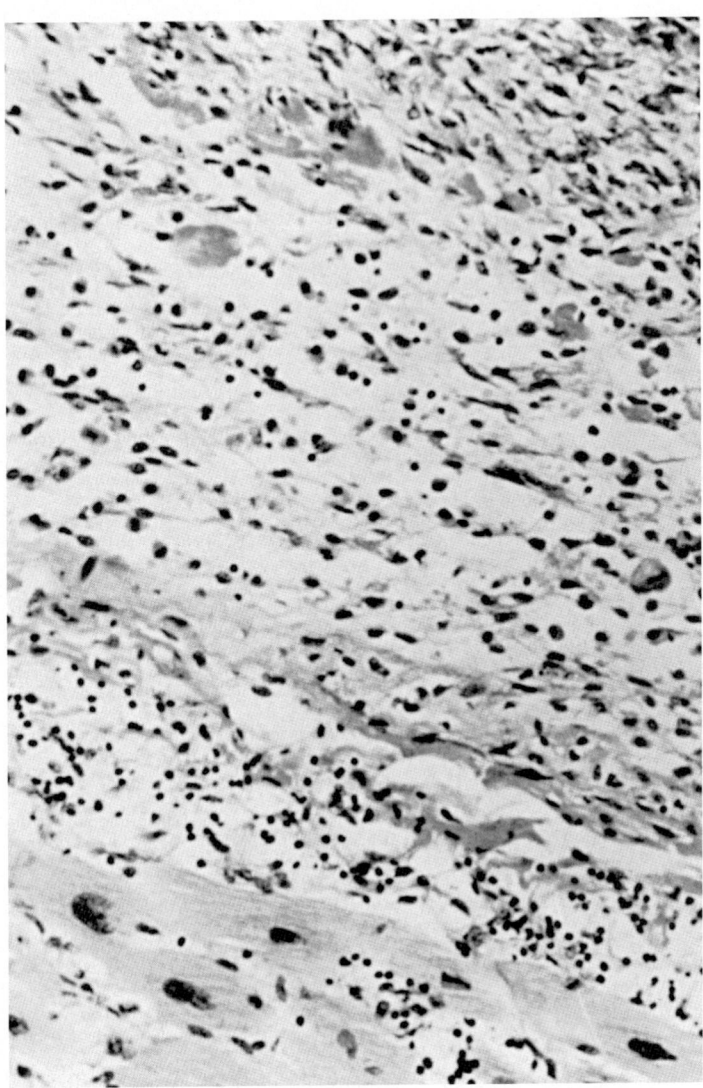

Figure 33–6 In this case of viral pericarditis, there is a layer of fibrin and fibroblasts along the pericardial surface. The mononuclear cell infiltrate in the epicardium extends into the outer myocardium (hematoxylin and eosin staining, ×400). *(Courtesy of Edith P. Hawkins, M.D., Texas Children's Hospital, Houston.)*

ETIOLOGY

The principal viruses implicated in pericarditis are the coxsackie-viruses.[65] Adenoviruses have been recovered less frequently.[49] Associations with varicella,[85] cytomegalovirus,[13] smallpox vaccinations, influenza,[43] influenza vaccinations,[83] and infectious mononucleosis[47,78] have been reported.

CLINICAL MANIFESTATIONS

In approximately 40 to 75 percent of cases, the patient has a history of upper respiratory tract infection for 10 days to 2 weeks preceding the onset of symptoms. Fever and chest and abdominal pain are the most common symptoms.[17] A friction rub may be heard in 50 to 80 percent of cases.[87] Children with viral pericarditis generally are less toxic and experience smaller elevations in body temperature than do children with purulent pericarditis. Some appear acutely ill, however. Large amounts of pericardial fluid accumulation and tamponade are rare findings.

INVESTIGATIVE TECHNIQUES

The electrocardiographic, radiographic, echocardiographic, and nuclear scanning findings described for patients with purulent pericarditis also are observed in patients with viral pericarditis. The peripheral leukocyte count may reveal fewer polymorphonuclear leukocytes than in patients with bacterial pericarditis. Mononuclear cell infiltrates in the pericardium with extension into the myocardium may be seen (Fig. 33–6).

If obtained, pericardial fluid should be sent for cell count and viral culture. Nasopharyngeal and rectal samples also should be obtained and cultured for viruses. Acute and convalescent sera should be obtained so that appropriate titers can be measured if a virus is isolated.

COURSE AND PROGNOSIS

Viral pericarditis generally resolves spontaneously over the course of 3 to 4 weeks.[65] Large pericardial effusions and tamponade are rare occurrences.[14] Generally, bed rest for approximately 1 week and analgesics for pain are the only therapy that is required. Constrictive pericarditis is a rare occurrence, but pericarditis may recur.[65]

REFERENCES

1. Ainger, L. E.: Diseases of the pericardium. *In* Kelley, V. C. (ed.): Practice of Pediatrics. Vol. III. New York, Harper Medical, Looseleaf Reference Services, 1969.

2. Altemeier, W. A., Tonelli, M. R., and Aitken, M. L.: Pseudomonal pericarditis complicating cystic fibrosis. Pediatr. Pulmonol. 27:62-65, 1999.

3. Baevsky, R. H.: Primary meningococcal pericarditis. Clin. Infect. Dis. 20:213-215, 1999.

4. Basher, H. E., Klaber, R., Baki, A. E., and Booy, R.: W135 meningococcal pericarditis: Report of two cases and review of the literature. Pediatr. Infect. Dis. J. 23:969-970, 2004.

5. Benzing, G., III, and Kaplan, S.: Purulent pericarditis. Am. J. Dis. Child. 106:287-294, 1963.

6. Boyd, G. L.: Tuberculous pericarditis in children. Am. J. Dis. Child. 86:293-300, 1953.

7. Boyle, J. D., Pearce, M. L., and Guze, L. B.: Purulent pericarditis: Review of literature and report of eleven cases. Medicine (Baltimore) 40:119-144, 1961.

8. Breen, J. F.: Imaging of the pericardium. J. Thorac. Imaging 16:47-54, 2001.

9. Brumund, M. R., Truemper, E. J., and Pearson-Shaver, A. L.: Disseminated varicella and staphylococcal pericarditis after topical steroids. J. Pediatr. 131:162-163, 1997.

10. Caird, R., Conway, N., and McMillan, I. K. R.: Purulent pericarditis followed by early constriction in young children. Br. Heart J. 35:201-203, 1973.

11. Cakir, Ö., Gurkan, F., Balci, A. E., et al.: Purulent pericarditis in childhood: Ten years of experience. J. Pediatr. Surg. 37:1404-1408, 2002.

12. Callanan, D. L., Morriss, M. J., Kaplan, S. L., et al.: Constrictive pericarditis due to *Streptococcus sanguis*. South. Med. J. 74:377-378, 1981.

13. Campbell, P. T., Li, J. S., Wall, T. C., et al.: Cytomegalovirus pericarditis: Case series and review of the literature. Am. J. Med. Sci. 309:229-234, 1995.

14. Cayler, G. G., and Riley, H. D.: Non-rheumatic inflammatory cardiovascular diseases. *In* Moss, A. J., and Adams, F. H. (eds.): Heart Disease in Infants, Children and Adolescents. Baltimore, Williams & Wilkins, 1968, p. 851.

15. Chapman, M. G., and Kaplan, L.: Cardiac involvement in coccidioidomycosis. Am. J. Med. 23:87-98, 1957.

16. Cheatham, J. E., Grantham, R. N., Peyton, M. D., et al.: *Haemophilus influenzae* purulent pericarditis in children. J. Thorac. Cardiovasc. Surg. 79:933-936, 1980.

17. Christian, H. A.: Nearly ten decades of interest in idiopathic pericarditis. Am. Heart J. 42:654, 1951.

18. Connolly, D. C., and Burchell, H. B.: Pericarditis: A ten-year survey. Am. J. Cardiol. 7:7-13, 1961.

19. Corachan, M., Poore, P., Hadley, G. P., et al.: Purulent pericarditis in Papua, New Guinea: Report of 12 cases and review of the literature in a tropical environment. Trans. R. Soc. Trop. Med. Hyg. 77:341-343, 1983.

20. Desai, H. N.: Tuberculous pericarditis: A review of 100 cases. S. Afr. Med. J. 55:877-880, 1979.

21. Dixon, L. M., and Sanford, H. S.: Meningococcal pericarditis in the antibiotic era. Milit. Med. 136:433-438, 1971.

22. Donnelly, L. F., Kimball, T. R., and Barr, L. L.: Purulent pericarditis presenting as acute abdomen in children: Abdominal imaging findings. Clin. Radiol. 54:691-693, 1999.

23. Dooley, D. P., Carpenter, J. L., and Rademacher, S.: Adjunctive corticosteroid therapy for tuberculosis: A critical reappraisal of the literature. Clin. Infect. Dis. 25:872-877, 1997.

24. Echeverria, P., Smith, E. W. P., Ingram, D., et al.: *Haemophilus influenzae* b pericarditis in children. Pediatrics 56:808-818, 1975.

25. Farraj, R. S., McCully, R. B., Oh, J. K., and Smith, T. F.: *Mycoplasma*-associated pericarditis. Mayo Clin. Proc. 72:33-36, 1997.

26. Farrow, C. D., Jr., Brom, A. G., and Nauta, J.: The surgical treatment of pericarditis: A follow-up study. Chest 48:478-483, 1965.

27. Feldman, W. E.: Bacterial etiology and mortality of purulent pericarditis in pediatric patients: Review of 162 cases. Am. J. Dis. Child. 133:641-644, 1979.

28. Fowler, N. O., and Manitasas, G. T.: Infectious pericarditis. Prog. Cardiovasc. Dis. 16:323-336, 1973.

29. Fredriksen, R. T., Cohen, L., and Mullins, C. B.: Pericardial window or pericardiocentesis for pericardial effusions. Am. Heart J. 82:158-162, 1971.

30. Friedland, I. R., du Plessis, J., and Cilliers, A.: Cardiac complications in children with *Staphylococcus aureus* bacteremias. J. Pediatr. 127:746-748, 1995.

31. Fyfe, D. A., Hagler, D. J., Puga, F. J., et al.: Clinical and therapeutic aspects of *Haemophilus influenzae* pericarditis in pediatric patients. Mayo Clin. Proc. 59:415-422, 1984.

32. Geggel, R. L.: Conditions leading to pediatric cardiology consultation in a tertiary academic hospital. Pediatrics 114:e409-e417, 2004.

33. Gersony, W. M., and McCracken, G. H.: Purulent pericarditis in infancy. Pediatrics 40:224-232, 1967.

34. Ginzton, L. E., and Laks, M. M.: The differential diagnosis of acute pericarditis from the normal variant: New electrocardiographic criteria. Circulation 65:1004-1009, 1982.

35. Go, C., Asnis, D. S., and Saltzman, H.: Pneumococcal pericarditis since 1980. Clin. Infect. Dis. 27:1338-1340, 1998.

36. Golinko, R. V., Kaplan, N., and Rudolph, A. M.: The mechanism of pulsus paradoxus during acute pericardial tamponade. J. Clin. Invest. 42:229, 1963.

37. Gore, I., and Kline, I. K.: Pericarditis and myocarditis: A. Pericarditis. *In* Gould, S. E. (ed.): Pathology of the Heart and Great Vessels. 3rd ed. Springfield, IL, Charles C Thomas, 1968, p. 724.

38. Greenberg, M. L., Niebulski, H. I. J., Uretsky, B. F., et al.: Occult purulent pericarditis detected by iridium-111 leukocyte imaging. Chest 85:701-703, 1984.

39. Gutgesell, H. P., and Paquet, M.: Atlas of Pediatric Echocardiography. Hagerstown, MD, Harper & Row, 1978, p. 161.

40. Hahn, R. S., Holman, E., and Fuerichs, J. B.: The role of the bronchial artery circulation in the etiology of pulmonary and pericardial suppuration. J. Thorac. Surg. 27:121, 1954.

41. Herman, G. R., Marchand, E. J., and Grur, G. H.: Pericarditis: Clinical and laboratory data of 130 cases. Am. Heart J. 43:641-652, 1952.

42. Herrick, W. W.: Meningococcal pericarditis. Med. Clin. North Am. 2:411, 1918.

43. Hildebrandt, H. M., Maassab, H. F., and Willis, P. W.: Influenza virus pericarditis. Am. J. Dis. Child. 104:579, 1962.

44. Hoffman, J. I. E., and Stanger, P.: Diseases of the pericardium. *In* Rudolph, A. (ed.): Pediatrics. New York, Appleton-Century-Crofts, 1977, pp. 1474-1477.

45. Horan, J. M.: Acute staphylococcal pericarditis. Pediatrics 19:36-43, 1957.

46. Horowitz, M. S., Schultz, C. S., Stinson, E. B., et al.: Sensitivity and specificity of echocardiography diagnosis of pericardial effusion. Circulation 50:239, 1974.

47. Hudgins, J. M.: Infectious mononucleosis complicated by myocarditis and pericarditis. J. A. M. A. 235:262, 1976.

48. Jaiyesimi, F., Abioye, A. A., and Antia, A. U.: Infective pericarditis in Nigerian children. Arch. Dis. Child. 54:384-390, 1979.

49. Johnson, R. T., Portnoy, B., Rodgers, N. G., et al.: Acute benign pericarditis: Virologic study of 34 patients. Arch. Intern. Med. 108:823, 1961.

50. Juneja, R., Kothari, S. S., Saxena, A., et al.: Intrapericardial streptokinase in purulent pericarditis. Arch. Dis. Child. 80:275-277, 1999.

51. Kanarek, K. S., and Coleman, J.: Purulent pericarditis in a neonate. Pediatr. Infect. Dis. J. 10:549-550, 1991.

52. Kaplan, S. L., Mason, E. O., Jr., Wald, E. R., et al.: Six-year multicenter surveillance of invasive pneumococcal infections in children. Pediatr. Infect. Dis. J. 21:141-147, 2002.

53. Kauffman, C. A., Watanakunakorn, C., and Phair, J. P.: Purulent pneumococcal pericarditis: A continuing problem in the antibiotic era. Am. J. Med. 54:743-750, 1973.

54. Kussmaul, A.: Ueber schwieglige mediastino-perikarditis und der paradoxen puls. Klin. Wochenschr. 10:443, 1873.

55. Lajos, T. Z., Black, H. E., Cooper, R. G., et al.: Pericardial compression. Ann. Thorac. Surg. 19:47-53, 1975.

56. Lane, E. J., and Carsky, E. W.: Epicardial fat: Lateral plain film analysis in normals and in pericardial effusion. Radiology 91:1-5, 1968.

57. Ledbetter, M. K.: Aortic aneurysm complicating staphylococcal pericarditis. Okla. State Med. Assoc. 74:222-225, 1981.

58. Levy, P. Y., Fournier, P. E., Charrel, R., et al.: Molecular analysis of pericardial fluid: A 7-year experience. Eur. Heart J. 27:1942-1946, 2006.

59. Lincoln, E. M., and Savell, E. M.: Tuberculosis in Children. New York, McGraw-Hill, 1963.

60. Mack, M. M., Acuff, T., Hazelrigg, S., and Landreneau, R.: Thoracoscopic approach for the pericardium. Endosc. Surg. Allied Technol. 1:271-274, 1993.

61. Mayosi, B. M., Burgess, L. J., and Doubell, A. F.: Tuberculous pericarditis. Circulation 112:3608-3616, 2005.

62. Morgan, R. J., Stephenson, L. W., Woolf, P. K., et al.: Surgical treatment of purulent pericarditis in children. J. Thorac. Cardiovasc. Surg. 85:527-531, 1983.

63. Mullen, D. C., Dillon, M. L., Young, W. G., Jr., et al.: Pericardiectomy in non-tuberculous pericarditis. J. Thorac. Cardiovasc. Surg. 58:517-529, 1969.

64. Nadas, A. S., and Levy, J. M.: Pericarditis in children. Am. J. Cardiol. 7:109-117, 1961.

65. Neill, C. A., and Harouturuan, L. M.: Diseases of the pericardium. *In* Watson, H. (ed.): Paediatric Cardiology. London, Lloyd-Luke, 1968, p. 703.

66. Nelson, C. T., and Taber, L. H.: Diagnosis of tuberculous pericarditis with a fluorochrome stain. Pediatr. Infect. Dis. J. 14:1004-1006, 1995.

67. O'Connell, B.: Pericarditis following meningococcal meningitis. Am. J. Dis. Child. 126:265-267, 1973.

68. Okoroma, E., Perry, L. W., and Scott, L. P.: Acute bacterial pericarditis in children: Report of 25 cases. Am. Heart J. 90:709-713, 1975.

69. Orbtals, D. W., and Avioli, L. V.: Tuberculous pericarditis. Arch. Intern. Med. 139:231-234, 1979.

70. Phillips, J. H., and Burch, G. E.: Selected clues in cardiac auscultation. Am. Heart J. 63:1, 1962.

71. Picardi, J. L., Kaufmann, C. A., Schwarz, J., et al.: Pericarditis caused by *Histoplasma capsulatum*. Am. J. Cardiol. 37:82-88, 1976.

72. Roodmeyma, S., and Sadeghian, N.: Acute pericarditis in childhood: A 10-year experience. Pediatr. Cardiol. 21:363-367, 2000.

73. Rubenstein, J. J., Goldblatt, A., and Daggett, W. M.: Acute constriction complicating purulent pericarditis in infancy. Am. J. Dis. Child. 124:591-594, 1972.

74. Schrank, J. H., Jr., and Dooley, D. P.: Purulent pericarditis caused by *Candida* species: Case report and review. Clin. Infect. Dis. 21:182-187, 1995.

75. Sethi, G. K., Nelson, R. M., and Jenson, C. B.: Surgical management of acute septic pericarditis. Chest 63:732-735, 1973.

76. Shreiner, D. P., Krishnaswami, V., and Murphy, J. H.: Unsuspected purulent pericarditis detected by gallium-67 scanning. Clin. Nucl. Med. 6:411-412, 1981.

77. Simon, H. B., Tarr, P. I., Hutter, A. M., et al.: Primary meningococcal pericarditis: Diagnosis by countercurrent immunoelectrophoresis. J. A. M. A. 235:278-280, 1976.

78. Smith, J. N., Jr.: Complications of infectious mononucleosis. Ann. Intern. Med. *44*:861, 1956.
79. Spodick, D. H.: Pericardial rub: Prospective multiple observer investigation of pericardial friction in 100 patients. Am. J. Cardiol. *35*:357, 1975.
80. Spodick, D. H.: Acute Pericarditis. New York, Grune & Stratton, 1959, p. 17.
81. Spodick, D. H.: Frequency of arrhythmias in acute pericarditis determined by Holter monitoring. Am. J. Cardiol. *53*:842-845, 1984.
82. Strauss, A. W., Santa-Maria, M., and Goldring, D.: Constrictive pericarditis in children. Am. J. Dis. Child. *129*:822-826, 1975.
83. Streifler, J. J., Dux, S., Garty, M., et al.: Recurrent pericarditis: A rare complication of influenza vaccination. B. M. J. *283*:526-527, 1981.

84. Tan, E. C., Rieu, P. N., Nijveld, A., et al.: Pericarditis as complication of appendicitis. Ann. Thorac. Surg. *78*:1086-1088, 2004.
85. Tatter, D., Gerard, P. W., and Silverman, A. H.: Fatal varicella pericarditis in a child. Am. J. Dis. Child. *108*:88, 1964.
86. Thebaud, B., Sisi, D., and Kachaner, J.: Purulent pericarditis in children: A 15-year experience. Arch. Pediatr. *3*:1084-1090, 1996.
87. Weir, E. K., and Joffe, H. S.: Purulent pericarditis in children: An analysis of 28 cases. Thorax *32*:438, 1977.
88. Wheat, J., Sarosi, G., McKinsey, D., et al.: Practice guidelines for the management of patients with histoplasmosis. Clin. Infect. Dis. *30*:688-695, 2000.
89. Wyler, F., Knulsi, D., Rutishauser, M., et al.: Pericarditis purulenta in children. Helv. Paediatr. Acta *32*:135-140, 1977.

MYOCARDITIS

Jesus G. Vallejo

Myocarditis is defined clinically and pathologically as inflammation of the myocardium. The clinical presentation and cause may be quite varied. This entity may go unrecognized in numerous patients whose illness may resolve spontaneously, or it may lead to significant morbidity and mortality.

In the early part of the 20th century, most cases of myocarditis were classified as idiopathic, and a diffuse or focal interstitial inflammation was identified on histologic examination. Rheumatic fever, diphtheria, and other bacterial infections were the only diseases recognized as associated with myocarditis, although some experts suspected that viruses might play a significant etiologic role in many cases.[157] After the discovery in 1947 of the coxsackievirus group and the subsequent isolation and identification of other viruses, the number of cases of myocarditis classified as idiopathic diminished rapidly.[35]

EPIDEMIOLOGY

The diverse clinical manifestations have made the true incidence of myocarditis difficult to determine. The clinical course of acute myocarditis can be insidious, with limited inflammation and cardiac dysfunction, or it can be overwhelming, leading to severe cardiac injury and cardiac failure. As a clinical entity, myocarditis is an uncommon occurrence in children. At Texas Children's Hospital, Houston, Texas, between 1954 and 1977, myocarditis represented 0.3 percent of the 14,322 patients seen by the Cardiology Service.

Because not all cases of myocarditis are recognized clinically, a much higher incidence is recorded in autopsy series. An autopsy incidence of 1.15 percent was found from 4343 studies performed between 1954 and 1977 at Texas Children's Hospital. This rate is considerably lower than the incidence of 6.83 percent reported by Saphir and Simon[157] in 1944 for 1420 autopsies performed on children. In Saphir's series, 32 of 97 cases had or probably had rheumatic carditis,[156] whereas only 2 cases occurred in the Texas Children's Hospital series. The discrepancy is even more pronounced when these observations are compared with those of Burch and colleagues,[26] who showed evidence of interstitial myocarditis in the hearts of 29 of 50 infants and young children undergoing routine postmortem studies.

Some of the discrepancies between the clinical and autopsy series may be explained by the fact that the manifestations of myocarditis are subclinical in many cases and may be recognized only by changes on electrocardiogram (ECG) or perhaps not at all. In many instances, myocarditis is only one component of a generalized illness, and the cardiac dysfunction, if mild, may be overlooked.

ETIOLOGIES

Myocarditis may occur with many common infectious illnesses that affect infants and children (Table 34–1). In most cases of myocarditis, the etiologic agent is never identified, however. In the United States and Western Europe, viruses are the most common causes of acute myocarditis. Myocarditis generally is a sporadic disease, but epidemics have been reported. Most epidemics have been caused by coxsackievirus group B and have affected infants in the newborn period.[46,52] Gear and Measroch[62] were the first to identify coxsackievirus B in association with myocarditis after an epidemic occurred in a nursery in a maternity home in southern Rhodesia.

The association between virus infection and the development of myocardial disease also was made by Grist and Bell,[70] who presented comprehensive serologic data correlating enterovirus infection with acute viral myocarditis. In the World Health Organization record during the 10-year period from 1975 through 1985, the coxsackieviruses B represented the most frequent inflammatory agents in cardiovascular disease (34.6/1000), followed by influenza B virus (17.4/1000), influenza A virus (11.7/1000), coxsackievirus A (9.1 per 1000), and cytomegalovirus (CMV) (8/1000).[27] Karjalainen and colleagues[90] prospectively examined 104 conscripts during the 1978 influenza A virus (H1N1) epidemic in Sweden. The incidence of myocarditis was 9 percent of the 67 verified cases of influenza virus infection.

The development of molecular techniques such as polymerase chain reaction (PCR) has improved the testing of endomyocardial biopsy specimens for potential viral pathogens. A study using PCR identified viral genome in 38 percent of endomyocardial biopsy specimens from patients diagnosed with acute myocarditis.[21] Of the positive PCR samples, 23 percent were positive for adenovirus, 14 percent for enterovirus, and 3 percent for CMV. Parvovirus B19, influenza A virus, Epstein-Barr virus, herpes simplex virus (HSV), and respiratory syncytial virus were detected in less than 1 percent of cases.

Investigators also have speculated for decades on the possibility that acute myocarditis is a common forerunner of idiopathic dilated cardiomyopathy (DCM). Evidence supporting this hypothesis was presented first by Orinius and Pernow,[136] who found cardiac disease in humans years after an apparent uncomplicated coxsackievirus infection. Subsequently, Bowles and colleagues,[22] using a slot-blot hybridization technique, provided conclusive evidence for the presence of enterovirus in endomyocardial biopsy samples from patients with DCM. In another study, Bowles and associates[21] detected viral genomes in 20 percent of 149 patients with the diagnosis of DCM. In these

TABLE 34–1   Causes of Myocarditis

Viruses	Coxsackieviruses A and B
	Echoviruses
	Polioviruses
	Rubella
	Measles
	Adenoviruses
	Vaccinia
	Mumps
	Herpes simplex
	Epstein-Barr
	Cytomegalovirus
	Rhinoviruses
	Hepatitis viruses
	Arboviruses
	Influenza viruses
	Varicella
Rickettsia	*Rickettsia rickettsii*
	Rickettsia tsutsugamushi
Bacteria	*Meningococcus*
	Klebsiella
	Leptospira
	Staphylococcus
	Treponema pallidum
	Haemophilus influenzae
	Hemolytic streptococci
	Mycobacterium tuberculosis
	Salmonella enterica subsp. *enterica* serovar Typhi (typhoid)
Mycoplasma	*Mycoplasma pneumoniae*
	Chlamydia psittaci
Protozoa	*Trypanosoma cruzi*
	African trypanosomiasis
	Toxoplasma
	Amebiasis
Other parasites	*Toxocara canis*
	Trichinella spiralis
Fungi and yeasts	*Actinomyces*
	Coccidioides
	Histoplasma
	Candida
Toxin	Diphtheria
	Scorpion
Drugs	Sulfonamides
	Phenylbutazone
	Cyclophosphamide
	Neo-mercazole
Hypersensitivity/ autoimmunity	Rheumatoid arthritis
	Rheumatic fever
	Ulcerative colitis
	Systemic lupus erythematosus
Other	Sarcoidosis
	Scleroderma
	Idiopathic
	Cornstarch

patients, adenovirus was identified in 12 percent and enterovirus in 8 percent of DCM cases. In all age groups, adenovirus and enterovirus were the viruses most commonly detected in acute myocarditis and DCM.

The discovery that coxsackievirus and adenovirus use the same receptor to infect host cells has provided an explanation for why these unrelated viruses account for most myocarditis cases. Bowles and colleagues[20] proposed that mutations in the coxsackie-adenovirus receptor could represent a host factor for the development of myocarditis or DCM. These investigators screened patients with myocarditis or DCM, including 24 patients in whom a viral etiology was identified by PCR and reverse transcription PCR. In addition, 50 patients who presented with heart failure and had echocardiograms diagnostic for DCM, but

in whom no etiology was identified, were screened. Three silent substitutions and an intronic substitution were detected, but no apparent disease-causing mutations were detected. These data suggested that mutations in the coxsackie-adenovirus receptor are unlikely to play an important role in the pathogenesis of viral myocarditis or DCM.

Myocarditis also has been reported as a complication of infection with many other viruses (see Table 34–1). The teratogenicity of the rubella virus in the first 4 months of pregnancy is well known. Ainger and colleagues[3] showed that, because of the persistence of the virus in the fetus, extensive involvement of the myocardium may lead to severe myocarditis. Of 47 infants with congenital rubella, 10 had myocarditis, and 4 died. Morbidity in the survivors was severe. Rubella immunization programs have succeeded in reducing the number of congenital cases, and since 2001, only five infants with congenital rubella syndrome have been reported. Three were born in 2001, one was born in 2003, and one was born in 2004. This epidemiologic evidence strongly suggests that rubella no longer is endemic in the United States.[146]

Osama and colleagues[137] prospectively evaluated 312 cases of varicella over a 1-year period. Eighteen (5.8%) of the 312 cases showed evidence of myocarditis. A statistically significant increase in myocarditis was found in patients who complained of skeletal myalgia.

Currently, neonatal HSV disease in the United States occurs in approximately 1 in 3200 deliveries, resulting in an estimated 1500 cases of neonatal HSV infection annually.[25] Most (85%) infected infants acquire their infections during birth, in the peripartum period. The spectrum of disease ranges from unapparent infection to a fatal encephalopathy. Myocardial involvement has been described, and herpesvirus has been isolated from the myocardium at autopsy.[48,197] Recognition of genital herpes and delivery of the infant by cesarean section reduce the incidence of myocarditis caused by this agent.

In December 2002, the U.S. Department of Defense began mandatory smallpox vaccination for select service members and employees without contraindications to vaccination, and in January 2003, the U.S. Department of Health and Human Services implemented a voluntary civilian smallpox vaccination program. As of June 15, 2003, the Department of Defense identified more than 50 cases of suspected, probable, or confirmed myopericarditis occurring within 30 days of vaccination in these individuals, based on clinical evaluation of symptoms, ECG, cardiac enzyme assays, echocardiography, and the exclusion of ischemic coronary artery disease. Myocarditis occurred in 7.8 per 100,000 primary vaccinees in the U.S. army, an incidence that was 3.6-fold more than that in unvaccinated individuals.[72]

Reports of respiratory diphtheria are rare in the United States in all age groups. The last culture-confirmed case of respiratory diphtheria in a U.S. adolescent was reported in 1996.[179] Acute mortality of this disease is due to toxin-mediated diphtheritic cardiomyopathy, suffocation by the pseudomembrane, disseminated intravascular coagulation, and renal failure. Approximately one third of cases have ECG findings suggesting myocardial involvement, although the rate of cardiac involvement may be 84 percent in severe cases.[15]

PATHOLOGY

Isolated or idiopathic myocarditis is a rare pathologic entity. The pathologic cardiac findings usually are nonspecific; similar gross and microscopic changes occur regardless of the causative agent.[66,132,142,150] Grossly, all four chambers of the heart are enlarged, and the cardiac weight is increased. The heart usually is flabby and pale. In some instances, especially with coxsackievirus B infections, petechial hemorrhages may be seen on the epicardial surfaces; pericardial fluid may be tinged with blood. On cut section, the ventricular muscle walls may be thinned. Occasionally, the ventricles are hypertrophied or increased in thickness because of edema. The valves are spared. The endocardial surface usually is unaffected but occasionally may be thickened and appear glistening white. This important observation suggested to some investigators that endocardial fibroelastosis, which manifests as congestive cardiomyopathy, represented a progression from acute viral myocarditis.[73,85]

In a study of 64 hearts of children who had myocarditis or endocardial fibroelastosis, Hutchins and Vie[85] found 18 with endocardial fibroelastosis only, five with myocarditis only, and 41 with features of both diseases. When time from onset of illness to death was 2 weeks or less, only myocarditis was evident. When the time interval was 2 weeks to 4 months, a combined picture was seen, whereas only endocardial fibroelastosis with trivial myocarditis was evident when the time from onset of disease to death was more than 4 months.

These findings were supported further by Hastreiter and Miller,[73] who found microscopic evidence of myocarditis after transthoracic needle biopsy of the myocardium in a child who had the classic clinical picture of endocardial fibroelastosis, including left ventricular hypertrophy on ECG. Fruhling and associates[58] extended these observations by showing coxsackievirus B3 in the myocardium of 13 of 28 infants with endocardial fibroelastosis. Ni and associates[130] analyzed 29 myocardial samples from patients with autopsy-proven endocardial fibroelastosis using specific PCR for enterovirus, adenovirus, mumps, CMV, parvovirus, influenza, and HSV. In 90 percent of samples, viral genome was amplified; more than 70 percent of the samples were positive for mumps viral RNA, whereas 28 percent amplified adenovirus. These data suggest that endocardial fibroelastosis also is a sequela of mumps virus infection.

Saphir and Field[156] observed mural thrombi in the left ventricular cavity in some patients with myocarditis and minute emboli in coronary and cerebral vessels. Coronary emboli, although rare, may play a role in the causation of cardiac dysrhythmias, which sometimes accompany myocarditis.

The microscopic picture of acute myocarditis typically shows a focal or diffuse interstitial collection composed predominantly of mononuclear cells, lymphocytes, plasma cells, and eosinophils. Polymorphonuclear leukocytes rarely are seen, unless the cause of the carditis is bacterial. Virus particles and inclusion bodies rarely are recognized.[144,150]

In severe infections caused by any agent, but especially coxsackieviruses and diphtheria, a loss of cross-striation in the muscle fibers, edema, and, sometimes, extensive necrosis of the myocardium occur. The diphtheria exotoxin has a particular affinity for conductive tissue; dysrhythmias, including complete heart block, are common findings in this form of myocarditis. The exotoxin interferes with protein synthesis by inhibiting a translocating enzyme in the delivery of amino acids.

Although the perivascular accumulation of lymphocytes and plasma cells is described in coxsackievirus B myocarditis, it is a minor finding. When myocarditis is caused by rickettsiae,[184] varicella,[123] trypanosomes,[138,141] or other parasites,[181] or when it occurs as a reaction to sulfonamide,[189] this pattern dominates.

Myocarditis seen with bacterial infections usually differs from that of presumed viral origin (Figs. 34–1 to 34–4). Microabscesses and patchy focal suppurative changes may be observed. Frequently, a perimyocarditis may be seen with concomitant bacterial infection of pericardium and myocardium.

Giant cells with or without granulomata are markers for the diagnosis of giant-cell myocarditis.[84] Granulomata have been observed in the myocardium of patients with tuberculosis, syphilis, rheumatoid arthritis, rheumatic heart disease, sarcoidosis, and certain fungal and parasitic infections. Occasionally, giant cells have been seen in interstitial myocarditis (idiopathic or Fiedler). In many cases, giant-cell myocarditis occurs, but no cause is found.

Two types of giant cells are recognized, one of which seems to be myogenic in origin and is thought to represent transitional forms of myocardial fibers. This type of cell has been found without granulomata. The second, more characteristic giant cell probably is derived from interstitial histiocytes. The latter type typically is seen in patients with myocarditis of nonviral cause, whereas the former is a response to viral infection. Hudson[84] described similar cells in an adult who had received neo-mercazole (carbimazole) therapy, and Hodge and Lawrence[79] reported two cases of granulomatous myocarditis associated with phenylbutazone therapy.

PATHOGENESIS

The pathogenesis of myocarditis is poorly understood, insofar as the disease progresses through different phases with distinctly different mechanisms and clinical manifestations. The

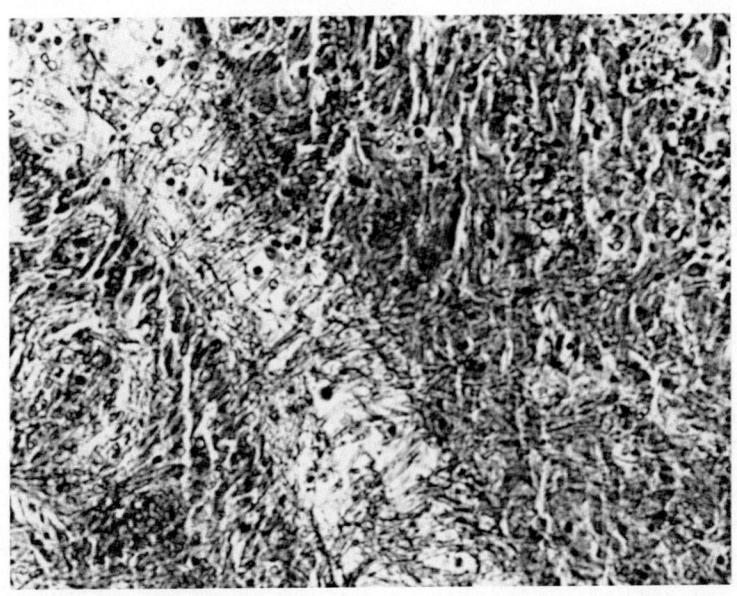

Figure 34–1 *Candida albicans* myocarditis. Notice the focal necrosis of the myocardium with central masses of hyphae and necrotic debris surrounded by mononuclear cell infiltrate (hematoxylin and eosin staining, ×160). *(Courtesy of Edith Hawkins, M.D., Houston, TX.)*

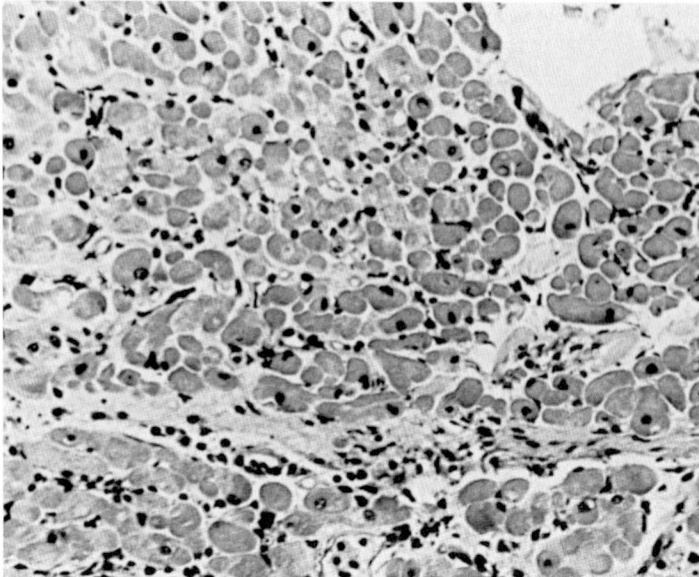

Figure 34–2 Right ventricular biopsy specimen. The presumed viral myocarditis is characterized by focal mononuclear cell infiltrates (hematoxylin and eosin staining, ×160). *(Courtesy of Edith Hawkins, M.D., Houston, TX.)*

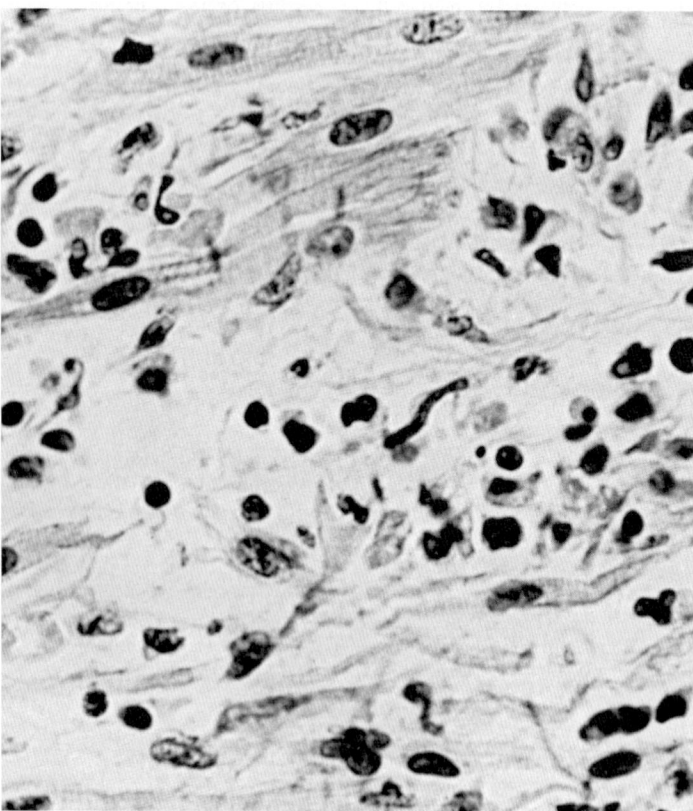

Figure 34–3 Picornavirus myocarditis characterized by interstitial edema, mononuclear cell infiltrates, and focal myofiber disruption (hematoxylin and eosin staining, ×400). *(Courtesy of Edith Hawkins, M.D., Houston, TX.)*

pathophysiology of myocarditis in humans was derived largely from experimental models of coxsackievirus infection. More recently, Liu and Mason[106] have suggested that myocarditis should be viewed as a continuum that comprises three separate phases: acute viral infection (phase I), autoimmunity (phase II), and DCM (phase III).

Phase I of the disease is triggered by the entry and proliferation in the myocardium of the causative virus. Impairment of left ventricular function in mice with histopathologically graded moderate cellular infiltration after coxsackievirus B3 infection

supports the important pathophysiologic role of direct viral damage of the myocardium.[173] Phase I concludes with activation of the cellular immune response, which attenuates viral proliferation but also may enhance cardiac injury. Ideally, the immune response should down-regulate to a resting state when viral proliferation is controlled. If immune activation continues unabated despite elimination of the virus, autoimmune disease may result, initiating phase II of the disease. The continuous activation of T cells long after viral clearance occurs is detrimental to the host because cytokine-mediated and direct T-cell–mediated myocyte

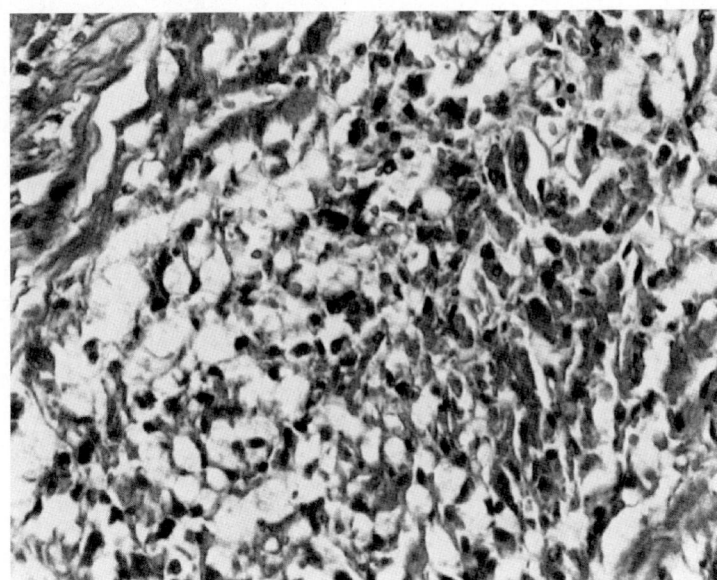

Figure 34–4 Section of myocardium. Vaccinia (smallpox vaccine) myocarditis. Note mononuclear cell infiltrates and fatty degenerative changes (hematoxylin and eosin staining, ×400). *(Courtesy of Edith Hawkins, M.D., Houston, TX.)*

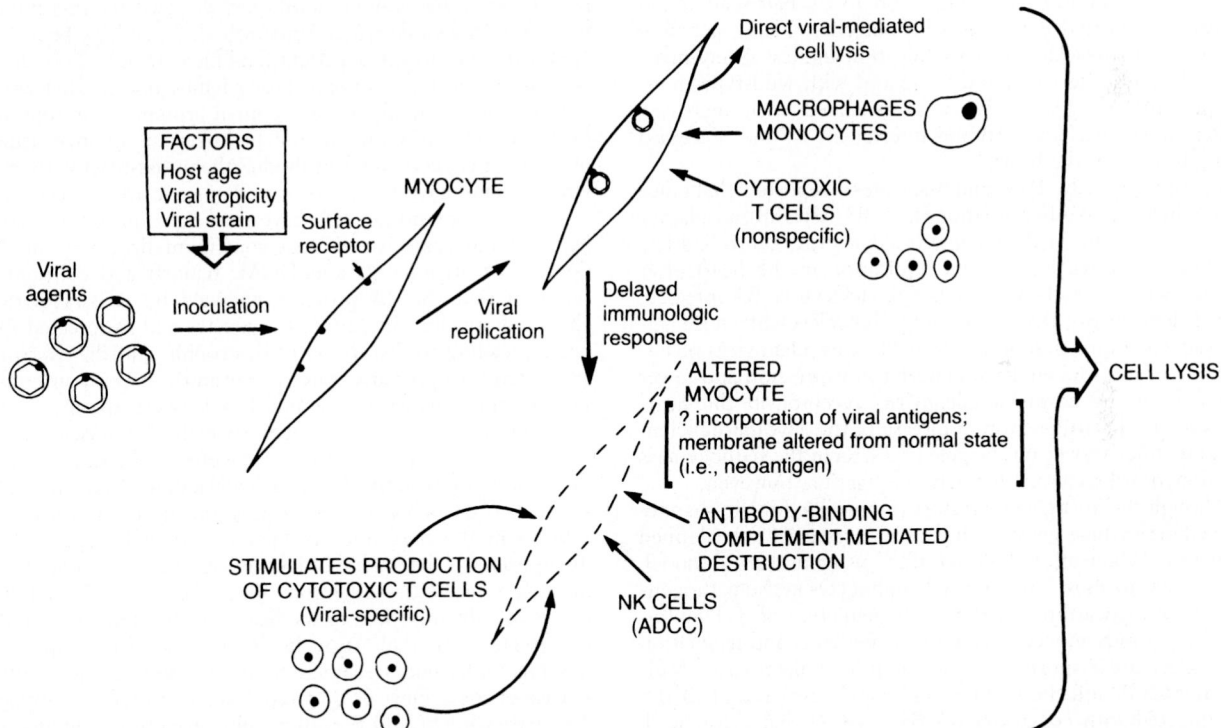

Figure 34–5 Schema for pathogenesis of myocarditis. Viral agents attach to cells by means of surface receptors. After a cell is infected, the cell cycle is changed. Direct virus-mediated cytolysis occurs. Cellular effectors of injury (i.e., macrophages, monocytes, and nonspecific cytotoxic T cells) are involved in the primary reaction. Myocytes that survive are altered in their structure. Cytotoxic T cells specifically targeted against the altered myocyte, natural killer (NK) cells, and complement-activated, antibody-mediated cardiocytolysis or antibody-dependent cellular cytotoxicity (ADCC) participate in the secondary reaction. *(Partially adapted from Maisch, B., Trostel-Soeder, R., Stechemesser, E., et al.: Diagnostic relevance of humoral and cell-mediated immune reactions in patients with acute viral myocarditis. Clin. Exp. Immunol. 48:533, 1982.)*

injury leads to impairment of contractile function (Fig. 34–5). Long-term remodeling and progression to DCM characterize phase III of the disease.[82]

The basic function of innate immunity is restriction of the early proliferation of infectious agents. Numerous effector cells and molecules work in concert to restrict this initial spread of an infectious focus. The responding cells include natural killer cells,

natural killer/T cells and γδ T cells. Several lines of evidence suggest that mediators of the innate immune system, such as tumor necrosis factor (TNF) and nitric oxide, play an important role in the pathogenesis of viral myocarditis.[115,198] Elevated levels of TNF have been reported in patients with viral myocarditis, and TNF mRNA and protein are consistently up-regulated in the hearts of these patients.[117,158] In mice, the exogenous administration of TNF aggravates myocarditis, and the neutralization of TNF by antibodies or soluble receptors attenuates the disease.[99,195] These data suggest that TNF production is detrimental in the setting of myocarditis.

More recent studies also have shown that TNF and nitric oxide are beneficial to the host by virtue of their antiviral effects. Mice with defective TNF or nitric oxide expression have increased myocardial injury, a significant increase in viral titers in the heart, and significantly higher mortality rates after infection with encephalomyocarditis virus or coxsackievirus B3.[183,198] These observations highlight the complexity of the innate immune response and suggest that innate immune mechanisms play a dual role in the setting of viral myocarditis. Although the prevailing notion has been that production of cytokine in the heart during viral infection is detrimental, the host-pathogen relationship is changed fundamentally when the host is unable to produce molecules such as TNF or nitric oxide.[183,198]

An important component of the innate immune system uses pattern recognition receptors, such as the Toll-like receptors (TLRs), to recognize pathogen-associated molecular patterns present in microbes.[4] TLRs induce the production of cytokines and interferons and modulate the adaptive immune response. The role of TLRs in the pathogenesis of viral myocarditis is still being explored. More recent studies suggest that cardiac inflammation during viral infection depends on TLRs. Fairweather and colleagues[53] reported that mice with defective TLR4 signaling had decreased coxsackievirus B3 replication and less severe myocarditis 12 days after infection compared with wild-type mice. The presence of TLR4 also was associated with increased production of interleukin-1β and interleukin-18 and increased viral replication in the heart.

In a similar study, Fuse and associates[59] reported that mice deficient in myeloid differentiation factor 88 (MyD88), an adapter protein involved in TLR signaling (except TLR3), also had less myocarditis and attenuated viral replication in the heart after infection with coxsackievirus B3. Coxsackievirus B3–infected, MyD88-deficient mice had significantly higher levels of interferon-β but reduced expression of the coxsackievirus-adenovirus receptor in the heart. The enhanced interferon expression and lower expression of the coxsackie-adenovirus receptor in the heart could explain the attenuation of disease in the MyD88-deficient mice. The final answer on the role of TLRs in the pathogenesis of viral myocarditis awaits further investigation, however.

Although the host genetic factors responsible for the changes observed in the three phases of myocarditis have yet to be defined completely, Woodruff and Woodruff,[192] using a murine model, were the first to show a role for T lymphocytes in the pathogenesis of viral myocarditis. In this study, depletion of T lymphocytes using antithymocyte serum or thymectomy and irradiation led to a decrease in mortality rates and in the inflammatory infiltrate after CVB3 infection. Huber and associates,[83] using BALB/c mice infected with coxsackievirus B3, showed that cytolytic T cells were the agents responsible for the major part of myocardial cell injury. In addition, proinflammatory mediators, such as TNF, released by infiltration cells also adversely affect cardiac function.

Opavsky and colleagues[135] defined the specific contributions of T-cell subsets (CD4 and CD8) and the T-cell receptor beta chain to the pathogenesis of viral myocarditis. When CD4$^{-/-}$ or CD8$^{-/-}$ mice were exposed to CVB3, loss of CD8$^{+/+}$ immune cells did not affect survival significantly, but viral proliferation was attenuated. In contrast, CD4$^{-/-}$ mice showed a trend toward an improvement in survival and a small but significant decrease in the inflammatory infiltrate at 14 days after infection. Mice deficient in CD4/CD8 immune cells and T-cell receptor beta had the best outcome in terms of decreased mortality. A marked decrease in inflammatory infiltrate was noted in CD4/CD8 double knockout mice. Although no significant change occurred in viral titers, a marked decrease in myocardial TNF mRNA 4 days after infection was seen in CD4/CD8 double knockout mice. These same investigators have shown that the T-cell receptor–associated tyrosine kinase p56^{lck} is crucial for coxsackievirus B3 proliferation in the heart and activation of T cells to target the heart.[105] Mice deficient in p56^{lck} were protected against the development of myocarditis, providing further support for the hypothesis that T-cell activation during viral myocarditis contributes to increased inflammation and myocyte destruction in the host.

The ongoing injury that persists may be considered an autoimmune process.[83,191] In murine models, cellular and humoral autoimmunity clearly are involved in the progression to chronic heart disease. Paque and colleagues[140] provide support for this concept. Using CD-1 mice infected with coxsackievirus B3, they found a potassium chloride–extractable antigen in the hearts of mice previously infected with a coxsackievirus B that was specifically immunoreactive with immune mouse peritoneal exudate cells (i.e., stimulated production of a migration inhibitory factor). No viral activity was detected in the animals that had this extractable antigen.

Similar experiments in a primate model confirmed earlier findings in mice and lent further support to similar circumstances in humans.[139] Experimental evidence also has shown that the antigen responsible for cytotoxic T-cell activity is not detectable by antiserum that contains antibodies directed at structural components of the viral capsid. Autoantibodies that have been associated with myocarditis in patients and mice include those directed at cardiac myosin, adrenoreceptor adenine nucleotide translocator, and sarcolemmal and myolemmal proteins. The role played by these autoantibodies in the pathogenesis of myocarditis is unclear; antisarcolemmal antibodies that cross-react with enteroviral epitopes have been shown to damage cardiac myocytes.

More recent studies also have shed light on the mechanisms by which coxsackievirus B3 may contribute directly to the development of myocarditis and DCM. Badorff and colleagues[10-12] reported that the 2A protease encoded by coxsackievirus B3 cleaves dystrophin in cultured myocytes and in infected mouse hearts, leading to disruption of dystrophin and the dystrophin-associated glycoprotein α-sarcoglycan and β-sarcoglycan complex. Dystrophin provides a structural link between the muscle cytoskeleton and extracellular matrix to maintain muscle integrity. Xiong and associates[194] compared the effects of coxsackievirus B3 infection in dystrophin-deficient (*mdx*) and wild-type mice. Coxsackievirus B3 infection significantly enhanced sarcolemmal disruption in the *mdx* mice compared with wild-type mice; the disruption was detectable 2 days postinfection and continued to increase after initial infection. Viral titers were higher in the hearts of *mdx* mice than in the hearts of wild-type mice, indicating greater viral replication in the absence of dystrophin. The observed differences seemed to be a result of more efficient release of coxsackievirus B3 from dystrophin-deficient myocytes. The expression of wild-type dystrophin in cultured cells decreased the cytopathic effect induced by coxsackievirus B3 and the release of virus from the cell. The expression of a cleavage-resistant mutant of the dystrophin protein inhibited coxsackievirus B3–mediated cytopathic effect and viral release further.

PATHOPHYSIOLOGY OF VENTRICULAR DYSFUNCTION IN MYOCARDITIS

With extensive interstitial inflammation, muscle-cell injury, or both, myocardial contractility is reduced. Consequently, the heart enlarges and the end-diastolic volume of the ventricle increases. In the normal heart, an increase in filling volume leads, by the Starling mechanism, to an increased force of contraction, ejection fraction, and cardiac output. In patients with myocarditis, the myocardium is unable to respond in this manner and cardiac output is reduced. Systemic blood flow may be maintained, however, by use of the cardiac reserve, mediated by the sympathetic nervous system and leading to vasoconstriction of the skin vessels and an increase in heart rate. With progressive disease or any stress (e.g., infection, anemia, fever), the heart may be unable to meet the oxygen demands of the tissues, and the clinical picture of congestive cardiac failure may become evident. Increased end-diastolic volume leads to progressive increase in ventricular end-diastolic pressure, which leads to increased filling pressure, and left atrial and pulmonary venous hydrostatic pressure may be elevated above the colloid osmotic pressure, which normally prevents transudation of fluid across the capillary membranes. Pulmonary congestion and edema and systemic venous engorgement (manifested in infants primarily as hepatic enlargement) are common findings in the more acute forms of myocarditis. In some infants and young children, the presentation is predominantly that of right-sided heart failure.[149]

An appreciation of the disturbance of myocardial function may be gained from the angiographic frames shown in Figure 34–6. The left ventricle is dilated considerably, and the outline is irregular in diastole and systole. The ejection fraction is reduced significantly at 35 percent instead of the normal 60 to 75 percent.

Another means of evaluating left ventricular function is the noninvasive technique of cardiac ultrasound. Gutgesell and colleagues[71] established normal standards for children. An example is shown in Figure 34–7A. The normal shortening fraction (i.e., percentage change in ventricular dimensions between end-diastole and end-systole) is 35 ± 4 percent, regardless of age (range 28–44%). Figure 34–7B illustrates the case of a 4-year-old child with idiopathic myocarditis and shows ventricular dilation with markedly reduced motion of the left ventricular posterior wall and septum, leading to a shortening fraction of only 12 percent. Further assessment of ventricular function can be achieved by measuring systolic time intervals obtained from simultaneous recording of the ECG and the semilunar valve opening and closing points on the echocardiogram.[71]

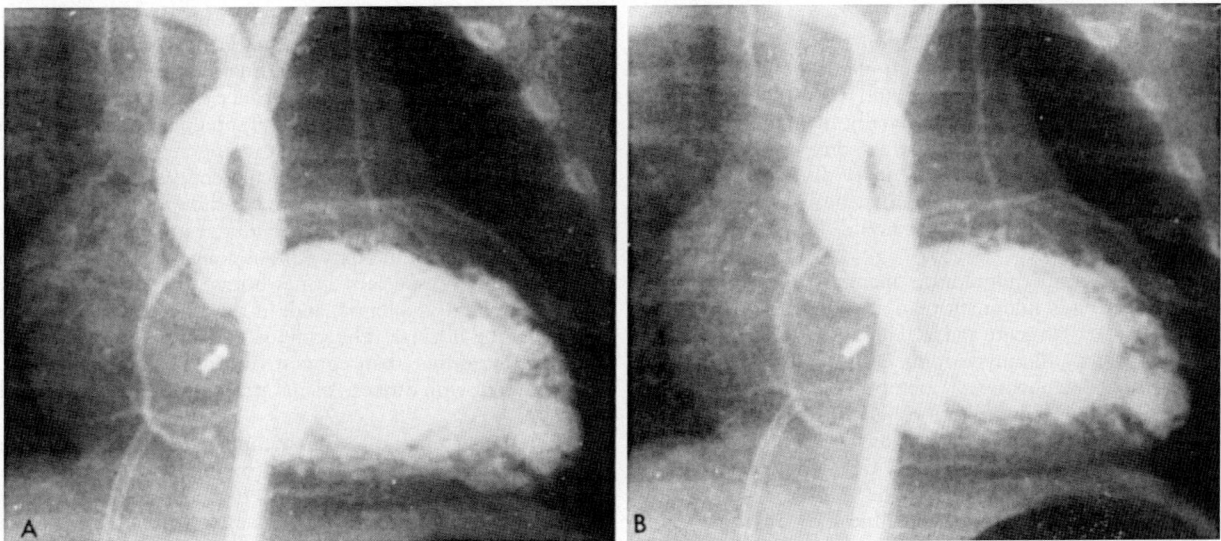

Figure 34–6 **A** and **B,** The end-diastolic (**A**) and end-systolic (**B**) frames from a left ventriculogram of a patient with idiopathic myocarditis show irregularity of the wall and poor contractility.

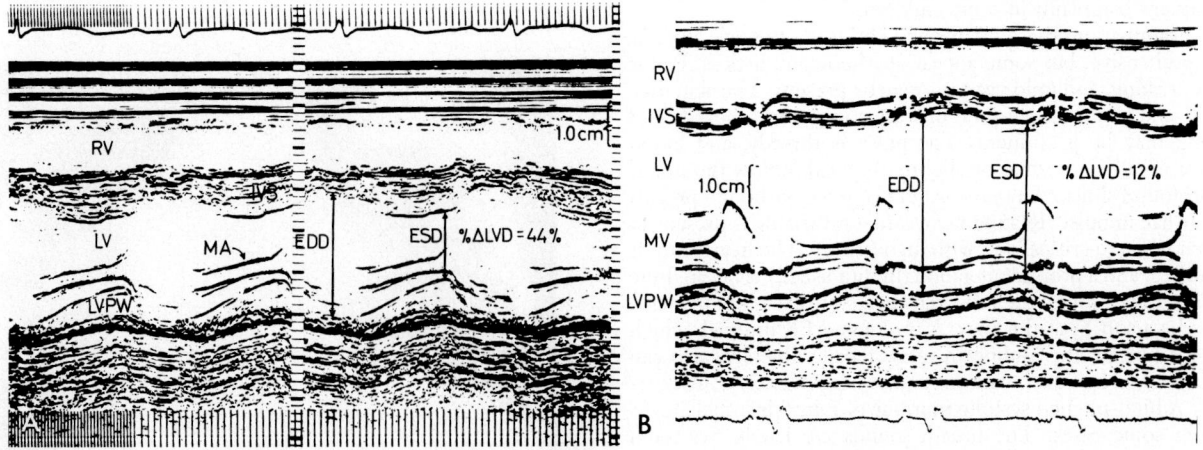

Figure 34–7 **A,** Normal echocardiogram of a 4-year-old child. **B,** Echocardiogram of a 4-year-old child with idiopathic myocarditis shows left ventricular dilation and severely reduced shortening fraction. EDD, end-diastolic dimension; ESD, end-systolic dimension; IVS, interventricular septum; LVPW, left ventricular posterior wall; MA, mitral apparatus; MV, mitral valve, %ΔLVD, percent change in left ventricular dimension (shortening fraction).

CLINICAL PRESENTATION

The clinical presentation of myocarditis varies with the age of the patient and the virulence of the organism. At one end of the spectrum is a fulminant, rapidly fatal illness, and at the other, no apparent clinical disturbance at all. A newborn especially is susceptible to the severe form of myocarditis usually caused by the coxsackieviruses B,[38,92] but it also is recognized with rubella[3] and HSV[193] infections and with toxoplasmosis.[84]

In many of these infections, myocarditis is only one component of a generalized illness, often with severe hepatitis and encephalitis.[17,92] In some instances, however, infections with these organisms may produce only a mild clinical disturbance.[24,86] In the report by Brightman and colleagues,[24] a nursery epidemic of coxsackievirus B5 infection in preterm infants was recognized only by chance because a virologic survey was in progress at the time in the institution. No cases of myocarditis were documented, and all the infants recovered. Findings included lethargy, failure to gain weight, and, in some infants, evidence of aseptic meningitis.

As described in the review by Kibrick and Benirschke[92] of 25 infants with coxsackievirus B myocarditis, vague symptoms such as lethargy and anorexia may herald the onset of the severe disease, emphasizing that close attention should be paid to all symptoms, especially in a newborn, no matter how nonspecific. Four infants had episodes of vomiting, and fever was documented for more than half of the cases; occasionally, the temperature was subnormal. Cyanosis; respiratory distress; and tachycardia, cardiomegaly, or ECG changes occurred in 19 of 23 infants. Tachypnea (a respiratory rate >60/min in a newborn) is an early sign of heart failure in a young infant and should alert the clinician to this diagnosis.

In older infants and children, the manifestations of myocarditis generally are less fulminant than are the manifestations in newborns.[149,154,185,190] An acute and fatal illness has been associated, however, with idiopathic myocarditis[104] and myocarditis caused by enteroviruses,[92] adenoviruses,[75] mumps,[100] chickenpox,[137] diphtheria,[15] CMV,[176] and many of the other causative agents listed in Table 34–1. Some older children have been reported with acute, substernal chest pain consistent with angina and have ECG changes of acute myocardial infarction.[81,119] The usual clinical picture is that of an acute or a subacute illness, which often begins with a mild upper respiratory infection and a low-grade fever.[9] Some infants have only vague, nonspecific suggestions of disease (e.g., irritability, periodic episodes of pallor) before the onset of cardiorespiratory symptoms, which begin a few days to 2 weeks after the onset of the initial symptoms. Abdominal pain may be a prominent complaint in some children.[185]

On examination, these infants and children often are anxious and apprehensive, but some appear apathetic and listless. Pallor may be striking, and mild cyanosis may be present. The skin may be cold and mottled. Respirations are rapid and labored, and grunting may be prominent. The pulse is thready, and blood pressure usually is normal or slightly reduced, unless the infant is in profound shock. The precordium is quiet, without a prominent cardiac impulse. Resting tachycardia invariably is present in children who are critically ill with myocarditis. The heart sounds are muffled, and a prominent gallop rhythm usually is heard. Fine and colleagues[55] found the most sensitive clinical sign of myocarditis to be a soft S_1 at the apex. A prolonged PR interval, which may be a nonspecific finding in many febrile illnesses, also can cause a soft S_1, however, without any other evidence of myocarditis.[162] A high-pitched systolic murmur of mitral insufficiency is heard in some cases. The breath sounds are harsh. Scattered rhonchi and, occasionally, fine crepitations in the lung bases may be detected.

Almost uniformly, the liver is enlarged; edema is a rare finding. Some infants are less distressed and have signs of only mild congestive cardiac failure, without the signs of peripheral circulatory failure. Other infants have no signs of cardiac compromise, and myocarditis is recognized only as part of a generalized illness by a disturbance in the ECG pattern.

DIAGNOSIS

CLINICAL CHARACTERISTICS AND RADIOGRAPHIC EVIDENCE

Myocarditis often is difficult to diagnose, but it should be suspected in any infant or child who presents with congestive heart failure and who has or recently has had a febrile illness. The history should include information regarding travel, exposure to tuberculosis, recent drug ingestion, and illnesses in other family members or schoolmates. A quiet precordium in the presence of a gallop rhythm and decreased intensity or muffling of the heart sounds are findings that strongly suggest the diagnosis. A tachycardia out of proportion to the level of fever also should be viewed with suspicion. A physiologic S_3 is a common finding in normal healthy children and in children with anemia and fever. Sometimes, as with fever and associated tachycardia, the cardiac rhythm may have a gallop cadence. In association with it, however, the precordium is hyperactive, and the heart sounds are crisp and have increased intensity. An unusually prominent S_3 suggests a disturbance of ventricular compliance without other evidence of compromised cardiac function and should be investigated further with an echocardiogram, a chest radiograph, and an ECG.

Chest radiographs of infants and children who have signs of congestive cardiac failure invariably show cardiomegaly, usually of a severe degree (Fig. 34–8). All four chambers may be enlarged, and evidence of pulmonary venous congestion often is found.

Sometimes, especially in newborns, the first sign of illness is acute circulatory collapse, and, in this circumstance, the cardiac size may be normal. The same is true of children who have an arrhythmia rather than congestive heart failure. Other patients may present with Stokes-Adams attacks caused by complete heart block.[103]

The occurrence of an arrhythmia, especially after a febrile illness, should alert the clinician to look for other signs of myocarditis.[33,165] Lind and Hulquist[104] detected significant dysrhythmias in five infants with isolated myocarditis. Four of the five infants died, and three of these infants had paroxysmal atrial tachycardia. Paroxysmal atrial tachycardia has been reported in patients with viral myocarditis[33,164] and has been described in patients with diphtheritic myocarditis.[15] Atrial ectopic tachycar-

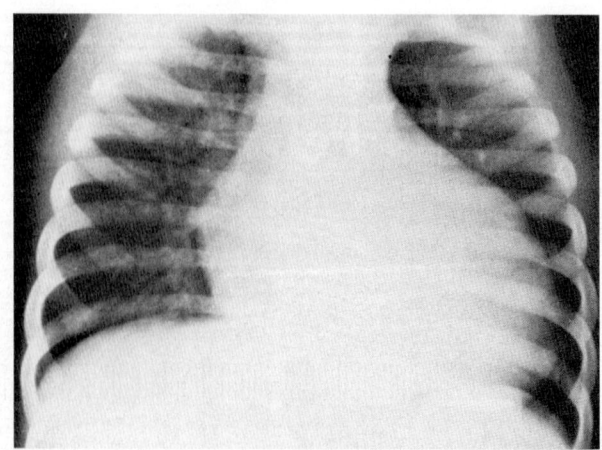

Figure 34–8 Marked cardiomegaly with a mild increase in the pulmonary venous pattern in the upper lobes.

dia may mimic sinus tachycardia and, if not carefully evaluated, may be the primary cause for significant myocardial dysfunction. Complete heart block has been described in children in association with acute idiopathic myocarditis[88,103] and with rubella,[107] coxsackievirus,[159] and respiratory syncytial virus[13,63] infections. In some instances, complete heart block is permanent, and in others, it is temporary.[13,64,88] The ECG is an essential diagnostic tool for all patients with suspected myocarditis.

The classic ECG pattern in myocarditis is one of diffuse low-voltage QRS complexes (<5 mm total amplitude) with low-amplitude or slightly inverted T waves and a small or absent Q wave in leads V_5 and V_6 (Fig. 34–9). The low-voltage signal may be present in the standard leads and the precordial leads. Figure 34–10 shows the ECG of an infant with acute myocarditis and shows a pattern of acute myocardial ischemia. Figure 34–11A shows multifocal extrasystoles and severe intraventricular conduction delay in a patient with diphtheritic myocarditis; the ECG of this child returned to normal over the course of 3 months (see Fig. 34–11B). The ECG from a 5-month-old infant who had mild fever, diarrhea, and vomiting for 3 to 4 days before admis-

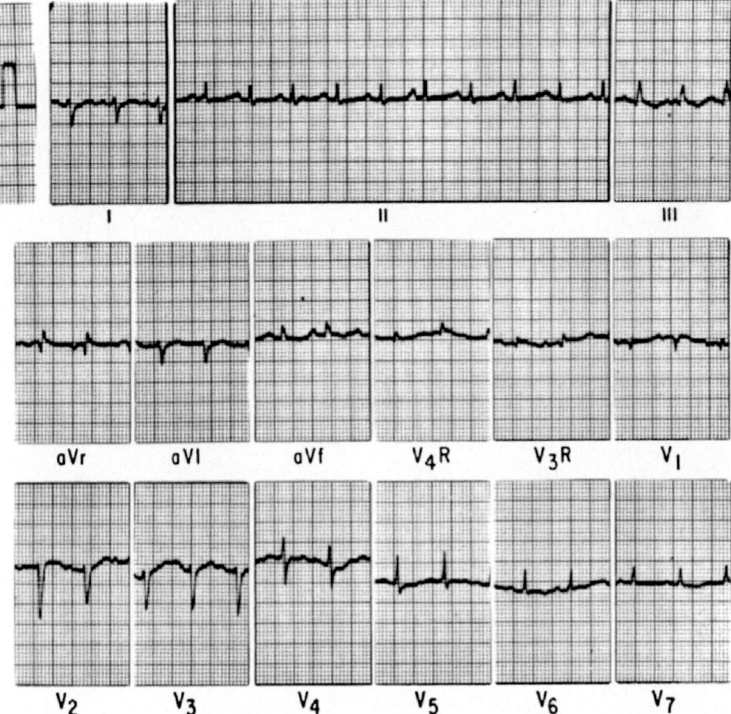

Figure 34–9 Diffuse low-voltage or QRS complexes with T-wave flattening and 1-mm Q waves in the lateral precordial leads represents the classic pattern in myocarditis.

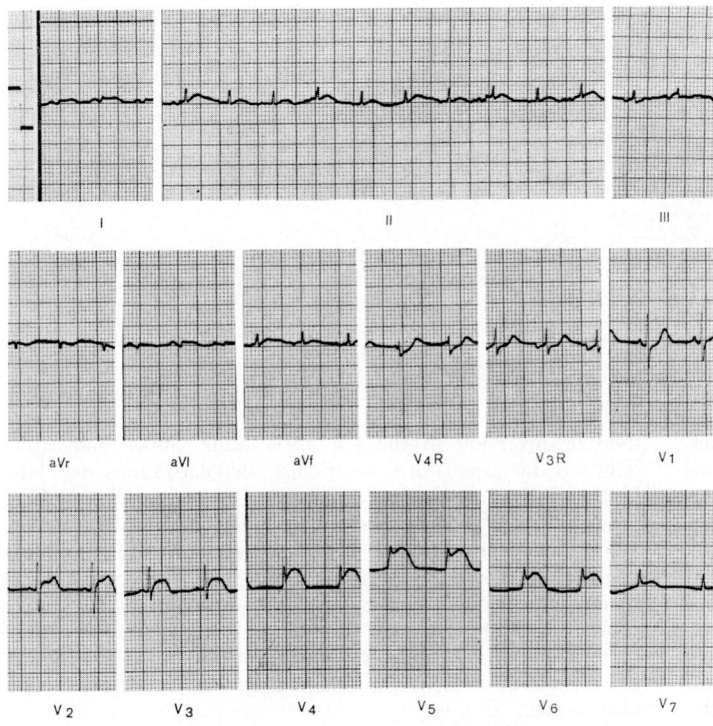

Figure 34–10 In addition to low voltage, there is evidence of acute myocardial ischemia with 4- to 5-mm ST-segment elevation dominantly in the middle and lateral precordial leads.

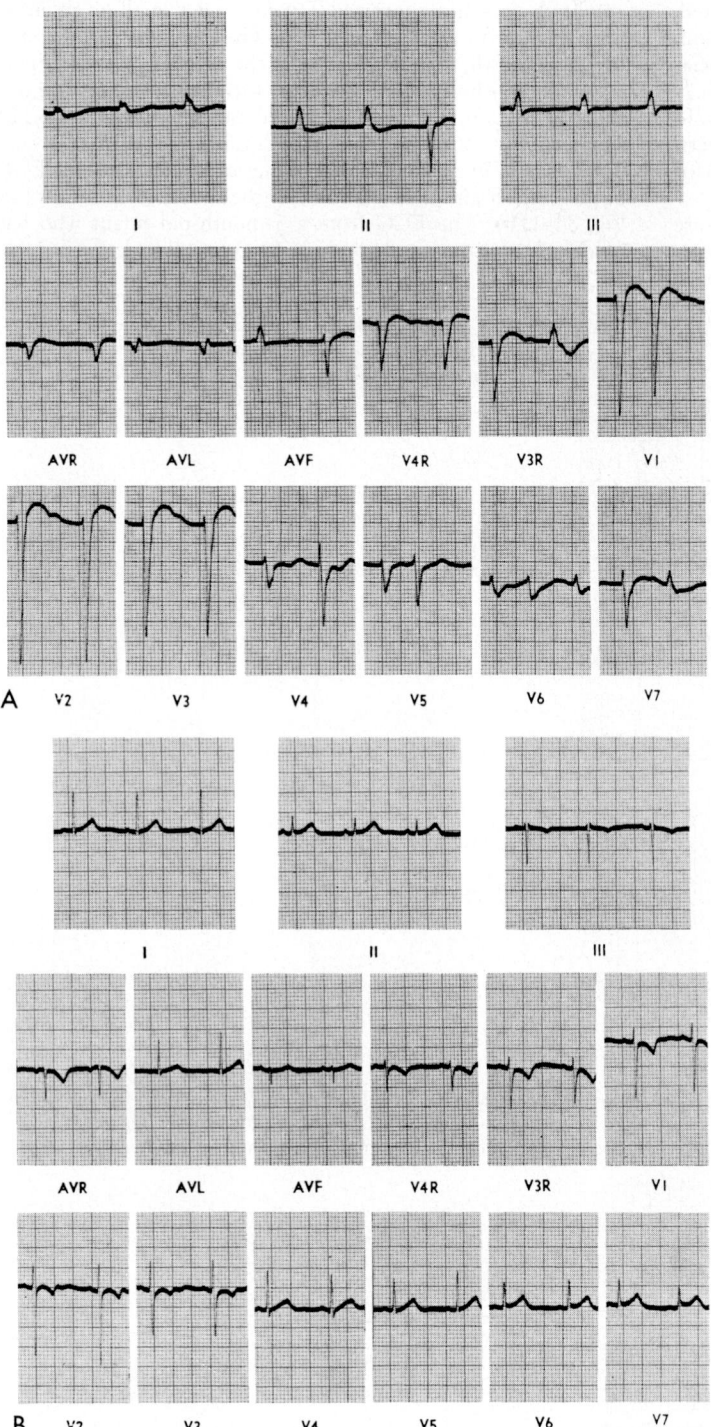

Figure 34–11 A, Multifocal premature beats are caused by atrioventricular dissociation and left bundle branch block resulting from diphtheritic myocarditis. **B,** A normal electrocardiogram is shown for the same patient 3 months after an episode of myocarditis.

sion is shown in Figure 34–12. The 2:1 atrioventricular block was associated with normal QRS complexes. This abnormality persisted in the absence of clinical symptoms for 1 year. Figure 34–13 shows a left bundle branch block that was identified in a 10-month-old infant with acute idiopathic myocarditis. Anomalous origin of the left coronary artery from the pulmonary artery was suspected but was excluded by catheterization. This ECG pattern persisted for at least 6 months.

Karjalainen and colleagues[90] studied the ECGs of 87 conscripts 18 and 30 years old, 28 of whom had myocarditis. The most frequent findings were T-wave changes of reduced ampli-

tude or inversion in the left chest leads. Sinus tachycardia followed by premature ventricular depolarizations was the most common dysrhythmia. Take and colleagues[171] examined serial ECGs of 16 patients with confirmed viral myocarditis. They found four patterns: (1) complete normalization in the presence of severe myocardial damage in the acute stage; (2) "pseudoinfarction" patterns with Q waves and poor R-wave progression; (3) permanent conduction disturbances that might require pacemaker support; and (4) chronic dysrhythmias, predominantly ventricular tachycardia and supraventricular tachycardia.

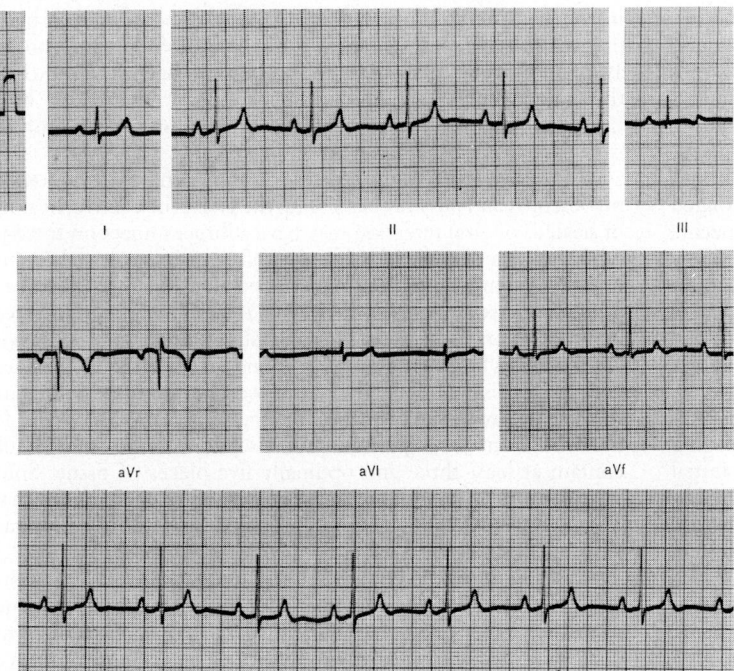

Figure 34–12 Second-degree atrioventricular block with an effective ventricular rate of 60 beats/min. The blocked P wave is placed on top of the T wave in each cycle.

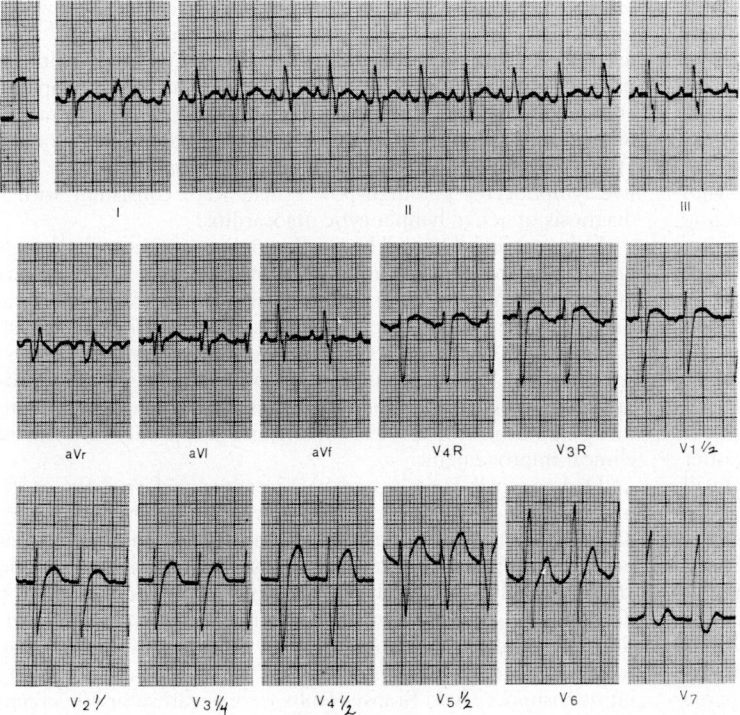

Figure 34–13 Sinus tachycardia (rate 150 beats/min) and left bundle branch block.

Hoshino and coworkers[80] induced coxsackievirus B3 myocarditis in Syrian golden hamsters and found that 80 percent of them had ST-segment or T-wave (or both) changes in the surface ECG. Most of the changes were seen between days 2 and 4, when mortality rates were highest. The endocardial third of the myocardium was most involved histologically, suggesting that the subendocardial myocardial injury corresponded to the observed ST-segment and T-wave changes. Kishimoto and coworkers,[97] using DBA/2 mice, induced myocarditis with encephalomyocarditis virus. Acute changes were correlated with advanced atrio-

ventricular block and with atrial and ventricular premature depolarizations. Sinus tachycardia and low voltage were seen in the late stages in the animals that survived. Over the long-term, the QRS voltages recovered toward normal, possibly reflecting loss of myocardial edema or development of ventricular hypertrophy, or both, as a compensatory mechanism for poor ventricular function.

Although T-wave and ST-segment changes are the most sensitive indices of myocardial ischemia, they also seem to be nonspecific. Prolongation of the PR interval is another nonspecific

ECG finding frequently noted in patients with febrile illnesses. Scott and colleagues[162] showed a 1.49 percent prevalence of these findings in a group of 737 infants and children with respiratory tract infections, but they also found a similar incidence among 108 control children without respiratory infection or other febrile illness. Abt and Vinnecour[1] recorded PR prolongation and T-wave changes in infants and children who had pneumonia without other signs of myocarditis. The QT interval has been prolonged in cases of acute myocarditis, but it also seems to be a nonspecific finding associated with certain infectious diseases, such as measles[151] and poliomyelitis.[89] A diagnosis of myocarditis cannot be established with certainty on the basis of these nonspecific changes.

Noninvasive diagnostic myocardial imaging techniques that are useful in the detection of myocarditis include echocardiography, nuclear imaging with gallium 67–labeled or indium 111–labeled antimyosin antibodies, and magnetic resonance imaging (MRI). Echocardiography is recommended currently in the initial diagnostic evaluation of all patients with suspected myocarditis.[153] The echocardiogram is useful in assessing ventricular function and helps to exclude pericardial effusion as the cause of the cardiomegaly.

Nuclear imaging has been advocated as a potentially helpful laboratory screening test. Some evidence suggests that using gallium 67 to screen patients with idiopathic DCM may select a subgroup of patients who could benefit from endomyocardial biopsy. The biopsy specimen could be used to confirm the presence of active inflammation. O'Connell and colleagues[131] studied 68 patients with DCM who underwent 71 parallel studies with endomyocardial biopsy and gallium scanning. For five of six patients, biopsy samples that showed myocarditis also showed dense gallium uptake, and only 9 of 65 negative biopsy specimens had "equivocally positive" gallium scans. A 36 percent incidence of myocarditis on biopsy was found for positive scans, and only a 1.8 percent incidence of myocarditis on biopsy was found for negative scans. No large studies enrolling children with viral myocarditis have been performed. The use of gallium imaging has diminished over time, mainly because of a lack of specificity.

Indium 111 antimyosin imaging[42] and the presence of major histocompatibility complex class I and II antigens measured by radioimmunoassay using monoclonal antibodies[76] can detect patients with active myocarditis. High titers (1 : 20) of an IgG antibody (i.e., heart-reactive antibodies) measured by indirect immunofluorescence have been reported in patients with biopsy-confirmed myocarditis.[129] Although none of the methods is yet clinically applicable to all patients, these noninvasive tests offer some hope that the diagnosis of inflammatory heart disease will become safer.

More recent studies suggest that contrast-enhanced cardiac MRI may be a promising technique for diagnosing myocardial inflammation and myocyte injury. Gagliardi and associates[60] reported the first case series on the use of cardiac MRI for the diagnosis of acute myocarditis in 11 infants and children. The authors reported 100 percent specificity and 100 percent sensitivity for T2-weighted spin echo cardiac MRI sequences compared with endocardial biopsy. Cardiac MRI may be a good tool for selecting patients for endomyocardial biopsy.

To undertake a hemodynamic study in patients with a classic picture of acute myocarditis, including an ECG that reveals low voltage, is unnecessary and potentially dangerous. If the clinical or ECG presentation is atypical (i.e., left ventricular hypertrophy with left axis deviation, infarction pattern, or left bundle branch block), the infant should be studied for exclusion of an anomalous origin of the left coronary artery or another unsuspected anomaly.

Endomyocardial biopsy has become a safe and effective means for sampling heart muscle.[5] The technique originally was introduced in 1962 in Japan by Sakakibara and Konno,[155] but it did not gain wide acceptance in the United States for another 10 or more years. Its widest application has been in monitoring the effectiveness of immunosuppressive therapy in heart transplant recipients who may undergo the procedure multiple times.

Endomyocardial biopsy used for establishing the diagnosis of myocarditis and possibly classifying the phase (i.e., active, healing, or healed) of viral infection may have a direct impact on the type of therapy employed. Classification of myocarditis based on histologic evidence found on biopsy specimens has proved to be a difficult and sometimes controversial task. No widespread agreement exists on the criteria for establishing the diagnosis of myocarditis from biopsy samples. Sampling error owing to the small amounts of tissue obtained and the focal nature of sampling and the disease process may lead to misdiagnosis. Samples usually are obtained from the right ventricular septum or apex and should contain at least three and optimally five pieces of tissue. Some investigators[180] have found sampling from other areas of the heart (e.g., left ventricle) to be more sensitive, but these techniques have not been applied widely.

Cases of "borderline myocarditis" (i.e., specimens containing increased numbers of inflammatory cells, but without evidence of myocyte necrosis) may require a repeat biopsy to confirm the diagnosis. Dec and colleagues[40] confirmed the diagnosis of myocarditis in four of six patients with an initial diagnosis of borderline myocarditis. These investigators did not show any significant advantage to sampling the left ventricle during the repeat study. Overinterpretation or misinterpretation has been cited as a major problem in the reading of biopsy specimens. Some studies[168,169,182] used this technique to establish a diagnosis of myocarditis in patients presenting with idiopathic congestive cardiomyopathy and in patients with serious ventricular dysrhythmias with otherwise structurally normal hearts. Edwards and associates[51] looked at 170 endomyocardial biopsy samples and found that more than five lymphocytes per high-power field were consistent with a diagnosis of active lymphocytic myocarditis.

Using endomyocardial biopsy, Fenoglio and coworkers[54] diagnosed myocarditis in 34 patients presenting with congestive heart failure of unknown origin. They classified these patients on the basis of clinical and histologic findings in an attempt to establish subgroups of patients who might benefit from immunosuppressive therapy. Three groups were established: acute, rapidly progressive, and chronic. Immunosuppressive therapy was thought to be significantly beneficial for the last group only in terms of clinical improvement.

Dec and colleagues[41] studied 27 patients referred for endomyocardial biopsy because of congestive heart failure of unknown origin. Two thirds of the patients had biopsy samples read as positive for myocarditis, but in contrast to the study of Fenoglio and coworkers,[54] in which the histologic grouping was slightly different, no correlation was found between histologic classification and outcome. Outcome did not differ between the group receiving immunosuppressives and the group not receiving immunosuppressives. Biopsy results were negative for 30 percent of the patients who already met all the clinical criteria of myocarditis and were positive for two of five patients without any clinical evidence of myocarditis (i.e., viral-like illness, pericarditis, or laboratory evidence of viral infection).

Olsen[134] reviewed 1200 biopsy specimens from patients with a clinical diagnosis of idiopathic DCM and found that slightly more than 25 percent had a diagnosis of myocarditis established on the basis of critical evaluation of their tissue specimens. No large study of pediatric patients has been conducted to confirm this finding in young patients.

Most physicians would agree that many cases of idiopathic DCM probably are the sequelae of unrecognized acute viral myocarditis. The role of endomyocardial biopsy in attempting to salvage patients by selecting them for specific therapy has some validity. The hope is that early intervention in some patients guided by this technique would prevent them from progressing to needing transplantation or to death from intractable heart failure.

MOLECULAR DIAGNOSTIC STUDIES

In Situ Hybridization

In 1986, Bowles and colleagues[22] showed the utility of molecular biologic analysis of tissue samples in establishing the diagnosis of myocarditis. Using in situ hybridization, they were able to show enteroviral RNA in the myocardium of patients suspected to have myocarditis. These investigators also showed that enteroviral RNA could be identified in the myocardial tissue samples obtained from patients with end-stage DCM, and the suggestion that some cases of DCM were caused by a previous episode of subclinical myocarditis gained scientific support. The ability to diagnose enteroviral myocarditis and the finding of enteroviral RNA in patients with DCM later were confirmed by other investigators.[9,23] Because of questions of excessive false-positive results, variations among laboratories, and the difficulty in performing the test routinely in hospital laboratories, this method never gained practical popularity.

Polymerase Chain Reaction

Jin and associates[87] first described the usefulness of PCR in identifying the viral genome in myocardial samples obtained from patients with suspected myocarditis. Using reverse transcription PCR, which employs RNA to amplify the corresponding complementary DNA before final DNA amplification, the researchers were able to identify an enteroviral genome from cardiac tissue samples. Patients with DCM were shown to harbor an enteroviral genome within myocardial specimens. Confirmation of the utility of PCR in the etiologic diagnosis of a viral genome in patients with clinical myocarditis and idiopathic DCM quickly followed.[32,50,67,77,127,145,186] Controversy existed, however, because reports of high levels of false-positive results,[50] contamination,[32] and low sensitivity[188] were published. The strength of this rapid (<5 hours) and powerful method of amplification of a specific viral genome is also its weakness. The method depends on the quality and quantity of nucleic acid extraction, but contamination may be commonplace in some laboratories. If any requirements are altered, amplification may not occur, leading to false-negative or false-positive (i.e., contamination) results.

Numerous publications have shown that PCR is a rapid and sensitive method for establishing the diagnosis of enteroviral myocarditis and that it is probably the test of choice in the diagnosis of all virus-induced cardiac disease. Towbin and colleagues[178] used PCR to diagnose adenoviral myocarditis in a fetus with nonimmune hydrops fetalis. In this case, the adenoviral genome was amplified from fetal blood and maternal blood at 29 weeks' gestation and again at delivery at 34 weeks' gestation using blood from the infant and mother and placental specimens. Treatment with digoxin in utero helped the fetus improve clinically, and the infant had normal cardiac function at delivery. Using viral primers designed to amplify enterovirus, adenovirus, CMV, and HSV nucleic acid, Martin and associates[111] reported 34 patients with suspected acute myocarditis, for whom 68 percent of samples analyzed were PCR-positive. In this report, samples from 17 control patients were PCR-negative. Adenovirus was the most common viral genome identified (58%), and enteroviruses were the second most common (29%). A few reported cases were PCR-positive for HSV and CMV.

Lozinski and coworkers[108] confirmed the importance of adenovirus in their study of cases of myocarditis for which no cause had been found previously; in this case, 66 percent of the previously unidentified cases were identified as adenovirus. In a more recent study by Bowles and colleagues,[21] viral genomes were detected in 20 percent of 149 patients with the diagnosis of DCM. In these patients, adenovirus was identified in 12 percent and enterovirus in 8 percent of DCM cases. In all age groups, adenovirus and enterovirus were the viruses most commonly detected in acute myocarditis and DCM.

Schowengerdt and colleagues[161] showed that a variety of viruses might be the inciting cause of rejection in patients after undergoing heart transplantation. Using PCR of endomyocardial biopsy specimens, the investigators showed a direct correlation between histologic rejection and PCR-positive viral study results. Studying patients undergoing serial endomyocardial biopsies, they found that the viral genome could be amplified in transplant-rejecting patients who previously had negative PCR analyses. In these cases, as the rejection grade improved, the PCR results again became negative. The most common viruses correlated with rejection were adenoviruses, CMV, and parvovirus. The researchers postulated that this form of rejection probably is another form of myocarditis, and this hypothesis has been supported by other clinical studies.[187]

VIROLOGIC AND BACTERIOLOGIC STUDIES

For each infant or child with a diagnosis of acute myocarditis, an attempt should be made to identify the offending organism. If the patient is seen early in the illness, isolation of the virus from throat washings, stool, blood, or the myocardium may be possible. Support for an active infection is obtained by showing a fourfold increase in antibody titer to the virus that has been isolated.[19,74,160]

Lerner and colleagues[102] suggested criteria that would help define an etiologic association between a coxsackievirus infection and myocarditis. High-order associations included isolation of the virus from the myocardium, the endocardium, or pericardial fluid and localization of type-specific virus in myocardium, endocardium, or pericardium at sites of pathologic change. Moderate-order associations are determined when virus is isolated from pharynx or feces, and a fourfold increase in type-specific, neutralizing, hemagglutination-inhibiting, or complement-fixing antibodies is shown, or when virus is isolated from pharynx or feces with a concurrent serum titer of 1 : 32 or greater of type-specific, IgM-neutralizing or hemagglutination-inhibiting antibodies. Schmidt and colleagues[160] stress the usefulness of the IgM-specific antibody titer. Coxsackieviruses B1, B3, B4, B5, and B6 are identifiable with this method. Immunofluorescent methods may be used during histologic analysis to identify specific antigens in the myocardium.[26] In chronic illness, attempts at virologic identification are less fruitful.[69]

Blood for aerobic and anaerobic cultures should be obtained from any infant with fever and signs of compromised cardiovascular function. The erythrocyte sedimentation rate and white blood cell count usually are elevated in acute myocarditis; occasionally a leukemoid reaction may be identified.[3] A normal value for these tests does not exclude myocarditis. Elevations of serum glutamic oxaloacetic and glutamic pyruvic transaminase levels have been detected, especially in diphtheritic myocarditis, but they may be elevated in any patient with acute myocardial damage. Although a high level of serum transaminase activity usually is an ominous prognostic sign, Tahernia[170] found the ECG to be a more sensitive indicator of the ultimate outcome in children with diphtheritic myocarditis. Creatine phosphokinase and lactate dehydrogenase enzymes also should be measured.

DIFFERENTIAL DIAGNOSIS

Any cause of circulatory failure, especially when acute in onset, may mimic myocarditis. In newborns, heart failure associated with hypoxia, hypoglycemia, and hypocalcemia is well recognized, whereas circulatory collapse may occur with any infection and without direct involvement of the myocardium. A careful history may help to elucidate possible precipitating factors. Biochemical investigations to exclude hypoglycemia and hypocalcemia always should be conducted in any newborn who has signs of heart failure. Blood cultures should be obtained when infection is suspected.

Many infants with structural cardiac defects (e.g., hypoplastic left heart syndrome, aortic valve stenosis) may not have audible murmurs when severely ill. Murmurs usually appear, however, with treatment and improvement in cardiac function. The precordium usually is hyperactive, rather than quiet, and the heart sounds are clear and increased in intensity, rather than muffled. The ECG usually shows severe right ventricular hypertrophy in the former condition and shows right ventricular or left ventricular hypertrophy in the latter; the ECG is useful in the differential diagnosis. The findings on an echocardiogram often are diagnostic.

Beyond the immediate neonatal period, the major disease entities that require differentiation from myocarditis are endocardial fibroelastosis, anomalous left coronary artery arising from the pulmonary artery, Cori type II glycogen storage disease (i.e., Pompe disease), medial necrosis of the coronary arteries, left atrial myxoma,[128] and other congestive cardiomyopathies of undetermined cause. Common to all of these disorders is moderate to severe cardiomegaly, usually associated with congestive cardiac failure, gallop rhythm, and the infrequent occurrence or absence of murmurs. The murmurs are associated primarily with an anomalous left coronary artery and endocardial fibroelastosis. They are not more than grade 3/6 in intensity, are high-pitched, are apically located, and represent some degree of mitral insufficiency. Idiopathic myocarditis occurs primarily in patients older than 6 months of age,[149,150] whereas most of the conditions described earlier manifest before the infant is 6 months old.

Endocardial fibroelastosis, a common cause of congestive cardiac failure in infants, is impossible to differentiate from acute myocarditis on the basis of clinical examination alone. An anomalous origin of the left coronary artery should be identified. The ECG usually shows left axis deviation of the QRS complex in the frontal plane, left ventricular hypertrophy, and a pattern of anterolateral myocardial infarction. It is recognized as a QR pattern with inverted T waves in standard leads I and AVL, a broad Q wave with inverted T waves in precordial leads V_5 and V_6, and loss of anterior forces in the mid-precordial leads. For definitive diagnosis, cardiac catheterization is essential.

Pericarditis, frequently caused by viruses, usually occurs in children rather than in infants. The clinical history may be identical to that of patients with myocarditis; however, considering the degree of cardiomegaly, cardiovascular function is compromised less than in patients with myocarditis, although cardiac tamponade may occur in some cases. Differentiation from myocarditis may be made clinically if the patient has a friction rub, no gallop rhythm, and a typical pattern of chest pain. Further studies may be required, however, to make a conclusive diagnosis. The echocardiogram is invaluable in establishing this diagnosis. It is the most sensitive and least traumatic technique available and easily identifies an effusion. Myocarditis and pericarditis may occur together. This combination is seen most frequently in the pancarditis of rheumatic fever, but it also may occur in coxsackievirus B infections and in many collagen vascular and autoimmune diseases. Myocarditis has been associated with rheumatoid arthritis,[120] systemic lupus erythematosus,[44] and ulcerative colitis.[56,126]

TREATMENT

STANDARD APPROACHES

Intensive medical care is required during the acute stage of the illness. Heart rate, respiratory rate, and blood pressure should be monitored frequently, and a careful assessment of urine output and fluid intake is mandatory. All patients require bed rest. Experimental studies in mice have shown that exercise increases replication of virus in the myocardium and increases the mortality rate from myocarditis by 100 percent.[61] Although extrapolating directly from experimental studies in animals to the human situation always is dangerous, suggesting strict bed rest during the early stages of acute myocarditis seems to be a prudent measure. For infants or children with signs of congestive cardiac failure or shock, oxygen should be administered to maintain a normal arterial blood oxygen tension.

No specific therapeutic modality is known that can reverse the myocardial injury directly, but much can be done to maintain adequate tissue perfusion, prevent metabolic disturbances, and support myocardial function. When congestive cardiac failure is identified, digitalis should be administered. This agent should be used with caution, given the increased expression of proinflammatory cytokine and increased mortality rates observed in murine myocarditis treated with high-dose digitalis.[116] Diuretics also are used frequently to treat cardiac failure. Diuretics have no direct beneficial effect on the myocardium; they should be used cautiously because rapid reduction in extracellular fluid volume may lead to shock, and the loss of potassium associated with vigorous diuresis may precipitate digitalis toxicity. The frequency of administration depends on the clinical state of the patient.

In some instances, especially in newborns, the primary presentation may be shock. The blood pressure usually is maintained close to normal levels until late in the course of disease; it cannot be a reliable index of the severity of the patient's condition. Cold extremities, increasing heart rate, and low urine output are much more sensitive indicators of a reduction in effective circulating blood volume. Although the hearts of these infants and children respond poorly to volume loading, a colloid transfusion may help in selected patients. Albumin as a 5 percent solution in Ringer's lactate or whole blood may be administered. The total amount administered should be guided by the response of the patient in terms of perfusion, urine output, heart rate, and central venous pressure.

These patients may require a high filling pressure (e.g., 12 to 18 mm Hg) to achieve any cardiac output, compared with 5 mm Hg, which would achieve sufficient filling in the normal heart. If the patient remains in shock despite administration of these high filling pressures, a positive inotropic agent is required. Dopamine exerts an inotropic effect on the heart and concomitantly dilates the renal vessels, improving urine output. The usual dose is 2 to 10 µg/kg/min. As the dose increases to 20 µg/kg/min, dopamine has a more dominant alpha-adrenergic effect and may increase systemic peripheral resistance; experts avoid doses greater than 15 µg/kg/min. Dobutamine, which is a sympathomimetic amine that stimulates beta$_1$-adrenergic, beta$_2$-adrenergic, and alpha-adrenergic receptors, may be useful when used in combination with dopamine. It has significant inotropic activity while decreasing left ventricular filling pressure. Dobutamine does not induce the positive chronotropic effect and increased ventricular irritability that are seen with dopamine. Used in combination with low doses of dopamine (<10 µg/kg/min), dobutamine (in doses ≤10 µg/kg/min) may result in significant positive inotropism, while preventing a sinus tachycardia that may compromise cardiac output further.

Isoproterenol, a commonly used inotropic agent, should be avoided because it causes a significant increase in heart rate and may affect cardiac function adversely. When these drugs are used, ensuring normal acid-base balance is important because action of the agents is decreased significantly by acidosis.

Sodium nitroprusside, phentolamine, and the nitrates have been used in adults. These agents have been used less extensively in children, primarily in the early postoperative period after open heart surgery, to improve cardiac function. They improve cardiac output by indirectly reducing systemic arterial resistance or venous filling pressure, or both. One study showed a marked improvement in the reduction of inflammation, necrosis, and dystrophic calcification in mice infected with coxsackievirus B3 when they were treated with captopril, an angiotensin-converting enzyme inhibitor, early after development of infection.[148] Besides its known afterload-reducing effects, this agent, which contains sulfhydryl groups in its chemical structure, is capable of scavenging oxygen free radicals in vitro. This ability may enable the drug to reduce myocyte damage by free radicals during the acute phase of the infection.

Another study failed to show any significant correlation between improved ventricular function and histologic improvement in patients with myocarditis treated with immunosuppressive therapy. Rather, an increase in the ejection fraction during the first 3 months of therapy seemed predictive of a good outcome.[39] Intravenously administered afterload-reducing agents should not be used, unless facilities are available for constant monitoring of the left ventricular filling pressure (i.e., mean wedge pressure) and unless that pressure is elevated.

Arrhythmias should be recognized and treated vigorously. Digitalis should be used with caution, and intravenous administration of this drug should be used only if the oral route is impossible. Rather than used as inotropic support, digitalis can be used to help control supraventricular arrhythmias. Levels must be monitored, especially when renal function is questionable. Lidocaine should be administered intravenously for acute treatment of complex ventricular arrhythmias, such as couplets and ventricular tachycardia. In cases of intractable ventricular arrhythmias, intravenously administered procainamide can be used. Monitoring the serum level on a daily basis beginning several hours after the drip is started is essential to prevent toxic side effects. Alternatively, amiodarone given intravenously can be used for life-threatening ventricular arrhythmias. Measures of contractility using echocardiographic techniques also are vital because procainamide is a negative inotrope.

A temporary pacing catheter should be inserted when complete heart block occurs. In many instances, the temporary pacing catheter allows time for spontaneous recovery of atrioventricular conduction. A permanent pacemaker may be required; if so, it should be inserted as an elective, rather than emergency, procedure. Only a demand pacemaker should be used because in most instances a return to normal rhythm is expected; use of this type of pacemaker avoids the risk of competition between the patient's inherent rhythm and the pacemaker, as would occur with a fixed-rate device. If infants or children experience Stokes-Adams attacks, a transthoracic pacing wire may have to be inserted as an emergency procedure.

Antibiotics should not be given routinely, unless a bacterial infection is suspected. Appropriate cultures need to be obtained before use of antibiotics.

The use of immunosuppressive agents in the treatment of viral or suspected viral myocarditis is controversial. Immunosuppressant therapy in animal models of viral myocarditis has not been shown to be beneficial. One reason for the lack of efficacy of immunosuppressant therapies may relate to the duality of the effects of the immune system. Corticosteroids enhanced viral titers in the early phase of viral murine myocarditis, whereas cyclosporine caused greater mortality and cardiac insufficiency in encephalomyocarditis virus myocarditis.[123,177] Other studies suggested an exacerbation of virus-induced cytotoxicity when such agents were given in the acute setting and possible interference

with the production of interferon.[93,94] A report of 13 children with biopsy-confirmed myocarditis treated with prednisone approximately 3 weeks after symptoms occurred showed a marked reduction in inflammation on the follow-up biopsy specimen.[31] This study was uncontrolled, however, and may not truly represent an accurate account of the role of immunosuppressive therapy.

Mason and colleagues[113] used endomyocardial biopsy as a means of diagnosing and following the effects of immunosuppressive therapy in 10 patients. Eight patients received a combination of prednisone and azathioprine, and two patients received prednisone alone. Four patients improved clinically and histologically while on therapy. Two patients who had medications discontinued had relapses, which were reversed with reinstitution of therapy. Only one patient worsened while on therapy, and that patient died. Although the study by Mason and colleagues[113] was uncontrolled, the reversal of congestive heart failure seen in the two patients who were restarted on therapy suggests the beneficial effect of these agents.

Daly and colleagues[36] treated nine patients using combined immunosuppressive therapy with prednisolone and azathioprine. Seven of the nine patients showed definite hemodynamic and histologic improvement after 2 months of therapy. After 4 months off therapy, only four of the seven patients still showed significant improvement, however. One patient improved with reinstitution of therapy, and two patients deteriorated.

Dec and colleagues[41] treated nine patients in their study with single or combined immunosuppressive therapy. They saw improvement in 4 of 9 patients; however, 6 of 18 patients not receiving immunosuppressive agents also improved, nullifying any statistically significant difference between the two groups. Lymphocytic myocarditis was found in 6 of 12 patients with no obvious cardiac disease, but with high-grade ventricular dysrhythmias, and who had undergone right ventricular endomyocardial biopsy.[182] All six patients received combined immunosuppressive therapy with prednisone and azathioprine. At follow-up, five of six patients had been cured of the dysrhythmia, and active myocardial inflammation had disappeared, as confirmed by repeat biopsy. Although this study was uncontrolled, the fact that none of the patients progressed to a cardiomyopathic state or died of his or her illness suggests a beneficial effect.

Kereiakes and Parmley[91] tabulated most of the studies showing the effects of immunosuppressive therapy in patients with myocarditis. Sixty percent of 82 biopsy-confirmed cases of myocarditis showed improvement with steroids alone or in combination with azathioprine. Patients with lower grade inflammatory changes seem to do better than did patients with higher grade changes. Complications of immunosuppressive therapy, including opportunistic infections and a cushingoid state, have been reported and may limit the amount and type of therapy.[113,168]

Hobbs and associates[78] used combined prednisone and azathioprine to treat 34 adults with biopsy-confirmed myocarditis. Survival was no better for patients with histologic improvement than for patients with persistent infiltrates. Most patients experienced side effects, some of them lethal, from the corticosteroids. The potential benefits of this type of therapy must be weighed against the risks of immunosuppression in each patient with myocarditis. This therapy apparently does not prevent the observed ECG changes seen in untreated patients or the associated neuritis.[175]

Although numerous anecdotal and small case series suggested that patients with viral myocarditis might benefit from early steroid or immunosuppressive therapy, the results of the Myocarditis Treatment Trial suggested that treating patients who received a histopathologic diagnosis of myocarditis with immunosuppressive therapy for 24 weeks (prednisone plus cyclosporine or prednisone plus azathioprine) did not lead to an improvement in ejection fraction compared with conventional therapy.[114] The major limitation of this study was the unexpectedly low rate of positive biopsy specimens (<10%) and the extension of enrollment to 2 years after the initial clinical presentation. For many patients, the disease possibly already had progressed from ongoing immune-mediated cardiac injury to DCM, and any form of therapy may have been ineffective in this setting.

Various immunomodulatory therapies have been proposed for the autoimmune phase of viral myocarditis. Kishimoto and colleagues[98] found that immunoglobulin therapy suppressed coxsackievirus B3-induced murine myocarditis and increased survival in C3H/He mice after infection with encephalomyocarditis virus. Intravenous immunoglobulin (IVIG) therapy reduced various proinflammatory markers, including TNF, interferon-γ, macrophage inflammatory protein-2, interleukin-6, plasma catecholamines, and soluble intercellular adhesion molecule-1.[98] Exogenous immunoglobulins modulate diverse immune response mechanisms; however, the exact mechanisms by which IVIG modifies myocarditis remains to be determined. Drucker and associates,[47] who investigated the use of IVIG in 21 of 46 children with myocarditis, showed that patients who received this drug had better left ventricular function at follow-up. Survival tended to be higher at 1 year, although the data did not reach statistical significance because of the small number of patients in the study. More recently, in a prospective placebo-controlled trial with IVIG in adult patients with recent-onset DCM or myocarditis, treatment with IVIG did not result in an improvement in left ventricular function compared with placebo-treated patients.[118]

At present, no form of immunosuppressant therapy has proved to be effective in the clinical setting. Routine immunosuppressive therapy no longer is recommended for patients with myocarditis and a stable clinical course. Many clinicians still recommend aggressive immunosuppressive therapy, however, for patients with fulminant myocarditis or a deteriorating clinical course or both.

PROGNOSIS

The prognosis of acute myocarditis caused by coxsackievirus B infection in a newborn is poor. Kibrick and Benirschke[92] reported a 75 percent mortality rate among 25 infants with coxsackievirus B myocarditis. The greatest number of deaths occurred in the first week of the illness. No apparent sequelae occurred in the six infants who survived, although no long-term follow-up data were available. The outlook in other infants and children with clinically recognized myocarditis is better, but mortality rates remain significant (10-25%). Hastreiter and Miller[73] observed complete recovery in 50 percent of patients. Another 25 percent became asymptomatic, but abnormal ECGs or chest radiographs persisted. An abnormality may not be evident on the ECG unless the patients are exercised.[16] Despite lack of symptoms, many adult patients have a reduced working capacity associated with exercise stress testing.[18]

The outcome of myocarditis is related partly to the cause. Patients with diphtheritic myocarditis who have arrhythmias or conduction abnormalities have a very poor prognosis. Tahernia[170] found in his study that all patients with disturbances of conduction died. Begg[15] also reported a 100 percent mortality rate for patients with diphtheritic myocarditis who developed supraventricular tachycardia.

Chronic arrhythmias may persist long after the acute disease has passed. Friedman and colleagues[57] performed a retrospective analysis of 12 patients with biopsy-confirmed myocarditis and complex ventricular arrhythmias at the time of presentation (11 with ventricular tachycardia). Five of the 12 patients still were receiving antiarrhythmic therapy at a median follow-up of 50 months. Complex ventricular arrhythmias still were present in these patients (three with ventricular tachycardia and two with couplets or multiforms), requiring ongoing therapy. The investigators concluded that although the arrhythmias were controlled more easily than at presentation of the patients, ongoing surveillance was essential in ensuring the suppression of these potentially life-threatening arrhythmias. Children who recover from myocarditis, regardless of cause, should be followed indefinitely.

MYOCARDITIS IN CASES OF HUMAN IMMUNODEFICIENCY VIRUS INFECTION

Infection with human immunodeficiency virus (HIV) may affect the heart adversely. Cardiac dysfunction, including congestive heart failure, may occur; many patients who have died and undergone autopsy are shown to have myocarditis. Anderson and associates[6] retrospectively analyzed 71 consecutive necropsy patients who died of acquired immunodeficiency syndrome (AIDS) and found that 52 percent had evidence of myocarditis. Opportunistic agents could account for only a few of the cases, and most were considered idiopathic.

Another study examined autopsy specimens of 26 consecutive cases. Lymphocytic myocarditis was seen in nine patients (35%), and another seven patients had lymphocytic infiltrates without myocytolysis.[14] Acierno[2] correctly pointed out that a distinction must be made between AIDS-associated myocarditis and secondary myocarditis caused by known pathogens or idiopathic myocarditis.

Reilly and colleagues[147] found a 45 percent incidence of myocarditis in 58 consecutive autopsy cases. Congestive heart failure, ventricular tachycardia, and other ECG abnormalities were seen in nearly 60 percent of the patients. Two patients died suddenly, both with myocarditis. In a prospective study of asymptomatic HIV-infected patients, the reported mean annual incidence of progression to DCM was 15.9 cases per 1000 patients. Endomyocardial biopsy specimens revealed myocardial inflammation in 63 of 76 (83%) of these high-risk patients. HIV-infected cardiac myocytes were detected by in situ hybridization in 58 of 76 (76%) patients.

In a prospective multicenter study of 205 vertically HIV-infected children enrolled at a median age of 1.9 years and 600 HIV-exposed children enrolled prenatally or as neonates, the 5-year cumulative incidence of cardiac dysfunction ranged from 18 to 39 percent in HIV-infected children.[167] Myocardial inflammation, with or without cell destruction, is a frequent finding in patients infected with HIV. Whether this response is due to the virus itself or to opportunistic agents or other toxic reactions is unclear. Specific therapy for myocarditis in these patients has not been elucidated, and no recommendations, other than inotropic support with anticongestive and afterload-reducing agents, can be made.

PARASITIC MYOCARDITIS

Parasitic myocarditis is an uncommon form of heart disease in the United States. Chagas disease is caused by infection with *Trypanosoma cruzi*, however, and it is a long-lived infection that affects approximately 17 million individuals in Latin America.[152] Although several countries in Latin America have well-established vector-control programs, contact with contaminated feces or urine from infected triatomine insects remains the main mode of infection.

The major cardiovascular manifestation of Chagas disease is an extensive myocarditis that typically becomes evident years or decades after the initial infection. The disease is transmitted to humans by various species of blood-sucking reduviid insects. After inoculation, the protozoa multiply and migrate widely throughout the body. Host control of this parasite has been shown to depend on humoral and cell-mediated adaptive responses and elements of the innate immune system.[65]

More recently, a role for TLR signaling in resistance to *T. cruzi* is suggested by the observations that mice deficient in MyD88, an adapter molecule required for signaling events by most TLRs, show enhanced susceptibility to infection with this protozoan parasite.[28] Acute Chagas disease usually is an illness of children, but it can occur at any age.[122] Histologic examination of the heart during the acute phase reveals intracellular parasites with a marked cellular infiltrate, particularly around myocytes that have ruptured and released the parasites.[138] A well-established fact is that intracellular parasites are found in cardiac myocytes only during the acute phase of illness.

Severe myocarditis develops in only a few acute cases, and most deaths are caused by the resultant congestive heart failure and pericardial effusion. Nonspecific ECG changes are seen, but the life-threatening arrhythmias that are frequent occurrences in chronic Chagas disease generally do not occur. In most patients with more acute disease (90% of cases), symptoms resolve gradually over weeks to months.

Chronic progressive Chagas disease develops in 10 to 20 percent of previously asymptomatically infected individuals.[49] It is manifested by a chronic, diffuse, progressive fibrosing myocarditis that involves the myocytes and the atrioventricular conduction system.[124,125] On gross examination, the heart usually is enlarged and flaccid. Thrombus formation frequently occurs, and thrombus may fill much of the apex of the left ventricle in some cases.

Immune-mediated cardiac injury, caused primarily by infiltrating mononuclear cells, probably is the main mechanism responsible for the development of chronic Chagas heart disease. This hypothesis is supported by several observations. Animal models of *T. cruzi* infection have shown lysis of nonparasitized cardiac myocytes by immune effector cells[8]; depletion of CD4+ T-lymphocyte subpopulations abrogates myocardial injury in a murine model of chronic Chagas disease; and myocardial damage can be induced in healthy animals by passive transfer of CD4+ T cells from *T. cruzi*–infected mice.[45] Although CD4+ T cells seem to be crucial in myocardial injury, CD8+ T cells may have a protective role. Mice depleted of CD8+ T cells have a robust parasitemia, but almost no inflammatory infiltrates are seen in the parasite-infected tissues.[172]

Histologic examination reveals focal but widespread areas of cellular infiltrates composed of plasma cells, eosinophils, mast cells, and macrophages.[124] Extensive fibrosis occurs, replacing previously damaged myocardial tissue. In contrast to the situation observed in acute disease, the presence of parasites (a rare finding) in tissue has little correlation with myocardial pathology. Inflammatory changes in the right bundle branch and the anterior fascicle of the left bundle branch explain the frequent occurrence of right bundle branch and left anterior fascicular block.[125]

The clinical manifestations of chronic Chagas disease range from isolated rhythm disturbances to advanced disease characterized by cardiomegaly, chronic congestive heart failure, and arrhythmias. Syncope also is a frequent problem of the disease. In one series of 53 patients with chronic Chagas disease, the most frequent causes of recurrent syncope were ventricular tachycardia (43%) with a poor prognosis and paroxysmal atrioventricular block (21%) with a favorable prognosis.[112] Sudden death caused by ventricular fibrillation is a constant threat and may develop before cardiomegaly or heart failure is diagnosed.[30]

The diagnosis of chronic Chagas disease cannot be made solely on the basis of histologic examination of the heart. Serologic testing is the method of choice for establishing the diagnosis of chronic Chagas disease. Several highly sensitive serologic tests

for the detection of anti–*T. cruzi* antibodies, such as indirect hemagglutination, complement fixation, indirect immunofluorescence, and enzyme-linked immunosorbent assay, are available.[95,163]

Benznidazole and nifurtimox are the only available drugs with activity against *T. cruzi*. Although these two drugs have been thought to be ineffective or too toxic, or both, for treating chronic infections, in one report a 60-day course of benznidazole therapy eliminated infection in more than 60 percent of chronically infected children.[7] The current emphasis on the management of Chagas disease is on prevention of infection. In 1991, the Latin American countries of Argentina, Bolivia, Brazil, Chile, Paraguay, and Uruguay initiated a program to decrease transmission of the parasite through vector control and the screening of blood donors. According to more recent studies, transmission has been virtually eliminated in much of the region.[196]

Myocarditis is one of the most serious complications of trichinosis. The disease develops when undercooked meat contaminated with infective larvae of *Trichinella* is eaten. Myocardial invasion by *Trichinella spiralis* has been well described, but encystment within the myocardium has been reported only rarely.[96] At autopsy, the heart may be dilated and a pericardial effusion may be identified. Histologically, a prominent focal infiltrate composed of lymphocytes and eosinophils with interstitial edema and scattered hemorrhages commonly is found.[165]

Myocarditis usually is mild, with few clinical signs and symptoms. This myocarditis may range from chest pain to fatal congestive heart failure, however, and may mimic acute myocardial infarction.[34,68] The frequencies of ECG abnormalities among 154 cases of trichinellosis were determined to be 56 percent.[143] The abnormalities on ECG most frequently observed were a nonspecific ventricular repolarization disturbance (with ST-T wave changes), followed by bundle branch conduction disturbances, and sinus tachycardia. Despite ECG evidence of myocardial involvement, less than 0.1 percent of patients with trichinosis die of this complication.[68]

The definitive diagnosis of trichinosis is based on the presence of the larval forms in tissue biopsy samples, usually from a large tender area such as the gastrocnemius muscle. Serologic testing is available through state laboratories and the Centers for Disease Control and Prevention. Typically, serum antibody titers become positive during or after the third week of illness. The efficacy of mebendazole or albendazole in the treatment of myocarditis caused by *Trichinella* infection has not been evaluated adequately.

Toxocara canis, the principal cause of visceral larva migrans, is a rare cause of myocarditis. Most reported cases have occurred in children younger than 3 years of age.[37,181] Children especially are susceptible to infection with *Toxocara* because of their habit of crawling on the ground and putting objects into their mouths. The myocardial lesions noted on histologic examination have included granulomata and extensive eosinophilic infiltrates with foci of muscle necrosis. The clinical presentation may be acute respiratory distress caused by congestive heart failure, requiring administration of oxygen and diuretic therapy. Asymptomatic infection involving the heart also has been reported.[37]

The definitive diagnosis of *T. canis* infection requires microscopic identification of the larvae in biopsy specimens of the liver or heart, but this finding is infrequent. An enzyme immunoassay for *Toxocara* serum antibodies, which is available at the Centers for Disease Control and Prevention, can provide presumptive evidence of toxocariasis.

Toxoplasma gondii may cause myocarditis as part of disseminated infection or, less frequently, as an isolated cardiac infection. In infants with congenital toxoplasmosis, the clinical manifestations usually are those of meningoencephalitis, but at autopsy, extensive myocardial involvement has been documented.[199] Outside the newborn period, infection with this intracellular parasite most commonly occurs in immunosuppressed patients with malignant diseases, patients with AIDS,[29] and patients who have undergone cardiac or bone marrow transplantation.[109] Histologic examination of the heart reveals focal interstitial infiltrates consisting of histiocytes, lymphocytes, plasma cells, eosinophils, and very few polymorphonuclear cells.[174] *Toxoplasma* is seen as basophilic masses within a pseudocyst in normal or damaged myocardial fibers.

Clinical manifestations may include arrhythmias (atrial and ventricular), atrioventricular block, atypical chest pain, pericarditis, and heart failure. The diagnosis of toxoplasmic myocarditis requires the exclusion of other specific forms of heart disease and the establishment of evidence of toxoplasmosis with serologic testing. The diagnosis may be aided by endomyocardial biopsy.[109] Treatment with pyrimethamine and sulfonamides (especially sulfadiazine) has been reported in patients with isolated toxoplasmic myocarditis, but the response to therapy has varied. In one series of toxoplasmic myocarditis, relapses occurred in 17 percent of cases after therapy.[101]

Myocardial disease also has been reported after infection with *Echinococcus granulosus* and *Plasmodium falciparum*.[96] Cardiac involvement is estimated to occur in less than 2 percent of cases of echinococcosis.[43] When it does occur, the cysts usually are located in the intramyocardial region and protrude into the adjacent cardiac chambers. The clinical manifestations depend primarily on the location and size of the cyst. Rupture of the cyst is the most dreaded complication because it may lead to pericarditis, anaphylactic shock, or pulmonary emboli. Two-dimensional echocardiography is the preferred imaging study to detect and localize cysts.[133] Myocardial changes also have been documented in fatal malaria, particularly when caused by *P. falciparum*. Histologically, blocking of the coronary arteries and capillaries with parasites, local hemorrhage, and deposit of pigment occurs. Clinical findings suggestive of cardiac involvement are rare, however. In a series of 49 patients with falciparum malaria, no ECG evidence of cardiac involvement was found.[166]

Myocarditis also has occurred in association with primary amebic meningoencephalitis caused by *Naegleria*. In a retrospective study, focal or diffuse myocarditis was documented in more than 40 percent of cases.[110] Myocardial involvement is not a clinically significant manifestation of this uniformly fatal central nervous system infection.

REFERENCES

1. Abt, A. F., and Vinnecour, M. I.: Electrographic studies during pneumonia in infants and children. Am. J. Dis. Child. 47:737, 1934.
2. Acierno, L. J.: Cardiac complications in acquired immunodeficiency syndrome (AIDS): A review. J. Am. Coll. Cardiol. 13:1144-1154, 1989.
3. Ainger, L. E., Lawyer, N. G., and Fitch, C. W.: Neonatal rubella myocarditis. Br. Heart. J. 28:691-697, 1966.
4. Akira, S.: Pathogen recognition and signaling pathways of toll-like receptors. J. Invest. Dermatol. 121:1234, 2003.
5. Ali, N., Ferrans, V. J., Roberts, W. C., and Massumi, R. A.: Clinical evaluation of transvenous catheter technique for endomyocardial biopsy. Chest 63:399-402, 1973.
6. Anderson, D. W., Virmani, R., Reilly, J. M., et al.: Prevalent myocarditis at necropsy in the acquired immunodeficiency syndrome. J. Am. Coll. Cardiol. 11:792-799, 1988.
7. Andrade, A. L., Martelli, C. M., Oliveira, R. M., et al.: Short report: Benznidazole efficacy among *Trypanosoma cruzi*-infected adolescents after a six-year follow-up. Am. J. Trop. Med. Hyg. 71:594-597, 2004.
8. Andrade, Z. A., Andrade, S. G., Correa, R., et al.: Myocardial changes in acute *Trypanosoma cruzi* infection: Ultrastructural evidence of immune damage and the role of microangiopathy. Am. J. Pathol. 144:1403-1411, 1994.
9. Archard, L. C., Richardson, P. J., Olsen, E. G., et al.: The role of Coxsackie B viruses in the pathogenesis of myocarditis, dilated cardiomyopathy and inflammatory muscle disease. Biochem. Soc. Symp. 53:51-62, 1987.
10. Badorff, C., Berkely, N., Mehrotra, S., et al.: Enteroviral protease 2A directly cleaves dystrophin and is inhibited by a dystrophin-based substrate analogue. J. Biol. Chem. 275:11191-11197, 2000.
11. Badorff, C., Fichtlscherer, B., Rhoads, R. E., et al.: Nitric oxide inhibits dystrophin proteolysis by coxsackieviral protease 2A through S-nitrosylation: A protective mechanism against enteroviral cardiomyopathy. Circulation 102:2276-2281, 2000.
12. Badorff, C., and Knowlton, K. U.: Dystrophin disruption in enterovirus-induced myocarditis and dilated cardiomyopathy: From bench to bedside. Med. Microbiol. Immunol. (Berlin) 193:121-126, 2004.
13. Bairan, A. C., Cherry, J. D., Fagan, L. F., et al.: Complete heart block and respiratory syncytial virus infection. Am. J. Dis. Child. 127:264-265, 1974.
14. Baroldi, G., Corallo, S., Moroni, M., et al.: Focal lymphocytic myocarditis in acquired immunodeficiency syndrome (AIDS): A correlative morphologic and clinical study in 26 consecutive fatal cases. J. Am. Coll. Cardiol. 12:463-469, 1988.
15. Begg, M. D.: Diphtheric myocarditis: EKG study. Lancet 1:857, 1937.
16. Bengtsson, E., and Lamberger, B.: Five-year follow-up study of cases suggestive of acute myocarditis. Am. Heart J. 72:751-763, 1966.
17. Benirschke, K., and Kibrick, S.: Acute aseptic myocarditis and meningoencephalitis in the newborn child infected with coxsackie virus group B, type 3. N. Engl. J. Med. 255:883-889, 1956.
18. Bergstrom, K., Erikson, U., Nordbring, F., et al.: Acute non-rheumatic myopericarditis: A follow-up study. Scand. J. Infect. Dis. 2:7-16, 1970.
19. Berkovich, S., Rodriguez-Torres, R., and Lin, J. S.: Virologic studies in children with acute myocarditis. Am. J. Dis. Child. 115:207-212, 1968.
20. Bowles, N. E., Fuentes-Garcia, F., Makar, K. A., et al.: Analysis of the coxsackievirus B-adenovirus receptor gene in patients with myocarditis or dilated cardiomyopathy. Mol. Genet. Metab. 77:257-259, 2002.
21. Bowles, N. E., Ni, J., Kearney, D. L., et al.: Detection of viruses in myocardial tissues by polymerase chain reaction: Evidence of adenovirus as a common cause of myocarditis in children and adults. J. Am. Coll. Cardiol. 42:466-472, 2003.
22. Bowles, N. E., Richardson, P. J., Olsen, E. G., et al.: Detection of Coxsackie-B-virus-specific RNA sequences in myocardial biopsy samples from patients with myocarditis and dilated cardiomyopathy. Lancet 1:1120-1123, 1986.
23. Bowles, N. E., Rose, M. L., Taylor, P., et al.: End-stage dilated cardiomyopathy: Persistence of enterovirus RNA in myocardium at cardiac transplantation and lack of immune response. Circulation 80:1128-1136, 1989.
24. Brightman, V. J., Scott, T. F., Westphal, M., et al.: An outbreak of coxsackie B-5 virus infection in a newborn nursery. J. Pediatr. 69:179-192, 1966.
25. Brown, Z. A., Wald, A., Morrow, R. A., et al.: Effect of serologic status and cesarean delivery on transmission rates of herpes simplex virus from mother to infant. J. A. M. A. 289:203-209, 2003.
26. Burch, G. E., Sun, S. C., Chu, K. C., et al.: Interstitial and coxsackievirus B myocarditis in infants and children: A comparative histologic and immunofluorescent study of 50 autopsied hearts. J. A. M. A. 203:1-8, 1968.
27. Calabrese, F., and Thiene, G.: Myocarditis and inflammatory cardiomyopathy: Microbiological and molecular biological aspects. Cardiovasc. Res. 60:11-25, 2003.
28. Campos, M. A., Closel, M., Valente, E. P., et al.: Impaired production of proinflammatory cytokines and host resistance to acute infection with *Trypanosoma cruzi* in mice lacking functional myeloid differentiation factor 88. J. Immunol. 172:1711-1718, 2004.
29. Cappell, M. S., Mikhail, N., and Ortega, A.: Toxoplasma myocarditis in AIDS. Am. Heart J. 123:1728-1729, 1992.
30. Carrasco, H. A., Parada, H., Guerrero, L., et al.: Prognostic implications of clinical, electrocardiographic and hemodynamic findings in chronic Chagas disease. Int. J. Cardiol. 43:27-38, 1994.
31. Chan, K. Y., Iwahara, M., Benson, L. N., et al.: Immunosuppressive therapy in the management of acute myocarditis in children: A clinical trial. J. Am. Coll. Cardiol. 17:458-460, 1991.
32. Chapman, N. M., Tracy, S., Gauntt, C. J., et al.: Molecular detection and identification of enteroviruses using enzymatic amplification and nucleic acid hybridization. J. Clin. Microbiol. 28:843-850, 1990.
33. Cherry, J. D., Jahn, C. L., and Meyer, T. C.: Paroxysmal atrial tachycardia associated with ECHO 9 virus infection. Am. Heart J. 73:681-686, 1967.
34. Compton, S. J., Celum, C. L., Lee, C., et al.: Trichinosis with ventilatory failure and persistent myocarditis. Clin. Infect. Dis. 16:500-504, 1993.
35. Dalldorf, G., and Gifford, R.: Clinical and epidemiologic observations of Coxsackie-virus infection. N. Engl. J. Med. 244:868-873, 1951.
36. Daly, K., Richardson, P. J., Olsen, E. G., et al.: Acute myocarditis: Role of histological and virological examination in the diagnosis and assessment of immunosuppressive treatment. Br. Heart J. 51:30-35, 1984.
37. Dao, A. H., and Virmani, R.: Visceral larva migrans involving the myocardium: Report of two cases and review of literature. Pediatr. Pathol. 6:449-456, 1986.
38. De Jager, H., and Van Creveld, S.: Myocarditis in newborns, caused by coxsackie virus; clinical and pathological data. Ann. Paediatr. 187:100-118, 1956.
39. Dec, G. W., Jr., Fallon, J. T., Southern, J. F., et al.: Relation between histological findings on early repeat right ventricular biopsy and ventricular function in patients with myocarditis. Br. Heart J. 60:332-337, 1988.
40. Dec, G. W., Fallon, J. T., Southern, J. F., et al.: "Borderline" myocarditis: An indication for repeat endomyocardial biopsy. J. Am. Coll. Cardiol. 15:283-289, 1990.
41. Dec, G. W., Jr., Palacios, I. F., Fallon, J. T., et al.: Active myocarditis in the spectrum of acute dilated cardiomyopathies: Clinical features, histologic correlates, and clinical outcome. N. Engl. J. Med. 312:885-890, 1985.

42. Dec, G. W., Palacios, I., Yasuda, T., et al.: Antimyosin antibody cardiac imaging: Its role in the diagnosis of myocarditis. J. Am. Coll. Cardiol. 16:97-104, 1990.
43. Dighiero, J., Canabal, E. J., Aguirre, C. V., et al.: Echinococcus disease of the heart. *Circulation* 17:127-132, 1958.
44. Doria, A., Iaccarino, L., Sarzi-Puttini, P., et al.: Cardiac involvement in systemic lupus erythematosus. Lupus 14:683-686, 2005.
45. dos Santos, R. R., Rossi, M. A., Laus, J. L., et al.: Anti-CD4 abrogates rejection and reestablishes long-term tolerance to syngeneic newborn hearts grafted in mice chronically infected with *Trypanosoma cruzi*. J. Exp. Med. 175:29-39, 1992.
46. Drew, J. H.: Echo 11 virus outbreak in a nursery associated with myocarditis. Aust. Paediatr. J. 9:90-95, 1973.
47. Drucker, N. A., Colan, S. D., Lewis, A. B., et al.: Gamma-globulin treatment of acute myocarditis in the pediatric population. Circulation 89:252-257, 1994.
48. Drut, R. M., and Drut, R.: Giant-cell myocarditis in a newborn with congenital herpes simplex virus (HSV) infection: An immunohistochemical study on the origin of the giant cells. Pediatr. Pathol. 6:431-437, 1986.
49. Dutra, W. O., Rocha, M. O., and Teixeira, M. M.: The clinical immunology of human Chagas disease. Trends Parasitol. 21:581-587, 2005.
50. Easton, A. J., and Eglin, R. P.: The detection of coxsackievirus RNA in cardiac tissue by in situ hybridization. J. Gen. Virol. 69(Pt. 2):285-291, 1988.
51. Edwards, W. D., Holmes, D. R., Jr., and Reeder, G. S.: Diagnosis of active lymphocytic myocarditis by endomyocardial biopsy: Quantitative criteria for light microscopy. Mayo Clin. Proc. 57:419-425, 1982.
52. Eichenwald, H. F., and Shinefield, H. R.: Viral infections of the fetus and of the premature and newborn infant. Adv. Pediatr. 12:249-305, 1962.
53. Fairweather, D., Yusung, S., Frisancho, S., et al.: IL-12 receptor beta 1 and Toll-like receptor 4 increase IL-1 beta- and IL-18-associated myocarditis and coxsackievirus replication. J. Immunol. 170:4731-4737, 2003.
54. Fenoglio, J. J., Jr., Ursell, P. C., Kellogg, C. F., et al.: Diagnosis and classification of myocarditis by endomyocardial biopsy. N. Engl. J. Med. 308:12-18, 1983.
55. Fine, I., Brainerd, H., and Sokolow, M.: Myocarditis in acute infectious diseases: A clinical and electrocardiographic study. Circulation 2:859-871, 1950.
56. Frid, C., Bjarke, B., and Eriksson, M.: Myocarditis in children with inflammatory bowel disease. J. Pediatr. Gastroenterol. Nutr. 5:964-965, 1986.
57. Friedman, R. A., Kearney, D. L., Moak, J. P., et al.: Persistence of ventricular arrhythmia after resolution of occult myocarditis in children and young adults. J. Am. Coll. Cardiol. 24:780-783, 1994.
58. Fruhling, L., Korn, R., Lavillaureix, J., et al.: Chronic fibroelastic myoendocarditis of the newborn and the infant (fibroelastosis): New morphological, etiological and pathogenic data: Relation to certain cardiac abnormalities. Ann. Anat. Pathol. 7:227-303, 1962.
59. Fuse, K., Chan, G., Liu, Y., et al.: Myeloid differentiation factor-88 plays a crucial role in the pathogenesis of Coxsackievirus B3-induced myocarditis and influences type I interferon production. Circulation 112:2276-2285, 2005.
60. Gagliardi, M. G., Bevilacqua, M., Di Renzi, P., et al.: Usefulness of magnetic resonance imaging for diagnosis of acute myocarditis in infants and children, and comparison with endomyocardial biopsy. Am. J. Cardiol. 68:1089-1091, 1991.
61. Gatmaitan, B. G., Chason, J. L., and Lerner, A. M.: Augmentation of the virulence of murine coxsackie-virus B-3 myocardiopathy by exercise. J. Exp. Med. 131:1121-1136, 1970.
62. Gear, J. H., and Measroch, V.: South African Institute for Medical Research Annual Report for 1952. South African Institute for Medical Research 38-39, 1953.
63. Giles, T. D., and Gohd, R. S.: Respiratory syncytial virus and heart disease: A report of two cases. J. A. M. A. 236:1128-1130, 1976.
64. Goldfinger, D., Schreiber, W., and Wosika, P. H.: Permanent heart block following German measles. Am. Heart J. 2:320, 1947.
65. Golgher, D., and Gazzinelli, R. T.: Innate and acquired immunity in the pathogenesis of Chagas disease. Autoimmunity 37:399-409, 2004.
66. Gore, I., and Saphir, O.: Myocarditis: A classification of 1402 cases. Am. Heart J. 34:827, 1947.
67. Grasso, M., Arbustini, E., Silini, E., et al.: Search for Coxsackievirus B3 RNA in idiopathic dilated cardiomyopathy using gene amplification by polymerase chain reaction. Am. J. Cardiol. 69:658-664, 1992.
68. Gray, D. F., Morse, B. S., and Phillips, W. F.: Trichinosis with neurologic and cardiac involvement: Review of the literature and report of three cases. Ann. Intern. Med. 57:230-244, 1962.
69. Grist, N. R., and Bell, E. J.: Coxsackie viruses and the heart. Am. Heart J. 77:295-300, 1969.
70. Grist, N. R., and Bell, E. J.: A six-year study of coxsackievirus B infections in heart disease. J. Hyg. (London) 73:165-172, 1974.
71. Gutgesell, H. P., Paquet, M., Duff, D. F., et al.: Evaluation of left ventricular size and function by echocardiography: Results in normal children. Circulation 56:457-462, 1977.
72. Halsell, J. S., Riddle, J. R., Atwood, J. E., et al.: Myopericarditis following smallpox vaccination among vaccinia-naive US military personnel. J. A. M. A. 289:3283-3289, 2003.
73. Hastreiter, A. R., and Miller, R. A.: Management of primary endomyocardial disease: The myocarditis-endocardial fibroelastosis syndrome. Pediatr. Clin. North Am. 11:401-430, 1964.
74. Haynes, R. E., Cramblett, H. G., Hilty, M. D., et al.: ECHO virus type 3 infections in children: clinical and laboratory studies. J. Pediatr. 80:589-595, 1972.
75. Henson, D., and Mufson, M. A.: Myocarditis and pneumonitis with type 21 adenovirus infection: Association with fatal myocarditis and pneumonitis. Am. J. Dis. Child. 121:334-336, 1971.
76. Herskowitz, A., Ahmed-Ansari, A., Neumann, D. A., et al.: Induction of major histocompatibility complex antigens within the myocardium of patients with active myocarditis: A nonhistologic marker of myocarditis. J. Am. Coll. Cardiol. 15:624-632, 1990.
77. Hilton, D. A., Variend, S., and Pringle, J. H.: Demonstration of Coxsackie virus RNA in formalin-fixed tissue sections from childhood myocarditis cases by in situ hybridization and the polymerase chain reaction. J. Pathol. 170:45-51, 1993.
78. Hobbs, R. E., Pelegrin, D., Ratliff, N. B., et al.: Lymphocytic myocarditis and dilated cardiomyopathy: Treatment with immunosuppressive agents. Cleve. Clin. J. Med. 56:628-635, 1989.
79. Hodge, P. R., and Lawrence, J. R.: Two cases of myocarditis associated with phenylbutazone therapy. Med. J. Aust. 44:640-641, 1957.
80. Hoshino, T., Matsumori, A., Kawai, C., et al.: Electrocardiographic abnormalities in Syrian golden hamsters with coxsackievirus B1 myocarditis. Jpn. Circ. J. 46:1305-1312, 1982.
81. Hoyer, M. H., and Fischer, D. R.: Acute myocarditis simulating myocardial infarction in a child. Pediatrics 87:250-253, 1991.
82. Huber, S. A.: Autoimmunity in myocarditis: Relevance of animal models. Clin. Immunol. Immunopathol. 83:93-102, 1997.
83. Huber, S. A., Job, L. P., and Woodruff, J. F.: Lysis of infected myofibers by coxsackievirus B-3-immune T lymphocytes. Am. J. Pathol. 98:681-694, 1980.
84. Hudson, R. E.: The cardiomyopathies: Order from chaos. Am. J. Cardiol. 25:70-77, 1970.
85. Hutchins, G. M., and Vie, S. A.: The progression of interstitial myocarditis to idiopathic endocardial fibroelastosis. Am. J. Pathol. 66:483-496, 1972.
86. Jahn, C. L., and Cherry, J. D.: Mild neonatal illness associated with heavy enterovirus infection. N. Engl. J. Med. 274:394-395, 1966.
87. Jin, O., Sole, M. J., Butany, J. W., et al.: Detection of enterovirus RNA in myocardial biopsies from patients with myocarditis and cardiomyopathy using gene amplification by polymerase chain reaction. Circulation 82:8-16, 1990.
88. Johnson, J. L., and Lee, L. P.: Complete atrioventricular heart block secondary to acute myocarditis requiring intracardiac pacing. J. Pediatr. 78:312-316, 1971.
89. Joos, H. A., and Yu, P. N.: Electrocardiographic observations in poliomyelitis: Changes of the Q-T interval in 23 cases. Am. J. Dis. Child. 80:22-33, 1950.
90. Karjalainen, J., Nieminen, M. S., and Heikkila, J.: Influenza A1 myocarditis in conscripts. Acta Med. Scand. 207:27-30, 1980.
91. Kereiakes, D. J., and Parmley, W. W.: Myocarditis and cardiomyopathy. Am. Heart J. 108:1318-1326, 1984.
92. Kibrick, S., and Benirschke, K.: Severe generalized disease (encephalohepatomyocarditis) occurring in the newborn period and due to infection with Coxsackie virus, group B: Evidence of intrauterine infection with this agent. Pediatrics 22:857-875, 1958.
93. Kilbourne, E. D., Smart, K. M., and Pokorny, B. A.: Inhibition by cortisone of the synthesis and action of interferon. Nature 190:650-651, 1961.
94. Kilbourne, E. D., Wilson, C. B., and Perrier, D.: The induction of gross myocardial lesions by a Coxsackie (pleurodynia) virus and cortisone. J. Clin. Invest. 35:362-370, 1956.
95. Kirchhoff, L. V., Gam, A. A., Gusmao, R. A., et al.: Increased specificity of serodiagnosis of Chagas' disease by detection of antibody to the 72- and 90-kilodalton glycoproteins of *Trypanosoma cruzi*. J. Infect. Dis. 155:561-564, 1987.
96. Kirchhoff, L. V., Weiss, L. M., Wittner, M., et al.: Parasitic diseases of the heart. Front. Biosci. 9:706-723, 2004.
97. Kishimoto, C., Matsumori, A., Ohmae, M., et al.: Electrocardiographic findings in experimental myocarditis in DBA/2 mice: Complete atrioventricular block in the acute stage, low voltage of the QRS complex in the subacute stage and arrhythmias in the chronic stage. J. Am. Coll. Cardiol. 3:1461-1468, 1984.
98. Kishimoto, C., Takada, H., Kawamata, H., et al.: Immunoglobulin treatment prevents congestive heart failure in murine encephalomyocarditis viral myocarditis associated with reduction of inflammatory cytokines. J. Pharmacol. Exp. Ther. 299:645-651, 2001.
99. Kubota, T., Bounoutas, G. S., Miyagishima, M., et al.: Soluble tumor necrosis factor receptor abrogates myocardial inflammation but not hypertrophy in cytokine-induced cardiomyopathy. Circulation 101:2518-2525, 2000.
100. Kussy, J. C.: Fatal mumps myocarditis. Minn. Med. 57:285-286, 1974.
101. Leak, D., and Meghji, M.: Toxoplasmic infection in cardiac disease. Am. J. Cardiol. 43:841-849, 1979.
102. Lerner, A., Wilson, F. M., and Reyes, M. P.: Enteroviruses and the heart (with special emphasis on the probable role of coxsackieviruses, group B, types 1-5), I: Epidemiological and experimental studies. Mod. Concepts Cardiovasc. Dis. 44:7-10, 1975.
103. Lim, C. H., Toh, C. C., and Chia, B. L.: Stokes-Adams attacks due to acute nonspecific myocarditis. Am. Heart J. 38:123, 1949.
104. Lind, J., and Hulquist, G. T.: Isolated myocarditis in newborn and young infants. Am. Heart J. 38:123, 1949.

105. Liu, P., Aitken, K., Kong, Y. Y., et al.: The tyrosine kinase p56(lck) is essential in coxsackievirus B3-mediated heart disease. Nat. Med. *6*:429-434, 2000.

106. Liu, P. P., and Mason, J. W.: Advances in the understanding of myocarditis. Circulation *104*:1076-1082, 2001.

107. Logue, B. L., and Hanson, J. L.: Complete heart block in German measles. Am. Heart J. *30*:205, 1945.

108. Lozinski, G. M., Davis, G. G., Krous, H. F., et al.: Adenovirus myocarditis: Retrospective diagnosis by gene amplification from formalin-fixed, paraffin-embedded tissues. Hum. Pathol. *25*:831-834, 1994.

109. Luft, B. J., Billingham, M., and Remington, J. S.: Endomyocardial biopsy in the diagnosis of toxoplasmic myocarditis. Transplant. Proc. *18*:1871-1873, 1986.

110. Markowitz, S. M., Martinez, A. J., Duma, R. J, et al.: Myocarditis associated with primary amebic (Naegleria) meningoencephalitis. Am. J. Clin. Pathol. *62*:619-628, 1974.

111. Martin, A. B., Webber, S., Fricker, F. J., et al.: Acute myocarditis: Rapid diagnosis by PCR in children. Circulation *90*:330-339, 1994.

112. Martinelli, F. M., Sosa, E., Nishioka, S., et al.: Clinical and electrophysiologic features of syncope in chronic chagasic heart disease. J. Cardiovasc. Electrophysiol. *5*:563-570, 1994.

113. Mason, J. W., Billingham, M. E., and Ricci, D. R.: Treatment of acute inflammatory myocarditis assisted by endomyocardial biopsy. Am. J. Cardiol. *45*:1037-1044, 1980.

114. Mason, J. W., O'Connell, J. B., Herskowitz, A., et al.: A clinical trial of immunosuppressive therapy for myocarditis. The Myocarditis Treatment Trial Investigators. N. Engl. J. Med. *333*:269-275, 1995.

115. Matsumori, A.: Molecular and immune mechanisms in the pathogenesis of cardiomyopathy—role of viruses, cytokines, and nitric oxide. Jpn. Circ. J. *61*:275-291, 1997.

116. Matsumori, A., Igata, H., Ono, K., et al.: High doses of digitalis increase the myocardial production of proinflammatory cytokines and worsen myocardial injury in viral myocarditis: A possible mechanism of digitalis toxicity. Jpn. Circ. J. *63*:934-940, 1999.

117. Matsumori, A., Yamada, T., Suzuki, H., et al.: Increased circulating cytokines in patients with myocarditis and cardiomyopathy. Br. Heart J. *72*:561-566, 1994.

118. McNamara, D. M., Holubkov, R., Starling, R. C., et al.: Controlled trial of intravenous immune globulin in recent-onset dilated cardiomyopathy. Circulation *103*:2254-2259, 2001.

119. Miklozek, C. L., Crumpacker, C. S., Royal, H. D., et al.: Myocarditis presenting as acute myocardial infarction. Am. Heart J. *115*:768-776, 1988.

120. Miller, J. J., III, and French, J. W.: Myocarditis in juvenile rheumatoid arthritis. Am. J. Dis. Child. *131*:205-209, 1977.

121. Monrad, E. S., Matsumori, A., Murphy, J. C., et al.: Therapy with cyclosporine in experimental murine myocarditis with encephalomyocarditis virus. Circulation *73*:1058-1064, 1986.

122. Montoya, R., Dias, J. C., and Coura, J. R.: Chagas disease in a community in southeast Brazil, I: A serologic follow-up study on a vector controlled area. Rev. Inst. Med. Trop. Sao Paulo *45*:269-274, 2003.

123. Moore, C. M., Henry, J., Benzing, G., et al.: Varicella myocarditis. Am. J. Dis. Child. *118*:899-902, 1969.

124. Morris, S. A., Tanowitz, H. B., Wittner, M., et al.: Pathophysiological insights into the cardiomyopathy of Chagas' disease. Circulation *82*:1900-1909, 1990.

125. Mott, K. E., and Hagstrom, J. W.: The pathologic lesions of the cardiac autonomic nervous system in chronic Chagas myocarditis. Circulation *31*:273-286, 1965.

126. Mowat, N. A., Bennett, P. N., Finlayson, J. K., et al.: Myopericarditis complicating ulcerative colitis. Br. Heart J. *36*:724-727, 1974.

127. Muir, P.: Enteroviruses and heart disease. Br. J. Biomed. Sci. *50*:258-271, 1993.

128. Neches, W. H., Park, S. C., Lenox, C. C., et al.: Left atrial myxoma: Clinical presentation suggesting acute myocarditis. J. A. M. A. *229*:1906-1907, 1974.

129. Neumann, D. A., Burek, C. L., Baughman, K. L., et al.: Circulating heart-reactive antibodies in patients with myocarditis or cardiomyopathy. J. Am. Coll. Cardiol. *16*:839-846, 1990.

130. Ni, J., Bowles, N. E., Kim, Y. H., et al.: Viral infection of the myocardium in endocardial fibroelastosis: Molecular evidence for the role of mumps virus as an etiologic agent. Circulation *95*:133-139, 1997.

131. O'Connell, J. B., Henkin, R. E., Robinson, J. A., et al.: Gallium-67 imaging in patients with dilated cardiomyopathy and biopsy-proven myocarditis. Circulation *70*:58-62, 1984.

132. Okuni, M., and Takamiya, Y.: Primary myocardial disease in children, with special references to idiopathic myocarditis. Jpn. Circ. J. *35*:771-776, 1971.

133. Oliver, J. M., Sotillo, J. F., Dominguez, F. J., et al.: Two-dimensional echocardiographic features of echinococcosis of the heart and great blood vessels: Clinical and surgical implications. Circulation *78*:327-337, 1988.

134. Olsen, E. G.: The role of biopsy in the diagnosis of myocarditis. Herz *10*:21-26, 1985.

135. Opavsky, M. A., Penninger, J., Aitken, K., et al.: Susceptibility to myocarditis is dependent on the response of αβ T lymphocytes to coxsackieviral infection. Circ. Res. *85*:551-558, 1999.

136. Orinius, E., and Pernow, B.: Primary cardiomyopathy: A prospective clinical and physiological study. Acta Med. Scand. *192*:55-66, 1972.

137. Osama, S. M., Krishnamurti, S., and Gupta, D. N.: Incidence of myocarditis in varicella. Ind. Heart J. *31*:315-320, 1979.

138. Palacios-Pru, E., Carrasco, H., Scorza, C., et al.: Ultrastructural characteristics of different stages of human chagasic myocarditis. Am. J. Trop. Med. Hyg. *41*:29-40, 1989.

139. Paque, R. E., Gauntt, C. J., and Nealon, T. J.: Assessment of cell-mediated immunity against coxsackievirus B3-induced myocarditis in a primate model (*Papio papio*). Infect. Immun. *31*:470-479, 1981.

140. Paque, R. E., Straus, D. C., Nealon, T. J., et al.: Fractionation and immunologic assessment of KCl-extracted cardiac antigens in coxsackievirus B3 virus-induced myocarditis. J. Immunol. *123*:358-364, 1979.

141. Poltera, A. A., Cox, J. N., and Owor, R.: Pancarditis affecting the conducting system and all valves in human African trypanosomiasis. Br. Heart J. *38*:827-837, 1976.

142. Pomerance, A.: Classification of the secondary cardiomyopathies: The pathologist's view. Postgrad. Med. J. *48*:714-721, 1972.

143. Puljiz, I., Beus, A., Kuzman, I., et al.: Electrocardiographic changes and myocarditis in trichinellosis: A retrospective study of 154 patients. Ann. Trop. Med. Parasitol. *99*:403-411, 2005.

144. Rantakallio, P., Lapinleimu, K., and Mantyjarvi, R.: Coxsackie B 5 outbreak in a newborn nursery with 17 cases of serous meningitis. Scand. J. Infect. Dis. *2*:17-23, 1970.

145. Redline, R. W., Genest, D. R., and Tycko, B.: Detection of enteroviral infection in paraffin-embedded tissue by the RNA polymerase chain reaction technique. Am. J. Clin. Pathol. *96*:568-571, 1991.

146. Reef, S. E., and Cochi, S. L.: The evidence for the elimination of rubella and congenital rubella syndrome in the United States: A public health achievement. Clin. Infect. Dis. *43*(Suppl. 3):S123-S125, 2006.

147. Reilly, J. M., Cunnion, R. E., Anderson, D. W., et al.: Frequency of myocarditis, left ventricular dysfunction and ventricular tachycardia in the acquired immune deficiency syndrome. Am. J. Cardiol. *62*:789-793, 1988.

148. Rezkalla, S., Kloner, R. A., Khatib, G., et al.: Beneficial effects of captopril in acute coxsackievirus B3 murine myocarditis. Circulation *81*:1039-1046, 1990.

149. Rosenbaum, H. D., Nadas, A. S., and Neuhauser, E. B.: Primary myocardial disease in infancy and childhood. Am. J. Dis. Child. *86*:28-44, 1953.

150. Rosenberg, H. S., and McNamara, D. G.: Acute myocarditis in infancy and childhood. Prog. Cardiovasc. Dis. *7*:179-197, 1964.

151. Ross, L. J.: Electrocardiographic findings in measles. Am. J. Dis. Child. *83*:282-291, 1952.

152. Rossi, M. A., Ramos, S. G., and Bestetti, R. B.: Chagas' heart disease: Clinical-pathological correlation. Front. Biosci. *8*:e94-e109, 2003.

153. Sahn, D. J., Vaucher, Y., Williams, D. E., et al.: Echocardiographic detection of large left to right shunts and cardiomyopathies in infants and children. Am. J. Cardiol. *38*:73-79, 1976.

154. Sainani, G. S., Dekate, M. P., and Rao, C. P.: Heart disease caused by Coxsackie virus B infection. Br. Heart J. *37*:819-823, 1975.

155. Sakakibara, S., and Konno, S.: Endomyocardial biopsy. Jpn. Heart J. *3*:537-543, 1962.

156. Saphir, O., and Field, M.: Complications of myocarditis in children. J. Pediatr. *45*:457-463, 1954.

157. Saphir, O., and Simon, W. A.: Myocarditis in children. Am. J. Dis. Child. *67*:294-312, 1944.

158. Satoh, M., Tamura, G., Segawa, I., et al.: Expression of cytokine genes and presence of enteroviral genomic RNA in endomyocardial biopsy tissues of myocarditis and dilated cardiomyopathy. Virchows Arch. *427*:503-509, 1996.

159. Schieken, R. M., and Myers, M. G.: Complete heart block in viral myocarditis. J. Pediatr. *87*:831-832, 1975.

160. Schmidt, N. J., Magoffin, R. L., and Lennette, E. H.: Association of group B coxsackie viruses with cases of pericarditis, myocarditis, or pleurodynia by demonstration of immunoglobulin M antibody. Infect. Immun. *8*:341-348, 1973.

161. Schowengerdt, K. O., Ni, J., Denfield, S. W., et al.: Diagnosis, surveillance, and epidemiologic evaluation of viral infections in pediatric cardiac transplant recipients with the use of the polymerase chain reaction. J. Heart Lung Transplant. *15*:111-123, 1996.

162. Scott, L. P., III, Gutelius, M. F., and Parrott, R. H.: Children with acute respiratory tract infections: An electrocardiographic survey. Am. J. Dis. Child. *119*:111-113, 1970.

163. Spencer, H. C., Allain, D. S., Sulzer, A. J., and Collins, W. E.: Evaluation of the micro enzyme-linked immunosorbent assay for antibodies to *Trypanosoma cruzi*. Am. J. Trop. Med. Hyg. *29*:179-182, 1980.

164. Spencer, M. J., Cherry, J. D., Adams, F. H., et al.: Letter: Supraventricular tachycardia in an infant associated with a rhinoviral infection. J. Pediatr. *86*:811-812, 1975.

165. Spink, W. W.: Cardiovascular complications of trichinosis. Arch. Intern. Med. *56*:238-245, 1935.

166. Sprague, W. W.: The effects of malaria on the heart. Am. Heart J. *31*:426-430, 1946.

167. Starc, T. J., Lipshultz, S. E., Easley, K. A., et al.: Incidence of cardiac abnormalities in children with human immunodeficiency virus infection: The prospective P2C2 HIV study. J. Pediatr. *141*:327-334, 2002.

168. Strain, J. E., Grose, R. M., Factor, S. M., et al.: Results of endomyocardial biopsy in patients with spontaneous ventricular tachycardia but without apparent structural heart disease. Circulation *68*:1171-1181, 1983.

169. Sugrue, D. D., Holmes, D. R., Jr., Gersh, B. J., et al.: Cardiac histologic findings in patients with life-threatening ventricular arrhythmias of unknown origin. J. Am. Coll. Cardiol. *4*:952-957, 1984.

170. Tahernia, A. C.: Electrocardiographic abnormalities and serum transaminase levels in diphtheritic myocarditis. J. Pediatr. 75:1008-1014, 1969.

171. Take, M., Sekiguchi, M., Hiroe, M., et al.: Long-term follow-up of electro-cardiographic findings in patients with acute myocarditis proven by endomyo-cardial biopsy. Jpn. Circ. J. 46:1227-1234, 1982.

172. Tarleton, R. L., Zhang, L., and Downs, M. O.: "Autoimmune rejection" of neonatal heart transplants in experimental Chagas disease is a parasite-specific response to infected host tissue. Proc. Natl. Acad. Sci. U. S. A. 94:3932-3937, 1997.

173. Taylor, L. A., Carthy, C. M., Yang, D. C., et al.: Host gene regulation during coxsackievirus B3 infection in mice—assessment by microarrays. Circ. Res. 87:328-334, 2000.

174. Theologides, A., and Kennedy, B. J.: Toxoplasmic myocarditis and pericardi-tis. Am. J. Med. 47:169-174, 1969.

175. Thisyakorn, U., Wongvanich, J., and Kumpeng, V.: Failure of corticosteroid therapy to prevent diphtheritic myocarditis or neuritis. Pediatr. Infect. Dis. J. 3:126-128, 1984.

176. Tiula, E., and Leinikki, P.: Fatal cytomegalovirus infection in a previously healthy boy with myocarditis and consumption coagulopathy as presenting signs. Scand. J. Infect. Dis. 4:57-60, 1972.

177. Tomioka, N., Kishimoto, C., Matsumori, A., et al.: Effects of prednisolone on acute viral myocarditis in mice. J. Am. Coll. Cardiol. 7:868-872, 1986.

178. Towbin, J. A., Griffin, L. D., Martin, A. B., et al.: Intrauterine adenoviral myocarditis presenting as nonimmune hydrops fetalis: Diagnosis by polym-erase chain reaction. Pediatr. Infect. Dis. J. 13:144-150, 1994.

179. Toxigenic Corynebacterium diphtheriae—Northern Plains Indian Community, August-October 1996. M. M. W. R. Morb. Mortal. Wkly. Rep. 46:506-510, 1997.

180. Unverferth, D. V., Fetters, K. K., and Uretsky, B.: Right versus left heart biopsies: Different information. Circulation 70(Suppl. II):402, 1984.

181. Vargo, T. A., Singer, D. B., Gillette, P. C., et al.: Myocarditis due to visceral larva migrans. J. Pediatr. 90:322-323, 1977.

182. Vignola, P. A., Aonuma, K., Swaye, P. S., et al.: Lymphocytic myocarditis presenting as unexplained ventricular arrhythmias: Diagnosis with endomyo-cardial biopsy and response to immunosuppression. J. Am. Coll. Cardiol. 4:812-819, 1984.

183. Wada, H., Saito, K., Kanda, T., et al.: Tumor necrosis factor-alpha (TNF-alpha) plays a protective role in acute viral myocarditis in mice: A study using mice lacking TNF-alpha. Circulation 103:743-749, 2001.

184. Walker, D. H., Paletta, C. E., and Cain, B. G.: Pathogenesis of myocarditis in Rocky Mountain spotted fever. Arch. Pathol. Lab. Med. 104:171-174, 1980.

185. Weber, M. W., Baldwin, J. S., and Hall, J. W.: Acute isolated myocarditis: Review of the literature and report of a case in a 10-year-old child. Pediatrics 6:829-836, 1949.

186. Weiss, L. M., Liu, X. F., Chang, K. L., et al.: Detection of enteroviral RNA in idiopathic dilated cardiomyopathy and other human cardiac tissues. J. Clin. Invest. 90:156-159, 1992.

187. Weiss, L. M., Movahed, L. A., Berry, G. J., et al.: In situ hybridization studies for viral nucleic acids in heart and lung allograft biopsies. Am. J. Clin. Pathol. 93:675-679, 1990.

188. Weiss, L. M., Movahed, L. A., Billingham, M. E., et al.: Detection of Coxsackievirus B3 RNA in myocardial tissues by the polymerase chain reac-tion. Am. J. Pathol. 138:497-503, 1991.

189. Well, A. H., and Sax, S. G.: Isolated myocarditis, probably of sulfonamide origin. Am. Heart J. 30:522, 1945.

190. Williams, H., O'Reilly, R. N., and Williams, A.: Fourteen cases of idiopathic myocarditis in infants and children. Arch. Dis. Child. 28:271-283, 1953.

191. Woodruff, J. F.: Viral myocarditis: A review. Am. J. Pathol. 101:425-484, 1980.

192. Woodruff, J. F., and Woodruff, J. J.: Involvement of T lymphocytes in the pathogenesis of coxsackie virus B3 heart disease. J. Immunol. 113:1726-1734, 1974.

193. Wright, H. T., Jr., and Miller, A.: Fatal infection in a newborn infant due to herpes simplex virus: Report of a case diagnosed before death. J. Pediatr. 67:130-132, 1965.

194. Xiong, D., Lee, G. H., Badorff, C., et al.: Dystrophin deficiency markedly increases enterovirus-induced cardiomyopathy: A genetic predisposition to viral heart disease. Nat. Med. 8:872-877, 2002.

195. Yamada, T., Matsumori, A., and Sasayama, S.: Therapeutic effect of anti-tumor necrosis factor-alpha antibody on the murine model of viral myocarditis induced by encephalomyocarditis virus. Circulation 89:846-851, 1994.

196. Yamagata, Y., and Nakagawa, J.: Control of Chagas disease. Adv. Parasitol. 61:129-165, 2006.

197. Young, E. J., Killam, A. P., and Greene, J. F., Jr.: Disseminated herpesvirus infection: Association with primary genital herpes in pregnancy. J. A. M. A. 235:2731-2733, 1976.

198. Zaragoza, C., Ocampo, C., Saura, M., et al.: The role of inducible nitric oxide synthase in the host response to Coxsackievirus myocarditis. Proc. Natl. Acad. Sci. U. S. A. 95:2469-2474, 1998.

199. Zwelzer, W. M.: Infantile toxoplasmosis. Arch. Pathol. 38:1-19, 1944.

CHAPTER 35

ACUTE RHEUMATIC FEVER

Diana R. Lennon

Acute rheumatic fever is an inflammatory disease of the heart, joints, central nervous system, and subcutaneous tissues that develops after a nasopharyngeal infection by one of the group A beta-hemolytic streptococci. The pathogenesis of this disease, a clinical syndrome without a specific diagnostic test, remains an enigma, and specific treatment is unavailable. Prevention of initial and recurrent attacks is possible, however, with penicillin prophylaxis. Rheumatic fever is especially important because of the heart disease that often ensues, and such disease may lead to chronic progressive damage and premature death. As succinctly stated by Lasegue many years ago, "Rheumatic fever licks the joints and bites the heart"[186]—a statement that holds true today.

The unexpected upsurge in this disease in the United States in the late 1980s and 1990s and reports of increasing numbers of invasive group A streptococcal infections have renewed interest in group A streptococci and their abilities. In addition, recogni-tion that rheumatic fever is the leading cause of acquired heart disease in children and young adults worldwide has led to action.[147]

EPIDEMIOLOGY

The overall incidence and severity of acute rheumatic fever have decreased in recent years in developed Western countries and in prosperous countries of Asia.[2] Reliable morbidity data on the occurrence of acute rheumatic fever in total populations are lacking because studies often consider only a segment of a popu-lation. The trend seems clear, however. Some of the best long-term data come from Denmark, where rheumatic fever has been a reportable disease for many years[201]; a steady decline has been occurring since 1900, except for a peak during World War II (Fig. 35–1). In the United States, rheumatic fever is not a report-able disease, but mortality rates (Fig. 35–2) and hospital discharge rates (Fig. 35–3 and Table 35–1) have shown a steady decline. Although this decline was already under way, it seems to have been accelerated by the introduction of penicillin.[126]

The dramatic decline in the incidence of rheumatic fever began in the United States in the late 1940s (see Fig. 35–2). During the late 1950s, the 1960s, and the early 1970s, studies in the United States showed annual rates of 13.5 to 62.5 first attacks per 100,000 children 5 to 14 years of age; however, these studies are not strictly comparable in design.[35,52,82,150,170,176] Some of them were conducted in low-income urban areas, locations in which the incidence of rheumatic fever was thought to be higher. Secondary prevention of rheumatic fever with penicillin prophylaxis to protect against recurrent attacks probably became widespread in the 1960s. Denny and colleagues[64] showed the possibility of pre-venting initial attacks with injectable penicillin in 1950 in military camps. Similar conclusive controlled studies were not repeated in the general or pediatric populations or with oral penicillin.

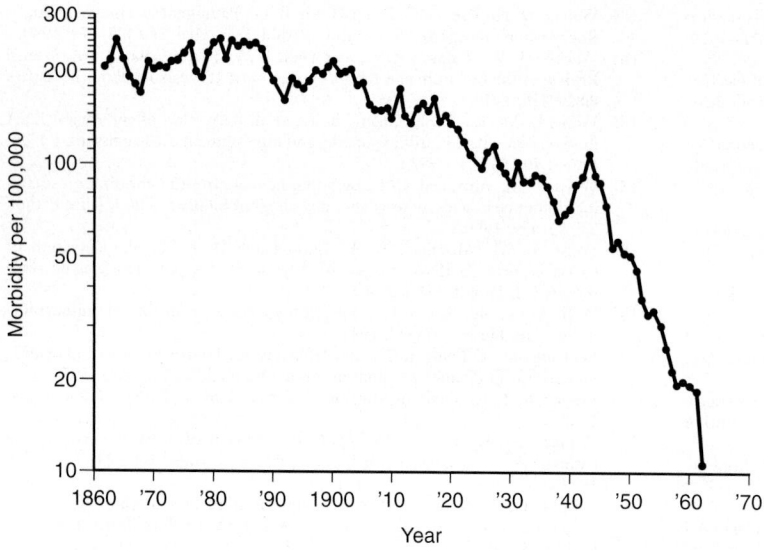

Figure 35–1 Reported annual incidence of acute rheumatic fever in Denmark, 1862 to 1962. (*Adapted from Public Health Board of Denmark: Reported rheumatic fever incidence in Denmark, 1862-1962. In Vendsborg, P., Fauerholdt, L., and Olsen, K. H.: Decreasing incidence of a history of acute rheumatic fever in chronic rheumatic heart disease. Cardiologica 53:332-340, 1968. Used with permission of S. Karger A. G., Basel.*)

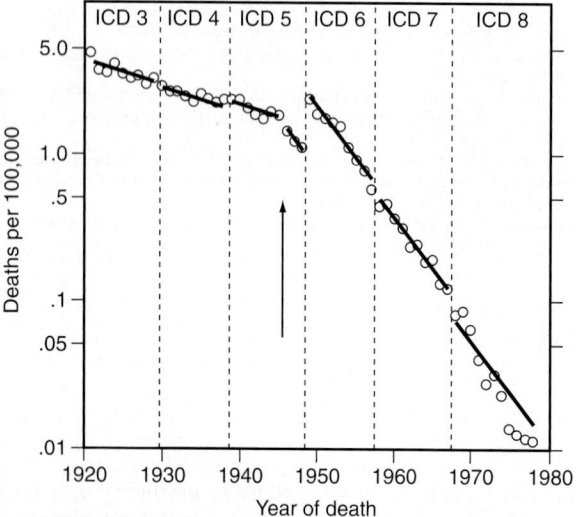

Figure 35–2 U.S. national mortality rates from rheumatic fever in individuals 5 to 19 years old, 1921 through 1978. Values are age-adjusted to the 1950 U.S. population. Trend lines are fitted for each era (1921 through 1945 and 1946 through 1978) separately and take International Classification of Diseases (ICD) revisions into account. The *arrow* separates the two eras. (*From Massell, B. F., Chute, C. G., Walker, A. M., et al.: Penicillin and the marked decrease in morbidity and mortality from rheumatic fever in the United States. N. Engl. J. Med. 318:280-286, 1988.*)

The most compelling evidence that appropriate medical intervention helps reduce the number of initial attacks of rheumatic fever comes from a study by Gordis[82] of health care availability in an inner-city Baltimore population at risk. The rate of acute rheumatic fever was reduced by 60 percent over the course of a decade in only the census tracts receiving a comprehensive care program, with that reduction occurring only in patients with an identifiable preceding clinical respiratory infection. A similar trend with small numbers of patients was seen for the Navajo and Papago Native American populations in school-based intervention programs[14,52] and in an Alaskan program.[33] Other school-based interventions[155] have reduced streptococcal prevalence rates but have not gone the necessary further step to show a

reduction in rheumatic fever morbidity in a controlled, carefully demarcated population.

An unexplained high incidence of acute rheumatic fever persists in Hawaii, especially in Polynesian and part-Polynesian children.[46] Similarly, rates are inexplicably higher in larger populations of Polynesian children in New Zealand.[113] In some areas of the continental United States, the rate of endemic rheumatic fever continues to exceed that of the general population in some children traditionally considered to be at risk (urban African-Americans), although not in others (recent Hispanic immigrants).[70] In contrast, in a hospital-based study in another urban area, Hispanic children, reflecting the pediatric population being served, were the most affected.[88]

Since the beginning of 1985, the number of patients with acute rheumatic fever in several centers on the U.S. mainland has increased.* Although these numbers are not large, they represent a definite increase in the outbreak areas (Table 35-2).[193] The resurgence in Utah since 1985 has led to more than 600 cases.[130] Nationally, the number of diagnoses of acute rheumatic fever may have continued to decline gradually from 1984 through 1990.[193] The populations (aside from clusters in military populations)[10,204] generally do not seem to be those considered to have been at risk in the past: Most patients are white and middle class and live in suburban or rural communities with ready access to medical care. In the Utah and Tennessee outbreaks,[200,210] the families were larger than the state average. The military outbreaks[10,205] were the first in 2 decades in U.S. military personnel. Factors other than the widespread use of antibiotics and improved availability of health care may be important. Overcrowded living circumstances long have been considered to be a risk factor,[153] although this hypothesis was not substantiated as an important risk factor by conditional logistic regression in a modern-day study.[202]

The disquieting feature in these more recent outbreaks was the severity of the illness, especially in the Salt Lake City, Utah, outbreak: 72 percent of patients had clinical carditis (Table 35-3), 19 percent had severe carditis with or without congestive heart failure, and three patients required mitral valve replacement. Because this report was from a cardiology center, however, it may reflect a referral bias. Earlier U.S. reports documented clinical carditis in initial attacks of rheumatic fever in 40 to 51 percent

---

*See references 27, 51, 66, 93, 109, 138, 199, 200, 204, 205, 220.

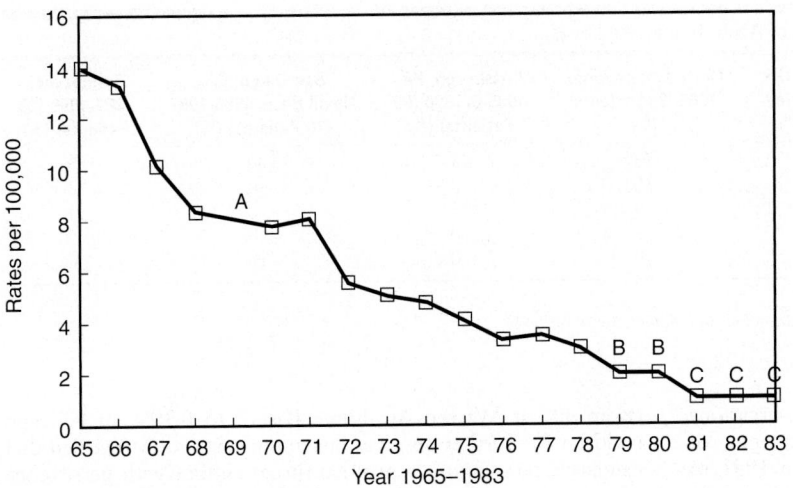

Figure 35-3 Annual rates (per 100,000) of discharge of patients with rheumatic fever from short-stay nonfederal hospitals in the United States, 1965 to 1983. *(From National Hospital Discharge Survey, NCHS. Adapted from Gordis, L.: The virtual disappearance of rheumatic fever in the United States: Lessons in the rise and fall of disease. Circulation 72:1155-1162, 1985.)*

A–Data not available
B–Average for 1979–80
C–Average for 1981–83

TABLE 35-1   Reported Incidence of Acute Rheumatic Fever in Studies in the United States, 1970 to 1981

Location	Years of Study	Rate/100,000	Age Range (yr)
Fairfax, VA	1970-1980	1.14	0-18
Rhode Island	1976-1980	0.23	5-17
Memphis, TN	1977-1981	1.88	5-17
Baltimore, MD	1977-1981	0.5	5-19
San Fernando, CA	1971-1980	0.63	5-17

Adapted from Veasy, L. G., Wiedmeier, S. E., Orsmond, G. S., et al.: Resurgence of acute rheumatic fever in the intermountain area of the U.S. N. Engl. J. Med. 316:421-427, 1987; and Markowitz M., and Kaplan, E. L.: Reappearance of rheumatic fever. Adv. Pediatr. 36:44, 1989.

TABLE 35-2   Reported Outbreaks of Acute Rheumatic Fever in the United States: Selected Epidemiologic Features

	Salt Lake City, UT[130,131]	Columbus, OH[60]	Akron, OH[32]	Pittsburgh, PA[132,144]	San Diego, CA[126]	Tennessee[139]*
Time	1985-1992	6/84-9/86	1986	1987-6/90	12/86-7/87	1/87-7/88
No. cases	274	40	23	60	50	26
White (%)	93	80	96	97	50	80
Family income	80% middle	73% middle	$20,000-$40,000	3 of 17 on assistance[132]	NA	$18,000
Suburban-rural residents	Most[130]	85%	Many	75%[137]	NA	20%
History of sore throat (n†)	77 (46)	22 (NA)	18 (NA)	4/17 (3/17)[132]; 28/43 (11/43)[144‡]	6 (3)	15 (7)
Family history of rheumatic fever (%)	NA	5	16	64[132]	NA	NA
Recurrences	27	1	0	2	1	0
M types of group A streptococci isolated from						
Patients	1 × M-1; 1 × M-5	NA	M-1, M-5, M-18	NA	§	Mucoid M-18/T-1; mucoid nontypeable
Families	3 × M-3; 1 × M-1; 1 × M-18; 1 × M-78	NA	M-6	NA	NA	NA
Community	9 × M-18 (8/9 mucoid); 1 × M-4, M-5, M-6, M-9, M-11, M-12; 6 nontypeable	Mucoid M-18	NA	NA	NA	Mucoid M-18

NA, not available.
*Family size greater than the state average.
†Number who sought treatment.
‡Respiratory illness.
§San Diego: five of seven available sera positive for antibodies to M-18; three of seven, positive for M-1 antibodies; two of seven, positive for M-5 and M-6 antibodies; and one of seven, positive for M-24 antibodies.
Adapted from Veasy, L. G., Wiedmeier, S. E., Orsmond, G. S., et al.: Resurgence of acute rheumatic fever in the intermountain area of the U.S. N. Engl. J. Med. 316:421-427, 1987; and Markowitz, M., and Kaplan, E. L.: Reappearance of rheumatic fever. Adv. Pediatr. 36:39-68, 1989.

TABLE 35-3 Clinical Manifestations in Four Outbreaks of Acute Rheumatic Fever

Manifestation	Salt Lake City, UT, 1985-1992 (274 Patients) (%)	Columbus, OH, 1984-1986 (40 Patients) (%)	Northeastern Ohio, 1986 (23 Patients) (%)	Pittsburgh, PA, 1985-6/1990 (60 Patients) (%)	San Diego, CA, Naval Base, 1986-1987 (10 Patients) (%)	Tennessee, 1987-1988 (26 Patients) (%)
Arthritis	36	62	78	43	100	58
Carditis	68*	50	30	52	30	73
Chorea	37	17	9	37	0	31
Erythema marginatum	4	12	1	0	0	4
Subcutaneous nodules	3	0	0	0	10	0

85 percent with Doppler ultrasound examination.
Adapted from Markowitz, M., and Kaplan, E. L.: Reappearance of rheumatic fever. Adv. Pediatr. 36:39-68, 1989.

of patients (1951 through 1965).[125] Longitudinal observations at the same institution suggest a decreasing frequency of clinical carditis (73% from 1921 to 1930; 51% from 1951 to 1960).[32,131]

Rheumatic fever in its milder form with arthritis is the sole major manifestation without a serologic search for other causes of polyarthritis, or echocardiography may cause difficulty in making a diagnosis, and the patient may not be admitted to the hospital, which could affect estimates of rates of carditis in studies that are not population-based. With the use of Doppler echocardiography, carditis rates in the Utah patients increased to 91 percent (see Table 35-3). The duration of secondary penicillin prophylaxis and endocarditis prophylaxis is an important consideration for patients with nonclinical carditis. The place of echocardiography in the diagnosis and management of rheumatic fever is evolving (see section on laboratory findings).

A more recent assessment of hospitalized acute rheumatic fever disease in the United States in children younger than 21 years of age found a low rate of 14.8/100,000 hospitalized children (503 cases).[138] The prevalence of rheumatic heart disease, which represents the result of many years of exposure to the risks of acquiring acute rheumatic fever, seems to have declined in the United States over the course of many years.[143]

Many different racial and ethnic groups have been deemed unusually susceptible to rheumatic fever. They usually have been minority groups within a given area who are of lower socioeconomic status than the general population (e.g., Malays in Singapore, Arabs in Israel, Bantus in South Africa, Maori in New Zealand, African-Americans in the United States, aborigines in Australia).[2,39,124] In the United States, when differences in socioeconomic status or degree of crowding were taken into account,[85] the differences in the incidence of rheumatic fever,[84] prevalence of rheumatic heart disease,[143] and mortality from acute rheumatic fever and rheumatic heart disease generally declined or disappeared,[162] at least in the population studied. Rates in African-Americans were slow to decline, however. Rates became very low in the 1970s, at least in some areas, but cases persisted in other areas.[70,108]

Gordis and associates[83] caution that some other socioeconomically determined factor closely paralleling crowding could be the actual determinant of rheumatic fever. Most authorities agree that the reduction in the incidence and severity of rheumatic fever that has been noted in the United States and Western Europe might be due partly to a higher standard of living and less crowding. In a case-control study in the former Yugoslavia, home dampness, change of place of residence during the last 5 years, low maternal education, body weight below normal, frequent sore throats, and a positive family history of rheumatic fever were found to be significant risk factors.[202]

A relationship between group A streptococcal throat infection and rheumatic fever was recognized following observations of the latter occurring after outbreaks of scarlet fever.[150] The attack rate noted after group A streptococcal throat infection varied widely

(from 3% at Warren Air Force Base[165] to 0.39% in Chicago children[178]). Further observations in the latter study revealed that exudative pharyngitis, a positive throat culture with persistence of group A streptococci beyond 21 days, and the development of significant antibody (antistreptolysin O [ASO]) responses were associated with a higher attack rate that approached 3 percent in the children studied.

Rheumatic fever, similar to streptococcal infection, occurs most commonly in children 5 to 15 years of age. First attacks of rheumatic fever rarely occur in children younger than 3 years of age or in adults older than 40 years because of the relative infrequency of streptococcal infection at these ages and perhaps other factors.

The incidence of acute rheumatic fever is highest in the spring and winter months in temperate zones and coincides with the seasonal variation in streptococcal pharyngitis. This incidence may be related to the greater tendency for spread of streptococcal infection by closer contact during the colder and damper months,[113,186,202] at least in some climates. In other climates, a seasonal peak for acute rheumatic fever is less pronounced.[31]

PATHOGENESIS

Evidence points toward acute rheumatic fever being preceded by a group A streptococcal upper respiratory tract infection. The events that occur after such infection and that culminate in rheumatic fever are poorly defined, suggesting a complex interaction of numerous factors. With the resurgence of interest in this disease after the outbreaks in the 1980s, laboratory data collected with the use of modern technologies have led to some new insights.[179,180] Pathogenesis involves the host, the environment (see section on epidemiology), and group A streptococci, individually and collectively.

So-called rheumatogenic strains of group A streptococci have been the subject of much discussion, more recently in relation to the latest focal upsurges in rheumatic fever.[25,29,97] Because no factor has been described or isolated, however, such strains remain a hypothesis. To date, rheumatic fever has been shown to occur only after nasopharyngeal infection,[206] although debate and research continue.[55,101] Why the site of infection seems to predispose individuals to the development of rheumatic fever remains an enigma, perhaps related to skin lipids.[100] Acute glomerulonephritis develops after skin or throat infections with a nephritogenic type of group A streptococci (e.g., M-49, M-12).[206]

Certain streptococcal M protein serotypes are implicated strongly and repetitively in epidemics of acute rheumatic fever. Serotypes M-3, M-5, M-14, M-18, and M-24 have been reported more than once in outbreaks, and M-1, M-6, M-19, M-27, and M-29 have been reported once only.[24] Distinct nucleotide sequences that determine different gene subfamilies encoding the M or M-like protein antigenic domain ("emm gene") may be the cause of these variations in streptococcal rheumatogenic potential, depending on the site of infection.[23] Other equally prevalent M types rarely, if ever, have been associated with epidemics of the disease[24] or have failed to cause recurrences in susceptible patients.[28] The current resurgence lends limited support for this concept: No predominance of a single serotype within a specific geographic zone was identified in any of the published outbreaks (Table 35-4; see Table 35-2). Specific M types and their production of mucoidal colonies (see Table 35-4), considered to be related to the amount of M protein and virulence,[207] may be more relevant to epidemic than to endemic rheumatic fever.

In Auckland, New Zealand, an average of 45 new cases of acute rheumatic fever occur annually in children (annual age-specific rate of 20/100,000/yr). Nine years (1984 to 1992) of surveillance of group A streptococcal isolates from hospitalized pediatric patients (one centralized children's facility for 8 of the 9 years in question) yielded 2410 isolates. Only 3 of 38 throat isolates (32 from well-documented cases of rheumatic fever, 6 from siblings) were strains described as possibly rheumatogenic (one each of M-1, M-3, and M-6).[129] None was described as mucoidal.[129] In that series, M types 6, 53, 55, and 66 (and NZ 1437, now known as M-89, when sibling isolates were included as cases) were statistically more likely to be associated with a case of acute rheumatic fever. Both streptococcal collections[97,129] (see Table 35-4) are limited samples and may not be representative. In addition, as in most series, group A streptococcal isolates are isolated from a few cases and are not supported by streptococcal or type-specific antibody data.

Strain selectivity is a further consideration. No documented evidence has shown that all members of an M type may be equally able to elicit acute rheumatic fever. Some streptococci from a particular serotype may be associated with acute rheumatic fever and acute poststreptococcal glomerulonephritis, although the two sequelae rarely occur simultaneously.[120,128,129] M types have been shown to be composed of genetically diverse streptococci, not all of which may be established within a community.[128] Genetic analysis of serotype M18 from acute rheumatic fever cases in Utah separated by 12 years showed strains nearly genetically identical.[179] The M type denotes possibly nothing more than

a shared type-specific marker, with the property of rheumatogenicity as yet remaining elusive. Streptococcal strains that are opacity factor–negative (a lipoprotein lipase) are unlikely to be rheumatogenic, according to some investigators (see Table 35-4).[97,210] This finding does not hold up in all geographic areas.[129] Surveillance of group A streptococci in different geographic zones must be encouraged to guide vaccine development.

Although current evidence strongly implicates an immunologic mechanism in the pathophysiology of rheumatic fever, the details of how the disease develops are unclear.[26,53,130,184] Evidence to date strongly suggests an abnormal cell-mediated and humoral immune response to cell membrane streptococcal antigens, which, because of molecular mimicry of human tissues, may result in continued damage to the cardiovascular and nervous systems.[36,184] The findings of circulating immune complexes in most patients[54] and the deposition of C3 and immunoglobulin in the myocardium of patients dying of acute rheumatic fever support an abnormal immune response in rheumatic fever.[102]

M proteins from some rheumatogenic group A streptococcal types share antigenic determinants with myosin, with the sarcolemma of cardiac muscle,[60,61] and with antigens of articular cartilage and synovium.[16] The immune response to streptococci may mistake the host antigens as foreign and result in tissue damage. Other streptococcal antigens, such as the group A carbohydrate component, are candidates for mistaken cross-reaction with a glycoprotein in human heart valves.[81] Group A streptococci have components that can amplify or down-regulate the immune response.[36] The mechanisms for molecular mimicry leading to central nervous system dysfunction are less defined.[130]

The site of the initial streptococcal infection may be important—lymphatic channels have been shown between the tonsils and the heart.[36] Unusual compartmentalization of rheumatic antigen–positive non–T cells has been shown in patients with acute rheumatic fever, with no positive cells detected in rheumatic tonsils but increased numbers in peripheral blood.[86]

Cell-mediated immunity to streptococcal antigens also is enhanced in patients with rheumatic fever.[184] The lymphocytic infiltrate of heart valves was found to be composed predominantly of CD4+ helper cells.[163] Increased expression of HLA-DR on fibroblasts, which can present antigens to CD4+ lymphocytes (cytotoxic/suppressor T cells), has been observed on the heart valves of patients with acute carditis.[66] The cytotoxicity induced in normal human helper and suppressor cells in vitro by purified protein from a type M-5 group A streptococcal organism has been shown to destroy several human cell types, including cultured myocardial cells.[62] T-cell subset study results are conflicting,[141,184] but production of interleukins is reported to be enhanced.[141,142,221] The role of M protein and streptococcal pyrogenic exotoxins as superantigens is being explored and perhaps might explain the exaggeration of the streptococcal immune response.[127,195]

The genetic background of the human host seems to influence susceptibility to rheumatic fever. Aggregation of rheumatic fever cases in families has been recognized for some time.[156] Low concordance for inheritance has been reported in monozygotic twins,[192] although affected siblings have significant concordance for arthritis, residual rheumatic heart disease, and chorea.[181] Patarroyo and associates[149] found that the B lymphocytes of patients with rheumatic fever have a specific marker (883 alloantigen) associated with host rheumatic susceptibility.[218,219] It seems to transcend ethnicity,[90,149] although studies in India were less supportive and may be similar to an immune response gene.[184] This work has been extended with the use of monoclonal antibodies to family members of patients with rheumatic fever.[69,168] Class I HLA molecules have not been associated with acute rheumatic fever. Many studies in different populations have shown an association with HLA-DR, but without a single HLA marker for susceptibility.[184] Genetic factors alone seem highly

TABLE 35-4 Group A Streptococci Isolated from Patients with Rheumatic Fever and from Their Siblings (1986 to May 1988)

Serotype	No. of Cases	No. of Siblings	No. of Total	No. (%) Mucoidal
OF-Negative				
M-1, T-1	6	2	8	7 (88)
M-3, T-3	3	6	9	1 (11)
M-18, T-18	6	2	8	7 (88)
M-5, T-5/27/44	1	3	4	1 (25)
M-6, T-6	3	0	3	2 (67)
M-41, T-13	1	0	1	0 (0)
Subtotal	20	13	33	18 (55)
OF-Positive				
OF-75, T-25	2	0	2	0 (0)
OF-77, T-13	2	0	2	0 (0)
OF-78, T-11	0	2	2	0 (0)
OF-48, T-28	1	0	1	1 (100)
M-2, T-2	1	0	1	0 (0)
M-4, T-4	1	0	1	0 (0)
Subtotal	7	2	9	1 (11)
Total	27	15	42	19 (45)

OF, opacity factor.
From Kaplan, E. L., Johnson, D. R., and Cleary, P. P.: Group A streptococcal serotypes isolated from patients and sibling contacts during the resurgence of rheumatic fever in the U.S. in the mid-1980s. J. Infect. Dis. 159:101-103, 1989.

unlikely to be responsible for susceptibility to rheumatic fever.[126] No predictive marker for susceptibility to rheumatic fever has been defined.

VACCINE DEVELOPMENT

Immunity to group A streptococci and to rheumatic fever is thought to depend largely on antibodies to M protein, a major virulence determinant; such antibodies can opsonize the bacteria in the presence of neutrophils.[107b] Immunity was thought to be strain-specific and to depend on antibodies to the variable sero-type-specific regions of the protein, and earliest vaccine development has followed this pathway.[19] Two early landmark studies showed that vaccines containing purified M protein evoked protective immune response in humans.[20,159] Antibodies against the variable amino-terminal end of the M protein opsonize streptococci in a type-specific manner, but the results of experiments in animals suggest that the conserved carboxyl-terminal end also may be an immune target. Some human evidence suggests that this conserved epitope acts as a subunit vaccine.[160] Complexities in this area include the risk of inducing cross-reacting antibodies that could injure rather than protect.[15,133] Separation of the peptide fragments of M proteins (epitopes) that evoke type-specific and not cross-reacting antibodies is an important step.[34,54]

With more than 120 different defined serotypes of group A streptococci, vaccine development[29,31a] falls into two broad approaches: vaccines based on common protective antigens of group A streptococci and multivalent vaccines based on type-specific N-terminal regions of the M protein. A 26-valent vaccine with components guided by North American surveillance of acute rheumatic fever, invasive infections, and pharyngitis has been shown to be safe and immunogenic in adults.[137] This vaccine includes 80 to 90 percent of important serotypes in North America, and epidemiologic studies indicate that vaccine coverage may be incomplete in other areas such as in Asia[161] or in New Zealand.[129] Information for serotype prevalence in many areas of high endemicity of acute rheumatic fever is urgently needed.

RHEUMATIC FEVER IN DEVELOPING COUNTRIES

Rheumatic heart disease is considered by some physicians to be one of the few preventable chronic diseases.[9] Despite impressive declines in incidence in developed countries (see Figs. 35–1 to 35–3), globally, rheumatic heart disease remains the most common form of acquired heart disease.[105,217] Four fifths of the world's population live in developing countries, where the prevalence of rheumatic heart disease suggests that the incidence of acute rheumatic fever remains at high levels in areas characterized by crowded living quarters and lower socioeconomic conditions. In Soweto, South Africa, the prevalence of rheumatic heart disease in the 1970s was estimated at 7.1 per 1000 schoolchildren.[136] A recent estimate using echocardiography in two developing country settings increased this estimate by nearly tenfold.[122]

Given the difference in medical care delivery, evaluation of the incidence of acute rheumatic fever must be viewed with caution. Estimates suggest, however, an annual incidence of 200 to 400 cases per 100,000 population in Soweto.[105] In India, the prevalence of rheumatic heart disease in school children has been estimated to be 1 to 5.4 cases per 1000.[148] The incidence of rheumatic fever (as judged by hospital admissions for rheumatic heart disease between 1966 and 1980) has remained stable in India during this period of rapid decline in the United States and the West.[2] Community-based secondary penicillin prophylaxis programs in developing countries are considered cost-

effective and more achievable than is primary prevention.[105] An estimate of the global burden of group A streptococcal diseases has been undertaken by the World Health Organization (www.who.int/ch-add-health).

PATHOLOGY

The unique pathologic lesion of rheumatic fever is the Aschoff body, which generally is considered to be a granuloma that results from injury to collagen fibers. Classically, Aschoff bodies are found in the heart, usually in the left atrial appendage, but similar foci can be found in the synovia of the joints and in and around joint capsules, tendons, and fascia.[171]

The early pathologic response to rheumatic fever may be an exudative reaction with Aschoff-like bodies as an inflammatory focus. They are cardiac or extracardiac, with a central area of fibrinoid necrosis surrounded mostly by polymorphonuclear leukocytes. Clinically, this condition may be manifested as arthritis and spontaneously subside in 2 to 4 weeks. No residual joint damage results. The proliferative phase of classic Aschoff nodules, which consists of central necrosis surrounded by a rosette of large mononuclear cells, giant multinuclear cells, and other cell types, is confined to the heart and usually causes pancarditis with simultaneous involvement of all three layers (the pericardium, the myocardium, and the endocardium). This event may result in permanent valvular damage in the following order of frequency: the mitral valve, the aortic valve, the tricuspid valve, and, rarely, the pulmonary valve.

The heart disease encountered clinically usually is mitral regurgitation, aortic regurgitation, or both. The scarring that leads to valvular stenosis (mitral or aortic) typically takes decades to develop but may occur much faster in hyperendemic areas. This process is not the full story, however, because although rheumatic mitral valve stenosis occurs more commonly in India[174] and occasionally in other less advantaged populations, it was never a common occurrence in the United States or the United Kingdom at the height of rheumatic fever incidence.[191]

The presence of Aschoff bodies is not evidence of rheumatic activity because these lesions are found in biopsy specimens of the left atrial appendage many years after an acute attack of rheumatic fever. Little is known about the pathology of Sydenham chorea, and the pathologic changes cannot be related to the clinical manifestations. Patients rarely die of this form of rheumatic fever.

CLINICAL COURSE

The stage is set for the development of rheumatic fever in a susceptible host after a pharyngeal infection by one of the types of group A beta-hemolytic streptococci.[115,125,182] If the infection is not treated, most individuals recover from the acute effects of the disease. Acute rheumatic fever develops in approximately 1 to 3 percent of children with known epidemic untreated exudative pharyngitis and a culture positive for group A streptococci. The frequency decreases to less than 1 percent, as shown in the one controlled study involving children,[178] when patients with less severe or less precisely diagnosed streptococcal infections are included.

This finding has been replicated more recently in a large community-based study in an endemic area in New Zealand. The attack rate observed was approximately 0.2 percent[114] with bacteriologic diagnosis and treatment of group A streptococcal throat infection and its effect on rheumatic fever.

The preceding pharyngitis is not recognized as an illness by the patient or parents in approximately 10 to 33 percent of cases of acute rheumatic fever, although 50 to 60 percent of patients remember having a sore throat.[82] In the New Zealand series, episodes of sore throat (with appropriately increased streptococcal serology) in this carefully monitored series preceded development of acute rheumatic fever cases in 14 of 19 (74%) of the cases enrolled in the program at the time of presentation.[114] In some series, this figure is lower (see Table 35–2). The infection is followed by a latent period that averages 19 days in duration,[164] during which time the patient seems well. The range seems to be between 1 and 5 weeks but has been difficult to establish.[41] In the New Zealand series, the average latent period was 27 days (range, 2 to 49 days) for seven rheumatic cases with proven group A streptococcal pharyngitis.[114] The average latent period is the same for recurrent attacks as for initial episodes.[41]

Acute rheumatic fever then begins. Table 35–3 suggests a clinical profile in the United States, although recurrent cases with their increased risk for carditis are included. In a prospective study in India, 67 percent of initial episodes were associated with migrating arthritis involving one or more of the large joints[173] accompanied by a fever of 38° C to 39° C, malaise, and anorexia. Just as the redness, swelling, and pain in a knee subside, the whole process may start again in the ankle. The elbows and wrists also are likely to be involved. Typically, multiple joints are involved, in tandem with overlap over the course of time, when symptoms are not suppressed by anti-inflammatory therapy. The whole polyarthritic episode usually subsides over 4 weeks, with no residua remaining.

Carditis generally appears early in the, illness (first 2 to 3 weeks) if it is going to occur.[1] The joint inflammation may be low-grade in some individuals, without limitation of motion or outward manifestations of redness and swelling (arthralgia). The literature supporting monarthritis that does not develop into migrating polyarthritis in acute rheumatic fever is unconvincing.[38,89,104,114,157,212] The clinician should act cautiously, however, in an area endemic for rheumatic fever in the early phase of presentation. The development of polyarthritis in a patient with a culture-negative monarthritis (e.g., a hip joint in a patient without prior antibiotic exposure) may be aborted by nonsteroidal anti-inflammatory drugs (NSAIDs). An early echocardiogram may assist in establishing the diagnosis.[3]

At examination, the striking findings are the patient's pallor and discomfort, especially on movement of the affected joints. The pulse is rapid. Examination of the heart may reveal in at least half of patients a grade II/IV apical pansystolic murmur that is transmitted to the axilla (mitral insufficiency) with or without an apical mid-diastolic flow murmur (Carey-Coombs murmur); half of these patients also may experience an early diastolic grade II/IV murmur at the left sternal edge (aortic insufficiency). In addition, less commonly, the child can have congestive heart failure or cardiac enlargement, indicative of active carditis. Carditis is more likely to occur in younger children. Pericarditis may be suspected with muffled heart sounds, a frictional rub, or chest pain. It becomes less common as acute rheumatic fever in a population becomes less severe. Death is a rare, but well-described, sequela of the acute phase of the disease. Murmurs of mitral and aortic stenosis are associated with chronic, but not with acute, rheumatic valve disease.

The distinctive rash, erythema marginatum, is observed in 10 percent of patients (Fig. 35–4). It is neither pruritic nor painful. The pink, slightly raised macules usually seen initially on the trunk and proximal ends of the extremities and never on the face fuse centrally and coalesce to form a serpiginous pattern. The lesions may disappear after a few hours or may reappear intermittently over the course of weeks, especially after a warm shower or bath. Subcutaneous nodules, usually associated with severe carditis, also occur uncommonly (<10% of patients). They are firm and painless and are found over bony surfaces or prominences and over tendons. Acute rheumatic fever is not likely to be diagnosed on the basis of the latter two major criteria without another major criterion.

Sydenham chorea, or St. Vitus' dance, may be the only manifestation of rheumatic fever, or it may be associated with other disease manifestations. It becomes less common as acute rheumatic fever becomes less severe in a population. Chorea is characterized by purposeless (most often bilateral, uncoordinated, involuntary) movements, mostly of the hands, feet, and face, which develop over the course of weeks and are accentuated by excitement and emotional stress. They disappear during sleep. Sensation remains intact. The speech can be explosive and indistinct, and the handwriting can be clumsy. Handwriting is a useful objective means of monitoring the course of the disease. The child has difficulty counting rapidly and holding the protruded tongue still. The fingers and wrists are hyperextended when the fingers are outstretched, and the palms usually are turned outward when the arms are held above the head. Handgrip generally is weak and may consist of spasmodic contractions followed by rapid relaxation.

The patient may be easily irritated and quarrelsome. Chorea typically is a delayed manifestation of rheumatic fever and may develop after other signs of the disease have subsided. Chorea commonly appears 2 to 6 months after the streptococcal infection. Most observers think that residual heart disease occurs less commonly when chorea is the only manifestation of rheumatic fever, but in the echocardiographic era this hypothesis may prove not to be the case.[3] The importance of prophylaxis to prevent recurrent attacks and possible subsequent carditis was reaffirmed in Kuwait.[119] Permanent serious residual neurologic deficits have

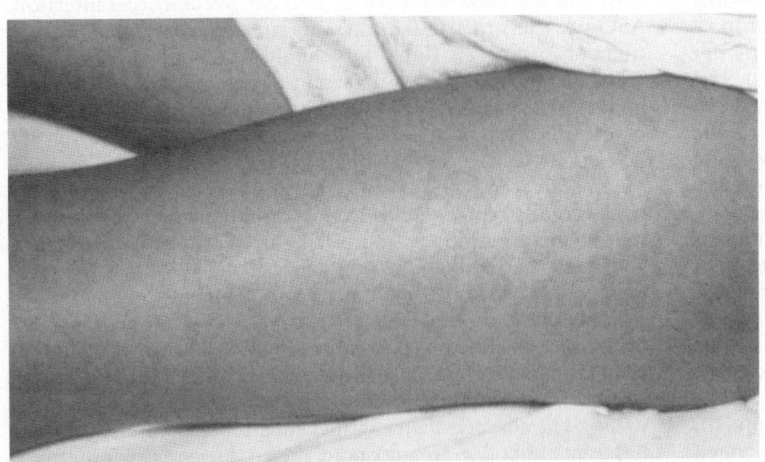

Figure 35–4 Erythema marginatum in an 8-year-old girl with acute rheumatic fever.

not been observed. A 25-year review found the duration of chorea to be 1 to 22 weeks, with a median of 12 weeks.[145] Rare cases may last 2 to 3 years.[4,13,37] Recurrent attacks are common and may occur despite faithful adherence to prophylaxis with intramuscular benzathine penicillin.[22,194] The neuropsychiatric sequelae of chorea were reviewed recently.[139]

Some cases of chorea are mild or atypical and may be confused with motor tics or the involuntary jerks of Tourette syndrome. Confusion may ensue between Sydenham chorea and these conditions. The term *pediatric autoimmune neuropsychiatric disorder associated with streptococcal infection (PANDAS)* refers to a subgroup of children with tic or obsessive-compulsive disorder, whose symptoms may develop or worsen after an episode of group A streptococcal infection. The following five criteria have been used to define the PANDAS subgroup[106,189]:

1. The presence of a tic disorder or obsessive-compulsive disorder or both
2. Prepubertal age of onset (usually between 3 and 12 years of age)
3. Abrupt onset of symptoms or episodic course of symptom severity, or both
4. Temporal association between exacerbations of symptoms and streptococcal infection (approximately 7 to 14 days)
5. Presence of neurologic abnormalities during periods of exacerbation of symptoms (typically adventitious movements or motoric hyperactivity)

The evidence supporting PANDAS as a distinct disease entity has been questioned.[106] In any population with a high prevalence of acute rheumatic fever, clinicians should rarely (if ever) make a diagnosis of PANDAS and rather should err on the side of overdiagnosis of acute rheumatic fever and secondary prophylaxis. If acute rheumatic fever is excluded, secondary prophylaxis is not needed, but such cases should be followed up carefully to ensure that they do not develop carditis in the long-term.

The average duration of an attack of acute rheumatic fever is approximately 3 months when unaltered by anti-inflammatory therapy.[125] Less than 5 percent of cases persist longer than 6 months with active symptoms, so-called chronic rheumatic fever.[191]

LABORATORY FINDINGS

The degree of inflammation in patients with acute rheumatic fever is measured by nonspecific indicators, such as the erythrocyte sedimentation rate (ESR) and C-reactive protein (CRP).[115,125,182] Unless the patient has taken corticosteroids or salicylates, these test results almost always are positive in patients with polyarthritis or acute carditis, whereas they often are normal in patients with chorea. The magnitude of the ESR is proportional to the intensity of the inflammatory reaction but is not site-specific (i.e., it can be high with polyarthritis or carditis). The ESR may be decreased in congestive heart failure, whereas CRP may be elevated in congestive heart failure attributable to any cause. The ESR may remain elevated for 6 weeks to 3 months in an untreated attack of acute rheumatic fever. Anti-inflammatory agents may reduce the ESR, but it rebounds if the drugs are stopped before the rheumatic process has run its course. Although chronic elevation of the ESR (>6 months) is not understood, it is not sufficient reason on its own to limit a patient's activities.[191] The CRP may reflect the patient's rheumatic activity more precisely than may the ESR.[125]

Chest radiographs are useful for detecting cardiomegaly, which may be caused by dilation, preexisting heart disease, or pericardial effusion. The degree of enlargement is helpful in judging severity. The electrocardiogram may show a prolonged

atrioventricular conduction time, usually evidenced by a prolonged PR interval or even greater degrees of heart block.[167] Generally, an increase in the PR interval in tracings with comparable rates is considered significant.[125] Upper limits of normal by age are available.[115] Atrioventricular conduction abnormalities per se bear no relation to the ultimate prognosis of patients. Changes of myocarditis and pericarditis also are seen.

The roles of two-dimensional and Doppler echocardiography in establishing the diagnosis and determining the prognosis of acute rheumatic fever are becoming clearer.[1,71,72,115,182,198-200,213] In a prospective blinded study using febrile controls and strict color and pulsed Doppler criteria, pathologic left-sided heart regurgitation could be differentiated from physiologic regurgitation.[1] Several centers using similar strict criteria have observed subclinical carditis in acute rheumatic fever.[73,74,199,200] The status of echocardiographic evidence as a major or minor Jones criterion remains to be settled by the American Heart Association.[71] It has important implications for patients with polyarthritis or chorea as a sole major criterion[3,182] or patients without major criteria and only echocardiographic evidence of mitral or aortic regurgitation. In an area of high endemicity (New Zealand), strict criteria have evolved and are incorporated into common usage.[115] In a prospective study of prevention of acute rheumatic fever, three additional cases (3 of 59 [5%]) met the case definition for acute rheumatic fever using the New Zealand Rheumatic Fever diagnostic criteria, which allows echocardiographic carditis to be a major or minor criterion in the presence of other major or minor criteria and evidence of preceding streptococcal infection.[114]

A positive throat culture for group A beta-hemolytic streptococci as evidence of a recent streptococcal infection seldom is found, and 50 percent of such patients could be carriers of the organism.[99] In the New Zealand prospective study of patients with sore throat episodes (*n* = 14) and enrolled in the program, 57 percent (8 of 14) had a positive throat culture and appropriately increased serology.[114] A positive culture may be helpful if it can be related to the time of the acute infection.

Corroboration of a previous streptococcal infection may be documented by numerous streptococcal antibody tests.[175,211] Antibody titers may be elevated in the absence of clinical or bacteriologic evidence of streptococcal pharyngitis (5 of 19 acute rheumatic fever cases in the New Zealand program).[114] The ASO titer is the most popular antibody test. It measures the inhibition of rabbit red blood cells by specific antibody to streptolysin O, an extracellular product of beta-hemolytic streptococci that in its reduced form hemolyzes red blood cells. The "normal" level for an ASO titer usually is defined as the highest titer exceeded by only 20 percent of a population, but it is influenced significantly by age, geography, season, and other factors.[98,175] ASO titers of 500 Todd units or greater are rare findings in normal schoolchildren and are good evidence of a recent streptococcal infection. ASO titers less than 250 Todd units could be considered normal; titers of 250 to 320 Todd units should be considered borderline elevated. Approximately 50 percent of patients with acute rheumatic fever have ASO titers in this range, and approximately 60 percent have titers of 500 Todd units or greater.[182] Conversely, ASO titers can be normal in 20 percent of patients with acute rheumatic fever.[185]

A recent streptococcal infection is more likely to be shown if more than one antibody titer is measured (e.g., antistreptokinase and antihyaluronidase).[185] Anti–deoxyribonuclease B is the most favored test because of its better reproducibility.

The Jones criteria (Table 35–5) call for an elevated or increasing titer of an antistreptococcal antibody.[182] The onset of clinical acute rheumatic fever usually coincides with the peak of the streptococcal antibody response. It may stay elevated for many weeks. The absence of an elevated antistreptococcal titer, if three different antibodies are measured, means, however, that the clini-

Major Manifestations†
Carditis
Polyarthritis
Chorea
Erythema marginatum
Subcutaneous nodules

Minor Manifestations†
Clinical findings
Arthralgia
Fever
Laboratory findings
Elevated acute-phase reactants
Elevated erythrocyte sedimentation rate
Elevated C-reactive protein
Prolonged PR interval

Supporting Evidence of Antecedent Group A Streptococcal Infection
Positive throat culture or rapid streptococcal antigen test
Elevated or rising streptococcal antibody titer

*If supported by evidence of a preceding group A streptococcal infection, the presence of two major manifestations or of one major and two minor manifestations indicates a high probability of acute rheumatic fever.
†See text for details.
From Guidelines for the diagnosis of rheumatic fever. Jones criteria, 1992 update. Special Writing Group of the Committee on Rheumatic Fever, Endocarditis, and Kawasaki Disease in the Young of the American Heart Association. J. A. M. A. 268:2069-2073, 1992. Copyright 1992, American Medical Association.

cian can be 95 percent certain that the patient has not had a streptococcal infection within the recent past. In patients with pure chorea, antibody levels may have declined to normal because of the length of the latent period between the development of streptococcal infection and the manifestation of this symptom. A slide agglutination test is available (Streptozyme antibody test; Wampole Laboratories, Stamford, CT). This test cannot be recommended at this time because of inconsistencies in results caused by variations in different lots of test material.[216]

The synovial fluid in joints affected by acute rheumatic fever contains 10,000 to 100,000 white blood cells/mm³, which are mostly neutrophils. The protein concentration is approximately 4 g/dL, glucose levels are normal, and a good mucin clot is present.[92] A more recent report corroborates the cellular findings and highlights similarities with septic arthritis.[89]

DIAGNOSIS

The signs and symptoms of rheumatic fever vary greatly, depending on the stage of the disease, the epidemiology of the rheumatic fever in that place at that time, the severity of the disease, and the sites of involvement. In the absence of a diagnostic test or pathognomonic sign, Jones suggested a series of criteria (major and minor) (see Table 35–5) that have stood the test of time, with ongoing modifications.[71,123]

The keystone on which the Jones criteria (1992 update[182]) rest is the demonstration of a recent streptococcal infection. Because few patients with acute rheumatic fever have positive throat cultures, demonstration of a previous streptococcal infection by a rising titer of one or more of the extracellular streptococcal antibodies is crucial confirmatory evidence to establish a recent streptococcal infection. The mere presence of an elevated titer to one or more of the streptococcal antibodies (see the section on laboratory findings) means only that the subject has had a recent group A beta-hemolytic streptococcal infection.

Clinical manifestations in outbreaks in the 1980s are summarized in Table 35–3. Before this time, during the period of declin-

ing incidence in the United States, carditis was found in fewer than half of rheumatic patients and generally was less severe.[131] Joint involvement alone was the most common manifestation, so arriving at a diagnostic certainty was difficult. A common avoidable error is the premature administration of salicylates or corticosteroids before the signs and symptoms become distinct; such therapy leaves in doubt the necessity of administering secondary prophylaxis without a firm diagnosis.

In contrast to the revised Jones criteria (1965), more updated criteria (1992)[182] are designed to establish a diagnosis of the initial attack of acute rheumatic fever; a previous attack of rheumatic fever or rheumatic heart disease no longer is a minor manifestation. Echocardiography currently is not a stand-alone criterion for the diagnosis of acute rheumatic fever in the United States using these criteria (see the section on laboratory findings); however, chorea and indolent carditis are considered stand-alone criteria for establishing the diagnosis of rheumatic fever. Recurrences of rheumatic fever in patients with a reliable past history of rheumatic fever or clear-cut rheumatic heart disease can be diagnosed by the demonstration of a single major or several minor criteria if supporting evidence of a recent group A streptococcal infection is present.

So-called poststreptococcal arthritis has been discussed as a possible entity when the initial symptoms and signs are atypical for acute rheumatic fever, fail to respond to salicylate therapy, or both. In some cases, rheumatic heart disease has ensued.[63a] In all such patients who fulfill the Jones criteria, a diagnosis of rheumatic fever should be considered, particularly for the purpose of administering secondary penicillin prophylaxis.[15]

Criteria have been proposed for establishing the diagnosis of poststreptococcal reactive arthritis that have yet to stand the test of time. A variable response to salicylates in series of this disease has not often been well documented with serum salicylate levels.[80] A shorter latent period is proposed, but the latent period between a group A streptococcal throat infection in original investigations of rheumatic fever varied (mean, 18.6 days), with 10 percent developing disease within 8 days (see the section on clinical course).[164] If this diagnosis is considered and rheumatic fever per se is not supported, vigilant follow-up for cardiac sequelae should ensue, and penicillin prophylaxis would be reconsidered. This diagnosis should be considered with caution in areas endemic for rheumatic fever. An atypical presentation of chorea (e.g., hemichorea) warrants consideration of neuroimaging.[222]

DIFFERENTIAL DIAGNOSIS

Many other diseases might be confused with acute rheumatic fever,[110] including rheumatoid arthritis, suppurative bacterial arthritis (especially gonococcal arthritis in adolescents), reactive arthritis (e.g., after Yersinia[107] or Mycoplasma[140] infection), infective endocarditis, sickle-cell anemia, leukemia, Lyme disease,[158] and poststreptococcal reactive arthritis (see earlier). In polyarthritis without clinical or echocardiographic evidence of carditis and fulfilling the Jones criteria, rheumatic fever is a diagnosis of exclusion. A follow-up echocardiogram after 2 to 3 weeks may reveal late presenting carditis.[1,203]

With the help of the Jones criteria and time, these diseases usually can be excluded. Heart involvement with rheumatoid arthritis is a rare occurrence. In suppurative arthritis, showing the infecting bacteria by smear and recovery by culture provide the answer. With sickle-cell disease, the bone is affected and not the joint, and a sickle-cell preparation helps establish the diagnosis. A blood smear usually establishes the diagnosis of leukemia.

The diagnosis of isolated Sydenham chorea based on presenting symptoms may be confirmed by an abnormal echocardiogram in the absence of clinical carditis. Other, much rarer considerations, especially in an area not endemic for rheumatic fever, include systemic lupus erythematosus (SLE), Wilson disease, juvenile Huntington chorea, and various medications.[40,110]

Common errors include diagnosing acute rheumatic fever and prescribing NSAIDs when a single joint is involved (see the section on clinical course)[212]; when an innocent murmur is present; when a nonspecific rash, especially an urticarial or an erythema multiforme rash, erroneously is called erythema marginatum; and when other symptoms similar to chorea (e.g., tics, phenothiazine-induced extrapyramidal syndrome) are misinterpreted.[95] Committing a child to many years of penicillin prophylaxis requires careful decision-making at the time of establishing the diagnosis.

TREATMENT

Therapy for acute rheumatic fever is symptomatic:[41,57,110,136,190] control the inflammation, decrease the fever, and keep cardiac failure in check. Neither salicylates nor corticosteroids are thought to affect severity or outcome.[7] Cardiac drugs (e.g., diuretics, angiotensin-converting enzyme inhibitors, beta blockers) may improve impaired function. The long-term benefits have not been studied systematically. If the physician thinks that a patient has acute rheumatic fever, a trial of salicylates may be useful as symptomatic therapy. If the diagnosis is uncertain, however, pain relief such as acetaminophen should be used as an interim measure to allow migrating polyarthritis to occur. This approach has not been evaluated critically.

Characteristically, the joint inflammation and fever subside in 24 to 48 hours with salicylate treatment if the serum level is 10 to 20 mg/dL, which usually is achieved by a dose of 60 to 100 mg/kg/24 hr (not exceeding 6 g/day in divided doses). This dose may be increased, but the clinician is advised to measure serum salicylate levels and adjust the dose regimen accordingly. A higher dose may result in the undesirable development of salicylism (tinnitus and hyperpnea). Except for occasional patients with rheumatoid arthritis, no other forms of arthritis respond in this dramatic way to aspirin. Salicylate therapy is recommended for 1 to 2 weeks and then can be reduced gradually, keeping in mind that inflammatory markers suggesting ongoing disease activity may persist 3 months or longer. Joint symptoms may recur, obviating a more gradual withdrawal of aspirin.

Most acute rheumatic fever episodes subside within 6 weeks, and 90 percent resolve within 12 weeks. Approximately 5 percent of cases require 6 months or more of salicylate therapy.[186] If lengthy therapy is required, influenza and varicella vaccines are important considerations to reduce the potential for developing Reye syndrome.[50] Newer NSAIDs for the treatment of acute rheumatic fever have been studied in limited fashion.[91,197] Naproxen (10 to 20 mg/kg/day given in two divided doses; maximum dose 1250 mg) had a dramatic effect similar to that of aspirin and is well-tolerated. Advantages are twice-daily administration, the availability of elixir, less hepatotoxicity, and no need to determine serum levels.

No evidence has substantiated that steroid therapy is superior or that treatment with steroid or aspirin decreases the severity or prevents the development of residual heart disease.[6,7,47] Both treatments are palliative and not curative. They are, however, effective anti-inflammatory agents for controlling the acute exudative manifestations of rheumatic fever. Steroids are more likely to reduce acute symptoms promptly and may be indicated for severely ill patients in whom inflammatory edema of the myocardium may be life-threatening during the acute stage of the illness.[8,115] The effect of NSAIDs has not been evaluated adequately.

A randomized controlled trial of intravenous immunoglobulin, a proven immunomodulator, in acute rheumatic fever failed to alter the natural history. No detectable difference was noted in the clinical, laboratory, or echocardiographic parameters found during the subsequent 12 months.[203]

Bed rest has not been studied critically.[125] Restriction of physical activity until the rheumatic process has become quiescent is a time-honored method of treatment. It has been based on the assumption that the workload of the inflamed heart is related to the degree of residual scarring. Suggested guidelines include 6 weeks of bed rest, depending on whether carditis is present, followed by gradual ambulation indoors over the course of a further 6 weeks before outside activity, in modified fashion, occurs.[169] Patients with severe carditis who have congestive heart failure are managed more conservatively.

All patients should receive intramuscular benzathine penicillin, even if the throat culture does not reveal group A beta-hemolytic streptococci. Patients then can be placed on the secondary preventive treatment regimen, which may be either oral penicillin V, 250 mg twice a day, or injections of benzathine penicillin, 1.2 million U every 4 weeks. The parenteral route has been shown to be more effective by the author's group[146] and others (Fig. 35–5).[75,215] In high-risk situations (e.g., after a recurrence in a compliant patient), administration of benzathine penicillin every 3 weeks has been advised (see the section on prevention for more detail).[117]

Rarely, a patient has congestive heart failure.[115] A diuretic or fluid restrictions or both are recommended for mild to moderate failure. Angiotensin-converting enzyme inhibitors should be considered for more severe failure, particularly if aortic regurgitation is present. Experience with beta blockers in acute rheumatic carditis is very limited, and their use is not recommended.

Chorea is benign and self-limited. Mild or moderate chorea does not require any specific treatment aside from rest and a calm environment, perhaps in the hospital. Overstimulation or stress can exacerbate the symptoms. The potential toxicity of recommended medication for severe distressing or limiting chorea should be taken into consideration. Aspirin does not have a significant treatment effect.[125] A randomized trial of prednisone in Sydenham chorea showed efficacy.[151] More studies are awaited to confirm this finding.

Small studies of intravenous immunoglobulin have suggested more rapid recovery from chorea,[188] but they have not shown reduced incidence of long-term valve disease in acute rheumatic fever without chorea.[203] Until more evidence is available, intravenous immunoglobulin is not recommended except for severe chorea refractory to other treatments.

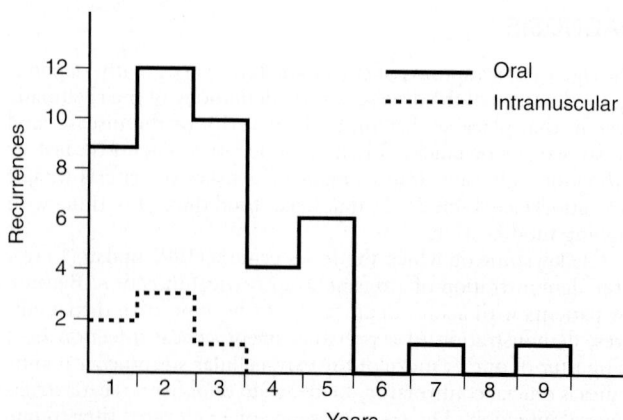

Figure 35–5 Influence of oral and intramuscular penicillin prophylaxis on the recurrence of rheumatic fever. Time is between the last attack and recurrence (years). (*From Newman, J. E., Lennon, D. R., and Wong-Toi, W.: Patients with rheumatic fever recurrences. N. Z. Med. J. 97:678-680, 1984.*)

Carbamazepine and valproic acid now are preferred to halo-peridol, which previously was considered the first-line medical treatment for chorea.[63,76] A small prospective comparison of these three agents concluded that valproic acid was the most effective.[152]

Other antichorea medications should be avoided because of potential toxicity. Because of the small potential for liver toxicity with valproic acid, the recommendation is that carbamazepine be used initially for severe chorea requiring treatment and that valproic acid be considered for refractory cases. A response may not be seen for 1 to 2 weeks, and successful medication may reduce, but not eliminate, the symptoms. Medication should be continued for 2 to 4 weeks after chorea has subsided and then withdrawn gradually. Recurrences of chorea usually are mild and can be managed conservatively, but in severe recurrences, the medication can be restarted if necessary.

CARDIAC SURGERY IN RHEUMATIC HEART DISEASE

Aggressive surgical therapy, with increasing acceptance that mitral repair rather than replacement is the treatment of choice for mitral regurgitation,[12] may be indicated in patients with severe active rheumatic heart disease. Extensive published experience in South Africa[17,44] and France[44] with excellent results has challenged the concept that congestive heart failure and death during active carditis are caused exclusively by myocarditis, rather than incompetence of the valve. Studies on left ventricular mechanics support this new evidence.[77] In addition, primary myocardial involvement as evidenced by histologic abnormalities of the myocardium has been well documented during acute rheumatic fever.[144,190] Careful postoperative management, including at least 4 months of physical rest, diuretics, and vasodilation with angiotensin-converting enzyme inhibitors, is thought to improve the long-term outcome by avoiding increased blood pressure and myocardial contractility before the repair has consolidated.

Surgery usually is deferred until active inflammation has subsided. Rarely, valve leaflet or chordae tendinae rupture leads to severe regurgitation; this event requires emergency surgery, which can be performed safely by experienced surgeons, although the risk seems to be slightly higher than when surgery is performed after active inflammation has resolved.[5] Valve replacement, rather than repair, usually is done during the acute episode because of the technical difficulties of repairing friable, inflamed tissue. Nonetheless, very experienced surgeons may achieve good results with repair in this situation.

PROGNOSIS

The prognosis for patients with acute rheumatic fever depends on the initial manifestations, as shown in the 20-year follow-up study from the pre-penicillin era by Bland and Jones.[32] A patient with marked cardiomegaly, congestive heart failure, or pericarditis had about a 70 to 80 percent chance of dying in the 10 years before the advent of secondary prevention programs, open heart surgery, and use of prosthetic valves. The prognosis today is not as poor, although the recurrence rates (with the attendant increased risk of carditis in individual patients) reported after some outbreaks[199,220] suggest a careful look at secondary prevention and its delivery. The risk of having rheumatic heart disease at 1-year[7] and 10-year[49] follow-up is 70 percent for patients with cardiomegaly or heart failure and who survive. Most of these patients have mitral insufficiency, and approximately 50 percent also have aortic insufficiency.

Approximately 50 percent of patients initially are left with residual heart disease after an attack of rheumatic fever. This rate is about the same as it was 25 to 30 years ago. Approximately 25 percent of these patients return to normal cardiac status, however, with a higher chance if the cardiac involvement is mild. Of patients with no or questionable carditis[7] during their attack of rheumatic fever, only 6 percent were found to have heart murmurs when re-examined 10 years later. Heart disease was present at follow-up in 30 percent of the patients initially found to have only apical systolic murmurs and in 40 percent of patients with basal diastolic murmurs during the acute phase. Patients with chorea may have a slightly lower incidence of residual heart disease.[118] More data from the echocardiographic era are required.

PREVENTION

Denny and associates[64,208] made one of the most important research contributions in the last 50 years when they showed that rheumatic fever can be prevented in most susceptible subjects if the preceding pharyngeal infection by one of the group A beta-hemolytic streptococci is treated adequately.[57] These studies used depot penicillin G. The effectiveness of other antimicrobial agents (benzathine penicillin, chlortetracycline, sulfadiazine, oxytetracycline) in the prevention of rheumatic fever also was studied. Eradication of the streptococcus was shown to be essential,[41] and a 10-day course of penicillin treatment was found to be more effective than a 5-day course.[208] From these studies, penicillin, a bactericidal agent with activity against streptococci, became the drug of choice.

Efficacy studies against rheumatic fever per se were performed, mainly in military populations with injectable penicillin. Only one inconclusive study was done in children.[178] These studies more recently have been subjected to meta-analysis,[172] with a relative risk of 0.20 (95% confidence interval 0.11, 0.36; $p < .00001$) favoring the intervention. The ability of oral penicillin to eradicate streptococci in throats is not equal to the ability of injectable penicillin to do so.[18] A school-based, randomized, controlled trial of sore throat clinics using oral penicillin in an area in New Zealand endemic for acute rheumatic fever (43,827 person-years of observation) revealed a clinically useful result, but with uncertainty about the effect size. A meta-analysis of published literature on community-based or school-based controlled studies to prevent first attacks of rheumatic fever revealed a risk of 0.62 (95% confidence interval 0.45, 0.85; $p = .003$), which favors these interventions, suggesting approximately 40 percent efficacy.[111] Our study used supervised oral penicillin treatment[114]; the treatment regimen was unclear in the other studies.[45,52,154] A complete explanation for the decline in rheumatic fever remains unclear.

Streptococcal pharyngeal infection should be identified before treatment is started. Guidelines using clinical parameters have evolved[43,116] and have been tested empirically to guide rational management.[134,135] Streptococcal pharyngeal infection can be diagnosed by throat culture or by using a rapid diagnostic antigen-detection kit.[30,57,79] Most tests have high specificity, so a patient with acute pharyngitis and a positive test result should be treated. Many of the tests have suboptimal sensitivity and should be confirmed by a throat culture. One study found that in one third of individuals with false-negative rapid antigen-detection test results, streptococcal antibody titers increased subsequently, suggesting infection.[78]

Military studies have shown that primary preventive treatment with penicillin is effective even if started 9 days after the infection develops,[42] so physicians can wait 24 to 48 hours for verification of infection by recovery of group A beta-hemolytic streptococci. A dose of 1.2 million U of benzathine penicillin intramuscularly (0.6 million U if weight is ≤27 kg) usually is adequate treatment. Because of the discomfort and a possible, but small, risk associated with intramuscular penicillin,[94] oral penicillin V (250 mg two or three times a day for children; 500 mg two or three times a day for adolescents and adults) may be preferred in areas in which the incidence of rheumatic fever is low. Erythromycin estolate (20 to 40 mg/kg/day in two to four divided doses; maximum 1 g/day) may be used in patients who are allergic to penicillin. Erythromycin ethyl succinate (40 mg/kg/day two to four times daily; maximum 1 g/day) is an alternative therapy. Accruing evidence supports the use of once-a-day amoxicillin.[48,67,112,177]

All oral treatments should be given for 10 days.[57] Although certain new wider spectrum agents have been administered in shorter courses with the desired streptococcal eradication, on the basis of penicillin's narrow spectrum of antimicrobial activity, the infrequency with which it produces adverse reactions, and its modest cost, it is the drug of choice for nonallergic patients.[30]

Reappearance of acute rheumatic fever in a specific geographic region should draw attention to therapeutic, preventive, and epidemiologic measures for control of the disease. A targeted approach to particularly high-risk population groups in schools may be cost-effective and efficacious.[9,33,52,155,170,196] Because treatment of pharyngitis seems likely to have contributed to the declining incidence of rheumatic fever, obtaining throat cultures (or a rapid antigen-detection test) and administering penicillin treatment, if positive for group A streptococci, still are recommended in low-risk populations, although this recommendation is being challenged by some physicians.[134,135] In addition, a negative culture avoids unnecessarily prescribing antibiotics in the 70 to 80 percent of children with a sore throat attributable to viral pharyngitis, although clinical assessment may obviate having to obtain a throat culture.[135,176]

Prompt administration of antibiotic therapy may shorten the duration of symptoms in patients with group A beta-hemolytic streptococcal pharyngitis.[166] Cultures should be used selectively in age groups in which rheumatic fever rarely occurs (e.g., <4 years of age or >20 years). Signs and symptoms usually not associated with streptococcal infection, such as simple coryza, hoarseness, cough, conjunctivitis, anterior stomatitis, and diarrhea,[58,135] may help target the approach in a low-risk population.

A follow-up throat culture taken after a course of treatment for streptococcal pharyngitis is not recommended routinely, unless the patient remains symptomatic or is from a family with a rheumatic member.[30] Such follow-up cultures probably identify long-term carriers for whom repeated courses of antibiotics generally are not indicated.[30] Streptococcal carriers seem to pose little threat to themselves regarding the development of sequelae from streptococcal infection or dissemination of the organism to people around them. When a symptomatic viral upper respiratory tract infection develops in such a carrier distinguishing whether the group A streptococci isolated indicate current streptococcal infection or identify that individual as a chronic carrier frequently is impossible. In one study, only 43 percent of children with paired sera from whom group A streptococci were recovered showed a significant antibody response to one of two different streptococcal antibodies.[99]

Often, a reasonable approach is to administer a single course of therapy. Indications for obtaining cultures from household contacts vary according to circumstances.[57] Family contacts of high-risk patients should have a culture performed and receive treatment if the culture is positive.

In the pre-penicillin era, 75 percent of individuals developed a recurrence of acute rheumatic fever.[32] Penicillin prophylaxis is well established in its ability to prevent recurrent attacks, with intramuscular long-acting preparations being superior to oral twice-daily delivery.[75,121] Persistent worsening rheumatic heart disease is prevented.[125] Secondary prophylaxis is considered the most cost-effective management of acute rheumatic fever and its sequelae.[187]

Recurrent attacks of rheumatic fever can be prevented by continuous penicillin prophylaxis, administered either orally or parenterally.[121] The parenteral route has been shown to be more effective (1.2 million U of benzathine penicillin intramuscularly at 28-day intervals).[214] In a comprehensive study, children experienced a recurrence rate of only 0.4/100 patient-years of observation (Table 35–6). A Cochrane systematic review found an 87 to 90 percent reduction with parenteral penicillin in four studies.[122] An international study of allergic reactions to long-term benzathine penicillin prophylaxis found that the benefits of preventing recurrence far outweighed the risk of development of a serious allergic reaction.[94] In areas of particularly high risk, administration of benzathine penicillin every 21 days may be more efficacious, although this study was not performed systematically.[118] Serum levels of penicillin toward the end of the time can be unreliable,[96] although this decision should be offset against practicability, cost, and probable compliance.

In a carefully monitored, community-based series with high compliance rates on four weekly injections of penicillin,[87] the penicillin failure rate per se was very low at 0.07/100 patient-years.[183] The program failure rate was 1.4/100 patient-years, with failure primarily resulting from nonadherence. This is in an environment endemic for rheumatic fever, where children had a 1:3 annual chance of having *Streptococcus pyogenes* detected in their throats.[114] A study in Egypt[103] showed that two weekly injections of penicillin resulted in an almost 50 percent reduction in recurrences. This result occurred, however, in an environment in which the rate of recurrences was approximately 45 percent of cases in the four-weekly penicillin comparison arm. A more recent publication supports the use of 1 percent lidocaine hydrochloride as a diluent for benzathine penicillin G to increase tolerability.[6a]

Patients allergic to penicillin may be given erythromycin (250 mg twice a day). Penicillin and sulfadiazine are oral regimens that have been studied for efficacy (see Table 35–6). Sulfadiazine is not readily available in the United States.[11] The lesser efficacy of oral regimens is related at least partly to compliance difficulties.

The risk of rheumatic fever occurring after a group A streptococcal infection increases from an attack rate of 1 to 3 percent with the first attack of streptococcal pharyngitis to 25 to 75 percent with subsequent attacks.[64] Patients who have had carditis are at increased risk for development of further carditis. Patients who have not had clinical carditis have considerably less risk of having cardiac involvement after a recurrence.[68,119] In the echocardiographic era, the dogma that a patient who escapes carditis in the first attack is highly likely to remain free of rheu-

TABLE 35–6   Prophylaxis and Attack Rates of Streptococcal Infection and Rheumatic Fever Recurrence

	Parenteral Benzathine Penicillin	Oral Penicillin	Oral Sulfadiazine
No. years	560	545	576
No./rate of all streptococcal infections, exclusive of carrier state	24/4.3	101/18.5	102/17.7
No./rate of rheumatic recurrences	2/0.4	30/5.5	16/2.8

Adapted from Wood, H. F., Feinstein, A. R., Taranta, A., et al.: Rheumatic fever in children and adolescents: A long-term epidemiologic study of subsequent prophylaxis, streptococcal infections, and clinical sequelae, III: Comparative effectiveness of three prophylaxis regimens in preventing streptococcal infections and rheumatic recurrences. Ann. Intern. Med. 60(Suppl. 5):31–45, 1964.

matic heart disease, even if prophylaxis fails in subsequent attacks, has been challenged.[68,183]

The risk of having a recurrence depends on several other factors, such as the length of time since the most recent attack, and the risk of acquiring streptococcal throat infections according to occupation or living circumstances. If possible, the length of prophylaxis should be individualized. The suggested length ranges from a minimum of 5 years of prophylaxis to a maximum of lifelong prophylaxis.[50] This approach has been validated in a study from Chile.[21]

A more recent publication supports the New Zealand approach.[115,169,183] All patients, regardless of cardiac status, receive at least 10 years of prophylaxis or until they reach 21 years of age (see earlier). Two recurrences in this series occurred in teenagers inadvertently discharged after at least 5 years of prophylaxis. Appropriate discharge of individuals as per the recommended parameters with mild or no carditis apparently was safe. Of equal importance is the prevention of infective endocarditis in patients with rheumatic heart disease or in patients who have had rheumatic fever by the administration of antimicrobial drugs before and after surgical procedures on the eyes, ears, mouth (dental extractions), nose, throat, and gastrointestinal and genitourinary tracts,[59] although opinions are changing on this subject.[213a]

CONCLUSION

Although having effective prophylaxis against a disease[132] for which the pathophysiology is understood incompletely and for which no pharmacologic cure exists is gratifying, rheumatic fever and its sequelae still occur in numerous young people, especially in the developing world and in disadvantaged populations in the developed world.[217] This rate is largely a reflection of complacency about rheumatic fever and rheumatic heart disease by physicians and health care funders, although it also is likely to reflect living conditions and health care access. Renewed educational efforts regarding prevention of rheumatic fever are needed by physicians and the public. The available preventive methods should be applied vigorously.

REFERENCES

1. Abernethy, M., Bass, N., Sharpe, N., et al.: Doppler echocardiography and the early diagnosis of carditis in acute rheumatic fever. Aust. N. Z. J. Med. 24:530-535, 1994.
2. Agarwal, B. L.: Rheumatic Fever and Rheumatic Heart Disease in Developing Countries. India, Arnold Publishers, 1988.
3. Agarwal, P. K., Misra, M., et al.: Usefulness of echocardiography in detection of subclinical carditis in acute rheumatic polyarthritis and rheumatic chorea. J. Assoc. Physicians India 46:937-938, 1998.
4. al-Eissa, A.: Sydenham's chorea: A new look at an old disease. Br. J. Clin. Pract. 47:14-16, 1993.
5. Al Kasab, S., Al Fabih, M., et al.: Valve surgery in acute rheumatic heart disease: One-to four-year follow-up. Chest 94:830-833, 1988.
6. Albert, D. A., Harel, L., et al.: The treatment of rheumatic carditis: A review and meta-analysis. Medicine 74:1-12, 1995.
6a. Amir, J., Ginat, S., Cohen, Y. H., et al.: Lidocaine as a diluent for administration of benzathine penicillin G. Pediatr. Infect. Dis. J. 17:890-893, 1998.
7. Anonymous: The natural history of rheumatic fever and rheumatic heart disease: Ten year report of a cooperative clinical trial of ACTH, cortisone and aspirin. Circulation 32:457-476, 1965.
8. Anonymous: Treatment of rheumatic fever (editorial). N. Engl. J. Med. 272:101-102, 1965.
9. Anonymous: Prevention of rheumatic heart disease. Lancet 143-144, 1982.
10. Anonymous: Acute rheumatic fever among army trainees—Fort Leonard Wood, Missouri 1987-1988. M. M. W. R. Morb. Mortal. Wkly. Rep. 37:519-522, 1988.
11. Anonymous: Availability of sulfadiazine—United States. M. M. W. R. Morb. Mortal. Wkly. Rep. 41:950-951, 1992.
12. Antunes, M. J.: Mitral valvuloplasty, a better alternative: Comparative study between valve reconstruction and replacement for rheumatic mitral valve disease. Eur. J. Cardiothorac. Surg. 4:257-264, 1990.
13. Aron, A. M., Freeman, J. M., et al.: The natural history of Sydenham's chorea. Am. J. Med. 38:83-95, 1965.

14. Atha, M., Enos, E., et al.: How an American Indian tribe controlled the streptococcus. World Health Forum 3:423-428, 1982.
15. Ayoub, E. M., and Majeed, H. A.: Poststreptococcal reactive arthritis. Curr. Opin. Rheumatol. 12:306-310, 2000.
16. Baird, R. W., Bronze, M. S., et al.: Epitopes of group A streptococcal M protein shared with antigens of articular cartilage and synovium. J. Immunol. 146:3132-3137, 1991.
17. Barlow, J. B.: Aspects of active rheumatic carditis. Aust. N. Z. J. Med. 22:592-600, 1992.
18. Bass, J. W., Crast, F. W., et al.: Streptococcal pharyngitis in children: A comparison of four treatment schedules with intramuscular penicillin G benzathine. J. A. M. A. 235:1112-1116, 1976.
19. Beachey, E. H., Bronze, M., et al.: Protective and autoimmune epitopes of streptococcal M proteins. Vaccine 6:192-196, 1988.
20. Beachey, E. H., Stollerman, G. H., et al.: Human immune response to immunization with a structurally defined polypeptide fragment of streptococcal M protein. J. Exp. Med. 150:862-877, 1979.
21. Berrios, X., del Campo, E., et al.: Discontinuing rheumatic fever prophylaxis in selected adolescents and young adults. Ann. Intern. Med. 118:401-406, 1993.
22. Berrios, X., Quesney, F., et al.: Are all recurrences of "pure" Sydenham chorea true recurrences of acute rheumatic fever? J. Pediatr. 107:867-872, 1985.
23. Bessen, D. E., Sotir, C. M., et al.: Genetic correlates of throat and skin isolates of group A streptococci. J. Infect. Dis. 173:896-900, 1996.
24. Bisno, A.: The concept of rheumatogenic and nephritogenic group A streptococci. In Read, S. E., and Zabriskie, J. B. (eds): Streptococcal Diseases and the Immune Response. New York, Academic Press, 1980, pp. 789-804.
25. Bisno, A.: Group A streptococcal infections and acute rheumatic fever. N. Engl. J. Med. 325:783-793, 1991.
26. Bisno, A., Brito, M., et al.: Molecular basis of group A streptococcal virulence. Lancet Infect. Dis. 3:191-200, 2003.
27. Bisno, A., and Land, M.: Incidence of acute rheumatic fever in Memphis and Shelby County, Tennessee, 1977-1981. In Shulman, A. (ed): Management of Pharngitis in an Era of Declining Rheumatic Fever. Columbus, OH, Ross Laboratories, 1984, pp. 13-24.
28. Bisno, A., Pearce, I., et al.: Streptococcal infections that fail to cause recurrences of rheumatic fever. J. Infect. Dis. 136:278-285, 1977.
29. Bisno, A. L., Brito, M. O., et al.: Molecular basis of group A streptococcal virulence. Lancet Infect. Dis. 3:191-200, 2003.
30. Bisno, A. L., Gerber, M. A., et al.: Practice guidelines for the diagnosis and management of group A streptococcal pharyngitis. Infectious Diseases Society of America. Clin. Infect. Dis. 35:113-125, 2002.
31. Bisno, A. L., Pearce, I. A., et al.: Contrasting epidemiology of acute rheumatic fever and acute glomerulonephritis. N. Engl. J. Med. 283:561-565, 1970.
31a. Bisno, A. L., Rubin, F. A., Cleary, P. P., et al.: Prospect for a group A streptococcal vaccine: Rationale, feasibility, and obstacles—report of a National Institute of Allergy and Infectious Diseases workshop. Clin. Infect. Dis. 41:1150-1156, 2005.
32. Bland, E. F., and Jones, T. D.: Rheumatic fever and rheumatic heart disease: A twenty year report on 1000 patients followed since childhood. Circulation 4:836-843, 1951.
33. Brant, L. J., Bender, T. R., et al.: Evaluation of an Alaskan streptococcal control program: Importance of the program's intensity and duration. Prev. Med. 15:632-642, 1986.
34. Bronze, M. S., Beachey, E. H., et al.: Protective and heart-crossreactive epitopes located within the NH_2 terminus of type 19 streptococcal M protein. J. Exp. Med. 167:1849-1859, 1988.
35. Brownell, K., and Bailen-Rose, F.: Acute rheumatic fever in children. J. A. M. A. 224:1593-1597, 1973.
36. Cairns, L. M.: Immunological studies in rheumatic fever: The immunology of rheumatic fever. N. Engl. J. Med. 101:388-391, 1988.
37. Carapetis, J., and Currie, B.: Rheumatic chorea in Northern Australia: A clinical and epidemiological study. Arch. Dis. Child. 80:353-358, 1999.
38. Carapetis, J., and Currie, B.: Rheumatic fever in a high incidence population: The importance of monoarthritis and low grade fever. Arch. Dis. Child. 223-227, 2001.
39. Carapetis, J., Wolff, D., et al.: Acute rheumatic fever and rheumatic heart disease in the Top End of Australia's Northern Territory. Med. J. Aust. 164:146-149, 1996.
40. Cardoso, F.: Chorea: Non-genetic causes. Curr. Opin. Neurol. 17:433-436, 2004.
41. Catanzaro, F., Rammelkamp, C., et al.: Prevention of rheumatic fever by treatment of streptococcal infections, II: Factors responsible for failures. N. Engl. J. Med. 259:51-57, 1958.
42. Catanzaro, F. J., Jetson, C. A., et al.: The role of the streptococcus in the pathogenesis of rheumatic fever. Am. J. Med. 17:749-756, 1954.
43. Centor, R. M., Witherspoon, J. M., Dalton, H. P., et al.: The diagnosis of strep throat in adults in the emergency room. Med. Decis. Making 1:239-246, 1981.
44. Chauvaud, S., Perier, P., et al.: Long-term results of valve repair in children with acquired mitral valve incompetence. Circulation 74(Suppl.):104-109, 1986.
45. Chun, L. T., Reddy, D. V., et al.: Occurrence and prevention of rheumatic fever among ethnic groups of Hawaii. Am. J. Dis. Child. 138:476-478, 1984.

46. Chun, L. T., Reddy, D. V., et al.: Rheumatic fever in children and adolescents in Hawaii. Pediatrics 79:549-552, 1987.

47. Cilliers, A. M., Manyemba, J., Saloojee, H.: Anti-inflammatory treatment for carditis in acute rheumatic fever (review). Cochrane Database Syst. Rev. 3, CD003176, 2003.

48. Clegg, H. W., Ryan, A. G., Dallas, S. D., et al.: Treatment of streptococcal pharyngitis with once-daily compared with twice-daily amoxicillin: A noninferiority trial. Pediatr. Infect. Dis. J. 25:761-767, 2006.

49. Combined Rheumatic Fever Study Group: A comparison of short-term, intensive prednisone and acetylsalicylic acid therapy in the treatment of acute rheumatic fever. N. Engl. J. Med. 272:63-70, 1965.

50. Committee on Infectious Diseases, American Academy of Pediatrics: Red Book: 2006 Report of the Committee on Infectious Diseases. Elk Grove, IL, American Academy of Pediatrics, 2006.

51. Congeni, B., Rizzo, C., et al.: Outbreak of acute rheumatic fever in northeast Ohio. J. Pediatr. 111:176-179, 1987.

52. Coulehan, J., Grant, S., et al.: Acute rheumatic fever and rheumatic heart disease on the Navajo Reservation, 1962-77. Public Health Rep. 95:62-68, 1980.

53. Cunningham, M.: Pathogenesis of group A streptococcal infections. Clin. Microbiol. Rev. 13:470-511, 2000.

54. Cunningham, M., and Russell, M.: Study of heart-reactive antibody in antisera and hybridoma culture fluids against group A streptococci. Infect. Immunity 42:531-538, 1983.

55. Currie, B. J.: Group A streptococcal infections of the skin: Molecular advances but limited therapeutic progress. Curr. Opin. Infect. Dis. 19:132-138, 2006.

56. Dajani, A., Bisno, A., et al.: Prevention of bacterial endocarditis: Recommendations by the American Heart Association. J. A. M. A. 264:2919-2922, 1990.

57. Dajani, A., Taubert, K., et al.: Treatment of acute streptococcal pharyngitis and prevention of rheumatic fever: A statement for health professionals. Pediatrics 96:758-764, 1995.

58. Dajani, A. S., Taubert, K., et al.: Treatment of acute streptococcal pharyngitis and prevention of rheumatic fever: A statement for health professionals. Pediatrics 96:758-764, 1995.

59. Dajani, A. S., Taubert, K. A., et al.: Prevention of bacterial endocarditis: Recommendations by the American Heart Association. J. A. M. A. 277:1794-1801, 1997.

60. Dale, J. B., and Beachey, E. H.: Protective antigenic determinant of streptococcal M protein shared with sarcolemmal membrane protein in human heart. J. Exp. Med. 156:1165-1176, 1982.

61. Dale, J. B., and Beachey, E. H.: Epitopes of streptococcal M proteins shared with cardiac myosin. J. Exp. Med. 162:583-591, 1985.

62. Dale, J. B., and Beachey, E. H.: Human cytotoxic T lymphocytes evoked by group A streptococcal M proteins. J. Exp. Med. 166:1825-1937, 1987.

63. Daoud, A. S., Zaki, M., et al.: Effectiveness of sodium valproate in the treatment of Sydenham's chorea. Neurology 40:1140-1141, 1990.

63a. De Cunto, C. L., Giannini, E. H., Fink, C. W., et al.: Prognosis of children with poststreptococcal reactive arthritis. Pediatr. Infect. Dis. J. 7:683-686, 1988.

64. Denny, F., Wannamaker, L., et al.: Prevention of rheumatic fever: Treatment of the preceding streptococcic infection. J. A. M. A. 143:151-153, 1950.

65. Denny, F. W.: A 45-year perspective on the streptococcus and rheumatic fever: The Edward H. Kass lecture in infectious disease history. Clin. Infect. Dis. 19:1110-1122, 1994.

66. Eckerd, J. M., and McJunkin, J. E.: Recent increase in incidence of acute rheumatic fever in southern West Virginia. W. Va. Med. J. 85:323-325, 1989.

67. Feder, H. M., Gerber, M. A., et al.: Once-daily therapy for streptococcal pharyngitis with amoxycillin. Pediatrics 103:47-51, 1999.

68. Feinstein, A. R., and Spagnuolo, M.: Mimetic features of rheumatic fever recurrences. N. Engl. J. Med. 262:533-540, 1960.

69. Feldman, B. M., Zabriskie, J. B., et al.: Diagnostic use of B-cell alloantigen D8/17 in rheumatic chorea. J. Pediatr. 123:84-86, 1993.

70. Ferguson, G. W., Shultz, J. M., et al.: Epidemiology of acute rheumatic fever in a multiethnic, multiracial urban community: The Miami-Dade County experience. J. Infect. Dis. 164:720-725, 1991.

71. Ferrieri, P., and Jones Criteria Working Group: Proceedings of the Jones Criteria workshop. Circulation 106:2521-2523, 2002.

72. Figueroa, F. E., Fernandez, M. S., et al.: Prospective comparison of clinical and echocardiographic diagnosis of rheumatic carditis: Long term follow up of patients with subclinical disease. Heart 85:407-410, 2001.

73. Folger, G. M., Hajar, R., et al.: Occurrence of valvular heart disease in acute rheumatic fever without evident carditis: Colour flow Doppler identification. Br. Heart J. 67:434-438, 1992.

74. Folger, G. M., Hajar, R., et al.: Doppler echocardiographic findings of mitral and aortic valve regurgitation in children manifesting only rheumatic arthritis. Am. J. Cardiol. 63:1278-1280, 1989.

75. Frankish, J. D.: Rheumatic fever prophylaxis: Gisborne experience. N. Z. Med. J. 97:674-675, 1984.

76. Genel, F., Arslanoglu, S., et al.: Sydenham's chorea: Clinical findings and comparison of the efficacies of sodium valproate and carbamazepine regimens. Brain Dev. 24:73-76, 2002.

77. Gentles, T. L., Colan, S. D., et al.: Left ventricular mechanics during and after acute rheumatic fever: Contractile dysfunction is closely related to valve regurgitation. J. Am. Coll. Cardiol. 37:201-207, 2001.

78. Gerber, M. A., Randolph, M. F., et al.: Antigen detection test for streptococcal pharyngitis: Evaluation of sensitivity with respect to true infections. J. Pediatr. 108:654-658, 1986.

79. Gerber, M. A., and Shulman, S. T.: Rapid diagnosis of pharyngitis caused by group A streptococci. Clin. Microbiol. Rev. 17:571-580, 2004.

80. Gibofsky, A., and Zabriskie, J.: Rheumatic fever: New insights into an old disease. Bull. Rheum. Dis. 42:5-7, 1994.

81. Goldstein, I., Halpern, B., et al.: Immunological relationship between streptococcus A polysaccharide and the structural glycoproteins of heart value. Nature 213:44-47, 1967.

82. Gordis, L.: Effectiveness of comprehensive-care programs in preventing rheumatic fever. N. Engl. J. Med. 289:331-335, 1973.

83. Gordis, L., Lilienfeld, A., et al.: A community-wide study of acute rheumatic fever in adults: Epidemiologic and preventive factors. J. A. M. A. 210:862-865, 1969.

84. Gordis, L., Lilienfeld, A., et al.: Studies in the epidemiology and preventability of rheumatic fever. II: Socio-economic factors and the incidence of acute attacks. J. Chron. Dis. 21:645-654, 1969.

85. Gordis, L., Lilienfeld, A., et al.: Studies in the epidemiology and preventability of rheumatic fever. II: Socio-economic factors and the incidence of acute attacks. J. Chron. Dis. 21:655-666, 1969.

86. Gray, E. D., Regelmann, W. E., et al.: Compartmentalisation of cells bearing "rheumatic" cell surface antigens in peripheral blood and tonsils in rheumatic heart disease. J. Infect. Dis. 155:247-252, 1987.

87. Grayson, S., Horsburgh, M., et al.: An Auckland regional audit of the nurse-led rheumatic fever secondary prophylaxis programme. N. Z. Med. J. 119:U2255, 2006.

88. Griffiths, S. P., and Gersony, W. M.: Acute rheumatic fever in New York City (1969-1988): A comparative study of two decades. J. Pediatr. 116:882-887, 1990.

89. Harlan, G. A., Tani, L. Y., et al.: Rheumatic fever presenting as monoarticular arthritis. Pediatr. Infect. Dis. J. 25:743-746, 2006.

90. Harrington, Z., Visvanathan, K., et al.: B-cell antigen D8/17 is a marker of rheumatic fever susceptibility in Aboriginal Australians and can be tested in remote settings. Med. J. Aust. 184:507-510, 2006.

91. Hashkes, P. J., Tauber, T., et al.: Naproxen as an alternative to aspirin for the treatment of arthritis of rheumatic fever: A randomized trial. J. Pediatr. 143:399-401, 2003.

92. Homer, C., and Shulman, S.: Clinical aspects of acute rheumatic fever. J. Rheumatol. 18:2-13, 1991.

93. Hosier, D., Craenen, J., et al.: Resurgence of acute rheumatic fever. Am. J. Dis. Child. 141:730-733, 1987.

94. International Rheumatic Fever Study Group: Allergic reactions to long-term benzathine penicillin prophylaxis for rheumatic fever. Lancet 337:1308-1310, 1991.

95. Kaplan, E.: Acute rheumatic fever. Pediatr. Clin. North Am. 25:817-829, 1978.

96. Kaplan, E., Berrios, X., et al.: Pharmacokinetics of benzathine penicillin G: Serum levels during the 28 days after intramuscular injection of 1,200,000 units. J. Pediatr. 115:146-151, 1989.

97. Kaplan, E., Johnson, D., et al.: Group A streptococcal serotypes isolated from patients and sibling contacts during the resurgence of rheumatic fever in the United States in the mid-1980s. J. Infect. Dis. 159:101-103, 1989.

98. Kaplan, E., Rothermel, C., et al.: Antistreptolysin O and anti-deoxyribonuclease B titers: Normal values for children ages 2 to 12 in the United States. Pediatrics 101:86-88, 1998.

99. Kaplan, E., Top, F., et al.: Diagnosis of streptococcal pharyngitis: Differentiation of active infection from the carrier state in the symptomatic child. J. Infect. Dis. 123:490-501, 1971.

100. Kaplan, E., and Wannamaker, L.: Streptolysin O: Suppression of its antigenicity by lipids extracted from skin. Proc. Soc. Exp. Biol. Med. 146:205-208, 1974.

101. Kaplan, E. L., and Bisno, A. L.: Antecedent streptococcal infection in acute rheumatic fever. Clin. Infect. Dis. 43:690-692, 2006.

102. Kaplan, M., Bolande, R., et al.: Presence of bound immunoglobulins and complement in the myocardium in acute rheumatic fever: Association with cardiac failure. N. Engl. J. Med. 271:637-645, 1964.

103. Kassem, A. S., Zaher, S. R., et al.: Rheumatic fever prophylaxis using benzathine penicillin G (BPG): Two-week versus four-week regimens: Comparison of two brands of BPG. Pediatrics 97(Pt. 2):992-925, 1996.

104. Khriesat, I., and Najada, A. H.: Acute rheumatic fever without early carditis: An atypical clinical presentation. Eur. J. Pediatr. 162:868-871, 2003.

105. Kumar, R.: Controlling rheumatic heart disease in developing countries. World Health Forum 16:47-51, 1995.

106. Kurlan, R., and Kaplan, E. L.: The pediatric autoimmune neuropsychiatric disorders associated with streptococcal infection (PANDAS) etiology for tics and obsessive-compulsive symptoms: Hypothesis or entity? Practical considerations for the clinician. Pediatrics 113:883-886, 2004.

107. Laitinen, O., Leirisalo, M., et al.: Rheumatic fever and Yersinia arthritis criteria and diagnostic problems in a changing disease pattern. Scand. J. Rheumatol. 4:145-157, 1975.

107a. Lancefield, R. C.: Current knowledge of type-specific Mantigens of group A streptococci. J. Immunol. 89:307-313, 1962.

108. Land, M., and Bisno, A.: Acute rheumatic fever: A vanishing disease in suburbia. J. A. M. A. 249:895-898, 1983.

109. Leggiadro, R., Birnbaum, S., et al.: A resurgence of acute rheumatic fever in a mid-South children's hospital. South. Med. J. *83*:1418-1420, 1990.

110. Lennon, D.: Acute rheumatic fever in children: Recognition and treatment. Pediatr. Drugs *6*:363-373, 2004.

111. Lennon, D., Arroll, B., et al.: Meta analysis of streptococcal throat treatment trials to prevent rheumatic fever primarily in a school-based setting supports this intervention for the control of acute rheumatic fever. Lancet 2007.

112. Lennon, D., Farrell, E., et al.: Once-daily amoxicillin versus twice-daily penicillin V in group A β-hemolytic streptococcal pharyngitis. 2006.

113. Lennon, D., Martin, D., et al.: Longitudinal study of poststreptococcal disease in Auckland: Rheumatic fever, glomerulonephritis, epidemiology and M typing 1981-86. N. Z. Med. J. *101*(Pt. 2):396-398, 1988.

114. Lennon, D., Stewart, J., et al.: A RCT of a school-based primary prevention programme for rheumatic fever. 2007.

115. Lennon, D., Wilson, N., et al.: New Zealand guidelines for rheumatic fever, 1: Diagnosis, management and secondary prophylaxis. 2006.

116. Lennon, D., Wilson, N., et al.: New Zealand guidelines for rheumatic fever, 2: Sore throat management. 2006.

117. Lue, H., Wu, M., et al.: Long-term outcome of patients with rheumatic fever receiving benzathine penicillin G prophylaxis every three weeks versus every four weeks. J. Pediatr. *125*(Pt. 1):812-817, 1994.

118. Lue, H. C., Wu, M. H., et al.: Three-versus four-week administration of benzathine penicillin G: Effects on incidence of streptococcal infections and recurrences of rheumatic fever. Pediatrics *97*(Pt. 2):984-988, 1996.

119. Majeed, H., Yousof, A., et al.: The natural history of acute rheumatic fever in Kuwait: A prospective 6-year follow-up report. J. Chron. Dis. *39*:361-369, 1986.

120. Majeed, H., Yousof, A., et al.: Group A streptococcal strains in Kuwait: A nine-year prospective study of prevalence and associations. Pediatr. Infect. Dis. J. *11*:295-300, 1992.

121. Manyemba, J., and Mayosi, B. M.: Penicillin for secondary prevention of rheumatic fever. Cochrane Database Syst. Rev. *3*:CD002227, 2002.

122. Marijon, E., Ou, P., Celermajer, D. S., et al.: Prevalence of rheumatic heart disease detected by echocardiographic screening. N. Engl. J. Med. *357*:470-476, 2007.

123. Markowitz, M.: Evolution and critique of changes in the Jones Criteria for diagnosis of rheumatic fever. N. Z. Med. J. *101*:392-394, 1988.

124. Markowitz, M.: Streptococcal disease in developing countries. Pediatr. Infect. Dis. J. *10*:S11-S38, 1991.

125. Markowitz, M., and Gordis, L.: Rheumatic Fever. Philadelphia, W. B. Saunders, 1972.

126. Markowitz, M., and Kaplan, E.: Reappearance of rheumatic fever. Adv. Pediatr. *36*:39-68, 1989.

127. Marrack, P., and Kappler, J.: The staphylococcal enterotoxins and their relatives. Science *248*:705-711, 1990.

128. Martin, D., and Single, L.: Molecular epidemiology of group A streptococcus M type 1 infections. J. Infect. Dis. *167*:1112-1117, 1993.

129. Martin, D. R., Voss, L. M., et al.: Acute rheumatic fever in Auckland, New Zealand: Spectrum of associated group A streptococci different from expected. Pediatr. Infect. Dis. J. *13*:264-269, 1994.

130. Martins, T. B., Veasy, L. G., et al.: Antibody responses to group A streptococcal infections in acute rheumatic fever. Pediatr. Infect. Dis. J. *25*:832-837, 2006.

131. Massell, B., Amezcuac, F., et al.: Evolving picture of rheumatic fever: Data from 40 years at the House of the Good Samaritan. J. A. M. A. *188*:287-294, 1964.

132. Massell, B., Chute, C., et al.: Penicillin and the marked decrease in morbidity and mortality from rheumatic fever in the United States. N. Engl. J. Med. *318*:280-286, 1988.

133. Massell, B. F., Honikman, L. H., et al.: Rheumatic fever following streptococcal vaccination: Report of three cases. J. A. M. A. *207*:1115-1119, 1969.

134. McIsaac, W. J., Goel, V., et al.: Reconsidering sore throats, Part 2: Alternative approach and practical office tool. Can. Fam. Physician *43*:495-500, 1997.

135. McIsaac, W. J., Kellner, J. D., et al.: Empirical validation of guidelines for the management of pharyngitis in children and adults. J. A. M. A. *291*:1587-1595, 2004.

136. McLaren, M. J., Hawkins, D. M., et al.: Epidemiology of rheumatic heart disease in black schoolchildren of Soweto, Johannesburg. B. M. J. *3*:474-478, 1975.

137. McNeil, S. A., Halperin, S. A., et al.: Safety and immunogenicity of 26-valent group A streptococcus vaccine in healthy adult volunteers. Clin. Infect. Dis. *41*:1114-1122, 2005.

138. Miyake, C. Y., Gauvreau, K., Tani, L. Y., et al.: Characteristics of children discharged from hospitals in the United States in 2000 with the diagnosis of acute rheumatic fever. Pediatrics *120*:503-508, 2007.

139. Moore, D.: Neuropsychiatric aspects of Sydenham's chorea: A comprehensive review. J. Clin. Psychiatry *57*:407-414, 1996.

140. Moore, P., and Mortland, T.: *Mycoplasma pneumoniae* infection mimicking acute rheumatic fever. Pediatr. Infect. Dis. J. *13*:81-82, 1994.

141. Morris, K., Mohan, C., et al.: Increased inactivated T cells and reduction in suppressor/cytotoxic T cells in acute rheumatic fever and active heart disease: A longitudinal study. J. Infect. Dis. *167*:3979-3983, 1993.

142. Morris, K., Mohan, C., et al.: Enhancement of IL-1, IL-2, production and IL-2 receptor generation in patients with acute rheumatic fever and active rheumatic heart disease: A prospective study. Clin. Exp. Immunol. *91*:429-436, 1993.

143. Morton, W., Huhn, L., et al.: Rheumatic heart disease epidemiology: Observations on 17,366 Denver schoolchildren. J. A. M. A. *199*:879-884, 1967.

144. Narula, J., Chopra, P., et al.: Does endomyocardial biopsy aid in the diagnosis of active rheumatic carditis? Circulation *88*(Pt. 1):2198-2205, 1993.

145. Nausieda, P., Grossman, B., et al.: Sydenham chorea: An update. Neurology *30*:331-334, 1980.

146. Newman, J., Lennon, D., et al.: Patients with rheumatic fever recurrences. N. Z. Med. J. *97*:678-680, 1984.

147. Nordet, P.: WHO/ISFC global programme for the prevention and control of RH/RHD. J. Infect. Cardiol. *3*:4-5, 1993.

148. Padmavati, S.: Rheumatic heart disease: Prevalence and preventive measures in the Indian Subcontinent (editorial). Heart J. *86*:127, 2001.

149. Patarroyo, M. E., Winchester, R. J., et al.: Association of a B-cell alloantigen with susceptibility to rheumatic fever. Nature *278*:173-174, 1979.

150. Paul, J. R.: Epidemiology of Rheumatic Fever. New York, American Heart Association, 1957.

151. Paz, J. A., Silva, C. A. A., et al.: Randomized double-blind study with prednisone in Sydenham's chorea. Pediatr. Neurol. *34*:264-269, 2006.

152. Pena, J., Mora, E., et al.: Comparison of the efficacy of carbamazepine, haloperidol and valproic acid in the treatment of children with Sydenham's chorea: Clinical follow-up of 18 patients. Arq. Neuro-Psiquiatr. *60*(2B):374-377, 2002.

153. Perry, C., and Roberts, J.: A study on the variability in the incidence of rheumatic heart disease within the city of Bristol. B. M. J. 154-158, 1937.

154. Phibbs, B.: Streptococcal control in school children: Is it worthwhile? Minn. Med. 607-610, 1975.

155. Phibbs, B., Lundin, S., et al.: Experience of a Wyoming County Streptococcal Control Project. West. J. Med. *148*:546-550, 1988.

156. Pickles, W.: A rheumatic family. Lancet *2*:241, 1943.

157. Pileggi, G. C. S., and Ferriani, P. L.: Atypical arthritis in children with rheumatic fever. J. Pediatr. 76:49-54, 2000.

158. Pinals, R.: Polyarthritis and fever. N. Engl. J. Med. *330*:769-774, 1994.

159. Polly, S. M., Waldman, R. H., et al.: Protective studies with a group A streptococcal M protein vaccine, II: Challange of volunteers after local immunization in the upper respiratory tract. J. Infect. Dis. *131*:217-224, 1975.

160. Pruksakorn, S., Currie, B., et al.: Towards a vaccine for rheumatic fever: Identification of a conserved target epitope on M protein of group A streptococci. Lancet *344*:639-642, 1994.

161. Pruksakorn, S., Sittisombut, N., et al.: Epidemiological analysis of non-M-typeable group A streptococcus isolates from a Thai population in Northern Thailand. J. Clin. Microbiol. *38*:1250-1254, 2000.

162. Quinn, R., and Federspiel, C.: The incidence of rheumatic fever in metropolitan Nashville, 1963-1969. Am. J. Epidemiol *99*:273-280, 1974.

163. Raizada, V., Williams, R., et al.: Tissue distribution of lymphocytes in rheumatic heart valves as defined by monoclonal anti-T cell antibodies. Am. J. Med. *74*:90-96, 1983.

164. Rammelkamp, C., and Stolzer, B.: The latent period before the onset of acute rheumatic fever. Yale J. Biol. Med. *34*:386-398, 1961.

165. Rammelkamp, C., Wannamaker, W., et al.: Studies on the epidemiology of rheumatic fever in the armed services. *In* Thomas, L. (ed.): Rheumatic Fever. Minneapolis, University of Minnesota Press, 1972, p. 72.

166. Randolph, M., Gerber, M., et al.: Effect of antibiotic therapy on the clinical course of streptococcal pharyngitis. J. Pediatr. *106*:870-875, 1985.

167. Reddy, D., Chun, L., et al.: Acute rheumatic fever with advanced degree AV block. Clin. Pediatr. *28*:326-328, 1989.

168. Regelmann, W., Talbot, R., et al.: Distribution of cells bearing "rheumatic" antigens in peripheral blood of patients with rheumatic fever/rheumatic heart disease. J. Rheumatol. *16*:931-935, 1989.

169. Atatoa-Carr, P., Lennon, D., and Wilson, N.: Rheumatic fever diagnosis, management, and secondary prevention: A New Zealand guideline. N. Z. Med. J. *121*:59-69, 2008.

170. Rhodes, P., and Jackson, H.: Rheumatic fever in Colorado: A conquered disease? J. A. M. A. *234*:157-158, 1975.

171. Robbins, S. L.: The Heart: Rheumatic Fever and Rheumatic Heart Disease. Philadelphia, W. B. Saunders, 1994.

172. Robertson, K. A., Volmink, J. A., et al.: Antibiotics for the primary prevention of acute rheumatic fever: a meta-analysis. B. M. C. Cardiovasc. Disord. *5*:1-9, 2005.

173. Sanyal, S., Berry, A., et al.: Sequelae of the initial attack of acute rheumatic fever in children from North India: A prospective 5 year follow-up study. Circulation *65*:375-379, 1982.

174. Sanyal, S., Thapar, M., et al.: The initial attack of acute rheumatic fever during childhood in North India: A prospective study of the clinical profile. Circulation *69*:7-12, 1974.

175. Shet, A., and Kaplan, E. L.: Clinical use and interpretation of group A streptococcal antibody tests: A practical approach for the pediatrician or primary care physician. Pediatr. Infect. Dis. J. *21*:420-426; quiz 427-430, 2002.

176. Shulman, S.: The decline of rheumatic fever: What impact on our management of pharyngitis? Am. J. Dis. Child. *138*:426-427, 1984.

177. Shvartzman, P., Tabenkin, H., et al.: Treatment of streptococcal pharyngitis with amoxycillin once a day. B. M. J. *306*:1170-1172, 1993.

178. Siegel, A., Johnson, E., et al.: Controlled studies of streptococcal pharyngitis in a pediatric population. N. Engl. J. Med. *265*:559-566, 1961.

179. Smoot, J. C., Barbian, K. D., et al.: Genome sequence and comparative microarray analysis of serotype M18 group A streptococcus strains associated with

acute rheumatic fever outbreaks. Proc. Natl. Acad. Sci. U. S. A. *99*:4668-4673, 2002.

180. Smoot, J. C., Korgenski, E. K., et al.: Molecular analysis of group A streptococcus type M18 isolates temporally associated with acute rheumatic fever outbreaks in Salt Lake City, Utah. J. Clin. Microbiol. *40*:1805-1810, 2002.
181. Spagnuolo, M., and Taranta, A.: Rheumatic fever in siblings: Similarity of its clinical manifestations. N. Engl. J. Med. *278*:183-188, 1968.
182. Special Writing Group of the Committee on Rheumatic Fever and Kawasaki Disease of the Council on Cardiovascular Disease in the Young of the American Heart Foundation: Guideline for the diagnosis of rheumatic fever: Jones Criteria 1992 update. J. A. M. A. *268*:2069-2073, 1992.
183. Spinetto, H., Lennon, D., et al.: Control of rheumatic fever recurrences in Auckland, New Zealand: Questions answered. 2007.
184. Stollerman, G.: Rheumatogenic streptococci and autoimmunity. Clin. Immunol. Immunopathol. *61*:131-142, 1991.
185. Stollerman, G., Lewis, A., et al.: Relationship of immune response to group A streptococci to the course of acute chronic and recurrent rheumatic fever. Am. J. Med. 163-169, 1956.
186. Stollerman, G. H.: Rheumatic Fever and Streptococcal Infection. New York, Grune & Stratton, 1975.
187. Strasser, T.: Cost-effective control of rheumatic fever in the community. Health Policy *5*:159-164, 1985.
188. Swedo, S.: Sydenham's chorea: A model for childhood autoimmune neuropsychiatric disorders. J. A. M. A. *272*:1788-1791, 1994.
189. Swedo, S., Leonard, H., et al.: Identification of children with pediatric autoimmune neuropsychiatric disorders associated with streptococcal infections by a marker associated with rheumatic fever. Am. J. Psychiatry *154*:110-112, 1997.
190. Taranta, A., and Markowitz, M.: Rheumatic Fever. 2nd ed. Boston, Kluwer Academic, 1989.
191. Taranta, A., Spagnuolo, M., et al.: "Chronic" rheumatic fever. Ann. Intern. Med. *56*:367-388, 1962.
192. Taranta, A., Spagnuolo, M., et al.: Rheumatic fever in monozygotic and dizygotic twins. Circulation *20*:778, 1959.
193. Taubert, K., Rowley, A.: Seven-year national survey of Kawasaki disease and acute rheumatic fever. Pediatr. Infect. Dis. J. *13*:704-708, 1994.
194. Terreri, M. T., Roja, S. C., Faustino, P. C., et al.: Sydenham's chorea—clinical and evolutive characteristics. Sao Paulo Med. J. (Rev. Paulista Med.) *120*:16-19, 2002.
195. Tomai, M., Kotb, M., et al.: Superantigenicity of streptococcal M protein. J. Exp. Med. *172*:359-362, 1990.
196. Tompkins, R., Burnes, D., et al.: An analysis of the cost-effectiveness of pharyngitis management and acute rheumatic fever prevention. Ann. Intern. Med. *86*:481-492, 1977.
197. Uziel, Y., Hashkes, P., et al.: The use of naproxen in the treatment of children with rheumatic fever. J. Pediatr. *137*:269-271, 2000.
198. Veasy, G.: Time to take soundings in acute rheumatic fever. Lancet *357*, 2001.
199. Veasy, L., Tani, L., et al.: Persistence of acute rheumatic fever in the intermountain area of the United States. J. Pediatr. *124*:9-16, 1994.
200. Veasy, L., Wiedmeier, S., et al.: Resurgence of acute rheumatic fever in the intermountain area of the United States. N. Engl. J. Med. *316*:421-427, 1987.
201. Vendsborg, P., Hansen, L., et al.: Decreasing incidence of a history of acute rheumatic fever in chronic rheumatic heart disease. Cardiologia *53*:332-340, 1968.

202. Vlajinac, H., Adanja, B., et al.: Influence of socio-economic and other factors on rheumatic fever occurrence. Eur. J. Epidemiol. 7:702-704, 1991.
203. Voss, L., Wilson, N., et al.: Intravenous immunoglobulin in acute rheumatic fever: A randomized controlled trial. Circulation 401-406, 2001.
204. Wald, E., Dashefsky, B., et al.: Acute rheumatic fever in western Pennsylvania and the tristate area. Pediatrics *80*:371-374, 1987.
205. Wallace, M., Garst, P., et al.: The return of acute rheumatic fever in young adults. J. A. M. A. *262*:2557-2561, 1989.
206. Wannamaker, L.: Differences between streptococcal infections of the skin and of the throat. N. Engl. J. Med. *282*:23-30, 78-85, 1970.
207. Wannamaker, L.: Virulence factors in streptococci. Scand. J. Infect. Dis. *31*(Suppl.):22-27, 1982.
208. Wannamaker, L., Denny, F., et al.: Effect of penicillin prophylaxis on streptococcal disease rates and the carrier state. N. Engl. J. Med. *249*:1-7, 1953.
209. Wannamaker, L., Rammelkamp, C., et al.: Prophylaxis of acute rheumatic fever: By treatment of the preceding streptococcal infection with various amounts of depot penicillin. Am. J. Med. *10*:673-695, 1951.
210. Westlake, R., Graham, T., et al.: An outbreak of acute rheumatic fever in Tennessee. Pediatr. Infect. Dis. J. *9*:97-100, 1990.
211. Widdowson, J. P., Maxted, W. R., et al.: The antibody responses in man to infection with different serotypes of group-A streptococci. J. Med. Microbiol. *7*:483-496, 1974.
212. Wilson, E., Wilson, N., et al.: Monoarthritis as a major criterion for acute rheumatic fever. Pediatr. Infect. Dis. J. 2007.
213. Wilson, N. J., and Neutze, J. M.: Echocardiographic diagnosis of subclinical carditis in acute rheumatic fever. Int. J. Cardiol. *50*:1-6, 1995.
213a. Wilson, W., Taubert, K. A., Gewitz, M., et al.: Prevention of infective endocarditis: Guidelines from the American Heart Association. Circulation *116*:1736-1754, 2007.
214. Wood, H., Feinstein, A., et al.: Rheumatic fever in children and adolescents: A long-term epidemiologic study of subsequent prophylaxis, streptococcal infections, and clinical sequelae, III: Comparative effectiveness of three prophylaxis regimens in preventing streptococcal infections and rheumatic recurrences. Ann. Intern. Med. *60*(Suppl.):31-45, 1964.
215. Wood, H. F., Feinstein, A. R., et al.: Rheumatic fever in children and adolescents: A long term epidemiologic study of subsequent prophylaxis, streptococcal infections and clinical sequelae, III: Comparative effectiveness of three prophylaxis regimens in preventing streptococcal infections and rheumatic recurrences. Ann. Intern. Med. *60*(Suppl. 5):31-46, 1964.
216. World Health Organization: WHO evaluation of the streptozyme test for streptococcal antibodies. Bull. W. H. O. *64*:504, 1986.
217. World Health Organization: The current evidence for the burden of Group A streptococcal diseases. 60, 2005.
218. Zabriskie, J., Lavenchy, D., et al.: Rheumatic fever-associated B cell alloantigens as identified by monoclonal antibodies. Arthritis Rheum. *28*:1047-1051, 1985.
219. Zabriskie, J. B.: Rheumatic fever: A model for the pathological consequences of microbial-host mimicry. Clin. Exp. Rheumatol. *4*:65-73, 1986.
220. Zangwill, K., Wald, E., et al.: Acute rheumatic fever in western Pennsylvania: A persistent problem into the 1990s. J. Pediatr. *118*:561-563, 1991.
221. Zedan, M., El-Shennawy, F., et al.: Interleukin-2 in relation to T cell subpopulations in rheumatic heart disease. Arch. Dis. Child. *67*:1373-1375, 1992.
222. Zomorrodi, M. D., and Wald, E. R.: Sydenham's chorea in western Pennsylvania. Pediatrics *117*:e675-e679, 2006.

CHAPTER 36

MEDIASTINITIS

Morven S. Edwards

The mediastinum is the extrapleural portion of the thoracic cavity situated between the two pleural sacs. The superior and inferior portions are separated arbitrarily by a line extending from the lower manubrium to the fourth thoracic vertebra. The superior mediastinum contains the thymus gland, trachea, esophagus, and aortic arch. The inferior mediastinum is divided into the anterior compartment, containing lymphatic tissue and fat; the middle compartment, containing the heart, pericardium, aorta, bifurcation of the trachea, main bronchi, and numerous lymph nodes; and the posterior compartment, containing the esophagus, thoracic duct, descending aorta, and vagus nerve. *Mediastinitis* refers to inflammation of the tissues located in the mediastinum. Infections of the mediastinum are uncommon occurrences, but often they pose a serious threat to vital structures and can prove extremely difficult to diagnose.

Acute mediastinitis is a fulminant, septic process, and chronic mediastinitis is an indolent infection that produces late symptoms caused by compression of adjacent structures. Acute mediastinitis is subclassified as (1) traumatic, occurring as a consequence of perforation of the esophagus; (2) infection extending to the mediastinum from adjacent structures; and (3) postoperative mediastinitis, usually occurring after thoracic surgery (Table 36-1).

ACUTE MEDIASTINITIS

ACUTE MEDIASTINITIS DUE TO ESOPHAGEAL PERFORATION

The esophagus is a thin-walled organ, and esophageal perforation is the most common cause of acute mediastinitis.[43] Perforation usually occurs at one of the three sites of anatomic narrowing of

TABLE 36-1   Classification of Mediastinitis

I. Acute mediastinitis
   A. Due to traumatic perforation of the esophagus
      1. Spontaneous or post-emetic
      2. Foreign body-associated
      3. Instrumentation or surgery
   B. Due to extension of infection from adjacent structures
      1. Infection of the head and neck
      2. Infections of lungs, pleura, lymph nodes, or pericardium
      3. Subphrenic infection
      4. Vertebral osteomyelitis
      5. Hematogenous dissemination
   C. Postoperative
II. Chronic mediastinitis

the esophagus: (1) the proximal end, located at the level of the cricopharyngeal muscle; (2) the midthoracic segment, where the aortic arch and left main stem bronchus indent the esophagus; or (3) the transdiaphragmatic segment. A correlation exists between the location of the perforation and the injury. Proximal perforations usually are caused by instrumentation or ingestion of a foreign body. The proximal segment is the narrowest, and perforations generally are located in the posterior wall, adjacent to the prevertebral and retrovisceral spaces. Perforations at the aortic arch usually are caused by ingested foreign bodies. Transdiaphragmatic perforations usually are spontaneous. In most such cases, a longitudinal tear occurs on the left posterolateral wall just above the cardia, where the esophagus has little connective tissue support and its intrinsic musculature is weak.

Retching or vomiting can generate sufficient force to cause esophageal perforation, also known as Boerhaave syndrome, but its occurrence is rare.[1] Traumatic perforation can occur after blunt trauma, from ingestion of a foreign body, or as a complication of endoscopic or open surgical procedures. In one large series of acute purulent mediastinitis, ingestion of a foreign body was a major cause of esophageal injury.[7] Children with mediastinitis from erosion of the esophagus caused by a foreign body tend to have small and well-contained perforations. Sharp objects, such as pins and bone fragments, can cause immediate transmural penetration. More commonly, and especially with blunt objects such as coins, teeth, and food particles (e.g., corn chips), the foreign body becomes impacted in the esophagus.[39] Eventually, suppurative necrosis of the wall occurs, with symptoms occurring days, weeks, or months after the ingestion.[22]

Perforations from instrumentation can produce precipitous clinical deterioration during the procedure from transmural laceration.[43] Alternatively, a superficial tear can occur from which infection subsequently extends, and several hours or days can elapse between instrumentation and the onset of symptoms. Repair of esophageal atresia is a common condition associated with a tear of the esophagus in childhood. In one review, 7 of 41 infants had a clinically significant esophageal disruption requiring reoperation 1 to 18 days after repair of esophageal atresia.[6] Mediastinitis complicated repair of esophageal atresia in 3.6 percent of 223 cases in another large series.[41] Postoperative perforations of the esophagus usually represent infectious complications of anastomotic leaks occurring after esophageal resection or of esophageal-pleural fistulas that develop after thoracic surgery. Most of these infections do not become apparent until weeks or months after surgery.

The predominant symptoms of acute mediastinitis after perforation of the esophagus are neck and chest pain, respiratory distress, and dysphagia. Chills, fever of 37.8° C to 39° C (100° F to 102° F), and leukocytosis also are common. Infants can present with tachypnea, tachycardia, stridor, or a supplemental oxygen requirement.[22] Some patients have a staccato breathing pattern characterized by an inspiratory halt with resumption of inspira-

tion after a brief rest.[12] The onset of symptoms usually is abrupt, and the course is fulminant. Approximately 20 to 30 percent of patients are comatose or hypotensive when first seen.[1] Physical examination often reveals cervical tenderness and subcutaneous emphysema in patients with proximal perforations, whereas patients with perforations of the lower esophagus are more likely to have signs suggesting an acute abdominal catastrophe. Examination of the lung fields often shows nonspecific abnormalities. The Hamman sign (a "crunching" sound heard in synchrony with the heartbeat along the left sternal border or cardiac apex) is observed in approximately 50 percent of cases of mediastinal emphysema, but it also occurs with left pneumothorax, dilated esophagus, gastric dilation, bullous emphysema, and pneumoperitoneum.

The principal findings on chest radiographs are a widened mediastinum, subcutaneous and mediastinal emphysema, and pleural effusions. Pleural effusions occur more commonly with perforations of the lower than the upper esophagus and usually involve the left side. Basilar or retrocardiac infiltrates ascribed to chemical pneumonitis can occur in the pulmonary segment adjacent to the site of perforation. Additional changes often include basilar atelectasis, pneumothorax, or a hydropneumothorax. Radiopaque foreign bodies can be detected with plain radiographs, but often they are seen better with mediastinal computed tomography (CT).

Gas in the soft tissues seen on radiography is highly suggestive of perforation of the esophagus if interpreted in the context of a compatible clinical presentation. Gas in the prevertebral tissue or superior mediastinum occurs most commonly with perforation of the upper esophagus. Other conditions, such as chest wall trauma or perforation of the trachea, also can cause mediastinal emphysema.

The diagnosis of acute mediastinitis caused by perforation of the esophagus often can be made on the basis of the clinical setting coupled with routine chest radiograph findings. Contrast-enhanced CT or magnetic resonance imaging (MRI) can provide additional anatomic detail and confirmation of the diagnosis.[47] The findings include esophageal thickening, fluid collections in the mediastinum adjacent to the perforation, and extraluminal air.[2] Other routine laboratory tests are not helpful. Analysis of pleural fluid usually shows a sterile exudate early in the disease course. Pleural fluid amylase levels often are normal within the first 24 hours after perforation. After 24 hours, the pleural fluid amylase level is elevated disproportionately compared with serum levels. Esophagoscopy is unnecessary and is contraindicated except for removing a foreign body.

The standard treatment comprises surgical drainage and repair and antimicrobial therapy and should be undertaken for large perforations, when there is communication with the pleural space or abdomen, when vascular erosion is a concern, and in the setting of underlying esophageal pathology. Nonsurgical management can be considered for children in whom the perforation is a small, well-contained lesion in the upper esophagus in the absence of underlying esophageal pathology.[10,22] Supportive measures include intravenous fluid support, maintenance of an adequate airway, esophageal rest (i.e., no food), and careful monitoring of vital functions.

Selection of antimicrobial treatment optimally is determined by bacteriologic studies. Blood and pleural fluid cultures should be obtained, but they usually are sterile except late in the course. Consequently, decisions with regard to antimicrobials necessarily are empiric and should be directed against oral anaerobic bacteria and streptococci.[5,8]

Mortality rates are 15 to 40 percent and are especially high when recognition of the infection in its early stages is delayed.[1,7,41,43] Mortality rates for children are lower than the rates for adults. An exception is postoperative perforation of the esophagus, which tends to follow a more indolent course.

ACUTE MEDIASTINITIS DUE TO EXTENSION OF INFECTION FROM ADJACENT STRUCTURES

The mediastinum is anatomically well situated for involvement when infection extends downward from the oropharynx. Fascial planes from the supraclavicular region and abdomen traverse the mediastinum, and the lymphatic duct is located in the mediastinum. The lung, situated laterally to the mediastinum, is a frequent locus of potentially serious infection. Despite its position as an anatomic crossroad, however, extension of infection to the mediastinum from adjacent structures occurs infrequently.

In the pre-antibiotic era, retropharyngeal or peritonsillar abscess, Ludwig angina, dental abscess, and other infections of the head and neck were common causes of acute mediastinitis.[8,14,46,51] Since the advent of penicillin, infections of the head and neck usually are contained at the site of origin. The principal spaces that serve as conduits to the mediastinum when these infections do spread are the visceral division of the deep cervical fascia that envelops the esophagus, trachea, larynx, and thyroid gland and the carotid sheath, which extends from the base of the skull, passes through the posterior pharyngomaxillary space along the prevertebral fascia, and enters the chest. Conditions other than pharyngitis and peritonsillar and dental abscesses that have preceded the development of mediastinitis include mastoiditis, laryngectomy, mediastinotomy, tracheostomy, and surgery or trauma of the oropharynx. Mediastinitis can complicate placement of airway stents for management of tracheal or bronchial stenoses in children.[21]

Children have developed mediastinitis after incurring intraoral injuries caused by falling with an object such as a toothbrush in their mouths.[25] Infection spreads to the mediastinum through the retropharyngeal space. Other sharp objects, such as fish bones, can perforate the esophagus, with resultant infection.[36] A penetrating wound to the oropharynx can be caused by falling on a sharp or pointed object such as a pencil. Occasionally, foreign bodies retained in the esophagus for months to years can have life-threatening complications, such as bronchoesophageal fistula or mediastinitis. Reported items causing such morbidity include coins, a heart pendant, a clothespin spring, and a toy soldier.[17] Mediastinitis rarely results in a complication of suppurative pleuropulmonary infection. Extension of infection from vertebrae, ribs, or sternum also is unusual. The main radiographic feature by plain chest radiograph is widening of the mediastinum. Contrast-enhanced cervicothoracic CT scan is crucial for establishing the diagnosis and can reveal heterogeneous infiltration, gas in tissues, abscesses, and fluid collections (Fig. 36–1).

The major bacteria responsible for suppurative infections that originate in the oral cavity and extend to the mediastinum are streptococci and anaerobic oral flora.[8,35] Mixed infection with aerobes and anaerobes should be anticipated when empiric therapy is initiated. Group A streptococcus is a common pathogen when the oropharynx is the original portal of entry. Other streptococci, including *Streptococcus milleri*, *Streptococcus anginosis*, and group F streptococcus, are common isolates. Anaerobic bacteria, principally *Prevotella* spp., *Bacteroides* spp., *Fusobacterium* spp., and peptostreptococci, are the major anaerobic pathogens. Gram-negative aerobic bacteria, including *Pseudomonas aeruginosa*, *Serratia* spp., and *Neisseria* spp., are isolated less often.[28] Clindamycin often is regarded as the agent of choice for streptococci and anaerobes, although some authorities prefer other regimens, including penicillin plus metronidazole, cefoxitin, cefotetan, meropenem, or a β-lactam–β-lactamase inhibitor.[8,13]

Surgical drainage combined with appropriate antibiotic therapy is the cornerstone of treatment. Transcervical incisions usually are employed when spread to the superior mediastinum has occurred. Extension of the infection below the level of the fourth thoracic vertebra requires a parasternal or paravertebral

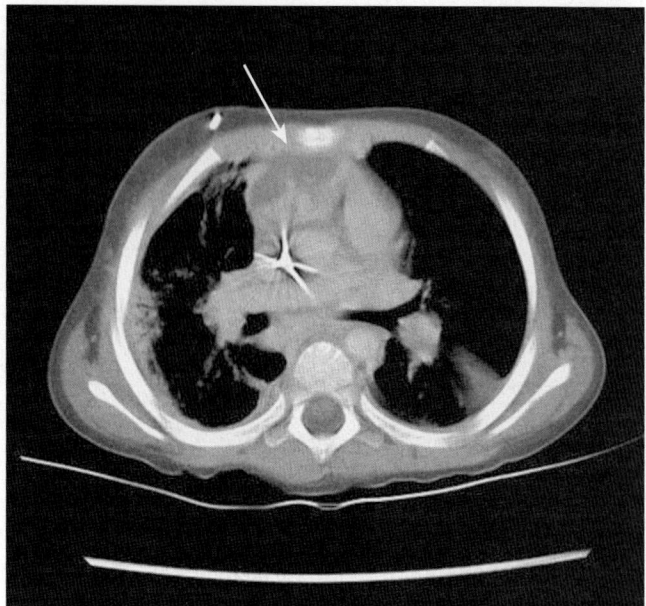

Figure 36–1 Contrast-enhanced computed tomography scan shows a 3 × 3 cm heterogeneous enhancing abscess *(arrow)* in the anterior mediastinum of a child acutely ill with *S. pneumoniae* bacteremia and pneumonia with empyema. Cultures from the mediastinal abscess at the time of surgical drainage were sterile.

TABLE 36–2 Risk Factors for Pediatric Poststernotomy Mediastinitis

Young age
Severe illness (assessed by high ASA score)
Asplenia
Prolonged duration of surgery
Cardiac transplantation
Delayed sternal closure

ASA, American Society of Anesthesiologists.
Data from references 3, 31, 48.

approach, depending on whether the anterior or posterior mediastinum is involved.

POSTOPERATIVE MEDIASTINITIS

Sternal wound infections are an uncommon complication of median sternotomy for cardiac surgery in children.[3,27,31,38,48] The Centers for Disease Control and Prevention classifies surgical site infections in cardiac patients as superficial or deep wound infection, sternal osteomyelitis, or mediastinitis.[20] Mediastinitis is a serious complication, with potential involvement of contiguous structures, including prosthetic valves, grafts, pericardium, lung, and chest wall. Contemporary incidence data for mediastinitis after median sternotomy in children is 0.2 to 1.4 percent of procedures.[3,27,31,48] The incidence is higher after cardiac transplantation.[27] Postoperative wound infection is more often a complication of double-outlet right ventricle repair, truncus repair, atrial switch, or valvulatory or conduit procedures than of repair of atrial septal defect, ventricular septal defect, or tetralogy of Fallot.[38] Mediastinal infection has developed from an infection of a retained epicardial pacemaker lead.[19]

Some of the well-established risk factors for development of poststernotomy mediastinitis in adults are not applicable to children. Table 36–2 lists factors that are linked to risk for development of poststernotomy mediastinitis in children. Obesity and diabetes mellitus, which are risk associations in adults, have not been assessed as potential risk factors in more recent pediatric series. Factors not associated with risk for infection include emergency surgery or prior infection.[31] Intraoperative introduction of organisms is considered the source of most infections. Outbreaks of mediastinitis with *Mycobacterium chelonei* or *Mycobacterium fortuitum* presumably reflect contact with nonsterile water.[23] Epidemics have been traced to operating room personnel who can serve as the source of *Staphylococcus aureus* or other bacteria.[15]

In three contemporary pediatric series, median age at diagnosis of mediastinitis after pediatric cardiac surgery ranged from 6 weeks to 3 years.[3,27,48] Median time to onset of infection after surgery was 10 to 14 days, with a range from 4 to 50 days. The time to infection after initial sternotomy was longer for infections caused by gram-positive bacteria than for infections caused by gram-negative bacteria or fungi in one report.[48] The presenting features include erythema, purulent drainage or tenderness of the sternal incision, wound dehiscence, sternal instability, persistent or recurrent postoperative fever, and leukocytosis. A common clinical sequence is fever and systemic toxicity followed by signs of a sternal wound infection with cellulitis or purulent drainage. The CT abnormalities include mediastinal soft tissue swelling, pleural effusion, and sternal dehiscence or erosion, but CT of the chest does not always reveal abnormalities.[33,50] Consideration should be given to use of alternative testing modalities, such as MRI, when infection is suspected. Lack of compelling radiographic evidence of infection should not delay surgical drainage when clinical signs are evident.

Empiric antibiotic treatment should be initiated based on the expected pathogens and modified according to the results of blood and wound cultures. Approximately two thirds of infections are caused by gram-positive bacteria, one fourth by gram-negative bacteria, and the remainder by yeasts and fungi. The most frequent pathogen is *S. aureus*, which accounts for more than half of infections; coagulase-negative staphylococci and enterococci (including vancomycin-resistant isolates) constitute the remainder of the gram-positive isolates.[3,27,48] In adults, methicillin-resistant *S. aureus* mediastinitis is associated with higher rates of overall mortality, mediastinitis-related mortality, and treatment failure than is infection caused by methicillin-sensitive *S. aureus*, but this association has not been reported for children.[32]

Approximately half of children have associated bacteremia, and infection with *S. aureus* is an independent risk factor for development of bacteremic postoperative mediastinitis.[44] Among gram-negative organisms, *Pseudomonas aeruginosa*, *Serratia* spp., and *Citrobacter* are common isolates. Infection is polymicrobial in one fourth of patients.[3,27,48] *Candida* spp. should be considered in any patient with infection of the mediastinum, particularly when broad-spectrum antimicrobials have been used.[9] Almost any microorganism gaining entry to the mediastinum theoretically can serve as the nidus for infection, and *Mycoplasma hominis*, *Ureaplasma urealyticum*, *Nocardia*, and *Aspergillus* all have been reported, albeit rarely.[16,26,30,49] Heart and lung transplant patients are prone to acquisition of infection with less common and more resistant pathogens, such as *Aspergillus fumigatus* and *Burkholderia cepacia*.[27] *M. fortuitum* can cause apparently culture-negative mediastinitis and has been reported in a child who had undergone a Fontan operation.[45]

Adequate surgical débridement is crucial to successful treatment of postoperative mediastinitis. The sternotomy wound should be reopened, and the sternum and mediastinum should be irrigated and débrided for removal of all devitalized tissue. Some wounds can be managed with direct sternal closure and mediastinal drain; open-wound packing and delayed rectus abdominis flap, pectoralis muscle flap, or omental reconstruction is required in some children.[4,37,48] Pectoralis muscle flap has been

an effective treatment even in neonates.[11,48] Early consultation with the hospital plastic surgery and reconstructive team is advisable in patients in whom sternal reconstruction is anticipated.[48] Infection superficial to the sternum can be treated simply with incision, packing, and a short course of antibiotics, usually for 10 to 14 days. Systemic antibiotics must be given for at least 3 to 6 weeks for children with postoperative mediastinitis.

CHRONIC MEDIASTINITIS

Chronic mediastinitis histologically can be fibrosing or granulomatous. Both are rare conditions in which a definite cause often remains elusive. The clinical presentations are identical, and considerable overlap can occur in histologic findings. Fibrosing mediastinitis, also known as *sclerosing mediastinitis*, can be focal or diffuse; calcification within the lesion is observed more often when the process is focal. Some authors propose that common etiologic mechanisms are responsible and that mediastinal fibrosis represents the end stage of mediastinal granuloma, whereas others suggest that the two are distinct entities.[42] Nonetheless, fibrosing mediastinitis stands apart in being associated sometimes with a fibrotic process at another anatomic site, such as the retroperitoneum.

Chronic mediastinitis occurs in virtually any age group. It is rare in very young children, but has been described in toddlers.[40] Many patients are asymptomatic, and the lesion initially is detected by routine chest radiographs showing a widened superior mediastinum near the tracheal bifurcation or the hilum with a lobulated configuration. Concomitant changes in the pulmonary parenchyma that are seen on chest radiograph vary. Symptoms, when manifested, usually reflect compression of adjacent structures, such as the superior vena cava, pulmonary vessels, esophagus, and tracheobronchial tree. The most common symptoms include cough, pleuritic chest pain, dyspnea, and pleuritic chest pain.[42] Low-grade fever, anemia, and weight loss can be present.

When an inciting cause for chronic mediastinitis can be identified, it usually is linked to infection with *Histoplasma capsulatum*. Two types of mediastinal fibrosis caused by histoplasmosis are recognized. Mediastinal granuloma is caused by coalescence of a cluster of mediastinal lymph nodes to form an encapsulated mass that may be large and compress adjacent structures, especially the superior vena cava or esophagus. Surgical resection often is feasible but is advocated only when the obstruction is significant. Fibrosing mediastinitis is thought to result from an exuberant inflammatory response to *H. capsulatum* and to represent a resolved, rather than an active, infectious process. Less common causes of fibrosing mediastinitis include tuberculosis, blastomycosis, cryptococcosis, aspergillosis, zygomycosis, autoimmune disease, nocardiosis, actinomycosis, and lymphoma.[18,24,29,34,40,42]

The diagnostic evaluation of patients with possible chronic mediastinitis should include a chest radiograph and contrast-enhanced CT or MRI. A vascular imaging study may be required if there is evidence of venous or vena caval obstruction or if arterial involvement is present. Tuberculin skin test and histoplasmosis serology should be obtained. Cultures of sputum for *Mycobacterium tuberculosis* and pathogenic fungi rarely are positive. Antigen assay for *H. capsulatum* using blood and urine usually is negative, and skin tests are not helpful. Complement-fixation titers usually exceed 1:8 in patients with chronic histoplasmosis.

Surgical resection of affected tissues can be associated with high morbidity rates, but can be curative. Biopsy of the lesion by mediastinoscopy provides a means to exclude a malignant process and obtain tissue for histopathologic evaluation. Antifungal therapy is not likely to affect resolution of the process when surgically excised tissue shows *H. capsulatum* in the setting of sterile cultures. Dense fibrosis of mediastinal structures without a granulomatous component does not respond to antifungal treatment. Newer agents used for histoplasmosis, such as fluconazole and itraconazole, also have an uncertain role in therapy.

REFERENCES

1. Abbott, O. A., Mansour, K. A., Logan, W. D., Jr., et al.: A traumatic so-called "spontaneous" rupture of the esophagus. J. Thorac. Cardiovasc. Surg. 59:67-83, 1970.
2. Akman, C., Kantarci, F., and Cetinkaya, S.: Imaging in mediastinitis: A systemic review based on aetiology. Clin. Radiol. 59:573-585, 2004.
3. Al-Sehly, A. A., Robinson, J. L., Lee, B. E., et al.: Pediatric poststernotomy mediastinitis. Ann. Thorac. Surg. 80:2314-2320, 2005.
4. Backer, C. L., Pensler, J. M., Tobin, G. R., et al.: Vascularized muscle flaps for life-threatening mediastinal wounds in children. Ann. Thorac. Surg. 57:797-801, 1994.
5. Brook, I.: The role of anaerobic bacteria in mediastinitis. Drugs 66:315-320, 2006.
6. Chavin, K., Field, G., Chandler, J., et al.: Save the child's esophagus: Management of major disruption after repair of esophageal atresia. J. Pediatr. Surg. 31:48-52, 1996.
7. Cherveniakov, A., and Cherveniakov, P.: Surgical treatment of acute purulent mediastinitis. Eur. J. Cardiovasc. Thorac. Surg. 6:407-410, 1992.
8. Civen, R., Vaisanen, M. L., and Finegold, S. M.: Peritonsillar abscess, retropharyngeal abscess, mediastinitis and nonclostridial anaerobic myonecrosis: A case report. Clin. Infect. Dis. 16(Suppl. 4):S299-S303, 1992.
9. Clancy, C. J., Nguyen, M. H., and Morris, A. J.: Candidal mediastinitis: An emerging clinical entity. Clin. Infect. Dis. 25:608-613, 1997.
10. Demirbag, S., Tiryaki, T., Atabek, C., et al.: Conservative approach to the mediastinitis in childhood secondary to esophageal perforation. Clin. Pediatr. 44:131-134, 2005.
11. Erez, E., Katz, M., Sharoni, E., et al.: Pectoralis major muscle flap for deep sternal wound infection in neonates. Ann. Thorac. Surg. 69:572-577, 2000.
12. Feldman, R., and Gromischm, D. S.: Acute suppurative mediastinitis. Am. J. Dis. Child. 121:79-81, 1971.
13. Finegold, S. M., and Wexler, H. M.: Therapeutic implications of bacteriologic findings in mixed aerobic-anaerobic infections. Antimicrob. Agents Chemother. 32:611-616, 1988.
14. Garatea-Crelgo, J., and Gay-Escoda, C.: Mediastinitis from odontogenic infection: Report of three cases and review of the literature. Int. J. Oral Maxillofac. Surg. 20:65-68, 1991.
15. Gaynes, R., Marosok, R., Mowry-Hanley, J., et al.: Mediastinitis following coronary artery bypass surgery: A 3-year review. J. Infect. Dis. 163:117-121, 1991.
16. Geers, T. A., Taege, A. J., Longworth, D. L., et al.: Ureaplasma urealyticum: Unusual cause of culture-negative mediastinitis. Clin. Infect. Dis. 29:949-950, 1999.
17. Gilchrist, B. F., Valerie, E. P., Nguyen, M., et al.: Pearls and perils in the management of prolonged, peculiar, penetrating esophageal foreign bodies in children. J. Pediatr. Surg. 32:1429-1431, 1997.
18. Goodwin, R. A., Nickell, J. A., and Des Prez, R. M.: Mediastinal fibrosis complicating healed primary histoplasmosis and tuberculosis. Medicine (Baltimore) 51:227-246, 1972.
19. Hachiro, Y., Kikuchi, S., Ito, M., et al.: Infection of a retained permanent epicardial pacemaker lead. Ann. Thorac. Surg. 71:2038-2039, 2001.
20. Horan, T. C., Gaynes, R. P., Martone, W. J., et al.: CDC definitions of nosocomial surgical site infections, 1992: A modification of CDC definitions of surgical wound infections. Am. J. Infect. Control 20:271-274, 1992.
21. Jacobs, J. P., Quintessenza, J. A., Botero, L. M., et al.: The role of airway stents in the management of pediatric tracheal, carinal, and bronchial disease. Eur. J. Cardiothorac. Surg. 18:505-512, 2000.
22. Kerschner, J. E., Beste, D. J., Conley, S. F., et al.: Mediastinitis associated with foreign body erosion of the esophagus in children. Int. J. Pediatr. Otorhinolaryngol. 59:89-97, 2001.
23. Kuritsky, J. N., Bullen, M. G., Broome, C. V., et al.: Sternal wound infections and endocarditis due to organisms of the Mycobacterium fortuitum complex. Ann. Intern. Med. 98:938-939, 1983.
24. Langerstrom, C. F., Mitchell, H. G., Graham, B. S., et al.: Chronic fibrosing mediastinitis and superior vena caval obstruction from blastomycosis. Ann. Thorac. Surg. 54:764-765, 1992.
25. Law, R. C., Fouque, C. A., Waddell, A., et al.: Penetrating intra-oral trauma in children. B. M. J. 314:50-51, 1997.
26. Lequier, L., Robinson, J., and Vaudry, W.: Sternotomy infection with Mycoplasma hominis in a neonate. Pediatr. Infect. Dis. J. 14:1010-1011, 1995.
27. Long, C. B., Shah, S. S., Lautenbach, E., et al.: Postoperative mediastinitis in children: Epidemiology, microbiology and risk factors for Gram-negative pathogens. Pediatr. Infect. Dis. J. 24:315-319, 2005.
28. Makeieff, M., Gresillon, N., Berthet, J. P., et al.: Management of descending necrotizing mediastinitis. Laryngoscope 114:772-775, 2004.
29. Mathisen, D. J., and Grillo, H. C.: Clinical manifestations of mediastinal fibrosis and histoplasmosis. Ann. Thorac. Surg. 54:1053-1057, 1992.
30. Mattila, P. S., Carlson, P., Sivonen, A., et al.: Life-threatening Mycoplasma hominis mediastinitis. Clin. Infect. Dis. 29:1529-1537, 1999.
31. Mehta, P. A., Cunningham, C. K., Colella, C. B., et al.: Risk factors for sternal wound and other infections in pediatric cardiac surgery patients. Pediatr. Infect. Dis. J. 19:1000-1004, 2000.
32. Mekontso-Dessap, A., Kirsch, M., Brun-Buisson, C., et al.: Poststernotomy mediastinitis due to Staphylococcus aureus: Comparison of methicillin-resistant and methicillin-susceptible cases. Clin. Infect. Dis. 32:877-883, 2001.
33. Misawa, Y., Fuse, K., and Hasegawa, T.: Infectious mediastinitis after cardiac operations: Computed tomographic findings. Ann. Thorac. Surg. 65:622-624, 1998.
34. Mole, T. M., Glover, J., and Sheppard, M. N.: Sclerosing mediastinitis: A report on 18 cases. Thorax 50:280-283, 1995.
35. Murray, P. M., and Finegold, S. M.: Anaerobic mediastinitis. Rev. Infect. Dis. 6:S123-S127, 1984.
36. Nozoe, T., Kitamura, M., Adachi, Y., et al.: Successful conservative treatment for esophageal perforation by a fish bone associated with mediastinitis. Hepatogastroenterology 45:2190-2192, 1998.
37. Ohye, R. G., Maniker, R. B., Graves, H. L., et al.: Primary closure for postoperative mediastinitis in children. J. Thorac. Cardiovasc. Surg. 128:480-486, 2004.
38. Pollock, E. M. M., Ford-Jones, E. L., Rebeyka, I., et al.: Early nosocomial infections in pediatric cardiovascular surgery patients. Crit. Care Med. 18:378-384, 1990.
39. Reino, A. J., Jahn, A. F., Parsons, J., et al.: Traumatic pneumomediastinum in a child secondary to corn chip perforation of the esophagus. Pediatr. Emerg. Care 9:211-215, 1993.
40. Robertson, B. D., Bautista, M. A., Russell, T. S., et al.: Fibrosing mediastinitis secondary to zygomycosis in a twenty-two-month-old child. Pediatr. Infect. Dis. J. 21:441-442, 2002.
41. Rokitansky, A. M., Kolankaya, V. A., Seidl, S., et al.: Recent evaluation of prognostic risk factors in esophageal atresia—a multicenter review of 223 cases. Eur. J. Pediatr. Surg. 3:196-201, 1993.
42. Rossi, S. E., McAdams, H. P., Rosado-de-Christenson, M. L., et al.: Fibrosing mediastinitis. RadioGraphics 21:737-757, 2001.
43. Salo, J. A., Isolauri, J. O., Heikkila, L. J., et al.: Management of delayed esophageal perforation with mediastinal sepsis. J. Thorac. Cardiovasc. Surg. 106:1088-1091, 1993.
44. Shah, S. S., Lautenbach, E., Long, C. B., et al.: Staphylococcus aureus as a risk factor for bloodstream infection in children with postoperative mediastinitis. Pediatr. Infect. Dis. J. 24:834-837, 2005.
45. Syed, A. U., Hussain, R., Bhat, A. N., et al.: Mediastinitis due to Mycobacterium fortuitum infection following Fontan operation in a child. Scand. Cardiovasc. J. 31:311-313, 1997.
46. Sztajnbok, J., Grassi, M. S., Katayama, D. M., et al.: Descending suppurative mediastinitis: Nonsurgical approach to this unusual complication of retropharyngeal abscesses in childhood. Pediatr. Emerg. Care 15:341-343, 1999.
47. Tecce, P. M., Fishman, E. K., and Kuhlman, J. E.: CT evaluation of the anterior mediastinum: Spectrum of disease. RadioGraphics 14:973-990, 1994.
48. Tortoriello, T. A., Friedman, J. D., McKenzie, E. D., et al.: Mediastinitis after pediatric cardiac surgery: A 15-year experience at a single institution. Ann. Thorac. Surg. 76:1655-1660, 2003.
49. Wenger, P. N., Brown, J. M., McNeil, M. M., et al.: Nocardia farcinica sternotomy site infections in patients following open heart surgery. J. Infect. Dis. 178:1539-1543, 1998.
50. Yamaguchi, H., Yamauchi, H., Yamada, T., et al.: Diagnostic validity of computed tomography for mediastinitis after cardiac surgery. Ann. Thorac. Cardiovasc. Surg. 7:94-98, 2001.
51. Zeitoun, I. M., and Dhanarajani, P. J.: Cervical cellulitis and mediastinitis caused by odontogenic infections: Report of two cases and review of the literature. J. Oral Maxillofac. Surg. 53:203-208, 1995.

CENTRAL NERVOUS SYSTEM INFECTIONS

BACTERIAL MENINGITIS BEYOND THE NEONATAL PERIOD

Ralph D. Feigin ⊙ William B. Cutrer

Bacterial meningitis is an inflammation of the meninges caused by bacterial infection. The term *leptomeningitis* denotes inflammation of the arachnoid and pia mater, the usual distribution of meningitis. Infections of neonates, including bacterial meningitis, are presented in Chapter 73, and infections of the central nervous system (CNS) caused by mycobacteria are discussed in Chapter 99.

INCIDENCE AND EPIDEMIOLOGY

Before the discovery and use of antibiotics, bacterial meningitis generally was fatal. Antibiotic therapy has improved dramatically the prognosis in patients with bacterial meningitis, although it continues to be a significant cause of morbidity and mortality in children. The number of deaths attributed to many other infectious diseases in the United States decreased by 10-fold to 200-fold between 1935 and 1968, whereas the number of reported deaths caused by bacterial meningitis decreased by only half during the same period.[379,380] In 1972, the Centers for Disease Control and Prevention (CDC) estimated that in the United States, 29,000 cases of meningitis were caused by *Haemophilus influenzae* type b, 4800 cases were caused by *Streptococcus pneumoniae*, and 4600 cases were caused by *Neisseria meningitidis*.

Population-based studies in South Carolina, Minnesota, Vermont, and New Mexico in the 1970s suggested that the actual incidence of bacterial meningitis ranged from 5.4 to 7.3 cases per 100,000 population.[63,130-133] Studies reported in 1995 suggested that the incidence in children aged 1 to 23 months ranged from 0.7 (for *H. influenzae* type b) to 6.6 (for *S. pneumoniae*) cases per 100,000 population.

Before the widespread use of conjugate *H. influenzae* type b vaccine, *H. influenzae* type b was the most common cause of bacterial meningitis in children in the United States, Canada, and Scandinavia, but this pattern was not universal.[162] Davey and associates[81] reported that between 1968 and 1977, *N. meningitidis* was the most common cause and *H. influenzae* type b was the second most common cause of bacterial meningitis for children and young adults in Great Britain. Data from 2001 showed that meningococcal meningitis accounted for 48 percent of meningitis in children in England.[82] Mortality rates in this group of patients were 3.5 percent for children with meningococcal meningitis, 7.7 percent for children with *H. influenzae* meningitis, and 30 percent for patients with pneumococcal meningitis.

By 1995 in the United States, the most frequent cause of bacterial meningitis in children aged 1 month to 24 months was *S. pneumoniae*, followed by *N. meningitidis*, group B streptococcus, and *H. influenzae* (Table 37–1). In children younger than 1 month, the most common cause of bacterial meningitis was group B streptococcus, followed by *S. pneumoniae*.[333] *Escherichia coli* and

Listeria monocytogenes are other common causes of meningitis in neonates 2 to 6 weeks of age.[7,35] *N. meningitidis* was the most common cause for individuals 2 to 29 years old, followed by *S. pneumoniae*.

Infants 6 to 12 months old seem to be at greatest risk for acquiring bacterial meningitis; 90 percent of reported cases occur in children between 1 month and 5 years of age.[130] The age distribution of patients with bacterial meningitis has not changed appreciably during the past 40 years.[285,349]

EPIDEMIOLOGY OF *HAEMOPHILUS INFLUENZAE* MENINGITIS

The most dramatic change in the epidemiology of bacterial meningitis since the advent of antibiotics has occurred in the past 2 decades as a result of licensure of conjugate vaccines against *H. influenzae* type b.[330] The first vaccine available was *H. influenzae* type b capsular polysaccharide (polyribosylribitol phosphate [PRP]), which was licensed in April 1985 for use in children 18 to 59 months of age. Newer vaccines with improved immunogenicity for children of younger ages were developed by covalently linking the capsular polysaccharide with protein antigens. In October 1990, the first conjugate, PRP diphtheria CRM$_{197}$ protein conjugate (HbOC), was approved for infant use, and in 1991, the Advisory Committee on Immunization Practices (ACIP) and the American Academy of Pediatrics (AAP) recommended universal infant immunization at 2, 4, and 6 months of age with either HbOC or PRP-meningococcal protein conjugate (PRP-OMP) vaccines.[12,64] Currently, four different conjugate vaccine preparations exist: PRP-T (tetanus toxoid), PRP-OMP, PRP-CRM$_{197}$, and PRP-D (diphtheria toxoid), which is not licensed in the United States.[395]

The *Haemophilus influenzae* Study Group[5] noted that the number of cases of *H. influenzae* meningitis in children younger than 5 years old reported through the National Bacterial Men-

TABLE 37–1 Age-Specific Incidence in 1995 of Bacterial Meningitis per 100,000 Population

Age	Haemophilus influenzae	Streptococcus pneumoniae	Neisseria meningitidis	Group B Streptococcus
<1 mo	0	15.7	0	125
1-23 mo	0.7	6.6	4.5	2.8
2-29 yr	0.1	0.5	1.1	0.1
30-59 yr	0.2	1	0.3	0.05
>60 yr	0.07	1.9	0.1	0.1

From Schuchat, A., Robinson, K., Wenger, J. D., et al.: Bacterial meningitis in the United States in 1995. N. Engl. J. Med. 337:970-976, 1997.

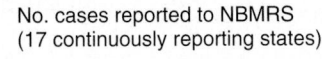

No. cases reported to NBMRS
(17 continuously reporting states)

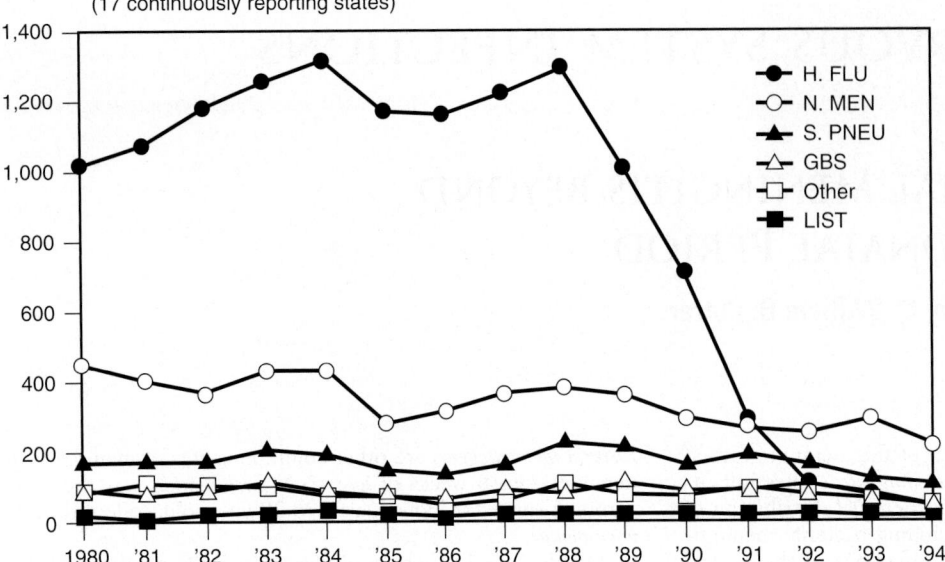

Figure 37–1 Incidence of bacterial meningitis in individuals from birth to 19 years of age. A marked decline in the incidence of *Haemophilus influenzae* type b meningitis is noted during the period between 1988 and 1994. GBS, group B streptococcus; H. FLU, *H. influenzae* type b; LIST, *Listeria monocytogenes*; NBMRS, National Bacterial Meningitis Reporting System; N. MEN, *Neisseria meningitidis*; S. PNEU, *Streptococcus pneumoniae*.

ingitis Reporting System began declining rapidly in 1988 (Fig. 37–1). In another CDC surveillance project conducted from 1989 to 1997, the race-adjusted incidence of invasive *H. influenzae* type b disease among children younger than 5 years declined from 34 to 0.4 per 100,000, a 99 percent reduction.[66] CDC data for 1998 to 2000 show that the incidence of *H. influenzae* infection remains low: 0.4, 0.4, and 0.3 per 100,000 children younger than 5 years in 1998, 1999, and 2000, respectively.[68] The average annual incidence of *H. influenzae* type b infection remains higher in select populations within the United States, including American Indians/Alaskan Natives (14 per 100,000), Hispanics (1 per 100,000), and nonblack Hispanics (0.6 per 100,000).[68]

Schoendorf and colleagues[332] evaluated national trends in mortality from meningitis from 1980 to 1991. From 1980 through 1987, mortality rates from *H. influenzae* meningitis decreased an average of 8.5 percent a year, from 1.72 per 100,000 children in 1980 to 0.94 per 100,000 children in 1987. From 1988 to 1991, mortality rates decreased an average of 48 percent a year, with a death rate of 0.11 per 100,000 children in 1991. The estimated case-fatality rate for *H. influenzae* meningitis was 3.3 percent from 1980 to 1987 and 2.3 percent from 1988 to 1991. In comparison, mortality rates from *S. pneumoniae* decreased 10 percent annually from 1980 to 1987 and 3 percent annually from 1988 to 1991. Similarly, mortality rates from meningococcal meningitis decreased by 13 percent annually from 1980 to 1987 and 12 percent annually from 1988 to 1991.

The dramatic decrease in the incidence of *H. influenzae* meningitis probably has been affected by several factors. The precipitous drop that occurred shortly after universal immunization of infants strongly suggests that this practice has affected the epidemiology of this disease. Conjugate vaccination protects against nasopharyngeal colonization,[268] decreasing the carriage rate of *H. influenzae* type b and diminishing the reservoir for transmission and providing immunity from infection. These factors would lessen the likelihood of development of infection in underimmunized children as well. Other changes in medical practice, such as the widespread use of outpatient antibiotics and improvements in supportive care, may have some effect, as shown by the decrease in case-fatality rates for *H. influenzae* meningitis, the steady decrease in mortality rates before vaccination, and the

decrease in instances of meningococcal and pneumococcal disease.

Before universal vaccination was initiated, the incidence of *H. influenzae* meningitis varied worldwide. The incidence of *H. influenzae* meningitis in Scandinavian children younger than 5 years averaged 16 to 28 cases per 100,000 children from 1975 to 1984.[288] The incidence of *H. influenzae* type b meningitis in three Pacific Island countries was 70 to 84 cases per 100,000 children younger than 5 years old in 2003[314] and 67 to 158 cases per 100,000 in Indonesian children younger than 5 years old in 1998 to 2002.[151] The incidence of *H. influenzae* meningitis in the Netherlands was 22 cases per 100,000 children younger than 5 years old.[381] A universal vaccination program in the Netherlands seems to have led to a marked decrease in the incidence, with six reported cases of meningitis caused by *H. influenzae* in a 1-year period after implementation of universal vaccination of infants compared with 34 cases per 100,000 children in a 1-year period before vaccination.

The incidence of *H. influenzae* meningitis is markedly higher in nonindustrialized populations. Before the vaccination era, Alaskan Eskimos had an annual incidence of 282 cases per 100,000 children younger than 5 years of age.[393] The Navajo and White Mountain Apache Native Americans had a much higher incidence compared with that of Native Americans in other regions of the United States,[77,242] and the incidence among Australian Aboriginals and among certain African populations, such as those in Gambia and Senegal, was 3 to 10 times higher than that of populations in the United States and Europe.[43,154,176] The incidence of *H. influenzae* meningitis was decreased in Gambia from more than 60 cases per 100,000 children to none per 100,000 in children younger than 5 years old after implementation of *H. influenzae* type b vaccination in May 1997.[6]

Good epidemiologic data concerning the incidence of *H. influenzae* infection are lacking in many other areas of the world. Measuring the extent of *H. influenzae* disease often is difficult, time-consuming, and expensive. In an attempt to decrease complexity, cost, and time required to collect data concerning the incidence of *H. influenzae* infection, the Hib Rapid Assessment Tool was developed. More and more countries are using such tools to estimate the local *H. influenzae* disease burden and to help determine the need for implementation of a local vaccination program.[395]

In one study, the incidence of *H. influenzae* meningitis was 3.5-fold higher in blacks than in whites, but this distribution of cases seemed to be related more closely to poverty than to race.[130] In whites, no increase in incidence occurred in overcrowded households, but the incidence was higher in rural than in urban areas. Fraser and associates[130] postulated that the increased incidence in rural whites and in blacks was related to lack of access to early medical care.

Ward and colleagues[391] studied prospective data obtained in 19 states to determine the risk of spread of severe *H. influenzae* illness among household contacts of patients with *H. influenzae* meningitis. The risk in children younger than 1 year of age was 6 percent; in children younger than 4 years, 2.1 percent; and in children younger than 6 years, 0.5 percent. The risk of *H. influenzae* disease occurring in household contacts younger than 6 years old is similar to the risk of secondary meningococcal disease occurring in all household contacts, indicating a need for effective antimicrobial prophylaxis.

Spread of *H. influenzae* disease in daycare centers also is well documented.[32,156,252,392] The precise risk of acquiring secondary *H. influenzae* type b infection in daycare centers is unclear.

Recurrent invasive *H. influenzae* type b disease has been reported. Detailed studies suggest that age and high incidence of disease alone are not the only factors contributing to the recurrence of the disease.[55] Patients who have recurrent disease caused by *H. influenzae* type b may represent a subset of a population with unusual disease susceptibility. In addition, children who develop invasive infection caused by *H. influenzae* type b after receiving appropriate conjugate vaccine frequently have subnormal immunoglobulin concentrations and should undergo immune evaluation.[186]

EPIDEMIOLOGY OF MENINGITIS CAUSED BY *STREPTOCOCCUS PNEUMONIAE*

The highest rate of invasive pneumococcal infection occurs in children younger than 2 years old. In a population-based surveillance study of invasive pneumococcal infection in southern California, the age-specific incidence of invasive pneumococcal disease for children 2 years or younger was 145 cases per 100,000. In the pre-vaccine era (before 2000 in the United States), for children 2 to 4 years old and 5 to 14 years old, the age-specific incidence decreased to 25 per 100,000 and 5 per 100,000, respectively.[406] The age-specific incidence for pneumococcal meningitis was 21, 12, 6, 2, and 0.5 cases per 100,000 for the age groups 0 to 6 months, 7 to 12 months, 13 to 24 months, 25 to 60 months, and older than 60 months, respectively. Since the initiation of *S. pneumoniae* vaccination, the incidence of invasive *S. pneumoniae* infections has declined. Data from CDC surveillance shows that from 1998-1999 to 2003, there has been a 94 percent decline in *S. pneumoniae* infection related to *S. pneumoniae* serotypes present in the vaccine (80 cases per 100,000 to 4.6 per 100,000 among children <5 years old).[69]

The risk for development of sepsis or meningitis caused by *S. pneumoniae* depends to some extent on the serotype with which the child is colonized. Although 90 pneumococcal serotypes have been identified, invasive disease, including sepsis and meningitis, in children younger than 6 years old is associated most commonly with serotypes 14, 6B, 19F, 18C, 23F, 4, and 9V.[58] The seven-valent pneumococcal conjugate vaccine (PCV7), added to the national vaccination schedule in 2000, contains each of the above-mentioned most common strains.

The risk of contracting pneumococcal meningitis is 5-fold to 36-fold greater among blacks than among whites and is independent of income or population density.[130] In one study, 11 percent of the black population with pneumococcal pneumonia had sickle-cell disease, a factor known to predispose an individual to development of pneumococcal disease.[130] On the basis of these data, Fraser and associates[130] suggested that 1 of every 24 children with sickle-cell disease may develop pneumococcal meningitis by the time they reach 4 years of age. This incidence is 36-fold greater than the incidence of pneumococcal meningitis in a normal black population and 314-fold greater than that in white children.

Daycare attendance, underlying disease, and lack of breast-feeding were risk factors for acquiring invasive pneumococcal infections in a large case-control study that included children from the United States and Canada.[237] Although cigarette smoking is a major risk factor for the development of invasive pneumococcal disease in adults, whether exposure to cigarette smoke increases the risk of developing systemic pneumococcal infection in children remains unclear.[162,280] The greatest mortality rate occurs in very old and very young patients and has been estimated to be 20 to 60 percent.[123,132,133,146]

Pneumococcal infections generally occur sporadically. Household contacts of a patient with pneumococcal disease are not considered to be at increased risk of acquiring secondary infection. The occurrence of concurrent pneumococcal disease (meningitis and bacteremia) in the household setting has been reported, however.[24,344] Although uncommon in the United States, *S. pneumoniae* has been associated with epidemics in locations such as Northern Ghana.[235]

The incidence of systemic infection with penicillin-resistant *S. pneumoniae* has been increasing steadily worldwide since it first was reported in Australia in the 1960s.[175] Systemic infection with penicillin-resistant pneumococci has become an increasing problem in the United States since the mid-1980s.[359,365,366] In 1995, a CDC multistate surveillance study showed that 35 percent of *S. pneumoniae* cerebrospinal fluid (CSF) isolates were resistant to penicillin.[333]

The first report of meningitis caused by resistant pneumococci was published in 1974,[274] and numerous case reports have appeared subsequently. Tan and colleagues[366] found that patients with systemic infections caused by penicillin-resistant pneumococci were more likely to have received a course of antibiotics within 1 month before acquiring their infection than were matched control subjects who had infections caused by pneumococci but whose isolates were susceptible to penicillin.

More recently, an increase has occurred in the number of cases of systemic infection and meningitis caused by *S. pneumoniae* organisms resistant to penicillin and third-generation cephalosporins. In 1998, CDC surveillance of multiple areas around the United States found that 24 percent of pneumococcal isolates associated with invasive infections were nonsusceptible to penicillin; 14 percent of isolates were nonsusceptible to cefotaxime.[398] As with many studies, rates of resistance were higher among children younger than 5 years old. In a prospective study involving eight children's hospitals nationwide during a 6-year period starting September 1993, a significant increase in the proportion of isolates nonsusceptible to penicillin or ceftriaxone was found. In the sixth year of the study ending August 1998, 37 percent and 11 percent of invasive isolates were nonsusceptible to penicillin and ceftriaxone.[203] Isolates of penicillin-resistant and third-generation cephalosporin–resistant *S. pneumoniae* have been recovered in other regions of the world as well.[136,139,305] Treatment failures in patients with *S. pneumoniae* meningitis resistant to penicillin and third-generation cephalosporins have led to changes in the empiric therapy of suspected bacterial meningitis, as discussed in the treatment section.[22,49,139,212,347]

Data from the Active Bacterial Core Surveillance of the Emerging Infections Program Network after introduction of the pneumococcal conjugate vaccine show an 87 percent decrease in rates of antibiotic-resistant disease by vaccine serotypes.[225] Their results show that rates of invasive pneumococcal disease with penicillin-nonsusceptible strains and strains nonsusceptible to multiple antibiotics "peaked in 1999 and decreased by 2004."[225] In children younger than 2 years old invasive pneumococcal disease with penicillin-nonsusceptible strains decreased from 70.3 to 13.1 cases per 100,000.[225] The proportion of disease caused by penicillin-nonsusceptible strains varied by location within the United States from 9.4 percent in California to 29.5 percent in Tennessee.[225] The incidence of invasive *S. pneumoniae* disease caused by cefotaxime-resistant *S. pneumoniae* strains has increased in children younger than 2 years of age however, in the post-vaccination period, from approximately 10 percent in 1999 to almost 15 percent in 2003.[225] The decreases in disease caused by vaccine-type *S. pneumoniae* strains were coupled with an increase in non-vaccine serotype *S. pneumoniae* strains, especially with serotype 19A (increased from 2 to 8.3 cases per 100,000).[225]

EPIDEMIOLOGY OF MENINGOCOCCAL MENINGITIS

The carriage rate for *N. meningitidis* in the civilian population has been estimated at various times to range from 1 to 15 percent. Carriage rates in military personnel during epidemic periods have been considerably greater. Meningococcal carriers generally are adults (>21 years old) who harbor the organism for months.

No correlation has been noted between meningococcal meningitis and crowding within households, but disease seems to be more prevalent in urban than in rural areas. In a civilian population, meningococcal meningitis generally is a disease of children and young adults who have been exposed to an adult carrier, usually in the same family, or to individuals with disease or who are carrying the organism in a daycare setting. The estimated likelihood of severe meningococcal disease in family contacts occurring simultaneously with the first case is 1 percent.[231] The rate is 1000-fold greater than the risk in the community. The risk of meningitis being acquired in daycare center contacts of children with meningococcal disease is 1 per 1000.

In a CDC surveillance study of invasive meningococcal disease in the United States, the average annual incidence of disease was 1.1 per 100,000 population for the years 1992 to 1996[310] and remained the same through 2002.[70] The highest age-specific incidence occurred in infants younger than 1 year old (9.2 cases per 100,000),[70] with the peak incidence occurring in infants 4 to 5 months old (15.9 cases per 100,000). The age-specific incidence declined sharply until the 10- to 14-year age range, at which point it began to increase again during the adolescent and early adult years. During the teenage range, the incidence peaked between 15 and 19 years of age (1.5 to 2.2 cases per 100,000). From 1990 to 2002 in the United States, mortality rates for meningococcal disease were 0.1 deaths per 100,000 population per year, with 58 percent of deaths occurring among individuals younger than 25 years old. Infants had a higher mortality rate than that of individuals in different age groups, but they experienced a decline from 1.3 deaths per 100,000 in 1990 to 0.42 deaths per 100,000 population in 2002.[339] Meningococcal disease mortality rates increased each year in individuals between the ages of 10 and 19 years, which was followed by a decline in mortality rates in the years following and throughout most of adulthood.[339]

In the United States, serogroups B, C, and Y account for most meningococcal disease. Meningococcal infections caused by serogroup B caused greater than 50 percent of infection in infants younger than 1 year. In the 1990s, serogroup Y became more common among older patients and caused more pneumonia than did the other serogroups. The overall incidence of serogroup Y infection increased from 2 percent during 1989 to 1991 to 37 percent during 1997 to 2002.[70] A study of the epidemiology of meningococcal disease in New York City from 1989 to 2000

revealed a threefold decrease in rates of serogroup B disease and almost no cases in children younger than 5 years old. The authors noted the coincident increase in the use of *H. influenzae* conjugate vaccine containing serogroup B meningococcal outer membrane protein and postulated the existence of a possible correlation.[263] CDC data reveal that 75 percent of meningococcal infections in individuals older than 11 years are caused by serogroups C, Y, and W-135, all of which are included in the newly available conjugate vaccine. An increased risk of contracting meningococcal infection also exists in college students, especially freshmen who reside on campus in dormitories.[179]

Another change in the epidemiology of meningococcal disease in the United States relates to the increasing number of outbreaks (>10 cases per 100,000 population during 3 months), generally caused by serogroup C. Although these outbreaks account for only 2 to 3 percent of the total number of cases, they cause tremendous public concern and anxiety, which frequently result in misunderstanding of the nature of an outbreak by the media and the public.[189]

An otherwise unprecedented outbreak of meningococcal disease occurred in a sixth-grade elementary school classroom.[106] Five children from a class of 24 developed meningococcal meningitis. In addition, two siblings of one of the index cases also developed meningococcal infection. Detailed epidemiologic investigation suggested that close contact in the classroom (nose-to-nose distances of ≤34 inches) correlated with an increased rate of carriage of *N. meningitidis* and with an increased risk for development of invasive meningococcal disease.

Major outbreaks of meningococcal meningitis have occurred worldwide. In the late 1980s and early 1990s, major epidemics of meningococcal meningitis caused by a specific clone (III-1) of serogroup A *N. meningitidis* occurred throughout sub-Saharan Africa.[2,168,172,292,318] The origins of a pandemic spread of clone III-1 were traced to epidemics in Asia in the early 1980s, with spread through the Near East.[1] An outbreak occurred during the annual pilgrimage to Mecca in 1987,[260,261] with pilgrims carrying clones back to their countries of origin, including the United States and the United Kingdom. Epidemics of closely related strains of clone III-1 serogroup A meningococcal meningitis occurred in the Sudan,[318] Ethiopia,[172] and Chad in 1988,[261] and in Kenya[292] in 1989. A report in 1992 described an epidemic of clone III-1 in the Central African Republic in an area traditionally outside the "meningitis belt."[168] These epidemics generally begin during the dry season and decline at onset of the rainy season. According to the World Health Organization, "in major African epidemics, attack rates range from 100 to 800 per 100,000 population, but individual communities have reported rates as high as 1000 per 100,000."[253] Major outbreaks have occurred in Brazil,[88] in Finland,[288] and at multiple sites in Africa.[399] A clonal outbreak of serogroup W135 (ET-37ST-11 clonal complex) occurred in 2000 among Hajj pilgrims returning to Europe from Saudi Arabia. In 2001, outbreaks with serogroup W135 also occurred in Niger and Burkina Faso.[364]

Shifts within a community or within a country as a whole from one serogroup to another also are associated with an increased incidence of disease for several years after the new serogroup is introduced into the community.[310] The mechanisms underlying the changing patterns of meningococcal serogroups that cause disease are unknown.

Meningococcal infections also occur more frequently in patients with a deficiency of the terminal components (C5-C8) of the complement system.[100,239,319] More recently, an increased risk for contracting meningococcal meningitis has been reported in individuals with an inherited deficiency of C9[273] and with properdin deficiency.[353] Individuals with a complement-depleting underlying illness also are at particular risk for acquiring invasive disease.[290] Screening for complement deficiency in pediatric patients with meningococcal disease is recommended.[232]

PATHOPHYSIOLOGY

ORGANISMS ENCOUNTERED

Any organism may produce meningitis in a susceptible individual. *S. pneumoniae* and *N. meningitidis* are the responsible agents in approximately 95 percent of healthy children older than 2 months. In compromised hosts, infection with other organisms may occur more frequently. The specific organism sometimes may be predicted on the basis of the type of deficit that is present in the host.

ROUTES OF INFECTION

Bacterial infection of the normally sterile leptomeningeal spaces can occur from a distant focus through the bloodstream or by direct invasion from a contiguous focus. Meningitis usually is the result of hematogenous dissemination of organisms from a distant site of infection,[349] often from the respiratory tract. The meninges are seeded with microorganisms during a bacteremic period. Bacterial meningitis in children with otitis media generally follows bacteremia, although direct invasion of the meninges may occur as a complication of otitis media.

The route of infection in bacterial meningitis has been studied by use of a variety of animal models, but the experimental infection was initiated in most cases in a manner that did not mimic human disease. Bacterial meningitis has been induced in rats[264] and monkeys[325] after intranasal inoculation of *H. influenzae* type b. Bacteremia developed hours before meningitis could be detected histologically, a finding that supports the concept that meningitis follows hematogenous dissemination from nasopharyngeal colonization or infection. Marginating bacteria could be detected by fluorescent staining initially in the lateral and dorsal longitudinal (sagittal) sinuses and subsequently spread to the leptomeninges. In the rat model, otitis media seemed to develop by spread of infection from the subarachnoid space to the inner ear and then to the middle ear.

Meningitis may develop after bacterial invasion from a contiguous focus of infection, as in infection of the mastoid or paranasal sinuses, or as a complication of otitis media. Fracture through the paranasal sinuses as a result of head trauma may precede development of meningitis caused by *S. pneumoniae* and *H. influenzae*, which may be recurrent. Direct invasion also may occur in individuals with dermoid sinus tracts or meningomyeloceles, when a direct communication between the skin and the meninges is present. In this setting, infection usually is produced by organisms found on the skin. Recurrent meningitis has been reported in patients with basiethmoidal encephaloceles[362] and a congenital defect in the stapedial footplate.[183] Surgical obliteration of the fistula with temporal muscle and fascia prevented the recurrence of meningitis. Meningitis also may develop subsequent to osteomyelitis of the skull or vertebral column. Rarely, meningitis may develop in the normal host with commensurate microorganisms after having a tooth extraction or getting dental fillings.[74,340]

Neurosurgical procedures, particularly procedures designed for diversion of CSF in children who have hydrocephalus, may lead to development of meningitis. A chemical meningitis also may occur after neurosurgical procedures, especially procedures involving the posterior fossa.[127] In these patients, evidence of inflammation develops rapidly, with elevation of temperature occurring on the first postoperative day.

Infection of the CNS may result from environmental contamination or manipulation. Meningeal infection may be acquired in utero transplacentally or during delivery through contact with the cervix or vaginal canal, which may be colonized with a variety of organisms, particularly group B streptococci and *L. monocytogenes*.[7,25] A newborn, a patient with cystic fibrosis, or a burned child may develop septicemia and meningitis as a result of persistent heavy colonization with *Staphylococcus aureus*. A humidified atmosphere promotes the colonization and growth of such organisms as *Serratia marcescens* and *Pseudomonas aeruginosa*. Placing a patient in this setting leads to an increased frequency of infection with these organisms. Indwelling catheters can predispose a patient to infection by bacterial (and fungal) organisms that generally are of low virulence in the normal host.

FACTORS PREDISPOSING THE HOST TO BACTERIAL MENINGITIS

Factors that predispose the host to the development of infection in other sites also predispose the host to the development of bacterial infection of the CNS. A strong interrelationship exists among factors relating to the host, the organism, and the environment with regard to the pathogenesis and outcome of meningitis. Although presented separately, they must be considered a complex interplay of factors that leads to infection.

An increased incidence of bacterial meningitis is observed in the very young; boys are affected more frequently than girls, and the severity of disease also is increased in these groups. Fraser and associates[133] reported that the greatest morbidity after bacterial meningitis occurred in children affected between birth and 4 years of age. A newborn is predisposed to development of septicemia and meningitis by factors that reflect physiologic deficiencies or immaturity of host defense mechanisms, including (1) decreased phagocytic and bactericidal activity of polymorphonuclear leukocytes, (2) defects in the response of neonatal leukocytes to chemotactic factors, (3) a deficiency in the capacity of leukocytes to support opsonization, and (4) defects in microtubular length and number that decrease the motility of the neonatal leukocytes compared with leukocytes from older children. Deficiencies in serum complement components (C1q, C3, and C5), low levels of serum properdin, and low concentrations of serum IgM and IgA have been documented repeatedly. Despite transplacental acquisition of IgG, antibodies against specific infective agents may be lacking. The precise age at which each of these factors reaches the concentration and functional activity noted in older children and adults is unclear and undoubtedly varies from individual to individual. In part, meningitis in children aged 1 month to 1 year may reflect qualitative or quantitative differences of the inflammatory and immunologic responses in older children compared with infants.

The increased risk for development of meningitis in the normal host with less than completely mature immunologic and inflammatory responses to infection may be attributable to age alone. This factor is exemplified in the report of Cole and associates,[72] who studied the risk of recurrent bacteremia in young children. Within 18 months of having bacteremic illness, none of 42 children older than 24 months had a documented additional episode of bacteremia or systemic infection. Fifteen of 135 children (11%) younger than 24 months at the time of the initial bacteremic disease had at least one additional documented bacteremic illness, however. Of these 15 children, 14 contracted both infections before reaching 2 years of age. Seven of these 15 children had meningitis. Only two patients had documented congenital or hereditary disorders of immunoglobulin or complement concentration or function.

A genetic determination for the predilection of some normal children for the development of bacteremia and meningitis has been suggested.[373] The ability of the host to produce, within the CSF, interleukin-12 (IL-12) and tumor necrosis factor-α (TNF-α)–induced interferon-γ is important in the natural immunity to various microorganisms that may cause meningitis.[223]

Congenital or acquired abnormalities of the immune system may predispose the host to the acquisition of bacterial infections. Congenital deficiency of the three major immunoglobulin classes may predispose the host to the acquisition of severe bacterial infection. Congenital defects of thymic-dependent, small lymphocyte function or combined T and B defects are detrimental to host defense. A deficiency of CD4+ helper-inducer T cells in patients with bacterial meningitis has been reported and may contribute to the impaired antibody synthesis to bacterial capsular polysaccharides in this disease.[303] Multiple studies have shown that deficiencies of various components of the complement system and increased consumption or loss of complement have been associated with increased risk for development of bacterial meningitis caused by encapsulated organisms.[319]

An increased incidence of overwhelming infection, including meningitis, occurs after splenectomy, but the likelihood of development of such infection depends on the age of the child at the time of splenectomy, the time since splenectomy, and the original indication for splenectomy.[101] Congenital asplenia or polysplenia also has been associated with an increased incidence of septicemia and meningitis caused by *S. pneumoniae*,[101] *H. influenzae* type b, and gram-negative enteric microorganisms. Children with sickle-cell disease and other hemoglobinopathies have meningitis caused by *S. pneumoniae*, *H. influenzae*, and *Salmonella* spp. more frequently than do normal children.

Children with malignant neoplasms with or without neutropenia seem to be susceptible to development of meningitis caused by organisms of low virulence that pose a minimal threat to healthy children, presumably because of abnormalities in immunologic function.[355] Decreased production of normal immunoglobulins, delayed and defective antibody responses to antigenic stimuli, production of abnormal immunoglobulins, depression in the clearance mechanisms of the reticuloendothelial system, and depression of cellular immunity have been documented in children with malignant neoplasms involving the reticuloendothelial system. In addition, the use of irradiation or immunosuppressive agents and antimetabolites predisposes the host to the development of infection in the CNS. Attributing the occurrence of bacterial meningitis in this population directly to these agents rather than to the disease for which this therapy has been provided may be difficult. Meningitis occurring after neurosurgical manipulation for tumors of the CNS in nonneutropenic children usually develops within 1 month of the neurosurgery.[355]

Malnutrition also predisposes children and adults to infectious disease. Impaired cellular immune responses, low levels of serum complement, impaired phagocytic activity of neutrophils, and decreased serum concentrations of transferrin have been documented in malnourished children.[114]

Patients with systemic diseases, such as diabetes mellitus, renal insufficiency, adrenal insufficiency, cystic fibrosis, hypoparathyroidism, and exudative enteropathy, have an increased frequency and severity of CNS infections.[47] Children with diabetes mellitus, coma caused by drug overdose, and Cushing syndrome have been shown to be at increased risk for development of bacteremia or meningitis caused by *H. influenzae* type b.[236] Some type of underlying condition was noted for 21 percent (37 of 181) of the children with pneumococcal meningitis in a multicenter surveillance study.[20] The most common of these conditions was some disorder of the CNS, which occurred in 16 children (9%). Defective chemotaxis, phagocytosis, and bactericidal function accompany these disorders and may explain in part the increased susceptibility of these individuals to infection.[114,115]

In the normal host, bacterial infections at sites other than the leptomeninges are associated with an increased incidence of CNS infection. Infection may spread hematogenously to the meninges in children with endocarditis, pneumonia, or thrombophlebitis or by direct extension from sinusitis, mastoiditis, or osteomyelitis

of the skull. Development of meningitis after lumbar puncture in children younger than 1 year has been described.[126,371]

An increased risk for development of meningitis also occurs in children after placement of cochlear implants. Reelhuis and colleagues[304] reported the incidence of meningitis caused by *S. pneumoniae* in patients after receiving cochlear implants to be 138.2 cases per 100,000 person-years, which represents a more than 30-fold increase over the age-controlled general population.[304] From 1999 to 2002, some children were implanted with cochlear devices, including a positioner, which were removed from the market subsequently as a result of an associated marked increase in incidence of pneumococcal meningitis. When removing the influence of cochlear devices containing a positioner, the incidence of pneumococcal meningitis among children with cochlear implants was still 16 times higher than that of an age-matched control population.

PATHOLOGY

The most detailed account in English of the pathologic changes occurring with meningitis was written in 1948 by Adams and colleagues.[4] They described the meningeal, cerebral, and vascular changes found post mortem in 14 patients who died of *H. influenzae* infection 14 hours to 76 days after the onset of disease. Although most patients in their series received inadequate treatment (effective antibiotic therapy was unavailable), the pathologic findings they describe differ little from the findings of subsequent reports by Smith and Landing,[350] Rorke and Pitts,[309] and Dodge and Swartz,[96] whose patients died despite administration of antibiotics. These descriptions are summarized later.

A meningeal exudate of variable thickness may be found (Fig. 37–2). Purulent material is distributed widely but may accumulate around the veins and venous sinuses, over the convexity of the brain, in the depths of the sulci, in the sylvian fissures, within the basal cisterns, and around the cerebellum. The spinal cord may be encased in pus. Ventriculitis (purulent material within the ventricles) has been noted repeatedly in children who died of their diseases. Subsequent experience suggests that ventriculitis may be a common finding in children with bacterial meningitis who survive, particularly neonates. Invasion of the ventricular wall with perivascular collections of purulent material has been noted. Loss of ependymal lining and subependymal gliosis may be seen. In some studies, purulent exudate tended to be thicker

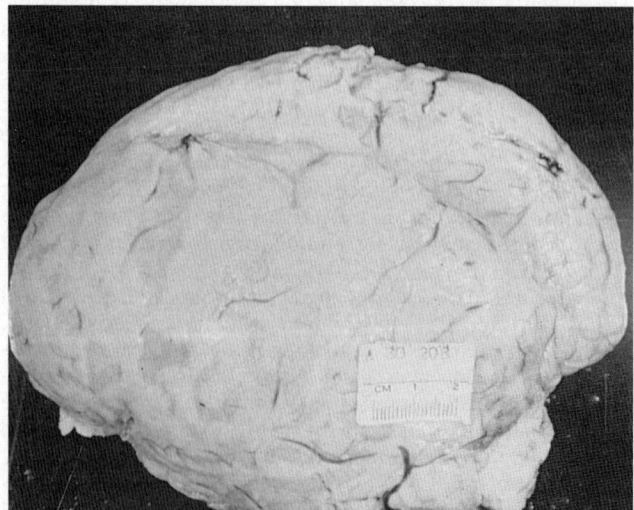

Figure 37–2 Note extensive purulent exudate over entire cerebral cortex in a patient who died as a result of bacterial meningitis.

over the convexity of the brain in patients with pneumococcal meningitis than in patients with other forms of meningitis.[96,309]

Vascular and parenchymatous changes have been shown at necropsy. Polymorphonuclear infiltrates extending to the subintimal region of small arteries and veins have been associated with the exudative meningeal process. Thrombosis of small cortical veins associated with necrosis of the cerebral cortex may be noted. Occlusion of one of the major venous sinuses, subarachnoid hemorrhage secondary to a necrotizing arteritis, and necrosis of the cerebral cortex in the absence of identifiable thrombosis of small vessels rarely may be observed. Reactive microglia and astrocytes may be identified in the cerebral cortex, particularly subadjacent to regions of heavy subarachnoid exudate. Because no bacteria are found in the cerebral cortex, these pathologic changes should be viewed as a noninfectious encephalopathy. "Toxic or circulatory factors" were suggested as possible causes by Adams and associates.[5] Dodge and Swartz[96] suggested systemic hypoxia and fever as additional possible causes. They also noted that an increase in intracranial pressure might interfere with cerebral circulation.

Impaired consciousness, deficits in motor and sensory functions, seizures, and retardation may be observed. Damage to the cerebral cortex, reflecting the effects of vascular occlusion, hypoxia, bacterial invasion, toxic encephalopathy, bacterial factors, inflammatory mediators, small molecule effectors, or some combination of these factors, provides an adequate explanation for these observations.

Hydrocephalus that develops in patients beyond the newborn period is an uncommon complication of meningitis. Most often, hydrocephalus is communicating and is the result of adhesive thickening of the arachnoid around the cisterns at the base of the brain. Less frequently, the aqueduct of Sylvius or the foramina of Magendie and Luschka are obstructed by fibrosis and reactive gliosis. The ensuing ventricular dilation may be coupled with coexistent necrosis of nervous tissue because of the meningitis itself or because of occlusion of cerebral veins and, rarely, arteries. Cerebral necrosis plus increased intraventricular pressure may result in total dissolution of the cerebrum.

Subdural effusions occur frequently during the course of meningitis. The exact pathogenesis is unknown. The high incidence of effusion and the fact that subdural fluid collections may be found early in the course of bacterial meningitis in children suggest, however, that subdural effusions should be considered a concomitant occurrence with meningeal inflammation rather than a complication of the disease. Numerous veins traverse the subdural space, and inflammation of these veins and of the dural capillaries could produce an increase in vascular permeability and loss of albumin-rich fluid into the subdural space. The ratio of albumin to gamma globulin is higher in the subdural fluid of children with meningitis than in serum.[159] When the inflammatory process subsides, formation of fluid generally ceases, but its presence may persist because of a continued transudation through newly formed vessels in the subdural membrane.

Subdural empyema, as opposed to subdural effusion, occurs rarely. It was observed in only 2 of the cases reported by Adams and associates,[5] in 1 of 34 patients examined by Smith and Landing,[350] and in 1 of the patients studied by Dodge and Swartz.[96]

Many factors contribute to the increase in intracranial pressure in patients with meningitis. Endotoxin and fragments of the cell wall of gram-positive organisms are capable of inducing the release of IL-1 and TNF from macrophages and other sources.[93,256] These substances, in addition to other interleukins and arachidonic acid metabolites, affect many systems, including endothelial cells, and profoundly affect the function of the vasculature and its interaction with neutrophils and other inflammatory cells. These substances play an important role in the pathogenesis of increased intracranial pressure and cerebral edema in patients

with meningitis by altering cerebral blood flow, intracranial blood volume, and permeability of the cerebral vasculature.[278] Experimentally, the main components of the blood-brain barrier, endothelial cells, astrocyte-end feet, and pericytes, have been found to be sensitive to the effects of such inflammatory mediators.[29] Intercellular junctions, which normally are tight, are open in experimental meningitis, which is associated with an increased permeability to circulating albumin.[298] Pinocytotic vesicles also are noted within the cytoplasm of endothelial cells. Swelling of cellular elements (cytotoxic edema) also has been noted.

Alterations in CSF resorption exacerbate cerebral edema and increased intracranial pressure further. In experimental meningitis, resorption of CSF is diminished as an accumulation of proteins, leukocytes, and other materials interferes with the function of the arachnoid villus.[329]

During the course of meningitis, excess secretion of antidiuretic hormone (ADH) occurs, which induces water retention and exacerbates electrolyte abnormalities already created secondary to the inflammatory processes occurring in the CNS. Cellular electrolyte disturbances may depolarize neuronal membranes, predisposing the host to seizure activity. Increased oxidation of glucose, increased lactate production, and depletion of high-energy compounds such as adenosine 5'-triphosphate and phosphocreatine are observed. Hypoglycorrhachia results primarily from decreased transport of glucose across the inflamed choroid plexus and from increased use of glucose by host tissues. Use of glucose by bacteria and polymorphonuclear leukocytes is of less relative importance.[96,328]

PATHOGENESIS

Most cases of bacterial meningitis progress through four steps: (1) infection or colonization of the upper respiratory tract, (2) invasion of the blood from a respiratory focus, (3) seeding of the meninges by a blood-borne organism, and (4) inflammation of the meninges and brain. Less commonly, infection of the leptomeninges can occur by contiguous spread or hematogenous dissemination from another remote site. The nasopharyngeal mucosa is colonized with *S. pneumoniae*, *N. meningitidis*, or other microorganisms, resulting most commonly in an asymptomatic carrier state or minor upper respiratory tract illness. This attachment is mediated by specific microbial cell surface components. *N. meningitidis* strains possess fimbriae that bind to cell surface receptors on nasopharyngeal mucosal cells[90] and apparently are transported across specialized cells within phagocytic vacuoles.[363]

When in the bloodstream, the common pathogenic organisms (*S. pneumoniae*, *H. influenzae*, *N. meningitidis*, *E. coli* K1, and group B streptococcus) are capable of evading host defense mechanisms through capsular polysaccharides, which inhibit neutrophil phagocytosis and classic complement-mediated bactericidal activity. These bacteria traverse the blood-brain barrier, most likely at the cerebral capillaries and choroid plexus. Fimbriae of *E. coli* have been shown to facilitate attachment in these regions.[286] *N. meningitidis* has been shown to invade via interaction of Opc membrane protein with serum fibronectin and an endothelial surface integrin, which leads to tyrosine kinase activation and subsequent intracellular signaling pathways.[354,378] *S. pneumoniae* has been shown to invade the blood-brain barrier via complex interaction of CbpA protein and platelet-activating factor on activated endothelial cells.[219] When in the CSF, and because of insufficient opsonic and phagocytic activity in the CSF, organisms multiply rapidly, liberating cell wall or membrane components (lipopolysaccharide, lipoteichoic acid, peptidoglycan, bacterial toxins).

Host defenses within the CSF before and after bacterial invasion seem to rely on two important mechanisms available to the host to clear bacteria.[343] One clearance system requires a type-specific antibody, a functional classic complement system for opsonization, and the presence of competent polymorphonuclear leukocytes for phagocytosis. A second system, which is independent of polymorphonuclear leukocytes, involves activation of the alternative complement cascade and other components of the innate immune system. This sequence begins with the recognition of a "pathogen-associated molecular pattern," such as bacterial lipopolysaccharide, peptidoglycan, or lipoteichoic acid. The pathogen-associated molecular patterns are recognized by host "pathogen recognition receptors," such as C-reactive protein (CRP), mannose-binding lectin, and Toll-like receptors (TLRs). Mannose-binding lectin and CRP can initiate the alternate complement pathway. TLRs (primarily TLR-2 and TLR-4), which can recognize different pathogen-associated molecular patterns, trigger an intracellular signaling pathway that leads to the production of proinflammatory transcription factors such as nuclear factor-κB and the subsequent gene transcription of proinflammatory cytokines such as TNF-α and interferon-β.[245]

Complement and opsonic proteins either are found at very low concentrations or are absent entirely within normal CSF.[128,343] The CSF is devoid of the factors required for bacterial clearance. When bacteria first invade the meninges, the lack of complement and opsonic proteins within the sanctuary of the CNS may permit the bacteria to multiply unrestrained for some time. The slow response of polymorphonuclear leukocytes and the lack of serum-specific antibody available during the initial inflammatory response enhance the probability that bacterial infection will be established.[41,103,152,389,408]

The specific pathophysiologic changes in bacterial meningitis are the result of the bacterial products and the inflammatory response of the host to those products. Initial bactericidal antibiotic therapy results in a rapid release of bacterial products, such as endotoxins, teichoic acid, and peptidoglycans. Augmented permeability of the blood-brain barrier can be induced by bacterial products alone, which cause disruption of the tight junctions between capillary endothelial cells and marked increase in pinocytotic activity within endothelial cells. An influx of serum albumin into the CSF is accompanied by other low-molecular-weight proteins, including components of the complement cascade.[193]

TNF-α and IL-1 seem to be key mediators in initiation of meningeal inflammation. Both proteins stimulate vascular endothelial cells to induce adhesion and passage of neutrophils into the CNS and trigger inflammatory processes. Astrocytes and microglia are capable of producing TNF-α.[374] TNF-α concentrations are elevated (1) in CSF, but not in serum; (2) in animal models of bacterial meningitis; and (3) in patients with bacterial meningitis caused by H. influenzae, N. meningitidis, S. pneumoniae, and Streptococcus agalactiae,[269] but not in patients with culture-proven viral meningitis.[301] A complete understanding of TNF-α and the precise role it plays in meningitis has not been achieved. TNF-α levels can be correlated with meningeal inflammation and severity of disease, but lack of TNF-α in the animal model is associated with "increased mortality and stronger deficits in spatial memory."[147]

IL-1 activity can be detected in infants and children with bacterial meningitis, and its presence is correlated significantly with CSF inflammatory abnormalities, TNF-α concentrations, and adverse outcome.[269] TNF-α and IL-1 are capable of inducing phospholipase A_2 activity, which triggers the production of platelet-activating factor and activates the arachidonic acid pathway. This process leads to the generation of prostaglandins, thromboxanes, and leukotrienes from membrane phospholipids of endothelial and polymorphonuclear cells, which modulate multiple aspects of the inflammatory process.

These cytokines activate adhesion-promoting receptors on cerebral vascular endothelial cells, resulting in attraction and attachment of leukocytes to sites of stimuli. These leukocytes release proteolytic compounds that allow intercellular junctions to be traversed. These enzymes in conjunction with platelet-activating factor and the arachidonic acid metabolites injure the vascular endothelium, resulting in increased permeability of the blood-brain barrier and activation of the coagulation cascade.

Superoxide and hydrogen peroxide are secreted by TNF-α-stimulated macrophages, including brain microglia, and leukocytes.[296,303] Hydrogen peroxide induces extensive neuronal damage.[281] In addition, macrophages secrete excitatory amino acids, such as glutamate, which potentially kill N-methyl-D-aspartate receptor–positive cells.[227]

For gram-positive bacterial meningitis, lipoteichoic acid peptidoglycans are the bacterial surface elements that induce inflammation.[376] The threshold concentration that triggers inflammation is approximately 10^5 bacterial cell equivalents of cell wall pieces.[376] For gram-negative meningitis, endotoxin is the major inflammatory component, with peptidoglycan serving as an important cofactor.[57] The inflammatory threshold is approximately 2 pg of endotoxin, or approximately 10^5 bacterial cell equivalents.[401]

Cytokines now seem to be the primary drivers of the inflammatory response. The following cytokines are involved in the inflammatory response noted in bacterial meningitis: IL-1, IL-3, IL-4, IL-6, IL-8, IL-10, IL-12, IL-18, interferon-γ, macrophage inflammatory protein, transforming growth factor-β, and TNF-α.[91,134,382,409]

The chemokines are a superfamily of small chemoattractant cytokines that play an important role in the initiation and modulation of inflammation in bacterial meningitis.[357] Complement factors are up-regulated in bacterial meningitis. The activated complement cascade in CSF, acting on up-regulated complement receptors on brain cells, potentially mediates direct brain damage.[53] Complement factors also are chemoattractants that enhance CSF leukocytosis and indirectly produce brain damage in patients with bacterial meningitis.[102]

The most potent final effectors of brain damage in bacterial meningitis seem to be host-derived, low-molecular-weight mediators, such as hydrogen peroxide, hydroxyl radicals, and hypochlorous acid.[299] Nitric oxide also can be induced in brain cells in response to bacterial products.[210] Nitric oxide and superoxide radicals react to form peroxynitrite anion, which decomposes and forms nitrogen dioxide, hydroxyl radicals, and strong oxidant compounds.[36] Peroxynitrite seems to be an important neuronal toxin.[218] Neuronal damage caused by reactive oxygen species and reactive nitrate species occurs via at least two separate pathways. Reactive oxygen species and reactive nitrate species lead to lipid peroxidation and subsequent cell membrane instability and via activation of poly(adenosine diphosphate ribose) polymerase and its subsequent cellular energy depletion.[219]

The various pathways to neuronal cell death are shown in Figure 37–3. Meningitis causes damage in the cortex and the hippocampal region via different mechanisms. Cortical damage is mainly via cellular necrosis surrounded by an area of caspase-3-dependent apoptosis. Damage in the hippocampus is mediated not only via the classic caspase-3-dependent pathway but also by caspase-independent apoptosis mediated by apoptosis-initiating factor.[40,42,257] The caspase-independent apoptotic pathway seems to be important earlier (by 18 hours after infection), whereas the classic caspase-dependent pathway assumes importance later.[257] Braun and Tuomanen[53] have provided a detailed review of the molecular mechanisms of brain damage in bacterial meningitis. In addition, a review by Scheld and coworkers[327] focuses specifically on neuronal injury. The role of inflammatory mediators and oxygen radicals in the pathogenesis of bacterial meningitis is described in detail in a review by Leib and Tauber.[234]

The increasing concentrations of chemotactic factors in the subarachnoid space lead to accumulation of large numbers of neutrophils in the CSF, and the growth of bacteria is not slowed

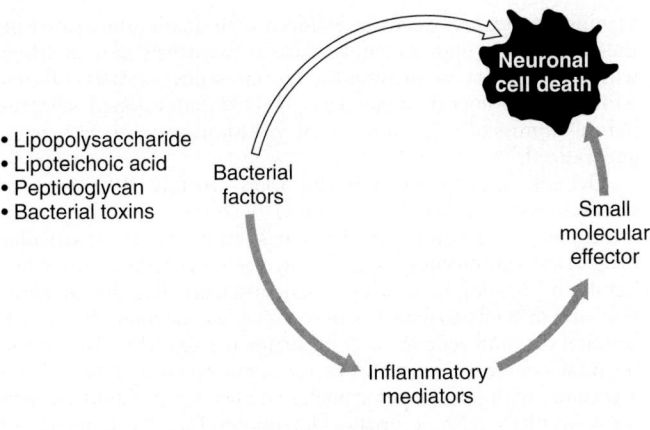

- Lipopolysaccharide
- Lipoteichoic acid
- Peptidoglycan
- Bacterial toxins

- Reactive oxygen species (superoxide, peroxynitrite)
- Reactive nitrogen species (nitric oxide)
- Excitatory amino acids (glutamate, aspartate, glycine, taurine, alanine)

- Cytokines (TNF, IL-1, IL-6, IL-8, IL-10, PAF, TGFβ)
- Arachidonic acid metabolites (prostaglandins, leukotrienes)
- Complement

Figure 37–3 Pathways to neuronal cell death. Although bacterial products can induce directly some neuronal toxicity, host-derived inflammatory agents are the primary source of final mediators of injury. IL, interleukin; PAF, platelet-activating factor; TGF, transforming growth factor; TNF, tumor necrosis factor. *(From Braun, J. S., and Tuomanen, E. I.: Molecular mechanisms of brain damage in bacterial meningitis. Adv. Pediatr. Infect. Dis. 14:49-71, 1999.)*

significantly by this response.[102] Impaired phagocytosis by neutrophils in the meningeal spaces may be related to weak activity in fluid medium, lack of complement activity and opsonization, and poor penetration of IgM and IgG through the blood-brain barrier, even during acute *H. influenzae* and *S. pneumoniae* meningitis.[153] Leukocyte entry into the CSF is still important, however. Brandt and colleagues[52] showed that blockage of leukocyte entry into the CSF was associated with poorer prognosis (likely secondary to an increase in bacterial counts in the blood) but did not affect the risk of brain damage.

Bacterial cell wall fragments, endotoxin, or both also contribute to vascular permeability. In experimental *E. coli* meningitis, the CSF endotoxin concentration increased markedly after treatment with β-lactam antibiotics. This increase was associated with an increase in brain water content. This effect could be blocked by polymyxin or a monoclonal antibody, both of which inactivate endotoxin.[368]

The inflammatory and vascular events described earlier act synergistically to produce the clinical symptoms and long-term sequelae that are noted in patients with bacterial meningitis. As described subsequently, altered vascular permeability leads to vasogenic edema, inflammatory and electrolyte changes lead to cytotoxic edema, and alterations in production and absorption of CSF lead to interstitial edema. The cytokines also trigger increased cerebral blood flow and further formation of edema, resulting in increased intracranial pressure.[23] The increased intracranial pressure and vasculitis lead to a subsequent decrease in cerebral blood flow, which does not seem to be caused by loss of autoregulation.[23] Activation of the coagulation cascade predisposes the patient to venous, microvascular, and, rarely, arterial thrombosis. Direct neurotoxic damage by inflammatory cells also may contribute to the neuropathologic changes seen in bacterial meningitis.

CLINICAL MANIFESTATIONS AND PATHOPHYSIOLOGIC RELATIONSHIPS

Inflammation of the meninges generally is associated with nausea, vomiting, irritability, anorexia, headache, confusion, back pain, and nuchal rigidity. In many cases, Kernig and Brudzinski signs are present. Kernig sign is present when the leg is flexed 90 degrees at the hips and cannot be extended more than 135 degrees. Brudzinski sign is present if the thighs and legs are flexed invol-

untarily when the neck is flexed. All of these findings suggest irritation of inflamed sensory nerves, which produces a reflex contraction of certain muscles in an attempt to minimize pain. These findings also can be the result of increased intracranial pressure and an associated distortion of nerve roots. These signs can be accompanied by hyperesthesia and photophobia. Currently, no satisfactory pathophysiologic explanation for photophobia exists. Signs of meningeal inflammation may be minimal in the infant, but irritability, restlessness, and poor feeding may be noted. Nuchal rigidity and Kernig and Brudzinski signs may occur late in a young child. Nuchal rigidity may not be elicited in comatose patients or when signs of focal or diffuse neurologic impairment are present. At the time of initial evaluation, 60 to 80 percent of children have a stiff neck.[195] A review of 1064 cases of bacterial meningitis in children beyond the neonatal period revealed that 16 (1.5%) had no meningeal signs during their entire period of hospitalization, despite the presence of CSF pleocytosis.[145] Fever, a hallmark of infection, generally is present; its absence in a patient with signs of meningeal inflammation, although infrequent, is not unusual.

Increased intracranial pressure is the rule; it may be reflected by complaints of headache in older children and by a bulging fontanelle and diastasis of sutures in infants. Papilledema is an uncommon finding in acute meningitis, presumably because of the brief duration of increased pressure at the time of diagnosis. When papilledema is observed, venous sinus occlusion, subdural empyema, or brain abscess should be sought.

Signs of cerebral edema may be present. Vasogenic edema occurs as a consequence of increased permeability of the blood-brain barrier. Interstitial edema may occur secondary to decreased clearance of CSF at the arachnoid villi and subsequent obstructive hydrocephalus. Cytotoxic cerebral edema mediated by the release of toxic factors from neutrophils and bacteria leads to increased concentration of intracellular water and sodium and loss of intracellular potassium. In many cases (88 percent in one prospective study[107]), meningitis is associated with the release of ADH, causing water retention and a relative dumping of sodium by the kidney. If the patient is given excessive free water during therapy, a further increase in intracranial pressure may be noted.

Transient or permanent paralysis of cranial nerves may be noted. Deafness or disturbances in vestibular function are common findings; optic nerve involvement with blindness rarely occurs. Involvement of the eighth cranial nerve may reflect disease at the level of the cochlear and vestibular end-organs, which may be related to concomitant infection of the inner ear. Paralysis of extraocular and facial nerves may be noted. Torticollis has been reported in two children with partially treated meningitis.[250] Obtundation, stupor, coma, and focal neurologic signs may be seen in children with bacterial meningitis.

The relative frequency with which these findings are noted is shown in Table 37–2, in which data for 235 children with bacterial meningitis who were enrolled prospectively have been analyzed according to the type of organism responsible for meningitis. Overall, 14.9 percent of children were semicomatose or comatose at the time of admission; rates for children with pneumococcal or meningococcal meningitis were higher than rates for children with *H. influenzae* disease. Focal neurologic signs were present at the time of admission in 16.5 percent of the total group (34.3% of children with pneumococcal meningitis). The presence of focal neurologic signs at the time of admission indicated a poor prognosis and could be correlated with persistent abnormal neurologic examinations at 1, 3, and 6 months ($p < .01$) and at 1 year after discharge ($p < .03$). The presence of focal signs at the time of admission also correlated with the presence of retardation ($p < .001$), as determined by detailed psychometric testing after discharge.

Generally, when focal signs are noted in the absence of seizures, cortical necrosis, occlusive vasculitis, or thrombosis of cortical veins has occurred. Thrombosis of meningeal vessels or cortical necrosis may be associated with hemiparesis or quadriparesis and with focal seizures. These signs may appear during the first 3 or 4 days of illness or, less commonly, may be noted after the first or second week of infection. A highly significant association ($p < .001$) between neurologic signs indicative of cerebral injury and late (1 to 15 years after the acute infection) afebrile seizures has been noted.[293] Ataxia has been a presenting sign of meningitis in numerous children and adults. Schwartz[336] described four children who presented with ataxia as an initial symptom. Adolescents with meningitis may present with behavioral abnormalities that may be confused with drug abuse or psychiatric disorders.[28]

Approximately 20 percent of children with bacterial meningitis experience seizures before admissions, and approximately 26 percent have them during the first or second day in the hospital. Green and colleagues[164] retrospectively examined the frequency of seizures before or at the time of presentation in children with meningitis. They found that 111 of 410 (27%) children with bacterial meningitis had seizures at or before the time of diagnosis; 88 of these children had complex seizures (focal, prolonged, or more than one in a 24-hour period). They found that all children with bacterial meningitis who presented with seizures had other signs or symptoms of meningitis, such as altered level of consciousness, nuchal rigidity, or complex seizures and petechial rash. The frequency of seizure activity is similar for children with *H. influenzae* type b or pneumococcal

meningitis; seizures occur in children with meningitis caused by these organisms approximately twice as frequently as in children with meningococcal meningitis. In one study of 181 children with pneumo-coccal meningitis, 41 (23%) developed seizures before admission; 75 percent of preadmission seizures were generalized.[20]

Overall, seizures are noted in approximately 30 percent of children with bacterial meningitis. Seizures noted before or during the first several days of hospitalization are of no particular prognostic significance. Specifically, their occurrence does not herald the development of a permanent seizure disorder. Seizures that are difficult to control or that persist beyond the fourth hospital day and seizures that occur for the first time late in the hospital course may be of greater significance and have been associated with permanent sequelae of meningitis. Children with focal seizures have a greater likelihood for development of sequelae of meningitis than do children with generalized seizure activity. Focal or prolonged seizures probably indicate serious cerebral vascular disturbances or cerebral infarction. Seizures that occur before admission have correlated positively with abnormal audiometric studies and permanent hearing handicaps. Seven percent of patients with bacterial meningitis have focal or generalized seizures 3 months to 15 years after recovery from bacterial meningitis.[293]

Collections of fluid in the subdural space can be shown in 50 percent of infants and children during acute illness.[96] In a prospective study of infants 1 to 18 months old with bacterial meningitis, subdural effusions were noted in 43 percent of infants with *H. influenzae* meningitis, 30 percent of infants with pneumococcal meningitis, and 22 percent of infants with meningococcal meningitis. Subdural effusions were found in 24 percent (25 of 103) of children undergoing neuroimaging in the multicenter pediatric surveillance study of pneumococcal meningitis.[20,351] No greater incidence of neurologic sequelae or developmental delay was found on long-term follow-up in patients with effusion compared with patients with bacterial meningitis who did not have effusion.[348,351]

Subdural effusions may cause enlargement in head circumference or may be responsible for abnormal transillumination of the skull. Vomiting, seizures, a full fontanelle, focal neurologic signs, or persistent fever may be noted sometimes, but these signs occur with such frequency in children with bacterial meningitis who do not have subdural effusions that it is difficult to attribute their occurrence to the subdural effusion.[110]

Blindness and optic atrophy may be related to optic arachnoiditis or infarction of the occipital lobe. Spastic paraparesis with sensory loss in the lower extremities may be secondary to meningomyelitis, spinal cord infarction, or both.

Arthralgia and myalgia are noted in many patients with bacterial meningitis, reflecting the systemic nature of the disease. Arthritis also may occur and does so most commonly during the course of meningococcal disease; generally, it is transient. Early

TABLE 37–2 Frequency of Selected Findings in Children with Bacterial Meningitis

	Total Group	*Haemophilus influenzae*	*Streptococcus pneumoniae*	*Neisseria meningitidis*	Others
No. patients	235	151	35	26	23
Level of consciousness (%)					
Irritable or lethargic	184 (78.3)	117 (77.5)	24 (68.6)	21 (80.8)	22 (95.7)
Somnolent	16 (6.8)	13 (8.6)	1 (2.8)	1 (3.8)	1 (4.3)
Obtunded-semicomatose	27 (11.5)	15 (9.9)	8 (22.9)	4 (15.4)	0 (0)
Comatose	8 (3.4)	6 (4)	2 (5.7)	0 (0)	0 (0)
Focal neurologic signs on admission (%)	37 (16.5)	22 (14.6)	12 (34.3)	2 (7.7)	1 (4.3)
Seizures before admission (%)	48 (20.4)	35 (23.2)	8 (23)	3 (11.5)	2 (8.7)
Seizures in hospital (%)	61 (26)	43 (28)	12 (34)	5 (19)	1 (4.5)

findings of arthritis may be related to direct invasion of the joint by the meningococcus. Arthritis that develops late in the course of meningococcal or *H. influenzae* meningitis may be an immune complex–mediated event. Petechial or purpuric lesions may be seen in 50 percent of patients with meningococcal meningitis[96] but also may accompany any infectious or noninfectious disease process in which vasculitis occurs. Purpura, shock, and hypothermia indicate a poor prognosis.

Pericardial effusions may be present; they generally resolve during the course of antibiotic therapy. In some cases, pericardial effusions are the cause of persistent fever, and pericardiocentesis or an open drainage procedure may be required.

Shock may be associated with any form of overwhelming bacteremia, but it occurs most often in patients with fulminant meningococcemia. In a prospective study, 3.8 percent of children with meningococcal meningitis developed profound hypotension. In the same study, shock occurred in 5.5 percent of children with *H. influenzae* meningitis. Endotoxin has been detected by Limulus lysate assay in the blood and CSF of children with meningococcal and *H. influenzae* meningitis.[311] Sixteen percent of the children in the multicenter pneumococcal meningitis study were in shock on admission.[20] Signs of disseminated intravascular coagulation may accompany hypotension in these patients.

Facial cellulitis (including buccal and periorbital cellulitis), pneumonia, epiglottitis, endophthalmitis, and other suppurative manifestations can manifest at the time of admission in any patient with bacterial meningitis. In one study of children with buccal cellulitis, less than 10 percent (7 of 73) had concomitant bacterial meningitis documented by lumbar puncture as part of their initial evaluation.[26] Five of the seven children had no clinical evidence of meningeal irritation. *H. influenzae* and *S. pneumoniae* were cultured from two patients with periorbital cellulitis, and no clinical evidence of meningeal irritation or abnormal CSF cell counts or chemistries was found.[320] In the largest review of facial cellulitis caused by *S. pneumoniae*,[160] 15 of 52 children had a lumbar puncture performed; 2 (13.3%) had a pleocytosis (18 white blood cells [WBCs]—52% polymorphonuclear leukocytes, and 9 WBCs—91% polymorphonuclear leukocytes). The Gram stain and cultures of the CSF specimens were negative. Lumbar puncture should be considered for children with facial cellulitis who are younger than 18 months and possibly bacteremic with *S. pneumoniae*.

DIFFERENTIAL DIAGNOSIS

The signs and symptoms described earlier suggest meningeal or intracranial pathologic processes but are not pathognomonic of acute bacterial infection. Tuberculous meningitis, fungal meningitis, aseptic meningitis, brain abscess, intracranial or spinal epidural abscesses, bacterial endocarditis with embolism, subdural empyema with or without thrombophlebitis, ruptured dermoid cysts, ruptured spinal ependymomas, and brain tumors may show similar signs and symptoms. Differentiation of these disorders depends on careful examination of CSF obtained by lumbar puncture and additional immunologic, radiographic, and isotopic studies as delineated later.

DIAGNOSIS

Early diagnosis and treatment of bacterial meningitis are imperative in reducing mortality rates and morbidity. Physicians must perform a lumbar puncture on any child in whom they suspect the diagnosis after a careful history and physical examination have been performed, unless specific contraindications to this procedure (e.g., clinical signs of increased intracranial pressure in a patient with a closed fontanelle and closed sutures) are present.

An association between performance of a lumbar puncture during bacteremia and the later development of meningitis has been reported.[126] This association was evident only in children younger than 1 year old. Perceptive physicians select children for lumbar puncture in whom clinical signs suggest developing meningitis before the CSF findings are diagnostic. These data suggest a need for careful observation and, if appropriate, hospitalization and antimicrobial therapy for infants younger than 1 year who undergo lumbar puncture and who concomitantly have risk factors (e.g., concurrent high temperature and WBC counts) for the development of bacteremia. Table 37–3 summarizes CSF findings characteristic of various inflammatory diseases of the CNS.

Measurement of pressure, often neglected in infants and young children, is an important component of each CSF examination. When the pressure is very high, only enough fluid to permit a careful examination should be removed. Compression of the jugular vein should be avoided unless compression of the spinal cord is suspected. Xanthochromic CSF derives its color primarily from bilirubin pigment. Hemorrhage, bilirubin staining in icteric patients who have meningitis (i.e., neonates, patients with leptospirosis), or an elevated protein concentration of CSF may be associated with xanthochromia.

CSF should be examined immediately. The total number of WBCs should be counted in a counting chamber, and after cytocentrifugation, a differential cell count should be done on a Wright-stained smear of the sediment. The normal CSF of children 3 months or older contains less than 6 WBCs/mm³. Ninety-five percent of children older than 3 months have no polymorphonuclear leukocytes in the CSF; the presence of a polymorphonuclear leukocyte in the CSF may be regarded as abnormal. When a lumbar puncture has been performed in a febrile child and a single polymorphonuclear leukocyte has been noted, careful clinical observation is imperative, and treatment should be considered until the results of the culture of the CSF are known.

If the lumbar puncture has been traumatic, a total cell count can be done in a counting chamber. The red blood cells (RBCs) can be lysed by acetic acid, and a cell count can be repeated. If the total number of WBCs compared with the number of RBCs is greater than that in whole blood, one can assume the presence of CSF pleocytosis. One simple way to estimate the WBC count in the presence of RBCs is to allow 1 WBC per 1000 RBCs/mm³. CSF protein should be measured (usually elevated in bacterial meningitis), and the CSF glucose concentration should be compared with the blood glucose concentration that has been obtained concomitantly. In patients with bacterial meningitis, depression of CSF glucose and of the ratio of CSF to blood glucose (normally approximately 66%) is the rule.

Separate smears should be made, and one smear should be Gram stained for bacteria. A Kinyoun stain for mycobacteria is performed if tuberculous meningitis is suspected. The probability of visualizing bacteria on a Gram stain of CSF depends on the number of organisms present. The percentage of positive smears is 25 percent with less than 10^3 colony-forming units (CFU)/mL, 60 percent in the range of 10^3 to 10^5 CFU/mL, and 97 percent with greater than 10^5 CFU/mL.[226] Quellung and agglutination reactions can provide immediate identification of various organisms if the appropriate type of specific antisera is available.

Treating a child with bacterial meningitis with an antibiotic before performing initial lumbar puncture usually does not alter markedly the morphologic or chemical results obtained (Table 37–4). In patients with *H. influenzae* meningitis (Table 37–5) who were pretreated, CSF cultures frequently grew *H. influenzae*; there is a tendency to pretreat children with pneumococcal or meningococcal disease to render the CSF sterile (see Table 37–4). Even when children received appropriate antibiotics for meningitis intravenously for 44 to 68 hours, the bacterial character

TABLE 37–3 Cerebrospinal Fluid Findings in Suppurative Diseases of the Central Nervous System and Meninges

Condition	Pressure (mm H₂O)	Leukocytes/mm³	Protein (mg/dL)	Sugar (mg/dL)	Specific Findings
Acute bacterial meningitis	Usually elevated; average 300	Several hundred to >60,000; usually a few thousand; occasionally <100 (especially meningococcal or early in disease); polymorphonuclears predominate	Usually 100-500, occasionally >1000	<40 in more than half the cases	Organism usually seen on smear or recovered on culture in >90% of cases
Subdural empyema	Usually elevated; average 300	<100 to a few thousand; polymorphonuclears predominate	Usually 100-500	Normal	No organisms on smear or by culture unless concurrent meningitis
Brain abscess	Usually elevated	Usually 10-200; fluid rarely is acellular; lymphocytes predominate	Usually 75-400	Normal	No organisms on smear or by culture predominate
Ventricular empyema (rupture of brain abscess)	Considerably elevated	Several thousand to 100,000; usually >90% polymorphonuclears	Usually several hundred	Usually <40	Organisms may be cultured or seen on smear
Cerebral epidural abscess	Slight to modest elevation	Few to several hundred or more cells; lymphocytes predominate	Usually 50-200	Normal	No organisms on smear or by culture
Spinal epidural abscess	Usually reduced with spinal block	Usually 10-100; lymphocytes predominate	Usually several hundred	Normal	No organisms on smear or by culture
Thrombophlebitis (often associated with subdural empyema)	Often elevated	Few to several hundred; polymorphonuclears and lymphocytes	Slightly to moderately elevated	Normal	No organisms on smear or by culture
Bacterial endocarditis (with embolism)	Normal or slightly elevated	Few to <100; lymphocytes and polymorphonuclears	Slightly elevated	Normal	No organisms on smear or by culture
Acute hemorrhagic encephalitis	Usually elevated	Few to >1000; polymorphonuclears predominate	Moderately elevated	Normal	No organisms on smear or by culture
Tuberculous infection	Usually elevated; may be low with dynamic block in advanced stages	Usually 25-100, rarely >500; lymphocytes predominate except in early stages when polymorphonuclears may account for 80% of cells	Nearly always elevated; usually 100-200; may be much higher if dynamic block	Usually reduced; <50 in 75% of cases	Acid-fast organisms may be seen on smear of protein coagulum (pellicle) or recovered from inoculated guinea pig or by culture
Cryptococcal infection	Usually elevated; average 225	Average 50 (0-800); lymphocytes predominate	Average 100; usually 20-500	Reduced in more than half of cases; average 30; often higher in patients with concomitant diabetes mellitus	Organisms may be seen in India ink preparation and on culture (Sabouraud medium); usually grow on blood agar; may produce alcohol in cerebrospinal fluid from fermentation of glucose
Syphilis (acute)	Usually elevated	Average 500; usually lymphocytes; rarely polymorphonuclears	Average, 100; gamma-globulin often high, with abnormal colloidal	Normal (rarely reduced)	Positive reagin test result for syphilis; spirochete not demonstrable by usual techniques of smear or by culture gold curve
Sarcoidosis	Normal to considerably elevated	0 to <100 mononuclear cells	Slight to moderate elevation	Normal	No specific findings

of the chemical and morphologic findings could be discerned in most cases.[46]

The CSF should be cultured on a blood agar plate and a chocolate agar plate. The CSF specimens always should be cultured, even when the fluid appears to be crystal-clear and acellular or nearly so.

In the 1970s, countercurrent immunoelectrophoresis was shown to be a useful technique for rapid diagnosis (within 1 hour) and management of bacterial meningitis caused by *H. influenzae* type b, *S. pneumoniae*, *N. meningitidis* (groups A, C, W135, and D), and group B streptococcus. It may be used to detect antigens from K1 strains of *E. coli* or *L. monocytogenes*.[117,248] The methodol-

TABLE 37-4 Comparison of Cerebrospinal Fluid Findings in Patients with Untreated and Pretreated Meningitis

	Untreated	Pretreated
No. patients	143	91
Total white blood cell count × 10³		
Mean ± 1 SD	4.9 ± 6.5	4.1 ± 5
Range	0-55	0.006-25.5
Percentage polys		
Mean ± 1 SD	84 ± 21	81 ± 25
Range	0-100	0-100
Glucose (mg/dL)		
Mean ± 1 SD	35 ± 28	32 ± 25
Range	0-109	0-100
CSF/blood glucose (%)		
Mean ± 1 SD	29 ± 21	29 ± 21
Range	0-78	0-94
Protein (mg/dL)		
Mean ± 1 SD	226 ± 228	174 ± 193
Range	13-2290	10-1640
Culture-positive	135	71
Gram stain–positive	114	62

CSF, cerebrospinal fluid; SD, standard deviation.

TABLE 37-5 Cerebrospinal Fluid Findings in Untreated and Pretreated Patients with *Haemophilus influenzae* Meningitis

	Untreated	Pretreated
No. patients	92	57
Total white blood cell count × 10³		
Mean ± 1 SD	5.6 ± 7.6	4 ± 4.8
Range	0.001-55	0.094-25
Percentage polys		
Mean ± 1 SD	91 ± 15	83 ± 22
Range	0-108	0-99
Glucose (mg/dL)		
Mean ± 1 SD	34 ± 27.5	29 ± 26
Range	0-109	0-99
CSF/blood glucose (%)		
Mean ± 1 SD	29 ± 21	24 ± 20
Range	0-78	0-82
Protein (mg/dL)		
Mean ± 1 SD	214 ± 129	187 ± 227
Range	25-752	29-1640
CIE (µg/mL)		
Mean ± 1 SD	1.83 ± 2.63	2.36 ± 4.73
Range	0-10.24	0-20.48
Culture-positive	91	51
Gram stain–positive	81	45
CIE-positive	77/88	50/55

CIE, counterimmunoelectrophoresis; CSF, cerebrospinal fluid; SD, standard deviation.

ogy is sensitive and can detect nonviable bacteria, permitting the detection of bacterial antigen, even in patients who have been pretreated with appropriate antibiotics. If this technique is employed, it is imperative to use antisera that have the greatest possible sensitivity and specificity.[187,338] Group B meningococcal antiserum, which is available commercially, is unreliable. When pneumococcal antisera are used, material obtained from the State Serum Institute in Copenhagen, Denmark, has proved to be highly efficacious; sensitivity is enhanced by using the various pools of pneumococcal antisera in addition to the omniserum. A negative result of countercurrent immunoelectrophoresis does not exclude the diagnosis of bacterial meningitis.

Latex particle agglutination commercial kits are available for detecting the polysaccharide antigens of *H. influenzae* type b, *S. pneumoniae*, *N. meningitidis*, and group B streptococcus. Latex

particle agglutination is superior to countercurrent immunoelectrophoresis in detecting PRP antigen of *H. influenzae* type b in CSF and serum. Nonspecific agglutination of latex particles in serum, urine, and other body fluids may result in an indeterminate test result.[80,188,326,394] A commercial latex particle agglutination kit containing antibody-coated latex particles for *H. influenzae* type b, *S. pneumoniae*, and *N. meningitidis* serogroups is available. The Food and Drug Administration does not recommend latex agglutination testing of urine of infants for group B streptococcus as a method for inferring invasive disease with this organism. Latex agglutination of urine for group B streptococcus or *N. meningitidis* should be avoided because of the high frequency of false-positive results.

The clinical utility of rapid antigen detection in CSF has been questioned in recent years since the decline in frequency of invasive infections caused by *H. influenzae* type b. A positive test response rarely alters the approach to therapy. Maxson and associates[247] examined this issue and suggested that bacterial antigen tests be reserved for patients with suspected bacterial meningitis whose initial CSF Gram stain was negative and whose culture was negative after 48 hours of incubation. Perkins and associates[289] reviewed all latex particle agglutination tests done during a 10-month period at two hospitals and reached the same conclusion. Finlay and colleagues[124] suggested that latex agglutination testing of CSF be used only when the Gram stain is negative when it is consistent with meningococci. In the latter case, clarifying the meningococcal serotype quickly may have implications in large outbreaks for recommending meningococcal vaccine for type A, C, Y, or W135 disease.

The rapidity with which results of bacterial antigen tests are obtained renders them tempting as a means to establish an early diagnosis. The degree to which they affect clinical decisions is unclear.[247] Performing these tests is unnecessary for every patient suspected to have bacterial meningitis, but they could play a role in certain circumstances, such as when a patient's clinical presentation suggests bacterial meningitis and pretreatment with antibiotics or with a traumatic lumbar puncture. Antigen detection is useful in developing countries, where CSF culture yields are lower.[85]

Polymerase chain reaction (PCR) analysis of CSF has been used to detect microbial DNA in patients with bacterial meningitis. Primers are available for the detection of *S. pneumoniae*, *N. meningitidis*, and *H. influenzae* type b simultaneously. Species-specific amplicons have been detected in 89 percent of patients with proven streptococcal, meningococcal, or *H. influenzae* type b meningitis.[300] No false-positive results were noted.

Kotilainen and associates[224] used PCR and DNA sequencing techniques in a prospective study of CSF from patients with suspected bacterial meningitis. The bacterial 23S rRNA gene was amplified from the CSF of 5 of 46 adults with possible infection of the CNS. After sequencing of the 16S or 23S rRNA gene PCR products, 98.3 to 100 percent homology with *N. meningitidis* was observed in all five patients. This PCR method was not timely enough for routine laboratory use because it required 2 to 5 days to obtain results that could be reported to the physician.

Dagan and associates[78] have described the use of PCR for detection of *S. pneumoniae* within CSF. du Plessis and associates[97] have developed a seminested PCR strategy based on the amplification of the pneumococcal penicillin-binding protein 2B gene to detect penicillin-susceptible or penicillin-nonsusceptible *S. pneumoniae* within CSF. PCR detected pneumococci in all of the 18 culture-positive CSF specimens (of 285 total specimens tested). No false-positive results were noted. This test required only a few hours to perform and used only 15 µL of CSF.

Advances in the field have made the use of PCR technology a more viable option in the diagnostic approach to meningitis. The use of real-time PCR has shortened the time needed for completion of specimen analysis from several days to several hours. PCR technology can be applied in a broad-spectrum manner, such as testing for amplification of bacterial 16s rRNA[334] or in a bacteria-specific manner using specific probes for *Neisseria* and *Streptococcus* spp.[78,262] or other bacterial pathogens. One diagnostic strategy combines the use of broad-range, real-time PCR for detection of bacterial presence in the CSF and is followed by bacterial identification after subsequent DNA sequencing.[89] The use of such PCR techniques is helpful in patients pretreated with antibiotics in whom the culture may be negative.[89,284] The possible addition of gene microarray technology offers the potential to probe for multiple different bacterial species simultaneously.[177]

PCR also is useful in rapidly documenting viral antigens within CSF, reducing the use of antibiotics in selected patients who are treated for presumptive bacterial disease but who may have viral meningitis.[312,331,385] Dicuonzo and associates[92] also documented the great sensitivity of oligoprobes on amplified DNA for the diagnosis of *H. influenzae*, streptococcal, and *Mycobacterium tuberculosis* meningitis. No false-negative results occurred in culture-positive CSF specimens.

Measurement of CRP has been proposed as a test that may be valuable in distinguishing bacterial from viral meningitis. In some studies, overlap in CRP determinations between these groups of patients has been observed. For this reason, we do not consider that one can rely on the CRP result to distinguish bacterial from viral meningitis with sufficient certainty.[112,150,191] Nonetheless, in the best study to date, serum CRP was superior to CSF parameters in distinguishing Gram stain–negative bacterial from viral meningitis.[356] Among 92 patients with viral meningitis, 93 percent had serum CRP levels within the normal range (<20 mg/L). Only one child with Gram stain–negative bacterial meningitis had a serum CRP value within the normal range.

Numerous metabolic changes have been reported to occur in the CSF and blood of patients with meningitis (Table 37–6). CSF lactate has been noted to be elevated significantly in patients with bacterial meningitis. The increase in CSF lactate apparently is related to decreased cerebral blood flow, cerebral hypoxia, and a change to anaerobic metabolism by the brain. Concentration of CSF lactate tends to parallel the CSF cellular response.[315] Although the concentration of CSF lactate in patients with bacterial meningitis generally is greater than that in patients with aseptic meningitis, such is not always the case. In some patients with aseptic meningitis, CSF lactate has been in the range generally observed in patients with bacterial infections. Conversely, in patients who proved to have bacterial meningitis but who had equivocal clinical and CSF findings, measurement of CSF lactate failed to differentiate bacterial from nonbacterial infection.[315] The determination of the concentration of CSF lactate cannot be used reliably to differentiate viral from bacterial meningitis in an individual patient.[220]

Depression of the pH of CSF also has been described in patients with bacterial meningitis. The depression of pH in CSF is more transient than is the elevation of CSF lactic acid, and its measurement is of even less value in the differential diagnosis.[397]

TABLE 37-6 Metabolic Changes Reported in Patients with Bacterial Meningitis

CSF lactate increased
CSF pH decreased
CSF lactate dehydrogenase increased
Creatine phosphokinase increased
Aspartate transaminase increased
CSF and blood elastase-α-proteinase inhibitor increased
CSF vasopressin increased

CSF, cerebrospinal fluid.

Lactate dehydrogenase, creatine phosphokinase, and aspartate transaminase may be elevated in patients with bacterial meningitis. In some cases, total lactate dehydrogenase activity within CSF may be similar in patients with bacterial and aseptic meningitis, but lactate dehydrogenase isoenzymic analysis may permit differentiation of bacterial from nonbacterial infection. This procedure is time-consuming and cumbersome and does not permit establishing a specific etiologic diagnosis in any patient.[198,276]

Despite the application of impeccable clinical judgment, examination of CSF, and use of one or more of the rapid diagnostic techniques, situations arise in which differentiation of bacterial from aseptic meningitis remains problematic. In these cases, a predominance of polymorphonuclear leukocytes generally is found in the CSF, the CSF cell count is less than 100 cells/mm³, the CSF glucose concentration is normal or nearly so, and the Gram stain result is negative. Most children with aseptic meningitis have a predominance of polymorphonuclear leukocytes on their initial CSF examination.[277] In addition, although patients exhibit signs and symptoms suggestive of meningitis, they do not appear acutely ill. Some investigators have advocated withholding antibiotic therapy in these patients and repeating the lumbar puncture after 6 to 12 hours of close observation.[3,113] Usually, the repeated examination of CSF either substantiates the impression of aseptic meningitis (a shift to a lymphocytic differential is noted) or points more conclusively to a bacterial process. This course of action is not recommended if the patient has been pretreated with antibiotics or is younger than 1 year old. Occasionally, children have a mild CSF pleocytosis, which may have a predominance of polymorphonuclear leukocytes, after they experience seizures.[403,405] Generally, CSF abnormalities should not be attributed to seizures, unless other causes of CNS inflammation have been excluded.

Other approaches to differentiate bacterial from viral meningitis have been suggested. Evaluation of CSF ferritin concentration has been proposed as a test with considerable predictive value. Kim and associates[209] showed in pediatric patients that CSF ferritin concentration is significantly elevated in bacterial meningitis compared with viral meningitis. Using a proposed cutoff of 15.6 ng/mL of CSF ferritin, the test had a sensitivity of 96.2 percent and a specificity of 96.6 percent in differentiating bacterial from viral meningitis.

Additional laboratory data are helpful and should be obtained. Blood cultures should be obtained in every patient suspected to have bacterial meningitis. In one prospective study in which blood was obtained for culture from every patient, the cultures were positive in 80 percent of children with *H. influenzae* meningitis, in 52 percent of children with pneumococcal meningitis, and in 33 percent of children with meningococcal meningitis.[108] Forty-four percent of the entire group had received some form of antibiotic therapy before admission to the hospital and before these blood cultures were performed. If these individuals were excluded, positive blood cultures were obtained from 90 percent, 80 percent, and 91 percent of children with meningitis caused by *H. influenzae*, *S. pneumoniae*, and *N. meningitidis*, respectively.

A thorough search for foci of infection adjacent to or remote from the meninges should be conducted. Repetitive neurologic evaluation also should be performed, and appropriate laboratory studies should be undertaken to define the extent of neurologic dysfunction.

When the concentration of bacteria within the blood is high, a Gram-stained smear of a buffy coat obtained from the blood may reveal the presence of microorganisms. If petechial lesions are present, a smear of the lesions after puncture with a small lancet may reveal microorganisms on Gram stain. A chest radiograph may be helpful in disclosing a focus of infection.

Radioisotope scanning may be helpful in selected patients, such as patients with a leak of CSF. The pattern of distribution of radioactivity recorded by gamma camera coincides with the accumulation of purulent material. Increased concentration of isotope may relate to the inflammatory response within the meninges or in the periventricular region or to alteration in the blood-brain barrier.[155] Localized concentrations of radionuclide may be seen in children with meningitis, most likely as a result of cerebral vasculitis or infarction.[96] Confirmation of impaired cerebral circulation, including occlusion and narrowing of arteries, sluggish circulation, and retrograde flow, has been provided by the studies of Gado and associates.[140] In these studies, resolution of the arterial lesions was shown in subsequent angiograms in two patients, despite the persistence of neurologic deficits; these findings prompted the authors to suspect vascular spasm at the earlier stage of disease. Hydrocephalus contributed to sluggish circulation through intracerebral vessels in two patients. Tyson and colleagues[377] showed at least transient disturbance in the circulation of CSF in 45 percent of patients with meningitis, but persistent hydrocephalus is a rare complication of purulent meningitis.

Computed tomography (CT) and magnetic resonance imaging (MRI) are noninvasive techniques that permit the prospective and repetitive assessment of children with meningitis. These techniques permit detection of ventricular dilation, subdural effusion, decrease in brain mass, and presence of vascular lesions or of brain infarcts (Fig. 37-4). With these procedures, ventricular dilation may be noted acutely in many children who never develop hydrocephalus after recovery from their disease.[108] Neuroimaging may be indicated in the following situations: (1) focal neurologic signs, (2) persistently positive CSF cultures despite administration of appropriate antibiotic therapy, (3) persistent elevation of CSF polymorphonuclear leukocytes (>30 to 40%) after more than 10 days of therapy, and (4) recurrent meningitis.[215]

Recurrent bacterial meningitis may be the result of a communication between the nasal passage or ear and the meninges. If rhinorrhea or otorrhea is present, a leak may be suspected, but documenting that CSF is present and locating the site of leakage are difficult when the sample is small or contaminated. Sectional (2 mm) coronal cranial CT has been reported to be an easy, noninvasive method for delineating anatomic abnormalities in children with recurrent meningitis.[362]

Meurman and associates[255] showed that an extra band of transferrin is located in the β_2-fraction after protein electrophoresis of CSF. This extra β_2-transferrin band could not be shown in serum, nasal secretions, saliva, tears, or perilymph and endolymph. The amount of sample required is small (<50 µL). We have applied this immunochemical method successfully in documenting that fluid found draining from the nose or ear was CSF. Differential suction may permit demonstration of the site of the anatomic communication among the nose, the ear, and the meninges. Moderate contamination with other body fluids does not invalidate the method. The method also is noninvasive and safe for the patient.

TREATMENT

ANTIMICROBIAL THERAPY

Prompt treatment of bacterial meningitis with an appropriate antibiotic is essential. Antibiotic selection should include consideration of such factors as the CSF penetration of the antibiotic, the activity of the drug in purulent CSF, the mode of administration of the drug, and the intrinsic pharmacodynamic relationships of CSF drug concentrations to bactericidal activity.[346] The initial selection always should be made before definitive cultures are available and ideally should be based on incidence and susceptibility patterns in the local community.[213]

For many years, ampicillin and chloramphenicol were preferred as the initial empirical therapy for children older than 3 months and thought to have bacterial meningitis. The development of newer cephalosporins and other antibiotics that have excellent bactericidal activity against *H. influenzae* type b, *N. meningitidis*, and *S. pneumoniae* within the CSF led to the current approaches to initial therapy of childhood meningitis. Cefotaxime and ceftriaxone are included in the empiric treatment regimen of choice in most centers.[211]

Cefotaxime is a third-generation cephalosporin that has a broad spectrum of activity against gram-positive and gram-negative organisms. It possesses a high level of resistance to hydrolysis by β-lactamase. Cefotaxime penetrates the blood-brain barrier and provides bactericidal activity in the CSF equivalent to or greater than that of antibiotics that have been used conventionally for treatment of bacterial meningitis in children.[265] It is an excellent choice for inclusion in empiric therapy in children 1 month or older but must be used with ampicillin for initial therapy in children younger than 1 month because *L. monocytogenes* and enterococci cannot be treated with cefotaxime but are sensitive to ampicillin. Vancomycin in a dose of 60 mg/kg/day in four divided doses is recommended in addition to cefotaxime for empiric therapy of children with meningitis because of the frequency with which penicillin-resistant and cephalosporin-resistant pneumococci have been isolated in recent years worldwide. Cefotaxime is given as a daily dose of 225 to 300 mg/kg/day in three or four divided doses intravenously. The higher dosage is preferred by some experts because the higher CSF concentrations achieved by high-dose therapy may be beneficial for patients whose disease may be caused by *S. pneumoniae* when the organisms are of intermediate susceptibility to third-generation cephalosporins.[75]

Ceftriaxone is another third-generation cephalosporin that possesses broad antimicrobial activity against the organisms that cause bacterial meningitis. Ceftriaxone readily penetrates the CSF of patients with inflamed meninges. In patients who receive adjunctive therapy with dexamethasone, meningeal inflammation

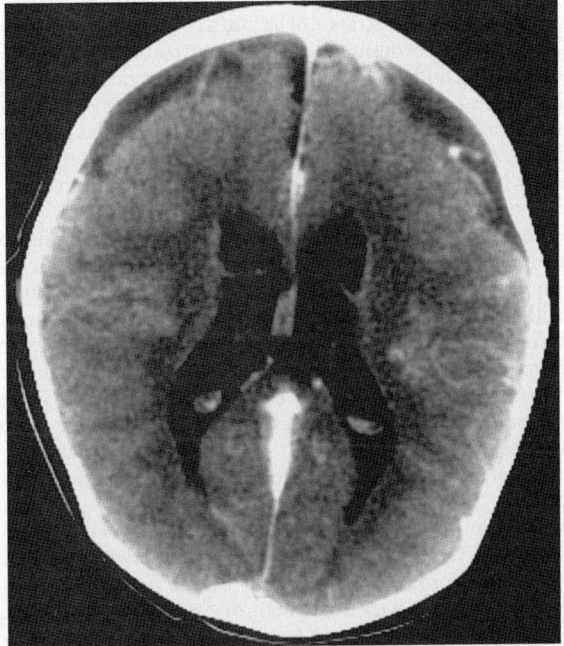

Figure 37-4 Computed tomography scan of a 2-year-old child with bacterial meningitis. Moderately severe ventricular dilation and the presence of bilateral extracerebral fluid collections overlying the convexities of the brain (subdural effusions) are noted. Note the several prominent vessels that run through the subdural space.

may be reduced, possibly decreasing the penetration of antibiotics into the CSF. Gaillard and colleagues[141] found that concentration of ceftriaxone in the CSF of children with bacterial meningitis treated with dexamethasone was similar to that found in children not treated with steroids. The half-life of ceftriaxone in serum is approximately 4 hours; a twice-daily dose regimen provides serum and CSF concentrations far in excess of the minimal bactericidal concentrations of most organisms that cause bacterial meningitis. Several prospective randomized studies have shown that ceftriaxone is comparable to ampicillin plus chloramphenicol for the treatment of bacterial meningitis in children.[21,33,56,76,87,157,361]

Ceftriaxone therapy has been associated with an increased incidence of diarrhea, which is mild and self-limited. An increased incidence of "gallbladder sludge," or precipitation of ceftriaxone salts in the gallbladder, diagnosed by ultrasound, also occurs and generally is asymptomatic but occasionally is associated with clinical symptoms of cholecystitis.[21,324] Ceftriaxone also has a high protein-binding capacity and can displace bilirubin from albumin in vitro[169] and needs to be used cautiously in neonates.

When ceftriaxone is used for the treatment of bacterial meningitis, it can be administered in a dose of 100 mg/kg/24 hours in two divided doses or one daily dose intravenously. Although a once-daily dose has proved to be effective,[49,135,167] is convenient, and lends itself particularly to home therapy for selected patients (after an initial period of hospitalization), we do not advocate single daily dosing; dosing errors, delayed doses, or missed doses undoubtedly occur, and inadequate treatment could result. Although ceftriaxone can be given intramuscularly, a single dose by this route may be impractical.[49] The solution used for intramuscular administration should contain no more than 250 mg/mL. A 15-kg child receiving a daily dose of 80 mg/kg would require 4.8 mL of fluid, a volume too large for injection in a single site in an infant. In addition, for penicillin-nonsusceptible but ceftriaxone-susceptible organisms, administration twice a day may be preferred.[75]

Ampicillin and chloramphenicol have been and continue to be effective as initial treatment of bacterial meningitis when organisms are susceptible to these agents, but they are used infrequently. Ampicillin may be provided intravenously in a dose of 300 mg/kg/24 hours in six divided doses. An initial bolus of 100 mg/kg is given. Chloramphenicol is administered intravenously in a dose of 100 mg/kg/24 hours in four divided doses. No loading dose of chloramphenicol is required.

An increasing number of strains of *S. pneumoniae* that are relatively or completely resistant to penicillin and third-generation cephalosporins have been identified.[54] Tan and coworkers[367] reported a retrospective analysis of five children who had pneumococcal meningitis caused by strains that were penicillin-resistant and that had minimal inhibitory concentrations (MICs) to cefotaxime or ceftriaxone of 0.5 to 2 μg/mL compared with strains that were penicillin-resistant but susceptible to cefotaxime or ceftriaxone (MIC ≥0.25 μg/mL); they found no difference in clinical outcome at the time of discharge. After publication of this report and others with similar findings, the National Committee for Clinical Laboratory Standards established the current guidelines for interpreting the MIC for cefotaxime or ceftriaxone for pneumococci isolated from patients with bacterial meningitis. The guidelines indicate that strains with an MIC of 2 μg/mL or greater are considered resistant, strains with an MIC of 1 μg/mL are intermediate, and strains with an MIC of 0.5 μg/mL or less are considered fully susceptible.[275]

Vancomycin has been used successfully to treat penicillin-resistant pneumococcal meningitis[50,137] and experimental models of cephalosporin-resistant pneumococcal meningitis.[139] In eight reports of treatment failures with third-generation cephalosporins, a variety of treatment regimens were used, all successfully. Vancomycin, alone or in combination with rifampin, chloramphenicol, or both, was used most frequently. The recommendation for empiric therapy of bacterial meningitis advocated by the AAP Committee on Infectious Diseases is to include vancomycin in addition to a third-generation cephalosporin in patients aged 1 month or older.[9] If nonsusceptibility to penicillin (MIC ≥0.1 μg/mL) and cephalosporins (MIC ≥0.1 μg/mL) is documented, treatment is continued with vancomycin plus cefotaxime or ceftriaxone (a synergistic effect is achieved when they are used together) with or without rifampin to complete an appropriate course. Vancomycin should be given at a dose of 60 mg/kg/24 hours in four divided doses. Peak serum concentrations of vancomycin in children whose renal function is normal should be 30 to 40 μg/mL.

Antibiotic tolerance is the ability of an organism to grow in the presence of antibiotics and frequently is a precursor phenotype to resistance. Clinical isolates of *S. pneumoniae* that are tolerant to vancomycin have been reported in the United States.[279] Meningitis caused by a vancomycin-tolerant organism in a patient was treated successfully with cefotaxime (300 mg/kg/day in four divided doses) plus vancomycin (60 mg/kg/day in four divided doses) and rifampin (20 mg/kg/day in two divided doses). Chloramphenicol also may be a suitable alternative for the treatment of these organisms if the pneumococcus proves to be sensitive to this antibiotic. Pneumococcal isolates resistant to penicillin or extended-spectrum cephalosporins frequently are nonsusceptible to chloramphenicol, however.

Cefuroxime is a second-generation cephalosporin that has been shown to be effective in vitro against *H. influenzae* type b, *S. pneumoniae*, and *N. meningitidis*. Initial clinical studies found that cefuroxime had equivalent effectiveness compared with ampicillin plus chloramphenicol. Subsequent studies showed delayed sterilization of the CSF, however; relapse during or after treatment was higher, and more frequent sensorineural hearing loss occurred than with use of ampicillin, chloramphenicol, cefotaxime, and ceftriaxone.[19,86,228,230,323] Cefuroxime *should not be used* to treat bacterial meningitis in children.

Ceftazidime has been efficacious in the treatment of meningitis caused by *P. aeruginosa*.[180,258,306,307] Cefoperazone and cefoxitin within CSF may fail to reach concentrations required to kill all susceptible strains of *H. influenzae* and *S. pneumoniae* and cannot be recommended for the treatment of bacterial meningitis in children.[59,121] Cefpirome concentrations in CSF of patients with bacterial meningitis were found to be significantly higher than the minimum bactericidal concentrations for *N. meningitidis*, *H. influenzae*, and *S. pneumoniae*,[402] but studies documenting its effectiveness in large numbers of children have not been done.

Cefepime is a fourth-generation cephalosporin that has been studied for the treatment of bacterial meningitis. In vitro, cefepime offers no advantage over cefotaxime or ceftriaxone for penicillin-resistant *S. pneumoniae*.[207] In addition, no in vitro data exist for the efficacy of cefepime against cefotaxime-resistant pneumococci. In two clinical trials, the efficacy of cefepime was found to be equivalent to the efficacy of either cefotaxime or ceftriaxone.[316,317] No penicillin-resistant or ceftriaxone-resistant pneumococci were encountered in either study, however. The role of cefepime for the treatment of bacterial meningitis is unclear.

Aztreonam is an antimicrobial agent that belongs to the monobactam family of antibiotics. It is effective against most gram-negative organisms, including *P. aeruginosa*. Limited data suggest its efficacy in the treatment of *Pseudomonas* and *H. influenzae* meningitis, suggesting a potential role for this agent in the treatment of patients who are allergic to penicillin and who are infected with these or other gram-negative organisms.[208,229,375]

If a history of *significant* allergy to penicillin or cephalosporin (anaphylaxis, urticaria, exfoliative dermatitis) is documented, vancomycin plus rifampin or chloramphenicol may be used. A cross-reactivity of approximately 10 to 15 percent has been noted for cephalosporins in penicillin-allergic patients.

When meningitis is caused by *Streptococcus pyogenes*, ampicillin or penicillin provides effective therapy. If meningitis is caused by a penicillin-resistant strain of *S. aureus*, oxacillin or nafcillin should be used, 200 mg/kg/24 hours intravenously in six divided doses. Vancomycin is effective against *S. aureus* strains resistant to penicillin and to semisynthetic penicillin derivatives[170] or *S. aureus* meningitis in patients who are penicillin allergic. Vancomycin also may be useful in treatment of meningitis caused by *Flavobacterium meningosepticum*.[94] Metronidazole is effective in treatment of anaerobic infection of the CNS when response to conventional therapy has been suboptimal. A dose of 40 mg/kg/24 hours in three or four divided doses results in CSF concentrations of greater than 10 µg/mL.[39]

Imipenem and meropenem have been evaluated for the treatment of meningitis. These carbapenems are active against the bacteria that cause meningitis, but the use of imipenem-cilastatin has been associated with drug-induced seizures.[404]

The safety and efficacy of meropenem and cefotaxime were compared in a prospective randomized trial of 190 children with bacterial meningitis.[216] Seizures occurred within 24 hours before administration of antibiotic therapy in 16 percent of patients randomly assigned to receive meropenem and in 7 percent of patients randomly assigned to receive cefotaxime. Seizures occurred in patients after administration of therapy in 6 percent of children receiving meropenem and in 1 percent of children receiving cefotaxime. None of these seizures could be attributed to drug therapy. All patients responded to therapy with clinical improvement, and bacterial eradication was proved by repeated lumbar puncture in 100 percent of patients in both groups. No significant difference in short-term outcomes occurred between the two groups.

Odio and associates[282] compared the efficacy and safety of meropenem with cefotaxime for the treatment of bacterial meningitis in 258 children who were randomly assigned to the meropenem or cefotaxime group. Clinical cure with or without sequelae was achieved in 97 percent and 96 percent of the meropenem-treated and cefotaxime-treated patients, respectively. At 7 weeks after treatment was concluded, 54 percent of patients treated with meropenem and 58 percent of patients treated with cefotaxime had no sequelae. Seizures were noted in 12 percent of the patients treated with meropenem and in 17 percent of patients treated with cefotaxime; none of the seizures was considered to be drug-related. These data suggest that meropenem is effective in the treatment of bacterial meningitis in children. Few children with pneumococcal meningitis in either study had isolates that were nonsusceptible to cefotaxime. No conclusions can be drawn regarding the usefulness of meropenem in treating pneumococcal meningitis caused by isolates with a cefotaxime or ceftriaxone MIC equal to or greater than 2 µg/mL. Meropenem should be studied further in children who may have meningitis that is caused by organisms resistant to extended-spectrum cephalosporins. For meropenem-susceptible isolates, meropenem alone or in combination with other drugs may provide a satisfactory alternative for patients who do not tolerate vancomycin.[75]

In animal models, the addition of bacterial protein-synthesis inhibitors, such as clindamycin[48] and rifampin,[149] has been associated with a neuroprotective effect, suggesting the possibility of their use as an adjunct therapy. Bottcher and associates[48] showed decreased bacterial cell wall release, a lessened pro-inflammatory response (including decreased leukocyte recruitment), less free radical formation, and decreased apoptosis and cellular damage after the addition of clindamycin to standard antibiotic therapy.

Table 37–7 provides current recommendations for antibiotic treatment of various microorganisms. An appropriate antibiotic should be continued until the patient is afebrile for 5 days, but for at least 7 to 10 days in every patient. Although some data

support a shorter course of therapy, we continue to recommend 10 days of treatment for pneumococcal and *H. influenzae* type b meningitis and 7 days for *N. meningitidis* meningitis.[190,240,246] If clinical improvement is noted within 24 hours, a repeated lumbar puncture is unnecessary, in most cases, during the course of treatment or after treatment has been completed. If infection is caused by *S. pneumoniae* that is resistant to penicillin and to third-generation cephalosporins, we recommend a repeated lumbar puncture at 48 to 72 hours to document bacterial sterilization of the CSF. If clinical improvement is slower than anticipated or is not noted, a repeated examination of the CSF is indicated at any time.

In the 1970s, lumbar puncture frequently was performed at the conclusion of therapy. Data from studies performed at that time (Table 37–8) reveal that WBC counts and protein concentrations within the CSF generally had not returned completely to normal and that the CSF-to-blood glucose ratio may have remained depressed. In every case, Gram stain of the CSF should reveal no organisms and cultures should be sterile. If a lumbar puncture is performed at the conclusion of therapy, we consider re-treatment to be mandatory if organisms are seen or grown. It also may be considered if more than 30 percent of the cells are polymorphonuclear leukocytes, or if the CSF glucose concentration is less than 20 mg/dL, and the CSF-to-blood glucose ratio is less than 20 percent.

Bacteriologic relapse after treatment of meningitis (particularly that caused by *H. influenzae* and treated with ampicillin) was highlighted in numerous reports.[27,71,73,173,174] Precise assessment of the frequency of relapse in children who have received an appropriate antibiotic to which the organism is sensitive or an appropriate dose intravenously and for an extended period has been difficult. The relapse rate is currently less than 1 percent.

Some physicians have discharged children with meningitis from the hospital before the conclusion of a course of therapy and prescribed home management. Benefits of home therapy include a decreased risk of acquiring nosocomial infection, a return of the child to his or her normal environment sooner, and a decrease in the total cost of therapy. Financial savings of outpatient, once-daily ceftriaxone for pediatric meningitis have been estimated to be $200 per day.[295]

Bradley and colleagues[49] reported the results of 54 children with bacterial meningitis treated as outpatients for 1 to 8 days (mean 4.6 days) with intramuscular ceftriaxone given once daily. Each dose was given in conjunction with a physician's examination. Each child had to be afebrile for 24 to 48 hours before initiation of home therapy, free of neurologic dysfunction except for auditory or vestibular dysfunction, and without evidence of inappropriate secretion of ADH before being considered for outpatient therapy. No child required readmission or developed neurologic sequelae or relapse. Powell and Mawhorter[295] reported a retrospective review of 26 patients with meningitis or other serious bacterial infections who received some portion of their therapy as an outpatient with ceftriaxone; none of the patients experienced relapse or recurrence.

Waler and Rathore[390] suggest 10 criteria for considering outpatient therapy for children with bacterial meningitis, as follows: (1) the child has received inpatient therapy for at least 6 days, (2) the child is afebrile for at least 24 to 48 hours before initiation of outpatient therapy, (3) the child has no significant neurologic dysfunction or focal findings, (4) the child has no seizure activity, (5) the child is clinically stable, (6) the child is taking all fluids by mouth, (7) the first dose of outpatient antibiotic is received in the hospital, (8) the antibiotic is administered in the office or emergency department setting or by qualified home health nursing, (9) daily examination is performed by a physician, and (10) parents are reliable and have transportation and a telephone. The dose of ceftriaxone of 80 to 100 mg/kg/24 hours intramuscularly may need to be aliquoted to account for the volume of diluent needed to achieve a concentration of no greater than 250 mg/mL. If oral

TABLE 37-7   Recommendations for Antibiotic Therapy

Organism	Antibiotic(s)	Recommended Dosages (IV)
Bacteroides fragilis	Chloramphenicol	100 mg/kg/day in 4 dd
	Metronidazole	30 mg/kg/day in 4 dd
Bacteroides other than *B. fragilis*	Penicillin G	300,000 U/kg/day in 6 dd
Clostridium	Penicillin G	300,000 U/kg/day in 6 dd
Corynebacterium	Penicillin G	300,000 U/kg/day in 6 dd
	Erythromycin	50 mg/kg/day in 4 dd
*Enterobacter, Klebsiella, Escherichia coli**	Ampicillin	300 mg/kg/day in 6 dd
	Gentamicin	7.5 mg/kg/day in 3 dd
	Amikacin	15 mg/kg/day in 3 dd
	Cefotaxime	200 mg/kg/day in 4 dd
	Ceftriaxone	100 mg/kg/day in 2 dd
	Ticarcillin	300 mg/kg/day in 4 dd
Haemophilus influenzae	Ampicillin	300 mg/kg/day in 6 dd
	Cefotaxime	200 mg/kg/day in 4 dd
	Ceftriaxone	100 mg/kg/day in 1 or 2 dd
	Chloramphenicol	100 mg/kg/day in 4 dd
Listeria monocytogenes	Ampicillin	300 mg/kg/day in 6 dd
	Gentamicin	7.5 mg/kg/day in 3 dd
	TMP-SMX	20 mg/kg/day in 4 dd (TMP component)
Neisseria meningitidis	Penicillin G	300,000 U/kg/day in 6 dd
Neisseria gonorrhoeae	Penicillin G (if sensitive to penicillin)	300,000 U/kg/day in 6 dd
	Ceftriaxone	100 mg/kg/day in 1 or 2 dd
Proteus mirabilis (indole-negative)	Ampicillin	300 mg/kg/day in 6 dd
P. mirabilis (indole-positive)	Cefotaxime	200 mg/kg/day in 4 dd
	Gentamicin	7.5 mg/kg/day in 3 dd
	Amikacin	22.5 mg/kg/day in 3 dd
	Ticarcillin	300 mg/kg/day in 4-6 dd
Pseudomonas	Gentamicin	7.5 mg/kg/day in 3 dd
	Ticarcillin	450 mg/kg/day in 4 or 6 dd
	Piperacillin	300 mg/kg/day in 4 or 6 dd
	Amikacin	15-20 mg/kg/day in 3 dd
	Ceftazidime	150-200 mg/kg/day in 3 dd
	Meropenem	120 mg/kg/day in 3 dd
Salmonella	Ampicillin	300 mg/kg/day in 6 dd
	Cefotaxime	200 mg/kg/day in 4 dd
	Gentamicin	7.5 mg/kg/day in 3 dd
	Chloramphenicol	100 mg/kg/day in 4 dd
Staphylococcus aureus (penicillinase-negative)[†]	Penicillin G	300,000 U/kg/day in 6 dd
S. aureus (penicillinase-positive)[†]	Oxacillin or nafcillin	200 mg/kg/day in 6 dd
S. aureus (resistant to semisynthetic penicillins)	Vancomycin *plus*	60 mg/kg/day in 4 dd
	Rifampin	20 mg/kg/day in 2 dd
Staphylococcus (coagulase-negative)	Vancomycin plus	60 mg/kg/day in 4 dd
	Rifampin	20 mg/kg/day in 2 dd
Streptococcus pneumoniae[†]	Penicillin G	300,000 U/kg/day in 6 dd
	Chloramphenicol	100 mg/kg/day in 4 dd
	Vancomycin	60 mg/kg/day in 4 dd
	Cefotaxime/ceftriaxone	225-300 mg/kg/day in 3 or 4 dd/100 mg/kg/day in 1 or 2 dd
	Rifampin[‡]	20 mg/kg/day in 2 dd
Unknown (<1 mo old)	Ampicillin *plus*	300 mg/kg/day in 6 dd
	Cefotaxime *plus*	200 mg/kg/day in 4 dd
	Vancomycin	60 mg/kg/day in 4 dd
Unknown (>1 mo old)	Cefotaxime *or*	225-300 mg/kg/day in 4 dd
	Ceftriaxone *plus*	100 mg/kg/day in 1 or 2 dd
	Vancomycin	60 mg/kg/day in 4 dd
	Nafcillin (if question of staphylococcal infection)	200 mg/kg/day in 6 dd
	Gentamicin (if question of *Pseudomonas*)	7.5 mg/kg/day in 3 dd

*TMP-SMX in a dose of 20 mg (TMP) and 100 mg (SMX) kg/day IV in 4 dd has been used successfully in selected patients with gram-negative enteric meningitis.
[†]Vancomycin may be provided in a dose of 60 mg/kg/day in 4 dd IV if patients are allergic to penicillin or penicillin derivatives or, in the case of Streptococcus pneumoniae, for multidrug-resistant pneumococci or pneumococci that are highly resistant to penicillin. In these cases, addition of rifampin may be considered.
[‡]Should never be used alone.
dd, divided doses; TMP-SMX, trimethoprim-sulfamethoxazole

chloramphenicol is used, therapeutic serum concentrations of 15 to 25 μg/mL must be documented before discharge and maintained.

H. influenzae type b organisms have been recovered from the throats of patients after completion of a course of treatment for *H. influenzae* type b meningitis. When members of a household to which the patient will return include children 4 years or younger, the patient should be given rifampin, 20 mg/kg once daily for 4 days, to prevent the occurrence of secondary cases. Children with meningococcal meningitis also should receive che-

TABLE 37–8   Cerebrospinal Fluid Findings at Conclusion of Antibiotic Treatment

	Total White Blood Cell Count		Polymorphonuclear Leukocytes (%)		CSF-to-Blood Protein (mg/dL)		Glucose (mg/dL)		Glucose Ratio	
	Mean ± 1 SD	Range	Mean ± 1 SD	Range	Mean ± 1 SD	Range	Mean ± 1 SD	Range	Mean ± 1 SD	Range
Total group	41 ± 80	0-850	5.5 ± 12	0-90	46 ± 72	7-970	47 ± 12.7	21-91	55.7 ± 17	23-156
Haemophilus influenzae	53 ± 98	0-850	5.5 ± 11	0-90	43 ± 37	10-334	47 ± 13	31-100	55 ± 17	31-100
H. influenzae (ampicillin)	56 ± 107	0-850	5.9 ± 12	0-90	44 ± 43	13-334	46 ± 14	21-91	53 ± 17	33-89
H. influenzae (chloramphenicol)	49 ± 83	0-325	5.1 ± 10.7	0-50	41 ± 26	7-127	48 ± 11	27-90	57 ± 13	30-100
Streptococcus pneumoniae	29 ± 30	0-110	5.5 ± 11.5	0-45	42 ± 39	7-211	48 ± 9	22-68	57 ± 13	22-91
Neisseria meningitidis	16 ± 27	0-132	3.4 ± 7.9	0-27	39 ± 46	7-188	47 ± 11	29-77	47 ± 19	23-100
Others	11 ± 18	0-77	7.3 ± 19	0-75	70 ± 197	10-970	48 ± 18	37-73	70 ± 28	44-156

CSF, cerebrospinal fluid; SD, standard deviation.

moprophylaxis to eradicate nasopharyngeal carriage before discharge, unless they were treated with cefotaxime or ceftriaxone.

ADJUNCTIVE THERAPY

As described earlier, the pathogenesis and subsequent sequelae of bacterial meningitis are as much a consequence of the host response to infection as of the bacterial organisms themselves. Anti-inflammatory agents used as adjuncts to antimicrobial therapy may decrease the degree of tissue injury during the course of the disease. Corticosteroids have been suggested as an adjunct to therapy of bacterial meningitis because they may (1) decrease intracranial pressure by decreasing meningeal inflammation and brain water content; (2) modulate the production of cytokines, which lessens the meningeal inflammatory response; and (3) decrease the incidence of sensorineural hearing loss or other neurologic complications of meningitis.[227,281]

Corticosteroids may play a role in acute management of increased intracranial pressure and cerebral herniation, although no data specifically indicate that corticosteroids decrease cerebral edema caused by bacterial meningitis. Odio and colleagues[281] found that dexamethasone therapy in children with bacterial meningitis decreased opening lumbar CSF pressure 12 hours after administration of the first dose, but this effect was lost by 24 hours of treatment. The significance of these findings is unclear because the steroids were not given as specific therapy for increased intracranial pressure, and most of the subjects were not showing signs of impending herniation.

In experimental *H. influenzae* meningitis, administration of dexamethasone 1 hour before, but not 1 hour after, administration of ceftriaxone was associated with significantly reduced TNF-α concentration and indices of inflammation in the CSF.[270] Administration of dexamethasone has been associated with decreased concentration in CSF of prostaglandin E$_2$ and decreased leakage of some proteins from serum into CSF in rabbits with experimental pneumococcal meningitis.[192] Among patients with bacterial meningitis, steroid-treated patients had significantly lower concentrations of IL-1β, TNF-α, platelet-activating factor, and prostaglandin E$_2$ in their CSF than those of patients who received antibiotics alone.[254,271,281] Patients tend to become afebrile sooner when they receive dexamethasone, but they have an increased incidence of secondary fevers.[388]

Although the understanding of the pathophysiologic events associated with initiation of the acute inflammatory response has been enhanced by more recent data, the ability of dexamethasone to reduce long-term complications of bacterial meningitis in pediatric patients remains controversial. In a prospective, randomized, double-blinded, placebo-controlled study evaluating adults in Europe with bacterial meningitis, de Gans and colleagues[84] showed a decrease in mortality rates in all patients and in unfavorable outcomes in patients with pneumococcal meningitis. By contrast, no pediatric studies of the use of dexamethasone for treatment of bacterial meningitis have shown an overall change in mortality rates.

In randomized, placebo-controlled trials of dexamethasone as adjunctive therapy in bacterial meningitis[227,281,322,388] and in retrospective studies[158,206] published since 1988, 68 percent (227 of 333) of steroid recipients in the six randomized trials had meningitis caused by *H. influenzae* type b; the remaining 32 percent had meningitis caused by *S. pneumoniae* (50 of 333) or *N. meningitidis* (56 of 333).[297] A meta-analysis of nine controlled trials published before 1991 failed to document a reduced risk of neurologic abnormality at hospital discharge or follow-up examination.[181] A more recent meta-analysis of randomized clinical trials of dexamethasone as adjunctive therapy for bacterial meningitis suggests a beneficial effect for *H. influenzae* meningitis and a possible beneficial effect in preventing severe hearing loss in *S. pneumoniae* meningitis, but only if it is given early.[251]

Most patients with *S. pneumoniae* meningitis in the studies that were reviewed were not treated with vancomycin. This issue is important because the penetrance of vancomycin across the blood-brain barrier is not optimal, and selected studies show that it is reduced further when dexamethasone is used concomitantly.[20,51,138,259] Despite the theoretical clinical concerns, CSF concentrations of vancomycin and ceftriaxone are adequate for treatment of penicillin-susceptible and penicillin-nonsusceptible *S. pneumoniae* when dexamethasone is given at recommended dosages.[104]

Odio and associates[281] found that the administration of dexamethasone immediately before the initiation of cefotaxime therapy was associated with a reduced incidence of neurologic sequelae (14% compared with 38% in patients receiving cefotaxime alone). They found no significant difference in auditory sequelae compared with control subjects. The frequency of neurologic sequelae in placebo-treated patients was significantly higher than that noted in other studies.[322,370,388]

Studies by Lebel and associates[227] and Schaad and colleagues[322] failed to show a significant reduction in the incidence of neurologic sequelae in comparisons of steroid-treated and placebo-treated patients. A prospective, multicenter, placebo-controlled study evaluated 143 children with bacterial meningitis caused by *H. influenzae* type b (58%), *S. pneumoniae* (23%), and *N. meningitidis* (17%).[388] Patients were treated with ceftriaxone and placebo or ceftriaxone and dexamethasone administered within 4 hours of the first dose of antibiotics. No significant difference in neurologic or developmental outcome was found between patients who received steroids or placebo.

Sensorineural hearing loss is a significant sequela of bacterial meningitis. In the two randomized studies by Lebel and associates,[227] patients treated with dexamethasone were significantly less likely to have moderate or severe bilateral sensorineural hearing loss; however, in one study, patients were treated with cefuroxime, which has been shown to result in delayed sterilization of the CSF and a higher rate of hearing loss compared with ceftriaxone.[323] An additional 100 infants and children with bacterial meningitis were treated with ceftriaxone for 10 days and either dexamethasone or placebo for 4 days. A significant reduction in moderate to severe hearing loss in children with *H. influenzae* type b meningitis ($p < .001$) was reported. No significant differences in other neurologic sequelae were found between the two groups. In addition, two patients receiving dexamethasone developed gastrointestinal bleeding severe enough to require transfusion, and two others developed heme-positive stools.[227] Odio and associates[281] found no significant difference in the incidence of moderate or severe hearing impairment between placebo and steroid groups (16% and 6%) respectively.

The Swiss Meningitis Group[322] found that treatment of children with dexamethasone 10 minutes before administration of ceftriaxone and then for 2 days subsequently resulted in persistent hearing loss in 5 percent (three) of children who had received dexamethasone and in 15 percent (eight) of children who received placebo, a difference that was not significant. One child treated with steroid and five children treated with placebo had unilateral hearing loss only. The group also documented a transient mild to moderate hearing impairment in five children treated with dexamethasone and four children treated with placebo; in six of the nine children, the impairment was caused by a conductive disturbance. Dexamethasone did not alter the incidence or natural history of the transient hearing impairment.

In a multicenter study,[388] audiologic measurements were made early in the course of the disease (within 24 hours of admission) and 6 weeks to 12 months after recovery from disease. The authors found no significant difference in the incidence of persistent moderate or severe hearing loss between children who received dexamethasone within 4 hours of antibiotics and children who received placebo, with the exception of bilateral deafness in children with *H. influenzae* type b meningitis (5 of 72 in the placebo-treated group versus 0 of 67 in the dexamethasone-treated group; $p = .02$). The overall incidence of moderate to severe hearing loss was 14.7 percent (10.3% unilateral and 4.4% bilateral) in the dexamethasone-treated group and 22.9 percent (13.5% unilateral and 9.4% bilateral; $p = .33$ for bilateral loss) in the placebo-treated group. These authors found that 22 children (8 in the dexamethasone-treated group and 14 in the placebo-treated group) had bilateral moderate or severe hearing loss at the initial evaluation. Only one child with *H. influenzae* meningitis and unilateral deafness at initial examination progressed to bilateral deafness. At follow-up, the resolution of hearing loss was nearly identical for each group, with 8 of the 22 children having normal hearing at follow-up, 5 having unilateral deafness, and 9 having bilateral deafness.

These results suggest that hearing loss occurs early in the course of meningitis and that early auditory brain stem response results need to be interpreted cautiously with regard to long-term audiologic sequelae. A strong relationship was noted between hearing loss early in the disease and a low concentration of CSF glucose at manifestation of meningitis, a finding that has been reported previously.[95]

Data from animal studies highlight a potential negative effect of dexamethasone therapy.[233,410] Leib and associates[233] examined infant rats with pneumococcal meningitis and found that the rats treated with dexamethasone had increased hippocampal apoptosis and deficiencies in learned behavior.

The AAP Committee on Infectious Diseases states that dexamethasone therapy should be considered for pneumococcal meningitis in infants and children 6 weeks and older.[9] Dexamethasone also is recommended for treatment of infants and children with *H. influenzae* type b meningitis by the Red Book Committee.[12] The reluctance on the part of some experts to recommend dexamethasone for pneumococcal meningitis is predicated on data that fail to show any diminution in morbidity or mortality rates from meningitis when meningitis is caused by *S. pneumoniae* and dexamethasone is used. The CSF concentrations of vancomycin, ceftriaxone, cefotaxime, and rifampin when they are given in dosages recommended for meningitis in children treated with dexamethasone *generally* are adequate to treat meningitis caused by most nonsusceptible strains of *S. pneumoniae*. Dexamethasone can lead to decreased fever and a misleading impression of clinical improvement, even though sterilization of the CSF has not been achieved.

Dexamethasone should not be used if aseptic or nonbacterial meningitis is suspected; if it is started before the diagnosis of nonbacterial meningitis is made, it should be discontinued immediately. It should not be used in "partially treated" meningitis. No data exist on which to base a recommendation for use of dexamethasone in the treatment of bacterial meningitis in infants younger than 6 weeks or in infants with congenital or acquired abnormalities of the CNS, with or without a prosthetic device. One prospective study in infants concluded that adjunctive dexamethasone therapy does not improve the outcome of neonatal bacterial meningitis.[79] Dexamethasone plus vancomycin may decrease the transport of vancomycin into the CSF of experimental animals with pneumococcal meningitis, but this finding was not observed in nine children who were treated with vancomycin and dexamethasone (0.6 mg/kg/day).[217] Dexamethasone should be used cautiously when vancomycin is used to treat meningitis caused by *S. pneumoniae* that may be resistant to penicillin, third-generation cephalosporins, or both.[51,201]

If dexamethasone is used, it should be used in all patients, regardless of disease severity, and it should be administered as early as possible in the course of treatment in a dose of 0.15 mg/kg/dose intravenously every 6 hours for no more than 4 days. One study[322] found no difference in children treated for 2 days instead of 4 days with 0.4 mg/kg/dose every 12 hours.

Except for hearing loss after *H. influenzae* type b meningitis, no clear evidence establishes that dexamethasone dramatically alters the long-term sequelae of meningitis, and its use is not without risk of causing adverse events. The markedly decreased frequency of meningitis caused by *H. influenzae* type b and the increased frequency of meningitis caused by *S. pneumoniae* nonsusceptible to penicillin (for which therapy with vancomycin may be necessary) suggest that initiation of dexamethasone should be considered carefully and that the clinician caring for the patient should evaluate the risk-to-benefit ratio of such therapy.

Research studies seek additional therapies that could be used to help reduce further mortality, morbidity, or both. Five main areas serve as the targets for therapeutic development: (1) bacterial killing and the release of bacterial products, (2) host recognition of bacteria or its products and the initiation of the inflammatory response, (3) modulation of the inflammatory response with adjuvant dexamethasone, (4) inhibition or interruption of the host inflammatory/neurotoxic mediators, and (5) modulation of the apoptotic pathways.[163] Inhibitors of inflammatory mediators and mediator effector molecules such as TNF-α, matrix metalloproteinases, and nitric oxide and antioxidants, neuroprotective factors (melatonin[148] and brain-derived neurotrophic factor[42]), and other anti-inflammatory therapies (triptans[184]) are being studied in experimental animal models of bacterial meningitis. Although their use is attractive theoretically because of the damage produced by the inflammatory cascade, none has emerged as a realistic potential candidate for general clinical use at present.

SUPPORTIVE CARE

In addition to antibiotic therapy, management of bacterial meningitis includes measures that apply generally to critically ill children.[215] Careful monitoring and attention to detail are essential. Pulse rate, blood pressure, and respiratory rate should be measured carefully every 15 minutes until stable and then every hour while the patient is in the intensive care unit. Temperature should be measured every 4 hours. A thorough neurologic examination should be done at the time of admission and at least daily thereafter. A rapid assessment of neurologic function should be done several times a day for the first several days of treatment. Body weight should be measured daily for at least the first 3 or 4 days. Head circumference should be measured in children younger than 18 months at the time of admission and repeated daily if concerns about increased intracranial pressure persist.

The following laboratory data are suggested if results of lumbar puncture indicate bacterial meningitis: (1) total peripheral WBC count and differential, (2) hemoglobin concentration, (3) hematocrit, (4) platelet count, and (5) serum electrolytes (serum and urine osmolalities may be useful in selected patients). Urine volume and specific gravity should be monitored. A low WBC count may suggest a poor prognosis. Anemia associated with *H. influenzae* type b septicemia has been reported[341,342] and has been attributed to immune hemolysis of RBCs that are coated with soluble bacterial antigens.[341]

Every child with meningitis should be evaluated carefully to identify inappropriate secretion of ADH, recognize seizure activity, and detect the development of subdural effusions. Determinations of body weight, serum electrolytes (serum and urine osmolalities in selected patients), urine volume, and specific gravity should be made at the time of admission and observed closely (every 6 to 12 hours) for the first 24 to 36 hours that the child is in the hospital and daily for several days thereafter. Initially, the child should receive nothing by mouth because of the risk of vomiting and aspiration. In addition, delivery of all fluid intravenously ensures greater accuracy in measurement of intake and output during the critical early days of therapy. Inappropriate secretion of ADH has been documented in 88 percent of children enrolled in a prospective study of bacterial meningitis.[107] Elevated serum concentrations of ADH in the presence of hyponatremia have been documented by direct measurement of ADH concentration in serum obtained from the same children.[111]

An electrolyte solution containing approximately 40 mEq/L of sodium and chloride, 35 mEq/L of potassium, and 20 mEq/L of acetate or lactate should be administered at a rate of 1000 to 1200 mL/m^2/24 hours in a patient without evidence of dehydration or shock. Fluid restriction is continued until it can be documented (frequently within 2 hours), on the basis of objective measures, that ADH secretion is not a factor or has resolved. The best indicators of retention of fluid in excess of solute are body weight and serum sodium concentration. As serum sodium concentration approaches normal (140 mEq/L), fluid administration may be liberalized progressively to normal maintenance levels of 1500 to 1700 mL/m^2/24 hours.

Powell and associates[296] found that elevated concentrations of arginine vasopressin in patients with bacterial meningitis who were clinically dehydrated responded to maintenance fluids plus deficit replacement with 0.9 percent saline. This study confirms that the syndrome of inappropriate secretion of ADH should not be diagnosed in the presence of dehydration. Decreased intravascular volume is a physiologic stimulus for the release of ADH, and its release is not inappropriate. Fluid restriction is not advocated for patients who are dehydrated; rehydration should be performed with careful and frequent assessment of fluid and electrolyte status.

Singhi and colleagues[345] examined the effect of fluid restriction on body water and outcome of 50 consecutive children who had been hospitalized with acute meningitis. These children were divided into two groups—patients with hyponatremia and patients without hyponatremia. Patients in both groups were randomly assigned to receive either normal maintenance or restricted fluids (65 to 70% of the volume of that received by the maintenance subgroup). Eleven to 15 patients were randomly assigned to any of the four subgroups in the study. No significant difference in overall outcome or intact survival was found when comparisons were made between fluid-restricted and non-fluid-restricted groups or within each group between the subgroups that received restricted fluids or maintenance fluids. After combination of the subgroups that received restricted fluids with the subgroups that received maintenance fluids, however, a trend toward higher intact survival and lower mortality rates was noted in the non-fluid-restricted groups. Nonetheless, children who had an extracellular water reduction of 10 mL/kg or greater in 48 hours had a significantly lower intact survival rate (10 of 28, 36%) than that of children with less than 10 mL/kg or no reduction of extracellular water (15 of 22, 64%). The mortality rate also was higher in the former group (7 of 28, 25%) than in the latter group (2 of 22, 9%). The authors concluded that fluid restriction did not improve the outcome of acute meningitis and that a decrease in extracellular water volume at 48 hours may increase the likelihood of having an adverse outcome.

This study is particularly difficult to interpret within the context of previous information in the literature. In studies of large numbers of children with bacterial meningitis, evidence of inappropriate secretion of ADH correlated significantly ($p < .01$) with abnormal neurologic findings, even 3 months after discharge, and with low IQ scores.[116] The original studies were in patients who were *not* fluid restricted.[110] As a result of these findings, coupled with documentation of inappropriate secretion of ADH, a recommendation was made to restrict fluids in patients who are hyponatremic at admission. Fluids are restricted only until evidence of inappropriate secretion of ADH can be excluded (usually within 2 hours).

The average patient in subsequent studies reported by Kaplan and Feigin[197] was fluid-restricted for only 0.75 days. The mortality rate in the largest single study reported by Feigin[105] of individuals who were fluid-restricted was 0.5 percent compared with 9 and 25 percent in the groups reported in the studies by Singhi and associates.[345] Singhi and associates[345] did not assess other important outcome variables, such as the number of patients with hearing loss or patients whose psychometric performance might or might not have been impaired. The total number of patients in any of their study groups was relatively small. Although their data are intriguing, other differences, either in the population studied or in the management of the patients, may have accounted for these differences.

In addition to the increased mortality rates of the patients studied by Singhi and associates[345] noted earlier, an extraordinarily high frequency of hydrocephalus and a very high frequency of seizures and status epilepticus were noted compared with groups of patients who have been studied in the United States. Because cerebral edema and increased intracranial pressure have been noted as major disturbances in seriously ill patients with meningitis and because many of the deaths and some of the sequelae have been related to the effects of cerebral edema and intracranial hypertension, we continue to recommend fluid restriction in patients with hyponatremia who are not dehydrated and liberalization of fluids as soon as the effects of excess ADH secretion have been dissipated (usually <1 day).

Meningitis complicated by shock creates a complex fluid management problem. Shock associated with meningitis is secondary to septicemia and generally is treated with intravenous infusion of large quantities of fluid to maintain blood pressure and adequate tissue perfusion (see Chapter 69). Patients with meningitis without shock or dehydration benefit from initial fluid restriction to avoid worsening of cerebral edema and severe hyponatremia with subsequent seizures. Children with meningitis and shock should receive sufficient quantities of isotonic fluid to maintain a systolic blood pressure of 80 to 90 mm Hg, a urine output equal to or greater than 500 mL/m^2/24 hours, and adequate cerebral perfusion as indicated by mental status. Central venous pressure monitoring is useful to guide fluid resuscitation and to prevent fluid overload. The addition of albumin (1 g/kg) to intravenously administered fluids may decrease the total volume of fluid needed to maintain adequate perfusion. Vasopressors, such as dopamine, dobutamine, and isoproterenol, also may provide support of blood pressure and perfusion and reduce requirements for intravenously administered fluids.

When increased intracranial pressure is suggested by such signs as progressive lethargy, increased muscle tone, or bulging anterior fontanelle, elevating the head approximately 30 degrees may be helpful. Increased intracranial pressure associated with deterioration in mental status or signs of cerebral herniation (Fig. 37–5) may be treated more vigorously with mannitol administered intravenously (0.5 g/kg) infused during 30 minutes and repeated as necessary. If steroids are used for this purpose, the recommended steroid is dexamethasone in a dose of 10 to 12 mg/m^2/day in four divided doses for no more than 4 or 5 days.[199] Other supportive measures to ensure appropriate delivery of oxygen and nutrients to the brain include a quiet environment, elective intubation, and the use of sedatives.[34]

Head circumference measurement and transillumination permit assessment of the development of subdural effusions or may suggest other causes for an enlarging head. CT may be helpful in detecting large subdural effusions or hydrocephalus. Because effusions can be considered part of the pathophysiologic changes that occur with bacterial meningitis, obtaining CT scans to evaluate effusions does not need to be part of the routine evaluation of a child with meningitis. Neuroimaging (CT or MRI) should be performed in children with focal neurologic signs. In children with hemiparesis or quadriparesis, CT or MRI may document cerebrovascular abnormalities. CT also should be performed in children with papilledema on an emergency basis before proceeding with the initial lumbar puncture. *Administration of antibiotics should not be delayed for diagnostic imaging in patients in whom bacterial meningitis is suspected.*

Subdural effusions should be treated with subdural paracentesis only when one suspects that the effusions are responsible for

seizures or for prolonged fever as a result of subdural empyema. Paracentesis also may be useful if the effusion is responsible for symptoms of increased intracranial pressure or is the cause of focal neurologic signs.[107,116] In most cases, subdural taps are not required.

Seizures, when noted, are treated expeditiously. A patent airway must be maintained, and appropriate anticonvulsants must be administered. Sodium phenobarbital (7 mg/kg loading dose) may be administered parenterally followed by a maintenance dose of 5 mg/kg/day in two divided doses. If necessary, diazepam (≤0.2 mg/kg) or lorazepam (0.05 mg/kg/dose, 4 mg maximum) infused intravenously for 1 to 2 minutes may be used. If prolonged seizure control is needed, phenytoin (5 mg/kg/day) in two divided doses may be used. Phenytoin generally does not depress the respiratory center to the same extent as phenobarbital does, and it may benefit the patient by inhibiting the secretion of ADH. If the seizure activity no longer is apparent after the second hospital day and the patient has no focal neurologic signs at the time of discharge from the hospital, anticonvulsants may be discontinued. Phenytoin and phenobarbital can induce hepatic microsomal enzymes; their use may increase the metabolism rate of chloramphenicol and possibly cause a significant decrease in the serum concentration of this antibiotic if it has been used for treatment of meningitis.[294]

An electroencephalogram is indicated in patients with meningitis and seizures when focal seizures are noted, seizures persist more than 72 hours after presentation, seizures occur after the third day of hospitalization, a subdural effusion is noted, or prolonged alteration in sensorium is present. An electroencephalogram may be valuable in distinguishing abnormal intermittent posturing from movements associated with seizure activity.

Persistent fever (>8 or 9 days' duration) has been noted.[27] In the multicenter pneumococcal study, the mean duration of fever was 4.4 ± 3.9 days.[19] Suppurative complications, including subdural or pleural empyema, septic arthritis, and pericarditis, should be sought carefully. The rare occurrence of brain abscess in association with bacterial meningitis also may lead to persistent fever. Nosocomial intercurrent infection, usually viral, may cause prolonged fever in a child with meningitis. Complications of therapy, such as suppurative thrombophlebitis or a urinary tract infection after prolonged catheterization, are additional considerations. Persistent fever may be related to the severity of the infection. Poor therapeutic response (especially in multidrug-resistant organisms) occurs, and repeated lumbar puncture must be considered on an individual basis. Drug fever often is cited, but rarely is the cause of persistent fever and remains a diagnosis of exclusion.

PROGNOSIS AND SEQUELAE

The prognosis in patients with bacterial meningitis depends on many factors, including the following: (1) the age of the patient, (2) the time course or progression of illness before antibiotic therapy is effective, (3) the specific microorganism causing the disease, (4) the number of organisms[119] or the quantity of capsular polysaccharide material present in the meninges and CSF at the time of diagnosis, (5) the rapidity with which CSF is sterilized after initiation of antibiotic therapy, and (6) the presence of disorders that may compromise host response to infection.[230]

The younger the patient and the greater the antigenic load at the time of admission, the worse the prognosis. Bacterial colony counts seem to be a more reliable indication of sequelae than is antigen concentration. Seizures, subdural effusions, bacteremia, and a more prolonged period of fever occur more frequently in children who have more than 10^7 CFU/mL of a particular organism in the CSF at the time of admission.[120] Children with colony counts equal to or greater than 10^7 CFU/mL

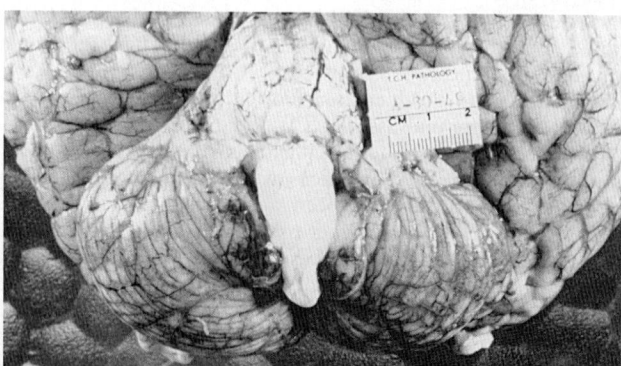

Figure 37–5 Inflammation and hemorrhage of cerebellar tonsils from a child with cerebellar herniation through the foramen magnum due to bacterial meningitis. (*From Kaplan, S.: Current management of common bacterial meningitides. Reproduced with permission of Pediatrics in Review 7:77, copyright 1985.*)

also are significantly more likely to experience hearing loss and speech disturbance than children with meningitis, but lower concentrations of bacteria within CSF specimens.[120] The presence of TNF in serum has been associated with a fatal outcome in patients with meningococcal meningitis.[386] Elevated concentrations of IL-1β and TNF within the CSF of patients with bacterial meningitis also have been correlated significantly ($p < .002$) with a higher incidence of neurologic sequelae of disease.[269]

The mortality rate for bacterial meningitis in children who are beyond the neonatal period has been reduced to 1 to 5 percent. Although antibiotic therapy has reduced the mortality rate, 50 percent of the survivors of meningitis have some sequelae of disease.[96,116,144,360] Most studies from which estimates of sequelae have been derived have been retrospective, and the patients were enrolled for many years (1951 to 1968). Although antibiotic treatment of these individuals may have been relatively standardized during this period, ancillary methods employed in their care were not controlled.

The frequency of complications of meningitis can be assessed most appropriately by prospective evaluation. In 1975, Sell[337] began a prospective study of 50 infants and children who recovered from H. influenzae meningitis. Fifty percent of this group were entirely normal, 9 percent were normal except for behavioral problems, and 28 percent had significant handicaps. The major handicaps noted included hearing loss (10-11%), language disorders or delayed language development (15%), impaired vision (2-4%), mental retardation (10-11%), motor abnormalities (3-7%), and seizures (2-8%).

Twenty-one postmeningitic children were paired with a sibling and tested by the Wechsler Intelligence Scale for Children. The mean IQ of the postmeningitic children was 86, and the mean IQ of control children was 97 ($p < .05$). Comparison of results for individual pairs revealed that 29 percent of postmeningitic children scored 1 full standard deviation below their siblings; no survivor had a score 1 standard deviation higher than a sibling. Feldman and Michaels[118] reported that children who recovered from meningitis caused by H. influenzae and who were evaluated 10 to 12 years later maintained grades and scores comparable with those of their siblings as they progressed to middle school. Their academic success may require more school and family support to compensate for the minor differences in IQs that had been noted.

A study by Taylor and associates[370] attempted to gain additional insight into the sequelae of H. influenzae meningitis, with particular emphasis placed on neuropsychologic function. Although the study was retrospective, it permitted a more detailed neuropsychologic assessment made at an earlier age than that

reported by investigators in previous studies. In addition, the index patients were compared with their siblings who were closest in age and the same sex, and the study was controlled for occupational and educational status. Only 14 percent of children who had had H. influenzae meningitis had any residual neurologic sequelae. Mean full-scale IQ was 102 for the index children and 109 for the control children.

The more recent results of our large prospective study of bacterial meningitis in children revealed that 32.8 percent of children had abnormalities detectable on neurologic examination at the time of discharge, but by 5 years after discharge, specific deficits were noted in only 11.1 percent of the total group.[109] As a result of the onset of late seizures in some of these patients, the frequency of neurologic sequelae 15 years after discharge was 14 percent.[293] Specific complications or sequelae of meningitis in these patients are shown in Table 37-9. Shortly after discharge, hemiparesis or quadriparesis was noted in 30 patients (12.4% of the total group), but at 1 year after discharge, paralysis was noted in only 5 patients. These data reflect the tendency for even major neurologic defects to clear unpredictably with time. This important observation suggests the need to maintain cautious optimism in discussing long-term complications of meningitis with parents.

In 1995, Grimwood and colleagues[166] reported the results of a prospective cohort study of 158 meningitis survivors, 3 months to 14 years old, who were treated in a single center between 1983 and 1986. Between 1991 and 1993, 130 children (82% of the original cohort) were evaluated at a mean age of 8.4 years and a mean of 6.7 years after their meningitis. Blended, audiologic, behavioral, neurologic, neuropsychologic, and sociodemographic assessments were compared with those of sex-matched and grade-matched control children. A systematic increase in the risk of abnormality or for poorer functioning was noted across all categories tested in children with meningitis versus control children. The differences reached statistical significance for tests of fine motor function, intelligence, neuropsychologic function, school behavior, and auditory figure-ground differentiation.

Eleven children who had experienced meningitis (8.5% of the cohort studied) had major deficits (hydrocephalus, persistent seizures, spasticity, blindness, IQ < 70, or profound hearing loss). Twenty-four (18.5%) of the survivors of meningitis and 14 (10.8%) of the control children had minor deficits (IQ of 70 to 80, inability to read, abnormalities in speech discrimination possibly referable to mild to moderate hearing loss, and school behavior problems). Overall, one in four of the children in this study had either a serious disabling sequela or a

TABLE 37-9   Complications or Sequelae of Meningitis

	Total	Haemophilus influenzae	H. influenzae (Ampicillin)	H. influenzae (Chloramphenicol)	Streptococcus pneumoniae	Neisseria meningitidis	Others
No.	235	151	90	61	35	26	23
Deaths <12 hr in hospital	4	4	3	1	0	0	0
Deaths >12 hr in hospital	1	0	0	0	0	1	0
Shock	8	6	5	1	1	1	0
Paralysis							
Early	30	18	7	11	7	3	2
Persistent	5	4	1	3	4	0	0
Persistent tone	5	4	1	3	1	2	0
Ataxia							
Early	7	5	2	3	2	0	0
Persistent	1	1	0	1	0	0	0
Visual problems	7	4	2	2	3	0	0
Clinically significant hearing deficit	25	17	6	11	5	2	1
Hydrocephalus	1	1	1	0	0	0	0

functionally important behavior disorder or neuropsychologic or auditory dysfunction that adversely affected academic performance.

This prospectively followed cohort was re-evaluated 12 years post-meningitis; impairment, although not severe, still persisted in the post-meningitis patients compared with controls.[18] Children post-meningitis were "more than twice as likely as controls to require special educational assistance" and "took longer to complete tasks, made more errors, were less organized, and struggled within problem-solving situations." Decreased performance in language tasks and executive skills also were seen in children whose age was less than 12 months at onset of meningitis.

Meta-analysis of 19 reports of prospectively enrolled and evaluated cohorts from developed countries published between 1980 and 1990[31] determined the mean probability of mortality to be 3.8 percent for *H. influenzae* type b, 7.5 percent for *N. meningitidis*, and 15.3 percent for *S. pneumoniae*, with an overall probability of 4.8 percent. The mean probabilities of sequelae in the survivors were deafness, 10.5 percent; mental retardation, 4.2 percent; spasticity, paresis, or both, 3.5 percent; and seizure disorder, 4.2 percent. The mean probability of no detectable sequelae was 83.6 percent.

Other specific sequelae or complications of bacterial meningitis that have been observed include cranial nerve involvement, hemiparesis or quadriparesis, muscle hypertonia, ataxia, permanent seizure disorders, and development of obstructive hydrocephalus. Subdural effusions (as noted earlier) are so frequent in young children that they can be considered a part of the general disease process, rather than a persistent or troublesome complication of the meningeal infection. Development of brain abscess after bacterial meningitis is exceedingly rare[122]; when it is found, the possibility that it preceded the development of meningeal infection must be considered, and a careful search for other sites of infections such as endocarditis should be initiated.

Arditi and associates[20] reviewed the outcomes of 180 children with 181 cases of pneumococcal meningitis who were enrolled in a prospective multicenter study between 1993 and 1996. Fourteen (7.7%) of 180 children died. No deaths were related to treatment failure caused by an antibiotic-resistant strain. Of the 166 surviving children, 41 (25%) developed motor defects, and 48 (32%) of 151 children had moderate to severe unilateral or bilateral hearing loss. By CT or MRI of 103 patients, brain infarcts were noted in 39 (38%); subdural effusions, in 25 (24%); hydrocephalus, in 22 (21%); cerebritis, in 12 (12%); and brain edema, in 6 (6%).

So far, the outcome of patients with pneumococcal meningitis caused by penicillin-nonsusceptible or cefotaxime-nonsusceptible isolates has not differed from that caused by susceptible strains.[20,125,205] This finding is explained in part because vancomycin has been administered empirically to most children with suspected bacterial meningitis since the mid-1990s in the United States and in other parts of the world where treatment failures have been reported as a result of antibiotic-resistant *S. pneumoniae*.[283]

Evoked response audiometry was used to detect hearing deficits in the patients described by Feigin and Dodge.[109] Some deficit in auditory nerve function was documented by this sensitive technique in 6 percent of children with *H. influenzae* meningitis, in 31 percent of children with pneumococcal meningitis, and in 10.5 percent of children with meningococcal disease.

Significant hearing loss after bacterial meningitis has been reported frequently. The mechanisms responsible for hearing deficits include spread of infection along the auditory canal and cochlear aqueduct, serous or purulent labyrinthitis, and, with time, replacement of the membranous labyrinth with fibrous tissue and new bone.[38,194,238,241,308] Damage to inner ear structures and subsequent hearing loss also is affected by the immune response of the host. TNF-α has been shown to produce cytolytic effects by the production of oxygen-free radicals. Animal studies have shown a decreased incidence of hearing loss when animals are treated with antibody blockade of TNF-α[16] and scavaging of oxygen-free radical by antioxidant therapy.[214]

Deafness generally is noted early in the course of bacterial meningitis and is independent of the therapy provided.[95,196,202,267,337,385] Ataxia has been reported as a presenting sign of bacterial meningitis in children with hearing loss noted at a later date.[200,336] Presumably, the insult to the vestibular and auditory systems occurred concomitantly in these children. The early loss of hearing noted by several investigators suggests that hearing loss is *not* associated specifically with the use of a particular antimicrobial agent. Early diagnosis and treatment apparently do not prevent the development of deafness in many children who develop hearing loss as a consequence of bacterial meningitis.

Estimates of the frequency of hearing loss in retrospective studies vary from 2.4 to 29 percent.[195,272] In our prospective studies, 7 percent of children have experienced marked to extensive (≥75-dB loss) hearing losses.[196,202] Overall, 48 of 151 (32%) of the children with pneumococcal meningitis in the multicenter study had unilateral or bilateral moderate to severe hearing loss.[20] Occasionally, hearing loss noted early may improve over weeks to months.[308]

In our studies, no correlation has been found between hearing loss and either the age of the patient at the onset of meningitis or the duration of illness before admission.[95,202] A significant correlation was noted between hearing loss and the presence of seizures before admission, the duration of fever in the hospital after therapy had been initiated (which presumably reflects more severe disease), treatment with antibiotics administered orally before a definitive diagnosis of bacterial meningitis was established, and a depressed CSF-to-blood glucose ratio at the time of admission.[95,202,204] Koomen and associates[221] developed a nomogram to predict the probability of development of hearing loss using five factors—duration of symptoms before admission, absence of petechiae, CSF glucose level, infection by *S. pneumoniae*, and ataxia—and were able to identify effectively patients at risk for developing hearing loss with excellent sensitivity (100%) using a cutoff of 0 on the point scale.

Because hearing deficits occur so commonly in patients with bacterial meningitis, hearing evaluation by evoked response audiometry in young, uncooperative children is recommended routinely at the time of or shortly after discharge from the hospital. Repeated audiometric evaluation is recommended after discharge if the results of the initial examination are abnormal. Pure tone audiometry can be used for older, cooperative children. Differentiation of hearing deficits resulting from conductive disturbances from deficits related to damage to the eighth cranial nerve is important. Some children who have repetitive episodes of otitis media may experience conductive loss that is unrelated to the meningitis.

In our studies, the mean IQ (±1 standard deviation) of the entire group of patients (235) after recovery was 94 (±23 standard deviations), with a range of 33 to 150. Twenty-nine children (17.3%) had IQs less than 80, and 22 (11.6%) had IQs less than 70. A comparison of these patients with their siblings and other control children revealed no significant difference in mean IQ. A significantly greater proportion ($p < .01$) of children who recovered from meningitis had IQs less than 80 compared with children from control groups. These results differ from those of Sell,[337] which were noted previously. Tejani and associates[372] also prospectively evaluated children who had recovered from bacterial meningitis using siblings as controls. They reported no significant differences in verbal performances or full-scale IQs between patients with meningitis and the sibling control population.

The prospective nature of these studies has permitted an assessment of factors that herald a poor prognosis and that may be discernible at or near the time of admission. Evidence of inappropriate secretion of ADH was correlated significantly ($p < .01$) with abnormal neurologic examinations at 3 months after discharge and with low IQs. The age of the child correlated inversely with the development of subdural effusion ($p < .01$), the occurrence of hearing deficits ($p < .02$), and low IQ ($p < .05$). The significantly increased impact of the disease on young children could be documented conclusively. The presence of focal neurologic findings in patients who were not postictal at the time of admission correlated significantly ($p < .001$) with abnormal neurologic examination, which was noted previously. Focal deficits indicating cerebral injury noted at admission or during the course of hospitalization were associated significantly ($p < .001$) with the development of late (1 to 15 years after discharge) afebrile seizures.[293] Focal neurologic findings at the time of admission proved to be a reliable predictor of permanent sequelae of bacterial meningitis. Focal deficits at admission also correlated significantly with low IQs ($p < .001$), even at 2 and 3 years after discharge from the hospital. The quantity of antigen in the initial CSF specimen and the number of organisms present also correlated significantly ($p < .01$) with sequelae of meningitis.[116]

Systematic review of neurocognitive impairment in children after CNS infection revealed deficits in cognition and motor function to be very common.[60] Koomen and associates[222] reported one third of Dutch children with non-*H. influenzae* type b meningitis were found on follow-up to have academic or behavioral limitations or both. Childhood meningitis survivors also were found to have a higher incidence of nonspecific symptoms, such as headaches, and significantly more symptoms of inattention, hyperactivity, and impulsiveness compared with nearest-age siblings.[37]

Only one study assessed the value of the Pediatric Risk of Mortality (PRISM) score in predicting outcomes of bacterial meningitis.[244] This study was done in a subgroup of children requiring mechanical ventilation. The best predictor of death and functional states on follow-up evaluation was the PRISM score. When the score was less than 20 within the first 24 hours of admission to the pediatric intensive care unit, a favorable outcome was noted in 82 percent. When the score was 20 or higher, a favorable outcome was noted in only 30 percent ($p < .009$).

CT has revealed evidence of cerebral infarction in children who had a diagnosis of bacterial meningitis established within 1 or 2 days of the onset of symptoms of a febrile illness.[352] In most of these cases, abnormalities in cerebrovascular dynamics (arteritis, thrombosis, thrombophlebitis), ventricular dilation, or both have been observed. In some of these cases, infarction has been associated with profound hypotension related to endotoxemia (personal experience). Brain infarction apparently is *not* related causally to a delay in diagnosis and therapy in many cases.

PREVENTION

HAEMOPHILUS INFLUENZAE MENINGITIS

Since the 1980s, methods of preventing meningitis caused by *H. influenzae* type b have improved. The dramatic decrease in the incidence of *H. influenzae* type b invasive disease and meningitis has been attributed to the introduction of vaccines that initially were found to be effective at 15 months of age[12] and then later found to be effective at 2 months of age.[332] Currently, three conjugate vaccines are approved for infants beginning at 2 months of age: HbOC, PRP-OMP, and PRP conjugated to tetanus toxoid (PRP-T). The ACIP and the AAP recommend universal infant immunization with HbOC or PRP-T at 2, 4, and 6 months of age or PRP-OMP at 2 and 4 months of age.[10,64]

Passive immunization of infants also has been studied with use of bacterial polysaccharide immunoglobulin.[8,321] This preparation given in a single intramuscular dose of 0.5 mL/kg provides significant protection for infants from *H. influenzae* type b disease for 3 or 4 months.

The most comprehensive study concerning the spread of *H. influenzae* type b infection among household contacts was coordinated by the CDC.[391] Data collected from 19 states were analyzed prospectively. *H. influenzae* meningitis was reported in 1403 patients. Eighty-two percent of exposed families were investigated for the occurrence of *H. influenzae* disease within 30 days of its onset in the index patient. Systemic disease caused by *H. influenzae* type b developed in 9 of 1687 contacts (0.5%) who were younger than 6 years. The risk of infection in patients younger than 4 years was 2.1 percent; the risk in children younger than 1 year was 6 percent. The risk of secondary infection of household contacts in the 30 days after onset of meningitis in the index case was 585 times greater than the age-adjusted risk in the general population and was similar to the risk of secondary meningococcal disease in household contacts. This nationwide study provided an important impetus for finding a chemoprophylactic regimen that could prevent secondary infection in household contacts.

A nationwide, collaborative, placebo-controlled trial was conducted subsequently among household (children <6 years old) and daycare center contacts of individuals with invasive *H. influenzae* type b disease.[30] Four of 765 placebo-treated contacts experienced secondary disease versus none of 1112 rifampin-treated contacts ($p = .027$).

The AAP Committee on Infectious Diseases recommends that rifampin be provided orally once each day for 4 days in a dose of 20 mg/kg (maximum dose 600 mg/day) to all household contacts (children and adults) regardless of age in households with at least one unvaccinated contact younger than 4 years.[10] The dose for infants younger than 1 month is not established, but it may be reduced to 10 mg/kg. Rifampin prophylaxis is not required, however, when all of the household contacts younger than 4 years have been fully immunized. All members of households with a fully immunized but immunocompromised child, regardless of age, should receive rifampin because of concern that the immunization may not have been effective.

When two or more cases of invasive disease have occurred within 60 days and unimmunized or incompletely immunized children attend a daycare facility, rifampin should be administered to all personnel and attendees. When a single case has been reported, the use of rifampin is controversial, and many experts recommend *no* prophylaxis.[10] Unimmunized or incompletely immunized children should receive a dose of vaccine and should be scheduled for completion of the recommended age-specific immunization schedule.

No data document the safety of rifampin administered during pregnancy. Prophylaxis with rifampin is not recommended for pregnant women who are contacts of infected infants.

Patients receiving rifampin should be advised routinely that their urine, sweat, and tears will be stained orange. Individuals should be advised to refrain from using contact lenses while receiving rifampin therapy because the lenses may be stained permanently.

PNEUMOCOCCAL INFECTION

In a large randomized trial conducted by Black and colleagues,[45] more than 37,000 infants received either the seven-valent pneumococcal vaccine containing polysaccharides of serotypes 4, 6B, 9V, 14, 18C, 19F, and 23F conjugated to CRM_{197} or meningococcal serogroup C oligosaccharide conjugated to the same protein. Vaccines were administered at 2, 4, 6, and 12 to 15 months of age. The pneumococcal conjugate vaccine was found to be 97.4 percent efficacious in preventing acquisition of invasive pneumococcal infections caused by vaccine serotype isolates. As a result of this study, the seven-valent pneumococcal protein conjugate vaccine is recommended by the ACIP and the AAP Committee on Infectious Diseases for all children younger than 24 months of age to prevent invasive pneumococcal infections.[14,67] Vaccine also is recommended for children 25 to 60 months of age with high risk of acquiring invasive disease and should be considered for otherwise normal children in this age range with other risk features that may increase their risk for development of systemic pneumococcal infection. Antibiotic chemoprophylaxis of children exposed to pneumococcal meningitis is not recommended regardless of immunization status.[9] In asplenic patients (functional and anatomic), daily chemoprophylaxis against pneumococcal infection is recommended with oral penicillin therapy.[9] The reader is referred to the CDC and AAP statements for the details of these recommendations.

MENINGOCOCCAL INFECTION

We advocate the use of chemoprophylaxis in all household members of a patient with meningococcal meningitis and in daycare and nursery school contacts, preferably within 24 hours of the diagnosis of the primary case.[11] Prophylaxis may be provided for individuals who had contact with the patient's oral secretions through kissing or sharing toothbrushes or eating utensils during the 7 days before onset of disease in the index case. Prophylaxis is not recommended routinely for health care personnel unless they have had close exposure through mouth-to-mouth resuscitation, intubation, or suctioning before antibiotic therapy was initiated. Schoolroom classmates and hospital contacts of patients usually are not given prophylactic treatment.

Minocycline and rifampin have proved to be 80 to 90 percent effective in eradicating carriage of meningococci.[171] Both drugs are secreted in the saliva in concentrations greater than the MICs for meningococci. The use of minocycline has been accompanied by frequent and significant vestibular reactions, even after a single dose of 100 mg, and, in our opinion, generally should not be used.[61-63,400]

Rifampin is the drug of choice in most instances and can be used in a dose of 600 mg twice daily for four doses in adults and in doses of 10 mg/kg/dose for four doses in children 1 to 12 years of age. A dose of 5 mg/kg every 12 hours for four doses can be used in children 3 months to 1 year of age.[266] The emergence of rifampin-resistant strains in treated meningococcal carriers has been reported to occur with a frequency of 0 to 27 percent.[83,99,396]

A single intramuscular dose of ceftriaxone has proved to be an effective alternative to rifampin for prophylaxis in meningococcal contacts.[335] This approach to prophylaxis may be particularly useful in circumstances in which compliance with the use of oral rifampin is considered questionable. The efficacy of ceftriaxone has been confirmed for only group A strains, but its effect is likely to be similar for other serogroups. Ceftriaxone has the advantage of easier dosage and administration and safety in pregnancy.[11] Ceftriaxone may be given intramuscularly in a dose of 125 mg for individuals younger than 12 years old and in a dose of 250 mg for individuals 12 years and older.

Ciprofloxacin given to adults in a single oral dose of 500 mg has been effective in eradicating meningococcal carriage.[11] Ciprofloxacin presently is not recommended for individuals younger than 18 years old or for pregnant women.

Because secondary cases may occur several weeks or more after onset of disease in the index case, meningococcal vaccine may be used as an adjunct to chemoprophylaxis when an outbreak is caused by a serogroup contained in the vaccine. The CDC has outlined recommendations for the administration of the meningococcal serogroup C vaccine to control outbreaks.[65]

A serogroup-specific quadrivalent polysaccharide meningococcal vaccine against group A, C, 4, and W135 N. meningitidis is approved for use in the United States in children 2 years old and older. The vaccine consists of 50 μg each of the respective purified bacterial polysaccharides. It may be given subcutaneously as a single 0.5-mL dose and can be given concurrently with other vaccines. Immunization with the meningococcal quadrivalent polysaccharide vaccine is recommended for children aged 2 to 10 years in high-risk groups, including children with anatomic or functional asplenia and children with terminal deficiencies of the complement system or with properdin deficiency.

In January 2005, the Food and Drug Administration approved a quadrivalent meningococcal conjugate vaccine, MCV4, which includes serotypes A, C, Y and W-135 for individuals 11 to 55 years old. Because of the conjugate vaccine's ability to induce a T-cell-dependent immune response and subsequently longer immunologic memory compared with polysaccharide vaccines, it is advantageous. The ACIP and the AAP made recommendations that the MCV4 vaccine be given to young adolescents at the 11- to 12-year visit, adolescents at high school entry or 15 years of age (whichever comes first), and students entering college planning to live in a dormitory,[15,44] with the goal of immunizing all adolescents by 2008. In addition to its use in the approved age group, MCV4 has been evaluated for use in the younger pediatric population. Pichichero and associates[291] showed an equivalent safety and tolerability profile of MCV4 compared with the quadrivalent polysaccharide vaccine and "significantly higher and more persistent serum bactericidal antibody responses against meningococcal serogroups A, C, Y, and W-135."

A single dose of serogroup C vaccine seems to be approximately 70 percent effective, for a period of 6 to 9 months, in preventing meningococcal disease in children who are older than 2 years.[369] Single 50-μg injections in children younger than 2 years of age do not produce adequate antibody responses.[369] A serogroup A polysaccharide vaccine has been field tested by the World Health Organization and is effective in children aged 3 months or older.[287,387] Serogroup-specific monovalent vaccines may be used to control outbreaks of disease caused by either type A or type C meningococci and may be valuable for travelers to countries with epidemic disease.[11,105] The vaccine is administered as a single dose parenterally in the volume specified by the package insert. Reactions noted after immunizations previously have been mild and infrequent; localized erythema of 1 or 2 days' duration is not unusual. The safety of the vaccine in pregnant women has not been established.

An effective serogroup B meningococcal vaccine has not been produced to date. The polysaccharide capsule cross-reacts with fetal neural tissues causing autoantibodies. Different strategies have been tried to develop a safe vaccine against serogroup B meningococcus, including use of outer membrane proteins (OMP) and lipopolysaccharide components.[182] Although OMP vaccines possess efficacy in older children and adults, the highest rates of serogroup B disease are in infants and young children, in which the OMP vaccines do not show efficacy.[70] Complete sequencing of the N. meningitidis serogroup B genome offers new membrane protein targets for vaccine targeting.[178] Similar to other protein conjugate vaccines, meningococcal C conjugate vaccines are more immunogenic than is the pure polysaccharide vaccine in infants younger than 2 years of age.[243] Because of a high incidence of meningococcal disease in the United Kingdom, a meningococcal serogroup C CRM$_{197}$ was administered in a phased program beginning November 1999 to all children younger than 18 years.[302] Surveillance studies to assess short-term efficacy have shown a 97 percent efficacy for teenagers and a 92 percent efficacy for toddlers in the prevention of meningococcal serogroup C infection.

REFERENCES

1. Achtman, M.: Molecular epidemiology of epidemic bacterial meningitis. Rev. Med. Microbiol. *1*:29-38, 1990.
2. Achtman, M.: Clonal properties of meningococci from epidemic meningitis. Trans. R. Soc. Trop. Med. Hyg. *85*(Suppl.):24-31, 1991.
3. Adair, C. V., Gould, R. L., and Smadel, J. E.: Aseptic meningitis, a disease of diverse etiology: Clinical and etiologic studies on 854 cases. Ann. Intern. Med. *39*:675-704, 1953.
4. Adams, R. D., Kubik, C. S., and Bonner, F. J.: The clinical and pathological aspects of influenzal meningitis. Arch. Pediatr. *65*:354-376, 1948.
5. Adams, W. G., Deaver, K. A., Cochi, S. L., et al.: Decline of childhood *Haemophilus influenzae* type b (Hib) disease in the Hib vaccine era. J. A. M. A. *269*:221-226, 1993.
6. Adegbola, R., Secka, O., Lahai, G., et al.: Elimination of *Haemophilus influenzae* type b (Hib) disease from The Gambia after introduction of routine immunization with Hib conjugate vaccine: A prospective study. Lancet. *366*:144-50, 2005.
7. Allbritton, W. L., Wiggins, G. L., and Feeley, J. C.: Neonatal listerioses: Distribution of serotypes in relation to age at onset of disease. J. Pediatr. *88*:481-483, 1976.
8. Ambrosino, D. M., Landesman, S. H., Gorham, C. C., et al.: Passive immunization against disease due to *Haemophilus influenzae* type b: Concentrations of antibody to capsular polysaccharide in high-risk children. J. Infect. Dis. *153*:1-7, 1986.
9. American Academy of Pediatrics: Pneumococcal Infections. *In* Pickering, L. K. (ed.): 2006 Red Book: Report of the Committee on Infectious Diseases. 27th ed. Elk Grove Village, IL, American Academy of Pediatrics, 2006, pp. 525-537.
10. American Academy of Pediatrics: *Haemophilus influenzae* infections. In Pickering, L. K. (ed.): 2006 Red Book: Report of the Committee on Infectious Diseases. 27th ed. Elk Grove Village, IL, American Academy of Pediatrics, 2006, pp. 310-318.
11. American Academy of Pediatrics: Meningococcal infections. In Pickering, L. K. (ed.): 2006 Red Book: Report of the Committee on Infectious Diseases. 27th ed. Elk Grove Village, IL, American Academy of Pediatrics, 2006, pp. 452-460.
12. American Academy of Pediatrics Committee on Infectious Diseases: *Haemophilus influenzae* type b conjugate vaccines: Recommendations for immunization of infants and children 2 months of age and older: Update. Pediatrics *88*:169-172, 1991.
13. American Academy of Pediatrics Committee on Infectious Diseases: Meningococcal disease prevention and control strategies for practice-based physicians (Addendum: Recommendations for college students). Pediatrics *106*:1500-1504, 2000.
14. American Academy of Pediatrics Committee on Infectious Diseases: Policy Statement: Recommendations for the prevention of pneumococcal infections, including the use of pneumococcal conjugate vaccine (Prevnar), pneumococcal polysaccharide vaccine, and antibiotic prophylaxis. Pediatrics *106*:362-366, 2000.
15. American Academy of Pediatrics Committee on Infectious Diseases: Prevention and control of meningococcal disease: Recommendations for use of meningococcal vaccines in pediatrics patients. Pediatrics *116*:155-157, 2005.
16. Aminpour, S., Tinling, S., and Brodie, H.: Role of tumor necrosis factor-α in sensorineural hearing loss after bacterial meningitis. Otol. Neurotol. *26*:602-609, 2005.
17. Anderson, G., Smithee, L., Rados, M., et al.: Progress toward elimination of *Haemophilus influenzae* type b disease among infants and children—United States, 1987-1993. M. M. W. R. Morb. Mortal. Wkly. Rep. *43*:144-148, 1994.
18. Anderson, V., Anderson, A., Grimwood, K., et al.: Cognitive and executive function 12 years after childhood bacterial meningitis: Effect of acute neurologic complications and age of onset. J. Pediatr. Psychol. *29*:67-81, 2004.
19. Arditi, M., Herold, B. C., and Yogev, R.: Cefuroxime treatment failure and *Haemophilus influenzae* meningitis: Case report and review of the literature. Pediatrics *84*:132-135, 1989.
20. Arditi, M., Mason, E., Jr., Bradley, J., et al.: Three-year multicenter surveillance of pneumococcal meningitis in children: Clinical characteristics, and outcome related to penicillin susceptibility and dexamethasone use. Pediatrics *102*:1087-1097, 1998.
21. Aronoff, S. C., Reed, M. O., O'Brien, C. A., et al.: Comparison of the efficacy and safety of ceftriaxone to ampicillin/chloramphenicol in the treatment of childhood meningitis. Antimicrob. Agents Chemother. *13*:143-151, 1984.
22. Asensi, F., Otero, M. C., Perez-Tamarit, D., et al.: Risk/benefit in the treatment of children with imipenem-cilastatin for meningitis caused by penicillin-resistant pneumococcus. J. Chemother. *5*:133-134, 1993.
23. Ashwal, S., Tomasi, L., Schneider, S., et al.: Bacterial meningitis in children: Pathophysiology and treatment. Neurology *42*:739-748, 1992.
24. Asmar, B. I., and Dajani, A. S.: Concurrent pneumococcal disease in two siblings. Am. J. Dis. Child. *136*:946-947, 1982.
25. Baker, C. J., and Barrett, F. F.: Transmission of group B streptococci among parturient women and their neonates. J. Pediatr. *83*:919-925, 1972.
26. Baker, R. C., and Bausher, J. C.: Meningitis complicating acute bacteremic facial cellulitis. Pediatr. Infect. Dis. *5*:421-423, 1986.
27. Balagtas, R. C., Levin, S., Nelson, K. E., et al.: Secondary and prolonged fevers in bacterial meningitis. J. Pediatr. *77*:957-964, 1970.
28. Baldwin, L. N., Henderson, A., Thomas, P., et al.: Acute bacterial meningitis in young adults mistaken for substance abuse. B. M. J. *306*:775-776, 1993.
29. Ballabh, P., Braun, A., and Nedergaard, M.: The blood-brain barrier: An overview: Structure, regulation, and clinical implications. Neurobiol. Dis. *16*:1-13, 2004.
30. Band, J., Fraser, D. W., and Ajello, G.: Prevention of *Hemophilus influenzae* type b disease. J. A. M. A. *25*:2381-2386, 1984.
31. Baraff, L. J., Lee, S., and Schriger, D. L.: Outcomes of bacterial meningitis in children: A meta-analysis. Pediatr. Infect. Dis. J. *12*:389-394, 1993.
32. Barenkamp, S. J., Granoff, D. M., and Munson, R. S., Jr.: Outer-membrane protein subtypes of *Haemophilus influenzae* type b and spread of disease in day-care centers. J. Infect. Dis. *144*:210-217, 1981.
33. Barson, W. J., Miller, M. A., Brady, M. T., et al.: Prospective comparative trial of ceftriaxone versus conventional therapy for treatment of bacterial meningitis in children. Pediatr. Infect. Dis. *4*:362-368, 1985.
34. Bashir, H., Laundy, M., and Booy, R.: Diagnosis and treatment of bacterial meningitis. Arch. Dis. Child. *88*:615-620, 2003.
35. Baumgartner, E. T., Augustine, A., and Steele, R. W.: Bacterial meningitis in older neonates. Am. J. Dis. Child. *137*:1052-1054, 1983.
36. Beckman, J. S., Beckman, T. W., Chen, J., et al.: Apparent hydroxyl radical production by peroxynitrite: Implications for endothelial injury from nitric oxide and superoxide. Proc. Natl. Acad. Sci. U. S. A. *87*:1620-1624, 1990.
37. Berg, S., Trollfors, B., Hugosson, S., et al.: Long-term follow-up of children with bacterial meningitis with emphasis on behavioral characteristics. Eur. J. Pediatr. *161*:330-336, 2002.
38. Berlow, S. J., Caldarelli, D. D., Matz, G. J., et al.: Bacterial meningitis: A prospective investigation. Laryngoscope *90*:1445-1452, 1980.
39. Berman, B. W., King, F. H., Jr., Rubenstein, D. S., et al.: *Bacteroides fragilis* meningitis in a neonate successfully treated with metronidazole. J. Pediatr. *93*:793-795, 1978.
40. Bermpohl, D., Halle, A., Freyer, D., et al.: Bacterial programmed cell death of cerebral endothelial cells involves dual death pathways. J. Clin. Invest. *115*:1607-1615, 2005.
41. Bernhardt, L. L., Semberkoff, M. S., and Rahal, J. J., Jr.: Deficient cerebrospinal fluid opsonization in experimental *Escherichia coli* meningitis. Infect. Immun. *32*:411-413, 1981.
42. Bifrare, Y., Kummer, J., Joss, P., et al.: Brain-derived neurotrophic factor protects against multiple forms of brain injury in bacterial meningitis. J. Infect. Dis. *191*:40-45, 2005.
43. Bijlmer, H. A.: World-wide epidemiology of *Haemophilus influenzae* meningitis: Industrialized versus non-industrialized countries. Vaccine *9*(Suppl.): S5-S9, 1991.
44. Bilukha, O., Rosenstein, N., and National Center for Infectious Diseases, Centers for Disease Control and Prevention: Prevention and control of meninogococcal disease. Recommendations of the Advisory Committee on Immunization Practices (ACIP). M. M. W. R. Recomm. Rep. *54*(RR-7):1-21, 2005.
45. Black, S., Shinfield, H., Fireman, B., et al.: Efficacy, safety and immunogenicity of heptavalent pneumococcal vaccine in children. Pediatr. Infect. Dis. J. *19*:187-195, 2000.
46. Blazer, S., Berant, M., and Alon, U.: Bacterial meningitis: Effect of antibiotic treatment on cerebrospinal fluid. Am. J. Clin. Pathol. *80*:386-387, 1983.
47. Bohr, V., Hansen, B., Jessen, O., et al.: Eight hundred and seventy-five cases of bacterial meningitis. Part I of a three-part series: Clinical data, prognosis, and the role of specialized hospital departments. J. Infect. *7*:21-30, 1983.
48. Bottcher, T., Ren, H., Goiny, M., et al.: Clindamycin is neuroprotective in experimental *Streptococcus pneumoniae* meningitis compared with ceftriaxone. J. Neurochem. *91*:1450-1460, 2004.
49. Bradley, J. S., Ching, D. K., and Phillips, S. E.: Outpatient therapy of serious pediatric infections with ceftriaxone. Pediatr. Infect. Dis. J. *7*:160-164, 1988.
50. Bradley, J. S., and Conner, J. D.: Ceftriaxone failure in meningitis caused by *Streptococcus pneumoniae* with reduced susceptibility to beta-lactam antibiotics. Pediatr. Infect. Dis. J. *10*:871-873, 1991.
51. Brady, M. T., Kaplan, S. L., and Taber, L. H.: Association between persistence of pneumococcal meningitis and dexamethasone administration. J. Pediatr. *99*:924-926, 1981.
52. Brandt, C., Lundgren, J., Frimolt-Moller, N., et al.: Blocking of leukocyte accumulation in the cerebrospinal fluid augments bacteremia and increased lethality in experimental pneumococcal meningitis. J. Neuroimmunol. *166*:126-131, 2005.
53. Braun, J. S., and Tuomanen, E. I.: Molecular mechanisms of brain damage in bacterial meningitis. Adv. Pediatr. Infect. Dis. *14*:49-71, 1999.
54. Breiman, R. F., Butler, J. C., Tenover, F. C., et al.: Emergence of drug-resistant pneumococcal infections in the United States. J. A. M. A. *271*:1831-1835, 1994.

55. Brenneman, G., Silimperi, D., and Ward, J.: Recurrent invasive *Haemophilus influenzae* type b disease in Alaskan natives. Pediatr. Infect. Dis. J. *6*:388-392, 1987.

56. Bryan, J. P., Rocha, H., da Silva, H. R., et al.: Comparison of ceftriaxone and ampicillin plus chloramphenicol for the therapy of acute bacterial meningitis. Antimicrob. Agents Chemother. *28*:361-368, 1985.

57. Burroughs, M., Cabellos, C., Prasad, S., et al.: Bacterial components and the pathophysiology of injury to the blood-brain barrier: Does cell wall add to the effects of endotoxin in gram-negative meningitis? J. Infect. Dis. *165*:S82-S85, 1992.

58. Butler, J. C., Breiman, R. F., and Lipman, H. B.: Serotype distribution of *Streptococcus pneumoniae* infections among preschool children in the United States, 1978-1994: Implications for development of conjugate vaccine. J. Infect. Dis. *171*:885-889, 1995.

59. Cable, D., Overturf, G., and Edralin, G.: Concentrations of cefoperazone in cerebrospinal fluid during bacterial meningitis. Antimicrob. Agents Chemother. *23*:688-691, 1983.

60. Carter, J., Neville, B., and Newton, C.: Neuro-cognitive impairment following acquired central nervous system infections in childhood: A systematic review. Brain Res. Rev. *43*:57-69, 2003.

61. Centers for Disease Control: Vestibular reactions to minocycline after meningococcal prophylaxis—New Jersey. M. M. W. R. Morb. Mortal. Wkly. Rep. *24*:9-11, 1975.

62. Centers for Disease Control: Vestibular reactions to minocycline follow-up—Georgia, New York, Vermont. M. M. W. R. Morb. Mortal. Wkly. Rep. *24*:55-56, 1975.

63. Centers for Disease Control: Bacterial meningitis and meningococcemia: United States—1978. M. M. W. R. Morb. Mortal. Wkly. Rep. *28*:277-278, 1979.

64. Centers for Disease Control: Haemophilus b conjugate vaccines for prevention of *Haemophilus influenzae* type b disease among infants and children two months of age and older: Recommendations of the Immunization Practices Advisory Committee (ACIP). M. M. W. R. Morb. Mortal. Wkly. Rep. *40*:1-7, 1991.

65. Centers for Disease Control and Prevention: Control and prevention of meningococcal disease and control and prevention of serogroup C meningococcal disease: Evaluation and management of suspected outbreaks. M. M. W. R. Morb. Mortal. Wkly. Rep. *46*(RR-5):1-21, 1997.

66. Centers for Disease Control and Prevention: Progress toward eliminating *Haemophilus influenzae* type b disease among infants and children—United States, 1987-1997. M. M. W. R. Morb. Mortal. Wkly. Rep. *47*:993-998, 1998.

67. Centers for Disease Control and Prevention: Recommendations of the Advisory Committee on Immunization Practices: Preventing pneumococcal disease among infants and young children. M. M. W. R. Morb. Mortal. Wkly. Rep. *49*(RR-9):1-35, 2000.

68. Centers for Disease Control and Prevention: Progress toward elimination of *Haemophilus influenzae* type b invasive disease among infants and children—United States 1998-2000. M. M. W. R. Morb. Mortal. Wkly. Rep. *51*:234-237, 2002.

69. Centers for Disease Control and Prevention: Direct and indirect effects of routine vaccination of children with 7-valent pneumococcal conjugate vaccine on incidence of invasive pneumococcal disease—United States, 1990-2003. M. M. W. R. Morb. Mortal. Wkly. Rep. *54*:893-897, 2005.

70. Centers for Disease Control and Prevention: Prevention and control of meningococcal disease recommendations of the Advisory Committee on Immunization Practices (ACIP). M. M. W. R. Morb. Mortal. Wkly. Rep. *54*(RR-7):1-17, 2005.

71. Cherry, J. D., and Sheenan, C. P.: Bacteriologic relapse in *Haemophilus influenzae* meningitis: Inadequate ampicillin therapy. N. Engl. J. Med. *278*:1001-1003, 1968.

72. Cole, F. S., Saryan, J. A., and Smith, A. L.: The risk of additional systemic bacterial illness in infants with systemic *Streptococcus pneumoniae* disease. J. Pediatr. *99*:91-94, 1981.

73. Coleman, S. J., Auld, E. B., Connor, J. D., et al.: Relapse of *Hemophilus influenzae* type b meningitis during intravenous therapy with ampicillin. J. Pediatr. *74*:781-784, 1969.

74. Colville, A., Davies, W., Heneghan, M., et al.: A rare complication of dental treatment: *Streptococcus oralis* meningitis. Br. Dent. J. *175*:133-134, 1993.

75. Committee on Infectious Diseases of the American Academy of Pediatrics: Therapy for children with invasive pneumococcal infections. Pediatrics *99*:289-299, 1997.

76. Congeni, B. L.: Comparison of ceftriaxone and traditional therapy of bacterial meningitis. Antimicrob. Agents Chemother. *25*:40-44, 1984.

77. Coulehan, J. L., Michaels, R. H., Hallowell, C., et al.: Epidemiology of *Haemophilus influenzae* type b disease among Navajo Indians. Public Health Rep. *99*:404-409, 1984.

78. Dagan, R., Shriker, O., Hazan, I., et al.: Prospective study to determine clinical relevance of detection of pneumococcal DNA in sera of children by PCR. J. Clin. Microbiol. *36*:669-673, 1998.

79. Daoud, A. S., Batieha, A., Al-Sheyyab, M., et al.: Lack of effectiveness of dexamethasone in neonatal bacterial meningitis. Eur. J. Pediatr. *158*:230-233, 1999.

80. Daum, R. S., Silber, G. R., Kamon, J. S., et al.: Evaluation of a commercial latex particle agglutination test for rapid diagnosis of *Haemophilus influenzae* type b infection. Pediatrics *69*:466-471, 1982.

81. Davey, P. G., Cruikshank, J. K., McManus, I. C., et al.: Bacterial meningitis—ten years' experience. J. Hyg. *88*:383-401, 1982.

82. Davison, K., and Ramsay, M.: The epidemiology of acute meningitis in England and Wales. Arch. Dis. Child. *88*:662-664, 2003.

83. Deal, W. B., and Sanders, E.: Efficacy of rifampin in treatment of meningococcal carriers. N. Engl. J. Med. *281*:641-645, 1969.

84. de Gans, J., and van de Beek, D., et al.: Dexamethasone in adults with bacterial meningitis. N. Engl. J. Med. *347*:1549-1556, 2002.

85. Deivanayagam, N., Ashaok, T. P., Nedunchelian, K., et al.: Evaluation of CSF variables as a diagnostic test for bacterial meningitis. J. Trop. Pediatr. *39*:284-287, 1993.

86. Del Rio, M. D. A., Chrane, D. F., Shelton, S., et al.: Pharmacokinetics of cefuroxime in infants and children with bacterial meningitis. Antimicrob. Agents Chemother. *22*:990-994, 1982.

87. Del Rio, M., Chrane, D., Shelton, S., et al.: Ceftriaxone versus ampicillin and chloramphenicol for treatment of bacterial meningitis in children. Lancet *1*:1241-1244, 1983.

88. de Morais, J. S., Munford, R. S., Rise, J. N., et al.: Epidemic disease due to serogroup L *Neisseria meningitidis* in São Paulo, Brazil. J. Infect. Dis. *129*:568-571, 1974.

89. Deutch, S., Pedersen, L., Podenphant, L., et al.: Broad-range real time PCR and DNA sequencing for the diagnosis of bacterial meningitis. Scand. J. Infect. Dis. *38*:27-35, 2006.

90. Devoe, I. W., and Gilchrist, J. E.: Pili on meningococci from primary cultures of nasopharyngeal carriers and cerebrospinal fluid of infants with acute disease. J. Exp. Med. *141*:297-305, 1975.

91. Diab, A., Zhu, J., Lindquist, L., et al.: *Haemophilus influenzae* and *Streptococcus pneumoniae* induce different intracerebral mRNA cytokine patterns during the course of experimental bacterial meningitis. Clin. Exp. Immunol. *109*:233-241, 1997.

92. Dicuonzo, G., Lorino, G., Lilli, D., et al.: Use of oligoprobes on amplified DNA in the diagnosis of bacterial meningitis. Eur. J. Clin. Microbiol. Infect. Dis. *18*:352-357, 1999.

93. Dinarello, C. A., and Mier, J. W.: Lymphokines. N. Engl. J. Med. *317*:940-945, 1987.

94. Di Pentima, M. C., Mason, E. O., Jr., and Kaplan, S. L.: In vitro antibiotic synergy against *Flavobacterium meningosepticum*: Implications for therapeutic options. Clin. Infect. Dis. *26*:1169-1176, 1998.

95. Dodge, P. R., Davis, H., Feigin, R. D., et al.: Prospective evaluation of hearing impairment as a sequela of acute bacterial meningitis. N. Engl. J. Med. *311*:869-874, 1984.

96. Dodge, P. R., and Swartz, M. N.: Bacterial meningitis: A review of selected aspects, II: Special neurologic problems, postmeningitic complications and clinicopathological correlations. N. Engl. J. Med. *272*:1003-1010, 1965.

97. du Plessis, M., Smith, A. M., and Klugman, K. P.: Rapid detection of penicillin-resistant *Streptococcus pneumoniae* in cerebrospinal fluid by a seminested-PCR strategy. J. Clin. Microbiol. *36*:453-457, 1998.

98. Edwards, K. M., Alford, R., Gewurz, H., et al.: Recurrent bacterial infections associated with C3 nephritic factor and hypocomplementemia. N. Engl. J. Med. *308*:1138-1141, 1983.

99. Eickhoff, T. C.: In-vitro and in-vivo studies of resistance to rifampin in meningococci. J. Infect. Dis. *123*:414-420, 1971.

100. Ellison, R. T., III, Kohler, P. F., Curd, J. G., et al.: Prevalence of congenital or acquired complement deficiency in patients with sporadic meningococcal disease. N. Engl. J. Med. *308*:913-916, 1983.

101. Eraklis, A. J., Kevy, S. V., Diamond, L. K., et al.: Hazard of overwhelming infection after splenectomy in childhood. N. Engl. J. Med. *276*:1225-1229, 1967.

102. Ernst, J. D., Decazes, J. M., and Sande, M. A.: Experimental pneumococcal meningitis: The role of leukocytes in pathogenesis. Infect. Immun. *41*:275-279, 1983.

103. Ernst, J. D., Hartiala, K. T., Goldstein, I. M., et al.: Complement (C5)-derived chemotactic activity accounts for accumulation of polymorphonuclear leukocytes in cerebrospinal fluid of rabbits with pneumococcal meningitis. Infect. Immun. *46*:81-86, 1984.

104. Feigin, R.: Use of corticosteroids in bacterial meningitis. Pediatr. Infect. Dis. J. *23*:355-357, 2004.

105. Feigin, R. D.: Bacterial meningitis beyond the newborn period. *In* Feigin, R. D., and Cherry, J. D. (eds.): Textbook of Pediatric Infectious Diseases. 2nd ed. Philadelphia, W. B. Saunders, 1987, pp. 439-465.

106. Feigin, R. D., Baker, C. J., Herwaldt, L. A., et al.: Epidemic meningococcal disease in an elementary-school classroom. N. Engl. J. Med. *307*:1255-1257, 1982.

107. Feigin, R. D., and Dodge, P. R.: Bacterial meningitis: Newer concepts of pathophysiology and neurologic sequelae. Pediatr. Clin. North Am. *23*:541-556, 1976.

108. Feigin, R. D., and Dodge, P. R.: Personal experience: Unpublished data for prospective studies of bacterial meningitis, 1974-1979.

109. Feigin, R. D., and Dodge, P. R.: Personal communications, 1974-1991.

110. Feigin, R. D., and Dodge, P. R.: Personal data.

111. Feigin, R. D., and Kaplan, S.: Inappropriate secretion of antidiuretic hormone (ADH) in children with bacterial meningitis. Am. J. Clin. Nutr. *30*:1482-1484, 1977.

112. Feigin, R. D., McCracken, G. H., and Klein, J. O.: Diagnosis and management of meningitis. Pediatr. Infect. Dis. J. *11*:785-814, 1992.

113. Feigin, R. D., and Shackelford, P. G.: Sequential lumbar puncture as a diagnostic aid in aseptic meningitis. N. Engl. J. Med. 289:571-574, 1973.
114. Feigin, R. D., and Shearer, W. T.: Opportunistic infection in children, Part I: In the compromised host. J. Pediatr. 87:507-514, 1975.
115. Feigin, R. D., and Shearer, W. T.: Opportunistic infection in children, Part II: In the compromised host. J. Pediatr. 87:677-694, 1975.
116. Feigin, R. D., Stechenberg, B. W., Chang, M. J., et al.: Prospective evaluation of treatment of Hemophilus influenzae meningitis. J. Pediatr. 88:773-775, 1976.
117. Feigin, R. D., Wong, M., Shackelford, P. G., et al.: Countercurrent immunoelectrophoresis of urine as well as CSF and blood for the diagnosis of bacterial meningitis. J. Pediatr. 89:773-774, 1976.
118. Feldman, H. M., and Michaels, R. H.: Academic achievement in children 10 to 12 years after Haemophilus influenzae meningitis. Pediatrics 81:339-344, 1988.
119. Feldman, W. E.: Concentrations of bacteria in cerebrospinal fluid of patients with bacterial meningitis. J. Pediatr. 88:549-552, 1976.
120. Feldman, W. E., Ginsburg, C. B., McCracken, G. H., et al.: Relation of concentrations of Haemophilus influenzae type b in cerebrospinal fluid to late sequelae of patients with meningitis. J. Pediatr. 100:209-218, 1982.
121. Feldman, W. E., Moffitt, S., and Manning, N. S.: Penetration of cefoxitin into cerebrospinal fluid of infants and children with bacterial meningitis. Antimicrob. Agents Chemother. 21:468-471, 1982.
122. Feldman, W. E., and Schwartz, J.: Haemophilus influenzae type b brain abscess complicating meningitis: Case report. Pediatrics 72:473-475, 1983.
123. Finland, M., and Barnes, M. W.: Acute bacterial meningitis at Boston City Hospital during 12 selected years, 1935-1972. J. Infect. Dis. 136:400-415, 1977.
124. Finlay, F. O., Witherow, H., and Rudd, P. T.: Latex agglutination testing in bacterial meningitis. Arch. Dis. Child. 73:160-161, 1995.
125. Fiore, A. E., Moroney, J. F., Farley, M. M., et al.: Clinical outcomes of meningitis caused by Streptococcus pneumoniae in the era of antibiotic resistance. Clin. Infect. Dis. 30:71-77, 2000.
126. Fischer, G. W., Brenz, R. W., Alden, E. R., et al.: Lumbar puncture and meningitis. Am. J. Dis. Child. 129:590-592, 1975.
127. Forgacs, P., Geyer, C. A., and Freidberg, S. R.: Characterization of chemical meningitis after neurological surgery. Clin. Infect. Dis. 32:179-185, 2001.
128. Franciosi, R. A., Knostman, J. D., and Zimmerman, R. A.: Group B streptococcal neonatal and infant infections. J. Pediatr. 82:707-718, 1973.
129. Frasch, C. E., Pepple, B. S., Cate, T. R., et al.: Immunogenicity and clinical evaluation of group B Neisseria meningitidis outer membrane protein vaccines. In Weinstein, L., and Fields, B. N. (eds.): Seminar in Infectious Diseases. Vol. 4. Bacterial Vaccines. New York, Thieme-Stratton, 1982, pp. 263-267.
130. Fraser, D. W., Darby, C. P., Koehler, R. E., et al.: Risk factors in bacterial meningitis: Charleston County, South Carolina. J. Infect. Dis. 127:271-277, 1973.
131. Fraser, D. W., Geil, C. C., and Feldman, R. A.: Bacterial meningitis in Bernalilla County, New Mexico: A comparison with three other American populations. Am. J. Epidemiol. 100:29-34, 1974.
132. Fraser, D. W., Henke, C. E., and Feldman, R. A.: Changing patterns of bacterial meningitis in Olmstead County, Minnesota, 1935-1970. J. Infect. Dis. 128:300-307, 1973.
133. Fraser, D. W., Mitchell, J. E., Silverman, L. P., et al.: Undiagnosed bacterial meningitis in Vermont children. Ann. J. Epidemiol. 102:394-399, 1975.
134. Frei, K., Piani, D., Pfister, H. W., et al.: Immune-mediated injury in bacterial meningitis. Int. Rev. Exp. Pathol. 34:183-192, 1993.
135. Frenkel, L. D., and the Multicenter Ceftriaxone Pediatric Study Group: Once-daily administration of ceftriaxone for the treatment of selected serious bacterial infections in children. Pediatrics 82:486-491, 1988.
136. Friedland, I. R., and Klugman, K. P.: Antibiotic-resistant pneumococcal disease in South African children. Am. J. Dis. Child. 146:920-923, 1992.
137. Friedland, I. R., Paris, M., Ehrett, S., et al.: Evaluation of antimicrobial regimens for treatment of experimental penicillin- and cephalosporin-resistant pneumococcal meningitis. Antimicrob. Agents Chemother. 37:1630-1636, 1993.
138. Friedland, I. R., Paris, M., Shelton, S., et al.: Time-kill studies of antibiotic combinations against penicillin-resistant and -susceptible Streptococcus pneumoniae. J. Antimicrob. Chemother. 34:231-237, 1994.
139. Friedland, I. R., Shelton, S., Paris, M., et al.: Dilemmas in diagnosis and management of cephalosporin-resistant Streptococcus pneumoniae meningitis. Pediatr. Infect. Dis. J. 12:196-200, 1993.
140. Gado, M., Axley, J., Appleton, D. B., et al.: Angiography in the acute and post-treatment phases of Haemophilus influenzae meningitis. Radiology 110:439-444, 1974.
141. Gaillard, J. L., Abadie, G., Cheron, J., et al.: Concentrations of ceftriaxone in cerebrospinal fluid of children with meningitis receiving dexamethasone therapy. Antimicrob. Agents Chemother. 38:1209-1210, 1994.
142. Garcia, H., Kaplan, S. L., and Feigin, R. D.: Cerebrospinal fluid concentration of arginine vasopressin in children with bacterial meningitis. J. Pediatr. 98:67-70, 1981.
143. Garred, P., Michaelsen, T. E., Bjune, G., et al.: A low serum concentration of mannan-binding protein is not associated with serogroup B or C meningococcal disease. Scand. J. Immunol. 37:468-470, 1993.
144. Gary, N., Powers, N., and Todd, J. K.: Clinical identification and comparative prognosis of high-risk patients with Haemophilus influenzae meningitis. Am. J. Dis. Child. 143:307-311, 1989.
145. Geiseler, P. J., and Nelson, K. E.: Bacterial meningitis without clinical signs of meningeal irritation. South. Med. J. 75:448-450, 1982.
146. Geiseler, P. J., Nelson, K. E., and Levin, S.: Community-acquired purulent meningitis: A review of 1,316 cases during the antibiotic era, 1954-1976. Rev. Infect. Dis. 2:725-744, 1980.
147. Gerber, J., Bottcher, T., Hahn, M., et al.: Increased mortality and spatial memory deficits in TNF-alpha-deficient mice in ceftriaxone-treated experimental pneumococcal meningitis. Neurobiol. Dis. 16:133-138, 2004.
148. Gerber, J., Lotz, M., Ebert, S., et al.: Melatonin is neuroprotective in experimental Streptococcus pneumoniae meningitis. J. Infect. Dis. 191:783-790, 2005.
149. Gerber, J., Pohl, K., Sander, V., et al.: Rifampin followed by ceftriaxone for experimental meningitis decreases lipoteichoic acid concentrations in cerebrospinal fluid and reduces neuronal damage in comparison to ceftriaxone alone. Antimicrob. Agents Chemother. 47:1313-1317, 2003.
150. Gerdes, L. U., Jorgensen, P. E., Nexo, E., et al.: C-reactive protein and bacterial meningitis: A meta-analysis. Scand. J. Clin. Lab. Invest. 58:383-393, 1998.
151. Gessner, B., Sutanto, A., Linehan, M., et al.: Incidences of vaccine-preventable Haemophilus influenzae type b pneumonia and meningitis in Indonesian children: Hamlet-randomised vaccine-probe trial. Lancet 365:43-52, 2005.
152. Giampaolo, C., Scheld, W. M., Boyd, J., et al.: Leukocyte and bacterial interrelationships in experimental meningitis. Ann. Neurol. 9:328-333, 1982.
153. Gigliotti, F., Lee, D., Insel, R. A., et al.: IgG penetration into the cerebrospinal fluid in a rabbit model of meningitis. J. Infect. Dis. 156:394-398, 1987.
154. Gilbert, G.: Epidemiology of Haemophilus influenzae type b disease in Australia and New Zealand. Vaccine 9(Suppl.):S10-S13, 1991.
155. Gilday, D. L.: Various radionuclide patterns of cerebral inflammation in infants and children. A. J. R. Am. J. Roentgenol. 120:247-253, 1974.
156. Ginsburg, C. M., McCracken, G. H., Jr., and Parke, J. J.: Haemophilus influenzae type b disease in a day-care center. Pediatr. Res. 11:435, 1977.
157. Girgis, N. I., Abu El Ella, A. H., Farid, Z., et al.: Intramuscular ceftriaxone versus ampicillin-chloramphenicol in childhood bacterial meningitis. Scand. J. Infect. Dis. 20:613-617, 1988.
158. Girgis, N. I., Farid, Z., Mikhail, I. A., et al.: Dexamethasone treatment for bacterial meningitis in children and adults. Pediatr. Infect. Dis. J. 5:210-215, 1989.
159. Gitlin, D.: Pathogenesis of subdural collections of fluid. Pediatrics 16:345-351, 1955.
160. Givner, L. B., Mason, E. O., Jr., Barson, W. J., et al.: Pneumococcal facial cellulitis in children. Pediatrics 106:e61, 2000.
161. Gold, R.: Bacterial meningitis—1982. Am. J. Med. 75:98-101, 1983.
162. Gold, R.: Epidemiology of bacterial meningitis. Infect. Dis. Clin. N. Am. 13:515-525, 1999.
163. Gradgirard, D., and Leib, S.: Strategies to prevent neuronal damage in pediatric bacterial meningitis. Curr. Opin. Pediatr. 18:112-118, 2006.
164. Green, S. M., Rothrock, S. G., Clem, K. J., et al.: Can seizures be the sole manifestation of meningitis in febrile children? Pediatrics 92:527-534, 1993.
165. Greenfield, S., and Feldman, H. A.: Familial carriers and meningococcal meningitis. N. Engl. J. Med. 277:487-502, 1967.
166. Grimwood, K., Anderson, V. A., Bond, L., et al.: Adverse outcomes of bacterial meningitis in school-age survivors. Pediatrics 95:646-656, 1995.
167. Grubbauer, H. M., Dornbusch, H. J., Dittrich, P., et al.: Ceftriaxone monotherapy for bacterial meningitis in children. Chemotherapy 36:441-447, 1990.
168. Guibourdenche, M., Caugant, D. A., Hervé, V., et al.: Characteristics of serogroup A Neisseria meningitidis strains isolated in the Central African Republic in February 1992. Eur. J. Clin. Microbiol. Infect. Dis. 13:174-177, 1994.
169. Gulian, J.-M., Gonard, V., Dalmasso, C., et al.: Bilirubin displacement by ceftriaxone in neonates: Evaluation by determination of "free" bilirubin and erythrocyte-bound bilirubin. J. Antimicrob. Chemother. 19:823-829, 1987.
170. Gump, D. W.: Vancomycin for treatment of bacterial meningitis. Rev. Infect. Dis. 3:S289-S292, 1981.
171. Guttler, R. B., Counts, G. W., Avent, C. K., et al.: Effect of rifampin and minocycline on meningococcal carrier rates. J. Infect. Dis. 124:199-205, 1971.
172. Haimanot, R. T., Caugant, D. A., Fekadu, D., et al.: Characteristics of serogroup A Neisseria meningitidis responsible for an epidemic in Ethiopia, 1988-89. Scand. J. Infect. Dis. 22:171-174, 1990.
173. Hall, B. D.: Failure of ampicillin in meningitis. Lancet 1:1033, 1968.
174. Haltalin, K. C., and Smith, J. B.: Reevaluation of ampicillin therapy for Haemophilus influenzae meningitis: An appraisal based on a review of cases of persistent or recurrent infection. Am. J. Dis. Child. 122:328-336, 1971.
175. Hansman, D., and Andrews, G. A.: A resistant pneumococcus. Lancet 2:264-265, 1967.
176. Hansman, D., Hanna, J., and Morey, F.: High prevalence of invasive Haemophilus influenzae disease in central Australia, 1986. Lancet 2:927, 1986.
177. Hanson, E. H., Niemeyer, D. M., Folio, L., et al.: Potential use of microarray technology for rapid identification of central nervous system pathogens. Milit. Med. 169:594-599, 2004.
178. Harrison, L.: Prospects for vaccine prevention of meningococcal infection. Clin. Microbiol. Rev. 19:142-164, 2006.
179. Harrison, L. H., Dwyer, D. M., Maples, C. T., et al.: Risk of meningococcal infection in college students. J. A. M. A. 281:1906-1910, 1999.
180. Hatch, D., Overturf, G. D., Kovacs, A., et al.: Treatment of bacterial meningitis with ceftazidime. Pediatr. Infect. Dis. 5:416-420, 1986.

181. Haven, P. L., Wendelgerger, K. J., Hoffman, G. M., et al.: Corticosteroids as adjunctive therapy in bacterial meningitis. Am. J. Dis. Child. *143*:1051-1055, 1989.
182. Healy, C., and Baker, C. The future of meningococcal vaccines. Pediatr. Infect. Dis. J. *24*:175-176, 2005.
183. Hirakawa, K., Kurokawa, M., Yajin, K., et al.: Recurrent meningitis due to a congenital fistula in the stapedial footplate. Arch. Otolaryngol. *109*:697-700, 1983.
184. Hoffmann, O., Keilwerth, N., Bille, M., et al.: Triptans reduce the inflammatory response in bacterial meningitis. J. Cereb. Blood Flow. Metab. *22*:988-996, 2002.
185. Hogasen, K., Michaelsen, T., Mellbye, O. J., et al.: Low prevalence of complement deficiencies among patients with meningococcal disease in Norway. Scand. J. Immunol. *37*:487-489, 1993.
186. Holmes, S. J., Lucas, A. H., Osterholm, M. T., et al.: Immunoglobulin deficiency and idiotype expression in children developing *Haemophilus influenzae* type b disease after vaccination with conjugate vaccine. The Collaborative Study Group. J. A. M. A. *266*:1960-1965, 1991.
187. Ingram, D. L., Anderson, P., and Smith, D. H.: Counter-current immunoelectrophoresis in the diagnosis of systemic disease caused by *Hemophilus influenzae*, type b. J. Pediatr. *81*:1156-1159, 1972.
188. Ingram, D. L., Pearson, A. W., and Occhiuti, A. R.: Detection of bacterial antigens in body fluids with the Wellcogen *Haemophilus influenzae* b, *Streptococcus pneumoniae*, and *Neisseria meningitidis* (ACYW135) latex agglutination tests. J. Clin. Microbiol. *18*:1119-1121, 1983.
189. Jackson, L. A., Schuchat, A., Reeves, M. W., et al.: Serogroup C meningococcal outbreaks in the United States: An emerging threat. J. A. M. A. *273*:383-389, 1995.
190. Jadavji, T., Biggar, W. D., Gold, R., et al.: Sequelae of acute bacterial meningitis in children treated for seven days. Pediatrics *78*:21-25, 1985.
191. Jaye, D. L., and Waites, K. B.: Clinical applications of C-reactive protein in pediatrics. Pediatr. Infect. Dis. J. *16*:735-746, 1997.
192. Kadurugamuwa, J. L., Hengstler, B., and Zak, O.: Effects of antiinflammatory drugs on arachidonic-acid metabolites and cerebrospinal fluid (CSF) proteins during infectious pneumococcal meningitis in rabbits. Pediatr. Infect. Dis. 6(Suppl.):1153-1154, 1987.
193. Kadurugamuwa, J. L., Hengstler, B., and Zak, O.: Cerebrospinal fluid protein profile in experimental pneumococcal meningitis and its alteration by ampicillin and anti-inflammatory agents. J. Infect. Dis. *159*:26-34, 1989.
194. Kaene, W. M., Postic, W. P., Rowe, L. D., et al.: Meningitis and hearing loss in children. Otolaryngology *105*:39-44, 1979.
195. Kaplan, S. L.: Clinical presentations, diagnosis, and prognostic factors of bacterial meningitis. Infect. Dis. Clin. N. Am. *13*:579-594, 1999.
196. Kaplan, S. L., Catlin, F. I., Weaver, T., et al.: Onset of hearing loss in children with bacterial meningitis. Pediatrics *73*:575-578, 1984.
197. Kaplan, S. L., and Feigin, R. D.: The syndrome of inappropriate secretion of antidiuretic hormone in children with bacterial meningitis. J. Pediatr. *92*:758-761, 1978.
198. Kaplan, S. L., and Feigin, R. D.: Rapid identification of the invading microorganism. Pediatr. Clin. North Am. *27*:783-803, 1980.
199. Kaplan, S. L., and Fishman, M. A.: Supportive therapy for bacterial meningitis. Pediatr. Infect. Dis. J. *6*:670-677, 1987.
200. Kaplan, S. L., Goddard, J., VanKleeck, M., et al.: Ataxia and deafness in children due to bacterial meningitis. Pediatrics *68*:8-13, 1981.
201. Kaplan, S. L., and Mason, E. O., Jr.: Management of infections due to antibiotic-resistant *Streptococcus pneumoniae*. Clin. Microbiol. Rev. *11*:628-644, 1998.
202. Kaplan, S. L., Mason, E. O., Jr., Mason, S. K., et al.: Prospective comparative trial of moxalactam versus ampicillin or chloramphenicol for treatment of *Haemophilus influenzae* type b meningitis. J. Pediatr. *104*:447-453, 1984.
203. Kaplan, S. L., Mason, E. O., Jr., Wald, E. R., et al.: Six-year multicenter surveillance of invasive pneumococcal infections in children. Pediatr. Infect. Dis. J. *21*:141-147, 2002.
204. Kaplan, S. L., Smith, E. O., Wills, C., et al.: Association between preadmission oral antibiotic therapy and cerebrospinal fluid findings and sequelae caused by *Haemophilus influenzae* type b meningitis. Pediatr. Infect. Dis. *5*:626-632, 1986.
205. Kellner, J., Scheifele, D., Halperin, S., et al.: Outcome of penicillin-non-susceptible *Streptococcus pneumoniae* meningitis: A nested case-control study. Pediatr. Infect. Dis. J. *21*:903-909, 2002.
206. Kennedy, W. A., Hoyt, M. J., and McCracken, G. H.: The role of corticosteroids in children with pneumococcal meningitis. Am. J. Dis. Child. *145*:1374-1478, 1991.
207. Kessler, R. E.: Cefepime microbiologic profile and update. Pediatr. Infect. Dis. J. *20*:331-336, 2001.
208. Kilpatrick, M., Girgis, N., Farid, Z., et al.: Aztreonam for treating meningitis caused by gram-negative rods. Scand. J. Infect. Dis. *23*:125-126, 1991.
209. Kim, Y. O., Kang, J. S., Youm, M. H., et al.: Diagnostic capability of CSF ferritin in children with meningitis. Pediatr. Neurol. *28*:271-276, 2003.
210. Kim, Y. S., and Tauber, M. G.: Neurotoxicity of glia activated by gram-positive bacterial products depends on nitric oxide production. Infect. Immun. *64*:3148-3153, 1996.
211. Klass, P. E., and Klein, J. O.: Therapy of bacterial sepsis, meningitis and otitis media in infants and children: 1992 poll of directors of programs in pediatric infectious diseases. Pediatr. Infect. Dis. J. *11*:702-705, 1992.
212. Kleiman, M. D., Weinberg, G. A., Reynolds, J. K., et al.: Meningitis with beta-lactam-resistant *Streptococcus pneumoniae*: The need for early repeat lumbar puncture. Pediatr. Infect. Dis. J. *12*:782-784, 1993.
213. Klein, J. O., Feigin, R. D., and McCracken, G. H., Jr.: Report of the Task Force on Diagnosis and Management of Meningitis. Pediatrics *78*:S959-S982, 1986.
214. Klein, M., Koedel, U., Pfister, H., and Kastenbauer, S.: Meningitis-associated hearing loss: Protection by adjunctive antioxidant therapy. Ann. Neurol. *54*:451-458, 2003.
215. Kline, M. W., and Kaplan, S. L.: Computed tomography in bacterial meningitis of childhood. Pediatr. Infect. Dis. J. *7*:855-857, 1988.
216. Klugman, K. P., Dagan, R., and The Meropenem Meningitis Study Group: Randomized comparison of meropenem with cefotaxime for treatment of bacterial meningitis. Antimicrob. Agents Chemother. *39*:1140-1146, 1995.
217. Klugman, K. P., Friedland, I. R., and Bradley, J. S.: Bactericidal activity against cephalosporin-resistant *Streptococcus pneumoniae* in cerebrospinal fluid of children with acute bacterial meningitis. Antimicrob. Agents Chemother. *39*:1988-1992, 1995.
218. Koedel, U., Bernatowicz, A., Paul, R., et al.: Experimental pneumococcal meningitis: Cerebrovascular alterations, brain edema, and meningeal inflammation are linked to the production of nitric oxide. Ann. Neurol. *37*:313-323, 1995.
219. Koedel, U., Scheld, W., and Pfister, H.: Pathogenesis and pathophysiology of pneumococcal meningitis. Lancet Infect. Dis. *2*:721-736, 2002.
220. Komorowski, R. N., Farmer, S. G., and Hause, L. L.: Cerebrospinal fluid lactic acid in diagnosis of meningitis. J. Clin. Microbiol. *8*:89-92, 1978.
221. Koomen, I., Grobbee, D., Roord, J., et al.: Hearing loss at school age in survivors of bacterial meningitis: Assessment, incidence and prediction. Pediatrics *112*:1049-1053, 2003.
222. Koomen, I., van Furth, A., Kraak, M., et al.: Neuropsychology of academic and behavioral limiations in school-age survivors of bacterial meningitis. Dev. Med. Child Neurol. *46*:724-732, 2004.
223. Kornelisse, R. F., Hack, C. E., Savelkoul, H. F., et al.: Intrathecal production of interleukin-12 and gamma interferon in patients with bacterial meningitis. Infect. Immun. *65*:877-881, 1997.
224. Kotilainen, P., Jalava, J., Meurman, O., et al.: Diagnosis of meningococcal meningitis by broad-range bacterial PCR with cerebrospinal fluid. J. Clin. Microbiol. *36*:2205-2209, 1998.
225. Kyaw, M., Lynfield, R., Schaffner, W., et al.: Effect of introduction of the pneumococcal conjugate vaccine on drug-resistant *Streptococcus pneumoniae*. N. Engl. J. Med. *354*:1455-1463, 2006.
226. LaScolea, L. J., Jr., and Dryja, D.: Quantitation of bacteria in cerebrospinal fluid and blood of children with meningitis and its diagnostic significance. J. Clin. Microbiol. *19*:187-190, 1984.
227. Lebel, M. H., Freij, B. J., Syrogiannopoulos, G. A., et al.: Dexamethasone therapy for bacterial meningitis: Results of two double-blind, placebo-controlled trials. N. Engl. J. Med. *319*:964-971, 1988.
228. Lebel, M. H., Hoyt, M. J., and McCracken, G. H.: Comparative efficacy of ceftriaxone and cefuroxime for treatment of bacterial meningitis. J. Pediatr. *114*:1049-1054, 1989.
229. Lebel, M. H., and McCracken, G. H., Jr.: Aztreonam: Review of the clinical experience and potential uses in pediatrics. Pediatr. Infect. Dis. J. *7*:331-339, 1988.
230. Lebel, M. H., and McCracken, G. H., Jr.: Delayed cerebrospinal fluid sterilization and adverse outcome of bacterial meningitis in infants and children. Pediatrics *83*:161-167, 1989.
231. Leedom, J. M., Ivler, D., Mathies, A. W., et al.: The problem of sulfadiazine-resistant meningococci. Antimicrob. Agents Chemother. *6*:281-292, 1966.
232. Leggiadro, R. J., and Winkelstein, J. A.: Prevalence of complement deficiencies in children with systemic meningococcal disease. Pediatr. Infect. Dis. J. *6*:75-76, 1987.
233. Leib, S., Heimgartner, C., Bifrare, Y., et al.: Dexamethasone aggravates hippocampal apoptosis and learning deficiency in pneumococcal meningitis in infant rats. Pediatr. Res. *54*:353-357, 2003.
234. Leib, S. L., and Tauber, M. D.: Pathogenesis of bacterial meningitis. Infect. Dis. Clin. N. Am. *13*:527-548, 1999.
235. Leimkugel, J., Adams Forgor, A., Gagneux, S., et al.: An outbreak of serotype 1 *Streptococcus pneumoniae* meningitis in northern Ghana with features that are characteristic of *Neisseria meningitides* meningitis epidemics. J. Infect. Dis. *192*:192-199, 2005.
236. Lerman, S. J.: Systemic *Hemophilus influenzae* infection: A study of risk factors. Clin. Pediatr. *21*:360-364, 1982.
237. Levine, O. S., Farley, M., Harrison, L. E., et al.: Risk factors for invasive pneumococcal disease in children: A population-based case-control study in North America. Pediatrics *103*:e28, 1999.
238. Liebman, E. P., Ronis, M. L., Loyrinic, J. H., et al.: Hearing improvement following meningitis deafness. Arch. Otolaryngol. *90*:470-473, 1969.
239. Lim, D., Gerurz, A., Lint, T. F., et al.: Absence of the sixth component of complement in a patient with repeated episodes of meningococcal meningitis. J. Pediatr. *89*:42-47, 1976.

240. Lin, T. Y., Chrane, D. F., Nelson, J. D., et al.: Seven days of ceftriaxone therapy is as effective as ten days' treatment for bacterial meningitis. J. A. M. A. *253*:3559-3563, 1985.
241. Lindsay, J.: Profound childhood deafness: Inner ear pathology. Ann. Otol. Rhinol. Laryngol. *82*(Suppl. 5):88-102, 1973.
242. Losonsky, G. A., Santosham, M., Sehgal, V. M., et al.: *Haemophilus influenzae* disease in the White Mountain Apaches: Molecular epidemiology of a high risk population. Pediatr. Infect. Dis. *3*:539-547, 1984.
243. MacLennan, J. M., Shackley, F., Heath, P. T., et al.: Safety, immunogenicity, and induction of immunologic memory by a serogroup C meningococcal conjugate vaccine in infants: A randomized controlled trial. J. A. M. A. *283*:2795-2801, 2000.
244. Madagame, E. T., Havens, P. L., Bresnahan, J. M., et al.: Survival and functional outcome of children requiring mechanical ventilation during therapy for acute bacterial meningitis. Crit. Care Med. *23*:1279-1283, 1995.
245. Mariscalco, M. M.: Innate immunity in critical care. Semin. Pediatr. Infect. Dis. *17*:25-35, 2006.
246. Marks, W. A., Stutman, H. R., Marks, M. I., et al.: Cefuroxime versus ampicillin plus chloramphenicol in childhood bacterial meningitis: A multicenter randomized controlled trial. J. Pediatr. *109*:123-130, 1986.
247. Maxson, S., Lewno, M. J., and Schutze, G. E.: Clinical usefulness of cerebrospinal fluid bacterial antigen studies. J. Pediatr. *125*:235-238, 1994.
248. McCracken, G. H., Sarff, L. D., Glode, M. P., et al.: Relation between *Escherichia coli* K1 capsular polysaccharide antigen and clinical outcome in neonatal meningitis. Lancet *2*:246-250, 1974.
249. McCracken, G. J., Jr., and Lebel, M. H.: Dexamethasone therapy for bacterial meningitis in infants and children. Am. J. Dis. Child. *143*:287-289, 1989.
250. McIntosh, D., Brown, J., Hanson, R., et al.: Torticollis and bacterial meningitis. Pediatr. Infect. Dis. J. *12*:160-161, 1993.
251. McIntyre, P. B., Berkey, C. S., King, S. M., et al.: Dexamethasone as adjunctive therapy in bacterial meningitis. J. A. M. A. *278*:925-931, 1997.
252. Melish, M. E., Nelson, A. J., Martin, T. E., et al.: Epidemic spread of *Hemophilus influenzae* type b disease in a day care center. Pediatr. Res. *10*:348, 1976.
253. Meningococcal Meningitis. Wkly. Epidemiol. Rec. *78*:292-296, 2003.
254. Mertsola, J., Kennedy, W. A., Waagner, D., et al.: Endotoxin concentrations in cerebrospinal fluid correlate with clinical severity and neurologic outcome of *Haemophilus influenzae* type b meningitis. Am. J. Dis. Child. *145*:1099-1103, 1991.
255. Meurman, O. H., Irjala, K., Suonpaa, J., et al.: A new method for the identification of cerebrospinal fluid leakage. Acta Otolaryngol. *87*:366-369, 1979.
256. Michie, H. R., Manogue, K. R., Spriggs, D. R., et al.: Detection of circulation tumor necrosis factor after endotoxin administration. N. Engl. J. Med. *318*:1481-1486, 1988.
257. Mitchell, L., Smith, S., Braun, J., et al.: Dual phases of apoptosis in pneumococcal meningitis. J. Infect. Dis. *190*:2039-2046, 2004.
258. Modai, J., Vittecoq, D., Decazes, J. M., et al.: Penetration of ceftazidime into cerebrospinal fluid of patients with bacterial meningitis. Antimicrob. Agents Chemother. *24*:126-128, 1983.
259. Moellering, R. C.: Pharmacokinetics of vancomycin. J. Antimicrob. Chemother. *14*:43-52, 1984.
260. Moore, P. S., Harrison, L. H., Telzak, E. E., et al.: Group A meningococcal carriage in travelers returning from Saudi Arabia. J. A. M. A. *260*:2686-2689, 1988.
261. Moore, P. S., Reeves, M. W., Schwartz, B., et al.: Intercontinental spread of an epidemic group A *Neisseria meningitidis* strain. Lancet *2*:260-263, 1989.
262. Mothershed, E. A., Sacchi, C. T., Whitney, A. M., et al.: Use of real-time PCR to resolve slide agglutination discrepancies in serogroup identification of *Neisseria meningitidis*. J. Clin. Microbiol. *42*:320-328, 2004.
263. Moura, A., Pablos-Mendez, A., Layton, M., and Weiss, D.: Epidemiology of meningococcal disease, New York City, 1989-2000. Emerg. Infect. Dis. *9*:355-361, 2003.
264. Moxon, E. R., Smith, A. L., Averill, D. R., et al.: *Hemophilus influenzae* meningitis in infant rats after intranasal inoculation. J. Infect. Dis. *129*:154-162, 1974.
265. Mullaney, D. T., and John, J. F.: Cefotaxime therapy: Evaluation of its effect on bacterial meningitis, CSF drug levels, and bactericidal activity. Arch. Intern. Med. *143*:1705-1708, 1983.
266. Mumford, R. J., deVasconelas, Z. J. S., Phillips, C. J., et al.: Eradication of carriage of *Neisseria meningitidis* in families: A study in Brazil. J. Infect. Dis. *129*:644-649, 1974.
267. Munoz, O., Benitez-Diaz, L., Martinez, M. C., et al.: Hearing loss after *Hemophilus influenzae* meningitis: Follow-up study with auditory brainstem potentials. Ann. Otol. Rhinol. Laryngol. *92*:272-275, 1983.
268. Murphy, T. V., Pastor, P., Medley, F., et al.: Decreased *Haemophilus* colonization in children vaccinated with *Haemophilus influenzae* type b conjugate vaccine. J. Pediatr. *122*:517-523, 1993.
269. Mustafa, M. M., Lebel, M. H., Ramilo, O., et al.: Correlation of interleukin 1β and cachectin concentrations in cerebrospinal fluid and outcome from bacterial meningitis. J. Pediatr. *115*:208-213, 1989.
270. Mustafa, M. M., Ramilo, O., Mertsola, J., et al.: Modulation of inflammation and cachectin activity in relation to treatment of experimental *Haemophilus influenzae* type b meningitis. J. Infect. Dis. *160*:818-825, 1989.
271. Mustafa, M. M., Ramilo, O., Saez-Llorens, X., et al.: Cerebrospinal fluid prostaglandins, interleukin 1β, and tumor necrosis factor in bacterial meningitis: Clinical and laboratory correlations in placebo and dexamethasone-treated patients. Am. J. Dis. Child. *144*:883-887, 1990.
272. Nadol, J. B., Jr.: Hearing loss as a sequela of meningitis. Laryngoscope *88*:739-755, 1978.
273. Nagata, M., Hara, T., Aoki, T., et al.: Inherited deficiency of ninth component of complement: An increased risk of meningococcal meningitis. J. Pediatr. *114*:260-264, 1989.
274. Naraqui, S., Kirkpatrick, G. P., and Kabins, S.: Relapsing pneumococcal meningitis: Isolation of an organism with decreased susceptibility to penicillin G. J. Pediatr. *85*:671-673, 1974.
275. National Committee for Clinical Laboratory Standards: Performance Standards for Antimicrobial Testing. Tenth informational supplement (aerobic dilution). M100-S10(M7) Table 2G. MIC Interpretive Standards (mg/mL) for *Streptococcus pneumoniae*. Wayne, PA, NCCLS, January 2000.
276. Neches, W., and Platt, M.: Cerebrospinal fluid LDH in 287 children including 53 cases of meningitis of bacterial and non-bacterial etiology. Pediatrics *41*:1097-1103, 1968.
277. Negrini, B., Kelleher, K. J., and Wald, E. R.: Cerebrospinal fluid findings in aseptic versus bacterial meningitis. Pediatrics *105*:316-319, 2000.
278. Niemoller, U. M., and Tauber, M. G.: Brain edema and increased intracranial pressure in the pathophysiology of bacterial meningitis. Eur. J. Clin. Microbiol. Infect. Dis. *8*:109-117, 1989.
279. Novak, R., Henriques, B., Charpentier, E., et al.: Emergency of vancomycin tolerance in *Streptococcus pneumoniae*. Nature *399*:590-593, 1999.
280. Nuorti, J. P., Butler, J. C., Farley, M. M., et al.: Cigarette smoking and invasive pneumococcal disease. N. Engl. J. Med. *342*:681-689, 2000.
281. Odio, C. M., Faingezicht, I., and Paris, M.: The beneficial effects of early dexamethasone administration in infants and children with bacterial meningitis. N. Engl. J. Med. *324*:1515-1531, 1991.
282. Odio, C. M., Puig, J. R., Feris, J. M., et al.: Prospective, randomized investigator-blinded study of the efficacy and safety of meropenem vs. cefotaxime therapy in bacterial meningitis in children. Pediatr. Infect. Dis. J. *18*:581-590, 1999.
283. Olivier, C., Cohen, R., Begue, P., et al.: Bacteriologic outcome of children with cefotaxime- or ceftriaxone-susceptible and -nonsusceptible *Streptococcus pneumoniae* meningitis. Pediatr. Infect. Dis. J. *19*:1015-1017, 2000.
284. Pandit, L., Kumar, S., Karunasagar, I., and Karunasagar, I.: Diagnosis of partially treated culture-negative bacterial meningitis using 16S rRNA universal primers and restriction endonuclease digestion. J. Med. Microbiol. *54*:539-542, 2005.
285. Parke, J. C., Jr., Schneerson, R., and Robbins, J. B.: The attack rate, age, incidence, racial distribution and case fatality rate of *Hemophilus influenzae*, type b meningitis in Mecklenburg County, North Carolina. J. Pediatr. *81*:765-769, 1972.
286. Parkkinen, J., Korhonen, T. K., Pere, A., et al.: Binding sites in the rat brain for *Escherichia coli* S fimbriae associated with neonatal meningitis. J. Clin. Invest. *81*:860-865, 1988.
287. Peltola, H., Makela, P. H., Kayhty, H., et al.: Clinical efficacy of meningococcus group A capsular polysaccharide vaccine in children three months to five years of age. N. Engl. J. Med. *297*:686-691, 1977.
288. Peltola, H., Rod, T. O., Jonsdottir, K., et al.: Life-threatening *Haemophilus influenzae* infections in Scandinavia: A five-country analysis of the incidence and the main clinical and bacteriologic characteristics. Rev. Infect. Dis. *12*:708-715, 1990.
289. Perkins, M. D., Mirrett, S., and Reller, R. B.: Rapid bacterial antigen detection is not clinically useful. J. Clin. Microbiol. *33*:1486-1491, 1995.
290. Peter, G., Weigart, M. B., Bissel, A. R., et al.: Meningococcal meningitis in familial deficiency of the fifth component of complement. Pediatrics *67*:882-886, 1981.
291. Pichichero, M., Casey, J., Blatter, M., et al.: Comparative trial of the safety and immunogenicity of quadrivalent (A, C, Y, W-135) meningococcal polysaccharide-diphtheria conjugate vaccine versus quadrivalent polysaccharide vaccine in two- to ten-year-old children. Pediatr. Infect. Dis. J. *24*:57-62, 2005.
292. Pinner, R. W., Onyango, F., Perkins, B. A., et al.: Epidemic meningococcal disease in Nairobi, Kenya, 1989. J. Infect. Dis. *166*:359-364, 1992.
293. Pomeroy, S. L., Holmes, S. J., Dodge, P. R., et al.: A prospective evaluation of the neurologic sequelae of bacterial meningitis in children with special emphasis on late seizures. N. Engl. J. Med. *323*:1651-1657, 1990.
294. Powell, D. A., Nahata, M. C., Durrell, D. C., et al.: Interactions among chloramphenicol, phenytoin and phenobarbital in a pediatric patient. J. Pediatr. *98*:1001-1003, 1981.
295. Powell, K. R., and Mawhorter, S.: Outpatient treatment of serious infections in infants and children with ceftriaxone. J. Pediatr. *110*:889-901, 1987.
296. Powell, K. R., Sugarman, L. I., Eskenazi, A. I., et al.: Normalization of plasma arginine vasopressin concentrations when children with meningitis are given maintenance plus replacement fluid therapy. J. Pediatr. *117*:515-522, 1990.
297. Prober, C. G.: The role of steroids in the management of children with bacterial meningitis. Pediatrics *95*:29-31, 1995.

298. Quagliarello, V. J., Long, W. J., and Scheld, W. M.: Morphologic alterations of the blood brain barrier with experimental meningitis in the rat: Temporal sequence and role of encapsulation. J. Clin. Invest. 77:1084-1095, 1986.

299. Quagliarello, V. J., and Scheld, W. M.: Bacterial meningitis: Pathogenesis, pathophysiology, and progress. N. Engl. J. Med. 327:864-872, 1992.

300. Radstrom, P., Backman, A., Qian, N., et al.: Detection of bacterial DNA in cerebrospinal fluid by an assay for simultaneous detection of Neisseria meningitidis, Haemophilus influenzae, and streptococci using a seminested PCR strategy. J. Clin. Microbiol. 32:1738-1744, 1994.

301. Ramilo, O., Mustafa, M. M., Porter, J., et al.: Detection of interleukin-1β but not tumor necrosis factor-alpha in cerebrospinal fluid of children with aseptic meningitis. Am. J. Dis. Child. 144:349-352, 1990.

302. Ramsay, M. E., Andrews, N., Kaczmarski, E. B., et al.: Efficacy of meningococcal serogroup C conjugate vaccine in teenagers and toddlers in England. Lancet 357:195-196, 2001.

303. Raziuddin, S., El-Awad, M. E., and Mir, N. A.: Bacterial meningitis: T cell activation and immunoregulatory CD4+ T cell subset alteration. J. Allergy Clin. Immunol. 87:1115-1120, 1991.

304. Reelhuis, J., Honein, M., Whitney, C., et al.: Risk of bacterial meningitis in children with cochlear implants. N. Engl. J. Med. 349:435-445, 2003.

305. Ridgway, E. J., Allen, K. D., Neal, T. J., et al.: Penicillin-resistant pneumococcal meningitis. Lancet 339:931, 1992.

306. Rodriguez, W. J., Khan, W. N., Gold, B., et al.: Ceftazidime in the treatment of meningitis in infants and children over one month of age. Am. J. Med. 79(Suppl. 2A):52-55, 1985.

307. Rodriguez, W. J., Puig, J. R., Khan, W. N., et al.: Ceftazidime vs. standard therapy for pediatric meningitis: Therapeutic, pharmacologic and epidemiologic observations. Pediatr. Infect. Dis. 5:408-415, 1986.

308. Roeses, R. J., and Campbell, J. C.: Recovery of auditory function following meningitis deafness. J. Speech Hear. Dis. 40:405-411, 1975.

309. Rorke, L. B., and Pitts, F. W.: Purulent meningitis: The pathological basis of clinical manifestations. Clin. Pediatr. 2:64-71, 1963.

310. Rosenstein, N. E., Perkins, B. A., Stephens, D. S., et al.: The changing epidemiology of meningococcal disease in the United States, 1992-1996. J. Infect. Dis. 180:1894-1901, 1999.

311. Ross, S., Rodriguez, W., Controni, G., et al.: Limulus lysate test for gram-negative bacterial meningitis: Bedside application. J. A. M. A. 233:1366-1369, 1975.

312. Rotbart, H. A.: Diagnosis of enteroviral meningitis with the polymerase chain reaction. J. Pediatr. 117:85-89, 1990.

313. Rowe, P. C., McLean, R. H., Wood, R. A., et al.: Association of homozygous C4B deficiency with bacterial meningitis. J. Infect. Dis. 160:448-451, 1989.

314. Russell, F., Carapetis, J., Mansoor, O., et al.: High incidence of Haemophilus influenzae type b infection in children in Pacific Island Countries. Clin. Infect. Dis. 37:1593-1599, 2003.

315. Rutledge, J., Benjamin, D., Hood, L., et al.: Is the CSF lactate measurement useful in the management of children with suspected bacterial meningitis? J. Pediatr. 98:20-24, 1981.

316. Saez-Llorens, X., Castano, E., Garcia, R., et al.: Prospective randomized comparison of cefepime and cefotaxime for treatment of bacterial meningitis in infants and children. Antimicrob. Agents Chemother. 39:937-940, 1995.

317. Saez-Llorens, X., and O'Ryan, M.: Cefepime in the empiric treatment of meningitis in children. Infect. Dis. 20:356-361, 2001.

318. Salih, M. A., Ahmed, H. S., Karrar, Z. A., et al.: Features of a large epidemic of group A meningococcal meningitis in Khartoum, Sudan, in 1988. Scand. J. Infect. Dis. 22:161-170, 1990.

319. Sanal, O., Loos, M., Ersoy, F., et al.: Complement component deficiencies and infection: C5, C8, C3. Eur. J. Pediatr. 151:676-679, 1992.

320. Sankrithi, U. M., and Lipuma, J. J.: Clinically inapparent meningitis complicating periorbital cellulitis. Pediatr. Emerg. Care 7:28-29, 1991.

321. Santhosham, M., Reid, R., and Ambrosino, D. M.: Prevention of Haemophilus influenzae type b infections in high-risk infants treated with bacterial polysaccharide immune globulin. N. Engl. J. Med. 317:923-929, 1987.

322. Schaad, U. B., Lips, U., Gnehm, H. E., et al.: Dexamethasone therapy for bacterial meningitis in children. Lancet 342:457-461, 1993.

323. Schaad, U. B., Suter, S., Gianella-Borradori, A., et al.: A comparison of ceftriaxone and cefuroxime for the treatment of bacterial meningitis in children. N. Engl. J. Med. 322:141-147, 1990.

324. Schaad, U. B., Wedgwood-Krucko, J., and Tschaeppeler, H.: Reversible ceftriaxone-associated biliary pseudolithiasis in children. Lancet 2:1411-1413, 1988.

325. Scheifele, D., Daum, R., Syriopoulou, V., et al.: A primate model of Hemophilus influenzae type b meningitis. 16th Interscience Conference on Antimicrobial Agents and Chemotherapy, Chicago, October 27-29, 1976. Abstract 238.

326. Scheifele, D. W., Ward, J. I., and Siber, G. R.: Advantage of latex agglutination over countercurrent immunoelectrophoresis in the detection of Haemophilus influenzae type b antigen in serum. Pediatrics 68:888-891, 1981.

327. Scheld, W., Koedel, U., Nathan, B.: Pathophysiology of bacterial meningitis: Mechanism(s) of neuronal injury. J. Infect. Dis. 186(Suppl 2):S225-S233, 2002.

328. Scheld, W. M.: Pathophysiological correlates in bacterial meningitis. J. Infect. 3(Suppl. 1):5-18, 1981.

329. Scheld, W. M.: Pathogenesis and pathophysiology of pneumococcal meningitis. In Sande, M. A., Smith, A. L., and Root, R. K. (eds.): Bacterial Meningitis. New York, Churchill Livingstone, 1985, pp. 37-69.

330. Schlech, W. F., Ward, J. L., Band, J. D., et al.: Bacterial meningitis in the United States, 1978-1981: The National Bacterial Meningitis Surveillance Study. J. A. M. A. 253:1749-1954, 1985.

331. Schlesinger, Y., Sawyer, M. H., and Storch, G. A.: Enteroviral meningitis in infancy: Potential role for polymerase chain reaction in patient management. Pediatrics 94:157-162, 1994.

332. Schoendorf, K. C., Adams, W. G., Kiely, J. L., et al.: National trends in Haemophilus influenzae meningitis mortality and hospitalization among children, 1980 through 1991. Pediatrics 93:663-668, 1994.

333. Schuchat, A., Robinson, K., Wenger, J. D., et al.: Bacterial meningitis in the United States in 1995. N. Engl. J. Med. 337:970-976, 1997.

334. Schuurman, T., de Boer, R. F., Kooistra-Smid, A. M. D., and van Zwet, A. A.: Prospective study of use of PCR amplification and sequencing of 16S ribosomal DNA from cerebrospinal fluid for diagnosis of bacterial meningitis in a clinical setting. J. Clin. Microbiol. 42:734-740, 2004.

335. Schwartz, B., Al-Tobaiqi, A., Al-Ruwais, A., et al.: Comparative efficacy of ceftriaxone and rifampin in eradicating pharyngeal carriage of group A Neisseria meningitidis. Lancet 1:1239-1242, 1988.

336. Schwartz, J. F.: Ataxia in bacterial meningitis. Neurology 22:1071-1074, 1972.

337. Sell, S. H.: Long-term sequelae of bacterial meningitis in children. Pediatr. Infect. Dis. 2:90-93, 1983.

338. Shackelford, P. G., Campbell, J., and Feigin, R. D.: Countercurrent immunoelectrophoresis in the evaluation of childhood infection. J. Pediatr. 85:478-481, 1974.

339. Sharip, A., Sorvillo, F., Redelings, M., et al.: Population-based analysis of meningococcal disease mortality in the United States: 1990-2002. Pediatr. Infect. Dis. J. 25:191-194, 2006.

340. Shetty, N., de Keyser, P., and Ridgway, G. L.: Acute bacterial meningitis after dental fillings. J. Infect. 37:89-90, 1998.

341. Shurin, S. B., and Anderson, P.: Anemia associated with H. influenzae b (Hib) septicemia is due to immune hemolysis of RBC coated with soluble bacterial antigens. Pediatr. Res. 17:932, 1983.

342. Sills, R. H., Caserta, M. T., and Landaw, S. A.: Decreased erythrocyte deformability in the anemia of bacterial meningitis. J. Pediatr. 101:395-398, 1982.

343. Simberkoff, M. D., Moldovec, N. H., and Rahal, J. J., Jr.: Absence of detectable bactericidal and opsonic activities in normal and infected human cerebrospinal fluids: A regional host defense deficiency. J. Lab. Clin. Med. 95:362-372, 1980.

344. Singer, J. I., and Berger, O. G.: Simultaneous occult pneumococcal bacteremia in identical twins. J. Pediatr. 98:250-251, 1981.

345. Singhi, S. C., Singhi, P. D., Srinivas, B., et al.: Fluid restriction does not improve the outcome of acute meningitis. Pediatr. Infect. Dis. J. 14:495-503, 1995.

346. Sinner, S., and Tunkel, A.: Antimicrobial agents in the treatment of bacterial meningitis. Infect. Dis. Clin. N. Am. 18:581-602, 2004.

347. Sloas, M. M., Barrett, F. F., Chesney, P. J., et al.: Cephalosporin treatment failure in penicillin- and cephalosporin-resistant Streptococcus pneumoniae meningitis. Pediatr. Infect. Dis. 11:662-666, 1992.

348. Smith, A. L.: Neurologic sequelae of meningitis. N. Engl. J. Med. 319:1012-1014, 1988.

349. Smith, D. H., Ingram, D. L., Smith, A. L., et al.: Bacterial meningitis. Pediatrics 52:586-600, 1973.

350. Smith, J. F., and Landing, B. H.: Mechanisms of brain damage in H. influenzae meningitis. J. Neuropathol. Exp. Neurol. 19:248-265, 1960.

351. Snedeker, J. D., Kaplan, S. L., Dodge, P. R., et al.: Subdural effusion and its relationship with neurologic sequelae of bacterial meningitis in infancy: A prospective study. Pediatrics 86:163-170, 1990.

352. Snyder, R. D., Stovring, J., Cushing, A. H., et al.: Cerebral infarction in childhood bacterial meningitis. J. Neurol. Neurosurg. Psychiatry 44:581-585, 1981.

353. Soderstrom, C., Sjoholm, A. G., Svensson, R., et al.: Another Swedish family with complete properdin deficiency: Association with fulminant meningococcal disease in one male family member. Scand. J. Infect. Dis. 21:259-265, 1989.

354. Sokolova, O., Heppel, N., Jagerhuber, R., et al.: Interaction of Neisseria meningitides with human brain microvascular endothelial cells: Role of MAP- and tyrosine kinases in invasion and inflammatory cytokine release. Cell Microbiol. 6:1153-1166, 2004.

355. Sommers, L. M., and Hawkins, D. S.: Meningitis in pediatric cancer patients: A review of forty cases from a single institution. Pediatr. Infect. Dis. J. 18:902-907, 1999.

356. Sormunen, P., Kallio, M. J. T., Kilpi, T., et al.: C-reactive protein is useful in distinguishing Gram stain-negative bacterial meningitis from viral meningitis. J. Pediatr. 134:725-729, 1999.

357. Spanaus, K. S., Nadal, D., Pfister, H. W., et al.: C-X-C and C-C chemokines are expressed in the cerebrospinal fluid in bacterial meningitis and mediate chemotactic activity on peripheral blood-derived polymorphonuclear and mononuclear cells in vitro. J. Immunol. 158:1956-1964, 1997.

358. Speer, C. P., Rethwilm, M., and Gahr, M.: Elastase-alpha 1-proteinase inhibitor: An early indicator of septicemia and bacterial meningitis in children. J. Pediatr. 111:667-671, 1987.

359. Spika, J. S., Facklam, R. R., Plikaytis, B. D., et al. (The Pneumococcal Surveillance Working Group): Antimicrobial resistance of *Streptococcus pneumoniae* in the United States, 1979-1987. J. Infect. Dis. *163*:1273-1278, 1991.
360. Sproles, E. T., III, Azerrad, J., Williamson, C., et al.: Meningitis due to *Hemophilus influenzae*: Long-term sequelae. J. Pediatr. *75*:782-788, 1969.
361. Steele, R. W., and Bradsher, R. W.: Comparison of ceftriaxone with standard therapy for bacterial meningitis. J. Pediatr. *103*:138-141, 1983.
362. Steele, R. W., McConnell, J. R., Jacobs, R. F., et al.: Recurrent bacterial meningitis: Coronal thin-section cranial computed tomography to delineate anatomic defects. Pediatrics 76:950-953, 1985.
363. Stephen, D. S., and McGee, Z. A.: Attachment of *Neisseria meningitidis* to human mucosal surfaces: Influence of pili and type of receptor cell. J. Infect. Dis. *143*:525-532, 1981.
364. Taha, M., Giorgini, D., Ducos-Galand, M., and Alonso, J.: Continuing diversification of *Neisseria meningitidis* W135 as a primary cause of meningococcal disease after emergence of the serogroup in 2000. J. Clin. Microbiol. *42*:4158-4163, 2004.
365. Tan, T. Q., Mason, E. O., Jr., and Kaplan, S. L.: Systemic infections due to *Streptococcus pneumoniae* relatively resistant to penicillin in a children's hospital: Clinical management and outcome. Pediatrics 90:928-933, 1992.
366. Tan, T. Q., Mason, E. O., Jr., and Kaplan, S. L.: Penicillin-resistant systemic pneumococcal infections in children: A retrospective case-control study. Pediatrics 92:761-767, 1993.
367. Tan, T. Q., Schutze, G. E., Mason, E. O., Jr., et al.: Antibiotic therapy and acute outcome of meningitis due to *Streptococcus pneumoniae* considered intermediately susceptible to broad-spectrum cephalosporins. Antimicrob. Agents Chemother. *38*:918-923, 1994.
368. Tauber, M. G., Shibl, A. M., Hackbarth, C. J., et al.: Antibiotic therapy endotoxin concentration in cerebrospinal fluid and brain edema in experimental *Escherichia coli* meningitis in rabbits. J. Infect. Dis. *156*:456-462, 1987.
369. Tauney, A. E., Galvao, P. A., DeMorais, J. S., et al.: Disease prevention by meningococcal serogroup C polysaccharide vaccine in pre-school children—São Paulo, Brazil. Unpublished.
370. Taylor, H. G., Mills, E. L., Ciampi, A., et al.: The sequelae of *Haemophilus influenzae* meningitis in school-age children. N. Engl. J. Med. *323*:1657-1663, 1990.
371. Teele, D. W., Dashefsky, B., Rakusan, T., et al.: Meningitis after lumbar puncture in children with bacteremia. N. Engl. J. Med. *305*:1079-1081, 1981.
372. Tejani, A., Dobias, B., and Sambursky, J.: Long-term prognosis after *H. influenzae* meningitis: Prospective evaluation. Dev. Med. Child. Neurol. *24*:338-343, 1982.
373. Tejani, A., Mahadevan, R., and Dobias, B.: Occurrence of HLA types in *H. influenzae* type b disease. Tissue Antigens *17*:205-211, 1981.
374. Tracey, K. J., Vlassara, J., and Cerami, A.: Cachectin/tumor necrosis factor. Lancet *1*:1122-1125, 1989.
375. Trujillo, H., Harry, N., Arango, A., et al.: Aztreonam in the treatment of aerobic, gram-negative bacillary infections in pediatric patients. Chemotherapy *35*(Suppl.):25-30, 1989.
376. Tuomanen, E., Liu, H., Hengstler, B., et al.: The induction of meningeal inflammation by components of the pneumococcal cell wall. J. Infect. Dis. *151*:859-868, 1985.
377. Tyson, J. E., Gilmartin, R. C., Jr., Friedman, B. I., et al.: 131I-HSA cisternography in children with meningitis. *In* Harbert, J. C. (ed.): Cisternography and Hydrocephalus. Springfield, IL, Charles C Thomas, 1972, pp. 413-432.
378. Unkmeir, A., Latsch, K., Dietrich, G., et al.: Fibronectin mediates Opc dependent internalization of *Neisseria meningitidis* by human brain microvascular endothelial cells. Mol. Microbiol. *46*:933-946, 2002.
379. U.S. Department of Commerce, Bureau of the Census: Mortality Statistics, 1935. Washington, D.C., Government Printing Office, 1937.
380. U.S. Department of Health, Education and Welfare, Public Health Service: Vital Statistics of the United States, 1968. Vol. II. Mortality. Washington, D.C., Government Printing Office, 1970.
381. van Alphen, L., Spanjaard, L., van der Ende, A., et al.: Predicted disappearance of *Haemophilus influenzae* type b meningitis in Netherlands. Lancet *344*:195, 1994.
382. van Furth, A. M., Roord, J. J., and van Furth, R.: Roles of proinflammatory and anti-inflammatory cytokines in pathophysiology of bacterial meningitis and effect of adjunctive therapy. Infect. Immun. *64*:4883-4890, 1996.
383. van Vliet, K. E., Glimaker, M., Lebon, P., et al.: Multicenter evaluation of the Amplicor Enterovirus PCR test with cerebrospinal fluid from patients with aseptic meningitis. J. Clin. Microbiol. *36*:2652-2657, 1998.
384. Veeder, M. H., Folds, J. D., Yount, W. J., et al.: Recurrent bacterial meningitis associated with C8 and IgA deficiency. J. Infect. Dis. *144*:399-402, 1981.
385. Vienny, H., Despland, P. A., Lutschg, J., et al.: Early diagnosis and evolution of deafness in childhood bacterial meningitis: A study using brainstem auditory evoked potentials. Pediatrics 73:579-586, 1984.
386. Waage, A., Halstensen, A., and Espevik, T.: Association between tumour necrosis factor in serum and fatal outcome in patients with meningococcal disease. Lancet *1*:355-357, 1987.
387. Wahden, M. H., Rizk, F., and El-Akkad, A. M.: A controlled field trial of a serogroup A meningococcal polysaccharide vaccine. Bull. World Health Organ. *48*:667-673, 1973.
388. Wald, E. R., Kaplan, S. L., Mason, E. O., Jr., et al.: Dexamethasone therapy for children with bacterial meningitis. Pediatrics 95:21-28, 1995.
389. Waldvogel, F. A.: Pathophysiological mechanisms in pneumococcal infection: Two examples—pleural empyema and acute bacterial meningitis. *In* Majno, G., Cotran, R. S., and Kaufman, N. (eds.): Current Topics in Inflammation and Infection. Baltimore, Williams & Wilkins, 1982, pp. 115-122.
390. Waler, J. A., and Rathore, M. H.: Outpatient management of pediatric bacterial meningitis. Pediatr. Infect. Dis. J. *14*:89-92, 1995.
391. Ward, J. I., Fraser, D. W., Baraff, L. J., et al.: *Hemophilus influenzae* meningitis: A national study of secondary spread in household contacts. N. Engl. J. Med. *19*:122-126, 1979.
392. Ward, J. I., Gorman, C., Philips, C., et al.: *Haemophilus influenzae* type b disease in a day care center. J. Pediatr. *92*:713-717, 1978.
393. Ward, J. I., Lum, M. K. W., Hall, D. B., et al.: Invasive *Haemophilus influenzae* type b disease in Alaska: Background epidemiology for a vaccine efficacy trial. J. Infect. Dis. *153*:17-26, 1986.
394. Ward, J. I., Siber, G. I., Scheifele, D. W., et al.: Rapid diagnosis of *Hemophilus influenzae* type b infections by latex particle agglutination and counterimmunoelectrophoresis. J. Pediatr. *93*:37-42, 1978.
395. Watt, J., Levine, O., Santosham, M.: Global reduction of Hib disease: What are the next steps? Proceedings of the meeting in Scottsdale, Arizona, September 22-25, 2002. J. Pediatr. *143*(6 Suppl):S163-S187, 2003.
396. Weidmer, C. E., Dunkel, T. B., Pettyjohn, F. S., et al.: Effectiveness of rifampin in eradicating the meningococcal carrier state in a relatively closed population: Emergence of resistant strains. J. Infect. Dis. *24*:172-178, 1971.
397. Weil, M. L.: Infections of the nervous system. *In* Menkes, J. H. (ed.): Textbook of Child Neurology. Philadelphia, Lea & Febiger, 1980, pp. 276-304.
398. Whitney, C. G., Farley, M. M., Hadler, J., et al.: Increasing prevalence of multi-drug resistant *Streptococcus pneumoniae* in the United States. N. Engl. J. Med. *343*:1917-1924, 2000.
399. Whittle, H. C., and Greenwood, B. M.: Meningococcal meningitis in the northern savanna of Africa. Trop. Doct. 6:99-104, 1976.
400. Williams, D. N., Laughlin, L. W., and Lee, Y. H.: Minocycline: Possible vestibular side-effects. Lancet *2*:744-746, 1974.
401. Wispelwey, B., Lesse, A. J., Hansen, E. J., et al.: *Haemophilus* lipopolysaccharide-induced blood brain barrier permeability during experimental meningitis in the rat. J. Clin. Invest. *82*:1339-1346, 1988.
402. Wolff, M., Chavanet, P., Kazmierczak, A., et al.: Diffusion of cefpirome into the cerebrospinal fluid of patients with purulent meningitis. J. Antimicrob. Chemother. *29A*:59-62, 1992.
403. Wong, M., Schlaggar, B. L., and Landt, M.: Postictal cerebrospinal fluid abnormalities in children. J. Pediatr. *138*:373-377, 2001.
404. Wong, V. K., Wright, H. T., Jr., Ross, L. A., et al.: Imipenem/cilastatin treatment of bacterial meningitis in children. Pediatr. Infect. Dis. J. *10*:122-125, 1991.
405. Woody, R. C., and Yamauchi, T.: Cerebrospinal fluid cell counts in childhood idiopathic status epilepticus. Pediatr. Infect. Dis. J. 7:298-299, 1988.
406. Zangwell, K. M., Vadheim, C. M., Vannier, A. M., et al.: Epidemiology of invasive pneumococcal disease in Southern California: Implications for the design and conduct of a pneumococcal conjugate vaccine efficacy trial. J. Infect. Dis. *174*:752-759, 1996.
407. Zollinger, W. D., Mandrell, R. E., Guffiss, J. M., et al.: Complex of meningococcal group B polysaccharide and type 2 outer membrane protein immunogenic in man. J. Clin. Invest. *63*:836-848, 1979.
408. Zwahlen, A., Nydegger, U. E., Vaudaux, P., et al.: Complement-mediated opsonic activity in normal and infected human cerebrospinal fluid: Early response during bacterial meningitis. J. Infect. Dis. *145*:635-646, 1982.
409. Zwijenburg, P., van der Poll, T., Florquin, S., et al.: Interleukin-18 gene-deficient mice show enhanced defense and reduced inflammation during pneumococcal meningitis. J. Neuroimmun. *138*:31-37, 2003.
410. Zysk, G., Bruck, W., Gerber, J., et al.: Anti-inflammatory treatment influences neuronal apoptotic cell death in the dentate gyrus in experimental pneumococcal meningitis. J. Neuropathol. Exp. Neurol. *55*:722-728, 1996.

PARAMENINGEAL INFECTIONS

Xavier Sáez-Llorens ☉ Javier Nieto Guevara

BRAIN ABSCESS

Brain abscess is an uncommon infection, but it remains a serious and life-threatening disease in children despite advances that have been made in diagnosis and management. Abscess formation may occur in the parenchyma of the central nervous system, in the subdural space, or in the epidural space. It can originate from contiguous site infections (e.g., skull osteomyelitis, chronic otitis), from underlying vascular anomalies (e.g., congenital cyanotic heart disease), after head trauma or neurosurgical procedures, or from cryptogenic sources. These conditions can alter neurologic function by direct destruction of nervous tissue, by infarction after inflammatory occlusion of veins and arteries, or by compression caused by mass effect.

Advances in diagnostic and therapeutic modalities since the 1990s have improved the prognosis of this serious disease. The mortality rate associated with brain abscesses seems to be decreasing. This reduction probably is the result of the advent of head imaging and its use to guide precise location and management, improvement in surgical techniques, and advances in antibiotic development. Goodkin and coworkers[43] identified 54 patients aged 5 days to 34 years of age who were diagnosed with a brain abscess at the Boston Hospital from 1945 to 1980 and 1981 to 2000. They found a reduction in the number of abscesses that occurred in the setting of sinus or middle ear infection (26% versus 11%, respectively) and an increase in the number of children who were treated with antibiotics alone (1% versus 22%). These investigators did not observe, however, any additional decline in the mortality rates in their institution between 1981 and 2000. Fischer and associates[17] found a reduction in mortality rate from 36 percent before 1970 to 14 percent after 1970. Tekkok and Erbengi[45] described a similar decline, from 30 percent in the era before the use of computed tomography (CT) to 6 percent in the last 5 years of their study and zero in the last 3 years of their study. Other case series also have reported a mortality rate of zero.[29]

Although the mortality rate seems to be decreasing, a significant percentage of children continue to have residual neurologic deficits, including epilepsy, permanent motor or sensory dysfunc-

tion, visual field defects, and personality changes.[17,20,25] Some children also require placement of a ventriculoperitoneal shunt.[10]

PATHOGENESIS AND PATHOLOGY

Brain abscess is a focal, intracerebral infection that begins as a localized area of cerebritis and eventually ends in a collection of pus surrounded by a well-vascularized capsule. For practical purposes, brain abscesses usually are classified according to the likely entry point of the infection (Table 38–1). Ear and mastoid infections are associated with formation of an abscess at the temporal or cerebellar locations; sinus and dental infections give rise to purulent collections in the frontal lobe; and metastatic spread from distant foci in children with congenital cardiac or pulmonary right-to-left shunts commonly results in involvement of any parenchymal area, including parietal or occipital regions.[17,28,41]

The most common origin of microbial infection in children remains direct or indirect cranial infection arising from the middle ear, paranasal sinuses, or teeth. Seeding of the brain presumably occurs via transit of infecting microbes through the valves and emissary veins that serve these regions. A direct erosion of skull and dura by osteomyelitis-induced sinus or middle ear infection can be another mechanism of bacterial spread.[7] Resulting abscesses tend to be solitary and superficial. Metastatic inoculation of the brain from distant extracranial sources (pulmonary infection, endocarditis) tends to provoke multiple cerebral abscesses, with a distribution that reflects the regional cerebral blood flow of the area affected, usually the middle cerebral artery network.[7]

In children with cyanotic congenital heart disease, bacteria are not filtered out by the pulmonary vascular bed, which allows for systemic spread.[10] This situation rarely occurs in patients younger than age 2 years, and the abscess or abscesses usually are in areas of brain perfused by the middle cerebral arteries. Evidence of associated endocarditis is rare in these cases, although acute bacterial endocarditis may be complicated by septic infarction of the brain and abscess formation.[36]

TABLE 38–1 Primary Source, Usual Location of Lesion, and Associated Neurologic Findings in Children with Brain Abscess

Primary Source	Location of Abscess	Associated Neurologic Findings
Upper respiratory site		
Sinusitis	Frontal lobe	Headache, behavioral changes, motor speech disorders, depressed consciousness, forced grasping and sucking, hemiparesis
Chronic otitis/mastoiditis	Temporal lobe	Dyspraxia and aphasia (dominant hemisphere), ipsilateral third cranial nerve palsy, ipsilateral headache, upper homonymous hemianopsia, motor dysfunction of face and arm
	Cerebellum	Dizziness, vomiting, ipsilateral ataxia and tremor, sixth cranial nerve palsy, nystagmus (toward lesion)
Dental infection	Frontal lobe	
Head trauma	Related to injured site	Variable by region involved
Postoperative	At operative site	Variable by region involved
Metastatic spread	Multiple lesions	Variable by region involved
	If parietal lobe involved	Visual field defects in inferior quadrant, homonymous hemianopsia, dysphasia (dominant hemisphere), dyspraxia and contralateral spatial neglect (no dominant hemisphere)

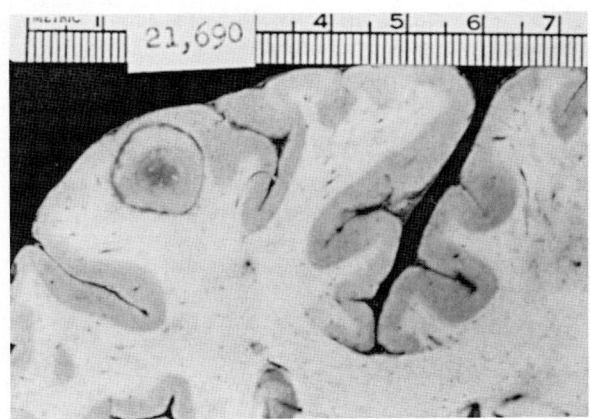

Figure 38–1 Circumscribed cerebral abscess of hematogenous origin.

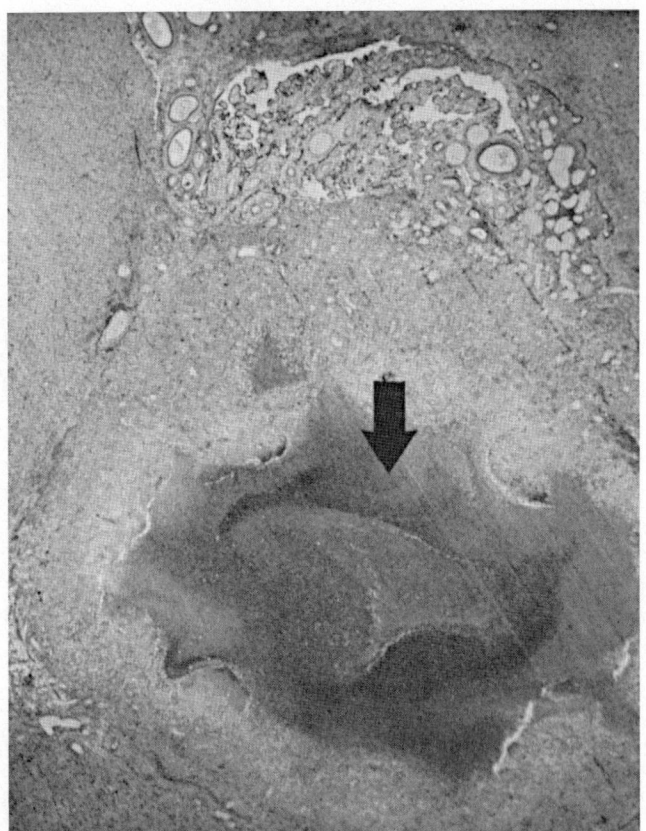

Figure 38–2 Area of necrosis and liquefaction in a cerebral abscess (*arrow*).

Formation of an abscess by direct bacterial implantation may complicate compound skull fractures, scalp wounds, anterior cranial fossa or temporal bone fractures, and chronic cerebrospinal fluid (CSF) fistula. Abscesses also rarely may develop during the course of bacterial meningitis.[40] Despite identification of all these potential routes, 20 to 30 percent of cases are classified as cryptic brain abscess for which no obvious predisposing factor can be identified.

The brain is remarkably resistant to microbial infection. Despite the common occurrence of occult bacteremia in infants and children, cerebral abscess is a quite rare disease. This resistance is attributable in part to the abundant blood supply of the brain and the relative impermeable blood-brain barrier.[1] Although certain underlying brain morbidities, such as previous stroke, intracerebral hematoma, or underlying neoplasm, may serve as a nidus of abscess formation in adults, affected children have no apparent predisposing brain lesion. In animal models of infection, induction of abscess usually requires direct inoculation of numerous organisms into the animal's cerebrum.[34]

Experimental animal studies and use of CT scanning techniques have provided evidence of the clinical evolution of a brain abscess.[2] In the early stage of cerebritis (days 1 to 3), a focal area of acute inflammation, vascular dilation, microthrombosis, rupture of small vessels, and edema are present. The center of the lesion then undergoes liquefaction. Expansion of the cerebritis and formation of a necrotic central focus are seen in the late cerebritis stage (days 4 to 9). Establishment of a ring-enhancing dense collagenous capsule of well-vascularized tissue with peripheral gliosis or fibrosis or both occurs at the early capsule stage (days 10 to 14). Finally, during the late capsule stage (>14 days), host defenses act to wall off the abscess, and a well-developed capsule results.

Death can occur if the volume of pus and surrounding edema induce a significant increase of intracranial pressure (ICP) leading to brain herniation. In addition, cerebral abscesses can rupture into the ventricular system or through the cortex into the subarachnoid space, resulting in acute deterioration and a life-threatening event.[10] Figure 38–1 shows the gross appearance of a well-defined abscess of hematogenous origin. Various microscopic features are illustrated in Figures 38–2, 38–3, and 38–4.

The spectrum of microorganisms cultured from brain abscesses has changed with time. This change reflects improved microbiologic isolation techniques, early and aggressive treatment of primary infections, and better neurosurgical procedures. In most more recent series, the predominance of *Staphylococcus aureus* has decreased, and identification of anaerobes has increased.[6,13,47]

Anaerobic bacteria isolated from brain abscesses include species of *Bacteroides*, *Peptostreptococcus*, *Fusobacterium*, *Veillonella*, *Propionibacterium*, *Prevotella*, and *Actinomyces*. Aerobic and microaerophilic streptococci, staphylococci, *Haemophilus* spp., gram-negative enteric bacilli, and *Pseudomonas aeruginosa* also are implicated frequently. In children with impaired host defenses, fungal etiology (*Candida*, *Aspergillus*, *Cryptococcus*, *Histoplasma*, *Coccidioides*, and *Mucor* spp.) or uncommon pathogens, such as *Toxoplasma*, *Nocardia*, *Mycobacterium*, and *Listeria* spp., can be identified.[17] Parasites such as amebae, *Cysticercus*, *Schistosoma*, or *Paragonimus* are very rare causative pathogens.[18] *Citrobacter koseri* (*diversus*) and *Enterobacter sakazakii* are particularly able to cause brain abscesses in neonates.

In order of etiologic importance, the predominant organisms causing brain abscess in children are aerobic and anaerobic streptococci (60-70% of cases), gram-negative anaerobic bacilli (20-40%), Enterobacteriaceae (20-30%), *S. aureus* (10-15%), and fungi (1-5%).[3-6,13,17,28,34,35,41,47] Multiple aerobic and anaerobic organisms are isolated in approximately one third of patients, especially in patients with chronic otitis. No growth is reported from 30 percent of properly handled purulent specimens. A reasonable speculation of the likely causative microbes can be made according to the predisposing source of infection (Table 38–2).

CLINICAL MANIFESTATIONS

The clinical presentation of a brain abscess depends on the size of the collection, its location, the multiplicity of lesions, the host's immune status, and the age of the patient. Generally, symptoms and signs can be related to the effect of a space-occupying mass, to the focal neuronal dysfunction of the parenchymal region

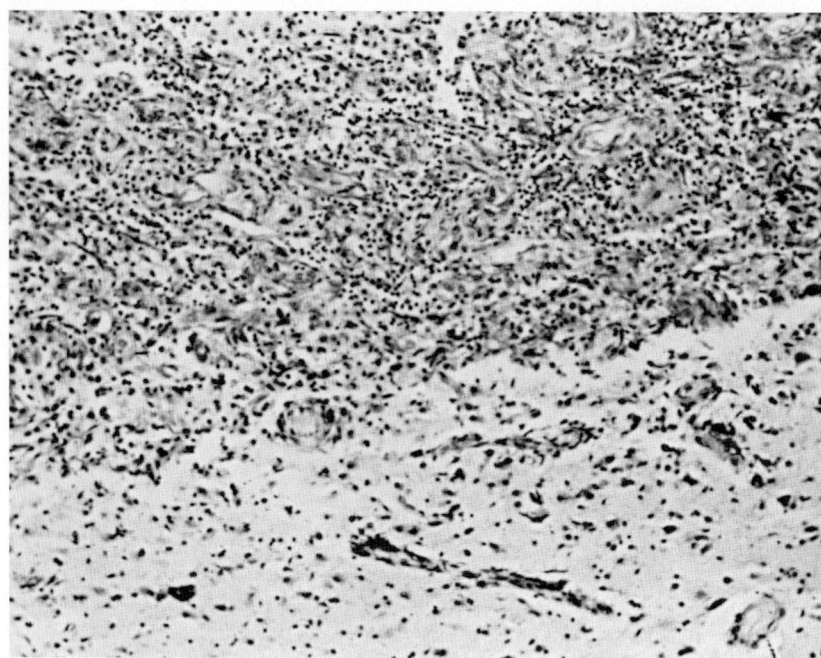

Figure 38–3 Astroglia and fibroblasts forming the capsule of a cerebral abscess.

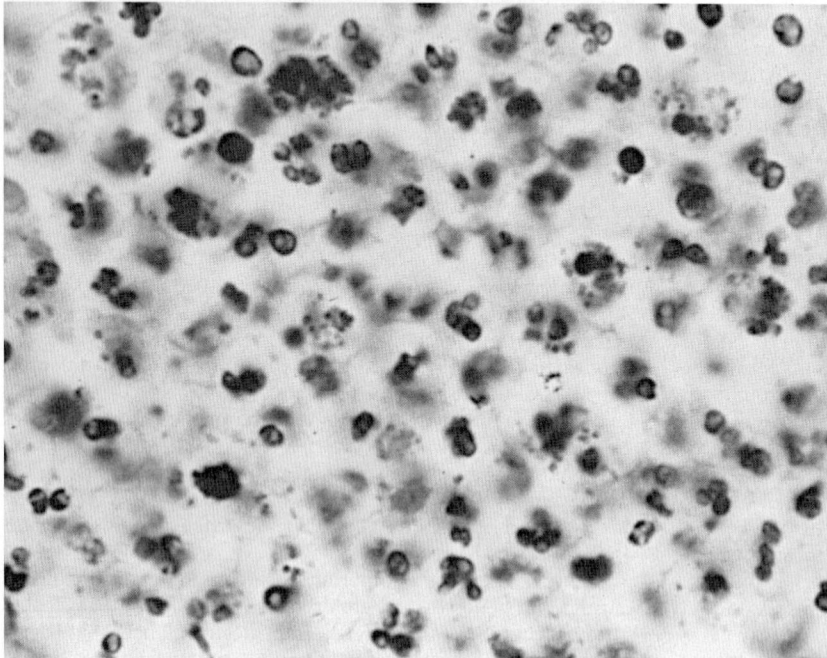

Figure 38–4 Mononuclear and polymorphonuclear leukocytes are in the center of a cerebral abscess.

involved (see Table 38–1), or to accompanying clinical findings of the underlying predisposing infection. Because on early evaluation most children with cerebral abscess present with vague or nonspecific signs and symptoms, the physician must have a high index of suspicion to recognize the condition as early as possible (Table 38–3). When a patient develops significant alterations in mental status, the prognosis is most ominous.[10,41]

In older children and adolescents, headache is the most common initial symptom. Irritability occurs more commonly in infants and small children. The nature of the headache has no particular distinguishing features and usually is poorly localized. A sudden worsening of a preexisting headache can indicate rupture of the brain abscess into the ventricular space, which has a poor prognosis.[8,16]

Absence of fever should not be used to exclude the diagnosis of brain abscess because this sign is detected in only approximately one half of affected children. Drowsiness, confusion, and vomiting occur frequently during the acute phase of disease. Lethargy, stupor, and coma usually are later events and potentially associated with adverse outcome. Papilledema is present in less than one fourth of the cases, but its presence requires immediate neurosurgical assessment and CT scanning.

Focal neurologic disturbances reflect the location of the abscess and can be detected in 30 to 50 percent of cases on presentation (see Tables 38–1 and 38–3).[48] Frontal location is characterized by development of motor speech disorders, memory deficits, personality changes, and depressed consciousness. Hemiparesis occurs with lesions in the postfrontal region or as a con-

TABLE 38–2 Primary Source, Usual Etiologic Pathogens, and Recommended Empiric Antibiotic Therapy in Children with Brain Abscess

Primary Source	Usual Etiologic Microorganisms	Recommended Empiric Antibiotic Combination
Upper respiratory infection		
Sinusitis/dental infection	Viridans and anaerobic streptococci, *Haemophilus* spp., *Fusobacterium* spp., *Bacteroides* spp. (non-*fragilis*)	Penicillin or cefotaxime/ceftriaxone + metronidazole or ampicillin + chloramphenicol or sulbactam
Chronic otitis/mastoiditis	Aerobic and anaerobic streptococci, gram-negative enteric bacilli, *Bacteroides* spp. (including *B. fragilis*), *Pseudomonas aeruginosa*	Penicillin + metronidazole + ceftazidime
Head trauma	*Staphylococcus aureus*, aerobic streptococci, gram-negative enteric bacilli	Oxacillin/nafcillin (vancomycin) + cefotaxime/ceftriaxone
Postoperative	*Staphylococcus epidermidis*, *S. aureus*, gram-negative rods, *P. aeruginosa*	Vancomycin + ceftazidime
Metastatic spread		
Endocarditis	*S. aureus*, viridans streptococci	Oxacillin/nafcillin (vancomycin) + cefotaxime/ceftriaxone + metronidazole
Pulmonary infection	Aerobic streptococci, *Actinomyces*, *Fusobacterium*	Oxacillin/nafcillin (vancomycin) + cefotaxime/ceftriaxone + metronidazole
Congenital heart disease	Viridans streptococci, *Haemophilus* spp., *Haemophilus aphrophilus*	Cefotaxime/ceftriaxone + metronidazole or ampicillin + chloramphenicol or sulbactam
Bacterial meningitis	*S. pneumoniae*, *Haemophilus influenzae* type b, *Salmonella* spp., *Citrobacter* (neonates)	Cefotaxime/ceftriaxone ± vancomycin (resistant pneumococcal strains)
Cryptogenic source and immunosuppression*	Any type of microorganisms	Oxacillin/nafcillin (vancomycin) + ceftazidime + metronidazole
	Nocardia, fungi, *Mycobacterium tuberculosis*	Oxacillin/nafcillin (vancomycin) + ceftazidime + metronidazole

*In areas with significant prevalence of methicillin-resistant staphylococcal strains or penicillin allergy, immunosuppressed children should be treated with broad coverage and with consideration of amphotericin B therapy. Antituberculous therapy should be considered for children with exposure to tuberculosis. Antibiotic regimens are likely to vary by geographic location based on resistant organisms.

TABLE 38–3 Frequency of Presenting Signs and Symptoms in Children with Brain Abscess

Symptoms	%	Signs	%
Headache	60–70	Focal neurologic deficits	35–50
Fever	50–80	Papilledema	30–40
Vomiting	35–55	Meningeal signs	25–35
Seizures	30–45	Hemiparesis	20–30
Mental changes	30–40	Nerve palsy	10–20
Coma	15–20	Ataxia	5–15

sequence of uncal herniation. Abscess in the temporal lobe is characterized by a contralateral homonymous upper quadrantopia. If the dominant hemisphere is affected, nominal dysphasia and aphasia are characteristic symptoms. Patients with cerebellar abscesses classically exhibit dizziness, nystagmus, defective conjugate eye movements, ataxia, tremor, and hypotonia. Seizures occur in at least 30 to 45 percent of patients, may be focal or generalized, and may occur at any time during the course of the disease. If the parietal region is involved, visual field defects, homonymous hemianopsia, dysphasia, and dyspraxia can be present.

The rapidity with which symptoms develop can vary substantially. Most patients are symptomatic within 1 week of the onset of formation of an abscess. Immunocompromised children can have a more insidious progression of clinical findings. The presentation of brain abscess in infancy can be suspected by bulging fontanelle, vomiting, irritability, and an enlarging head circumference. Seizures occur commonly, particularly in small infants, and at any time during the course of the disease.[14] School-aged children with cyanotic congenital heart disease, notably tetralogy of Fallot or transposition of the great vessels, also can exhibit symptoms and signs related to their chronic cardiac disease.

RUPTURE OF BRAIN ABSCESS INTO THE VENTRICULAR SYSTEM

Rupture of an abscess into the ventricle with consequent ventricular empyema is a dreaded complication because the mortality rate is greater than 50 percent, and residual neurologic deficits, including hydrocephalus, are the rule in patients who survive. Frequently, rupture occurs before the diagnosis of abscess has been established and surgical removal can occur. A sudden worsening in the patient's clinical state heralds this event. High fever, shock, meningismus, and altered consciousness are prominent clinical signs.

Rupture of the abscess into the ventricle is seen more frequently in patients with deep-seated abscesses or in immunocompromised patients.[44] Although a modest pleocytosis and elevated protein concentration in CSF may have been identified earlier, the findings of 50,000 to 100,000 polymorphonuclear leukocytes and markedly reduced glucose concentration in the CSF are usual findings. Organisms may be seen on smear of the CSF and cultured from the fluid. In other words, the patient has developed purulent meningitis, and treatment must include high doses of antibiotics and surgery (see the treatment section).

The concurrence of abscess and meningitis in the past has led to the assumption that brain abscess can be a complication of meningitis; this rarely, if ever, is the case, although meningitis may develop during the incipient stages of abscess formation after intracranial invasion of organisms from a contiguous extracranial source. In such circumstances, the abscess may seem to be a consequence of the leptomeningitis. Given a potential source of infection in the ear or paranasal sinuses, the clinician must be wary and appreciate the possibility of this sequence of events. Abscess has been reported to complicate *Citrobacter* meningitis in infants, but careful pathologic study has shown vasculitis and liquefaction necrosis of the white matter without capsule formation.[47]

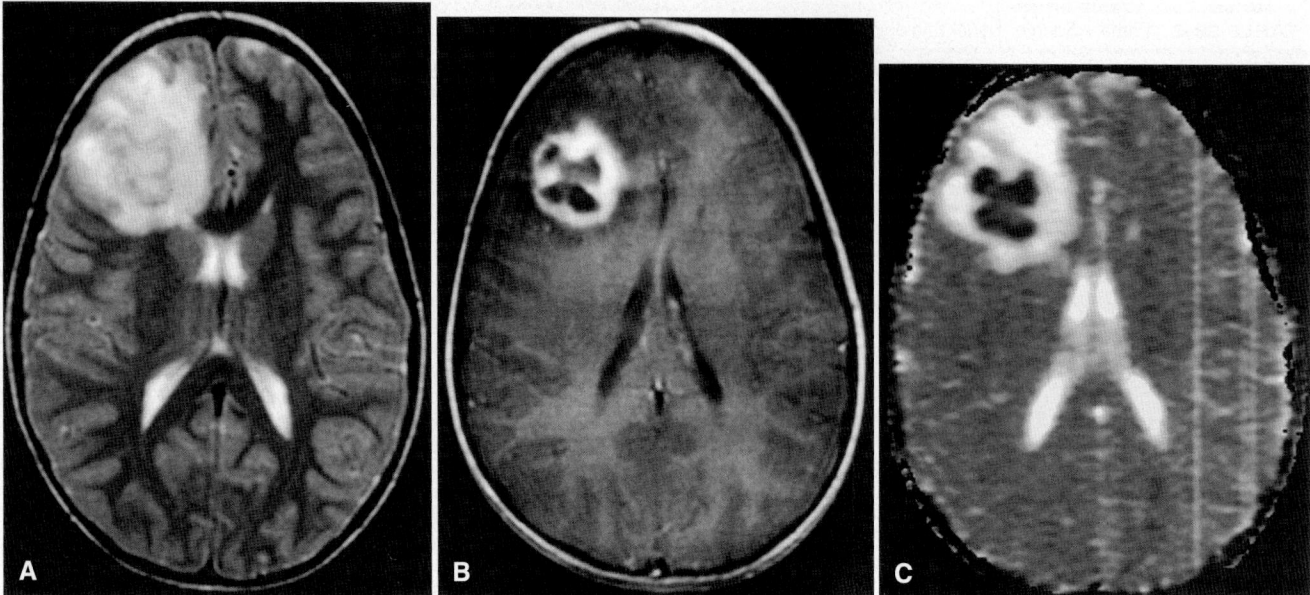

Figure 38–5 Bacterial abscess in a 10-year-old girl. **A,** Axial T2-weighted magnetic resonance (MR) image shows an irregular mass in the right frontal lobe with a hypointense wall *(arrows)* and surrounding vasogenic edema. **B,** Gadolinium-enhanced T1-weighted MR image shows intense, smooth enhancement of the capsule. **C,** Apparent diffusion coefficient map from a line-scan, diffusion-weighted study shows decreased signal within the cavity, compatible with restricted diffusion and suggesting an abscess cavity rather than tumor necrosis. *(Courtesy of F. Kim, M.D., Northwestern University School of Medicine, Chicago.)*

LABORATORY DIAGNOSIS

Laboratory tests frequently are not helpful in supporting the clinical diagnosis of brain abscess.[10,33,41] Children usually have unremarkable leukocyte counts, and the erythrocyte sedimentation rate can be normal. Blood cultures rarely are positive. Performance of a lumbar puncture is potentially dangerous because it can be associated with brain stem herniation.[9] In addition, CSF analysis uncommonly provides useful clinical information. Usual CSF findings include an elevated protein, mild mononuclear pleocytosis, and hypoglycorrhachia. CSF cultures usually are negative, unless the abscess has drained into the ventricular system or has been a complication of meningitis.

Culturing abscess material obtained at the time of surgical drainage provides the best opportunity to make a microbiologic diagnosis. Proper handling and processing, with attention given to optimal anaerobic and aerobic isolation techniques, can identify the causative organism in most cases, especially when antimicrobial therapy has not been instituted previously.[33] When the clinical condition warrants immediate use of empiric antibiotics, Gram stain of the purulent material frequently can help direct selection of the appropriate antibiotic.

DIAGNOSIS

Magnetic resonance imaging (MRI) is the modality of choice for the diagnosis and localization of cerebral abscesses. Similar MRI findings can be observed in infarction, demyelinating disorders, and neoplastic processes. Diffusion-weighted MRI and magnetic resonance spectroscopy have been shown to be effective methods in differentiating cerebral abscesses from tumors.[5,34] Figure 38–5 illustrates the appearance on MRI of a right frontal cerebral abscess in a 10-year-old girl. CT scanning remains an excellent alternative, however, if MRI is unavailable (Fig. 38–6). Intrave-

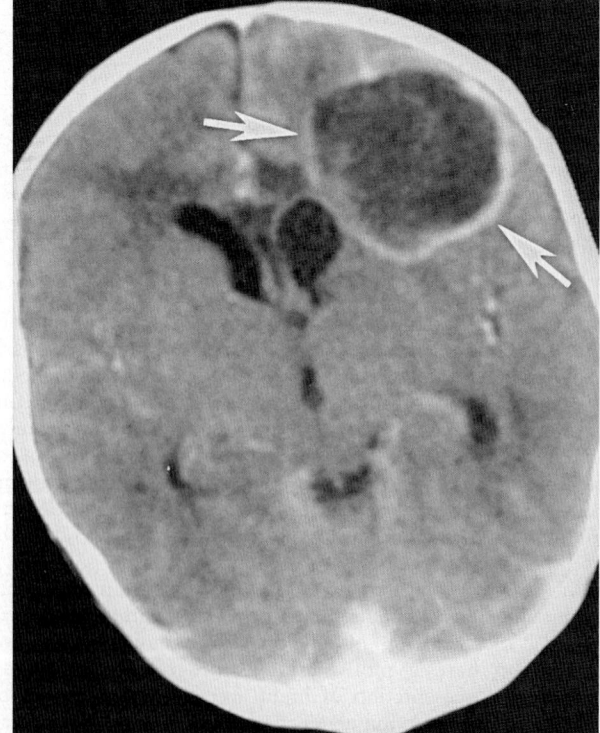

Figure 38–6 Contrast-enhanced computed tomography (CT) scan shows a ring-enhancing left frontal cerebral abscess *(arrows)* in a 3-week-old boy with concurrent *Enterobacter* meningitis. *(Courtesy of C. D. Robson, M.D., Harvard Medical School, Boston, MA, and P. D. Barnes, M.D., Stanford University School of Medicine, Stanford, CA.)*

nous administration of contrast material is advised because the abscess may be missed otherwise.[12,26] Serial CT or MRI scanning, performed weekly or biweekly, provides evaluation of the response to therapy and of the need for repeating the surgical procedure. MRI is more accurate than is CT for establishing the diagnosis of cerebritis, cerebellar, edema formation, and brain stem purulent collections.[19,24] On T1-weighted sequences, brain abscesses appear hypointense and show ring enhancement after administration of intravenous gadolinium. In contrast, on T2-weighted images, the typical mature abscess has a hyperintense central area of pus surrounded by a well-defined hypointense capsule and surrounding edema.

Because specific images allow precise lesion staging, this information provides important clues for the surgeon to suspect the likelihood of encountering purulent material of a well-developed abscess at the moment of drainage. The presence of gas within the abscess cavity on head imaging suggests communication of the abscess with air outside the skull, although gas-forming bacteria in the abscess cavity rarely may be responsible.[49]

Plain skull films generally are normal in children with brain abscess. In small infants, separation of cranial sutures indicates intracranial hypertension. Radionuclide brain scan, arteriography, and ventriculography have been replaced largely by CT and MRI for the diagnosis of brain abscess. Indium-labeled leukocyte scans and thallium-brain single photon emission computed tomography (SPECT) to differentiate brain abscess from tumor in questionable cases have not been studied adequately in the pediatric population, but these methods seem promising in affected adults.[39]

Abnormalities on electroencephalography may be localized and can help in excluding a more generalized, bilateral intracranial disease, such as encephalitis. Unilateral slow waves (delta, 1 to 3/sec) characterize the usual electroencephalographic findings in cases of cerebral abscess.

After the diagnosis of brain abscess has been established, a careful search should be made for a source of infection serving as a site of origin for hematogenous spread or direct inoculation of organisms into the central nervous system. In addition to obtaining data from the history and physical examination, the physician should extend the MRI or CT evaluation to include the mastoids and paranasal sinuses. An echocardiogram should be obtained to assess for concurrent endocarditis. Other testing should be guided by the history and physical examination findings.

TREATMENT

No prospective clinical trials have compared various surgical and medical treatment strategies available to guide the management of cerebral abscesses in children. Most surgical and medical treatment guidelines are based on populations consisting primarily of adult patients. Appropriate management of brain abscesses apparently requires a combined surgical and medical approach,[31] with isolated medical management limited to patients who are neurologically intact and in whom the abscess is in the cerebritis stage[21] or the abscess or abscesses are small,[38] or to patients who are too unstable to undergo a surgical procedure.

The initial treatment of solitary and multiple brain abscesses relies on the aspiration of the cavity contents followed by the initiation of empiric antibiotic coverage while the cultures are processing. CT-guided or MRI-guided stereotactic aspiration is accurate, minimally invasive, and associated with few complications. Mamelak and colleagues[32] suggested performing head imaging biweekly or on any sign of clinical deterioration, with further aspiration if the cavity enlarges or fails to diminish in size after 3 to 4 weeks. Because excisions may be associated with

increased risk of developing neurologic sequelae, surgery should be reserved for patients who do not respond to the strategy of repeated aspiration and medical management, and when an abscess results in a significant mass effect.

While results of cultures are pending, the selection of antibiotics should be guided by the primary source of infection, pertinent patient history, and results of microscopic examination of the pus (see Table 38–3). The appropriate duration of antimicrobial therapy for brain abscess is unclear. A 6- to 8-week course of parenteral antibiotics has been recommended traditionally, provided that the etiologic organisms are susceptible and adequate surgical drainage is achieved.[33] In selected cases with uncomplicated infection and complete surgical removal of a well-delineated abscess, shorter courses of treatment (3 to 4 weeks) are likely to be sufficient.[42] Nonetheless, many authorities recommend 2 to 3 months of additional oral antimicrobial therapy to prevent relapses.[10] In fungal, nocardial, and helminthic infection, surgical intervention frequently is required because of failure of medical treatment. Surgical procedures can be used to reduce increased ICP, obtain pus for microbiologic diagnosis, and enhance the antibiotic efficacy. In carefully selected patients (illness duration ≤2 weeks, neurologically intact, no signs of increased ICP, and abscess ≤3 cm in diameter), medical therapy alone can be successful.

With the advent of head imaging and the current methods of treatment employing head imaging, an overall reduction in the mortality rate has occurred; however, a high proportion of children with cerebral abscesses develop neurologic deficits. Eradication of potential sources of infection before the abscess has developed is logical preventive medicine. Early diagnosis and treatment are imperative and can be facilitated by the liberal use of MRI or CT scanning when this diagnosis is even a remote consideration.

ADJUNCTIVE AGENTS

The use of corticosteroids for treatment of brain abscess is controversial. These agents usually are indicated to control life-threatening intracranial hypertension that is associated with risk of herniation or when significant symptoms and signs are presumed to be the result of cerebral edema. Severe brain edema may necessitate the additional administration of intravenous mannitol. Steroids interfere with the inflammatory response, retard the encapsulation process, increase development of necrosis, potentially reduce antibiotic concentrations inside the purulent collection, and alter CT images.[37]

Anticonvulsants are recommended in children who have developed seizures potentially to prevent further episodes. Duration of anticonvulsant therapy should be individualized and guided by an electroencephalographic study in the follow-up phase of disease. Most authors recommend providing at least 3 months of prophylaxis if no more seizures have occurred.[10]

SUBDURAL EMPYEMA

Pyogenic infection in the subdural space is designated as subdural empyema or sometimes, but less correctly, as subdural abscess. The sources of infection and microorganisms responsible are the same as those encountered in brain abscess. It is a rare disease; only 1 case was seen at St. Louis Children's Hospital during a period when 122 patients with bacterial meningitis and 3 patients with cerebral abscess were treated. The primary source of subdural empyema in this single case was not found, which increasingly is true for the pediatric experience. Farmer and Wise[15] and Jacobson and Farmer[27] found associated meningitis in six of eight infants with subdural empyema (seen over a 16-year period), suggesting that the latter was a complication of the former. We also have encountered this situation, albeit rarely, and the subdural fluid usually is turbid, rather than frankly purulent.

In older children, the infection apparently does not follow leptomeningitis. Although leptomeningitis may complicate subdural empyema, infections of the paranasal sinuses and mastoid region, usually chronic, spread to the subdural space directly because of osteomyelitis or by way of infected veins that penetrate the skull. Extension to cortical veins and to major venous sinuses frequently is associated with subdural empyema, as discussed elsewhere in this section. Why in some cases the infection is restricted to one or another anatomic site or sites (e.g., epidural space, subdural space, parenchyma of the brain or blood vessels) is unknown. Subdural empyema may be hematogenous in origin. It is an infrequent but recognized complication of intracranial surgery. The anatomy of the subdural space is such that the infection often extends widely over one or both cerebral hemispheres, and accumulation of pus in the parafalcine region occurs commonly.

CLINICAL MANIFESTATIONS

The symptoms and signs of the primary source of infection may be prominent, subtle, or absent. Increasingly severe headache, high fever, signs of meningeal irritation, and progressive neurologic deficits referable to the site of the lesion are reported in the typical untreated case. Focal or generalized seizures are prominent, especially in cases of cortical injury from associated vasculitis. Signs of increased ICP become prominent as the mass of pus enlarges. In infants, a fullness of fontanelle, vomiting, and depressed responsiveness are seen. Transillumination of the skull can be positive. Older children also may develop papilledema. As the ICP increases, symptoms and signs progress, ultimately leading to temporal lobe or cerebellar herniation and the characteristic syndromes of these complications.

DIAGNOSIS

The laboratory findings reflect the active infectious process. Peripheral leukocytosis and a predominance of polymorphonuclear leukocytes with immature cells frequently are seen. The CSF in infants reflects the common association with leptomeningitis, and the findings depend on when the fluid is examined. Before the meningitis has been treated adequately, organisms may be cultured; the glucose concentration may be low and the protein concentration high in the CSF. Later, the CSF findings are the same as those for treated meningitis, but viable organisms can be recovered from the subdural collections when the CSF is sterile. Specific antigens may be shown in subdural collections by tests such as countercurrent immunoelectrophoresis in the absence of viable organisms. In older children, the characteristic CSF findings include elevated pressure with a few to a few hundred or more leukocytes, with polymorphonuclear leukocytes predominating. The protein concentration frequently is elevated, the glucose concentration is normal, and the fluid is sterile.

In the past 2 or more decades, subdural empyema in children has become more difficult to diagnose clinically because of antimicrobial therapy. When initiated early, antimicrobial therapy may attenuate the dramatic nature of the disease, especially the symptoms and signs of acute infection. Because the diagnosis of subdural empyema often is confused with that of brain abscess, radiographic studies are necessary to establish the correct diagnosis. CT scanning (Fig. 38–7) and MRI are effective noninvasive techniques, as previously discussed in relation to brain abscess.

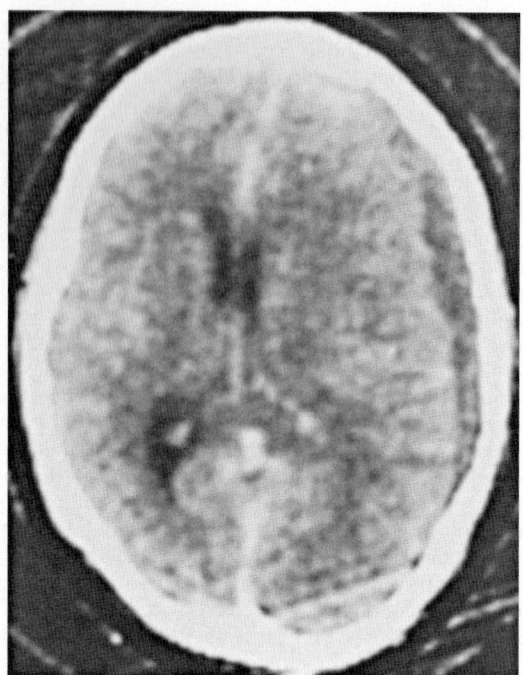

Figure 38–7 CT scan shows a subdural empyema with marked displacement of the ventricular system.

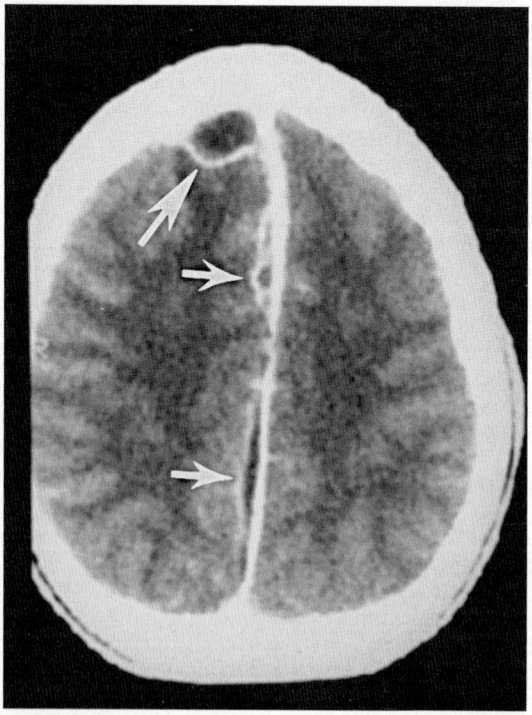

Figure 38–8 Contrast-enhanced CT scan shows a right frontal epidural abscess *(large arrow)* concurrent with an interhemispheric subdural abscess *(small arrows)* in a 13-year-old boy who developed headache, fever, and vomiting after fracture of the right frontal sinus. *(Courtesy of C. D. Robson, M.D., Harvard Medical School, Boston, MA, and P. D. Barnes, M.D., Stanford University School of Medicine, Stanford, CA.)*

Cerebral CT can show a failure of the cerebral vessels to approximate the inner surface of the skull. These studies reveal the extent of subdural disease and may define an epidural abscess or other infectious exudate collection concurrent with subdural empyema (Fig. 38–8).

TREATMENT

Until a causative organism is identified, the patient should receive broad-spectrum antibiotics intravenously in dosages appropriate for bacterial meningitis. After the offending organism is identified, the sensitivities of that organism to specific medications dictate selection of more precise antibiotic therapy. In infants, antibiotic therapy may be sufficient when the fluid is cloudy only, but if thick, purulent material is obtained by subdural paracentesis or, in older children, if the clinical and radiographic evidence indicates a subdural empyema, surgery is requisite. Depending on individual circumstances, craniotomy or multiple burr holes with irrigation of the subdural space should be accomplished.

Mortality and morbidity rates are high (20-40%) in most series but lower in some.[43,50] Early diagnosis and treatment are imperative. The early use of CT scanning seems to be responsible for improved therapeutic results.[50]

EPIDURAL ABSCESS

Because the dura mater is adherent to the inner aspect of the cranium, epidural abscesses rarely attain a large size, and they consequently do not exert significant pressure on the brain. They are important because they can serve as a focus for spread of infection into the subdural space, leptomeninges, or brain. The infection may involve local penetrating vessels and lead to their occlusion, with extension to venous sinuses and other vessels. Infection of the middle ear, mastoid bone, or ancillary air sinuses may lead to epidural abscess, as in the case of subdural empyema and brain abscess. Often, epidural abscess coexists with the other lesions and presumably develops first. Osteomyelitis may be evident, which usually is the case with mastoiditis and often is evident after head injury with comminuted fracture of the skull or after intracranial surgery. A case of an adolescent boy with osteomyelitis and epidural abscess complicating a wrestling injury was reported.[46]

Local pain, tenderness, and fever may be the only signs. Treatment usually includes antibiotic drugs and surgery in the presence of osteomyelitis. Exclusion of associated intracranial infections is mandatory; the epidural infection serves to raise these diagnostic possibilities.

SPINAL EPIDURAL INFECTIONS

Spinal epidural infections may be acute or chronic, and they may be restricted in their extent or extend longitudinally over many segments of the spinal cord because the epidural space offers no resisting structures. Most often, the process affects the posterior region of the spine, with maximal pus or granulomatous tissue found over the dorsal aspect of the cord or spinal roots. In Danner and Hartman's[11] series from the New York Hospital, however, in approximately half of the patients, the pus primarily was anterior to the cord. In the case of spinal osteomyelitis, the pus may be more viscous ventrally. Occasionally, the purulent material may encircle the neural elements. In infants and children, this condition is rare; no case was encountered at the St. Louis Children's Hospital during the 39 months in which 122 cases of bacterial meningitis were seen. In an extensive report by Baker and colleagues[4] covering a 27-year period at the Massachusetts General Hospital, only 6 of 39 patients were younger than 20 years of age, and the youngest was 11 years old. The incidence ranged from 0.2 to 1.2 hospital admissions each year. In approximately half of the patients in this series, acute purulent material was discovered at operation or autopsy, with *S. aureus* incriminated in more than half of the cases. In the remainder, a granulomatous process was found, associated with a wide variety

of bacteria. No instance of tuberculous infection occurred, although in many regions of the world, this organism remains an important consideration. Nonbacterial infective agents may include fungi or parasites.

The neural dysfunction probably results from direct compression of the spinal cord, roots, and nerves, but impaired circulation from associated inflammation and occlusion of vessels is at least a contributory factor in some cases. Determining with certainty the extent to which each of the previous mechanisms contributes to neural dysfunction often is difficult. Extensive necrosis of the cord may result in advanced cases in which a prompt diagnosis has not been made.

SOURCES OF INFECTION

In tuberculous and other chronic infections, osteomyelitis and intervertebral disk infection are common occurrences, but adults primarily are affected. Acute spinal epidural infections usually occur after hematogenous spread from furuncles, pharyngitis, dental abscesses, decubitus ulcers, and urinary tract and wound infections.[30] They may complicate spinal surgery, and lumbar puncture rarely has been implicated as a source.[6] Osteomyelitis seldom occurs. The patient may have a history of minor trauma to the back. Presumably, trauma results in local tissue injury or hemorrhage, forming a nidus for the developing infection.

CLINICAL MANIFESTATIONS

Fever is the rule, and the temperature is higher in patients with acute infections. Patients appear septic, and toxic delirium occurs frequently. Heusner,[22] in his classic article dealing primarily with acute epidural abscesses, divided the clinical phases as follows: (1) spinal ache, (2) root pain, (3) weakness, and (4) paralysis. Although certain therapeutic implications render this separation a useful way to consider the disorder, phases 3 and 4 are combined in the following discussion. That the various stages often overlap is axiomatic.

Phase 1: Spinal Ache

Spinal ache was a universal finding in Heusner's experience.[22] In a report from Baker and associates,[4] all 39 patients had backache of various degrees of severity. Local tenderness was absent in only two of their patients and should be searched for by carefully tapping over the spine.

Phase 2: Root Pain

Root pain is characteristic and is an early symptom that may assist in localization of the pathologic process. Root pain especially is prominent with lumbosacral disease in which roots are implicated without involvement of the spinal cord. The diagnosis is suspected infrequently until functional motor and sensory losses occur, which is unfortunate because therapy is most effective during the early stages. Progression to symptoms and signs of spinal cord involvement usually occurs within a few days except when the process is granulomatous, in which case the course tends to be prolonged, extending over several or more weeks.

Phases 3 and 4: Weakness and Paralysis

After weakness and impaired sensation referable to disease of the spinal cord appear, the progression to paralysis can be rapid, and immediate surgical treatment is imperative to maximize the likelihood of reasonable functional recovery. Even appropriate therapy at this stage often is ineffective, however, in restoring normal neurologic functions. Death occurs in at least 20 percent of cases; this rate has not changed significantly since 1948, despite the availability of a wide range of antibiotic agents.

DIAGNOSIS

The diagnosis of spinal epidural infection is established by MRI of the spine (Fig. 38–9). Imaging also may reveal evidence of concurrent osteomyelitis of the spine, which is found in approximately 20 percent of chronic lesions. After epidural abscess is discovered, immediate neurosurgical intervention is necessary to prevent long-term neurologic sequelae. At the time of surgery, stains and cultures for aerobic and anaerobic bacteria, mycobacteria, and fungi should be obtained. If lumbar puncture is attempted when epidural abscess is suspected, the spinal needle (with stylet) is advanced slowly into the lumbar region, with periodic removal of the stylet and with suction applied gently *before* the thecal sac is entered.

If purulent material is obtained, the diagnosis is established, and the pus must be examined by a Gram-stained smear and cultured on various media under aerobic and anaerobic conditions. The leptomeninges should not be penetrated if purulent material is encountered; otherwise, CSF should be obtained. Characteristically, the CSF is clear or slightly opalescent and yellow if there is a block. Pleocytosis with a few too many hundred cells (with lymphocytes predominating) reflects a contiguous infectious process, but in the absence of meningitis, no organisms can be identified and the CSF glucose concentration should be

normal. The protein concentration always is elevated, and the level may be very high (several hundred to 2000 mg/dL) in the case of a partial or total manometric block.

The differential diagnosis includes myelitis caused by bacterial meningitis, syphilis, viruses, and a parainfectious process and by the syndrome of acute transverse myelopathy of unknown cause. Spinal ache is most prominent in acute transverse myelopathy, but as a general rule, the entire illness is compressed in time, with paresis or paralysis evolving over the course of hours or a few days from the onset of disease. Impaired circulation of CSF does not occur in this or the aforementioned disorders. Rarely, a lymphoma may mimic a spinal epidural abscess. Spinal cord tumors, vascular malformations, and arachnoiditis are considerations when the course of disease is prolonged and evidence of sepsis is minimal or absent, as occurs with chronic epidural infections.

TREATMENT

Prompt surgical removal of purulent or granulomatous material is essential. Surgery should be combined with intravenous administration of an appropriate antibiotic. Initial empiric antibiotic coverage is similar to that for brain abscess, although antifungal therapy need not be included, unless cultures or stains are positive for fungi. Treatment typically should be continued for 3 to 4 weeks, but it should be prolonged for twice this period if the patient has osteomyelitis. Despite advances, the morbidity and mortality rates for spinal epidural abscess remain high. One third of children with the disease die, and another third are left with permanent neurologic sequelae, including weakness, incontinence, and sensory abnormalities. Rapid diagnosis and treatment are essential to ensure a successful outcome.

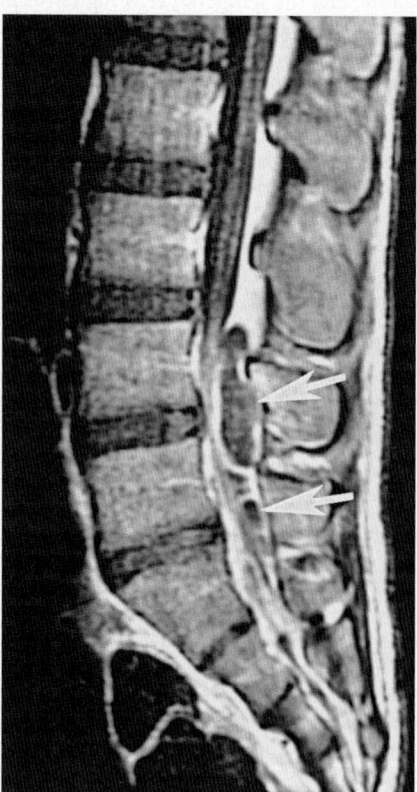

Figure 38–9 Gadolinium-enhanced, sagittal, T1-weighted MR image shows a rim-enhancing lumbar spinal epidural abscess *(arrows)* in a 15-year-old boy with a 3-week history of lower back pain, followed by rapidly progressing left leg numbness and decreased bowel and bladder function. *Staphylococcus aureus* was cultured from purulent fluid removed after L4-L5 laminectomy was performed. *(Courtesy of C. D. Robson, M.D., Harvard Medical School, Boston, MA, and P. D. Barnes, M.D., Stanford University School of Medicine, Stanford, CA.)*

REFERENCES

1. Amano, K., and Kamano, S.: Cerebellar abscess due to penetrating orbital wound. J. Comput. Assist. Tomogr. 6:1163-1166, 1982.
2. Armstrong, D.: Central nervous system infections in the immunocompromised host. Infection 12:58-63, 1984.
3. Arseni, C., Horvath, L., and Dumitrescu, L.: Cerebral abscess in children. Acta Neurochirurg. 14:197-224, 1966.
4. Baker, A. S., Ojemann, R. G., Swartz, M. N., and Richardson, E. P., Jr.: Spinal epidural abscess. N. Engl. J. Med. 293:463-468, 1975.
5. Barlas, O., Sencer, A., Erkan, K., et al.: Stereotactic surgery in the management of brain abscess. Surg. Neurol. 52:404-410, 1999.
6. Bergman, I., Wald, E. R., Meyer, J. D., and Painter, M. J.: et al.: Epidural abscess and vertebral osteomyelitis following serial lumbar punctures. Pediatrics 72:476-480, 1983.
7. Brook, I.: Brain abscess in children: Microbiology and management. J. Child Neurol. 10:283-288, 1995.
8. Choudhari, K. A.: Prodromal signs and clinical factors influencing outcome in patients with intraventricular rupture of purulent brain abscess. Neurosurgery 49:481-483, 2001.
9. Chun, C. H., Johnson, J. D., Hofstetter, M., et al.: Brain abscess. Medicine 65:415-431, 1986.
10. Cochrane, D. D.: Brain abscess. Pediatr. Rev. 20:209-214, 1999.
11. Danner, R. L., and Hartman, B. J.: Update on spinal epidural abscess: 35 cases and review of the literature. Rev. Infect. Dis. 9:265-274, 1987.
12. De Louvois, J., Gortvai, P., and Hurley, R.: Antibiotic treatment of abscess of the central nervous system. B. M. J. 2:985-987, 1977.
13. Domingo, Z., and Peter, J. C.: Brain abscess in childhood. S. Afr. Med. J. 84:13-15, 1994.
14. Ersahin, Y., Mutluer, S., and Guzelbag, E.: Brain abscess in infant and children. Childs Nerv. Syst. 10:185-189, 1994.
15. Farmer, T. W., and Wise, G. R.: Subdural empyema in infants, children and adults. Neurology 23:254-261, 1973.
16. Ferre, C., Ariza, J., Viladrich, P. F., et al.: Brain abscess rupturing into the ventricles or subarachnoid space. Am. J. Med. 106:254-257, 1999.
17. Fischer, E. G., McLennan, J. E., Suzuki, Y., et al.: Cerebral abscess in children. Am. J. Dis. Child. 135:746-749, 1981.
18. Molinari, G. F., Smith, L., Goldstein, M. N., and Satran, R.: Brain abscess from septic cerebral embolism: An experimental model. Neurology 23:1205-1210, 1973.

19. Haimes, A. B., Zimmerman, R. D., Morgello, S., et al.: MR imaging of brain abscesses. A. J. R. Am. J. Roentgenol. *152*:1073-1085, 1989.
20. Hegde, A. S., et al.: Brain abscess in children. Childs Nerv. Syst. *2*:90-92, 1986.
21. Heineman, H. S., et al.: Intracranial suppurative disease: Early presumptive diagnosis and successful treatment without surgery. J. A. M. A. *218*:1542-1547, 1971.
22. Heusner, A. P.: Nontuberculous spinal epidural infections. N. Engl. J. Med. *239*:845-854, 1948.
23. Goodkin, H. P., Harper, M. B., and Pomeroy, S. L.: Intracranial abscess in children: Historical trends at Children's Hospital Boston. Pediatrics *113*:1765-1770, 2004.
24. Hunter, J. V.: Neuroimaging of central nervous system infections. Semin. Pediatr. Infect. Dis. *14*:140-164, 2003.
25. Idriss, Z. H., Gutman, L. T., and Kronfol, N. M.: Brain abscesses in infants and children: Current status of clinical findings, management and prognosis. Clin. Pediatr. (Phila.) *17*:738-740, 745-746, 1978.
26. Itakura, T., Yokote, H., Osaki, F., et al.: Stereotactic operation of brain abscess. Surg. Neurol. *28*:196-200, 1987.
27. Jacobson, P. L., and Farmer, T. W.: Subdural empyema complicating meningitis in infants: Improved prognosis. Neurology *31*:190-193, 1981.
28. Jadavji, T., Humphreys, R. P., and Prober, C. G.: Brain abscesses in infant and children. Pediatr. Infect. Dis. J. *4*:394-398, 1985.
29. Jamjoom, A.: Childhood brain abscess in Saudi Arabia. Ann. Trop. Paediatr. *17*:95-99, 1997.
30. Kaufman, D. M., Kaplan, J. G., and Litman, N.: Infectious agents in spinal epidural abscesses. Neurology *30*:844-850, 1980.
31. Leys, D., Christiaens, J. L., Derambure, P., et al.: Management of focal intracranial infections: Is medical treatment better than surgery? J. Neurol. Neurosurg. Psychiatry *53*:472-475, 1990.
32. Mamelak, A. N., Mampalam, T. J., Obana, W. G., and Rosenblum, M. L.: Improved management of multiple brain abscesses: A combined surgical and medical approach. Neurosurgery *36*:76-85, 1995.
33. Mathisen, G. E., and Johnson, J. P.: Brain abscess. Clin. Infect. Dis. *25*:763-781, 1997.
34. Molinari, G. F., Smith, L., Golstein, M. N., et al.: Brain abscess from septic cerebral embolism: An experimental model. Neurology *23*:1205-1210, 1973.
35. Nielsen, H.: Cerebral abscess in children. Neuropediatrics *14*:76-80, 1983.
36. Pruitt, A. A., Rubin, R. H., Karchmer, A. W., and Duncan, G. W.: Neurologic complications of bacterial endocarditis. Medicine (Baltimore) *57*:329-343, 1978.
37. Quartey, G. R. C., Johnston, J. A., and Rozdilsky, B.: Decadron in the treatment of cerebral abscess. J. Neurosurg. *45*:301-310, 1976.
38. Rosenblum, M. L., Hoff, J. T., Norman, D., et al.: Nonoperative treatment of brain abscesses in selected high-risk patients. J. Neurosurg. *52*:217-225, 1980.
39. Ruiz, A., Ganz, W. I., Post, J. D., et al.: Use of thallium-201 brain SPECT to differentiate cerebral lymphoma from toxoplasma encephalitis in AIDS patients. A. J. N. R. Am. J. Neuroradiol. *15*:1885-1894, 1994.
40. Sáez-Llorens, X., and McCracken, G. H.: Bacterial meningitis in neonates and children. Infect. Dis. Clin. N. Am. *4*:623-644, 1990.
41. Sáez-Llorens, X., Umaña, M. A., Odio, C. M., et al.: Brain abscess in infants and children. Pediatr. Infect. Dis. J. *8*:449-458, 1989.
42. Skoutelis, A. T., Gogos, C. A., Maraziotis, T. E., et al.: Management of brain abscess with sequential intravenous/oral antibiotic therapy. Eur. J. Clin. Microbiol. Infect. Dis. *19*:332-335, 2000.
43. Smith, H. P., and Hendrick, E. B.: Subdural empyema and epidural abscess in children. J. Neurosurg. *58*:392-397, 1983.
44. Takeshita, M., Kagawa, M., Izawa, M., and Takakura, K.: Current treatment strategies and factors influencing outcome in patients with bacterial brain abscess. Acta Neurochir. *140*:1263-1270, 1998.
45. Tekkok, I. H., and Erbengi, A.: Management of brain abscess in children: Review of 130 cases over a period of 21 years. Childs Nerv. Syst. *8*:411-416, 1992.
46. Tudor, R. B., Carson, J. P., Pulliam, M. W., and Hill, A.: Pott's puffy tumor, frontal sinusitis, frontal bone osteomyelitis, and epidural abscess secondary to a wrestling injury. Am. J. Sports. Med. *9*:390-391, 1981.
47. Woods, C. R.: Brain abscess and other intracranial suppurative complications. Adv. Pediatr. Infect. Dis. *10*:41-79, 1995.
48. Yogev, R.: Focal suppurative infections of the central nervous system. *In* Long, S. S., Pickering, L. K., and Prober, C. G. (eds.): Principles and Practice of Pediatric Infectious Diseases. 2nd ed., Vol. 1. New York, Churchill Livingstone, 2003, pp. 302-212.
49. Young, R. F., and Frazee, J.: Gas within intracranial abscess cavities: An indication for surgical excision. Ann. Neurol. *16*:35-39, 1984.
50. Zimmerman, R. D., Leeds, N. E., and Danziger, A.: Subdural empyema: CT findings. Radiology *150*:417-422, 1984.

FUNGAL MENINGITIS

CHAPTER 39

J. Thomas Cross, Jr. ⊛ Richard F. Jacobs

Fungi are rare causes of meningitis in children. *Candida albicans*, *Cryptococcus neoformans*, and *Coccidioides immitis* are the isolates found most commonly in pediatric patients. Making a diagnosis can be difficult. Fungal meningitis frequently is chronic, and patients may have few symptoms. The lack of obvious meningeal signs and symptoms and the uncommon incidence of a fungal cause often delay establishing the diagnosis. Inherent problems with the diagnosis of fungal infections of the central nervous system (CNS) begin with the basic microbiology of the organisms. Their fastidious growth, the prolonged time needed for culture, and the requirement of special media can render making a diagnosis of meningitis difficult.

Because cultivating many fungi from the cerebrospinal fluid (CSF) frequently is difficult, the use of serologic tests for antibodies and antigens helps define the infection more quickly and with more sensitivity. These tests can be done on CSF, serum, and, in some instances, urine.[177] For most infections, amphotericin B is the drug of choice, although its supremacy is being tested by some of the newer azoles and the introduction of lipid formulations of amphotericin B. Namdar and colleagues[113] compared Abelcet, Amphotec, and AmBisome in neonatal and pediatric patients. CNS disease caused by fungi generally has high morbidity and mortality rates.

EPIDEMIOLOGY

The epidemiology of fungal meningitis depends on many factors. The geographic location of the patient or travel to an endemic area can be an important clue to defining the cause of the infection. The geographic distribution of fungal meningitis varies in the United States and worldwide. Histoplasmosis generally occurs in endemic areas of the Mississippi River valley.[176] Coccidioidomycosis occurs in the San Joaquin Valley and the desert Southwest of the United States and in Mexico.[3,118] Cryptococcosis distribution is worldwide, rather than in discrete endemic areas, but it seems to be associated with pigeon droppings and nesting areas of other birds.[98] Blastomycosis has a sporadic pattern of infectivity but generally occurs in states bordering the Mississippi and Ohio River basins, with occasional outbreaks occurring in the Great Lakes region and Canada.[50,83,143] *Candida* spp., *Aspergillus* spp., *Sporothrix schenckii*, and other fungal pathogens generally are not defined by geographic boundaries but depend more on environmental exposures and the immunocompetence of the individual. Uncommon species of yeasts and fungi, including *Rhodotorula rubra*, *Aureobasidium mansoni*, *Clavispora lusitaniae*, and *Bipolaris spicifera*, have been reported in nosocomial cases of meningitis.[68,89]

Many fungal infections (particularly infections caused by *Candida* spp. and *Histoplasma*) do not usually cause meningitis, unless the host is immunocompromised. The number of cases of cryptococcal meningitis has increased dramatically in association with the acquired immunodeficiency syndrome (AIDS) epidemic. A review from the mid-1980s by the Centers for Disease Control and Prevention showed an incidence rate of 6.8 percent for cryptococcal meningitis in patients with AIDS; however, the rate in pediatric patients with AIDS was 10 times lower (0.6%).[140] In the pre-AIDS era, patients known to be at risk for acquiring disseminated cryptococcosis included patients with lymphoma, patients on high-dose corticosteroid therapy, and patients with underlying cellular immune dysfunction.[23] Risk factors for developing *Candida* meningitis are similar to those for candidemia and include prolonged antimicrobial therapy, indwelling venous catheters, hyperalimentation, corticosteroid use, recent intra-abdominal surgery, and intravenous drug abuse.[137,157] Pediatric cases occur most commonly in neonates, particularly in very-low-birth-weight newborns.[9,58,70,73,149] In the early 1980s, 3.8 percent of infants weighing less than 1500 g in a large pediatric teaching hospital developed systemic fungal infections, most of which were caused by *Candida* spp. The mean birth weight was 809 g, with 86 percent of the infants weighing less than 1000 g.

Inhalation is the most common means by which many fungi infect the host. Other fungi can be inoculated directly into the skin; this inoculation can occur in the outdoor environment or in the hospital setting (e.g., intravenous catheters), especially in very-low-birth-weight infants.[9]

CLINICAL MANIFESTATIONS

Infections caused by *Candida* spp. in very-low-birth-weight newborns can be particularly difficult to diagnose because of the broad range of symptoms. Most infants with disseminated candidiasis with meningitis present with respiratory distress and a supplemental oxygen requirement, and most progress to require mechanical ventilation.[9] *Candida* usually is identified in endotracheal washings, urine, and blood in patients with *Candida* meningitis, but infants have symptoms on average 11 days before the diagnosis is made. Ophthalmologic examinations may be very important in identifying disseminated *Candida* infections.[28] A careful funduscopic examination also can help determine if increased intracranial pressure is present with papilledema. Marked abdominal distention also occurs commonly in disseminated *Candida* infections in low-birth-weight infants and frequently is associated with guaiac-positive stools. Most patients also have temperature instability, elevated white blood cell counts, and feeding intolerance. Hepatomegaly may indicate the presence of systemic infection.

Physical manifestations that are diagnostic for other causes of fungal meningitis (e.g., *Cryptococcus, Blastomyces, Histoplasma*) rarely are found because the infections usually are chronic. Looking carefully for other manifestations of fungal infections, especially the presence of skin lesions, is very important, however. All superficial lesions, nodules, and draining abscesses should be investigated because they may give a clue to the cause of subacute and chronic infections (e.g., *Coccidioides, Blastomyces, Cryptococcus*).[62] Fungal stains, including India ink, should be performed on all biopsy specimens and drainage material, and all specimens should be processed for culture. Bone involvement is a common occurrence with certain fungal infections (e.g., *Cryptococcus, Blastomyces*).

The significance of isolating a fungus from CSF cannot be overemphasized. The finding of fungal organisms should be considered a true infection, and appropriate antifungal therapy should be initiated. A single CSF culture for *Candida* or an unlikely meningeal pathogen (*Paecilomyces*) with an otherwise normal CSF should lead the physician to consider the possibility of contamination.[5] Repeat CSF cultures should be sought in such patients.

INFECTION WITH SPECIFIC ORGANISMS

Candidal Meningitis

Candidal meningitis is rare in children. Arisoy and associates[5] reported that 2 percent of all positive CSF cultures were fungal

organisms. *Candida* spp. accounted for 94.5 percent of the fungal isolates. Nine of 23 patients were newborns, 8 of whom were very-low-birth-weight infants. Risk factors for positive CSF fungal cultures from neonates included antimicrobial therapy, umbilical catheterization, total parenteral nutrition, intubation, and prematurity.[43,44] Risk factors in children beyond the neonatal period included concurrent bacterial infection, chronic systemic or CNS disease, and the presence of central venous catheters. Histopathology models in animals have revealed hyphal invasion, vasculitis, abscesses, and acute and chronic inflammatory infiltration of meninges and brain parenchyma.[72]

Children with human immunodeficiency virus (HIV) infection are at risk for acquiring disseminated *Candida* infections, including meningitis. In one study, 27 percent of HIV-infected patients with disseminated *Candida* infections had CNS involvement.[95] Nearly all HIV-infected patients who develop *Candida* infection do so as a result of nosocomial infection. Predisposing factors include oral candidiasis, central venous catheters, prolonged antibiotic therapy, and total parenteral nutrition. In HIV-infected patients, neutropenia is not a major risk factor. Simultaneous pulmonary disease, particularly viral, bacterial, or *Pneumocystis carinii* pneumonias, exists in most HIV-infected patients with disseminated *Candida* infection. Most patients are febrile for more than 14 days, with peak temperatures greater than 39° C before the diagnosis is established.

The incidence of infection with *Candida* spp. other than *C. albicans* has increased dramatically in immunocompromised children, particularly children with malignancies. In a case series of children with leukemia, *Candida tropicalis* meningitis was uniformly fatal.[47] In addition to patients with malignancies and HIV infections, other children at risk for developing infection have been reported, including a child with myeloperoxidase deficiency.[97]

Candida spp. have become another concern because of the development of resistance. Intensive efforts to develop standardized, reproducible, and clinically relevant susceptibility testing methods for the fungi have resulted in the development of the NCCLS M27-A methodology for susceptibility testing of yeasts for the azole agents.[131] Reliable breakpoints are unavailable for amphotericin B. Isolates of *Candida glabrata* and *Candida krusei* with increasing resistance to amphotericin B have been described.[175] *Candida lusitaniae* has shown resistance to amphotericin B, and meningitis in an adult patient with a resistant strain has been reported.[138] *C. krusei* has been noted to have azole resistance, particularly in immunocompromised patients receiving suppressive azole therapy. These fungal infections already are difficult to treat, without the added burden of drug resistance. If patients with *Candida* spp. (including *C. albicans*) meningitis are slow to clear infection, or unexpected relapse occurs, susceptibility testing is recommended.

Candida meningitis usually responds to therapy with intravenous amphotericin B alone or in combination with oral flucytosine. The use of flucytosine is controversial; however, most reports support its use in meningitis. Flucytosine has been difficult to use in low-birth-weight infants because of the immaturity of their gastrointestinal tracts and the risks of their developing necrotizing enterocolitis. Amphotericin alone for systemic candidiasis, including meningitis, in neonates has been used successfully in patients who could not tolerate oral medication.[22] The *most* important factor in successful treatment was the initiation of therapy quickly, as soon as systemic *Candida* infection was suspected and frequently before the organism was isolated. Prolonged delays in initiating therapy result in high mortality rates.

Amphotericin B initiated at a dose of 0.25 mg/kg body weight diluted in 5 percent or 10 percent dextrose-water can be infused over 2 to 4 hours. In most neonates, the dose can be increased in 0.25-mg/kg increments at 6- to 12-hour intervals until the desired 1-mg/kg daily dose is attained. In older children and adolescents, a test dose may be given, with an initial dose of 0.1 mg/kg (1 mg maximum). If this dose is tolerated, the initial dose of therapy (0.25 mg/kg) is given. Many authorities now believe that a test dose is unnecessary and that cautious infusion of the first dose is adequate.[39] In severely ill patients, the dose can be increased rapidly in 6- to 12-hour intervals to 1 mg/kg/dose. Flucytosine generally is recommended in a dose of 150 mg/kg/day, divided every 6 hours. The use of flucytosine often requires monitoring and adjustment of the dosage based on serum determinations.

Large, controlled trials using the azoles and newer agents for *Candida* meningitis are lacking. Huttova and coworkers[67] reported eight neonates with candidal meningitis treated with intravenous fluconazole with and without amphotericin B. Numbers from the study were too small to make conclusive recommendations. Lipid formulations of amphotericin B increasingly are preferred in adults, and liposomal amphotericin B was used successfully in five of six cases of *Candida* meningitis in newborns.[139] Optimal dosing is unknown, but many physicians prescribe liposomal amphotericin B or amphotericin B lipid complex at a dose of 5 mg/kg daily. Marr and associates[104] reported on the use of fluconazole plus flucytosine for the treatment of *Candida* meningitis in a very-low-birth-weight infant. Voriconazole has excellent penetration of the CNS and is active against most *Candida* isolates causing CNS infections; however, the clinical experience with voriconazole is too limited to recommend its use at this time.[74] Caspofungin and the other echinocandins do not achieve adequate CSF concentrations for treatment of *Candida* meningitis.[35,127]

Cryptococcosis

Cryptococcal meningitis was rare in the United States in the pre-HIV era. With the growth of the AIDS epidemic, however, this infection has become a common cause of meningitis in adults in certain areas of the United States and infects 2 to 9 percent of adults with AIDS.[29,38,85,183] It remains an uncommon finding in pediatric patients.[114,132] Cryptococcosis is a systemic fungal infection, and meningitis is its most serious manifestation. Patients with initial pulmonary involvement may have few symptoms but can present with fever, cough, weight loss, and dyspnea on exertion.[105] In adult studies, progressively severe headaches without the presence of fever were common manifestations.[159] Patients with cryptococcal meningitis frequently have few symptoms but can present with nausea, dizziness, and irritability. Nuchal rigidity usually is absent. Careful examination for cranial nerve palsies, which are found in approximately one fifth of adult patients, should be performed. Diplopia, in particular, is one of the most common manifestations of cryptococcal meningitis. Papilledema is seen in nearly one third of patients with cryptococcal meningitis.[37] Patients with coexistent AIDS frequently have very few symptoms.[38]

Pediatric patients with cryptococcal meningitis usually present with signs and symptoms not referable to the CNS.[148] Leggiadro and associates[94] reported on 13 children with AIDS, compiled from 11 institutions, who were diagnosed with extrapulmonary cryptococcosis. Meningitis was diagnosed in 62 percent of these patients and was the most common clinical manifestation of extrapulmonary disease. Patients who initially responded to antifungal therapy did not die of the fungal infection but died of other illnesses related to their immunodeficiency. Death can occur, however, even in an immunocompetent child receiving effective therapy.[135]

Leggiadro and associates[93] reported on eight children with acute lymphoblastic leukemia who developed extrapulmonary cryptococcosis. Of these immunocompromised children, 63 percent had meningitis. Fever was the most common symptom, occurring in 60 percent of the children with meningitis. Headache was present in only 40 percent. A significant number of the children (40%) were completely asymptomatic and had lumbar punctures performed as routine management of acute lymphoblastic leukemia, with the subsequent unexpected growth of *C. neoformans* on culture. One child had cutaneous lesions, and another had ptosis and an unsteady gait. Treatment in this series of patients included amphotericin B (intravenous, intrathecal, or both), alone or combined with oral flucytosine. In these patients with acute lymphoblastic leukemia, relapse was a major complication, occurring in 60 percent of patients thought to have been treated successfully. The relapses occurred within 2 to 6 months of completing therapy. Treatment of the relapses generally included combination therapy of amphotericin B and flucytosine, with the occasional use of intrathecal amphotericin B.

Other illnesses that may lead to cryptococcal meningitis include systemic lupus erythematosus being treated with corticosteroids alone or in combination with azathioprine,[2,93,97,129] chronic mucocutaneous candidiasis,[69,170] and hyper-IgE syndrome.[154] Zoonotic transmission from a pet cockatoo was described in an immunocompromised adult.[115]

Direct examination of the CSF using the India ink test can provide an immediate presumptive diagnosis of cryptococcal meningitis. The sensitivity of this test varies, but in studies of adult patients with AIDS, positive results with the stain approached 75 percent.[29] Other useful stains include silver, periodic acid–Schiff, and mucicarmine. Gram stain of CSF is insensitive and unreliable.

Diagnosis of cryptococcal meningitis is aided by the use of serologic tests. The most common test is the cryptococcal capsular polysaccharide antigen test, which can be performed on serum, CSF, or other sterile body fluids. The sensitivity of this test is nearly 100 percent for the serum of patients who are HIV-positive.[30,85,183] The CSF antigen test in some studies seems to be less sensitive, with a 91 percent sensitivity.[29] False-positive results caused by cross-reactions of antigens in disseminated infections with *Trichosporon beigelii* have been reported.[107] Culture still is the gold standard for establishing the diagnosis and monitoring the success of therapy.

Treatment of cryptococcal meningitis is prolonged and, in immunocompromised patients, frequently requires lifelong maintenance therapy. In adults with HIV infection, multiple regimens have been suggested. Practice guidelines have been published for patients with cryptococcal meningitis who are HIV-negative or HIV-positive.[136] For HIV-negative patients, amphotericin B (0.7 to 1 mg/kg/day) plus flucytosine (100 mg/kg/day in four divided doses) for 2 weeks and then fluconazole (400 mg) for a minimum of 10 weeks, or, alternatively, amphotericin B (0.7 to 1 mg/kg day) plus flucytosine (100 mg/kg/day) for 6 to 10 weeks, is recommended. A repeat lumbar puncture is recommended at 2 weeks. If cultures still are positive, prolonged induction therapy should be continued, and fluconazole when started for therapy should be continued for 6 to 12 months. The investigators who proposed the guidelines do not recommend initiating therapy with fluconazole alone. The use of AmBisome (4 mg/kg) for 6 to 10 weeks is a possible alternative if the patient cannot tolerate amphotericin B or azole therapy.

For HIV-infected patients, the practice guideline study group recommends induction therapy of amphotericin B (0.7 to 1 mg/kg/day) plus flucytosine (100 mg/kg/day in four divided doses) for 2 weeks and then fluconazole (400 mg/day) for a minimum of 10 weeks.[136] When flucytosine cannot be administered, amphotericin B is an acceptable alternative; however, a trial from Thailand evaluated sterilization of the CSF in 64 patients and revealed that the combination of amphotericin B plus flucytosine was the most rapidly fungicidal regimen.[20] The use of lipid formulations of amphotericin B may be helpful in patients who cannot tolerate amphotericin B because of renal toxicity.[33] AmBisome has been effective at doses of 4 mg/kg/day.[92]

In patients with renal compromise associated with amphotericin B, flucytosine levels must be monitored carefully. The recommendation is that the dose of flucytosine be reduced to 75 to 100 mg/kg/day and continuing doses be adjusted to maintain serum flucytosine levels of 25 to 60 μg/mL.[6,48] Serum cryptococcal antigens are not useful in monitoring response to therapy, and the use of CSF cryptococcal antigens to monitor response to therapy also is controversial. Therapy is best judged to be successful by the demonstration of sterility of CSF fungal cultures.

In pediatric patients, a combination of amphotericin B and flucytosine has been used most frequently. In children with AIDS, amphotericin B in a dose of 0.5 to 1 mg/kg/day with or without flucytosine (150 mg/kg/day in four divided doses) is recommended for 4 to 8 weeks, followed by maintenance therapy with fluconazole (3 to 6 mg/kg/day) indefinitely.[174] HIV and AIDS guidelines change frequently, and the physician should consult the most recent guidelines for changes, particularly with regard to need for maintenance therapy.

Histoplasmosis

Infection with *Histoplasma capsulatum*, usually a benign and self-limited disease, is endemic in many parts of the United States. Disseminated disease, including meningitis, is a rare occurrence in children.[80] Case reports of adults generally describe immunocompromised individuals.[54,164] Clinical presentations reported in the literature show a wide variability in the manifestation of meningitis. In these cases, 39 percent of patients presented with meningitis associated with acute dissemination, 25 percent presented with single histoplasmoma that manifested as symptomatic mass lesions alone or with dissemination, 25 percent presented with chronic meningitis without evidence of dissemination, and the remaining patients presented with meningitis as a manifestation of recurrent disease. Rarely, embolization to the brain caused by *Histoplasma* endocarditis has been associated with meningitis.[176]

Meningitis occurring in patients with AIDS has become common in endemic areas. In one report, disseminated histoplasmosis caused 8 percent of the AIDS-defining illnesses in children.[141] The duration of symptoms varies. In patients who do not have AIDS, the symptoms generally last longer than 6 months and can last 7 years.[41,54,122,171] In patients with AIDS, symptoms usually manifest more acutely and in a much shorter time-frame.[176] In this series, neurologic findings occurred in all but 6 percent of the patients.[176] The most common signs and symptoms include depressed consciousness (29%), headaches (24%), confusion (22%), cranial nerve deficits (19%), other focal deficits (16%), seizures (14%), personality changes (12%), and ataxia (11%). Findings more commonly observed with acute bacterial meningitis, such as meningismus, a Babinski sign, or papilledema, were seen in fewer than 8 percent of the cases. In adult patients who do not have AIDS, the death rate is approximately 12 percent, with a relapse rate of 44 percent. In adult patients with AIDS, the death rate is 100 percent in some series.[4,176]

Diagnosis can be aided by serologic testing. High levels of anti-*H. capsulatum* antibodies were detected in the serum of 70 percent of patients tested. CSF serology was helpful in 75 percent of patients who were tested. Culture of the CSF was positive for fewer than half of the cases in one review.[80] In a second series in patients with AIDS, blood cultures were positive for 49 percent, bone marrow cultures were positive for 53 percent, respiratory secretions cultures were positive for 58 percent, and brain or meninges cultures were positive for 75 percent of those tested. Serologic testing can be negative because 10 to 25 percent of patients with disseminated disease lack a positive antibody response. The serology also can be false-positive in patients with other fungal diseases or tuberculosis. The antibody response to

acute *Histoplasma* infection may remain elevated for years, without evidence of dissemination or meningeal disease. The use of *Histoplasma* antigen has become widely held as a useful test in immunocompromised patients with disseminated *Histoplasma*. Data from Wheat and associates[176] showed that antigen was found in the urine of six of seven patients with AIDS and meningitis.

Treatment with liposomal amphotericin B (3 to 5 mg/kg/day for a total dose of 100 to 150 mg/kg for 6 to 12 weeks) is considered standard therapy in adults.[178] The liposomal form provides higher CNS levels than does the deoxycholate form. For the deoxycholate form, a total dose of at least 30 mg/kg is considered by many physicians to be necessary to ensure a cure. The use of intrathecal amphotericin B is not recommended for *H. capsulatum* meningitis. A practice guideline for adults written before the previous article recommends that liposomal amphotericin B (3 to 5 mg/kg/day or every other day for 3 to 4 months) be considered for patients who have failed therapy with amphotericin B followed by fluconazole.[179] Johnson and colleagues[75] reported on a trial comparing amphotericin B with liposomal amphotericin B (AmBisome, LAmB) as induction therapy and showed the agents had similar efficacy for treating disseminated histoplasmosis. LeMonte and associates[96] found that amphotericin B combined with fluconazole might have antagonistic effects for treatment of histoplasmosis, but data are needed to determine the efficacy of combination therapy for meningitis.

Patients with AIDS for whom induction therapy was successful must remain on an anti-*Histoplasma* agent indefinitely. A few cases of children with disseminated histoplasmosis and AIDS have been reported, but none with meningitis, and in these children, antifungal therapy must be continued indefinitely.[25,141] The case report by Schutze and associates[141] showed that ketoconazole was ineffective for preventing recurrence of nonmeningeal disseminated disease, and because ketoconazole has poor CNS penetration, it is likely to be ineffective for prophylaxis of meningitis. In patients with AIDS, some success has been achieved with the use of itraconazole for suppressive therapy in disseminated disease. Few data exist, however, on the use of itraconazole for suppressive therapy for meningitis or other CNS lesions caused by *Histoplasma*. For maintenance therapy, fluconazole (high-dose), itraconazole, or intravenous amphotericin B in a weekly dose of 1 mg/kg are available. In one case report, fluconazole was effective in an adult with *Histoplasma* meningitis refractory to amphotericin B therapy.[158]

Coccidioidomycosis

C. immitis (*C. posadasii* in Texas and Central and South America) meningitis is a more common cause of chronic meningitis than is *Histoplasma*.[76] Approximately 1 percent of children with symptomatic pulmonary disease develop disseminated disease.[77] Of patients with disseminated coccidioidomycosis, 15 to 20 percent develop meningitis.[77,82] History of exposure is a crucial factor in diagnosing this disease and relies on careful questioning of the patient about travel to or residence in an endemic area.[155,156] Exposure of wounds to colonized soil has been implicated in at least one pediatric case.[112] An association between facial cutaneous coccidioidomycosis and meningitis has been described.[7]

CSF shows a mononuclear pleocytosis with an elevated protein and decreased glucose concentration. Diagnosing coccidioidal meningitis is made easier by the availability of reliable serologic tests. Smith and associates[150] showed that complement-fixing antibodies appeared in the CSF only in patients with meningitis and provided a sensitivity of 76 percent. Ninety-six percent sensitivity was seen when the complement-fixation test was incubated at 4° C.[119] McGinnis,[106] in his review of the literature based on pooling five studies, showed that *Coccidioides* could be cultured from the CSF in 76 percent of patients with meningitis and was seen on direct examination of the CSF in only 8 percent of the cases. He concluded that these values were too high and were likely skewed because of reporting bias. Other experts in the field also consider that the rate of positive CSF cultures is much lower (approximately 33%), and that finding the organism in the CSF by direct examination rarely occurs.[153]

Coccidioidomycosis in infancy was described more than 40 years ago and continues to be a problem today.[160] Infants usually have severe disease with high mortality rates and morbidity. In the 1980s, two studies described children with *Coccidioides* spp. meningitis who were treated with oral, intravenous, or intrathecal imidazoles.[64,145] The authors reported promising results with the use of ketoconazole and imidazole therapy compared with standard intravenous or intrathecal amphotericin B.

If untreated, *Coccidioides* meningitis is uniformly fatal. Therapy with intravenous and intrathecal amphotericin B reduced the mortality rate to 30 percent.[119] The use of fluconazole has been found in adult studies to have a success rate of 79 percent.[52] It seems to be safe in clinical use, despite a case report of a pregnant woman with *Coccidioides* meningitis treated with fluconazole who delivered an infant with congenital malformations. The infant was thought to have an autosomal recessive disorder (Antley-Bixler syndrome), however, and not teratogenic malformations caused by fluconazole.[91] Fluconazole may be the superior agent for sustaining remission of meningitis caused by *Coccidioides* because of its oral bioavailability, the toxicity associated with amphotericin B, and the elimination of the need for intrathecal administration.[125]

Galgiani and coworkers[51] have written practice guidelines for the treatment of coccidioidomycosis in adults. Therapy with oral fluconazole is preferred, with most authorities recommending 400 mg/day orally, although some physicians begin with higher doses of 800 to 1000 mg/day. Fluconazole in a dose of 400 to 600 mg/day for 9 to 12 months has been shown to be effective in adults.[52,162] A corresponding dose of 6 mg/kg/day in pediatric patients also has been used, but no controlled studies using this agent in pediatric patients have been published. If treatment is begun with azole therapy, it should be continued for life.[36]

Itraconazole has proven efficacy in nonmeningeal coccidioidomycosis, with 63 percent of adult patients treated showing a complete response.[163] Doses of itraconazole of 400 to 600 mg/day have been reported to be effective in adults. Because itraconazole has variable oral bioavailability, many authorities recommend monitoring for adequate serum drug levels.[169] The use of itraconazole for meningeal involvement led to great hope for the use of an oral agent in this disease.[161] Adult patients with *Coccidioides* meningitis had high relapse rates (40-50%), which rendered them dependent on lifelong therapy with itraconazole.[60] The alternative of continued intrathecal amphotericin B renders this treatment much more appealing.

Well-developed, controlled clinical trials with large numbers of children do not exist for the azoles; some authorities consider intravenous and intrathecal amphotericin B to be the standard therapy for coccidioidal meningitis. It also is recommended for patients who do not respond to fluconazole or itraconazole treatment. Some experts initially use a combination of oral azole with intrathecal amphotericin B with the thought that responses are more prompt with this approach. Amphotericin B can be administered intrathecally into the lumbar area or into the cisterna magna, or by using an Ommaya reservoir.[34,53,87,182] In younger children, intraventricular or intracisternal therapy using the Ommaya reservoir allows ease of administration but has the disadvantage of increasing susceptibility to secondary bacterial infection.

The initial dose of amphotericin B administered into the CSF is 0.025 mg. The dose is increased by doubling until a maintenance dose of 0.1 to 0.5 mg is attained. After this dose has been achieved, therapy can be given every other day, alternating with the intravenous administration of amphotericin B. Therapy is continued until the child's condition has stabilized, at which point intrathecal therapy gradually can be stretched out to every 3 weeks. This program is continued until the CSF indices are normal and culture results have been negative for at least 1 year.

Use of voriconazole has been successful in two case reports, and other similar anecdotal references have been reported at referral centers; some centers use voriconazole, 4 mg/kg every 12 hours orally, for salvage therapy.[32,51,128] Miconazole, an imidazole compound that no longer is commercially available, was used in the treatment of *Coccidioides* meningitis and, in combination with oral ketoconazole, had good results in nine children.[145]

Blastomycosis

Blastomyces dermatitidis is an uncommon cause of chronic meningitis and is difficult to diagnose premortem unless the patient has other signs of systemic blastomycosis. When systemic blastomycosis occurs, it can involve the CNS in 5 percent of cases.[18] Common sites for this organism include bone, genitourinary tract, and skin.[10,19] Although examination of CSF obtained by lumbar puncture usually is negative (9% sensitivity), ventricular fluid (four of four patients tested) seems to have a higher yield.[86] Typically, fungal meningitis is associated with a lymphocytic pleocytosis; however, meningitis caused by *B. dermatitidis* frequently has a neutrophilic predominance.[63] Previously, blastomycosis most often affected patients who were immunocompetent. Patients with AIDS are at a high risk for developing chronic infection.[63] Because of the difficulty in diagnosing meningitis caused by *B. dermatitidis* and its similarities to tuberculous meningitis, patients usually are treated for presumptive tuberculous meningitis.[57,111] Although meningitis is the most common form of CNS blastomycosis, solitary mass lesions also can occur.[133]

Diagnosis relies on the characteristic histopathologic appearance in tissues and occasionally on culture of CSF obtained from the ventricles. If the difficulty in performing these procedures is prohibitive, looking for other sources of blastomycosis, including sputum and urine, is indicated. A study in patients with AIDS showed that examination of sputum was useful for establishing the diagnosis of disseminated blastomycosis.[120]

Treatment of systemic blastomycosis, including meningitis, relies on amphotericin B in a dose of 1 mg/kg/day.[152] The duration of therapy is unknown, but adults with systemic disease usually require a minimum of 2 g to prevent relapse of nonmeningeal disease.[121] In adult patients who have been "cured" of their meningitis, doses of 2400 to 3150 mg were required, which would correspond to a total dose of 35 to 45 mg/kg in a child. The use of lipid formulations of amphotericin B has not been reported for CNS blastomycosis, but this treatment according to current practice guidelines of the Mycoses Study Group may be an alternative for patients unable to tolerate amphotericin B because of toxicity.[27] Azoles should not be considered for primary treatment of CNS blastomycosis. Schutze and colleagues[140] reported that children respond less satisfactorily to oral azole therapy than do adults.

Aspergillosis

CNS infections with *Aspergillus fumigatus* and other *Aspergillus* spp. in immunocompromised patients usually are fatal. Conditions that place the patient at risk include organ transplantation, malignancies, and neutropenia. In most reported cases, patients were receiving high-dose corticosteroid therapy in addition to broad-spectrum antibiotics.[11,88] Many patients had fever, and pulmonary findings preceded neurologic manifestations. *Aspergillus* infection of the CNS usually is acquired by hematogenous spread from the lungs. Other modes of acquisition include extension from a contiguous focus (sinuses) and intravenous drug abuse.[110]

Brain abscesses are the most typical manifestation of *Aspergillus* spp. infection in the CNS, but meningoencephalitis, isolated spinal cord lesions, aqueductal stenosis, and mycotic aneurysms also have been described.[26,45,168,172,181] Magnetic resonance imaging has been suggested to be superior to computed tomography for the delineation of CNS lesions in patients with bone marrow transplantation.[108] The lesions are consistent with acute infarcts.

Some early reports of CNS aspergillosis were in infants who appeared to be normal.[1,101] The diagnosis of meningitis relies on CSF cultures, but the results of a bronchoscopy or biopsy frequently are more helpful and provide a more expedient diagnosis. Use of *Aspergillus* antigen in the CSF has been helpful, and it may be used for serial observations during the course of therapy.[173] Because the disease is uniformly fatal, the importance of treating pulmonary aspergillosis before the development of meningeal involvement cannot be overemphasized. Amphotericin B in doses of 1 to 1.5 mg/kg/day is recommended, with or without the addition of flucytosine, rifampin, or both agents.[58,167] Itraconazole has been used successfully in one case report, as has voriconazole.[109,173]

Sporotrichosis

Sporothrix schenckii, although primarily a lymphocutaneous disease, has been reported to cause meningitis.[42,49,84,123,147] Many of the cases described more recently have occurred in adults with AIDS as an underlying risk factor.[40,134] Meningeal seeding may occur through hematogenous spread from the lungs, as is seen in most other fungal infections.[42] Meningeal involvement with sporotrichosis produces CSF indices and abnormalities similar to those seen with the other fungal meningitides.[41] CSF fungal culture is insensitive for the diagnosis of meningitis caused by sporotrichosis. The use of *S. schenckii* antibody in the CSF has been effective in diagnosing meningitis in patients without other overt signs of this infection.[142]

Treating this infection is very difficult. Amphotericin B alone has been successful occasionally.[81] Some experts recommend the addition of flucytosine, but no studies have evaluated the efficacy of this combination. The azoles, particularly itraconazole, had excellent results in nonmeningeal disease, but successful treatment of meningitis with this agent has not been proved.

Mucormycosis

Meningitis caused by *Mucor* spp. or other Zygomycetes usually occurs as a result of direct extension from paranasal sinus disease.

Infection with these organisms most commonly is seen in the immunocompromised host and particularly in patients with diabetes mellitus or patients receiving high doses of corticosteroids. Patients (particularly dialysis patients) undergoing chelation therapy with deferoxamine are at risk for developing infection.[16,17,79,180] The association with deferoxamine therapy is seen with *Cunninghamella*.[130] *Mucor* spp. have been reported as a cause of CNS disease in children but very rare rarely.[61,71] Treatment employs amphotericin B in doses of 1 to 1.5 mg/kg/day, but it usually is unsuccessful. Surgical excision of rhinocerebral infection is recommended along with antifungal therapy.

Other Fungal Infections

Acremonium spp. are common soil fungi that may cause chronic meningitis in humans.[117] *Xylohypha bantiana*, an uncommon dematiaceous fungus, caused a fungal brain abscess in an adolescent girl; this report increases the number of cases reported in the literature to nearly 40.[116] Cerebral chromoblastomycosis also has been reported.[146] Other fungal organisms causing CNS infection include *Paracoccidioides brasiliensis* (i.e., South American blastomycosis),[124] *Prototheca wickerhamii*,[78] *Blastoschizomyces capitatus*,[55] *Rhodotorula* spp.,[103,126] *Pseudallescheria boydii*,[13] *Aureobasidium mansoni*,[68] *Clavispora lusitaniae*,[68] and *Bipolaris spicifera*.[89]

DIAGNOSIS

Specific information about the diagnosis of individual organisms is provided in the previous sections. Table 39–1 provides specific data for some fungal meningitides. Overall, the problem with diagnosing many of these infections is that most patients have nonspecific signs and symptoms without reference to the CNS. Standard culture media may not be useful for these organisms, and it can take weeks before an organism is identified on culture. The use of antigen and antibody testing has proved quite useful for the diagnosis of *Cryptococcus*, *Coccidioides*, and *Histoplasma* infections. The hope is that polymerase chain reaction technology may be helpful in the future, as it has been for bacterial and mycobacterial diagnoses. Neonates may have only a mild CSF pleocytosis. In one series of 16 neonates with definite *Candida* meningitis, the median CSF white blood cell count was 53 cells/mm³ (range, 0 to 1120 cells/mm³).[46]

CSF examination may be helpful in some instances. As much CSF as can be removed safely should be obtained, especially at the time of ventriculography or pneumoencephalography.[41] A minimum of 5 mL of spinal fluid has been suggested, based on

TABLE 39–1 Fungal Cerebrospinal Fluid Characteristics

Organism	WBCs	Protein	Glucose	Smears	Serology	Cultures
Blastomyces	Variable up to 15,000 cells/mm³ with PMNs or lymphocytes	Elevated up to 300 mg/dL	Normal or low	Rare on smear	No good serology	CSF cultures rarely positive; increased yield with ventricular taps
Candida	Mean 600 cells/mm³ up to 1900 cells/mm³ with lymphocytes or PMNs	Elevated	Low or normal	40% positive on smears	Serology not helpful	CSF cultures useful
Coccidioides	100-750 WBCs, mostly lymphocytes	150-2000 mg/dL	21-62% serum	Rare on smear	CSF CF antibody positive in 75-95%	CSF cultures positive in 33-60%
Cryptococcus	40-400 WBCs, mostly lymphocytes	High	Low	India ink positive in 25-50%	CSF and serum cryptococcal antigen positive in 85-90%	CSF cultures positive in 75%
Histoplasma	0-300 WBCs, lymphocytes, or PMNs; most 11-101/mm³	Usually elevated, but can be normal	Usually low (<40 mg/dL) to normal	Rare on smear	Polysaccharide antigen in urine, blood, CSF positive in 61%	CSF cultures positive in 27-65%

CF, complement fixation; CSF, cerebrospinal fluid; PMNs, polymorphonuclear leukocytes; WBCs, white blood cells.
Data from references 57, 64, 106, 175.

experimental work.[99] Repeated cultures of large volumes of CSF may be helpful.[41] The fluid obtained should be centrifuged and the sediment saved for culture and India ink preparation. The supernatant is sent for serologic tests. The India ink test should be interpreted with caution and must be followed with cultures because artifacts frequently can cause misinterpretation.[41] The cumulative efficacy of repeated lumbar punctures for cryptococcal meningitis improved the sensitivity of the India ink smear from 26 percent in one lumbar puncture to 52.6 percent with the second.[106] If large volumes are available, membrane filtration may be used to concentrate the fungal elements. The membrane containing the fungi is placed aseptically on isolation media and incubated at 30° C for 4 weeks. The CSF that passes through the membrane can be used for serology or chemistry determinations.[106] The remaining CSF can be inoculated onto Sabouraud glucose agar, blood agar, and brain-heart infusion agar or into broth media or into both types of media. CSF cultures generally are unhelpful for *Histoplasma, Blastomyces,* and other dimorphic fungi.

Serologic techniques are extremely useful for *Cryptococcus* and *Coccidioides.* Approximately 100 percent sensitivity is seen with serum cryptococcal antigen tests in HIV-positive patients.[30,85,183] The CSF antigen test in HIV-positive patients seems to be less sensitive (91%) in some studies.[29] In patients not infected with HIV, the sensitivity of the serologic test in the CSF approaches 90 percent.[65] For coccidioidal meningitis, the sensitivity rate is greater than 76 percent.[119,150]

Candida can be cultured but may require a prolonged incubation period, necessitating institution of empiric therapy while awaiting results of cultures. For other organisms, such as *Histoplasma, Blastomyces,* and *Coccidioides,* culturing other body fluids, such as blood, urine, sputum, or draining wounds, can be helpful.

ANTIFUNGAL AGENTS AND TREATMENT GUIDELINES

Amphotericin B remains the treatment of choice for most CNS fungal infections in children. Amphotericin B has less than 5 percent oral bioavailability and is more than 90 percent protein-bound.[14] It has a prolonged terminal elimination half-life of 15 days, with only approximately 3 percent of the parent compound found unchanged in the urine.[8] CSF concentrations are approximately 2 to 4 percent of those found in serum.[53,166] The recommended dose varies depending on the organism and the severity of the illness. In most children and infants, a dose of 1 mg/kg/day seems to be satisfactory, particularly in view of the increased clearance of the drug compared with clearance in adults.[12,151]

Toxicity and adverse effects are universal with the use of amphotericin B. Acetaminophen and diphenhydramine may be helpful in reducing the incidence of fever, nausea, and chills. The effective use of hydrocortisone to reduce febrile reactions has been documented.[165] Great variability in patient responses to this treatment occurs, however. The use of corticosteroids can potentiate water retention and amphotericin B–induced hypokalemia; the dosage of corticosteroids should be kept to a minimum.[53] If chills occur, they can be stopped with the use of meperidine.[21]

Amphotericin B induces reversible impairment of renal function in 80 percent of patients during the first 2 weeks of therapy.[24] In most cases, renal function returns to normal after cessation of administration of the drug. The manifestations of toxicity include renal tubular acidosis, azotemia, oliguria, and potassium-magnesium wasting. Other nephrotoxic drugs worsen the azotemia. Renal failure in adult studies has been shown to be ameliorated by the use of salt loading.[66] The adult studies used 500 mL of a 0.9 percent sodium chloride solution as prehydration and posthydration therapy; in children, 10 mL/kg seems to work

as well. Hypokalemia along with hypomagnesemia occurs frequently and may require supplementation. A normocytic, normochromic anemia occurs in many patients who receive amphotericin B, with an 18 to 35 percent decrease in hemoglobin seen after 10 weeks of therapy; this anemia seems to be related partly to changes in erythropoietin levels.[102]

One approach to minimize amphotericin B toxicity while maintaining the drug's pharmacologic spectrum and clinical utility is the use of liposomal and lipid-complexed formulations. The three formulations approved for clinical use include amphotericin B lipid complex (Abelcet; Liposome Company, Princeton, NJ), amphotericin B colloidal dispersion (Amphotec, Amphocil; Sequus Pharmaceuticals, Menlo Park, CA), and liposomal amphotericin B (AmBisome; NeXstar Pharmaceuticals, Boulder, CO; Fujisawa USA, Deerfield, IL). Although each of these lipid delivery systems is unique and has different pharmacokinetic and pharmacodynamic profiles, no clinical comparisons of lipid formulations have been done in children. Their use is discussed briefly in the case reports that exist for the individual infections listed previously. Most of the published pediatric literature describes cases in which AmBisome has been used.

Ketoconazole has not been an effective agent for treating most fungal CNS disease processes. It has been supplanted by the newer azoles, fluconazole and itraconazole, because of their better bioavailability and more favorable results in clinical trials.

Fluconazole is a very effective agent for the suppression of cryptococcal meningitis in patients with AIDS and immunocompetent patients and seems to be superior to amphotericin B for prolonged maintenance therapy in patients with AIDS. Fluconazole absorption by the gastrointestinal tract is not affected by the presence of food or gastric acidity.[15] Fluconazole is highly water soluble and minimally bound to plasma proteins.[90] The terminal elimination half-life of fluconazole is 22 to 31 hours, with 80 percent of the drug excreted unchanged in the urine.[31] Fluconazole readily penetrates into CSF in inflamed or noninflamed meninges, achieving levels that are 60 to 80 percent of serum levels. Rifampin, cyclosporine, and phenytoin have significant interactions with fluconazole. Adverse effects are uncommon, especially compared with the effects associated with amphotericin B. Less than 5 percent of patients have nausea and vomiting. Asymptomatic elevations of plasma aminotransferases occur in less than 1 to 7 percent of patients.[31]

Data for itraconazole use in pediatrics are limited, and itraconazole is not recommended at this time for CNS fungal infections in children. Itraconazole has increased absorption when taken with food.[168] Itraconazole is highly protein-bound (>99 percent); less than 1 percent is excreted unchanged in urine.[59] CSF concentrations are low compared with those of fluconazole; however, itraconazole is much more lipophilic, allowing it to show efficacy in treatment of some fungal meningitides. Additional data on it and the other azoles, particularly for treatment of coccidioidal meningitis in children, should be forthcoming in the next several years,. Promising results from an adult study have been published.[161]

CONCLUSION

With the large increase in the number of immunocompromised children caused by the epidemic of HIV, the advent of new antineoplastic agents, the growth of organ transplantation, and the increased use of corticosteroids, the relative rarity of fungal meningitides has been replaced by a burgeoning upswing in the incidence and prevalence of these infections. New modalities for diagnosis are needed because many of these fungal infections still require weeks for identification. We expect that trials in progress will help determine the role of azoles, amphotericin B, lipid formulations of amphotericin B, or combinations of these drugs as the optimal treatment of many fungal meningitides.

REFERENCES

1. Allan, G. W., and Anderson, D. H.: Generalized aspergillosis in an infant 18 days of age. Pediatrics 26:432-440, 1960.
2. al-Rasheed, S. A., and al-Fawaz, I. M.: Cryptococcal meningitis in a child with systemic lupus erythematosus. Ann. Trop. Paediatr. 10:323-326, 1990.
3. Ampel, N. M., Wieden, M. A., and Galgiani, J. N.: Coccidioidomycosis: Clinical update. Rev. Infect. Dis. 11:897, 1989.
4. Anaissie, E., Fainstein, V., Samo, T., et al.: Central nervous system histoplasmosis: An unappreciated complication of the acquired immunodeficiency syndrome. Am. J. Med. 84:215-217, 1988.
5. Arisoy, E. S., Arisoy, A. E., and Dunne, W. M., Jr.: Clinical significance of fungi isolated from cerebrospinal fluid in children. Pediatr. Infect. Dis. J. 13:128-133, 1994.
6. Armstrong, D.: Treatment of opportunistic fungal infections. Clin. Infect. Dis. 16:1-9, 1993.
7. Arsura, E. L., Kilgore, W. B., Caldwell, J. W., et al.: Association between facial cutaneous coccidioidomycosis and meningitis. West. J. Med. 169:13-16, 1998.
8. Atkinson, A. J., and Bennett, J. E.: Amphotericin B pharmacokinetics in humans. Antimicrob. Agents Chemother. 13:271, 1978.
9. Baley, J. E., Kliegman, R. M., and Fanaroff, A. A.: Disseminated fungal infections in very low-birth-weight infants: Clinical manifestations and epidemiology. Pediatrics 73:144-152, 1984.
10. Baumgardner, D. J., Buggy, B. P., Mattson, B. J., et al.: Epidemiology of blastomycosis in a region of high endemicity in north central Wisconsin. Clin. Infect. Dis. 15:629-635, 1992.
11. Beal, M. F., O'Carroll, C. P., Kleinman, G. M., et al.: Aspergillosis of the central nervous system. Neurology 32:473-479, 1982.
12. Benson, J. M., and Nahata, M. C.: Pharmacokinetics of amphotericin B in children. Antimicrob. Agents Chemother. 33:1989-1993, 1989.
13. Berenguer, J., Diaz-Mediavilla, J., Urra, D., et al.: Central nervous system infection caused by Pseudallescheria boydii: Case report and review. Rev. Infect. Dis. 11:890-896, 1989.
14. Block, E. R., Bennett, J. E., Livoti, L. G., et al.: Flucytosine and amphotericin B: Hemodialysis effects on the plasma concentration and clearance. Ann. Intern. Med. 80:613-617, 1974.
15. Blum, R., A., D'Andrea, D. T., Florentino, B. M., et al.: Increased gastric pH and the bioavailability of fluconazole and ketoconazole. Ann. Intern. Med. 114:755-757, 1991.
16. Boelaert, J. R., de Locht, M., Van Cutsem, J., et al.: Mucormycosis during deferoxamine therapy is a siderophore-mediated infection: In vitro and in vivo animal studies. J. Clin. Invest. 91:1979-1986, 1993.
17. Boelaert, J. R., Vergauwe, P. L., and Vandepitte, J. M.: Mucormycosis infection in dialysis patients. Ann. Intern. Med. 107:782-783, 1987.
18. Bradsher, R. W.: Blastomycosis. Clin. Infect. Dis. 14(Suppl. 1):S582-S590, 1992.
19. Bradsher, R. W., Rice, D. C., and Abernathy, R. S.: Ketoconazole therapy for endemic blastomycosis. Ann. Intern. Med. 103:872-879, 1985.
20. Brouwer, A. E., Rajanuwong, A., Chierakul, W., et al. Combination antifungal therapies for HIV-associated cryptococcococal meningitis: A randomized trial. Lancet 363:1764-7, 2004.
21. Burks, L. C., Aisner, J., Fortner, C. L., et al.: Meperidine for the treatment of shaking chills and fever. Arch. Intern. Med. 140:483-484, 1980.
22. Butler, K. M., Rench, M. A., and Baker, C. J.: Amphotericin B as a single agent in the treatment of systemic candidiasis in neonates. Pediatr. Infect. Dis. J. 9:51-56, 1990.
23. Butler, W. T., Alling, D. W., Spickard, A., et al.: Diagnostic and prognostic value of clinical and laboratory findings in cryptococcal meningitis: A follow-up study of forty patients. N. Engl. J. Med. 270:59-66, 1964.
24. Butler, W. T., Bennett, J. E., Alling, D. W., et al.: Nephrotoxicity of amphotericin B: Early and late effects in 81 patients. Ann. Intern. Med. 61:175-187, 1964.
25. Byers, M., Feldman, S., and Edwards, J.: Disseminated histoplasmosis as the acquired immunodeficiency syndrome-defining illness in an infant. Pediatr. Infect. Dis. J. 11:127-128, 1992.
26. Casey, A. T., Wilkins, P., and Uttley, D.: Aspergillosis infection in neurosurgical practice. Br. J. Neurosurg. 8:31-39, 1994.
27. Chapman, S. W., Bradsher, R. W., Campbell, G. D., et al.: Practice guidelines for the management of patients with blastomycosis. Clin. Infect. Dis. 30:679-683, 2000.
28. Chen, J. Y.: Neonatal candidiasis associated with meningitis and endophthalmitis. Acta Pediatr. Jpn. 36:261-265, 1994.
29. Chuck, S. L., and Sande, M. A.: Infections with Cryptococcus neoformans in the acquired immunodeficiency syndrome. N. Engl. J. Med. 321:794-799, 1989.
30. Clark, R. A., Greer, D., Atkinson, W., et al.: Spectrum of Cryptococcus neoformans infection in 68 patients infected with human immunodeficiency virus. Rev. Infect. Dis. 12:768-777, 1990.
31. Como, J. A., and Dismukes, W. E.: Oral azole drugs as systemic antifungal therapy. N. Engl. J. Med. 330:263-272, 1994.
32. Cortez, K. J., Walsh, T. J., Bennett, J. E.: Successful treatment of coccidioidal meningitis with voriconazole. Clin. Infect. Dis. 36:1619-1622, 2003.
33. Coukell, A. J., and Brogden, R. N.: Liposomal amphotericin B: Therapeutic use in the management of fungal infections and visceral leishmaniasis. Drugs 55:585-612, 1998.
34. Dennis, M., and Rasch, J. R.: The Ommaya reservoir in fungal meningitis: A case report. In Ajello, L. (ed.): Coccidioidomycosis. Tucson, AZ, University of Arizona Press, 1967, pp. 119-122.
35. Deresinski, S. C., and Stevens, D. A.: Caspofungin. Clin. Infect. Dis. 36:1445-1457, 2003.
36. Dewsnup, D. H., Galgiani, J. N., Graybill, J. R., et al.: Is it ever safe to stop azole therapy for Coccidioides immitis meningitis? Ann. Intern. Med. 124:305-310, 1996.
37. Diamond, R. D.: Cryptococcus neoformans. In Mandell, G. L., Bennett, J. E., and Dolin, R. (eds.): Principles and Practice of Infectious Diseases. 4th ed. New York, Churchill Livingstone, 1995, pp. 2331-2340.
38. Dismukes, W. E.: Cryptococcal meningitis in patients with AIDS. J. Infect. Dis. 157:624-628, 1988.
39. Dismukes, W. E.: Introduction to antifungal drugs. Clin. Infect. Dis. 30:653-657, 2000.
40. Donabedian, H., O'Donnell, E., Olszewski, C., et al.: Disseminated cutaneous and meningeal sporotrichosis in an AIDS patient. Diagn. Microbiol. Infect. Dis. 18:111-115, 1994.
41. Ellner, J. J., and Bennett, J. E.: Chronic meningitis. Medicine (Baltimore) 55:341-396, 1976.
42. Ewing, G. E., Bosl, G. J., and Peterson, P. K.: Sporothrix schenckii meningitis in a farmer with Hodgkin's disease. Am. J. Med. 68:455-457, 1980.
43. Faix, R. G.: Systemic Candida infections in infants in intensive care nurseries: High incidence of central nervous system involvement. J. Pediatr. 105:616-622, 1984.
44. Faix, R. G., Kovarik, S. M., Shaw, T. R., et al.: Mucocutaneous and invasive candidiasis among very low birth weight (<1500 grams) infants in intensive care nurseries: A prospective study. Pediatrics 83:101-107, 1989.
45. Feely, M., and Steinberg, M.: Aspergillus infection complicating transsphenoidal yttrium-90 pituitary implant. J. Neurosurg. 46:530-532, 1977.
46. Fernandez, M., Moylett, E. H., Noyala, D. E., et al.: Candida meningitis in neonates. Clin. Infect. Dis. 31:458-463, 2000.
47. Flynn, P. M., Marina, N. M., Rivera, G. K., et al.: Candida tropicalis infections in children with leukemia. Leuk. Lymphoma 10:369-376, 1993.
48. Francis, P., and Walsh, T. J.: Evolving role of flucytosine in immunocompromised patients: New insights into safety, pharmacokinetics, and antifungal therapy. Clin. Infect. Dis. 15:1003-1008, 1992.
49. Freeman, J. W., and Ziegler, D. K.: Chronic meningitis caused by Sporotrichum schenckii. Neurology 27:989-992, 1977.
50. Furcolow, M. L., Chick, E. W., Busey, J. F., et al.: Prevalence and incidence studies of human and canine blastomycosis, I: Cases in the United States, 1885-1968. Am. Rev. Respir. Dis. 102:60-67, 1970.
51. Galgiani, J. N., Ampel, N. M., Blair, J. E., et al.: Practice guidelines for treatment of coccidioidomycosis. Clin. Infect. Dis. 41:1217, 2005.
52. Galgiani, J. N., Catanzaro, A., Cloud, G. A., et al.: Fluconazole therapy for coccidioidal meningitis: The NIAID-Mycoses Study Group. Ann. Intern. Med. 119:28-35, 1993.
53. Gallis, H. A., Drew, R. H., and Pickard, W. W.: Amphotericin B: 30 years of clinical experience. Rev. Infect. Dis. 12:308-329, 1990.
54. Gelfand, J. A., and Bennett, J. E.: Active Histoplasma meningitis of 22 years duration. J. A. M. A. 233:1294-1295, 1975.
55. Girmenia, C., Micozzi, A., Venditti, M., et al.: Fluconazole treatment of Blastoschizomyces capitatus meningitis in an allogeneic bone marrow recipient. Eur. J. Clin. Microbiol. Infect. Dis. 10:752-756, 1991.
56. Glick, C., Graves, C. R., and Feldman, S.: Neonatal fungemia and amphotericin B. South. Med. J. 86:1368-1371, 1993.
57. Gonyea, E. F.: The spectrum of primary blastomycotic meningitis: A review of central nervous system blastomycosis. Ann. Neurol. 3:26-39, 1978.
58. Gordon, M. A., Holzman, R. S., Senter, H., et al.: Aspergillus oryzae meningitis. J. A. M. A. 235:2122-2123, 1976.
59. Grant, S. M., and Clissold, S. P.: Itraconazole: A review of its pharmacodynamic and pharmacokinetic properties and therapeutic use in superficial and systemic mycoses. Drugs 37:310-344, 1989.
60. Graybill, J. R.: Future directions of antifungal chemotherapy. Clin. Infect. Dis. 14 (Suppl. 1):S170-S181, 1992.
61. Hale, L. M.: Orbital-cerebral phycomycosis: Report of a case and a review of the disease in infants. Arch. Ophthalmol. 86:39-43, 1971.
62. Hamner, R. W., Baum, E. W., and Pritchett, P. S.: Coccidioidal meningitis diagnosed by skin biopsy. Cutis 29:603-610, 1982.
63. Harley, W. B., Lomis, M., and Haas, D. W.: Marked polymorphonuclear pleocytosis due to blastomycotic meningitis: Case report and review. Clin. Infect. Dis. 18:816-818, 1994.
64. Harrison, H. R., Galgiani, J. N., Reynolds, A. F., Jr., et al.: Amphotericin B and imidazole therapy for coccidioidal meningitis in children. Pediatr. Infect. Dis. 2:216-221, 1983.
65. Hay, R. J., Mackenzie, D. W. R., Campbell, C. K., et al.: Cryptococcosis in the United Kingdom and the Irish Republic: An analysis of 69 cases. J. Infect. 2:13-22, 1980.

66. Heidemann, H. T., Gerkens, J. F., Spickard, W. A., et al.: Amphotericin B nephrotoxicity in humans decreased by salt repletion. Am. J. Med. 75:476-481, 1983.

67. Huttova, M., Hartmanova, I., Kralinsky, K., et al.: *Candida* fungemia in neonates treated with fluconazole: Report of forty cases, including eight with meningitis. Pediatr. Infect. Dis. J. 17:1012-1015, 1998.

68. Huttova, M., Kralinsky, K., Horn, J., et al.: Prospective study of nosocomial fungal meningitis in children—report of 10 cases. Scand. J. Infect. Dis. 30:485-487, 1998.

69. Imperato, P. J., Buckley, C. E., and Callaway, J. L.: *Candida* granuloma. Arch. Dermatol. 97:139-146, 1968.

70. Isaacs, D., Barfield, C. P., Grimwood, K., et al.: Systemic bacterial and fungal infections in infants in Australian neonatal units. Australian Study Group for Neonatal Infections. Med. J. Aust. 162:198-201, 1995.

71. Isaacson, C., and Levin, S. E.: Gastrointestinal mucormycosis in infancy. S. Afr. Med. J. 35:581-584, 1961.

72. Jafari, H. S., Saez-Llorens, X., Grimprel, E., et al.: Characteristics of experimental *Candida albicans* infection of the central nervous system in rabbits. J. Infect. Dis. 164:389-395, 1991.

73. Johnson, D. E., Thompson, T. R., Green, T. P., et al.: Systemic candidiasis in very-low-birth-weight infants (<1500 grams). Pediatrics 73:138-143, 1984.

74. Johnson, L. B., and Kauffman, C. A.: Voriconazole: A new triazole antifungal agent. Clin. Infect. Dis. 36:630-637, 2003.

75. Johnson, P., Wheat, L. J., Cloud, G., et al.: A multicenter randomized trial comparing amphotericin B (AmB) and liposomal amphotericin B (AmBisome, LAmB) as induction therapy of disseminated histoplasmosis (DH) in AIDS patients. Abstract L40e. *In*: Proceedings of the 7th Conference on Retroviruses and Opportunistic Infections, San Francisco, January 30-February 2, 2000. San Francisco, Foundation for Retrovirology and Human Health, 2000.

76. Johnson, R. H., and Einstein, H. E.: Coccidioidal meningitis. Clin. Infect. Dis. 42:103-107, 2006.

77. Kafka, J. A., and Catanzaro, A.: Disseminated coccidioidomycosis in children. J. Pediatr. 98:355-361, 1981.

78. Kaminski, Z. C., Kapila, R., Sharer, L. R., et al.: Meningitis due to *Prototheca wickerhamii* in a patient with AIDS. Clin. Infect. Dis. 15:704-706, 1992.

79. Kaneko, T., Abe, F., Ito, M., et al.: Intestinal mucormycosis in a hemodialysis patient treated with desferrioxamine. Acta. Pathol. Jpn. 41:561-566, 1991.

80. Karalakulasingam, R., Arora, K. K., and Adams, G.: Meningoencephalitis caused by *Histoplasma capsulatum*: Occurrence in a renal transplant and review of the literature. Arch. Intern. Med. 136:217-220, 1976.

81. Kauffman, C. A.: Old and new therapies for sporotrichosis. Clin. Infect. Dis. 21:981-985, 1995.

82. Kelly, P. C.: Coccidioidal meningitis. *In* Stevens, D. A. (ed.): Coccidioidomycosis: A Text. New York, Plenum Medical Book, 1980, pp. 163-194.

83. Klein, B. S., Vergeront, J. M., Weeks, R. J., et al.: Isolation of *Blastomyces dermatitidis* in soil associated with a large outbreak of blastomycosis in Wisconsin. N. Engl. J. Med. 314:529-534, 1986.

84. Klein, R. C., Ivens, M. S., Seabury, J. H., et al.: Meningitis due to *Sporotrichum schenckii*. Arch. Intern. Med. 118:145-149, 1966.

85. Kovacs, J. A., Kovacs, A. A., Polis, M., et al.: Cryptococcosis in the acquired immunodeficiency syndrome. Ann. Intern. Med. 103:533-538, 1985.

86. Kravitz, G. R., Davies, S. F., Eckman, M. R., et al.: Chronic blastomycotic meningitis. Am. J. Med. 71:501-505, 1981.

87. Kucers, A., and Bennett, N. McK.: Amphotericin B. *In* Kucers, A., and Bennett, N. McK. (eds.): The Use of Antibiotics. 4th ed. Philadelphia, J. B. Lippincott, 1987, pp. 1441-1477.

88. Lammens, M., Robberecht, W., Waer, M., et al.: Purulent meningitis due to aspergillosis in a patient with systemic lupus erythematosus. Clin. Neurol. Neurosurg. 94:39-43, 1992.

89. Latham, R. H.: *Bipolaris spicifera* meningitis complicating a neurosurgical procedure. Scand. J. Infect. Dis. 32:102-103, 2000.

90. Lazar, J. D., and Hilligoss, D. M.: The clinical pharmacology of fluconazole. Semin. Oncol. 17(Suppl. 6):14-18, 1990.

91. Lee, B. E., Feinberg, M., Abraham, J. J., et al.: Congenital malformations in an infant born to a woman treated with fluconazole. Pediatr. Infect. Dis. J. 11:1062-1064, 1992.

92. Leenders, A. C., Riss, P., Portegies, P., et al.: Liposomal amphotericin B (AmBisome) compared with amphotericin B followed by oral fluconazole in the treatment of AIDS-associated cryptococcal meningitis. AIDS 11:1463-1471, 1997.

93. Leggiadro, R. J., Barrett, F. F., and Hughes, W. T.: Extrapulmonary cryptococcosis in immunocompromised infants and children. Pediatr. Infect. Dis. J. 11:43-47, 1992.

94. Leggiadro, R. J., Kline, M. W., and Hughes, W. T.: Extrapulmonary cryptococcosis in children with acquired immunodeficiency syndrome. Pediatr. Infect. Dis. J. 10:658-662, 1991.

95. Leibovitz, E., Rigaud, M., Chandwani, S., et al.: Disseminated fungal infections in children infected with human immunodeficiency virus. Pediatr. Infect. Dis. J. 10:888-894, 1991.

96. LeMonte, A. M., Washum, K. E., Smedema, M. L., et al.: Amphotericin B combined with itraconazole or fluconazole for treatment of histoplasmosis. J. Infect. Dis. 182:545-550, 2000.

97. Lesser, R. L., Simon, R. M., Leon, H., et al.: Cryptococcal meningitis and internal ophthalmoplegia. Am. J. Ophthalmol. 87:682-687, 1979.

98. Littman, M. L., and Walter, J. E.: Cryptococcosis: Current status. Am. J. Med. 45:922-932, 1968.

99. Louria, D. B., Feder, N., Mitchell, W., et al.: Influence of fungus strain and lapse on time in experimental histoplasmosis and of volume of inoculum in cryptococcosis upon recovery of the fungi. J. Lab. Clin. Med. 53:311-317, 1959.

100. Ludviksson, B. R., Thorarensen, O., Gudnason, T., et al.: *Candida albicans* meningitis in a child with myeloperoxidase deficiency. Pediatr. Infect. Dis. J. 12:162-164, 1993.

101. Luke, J. L., Bolande, R. P., and Gross, S.: Generalized aspergillosis and *Aspergillus endocarditis* in infancy. Pediatrics 31:115-122, 1963.

102. MacGregor, R. R., Bennett, J. E., and Erslev, A. J.: Erythropoietin concentration in amphotericin B-induced anemia. Antimicrob. Agents Chemother. 14:270-273, 1978.

103. Marinova, I., Szabadosova, V., Brandeburova, O., et al.: *Rhodotorula* spp. fungemia in an immunocompromised boy after neurosurgery successfully treated with miconazole and 5-flucytosine: Case report and review of the literature. Chemotherapy 40:287-289, 1994.

104. Marr, B., Gross, S., Cunningham, C., and Weiner, L.: Candidal sepsis and meningitis in a very-low-birth-weight infant successfully treated with fluconazole and flucytosine. Clin. Infect. Dis. 19:795-796, 1994.

105. McDonald, R., Greenberg, E. N., and Kramer, R.: Cryptococcal meningitis. Arch. Dis. Child. 45:417-420, 1970.

106. McGinnis, M. R.: Detection of fungi in cerebrospinal fluid. Am. J. Med. 75:129-138, 1983.

107. McManus, E. J., and Jones, J. M.: Detection of a *Trichosporon beigelii* antigen cross-reactive with *Cryptococcus neoformans* capsular polysaccharide in serum from a patient with disseminated *Trichosporon* infection. J. Clin. Microbiol. 21:681-685, 1985.

108. Miaux, Y., Ribaud, P., Williams, M., et al.: MR of cerebral aspergillosis in patients who have had bone marrow transplantation. A. J. N. R. Am. J. Neuroradiol. 16:555-562, 1995.

109. Mikolich, D. J., Kinsella, L. J., Skowron, G., et al.: *Aspergillus* meningitis in an immunocompetent adult successfully treated with itraconazole. Clin. Infect. Dis. 23:1318-1319, 1996.

110. Morrow, R., Wong, B., Finkelstein, W. E., et al.: Aspergillosis of the cerebral ventricles in a heroin abuser: Case report and review of the literature. Arch. Intern. Med. 143:161-164, 1983.

111. Morse, H. G., Nichol, W. P., Cook, D. M., et al.: Central nervous system and genitourinary blastomycosis: Confusion with tuberculosis. West. J. Med. 139:99-103, 1983.

112. Morwood, D. T., Nichter, L. S., and Wong, V.: An unusual complication of an open-head injury: Coccidioidal meningitis. Ann. Plast. Surg. 23:437-441, 1989.

113. Namdar, R., Anderson, J. D., and Kline, S. S.: Abelcet, Amphotec, and AmBisome in the neonatal and pediatric populations: A literature review. J. Pediatr. Pharm. Pract. 3:13-28, 1998.

114. Nicholas, S. W., Dondheimer, D. L., Willoughby, A. D., et al.: Human immunodeficiency virus infection in childhood, adolescence, and pregnancy: A status report and national research agenda. Pediatrics 83:293-308, 1989.

115. Nosanchuk, J. D., Shoham, S., Fries, B. C., et al.: Evidence of zoonotic transmission of *Cryptococcus neoformans* from a pet cockatoo to an immunocompromised adult. Ann. Intern. Med. 132:205-208, 2000.

116. Palaoglu, S., Sav, A., Basak, T., et al.: Cerebral phaeohyphomycosis. Neurosurgery 33:894-897, 1993.

117. Papadatos, C., Pavatou, M., and Alexiou, D.: *Cephalosporium* meningitis. Pediatrics 44:749-751, 1969.

118. Pappagianis, D.: Epidemiology of coccidioidomycosis. *In* Stevens D. A. (ed.): Coccidioidomycosis: A Text. New York, Plenum Medical, 1980, p. 63.

119. Pappagianis, D., and Crane, R.: Survival in coccidioidal meningitis since introduction of amphotericin B. *In* Ajello, L. (ed.): Coccidioidomycosis: Current Clinical and Diagnostic Status. Miami, Symposia Specialists Medical Books, 1977, pp. 223-237.

120. Pappas, P. G., Pottage, J. C., Powderly, W. G., et al.: Blastomycosis in patients with the acquired immunodeficiency syndrome. Ann. Intern. Med. 116:847-853, 1992.

121. Parker, J. D., Doto, I. L., and Tosh, F. E.: A decade of experience with blastomycosis and its treatment with amphotericin B. Am. Rev. Respir. Dis. 99:895-902, 1969.

122. Parsons, R. J., and Zarafonetis, C. J. D.: Histoplasmosis in man: Report of seven cases and a review of seventy-one cases. Arch. Intern. Med. 75:1-23, 1945.

123. Penn, C. C., Goldstein, E., and Bartholomew, M. R.: *Sporothrix schenckii* meningitis in a patient with AIDS. Clin. Infect. Dis. 15:741-743, 1992.

124. Pereira, W. C., Tenuto, R. A., Raphael, A., et al.: Localizacao encefalica da blastomicose Sul-Americana. Arq. Neuro-Psiquiat. (Sao Paulo) 23:113-126, 1965.

125. Perez, J. A., Jr., Johnson, R. A., Caldwell, J. W., et al.: Fluconazole therapy in coccidioidal meningitis maintained with intrathecal amphotericin B. Arch. Intern. Med. 155:1665-1668, 1995.

126. Pore, R. S., and Chen, J.: Meningitis caused by *Rhodotorula*. Sabouraudia. 14:331-335, 1976.

127. Prabhu, R. M., and Orenstein, R.: Failure of caspofungin to treat brain abscesses secondary to *Candida albicans* prosthetic valve endocarditis. Clin. Infect. Dis. 39:1253-1254, 2004.

128. Proia, L. A., and Tenorio, A. R.: Successful use of voriconazole for treatment of *Coccidioides* meningitis. Antimicrob. Agents Chemother. *48*:2341, 2004.

129. Rapaport, S. I., Ames, S. B., and Duvall, B. J.: A plasma coagulation defect in systemic lupus erythematosus arising from hypoprothrombinemia combined with antiprothrombinase activity. Blood *15*:212-227, 1960.

130. Rex, J. H., Ginsberg, A. M., Fries, L. F., et al.: *Cunninghamella bertholetiae* infection associated with deferoxamine therapy. Rev. Infect. Dis. *10*:1187-1194, 1988.

131. Rex, J. H., Pfaller, M. A., Galgiani, J. N., et al.: Development of interpretive breakpoints for antifungal susceptibility testing: Conceptual framework and analysis of in vitro-in vivo correlation data for fluconazole, itraconazole, and *Candida* infections. Clin. Infect. Dis. *24*:235-247, 1997.

132. Rogers, M. F., Thomas, P. A., Starcher, E. T., et al.: Acquired immunodeficiency syndrome in children: Report of the Centers for Disease Control national surveillance, 1982-1985. Pediatrics *79*:1008-1014, 1987.

133. Ross, K. L., Bryan, J. P., Maggio, W. W., et al.: Intracranial blastomycoma. Medicine (Baltimore) *66*:224-235, 1987.

134. Rotz, L. D., Slater, L. N., Wack, M. F., et al.: Disseminated sporotrichosis with meningitis in a patient with AIDS. Infect. Dis. Clin. Pract. *5*:566-568, 1996.

135. Ruggierei, M., Polizzi, A., Vitaliti, M. C., et al.: Fatal biphasic brainstem and spinal leptomeningitis with *Cryptococcus neoformans* in a non-immunocompromised child. Acta Paediatr. *88*:671-674, 1999.

136. Saag, M. S., Graybill, R. J., Larsen, R. A., et al.: Practice guidelines for the management of cryptococcal disease. Clin. Infect. Dis. *30*:710-718, 2000.

137. Salaki, J. S., Louria, D. B., and Chmel, H.: Fungal and yeast infections of the central nervous system: A clinical review. Medicine (Baltimore) *63*:108-132, 1984.

138. Sarma, P. S., Durairaj, P., and Padhye, A. A.: *Candida lusitaniae* causing fatal meningitis. Postgrad. Med. J. *69*:878-880, 1993.

139. Scarcella, A., Pasquariello, M. B., Guigliano, B., et al.: Liposomal amphotericin B treatment for neonatal fungal infections. Pediatr. Infect. Dis. J. *17*:146-148, 1998.

140. Schutze, G. E., Hickerson, S. L., Fortin, E. M., et al.: Blastomycosis in children. Clin. Infect. Dis. *22*:496-502, 1996.

141. Schutze, G. E., Tucker, N. C., and Jacobs, R. F.: Histoplasmosis and perinatal human immunodeficiency virus. Pediatr. Infect. Dis. J. *11*:501-502, 1992.

142. Scott, E. N., Kaufman, L., Brown, A. C., et al.: Serologic studies in the diagnosis and management of meningitis due to *Sporothrix schenckii*. N. Engl. J. Med. *317*:935-940, 1987.

143. Sekshon, A. S., Borgorus, M. S., and Sims, H. V.: Blastomycosis: Report of three cases from Alberta with a review of Canadian cases. Mycopathologia *1*:53-63, 1979.

144. Selik, R., Starcher, E., and Curran J.: Opportunistic diseases reported in AIDS patients: Frequencies, associations, and trends. AIDS *1*:175-182, 1987.

145. Shehab, Z. M., Britton, H., and Dunn, J. H.: Imidazole therapy of coccidioidal meningitis in children. Pediatr. Infect. Dis. J. *7*:40-44, 1988.

146. Shimosaka, S., and Waga, S.: Cerebral chromoblastomycosis complicated by meningitis and multiple fungal aneurysms after resection of a granuloma: Case report. J. Neurosurg. *59*:158-161, 1983.

147. Shoemaker, E. H., Bennett, H. D., Fields, W. S., et al.: Leptomeningitis due to *Sporotrichum schenckii*. Arch. Pathol. *64*:222, 1957.

148. Siewers, C. M. F., and Cramblett, H. G.: Cryptococcosis (torulosis) in children: A report of four cases. Pediatrics *34*:393-400, 1964.

149. Smego, R. A., Perfect, J. R., and Durack, D. T.: Combined therapy with amphotericin B and 5-fluorocytosine for *Candida* meningitis. Rev. Infect. Dis. *6*:791-801, 1984.

150. Smith, C. E., Saito, M. T., and Simons, S. A.: Pattern of 39,500 serologic tests in coccidioidomycosis. J. A. M. A. *160*:546-552, 1956.

151. Starke, J. R., Mason, E. O., Jr., Kramer, W. G., et al.: Pharmacokinetics of amphotericin B in infants and children. J. Infect. Dis. *155*:766-774, 1987.

152. Steele, R. W., and Abernathy, R. S.: Systemic blastomycosis in children. Pediatr. Infect. Dis. J. *2*:304-307, 1983.

153. Stevens, D.: *Coccidioides immitis. In* Mandell, G. L., Bennett, J. E., and Dolin, R. (eds.): Principles and Practice of Infectious Diseases. 4th ed. New York, Churchill Livingstone, 1995, pp. 2365-2375.

154. Stone, B. D., and Wheeler, J. G.: Disseminated cryptococcal infection in a patient with hyperimmunoglobulinemia E syndrome. J. Pediatr. *117*:92-95, 1990.

155. Takeda, K., Oritsu, M., and Sakuta, M.: A case of coccidioidomycosis with central nervous system involvement. Rinsho Shinkeigaku *33*:1184-1187, 1993.

156. Taylor, G. D., Boettger, D. W., Miedzinski, L. J., et al.: Coccidioidal meningitis acquired during holidays in Arizona. Can. Med. Assoc. J. *142*:1388-1390, 1990.

157. Taylor, G. D., Buchanan-Chell, M., Kirkland, T., et al.: Trends and sources of nosocomial fungaemia. Mycoses *37*:187-190, 1994.

158. Tiraboschi, I., Parera, I. C., Pikielny, R., et al.: Chronic *Histoplasma capsulatum* infection of the central nervous system successfully treated with fluconazole. Eur. Neurol. *32*:70-73, 1992.

159. Tjia, T. L., Yeow, Y. K., and Tan, C. B.: Cryptococcal meningitis. J. Neurol. Neurosurg. Psychiatry *48*:853-858, 1985.

160. Townsend, T. E., and McKay, R. W.: Coccidioidomycosis in infants. Am. J. Dis. Child. *86*:51-53, 1953.

161. Tucker, R. M., Denning, D. W., Dupont, B., et al.: Itraconazole therapy for chronic coccidioidal meningitis. Ann. Intern. Med. *112*:108-112, 1990.

162. Tucker, R. M., Galgiani, J. N., Denning, D. W., et al.: Treatment of coccidioidal meningitis with fluconazole. Rev. Infect. Dis. *12*(Suppl. 3):S390-S399, 1990.

163. Tucker, R. M., Williams, P. L., Arathoon, E. G., et al.: Treatment of mycoses with itraconazole. Ann. N. Y. Acad. Sci. *544*:451-470, 1988.

164. Tynes, B. S., Crutcher, J. C., and Utz, J. P.: Histoplasma meningitis. Ann. Intern. Med. *59*:615-621, 1963.

165. Tynes, B. S., Utz, J. P, Bennett, J. E., et al.: Reducing amphotericin B reactions: A double-blind study. Am. Rev. Respir. Dis. *87*:264-268, 1963.

166. Utz, J. P., Garriques, I. L., Sande, M. A., et al.: Therapy of cryptococcosis with a combination of flucytosine and amphotericin B. J. Infect. Dis. *132*:368-373, 1975.

167. Van de Wyngaert, F. A., Sindic, C. J., Rousseau, J. J., et al.: Spinal arachnoiditis due to *Aspergillus meningitis* in a previously healthy patient. J. Neurol. *233*:41-43, 1986.

168. van Landeghem, F. K., Stiller, B., Lehmann, T. N., et al.: Aqueductal stenosis and hydrocephalus in an infant due to aspergillus infection. Clin. Neuropathol. *19*:26-29, 2000.

169. Van Peer, A., Woestenborghs, R., Heykants, J., et al.: The effects of food and dose on the oral systemic availability of itraconazole in healthy subjects. Eur J. Clin. Pharmacol. *36*:423-426, 1989.

170. Van't Wout, J. W., DeGraeff-Meeder, E. R., Paul, L. C., et al.: Treatment of two cases of cryptococcal meningitis with fluconazole. Scand. J. Infect. Dis. *20*:193-198, 1988.

171. Venger, B. H., Landon, G., and Rose, J. E.: Solitary histoplasmoma of the thalamus: Case report and literature review. Neurosurgery *20*:784-787, 1987.

172. Venugopal, P. V., Venugopal, T. V., Thiruneelakantan, D., et al.: Cerebral aspergillosis: Report of two cases. Sabouraudia *15*:225-230, 1977.

173. Verweij, P. E., Brinkman, K., Kremer, H. P. H., et al.: *Aspergillus* meningitis: Diagnosis by nonculture-based microbiological methods and management. J. Clin. Microbiol. *37*:1186-1189, 1999.

174. Walsh, T. J.: Fungal infections complicating pediatric HIV infection. *In* Pizzo, P. A., and Wilfert, C. M. (eds.): Pediatric AIDS: The Challenge of HIV Infection in Infants, Children, and Adolescents. 2nd ed. Baltimore, Williams & Wilkins, 1994, pp. 321-343.

175. Wanger, A., Mills, K., Nelson, P. W., and Rex, J. H.: Comparison of Etest and National Committee for Clinical Laboratory Standards broth microdilution method for antifungal susceptibility testing: Enhanced ability to detect amphotericin B-resistant isolates. Antimicrob. Agents. Chemother. *39*:2520-2522, 1995.

176. Wheat, L. J., Batteiger, B. E., and Sathapatayavongs, B.: *Histoplasma capsulatum* infections of the central nervous system: A clinical review. Medicine (Baltimore) *69*:244-260, 1990.

177. Wheat, L. J., Connolly-Stringfield, P. A., Baker, R. L., et al.: Disseminated histoplasmosis in the acquired immune deficiency syndrome: Clinical findings, diagnosis and treatment and review of the literature. Medicine (Baltimore) *69*:361-374, 1990.

178. Wheat, L. J., Musial, C. E., and Jenny-Avital, E.: Diagnosis and management of central nervous system histoplasmosis. Clin. Infect. Dis. *40*:844-852, 2005.

179. Wheat, J., Sarosi, G., McKinsey, D., et al.: Practice guidelines for the management of patients with histoplasmosis. Clin. Infect. Dis. *30*:688-695, 2000.

180. Windus, D. W., Stokes, J. J., Julian, B. A., et al.: Fatal *Rhizopus* infections in hemodialysis patients receiving deferoxamine. Ann. Intern. Med. *107*:678-680, 1987.

181. Young, R. C., Bennett, J. E., Vogel C. L., et al.: Aspergillosis: The spectrum of the disease in 98 patients. Medicine (Baltimore) *49*:147-173, 1970.

182. Zealear, D. S., and Winn, W. A.: The neurosurgical approach in the treatment of coccidioidal meningitis: Report of ten cases. *In* Ajello, L. (ed.): Coccidioidomycosis. Tucson, AZ, University of Arizona Press, 1967, pp. 43-53.

183. Zuger, A., Louie, E., Holzman, R. S., et al.: Cryptococcal disease in patients with the acquired immunodeficiency syndrome: Diagnostic features and outcome of treatment. Ann. Intern. Med. *104*:234-240, 1986.

EOSINOPHILIC MENINGITIS

Barbara W. Stechenberg

Eosinophilic meningitis may include any meningitis, infectious or noninfectious, in which one finds a cerebrospinal fluid (CSF) pleocytosis with a significant percentage of eosinophils. The diagnosis of eosinophilic meningitis can be made by the presence of 10 or more eosinophils in the CSF or if at least 10 percent of the CSF leukocytes are eosinophils.[18] Such a finding strongly suggests invasion of the central nervous system (CNS) by a helminthic parasite. In the last 20 years, the term *eosinophilic meningitis* has been applied more specifically to a typical form of meningitis caused by *Angiostrongylus cantonensis*, a rat lungworm found primarily in the Pacific Islands and Southeast Asia. *Gnathostoma spinigerum* and *Baylisascaris procyonis* also may be considered in particular circumstances.

The first documented case of eosinophilic meningitis was reported from Taiwan in 1945.[1] The patient was a 15-year-old boy who developed severe headache and vomiting. Examination of the CSF revealed 528 leukocytes, of which 50 percent were eosinophils. Ten actively moving nematodes also were recovered from the specimen. Since the early 1960s, many new cases have been reported, with particularly large numbers coming from Thailand,[26,27] Tahiti,[32] Taiwan,[47] and Hawaii.[12a,15]

ETIOLOGIC AGENTS

The organism that presumably is involved in most cases is the rodent lungworm. *A. cantonensis*, which as an adult is 17 to 25 mm long and 0.25 to 0.36 mm at its maximum width, has a smooth cuticle, and has three minute lips at the cephalic end. The male has a copulatory bursa supported by bursal rays.

In its life cycle, rodents such as *Rattus rattus* are the principal hosts. These rodents ingest mollusks containing third-stage larvae, which travel from the liver and lung into the general circulation. The larvae selectively leave the circulation to enter the CNS within the first 48 hours. There they develop into young adults in approximately 2 weeks.[44] From the brain, they travel to the pulmonary arteries, where their eggs are laid. The eggs hatch in the pulmonary capillaries; the first-stage forms then travel from the alveolar spaces up the rat trachea to the gastrointestinal tract, from which they are eliminated in the feces. The larvae can survive for approximately 2 weeks under humid conditions. The third-stage larvae develop in the intermediate hosts in approximately 2 weeks.

Another form of eosinophilic meningitis has been attributed to the nematode *G. spinigerum*. The adult *G. spinigerum* is stout and reddish and has a globose cephalic bulb that is separated from the body by a slight constriction. The head and anterior part of the body have spines. Males may be 11 to 25 mm long, and females may be 25 to 54 mm long. The adults lie coiled in lesions along the alimentary canal, from which they release eggs into the feces, where they become embryonated. The eggs hatch on reaching water, releasing a larva that is ingested by a copepod (*Cyclops*) and continues to develop. When the infected copepod is eaten by a fish, frog, snake, or bird, a third-stage larva develops and becomes encapsulated in the intermediate host. When it is ingested by the definitive host (cats, dogs, hogs, mink, humans), the parasite localizes in the stomach wall.[35]

The adult worms of *Baylisascaris procyonis*, the raccoon ascarid, reside in the intestines. They are large, tan-colored roundworms;

the female is 20 to 22 cm long, and the male is 9 to 11 cm long. Infection in raccoons usually is subclinical, with the adult female worm producing 115,000 to 179,000 eggs/worm/day, most of which are shed in feces.[12] Young raccoons have a higher prevalence of infection and higher parasitic burden; in their first few months of life, they ingest eggs that are in their environment or sticking to their mothers' fur.

EPIDEMIOLOGY

The geographic distribution of eosinophilic meningitis depends on the distribution of *A. cantonensis*. Many cases have been reported from Taiwan and Thailand. Other areas include Vietnam, the Society Islands (especially Tahiti), Hawaii, the Marshall Islands, and Ponape. Rodents infected with the worm have been documented in other areas of the Pacific Islands and Asia. Disease has been reported from Cuba, Egypt, and many other countries. As infected rodents are carried to other countries on cargo ships, spread of these organisms will continue to increase. Two cases have been diagnosed in the continental United States in travelers from endemic regions.[10,14] An outbreak was described in 12 of 23 young adults who had traveled together to Jamaica.[17,38]

The seasonal incidence of the disease varies in different areas. The months of highest prevalence usually correspond with the more humid periods in each country.

Patients with eosinophilic meningitis have eaten terrestrial snails, slugs, fish, or fresh-water shrimp, all of which can serve as intermediate hosts for the parasites.[41-43] In Thailand, the most common source is the *Pila* snails, which are eaten raw or pickled.[25] They may be served as an appetizer with alcoholic beverages, which may explain partly the increased incidence of the disease in men.[26] The giant African snail *Achatina fulica* is found commonly in Taiwan and may carry thousands of roundworm larvae, explaining the higher incidence of recovery of organisms from the patients in Taiwan.[43] The larvae also may remain infective in water for approximately 60 hours. Cases have been associated with the ingestion of leafy vegetables, presumed to be contaminated by slugs or snails.[15]

The distribution of disease among age groups varies. In Thailand, most of the cases occur in the third to fourth decades of life, but in Taiwan and Hawaii, most cases occur in children younger than 15 years old.[26,47] Although eosinophilic meningitis rarely occurs in very young children, one report documented disease in five children younger than 2 years.[37]

The first confirmed cases of *B. procyonis* neural larva migrans were described in the 1980s in 10-month-old and 18-month-old boys from Pennsylvania and Illinois, respectively.[11,13] Both boys had rapidly progressive, fatal eosinophilic meningoencephalitis. Subsequent reports of fatal and nonfatal disease have been reported from areas with large raccoon populations. They have occurred in rural, urban, and suburban areas. Two risk factors for acquisition of severe infection are contact with raccoons, particularly baby or young animals, or their feces or a contaminated environment, and pica or geophagia. Outdoor contamination of children's play areas by raccoons and proximity of raccoon communal latrines to human habitation may contribute to risk.[33]

PATHOGENESIS

The pathogenesis of this disease in humans has not been studied rigorously but is presumed to parallel the pathogenesis in the rodent host. The larvae are ingested, make their way into the general circulation, and selectively enter the CNS. The number of nematodes found on autopsy specimens has varied. In a 5-year-old Taiwanese girl, 150 nematodes were found on the surface of the cerebrum and cerebellum and in the subarachnoid spaces, and more than 500 were recovered from the normal saline in which the spinal cord and meninges were placed. *A. cantonensis* also were found in the pulmonary arteries.[47]

Pathologic specimens have shown a leptomeningitis in which plasma cells and eosinophils predominate. Tortuous tracks of variable size in the brain and spinal cord parenchyma surrounded by variable reaction and degenerating neurons may be present. Granulomata may form around dead *A. cantonensis*.[24,31]

Hemorrhagic, necrotic tracks caused by the organisms have been associated more commonly with *G. spinigerum* infection.[4] *Angiostrongylus* is capable of causing a vascular reaction, however, including thrombosis and rupture of vessels and arteritis, leading to formation of an aneurysm.[24] The tracks caused by *G. spinigerum* may be larger and more necrotic.

In baylisascariasis, information about the pathology is based on a few fatal cases with massive larvae invasion of the CNS.[12] Swelling of the brain, leptomeningeal congestion, and evidence of herniation have been seen. Necrosis is most marked in the periventricular white matter. Large deposits of eosinophils are present along necrotic migration tracks.

CLINICAL MANIFESTATIONS

On the basis of information obtained from patients with a history of ingestion of the intermediate hosts, the incubation period is 7 to 30 days. Most patients with typical eosinophilic meningitis have an abrupt onset of disease; a more insidious onset may be noted in 20 percent of cases. Headache is the most common and distressing symptom. It usually is intermittent but is frequent and severe. Other common symptoms are nausea, vomiting (often projectile), intermittent somnolence, malaise, anorexia, constipation, and fever with temperatures usually reaching a maximum of 38° C to 39° C in the early phase of the disease, although many patients have no documented fever. Nuchal rigidity is seen more commonly in older patients, often in association with severe headache. Paresthesias occur in a large variety of locations and are expressed as pain, numbness, itching, or a sense of worms crawling on the skin. Some patients also note diplopia with or without strabismus. Convulsions are unusual occurrences.

The findings on physical examination are normal in half the patients. Physical findings may include mild hepatomegaly, mild changes in deep tendon reflexes (usually decreased), nuchal rigidity, absent abdominal wall reflexes, and, less commonly, ophthalmoplegia or facial paralysis. Twelve percent of Thai patients had abnormal ophthalmoscopic examinations.[14]

Examination of the CSF reveals grossly turbid or opalescent fluid in most patients, with leukocyte counts usually 100/mm³ to 5000/mm³. All counts usually reach their maximum in the first 3 weeks of disease, decreasing sharply thereafter. Generally, the percentage of eosinophils in the CSF is high, often greater than 50 percent. Fluids with higher cell counts tend to have a higher percentage of eosinophils.[27,47] The proportion of eosinophils may decrease after the first 4 weeks. CSF protein concentration is moderately high (often 50 to 200 mg/dL), but the glucose concentration usually is normal.

Peripheral white blood cell count varies, but the differential cell count often shows striking eosinophilia. Examination of the feces may reveal concurrent infestation with other parasites, such as *Ascaris* or *Trichuris*.

The clinical manifestations of the eosinophilic radiculomyeloencephalitis thought to be associated with *G. spinigerum* overlap to some degree with the manifestations of typical eosinophilic meningitis. Headache is less prominent, however. Many patients report sharp, shooting pains of the trunk or limbs, flaccid paralyses, and impairment of superficial sensation.[28] Impairment of the sensorium may be sudden in association with cerebral hemorrhage. Grossly bloody spinal fluid is a common finding when myeloencephalitis is present, but it is extremely rare in typical eosinophilic meningitis.

Patients with baylisascariasis develop an acute fulminant eosinophilic meningoencephalitis; early features include low-grade fever, increasing lethargy, ataxia, somnolence, and irritability. There is progression to posturing, spasticity, and ocular or cranial nerve involvement. Seizures are common occurrences. Continued deterioration to coma and death, or, with survival, to a persistent vegetative state or severe deficits, may occur.

DIAGNOSIS

The diagnosis of cerebral angiostrongyliasis usually is based on the clinical presentation with associated CSF eosinophilia and an epidemiologic history consistent with possible exposure to the *A. cantonensis* larvae. Rarely, larvae may be recovered from the CSF. Two thirds of patients also have peripheral eosinophilia. Enzyme-linked immunosorbent assay helps to confirm the diagnosis.[39] The absence of focal findings on computed tomography and abnormal enhancement in the globus pallidus may be valuable in establishing a diagnosis.

Gnathostomiasis often is associated with xanthochromic or bloody CSF with an eosinophilic pleocytosis. Peripheral eosinophilia often is pronounced. Computed tomography and magnetic resonance imaging show areas of hemorrhage.[35] Western blot serologies are available,[9] but definitive diagnosis is by recovery of the pathogen, which may be found in subcutaneous tissue.

Baylisascariasis should be suspected in a child with CSF and peripheral eosinophilia, with severe encephalopathy with diffuse white matter disease on neuroimaging,[34] and with or without eye disease in North America or Europe. A history of exposure to raccoons or their feces would strongly suggest the diagnosis. In the absence of brain biopsy, the diagnosis is made serologically.[13]

DIFFERENTIAL DIAGNOSIS

Other helminths may invade the CNS of humans and may be associated with an eosinophilic pleocytosis,[45] including *Taenia solium*, the pork tapeworm causing cerebrospinal cysticercosis; *Schistosoma* spp.; *Paragonimus westermani*; and *Echinococcus*. The diseases produced generally have a chronic and intermittent course. Signs of a space-occupying lesion and convulsions are found frequently. Visceral myiasis with invasion of the CNS by botfly larvae may cause CSF eosinophilia.[3] The larvae of *Trichinella spiralis* can invade the CNS, but pleocytosis seems to be an unusual occurrence.[3] Neurologic involvement in visceral larva migrans caused by *Toxocara canis* rarely occurs; it may occur in association with CSF pleocytosis and eosinophilia.[21,40]

Coccidioidomycosis is the one fungal infection that may be associated with CSF eosinophilia when infection involves the meninges.[30,36] In one series, 30 percent of cases with coccidioidal meningitis had significant CSF eosinophilia.[30] Neurosyphilis and tuberculous meningitis rarely have been associated with eosinophils in the CSF, as have several malignant neoplasms, particularly lymphomas, involving the CNS.[16,22] Other known causes of significant eosinophilic pleocytosis include intrathecal injection of various foreign proteins, rabies vaccination, the insertion of rubber tubing into the CNS during neurosurgery, lymphocytic choriomeningitis,[14] and Rocky Mountain spotted fever.[8] Eosinophilic pleocytosis has been documented in infants with congenital toxoplasmosis and late-onset group B streptococcal meningitis.[20,46]

Eosinophilia in the CSF indicating hypersensitivity has been difficult to document, although one case report described the association of eosinophilic meningitis and ibuprofen therapy.[29] Eosinophilic meningitis developing after implantation of a ventriculostomy catheter impregnated with rifampin and minocycline has been reported.[2] A study documented more than 5 percent eosinophils in the ventricular fluid of patients with shunt-associated pathology, particularly malfunction.[19]

TREATMENT

In a study in Thailand in which the disappearance of headache was used as the criterion for improvement in patients with *A. cantonensis* meningitis, no significant differences were noted among groups when 284 patients were treated with analgesics alone, 96 patients were treated with analgesics and steroids (30 to 60 mg of prednisone daily for 5 days), and 56 patients were treated with analgesics and antibiotics (penicillin or tetracycline).[23] A study that compared adult patients given a 2-week course of prednisolone (60 mg/day) with patients treated with a placebo showed a significant decrease in the number of patients with headache and in the duration of headache in the prednisolone-treated group.[6] Treatment with thiabendazole also has been tried without significant benefit. The combination of albendazole or mebendazole with prednisolone has shown promise.[5,7] Treatment of gnathostomiasis is supportive, although steroids have been used to decrease meningeal inflammation. Baylisascariasis has no effective antihelminthic therapy.

COURSE AND PROGNOSIS

In most patients, eosinophilic meningitis is a self-limited disease characterized by repeated attacks of severe headache, vomiting, intermittent fever, and somnolence. Many patients experience a dramatic improvement soon after undergoing a lumbar puncture, so repeated lumbar punctures may be performed at weekly intervals to relieve the headache. In most patients, most symptoms disappear within 4 weeks of onset, often within a few days after the first lumbar puncture is performed, leaving no sequelae. The mortality rate in large series from Thailand and Taiwan has been less than 5 percent; the incidence of permanent sequelae also has been less than 5 percent for *Angiostrongylus* infection.[27,46] The mortality in gnathostomiasis is higher, ranging from 7.7 to 25 percent.[35] No evidence suggests that immunity develops after recovery from infection; many recurrences have been reported.[27,32,47] In baylisascariasis, the mortality rate is high, and survivors often have severe sequelae.

PREVENTION

Disease can be prevented only by control of rodents and proper cooking of mollusks, shrimp, fish, and other intermediate hosts. Careful washing of fruits and vegetables that may be contaminated by rodent feces also is important. The larvae may remain infective in water for 60 hours, so protection of the water supply should be attempted. Prevention of baylisascariasis depends on eliminating exposure to raccoon feces.

REFERENCES

1. Beaver, P. C., and Rosen, L.: Memorandum on the first report of *Angiostrongylus* in man by Nomura and Lin, 1945. Am. J. Trop. Med. Hyg. *13*:589-590, 1964.
2. Bell, R. S., Vo, A. H., Cooper, P. B., et al.: Eosinophilic meningitis after implantation of a rifampin and minocycline-impregnated ventriculostomy catheter in a child: Case report. J. Neurosurg. *104*(Suppl.):50-54, 2006.
3. Char, D. F. B., and Rosen, L.: Eosinophilic meningitis among children in Hawaii. J. Pediatr. *70*:28-35, 1967.
4. Chitanondh, H., and Rosen, L.: Fatal eosinophilic encephalomyelitis caused by the nematode *Gnathostoma spinigerum*. Am. J. Trop. Med. Hyg. *16*:638-645, 1967.
5. Chotmongkol, V., Sawadpanitch, K., Sawanyawisuth, K., et al.: Treatment of eosinophilic meningitis with a combination of prednisolone and mebendazole. Am. J. Trop. Med. Hyg. *74*:1122-1124, 2006.
6. Chotmongkol, V., Sawanyawisuth, K., and Thavornpirak, Y.: Corticosteroid treatment of eosinophilic meningitis. Clin. Infect. Dis. *31*:660-662, 2000.
7. Chotmongkol, V., Wongjitrat, C., Sawadpanit, K., et al.: Treatment of eosinophilic meningitis with a combination of albendazole and corticosteroid. Southeast Asian J. Trop. Med. Public Health. *35*:172-174, 2004.
8. Crennan, J. M., and VanScoy, R. E.: Eosinophilic meningitis caused by Rocky Mountain spotted fever. Am. J. Med. *80*:288-289, 1986.
9. Eamsobhana, P., Ongrotchanakun, J., Yoolek, A., et al.: Multi-immunodot for rapid differential diagnosis of eosinophilic meningitis due to parastic infections. J. Helminthol. *80*:249-254, 2006.
10. Fischer, P. R.: Eosinophilic meningitis. West. J. Med. *139*:372-373, 1983.
11. Fox, A. S., Kazacos, K. R., Gould, N. S., et al.: Fatal eosinophilic meningoencephalitis and visceral larva migrans caused by the raccoon ascarid *Baylisascaris procyonis*. N. Engl. J. Med. *312*:1619-1623, 1985.
12. Gavin, P. J., Kazacos, K. R., and Shulman, S. T.: Baylisascariasis. Clin. Microbiol. Rev. *18*:703-718, 2005.
12a. Hochberg, N. S., Park, S. Y., Blackborn, B. G., et al.: Distribution of eosinophilic meningitis cases attributable to *Angiostrongylus cantonensis*, Hawaii. Emerg. Infect. Dis. *13*:1675-1680, 2007.
13. Huff, D. S., Neatie, R. C., Binder, M. J., et al.: Case 4: The first fatal *Baylisascaris* infection in humans: An infant with eosinophilic meningoencephalitis. Pediatr. Pathol. *2*:345-352, 1984.
14. Kanchanaranya, C., and Punyagupta, S.: Case of ocular angiostrongyliasis associated with eosinophilic meningitis. Am. J. Ophthalmol. *71*:931-934, 1971.
15. Koo, J., Pien, F., and Kliks, M. M.: *Angiostrongylus* (parastrongylus) eosinophilic meningitis. Rev. Infect. Dis. *10*:1155-1162, 1988.
16. Kuberski, T.: Eosinophils in the cerebrospinal fluid. Ann. Intern. Med. *91*:70-75, 1979.
17. Lo Re, V., and Glickman, S. J.: Eosinophilic meningitis due to *Angiostrongylus cantonensis* in a returned traveler: Case report and review of the literature. Clin. Infect. Dis. *33*:e112-115, 2001.
18. Lo Re, V., and Glickman, S. J.: Eosinophilic meningitis. Am. J. Med. *114*:217-223, 2003.
19. McClinton, D., Caraccio, C., and Englander, R.: Predictors of ventriculoperitoneal shunt pathology. Pediatr. Infect. Dis. J. *20*:593-597, 2001.
20. Miron, D., Snelling, L. K., Josephson, S. L., et al.: Eosinophilic meningitis in a newborn with group B streptococcal infection. Pediatr. Infect. Dis. J. *12*:966-967, 1993.
21. Moreira-Silva, S. F., Rodrigues, M. G., Pimenta, J. L., et al.: Toxocariasis of the central nervous system: With report of two cases. Rev. Soc. Brasil. Med. Trop. *37*:169-174, 2004.
22. Mulligan, M. J., Vasu, R., Grossi, C. E., et al.: Case report: Neoplastic meningitis with eosinophilic pleocytosis in Hodgkin's disease: A case with cerebellar dysfunction and a review of the literature. Am. J. Med. Sci. *296*:322-326, 1988.
23. Noskin, G. A., McMenamin, M. B., and Grohmann, S. M.: Eosinophilic meningitis due to *Angiostrongylus cantonensis*. Neurology *42*:1423-1424, 1992.
24. Nye, S. W., Tangchai, P., and Sundarakiti, S.: Lesion of the brain in eosinophilic meningitis. Arch. Pathol. *89*:9-19, 1970.
25. Punyagupta, S.: Eosinophilic meningoencephalitis in Thailand: Summary of nine cases and observations on *Angiostrongylus cantonensis* as a causative agent and *Pila ampullacea* as a new intermediate host. Am. J. Trop. Med. Hyg. *14*:370-374, 1965.
26. Punyagupta, S., Bunnag, T., Juttijudata, P., et al.: Eosinophilic meningitis in Thailand: Epidemiologic studies of 484 typical cases and the etiologic role of *Angiostrongylus cantonensis*. Am. J. Trop. Med. Hyg. *19*:950-958, 1970.
27. Punyagupta, S., Juttijudata, P., and Bunnag, T.: Eosinophilic meningitis in Thailand: Clinical studies of 484 typical cases probably caused by *Angiostrongylus cantonensis*. Am. J. Trop. Med. Hyg. *24*:921-931, 1975.
28. Punyagupta, S., Limtrakul, C., Vichipanthu, P., et al.: Radiculomyeloencephalitis associated with eosinophilic pleocytosis: Report of nine cases. Am. J. Trop. Med. Hyg. *17*:551-560, 1968.
29. Quinn, J. P., Weinstein, R. A., and Caplan, L. R.: Eosinophilic meningitis and ibuprofen therapy. Neurology *34*:108-109, 1984.
30. Ragland, A. S., Arsura, E., Ismail, Y., et al.: Eosinophilic pleocytosis in coccidioidal meningitis: Frequency and significance. Am. J. Med. *95*:254-256, 1993.
31. Rosen, L., Chappel, R., Laqueur, G. L., et al.: Eosinophilic meningoencephalitis caused by a metastrongylid lungworm of rats. J. A. M. A. *179*:620-624, 1962.

32. Rosen, L., Loison, G., Laigret, J., et al.: Studies on eosinophilic meningitis, 3: Epidemiologic and clinical observations on Pacific Islands and the possible etiologic role of *Angiostrongylus cantonensis*. Am. J. Epidemiol. *85*:17-44, 1967.

33. Roussere, G. P., Murray, W. J., Raudenbush, C. B., et al.: Raccoon roundworm eggs near homes and risk for larva migrans disease, California communities. Emerg. Infect. Dis. *9*:1516-1522, 2003.

34. Rowley, H. A., Uht, R. M., Kazacos, K. R., et al.: Radiologic-pathologic findings in raccoon roundworm (*Baylisascaris procyonis*) encephalitis. A. J. N. R. Am. J. Neuroradiol. *21*:415-420, 2000.

35. Rusnak, J. M., and Lucey, D. R.: Clinical gnathostomiasis: Case report and review of the English language literature. Clin. Infect. Dis. *16*:33-50, 1993.

36. Schermoly, M. J., and Hinthorn, D. R.: Eosinophilia in coccidioidomycosis. Arch. Intern. Med. *148*:895-896, 1988.

37. Shih, S.-L., Hsu, C.-H., Huanig, F.-Y., et al.: *Angiostrongylus cantonensis* infection in infants and young children. Pediatr. Infect. Dis. J. *11*:1064-1065, 1992.

38. Slom, T. J., Cortese, M. M., Gerber, S. I., et al.: An outbreak of eosinophilic meningitis caused by *Angiostrongylus cantonensis* in travelers returning from the Caribbean. N. Engl. J. Med. *346*:668-675, 2002.

39. Tsai, H. C., Liu, Y. C., Kunin, C. M., et al.: Eosinophilic meningitis caused by *Angiostrongylus cantonensis*: Report of 17 cases. *111*:318-320, 2001.

40. Vidal, J. E., Sztanjbok, J., and Seguro, A. C.: Eosinophilic meningoencephalitis due to *Toxacara canis*: Case report and review of the literature. Am. J. Trop. Med. Hyg. *69*:341-343, 2003.

41. Wallace, G. D., and Rosen, L.: Studies on eosinophilic meningitis, 2: Experimental infection of shrimp and crabs with *Angiostrongylus cantonensis*. Am. J. Epidemiol. *84*:120-131, 1966.

42. Wallace, G. D., and Rosen, L.: Studies on eosinophilic meningitis, 4: Experimental infection of freshwater and marine fish with *Angiostrongylus cantonensis*. Am. J. Epidemiol. *85*:395-402, 1967.

43. Wallace, G. D., and Rosen, L.: Studies on eosinophilic meningitis, V: Molluscan hosts of *Angiostrongylus cantonensis* on Pacific Islands. Am. J. Trop. Med. Hyg. *18*:206-216, 1969.

44. Wallace, G. D., and Rosen, L.: Studies on eosinophilic meningitis, VI: Experimental infection of rats and other homoiothermic vertebrates with *Angiostrongylus cantonensis*. Am. J. Epidemiol. *89*:331-344, 1969.

45. Weller, P. F.: Eosinophilic meningitis. Am. J. Med. *95*:250-253, 1993.

46. Woods, C. R., and Englund, J.: Congenital toxoplasmosis presenting with eosinophilic meningitis. Pediatr. Infect. Dis. J. *12*:347-348, 1993.

47. Yii, C.: Clinical observations on eosinophilic meningitis and meningoencephalitis caused by *Angiostrongylus cantonensis* on Taiwan. Am. J. Trop. Med. Hyg. *25*:233-249, 1976.

CHAPTER
41   ASEPTIC MENINGITIS AND VIRAL MENINGITIS

James D. Cherry ☙ David E. Bronstein

Aseptic meningitis is an inflammatory process of the meninges. It is relatively common and is caused by many different etiologic factors. The cerebrospinal fluid (CSF) is characterized by pleocytosis, increased protein, and the absence of microorganisms on Gram stain and on routine culture. Usually, the illnesses are self-limited; with some etiologies, however, the resulting diseases may be severe, protracted, recurrent, or progressive, and lead to disability and death.

Serous meningitis, lymphocytic meningitis, and *nonparalytic poliomyelitis* are terms that were used in the past to denote aseptic meningitis. Viral meningitis is an inflammation of the leptomeninges caused by infections with many different viruses. Viruses are the causes of most cases of aseptic meningitis.

HISTORY

Aseptic meningitis is a syndrome that first was described by Wallgren in 1925.[289] Wallgren's criteria for this diagnosis included (1) an acute onset with obvious signs and symptoms of meningeal involvement; (2) alteration of CSF typical of meningitis, which may show a small or large number of cells; (3) absence of bacteria in the CSF, as shown by appropriate culture; (4) a relatively short, benign course of illness; (5) absence of local parameningeal infection (e.g., otitis, sinusitis, trauma) or a general disease that might have meningitis as a secondary manifestation; and (6) absence from the community of epidemic disease, of which meningitis is a feature. In 1951, Wallgren[290] redefined aseptic meningitis as a syndrome likely to be encountered in many different infectious diseases.

The clinical occurrence of aseptic meningitis first was recognized in epidemic poliomyelitis and in mumps at the beginning of the 20th century.[93,296] Rivers and Scott[225] reported the recovery of lymphocytic choriomeningitis (LCM) virus from the CSF of several patients with aseptic meningitis in 1935, and in 1934, Johnson and Goodpasture[148] proved that mumps was caused by a virus. The discovery of coxsackieviruses in 1948 by Dalldorf and Sickles[74] and the introduction of tissue culture in 1949 by Enders and colleagues,[94] which resulted in the discovery of echoviruses, paved the way for the widespread investigation into the etiology of aseptic meningitis.

Rasmussen[220] reported on 374 cases evaluated at the Walter Reed Army Institute of Research laboratory between 1941 and 1946 and found the probable or definite etiology in 26 percent of "viral" disease of the central nervous system (CNS). Mumps and LCM viruses were the two etiologic agents identified in his study.

In 1953, Adair and associates[5] reviewed 480 additional cases of aseptic meningitis occurring in military personnel and their dependents from 1947 through 1952 and were able to confirm the etiology in 25 percent of those patients. Herpes simplex virus (HSV) and *Leptospira* spp. were added to the previously identified mumps and LCM viruses as causes of aseptic meningitis. Meyer and associates[188] extended these studies to include 713 more children and adults with acute CNS syndromes of "viral" etiology admitted to military and Veterans Administration hospitals between 1953 and 1958. Of these 713 patients, 430 had the clinical syndrome of aseptic meningitis. Approximately 80 percent of these patients were hospitalized in the United States. An etiologic diagnosis was determined in 71 percent of patients with aseptic meningitis. In addition to the agents identified earlier, poliovirus, coxsackieviruses of groups A and B, echoviruses, and arthropod-borne viruses were identified as causes of aseptic meningitis.

Lepow and colleagues[174,175] reported the probable viral etiology in 54 percent of the 407 patients they studied in Cleveland between 1955 and 1958. In 1958, Lennette and associates[173] determined a viral etiology in 65 percent of 511 children and adults with presumed viral CNS disease in Los Angeles; 368 of these patients were diagnosed as having aseptic meningitis. Sköldenberg[253] analyzed 3117 patients admitted to the Hospital for Infectious Diseases in Stockholm between 1955 and 1964 with the diagnosis of aseptic meningitis, with or without encephalitis or myelitis, and a virologic or clinical diagnosis (or both) of an associated viral infection was established in 72.6 percent. Berlin and associates[25] performed a surveillance study of aseptic meningitis in pediatric ambulatory clinics and emergency departments of three Baltimore hospitals between July 1986 and December 1990. They identified a single viral agent in 169 (62%) of the 274 cases with laboratory study; 168 enteroviruses and 1 adenovirus were identified. Today, with the use of polymerase chain reaction (PCR) and culture and appropriate serologic study,

TABLE 41–1 Etiologic Agents, Factors, and Diseases Associated with Aseptic Meningitis

Viruses
Arboviruses (in the United States: West Nile, St. Louis, California, Colorado tick fever, Eastern equine, Western equine, Venezuelan equine, and Powassan)*
Coronaviruses
Cytomegalovirus
Encephalomyocarditis
Enteroviruses (echoviruses, coxsackieviruses A and B, polioviruses, enteroviruses) and parechoviruses
Epstein-Barr
Hendra and Nipah
Herpes simplex type 1
Herpes simplex type 2
Human herpesvirus-6
Human herpesvirus-7
Human immunodeficiency virus (HIV-1)
Human T-cell lymphotrophic virus (HTLV-1)
Influenza A and B
Lymphocytic choriomeningitis
Measles
Mumps
Parainfluenza
Parvovirus B19
Rhinoviruses
Rotaviruses
Rubella
Varicella-zoster
Variola

Postvaccine
Measles
Mumps
Polio
Rabies
Vaccinia

Bacteria
Atypical mycobacteria
Bartonella henselae
Borrelia spp. (relapsing fever)
Borrelia burgdorferi (Lyme disease)
Brucella spp.
Leptospira spp. (leptospirosis)
Mycobacterium tuberculosis
Nocardia spp. (nocardiosis)
Pyogenic—partially treated
Treponema pallidum (syphilis)

Rickettsia
Coxiella burnetii
Ehrlichia canis
Rickettsia rickettsii (Rocky Mountain spotted fever)
Rickettsia prowazekii (typhus)

Mycoplasma
Mycoplasma hominis
Mycoplasma pneumoniae

Chlamydia
Chlamydia pneumoniae
Chlamydia psittaci

Ureaplasma
Ureaplasma urealyticum

Fungi
Blastomyces dermatitidis
Candida spp.
Coccidioides immitis
Cryptococcus neoformans
Histoplasma capsulatum
Other: *Acremonium* spp., *Alternaria* spp., *Aspergillus* spp., *Blastoschizomyces capitus*, *Cephalosporium* spp., *Cladosporium trichoides*, *Drechslera hawaiiensis*, *Fusarium* spp., *Paecilomyces* spp., *Paracoccidioides brasiliensis*, *Penicillium marneffei*, *Phaeohyphomycosis*, *Pseudallescheria boydii*, *Sporothrix schenckii*, *Trichosporon beigelii*, *Ustilago* spp., *Zygomycetes* spp.

Parasites (Eosinophilic Meningitis)
Flukes: *Paragonimus westermani*, schistosomiasis, fascioliasis
Roundworms: *Angiostrongylus cantonensis*, *Gnathostoma spinigerum*, *Baylisascaris procyonis*, *Strongyloides stercoralis*, *Trichinella spiralis*, *Toxocara canis*
Tapeworms: cysticercosis

Parasites (Noneosinophilic Meningitis)
Acanthamoeba
Naegleria fowleri
Toxoplasma gondii (toxoplasmosis)

Parameningeal Infections
Malignancy
Central nervous system tumor
Leukemia

Immune Diseases
Behçet syndrome
Lupus erythematosus
Sarcoidosis

Miscellaneous
Antimicrobial agents
Epidermoid, dermoid, other cysts
Foreign bodies (shunt, reservoir)
Heavy metal poisoning
Intrathecal injections (e.g., contrast media, antibiotics)
Kawasaki disease
Other drugs

In other areas of the world, many other arboviruses are important.

the etiology of most cases of aseptic meningitis can be determined.

ETIOLOGY

Table 41–1 lists etiologic agents and factors in aseptic meningitis. At present, the diagnostic work-up of aseptic meningitis usually is not undertaken vigorously, and the etiologic agent is identified in only approximately 10 percent of all cases. Epidemiologic study and intensive investigations at some centers indicate, however, that most cases result from viral infections. Enteroviruses account for approximately 85 percent of all cases of aseptic meningitis.[44,78-80,195] The following enteroviruses have been asso-

ciated with aseptic meningitis: polioviruses 1 to 3; coxsackieviruses A 1 to 14, 16 to 18, 21, 22, and 24; coxsackieviruses B 1 to 6; echoviruses 1 to 9, 11 to 21, 24 to 27, and 29 to 33; enterovirus 71; and parechoviruses 1 and 2.

In recent years, multiple outbreaks of aseptic meningitis caused by enteroviruses have been described, including outbreaks caused by echovirus 30 in several countries throughout Eastern and Western Europe, China, Japan, Australia, the Arabian Gulf, the United States, and Brazil.* Echovirus 13 was responsible for reported outbreaks of aseptic meningitis in the United States,

*See references 9, 19, 26, 51, 54, 58, 88, 99, 119, 132, 152, 161, 204, 223, 245, 275, 283, 284, 292, 310.

England, Wales, Germany, Belgium, Spain, France, Lithuania, Israel, Japan, Korea, and Australia.* Enterovirus 71 caused a major epidemic in Taiwan from 1998 to 1999, with multiple cases of hand, foot, and mouth syndrome associated with aseptic meningitis and other neurologic manifestations.[142,177,178,181,249,291,292,304,306] Similar outbreaks of aseptic meningitis caused by enterovirus 71 were reported in Malaysia, Japan, and Australia.[59,106,140,187,248-250] Other enteroviruses involved in more recent outbreaks include echovirus 4 in Italy and Israel/Palestine,[129,217] echovirus 9 in Japan and regions of the United States,[8,57] echovirus 11 among institutionalized children in Israel,[218] echovirus 16 in Cuba,[241] and echovirus 33 in New Zealand.[144] In the United States, the most common specific enteroviral types in the vaccine era are coxsackievirus B5 and echoviruses 4, 6, 9, and 11, with echoviruses 9 and 30 being the most frequently identified etiologies of aseptic meningitis since 2003.[54,56,226]

Sharing seasonality with the enteroviruses, several arboviruses cause CNS disease in North America. Although encephalitis is the most recognizable manifestation of many of these infections, some arboviruses commonly are associated with aseptic meningitis as well.[117,226,230] Since the mid-1990s, outbreaks of West Nile virus meningitis and encephalitis have occurred in Romania, Russia, and Israel.[63,214,278] First detected in the Western Hemisphere in 1999 in New York City, West Nile virus subsequently spread across North America from the Atlantic to the Pacific coasts and into Canada and Mexico.[35,96,145,201,212] Between 1999 and 2005, greater than 18,000 cases were reported in the United States, with more than 700 deaths.[55,134] An estimated 1 in 150 infections results in severe neurologic illness, with meningitis as the primary manifestation in 16 to 40 percent of hospitalized patients.[150] Although the incidence of neuroinvasive disease increases with age, West Nile virus has been responsible for meningitis in young children and adolescents, occurring in at least one quarter of the 150 pediatric cases diagnosed in the United States in 2002.[65,103,133] Even in regions with increased incidence of West Nile virus, episodes of meningitis caused by enterovirus greatly outnumber those caused by West Nile virus.[150]

Before the introduction of West Nile virus, arboviruses accounted for approximately 5 percent of cases of aseptic meningitis in North America, with St. Louis encephalitis virus being the most common.[36,41,46,48] Infection with La Crosse encephalitis virus (a California encephalitis virus subtype) often resembles herpes encephalitis, but it may manifest as aseptic meningitis in children. In a study of 127 patients, mainly children, hospitalized in the southern United States with La Crosse virus infection, headache, fever, vomiting, and seizures were predominant findings. Thirteen percent of these patients had aseptic meningitis.[186] Other California serogroup viruses, such as Jamestown Canyon virus and snowshoe hare virus, and other arboviruses, such as Colorado tick fever, result in aseptic meningitis more frequently than encephalitis.[117,226,262] Tick-borne encephalitis can manifest as aseptic meningitis in endemic areas. Tick-borne encephalitis virus cases were reported more recently in studies conducted in Slovenia and Sweden, and in mild cases, the clinical presentation was that of aseptic meningitis.[125,176,182]

Aseptic meningitis is an occasional manifestation of acute and recurrent genital infections with HSV-2.[15,24,71,87,254,274] In contrast to HSV-1 CNS infections, which without treatment usually are fatal, HSV-2 aseptic meningitis in otherwise immunocompetent patients is a benign, self-limited illness. Herpes family viruses other than HSV-1 and HSV-2 also are potential causes of aseptic meningitis. Although neurologic involvement in primary varicella-zoster viral infections usually is an encephalitis rather than a benign meningitis, pleocytosis is noted occasionally in herpes

zoster.[78,218,222,295] Varicella-zoster virus has been identified by PCR in the CSF of patients who had acute aseptic meningitis but no cutaneous lesions.[1,92,147] A variety of neurologic disorders, including aseptic meningitis, are rare complications of Epstein-Barr virus infection.[97,105,121,266,280] Most noncongenital infections with cytomegalovirus in nonimmunocompromised patients are unrecognized; however, occasional instances of aseptic meningitis have been noted.[78-80]

The role of human herpesvirus-6 (HHV-6) in causing meningitis is unclear; although HHV-6 has been found in CSF samples from infants with meningitis, the virus also is detectable in the CSF of asymptomatic individuals.[11,38,305,308] Similarly, PCR identified HHV-7 in the CSF of six children with neurologic diseases, including aseptic meningitis, meningoencephalitis, facial palsy, vestibular neuritis, and febrile seizures.[215] The role of HHV-7 as a causative agent in aseptic meningitis remains to be determined.

Occasionally, meningitis or meningoencephalitis occurs as a manifestation of acute illness with HIV-1 infection.[16,128] Neurologic manifestations develop 3 to 6 weeks after primary infection at the same time as an infectious mononucleosis–like illness.

Although LCM virus was an important historical cause of aseptic meningitis, it rarely is recognized today as a cause of meningitis except in animal-exposure outbreak situations.[17,21,28,81,188] In 1974, eight cases of aseptic meningitis caused by LCM virus were found in New York State.[81] Many sporadic instances of LCM virus infection probably go unrecognized. Physicians should be alert to the possibility in all situations of rodent (pet or wild) exposure. Encephalomyocarditis virus is another rodent virus that rarely is recognized in humans.[293] It is associated with a variety of neurologic manifestations, including aseptic meningitis.[107]

Adenoviral types 1, 2, 3, 5, 6, 7, 12, 14, and 32 have been associated with meningitis and meningoencephalitis.[25,69,78-80,98,159,210,251,257] Although they occur infrequently, adenoviral CNS infections tend to be more severe than are enteroviral infections. Rarely, aseptic meningitis has been noted during illnesses caused by rhinoviruses, influenza A and B viruses, parainfluenza viruses, parvovirus B19 virus, rotaviruses, and coronaviruses.* Most infections with measles, rubella, and variola viruses that involve the CNS are encephalitic.[42,43,45,192]

In the pre-vaccine era, mumps virus was the agent responsible for the greatest number of cases of aseptic meningitis; today in the United States, use of vaccine has rendered mumps rare, although mumps outbreaks with associated cases of aseptic meningitis occur occasionally.[47,57] Aseptic meningitis and encephalitis resulting from administration of mumps vaccine have been noted in Canada, Brazil, Japan, and Europe.[†] The Leningrad 3, Urabe Am 9, and three Japanese strains of vaccine viruses have been implicated. In the United States, where the Jeryl Lynn vaccine strain has been used exclusively, the rate of encephalitis in vaccinees has been no higher than that of the observed background incidence of similar illness in the population.[47] More recently, a preliminary analysis of the Vaccine Safety Datalink project showed a possible increased risk of developing aseptic meningitis 8 to 14 days after receiving immunization with Jeryl Lynn mumps vaccine strain. A follow-up case-control evaluation of hospitalized cases failed to show an increased risk, however.[30]

Neurologic illness is a rare complication of measles, smallpox, polio, and rabies viral vaccines. In most instances, the illnesses are complex and severe, but occasionally, aseptic meningitis is the only manifestation.[25,42,45,53,191,246,261] A case of aseptic meningitis caused by vaccine-derived poliovirus was reported in the Philippines in 2001.[53] It was in association with two pediatric cases of acute flaccid paralysis that occurred during the same time period.

---

*See references 52, 61, 62, 85, 151, 158, 162, 198, 200, 258, 275, 277.

*See references 13, 40, 72, 78-80, 141, 157, 203, 205, 209, 224, 285, 301.
†See references 10, 14, 66, 67, 73, 75, 89, 185, 190, 199.

Viral isolates from all three patients revealed type 1 poliovirus derived from the Sabin vaccine strain.

Certain bacteria are important to recognize as etiologic agents in aseptic meningitis because the illnesses are treatable and early initiation of therapy is crucial. Of greatest importance is tuberculous meningitis. Early treatment of this illness nearly always results in complete cure, whereas diagnostic delay or inadequate treatment frequently results in permanent neurologic sequelae. Lyme disease, relapsing fever, brucellosis, leptospirosis, and rickettsial infections are illnesses acquired either directly or indirectly from animals, in which aseptic meningitis may be a part of the disease process.* *Mycoplasma pneumoniae* is an important cause of neurologic illness.[89,124,215,279] Pönkä[216] noted that 8 of 560 hospitalized patients with *M. pneumoniae* infections had aseptic meningitis, and 18 had encephalitis or meningoencephalitis. *Mycoplasma hominis* and *Ureaplasma urealyticum* are rare causes of neonatal meningitis.[108,183,286,287] Meningitis and meningoencephalitis have been associated with *Chlamydia pneumoniae* infections.[12,123,255,267] Partially treated common bacterial meningitides are a common cause of meningitis in which cultures of CSF fail to grow organisms. Antigen detection systems, such as latex agglutination, can be useful in identifying the causative agents in some of these cases.

Numerous fungi and yeasts cause meningitis.[238] Although many fungal meningitides occur almost exclusively in immunocompromised patients, children and adults with normal immune status experience meningitis most commonly caused by the following: *Blastomyces dermatitidis, Coccidioides immitis, Cryptococcus neoformans, Cladosporium* spp., *Histoplasma capsulatum*, and *Paracoccidioides brasiliensis*. In infants who are premature or younger than 1 month of age, *Candida albicans* is an important cause of meningitis, associated with significant morbidity and mortality.[22,120,196]

Parasites occasionally cause aseptic meningitis. Eosinophilic meningitis is caused by *Angiostrongylus cantonensis*, a rat lungworm.[60,128,228,294] Aseptic meningitis caused by *A. cantonensis* has been observed on several islands in the Pacific, and the infection may be acquired by the consumption of freshwater shrimp. *Baylisascaris procyonis*, the intestinal roundworm of raccoons, is a rare cause of neural larva migrans in infants and young children and manifests as acute fulminant eosinophilic meningoencephalitis.[109,110,300] Between 1973 and 2002, 14 probable or confirmed cases were described in eight states throughout the United States, reported approximately once every 1 to 2 years. The infection was fatal in 6 of the 14 children, and all documented survivors were neurologically devastated.[300]

A sterile CSF pleocytosis occurs in 12 to 13 percent of young infants with bacterial urinary tract infections[6,100,269] and in approximately one third of patients with Kawasaki disease who undergo lumbar puncture.[82,116] Numerous drugs and biologicals have been implicated in aseptic meningitis.† Of most importance in pediatrics are trimethoprim-sulfamethoxazole and intravenous immunoglobulin. Other causes of aseptic meningitis are listed in Table 41-1.‡

EPIDEMIOLOGY

Because many different types of organisms cause aseptic meningitis, no unified epidemiologic pattern exists. The epidemiology of the specific individual infectious agents or diseases is presented in detail in the various chapters of this book, and only a brief overview is presented here.

Because approximately 85 percent of all cases of aseptic meningitis are caused by enteroviral infections, the basic epidemiologic pattern of aseptic meningitis reflects these agents. In temperate climates, most cases occur in the summer and fall; infection with enteroviruses is spread directly from person to person, and the incubation period usually is 4 to 6 days. Epidemiologic considerations in aseptic meningitis caused by agents other than enteroviruses depend markedly on season, geography, climatic conditions, animal exposures, and many other factors related to the specific pathogens.

CLINICAL MANIFESTATIONS

Aseptic meningitis has many different causes (see Table 41-1), and clinical manifestations vary with the different diseases. In some instances, the signs and symptoms resulting from meningeal inflammation dominate the clinical illness, whereas in other instances, the main signs and symptoms reflect other organ system involvement. Clinical manifestations in aseptic meningitis, regardless of etiology, also vary markedly by patient age.

ENTEROVIRUSES

Enteroviruses are the most common cause of aseptic meningitis, and they can be considered the prototype for a description of general clinical manifestations of aseptic meningitis.* Even among the enteroviruses, however, significant differences in clinical manifestations exist among the different viral types. Some general aspects of epidemic enteroviral aseptic meningitis are presented by viral type in Chapter 178.

The onset of illness generally is acute, although it may be insidious over the course of a week or so, or may be preceded by a nonspecific acute febrile illness of a few days' duration. Almost all children have fever, and most older children have headache, which most often is retro-orbital or frontal in location. Photophobia is common. Temperature elevation varies, ranging from 38° C to 40.5° C (100.4° F to 105° F), and usually lasts approximately 5 days. Occasionally, fever is biphasic, with the initial elevation occurring before the onset of neurologic signs and symptoms. Anorexia, nausea, and vomiting are common, and abdominal pain and diarrhea also are reported frequently.

Meningeal signs (stiff neck and back, tightness of the hamstring muscles, Brudzinski and Kernig signs) usually are present, but deep tendon reflexes usually are normal or hyperactive. Seizures occur occasionally, usually when concomitant high fever is present. Muscle weakness rarely is reported, but myalgia occasionally is noted. In young children, fever, irritability, and lethargy are the most common findings. Infants may be irritable and show resentment to handling, and the fontanelle may be tense.

Other manifestations of enteroviral infections also occur in children with aseptic meningitis. Most common is pharyngitis, which may occur during infection with all of the neurotropic enteroviral types. Rash occurs commonly, but varies by viral type. With echovirus 9 meningitis, 30 to 50 percent of children have rashes, whereas with echovirus 6, exanthem is rare. Cases of meningitis caused by enterovirus 71 frequently are accompanied by hand, foot, and mouth syndrome. Enanthem, pleurodynia, pericarditis, myocarditis, and conjunctivitis are other findings noted in children with enteroviral aseptic meningitis. Illness often is biphasic with fever, an interlude, then return of fever and neurologic manifestations.

*See references 27, 29, 31, 33, 95, 115, 146, 149, 154, 164, 171, 206, 211, 260, 273, 288, 299, 303, 309.
†See references 17, 37, 83, 101, 118, 127, 184, 187, 197, 219, 302.
‡See references 49, 86, 104, 114, 136, 139, 163, 164, 166, 172, 184, 247, 268.

*See references 3, 8, 9, 32, 50-53, 58, 76, 85, 102, 111, 122, 126, 129, 130, 135, 137, 142, 152, 155, 156, 169, 178, 221, 229, 234, 235, 237, 239, 252, 265, 270, 297.

CSF leukocyte counts vary from a few cells to a few thousand cells; the median is in the range of 100 to 500 cells/mm⁴. The percentage of neutrophils also varies greatly. Initially, a predominance of neutrophils commonly occurs, but later, CSF examinations show a decline in the percentage of neutrophils. The CSF protein usually is elevated mildly, and the glucose concentration usually is normal; rarely, hypoglycorrhachia is noted.

The duration of illness varies. Usually, disability because of neurologic involvement lasts 1 to 2 weeks.

ASEPTIC MENINGITIS CAUSED BY OTHER AGENTS

In meningitis caused by arboviruses, involvement of the brain often occurs as well (meningoencephalitis). With St. Louis and California viral infections in children, the illness commonly is benign, without changes in sensorium or other findings indicative of brain involvement. Similarly, meningitis without encephalitis is present in a significant proportion of patients with neuroinvasive West Nile virus infections.[133,212] Seizures occur more commonly in arboviral meningitides than in enteroviral illnesses of otherwise comparable severity.[131] When neurologic disease caused by mumps is recognized, usually evidence of brain involvement is present. Examination of the CSF in mild cases of mumps often reveals pleocytosis.

Tuberculous meningitis usually has a gradual onset over the course of 2 to 3 weeks.[160,193,227] Initially, personality changes, irritability, anorexia, listlessness, and low-grade fever may be present, followed by signs of increased intracranial pressure, such as drowsiness, stiff neck, cranial nerve palsies, inequality of the pupils, vomiting, and convulsions. Finally, coma, irregular pulse and respirations, and high fever occur. In fungal diseases, the course of meningitis is similar to the course of tuberculosis. In tuberculosis and several fungal meningitides, such as those caused by *C. immitis*, *H. capsulatum*, and *C. neoformans*, historical and radiographic evidence of pulmonary disease may be present.

Aseptic meningitis caused by *M. pneumoniae* is unique in that it frequently occurs a few days to 3 weeks after a respiratory illness (pharyngitis, bronchitis, or pneumonia).[124,179,256,279] In non-enteroviral aseptic meningitides, the CSF findings generally are similar to those in enteroviral disease. Generally, the likelihood of a predominance of neutrophils is less in other aseptic meningitides, and low glucose levels are likely in parameningeal bacterial infections, partially treated bacterial meningitides, brain tumors, leukemic infiltration, *M. pneumoniae* infections, fungal infections, and tuberculosis.

RECURRENT ASEPTIC MENINGITIS (MOLLARET MENINGITIS)

In 1944, Mollaret[194] described three patients with recurrent aseptic meningitis whom he had observed over the course of 15 years. Subsequently, many other cases have been reported, and some cases have been noted in children.[34,67,68,138,213,263,272] The illness is characterized by recurrent attacks of fever with meningeal signs and symptoms. The attacks last several days and are separated by symptom-free periods lasting weeks or months. In addition to a lymphocyte predominant pleocytosis, CSF samples obtained from certain patients contain large mononuclear cells (Mollaret cells). The disease remits spontaneously. HSV-2 has been identified by PCR or DNA probes in the CSF of most patients with recurrent meningitis.[18,67,91,167,213,271,272,242,281] Other viruses, such as HSV-1 and Epstein-Barr virus, and noninfectious causes, such as systemic lupus erythematosus, intracranial cysts, and environmental exposures, also have been identified as less frequent etiologies of recurrent meningitis.[121,163,236,240,263]

DIFFERENTIAL DIAGNOSIS

Careful analysis of the history and epidemiologic circumstances may point toward one of the specific causes listed in Table 41–1. During the summer and autumn, the presence of pleurodynia, herpangina, or unexplained febrile eruptions in the community suggests the possibility of enteroviral infections. Acute paralytic disorders in other patients suggests poliomyelitis or West Nile virus. Exposure to mosquitoes and encephalitis in horses implicates certain arboviruses, and exposure to ticks may be suggestive of Lyme disease, relapsing fever, or rickettsial disease, depending on the geographic location and other symptoms of the illness. A history of swimming in waters contaminated by urine from infected animals and exposure to rats in urban slums suggest leptospiral infection. Knowledge of clear-cut exposure to or concurrent evidence of mumps or of one of the common exanthems is helpful in delineating the differential diagnosis. The association of pneumonia or other respiratory illness preceding aseptic meningitis strongly suggests the possibility of *M. pneumoniae* as the etiologic agent.

Most difficult from the diagnostic, therapeutic, and prognostic points of view are instances of incipient or partially treated bacterial (especially when caused by *Haemophilus influenzae*) or mycobacterial meningitis. The clinical findings; the dosage of antibiotic previously used; the spinal fluid smear, latex agglutination, or other rapid antigen identification test; the culture; and the glucose level may be helpful in diagnosing bacterial meningitis. The quantitative determination of C-reactive protein in the CSF also may be useful in differentiating bacterial from viral meningitis.[2,70,77,207,208] Lindquist and associates[180] found that the determination of CSF concentrations of lactate was the most useful test in differentiating bacterial from nonbacterial causes of meningitis. Studies suggest that the presence of tumor necrosis factor-α in the CSF is rare in viral infections, but common in bacterial disease.[7,90,113] When tuberculous meningitis is suspected, a careful evaluation of contacts, a careful examination of an appropriately stained smear from the pellicle of the CSF that was allowed to settle, and a positive tuberculin reaction may confirm the diagnosis. Because combined bacterial and viral infection has occurred, examinations of CSF should be repeated if any doubt exists. The possibility that the observed meningeal reaction is of neither viral nor bacterial origin must be considered. Finally, CNS tumor must be considered in the differential diagnosis, particularly if hypoglycorrhachia and prominent signs of increased intracranial pressure are present.[166]

SPECIFIC DIAGNOSIS

Obtaining a meticulous history is essential. The clinician must evaluate exposure of the patient in the past 2 to 3 weeks to illness in contacts; exposure to mosquitoes, ticks, and animals during recent vacations, picnics, and so on; awareness of illness in animals, especially horses and other Equidae, in the patient's environment; recent travel from the home area; recent injections or medications of any kind; and the possibility of accidental exposure to heavy metals.

The CSF must be examined carefully to exclude disorders that respond to specific therapy. Smears for bacteria, appropriate rapid antigen identification tests, and cultures of the CSF are mandatory; the history and clinical findings may indicate the need for performing acid-fast stain and culture of the sediment for mycobacteria. Other circumstances may indicate the need for excluding fungal or protozoal infection; atypical cells may require cytopathologic study to exclude neural neoplasms, which may manifest acutely.

In any patient suspected to have viral meningitis, spinal fluid, blood, feces, and throat swabs should be collected and sent to a laboratory offering viral diagnostic services. An additional serum specimen should be collected 10 to 21 days later so that paired sera can be examined for antibody titer increases. This pairing is particularly useful in arboviral, LCM viral, encephalomyocarditis viral, leptospiral, borrelial, rickettsial, mycoplasmal, and toxoplasmal infections. Although these studies may not provide an immediate diagnosis, they may give early warning of a specific epidemic, and they are useful for prognostication, particularly in very young infants.

The introduction of PCR has facilitated the etiologic diagnosis of CNS viral infections, particularly infections caused by enteroviruses and herpesviruses.* PCR detects enterovirus in the CSF more rapidly than does cell culture and has been shown to shorten the duration of hospitalization for children with meningitis, reducing costs.[202,264] PCR is the test of choice for detecting CNS infections caused by HSV, and molecular techniques also have been used to identify in CSF such rare causes of meningitis and meningoencephalitis as varicella-zoster virus, HHV-6, parvovirus B19, and rotavirus.[20,147,165,282] Although such techniques are of limited value for many arboviruses with short periods of viremia and presence in the CSF, real-time PCR analysis of CSF samples used during the 1999 West Nile encephalitis outbreak in New York had 57 percent sensitivity and 100 percent specificity.[64,170]

TREATMENT

Hospitalization usually is necessary because of the possibility of treatable bacterial disease and the frequent need for fluid therapy for dehydration. Treatment is symptomatic. Headache and hyperesthesia are treated with rest; analgesics; and a reduction in room light, noise, and visitors. Antipyretics are recommended for fever. Using acetaminophen rather than aspirin is prudent because of the risk for developing Reye syndrome associated with the latter antipyretic. Codeine, morphine, and the phenothiazine derivatives often are used for pain and vomiting, but they rarely are necessary in children, and they should be avoided because they may induce misleading signs and symptoms. The investigational antiviral drug pleconaril has been shown to be effective in the treatment of enteroviral meningitis; however, this drug presently is unavailable.[84,231,233] Treatment for such illnesses as tuberculous meningitis, fungal meningitides, and other illnesses for which specific therapies are available is covered in specific chapters of this book.

Several weeks after the patient has apparently recovered, a careful neuromuscular assessment should be conducted to ensure that muscular weakness is not a sequela. Bilateral audiometry is recommended, especially when mumps virus was involved.

PROGNOSIS

The prognosis in aseptic meningitis depends on the etiology. Some illnesses have an ominous prognosis (tuberculous meningitis, parameningeal infections, rickettsial infections), but patients usually do well if appropriate specific therapy is instituted early in the course of the illness. In *C. immitis* meningitis, the prognosis for cure is guarded even with early optimal therapy.

In enteroviral and other viral meningitides, children usually recover completely. Some patients complain of fatigue, irritability, decreased ability to concentrate, muscle pain, muscle weakness and spasm, and incoordination for several weeks after an acute illness. Although the outcome of enteroviral meningitis most often is without residual, some infants who have enteroviral

meningitis in the first few months of life have an increased risk for altered language development.[23,298] Formally evaluating such children at age 3 to 6 years is important.

PREVENTION

The universal use of polio and mumps vaccines in children clearly is effective in controlling these two diseases. Control of insect vectors by suitable spraying methods and eradication of insect breeding sites is important in the control of many arboviruses. The control of animal vectors such as mice and rats alters the incidence of infections with LCM and encephalomyocarditis viruses.

REFERENCES

1. Aberle, S. W., Aberle, J. H., Steininger, C., and Puchhammer-Stockl, E.: Quantitative real time PCR detection of varicella-zoster virus DNA in cerebrospinal fluid in patients with neurological disease. Med. Microbiol. Immunol. *194*:7-12, 2005.
2. Abramson, J. S., Hampton, K. D., Babu, S., et al.: The use of C-reactive protein from cerebrospinal fluid for differentiating meningitis from other central nervous system diseases. J. Infect. Dis. *151*:854-858, 1985.
3. Abzug, M. J., Levin, M. J., and Rotbart, H. A.: Profile of enterovirus disease in the first two weeks of life. Pediatr. Infect. Dis. J. *12*:820-824, 1993.
4. Abzug, M. J., Loeffelholz, M., and Rotbart, H. A.: Clinical and laboratory observations: Diagnosis of neonatal enterovirus infection by polymerase chain reaction. J. Pediatr. *126*:447-450, 1995.
5. Adair, C. V., Gauld, R. L., and Smadel, J. E.: Aseptic meningitis, a disease of diverse etiology: Clinical and etiologic studies on 854 cases. Ann. Intern. Med. *39*:675-704, 1953.
6. Adler-Shohet, F. C., Cheung, M. M., Hill, M., and Lieberman, J. M.: Aseptic meningitis in infants younger than six months of age hospitalized with urinary tract infections. Pediatr. Infect. Dis. J. *22*:1039-1042, 2003.
7. Akalin, H., Akdis, A. C., Mistik, R., et al.: Cerebrospinal fluid interleukin-1 beta/interleukin-1 receptor antagonist balance and tumor necrosis factor concentrations in tuberculous, viral and acute bacterial meningitis. Scand. J. Infect. Dis. *26*:667-674, 1994.
8. Akasu, Y.: Outbreak of aseptic meningitis due to ECHO-9 in northern Kyushu island in the summer of 1997. Kurume Med. J. *46*:97-104, 1999.
9. Amvrosiena, T. V., Titov, L. P., Mulders, M., et al.: Viral water contamination as the cause of aseptic meningitis outbreak in Belarus. Cent. Eur. J. Public Health. *9*:154-157, 2001.
10. Anonymous: Mumps meningitis and MMR vaccination. Lancet *2*:1015-1016, 1989.
11. Ansari, A., Li, S., Abzug, M. J., and Weinberg, A.: Human herpesviruses 6 and 7 and central nervous system infection in children. Emerg. Infect. Dis. *10*:1450, 2004.
12. Anton, E., Otegui, A., and Alonso, A.: Meningoencephalitis and *Chlamydia pneumoniae* infection. Eur. J. Neurol. 7:586, 2000.
13. Arisoy, E. S., Demmler, G. J., Thakar, S., et al.: Meningitis due to parainfluenza virus type 3: Report of two cases and review. Clin. Infect. Dis. *17*:995-997, 1993.
14. Arruda, W. O., and Kondageski, C.: Aseptic meningitis in a large MMR vaccine campaign (590,609 people) in Curitiba, Parana, Brazil, 1998. Rev. Inst. Med. Trop. Sao Paulo *43*:301-302, 2001.
15. Atia, W. A., Ratnatunga, C. S., Greenfield, C., et al.: Aseptic meningitis and herpes simplex proctitis: A case report. Br. J. Vener. Dis. *58*:53-58, 1982.
16. Atwood, W. J., Berger, J. R., Kaderman, R., et al.: Human immunodeficiency virus type 1 infection of the brain. Clin. Microbiol. Rev. *6*:339-366, 1993.
17. Auxier, G. G.: Aseptic meningitis associated with administration of trimethoprim and sulfamethoxazole. Am. J. Dis. Child. *144*:144-145, 1990.
18. Bachmeyer, C., de la Blanchardière, A., Lepercq, J., et al.: Recurring episodes of meningitis (Mollaret's meningitis) with one showing an association with herpes simplex virus type 2. J. Infect. *32*:247-248, 1996.
19. Bailly, J. L., Brosson D., Archimbaud C., et al.: Genetic diversity of echovirus 30 during a meningitis outbreak, demonstrated by direct molecular typing from cerebrospinal fluid. J. Med. Virol. *68*:558-567, 2002.
20. Barah, F., Vallely, P. J., Chiswick, M. L., et al.: Association of human parvovirus B19 infection with acute meningoencephalitis. Lancet *358*:729-730, 2001.
21. Barton, L. L., and Hyndman, N. J.: Lymphocytic choriomeningitis virus: Reemerging central nervous system pathogen. Pediatrics *105*:835, 2000.
22. Benjamin, D. K., Stoll, B. J., Fanaroff, A. A., et al.: Neonatal candidiasis among extremely low birth weight infants: risk factors, mortality rates, and neurodevelopmental outcomes at 18 to 22 months. Pediatrics *117*:84-92, 2006.

---

*See references 4, 8, 64, 112, 129, 143, 153, 161, 167, 232, 243, 244, 276, 307.

23. Bergman, I., Painter, M. J., Wald, E. R., et al.: Outcome in children with enteroviral meningitis during the first year of life. J. Pediatr. *110*:705-709, 1987.

24. Bergstrom, T., Vahlne, A., Alestig, K., et al.: Primary and recurrent herpes simplex virus type 2-induced meningitis. J. Infect. Dis. *162*:322-330, 1990.

25. Berlin, L. E., Rorabaugh, M. L., Heldrich, F., et al.: Aseptic meningitis in infants <2 years of age: Diagnosis and etiology. J. Infect. Dis. *168*:888-892, 1993.

26. Bernit, E., de Lamballerie, X., Zandotti, et al.: Prospective investigation of a large outbreak of meningitis due to echovirus 30 during summer 2000 in Marseilles, France. Medicine *83*:245-253, 2004.

27. Bharti, A. R., Nally, J. E., Ricaldi, J. N., et al.: Leptospirosis: A zoonotic disease of global importance. Lancet Infect. Dis. *3*:757-771, 2003.

28. Biggar, R. J., Woodall, J. P., Walter, P. D., et al.: Lymphocytic choriomeningitis outbreak associated with pet hamsters: Fifty-seven cases from New York State. J. A. M. A. *232*:494-500, 1975.

29. Bingham, P. M., Galetta, S. L., Athreya, B., et al.: Neurologic manifestations in children with Lyme disease. Pediatrics *96*:1053-1056, 1995.

30. Black, S., Shinefield, H., Ray, P., et al.: Risk of hospitalization because of aseptic meningitis after measles-mumps-rubella vaccination in one- to two-year-old children: An analysis of the Vaccine Safety Datalink (VSD) Project. Pediatr. Infect. Dis. *16*:500-503, 1997.

31. Bowen, A. P.: A cluster of children with Lyme meningitis presenting to one emergency department in a Boston suburb. J. Emerg. Nurs. *28*:355-357, 2002.

32. Bowen, G. S., Fisher, M. C., DeForest, A., et al.: Epidemic of meningitis and febrile illness in neonates caused by echo type 11 virus in Philadelphia. Pediatr. Infect. Dis. *2*:359-363, 1983.

33. Bruhn, F. W.: Lyme disease. Am. J. Dis. Child. *138*:467-470, 1984.

34. Bruyn, G. W., Straathof, L. J. A., and Raymakers, G. M. J.: Mollaret's meningitis: Differential diagnosis and diagnostic pitfalls. Neurology *12*:745-753, 1962.

35. Buck, P. A., Sockett, P., Barker, I. K., et al.: West Nile virus: Surveillance activities in Canada. Ann. Epidemiol. *13*:582, 2003.

36. Calisher, C. H.: Medically important arboviruses of the United States and Canada. Clin. Microbiol. Rev. *7*:89-116, 1994.

37. Carlson, J., and Wiholm, B. E.: Trimethoprim-associated aseptic meningitis. Scand. J. Infect. Dis. *19*:687-691, 1987.

38. Caserta, M. T., Hall, C. B., Schnabel, K., et al.: Neuroinvasion and persistence of human herpesvirus 6 in children. J. Infect. Dis. *170*:1586-1589, 1994.

39. Cassell, G. H., and Cole, B. C.: Mycoplasmas as agents of human disease. N. Engl. J. Med. *304*:80-89, 1981.

40. Cassinotti, P., Schultze, D., Schlageter, P., et al.: Persistent human parvovirus B19 infection following an acute infection with meningitis in an immunocompetent patient. Eur. J. Clin. Microbiol. Infect. Dis. *12*:701-704, 1993.

41. Centers for Disease Control: Neurotropic viral diseases surveillance: Aseptic meningitis, annual summary 1975. Issued July 1977.

42. Centers for Disease Control: Neurotropic diseases surveillance, summary 1974-1976. Issued October 1977.

43. Centers for Disease Control: Encephalitis surveillance, annual summary 1978. Issued May 1981.

44. Centers for Disease Control: Enterovirus surveillance, summary 1970-1979. Issued November 1981.

45. Centers for Disease Control: Measles surveillance, 1977-1981. Issued September 1982.

46. Centers for Disease Control: Arboviral infections of the central nervous system: United States, 1985. M. M. W. R. Morb. Mortal. Wkly. Rep. *35*:341-350, 1986.

47. Centers for Disease Control: ACIP: Mumps prevention. M. M. W. R. Morb. Mortal. Wkly. Rep. *38*:388-400, 1989.

48. Centers for Disease Control: Arboviral surveillance: United States, 1990. M. M. W. R. Morb. Mortal. Wkly. Rep. *39*:593-598, 1990.

49. Centers for Disease Control: Outbreak of Hendra-like virus—Malaysia and Singapore, 1998-1999. M. M. W. R. Morb. Mortal. Wkly. Rep. *48*:265-269, 1999.

50. Centers for Disease Control: Enterovirus surveillance—United States, 1997-1999. M. M. W. R. Morb. Mortal. Wkly. Rep. *49*:913-916, 2000.

51. Centers for Disease Control: Outbreak of aseptic meningitis associated with multiple enterovirus serotypes—Romania, 1999. M. M. W. R. Morb. Mortal. Wkly. Rep. *49*:669-671, 2000.

52. Centers for Disease Control: Echovirus type 13—United States, 2001. M. M. W. R. Morb. Mortal. Wkly. Rep. *50*:777-780, 2001.

53. Centers for Disease Control: Acute flaccid paralysis associated with circulating vaccine-derived poliovirus—Philippines, 2001. M. M. W. R. Morb. Mortal. Wkly. Rep. *50*:874-875, 2001.

54. Centers for Disease Control and Prevention: Outbreaks of aseptic meningitis associated with echoviruses 9 and 30 and preliminary surveillance reports on enterovirus activity—United States, 2003. M. M. W. R. Morb. Mortal. Wkly. Rep. *52*:761-764, 2003.

55. Centers for Disease Control and Prevention: West Nile virus activity—United States, January 1-December, 2005. M. M. W. R. Morb. Mortal. Wkly. Rep. *54*:1253-1256, 2005.

56. Centers for Disease Control and Prevention: Enterovirus surveillance—United States, 2002-2004. M. M. W. R. Morb. Mortal. Wkly. Rep. *55*:153-156, 2006.

57. Centers for Disease Control and Prevention: Update: multistate outbreak of mumps—United States, January 1-May 2, 2006. M. M. W. R. Morb. Mortal. Wkly. Rep. *55*:559-563, 2006.

58. Cernescu, C., Tardei, G., Ruta, S., et al.: An outbreak of aseptic meningitis due to Echo 30 virus in Romania during the 1999 summer. Rom. J. Virol. *50*:99-106, 1999.

59. Chan, L. G., Parashar, U. D., Lye, M. S., et al.: Deaths of children during an outbreak of hand, foot and mouth disease in Sarawak, Malaysia: Clinical and pathological characteristics of the disease. Clin. Infect. Dis. *31*:678-683, 2000.

60. Char, D. F. B., and Rosen, L.: Eosinophilic meningitis among children in Hawaii. J. Pediatr. *70*:28-35, 1967.

61. Cheon, D. S., Lee, J., Lee, K., et al.: Isolation and molecular identification of echovirus 13 isolated from patients of aseptic meningitis in Korea, 2002. J. Med. Virol. *73*:439-442, 2004.

62. Chomel, J. J., Antona, D., Thouvenot, D., and Lina, B.: Three ECHOvirus serotypes responsible for outbreak of aseptic meningitis in Rhone-Alpes region, France. Eur. J. Clin. Microbiol. Infect. Dis. *22*:191-193, 2003.

63. Chowers, M. Y., Lang, R., Nassar, F., et al.: Clinical characteristics of the West Nile fever outbreak, Israel, 2000. Emerg. Infect. Dis. *7*:675-678, 2001.

64. Cinque, P., Bossolasco, S., and Lundkvist, A.: Molecular analysis of cerebrospinal fluid in viral diseases of the central nervous system. J. Clin. Virol. *26*:1-28, 2003.

65. Civen, R., Villacorte, F., Robles, D., et al.: West Nile virus infection in the pediatric population. Pediatr. Infect. Dis. J. *25*:75-78, 2006.

66. Cizman, M., Mozetic, M., Radescek-Rakar, R., et al.: Aseptic meningitis after vaccination against measles and mumps. Pediatr. Infect. Dis. *8*:302-308, 1989.

67. Cohen, B. A., Rowley, A. H., and Long, C. M.: Herpes simplex type 2 in a patient with Mollaret's meningitis: Demonstration by polymerase chain reaction. Ann. Neurol. *35*:112-116, 1994.

68. Coleman, W. S., Lischner, H. W., and Grover, W. D.: Recurrent aseptic meningitis without sequelae. J. Pediatr. *87*:89-91, 1975.

69. Connor, J. D., Buchta, R. M., DeGenaro, F., Jr., et al.: Potpourri of adenoviral infections. West. J. Med. *120*:55-61, 1974.

70. Corrall, C. J., Pepple, J. M., Moxon, E. R., et al.: C-reactive protein in spinal fluid of children with meningitis. J. Pediatr. *99*:365-369, 1981.

71. Craig, C. P., and Nahmias, A. J.: Different patterns of neurologic involvement with herpes simplex virus types 1 and 2: Isolation of herpes simplex virus type 2 from the buffy coat of two adults with meningitis. J. Infect. Dis. *127*:365-372, 1973.

72. Craver, R. D., Gohd, R. S., Sundin, D. R., et al.: Isolation of parainfluenza virus type 3 from cerebrospinal fluid associated with aseptic meningitis. Clin. Microbiol. Infect. Dis. *99*:705-707, 1993.

73. DaCunha, S. S., Rodrigues, L. C., Barreto, M. L., and Dourado, I.: Outbreak of aseptic meningitis and mumps after mass vaccination with MMR vaccine using the Leningrad-Zagreb mumps strain. Vaccine *20*:1106-1112, 2002.

74. Dalldorf, G., and Sickles, G. M.: An unidentified, filtrable agent isolated from the feces of children with paralysis. Science *108*:61-62, 1948.

75. DaSilveira, C. M., Kmetzsch, C. I., Mohrdieck, R., et al.: The risk of aseptic meningitis associated with the Leningrad-Zagreb mumps vaccine strain following mass vaccination with measles-mumps-rubella vaccine, Rio Grande do Sul, Brazil, 1997. Int. J. Epidemiol. *31*:978-982, 2002.

76. Davies, J. W., McDermott, A., and Severs, D.: Epidemic virus meningitis due to echo 9 virus in Newfoundland. Can. Med. Assoc. J. *79*:162-167, 1958.

77. DeBeer, F. C., Kirsten, G. F., Gie, R. P., et al.: Value of C reactive protein measurement in tuberculous, bacterial, and viral meningitis. Arch. Dis. Child. *59*:653-656, 1984.

78. Deibel, R., and Flanagan, T. D.: Central nervous system infections: Etiologic and epidemiologic observations in New York State, 1976-1977. N. Y. State J. Med. *79*:689-695, 1979.

79. Deibel, R., Flanagan, T. D., and Smith, V.: Central nervous system infections in New York State: Etiologic and epidemiologic observations, 1974. N. Y. State J. Med. *75*:2337-2342, 1975.

80. Deibel, R., Flanagan, T. D., and Smith, V.: Central nervous system infections: Etiologic and epidemiologic observations in New York State, 1975. N. Y. State J. Med. *77*:1398-1404, 1977.

81. Deibel, R., Woodall, J. P., Decher, W. J., et al.: Lymphocytic choriomeningitis virus in man: Serologic evidence of association with pet hamsters. J. A. M. A. *232*:501-504, 1975.

82. Dengler, L. D., Capparelli, E. V., Bastian, J. F., et al.: Cerebrospinal fluid profile in patients with acute Kawasaki disease. Pediatr. Infect. Dis. J. *17*:478-481, 1998.

83. Derbes, S. J.: Trimethoprim-induced aseptic meningitis. J. A. M. A. *252*:2865-2866, 1984.

84. Desmond, R. A., Accortt, N. A., Talley, L., et al.: Enteroviral meningitis: Natural history and outcome of pleconaril therapy. Antimicrob. Agents Chemother. *50*:2409-2414, 2006.

85. Diedrich, S., and Schreier, E.: Aseptic meningitis in Germany associated with enterovirus type 13. B. M. C. Infect. Dis. *1*:14, 2001.

86. Dimmitt, D. C., Fishbein, D. B., and Dawson, J. E.: Human ehrlichiosis associated with cerebrospinal fluid pleocytosis: A case report. Am. J. Med. *87*:677-678, 1989.

87. Do, A. N., Green, P. A., and Demmler, G. J.: Herpes simplex virus type 2 meningitis and associated genital lesions in a three-year-old child. Pediatr. Infect. Dis. J. *13*:1014-1016, 1994.

88. Dos Santos, G. P. L., Skraba, I., Oliveira, D., et al.: Enterovirus meningitis in Brazil, 1998-2003. J. Med. Virol. *78*:98-104, 2006.

89. Dourado, I., Cunha, S., Teixeira, M. G., et al.: Outbreak of aseptic meningitis associated with mass vaccination with a urabe-containing measles-mumps-rubella vaccine: Implications for immunization program. Am. J. Epidemiol. *151*:524-530, 2000.

90. Dulkerian, S. J., Kilpatrick, L., Costarino, A. T., Jr., et al.: Cytokine elevations in infants with bacterial and aseptic meningitis. J. Pediatr. *126*:872-876, 1995.

91. Dylewski, J. S., and Bekhor, S.: Mollaret's meningitis caused by herpes simplex virus type 2: Case report and literature review. Eur. J. Clin. Microbiol. Infect. Dis. *23*:560-562, 2004.

92. Echevarria, J. M., Casas, I., Tenorio, A., et al.: Detection of varicella-zoster virus-specific DNA sequences in cerebrospinal fluid from patients with acute aseptic meningitis and no cutaneous lesions. J. Med. Virol. *43*:331-335, 1994.

93. Enders, J. F.: Mumps. *In* Rivers, T. M., and Horsfall, F. L. (eds.): Viral and Rickettsial Infections of Man. Philadelphia, J. B. Lippincott, 1959, pp. 780-789.

94. Enders, J. R., Weller, T. H., and Robbins, F. C.: Cultivation of the Lansing strain of poliomyelitis virus in cultures of various human embryonic tissues. Science *109*:85-87, 1949.

95. Eppes, S. C., Nelson, D. K., Lewis, L. L., and Klein, J. D.: Characterization of Lyme meningitis and comparison with viral meningitis in children. Pediatrics *103*:957-960, 1999.

96. Estrada-Franco, J. G., Navarro-Lopez, R., Beasely, D. E., et al.: West Nile virus in Mexico: Evidence of widespread circulation since July 2002. Emerg. Infect. Dis. *9*:1604-1608, 2003.

97. Evans, A. S., and Niederman, J. C.: Epstein-Barr virus. *In* Evans, A. S. (ed.): Viral Infections of Humans: Epidemiology and Control. 2nd ed. New York, Plenum Medical, 1982, pp. 253-281.

98. Faulkner, R., and Van Rooyen, C. E.: Adenoviruses types 3 and 5 isolated from the cerebrospinal fluid of children. Can. Med. Assoc. J. *87*:1123-1125, 1962.

99. Faustini, A., Fano, V., Muscillo, M., et al.: An outbreak of aseptic meningitis due to echovirus 30 associated with attending school and swimming in pools. Int. J. Infect. Dis. *10*:291-297, 2006.

100. Finkelstein, Y., Mosser, R., and Garty, B. Z.: Concomitant aseptic meningitis and bacterial urinary tract infection in young febrile infants. Pediatr. Infect. Dis. J. *20*:630-632, 2001.

101. Fobelo, M. J., Corzo Delgado, J. E., Romero Alonso, A., et al.: Aseptic meningitis related to valacyclovir. Ann. Pharmacother. *35*:128-129, 2001.

102. Forbes, J. A.: Meningitis in Melbourne due to ECHO virus, Part I: Clinical aspects. Med. J. Aust. *1*:246-248, 1958.

103. Francisco, A. M., Glaser, C., Frykman, E., et al.: 2004 California pediatric West Nile virus case series. Pediatr. Infect. Dis. J. *25*:81-84, 2006.

104. Fryden, A., Kihlstrom, E., Maller, R., et al.: A clinical and epidemiological study of "ornithosis" caused by *Chlamydia psittaci* and *Chlamydia pneumoniae* (strain TWAR). Scand. J. Infect. Dis. *21*:681-691, 1989.

105. Fujimoto, H., Asaoka, K., Imaizumi, T., et al.: Epstein-Barr virus infections of the central nervous system. Intern. Med. *42*:33-40, 2003.

106. Fujimoto, T., Chikahira, M., Yoshida, S., et al.: Outbreak of central nervous system disease associated with hand, foot, and mouth disease in Japan during the summer of 2000: Detection and molecular epidemiology of enterovirus 71. Microbiol. Immunol. *46*:621-627, 2002.

107. Gajdusek, D. C.: Review article: Encephalomyocarditis virus infection in childhood. Pediatrics *16*:902-906, 1955.

108. Garland, S. M., and Murton, L. J.: Neonatal meningitis caused by *Ureaplasma urealyticum*. Pediatr. Infect. Dis. *6*:868-870, 1987.

109. Gavin, P. J., Kazacos, K. R., and Shulman, S. T.: Baylisascaris. Clin. Microbiol. Rev. *18*:703-718, 2005.

110. Gavin, P. J., and Shulman, S. T.: Raccoon roundworm (*Baylisascaris procyonis*). Pediatr. Infect. Dis. J. *22*:651-652, 2003.

111. Gilbert, G. L., Dickson, K. E., Waters, M. J., et al.: Outbreak of enterovirus 71 infection in Victoria, Australia, with a high incidence of neurologic involvement. Pediatr. Infect. Dis. J. *7*:484-488, 1988.

112. Glimaker, M., Johansson, B., Olcen, P., et al.: Detection of enteroviral RNA by polymerase chain reaction in cerebrospinal fluid from patients with aseptic meningitis. Scand. J. Infect. Dis. *25*:547-557, 1993.

113. Glimaker, M., Kragsbjerg, P., Forsgren, M., et al.: Tumor necrosis factor-alpha in cerebrospinal fluid from patients with meningitis of different etiologies: High levels of TNF-alpha indicate bacterial meningitis. J. Infect. Dis. *167*:882-889, 1993.

114. Golden, S. E.: Aseptic meningitis associated with *Ehrlichia canis* infection. Pediatr. Infect. Dis. *8*:335-337, 1989.

115. Gonzalez Garcia, H., Ernandez Alonso, J. F., de Paz Garcia, M., et al.: Meningitis as the first and only manifestation of brucellosis. An. Esp. Pediatr. *53*:280-282, 2000.

116. Gonzalez Pascual, E., Villanueva Lamas, J., Ros Viladoms, J., et al.: Kawasaki disease: A report of 50 cases. An. Esp. Pediatr. *50*:39-43, 1999.

117. Goodpasture, H. C., Poland, J. D., Francy, D. B., et al.: Colorado tick fever: Clinical, epidemiologic, and laboratory aspects of 228 cases in Colorado in 1973-1974. Ann. Intern. Med. *88*:303-310, 1978.

118. Gordon, M. F., Allon, M., and Coyle, P. K.: Drug-induced meningitis. Neurology *40*:163-164, 1990.

119. Gosbell, I., Robinson, D., Chant, K., et al.: Outbreak of echovirus 30 meningitis in Wingecaribee Shire, New South Wales. Commun. Dis. Intell. *24*:121-124, 2000.

120. Gottfredsson, M., and Perfect, J. R.: Fungal meningitis. Semin. Neurol. *20*:307-322, 2000.

121. Graman, P. S.: Mollaret's meningitis associated with acute Epstein-Barr virus mononucleosis. Arch. Neurol. *44*:1204-1205, 1987.

122. Grist, N. R., Bell, E. J., and Assaad, F.: Enteroviruses in human disease. Prog. Med. Virol. *24*:114-157, 1978.

123. Guglielminotti, J., Lellouche, N., Maury, E., et al.: Severe meningoencephalitis: An unusual manifestation of *Chlamydia pneumoniae* infection. Clin. Infect. Dis. *30*:209-210, 2000.

124. Guleria, R., Nisar, N., Chawla, T. C., and Biswas, N. R.: *Mycoplasma pneumoniae* and central nervous system complications: a review. J. Lab. Clin. Med. *146*:55-63, 2005.

125. Gunther, G., Haglund, M., Lindquist, L., et al.: Tick-borne encephalitis in Sweden in relation to aseptic meningo-encephalitis of other etiology: A prospective study of clinical course and outcome. J. Neurol. *244*:230-238, 1997.

126. Guthrie, N.: Coxsackie B5 meningitis: Report of an outbreak in a high school football squad. J. Tenn. State Med. Assoc. *55*:355-356, 1962.

127. Haase, S. K., Lapointe, M., and Haines, S. J.: Aseptic meningitis after intraventricular administration of gentamicin. Pharmacotherapy *21*:103-107, 2001.

128. Hammer, S. M., and Connolly, K. J.: Viral aseptic meningitis in the United States: Clinical features, viral etiologies, and differential diagnosis. Curr. Clin. Top. Infect. Dis. *12*:1-25, 1992.

129. Handsher, R., Shulman, L. M., Abramovitz, B., et al.: A new variant of echovirus 4 associated with a large outbreak of aseptic meningitis. J. Clin. Virol. *13*:29-36, 1999.

130. Hanninen, P., and Pohjonen, R.: Echovirus type 6 meningitis: Clinical and virological observations during an epidemic in Turku in 1968. Scand. J. Infect. Dis. *3*:121-125, 1971.

131. Hardin, S. G., Erwin, P. C., Patterson, L., et al.: Clinical comparisons of La Crosse encephalitis and enteroviral central nervous system infections in a pediatric population: 2001 surveillance in east Tennessee. Am. J. Infect. Control *31*:508-510, 2003.

132. Hauri, A. M., Schimmelpfennig, M., Walter-Domes, M., et al.: An outbreak of viral meningitis associated with a public swimming pond. Epidemiol. Infect. *133*:291-298, 2005.

133. Hayes, E. B., and O'Leary, D. R.: West Nile virus infection: A pediatric perspective. Pediatrics *113*:1375-1381, 2004.

134. Hayes, E. B., Sejvar, J. J., Zaki, S. R., et al.: Virology, pathology, and clinical manifestations of West Nile virus disease. Emerg. Infect. Dis. *11*:1174-1179, 2005.

135. Haynes, R. E., Cramblett, H. G., and Kronfol, H. J.: Echovirus 9 meningoencephalitis in infants and children. J. A. M. A. *208*:1657-1660, 1969.

136. Haynes, R. E., Sanders, D. Y., and Cramblett, H. G.: Rocky Mountain spotted fever in children. J. Pediatr. *76*:685-693, 1970.

137. Helin, I., Widell, A., Borulf, S., et al.: Outbreak of coxsackievirus A-14 meningitis among newborns in a maternity hospital ward. Acta Paediatr. Scand. *76*:234-238, 1987.

138. Hermans, P. E., Goldstein, N. P., and Wellman, W. E.: Mollaret's meningitis and differential diagnosis of recurrent meningitis. Am. J. Med. *52*:128-140, 1972.

139. Heusner, A. P.: Nontuberculous spinal epidural infections. N. Engl. J. Med. *239*:845-854, 1948.

140. Ho, M.: Enterovirus 71: The virus, its infections and outbreaks. J. Microbiol. Immunol. Infect. *33*:205-216, 2000.

141. Holzel, A., Smith, P. A., and Tobin, J. O. H.: A new type of meningoencephalitis associated with a rhinovirus. Acta Paediatr. Scand. *54*:168-174, 1965.

142. Huang, C. C., Liu, C. C., Chang, Y. C., et al.: Neurologic complications in children with enterovirus 71 infection. N. Engl. J. Med. *341*:936-942, 1999.

143. Huang, C., Morse, D., Slater, B., et al.: Multiple-year experience in the diagnosis of viral central nervous system infections with a panel of polymerase chain reaction assays for detection of 11 viruses. Clin. Infect. Dis. *39*:630-635, 2004.

144. Huang, Q. S., Carr, J. M., Nix, W. A., et al.: An echovirus type 33 winter outbreak in New Zealand. Clin. Infect. Dis. *37*:650-657, 2003.

145. Huhn, G. D., Sejvar, J. J., Montgomery, S. P., and Dworkin, M. S.: West Nile virus in the United States: An update on an emerging infectious disease. Am. Fam. Physician *68*:653-660, 2003.

146. Jhaveri, R., Cherry, J. D., Phillips, S., et al.: Erythema migrans after ceftriaxone treatment of aseptic meningitis caused by *Borrelia burgdorferi*. Pediatr. Infect. Dis. J. *20*:1010-1012, 2001.

147. Jhaveri, R., Sankar, R., Yazdani, S., and Cherry, J. D.: Varicella-zoster virus: An overlooked cause of aseptic meningitis. Pediatr. Infect. Dis. J. *22*:96-97, 2003.

148. Johnson, C. D., and Goodpasture, E. W.: An investigation of the etiology of mumps. J. Exp. Med. *59*:1-20, 1934.

149. Jorbeck, H. J. A., Guftafsson, P. M., Lind, H. C. F., et al.: Tick-borne *Borrelia* meningitis in children. Acta Paediatr. Scand. *76*:228-233, 1987.

150. Julian, K. G., Mullins, J. A., Olin, A., et al.: Aseptic meningitis epidemic during a West Nile virus avian epizootic. Emerg. Infect. Dis. *9*:1082-1088, 2003.

151. Kaida, A., Kubo, H., Iritani, N., et al.: Isolation of echovirus type 13 in Osaka City during 2001-2002. Jpn. J. Infect. Dis. 57:127-128, 2004.

152. Kajiwara, I., Kusaba, T., Hayashida, I., et al.: Clinical study of an outbreak of aseptic meningitis due to echovirus type 30 in Munakata City in 1997-1998. Kansenshogaku Zasshi 74:231-236, 2000.

153. Kammerer, U., Kunkel, B., and Korn, K.: Nested PCR for specific detection and rapid identification of human picornaviruses. J. Clin. Microbiol. 32:285-291, 1994.

154. Karande, S., Patil, S., Kulkarni, M., et al.: Acute aseptic meningitis as the only presenting feature of leptospirosis. Pediatr. Infect. Dis. J. 24:390, 2005.

155. Karzon, D. T., and Barron, A. L.: An epidemic of aseptic meningitis syndrome due to echo virus type 6. I. Correlation of enterovirus isolation with illness. II. Clinical study. III. Sequelae. Pediatrics 29:409-417, 418-431, 432-437, 1962.

156. Karzon, D. T., Eckert, G. L., Barron, A. L., et al.: Aseptic meningitis epidemic due to echo 4 virus. Am. J. Dis. Child. 101:610-622, 1961.

157. Kehle, J., Metzger-Boddien, C., Tewald, F., et al.: First case of confirmed rotavirus meningoencephalitis in Germany. Pediatr. Infect. Dis. J. 22:468-470, 2003.

158. Keino, M., Kanno, M., Hirasawa, K., et al.: Isolation of echovirus type 13 from patients of aseptic meningitis. Jpn. J. Infect. Dis. 54:249-250, 2001.

159. Kelsey, D. S.: Adenovirus meningoencephalitis. Pediatrics 61:291-293, 1978.

160. Kennedy, D. H., and Fallon, R. J.: Tuberculous meningitis. J. A. M. A. 241:264-268, 1979.

161. Khalfan, S., Aymaard, M., Lina, B., et al.: Epidemics of aseptic meningitis due to enteroviruses following national immunization days in Bahrain. Ann. Trop. Paediatr. 18:101-109, 1998.

162. Kirschke, D. L., Jones, T. F., Buckingham, S. C., et al.: Outbreak of aseptic meningitis associated with echovirus 13. Pediatr. Infect. Dis. J. 21:1034-1038, 2002.

163. Kitai, I., Navas, L., Rohlicke, C., et al.: Recurrent aseptic meningitis secondary to an intracranial cyst: A case report and review of clinical features and imaging modalities. Pediatr. Infect. Dis. J. 11:671-675, 1992.

164. Kochar, D. K., Agarwal, N., Jain, N., et al.: Clinical profile of neurobrucellosis: A report on 12 cases from Bikar (north-west India). Assoc. Physicians India 48:376-380, 2000.

165. Kondo, K., Nagafuji, H., Hata, A., et al.: Association of human herpesvirus 6 infection of the central nervous system with recurrence of febrile convulsions. J. Infect. Dis. 167:1197-1200, 1993.

166. Kriss, T. C., Kriss, V. M., and Warf, B. C.: Recurrent meningitis: The search for the dermoid or epidermoid tumor. Pediatr. Infect. Dis. J. 14:697-700, 1995.

167. Kupila, L., Vainionpaa, R., Vuorinem, T., et al.: Recurrent lymphocytic meningitis: The role of herpesviruses. Arch. Neurol. 61:1553-1557, 2004.

168. Kupila, L., Vuorinen, T., Vainionpaa, R., et al.: Etiology of aseptic meningitis and encephalitis in an adult population. Neurology 66:75-80, 2006.

169. LaForest, R. A., McNaughton, G. A., Beale, A. J., et al.: Outbreak of aseptic meningitis (meningoencephalitis) with rubelliform rash: Toronto, 1956. Can. Med. Assoc. J. 77:1-4, 1957.

170. Lanciotti, R. S., Kerst, A. J., Nasci, R. S., et al.: Rapid detection of West Nile virus from human clinical specimens, field-collected mosquitoes, and avian samples by a TaqMan reverse transcriptase-PCR assay. J. Clin. Microbiol. 38:4066-4071, 2000.

171. Lecour, H., Miranda, M., Magro, C., et al.: Human leptospirosis: A review of 50 cases. Infection 16:8-12, 1989.

172. Lee, K. E., Umapathi, T., Tan, C. B., et al.: The neurological manifestations of Nipah virus encephalitis, a novel paramyxovirus. Ann. Neurol. 46:428-432, 1999.

173. Lennette, E. H., Magoffin, R. L., and Knouf, E. G.: Viral central nervous system disease: An etiologic study conducted at the Los Angeles County General Hospital. J. A. M. A. 179:687-695, 1962.

174. Lepow, M. L., Carver, D. H., Wright, H. T., Jr., et al.: A clinical, epidemiologic and laboratory investigation of aseptic meningitis during the four-year period 1955-1958, I: Observations concerning etiology and epidemiology. N. Engl. J. Med. 266:1181-1187, 1962.

175. Lepow, M. L., Coyne, N., Thompson, L. B., et al.: A clinical, epidemiologic and laboratory investigation of aseptic meningitis during the four-year period 1955-1958, II: The clinical disease and its sequelae. N. Engl. J. Med. 266:1188-1193, 1962.

176. Lesnicar, G., Poljak, M., Seme, K., and Lesnicar, J.: Pediatric tick-borne encephalitis in 371 cases from an endemic region in Slovenia, 1959 to 2000. Pediatr. Infect. Dis. J. 22:612-617, 2003.

177. Li, C. C., Yang, M. Y., Chen, R. F., et al.: Clinical manifestations and laboratory assessment in an enterovirus 71 outbreak in southern Taiwan. Scand. J. Infect. Dis. 34:104-109, 2002.

178. Liao, H. T., and Hung, K. L.: Neurologic involvement in an outbreak of enterovirus 71 infection: A hospital-based study. Acta Paediatr. Taiwan 42:27-32, 2001.

179. Lin, W. C., Lee, P. I., and Lu, C. Y.: Mycoplasma pneumoniae encephalitis in childhood. J. Microbiol. Immunol. Infect. 35:173-178, 2002.

180. Lindquist, L., Linne, T., Hansson, L. O., et al.: Value of cerebrospinal fluid analysis in the differential diagnosis of meningitis: A study in 710 patients with suspected central nervous system infection. Eur. J. Clin. Microbiol. Infect. Dis. 7:374-380, 1988.

181. Liu, C. C., Tseng, H. W., Wang, S. M., et al.: An outbreak of enterovirus 71 infection in Taiwan, 1998: Epidemiologic and clinical manifestations. J. Clin. Virol. 177:23-30, 2000.

182. Logar, M., Arnez, M., Kolbl, J., et al.: Comparison of the epidemiological and clinical features of tick-borne encephalitis in children and adults. Infection 28:74-77, 2000.

183. Mardh, P. A.: Mycoplasma hominis infection of the central nervous system in newborn infants. Sex. Transm. Dis. 10:331-334, 1983.

184. Martin, M. A., Massanari, R. M., Nghiem, D. D., et al.: Nosocomial aseptic meningitis associated with administration of OKT3. J. A. M. A. 259:2002-2005, 1988.

185. McDonald, J. C., Moore, D. L., and Quennec, P.: Clinical and epidemiologic features of mumps meningoencephalitis and possible vaccine-related disease. Pediatr. Infect. Dis. 8:751-755, 1989.

186. McJunkin, J. E., de los Reyes, E. C., Irazuzta, J. E., et al.: La Crosse encephalitis in children. N. Engl. J. Med. 345:148-149, 2001.

187. McMinn, P., Stratov, I., Nagarajan, L., et al.: Neurological manifestations of enterovirus 71 infection during an outbreak of hand, foot and mouth disease in Western Australia. Clin. Infect. Dis. 32:236-242, 2001.

188. Meyer, H. M., Jr., Johnson, R. T., Crawford, I. P., et al.: Central nervous system syndromes of "viral" etiology: A study of 713 cases. Am. J. Med. 29:334-347, 1960.

189. Mifsud, A. J.: Drug-related recurrent meningitis. J. Infect. 17:151-153, 1988.

190. Miller, E., Goldacre, M., Pugh, S., et al.: Risk of aseptic meningitis after measles, mumps, and rubella vaccine in UK children. Lancet 341:979-982, 1993.

191. Miller, H. G., and Stanton, J. B.: Neurological sequelae of prophylactic inoculation. Q. J. M. 89:1-27, 1954.

192. Miller, H. G., Stanton, J. B., and Gibbons, J. L.: Parainfectious encephalomyelitis and related syndromes: A critical review of the neurological complications of certain specific fevers. Q. J. M. 100:427-505, 1956.

193. Molavi, A., and LeFrock, J. L.: Tuberculous meningitis. Med. Clin. North Am. 69:315-331, 1985.

194. Mollaret, P.: La meningite endothelio-leukocytaire multirecurrente benigne: Syndrome nouveau ou maladie nouvelle? Rev. Neurol. 72:57-76, 1944.

195. Moore, M.: Enteroviral disease in the United States, 1970-1979. J. Infect. Dis. 146:103-108, 1982.

196. Moylett, E. H.: Neonatal Candida meningitis. Semin. Pediatr. Infect. Dis. 14:115-122, 2003.

197. Muller, M. P., Richardson, D. C., and Walmsley, S. L.: Trimethoprim-sulfamethoxazole induced aseptic meningitis in a renal transplant patient. Clin. Nephrol. 55:80-84, 2001.

198. Mullins, J. A., Khetsuriani, N., Nix, W. A., et al.: Emergence of echovirus type 13 as a prominent Enterovirus. Clin. Infect. Dis. 38:70-77, 2004.

199. Nagai, T., Okafuji, T., Miyazaki, C., et al.: A comparative study of the incidence of aseptic meningitis in symptomatic natural mumps patients and monovalent mumps vaccine recipients in Japan. Vaccine 25:2742-2747, 2006.

200. Narkeviciute, I., and Vaiciuniene, D.: Outbreak of echovirus 13 infection among Lithuanian children. Clin. Microbiol. Infect. 10:1023-1025, 2004.

201. Nash, D., Mostashari, F., Fine, A., et al.: The outbreak of West Nile virus infection in the New York City area in 1999. N. Engl. J. Med. 344:1807-1814, 2001.

202. Nigrovic, L. E., and Chiang, V. W.: Cost analysis of enteroviral polymerase chain reaction in infants with fever and cerebrospinal fluid pleocytosis. Arch. Pediatr. Adolesc. Med. 154:817-821, 2000.

203. Okumura, A., and Ichikawa, T.: Aseptic meningitis caused by human parvovirus B19. Arch. Dis. Child. 68:784-785, 1993.

204. Ozkaya, E., Hizel, K., Uysal, G., et al.: An outbreak of aseptic meningitis due to echovirus type 30 in two cities of Turkey. Eur. J. Epidemiol. 18:823-826, 2003.

205. Paisley, J. W., Bruhn, F. W., Lauer, B. A., et al.: Type A2 influenza viral infections in children. Am. J. Dis. Child. 132:34-36, 1978.

206. Panicker, J. N., Mammachan, R., and Jayakumar, R. V.: Primary neuroleptospirosis. Postgrad. Med. J. 77:589-590, 2001.

207. Peltola, H. O.: C-reactive protein for rapid monitoring of infections of the central nervous system. Lancet 1:980-983, 1982.

208. Peltola, H., and Valmari, P.: Serum C-reactive protein as detector of pretreated childhood bacterial meningitis. Neurology 35:251-253, 1985.

209. Pereira, A. C., Barros, R. A., do Nascimento, J. P., et al.: Two family members with a syndrome of headache and rash caused by human parvovirus B19. Braz. J. Infect. Dis. 5:37-39, 2001.

210. Pereira, M. S., and MacCallum, F. O.: Infection with adenovirus type 12. Lancet 1:198-199, 1964.

211. Peter, G.: Leptospirosis: A zoonosis of protean manifestations. Pediatr. Infect. Dis. 1:282-288, 1982.

212. Petersen, L. R., and Marfin, A. A.: West Nile virus: A primer for the clinician. Ann. Intern. Med. 137:E173-E179, 2002.

213. Picard, F. J., Dekaban, G. A., Silva, J., et al.: Mollaret's meningitis associated with herpes simplex type 2 infection. Neurology 43:1722-1727, 1993.

214. Platonov, A. E., Shipulin, G. A., Shipulina, O. Y., et al.: Outbreak of West Nile virus infection, Volgograd region, Russia, 1999. Emerg. Infect. Dis. 7:128-132, 1999.

215. Pohl-Koppe, A., Blay, M., Jager, G., et al.: Human herpes virus type 7 in the cerebrospinal fluid of children with central nervous system disease. Eur. J. Pediatr. 160:351-358, 2001.

216. Pönkä, A.: Central nervous system manifestations associated with serologically verified *Mycoplasma pneumoniae* infection. Scand. J. Infect. Dis. *12*:175-184, 1980.

217. Portolani, M., Pecorari, M., Pietrosemoli, P., et al.: Outbreak of aseptic meningitis by echo 4: Prevalence of clinical cases among adults. New Microbiol. *24*:11-15, 2001.

218. Preblud, S. R.: Age-specific risks of varicella complications. Pediatrics *68*:14-17, 1981.

219. Rao, S. P., Teitlebaum, J., and Miller, S. T.: Intravenous immune globulin and aseptic meningitis. Am. J. Dis. Child. *146*:539-540, 1992.

220. Rasmussen, A. F.: The laboratory diagnosis of lymphocytic choriomeningitis and mumps. *In*: Rocky Mountain Conference on Infantile Paralysis. Denver, University of Colorado School of Medicine, 1946, p. 45.

221. Reeves, W. C., Quiroz, E., Brenes, M. M., et al.: Aseptic meningitis due to echovirus 4 in Panama City, Republic of Panama. Am. J. Epidemiol. *125*:562-575, 1987.

222. Reimer, L. G., and Reller, L. B.: CSF in herpes zoster meningoencephalitis. Arch. Neurol. *38*:668, 1981.

223. Reintjes, R., Pohle, M., Vieth, U., et al.: Community-wide outbreak of enteroviral illness caused by echovirus 30: A cross-sectional survey and a case-control study. Pediatr. Infect. Dis. J. *18*:104-108, 1999.

224. Riski, H., and Hovi, T.: Coronavirus infections of man associated with diseases other than the common cold. J. Med. Virol. *6*:259-265, 1980.

225. Rivers, T. M., and Scott, T. F. M.: Meningitis in man caused by a filterable virus. Science *81*:439-440, 1935.

226. Romero, J. R., and Newland, J. G.: Viral meningitis and encephalitis: Traditional and emerging viral agents. Semin. Pediatr. Infect. Dis. *14*:72-82, 2003.

227. Roos, K. L.: *Mycobacterium tuberculosis* meningitis and other etiologies of the aseptic meningitis syndrome. Semin. Neurol. *20*:329-335, 2000.

228. Rosen, L., Loison, G., Laigret, J., et al.: Studies on eosinophilic meningitis, 3: Epidemiologic and clinical observations on Pacific islands and the possible etiologic role of *Angiostrongylus cantonensis*. Am. J. Epidemiol. *85*:17-44, 1967.

229. Rotbart, H. A.: Enteroviral infections of the central nervous system. Clin. Infect. Dis. *20*:971-981, 1995.

230. Rotbart, H. A.: Viral meningitis. Semin. Neurol. *20*:277-292, 2000.

231. Rotbart, H. A., O'Connell, J. F., and McKinlay, M. A.: Treatment of human enterovirus infections. Antiviral Res. *38*:1-14, 1998.

232. Rotbart, H. A., Sawyer, M. H., Fast, S., et al.: Diagnosis of enteroviral meningitis by using PCR with a colorimetric microwell detection assay. J. Clin. Microbiol. *32*:2590-2592, 1994.

233. Rotbart, H. A., and Webster, A. D.: Treatment of potentially life-threatening enterovirus infections with pleconaril. Clin. Infect. Dis. *32*:228-235, 2001.

234. Rotem, C. E.: Meningitis of virus origin. Lancet *1*:502-504, 1957.

235. Rothenberg, R., Murphy, W., O'Brien, C. L., et al.: Aseptic meningitis associated with ECHO virus type 9: An outbreak in Norfolk, Va. South. Med. J. *63*:280-285, 1970.

236. Rottach, K.: Mollaret's meningitis: A new aetiologic feature. Eur. Neurol. *36*:172-173, 1996.

237. Sabin, A. B., Krumbiegel, E. R., and Wigand, R.: ECHO type 9 virus disease: Virologically controlled clinical and epidemiologic observations during a 1957 epidemic in Milwaukee with notes on concurrent similar diseases associated with coxsackie and other ECHO viruses. Prog. Pediatr. *96*:197-219, 1958.

238. Salaki, J. S., Louria, D. B., and Chmel, H.: Fungal and yeast infections of the central nervous system: A clinical review. Medicine *63*:108-132, 1984.

239. Samuda, G. M., Chang, W. K., Yeung, C. Y., et al.: Monoplegia caused by enterovirus 71: An outbreak in Hong Kong. Pediatr. Infect. Dis. *6*:206-208, 1987.

240. Sands, M. L., Ryczak, M., and Brown, R. B.: Recurrent aseptic meningitis followed by transverse myelitis as a presentation of systemic lupus erythematosus. J. Rheumatol. *15*:862-864, 1988.

241. Sarmiento, L., Mas, P., Goyenechea, et al.: First epidemic of echovirus 16 meningitis in Cuba. Emerg. Infect. Dis. *7*:887-889, 2001.

242. Sato, R., Ayabe, M., Shoji, H., et al.: Herpes simplex virus type 2 recurrent meningitis (Mollaret's meningitis): A consideration for the recurrent pathogenesis. J. Infect. *51*:e217-e220, 2005.

243. Sawyer, M. H., Holland, D., Aintablian, N., et al.: Diagnosis of enteroviral central nervous system infection by polymerase chain reaction during a large community outbreak. Pediatr. Infect. Dis. J. *13*:177-182, 1994.

244. Schlesinger, Y., Sawyer, M. H., and Storch, G. A.: Enteroviral meningitis in infancy: Potential role for polymerase chain reaction in patient management. Pediatrics *94*:157-162, 1994.

245. Schumaker, J. D., Chuard, C., Renevey, F., et al.: Outbreak of echovirus type 30 meningitis in Switzerland. Scand. J. Infect. Dis. *31*:539-542, 1999.

246. Sejvar, J. J., Labutta, R. J., Chapman, L. E., et al.: Neurologic adverse events associated with smallpox vaccination in the United States, 2002-2004. J. A. M. A. *294*:2744-2750, 2003.

247. Shaked, Y., and Samra, Y.: Q fever meningoencephalitis associated with bilateral abducens nerve paralysis, bilateral optic neuritis and abnormal cerebrospinal fluid findings. Infection *17*:394-396, 1989.

248. Shekhar, K., Lye, M. S., Norlijah, O., et al.: Deaths in children during an outbreak of hand, foot and mouth disease in Peninsular Malaysia—clinical and pathological characteristics. Med. J. Malay. *60*:297-304, 2005.

249. Shimizu, H., Utama, A., Yoshii, K., et al.: Enterovirus 71 from fatal and non-fatal cases of hand, foot and mouth disease epidemics in Malaysia, Japan and Taiwan in 1997-1998. Jpn. J. Infect. Dis. *52*:12-15, 1999.

250. Shinora, M., Uchida, K., Shimada, S., et al.: Characterization of enterovirus type 71 isolated in Saitama Prefecture in 2000. Kansenshogaku Zasshi *75*:490-494, 2001.

251. Simila, S., Jouppila, R., Salmi, A., et al.: Encephalomeningitis in children associated with an adenovirus type 7 epidemic. Acta Paediatr. Scand. *59*:310-316, 1970.

252. Singer, J. I., Maur, P. R., Riley, J. P., et al.: Management of central nervous system infections during an epidemic of enteroviral aseptic meningitis. J. Pediatr. *96*:559-563, 1980.

253. Sköldenberg, B.: On the role of viruses in acute infectious diseases of the central nervous system: Clinical and laboratory studies on hospitalized patients. Scand. J. Infect. Dis. *3*(Suppl.):5-95, 1975.

254. Sköldenberg, B., Jeansson, S., and Wolontis, S.: Herpes simplex virus type 2 and acute aseptic meningitis. Scand. J. Infect. Dis. *7*:227-232, 1975.

255. Socan, M., Beovic, B., and Kese, D.: *Chlamydia* pneumonia and meningoencephalitis. N. Engl. J. Med. *331*:406, 1994.

256. Socan, M., Ravnik, I., Bencina, D., et al.: Neurological symptoms in patients whose cerebrospinal fluid is culture—and/or polymerase chain reaction—positive for *Mycoplasma pneumoniae*. Clin. Infect. Dis. *32*:E31-35, 2001.

257. Sohier, R., Chardonnet, Y., and Prunieras, M.: Adenoviruses: Status of current knowledge. Prog. Med. Virol. *7*:253-325, 1965.

258. Somekh, E., Cesar, K., Handsher, R., et al.: An outbreak of echovirus 13 meningitis in central Israel. Epidemiol. Infect. *130*:257-262, 2003.

259. Somekh, E., Shobat, T., Hansher, R., et al.: An outbreak of echovirus 11 in a children's home. Epidemiol. Infect. *126*:441-444, 2001.

260. Southern, P. M., Jr.: Relapsing fever. *In* Tice, F. (ed.): Practice of Medicine. Vol. 3. Scranton, PA, Hoeber Medical Div., Harper & Row, 1969, pp. 1-19.

261. Spillane, J. D., and Wells, C. E. C.: The neurology of Jennerian vaccination: A clinical account of the neurological complications which occurred during the smallpox epidemic in South Wales in 1962. Brain *87*:1-44, 1964.

262. Srihongse, S., Grayson, M. A., and Deibel, R.: California serogroup viruses in New York State: The role of subtypes in human infections. Am. J. Trop. Med. Hyg. *33*:1218-1227, 1984.

263. Steel, J. G., Dix, R. D., and Baringer, J. R.: Isolation of herpes simplex virus type 1 in recurrent (Mollaret) meningitis. Ann. Neurol. *11*:17-21, 1982.

264. Stellrecht, K. A., Harding, I., Woron, A. M., et al.: The impact of an enteroviral RT-PCR assay on the diagnosis of aseptic meningitis and patient management. J. Clin. Virol. *25*:S19-S26, 2002.

265. Sumaya, C. V., and Corman, L. I.: Enteroviral meningitis in early infancy: Significance in community outbreaks. Pediatr. Infect. Dis. *1*:151-154, 1982.

266. Sumaya, C. V., and Ench, Y.: Epstein-Barr virus infectious mononucleosis in children, I: Clinical and general laboratory findings. Pediatrics *75*:1003-1010, 1985.

267. Sundelof, B., Gnarpe, H., and Gnarpe, J.: An unusual manifestation of *Chlamydia pneumoniae* infection: Meningitis, hepatitis, iritis and atypical erythema nodosum. Scand. J. Infect. Dis. *25*:259-261, 1993.

268. Suzuki, N., Terada, S., and Inoue, M.: Neonatal meningitis with human parvovirus B19 infection. Arch. Dis. Child. Fetal Neonatal Ed. *73*:F196-F197, 1995.

269. Syrogiannopoulos, G. A., Grivea, I. A., Anastassiou, E. D., et al.: Sterile cerebrospinal fluid pleocytosis in young infants with urinary tract infection. Pediatr. Infect. Dis. J. *20*:927-930, 2001.

270. Syverton, J. T., McLean, D. M., daSilva, M. M., et al.: Outbreak of aseptic meningitis caused by coxsackie B5 virus: Laboratory, clinical and epidemiologic study. J. A. M. A. *164*:2015-2019, 1957.

271. Tang, Y., Cleavinger, P. J., Li, H., et al.: Analysis of candidate-host immunogenetic determinants in herpes simplex virus-associated Mollaret's meningitis. Clin. Infect. Dis. *30*:176-178, 2000.

272. Tedder, D. G., Ashley, R., Tyler, K. L., et al.: Herpes simplex virus infection as a cause of benign recurrent lymphocytic meningitis. Ann. Intern. Med. *121*:334-338, 1994.

273. Tena, D., Gonzalez-Praetorius, A., Lopez-Alonso, A., et al.: Acute meningitis due to *Brucella* spp. Eur. J. Pediiatr. *165*:726-727, 2006.

274. Terni, M., Caccialanza, P., Cassai, E., et al.: Aseptic meningitis in association with herpes progenitalis. N. Engl. J. Med. *285*:503-504, 1971.

275. Thoelen, I., Lemey, P., Van der Donck, I., et al.: Molecular typing and epidemiology of enteroviruses identified from an outbreak of aseptic meningitis in Belgium during the summer of 2000. J. Med. Virol. *70*:420-429, 2003.

276. Thoren, A., and Widell, A.: PCR for the diagnosis of enteroviral meningitis. Scand. J. Infect. Dis. *26*:249-254, 1994.

277. Trallero, G., Casas, I., Avellon, A., et al.: First epidemic of aseptic meningitis due to echovirus type 13 among Spanish children. Epidemiol. Infect. *130*:251-256, 2001.

278. Tsai, T. F., Popovici, F., Cernescu, C., et al.: West Nile encephalitis epidemic in southeastern Romania. Lancet *352*:767-771, 1998.

279. Tsiodras, S., Kelesidis, I., Kelesidis, T., et al.: Central nervous system manifestations of *Mycoplasma pneumoniae* infections. J. Infect. *51*:343-354, 2005.

280. Tsutsumi, H., Kamazaki, H., and Nakata, S.: Sequential development of acute meningoencephalitis and transverse myelitis caused by Epstein-Barr virus during infectious mononucleosis. Pediatr. Infect. Dis. J. *13*:665-667, 1994.

281. Tyler, K. L.: Herpes simplex virus infections of the central nervous system: Encephalitis and meningitis, including Mollaret's. Herpes *11*:57A-64A, 2004.

282. Ushijima, H., Xin, K. Q., Nishimura, S., et al.: Detection and sequencing of rotavirus YP7 gene from human materials (stools, sera, cerebrospinal fluids, and throat swabs) by reverse transcription and PCR. J. Clin. Microbiol. 32:2893-2897, 1994.

283. Uysal, G., Ozkaya, E., and Guven, A.: Echovirus 30 outbreak of aseptic meningitis in Turkey. Pediatr. Infect. Dis. J. 19:490, 2000.

284. Vieth, U. C., Kunzelmann, M., Diedrich, S., et al.: An echovirus 30 outbreak with high meningitis attack rate among children and household members at four day-care centers. Eur. J. Epidemiol. 15:655-658, 1999.

285. Vreede, R. W., Schellekens, H., and Zuijderwijk, M.: Isolation of parainfluenza virus type 3 from cerebrospinal fluid. J. Infect. Dis. 165:1166, 1992.

286. Waites, K. B., Duffy, L. B., Crouse, D. T., et al.: Mycoplasmal infections of cerebrospinal fluid in newborn infants from a community hospital population. Pediatr. Infect. Dis. 9:241-245, 1990.

287. Waites, K. B., Rudd, P. T., Crouse, D. T., et al.: Chronic *Ureaplasma urealyticum* and *Mycoplasma hominis* infections of central nervous system in preterm infants. Lancet 1:17-21, 1988.

288. Wallach, J. C., Baldi, P. C., and Fossati, C. A.: Clinical and diagnostic aspects of relapsing meningoencephalitis due to *Brucella suis*. Eur. J. Clin. Microbiol. Infect. Dis. 21:760-762, 2002.

289. Wallgren, A.: Une nouvelle maladie infectieuse du système nerveux central? Acta Paediatr. Scand. 4(Suppl.):158-182, 1925.

290. Wallgren, A.: Die ätiologie der enzephalomeningitis bei kindern, besonders des syndromes der akuten abakteriellen (aseptichen) meningitis. Acta Paediatr. Scand. 40:541-565, 1951.

291. Wang, J. R., Tsai, H. P., Chen, P. F., et al.: An outbreak of enterovirus 71 infection in Taiwan, 1998, II: Laboratory diagnosis and genetic analysis. J. Clin. Virol. 17:91-99, 2000.

292. Wang, J. R., Tsai, H. P., Huang, S. W., et al.: Laboratory diagnosis and genetic analysis of an echovirus 30-associated outbreak of aseptic meningitis in Taiwan in 2001. J. Clin. Microbiol. 40:4439-4444, 2002.

293. Warren, J.: Encephalomyocarditis viruses. *In* Horsfall, F. L., and Tamm, I. (eds.): Viral and Rickettsial Infections of Man. Philadelphia, J. B. Lippincott, 1965, pp. 562-568.

294. Weller, P. F.: Eosinophilic meningitis. Am. J. Med. 95:250-253, 1993.

295. Weller, T. H.: Varicella-Herpes zoster virus. *In* Evans, A. S. (ed.): Viral Infections of Humans: Epidemiology and Control. 2nd ed. New York, Plenum Medical, 1982, pp. 569-595.

296. Wickman, I.: Studien über poliomyelitis acuta: Zugleich ein beitrag zur kenntnis der myelitis acuta. Berlin, S. Karger, Engl. Trans. Nev. and Ment. Dis. Monog. Ser. No. 16, 1905, p. 1913,

297. Wilfert, C. M., Lehrman, S. N., and Katz, S. L.: Enteroviruses and meningitis. Pediatr. Infect. Dis. 2:333-341, 1983.

298. Wilfert, C. M., Thompson, R. J., Jr., Sunder, T. R., et al.: Longitudinal assessment of children with enteroviral meningitis during the first three months of life. Pediatrics 67:811-815, 1981.

299. Williams, C. L., Strobino, B., Lee, A., et al.: Lyme disease in childhood: Clinical and epidemiologic features of ninety cases. Pediatr. Infect. Dis. 9:10-14, 1990.

300. Wise, M. E., Sorvillo, F. J., Shafir, S. C., et al.: Severe and fatal central nervous system disease in humans caused by *Baylisascaris procyonis*, the common roundworm of raccoons: A review of current literature. Microbes Infect. 7:317-323, 2005.

301. Wong, C. J., Price, Z., and Bruckner, D. A.: Aseptic meningitis in an infant with rotavirus gastroenteritis. Pediatr. Infect. Dis. 3:244-246, 1984.

302. Wong, J. G., Hathaway, S. C., Paat, J. J., et al.: Drug-induced meningitis: A case involving trimethoprim-sulfamethoxazole. Postgrad. Med. 96:117-124, 1994.

303. Wong, M. L., Kaplan, S., Dunkle, L. M., et al.: Leptospirosis: A childhood disease. J. Pediatr. 90:532-537, 1977.

304. Yan, J. J., Wang, J. R., Liu, C. C., et al.: An outbreak of enterovirus 71 infection in Taiwan 1998: A comprehensive pathological, virological, and molecular study on a case of fulminant encephalitis. J. Clin. Virol. 17:13-22, 2000.

305. Yanagihara, K., Tanaka-Taya, K., Itagaki, Y., et al.: Human herpesvirus 6 meningoencephalitis with sequelae. Pediatr. Infect. Dis. J. 14:240-242, 1995.

306. Yang, T. T., Huang, L. M., Lu, C. Y., et al.: Clinical features and factors of unfavorable outcomes for non-polio enterovirus infection of the central nervous system in northern Taiwan, 1994-2003. J. Microbiol. Immunol. Infect. 38:417-424, 2005.

307. Yerly, S., Gervaix, A., Simonet, V., et al.: Rapid and sensitive detection of enteroviruses in specimens from patients with aseptic meningitis. J. Clin. Microbiol. 34:199-201, 1996.

308. Yoshikawa, T., Ihira, M., Suzuki, K., et al.: Invasion by human herpesvirus 6 and human herpesvirus 7 of the central nervous system in patients with neurological signs and symptoms. Arch. Dis. Child. 83:170-171, 2000.

309. Young, E. J.: Human brucellosis. Rev. Infect. Dis. 5:821-842, 1983.

310. Zhao, Y. N., Jiang, Q. W., Jiang, R. J., et al.: Echovirus 30, Jiangsu Province, China. Emerg. Infect. Dis. 11:562-567, 2005.

CHAPTER 42

ENCEPHALITIS AND MENINGOENCEPHALITIS

James D. Cherry ❂ W. Donald Shields ❂ David E. Bronstein

Encephalitis is an inflammation of the brain, and meningoencephalitis is a similar inflammatory illness in which the brain and the meninges are involved. The diagnosis of encephalitis can be established with absolute certainty only by the microscopic examination of brain tissue, and, similarly, the etiology is established only by the recovery from or the demonstration in brain tissue of an infectious agent. In clinical practice, the diagnosis frequently is based on neurologic manifestations, the recovery of infectious agents from other sites in the body, the serologic evidence of a specific infection, and relevant epidemiologic findings.

Encephalitis frequently is classified as primary or as postinfectious or parainfectious. Primary encephalitis is an illness in which encephalitis is the major manifestation. Symptoms are caused by direct invasion and replication of an infectious agent in the central nervous system (CNS), resulting in objective clinical evidence of cerebral or cerebellar dysfunction. Postinfectious or parainfectious encephalitis occurs after or in combination with other illnesses that are not CNS illnesses, or after a vaccine or other product has been administered. Manifestations may be mediated immunologically.

When neurologic clinical findings suggest encephalitis but inflammation of the brain has not occurred (e.g., in Reye syndrome), the condition is identified by the less specific term *encephalopathy*. Frequently, when encephalitis or meningoencephalitis occurs, other areas of the nervous system, such as the spinal cord (myelitis), nerve roots (radiculitis), and nerves (neuritis), also are involved.

HISTORY

Rabies encephalitis was recognized in ancient times in Europe and Asia.[169] In 100 CE, Celsus noted the relationship of animal rabies to human disease. "Sleeping sickness" associated with epidemic influenza was noted early in the 18th century.[345] For the past 100 years, epizootics of encephalitis in equine animals have been observed in the United States, and in 1933, St. Louis encephalitis virus was isolated from the brains of humans dying from epidemic encephalitis.[230,251] Meningoencephalitis was recognized at the beginning of the 20th century as a complication of mumps.[103] Nonpolio enteroviruses have been known for the past 55 years to be a cause of encephalitis; during the same period, more than 400 zoonotic arthropod-borne viruses have been discovered, and of these, 100 or more cause encephalitis in humans.[26]

ETIOLOGY

Table 42–1 presents etiologic agents in acute encephalitis, meningoencephalitis, and acute illnesses with an encephalitic component. All of the infectious agents or diseases are presented more fully and are referenced more completely elsewhere in this book (see Index).

Despite extensive testing and evaluation, the etiology of most cases of encephalitis remained unexplained in more recent prospective studies.[121,193] During the first 2.5 years of the California Encephalitis Project, 334 immunocompetent patients older than 6 months of age were identified who met the case definition of encephalopathy requiring hospitalization and having at least one other sign or symptom, including fever, seizure, focal neurological findings, cerebrospinal fluid (CSF) pleocytosis, or electroencephalography (EEG) or neuroimaging findings consistent with encephalitis.[121] Of these cases, a confirmed or probable viral agent was identified in only 9 percent of cases, and bacterial and parasitic agents were found in only 3 percent and 1 percent, respectively; an etiology was not discovered for 62 percent of the cases. A possible etiology was noted in 12 percent, a noninfectious cause was identified in 10 percent, and a nonencephalitis infection was identified in 3 percent.

VIRUSES

As a group, the herpesviruses are the most frequently identified agents responsible for viral encephalitis. Herpes simplex encephalitis is the most common cause of sporadic fatal encephalitis in the United States, with approximately one third of cases occurring in patients younger than age 20 years but older than 6 months and approximately half occurring in patients older than 50 years.[230,281,335,351] Molecular analyses of paired oral or labial and brain sites have indicated that herpes simplex encephalitis can be the result of a primary infection, a reactivation of latent herpes simplex virus (HSV), or a reinfection by a second HSV.[348] Although in neonates HSV type 2 (HSV-2) is a leading cause of severe and frequently fatal encephalitis,[352] in older children, the usual cause is HSV-1.[71,164,183,219,231,263,273,337] Recurrent genital infection with HSV-2 occasionally is associated with an aseptic meningitis, but this type 2 virus rarely causes encephalitis outside the newborn period except in immunocompromised individuals.

Encephalitis can occur in association with primary infection with varicella-zoster virus (VZV) (chickenpox) and with endogenous recurrent disease (herpes zoster).* In a study in Finland of more than 3000 patients with acute CNS infections of suspected viral origin, VZV constituted 29 percent of all confirmed or probable etiologic agents.[187] In chickenpox, the rate of encephalitis is approximately 0.3/1000 cases,[49] and the case-fatality rate is approximately 17 percent.[265] Of patients with herpes zoster, 0.5 to 5 percent have encephalitis.[168] This complication occurs more commonly in immunocompromised patients.

In infectious mononucleosis, encephalitis occurs in less than 1 percent of cases. Most patients with Epstein-Barr virus encephalitis are adolescents and young adults, and although patients typically present 1 to 3 weeks after the onset of mononucleosis syndrome, encephalitis may be the presenting complaint in Epstein-Barr virus infection.[79,82,96,153,207,335] Caruso and associates[45] reported five children with subacute and chronic neurologic deficits associated with apparent primary Epstein-Barr virus infections. Severe chronic involvement of the brain is a common finding in congenital cytomegalovirus (CMV) infection.[143] Encephalitis caused by acquired CMV infection is uncommon

---

*See references 1, 42, 74, 84, 101, 148, 167, 188, 189, 271, 305.

TABLE 42–1 Etiologic Agents in Acute Encephalitis and Acute Meningoencephalitis

Etiologic Agents	Frequency*
Viruses	
Spread person-to-person only	
Herpes simplex types 1 and 2	+++
Varicella zoster	++
Epstein-Barr	+
Cytomegalovirus	++
Human herpesvirus type 6	++
Human herpesvirus type 7	+
Enteroviruses	++
Reoviruses	+
Influenza A and B	++
Respiratory syncytial	+
Parainfluenza 1-3	+
Adenovirus	+
Rubella	++
Human Coronavirus	+
Mumps	+++
Measles	++
Variola	+
Hepatitis A, B, C	+
Human parvovirus	+
Rotavirus	+
BK and JC	+
Spread to humans by mosquitoes or ticks	++
Arboviruses†—those that occur in the United States are the following: St. Louis, West Nile, Eastern equine, Western equine, Venezuelan equine, California, Powassan, and Colorado tick fever	
Spread by warm-blooded mammals	
Rabies	+++
Simian herpesvirus (herpesvirus B)	+
Lymphocytic choriomeningitis	++
Encephalomyocarditis	+
Vesicular stomatitis	+
Equine Morbillivirus (Hendra virus)	+
Nipah	+
Monkeypox	+
Bacteria	
Haemophilus influenzae, Neisseria meningitidis, Streptococcus pneumoniae, Mycobacterium tuberculosis, and other bacterial meningitides often have an encephalitic component	+++
Spirochetal infections: *Treponema pallidum, Leptospira, Borrelia burgdorferi,* and other *Borrelia* spp. infections	+++
Brucella spp.	+
Actinomyces and *Nocardia*	+
Bartonella henselae	+
Listeria monocytogenes	+
Other	
Chlamydia psittaci, Chlamydia pneumoniae	+
Rickettsial infections: Rocky Mountain spotted fever, ehrlichiosis, Q fever, and typhus	+++
Mycoplasma infections: *Mycoplasma pneumoniae* and *Mycoplasma hominis*	++
Fungal: *Coccidioides immitis, Cryptococcus neoformans,* and other fungal meningitides often have an encephalitic component	++
Protozoal: *Plasmodium* spp., *Trypanosoma* spp., *Naegleria* spp., *Acanthamoeba* spp., *Balamuthia mandrillaris,* and *Toxoplasma gondii*	+++
Helminths: *Trichinella spiralis, Schistosoma* spp., *Strongyloides stercoralis, Baylisascaris procyonis*	++
Drug: trimethoprim	+

Frequency refers to the rate of occurrence of encephalitis or encephalitis component in the particular disease cited and not its relative overall occurrence; +++ = frequent, ++ = infrequent; + = rare.

†*See Chapters 184, 187, 188, 202 and 203 for viral diseases in other countries transmitted by arthropods.*

and usually occurs in immunocompromised children.[135,153,304] Several cases have been described in previously healthy patients, however.

Human herpesvirus type 6 (HHV-6) is an important cause of acute febrile illness and roseola infantum in young children, commonly associated with febrile convulsions.[100] Encephalitis is a rare complication of HHV-6 infection in children with and without roseola.[8,46,164-166,221,247,361] HHV-6 increasingly has become recognized as an important cause of encephalitis in immunocompromised, post-transplantation patients, occasionally manifesting as severe amnesia after they have undergone bone marrow transplantation.[35,70,76,115,213,290,306,338] HHV-7 also they have undergone has been implicated as a causative agent in encephalitis.[263,328,344]

Enteroviruses now are the leading viral cause of neurologic disease in children in the United States, and they are a major cause of encephalitis.* The following viral types have been associated with encephalitis: coxsackieviruses A2, 4 to 7, 9, 10, 16, and B1-5; echoviruses 1 to 9, 11 to 25, 27, 30, and 33; and enterovirus 71. In 1998, an extensive epidemic of enterovirus 71 disease occurred in Taiwan.[64,154,157,208,211,342,357,358] Manifestations of illness in this epidemic varied, and many children had severe neurologic events, including meningitis, meningoencephalitis, encephalitis, cerebellitis, and polio-like syndrome. In particular, numerous children had brain stem encephalitis, with many fatalities occurring. A variety of neurologic illnesses, including encephalitis, have occurred rarely in reoviral infections.[102,173,188,190,364]

Encephalitis occurs with some regularity as a manifestation of influenza viral infection,† more often described in children than in adults. Although particularly notable during 1997 to 2001 influenza A epidemics in Japan, cases of influenza-associated encephalitis and encephalopathy also have been described in North America and Europe, and influenza B has been implicated as well.[237,240,318,326,360] Numerous other clinical CNS manifestations have been shown to occur during the course of influenza infection, including Reye syndrome (see Chapter 56), acute necrotizing encephalopathy, and myelitis.[160,250,289,317] Rarely, encephalitis occurs during the course of respiratory infections with respiratory syncytial virus, human coronavirus, and parainfluenza virus infections.‡

Adenoviruses are uncommon, but not rare, causes of encephalitis and meningoencephalitis.[50,88,89,97,186,244,252] Adenoviral types 1 to 3, 5 to 7, 11, 12, and 32 have been recovered from either the brain or the CSF in affected patients. More recently, a syndrome of transient encephalopathy associated with adenovirus type 3 has been described.[316]

Neurologic involvement is a common manifestation of congenital rubella virus infection,[144] and encephalitis is a rare complication of noncongenital disease.[63,201,232] Some data suggest a rate of encephalitis in rubella between 1/5000 and 1/10,000 cases.[50] In the pre-vaccine era, the encephalitis rate in one epidemic in 1964 was 1/5000 cases, and in another epidemic in 1942, it was 1/6000 cases.[217,301]

Before the use of mumps vaccine became widespread, this virus was the leading cause of meningoencephalitis in the United States. Today, mumps is rare, although extensive mumps outbreaks with associated cases of encephalitis occurred in 2006.[60] The incidence of encephalitis among individuals with mumps is approximately three episodes per 1000 cases, and the case-fatality rate is 1.4 percent.[53] In the pre-vaccine era, measles was an important cause of severe encephalitis in children.[49,51] Measles is a rare occurrence in the United States, and encephalitis occurs uncommonly, at a rate of 0.74/1000 cases of measles; the case-fatality

rate is 14 percent. Smallpox (variola virus infection), before its worldwide eradication, was a rare cause of encephalitis.

Hepatitis B virus and potentially hepatitis C virus are rare causes of encephalitis, and encephalitis has been reported as a complication of erythema infectiosum (human parvovirus infection).[16,17,34,141,246,315] Encephalitis and cerebellitis have been noted in association with rotavirus gastroenteritis,[126,212,242] and BK and JC viruses have been detected in the CSF of patients with suspected encephalitis.[23,24,340] A case of encephalitis in a 3-year-old boy caused by vesicular stomatitis virus has been described.[270] This virus can be spread by direct contact with infected animals or by insects.

Arboviruses are the most important worldwide cause of severe encephalitis. The occurrence of specific arboviruses is seasonal and highly geographic. More than 400 different arboviruses exist, and detailed information about illnesses caused by specific types in various areas of the world is provided in Chapters 184, 187, 188, 202 and 203.[26,153,176] In the United States, eight arboviruses (eastern equine, western equine, Venezuelan equine, St. Louis, Powassan, West Nile, California, and Colorado tick fever) that cause encephalitis have been isolated.

First detected in the Western Hemisphere in 1999 in New York City, West Nile virus subsequently spread across North America from the Atlantic to the Pacific coasts, and into Canada and Mexico.[39,55,104,216,162,239,261] Between 1999 and 2005, greater than 18,000 cases were reported in the United States, with more than 700 deaths.[57,150] An estimated 1 in 150 infections results in severe neurologic illness, and, although the incidence of neuroinvasive disease increases with age, West Nile virus has been responsible for encephalitis in young children and adolescents, occurring in approximately one fifth of the 150 pediatric cases diagnosed in the United States in 2002.[73,113,149] Before the introduction of West Nile virus, La Crosse encephalitis virus was the most common cause of pediatric arboviral encephalitis in the United States.[225,294] Of all North American causes of arboviral encephalitis, eastern equine encephalitis virus results in the most severe disease and has the highest case-fatality rate, particularly among infants and children.[280]

Human rabies is uncommon in the United States, but more than 20,000 cases and deaths occur worldwide every year.[356] Since the early 1970s, approximately two cases of rabies have occurred per year in the United States, and approximately 50 percent of the cases have occurred in children and teenagers.[6,52] Although rabies previously was considered to be universally fatal, a 15-year-old girl with clinical rabies survived after induction of coma and administration of antiviral therapy.[353] Encephalitis caused by herpesvirus B is rare; it occurs predominantly in monkey handlers and usually after monkey bites.[163] Except in outbreak situations, lymphocytic choriomeningitis virus rarely is recognized as a cause of encephalitis.[28] Serologic surveys have indicated, however, that neurologic disease caused by this virus is not rare in the United States,[89-91,170,230] and clusters of lymphocytic choriomeningitis virus cases were identified among recipients of solid organ transplants in 2003 and 2005.[108] Rare cases of encephalitis are caused by encephalomyocarditis virus; infection of humans with this virus is common, but most infections go unrecognized.[324]

Since its emergence in Japan in the 1870s, Japanese encephalitis virus, a mosquito-borne flavivirus, has spread across Asia to become the most important cause of epidemic encephalitis worldwide, with an estimated 35,000 to 50,000 cases and 10,000 deaths annually.[309,310,332] Nipah virus, a new paramyxovirus, is the first wide-scale epizoonotic encephalitis with direct animal-to-human, rather than vectorial, transmission.[66] The initial outbreak of Nipah virus encephalitis occurred among pig farmers in Malaysia and Singapore in 1999, and subsequently outbreaks have been identified in Bangladesh and India.[25,62,124,145,156,195,204,321,322] A fatal case of encephalitis caused by Hendra virus (equine morbillivirus), another novel paramyxovirus, was reported in an adult[253];

---

*See references 22, 50, 58, 59, 71, 88, 89, 91, 97, 136, 153, 175, 179, 186, 198, 230, 234, 236, 244.

†See references 22, 50, 74, 88, 89, 91, 109, 122, 123, 188, 244, 255, 271, 317, 343, 366.

‡See references 16, 29, 49, 88, 91, 188, 241, 319, 341, 359.

previously, this virus had been noted in association with fatal respiratory infections in horses and humans.

In 2003, another emerging pathogen, Chandipura virus, was responsible for a large outbreak of acute encephalitis in 329 children in southern India, with a case-fatality rate of 56 percent.[272] This rhabdovirus transmitted to humans by sandflies was responsible for a second outbreak in western India in 2004, with an even higher case-fatality rate of 78 percent.[61] During the 2003 monkeypox outbreak in the midwestern United States, one child developed severe acute encephalitis and seizures; no additional encephalitis cases were identified.[295]

BACTERIA

Signs and symptoms of acute encephalitis (drowsiness, coma, convulsions, mental confusion) commonly occur in *Haemophilus influenzae*, *Neisseria meningitidis*, and *Streptococcus pneumoniae* bacterial meningitides, but the true etiology usually is established easily by the examination of the CSF. Spirochetal infections are a more common cause of nervous system disease, specifically encephalitis, than generally is appreciated. Encephalitis is a recognized complication of leptospirosis, Lyme disease, and relapsing fever.[29,38,95,257,260,311] *Brucella* spp. are infrequent causes of meningoencephalitis, and *Bartonella henselae* encephalitis is an uncommon complication of cat-scratch disease.[43,120,227,228,245,314,362] Infection with *Listeria monocytogenes* has been shown to mimic herpetic and West Nile virus encephalitis.[81,266]

Neurologic disease is a common complication of pertussis. A 10-year study in the United States indicated a rate of neurologic disease in infants of approximately 9 per 1000 cases.[105] An extensive review by Miller and associates[232] suggested that the neurologic disease occurring with pertussis rarely, if ever, is inflammatory, and it is better classified as an encephalopathy.

OTHER AGENTS

Encephalitis is an uncommon occurrence in psittacosis, occurring in 1 to 3 percent of cases.[44,114] It can be caused by *Chlamydia psittaci* and *Chlamydia pneumoniae*. Neurologic involvement commonly occurs in Rocky Mountain spotted fever.[151,178] In one study, two thirds of the ill children had evidence of encephalitis. Neurologic sequelae are common.[127] Neurologic involvement also occurs in nonspotted fever rickettsial infections.[98,125,191,210,258,273,299] *Coxiella burnetii*, *Ehrlichia canis*, *Rickettsia typhi*, *Rickettsia canada*, and *Rickettsia conorii* all have been implicated.

Mycoplasma pneumoniae is an important cause of encephalitis.* Pönkä[264] noted that 4.8 percent of hospitalized patients with *M. pneumoniae* infections had CNS manifestations, and most of them had encephalitis or meningoencephalitis. *Mycoplasma hominis* is a rare cause of neonatal meningoencephalitis.[215]

Numerous fungi cause neurologic illness.[287] These illnesses occur most commonly in immunocompromised patients, but some infections occur in apparently normal individuals. Meningitis and brain abscess are the most common pathologic events, but encephalitis is associated commonly with meningitis. The following fungal agents are the most common causes of meningoencephalitis in children and adults with normal immunologic status: *Blastomyces dermatitidis*, *Coccidioides immitis*, *Cryptococcus neoformans*, *Cladosporium* spp., *Histoplasma capsulatum*, and *Paracoccidioides brasiliensis*.

Involvement of the brain in parasitic infections is common, and the reader is referred to Section XXII for a complete review.

---

*See references 30, 31, 47, 77, 85, 86, 140, 185, 209, 264, 302, 308, 331.

Cerebral malaria is a common complication of *Plasmodium falciparum* infection. Meningoencephalitis and enlarging cerebral mass lesions rarely occur in acute acquired toxoplasmosis.[330] The free-living ameba *Naegleria fowleri* is a rare cause of encephalitis, but infection with this agent usually is fatal.[293,325] Most cases occur in children and young adults and are caused by swimming or playing in contaminated water. Fatal encephalitis also has resulted from infection with *Balamuthia mandrillaris*, a soil ameba formerly thought to be innocuous.[132,339] *Baylisascaris procyonis*, a raccoon roundworm, has been associated with severe and often fatal encephalitis in children.[56,117,118,354] A recurrent encephalitis caused by administration of trimethoprim has been reported.[152]

POSTIMMUNIZATION

Neurologic disease, including encephalitis and meningoencephalitis, has occurred after immunization with a variety of prophylactic and therapeutic preparations. Depending on the type of immunizing agent, the encephalitis can be the result of an immunologic reaction, a CNS infection with the vaccine virus, or a combination of infection and immunologic reaction. Historically, many of the observed neurologic reactions occurred after the administration of antisera prepared in animals in the treatment of specific diseases. Antisera to the following diseases or infectious agents have been noted in association with neurologic illness: tetanus, diphtheria, scarlet fever, tuberculosis, gas gangrene, pneumococcus, gonococcus, meningococcus, and streptococci.[3,161,180,231,279] Of 100 neurologic syndromes complicating administration of serum reviewed by Miller and Stanton,[231] only 10 percent were of a cerebral or meningeal type.

Neurologic disease was a common complication of rabies vaccine derived from animal nervous tissue.[231] The incidence of complication was between 3/1000 and 1/6000 cases.[32,231] Approximately 10 percent of the neurologic disease attributed to this rabies vaccine was meningoencephalitic or encephalomyelitic. Five cases of CNS disease (Guillain-Barré syndrome, demyelination, meningoradiculitis) have been reported in temporal association with the administration of human diploid cell rabies vaccine.[262] This occurrence is so rare that a causal relationship with vaccine is uncertain.

Encephalitis was an important complication of smallpox vaccination.[7,37,110,130,175,199,238,312] The rate of encephalitis varied markedly from one study to another, from 1 in 4000 primary vaccinations in the Netherlands[238] to approximately 1 in 80,000 primary vaccinations in the United States.[200] After reinstatement of the vaccination among military personnel and selected civilian groups in the United States, three cases of suspected encephalitis or myelitis were identified among 665,000 individuals vaccinated from 2002 to 2004.[296]

Neurologic disease, including encephalitis, occurs rarely after the administration of typhoid-paratyphoid vaccine.[231] Neurologic disease also rarely has been attributed to administration of tetanus toxoid and diphtheria toxoid, but the manifestations seldom are central.

Encephalitis and encephalopathy have been observed after the administration of influenza immunization.[119,131,282,355] In the extensive surveillance that occurred in the United States during the period October 1, 1976, to December 16, 1976, when 45,651,113 people received the A/New Jersey/76 influenza vaccine, no epidemiologic evidence of an association between vaccine and encephalitis was noted.[139] Two children who developed acute disseminated encephalomyelitis after receiving Japanese B encephalitis vaccination have been reported.[248]

Neurologic disease developing after administration of a whole-cell pertussis vaccine is a well-known event.[67-69] Pathologic evidence in fatal cases suggests encephalopathy rather than encephalitis.[80] Because neurologic illness similar to that which occurs after the administration of pertussis vaccination is a frequent development in infants who have not been vaccinated, establishing a true rate of pertussis vaccine encephalopathy, or that such an entity exists at all, has been difficult. The analysis of studies suggests that encephalopathy caused by pertussis vaccine does not occur.[68,69,134,280]

Neurologic disease, including encephalitis, is a rare complication of measles immunization.[48,51,111,197] The rate in vaccinees in the United States is less than 1/1 million. In contrast, the finding in the National Childhood Encephalopathy Study in England, Scotland, and Wales indicated a rate of 1/87,000 immunizations.[2] This high rate of encephalopathy may be an artifact due to the misclassification of complicated febrile convulsions as encephalopathy. Meningoencephalitis has been shown to be a rare complication of mumps immunization with some vaccine virus strains,[222] although it has not been a problem in the United States. More recent studies in the United States and Finland have failed to show an association between measles-mumps-rubella vaccination and encephalitis or encephalopathy.[214,275] A fatal encephalitis occurred in a 3-year-old child after receiving 17D yellow fever vaccine.[268]

POSTINFECTIOUS ENCEPHALITIS

Postinfectious or parainfectious encephalitis occurs after a demonstrated or presumed viral infection and is thought to be immune-mediated rather than due to a direct effect of the virus in nerve cells.[133,170-172,285] This theory has been studied extensively by Johnson[171,172] and Griffin[133] in encephalitis associated with measles. They have described a periventricular demyelinating disease and have not been able to isolate measles virus or identify measles antigens in nervous tissue. Other investigators, including one of us (J. D. C.), have recovered measles virus, however, from the CSF and brain of affected patients.[111,226,229,269,298] We suggest that immune mechanisms play a role in the pathogenesis of measles and perhaps other postinfectious neurologic illnesses, but the process is stimulated by the direct presence of the antigen in the nervous system. The mechanism of disease is important regarding possible treatment: steroids might be useful in immune-mediated disease but could be detrimental in an acute viral infection.

In contrast to measles, other apparent postinfectious encephalitides that usually have a subacute onset are immune mediated and have multifocal white-matter lesions.* Specifically, acute demyelinating encephalomyelitis (ADEM) usually is subacute in onset and is characterized by optic neuritis, myelitis, ataxia, hemiparesis, cranial nerve palsies, and multifocal white-matter lesions that are easily confused with multiple sclerosis. Subtle features help distinguish between the two disorders, however.[307] If solitary or unilateral lesions are present, it most likely is ADEM, whereas lesions in the corpus callosum are much more common in multiple sclerosis. Lesions greater than 4 cm diameter suggest ADEM, and ADEM lesions generally have indistinct borders compared with multiple sclerosis lesions, which generally have sharp borders. Patients with ADEM may respond dramatically to treatment with steroids and perhaps intravenous immunoglobulin or plasmapheresis.

CHRONIC ENCEPHALITIC OR ENCEPHALOPATHIC ILLNESSES

"Slow infections" that cause encephalitic and encephalopathic illness in humans have been recognized for many years. Many of

these illnesses now are recognized as viral infections or caused by prions. Viral illnesses include progressive multifocal leukoencephalopathy (JC, SV40, and BK viruses), subacute sclerosing panencephalitis (measles virus), and acquired immunodeficiency syndrome (AIDS) (human immunodeficiency virus [HIV] type 1 [HIV-1] and HIV-2). Prion diseases, termed *transmissible spongiform encephalopathies*, include kuru, Jakob-Creutzfeldt disease, and Gerstmann-Sträussler-Scheinker disease.[267] Prion diseases are related to scrapie of sheep and bovine spongiform encephalopathy (mad cow disease), which are prion diseases of animals. These chronic illnesses are discussed in Chapter 205.

EPIDEMIOLOGY

Because encephalitis has many different causes, no unified epidemiologic pattern exists. The specific epidemiology of each infectious agent or disease is presented in detail in the respective chapters of this book; only a brief overview is presented here. Most cases occur in the summer and fall, reflecting arboviral and enteroviral etiologies. Encephalitis caused by arboviruses occurs in localized outbreaks and epidemics, with boundaries determined by the range of particular mosquito vectors and the prevalence of natural reservoir animals.

Arboviruses are zoonoses in which humans are infected accidentally by an arthropod vector, humans not being essential in the life cycle of arboviruses. Most commonly, mosquitoes or other insects acquire arboviruses by biting infected birds, which often have prolonged viremia without illness. The insect vectors, although preferring birds, bite other vertebrates, including humans and horses. Encephalitis in horses and mules may be the first indication of incipient trouble in an area; veterinarians often are the first to detect an impending epidemic. Rural exposure is not a sine qua non; urban and suburban outbreaks are frequent.

Although enteroviral disease, including aseptic meningitis, occurs in epidemics, severe encephalitis caused by these agents usually is a sporadic event. Sporadic cases of encephalitis occur in any season; epidemiologic considerations that must be reviewed in a search for the causative agent include geographic area; climatic conditions; animal, water, food, soil, and personal exposures; and host factors.

PATHOGENESIS

Because encephalitis and meningoencephalitis have multiple causes, the lack of a unified pathogenesis is not surprising.* Clinical manifestations of encephalitis can result from a direct or an indirect effect of an infectious agent on the brain. Rabies, arbovirus, herpes simplex, and enteroviral encephalitides are examples in which the viral infections directly involve tissue cells within the brain. In contrast, encephalitic symptoms in bacterial meningitides and in rickettsial infections may be caused by the vasculitis and liberated toxins of the surrounding infection. In addition, in many postinfectious or parainfectious encephalitides, immunologic events clearly are important in the pathogenesis. Measles and *M. pneumoniae* infections are in this category.

Postinfectious or parainfectious encephalitis is an acute demyelinating disease of the brain in which the findings suggest an autoimmune process. Usually, little evidence of an active infectious process is present when symptoms occur. Viral or other agents probably invaded the CNS initially and then were cleared but were a trigger for the subsequent development of disease. An immune (T-cell) response to myelin basic protein occurs.

---

*See references 4, 11, 15, 36, 83, 138, 181, 202, 224, 227, 238, 323, 359.

*See references 7, 27, 47, 77, 99, 107, 111, 127, 133, 137, 144, 153, 168, 170, 230-232, 235, 349.

In most encephalitides, such as those caused by arboviruses, mumps, and enteroviruses, the CNS infection is secondary to a primary viral infection elsewhere in the body. Generally, the infectious agents, whether from ingestion, as in enteroviral infections, or from the bite of a mosquito, as in an arboviral infection, enter the lymphatic system. In the lymphatics, viral multiplication occurs, which results in seeding of the bloodstream and infection of other organs in the body. Viral multiplication occurs at these secondary infection sites, extensive secondary viremia occurs, and then the CNS becomes infected. Actual involvement of nervous tissue may result from growth across or passive diffusion through brain capillaries or centripetal axonal transport of virus from the olfactory neuroepithelium to the olfactory bulb.[235]

Infection of the brain also may occur through the peripheral nerves. This retrograde spread of virus is important in rabies and HSV encephalitis.

PATHOLOGY

Determining the etiology of encephalitis at autopsy is difficult, although morphologic identification of falciparum malaria, trypanosomiasis, and fungal encephalitis is possible.[80,170,231,232,312] In viral encephalitides, the histopathologist may recognize rabies (Negri bodies) or an agent of the herpesvirus group (intranuclear inclusion bodies).

Tissue sections of the brain generally reveal meningeal congestion and mononuclear infiltration, perivascular cuffs of lymphocytes and plasma cells, some perivascular tissue necrosis with myelin breakdown, neuronal disruption in various stages (including ultimately neuronophagia), and endothelial proliferation or necrosis. A marked degree of demyelination with preservation of neurons and their axons is considered to be predominantly postinfectious or parainfectious (autoimmune) encephalitis. The severity and the extent of observed lesions vary with the infectious agent and with the degree of reaction of the host. The cerebral cortex, especially the temporal lobe, often is affected severely by HSV; the arboviruses tend to affect the entire brain; and rabies has a predilection for the basal structures. Involvement of the spinal cord, nerve roots, and peripheral nerves varies.

CLINICAL MANIFESTATIONS

The clinical findings in encephalitis are determined by the severity of involvement and anatomic localization of the affected portions of the nervous system, the inherent pathogenicity of the offending agent, and the immune and other reactive mechanisms of the patient ("host factors"). A wide range of severity of clinical manifestations exists even with the same etiologic agent. Evidence of brain parenchymal involvement is the hallmark of encephalitis. Children with encephalitis may show evidence of diffuse disease, such as behavioral or personality changes; decreased consciousness; and generalized seizures or localized changes, such as focal seizures, hemiparesis, movement disorders, cranial nerve defects, and ataxia. Some children may seem to be mildly affected initially only to lapse into coma and sudden death. In others, the illness is ushered in by high fever, violent convulsions interspersed with bizarre movements, and hallucinations alternating with brief periods of clarity, and the children emerge with relatively few sequelae.

Most commonly, the initial manifestations resemble an undifferentiated acute systemic illness with fever, headache, or, in infants, screaming spells, abdominal distress, nausea, and vomiting. Signs of an associated mild nasopharyngitis may suggest a respiratory infection. As the temperature increases, new findings direct attention to the nervous system: mental dullness eventuating in stupor; bizarre movements; convulsions; nuchal rigidity, often not as pronounced as in purely meningitic illness; and focal neurologic signs, which may be stationary, progress, or fluctuate. Loss of bowel and bladder control and unprovoked emotional outbursts may occur.

SPECIFIC FORMS OF ENCEPHALITIS

Specific forms of encephalitis or complicating manifestations of encephalitis include Guillain-Barré syndrome and related syndromes, acute transverse myelitis, acute hemiplegia, brain stem encephalitis, and acute cerebellar ataxia. Acute cerebellar ataxia is characterized by an abrupt onset of truncal ataxia resulting in varying degrees of gait disturbance and balance abnormalities. Children with this illness have tremulousness of the head and trunk when in the upright position and of the extremities when attempting to move them against gravity. The duration of illness varies from 3 to 4 days to several weeks. Acute cerebellar ataxia often follows chickenpox or other viral illnesses. In one study, 3 percent were related to immunization.[78] Approximately 90 percent of patients recovered completely from the ataxia, but 20 percent had transient behavioral or intellectual disturbances. Five percent had persistent learning problems.

Brain stem encephalitis (Bickerstaff encephalitis) is a rare disorder, but it is important because clinical signs appear similar to those of a brain stem glioma. The differentiation is important because treatment is radically different. The differentiation is made by the time of onset of symptoms and by the course. Brain stem glioma usually has slowly progressive symptoms developing over the course of several weeks or months. Brain stem encephalitis evolves over 1 to 7 days. Both disorders may be associated with radiographic evidence of brain stem enlargement. Brain stem encephalitis resolves after 1 to 4 weeks, whereas a tumor continues to progress until radiation therapy is given.

Most cases of brain stem encephalitis seem to be postinfectious and are similar to postinfectious cerebellar ataxia, Miller-Fisher syndrome, or Guillain-Barré syndrome. The conditions often overlap.[12] In postinfectious cases, the onset of brain stem encephalitis begins 1 to 3 weeks after a nonspecific viral infection. Brain stem encephalitis has been reported to occur, however, as a result of specific, identifiable, and possibly treatable infectious agents, including HSV,[278,292] VZV,[283,320] CMV,[116,174] and enterovirus 71[157,159] and M. pneumoniae,[196,313] L. monocytogenes,[5,9,10,13,19] Propionibacterium acnes,[41] and Campylobacter jejuni.[363]

Some patients with a typical clinical picture of brain stem encephalitis have had anti-GQ1b antibodies in the serum,[65] which may represent a subgroup of postinfectious brain stem encephalitis. Brain stem encephalitis may arise in HIV-infected patients and may be due to a treatable cause, such as herpes simplex encephalitis.[116,143,282] Brain stem encephalitis caused by viral infections may resolve similar to the typical postinfectious type, but some viral infections may lead to permanent neurologic sequelae. In an enterovirus outbreak in Taiwan, the most common neurologic complication was rhombencephalitis, and a 14 percent mortality rate was reported.[157,159] More recent reports suggest that intravenous immunoglobulin may be an effective therapy in some patients.[112] In a Cochrane review, this therapy remains unproven, however.[254]

DIFFERENTIAL DIAGNOSIS

The evaluation of a patient with an acute CNS illness (encephalopathy) must be considered carefully, and the sequence of tests should be dictated by the specific circumstances of the individual patient. Several disease processes may have a presentation similar to that of encephalitis or meningoencephalitis. The differential diagnosis of acute encephalopathy includes the following:

1. Metabolic diseases, such as hypoglycemia, uremic encephalopathy, hepatic encephalopathy, and rare genetic inborn errors of metabolism, including disorders of glucose or ammonia metabolism

2. Toxic disorders, such as drug ingestion or Reye syndrome

3. Mass lesions, such as tumor or abscess

4. Subarachnoid hemorrhage from arteriovenous malformation or aneurysm

5. Embolic lesions caused by bacterial endocarditis

6. Acute demyelinating disorders, including acute multiple sclerosis, ADEM, and acute hemorrhagic leukoencephalitis

7. Status epilepticus, especially nonconvulsive status epilepticus, such as complex-partial status or absence status

8. Infectious diseases, including viral, bacterial, fungal, chlamydial, mycoplasmal, and parasitic

9. Postinfectious diseases, including Guillain-Barré syndrome, brain stem encephalitis, Miller-Fisher syndrome, and acute cerebellar ataxia

10. Acute confusional migraine

EVALUATION OF A PATIENT WITH ENCEPHALOPATHY OR POSSIBLE ENCEPHALITIS

Obtaining a careful history and performing a physical and neurologic examination are essential in all patients who present with a history consistent with encephalitis. The differential diagnosis previously presented indicates that encephalitis is only one of many disorders that can manifest with an acute or subacute picture of encephalopathy. Although the diagnosis of encephalitis may be determined best with a lumbar puncture and evaluation of the CSF, lumbar puncture may be contraindicated in some disorders and, if performed inappropriately, may lead to serious complications and even death. A child who has a cerebellar tumor with acute obstruction of the fourth ventricle may present with a decreasing level of consciousness caused by the rapidly increasing intracranial pressure (ICP). Nuchal rigidity may be present. The family may not have recognized the more subtle changes in cerebellar functions for the months before the acute obstruction developed and may give a history of acute encephalopathy. In that case, a lumbar puncture could result in herniation through the foramen magnum. It is essential that the patient be assessed for the possibility of increased ICP and the potential for herniation.

The history should be reviewed carefully, questioning specifically for symptoms of neurologic problems that manifested in the days or weeks before the acute disorder occurred. The physical examination must be performed with special attention given to focal neurologic abnormalities, cerebellar signs, and evidence of increased ICP. Conducting a careful funduscopic examination is important but may be impossible in an agitated patient or young child. The presence of papilledema indicates that neuroimaging should be performed before doing the lumbar puncture. If spontaneous venous pulsations are noted on funduscopic examination, ICP is not increased, and the lumbar puncture can be done without imaging the patient.

In addition to lumbar puncture, neuroimaging and EEG can help in determining the cause of the encephalopathy and in determining the most appropriate course of therapy. The history and physical examination are a guide to the most appropriate first test to perform, but generally neuroimaging is the most likely to be helpful. The exception would be a child in nonconvulsive status epilepticus. The history may suggest encephalitis as the most likely diagnosis, but in some patients, nonconvulsive status epilepticus may be clinically indistinguishable from encephalitis.

NEUROIMAGING

Most patients with encephalopathy should undergo neuroimaging to aid diagnosis of treatable conditions, such as HSV encephalitis. Computed tomography (CT) is helpful in the acute setting to identify abnormalities such as tumor or abscess and to decide whether performing a lumbar puncture is safe. CT is not as helpful, however, as is magnetic resonance imaging (MRI) in detecting the subtle changes associated with encephalitis.[40,206,300] In many cases of viral encephalitis, CT and MRI yield normal results or only nonspecific changes, such as swelling[347] or edema.[206] An important exception is herpes simplex encephalitis.

As previously noted, MRI is more sensitive than is CT. In one study, CT initially was positive in only 42 percent of cases, whereas MRI was positive in all cases.[182] MRI in HSV characteristically shows abnormalities in the medial temporal lobes, inferior frontal cortex, and insula.[205,350] The likelihood of finding the abnormalities may be increased by using T2-weighted imaging and fluid attenuated inversion recovery (FLAIR) sequences[14,177] or diffusion-weighted imaging.[297,327] Diffusion-weighted MRI seems to be more sensitive than is FLAIR or T2-weighted sequences in the detection of HSV or other encephalitides.[334] The localization of abnormalities may differ, however, from the classic pattern in young children. In neonatal herpes encephalitis, widespread changes occur in the periventricular white matter, often sparing the medial temporal and inferior frontal lobes. Another pattern has been described in children aged 4 to 13 months in whom the cortex and adjacent white matter of the hemispheres were abnormal.[205]

In addition to herpes, other encephalitides may yield abnormal neuroimaging. CT and MRI results often are abnormal with disorders caused by arbovirus or enterovirus infections. When imaging is abnormal, it usually is nonspecific, showing areas of decreased density (with CT) or increased signal intensity (with MRI) in the gray or white matter. A variety of MRI abnormalities with certain viral encephalitides have been reported. The basal ganglia, brain stem, and thalami have been reported to be abnormal on MRI of patients with eastern equine encephalitis,[93] Japanese encephalitis,[158,192] and enterovirus 71.[157,159] These differences help to distinguish HSV from other, nontreatable causes of viral encephalitis.

Postinfectious disorders most often are associated with selective oligodendrocyte involvement.[21] Imaging shows increased signal in white matter with T2-weighted MRI or low-density white matter with CT.[18,35,147,181,249] Patients with acute hemorrhagic leukoencephalitis, a rare disease that is rapidly progressive and often fatal, may present with a clinical picture similar to that of herpes simplex encephalitis. In contrast to HSV infection, the CT results often are abnormal within the first 1 or 2 days.[284,346] If a patient with suspected herpes simplex encephalitis has abnormal CT results early in the course, acute hemorrhagic leukoencephalitis should be considered.

Another imaging technique that has been reported to be helpful in establishing the diagnosis of encephalitis is single photon emission computed tomography (SPECT). Initial reports suggest that SPECT is more sensitive than is CT. Ackerman and colleagues[2] found that SPECT showed greater sensitivity and more precise localization than did conventional radionuclide scanning and CT. Laures and associates[202] studied 14 encephalitis patients and found that SPECT detected temporal lobe abnormalities in all six of the patients with HSV encephalitis and yielded normal results in the remaining eight who had other etiologies. A few cases of normal MRI scans but abnormal SPECT in patients with herpes simplex encephalitis have been reported[146,218]; this is less likely to occur with newer MRI sequences such as diffusion weighted imaging. If SPECT is performed, Tc 99 m hexamethylpropyleneamine oxime seems to be superior to Tc 99 m ethyl cysteinate dimer.[87,106] Generally, SPECT should be reserved for cases with normal MRI and a nondiagnostic EEG in which herpes simplex encephalitis is still strongly suspected. Intracranial ultrasonography in neonates has been shown to be helpful in establishing the diagnosis and in follow-up of infants with HSV or CMV infections.[219]

ELECTROENCEPHALOGRAM

Generally, an EEG should be performed in most patients with encephalitis. EEG results of patients with encephalitis generally are normal or nonspecifically abnormal, showing diffuse slowing. Crucial exceptions to the general rule exist, however.

In acute encephalopathy, comatose patients may be in nonconvulsive status epilepticus,[328] which requires immediate and appropriate intervention. The presence of periodic lateralized epileptiform discharges (PLEDs) on EEG strongly suggests the possibility of herpes simplex encephalitis but also may be an indication of seizures.[20] Early in the course of herpes encephalitis, generalized slowing of the background frequencies and focal slowing over the affected temporal lobe may occur. Within a few days, the characteristic PLEDs pattern develops in most cases. Later in the course, the background activity between the bursts of PLEDs gradually may flatten. Occasionally, other areas of the brain seem to be involved, primarily with HSV. PLEDs, although strongly suggestive of HSV encephalitis, are not diagnostic. PLEDs have been reported with stroke and infectious mononucleosis encephalitis,[129] and periodic complexes are characteristic of the slow virus and prion disorders, including Jakob-Creutzfeldt disease and subacute sclerosing panencephalitis.

The EEG abnormalities in neonatal herpes encephalitis are similar. The characteristic EEG results yield periodic or pseudoperiodic complexes, usually triangular or sharp waves, occurring in a multifocal pattern.[233] In one study of 34 infants with herpes encephalitis, 21 underwent EEG; the results of 19 of the 21 were abnormal. The results of three showed only focal slowing, but the other 16 showed the characteristic periodic or pseudoperiodic complexes.[286] The authors reviewed 500 other neonatal EEG records and found 20 with similar complexes; 11 patients had meningoencephalitis of unknown etiology, 3 had hemorrhage, and 2 had asphyxia. Four were placed in a miscellaneous category. Periodic or pseudoperiodic complexes in neonatal EEG results strongly suggest HSV encephalitis, but they are not diagnostic.

SPECIFIC DIAGNOSIS

A meticulous history is essential and must evaluate exposure in the previous 2 to 3 weeks to illness in contacts; exposure to mosquitoes, ticks, and animals during recent vacations or picnics or other outdoor activities; awareness of illness in animals, especially horses and other Equidae, in the patient's environment; recent travel from the home area; recent injections of any kind; and the possibility of accidental exposure to heavy metals, pesticides, or other questionable substances. The CSF must be examined carefully to exclude other disorders that respond to specific therapy. Smears for bacteria, appropriate rapid antigen-identification tests, and cultures of the CSF are mandatory; the history and clinical findings may indicate the need for acid-fast stain and

culture of the sediment for mycobacteria. Other circumstances may indicate the need for excluding fungal or protozoal infection; atypical cells may require cytopathologic study to exclude neural neoplasms that may manifest acutely.

The availability of polymerase chain reaction has allowed the definitive and rapid diagnosis of HSV encephalitis to be established, eliminating the need for brain biopsy.[94,194,291,337,352] HSV DNA was detected in the CSF of 53 of 54 patients with biopsy-proven herpes simplex encephalitis.[194] The etiology of encephalitis caused by other herpesviruses also has been determined by polymerase chain reaction assay of CSF.[84,221,335] In addition to its use in herpesvirus infections, polymerase chain reaction is useful in neurologic illnesses caused by enteroviruses and *M. pneumoniae* and in the future is likely to be useful in other encephalitides.[31,184,256,276]

In viral encephalitis, the CSF frequently is clear; the leukocyte count ranges from none to several thousand, often with a significant percentage of polymorphonuclear cells initially, moderate or no elevation of protein, and an initially normal level of glucose relative to the simultaneously determined blood glucose level. In any patient suspected to have viral meningoencephalitis, spinal fluid, blood, feces, and throat swabs should be collected and sent to a laboratory offering viral diagnostic services. An additional serum specimen should be collected 10 to 21 days later. Although these studies may not provide an immediate diagnosis, they may give early warning of a specific epidemic, and the use of specific antiviral chemotherapy may be indicated by the preliminary culture results.

Inquiry regarding recent illness, recent injections, and, especially, recent exposures away from the home environment sometimes is helpful. The incubation periods of some arboviruses are such that mosquito bites acquired at least 1 week earlier or insect bites now healed may give a clue. Occasionally, patients who have traveled to Africa or Asia in preceding weeks present with encephalitis caused by viruses, trypanosomiasis, or falciparum malaria with bizarre systemic and CNS signs and symptoms.

TREATMENT

Acyclovir should be used to treat herpes simplex and VZV encephalitis and perhaps encephalitis caused by Epstein-Barr virus. CMV encephalitis should be treated with ganciclovir. Pleconaril (if it becomes available) should be considered for treatment of enteroviral encephalitis, and oseltamivir should be considered for treatment of encephalitis caused by influenzaviruses A or B. Specific antimicrobial treatment should be used for infections caused by spirochetes, *Chlamydia*, *Mycoplasma*, fungi, and parasites.

General treatment is nonspecific and empiric, aimed at maintaining life and supporting each involved organ system. The effectiveness of various recommended regimens in most instances has not been evaluated objectively. Until a bacterial etiology and, in particular, a brain abscess are excluded substantially, parenteral antibiotic therapy should be administered.

Anticipating and being prepared for convulsions, cerebral edema, hyperpyrexia, inadequate respiratory exchange, disturbed fluid and electrolyte balance, aspiration and asphyxia, abrupt cardiac and respiratory arrest of central origin, cardiac decompensation, and gastrointestinal bleeding are crucial. The syndrome of disseminated intravascular coagulation may be an additional complication.

For these reasons, all patients with severe encephalitis should receive care in intensive care units. Cardiac monitoring should be maintained. Repeat CT and MRI scans are helpful in following comatose patients and often show signs of brain swelling before the patient has the typical clinical indicators of

ICP, such as Cushing triad (systolic hypertension, bradycardia, and slowing of respirations), dilated pupils, and decorticate or decerebrate posturing. The Cushing triad is an unreliable indicator of increased ICP, and, when the other signs of increased ICP occur, they often do so late in the course, when the patient's cerebral perfusion already is at risk.[223] If brain swelling becomes a problem, placing an ICP monitor may be necessary. The ICP should be maintained at less than 15 mm Hg if possible using the standard techniques for reduction of ICP, including hyperventilation, osmotic diuretics, and removal of CSF. As a last resort, inducing a barbiturate coma may be necessary. A related consequence of ICP is the syndrome of inappropriate antidiuretic hormone secretion. Careful monitoring of the fluid and electrolyte balance is essential in all seriously ill patients with encephalitis.

All fluids, electrolytes, and medications initially are given parenterally. In patients with prolonged coma, parenteral hyperalimentation is indicated. Normal blood levels of glucose, magnesium, and calcium must be maintained to minimize the threat of convulsions.

Status epilepticus caused by encephalitis should be treated vigorously using a structured protocol to ensure optimal control.[303,331] The current standard initial therapy is intravenous lorazepam, 0.1 to 0.2 mg/kg, up to 4 mg maximum. Seizures associated with encephalitis may be refractory to the usual therapy, and other anticonvulsants may be required to achieve and maintain control of seizures. In patients who fail initial therapy and are in medically refractory status epilepticus, continuous EEG monitoring usually is recommended to monitor the efficacy of the therapy, especially when the patient is in nonconvulsive status epilepticus.[92,329]

If after a second attempt, lorazepam fails to control the seizures, intravenous phenytoin (preferably phosphenytoin in children) is the next drug of choice. The dose is 18 to 20 mg/kg, maximum 1000 mg, given over 20 minutes. Phosphenytoin is preferred because it can be administered faster and does not cause sclerosis of the veins as does phenytoin and is not as likely to cause cardiac arrhythmias. Virtually all patients who require therapy beyond lorazepam need to be intubated to prevent respiratory embarrassment. If phosphenytoin is unsuccessful, or as an alternative to phosphenytoin, intravenous midazolam has gained favor in recent years.[75,258] The initial dose is 0.1 to 0.2 mg/kg over 5 minutes, with a maintenance infusion starting at 0.05 mg/kg/hr up to a maximum of 0.4 mg/kg/hr. Another alternative therapy is propofol, which generally is administered by an anesthesiologist.

Many methods have been proposed to minimize cerebral edema and to diminish the consequences of cerebral anoxia. The following measures are difficult to evaluate and generally are reserved for patients with severe illness whose condition apparently is desperate.

1. Dexamethasone, 0.1 to 0.2 mg/kg intravenously in an initial dose followed by 0.05 to 0.1 mg/kg intravenously every 4 to 6 hours, is given. This large dose should be reduced gradually after a few days if recovery or improvement is evident. Dexamethasone probably should not be used in acute viral diseases because steroids may potentiate the viral infection.

2. Other substances employed in an effort to reduce elevated ICP include (a) mannitol, given intravenously, as a 20 percent solution in a dose of 0.25 to 1 g/kg over a 30- to 60-minute period (this may be repeated every 8 to 12 hours), and (b) glycerol, by nasogastric tube, using 0.5 to 1 mL/kg diluted with twice that volume of orange juice. This regimen is nontoxic and may be repeated every 6 hours for an extended period.

For more than 40 years, steroids and adrenocorticotropic hormone frequently have been used as empiric therapy for encephalitis. No controlled studies have shown any efficacy, however. In two comparative studies of measles encephalitis, steroids were found to offer no benefit, and in both studies, the steroid recipients seemed to have had worse outcomes.[33,365] More recently, in a carefully controlled study, no benefit of high-dose dexamethasone was found in the treatment of acute encephalitis caused by Japanese encephalitis virus.[155]

In contrast to these investigations are more recent clinical experiences in the treatment of acute disseminated encephalomyelitis, in which MRI studies have indicated multifocal white-matter lesions.[36,138,181,224] Patients treated with steroids often have responded dramatically, with clinical improvement and resolution of the lesions as shown by MRI. Steroids, along with specific antibiotic therapy, also may be beneficial in the treatment of encephalitis caused by *M. pneumoniae* infection.[185,302]

In our opinion, steroids should not be used to treat encephalitis if the patient has an active infection, unless the infection can be treated concomitantly with an effective antimicrobial agent. Plasmapheresis and intravenous immunoglobulin have been used empirically to treat brain stem encephalitis and other encephalitides, but no studies have been done that indicate such therapies are helpful.[243]

Equipment and personnel for handling emergencies such as cardiac and respiratory arrest must be on hand constantly. Early consultation with an anesthesiologist or intensive care specialist is useful in anticipating the need for artificially assisted respiration.

Supportive and rehabilitative efforts are important after the patient recovers. Motor incoordination, convulsive disorders, squint, total or partial deafness, or behavioral disturbances may appear only after some time. Visual disturbances caused by chorioretinopathy and perceptual amblyopia also may make a delayed appearance. Special facilities and sometimes institutional placement may become necessary.

PROGNOSIS

The prognosis in all encephalitides is guarded with respect to immediate outcome and sequelae. Sequelae involving the CNS may be intellectual, motor, psychiatric, epileptic, visual, or auditory. Cardiovascular, intraocular, pulmonary, hepatic, and other systems sometimes are affected permanently. The short-term and long-term prognoses depend to some extent on etiology and age. Young infants usually have severe disease and sequelae. Generally, HSV carries a worse prognosis for survival and residual disability than do the enteroviruses.

Rautonen and associates[274] examined prognostic factors in childhood acute encephalitis at the Children's Hospital, University of Helsinki, during a 20-year period from 1968 to 1987. This study comprised 462 cases with the following etiologies: mumps virus, measles virus, rubella virus, VZV, HSV, enteroviruses, respiratory viruses, *M. pneumoniae*, other agents, and cause undetermined. The investigators found that mortality was fivefold greater in infants compared with older children. Children who were disorientated or unconscious before admission had 4-fold and 25-fold greater risks for death and severe damage than did children whose level of consciousness had been normal. Patients with HSV or *M. pneumoniae* infection had the greatest risks for death or serious residual damage compared with children with encephalitis of other etiologies.

California encephalitis has a low mortality rate but occurs most frequently in the pediatric age group. Of patients who experience seizures in the acute phase of their disease, 25 percent have a permanent seizure disorder.[128] Psychological sequelae were present in 15 percent in one series but were not found to be significant in several series if the children were evaluated several years after their illnesses.[72,220,277]

Prognosis in encephalitis caused by western equine virus is guarded; 56 percent of infants younger than 1 month of age have had recurring seizures with marked motor and behavioral changes. After they reach 1 year of age, the sequelae appear to diminish; only 5 percent of adults have neurologic sequelae. Fifty-seven percent of infants who survived western equine virus infection and who were younger than 1 year of age at the time of infection had major neurologic sequelae requiring either a special school or institutionalization late in life. Severe retardation, paralysis, spasticity, recurrent convulsions, hearing deficits, and speech difficulties all were reported as complications.[100,107]

Eastern equine encephalitis has a high mortality rate. Infants and children younger than 5 years of age who survive usually have severe sequelae consisting of mental retardation, convulsions, and paralysis. These consequences are in contrast to adults older than 40 years of age who survive, who recover completely or have only slight damage.

St. Louis encephalitis has a low mortality rate. Although neurologic sequelae are reported, their incidence is low in the pediatric age group.

PREVENTION

The widespread use of effective attenuated viral vaccines for measles, mumps, and rubella almost has eliminated CNS complications from these diseases in the United States. The control of encephalitis caused by arboviruses has been less successful because specific vaccines for the arbovirus diseases that occur in North America are unavailable. Control of insect vectors by suitable spraying methods and eradication of insect breeding sites is useful.

REFERENCES

1. Aberle, S. W., Aberle, J. H., Steininger, C., et al.: Quantitative real time PCR detection of varicella-zoster virus DNA in cerebrospinal fluid in patients with neurological disease. Med. Microbiol. Immunol. 194:7-12, 2005.
2. Ackerman, E. S., Tumeh, S. S., Charron, M., et al.: Viral encephalitis: Imaging with SPECT. Clin. Nucl. Med. 13:640-643, 1988.
3. Allen, I. M.: The neurological complications of serum treatment: With report of a case. Lancet 2:1128-1131, 1931.
4. Alper, G., and Schor, N. F.: Toward the definition of acute disseminated encephalitis of childhood. Curr. Opin. Pediatr. 16:637-640, 2004.
5. Alstadhaug, K. B., Antal, E. A., Nielsen, E. W., et al.: Listeria rhombencephalitis—a case report. Eur. J. Neurol. 13:93-102, 2006.
6. Anderson, L. J., Nicholson, K. G., Tauxe, R. V., et al.: Human rabies in the United States, 1960 to 1979: Epidemiology, diagnosis and prevention. Ann. Intern. Med. 100:728-735, 1984.
7. Angulo, J. J., Pimenta-de-Campos, E., and de Salles-Gomes, L. F.: Postvaccinial meningo-encephalitis: Isolation of the virus from the brain. J. A. M. A. 187:151-153, 1964.
8. Ansari, A., Li, S., Abzug, M. J., et al.: Human herpesviruses 6 and 7 and central nervous system infection in children. Emerg. Infect. Dis. 10:1450-1454, 2004.
9. Antal, E. A., Dietrichs, E., Loberg, E. M., et al.: Brain stem encephalitis in listeriosis. Scand. J. Infect. Dis. 37:190-194, 2005.
10. Antal, E. A., Loberg, E. M., Dietrichs, E., et al.: Neuropathological findings in 9 cases of Listeria monocytogenes brain stem encephalitis. Brain Pathol. 15:187-191, 2005.
11. Apak, R. A., Köse, G., Anlar, B., et al.: Acute disseminated encephalomyelitis in childhood: Report of 10 cases. J. Child. Neurol. 14:198-201, 1999.
12. Arai, M., Odaka, M., Yuki, N., et al.: A patient with overlapping Bickerstaff's brainstem encephalitis, Miller Fisher syndrome and Guillain-Barré syndrome during the clinical course. Eur. J. Neurol. 9:115-116, 2002.
13. Armstrong, R. W., and Fung, P. C.: Brainstem encephalitis (rhombencephalitis) due to Listeria monocytogenes: Case report and review. Clin. Infect. Dis. 16:1089-1093, 1993.
14. Ashikaga, R., Araki, Y., and Ishida, O.: MR FLAIR imaging of herpes simplex encephalitis. Radiat. Med. 14:349-352, 1996.
15. Assa, A., Watemberg, N., Bujanover, Y., et al.: Demyelinative brainstem encephalitis responsive to intravenous immunoglobulin therapy. Pediatrics 104:301-303, 1999.
16. Assaad, F., and Borecka, I.: Nine-year study of WHO virus reports on fatal viral infections. Bull. W. H. O. 55:445-453, 1977.
17. Balfour, H. H., Jr., Schiff, G. M., and Bloom, J. E.: Encephalitis associated with erythema infectiosum. J. Pediatr. 77:133-136, 1970.
18. Barnes, P. D., Poussaint, T. Y., and Burrows, P. E.: Imaging of pediatric central nervous system infections. Neuroimaging Clin. North Am. 4:367-391, 1994.
19. Barontini, F., and Leoncini, F.: Brainstem encephalitis due to Listeria monocytogenes: Favourable outcome after early antibiotic therapy. Ital. J. Neurol. Sci. 10:85-87, 1989.
20. Baykan, B., Kinay, D., Gokyigit, A., et al.: Periodic lateralized epileptiform discharges: Association with seizures. Seizure 9:402-406, 2000.
21. Becker, L. E.: Infections of the developing brain. A. J. N. R. Am. J. Neuroradiol. 13:537-550, 1992.
22. Beghi, E., Nicolosi, A., Kurland, L. T., et al.: Encephalitis and aseptic meningitis, Olmsted County, Minnesota, 1950-1981, I: Epidemiology. Ann. Neurol. 16:283-294, 1984.
23. Behzad-Behbahani, A., Klapper, P. E., Vallely, P. J., et al.: BK virus DNA in CSF of immunocompetent and immunocompromised patients. Arch. Dis. Child. 88:174-175, 2003.
24. Behzad-Behbahani, A., Klapper, P. E., Vallely, P. J., et al.: BKV-DNA and JCV-DNA in CSF of patients with suspected meningitis or encephalitis. Infection 31:374-378, 2003.
25. Bellini, W. J., Harcourt, B. H., Bowden, N., et al.: Nipah virus: An emergent paramyxovirus causing severe encephalitis in humans. J. Neurovirol. 11:481-487, 2005.
26. Berge, T. O. (ed.): International Catalogue of Arboviruses including Certain Other Viruses of Vertebrates. 2nd ed. Atlanta, U.S. Dept. of Health, Education and Welfare, Public Health Service, No. (CDC) 75-8301, 1975.
27. Bergey, G. K., Coyle, P. K., Kromholz, A., et al.: Herpes simplex encephalitis with occipital localization. Arch. Neurol. 39:312-313, 1982.
28. Biggar, R. J., Woodall, J. P., Walter, P. D., et al.: Lymphocytic choriomeningitis outbreak associated with pet hamsters: Fifty-seven cases from New York State. J. A. M. A. 232:494-500, 1975.
29. Bingham, P. M., Galetta, S. L., Athreya, B., et al.: Neurologic manifestations in children with Lyme disease. Pediatrics 96:1053-1056, 1995.
30. Bitnum, A., Ford-Jones, E., Blaser, S., et al.: Mycoplasma pneumoniae encephalitis. Semin. Pediatr. Infect. Dis. 14:96-107, 2003.
31. Bitnum, A., Lee Ford-Jones, E., Petric, M., et al.: Acute childhood encephalitis and Mycoplasma pneumoniae. Clin. Infect. Dis. 32:1674-1684, 2001.
32. Blatt, N. H., and Lepper, M. H.: Reactions following antirabies prophylaxis: Report on sixteen patients. Am. J. Dis. Child. 86:395-402, 1953.
33. Boe, J., Solberg, C. O., and Saeter, T.: Corticosteroid treatment for acute meningoencephalitis: A retrospective study of 346 cases. B. M. J. 1:1094-1095, 1965.
34. Bolay, H., Soylemezoglu, F., Nurlu, G., et al.: PCR detected hepatitis C virus genome in the brain of a case with progressive encephalomyelitis with rigidity. Clin. Neurol. Neurosurg. 98:305-308, 1996.
35. Bollen, A. E., Wartan, A. N., Krikke, A. P., et al.: Amnestic syndrome after lung transplantation by human herpes virus-6 encephalitis. J. Neurol. 248:619-620, 2001.
36. Boulloche, J., Parain, D., Mallet, E., et al.: Postinfectious encephalitis with multifocal white matter lesions. Neuropediatrics 20:173-175, 1989.
37. Brown, E. H.: Complications of smallpox vaccination. Postgrad. Med. J. 41:634-635, 1965.
38. Bruhn, F. W.: Lyme disease. Am. J. Dis. Child. 138:467-470, 1984.
39. Buck, P. A., Sockett, P., Barker, I. K., et al.: West Nile Virus: Surveillance activities in Canada. Ann. Epidemiol. 13:582, 2003.
40. Cakmakci, H., Kovanlikaya, A., Obuz, F., et al.: Herpes encephalitis in children, MRI assessment. Turkish J. Pediatr. 40:559-566, 1998.
41. Camarata, P. J., McGeachie, R. E., and Haines, S. J.: Dorsal midbrain encephalitis caused by Propionibacterium acnes: Report of two cases. J. Neurosurg. 72:654-659, 1990.
42. Carithers, H. A., and Margileth, A. M.: Cat-scratch disease: Acute encephalopathy and other neurologic manifestations. Am. J. Dis. Child. 145:98-101, 1991.
43. Carmack, M. A., Twiss, J., Enzmann, D. R., et al.: Multifocal leukoencephalitis caused by varicella-zoster virus in a child with leukemia: Successful treatment with acyclovir. Pediatr. Infect. Dis. J. 12:402-406, 1993.
44. Carr-Locke, D. L., and Mair, H. J.: Neurological presentation of psittacosis during a small outbreak in Leicestershire. B. M. J. 3:853-854, 1976.
45. Caruso, J. M., Tung, G. A., Gascon, G. G., et al.: Persistent preceding focal neurologic deficits in children with chronic Epstein-Barr virus encephalitis. J. Child. Neurol. 15:791-796, 2000.
46. Caserta, M. T., Hall, C. B., Schnabel, K., et al.: Neuroinvasion and persistence of human herpesvirus 6 in children. J. Infect. Dis. 170:1586-1589, 1994.
47. Cassell, G. H., and Cole, B. C.: Mycoplasmas as agents of human disease. N. Engl. J. Med. 304:80-89, 1981.
48. Centers for Disease Control: Measles surveillance: 1973-1976. Issued July 1977.
49. Centers for Disease Control: Encephalitis surveillance: Annual summary 1977. Issued December 1979.
50. Centers for Disease Control: Encephalitis surveillance: Annual summary 1978. Issued May 1981.

51. Centers for Disease Control: Measles surveillance: Annual report 1977-1981. Issued September 1982.

52. Centers for Disease Control: Rabies surveillance: Annual summary 1980-1982. Issued August 1983.

53. Centers for Disease Control: Mumps surveillance, January 1977-December 1982. Issued September 1984.

54. Centers for Disease Control: Rabies prevention: United States, 1984. M. M. W. R. Morb. Mortal. Wkly. Rep. 33:393-408, 1984.

55. Centers for Disease Control: West Nile virus activity—eastern United States, 2001. M. M. W. R. Morb. Mortal. Wkly. Rep. 50:617-619, 2001.

56. Centers for Disease Control: Raccoon roundworm encephalitis—Chicago, Illinois, and Los Angeles, California, 2000. M. M. W. R. Morb. Mortal. Wkly. Rep. 50:1153-1155, 2002.

57. Centers for Disease Control and Prevention: West Nile virus activity—United States, January 1-December, 2005. M. M. W. R. Morb. Mortal. Wkly. Rep. 54:1253-1256, 2005.

58. Centers for Disease Control and Prevention: Enterovirus surveillance—United States, 1970-2005. M. M. W. R. Morb. Mortal. Wkly. Rep. 55:1-20, 2006.

59. Centers for Disease Control and Prevention: Enterovirus surveillance—United States, 2002-2004. M. M. W. R. Morb. Mortal. Wkly. Rep. 55:153-156, 2006.

60. Centers for Disease Control and Prevention: Update: multistate outbreak of mumps—United States, January 1-May 2, 2006. M. M. W. R. Morb. Mortal. Wkly. Rep. 55:559-563, 2006.

61. Chadha, M. S., Arankalle, V. A., Jadi, R. S., et al.: An outbreak of chandipura virus encephalitis in the eastern districts of Gujarat State, India. Am. J. Trop. Med. Hyg. 73:566-570, 2005.

62. Chadha, M. S., Comer, J. A., Lowe, L., et al.: Nipah virus-associated encephalitis outbreak, Siliguri, India. Emerg. Infect. Dis. 12:235-240, 2006.

63. Chang, D. I., Park, J. H., and Chung, K. C.: Encephalitis and polyradiculoneuritis following rubella virus infection. J. Korean Med. Sci. 12:168-170, 1997.

64. Chang, L. Y., Lin, T. Y., Huang, Y. C., et al.: Comparison of enterovirus 71 and coxsackie-virus A16 clinical illnesses during the Taiwan enterovirus epidemic, 1998. Pediatr. Infect. Dis. J. 18:1092-1096, 1999.

65. Chataway, S. J. S., Larner, A. J., Kapoor, R.: Anti-GQ1b antibody status, magnetic imaging, and the nosology of Bickerstaff's brainstem encephalitis. Eur. J. Neurol. 8:355-357, 2001.

66. Chaudhuri, A., and Kennedy, P. G. E.: Diagnosis and treatment of viral encephalitis. Postgrad. Med. J. 78:575-583, 2002.

67. Cherry, J. D.: The epidemiology of pertussis and pertussis immunization in the United Kingdom and the United States: A comparative study. Curr. Probl. Pediatr. 14:1-78, 1984.

68. Cherry, J. D.: "Pertussis vaccine encephalopathy": It is time to recognize it as the myth that it is. J. A. M. A. 263:1679-1680, 1990.

69. Cherry, J. D., Brunell, P. A., Golden, G. S., et al.: Report of the Task Force on Pertussis and Pertussis Immunization—1988. Pediatrics 81:939-984, 1988.

70. Chik, K. W., Chan, P. K. S., Li, C. K., et al.: Human herpesvirus-6 encephalitis after unrelated umbilical cord blood transplant in children. Bone Marrow Transplant. 29:991-994, 2002.

71. Chonmaitree, T., Menegus, M. A., Schervish-Swierkosz, E. M., et al.: Enterovirus 71 infection: Report of an outbreak with two cases of paralysis and a review of the literature. Pediatrics 67:489-493, 1981.

72. Chun, R. W. M., Thompson, W. H., Grabow, J. D., et al.: California arbovirus encephalitis in children. Am. J. Dis. Child. 124:530-533, 1968.

73. Civen, R., Villacorte, F., Robles, D., et al.: West Nile virus infection in the pediatric population. Pediatr. Infect. Dis. J. 25:75-78, 2006.

74. Cizman, M., and Jazbec, J.: Etiology of acute encephalitis in childhood in Slovenia. Pediatr. Infect. Dis. J. 12:903-908, 1993.

75. Claassen, J., Hirsch, L. J., Emerson, R. G., et al.: Continuous EEG monitoring and midazolam infusion for refractory nonconvulsive status epilepticus. Neurology 57:1036-1042, 2001.

76. Clark, D. A.: Human herpesvirus 6 and human herpesvirus 7: Emerging pathogens in transplant patients. Int. J. Hematol. 76:246-252, 2002.

77. Clyde, W. A., Jr.: Neurological syndromes and mycoplasmal infections. Arch. Neurol. 37:65-66, 1980.

78. Connelly, A. M., Dodson, W. E., Prensky, A. L., et al.: Course and outcome of acute cerebellar ataxia. Ann. Neurol. 35:673-679, 1994.

79. Connelly, K. P., and DeWitt, L. D.: Neurologic complications of infectious mononucleosis. Pediatr. Neurol. 10:181-184, 1994.

80. Corsellis, J. A. N., Janota, I., and Marshall, A. K.: Immunization against whooping cough: A neuropathological review. Neuropathol. Appl. Neurobiol. 9:261-270, 1983.

81. Cunha, B. A., Filoxov, A., Reme, P., et al.: Listeria monocytogenes encephalitis mimicking West Nile encephalitis. Heart Lung 33:61-64, 2004.

82. Dagan, R., and Shahak, E.: Prolonged meningoencephalitis due to Epstein-Barr virus with favorable outcome in a young infant. Infection 21:400-402, 1993.

83. Dale, R. C.: Acute disseminated encephalomyelitis. Semin. Pediatr. Infect. Dis. 14:90-95, 2003.

84. Dangond, F., Engle, E., Yesseyan, L., et al.: Pre-eruptive varicella cerebellitis confirmed by PCR. Pediatr. Neurol. 9:491-493, 1993.

85. Daxboeck, F.: Mycoplasma pneumoniae central nervous system infections. Curr. Opin. Neurol. 19:374-378, 2006.

86. Daxboeck, F., Blacky, A., Seidl, R., et al.: Diagnosis, treatment, and prognosis of Mycoplasma pneumoniae childhood encephalitis: Systematic review of 58 cases. J. Child Neurol. 19:865-871, 2004.

87. DeDeyn, P. P., Van den Broucke, P. W., Pickut, B. A., et al.: Perfusions and thallium single photon emission computed tomography in herpes simplex encephalitis. J. Neurol. Sci. 157:96-99, 1998.

88. Deibel, R., and Flanagan, T. D.: Central nervous system infections: Etiologic and epidemiologic observations in New York State, 1976-1977. N. Y. State J. Med. 79:689-695, 1979.

89. Deibel, R., Flanagan, T. D., and Smith, V.: Central nervous system infections: Etiologic and epidemiologic observations in New York State, 1975. N. Y. State J. Med. 77:1398-1404, 1977.

90. Deibel, R., Flanagan, T. D., and Smith, V.: Central nervous system infections in New York State: Etiologic and epidemiologic observations, 1974. N. Y. State J. Med. 75:2337-2342, 1975.

91. Deibel, R., Woodall, J. P., Decher, W. J., et al.: Lymphocytic choriomeningitis virus in man: Serologic evidence of association with pet hamsters. J. A. M. A. 232:501-504, 1975.

92. DeLorenzo, R. J., Waterhouse, E. J., Towne, A. R., et al.: Persistent nonconvulsive status epilepticus after the control of convulsive status epilepticus. Epilepsia 39:833-840, 1998.

93. Deresiewicz, R. L., Thaler, S. J., Hsu, L., et al.: Clinical and neuroradiologic manifestations of eastern equine encephalitis. N. Engl. J. Med. 336:1867-1874, 1997.

94. DeVincenzo, J. P., and Thorne, G.: Mild herpes simplex encephalitis diagnosed by polymerase chain reaction: A case report and review. Pediatr. Infect. Dis. J. 13:662-664, 1994.

95. Dimopoulou, I., Politis, P., Panagyiotakopoulos, G., et al.: Leptospirosis presenting with encephalitis-induced coma. Intensive Care Med. 28:1682, 2002.

96. Doja, A., Bitnun, A., Jones, E. L., et al.: Pediatric Epstein-Barr virus-associated encephalitis: 10-year review. J. Child Neurol. 21:384-391, 2006.

97. Donat, J. F., Rhodes, K. H., Groover, R. V., et al.: Etiology and outcome in 42 children with acute nonbacterial meningoencephalitis. Mayo Clin. Proc. 55:156-160, 1980.

98. Drancourt, M., Raoult, D., Xeridat, B., et al.: Q fever meningoencephalitis in five patients. Eur. J. Epidemiol. 7:134-138, 1991.

99. Dutt, M. K., and Johnston, I. D. A.: Computed tomography and EEG in herpes simplex encephalitis. Arch. Neurol. 39:99-102, 1982.

100. Earnest, M. P., Goolishian, H. A., Calverley, J. R., et al.: Neurologic, intellectual, and psychologic sequelae following western equine encephalitis: A study of 35 cases. Neurology 21:969-974, 1971.

101. Elliott, K. J.: Other neurological complications of herpes zoster and their management. Ann. Neurol. 35:S57-S61, 1994.

102. El-Rai, F. M., and Evans, A. S.: Reovirus infections in children and young adults. Arch. Environ. Health 7:700-704, 1963.

103. Enders, J. F.: Mumps. In Rivers, T. M., and Horsfall, F. L., Jr. (eds.): Viral and Rickettsial Infections of Man. Philadelphia, J. B. Lippincott, 1959, pp. 780-789.

104. Estrada-Franco, J. G., Navarro-Lopez, R., Beasely, D. E., et al.: West Nile virus in Mexico: Evidence of widespread circulation since July 2002. Emerg. Infect. Dis. 9:1604-1608, 2003.

105. Farizo, K. M., Cochi, S. L., Zell, E. R., et al.: Epidemiological features of pertussis in the United States, 1980-1989. Clin. Infect. Dis. 14:708-719, 1992.

106. Fazekas, F., Roob, G., Payer, F., et al.: Technetium-99 m-ECD SPECT fails to show focal hyperemia of acute herpes encephalitis. J. Nucl. Med. 39:790-792, 1998.

107. Finlay, K. H., Fitzgerald, L. H., Richter, R. W., et al.: Western encephalitis and cerebral ontogenesis. Arch. Neurol. 16:140-167, 1967.

108. Fischer, S. A., Graham, M. B., Kuehnert, M. J., et al.: Transmission of lymphocytic choriomeningitis virus by organ transplantation. N. Engl. J. Med. 25:2235-2249, 2006.

109. Flewett, T. H., and Hoult, J. G.: Influenzal encephalopathy and postinfluenzal encephalitis. Lancet 2:11-15, 1958.

110. Flexner, S.: Postvaccinal encephalitis and allied conditions. J. A. M. A. 94:305-311, 1930.

111. Forman, M. L., and Cherry, J. D.: Isolation of measles virus from the cerebrospinal fluid of a child with encephalitis following measles vaccination. Evanston, IL, The Program for the American Pediatric Society, 1967.

112. Fox, R. J., Kasner, S. E., Galetta, S. L., et al.: Treatment of Bickerstaff's brainstem encephalitis with immune globulin. J. Neurol. Sci. 15:88-90, 2000.

113. Francisco, A. M., Glaser, C., Frykman, E., et al.: 2004 California pediatric West Nile virus case series. Pediatr. Infect. Dis. J. 25:81-84, 2006.

114. Fryden, A., Kihlstrom, E., Maller, R., et al.: A clinical and epidemiological study of "ornithosis" caused by Chlamydia psittaci and Chlamydia pneumoniae (strain TWAR). Scand. J. Infect. Dis. 21:681-691, 1989.

115. Fujimaki, K., Mori, T., Kida, A., et al.: Human herpesvirus 6 meningoencephalitis in allogeneic hematopoietic stem cell transplant recipients. Int. J. Hematol. 84:432-437, 2006.

116. Fuller, G. N., Guiloff, R. J., Scaravilli, F., et al.: Combined HIV-CMV encephalitis presenting with brainstem signs. J. Neurol. Neurosurg. Psychiatry 52:975-979, 1989.

117. Gavin, P. J., Kazacos, K. R., and Shulman, S. T.: Baylisascaris. Clin. Microbiol. Rev. *18*:703-718, 2005.

118. Gavin, P. J., and Shulman, S. T.: Raccoon roundworm (*Baylisascaris procyonis*). Pediatr. Infect. Dis. J. *22*:651-652, 2003.

119. Genz, R. D., and Beecham, H. J.: Meningoencephalitis after influenza inoculation. N. Engl. J. Med. *299*:721-722, 1978.

120. Gerber, J. E., Johnson, J. E., Scott, M. A., et al.: Fatal meningitis and encephalitis due to *Bartonella henselae* bacteria. J. Forensic Sci. *47*:640-644, 2002.

121. Glaser, C. A., Gilliam, S., Schnurr, D., et al.: In search of encephalitis etiologies: Diagnostic challenges in the California Encephalitis Project, 1998-2000. Clin. Infect. Dis. *36*:731-742, 2003.

122. Glezen, W. P.: Consideration of the risk of influenza in children and indications for prophylaxis. Rev. Infect. Dis. *2*:408-420, 1980.

123. Glezen, W. P., Paredes, A., and Taber, L. H.: Influenza in children: Relationship to other respiratory agents. J. A. M. A. *243*:1345-1349, 1980.

124. Goh, K. J., Tan, C. T., Chew, N. K., et al.: Clinical features of Nipah virus encephalitis among pig farmers in Malaysia. N. Engl. J. Med. *342*:1229-1235, 2000.

125. Golden, S. E.: Aseptic meningitis associated with *Ehrlichiae canis* infection. Pediatr. Infect. Dis. *8*:335-337, 1989.

126. Goldwater, P. N., Rowland, K., Power, R., et al.: Rotavirus encephalopathy: Pathogenesis reviewed. J. Paediatr. Child Health *37*:206-209, 2001.

127. Gorman, R. J., Saxon, S., and Snead, O. C.: Neurologic sequelae of Rocky Mountain spotted fever. Pediatrics *67*:354-357, 1981.

128. Grabow, J. D., Matthews, G. G., Chun, R. W. M., et al.: The electroencephalogram and clinical sequelae of California arbovirus encephalitis. Neurology *19*:394-404, 1969.

129. Greenberg, D. A., Weinkle, D. J., and Aminoff, M. J.: Periodic EEG complexes in infectious mononucleosis encephalitis. J. Neurol. Neurosurg. Psychiatry *45*:648-651, 1982.

130. Greenberg, M.: Complications of vaccination against smallpox. Am. J. Dis. Child. *76*:492-502, 1948.

131. Greenberg, S. B., Taber, L., Septimus, E., et al.: Computerized tomography in brain biopsy proven herpes simplex encephalitis. Arch. Neurol. *38*:58-59, 1981.

132. Griesemer, D. A., Barton, L. L., Reese, C. M., et al.: Amebic meningoencephalitis caused by *Balamuthia mandrillaris*. Pediatr. Neurol. *10*:249-254, 1994.

133. Griffin, D. E.: Post-infectious and post-vaccinal disorders of the central nervous system. Immunol. Allergy Clin. North Am. *8*:239-249, 1988.

134. Griffith, A. H.: Permanent brain damage and pertussis vaccination: Is the end of the saga in sight? Vaccine *7*:199-210, 1989.

135. Griffiths, P.: Cytomegalovirus infection of the central nervous system. Herpes *11*(S2):95A-103A, 2004.

136. Grist, N. R., Bell, E. J., and Assaad, F.: Enteroviruses in human disease. Prog. Med. Virol. *4*:114-157, 1978.

137. Gross, W. L., Ravens, K. G., and Hansen, H. W.: Meningoencephalitic syndrome following influenza vaccination. J. Neurol. *217*:219-222, 1978.

138. Grossman, M., and Azimi, P. H.: An encephalitis syndrome in a seven-year-old. Pediatr. Infect. Dis. J. *14*:550-555, 1995.

139. Guerrero, I. C., Retailliau, H. F., Brandling-Bennett, A. D., et al.: No increased meningoencephalitis after influenza vaccine. N. Engl. J. Med. *300*:565, 1979.

140. Guleria, R., Nisar, N., Chawla, T. C., and Biswas, N. R.: *Mycoplasma pneumoniae* and central nervous system complications: A review. J. Lab. Clin. Med. *146*:55-63, 2005.

141. Hall, C. B., and Horner, F. A.: Encephalopathy with erythema infectiosum. Am. J. Dis. Child. *131*:65-67, 1977.

142. Hall, C. B., Long, C. E., Schnabel, K. C., et al.: Human herpesvirus-6 infection in children: A prospective study of complications and reactivation. N. Engl. J. Med. *331*:432-438, 1994.

143. Hamilton, R. L., Achim, C., Grafe, M. R., et al.: Herpes simplex virus brainstem encephalitis in an AIDS patient. Clin. Neuropathol. *14*:45-50, 1995.

144. Hanshaw, J. B., Dudgeon, J. A., and Marshall, W. C.: Congenital cytomegalovirus. *In* Hanshaw, J. B., Dudgeon, J. A., and Marshall, W. C. (eds.): Viral Diseases of the Fetus and Newborn. 2nd ed. Philadelphia, W. B. Saunders, 1985, pp. 92-131.

145. Harit, A. K., Ichhpujani, R. L., Gupta, S., et al.: Nipah/Hendra virus outbreak in Siliguri, West Bengal, India in 2001. Indian J. Med. Res. *123*:553-560, 2006.

146. Hasegawa, Y., Morishita, M., Ikeda, T., et al.: Early diagnosis of herpes simplex virus encephalitis by single photon emission computed tomography (SPECT) in patients with normal MRI. Rinsho Shinkeigaku Clin. Neurol. *36*:475-480, 1996.

147. Hattori, H., Kawamori, J., Takao, T., et al.: Computed tomography in postinfluenzal encephalitis. Brain Dev. *5*:564-567, 1983.

148. Hausler, M., Schaade, L., Kemeny, M., et al.: Encephalitis related to primary varicella-zoster virus infection in immunocompetent children. J. Neurol. Sci. *195*:111-116, 2002.

149. Hayes, E. B., and O'Leary, D. R.: West Nile virus infection: A pediatric perspective. Pediatrics *113*:1375-1381, 2004.

150. Hayes, E. B., Sejvar, J. J., Zaki, S. R., et al.: Virology, pathology, and clinical manifestations of West Nile virus disease. Emerg. Infect. Dis. *11*:1174-1179, 2005.

151. Haynes, R. E., Sanders, D. Y., and Cramblett, H. G.: Rocky Mountain spotted fever in children. J. Pediatr. *76*:685-693, 1970.

152. Hedlund, J., Aurelius, E., and Andersson, J.: Recurrent encephalitis due to trimethoprim intake. Scand. J. Infect. Dis. *22*:109-112, 1990.

153. Ho, D. D., and Hirsch, M. S.: Acute viral encephalitis. Med. Clin. North Am. *69*:415-429, 1985.

154. Ho, M.: Enterovirus 71: The virus, its infections and outbreaks. J. Microbiol. Immunol. Infect. *33*:205-216, 2000.

155. Hoke, C. H., Jr., Vaughn, D. W., Nisalak, A., et al.: Effect of high-dose dexamethasone on the outcome of acute encephalitis due to Japanese encephalitis virus. J. Infect. Dis. *165*:631-637, 1992.

156. Hsu, V. P., Hossain, M. J., Parashar, U. D., et al.: Nipah virus encephalitis reemergence, Bangladesh. Emerg. Infect. Dis. *10*:2082-2087, 2004.

157. Huang, C. C., Liu, C. C., Chang, Y. C., et al.: Neurologic complications in children with enterovirus 71 infection. N. Engl. J. Med. *341*:936-942, 1999.

158. Huang, C. R., Chang, W. N., Lui, C. C., et al.: Neuroimages of Japanese encephalitis: Report of three patients. Ching-Hua I Hseuh Tsa Chih *60*:105-108, 1997.

159. Huang, M. C., Wang, S. M., Hsu, Y. W., et al: Long-term cognitive and motor deficits after enterovirus 71 brainstem encephalitis in children. Pediatrics *118*:e1785-e1788, 2006.

160. Huang, Y., Lin, T., Wu, S., and Tsao, K.: Influenza A-associated central nervous system dysfunction in children presenting as transient visual hallucination. Pediatr. Infect. Dis. J. *22*:366-368, 2003.

161. Hughes, R. R.: Neurological complications of serum and vaccine therapy. Lancet *2*:464-467, 1944.

162. Huhn, G. D., Sejvar, J. J., Montgomery, S. P., et al.: West Nile virus in the United States: An update on an emerging infectious disease. Am. Fam. Physician *68*:653-660, 2003.

163. Hummeler, K., Davidson, W. L., Henle, W., et al.: Encephalomyelitis due to infection with *Herpesvirus simiae* (herpes B virus): A report of two fatal, laboratory-acquired cases. N. Engl. J. Med. *261*:64-67, 1959.

164. Irving, W. L., Chang, J., Raymond, D. R., et al.: Roseola infantum and other syndromes associated with acute HHV-6 infection. Arch. Dis. Child. *65*:297-300, 1990.

165. Isaacson, E., Glaser, C. A., Forghani, B., et al.: Evidence of human herpesvirus 6 infection in 4 immunocompetent patients with encephalitis. Clin. Infect. Dis. *40*:890-893, 2005.

166. Ishiguro, N., Yamada, S., Takahashi, T., et al.: Meningoencephalitis associated with HHV-6 related exanthem subitum. Acta Paediatr. Scand. *79*:987-989, 1990.

167. Jackson, M. A., Burry, V. F., and Olson, L. C.: Complications of varicella requiring hospitalization in previously healthy children. Pediatr. Infect. Dis. J. *11*:441-445, 1992.

168. Jemsek, H., Greenberg, S. B., Taber, L., et al.: Herpes zoster-associated encephalitis: Clinicopathologic report of 12 cases and review of the literature. Medicine *62*:81-97, 1983.

169. Johnson, H. N.: Rabies. *In* Rivers, T. M., and Horsfall, F. J., Jr. (eds.): Viral and Rickettsial Infections of Man. 3rd ed. Philadelphia, J. B. Lippincott, 1959, pp. 405-431.

170. Johnson, R. T.: Viral Infections of the Nervous System. New York, Raven Press, 1982, pp. 87-128.

171. Johnson, R. T.: The pathogenesis of acute viral encephalitis and postinfectious encephalomyelitis. J. Infect. Dis. *155*:359-364, 1987.

172. Johnson, R. T.: The virology of demyelinating diseases. Ann. Neurol. *36*:S54-S60, 1994.

173. Joske, R. A., Keall, D. D., Leak, P. J., et al.: Hepatitis-encephalitis in humans with reovirus infection. Arch. Intern. Med. *113*:811-816, 1964.

174. Kanzaki, A., Yubuki, S., and Yuki, N.: Bickerstaff's brainstem encephalitis associated with cytomegalovirus infection. J. Neurol. Neurosurg. Psychiatry *58*:260-261, 1993.

175. Kaplan, M. H., Klein, S. W., McPhee, J., et al.: Group B coxsackievirus infections in infants younger than three months of age: A serious childhood illness. Rev. Infect. Dis. *5*:1019-1032, 1983.

176. Kappus, K. D., Sather, G. E., Kaplan, J. E., et al.: Human arboviral infections in the United States in 1980. J. Infect. Dis. *145*:283-286, 1982.

177. Kato, T., Ishii, C., Furusho, J., et al.: Early diagnosis of herpes encephalopathy using fluid-attenuated inversion recovery pulse sequences. Pediatr. Neurol. *19*:58-61, 1998.

178. Katz, D. A., Dworzack, D. L., Horowitz, E. A., et al.: Encephalitis associated with Rocky Mountain spotted fever. Arch. Pathol. Lab. Med. *109*:771-773, 1985.

179. Kennedy, C.: Acute viral encephalitis in childhood. B. M. J. *310*:139-140, 1995.

180. Kennedy, F.: Certain nervous complications following the use of therapeutic and prophylactic sera. Am. J. Med. Sci. *177*:555-559, 1929.

181. Kesselring, J., Miller, D. H., Robb, S. A., et al.: Acute disseminated encephalomyelitis: MRI findings and the distinction from multiple sclerosis. Brain *113*:291-302, 1990.

182. Koelfen, W., Freund, M., Guckel, F., et al.: MRI of encephalitis in children: Comparison of CT and MRI in the acute stage with long-term follow-up. Neuroradiology *38*:73-79, 1996.

183. Kohl, S., and James, A. R.: Herpes simplex virus encephalitis during childhood: Importance of brain biopsy diagnosis. J. Pediatr. *107*:212-215, 1985.

184. Kolski, H., Ford-Jones, E. L., Richardson, S., et al.: Etiology of acute childhood encephalitis at The Hospital for Sick Children, Toronto, 1994-1995. Clin. Infect. Dis. 26:398-409, 1998.
185. Koskiniemi, M.: CNS manifestations associated with *Mycoplasma pneumoniae* infections: Summary of cases at the University of Helsinki and review. Clin. Infect. Dis. 17:S52-S57, 1993.
186. Koskiniemi, M., Manninen, V., Vaheri, A., et al.: Acute encephalitis: A survey of epidemiological, clinical and microbiological features covering a twelve-year period. Acta Med. Scand. 209:115-120, 1981.
187. Koskiniemi, M., Rantalaiho, T., Piiparinen, H., et al.: Infections of the central nervous system of suspected viral origin: a collaborative study from Finland. J. Neurovirol. 7:400-408, 2001.
188. Koskiniemi, M., and Vaheri, A.: Effect of measles, mumps, rubella vaccination on pattern of encephalitis in children. Lancet 1:31-34, 1989.
189. Kovacs, S. O., Kuban, K., and Strand, R.: Lateral medullary syndrome following varicella infection. Am. J. Dis. Child. 147:823-825, 1993.
190. Krainer, L., and Aronson, B. E.: Disseminated encephalomyelitis in humans with recovery of hepato-encephalitis virus (HEV). J. Neuropathol. Exp. Neurol. 18:339-342, 1969.
191. Kubota, H., Tanabe, Y., Komiya, T., et al.: Q fever encephalitis with cytokine profiles in serum and cerebrospinal fluid. Pediatr. Infect. Dis. J. 20:318-319, 2001.
192. Kumar, S., Misra, U. K., Kalita, J., et al.: MRI in Japanese encephalitis. Neuroradiology 39:180-184, 1997.
193. Kupila, L., Vuorinen, T., Vainionpaa, R., et al.: Etiology of aseptic meningitis and encephalitis in an adult population. Neurology 66:75-80, 2006.
194. Lakeman, F. D., Whitley, R. J., and the NIAID Collaborative Antiviral Study Group: Diagnosis of herpes simplex encephalitis: Application of polymerase chain reaction to cerebrospinal fluid from brain-biopsied patients and correlation with disease. J. Infect. Dis. 171:857-863, 1995.
195. Lam, S. K., and Chua, K. B.: Nipah virus encephalitis outbreak in Malaysia. Clin. Infect. Dis. 34:S48-51, 2002.
196. Lanczik, O., Lecei, O., Schwarz, S., et al.: *Mycoplasma pneumoniae* infection as a treatable cause of brainstem encephalitis. Arch. Neurol. 60:1813, 2003.
197. Landrigan, P. J., and Witte, J. J.: Neurologic disorders following live measles virus vaccination. J. A. M. A. 223:1459-1462, 1973.
198. Landry, M. L., Ponseca, S. S., Cohen, S., et al.: Fatal enterovirus type 71 infection: Rapid detection and diagnostic pitfalls. Pediatr. Infect. Dis. J. 14:1095-1100, 1995.
199. Lane, J. M., Ruben, R. L., Neff, J. M., et al.: Complications of smallpox vaccination, 1968: National surveillance in the United States. N. Engl. J. Med. 281:1201-1208, 1969.
200. Lane, J. M., Ruben, F. L., Neff, J. M., et al.: Complications of smallpox vaccination, 1968: Results of ten statewide surveys. J. Infect. Dis. 122:303-309, 1970.
201. Lau, K. K., Lai, S. T., Lai, J. Y., et al.: Acute encephalitis complicating rubella. Hong Kong Med. J. 4:325-328, 1998.
202. Launes, J., Nikkinen, P., Lindroth, L., et al.: Diagnosis of acute herpes simplex encephalitis by brain perfusion single photon emission computed tomography. Lancet 1:1188-1191, 1988.
203. Leake, J. A. D., Albani, S., Kao, A. S., et al.: Acute disseminated encephalomyelitis in childhood: Epidemiologic, clinical, and laboratory features. Pediatr. Infect. Dis. J. 23:756-764, 2004.
204. Lee, K. E., Tan, C. B., Tjia, H. T. L., et al.: The neurological manifestations of Nipah virus encephalitis, a novel paramyxovirus. Ann. Neurol. 46:428-432, 1999.
205. Leonard, J. R., Moran, C. J., Cross, D. T., et al.: MR imaging of herpes simplex type 1 encephalitis in infants and young children: A separate pattern of findings. A. J. R. Am. J. Roentgenol. 174:1651-1655, 2000.
206. Lester, J. W., Carter, M. P., and Reynolds, T. L.: Herpes encephalitis: MR monitoring of response to acyclovir therapy. J. Comput. Assist. Tomogr. 12:941-943, 1988.
207. Lewis, P., and Glaser, C. A.: Encephalitis. Pediatr. Rev. 25:353-363, 2005.
208. Li, C. C., Yang, M. Y., Chen, R. F., et al.: Clinical manifestations and laboratory assessment in an enterovirus 71 outbreak in southern Taiwan. Scand. J. Infect. Dis. 34:104-109, 2002.
209. Lin, W. C., Lee, P. I., and Lu, C. Y.: *Mycoplasma pneumoniae* encephalitis in childhood. J. Microbiol. Immunol. Infect. 35:173-178, 2002.
210. Linnemann, C. C., Jr., Pretzman, C. I., and Peterson, E. D.: Acute febrile cerebrovasculitis: A non-spotted fever group rickettsial disease. Arch. Intern. Med. 149:1682-1684, 1989.
211. Liu, C. C., Tseng, H. W., Wang, S. M., et al.: An outbreak of enterovirus 71 infection in Taiwan, 1998: Epidemiologic and clinical manifestations. J. Clin. Virol. 17:23-30, 2000.
212. Lynch, M., Lee, B., Azimi, P., et al.: Rotavirus and central nervous system symptoms: Cause or contaminant? Case reports and review. Clin. Infect. Dis. 33:932-938, 2001.
213. MacLean, H. J., and Douen, A. G.: Severe amnesia associated with human herpesvirus 6 encephalitis after bone marrow transplantation. Transplantation 73:1086-1089, 2002.
214. Makela, A., Nuorti, P., and Peltola, H.: Neurologic disorders after measles-mumps-rubella vaccination. Pediatrics 110:957-963, 2002.
215. Mardh, P. A.: *Mycoplasma hominis* infection of the central nervous system in newborn infants. Sex. Transm. Dis. 10:331-334, 1983.
216. Marfin, A. A., and Gubler, D. J.: West Nile encephalitis: An emerging disease in the United States. Clin. Infect. Dis. 33:1713-1719, 2001.
217. Margolis, F. J., Wilson, J. L., and Top, F. H.: Postrubella encephalomyelitis: Report of cases in Detroit and review of literature. J. Pediatr. 23:158-165, 1943.
218. Masdeu, J. C., VanHeertum, R. L., and Abdel-Dayem, H.: Viral infections of the brain. J. Neuroimaging Suppl. 1:S40-S44, 1995.
219. Matsumoto, N., Yano, S., Miyao, M., et al.: Two-dimensional ultrasonography of the brain: Its diagnostic usefulness in herpes simplex encephalitis and cytomegalic inclusion disease. Brain Dev. 5:327-333, 1983.
220. Matthews, C. G., Chun, R. W. M., Grabow, J. D., et al.: Psychological sequelae in children following California arbovirus encephalitis. Neurology 18:1023-1030, 1968.
221. McCullers, J. A., Lakeman, F. D., and Whitley, R. J.: Human herpesvirus 6 is associated with focal encephalitis. Clin. Infect. Dis. 21:571-576, 1995.
222. McDonald, J. C., Moore, D. L., and Quennec, P.: Clinical and epidemiologic features of mumps meningoencephalitis and possible vaccine-related disease. Pediatr. Infect. Dis. 8:751-755, 1989.
223. McDowall, D. G.: Monitoring the brain. Anesthesiology 45:117-134, 1976.
224. McHugh, K., and McMenamin, J. B.: Acute disseminated encephalomyelitis in childhood. Irish Med. J. 80:412-414, 1987.
225. McJunkin, J. E., De Los Reyes, E. C., Irazuzta, J. E., et al.: La Crosse encephalitis in children. N. Engl. J. Med. 344:801-807, 2001.
226. McLean, D. M., Best, J. M., Smith, P. A., et al.: Viral infections of Toronto children during 1965, II: Measles encephalitis and other complications. Can. Med. Assoc. J. 94:905-910, 1966.
227. Melis, K., Bochner, A., Vandenberghe, P., et al.: Cat-scratch disease with reversible encephalopathy. Eur. J. Pediatr. 149:2-25, 1989.
228. Menge, T., Hemmer, B., Nessler, S., et al.: Acute disseminated encephalomyelitis: An update. Arch. Neurol. 62:1673-1680, 2005.
229. Meulin, V. T., Kackell, Y., Muller, D., et al.: Isolation of infectious measles virus in measles encephalitis. Lancet 2:1172-1175, 1972.
230. Meyer, H. M., Jr., Johnson, R. T., Crawford, I. P., et al.: Central nervous system syndromes of "viral" etiology: A study of 713 cases. Am. J. Med. 2:334-347, 1960.
231. Miller, H. G., and Stanton, J. B.: Neurological sequelae of prophylactic inoculation. Q. J. M. 89:1-27, 1954.
232. Miller, H. G., Stanton, J. B., and Gibbons, J. L.: Parainfectious encephalomyelitis and related syndromes. Q. J. M. 100:427-505, 1956.
233. Mizrahi, E. M., and Tharp, B. R.: A characteristic EEG pattern in neonatal herpes simplex encephalitis. Neurology 32:1215-1220, 1982.
234. Modlin, J. F., Dagan, R., Berlin, L. E., et al.: Focal encephalitis with enterovirus infections. Pediatrics 88:841-845, 1991.
235. Monath, T. P., Cropp, C. B., and Harrison, A. K.: Mode of entry of a neurotropic arbovirus into the central nervous system: Reinvestigation of an old controversy. Lab. Invest. 48:399-410, 1983.
236. Moore, M.: Enteroviral disease in the United States, 1970-1979. J. Infect. Dis. 146:103-108, 1982.
237. Morishima, T., Togashi T., Yokota, S., et al.: Encephalitis and encephalopathy associated with an influenza epidemic in Japan. Clin. Infect. Dis. 35:512-517, 2002.
238. Nanning, W.: Prophylactic effect of antivaccinia gammaglobulin against postvaccinal encephalitis. Bull. W. H. O. 27:317-324, 1962.
239. Nash, D., Mostashari, F., Fine, A., et al.: The outbreak of West Nile virus infection in the New York City area in 1999. N. Engl. J. Med. 344:1807-1814, 2001.
240. Newland, J. G., Romero, J. R., Varman, M., et al.: Encephalitis associated with influenza B virus infection in 2 children and a review of the literature. Clin. Infect. Dis. 36:e87-e95, 2003.
241. Ng, Y. T., Cox, C., Atkins, J., et al.: Encephalopathy associated with respiratory syncytial virus bronchiolitis. J. Child Neurol. 16:105-108, 2001.
242. Nigrovic, L. E., Lumeng, C., Landrigan, C., et al.: Rotavirus cerebellitis? Clin. Infect. Dis. 34:130, 2002.
243. Nishikawa, M., Ichiyama, T., Hayashi, T., et al.: Intravenous immunoglobulin therapy in acute disseminated encephalomyelitis. Pediatr. Neurol. 21:583-586, 1999.
244. Noah, N. D., and Urquhart, A. M.: Virus meningitis and encephalitis in 1979. J. Infect. 2:379-383, 1980.
245. Noah, R. L., Bresee, J. S., Gorensek, M. J., et al.: Cluster of five children with acute encephalopathy associated with cat-scratch disease in South Florida. Pediatr. Infect. Dis. J. 14:866-869, 1995.
246. Nolan, R. C., Chidlow, G., French, M. A.: Parvovirus B19 encephalitis presenting as immune restoration disease after highly active antiretroviral therapy for human immunodeficiency virus infection. Clin. Infect. Dis. 36:1191-1194.
247. Ohsaka, M., Houkin, K., Takigami, M., et al.: Acute necrotizing encephalopathy associated with human herpesvirus-6 infection. Pediatr. Neurol. 34:160-163, 2006.
248. Ohtaki, E., Murakami, Y., Komori, H., et al.: Acute disseminated encephalomyelitis after Japanese B encephalitis vaccination. Pediatr. Neurol. 8:137-139, 1992.

249. Okuno, T., Takao, T., Ito, M., et al.: Contrast-enhanced hypodense areas in a case of acute disseminated encephalitis following influenza A virus. Comput. Radiol. 6:215-217, 1982.

250. Olgar, S., Ertugrul, T., Nisli, K., et al.: Influenza A-associated acute necrotizing encephalopathy. Neuropediatrics 37:166-168, 2006.

251. Olitsky, P. K., and Casals, J.: Arthropod-borne group A virus infections of man. In Rivers, R. M., and Horsfall, F. L., Jr. (eds.): Viral and Rickettsial Infections of Man. Philadelphia, J. B. Lippincott, 1959, pp. 286-304.

252. Osamura, T., Mizuta, R., Yoshioka, H., et al.: Isolation of adenovirus type 11 from the brain of a neonate with pneumonia and encephalitis. Eur. J. Pediatr. 152:496-499, 1993.

253. O'Sullivan, J. D., Allworth, A. M., Peterson, D. L., et al.: Fatal encephalitis due to novel paramyxovirus transmitted from horses. Lancet 349:93-95, 1997.

254. Overell, J. R., Hsieh, S. T., Odaka, M., et al.: Treatment for Fisher syndrome, Bickerstaff's brainstem encephalitis and related disorders. Cochrane Database Syst. Rev. 2007, Issue 1. Art. No.: CD004761. DOI: 10.1002/14651858.CD004761.pub2.

255. Paisley, J. W., Bruhn, F. W., Lauer, B. A., et al.: Type A2 influenza viral infections in children. Am. J. Dis. Child. 132:34-36, 1978.

256. Palacios, G., Quan, P., Jabado, O. J., et al.: Panmicrobial oligonucleotide array for diagnosis of infectious diseases. Emerg. Infect. Dis. 13:73-81, 2007.

257. Panicker, J. N., Mammachan, R., and Jayakumar, R. V.: Primary neuroleptospirosis. Postgrad. Med. J. 77:589-590, 2001.

258. Parent, J. M., and Lowenstein, D. H.: Treatment of refractory generalized status epilepticus with continuous infusion of midazolam (abstract). Neurology 4:1837-1840, 1994.

259. Parra-Martinez, J., Sancho-Rieger, J., Ortiz-Sanchez, P., et al.: Encephalitis caused by *Rickettsia conorii* without exanthema. Rev. Neurol. 35:731-734, 2002.

260. Peter, G.: Leptospirosis: A zoonosis of protean manifestations. Pediatr. Infect. Dis. 1:282-288, 1982.

261. Petersen, L. R., and Marfin, A. A.: West Nile virus: A primer for the clinician. Ann. Intern. Med. 137:E173-E179, 2002.

262. Plotkin, S. A., Rupprecht, C. E., and Koprowski, H.: Rabies vaccine. In Vaccines. 4th ed. Philadelphia, W. B. Saunders, 2004, pp.1017-1038.

263. Pohl-Koppe, A., Blay, M., Jäger, G., et al.: Human herpes virus type 7 DNA in the cerebrospinal fluid of children with central nervous system diseases. Eur. J. Pediatr. 160:351-358, 2001.

264. Pönkä, A.: Central nervous system manifestations associated with serologically verified *Mycoplasma pneumoniae* infection. Scand. J. Infect. Dis. 12:175-184, 1980.

265. Preblud, S. R.: Age-specific risks of varicella complications. Pediatrics 68:14-17, 1981.

266. Protopsaltis, J., Kokkoris, S., Brestas, P. S., et al.: Neurolisteriosis mimicking herpes simplex encephalitis ain an immunocompromised patient. Scand. J. Infect. Dis. 38:825-828, 2006.

267. Prusiner, S. B., and Hsiao, K. K.: Human prion diseases. Ann. Neurol. 35:385-395, 1994.

268. Public Health Service, U.S. Dept. Health, Education and Welfare, joint statement: Fatal viral encephalitis following 17D yellow fever vaccine inoculation: Report of a case in a 3-year-old child. J. A. M. A. 198:203-204, 1966.

269. Purdham, D. R., and Batty, P. F.: A case of acute measles meningoencephalitis with virus isolation. J. Clin. Pathol. 27:994-996, 1974.

270. Quiroz, E., Moreno, N., Peralta, P. H., et al.: A human case of encephalitis associated with vesicular stomatitis virus (Indiana serotype) infection. Am. J. Trop. Med. Hyg. 39:312-314, 1988.

271. Rantala, H., and Uhari, M.: Occurrence of childhood encephalitis: A population-based study. Pediatr. Infect. Dis. J. 8:426-430, 1989.

272. Rao, B. L., Basu, A., Wairagkar, N. S., et al.: A large outbreak of acute encephalitis with high fatality rate in children in Andhra Pradesh, India, in 2003, associated with Chandipura virus. Lancet 364:869-874, 2004.

273. Raoult, D., and Marrie, T.: Q fever. Clin. Infect. Dis. 20:489-496, 1995.

274. Rautonen, J., Koskiniemi, M., and Vaheri, A.: Prognostic factors in childhood acute encephalitis. Pediatr. Infect. Dis. J. 10:441-446, 1991.

275. Ray, P., Hayward, J., Michelson, D., et al.: Encephalopathy after whole-cell pertussis or measles vaccination: Lack of evidence for a causal association in a retrospective case-control study. Pediatr. Infect. Dis. J. 25:768-773, 2006.

276. Read, S. J., Jeffery, K. J., and Bangham, C. R.: Aseptic meningitis and encephalitis: The role of PCR in the diagnostic laboratory. J. Clin. Microbiol. 35:691-696, 1997.

277. Rie, H. E., Hilty, M. D., and Cramblatt, H. G.: Intelligence and coordination following California encephalitis. Am. J. Dis. Child. 125:824-827, 1973.

278. Robb, L., and Butt, W.: Brain stem encephalitis due to herpes simplex virus. Aust. Paediatr. J. 25:246-247, 1989.

279. Robinson, L. J.: Neurologic complications following the administration of vaccines and serums: Report of a case of peripheral paralysis following the injection of typhoid vaccine. N. Engl. J. Med. 216:831-837, 1937.

280. Romero, J. R., and Newland, J. G.: Viral meningitis and encephalitis: Traditional and emerging viral agents. Semin. Pediatr. Infect. Dis. 14:72-82, 2003.

281. Roos, K.: Encephalitis. Neurol. Clin. 17:813-833, 1999.

282. Rosenberg, G. A.: Meningoencephalitis following an influenza vaccination. N. Engl. J. Med. 283:1209-1210, 1970.

283. Rosenblum, M. K.: Bulbar encephalitis complicating trigeminal zoster in the acquired immune deficiency syndrome. Hum. Pathol. 20:292-295, 1989.

284. Rothstein, T., and Shaw, C. M.: Computerized tomography as a diagnostic aid in acute hemorrhagic leukoencephalitis. Ann. Neurol. 13:331-333, 1983.

285. Rubeiz, H., and Roos, R. P.: Viral meningitis and encephalitis. Semin. Neurol. 12:165-177, 1992.

286. Sainio, K., Granstrom, M. L., Pettay, O., et al.: EEG in neonatal herpes simplex encephalitis. Electroencephalogr. Clin. Neurophysiol. 56:556-561, 1983.

287. Salaki, J. S., Louria, D. B., and Chmel, H.: Fungal and yeast infections of the central nervous system: A clinical review. Medicine 63:108-132, 1984.

288. San Miguel, P., Fernandez, G., Vasallo, F. J., et al.: Neurobrucellosis mimicking cerebral tumor: Case report and literature review. Clin. Neurol. Neurosurg. 108:404-406, 2006.

289. Sato, S., Kumada, S., Koji, T., et al.: Reversible frontal lobe syndrome associated with influenza virus infection in children. Pediatr. Neurol. 22:318-321, 2000.

290. Savolainen, H., Lautenschlager, I., Piiparinen, H., et al.: Human herpesvirus-6 and -7 in pediatric stem cell transplantation. Pediatr. Blood Cancer 45:820-825, 2005.

291. Schlesinger, Y., Butler, R. S., and Brunstrom, J. E.: Expanded spectrum of herpes simplex encephalitis in childhood. J. Pediatr. 126:234-241, 1995.

292. Schmidbauer, M., Budka, H., and Amros, P.: Herpes simplex virus (HSV) DNA in microglial nodular brainstem encephalitis. J. Neuropathol. Exp. Neurol. 48:645-652, 1989.

293. Seidel, J. S., Harmatz, P., Visvesvara, G. S., et al.: Successful treatment of primary amebic meningoencephalitis. N. Engl. J. Med. 306:346-348, 1982.

294. Sejvar, J. J.: The evolving epidemiology of viral encephalitis. Curr. Opin. Neurol. 19:350-357, 2006.

295. Sejvar, J. J., Chowdary, Y., Schomogyi, M., et al.: Human monkeypox infection: A family cluster in the midwestern United States. J. Infect. Dis. 190:1833-1840, 2004.

296. Sejvar, J. J., Labutta, R. J., Chapman, L. E., et al.: Neurologic adverse events associated with smallpox vaccination in the United States, 2002-2004. J. A. M. A. 294:2744-2750, 2005.

297. Sener, R. N.: Herpes simplex encephalitis: Diffusion MR imaging findings. Comput. Med. Imaging Graph. 25:391-397, 2001.

298. Shaffer, M. F., Rake, G., and Hodes, H. L.: Isolation of virus from a patient with fatal encephalitis complicating measles. Am. J. Dis. Child. 64:815-819, 1942.

299. Shaked, Y., and Samra, Y.: Q fever meningoencephalitis associated with bilateral abducens nerve paralysis, bilateral optic neuritis and abnormal cerebrospinal fluid findings. Infection 17:394-395, 1989.

300. Shaw, D. W. W., and Cohen, W. A.: Viral infections of the CNA in children: Imaging features. A. J. R. Am. J. Roentgenol. 160:125-133, 1993.

301. Sherman, F. E., Michaels, R. H., and Kenny, F. M.: Acute encephalopathy (encephalitis) complicating rubella. J. A. M. A. 192:675-681, 1965.

302. Sheth, R. D., Goulden, K. J., and Pryse-Phillips, W. E.: The focal encephalopathies associated with *Mycoplasma pneumoniae*. Can. J. Neurol. Sci. 20:319-323, 1993.

303. Shields, W. D.: Status epilepticus. Pediatr. Clin. North Am. 36:383-393, 1989.

304. Siegman-Igra, Y., Michaeli, D., Doron, A., et al.: Cytomegalovirus encephalitis in a noncompromised host. Isr. J. Med. Sci. 20:163-166, 1984.

305. Sillimsan, C. C., Tedder, D., Ogle, J. W., et al.: Unsuspected varicella-zoster virus encephalitis in a child with acquired immunodeficiency syndrome. J. Pediatr. 123:418-422, 1993.

306. Singh, N., and Paterson, D. L.: Encephalitis caused by human herpesvirus-6 in transplant recipients: relevance of a novel neurotropic virus. Transplantation 69:2474-2479, 2000.

307. Singh, S., Prabhankar, S., Korah, I. H., et al.: Acute disseminated encephalomyelitis and multiple sclerosis: Magnetic resonance imaging differentiation. Aust. Radiol. 44:404-411, 2000.

308. Socan, M., Ravnik, I., Bencina, D., et al.: Neurological symptoms in patients whose cerebrospinal fluid is culture—and/or polymerase chain reaction—positive for *Mycoplasma pneumoniae*. Clin. Infect. Dis. 32:E31-E35, 2001.

309. Solomon, T.: Control of Japanese encephalitis—within our grasp? N. Engl. J. Med. 355:869-871, 2006.

310. Solomon, T., Ni, H., Beasley, D. W. C., et al.: Origin and evolution of Japanese encephalitis virus in Southeast Asia. J. Virol. 77:3091-3098, 2003.

311. Southern, P. M., Jr.: Relapsing fever. In Tice, F. (ed.): Practice of Medicine. Vol. 3. Scranton, PA, Hoeber Medical Division, Harper & Row, 1969, pp. 1-19.

312. Spillane, J. D., and Wells, C. E. C.: The neurology of Jennerian vaccination: A clinical account of the neurological complications which occurred during the smallpox epidemic in South Wales in 1962. Brain 87:1-44, 1964.

313. Steer, A. C., Starr, M., and Kornberg, A. J.: Bickerstaff brainstem encephalitis associated with *Mycoplasma pneumonia* infection. J. Child Neurol. 21:533-554, 2006.

314. Steiner, M. M., Vuckovitch, D., and Hadawi, S. A.: Cat-scratch disease with encephalopathy: Case report and review of the literature. J. Pediatr. 62:514-520, 1963.

315. Steinfort, D. P., and Dixon, B.: Parvovirus encephalitis and pneumonia in an immunocompetent adult. Intern. Med. J. 36:209-210, 2006.

316. Straussberg, R., Harel, L., Levy, Y., et al.: A syndrome of transient encephalopathy associated with adenovirus infection. Pediatrics 107:E69, 2001.

317. Studahl, M.: Influenza virus and CNS manifestations. J. Clin. Virol. 28:225-232, 2003.

318. Surtees, R., and DeSousa, C.: Influenza virus associated encephalopathy. Arch. Dis. Child. 91:455-456, 2006.
319. Sweetman, L. L., Ng, Y., Butler, I. J., and Bodensteiner, J. B.: Neurologic complications associated with respiratory syncytial virus. Pediatr. Neurol. 32:307-310, 2005.
320. Tagawa, Y., and Nobuhiro, Y.: Bickerstaff's brainstem encephalitis associated with shingles. J. Neurol. 247:218-219, 2000.
321. Tambyah, P. A., Tan, J. H., Ong, B. K. C., et al.: First case of Nipah virus encephalitis in Singapore. Intensive Med. J. 31:132-133, 2001.
322. Tan, C. T., Goh, K. J., Wong, K. T., et al.: Relapsed and late-onset Nipah encephalitis. Ann. Neurol. 51:703-708, 2002.
323. Tenembaum, S., Chamoles, N., and Fejerman, N.: Acute disseminated encephalomyelitis: A long-term follow-up study of 84 pediatric patients. Neurology 59:1224-1231, 2002.
324. Tesh, R. B.: The prevalence of encephalomyocarditis virus neutralizing antibodies among various human populations. Am. J. Trop. Med. Hyg. 27:144-149, 1978.
325. Thong, T. H.: Primary amoebic meningoencephalitis: Fifteen years later. Med. J. Aust. 1:352-354, 1980.
326. Togashi, T., Matsuzono, Y., Narita, M., et al.: Influenza-associated acute encephalopathy in Japanese children in 1994-2002. Virus Res. 103:75-78, 2004.
327. Tokunaga, K., Kira, R., Takemoto, M., et al.: Diagnostic usefulness of diffusion-weighted magnetic resonance imaging in influenza-associated encephalopathy or encephalitis. Brain Dev. 22:451-453, 2000.
328. Torigoe, S., Koide, W., Yamada, M., et al.: Human herpesvirus 7 infection associated with central nervous system manifestations. J. Pediatr. 129:301-305, 1996.
329. Towne, A. R., Waterhouse, E. J., Boggs, J. G., et al.: Prevalence of nonconvulsive status epilepticus in comatose patients. Neurology 54:340-345, 2000.
330. Townsend, J. J., Wolinsky, J. S., Baringer, J. R., et al.: Acquired toxoplasmosis: A neglected cause of treatable nervous system disease. Arch. Neurol. 32:335-343, 1975.
331. Treatment of convulsive status epilepticus. Recommendation of the Epilepsy Foundation of America's Working Group on Status Epilepticus. J. A. M. A. 270:854-859, 1993.
332. Tsai, T. F.: New initiatives for the control of Japanese encephalitis by vaccination: Minutes of a WHO/CVI meeting, Bangkok, Thailand, 13-15 October 1998. Vaccine 18:1-24, 2000.
333. Tsiodras, S., Kelesidis, I., Kelesidis, T., et al.: Central nervous system manifestations of Mycoplasma pneumoniae infections. J. Infect. 51:343-354, 2005.
334. Tsuchiya, K., Katase, S., Yoshino, A., et al.: Diffusion-weighted MR imaging of encephalitis. A. J. R. Am. J. Roentgenol. 173:1097-1099, 1999.
335. Tsutsumi, H., Kamazaki, H., Nakata, S., et al.: Sequential development of acute meningoencephalitis and transverse myelitis caused by Epstein-Barr virus during infectious mononucleosis. Pediatr. Infect. Dis. J. 13:665-667, 1994.
336. Tyler, K. L.: Herpes simplex virus infections of the central nervous system: Encephalitis and meningitis, including Mollaret's. Herpes 11(S2):57A-64A, 2004.
337. Uren, E. C., Johnson, P. D. R., Montanaro, J., et al.: Herpes simplex virus encephalitis in pediatrics: Diagnosis by detection of antibodies and DNA in cerebrospinal fluid. Pediatr. Infect. Dis. J. 12:1001-1006, 1993.
338. Visser, A. M., van Doornum, G. J. J., Cornelissen, J. J., et al.: Severe amnesia due to HHV-6 encephalitis after allogenic stem cell transplantation. Eur. Neurol. 54:233-234, 2005.
339. Visvesvara, G. S., Martinez, A. J., Schuster, F. L., et al.: Leptomyxid ameba, a new agent of amebic meningoencephalitis in humans and animals. J. Clin. Microbiol. 28:2750-2756, 1990.
340. Voltz, R., Gundula, J., Seelos, K., et al.: BK virus encephalitis in an immunocompetent patient. Arch. Neurol. 53:101-103, 1996.
341. Wallace, S. J., and Zealley, H.: Neurological, electroencephalographic, and virological findings in febrile children. Arch. Dis. Child. 45:611-623, 1970.
342. Wang, S. M., Liu, C. C., Tseng, H. W., et al.: Clinical spectrum of enterovirus 71 infection in children in southern Taiwan, with an emphasis on neurological complications. Clin. Infect. Dis. 29:184-190, 1999.
343. Wang, Y., Huang, Y., Chang, L., et al.: Clinical characteristics of children with influenza A virus infection requiring hospitalization. J. Microbiol. Immunol. Infect. 36:111-116, 2003.
344. Ward, K. N., Kalima, P., MacLeod, K. M., et al.: Neuroinvasion during delayed primary HHV-7 infection in an immunocompetent adult with encephalitis and flaccid paralysis. J. Med. Virol. 67:538-531, 2002.
345. Warren, J.: Encephalitis lethargica. In Rivers, T. M., and Horsfall, F. L., Jr. (eds.): Viral and Rickettsial Infections of Man. Philadelphia, J. B. Lippincott, 1959, pp. 914-915.
346. Watson, R. T., Ballinger, W. E., and Quisling, R. G.: Acute hemorrhagic leukoencephalitis: Diagnosis by computed tomography. Ann. Neurol. 15:611-612, 1984.
347. Weisberg, L. A.: The role of CT in the evaluation of patients with intracranial CNS infectious-inflammatory disorders. Comput. Radiol. 8:29-36, 1984.
348. Whitley, R., Laeman, A. D., Nahmias, A., et al.: DNA restriction enzyme analysis of herpes simplex virus isolates obtained from patients with encephalitis. N. Engl. J. Med. 307:1060-1062, 1982.
349. Whitley, R. J.: Viral encephalitis. N. Engl. J. Med. 323:242-250, 1990.
350. Whitley, R. J., Cobbs, C. G., Alford, C. A., Jr., et al.: Diseases that mimic herpes simplex encephalitis: Diagnosis, presentation and outcome. J. A. M. A. 262:234-239, 1989.
351. Whitley, R. J., and Kimberlin, D. W.: Herpes simplex encephalitis: Children and adolescents. Semin. Pediatr. Infect. Dis. 16:17-23, 2005.
352. Whitley, R. J., and Lakeman, F.: Herpes simplex virus infections of the central nervous system: Therapeutic and diagnostic considerations. Clin. Infect Dis. 20:414-420, 1995.
353. Willoughby, R. E., Jr., Tieves, K. S., Hoffman, G. M., et al.: Survival after treatment of rabies with induction of coma. N. Engl. J. Med. 352:2508-2514, 2005.
354. Wise, M. E., Sorvillo, F. J., Shafir, S. C., et al.: Severe and fatal central nervous system disease in humans caused by Baylisascaris procyonis, the common roundworm of raccoons: A review of current literature. Microbes Infect. 7:317-323, 2005.
355. Woods, C. A., and Ellison, G. W.: Encephalopathy following influenza immunization. J. Pediatr. 65:745-748, 1964.
356. World Health Organization: World Health Statistics Annual. Vol. 11, Infectious Diseases: Cases and Deaths. Geneva, World Health Organization, 1978.
357. Yan, J. J., Wang, J. R., Liu, C. C., et al.: An outbreak of enterovirus 71 infection in Taiwan 1998: A comprehensive pathological, virological, and molecular study on a case of fulminant encephalitis. J. Clin. Virol. 17:13-22, 2000.
358. Yang, T. T., Huang, L. M., Lu, C. Y., et al.: Clinical features and factors of unfavorable outcomes for non-polio enterovirus infection of the central nervous system in northern Taiwan, 1994-2003. J. Microbiol. Immunol. Infect. 38:417-424, 2005.
359. Yeh, E. A., Collins, A., Cohen, M. E., et al.: Detection of coronavirus in the central nervous system of a child with acute disseminated encephalomyelitis. Pediatrics 113:e73-e76, 2004.
360. Yoshikawa, H., Yamaszaki, S., Watanabe, T., et al.: Study of influenza-associated encephalitis/encephalopathy in children during the 1997 to 2001 influenza seasons. J. Child Neurol. 16:885-890, 2001.
361. Yoshikawa, T., Nakashima, T., Suga, S., et al.: Human herpesvirus-6 DNA in cerebrospinal fluid of a child with exanthem subitum and meningoencephalitis. Pediatrics 89:888-890, 1992.
362. Young, E. J.: Human brucellosis. Rev. Infect. Dis. 5:821-842, 1983.
363. Yuki, N., Odaka, M., and Hirata, K.: Bickerstaff's brainstem encephalitis subsequent to Campylobacter jejuni enteritis. J. Neurol. Neurosurg. Psychiatry 68:680-681, 2000.
364. Zalan, E., Leers, W. D., and Labzoffsky, N. A.: Occurrence of reovirus infection in Ontario. Can. Med. Assoc. J. 87:714-715, 1962.
365. Ziegra, S. R.: Corticosteroid treatment for measles encephalitis. J. Pediatr. 39:322-323, 1961.
366. Zinserling, A. V., Aksenov, O. A., Melnikova, V. F., et al.: Extrapulmonary lesions in influenza. Tohoku J. Exp. Med. 140:259-272, 1983.

PARAINFECTIOUS AND POSTINFECTIOUS DISORDERS OF THE NERVOUS SYSTEM

CHAPTER **43a**

PARAINFECTIOUS AND POSTINFECTIOUS DEMYELINATING DISORDERS OF THE CENTRAL NERVOUS SYSTEM

Timothy Edward Lotze

ACUTE DISSEMINATED ENCEPHALOMYELITIS

Acute disseminated encephalomyelitis (ADEM) is a monophasic demyelinating disease of the central nervous system (CNS) that results in acute, polysymptomatic neurologic disability. It also has been termed *postinfectious encephalomyelitis*. It is related to other central inflammatory demyelinating conditions of childhood, including optic neuritis, transverse myelitis, neuromyelitis optica (Devic disease), and multiple sclerosis. Although no single diagnostic test can be used to distinguish among these conditions at the initial presentation, certain clinical features, laboratory results, and imaging findings can be used to ensure a correct diagnosis. Most of these conditions are thought to be caused by autoimmune dysregulation triggered by an infectious agent in a genetically susceptible host.

DIAGNOSTIC CRITERIA

The term *acute disseminated encephalomyelitis* has been used variably in the literature in describing clinical characteristics of this disease. Discrepancies exist among descriptive studies regarding (1) the occurrence of encephalopathy, (2) the association with preceding infection, (3) symptoms that are monofocal or multifocal, and (4) the possibility for recurrence. Lack of standardized diagnostic criteria for ADEM has impeded the ability to understand this distinct disease better as part of the spectrum of demyelinating conditions occurring in childhood.

More recently, the International Pediatric Multiple Sclerosis Study Group developed diagnostic criteria for ADEM.[32] The group created working definitions for monophasic ADEM and for recurrent forms of the disease. Table 43–1 lists the diagnostic criteria. An absolute criterion for a diagnosis of ADEM is the presence of encephalopathy. This criterion is defined to include either behavioral changes, such as lethargy or irritability, or more severe alterations in level of consciousness, such as coma. The onset of the encephalopathy must correspond with the occurrence of the disease state. Premorbid cognitive difficulties, such as learning difficulties or mental retardation, would not be included in this definition. Magnetic resonance imaging (MRI) shows multiple lesions in both hemispheres distributed throughout the white matter (Fig. 43–1). A distinguishing characteristic

of ADEM is prominent involvement of the cortical gray matter and deep gray nuclei (basal ganglia and thalamus). Such involvement is atypical for multiple sclerosis and other demyelinating conditions. The lesions of ADEM are asymmetric, showing variable size, shape, and distribution between the hemispheres. MRI showing symmetric and confluent lesions should prompt the clinician to consider other diagnoses, such as leukodystrophies and inborn errors of metabolism. If MRI shows evidence of previous demyelination, the clinician should query the history further for previous attacks, which would suggest either a recurrent form of the disease or a chronic demyelinating condition. Cerebrospinal fluid (CSF) analysis may show a pleocytosis of greater than 50 cells, in contrast to pediatric multiple sclerosis, in which only a slight pleocytosis (<50 cells) is observed.

The International Pediatric Multiple Sclerosis Study Group has defined criteria to distinguish between an evolving pattern for the initial event and for recurrent forms of ADEM. Any new and fluctuating symptoms occurring within 3 months of the initial event are considered to be part of the same inciting event. In addition, symptoms that occur during steroid taper or within 1 month of the patient's completing a steroid taper are considered to be part of the same inciting event. Relapsing ADEM and multiphasic ADEM are the two recurrent forms of the disease. Both forms are defined to occur more than 3 months after the initial event and more than 1 month after completion of steroids. By definition for ADEM, both forms must include a clinical

TABLE 43–1 Diagnostic Criteria of Acute Disseminated Encephalomyelitis

Clinical Features
First clinical attack of demyelinating disease in CNS
Acute or subacute onset
Polysymptomatic presentation
Must include encephalopathy
    Acute behavioral change (e.g., irritability, lethargy)
    Alteration in consciousness (e.g., somnolence, coma)
Attack should be followed by improvement

Lesion Characteristics on MRI FLAIR and T2-Weighted Images
Multifocal, hyperintense, bilateral, asymmetric lesions in the white matter
At least one or more lesions >1-2 cm
Gray matter, especially basal ganglia and thalamus, may be involved
Spinal cord MRI may show confluent intramedullary lesions
No radiologic evidence of previous destructive white matter changes

Cerebrospinal Fluid
Pleocytosis ≥50 WBCs can be observed

Other
No other etiologies can explain the event
New or fluctuating symptoms and signs occurring within 3 mo of the inciting ADEM event are part of the same acute event

Note: *Symptoms that vary during periods of steroid taper within 3 mo of the inciting event or occur <30 days after discontinuation of all steroids are considered part of the initial inciting event.*
ADEM, acute disseminated encephalomyelitis; CNS, central nervous system; FLAIR, fluid-attenuated inversion recovery; MRI, magnetic resonance imaging; WBCs, white blood cells.

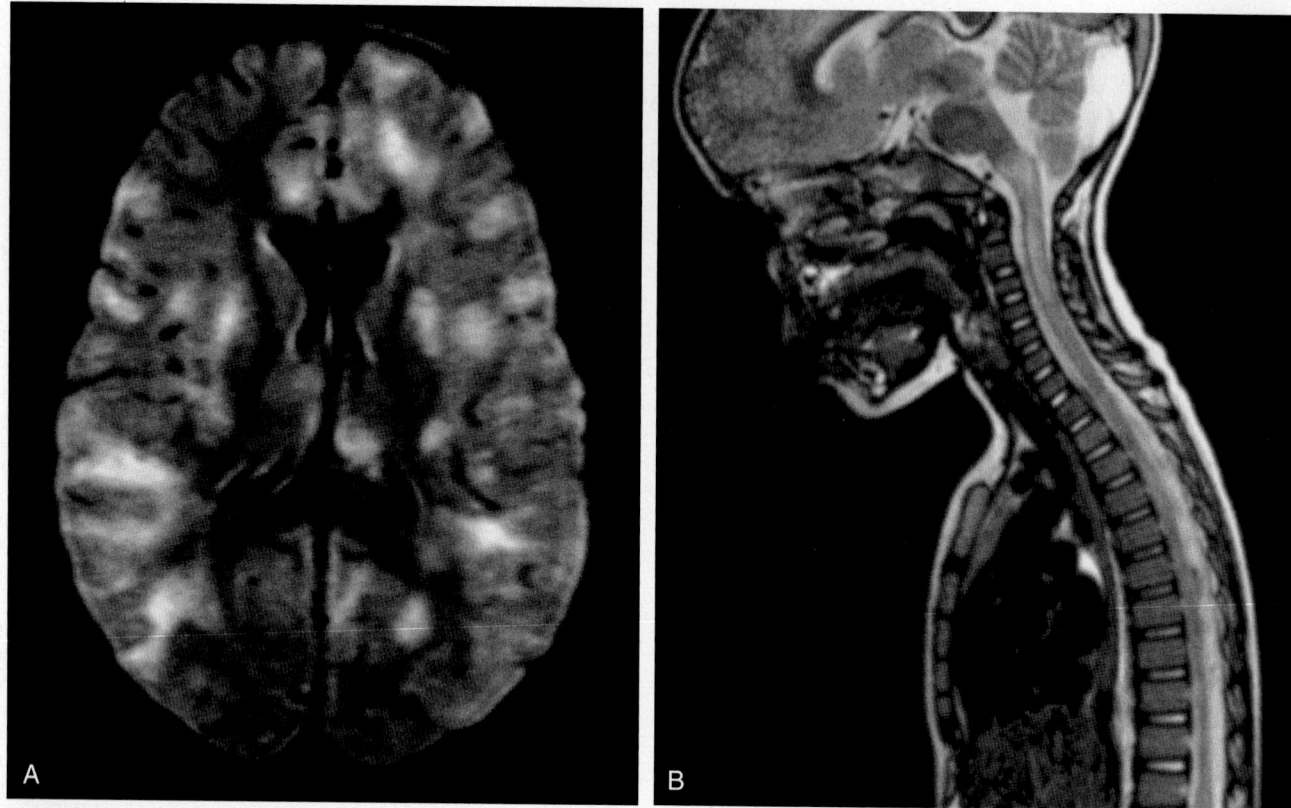

Figure 43–1 A, Axial fluid-attenuated inversion recovery (FLAIR) image showing multifocal areas of hyperintensity in both cerebral hemispheres involving cortical gray matter, centrum semiovale, and deep gray nuclei. **B,** Sagittal T2-weighted spine image with increased intrinsic signal consistent with longitudinally extensive transverse myelitis in the same patient. (*Courtesy of Tim Lotze, M.D.*)

presentation with encephalopathy. Relapsing ADEM describes the recurrence of the same symptoms that occurred at the time of the initial presentation. The MRI findings also are similar to the initial event, although they may show enlargement of the previous lesions. Multiphasic ADEM describes children with recurrent disease characterized by symptoms that differ from the initial event. MRI likewise shows development of new lesions different from those seen with the first attack.

CLINICAL MANIFESTATIONS

A febrile illness occurs in 50 to 75 percent of children in the 4 weeks before the onset of typical neurologic symptoms.[38] Preceding vaccinations have been associated with the occurrence of ADEM, but this is less common.[13,47] Fever, headache, vomiting, and meningismus often are present at the time of initial presentation and may persist during the hospitalization.[8,23] Neurologic symptoms typically appear 4 to 13 days after the infection develops or vaccination is administered.[13,23,40,47] New clinical symptoms may continue during hospitalization, and they may alter the treatment for the patient. As per current diagnostic criteria, all children with ADEM have an encephalopathy at the time of presentation.[32] The degree of altered mental status varies, ranging from irritability to somnolence to coma. Encephalopathy may be the initial symptom that brings the child to medical attention. Although alteration in mental state often raises concern for the possibility of seizures, they occur in only one third of patients.[15,47] In addition to having encephalopathy, patients exhibit various other neurologic features. The most common of these are long tract signs, acute hemiparesis, cerebellar ataxia, and cranial neuropathy.[8,15,23,40,47] Aphasia, movement disorders, and sensory deficits occur less commonly.

Demyelination of the optic nerves (optic neuritis) or spinal cord (transverse myelitis) may occur. Symptoms of optic neuritis include vision loss, pain with eye movement, and an afferent papillary defect. Inflammation of the optic disk may be seen on direct funduscopic examination if there is extensive involvement of the optic nerve. Patients with retrobulbar optic neuritis typically have a normal funduscopic examination. Optic neuritis may occur in one or both eyes, with differing degrees of involvement. Symptoms of transverse myelitis include flaccid paralysis of the legs, with a sensory level on examination. The arms can be involved as well if the demyelinating lesion is in the cervical cord. Respiratory failure may occur with high cervical lesions that extend into the brain stem. Bowel and bladder involvement secondary to spinal cord disease results in constipation and urinary retention.

The extent of demyelination in the CNS may not be recognized fully at the time of initial presentation, particularly if the patient has a severe encephalopathy. Imaging of the entire CNS to include the brain, orbits, and spinal cord should be done in all patients meeting diagnostic criteria for ADEM because co-occurrence of transverse myelitis or optic neuritis can have a significant impact on rehabilitation needs and long-term outcome.

CLINICAL VARIANTS

Relapsing ADEM and multiphasic ADEM are the two recurrent forms of the disease. Both forms are defined by reoccurrence of neurologic symptoms more than 3 months after the initial event and more than 1 month after completion of steroids. Most often, recurrence of disease is singular. Repeated events are unusual and should prompt assessment for a different underlying disease process, including metabolic disorders or primary inflammatory diseases such as multiple sclerosis.

Acute hemorrhagic leukoencephalitis is considered to be a severe variant of ADEM. It accounts for 2 percent of patients with ADEM.[47] Clinical presentation is similar to that of ADEM, including an acute onset of neurologic deficits 1 to 3 weeks after an upper respiratory infection or vaccination. Seizures and coma ensue within hours. The mortality rate is extremely high with fulminant disease. Survivors often have severe residual neurologic deficits. The clinical presentation and imaging features mimic those typically seen in herpes simplex virus encephalitis. Evidence of inflammatory changes and hemorrhage on MRI often is not present for the first few days in herpes simplex virus encephalitis, which may help to distinguish the two conditions.[18] Early recognition with prompt institution of steroids or other immunosuppressive agents can be lifesaving.

Historically, site-restricted forms of demyelination, such as optic neuritis or transverse myelitis, have been included as part of the spectrum of ADEM. Although these conditions share similar underlying pathology, clinical presentations and prognosis are different, and they should be considered to be separate entities. They are considered to be clinically isolated syndromes by the current consensus definitions for demyelinating disease.[32] Clinically isolated syndromes may carry a greater risk for the development of multiple sclerosis or other recurrent forms of demyelinating disease.[49] *Neuromyelitis optica*, also known as *Devic disease*, describes coincident or sequential optic neuritis and longitudinally extensive myelitis. It is not always periinfectious in onset and is associated with antibodies directed against aquaporin-4 water channels in the CNS.[50]

Multiple sclerosis is the second most common cause of acquired neurologic disability in adults. It is an uncommon finding in pediatric patients. Five percent of adults with multiple sclerosis had onset of disease before reaching 18 years of age.[4] Clinical phenotypes consistent with ADEM, relapsing ADEM, and multiphasic ADEM should not be confused with multiple sclerosis. Although they may share some of the same initiating pathologic mechanisms, they are different diseases.[10] The diagnosis of multiple sclerosis requires clinical or radiographic evidence for demyelinating events separated in space and time in the CNS. Patients typically follow a relapsing course of neurologic attacks with resolution or remission of disability between attacks. Evolution into a course of progressive disability occurs in 50 percent of patients who have had the disease for more than 15 years.[7] Treatment consists of medications that modulate the immune response by decreasing migration into the CNS, altering cytokine profiles, and interrupting antigen presentation.

EPIDEMIOLOGY

The estimated incidence of ADEM is 0.8 per 100,000 population per year.[34] ADEM occurs just as frequently in children as it does in adults.[10] It has no specific gender predilection or ethnic distribution.[13,14] In contrast to multiple sclerosis, which generally has a higher incidence at more northern latitudes, ADEM has no appreciable geographic distribution.

PATHOLOGY AND PATHOGENESIS

ROLE OF INFECTION

ADEM is preceded by a viral or bacterial infection in 75 percent of the cases. This infection usually is in the form of a nonspecific upper respiratory infection. Many different pathogens have been identified in association with the illness (Table 43–2). No well-defined latency period has been identified in which an infection

TABLE 43–2 Infectious Pathogens Associated with Acute Disseminated Encephalomyelitis

Viral
Coxsackie
Cytomegalovirus
Epstein-Barr
Hepatitis A or B
Herpes simplex
HHV-6
HTLV-1
Human immunodeficiency virus
Influenza A or B
Measles
Mumps
Rocky Mountain spotted fever
Rubella
Vaccinia
Varicella

Bacterial
Borrelia burgdorferi
Campylobacter
Chlamydia
Legionella
Leptospira
Mycoplasma pneumoniae
Rickettsia rickettsii
Streptococcus

HHV-6, human herpesvirus-6; HTLV-1, human T-cell lymphotrophic virus-1.

can be related to ADEM. Generally, patients present within 1 month of their illness. Correlation between ADEM and an infection occurring more than 30 days prior is more difficult because children are diagnosed with a viral infection four to six times per year, resulting in a positive infectious history in 33 to 50 percent of patients.[38]

The phenotypic presentation for ADEM varies depending on the infectious agent. Some organisms have been associated with typical clinical features. Measles virus infection is associated with ADEM in 1 in 1000 cases. The clinical course often is fulminating, with severe neurological sequelae or death in most patients. Introduction of vaccination has reduced markedly the occurrence of measles in developed countries, although vaccine-associated ADEM is described in 2 cases per 1 million.[6]

Post-varicella ADEM is characterized by ataxia in more than 90 percent of patients, occasionally with an explosive onset.[24] Headache and meningismus are typical constitutional signs. Pyramidal symptoms include bilateral symmetric upper motor neuron weakness. Patients also may have mood disturbances with a depressed affect or irritability.

ADEM that develops after a rubella infection is similar to measles, with an explosive onset in most children.[24] There is often profound lethargy and coma and generalized seizures. Most patients with explosive onset of disease have pyramidal signs and myelitis, whereas a milder phenotype is more likely to have ataxia. Both forms also have been associated with brain stem signs.

Group A beta-hemolytic streptococcal infection has been associated with a dystonic extrapyramidal syndrome. Abnormal movements include dystonia, tremor, and parkinsonism. Tics and chorea have not been associated with this condition. Similar to Sydenham chorea and pediatric autoimmune neuropsychiatric disorders associated with streptoccocal infection (PANDAS), behavioral disturbances, such as emotional lability, obsessive-compulsive tendencies, and inappropriate speech, can occur. Changes in mental status can vary from irritability to coma. MRI shows a predilection for demyelination within the basal ganglia, which includes the caudate, putamen, and globus pallidus. Other deep gray structures, including the thalamus, subthalamus, and substantia nigra, may be affected as well. This finding is distinct from Sydenham chorea and PANDAS, in which imaging is unremarkable. It has been associated with anti–basal ganglia antibodies that cross-react with certain strains of streptococcus.[14]

ROLE OF IMMUNIZATION

Vaccine-associated ADEM has been described with nearly every immunization (Table 43–3). The Collaborating Center for Reference and Research on Viral Hepatitis of the World Health Organization has suggested a maximal period of 3 months to diagnose vaccination-associated ADEM. Post-vaccination ADEM accounts for less than 5 percent of ADEM cases.

Historically, Pasteur rabies vaccination was associated with prototypic ADEM in approximately one in 1000 individuals.[6] The inoculum was derived from rabbit spinal cord injected with fixed rabies virus. The disease was thought to result principally from the neural tissue contaminating the vaccine, rather than the virus itself. This suggestion is supported further by the continued higher incidence of vaccine-associated encephalomyelitis in patients receiving the Semple or duck embryo vaccinations, both of which contain neural tissue. These forms of the vaccination usually are found in developing countries. Experimental allergic encephalomyelitis, the animal model of demyelinating disease, is induced by inoculating myelin or myelin antigens into a suitable experimental animal, further supporting a role of CNS tissue as the causal agent.

Currently, measles, mumps, and rubella vaccination is associated most often with post-vaccination encephalomyelitis. There is a significant difference between the incidence of live-measles vaccination associated ADEM (1 to 2 per 1 million) and the incidence of ADEM previously associated with the measles virus infection (1 in 1000).

Smallpox was eradicated in 1980 following a successful vaccination program that was discontinued in the United States in 1971.[11] The World Health Organization has allowed retention of the variola virus at a designated laboratory in the United States and Russia for the purpose of creating a safer vaccination than the presently available live vaccinia virus. More recent concerns for bioterrorism have resulted in the reinstitution of smallpox vaccination to certain identified groups within the United States that might come into contact with the virus as first responders to a possible smallpox outbreak. The previously reported incidence of ADEM associated with smallpox vaccination was 10 to 300 cases for every 1 million vaccinations. It is estimated, based on these figures, that vaccination of the entire British population would result in approximately 600 cases of vaccine-associated ADEM. Administration of anti-vaccinia gamma-globulin at the time of vaccination can help to prevent this complication.[44]

TABLE 43–3 Vaccines Associated with Acute Disseminated Encephalomyelitis

Diphtheria-tetanus-polio
Hepatitis B
Hog vaccine
Japanese B encephalitis
Measles
Mumps
Polio
Rabies
Smallpox
Tetanus
Tick-borne encephalitis

IMMUNOLOGIC FACTORS

A review of the normal process of immune system regulation and surveillance of the CNS is useful when discussing immune dysfunction in the pathogenesis of ADEM. Similar to other disorders of immune dysfunction, activated $CD4^+$ T cells play a principal role in the disease process. T cells reactive against self-antigens, including myelin components, are present in the normal immune system. Several regulatory mechanisms are thought to prevent activation of these lymphocytes, and failure of such processes results in autoimmune conditions. The thymus plays a crucial role in normal T-cell development by deleting many autoreactive lymphocytes from the immune system. Other peripheral mechanisms also are needed because this thymic depletion often is incomplete. Clonal anergy describes the unresponsive state of T cells that have encountered their antigen without costimulatory factors.[41] A risk for failure of this mechanism exists through release of nonspecific, costimulatory factors from damaged tissue. Another peripheral process is immunologic ignorance, in which no productive reaction exists between the T cell and its corresponding peptide/MHC complex on an antigen-presenting cell. Changes in antigen availability, such as through increased antigen presentation by an invading microorganism, can disrupt this safeguard.[26]

Active regulation is a third process by which regulatory T cells prevent expansion of self-reactive lymphocytes.[31] Regulatory T cells exert their suppressive effects through direct cell-to-cell contact with membrane-bound molecules (CTLA-4) or indirectly through soluble suppressive cytokines, such as interleukin-10 and transforming growth factor-β.[25] Natural killer cells expressing a T-cell receptor also can regulate autoimmune diseases.[37] The presence of such cells within demyelinating regions suggests that some of the inflammation associated with ADEM may have a protective effect.

Although failure of these mechanisms may result in the activation of T cells reactive against myelin antigens, migration of lymphocytes into the CNS is required to produce disease. The CNS has been considered to be a site of limited immunologic surveillance because of the blood-brain barrier and lack of classic lymph vessels. The blood-brain barrier is principally a mechanical diffusion barrier, however, for hydrophilic molecules formed by specialized endothelial cells at the level of the capillaries. Leukocytes readily cross through endothelial cells in post-capillary venules to occupy the perivenular spaces or move on to the neuropil.[21] In addition, antigens and antigen-presenting cells drain from the brain into cervical lymph nodes via the cribriform plate and perineural sheath of the cranial nerves.[12,28] As discussed later, these factors allow for the presentation of antigen in the systemic immune compartment and passage of leukocytes into the CNS for production of disease.

Children with demyelinating disease of the CNS are thought to have a genetic predisposition for such conditions. The strongest data relate to susceptibility genes on chromosome 6p21 in the area of the histocompatibility leukocyte antigen (HLA). Much of the research into these genetic determinants has been related to adult-onset multiple sclerosis.[46] Limited research is available for pediatric demyelinating diseases. Some of the findings show similarities, however, among age groups and various demyelinating diseases. Linkage studies in Russian children found an association between ADEM and HLA-DRB1*01 and HLA-DRB1*017(03) alleles.[24] Korean children with ADEM were found to have higher frequencies of HLA-DRB4*0101 and HLA-DRB1*1501 compared with controls. In adults with multiple sclerosis, the specific genes that confer the highest risk include HLA-DRB1*1501 and HLA-DRB5*0101 among others. In multiple sclerosis, these genes have been linked to earlier disease onset, female gender, a relapsing remitting course, and optic neuritis or spinal involvement as the initial symptom. In addition, genes associated with this haplotype include transforming growth factor-β family members, CTLA-4, the tumor necrosis factor cluster, interleukin-1 receptor antagonist, interleukin-1, and estrogen receptor. Polymorphisms in these genes also have been associated with increased risk for development of demyelinating disease.[16]

The precise mechanism by which these HLA class II genes confer risk for development of demyelinating disease is unclear. Possibilities include (1) preferential binding of self-antigens by these peptides, (2) preferential linkage of autoreactive T cells to the antigen-presenting cell expressing these peptides, (3) abnormal antigen presentation by certain DR molecules, and (4) engagement of HLA class II molecules leading to intracellular signaling events.[46]

Humoral factors also play a role in the production of demyelinating disease. This finding is based on disease-associated laboratory findings and treatment responses. Analysis of CSF in one third of patients with ADEM shows production of oligoclonal bands, which are not found to be present in the serum.[13] In addition, some patients with post-rabies inoculation ADEM have been found to have positive serum antibodies against myelin basic protein and galactocerebroside.[33]

PATHOGENESIS

ADEM is considered to occur in genetically susceptible individuals prone to immune system dysregulation after an encounter with an appropriate environmental stimulus. Mechanisms of disease production are based principally on two animal models that closely resemble the disease. The first is experimental autoimmune encephalomyelitis.[43] In this model, animals develop monophasic neurologic disease similar to ADEM after receiving immunization with CNS homogenate or encephalitogenic myelin peptides emulsified in Freund complete adjuvant. The second model is Theiler murine encephalomyelitis, in which susceptible mouse strains develop disease after receiving direct injection of Theiler murine encephalomyelitis virus into the cerebrum.[22] In both of these models, increased exposure of the immune system to myelin proteins produces disease.

By comparing these models with ADEM in humans, two pathogenetic concepts have been developed. The inflammatory cascade concept implies a direct CNS infection with a neurotropic pathogen, which results in CNS tissue damage and systemic leakage of CNS-confined autoantigens through a damaged blood-brain barrier into the systemic circulation. Presentation of these antigens within systemic lymphatic organs leads to tolerance breakdown and a self-reactive encephalitogenic T-cell response. The molecular mimicry concept suggests structural amino acid homology between the invading pathogen and myelin basic protein in the host.[17] Although similar to myelin peptides, the amino acid sequence contains subtle differences that fail to prevent immune tolerance and result in activation of myelin-reactive T cells against similar "self" myelin antigens. Epstein-Barr virus provides an example of this. The virus contains a pentapeptide sequence in its nuclear antigen (EBNA) that shares sequence homology with an epitope of myelin basic protein, a major protein of the myelin sheath.[9] Epstein-Barr virus has been implicated in the pathogenesis of multiple sclerosis partly based on this concept of molecular mimicry.[1]

The immunopathologic events leading to ADEM can be divided into two major phases: (1) initial T-cell priming and activation and (2) subsequent recruitment and effector phase.[5] The priming phase occurs in systemic secondary lymphoid organs, where the antigen-presenting cell presents myelin protein antigen and peptides to neuroantigen-reactive T cells. The activated T cells expand and then migrate to the CNS via the postcapillary venules into the perivascular space. In the Virchow-Robin space, the T cells re-encounter their cognate antigen, in the context of HLA class II molecules expressed by dendritic cells.[19] This reactivation allows the T cells to migrate through the glial limitans and enter the brain parenchyma.

Further recruitment occurs through the production of cytokines and chemokines by antigen-presenting cells and activated T cells, promoting migration into the CNS of additional T cells and other leukocytes, such as polymorphonuclear and monomorphonuclear phagocytes.[46] Breakdown of the blood-brain barrier occurs by release of proteases from recruited mast cells, T cells, and monocytes. In addition, production of reactive oxygen radicals occurs, causing further endothelial injury, which leads to the effector phase in which T cells have more of a secondary role to other inflammatory processes that cause demyelination and axonal injury. These inflammatory processes include oxygen and nitrogen radicals, tumor necrosis factor-α, direct and indirect complement activation, antibody-dependent cellular toxicity, myelin phagocytosis, direct axonal injury by CD8+ cytotoxic T lymphocytes, protease secretion, and oligodendrocyte apoptosis.[46] Glutamate-mediated excitotoxic injury of the oligodendrocytes also occurs.[42] The inflammatory process continues for a few days to 2 weeks, resulting in stretches of demyelinated axons, some of which may be transected.

The repair process begins with activation and proliferation of astrocytes. Clearing of debris by macrophages and increased production of anti-inflammatory cytokines and various growth factors by resident cells and T cells occur. Oligodendrocyte precursors become activated and, along with surviving oligodendrocytes, begin the process of remyelination. The clinical and imaging outcome of ADEM most often shows complete recovery. Subtle differences in repaired myelin, including altered thickness and redistribution of sodium channels, may occur, however. In addition, the relative composition of myelin peptides is altered to forms that may have increased vulnerability to further damage[48] and may explain recurrent forms of ADEM.

CLINICAL EVALUATION

ADEM should be considered in a child presenting several days after a febrile illness with subacute onset of encephalopathy and polysymptomatic neurologic deficits. The clinical features require ruling out other possible diagnoses, however, through additional diagnostic tests.

Diagnostic imaging is the most useful tool in establishing the diagnosis. Computed tomography (CT) scans usually are done on an emergent basis for encephalopathic patients. Areas of demyelination may appear as darker areas of hypodensity, with any hemorrhagic component being hyperdense. CT does not adequately show the full burden of disease, however, and may be completely normal. MRI is the most sensitive means for showing the widespread demyelination typical of the disease (see Fig. 43-1). T2-weighted sequences provide the best assessment of the disease, with demyelinating areas being hyperintense and accompanied by surrounding edema. Administration of gadolinium contrast material may show breakdown of the blood-brain barrier with areas of enhancement. This enhancement may appear homogeneous throughout the lesion or show a "broken ring" appearance, with the open edge pointing toward the cortex. Lesions may be large, measuring more than 1 cm in diameter. They typically are rounded with poorly defined margins.

Of most common concern in children presenting with a febrile encephalopathy is the possibility of an underlying CNS infection. A lumbar puncture often is done to investigate this possibility. A lymphocytic pleocytosis may occur (commonly >50 cells). Elevated albumin levels also may be present. Findings of neutrophils and elevated red blood cells alternatively would raise concern for the possibility of herpes encephalitis.

Intrathecal oligoclonal bands may be positive, and IgG synthesis may be increased in 30 percent of patients with ADEM. These abnormalities usually are associated with multiple sclerosis. In ADEM, convalescent testing for both should normalize, whereas tests remain positive in multiple sclerosis. Their relationship to the underlying disease pathophysiology is unclear but is thought to represent a response of B cells within the CNS to the inflammatory process.[3] Serologic studies of the CSF may be useful to uncover the causal agent, although results should be interpreted with caution because many neurotropic viruses have a high prevalence in the general population.

Rarely, patients may present with very large demyelinating lesions, characteristically described as *tumefactive*. In such circumstances, a biopsy may be needed to determine the underlying etiology. Findings typical of demyelination help to rule out a CNS malignancy. Before a biopsy is done, the clinician should investigate for other evidence of demyelinating disease, including imaging of the spinal cord. A comorbid transverse myelitis would provide more evidence of a demyelinating condition and reduce the need for a biopsy. In addition, normal CSF cytology helps to discount an underlying malignancy.

Either a primary or a secondary CNS vasculitis associated with collagen vascular diseases, such as systemic lupus erythematosus or antiphospholipid antibody syndrome, may manifest with a similar clinical and radiologic picture. These diseases are typified by recurrent ischemic strokes. Distinguishing features for antiphospholipid antibody syndrome include a family history of strokes or other thromboses at a young age and fetal loss. Testing for antiphospholipid antibody and lupus anticoagulant is positive. A primary CNS vasculitis with strokes is best investigated through conventional angiography showing an irregular vessel lumen. Leptomeningeal biopsy is considered the gold standard to confirm the diagnosis.

A severe course that principally affects the optic nerves and spinal cord should raise concern for neuromyelitis optica. Serum or CSF testing for the aquaporin-4 water channel antibody that is associated with this disease is clinically available. The test is greater than 90 percent specific for neuromyelitis optica.[50]

Neurophysiologic studies can be useful to evaluate comorbidities and burden of disease. An electroencephalogram should be obtained in patients with seizures and severe encephalopathy to characterize the seizure focus and to investigate for subclinical seizures. Findings often are consistent with a diffuse disturbance in brain function noting slowing of the normal electric rhythms. Visual evoked potentials can evaluate for demyelination of the optic nerves, which may not be appreciated on imaging. The examination measures the time for an electric impulse to travel from the retina to the occipital lobe, with delays suggesting a demyelinating lesion. The patient needs to be attentive to a flashing light stimulus, rendering this test difficult to perform in patients with severe encephalopathy.

TREATMENT

To date, no controlled clinical trials have been conducted regarding the optimal treatment for ADEM. Based on empiric evidence, intravenous high-dose corticosteroids are accepted as first-line treatment.[45] Methylprednisolone is given at 30 mg/kg per dose (maximum 1000 mg) for a total of five doses. Alternatively, dexamethasone, 1 mg/kg per dose for five doses, may be used. A prednisone taper typically is instituted on completion of this regimen with an initial dosing of 1 mg/kg/day and tapering by 5 mg every 5 days. Alternative anti-inflammatory and immunosuppressive therapies may be used depending on the response to the initial steroid treatment. Intravenous immunoglobulin (IVIG) has been found to be beneficial in some patients.[45] IVIG is given 2 g/kg divided over 2 to 5 days.

Plasmapheresis also may be used.[29,30] The patient receives a total of seven treatments consisting of 1.1 to 1.4 plasma volume exchanges over a 14-day course. IVIG and plasmapheresis typically are not considered as first-line treatment for ADEM, partly related to availability of IVIG or pheresis units, cost of treatment compared with steroids, prolonged hospitalization, and need for adequate venous access. Nonetheless, they should be considered as secondary treatment options, especially in the occasional patient who continues to deteriorate during steroid treatment or who fails to show adequate recovery 7 days after completing intravenous steroids. The choice between the two agents is arbitrary. Particular consideration for plasmapheresis might be given in the setting of a comorbid myelopathy because this has been noted to be beneficial in patients presenting with transverse myelitis.[27] Severe cases failing to respond to any of these measures may require immunosuppressive agents, such as cyclophosphamide.[36]

Additional treatment that may be needed for patients depends on the nature of their neurologic deficits. Anticonvulsants should be given for management of seizures. Attention given to bowel and bladder care is important to avoid secondary complications of retention. Impaired swallowing requires adequate nutrition to be provided by gavage feedings. Transverse myelopathy can be associated with autonomic dysfunction, including orthostatic hypotension, necessitating the use of an abdominal binder. Rehabilitation should begin at the time of admission with the assistance of physical medicine and rehabilitation specialists. During the long-term recovery period, modifications to the home and school environment may be needed depending on residual deficits.

OUTCOME AND PROGNOSIS

Historically, ADEM was associated with high morbidity and mortality rates principally related to disease associated with the measles virus. Measles-associated ADEM was associated with death in 25 percent of affected patients, with an additional 30 percent of patients having severe neurologic sequelae.[35] This dismal outcome has improved dramatically with institution of measles vaccination. The introduction of high-dose steroid treatment in modifying the disease course also may have improved the current outcome findings. A 5 percent mortality rate remains associated with this disease.

Currently, 80 to 90 percent of patients show excellent recovery of functional and cognitive deficits.[2,13,24,47] Mild neurologic disabilities, weakness and fine motor difficulties being the most common ones, may be present in some patients. Epilepsy may occur in 6 percent of patients after an episode of ADEM.[13] Neurocognitive testing of children recovering from ADEM has shown mild impairments in attention and executive function and reduced visuospatial and visuomotor skills.[20] The greatest risk for development of neurologic sequelae may be in older patients with sudden onset of severe neurologic symptoms.

Recurrent forms of the disease often raise concern for pediatric multiple sclerosis. The exact relationship between ADEM and multiple sclerosis remains to be better defined. The conditions are distinct, however, based on the clinical presentations, imaging, and clinical courses. Studies investigating risk for disease recurrence or evolution into multiple sclerosis have been limited and do not adequately define ADEM in the context of the current definition, and they do not distinguish between recurrent forms of the disease and multiple sclerosis. Disease recurrence occurs in 30 percent of patients.[38] Most patients have their second attack within the first year after their initial event.[2,39] It often occurs soon after discontinuation of steroid taper, or after an infection or vaccination encountered shortly after the initial event. Treatment and outcome for recurrences are not different from those described for the initial event.

REFERENCES

1. Alotaibi, S., et al.: Epstein-Barr virus in pediatric multiple sclerosis. J. A. M. A. *291*:1875-1879, 2004.
2. Anlar, B., et al.: Acute disseminated encephalomyelitis in children: Outcome and prognosis. Neuropediatrics *34*:194-199, 2003.
3. Antel, J., and Bar-Or, A.: Roles of immunoglobulins and B cells in multiple sclerosis: From pathogenesis to treatment. J. Neuroimmunol. *180*:3-8, 2006.
4. Banwell, B. L.: Pediatric multiple sclerosis. Curr. Neurol. Neurosci. Rep. *4*:245-252, 2004.
5. Becher, B., Bechmann, I., and Greter, M.: Antigen presentation in autoimmunity and CNS inflammation: How T lymphocytes recognize the brain. J. Mol. Med. *84*:532-543, 2006.
6. Bennetto, L., and Scolding, N.: Inflammatory/post-infectious encephalomyelitis. J. Neurol. Neurosurg. Psychiatry 75(Suppl. 1): i22-i28, 2004.
7. Boiko, A., et al.: Early onset multiple sclerosis: A longitudinal study. Neurology *59*:1006-1010, 2002.
8. Brass, S. D., et al.: Multiple sclerosis vs acute disseminated encephalomyelitis in childhood. Pediatr. Neurol. *29*:227-231, 2003.
9. Bray, P. F., et al.: Antibodies against Epstein-Barr nuclear antigen (EBNA) in multiple sclerosis CSF, and two pentapeptide sequence identities between EBNA and myelin basic protein. Neurology *42*:1798-1804, 1992.
10. Brinar, V. V., and Poser, C. M.: The spectrum of disseminated encephalitis. Clin. Neurol. Neurosurg. *108*:295-310, 2006.
11. Casey, C. G., et al.: Adverse events associated with smallpox vaccination in the United States, January-October 2003. J. A. M. A. *294*:2734-2743, 2005.
12. Cserr, H. F., and Knopf, P. M.: Cervical lymphatics, the blood-brain barrier and the immunoreactivity of the brain: A new view. Immunol. Today *13*:507-512, 1992.
13. Dale, R. C., et al.: Acute disseminated encephalomyelitis, multiphasic disseminated encephalomyelitis and multiple sclerosis in children. Brain *123*(Pt. 12):2407-2422, 2000.
14. Dale, R. C., et al.: Poststreptococcal acute disseminated encephalomyelitis with basal ganglia involvement and auto-reactive antibasal ganglia antibodies. Ann. Neurol. *50*:588-595, 2001.
15. Davis, L. E., and Booss, J.: Acute disseminated encephalomyelitis in children: A changing picture. Pediatr. Infect. Dis. J. *22*:829-831, 2003.
16. Dyment, D. A., Ebers, G. C., and Sadovnick, A. D.: Genetics of multiple sclerosis. Lancet Neurol. *3*:104-110, 2004.
17. Fujinami, R. S., and Oldstone, M. B.: Amino acid homology between the encephalitogenic site of myelin basic protein and virus: Mechanism for autoimmunity. Science *230*:1043-1045, 1985.
18. Gibbs, W. N., et al.: Acute hemorrhagic leukoencephalitis: Neuroimaging features and neuropathologic diagnosis. J. Comput. Assist. Tomogr. *29*:689-693, 2005.
19. Greter, M., et al.: Dendritic cells permit immune invasion of the CNS in an animal model of multiple sclerosis. Nat. Med. *11*:328-334, 2005.
20. Hahn, C. D., et al.: Neurocognitive outcome after acute disseminated encephalomyelitis. Pediatr. Neurol. *29*:117-123, 2003.
21. Hickey, W. F.: Basic principles of immunological surveillance of the normal central nervous system. Glia *36*:118-124, 2001.
22. Humphries, J. M.: Encephalitis complicating measles. J. Med. Assoc. State Ala. *25*:113-116, 1955.
23. Hynson, J. L., et al.: Clinical and neuroradiologic features of acute disseminated encephalomyelitis in children. Neurology *56*:1308-1312, 2001.
24. Idrissova, Z. R., et al.: Acute disseminated encephalomyelitis in children: Clinical features and HLA-DR linkage. Eur. J. Neurol. *10*:537-546, 2003.
25. Jonuleit, H., and Schmitt, E.: The regulatory T cell family: Distinct subsets and their interrelations. J. Immunol. *171*:6323-6327, 2003.
26. Kamradt, T., and Mitchison, N. A.: Tolerance and autoimmunity. N. Engl. J. Med. *344*:655-664, 2001.
27. Kaplin, A. I., et al.: Diagnosis and management of acute myelopathies. Neurologist *11*:2-18, 2005.
28. Karman, J., et al.: Initiation of immune responses in brain is promoted by local dendritic cells. J. Immunol. *173*:2353-2361, 2004.
29. Keegan, M., et al.: Plasma exchange for severe attacks of CNS demyelination: Predictors of response. Neurology *58*:143-146, 2002.
30. Khurana, D. S., et al.: Acute disseminated encephalomyelitis in children: Discordant neurologic and neuroimaging abnormalities and response to plasmapheresis. Pediatrics *116*:431-436, 2005.
31. King, C., et al.: Homeostatic expansion of T cells during immune insufficiency generates autoimmunity. Cell *117*:265-277, 2004.
32. Krupp, L. B., Banwell, B., and Tenembaum, S.: Consensus definitions proposed for pediatric multiple sclerosis and related childhood disorders. Neurology *68*:57-512, 2008.
33. Laouini, D., et al.: Antibodies to human myelin proteins and gangliosides in patients with acute neuroparalytic accidents induced by brain-derived rabies vaccine. J. Neuroimmunol. *91*(1-2):63-72, 1998.
34. Leake, J. A., et al.: Acute disseminated encephalomyelitis in childhood: Epidemiologic, clinical and laboratory features. Pediatr. Infect. Dis. J. *23*:756-764, 2004.
35. Lipton, L. H.: Theiler's virus infection in mice: An unusual biphasic disease process leading to demyelination. Infect. Immun. *11*:1147-1155, 1975.
36. Markus, R., et al.: Successful outcome with aggressive treatment of acute haemorrhagic leukoencephalitis. J. Neurol. Neurosurg. Psychiatry *63*:551, 1997.
37. McHugh, R. S., and Shevach, E. M.: Cutting edge: depletion of CD4+CD25+ regulatory T cells is necessary, but not sufficient, for induction of organ-specific autoimmune disease. J. Immunol. *168*:5979-5983, 2002.
38. Menge, T., et al.: Acute disseminated encephalomyelitis: An update. Arch. Neurol. *62*:1673-1680, 2005.
39. Mikaeloff, Y., et al.: First episode of acute CNS inflammatory demyelination in childhood: Prognostic factors for multiple sclerosis and disability. J Pediatr. *144*:246-252, 2004.
40. Murthy, S. N., et al.: Acute disseminated encephalomyelitis in children. Pediatrics *110*(2 Pt. 1):e21, 2002.
41. Nossal, G. J. V.: A purgative mastery. Nature *412*:685-686, 2001.
42. Pitt, D., Werner, P., and Raine, C. S.: Glutamate excitotoxity in a model of multiple sclerosis. Nat. Med. *6*:67-70, 2000.
43. Rivers, T. M., McNair-Scott, T. F.: Meningitis in man caused by a filterable virus. Science *31*:439-440, 1935.
44. Sejvar, J. J., et al.: Neurologic adverse events associated with smallpox vaccination in the United States, 2002-2004. J. A. M. A. *294*:2744-2750, 2005.
45. Shahar, E., et al.: Outcome of severe encephalomyelitis in children: Effect of high-dose methylprednisolone and immunoglobulins. J. Child Neurol. *17*:810-814, 2002.
46. Sospedra, M., and Martin, R.: Immunology of multiple sclerosis. Annu. Rev. Immunol. *23*:683-747, 2005.
47. Tenembaum, S., Chamoles, N., and Fejerman, N.: Acute disseminated encephalomyelitis: A long-term follow-up study of 84 pediatric patients. Neurology *59*:1224-1231, 2002.
48. Whitaker, J. N., et al.: An immunochemical comparison of human myelin basic protein and its modified, citrullinated form, C8. J. Neuroimmunol. *36*(2-3):135-146, 1992.
49. Wilejto, M., et al.: The clinical features, MRI findings, and outcome of optic neuritis in children. Neurology *67*:258-262, 2006.
50. Wingerchuk, D. M., et al.: Revised diagnostic criteria for neuromyelitis optica. Neurology *66*:1485-1489, 2006.

CHAPTER **43b**

INFECTION-ASSOCIATED MYELITIS AND MYELOPATHIES OF THE SPINAL CORD

Mark P. Gorman ● Scott L. Pomeroy

ACUTE TRANSVERSE MYELITIS

The rapid onset of paraplegia and bowel and bladder dysfunction that characterizes acute transverse myelitis (ATM) terrifies affected children and their families. Successful management requires prompt diagnosis and treatment. Because of the association of ATM with numerous infections, specialists in infectious diseases frequently participate in the care of children with ATM. The clinical presentation, radiologic features, differential diagnosis, pathophysiology, treatment, and prognosis of pediatric ATM are reviewed here.

TERMINOLOGY

ATM is a clinical syndrome consisting of progressive symptoms and signs reflecting bilateral sensory, motor, or autonomic dysfunction attributable to the spinal cord. This constellation of symptoms and signs can be caused by a heterogeneous group of disorders, including ATM. Several disorders, including direct infections of the spinal cord, can mimic ATM.

ATM can be associated with more widespread central nervous system (CNS) demyelinating disorders or systemic autoimmune disorders; in such cases, the term *disease-associated transverse myelitis* has been used. Isolated ATM can be triggered by identifiable preceding infections. Alternatively, ATM can be associated with a nonspecific preceding infection or have no apparent cause; for both of these subgroups, the term *idiopathic ATM* has been used. This last group constitutes the most common category in pediatric ATM. Although the precise pathophysiology of idiopathic ATM is uncertain, the frequent association with preceding infections and vaccinations and accumulating immunologic data suggest an inflammatory cause for the disorder.[12,18,37,56]

CLINICAL PRESENTATION

Idiopathic ATM affects approximately 1.34 persons per 1 million.[12] Six published case series ranging in size from 9 to 50 patients report common symptoms in pediatric patients with ATM. Patients present at a mean age of 8 years, with a slight female predominance.[18,19,25,39,57,59] Patients universally report acute to subacute, bilateral leg weakness, which is symmetric in approximately 67 percent of patients.[18] Involvement of the arms occurs in approximately 40 percent of patients. Approximately 90 percent of patients complain of bowel and bladder dysfunction, ranging from urinary retention and constipation to incontinence. A similar percentage of patients report sensory symptoms, including paresthesias and numbness. Back pain and fever affect nearly 50 percent of patients and may prompt consideration of primary infectious etiologies, such as an epidural abscess. The symptoms of ATM develop rapidly. In one study, the constellation of weakness, sensory changes, bowel and bladder dysfunction, and back pain reached a peak at an average of 5 days (range, 1 to 14 days).[18]

The general examination, although usually unremarkable, may reveal signs suggestive of an underlying systemic infection or autoimmune disorder. Abdominal examination may reveal a distended bladder. A diffuse or dermatomal vesicular rash or its sequelae suggest concurrent or preceding chickenpox or shingles.

On the neurologic examination, the presence of any mental status changes suggests that the myelitis is a component of a more diffuse process (i.e., acute disseminated encephalomyelitis). In the acute stages, muscle tone is flaccid in affected limbs. Detailed muscle strength testing with objective grading serves as a crucial baseline to compare with serial examinations to determine whether the patient is improving. All sensory modalities should be assessed carefully. In one series, preferential involvement of pain and temperature sensation with sparing of vibration sense and proprioception led the authors to speculate that thrombosis of the anterior spinal artery led to most cases of ATM (Fig. 43–2).[59] This series was limited, however, by its retrospective nature and lack of available neuroimaging. In addition, most patients in subsequent series have had involvement of all sensory modalities.[18,25,39,57] A spinal cord sensory level usually is located in the thoracic region (80%) and less commonly in the cervical (10%) or lumbar (10%) area.[12] In the acute phase, deep tendon reflexes are depressed in approximately 70 percent of patients and later become hyperactive. Similarly, Babinski responses may be negative early in the acute phase but soon become positive, indicating upper motor neuron dysfunction.

RADIOLOGIC FEATURES

Every patient with suspected ATM should undergo emergent gadolinium-enhanced magnetic resonance imaging (MRI) of the entire spine to confirm the diagnosis and rule out alternative diagnoses, particularly compressive lesions, such as epidural abscess, epidural hematoma, and extramedullary tumors. T1-

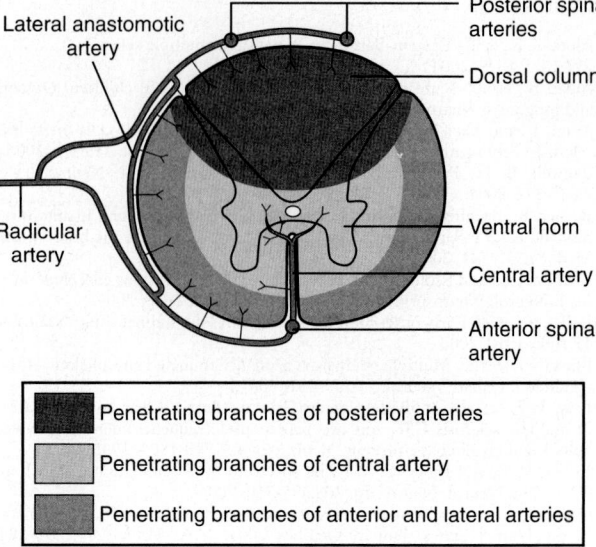

Figure 43–2   The ventral horns, which contain the lower motor neurons, and the lateral spinothalamic tract, which carries pain and temperature sensation, are supplied by the anterior spinal artery. The dorsal columns, which mediate vibration and joint position sense, are supplied by the posterior spinal arteries.

weighted and T2-weighted sagittal imaging of the entire spine can serve as an initial screen, followed by axial imaging in areas of suspected pathology.[3]

Spinal MRI in ATM typically reveals T1-isointense and T2-hyperintense signals over several contiguous spinal cord segments[18] and may involve the entire spine (Fig. 43–3).[3] This "longitudinally extensive" subtype (extending over three or more vertebral segments) seems to occur more commonly in children than in adults.[3,63] The hyperintense signal can extend into the lower brain stem.[3] Spinal cord swelling with effacement of the surrounding cerebrospinal fluid (CSF) spaces may be present in severe cases (Fig. 43–4). Axial imaging can determine whether gray or white matter or both are affected. Contrast enhancement is variably present and may appear diffuse, patchy, or nodular. In some patients with very suggestive clinical features, initial spine MRI may be normal and should be repeated several days later.[18,39,57] In rare cases, the MRI remains normal but does not rule out the diagnosis.

LUMBAR PUNCTURE

Approximately 50 percent of pediatric patients with ATM have CSF pleocytosis, typically with a lymphocytic predominance. Elevated CSF protein levels, either in isolation or in conjunction with pleocytosis, also are detected in approximately 50 percent of patients. Glucose typically is normal. A normal CSF profile does not rule out ATM because this pattern is seen in approximately 25 percent of patients. CSF cytology should be sent on all patients to assess for the possibility of neoplasm. Additional CSF testing is discussed further subsequently.

DIFFERENTIAL DIAGNOSIS

CONDITIONS THAT MIMIC ACUTE TRANSVERSE MYELITIS

Numerous disorders can affect the spinal cord and produce identical symptoms and signs that mimic idiopathic ATM (Table 43–4). Such conditions must be ruled out through a combination

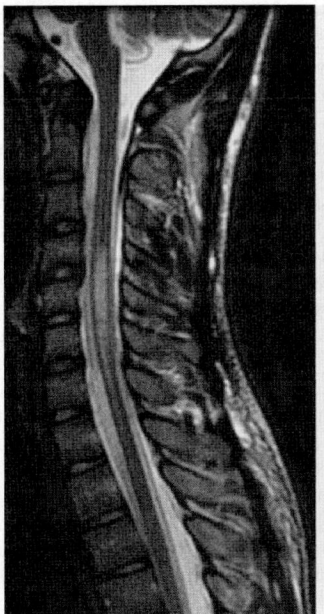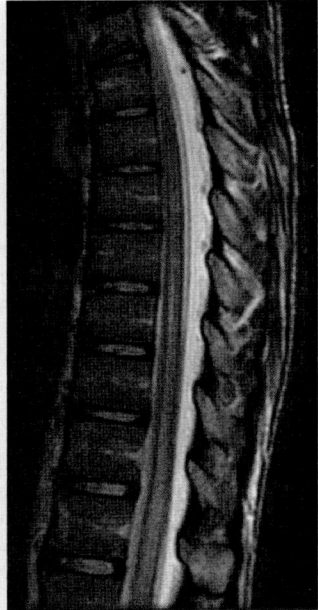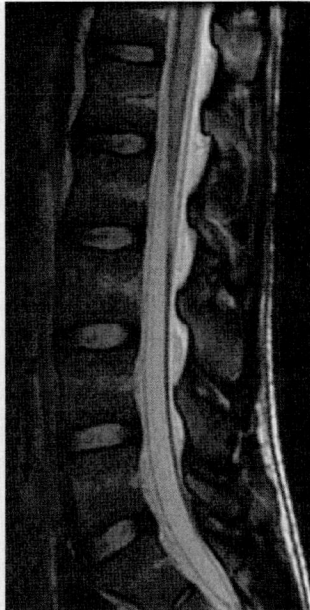

Figure 43-3 Sagittal T2-weighted MR image of the spine of a 16-year-old boy who presented with bilateral leg paresthesias that progressed to paraplegia and urinary and bowel retention. MRI shows diffuse T2-hyperintense signal extending from C4 through the thoracic region to the conus medullaris. The boy's symptoms resolved with administration of high-dose steroids.

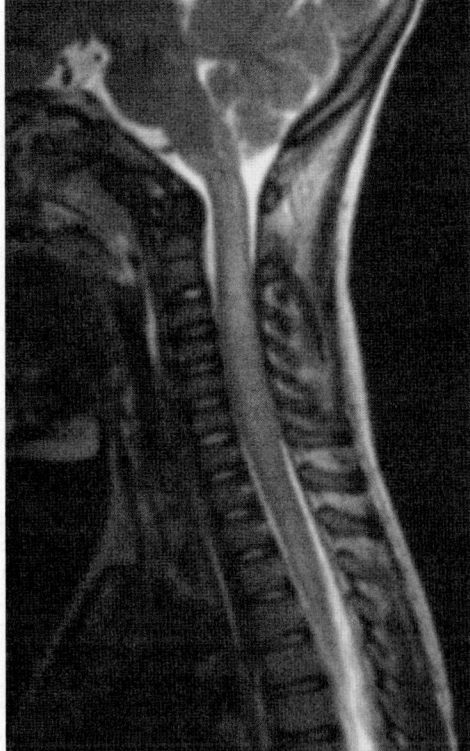

Figure 43-4 Sagittal T2-weighted MR image of a 7-year-old boy with transverse myelitis in the setting of acute disseminated encephalomyelitis. There is T2-hyperintense signal in the cervical cord with associated swelling and effacement of the cerebrospinal fluid spaces. The abnormal signal also extends into the lower brain stem.

of history, physical examination, neuroimaging, and laboratory evaluation.

Extramedullary compressive lesions are neurosurgical emergencies that must be diagnosed rapidly for effective treatment. Spinal epidural abscesses are rare in children. In one series of

TABLE 43-4   Conditions That Mimic Idiopathic Acute Transverse Myelitis

Direct infectious myelopathies
Extramedullary compressive lesions
Epidural abscess
Epidural hematoma
Extramedullary tumors
Guillain-Barré syndrome
Intramedullary spinal cord tumors
Astrocytomas
Ependymomas
Ischemia/infarction
Radiation injury
Traumatic spinal cord injury
Vascular malformations

eight children compiled over a 15-year period at a major children's hospital, seven had fever, and all eight had back pain.[8] *Staphylococcus aureus*, some of which were methicillin-resistant, were the most common isolates in this and other series. Spinal epidural hematomas also are rare occurrences in children. They can occur spontaneously or may be associated with anticoagulant use, clotting disorders, trauma, or lumbar puncture.[61] Spinal epidural hematomas usually are located in the lower cervical region and extend over two to three vertebral segments, much fewer than in ATM. In one series of 1147 children with cancer, 70 (6%) developed spinal cord compression at some point during their course.[64] The most common responsible tumor types were primitive neuroectodermal tumor, soft tissue sarcoma, and neuroblastoma. When spinal cord compression is the initial manifestation of cancer, as was the case for 67 percent of the patients in this series, it can mimic ATM. Spinal MRI readily distinguishes each of these disorders from ATM.

The initial clinical presentation of ATM can be quite similar to that of Guillain-Barré syndrome. Both disorders can manifest with back pain, paraparesis, and sensory abnormalities. Although typically absent in both disorders, the presence of deep tendon reflexes would point strongly toward ATM. When deep tendon reflexes are absent, the presence of a spinal cord sensory level and bowel and bladder involvement suggests ATM. Some patients have albuminocytologic dissociation, which is indistinguishable from Guillain-Barré syndrome. In some cases, ATM and Guillain-Barré syndrome can be distinguished only with MRI. Spinal cord, nerve root, and peripheral nerve pathology can coexist in myeloradiculoneuritis, suggesting that ATM and Guillain-Barré syndrome may share a common pathophysiologic mechanism in some cases.[48]

The most common intramedullary spinal cord tumors in children are astrocytomas (60%), followed by ependymomas (30%).[7,22,35] Although biopsy of the tumors is necessary to establish the exact histologic diagnosis, biopsy of the spinal cord rarely is needed to distinguish tumor from ATM. Despite similarities in presenting symptoms, clinical features can help to distinguish intramedullary tumors from ATM. Intramedullary spinal cord tumors manifest more subacutely or chronically than does ATM, reflecting their low cellular growth rate.[35] In one study, the mean duration of symptoms before presentation of children with intramedullary spinal cord tumors was 254 days.[22] In ATM, the symptoms peak much earlier from onset, with a mean duration of 5 days in one study.[18] On examination, the presence of scoliosis or torticollis suggests the presence of longer standing tumors rather than ATM.[22]

ATM and spinal cord tumors typically are isointense on T1-weighted MR images and hyperintense on T2-weighted images. Although intramedullary tumors display swelling, contrast enhancement, and associated syrinxes more frequently than does ATM, these features also can be seen in the latter (Fig. 43–5; see Fig. 43–4). Other radiographic features may be used to distinguish the two entities. The eccentric location of astrocytomas within the spinal cord[7] can be used to differentiate them from ATM, which usually produces symmetric findings. Although ependymomas can produce symmetric spinal cord expansion because of their origin from the central canal, these tumors usually span three to four vertebral segments,[7] whereas pediatric ATM typically involves longer areas of the spinal cord. In addition, an area of low signal intensity reflecting hemosiderin deposits from chronic hemorrhage at the edge of ependymomas also can serve as a radiographic clue.[7] Because patients with intramedullary spinal cord tumors may be diagnosed on the basis of CSF cytology, this test should be sent on all patients with suspected ATM.

Clinical features and neuroimaging also can be used to distinguish ATM from spinal cord infarction, which is an exceedingly rare finding in children. The latter diagnosis typically manifests in a hyperacute fashion with dissociated sensory loss (absent temperature and pain sensation with preserved vibration and proprioception) from thrombosis of the anterior spinal artery (see Fig. 43–2). Accompanying MRI signal abnormality in the adjacent vertebral body is highly suggestive of the diagnosis.[60] Diffusion-weighted MRI also may reveal the presence of ischemia and aid in making the differential diagnosis.

The clinical presentation of spinal cord dysfunction in the setting of prior irradiation suggests radiation-induced transverse myelitis as the most likely diagnosis. This entity typically manifests 9 to 18 months after radiotherapy, but it can occur earlier in children.[76]

Although they typically cause slowly progressive symptoms, spinal arteriovenous malformations can manifest acutely as a result of hemorrhage or venous congestion.[71] These lesions usually can be detected as abnormal, dilated vasculature on MRI of the spine; subsequent spinal angiography can confirm the diagnosis.

DISEASE-ASSOCIATED ACUTE TRANSVERSE MYELITIS

ATM with a presumed inflammatory basis can be associated with recurrent CNS demyelinating disorders and systemic autoimmune disorders. In these cases, the term *disease-associated ATM* can be applied (Table 43–5).[5,20]

The presence of changes in mental status and MRI abnormalities of cerebral white matter points toward acute disseminated encephalomyelitis as the correct diagnosis (Fig. 43–6). Spinal cord demyelination in multiple sclerosis tends to be limited to fewer than two vertebral segments and partial in the transverse plane, resulting in mild, asymmetric symptoms compared with the typically severe, symmetric symptoms in ATM.[67] In addition, the recurrence of lesions over the course of time and in different parts of the CNS is required for establishing the diagnosis of

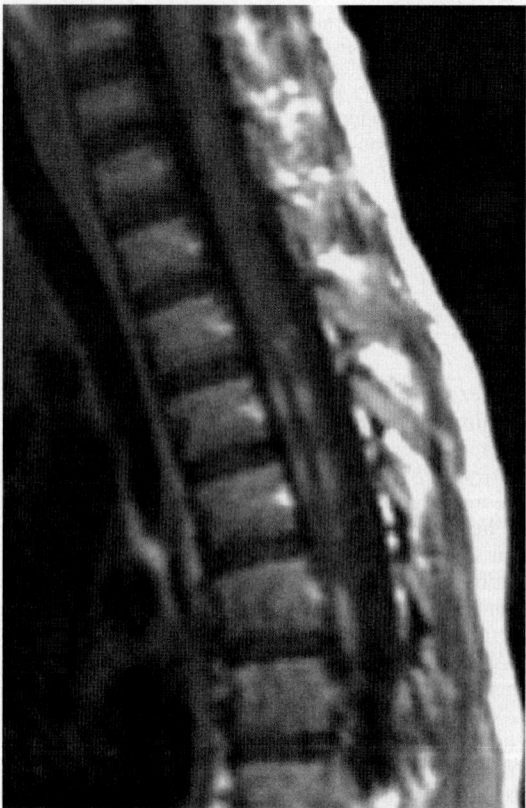

Figure 43–5 Sagittal post-gadolinium T1-weighted MR image of the thoracic spinal cord of a 9-year-old girl who presented with bilateral leg weakness and urinary retention, showing patchy enhancement and a small syrinx. Although these findings raised concern for an intramedullary tumor, her spontaneous improvement and the resolution of enhancement without treatment favored a diagnosis of transverse myelitis.

TABLE 43–5 Central Nervous System and Systemic Autoimmune Disorders Associated with Acute Transverse Myelitis

Central Nervous System Disorders
Acute disseminated encephalomyelitis
Multiple sclerosis
Neuromyelitis optica

Systemic Autoimmune Disorders
Antiphospholipid antibody syndrome
Behçet disease
Mixed connective tissue disorder
Neurosarcoidosis
Sjögren syndrome
Systemic lupus erythematosus

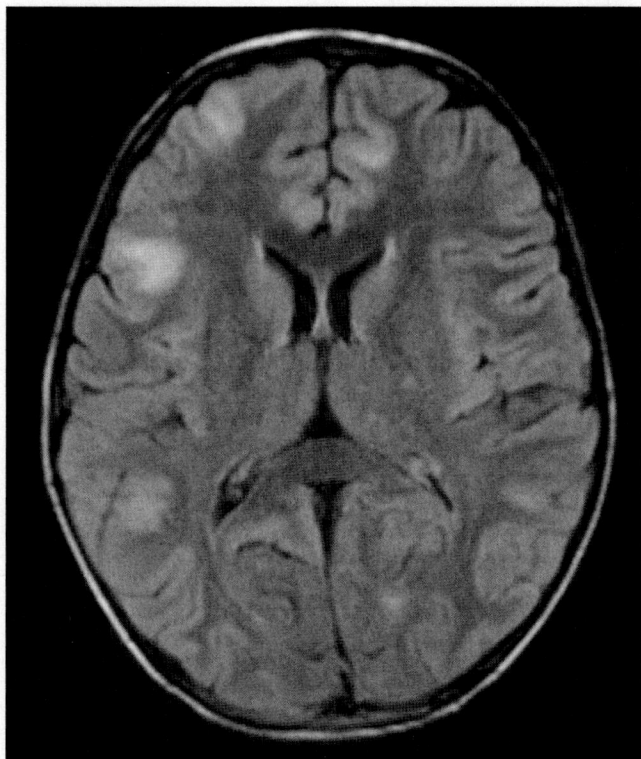

Figure 43–6 Fluid-attenuated inversion recovery (FLAIR) sequence of a brain MR image of the same patient from Figure 43–3, showing multifocal areas of hyperintense signal in the subcortical white matter consistent with acute disseminated encephalomyelitis.

TABLE 43–6   Distinguishing Acute Transverse Myelitis from Other Central Nervous System Demyelinating Disorders

Finding	ATM	ADEM	MS	NMO
Myelitis	+	+/–	+/– (partial)	+
Acute mental status changes	–	+	–	–
Optic neuritis	–	+/–	+/–	+
Abnormal brain MRI	–	+	+	+/–
CSF oligoclonal bands	–	+/–	+	–
Serum NMO-IgG	–	–	–	+/–
Recurrences	+/–	+/–	+	+

+, *always present;* +/–, *variably present;* –, *usually absent.*
ADEM, *acute disseminated encephalomyelitis;* ATM, *acute transverse myelitis;* CSF, *cerebrospinal fluid;* MRI, *magnetic resonance imaging;* MS, *multiple sclerosis;* NMO, *neuromyelitis optica.*

TABLE 43–7   Suggested Diagnostic Work-up for Recurrent Central Nervous System Demyelinating Disorders and Systemic Autoimmune Disorders Associated with Acute Transverse Myelitis

All Patients	Suggestive of Neuromyelitis Optica	Also Consider
Brain MRI with gadolinium	Ophthalmology consultation	Angiotensin-converting enzyme (serum, CSF)
CSF oligoclonal bands	Visual evoked potentials	Other autoantibodies
Antinuclear antibodies	Formal visual field testing	Anti-dsDNA
Antiphospholipid antibodies	Serum NMO-IgG	Anti-La
		Anti-Ro Anti-Smith

CSF, cerebrospinal fluid; MRI, magnetic resonance imaging; NMO, neuromyelitis optica.

multiple sclerosis. Previous subtle visual or sensory symptoms suggestive of a recurrent demyelinating disorder may be elicited only with detailed questioning. Oligoclonal bands are present more commonly in multiple sclerosis-related myelitis,[67] but they also have been reported in idiopathic ATM (Table 43–6).[57]

ATM is a necessary feature of neuromyelitis optica (NMO), a severe, relapsing demyelinating disorder restricted mainly to the spinal cord and optic nerves. Specific diagnostic criteria for NMO have been developed.[80] Concurrent or preceding optic neuritis suggests NMO as the correct diagnosis. NMO may manifest initially as ATM, with a future episode of optic neuritis leading to the reclassification of ATM as NMO. Some patients also can have recurrent episodes of idiopathic ATM without optic neuritis; in the literature, such patients have been considered to have a "restricted" or "limited" form of NMO.[63]

A novel biomarker (NMO-IgG) targeting the predominant CNS water channel protein aquaporin-4, which is concentrated in astrocytic foot processes in the blood-brain barrier, has been detected in 73 percent of adult patients with NMO and 52 percent of adult patients with recurrent longitudinally extensive ATM.[44,45] This antibody also has been detected in several pediatric patients with NMO.[52]

ATM also can occur secondary to a variety of systemic autoimmune disorders. Involvement of other organ systems, particularly the skin, lungs, kidneys, and joints, may point to a particular diagnosis, including systemic lupus erythematosus, sarcoidosis, and Sjögren syndrome. A personal or family history of recurrent miscarriages or hypercoagulability is suggestive of antiphospholipid antibody syndrome.

The long list of demyelinating and rheumatologic disorders potentially associated with ATM precludes diagnostic testing for every possible disorder. Table 43–7 presents a schema to guide which tests should be obtained in patients with ATM.

IDIOPATHIC ACUTE TRANSVERSE MYELITIS

Because of the numerous conditions that mimic or are associated with idiopathic ATM, establishing the diagnosis requires a systematic approach. Although all case series have emphasized the presence of bilateral lower extremity motor dysfunction and loss of voluntary bowel/bladder control, definitions of ATM have varied in the literature regarding the duration of symptoms and the necessary diagnostic testing.[18,39] To address this nonuniformity, the criteria proposed by the Transverse Myelitis Consortium Working Group[5] should be used to secure the diagnosis and guide the differential diagnosis and work-up (Table 43–8).

ROLE OF INFECTIONS IN TRANSVERSE MYELITIS

Infectious agents can cause spinal cord dysfunction by directly infecting the spinal cord parenchyma (infectious myelopathy) or by triggering postinfectious, immune-mediated processes (postinfectious ATM). In some cases, such as human T-cell lymphotrophic virus (HTLV)–associated myelitis, damage to the spinal cord may be produced by direct infection and by the immune response to the agent. Several agents, including cytomegalovirus (CMV) and varicella-zoster virus (VZV), are associated with direct CNS infection in certain patients (many of whom are

TABLE 43-8   Transverse Myelitis Consortium Working Group Diagnostic Criteria

Inclusion Criteria	Exclusion Criteria
Development of sensory, motor, or autonomic dysfunction attributable to spinal cord	History of previous radiation to spine within last 10 yr
	Clear arterial distribution clinical deficit consistent with thrombosis of anterior spinal artery
Bilateral signs/symptoms (not necessarily symmetric)	
Clearly defined sensory level	Abnormal flow voids on surface of the spinal cord consistent with AVM
	Serologic or clinical evidence of connective tissue disease (sarcoidosis, Behçet disease, Sjögren syndrome, SLE, mixed connective tissue disorder)*
Exclusion of extra-axial compressive etiology by neuroimaging (MRI or myelography; CT of spine inadequate)	
Inflammation within spinal cord shown by CSF pleocytosis or elevated IgG index or gadolinium enhancement. If no inflammatory criteria are met at symptom onset, repeat MRI and lumbar puncture evaluation 2-7 days after symptom onset meet criteria	CNS manifestations of syphilis, Lyme disease, HIV, HTLV-1, *Mycoplasma*, other viral infection (e.g., HSV-1, HSV-2, VZV, EBV, CMV, HHV-6, enteroviruses)*
	Brain MRI abnormalities suggestive of MS*
	History of clinically apparent optic neuritis*
Progression to nadir 4 hr to 21 days after onset of symptoms (if patient awakens with symptoms, symptoms must become more pronounced from point of awakening)	

Do not exclude disease-associated acute transverse myelitis.
AVM, arteriovenous malformation; CMV, cytomegalovirus; CNS, central nervous system; CSF, cerebrospinal fluid; CT, computed tomography; EBV, Epstein-Barr virus; HIV, human immunodeficiency virus; HHV-6, human herpesvirus-6; HSV, herpes simplex virus; HTLV-1, human T-cell lymphotrophic virus-1; MRI, magnetic resonance imaging; MS, multiple sclerosis; SLE, systemic lupus erythematosus; VZV, varicella-zoster virus.
Data from Transverse Myelitis Working Group: Proposed diagnostic criteria and nosology of acute myelitis. Neurology 59:499-505, 2002.

immunocompromised) and postinfectious ATM in others. When a specific agent is identified as a trigger of ATM, it should be indicated in the diagnostic terminology (i.e., post-varicella ATM).

Within the postinfectious category of ATM, the preceding infection usually is a nonspecific upper respiratory tract infection without an identifiable, specific microbe.[12,18,59] Approximately 50 percent of patients report having had such an infection with an intervening symptom-free interval of 5 to 10 days.[12,18,59] In instances in which the specific microbe is not identified and in cases in which no associated infection, systemic disorder, or recurrent demyelinating disorder is identified, the term *idiopathic ATM* has been applied.

Clues in the history can suggest the involvement of specific microbes. Immune status should be determined because immunocompromised patients are more susceptible to particular agents, such as CMV.[27] A history of exposure to cats or parakeets may point to *Bartonella henselae* (cats)[66] or *Chlamydia psittaci* (parakeets)[79] as rare causes of ATM. A detailed travel history may lead to the consideration of agents not typically encountered in the patient's primary residence, such as *Schistosoma*.[4]

Vaccination status also should be determined. Some cases of ATM seem to be related to recent vaccination, although causality usually is difficult to prove, given the paucity of reported cases.[18,26,38,57,81] Alternatively, unimmunized children are susceptible to particular agents, such as measles, mumps, and rubella, which have been associated with ATM.[24]

INFECTIOUS MYELOPATHIES

The etiology of an infectious myelopathy usually is established by positive CSF culture or polymerase chain reaction (PCR) results. Biopsy or autopsy results also have provided evidence of direct CNS infection in some patients. Some authors consider elevated CSF titers without positive culture or PCR results to be sufficient evidence of direct CNS infection, but this issue has not been resolved. Viruses constitute the most frequently reported category of infectious myelopathies, with bacteria and parasitic causes being less frequent (Table 43-9).

TABLE 43-9   Partial Listing of Microbes That Cause Infectious Myelopathies

Cytomegalovirus[49]
Epstein-Barr virus[48]
Echinococcus granulosus[11]
Enteroviruses[11]
    Coxsackieviruses
    Echoviruses[77]
    Enterovirus 71[53]
    Polioviruses (vaccine associated and wild-type)
Herpes simplex virus-1[54]
Herpes simplex virus-2[31]
Human immunodeficiency virus[10,62]
Human T-cell lymphotrophic virus-1 and -2[10]
Mycobacterium tuberculosis[13]
Mycoplasma pneumoniae[5]
Schistosoma haematobium and *Schistosoma mansoni*[4]
Taenia solium (neurocysticercosis)[11]
Treponema pallidum[13,29]
Varicella-zoster virus[29]
West Nile virus[65]

POSTINFECTIOUS ACUTE TRANSVERSE MYELITIS

In postinfectious cases, a specific etiology can be suggested by elevated acute or rising convalescent serum titers, isolation of the agent from systemic sources in the setting of a suggestive clinical picture, or both. In such cases, the presumptive pathophysiology entails an aberrant autoimmune response to the spinal cord via mechanisms such as molecular mimicry, rather than direct CNS invasion by the microbe. A variety of bacterial and viral pathogens and vaccinations have been associated with postinfectious ATM (Table 43-10). Microbes that have been reported to cause infectious and postinfectious myelitis are listed in both Tables 43-9 and 43-10.

TABLE 43–10 Partial Listing of Microbes and Vaccines Associated with Postinfectious or Postvaccinial Acute Transverse Myelitis

Bacteria/Spirochetes	Viruses	Vaccinations
Bartonella henselae[66]	Adenovirus[47]	Hepatitis B[73]
Borrelia burgdorferi[46]	Cytomegalovirus[27]	Influenza[26]
Brucellosis[40]	Coxsackieviruses[56]	Measles, mumps,
Chlamydia psittaci[79]	Enterovirus 71[33,53]	and rubella[81]
Mycoplasma	Epstein-Barr virus[33]	Poliovirus[38]
pneumoniae[74]	Hepatitis A[15,75]	Rabies[26]
	Hepatitis B[50]	Smallpox[26]
	Hepatitis C[32]	
	Herpes simplex virus-1[28]	
	Herpes simplex virus-2[31]	
	Human herpesvirus-6[34]	
	Mumps[58]	
	Rubella[24]	
	Varicella-zoster virus[51]	

TABLE 43–11 Suggested Diagnostic Work-up for Infections Associated with Acute Transverse Myelitis

Blood	Cerebrospinal Fluid	Other
Blood cultures	Bacterial culture	Viral culture of stool
Acute and	Viral culture	and respiratory
convalescent titers	PCR testing for	secretions
to	CMV	Consider stool ova
Borrelia burgdorferi	EBV	and parasite testing
EBV	Enterovirus	and serum titers if
Mycoplasma	HSV	parasitic infection is
pneumoniae	M. pneumoniae	suspected
	VZV	

CMV, cytomegalovirus; EBV, Epstein-Barr virus; HSV, herpes simplex virus; PCR, polymerase chain reaction; VZV, varicella-zoster virus.

TABLE 43–12 Additional Diagnostic Work-up for Infections Associated with Acute Transverse Myelitis

Blood	Cerebrospinal Fluid	Other
Bartonella titers	Cryptococcal antigen	PPD placement
HIV antibody	HTLV antibody	Stool ova and parasite
HTLV-1 antibody	Fungal culture	testing
Parasitic infection	VDRL	
titers		
RPR		

HIV, human immunodeficiency virus; HTLV, human T-cell lymphotrophic virus; PPD, purified protein derivative; RPR, rapid plasma reagin; VDRL, Venereal Disease Research Laboratory.

The long list of potential pathogens precludes performing diagnostic testing for every possible agent. The work-up instead should focus on the pathogens that are common, treatable, or suggested by particular clues in the history or examination. Table 43–11 lists the infectious disease tests that should be sent for every patient with ATM. Additional infectious disease tests that should be considered depending on the clinical scenario and immune status are listed in Table 43–12. Although a detailed description of every infectious cause of transverse myelitis is beyond the scope of this discussion, several examples of the most commonly reported entities in the literature that highlight general features of the infectious disease aspects of ATM are described subsequently.

CYTOMEGALOVIRUS

Although reported more frequently in immunocompromised patients, CMV myelitis also may affect immunocompetent individuals.[27,75] CMV can infect the spinal cord directly and can produce secondary vasculitis in immunocompromised patients. In such cases, CSF PCR testing frequently is positive.[27] In other cases of reported CMV-associated myelitis, evidence for concurrent or recent infection has included isolation of the virus from blood or urine, detection of anti-CMV IgM in the serum, or significant increases in convalescent CMV serum titers in the absence of viral detection by CSF viral cultures or PCR.[27,75] The inflammatory process in CMV myelitis extends into the brain stem or nerve roots in some cases.[75] Treatment with ganciclovir or foscarnet should be considered.[11] The combined treatment of CMV-associated myelitis with ganciclovir and methylprednisolone was associated with marked recovery in an immunocompetent adult.[27] As illustrated by CMV, myelitis associated with viral infections may be produced by direct infection, accompanying secondary processes such as vasculitis, or postinfectious immune-mediated mechanisms. Whether optimal treatment requires antiviral agents or immunomodulation or both is uncertain.

HUMAN IMMUNODEFICIENCY VIRUS-ASSOCIATED MYELOPATHY

Infections such as HTLV, herpes simplex virus, syphilis, tuberculosis, and VZV can cause myelopathies in patients with acquired immunodeficiency syndrome (AIDS) and seem to be particularly important in developing countries.[13] In addition, human immunodeficiency virus (HIV) itself has been linked to a particular form of myelopathy termed *vacuolar myelopathy*, which is the most common cause of paraparesis in adults with HIV infection in developed countries.[62] Typically occurring in the setting of advanced disease, vacuolar myelopathy has been detected in pathologic series in 22 percent of patients with AIDS.[62] Myelopathy also can occur acutely in conjunction with seroconversion, but this form is less common than vacuolar myelopathy.[11]

In vacuolar myelopathy, spinal cord pathology reveals noninflammatory myelin loss and spongy degeneration affecting mainly the lateral and posterior columns and producing vacuolization of the white matter, which provides the disorder its name.[62] HIV can be cultured from affected spinal cords, but the exact role of the virus in causing the disorder is unclear. The description of similar vacuolar myelopathies in patients with cancer or other immunocompromising conditions without HIV infection has cast some doubt on the central role of HIV in the disorder. Nutritional or metabolic factors in the vitamin B_{12} pathway may play a central or contributing role.[11]

The clinical presentation is similar to the presentation of other causes of chronic progressive myelopathy, and HIV-associated myelopathy may be underrecognized.[11,23] The diagnosis relies on determining a patient's HIV status and ruling out other bacterial, viral, fungal, and parasitic causes of myelopathy. No specific, effective treatments are available for vacuolar myelopathy.

Children with AIDS encephalopathy frequently develop upper motor neuron symptoms and signs, with resultant delay or regression in motor development.[23] In one series of 15 children with AIDS, only one patient had evidence of vacuolar myelopathy.[23] The most common finding in this series was demyelination with or without axonal loss in the lateral corticospinal tracts in the spinal cord. The pathologic expression of HIV-associated spinal cord damage seems to be age-dependent.

As illustrated by HIV myelopathy, the existence of co-infections or accompanying systemic illnesses or both may confound the association of particular infectious agents with myelitis. Distinguishing these different causes clinically may be impossible, or they all may contribute to the disorder in some cases; treatment directed at multiple possible mechanisms may be warranted.

MYELOPATHY ASSOCIATED WITH HUMAN T-CELL LYMPHOTROPHIC VIRUS-1 AND HUMAN T-CELL LYMPHOTROPHIC VIRUS-2

The retrovirus HTLV-1 can cause a chronic, progressive myelopathy in immunocompromised and immunocompetent patients. Although reported less frequently, HTLV-2 infection can produce an identical clinical picture.[6] Risk factors for the acquisition of HTLV-1 and HTLV-2 include blood transfusions, intravenous drug use, and multiple sexual partners.[10] HTLV also can be transmitted from mother to infant, usually via breast-feeding. HTLV-1 is endemic to regions closer to the equator, including the Caribbean and southeastern United States.[70] Although the average age of onset is approximately 40 years,[16] rare pediatric cases have been reported.

Approximately 1 of 250 patients with HTLV-1 infection develops myelopathy.[11] Differences in the immune response to HTLV-1 seem to play a role in determining whether an infected individual develops myelopathy. Patients who also are infected with HIV seem to be at higher risk for the development of HTLV-associated myelopathy compared with other patient groups.[10]

The presence of serum and CSF antibodies to HTLV-1/HTLV-2 and of CSF HTLV-1/HTLV-2 DNA (detected by PCR) confirms the diagnosis. Immunomodulation, particularly corticosteroids, may be transiently beneficial early in the course of the disorder, but the progressive nature of the disorder nonetheless ensues.[10,11]

Pathologic specimens of HTLV-associated myelopathy reveal demyelination and degeneration of the long tracts with perivascular T-cell–predominant infiltrates and gliosis.[11] HTLV-infected CD4[+] and CD8[+] lymphocytes can be detected in the blood, CSF, and white matter of patients with HTLV-associated myelopathy.[9] Although the pathophysiology is uncertain, the evolution of an initially beneficial immune response into a self-destructive autoimmune process has been emphasized in the literature.[9] Possible mechanisms include cytotoxic T-lymphocyte–mediated killing of infected cells, bystander damage from enhanced cytokine production, and cross-reacting autoantibodies directed against CNS autoantigens via molecular mimicry. The example of HTLV-associated myelitis reveals that the boundaries between infectious and postinfectious myelitis may be unclear.

MYCOPLASMA PNEUMONIAE

Antimyelin antibodies reactive against glycolipid components have been detected in patients with *Mycoplasma*-associated inflammatory nervous system disorders, including one patient with ATM.[17,42,74] Such antibodies may be induced via molecular mimicry because of similarities in the glycolipid components of myelin and *Mycoplasma pneumoniae*.[42] Although the specificity of *M. pneumoniae* serologic testing has been questioned,[14] *Mycoplasma*-associated ATM seems to be a true entity based on the available literature, which includes cases of infectious myelopathy with positive CSF *Mycoplasma* PCR results and postinfectious cases.[1,74]

VARICELLA-ZOSTER VIRUS

After producing chickenpox, VZV survives in a latent form in cranial nerve and dorsal root ganglia, particularly in the trigeminal and thoracic regions.[30] Reactivation of the virus increases with immunosuppression and advancing age. Myelitis can occur in immunocompetent patients, often 1 to 2 weeks after the rash of varicella or zoster occurs, but it also can occur without a preceding rash.[30] In such cases, VZV DNA or antibodies can be detected in the CSF, but the virus cannot be cultured. In immunocompromised patients, invasion of the spinal cord by VZV has been described. Treatment with acyclovir or corticosteroids or both in combination may be effective.[21,29]

ROLE OF THE IMMUNE SYSTEM IN IDIOPATHIC ACUTE TRANSVERSE MYELITIS

In cases of idiopathic ATM, infections seem to provoke spinal cord dysfunction via secondary, immune-mediated mechanisms, rather than via CNS invasion. In such cases, a specific triggering agent usually is not identified. Increased peripheral blood lymphocyte responses to myelin basic protein have been shown in the research setting in patients with ATM, three of whom had a preceding viral illness.[2] The patients in this study who did not show increased lymphocyte responses were receiving steroids; reduction of autoimmune cell–mediated responses to CNS myelin antigens may underlie the beneficial effect of these medications in ATM (discussed further subsequently). None of the six patients who were tested in the recovery stage showed significant responses to myelin basic protein, suggesting that the cellular autoimmune reaction is short-lived.

In addition, the production of interleukin-6 by astrocytes seems to lead to nitric oxide–induced injury to spinal cord oligodendrocytes and axons in patients with idiopathic ATM. Interleukin-6 levels are markedly elevated in the CSF of patients with ATM and correlate with long-term disability.[37] The efficacy of corticosteroids in ATM may be due partially to their reduction of interleukin-6 production.[68]

TREATMENT

All patients with ATM should be hospitalized for further monitoring and treatment. Most patients can receive care on the regular ward, although the approximately 5 percent of patients with respiratory involvement from cervical myelitis require intensive care monitoring and may need endotracheal tube placement and mechanical ventilation.

No randomized, controlled treatment trials in ATM have been done. Based on case reports and series that have suggested a beneficial effect,[19,43,68] high-dose corticosteroids have become the standard of care in ATM. In one series of 12 children with severe ATM compared with a historical control group of 17 patients, the use of high-dose intravenous methylprednisolone (IVMP) significantly increased the proportion of children walking independently at 1 month (66% compared with 18%) and with full recovery at 1 year (55% compared with 12%).[19] Although a variety of agents and courses have been used, we use IVMP, 30 mg/kg per dose for 5 maximum 1 g. The need for a prednisone taper is controversial and may be based on whether full or partial recovery is achieved with the intravenous steroids. Most patients improve, often dramatically, with intravenous steroid treatment. Although some patients may improve spontaneously,[59] the collective data suggest that high-dose IVMP should be used in all patients with ATM. For the rare patient who does not improve with IVMP, intravenous immunoglobulins[69] or plasmapheresis can be used.

The use of antimicrobial agents in patients with ATM is controversial. Because most cases are caused by secondary, immune-mediated mechanisms, such treatment may not have significant benefit. Antimicrobial therapy is indicated, however, in cases with highly suspected or proven direct or associated infections, such as doxycycline for *Mycoplasma*,[74] ganciclovir for CMV,[27] and acyclovir for herpes simplex virus and VZV.[29] When antimicrobials are used, agents with good CSF penetration are preferred because direct invasion of the CNS may be present in some cases.

Additional treatment includes pain management, urinary bladder catheterization, bowel regimens, and peptic ulcer and deep venous thrombosis prophylaxis. The early institution of clean intermittent catheterization may improve long-term neurourologic outcomes in children with ATM.[72] Physical therapy should be instituted early to maximize the chance for recovery and continued in inpatient rehabilitation or an outpatient setting after the patient has been discharged from the acute care hospital.

Patients with ATM usually are fearful that they will not recover control of their legs or of their bowel or bladder, or that they will have a recurrence. Clinicians caring for patients with ATM must be attuned to their psychosocial needs. Psychiatric consultation may be necessary in some cases. Patients and their families may find the resources of the patient support group Transverse Myelitis Association (www.myelitis.org) helpful.

PROGNOSIS

DISABILITY

Although the variable definitions of recovery reported in the literature preclude a definitive assessment, the prognosis for pediatric patients with ATM generally is favorable and is better than their adult counterparts.[63] Paine and Byers'[59] degree of recovery categories have been the most widely reported outcome scale but are limited by vague terminology. Based on this scale, approximately 80 percent of pediatric patients who receive high-dose IVMP achieve full or good recovery, and 20 percent have a fair or poor outcome.[19,43] Among patients not treated with high-dose IVMP, 60 percent have a full or good recovery, whereas 40 percent have a fair or poor outcome.[59] In one series comprising 33 percent children and 67 percent adults who were not treated with steroids, approximately 33 percent each achieved good, fair, and poor recovery.[12] In a study of adult patients with ATM who were treated with high-dose IVMP and additional immunosuppressive agents if needed, approximately 67 percent were reported to have a good outcome, and 33 percent had a poor outcome. Comparisons with the aforementioned studies are difficult to make because a different outcome scale was used. Future studies in pediatric ATM may be improved by the use of the Extended Disability Status Scale, which has been used widely to assess outcomes in the adult and pediatric multiple sclerosis literature.[41]

During recovery, motor function returns first, with an average time to independent ambulation of 56 days in one study[18] and 25 days in a group of patients treated with high-dose IVMP.[19] Bowel and bladder control recovers more slowly, with an average time to recovery of normal urinary function of 7 months.[18] In one study, 86 percent of children with ATM showed evidence of bladder dysfunction on long-term follow-up.[72] Although these results likely were affected by selection bias for more severely affected patients, this study suggests that urodynamic studies should be considered in all patients after the acute phase has resolved. Based on these results, clean intermittent catheterization and anticholinergic medications may be required.[72]

Patients with hyperreflexia at presentation[57] and independent ambulation at 1 month[18] have a better prognosis. Complete paraplegia, time to maximal deficit of less than 24 hours, and younger age of onset are associated with a poor prognosis.[18,57] Levels of the intracellular neuronal 14-3-3 protein in the CSF of patients with ATM may reflect the extent of neuronal injury and correlate with outcome.[36,37]

RECURRENCES

In contrast to adult patients with idiopathic ATM, who have an approximately 25 percent likelihood of experiencing relapses,[20] most pediatric patients with idiopathic ATM do not have any recurrences. In a series of 24 pediatric patients with a mean follow-up of 7 years, there were no recurrences.[18] In another study of children with a variety of initial acute demyelinating events, only 2 of 29 patients with transverse myelitis had a later demyelinating event.[55,78] In this same study, the presence of myelitis for all patients with acute demyelinating disorders was negatively correlated with recurrence.

The detection of NMO-IgG is predictive of later recurrences and conversion to a diagnosis of NMO.[78] In adult patients with longitudinally extensive ATM, 56 percent of seropositive patients had relapses of either transverse myelitis or optic neuritis within 1 year; none of the seronegative patients had relapses.[78] Some researchers have suggested that NMO-IgG should be checked in all patients with longitudinally extensive ATM to predict more accurately the possibility of relapses.[63] In our anecdotal experience, NMO-IgG usually is not present in the serum of pediatric patients with ATM, even patients with a longitudinally extensive pattern. This finding suggests that NMO-IgG may not play a major role in idiopathic pediatric ATM and may partially explain the differential recurrence rates in pediatric and adult ATM.

REFERENCES

1. Abele-Horn, M., Franck, W., Busch, U., et al.: Transverse myelitis associated with *Mycoplasma pneumoniae* infection. Clin. Infect. Dis. *26*:909-912, 1998.
2. Abramsky, O., and Teitelbaum, D.: The autoimmune features of acute transverse myelopathy. Ann. Neurol. *2*:36-40, 1977.
3. Andronikou, S., Albuquerque-Jonathan, G., Wilmshurst, J., et al.: MRI findings in acute idiopathic transverse myelopathy in children. Pediatr. Radiol. *33*:624-629, 2003.
4. Anonymous: Acute schistosomiasis with transverse myelitis in American students returning from Kenya. M. M. W. R. Morb. Mortal. Wkly. Rep. *33*:445-447, 1984.
5. Anonymous: Proposed diagnostic criteria and nosology of acute transverse myelitis. Neurology *59*:499-505, 2002.
6. Araujo, A., and Hall, W. W.: Human T-lymphotropic virus type II and neurological disease. Ann. Neurol. *56*:10-19, 2004.
7. Auguste, K. I., and Gupta, N.: Pediatric intramedullary spinal cord tumors. Neurosurg. Clin. N. Am. *17*:51-61, 2006.
8. Auletta, J. J., and John, C. C.: Spinal epidural abscesses in children: A 15-year experience and review of the literature. Clin. Infect. Dis. *32*:9-16, 2001.
9. Barmak, K., Harhaj, E. W., and Wigdahl, B.: Mediators of central nervous system damage during the progression of human T-cell leukemia type I-associated myelopathy/tropical spastic paraparesis. J. Neurovirol. *9*:522-529, 2003.
10. Berger, J. R., Raffanti, S., Svenningsson, A., et al.: The role of HTLV in HIV-1 neurologic disease. Neurology *41*:197-202, 1991.
11. Berger, J. R., and Sabet, A.: Infectious myelopathies. Semin. Neurol. *22*:133-142, 2002.
12. Berman, M., Feldman, S., Alter, M., et al.: Acute transverse myelitis: Incidence and etiologic considerations. Neurology *31*:966-971, 1981.
13. Bhigjee, A. I., Madurai, S., Bill, P. L., et al.: Spectrum of myelopathies in HIV seropositive South African patients. Neurology *57*:348-351, 2001.
14. Bitnun, A., Ford-Jones, E., Blaser, S., et al.: *Mycoplasma pneumoniae* encephalitis. Semin. Pediatr. Infect. Dis. *14*:96-107, 2003.
15. Breningstall, G. N., and Belani, K. K.: Acute transverse myelitis and brainstem encephalitis associated with hepatitis A infection. Pediatr. Neurol. *12*:169-171, 1995.
16. Cabre, P., Smadja, D., Cabie, A., et al.: HTLV-1 and HIV infections of the central nervous system in tropical areas. J. Neurol. Neurosurg. Psychiatry *68*:550-557, 2000.

17. Cotter, F. E., Bainbridge, D., and Newland, A. C.: Neurological deficit associated with *Mycoplasma pneumoniae* reversed by plasma exchange. B. M. J. (Clin. Res. Ed.) *286*:22, 1983.

18. Defresne, P., Hollenberg, H., Husson, B., et al.: Acute transverse myelitis in children: Clinical course and prognostic factors. J. Child. Neurol. *18*:401-406, 2003.

19. Defresne, P., Meyer, L., Tardieu, M., et al.: Efficacy of high dose steroid therapy in children with severe acute transverse myelitis. J. Neurol. Neurosurg. Psychiatry *71*:272-274, 2001.

20. de Seze, J., Lanctin, C., Lebrun, C., et al.: Idiopathic acute transverse myelitis: Application of the recent diagnostic criteria. Neurology *65*:1950-1953, 2005.

21. de Silva, S. M., Mark, A. S., Gilden, D. H., et al.: Zoster myelitis: Improvement with antiviral therapy in two cases. Neurology *47*:929-931, 1996.

22. DeSousa, A. L., Kalsbeck, J. E., Mealey, J., Jr., et al.: Intraspinal tumors in children: A review of 81 cases. J. Neurosurg. *51*:437-445, 1979.

23. Dickson, D. W., Belman, A. L., Kim, T. S., et al.: Spinal cord pathology in pediatric acquired immunodeficiency syndrome. Neurology *39*:227-235, 1989.

24. Dubnov, G., and Constantini, N. W.: Rapid recovery from acute transverse myelitis in an elite female swimmer. Br. J. Sports Med. *40*:e8; discussion e8, 2006.

25. Dunne, K., Hopkins, I. J., and Shield, L. K.: Acute transverse myelopathy in childhood. Dev. Med. Child Neurol. *28*:198-204, 1986.

26. Fenichel, G. M.: Neurological complications of immunization. Ann. Neurol. *12*:119-128, 1982.

27. Fux, C. A., Pfister, S., Nohl, F., et al.: Cytomegalovirus-associated acute transverse myelitis in immunocompetent adults. Clin. Microbiol. Infect. *9*:1187-1190, 2003.

28. Galanakis, E., Bikouvarakis, S., Mamoulakis, D., et al.: Transverse myelitis associated with herpes simplex virus infection. J. Child Neurol. *16*:866-867, 2001.

29. Gilden, D. H., Beinlich, B. R., Rubinstien, E. M., et al.: Varicella-zoster virus myelitis: An expanding spectrum. Neurology *44*:1818-1823, 1994.

30. Gilden, D. H., Kleinschmidt-DeMasters, B. K., LaGuardia, J. J., et al.: Neurologic complications of the reactivation of varicella-zoster virus. N. Engl. J. Med. *342*:635-645, 2000.

31. Gobbi, C., Tosi, C., Stadler, C., et al.: Recurrent myelitis associated with herpes simplex virus type 2. Eur. Neurol. *46*:215-218, 2001.

32. Grewal, A. K., Lopes, M. B., Berg, C. L., et al.: Recurrent demyelinating myelitis associated with hepatitis C viral infection. J. Neurol. Sci. *224*:101-106, 2004.

33. Grose, C., and Feorino, P. M.: Epstein-Barr virus and transverse myelitis. Lancet *1*:892, 1973.

34. Hill, A. E., Hicks, E. M., and Coyle, P. V.: Human herpes virus 6 and central nervous system complications. Dev. Med. Child Neurol. *36*:651-652, 1994.

35. Innocenzi, G., Raco, A., Cantore, G., et al.: Intramedullary astrocytomas and ependymomas in the pediatric age group: A retrospective study. Childs Nerv. Syst. *12*:776-780, 1996.

36. Irani, D. N., and Kerr, D. A.: 14-3-3 protein in the cerebrospinal fluid of patients with acute transverse myelitis. Lancet *355*:901, 2000.

37. Kaplin, A. I., Deshpande, D. M., Scott, E., et al.: IL-6 induces regionally selective spinal cord injury in patients with the neuroinflammatory disorder transverse myelitis. J. Clin. Invest. *115*:2731-2741, 2005.

38. Kelly, H.: Evidence for a causal association between oral polio vaccine and transverse myelitis: A case history and review of the literature. J. Paediatr. Child Health. *42*:155-159, 2006.

39. Knebusch, M., Strassburg, H. M., and Reiners, K.: Acute transverse myelitis in childhood: Nine cases and review of the literature. Dev. Med. Child Neurol. *40*:631-639, 1998.

40. Krishnan, C., Kaplin, A. I., Graber, J. S., et al.: Recurrent transverse myelitis following neurobrucellosis: Immunologic features and beneficial response to immunosuppression. J. Neurovirol. *11*:225-231, 2005.

41. Kurtzke, J. F.: Rating neurologic impairment in multiple sclerosis: An Expanded Disability Status Scale (EDSS). Neurology *33*:1444-1452, 1983.

42. Kusunoki, S., Shiina, M., and Kanazawa, I.: Anti-Gal-C antibodies in GBS subsequent to mycoplasma infection: Evidence of molecular mimicry. Neurology *57*:736-738, 2001.

43. Lahat, E., Pillar, G., Ravid, S., et al.: Rapid recovery from transverse myelopathy in children treated with methylprednisolone. Pediatr. Neurol. *19*:279-282, 1998.

44. Lennon, V. A., Kryzer, T. J., Pittock, S. J., et al.: IgG marker of optic-spinal multiple sclerosis binds to the aquaporin-4 water channel. J. Exp. Med. *202*:473-477, 2005.

45. Lennon, V. A., Wingerchuk, D. M., Kryzer, T. J., et al.: A serum autoantibody marker of neuromyelitis optica: Distinction from multiple sclerosis. Lancet *364*:2106-2112, 2004.

46. Lesca, G., Deschamps, R., Lubetzki, C., et al.: Acute myelitis in early *Borrelia burgdorferi* infection. J. Neurol. *249*:1472-1474, 2002.

47. Linssen, W. H., Gabreels, F. J., and Wevers, R. A.: Infective acute transverse myelopathy: Report of two cases. Neuropediatrics *22*:107-109, 1991.

48. Majid, A., Galetta, S. L., Sweeney, C. J., et al.: Epstein-Barr virus myeloradiculitis and encephalomyeloradiculitis. Brain *125*:159-165, 2002.

49. Marriage, S. C., Booy, R., Hermione Lyall, E. G., et al.: Cytomegalovirus myelitis in a child infected with human immunodeficiency virus type 1. Pediatr. Infect. Dis. J. *15*:549-551, 1996.

50. Matsui, M., Kakigi, R., Watanabe, S., et al.: Recurrent demyelinating transverse myelitis in a high titer HBs-antigen carrier. J. Neurol. Sci. *139*:235-237, 1996.

51. McCarthy, J. T., and Amer, J.: Postvaricella acute transverse myelitis: A case presentation and review of the literature. Pediatrics *62*:202-204, 1978.

52. McLinskey, N. A., Belman, A., MacAllister, W., Milazzo, M., and Krupp, L.: Neuromyelitis optica in childhood. Neuropediatrics *26*:S85, 2006.

53. McMinn, P. C.: An overview of the evolution of enterovirus 71 and its clinical and public health significance. F. E. M. S. Microbiol. Rev. *26*:91-107, 2002.

54. Mewasingh, L. D., Christiaens, F. J., Dachy, B., et al.: Cervical myelitis from herpes simplex virus type 1. Pediatr. Neurol. *30*:54-56, 2004.

55. Mikaeloff, Y., Suissa, S., Vallee, L., et al.: First episode of acute CNS inflammatory demyelination in childhood: Prognostic factors for multiple sclerosis and disability. J. Pediatr. *144*:246-252, 2004.

56. Minami, K., Tsuda, Y., Maeda, H., et al.: Acute transverse myelitis caused by coxsackie virus B5 infection. J. Paediatr. Child Health. *40*:66-68, 2004.

57. Miyazawa, R., Ikeuchi, Y., Tomomasa, T., et al.: Determinants of prognosis of acute transverse myelitis in children. Pediatr. Int. *45*:512-516, 2003.

58. Nussinovitch, M., Brand, N., Frydman, M., et al.: Transverse myelitis following mumps in children. Acta Paediatr. *81*:183-184, 1992.

59. Paine, R. S., and Byers, R. K.: Transverse myelopathy in childhood. A. M. A. Am. J. Dis. Child. *85*:151-163, 1953.

60. Parazzini, C., Rossi, L., Righini, A., et al.: Spinal cord and vertebral stroke: A paediatric case. Neuropediatrics *37*:107-109, 2006.

61. Patel, H., Boaz, J. C., Phillips, J. P., et al.: Spontaneous spinal epidural hematoma in children. Pediatr. Neurol. *19*:302-307, 1998.

62. Petito, C. K., Navia, B. A., Cho, E. S., et al.: Vacuolar myelopathy pathologically resembling subacute combined degeneration in patients with the acquired immunodeficiency syndrome. N. Engl. J. Med. *312*:874-879, 1985.

63. Pittock, S. J., and Lucchinetti, C. F.: Inflammatory transverse myelitis: Evolving concepts. Curr. Opin. Neurol. *19*:362-368, 2006.

64. Pollono, D., Tomarchia, S., Drut, R., et al.: Spinal cord compression: A review of 70 pediatric patients. Pediatr. Hematol. Oncol. *20*:457-466, 2003.

65. Roos, K. L.: West Nile encephalitis and myelitis. Curr. Opin. Neurol. *17*:343-346, 2004.

66. Salgado, C. D., and Weisse, M. E.: Transverse myelitis associated with probable cat-scratch disease in a previously healthy pediatric patient. Clin. Infect. Dis. *31*:609-611, 2000.

67. Scott, T. F., Bhagavatula, K., Snyder, P. J., et al.: Transverse myelitis: Comparison with spinal cord presentations of multiple sclerosis. Neurology *50*:429-433, 1998.

68. Sebire, G., Hollenberg, H., Meyer, L., et al.: High dose methylprednisolone in severe acute transverse myelopathy. Arch. Dis. Child. *76*:167-168, 1997.

69. Shahar, E., Andraus, J., Savitzki, D., et al.: Outcome of severe encephalomyelitis in children: Effect of high-dose methylprednisolone and immunoglobulins. J. Child Neurol. *17*:810-814, 2002.

70. Sheremata, W. A., Berger, J. R., Harrington, W. J., Jr., et al.: Human T lymphotropic virus type I-associated myelopathy: A report of 10 patients born in the United States. Arch. Neurol. *49*:1113-1118, 1992.

71. Sure, U., Wakat, J. P., Gatscher, S., et al.: Spinal type IV arteriovenous malformations (perimedullary fistulas) in children. Childs Nerv. Syst. *16*:508-515, 2000.

72. Tanaka, S. T., Stone, A. R., and Kurzrock, E. A.: Transverse myelitis in children: Long-term urological outcomes. J. Urol. *175*:1865-1868; discussion 1868, 2006.

73. Tartaglino, L. M., Heiman-Patterson, T., Friedman, D. P., et al.: MR imaging in a case of postvaccination myelitis. A. J. N. R. Am. J. Neuroradiol. *16*:581-582, 1995.

74. Tsiodras, S., Kelesidis, T., Kelesidis, I., et al.: Mycoplasma pneumoniae-associated myelitis: A comprehensive review. Eur. J. Neurol. *13*:112-124, 2006.

75. Tyler, K. L., Gross, R. A., and Cascino, G. D.: Unusual viral causes of transverse myelitis: Hepatitis A virus and cytomegalovirus. Neurology *36*:855-858, 1986.

76. Ullrich, N. J., Marcus, K., Pomeroy, S. L., et al.: Transverse myelitis after therapy for primitive neuroectodermal tumors. Pediatr. Neurol. *35*:122-125, 2006.

77. Unay, B., Kendirli, T., Meral, C., et al.: Transverse myelitis due to echovirus type 30. Acta Paediatr. *94*:1863-1864, 2005.

78. Weinshenker, B. G., Wingerchuk, D. M., Vukusic, S., et al.: Neuromyelitis optica IgG predicts relapse after longitudinally extensive transverse myelitis. Ann. Neurol. *59*:566-569, 2006.

79. Williams, W., and Sunderland, R.: As sick as a pigeon—psittacosis myelitis. Arch. Dis. Child. *64*:1626-1628, 1989.

80. Wingerchuk, D. M., Lennon, V. A., Pittock, S. J., et al.: Revised diagnostic criteria for neuromyelitis optica. Neurology *66*:1485-1489, 2006.

81. Zanoni, G., Nguyen, T. M., Destefani, E., et al.: Transverse myelitis after vaccination. Eur. J. Neurol. *9*:696-697, 2002.

PARAINFECTIOUS AND POSTINFECTIOUS DISORDERS OF THE PERIPHERAL NERVOUS SYSTEM

Benjamin A. Ross ● Daniel G. Glaze

GUILLAIN-BARRÉ SYNDROME

Guillain-Barré syndrome (GBS) encompasses a spectrum of acute-onset, flaccid paralytic disease involving the peripheral nervous system. The classic form now generally is referred to as *acute inflammatory demyelinating polyradiculoneuropathy* (AIDP). With the decline in the incidence of poliomyelitis, GBS emerged as the most frequent cause of acute, severe generalized human paralytic disease.[195] GBS typically occurs several weeks after an upper respiratory or gastrointestinal tract illness, but it has been associated with other factors, including immunization and surgery. It is characterized by progressive ascending motor weakness, hyporeflexia, and minor sensory disturbances.

No specific diagnostic test for GBS exists; the diagnosis is based on the clinical features supported by other data, including cerebrospinal fluid (CSF) protein elevation, electrophysiologic changes, and pathologic changes of the peripheral nerves. The consensus is that GBS is mediated immunologically; however, the specific immunologic alterations necessary to initiate the events that result in demyelination of human peripheral nerves are unclear. The primary treatment is supportive care, but the efficacy of other therapies, such as plasma exchange transfusion and intravenous immunoglobulin (IVIG) therapy, in shortening the duration of the illness has been shown.[87,96,207,208] Following is an overview of GBS and its variants, including diagnostic criteria, the role of preceding infection and immunization, immunologic aspects, and treatment modalities.

HISTORY

Although bearing the names of Guillain and Barré, GBS was recognized first by Landry in 1859.[114] Landry described 10 patients who presented first with generalized weakness, followed by paresthesia and transitory muscle cramps, and then a rapidly ascending paralysis that involved the respiratory muscles last. He named this disorder *acute ascending paralysis*, postulated that it occurred after another illness, and considered it to be a severe disease because 2 of the 10 patients died. Other reports of this disorder appeared, but in 1916, Guillain, Barré, and Strohl[72] clearly characterized it and were the first to call attention to the "albuminocytologic dissociation," or increased CSF protein with absence of cells. Barré and Guillain favored an infectious cause for the disease.

In 1955, Waksman and Adams[215] pointed out the similarity in the clinical and pathologic pictures between GBS and experimental allergic neuritis in rabbits. In 1963, Melnick[131] found antibodies to nervous tissue in 19 of 38 patients with GBS. In 1960, Osler and Sidell[149] indicated the need for exact diagnostic criteria for GBS and presented 12 diagnostic criteria restricting the definition of the disorder. Most subsequent studies arrived at a broader concept of the disorder, however.[9,13,54] After reports of an increased incidence of GBS in association with the 1976 inocula-

tion program for swine influenza, the National Institute of Neurological and Communicative Disorders and Stroke (NINCDS) proposed a standardized inclusion and exclusion diagnostic criteria.[12,13,14]

DIAGNOSTIC CRITERIA

The diagnosis of GBS is based on the clinical history and examination and supported by clinical laboratory (i.e., CSF) and electrodiagnostic (i.e., nerve conduction velocities) evaluations. The "typical" case of GBS often occurs a few days or weeks after a recognizable, nonspecific infection that is more often viral than bacterial in origin. The paralytic stage usually begins with pain or paresthesia, followed by hypotonia, ascending paralysis without pyramidal tract involvement, and loss of deep tendon reflexes rather than hyperreflexia or pathologic reflexes. Initial weakness usually is noted in the lower extremities and less commonly in the upper extremities or the face. Many patients experience minimal to moderate sensory loss in a glove-stocking distribution. Maximal paralysis is reached in approximately 3 weeks. In 46 to 75 percent of patients, cranial nerves, including VII, IX/X, or both, may be affected, giving rise to facial weakness and difficulties in swallowing. Respiratory weakness occurs in 12 to 20 percent of patients, and some may require mechanical ventilation.

Although not part of any diagnostic criteria, pain has been reported to occur in 55 to 90 percent of patients with GBS, and it may precede weakness in some patients.[176] Approximately 79 percent of children with GBS who are younger than 6 years of age present with pain that may be present for longer than 1 week before the correct diagnosis is made.[140] Multiple pain syndromes that have been described include (1) deep, aching throbbing discomfort in the lower back that radiates to the buttock, thighs, or calves (67%); (2) dysesthesias, described as burning, tingling, or shock-like pain (20%); and (3) myalgias or muscle aches (9%). Severity of pain has not been found to be a predictor of the clinical course.[136]

Routine laboratory tests are unremarkable except for characteristic elevation of CSF protein (typical values of 50 to 200 mg/dL) without appearance of cells. The CSF protein concentration usually peaks between the second and eighth week of illness, with a slow decline occurring thereafter. Although most patients experience "complete" recovery, 20 percent have permanent residual disease (weakness, muscle atrophy), and approximately 1 to 4 percent die of respiratory failure.[19,130]

As Asbury[12] has emphasized, the problem is not with recognition of a typical case but with knowing the boundaries of the disorder. To define those limits, specific criteria were created in 1978 (Table 43–13).[14,15] These criteria consist of specific features required for establishing the diagnosis and additional features that strongly support, cast doubt on, or rule out the diagnosis entirely. The two features required for establishing the diagnosis are progressive motor weakness involving more than one limb and areflexia.

Clinical features supporting the diagnosis include the following: (1) progression of symptoms with signs of motor weakness that cease to progress after 4 weeks; (2) symmetry of symptoms; (3) sensory, cranial nerve, and autonomic dysfunction; (4) recovery; and (5) absence of fever. Laboratory features supporting the diagnosis include CSF protein elevation after the first week of symptoms or an increase in protein on serial lumbar punctures and less than 10 mononuclear leukocytes/mm³.

Electrodiagnostic studies in GBS show evidence of an axonal, a demyelinating, or a mixed neuropathy. Features suggestive of demyelination include slowing of conduction velocity, prolongation of distal compound motor action potential latencies, prolonged or absent F-wave response, and a partial conduction block

TABLE 43–13   Criteria for Diagnosis of Guillain-Barré Syndrome

Required
Progressive motor weakness in more than one extremity
Areflexia (at least distal with hyporeflexia of the biceps and knee jerks)

Strongly Supportive
Clinical features (in order of importance)
Progression—ceases by 4 wk
Relative symmetry
Mild sensory symptoms or signs
Cranial nerve involvement
Recovery—usually 2-4 wk after progression ceases
Autonomic dysfunction
Absence of fever at onset of neurologic symptoms

CSF Features
Protein—elevated after first week of symptoms, or increasing on serial lumbar punctures
Cells—≤10 mononuclear leukocytes/mm³

Electrodiagnostic Features
Nerve conduction slowing

Casting Doubt
Marked, persistent asymmetry of weakness
Persistent bladder or bowel dysfunction
Bowel or bladder dysfunction at onset
>50 mononuclear leukocytes/mm³ in CSF
Presence of polymorphonuclear leukocytes in CSF
Sharp sensory level

Rule Out the Diagnosis
Current history of hexacarbon abuse
Abnormal porphyrin metabolism
Recent diphtheria infection
Evidence of lead neuropathy or intoxication
Purely sensory syndrome
Definite diagnosis of poliomyelitis, botulism, hysterical paralysis, or toxic neuropathy

CSF, cerebrospinal fluid.
Data from references 14 and 15.

TABLE 43–14   New Diagnostic Criteria for Guillain-Barré Syndrome

Necessary Criteria for Diagnosis
1. Subacutely developing flaccid paralysis
2. Weakness is bilateral at onset with a strong tendency toward symmetry
3. Myotatic reflexes decrease and usually disappear entirely
4. Other causes for rapidly developing flaccid weakness are highly unlikely based on history or additional tests

Other Characteristics with Limited Diagnostic Value but May Add to the Diagnosis if No. 4 is Uncertain
Elevated CSF protein with normal (or slightly increased) cell count
Electrophysiologic testing supports a polyneuropathy

Subclassifications (Criteria 1-4 Should Be Met)
Motor-sensory GBS—sensory deficit is present
Pure motor GBS—sensory deficit is not present
Miller Fisher syndrome—requires weakness to begin in the external eye muscles and either ataxia or anti-GQ1b antibodies (diagnosis is probable if only ophthalmoplegia is present)
Bulbar (pharyngocervicobrachial) variant—onset of weakness is in muscles of the face, pharynx, or tongue
Demyelinating or primary axonal—based solely on electrophysiologic or pathologic features, or both (there are no clinical criteria)

CSF, cerebrospinal fluid; GBS, Guillain-Barré syndrome.
From Van der Meche, F. G. A., et al.: Diagnostic and classification criteria for the Guillain-Barré syndrome. Eur. Neurol. 45:133-139, 2001.

or evidence of temporal dispersion (broadening of the compound motor action potential response). Signs of axonal neuropathy include absent or significantly reduced compound motor action potential amplitudes and absence of the features suggestive of demyelination.[87] Early in the course of the disease, many of these findings may not be present, and findings may remain normal in 20 percent of cases.[12,13] The earliest electrodiagnostic signs of GBS are most likely to be decreased or absent F waves, absent h reflex, and the presence of A waves.[5,67,213]

Certain features, including persistent asymmetry of weakness, bowel or bladder dysfunction at onset or a persistence of dysfunction, elevation of cells in the CSF, or a discrete sensory level, cast doubt on the diagnosis. Features that can rule out the diagnosis entirely include (1) a purely sensory syndrome; (2) a current history of hexacarbon abuse; (3) abnormal porphyrin metabolism (increased excretion of porphobilinogen and δ-minolevulinic acid in the urine); (4) evidence of recent diphtheritic infection; (5) lead neuropathy or intoxication; or (6) a definite diagnosis of a condition such as poliomyelitis, botulism, hysterical paralysis, or toxic neuropathy (nitrofurantoin, dapsone, or organophosphorus).[12,13]

A diagnostic process has been suggested.[12] If the clinical features and temporal evolution are typical and without variant features or features that rule out GBS, the diagnosis may be made on clinical grounds alone. Laboratory findings, such as CSF protein elevation, may not appear until after 1 week, and electro-

diagnostic findings may never occur. If clinical features are unusual, however, laboratory studies may provide important supportive information, and a diagnosis of GBS may have to be delayed to evaluate these test results fully. Asbury and Cornblath[15] reported that certain variant features are seen occasionally in otherwise typical cases of GBS. These variant features include fever at onset of neuritic symptoms, severe sensory loss with pain, progression beyond 4 weeks, cessation of progression without recovery or with major permanent residual deficit, sphincter dysfunction, central nervous system involvement, no increase in CSF protein 1 to 10 weeks after onset of symptoms, and cell counts of 11 to 50 mononuclear leukocytes/mm³ in CSF.

Asbury and Cornblath[15] suggested that the presence of one of these symptoms, signs, or laboratory results should raise doubt about the validity of the diagnosis and that the presence of two or more suggest the diagnosis of GBS is incorrect. Manifestations of systemic illness or constitutional symptoms (or both) preceding or coinciding with signs and symptoms of involvement of the peripheral nervous system suggest a diagnosis of a systemic illness or intoxication and not GBS. In patients who have features consistent with GBS and who also have human immunodeficiency virus (HIV) seropositivity, CSF cell counts frequently are elevated.[15,41]

To facilitate use for poliomyelitis surveillance, the diagnostic criteria were simplified by the World Health Organization in 1993 to involve solely clinical features. Cases that fulfilled the aforementioned clinical criteria were diagnosed as GBS. If further electrodiagnostic or pathologic data were obtained, however, the terms *demyelinating* or *axonal* could be applied, and all subtypes were described independently.[219]

With further advancement in diagnostic techniques and identification of additional variant syndromes, a new set of criteria has been proposed to include a systematic approach for further subclassifications and to support future research (Table 43–14).[209] This new classification is based on four main criteria necessary for establishing the clinical diagnosis of GBS: (1) flaccid paralysis that develops subacutely, (2) bilateral onset of weakness (with a tendency for symmetry), (3) loss of reflexes, and (4) other causes being highly unlikely (ruled out with additional testing as necessary). Electrodiagnostic studies and CSF analysis (as previously discussed) can assist in the diagnosis if the fourth criterion is in question. For all subclassifications, the main criteria first must be met.

Motor-sensory GBS requires the presence of a sensory deficit at some point during the course of the disease. In pure motor GBS, paresthesias may be present, but no sensory deficit at anytime. Miller Fisher syndrome requires weakness of the external ocular muscles and either ataxia or positive anti-G_{Q1b} antibodies in the serum. The bulbar variant requires the onset of weakness to be within the bulbar musculature: facial muscles, tongue, or muscles of deglutition. Lastly, electrodiagnostic or pathologic studies or both can be used to distinguish between the primary axonal and demyelinating forms because this determination cannot be made by clinical signs and symptoms alone.[209]

CLINICAL VARIANTS

GBS typically has an acute onset followed by rapidly ascending weakness. In some patients, the onset is stuttering with periods of progression and plateaus before reaching a nadir of involvement. In other patients, the onset is subacute, with a slow progression that can occur over a few weeks.[123] In addition to weakness and areflexia, other individual features may be observed in patients with GBS, such as total and incomplete external ophthalmoplegia[65,70]; papilledema[42]; and autonomic dysfunction, including hypertension, postural hypotension, and cardiovascular disturbances.[38,42,43,196] Hypertension may be a consequence of sympathetic nervous system hypersensitivity and increased excretion of catecholamines,[42] but it also has been associated with increased renin-angiotensin activity.[183] Cardiovascular disturbances have been reported to be more prevalent in patients with GBS who are severely paralyzed and require mechanical ventilation.[38] Autonomic dysfunction in GBS, including tachycardia and other arrhythmias, may contribute to morbidity.[43]

An axonal form of GBS was described first in 1986. This new variant syndrome seemed to have a more severe disease course with poorer recovery.[58] The pure motor axonal form, termed *acute motor axonal neuropathy* (AMAN), initially was characterized in north China[129] as a summertime epidemic pattern mostly in children and young adults after they experienced an acute diarrheal illness. When sensory symptoms are present, it is called *acute motor-sensory axonal neuropathy*. Although these axonal subtypes tend to have a more severe and rapidly progressive clinical course, the diagnosis can be made only by electrodiagnostic studies or by pathologic examination of peripheral nerves. Despite some initial conflicting reports, recovery can be either rapid or quite prolonged; however, the long-term recovery potential is similar to that of classic demyelinating GBS (AIDP).[83,152,202]

One criticism of the NINCDS Ad Hoc Committee criteria is that they are too restrictive.[12,14] The criteria initially were designed for use during field studies of GBS, and certain variants are allowed: fever at onset of neuritic symptoms; severe sensory loss with pain; occasional progression beyond 4 weeks; major permanent residual deficits; transient bladder paralysis; and, possibly, central nervous system involvement, such as ataxia (cerebellar), dysarthria, extensor plantar responses, and ill-defined sensory levels. These features need not exclude the diagnosis of GBS.[12,13]

Specific variants in which the clinical features are atypical but fall in the spectrum of GBS have been described.[12,13] Findings of ophthalmoplegia, ataxia, and areflexia were described initially by Fisher in 1956, and he postulated that it was a variant of GBS because of the areflexia and CSF findings of cytoalbuminologic dissociation. This clinical syndrome now is referred to as *Miller*

Fisher syndrome.[61,172] The rapid onset of these symptoms usually indicates a benign course with fairly complete recovery occurring within weeks to months.[12,13] According to new diagnostic criteria, Miller Fisher syndrome must meet general criteria for GBS and in addition requires onset of weakness in the extraocular muscles and either ataxia or positive anti-G_{Q1b} IgG antibodies (present in 85%).[209]

Similarities with Miller Fisher syndrome occur in a subgroup of patients with Bickerstaff brain stem encephalitis. Bickerstaff and Cloake first described a syndrome of altered mental status, ophthalmoplegia, and ataxia in 1951. This syndrome was termed *Bickerstaff brain stem encephalitis* when Bickerstaff reviewed his collection of cases for the *Handbook of Clinical Neurology* in 1978. Bickerstaff's clinical criteria for Bickerstaff brain stem encephalitis include progressive external ophthalmoplegia and ataxia along with either alteration of consciousness or hyperreflexia. More recent studies have questioned these strict criteria because a subgroup of these patients may have normal or absent reflexes and varying degrees of weakness and cytoalbuminologic dissociation, indicating an overlap with GBS. In addition, 65 percent of patients with a diagnosis of Bickerstaff brain stem encephalitis have positive anti-G_{Q1b} antibodies, which suggests that all of these syndromes may be part of a clinical spectrum of disease.[145]

A rarer form of GBS, pharyngeal-cervical-brachial or bulbar, has been described in adults, and even fewer reports exist in children. This subtype has predominant weakness of the facial and bulbar musculature and weakness in the neck and upper extremities.[134] Sensory loss and areflexia without motor weakness or simultaneous onset of symmetric cranial nerve dysfunction (cranial polyneuritis) also may be accepted as variants of GBS if they are characterized by rapid onset with recovery, elevation of CSF protein, and the typical electrodiagnostic pattern of demyelination.[12,13,147] The presentation of acute sensory neuropathy characterized by symmetric glove-and-stocking sensory loss for pain and temperature (acute numbness) with normal muscle strength and tendon reflexes (acute small fiber sensory neuropathy 1) also is suggested as a variant of GBS.[5,188]

EPIDEMIOLOGY

Worldwide, the incidence of GBS has been reported to range from 0.4 to 4 cases per 100,000, with a median value of 1.3.[110,173,178] GBS can occur at any age; however, peaks occur in older adolescents or young adults and in the elderly. Overall, men tend to be affected more often than are women, at a ratio of approximately 1.25 : 1. Specific incidence rates do not exist for the various subtypes, although AIDP accounts for approximately 90 percent of cases compared with only 10 percent in Western countries. Approximately two-thirds of patients have had a preceding illness, typically involving the upper respiratory or gastrointestinal tracts, within 6 weeks of diagnosis.[39,100,173,178] No clear seasonal or geographic clustering of GBS has been observed, with the exception of the increased incidence of AMAN related to *Campylobacter jejuni* infection observed in children and young adults in China during the summer months.[129]

Age-related differences in the expression of GBS in children have been observed.[183] In children younger than 5 years old, a greater incidence of bulbar nerve (cranial nerves IX, X, and XII) dysfunction occurs, and muscle weakness is the most frequent initial symptom (72%). In children older than 5 years, limb pain is the most frequent initial symptom (53.4%). The interval between previous illness and onset of GBS is shorter for children older than 5 years and typically is 2 to 14 days. No statistically significant differences occurred in respiratory complications or fatal outcomes between the older and younger children with GBS.

PATHOLOGY AND PATHOGENESIS

GBS has been described as a distinctive neuropathy characterized pathologically by inflammatory lesions scattered throughout the peripheral nervous system.[143,161] Asbury and associates[13,14] studied 19 fatal cases and observed that the pathologic hallmark of this disorder is perivenular mononuclear inflammatory infiltrates, which occurs throughout the peripheral nervous system, even in cases with a short clinical course (1 to 4 days). These authors observed that the lesions were predominantly lymphocytic and that the inflammatory infiltrates tended to cluster about small endoneural and epineural vessels, particularly veins, in a seemingly random, multifocal distribution. All levels, including anterior and posterior roots, ganglia, proximal and distal nerve trunks, terminal twigs, cranial nerves, and sympathetic chains and ganglia, seemed vulnerable to attack. The site of maximal involvement correlated with the degree of premorbid clinical findings. Segmented demyelination was the predominant form of nerve fiber damage, with myelin destruction restricted to the regions of nerve trunks that were infiltrated by inflammatory cells.

Subsequent reports have confirmed the observation that primary demyelination occurs only in tissue infiltrated by inflammatory cells. These studies have shown that the destructive process is affected by macrophages in the presence of lymphocytes and directed only at the part of the Schwann cell plasma membrane forming the myelin sheath.[27,160,161,218,224] Kanda and associates[99] reported the findings of a necropsy of early fulminant GBS in an adult, however. Using semi-thin sections, they observed less extensive mononuclear infiltration than expected and found nerve fibers with myelin splitting, even in regions where inflammatory cell reaction was inconspicuous. Small myelinated fibers were involved preferentially, and no abnormalities of unmyelinated fibers occurred. Sensory roots were involved as severely as motor roots. These authors concluded that the underlying pathologic mechanism of GBS is heterogeneous. They suggested that some cases are cell-mediated, with predominant perivascular infiltration, whereas other cases are humorally mediated, with predominant demyelination without lymphocytic infiltration.

We now know that demyelinating and axonal forms of GBS exist and, as one would expect, that their mechanisms of injury to the nervous system differ. As a result of molecular mimicry, an immune attack is generated against the peripheral nerves and is mediated by immunoglobulins, macrophages, and complement factors. In AIDP, the initial target is the Schwann cell, which is responsible for myelination of the peripheral nervous system. In the axonal forms of GBS, the initial attack is targeted at the nodes of Ranvier, which allows macrophages to penetrate the basal lamina and enter the periaxonal space, causing subsequent axonal degeneration to ensue.[227]

ROLE OF INFECTION

The onset of GBS frequently follows an acute febrile infectious illness. GBS has been reported to occur after childhood illnesses such as mumps,[31] varicella,[23,44,216] measles,[50,116,156] and rubella.[48,180] These childhood illnesses rarely are associated with GBS, however.[48] Epidemiologic studies have indicated the significant occurrence of upper respiratory or gastrointestinal tract illnesses before the onset of GBS and support the concept that both of these categories of illness constitute important risk factors for GBS.[101,132] One case-control study[132] reported a higher incidence of elevated specific complement-fixation antibody titers in GBS cases compared with control cases for infectious mononucleosis and parainfluenza. Although influenza A and B infections have been observed in patients with GBS,[22,141,142,217]

this case-control study found no significantly higher incidence of elevated complement-fixation titers in patients with GBS compared with control subjects for influenza A or B.[132] During outbreaks of influenza A2 in 1960 to 1961 and influenza B in 1961 to 1962, the prevalence of GBS was high; however, the greatest number of cases occurred from November 1959 to October 1960, when the prevalence of influenza was comparatively low.[132]

Infectious hepatitis has been reported in association with GBS,[154,158] and four case reports have observed hepatitis B antigenemia in patients with GBS.[60,128,139,140] Acute viral hepatitis rarely is complicated by GBS. GBS has been associated with serologically documented cases of acute A, B, non-A/non-B, and delta hepatitis.[117,199,204] Immune complexes containing hepatitis B surface antigen in the serum and CSF were found in patients with GBS. These complexes were present with acute hepatitis B during the acute phase of GBS and disappeared when the neurologic symptoms resolved.[124,199,204] A causal association has not been established, however, and the fact that many of the populations at risk for hepatitis B and A also are at risk for other acquired viral infections, such as Epstein-Barr virus and cytomegalovirus (CMV), has been emphasized.[199]

Echoviruses and various serotypes of coxsackievirus A and B isolates have been observed in patients with GBS.[17,56,63,94,102,132,153,206] Most isolates were obtained from stool, although some were obtained from CSF in a few cases.[48] Recovery of virus does not prove causation, however; some isolates were recovered when enterovirus was prevalent in the community and in one instance equaled the frequency from control subjects.[48,122] In one series investigating West Nile virus, 1 patient of 224 had a clinical diagnosis of GBS.[126] Direct isolation of coxsackievirus A4 from nerve roots and dorsal root ganglia has been reported.[56] GBS also has been reported to occur after herpes simplex virus type 2 encephalitis,[133,194] in association with HIV infection,[41] and during rabies infection.[210]

Laboratory research has suggested that an important association exists between herpesviruses and GBS. Dowling and Cook[48] reported that 15 percent of patients tested with GBS had high titers of IgM antibodies against CMV antigen in tissue culture cells. Other studies also have observed an association between CMV and GBS.[11,35,45,97,137,157,185] Dowling and Cook[48] reported a wide spectrum of antecedent illness, ranging from asymptomatic infection to typical respiratory tract and gastrointestinal tract symptoms, in CMV-positive patients. A predilection for CMV-positive GBS was found to occur in patients younger than 30 years, corresponding to the age incidence described in heterophil-negative, CMV-induced, mononucleosis-like illness.[48] Time clustering of cases was observed, with CMV antibody–positive cases appearing in 10- to 16-week clusters. Dowling and Cook[48] suggested that in cases associated with preceding surgery, GBS may be consequent to CMV, either acquired during transfusion or caused by activation of latent virus, or occurrence of nontransfusion, non-A/non-B hepatitis.

Dowling and Cook[47] also observed the frequent (8%) occurrence of IgM antibodies to Epstein-Barr virus in GBS. In contrast, less than 2 percent (1 of 75) of GBS patients showed IgM herpes simplex virus–specific antibody.[21] These studies indicate that two herpesviruses are common antecedents of the syndrome, but the precise mechanism by which they initiate destruction of myelin is unknown.

Hart and Kennedy[74] emphasized the difficulty of establishing CMV as a cause of GBS. Using serologic tests, they confirmed active CMV infection in three patients with GBS. They reported that CMV could be isolated in 1 percent of asymptomatic individuals and in 10 percent of pregnant women; hence, isolation may be coincidental. These authors suggested that other viruses may activate latent CMV, and isolation may reflect such a nonspecific phenomenon. GBS also has been observed in association with HIV infection.[41] Elevated levels of circulating antibody to Epstein-Barr virus, CMV, and other infectious agents are common findings in these patients and may be directly responsible for some cases of GBS occurring in association with HIV infection.

Nonviral infectious agents also may precede occurrence of GBS. A preceding infection with *C. jejuni* associated with a diarrheal illness commonly occurs.[168,169,171] After two case reports,[33,162] a retrospective study was conducted to determine serologic evidence of recent *C. jejuni* infection in GBS.[98] Of 56 GBS patients, 38 percent (20 patients) were found to have serum evidence, CSF serologic evidence (including documentation of increase in titer, two or more elevated antibody titers, or positive CSF titer), or both. Preceding diarrheal illnesses were documented in 20 percent of these patients with GBS. Groups of normal control subjects and subjects with other neurologic disorders had no evidence of having had a recent *C. jejuni* infection. IgA-specific and IgM-specific antibody was found only in the CSF of patients with recent *C. jejuni* infection, suggesting production of specific antibodies by the central nervous system because passive diffusion into the CSF is unlikely.

Patients with GBS who also showed serologic evidence of *C. jejuni* seemed to have a significantly more severe illness; 90 percent of these patients required mechanical ventilation. Electrodiagnostically, GBS preceded by *C. jejuni* selectively elicits the AMAN subtype rather than AIDP.[112] One report noted mild illness in patients with GBS and positive serology and stool culture for *C. jejuni*.[162] Rees and associates,[169] in a prospective, case-controlled study in a cohort of patients with GBS (96 patients) or Miller Fisher syndrome (7 patients) who were admitted to hospitals throughout England and Wales between November 1992 and April 1994, found evidence of recent *C. jejuni* infection in 26 percent of the patients with GBS or Miller Fisher syndrome compared with 16 percent of household controls and 1 percent of age-matched hospital controls. A study in Japan has shown the *C. jejuni* serotype HS:19 to be more common in patients with GBS (67%) than in control patients with enteritis (5%).[200] Seventy percent of the patients with *C. jejuni* infection reported having had a diarrheal illness within 12 weeks before the onset of the neurologic illness. *C. jejuni* was associated with axonal degeneration, slow recovery, and greater disability after 1 year. The median interval from onset of diarrhea to the onset of symptoms for all *C. jejuni*–positive patients was 9 days, suggesting that GBS is a consequence of an immune response to *C. jejuni*, rather than a direct effect of the organism or one of its toxins.[95]

Mycoplasma pneumoniae is the second most prominent nonviral agent reported in association with GBS. One report observed that 5 percent of patients with GBS had serologic evidence of active *Mycoplasma* infection.[66] GBS has been reported rarely after infection with *Haemophilus influenzae*, *Francisella tularensis* (tularemia), *Chlamydia* (psittacosis), *Plasmodium* (malaria), *Mycobacterium tuberculosis*, *Bartonella henselae*, and *Toxoplasma gondii*.[24,69,125,132,135,138,148,184,214]

Patients with GBS frequently give a history of prodromal symptoms. An association between GBS and an infectious agent long has been considered. Isolation of a pathogen in a patient with GBS does not confer a direct correlation, however. McFarlin[127] has suggested that demyelination of peripheral nerves may result from direct infection of Schwann cells by the infectious agent, producing prodromal symptoms, or from immunologic mechanisms triggered by the infection. The second possibility is favored because epidemiologic and virologic surveys of patients with GBS have failed to identify reactivity with a single infectious agent and because the disorder can be triggered by other events, including surgery and immunizations. In addition, the clinical course may be shortened by plasmapheresis.

ROLE OF IMMUNIZATION

GBS occurs infrequently after immunization, including smallpox, diphtheria, tetanus, pertussis, combined mumps-rubella, hepatitis B, rabies, *H. influenzae* type b, and polyvalent pneumococcal vaccines.[40,64,73,92,104] A nationwide GBS surveillance conducted from December 16, 1976, until January 31, 1977, suggested that an excess risk of developing GBS was related to A/New Jersey influenza vaccine for adults 18 years or older.[28] The peak time of onset of GBS was 2 to 3 weeks after the vaccine was given. For the 10 weeks after vaccination with A/New Jersey vaccine, the risk was approximately 13.3 cases per 100,000 for vaccine recipients, which was five to six times higher than that in unvaccinated individuals (2.6 per 100,000).[186,187]

A subsequent survey of adults older than 18 years of age vaccinated in the 1978 to 1979 influenza campaign revealed that the relative risk of developing vaccine-associated GBS (individuals vaccinated within 8 weeks before the onset of GBS) was 1.4, which was significantly below the risk (6.2) associated with A/New Jersey vaccine for the equivalent 8-week period.[28,92,187] The survey of 1979 to 1980 also did not reveal an increased incidence of GBS for vaccinated versus nonvaccinated individuals.[92,100,187] The clustering of onset of GBS in the second and third weeks after the influenza vaccinations were administered in 1976 was not observed after administration of vaccinations in either 1978 to 1979 or 1979 to 1980.[187] These results suggested that A/New Jersey influenza vaccine differed from subsequent influenza vaccines in its ability to trigger GBS.[187] The neurotigenic P2 protein of peripheral nerve myelin has been shown to have been present and biologically active in the 1976 influenza vaccine.[193] P2 may have been a factor in the production of GBS after administration of the A/New Jersey influenza vaccination in susceptible individuals.[192]

Asbury[12] concluded that an "epidemic" of GBS actually occurred, but the precise cause of the illness remains undetermined. Whether a special antigenic site was present on the A/New Jersey viral product remains unknown. Patients with GBS who were vaccinated were spread throughout all 141 lots, and the problem could not be traced to individual lots or a single manufacturer. Surveillance for GBS in the subsequent (1979) influenza programs did not show any excess number of cases of GBS.[12]

GBS has occurred after the administration of rabies vaccine prepared in suckling mouse brain.[26,80] A severe protracted course with involvement of cranial nerves, increased mortality rate (20%), and increased long-term sequelae were observed. GBS occurs less commonly after immunization with sample-type vaccine prepared in brain and spinal cord of mature animals.

The prevalence of GBS cases was increased in children and adults in Finland in 1985 after institution of a mass vaccination program with oral polio vaccine.[103,205] This one-time campaign involved the entire Finnish population, and further study of the association between oral polio vaccine and GBS in Finland was impossible. This potential relationship was examined further during a retrospective epidemiologic survey in southern California.[165] No apparent temporal association between GBS and oral polio vaccine was noted. The frequency of GBS was low in the age groups during which children usually are immunized (before 2 years old and 5 years old). Researchers concluded that the failure to find a correlation between the usual age of oral polio vaccine immunization and the incidence of GBS by age coupled with the failure to find any children with GBS with onset within 1 month of receiving oral polio vaccine immunization provided strong evidence against a causal relationship between administration of oral polio vaccine and development of GBS. They suggested that the differences noted in the outcomes of these studies may be related to the fact that the entire population in the study in Finland already was vaccinated with inactivated polio vaccine and that different types of oral polio vaccine were used in Finland and California.

In October 2005, five cases of GBS occurring after the administration of the meningococcal polysaccharide diphtheria toxoid conjugate vaccine (Menactra, MCV4) in the United States were reported to the Vaccine Adverse Events Reporting System. Following a heightened awareness, three additional cases were reported. A subsequent investigation determined that the occurrence of eight cases of GBS out of the total number of vaccines given within the time period reported is similar to what might be expected on chance alone, based on an average annual incidence rate of 1.4 per 100,000 per year. The Centers for Disease Control and Prevention and the Global Advisory Committee on Vaccine Safety (World Health Organization) have concluded that no change should be made in vaccine policies, with the exception that individuals with a history of GBS not be vaccinated unless they are thought to have an elevated risk of contracting meningococcal infection.[29]

IMMUNOLOGIC FACTORS

Current opinion strongly favors the hypothesis that GBS is an autoimmune disease. Much evidence suggests that GBS represents an aberrant immune response to peripheral nerve components.[9] McFarlin[127] suggested that the following factors support an autoimmune mechanism in GBS: (1) plasmapheresis shortens the clinical course of GBS; (2) sera from patients with GBS contain IgM antibodies against a component of peripheral nerve myelin; (3) lipid antigen reacts with these antibodies; and (4) at least one lipid, sulfate-3-glucuronyl paragloboside (SGPG), can produce an experimental disease similar to GBS. This hypothesis is supported by the similarities of GBS, experimental allergic neuritis, and Marek disease.[203,215] Serum antibodies or antibody-like factors have been shown in peripheral nervous system tissues in experimental allergic neuritis and in GBS.[28,110,115,137,167,168,190,193,199] P2, a neurotigenic component of peripheral nervous system myelin administered in complete Freund adjuvant, has been shown to induce experimental allergic neuritis,[217] and sensitization to P2 has been reported in GBS.[2-4,192] Sensitized lymphocytes capable of producing demyelination have been found in experimental allergic neuritis and GBS.[10,59,68,222] Evidence of hypersensitization to peripheral nervous system antigens by use of the technique of macrophage migration inhibition factor assay has been reported in experimental allergic neuritis[191] and GBS.[68,106,119,174]

The cause of GBS and the nature of the antigen or antigens against which the immune response is directed are not known precisely. Studies have provided evidence that an intense immunologic response is an invariable accompaniment of the disease.[4,36,93,179,181] Cell-mediated and humoral immunity have been found to be altered in GBS and may contribute to the pathogenesis and pathology of GBS.

Several lines of investigation have implicated a cell-mediated immunologic reaction to the constituent of myelin as being of primary importance in the pathogenesis of GBS.[3,4,9,68,93,106,181] Activated lymphocytes can be identified in early phases of GBS.[46] Secretion of mediators, such as macrophage migration inhibitory factor (a measure of T-cell sensitization), in the presence of P2 protein has been shown during the acute phase of GBS.[20,68,106,174,192] By means of in vitro lymphocytic transformation technique, some researchers found lymphocytes sensitized to P2 in GBS,[4] whereas others have not confirmed these results and suggest that P2 may not be the antigen in GBS.[93] Goust and associates[68] reported finding circulating immune complexes in GBS and an association between increased immune complex and decreased suppressor

cell function. Abnormal T-cell subsets have been reported,[120] but other investigators have not reproduced this finding.[86,93] Additional evidence of cell-mediated immunity in GBS is suggested by studies observing demyelinization of rat peripheral nerves in tissue culture by circulating immunocytes from patients with GBS or lymph node cells from animals with experimental allergic neuritis.[10,93,182]

Activation of T cells has been reported in GBS.[4,77,78,201] Alterations in T-cell subsets, including decreased numbers of CD3+ and CD4+ and increased CD19, have been observed.[225] These changes normalized after plasmapheresis occurred in patients who improved. Taylor and Hughes[201] observed an increase in the levels of T cells bearing activator markers (interleukin-2 receptor and transferrin receptor) in the serum of GBS patients compared with normal control subjects. Hartung and associates[77,78] showed T-cell activation in the acute phase of GBS, as evidenced by increased interleukin-2 receptor expression on T cells, increased serum concentrations of interleukin-2 and soluble interleukin-2 receptor, and increased numbers of DR-positive circulating T cells. They reported that increased soluble interleukin-2 receptor concentrations that were found in several samples decreased with clinical improvement. The suggested role of activated T cells in GBS could include cytotoxic effect on Schwann cells, myelinotoxic effects, recruitment of macrophages in a delayed hypersensitivity reaction, or helping B cells to produce antibody against myelin. Activated T cells also may play a role in recovery.[77,78]

Protective and destructive roles have been ascribed to antibodies in GBS.[10,223] One suggestion is that the destructive effects of antibodies are mediated either directly by lysis of peripheral myelin with or without a requirement for complement or indirectly by opsonizing myelin, which then is attacked by macrophages.[93] Serum and CSF immunoglobulins of restricted electrophoretic heterogenicity have been reported to be increased in GBS, and these increased levels return toward normal with clinical improvement.[34,36,118] Autoantibodies to erythrocytes and circulating antigen-antibody complexes have been found in GBS.[34,37,46,49,68] Melnick[131] first showed anti-neural antibody in GBS sera, and anti-neural antibodies also have been reported in the CSF of patients with GBS.[179] The cytotoxic effect of GBS serum in vitro has been reported.[36,38,51] Several studies have suggested the presence of anti-neuronal antibodies in GBS patients. Indirect immunofluorescence has been used to show that sera of patients with GBS have IgG antibody to monkey dorsal root ganglia.[47]

Some findings indicate that sera from patients with GBS react with multiple antigens in peripheral nerve myelin.[49,110,163,226] Complement-fixing antibodies to peripheral nerve myelin have been detected in the sera of patients with GBS.[108,131] Increasing titers of complement-fixing antiperipheral nerve myelin antibodies (IgM) have been found during the acute phase of GBS, and decreasing titers have been observed during convalescence.[108] Koski and associates[108,109] found that some of the antiperipheral nerve myelin antibody in sera from patients with GBS binds a neutral glycolipid of human peripheral nerve myelin and cross-reacts with Forssman antigen, a cross-species antigen found in many infectious diseases. These investigators suggested that IgM antibodies, triggered by multiple infectious agents in patients with GBS, can bind to a glycolipid surface determinant of human peripheral nerve myelin and, after penetration of the damaged blood-nerve barrier, participate in the demyelination of peripheral nerves through activation of complement. Yu and associates[226] found that sera from patients with GBS reacted with antigens in peripheral nerve myelin, including one lipid, SGPG. In rabbits, immunization with SGPG produced weakness and physiologic abnormalities consistent with a demyelinating neuropathy.

PATHOGENESIS

GBS is regarded as an autoimmune disorder involving cellular and humoral immune mechanisms.[209] Immunologic studies have not resulted in a simple concept of the pathogenesis of GBS. The animal model of GBS, experimental allergic neuritis, has allowed researchers to analyze the pathogenetic mechanisms involved in the demyelinating process.[209] In the Lewis rat, GBS can be transferred by CD4$^+$ T cells reactive to neuroautoantigens P2 and P0. In the rabbit, experimental allergic neuritis serum injected intraneurally demyelinates rat nerve largely because of antigalactocerebroside antibody.[159] In humans, no peripheral nerve antigen has been identified as the responsible target.[208] Involvement of the cellular immune system also has been implicated. T and B cells become activated at the onset of GBS, as indicated by an increase of activation markers, including interleukin-2, soluble interleukin-2 receptor, and tumor necrosis factor-α, in serum and CSF.[18,76,189,208] The serum levels of these markers decrease with recovery.[18,189]

Disruption of myelin has been reported secondary to increased serum concentrations of the cytokine tumor necrosis factor-α.[189] Increased serum concentrations of tumor necrosis factor-α are detected in 50 percent of patients with GBS and in 26 percent of patients with unrelated neuropathies and other neurologic disorders. Increased serum concentrations of tumor necrosis factor-α are not specific for GBS, however. Tumor necrosis factor-α serum concentrations correlate with clinical severity, decrease as patients recover,[189] and are similar in patients with GBS whether or not preceding infections were noted. These elevations likely are not merely secondary to the antecedent infection. In contrast, soluble concentrations of interleukin-2 receptor are elevated in healthy relatives of patients with GBS and in patients with GBS. These data suggest that these concentrations may be secondary to environmental or infectious factors, rather than related to the pathogenic mechanism responsible for GBS.[189]

The involvement of complement is suggested by findings that include increased concentrations of the soluble terminal complement in serum and CSF and increases of C3a and C5a in CSF alone.[76,159,208] One study showed a breakdown of the blood-nerve barrier by activated T cells, allowing the development of focal conduction block and demyelinization in the presence of circulating anti-myelin antibodies.[159] Elevated serum concentrations of endothelial leukocyte adhesion molecule-1 have been shown in GBS during the acute phase, with serum concentrations returning to normal by 14 days. Endothelial leukocyte adhesion molecule-1 may be important by virtue of breakdown of the blood-nerve barrier.[148]

The diversity of preceding infectious factors and the observation that GBS may occur after noninfectious factors, such as surgery, trauma, epidural anesthesia, drug administration, and immunizations (Table 43-15),[9,28,57,198] have suggested that infection is not a necessary precondition for the development of GBS. A single factor, such as the release of antigen, may be the common mechanism leading to nerve damage. Also, the peripheral nervous system may possess a limited repertoire of pathologic responses and may react to diverse insults in a restricted fashion.[191] As noted, numerous reports have indicated alterations of cell-mediated immunity and humoral immunity in GBS and have suggested an immunologic basis for the demyelination in GBS. The exact mechanism and precise interaction of a preceding event and the patient's cell-mediated and humoral immune responses in causing demyelination are unknown. Whether GBS is the result of an autoimmune process or represents neural injury from an immune response to viral antigen that might be present in neural tissue is unclear.[36] Proposed mechanisms for the immunopathogenesis of GBS lesions have included antibody or cell-mediated immunity to an infectious agent with secondary neural

TABLE 43–15 Antecedent Factors

Strongly Suggestive Evidence
Cytomegalovirus
Epstein-Barr virus
Coxsackieviruses A
Campylobacter jejuni
Mycoplasma pneumoniae

Suggestive Evidence
A/New Jersey 1976 influenza immunization
Survey study or anecdotal reports

Viral Agents
Echoviruses
Coxsackieviruses A and B
Influenza viruses A and B
Measles
Varicella virus
Rubella
Mumps
Hepatitis viruses
Herpes simplex viruses
Rabies
Human immunodeficiency virus

Nonviral Agents
Francisella (Pasteurella) tularensis (tularemia)
Chlamydia
Plasmodium (malaria)
Toxoplasma gondii
Mycobacterium tuberculosis

Noninfectious Agents
Immunizations
  Trivalent oral poliovirus
  Diphtheria-tetanus-pertussis
  Measles-mumps-rubella
  Rabies
  Influenza, other than A/New Jersey
  Polyvalent pneumococcal
  Hepatitis
  Haemophilus influenzae type b
Surgery
Trauma
Epidural anesthesia
Neoplasm (Hodgkin)
Vasculitides (systemic lupus erythematosus)
Drug hypersensitivities
Heroin addiction
Drug (zimeldine)

injury, autoantibody or cell-mediated immunity to peripheral nervous system tissue, and demyelinization caused by deposition of circulatory antigen-antibody complexes in blood vessels of peripheral nerves.[36] One suggestion is that GBS is a syndrome and not a disease and that it may have several different causes.[197]

Increasingly, researchers have noted that the expression of GBS varies considerably.[52,208] Although the NINCDS Ad Hoc Committee proposed criteria for the research diagnosis of GBS, this committee recognized the occurrence of the many variant subtypes previously discussed. GBS could be viewed as a family of closely related diseases that can be categorized by class of axon (motor, sensory, autonomic, or mixtures), pathologic process (inflammatory-demyelinating, antibody attack), preceding infection, associated antibody, underlying disease mechanism, or response to treatment.[208]

The clinical variability of GBS may reflect different pathogenetic mechanisms. Pathology results suggest the heterogeneity of GBS. Studies by Asbury and coworkers[12,13,15] indicated the early occurrence of inflammatory cells as the primary mechanism resulting in demyelination. The lesions were found along the entire length of the nerve, but with variable expression among patients corresponding to their clinical deficits. The role of lymphocytic infiltration has been reappraised. Lymphocytic infiltration varies widely among patients with GBS, and severe demyelination can occur without lymphocytic infiltration. Heterogeneity is suggested further by experimental allergic neuritis models.[208] The rat experimental allergic neuritis model is a T-cell–dependent response to the antigen P2. In the rabbit model, demyelination results from a B-cell–dependent response to galactocerebroside. These models suggest that the variability of GBS may depend on the relative contribution of T-cell and B-cell responses.

Serum antibodies against such glycolipids as G_{M1}, G_{M1b}, G_{M2}, GALNAc-GD$_{1a}$, G_{D1a}, G_{D1b}, G_{D3}, G_{T1a}, G_{T1b}, G_{Q1b}, and L_{M1} have been reported in the acute phase of GBS.[55,75,144,211,227,228] In GBS, the specificity of anti-ganglioside antibodies varies.[31,220] The presence of anti–G_{M1} ganglioside IgG antibodies may be associated with a more severe and predominantly motor form of GBS (AMAN). Among 132 patients with GBS participating in the Dutch GBS trial and for whom suitable pretreatment serum was available, 25 (19%) showed high anti-G_{M1b} antibody titers of the IgG ($n = 15$) or IgM ($n = 14$) class or both ($n = 4$). Patients who were antibody-positive more frequently experienced preceding diarrhea and had serologic evidence of recent *C. jejuni* infection without antecedent evidence of CMV, Epstein-Barr virus, or *M. pneumoniae* infection than did patients who were antibody-negative. In the patients who were antibody-positive, the onset was more rapid, limb weakness was more severe, distal weakness was more prominent, and recovery time was more prolonged. These patients had less frequent sensory deficit or cranial nerve involvement.[229]

Serum anti–G_{Q1b} ganglioside antibodies have been observed in the Miller Fisher (and Bickerstaff brain stem encephalitis) variant of GBS.[31,95,220] Eighty-two percent of patients with the Miller Fisher variant of GBS may have IgG antibodies to G_{Q1b}. The circulating anti-G_{Q1b} IgG antibodies induce presynaptic and postsynaptic blockade. After the patients recovered, this blocking activity was lost, and sera became negative for anti-G_{Q1b} antibodies. These IgG antibodies may play a pathogenic role in the Miller Fisher variant of GBS.[25] In addition, the G_{Q1b} epitope is expressed preferentially on the paranodal regions of the oculomotor, trochlear, and abducens nerves, which correlates with the clinical picture of ophthalmoplegia.[227] Researchers also have hypothesized that the anti-G_{Q1b} antibodies may bind to 1a afferent nerve fibers within the spinocerebellar tract, leading to ataxia.[227]

These findings suggest that some association exists between antigenic specificities of anti-glycolipid antibodies and clinical forms of GBS. The exact role of these antibodies as either neurotoxic and directly responsible for the symptoms or incidental by-products is not clearly established, however.[31,208,220] A decline in anti–G_{D1b} ganglioside titers in relation to clinical recovery has been reported in patients with GBS after receiving plasma exchange.[170] Although studies confirm the activation of the immune system in GBS, whether the increase in activation markers is caused by preceding infection, why they are found only in some and not all patients with GBS, and what their role is in destruction of myelin remain unknown.

Evidence for shared antigenic determinants among certain infective agents associated with GBS and various antigens within peripheral nerve includes the following: (1) shared antigenic determinants between herpes simplex virus ribonucleotide reductase and peripheral nerve P0 glycoprotein have been shown, (2) amino acid sequence homology between CMV and varicella-zoster virus and P0 glycoprotein has been observed, and (3) antibodies to ganglioside have been detected in patients with GBS after they have had an infection caused by *C. jejuni* or *M.*

pneumoniae.[7,159] Some studies indicate that molecular mimicry may contribute to the presence of antiganglioside antibodies after infection with *C. jejuni* has occurred.[55,144,228] Humoral immune mechanisms directed at an infectious agent may cross-react with antigens of the peripheral nervous system and cause an immunopathologic disease. The family of glycoconjugates, which includes gangliosides, is one of the myelin antigenic groups with which antibodies have been identified in GBS. The frequency of these antibodies may be 35 percent of patients with GBS. Nonetheless, the presence of high titers of anti-glycoconjugate antibodies is not correlated with the more severe course of this disease.[55,71,98,211]

The association of *C. jejuni* infection preceding presentation of GBS and the occurrence of antiganglioside antibodies may contribute to an understanding of pathogenesis of GBS. *C. jejuni* has a lipopolysaccharide capsule that is rich in glycoconjugates containing sialic acid that resemble human glycoconjugates.[71] A terminal tetrasaccharide immunogenically identical to the ganglioside G_{M1} in human peripheral nerve has been shown on the outer membrane of a *Campylobacter* strain cultured from a patient with GBS.[17] Serologic evidence of an antecedent *C. jejuni* infection has been shown to correlate with the presence of anti-G_{M1} antibodies.[55,95,211,228] Anti-G_{M1} IgG antibodies in GBS sera recognize surface epitopes on whole *Campylobacter* bacteria, and this recognition is strain-specific. *Campylobacter* isolated from patients with GBS and with enteritis have been found to have similar ganglioside-like moieties. This finding indicates that patients who develop GBS respond differently to the ganglioside-like epitopes on *Campylobacter* than do patients with non-GBS diarrhea.[95] The finding also suggests a role for host susceptibility as a determinant for outcome after *Campylobacter* infection.[190]

C. jejuni, but not *Escherichia coli*, bacteria can absorb G_{M1} antibodies of the IgG class.[144] Studies suggest that molecular mimicry might play a role in the pathogenesis of GBS. Molecular mimicry is suggested further by the observation that the G_{Q1b} epitope is present in the lipopolysaccharide fractions of *C. jejuni* isolated from patients with the Miller Fisher variant.[220,228] Direct infection of cells of the peripheral nervous system leading to an immune attack seems unlikely in the case of *C. jejuni* because extraintestinal infection, especially peripheral nervous system infection, probably is irrelevant. *C. jejuni* may generate toxins that directly damage peripheral nerves. Although strain-specific toxins may play a role in post–*C. jejuni* GBS, an immune mechanism remains most likely.[71] Especially appealing is that the association with *C. jejuni* provides indirect support for the shared epitope or molecular mimicry model of the immunopathogenesis of GBS.[190] One hypothesis is that an infectious agent with a specific antigenetic repertoire induces an immune response involving T-cell activation and antibodies that cross-react with gangliosides in peripheral nerves.[55]

In the motor axonal form of GBS, the nodes of Ranvier of the motor fibers are the primary targets. The earliest changes seem to be antibody-mediated and complement-mediated, and T lymphocytes are a rare finding in nerve. The axonal form of GBS has been associated with antiganglioside G_{M1}, G_{M1b}, G_{D1a}, and GalNAc-G$_{D1a}$, antibodies, and *C. jejuni* infection.[75,227] The epitopes for the aforementioned antibodies have been shown to be located on the nodal axolemma of motor nerves. Most of the Chinese cases are reported to be triggered by recent *C. jejuni* infection in the gut. Surface lipopolysaccharides of *C. jejuni* strains associated with GBS contain epitopes that are similar or identical to G_{M1} ganglioside that is concentrated at the nodes of Ranvier. This finding supports the role of molecular mimicry for inducing GBS.[16]

Conflicting results have been reported concerning the relationship of G_{M1} antibody to axonal degeneration.[113] Antibodies to other gangliosides have been reported to be elevated in sera of patients with GBS during the acute phase. Only a 50 percent concordance between serologic evidence of *C. jejuni* infection and the presence of anti-G_{M1} antibody was found during large studies. GBS patients with anti-G_{M1} antibodies have had identified infections that included *C. jejuni* (23%), CMV (10%), *M. pneumoniae* (6%), and Epstein-Barr virus (3%).[146] Microorganisms other than *C. jejuni* may trigger an anti-ganglioside response and elicit axonal GBS. Whether the presence of anti-G_{M1} antibodies is associated with extensive axonal loss and poor outcome is controversial. Some patients with GBS and anti-G_{M1} antibodies recover quickly or have conduction abnormalities suggestive of demyelination.[85,113,167,212]

OUTCOME

Most patients with GBS recover spontaneously. Epidemiologic studies have indicated, however, that 10 to 23 percent of patients may require mechanical ventilation, 7 to 22 percent have some residual disability, 3 to 10 percent relapse, and 2 to 5 percent die.[12,30,62,85,105,121,164,221] Patients may be left with residual symptoms, such as facial weakness, weakness in the lower extremities with footdrop, weakness and atrophy of hands, and autonomic dysfunction (impotence and urinary retention).[123] In the North American study of the effect of plasmapheresis,[87] the median time to recovery of independent walking was 85 days for control subjects compared with 169 days for patients who received mechanical ventilation. This same study indicated that children walked at 52 days. Five prognostic factors were identified: age, requirement for respiratory support, rate of progress, abnormal physiologic characteristics of peripheral nerve function, and plasmapheresis. In children, the overall recovery and outcome generally is better than that seen in adults. Much of the literature now uses the Hughes functional disability rating scale in assessing outcome measures. This is a scale from 0 to 6: 0—healthy, 1—minor symptoms and able to run, 2—able to walk 5 m independently, 3—able to walk 5 m with assistance, 4—confined to bed (or chair), 5—requiring assisted ventilation, 6—death.[87]

Complete recovery from motor or sensory deficits after an episode of GBS has been reported in 70 percent of cases after 12 months and in 82 percent after 15 years.[177] Kleyweg and associates[105] compared the outcome of GBS in groups of children and adults. They observed that 22 percent of children compared with 30 percent of adults required mechanical ventilation, with a median duration of 21.5 days in children and 32 days in adults. Mean duration of hospitalization was 84 days for children and 86 days for adults. Two of 18 children died. At 1 year, 77 percent of children had a good outcome, and at 2 years, 83 percent had a good outcome. For adults, good outcomes at 1 and 2 years were observed in 86 percent and 92 percent. Significant slowing of motor and sensory nerve conduction or electromyographic abnormalities may persist for weeks to years after recovery.[164,177] Reported unfavorable signs for complete recovery in children included a period longer than 18 days of plateau between onset of weakness and time of greatest weakness, weakness and maximum motor deficit of greater than 3 weeks, or marked paralysis alone (need for assisted ventilation).[53,177,221]

There are different recovery patterns for demyelinating forms of GBS compared with axonal variants. The axonal varieties overall have a more aggressive and progressive course, reaching their nadir much earlier than do AIDP variants. Demyelinating or AIDP syndromes tend to have a uniform recovery, with most patients having a complete or near-complete recovery over the course of several weeks to months, as previously described. Patients with axonal subtypes (specifically AMAN) seem to have two distinct recovery patterns: a rapid recovery observed within the first few weeks or a prolonged recovery period lasting several months or longer (more often seen with acute motor-sensory axonal neuropathy). Some patients have shown improvements

and regained the ability to walk years later,[81,82] which may explain earlier studies that predicted a worse outcome overall for the axonal subtypes because the evaluation period was too brief to measure their long-term recovery potential accurately. The recovery and outcome have been shown to be better and faster in children. One study in children showed similar outcomes at 1 year, regardless of subtype; however, the axonal subtypes had a more protracted course.[202]

TREATMENT

The mainstay of treatment of GBS is supportive care because there is no known cure. Intensive nursing and medical care are essential for proper management. Most deaths are related to respiratory failure, pulmonary embolism, and autonomic dysfunction.[88] Respiratory function must be monitored closely, especially during the acutely progressive phase. The need for endotracheal intubation and mechanical ventilation has been suggested if vital capacity decreases to less than 12 to 15 mL/kg, arterial Po_2 decreases to less than 70 mm Hg, or clinical signs of fatigue develop. Tracheostomy may be indicated if paralysis is prolonged.[175] Physiotherapy and preventive measures for pulmonary embolism are indicated. Because of autonomic dysfunction, electrocardiogram and blood pressure monitoring are essential. Hyponatremia is a reported complication and probably is caused by inappropriate secretion of antidiuretic hormone[155]; fluid and sodium balance and adequate nourishment must be maintained. Reassurance and attention to anxiety, anger, and depression are important during the progressive phase of GBS, especially for patients being ventilated.[88]

Pain is a very common feature of GBS, especially in children, and may be the earliest and most common symptom, occurring in as many as 90 percent of cases. Pain often is either underrecognized or underappreciated and undertreated. Although nonsteroidal anti-inflammatory drugs and opioids can be effective in pain management, they may not be optimal treatment options because of side effects or relative ineffectiveness for neuropathic pain. Gabapentin and carbamazepine have proven efficacy in a variety of neuropathic pain syndromes and in GBS as measured by a reduction in use of intravenous opiates and subjective patient reporting.[136,150,151] Carbamazepine and gabapentin were compared head to head in a randomized, prospective, double-blind, placebo-controlled study. Although both treatments were effective, gabapentin showed earlier and more profound pain relief and less sedation compared with carbamazepine.[151]

A variety of treatment modalities have been used in an attempt to hasten recovery, shorten the duration of time on a ventilator or in an intensive care unit, and decrease the incidence of residual neurologic deficits. These treatments include steroids, plasmapheresis or plasma exchange, CSF filtration, immunoadsorption, and IVIG. The Cochrane Collaboration has published separate systematic reviews of corticosteroids, plasma exchange, and IVIG therapy for GBS.[89,90,166] In 2003, the American Academy of Neurology (AAN) published practice guidelines with regard to immunotherapy in GBS, largely based on the Cochrane systematic reviews of the literature.[91]

The earliest studies investigated the effects of steroids on GBS. Limited evidence suggests that oral steroids slow the recovery process. Intravenous steroids have shown a trend toward a more rapid recovery that is not statistically significant. No effects of intravenous steroids on long-term outcome have been reported, and no significant adverse effects from intravenous steroids have been reported. Currently, corticosteroids are not recommended in the treatment of GBS.[90,91]

Plasma exchange has been shown to be beneficial in the treatment of GBS by shortening recovery time and duration of mechanical ventilation and reducing medical costs. Plasmapheresis may be beneficial in patients treated 30 days after the onset of disease, although it is more beneficial when started within 7 days of onset.[166] Studies in children also have shown the efficacy of plasmapheresis for treatment of GBS. In children, the benefits have included decrease in the number of days of mechanical ventilation and time to motor recovery and a decrease in the overall cost of care.[96,207] A further study suggested that two exchanges are better than none for mild GBS, four exchanges are more beneficial than are two for moderate GBS, and six exchanges are no more beneficial than are four in severe GBS.[16]

Although plasmapheresis can be a cumbersome procedure with many technical difficulties, it has been used safely in critically ill children 8 months old. Mild hypotension related to rapid fluid removal has been reported, but no major complications or deaths related to plasmapheresis have been reported in pediatric patients with GBS. Reported complications in adults include hypotension, transfusion reactions, hypocalcemia, arrhythmias, cardiopulmonary arrest, and infection caused by transmitted blood products or sepsis secondary to indwelling catheters. As the only treatment with proven benefit in randomized placebo-controlled trials, plasma exchange is the standard against which all subsequent treatments will be compared. Based on the evidence, current AAN guidelines recommend plasma exchange for nonambulatory patients within 4 weeks of onset of symptoms and for ambulatory patients within 2 weeks of onset.[91,166]

Immunoadsorption has been tried as an alternative to plasma exchange to remove immunoglobulins; however, only one small nonrandomized, unblinded trial and case reports exist suggesting efficacy. Also, CSF filtration has been used in some small studies, but no good large, randomized trials have been done. Currently, the evidence is insufficient to suggest whether or not either of these options is a valid treatment in GBS.[8,79,84,91]

Contraindications to the use of plasmapheresis in some patients with GBS, complications, and lack of universal availability led to the initial studies of IVIG as an alternative therapy to plasmapheresis. Because plasma exchange has proven efficacy in the treatment of GBS, no placebo-controlled trials have been performed of IVIG, only trials comparing IVIG with plasma exchange. IVIG has been shown to have equal efficacy to plasma exchange in speeding recovery in GBS.[89] In addition, some reports indicate that certain GBS subtypes (anti-G_{M1} or anti-G_{M1b}) may respond more favorably to IVIG than to plasma exchange.[111,229] Advantages of IVIG therapy for GBS include its wide availability, ease of administration, safety, and absence of serious complications. Therapy with IVIG generally is less expensive than is plasmapheresis.[207] Current AAN guidelines recommend IVIG for patients with GBS who lose independent ambulation within 2 to 4 weeks of onset of symptoms.[91]

No large trials of IVIG therapy have been performed exclusively in children. Small studies indicate improvement in children similar to that in adults when plasmapheresis or IVIG therapy is used. Plasma exchange and IVIG are treatment options for children with severe GBS (mostly derived from evidence in adult populations). A more recent multicenter, randomized trial[107] investigated the use of IVIG in children and compared IVIG, 2 g/kg (total dose) given over 2 days versus over 5 days, with the primary outcome measure being time required to regain ability to walk unassisted. No statistically significant difference was found between the two groups on the primary outcome measure (19 days versus 13 days). In the 2-day treatment group, early transient deterioration in the disability score before recovery occurred more often. Generally, in centers where it is available, IVIG has emerged as the treatment of choice for moderate to severe GBS in children because of its relative ease of administration, lower incidence of side effects, and overall cost-effectiveness.

REFERENCES

1. Abd-Allah, S. A., Jansen, P. W., Ashwal, S., et al.: Intravenous immunoglobulin as therapy for pediatric Guillain-Barré syndrome. J. Child Neurol. 12:376-380, 1997.
2. Abramsky, O., and Korn-Luhetzky, I.: Association with autoimmune diseases and cellular immune response to the neurotigenic protein in Guillain-Barré syndrome. Trans. Am. Neurol. Assoc. 105:350-354, 1980.
3. Abramsky, O., Teitelbaum, D., and Arnon, R.: Experimental allergic neuritis induced by a basic neurotigenic protein (P1L) of human peripheral nerve origin. Eur. J. Immunol. 7:213-217, 1977.
4. Abramsky, O., Webb, C., Teitelbaum, D., et al.: Cell mediated immunity to neural antigens in idiopathic polyneuritis and myeloradiculitis. Neurology 25:1154-1159, 1975.
5. Alaedini, A., Briana, C., Wirguin, I., et al.: Detection of anti-ganglioside antibodies in Guillain-Barré syndrome. Indian J. Med. Res. 113:234-238, 2001.
6. Al-Shekhlee, A., Hackwi, R., Preston, D., et al.: New criteria for early electrodiagnosis of acute inflammatory demyelinating polyneuropathy. Muscle Nerve 32:66-72, 2005.
7. Ang, C., Tio-Gillen, A., Groen, J., et al.: Cross-reactive antigalactocerebroside antibodies and *Mycoplasma pneumoniae* infections in Guillain-Barré syndrome. J. Neuroimmunol. 130:179, 2002.
8. Arakawa, H., Yuhara, Y., Todokoro, M., et al.: Immunoadsorption therapy for a child with Guillain-Barré syndrome subsequent to *Mycoplasma* infection: A case study. Brain Dev. 27:431-433, 2005.
9. Arnason, B. G. W.: Inflammatory polyradiculoneuropathies. In Dyck, P. J., Thomas, P. K., and Lambert E. H. (eds.): Peripheral Neuropathy. Philadelphia, W.B. Saunders, 1975.
10. Arnason, B. G. W., Winkler, G. F., and Hadler, N. M.: Cell mediated demyelination of peripheral nerve in tissue culture. Lab. Invest. 21:1-10, 1969.
11. Arnold, A. G., Lawrence, D. S., and Corbitt, G.: Cytomegalovirus infection and the Guillain-Barré syndrome. Postgrad. Med. J. 54:112-114, 1978.
12. Asbury, A. K.: Diagnostic considerations in Guillain-Barré syndrome. Ann. Neurol. 9(Suppl.):1-5, 1981.
13. Asbury, A. K.: Guillain-Barré syndrome: Historical aspects. Ann. Neurol. 27(Suppl.):S2-S6, 1990.
14. Asbury, A. K., Arnason, B. G., Karp, H. R., et al.: Criteria for diagnosis of Guillain-Barré syndrome. Ann. Neurol. 3:565-566, 1978.
15. Asbury, A. K., and Cornblath, D. R.: Assessment of current diagnostic criteria for Guillain-Barré syndrome. Ann. Neurol. 27(Suppl.):S21-S24, 1990.
16. Asbury, A. K., and McKhann, G. M.: Changing views of Guillain-Barré Syndrome. Ann. Neurol. 41:287-288, 1997.
17. Banerjii, N. K., and Miller, J. H. D.: Guillain-Barré syndrome in children with special reference to serial nerve conduction studies. Dev. Med. Child Neurol. 14:56-63, 1972.
18. Bansil, S., Mithen, F. A., Cook, S. D., et al.: Clinical correlation with serum-soluble interleukin-2 receptor levels in Guillain-Barré syndrome. Neurology 41:1302-1305, 1991.
19. Beghi, E., Kurland, L. T., Mulder, D. W., et al.: Guillain-Barré syndrome: Clinicoepidemiologic features and effect of influenza vaccine. Arch. Neurol. 42:1053-1057, 1985.
20. Behan, P. O., Lamarche, J. B., Feldman, R. G., et al.: Lymphocyte transformation in the Guillain-Barré syndrome. Lancet 1:421, 1970.
21. Bernsen, H. J., Van-Loon, A. M., Poels, R. F., et al.: Herpes simplex virus specific antibody determined by immunoblotting in cerebrospinal fluid of a patient with the Guillain-Barré syndrome. J. Neurol. Neurosurg. Psychiatry 52:788-791, 1989.
22. Bertrand, A., Janbon, F., Clot, J., et al.: Guillain-Barré polyradiculoneuritis and influenza virus. Presse Med. 79:2328, 1971.
23. Boucharlat, J., Groslambert, R., and Chateau, R.: Polyradiculoneuritis as a symptom of varicella (a case report). J. Med. Lyon 49:1443-1445, 1968.
24. Bouchez, B., Poirriez, J., Arnott, G. E., et al.: Acute polyradiculoneuritis during toxoplasmosis. J. Neurol. 231:347, 1985.
25. Buchwald, B., Bufler, J., Carpo, M., et al.: Combined pre- and post-synaptic action of IgG antibodies in Miller Fisher syndrome. Neurology 56:67-74, 2001.
26. Cabrera, J., Griffin, D. E., and Johnson, R. T.: Unusual features of the Guillain-Barré syndrome after rabies vaccine prepared in suckling mouse brains. J. Neurol. Sci. 81:239-245, 1987.
27. Carpenter, S.: An ultrastructural study of an acute fatal case of the Guillain-Barré syndrome. J. Neurol. Sci. 15:125-140, 1972.
28. Centers for Disease Control: National surveillance for Guillain-Barré syndrome. January 1978-March 1979. M. M. W. R. Morb. Mortal. Wkly. Rep. 28:547-548, 1979.
29. Centers for Disease Control and Prevention: Update: Guillain-Barré syndrome among recipients of Menactra meningococcal conjugate vaccine—United States, October 2005-February 2006. M. M. W. R. Morb. Mortal. Wkly. Rep. 55:364-366, 2006.
30. Cheng, Q., Jian, G. X., Press, R., et al.: Clinical epidemiology of Guillain-Barré syndrome in adults in Sweden 1996-1997: A prospective study. Eur. J. Neurol. 7:685-692, 2000.
31. Chiba, A., Kusunoki, S., Shimizu, T., et al.: Serum IgG antibody to ganglioside GQ1b is a possible marker of Miller Fisher syndrome. Ann. Neurol. 31:677-679, 1992.

32. Collens, W. S., and Rabinowitz, M. A.: Mumps polyneuritis: Quadriplegia with bilateral facial paralysis. Arch. Intern. Med. 41:61-65, 1928.

33. Constantino, T., and Weintraub, A.: The Guillain-Barré syndrome as a complication of the postperfusion syndrome. Am. Heart J. 84:678-680, 1972.

34. Cook, S., Murray, M. R., Whitaker, J. N., et al.: Myelinotoxic antibody in the Guillain-Barré syndrome. Neurology 19:284, 1969.

35. Cook, S. D., and Dowling, P. C.: The role of autoantibody and immune complexes in the pathogenesis of Guillain-Barré syndrome. Ann. Neurol. 9(Suppl.):70-79, 1981.

36. Cook, S. D., Dowling, P. C., Murray, M. R., et al.: Circulating demyelinating factors in acute idiopathic polyneuropathy. Arch. Neurol. 24:136-144, 1971.

37. Cook, S. D., Dowling, P. C., and Whitaker, J. N.: Serum immunoglobulins in the Guillain-Barré syndrome. Neurology 20:403, 1970.

38. Cooper, W. O., Daniels, S. R., and Loggie, J. M.: Prevalence and correlates of blood pressure elevation in children with Guillain-Barré syndrome. Clin. Pediatr. (Phila.) 37:621-624, 1998.

39. Cosi, V., Versino, M.: Guillain-Barré syndrome. Neurol. Sci. 27:S47-S51, 2006.

40. D'Cruz, O. F., Shapiro, E. D., Spiegelman, K. N., et al.: Acute inflammatory demyelinating polyradiculoneuropathy (Guillain-Barré syndrome) after immunization with *Haemophilus influenzae* type b conjugate vaccine. J. Pediatr. 115:743-746, 1989.

41. Dalakas, M. C., and Pezeshkpour, G. H.: Neuromuscular disease associated with human immunodeficiency virus infection. Ann. Neurol. 23(Suppl.):S38-S48, 1988.

42. Davidson, D. L. W., and Jellinek, E. H.: Hypertension and papilloedema in the Guillain-Barré syndrome. J. Neurol. Neurosurg. Psychiatry 40:144-148, 1977.

43. Davies, A. G., and Dingle, H. R.: Observations on cardiovascular and neuro-endocrine disturbance in the Guillain-Barré syndrome. J. Neurol. Neurosurg. Psychiatry 35:176-179, 1972.

44. Davis, J., and Rowlatt, R. J.: Transient severe hypertension and polyradiculitis after chickenpox. B. M. J. 2:1608, 1978.

45. Dowling, P., Menonna, J., and Cook, S.: Cytomegalovirus complement fixation antibody in Guillain-Barré syndrome. Neurology 27:1153-1156, 1977.

46. Dowling, P. C., and Cook, S. D.: Circulating complexes in neurologic disease. J. Neuropathol. Exp. Neurol. 1:161, 1972.

47. Dowling, P. C., and Cook, S. D.: Antibodies to dorsal root ganglia in Guillain-Barré syndrome. Neurology 23:423, 1973.

48. Dowling, P. C., and Cook, S. D.: Role of infection in Guillain-Barré syndrome: Laboratory confirmation of herpesviruses in 41 cases. Ann. Neurol. 9(Suppl.):44-55, 1981.

49. Dowling, P. C., Cook, S. D., and Whitaker, J. N.: Cold agglutinin positive Guillain-Barré syndrome. Trans. Am. Neurol. Assoc. 95:234-235, 1970.

50. Drueke, T. B., Pujade-Lauraine, E., Poisson, M., et al.: Measles virus and Guillain-Barré syndrome during long-term hemodialysis. Am. J. Med. 60:444-446, 1976.

51. Dubois-Dalcq, M., Buyse, M., Buyse, G., et al.: The action of Guillain-Barré syndrome serum on myelin: A tissue culture and electronmicroscopic analysis. J. Neurol. Sci. 13:67-83, 1971.

52. Dyck, P. J.: Is there an axonal variety of GBS? Neurology 43:1277-1280, 1993.

53. Eberle, E., Brink, S., Azen, S., et al.: Early predictors of incomplete recovery in children with Guillain-Barré polyneuritis. J. Pediatr. 86:356-359, 1975.

54. Eiben, R. M., and Gersiny, W. M.: Recognition, prognosis and treatment of the Guillain-Barré syndrome (acute idiopathic polyneuritis). Med. Clin. North Am. 47:1371-1380, 1963.

55. Enders, U., Karch, H., Toyka, K. V., et al.: The spectrum of immune responses to *Campylobacter jejuni* and glycoconjugates in Guillain-Barré syndrome and in other neuroimmunological disorders. Ann. Neurol. 34:136-144, 1993.

56. Estrada-Gonzales, R., and Mas, P.: Virological studies in acute polyradiculo-neuritis-Landry-Guillain-Barré syndrome: Various findings in relation to cox-sackie A4 virus. Neurol. Neurocir. Psiquiatr. 18(Suppl. 2-3):527-531, 1977.

57. Fagius, J., Osterman, P. O., and Siden, A.: Guillain-Barré syndrome following zimeldine treatment. J. Neurol. Neurosurg. Psychiatry 48:65-69, 1985.

58. Feasby, T. E., Gilbert, J. J., Brown, W. F., et al.: An acute axonal form of Guillain-Barré polyneuropathy. Brain 109:1115-1126, 1986.

59. Feasby, T. E., Hahn, A. F., and Gilbert, J. J.: Passive transfer of demyelinating activity in Guillain-Barré polyneuropathy. Neurology 30:363, 1980.

60. Feutren, G., Gerbal, J.-L., Allinquant, B., et al.: Association of Guillain-Barré syndrome and B-virus hepatitis: Simultaneous presence of anti-DS-DNA antibodies and HBs antigen in cerebrospinal fluid. J. Clin. Lab. Immunol. 11:161-164, 1983.

61. Fisher, M.: An unusual variant of acute idiopathic polyneuritis syndrome of ophthalmoplegia, ataxia and areflexia. N. Engl. J. Med. 255:57-65, 1956.

62. Fletcher, D. D., Lawn, N. D., Wolter, T. D., et al.: Long-term outcome in patients with Guillain-Barré syndrome requiring mechanical ventilation. Neurology 54:2311-2315, 2000.

63. Forbes, F. J., Brumlik, J., and Harding, H. B.: Acute ascending polyradiculo-myelitis associated with Echo 9 virus. Dis. Nerv. Syst. 28:537-540, 1967.

64. Friedland, M. L., and Wittels, E. G.: An unusual neurologic reaction following polyvalent pneumococcal vaccine in a patient with hairy cell leukemia. Am. J. Hematol. 14:189, 1983.

65. Gibberd, F. B.: Ophthalmoplegia in acute polyneuritis. Arch. Neurol. 23:161-164, 1970.

66. Goldschmidt, B., Menonna, J., Fortunato, T., et al.: *Mycoplasma* antibody in Guillain-Barré syndrome and other neurological disorders. Ann. Neurol. 7:108-112, 1980.

67. Gordon, P. H., Wilbarn, A. J., Early electrodiagnostic findings in Guillain-Barré syndrome. Arch. Neurol. 58:913-917, 2001.

68. Goust, J. M., Chenais, F., Carnes, J. E., et al.: Abnormal T cell subpopulations and circulating immune complexes in the Guillain-Barré syndrome and multiple sclerosis. Neurology 28:421-425, 1978.

69. Grattan, C. E. H., and Berman, P.: Chlamydial infection as a possible aetiological factor in the Guillain-Barré syndrome. Postgrad. Med. J. 58:776-777, 1982.

70. Green, S. H.: Polyradiculitis (Landry-Guillain-Barré syndrome) with total external ophthalmoplegia: Encephalo-myelo-radiculo-neuropathy. Dev. Med. Clin. Neurol. 13:369-373, 1976.

71. Griffin, J. W., and Ho, T. W. H.: The Guillain-Barré syndrome at 75: The *Campylobacter* connection. Ann. Neurol. 34:125-127, 1993.

72. Guillain, G., Barré, J. A., and Strohl, A.: Sur un syndrome de radiculonevrite avec hyperalbuminose du liquide cephalo-rachidien sans regraphiques des reflexes tendineux. Bull. Soc. Med. Hop. Paris 40:1462-1470, 1916.

73. Gunderman, J. R.: Guillain-Barré syndrome: Occurrence following combined mumps-rubella vaccine. Am. J. Dis. Child. 125:834-835, 1973.

74. Hart, I. K., and Kennedy, P. G.: Guillain-Barré syndrome associated with cytomegalovirus infection. Q. J. M. 67:425-430, 1988.

75. Hartung, H., Willison, H., and Kieseier, B.: Acute immunoinflammatory neuropathy: Update on Guillain-Barré. Curr. Opin. Neurol. 15:571-577, 2002.

76. Hartung, H. P.: Immune-mediated demyelination. Ann. Neurol. 33:563-567, 1993.

77. Hartung, H. P., Hughes, R. A., Taylor, W. A., et al.: T-cell activation in Guillain-Barré syndrome and in MS: Elevated serum levels of soluble IL-2 receptors. Neurology 40:215-218, 1990.

78. Hartung, H. P., and Toyka, K. V.: T-cell and macrophage activation in experimental autoimmune neuritis and Guillain-Barré syndrome. Ann. Neurol. 27(Suppl.):S57-S63, 1990.

79. Haupt, W. F., Rosenow, F., van der Ven, C., et al.: Sequential treatment of Guillain-Barré syndrome with extracorporeal elimination and intravenous immunoglobulin. J. Neurol. Sci. 137:145-149, 1996.

80. Hemachudha, T., Griffin, D. E., Chen, W. W., et al.: Immunologic studies of rabies vaccination-induced Guillain-Barré syndrome. Neurology 38:375-378, 1988.

81. Hiraga, A., Mori, M., Ogawara, K., et al.: Differences in patterns of progression in demyelinating and axonal Guillain-Barré syndrome. Neurology 61:471-474, 2003.

82. Hiraga, A., Mori, M., Ogawara, K., et al.: Recovery patterns and long term prognosis for axonal Guillain-Barré syndrome. J. Neurol. Neurosurg. Psychiatry 76:719-722, 2005.

83. Higara, A., Kuwabara, S., Ogawara, K., et al.: Patterns and serial changes in electrodiagnostic abnormalities of axonal Guillain-Barré syndrome. Neurology 64:656-660, 2005.

84. Hirai, K., Kihara, M., Nakajima, F., et al.: Immunoadsorption therapy in Guillain-Barré syndrome. Pediatr. Neurol. 19:55-57, 1998.

85. Ho, T. W., Li, C. Y., Cornblath, D. R., et al.: Patterns of recovery in the Guillain-Barré syndromes. Neurology 48:695-700, 1997.

86. Hughes, R. A. C., Aslan, S., and Gray, I. A.: Lymphocyte subpopulations and suppression cell activity in acute polyradiculoneuritis (Guillain-Barré syndrome). Clin. Exp. Immunol. 51:448-454, 1983.

87. Hughes, R. A. C., Guillain-Barré Syndrome Steroid Trial Group: Double-blind trial of intravenous methylprednisolone in Guillain-Barré syndrome. Lancet 341:586-590, 1993.

88. Hughes, R. A. C., Kadlubowski, M., and Hufschmidt, A.: Treatment of acute inflammatory polyneuropathy. Ann. Neurol. 9(Suppl.):125-133, 1981.

89. Hughes, R. A. C., Raphael, J. C., and van Doorn, P. A.: Intravenous immunoglobulin for Guillain-Barré syndrome. Cochrane Database Syst. Rev. CD002063, 2006.

90. Hughes, R. A. C., Swan, A. V., van Koningsveld, R., and van Doorn, P. A.: Corticosteroids for Guillain-Barré syndrome. Cochrane Database Syst. Rev. CD001446, 2006.

91. Hughes, R. A., Wijdicks, E. F., Barohn, R., et al.: Practice parameter: Immunotherapy for Guillain-Barré syndrome. Neurology 61:736-740, 2003.

92. Hurwitz, E. S., Schonberger, L. B., Nelson, D. B., et al.: Guillain-Barré syndrome and the 1978-1979 influenza vaccine. N. Engl. J. Med. 304:1557-1561, 1981.

93. Iqbal, A., Oger, J. J.-F., and Arnason, B. G.: Cell-mediated immunity in idiopathic polyneuritis. Ann. Neurol. 9(Suppl.):65-68, 1981.

94. Jackson, A. L.: A clinical study of the Landry-Guillain-Barré syndrome with reference to aetiology, including the role of coxsackie virus infections. S. Afr. J. Lab. Clin. Med. 7:121-137, 1961.

95. Jacobs, B. C., Endtz, H., van der Meche, F. G., et al.: Serum anti-GQ1b IgG antibodies recognize surface epitopes on *Campylobacter jejuni* from patients with Miller Fisher syndrome. Ann. Neurol. 37:260-264, 1995.

96. Jansen, P. W., Perkin, R. M., and Ashwal, S.: Guillain-Barré syndrome in childhood: Natural course and efficacy of plasmapheresis. Pediatr. Neurol. 9:16-20, 1993.

97. Kabins, S., Keller, R., Peitchel, R., et al.: Acute idiopathic polyneuritis caused by cytomegalovirus. Arch. Intern. Med. 136:100-101, 1976.

98. Kaldor, J., and Speed, B. R.: Guillain-Barré syndrome and *Campylobacter jejuni*: A serological study. B. M. J. 288:1867-1870, 1984.

99. Kanda, T., Hayashi, H., Tanabe, H., et al.: A fulminant case of Guillain-Barré syndrome: Topographic and fibre size related analysis of demyelinating changes. J. Neurol. Neurosurg. Psychiatry 52:857-864, 1989.

100. Kaplan, J. E., Katona, P., Hurwitz, E. S., et al.: Guillain-Barré syndrome in the United States, 1979-1980 and 1980-1981: Lack of an association with influenza vaccination. J. A. M. A. 248:696-700, 1982.

101. Kennedy, R. H., Danielson, M. A., Mulder, D. W., et al.: Guillain-Barré syndrome: A 42 year epidemiologic and clinical study. Mayo Clin. Proc. 53:93-99, 1978.

102. Kibrich, S.: Current status of coxsackie and Echo viruses in human disease. Prog. Med. Virol. 6:27-70, 1964.

103. Kinnunen, E., Färkkilä, M., Hovi, T., et al.: Incidence of Guillain-Barré syndrome during a nationwide oral poliovirus vaccine campaign. Neurology 39:1034-1036, 1989.

104. Kisch, A. L.: Guillain-Barré syndrome following smallpox vaccination: Report of a case. N. Engl. J. Med. 258:83, 1958.

105. Kleyweg, R. P., van der Meche, F. G., Loonen, M. C., et al.: The natural history of the Guillain-Barré syndrome in 18 children and 50 adults. J. Neurol. Neurosurg. Psychiatry 52:853-856, 1989.

106. Knowles, M., Saunders, M., Currie, S., et al.: Lymphocyte transformation in the Guillain-Barré syndrome. Lancet 2:1168-1170, 1969.

107. Korinthenberg, R., Schessl, J., Kirschner, J. Mönting, J. S.: Intravenously administered immunoglobulin in the treatment of childhood Guillain-Barré syndrome: A randomized trial. Pediatrics 116:8-14, 2005.

108. Koski, C. L.: Characterization of complement-fixing antibodies to peripheral nerve myelin in Guillain-Barré syndrome. Ann. Neurol. 27(Suppl.):S44-S47, 1990.

109. Koski, C. L., Chou, D. K., and Jungalwala, F. B.: Anti-peripheral nerve myelin antibodies in Guillain-Barré syndrome bind a neutral glycolipid of peripheral myelin and cross-react with Forssman antigen. J. Clin. Invest. 84:280-287, 1989.

110. Kuwabara, S.: Guillain-Barré syndrome: Epidemiology, pathophysiology and management. Drugs 64:597-610, 2004.

111. Kuwabara, S., Mori, M., Ogawara, K., et al.: Intravenous immunoglobulin therapy for Guillain-Barré syndrome with IgG anti-GM1 antibody. Muscle Nerve 24:54-58, 2001.

112. Kuwabara, S., Ogawa, K., Misawa, S., et al.: Does Campylobacter jejuni infection elicit "demyelinating" Guillain-Barré syndrome? Neurology 63:529-533, 2004.

113. Kuwabara, S., Yuki, N., Koga, M., et al.: IgG anti-GM1 antibody is associated with reversible conduction failure and axonal degeneration in Guillain-Barré syndrome. Ann. Neurol. 44:202-208, 1998.

114. Landry, O.: Note sur la paralysis ascendante aique. Gaz. Hebdom. Med. Chir. 6:472-474, 486-488, 1859.

115. Leneman, F.: The Guillain-Barré syndrome. Arch. Intern. Med. 118:139-144, 1966.

116. Lidin-Janson, G., and Strannegard, O.: Two cases of Guillain-Barré syndrome and encephalitis after measles. B. M. J. 2:572, 1972.

117. Lin, S. M., Ryu, S. T., and Liaw, Y. F.: Guillain-Barré syndrome associated with acute delta-hepatitis virus superinfection. J. Med. Virol. 28:144-145, 1989.

118. Link, H.: Immunoglobulin abnormalities in Guillain-Barré syndrome. J. Neurol. Sci. 18:11-23, 1973.

119. Lisak, R. P., Kuchmy, D., Armati-Gulsin, P. J., et al.: Serum-mediated Schwann cell cytotoxicity in the Guillain-Barré syndrome. Neurology 34:1240-1243, 1984.

120. Lisak, R. P., Zweiman, B., Guerrero, F., et al.: Circulating T-cell subsets in Guillain-Barré syndrome. J. Neuroimmunol. 8:93-101, 1985.

121. Loffel, N. B., Rossi, L. W., Mumenthaler, M., et al.: The Landry-Guillain-Barré syndrome: Complications, prognosis, and natural history in 123 cases. J. Neurol. Sci. 33:71-79, 1977.

122. Lopez, F., Lopez, J. H., Holquin, H., et al.: An outbreak of acute polyradiculoneuropathy in Columbia in 1968. Am. J. Epidemiol. 98:226-230, 1973.

123. Marshall, J.: The Landry-Guillain-Barré syndrome. Brain 86:55-66, 1963.

124. Marti-Masso, J. F., Obeso, J. A., Cosme, A., et al.: Guillain-Barré syndrome associated with a type B acute hepatitis. Med. Clin. (Barc.) 73:447-450, 1979.

125. Massei, F., et al.: Bartonella henselae infection associated with Guillain-Barré syndrome. Pediatr. Infect. Dis. J. 25:90-91, 2006.

126. Mazurek, J. M., et al.: The epidemiology and early clinical features of West Nile virus infection. Am. J. Emerg. Med. 23:536-543, 2005.

127. McFarlin, D. E.: Immunological parameters in Guillain-Barré syndrome. Ann. Neurol. 27(Suppl.):S25-S29, 1990.

128. McKhann, G. M.: Guillain-Barré syndrome: Clinical and therapeutic observations. Ann. Neurol. 27(Suppl.):S13-S16, 1990.

129. McKhann, G. M., Cornblath, D. R., Griffin, J. W., et al.: Acute motor axonal neuropathy: A frequent cause of acute placid paralysis in China. Ann. Neurol. 33:333-342, 1993.

130. McLeod, J. G., Walsh, J. C., Prineas, J. W., et al.: Acute idiopathic polyneuritis: A clinical and electrophysiological follow-up study. J. Neurol. Sci. 27:145-162, 1976.

131. Melnick, S. C.: Thirty-eight cases of the Guillain-Barré syndrome: An immunological study. B. M. J. 1:368-373, 1963.

132. Melnick, S. C., and Flewelt, T. H.: Role of infection in the Guillain-Barré syndrome. J. Neurol. Neurosurg. Psychiatry 27:385-407, 1964.

133. Menonna, J., Goldschmidt, B., Haidri, N., et al.: Herpes simplex virus IgM specific antibodies in Guillain-Barré syndrome and encephalitis. Acta Neurol. Scand. 56:223-231, 1977.

134. Mogale, K., Antony, J., and Ryan, M.: The pharyngeal-cervical-brachial form of Guillain-Barré syndrome in childhood. J. Pediatr. Neurol. 33:285-288, 2005.

135. Mori, M., Kuwabara, S., Miyake, M., et al.: Haemophilus influenzae infection and Guillain-Barré syndrome. Brain 123:2171-2178, 2000.

136. Moulin, D. E., Hagen, N., Hahn, A., et al.: Pain in Guillain-Barré syndrome. Neurology 48:328-331, 1997.

137. Mozes, B., Pines, A., Sayar, Y., et al.: Guillain-Barré syndrome associated with acute cytomegalovirus mononucleosis syndrome. Eur. Neurol. 23:237-239, 1984.

138. Mushinski, J. F., Taniguchi, R. M., and Stiefel, J. W.: Guillain-Barré syndrome associated with ulceroglandular tularemia. Neurology 14:877-879, 1964.

139. Ng, P. L., Powell, I. W., and Campbell, C. P.: Guillain-Barré syndrome during the pre-icteric phase of acute type B viral hepatitis. Aust. N. Z. J. Med. 5:367-369, 1975.

140. Nguyen, D. K., Agenarioti-Belanger, S., and Vanasse, M.: Pain and the Guillain-Barré syndrome in children under 6 years old. J. Pediatr. 134:773-776, 1999.

141. Novak, M.: Guillain-Barré syndrome as a sequela of influenza. Cesk. Neurol. Neurochir. 38:314-316, 1975.

142. Nowicki, J.: Neurological syndromes occurring in the course of influenza. Neurol. Neurochir. Pol. 7:695-699, 1973.

143. Nyland, H., Matre, R., and Mork, S.: Immunological characterization of sural nerve biopsies from patients with Guillain-Barré syndrome. Ann. Neurol. 9(Suppl.):80-86, 1981.

144. Oames, P. G., Jacobs, B. C., Hazenberg, M. P. H., et al.: Anti-GM1 IgG antibodies and Campylobacter bacteria in Guillain-Barré syndrome: Evidence of molecular mimicry. Ann. Neurol. 38:170, 1995.

145. Odaka, M., Yuki, N., Kuwabara, S., et al.: Bickerstaff's brainstem encephalitis: Clinical features of 62 cases and a subgroup associated with Guillain-Barré syndrome. Brain 126:2279-2290, 2003.

146. Ogawara, K., Kuwabara, S., Mori, M., et al.: Axonal Guillain-Barré syndrome: Relation to anti-ganglioside antibodies and Campylobacter jejuni infection in Japan. Ann. Neurol. 48:624-631, 2000.

147. Oh, S. J., LaGanke, C., and Claussen, G. C.: Sensory Guillain-Barré syndrome. Neurology 56:82-86, 2001.

148. Oka, N., Akiguchi, I., Kawasaki, T., et al.: Elevated serum levels of endothelial leukocyte adhesion molecules in Guillain-Barré syndrome and chronic inflammatory demyelinating polyneuropathy. Ann. Neurol. 35:621-624, 1994.

149. Osler, L. D., and Sidell, A. D.: The Guillain-Barré syndrome: The need for exact diagnostic criteria. N. Engl. J. Med. 262:964-969, 1960.

150. Pandey, C. K., Bose, N., Garg, G., et al.: Gabapentin for the treatment of pain in Guillain-Barré syndrome: A double blinded, placebo controlled, crossover study. Anesth. Analg. 95:1719-1723, 2002.

151. Pandey, C. K., Raza, M., Tripathi, M., et al.: The comparative evaluation of gabapentin and carbamazepine for pain management in Guillain-Barré syndrome patients in the ICU. Anesth. Analg. 101:220-225, 2005.

152. Paradiso, G., Tripoli, J., Galicchio, S., et al.: Epidemiological, clinical and electrodiagnostic findings in childhood Guillain-Barré syndrome: A reappraisal. Ann. Neurol. 46:701-707, 1999.

153. Parker, W., Witt, J. C., Dawson, J. W., et al.: Landry-Guillain-Barré syndrome: The isolation of an Echovirus type 6. Can. Med. Assoc. J. 82:813-815, 1960.

154. Partnow, M. J., Devereaux, M. W., and Humphries, T. S.: Infectious hepatitis and the Guillain-Barré syndrome. J. Med. Soc. N. J. 77:118-120, 1980.

155. Penney, M. D., Murphy, D., and Walters, G.: Resetting of osmoreceptor response as cause of hyponatremia in acute idiopathic polyneuritis. B. M. J. 2:1474-1476, 1979.

156. Phillips, P. E.: Guillain-Barré syndrome after measles. B. M. J. 4:50-57, 1972.

157. Plachy, U., Lichy, J., Horacek, J., et al.: Polyradiculoneuritis syndrome in cytomegalovirus infection. Cesk. Neurol. Neurochir. 42:396-401, 1979.

158. Plough, J. C., and Ayerle, R. S.: The Guillain-Barré syndrome associated with acute hepatitis. N. Engl. J. Med. 249:61-62, 1953.

159. Pollard, J. D., Westland, K. W., Harvey, G. K., et al.: Activated T cells of non-neural specificity open the blood-nerve barrier to circulating antibody. Ann. Neurol. 37:467-475, 1995.

160. Prineas, J. W.: Acute idiopathic polyneuritis: An electron microscopic study. Lab. Invest. 26:133-146, 1972.

161. Prineas, J. W.: Pathology of the Guillain-Barré syndrome. Ann. Neurol. 9(Suppl.):6-19, 1981.

162. Pryor, W. M., Freiman, J. S., Gillies, M. A., et al.: Guillain-Barré syndrome associated with Campylobacter infection. Aust. N. Z. J. Med. 14:687, 1984.

163. Quarles, R. H., Ilyas, A. A., and Willison, H. J.: Antibodies to gangliosides and myelin proteins in Guillain-Barré syndrome. Ann. Neurol. 27(Suppl.):S48-S52, 1990.

164. Raman, P. T., and Taori, G. M.: Prognostic significance of electrodiagnostic studies in the Guillain-Barré syndrome. J. Neurol. Neurosurg. Psychiatry 39:163-170, 1976.

165. Rantala, H., Cherry, J. D., Shields, W. D., et al.: Epidemiology of Guillain-Barré syndrome in children: Relationship of oral polio vaccine administration to occurrence. J. Pediatr. *124*:220-223, 1994.
166. Raphael, J. C., Chevret, S., Hughes, R. A., and Annane, D.: Plasma exchange for Guillain-Barré syndrome. Cochrane Database Syst. Rev. CD001798, 2002.
167. Rees, J. H., Gregson, N. A., and Hughes, R. A. C.: Anti-ganglioside GM1 antibodies in Guillain-Barré syndrome and their relationship to *Campylobacter jejuni* infection. Ann. Neurol. *38*:809-816, 1995.
168. Rees, J. H., and Hughes, R. A. C.: *Campylobacter jejuni* and Guillain-Barré syndrome. Ann. Neurol. *35*:248-249, 1994.
169. Rees, J. H., Soudain, S. E., Gregson, N. A., et al.: *Campylobacter jejuni* infection and Guillain Barré syndrome. N. Engl. J. Med. *333*:1374-1379, 1995.
170. Reuben, S., Mathai, A., Sumi, M. G., et al.: Significance of serum antibody to GD1b ganglioside in patients with Guillain-Barré syndrome. Indian J. Med. Res. *113*:234-238, 2001.
171. Rhodes, K. M., and Tattersfield, A. E.: Guillain-Barré syndrome associated with *Campylobacter* infection. B. M. J. *285*:173-174, 1982.
172. Richter, R. B.: The ataxic form of polyradiculoneuritis (Landry-Guillain-Barré syndrome). J. Neuropathol. Exp. Neurol. *21*:171-184, 1962.
173. Rocha, M. S. G., et al.: Epidemiologic features of Guillain-Barré syndrome in Sao Paulo, Brazil. Arq. Neuro-Psiq. *62*:33-37, 2004.
174. Rocklin, R. E., Sheremata, W. A., Feldman, R. G., et al.: The Guillain-Barré syndrome and multiple sclerosis: In vitro cellular responses to nervous tissue antigens. N. Engl. J. Med. *284*:803-808, 1971.
175. Ropper, A. H., and Kehne, S. M.: Guillain-Barré syndrome: Management of respiratory failure. Neurology *35*:1662-1665, 1985.
176. Ropper, A. H., and Shahani, B. T.: Pain in Guillain-Barré syndrome. Arch. Neurol. *41*:511-514, 1984.
177. Rossi, L. N., Mumenthaler, M., Lutschg, J., et al.: Guillain-Barré syndrome in children with special reference to the natural history of 38 personal cases. Neuropadiatrie 7:42-51, 1976.
178. Ryan, M.: Guillain-Barré syndrome in childhood. J. Pediatr. Child Health *41*:237-241, 2005.
179. Ryberg, B.: Extra- and intrathecal production of antinerve and antibrain antibodies in Guillain-Barré syndrome: Evaluation by an antibody index. Neurology *34*:1378-1381, 1984.
180. Saeed, A. A., and Lange, L. S.: Guillain-Barré syndrome after rubella. Postgrad. Med. J. *54*:333-334, 1978.
181. Saida, T., Saida, K., Lisak, R. P., et al.: In vivo demyelinating activity of sera from patients with Guillain-Barré syndrome. Ann. Neurol. *11*:69-75, 1982.
182. Saida, T., Saida, K., Silbergerg, D. H., et al.: Transfer of demyelination by intraneural injection of experimental allergic neuritis serum. Nature *272*:639-641, 1978.
183. Sakakihara, Y., and Kamoshita, S.: Age-associated changes in the symptomatology of Guillain-Barré syndrome in children. Dev. Med. Child Neurol. *31*:611-616, 1991.
184. Samantray, S. K., Johnson, S. C., Mathai, K. V., et al.: Landry-Guillain-Barré-Strohl syndrome: A study of 302 cases. Med. J. Aust. 2:84-91, 1977.
185. Schmitz, H., and Enders, G.: Cytomegalovirus as a frequent cause of Guillain-Barré syndrome. J. Med. Virol. *1*:21-27, 1977.
186. Schonberger, L. B., Bergman, D. J., Sullivan-Bolyai, J. Z., et al.: Guillain-Barré syndrome following vaccination in the national influenza immunization program, United States, 1976-1977. Am. J. Epidemiol. *110*:105-123, 1979.
187. Schonberger, L. B., Hurwitz, E. S., Katona, P., et al.: Guillain-Barré syndrome: Its epidemiology and associations with influenza vaccination. Ann. Neurol. *9*(Suppl.):31-38, 1981.
188. Seneviratne, U., and Gunasekera, S.: Acute small fibre sensory neuropathy: Another variant of Guillain-Barré syndrome? J. Neurol. Sci. *196*:41-44, 2002.
189. Sharief, M. K., McLean, B., Thompson, E. J.: Elevated serum levels of tumor necrosis factor in Guillain-Barré syndrome. Ann. Neurol. *33*:591-596, 1993.
190. Sheikh, K. A., Nachamkin, I., Ho, T. W., et al.: *Campylobacter jejuni* lipopolysaccharides in Guillain-Barré syndrome: Molecular mimicry and host susceptibility. Neurology *51*:371-378, 1998.
191. Shermata, W., and Behan, P. O.: Experimental allergic neuritis: A new experimental approach. J. Neurol. Neurosurg. Psychiatry *36*:139-145, 1973.
192. Sheremata, W., Colby, S., Lusky, G., et al.: Cellular hypersensitization to peripheral nervous antigens in the Guillain-Barré syndrome. Neurology *25*:833-839, 1975.
193. Sheremata, W., Eylar, E. H., Szymanska, I., et al.: Peripheral nerve myelin P2 protein in influenza vaccine. Ann. Neurol. *10*:91-92, 1981.
194. Siebert, D. G., and Seals, J. E.: Polyneuropathy after herpes simplex type 2 meningitis. South. Med. J. 77:1476, 1984.
195. Soffer, D., Feldman, S., and Alter, M.: Epidemiology of Guillain-Barré syndrome. Neurology *28*:686-690, 1978.
196. Stapleton, F. D., Skoglund, R. R., and Daggett, R. B.: Hypertension associated with the Guillain-Barré syndrome. Pediatrics *62*:588-590, 1978.
197. Steinberg, A. D.: Modulation of a complex immune system. Ann. Neurol. *9*(Suppl.):117-124, 1981.
198. Steiner, I., Argov, Z., Cahan, C., et al.: Guillain-Barré syndrome after epidural anesthesia: Direct nerve root damage may trigger disease. Neurology *35*:1473-1475, 1985.
199. Tabor, E.: Guillain-Barré syndrome and other neurologic syndromes in hepatitis A, B, and non-A, non-B. J. Med. Virol. *21*:207-216, 1987.
200. Takahashi, M., Koga, M., Yokoyama, K., and Yuki, N.: Epidemiology of *Campylobacter jejuni* isolated from patients with Guillain-Barré and Fisher syndromes in Japan. J. Clin. Microbiol. *43*:335-339, 2005.
201. Taylor, W. A., and Hughes, R. A.: T lymphocyte activation antigens in Guillain-Barré syndrome and chronic idiopathic demyelinating polyradiculoneuropathy. J. Neuroimmunol. *24*:33-39, 1989.
202. Tekgul, H., Serdaroglu, G., and Tutuncuoglu, S.: Outcome of axonal and demyelinating form of Guillain-Barré syndrome in children. Pediatr. Neurol. *28*:295-299, 2003.
203. Tindall, R. S. A., Zinn, P., and Rosenberg, R. N.: Humoral immunity in the Guillain-Barré syndrome: Evidence for circulating IgG and IgM. Neurology *30*:362-363, 1980.
204. Tsukada, N., Koh, C. S., Inoue, A., et al.: Demyelinating neuropathy associated with hepatitis B virus infection: Detection of immune complexes composed of hepatitis B virus surface antigen. J. Neurol. Sci. 77:203-216, 1987.
205. Uhari, M., Rantala, H., and Niemela, M.: Cluster of childhood Guillain-Barré cases after an oral polio vaccine campaign. Lancet 2:440-441, 1989.
206. Usui, T., Hammada, Y., and Anta, M.: A case of Guillain-Barré associated with coxsackie. Tok. J. Exp. Med. *21*:17-19, 1974.
207. Vajsar, J., Sloane, A., Wood, E., et al.: Plasmapheresis vs. intravenous immunoglobulin treatment in childhood Guillain-Barré syndrome. Arch. Pediatr. Adolesc. Med. *148*:1210-1212, 1994.
208. Van der Meche, F. G., and van Doorn, P. A.: Guillain-Barré syndrome and chronic inflammatory demyelinating polyneuropathy: Immune mechanisms and update on current therapies. Ann. Neurol. *37*(Suppl. 1):S14-S31, 1995.
209. Van der Meche, F. G. A., et al.: Diagnostic and classification criteria for the Guillain-Barré syndrome. Eur. Neurol. *45*:133-139, 2001.
210. Verma, A. K., Maheshwari, M. C., Chardhary, C., et al.: Acute ascending motor paralysis due to rabies: A clinicopathological report. Eur. Neurol. *24*:160-162, 1985.
211. Vriesendorp, F. J., Mishu, B., Blasher, M. J., et al.: Serum antibodies to GM1, GD1b, peripheral nerve myelin, and *Campylobacter jejuni* in patients with Guillain-Barré syndrome and controls: Correlation and prognosis. Ann. Neurol. *34*:130-135, 1993.
212. Vriesendorp, F. J., Triggs, W. J., Mayer, R. F., et al.: Electrophysiological studies in Guillain-Barré syndrome: Correlation with antibodies to GM1, GD1b and *Campylobacter jejuni*. J. Neurol. *242*:460-465, 1995.
213. Vucic, S., Cairns, K. D., Black, K. R., et al.: Neurophysiologic findings in early acute inflammatory demyelinating polyradiculoneuropathy. Clin. Neurophysiol. *115*:2329-2335, 2004.
214. Vyravanathan, S., and Senanayake, N.: Guillain-Barré syndrome associated with tuberculosis. Postgrad. Med. J. *59*:516-517, 1983.
215. Waksman, B. H., and Adams, R. D.: Allergic neuritis: An experimental disease of rabbits induced by the injection of peripheral nervous tissue and adjuvants. J. Exp. Med. *102*:213-235, 1955.
216. Welch, R. G.: Chickenpox and the Guillain-Barré syndrome. Arch. Dis. Child. *37*:557-559, 1962.
217. Wells, C. E. C., James, W. R. I., and Evans, A. D.: Guillain-Barré syndrome and virus of influenza A (Asian strain): Report of two fatal cases during the 1957 epidemic in Wales. Arch. Neurol. Psychiatry *81*:699-705, 1959.
218. Whitaker, J. N., Hirano, A., Cook, S. D., et al.: The ultrastructure of circulating immunocytes in Guillain-Barré syndrome. Neurology *20*:765-770, 1970.
219. WHO—World Health Organization, and Arien, A. H. C.: Acute onset flaccid paralysis. Geneva, World Health Organization, 1993.
220. Willison, H. J., Veitch, J., Paterson, G., et al.: Miller Fisher syndrome is associated with serum antibodies to GQ1b ganglioside. J. Neurol. Neurosurg. Psychiatry *56*:204-206, 1993.
221. Winer, J. B., Hughes, R. A. C., Greenwood, R. J., et al.: Prognosis in Guillain-Barré syndrome. Lancet *1*:1202-1203, 1985.
222. Winkler, G. F.: In vitro demyelination of peripheral nerve induced with sensitized cells. Ann. N. Y. Acad. Sci. *122*:287-296, 1965.
223. Winkler, G. F., and Arnason, B. G. W.: Antiserum to immunoglobulin A: Inhibition of cell mediated demyelination in tissue culture. Science *153*:75-76, 1966.
224. Wisniewski, H., Terry, R. D., Whitaker, J. N., et al.: The Landry-Guillain-Barré syndrome: A primary demyelinating disease. Arch. Neurol. *21*:269-276, 1969.
225. Yoshii, F., and Shinohara, Y.: Lymphocyte subset proportions in Guillain-Barré syndrome patients treated with plasmapheresis. Eur. Neurol. *44*:162-167, 2000.
226. Yu, R. K., Ariga, T., Kobriyama, T., et al.: Autoimmune mechanisms in peripheral neuropathies. Ann. Neurol. *27*(Suppl.):S30-S35, 1990.
227. Yuki, N.: Infectious origins of, and molecular mimicry in, Guillain-Barré and Fisher syndromes. Lancet Infect. Dis. *1*:29-37, 2001.
228. Yuki, N., Taki, T., Takahasi, M., et al.: Molecular mimicry between GQ1b ganglioside and lipopolysaccharides of *Campylobacter jejuni* isolated from patients with Fisher's syndrome. Ann. Neurol. *36*:791-793, 1994.
229. Yuki, N., Wim-Ang, C., Koga, M., et al.: Clinical features and response to treatment in Guillain-Barré syndrome associated with antibodies to GM1b ganglioside. Ann. Neurol. *47*:314-321, 2000.

GENITOURINARY TRACT INFECTIONS

URETHRITIS

Ellen R. Wald

Urethritis refers to inflammation of the urethra and periurethral tissues in males and females. It may be associated with a variety of infectious and noninfectious disorders.

EPIDEMIOLOGY

The cause of urethritis varies with the age of the patient, sexual practices, and hygienic standards.[10,45] *Chlamydia* infections and gonorrhea are common occurrences in adolescents; fecal contamination or irritation caused by physical or chemical substances is a more usual occurrence in preschool-aged children. Transmission during sexual activity is the usual means of spread of *Neisseria gonorrhoeae* and *Chlamydia trachomatis* in teenagers and in sexually abused patients; nonvenereal transmission has been described in prepubertal children.[46] Manifestations after nonvenereal spread has occurred may include vaginitis, balanitis, and conjunctivitis in addition to urethritis.[13,46]

The home and social environments of prepubertal children must be examined to identify fully the pattern of spread and infection in the patient and contacts because complex psychosocial diagnoses and therapies often are involved.[38] Children with gonorrhea and chlamydial infections are concentrated in large urban centers, usually in poor socioeconomic environments.

Gonococcal infections in children 2 to 10 years of age should be considered evidence of probable sexual abuse.[1,19,21-23] Household contacts have been found to have positive cultures in 27 to 63 percent of such cases. Prepubertal girls infected with *N. gonorrhoeae* as a result of sexual abuse outnumber boys by a ratio of at least 3 : 1 and in one report 8 : 1.[15]

PATHOPHYSIOLOGY

Infection caused by *N. gonorrhoeae* usually is localized to the urethra in boys and to the vagina in girls; however, rectal carriage sometimes occurs in the absence of urethral colonization. Gonococcal virulence factors include pili, the ability to attach to urethral epithelial cells, and production of extracellular proteases that cleave IgA. Initial attachment of gonococci to the surface of columnar epithelial cells is mediated by pili, which are filamentous outer membrane appendages composed of multiple subunits, the most important of which is pilin.[44] Local invasion involves multiple adhesins interacting with host receptors at the mucosal cell level. After attachment occurs, gonococci become engulfed in a process known as parasite-directed endocytosis.[16] The organisms are able to undergo intracellular replication within phagocytic vacuoles and columnar epithelial cells, which is a successful adaptive response promoting survival.

Chlamydia infections are the most frequent cause of sexually transmitted disease in the United States.[6,9,51] Chlamydiae are structurally complex organisms that are obligate intracellular parasites and contain DNA and RNA. Attachment, which is not understood completely, is the first step in the infectious process of the susceptible host cell. It is followed by phagocytosis and then the failure of cellular lysosomes to fuse with the phagosome containing the elementary body, which may be mediated partly by macromolecules in the chlamydial cell envelope. After these two crucial events occur, the elementary bodies undergo biologic changes, and after approximately 72 hours, they are released from the host cell as new infective elementary bodies (Fig. 44–1).

Urethritis in younger children also may be caused by the introduction of fecal bacteria or pinworms into the urethra during the early years of toilet training, particularly in girls. Inflammation may be related to bubble baths and other chemical and physical irritants. Edema of the mucosa and the presence of inflammation and red blood cells are common histopathologic features of urethritis that lead to dysuria, hematuria, and microscopic pyuria.

CLINICAL PRESENTATION

Gonococcal urethritis is characterized by a 2- to 8-day incubation period after sexual intercourse. The onset often is sudden, with dysuria and copious urethral discharge in boys and leukorrhea in girls. The urethral discharge often is thick, profuse, and yellow. The patient usually has no fever. In prepubertal girls, leukorrhea is more prominent as a sign of gonococcal infection, and urethritis occurs less commonly. This difference may be related to the method of infection and to the different sensitivity of the vaginal epithelial surface to infection in a prepubertal child. Leukorrhea may be minimal in adolescent girls, and dysuria may be absent.[1]

Diagnosis often is made earlier in adolescent boys than in girls, perhaps because of the prominence of urethral discharge in boys and misinterpretation of the significance of leukorrhea in girls. Gonococcal urethritis also may cause asymptomatic pyuria in boys. Occasionally, prepubertal patients have conjunctivitis or balanitis without significant urethritis. Clinical presentations include systemic illness with fever, arthritis, and skin lesions secondary to bacteremia in 3 percent of untreated individuals with mucosal gonorrhea.[1] These lesions often begin on the extremities as small erythematous macules that progress to circular papules with an area of central necrosis.

The clinical presentation of nongonococcal urethritis may be similar to that described for gonorrhea, but it more commonly has a longer incubation period (often 8 to 14 days after sexual intercourse) and a scanty exudate, which may be clear in character and intermittent. This condition also is called nonspecific urethritis and may be present in association with or subsequent to gonococcal urethritis. In the latter case, the scant urethral discharge may persist after the patient has been treated for

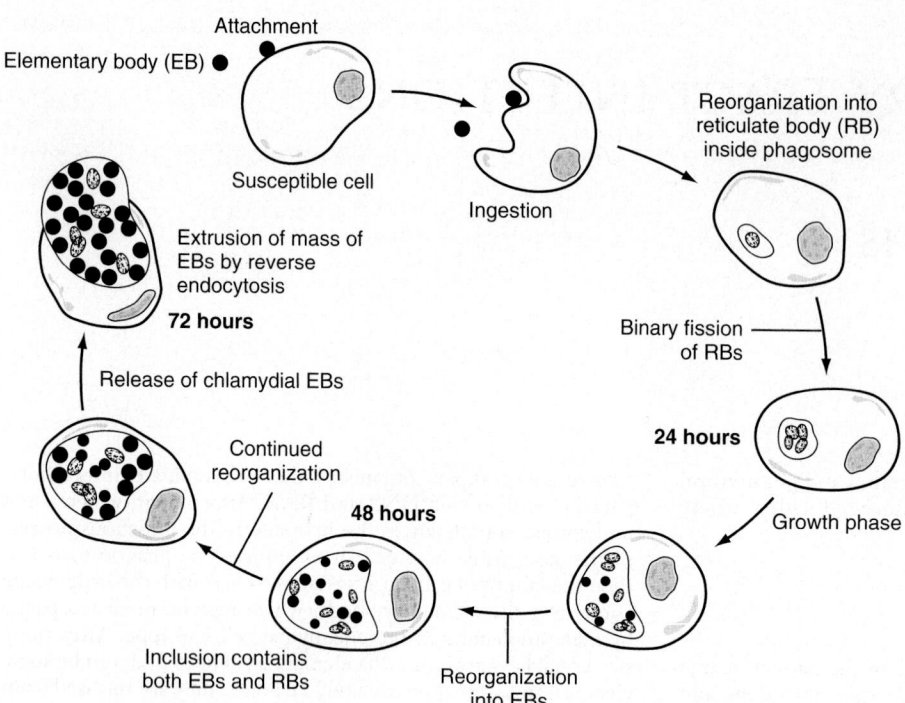

Figure 44–1 Schematic description of the growth cycle of *Chlamydia trachomatis*. (From Batteiger, B. E., and Jones, R. B.: Chlamydial infections. Infect. Dis. Clin. North Am. 1:55-81, 1987.)

gonorrhea. Asymptomatic urethral colonization with *C. trachomatis* also is reported in males.[49]

An equivalent syndrome, acute urethral syndrome, has been described in sexually active females. The patient experiences an acute onset of dysuria and increased frequency, and pyuria ($\geq$8 white blood cells/mm^3 of midstream urine) is a common finding. Bacterial cultures of the urine often are sterile or show less than 10^5 bacteria/mL; coliform bacteria, *Staphylococcus saprophyticus*, and *C. trachomatis* are the most common causes. Clinical expression of infection with *C. trachomatis* in adolescent girls is characterized by a yellowish, mucopurulent secretion at the cervical os.[7] However, infection with *C. trachomatis* may be asymptomatic in both sexes, an important consideration in designing effective strategies for diagnosis and management of sexual contacts.

A patient with urethritis caused by trauma may have hematuria and dysuria without fever. The trauma may be obvious or related to masturbation or introduction of foreign bodies into the urethra. Patients with urethritis secondary to bubble bath or soap usually have transient dysuria and no systemic signs. Fecal contamination of the urethra may be accompanied by hematuria, dysuria, and pyuria.

DIFFERENTIAL DIAGNOSIS

Table 44–1 lists the differential diagnoses for urethritis.

NONINFECTIOUS

Trauma, bubble bath, detergents found in shampoos, masturbation, radiation, dysfunctional elimination syndrome, and caustic substances may lead to the development of urethritis.[26] Urethritis also may be a component of several systemic syndromes, including erythema multiforme (Stevens-Johnson syndrome), Kawasaki disease, and occasionally other forms of allergy. Reiter syndrome denotes the association of nongonococcal urethritis with conjunctivitis and arthritis.

TABLE 44–1   Etiology of Urethritis

Infectious	Noninfectious
Sexually transmitted infections	**Vasculitides**
Neisseria gonorrhoeae	Reiter syndrome
Chlamydia trachomatis	Erythema multiforme
Trichomonas vaginalis	Kawasaki disease
Herpes simplex virus type 2	
Mycoplasma spp.	**Mechanical**
	Masturbation
Non–sexually transmitted infections	Foreign body
Staphylococcus saprophyticus	Trauma
Enterobacteriaceae	
Gardnerella vaginalis	**Chemical**
Streptococcus spp.	Soaps
Enterobius vermicularis	Detergents
	Drugs

INFECTIOUS

The most common forms of urethritis in sexually active adolescents and young adults are gonococcal and so-called nongonococcal urethritis. They may occur together or sequentially. Nongonococcal urethritis has been related causally to infections with *C. trachomatis* in approximately 30 to 50 percent of cases and with *Ureaplasma urealyticum* (T-strain mycoplasma) in approximately 25 percent of cases of nongonococcal, nonchlamydial urethritis in males.[7,50] The remaining cases of infectious urethritis in postpubescent, sexually active patients may be caused by a variety of pathogenic microorganisms, including *Gardnerella vaginalis*, *Mycoplasma hominis*, *Trichomonas vaginalis*, *Candida albicans*, herpes simplex virus type 2, *Treponema pallidum* (syphilis), and other bacteria, such as staphylococci, Enterobacteriaceae, and occasionally streptococci including group B.[18]

Mycoplasma genitalium is a newer species, first isolated from males with urethritis.[8,28] Studies also have implicated a causative role in *Chlamydia*-negative nongonococcal urethritis for anaerobic organisms of the *Bacteroides* spp., in particular *Bacteroides urealyticus*.

In younger children, urethritis usually has noninfectious causes as outlined earlier. Gonorrhea, *Chlamydia*, and fecal bacteria may be important as well.

SPECIFIC DIAGNOSIS

A standard method for diagnosing gonorrhea in a sexually active male is to obtain urethral discharge by manually stripping the urethra or, if that is unproductive, by gently inserting a swab 2 to 3 cm into the distal urethra. The best culture technique for isolating *N. gonorrhoeae*, a fastidious organism, is immediate inoculation of this material onto a selective growth medium, such as regular or modified Thayer-Martin agar. Any delay in inoculation of the plates necessitates the use of a transport method with growth media in a carbon dioxide environment that support the gonococcus at ambient temperatures. These media protect the organism from its marked susceptibility to the effects of drying, cold, and overgrowth by other bacteria. Urethral exudate from a male patient should be Gram-stained at the same time; typical kidney bean–shaped, gram-negative, intracellular diplococci are presumptively diagnostic, with a sensitivity and specificity approaching 100 percent (Fig. 44–2).

Putative gonococcal colonies should be confirmed by oxidase reaction, Gram staining, sugar use tests, rapid enzyme tests, nucleic acid probes, or agglutination reactions with antibodies specific for *N. gonorrhoeae*. The last four tests are especially important in evaluating sites of infection (e.g., the pharynx) or populations of patients with a low prevalence of gonorrhea.

Sexually active females with urethritis also should undergo urethral culture. Although the Gram stain of cervical secretions is only 66 percent sensitive in detecting *N. gonorrhoeae* in adolescent girls, the finding of kidney bean–shaped, intracellular gram-negative diplococci is highly specific and helpful.[52] Vaginal, cervical, and rectal swabs are recommended. Asymptomatic colonization with gonococci seems to occur most commonly in female patients, although it has been described in adolescent boys.[1,25] Pharyngitis, conjunctivitis, balanitis, and other, less common, manifestations of gonorrhea may coexist with urethritis. Samples obtained from these sites should be handled as described earlier. Blood agar and other specialized media may be indicated to identify nongonococcal causes of urethritis.

Nucleic acid amplification (NAA) tests are highly sensitive and specific when used on urethral (males), endocervical swab, and urine specimens.[9] These tests include polymerase chain reaction, transcription-mediated amplification (TMA), and strand displacement assays. Only the TMA assay is approved by the U.S. Food and Drug Administration for testing vaginal swabs from postmenarcheal females. Use of urine specimens increases the feasibility of initial testing and follow-up of hard-to-access populations such as adolescents.[1] These techniques also permit dual testing of urine for *C. trachomatis* and *N. gonorrhoeae*. NAA tests are not recommended for rectal and pharyngeal swabs.[1] Although none of these tests is superior to culture, their ease of use (for urine or self-obtained specimens) renders them extremely attractive.

Gonococcal urethritis in prepubescent boys is diagnosed as described earlier for adolescent boys. Vaginal swabs are most useful in female patients, although vaginal discharge may not be prominent. Endocervical cultures are not recommended for the diagnosis of gonorrhea in prepubescent girls. The yield of vaginal swabs seems to be adequate for most diagnostic purposes; rectal swabs also may be useful in female patients. Showing kidney bean–shaped, gram-negative, intracellular diplococci in a prepubescent boy and girl is useful for establishing a presumptive diagnosis and instituting therapy. Confirmation by culture as described for a sexually active male is necessary.

Other infectious causes of urethritis may be diagnosed by specific techniques, including wet mount for *Trichomonas*, Gram stain and culture on Sabouraud dextrose agar for *C. albicans*, and culture for herpes simplex virus, used in the patients and their contacts. New culture techniques for *Chlamydia*, such as the use of microtiter cell monolayers, have increased the recovery rates, decreased the cost, and shortened the turn-around time for the isolation of *C. trachomatis*.[3] The rigorous transport conditions and the small number of laboratories with cell culture techniques have limited the availability of *Chlamydia* cultures; however, noncultural methods, including direct immunofluorescence staining of smears with use of monoclonal antibodies,[3,20,27,34,47] enzyme-linked immunosorbent assay (ELISA) techniques, and NAA testing, are available.

The use of immunofluorescence and ELISA techniques has been surpassed in sensitivity and ease of use by NAA testing.

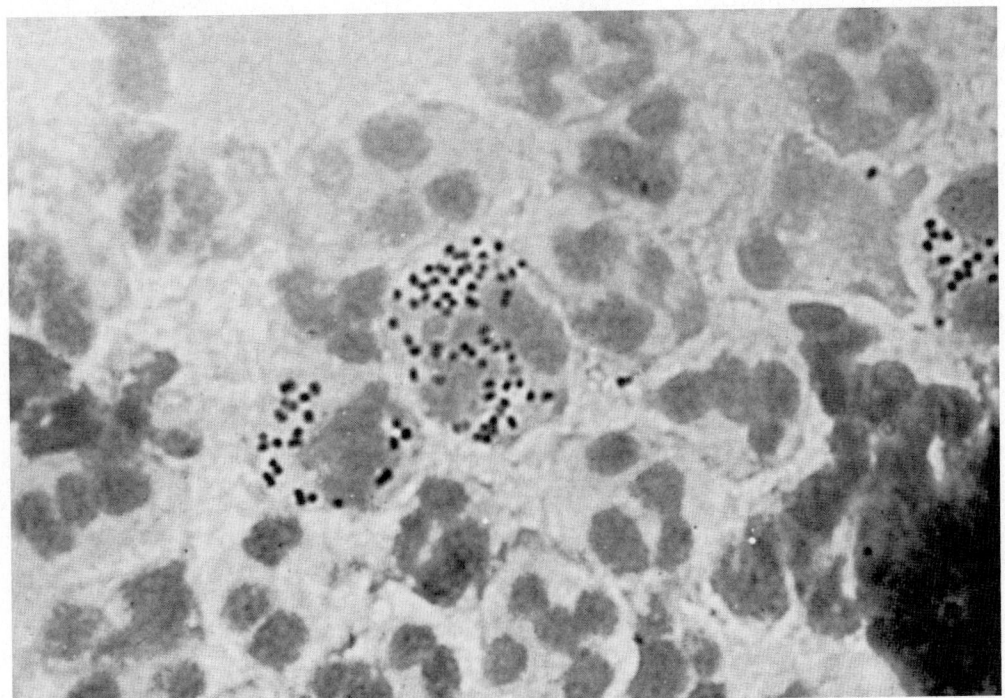

Figure 44–2 Gram-stained smear of urethral discharge from a teenage boy with gonorrhea.

NAA tests such as polymerase chain reaction, TMA, and strand displacement assays are available and are more sensitive than cell culture, DNA probe, direct fluorescent antibody tests, or ELISAs, although specificity varies compared with culture.[1] Polymerase chain reaction, strand displacement assay, and TMA are useful for evaluating urine specimens from either sex. The Food and Drug Administration has approved TMA for testing vaginal swabs from postmenarcheal adolescents. NAA tests are not recommended for specimens obtained from rectal or pharyngeal swabs or for urethral swabs from females.

When documentation of infection is being sought in cases of suspected child abuse, the performance of cultures is strongly preferred and may be the only acceptable test in certain jurisdictions.[1] When culture is unavailable, some experts support using NAA testing if a positive result can be verified by another NAA test. ELISA and fluorescent antibody tests should not be used for testing rectal, vaginal, or urethral specimens from infants and children because of low sensitivity and specificity.[1] Ligase chain reaction seems to be substantially more sensitive in children than is culture for *Chlamydia*.[17,31]

Ureaplasma and other genital *Mycoplasma* spp. can be identified only by culture at this time. This test should be reserved for the evaluation of recurrent cases of urethritis with poor response to treatment.[8,27] Specimens of urethral and vaginal discharge secondary to fecal contamination and foreign bodies can be examined by conventional diagnostic bacterial techniques.

TREATMENT

Table 44–2 presents antibiotic regimens for treatment of urethritis. The treatment of urethritis should include treatment of the sexual partners of the index case to avoid reinfection and further spread of infection. Patients with urethritis frequently have mixed infections with *N. gonorrhoeae* and the pathogens linked with nongonococcal urethritis, such as *C. trachomatis* and *U. urealyticum*. Concurrent infection with *N. gonorrhoeae* and *C. trachomatis* is documented frequently. In a survey of adolescents admitted to juvenile detention centers throughout the United States, screening for sexually transmitted infections was performed on adolescent girls with gonorrhea. Fifty-four percent were coinfected with chlamydia; of adolescent boys infected with gonorrhea, 51 percent were coinfected with *Chlamydia*.[30] A study determining chlamydia and gonorrhea co-occurrence in a high school population showed similar results: of 117 students with gonorrhea, 50 (42.7%) had chlamydia; of 451 with chlamydia, 50 (11.1%) had gonorrhea.[39] Patients with gonococcal urethritis also are at risk for development of early incubating syphilis. One must consider these factors and the possibility of systemic infection when choosing a treatment regimen for urethritis.[36]

Sexual abuse is the most common cause of gonococcal infection among children 2 to 10 years of age. Anorectal and pharyngeal infections with *N. gonorrhoeae* are common and frequently asymptomatic occurrences among these patients.[37]

In 2006, the Centers for Disease Control and Prevention (CDC) published treatment guidelines for sexually transmitted diseases, including urethritis (see Table 44–2). Every attempt should be made to ascertain the specific diagnosis. If doing so is impossible, the treatment regimen chosen always should be appropriate for nongonococcal urethritis and gonococcal infection. The emergence of penicillin-resistant and tetracycline-resistant strains of *N. gonorrhoeae* has led to the abandonment of penicillin and tetracycline for the treatment of gonorrhea.[14]

Single-dose azithromycin for nongonococcal urethritis and either intramuscular or oral single-dose regimens for uncomplicated gonococcal infections are likely to increase compliance.[23,24,32,35,40,41,48,53] Test of cure is not indicated for uncomplicated gonococcal or chlamydial infection when single-dose treatment

TABLE 44–2   Antibiotic Regimen for Urethritis

Nongonococcal Urethritis	
Recommended regimen	Azithromycin 1 g orally in a single dose
	or
	Doxycycline 100 mg orally bid for 7 days
Alternative regimen	Erythromycin base 500 mg qid for 7 days
	or
	Erythromycin ethylsuccinate 800 mg qid for 7 days
	or
	Ofloxacin 300 mg bid for 7 days
	or
	Levofloxacin 500 mg once daily for 7 days
Chlamydial Infection	
Recommended regimen (adults and adolescents)	Azithromycin 1 g orally in a single dose
	or
	Doxycycline 100 mg orally bid for 7 days
Alternative regimens	Erythromycin base 500 mg qid for 7 days
	or
	Erythromycin ethylsuccinate 800 mg qid for 7 days
	Ofloxacin 300 mg bid for 7 days
	or
	Levofloxacin 500 mg once daily for 7 days
Children	
<45 kg	Erythromycin 50 mg/kg/day qid for 14 days
≥45 kg and <8 years old	Azithromycin 1 g orally in a single dose
>8 years old	Use same regimen as for adults
Gonococcal Infection	
Recommended regimen (adults and adolescents)	Ceftriaxone 125 mg IM in a single dose
	or
	Cefixime 400 mg orally in a single dose
	plus
	Regimen effective for *Chlamydia*
Children	
<45 kg	Ceftriaxone 125 mg IM in a single dose
If bacteremia, arthritis, or meningitis	Ceftriaxone 50-100 mg/kg/day (maximum 2 g/day) IV for 7-14 days
≥45 kg	Use adult regimen

bid, twice a day; IM, intramuscularly; IV, intravenously; qid, four times a day.

regimens are used.[9] Emergence of resistance to quinolones initially restricted the use of these drugs in cases of gonorrhea that originated from California, Hawaii, and Asia,[1,4,9] However, in 2007, the CBC recommended that fluoroquinolones no longer be used for treatment of gonorrhea.[9a] If these regimens fail, infections with other pathogens, such as herpes simplex virus or *T. vaginalis*, or bacterial urethritis should be considered. Appropriate testing and specific treatment should be provided when indicated.

PROGNOSIS

Gonococcal urethritis may subside and lead to asymptomatic carriage in female patients. Carriage may last for weeks to months in adults; this period is undefined in children. Untreated gonococcal urethritis also may lead to prostatitis and epididymitis in male patients and urethral stricture. Asymptomatic genital infections in women can progress to pelvic inflammatory disease with tubal scarring and infertility. Systemic complications of asymptomatic gonorrheal infections include arthritis, endocarditis, and necrotic skin lesions.

Chlamydial infections frequently have been associated with pelvic inflammatory disease in women, resulting sometimes in infertility or ectopic pregnancy. *Chlamydia* can be transmitted to a newborn in the birth canal, which can result in conjunctivitis, pneumonia, or both.

The frequency of *U. urealyticum* is higher in sperm samples from men of infertile couples. It also has been associated in women with premature delivery and postpartum fever. In a newborn, this organism might be linked with the development of bronchopulmonary dysplasia. *Ureaplasma* infection of the central nervous system occasionally is reported in newborns.

PREVENTION

Despite substantial efforts, a specific gonococcal vaccine has not been developed. The mainstays of prevention continue to be education and screening. Prepubescent gonorrhea can be prevented from recurring only by careful family counseling and psychosocial therapy; legal intervention may be necessary.

The availability of diagnostic tests performed on urine (a noninvasive alternative to specimens obtained from the urethra or endocervix) renders extensive screening possible in nontraditional settings such as schools and recreation centers.[22] Large-scale efforts that have implemented screening for all sexually active teens attending school-based clinics have been successful in reducing the prevalence of *Chlamydia* infection in boys.[11]

Prevention of noninfectious causes of urethritis usually depends on education and specific counseling of the family. Physical agents or allergens identified as a cause of urethritis must be removed.

Acknowledgments

The author acknowledges the contribution of Dr. Melvin I. Marks and Dr. Antonio C. Arrieta to the previous edition of this chapter. Many sections required minimal changes apart from addition of more recently published information.

REFERENCES

1. American Academy of Pediatrics: Gonococcal infections. *In* Pickering, L. K. (Baker, C. J., Long, S. S., and McMillan, J. A. [eds.]): 2006 Red Book: Report of the Committee on Infectious Diseases. 27th ed. Elk Grove Village, IL, American Academy of Pediatrics, 2006, p. 254.
2. Arnold, A. J., and Kleris, G. S.: The "borderline" smear in men with urethritis. J. A. M. A. *244*:157-159, 1980.
3. Batteiger, B. E., and Jones, R. B.: Chlamydial infections. Infect. Dis. Clin. North Am. *1*:55-81, 1987.
4. Bauer, H. M., Mark, K. E., Samuel, M., et al.: Prevalence of and associated risk factors for fluoroquinolone-resistant *Neisseria gonorrhoeae* in California, 2000-2003. Clin. Infect. Dis. *41*:795-803, 2005.
5. Bowie, W. R., Alexander, E. R., Floyd, J. F., et al.: Differential responses of chlamydial and ureaplasma-associated urethritis to sulphafurazole (sulfisoxazole) and aminocyclitols. Lancet *2*:1276-1278, 1976.
6. Braverman, P. K.: Sexually transmitted diseases in adolescents. Med. Clin. North Am. *84*:869-890, 2000.
7. Brunham, R. C., Paavonen, J., Stevens, C. E., et al.: Mucopurulent cervicitis: The ignored counterpart in women of urethritis in men. N. Engl. J. Med. *311*:1-6, 1984.
8. Cassell, G. H., Davis, J. K., Waites, K. B., et al.: Pathogenesis and significance of urogenital mycoplasmal infections. Adv. Exp. Med. Biol. *224*:93-115, 1987.
9. Centers for Disease Control and Prevention: 2002 Guidelines for treatment of sexually transmitted diseases. M. M. W. R. Morb. Mortal. Wkly. Rep. *51*:1-136, 2002.
9a. Centers for Disease Control and Prevention: Updated recommended treatment regiments for gonococcal infections and associated conditions—United States. M. M. W. R. *56*:332-336, 2007.
10. Chacko, M. R., and Lovchik, J. C.: *Chlamydia trachomatis* infection in sexually active adolescents: Prevalence and risk factors. Pediatrics *73*:836-840, 1984.
11. Cohen, D. A., Nsaumi, M., Martin, D. H., and Farley, T. A.: Repeated school-based training for sexually transmitted disease: A feasible strategy for reaching adolescents. Pediatrics *104*:1281-1285, 1999.
12. Dallabetta, G., and Hook, E. W., III: Gonococcal infections. Infect. Dis. Clin. North Am. *1*:25-54, 1987.
13. Dayan, L.: Transmission of *Neisseria gonorrhoeae* from a toilet seat. www. st.journal.com Sex. Transm. Infect. *80*:327, 2004.
14. De Maria, A., Jr.: Challenges of sexually transmitted disease prevention and control: No magic bullets, but some bullets would be appreciated. Clin. Infect. Dis. *41*:804-807, 2005.
15. Folland, D. S., Burke, R. E., Hinman, A. R., et al.: Gonorrhea in preadolescent children: An inquiry into source of infection and mode of transmission. Pediatrics *60*:153-156, 1977.
16. Fox, K. K., and Leone, P. A.: Epidemiology and pathogenesis of *Neisseria gonorrhoeae* infection. UpToDate 2008.
17. Girardet, R. G., McLain, N., Laoti, S., et al.: Comparison of urine-based ligase chain reaction test to culture for detection of *Chlamydia trachomatis* and *Neisseria gonorrhoeae* in pediatric sexual abuse victims. Pediatr. Infect. Dis. J. *20*:144-147, 2001.
18. Greenberg, R. N., Rein, M. F., Sanders, C. V., et al.: Urethral syndrome in women. J. A. M. A. *245*:923, 1981.
19. Hadlich, S., and Kohl, P. K.: Sexually transmitted diseases in children: A practical approach. Dermatol. Clin. *16*:859-861, 1998.
20. Hagay, Z. J., Sarov, B., and Sachs, J.: Detecting *Chlamydia trachomatis* in men with urethritis: Serology v isolation in cell culture. Genitourin. Med. *65*:166-170, 1988.
21. Hammershlag, M. R.: The transmissibility of sexually transmitted diseases in sexually abused children. Child Abuse Neglect *22*:623-635, 1998.
22. Hammershlag, M. R.: Appropriate use of non-culture tests for the detection of sexually transmitted diseases in children and adolescents. Semin. Pediatr. Infect. Dis. *14*:54-59, 2003.
23. Hammerschlag, M. R., Golden, N. H., Oh, M. K., et al.: Single dose of azithromycin for the treatment of genital chlamydial infections in adolescents. J. Pediatr. *122*:961-965, 1993.
24. Handsfield, H. H., McCormack, W. M., Hook, E. W., et al.: A comparison of single-dose cefixime with ceftriaxone as treatment for uncomplicated gonorrhea. N. Engl. J. Med. *325*:1337-1340, 1991.
25. Hein, K., Marks, A., and Cohen, M.: Asymptomatic gonorrhea: Prevalence in a population of urban adolescents. J. Pediatr. *90*:634-635, 1977.
26. Herz, D., Weiser, A., Collette, T., et al.: Dysfunctional elimination syndrome as an etiology of idiopathic urethritis in childhood. J. Urol. *173*:2132-2137, 2005.
27. Hooton, T. M., and Barnes, R. C.: Urethritis in men. Infect. Dis. Clin. North Am. *1*:165-178, 1987.
28. Horner, P., Gilroy, C. B., Naidoo, B. J., and Taylor-Robinson, D.: Association of *Mycoplasma genitalium* with acute non-gonococcal urethritis. Lancet *342*:582-585, 1993.
29. Ingram, D. L., Runyan, D. K., Collins, A. D., et al.: Vaginal *Chlamydia trachomatis* infection in children with sexual contact. Pediatr. Infect. Dis. *3*:97-99, 1984.
30. Kahn, R. H., Mosure, D. J., Blank, S., et al.: *Chlamydia trachomatis* and *Neisseria gonorrhoeae* prevalence and coinfection in adolescents entering selected U.S. juvenile detention centers, 1997-2002. Sex. Transm. Dis. *32*:255-259, 2005.
31. Kellogg, N. D., Baillargeon, J., Lukefahr, J. L., et al.: Comparison of nucleic acid amplification tests and culture techniques in the detection of *Neisseria gonorrhoeae* and *Chlamydia trachomatis* in victims of suspected child sexual abuse. J. Pediatr. Adolesc. Gynecol. *17*:331-339, 2004.
32. Lauharanta, J., Saarinen, K., Mustonen, M. T., et al.: Single-dose oral azithromycin versus seven-day doxycycline in treatment of non-gonococcal urethritis and cervicitis. J. Antimicrob. Chemother. *31*(Suppl.):177-183, 1993.
33. Lee, H. H., Chernesky, M. A., Schachter, J., et al.: Diagnosis of *Chlamydia trachomatis* genitourinary infection in women by ligase chain reaction assay of urine. Lancet *345*:213-216, 1995.
34. Mahony, J., Castriciano, S., Sellors, J., et al.: Diagnosis of *Chlamydia trachomatis* genital infections by cell culture and two enzyme immunoassays detecting different chlamydial antigens. J. Clin. Microbiol. *27*:1934-1938, 1989.
35. Martin, D. H., Mroczkowski, T. F., Dalu, Z. A., et al.: A controlled trial of single dose of azithromycin for the treatment of chlamydial urethritis and cervicitis. N. Engl. J. Med. *327*:921-925, 1992.
36. Moran, J. S., and Levine, W. C.: Drugs of choice for the treatment of uncomplicated gonococcal infections. Clin. Infect. Dis. *20*(Suppl.):S47-S65, 1995.
37. Nair, P., Glazer-Semmel, E., Gould, C., and Ruff, E.: *Neisseria gonorrhoeae* in asymptomatic prepubertal household contacts of children with gonococcal infection. Clin. Pediatr. *25*:160-163, 1986.
38. Neinstein, L. S., Goldenring, J., and Carpenter, S.: Non-sexual transmission of sexually transmitted diseases: An infrequent occurrence. Pediatrics *74*:67-76, 1984.

39. Nsaumi, M., Cammarata, C. L., Brooks, B. N., et al.: Chlamydia and gonorrhea co-occurrence in a high school population. Sex. Transm. Dis. *31*:424-427, 2004.
40. Odugbemi, T., Oyewold, F., Isichei, C. S., et al.: Single oral dose of azithromycin for therapy of susceptible sexually transmitted diseases: A multicenter open evaluation. W. Afr. J. Med. *12*:136-140, 1993.
41. Plourde, P. J., Tyndall, M., Agoki, E., et al: Single-dose cefixime versus single-dose ceftriaxone in the treatment of antimicrobial-resistant *Neisseria gonorrhoeae* infection. J. Infect. Dis. *166*:919-922, 1992.
42. Rasmussen, S. J., Smith-Vaughan, H., Nelson, M., et al.: Detection of *Chlamydia trachomatis* in urine using enzyme immunoassay and DNA amplification. Mol. Cell. Probes 7:425-430, 1993.
43. Richmond, S. J., and Sparling, P. F.: Genital chlamydial infections. Am. J. Epidemiol. *103*:428-435, 1976.
44. Scheuerpflug, I., Rudel, T., Ryll, R., et al.: Roles of PilC and pilE proteins in pilus-mediated adherence of *Neisseria gonorrhoeae* and *Neisseria meningitidis* to human erythrocytes and endothelial and epithelial cells. Infect. Immun. 67:834-843, 1999.
45. Shafer, M. A., Beck, A., Blain, B., et al.: *Chlamydia trachomatis*: Important relationships to race, contraception, lower genital tract infection, and Papanicolaou smear. J. Pediatr. *104*:141-146, 1984.
46. Shore, W. B., and Winkelstein, J. A.: Nonvenereal transmission of gonococcal infections to children. J. Pediatr. 79:661-663, 1971.
47. Stamm, W. E.: Diagnosis of *Chlamydia trachomatis* genitourinary infections. Ann. Intern. Med. *108*:710-717, 1988.
48. Stamm, W. E.: Azithromycin in the treatment of uncomplicated genital chlamydial urethritis and cervicitis. Am. J. Med. *9*:195-225, 1991.
49. Stamm, W. E., Koutsky, L. A., Benedetti, J. K., et al.: *Chlamydia trachomatis* urethral infections in men: Prevalence, risk factors, and clinical manifestations. Ann. Intern. Med. *100*:47-51, 1984.
50. Steele, R. W.: Prevention and management of sexually transmitted diseases in adolescents. Adolesc. Med. *11*:315-326, 2000.
51. U.S. Preventive Services Task Force: USPSTF Guidelines: Screening for gonorrhea: Recommendation statement. Ann. Fam. Med. 3:263-267, 2005.
52. Wald, E. R.: Gonorrhea: Diagnosis by Gram stain in the female adolescent. Am. J. Dis. Child. *131*:1094-1096, 1977.
53. Weber, J. T., and Johnson, R. E.: New treatments for *Chlamydia trachomatis* genital infection. Clin. Infect. Dis. *20*(Suppl.):S66-S71, 1995.
54. Wilkinson, A. E., Seth, A. D., and Rodin, P.: Infection with penicillinase-producing gonococcus. B. M. J. 2:1233-1235, 1976.

CHAPTER 45

CYSTITIS AND PYELONEPHRITIS

Ellen R. Wald

Urinary tract infections (UTIs) are the most common serious bacterial infections in children. In several series of children evaluated for fever, UTIs accounted for 5 to 6 percent of infections. They are more common than occult bacteremia, bacterial pneumonia, and bacterial meningitis. UTI is especially common as a cause of infection in white infant girls; UTI may explain febrile episodes in nearly 20 percent of such infants.

EPIDEMIOLOGY

UTIs occur in all age groups and may be symptomatic or asymptomatic. Factors that affect the incidence of UTIs are associated with gender, age, race, circumcision status, and general health.[93] The site of infection may be the bladder (cystitis), ureters (ureteritis), pelvis (pyelitis), and renal parenchyma (pyelonephritis). Infections in neonates and infants are common occurrences. In the first 3 months of life, infections in uncircumcised boys are most common.[116,123] Beyond 6 months, infections in infant girls are substantially more common than are infections in boys; the female predominance of UTIs is maintained throughout the remainder of childhood and adolescence.[31]

RISK OF URINARY TRACT INFECTION

The risk of developing a UTI during childhood seems to have increased since early studies by Winberg and colleagues[159] in 1960. These investigations showed that the risk of developing a UTI during the first 10 years of life was 3 percent in girls and 1.1 percent in boys. In a more recent retrospective study of a cohort of 3556 school entrants, 7.8 percent of girls and 1.6 percent of boys were found to have had symptomatic UTIs as confirmed by significant bacteriuria.[47] In approximately half of these cases, the clinical presentation was consistent with acute pyelonephritis (APN).[42] Another population-based study was performed in Göteborg, Sweden, to describe the incidence rate of first-time symptomatic UTI in children younger than 6 years old. The cumulative incidence rate during the first 6 years of life was 6.6 percent for girls and 1.8 percent for boys.[94] The apparent increase in risk most likely relates to an increased awareness of the diagnosis of UTI as an explanation for fever in children and the more frequent practice of culturing the urine of children who are ill.

Several studies have investigated systematically the prevalence of UTI as the explanation for fever in febrile young children presenting to the emergency department. Although the definition of significant bacteriuria has varied among studies, the overall prevalence of UTI is 3.3 to 5.3 percent.[52,128] White infant girls had significantly more UTIs than did black boy infants. Higher prevalences occurred in uncircumcised boys or boys with abdominal or suprapubic tenderness on examination.[128] White girls with a temperature of 39° C or greater had a prevalence of UTIs of 17 percent.[52] In a large prospective study of febrile (temperature ≥38° C) infants 3 months or younger evaluated in pediatric office settings, 54 percent of infants had urine tested, and 10 percent had UTIs.[99]

RISK FACTORS FOR URINARY TRACT INFECTION

Uncircumcised Boys

The common problem of UTIs in uncircumcised boys, although suspected in the 1970s, was first documented in the 1980s by Ginsburg and McCracken.[35] The strongest evidence of a causal link between an intact foreskin and a UTI comes from several studies conducted by Wiswell and colleagues.[161] In their series, an overall 10-fold increased incidence of UTI was found in uncircumcised compared with circumcised male infants (1.12% versus 0.11%; *p* < .001).[161] Wiswell and other investigators have continued to document this problem.[123,129,160] Where and when rates of circumcision have decreased, the frequency of UTIs in boys has increased. The presence of preputial folds in uncircumcised boys encourages a high density of bacterial growth and contamination of the urethral opening.[14] Circumcision reduces meatal contamination, decreasing the ascent of bacteria into the bladder.[160] The high risk of acquiring UTIs in uncircumcised boys diminishes with age (as the foreskin becomes more retractable) but is still present in the toddler age group.[19]

Dysfunctional Voiding

Dysfunctional voiding is a risk factor for the development of a UTI and an occasional consequence of UTI. Dysfunctional voiding refers to a lack of coordination between the two functions that are essential for normal voiding to occur—relaxation of the urethral sphincter and contraction of the detrusor muscle of the bladder. Ordinarily, the sphincter must relax as the detrusor contracts.[5] The failure of the sphincter to relax causes an obstruction to the outflow of urine. Consequently, voiding pressures and intravesicular pressure are high, the bladder becomes overdistended, dribbling instead of a good flow occurs, and residual urine remains in the bladder after the void. This dyscoordination is termed *dyssynergia*.[5]

Clinical manifestations typically appear after toilet training and include incontinence, enuresis, urinary urgency, and UTI.[29] Constipation is a common occurrence because of the inability to relax the pelvic floor musculature. The presence of dysfunctional voiding also may promote the persistence of vesicoureteral reflux (VUR) and lead to recurrence or contralateral reflux after attempts are made at surgical correction of reflux.[72]

Constipation

The distended rectum in constipated children has been suggested to press on the bladder wall and produce an obstruction to bladder outflow that may cause dysfunctional voiding. Urodynamic studies have shown instability of the detrusor muscle in patients with functional constipation and associated enuresis or UTI.[162] Loening-Baucke[86] studied a group of children referred with encopresis and constipation. The history indicated that many were incontinent of urine, and 11 percent had histories of UTIs. When a vigorous regimen to alleviate the constipation was prescribed, a dramatic improvement occurred in the enuresis and the frequency of recurrent UTI.

Wan and colleagues[151] prospectively evaluated the toilet habits of 77 girls and 24 boys diagnosed with UTIs. Parents were instructed to use a "toilet diary" to record the frequency of voiding and stooling. An abnormal voiding habit was defined as infrequent urination (four times or fewer daily when awake), an abnormal voiding pattern (>4 hours between voidings), or the practice of avoidance maneuvers (repetitive habitual squirming, crossing of legs, or sitting on heels).[149] Constipation was defined as stooling less frequently than every third day. Children with and without abnormal imaging studies were compared. Although abnormal voiding patterns and constipation were identified in both groups, only 10 percent of children with normal images were without constipation or abnormal voiding compared with 60 percent of the group with abnormal images ($p = .0001$). These data strongly suggest that evaluation of children with UTIs should include inquiry into these functional matters, especially when imaging study results are normal.

Sexual Activity

The well-recognized association in women of acute cystitis with sexual intercourse is reflected in the popular, now perhaps outdated, term *honeymoon cystitis*.[101] This phenomenon usually is related to the new onset of sexual activity or a recent change in sexual partners. A novel study of 15 patients with a history of recurrent UTIs involved daily monitoring for the presence of UTI with dipslides and calendars that recorded episodes of intercourse, menses, and the occurrence of symptoms.[101] Eleven patients experienced 16 infections; 12 infections occurred within 24 hours of engaging in intercourse. In 12 control subjects, three infections occurred, all within 24 hours of having intercourse. The authors concluded that in sexually active women, most UTIs are related to intercourse.

These results were reinforced by a large prospective study from Seattle, Washington, which confirmed that the incidence of symptomatic UTI is high in sexually active young women and that a strong and independent association exists between UTI and recent sexual intercourse, recent use of a diaphragm with spermicide, and a history of recurrent UTIs.[59] Most of these same risk factors, including frequency of sexual intercourse and use of spermicide, were documented as risk factors associated with development of APN in healthy women.[124]

Catheters

In the hospital, urinary catheters are major risk factors for acquisition of nosocomial infection. In adults, the risk of developing an infection is approximately 5 percent per day of catheterization.[100] The usual infecting strains include *Escherichia coli*, *Proteus*, *Pseudomonas*, *Klebsiella*, and *Serratia*. Many strains of bacteria that cause infection display antibiotic susceptibilities that are more resistant than usual. The route of infection may be either intraluminal or periurethral. Bacteremia is an unusual complication of nosocomial UTI. In a study of nosocomial infections in a children's hospital, catheter-associated UTI accounted for 48 percent of the UTIs. Secondary bacteremia occurred rarely, with an incidence of 2.9 percent.[21]

PATHOGENESIS

BACTERIOLOGY

Most uncomplicated UTIs are caused by members of a large family of gram-negative bacteria known as Enterobacteriaceae. In most instances, the urinary tract becomes infected by the ascending route. Bacteria derived from the fecal flora colonize the periurethral area and gain access to the urethra. The most common bacterial species in primary and recurrent infections is *E. coli*. Other gram-negative species that commonly cause UTI are *Klebsiella*, *Proteus*, *Enterobacter*, and *Citrobacter*, although virtually any enteric organism can cause UTI. Gram-positive bacterial species account for approximately 5 percent of UTIs and primarily include *Staphylococcus saprophyticus* and enterococcal species. After *E. coli*, *S. saprophyticus* is the most common cause of uncomplicated UTIs in teenagers and young adults of both sexes.

Rarely, the urinary tract may become infected hematogenously in the course of a bacteremic infection. This mechanism is thought to account for at least some cases of neonatal UTI. Increasingly, evidence indicates that even in neonates, most infections occur by the ascending route.

VIRULENCE FACTORS

The key virulence factor for isolates of *E. coli* is the mechanism by which they attach or adhere to the uroepithelial cell.[62] Bacterial adherence is an essential initiating step in all infections. So-called uropathogenic bacteria, derived from the numerous species found in the fecal flora, can attach to specific receptor sites on the uroepithelium and can bind in a nonspecific manner by electrostatic and hydrophobic bonds.[118] A principal means of attachment is through adhesins localized on specialized pili of the *E. coli*. These pili are referred to as *P fimbriae* because they can recognize and agglutinate erythrocytes of the P1 blood group; this P blood group antigen also is present on human uroepithelial cells.

Evidence to support the notion of the increased pathogenicity or virulence of the P fimbriae comes from studies of *E. coli* recovered from children with infection at different levels of the urinary tract. When *E. coli* strains recovered from patients with pyelonephritis are examined, 76 to 94 percent are P fimbriated; in contrast, strains of *E. coli* recovered from patients with cystitis or asymptomatic bacteriuria are 19 to 23 percent and 14 to 18 percent P fimbriated, respectively.[69,147] Although P fimbriated strains of *E. coli* are common findings in patients with pyelonephritis whose urinary tracts are completely normal, their frequency decreases considerably when strains of *E. coli* are examined from patients with pyelonephritis associated with VUR. Apparently, this virulence characteristic (and others described later) is unnecessary when reflux is present.[89]

The principal adhesin on the tip of the P fimbriae that fosters adherence to the uroepithelial cell is known as the *PapG adhesin*. More recently, 153 *E. coli* organisms recovered from the urinary tracts of infants and children with pyelonephritis were analyzed by polymerase chain reaction for class I, II, and III alleles of the pyelonephritis-associated adhesin gene *papG*. Strains with any class II *papG* alleles were found significantly more often in infants with normal anatomy and function or in infants with clinically insignificant abnormalities than in infants with significant abnormalities (90 of 119 versus 14 of 34 infants; *p* < .001).[63] This virulence factor is more important when the urinary tract is structurally normal than when anatomic features predispose the individual to infection.

Other virulence factors related to the bacterial species causing UTIs are the K antigen, lipopolysaccharides, hemolysins, colicins, resistance to the bactericidal action of serum, and increased iron-binding capacity. In addition to the immunogenic activity of lipopolysaccharides (activating an intense host response), they have been shown to have direct toxic effects on renal cells via their biologically active component lipid A.[144] The K antigen is a capsular polysaccharide that constitutes an outer surface of the *E. coli* organism. The capsule has the capacity to impede phagocytosis and to shield the bacteria from lysis induced by complement.[60] Hemolysins are cytotoxic proteins that can damage renal tubular cells in vitro.

Approximately 50 percent of the types of *E. coli* isolated from the urine of patients with APN produce a pore-forming toxin, alpha-hemolysin. Alpha-hemolysin damages the cell membrane and may activate apoptosis in renal tubular cells.[16] Colicins, elaborated by "uropathogenic" strains of *E. coli*, kill other bacteria that are in their vicinity. In the presence of human serum, many bacteria are killed after activation of complement. Virulent *E. coli* organisms have the capacity to resist this bactericidal effect of serum. Another virulence factor found in bacteria is their ability to acquire and bind iron. Most bacteria require iron for optimal growth and metabolism and have developed mechanisms to acquire iron when the supply is limited. Increased iron-binding capacity, mediated by proteins such as aerobactin, which are made by some *E. coli* strains, provides additional pathogenic potential.

After reaching the bladder, P fimbriated *E. coli* organisms can colonize the ureter even in the absence of VUR.[116] Bacterial colonization of the ureter affects ureteral peristalsis, leading to dilation and a physiologic obstruction. This dilation of the ureter and calyces favors a change in the shape of the renal papillae, which facilitates intrarenal reflux of colonizing bacteria at low pressure. APN develops because the receptors for the P fimbriated *E. coli* are present in the collecting duct and proximal tubules.[102,116]

Experimental studies conducted by Roberts[116] have led to a theory of the chain of events involved in the process that ultimately leads to renal scarring. The initial event is the inoculation of the renal parenchyma with bacteria, which leads to an intense inflammatory response. Liberation of proinflammatory cytokines (interleukin-1, interleukin-6, and interleukin-8) is followed by recruitment of inflammatory cells and a second cytokine burst.[67] This inflammation results in the release of toxic enzymes within the granulocytes and tubular lumen. Superoxide is released simultaneously, generating oxygen radicals that are toxic to the

bacteria and to the tubular cells.[117] The resultant death of the tubules intensifies and extends the inflammatory process into the interstitium. At the same time, focal ischemia results from the intravascular aggregation of granulocytes and edema.[66] The tissue damage that results from the toxic enzymes, oxygen radicals, inflammatory response, and ischemia culminates in the creation of renal scars.[62,116]

CLINICAL PRESENTATION

CYSTITIS

Most children with cystitis present with urgency, frequency, or dysuria. Children who have the urge to urinate may have a history of difficulty in initiating the urinary stream. Occasionally, children may complain of abdominal or suprapubic pain. If fever is present, it is low-grade. Suprapubic tenderness may be present on palpation. The urine may be foul-smelling and cloudy in appearance.

PYELONEPHRITIS

Many children who present with APN have impressive chills, spiking fevers, and complaints of back pain. They may have associated gastrointestinal complaints of vomiting and diarrhea, especially vomiting. Lower urinary tract symptoms, such as frequency, urgency, dysuria, and suprapubic discomfort, may or may not be present.

Other findings, such as irritability, poor feeding, vomiting, decreased urinary output, and clinical evidence of dehydration, vary. The youngest children with APN usually present with high fever without other localizing features.[54,93,164]

PHYSICAL EXAMINATION

Features of the physical examination that should be emphasized include (1) an accurate measurement of blood pressure (hypertension may be present in patients who have chronic renal disease), (2) general growth and development (failure to thrive may be a sign of more chronic or recurrent UTI), and (3) a careful abdominal examination (which might reveal tenderness or a mass caused by either an enlarged bladder or an obstructed urinary tract).[142] An effort should be made to elicit the finding of costovertebral angle tenderness in children of all ages. The perineum should be inspected carefully to search for signs of irritation, scars, tears, signs of trauma, labial adhesions, or evidence of vulvovaginitis. In uncircumcised infants, the foreskin may not be retractable, leading to phimosis. A rectal examination should be considered to detect masses or poor sphincter tone, which might be associated with a neurogenic bladder.[142] The lower back should be observed for any lipoma, sinus, pigmentation, or tufts of hair that may be signs of an occult myelodysplasia.

Neurologic examination of the lower extremities and evaluation of the bulbocavernosal reflex often reflect the neurologic integrity of the lower motor neuron reflex arcs. The bulbocavernosus reflex is elicited by squeezing the glans penis or clitoris and observing or feeling a reflex contraction at the external anal sphincter. Absence of this reflex suggests a possible sacral lesion.[5]

ASYMPTOMATIC BACTERIURIA

A large body of work has been produced dealing with the issue of asymptomatic bacteriuria. Data were accumulated during a long-term study by Kunin[73] of the natural history of recurrent bacteriuria among school-age girls in a well-defined community in central Virginia. Girls were identified in the first grade and were observed prospectively for 10 years. Each year, approximately 0.5 percent of school-aged girls developed asymptomatic bacteriuria. The overall prevalence was 5 percent for the years between entrance to grade school and graduation from high school. Although it was billed as asymptomatic bacteriuria, approximately one third of the girls did have symptoms, and some were known to have had infection or, rarely, abnormalities of the urinary tract before the first screening.

Just a few years after Kunin[73] began his investigations, a similar study was conducted in Göteborg, Sweden. Beginning in 1970, 19,000 girls a year were screened routinely for bacteriuria in Göteborg schools at ages 7, 11, 14, and 16 years.[84] A significant minority had a history of previous infection or symptoms that were referable to the urinary tract.

Savage and colleagues[120] also studied covert bacteriuria in school-age girls. In the three studies, the prevalence of bacteriuria ranged from 0.7 percent[84] to 1.1 percent[73] to 1.6 percent.[120] The risks associated with asymptomatic bacteriuria are difficult to assess from these studies because patients who were truly asymptomatic were difficult to separate from patients with symptoms.

Several prospective studies of infants and school-aged girls from Scandinavia have provided important information regarding the natural history of asymptomatic bacteriuria.[42,154] Most children identified as having asymptomatic bacteriuria among a large cohort of infants ($N = 3581$) spontaneously cleared the bacteriuria within months. Only 2 of 45 went on to develop symptomatic bacteriuria. In contrast, none of 42 infants who developed symptomatic UTIs had been identified previously as having asymptomatic bacteriuria, suggesting that asymptomatic bacteriuria rarely is a precursor to symptomatic UTI. In addition, prophylactic antibiotics used to treat children with asymptomatic bacteriuria seemed to predispose them to the development of pyelonephritis, usually with microorganisms that had not been present at the outset.[42]

Currently, physicians have little enthusiasm for screening children of any age to discover the presence of asymptomatic bacteriuria. The absence of pyuria in these specimens of urine provides additional evidence that the host is not perturbed by the presence of asymptomatic bacteriuria. The presence of bacteria of low virulence in the urine in asymptomatic patients seems to be protective. These strains apparently prevent invasion by other bacteria and provide a kind of biologic prophylaxis.[42,70]

Rather than screening asymptomatic populations of children, an appropriate approach is vigorous evaluation for the presence of UTIs in febrile children without an obvious focus of infection. In addition, health maintenance examinations should be used as an opportunity to screen for historical information that might suggest the need to collect a urine specimen for culture (Table 45–1). Important items include frequent episodes of unexplained fever, dribbling when urinating, enuresis, encopresis, constipation, urgency, frequency, and dysuria. In addition, it is valuable to know when toilet training was accomplished; frequency of voiding; frequency of stooling; and any apparent difficulties associated with voiding, such as in initiating the urinary stream. The practitioner also should inquire about so-called avoidance maneuvers (e.g., repetitive habitual squirming, crossing of legs, or sitting on heels)[151] and family history of UTI.

DIFFERENTIAL DIAGNOSIS

INFECTIOUS

E. coli is the most common cause of infection in the urinary tract for primary infections (in which *E. coli* causes 85 to 90% of

TABLE 45–1 Renal-Focused History and Physical Examination

History
Age of toilet training
Characteristics and frequency of voiding (urgency, dysuria, dribbling)
Frequency and characteristics of stooling
Family history of renal disease
Habitual squirming
Color and odor of urine
Unexplained episodes of fever

Physical Examination
Temperature
Blood pressure
Abdominal tenderness
Costovertebral angle tenderness
Suprapubic tenderness
Genital examination (irritation, scars, tears)
Rectal examination (sphincter tone, bulbocavernosus reflex)
Lower back (sinus, pigmentation, lipoma, tufts of hair)

infections) and recurrent infections (in which *E. coli* causes approximately 75% of infections). Virtually any other gram-negative enteric bacteria may cause infection. Common etiologic agents include *Klebsiella, Proteus, Enterobacter, Serratia,* and *Pseudomonas. Proteus mirabilis* is a common cause of UTIs in some series of boys and in nosocomial UTIs associated with catheterization.[71,105] In young women, *S. saprophyticus* is second only to *E. coli* as a cause of cystitis. Rarely, *Staphylococcus epidermidis* has been reported as a cause of pyelonephritis in young boys with anatomic abnormalities of the urinary tract.[40]

In the context of bacteremia or septicemia, occasionally the blood culture and the urine culture are positive for the same bacterial species. In these instances, the kidney has been seeded as part of a hematogenous dissemination. Any organism that is responsible for sepsis, such as *Haemophilus influenzae* type b, *Neisseria meningitidis, Neisseria gonorrhoeae, Staphylococcus aureus, Streptococcus pneumoniae,* or *Streptococcus pyogenes,* may be found in the urine.

Anaerobic infections of the urinary tract are rare occurrences in children despite the high density of gram-positive and gram-negative anaerobes in the fecal flora; this fact relates to the probable lack of adherence of these bacterial species to the uroepithelium. Anaerobic infections of the urinary tract should be suspected when organisms are seen on Gram stain but do not grow in conventional culture, or when the urine of symptomatic children shows no bacterial growth.[13] Another unusual infecting agent that should be suspected in instances in which the Gram stain of the urine shows gram-negative rods but the urine culture is negative is *H. influenzae.*[97]

Fungal infections of the urinary tract usually are caused by *Candida* spp., but they also may be caused by *Cryptococcus neoformans, Aspergillus* spp., and the endemic mycoses.[139] Candiduria is an increasingly common form of nosocomial infection that may involve any level of the urinary tract.[50,109] It often occurs in immunosuppressed patients, especially patients who are receiving broad-spectrum antibiotics for treatment of documented or undocumented systemic infections. In many immunosuppressed patients, the infection is complicated by the presence of an indwelling urinary catheter.

Viruses also may cause infection of the urinary tract. For the most part, these infections involve the bladder rather than the kidney, although infection of any part of the urinary tract may occur. The principal etiologic agents are adenoviruses, enteroviruses, coxsackieviruses, and echoviruses. Mumps virus and hepatitis viruses occasionally have been implicated. Type 11 adenovirus has been the most common cause of acute hemorrhagic cystitis in school-age boys; type 21 also has been documented to be a cause of infection in this age group. In immunosuppressed patients, especially children who have undergone bone marrow transplantation or are recipients of kidney transplants, BK polyomavirus and adenovirus may cause hemorrhagic cystitis.[17,81]

Granulomatous cystitis is the histopathologic description of cystitis caused by *Mycobacterium tuberculosis* and by schistosomiasis and other parasitic infections. Granulomata formed in response to certain parasites, such as *Toxocara* and microfilariae, also may contain numerous eosinophils. *Enterobius vermicularis* infection occasionally leads to signs and symptoms of cystitis and inflammatory changes of the bladder wall.

Xanthogranulomatous pyelonephritis is a rare, chronic, suppurative renal infection. Although it can occur at any age, it typically involves middle-aged women. Cases in children have been reported across all age groups, including infants.[1,114] The patient usually presents with what appears to be an acute UTI, caused most often by *E. coli* or *Proteus* spp. Evaluation of the patient usually reveals a unilateral enlargement of the kidney, often accompanied by urolithiasis and sometimes a staghorn calculus. The differential diagnosis of the mass lesion includes neuroblastoma, Wilms tumor, tuberculosis, and renal carcinoma. The lesion is characterized histologically by granulomata, abscesses, and lipid-laden foam cells. Nephrectomy is the usual means of management.

Infectious urethritis caused by *N. gonorrhoeae* or *Chlamydia trachomatis* is a common cause of symptoms suggestive of UTI. In addition, any etiologic agents of vulvovaginitis may cause inflammation of the distal urethra, with urgency, frequency, or dysuria; they include *Candida* spp., *Gardnerella vaginalis*, *Trichomonas vaginalis*, *S. pyogenes*, *S. pneumoniae*, *H. influenzae*, *C. trachomatis*, *Shigella* spp., and *Yersinia enterocolitica*.

NONINFECTIOUS

Urethral symptoms, such as urgency, frequency, and dysuria, may be caused by any factor or process that gives rise to inflammation in the lower urinary tract. Examples include mechanical irritation (which might result from insertion of foreign bodies, migration of pinworms, or masturbation) and chemical irritation (which might arise from bubble baths or shampoos). Chemical cystitis has been reported from the inadvertent insertion of a vaginal contraceptive suppository (nonoxinol 9) into the bladder. Pharmacologic causes of urethral symptoms include cyclophosphamide and methenamine mandelate, both of which can lead to inflammatory changes in the urinary bladder. Several other agents used in the topical treatment of bladder cancer have been noted to cause cystitis.

SPECIFIC DIAGNOSIS

COLLECTION OF A URINE SPECIMEN

Proper collection of a urine specimen is crucial to facilitate interpretation of the culture. In toilet-trained children, a midstream clean-catch specimen is appropriate for evaluation. When this specimen is used, the definition of significant bacteriuria is 10^5 colony-forming units (CFU)/mL or more. The child is asked to void into the toilet. Straddling the commode in a reverse position creates a natural separation between the urethra and the vulva. Cleansing of the perineum does not result in less contamination of the specimen and is no longer encouraged.[122] The child is asked to begin voiding. A second or two after the void has been initiated, a sterile cup is passed into the stream. The hope is that the initial void succeeds in washing out the distal urethra, the

site from which the urine specimen is most likely to be contaminated.

If the child is not toilet-trained, a specimen may be collected by urethral catheterization or suprapubic aspiration. When the urine is collected by urethral catheterization, the perineum is cleaned with 1 percent iodine. A properly sized catheter (10 or 12 French) or a size 5 feeding tube may be used. The catheter is lubricated and inserted into the urethra and threaded a short distance. The first few drops of urine should not be collected in the sterile container. This part of the specimen is the most likely to be contaminated with fecal flora from the distal urethra; these bacteria are not eliminated by the process of perineal cleansing. The remaining urine is collected in a sterile container and sent to the laboratory. When a urine specimen is collected by urethral catheterization, significant bacteriuria is defined as 50,000 CFU/mL or more.[57] This method is preferred when a small volume of urine in the bladder is anticipated and collecting a specimen of urine is necessary so that antibiotics can be initiated.

An alternative to urethral catheterization is suprapubic aspiration. Although some physicians might contend that catheterization is less traumatic than suprapubic aspiration,[142] little evidence supports this notion. The procedure can be done in children of any age; it has been used to obtain specimens of urine in pregnancy.[96] Urine culture specimens obtained by suprapubic aspiration are easy to interpret because the usual source of contamination, the distal urethra, has been bypassed. The presence of any bacteria in a specimen collected by suprapubic aspiration is significant, although most samples contain 10^5 CFU/mL or more.

The patient is in a supine position with the lower extremities flexed (Fig. 45–1 and Table 45–2). The suprapubic area is cleaned with iodine and alcohol. The symphysis pubis is located with the index finger. A 3-mL syringe is attached to a $1\frac{1}{2}$-inch, 22-gauge needle. A spinal needle (21-gauge, $2\frac{1}{2}$- or 3-inch) can be used in older patients. The needle is passed in the midline about 1.5 cm above the symphysis pubis. It is angled about 10 to 20 degrees from the vertical, pointing in a slightly cephalad direction (Fig. 45–2). Negative pressure is applied while the needle is inserted. The procedure is most likely to be successful when the infant can be encouraged to drink and the diaper has been dry for at least 60 minutes before the procedure is done. The success rate of suprapubic aspiration can be improved with the use of a portable ultrasound device.[36] If the suprapubic aspiration is unsuccessful,

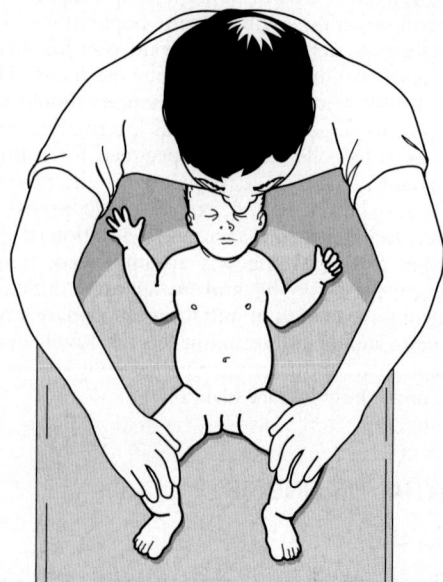

Figure 45–1 Suprapubic aspiration technique, position of patient.

TABLE 45-2 Suprapubic Aspiration Technique

Step 1	Child should not have voided within 1 hr of the procedure
Step 2	Restrain the infant in a supine, frog leg position
Step 3	Clean the suprapubic area with povidone-iodine and alcohol
Step 4	Identify the site of puncture at 1-2 cm above the symphysis pubis in the midline
Step 5	Use a 22-gauge, 1½-inch needle (with 3-mL syringe attached to it) and puncture at 10- to 20-degree angle of the true vertical aiming cephalad; a second attempt can be made at a similar angle aiming caudad
Step 6	Exert suction gently as the needle is advanced until urine enters syringe; aspirate urine with gentle suction. If urine is not obtained, further trials are unlikely to be successful

TABLE 45-3 Urinary Tract Infection—Definitions

Method of Collection	Colony Count (CFU/mL)
Clean catch	$\geq 10^5$
Catheter	$\geq 5 \times 10^4$
Suprapubic	Any

CFU, colony-forming unit.

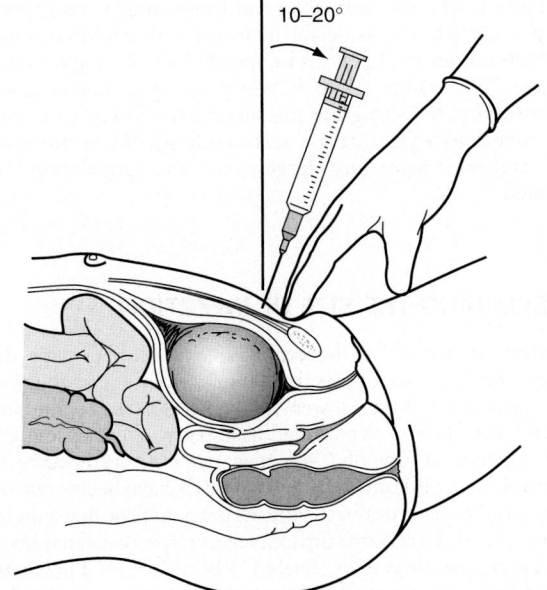

Figure 45-2 Suprapubic aspiration technique, position of needle.

a catheterized specimen should be obtained. Complications of suprapubic aspiration are rare and include formation of a hematoma, perforation of the bowel, and formation of a suprapubic abscess.[111] Suprapubic aspiration is contraindicated if the patient has a bleeding diathesis.

The last method of urine collection is the bag technique. The perineum is washed with soap and water and allowed to dry. A sterile plastic bag is attached. The bag is removed as soon as the patient voids. If the patient has not voided in 20 minutes, the bag is removed, the perineum is cleaned again, and a new bag is attached. If this procedure is followed meticulously, a reasonable specimen can be collected. This specimen is susceptible to contamination from periurethral flora,[121] however, and the technique is not recommended if the patient appears ill and antibiotics need to be started immediately after the specimen of urine is collected. The results of the culture of a bagged specimen are useful only if they are negative. If the culture is positive, a second specimen must be collected by a more reliable method.[3]

DIAGNOSIS OF URINARY TRACT INFECTION

The diagnosis of UTI hinges on the results of culture of a properly collected urine specimen. Disagreement within the literature

is substantial regarding the definition of significant bacteriuria.[38] As indicated in the previous section, the definition of UTI varies according to the method by which the urine is collected. This variability in definition acknowledges that although the bladder urine is regarded as a sterile body fluid, contamination of the urine specimen may occur as it passes through the urethra. The distal urethra frequently is colonized with coliforms derived from the gastrointestinal tract. The only urine specimen that bypasses the urethra and is free of contamination is obtained by suprapubic aspiration. When a specimen is collected by this technique, any colony count of coliforms is significant.[164]

In urine that is collected by a midstream clean-catch method, significant bacteriuria is defined, most stringently, by the recovery of 100,000 CFU/mL or more (Table 45-3). For specimens of urine obtained by catheter, significant bacteriuria is defined as 50,000 CFU/mL or more. In each of these instances, physicians recognize that although urine specimens containing lower colony counts rarely may represent true infection, for the most part, lower colony counts usually are the result of contamination of the specimen.[57]

Specimens of urine usually are inoculated onto two different kinds of solid media—one that supports the growth of only gram-negative enteric bacteria (e.g., MacConkey agar) and another that supports gram-positive and gram-negative bacteria (e.g., 5 percent sheep blood agar), with use of a 0.001 calibrated loop. Colonies are counted the next day (18 hours later), and the total is multiplied by 1000 to determine the colony count. The results of the urine culture are unavailable during the practitioner's first encounter with the ill child. Consequently, there is great interest in the development of a method that would predict the results of the urine culture so that appropriate antimicrobial therapy could be initiated presumptively at the time of the initial encounter. Microscopic methods (to evaluate pyuria and bacteriuria) and biochemical tests (which can be evaluated with a dipstick) have been evaluated.

Microscopy

Two surrogate markers for UTI on microscopic assessment are pyuria and bacteriuria. A problem in assessing pyuria and bacteriuria has been the issue of the definition of significant microscopic pyuria and bacteriuria. How many white blood cells (WBCs) in the urine are too many? Should the specimen of urine that is examined be centrifuged or uncentrifuged? How should the WBCs in a specimen of urine be enumerated? Should the number of WBCs on a centrifuged specimen be enumerated as the number per high-power field, or should they be enumerated on a counting chamber as the number of cells per cubic millimeter, as they would be in a sample of cerebrospinal fluid? If the urine is centrifuged, additional variables are introduced: the initial volume of urine, the duration of the spin, and the volume of urine used to resuspend the sediment. All of these variables influence substantially the enumeration of WBCs per high-power field, especially the volume used to resuspend the sediment.

Methods to assess bacteriuria also have raised issues of definition. Should bacteriuria be assessed on a centrifuged specimen or an uncentrifuged specimen, and should the bacteria be evaluated on a wet mount or a Gram-stained specimen? Should bacteria be enumerated as the number per high-power field?

The standard definition of pyuria in the pediatric literature has been 5 WBCs per high-power field on a centrifuged specimen. Traditionally, microscopic bacteriuria has been expressed as the number of bacteria per high-power field on a Gram stain of a centrifuged specimen of urine. Several investigations undertaken by Hoberman and colleagues[56] have shown, however, that a so-called enhanced urinalysis has greater sensitivity, specificity, and positive predictive value than the standard urinalysis. An enhanced urinalysis is performed on an uncentrifuged sample of urine that has been obtained by catheter. The urine is placed on a counting chamber, and the cells are enumerated as the number per cubic millimeter. A Gram stain is performed in a manner that standardizes the number of drops of urine that are assessed and the number of oil immersion fields that are reviewed.

An enhanced urinalysis is considered to be positive when 10 WBCs/mm^3 or more are present and at least one gram-negative rod in 10 oil immersion fields is present. This definition of significant pyuria is much more sensitive than were previous definitions, and it has performed well for numerous investigators and in neonates and in older infants.[49,82,84,164] A systematic review of the existing literature to assess the performance of rapid diagnostic tests for UTI concluded that use of the traditional definition of pyuria (>5 WBCs per high-power field on a centrifuged specimen) is sufficiently poor that it cannot be recommended for making a presumptive diagnosis of UTI.[38] Huicho and coworkers[61] also performed a meta-analysis of urine screening tests to determine the risk of UTI in children. This more recent study concluded that pyuria of at least 10 WBCs/mm^3 and bacteriuria are best suited for assessing the risk of UTIs in children.

Automated methods to perform urinalysis are being used in many hospitals and laboratories. The most updated automated image-based urinalysis system, the iQ200 (Iris Diagnostics, Chatsworth, CA) received clearance from the Food and Drug Administration more recently. The system uses flow imaging analysis technology and so-called Auto Particle Recognition (APR; Iris Diagnostics) software to classify particles found in an uncentrifuged urine specimen based on multiple parameters. Images are stored and can be viewed later on the workstation screen, eliminating the need for manual microscopy in most cases.[148] The iQ200 provides for a rapid turn-around time, and results correlate well with manual methods, especially for red blood cells, WBCs, and squamous epithelial cells.[74,85]

Pyuria is not specific for UTI. In numerous other conditions, including fever, streptococcal infections, and Kawasaki disease, and after exercise, WBCs are found in the urine. Finding pyuria does not ensure that an infection of the urinary tract is present. Despite reports to the contrary, finding true UTI without pyuria is unusual.[150] Generally, inflammation is expected to accompany infection. The absence of pyuria in children with UTIs is rare; it may occur when a child is being evaluated so early in the clinical course of the infection that the inflammatory response has not yet developed. It also may occur when a child is experiencing an episode of asymptomatic bacteriuria.

The most likely explanation for significant bacteriuria by culture in the absence of pyuria is a contaminated specimen. In most cases when UTI has been reported to occur in the absence of pyuria, the definition of pyuria has been at fault. The requirement for 5 WBCs per high-power field on a centrifuged specimen corresponds to approximately 25 WBCs/mm^3; it is too stringent a requirement, with a low sensitivity for the detection of UTIs in infants and children.

Urine Dipsticks

Urine dipsticks (or reagent strips) have been used to indicate the presence of leukocyte esterase (as a surrogate marker for pyuria) and urinary nitrite (which is converted from dietary nitrates by the presence of gram-negative bacteria in the urine). The conversion of dietary nitrates to nitrites by bacteria takes approximately 4 hours. The test result is most likely to be positive when the urine tested is the first morning void (representing a urine that has incubated in the bladder overnight) or a urine that has been in the bladder for at least 4 hours (e.g., obtained from an older child who may hold urine in the bladder for several hours at a time).

The performance characteristics of leukocyte esterase and nitrites vary according to the definition used for a positive urine culture, the age and symptoms of the population being studied, and the method of urine collection. A nitrite test, although not a sensitive marker in children, is helpful when the result is positive because it is highly specific. A negative nitrite test result has little value in ruling out UTI, however.[25] The leukocyte esterase test has an average sensitivity of 83 percent.[26] It can have a sensitivity of 94 percent in settings in which UTIs are suspected clinically and a sensitivity of 52.9 percent when it is performed on febrile children, most of whom do not have a UTI.[57] The specificity of leukocyte esterase (average 72%; range 64 to 92%) generally is not as good as the sensitivity, reflecting the nonspecificity of pyuria in general. A positive leukocyte esterase test result should be interpreted with caution, depending largely on the population being evaluated.[25]

DETERMINING THE SITE OF INFECTION

Urinalysis is useful for detecting infection but not for determining the location of the infection within the urinary tract (i.e., upper tract versus lower tract). To determine the site of infection (i.e., kidney versus bladder), many investigations of the discriminatory ability of C-reactive protein, erythrocyte sedimentation rate, and total peripheral WBCs have been performed. Several studies have evaluated the accuracy of procalcitonin levels compared with C-reactive protein levels to predict renal involvement among children with febrile UTIs.[8,34,107,112,138] These studies showed that serum procalcitonin concentrations, measured with either an immunoluminetric quantitative test or a rapid semiquantitative test, diagnosed APN with a sensitivity of 70.3 to 94.1 percent and a specificity of 82.6 to 93.6 percent. The specificity of procalcitonin was always higher than that of C-reactive protein, and a highly significant correlation was noted between elevated procalcitonin levels and severity of renal involvement as measured by dimercaptosuccinic acid (DMSA) scintigraphic scores.[107]

IMAGING

The current standard of care is to perform imaging procedures on children with a diagnosis of UTI. The categories of children for whom imaging generally is recommended are (1) any child who experiences an episode of APN, (2) boys of any age with a first UTI, (3) girls younger than 3 years old with a first UTI, (4) girls older than 3 years of age with a second UTI, and (5) girls older than 3 years old with a first UTI if an extenuating circumstance exists (Table 45–4). The extenuating circumstances include a family history of renal disease, recognition of abnormal voiding patterns, poor growth, hypertension, known abnormalities of the urinary tract, and failure to respond promptly to therapy. The imaging studies that usually are considered are renal ultrasonography, contrast voiding cystourethrography (VCUG) to detect VUR, renal cortical scintigraphy, and magnetic resonance imaging (MRI).

TABLE 45–4 Indications for Imaging Procedures in Children with Urinary Tract Infection

Any episode of acute pyelonephritis
Boys with first UTI
Girls <3 years old with first UTI
Girls ≥3 years old with second UTI
Girls ≥3 years old with first UTI if
    Positive family history
    Abnormal voiding patterns
    Poor growth
    Hypertension
    Abnormalities of urinary tract
    Failure to respond promptly to treatment

UTI, urinary tract infection.

RENAL ULTRASONOGRAPHY

The renal ultrasound examination has replaced completely intravenous pyelography as a means to assess the gross anatomy of the urinary tract. Generally, ultrasonography has been performed promptly after diagnosis of the UTI has been made. It is a noninvasive test that can describe the size and shape of the urinary tract, the presence of duplication and dilations of the ureters, the presence of ureteroceles, and the existence of gross anatomic abnormalities such as a horseshoe kidney.[3] It is not sensitive enough, however, to signal consistently the presence of hydronephrosis, hydroureter, VUR, or renal scarring.[30] When ultrasonography was compared with intravenous pyelography for the detection of renal scars, wide interobserver variations were noted, with sensitivity ranging from 40 to 90 percent.[42]

Some investigators have questioned whether routine performance of renal ultrasonography is essential.[54] Given the current frequency with which fetal ultrasound examinations are performed during gestation, the likelihood that ultrasonography would disclose information that is not already known is small. In a study of 306 children younger than 2 years old with UTIs, only 1 child had a clinically important finding discovered by the routine performance of renal ultrasonography.[55] In a more recent study of 255 children younger than 5 years old with a first diagnosed uncomplicated febrile UTI, abnormalities were found on ultrasonography in 14 percent of patients; in none of these patients did the ultrasonography findings influence management.[163]

Most obstructions of the urinary tract are diagnosed in utero. Selective performance of renal ultrasonography is recommended for children with UTIs who do not respond promptly to antibiotic therapy (i.e., have persistent fever or abdominal findings) and in children who did not have a prenatal ultrasound examination performed beyond 30 weeks of gestation at a reliable center.

RENAL SCINTIGRAPHY

In patients with presumed APN, renal scintigraphy with Tc 99m DMSA or Tc 99m glucoheptonate has been shown to be the most practical and reliable method for detecting APN.[126] DMSA and glucoheptonate are amino acids that are cleared by the renal tubules. When these amino acids are labeled with technetium and injected intravenously, they can be used to create an image of the kidney, which reflects vascular flow and tubular function (Fig. 45–3). In experimentally induced APN in piglets, the DMSA scan had a sensitivity of 87 percent and a specificity of 100 percent in showing lesions consistent with APN compared with histology as the gold standard.[119]

In most patients with APN, renal scintigraphy performed during the acute phase of the illness shows a decreased uptake of DMSA (Fig. 45–4). High-resolution pinhole images of the kidney

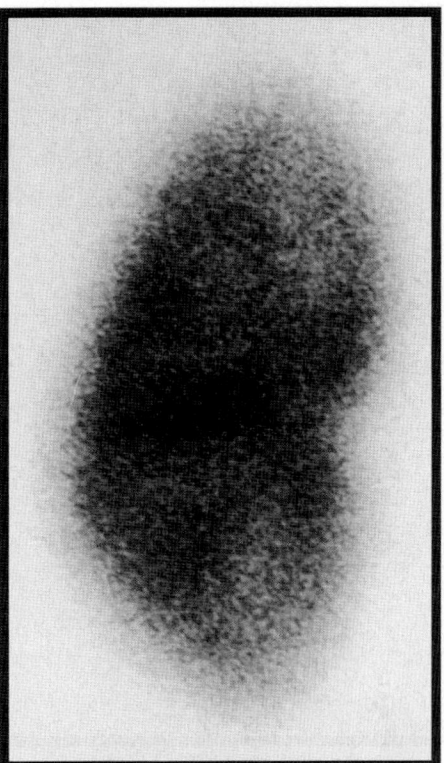

Figure 45–3 Normal renal scintigram.

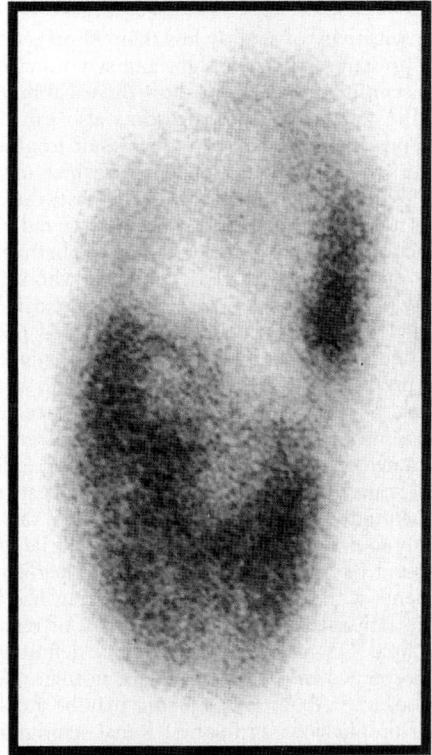

Figure 45–4 Scintigram showing acute pyelonephritis, manifesting as a photon-deficient area in the upper pole.

reveal focal, multifocal, or diffuse areas of decreased uptake of isotope in the kidney without loss of volume and with maintenance of the contour of the kidney.[126] DMSA renal scintigraphy can be used to localize the level at which the urinary tract is infected, specifically distinguishing between acute cystitis and

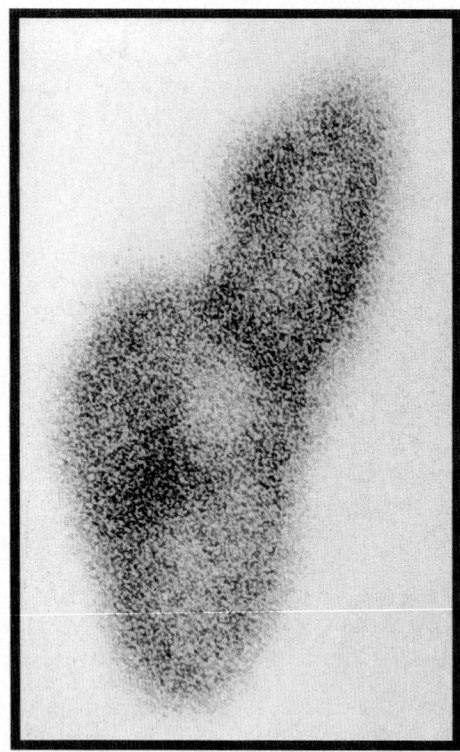

Figure 45–5 Scintigram showing a renal scar with loss of the normal contour.

APN with a sensitivity of slightly less than 90 percent. Rarely, a patient may present with classic signs and symptoms of APN in whom renal scintigraphy does not show the usual findings.[32]

The DMSA and glucoheptonate scans also can be used to indicate the presence of renal scars that result from an episode of APN. The scar is indicated by an area in which uptake of the radioisotope is decreased (Fig. 45–5). In this case, the contour of the kidney is not preserved. Scarring also may be indicated by an overall reduction of the size of the kidney. Hoberman and colleagues[53] prospectively evaluated 309 children who were 1 to 24 months old with their first febrile UTI. An initial DMSA scan was performed on all children and showed that 61 percent (190 of 309) had findings compatible with APN, and only 1 child had evidence of previous scars. Repeated scintigraphic scanning was done 6 months after entry in 89 percent to detect renal scarring. A small percentage of renal parenchymal involvement (mean 8.2%) was noted in 9.6 percent of the children. All children whose initial scans were normal had normal scans at follow-up.

DMSA scintigraphy has been suggested as the preferred imaging study to evaluate a child with a first febrile UTI rather than ultrasound or VCUG.[41,46] A strategy to perform VCUG only in patients with an abnormal DMSA scan has been proposed.[41] The rationale is based on the rarity of renal scarring when the initial DMSA is normal. Reflux definitely may be present, however, when DMSA scans are normal (30 of 99 in Hoberman's data).[53] Absence of scarring may be attributable to the effect of prophylactic antibiotics. Renal scintigraphy is the most sensitive study to indicate the presence of small renal scars that may occur after APN.

MAGNETIC RESONANCE IMAGING

MRI can be used to detect the presence of APN. Two studies by Lonergan and colleagues[91,108] showed a sensitivity and a specificity of MRI that are equal to and perhaps even greater than those of renal scintigraphy with DMSA. In both instances, the best pulse sequence to show areas of APN with MRI was gadolinium-enhanced, fast spin-echo inversion recovery. These results have been confirmed by others.[78] Several investigators have urged, however, that MRI not become a screening test for children with UTIs until the detection of minor changes in the renal parenchyma (by either DMSA or MRI) has been proved to be of clinical importance.[78,90] The time and sedation requirements for MRI render it an unattractive choice for routine management.

VOIDING CYSTOURETHROGRAPHY

Two types of cystography are available for the diagnosis of VUR—fluoroscopic contrast VCUG and radionuclide cystography. Contrast VCUG has excellent anatomic resolution and provides detailed images of the bladder and the urethra. It can be used specifically to label the degree of reflux (according to the international classification);[75] to look for trabeculations, diverticula, or ureteroceles of the bladder; and to outline the urethra (which is essential to identify posterior urethral valves causing obstruction). Radionuclide cystography provides less anatomic detail and is most useful when urethral disease is not suspected and when the patient has no history of voiding dysfunction. It is used to observe patients who are known to have reflux (to assess whether reflux is still present) and can be used for screening purposes in siblings of children with reflux and in children of adults known to have had reflux. Compared with conventional contrast VCUG, the amount of radiation exposure is reduced substantially when the radioisotope is used.

The international classification of reflux is a universally used system involving five degrees of reflux.[75] Grade I is reflux into the distal ureter; grade II is reflux into the pelvis; and grades III, IV, and V are reflux with mild, moderate, and severe dilation of the pelvis and calyces (Fig. 45–6).

VCUG is performed on children who have experienced a symptomatic UTI to determine the presence of VUR. Children who have VUR are at risk for developing reflux nephropathy—permanent renal damage secondary to the reflux of infected urine into the kidney. Because reflux often resolves spontaneously over the course of several years, the purpose of identifying a child with VUR is to recommend antibiotic prophylaxis until the reflux either has resolved spontaneously or, in cases of high degrees of reflux, has been corrected surgically.

Although imaging of children with UTI is routine, little evidence exists that diagnostic imaging of children after their first UTI results in prevention of renal scarring, hypertension, or renal failure.[23] In a systematic overview of the literature using the MEDLINE database, no controlled trials or analytic studies evaluating or comparing different management strategies with regard to imaging were discovered.[23] If studies can show with certainty that antibiotic prophylaxis to prevent UTIs in children with VUR is superior to placebo in the prevention of renal scarring, the necessity and importance of performing VCUG would be established. Such a study was funded by the National Institutes of Health to begin in 2007[39a] (see the section on management of VUR).

TREATMENT

ANTIBIOTICS FOR TREATMENT OF ACUTE INFECTION

The treatment of UTI is influenced by the age of the patient, the probable site of infection (cystitis or APN), the degree of toxicity, and the likelihood of adherence to the treatment regimen. Oral antimicrobial therapy is appropriate for children with cystitis and for older children with suspected APN who are neither toxic nor

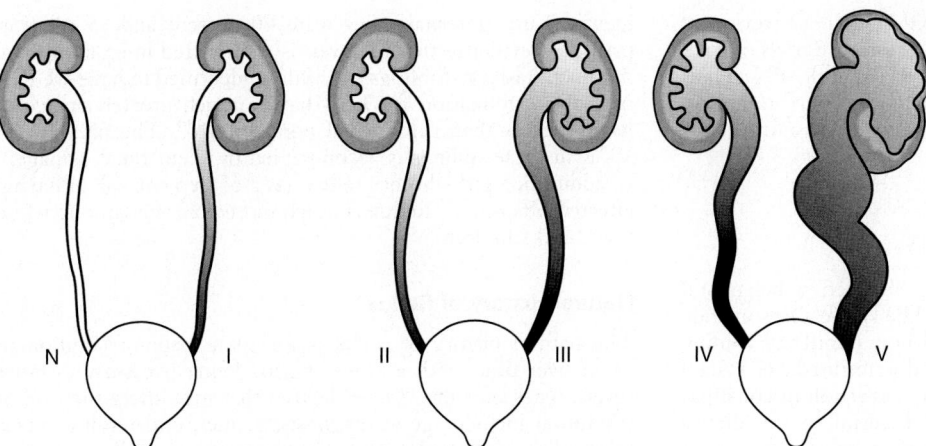

Figure 45–6 Vesicoureteral reflux, international classification.

N   I   II   III   IV   V

TABLE 45–5 Antibiotic Treatment

Oral

Amoxicillin + potassium clavulanate	45 mg/kg/day in 2 divided doses
Cefuroxime	30 mg/kg/day in 2 divided doses
Cefprozil	30 mg/kg/day in 2 divided doses
Cefixime	10 mg/kg/day in 1 dose
Cefpodoxime	9 mg/kg/day in 1 dose
Ceftibuten	10 mg/kg/day in 1 dose
Cefdinir	14 mg/kg/day in 1 dose
Trimethoprim-sulfamethoxazole	10 mg/kg/day (trimethoprim) in 2 divided doses

Parenteral

Ampicillin + sulbactam	200 mg/kg/day in 4 divided doses
Cefuroxime	150 mg/kg/day in 3 divided doses
Cefotaxime	200 mg/kg/day in 4 divided doses
Ceftriaxone	80 mg/kg/day in 1 dose
Ceftazidime	150 mg/kg/day in 3 divided doses
Cefipime	100 mg/kg/day in 2 divided doses
Gentamicin	7.5 mg/kg/day in 3 divided doses

vomiting. The more complex issue is the management of a young infant with high fever in whom the likely diagnosis is APN. These children traditionally have been admitted to the hospital for parenteral administration of antibiotics.

Numerous choices of oral antimicrobials are available for patients who present with presumed cystitis (Table 45–5). Alternatives include amoxicillin-potassium clavulanate; second-generation cephalosporins, such as cefuroxime and cefprozil; third-generation cephalosporins, such as cefixime, cefpodoxime, ceftibuten, and cefdinir; and the combination agent trimethoprim-sulfamethoxazole. Generally, neither amoxicillin nor first-generation cephalosporins are recommended for first-line therapy because 30 to 50 percent of *E. coli* now are inherently resistant to these agents. Because of some geographic variability in the prevalence of resistance, the practitioner should check with local infectious disease specialists to verify these susceptibility patterns.

In an older patient who appears ill but is not toxic, a repeated visit or telephone follow-up is indicated to ensure that recovery is progressing as predicted. If fever is present, the patient generally becomes afebrile within 1 or 2 days, although occasionally it may take longer. If other indices of recovery, such as general well-being, appetite, and playfulness, are improving appropriately, the persistence of fever is not alarming. If susceptibility test results are available and the organism causing infection is susceptible to the antimicrobial being used, repeating the urine culture after 24 hours is unnecessary.[55] The rapid sterilization of urine is a testimony to the fact that virtually all the antibiotics that are used to treat UTIs are concentrated in the kidney and excreted in the urine.

Duration of treatment for patients who are presumed to have cystitis has been controversial. Conventional recommendations are for 7 to 10 days of antimicrobial therapy. Short courses of therapy, varying from single-dose regimens to 3- or 4-day courses, have been evaluated with mixed results. The potential advantages of short-course therapy include the likelihood of improved adherence to the drug regimen; lower cost of drug; and fewer undesirable side effects, including less alteration of normal flora.[127] A meta-analysis (and the most comprehensive review of the data) was performed by Tran and coworkers[143] after review of 22 published trials and a total of 1279 patients. Amoxicillin in a single dose and trimethoprim-sulfamethoxazole as either a single dose or a 3-day regimen were the short-course regimens most commonly evaluated. The authors found that short-course antimicrobial therapy is less effective than therapy of conventional duration, largely because of the ineffectiveness of single-dose amoxicillin. A 3-day course of trimethoprim-sulfamethoxazole was an effective alternative to the standard course of treatment.

A more recent meta-analysis evaluated 10 trials in 652 children with lower tract UTIs.[58] No significant difference was found in the frequency of positive urine cultures between short-duration (2 to 4 days) and standard-duration (7 to 14 days) oral antibiotic therapy for UTIs in children 1 to 15 months after treatment. In children with clear evidence of cystitis without APN, short-course therapy may be acceptable.[149]

Management of a young infant with presumed APN has been controversial. A study conducted by Hoberman and colleagues[55] compared oral therapy with cefixime (for 14 days) with a combination of intravenous therapy with cefotaxime (for 3 or 4 days) plus oral cefixime for 9 to 10 days. Children were eligible for this study if they were 1 to 24 months of age and presented to the physician with temperature greater than 38.3° C, and were found to have a positive enhanced urinalysis (≥10 WBCs/mm³ and 1 organism per 10 oil immersion fields). After blood and urine cultures, complete blood count, C-reactive protein determination, and erythrocyte sedimentation rate were performed, the children were randomly assigned to treatment groups. Outcome was evaluated with regard to the short-term measures of sterilization of the urine and time to defervescence and the long-term measures of reinfection and scarring 6 months after the initial infection. No statistically significant differences in any outcome were found.

Bloomfield and colleagues[12] performed a systematic review of the treatment of APN in children. They assessed 18 trials of 2612 children aged 0 to 18 years with proven UTIs and APN. Their results suggested that children with APN could be treated effectively with oral cefixime or with a short course of intravenous therapy followed by oral therapy.[58]

MANAGEMENT OF DYSFUNCTIONAL VOIDING

If a history of dysfunctional voiding is obtained, a behavioral modification approach may be helpful. The key features include frequent volitional voiding every 2 to 3 hours until the voiding pattern has been re-established, increased water intake (1 L/day) in addition to all other fluids consumed, correction of constipation, and adequate perineal hygiene.[28] Referral to a pediatric urologist may be necessary. Children who exhibit persistent inability to relax their sphincters may require training that involves relaxation techniques reinforced with biofeedback. Pharmacologic treatment with anticholinergics may be necessary if uninhibited bladder contractions are shown with urodynamic studies.[28] Special attention must be paid to the management of constipation if anticholinergics are initiated because they would exaggerate the problem.

ANTIBIOTIC PROPHYLAXIS

Although antibiotic prophylaxis commonly is recommended for children with recurrent UTIs,[79] only limited data support this position. In a review of the literature, Le Saux and colleagues[79] found sparse data of low quality to support the use of antibiotic prophylaxis in children with a normal urinary tract. A meta-analysis by Williams and associates[156] revealed five randomized controlled trials assessing the use of prophylactic therapy. Of these, only two trials with 71 children evaluated the effectiveness of long-term, low-dose antibiotics to prevent UTIs.[87,134] The authors concluded that well-designed, randomized, placebo-controlled trials still are required to evaluate this commonly used intervention.

MANAGEMENT OF VESICOURETERAL REFLUX

The clinical significance of VUR as a predisposing factor for UTIs in general or APN in particular and its contribution to the formation of renal scarring have been questioned more recently. As a corollary to the latter, the question also has been framed as to whether long-term antibiotic prophylaxis would prevent renal damage in patients with VUR.[32] The authors concluded that the role of VUR in UTIs needs to be redefined through well-designed, multicenter, prospective, randomized, controlled studies using state-of-the-art renal imaging techniques.

Epidemiology

The incidence of VUR in the general population is thought to be approximately 1 percent.[22] Children usually are tested for the possibility of VUR in one of two clinical situations—during the assessment of prenatally diagnosed hydronephrosis and in the evaluation of a UTI. Reflux is diagnosed in approximately 10 to 20 percent of cases of prenatally identified hydronephrosis; it often is high-grade and occurs more frequently in boys than in girls in this situation.[48,146] The incidence of reflux in girls evaluated after a first UTI is 25 to 40 percent.[26]

An increased incidence of VUR within families suggests a genetic mode of transmission.[68] Rates for prevalence of VUR in identical and fraternal twins were 80 percent and 35 percent, providing evidence that this trait is transmitted in an autosomal dominant fashion. Siblings of children identified to have VUR as part of an evaluation for UTI have a much greater chance of having reflux than the normal population.[4,106] The presence of VUR in these siblings is accompanied by silent renal damage.[15] In addition, a girl who has reflux has a 65 percent risk of having affected offspring.[22] Reflux is much more common among white than black children.

Natural History of Reflux

The natural history of reflux is for spontaneous resolution to occur over time, with a longer period being necessary in more severe types of reflux. Other factors that may affect the rate of resolution include age at diagnosis, gender, unilaterality versus bilaterality, and whether there is dysfunctional voiding. Average figures for spontaneous resolution are 80 to 86 percent for grade II reflux and 40 to 46 percent for grade III reflux during a 5-year period.

In a report from Skoog and associates,[130] spontaneous resolution occurred within 1.65 years of diagnosis in patients with grade II reflux, but 1.97 years was required for resolution in patients with grade III reflux ($p < .04$). Ninety percent of patients with reflux grades between I and III who ultimately had resolution of reflux experienced this result within 5 years. The rate of resolution was approximately 30 to 35 percent per year, although the duration of reflux was shorter for patients in whom the diagnosis was made before they reached 1 year of age compared with patients who were older at the time of diagnosis.[7]

In another study of the natural history of reflux, Schwab and coworkers[125] determined the resolution rate by patient for 179 girls and 35 boys with UTIs and diagnoses of primary VUR between 1981 and 1984. Reflux spontaneously resolved in 68 percent of patients during the study. Grades I to III reflux resolved at a rate of 13 percent per year for the first 5 years of follow-up and then at a rate of 3.5 percent per year during subsequent follow-up. Grades IV and V reflux resolved at a rate of 5 percent per year. Bilateral reflux resolved more slowly than unilateral reflux and more rapidly in boys than in girls. There is no specific age in adolescence at which one can assume reflux will not resolve. Leneghan and colleagues[76] reported cessation of reflux after 14 years of age in 27 percent of patients observed without surgical intervention.

Management of Reflux

The optimal management of children with high grades of reflux (grades III to V) has been the subject of numerous retrospective and prospective studies.[64] Since 1970, two large prospective randomized trials, the Birmingham Reflux study[9-11] and the International Reflux Study in Children,[115] have been performed to compare medical therapy (antibiotic prophylaxis) with surgical therapy (reimplantation of ureters). The International Reflux Study in Children reported results from Europe and the United States. Because entry criteria were different, the results have been reported separately.

In Europe and the United States, the surgical management of VUR is neither superior nor inferior to medical treatment. In both groups, new scars were acquired during the 5-year follow-up period, some in patients who did not show scarring at the time of entry. In other children, scars present at entry worsened.[110] No detectable differences were found between study groups in either renal function or renal growth. The number of episodes of infection also was similar in both groups. The only exception was a greater frequency of episodes of febrile UTIs (presumed pyelonephritis) in children receiving medical therapy.

Wheeler and colleagues[155] conducted a systematic review of randomized trials of the effects of various interventions in patients with VUR on the development of subsequent UTI and renal parenchymal injury. The aim was to evaluate whether any intervention for reflux (surgical) is better than nonsurgical treatment. Eight trials involving 859 evaluable children were reviewed. Seven trials compared antimicrobials alone with surgery plus antimicrobial propylaxis. The risk of a UTI developing by 1 or 2 and 5 years was not significantly different between surgical and medical groups, and the risk of renal scarring or progressive renal damage occurring was similar. The choice of treatment remains a value judgment governed by such local factors as preference of the parents, availability of skilled surgeons, availability of closely supervised medical treatment, and willingness to comply with prolonged periods of prophylaxis.

Does VUR predispose to pyelonephritis? Garin and associates[32] reviewed 10 studies of children with acute UTIs who underwent DMSA scanning and VCUG. Selection of patients in at least one of the studies was biased toward the association between reflux and APN because the VCUG often was performed after the DMSA scan was reported to be abnormal. Six of 10 studies showed statistically significant results indicating that the presence of reflux definitely was associated with the occurrence of APN; all 4 of the remaining studies showed a trend in the same direction.

Antimicrobial Prophylaxis

Although the use of antimicrobial prophylaxis has become routine in the management of children with VUR, substantial controversy currently surrounds this approach, and an increasing literature challenges its benefit. In 2003, a Cochrane Review of the effectiveness of long-term antibiotics for preventing recurrent UTIs in children indicated that most studies published before this date were poorly designed without proper blinding.[157] Although Garin and colleagues[33] contributed a large study suggesting that antibiotic prophylaxis is not an effective intervention compared with no treatment in children with VUR, this study also had many methodologic flaws.[150]

Accepting for the moment that prophylaxis is the most effective medical therapy that can be offered to children with mild to moderate degrees of reflux, the duration of prophylaxis also is an issue. VUR spontaneously remits in most cases during the first 3 to 5 years of life. Conventional wisdom is that prophylaxis should be maintained until reflux ceases, either spontaneously or with surgical intervention. Greenfield and colleagues[39] suggested that two normal VCUGs performed 12 months apart are necessary before prophylactic antibiotics are discontinued. This recommendation is based on the observation that 27 percent of children exhibit VUR again after a single normal study.

Greenfield and colleagues[39] maintained that administration of prophylactic antibiotics should continue until reflux resolves, no matter what the age. They supported this position by noting that older children with reflux may have new scars evolve when they become infected. In contrast, other authors suggest that prophylaxis should be discontinued in older children, even if reflux persists.[2,7,18,141,158] The only two antimicrobial agents that are recommended for prophylaxis of the urinary tract are nitrofurantoin and trimethoprim-sulfamethoxazole. Each agent is used in half the usual therapeutic dose and given before bedtime. These two agents can be used for months to years without the emergence of antibiotic resistance. In contrast, most other agents that are used for treatment of UTIs are not recommended for prophylaxis. Invariably, if agents such as amoxicillin, cephalexin, and second-generation and third-generation cephalosporins are used for prophylaxis, infection with resistant strains emerges within weeks.

Surgery

When antireflux surgery is undertaken, a variety of approaches are available, no one of which seems to be superior. In most cases, the surgical approach is intravesicular. Interest has been gaining in evaluation of an extravesicular approach to reimplantation of the ureters.[95] The advantage of extravesicular approaches seems to be a diminution of the intensity and frequency of bladder spasms and less requirement for postoperative analgesia. This technique is indicated primarily in unilateral VUR.[44] When experienced senior surgeons embark on reimplantation of ureters, the outcome generally is successful.[22] Generally, all surgical techniques have a high success rate of 92 to 98 percent.[44] Repeated operation for persistence or recurrence of reflux seldom is required. Rarely, when children younger than 2 years old undergo surgery, ureteral obstruction may result; its persistence mandates a second operation.[115]

A newer technique for the management of VUR is endoscopic injection therapy using a variety of materials. Developed as a minimally invasive approach to the treatment of VUR in 1984, dextranomer/hyaluronic acid copolymer has emerged as the favored bulking agent since its approval by the Food and Drug Administration.[43,92] Although success is defined differently from after surgery, overall success rates range from 82 to 89 percent with initial injections of dextranomer/hyaluronic acid. The bulking agent is injected beneath the ureteral orifice and effectively closes the distal ureter. The procedure is done in the outpatient setting and is associated with less pain and a quicker recovery compared with traditional reimplantation procedures.[92] The success rates are lower, however, than those of traditional therapy, and the results have questionable durability. Long-term prospective studies are necessary to evaluate endoscopic treatments critically.

PROGNOSIS

Generally, a review of reports suggests that the short-term prognosis for previously normal children who experience an episode of UTI is excellent. In a large cohort of 306 children experiencing their first febrile episode of UTI, 40 percent were found to have reflux.[55] Only five (1.6%) of the children had grade IV reflux; none had grade V reflux. Most of the children with grades I, II, and III reflux can be expected to have spontaneous resolution of the process during the subsequent several years. Although many reports indicate that recurrent UTIs are common occurrences in children who have recovered from UTIs, recurrence during the first 6 months after recovery from the index episode of UTI was an infrequent event in this cohort of children.

Recurrence is seen most commonly in the early months after a symptomatic or asymptomatic UTI has occurred. Symptomatic reinfections (fever, pyuria, and positive urine culture) occurred in 7 children treated orally and in 11 children treated intravenously (for a total of 5.9% of children) during the 6-month follow-up period.[55] Asymptomatic bacteriuria (positive urine culture in the absence of fever and pyuria) occurred in one child treated orally and in two children treated intravenously (1%). Renal scarring occurred in 9.5 percent of all children; the average percentage of renal parenchymal involvement was 8.2 percent. In children who had an abnormal renal scintigram at the time of diagnosis, the frequency of scarring was 15.3 percent. None of the children with a normal renal scintigram at the time of diagnosis developed scars. This experience, reflecting an aggressive approach to the early diagnosis of UTI in infancy, is encouraging with regard to outcome.

When children with a diagnosis of UTI are found to have anomalies of the urinary tract, congenital dysplasias, or massive degrees of reflux, the prognosis is less optimistic. The most profound degrees of scarring are associated with advanced degrees of reflux. Reflux nephropathy is a major cause of severe hypertension in children and young adults. It occasionally progresses to chronic renal failure,[136] which accounts for approximately 25 percent of the children in the United Kingdom with end-stage renal failure requiring regular dialysis or transplantation.[80] Although surgical correction may relieve the reflux, the overall outcome for children with reflux who have undergone surgical correction has not been shown to be materially better than that for children who have been managed medically.[103,104,137]

Smellie and colleagues[133] undertook a randomized trial of medical management versus surgical correction in 53 children with bilateral severe VUR and bilateral nephropathy. The glomerular filtration rate of the children at enrollment was 20 mL/min/1.73 m² body surface area. Children with this degree of severity of renal impairment are rare; recruitment to this study took 5 years. No significant differences were observed in glomerular filtration rate, renal growth, or scarring during a 10-year follow-up period. The failure to find differences may be due to the small sample size and broad heterogeneity of the study group. Nonetheless, no convincing evidence that outcome for renal function is improved by surgical correction of VUR in children with bilateral disease exists.

PREVENTION

Primary prevention of UTI can be accomplished in infant boys by promoting the practice of circumcision. Whether this procedure can be justified simply to prevent UTIs in the context of social rituals is uncertain. Circumcision should be recommended, however, for selected groups of patients, including newborns with prenatal hydronephrosis who are found to have VUR in the neonatal period, boys with high grades of VUR, and boys in whom VUR is associated with unilateral renal agenesis or multicystic kidney.[14]

Other commonly recommended strategies to prevent UTI, such as the avoidance of bathing in tubs or swimming and the instruction in correct wiping techniques, are not accompanied by convincing evidence.[45] The relationship between constipation and UTI is well known. Effective treatment of constipation results in normalization of bladder function and cessation of UTIs.[86]

The role of prophylactic antibiotics for patients with VUR is discussed in the section on treatment. Prophylaxis has not been shown in large, prospective, placebo-controlled, randomized trials to reduce effectively the frequency of UTI and subsequent renal scarring either in patients with reflux or in patients who have experienced an episode of APN.[33,157] Although definite biologic plausibility to this likelihood exists, strong evidence is lacking.

An additional preventive strategy for UTI is immunization. A small pilot study was reported from Turkey.[98] Ten otherwise healthy girls aged 5 to 11 years old with recurrent UTIs were immunized with inactivated uropathogenic bacteria intramuscularly once a week for 3 consecutive weeks. A booster injection was given after 6 months. The frequency of infection was compared with that in a group of 10 age-matched girls with UTIs who were not immunized. Immunization therapy caused a significant reduction in the frequency of infection and an increase in the concentration of the secretory component of IgA in the urine. Other mucosa, such as vaginal and oral surfaces, are alternative targets for vaccine delivery.

A vaginal mucosal vaccine composed of a mixture of heat-killed bacteria from 10 human uropathic strains (6 *E. coli* and 4 other gram-negative enteric bacteria) was developed for women with recurrent UTIs.[145] Fifty-four women completed a double-blind, placebo-controlled, phase 2 trial. Time until reinfection was longest for women who received primary and booster immunization compared with women receiving a placebo. This strategy has potential for further development.

REFERENCES

1. Aia-ul-Miraj, M., and Cheema, M. A.: Xanthogranulomatous pyelonephritis presenting as a pseudotumor in a 2 month old boy. J. Pediatr. Surg. 35:1256-1258, 2000.
2. Al-Sayyad, A. J., Pike, J. G., and Leonard, M. P.: Can prophylactic antibiotics safely be discontinued in children with vesicoureteral reflux? J. Urol. 174:1587-1588, 2005.
3. American Academy of Pediatrics, Committee on Quality Improvement, Subcommittee on Urinary Tract Infection: Practice parameter: The diagnosis, treatment, and evaluation of the initial urinary tract infection in febrile infants and young children. Pediatrics 103:843-853, 1999.
4. Ataei, N., Madani, A., Esfahani, S. T., et al.: Screening for vesicoureteral reflux and renal scars in siblings of children with known reflux. Pediatr. Nephrol. 19:1127-1131, 2004.
5. Austin, P. F., and Ritchey, M. L.: Dysfunctional voiding. Pediatr. Rev. 21:336-340, 2000.
6. Belman, A. B.: A perspective on vesicoureteral reflux. Urol. Clin. North Am. 22:139-150, 1995.
7. Belman, A. B.: Vesicoureteral reflux. Pediatr. Clin. North Am. 44:1171-1190, 1997.
8. Benador, N., Siegrist, C. A., Gendrel, D., et al.: Procalcitonin is a marker of severity of renal lesions in pyelonephritis. Pediatrics 102:1422-1425, 1998.
9. Birmingham Reflux Study Group: Prospective trial of operative versus nonoperative treatment of severe vesicoureteric reflux: Two years' observation in 96 children. B. M. J. 287:171-174, 1983.
10. Birmingham Reflux Study Group: A prospective trial of operative versus non-operative treatment of severe vesicoureteric reflux: 2 years' observation in 96 children. Contrib. Nephrol. 39:169-185, 1984.
11. Birmingham Reflux Study Group: Prospective trial of operative versus non-operative treatment of severe vesicoureteric reflux in children: Five years' observation. B. M. J. 295:237-241, 1987.
12. Bloomfield, P., Hodson, E. M., and Craig, J. C.: Antibiotics for acute pyelonephritis in children. Cochrane Database Syst. Rev. 2006. Jan 25(1): CD003772, 2005, DOI: 10.1002/14651858 CD003772.pub2
13. Brook, I.: Urinary tract infection caused by anaerobic bacteria in children. Urology 16:596-598, 1980.
14. Cascio, S., Colhoun, E., and Puri, P.: Bacterial colonization of the prepuce in boys with vesicoureteral reflux who receive antibiotic prophylaxis. J. Pediatr. 139:160-162, 2001.
15. Cascio, S., Yoneda, A., Chertin, B., et al.: Renal parenchymal damage in sibling vesicoureteric reflux. Acta Pediatr. 92:17-20, 2003.
16. Chen, M., Bao, W., Aizman, R., et al.: ERK activation mediates apoptosis induced by uropathogenic *Escherichia coli* toxins via nitric oxide synthesis: Protective role of heme-oxygenase-1. J. Infect. Dis. 190:127-135, 2004.
17. Childs, R., Sanchez, C., Engler, H., et al.: High incidence of adeno- and polyomavirus-induced hemorrhagic cystitis in bone marrow allotransplantation for hematological malignancy following T cell depletion and cyclosporine. Bone Marrow Transplant. 22:889-893, 1998.
18. Cooper, C. S., Chung, B. I., Kirsch, A. J., et al.: The outcome of stopping prophylactic antibiotics in older children with vesicoureteral reflux. J. Urol. 163:269-272, 2000.
19. Craig, J. C., Knight, J. F., Sureshkumar, P., et al.: Effect of circumcision on incidence of urinary tract infection in preschool boys. J. Pediatr. 128:23-27, 1996.
20. Crain, E., and Gershel, J. C.: Urinary tract infections in febrile infants younger than 8 weeks of age. Pediatrics 86:363-367, 1990.
21. Davies, H. D., Jones, E. L., Sheng, R. Y., et al.: Nosocomial urinary tract infections at a pediatric hospital. Pediatr. Infect. Dis. J. 11:349-354, 1992.
22. Decter, R. M.: Vesicoureteral reflux. Pediatr. Rev. 22:205-210, 2001.
23. Dick, P. T., and Feldman, W.: Routine diagnostic imaging for childhood urinary tract infections: A systematic overview. J. Pediatr. 128:15-22, 1996.
24. Djojohodipringgo, R., Abdulhamed, R. H., Thahir, S., et al.: Bladder puncture in newborns: A bacteriologic study. Paediatr. Indones. 16:527-534, 1976.
25. Downs, S. M.: Diagnostic testing strategies in childhood urinary tract infections. Pediatr. Ann. 28:670-676, 1999.
26. Downs, S. M.: Technical report: Urinary tract infections in febrile infants and young children. The Urinary Tract Subcommittee of the American Academy of Pediatrics Committee on Quality Improvement. Pediatrics 103:e54, 1999.
27. Duckett, J. W., Walker, R. D., and Weiss, R.: Surgical results: International Reflux Study in Children—United States branch. J. Urol. 148:1674-1675, 1992.
28. Farhat, W., and McLorie, G.: Urethral syndromes in children. Pediatr. Rev. 22:17-20, 2001.
29. Feldman, A. S., and Bauer, S. B.: Diagnosis and management of dysfunctional voiding. Curr. Opin. Pediatr. 18:139-147, 2006.

30. Foresman, W. H., Hulbert, W. C., Jr., and Rabinowitz, R.: Does urinary tract ultrasonography at hospitalization for acute pyelonephritis predict vesicoureteral reflux? J. Urol. *165*:2232-2234, 2001.

31. Foxman, B.: Epidemiology of urinary tract infections: Incidence, morbidity and economic costs. Am. J. Med. *113*:5S-13S, 2002.

32. Garin, E. H., Campos, A., and Homsy, Y.: Primary vesicoureteral reflux: Review of current concepts. Pediatr. Nephrol. *12*:249-256, 1998.

33. Garin, E. H., Olavarria, F., Garcia-Nieto, V., et al.: Clinical significance of primary vesicoureteral reflux and urinary antibiotic prophylaxis after acute pyelonephritis: A multicenter, randomized, controlled study. Pediatrics *117*:626-632, 2006.

34. Gervaix, A., Galletto-Lacour, A., Gueron, T., et al.: Usefulness of procalcitonin and C-reactive protein rapid tests for the management of children with urinary tract infection. Pediatr. Infect. Dis. J. *20*:507-511, 2001.

35. Ginsburg, C. M., and McCracken, G. H., Jr.: Urinary tract infections in young infants. Pediatrics *69*:409-412, 1982.

36. Gochman, R. F., Karasic, R. B., and Heller, M. B.: Use of portable ultrasound to assist urine collection by suprapubic aspiration. Ann. Emerg. Med. *20*:631-635, 1991.

37. Gordon, A. C., Thomas, D. F. M., Arthur, R. J., et al.: Prenatally diagnosed reflux: A follow up study. Br. J. Urol. *65*:407-412, 1990.

38. Gorelick, M. H., and Shaw, K. N.: Screening tests for urinary tract infection in children: A meta-analysis. Pediatrics *104*:e54, 1999.

39. Greenfield, S. P., Ng, M., and Wan, J.: Experience with vesicoureteral reflux in children: Clinical characteristics. J. Urol. *158*:574-577, 1997.

39a. Greenfield, S. P., Cherry, R. W., Carpenter, M., et al.: Vesicoureteral reflux: The RIVUR study and the way forward. J. Urol. *179*:405-407, 2008.

40. Hall, D. E., and Snitzer, J. A., III: *Staphylococcus epidermidis* as a cause of urinary tract infections in children. J. Pediatr. *124*:437-438, 1994.

41. Hansson, S., Dhamey, M., Sigstrom, O., et al.: Dimercapto-succinic acid scintigraphy instead of voiding cystourethrography for infants with urinary tract infection. J. Urol. *172*:1071-1074, 2004.

42. Hansson, S., Martinell, J., Stokland, E., et al.: The natural history of bacteriuria in childhood. Infect. Dis. Clin. North Am. *11*:499-512, 1997.

43. Harrell, W. B., and Snow, B. W.: Endoscopic treatment of vesicoureteral reflux. Curr. Opin. Pediatr. *17*:409-411, 2005.

44. Heidenreich, A., Ozgur, E., Becker, T., and Haupt, G.: Surgical management of vesicoureteral reflux in pediatric patients. World J. Urol. *22*:96-106, 2004.

45. Hellerstein, S.: Urinary tract infections in children: Why they occur and how to prevent them. Am. Fam. Physician *57*:2440-2446, 1998.

46. Hellerstein, S.: Acute urinary tract infection—evaluation and treatment. Curr. Opin. Pediatr. *18*:134-138, 2006.

47. Hellstrom, A., Hanson, E., Hansson, S., et al.: Association between urinary symptoms at 7 years old and previous urinary tract infection. Arch. Dis. Child. *66*:232-234, 1991.

48. Herndon, A. C. D., McKenna, P. H., and Kolon, T. F.: A multicenter outcomes analysis of patients with neonatal reflux presenting with prenatal hydronephrosis. J. Urol. *162*:1203-1208, 1999.

49. Herr, S. M., Wald, E. R., Pitetti, R. D., and Choi, S. S.: Enhanced urinalysis improves identification of febrile infants ages 60 days and younger at low risk for serious bacterial illness. Pediatrics *108*:866-871, 2001.

50. Hitchcock, R. J., Pallett, A., Hall, M. A., et al.: Urinary tract candidiasis in neonates and infants. Br. J. Urol. *76*:252-256, 1995.

51. Hjalmas, K., Lohr, G., Tamminen-Mobius, T., et al.: Surgical results in the international reflux study in children (Europe). J. Urol. *148*:1657-1661, 1992.

52. Hoberman, A., Chao, H. P., Keller, D. M., et al.: Prevalence of urinary tract infection in febrile infants. J. Pediatr. *123*:17-23, 1993.

53. Hoberman, A., Charron, M., Hickey, R. W., et al.: Imaging studies after a first febrile urinary tract infection in young children. N. Engl. J. Med. *248*:195-202, 2003.

54. Hoberman, A., and Wald, E. R.: Urinary tract infections in young febrile children. Pediatr. Infect. Dis. J. *16*:11-17, 1997.

55. Hoberman, A., Wald, E. R., Hickey, R. W., et al.: Oral versus initial intravenous therapy for urinary tract infections in young febrile children. Pediatrics *104*:79-86, 1999.

56. Hoberman, A., Wald, E. R., Penchansky, L., et al.: Enhanced urinalysis as a screening test for urinary tract infection. Pediatrics *91*:1196-1199, 1993.

57. Hoberman, A., Wald, E. R., Reynolds, E. A., et al.: Pyuria and bacteriuria in urine specimens obtained by catheter from young children with fever. J. Pediatr. *124*:513-519, 1994.

58. Hodson, M. M., Craig, E. M., Martin, S., et al.: Short versus standard duration oral antibiotic therapy for acute urinary tract infection in children. Cochrane Database Syst. Rev. (1): CD003966, 2003.

59. Hooten, T. M., Scholes, D., Hughes, J. P., et al.: A prospective study of risk factors for symptomatic urinary tract infection in young women. N. Engl. J. Med. *335*:468-474, 1996.

60. Horwitz, M. A., and Silverstein, S. C.: Influence of *Escherichia coli* capsule on complement fixation and on phagocytosis and killing by human phagocytes. J. Clin. Invest. *65*:82-94, 1980.

61. Huicho, L., Campos-Sanchez, M., and Alamo, C.: Meta-analysis of urine screening tests for determining the risk of urinary tract infection in children. Pediatr. Infect. Dis. J. *21*:1-11, 2002.

62. Jahnukainen, T., Chen, M., and Celsi, G.: Mechanism of renal damage owing to infection. Pediatr. Nephrol. *20*:1043-1053, 2005.

63. Jantunen, M. E., Siitonen, A., Koskimies, O., et al.: Predominance of class II *papG* allele of *Escherichia coli* in pyelonephritis in infants with normal urinary tract anatomy. J. Infect. Dis. *181*:1822-1824, 2000.

64. Jodal, U., Hansson, S., and Hjalmas, K.: Medical or surgical management for children with vesicoureteric reflux? Acta Paediatr. *431*(Suppl.):53-61, 1999.

65. Jodal, U., Koskimies, O., Hanson, E., et al.: Infection pattern in children with vesicoureteral reflux randomly allocated to operation or long term antibacterial prophylaxis. J. Urol. *148*:1650-1652, 1992.

66. Kaack, M. B., Dowling, K. J., Patterson, G. M., et al.: Immunology of pyelonephritis, VIII: *E. coli* causes granulocytic aggregation and renal ischemia. J. Urol. *136*:1117-1122, 1986.

67. Kabore, A. F., Simord, M., and Bergeron, M. G.: Local production of inflammatory mediators in an experimental model of acute obstructive pyelonephritis. J. Infect. Dis. *179*:1162-1172, 1999.

68. Kaefer, M., Curran, M., Treves, S. T., et al.: Sibling vesicoureteral reflux in multiple gestation births. Pediatrics *105*:800-804, 2000.

69. Kallenius, G., Mollby, R., Svensson, S. B., et al.: The pK antigen as receptor for the hemagglutination of pyelonephritogenic *Escherichia coli*. FEMS Microbiol. Lett. 7:297, 1980.

70. Kemper, K. J., and Avner, E. D.: The case against screening urinalyses for asymptomatic bacteriuria in children. Am. J. Dis. Child. *146*:343-346, 1992.

71. Khan, A. J., Ubriani, R. S., Bombach, E., et al.: Initial urinary tract infection caused by *Proteus mirabilis* in infancy and childhood. J. Pediatr. *93*:791-793, 1978.

72. Koff, S. A., Wagner, T. T., and Jayanthi, V. R.: The relationship among dysfunctional elimination syndromes, primary vesicoureteral reflux and urinary tract infections in children. J. Urol. *160*:1019-1022, 1998.

73. Kunin, C. M.: A ten-year study of bacteriuria in schoolgirls: Final report of bacteriologic, urologic and epidemiologic findings. J. Infect. Dis. *122*:382-393, 1970.

74. Lamchiogdhase, P., Preechaborisutkul, K., Lomsomboon, P., et al.: Urine sediment examination: A comparison between manual method and the iQ200 automated urine microscopy analyzer. Clin. Chim. Acta *359*:167-174, 2005.

75. Lebowitz, R. L., Olbing, H., Parkkulainen, K. V., et al.: International system of radiographic grading of vesicoureteral reflux: International reflux study in children. Pediatr. Radiol. *15*:105-109, 1985.

76. Leneghan, D., Whitaker, J. G., Jensen, F., and Stephens, F. D.: The natural history of reflux and long term effects of reflux on the kidney. J. Urol. *115*:728-730, 1976.

77. Leong, Y. Y., and Tan, K. W.: Bladder aspiration for diagnosis of urinary tract infection in infants and young children. J. Singapore Paediatr. Soc. *18*:43-47, 1976.

78. Leonidas, J. C., and Berdon, W. E.: MR imaging of urinary tract infections in children. Radiology *210*:582-583, 1999.

79. Le Saux, N., Pham, B. A., and Moher, D.: Evaluating the benefits of antimicrobial prophylaxis to prevent urinary tract infections in children: A systematic review. Can. Med. Assoc. J. *163*:523-529, 2000.

80. Lewis, M.: Report of the Paediatric Renal Registry 1999. *In* Ansell, D., and Feest, T. (eds.): The Second Annual Report of the UK Renal Registry. Bristol, U.K., Renal Association, 1999, pp. 175-187.

81. Liles, W. C., Cushing, H., Holt, S., et al.: Severe adenoviral nephritis following bone marrow transplantation: Successful treatment with intravenous ribavirin. Bone Marrow Transplant. *12*:409-412, 1993.

82. Lin, D. S., Huang, F. Y., Chiu, N. C., et al.: Comparison of hemocytometer leukocyte counts and standard urinalyses for predicting urinary tract infections in febrile infants. Pediatr. Infect. Dis. J. *19*:223-227, 2000.

83. Lin, D. S., Huang, S., Lin, C., et al.: Urinary tract infection in febrile infants younger than eight weeks of age. Pediatrics *105*:e20, 2000.

84. Lindberg, U., Claesson, I., Hanson, L. A., et al.: Asymptomatic bacteriuria in schoolgirls: Clinical and laboratory findings. Acta Paediatr. Scand. *64*:425-431, 1975.

85. Linko, S., Kauri, T. K., Toivonen, E., et al.: Analytic performance of the Iris iQ200 automated urine microscopy analyzer. Clin. Chim. Acta *372*:54-56, 2006.

86. Loening-Baucke, V.: Urinary incontinence and urinary tract infection and their resolution with treatment of chronic constipation of childhood. Pediatrics *100*:228-232, 1997.

87. Lohr, J. A., Nunley, D. H., Howards, S. S., et al.: Prevention of recurrent urinary tract infections in girls. Pediatrics *59*:562-565, 1977.

88. Lohr, J. A., Portilla, M. G., Geuder, T. G., et al.: Making a presumptive diagnosis of urinary tract infection by using a urinalysis performed in an on-site laboratory. J. Pediatr. *122*:22-25, 1993.

89. Lomberg, L., Hellstrom, M., Jodal, U., et al.: Virulence-associated traits in *Escherichia coli* causing first and recurrent episodes of urinary tract infection in children with or without vesicoureteral reflux. J. Infect. Dis. *150*:561-569, 1984.

90. Lonergan, D. J., and Pennington, D. J.: MR imaging of urinary tract infections in children. Reply. Radiology *210*:583-584, 1999.

91. Lonergan, G. J., Pennington, D. J., Morrison, J. C., et al.: Childhood pyelonephritis: Comparison of gadolinium-enhanced MR imaging and renal cortical scintigraphy. Radiology *207*:377-384, 1998.

92. Lorenzo, A. J., and Khoury, A. E.: Endoscopic treatment of reflux: Management of pros and cons. Curr. Opin. Urol. *16*:299-304, 2006.

93. Ma, J. F., and Shortliffe, L. M. D.: Urinary tract infection in children: Etiology and epidemiology. Urol. Clin. North Am. *31*:517-526, 2004.

94. Marild, S., and Jodal, U.: Incidence rate of first-time symptomatic urinary tract infection in children under 6 years of age. Acta Paediatr. *87*:549-552, 1998.

95. Marotte, J. B., and Smith, D. P.: Extravesical ureteral reimplantations for the correction of primary reflux can be done as outpatient procedures. J. Urol. *165*:2228-2231, 2001.

96. McFadyen, I. R., and Eykyn, S. J.: Suprapubic aspiration of urine in pregnancy. Lancet *1*:1112-1114, 1968.

97. Morgan, M. G., and Hamilton-Miller, J. M.: *Haemophilus influenzae* and *H. parainfluenzae* as urinary pathogens. J. Infect. *20*:143-145, 1990.

98. Nayir, A., Emre, S., Sirin, A., et al.: The effects of vaccination with inactivated uropathogenic bacteria in recurrent urinary tract infections of children. Vaccine *13*:987-990, 1995.

99. Newman, T. B., Bernzweig, J. A., Takayama, J. I., et al.: Urine testing and urinary tract infections in febrile infants seen in office settings: The pediatric research in office settings febrile infant study. Arch. Pediatr. Adolesc. Med. *156*:44-54, 2002.

100. Nicolle, L. E.: Catheter-related urinary tract infection. Drugs Aging *22*:627-639, 2005.

101. Nicolle, L. E., Harding, G. K. M., Preiksaitis, J., et al.: The association of urinary tract infection with sexual intercourse. J. Infect. Dis. *146*:579-583, 1982.

102. Nowicki, B., Holthofer, H., Saraneva, T., et al.: Location of adhesion sites for P-fimbriated and for O75X-positive *Escherichia coli* in the human kidney. Microb. Pathog. *1*:169-180, 1986.

103. Olbing, H., Claesson, I., Ebel, K. D., et al.: Renal scars and parenchymal thinning in children with vesicoureteral reflux: A 5-year report of the International Reflux Study in Children (European branch). J. Urol. *148*:1653-1656, 1992.

104. Olbing, H., Hirche, H., Koskimies, O., et al.: Renal growth over 10 years in a prospective study of medical or surgical treatment in children with severe vesicoureteral reflux: 10-year prospective study of medical and surgical treatment. Radiology *216*:731-737, 2000.

105. Orrett, F. A., Brooks, P. J., Richardson, E. G., et al.: Paediatric nosocomial urinary tract infection at a regional hospital. Int. Urol. Nephrol. *31*:173-179, 1999.

106. Parekh, D. J., Pope, J. C., Adams, M. C., and Brock, J. W.: Outcome of sibling vesicoureteral reflux. J. Urol. *167*:283-284, 2002.

107. Pecile, P., Miorin, E., Romanello, C., et al.: Procalcitonin: A marker of severity of acute pyelonephritis among children. Pediatrics *114*:e249-e254, 2004.

108. Pennington, D. J., Lonergan, G. J., Flack, C. E., et al.: Experimental pyelonephritis in piglets: Diagnosis with MR imaging. Radiology *201*:199-205, 1996.

109. Phillips, J. R., and Karlowicz, M. G.: Prevalence of *Candida* species in hospital-acquired urinary tract infections in a neonatal intensive care unit. Pediatr. Infect. Dis. J. *16*:190-194, 1997.

110. Piepsz, A., Tamminen-Mobius, T., Reiners, C., et al.: Five-year study of medical or surgical treatment in children with severe vesicoureteral reflux dimercaptosuccinic acid findings. Eur. J. Pediatr. *157*:753-758, 1998.

111. Polnay, L., Fraser, A. M., and Lewis, J. M.: Complication of suprapubic bladder aspiration. Arch. Dis. Child. *50*:80-81, 1975.

112. Prat, C., Dominguez, J., Rodrigo, C., et al.: Elevated serum procalcitonin values correlate with renal scarring in children with urinary tract infection. Pediatr. Infect. Dis. J. *22*:438-442, 2003.

113. Pryles, C. V., Atkins, M. D., Morse, T. S., et al.: Comparative bacteriologic study of urine obtained from children by percutaneous suprapubic aspiration of the bladder and by catheter. Pediatrics *24*:983-991, 1959.

114. Quinn, F. M. J., Dick, A. C., Corbally, M. T., et al.: Xanthogranulomatous pyelonephritis in childhood. Arch. Dis. Child. *81*:483-486, 1999.

115. Report of the International Reflux Study Committee: Medical versus surgical treatment of primary vesicoureteral reflux: A prospective international reflux study in children. Pediatrics *67*:392-400, 1981.

116. Roberts, J. A.: Etiology and pathophysiology of pyelonephritis. Am. J. Kidney Dis. *17*:1-9, 1991.

117. Roberts, J. A., Angel, J. R., and Roth, J. K., Jr.: The hydrodynamics of pyelo-renal reflux, II: The effect of chronic obstructive changes on papillary shape. Invest. Urol. *18*:296-301, 1981.

118. Rushton, H. G.: Urinary tract infections in children: Epidemiology, evaluation, and management. Pediatr. Clin. North Am. *44*:1133-1169, 1997.

119. Rushton, H. G., Majd, M., Chandra, R., et al.: Evaluation of 99m technetium-dimercaptosuccinic acid in renal scans in experimental acute pyelonephritis in piglets. J. Urol. *140*:1169-1174, 1988.

120. Savage, D. C. L., Wilson, M. I., McHardy, M., et al.: Covert bacteriuria of childhood: A clinical and epidemiological study. Arch. Dis. Child. *48*:8-20, 1973.

121. Schlager, T. A., Hendley, J. O., Dudley, S. M., et al.: Explanation for false-positive urine cultures obtained by bag technique. Arch. Pediatr. Adolesc. Med. *149*:170-173, 1995.

122. Schlager, T. A., Smith, D. E., and Donowitz, L. G.: Perineal cleansing does not reduce contamination of urine samples from pregnant adolescents. Pediatr. Infect. Dis. J. *14*:909-911, 1995.

123. Schoen, E. J., Colby, C. J., and Ray, G. T.: Newborn circumcision decreases incidence and cost of urinary tract infections during the first year of life. Pediatrics *105*:789-793, 2000.

124. Scholes, D., Hooton, T. M., Roberts, P. L., et al.: Risk factors associated with acute pyelonephritis in healthy women. Ann. Intern. Med. *142*:20-27, 2005.

125. Schwab, C. W., Wu, H., Selman, H., et al.: Spontaneous resolution of vesicoureteral reflux: A 15-year perspective. J. Urol. *168*:2594-2599, 2002.

126. Shalaby-Rana, E., Lowe, L. H., Blask, A. N., et al.: Imaging in pediatric urology. Pediatr. Clin. North Am. *44*:1065-1089, 1997.

127. Shapiro, E. D.: Short course antimicrobial treatment of urinary tract infections in children: A critical analysis. Pediatr. Infect. Dis. J. *1*:294-297, 1982.

128. Shaw, K. N., Gorelick, M., McGowan, K. L., et al.: Prevalence of urinary tract infection in febrile young children in the emergency department. Pediatrics *102*:e16, 1998.

129. Singh-Grewal, D., Macdessi, J., and Craig, J.: Circumcision for the prevention of urinary tract infection in boys: A systematic review of randomized trials and observational studies. Arch. Dis. Child. *90*:853-858, 2005.

130. Skoog, S. J., Belman, A. B., and Majd, M.: A nonsurgical approach to the management of primary vesicoureteral reflux. J. Urol. *138*:941, 1987.

131. Smellie, J. M.: Commentary: Management of children with severe vesicoureteral reflux. J. Urol. *148*:1676-1678, 1992.

132. Smellie, J. M.: Vesicoureteric reflux. Acta Paediatr. *88*:1182-1183, 1999.

133. Smellie, J. M., Barratt, T. M., Chantler, C., et al.: Medical versus surgical treatment in children with severe bilateral vesicoureteric reflux and bilateral nephropathy: A randomised trial. Lancet *357*:1329-1333, 2001.

134. Smellie, J. M., Katz, G., and Gruneberg, R. N.: Controlled trial of prophylactic treatment in childhood urinary tract infection. Lancet *2*:175-178, 1978.

135. Smellie, J. M., Poulton, A., and Prescod, N. P.: Retrospective study of children with renal scarring associated with reflux and urinary infection. B. M. J. *308*:1193, 1994.

136. Smellie, J. M., Prescod, N. P., Shaw, P. J., et al.: Childhood reflux and urinary infection: A follow-up of 10-41 years in 226 adults. Pediatr. Nephrol. *12*:727-736, 1998.

137. Smellie, J. M., Tamminen-Mobius, T., Olbing, H., et al.: Five year study of medical or surgical treatment in children with severe reflux: Radiological renal findings. Pediatr. Nephrol. *6*:223-230, 1992.

138. Smolken, V., Koren, A., Raz, R., et al.: Procalcitonin as a marker of acute pyelonephritis in infants and children. Pediatr. Nephrol. *17*:409-412, 2002.

139. Sobel, J. D., and Vasquez, J. A.: Fungal infections of the urinary tract. World J. Urol. *17*:410-414, 1999.

140. Tamminen-Mobius, T., Brunier, E., Ebel, K. D., et al.: Cessation of vesicoureteral reflux for 5 years in infants and children allocated to medical treatment. J. Urol. *148*:1662-1666, 1992.

141. Thompson, R. H., Chen, J. J., Pugach, J., et al.: Cessation of prophylactic antibiotics for managing persistent vesicoureteral reflux. J. Urol. *161*:1465-1469, 2001.

142. Todd, J. K.: Management of urinary tract infections: Children are different. Pediatr. Rev. *16*:190-196, 1995.

143. Tran, D., Muchant, D. G., and Aronoff, S. C.: Short-course versus conventional length antimicrobial therapy for uncomplicated lower urinary tract infections in children: A meta-analysis of 1279 patients. J. Pediatr. *139*:93-99, 2001.

144. Traylor, L. A., and Mayeux, P. R.: Nitric oxide generation mediates lipid-A-induced oxidant injury in renal proximal cells. Arch. Biochem. Biophys. *338*:129-135, 1997.

145. Uehling, D. T., Hopkins, W. J., Elkahwaji, J. E., et al.: Phase 2 clinical trial of a vaginal mucosal vaccine for urinary tract infections. J. Urol. *170*:867-869, 2003.

146. Upadhyaj, J., McLorie, G. A., Bolduc, S., et al.: Natural history of neonatal reflux associated with prenatal hydronephrosis: Long-term results of a prospective study. J. Urol. *69*:1837-1841, 2003.

147. Vaisanen-Rhen, V., Elo, J., Vaisanen, E., et al.: P-fimbriated clones among uropathogenic *Escherichia coli* strains. Infect. Immun. *43*:149-155, 1984.

148. Wah, D. T., Wises, P. K., and Butch, A. W.: Analytic performance of the iQ200 automated urine microscopy analyzer and comparison with manual counts using Fuchs-Rosenthal cell chambers. Am. J. Clin. Pathol. *123*:290-296, 2005.

149. Wald, E.: Urinary tract infections in infants and children: A comprehensive review. Curr. Opin. Pediatr. *16*:85-88, 2004.

150. Wald, E.: Vesicoureteral reflux: The role of antibiotics. Pediatrics *117*:919-922, 2006.

151. Wan, J., Kaplinsky, R., and Greenfield, S.: Toilet habits of children evaluated for urinary tract infection. J. Urol. *154*:797-799, 1995.

152. Weiss, R., Duckett, J., and Spitzer, A.: Results of a randomized clinical trial of medical versus surgical management of infants and children with grades III and IV primary vesicoureteral reflux (United States). J. Urol. *148*:1667-1673, 1992.

153. Weiss, R., Tamminen-Mobius, T., Koskimies, O., et al.: Characteristics at entry of children with severe primary vesicoureteral reflux recruited for a multicenter, international therapeutic trial comparing medical and surgical management. J. Urol. *148*:1644-1649, 1992.

154. Wettergren, B., and Jodal, U.: Spontaneous clearance of asymptomatic bacteriuria in infants. Acta Paediatr. Scand. *79*:300-304, 1990.

155. Wheeler, D., Vimalachendra, D., Hodson, E. M., et al.: Antibiotics and surgery for vesicoureteric reflux: A meta-analysis of randomized controlled trials. Arch. Dis. Child. *88*:688-694, 2003.

156. Williams, G., Lee, A., and Craig, J.: Antibiotics for the prevention of urinary tract infection in children: A systematic review of randomized controlled trials. J. Pediatr. *138*:868-874, 2001.

157. Williams, G. J., Lee, A., and Craig, J. C.: Long-term antibiotics for preventing recurrent urinary tract infection in children. Cochrane Database of Syst. Rev. 2001(4)CD001534 updated 2006, 3;CD001534.

158. Winberg, J.: Management of primary vesicoureteric reflux in children—operation ineffective in preventing progressive renal damage. Infection 22(Suppl. 1):S4-S7, 1994.

159. Winberg, J., Andersen, H. J., Bergstrom, T., et al.: Epidemiology of symptomatic urinary tract infection in childhood. Acta Paediatr. Scand. 252(Suppl.):1-20, 1974.

160. Wiswell, T. E., and Roscelli, J. D.: Corroborative evidence for the decreased incidence of urinary tract infections in circumcised male infants. Pediatrics 78:96-99, 1986.

161. Wiswell, T. E., Smith, F. R., and Bass, J. W.: Decreased incidence of urinary tract infections in circumcised male infants. Pediatrics 75:901-903, 1985.

162. Yazbeck, S., Schick, E., and O'Regan, S.: Relevance of constipation to enuresis, urinary tract infection and reflux: A review. Eur. Urol. 13:318-321, 1987.

163. Zamir, G., Sakran, W., Horowitz, Y., et al.: Urinary tract infection: Is there a need for routine renal ultrasonography? Arch. Dis. Child. 89:466-468, 2004.

164. Zorc, J. J., Kiddoo, D. A., and Shaw, K. N.: Diagnosis and management of pediatric urinary tract infections. Clin. Microbiol. Rev. 18:417-422, 2005.

CHAPTER 46

RENAL ABSCESS

Edmond T. Gonzales, Jr. ☻ Sheldon L. Kaplan

Although acute pyelonephritis is a common infection in children, the primary development of a renal abscess or progression of pyelonephritis to a renal or perinephric abscess is an uncommon occurrence. In one study conducted over a 10-year period, 8 children with a renal abscess were found among 43,224 discharge diagnoses—approximately 1 case per 5400 pediatric admissions.[5] Six of the eight children were 11 years or older. Although rare, renal abscesses have been reported in neonates.[8] Renal abscess may be a primary problem—that is, one that develops in a kidney without an antecedent infection or underlying anatomic abnormality—or it may occur secondarily in a patient with previously recognized acute pyelonephritis or in a child with congenital urologic abnormalities known to predispose one to the development of pyelonephritis.

A primary renal abscess is thought to develop most often after an episode of bacteremia and frequently occurs in younger children. Hematogenous spread of bacteria to the kidney usually results in a cortical abscess.[5] The most common organisms involved in these abscesses are gram-positive cocci, primarily *Staphylococcus aureus*, and less often a streptococcus. In some cases, a cutaneous infection might have been present before development of the renal abscess, and this infection is thought to be the primary source for the bacteremia.[14] Most children in whom a renal abscess develops hematogenously are normal hosts.[5,10,18,20]

In older children and teenagers, tuberculous abscesses and caseous necrosis of the renal parenchyma also should be included in this primary classification. These infections tend to be indolent, although renal tuberculosis may be complicated by bacterial infection because of associated ureteral strictures and severe tuberculous cystitis. Pediatricians should become familiar with this "adult" malady because of the resurgence of tuberculosis and the generally older age group for which many pediatricians now provide care.

When a renal abscess occurs in association with a recognized urologic disorder, the organism responsible most often is a gram-negative bacillus or an enterococcus, bacteria usually seen in simple urinary tract infections and pyelonephritis.[17] Examples of urologic disorders that one might encounter with these infections include congenital and acquired obstructions (e.g., ureteropelvic and ureterovesical obstruction, retrocaval ureter, ureteral stricture after surgical intervention), calculous disease (obstructing and nonobstructing), infundibular stenosis, and renal dysplasia with cystic changes. Abscesses that occur as a result of infection of the urinary tract generally are found in a corticomedullary location.[5]

Anaerobic organisms also have been implicated as a cause of renal abscess. They often are present simultaneously with the more usual aerobic bacteria, but they can cause infections and abscesses alone. These anaerobic renal infections develop most commonly in association with infections complicating bowel injury or surgery, renal transplantation, malignancy, and orodental infections.[4] The genus of the anaerobic organism may provide a clue to its source. *Bacteroides fragilis* is likely to arise from an intra-abdominal source, whereas an oral site is more common for *Prevotella oralis*.[4]

Children with human immunodeficiency virus infection seem to have an increased risk for development of renal abscesses from the more common traditional organisms[3] and from unusual opportunistic fungal organisms, especially *Aspergillus*.[12] As expected, these children also tend to have a more fulminant course that often requires extensive surgical intervention and drainage.

The presence of a renal abscess implies the destruction and liquefaction of tissue in a confined space. Two other infectious disorders of the kidney, xanthogranulomatous pyelonephritis and acute lobar nephropathy (acute focal bacterial nephritis), frequently are included in this general category, although technically, true abscesses do not always develop in these disorders. Acute lobar nephropathy may progress to renal abscess, however, if not treated appropriately.

Xanthogranulomatous pyelonephritis describes a more chronic form of severe renal parenchymal destruction that often is associated with chronic stone disease. The process may involve the whole kidney or may be focal. In children, the focal form occurs more commonly. The pathognomonic histologic finding is an accumulation of lipid-laden macrophages that coalesce into discrete yellow nodules. Small abscess cavities often are studded throughout the kidney. The organism most frequently recovered from the kidney is *Proteus*, and urinary calculi are common findings. Although these patients often have acute symptoms, the symptoms frequently are superimposed on more chronic manifestations, such as weight loss, failure to thrive, and anemia. Treatment is complete or partial nephrectomy because the renal destruction generally is severe.[19]

Acute lobar nephropathy describes a focal area of intense edema at the site of infection in acute pyelonephritis.[2] It usually is recognized as a mass effect on an initial screening renal ultrasonogram. Severe nephromegaly (renal length >3 standard deviations above the mean for age) is another finding on renal ultrasound suggestive of acute lobar nephropathy.[6] Computed tomography (CT) of the kidney shows poor uptake in the involved segment, but no well-defined liquefaction (Fig. 46–1). Whether this edema is just an exaggerated response to infection or represents a pre-abscess change is unknown. Klar and colleagues[11] described 13 children, 4 months to 8 years of age, with acute lobar nephropathy in a prospective study during a 4-year period. Bacteremia was documented in only one child. Evolution to abscess formation occurred in four (31%). In another prospective study, Cheng and associates[7] found bacteremia occurred in 4 of 80 children (5%) with acute lobar nephropathy. These lesions

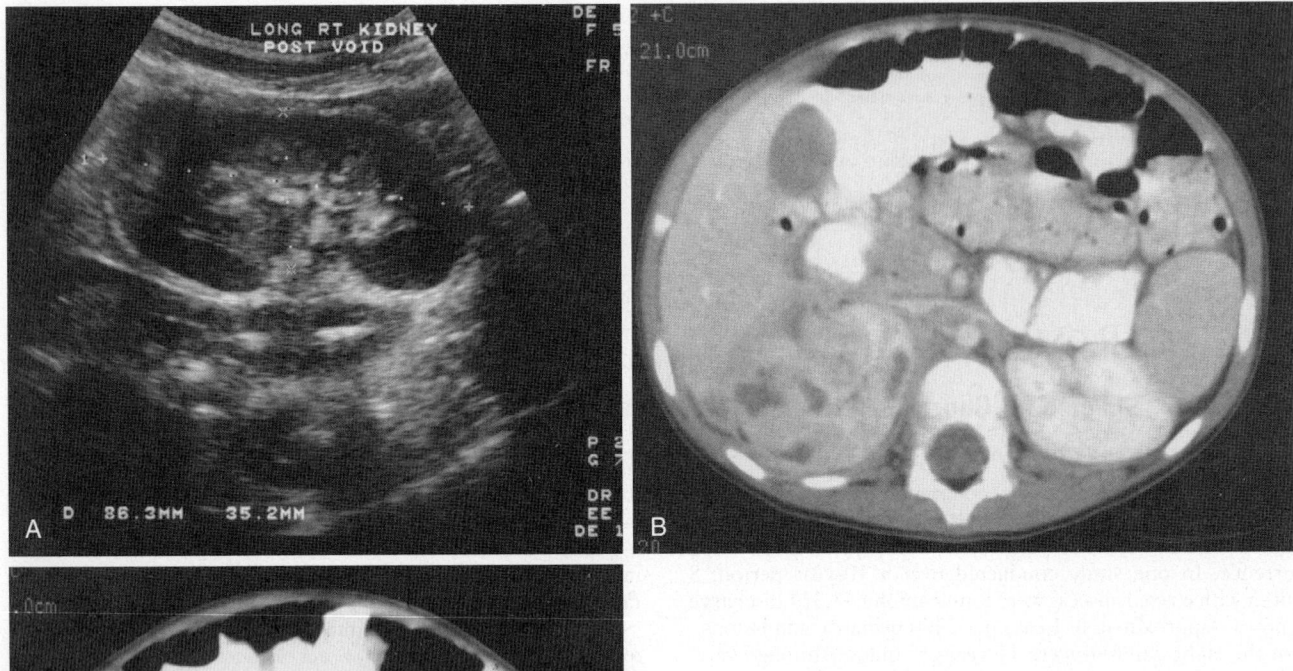

Figure 46–1 Acute lobar nephropathy in a 3-year-old girl with fever, right flank pain, and urinary tract infection. **A,** Initial renal ultrasonogram shows enlargement and swelling of the right upper pole. **B,** Initial upper pole cuts by computed tomography show poor uptake of contrast media and differing tissue densities. **C,** More caudal cuts reveal better function in the right lower pole. The infection and swelling resolved completely with antibiotics alone, with no evidence of postinfectious atrophy. This case was thought to represent acute lobar nephropathy.

generally heal satisfactorily with administration of antibiotics alone.

CLINICAL FINDINGS

Children with acute renal abscess are febrile and have localized pain in the costovertebral location. Prolonged fever is a common finding, especially in older children. Most patients are febrile for longer than 7 days before the diagnosis is established. The initial findings generally do not differentiate, however, between acute pyelonephritis with and without an abscess. If the abscess has spread into the perinephric region, one might be able to recognize psoas muscle irritation in the patient—that is, the patient is more comfortable with the ipsilateral leg in a position of flexion and experiences pain with full extension. A large abscess may be palpable as a flank mass.

Findings on urinalysis can be confusing. With a primary (hematogenous) abscess, the urine may be deceptively benign, and culture generally is negative.[14] Blood cultures may be positive, depending on the duration of the illness when blood is obtained for culture. Abscesses associated with underlying uro-

logic disorders can be expected to contain organisms and pyuria. Generally, severe leukocytosis is present. The erythrocyte sedimentation rate typically is elevated; the same probably is true for C-reactive protein.[20] All these findings are nonspecific, however, and often further studies are needed to establish the diagnosis. If a more indolent process is encountered, one should consider performing appropriate staining and cultures for tuberculosis.

DIAGNOSTIC EVALUATION

All children admitted to the hospital with a febrile urinary tract infection should undergo renal ultrasonography as soon as is reasonable after admission. The findings on this initial study can have a significant effect on the choice of therapeutic options. If both kidneys are normal and unobstructed, organism-specific therapy is satisfactory in most patients. If significant obstruction or stones are present, antibiotic therapy may not be as effective, and interventional drainage may become necessary if the response to antibiotics is inadequate. At the time of this initial screening study, findings may suggest the presence of a renal abscess. Such findings include a mass effect within the margins of the kidney along with a thickened wall and material of varying sonographic density within the mass (Fig. 46–2). Similar findings can be seen in infections accompanied by severe ureteropelvic junction obstruction or infundibular stenosis with isolated calyceal dilation, in which case purulent material within the dilated collecting system layers out and can mimic a renal abscess (Figs. 46–3 and 46–4).

When the diagnosis of an abscess is suspected on ultrasonography, performing CT of the involved kidney is in order.[9] CT more clearly defines the margins of the abscess, assesses whether loss of function is significant, and can screen the remainder of the kidney for small satellite abscesses.[16] If loss of function in the affected kidney seems to be significant, a dimercaptosuccinic acid renal scan should be done because it is an even more sensitive test to quantitate overall renal function. Currently, gallium 67 scintigraphy is not used frequently to diagnose an obscure inflammatory mass. If CT suggests the diagnosis, percutaneous aspiration can confirm clearly whether an abscess is present, without having to perform additional studies, and, at the same time, provide material for culture.

If a child with a urinary tract infection and a previously normal result on renal ultrasonogram is taking culture-specific antibiotics and a new fever subsequently develops, ultrasonography should be repeated. A previously small, unrecognized abscess

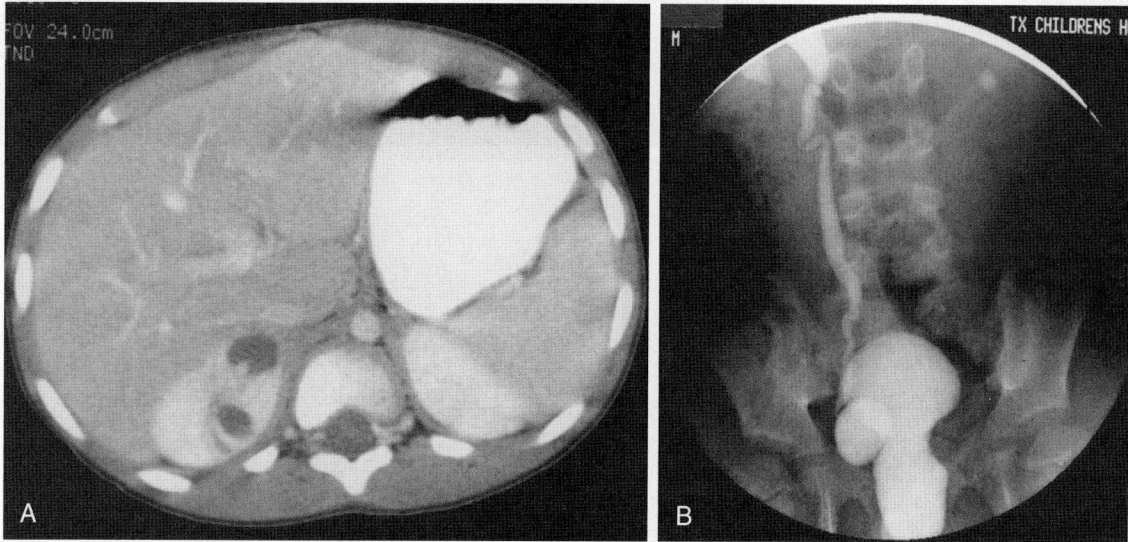

Figure 46–2 Renal abscess (secondary) in a 6-month-old boy with urinary tract infection. A screening renal ultrasonogram showed a small mass in the right kidney. **A,** Computed tomography shows two clearly defined cystic areas consistent with small parenchymal abscesses. Treatment consisted of intravenous antibiotics only. **B,** Voiding cystogram revealed the presence of vesicoureteral reflux.

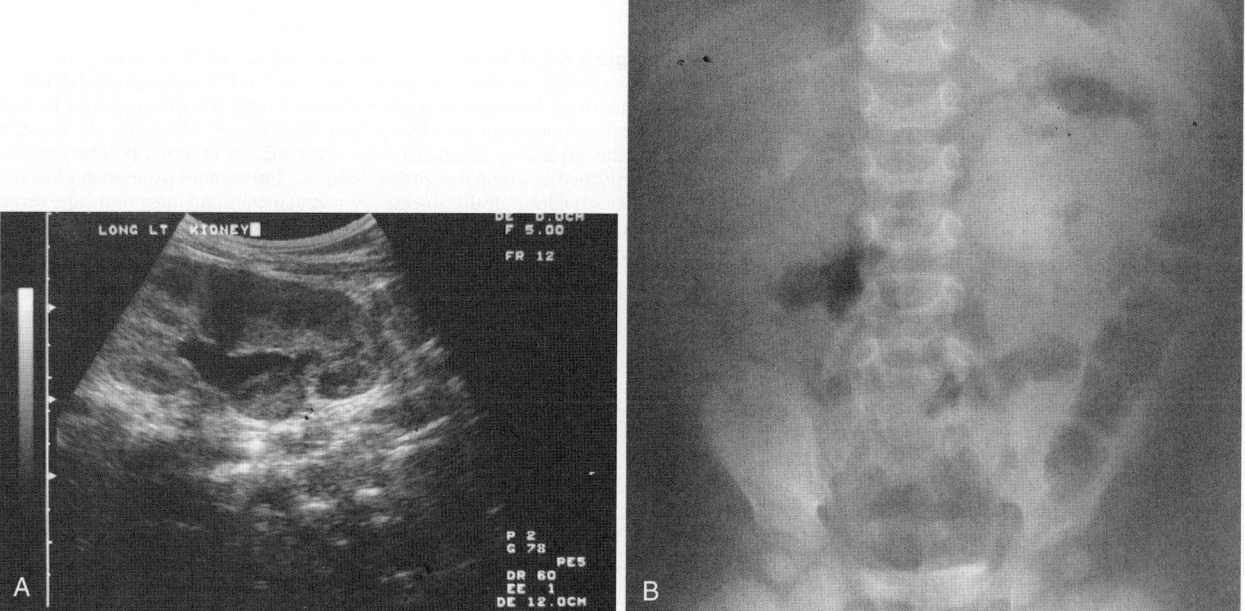

Figure 46–3 Pyonephrosis associated with ureteropelvic junction obstruction in a 3-month-old boy with fever, left abdominal and flank tenderness, and urinary tract infection. **A,** Renal ultrasonogram shows a medially placed cystic mass with layered fluids of different density consistent with purulent material. The position of the mass is most consistent with the renal pelvis. **B,** Intravenous pyelogram confirms ureteropelvic junction obstruction. This infant was treated initially with percutaneous nephrostomy drainage in addition to appropriate antibiotics.

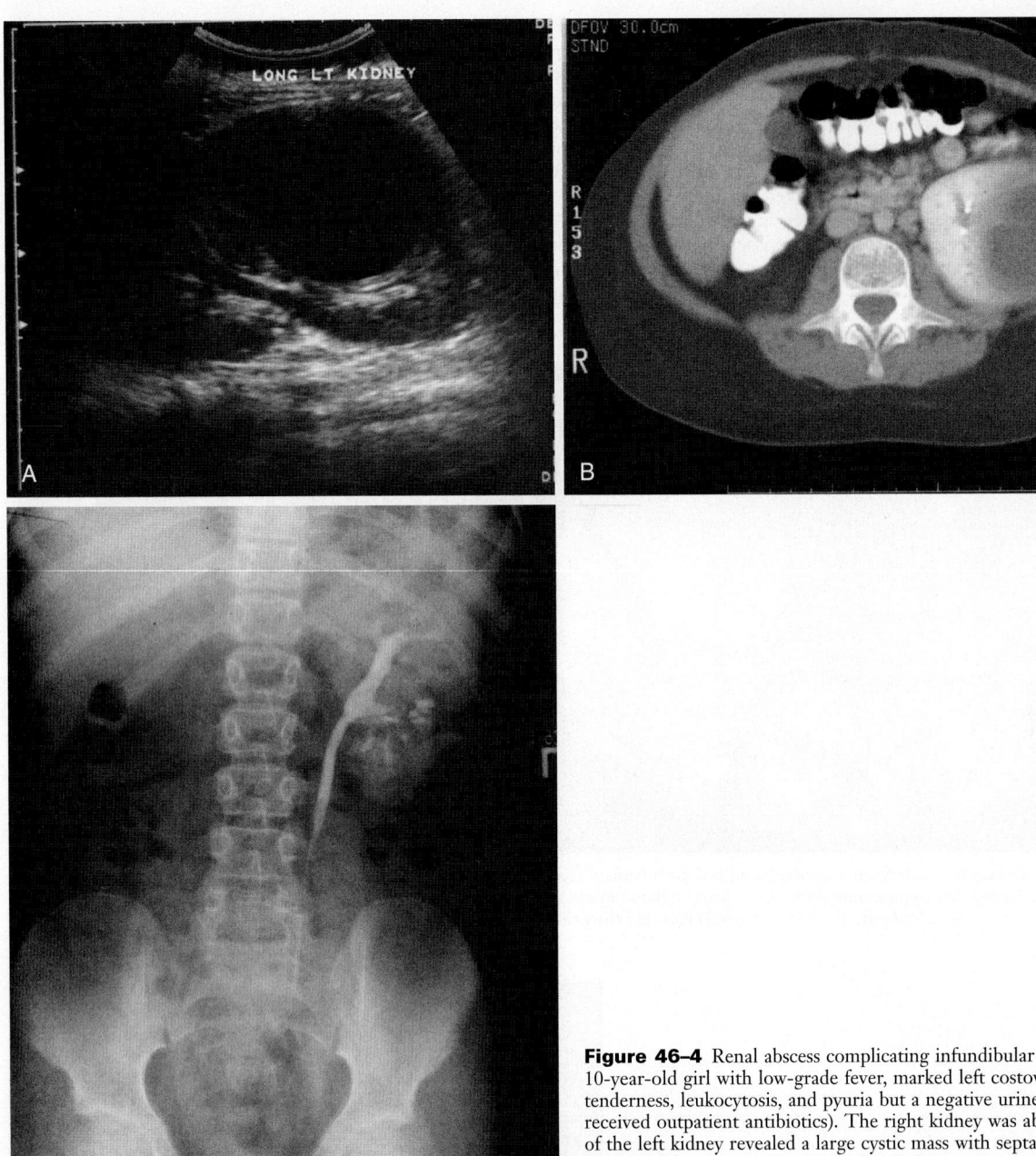

Figure 46–4 Renal abscess complicating infundibular stenosis in a 10-year-old girl with low-grade fever, marked left costovertebral angle tenderness, leukocytosis, and pyuria but a negative urine culture (she had received outpatient antibiotics). The right kidney was absent. **A,** Sonogram of the left kidney revealed a large cystic mass with septa. **B,** The mass was confirmed by computed tomography. **C,** Intravenous pyelogram obtained after resolution of the abscess (by percutaneous and open drainage) reveals anomalous development of the lower infundibulum and calyces.

may have been treated inadequately and now may be more apparent.

Occasionally, imaging studies cannot distinguish between a renal abscess and severe acute lobar nephropathy. The latter condition also may show tissues of differing density by ultrasonography or CT. In these situations, ultrasonography-guided or CT-guided percutaneous aspiration of the lesion may be necessary to determine whether purulent material can be obtained.

THERAPEUTIC CONSIDERATIONS

When the diagnosis of an abscess is confirmed, the choice of therapeutic options is dictated by several factors, including the overall status of the patient, the size and number of abscesses,

whether the abscess appears to be unilocular or septate, associated uropathies, and the extent of renal function in the involved kidney. Included in these considerations is some insight into the responsible organism. If it is a solitary abscess in a child with unimpressive urinalysis findings and an otherwise normal kidney, one should suspect a staphylococcal abscess, which can be confirmed by percutaneous aspiration, Gram stain, and culture. If bacteremia caused by *S. aureus* possibly was nosocomial in origin, or if methicillin-resistant *S. aureus* isolates are found commonly in the community, antibiotics such as vancomycin or clindamycin should be included in the initial empiric regimen.

Subsequent therapy is based on the antibiotic susceptibility pattern of the organism isolated. If urinalysis reveals an obvious infection, one can assume that the urine culture reflects the organism responsible for the abscess. In this situation, empiric therapy is directed against gram-negative enteric organisms. Cefotaxime, ceftriaxone, or ceftazidime plus an aminoglycoside would be suggested. The only caution is if the abscess is complicated by significant stone disease. In this situation, more than one organism may be in the urinary tract, and urine culture alone may be misleading. Percutaneous aspiration can identify accurately the organism responsible for the abscess. The optimal duration of antibiotic therapy for treatment of a renal abscess is not established, but 3 weeks of treatment is superior to 2 weeks for acute lobar nephropathy.[7]

Renal abscesses traditionally have been managed by open surgical drainage. With the introduction of safe percutaneous access, particularly when used with ultrasonography or CT guidance, single, unilocular lesions now can be managed effectively with percutaneous placement of an indwelling catheter that allows not only for primary drainage but also for irrigation of the cavity with appropriate antibiotic solutions.[1,11] Small renal abscesses have been treated successfully with antibiotics alone.[13,18] If the child does not improve with medical therapy alone, some type of drainage procedure is indicated. When function is insufficient to justify renal salvage and ultimate nephrectomy is planned, a short course of specific antibiotics and percutaneous drainage is initiated, if the abscess is large, to decrease inflammation in the perinephric tissues and to reduce the possibility of causing bacteremia at the time of surgery.

When required, surgical repair of associated congenital anomalies of the urinary tract generally is performed at a separate session after the abscess has resolved. Reconstructive surgery in the presence of active infection significantly increases the risk of development of surgical complications and the possibility that additional surgical procedures might be required.

CONCLUSION

Treatment of renal abscess today is multifaceted, and each case must be individualized. In addition to culture-specific antibiotics, treatment may include observation only, percutaneous drainage, or open surgical drainage. Diagnostic evaluation, including renal ultrasonography, CT, and percutaneous aspiration, generally can confirm that an abscess is present and assist in the decision regarding therapeutic options.

REFERENCES

1. Barker, A. P., and Ahmed, S.: Renal abscess in childhood. Aust. N. Z. J. Surg. *61*:217-221, 1991.
2. Boam, W. D., and Miser, W. F.: Acute focal bacterial pyelonephritis. Am. Fam. Physician *52*:919-924, 1995.
3. Brandels, J. M., Baskin, L. S., Kogan, B. A., et al.: Recurrent *Staphylococcus aureus* renal abscess in a child positive for the human immunodeficiency virus. Urology *46*:246-248, 1995.
4. Brook, I.: The role of anaerobic bacteria in perinephric and renal abscesses in children. Pediatrics *92*:261-264, 1994.
5. Casullo, V. A. M. C., Bottone, E., and Herold, B. C.: *Peptostreptococcus asaccharolyticus* l abscess: A rare cause of fever of unknown origin. Pediatrics *107*:E11, 2001.
6. Cheng, C.-H., Tsau, Y.-K., Hsu, S.-Y., and Lee, T.-L.: Effective ultrasonographic predictor for the diagnosis of acute lobar nephronia. Pediatr. Infect. Dis. J. *23*:11-14, 2004.
7. Cheng, C.-H., Tsau, Y.-K., and Lin, T.-Y.: Effective duration of antimicrobial therapy for the treatment of acute lobar nephronia. Pediatrics *117*:e84-e89, 2006.
8. Dougherty, F. E., Gottlieb, R. P., Gross, G. W., and Denison, M. R.: Neonatal renal abscess caused by *Staphylococcus aureus*. Pediatr. Infect. Dis. J. *10*:463, 1991.
9. Gerzof, S. G., and Gale, M. E.: Computer tomography and ultrasonography for diagnosis and treatment of renal and retroperitoneal abscesses. Urol. Clin. North Am. *9*:185-193, 1982.
10. Higham, M., Santos, J. I., Grodin, M., and Klein, J. O.: Renal abscess without preexisting structural abnormality. Pediatr. Infect. Dis. J. *3*:138-141, 1984.
11. Klar, A., Hurvitz, H., Berkun, Y., et al.: Focal bacterial nephritis (lobar nephronia) in children. J. Pediatr. *128*:850-853, 1996.
12. Martinez-Jabalonas, J., Osca, J. M., Ruiz, J. L., et al.: Renal aspergillosis and AIDS. Eur. Urol. *27*:167-169, 1995.
13. Pedersen, J. F., Hancke, S., and Kristensen, J. V.: Renal carbuncle: Antibiotic therapy governed by ultrasonically guided aspiration. J. Urol. *109*:777-778, 1973.
14. Rote, A. R., Bauer, S. B., and Retik, A. B.: Renal abscess in children. J. Urol. *119*:254-258, 1978.
15. Schiff, M., Glickman, M., Weiss, R. M., et al.: Antibiotic treatment of renal carbuncle. Ann. Intern. Med. *8*:305, 1977.
16. Thornbury, J. R.: Acute renal infections. Urol. Radiol. *12*:209-213, 1991.
17. Timmons, J. W., and Perlmutter, A. D.: Renal abscess: A changing concept. J. Urol. *115*:299-301, 1976.
18. Vachvanichsanong, P., Dissaneewate, P., Patrapinyokul, S., et al.: Renal abscess in healthy children: Report of three cases. Pediatr. Nephrol. *6*:273-275, 1992.
19. Watson, A. R., Marsden, H. B., Cendon, M., et al.: Renal pseudotumors caused by xanthogranulomatous pyelonephritis. Arch. Dis. Child. *57*:635, 1982.
20. Wippermann, C. F., Schofer, O., Beetz, R., et al.: Renal abscess in childhood: Diagnostic and therapeutic progress. Pediatr. Infect. Dis. J. *10*:446-450, 1991.

PROSTATITIS

47

Edmond T. Gonzales, Jr. ⊙ Sheldon L. Kaplan

Prostatitis, a major source of chronic infection and symptoms in men, occurs rarely in prepubertal children. Although prostatitis may develop in postpubertal teenagers, even in this age group the diagnosis is recognized infrequently. The disorder commonly called prostatitis generally is divided into three separate clinical problems: acute prostatitis, chronic prostatitis, and prostatodynia.

Acute prostatitis is a severe infection generally associated with significant toxicity (high fever, elevated white blood cell count, systemic symptoms). Marked urinary symptoms, such as frequency, dysuria, and urinary retention, may be present. The urine usually is infected. On rectal examination, the prostate is enlarged, boggy (edematous), and exquisitely tender. Care must be taken when performing the rectal examination or

when inserting a transurethral catheter because bacteremia can result.

The organism responsible usually is one of the gram-negative pathogens that commonly causes urinary tract infection (UTI). The virulence factors of *Escherichia coli* strains recovered from men with acute prostatitis and women with UTIs, such as adhesins and cytotoxins, were similar in one study.[13] Johnson and colleagues[6] found, however, that prostatitis *E. coli* isolates differed significantly from *E. coli* associated with cystitis or pyelonephritis by having a higher prevalence of the genes encoding P fimbriae structural subunits, P fimbriae assembly, fimbriae tip pilins, hemolysin, and cytotoxic necrotizing factor, and a lower prevalence of the gene encoding invasion of brain endothelium virulence factor. Rarely, *Trichomonas vaginalis* can cause prostatitis.

Treatment generally begins with administration of broad-spectrum parenteral antibiotics, such as cefotaxime, and aminoglycosides that are effective against gram-negative enteric organisms, pending the availability of culture-proven sensitivity results and a satisfactory clinical response. In patients older than 17 years of age, a fluoroquinolone also is recommended.

Chronic prostatitis is a more indolent infection associated with intermittent UTI, bladder irritative symptoms, and perineal discomfort. Ejaculation may be painful. Expressed prostatic secretions usually show an increase in the white blood cell count. Chronic prostatitis generally is recognized to occur in two different patterns: bacterial and nonbacterial. The clinical features of the two disorders are remarkably similar, including an increase in the white blood cell count in expressed prostatic secretions, but patients with chronic bacterial prostatitis usually also have recurring episodes of UTI with the same organism, most often one of the gram-negative pathogens.

The diagnosis of chronic prostatitis is related partly to detecting inflammation in expressed prostatic secretions. More precise methods of determining inflammatory parameters, such as counting the white blood cells per cubic millimeter with a hemocytometer, have been proposed.[14] In a large cohort study, the severity of symptoms in men with chronic prostatitis did not correlate with leukocyte or bacterial counts, however.[17] This study suggested that the symptoms associated with chronic pelvic pain syndrome were related to factors other than leukocytes and bacteria.

E. coli isolates associated with chronic prostatitis possess urovirulence profiles similar to those of strains from women with acute uncomplicated pyelonephritis.[1] In most studies, chronic nonbacterial prostatitis occurs more commonly than chronic bacterial prostatitis.

The cause of nonbacterial prostatitis remains enigmatic. Prostatic secretions do not show a common organism consistently, and UTI does not recur. Culture of prostatic secretions is notoriously unreliable, because of the means by which this material is collected; these secretions are contaminated easily as they pass through the urethra.[12] A specific causal relationship in nonbacterial prostatitis has not been found for either *Ureaplasma urealyticum* or *Chlamydia trachomatis*, two organisms commonly implicated in urethritis.[18] Molecular studies using polymerase chain reaction have shown DNA evidence of the presence of bacteria despite negative cultures for the typical bacteria associated with prostatitis.[5] Using these new techniques may lead to greater understanding of the role of infection in the pathogenesis of prostatitis.

Treatment of chronic bacterial prostatitis is frustrating because few patients truly are cured, and relapse occurs commonly after discontinuation of antibiotic therapy. Several studies have confirmed satisfactory concentrations of most common antibiotics in prostatic tissues,[5,8,10] but no study has provided a convincing explanation for the high treatment failure rate. Levofloxacin and other fluoroquinolones penetrate well into seminal and prostatic fluids and reach concentrations equivalent to corresponding plasma levels.[3] Researchers have postulated that antibiotic concentrations may be inadequate within the acini of the prostatic glands and their secretions, but this theory has not been proved.[15]

Normal prostatic secretions exhibit an antibacterial effect that is not present in men with chronic bacterial prostatitis. Several investigators have shown this factor to be free zinc or a zinc-based compound.[16] This antibacterial factor is depressed or absent in men with chronic prostatitis, but whether it causes or results from prostatitis is unknown. The most successful antibiotic therapy has been with trimethoprim-sulfamethoxazole or one of the fluoroquinolones.[9] In many instances, low-dose maintenance chemoprophylaxis with trimethoprim-sulfamethoxazole or nitrofurantoin is the most effective means of controlling symptoms.

A final population of patients have all the symptoms described in patients with chronic (bacterial) prostatitis but no history of UTI and microscopically normal prostatic secretions. To distinguish this group of patients from patients with prostatic infection, the term *prostatodynia* is used. The etiology of prostatodynia is unknown, but most investigators think that the disorder is a form of perineal and urethral muscle dysfunction with sphincter spasm, high voiding pressure within the prostatic urethra, reflux of urine into the prostatic ducts, and, ultimately, the development of chemical prostatitis.[4,11] Treatment generally consists of the use of alpha-adrenergic blocking agents to relax the bladder neck and proximal prostatic urethra and diazepam to relax the striated muscle of the perineum. Although most patients seem to experience some benefit, the results of therapy are difficult to quantitate, and underlying psychosocial issues are thought to be responsible for the symptoms of many patients. Psychological assessment and indicated treatment are essential parts of the total management of these patients.

In the older age group still seen in a pediatric practice, symptoms similar to those of the chronic form of prostatitis also might occur with urethritis. As noted earlier, *Chlamydia* and *Ureaplasma* spp. commonly are found in the urethral discharge in these patients[2] and are thought to be responsible for these specific symptoms. These organisms also have been implicated as a cause of epididymitis in young men. The organisms are transmitted sexually and are treated effectively with a tetracycline (minocycline or doxycycline) or a macrolide (erythromycin or azithromycin).[19] To prescribe these drugs empirically for sexually active young adults with lower tract irritative symptoms and clinical findings consistent with urethritis while awaiting culture results seems reasonable.

Nonspecific urethritis is the term commonly used for the infection in men with irritative voiding symptoms and a clear mucoid discharge and in whom culture of the discharge reveals a mixture of common perineal and gram-negative organisms but without a predominant organism thought to be responsible for the infection. Some of these patients likely have undiagnosed *Chlamydia* or *Ureaplasma* infection. Although specific treatment is empiric, a tetracycline or erythromycin seems to be a prudent first choice in most cases. Finally, one must not overlook the possibility of gonococcal urethritis.

In males, ectopic ureters can drain into the prostatic urethra or the seminal vesicle. With this anomaly, the ipsilateral renal parenchyma generally is dysplastic, the ureter is highly dilated, and the seminal vesicle may be distended markedly and form a large cystlike structure behind the prostate, the bladder neck, and the trigone. If this anomaly becomes infected, pain in the perineum and on rectal examination generally is significant. Occasionally, frankly purulent material is passed at the urethral meatus or expressed from the urethra after rectal examination.

In most cases, the kidney drained by the ectopic ureter is highly dysplastic and shows little or no function. Ultimate management usually consists of nephroureterectomy (ureteroneocystostomy if the kidney works) and, if the seminal vesicle is unusually large, partial excision and decompression of the seminal vesicle. Although these abnormalities are congenital and recognized easily by fetal ultrasonography, they can occur at almost any age if not identified before birth. Unless a palpable flank or lower abdominal mass is felt, infection usually is the initial symptom. Despite the severe degree of abnormality and ureteral and seminal vesicle dilation, the development of infection can be delayed well into the adult years. Infrequently, distortion at the bladder neck can result in obstruction to urinary flow.

SUMMARY

Prostatitis as it is seen and described in adults is a rare event in pediatric patients. When it does occur, it affects pubertal adolescents. Even in these patients, distinguishing true prostatitis from simple urethritis may be difficult.

Appropriate evaluation of an adolescent boy with a lower tract urinary infection generally begins with renal ultrasonography. Special attention should be directed to the region of the bladder and prostate. With this imaging modality, one can assess the presence and normalcy of both kidneys, the degree of thickening of the bladder wall, the ability of the bladder to empty, and whether any cystic masses are located behind the bladder or prostate. Any obvious abnormality justifies obtaining a voiding cystourethrogram. A thickened detrusor or recurrence of infection suggests the possibility of urethral obstruction. Although properly performed voiding cystourethrography does image the entire urethra, other diagnostic tests might include retrograde urethrography or determination of the urinary flow rate, especially if one suspects a urethral stricture. Performing cystoscopy usually is unnecessary if all imaging study results are normal, although cystoscopy may be used to confirm, and sometimes manage, obvious urethral obstruction.

REFERENCES

1. Andreu, A., Stapleton, A. E., Fennell, C., et al.: Urovirulence determinants in *Escherichia coli* strains causing prostatitis. J. Infect. Dis. *176*:464-469, 1997.
2. Bowie, W. R., Wang, S. P., Alexander, E. R., et al.: Etiology of nongonococcal urethritis: Evidence for *C. trachomatis* and *U. urealyticum*. J. Clin. Invest. *59*:735-742, 1977.
3. Bundrick W., Heron S. P., Ray, P., et al.: Levofloxacin versus ciprofloxacin in the treatment of chronic bacterial prostatitis: A randomized double-blind multicenter study. Urology *62*:537-541, 2003.
4. Hellstrom, W. J., Schmidt, R. A., Lue, T. F., et al.: Neuromuscular dysfunction in non-bacterial prostatitis. Urology *30*:183-188, 1987.
5. Hensle, T. W., Prout, G. R., Jr., and Griffin, P.: Minocycline diffusion into benign prostatic hyperplasia. J. Urol. *118*:609-611, 1977.
6. Johnson, J. R., Kuskowski, M. A., Gajewski, A., et al.: Extended virulence genotypes and phylogenetic background of *Escherichia coli* isolates from patients with cystitis, pyelonephritis, or prostatitis. J. Infect. Dis. *191*:46-50, 2005.
7. Krieger, J. N., and Riley, D. E.: Prostatitis: What is the role of infection? Int. J. Antimicrob. Agents *19*:475-479, 2002.
8. Larsen, E. H., Grasser, T. C., Dorflinger, T., et al.: The concentration of various quinolone derivatives in the human prostate. *In* Weidner, W., Brunner, H., Krause, W., et al. (eds.): Therapy of Prostatitis. Munich, W. Zucksweidt Verlag, 1986, pp. 40-44.
9. Meares, E. M., Jr.: Prostatitis syndromes: New perspectives about old woes. J. Urol. *123*:141-147, 1980.
10. Meares, E. M., Jr.: Prostatitis: Review of pharmacokinetics and therapy. Rev. Infect. Dis. *4*:475-483, 1982.
11. Meares, E. M., Jr.: Prostatodynia: Clinical findings and rationale for treatment. *In* Weidner, W., Brunner, H., Krause, W., et al. (eds.): Therapy of Prostatitis. Munich, W. Zucksweidt Verlag, 1986, pp. 207-212.
12. Meares, E. M., Jr., and Stamey, T. A.: Bacteriologic localization patterns in bacterial prostatitis and urethritis. Invest. Urol. *5*:492-518, 1968.
13. Mistumori, K., Terai, A., Yamamoto, S., et al.: Virulence characteristics of *Escherichia coli* in acute bacterial prostatitis. J. Infect. Dis. *180*:1378-1381, 1999.
14. Muller, C. H., Berger, R. E., Mohr, L. E., and Krieger, J. N.: Comparison of microscopic methods for detecting inflammation in expressed prostatic secretions. J. Urol. *166*:2518-2524, 2001.
15. Nielsen, O. S., Frimodt-Moeller, N., Maiqaard, S., et al.: Penicillanic acid derivatives in the canine prostate. Prostate *1*:79-85, 1980.
16. Parrish, R. F., Perinette, E. P., and Fair, W. R.: Evidence against a zinc binding peptide in pilocarpine-stimulated canine prostatic secretions. Prostate *4*:189-193, 1983.
17. Schaeffer, A. J., Knauss, J. S., Landis, J. R., et al.: Leukocyte and bacterial counts do not correlate with severity of symptoms in men with chronic prostatitis. The National Institutes of Health Chronic Prostatitis Cohort Study. J. Urol. *168*:1048-1053, 2002.
18. Shortliffe, L. M., and Wehner, N.: The characterization of bacterial and non-bacterial prostatitis by prostatic immunoglobulins. Medicine (Baltimore) *65*:399-414, 1986.
19. Skerk, V., Markekovic, I., Markovinovic, L., et al.: Comparative randomized study of azithromycin and doxycycline efficacy and tolerability in the treatment of prostate infection caused by *Ureaplasma urealyticum*. Chemotherapy *52*:9-11, 2006.

CHAPTER

48 GENITAL INFECTIONS

Mariam R. Chacko ✪ Mary Allen Staat ✪ Charles R. Woods, Jr.

This chapter reviews the clinical aspects of genital tract infections in children and adolescents. Genital infection in boys is limited to balanoposthitis. For details on other genital infections in boys, such as urethritis, epididymitis, and orchitis, refer to the other chapters in this section. Genital tract infections in premenarcheal girls are limited mostly to the vulva and vagina. The clinical presentations and management differ from those of similar infections in older patients. Genital infections in postmenarcheal girls include all the infections found in women; the symptoms accompanying them are similar to those in adults, and their treatment essentially is the same. Genital infections associated with pregnancy are not addressed in this chapter.

GENITAL TRACT INFECTIONS IN BOYS

Genital tract infections in boys are uncommon at any age but can be serious when they occur. Group A streptococcal proctitis and perianal skin infections have been reported.[154,180,261] Perianal pruritus, erythema, and tenderness occur commonly, and abdominal pain and rectal bleeding may be present. Penile involvement occurs rarely if at all.[261]

Balanoposthitis is a condition characterized by inflammation of the prepuce[210] and glans penis.[53] Causes of this condition have been described poorly in the literature; however, researchers have suggested that balanoposthitis results from trauma, irritation, or infection. A few cases of balanitis caused by *Streptococcus pyogenes* and *Staphylococcus aureus* have been reported.[53,60,69,105,160,205,210]

Balanoposthitis occurs more commonly in uncircumcised boys compared with circumcised boys. In one survey, the frequency of balanitis and penile irritation was determined in 272 uncircumcised and 273 circumcised boys.[124] Balanitis was defined as redness or swelling of the entire foreskin or glans, with or without pus, and irritation was defined as redness without swelling or pus. Six percent of uncircumcised and 3 percent of circumcised boys had balanitis. Four percent of the uncircumcised boys were found to have irritation alone compared with 1 percent of the circumcised boys. In another study examining penile problems in boys from birth to 8 years of age, penile inflammation developed in 8 percent of circumcised and 14 percent of uncircumcised boys.[78]

The diagnosis of balanoposthitis is made on clinical grounds. A boy may complain of soreness, swelling, and discharge around the penis. Examination reveals redness, swelling, and discharge of the prepuce or glans penis, or both. The discharge originates from the area under the foreskin or around the glans penis and not from the urethra. Urethritis may be associated with urethral discharge, but it is not seen commonly. In a case series of 100 boys with balanitis, 100 percent had redness, 91 percent had swelling, and 73 percent had discharge on examination.[75] If an infectious etiology is suspected, Gram stain and culture of the discharge can be performed to determine the cause and guide therapy.

For nonspecific balanoposthitis, local therapy, including sitz baths, gentle cleansing, and application of hydrocortisone cream, is suggested.[244] In cases in which an infectious etiology is suspected, or local therapy has not been effective, a topical or oral antibiotic with coverage against *S. pyogenes* and *S. aureus* can be used.

Circumcision or a dorsal slit procedure may be necessary for recalcitrant or recurrent balanoposthitis. In a study reviewing the reasons for circumcision beyond the neonatal period, 23 percent of 476 boys underwent the procedure for recurrent balanoposthitis.[290] Aside from the need for circumcision, most cases of balanoposthitis seem to be uncomplicated. Cases resulting in necrotizing fasciitis and *Staphylococcus*-induced toxic shock have been reported, however.[53,132]

GENITAL TRACT INFECTIONS IN GIRLS

In this section on genital infections in girls, the normal vaginal microenvironment is reviewed first, followed by specific and nonspecific premenarcheal bacterial and fungal causes for vulvovaginitis. Issues of sexual abuse in children with genital tract infections also are addressed. The section on sexual abuse in children with genital tract infections addresses bacterial and viral sexually transmitted diseases (STDs) in sexually abused children. These sections are followed by postmenarcheal lower genital tract infections of the external genitalia, including clitoris and Bartholin ducts and glands, and bacterial, protozoal, and fungal vulvovaginitis. Vulvovaginal viral infections, granulomatous and ulcerative vulvovaginal disorders, infections of the cervix, and upper genital tract infections are reviewed for premenarcheal and postmenarcheal girls.

These sections provide information regarding infections by specific microbes and syndromes, including trichomoniasis, candidiasis, gonorrhea, syphilis, chlamydial infections, bacterial vaginosis, genital herpes, condyloma acuminatum, molluscum contagiosum, lymphogranuloma venereum, granuloma inguinale, chancroid, tuberculosis, Behçet syndrome, and vulvar vestibulitis, and infections caused by group A streptococci, *Shigella*, and other agents that occasionally cause genital tract disease. Additional information on the microbes can be found in the respective chapters.

Supplemental information concerning the principles of gynecologic infections in children and adolescents can be found in referenced sources.[22,28,29,62,73,129,234] Although the infectious complications of pregnancy are not discussed, pregnancy is a common occurrence in teenage girls. Pregnancy-related infection should be considered when confronted with a septic state in an adolescent girl.

NORMAL VAGINAL FLORA

The lower female genital tract is colonized by nonpathogenic bacteria from birth. Throughout life, this colonization is dynamic

and complex. A wide range of aerobic and anaerobic species have been cultured from asymptomatic girls. The results of several modern series are summarized in Table 48–1.

Most girls harbor several organisms in the vagina at any given time. Vaginal specimens obtained for culture during anesthesia for elective surgery from 19 healthy girls aged 3 months to 5.7 years old yielded a mean of 12 bacterial species.[127] Anaerobes predominated, with a mean of 8.7 species versus 3.4 aerobic species. In a series of 25 asymptomatic girls aged 2 months to 15 years, a mean of 8.7 different species (approximately 4 aerobes and 5 anaerobes) per vaginal specimen were detected.[114] Another series of adolescents and young adults aged 13 to 21 years in which only aerobic flora were evaluated noted a mean of approximately three organisms in non-sexually active subjects versus six in sexually active patients.[249] This heterogeneity in vaginal microflora during childhood and adolescence is similar to that found in women.[164]

TABLE 48–1 Vaginal Organisms Isolated from Asymptomatic Girls 2 Months to 16 Years of Age

Organism	%*
Coagulase-negative staphylococci	35-73
Diphtheroids	14-78
Streptococcus viridans	13-39
Enterococci	29-62
Group B streptococcus	5-11
Group D streptococcus	
Staphylococcus epidermidis	
Staphylococcus aureus	
Streptococcus pneumoniae	
Micrococcus spp.	
Gaffkya (Aerococcus) spp.	
Lactobacillus spp.	10-39†
Escherichia coli	12-67
Klebsiella spp.	15-52
Enterobacter spp.	
Proteus spp.	3-5
Pseudomonas aeruginosa	5-6.5
Citrobacter spp.	
Haemophilus influenzae	
Neisseria spp. other than gonococci	
Moraxella (Branhamella) catarrhalis	
Flavobacterium spp.	
Alcaligenes spp.	
Acinetobacter spp.	
Mycoplasma hominis	
Ureaplasma urealyticum	
Gardnerella vaginalis‡	
Peptostreptococcus spp.	29-56
Peptococcus spp.	39-76
Veillonella spp.	
Eubacterium spp.	
Propionibacterium acnes	
Bacteroides fragilis	
Bacteroides melaninogenicus	
Other *Bacteroides* spp.	
Prevotella spp.	
Bifidobacterium spp.	
Clostridium perfringens	
Other *Clostridium* spp.	
Fusobacterium spp.	
Candida spp.	3-18
Other yeasts	
Actinomyces spp.	

*Percentage range when the organism was isolated from patients in at least two studies. If no range is present, the organism was isolated from 3 to 33% of patients in a single study.
†In one series, 88% of girls were older than 11 years.
‡Isolated in numerous cases without discharge.
Data from references 72, 95, 114, 120, 127, 164, 165, 177, 230.

Different types of bacteria are isolated at various ages. The vagina and its microbial flora form an ecosystem that changes over time from infancy to childhood to adolescence and adulthood.[126] The major forces that influence these changes are fluctuations in estrogen levels and the advent of sexual activity. Hygienic practices and medications, including oral contraceptives and antimicrobial agents, also affect the complex interactions among the various flora present in the vagina in terms of persistence, predominance, and overgrowth. The vaginal flora of most healthy women is dominated by one or more *Lactobacillus* spp., but a substantial minority may harbor other predominant flora, including *Bifidobacterium*, *Gardnerella*, *Prevotella*, *Pseudomonas*, or streptococci, in the absence of lactobacilli.[135]

Gram-negative enteric bacteria and enterococci commonly are encountered in infants and toddlers before completion of toilet training, but less frequently thereafter.[114,127] Younger adolescents have a greater prevalence of anaerobic bacteria than do women. From puberty, aerobic colonization increases with age, onset of sexual activity, and parity.[165] Lactobacilli are the predominant flora in most girls by the end of adolescence and may play a protective role in limiting the overgrowth of other flora.[126] In children, lactobacilli are present more often in girls younger than 2 years than in older prepubertal girls. The increasing presence of yeast and *Gardnerella vaginalis* from puberty to adulthood, although much less common in all ages, parallels that of lactobacilli.[114]

Mycoplasma hominis and *Ureaplasma urealyticum* are present more commonly in sexually active adolescents and in girls of any age who have been sexually abused than in nonsexually active girls. Genital mycoplasmas were found in 17 percent of one series of young girls who were not known to have undergone any sexual abuse.[108,249]

Microbes that usually behave as commensals sometimes are associated with vulvovaginitis. The difference between colonization and disease is at least partially a function of the magnitude of the replication and the quantity of a given bacterial species. In women with bacterial vaginosis in which *G. vaginalis* is a predominant microbe, colony counts generally are greater than 10^7 colony-forming units/g of vaginal fluid. Asymptomatic colonization with *G. vaginalis* usually is associated with colony counts of less than 10^5 colony-forming units/g of vaginal fluid.[165] Alteration in the vaginal microenvironment by factors such as poor hygiene, foreign bodies, or hormonal fluctuations results in loss of environmental constraints on bacterial replication and facilitates the overgrowth of one or more commensals.

When bacterial vaginosis occurs, typically the numbers of lactobacilli, which produce hydrogen peroxide, are decreased. When such a decrease occurs, catalase-negative microbes, such as *G. vaginalis*, *Mobiluncus* spp., and other anaerobes, can increase in number. Lactobacilli probably have mechanisms other than hydrogen peroxide production that may help restrain the growth of other microbes present on the surfaces of the lower genital tract.[165,258]

PREMENARCHEAL VULVOVAGINITIS

Infections and inflammation of the vulva and vagina account for 85 to 90 percent of all genital problems in premenarcheal girls. These conditions are encountered most commonly in children 2 to 7 years old.[213,226] Infections of the vulva and vagina usually occur together and generally are discussed as one entity, vulvovaginitis. The various types of vulvovaginitis are differentiated by determining the presence or absence of specific agents associated with the inflammation in a particular case.

Genital discharge and perineal or vulvar discomfort are the most common symptoms that bring a child with vulvovaginitis to the physician.[133,213] The discomfort may be only minor pain or

soreness, or it may be intense perineal burning or pruritus. Genital erythema is the most common sign in girls with vulvovaginitis and is noted in more than 80 percent of cases. Visible discharge is present in one third of cases.[213] The discharge may be scanty serous fluid, bloody, or profuse and purulent. Infections of the vulva and vagina are more likely to be accompanied by moderate or severe inflammation and prominent discharge than is nonspecific vulvovaginitis.[142] Infection can be present at times, however, with neither discomfort nor discharge.

In a series of 80 prepubertal girls aged 2 to 12 years old with vulvovaginitis and no suspicion of sexual abuse, probable bacterial pathogens were found in cultures of 36 percent. Group A streptococci, *S. aureus*, and *Haemophilus influenzae* (non–type b) were the most common isolates.[266] In another series of 74 girls, group A streptococci and *H. influenzae* were isolated in 47 percent and 12 percent. Most of these girls had had symptoms for 7 days or less at the time treatment was sought.[51] These bacteria, especially group A streptococci, causing vulvovaginitis may lead to more severe symptoms that result in care being sought soon after onset, whereas pathogenic bacteria generally are less likely to be found when girls present for care after several weeks of symptoms.

Genital discharge does not always indicate infection or inflammation. Most female infants have a grayish white, mucoid discharge from the vagina during the newborn period. This discharge consists of desquamated vaginal mucosa and cervical epithelium that has undergone hypertrophy because of prenatal stimulation by placental and maternal hormones. Microscopic examination of the material reveals masses of large, superficial vaginal epithelial cells (Fig. 48–1). The condition may last for several weeks, is not pathogenic, and does not require treatment. Urinary leakage from an ectopic ureter opening into the genital tract may mimic a vaginal discharge.

A pubertal girl nearing menarche may have a copious viscous, transparent secretion that fills the vagina, bathes the vulvar tissues, and soils underclothing. The parents of such a girl may be concerned that she has a vaginal infection. In this case, the vulvar and vaginal tissues are thick and moist, a sign of increased estrogen stimulation. Microscopic examination of the vaginal fluid reveals masses of estrogenized superficial vaginal epithelial cells and few leukocytes (Fig. 48–2). Test results for pathogenic bacteria are negative. The parents should be reassured that the girl does not have an infection. Frequent bathing and changes of underclothing are all that is needed.

Poor hygiene with subsequent overgrowth of a mixed aerobic and anaerobic bacterial flora is the most common cause of pre-

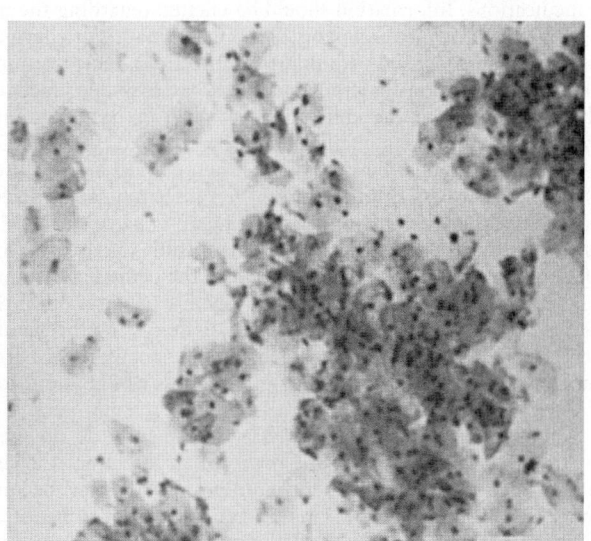

Figure 48–1 Cytosmear from the vaginal discharge of a newborn.

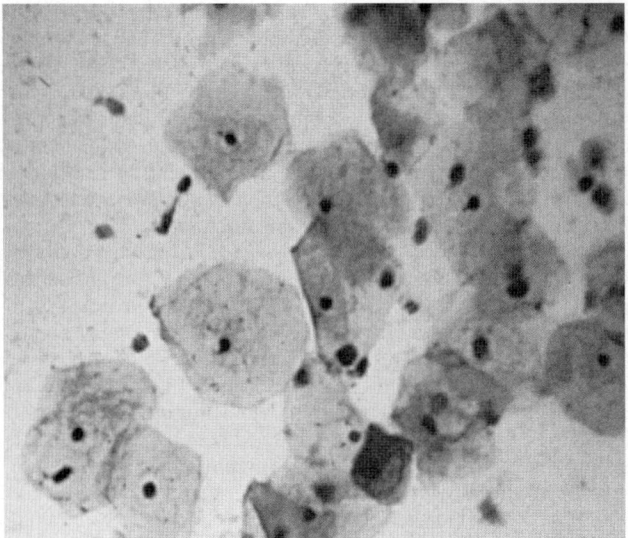

Figure 48–2 Cytosmear from the vaginal secretion of a pubertal girl. Masses of epithelial cells and few bacteria or leukocytes attest to its nonpathologic character.

menarcheal vulvovaginitis.[209] Inflammation of the lower genitourinary tract also may be caused by a variety of specific microorganisms, chemicals, and other physical agents. Contact irritation and allergic reactions induced by soaps, detergents, and medications are frequent causes of vulvovaginitis. Some systemic diseases and focal skin disorders may mimic vulvovaginitis or allow it to develop as a secondary process when these conditions involve the vulvar or perineal tissues.[80,90] Anatomic abnormalities also may be associated with vulvovaginitis. An increased incidence of vulvovaginitis and urinary tract infections has been reported in girls with high posterior commissures.[287] Drainage from an ectopic ureter into the vagina can cause chronic vulvovaginitis and lead to the formation of vaginal calculus. Labial adhesions were present in 7 percent of girls with vulvovaginitis in one series.[213] Table 48–2 outlines the causes of vulvovaginitis in premenarcheal girls.

The history should include information about the manner and circumstances surrounding the onset of the complaint, the characteristics of any discharge, the duration of symptoms, whether the problem is recurrent, and the nature of any recent treatments or medications. Information should be elicited regarding the use of bubble baths, enuresis, history of atopic dermatitis or allergies, anal pruritus (associated with pinworm infection), recent respiratory or skin infections in family members, and hygienic practices. The possibility that the child may have had or has a systemic disorder affecting the genitalia should be explored.

Sexual abuse must be considered when a child has a genital infection, regardless of the nature of the infection or the socioeconomic status of the family. This concern is particularly relevant when the child has a sexually transmissible disease, but any infectious organism can be transmitted to the genitalia by digital contact. Sexual abuse does not require penile penetration of the vagina. The history of vaginal or penile discharge in other family members should be ascertained. Behavioral changes, nightmares, fears, abdominal pain, headaches, and enuresis can be indicators of abuse or other psychosocial stressors.

The characteristics of the discharge frequently do not help identify a specific cause. At the onset of an infection, the discharge likely is thick, purulent, and profuse. It may become scanty and seropurulent in later chronic stages of infection.[133] Discharges that are odorless and bloody or serosanguineous may result from noninfectious conditions, such as vulvar irritation,

trauma, precocious puberty, foreign body, urethral prolapse, or tumor. Vulvovaginitis caused by *Shigella* or group A streptococci also can cause bleeding, as can an eroding foreign body. Foulsmelling discharge suggests a foreign body but also may result from a necrotic tumor. Specific diagnoses are made more often when symptoms have been present for less than 1 month.[279]

A general physical examination should precede assessment of the genital tract. The gynecologic examination begins with abdominal inspection and palpation followed by external examination of the perineum and genitalia, including the vulva, urethral meatus, clitoris, hymen, and anus. The examination should be done with the child in a supine, frog leg position. The labia can be retracted gently to visualize the anterior of the vagina. Speculum and bimanual examinations generally are inappropriate in prepubertal children.[214] Note should be made of structural abnormalities, inflammation, sores and ulcerations, and excoriations. If complaints consist only of vulvitis, and findings on external examination are limited to a scanty mucoid discharge and an erythematous introitus, further examination generally is unnecessary.[72]

If the vaginal discharge is purulent, persistent, or recurrent, a thorough gynecologic assessment is warranted. Visualization of the vagina and cervix without instrumentation is possible with the child in the prone knee-chest position.[74] This method is useful in children older than 2 years. In this position, with labial traction, the vaginal muscles relax and stretch the hymenal membrane open. An otoscope head or a magnifying lens with a good wall light is used to visualize the cervix. Because the vagina of a prepubertal child is short, a foreign body or a lesion may be seen.[71]

A rectal examination may be important when persistent discharge, bleeding, or pelvic or abdominal pain is present. The rectal examination may help express discharge from the vagina that previously was not recognized and can permit palpation of hard foreign bodies or abnormal masses.

Visualization with instrumentation (vaginoscopy) is required in some situations. General anesthesia may be required for girls who are small or unable to cooperate, or who may experience significant anxiety or discomfort during the procedure. Conscious sedation for the procedure may be an option in some situations. When a purulent, persistent, or recurrent vaginal discharge is present, samples should be obtained for culture and Gram stain. Gram stain of exudates may provide information rapidly that points toward a specific pathogen and may indicate the need for additional evaluations or interventions. Wet mount preparations may be useful if fungal infection (potassium hydroxide preparations) or pinworms are suspected. Saline wet mount may be indicated for trichomoniasis if sexual abuse is suspected. Urinalysis with microscopic examination should be performed. A complete blood cell count may be useful when pyogenic infection is suspected or bleeding has occurred.

When cultures are indicated, separate vulvar and vaginal specimens may be necessary. The type and duration of discharge and considerations of potential sexual abuse influence this decision. Vulvar specimens alone may be appropriate when etiologies such as group A streptococci are suspected. Exudates emanating from the vagina in prepubertal girls also are adequate specimens for evaluation for gonorrhea, such that vaginal swabs or aspirates are not required. Further information on types of specimens required for specific sexually transmitted infections such as gonorrhea or *Chlamydia trachomatis* is provided in Chapters 100 (gonorrhea) and 206 (*C. trachomatis*).

Options for obtaining vaginal specimens in young girls, when needed, include use of (1) a nasopharyngeal Dacron swab moistened in nonbactericidal saline, inserted carefully through the hymenal opening; (2) a catheter-within-a-catheter technique (Fig. 48–3)[214]; or (3) a sterile newborn suction catheter, with insertion 2 to 3 cm into the vagina.[266] For the catheter-within-a-

TABLE 48–2   Etiologic Factors in Premenarcheal Vulvovaginitis

Bacterial Infections
Nonspecific mixed infections secondary to
  Poor perineal hygiene
  Foreign body in vagina
  Respiratory tract infections
  Skin infections (impetigo)
  Urinary tract infection
Specific nonvenereal infection
  Hemolytic streptococci (groups A, B, F)
  Escherichia coli
  Shigella flexneri, Shigella sonnei
  Neisseria meningitidis, Neisseria sicca
  Haemophilus influenzae type b, nontypeable strains
  Streptococcus pneumoniae
  Corynebacterium diphtheriae
  Yersinia enterocolitica
  Mycobacterium tuberculosis
  Moraxella (Branhamella) catarrhalis
  Staphylococcus aureus
Specific venereal infections
  Neisseria gonorrhoeae
  Treponema pallidum
  Chlamydia trachomatis
  Chancroid (*Haemophilus ducreyi*)
  Granuloma inguinale
Bacterial vaginosis
  Gardnerella vaginalis
  Mobiluncus species

Fungal Infections
Candida albicans
Other yeasts
Dermatophytes

Protozoan and Parasitic Infections
Trichomoniasis
Amebiasis
Enterobius vermicularis
Hirudiniasis
Schistosomiasis
Other parasitic infections (ascariasis, trichuriasis)

Viral Infections
Venereal
  Herpes simplex
  Condyloma acuminatum (papillomavirus)
  Molluscum contagiosum
Involvement as part of systemic infection
  Measles
  Varicella
  Mononucleosis (Epstein-Barr virus)
  Coxsackievirus
  Smallpox

Infestations
Pediculosis
Scabies

Contact Irritation or Allergic Reactions
Bubble bath preparations
Hair shampoos
Vulvar deodorant sprays
Soaps, laundry detergents
Other medications

Vulvar or Perineal Skin Diseases
Local
  Seborrhea
  Lichen sclerosus et atrophicus
  Lichen planus
  Lichen simplex chronicus
  Premalignant leukoplakia
  Erythrasma (*Corynebacterium minutissimum*)
  Bartholinitis
  Skenitis
Involvement as part of a systemic disorder
  Psoriasis
  Bullous pemphigoid
  Atopic dermatitis
  Drug eruption
  Generalized pruritus with excoriation
  Chronic liver disease
  Chronic renal disease
  Metabolic errors
  Psychosomatic
  Crohn disease
  Sjögren syndrome
  Henoch-Schönlein purpura
  Histiocytosis
  Kawasaki disease
  Stevens-Johnson syndrome
  Typhoid
  Zinc deficiency

Physical Factors
Sand (sandbox)
Chemical or thermal trauma
Physical trauma (accidents, abuse, masturbation)
Nylon, rayon underclothing
Tight garments (maceration in warm climates)
Anatomic abnormalities
  Neoplasms (sarcoma botryoides)
  Polyps
  Labial agglutination, adhesion
  Prolapsed urethra
  Ectopic ureter
  Rectal fistula
  Draining pelvic abscess via fistula

Data from references 11, 12, 72, 80, 81, 134, 163, 183, 250.

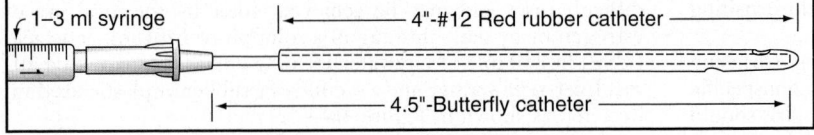

Figure 48–3 Assembled catheter-within-a-catheter for obtaining specimens from a prepubertal child. (*From Pokorny, S. F., and Stormer, J: A traumatic removal of secretions from the prepubertal vagina. Am. J. Obstet. Gynecol. 156:581, 1987.*)

catheter technique, the distal 4 inches of a soft, size 12 bladder catheter and the proximal 4 inches of butterfly needle intravenous tubing are excised from their parent devices by sterile technique. The catheter-within-a-catheter is inserted into the vagina, and fluid is flushed in and out of the upper part of the vagina several times before final aspiration into the syringe and removal of the device.

Nonspecific Vulvovaginitis

Nonspecific vulvovaginitis is identified by vaginal cultures that yield a growth of mixed bacteria not related etiologically to a specific disease. Nonspecific vulvovaginitis is the premenarcheal genital disorder most frequently encountered[133] and is responsible for 25 to 75 percent of cases of vulvovaginitis diagnosed in this age group in referral centers.[279] In most cases, as noted in Table 48–2, identifiable secondary factors contribute to non-specific vulvovaginitis.

Several factors other than those listed in Table 48–2 contribute to the occurrence of vulvovaginal infections in young children. The developing immature labia minora and majora flare outward as a young girl squats or sits. As a result, they do not protect the vestibular and vulvar mucosae from contamination, as occurs later in life. The nonestrogenized, prepubertal vulvar and vaginal epithelium, which consists of only a few layers of cells, is traumatized easily and infected readily; however, no evidence suggests that estrogen deficiency is a causative factor in premenarcheal vulvovaginitis. The alkaline vaginal reaction during childhood also is not as resistant to infection as is the acidic vaginal secretion of postmenarcheal girls and women. Because children frequently do not cleanse themselves properly after defecation, the perineum and vulva often are contaminated by fecal material. Nonabsorbent nylon garments or other tight-fitting clothes can lead to maceration, which predisposes to the development of infection.

VULVOVAGINITIS SECONDARY TO POOR PERINEAL HYGIENE

A vulvovaginal infection is considered to be secondary to poor perineal hygiene when bacteria native to the lower gastrointestinal tract are found in properly obtained cultures from the vagina. In a large series of cases of vulvovaginitis subjected to culture, *Escherichia coli* or other coliform organisms were found in 70 percent of patients in the series.[120] Other studies also have found a higher prevalence of *E. coli* in vaginal cultures from girls with vulvovaginitis than in asymptomatic controls.[72] The reappearance and disappearance of premenarcheal vulvovaginitis secondary to poor perineal hygiene are related directly to the appearance and disappearance of coliform organisms in vulvovaginal cultures. The primary role of vulvar and vaginal contamination with fecal material as a result of inadequate cleansing after defecation is supported by the observation that symptoms resolve in most cases when proper perineal hygiene is the only treatment recommended. Fifteen to 20 percent of children have recurrences, usually 1 month or more after resolution of the initial episode. In most instances, recurrences can be attributed to poor perineal hygiene.[120]

Children with nonspecific vulvovaginitis secondary to poor perineal hygiene do not have any uniform historical findings. If asked, the parent may be able to describe the way that the child cleanses herself after defecation. Many children wipe themselves from back to front after defecation. In girls, this practice easily results in fecal contamination of the vulvar area.

On examination, the vulvar mucosa and outer third of the vagina usually are hyperemic and covered with a scant, light gray mucoid discharge. Frequently, a clue to the cause of the infection is fecal soiling around the anus or on the perineum. Inspection of the undergarments may show fecal material in the area that comes in contact with the vulva, unless, as often is the case, the girl has been bathed and dressed in clean clothes before visiting the physician.

Instructing parents regarding perineal and vulvar cleansing when girls are bathed decreases the likelihood that nonspecific vulvovaginitis will develop in their daughters. Young girls should be taught proper hygiene and that they should wash their hands before and after urinating and defecating. Routine inspection of the perineum, vulva, hymen, and clitoris should be a part of routine physical examinations, including well-child checkups.[133]

Proper cleansing of the perineum and anus after defecation and sitz baths leads to the resolution of symptoms and infection in most cases. Sitz baths (warm water with or without Aveeno colloidal oatmeal or baking soda) 10 to 15 minutes in duration should be taken two to six times per day, depending on the

severity of the vulvovaginal inflammation.[72] For intense, oozing inflammation, wet compresses with Burow's solution (1:40) or plain water applied every 3 to 4 hours may be used instead of sitz baths.[11] In mild cases, the vulva may be washed twice a day with water or a mild, unscented, nonmedicated soap (e.g., Basis, unscented Dove, Neutrogena). The perineum should be patted dry gently after baths or treatments. Complete drying may be facilitated by sitting for 10 minutes with the legs spread apart. Urinating with the labia and legs spread apart to minimize urinary reflux into the vagina may be helpful. Witch hazel pads (Tucks) may be used for cleansing after defecating and to provide mild analgesia.[252]

White cotton underpants, changed frequently to absorb discharge, and loose-fitting clothing should be worn for several days to a few weeks after the symptoms resolve. Continued wearing of such clothing also may be helpful in preventing recurrences of vulvovaginitis, especially in girls living in warmer climates.

As the inflammation and exudate subside over 1 to 2 days, sitz baths may be reduced in frequency and alternated two to four times a day with the application of either calamine lotion or protective ointments, such as zinc oxide, Desitin, Vaseline, and A and D ointment. If pruritus is a significant symptom, an oral agent such as hydroxyzine hydrochloride (Atarax) or diphenhydramine hydrochloride (Benadryl) may be administered. Topical application of 1 percent hydrocortisone cream or triamcinolone acetonide (Mycolog) cream may be used as the inflammation resolves but should be avoided in the acute phase.[252]

Shampooing the hair while sitting in a bathtub and using harsh soaps, bubble baths, or other preparations that might lead to chemical irritation of the vulvar skin and vaginal mucosa should be avoided throughout the course of vulvovaginitis.[19,32,39] The application of powders should be avoided, at least until the acute symptoms have resolved.

Patients who do not improve after 2 to 3 days of hygienic measures should be re-evaluated. Specimens taken from the vagina should be sent for aerobic and anaerobic bacterial cultures, if these were not done initially. An intravaginal triple-sulfa medication such as Sultrin vaginal cream, which consists of sulfathiazole, sulfacetamide, and sulfabenzamide, may be given.[2,90] Approximately 1 mL is inserted into the vagina with a 5-mL Luer syringe each night for 7 nights (the applicator that comes with the tube of cream is too large to insert into the immature vagina). A 5-cm piece of 12 or 14 French urethral catheter attached to the syringe facilitates application of the cream, if the patient is cooperative (Fig. 48–4). Parents must be warned against and instructed on how to avoid inserting the cream into the child's urethra and bladder.[120] Alternatively, the vagina may be irrigated with a 1 percent povidone-iodine (Betadine) solution with this same method and caveat.[72]

Intractable nonspecific vulvovaginal infections that are not caused by foreign bodies, intestinal parasites, or poor perineal hygiene are encountered occasionally. They are resistant to hygienic measures and topical antibiotics. Reducing vaginal pH from an alkaline or neutral to an acid reaction often helps in these difficult cases and may be achieved either by the local use of estrogen or by daily flushing of a solution of 1 mL of lactic acid (USP) in 250 mL of tap water into the child's vagina with a 10-mL Luer-type syringe and a section of a rubber or plastic urethral catheter, as shown in Figure 48–4.[120]

Estrogens cause thickening of the thin prepubertal vaginal mucosa, which reduces vaginal pH. These events generally are therapeutic. Estrogens are not recommended for the treatment of routine cases of premenarcheal vulvovaginitis for two reasons: the results do not seem to be superior to nonhormonal therapies in these cases,[120] and prolonged administration of topical estrogens may cause isosexual pseudoprecocity. For intractable cases, estrogen should be applied topically and not orally. A globule of estrogen cream (Premarin vaginal cream) measuring not more

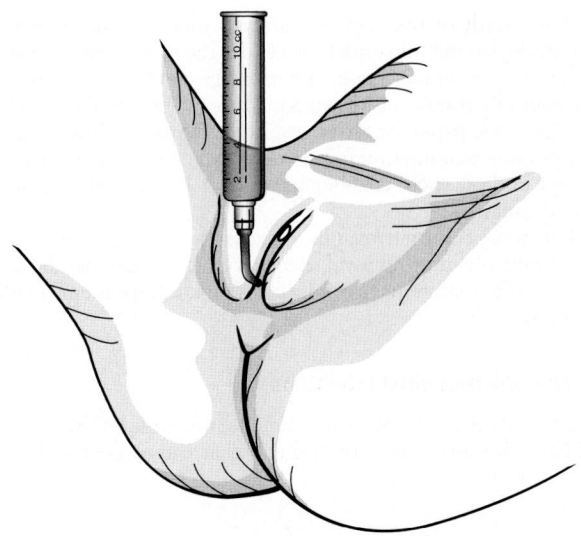

Figure 48–4 The barrel of a Luer-type syringe and attached piece of urethral catheter are used for vaginal lavage in an older child with a vaginal infection.

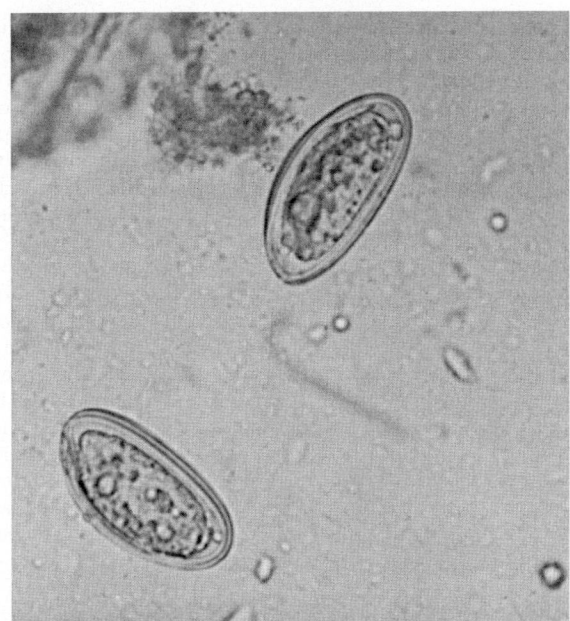

Figure 48–5 Pinworm ova discovered in a vaginal smear from a child with intractable vulvovaginitis.

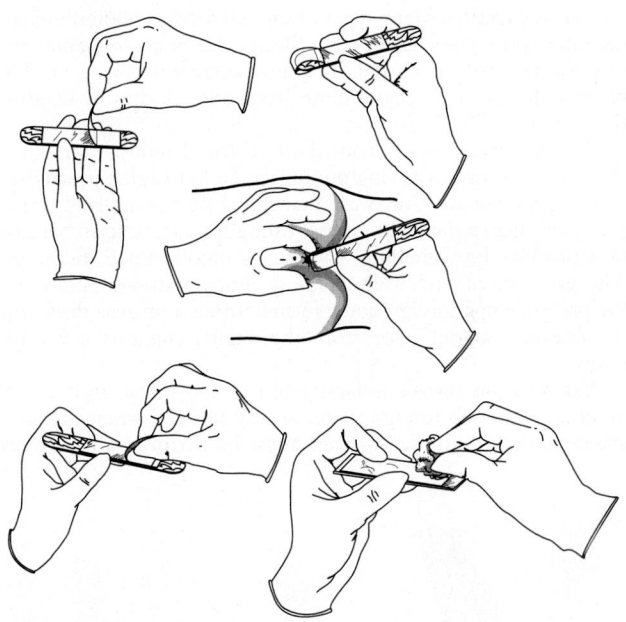

Figure 48–6 Technique for obtaining a perianal smear for detection of pinworm ova, using Scotch tape and a tongue depressor.

than 5 mm in diameter should be rubbed gently onto the inner surfaces of the labia minora and external surface of the hymen. This procedure is repeated daily for 2 to 4 weeks. After 7 to 10 days, the vulvar and vaginal tissues usually thicken, and a mucoid vaginal secretion may appear. The parents must understand clearly that the cream must be used for no longer than instructed. The cream should be discontinued if thelarche occurs.

Oral or parenteral antibiotics may be indicated if symptoms persist for 2 to 3 weeks, or if a specific pathogen that requires antibiotic treatment is isolated. When possible, selection of antibiotic agents and the route of administration should be based on susceptibility testing of organisms isolated from vaginal cultures. Nonspecific vulvovaginal infections are benign, superficial, localized mucosal inflammations that usually respond to less potent chemotherapeutic agents when they are needed. Many antibiotics are absorbed through the vaginal mucosa. The indiscriminate use of vaginal, oral, or parenteral antibiotics may result in the child becoming sensitized to them.

NONSPECIFIC VULVOVAGINITIS SECONDARY TO INTESTINAL PARASITES

Pinworms (*Enterobius vermicularis*) are the causative factor in many cases of recurrent or intractable nonspecific vulvovaginitis in children.[72] Infection occurs when the worms in the lower bowel crawl out of the anus onto the perineum and migrate into the vagina, where they deposit ova. The pinworms may carry *E. coli* and other coliform bacteria into the vagina, which may lead to vulvovaginitis. Other intestinal parasites seldom invade the vagina, although in one case *Ascaris lumbricoides* was discovered in the vagina of a child.[133]

Infestation with pinworms occurs commonly and does not indicate poor hygiene. Pinworm ova may be deposited in playground soil, on toys or books, and on the hands of infected individuals. Infection frequently is asymptomatic.

A child with a pinworm infection and vulvovaginitis usually has a history of a chronic vaginal discharge that has recurred despite repeated attempts to eradicate it. Parents may note worms on the perineum of the child and that she awakens at night because of perineal itching. Other family members or the girl herself may have had pinworms previously.

Examination reveals a low-grade inflammation of the vulva and vagina. Excoriations from scratching may be seen on the perineum. Vaginoscopy (if indicated) shows an inflammatory reaction extending to, but not including, the cervix. Vaginal cultures produce a mixed growth of nonpathogenic bacteria, with *E. coli* and other coliform bacteria generally predominating.

The diagnosis depends on finding pinworm ova on smears from the perineum or in the vaginal discharge or a report from parents that worms are visible on the child's perianal skin. A perineal smear is most likely to show the presence of pinworms, but pinworm ova may be detected in a wet smear of vaginal secretions (Fig. 48–5).

When a perineal smear for the ova of *E. vermicularis* is to be obtained, the parent is given a wooden tongue blade, a piece of Scotch tape, and a glass microscopic slide. The tape is attached to the tongue blade, adhesive side out (Fig. 48–6), and applied firmly to several areas around the anus. It is removed and applied, adhesive side down, to the glass slide, which is sent to the laboratory for examination.

The type of discharge, the appearance of the vaginal mucosa, or the presence or absence of pruritus does not aid in establishing a diagnosis. A history of a previous pinworm infection in the patient, a member of the family, or a playmate is significant. Pinworms should be suspected when a child has recurrent episodes of intractable nonspecific vulvovaginitis.

Treatment consists of eradicating the pinworms. All members of the family are presumed to be infected and must be treated. Several highly effective drugs are available for this purpose; among them are pyrantel pamoate, given as a single dose of 11 mg/kg, not to exceed 1 g, and mebendazole, 100 mg given orally as a single dose. Either treatment should be repeated after 2 weeks. Three negative perianal smears, taken at weekly intervals, should be obtained before one can assume that the worms have been eradicated. The vulvovaginitis caused by coliform organisms carried on pinworms is treated the same as other cases of nonspecific vulvovaginitis caused by poor perineal hygiene (see earlier).

NONSPECIFIC VULVOVAGINITIS SECONDARY TO VAGINAL FOREIGN BODIES

Foreign bodies account for approximately 4 percent of cases of vaginal discharge in premenarcheal girls.[11] When a foreign body remains in the vagina for some time, it inevitably causes nonspecific vulvovaginitis. Many types of vaginal foreign bodies, including safety pins, glass beads, coins, beans, bits of crayon, and parts of toys, have been reported. The most common objects are bits of toilet paper or shreds of cloth from nightclothes or bedding (Fig. 48–7).[122,134]

The history does not contribute to the diagnosis unless the child has a record of having put objects in her vagina previously. Usually, the parent is unaware that the child has inserted something into her vagina. The child is brought to a physician because of a profuse, foul-smelling, sometimes blood-tinged discharge. The presence of such a discharge is almost pathognomonic for the presence of a foreign body. Even without a profuse discharge or bleeding, a foul odor from the vagina suggests a foreign body.

Examination reveals inflammation of the vulvar and vaginal mucosa. Although foreign material may be seen when the labia are separated, vaginoscopy often must be performed to explore

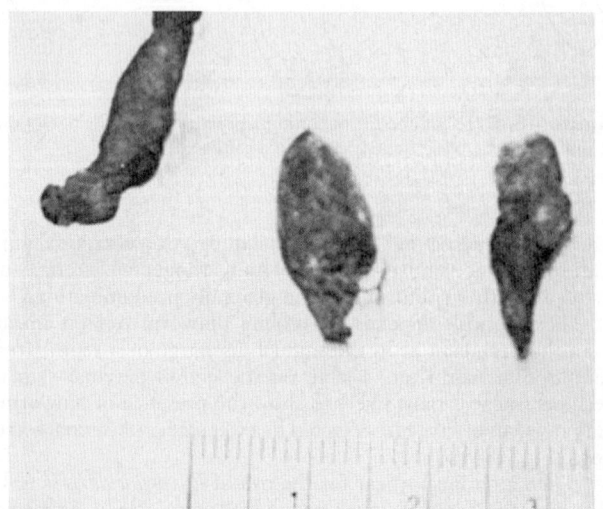

Figure 48–7 Bits of paper or cloth are the vaginal foreign bodies most frequently found in children.

the full length of the vagina. Rarely, a metallic object that has been in the vagina for some time erodes the mucosa and becomes hidden in granulation tissue. When such a condition is suspected, a radiograph should be obtained. Most foreign bodies, such as glass, plastics, paper, or cloth, are not radiopaque, however, and radiographic examination fails to detect the foreign material. Soft foreign bodies, such as toilet paper, can be flushed out of the vaginal canal.

The nonspecific vulvovaginitis caused by a foreign body disappears gradually after removal. Recovery can be hastened by using the hygienic treatments previously described. Repeat episodes are common.

Specific Vulvovaginal Infections

Specific vulvovaginal infections include infections of the premenarcheal vulva and vagina by bacteria that cause specific diseases in other sites.

GONORRHEAL VULVOVAGINITIS

Gonococcal infections of the prepubertal genital tract are manifested as vulvovaginitis and not the endocervicitis seen in postmenarcheal girls and women.[40,72,121,247,277,293] The alkaline environment of the unestrogenized vaginal tissues of young girls apparently limits spread of infection to the upper genital tract. Gonorrhea is found less commonly in children now than in the past but must be considered whenever a girl has vulvovaginitis.

Sexual contact should be suspected strongly and almost always is the source when a child has a gonococcal infection. Whether gonococcal infection is transmitted through nonsexual contact is controversial. Researchers have suggested that transmission may occur from freshly infected bedding, towels, or a toilet seat, or digital transmission from an infected adult. No absolute evidence exists, however, for any of these sources of infection. Gonococcal infections in nurseries have been traced to rectal thermometers, other instruments, fomites, and attendants, but before attributing a gonococcal infection to an environmental source, the possibility of sexual transmission must be considered strongly and investigated, and supportive epidemiologic evidence should be sought (e.g., cultures of potential reservoirs).

Neisseria gonorrhoeae was the most common cause of vulvovaginal discharge among prepubertal girls in Rwanda in the late 1980s. Sexual contact was considered likely in all cases because of a cultural belief that a man with a purulent urethral discharge could be cured by rubbing his penis on the external genitalia of a prepubertal girl.[25] In a prospective study of girls 12 months to 12 years of age in the mid-1990s in Cincinnati, Ohio, who had vaginal discharge and no suspicion of sexual abuse, 4 of 43 had positive cultures for *N. gonorrhoeae.*[250] Such cases should lead to investigation for probable sexual abuse.

The acute stage of gonorrheal vulvovaginitis is characterized by inflammation and a purulent discharge. The child may complain of vulvar discomfort, dysuria, frequent urination, and pain on walking. The child usually is well otherwise. Asymptomatic vaginal infection is rare. On examination, the vulvar tissues are edematous; hyperemic; and covered by a profuse, thick, yellowish discharge that exudes from the vagina. The entire vaginal mucosa is inflamed.

The urethra, paraurethral glands, and the major vestibular (Bartholin) glands rarely are involved in a premenarcheal gonorrheal infection. Vulvovaginal infections, including gonorrhea, in prepubertal children rarely, if ever, affect the upper genitalia (uterus, uterine tubes, ovaries, or pelvic peritoneum). Symptoms suggestive of pelvic peritonitis have been reported in premenarcheal children who had gonorrheal vulvovaginitis; all the patients recovered promptly after the administration of penicillin.[40,88]

The acute phase of infection lasts for a few weeks, after which most of the symptoms disappear except the discharge. The vulvar and vaginal tissues may remain hyperemic and macerated in some cases. The discharge becomes scanty and seropurulent, which may persist chronically.

The diagnosis of gonorrheal vulvovaginitis and its differentiation from other types of vulvovaginitis are established by vaginal smears and cultures. Specimens from the pharynx and rectum to test for *N. gonorrhoeae* also should be obtained. Because of the potential medicolegal use of the test results for *N. gonorrhoeae* among children, standard culture systems should be used for the diagnosis of *N. gonorrhoeae* in children. DNA probes (available for vaginal and urine specimens) and other rapid tests can be used as adjunctive evidence, but they should not be done in place of culture for the diagnosis of gonococcal infection in children. The presence of gram-negative intracellular diplococci in vaginal smears from a child with a history of exposure or with typical clinical findings is sufficient reason to start treatment, but it does not establish a definitive diagnosis. Other related species, particularly *Moraxella (Branhamella) catarrhalis* and *Neisseria sicca*, may be found in association with vulvovaginitis. A definitive diagnosis of gonorrhea is made only when *N. gonorrhoeae* is differentiated from other *Neisseria* spp. on the basis of glucose use. Additional confirmation of *N. gonorrhoeae* is recommended in children. Monoclonal fluorescent antibody tests or DNA probe confirmation tests are available. Isolates should be preserved to permit repeated or additional analyses.

Children weighing less than 45 kg with uncomplicated gonococcal vulvovaginitis and urethritis, pharyngitis, or proctitis are treated with a single dose of 125 mg of intramuscular ceftriaxone. An alternative is a single dose of intramuscular spectinomycin, 50 mg/kg (maximum 2 g), if ceftriaxone is contraindicated. Spectinomycin is not recommended for the treatment of gonococcal pharyngitis. Presently, spectinomycin is unavailable in the United States.[43] Treatment of children who are 8 years or older and weigh more than 45 kg follows the guidelines for postmenarcheal girls. In addition to ceftriaxone, 125 mg intramuscularly, single oral doses of cefixime (400 mg), ciprofloxacin (500 mg), or ofloxacin (400 mg) can be given to these girls. Local treatment is limited to gentle cleansing of the vulva and perineum. For hospitalized children, standard isolation precautions are recommended until 24 hours after effective parenteral therapy has been administered. Empiric therapy with erythromycin, azithromycin, or doxycycline to treat potential concomitant infection with *C. trachomatis* is given routinely to individuals with gonococcal infection.[42]

Follow-up cultures should be obtained from all infected sites 2 weeks after treatment to ensure that it has been effective. If not done as part of the initial evaluation, children confirmed as having gonorrhea should be evaluated for co-infection with *C. trachomatis*, *Treponema pallidum*, *Trichomonas*, human immunodeficiency virus (HIV), and hepatitis B virus.

PREMENARCHEAL CHLAMYDIAL VAGINITIS

Although *C. trachomatis* apparently is an uncommon cause of vaginitis in prepubertal girls, vaginal infection with *C. trachomatis* can occur in children with or without a known history of sexual activity and should be considered in the evaluation of a child with vaginal symptoms. Only a few studies have evaluated young children for *C. trachomatis*. These studies have involved mostly children being evaluated for sexual abuse or vulvovaginal symptoms, or both, and some have included a control group in an attempt to control either for a history of sexual activity or for vaginal symptoms.

In studies evaluating premenarcheal children with vulvovaginitis, recovery of *C. trachomatis* has been low in children with symptoms and healthy control groups. In one study, none of the 35 children with symptoms had *C. trachomatis*, whereas 1 of 35 without symptoms had *C. trachomatis* isolated.[209] In another study conducted in a pediatric gynecology clinic, 4 of 29 (14%) premenarcheal girls were found to have *C. trachomatis*.[37] All four had a homogeneous white discharge, and one had a bloody discharge. Sexual abuse occurred in two of the children and was considered possible in another. In a Cincinnati study evaluating vaginitis in girls younger than 12 years in whom sexual abuse was not suspected, none of the 87 children had a positive culture for *C. trachomatis*.[250] Similarly, in a smaller study of 11 girls with vaginitis, none was found to have *C. trachomatis*.[225]

In studies evaluating children suspected of being sexually abused, rates of recovery tend to be higher than those seen in children with vaginitis. In one study, a history of sexual abuse was discovered in two control children only after *C. trachomatis* was identified.[109] Initially, 2 percent of children with a history of sexual abuse versus 4 percent of healthy controls had positive vaginal cultures for *Chlamydia*. On further questioning, however, the two children in the control group with *C. trachomatis* were siblings who were sexually abused 3 years earlier, changing the rate of *C. trachomatis* vaginal infection in the sexual abuse group to 6 percent and decreasing the rate in the control group to 0 percent. This misclassification, if not discovered, would have changed the conclusion of the study, which suggested that similar rates of *C. trachomatis* infection occur in children with and without a history of sexual contact. This incidence illustrates the importance of thoroughly investigating the possibility of sexual abuse whenever a sexually transmitted pathogen is isolated in a young child. In a Cincinnati study evaluating children for sexual abuse, rates were low in prepubertal girls compared with pubertal girls (0.8% versus 7%),[253] whereas in a study in Raleigh, North Carolina, 6 percent of sexually abused girls younger than 12 years versus 0 percent of control children had *C. trachomatis* isolated from their vagina.[140] Four of the 10 children in the latter study had a vaginal discharge.

The highest rates of *C. trachomatis* infection were seen in a Los Angeles study, in which 47 prepubertal girls were examined for alleged sexual abuse and 17 percent had *C. trachomatis* isolated from vaginal specimens.[89] The variation in rates among studies may reflect differences in the prevalence of *C. trachomatis* in different communities. Although co-infection with *C. trachomatis* has not been studied well in prepubertal children, experience from adult populations has shown that it should be suspected in children with *N. gonorrhoeae* infection. In one study in prepubertal girls, 30 percent with *N. gonorrhoeae* also tested positive for *C. trachomatis*.[225]

One possibility is that a positive chlamydial culture in a young child, especially a child younger than 3 years, may be due to persistence of perinatal infection. Subclinical infections have been reported in 14 percent of infants of mothers with active *C. trachomatis* infection.[238] Many infants infected with *C. trachomatis* at birth remain infected for 372 days in the vagina; 383 days in the rectum; and 866 days in the conjunctiva, nasopharynx, and oropharynx.[21] Persistence of perinatal infection for 18 months and for 6 years has been reported in other studies as well.[172,237,275] Although persistence of perinatal infection can occur, when *C. trachomatis* is identified in vaginal specimens, sexual abuse still must be suspected strongly.

In contrast to premenarcheal gonorrhea infections, chlamydial vaginitis in children often seems to be asymptomatic. Because of study design issues in evaluating children with *C. trachomatis* infection, in which only children with a history of sexual abuse or vaginal symptoms, or both, are included, fully understanding the spectrum of symptoms seen in young children is difficult. In one study evaluating symptomatic children with *C. trachomatis* vaginal infection, 25 percent had a vaginal discharge and 12 percent had vaginal bleeding.[89]

Numerous diagnostic methods for *Chlamydia* are available.[23] Direct tissue culture isolation of *C. trachomatis* remains the gold standard and is the only test that should be used in prepubertal children or in cases in which sexual abuse is under consideration.[42] Culturing for chlamydiae requires isolation of the organism in tissue culture and confirmation of the characteristic intracytoplasmic inclusions by fluorescent monoclonal antibody staining.[42] Although the specificity of tissue culture approaches 100 percent, tissue culture is only 70 to 85 percent sensitive compared with DNA amplification techniques.[23] The low recovery rate in studies of prepubertal children may be due to the low sensitivity of tissue culture or the use of vaginal cultures in young children. Isolation rates from the vagina usually are lower than rates of recovery from the endocervix.[176]

Nonculture chlamydia tests, including enzyme immunoassays, direct fluorescent antibody tests,[1] DNA hybridization, and DNA amplification tests, are available and have been investigated in cervical and urine specimens and approved for use in sexually active postmenarcheal adolescents and adults. These tests have not been field-tested for large numbers of vaginal specimens from premenarcheal girls. In addition, rectal or pharyngeal specimens have not been tested. False-positive results have been reported in vaginal specimens for some of these tests in children, and these tests should not be used in premenarcheal children.[112,215] False-positive results probably are caused by cross-reactivity with common anogenital organisms, such as group A and B streptococci, *Acinetobacter* spp., *N. gonorrhoeae, G. vaginalis, E. coli, Proteus* spp., and *Staphylococcus* spp.[156,228,231,232,274]

The treatment of choice for chlamydial infection, including vaginitis in children weighing less than 45 kg, is erythromycin, 50 mg/kg/day in four divided doses for 10 to 14 days.[42] Because erythromycin base or ethyl succinate is only 80 percent efficacious, a test of cure should be considered 3 weeks after completion of treatment. A second course of therapy is recommended if the repeat culture is positive. Children weighing 45 kg or more but who are younger than 8 years of age should be treated with azithromycin as a single 1-g oral dose. For children 8 years and older, two regimens are recommended: azithromycin as a single 1-g dose or doxycycline at a dose of 100 mg twice a day for 7 days.[42] Because these two regimens are highly efficacious, a test of cure is recommended only if symptoms persist or re-infection is suspected.

PREMENARCHEAL VAGINAL TRICHOMONIASIS

Vaginal trichomoniasis is reported infrequently in prepubertal children. This low prevalence may be accurate or could be due to lack of appropriate testing or limitations of the diagnostic techniques used in studies in prepubertal children. Many diagnostic techniques are available; however, the diagnosis of *Trichomonas vaginalis* infection typically is made by identifying the motile, triflagellated trichomonads in urine or wet preparations of vaginal secretions or through culture of vaginal secretions (see Chapter 226).[42,72] Stained smears of vaginal discharge may reveal trichomonads, but this method is the least sensitive of the available methods. The sensitivity of wet-mount examination of vaginal secretions depends on prompt transport of the specimen to the laboratory before the organisms lyse or lose motility and on the expertise of the individual examining the specimen.[157]

Although culturing of vaginal specimens is more sensitive, this method is not widely available. More sensitive techniques have allowed for the evaluation of culture and wet-mount methods. In a study examining vaginal swab samples using polymerase chain reaction (PCR), culture and wet-mount evaluations were found to have sensitivities of 70 percent and 36 percent.[72] A urine-based PCR enzyme-linked immunosorbent assay had a sensitivity and specificity of 91 percent and 93 percent compared with wet mount or culture.[147] Such techniques may be promising for detec-

tion of *T. vaginalis* when vaginal specimens are unavailable and culture of specimens is not feasible. Because of a lower specificity than that of culture, however, these techniques probably never will be recommended for use in prepubertal children in whom sexual abuse would need to be considered.

Trichomoniasis in newborns through the acquisition of *T. vaginalis* from the mother's vagina during delivery, with recovery of *T. vaginalis* from urine, vaginal, and respiratory tract specimens, has been described in several case reports.[5,50,54,169,178,216,260] The prevalence of *T. vaginalis* in healthy, vaginally delivered infants of mothers with *T. vaginalis* is unknown. In one study, *T. vaginalis* could not be identified in any of the 14 female infants of mothers in whom *T. vaginalis* was diagnosed.[34] The overall prevalence of *T. vaginalis* in the 868 mothers was 4 percent, but the denominator of mothers of female infants was not described. In another study of 984 female infants, direct smear or culture (or both) of infant vaginal specimens identified 3 infants with *T. vaginalis*, a prevalence of 0.3 percent.[9] Two of the three infants had a vaginal discharge. The overall prevalence of infection in the mothers of the 984 infants was not reported. Of the three infants with *T. vaginalis*, one mother had a history of vaginal discharge and a negative direct smear for *T. vaginalis*, and the other two mothers had no history of *T. vaginalis*.

Numerous reports in the literature confirm the occurrence of *T. vaginalis* outside the newborn period in prepubertal girls evaluated for vaginitis. The prevalence of *T. vaginalis* in prepubertal girls with vaginitis but no history of sexual abuse ranged from 0 to 4 percent.[102,120,142,209,250] In studies with a healthy control population,[101,120,142] *T. vaginalis* was not identified in any of the children in the asymptomatic control group.

T. vaginalis has been described in varying frequency in sexually abused prepubertal girls. A case report described *Trichomonas* vaginitis in two sexually abused children with vaginal discharge.[143] In two studies conducted in Raleigh, North Carolina, which described isolated pathogens in sexually abused children with a vaginal discharge, 19 percent of 52 children at risk for being sexually abused had positive wet mounts for *T. vaginalis* in one study, whereas only 2 percent of 141 children had *T. vaginalis* in the second study.[140] The variation in detection in this high-risk population cannot be explained easily. In studies systematically evaluating children for sexual abuse regardless of symptoms, *T. vaginalis* has not been recovered. In an Australian study evaluating 160 children younger than 10 years and 95 healthy age-matched controls, none of the children had *T. vaginalis* isolated from vaginal cultures.[93] Similarly, none of the 119 prepubertal girls evaluated for sexual abuse in a Cincinnati, Ohio, study had *T. vaginalis* identified by urinalysis or wet mount of vaginal secretions.[253] Without additional studies using culture techniques and conducted in diverse populations of prepubertal girls, determining the true prevalence of *T. vaginalis* in prepubertal girls who have vaginitis, with or without a history of sexual abuse, is difficult.

A more recent case report suggests that *T. vaginalis* could be transmitted within a family without sexual abuse or contact.[3] In this report, *Trichomonas* vaginitis was diagnosed in the mother, and her three prepubertal daughters were symptomatic with a vaginal discharge. Two of the three girls had *T. vaginalis* identified on wet-mount evaluation of their vaginal specimens. They had no history or evidence of sexual abuse, the father was asymptomatic, and microscopy of an early morning urine specimen was negative for *T. vaginalis*. Although these cases may have resulted from transmission within a family without sexual abuse, identification of *T. vaginalis* in a prepubertal child outside the newborn period should prompt further medical and social evaluation for sexual abuse. Additionally, if *T. vaginalis* is recovered from a child, the child should be evaluated for other sexually transmitted infections, including syphilis, *N. gonorrhoeae, C. trachomatis*, hepatitis B, and HIV infection.[72]

Metronidazole (Flagyl) is effective in the treatment of vaginal trichomoniasis in premenarcheal children. The recommended dose for prepubertal girls is 15 mg/kg/day in three divided doses (maximal dose 250 mg three times a day for 7 days), 500 mg twice a day for 7 days, or 40 mg/kg (maximum 2 g) in a single dose.[72] Metronidazole can be made into a suspension for young children and has a low level of toxicity. Possible side effects are described in the discussion of trichomoniasis in adolescent girls. Metronidazole is very effective, with cure rates of 90 to 95 percent; however, if the infection does not respond to treatment, prepubertal children should be re-treated with a 7-day course as described.[4,42] A vaginal preparation of metronidazole is available, but it is not recommended for the treatment of *T. vaginalis* infection.[42]

BACTERIAL VAGINOSIS

Bacterial vaginosis is a cause of vaginal discharge in adolescent girls and women and may be seen in premenarcheal girls. Bacterial vaginosis is caused by a change in the relative proportions of bacteria in the vaginal flora: an overgrowth of anaerobes and *G. vaginalis* and a decrease in hydrogen peroxide-producing lactobacilli.[12] Although overgrowth of *G. vaginalis* often is found in bacterial vaginosis, identification of *G. vaginalis* by culture of the vaginal discharge is not diagnostic because *G. vaginalis* may be present in girls with or without bacterial vaginosis.[42]

Two methods are used to establish the diagnosis of bacterial vaginosis—Gram stain of vaginal discharge and clinical criteria,[42,72] with clinical criteria being used more commonly. The Gram stain method is used to determine the relative concentrations of bacterial morphotypes and evaluate for the overgrowth of anaerobes. This method requires an examiner with expertise in evaluating specimens for bacterial vaginosis and is less practical than is the use of clinical criteria; thus, clinical criteria are used more widely. The clinical criteria used for establishing the diagnosis of bacterial vaginosis are the presence of three of four findings: a grayish homogeneous discharge, the presence of clue cells on a wet-mount evaluation, a pH greater than 4.5, and a positive amine test result (amine or fishy odor when vaginal secretions are mixed with 10% potassium hydroxide). Although these criteria have been used routinely in studies in postmenarcheal women, use of these criteria in premenarcheal girls has been inconsistent, rendering assessment of the prevalence of bacterial vaginosis in this population difficult.

Despite the fact that the presence of *G. vaginalis* is not diagnostic of bacterial vaginosis, studies in premenarcheal girls have examined the presence of *G. vaginalis* in vaginal secretions.[18,93,114,142] In a survey of vaginal flora in children without a vaginal discharge, *G. vaginalis* was isolated from 14 percent.[114] In another study, prepubertal girls with a history of sexual abuse were more likely to have *G. vaginalis* isolated from vaginal specimens (15%) than were girls with no history of sexual abuse and either genitourinary complaints (4%) or no genitourinary complaints (4%).[18] In girls with a vaginal discharge, *G. vaginalis* was isolated from 20 percent of 25 sexually abused girls versus none of 11 girls with no history of sexual abuse. In a study examining the vaginal flora of sexually abused and nonabused 3- to 10-year-old girls, 6 percent of abused versus 1 percent of nonabused girls had *G. vaginalis* in their vaginal secretions.[93] In a study of premenarcheal girls older than 2 years with vulvovaginitis, none of the 50 girls or their age-matched controls had *G. vaginalis* isolated from vaginal specimens.[142] Because *G. vaginalis* has been isolated from symptomatic and asymptomatic girls and from girls with and without a history or evidence of sexual abuse, culture for *G. vaginalis* should not be done in the evaluation of a child with a vaginal discharge or to determine whether sexual contact has occurred.

Bacterial vaginosis is defined poorly in premenarcheal girls. No published studies using the recommended criteria to make the

diagnosis exist. Some studies have used some of the criteria, however, in an attempt to examine bacterial vaginosis in premenarcheal girls. In a study examining sexually transmitted infections in girls aged 1 to 12 years who were evaluated for possible sexual abuse, 99 of the 245 girls with a vaginal discharge had an amine test and were examined for clue cells.[139] Seven of the 99 girls (7%) had clue cells or a positive amine test, or both. In a similar study, 22 of 51 girls with a history of sexual contact and a vaginal discharge had an amine test performed and were evaluated for clue cells; all of them were negative for both tests.[140] In the same study, in a second group of girls defined as being at risk for having had undetected previous sexual contact, 30 girls had a vaginal discharge, and 10 had wet-mount preparations performed. One had a positive amine test and clue cells, and one had a positive amine test only. In both of these studies, the full criteria were not used, and only subgroups of girls with vaginal discharge were evaluated.

In another study, 31 abused and 23 nonabused girls aged 2.5 to 13 years had vaginal washes performed along with amine tests and testing for clue cells.[110] The abused girls had an initial visit and a follow-up visit more than 7 days after the abuse occurred. The nonabused girls had only an initial evaluation. One of the 23 nonabused girls had a positive amine test with normal examination results and was asymptomatic. Similarly, 1 of the 31 abused girls had a positive amine test on the initial visit. On follow-up evaluation, clue cells and a positive amine test developed in 4 of the 31 abused girls, and either clue cells or a positive amine test was noted in another 4 of the 31 girls. Either a new vaginal discharge or dysuria developed in five of these eight girls. Three of the eight girls were postmenarcheal. Whether the testing itself could have been responsible for the positive results is unclear because the control group did not undergo the follow-up evaluation.

Until studies using the proper and complete criteria are done in young girls with and without a vaginal discharge, the prevalence of bacterial vaginosis will be unknown and the significance of bacterial vaginosis as a cause of vaginal discharge in premenarcheal girls will remain unclear. At this time, the presence of manifestations of bacterial vaginosis should prompt the health care provider to consider treatment of bacterial vaginosis. In addition, the possibility of sexual abuse should be contemplated because a diagnosis of bacterial vaginosis does not provide evidence of sexual abuse. Because bacterial cultures may be performed in the evaluation of a vaginal discharge in a premenarcheal girl and *G. vaginalis* may be identified, identification of *G. vaginalis* should not be considered evidence of sexual abuse or diagnostic of bacterial vaginosis.

Numerous regimens for the treatment of bacterial vaginosis exist, but no specific recommendations are available for premenarcheal girls. Probably because bacterial vaginosis is diagnosed infrequently, clinical trials evaluating treatment of bacterial vaginosis in premenarcheal girls are lacking. The drugs recommended for use in young girls are those recommended for postmenarcheal women, with dosages based on the child's body weight. In small children (<45 kg), metronidazole can be given at 15 mg/kg/day divided two times a day for 7 days (maximum dose 1 g/day).[42,72] Two intravaginal preparations also are available as alternative regimens for adolescents. Two percent clindamycin given once a day for 7 days or 0.75 percent metronidazole gel given twice a day for 5 days can be used to treat bacterial vaginosis.[42] An alternative regimen for younger girls is oral clindamycin; a dose of 10 to 20 mg/kg/day divided three times a day for 7 days is suggested.[197]

MYCOTIC (FUNGAL) VULVOVAGINITIS

Candida albicans and other fungi can cause vulvovaginitis in infants and children. Although these infections can occur in any child, children with a history of recent antibiotic use, uncontrolled

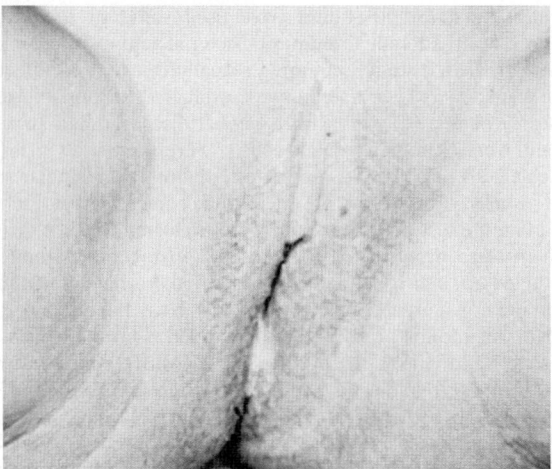

Figure 48–8 Mycotic vulvovaginitis. The child is a diabetic.

diabetes mellitus, or immunosuppression are at an increased risk for development of fungal vulvovaginitis. In children with recurrent or persistent infection, especially with no history of antibiotic use, immunosuppressive conditions, such as diabetes or HIV infection, should be considered. Mycotic infections are not considered sexually transmitted infections, but they are discussed in this section because they can cause genital infections in young children.

Children with fungal vulvovaginitis usually complain of vulvar pruritus and burning. The burning results from urine coming in contact with desquamated or excoriated areas of the vulva. A vaginal discharge also may be present. In diapered children, an erythematous rash in the child's diaper area may be noticed.

Examination reveals findings of diffuse erythema of the vulvar mucosa that may extend onto the perineal area. The involved areas are red and shiny, and whitish plaques and edema may be found. Excoriated areas, caused by scratching, can be seen as well. If the condition has been long-standing, the edema, secondary infection, and repeated scratching may produce thickened and fissured lesions closely resembling chronic eczema or lichen sclerosus et atrophicus (Fig. 48–8). If the vagina is involved, the mucosa is dusky red, and small, whitish plaques on the vaginal surface or a scant white curdled discharge may be noted. The discharge, when present, is odorless.

The diagnosis of fungal vulvovaginitis is made by finding yeast and pseudohyphae on examination of the vaginal discharge or scraped material from the vulvar skin by Gram stain or wet preparation suspended in 10 to 20 percent potassium hydroxide (Fig. 48–9).[72] Further confirmation can be obtained by identifying fungus by culture of material from the vagina or vulva on Sabouraud or Nickerson media.

C. albicans and other fungi have been isolated from the vagina in asymptomatic and symptomatic girls. In a study examining the microbiology of the vagina, yeast was cultured from 48 percent of girls aged 2 months to 2 years, from 12.5 percent of girls aged 3 to 10 years, and from 35 percent of girls aged 11 to 15 years.[122] *C. albicans* (37%) and *Candida tropicalis* (26%) were the species most frequently isolated, but *Candida parapsilosis*, *Torulopsis glabrata*, non-*Candida* yeast species, and other *Candida* spp. were isolated as well.

In studies evaluating prepubertal girls with vulvovaginitis, fungi have been recovered at varying rates. In one study, *C. albicans* was isolated from 25 percent of 31 symptomatic prepubertal girls with an abnormal vaginal discharge or vulvovaginitis, whereas only 3 percent of asymptomatic girls had *C. albicans* isolated.[95] Another study found different results, with none of the

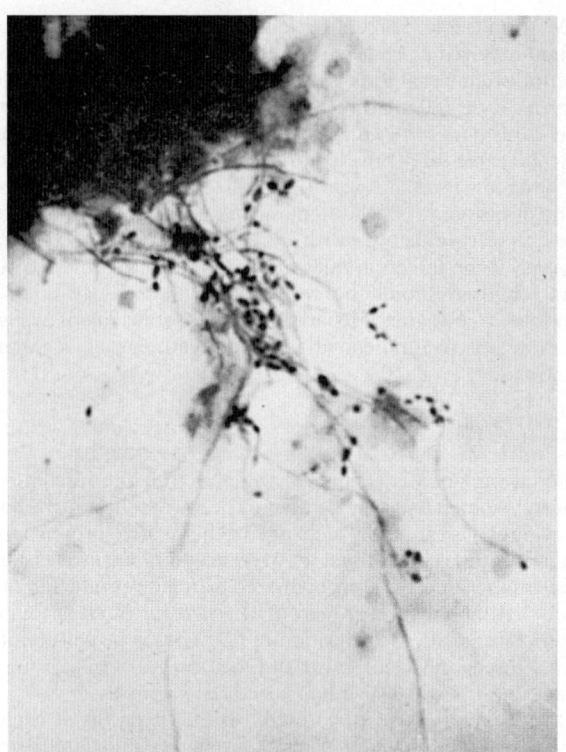

Figure 48–9 Hyphae of *Candida albicans* discovered on a wet smear of vaginal discharge.

50 asymptomatic girls and only 2 percent of the 50 girls with vulvovaginitis having *C. albicans*.[142] Similarly, in a study evaluating girls younger than 12 years with vaginal complaints, only 3 percent of the 74 girls had *C. albicans* isolated.[250] Neither of these groups of girls had a discharge on examination, and both had been treated recently with antibiotics. In a study that examined recovery of microorganisms from girls with vaginitis, 8 percent of the vaginal cultures of the 35 girls evaluated grew yeast.[101] In these latter two studies, assessing the role of yeast in the disease is difficult because there was no control population for comparison.

Several modes of therapy can be used for the management of fungal vulvovaginitis.[72] Numerous antifungal creams, including nystatin, miconazole, clotrimazole, or terconazole, are available. The creams should be applied as prescribed to the affected area after cleansing. In diapered children, the cream should be applied with each diaper change.

Curing fungal infections often is difficult in children who are taking antibiotics or who receive repeated courses of antibiotic therapy. In such cases, a 1-mL dose of nystatin suspension (Mycostatin), 100,000 U/mL, can be injected into the vagina three times a day for 10 days in infants and small children. In addition, the suspension should be administered at the same dose orally four times daily. Fluconazole (Diflucan) also can be administered as a one-time oral dose. A second dose may need to be administered for severe infections.[72] In older girls, vulvovaginal fungal infections can be treated with fungicidal vaginal creams, suppositories, or oral fluconazole as described in the section on vaginal infections in adolescent girls.[42]

NONGONORRHEAL NEISSERIAL VULVOVAGINITIS

Occasionally, other species of *Neisseria* are the causative agents in cases of premenarcheal vulvovaginitis. These gram-negative, intracellular and extracellular diplococci resemble *N. gonorrhoeae* on stained smears. *M. catarrhalis* also is identical on Gram stain. Gram-negative diplococci should be speciated completely by the microbiology laboratory to avoid misidentifying of nongonococcal diplococci as gonococci and vice versa. Especially for pediatric patients, misidentification can result in serious medicolegal consequences for the family when unwarranted intervention is initiated, or it can result in failure to protect the child's welfare when appropriate measures are deemed unnecessary.[9]

N. sicca, generally considered nonpathogenic, has been isolated from children with vulvovaginal infections that clinically resembled gonorrhea.[283] *Neisseria meningitidis* also has been reported as a cause of vulvovaginitis.[77,102] Nongonococcal *Neisseria* spp. may be considered the cause of vulvovaginal infections when isolated as the predominant flora in the setting of vaginal inflammation and discharge.

Treatment of vulvovaginitis caused by nongonococcal *Neisseria* spp. or *M. catarrhalis* is the same as for *N. gonorrhoeae*. Most nongonococcal *Neisseria* spp. are not resistant to penicillin, but the need for therapy generally is based on the Gram stain finding of gram-negative diplococci, which for therapeutic purposes should be considered gonococci pending culture results. Although data are unavailable, a single dose of ceftriaxone probably should be as effective for these noninvasive *Neisseria* infections as it is for gonorrhea. Chemoprophylaxis, generally with rifampin, should be considered for family members and other contacts in cases of meningococcal vulvovaginitis.

GROUP A STREPTOCOCCAL VULVOVAGINITIS

Group A streptococci are a frequent cause of vulvovaginitis in premenarcheal girls and accounted for 9 to 20 percent of cases in several series.[64,67,120,265,279] Most cases occur in girls aged 2 to 7 years, but cases in infants and teenagers have been reported.[26,64,97,265] A marked seasonal variation in incidence in some geographic regions, with peak rates occurring in late fall and winter, may explain the low number of cases of vulvovaginitis caused by group A streptococci in some series.[79,182] The nasopharynx seems to be the primary reservoir for group A streptococci in these girls. Infection may occur from self-inoculation by hand to nose to the vulvovaginal area.[245] The skin also may serve as the source of group A streptococcal vulvovaginitis.[97,265] Preceding or concurrent symptoms of upper respiratory tract infection are uncommon findings, but many girls with group A streptococcal vulvovaginitis have throat cultures positive for *S. pyogenes*.[97,265] Perineal symptoms have preceded pharyngeal symptoms in some patients.[79] Group A streptococcal vulvovaginitis may occur during the course of scarlet fever.[26,119,120]

The signs and symptoms of group A streptococcal vulvovaginitis often overlap those caused by other bacterial infections, but symptoms usually are abrupt in onset. Most patients seek medical care within 1 week of onset. Vaginal discharge and dysuria are the most common complaints. These girls usually are afebrile. Localized tenderness and an intense, fiery red erythema of the vulvar tissues are frequent findings, but some cases have only mild erythema. Pruritus and excoriation may be present. The discharge usually is seropurulent but may be serosanguineous. The color may be white or green. Petechiae may be present on the vaginal mucosa, and regional papular or scarlatiniform rashes can occur.[79,97,245,265] Acute poststreptococcal glomerulonephritis has been reported in association with group A streptococcal vulvovaginitis.[193] Labial abscesses caused by *S. pyogenes* have been noted rarely in prepubertal girls.[279]

Concomitant streptococcal proctitis and perianal skin infections have been reported.[79,154,261] Perianal pruritus, erythema, and tenderness are common findings. Abdominal pain and rectal bleeding may be present. Penile involvement occurs rarely if at all.[181]

The diagnosis of *S. pyogenes* infection may be missed if vaginal secretions are not plated onto sheep blood agar or other media that readily support the growth of streptococci.[265] The vulvovaginitis caused by group A streptococci usually shows initial response to oral antimicrobial therapy within 24 hours. A 10-day course of oral penicillin, amoxicillin, or erythromycin generally is sufficient. A second course sometimes is necessary when perianal disease is present.[261] Adjunctive use of the hygienic measures discussed for nonspecific vulvovaginitis hastens clinical improvement. Group B and group F streptococci also have been isolated from girls with acute vulvovaginitis.[250]

VULVOVAGINITIS SECONDARY TO BACTERIA THAT COLONIZE THE NASOPHARYNX

Often, a history of an upper respiratory tract infection precedes the onset of vulvovaginitis by a few days. Suspicion that the two conditions are related is strengthened when vaginal cultures yield organisms that commonly colonize the nasopharynx. Vulvovaginitis is assumed to result from autoinoculation of microbes from the nasopharynx to the genitalia. The onset of vulvovaginal symptoms in these infections tends to be more acute, the inflammation and discomfort more marked, and the discharge less profuse and less purulent than in nonspecific vulvovaginitis.[133]

H. influenzae and *S. aureus* are the species isolated most frequently from cultures in this setting. *Streptococcus pneumoniae* is seen occasionally. *H. influenzae* was the organism isolated most frequently in a series of 200 girls with vulvovaginitis.[213] Acute and chronic cases of *H. influenzae* vulvovaginitis do occur, and the discharge usually is mucoid or mucopurulent, yellow, and odorless. Vulvovaginitis can be caused by serotypes a, b, and c and by nontypeable strains.[120,179] Concurrent otitis media or urinary tract infection may be present. All three of these species occasionally are found in vaginal cultures from asymptomatic children. Their isolation in pure culture from symptomatic girls is what leads to the clinical conclusion of cause and effect.

Vulvovaginitis caused by these organisms often responds to the treatment described earlier for nonspecific vulvovaginitis secondary to poor perineal hygiene. Systemic antibiotics may be required for persistent cases or may be helpful early in severely symptomatic cases. The choice of agent depends on the anticipated or known antimicrobial susceptibilities of the specific organism. The vagina is a well-recognized source of *S. aureus* colonization in cases of toxic shock syndrome (TSS) associated with this organism. Such cases generally have occurred in adolescent girls and women in association with the use of tampons. Vulvovaginitis caused by *S. aureus* in prepubertal girls has not been reported in connection with TSS. Labial abscesses caused by *S. aureus* have been described in prepubertal girls.[72]

VULVOVAGINITIS SECONDARY TO SKIN INFECTIONS

Similar to a child with an upper respiratory tract infection, a child with impetigo or an infected superficial wound may transmit bacteria from the wound to the genitalia by hand contamination. Cultures in such cases usually yield hemolytic streptococci or *S. aureus*. Treatment is the same as that described for nonspecific vulvovaginitis secondary to respiratory tract infections.

SHIGELLA VULVOVAGINITIS

Vulvovaginitis may be caused by infection with pathogens from the intestinal tract, especially when the organisms are endemic in a community. *Shigella* spp., mainly *Shigella flexneri* and *Shigella sonnei*, seem to account for most of these cases.[25,28,29,59,189] Vaginal discharge without pain, pruritus, or dysuria is the most frequent manifestation of *Shigella* vulvovaginitis. The course can be acute, but discharge that persists for 4 weeks to several months before the diagnosis is made is common. Bloody discharge has been observed in approximately half the cases reported from developed countries, but it was not seen in any of 27 girls with *Shigella* vulvovaginitis in Rwanda between 1988 and 1991.[25] The discharge may be purulent and heavy; occasionally, it is absent. The vulvar tissues usually appear inflamed.

In most instances, *Shigella* vulvovaginitis is not associated with current or recent diarrhea.[25,189] The clinical presentation can be very similar to that of a vaginal foreign body. Local application of triple-sulfa cream (Sultrin) may clear the infection in some cases. Refractory cases have been described, however.[59,189] Systemic treatment with an antibiotic to which the *Shigella* isolate is susceptible is recommended. Single-dose therapy with third-generation cephalosporins is ineffective; 5-day courses of oral agents generally are required.[25] Amoxicillin, trimethoprim-sulfamethoxazole, and cefixime are reasonable choices for susceptible isolates; however, most *Shigella* isolates are resistant to ampicillin and trimethoprim-sulfamethoxazole. Ciprofloxacin use has been described in one case.[18] Azithromycin also may be an effective treatment option.[153] As with other causes of vulvovaginitis, adjunctive use of hygienic measures may help resolve the process and prevent recurrence.

OTHER SPECIFIC CAUSES OF PREMENARCHEAL VULVOVAGINITIS

Diphtheritic, amebic, and other types of specific vulvovaginitis in children have been reported in the literature.[84,163,212] Most such cases have had associated primary disease elsewhere.

Diphtheritic vulvovaginitis can be the primary site of infection, but most reported cases have been secondary to nasopharyngeal infection. Although diphtheria seldom occurs today, sporadic cases occasionally appear in areas where immunization coverage is inadequate. The vulva is the most common genital site involved in diphtheria,[212] but diphtheritic lesions may occur in the vagina without vulvar involvement. The diagnosis is suspected when a child has the severe systemic symptoms produced by upper respiratory tract diphtheria and a local ulceration covered by a gray adherent membrane; it is confirmed by finding *Corynebacterium diphtheriae* in discharge from the lesion.[70] Treatment of diphtheria is the same regardless of the site of the infection and is discussed in Chapter 101.

One case of vulvovaginitis with *Yersinia enterocolitica* isolated as the predominant organism was reported in a 4-year-old girl who also had a positive stool culture and associated fever and abdominal pain but no diarrhea.[281] In other members of the community in which she lived, diarrhea developed with cultures positive for *Y. enterocolitica.* The outbreak was linked to contaminated food. Infections with this organism may be missed because special culture techniques are required for isolation.

Rarely, ulcerative vulvovaginitis caused by *Entamoeba histolytica* or related to typhoid fever has been reported. Generally, specific genital infections with pathogenic organisms usually found in the gastrointestinal tract are the result of fecal contamination of the vulva and vagina. Treatment of infections caused by *E. histolytica* is described in Chapter 221.

OTHER LOWER AND UPPER GENITAL TRACT INFECTIONS OF PREMENARCHEAL GIRLS

Other specific and nonspecific infections of the premenarcheal female lower and upper genital tract genitalia, including genital herpes, condylomata acuminata, molluscum contagiosum, granulomatous and ulcerative disorders, cervicitis, and pelvic inflammatory disease (PID), are discussed in the section on genital infections in adolescents.

SEXUALLY TRANSMITTED DISEASES IN SEXUALLY ABUSED CHILDREN

Isolation of an STD in a child (especially a prepubertal child) places a health care provider in an awkward position of having to report the case to a children's protective service agency for investigation of sexual abuse. Management of children who have sexually transmitted infections requires close cooperation among clinicians, laboratories, and child protection agencies. The possibility of nonsexual transmission of these diseases often is raised, particularly when a preliminary investigation cannot elicit a history of sexual abuse. The rate of eliciting evidence of sexual abuse in prepubertal children can be 67 percent, however, in children with STDs.[15] Bacterial sexually transmitted infections are isolated more frequently than are viral infections in sexually abused children. Many challenges are involved in eliciting and validating sexual abuse in children. Verbal communication in children younger than 2 to 3 years old is impossible or difficult to interpret. Fear of disclosure by children or family members because of threats of violence may be a major barrier to validating a case in an older child.[179]

The first step in managing such situations is for a physician to assess critically the type of diagnostic test used to detect the infection. A major problem exists with inappropriate use of nonculture tests for testing for chlamydia.[8,107] The second step is for a physician to perform a genital examination on the child to look for evidence of acute or chronic vulvar and hymeneal trauma. Referral to a physician with expertise in this field is appropriate. A brief interview of the child in a nondirected manner with open-ended questions also should be done. Regardless of whether the child divulges any information, the case should be reported to the local children's protective service agency. The objective is for an agency caseworker to interview the child also in a nonthreatening manner. In addition, the caseworker should request that all household members be tested for STDs. More than one visit and interview by the caseworker may be necessary for such testing to be accomplished. Based on a review of the literature, common STDs in prepubertal children and their potential mode of transmission are summarized in Table 48–3 and discussed in this section.

GONOCOCCAL INFECTION

In infants, perinatal nonsexual transmission is considered the most likely cause of gonococcal infection. Branch and Paxton[27] found that in 1- to 11-month-old infants, all the mothers were found to have gonococcal infection, and no history of sexual contact could be elicited. The authors concluded that transmission of the infection was perinatal, from freshly contaminated hands, or through fomites.

Prepubertal children with gonococcal infection frequently are found to have a history of sexual contact.[139] The rate of eliciting a history of sexual contact in prepubertal children with gonorrhea ranges from 36 to 93 percent.[27,83,136,138] Branch and Paxton[27] reported that 93 percent of children aged 1 to 9 years with gonorrhea had sexual contact with relatives in the household. Ingram and colleagues[136,138] found that 35 percent of 1- to 4-year-old children and 100 percent of children older than 4 years with gonorrhea reported having sexual contact with an older male family member. Folland and coworkers[83] elicited a history of sexual contact from 34 percent of children with gonococcal urethritis and vaginitis.

Other infected adults and children often are found in an infected child's environment.[217] Testing of household members can detect infected adults at a rate of 18 to 29 percent.[8,192] In a retrospective study of 14 Native Alaskan children with

TABLE 48-3 Sexually Transmitted Diseases (STDs) in Prepubertal Children: Modes of Transmission and Implications for Child Sexual Abuse

Infectious Agent	Persistence after Perinatal Acquisition	STD Rate in Alleged Sexual Abuse Cases	Alleged Sexual Abuse Rate in STD Cases	Infection in Household Members of Infected Children	Survival on Fomites	AAP CCAN 2005 Guideline Recommendations for Abuse Reports	Other Comments
Neisseria gonorrhoeae	Up to 1 yr old[27]	5-7%[59]	35%, 1-4 yr old[40] 100%, >4 yr old[136] 93%, 1-9 yr old[27]	18-29% of adults in household[8,192] (abuse was thought unlikely in these series)	24 hr on wet fomites; 2 hr on dry fomites. None from public toilet seats[96,214]	Diagnostic for abuse. Report to Child Protective Services*	Although fomite transmission can occur, sexual transmission must be considered the likely mode, unless strong evidence of an alternative mode is found. Fomite or maternal nonsexual transmission plausible <1 yr old[27]
Chlamydia trachomatis	Up to 3 yr old[238] Rectal and vaginal sites up to 54 wk	6-8%[20,45,137,140] 4% cases vs. 9% controls[111]	75%		No data	Diagnostic for abuse. Report to Child Protective Services*	Perinatal acquisition likely <1 yr old; if >1 yr old, genital infection strongly suggests sexual transmission[137]
Trichomonas vaginalis	Up to 1 yr old	No data	Case report[143]	43% fathers, 72% mothers, with no history of sexual abuse elicited (Poland)[159]	Up to 6 hr on wood surface and in discharge.[149] Isolated from bathing implements[196]	Highly suspicious for abuse. Report to Child Protective Services*	If >1 yr old, genital infection strongly suggests sexual transmission. Bathing in tanks or rivers may increase infection risk in girls (India).[196] Has been isolated from mud baths, warm mineral waters, water from toilets[59,159]
Syphilis	Months to years if untreated	0-5%[59,139]	Case reports		Unlikely, based on difficulty in culturing the microbes, but no data	Diagnostic for abuse. Report to Child Protective Services*	Infection not known to be congenital should be considered sexually transmitted. Clinical manifestations (e.g., late congenital syphilis) may be helpful in discerning mode in some cases[42]
Bacterial vaginosis (Gardnerella vaginalis)	No systematic studies; colonization at birth potentially persists for years	7-13%[110]	28%[4]			Inconclusive; conduct medical follow-up	G. vaginalis can be found as part of normal flora in nonabused virginal children. Presence of clue cells in a vaginal wet mount, not culture results, is diagnostic.[42]
Haemophilus ducreyi (chancroid)	Asymptomatic persistence unlikely						Should be considered sexually transmitted

TABLE 48-3 Sexually Transmitted Diseases (STDs) in Prepubertal Children: Modes of Transmission and Implications for Child Sexual Abuse—cont'd

Infectious Agent	Persistence after Perinatal Acquisition	STD Rate in Alleged Sexual Abuse Cases	Alleged Sexual Abuse Rate in STD Cases	Infection in Household Members of Infected Children	Survival on Fomites	AAP CCAN 2005 Guideline Recommendations for Abuse Reports	Other Comments
Calymmatobacterium (Klebsiella) granulomatis (granuloma inguinale)							Should be considered sexually transmitted[42]
Herpes simplex virus (genital sites)	Symptomatic congenital infection usually develops within first 6 wk of life		Case reports only	Case report only (mother with an infected finger)[146]	2 hr on latex gloves, toilet seats; 24 hr on speculum; 72 hr on gauze[167]	Suspicious for abuse. Report to Child Protective Services*†	Autoinoculation from oral lesions is possible,[191] but fomite transmission is unlikely because it requires direct contact of viable virus with broken skin or mucous membranes
Human papillomavirus‡ (anogenital warts)	Up to at least 3 yr old and probably years longer[57]		27-90%[47]			Suspicious for abuse. Report to Child Protective Services*§	The possibility of sexual abuse should be considered when oral warts or laryngeal papillomas are found in older children
Human immunodeficiency virus (HIV)	Perinatal acquisition may not become evident for many years in slowly progressive cases	Very low in the U.S.; higher in countries with higher prevalences of HIV infection	26 of 9136 HIV cases in children were associated with sexual abuse by individuals with confirmed or suspected HIV infection[168a]	Common¶	Exposure to infected blood can lead to infection. Casual household contact alone has not been associated with transmission	Diagnostic for abuse if not perinatally or transfusion acquired. Report to Child Protective Services if mother is HIV-negative and child has no transfusion exposure*	History of maternal HIV infection suggests perinatal acquisition unless the child's presentation suggests acute HIV infection or perinatal transmission was reasonably excluded during infancy
Hepatitis B virus	Perinatal transmission can be asymptomatic for years to decades			Household transmission can occur			Nonsexual transmission can occur, so positive HBsAg tests do not necessarily indicate sexual abuse. Vaccination history for hepatitis B virus should be reviewed
Hepatitis C virus	Perinatal transmission can be asymptomatic for years to decades						Sexual transmission has been thought possible, but is currently uncertain. Maternal history may be helpful

*Or other local agency mandated to receive reports of suspected child sexual abuse.

†Report unless there is a clear history of autoinoculation. Type of herpes simplex virus (1 versus 2) is generally not helpful in determining whether acquisition was by abuse or autoinoculation, although presence of type 1 may increase the likelihood of nonsexual transmission.

‡Laryngeal papillomas in young children are likely perinatally acquired.

§Some experts do not believe reporting is warranted in all cases. In children <3 or 4 years old for whom a thorough evaluation by an experienced child sexual abuse investigator reveals no concerns of abuse, reporting to Child Protective Services may be unnecessary. Close medical follow-up may be appropriate. Physicians must be clear when reporting that anogenital human papillomavirus is not always acquired by sexual abuse even in older children.

¶All siblings should be tested, whether perinatal or postnatal acquisition is suspected, unless perinatal infection is the known route and an older child was born during a time period in which the mother was known to be HIV-negative.

HBsAg, hepatitis B surface antigen.

Modified from Chacko, M., Staat, M. A., and Woods, C. R.: Genital infections in childhood and adolescence. In Feigin, R. D., Cherry, J. D., Demmler, G. J., and Kaplan, S. L. (eds.): Textbook of Pediatric Infectious Diseases. 5th ed. Philadelphia, W. B. Saunders, 2004, p. 577; and Committee on Child Abuse and Neglect.

gonococcal infection, 3 reported having sexual contact. Seven children slept with their parents, one or both of whom had gonorrhea; the authors assumed that these children acquired the infection by nonsexual means.[251]

N. gonorrhoeae has been shown to survive for 20 to 24 hours in infected secretions on towels and handkerchiefs.[263] Although N. gonorrhoeae has survived on toilet seats for 2 hours, no gonococci were recovered from toilet seats in public restrooms or in a clinic for STDs.[96,224] Nonsexual transmission to adults is rare.

Nonsexual transmission conceivably occurs in children who sleep and bathe with their parents. Sexual transmission is the more common and most likely mode of transmission, however.[112] The presence of gonorrhea should be considered diagnostic of sexual abuse. An investigation for sexual abuse must be pursued in a child with gonorrhea by reporting the case to the appropriate legal authority.[42]

CHLAMYDIAL INFECTION

C. trachomatis can be transmitted to an infant from an infected mother during the perinatal period. C. trachomatis has been isolated from the conjunctiva, nasopharynx, vagina, and rectum of infants born to infected mothers.[238] Perinatally acquired rectal and vaginal chlamydial infection in infants can persist for 372 and 383 days, respectively. Persistent chlamydial infection of the pharynx in infants can persist for 2 years.[21]

Sexual abuse as a potential mode of transmission of C. trachomatis infection should be considered in children older than 1 year.[89,111] In a retrospective study, Ingram and associates[137] found that 6 percent of girls who allegedly were sexually abused and no girls who denied sexual abuse had C. trachomatis infection. Except for one child, all the children in the control group were determined later to have been sexually abused. In a prospective study, Ingram and associates[139,140] found C. trachomatis in 8 percent of girls with a history of sexual abuse compared with 0 percent in girls with no history of sexual abuse. In the former group, three girls also were found to have rectal infection and one to have pharyngeal infection.

Perinatally acquired genital chlamydial infection is a strong possibility in children younger than 1 year. Perinatal transmission is possible in children aged 3 years. After 1 year of age, however, sexual transmission should be considered diagnostic of sexual abuse in children with genital chlamydial infection.[42] An investigation for sexual abuse must be pursued in a child in whom genital chlamydial infection is diagnosed.[42,107] Studies have evaluated the presence of C. trachomatis on fomites and its coexistence in family members of infected children.

SYPHILIS

The prevalence of syphilis in children suspected of having been sexually abused is lower than that of gonorrhea or chlamydia. Syphilis infections not found to be acquired congenitally should be considered sexually transmitted. Sexually acquired infection is a strong possibility in all prepubertal children with syphilis. Syphilitic lesions and positive serologic results have been detected in alleged sexual abusers of children with syphilis.[1] No data are available on the survival of T. pallidum on fomites. The presence of syphilis should be considered diagnostic of sexual abuse, and an investigation must be pursued.

TRICHOMONAS VAGINALIS INFECTION

T. vaginalis has been found in the nasopharynx and vagina of newborns of infected mothers. Transmission of T. vaginalis in infants aged 1 year probably is perinatal. The mode of transmission in children older than 1 year is controversial. Two cases of T. vaginalis infection in premenarcheal girls who were sexually abused have been reported.[143] Prevalence studies either do not address the mode of transmission at all or, if they do, do not address the possibility of sexual abuse. In addition, a vaginal wet mount for trichomonads is not performed routinely in children assessed for possible sexual abuse. A survey from Poland found one case of T. vaginalis infection in children aged 2 to 7 years and a significantly higher number of cases in 8- to 10-year-old girls. The numbers increased even further for children older than 10 years, suggesting a strong association between T. vaginalis and the presence of an estrogenic environment, which promotes glycogen production and decreases vaginal pH.[159]

The Polish survey tested families of women infected with T. vaginalis and found that almost a third of their sexual partners and 8 percent of the children (mostly girls) had T. vaginalis. When families of men infected with T. vaginalis were tested, 91 percent of their sexual partners and 13 percent of the children had T. vaginalis. When families of children (mostly girls) infected with T. vaginalis were tested, 72 percent of the mothers and 43 percent of the fathers had the infection. The investigators considered that the infection in the latter group originated from mothers and that the primary mode of transmission was nonsexual (beds, sponges, towels, overcrowding). Information regarding sharing of potentially infected fomites, sexual abuse, or physically intimate behavior between parents and children was not gathered in these cases.[159]

Although T. vaginalis has been known to survive on fomites in controlled experiments, its ability to spread by these means is unknown. No cases of adults being infected by fomites have been documented. T. vaginalis has been found to survive for 6 hours on droplets of discharge and enameled surfaces of wood blocks.[149] It has been isolated from droplets of water splashed from toilets containing the urine of an infected individual.[39] T. vaginalis also has been found to survive in mud baths, bathing waters, and warm mineral waters and on moist bathing implements.[159,196] In rural India, a survey found that young girls who bathed in tanks or rivers had a significantly higher risk of acquiring T. vaginalis than did girls who used pipe or well water.[46]

T. vaginalis conceivably is transmitted to children nonsexually. The likelihood of perinatal transmission is high in infants younger than 1 year. A child or an infant younger than 1 year with T. vaginalis also may have been sexually abused. In a child older than 1 year, the probability of sexual abuse must be considered highly suspicious, and the case must be investigated and reported. Perinatal transmission and transmission of infection through fomites should not be assumed without an investigation for sexual abuse.[42]

BACTERIAL VAGINOSIS

The significance of bacterial vaginosis and G. vaginalis and their relationship to sexual abuse in prepubertal girls are unclear and inconclusive. Data on the prevalence of bacterial vaginosis in children with vaginal discharge and suspected sexual abuse are limited. Based on the presence of clue cells and a positive amine test result in vaginal secretions, bacterial vaginosis has been diagnosed in 13 percent of sexually abused children versus 4 percent of girls who denied sexual abuse.[110,139] Similar prevalence rates for G. vaginalis have been reported in children who have and have not been sexually abused.[21] No data are available regarding the survival of G. vaginalis on fomites.

Although the prevalence of G. vaginalis and bacterial vaginosis is higher in sexually abused children than in nonabused children, their significance as a marker for sexual abuse is unclear. G. vaginalis is not the sole cause of bacterial vaginosis and is not a suitable marker of sexual activity. The recommendation is that a child with a vaginal discharge, the presence of clue cells, and a positive amine test be questioned about sexual abuse and be followed medically. An investigation by a children's protective service agency is unnecessary, however.[42]

GENITAL HERPES

Perinatal transmission of herpes simplex virus (HSV) types 1 and 2 in the form of stomatitis occurs in infants. HSV type 2 is an uncommon finding. HSV types 1 and 2 have been isolated in the genital area in children alleging sexual abuse.[94,139] No studies have reported the coexistence of HSV genital infection in household members and infected children, however. Physical contact by a mother's infected finger has been reported.[146] Autoinoculation from the mouth to the genitals as a mode of transmission is possible, especially when oral HSV infection precedes genital herpes lesions.[191] HSV has been known to survive for 2 hours on latex gloves and toilet seats, 24 hours on a speculum, and 72 hours on gauze.[167] Transmission of HSV from fomites requires direct contact of viable virus with either a mucous membrane or a break in the skin, however, rendering fomite transmission unlikely. A child with genital herpes infection should be considered suspicious and evaluated for sexual abuse, and the case should be reported to the authorities.[42]

GENITAL WARTS (CONDYLOMATA ACUMINATA)

Perinatal transmission of human papillomavirus (HPV) from an infected mother to her infant is well-documented. The incubation period after exposure to the virus may range from 1 to 20 months.[57] Data on the presence of HPV DNA in children beyond the neonatal period are inconsistent—1.2 to 27 percent in three different studies.[166,219,282] In addition, the relationship between the presence of HPV DNA and the ultimate development of disease in children is unclear. Because the exact incubation period for the development of genital lesions is unknown, perinatal transmission has been found to be the most likely cause of genital warts in almost 96 percent of patients younger than 3 years.[57] In children 3 years or older, a history of sexual abuse has been elicited in 27 to 90 percent with venereal warts.[47,123]

Condylomata acuminata are acquired by children as a result of close physical contact with an infected individual, by digital infection of the child's genitalia by an infected individual, or by sexual contact with an infected individual.[246] A history of condylomata in other members of the family, particularly the mother or older sisters who care for the child, sometimes may be elicited. Perinatal exposure, poor hygiene, and shared bathing have been suggested sources of infection.[267,268] HPV types 6, 11, 16, and 18 are seen in adults with anogenital warts and are the most common genital types detected in children. This finding has raised questions about warts in children resulting from sexual abuse. In many cases, however, the mode of transmission is unknown.[57] Based on failure to identify sexual abuse, a report from a dermatology clinic concluded that transmission of HPV possibly occurs by fomites.[47] No reports in the literature address survival of the virus on fomites.

Sexual abuse is the most common means of acquiring anogenital HPV infection and should be considered suspicious for sexual abuse and investigated and reported in all prepubertal children older than 3 years who are infected. In children younger than 3 years, although perinatal transmission is likely, sexual abuse should be suspected and investigated.[42]

As recommended by the Centers for Disease Control and Prevention,[42] the possibility of sexual abuse should be considered strongly if no conclusive explanation for nonsexual transmission of a sexually transmitted infection has been identified. When the only evidence of sexual abuse is the isolation of an organism or the detection of antibodies to a sexually transmitted agent, findings should be confirmed, and implications should be considered carefully.

POSTMENARCHEAL LOWER GENITAL TRACT INFECTIONS

Infections of the postmenarcheal female clitoris, urinary tract, vulva, vagina, and cervix produce a variety of overlapping symptoms, including vulvar pruritus, dysuria, and increased or altered vaginal discharge and spotting.[87,175] As a result, distinguishing among various lower genital tract infections based solely on symptoms is difficult. The history, physical examination, and laboratory tests play an important role in assisting the clinician in diagnosing urethritis, vaginitis, or cervicitis.

DISORDERS OF THE CLITORIS

Cellulitis with induration, edema, and erythema, analogous to posthitis in boys, occasionally develops in the clitoral hood. Staphylococci and streptococci are the most common etiologies. Oral antibiotics with efficacy against these organisms usually are effective. Warm soaks or sitz baths also may provide symptomatic relief.[72]

Clitorimegaly with erythema can occur with vulvovaginitis of any etiology but usually is associated with HSV infections.[67] Edematous enlargement of the clitoris and the labia without erythema has been reported in patients with Crohn disease.[188]

POSTMENARCHEAL URETHRITIS

Urethritis is manifested clinically by dysuria or urinary urgency or both. Attempting to differentiate external from internal dysuria is important. External dysuria is pain from urine flowing over the vulva. Such a history suggests vulvitis and vaginitis. Internal dysuria is pain with initiation of urination and is not associated with urine flowing over the vulva. It indicates urethritis or a urinary tract infection. A careful history and examination assist the physician in differentiating urethritis from vaginitis.

Urethritis occurs commonly, particularly in sexually active postmenarcheal girls. Urethritis with internal dysuria can occur as a result of sexually transmitted infections, such as *T. vaginalis*, *N. gonorrhoeae*, and *C. trachomatis*, and has been implicated as an important cause of dysuria in sexually active girls. It is called *acute urethral syndrome*, and clinical features include dysuria, frequency, and pyuria with significant bacteriuria.[264] Urethral infection by *C. trachomatis* may occur with or without cervical infection; such infection was associated with sterile pyuria in 50 percent of girls with acute-onset dysuria and frequency, and *C. trachomatis* was isolated in 31 percent of these cases.[264]

When a sexually active adolescent girl has internal dysuria, in addition to being tested for conventional uropathogens, she should be screened for common STDs, such as gonorrhea and *Chlamydia* and *Trichomonas* infection.[61] Urinalysis and microscopy for the presence of leukocytes and bacteria should be done in these patients as well. For treatment of urethritis caused by sexually transmitted organisms, the sections in this chapter on trichomoniasis, gonorrhea, and chlamydial infections should be reviewed.

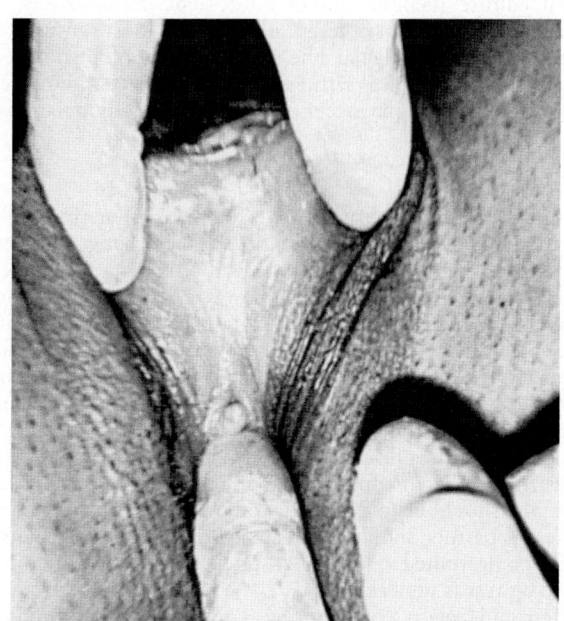

Figure 48–10 Urethral and paraurethral duct discharge is obtained by placing downward and outward digital pressure on the distal urethrovaginal septum.

PARAURETHRAL DUCT ABSCESS, BARTHOLINITIS, AND BARTHOLIN ABSCESS

The paraurethral ducts lie on each side of the urethral meatus. The Bartholin glands are small, bean-shaped glands that lie on each side of the vaginal opening, behind the hymen. Each gland opens by means of a long single duct immediately external to the hymen. Infections of the paraurethral and Bartholin ducts are found more commonly in women but occasionally occur in adolescent girls.

A paraurethral duct abscess creates a small, exquisitely painful swelling in the urethrovaginal septum. If the abscess is not incised and drained, it may rupture into the urethra and create a urethral diverticulum. Discharge for Gram stain should be obtained from the urethral lumen and the paraurethral ducts by downward and outward pressure on the urethrovaginal septum (Fig. 48–10).

Bartholinitis, or inflammation of the Bartholin ducts, causes pain, tenderness, and a linear rope-shaped swelling, best palpated by holding the vulvar mucosa and labia majora between the fingers. Purulent or mucoid exudate can be expressed occasionally from the Bartholin duct.

N. gonorrhoeae and *C. trachomatis* have been isolated from ductal exudates in women with bartholinitis.[56,223] This condition should be treated with antibiotics that provide coverage for *N. gonorrhoeae*, *C. trachomatis*, and anaerobes. Symptomatic relief may be achieved with sitz baths.

Although a Bartholin abscess is seen most often in women 20 to 29 years old, it does occur in sexually active adolescent girls. It also is the second most common urogenital complication of gonorrhea, after PID, in women. Risk factors for development of Bartholin abscess are similar to those for STDs.[4]

Infection of a Bartholin cyst results in a markedly tender abscess (Fig. 48–11). The abscess can rupture spontaneously and drain foul-smelling, purulent material externally through the skin. Multiple organisms are isolated from Bartholin abscesses. An early study using percutaneous aspirates from abscesses showed predominantly anaerobes and facultative organisms. *N. gonorrhoeae* was isolated in 8 percent of cases, and gram-negative

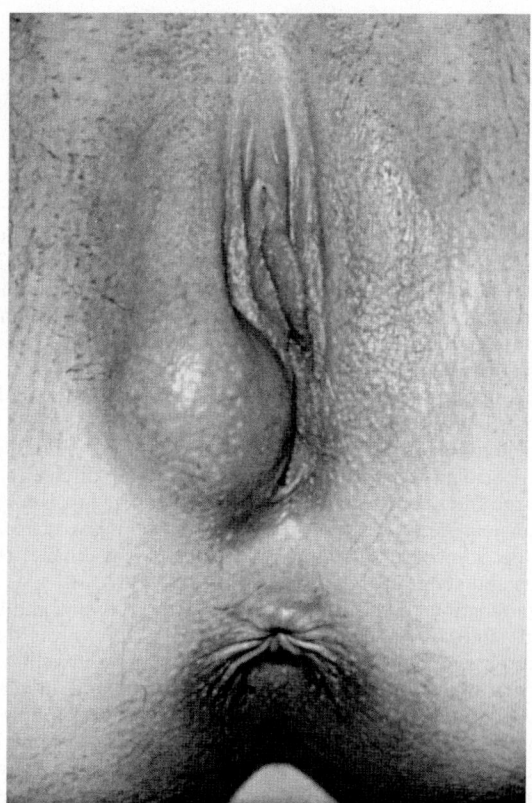

Figure 48–11 Acute Bartholin duct abscess.

bacilli were isolated in 16 percent. Although genital Mycoplasmataceae organisms were isolated from the duct secretions, they were not isolated directly from abscesses.[168] *Porphyromonas asaccharolytica* (a black-pigmented, gram-negative anaerobe) and *Salmonella panama* (after an attack of *Salmonella* enteritis) have been isolated from a Bartholin abscess.[52,68] Tuberculosis of the Bartholin gland has been reported.[63,133,134] Huffman[133] encountered tuberculosis of the Bartholin gland in a 14-year-old, sexually inactive girl with pulmonary tuberculosis. She had painless, unilateral swelling of the left labium majus with a brown discharge exuding from a small sinus. *Mycobacterium tuberculosis* was isolated in the discharge.

A Bartholin abscess should be incised and drained by applying a surface anesthetic, ethyl chloride, and making a 1- to 1.5-cm, full-thickness incision on the medial aspect of the labium majus. The cavity should be probed with a sterile cotton-tipped swab to break up loculations within the abscess. To allow for further drainage, one should pack the abscess cavity with sterile gauze. Alternatively, a Word catheter, a small rubber catheter with an inflatable balloon tip, can be inserted into the cavity and the balloon inflated with water. Clinical experience indicates that the packing method is far more painful to the patient, and healing takes longer.

Antibiotic coverage for anaerobes, *N. gonorrhoeae*, and *C. trachomatis* should be provided for at least 2 weeks, and a nonsteroidal medication is recommended for inflammation and pain. Frequent sitz baths help further with drainage and healing. Close follow-up during the first week is advised. The packing or the catheter may be removed after 4 days of antibiotics. Although marsupialization frequently was used to treat recurrent Bartholin abscesses, incision plus drainage and primary suture of the abscess cavity along with administration of an antibiotic (clindamycin) has been found to lead to more rapid healing and to decrease significantly the incidence of recurrent abscesses.[13]

POSTMENARCHEAL VULVOVAGINITIS

The most common types of vulvovaginitis in postmenarcheal girls are *T. vaginalis* vaginitis, vulvovaginal candidiasis, and bacterial vaginosis.

Postmenarcheal Vaginal Trichomoniasis

T. vaginalis is a triflagellated protozoan (Fig. 48–12). The organism, which is larger than a polymorphonuclear leukocyte, has a distinctive vibrating or whiplike movement when seen microscopically in fresh wet smears taken from the vagina. It quickly succumbs to reduction of the pH, drying, cooling, and changing the osmotic pressure of the fluid surrounding it. Most infections are encountered in sexually active young women; the incidence increases during the early reproductive years.

Trichomoniasis frequently is asymptomatic. When it is symptomatic, patients complain of a profuse, irritating discharge. The discharge and the pruritus tend to be more severe just before and immediately after a menstrual period. Recurrent exacerbations of the infection occur commonly. Patients occasionally report dysuria and abdominal pain.

Examination reveals diffuse vulvitis with erythema and excoriations and copious leukorrhea that covers the vulvar tissues. The discharge typically is frothy or bubbly, grayish yellow, and watery or mucopurulent. It has a pH of 5 to 7 and an acrid or musty odor. A "strawberry" or punctate vaginal eruption with hemorrhagic spots has been described as being typical of trichomoniasis. Such eruptions frequently are not present, however, even in severe cases. More often, diffuse inflammation causes the vaginal mucosa to be brilliant red.

The diagnosis of trichomoniasis usually is confirmed clinically by finding trichomonads in a wet smear of vaginal fluid. The vaginal specimen is obtained on a cotton-tipped swab and dipped into a small test tube with saline. After the solution has been stirred with the swab, one or two drops of the solution are placed with the swab on a slide. It is important that the slide be viewed under the microscope (dry high power) promptly because the organisms do not remain viable for long outside the vagina and are difficult to detect when they cease to be motile. The observer sees numerous ovoid-shaped, motile organisms. The sensitivity of this test with immediate evaluation is 60 to 70 percent. A vaginal cytosmear including a Papanicolaou (Pap) smear to detect trichomoniasis is not recommended because of the high rate of error in identifying trichomonads in stained smears. Other methods used to diagnose trichomoniasis include isolation by

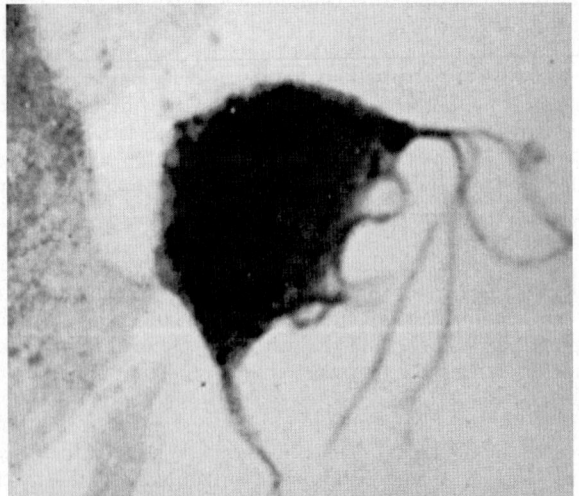

Figure 48–12 *Trichomonas vaginalis* is a triflagellated protozoan that, when motile, is identified easily in wet smears of vaginal discharge.

special culture medium, direct fluorescent immunoassay, and nucleic acid amplification test. Culture is the most sensitive, but it is not routinely available. The nucleic acid amplification test is available in some clinical settings (point-of-care test); however, a false-positive result may occur in low-prevalence populations.[42]

TREATMENT

A single 2-g oral dose of metronidazole (Flagyl) or tinidazole is the recommended treatment of choice. An alternative regimen is metronidazole, 500 mg orally twice daily for 7 days.[42] The cure rate is 95 percent in girls. If symptoms persist and wet smears from the vagina still show trichomonads, the treatment is repeated. Only in unusually persistent cases is a third course necessary. Strains resistant to metronidazole are rare. The patient should be warned of possible gastrointestinal side effects (nausea, diarrhea). Alcohol can aggravate the side effects of metronidazole therapy and cause a disulfiram-like reaction. The patient should be instructed not to consume alcoholic beverages during treatment. She should be told that trichomoniasis is an STD and that her sexual partner should be treated. Reacquisition of infection should be prevented via sexual abstinence or use of condoms. A follow-up test is unnecessary.

Metronidazole is a pregnancy category B drug, and tinidazole is a pregnancy category C drug; its safety in pregnant females has not been well evaluated. Multiple studies and data analysis subsequently have not shown a consistent association between metronidazole and teratogenic or mutagenic effects in infants.[42] Metronidazole can be given during the first trimester of pregnancy in adolescents.[42] Gentle vaginal douching with vinegar and water may relieve some symptoms but should not be encouraged during pregnancy.[134] Metronidazole gel is less effective in the treatment of trichomoniasis (<50%) and should not be used.[42] During lactation, breast-feeding can be withheld for 12 to 24 hours to reduce the exposure of metronidazole to the infant. Lactation should be withheld for 3 days when using tinidazole.

Postmenarcheal Mycotic Vulvovaginitis

Several factors play roles in causing the increased incidence of vaginal candidiasis after menarche. Menstruation, by altering vaginal pH, may offer a favorable medium for the growth of mycotic organisms. *Candida* spp. are found commonly in the intestinal tract and frequently are detected in stool cultures. Fecal contamination of the vulva during cleansing after defecation at a time when the normal vulvar and vaginal flora are depleted and not able to inhibit fungal growth would permit the development of symptomatic vulvovaginal candidiasis. Wearing tight-fitting underclothes (which keep the perineum warm and moist) is a factor that contributes to the growth of mycotic organisms. Female athletes and ballet dancers seem to be predisposed to development of candidiasis from wearing tight-fitting clothing and from increased sweating. The widespread use of antibiotics that disturb the vaginal flora and the use of oral contraceptives are additional factors that increase the incidence of candidal infection. Other predisposing factors include pregnancy, obesity, uncontrolled diabetes mellitus, immunosuppressive therapy, and heroin or other drug addiction. If a patient has a recurrent unexplainable or resistant infection, a glucose tolerance test should be done to rule out diabetes mellitus.

C. albicans and *Torulopsis glabrata* are the yeastlike fungi found most often in the vagina. *C. albicans* is responsible for 80 to 95 percent and *T. glabrata* for 3 to 16 percent of fungal infections. Other *Candida* spp. are detected less often in the vagina but can be pathogenic. *C. tropicalis*, similar to *C. albicans*, produces systemic infection in immunosuppressed hosts. Mycotic vulvovaginitis causes severe vulvar and vaginal itching; usually, the patient does not have an excessive discharge. The discharge is white, thick, and curdled and has a yeasty sour odor. The patient may have pain during and after voiding or external dysuria as a result of urine coming in contact with excoriated areas on the urethra and vulva.

Examination in the acute stage reveals intense inflammation of the vulva and vagina that may extend to the perineal skin. Long-standing infection can cause lichenification and hyperpigmentation of the perineal skin. During acute infection, the involved areas are shiny and beefy red with linear excoriations and edema. *C. albicans* typically forms patches of mycelia that create adherent white plaques scattered over the inflamed surfaces. Superficial, red, weeping areas remain after the plaques are pulled away. Other *Candida* spp., notably *C. tropicalis*, do not form adherent plaques but produce a cottage cheese–like discharge similar to that found with *C. albicans*. Vaginal pH usually is normal (<4.5).

The diagnosis is established by wet preparation under microscopy and by finding hyphae and buds of the fungus in vaginal fluid (see Fig. 48–9), in the curdled discharge, in material scraped from the vulvar mucosa, or on the perineal skin. A wet preparation in normal saline may suffice, but debris and cellular material may render identifying the fungus difficult. If so, a smear using 10 percent potassium hydroxide solution is helpful. After one drop of potassium hydroxide has been added to one to two drops of vaginal fluid on a slide, the slide is heated gently until bubbles appear under the coverslip. The potassium hydroxide solution dissolves other extraneous material without affecting the fungus. With an experienced microscopist, this method yields a sensitivity of 86 percent in symptomatic girls; however, the yield may be only 40 percent. The diagnosis frequently is based on clinical findings, and cultural confirmation is unnecessary.

TREATMENT

Several vaginal preparations can be used. The antifungal creams commonly used are imidazoles (clotrimazole and miconazole) and polyenes (nystatin), but the polyenes should not be used because of increasing resistance of fungi to these compounds. A variety of imidazoles are available as over-the-counter vaginal creams, tablets, and coated tampons. Such agents include clotrimazole, miconazole, and terconazole. Intravaginal treatment with one 100-mg vaginal tablet of clotrimazole every night for 7 days produces a cure rate of 90 percent. Comparable cure rates are observed with 100 to 200 mg of clotrimazole or miconazole (2 tablets) for 3 days. The shorter regimen may result in better compliance. Creams and tablets are equally effective.[42]

Oral fluconazole, 150 mg as a single dose, is an effective preparation for the treatment of uncomplicated vulvovaginal candidiasis.[42] Low-dose prophylactic treatment also may be appropriate in these cases. Gentian violet, which has been used for many years, is considered an effective cheap treatment for vulvovaginal candidiasis in countries where the recommended pharmaceutical agents are unavailable.[133] Huffman[133] described painting the cervix and the vaginal and vulvar mucosa with a 1 percent aqueous solution. Care is taken to rotate the speculum so that the anterior and posterior vaginal walls are treated. The creases between the folds of the vulvar mucosa also are covered with the dye. The speculum is reinserted, opened, and left in place for 5 minutes so that all painted surfaces become dry. Treatment with gentian violet is repeated once weekly for 3 weeks and should include one treatment during a menstrual period. According to Huffman, gentian violet can cause herpes-like lesions on the vulva of some patients, and it is extremely messy.

Postmenarcheal Bacterial Vaginosis

Bacterial vaginosis is a noninflammatory polymicrobial condition caused by an ecologic change in the vagina; an overgrowth of anaerobes, especially *Bacteroides* and *Mobiluncus* spp., *G. vaginalis*, and *M. hominis*; and a decrease in the concentration of lactobacilli.[12,90,91,92,207] Bacterial vaginosis is considered an STD based on the occurrence of bacterial vaginosis with other STDs and in male partners of women with this condition. Bacterial vaginosis also has been described in adolescent girls who are not sexually active.[38]

Bacterial vaginosis has been associated with vaginal douching. It also has been noted in connection with postpartum endometritis, premature rupture of membranes, and PID.[131]

The primary complaint is an offensive odor with moderately profuse, gray-colored leukorrhea that stains the underwear. A mild pruritus or dyspareunia may be reported. A clinician often is able to identify this condition simply by the odor of the discharge. Examination shows little or no vulvar or vaginal erythema. The urethral and vulvar glands are not involved. The vagina contains a thick, homogeneous, grayish white discharge. The pH of vaginal secretions in bacterial vaginosis is 5 to 6. *T. vaginalis* tends to be associated with a vaginal pH of 6 to 8.

The diagnosis is made by the presence of any three of the following four criteria: (1) a homogeneous, gray-white malodorous discharge that smoothly coats the vaginal walls[73]; (2) a pH of nonbloody vaginal secretions greater than 4.5; (3) a fishy odor caused by the release of amines when 10 percent potassium hydroxide is added to a nonbloody vaginal specimen (whiff test); and (4) the presence of clue cells in a nonbloody specimen.[12] Microscopic examination of some of the discharge mixed with normal saline solution in a wet-mount preparation shows masses of desquamated vaginal epithelial cells and cellular debris. Clusters of bacteria adhere to the surface of many of the vaginal cells; these "clue cells" (Fig. 48–13) are characteristic of the condition.

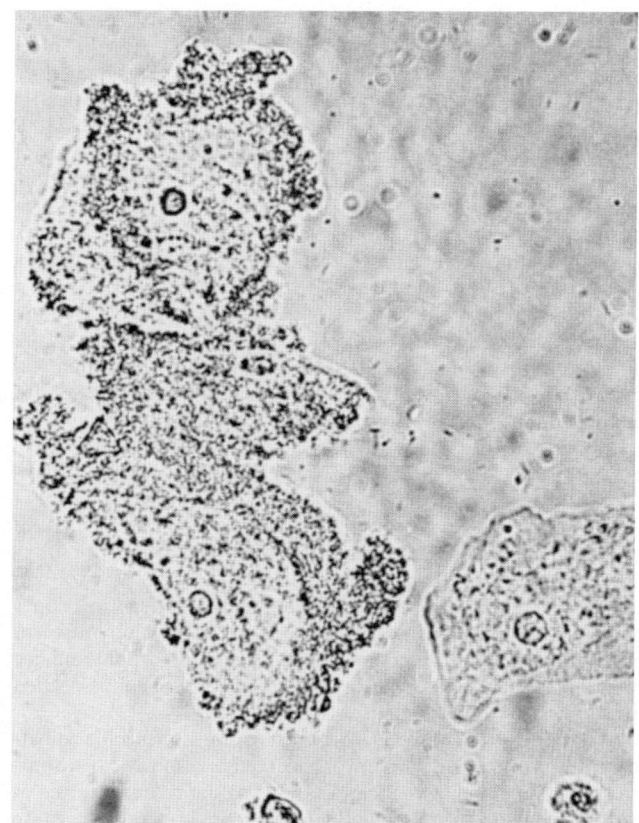

Figure 48–13 The finding of bacteria clinging to the sides of a vaginal epithelial cell ("clue cell") is significant in bacterial vaginosis. (*Courtesy of Dr. Herman L. Gardner.*)

Absence of erythrocytes and leukocytes in the discharge is another characteristic finding.

A Gram stain of vaginal secretions is considered the most reliable diagnostic test for bacterial vaginosis. A predominance of gram-variable cocci and curved rods (anaerobes) and occasional long gram-positive rods (lactobacilli) is seen.[12] A wet mount of vaginal secretions is a rapid and helpful test for clue cells in a busy clinical setting. Cultures for *G. vaginalis* and anaerobes are not useful clinically and are not recommended; Pap tests have no clinical utility for the diagnosis of bacterial vaginosis.

TREATMENT

The goal of therapy for symptomatic bacterial vaginosis is to relieve vaginal symptoms and prevent an ecologic environment that predisposes to the development of PID. Treatment of asymptomatic bacterial vaginosis may be considered before performing a surgical abortion procedure to prevent postpartum PID. In most cases, bacterial vaginosis responds to metronidazole, 500 mg given orally twice daily for 7 days,[42] or 2 percent clindamycin cream intravaginally every night for 7 days or 0.75 percent metronidazole gel intravaginally once a day for 5 days. Alternative regimens include clindamycin, 800 mg orally twice a day for 7 days, or clindamycin ovules, 100 mg intravaginally once a day for 3 days. These regimens provide effective coverage of anaerobes and *G. vaginalis*. Bacterial vaginosis that occurs during pregnancy generally is treated during the first trimester with clindamycin cream. During the second and third trimesters of pregnancy, it can be treated with clindamycin cream or metronidazole gel. Treatment of the sexual partner has not proved to be beneficial.[42]

Postmenarcheal Nonspecific Vulvovaginitis

Nonspecific vulvovaginitis has several contributory factors.[73,133] Vaginal foreign bodies cause discharges that are profuse, extremely malodorous, and sometimes bloody. The most frequent offender is a forgotten menstrual tampon, toilet paper, or a piece of condom. Improper or inadequate cleansing of the perineum after defecation also is responsible for many cases of chronic nonspecific vulvovaginitis, especially in mentally handicapped adolescent girls. If a male partner inserts his penis into the rectum first and then into the vagina or inadvertently touches the anal area before having vaginal intercourse, coliform organisms are carried into the vagina.

A tumor as the cause of a vaginal discharge is a very rare possibility. A discharge, with or without bleeding, may be one of the first symptoms of adenosis or adenocarcinoma of the vagina and cervix. These neoplasms are associated with prenatal exposure to diethylstilbestrol and related synthetic estrogens.

TREATMENT

Treating nonspecific vulvovaginitis in a postmenarcheal girl can be frustrating when no causative agent is found. Often, identifying the causative agent is impossible. In the case of a foreign body, it should be removed. Instructing the patient in proper perineal cleansing after defecation eradicates a major source of nonspecific vaginal infection in teenagers. Providing advice regarding sexual habits is necessary in some cases if coitus-related infections are to be avoided.

According to Huffman,[133] in most cases, nonspecific vulvovaginitis unassociated with chronic cervicitis responds to antimicrobial creams such as Sultrin or AVC vaginal cream inserted at bedtime for 14 days. Generally, creams are preferable because they spread over a larger area of the vaginal mucosa than is treatable with suppositories. Vaginal douching sometimes may be considered helpful in the treatment of nonspecific vulvovaginitis.

More recent data suggest, however, that a causative relationship exists between vaginal douching and PID in inner-city populations at high risk for acquiring STDs.[291] Vaginal douching should be discouraged strongly.

Toxic Shock Syndrome

First recognized in the late 1970s, TSS is an uncommon, serious, sometimes fatal acute infection caused by toxin-producing *S. aureus* infection. TSS can occur in males and females of all ages; this entity is discussed fully in Chapter 71. With regard to the genital tract, more than 800 TSS cases occurred in women in 1980 in association with use of a very high absorbency tampon. This type of tampon is no longer marketed. Prolonged retention of currently marketed tampons could be a predisposing factor for TSS or other local infections, but TSS associated with tampon use is now a rare event.

VULVOVAGINAL VIRAL INFECTIONS

GENITAL HERPES

Premenarcheal Patient

HSV infection of the genitalia rarely occurs in children.[116] The mode of acquisition of the infection is not always known, but case reports describe the possibility of autoinoculation from oral lesions, physical contact by a mother's infected finger, and sexual abuse.[146] The presence of genital herpes lesions in a child or any disease that is known to be sexually transmitted in an adult should raise a question about whether the child has been subjected to some type of sexual molestation. The virus can be isolated from the pharynx or vagina of approximately 5 percent of asymptomatic adults. Such individuals are carriers and may transmit the infection to susceptible contacts. That children would have either HSV type 1 or HSV type 2 genital lesions is not surprising.[191]

Herpetic lesions on the vulva begin as small, erythematous spots. Papules quickly develop on the inflamed areas. The papules become serum-filled vesicles that rupture and leave slightly eroded red areas. The latter become covered with crusts, which remain for a few days. The lesions typically cause pruritus and burning. If they do not become secondarily infected, they heal within 2 weeks.

Herpes limited to the genitalia of a healthy child is a painful but relatively benign disease. An infection in a poorly nourished child may spread beyond the vulva and become a serious, life-threatening matter. Treatment of genital herpes is discussed later.

Adolescent Patient

HSV is the most common cause of vesiculoulcerative disease of the adult genitalia.[190] It is sexually transmitted, and its increasing frequency in teenage girls is related to their sexual activity. As noted in Chapter 170, two types of HSV exist and can be antigenically and culturally distinguished from each other. Type 1 is the causative agent in oronasal cold sores. Type 2 is responsible for 70 to 95 percent of genital herpes, but genital infections with type 1 have become more common (5 to 30%), probably related to increasing engagement in genital-oral sex play.[45]

Seroprevalence studies show that type 2 antibodies do not begin to appear until the early teens. The frequency gradually increases through late adulthood and is related to sexual activity, especially with multiple partners. Most individuals with type 2 antibodies are not diagnosed with genital herpes. Type 2 infections are highly contagious and may be transmitted by carriers who are asymptomatic. Because of its frequency and diverse clinical appearance, it should be considered in the differential diagnosis of all vulvar vesiculoulcerative lesions. Because of its acute symptoms, it may mask the presence of other venereal disease acquired concurrently; a patient with genital herpes always should be examined for gonorrhea and syphilis.

Three manifestations of genital disease are recognized: primary initial, nonprimary initial, and recurrent infection. Primary initial genital herpes infection develops with no preexisting herpes antibody. A nonprimary initial infection develops in an individual for the first time with preexisting herpes antibody. Recurrent infection is diagnosed when an individual has a history of previous similar genital infection. Patients with nonprimary initial infection have fewer lesions, less pain, fewer constitutional symptoms, shorter duration of viral shedding, and an overall shorter course of illness.[48]

A primary infection begins with sexual contact with an infected individual 2 to 8 days before the onset of symptoms. The individual probably has a prodromal episode of fever, malaise, and myalgia, often accompanied by vulvar paresthesia and burning, dysuria, and tender nonsuppurative inguinal lymphadenopathy.

Primary lesions, which often involve all the vulvar tissues, the vaginal mucosa, and the cervix, occur during a 2-week period. They first appear as papules surrounded by an erythematous zone and subsequently become vesiculopustular lesions. The vesicles enlarge and rupture, and shallow ulcerations are exposed. During the acute phase of a severe infection, more or less edema and generalized erythema of the vulvar mucosa are present (Fig. 48–14).

The ulcers generally become covered with a firm yellow crust that drops off after a week or so, with a smooth, red area left behind that eventually disappears. The lesions usually are asymptomatic for 10 to 21 days, depending on the severity of the infection. Secondary bacterial infection and a coexisting immunodeficiency state, such as HIV infection, delay healing. Urethral and vesical involvement may cause severe dysuria leading to retention of urine. Proctitis may occur in adolescent

girls who engage in anal intercourse, although perianal ulcers also may occur without anal intercourse. The cervical lesions are ulcerations on the exocervix and may range from erythema to severe necrotic cervicitis. Acute cervicitis may be the only manifestation of primary HSV infection.

Inguinal lymphadenopathy and moderate lower abdominal pain may be present; if so, they usually occur only with the more severe first eruption. Tender inguinal lymphadenopathy is the last to resolve. If the urethra is involved, the dysuria may be sufficiently severe to cause urinary retention. Insertion of a vaginal speculum may be exquisitely painful. Extension to the perianal area may cause severe discomfort on defecation. Complete healing of lesions at all sites occurs in approximately 3 weeks. When healed, herpetic lesions rarely leave scars.

The diagnosis of genital herpes usually is not difficult to establish. The intense pain and the superficial vesiculoulcerative lesions with their irregular margins and red areolae are sufficiently characteristic to render clinical identification easy in a typical case. Laboratory confirmation should be attempted for all children and adolescents. Direct isolation of HSV by tissue culture is the preferred diagnostic method and is best when the specimen is taken from a lesion within the first 48 hours of the onset of symptoms. The virus can be cultured from the cervix in 90 percent of girls with primary type 2 infections, and the cervix appears abnormal in almost 90 percent of cases with positive cervical cultures. PCR assays for HSV DNA are more sensitive than is culture and are used in settings when available. PCR testing of genital secretions has not been approved by the U.S. Food and Drug Administration (FDA), however.[42]

Type-specific and non–type-specific antibodies to HSV develop during the first several weeks after infection occurs and persist indefinitely. Commonly available serologic tests cannot differentiate type 1 from type 2 virus. Type-specific antisera using glycoprotein G–based assays showing an increase in anti-HSV titer are useful in identifying primary type 2 infections. These tests have limited usefulness for recurrent infection, however. A variety of glycoprotein G–based assays (enzyme-linked immunosorbent assay) are available and have to be specifically requested. Point-of-care HSV tests using glycoprotein G also are available for immediate office-based testing and work best in settings with high prevalence of infection. False-positive results have been reported in individuals with low likelihood of infection.[42]

The presence of multinucleated giant cells in a Pap smear (Fig. 48–15) or in a herpetic fluid smear with a Tzanck preparation is only 40 to 50 percent sensitive compared with culture. These tests may be useful in settings where other diagnostic tests are unavailable but should not be relied on.[42]

For many weeks after the infection has subsided clinically and the patient seems to be cured, type 2 virus can be recovered from the cervix and vagina. The latent virus may infect others or cause recurrent infections in the host. Although the recurrence rate of genital herpes is unknown, recurrent episodes develop in 80 percent of patients with type 2 infection; clinical recurrence of type 1 genital infection is much less common.[48] Factors influencing recurrence rates are the severity of the initial episode and the host immune response to the disease. Emotional stress, heat, moisture, climate change, menstruation, pregnancy, oral contraceptive use, anesthesia, and trauma seem to be triggering factors. The median time from a primary infection to development of a secondary or recurrent infection is approximately 120 days.[48,256,284] Such recurrent episodes, although painful, usually are less severe than are primary infections. Some patients have recurrences immediately preceding or at the time of each menstrual period. Researchers have suggested that genital herpes and squamous cell carcinoma of the cervix are related.[36] Most of the evidence favoring this association originally came from seroepidemiologic studies. A much stronger association now has been observed

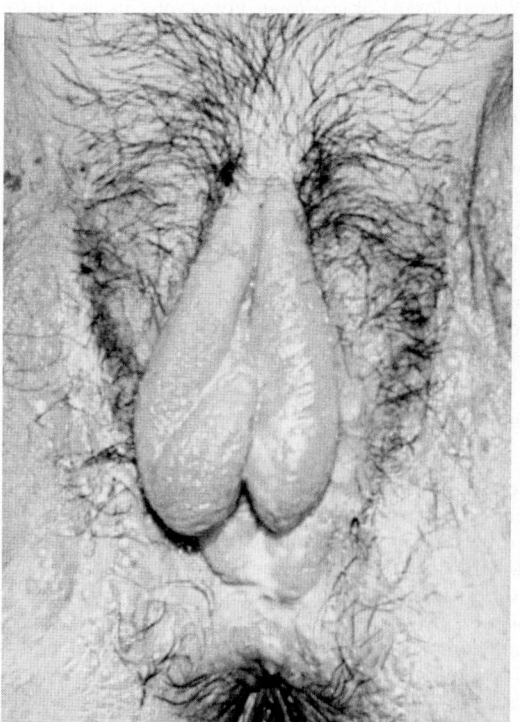

Figure 48–14 Genital herpes in an adolescent patient.

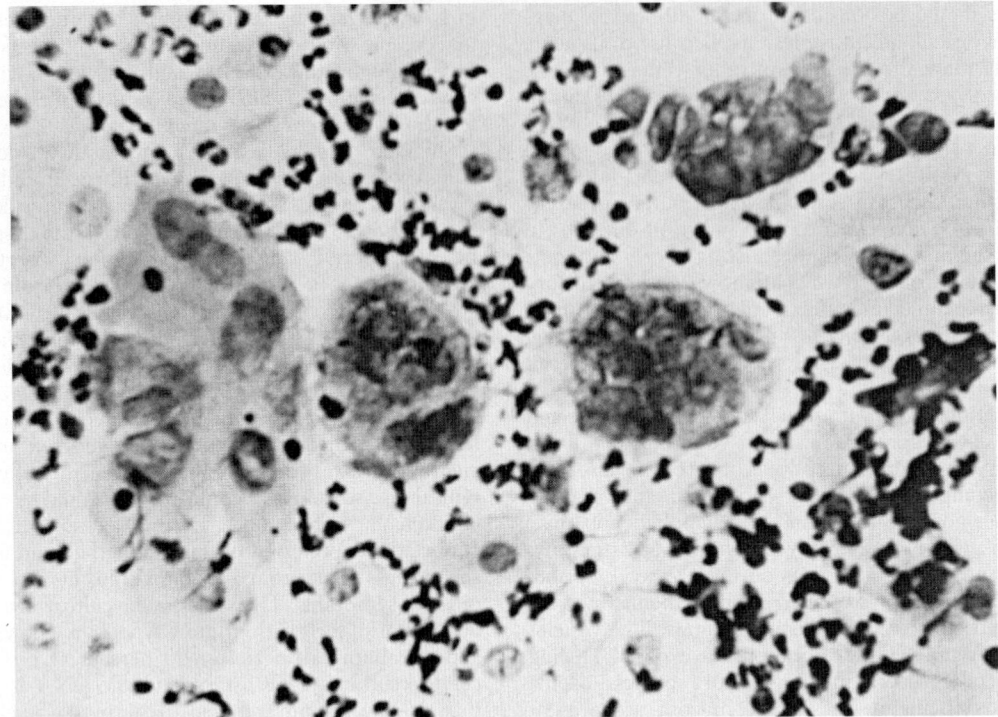

Figure 48–15 Multinucleated giant cells in a vaginal smear are characteristic of genital herpes. *(Courtesy of Dr. Herman L. Gardner.)*

between HPV and cervical cancer. At most, HSV may be causative or may be a cofactor in some cases of cervical cancer.[48]

Treatment

Several medications are available today for the treatment of genital herpes.[42] Acyclovir is the most affordable current drug on the market. For the treatment of initial genital herpes, acyclovir, one 400-mg capsule orally three times a day or one 200-mg capsule five times a day, is administered for 7 to 10 days until clinical resolution. Alternative drugs include famciclovir, one 250-mg capsule three times a day, or valacyclovir, one 1-g capsule twice a day for 7 to 10 days. These drugs are reported to shorten the time that the patient has pain, decrease the number of new lesions, hasten crusting, and reduce the time that the virus can be found in the lesions. The earlier treatment is started after the initial lesions appear, the sooner patients obtain relief.

In severe primary herpes infection with marked systemic symptoms, intravenous acyclovir, 5 to 10 mg/kg/day every 8 hours for 5 to 7 days or until clinical resolution occurs, is recommended. Frequent or severe recurrent disease may benefit from medication if it is started within 2 days of the onset of lesions or at the beginning of the prodrome. Oral acyclovir may be given at 800 mg twice a day, 400 mg three times a day for 5 days, or acyclovir 800 mg three times a day for 2 days. Alternatively, famciclovir, 125 mg twice a day, or valacyclovir, 500 mg twice a day for 3 days, or valacyclovir 1000 mg once a day for 5 days, may be prescribed. Daily suppressive treatment reduces recurrence by at least 75 percent in patients with frequent recurrences. Because of adherence problems, daily suppressive therapy may not be a practical treatment approach for adolescents. The recommended treatment is oral acyclovir, 400 mg twice a day; famciclovir, 250 mg twice a day; or valacyclovir, 500 or 1000 mg once a day for 1 year. Medication should be discontinued after 1 year to reassess the recurrence rate. The dosage regimen of medications for treating prepubertal genital herpes is unknown, and such medications are not used commonly in this age group for mild cases. In moderate to severe cases, clinicians have prescribed approximately 50 percent of the adult dose.[42]

Recurrences can be reduced in frequency in some cases if the patients can avoid stress-inducing situations. Topical anesthetics, cold wet compresses, and sitz baths with 1:40 Burow's solution frequently reduce local discomfort. Severe dysuria may be relieved by urinating when sitting in water. Local therapies used in the past, such as povidone-iodine solutions, photodynamic dye light therapy, and topical surfactant, have not been found to be beneficial and are messy and potentially toxic.

Lesions caused by HSV are common manifestations in patients with HIV infection. Immunocompromised patients benefit from an increased dosage of acyclovir. For severe disease, hospitalization may be required for intravenous acyclovir treatment.[42]

CONDYLOMATA ACUMINATA AND HUMAN PAPILLOMAVIRUS

Condylomata acuminata are encountered in premenarcheal and teenage girls. The agent causing them is HPV, a small, slow-growing virus of the papovavirus group. HPV types 6 and 11 are responsible for low-grade lesions and for 90 percent of genital warts. HPV types 16, 18, and 31 are associated with premalignant and malignant cervical carcinoma in women,[252] with HPV types 16 and 18 causing 70 percent of premalignant and malignant lesions.

Premenarcheal Patient

Warts in premenarcheal children may cover the entire vulva. Most often, however, warts in this population are single or scattered, cauliflower-like lesions (Fig. 48–16). They have a predilection for the smooth, moist mucosa covering the inner surfaces of the labia minora and for the mucosa around the urethral meatus. The vestibular mucosa may be studded with innumerable minute excrescences as well.

Condylomata in children seldom become ulcerative, but sessile condylomata arising within the vagina may become necrotic; produce a bloody vaginal discharge; and resemble, on cursory examination, a mixed mesodermal tumor (sarcoma botryoides) of the vagina. Although not tumors, condylomata acu-

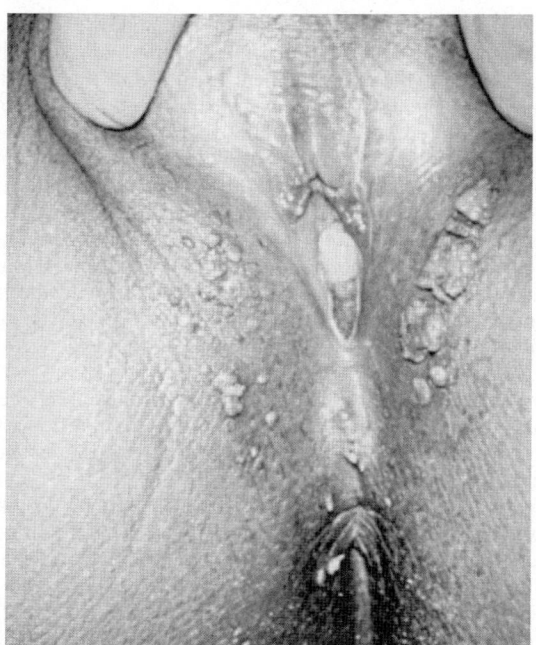

Figure 48–16 Condylomata acuminata usually are single or scattered, small warts in premenarcheal children.

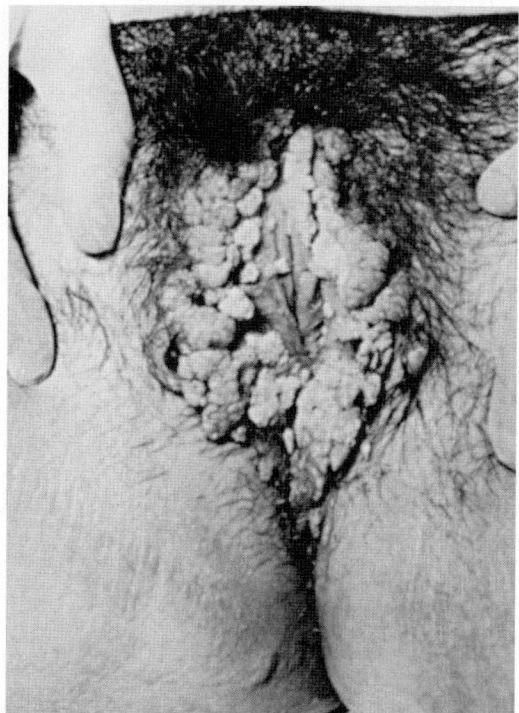

Figure 48–17 Condylomata acuminata may form large masses covering the vulva in postmenarcheal patients.

minata should be considered in the differential diagnosis of vaginal neoplasms. HIV infection should be considered in infants and children with severe, extensive warts.[47,57,100,252]

Adolescent Patient

Condylomata acuminata develop in adolescent girls by sexual transmission. The prevalence of HPV in adolescent girls and young women is 11 to 46 percent, depending on the method of HPV DNA detection used.[229,252] The PCR technique is more sensitive than is the dot-blot hybridization method (ViraPap; Life Technologies, Gaithersburg, MD). The prevalence of HPV in adolescents as detected by DNA isolation techniques is far higher than the prevalence of active disease. The cell-mediated or T-cell immune system seems to play an important role in whether the presence of virus results in clinically manifested disease. Cofactors of HPV infection are herpes, cervicitis, and tobacco use. Immunosuppression from a variety of conditions, including renal transplantation, Hodgkin disease, and HIV infection, is associated with a greater likelihood of development of HPV disease.[229] With regard to the natural history of HPV infection, Moscicki and colleagues[184,185] found that during the course of a 2-year period, 70 percent of cases showed regression, and low-grade squamous intraepithelial lesions (LSIL) did not develop. Daily cigarette smoking was strongly linked to the development of LSIL.[185] Regression was more likely to be seen in young women with LSIL as opposed to high-grade squamous intraepithelial lesions (HSIL). HSIL was more likely to develop in individuals with persistent positive tests showing oncogenic HPV types.

In postmenarcheal girls, condylomata usually form discrete, sessile, vegetative, wartlike growths covered with folded grayish pink epithelium. They are found most frequently on the smooth mucosa of the vulvar vestibule. Usually, they are accompanied by more or less vaginal discharge, which is increased by moisture that exudes from between the leaflike folds of the warty masses. Most often, associated pruritus and secondary infection are present. Warts are more likely to become necrotic in adults than in children. Contact lesions frequently appear on contiguous

surfaces. Huge condylomatous masses (Fig. 48–17) that completely hide the introitus are common findings in adolescent patients; if not treated, these huge growths may invade the rectum. Vaginal and cervical lesions commonly accompany the lesions on the vulva.

Treatment

The goal of treatment is removal of warts and amelioration of symptoms, not eradication of HPV. No therapy has been shown to eradicate HPV. When only a few lesions are present, they can be treated in the outpatient setting with 85 percent trichloracetic acid. In infants and children with extensive lesions, Emans and colleagues[74] recommend carbon dioxide laser treatment with general anesthesia. It may be performed in an outpatient surgical setting when few lesions are present. Electrocautery, electrocoagulation, or laser treatment may result in deep scarring and distortion of the vulva. Older children and adolescents usually tolerate cryotherapy without general anesthesia if they know that some tingling or burning sensation is associated with it. Liquid nitrogen may be used in the same manner as solid carbon dioxide.

The therapeutic methods available are 22 to 94 percent effective in clearing exophytic genital warts, but recurrence rates are high, at least 25 percent within 3 months. Treatment seems to be more successful for genital warts that are small and present for less than 1 year.[42] Self-application of medication may be considered in young adults but should be discouraged for adolescents because of the risk of causing dermatologic side effects. When a few lesions are present, they can be treated with 10 to 25 percent podophyllin resin or a solution of 85 percent trichloroacetic acid. The lesions that are treated should be less than 1 cm in diameter and should not be in a confluent mass. Four hours after podophyllin has been applied, the treated area should be washed off with soap and water. The medication is applied to the wart only (not to the surrounding skin), and treatment is

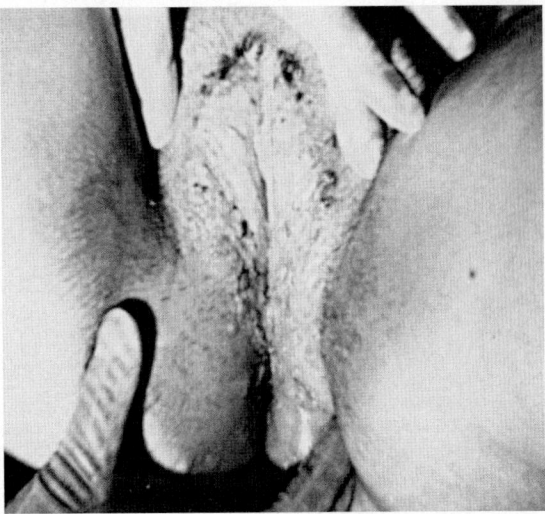

Figure 48–18 The appearance of the vulva 10 days after electrocoagulation and surgical excision of the condylomatous mass shown in Figure 48–17.

repeated once weekly until the lesions have disappeared (usually 3 to 4 weeks).

Urethral, anal, vaginal, and cervical lesions should not be treated with podophyllin. Podophyllin and trichloracetic acid can cause severe irritation of normal skin and can cause ulcerations. Before application, the normal skin around a wart should be covered with K-Y jelly, and a thin or narrow swab should be used for small warts. If excessive medication has been applied, the area should be washed immediately with soap and water, followed by the application of talcum powder or bicarbonate of soda to soothe the area. Imiquimod 5 percent cream also is recommended for the treatment of warts in patients older than 18 years.[41] This medication is self-applied to the lesions, three times a week for 16 weeks. There are reports in the international literature regarding the successful treatment of extensive warts in children using imiquimod 5 percent cream.[171] Laser treatment or cryocautery is recommended if the lesions do not respond to chemical cautery or if they progressively increase in size. Large perianal warts may need to be removed surgically if cryotherapy does not work (Fig. 48–18). Alternative treatments for adolescents are topical 5-fluorouracil in 5 percent creams and intralesional interferon. 5-Fluorouracil is preferable for vaginal and intraurethral warts because it causes erosive dermatitis of normal surrounding skin. The use of 5-fluorouracil seems to be more effective than is the laser in treating exophytic warts in the vagina.[42,57]

An annual Pap smear is recommended in all adolescent girls 3 years after the onset of sexual activity. In an adolescent girl who has not had sex, the first Pap smear is recommended at age 21 years.[294] The quadrivalent HPV vaccine contains HPV types 6, 11, 16, and 18 and has been approved by the FDA to prevent genital warts and cervical cancer. It is recommended that females 9 to 26 years old receive the vaccine at age 11 to 12 years during their routine immunization visit. Catch-up vaccination is recommended for females 13 to 26 years old who have not been vaccinated previously, regardless of their sexual history.[174] FDA approval for a bivalent HPV vaccine containing HPV types 16 and 18, to prevent cervical cancer for a broader age range of women, is in progress.

MOLLUSCUM CONTAGIOSUM

Molluscum contagiosum is a viral infection of the skin characterized by small, discrete, translucent, grayish pink, umbilicated,

wartlike papules that sometimes are surrounded by a narrow ring of erythema. The lesions, which are asymptomatic, usually are less than 5 mm in diameter and may be missed by the patient and the examiner. The disease is transmitted by close physical contact and is encountered most often in postmenarcheal patients on the inner surfaces of the thighs and perineum. Although lesions on the lower part of the abdomen and thighs have caused this infection to be classed with venereal diseases, coitus is not necessary for transmission. Pediatricians frequently encounter molluscum contagiosum on the nongenital skin of children. It can be contracted from contaminated towels, bedding, and garments. Lesions of molluscum contagiosum on the lower part of the abdomen, pubis, thighs, or perineum of a child are tacit evidence of sexual contact.[129,170]

The appearance of the lesions usually is sufficient to establish the diagnosis. It can be confirmed by finding large, intracytoplasmic inclusion bodies in a smear or biopsy specimen from a lesion.

Treatment consists of lifting off the roof of each lesion and lightly curetting its base. Cryotherapy and topical imiquimod also give good results.[129,170] A variety of treatment approaches are available for children and adolescents. Curettage is the most efficacious treatment, with a low rate of side effects; however, the procedure requires anesthesia and is time-consuming. The roof of each lesion is lifted off, and the base is lightly curetted. Cryotherapy gives good results. Cantharadin is another useful bloodless alternative, but it can cause blisters. Topical imiquimod holds promise, but an optimal treatment schedule has not been determined.[42]

VULVOVAGINAL GRANULOMATOUS AND ULCERATIVE DISORDERS

Sexually transmitted genital ulcerative diseases occur throughout the world but are found most frequently in tropical countries. Genital ulcers are a common finding on evaluation of adolescent and adult patients with genital symptoms. They are less common findings in young children. Ulcers usually are secondary lesions that result from the breakdown of vesicles, papules, or pustules. By the time that many patients with genital infections seek medical attention for their symptoms, the primary lesion has proceeded to ulceration.[254] Microbial causes vary by geographic region and socioeconomic status: HSV is the most common cause in Western Europe and North America, whereas chancroid is the most common one in the tropics; in the United States, syphilis and chancroid are more common occurrences in urban minority groups, whereas HSV is found more commonly in more affluent groups. Complications of sexually transmitted genital ulcerative diseases also occur more commonly in developing countries and often are the reason for seeking medical care.[187]

HSV infection, syphilis, chancroid, lymphogranuloma venereum, granuloma inguinale, and tuberculosis all may have genital ulcers as a major clinical finding (Table 48–4). Although each of these diseases has a characteristic lesion and course, considerable overlap exists, so a diagnosis based on the history and physical appearance alone often is inaccurate. Herpetic ulcers, contrary to classic manifestations, can be painless, and syphilis chancres can be painful at times. Secondary infection of an ulcerated area may cause pain in lesions that characteristically are painless. In addition, more than one STD may be present in at least 3 to 10 percent of patients with genital ulcers.

Genital ulcers also may result from infestation, fixed drug eruption, mechanical or chemical trauma, autoimmune processes (e.g., Behçet syndrome and Crohn disease), and neoplasia. The presence of ulcers in sites other than the genital regions or oropharynx suggests a noninfectious etiology.

TABLE 48–4   Diagnostic Features of Genital Ulcerations Caused by Sexually Transmitted Diseases

Feature	Primary Syphilis	Genital Herpes	Chancroid	Lymphogranuloma Venereum	Granuloma Inguinale
Incubation period	9-90 days; avg., 2-4 wk	2-7 days	1-35 days; avg., 3-7 days	3 days to 3 wk; avg., 10-14 days	Precise data unavailable; probably a few days to several months
No. lesions	Usually one; may be multiple	Multiple; may coalesce, more with primary episodes than with recurrences	Usually one to three, may be multiple	Usually single	Single or multiple
Description of genital ulcers	Sharply demarcated, round or oval ulcer with slightly elevated edges; may be irregular, symmetric "kissing chancre"	Small, superficial, grouped vesicles, erosions, or both; lesions may coalesce and form bullae or large areas of ulceration; lesions have irregular borders	Superficial, shallow, sharply demarcated ulcer; irregular, ragged, undermined edge; a few millimeters to 2 cm in diameter	Papule, pustule, vesicle, or ulcer discrete and transient; frequently overlooked	Sharply defined, irregular ulcerations or hypertrophic, verrucous, necrotic, or cicatricial granulomata
Base	Red, smooth, and shiny or crusty; oozing serous exudate when squeezed	Bright red and smooth	Rough, uneven, yellow to gray	Variable	Usually friable, rough, beefy granulations; can be necrotic, verrucous, or cicatricial
Induration	Firm; does not change shape with pressure	None	Soft; changes shape with pressure	None	Firm granulation tissue
Pain	Painless; may become tender if secondarily infected	Common; more prominent with initial infection than with recurrences	Common	Variable	Rare
Inguinal lymphadenopathy	Unilateral or bilateral, firm, movable, and nontender; does not suppurate	Usually bilateral, firm, and tender; more common in primary episodes than in recurrences	Unilateral; bilateral rarely occurs; overlying erythema; matted, fixed, and tender; suppuration may occur	Unilateral or bilateral; initially movable, firm, and tender; later indolent; fixed and matted; "sign of groove" may suppurate; fistulas	Pseudobuboes; subcutaneous perilymphatic granulomatous lesions that produce inguinal swellings
Constitutional symptoms	Rare	Common in primary episode; less likely in recurrences	Rare	Frequent	Rare
Course of untreated disease	Slowly (2-6 wk) resolves to latency	Recurrence is the rule	May progress to erosive lesions	Local lesions heal; systemic disease may progress; disfiguring; late complications	Worsens slowly
Diagnostic tests	Darkfield examination, direct immunofluorescence, FTA-ABS, VDRL	Tzanck smear, culture, Pap smear, direct immunofluorescence, electron microscopy, direct immunoperoxidase staining, serology	Culture, biopsy (rarely used), Gram-stained smears have low specificity	Complement fixation, isolation of microorganism by culture	"Donovan bodies" in tissue smears; biopsy

FTA-ABS, fluorescent treponemal antibody absorption test; VDRL, Venereal Disease Research Laboratory.
From Mroczkowski, T. R., and Martin, D. H.: Genital ulcer disease. Dermatol. Clin. North Am. 12:753-764, 1994.

In the United States, most patients with genital ulcers have genital herpes, syphilis, chancroid, or a combination thereof. Empiric treatment often must be given before diagnostic test results are available, and laboratory confirmation of a specific diagnosis is lacking in at least a quarter of patients with genital ulcer disease. Treatment of syphilis and chancroid should be considered in such circumstances, especially in geographic regions where chancroid morbidity is notable (see later).[41,203] Diagnosis and treatment of the listed infectious etiologies of genital ulcers and Behçet syndrome are discussed in this chapter and elsewhere in this text.

Genital ulcers of any etiology, but especially those caused by herpes, syphilis, chancroid, and granuloma inguinale, are associated with an increased risk of acquiring HIV infection. Serologic testing for HIV infection should be considered in the management of patients with genital ulcers.[41,188] Improved treatment of STDs can affect the rate of HIV seroconversion in a population: HIV seroconversion was reduced by 40 percent over the course of a 2-year follow-up period in rural communities in Tanzania where treatment programs were instituted compared with control communities with no programs.[103]

LYMPHOGRANULOMA VENEREUM

Lymphogranuloma venereum is an STD characterized by chronicity, indolent inflammatory infiltration, granulomatous ulceration, formation of abscesses, and fibrotic cicatrization of the inguinal, perineal, and rectal lymphatics. The infecting agent is *C. trachomatis*, subtypes L1 to L3. It occurs more often in tropical than temperate climates.

Premenarcheal Patient

Lymphogranuloma venereum has been reported in children.[17,98,285] The disease usually is acquired in childhood as a result of sexual contact, but transmission also may occur by accidental inoculation of infected material from family members, such as by handling of garments or towels that have been contaminated by drainage from ulcerative lesions or buboes. Sexual abuse always should be considered, however. Some evidence suggests that transplacental or perinatal transmission of the lymphogranuloma venereum serovars of *C. trachomatis* can occur.[98]

The primary lesion, a small papule or superficial and relatively asymptomatic ulcer, seldom is seen in either children or older patients. A prodromal episode of fever, malaise, and joint pain accompanied by leukocytosis, anemia, and an increased erythrocyte sedimentation rate may precede the local signs. These symptoms often are mild and not diagnostically significant.

The most common manifestations in prepubertal children are inguinal lymphadenopathy and proctitis. The glands may be swollen and tender for a while, and then regress spontaneously. More often, if treatment is not initiated, the lesions progress to formation of an abscess and then rupture, with the development of draining sinuses. Rectal, anal, and deep pelvic tissue infiltration with rectal and colonic strictures is an uncommon finding in children. Arthritis, usually of the knees, and erythema nodosum occasionally occur in children, as they do in older patients.[98]

Adolescent Patient

Adolescents usually acquire lymphogranuloma venereum through sexual activity. The primary lesion—a small papule, vesicle, or shallow ulcer on the vulva (Fig. 48–19), vaginal wall, or cervix—seldom is seen. Cervicitis is a more common finding in primary lymphogranuloma venereum, and the primary lesion often is asymptomatic, heals rapidly, and leaves no scar. The incubation period usually is 2 to 5 days after exposure, but several weeks may elapse before the primary lesion appears.[98,133]

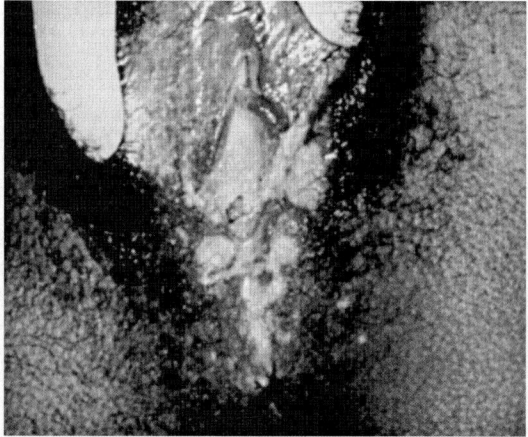

Figure 48–19 Early lesions of lymphogranuloma venereum in the form of herpetic-like ulcers in an adolescent. The diagnosis was confirmed serologically.

Painful enlargement of the inguinal lymph nodes generally occurs after the manifestation of the initial lesions. Inguinal adenitis usually is unilateral in the early stages of infection. The perirectal lymph nodes occasionally are the first to be involved; pain on defecation is an early symptom when this condition occurs. The rectovaginal septum may become involved when the posterior vaginal area is a primary site of infection.

If the disease goes untreated, it may enter a secondary stage called the *inguinal syndrome*, in which the inguinal glands and the surrounding subcutaneous tissues become a brawny mass that adheres to the indurated, purplish red overlying skin. The nodes increase in size and form abscesses (buboes). Unless aspirated, the buboes rupture and create chronically draining sinuses.[133] Enlargement of lymph nodes above and below the inguinal ligament may lead to the "groove" sign.[98] Complaints of lower abdominal pain and backache may indicate concurrent proctitis. The deep iliac nodes may be enlarged in 75 percent of cases; rupture of these nodes may cause large pelvic abscesses.

Healing of draining buboes is slow, and severe scarring occurs. In most cases, healing of buboes indicates the end of the disease, but relapses have been reported in 20 percent of untreated cases. Disseminated disease, hepatitis, pneumonia, arthritis, erythema nodosum, erythema multiforme, and ocular infection can occur in association with the inguinal syndrome.

The anogenitorectal syndrome is a subacute manifestation of lymphogranuloma venereum. It includes proctocolitis and hyperplasia of intestinal and perirectal lymphatic tissue. Perirectal abscesses often develop and lead to ischiorectal and rectovaginal fistulas, anal fistulas, and rectal stricture or stenosis. The clinical findings consist of fever, rectal pain, and abdominal cramping. Progression of the disease causes rectal bleeding and a purulent rectal discharge. Rectal strictures lead to constipation and "pencil stools." Weight loss, bowel perforation, and peritonitis may occur. Genital elephantiasis (esthiomene), a primary infection affecting the lymphatics of the scrotum, penis, or vulva, may occur with chronic infection.

The diagnosis of lymphogranuloma venereum should be considered whenever a patient has a tender, enlarged inguinal gland or an ulcerative or granulomatous lesion of the vulva, perineum, vagina, or cervix. Acutely painful, unilateral inguinal lymphadenitis strongly suggests lymphogranuloma venereum. A definitive diagnosis is made by identification of *C. trachomatis* serotype L1, L2, or L3 in tissue cultures of material from buboes or ulcerative lesions. The sensitivity of culture for lymphogranuloma venereum is only approximately 50 percent, however.[145] Serologic tests may be used when cultures are negative or buboes are not present. Complement fixation has been available since the 1930s and 1940s. In clinical settings suggestive of lymphogranuloma venereum, a complement-fixation antibody titer of 1:64 or higher is considered diagnostic. Most patients with lymphogranuloma venereum have titers of 1:128 or higher. Titers between acute and convalescent specimens may not increase because most patients seek care well after the acute phase of the infection has developed. Cross-reaction with other chlamydial serotypes does occur, but titers higher than 1:6 rarely are seen with chlamydial urethritis. Microimmunofluorescence is more specific than is complement fixation and can detect IgM and IgG titers. This test is not widely available.[145]

Complement fixation remains the recommended test for diagnosis when the clinical findings lead to a presumptive diagnosis of lymphogranuloma venereum. If complement-fixation titers are negative, repeat testing in a few weeks may be helpful in patients who happen to be evaluated first early in the course of illness. DNA probes or monoclonal antibodies specific for lymphogranuloma venereum serovars may become available in the near future.

Lymphogranuloma venereum must be differentiated from syphilis, with which it may coexist. False-positive Venereal Disease Research Laboratory test results may occur in 20 percent of patients with lymphogranuloma venereum. When the diagnosis is in doubt, specific tests for antitreponemal antibodies must be used to rule out syphilis. The disease is differentiated from other granulomatous and ulcerative disorders by specific tests for each, by biopsy, and by the clinical appearance of the lesions (see Table 48–3).

Treatment

The earlier the diagnosis is made and treatment is started, the better the response to therapy and the less serious the tissue destruction. Fluctuant buboes are aspirated, not incised, before they rupture. The discharge from the ulcerated areas and buboes is infectious, so precautions against transmission of the disease must be taken. The patient would be more comfortable if kept in bed. Ice-cold compresses may be applied to the inguinal areas. The vulva is cleansed gently twice daily.

The preferred treatment of lymphogranuloma venereum is doxycycline, 100 mg orally twice a day for 21 days.[42] The latter is preferred in pediatric patients younger than 8 years. The alternative regimen is erythromycin base 500 mg orally four times a day for 21 days. Either of these medications also should be given for 21 days. Because of the potential for shorter treatment courses and improved compliance, azithromycin may become a treatment option for lymphogranuloma venereum in the future. It cannot be recommended now because data are insufficient.

After treatment is initiated, patients should be monitored clinically until the signs and symptoms have resolved. Individuals who have had sexual contact with a patient during the 30 days before the onset of symptoms of lymphogranuloma venereum should be examined, tested for chlamydial infection, and treated.[41] Adolescents are likely to be treated before development of the extensive anal and rectal strictures and distorting vulvar cicatrizations occur, for which extensive surgery is sometimes necessary in older patients.

GRANULOMA INGUINALE

Granuloma inguinale is a chronic disease characterized by ulcerative granulomatous lesions of the skin and subcutaneous tissues (Fig. 48–20; see Table 48–4). Common synonyms for the infec-

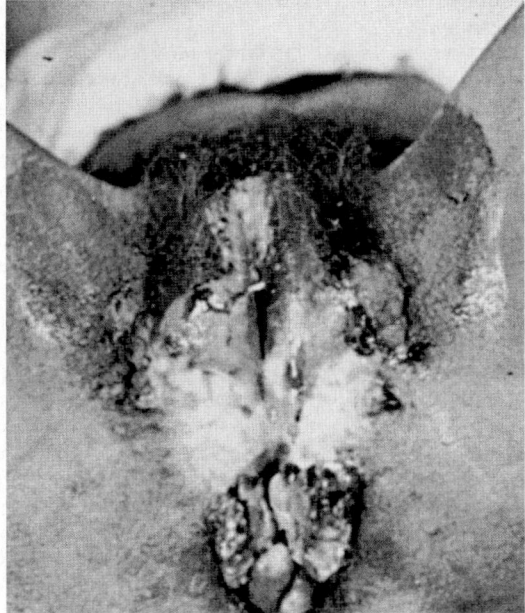

Figure 48–20 Granuloma inguinale.

tion include granuloma venereum and donovanosis. The disease most often affects the external genitalia, perineum, and inguinal regions, but the vagina, cervix, and, rarely, distant extragenital sites may be involved. The disease is caused by *Klebsiella granulomatis* (formerly known as *Calymmatobacterium granulomatis*, *Donovania granulomatis*, Donovan bodies), an encapsulated, gram-negative bacillus.[30,65,161,200] Granuloma inguinale occurs commonly in tropical and subtropical regions of the world.[191,201,203] It is relatively rare in the United States and other developed countries.[41,104] The male-to-female ratio seems to be at least 2:1. The disease rarely occurs in premenarcheal children, but it should be considered in the differential diagnosis of granulomatous lesions of the genitalia in adolescents.

The disease is transmitted to adolescents and adults during sexual intercourse. The close physical contact of the inguinal, perineal, and genital regions that occurs during sexual activity, and not intercourse per se, probably is more important for transmission of the infection. The organism is not highly contagious; sexual partners of patients with granuloma inguinale often do not become infected. Breaches in the integrity of the skin or mucous membranes, such as with minor trauma, may be required for an inoculum to establish a successful infection.[202] The disease apparently can be transmitted to young children by contaminated clothing or towels. Close physical contact, such as sitting on the lap of an infected parent, also has been reported as a mode of transmission to young children.[295]

The incubation period usually is less than 2 weeks but may be 3 months.[202] The first manifestation of infection usually is single or multiple small, painless hard nodules on the vulva or perineum that erode the skin and form ulcers. Genital tract bleeding is the next most common finding. Ulcers are shallow and have a beefy, granular base that is friable and bleeds easily. The edges are nodular, raised, and undermined. These ulcers usually are painless, unless they become infected secondarily. Regional (inguinal) lymphadenopathy is not associated with granuloma inguinale.[200]

If left untreated, lesions progress slowly outward by eccentric expansion of the leading edge. Over time, this ulcerative stage involves large areas of the perineum, external genitalia, and surrounding skin surfaces. The central areas usually remain ulcerative but may become hypertrophic. Hypertrophic lesions consist of large, vegetating masses with overgrowth of granulation tissue. Less frequently, extensive, destructive necrosis develops in the lesions, or they are dry with sclerotic scarring, which distorts the tissues. Lymphedema of distal tissues occurs commonly during the course of the disease. Lymphatic obstruction or elephantiasis occasionally results in enlargement of the clitoris or labia.[93,149] Subcutaneous granulation develops in approximately 5 percent of cases and may mimic the appearance of bubo formation, termed *pseudobuboes*. When true regional adenopathy occurs in granuloma inguinale, it generally represents a response to a secondary infection or another associated sexually transmitted infection.

Extragenital disease may occur in 6 percent of cases and usually involves the head and neck. Autoinoculation is postulated as the means of transmission of infection of these sites.[86] Occasional involvement of the liver, thorax, and bones remote from the primary genital site suggests that hematogenous spread can occur. Systemic disease is encountered more frequently in girls with cervical lesions and is associated with prolonged spiking fever, anemia, and weight loss.[31,151,220]

Successful isolation of *K. granulomatis* rarely has proved feasible. Reliable culture techniques are unavailable. The diagnosis of granuloma inguinale is based on the presence of Donovan bodies in large, histiocytic cells on crush preparations from lesions (Fig. 48–21). A portion of the granulation tissue is removed and pressed onto a clean slide, which is allowed to air-dry. The slide then is stained with Giemsa, Wright, or Warthin-Starry

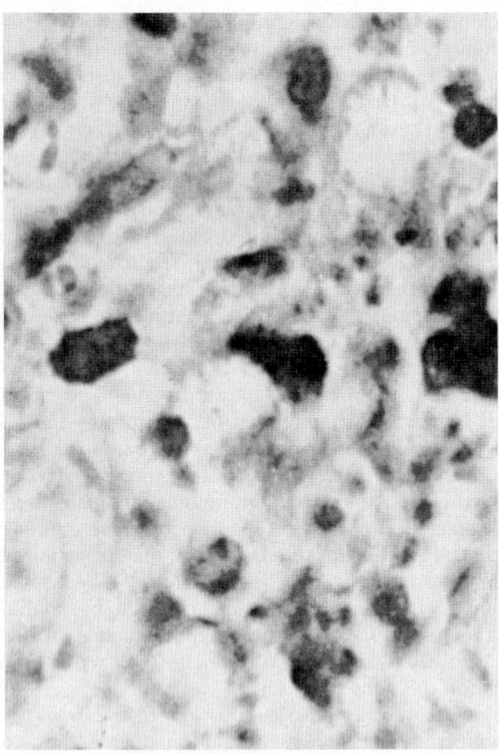

Figure 48–21 Donovan bodies.

stain. Donovan bodies, which are pathognomonic for granuloma inguinale, are vacuolar compartments within the cytoplasm that contain 20 to 30 viable organisms.[65] Histopathologic study of biopsy specimens sometimes is required for establishing a diagnosis. Biopsy specimens should be very early, very sclerotic, or heavily superinfected lesions. Specimens with a scarcity of organisms and smear or crush specimens are likely to be nondiagnostic in such circumstances. Biopsy also should be performed when malignancy is thought possible, or when antibiotic therapy does not lead to improvement.[145]

Complement-fixation and indirect immunofluorescence serologic tests have been developed but have limited specificity.[145] There are no FDA-approved, PCR-based tests for chancroid, but such testing can be performed by commercial laboratories that have developed their own test and conducted a Clinical Laboratory Improvement Act (CLIA) verification study.[41] The differential diagnosis of granuloma inguinale includes carcinoma, syphilis, tuberculosis, chancroid, lymphogranuloma venereum, condyloma acuminatum, blastomycosis, schistosomiasis, and other granulomatous diseases.[20,200,202] STDs such as syphilis may coexist with granuloma inguinale. Darkfield examination of tissue specimens and serologic tests for syphilis should be done. Biopsy may be required to rule out neoplasia or tuberculosis.[86] Chancroid ulcers tend to be deeper and more ragged and often have associated bubo formation. Physical examination alone often is insufficient to distinguish any of these processes from the others (see Table 48–4). Granuloma inguinale also is associated with the development of carcinoma within areas that have been involved in the ulcerative process.

Treatment

Doxycycline, 100 mg orally twice a day for at least 3 weeks and until all lesions have completely healed, is the recommended treatment. Alternatives include azithromycin, 1 g orally once weekly; ciprofloxacin, 750 mg orally twice a day; erythromycin base, 500 mg orally four times a day; or trimethoprim-

sulfamethoxazole, one double-strength tablet orally twice a day. Each regimen should be continued until all lesions have healed completely, with a minimum course of 3 weeks.[47] Chloramphenicol and gentamicin also have been used.[227]

Vulvar lesions usually heal within 2 weeks of therapy, but cervical and pelvic lesions may require longer than 3 months. Incomplete treatment can result in recurrence with extensive fibrosis and scarring.[20] The disease recurs in approximately 10 percent of cases. Surgery may be required for complications of granuloma inguinale, such as elephantiasis, strictures, and pelvic abscesses.

Precautions regarding infections should be taken in the home or hospital until the lesions have healed. Sexual contacts of patients with granuloma inguinale within 60 days before onset of the index patient's symptoms should be evaluated and offered therapy, even if no lesions are present. The value of empiric therapy in the absence of overt clinical signs and symptoms has not been determined, however.[41] Adolescent girls who have had granuloma inguinale should be kept under clinical surveillance for many years for the potential development of carcinoma in the perineum and genital tract.

CHANCROID

Chancroid is an acute, ulcerative disease that involves primarily the external genitalia.[7,289] The causative agent, *Haemophilus ducreyi*, is a fastidious, gram-negative coccobacillus. It is a strict human pathogen, and the only known route of transmission is sexual contact. The incubation period usually is 3 to 7 days, but it may be longer. Chancroid rarely is encountered in young children, but occasionally is seen in sexually active adolescents. It occurs far more commonly in boys than in girls for reasons that are unclear, although asymptomatic carriage in girls has been hypothesized.[24,115,206,278]

Chancroid is well established as a cofactor for transmission of HIV infection.[41,42] Ten percent of patients with chancroid may be infected with HIV. Chancroid is found more commonly in tropical and subtropical regions than in developed countries, but its frequency is increasing in many parts of the world.[206] Chancroid is endemic in the United States and occurs primarily in discrete occasional outbreaks. Outbreaks caused by unrelated strains occurred in New Orleans, Louisiana, and Jackson, Mississippi, in the 1990s.[118] The disease probably is underrecognized and underreported.[41]

A recent case series described three girls 5 to 9 years old with chronic skin ulcerations on their lower legs after visiting Samoa. *H. ducreyi* was found in specimens from each child. No evidence of acquisition by sexual contact was found. Lower limb ulcerations were present among household contacts while the girls were in Samoa. Autoinoculation leading to nongenital skin lesions has been described.[278] Although the potential for nongenital transmission of *H. ducreyi* to nongenital sites exists, chancroid lesions in the genital area should be considered the result of sexual contact.

The first sign of chancroid infection of the genital tract is a small, hyperemic macule. The macule becomes a papule and then a pustule before ulceration occurs. The ulcer is painful and usually deep, with irregular borders and undermined edges. The base is gray and covered with purulent exudate laden with the *H. ducreyi* bacillus. Ulcers may occur on the vulva, vaginal mucosa, cervix, or anus but usually are found on the labia minora. Dysuria is a frequent complaint. Tenesmus and rectal bleeding may be associated with anal lesions. Single ulcers are found frequently, but multiple ulcers occur more often. They may become contiguous and form large, eroded areas. Phagedenic destruction of the external genitalia may occur when treatment is not sought early, or a secondary infection develops in the ulcers. In such cases, scarring persists despite successful eradication of the microbe. Infection, at least experimentally, does not seem to confer protection on re-exposure to the microbe.[6]

Associated, painful inguinal adenitis occurs in 25 to 50 percent of cases. Adenitis occurs more commonly when genital ulcers have been present for more than 10 days. The skin overlying the nodes frequently is erythematous. Discharge from buboes and vulvar lesions is highly infectious. Constitutional symptoms are unusual, and invasiveness beyond regional lymph nodes does not seem to occur even in immunocompromised hosts.

Many patients with chancroid have concurrent infections with other STDs. Patients should be tested for HIV infection and syphilis when chancroid is diagnosed. Testing for both diseases should be repeated in 3 months if the initial results are negative.[42]

In the United States, a probable diagnosis of chancroid is made clinically if (1) one or more painful genital ulcers are present; (2) the individual has no evidence of *T. pallidum* infection by either darkfield examination of ulcer exudate or a serologic test for syphilis performed at least 7 days after the onset of ulcers; (3) the clinical findings, appearance of the genital ulcers, and regional lymphadenopathy, if present, are typical for chancroid; and (4) a test for HSV done on ulcer exudate is negative. When present, the combination of a painful ulcer with tender inguinal adenopathy suggests chancroid. A painful genital ulcer accompanied by suppurative inguinal adenopathy is almost pathognomonic for chancroid.[42]

Definitive diagnosis of chancroid requires isolation of *H. ducreyi* on special culture media. The sensitivity of culture is at best 80 percent.[42] When culture is performed, exudate from the purulent base of the ulcer or material aspirated from buboes should be inoculated onto appropriate media. Gram-negative coccobacilli in a "school-of-fish" grouping on Gram stain suggests *H. ducreyi*, but this pattern often is absent. The diagnosis also can be based on the histologic appearance of tissue obtained by biopsy. There are no FDA-approved, PCR-based tests for chancroid, but such testing can be done by commercial laboratories that have developed their own test and conducted a CLIA verification study.[8,243]

Treatment

Effective agents for the treatment of chancroid in adolescents and adults include azithromycin, 1 g orally in a single dose; ceftriaxone, 250 mg intramuscularly in a single dose; ciprofloxacin, 500 mg orally twice a day for 3 days; and erythromycin base, 500 mg orally three times a day for 7 days.[42] Trimethoprim-sulfamethoxazole no longer is recommended because of the frequency of resistant isolates of *H. ducreyi*. Isolates typically are resistant to penicillin and tetracyclines.

Patients should be re-examined 3 to 7 days after therapy has been initiated. If treatment is effective, ulcers should improve symptomatically within 3 days and show objective improvement within 7 days. If no clinical improvement occurs, one or more of the following should be considered: (1) the diagnosis may be incorrect, (2) co-infection with another sexually transmitted agent may be present, (3) the infecting strain may be resistant to the prescribed antimicrobial agent, (4) compliance with multiple-dose regimens may have been poor, or (5) the patient may have HIV infection. The time required for complete healing of ulcers to occur is related to their size. Large ulcers may require 2 weeks or more.[42]

Resolution of fluctuant lymphadenopathy (buboes) is slower than that of ulcers. Drainage of buboes, when present, usually is required for resolution. Needle aspiration, if adequate drainage can be accomplished, is preferred over surgical incision because it results in less cicatricial scarring. Healed ulcers frequently leave significant scarring.

Individuals who have had sexual contact with an individual who has chancroid during the 10 days before the onset of symptoms should be examined and treated for chancroid, even in the absence of symptoms. Patients co-infected with HIV should be monitored closely. Longer courses of therapy may be required, and healing may be slower. The optimal duration of therapy in these patients is unknown.[42]

TUBERCULOSIS

Even before the advent of chemotherapy for the treatment of tuberculosis, tuberculous disease of the lower genital tract was uncommon.[240,269] The lower genital tract can be affected by primary local infection of the vulvar and vaginal tissues or by scrofulous tuberculosis. Both manifestations of tuberculosis are now exceedingly rare findings. Most such cases occur in young women in developing countries. Tuberculosis of the upper genital tract also is an uncommon occurrence but frequently leads to infertility when it does occur, probably because of scarring of the uterine tubes.[235]

The primary lesions of vulvar tuberculosis may appear as painless, slowly developing, localized, nodular thickening of the skin and subcutaneous tissues or as ulcerative lesions that begin as firm, slightly raised, reddish areas. The ulcers are demarcated sharply and with progression develop undermined edges and granular, grayish brown bases with tubercles and areas of caseation studding their bases.

The scrofulous type is characterized by fistulous tracts and burrowing sinuses that extend from underlying tuberculous infection in the bowel, bladder, or pelvic viscera. Drainage from the ulcers and sinuses keeps the surrounding skin macerated and can lead to extension of the disease.

The diagnosis is straightforward if the patient is known to have visceral tuberculosis, as most often is the case. Isolation of *M. tuberculosis* from the discharge or from lesions or examination of a biopsy specimen from the base of an ulcer is confirmatory. Primary tuberculosis of the vulva must be differentiated from other granulomatous diseases, and the scrofulous type must be distinguished from syphilis, lymphogranuloma inguinale, and Crohn disease.

Treatment

The chemotherapeutic agents used to treat pulmonary and other types of systemic tuberculosis also are effective in treating the disease when it affects the genitalia. Treatment of tuberculosis is described in Chapter 107.

VULVOVAGINAL ULCERATIVE INFECTIONS

BEHÇET DISEASE

In 1937, Behçet described a syndrome characterized by recurrent genital ulcers, aphthous stomatitis, and ocular inflammation.[125,150,181,199,221] Clinical manifestations are not due directly to infection but may result from immunologic events triggered by one or more infections.[204] Arthritis, abnormalities of the central nervous system, a variety of skin lesions including erythema nodosum, and other systemic symptoms also may be associated with the disease. Ocular inflammation frequently is sight-threatening when it occurs. Deep vein thrombosis and arterial occlusion or aneurysms can develop. The onset usually is in patients who are 20 to 30 years old and more frequently in men than in women. Behçet disease is rare in children and may develop more often in girls than in boys.[150] In an international series, 15 percent of children had a family history of Behçet disease.[155]

The cause of Behçet disease is unknown, but an autoimmune basis is suspected. The HLA-B51 phenotype, and especially the B*5101 allele, is associated with Behçet disease in countries with higher prevalences of HLA-B51. Other factors also are involved because a substantial proportion of cases occur in individuals without HLA-B51. Lymphocyte reactivity with peptides derived from human heat shock protein-60 (HSP-60) has been shown. Human HSP-60 is a homologue of streptococcal HSP-65. Aberrant expression of HSP-60 has been found in oral mucosa, skin, and circulating lymphocytes in patients with Behçet disease. In addition to streptococcal species, HSV and *E. coli* antigens have been implicated as potential triggers of Behçet disease.[155,204]

The vulvar lesions take the form of destructive, deep ulcerations that, on recurrence, result in marked scarring and distortion with progressive loss of vulvar tissue (Fig. 48–22). Despite their destructiveness, the lesions are relatively painless. The oral lesions resemble common aphthous ulcers and may precede all other manifestations of Behçet syndrome by 5 to 10 years or longer. Ocular inflammation may be manifested as iridocyclitis, chorioretinitis, or other lesions of the posterior segment. Hypopyon may be seen in some cases.

The vulvar lesions of Behçet syndrome are nonspecific. Diagnosis is based on associated findings and negative test results for diseases that might resemble the vulvar ulcers, notably syphilis, herpes, granulomatous disorders, and Crohn's disease. Histologic study of a biopsy specimen from an ulcer shows only obliterative vasculitis and chronic inflammation.

Many agents have been used to treat Behçet syndrome in the past. Few have been evaluated in controlled trials. Modern treatment regimens usually have used systemic corticosteroids, with or without chlorambucil, colchicine, azathioprine, or thalidomide. More recent studies have suggested that cyclosporine and interferon α-2a may be effective.[10,208] A randomized trial reported in 1998 of the use of colchicine plus benzathine penicillin, with or without interferon α, for the treatment of adults with Behçet disease showed a decrease in the frequency of eye involvement, episodes of arthritis, vascular events, and mucocutaneous lesions in patients treated with all three agents.[155] Infliximab, a humanized monoclonal antibody against tumor necrosis factor-α, may be effective in diminishing new ocular attacks. Etanercept, a tumor necrosis factor receptor analogue, may have an impact on mucocutaneous manifestations.[204] Plastic surgery for correction of vaginal distortions is contraindicated because trauma may be followed by an exacerbation of the disease.

VULVAR VESTIBULITIS

The vulvar vestibulitis syndrome is the most common type of chronic vulvovaginal pain. Approximately 10 percent of women are affected at some point in their lives. Onset in adolescence can occur, and complaints sometimes may mimic those of sexually transmitted infections. The etiology is unknown and probably multifactorial. An exaggerated inflammatory response of the vestibule (vulvar mucosa) to injury may be involved. Vestibulitis clinically is defined by three signs and symptoms: (1) dyspareunia during intercourse, (2) vestibular tenderness to light touch (e.g., gentle palpation with a cotton swab), and (3) the presence of vestibular erythema. Pain and tenderness are distinctly limited to the vulvar vestibule. Exudates indicate another disease process. Minor ulcerations have been described, but ulceration is not a prominent feature.[27,58,182,220,230]

Debate is ongoing as to the organic versus functional nature of vulvar vestibulitis. Symptoms sometimes respond to biofeedback or cognitive behavioral therapy. Chronic inflammatory changes can be found in the vulvar mucosa of affected women, and surgical resection relieves pain in some patients. Organic and functional components seem to exist, with one or the other predominating in a particular patient.[55,173,296]

Patients with acute vulvar vestibulitis should be evaluated for STDs and treated for any that are found. A history of all medicinal agents or other treatment modalities used by the patient should be obtained. Any agent that might be contributing to the problem should be discontinued if possible. Adolescent girls who have symptoms and signs suggestive of vulvar vestibulitis should be referred for gynecologic evaluation.

CERVICITIS

PREMENARCHEAL

The cervix is not involved when a premenarcheal child has vaginitis because most vaginal infections affect only the distal half of the vagina in children; the exception is gonococcal vaginitis, which in addition usually involves the squamous epithelium over the external cervix. Cervicitis also may occur when a vaginal foreign body is present. Endocervicitis is an unusual finding in premenarcheal girls because the endocervical glands and mucosa are developed poorly before menarche, providing a poor environment for invading organisms.

Erosions of the cervix seldom are seen in children older than 1 year. So-called congenital ectopy is not the result of infection; rather, it is persistence of the fetal paramesonephric (müllerian) glandular epithelium on the outer cervix. This epithelium normally recedes into the endocervical canal as the cervix develops postnatally. Inflammation of the external cervix, which occasionally occurs with vaginitis in a premenarcheal child, need not be treated; it heals as the vaginitis improves.[133]

POSTMENARCHEAL

The structure of the cervix during the reproductive years renders it vulnerable to infections induced by numerous factors. The

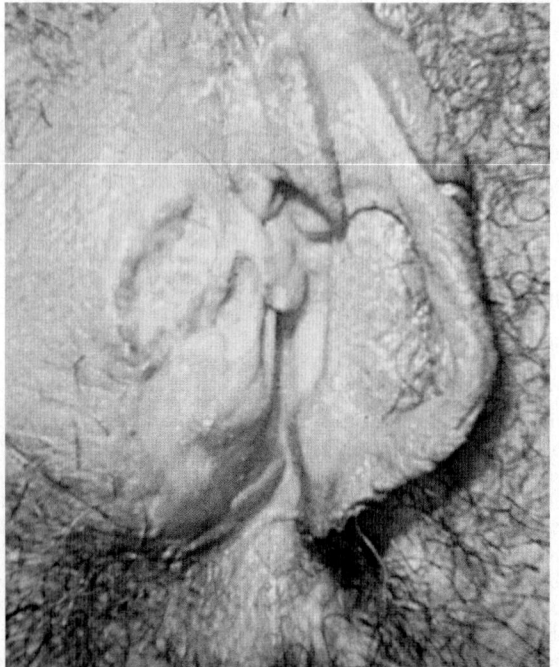

Figure 48–22 Vulvar lesions in Behçet syndrome. (*From Friedrich, E. G., Jr.: Vulvar Disease. Philadelphia, W. B. Saunders, 1976. Reproduced by permission of the author.*)

long, narrow, deeply pocketed cervical canal, which is lined by open cryptic glands bathed in alkaline secretion and washed periodically by menstrual blood, is an excellent nidus for the growth of bacteria. Pathogenic bacteria in the vagina find ready access to the cervical canal. The use of oral contraceptive pills promotes cervical ectopy, increasing the vulnerability of endocervical cells to chlamydial infection.[130,229]

Early recognition and aggressive treatment of cervicitis in sexually active adolescents are important to prevent serious complications, including PID and tubo-ovarian abscess. Some confusion tends to occur, however, with regard to differentiating normal ectopic columnar epithelium on the exocervix (ectopy) from cervicitis. Ectopy is not an abnormal finding. When the squamocolumnar junction is exposed on the exocervix, it is called *ectopy*. It appears bright shiny red, in contrast to the dull pearly pink appearance of the exocervix. This area does not bleed easily when touched with a swab. During adolescence, the normal cervix may exhibit no ectopy, a small area of ectopy, or sometimes 50 percent ectopy. When the ectopy appears edematous, raised, and friable (often with marked bleeding when touched lightly with a swab), cervicitis should be suspected.[130,229]

Mucopurulent cervicitis primarily is endocervicitis associated with *C. trachomatis, M. hominis, U. urealyticum, N. gonorrhoeae, G. vaginalis,* and group B streptococci. In contrast, *T. vaginalis* causes an exocervicitis by extension of vaginitis. Because of the high prevalence of coexisting infections of the cervix, associating any one organism with the clinical signs and symptoms of cervicitis often is difficult. Although studies have shown a strong association between mucopurulent cervicitis and *C. trachomatis,* in most cases no organism is isolated.[130,230,248]

Cervicitis often is asymptomatic, but it should be clinically suspected if an adolescent reports a vaginal discharge and bleeding, especially after having sexual intercourse. Criteria for a clinical diagnosis of mucopurulent cervicitis include the presence of mucopurulent secretion from the endocervix, erythema of the cervix, friable ectopy, and bleeding from the cervix.[34] The mucopurulent secretion in chlamydial cervicitis is tenacious mucoid material mixed with yellow exudate and is difficult to remove from the endocervix. The ectopic area on the cervix may appear erythematous and friable. In chronic chlamydial cervicitis, the ectopic area may be swollen and irregular with a cobblestone appearance, a condition called *hypertrophic cervicitis.* In gonococcal cervicitis, the endocervical mucosa is swollen, intensely inflamed, and often friable as well. In contrast to the mucopurulent discharge present in chlamydial cervicitis, a profuse, yellowish green acrid discharge is present in gonococcal cervicitis.

Cervical erosions occur in sexually active adolescents. Infections other than those listed earlier as causing mucopurulent cervicitis also can involve the cervix. A chancre, the primary lesion of syphilis, may appear on the cervix, where it forms an irregularly shaped ulcer that only remotely resembles a chancre on the vulva. Tuberculosis, HSV, granuloma inguinale, lymphogranuloma venereum, chancroid, schistosomiasis, and actinomycosis also may affect the cervix. The cervical lesions of most of these infections are altered by the warmth and moisture of the vagina and are atypical in appearance. None of these lesions is a common finding, but all of them should be considered in the differential diagnosis when a patient has an unusual ulcerative or fungating lesion of the cervix.[133]

Treatment

The first step is to obtain good specimens from the endocervix. The cervix should be wiped with a large swab to remove vaginal secretions. Endocervical specimens then are obtained for detection of *C. trachomatis* and *N. gonorrhoeae* and a vaginal specimen for a saline wet-mount preparation and potassium hydroxide preparation under microscopy. The types of tests available for

chlamydial and gonococcal infection are described in this section under chlamydial and gonococcal cervicitis. If an endocervical Gram stain can be performed, an endocervical specimen should be obtained. This test is useful in a clinical setting. Cervicitis is suspected when an endocervical Gram-stained smear shows more than 5 to 10 polymorphonuclear cells per field under oil immersion. The presence of at least eight pairs of gram-negative intracellular diplococci in at least three polymorphonuclear cells strongly suggests the presence of gonococcal cervicitis. The absence of gram-negative intracellular diplococci, but the presence of more than 5 to 10 polymorphonuclear cells per oil immersion field suggests nongonococcal cervicitis.[34,186] When cervical erosions or ulcers are seen, a specimen for culture of HSV should be obtained. *T. vaginalis* is identified by microscopic examination of vaginal secretions in saline.

The same guidelines for the treatment of gonococcal and chlamydial cervicitis are used for the treatment of cervicitis in nonpregnant adolescent girls or women. Current treatment of gonococcal infection is influenced by the emergence of antibiotic-resistant strains, including penicillinase-producing *N. gonorrhoeae,* fluoroquinolone-resistant strains, tetracycline-resistant strains, and chromosomally resistant strains.[42] The high frequency of chlamydial infection in individuals with gonorrhea (45% in certain populations) and the serious complications resulting from untreated gonorrhea and chlamydial infections also have influenced the treatment approach. Treatment options include intramuscular ceftriaxone, 125 mg in a single dose, cefixime, 400 mg orally in a single dose; plus azithromycin, 1 g orally in a single dose; or doxycycline, 100 mg orally twice a day for 7 days.[42]

In the case of penicillin allergy, a single dose of intramuscular spectinomycin, 2 g, instead of cephalosporins is recommended. Spectinomycin is unavailable in the United States, however.[43] Azithromycin, 2 g, can be used instead of cefixime or ceftriaxone to treat gonococcal cervicitis; however, its cost and severe gastrointestinal side effects need to be considered.[42] Pregnant adolescent girls or women should not be treated with doxycycline. Azithromycin, 1 g orally in a single dose, or erythromycin base, 500 mg orally four times a day for 7 days, is recommended for presumptive *C. trachomatis* cervicitis.[42] If pharyngeal gonorrhea is suspected, the recommended treatment is intramuscular ceftriaxone. When *T. vaginalis* vaginitis is diagnosed, or HSV is suspected strongly, the appropriate treatment for these infections should be given (see sections on trichomoniasis and genital herpes).

Integral to treating the patient is notification, examination, and treatment of the patient's sexual partners if gonococcal or chlamydial infection (or both) is confirmed. Direct notification by the patient should be encouraged, and, based on state laws, a prescription for partner therapy can be given. Written information should be provided with names of diseases and medication side effects to assist with this process. When tests are positive for gonorrhea or chlamydial infection, retesting for these infections is recommended: in 3 weeks if treated with erythromycin or if symptoms persist, and in 3 months if treated with other regimens to detect re-infection from an untreated or new partner.[42]

CHLAMYDIAL

Some of the highest rates of chlamydial cervicitis (8-25%) have been reported in adolescents.[44,82,85,233] It is three to four times more common than gonococcal cervicitis. *C. trachomatis* causes cervicitis by infecting the columnar and transitional epithelium of the cervix. Cervical ectopy seems to be a predisposing factor for acquisition of *C. trachomatis* infection.[16]

C. trachomatis cervicitis is predominantly an asymptomatic disease in adolescent girls.[44] A clinical diagnosis is made when friable ectopy with a mucopurulent cervical discharge (mucopus) is noted. Chlamydial cervicitis is suspected when a Gram stain of an adequate endocervical smear shows more than 5 to 10 polymorphonuclear cells per oil immersion field in the absence of gram-negative intracellular diplococci.[34,185]

Numerous tests, including culture, direct fluorescent antibody tests, enzyme immunoassay, nucleic acid hybridization tests, enhanced optical immunoassays, and nucleic acid amplification tests, are available today to diagnose *C. trachomatis* infection. Material from the cervix must be obtained directly from the endocervix with a sterile swab. The tissue culture method was considered the gold standard,[236] but because of the high cost of this technique, it is not used widely for adolescents and adults. It continues to be the gold standard, however, for prepubertal children suspected of being infected. Overall, amplification tests are considered the most sensitive and specific tests today, and testing of urine specimens is expected to revolutionize screening and diagnosis. Presently, amplification tests are being used predominantly for research purposes because of their high cost, but gradually they may become available for clinical use.

In large-volume, community-based clinics, the DNA hybridization assay or DNA probe (Gen-Probe) and enzyme immunoassay (Abbot, Wampole, Kodak, Gen-Probe) can be used.[158,242] Both tests perform best in clinic populations with high prevalence rates of *C. trachomatis* infection; however, the DNA probe seems to have greater sensitivity for detection and is simple to perform. The Gen-Probe is approximately 80 percent sensitive and 100 percent specific detecting *C. trachomatis* in girls and women. It can be used as a "mail-out" specimen as well.[242,252] The direct fluorescent antibody test or MicroTrak is considered to be suited best for low-volume laboratories and requires technical expertise. It continues to be used in some hospital-based settings. This test detects *Chlamydia* elementary bodies in cervical secretions and takes 15 to 20 minutes to perform. It has a sensitivity of 75 to 90 percent and specificity of 95 to 97 percent compared with the culture method.[74,242]

The reliability of amplification tests such as PCR, strand displacement amplification, and transcription-mediated amplification in detecting *C. trachomatis* seems to be equivalent for vaginal, cervical, and urine specimens as long as the urine collected is a first-catch specimen. The sensitivity of PCR, ligase chain reaction, strand displacement amplification, and transcription-mediated amplification ranges from 87 to 99 percent, and specificity ranges from 97 to 100 percent.[23,239,252] Treatment of chlamydial cervicitis was discussed in the earlier section on cervicitis.

GONOCOCCAL

Gonococcal cervicitis may be symptomatic or asymptomatic. The risk of acquiring infection varies with the population. Adolescents seen in private practices in the suburbs have a significantly lower rate of gonococcal cervicitis than that noted in adolescents seen in large outpatient hospital clinics or community clinics serving inner-city populations. The rate of asymptomatic endocervical infection in adolescent girls seen in urban settings ranges from 3 to 12 percent. Anal gonorrhea usually is secondary to discharge from gonococcal cervicitis infecting the anus. Primary anal gonorrhea as a result of anal intercourse should be suspected in a sexually active adolescent with anal discomfort. In addition, gonococcal infection should be considered in the differential diagnosis of pharyngitis in sexually active adolescents.[218] Gonococcal endocarditis, arthritis, and dermal abscesses occur, but they are beyond the scope of this chapter.

The initial complaints in gonococcal cervicitis include vaginal discharge, dysuria, urinary frequency, and dyspareunia. Although gonococcal cervicitis is reported to be predominantly an asymptomatic condition in girls and women, many patients, after careful questioning, are found to have symptoms. The discharge is profuse and prevalent. On examination, the vulvar tissues may be inflamed and edematous. Discharge also may be seen exuding out of the urethra and paraurethral ducts in severe cases. On speculum examination, the patient has a normal-appearing cervix, or the cervix appears erythematous and friable, with a foul-smelling purulent discharge draining from the cervical os.

Laboratory diagnosis is made by detecting *N. gonorrhoeae* by culture technique, a DNA hybridization test or DNA probe (Gen-Probe), or an amplification test. Material from the cervix must be obtained directly from the endocervix with a sterile swab. Vaginal swabs that can be obtained by the adolescent also are a recommended method for amplification tests. Although the reliability of detecting gram-negative intracellular diplococci on a Gram stain of cervical secretions is low, this test can be useful in areas where more sophisticated tests are unavailable. The presence of at least eight pairs of gram-negative intracellular diplococci in at least three polymorphonuclear cells strongly suggests gonococcal cervicitis.

Hospital-based settings should continue to use the culture method in children and adolescents for medicolegal cases. The DNA probe (Gen-Probe) can be used in hospital and community-based clinics for the reasons described in the section on chlamydial cervicitis. This test has sensitivities ranging from 90 to 97 percent and a specificity of 99 percent. Amplification tests such as PCR and strand displacement amplification for *N. gonorrhoeae* from vaginal, cervical, and first-catch urine specimens have a sensitivity of 95 to 97 percent and a specificity of 99 to 100 percent.[252,257] The sensitivity of the transcription-mediated amplification test in detecting *N. gonorrhoeae* from urine specimens is poor. Treatment of gonococcal cervicitis was discussed in the earlier section on cervicitis.

UPPER GENITAL TRACT INFECTIONS

PELVIC INFLAMMATORY DISEASE

PID (i.e., infection of the uterine tubes, ovaries, and pelvic peritoneum) is an extremely rare finding in premenarcheal girls and often is undiagnosed until advanced infection occurs.[33,66,133] With the exception of gonorrhea and the inflammation caused by a foreign body, most vulvar and vaginal infections do not involve the upper third of the vagina and do not approach the cervix of premenarcheal patients. The premenarcheal cervix and endometrium apparently are barriers rather than passageways for bacteria causing all types of vulvovaginitis in children.

The causative organisms are diverse. Gonococcal pelvic infection has been reported after sexual abuse has occurred. *S. pneumoniae* serotypes 1 and 2 and *E. coli* also have been reported in pubertal girls with salpingitis and peritonitis and tubo-ovarian abscess.[33]

When intrapelvic infection has been reported in premenarcheal girls, it usually has been part of either generalized primary peritonitis or peritonitis secondary to a ruptured appendix or some other intra-abdominal infection.[72,241] Pelvic infection that is part of an intra-abdominal infection characteristically affects the surfaces of the uterine tubes, uterus, and ovaries and produces perisalpingitis and periovaritis; periappendicitis also is present even if the infection did not begin as appendicitis. An ascending infection from the lower genital tract, such as that caused by gonorrhea, involves the tubal mucosa and produces endosalpingitis and pyosalpingitis. Identical bacteria should be isolated in cultures from the lower genitalia and from the pelvic exudate before an ascending infection is considered to be the cause of a pelvic infection in a specific case in which the patient is a premenarcheal child.

PID in postmenarcheal girls is a common problem. Salpingitis has been reported in virgins, and, although the etiology is unknown, the organisms are thought to spread hematogenously, lymphatically, or transmurally from intestines or ascending infection from the vagina.[66,74,133] PID occurs primarily in sexually active adolescents at risk for developing ascending infection acquired from STDs.[76,252]

PID is defined as an acute clinical syndrome (unrelated to pregnancy or surgery) attributed to the ascent of microorganisms from the vagina and endocervix to the endometrium, fallopian tubes, or contiguous structures that result in pelvic and generalized peritonitis. The use of terms specifically describing the anatomic sites involved is preferable (e.g., endometritis, salpingitis, salpingo-oophoritis, tubo-ovarian abscess). In most adolescents with acute severe infection, however, differentiating some of these entities is difficult; the term *PID* is used commonly.

Reasons for the development of PID are physiologic and social and include alterations in cervical mucus caused by immature and anovulatory menstrual cycles, onset of sexual activity during early puberty, and multiple sexual partners. Cervical mucus is less viscous during menses and at midcycle, rendering it more permeable to ascending infection. In vitro experiments show that *N. gonorrhoeae*, *C. trachomatis*, *U. urealyticum*, and other aerobic and anaerobic agents can adhere to spermatozoa and migrate with them.[276] Whether this event can occur in vivo is unknown. Most organisms found in nongonococcal and nonchlamydial PID also are found in bacterial vaginosis, suggesting that bacterial vaginosis may be a predisposing or a precipitating factor for the development of PID. In addition, researchers have suggested that *T. vaginalis* can act as a vector for transporting bacteria.[148] Another possible factor is upward transport of bacteria from orgasmic myometrial contractions.[288] Lastly, vaginal douching has been reported to be a risk factor in promoting ascending infection.[198,288,291]

Other factors influencing the risk of acquiring PID are the method of contraception and a history of gonococcal or chlamydial lower genital tract infection, with or without uterine instrumentation, such as the use of an intrauterine device or dilation and curettage. Oral contraceptives are used commonly by adolescents. Their possible protective effect on the development of PID has been reported. Laparoscopic studies also have shown that women with PID who were using oral contraceptive pills have significantly milder degrees of fallopian tube inflammation than those of women who do not use the pills. This finding suggests that the oral contraceptive pill may reduce potential tubal damage. Other studies report, however, that by promoting cervical ectopy, oral contraceptives are a potential risk factor for acquiring chlamydial PID.[248,273,292] In contrast, compared with other methods of contraception, women using depot medroxyprogesterone acetate (Depo-Provera) had a significantly decreased risk of developing PID.[19,292] Risk for acquiring a PID with the intrauterine device seems to be related to the individual's background risk for acquiring sexually transmitted infection.[252]

Women who have had one episode of PID have a 20 to 25 percent chance of having subsequent ones. Reasons for this susceptibility may be re-infection from untreated sexual partners, an inadequately treated first infection, or increased susceptibility of the tubal epithelium to infection.[76,288]

Endometritis

Infections of the endometrium in postmenarcheal girls and women are as rare as previously thought. The gonococcus, on its way upward to the uterine tubes, produces a fleeting asymptomatic infection of the endometrium, or the symptoms produced are overshadowed by those of the vulvar and cervical infections. Evidence also suggests that endometritis occurs in 40 percent of patients with asymptomatic endocervical chlamydial infection.[144] It also is called *subclinical PID*, and repeated episodes have been linked to infertility.[144,286] The role of HIV infection in the development of PID is unclear. An increased prevalence of endometritis in HIV-infected women compared with uninfected women has been noted, and altered immune function might contribute to difficulty clearing endometritis in these cases.[35]

Symptoms specific to endometritis are uncommon. It is commonly an asymptomatic condition. Symptoms include recurrent intermittent or acute suprapubic pain and tenderness with vaginal bleeding or spotting. On bimanual examination, the uterus is tender, and cervical motion tenderness may or may not be present. Endometritis in adolescent girls and young women also has been associated with postabortive and puerperal endometritis. Poor compliance with prophylactic antibiotics places an adolescent at an increased risk for development of endometritis after having an abortion. Young women who engage in high-risk sexual behaviors and use intrauterine devices are likely to have asymptomatic, low-grade, chronic endometritis.

Endometrial tuberculosis is a rare occurrence in the United States and is encountered most often in patients with pulmonary tuberculosis. This entity needs to be considered in HIV-infected girls and women and in geographic areas and regions where tuberculosis is endemic. In a study from a province in Iran, tuberculous endometritis was detected in 72 percent of genital tuberculosis cases in women.[194] The disease may not manifest for years after initial seeding, and the infection is thought to reach the uterus via the gastrointestinal tract through hematogenous seeding and by lymphatic spread. It is not acquired as a result of an ascending infection or through coitus with an infected man. The symptoms of endometrial tuberculosis vary from none to amenorrhea, pelvic pain, dysmenorrhea, abnormal uterine bleeding, and tuberculosis. Often, the patient has a history of healed or active pulmonary disease. Overall, 60 percent of patients with pelvic tuberculosis have tuberculous endometritis.[5,117]

Endometrial tuberculosis is diagnosed by endometrial biopsy and demonstration of acid-fast *M. tuberculosis* in cultures of curettage material or menstrual blood. Menstrual fluid has been reported to be culture-positive more frequently than are biopsy specimens.[117] Endometrial tuberculosis and the management of tuberculosis are described further in Chapter 107.

Salpingitis

The pathogenesis of salpingitis has been studied best with *N. gonorrhoeae* and *C. trachomatis*. In the fallopian tube, gonococci attach to nonciliated epithelial cells and induce sloughing of ciliated epithelial cells into the lumen.[271,288] Gonococci also enter the subepithelial space, where a local inflammatory response, predominantly polymorphonuclear leukocytic infiltrate and anaerobic bacteria, is produced and may reach the bloodstream. A purulent exudate is produced within the tube and may cause pelvic peritonitis. Chlamydial infection produces a similar picture except that it causes a predominantly lymphocytic infiltrate in the submucosa.[211,271,288]

Salpingitis also is caused by several other microbial agents that have been isolated directly from the fallopian tubes. The organisms most commonly recovered from the upper tract in salpingitis are mixed anaerobes (25-84%), followed by *N. gonorrhoeae* (25-40%) and *C. trachomatis* (25-40%). Mixed aerobic and anaerobic infections, including *Bacteroides* and *Peptostreptococcus* spp., account for 25 to 60 percent of cases. These mixed infections occur more frequently in girls and women with severe PID, chronic PID, and recurrent PID. PID develops in approximately 10 to 17 percent of girls and women with endocervical *N. gonorrhoeae* and in 10 to 30 percent with endocervical *C. trachomatis*. At first, researchers thought that *N. gonorrhoeae* initiated the infection and that superinfection with anaerobes followed. They now realize that apparently anaerobes and aerobes can initiate PID without *C. trachomatis* or *N. gonorrhoeae*.[73,74,76,252,288]

Differentiating salpingitis caused by different microbiologic organisms is difficult. *N. gonorrhoeae* has been identified most frequently within the initial 24 hours of development of symptoms. Beyond 48 hours, the most frequent isolates are anaerobes. Gonococcal and chlamydial salpingitis seem to occur most often within 1 week of menstruation.[272] The clinical presentation varies from asymptomatic to severe disease. The severity of infection depends on duration of symptoms and the etiologic agent. Chlamydial PID tends to be less symptomatic than infection from *N. gonorrhoeae*.

Diagnosis

The classic manifestation of acute PID is lower abdominal pain, which usually is bilateral and continuous and may worsen with movement. After the onset of abdominal pain, fever, nausea, and vomiting develop. The temperature may reach 39°C to 39.5°C (102°F-103°F). A chill seldom precedes the fever. Other common initial symptoms include vaginal discharge, irregular vaginal bleeding, and urinary symptoms.

On physical examination, the patient usually looks sick and uncomfortable. Abdominal examination reveals a markedly tender and often tense lower part of the abdomen. Rebound tenderness indicates generalized peritonitis. The genital examination may show a purulent vaginal discharge in the vaginal vault. Even gentle bimanual rectovaginal abdominal palpation causes great distress. Attempted mobilization of the cervix is extremely painful. The uterus is tense and tender. The adnexa may not be outlined because of discomfort produced by the examination. Palpation of the adnexa unilaterally or bilaterally may be exceptionally painful. An adnexal swelling may be palpated, but this finding is unreliable in diagnosing an adnexal mass. In a less acutely tender patient, the examination may reveal a thickened, tender tube.

Common laboratory findings in patients with PID include a peripheral white blood cell count greater than 10,000/mm³ and an erythrocyte sedimentation rate greater than 15 mm/hr. In addition, endocervical gonorrhea and chlamydial infection may be present simultaneously in 10 to 30 percent of cases. Ultrasonography of the pelvic cavity helps exclude adnexal masses and may detect pelvic abscesses. A study involving the use of pelvic ultrasonography in adolescents with PID showed that the presence of fluid in the cul-de-sac was not helpful in differentiating patients with and without PID.[99] Almost 20 percent of patients with PID had a tubo-ovarian abscess; in the absence of a tuboovarian abscess, adnexal volume was significantly larger in adolescents with PID than in adolescents without it.[99] Ultrasonography (transvaginal) can be very useful in ruling out other diagnoses and defining adnexal masses.

The clinical diagnosis of PID is made by having a high index of suspicion of this entity. The clinical criteria for the diagnosis of PID were developed originally by Jacobsen and Westrom.[141] The benefits of using laparoscopy are that an accurate diagnosis can be made rapidly by direct visualization of the fallopian tubes and adjacent structures,[141] tubal exudate can be obtained for culture, and the outcome of therapy can be evaluated.[292] This diagnostic method, however, is not without risks, is not a sensitive diagnostic tool, and adds to the cost of care.[81] For practical reasons, the clinical criteria developed by Jacobsen and Westrom[141] and revised by the Centers for Disease Control and Prevention[42] are recommended to aid in making the diagnosis and subsequently to increase the index of suspicion for PID (Table 48–5). When comparing the reliability of clinical criteria using endometrial sampling as the reference test,[42] the sensitivity of using one criterion—adnexal tenderness—was 95 percent, and the sensitivity of using three criteria—abdominal pain, cervical motion tenderness, and adnexal tenderness—was 83 percent.

The minimum criteria recommended for empiric treatment include abdominal pain with uterine tenderness or cervical

TABLE 48–5 Clinical Criteria for the Diagnosis of Acute Pelvic Inflammatory Disease

Minimal Criteria
Lower abdominal or pelvic pain with one or more of the following: uterine or adnexal tenderness or cervical motion tenderness

Additional Criteria to Enhance Specificity
Temperature >38.3°C (>101°F)
Abnormal cervical or vaginal mucopurulent discharge
Presence of white blood cells on saline microscopy of vaginal secretions
Elevation of erythrocyte sedimentation rate
Elevated C-reactive protein
Laboratory documentation of cervical infection with *Neisseria gonorrhoeae* or *Chlamydia trachomatis* or both

Specific Criteria
Endometrial biopsy specimen with histopathologic evidence of endometritis
Transvaginal sonography or magnetic resonance imaging technique showing thickened fluid-filled or tubo-ovarian complex
Laparoscopic abnormalities consistent with pelvic inflammatory disease

From Centers for Disease Control and Prevention: Sexually transmitted disease treatment guidelines 2006. M. M. W. R. Recomm. Rep. 55(RR-11):1-93, 2006.

motion tenderness or adnexal tenderness.[42] The more criteria that can be met, the more likely that a tubal infection is present. Clinicians who use only the criteria listed in Table 48–5 to treat would miss adolescents with mild disease, however.[42,106,141,280] The differential diagnosis of PID is an acute abdomen. Conditions of the urinary tract that should be considered include cystitis, pyelonephritis, and urethritis. Gastrointestinal tract conditions include appendicitis, constipation, diverticulitis, gastroenteritis, inflammatory bowel disease, and irritable bowel syndrome. Gynecologic conditions include dysmenorrhea, ectopic pregnancy, endometriosis, endometritis, mittelschmerz, torsion or rupture of an ovarian cyst, ruptured follicle, septic abortion, threatened abortion, and pyogenic sacroiliitis. Although pyogenic sacroiliitis is very rare, it was reported in a 13-year-old girl secondary to an infected umbilical ring.[152]

As in PID, establishing an early diagnosis of acute appendicitis and ectopic pregnancy is important. In acute appendicitis, an adolescent is more likely to have nausea, vomiting, a short history of right lower quadrant abdominal pain, lower grade fever, a higher leukocyte count in relation to the fever, and little discomfort during pelvic examination. Occasionally, the appendix hangs over the pelvic brim and causes pelvic tenderness. A ruptured appendix and peritonitis may simulate PID closely. Differentiating PID from ectopic pregnancy is less difficult if the history suggests pregnancy. PID can occur during the first trimester of pregnancy. In ectopic pregnancy, the patient does not have fever or leukocytosis. The symptoms almost always are unilateral, and signs of hemoperitoneum are present if the tube is ruptured.[288] If ectopic pregnancy is suspected, a serum pregnancy test and pelvic ultrasonography (transvaginal) for detection of a gestational sac should be performed immediately.

Treatment

The major goals of treatment of PID are preservation of fertility and prevention of other long-term sequelae, including ectopic pregnancy. Although some data suggest that women younger than 25 years old have a better fertility prognosis overall after having PID and ectopic pregnancy, no difference exists among age groups regarding tubal infertility specifically after PID.[288] The earlier the treatment is initiated, the lower the risk of developing infertility. Girls and women initially evaluated after more than 3 days of abdominal pain are found to have a 2.8-fold increased risk of having impaired fertility (tubal infertility or ectopic pregnancy) compared with those evaluated within 3 days of the onset of abdominal pain.[128] Generally, the more severe the PID, the higher the risk of future infertility occurring. In addition, the more episodes of PID, the higher the risk of future infertility occurring. After one episode, the risk of infertility ranges from 8 to 13 percent; after two episodes, the risk is 20 to 35 percent; and after three or more episodes, it is 40 to 75 percent.[252,270]

To reduce the incidence of sequelae associated with this condition, early recognition of PID, the use of broad-spectrum antibiotics to treat polymicrobial disease, careful clinical re-evaluation 48 hours after initiating antibiotic treatment to assess antibiotic response, and evaluation and treatment of sexual partners are important. Screening the patient for other STDs, such as trichomoniasis, bacterial vaginosis, and syphilis, also is important.

Patients with PID often are treated on an ambulatory basis. The primary reason to hospitalize an adolescent with PID is to ensure compliance with medication when she is unable to follow or tolerate an outpatient oral regimen because of the seriousness of the sequelae and problems with compliance in this age group. Other reasons for hospitalization are an uncertain diagnosis, the presence of a tubo-ovarian abscess, pregnancy, infection with HIV, temperature greater than 38.5° C, nausea and vomiting precluding the use of oral medications, and lack of improvement after 48 hours of oral antibiotic treatment.

The recommendations of the Centers for Disease Control and Prevention for treating PID in ambulatory and hospitalized patients address antibiotic coverage for the polymicrobial etiology of this condition (Tables 48–6 and 48–7).[42] In addition to antibiotic treatment, bed rest is recommended. Intravenous fluids are administered for hydration when necessary. When the diagnosis of PID is certain, oral analgesic agents may be prescribed. Close follow-up is recommended, with a bimanual examination performed after 48 hours of antibiotic treatment to assess the patient's response to treatment.[42] Overall, most studies show that response to antibiotic regimens is similar between HIV-positive and HIV-negative patients. The treatment recommendations for HIV-positive patients are no different.[259] Complications associated with PID are perihepatitis, tubo-ovarian abscess, hydrosalpinx (obstruction of the tube caused by scarring [Fig. 48–23]), chronic abdominal pain from adhesions surrounding the fallopian tubes and ovaries, recurrent PID, ectopic pregnancy, and infertility.[106,252]

PERIHEPATITIS

The classic manifestation of perihepatitis, or Fitz-Hugh–Curtis syndrome,[288] is severe right upper abdominal pain that often radiates to the shoulder. Concurrent left upper abdominal pain also may be present. Lower abdominal pain and evidence of acute or subacute PID are frequent findings. The right upper quadrant pain lasts about 48 hours. Nausea, fever, and leukocytosis are common manifestations. Elevation of the erythrocyte sedimentation rate and liver enzymes may be present. The pathogenesis of perihepatitis is thought to be from direct spread of *N. gonorrhoeae* and *C. trachomatis* from the fallopian tubes into the peritoneal cavity, along the paracolic sulci. From there, they reach the subphrenic space and hepatic surface. Spread from the reproductive tract also is possible via the retroperitoneal lymphatics.[288]

The diagnosis is made by having a high index of suspicion. Perihepatitis frequently mimics cholelithiasis, hepatitis, pleuritis, subphrenic abscess, perforated peptic ulcer, nephrolithiasis, appendicitis, ectopic pregnancy, abdominal trauma, and pancreatitis. Treatment of this condition is similar to treatment of PID.

TUBO-OVARIAN ABSCESS

The formation of a tubo-ovarian abscess is a late manifestation of PID. The incidence of tubo-ovarian abscess ranges from 14 to 38 percent in hospital-based adolescents and adults with salpingitis.[99,106,162,195,255] Although tubo-ovarian abscesses rarely are seen in adolescents and young women who are not sexually active,

TABLE 48–6   Ambulatory Management of Pelvic Inflammatory Disease

Ceftriaxone 250 mg IM in a single dose *or* cefoxitin 2 g IM in a single dose *plus* probenecid 1 g orally in a single dose *or* other parenteral third-generation cephalosporins (e.g., ceftizoxime or cefotaxime)
plus
Doxycycline 100 mg PO two times a day for 14 days
with or without
Metronidazole 500 mg PO twice a day for 14 days

From Centers for Disease Control and Prevention: Sexually transmitted disease treatment guidelines 2006. M. M. W. R. Recomm. Rep. 55(RR-11):1-93, 2006.

TABLE 48–7   Inpatient Treatment of Pelvic Inflammatory Disease

Regimen A
Cefoxitin 2 g IV every 6 hr *or* cefotetan 2 g IV every 12 hr
plus
Doxycycline 100 mg every 12 hr PO or IV

Regimen B
Clindamycin 900 mg IV every 8 hr
plus
Gentamicin loading dose IV or IM (2 mg/kg) followed by a maintenance dose (1.5 mg/kg) every 8 hr

Note: The above regimens are given for at least 24 hr after the patient improves. After discharge from the hospital, the patient is continued on doxycycline at 100 mg PO two times a day for a total of 14 days.
From Centers for Disease Control and Prevention: Sexually transmitted disease treatment guidelines 2002. M.M.W.R. Recomm. Rep. 55(RR-11): 1-93, 2006.

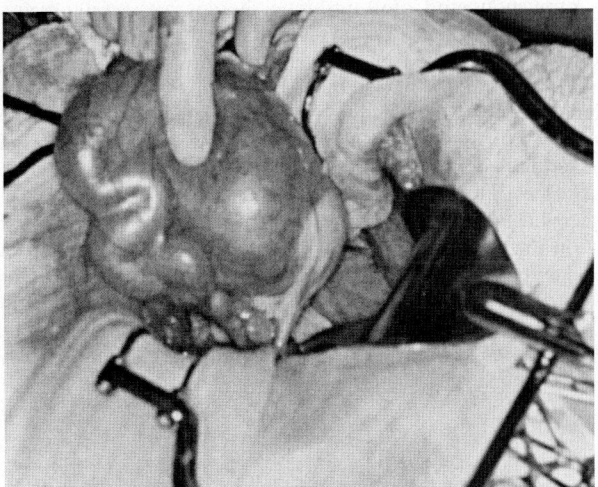

Figure 48–23 Large hydrosalpinx, the result of gonorrheal salpingitis in an older teenage girl who had repeated gonorrheal infections. The other tube also was diseased.

three case reports are in this group.[66] In two cases, *E. coli* and alpha-hemolytic streptococci were isolated, and in one case, *Pasteurella multocida* was isolated. The actual cause for ascending infection in these cases is unknown. Alterations in cervical secretions, which usually serve as a barrier, have been hypothesized. The abscess typically results from a mixture of facultative and anaerobic bacteria, with facultative bacteria dominating the early phase of infection, and bacterial metabolic products producing an environment of low oxygen tension that favors the growth of anaerobic bacteria.[288]

The most common organisms recovered from tubo-ovarian abscesses are *E. coli*, *Bacteroides fragilis*, other *Bacteroides* spp., *Peptostreptococcus*, *Peptococcus*, and aerobic streptococci.[222] Diagnosing the presence of a tubo-ovarian abscess clinically usually is difficult. Adolescents with a tubo-ovarian abscess tend to seek care later in their menstrual cycle (>18 days from the last menstrual period) than do girls without a tubo-ovarian abscess.[255] Bimanual examination frequently does not reveal a pelvic mass.[49] Four potentially useful clinical features that suggest the presence of a pelvic abscess are pain, persistent fever, adnexal tenderness (for >7 days), and an erythrocyte sedimentation rate greater than 30 mm/hr.[49] Ultrasonography of the pelvis is valuable in confirming the presence of an abscess.[99]

The prompt administration of antibiotics has reduced greatly the incidence of pelvic abscess. Most of those encountered today are in adolescents who have not had adequate care and have delayed seeking treatment.[106] Adolescents are far more likely to delay seeking treatment than are young women.[262]

A conservative approach is favored for the treatment of a tubo-ovarian or ovarian abscess (i.e., bed rest, supportive care, intravenous antibiotics).[252] The choice of antibiotics for treating tubo-ovarian abscess should include the following considerations: effectiveness against β-lactamase–producing anaerobes, adequate coverage against resistant *Bacteroides* spp., penetration into the abscess, and ability to remain stable in an abscess environment. The antibiotic regimens for inpatient treatment of PID fulfill these considerations and are appropriate for the treatment of tubo-ovarian abscess (see Table 48–7). As is the case with cefoxitin, cefotetan, and clindamycin, metronidazole provides good activity against anaerobes.[222] Many hospitals prefer the use of triple antibiotics: cefoxitin and gentamicin plus clindamycin or metronidazole.

A clinical response to treatment consisting of a decrease in pain, fever, and total leukocyte count should be noted in 72 hours. Pelvic ultrasonography should be repeated at this time to note any further increase in the size of the abscess. The duration of intravenous and oral antibiotic therapy for a tubo-ovarian abscess should be at least 21 days. The patient may begin oral antibiotics when she is afebrile and asymptomatic and when the size of the abscess has stabilized. The abscess either resolves without drainage or becomes an encapsulated pool of pus. The latter eventually "points" either in the cul-de-sac or anteriorly in the abdominal wall.

Surgical intervention may be needed in 25 percent of cases, either during the initial period or within a year, usually depending on the size of the abscess. An abscess larger than 10 cm has a 60 percent chance, a 7- to 9-cm abscess has a 35 percent chance, and a 4- to 6-cm abscess has a 20 percent chance of requiring surgical intervention. The fertility rate after treatment of tubo-ovarian abscesses may be 20 to 50 percent with conservative medical and surgical approaches.

OVARITIS AND OOPHORITIS

Ovaritis generally refers to inflammation of the ovaries, and *oophoritis* refers to inflammation of the substance of the ovaries, the oocytes in particular. Viral exanthems such as mumps and cytomegalovirus are complicated most frequently by ovaritis or oophoritis. Immunosuppressed children and adolescents are at risk for development of ovaritis and oophoritis. Improved immunization practices have decreased the prevalence of mumps ovaritis. The presence of an enlarged, tender, boggy, smooth mobile ovary in a child with mumps or one of the exanthems is an indication for repeated examinations and watchfulness. The ovary becomes less tender and gradually shrinks. Mumps ovaritis, in particular, may convert one or both ovaries into swellings that are 6 to 8 cm in diameter. The enlargement may persist for several months. Treatment is palliative, with analgesics given for discomfort and fever.[133]

REFERENCES

1. Ackerman, A. B., Goldfaden, G., and Cosmides, J. C.: Acquired syphilis in prepubertal children. Arch. Dermatol. *106*:92, 1972.
2. Adams, R.: A Formulary for Pediatric Skin Disease. Vol. 3. Philadelphia: W. B. Saunders, 1976.
3. Adu-Sarkodie, Y.: *Trichomonas vaginalis* transmission in a family. Genitourin. Med. *71*:199, 1995.
4. Aghajanian, A., Bernstein, L., and Grimes, D. A.: Bartholin's duct abscess and cyst: A case-control study. South. Med. J. *87*:26, 1994.
5. Al-Salihi, F. L., Curran, J. P., and Wang, J.: Neonatal *Trichomonas vaginalis*: Report of three cases and review of the literature. Pediatrics *53*:196, 1974.
6. Al-Tawfiq, J. A., Palmer, K. L., Chen, C.-Y., et al.: Experimental infection of human volunteers with *Haemophilus ducreyi* does not confer protection against subsequent challenge. J. Infect. Dis. *179*:1283, 1999.
7. Alergant, C.: Chancroid. Practitioner *209*:624, 1972.
8. Alexander, E. R.: Misidentification of sexually transmitted organisms in children: Medicolegal implications. Pediatr. Infect. Dis. *7*:1, 1988.
9. Alexander, W. J., Griffith, H., Housch, J. G., et al.: Infections in sexual contacts and associates of children with gonorrhea. Sex. Transm. Dis. *11*:156, 1983.
10. Alpsoy, E., Yilmaz, E., and Basaran, E.: Interferon therapy for Behcet disease. J. Am. Acad. Dermatol. *31*:617, 1994.
11. Altchek, A.: Vulvovaginitis, vulvar skin disease, and pelvic inflammatory disease. Pediatr. Clin. North Am. *28*:397, 1981.
12. Amsel, R., Totten, P. A., Speigel, C. A., et al.: Nonspecific vaginitis: Diagnostic criteria, microbial and epidemiologic assocations. Am. J. Med. *74*:14, 1983.
13. Andersen, P. G., Christensen, S., Detlefsen, G. J., et al.: Treatment of Bartholin's abcess: Marsupialization versus incision, curretage and suture under antibiotic cover: A randomized study with 6 months' follow up. Acta Obstet. Gynaecol. Scand. *71*:59, 1992.
14. Andrew, D., and Bumstead, E.: The role of fomites in the transmission of vaginitis. Can. Med. Assoc. J. *112*:1181, 1975.
15. Argent, A. C., Lachman, P. I., Hanslo, D., and Bass, D.: Sexually transmitted diseases in children and evidence of sexual abuse. Child Abuse Negl. *19*:1303, 1995.
16. Arya, O. P., Mallinson, H., and Goddard, A. D.: Epidemiological and clinical correlates of chlamydial infection of the cervix. Br. J. Vener. Dis. *57*:118, 1981.
17. Banov, L., Jr.: Rectal lesions of lymphogranuloma venereum in childhood. Am. J. Dis. Child. *83*:600, 1952.
18. Bartley, D. L., Morgan, L., and Rimsza, M. E.: *Gardnerella vaginalis* in prepubertal girls. Am. J. Dis. Child. *141*:1014, 1987.
19. Bass, H. N.: "Bubble bath" as an irritant to the urinary tract of children. Clin. Pediatr. *7*:174, 1968.
20. Bassa, A. G., Hoosen, A. A., Moodley, J.: Granuloma inguinale (donovanosis) in women: An analysis of 61 cases from Durban, South Africa. Sex. Transm. Dis. *20*:164, 1993.
21. Bell, T. A., Stamm, W. E., Wang, S. P., et al.: Chronic *Chlamydia trachomatis* infections in infants. J. A. M. A. *267*:400, 2001.
22. Berenson, A. B.: Adolescent gynecology. Obstet. Gynecol. Clin. North Am. *27*:1, 2000.
23. Black, C. M.: Current methods of laboratory diagnosis of *Chlamydia trachomatis* infections. Clin. Microbiol. *10*:160, 1997.
24. Blackmore, C. A., Limpakarnjanarat, K., Rigau-Perez, J. G., et al: An outbreak of chancroid in Orange County, California: Descriptive epidemiology and disease-control measures. J. Infect. Dis. *151*:840, 1985.
25. Bogaerts, J., Leparge, P., De Clercq, A., et al.: *Shigella* and gonococcal vulvovaginitis in prepubertal Central African girls. Pediatr. Infect. Dis. *11*:890, 1992.
26. Boisvert, P., and Walcher, D.: Hemolytic streptococcal vaginitis in children. Pediatrics *2*:24, 1948.
27. Branch, G., and Paxton, R.: A study of gonococcal infections among infants and children. Public Health Rep. *80*:347, 1965.
28. Braverman, P., and Polaneczky, M.: Adolescent gynecology, part I: Common disorders. Pediatr. Clin. North Am. *46*:489, 1999.
29. Braverman, P., and Polaneczky, M.: Adolescent gynecology, part II: The sexually active adolescent. Pediatr. Clin. North Am. *46*:649, 1999.

30. Breschi, L. C., Goldman, G., and Shapiro, S. R.: Granuloma inguinale in Vietnam. J. Am. Vener. Dis. Assoc. *1*:118, 1975.

31. Bridgen, M., and Guard, R.: Extragenital granuloma inguinale in North Queensland. Med. J. Aust. *2*:565, 1980.

32. Brown, J. L.: Hair shampooing technique and pediatric vulvovaginitis. Pediatrics *83*:146, 1989.

33. Brown-Harrison, M. C., Christenson, J. C., Harrison, A. M., and Matlak, M. E.: Group A streptococcal salpingitis in a prepubertal girl. Clin. Pediatr. (Phila.) *34*:556, 1995.

34. Brunham, R. C., Paavonen, J., Stevens, C. E., et al.: Mucopurulent cervicitis: The ignored counterpart in women of urethritis in men. N. Engl. J. Med. *311*:1, 1984.

35. Bukusi, E. A., Cohen, C. R., Stevens, C. E., et al.: Effects of human immunodeficiency virus 1 infection on microbial origins of pelvic inflammatory disease and on efficacy of ambulatory oral therapy. Am. J. Obstet. Gynecol. *181*:1374, 1999.

36. Bulletin: Oncogenic potential of new herpes simplex therapy in FDA. F. D. A. Drug Bull. *5*:3, 1975.

37. Bump, R. C.: *Chlamydia trachomatis* as a cause of prepubertal vaginitis. Obstet. Gynecol. *65*:384, 1985.

38. Bump, R. C., and Buesching, W. J.: Bacterial vaginosis in virginal and sexually active adolescent females: Evidence against exclusive sexual transmission. Am. J. Obstet. Gynecol. *158*:935, 1988.

39. Burgess, J. A.: *Trichomonas vaginalis* infection from splashing in water closets. Br. J. Vener. Dis. *39*:248, 1963.

40. Burry, V.: Gonococcal vulvovaginitis and possible peritonitis in prepubertal girls. Am. J. Dis. Child. *121*:536, 1971.

41. Centers for Disease Control and Prevention: Division of STD/HIV Prevention: Sexually Transmitted Disease Surveillance. Atlanta, U.S. Department of Health and Human Services, Public Health Service, 1994.

42. Centers for Disease Control and Prevention: Sexually transmitted disease treatment guidelines 2006. M. M. W. R. Recomm. Rep. *55*(RR-11):1-93, 2006.

43. Centers for Disease Control and Prevention: Updated recommended treatment regimens for gonococcal infections and associated conditions—United States. April 2007. Available at www.cdc.gov/std/treatment/2006/updated-regimens.htm.

44. Chacko, M. R., and Lovchik, J. C.: *Chlamydia trachomatis* infection in sexually active adolescents: Prevalence and risk factors. Pediatrics *73*:836, 1984.

45. Chang, T.: Genital herpes, the source of infection. Int. J. Dermatol. *14*:201, 1975.

46. Charles, S. X.: Epidemiology of *Trichomonas vaginalis* in rural adolescent and juvenile children. J. Trop. Pediatr. *37*:90, 1991.

47. Cohen, B. A., Honig, P., and Androphy, E.: Anogenital warts in children. Arch. Dermatol. *126*:1575, 1990.

48. Corey, L., and Ward, A.: Genital herpes. *In* Holmes, K. K., Sparling, P. F., Mardh, P. A., et al. (eds.): Sexually Transmitted Diseases. New York, McGraw-Hill, 1999.

49. Cromer, B. A., Brandstaetter, L. A., Fischer, R. A., et al.: Tubo-ovarian abscess in adolescents. Adolesc. Pediatr. Gynecol. *3*:21, 1990.

50. Crowther, I.: Trichomonas vaginitis in infancy. Lancet *1*:1074, 1962.

51. Cuadros, J., Mazon, A., Martinez, R., et al.: The aetiology of paediatric inflammatory vulvovaginitis. Eur. J. Pediatr. *163*:105, 2004.

52. Cummins, A. J., and Atia, W. A.: Bartholin's abscess complicating food poisoning with *Salmonella panama*: A case report. Genitourin. Med. *70*:46, 1994.

53. Daher, A., and Fortenberry, J. D.: *Staphylococcus*-induced toxic shock following balanitis. Clin. Pediatr. *34*:172, 1995.

54. Danesh, I. S., Stephen, J. M., and Gorbach, J.: Neonatal *Trichomonas vaginalis* infection. J. Emerg. Med. *13*:51, 1995.

55. Danielsson, I., Sjoberg, I., and Wikman, M.: Vulvar vestibulitis: Medical, psychosexual and psychosocial aspects, a case control study. Acta Obstet. Gynecol. Scand. *79*:872, 2000.

56. Davies, J. A., Res, E., and Hobson, D.: Isolation of *Chlamydia trachomatis* from Bartholin's ducts. Br. J. Vener. Dis. *54*:409, 1978.

57. Davis, A. M., and Emans, S. J.: Human papilloma virus in the pediatric and adolescent patients. J. Pediatr. *115*:1, 1989.

58. Davis, B.: Deodorant vulvitis. Obstet. Gynecol. *36*:812, 1970.

59. DeJong, A. R.: Sexually transmitted diseases in sexually abused children. Sex. Transm. Dis. *13*:123, 1986.

60. Deliyanni, V. A., Boniastsi, L. S., and Photinou, A. S.: Balanitis caused by group A beta-hemolytic streptococcus in an 8-year-old boy. Pediatr. Infect. Dis. J. *8*:61, 1989.

61. Demetriou, E., Emans, S. J., and Masland, R. P.: Dysuria in adolescent girls: Urinary tract infection or vaginitis? Pediatrics *70*:299, 1982.

62. Dewhurst, C. J.: Practical Pediatric and Adolescent Gynecology. New York, Marcel Dekker, 1980.

63. Dhall, K., Das, S. S., and Dey, P.: Tuberculosis of Bartholin's gland. Int. J. Gynaecol. Obstet. *48*:223, 1995.

64. Dhar, V., Roker, K., Adhami, Z., et al.: Streptococcal vulvovaginitis in girls. Pediatr. Dermatol. *10*:366, 1993.

65. Dodson, R. F., Fritz, G. S., Hubler, W. R., et al.: Donovanosis: A morphologic study. J. Invest. Dermatol. *62*:611, 1974.

66. Dogan, E., Altuyurt, S., Altindog, T., et al.: Tubo-ovarian abscess mimicking ovarian tumor in a sexually inactive girl. J. Pediatr. Adolesc. Gynecol. *17*:351, 2004.

67. Donald, F. E., Slack, D. B., and Colman, G.: *Streptococcus pyogenes* vulvovaginitis in children in Nottingham. Epidemiol. Infect. *106*:459, 1991.

68. Duerden, B. I.: Black-pigmented gram-negative anaerobes in genito-urinary tract and pelvic infections. F. E. M. S. Immunol. Med. Microbiol. *6*:223, 1993.

69. Duhra, P., and Ilchyshyn, A.: Perianal streptococcal cellulitis with penile involvement. Br. J. Dermatol. *123*:793, 1990.

70. Eigen, L.: Vaginal diphtheria. J. Med. Assoc. N. J. *29*:778, 1932.

71. Emans, S. J.: Office evaluation of the child and adolescent. *In* Emans, S. J. H., Laufer, M. R., and Goldstein, D. P. (eds.): Pediatric and Adolescent Gynecology. 5th ed. Philadelphia, Lippincott-Raven, 2005.

72. Emans, S. J.: Vulvovaginal problems in the prepuberatal child. *In* Emans, S. J. H., Laufer, M. R., and Goldstein, D. P. (eds.): Pediatric and Adolescent Gynecology. 5th ed. Philadelphia, Lippincott-Raven, 2005.

73. Emans, S. J. H., Laufer, M. R., and Goldstein, D. P. (eds.): Pediatric and Adolescent Gynecology. 5th ed. Philadelphia, Lippincott-Raven, 2005.

74. Emans, S. J. H., Laufer, M. R., and Goldstein, D. P.: The gynecologic examination of the prepubertal child with vulvovagintis: Use of the knee-chest position. Pediatrics *65*:758, 1980.

75. Escala, J. M., and Rickwood, A. M.: Balanitis. Br. J. Urol. *63*:196, 1989.

76. Eschenbach, D. A.: Acute pelvic inflammatory disease. Urol. Clin. North Am. *11*:65, 1984.

77. Fallon, P., and Robinson, E. T.: Meningococcal vulvovaginitis. Scand. J. Infect. Dis. *6*:295, 1974.

78. Fergusson, D. M., Lawton, J. M., and Shannon, F. T.: Neonatal circumcision and penile problems: An 8-year longitudinal survey. Pediatrics *81*:537, 1988.

79. Figueroa-Colon, R., Grunow, J. E., Torres-Pinedo, T., et al.: Group A streptococcal proctitis and vulvovaginitis in a prepubertal girl. Pediatr. Infect. Dis. J. *3*:439, 1984.

80. Fink, C. W.: A perineal rash in Kawasaki disease. Pediatr. Infect. Dis. J. *2*:140, 1983.

81. Fischer, G., and Rogers, M.: Vulvar disease in children: A clinical audit of 130 cases. Pediatr. Dermatol. *17*:1, 2000.

82. Fisher, M., Swenson, P. D., Risucci, D., et al.: *Chlamydia trachomatis* in suburban adolescents. J. Pediatr. *111*:617, 1987.

83. Folland, D. S., Burke, R. E., Hinman, A. R., et al.: Gonorrhea in preadolescent children: An inquiry into source of infection and mode of transmission. Pediatrics *60*:153, 1977.

84. Forssner, H.: Vaginaltresia mit diptherischer pathogenese. Acta Med. Scand. *59*:690, 1923.

85. Frazer, J. J., Rettig, P. J., and Kaplan, D. W.: Prevalence of cervical *Chlamydia trachomatis* and *Neisseria gonorrhoeae* in female adolescents. Pediatrics *71*:333, 1983.

86. Freinkel, A. L.: Granuloma inguinale of cervical lymph nodes simulating tuberculous lymphadenitis: Two case reports and review of published reports. Genitourin. Med. *64*:339, 1988.

87. Friedrich, E.: Vulvar Disease: Recognition and Treatment (Major Problems in Obstetrics and Gynecology). Philadelphia: W. B. Saunders, 1976.

88. Fuld, G.: Gonococcal peritonitis in a prepubertal child. Am. J. Dis. Child. *115*:621, 1968.

89. Fuster, C., and Neinstein, L. S.: Vaginal *Chlamydia trachomatis*: Prevalence in sexually abused pubertal girls. Pediatrics *79*:235, 1987.

90. Gardner, H.: The vulvovaginitides (new interpretation and treatment methods). *In* Traymor, M., and Green, T., Jr. (eds.): Progress in Gynecology, Vol. 6. New York, Grune & Stratton, 1975.

91. Gardner, H., and Dukes, C.: A newly defined specific infection previously classified "non-specific" vaginitis. Am. J. Obstet. Gynecol. *69*:962, 1955.

92. Gardner, H. L.: Hemophilus vaginalis after twenty-five years. Am. J. Obstet. Gynecol. *137*:385, 1980.

93. Gardner, J. J.: Comparison of the vaginal flora in sexually abused and non-abused girls. J. Pediatr. *120*:872, 1992.

94. Gardner, M., and Jones, J. G.: Genital herpes acquired by sexual abuse of children. J. Pediatr. *104*:243, 1984.

95. Gerstner, G. J., Grunberger, W., Boschitsch, E., et al.: Vaginal organisms in prepubertal children with and without vulvovaginitis. Arch. Gynecol. *231*:247, 1982.

96. Gilbaugh, J. H., and Fuchs, P. C.: The gonococcus and the toilet seat. N. Engl. J. Med. *301*:91, 1979.

97. Ginsberg, C. M.: Group A stretococcal vaginitis in children. Pediatr. Infect. Dis. J. *1*:36, 1982.

98. Goh, B. T., and Forster, G. E.: Sexually transmitted diseases in children: *Chlamydia* oculo-genital infection. Genitourin. Med. *69*:213, 1993.

99. Golden, N., Cohen, H., Gennari, G., et al.: The use of pelvic ultrasonography in evaluation of adolescents with pelvic inflammatory disease. Am. J. Dis. Child. *141*:1235, 1987.

100. Grace, D. A., Ochsner, J. A., McLain, C. R., et al.: Vulvar condylomata acuminata in prepubertal females. J. A. M. A. *201*:151, 1967.

101. Gray, L. A., and Kutcher, E.: Vulvovaginitis in childhood. Clin. Obstet. Gynecol. *3*:165, 1960.

102. Gregory, J. E., and Abramson, E.: Meningococci in vaginitis. Am. J. Dis. Child. *121*:423, 1971.

103. Grosskurth, H., Mosha, F., Todd, J., et al.: Impact of improved treatment of sexually transmitted diseases on HIV infection in rural Tanzania: Randomised controlled trial. Lancet *346*:530, 1995.

104. Growden, W., Lebherz, T. B., and Moore, J. G.: Granuloma inguinale in a white teenager: A diagnosis easily forgotten, poorly pursued. West. J. Med. *143*:105, 1985.
105. Guerrero-Vasquez, J., Sebastian-Planes, M., and Olmedo-Sanlaureno, S.: Group A streptococcal proctitis and balantitis. Pediatr. Infect. Dis. J. *9*:223, 1990.
106. Hager, W. D.: Followup of patients with tubo-ovarian abcess(es) in association with salpingitis. Obstet. Gynecol. *61*:680, 1983.
107. Hammerschlag, M.: Sexually transmitted diseases in sexually abused children: Medical and legal implications. Sex. Transm. Infect. *74*:167, 1998.
108. Hammerschlag, M. R., Doraiswamy, B., Cox, P., et al.: Colonization of sexually abused children with genital mycoplasmas. Sex. Transm. Dis. *14*:23, 1987.
109. Hammerschlag, M. R.: *Chlamydia trachomatis* in children. Pediatr. Ann. *23*:349, 1994.
110. Hammerschlag, M. R., Cummings, M., Doraiswamy, B., et al.: Nonspecific vaginitis following sexual abuse in children. Pediatrics *75*:1028, 1985.
111. Hammerschlag, M. R., Doraiswamy, B., Alexander E. R., et al.: Are rectogenital chlamydial infections a marker of sexual abuse in children? Pediatr. Infect. Dis. J. *3*:100, 1984.
112. Hammerschlag, M. R., Rettig, P. J., and Shields, M. E.: False-positive results with the use of chlamydial antigen detection tests in the evaluation of suspected sexual abuse in children. Pediatr. Infect. Dis. J. *7*:11, 1988.
113. Hammerschlag, M. R., Alpert, S., Onderdonk, A. B., et al.: Anaerobic microflora of the vagina in children. Am. J. Obstet. Gynecol. *131*:853, 1978.
114. Hammerschlag, M. R., Alpert, S., Rosner, I., et al.: Microbiology of the vagina in children: Normal and potentially pathogenic organisms. Pediatrics *62*:57, 1978.
115. Hammond, G. W., Slutchuk, M., Scatliff, J., et al.: Epidemiologic, clinical, laboratory, and therapeutic features of an urban outbreak of chancroid in North America. Rev. Infect. Dis. *2*:867, 1980.
116. Hare, M., and Mowla, A.: Genital herpesvirus infection in a prepubertal girl. Br. J. Dermatol. Gynaecol. *84*:141, 1977.
117. Hassoun, A., Jacquette, G., Huang, A., et al.: Female genital tuberculosis: Uncommon presentation of tuberculosis in the United States. Am. J. Med. *118*:1295, 2005.
118. Haydock, A. K., Martin, D. H., Morse, S. A., et al.: Molecular characterization of *Haemophilus ducreyi* strains from Jackson, Mississippi, and New Orleans, Louisiana. J. Infect. Dis. *179*:1423, 1999.
119. Hedlund, P.: Acute vulvovaginitis in patients with streptococcal infections. Nord. Med. *49*:566, 1953.
120. Heller, R. H., Joseph, J. M., and Davis, H. J.: Vulvovaginitis in the premenarcheal child. J. Pediatr. *74*:370, 1969.
121. Hellgren, L.: Gonorre-tonsillit efter genitooral kontakt. Lakartidningen *68*:569, 1971.
122. Henderson, P., and Scott, R.: Foreign body vaginitis caused by toilet tissue. Am. J. Dis. Child. *111*:529, 1966.
123. Herman-Giddens, M. E., Gutman, L. T., and Berson, N. L.: Association of coexisting vaginal infections and multiple abusers in female children with genital warts. Sex. Transm. Dis. *1*:63, 1987.
124. Herzog, L. W., and Alvarez, S. R.: The frequency of foreskin problems in uncircumcised children. Am. J. Dis. Child. *140*:254, 1986.
125. Hewitt, A. B.: Behcet's disease. Br. J. Vener. Dis. *47*:52, 1971.
126. Hill, G. B., Eschenbach, D. A., and Holmes, K. K.: Bacteriology of the vagina. Scand. J. Urol. Nephrol. *86*(Suppl.):23, 1984.
127. Hill, G. B., St. Claire, K. K., and Gutman, L. T.: Anaerobes predominate among the vaginal microflora of prepubertal girls. Clin. Infect. Dis. *20*(Suppl. 2):269, 1995.
128. Hillis, S. D., Joesoef, R., Marchbanks, P. A., et al.: Delayed care of pelvic inflammatory disease as a risk factor for impaired fertility. Am. J. Obstet. Gynecol. *168*:1503, 1993.
129. Holmes, K. K., Sparling, P. F., Stamm, W. E., et al.: Sexually Transmitted Diseases. New York, McGraw-Hill Medical, 2008.
130. Holmes, K. K., and Stamm, W. E.: Lower genital tract infection syndromes in women. *In* Holmes, K. K., Sparling, P. F., Stamm, W. E., et al.: Sexually Transmitted Diseases. New York, McGraw-Hill Medical, 2008.
131. Holzman, C., Levnthal, J. M., Qiu, H., et al.: Factors linked to bacterial vaginosis in nonpregnant women. Am. J. Public Health *91*:1664, 2001.
132. Hsieh, W. S., Yang, P. H., Chao, H. C., and Lai, J. Y.: Neonatal necrotizing fasciitis: A report of three cases and review of the literature. Pediatrics *103*:e53, 1999.
133. Huffman, J. W.: Gynecologic infections in childhood and adolescence. *In* Feigin, R. D., and Cherry, J. D. (eds.): Textbook of Pediatric Infectious Diseases. Vol. 2. Philadelphia, W. B. Saunders, 1987.
134. Huffman, J. W., Dewhurst, C. J., and Capraro, V. J.: The Gynecology of Childhood and Adolescence. Vol. 2. Philadelphia, W. B. Saunders, 1981.
135. Hyman, R., Fukushima,. M., Diamond, L., et al.: Microbes on the human vaginal epithelium. Science *102*:7952, 2005.
136. Ingram, D., Runyan, D. K., Collins, A. D., et al.: Sexual contact in children with gonorrhea. Am. J. Dis. Child. *136*:994, 1982.
137. Ingram, D., Runyan, D. K., Collins, A. D., et al.: Vaginal *Chlamydia trachomatis* infection in children with sexual contact. Pediatr. Infect. Dis. J. *3*:97, 1984.
138. Ingram, D. L.: *Neisseria gonorrhoeae* in children. Pediatr. Ann. *23*:341, 1994.
139. Ingram, D. L., Everett, V. D., Lyna, P. R., et al.: Epidemiology of adult sexually transmitted disease agents in children being evaluated for sexual abuse. Pediatr. Infect. Dis. J. *11*:945, 1992.
140. Ingram, D. L., White, S. T., Occhiuti, A. R., et al.: Childhood vaginal infections: Association of *Chlamydia trachomatis* with sexual contact. Pediatr. Infect. Dis. J. *5*:226, 1986.
141. Jacobsen, L., and Westrom, L.: Objectivized diagnosis of acute pelvic inflammatory disease. Am. J. Obstet. Gynecol. *105*:1088, 1969.
142. Jaquiery, A., Stylianopoulos, A., Hogg, G., et al.: Vulvovaginitis: Clinical features, aetiology, and microbiology of the genital tract. Arch. Dis. Child. *81*:64, 1999.
143. Jones, J. G., Yamauchi, T., and Lambert, B.: *Trichomonas vaginalis* infestation in sexually abused girls. Am. J. Dis. Child. *139*:846, 1985.
144. Jones, R. B., Mammel, J. B., Shepard, M. K., et al.: Recovery of *Chlamydia trachomatis* from the endometrium of women at risk for chlamydial infection. Am. J. Obstet. Gynecol. *155*:35, 1986.
145. Joseph, A. K., and Rosen, T.: Laboratory techniques used in the diagnosis of chancroid, granuloma inguinale, and lymphogranuloma venereum. Dermatol. Clin. *12*:1, 1994.
146. Kaplan, K. M., Fleisher, G. R., Paradise, J. E., et al.: Social relevance of genital herpes simplex in children. Am. J. Dis. Child. *138*:872, 1984.
147. Kaydos, S. C., Swygard, H., Wise, S. L., et al.: Development and validation of a PCR-based enzyme-linked immunosorbent assay with urine for use in clinical research settings to detect *Trichomonas vaginalis* in women. J. Clin. Microbiol. *40*:89, 2002.
148. Keith, L. G., Berger, G. S., Edelman, D. A., et al.: On the causation of pelvic inflammatory disease. Am. J. Obstet. Gynecol. *149*:215, 1984.
149. Kessel, J. F., and Thomspon, C. F.: Survival of *Trichomonas vaginalis* infestation in vaginal dischare. Proc. Soc. Exp. Biol. Med. *74*:755, 1950.
150. Kim, D. K., Chang, S. N., Bang, D., et al.: Clinical analysis of 40 cases of childhood-onset Behcet's disease. Pediatr. Dermatol. *11*:95, 1994.
151. Kirkpatrick, D.: Donovanosis (granuloma inguinale): A rare cause of osteolytic bone lesions. Clin. Radiol. *21*:101, 1970.
152. Kives, S., and Lara-Torre, E.: Pyogenic sacroiliitis following an infected umbilical ring. Pediatr. Adolesc. Gynecol. *17*:125, 2004.
153. Klebanoff, M. A., Carey, C. J., Hauth, J. C., et al.: Failure of metronidazole to prevent preterm delivery among pregnant women wih asymptomatic *Trichomonas vaginalis* infection. N. Engl. J. Med. *345*:487, 2001.
154. Kokx, N., Comstock, J. A., and Facklam, R. R.: Streptococcal perianal disease in children. Pedatrics *80*:659, 1987.
155. Kone-Paut, I., Yurdakul, S., Bahabri, S. A., et al.: Clinical features of Behcet disease in children: An international collaborative study of 86 cases. J. Pediatr. *132*:721, 1998.
156. Krech, T., Gerhard-Fsadni, D., Hoffman, N., et al.: Interference of *Staphylococcus aureus* in the detection of *Chlamydia trachomatis* by monoclonal antibodies. Lancet *1*:1161, 1985.
157. Krieger, J. N., Tam, M. R., and Stevens, C. E.: Diagnosis of trichomoniasis: Comparison of conventional wet-mount examination with cytologic studies, cultures, and monoclonal antibody staining of direct specimens. J. A. M. A. *259*:1223, 1988.
158. Krowchuk, D., Anglin, T. M., Lembo, R. M., et al.: Use of enzyme immunoassay for the rapid diagnosis of *Chlamydia trachomatis* endocervical infection in female adolescents. J. Adolesc. Health Care *9*:296, 1988.
159. Kurnatowska, A., and Komorowska, A.: Urogenital trichomoniasis in children. *In* Honigsberg, B. M. (ed.): Trichomonads Parasites in Humans. New York, Springer-Verlag, 1989.
160. Kyriazi, N., and Costenbader, C. L.: Group A beta-hemolytic streptococcal balanitis: It may be more common than you think. Pediatrics *88*:154, 1991.
161. Lal, S., and Nicholas, C.: Epidemiological and clinical features in 165 cases of granuloma inguinale. Br. J. Vener. Dis. *465*:461, 1970.
162. Landers, D., and Sweet, R. L.: Tubo-ovarian abcess: Contemporary approach to management. Rev. Infect. Dis. *5*:876, 1983.
163. Lang, W.: Pediatric vaginitis. N. Engl. J. Med. *253*:1153, 1955.
164. Larsen, B., and Galask, R. P.: Vaginal microbial flora: Composition and influences of host physiology. Ann. Intern. Med. *96*:926, 1982.
165. Larsen, B., and Monif, G. R. G.: Understanding the bacterial flora of the female genital tract. Clin. Infect. Dis. *32*:e69, 2001.
166. Larson, J., Kaye, J. M., Jewers, R. J., et al.: Perinatal transmission and persistence of human papillomavirus types 16 and 18 in infants. J. Med. Virol. *47*:209, 1995.
167. Larson, T., and Bryson, Y. J.: Fomites and herpes simplex virus. J. Infect. Dis. *151*:746, 1985.
168. Lee, Y.-H., Rankin, J. S., Alpert, S., et al.: Microbiological investigation of Bartholin's gland abscesses and cysts. Am. J. Obstet. Gynecol. *129*:150, 1977.
168a. Lindegren, M. L., Hanson, C., Hammett, T. A., et al.: Sexual abuse of children. Intersection with HIV epidemic. Pediatrics *102*:e46, 1998.
169. Littlewood, J. M., and Kohler, H. G.: Urinary tract infection by *Trichomonas vaginalis* in a newborn baby. Arch. Dis. Child. *41*:693, 1966.
170. Lynch, P.: Molluscum contagiosum venereum. Clin. Obstet. Gynecol. *15*:966, 1972.
171. Majewski, S., Pniewski, T., Malejczyk, M., and Jablonska, S.: Imiquimod is highly effective for extensive, hyperproliferative condyloma in children. Pediatr. Dermatol. *20*:440, 2003.
172. Mardh, P.-A., and Stenberg, K.: Long-term vaginal carriage of chlamydia? Lancet *1*:804, 1987.
173. Marinoff, S. C., and Turner, M. L. C.: Vulvar vestibulitis syndrome: An overview. Am. J. Obstet. Gynecol. *165*:1228, 1991.

174. Markowitz, L. E., Dunne, E. F., Saraiya, M., et al.: Centers for Disease Control and Prevention (CDC); Advisory Committee on Immunization Practices (ACIP): Quadrivalent human papillomavirus vaccine: Recommendations of the Advisory Committee on Immunization Practices (ACIP). M. M. W. R. Morb. Mortal. Wkly. Rep. 56:1, 2007.

175. McCormack, W. M.: Clinical spectrum of gonococcal infection in women. Lancet 2:1182, 1977.

176. McCormack, W. W., Alpert, S. A., McComb, D. E., et al.: Fifteen-month follow-up study of women infected with Chlamydia trachomatis. N. Engl. J. Med. 300:123, 1979.

177. McFarlane, D. E., and Sharma, D. P.: Haemophilus influenzae and genital tract infections in children. Acta Paediatr. Scand. 76:363, 1987.

178. McLaren, L. C., Davis, L. E., Healy, G. R., and James, C. G.: Isolation of Trichomonas vaginalis from the respiratory tract of infants with respiratory disease. Pediatrics 71:888, 1983.

179. Mishaw, C. O.: Sexual abuse and sexually transmitted diseases in prepubertal children. Semin. Pediatr. Infect. Dis. 4:131, 1993.

180. Mogielnicki, N. P., Schwartzman, J. D., and Elliott, J. A.: Perineal group A streptococcal disease in a pediatric practice. Pediatrics 106:276, 2000.

181. Monacelli, M., and Nazzaro, P.: Behcet's Disease. New York, S. Karger, 1966.

182. Morris, C. A.: Seasonal variation of streptococcal vulvo-vaginitis in an urban community. J. Clin. Pathol. 24:805, 1971.

183. Morrison, J. C., and Fish, S. A.: Adolescent genital dermatoses. South. Med. J. 69:1136, 1976.

184. Moscicki, A. B., Hills, N., Shiboski, S., et al.: Risks for incident human papilloma virus infection and low-grade squamous intraepithelial lesion development in young females. J. A. M. A. 285:2995, 2001.

185. Moscicki, A. B., Shiboski, S., Broering, J., et al.: The natural history of human papillomavirus infection as measured by repeated DNA testing in adolescent and young women. J. Pediatr. 132:277, 1998.

186. Moscicki, B., Shafer, M. A., Millstein, S. G., et al.: The use and limitations of endocervical gram stains and mucopurulent cervicitis as predictors for Chlamydia trachomatis in female adolescents. Am. J. Obstet. Gynecol. 157:65, 1987.

187. Mroczkowski, T., and Martin, D. H.: Genital ulcer disease. Dermatol. Clin. 12:753, 1994.

188. Muram, D., Savage, M. O., Harries, J. T., et al.: Crohn's disease of the vulva in a prepubertal girl. Pediatr. Adolesc. Gynecol. 1:189, 1983.

189. Murphy, T. V., and Nelson, J. D.: Shigella vaginitis: Report of 38 patients and review of the literature. Pediatrics 63:511, 1979.

190. Nahamias, A.: Herpes simplex infection. In Gellis, S., and Kagan, B. (eds.): Current Pediatric Therapy 7. Philadelphia, W. B. Saunders, 1976.

191. Nahamias, A., Dowdle, W. R., Naib, Z. M., et al.: Genital infection with herpes virus hominis types 1 and 2 in children. Pediatrics 42:659, 1968.

192. Nair, P., Glazer-Semmel, E., Gould, C., et al.: Neisseria gonorrhoeae in asymptomatic prepubertal household contacts of children with gonococcal infection. Clin. Pediatr. 25:160, 1986.

193. Nair, S., and Schoeneman, M. J.: Acute glomerulonephritis with group A streptococcal vulvovaginitis. Clin. Pediatr. 39:721, 2000.

194. Namavar, J. B., Parsanezhad, M. E., and Grane-Shirazi, R.: Female genital tuberculosis and infertility. Int. J. Gynaecol. Obstet. 75:269, 2001.

195. Nebel, W. A., and Lucas, W. E.: Management of tubo-ovarian abcess. Obstet. Gynecol. 32:382, 1968.

196. Neinstein, L. S., Goldenring, J., and Carpenter, S.: Nonsexual transmission of sexually transmitted diseases: An infrequent occurrence. Pediatrics 74:67, 1984.

197. Nelson, J. D., and Bradley, J. S. (eds.): Nelson's Pocket Book of Pediatric Antimicrobial Therapy. 15th ed. Philadelphia, Lippincott Williams & Wilkins, 2002.

198. Ness, R. B., Soper, D. E., Holley, R. L., et al.: Douching and endometritis: Results from the PID Evaluation And Clinical Health (PEACH) study. Sex. Transm. Dis. 28:240, 2001.

199. O'Duffy, J. D., Carney, J. A., and Deodhar, S.: Behcet's disease. Ann. Intern. Med. 75:561, 1971.

200. O'Farrell, N.: Clinico-epidemiological study of donovanosis in Durban, South Africa. Genitourin. Med. 69:108, 1993.

201. O'Farrell, N.: Global eradication of donovanosis: An opportunity for limiting the spread of HIV-1 infection. Genitourin. Med. 71:27, 1995.

202. O'Farrell, N.: Donovanosis. In Holmes, K., Sparling, P. F., and Mardh, P. A. (eds.): Sexually Transmitted Disease. New York, McGraw-Hill, 1999.

203. O'Farrell, N., Hoosen, A. A., and Coetzee, K. D.: Genital ulcer disease: Accuracy of clinical diagnosis and strategies to improve control in Durban, South Africa. Genitourin. Med. 70:7, 1994.

204. Okada, A.: Behcet's disease: General concepts and recent advances. Curr. Opin. Ophthalmol. 17:551, 1996.

205. Orden, B., Martin, R., Franco, A., et al.: Balanitis caused by group A beta-hemolytic streptococci. Pediatr. Infect. Dis. J. 15:920, 1984.

206. Orellana-Diaz, O., and Hernandez-Perez, E.: Chancroid in El Salvador. Int. J. Dermatol. 27:243, 1988.

207. Owen, R., Christiansen, G., Hansen, E., et al.: Reports from the working groups at the Symposium on Bacterial Vaginosis: Taxonomy of anaerobic curved rods. Scand. J. Urol. Nephrol. 86(Suppl.):259, 1984.

208. Pacor, M. L., Biasi, D., Lundardi, C., et al.: Cyclosporin in Behcet's disease: Results in 16 patients after 24 months of therapy. Clin. Rheumatol. 13:224, 1994.

209. Paradise, J. E., Campos, J. M., and Friedman, H. M.: Vulvovaginitis in premenarcheal girls: Clinical features and diagnostic evaluation. Pediatrics 70:193, 1982.

210. Patrizi, A., Costa, A. M., Fiorillo, L., et al.: Perianal stretococcal dermatitis associated with guttate psoriasis and/or balanoposthitis: A study of five cases. Pediatr. Dermatol. 11:168, 1994.

211. Patton, D. C.: Immunopathology and histopathology of experimental chlamydial salpingitis. Rev. Infect. Dis. 7:746, 1985.

212. Peter, R., and Vesely, K.: Kindergynakologie. Leipzig, Germany, Georg Thieme, 1966.

213. Pierce, A. M., and Hart, C. A.: Vulvovaginitis: Causes and management. Arch. Dis. Child. 67:509, 1992.

214. Pokorny, S.: Prepubertal vulvovaginopathies. Obstet. Gynecol. Clin. North Am. 19:39, 1992.

215. Porder, K., Sanchez, N., Roblin, P. M., et al.: Lack of specificity of Chlamydiazyme for detection of vaginal chlamydial infection in prepubertal girls. Pediatr. Infect. Dis. J. 8:385, 1989.

216. Postlethwaite, R.: Trichomonas vaginalis and Escherichia coli urinary tract infection in a newborn infant. Clin. Pediatr. (Phila.) 14:866, 1975.

217. Potterat, J. J., Markewich, G. S., King, R. D., et al.: Child-to-child transmission of gonorrhea: Report of asymptomatic genital infection in a boy. Pediatrics 60:153, 1977.

218. Prayson, R. A., Stoler, M. H., and Hart, W. R.: Vulvar vestibulitis: A histopathologic study of 36 cases, including human papillomavirus in a situ hybridization analysis. Am. J. Surg. Pathol. 19:154, 1995.

219. Puranen, M., Yliskoski, M., Saarikoski, S., et al.: Vertical transmission of human papilloma virus from infected mothers to their newborn babies and persistence of the virus in childhood. Am. J. Clin. Oncol. 174:694, 1996.

220. Rajam, R. V., Rangiah, P. N., and Anguli, V. C.: Systemic donovanasis. Br. J. Vener. Dis. 30:73, 1954.

221. Rakover, Y., Ada, H., Tal, I., et al.: Behcet disease: Long-term follow-up of three children and review of the literature. Pediatrics 83:986, 1989.

222. Reed, S. D., Landers, D. V., and Sweet, R. L.: Antibiotic treatment of tubo-ovarian abscess: Comparison of broad-spectrum beta-lactam agents versus clindamycin-containing regimens. Am. J. Obstet. Gynecol. 164:1556, 1991.

223. Rees, E.: Gonococcal bartholinitis. Br. J. Vener. Dis. 43:150, 1967.

224. Rein, M. F.: Survival of gonococci outside the body. N. Engl. J. Med. 301:1347, 1979.

225. Rettig, P. J., and Nelson, J. D.: Genital tract infection with Chlamydia trachomatis in prepubertal children. J. Pediatr. 99:206, 1981.

226. Rey-Stocker, I.: Vulvitis and vaginitis in the infant. Gynaecologia 168:413, 1969.

227. Richens, J.: The diagnosis and treatment of donovanosis (granuloma inguinale). Genitourin. Med. 67:441, 1991.

228. Riordon, T., Ellis, D. A., Mathews, P. I., et al.: False positive results with an ELISA for detection of Chlamydia antigen. J. Clin. Pathol. 39:1276, 1986.

229. Rosenfeld, W., Vermund, S., Wentz, S., et al.: High prevalence rate of human papilloma virus infection and association with abnormal Papanicolaou smears in sexually active adolescents. Am. J. Dis. Child. 143:1443, 1989.

230. Rosenfeld, W. D., and Clark, J.: Vulvovaginitis and cervicitis. Pediatr. Clin. North Am. 36:489, 1989.

231. Rothburn, M. M., Mallinson, H., and Mutton, K. J.: False-positive EIA for Chlamydia trachomatis recognized by atypical morphology on fluorescent staining. Lancet 2:982, 1986.

232. Saikku, P., Puolakkainen, M., and Nissinen, A.: Cross reactivity between Chlamydiazyme and Acinetobacter strains. N. Engl. J. Med. 314:922, 1986.

233. Saltz, G. F., Linneman, C. C., Brookman, R. R., et al.: Chlamydia trachomatis cervical infections in female adolescent. J. Pediatr. 98:981, 1981.

234. Sanfilippo, J.: Pediatric and adolescent gynecology. Obstet. Gynecol. Clin. North Am. 19:1, 1992.

235. Saracoglu, O., Mungan, T., and Tanzer, F.: Pelvic tuberculosis. Int. J. Gynecol. Obstet. 37:115, 1992.

236. Schachter, J., and Stephens, R. S.: Biology of Chlamydia trachomatis. In Holmes, K. K., Sparling, P. F., Stamm, W. E., et al. (eds.): Sexually Transmitted Diseases. New York, McGraw-Hill Medical, 2008.

237. Schachter, J., and Dattel, B. J.: Sexually transmitted diseases in victims of sexual assault. N. Engl. J. Med. 316:1023, 1987.

238. Schachter, J., Grossman, M., Sweet, R. L., et al.: Prospective study of perinatal transmission of Chlamydia trachomatis. J. A. M. A. 255:3374, 1986.

239. Schachter, J., Stamm, W. E., Quinn, T. C., et al.: Ligase chain reaction to detect C. trachomatis infection of the cervix. J. Clin. Microbiol. 32:2540, 1994.

240. Schaefer, G.: Tuberculosis of the female genital tract. Clin. Obstet. Gynecol. 13:965, 1970.

241. Scheid, F.: Diseases of adnexa in children and their differentiation from appendicitis. Med. Klin. 18:1277, 1922.

242. Schubiner, H., Lebar, W., Jemal, C., et al.: Comparison of three new nonculture tests in the diagnosis of Chlamydia genital infections. J. Adolesc. Health Care 11:505, 1990.

243. Schulte, J. M., and Schmid, G. P.: Recommendations for treatment of chancroid. Clin. Infect. Dis. 15:176, 1995.

244. Schwartz, R. H., and Rushton, H. G.: Acute balanoposthitis in young boys. Pediatr. Infect. Dis. J. 15:176, 1996.

245. Schwartz, R. H., Wientzen, R. L., and Barsanti, R. G.: Vulvovaginitis in prepubertal girls: The importance of group A Streptococcus. South. Med. J. 75:446, 1982.

246. Seidel, J., Zonang, J., and Totten, E.: Condylomata acuminata as a sign of sexual abuse in children. J. Pediatr. *95*:553, 1979.
247. Sgroi, S.: Pediatric gonorrhea beyond infancy. Pediatr. Ann. *8*:326, 1979.
248. Shafer, M. A., Beck, A., Blain, B., et al.: *Chlamydia trachomatis*: Important relationships to race, contraception, lower genital tract infection, and Papanicolaou smear. J. Pediatr. *104*:141, 1984.
249. Shafer, M. A., Sweet, R. L., Ohm-Smith, M. J., et al.: Microbiology of the lower genital tract in postmenarcheal adolescent girls: Differences by sexual activity, contraception, and presence of nonspecific vaginitis. J. Pediatr. *107*:974, 1985.
250. Shapiro, R. A., Schubert, C. J., and Siegel, R. M.: *Neisseria gonorrhoeae* infection in girls younger than 12 years of age evaluated for vaginitis. Pediatrics *104*:e72, 1999.
251. Shore, W. B., and Winkelstein, J. A.: Nonvenereal transmission of gonococcal infections to children. J. Pediatr. *79*:661, 1971.
252. Shrier, L. A.: Bacterial sexually transmitted infections: Gonorrhea, chlamydia, pelvic inflammatory disease and syphilis. *In* Emans, S. J., Laufer, M. R., and Goldstein, D. R. (eds.): Pediatric and Adolescent Gynecology. 5th ed. Philadelphia, Lippincott Williams & Wilkins, 2005.
253. Siegel, R. M., Schubert, C. J., Myers, P. A., and Shapiro, R. A.: The prevalence of sexually transmitted diseases in children and adolescents evaluated for sexual abuse in Cincinnati: Rationale for limited STD testing in prepubertal girls. Pediatrics *96*:1090, 1995.
254. Silber, T.: Genital ulcer syndrome. Semin. Adolesc. Med. *2*:155, 1986.
255. Slap, G. B., Forke, C. M., Cnaan, A., et al.: Recognition of tubo-ovarian abscess in adolescents with pelvic inflammatory disease. J. Adolesc. Health *18*:397, 1996.
256. Smith, E. W., Peutherer, J. F., Robertson, D. H., et al.: Virological studies in genital herpes. Lancet *2*:1089, 1976.
257. Smith, K. R., Ching, S., and Lee, M.: Evaluation of ligase, chain reaction for use with urine for identification of *N. gonorrhoeae* in females attending a sexually transmitted disease clinic. J. Clin. Microbiol. *33*:455, 1995.
258. Sobel, J. D.: Vaginitis. N. Engl. J. Med. *337*:1896, 1997.
259. Sobel, J. D.: Gynecologic infections in human immunodeficiency virus-infected women. Clin. Infect. Dis. *31*:1225, 2000.
260. Sokol, A. B., and Min, D. S.: Trichomonas cystitis in a six-week old infant—effective treatment with metronidazole. J. Indiana State Med. Assoc. *65*:1084, 1972.
261. Spear, R. M., Rothbaum, R. J., Keating, J. P., et al.: Perianal streptococcal cellulitis. J. Pediatr. *107*:557, 1985.
262. Spence, M. R., Adler, J., and McLellan, R.: Pelvic inflammatory disease. J. Adolesc. Health Care *11*:304, 1990.
263. Srivastava, A.: Survival of gonococci in urethral secretions with reference to the nonsexual transmission of gonococcal infection. J. Med. Microbiol. *13*:593, 1980.
264. Stamm, W. E., Wagner, K. F., Amsel, R., et al.: Causes of acute urethral syndrome in women. N. Engl. J. Med. *303*:409, 1980.
265. Straumanis, J. P., and Bocchini, J. A.: Group A beta-hemolytic streptococcal vulvovaginitis in prepubertal girls: A case report and review of the past twenty years. Pediatr. Infect. Dis. J. *9*:845, 1990.
266. Stricker, T., Navratil, F., and Sennhauser, F. H.: Vulvovaginitis in prepubertal girls. Arch. Dis. Child. *88*:324, 2003.
267. Stringel, G., Spence, J., and Corsini, L.: Genital warts in children. Can. Med. Assoc. J. *132*:1397, 1985.
268. Stumpf, P. G.: Increasing occurrence of condyloma acuminata in premenarcheal children. Obstet. Gynecol. *56*:262, 1980.
269. Swain, V.: Tuberculous vulvovaginitis: Report of a case in infancy. Lancet *1*:868, 1937.
270. Sweet, R. L.: Pelvic inflammatory disease and infertility in women. Infect. Dis. Clin. North Am. *1*:199, 1987.
271. Sweet, R. L., Banks, J., Sung, M., et al.: Experimental chlamydial salpingitis in the guinea pig. Am. J. Obstet. Gynecol. *138*:952, 1980.
272. Sweet, R. L., Banks, J., Sung, M., et al.: The occurrence of chlamydial and gonococcal salpingitis during the menstrual cycle. J. A. M. A. *255*:2062, 1986.
273. Swensson, L., Westrom, T., and Mardh, P.-A.: Contraceptives and acute salpingitis. J. A. M. A. *251*:2553, 1984.
274. Taylor-Robinson, D., Thomas, B. J., and Osborn, M. F.: Evaluation of enzyme immunoassay (Chlamydiazyme) for detecting *Chlamydia trachomatis* in genital tract specimens. J. Clin. Pathol. *40*:194, 1987.
275. Thompson, C., Macdonal, A., and Sutherland, A.: A family cluster *of Chlamydia trachomatis* infection. B. M. J. *322*:1473, 2001.
276. Toth, A., O'Leary, W. M., and Ledger, W.: Evidence for microbial transfer by spermatozoa. Obstet. Gynecol. *59*:556, 1982.
277. Tunnessen, W. W., Jr., and Jastermski, M.: Prepubescent gonococcal vulvovaginitis. Clin. Pediatr. (Phila.) *13*:675, 1974.
278. Ussher, J. E., Wilson, E., Campanella, S., et al.: *Haemophilus ducreyi* causing chronic skin ulceration in children visiting Samoa. Clin. Infect. Dis. *44*:e85, 2007.
279. Vandeven, A. M., and Emans, J.: Vulvovaginitis in the child and adolescent. Pediatr. Rev. *14*:141, 1993.
280. Washington, A E., Sweet, R. L., and Shafer, M. B.: Pelvic inflammatory disease and its sequelae in adolescents. J. Adolesc. Health Care *6*:298, 1985.
281. Watkins, S., and Quan, L.: Vulvovaginitis caused by *Yersinia enterocolitica*. Pediatr. Infect. Dis. J. *3*:444, 1984.
282. Watts, D. M., Koustdky, L. A., Holmes, K. K., et al.: Low risk of perinatal transmission of human papillomavirus: Results from a prospective cohort study. Am. J. Obstet. Gynecol. *178*:365, 1998.
283. Weaver, J.: Non-gonorrheal vulvovaginitis due to gram-negative intracellular diplococci. Am. J. Obstet. Gynecol. *60*:257, 1950.
284. Webb, D. H., and Fife, K. H.: Genital herpes simplex virus infection. Infect. Dis. Clin. North Am. *1*:97, 1987.
285. Weinstock, H., and Keesol, S.: Lymphogranuloma venereum: Report of 24 cases in children. Urol. Cutan. Rev. *50*:520, 1946.
286. Weisenfeld, H. C., Hillier, S. L., Krohn, M. A., et al.: Lower genital tract infection and endometritis: Insight into subclinical pelvic inflammatory disease. Obstet. Gynecol. *100*:456, 2002.
287. Weissenbacher, G., and Wiltschke, H.: Chronic urinary tract infections and vulvitis in girls with high posterior commissures. Paediatr. Padol. *9*:60, 1974.
288. Westrom, L., and Eschenbach, D.: Pelvic inflammatory disease. *In* Holmes, K. K., Sparling, P. F., and Mardh, P. A., et al. (eds.): Sexually Transmitted Diseases. New York, McGraw-Hill, 1999.
289. Willcox, R.: Chancroid. *In* Morton, R. S., and Harris, J. R. (eds.): Recent Advances in Sexually Transmitted Diseases. New York, Longman, 1975.
290. Wiswell, T. E., Tencer, H. L., Welch, C. A., et al.: Circumcision in children beyond the neonatal period. Pediatrics *92*:971, 1993.
291. Wolner-Hanssen, P., Eschenbach, D. A., Paavonen, J., et al.: Association between vaginal douching and acute pelvic inflammatory disease. J. A. M. A. *263*:1936, 1990.
292. Wolner-Hanssen, P., Sensoon, L., and Mardh, P.-A.: Laparoscopic findings and contraceptive use in women with signs and symptoms suggestive of acute salpingitis. Obstet. Gynecol. *66*:233, 1985.
293. Woods, C. R.: Gonococcal infections in children and adolescents. Semin. Pediatr. Rev. *14*:141, 1993.
294. Wright, T. J., Cox, J. T., Massad, L. S., et al.: 2001 Consensus Guidelines for the management of women with cervical cytological abnormalities. J. A. M. A. *287*:2120, 2002.
295. Zigas, V.: Donovanosis project in Goilala (1951-1954). Papua New Guinea Med. J. *14*:148, 1971.
296. Zolnoun, D., Hartmann, K., Lamvu, G., et al.: A conceptual model for the pathophysiology of vulvar vestibulitis syndrome. Obstet. Gynecol. Surv. *61*:395, 2006.

GASTROINTESTINAL TRACT INFECTIONS

ESOPHAGITIS

Paul Krogstad ☉ Marvin E. Ament

Infectious esophagitis is distinct from other gastrointestinal infections in that it is a rare finding in previously healthy individuals, is predominantly of fungal and viral etiology, and usually is an indicator of a primary or secondary immunodeficiency state. In normal children, infectious esophagitis frequently is associated with conditions that compromise esophageal defense mechanisms.[46]

In view of the numerous predisposing conditions, the incidence of infectious esophagitis in children is difficult to quantify. It has been reported frequently after patients have undergone chemotherapy for hematologic malignancies and after solid organ and hematopoietic stem cell transplantation. Infectious esophagitis has been reported in 3 percent of patients with ataxia-telangiectasia.[29] Before the availability of highly active antiretroviral therapy (HAART), 8 to 10 percent of children infected with human immunodeficiency virus (HIV) developed Candida esophagitis.[4,7,37] Despite the availability of HAART, Candida esophagitis remains one of the most common opportunistic infections in HIV-infected children and generally is associated with low CD4+ T-cell count (<100/μL), prior episodes of oropharyngeal candidiasis, high plasma HIV-1 load, and neutropenia (<500/μL).[7,8,45]

PATHOPHYSIOLOGY AND CAUSATIVE ORGANISMS

The defense mechanisms of the esophagus against infection include motility (continuous flow of luminal contents, which discourages colonization by microbes), a mucosal lining of stratified squamous epithelium that is resistant to microbial invasion, and local and systemic immune responses. Disruption of any of these protective factors may lead to esophageal infections. Immunosuppression (as seen in patients with acquired immunodeficiency syndrome [AIDS] or after organ transplantation), chronic mucocutaneous candidiasis, malignancy, cancer chemotherapy, and prolonged corticosteroid treatment are the most common underlying etiologic factors for fungal and viral infection of the esophagus.[6-8,19,27,37] In immunocompetent children, dysmotility of the esophagus, in addition to mucosal injury secondary to gastroesophageal reflux, can render the esophagus vulnerable to infections.

Most esophageal infections are caused by fungi and viruses.[3] The esophagus can be infected by local invasion (Candida, herpes simplex virus [HSV], bacteria), as a result of systemic infection (cytomegalovirus [CMV], Candida, Pneumocystis), or by contiguous spread from the mediastinum or neck (tuberculosis, retropharyngeal abscess). Candida spp. (especially Candida albicans), HSV, and CMV are the major pathogens.[4,37,46] Infections with fungi such as Pneumocystis, Aspergillus, and Histoplasma spp.; viruses such as varicella-zoster virus (VZV), papillomavirus, Epstein-Barr virus, and HIV; and protozoa such as Cryptosporid-

ium and Leishmania donovani are frequent, well-documented causes of esophagitis.[9,14,15,17,18,23,30,34,41] Bacterial infections of the esophagus probably are under-reported. Of esophageal infections, 10 to 16 percent can have a bacterial etiology, mostly in granulocytopenic patients and as secondary infection in fungal or viral esophagitis. Gram-positive and gram-negative oropharyngeal bacterial flora and Mycobacterium tuberculosis are the common pathogens causing esophagitis.[13,44] Helicobacter pylori has been isolated from involved tissue in Barrett esophagitis. This "infection" seems, however, to be related to gastroesophageal reflux disease, rather than to direct invasion of the esophagus by H. pylori.[31]

CLINICAL FEATURES

Patients with infectious esophagitis can present with esophageal, abdominal, or systemic symptoms (Table 49–1). Odynophagia and dysphagia are the most common symptoms of esophagitis, but they may not be apparent in small children.[7,8,35] In adults, only 59 to 79 percent of patients with documented esophageal infection had these symptoms.[3] Children also may describe a sensation of food "sticking" behind the sternum or a feeling of a food or liquid bolus passing through the chest.

Nearly all patients with AIDS and oral candidiasis and odynophagia have endoscopic evidence of esophageal candidiasis.[5,7,39] Some patients ultimately proven to have esophagitis have no signs or symptoms at presentation, however. Children who develop esophageal candidiasis despite being treated with HAART are less likely to have typical symptoms (e.g., odynophagia and retrosternal pain) or to have concomitant oropharyngeal candidiasis.[8] Similarly, approximately a fourth of adult patients with esophageal candidiasis are asymptomatic.[3]

Drooling is an unusual manifestation in esophagitis per se but may be present with pharyngeal involvement. Fever is caused mostly by systemic or secondary infection, such as disseminated CMV disease or tuberculosis, or complications that occur after esophageal perforation. Fever does not occur commonly in bacterial esophagitis. Cough is characteristic of tuberculosis, tracheobronchial fistulas, or high-grade esophageal obstruction.

Nausea and vomiting are associated more commonly with CMV esophagitis. The abdominal pain in esophagitis may be caused by referred pain from the distal end of the esophagus, associated gastritis (as in CMV infection), or concomitant intra-abdominal infections in immunocompromised hosts. A maculopapular truncal rash and fever may be present in patients with idiopathic esophageal ulceration during acute HIV seroconversion.[34] Diarrhea can be present in CMV infection (diffuse involvement of the gastrointestinal tract) or HIV infection (opportunistic enteral infections, HIV enteropathy). In one report of fungal esophagitis in children, hematemesis was the most common initial symptom.[46] Finally, because physicians seldom seek evi-

TABLE 49–1 Signs and Symptoms of Infectious Esophagitis

Dysphagia
Odynophagia
Oral lesions
Nausea/vomiting
Abdominal pain
Fever
Diarrhea
Cough
Rash
Hematemesis

dence of esophagitis in the absence of dysphagia or odynophagia, infectious esophagitis may be under diagnosed in infants and children.

Oral lesions are seen in patients with *Candida*, HSV, or HIV esophagitis, but they rarely are present with CMV infection and tuberculosis. Oral thrush is a common occurrence, however, in infants and immunocompromised patients. The frequency of *Candida* esophagitis in infants with oral thrush is unknown. The presence of oral thrush and esophageal symptoms does not exclude concomitant esophageal infection with pathogens other than *Candida* or the esophageal ulcerations associated with acute HIV infection. Oropharyngeal lesions are less common findings in HSV esophagitis than in *Candida* esophagitis. Recurrent cold sores, vesicular lesions on the nasolabial folds, and esophageal symptoms sometimes are seen as initial features of HSV esophagitis in immunocompetent adults and children, but their absence does not exclude HSV infection.[3,35]

DIFFERENTIAL DIAGNOSIS

"Pill" esophagitis may be identified by history. Pathologic gastroesophageal reflux is the most common cause of esophagitis in children. In previously healthy children, esophageal symptoms are likely to be caused by reflux esophagitis, whereas in immunocompromised patients, the physician needs to rule out infectious esophagitis. Secondary bacterial or fungal infections can be present in reflux esophagitis and Chagas disease, especially with severe inflammation and obstruction. Absence of reflux symptoms (long-standing heartburn, a water brash taste in the mouth, vomiting, spitting up [in infants], pillow wetting, or coughing) does exclude reflux esophagitis. Achalasia, diffuse esophageal spasm, foreign body impaction, and mediastinal or retropharyngeal abscesses can cause esophageal symptoms and may result in secondary infection.

DIAGNOSIS

Establishing a specific diagnosis is essential for management of infectious esophagitis, particularly because fungal and bacterial superinfections occur commonly in viral esophagitis. Although the clinical profile, barium esophagogram, and endoscopic appearance can provide some clue to the etiology of esophagitis, histopathology, immunohistochemistry, and culture of endoscopic and brush biopsy specimens are essential for confirmation of specific pathogens. Serology for HSV, CMV, or Epstein-Barr virus may help establish the diagnosis in some cases by providing evidence of acute infection. DNA detection methods also may provide evidence of viremia with these herpesviruses. Detection of fungal or viral esophagitis in an ostensibly healthy host should prompt an evaluation for the presence of primary or secondary immunodeficiency states, including HIV infection.

BARIUM ESOPHAGOGRAPHY

The usefulness of an esophagogram in diagnosing infectious esophagitis is limited because it does not provide an etiologic diagnosis; normal or nonspecific findings also are found in some cases of esophagitis. These studies are useful for assessing motility and for excluding obstruction, perforation, and fistulas of the esophagus. Barium studies are not indicated if endoscopy is planned. Double-contrast barium esophagography with air and barium, which details the mucosal lining, is the radiologic investigation of choice. Children may not tolerate this procedure well, however.[25]

Candida esophagitis generally is diffuse, whereas HSV or CMV lesions are found more frequently in the mid to distal portion of the esophagus. Discrete longitudinal plaques, a grossly irregular or "shaggy" appearance, or tiny nodular lesions with a granular appearance are characteristic of *Candida* esophagitis (Fig. 49–1). The presence of discrete superficial stellate ulcers in the mid esophagus with normal-appearing surrounding mucosa is characteristic of HSV esophagitis. CMV lesions may mimic HSV lesions on barium esophagography. Oval or elongated large ulcers are found mostly in CMV infection, however, and idiopathic esophageal ulceration is found in HIV infection.[24,43] Esophagograms of patients with tuberculosis can show intramural pseudodiverticula, extrinsic compression, or esophageal displacement by mediastinal lymph nodes and sinus tracts.[10]

ESOPHAGOSCOPY

The technique for performing endoscopy with videoendoscopes miniaturized to a diameter of 4.8 mm has made the procedure far more tolerable in immunocompromised patients, requiring less sedation and anesthesia and allowing the procedure to be performed even in newborns. These new instruments have biopsy capabilities comparable to older, wider endoscopes.

Characteristic macroscopic lesions are associated with some infectious agents. Macroscopic appearances overlap considerably, however, and histopathologic or immunohistochemical analysis (or both) of endoscopic and brush biopsy specimens is essential for diagnosis. A diffuse esophageal lesion is characteristic of *Candida* infection, whereas CMV and HSV infections mainly involve the distal part of the esophagus. White, longitudinal plaques adhering to the mucosa are characteristic of *Candida* infection.[20] Plaques from oral thrush, common findings in infants and immunocompromised children, can be washed away and reveal a nonulcerated underlying mucosa. Similar-appearing plaques also may be seen in CMV, HSV, bacterial, and "pill" esophagitis, and after sucralfate ingestion.

Small, 1- to 3-mm vesicles are characteristic of HSV esophagitis, but by the time endoscopy is done, these vesicles usually slough off and reveal sharply demarcated ulcers with a raised edge, necrotic base, and normal-appearing surrounding mucosa.[35] In progressive disease, these ulcers may coalesce to resemble *Candida* esophagitis.[1] Multiple superficial ulcers in the distal portion of the esophagus often are seen in CMV esophagitis. Large elongated ulcers also are typical manifestations of CMV infection, but they may occur in idiopathic esophageal ulcerations in HIV infection as well.[24] Complete denudation of the mucosa is an unusual finding with CMV infection.[40] Endoscopy done in patients with VZV esophagitis can show vesicles, discrete ulcers, or necrotizing esophagitis, depending on the stage of the disease. Tubercular ulcers of the esophagus usually are of varying size, distinct, and shallow with a necrotic base.

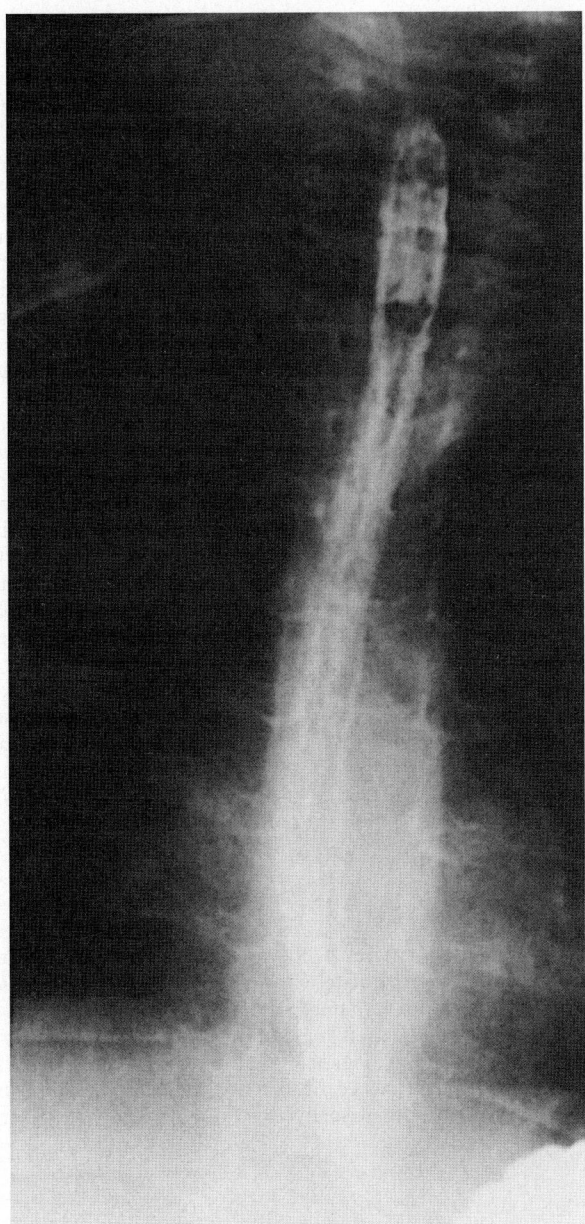

Figure 49–1 *Candida* esophagitis. Barium esophagogram shows diffuse mucosal irregularity suggestive of inflammation and longitudinal filling defects suggestive of plaques. *(Courtesy of Sjirk Westra, M.D., Division of Pediatric Radiology, UCLA Medical Center, Los Angeles.)*

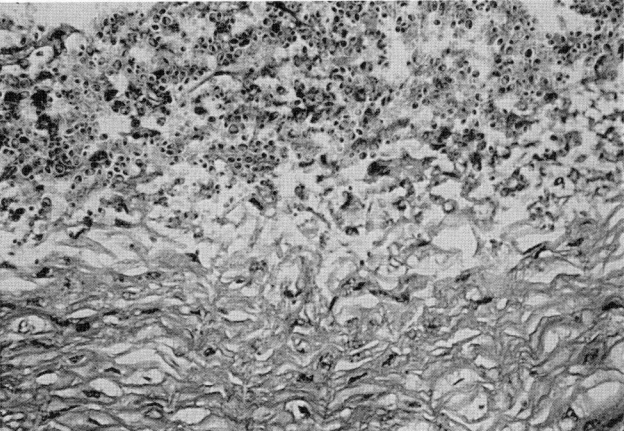

Figure 49–2 *Candida* esophagitis. Photomicrograph shows yeastlike organisms in the esophageal mucosa. Methenamine silver stain. *(Courtesy of Klaus Lewin, M.D., Department of Pathology, UCLA Medical Center, Los Angeles.)*

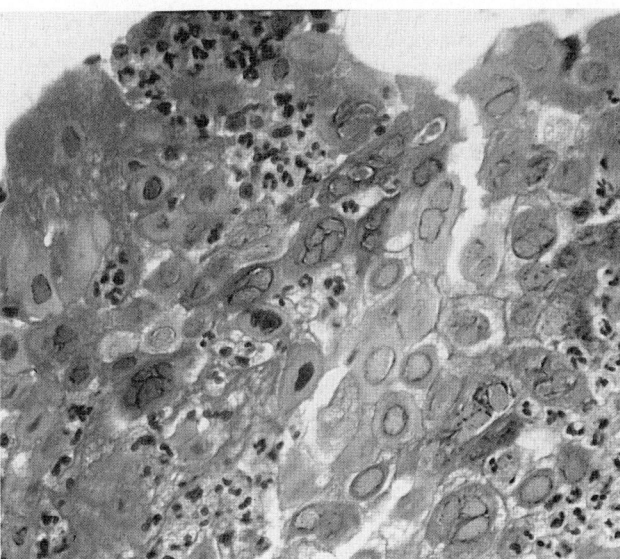

Figure 49–3 Herpes simplex virus esophagitis. Photomicrograph shows viral inclusions in squamous epithelium. Hematoxylin and eosin stain. *(Courtesy of Klaus Lewin, M.D., Department of Pathology, UCLA Medical Center, Los Angeles.)*

BIOPSY AND BRUSHING

Endoscopic biopsy specimens should be obtained from the edge and the base of the lesions. In CMV infection, specimens from the edge do not yield diagnostic information.[40] The pathologist should be alerted to the possibility of fungal, viral, and polymicrobial infection. Appropriate fixatives should be used for routine hematoxylin and eosin stain, Gram stain, and special stains for fungi and bacteria such as *Mycobacterium. Candida* and *Aspergillus* can be shown by silver stain, periodic acid–Schiff stain, or Gram stain (Fig. 49–2). Diagnostic histopathologic changes, such as multinucleated giant cells, ballooning degeneration, intranuclear Cowdry type A inclusion bodies, and margination of chromatin in HSV infection (Fig. 49–3), and amphophilic intranuclear inclusions and small multiple cytoplasmic inclusion bodies in CMV infection (Fig. 49–4), can be diagnostic. Immunohisto-

chemical studies and DNA hybridization techniques often are required to establish the diagnosis, however.

Viral culture, with or without immunohistochemical techniques, may aid in confirmation. Material obtained by endoscopy-guided brush biopsy can reveal the features of *Candida* or viral infection described earlier. Blind brushings of the esophagus may be useful for *Candida* infection when endoscopy is impossible or is unavailable.[5] If abdominal pain, fever, or other unusual symptoms are present, the possibility of disseminated or abdominal infection should be excluded by appropriate investigations.

TREATMENT

CANDIDA ESOPHAGITIS

Treatment of esophageal candidiasis requires systemic antifungal therapy. Topical therapy may produce an initial response, but early treatment failures are more common occurrences.[33] Sys-

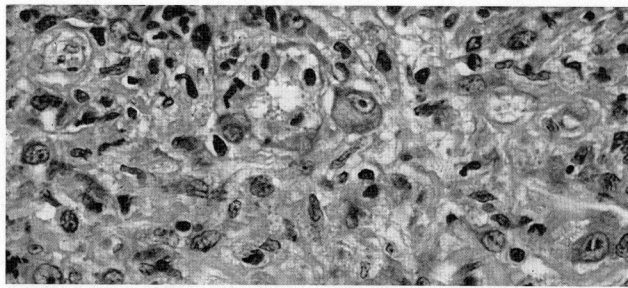

Figure 49–4 Cytomegalovirus esophagitis. Photomicrograph shows intracytoplasmic inclusion bodies in the lamina propria. Hematoxylin and eosin stain. (*Courtesy of Klaus Lewin, M.D., Department of Pathology, UCLA Medical Center, Los Angeles.*)

temic therapy with newer azole medications (fluconazole, itraconazole solution, or voriconazole) is now the preferred approach.[32] Numerous trials have been done comparing the azole agents, most often in adults with AIDS. Patients are less likely to respond and more likely to experience drug-related toxicity when treated with ketoconazole compared with fluconazole.[11] Oral fluconazole and itraconazole suspension seem comparable in efficacy for initial therapy, and some patients whose disease fails to respond to fluconazole may see improvement with subsequent itraconazole therapy.[12,36,44] Regardless of the initial severity of esophagitis, voriconazole and fluconazole seemed comparable in efficacy in one study, although toxicity occurred more commonly with voriconazole.[2,8]

Overall, experience with the azole medications supports recommendations for the initial use of oral fluconazole therapy for *Candida* esophagitis. Therapy generally is given for 14 to 21 days. Intravenous administration of azole medications may be used for patients with severe dysphagia.[26,32]

Infection with azole-resistant variants of *Candida*, including species with intrinsic or acquired resistance to fluconazole (e.g., *Candida krusei*), may occur.[2,8] Although pediatric data currently are limited, large-scale studies in adults have shown that intravenous therapy with echinocandin agents (caspofungin, anidulafungin, or micafungin) is an alternative to azole therapy.[26,32,42]

Intravenous amphotericin B deoxycholate remains an alternative for patients with disease that is refractory to treatment with azole medications.[21,32] Nephrotoxicity is a major toxic effect of amphotericin B, but brief, low-dose therapy (7 to 14 days, 0.3 to 0.7 mg/kg/day) generally is sufficient to treat esophagitis. Lipid formulations of amphotericin B also may be useful for treating refractory disease, but they are not known to be superior in efficacy or lower in toxicity than is the low-dose deoxycholate formulation for the treatment of *Candida* esophagitis.

OTHER CAUSES OF FUNGAL ESOPHAGITIS

Cases of esophagitis caused by *Aspergillus*, *Mucor*, *Cryptococcus*, and *Histoplasma* spp. have been described. Optimal therapy has not been established, but systemic therapy, as for other manifestations of invasive infection with these organisms, has been successful. Currently, this approach would involve the use of intravenous or oral azole agents or an amphotericin B preparation. Echinocandins (micafungin, caspofungin, or anidulafungin) may be useful for *Aspergillus* or *Histoplasma* infections, but they have no activity against cryptococci.

VIRAL ESOPHAGITIS

Although spontaneous resolution of HSV esophagitis may occur in some individuals, antiviral therapy for HSV esophagitis gener-

ally is advised. Immunocompromised patients usually are treated with intravenous acyclovir, but in older patients, valacyclovir and famciclovir may be useful alternatives, in view of their clinical efficacy and convenient dosing schedule.[28] Ganciclovir is used for CMV infection.[3,38] Acyclovir is the treatment of choice for VZV, and prophylaxis has reduced effectively the rate of VZV infection in post-transplantation patients. Foscarnet is an alternative treatment for patients with HSV, VZV, or CMV who cannot tolerate or do not respond to initial therapy with acyclovir or ganciclovir therapy. Therapy for 14 to 21 days usually is recommended for esophagitis caused by these herpesviruses. HIV-associated idiopathic ulcers do not respond to empiric antiviral or antifungal therapy, but they may respond to treatment with thalidomide.[16]

BACTERIAL ESOPHAGITIS

Bacterial esophagitis typically occurs in immunocompromised hosts and may involve gram-positive or gram-negative bacteria, or a mixture of both. In immunocompromised hosts, esophagitis may be associated with bacteremia. Consequently, empiric therapy should include broad-spectrum antibacterial agents active against *Staphylococcus aureus*, viridans streptococci, and aerobic gram-negative organisms. Blood cultures always should be performed to exclude bacteremia.[44]

Esophageal infections with *M. tuberculosis* or atypical mycobacteria are treated with regimens appropriate for other systemic infections with these organisms. Lack of response to appropriate therapy may indicate concomitant superinfection by other organisms or resistance to the drugs used. Repeat endoscopy is indicated for documenting eradication of infection.

PROGNOSIS

Candida esophagitis carries a poor prognosis for patients with AIDS. Survival is approximately 1 year after an episode of *Candida* esophagitis in children with untreated HIV infection, and *Candida* esophagitis is an indication for administration of antiretroviral therapy.[4,34] Fungal esophagitis, if not treated successfully, can lead to esophageal strictures, obstruction, perforation, and fistulas.[22,27] Viral esophagitis usually does not have any long-term sequelae.

REFERENCES

1. Agha, F. P., Lee, H. H., and Nostrant, T. T.: Herpetic esophagitis: A diagnostic challenge in immunocompromised patients. Am. J. Gastroenterol. 81:246-253, 1986.
2. Ally, R., Schurmann, D., Kreisel, W., et al.: A randomized, double-blind, double-dummy, multicenter trial of voriconazole and fluconazole in the treatment of esophageal candidiasis in immunocompromised patients. Clin. Infect. Dis. 33:1447-1454, 2001.
3. Baehr, P. H., and McDonald, G. B.: Esophageal infections: Risk factors, presentation, diagnosis, and treatment. Gastroenterology 106:509-532, 1994.
4. Blanche, S., Tardieu, M., Duliege, A., et al.: Longitudinal study of 94 symptomatic infants with perinatally acquired human immunodeficiency virus infection: Evidence for a bimodal expression of clinical and biological symptoms. Am. J. Dis. Child. 144:1210-1215, 1990.
5. Bonacini, M., Laine, L., Gal, A. A., et al.: Prospective evaluation of blind brushing of the esophagus for *Candida* esophagitis in patients with human immunodeficiency virus infection. Am. J. Gastroenterol. 85:385-389, 1990.
6. Brouillette, D. E., Alexander, J., Yoo, Y. K., et al.: T-cell populations in liver and renal transplant recipients with infectious esophagitis. Dig. Dis. Sci. 34:92-96, 1989.
7. Chiou, C. C., Groll, A. H., Gonzalez, C. E., et al.: Esophageal candidiasis in pediatric acquired immunodeficiency syndrome: Clinical manifestations and risk factors. Pediatr. Infect. Dis. J. 19:729-734, 2000.
8. Chiou, C. C., Groll, A. H., Mavrogiorgos, N., et al.: Esophageal candidiasis in human immunodeficiency virus-infected pediatric patients after the introduction of highly active antiretroviral therapy. Pediatr. Infect. Dis. J. 21:388-392, 2002.

9. Datry, A., Similowski, T., Jais, P., et al.: AIDS-associated leishmaniasis: An unusual gastro-duodenal presentation. Trans. R. Soc. Trop. Med. Hyg. *84*:239-240, 1990.

10. de Silva, R., Stoopack, P. M., and Raufman, J. P.: Esophageal fistulas associated with mycobacterial infection in patients at risk for AIDS. Radiology *175*:449-453, 1990.

11. De Wit, S., Weerts, D., Goossens, H., et al.: Comparison of fluconazole and ketoconazole for oropharyngeal candidiasis in AIDS. Lancet *1*:746-748, 1989.

12. Eichel, M., Just-Nubling, G., Helm, E. B., et al.: [Itraconazole suspension in the treatment of HIV-infected patients with fluconazole-resistant oropharyngeal candidiasis and esophagitis]. Mycoses *39*(Suppl. 1):102-106, 1996.

13. Eng, J., and Sabanathan, S.: Tuberculosis of the esophagus. Dig. Dis. Sci. *36*:536-540, 1991.

14. Grimes, M. M., LaPook, J. D., Bar, M. H., et al.: Disseminated *Pneumocystis carinii* infection in a patient with acquired immunodeficiency syndrome. Hum. Pathol. *18*:307-308, 1987.

15. Hirsch, M. S.: Herpes group virus infections in the compromised host. *In* Rubin, R. H., and Young, L. S. (eds): Clinical Approach to Infections in the Compromised Host, 2nd ed. New York, Plenum, 1988, pp. 347-366.

16. Jacobson, J. M., Spritzler, J., Fox, L., et al.: Thalidomide for the treatment of esophageal aphthous ulcers in patients with human immunodeficiency virus infection. National Institute of Allergy and Infectious Disease AIDS Clinical Trials Group. J. Infect. Dis. *180*:61-67, 1999.

17. Javdan, P., and Pitman, E. R.: Squamous papilloma of esophagus. Dig. Dis. Sci. *29*:317-320, 1984.

18. Kazlow, P. G., Shah, K., Benkov, K. J., et al.: Esophageal cryptosporidiosis in a child with acquired immune deficiency syndrome. Gastroenterology *91*:1301-1303, 1986.

19. Kesten, S., Hyland, R. H., Pruzanski, W. R., et al.: Esophageal candidiasis associated with beclomethasone dipropionate aerosol therapy. Drug Intell. Clin. Pharm. *22*:568-569, 1988.

20. Kodsi, B. E., Wickremesinghe, C., Kozinn, P. J., et al.: *Candida* esophagitis: A prospective study of 27 cases. Gastroenterology *71*:715-719, 1976.

21. Lake, D. E., Kunzweiler, J., Beer, M., et al.: Fluconazole versus amphotericin B in the treatment of esophageal candidiasis in cancer patients. Chemotherapy *42*:308-314, 1996.

22. Lal, D. R., Foroutan, H. R., Su, W. T., et al.: The management of treatment-related esophageal complications in children and adolescents with cancer. J. Pediatr. Surg. *41*:495-499, 2006.

23. Lee, J. H., Neumann, D. A., and Welsh, J. D.: Disseminated histoplasmosis presenting with esophageal symptomatology. Am. J. Dig. Dis. *22*:831-834, 1977.

24. Levine, M. S., Loercher, G., Katzka, D. A., et al.: Giant, human immunodeficiency virus-related ulcers in the esophagus. Radiology *180*:323-326, 1991.

25. Levine, M. S., Macones, A. J., Jr., and Laufer, I.: *Candida* esophagitis: Accuracy of radiographic diagnosis. Radiology *154*:581-587, 1985.

26. Mofenson, L. M., Oleske, J., Serchuck, L., et al.: Treating opportunistic infections among HIV-exposed and infected children: Recommendations from CDC, the National Institutes of Health, and the Infectious Diseases Society of America. Clin. Infect. Dis. *40*(Suppl. 1):S1-S84, 2005.

27. Naito, Y., Yoshikawa, T., Oyamada, H., et al.: Esophageal candidiasis. Gastroenterol. Jpn. *23*:363-370, 1988.

28. Nassar, N. N., and Gregg, C. R.: Esophageal infections. Curr. Treat. Options Gastroenterol. *1*:56-63, 1998.

29. Nowak-Wegrzyn, A., Crawford, T. O., Winkelstein, J. A., et al.: Immunodeficiency and infections in ataxia-telangiectasia. J. Pediatr. *144*:505-511, 2004.

30. Obrecht, W. F., Jr., Richter, J. E., Olympio, G. A., et al.: Tracheoesophageal fistula: A serious complication of infectious esophagitis. Gastroenterology *87*:1174-1179, 1984.

31. O'Connor, H. J., and Cunnane, K.: *Helicobacter pylori* and gastro-oesophageal reflux disease—a prospective study. Irish J. Med. Sci. *163*:369-373, 1994.

32. Pappas, P. G., Rex, J. H., Sobel, J. D., et al.: Guidelines for treatment of candidiasis. Clin. Infect. Dis. *38*:161-189, 2004.

33. Pons, V., Greenspan, D., and Debruin, M.: Therapy for oropharyngeal candidiasis in HIV-infected patients: A randomized, prospective multicenter study of oral fluconazole versus clotrimazole troches. The Multicenter Study Group. J. Acquir. Immune Defic. Syndr. *6*:1311-1316, 1993.

34. Rabeneck, L., Popovic, M., Gartner, S., et al.: Acute HIV infection presenting with painful swallowing and esophageal ulcers. J. A. M. A. *263*:2318-2322, 1990.

35. Rodrigues, F., Brandao, N., Duque, V., et al.: Herpes simplex virus esophagitis in immunocompetent children. J. Pediatr. Gastroenterol. Nutr. *39*:560-563, 2004.

36. Saag, M. S., Fessel, W. J., Kaufman, C. A., et al.: Treatment of fluconazole-refractory oropharyngeal candidiasis with itraconazole oral solution in HIV-positive patients. AIDS Res. Hum. Retroviruses *15*:1413-1417, 1999.

37. Scott, G. B., Hutto, C., Makuch, R. W., et al.: Survival in children with perinatally acquired human immunodeficiency virus type 1 infection. N. Engl. J. Med. *321*:1791-1796, 1989.

38. Stratta, R. J., Shaefer, M. S., Cushing, K. A., et al.: Successful prophylaxis of cytomegalovirus disease after primary CMV exposure in liver transplant recipients. Transplantation *51*:90-97, 1991.

39. Tavitian, A., Raufman, J. P., and Rosenthal, L. E.: Oral candidiasis as a marker for esophageal candidiasis in the acquired immunodeficiency syndrome. Ann. Intern. Med. *104*:54-55, 1986.

40. Theise, N. D., Rotterdam, H., and Dieterich, D.: Cytomegalovirus esophagitis in AIDS: Diagnosis by endoscopic biopsy. Am. J. Gastroenterol. *86*:1123-1126, 1991.

41. Tilbe, K. S., and Lloyd, D. A.: A case of viral esophagitis. J. Clin. Gastroenterol. *8*:494-495, 1986.

42. Wagner, C., Graninger, W., Presterl, E., et al.: The echinocandins: Comparison of their pharmacokinetics, pharmacodynamics and clinical applications. Pharmacology *78*:161-177, 2006.

43. Wall, S. D., and Jones, B.: Gastrointestinal tract in the immunocompromised host: Opportunistic infections and other complications. Radiology *185*:327-335, 1992.

44. Walsh, T. J., Belitsos, N. J., and Hamilton, S. R.: Bacterial esophagitis in immunocompromised patients. Arch. Intern. Med. *146*:1345-1348, 1986.

45. Ylitalo, N., Brogly, S., Hughes, M. D., et al.: Risk factors for opportunistic illnesses in children with human immunodeficiency virus in the era of highly active antiretroviral therapy. Arch. Pediatr. Adolesc. Med. *160*:778-787, 2006.

46. Young, C., Chang, M. H., and Chen, J. M.: Fungal esophagitis in children. Zhonghua Min Guo Xiao Er Ke Yi Xue Hui Za Zhi *34*:436-442, 1993.

CHAPTER 50

APPROACH TO PATIENTS WITH GASTROINTESTINAL TRACT INFECTIONS AND FOOD POISONING

Larry K. Pickering

The approach to treatment of patients with gastrointestinal (GI) tract infections begins with obtaining a thorough medical history including information about epidemiologic factors, a physical examination, and knowledge of the pathophysiologic process and clinical manifestations of various enteropathogens. GI tract infections result in a wide range of symptom complexes and can be produced by a variety of enteropathogens. Most infectious diarrheal illness can be classified into one of several categories based on the causative agent, the pathophysiologic mechanism of the agent, and the clinical response. This information then can be used to determine appropriate laboratory evaluation and therapy. All patients with diarrhea require some degree of fluid and electrolyte therapy; a few need other nonspecific support; and for some, specific antimicrobial therapy is indicated to shorten the duration of the illness and to eradicate fecal excretion of the organism. Practice guidelines for management of infectious diarrhea have been developed by the Infectious Diseases Society of America.[163] Other recommendations include a primer for physicians dealing with diagnosis and management of food-borne illnesses developed jointly by the American Medical Association, Centers for Disease Control and Prevention (CDC), U.S. Food and Drug Administration (FDA), and United States Department of Agriculture[62]; surveillance of food-borne disease outbreaks in the United States by the CDC[245]; guidelines for prevention of

All material in this chapter is in the public domain, with the exception of any borrowed figures or tables.

opportunistic infections in patients with human immunodeficiency virus (HIV) developed by the U.S. Public Health Service and the Infectious Diseases Society of America[71]; management of acute gastroenteritis in young children developed by the CDC[66]; and guidelines on acute diarrhea in adults.[111]

EPIDEMIOLOGY AND ETIOLOGY

Establishing the cause of diarrhea often is difficult because of variations in host susceptibility and response to infection, geographic location, season, and complexity of laboratory techniques necessary to identify the wide array of causative agents. In the United States and other parts of the world, acute infectious diarrhea is caused by many enteropathogens; but on the basis of epidemiologic and etiologic considerations, major categories can be differentiated (Table 50–1): diarrhea in childcare centers, hospitals, or other institutional settings and in family members or other close contacts; food- or water-associated diarrhea; antimicrobial-associated diarrhea; diarrhea of travelers; diarrhea in immunosuppressed hosts, including patients with primary and secondary immune deficiencies; and others, which include sporadic episodes in which these categories do not apply. In addition, history of chronic diarrhea or other GI tract diseases should be obtained.

When a patient complains of moderate or severe diarrhea, a decision should be made as to whether he or she should be hospitalized or treated as an outpatient. The following patients with diarrhea should be considered for hospitalization: infants and elderly people who appear toxic, are lethargic, or have high temperatures; patients with excessive loss of fluid and electrolytes through stools, especially in association with vomiting; patients with grossly bloody stools; and patients who are immunosuppressed, including people with acquired immunodeficiency syndrome (AIDS). Once the decision has been made either to hospitalize or to treat on an outpatient basis, appropriate diagnostic procedures and therapy can be instituted.

OUTBREAKS IN CHILDCARE CENTERS

The risk for a person to acquire a GI tract infection varies with age, environment, season, exposure, and immune status. Clinical and epidemiologic data often guide classification of an episode of acute infectious diarrhea into one of the categories mentioned earlier. If predisposing factors are not present, the episode can be classified as sporadic. Most cases of sporadic diarrhea occur in children younger than 5 years old, although all age groups are affected. Infants who are breast-fed are relatively protected from contaminated food and water. Protection also is afforded by factors present in human milk.[310] During and after weaning, the risk for development of diarrhea increases. When an episode of acute infectious diarrhea occurs, an association with other cases should be sought, especially when highly contagious organisms, such as *Shigella* spp., *Escherichia coli* O157:H7, *Giardia lamblia*, *Cryptosporidium* spp., rotavirus, astrovirus, enteric adenovirus, and calicivirus, are isolated and in conditions in which close contact is facilitated, such as institutions for mentally impaired people, childcare centers, hospitals, and other institutional settings.[188,263,289,311,314,412] After respiratory tract illness, diarrhea is the second most common disease among children in childcare facilities,[188] occurring most frequently in children younger than 3 years.

FOOD-BORNE OR WATER-BORNE DIARRHEA

Reporting of food-borne and water-borne diseases in the United States began in 1923 because of concern about typhoid fever and infantile diarrhea.[245] Since 1978, food-borne and water-borne outbreaks have been published in separate annual summaries. The purposes of the outbreak surveillance include disease prevention and control, knowledge of disease causation, and administrative guidance. In 1996, the CDC established the Foodborne Disease Active Surveillance Network (FoodNet) for population-based, active surveillance investigation of food-borne disease in the United States.[362] The active surveillance includes laboratory-confirmed infections for nine pathogens (*Campylobacter* spp., *Listeria* spp., *Salmonella* spp., *Shigella* spp., Shiga toxin–producing *Escherichia coli*, *Vibrio* spp., *Yersinia* spp., *Cryptosporidium* spp., and *Cyclospora* spp.).

An outbreak of food-borne or water-borne disease is defined as an incident in which two or more people experience a similar illness, usually involving the GI tract, after ingesting common food or water.[120,236,245] Surveillance for water-borne disease and outbreaks in the United States is characterized by disease associated with recreational water and disease associated with drinking water and water not intended for drinking.[120,236] Food-borne or water-borne disease can result from ingestion of food or water contaminated with bacteria or a bacterial toxin, a chemical, a virus, or a parasite.[62,236,245] Table 50–2 outlines characteristics of food-borne and water-borne outbreaks, including outbreaks not characterized by diarrhea. Although most enteropathogens can be spread by either food or water, the epidemiology of outbreaks often suggests specific etiologic agents. A determination of the incubation period and the presence or absence of selected clinical findings (especially fever, vomiting, and bloody diarrhea) often leads a physician or other health care professional toward establishing the correct diagnosis in outbreaks of food-borne or water-borne disease.[62] As a general rule, when outbreaks are

TABLE 50–1   Major Categories of Acute Infectious Diarrhea

Category of Diarrhea	Epidemiologic Considerations	Most Commonly Involved Enteropathogens
Outbreaks usually due to person-to-person transmission	Childcare centers, hospitals, and other institutional settings	Enteric viruses, *Cryptosporidium*, *Giardia lamblia*, occasionally bacteria
Food-borne or water-borne	Other people involved after common food or water exposure	See Tables 50–2 and 50–3
Antimicrobial-associated	Recent administration of an antimicrobial agent	*Clostridium difficile*
Travelers	Recent travel to a developing country	Enterotoxigenic *Escherichia coli*, *Campylobacter*, *Shigella*, *Salmonella*, other organisms
Immunosuppressed hosts	Primary or secondary (underlying disease, including HIV infection; recent administration of an immunosuppressive drug or radiation therapy) immune deficiencies	See Table 50–4

divided by an incubation period, illnesses manifesting in less than 1 hour usually are caused by chemical poisoning; illness of 1 to 7 hours, by either *Staphylococcus aureus* or *Bacillus cereus* preformed toxins; illness of 8 to 14 hours, by *Clostridium perfringens* or *B. cereus* enterotoxins; and illness of more than 14 hours, by other infectious or toxic agents (see Table 50–2). Clinical manifestations can involve the central nervous system or be systemic with little or no intestinal tract involvement.

During the period from 1998 through 2002, a total of 6647 outbreaks of food-borne disease, which included 128,370 cases, were reported to the CDC from various regions of the United States.[245] Since 2001, reports of food-borne disease outbreaks have been submitted by state, local, and territorial public health departments through a Web application on the Internet called the electronic Food-borne Outbreak Reporting System.[245] This surveillance system has resulted in an increase in the number of reported outbreaks. Among outbreaks in which the cause was determined (33%), bacterial pathogens caused the largest percentage of outbreaks (55%) and cases (55%), with *Salmonella* serotype Enteritidis accounting for the largest number of

outbreaks and outbreak-related cases.[245] *Listeria monocytogenes* accounted for most deaths from any pathogen, followed by *Salmonella* spp. Outbreaks with a known cause accounted for 54 percent of illnesses. Viruses caused 33 percent of outbreaks and 41 percent of cases, predominantly due to noroviruses, with hepatitis A being the second most common viral cause. Parasites caused 1 percent of outbreaks and 1 percent of cases, with anisakis, cryptosporidium, cyclospora, *Giardia*, and trichinella reported as causing outbreaks. Chemical agents caused 10 percent of outbreaks and 2 percent of cases, with ciguatoxin, heavy metals, mushrooms, paralytic shellfish, and scombrotoxin accounting for outbreaks caused by chemical agents (Table 50–3). The etiologic agent was not detected in 67 percent of outbreaks, indicating the need for improved epidemiologic and laboratory investigations. Factors contributing to outbreaks were classified as those that are thought to have led to contamination of a food and those that allowed proliferation of the pathogen in the food. At least one contributing factor was reported in 46 percent of outbreaks reported from 1998 through 2002.[245,438] Major contaminating factors that contributed to outbreaks were bare-handed contact

TABLE 50–2 Characteristics of Food-Borne or Water-Borne Outbreaks of Diarrhea

Usual Incubation Periods	Clinical Illness			Causative Agent	Epidemiologic and Laboratory Diagnosis
	Fever	Diarrhea	Vomiting		
5 minutes–6 hours (usually <3 hours)	Rare	Occasional (see Table 50–3)	Common	Chemical or toxin	Demonstration of toxin or chemical from food or epidemiologic incrimination of food
1–6 hours (usually <1 hour)	Rare	Occasional	Profuse	*Staphylococcus aureus* enterotoxin *Bacillus cereus* emetic toxin	Detection of toxin in food, isolation of organisms in food (>10⁵/g) or in vomitus or stool
8–16 hours	Rare	Typical	Occasional	*Clostridium perfringens* enterotoxin *B. cereus* enterotoxin	Isolation of organisms or toxin from food (>10⁵g) or stools of ill persons, epidemiologic incrimination of food
16–96 hours	Common	Typical	Occasional	*Shigella* *Salmonella* *Vibrio parahaemolyticus* Enteroinvasive *Escherichia coli* *Yersinia enterocolitica*	Isolation of organisms from food or stools of ill persons
12–72 hours	Clinical syndrome compatible with botulism			*Clostridium botulinum*	Isolation of organism or toxin from food (10⁵/g) or stools Demonstration of toxin in serum or food
16–96 hours	Occasional	Typical	Occasional	*E. coli* enterotoxin *V. parahaemolyticus* enterotoxin *Vibrio cholerae* enterotoxin *Y. enterocolitica* enterotoxin *Listeria monocytogenes*	Isolation of organism from food and stools of ill persons Identification of toxin Epidemiologic incrimination of food Blood or cerebrospinal fluid cultures; stool culture usually not helpful
1–11 days	Occasional	Common	Occasional	*Cryptosporidium parvum* *Cyclospora cayetanensis*	Request special stool examination; may need to examine water or food
2 days–weeks	Common	Typical	Frequent	*Bacillus anthracis*	Isolation of organism from blood or contaminated meat
1–7 days	Uncommon	Typical	Frequent	*E. coli* O157:H7 and other Shiga toxin-producing *E. coli*	Isolation of organism from food or stool or identification of toxin in stools of ill persons Epidemiologic incrimination of food
1–3 days	Occasional	Typical	Common	Caliciviruses (noroviruses) Rotavirus	Antigen detection (enzyme immunoassay) in stool Immune electron microscopy of stool Serology
2–5 days	Occasional	Typical	Occasional	*Campylobacter jejuni*	Isolation of organisms from food or stools of ill persons Epidemiologic incrimination of food
7–21 days	Common	Common	Rare	*Brucella abortus*, *Brucella melitensis*, and *Brucella suis*	Blood culture and positive serology
1–4 weeks	Rare	Common	Rare	*Giardia lamblia*	Stool for ova and parasite examination enzyme immunoassay
2 days–8 weeks	Common	Common	Common	*Trichinella spiralis*	Serology, muscle biopsy

TABLE 50-3 Chemical Causes of Food Poisoning

Type of Chemical, Toxin, or Poison	Food	Clinical Symptoms	Onset of Symptoms (hr)
Heavy metals*	Water (through metallic container) and food	Gastrointestinal	1
Scombrotoxin	Fish (tuna, mackerel, marlin, mahi-mahi, bluefish)	*Due to histamine:* flushing, headache, burning of mouth and throat, urticaria, rash, paresthesia	1
Ciguatera	Fish (barracuda, amberjack, snapper, grouper)	*Neurologic:* paresthesia, reversal of cold-hot sensations *Gastrointestinal:* nausea, abdominal pain, vomiting, diarrhea	1-6
Tetrodotoxin	Puffer fish	*Neurologic:* paresthesia, numbness, loss of proprioception, ascending paralysis, death	<1
Paralytic or neurotoxic compounds	Shellfish (clams, oysters, scallops, mussels, other mollusks)	Paresthesia, weakness, respiratory difficulties, dysphasia, dysphonia, gastrointestinal	1-4
Domoic acid	Shellfish (mussels)	Gastrointestinal *Acute CNS:* headache, seizures, hemiparesis, ophthalmoplegia, abnormalities of arousal *Chronic CNS:* memory deficits, motor neuropathy or axonopathy	Within 24
Monosodium glutamate	Chinese food	Burning sensation, heavy feeling in chest, pressure over face, flushing, gastrointestinal	1
Ibotenic acid, muscimol	Mushroom	*CNS:* confusion, delirium, visual disturbances, lethargy	2
Coprine	Mushroom	*Disulfiram-like effect:* nausea, vomiting, headache, hypotension, flushing, paresthesia and tachycardia	2
Muscarine	Mushroom	*Parasympathetic:* sweating, salivation, lacrimation, blurred vision, diarrhea, bradycardia, hypotension	2
Psilocybin, psilocin	Mushroom	*CNS:* hallucinations, anxiety, mood elevation, weakness	2
Diverse, mostly unknown	Mushroom	Gastrointestinal	2
Monomethylhydrazine, gyromitrin	Mushroom	Cellular destruction, gastrointestinal, loss of coordination, convulsion, coma, death	6-12
Amatoxins, phallotoxins	Mushroom	Cellular destruction, gastrointestinal, hepatic and renal necrosis	6-24
Vomitoxin (deoxynivalenol)	Cereals contaminated with *Fusarium* species	Vomiting acutely Altered mucosal immunity with chronic exposure	<3

Includes antimony, arsenic, cadmium, copper, mercury, thallium, tin, and zinc.
CNS, central nervous system.

by a food handler or preparer (e.g., ready-to-eat food), inadequate cleaning of processing or preparation equipment or utensils (e.g., cutting board), handling by an infected person or carrier of a pathogen (*Salmonella* spp. or norovirus), and cross-contamination from a raw ingredient of animal origin (e.g., raw poultry on preparatory surface). Factors associated with proliferation of a pathogen in food include allowing foods to remain at room or warm outdoor temperature for several hours, inadequate cold-holding temperatures, slow cooking, insufficient time or temperature during hot holding, and preparation of foods a half day or more before serving. Most of the proliferation factors are associated with outbreaks due to bacteria. The major places where food associated with outbreaks was eaten are restaurants and delicatessens (50%) and private residences (20%); a variety of other or unknown places account for the remainder.[245]

Outbreaks of gastroenteritis caused by caliciviruses have been associated with consumption of contaminated oysters, salads, and bakery products and with transmission of the virus by food handlers.[229,272] The major causes of reported food-borne disease outbreaks due to bacteria are *Salmonella* spp., Shiga toxin–producing *E. coli*, *C. perfringens*, *S. aureus*, *Shigella* spp., and *Campylobacter jejuni*. Bacterial diseases associated with ingestion of unpasteurized milk include salmonellosis and campylobacteriosis and, less frequently, infection with *Brucella* spp., *E. coli*, *L. monocytogenes*, *Mycobacterium* spp., *S. aureus*, *Streptococcus* spp., *Streptobacillus moniliformis*, and *Yersinia enterocolitica*.[245] A nationwide outbreak of *Salmonella enteritidis* gastroenteritis involved 224,000 people in the United States and was associated with ingestion of contaminated ice cream. The origin of the outbreak was pasteurized ice cream premix that was contaminated in tanker trailers that previously had carried nonpasteurized liquid eggs containing *S. enteritidis*.[171] Consumption of raw milk has been associated with a chronic diarrhea syndrome of unknown cause,[294] initially identified in Minnesota and referred to as *Brainerd diarrhea*. It is manifested by acute onset with marked urgency and a lack of systemic symptoms. The duration of illness is at least 9 months and generally has involved adults. Clinical and laboratory data indicate that diarrhea is caused by a secretory mechanism. No evidence of secondary transmission exists. Antimicrobial therapy has not been successful.[294] In addition, an outbreak of chronic diarrhea involving 72 people who ingested untreated drinking water was reported.[297] The cause and pathophysiologic mechanism of the illness remain unknown.

Ingestion of raw fish (sushi or sashimi) has led to infection with *Vibrio parahaemolyticus* and various parasites from infected fish.[87,245] Parasites acquired through ingestion of raw fish include larval nematodes of the family Anisakidae, fish tapeworm of the species *Diphyllobothrium*, the fluke *Nanophyetus salmincola* from salmon, and many other helminths.[363,436] Most worm infections acquired from raw fish in the United States have been acquired from dishes prepared at home and not from sushi restaurants.

Symptoms in patients with chemical poisoning generally begin within 1 to 2 hours after ingestion, although certain mushroom toxins may produce symptoms for up to 24 hours (see Table 50-3). Heavy metals, such as antimony, arsenic, cadmium, copper, mercury, thallium, tin, and zinc, cause irritation of the gastric mucosa, with nausea, vomiting, and abdominal cramps, which usually resolve 2 to 3 hours after the offending agent has been removed.[62]

The toxic syndromes acquired from fish and shellfish can be grouped clinically into two categories: the histamine-like syndrome of scombroid poisoning and the neurotoxic syndrome, which includes ciguatera, paralytic shellfish poisoning, neurotoxic shellfish poisoning, and puffer fish poisoning caused by tetrodotoxin.[121] The neurologic symptoms produced by fish, shellfish, and the Chinese restaurant syndrome agent include paresthesia, reversal of hot-cold sensations, loss of proprioception, flushing, weakness, and burning sensations. Chinese restaurant syndrome appears to be caused by excessive amounts of monosodium glutamate in foods. Fish poisoning may be caused by scombrotoxin, ciguatoxin, or tetrodotoxin. Scombroid fish poisoning is characterized by symptoms resembling those of histamine release. Shellfish poisoning can be of two types: paralytic, caused by neurotoxins including saxitoxin, and neurotoxic, caused by several poorly characterized neurotoxins. Domoic acid from contaminated mussels causes acute widespread neurologic dysfunction and GI tract manifestations followed by chronic residual memory deficits and motor neuropathy or axonopathy.[303,400]

Infectious diseases associated with consumption of raw and lightly cooked shellfish (mussels, clams, oysters, lobsters, and other mollusks) are caused by bacterial agents that are native to the marine environment and by viral and bacterial agents from sewage effluents and other sources that contaminate environmental waters. As filter-feeding organisms, shellfish amplify public health problems associated with environmental contamination because they accumulate microbial pathogens at densities many times those found in overlying waters.

Public health problems of greatest concern to consumers of molluscan shellfish are associated with viral pathogens. The numbers of cases and outbreaks caused by these pathogens far exceed those of all other infectious causes.[245] The *Vibrio* genus (specifically *Vibrio vulnificus*) presents the most serious problem in terms of the severity of human illness and death, especially in people with liver disease.[180]

Mushrooms produce several clinical syndromes, generally within 2 hours of ingestion (see Table 50–3),[167] except for poisoning caused by amatoxins, phallotoxins, amantin, monomethylhydrazine, and gyromitrin, which may produce symptoms, including death, up to 24 hours after ingestion.[167] Mushrooms also can be contaminated with other agents, including *S. aureus* enterotoxin A.[235]

PulseNet is a national network of public health laboratories that perform pulsed-field gel electrophoresis analysis on bacteria that might be food-borne.[362] This network provides rapid comparison of pulsed-field gel electrophoresis patterns through an electronic database at the CDC. PulseNet has assisted in detecting food-borne outbreaks, especially those that involve multiple states.[362] An annual listing of food-borne disease outbreaks reported to the CDC is available at *www.cdc.gov/foodborneoutbreaks/outbreak_data.htm.*

Since 1971, the number of reported water-borne outbreaks in the United States has averaged 30 per year (range, 13 to 53 years), involving approximately 7600 people annually (range, 1569 to 21,149 people).[120,236] The CDC has published recommendations for management of fecal accidents in disinfected recreational water venues contaminated with formed or liquid stool.[72]

Water-borne disease and outbreaks are reported as those associated with drinking water and water not intended for drinking and those associated with recreational water.[120,236] During 2003 through 2004, 36 water-borne disease outbreaks associated with drinking water were reported; 30 were associated with water intended for drinking, 3 with water not intended for drinking, and 3 with water of unknown source.[236] In the 30 outbreaks associated with drinking water, 4 deaths occurred among the 2760 people who became ill. Etiologic agents were identified in 25, with 68 percent involving pathogens (13 bacterial, 1 parasitic, 1 viral, and 2 mixed organisms) and 32 percent involving chemical or toxin poisonings. The major clinical manifestations in these outbreaks were gastroenteritis (68%), acute respiratory tract illness (26%), and dermatitis (7%). Organisms associated with gastroenteritis were *Campylobacter* spp., *Shigella* spp., *Salmonella typhimurium*, *Giardia*, *Cryptosporidium*, and norovirus. *Legionella* spp. were associated with all of the respiratory tract outbreaks.

Types of water systems involved community, noncommunity, individual, and mixed systems. Types of deficiencies associated with outbreaks included untreated surface water intended for drinking, untreated ground water intended for drinking, water treatment deficiencies, and deficiencies in distribution systems including storage. All water-borne disease outbreaks should be reported to the state health department.

During 2003 through 2004, there were 62 reported water-borne disease outbreaks associated with recreational water that involved 2698 people, resulting in 58 hospitalizations and one death.[120] Of the 62 outbreaks (1945 people), 48 percent were gastroenteritis outbreaks associated with enteric pathogens, chemicals, or toxins (*Cryptosporidium*, *Giardia*, *Shigella* spp., norovirus, *Plesiomonas shigelloides*, and microcystin toxin from blue-green algae); 21 percent were dermatitis; 11 percent were respiratory illness; and 13 percent were other illnesses.

Recreational water–associated outbreaks of gastroenteritis followed exposure to both treated (60%) and untreated (40%) water. In outbreaks that occurred after exposure to treated water, *Cryptosporidium* was associated with 56 percent; in exposure to untreated water, *Cryptosporidium* accounted for 8 percent of outbreaks. There also were 142 *Vibrio* illnesses associated with recreational water exposure.

The main therapeutic modality in most patients with food poisoning is supportive care because most of these illnesses are self-limited. Exceptions include botulism, paralytic shellfish poisoning, tetrodotoxin, long-acting mushroom poisoning, and Shiga toxin–producing *E. coli* (STEC) infection, all of which may be fatal in previously healthy people. Food-borne disease caused by any agent can produce fatalities in infants, elderly people, debilitated people, or people with primary or secondary immune deficiencies. Food irradiation is an important technology that can protect the public against food-borne diseases.[395] Several Web sites that provide information about food-borne disease include *www.ama-assn.org/foodborne, www.cdc.gov/foodnet, www.cdc.gov/foodsafety,* and *www.fightbac.org.*

ANTIMICROBIAL-ASSOCIATED DIARRHEA

Diarrhea associated with use of an antimicrobial agent is a common occurrence. Changes in bowel flora may result in abnormal stools in the absence of a documented enteropathogen, and discontinuation of the medication may be sufficient to eliminate symptoms. In some patients with antibiotic-induced diarrhea, a severe and potentially fatal form of colitis may develop.[31,44,184,249]

Pseudomembranous or antimicrobial-associated colitis (AAC) refers to the presence of a pseudomembrane or of multiple plaquelike lesions in the colon induced by administration of an antimicrobial agent within the preceding 8 weeks. Pseudomembranous colitis not associated with use of antibiotics also may occur with *Shigella dysenteriae* serotype 1 and STEC.[214] Toxins produced by *Clostridium difficile* are the specific cause of essentially all cases of AAC.[365] Since 2005, an epidemic of *C. difficile* infection that is more serious and more refractory to therapy has been reported.[192,241,256,424] These studies have reported a highly characterized strain designated BI/NAP1, which is responsible for most of these outbreaks. The strain is a hypersecretor of the classic toxins A and B associated with *C. difficile*, possesses an additional toxin known as binary toxin, manifests deletion of an 18–base pair sequence in the pathogenicity locus responsible for down-regulation of toxin production, and has in vitro resistance to fluoroquinolones.[31,302]

Disease associated with *C. difficile* encompasses a range of severity from colitis, which often manifests as diarrhea, to toxic megacolon, requirement for colectomy, leukemoid reaction, and severe hypoalbuminemia that may result in sepsis, shock, and death.[44,88,134] These complications occur more commonly in older adults. In addition, nosocomial infection with *C. difficile* occurs and can result in asymptomatic carriage or diarrhea.[257] Most antimicrobial agents have been reported to cause this condition; broad-spectrum cephalosporins and clindamycin are implicated most commonly. Fluoroquinolones have emerged as a predominant risk for development of *C. difficile*–associated diarrhea.[302] Cancer chemotherapeutic agents also have been associated with AAC.

The diagnosis of AAC in a patient with diarrhea is supported by the following[29]:

1. A history of ongoing or recent antimicrobial therapy. Twenty to 40 percent of episodes occur after the drug has been discontinued.

2. Finding of leukocytes on a stain of fecal material.

3. Exclusion of other agents known to cause fecal leukocytes.

4. Identification of *C. difficile* toxins in stool specimens.

5. Endoscopy with rectal biopsy to identify pseudomembranes or plaques that contain mucin, fibrin, leukocytes, and sloughed epithelial cells.

Plaque and pseudomembranes not always are present in patients with AAC, but when they are, *C. difficile* usually can be presumed to be the cause of disease. The finding of *C. difficile* in feces suggests but does not confirm that *C. difficile* is the cause of the diarrhea. The finding of fecal toxin is a more useful method of diagnosing *C. difficile*–induced disease than is bacterial culture.[288] The enzyme immunoassay is used now by most laboratories because of ease of processing, cost, and speed of results.[31] This organism and the toxins may be found in the GI tract of some healthy people.[257,265] Approximately 15 to 63 percent of neonates, as many as 50 percent of infants younger than 1 year, and as many as 8 percent of children are asymptomatic carriers.[76,103]

The most important aspect of therapy in patients with AAC is discontinuation of the antimicrobial agent, after which symptoms usually resolve within 1 to 2 weeks; however, if symptoms persist or worsen or if the patient has severe diarrhea, specific therapy with metronidazole or oral vancomycin should be instituted.[169,260,301,399] Rifampin has been used as an adjunct to treatment with metronidazole, but it is not recommended.[230] Teicoplanin, fusidic acid, bacitracin, and nitazoxanide also have been used.[184,277,429] Metronidazole is preferred in guidelines, but vancomycin appears to be more effective in patients with severe disease.[31,276,300,441] After therapy has been initiated, symptoms generally resolve within several days, and fecal toxin disappears. Relapse of colitis after discontinuation of metronidazole or vancomycin has been documented in 10 to 20 percent of patients, generally 1 to 4 weeks after treatment has been discontinued.[32,301,399] Relapses are caused by germination of *C. difficile* spores that persist despite treatment and are not due to development of resistance. Relapses can be treated with a second course of metronidazole. Other modes of therapy include dietary reduction of carbohydrates and administration of probiotics to allow normal intestinal flora to be re-established.[184] Two meta-analyses demonstrated the benefit of probiotics in preventing antibiotic-associated diarrhea and treating *C. difficile* disease.[256,390] One study evaluated a variety of different types of probotics[256]; the other

evaluated *Saccharomyces boulardii*.[390] Further research is needed to determine the optimal probiotic, the best dose and duration of treatment, and the effectiveness against specific antimicrobial agents.

TRAVELER'S DIARRHEA

Traveler's diarrhea is the most common illness encountered by people from the United States, northern Europe, Canada, or Australia who travel to Latin America, Asia, the Middle East, or Africa, where diarrhea is hyperendemic.[113,115-117,160] Half of these travelers experience diarrhea within the first few weeks after arrival. Enterotoxigenic *E. coli* (ETEC) is the most commonly identified cause of traveler's diarrhea, but the illness can be caused by a variety of bacteria, viruses, and parasites,[115,116,290,364] including *Shigella* spp., *C. jejuni*, *Aeromonas* spp., *P. shigelloides*, *Salmonella* spp., *V. parahaemolyticus* (in Asia), *G. lamblia*, enteroaggregative *E. coli*, and enteric viruses, specifically norovirus. Information from existing studies concerning pathogens associated with diarrhea among children or elderly people who travel is limited. Studies of diarrhea in travelers visiting the United States and Great Britain from developed and developing countries showed attack rates of 2 and 0.6 percent, respectively.[346]

Clinical illness varies, reflecting the diversity of causative agents. Typically, illness occurs within several weeks of arrival in a foreign country and is defined as passage of at least three unformed stools in a 24-hour period, together with cramps, nausea, fecal urgency, tenesmus, or a combination thereof. Bloody diarrhea, vomiting, and documented elevation of temperature are less frequent signs and symptoms. Approximately 50 percent of people who become ill have mild disease, 15 to 40 percent are forced to alter their scheduled activities, and 15 to 30 percent are confined to bed. Because traveler's diarrhea is caused by a variety of enteropathogens, travelers may experience more than one episode. Traveler's diarrhea is spread by many fecally contaminated vehicles; most studies implicate food, particularly uncooked food,[128,405] and untreated water and ice.[174] Careful attention given to food consumption with avoidance of foods that are not steaming hot, raw vegetables, fruit not peeled by the traveler, tap water, and ice is critical to prevention of disease.[128,174] Predisposing factors and host factors that increase susceptibility to traveler's diarrhea or complicate its course include young age, short duration of travel, eating in restaurants, season, reduced gastric acidity, chronic and active GI tract disease, and immunodeficiency disorders.[128,183]

Several studies have evaluated prevention and treatment of traveler's diarrhea in adults using either antidiarrheal compounds or antimicrobial agents.[117] Compounds that have been shown to be effective chemoprophylactic agents include doxycycline, bismuth subsalicylate, trimethoprim-sulfamethoxazole (TMP-SMX), fluoroquinolones, and nonabsorbable antibiotics including rifaximin.[4,108,113,114,117] These compounds have been shown to offer 50 to 100 percent protection against traveler's diarrhea.[4,117] Potential problems with antibiotic regimens include development of resistance against certain agents, including ETEC, *Salmonella* spp., *Shigella* spp., and *C. jejuni*, and side effects, such as nausea, diarrhea, and photosensitivity reactions. Large doses of bismuth subsalicylate can result in significant concentrations of serum salicylate.[135,316] The bioavailability of salicylate in 1 ounce of Pepto-Bismol is equivalent to that of one 325-mg adult aspirin tablet.[135] Probiotics have been shown to be only minimally effective in prevention of diarrhea.[117]

Because of the uncertain risk of widespread prophylactic administration of these antimicrobial agents, including development of resistance among enteric bacteria, and the mildness of most cases of traveler's diarrhea, prophylactic use of antimicrobial agents is not recommended in children and has limited use in adults.[117,160] Instructing travelers with regard to appropriate dietary practices as a prophylactic measure is recommended.[128,405] If a person becomes ill in a locale where medical facilities are inadequate, self-treatment may be indicated.[4,117] Antidiarrheal compounds as therapy for traveler's diarrhea have been used in people with nondysenteric disease. Bismuth subsalicylate has been shown to be effective in decreasing the incidence of diarrhea by up to 60 percent.[116] Loperamide should not be used in infants or older children with bloody diarrhea or fever, although it may benefit older children and adults with watery diarrhea, especially when it is given in combination with an antimicrobial agent.[18,107,125] Other nonantimicrobial compounds have been shown to be ineffective or even dangerous or have not been evaluated.[18]

For self-treatment of diarrhea that occurs during travel in areas where medical care may not be available, travelers should take with them medication with expected activity against the prevalent bacteria. A 3- to 5-day antibiotic course may help children who develop diarrhea with three or more loose stools in an 8-hour period, especially if associated symptoms such as nausea, vomiting, abdominal cramps, fever, and blood in stools are present. A fluoroquinolone, azithromycin, or rifaximin for adults and azithromycin for children should be considered.[4,5,106,107,117,125,307] Problems with development of resistance by *C. jejuni* to fluoroquinolones may preclude their use in certain areas.

Approximately 3 percent of people develop persistent diarrhea after an episode of traveler's diarrhea.[109] The differential diagnosis should include persistent infection, particularly with *Giardia*, *Cryptosporidium*, *Cyclospora*, or *Isospora* spp.; antibiotic-associated colitis; small intestinal bacterial overgrowth; transient disaccharidase deficiency; initial manifestation of ulcerative colitis or regional enteritis; postdysenteric colitis; irritable bowel syndrome; and tropical sprue.[109] An underlying immune system defect, such as occurs with AIDS, also should be considered.

HUMAN IMMUNODEFICIENCY VIRUS INFECTION

Diarrheal disease often is a major problem in people with primary and secondary immunologic disorders.[22,356,439] The GI tract must act as the first line of defense against a wide variety of potentially harmful organisms and toxins. Immune deficiencies can result in an increased host susceptibility to intestinal tract infections or an atypical, prolonged, or disseminated course once an organism is established.

Causes of GI tract disease in children with AIDS can be grouped under the major headings of infection, malignant disease, and HIV enteropathy. The location of GI tract involvement by infectious agents determines the clinical symptoms and the ease with which these organisms can be diagnosed and treated (Table 50–4). Organisms and diseases of the GI tract that fulfill the CDC surveillance case definition of AIDS[59] are candidiasis, cryptosporidiosis, cytomegalovirus, herpes simplex, *Mycobacterium avium* complex, *Microsporidium*, isosporiasis, and *Salmonella* spp.[21,225,264] In addition, the AIDS wasting syndrome (HIV infection without superimposed opportunistic enteric infection of known cause) is part of the CDC case definition for AIDS.[59] Infection with any organism requires more attention because of malnutrition and co-morbidity.[203] Patients with AIDS have been shown to have D-xylose malabsorption and steatorrhea, and on jejunal and rectal biopsy specimens, a specific pathologic process can be demonstrated in the lamina propria of the small intestine and colon.[225] Before institution of highly active antiretroviral therapy (HAART), a significant proportion of patients with AIDS and severe small intestinal injury had enterocyte infection,[224] and infections occurred more frequently and were more likely to be severe, recurrent, persistent, or associated with extraintestinal disease.

TABLE 50–4   Organisms That Cause Gastrointestinal Tract Infections in Patients with AIDS

Area	Organisms
Esophagus	*Candida albicans** Cytomegalovirus* Herpes simplex virus*
Hepatobiliary	Cytomegalovirus *Cryptosporidium** Hepatotropic viruses *Mycobacterium avium* complex*
Small intestine	*Campylobacter* species Cytomegalovirus* *Cryptosporidium** *Giardia lamblia** *Isospora belli** *Mycobacterium avium* complex* *Microsporidium** (*Enterocytozoon bieneusi* and *Encephalitozoon intestinalis*) *Salmonella* species* *Strongyloides stercoralis*
Large intestine	*Campylobacter* species *Clostridium difficile* Cytomegalovirus* *Entamoeba histolytica* Herpes simplex virus* *Salmonella* species* *Shigella* species

Diseases of the gastrointestinal tract that fulfill the Centers for Disease Control and Prevention surveillance case definition of AIDS.

The occurrence of opportunistic infections in people infected with HIV should be considered as infections that occurred before and those since the advent of HAART. In 1993, 11,285 HIV-infected children aged 18 years or younger in the United States were hospitalized, compared with an estimated 3419 in 2003 (a 71% decrease).[227] The inpatient fatality rate also decreased from 5 percent in 1994 to 1.8 percent in 2003. In Thailand, the hospitalization rate in children decreased from 31 percent during the first 24-week period to 2 percent during weeks 120 to 144 after initiation of HAART.[327] The mortality rate also decreased from 5.7 percent in the first 24 weeks to 0 to 0.6 percent in the subsequent weeks of HAART therapy.[327] In another study in the United States, the impact of HAART on the overall incidence of opportunistic infection was significant, with a decline in incidence from 14.4 to 1.1 cases per 100 patient-years.[285] A study in adults examined the annual incidence of bacterial diarrhea before and during the HAART era in a large cohort of people with HIV infection.[285] Between 1992 and 2002, the overall rate of bacterial diarrhea in people with clinical AIDS decreased (odds ratio, 0.4; 95% confidence interval, 0.2 to 0.6). *C. difficile* was the most common cause of bacterial diarrhea. HAART can result in complete clinical, microbiologic, and histologic responses in patients with AIDS infected with *Cryptosporidium parvum* and *Enterocytozoon bieneusi*[56] and in patients with HIV enteropathy.[225] Guidelines for prevention of opportunistic infections, including those involving the GI tract, have been published.[64]

ORGANISMS THAT CAUSE ACUTE GASTROENTERITIS

BACTERIA

Many bacterial, viral, and parasitic organisms produce diarrhea in humans. Tables 50–5 and 50–6 show the major bacterial enteric pathogens associated with acute infectious diarrhea.[80] These organisms are discussed here in alphabetical order for ease

TABLE 50-5 Pathogenic Bacteria Associated with Acute Infectious Diarrhea

Agent	Epidemiologic Considerations
Aeromonas hydrophila	Water, food, or animal exposure
Bacillus cereus	Food exposure
Campylobacter jejuni	Animal or food exposure
Clostridium difficile	Exposure to antimicrobial agents
Clostridium perfringens	Food exposure
Listeria monocytogenes	Food exposure
Plesiomonas shigelloides	Water, fish, or animal exposure
Salmonella species	Exposure to carrier; food and reptile exposure
Shigella species	Exposure to an infected person or to contaminated food
Staphylococcus aureus	Food exposure
Vibrio cholerae O1	Food or water exposure
Vibrio cholerae O139	Food or water exposure
Vibrio parahaemolyticus	Seafood exposure
Yersinia enterocolitica	Food or animal exposure

TABLE 50-6 Pathogenic *Escherichia coli* Associated with Acute Infectious Diarrhea

Class of *E. coli*	Abbreviation	Usual Presentation of Disease
Shigatoxigenic	STEC	Bloody diarrhea, water- and food-borne outbreaks, associated with hemorrhagic colitis and hemolytic-uremic syndrome
Enterotoxigenic	ETEC	Watery diarrhea in children living in and travelers visiting developing countries
Enteroinvasive	EIEC	Dysentery in adults and watery diarrhea, occasionally food-borne outbreaks
Enteropathogenic	EPEC	Acute and chronic watery diarrhea in infants in nurseries, diarrhea in children younger than 1 year in developing countries
Enteroaggregative	EAEC	Acute and chronic watery diarrhea in children

of reference. The relative importance of each organism as a cause of diarrhea varies in different populations.

Aeromonas hydrophila

Aeromonas spp. are gram-negative bacteria found in soil and fresh and brackish water worldwide. *Aeromonas* spp. are recognized as colonizers and pathogens of cold-blooded animals, including fish, reptiles, and amphibians.[16] *Aeromonas* spp. have been associated with a wide spectrum of human disease, most frequently gastroenteritis, soft tissue infection, and bacteremia, especially in immunocompromised hosts.[16,196] Of the 14 species in the genus, *Aeromonas hydrophila*, *Aeromonas veronii*, *Aeromonas caviae*, *Aeromonas jandaei*, and *Aeromonas schubertii* have been associated with human disease; the first three are defined as major pathogens and the species associated with gastroenteritis.[196] Because many clinical laboratories cannot perform precise identification, most species isolated are reported as *A. hydrophila*.

The role of *A. hydrophila* in human diarrhea remains uncertain. Despite the association of this organism with acute gastroenteritis and in some studies its more frequent isolation from patients with diarrhea than from healthy controls,[196] volunteers

who have been fed the organism have not become ill.[270] *A. hydrophila* has been isolated from stools of less than 3 percent of healthy humans[16]; however, in Thailand, the isolation rate from healthy controls increased with age, up to 27 percent in adults.[16] *A. hydrophila* strains have been shown to produce both cytotoxin and enterotoxin, including heat-labile (cholera-like) enterotoxin and heat-stable enterotoxins.[365] Children with watery diarrhea associated with *Aeromonas* are significantly more likely to have organisms that possess genes for both a heat-labile cytotonic enterotoxin and the heat-stable cytotonic enterotoxin than are control children.[11] Other toxic or invasive properties may be important in production of disease because a fourth of patients have a dysentery-like illness.[196]

Bacillus cereus

Bacillus cereus is an aerobic, spore-forming, gram-positive bacillus that is a rare cause of food poisoning in the United States.[60,244] Although frequently present in food, *B. cereus* should be suspected as the cause of GI tract illness if appropriate symptoms are present and if incriminated food, particularly fried rice, contains 10^5 or more *B. cereus* organisms per gram.[62] Two distinct forms of GI tract illness can be produced by this organism. One is caused by production of a low-molecular-weight (1.2-kd) preformed emetic toxin, cereulide, that survives high temperatures, exposure to trypsin, and pH extremes. The other is caused by a group of three enterotoxins sensitive to high temperatures, proteolytic enzymes, and acids and is formed in vivo.[365] If the strain causing illness produces the emetic toxin, a syndrome occurs that resembles illness produced by staphylococcal enterotoxin, with nausea, vomiting, and abdominal cramps that begin within 1 to 6 hours of ingestion. Rarely, illness associated with the emetic toxin is followed by fulminant liver failure.[97] The diagnosis may be difficult to confirm because heating may kill the organism but leave the toxin intact. If the strain produces enterotoxins, profuse watery diarrhea and abdominal pain begin within 6 to 24 hours, with minimal or no vomiting. Some strains produce both toxins, whereas others produce only one toxin. Symptoms caused by either toxin usually resolve in less than 24 hours, and fever rarely occurs. Spores of *B. cereus* are resistant to heat and, therefore, may withstand a brief period of cooking or boiling. *B. cereus* can grow in temperatures ranging from 25° C to 40° C. *B. cereus* also has been associated with panophthalmitis, endophthalmitis, pneumonia, bacteremia, endocarditis, and meningitis.[105]

Campylobacter

Campylobacter spp. are recognized as one of the most important causes of acute diarrheal disease in humans throughout the world[15,55,202] and are a major bacterial cause of diarrhea in the United States.[15,70] Most diarrheal illness in the United States caused by *Campylobacter jejuni* is food-borne.[245] Currently, 18 *Campylobacter* spp. and subspecies are recognized. *C. jejuni* and *Campylobacter coli* are the two predominant species, although use of selective media and lack of use of stool filtration techniques may preclude isolation of other *Campylobacter* spp.[202,231,411] Many clinical microbiology laboratories do not differentiate *C. jejuni* and *C. coli*. *Campylobacter fetus*, recognized as a cause of fever, bacteremia, and meningitis in immunocompromised hosts and of abortion, rarely causes diarrhea. People infected with *C. jejuni* may develop diarrhea, cramping abdominal pain, chills, and fever. Gross rectal bleeding may occur, and mucus and fecal leukocytes may be present, resembling the illness produced by *Shigella*. The clinical presentation also may mimic that of inflammatory bowel disease. Both a heat-labile enterotoxin and mucosal invasion have been incriminated in the pathogenesis. *C. jejuni* also has been associated with reactive arthritis and Guillain-Barré syndrome.[278,393]

Phylogenetic trees have been established for *Campylobacter* and contain three distinct clades (species groups). The first consists of *C. fetus*, *Campylobacter hyointestinalis*, and *Campylobacter mucosalis*, all generally associated with disease in farm animals, although *C. fetus* and *C. hyointestinalis* produce human disease. The second clade consists of *C. coli*, *C. jejuni*, *Campylobacter helveticus*, *Campylobacter lari*, and *Campylobacter upsaliensis*; all (except *C. helveticus*) have been associated with gastroenteritis in humans. The third clade contains *Campylobacter curvus*, *Campylobacter concisus*, *Campylobacter gracilis*, *Campylobacter rectus*, *Campylobacter showae*, and *Campylobacter sputorum*, organisms generally associated with the periodontal cavity of humans and animals.

Helicobacter pylori (formerly *Campylobacter pylori*) has been isolated from the stomach and duodenum of patients with histologically confirmed type B antral gastritis, peptic ulcer disease, duodenal ulcers, and gastric lymphoma.[46] This organism is not associated with diarrhea. *Helicobacter cinaedi* and *Helicobacter fennelliae* were identified previously as *Campylobacter* spp. but have been reclassified.

Clostridium perfringens

Clostridium perfringens types A, C, and D produce an enterotoxin that is implicated in the pathogenesis of disease caused by this organism.[365] Most food-borne outbreaks are caused by type A strains. *C. perfringens* causes a short-duration food poisoning syndrome.[251] After contaminated meat or poultry products have been ingested, in vivo sporulation occurs in the small intestine, with release of a structural spore protein that has enterotoxic and cytotoxic properties. The heat-labile, 35-kd, single-polypeptide enterotoxin induces fluid accumulation in ileal loops in animals and produces diarrhea in humans. Within 14 hours after ingesting contaminated food, patients experience watery diarrhea and abdominal pain with minimal nausea, vomiting, or fever ensuing. Illness resolves in less than 24 hours. Less than 5 percent of *C. perfringens* isolates contain the chromosomal *cpe* gene encoding this toxin. *C. perfringens* type C also is associated with a rare destructive intestinal disease called *enteritis necroticans* or *pigbel*. These strains produce three toxins (alpha-toxin, beta-toxin, and an enterotoxin) of potential pathogenetic significance.[365] Enteritis necroticans occurs after ingestion of undercooked pig at pork feasts in Papua, New Guinea. It is characterized by vomiting, abdominal pain, bloody diarrhea, and small bowel necrosis, with peritonitis, shock, and death.[275]

Escherichia coli

Several recognized categories of *Escherichia coli* produce diarrhea (see Table 50–6).[279,365] *E. coli* is among the most common cause of bacterial diarrhea in humans worldwide.[315]

Shiga toxin–producing *E. coli* (STEC) produces bloody diarrhea, usually without fever. This hemorrhagic colitis syndrome has been recognized to be caused most often by *E. coli* O157:H7 and other STEC strains, which produce large quantities of a potent cytotoxin[65,210,279,365] similar or identical to the cytotoxin produced by *S. dysenteriae* serotype 1.[210] STEC also is referred to as enterohemorrhagic *E. coli* (EHEC) and verotoxin *E. coli* (VTEC).[323] Several closely related toxins are recognized. The *E. coli* toxin that essentially is identical to Shiga toxin made by *S. dysenteriae* is called Shiga toxin 1 (Stx1, also called verotoxin 1). A structurally and functionally related toxin that is distinct immunologically is called Stx2 (or verotoxin 2). Both toxins are encoded by bacteriophages. Multiple additional variants exist that are more closely related to the second toxin. *E. coli* organisms that produce high levels of cytotoxin are important clinically because, like *S. dysenteriae* 1, they have been incriminated as etiologic agents of hemolytic-uremic syndrome.[317] Most reported outbreaks result after ingestion of contaminated food or water.

Healthy cattle harbor the organism as part of their intestinal flora and are the main animal reservoir for STEC. Direct transmission from animals and their environments to humans in public settings where children come in contact with farm animals, such as petting zoos, represents a public health concern.[319] Hemolytic-uremic syndrome is characterized by the triad of hemolytic anemia, thrombocytopenia, and renal insufficiency and is associated most frequently with *E. coli* O157:H7. Approximately 8 percent of people infected with *E. coli* O157:H7 develop hemolytic-uremic syndrome; most reported cases occur in children younger than 5 years old.

Enterotoxigenic *E. coli* (ETEC) disease is caused by heat-stable (ST) and heat-labile (LT) enterotoxins.[279,328,365,398] STa and LT-I are associated with disease in humans and other animals, whereas STb is associated primarily with disease in piglets, and LT-II has been associated only with animal disease. ETEC strains from humans with diarrhea produce STa only, LT-I only, or both together. These toxins often are produced by strains that have colonization factor antigens, which are important in adherence of the organism to the GI tract.[279] ETEC strains belong to many different serogroups and cause disease in patients of all ages, especially infants and children living in developing countries and travelers from developed to developing countries, and outbreaks of food-borne disease in the United States.[328,398]

Enteroinvasive *E. coli* (EIEC) is related antigenically and biochemically to *Shigella* and causes either a dysentery-like illness or watery diarrhea. EIEC possesses 140-Md plasmids that encode invasiveness and contribute to dysenteric illness. This plasmid is related closely to the plasmids that are associated with *Shigella* virulence.[279] The watery diarrhea may be due to an enterotoxin referred to as *EIEC enterotoxin*. Infections generally occur in adults; food-borne outbreaks have been reported.

Enteropathogenic *E. coli* (EPEC) has been incriminated as a cause of both sporadic and epidemic diarrhea in infants, especially in developing countries.[100] Originally, EPEC was a term used to describe all *E. coli* organisms associated with diarrheal syndromes. Currently, the term EPEC is defined more narrowly. Volunteer studies[100] and studies comparing rates of isolation from sick and healthy infants[279] have demonstrated that EPEC organisms are pathogens, although these strains rarely cause diarrhea in older children and adults. The specific mechanisms involved in production of disease may be related to adherence, which can be demonstrated in HEp-2 cells.[101,279] The proposed three stages of EPEC infection include (1) intestinal colonization mediated by the bundle-forming pilus; (2) induction of the attaching and efficacy lesion through intimin and other secreted proteins; and (3) signal transduction, resulting in induction of a net secretory state.[95,100,102,365]

Enteroaggregative *E. coli* (EAEC) is a cause of acute diarrheal illness among many different subpopulations in both developing and industrial regions of the world,[191,192] including the United States. EAEC also has been associated with chronic diarrhea in developing countries[39,156,364] and in adults with traveler's diarrhea.[3,156] Bloody diarrhea has been described in approximately a third of patients. Chronic persistent diarrhea is especially likely to be caused by EAEC.[361,364] Pathogenicity of EAEC in humans has been confirmed in volunteer studies and outbreak investigations.[252,376] EAEC is defined by its aggregative or stacked brick pattern of adherence in HEp-2 cell assays,[279] the "gold standard" for identification. Some strains elaborate an enterotoxin (EAEC ST enterotoxin 1 [EAST1]).[279,359] However, this toxin is not uniquely present in EAEC, nor is it found consistently (only 40-45% of EAEC pathogens are EAST1-positive in some series).[279,361] A plasmid-encoded enterotoxin may be important, but its role is not fully defined.[124,282] Many EAEC pathogens have genes for aggregative adherence fimbriae (*AAF/I* or *AAF/II*).[85,334] A gene probe that appeared in initial studies to be both sensitive and specific appears to be less useful than is the original HEp-2 cell assay.[131,334]

Listeria monocytogenes

The genus *Listeria* includes six species, of which two are potentially pathogenic, *Listeria monocytogenes* and *Listeria ivanovii*.[410] *L. monocytogenes* is a rare but serious localized and generalized infection in humans. Listeriosis is primarily food-borne. Acute febrile gastroenteritis caused by *L. monocytogenes* contamination of a variety of foods has been described.[28,67,86,161] The foods most frequently implicated are soft cheeses and dairy products; pâtés and sausages; smoked fish; and industrially produced, refrigerated, ready-to-eat products that are eaten without cooking or reheating. *L. monocytogenes* tolerates high concentrations of salt and relatively low pH and is able to multiply at refrigerator temperatures. Bacteremia may complicate diarrheal illness caused by this organism,[28,67,352] especially in immunocompromised hosts, during pregnancy, and in older people. Symptoms include fever (temperature as high as 40.3° C), chills, headache, cramps, myalgia, and diarrhea.[28,291]

Plesiomonas shigelloides

Plesiomonas shigelloides is a gram-negative bacillus that has been associated with opportunistic infections in immunocompromised hosts and with sporadic cases of diarrhea in immunocompetent hosts in a variety of countries.[187,208] In some case-control studies, the organism has been found to be associated with diarrhea, whereas in others, it has not.[12] Whether a subset of *P. shigelloides* has virulence genes that make them pathogens, whereas other members of this species do not have such genes, is unclear. Organisms produce ST and HL enterotoxins, but their associations with disease are unknown.[365] The organism has been isolated from surface water and the intestines of freshwater fish and many animals, including dogs and cats.[404] *Plesiomonas* occurs commonly in tropical and subtropical areas from which most stool isolates have been reported.[187] Patients with *P. shigelloides* infection describe self-limited diarrhea, occasionally characterized by blood and mucus. The organism is a rare cause of extraintestinal illness, such as meningitis or bacteremia.[208] Appropriate antimicrobial therapy appears to shorten the duration of diarrheal illness.[196,208] The organism has failed to produce illness when fed to volunteers, and its role as an enteric pathogen remains unknown.[173]

Salmonella

Identification of *Salmonella* spp. in the laboratory is not difficult, but the various terminologies used to classify *Salmonella* spp. is confusing. Most hospital laboratories biochemically differentiate *Salmonella* ser. Enterica and *Salmonella* ser. Typhi, although other nomenclature schemes may be used.[51] Since 1993, the *Salmonella* isolates most frequently reported have been *S. enterica* serotype Typhimurium and *S. enterica* serotype Enteritidis.[58,73] Several clinical syndromes are caused by *Salmonella*: the carrier state; acute gastroenteritis; bacteremia, enteric fever, or both; and dissemination with localized suppuration, such as abscess, osteomyelitis, or meningitis. Although *S.* ser. Typhi is the prototype of *Salmonella* able to penetrate intestinal mucosa, reach intestinal lymphatic tissue, and disseminate, other *Salmonella* organisms, particularly *Salmonella* Paratyphi A, occasionally behave in this manner.[73,185] Invasion of intestinal epithelium by *S.* ser. Typhi and occasionally by nontyphoidal *Salmonella* strains is a well-known virulence trait of *Salmonella* spp. Most nontyphoidal *Salmonella* serotypes are associated with watery diarrhea. *Salmonella* rarely causes an illness similar to pseudomembranous colitis.[190] *Salmonella* gastroenteritis occurs throughout life but

most commonly in the first 5 years of life, decreases during childhood, and remains relatively constant throughout the adult years.[73] Although most episodes of *Salmonella* infection are food-borne, reptiles, including turtles, snakes, lizards, and iguanas, carry certain serotypes of *Salmonella* in their intestinal tracts and have been associated with episodes of salmonellosis.[281,319,387] Numerous outbreaks of disease caused by *Salmonella* after ingestion of contaminated food products, including eggs, milk, ice cream, peanut butter, and fresh produce, have been reported.[48,68,171,245,326] Food-borne outbreaks associated with *Salmonella* have been reported from fairs or festivals, hospitals, nursing homes, and prisons.[73]

Shigella

Four serogroups of *Shigella*, containing more than 40 serotypes and subtypes, exist.[215] *Shigella sonnei* accounts for more than 75 percent of shigellosis in the United States. *Shigella boydii* and *Shigella dysenteriae* are uncommon causes of diarrhea in the United States. In 2005, a strain of *S. sonnei* resistant to ampicillin and TMP-SMX emerged as a cause of prolonged community-wide outbreaks of shigellosis associated with childcare centers in three states.[368] In addition to person-to-person spread, shigellae can be transmitted through contaminated foods, sexual contact, and water used for drinking or recreational purposes.[120,245] Patients with *Shigella* isolated from stool may present with several clinical patterns: asymptomatic excretion,[312] enterotoxin-like watery diarrhea, bacillary dysentery,[385] arthritis similar to that seen in Reiter syndrome,[9] and hemolytic-uremic syndrome occurring after infection with *S. dysenteriae* 1. The arthritis occurs 2 to 5 weeks after the dysenteric illness, characteristically in patients with histocompatibility antigen HLA-B27. Postinfectious arthritis also occurs in patients after they have had *Salmonella*, *Campylobacter*, and *Y. enterocolitica* infections.[119] *S. dysenteriae* 1 produces Shiga toxin in high levels.[385] Infection by *Shigella* spp. rarely occurs in the first few months of life but is a common occurrence in children between the ages of 6 months and 10 years.[73]

Staphylococcus aureus

Two enteric syndromes have been associated with *Staphylococcus aureus*. Although previously it was considered a cause of AAC, whether antibiotic-associated staphylococcal enteritis actually exists as a disease entity is unclear because most antibiotic-associated colitis is associated with *C. difficile*.[33] The existence of the other major staphylococcal enteric syndrome is well established. Staphylococcal food poisoning is caused by ingestion of food contaminated with preformed *S. aureus* ST enterotoxin.[123,235] Illness usually occurs within 2 to 4 hours after ingestion of contaminated food[244] and is manifested by vomiting and diarrhea. Although multiple enterotoxins (A to F) have been described, only enterotoxin types A to E cause enteric disease. Type A has been responsible for more than half of the reported outbreaks of staphylococcal food poisoning in the United States.[186,235] All toxins are antigenically related, low-molecular-weight proteins. Illness caused by these preformed toxins begins within 1 to 6 hours after ingestion and lasts less than 12 hours. Nausea, vomiting, abdominal pain, and diarrhea occur without fever.

Vibrio cholerae

Strains of *Vibrio cholerae* are classified according to somatic or O groups. *V. cholerae* strains are separated further into two main serotypes (Ogawa and Inaba) and two biotypes (classic and El Tor).[209] *V. cholerae* responsible for epidemic cholera belong to serogroups O1 and O139; all other *V. cholerae* strains belong to serogroups other than O1 and O139 and occasionally cause diarrhea or extraintestinal infections.[197] Cholera affects people of all ages, but children are involved disproportionately. *V. cholerae* O139 infection occurs primarily in Southeast Asia. *V. cholerae* O1 infection occurs primarily in Asia, Africa, and South America, although a focus is present in the Gulf Coast of the United States.[209,243,271] Most clinical isolates of *V. cholerae* O1 in the United States are associated with foreign travel and with ingestion of undercooked seafood,[73,271] and many are resistant to antimicrobial agents.[386] Crabs harvested from the U.S. Gulf coast are a common source of cholera.[73] After Hurricane Katrina in 2005, crabs were the source of illness for certain cases of cholera.[73,74] Epidemic cholera appeared in Peru in January 1991 and subsequently spread throughout the Americas, including the United States.[209] The epidemic strain is biotype El Tor, serotype Inaba. This strain can be differentiated from the strain of *V. cholerae* that is endemic to the U.S. Gulf coast by production of hemolysin and by molecular subtyping techniques.

V. cholerae O1 adheres to and multiplies on small intestinal mucosa. Diarrhea occurs after elaboration of several toxins, the most important of which is cholera toxin, an HL enterotoxin composed of one A and five B subunits.[365] The B subunits bind the toxin to the terminal galactose of the G_{M1} ganglioside receptors present on intestinal mucosal cells. The A subunit adenosine 5′-diphosphate ribosylates the guanosine 5′-triphosphate–binding regulatory protein of adenylate cyclase in gut epithelium.[365] The resulting intracellular increase in cyclic adenosine monophosphate causes inhibition of sodium absorption and causes chloride and fluid secretion in the small intestine. Most non-O1 strains isolated from ill people in the United States lack cholera toxin–like activity[197] and, when tested with gene probes, are found not to possess gene sequences homologous to those of cholera toxin.[209] Two additional toxins are produced by *V. cholerae*, Zot (zonula occludens toxin) and Ace (accessory cholera enterotoxin). Strains of *V. cholerae* belonging to serotypes other than O1 and O139 are much less significant pathogens, although they can cause mild and occasionally profuse, watery diarrhea. Other *Vibrio* spp., including *Vibrio fluvialis*, *Vibrio mimicus*, *Vibrio hollisae*, and *Vibrio furnissii*, have been shown occasionally to cause GI tract disease.[197]

Vibrio parahaemolyticus

Vibrio parahaemolyticus is a gram-negative, halophilic bacterium that inhabits warm estuarine waters worldwide. The organism has been found in water, shellfish, fish, and plankton[180] and has caused outbreaks of gastroenteritis after ingestion of contaminated seafood.[258,271] Although widely distributed in coastal waters, *V. parahaemolyticus* is an uncommon cause of diarrhea where consumption of raw seafood is common. Clinical manifestations of infection with *V. parahaemolyticus* are gastroenteritis in 59 percent of cases and include abdominal cramps, nausea, and, less frequently, vomiting, headache, low-grade fever, and chills; wound infections, including hemorrhagic cellulitis in 34 percent; and septicemia in 5 percent.[87] A dysentery-like syndrome has been described in India and Bangladesh.[193] Preexisting liver disease predisposes infected patients to development of septicemia and death.[180] A selective culture medium is required for isolation of the organism from stool cultures.

Yersinia enterocolitica

Yersinia enterocolitica is a gram-negative bacillus that appears to be a common cause of gastroenteritis among children in Europe and Canada but is a relatively uncommon cause of enteritis in the United States, where *Y. enterocolitica* O8 has been the predominant clinical serotype.[45] The ingestion of contaminated milk or food such as chitterlings[206,232] has been implicated as the mode of transmission in reported outbreaks. The clinical manifestations vary according to the age of the person involved. Illness in chil-

dren younger than 5 years usually is self-limited gastroenteritis. Stools may contain blood and mucus or be watery. Associated symptoms consist of fever, vomiting, and abdominal pain. Older children may present with abdominal pain associated with mesenteric adenitis that mimics acute appendicitis. Adults develop diarrhea and abdominal pain less frequently than do children but may present with polyarthritis, arthralgia, or erythema nodosum. Patients with beta-thalassemia and iron overload are at an increased risk for development of severe yersiniosis.[6]

VIRUSES

Acute infectious diarrhea of viral origin generally is a self-limited disease characterized by various combinations of diarrhea, nausea, vomiting, abdominal cramps, headaches, myalgias, and low-grade fever.[254,263,289,412] Bowel movements are watery and generally do not contain mucus or blood. Vomiting is the most common manifestation of this condition. Rotavirus, enteric adenovirus, astrovirus, and norovirus are common causes of viral gastroenteritis (Table 50–7). Other viruses, including coronaviruses, Breda virus, parvoviruses, pestiviruses, picobirnaviruses, and toroviruses, have been linked to gastroenteritis in humans with varying degrees of certainty.[34,222,440]

Rotaviruses

Rotavirus is a 70-nm particle that on electron microscopy resembles a wheel with radiating spokes (Fig. 50–1). Rotavirus was associated with diarrhea in children first by Bishop and associates in 1973.[42] Since then, human rotavirus has been established as a

TABLE 50–7   Viruses Associated with Gastroenteritis

Virus	Approximate Size (nm)
Rotavirus	70
Enteric adenovirus (types 40 and 41)	70-80
Astrovirus	20-30
Calicivirus (noroviruses)	35-39
Parvovirus	20-30
Coronavirus	80-180
Pestivirus	40-60
Breda virus	100

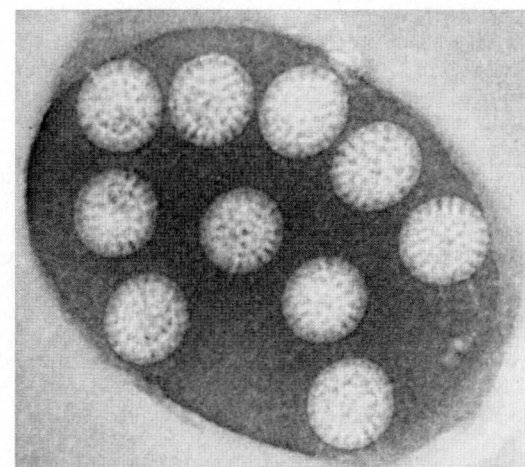

Figure 50–1 Electron micrograph of rotavirus particles in a fecal specimen from an infant with diarrhea. (Phosphotungstic acid, ×238,000.)

major cause of acute gastroenteritis in infants, children, and various animal species worldwide. Six antigenically distinct groups of rotavirus (A through F) have been recognized. Three of these groups (A, B, and C) have been identified in humans. The group A rotaviruses are those associated with infantile diarrhea.[130] Group B rotaviruses have caused epidemics of cholera-like illness in China and sporadic cases elsewhere.[279,366] Group C rotaviruses have caused outbreaks of diarrhea in children in many countries.[286]

Group A rotaviruses have two outer capsid proteins, a hemagglutinin (VP4) and a glycoprotein (VP7), each of which induces neutralizing antibodies.[130] Fourteen different antigenic types of VP7 (which define serotype) and seven human serotypes of VP4 (also designated P serotypes because VP4 is protease sensitive), including two subtypes, are known. This number, combined with the ability of the gene segments to reassort independently, indicates that rotaviruses are complex antigenically.[130] VP7 (also designated G serotype) serotypes 1, 2, 3, 4, and 9 are of epidemiologic importance. Epidemiologic studies indicate that these serotypes are endemic in most regions, that one serotype tends to be predominant at any particular time, that predominant serotypes differ among regions in the same country, and that predictable cycles of change of the predominant serotype may occur.[254]

Rotavirus gastroenteritis affects more than 90 percent of children by the time they are 3 years of age and may cause moderate to severe vomiting that precedes diarrhea. It accounts for 10 to 50 percent of the cases of diarrhea in children and is the most common cause of diarrhea in infants and children during winter months in colder climates. Rotavirus accounts for 35 to 50 percent of infants and young children hospitalized for acute diarrhea. In the United States, rotavirus accounts for 60,000 hospitalizations per year and 37 deaths.[140] Stools usually are watery or soft, and the presence of blood or leukocytes is rare. Asymptomatic rotavirus infections occur frequently,[289,311] and re-infection appears to be a common event.[415,416] The mechanism of spread is fecal-oral; whether respiratory transmission occurs is uncertain. Shedding of virus most frequently occurs from a few days before to 10 days after the onset of illness.[311] Before licensure of the rotavirus vaccine in 2006, outbreaks of rotavirus in childcare centers occurred commonly (usually in the colder months), were caused by a single serotype,[289] and were manifested by the fact that half the infected children were asymptomatic.[30]

The incubation period of human rotavirus infection ranges from 2 to 4 days. Animal models suggest that whereas morphologic changes in the villous tip cells contribute to malabsorption and diarrhea, altered cell function, resulting in enzyme deficiencies, results from enterocyte immaturity and may account for the major part of the disordered physiologic findings. Adults with rotavirus gastroenteritis treated with nitazoxanide showed a significant reduction in time to resolution of symptoms compared with controls (1.5 versus 2.5 days).[341] In hospitalized children, nitazoxanide reduced the duration of rotavirus infection.[338]

The first rotavirus vaccine licensed in the United States was associated with an increased rate of intussusception, resulting in its withdrawal from the market within 14 months of being licensed.[274,332] In February 2006, a bovine-based pentavalent rotavirus vaccine was licensed by the FDA for use in infants in the United States[19,71] as a three-dose vaccine administered orally at 2, 4, and 6 months of age, with all doses administered by the time the child reaches 32 weeks of age. A two-dose orally administered, attenuated monovalent G1 (P8) human rotavirus vaccine is available in many countries throughout the world and is being reviewed by the FDA for licensing in the United States.[343]

Astroviruses

Astroviruses, identified in 1975, are 20 to 30 nm in diameter and have a characteristic five- to six-pointed star. The virus genome is a positive-stranded RNA of about 7500 nucleotides that encodes four structural proteins.[157,422] Eight different antigenic types have been described. Astrovirus gastroenteritis occurs worldwide and has been associated with outbreaks of mild gastroenteritis in schools, childcare centers, pediatric wards, and nursing homes.[94,157,164,263] Illness is restricted primarily to children and elderly people; 80 percent or more of adults have antibodies against the virus. The incubation period is 3 to 4 days.[157] Symptoms include fever and malaise, followed by watery diarrhea that may last approximately 3 days. Vomiting is an uncommon symptom. Short-term intolerance of monosaccharides and more prolonged intolerance of cow's milk protein have been reported after astrovirus infection.[157]

Noroviruses

Members of the genus *Norovirus* in the family *Caliciviridae* have been identified as the most common viral cause of acute gastroenteritis in humans, with an estimated 23 million cases occurring annually.[43,407] The mean incubation period for norovirus is 24 to 48 hours. The primary routes of transmission are fecal-oral, including consumption of fecally contaminated food or water; direct person-to-person contact, especially in schools, childcare centers, restaurants, summer camps, hospitals, nursing homes, and cruise ships[10,69,200,201,221,330]; and through contaminated objects or environments. A low inoculum dose is required for infection, and prolonged, asymptomatic shedding can occur in infected people. Clinical manifestations include acute onset of vomiting, nonbloody diarrhea, or both lasting 12 to 60 hours. Molecular epidemiology techniques have identified substantial diversity in strains, indicating that epidemic strains of norovirus might be more virulent or more environmentally persistent than are nonepidemic strains.[43] The identification of human histo-blood group antigens as norovirus receptors opens a new approach for evaluation of susceptibility and therapy of norovirus infection.[136] The demonstration of an in vitro cell culture infectivity assay for human norovirus may improve understanding of the pathogenesis of human norovirus infections.[389]

Enteric Adenoviruses

Human adenoviruses of subgroups A to F have been identified as etiologic agents in a wide range of human diseases, including conjunctivitis, upper respiratory tract infections, and pneumonia. A subgroup of fastidious adenoviruses (group F) with a distinct set of antigenic determinants and specific tissue culture growth characteristics have been shown to be associated with acute gastroenteritis and are referred to as *enteric adenoviruses*.[50,226,412] These agents fail to propagate in conventional cell lines used to grow adenoviruses but grow readily in 293 cells, an adenovirus type 5 transformed line.

The enteric adenoviruses in group F include serotypes 40 and 41.[226] Types 40 and 41 both appear to be widespread and endemic causes of diarrhea in children. Antibody prevalence to enteric adenovirus increases from 20 percent during the first 6 months of life to 50 percent or greater by the third or fourth year of life.[372] Seasonal shifts in the predominance of types 40 and 41, similar to those described for rotavirus, may occur. A 9-year study in Washington, DC, found that enteric adenovirus types 40 and 41 circulate simultaneously all year.[50] Infection with enteric adenovirus appears to increase in the summer, although with a less marked seasonal variation than that exhibited by rotavirus, which peaks in the winter.[50] Outbreaks of enteric adenovirus diarrhea have been described in childcare centers, where asymptomatic excretion is a common occurrence.[412]

PARASITES

The most important protozoa known to cause diarrhea in various populations in the United States are *Entamoeba histolytica*, *G. lamblia*, and spore-forming protozoa: *Cryptosporidium parvum*, *Isospora belli*, *Microsporidium* spp. (*Encephalitozoon intestinalis* and *Enterocytozoon bieneusi*), and *Cyclospora cayetanensis*. Among helminths, *Strongyloides stercoralis* and *Trichuris trichiura* may produce diarrhea. Data associating *Ascaris* and hookworm with diarrhea are lacking, but both cause abdominal pain. HIV infections stimulated renewed interest in several of these organisms, including various *Microsporidium* spp., *C. parvum*, and *I. belli*.[159] *Balantidium coli* is a cause of bloody diarrhea in humans. The roles of *Blastocystis hominis* and *Dientamoeba fragilis* as causes of diarrhea are not known.

Cryptosporidium

Cryptosporidium organisms are coccidian protozoa that invade and replicate within the microvillous region of epithelial cells lining the digestive and respiratory tracts of vertebrates.[79] *Cryptosporidium* spp. are related taxonomically to *Toxoplasma*, *Sarcocystis*, *Isospora*, and *Plasmodium* spp. Fecal-oral transmission of *Cryptosporidium* oocysts occurs from person to person, through ingestion of contaminated drinking water or recreational water, through consumption of contaminated food, or by contact with infected animals (cattle and sheep).[61,73,120,181,236] Unlike bacterial pathogens, *Cryptosporidium* are resistant to chlorine disinfection and can survive for days in treated recreational water, including swimming pools and recreational water parks.[120] Children aged 4 years old and younger appear to be at a particularly high risk for acquiring this organism.[73] Cryptosporidia have been implicated as a cause of diarrhea in travelers and of epidemics in hospitals, childcare centers, and other institutional settings worldwide. Other groups at risk include animal handlers, travelers to foreign countries with a high prevalence of *Cryptosporidium*, and hospital personnel. The largest water-borne outbreak of diarrhea documented in the United States was caused by *Cryptosporidium*.[246] Volunteer studies in adults showed that 132 oocysts cause disease.[112] The incubation period in humans has been estimated to be 2 to 14 days.

Cryptosporidiosis can be manifested with a wide spectrum of symptoms, including asymptomatic excretion, acute diarrhea, chronic diarrhea, epidemic diarrhea, severe life-threatening watery diarrhea, and biliary tract disease.[79] Watery diarrhea is the hallmark of symptomatic infections, but few if any features distinguish gastroenteritis caused by *Cryptosporidium* in the immunocompetent patient from other enteric infections. Stools do not contain blood or leukocytes. Vomiting, flatulence, abdominal pain, and low-grade fever routinely accompany diarrhea.[168] Symptoms usually subside in an average of 9 days. Patients may have cholera-like illness, transient diarrhea, relapsing episodes, or a protracted clinical course with unremitting, profuse diarrhea lasting for months accompanied by profound malabsorption and weight loss. Before HAART was instituted, enteritis caused by *Cryptosporidium* occurred in 10 to 15 percent of patients with AIDS in the United States and approximately 15 percent of patients with AIDS in the developing world.[248] The frequency with which *Cryptosporidium* and microsporidia are identified in stools of patients with AIDS is a reflection of the CD4 count; identification of the organisms and symptoms is more frequent when the count is less than 100 cells/μL.[141] Antiretroviral therapy is protective against disease.[56,248] Biliary tract infection with *Cryptosporidium* produces two syndromes: sclerosing cholangitis–type lesions, which cause progressive, irregular obstruction and dilation of the intrahepatic and extrahepatic bile ducts,[37] and acalculous cholecystitis, caused by infection of the wall of the gallbladder. Symptoms have been characterized by right upper quadrant pain, nausea, and vomiting.

Entamoeba histolytica

The life cycle of *Entamoeba histolytica* involves encystment of a trophozoite, followed by release of the trophozoite from the cyst under appropriate conditions in the GI tract (Fig. 50–2).[129] Trophozoites vary in size and are found in stools of patients with dysentery or diarrhea. The cyst is more resistant to environmental stresses and is the infective stage. Cysts are found more frequently in formed stools. The minimum period between ingestion of cysts and development of symptoms is 8 days. The incubation period ranges up to 95 days.

The genus *Entamoeba* contains many species, six of which can reside in the human intestinal lumen. *E. histolytica* is the only species definitely pathogenic. *Entamoeba dispar* and *Entamoeba moshkovskii* do not appear to be pathogenic. New approaches to identifying *E. histolytica* are based on detection of *E. histolytica*–specific antigen and DNA in stool and other clinical specimens.[142] Several molecular techniques, including polymerase chain reaction (PCR), have been developed for detection and differentiation of *E. histolytica*, *E. dispar*, and *E. moshkovskii*.

Clinical patterns that occur in patients with amebiasis consist of intestinal amebiasis, with the gradual onset of colicky abdominal pain and frequent bowel movements, tenesmus, and little or no constitutional disturbance; amebic dysentery, characterized by profuse diarrhea containing blood and mucus and the presence of constitutional signs, such as fever, dehydration, and electrolyte alterations; hepatic amebiasis, which usually presents as abscess formation without GI tract symptoms[8]; and asymptomatic

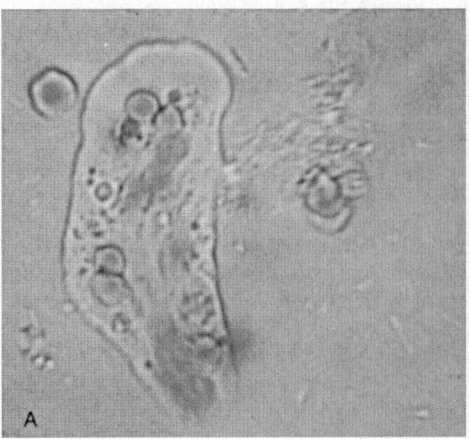
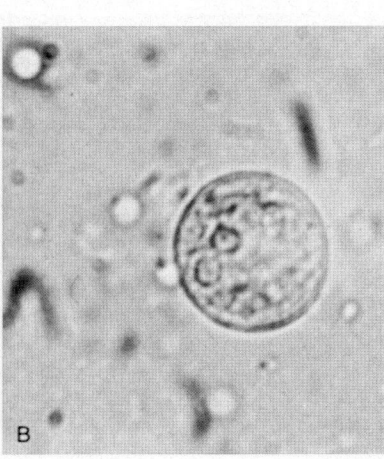

Figure 50–2 A, Trophozoite of *Entamoeba histolytica* with ingested material in the cytoplasm. **B,** Cyst of *E. histolytica* seen in a merthiolate-iodine-formalin–stained preparation from a stool specimen. Note two visible nuclei (×1000). (*From DuPont, H. L., and Pickering, L. K.: Infections of the Gastrointestinal Tract. New York, Plenum Publishing, 1980.*)

colonization. Patients may experience tender hepatomegaly, jaundice, weight loss, fever, and anorexia. The frequency of liver abscess in patients with amebiasis is between 1 and 5 percent. The complications of intestinal amebiasis include perforation, ameboma, stricture, hemorrhage secondary to erosion into a blood vessel, intussusception, ischiorectal abscess, fistulas, and rectal prolapse. People in the third through fifth decades of life have the highest incidence of infection and clinical symptoms, although people of all ages are susceptible.

Giardia intestinalis

Giardia intestinalis (formerly *G. lamblia*), a flagellated protozoan, is the most common intestinal parasite identified by public health laboratories in the United States.[63,146] Giardia infection is transmitted by the fecal-oral route and occurs after ingestion of *Giardia* cysts in fecally contaminated food or water or through person-to-person transmission.[120,236,245] The low infectious dose of 10 cysts places people in close contact, including children in childcare, at risk of acquiring infection.[331] The relative contribution of person-to-person, animal-to-person, water-borne, and food-borne transmission to sporadic human disease is unknown. Children appear to be more susceptible to *Giardia* than are adults. Specific conditions that predispose to giardiasis are hypogammaglobulinemia, secretory immunoglobulin A (IgA) deficiency, peptic ulcer disease, biliary tract disease, and pancreatitis. The parasite may exist in two forms: cyst and trophozoite (Fig. 50–3). After being ingested, each cyst divides into two trophozoites,

which subsequently mature. The trophozoites usually are seen in duodenal aspirates and loose stools, whereas cysts can be found in formed stools and can remain viable and infectious in water for longer than 3 months. Scanning electron micrographic examination of *Giardia* reveals firm attachment to the intestine (Fig. 50–4).

People vary in their response to infection with *Giardia*, with the following clinical manifestations: asymptomatic; an acute illness with a sudden onset of explosive, watery, foul-smelling stools and flatulence, abdominal distention, nausea, and anorexia, with the absence of blood and mucus; and chronic diarrhea and malabsorption, with exacerbations and remissions of flatulence, abdominal distention, and abdominal pain often lasting for months.[309]

Strongyloides stercoralis

Strongyloides stercoralis is a nematode that infects humans through the intestinal tract or through skin if either comes in contact with soil that contains larvae. About one third of people with strongyloidiasis are asymptomatic, and the remainder may have skin, pulmonary, or, more frequently, GI tract involvement.[373] People at risk include residents and travelers to endemic areas; natives and residents of the Appalachian region in the United States; institutionalized patients; and people treated with corticosteroids, cimetidine, and antacids.[152] Epigastric abdominal pain occurs and is associated with diarrhea that contains mucus and blood. Some patients may complain of nausea, vomiting, and weight loss with

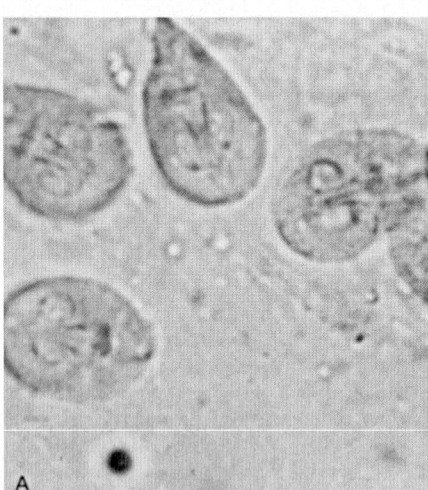
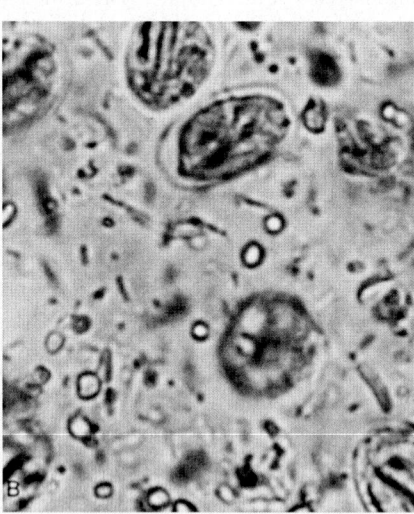

Figure 50–3 A. Trophozoites of *Giardia lamblia* seen in a merthiolate-iodine-formalin–stained preparation of stool from a patient with diarrhea (×1000). **B.** Cysts of *G. lamblia* seen in a merthiolate-iodine-formalin–stained preparation of stool from a patient without diarrhea (×1000).

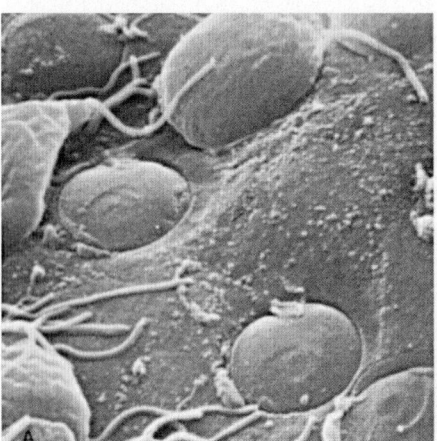
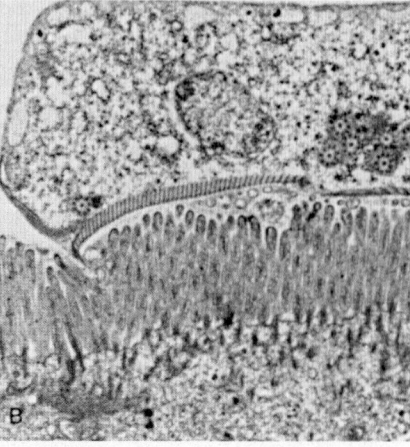

Figure 50–4 A. Scanning electron micrograph of an intestinal villus revealing firm attachment of *Giardia muris* trophozoites to the microvillous border. Circular dome-shaped lesions in the microvillous border are produced by attachment of the adhesive disk of trophozoite (×4600). **B.** Transmission electron micrograph of a *G. muris* trophozoite illustrating how lesions in the microvillous border are produced. Note that the edges of the adhesive disk penetrate the microvillous border and compress the microvilli centrally. The microvilli also show some vesiculation under the adhesive disk (×20,000). *(A, B, Courtesy of Dr. S. L. Erlandsen.)*

evidence of malabsorption. Eosinophilia and an urticarial rash are prominent features of infection. *S. stercoralis* hyperinfection syndrome can present in immunocompromised patients years after exposure and can result in multisystem organ involvement culminating in sepsis.[213] People infected with *S. stercoralis* should be treated with ivermectin or albendazole in an attempt to eradicate the infection.[259]

Isospora belli

Isospora was established as a cause of diarrhea in humans in the early 1900s, when sporadic cases of isosporiasis and a few clinical series were reported in the medical literature.[99] *Isospora belli* gained importance with the advent of AIDS and before HAART was shown to be an important cause of severe and prolonged gastroenteritis.[295] Humans are the only known host for *I. belli*, but the actual prevalence of this parasite is unknown. Infection can occur in adults and children and has been reported in infants with severe diarrhea.[239] This organism also has been implicated as a cause of traveler's diarrhea.[154]

Transmission is fecal-oral from one human to another, but the infective dose in humans is unknown. Oocysts may be present in stools for as long as 120 days after infection occurs. No animal reservoir of *I. belli* has been documented. Transmission is thought to occur by ingestion of oocysts contaminating food, water, or environmental surfaces.[239] *I. belli* oocysts are resistant to commonly used disinfectants and may remain viable for months in a cool, moist environment.

The clinical spectrum of disease caused by *Isospora* is indistinguishable from that described for *Cryptosporidium*. The spectrum includes asymptomatic infection, acute diarrhea in children in developing countries, and chronic diarrhea or severe protracted life-threatening diarrhea in patients with AIDS. Infection of the biliary tract in patients with AIDS by *Isospora* has been associated with acalculous cholecystitis.[36] The incubation period was 8 to 14 days in four subjects who had been exposed to the organism in the laboratory.[170] Fever, malaise, abdominal pain, and headache have been reported. Stools are watery and do not contain blood or leukocytes. Malabsorption, steatorrhea, severe weight loss, and chronic diarrhea lasting months to years are most likely occurrences in immunocompromised hosts.[92]

Microsporidia

Microsporidia are unicellular, spore-forming, obligate intracellular protozoal parasites that cause disease in a wide range of vertebrate and invertebrate hosts.[223,253] Of the more than 100 genera of microsporidia that have been identified, six cause disease in humans. The nontaxonomic term *human microsporidia* can refer to any of the microsporidia known to cause disease in humans: *Enterocytozoon* spp., *Encephalitozoon* spp., *Pleistophora* spp., and *Nosema* spp. Of these, *Enterocytozoon bieneusi* and *Encephalitozoon intestinalis* (formerly *Septata intestinalis*) are the most important in GI tract disease of humans.[26,426] These organisms emerged as important opportunistic pathogens when AIDS became pandemic. Infections with these organisms have been documented in immunocompetent and immunosuppressed people from Africa, Asia, Europe, and North and South America.[367]

In animals, transmission occurs by ingestion of environmentally resistant, infective spores shed into the environment.[253] The person-to-person, fecal-oral route may play a role in transmission, and water-borne disease occurs.[84] The zoonotic potential has been documented for several *Encephalitozoon* species.[253] The clinical spectrum appears to depend on the immune status of the host. *E. bieneusi* and *E. intestinalis* have been detected in intestinal biopsy specimens of patients with AIDS, with a clinical picture of prolonged diarrhea and weight loss.[84] The primary location of all intestinal spore-forming protozoal infection is the small intestine, but colonic infection has been reported with *E. bieneusi*.[159] Infection of the biliary tract with *E. bieneusi* and *E. intestinalis* in patients with AIDS can cause sclerosing cholangitis–type lesions[322,371,434] and acalculous cholecystitis caused by infection of the wall of the gallbladder. *E. intestinalis* can infect lamina propria macrophages, fibroblasts, and endothelial cells and can disseminate to other organs, including liver, respiratory tract, and kidney.[159,434] Extraintestinal infection develops after infection with other species of microsporidia occurs.

Cyclospora

Cyclospora cayetanensis (formerly cyanobacteria or blue-green algae–like bodies) is a coccidian protozoon that first was diagnosed as causing infection in humans in 1977.[293] *Cyclospora* is transmitted by the fecal-oral route; direct person-to-person transmission is unlikely to occur because excreted oocysts require days to weeks under favorable environmental conditions to sporulate and to become infectious. An animal reservoir has not been described. Outbreaks of diarrhea caused by consumption of water and fresh fruits contaminated with *Cyclospora* have been described,[175,245,247] and travelers to developing countries are at increased risk for development of diarrhea caused by *Cyclospora*.[292] Most of the reported cases have occurred during the spring and summer. The mean incubation period appears to be 7 days. Clinical manifestations include asymptomatic excretion, acute watery diarrhea, and diarrhea that may be protracted for days to weeks with frequent, watery stools, which may remit and relapse.

DIAGNOSIS

Determination of the cause of an episode of acute infectious diarrhea depends on epidemiologic information, the clinical syndrome, laboratory tests, and knowledge or assessment of an organism for virulence factors. Because virulence properties determine clinical manifestations of disease, an understanding of pathophysiologic mechanisms guides the laboratory evaluation and empiric therapy. The major virulence properties of enteropathogens include adherence; production of enterotoxin, cytoskeleton-altering toxin, cytotoxin, and toxins with neural activity; and epithelial cell invasion.[365] Certain enteropathogens may produce diarrhea by other mechanisms, and enteric pathogens may possess one or several of these virulence properties. Both host and microbiologic factors ultimately determine clinical expression in the individual patient. Not all of the recognized virulence properties of a given species are obvious clinically in each episode of disease. Virulence properties of individual bacterial, viral, and parasitic enteropathogens are discussed in specific chapters.

LABORATORY EVALUATION

Proper identification of the causative agent of an episode of acute infectious diarrhea will help facilitate initiation of appropriate therapy. A gross examination of the stool specimen should be routine in all patients with diarrhea, even if no laboratory studies are performed. Diarrheal stool that is watery and without mucus or blood usually is caused by an enterotoxin, virus, or protozoan organism, or it may be caused by infection outside the GI tract. The color of stools generally conveys little information if the stool does not contain blood. Infectious causes to be considered when stools contain blood or mucus include a cytotoxin-producing bacterium; an enteroinvasive bacterium causing mucosal inflammation; and an enteric parasite associated with blood in stools, such as *E. histolytica*, *B. coli*, and *T. trichiura*.

TABLE 50-8   Laboratory Tests Used to Detect Enteropathogens

Laboratory Tests	Organisms Suggested or Identified
Microscopic examination of stool	
Fecal leukocytes	Invasive or cytotoxin-producing bacteria
Trophozoites, cysts, oocysts, or spores	*Giardia lamblia, Entamoeba histolytica, Cryptosporidium, Isospora belli, Cyclospora, Enterocytozoon bieneusi, Encephalitozoon intestinalis*
Rhabditiform larva	*Strongyloides*
Spiral or S-shaped gram-negative bacilli	*Campylobacter jejuni/coli*
Stool culture	
Standard	*Escherichia coli, Shigella, Salmonella, Campylobacter jejuni*
Special	*Yersinia enterocolitica, Vibrio cholerae, Vibrio parahaemolyticus, Clostridium difficile, E. coli* O157:H7, *Listeria monocytogenes*
Stool cytotoxicity assay	*C. difficile*
Enzyme immunoassay or latex agglutination	Rotavirus, *G. lamblia, Cryptosporidium*, enteric adenovirus, *C. difficile*, STEC, *E. histolytica*
Serotyping	*E. coli* O157:H7 and other STEC, enteropathogenic *E. coli*
Latex agglutination after broth enrichment	*Salmonella, Shigella*
Tests performed in research or reference laboratories	Toxin-producing bacteria, small round viruses, invasive *E. coli*, EAEC, gene probe or polymerase chain reaction for virulence genes

STEC, Shiga toxin–producing E. coli; EAEC, enteroaggregative E. coli.

When it is present, blood usually is mixed evenly into the stool, except in the case of *E. histolytica* infections, in which blood often is on the surface of the stool, and some STEC infections, in which the stool may be blood streaked. Stools that are particularly foul smelling are consistent with *Salmonella* and other bacteria as well as *Giardia, Cryptosporidium*, and *Strongyloides* spp. Stools with little odor suggest an enterotoxin, such as cholera toxin or ETEC, or a viral enteropathogen. Laboratory tests used to detect enteropathogens are listed in Tables 50–8 and 50–9.

MICROSCOPIC EXAMINATION

Microscopic examination of stool specimens for evidence of fecal leukocytes provides information about the cause of diarrhea and helps determine the anatomic location and presence of mucosal inflammation.[313] Fecal leukocytes are produced in response to bacteria that diffusely invade the colonic mucosa and indicate that the patient has colitis. No inflammatory bacterial enteritis exists in which results of the fecal leukocyte examination are uniformly positive.[178] Thus, results of examination are more helpful when they are positive than when negative. When results are positive, the patient probably has an invasive or cytotoxin-producing organism, such as *Shigella* spp., *Salmonella* spp., *Campylobacter* spp., invasive *E. coli*, STEC, *C. difficile*, or *Y. enterocolitica*, although ulcerative colitis and Crohn disease also are associated with fecal leukocytes. Fecal leukocytes generally are not present in stools from patients with diarrhea secondary to viruses, enterotoxin-producing bacteria, or parasites. The leukocytes seen in cytotoxin-associated and invasive bacterial diarrhea syndromes are polymorphonuclear leukocytes. The exception is infection by *S. typhi*, in which the leukocytes are mononuclear. If the fecal leukocyte examination shows evidence of inflammatory enteritis,

further laboratory evaluation is indicated. The fecal lactoferrin assay has been shown to be a more accurate test than are fecal leukocytes or occult blood in patients with inflammatory diarrhea.[194]

Normally, examination of stools for ova and parasites is unnecessary unless the patient has a history of recent travel to high-risk areas, stool cultures are negative for other enteropathogens, the patient is involved in an outbreak of diarrhea, diarrhea persists for longer than 1 week, or the patient is immunosuppressed. *G. lamblia* and *S. stercoralis* can be visualized microscopically in stools, duodenal fluid, and small intestinal biopsy material. Both trophozoites and cysts of *G. lamblia* and larvae of *Strongyloides* spp. can be identified on direct smears of stool specimens (see Fig. 50–3); however, the sensitivity of stool examination for most parasites can be improved by use of a concentration technique and by placement of stools in vials containing a stool preservative. Trichrome and iron hematoxylin both are useful as permanent stains for *Giardia* spp. Pooling of preserved fecal samples is an efficient and economical procedure for detecting ova and parasites.[13] Rational use of the stool ova and parasite examination relies on communication between the clinician and laboratory personnel.[49]

For patients in whom giardiasis, cryptosporidiosis, isosporiasis, or strongyloidiasis is considered and in whom stool cultures are negative, aspiration or biopsy of the duodenum or upper jejunum may be indicated. Because these organisms live in the upper intestine, this procedure is more reliable than is examination of stool specimens.[336] Duodenal biopsy is a sensitive and specific method for diagnosing giardiasis, strongyloidiasis, and spore-forming protozoa. Small intestinal biopsy should be considered in patients with characteristic clinical symptoms, negative stool and duodenal fluid specimens, and one of the following: abnormal radiographic findings such as edema and segmentation in the small intestine, abnormal lactose tolerance test results, absent secretory IgA, hypogammaglobulinemia, achlorhydria, AIDS, or severe malabsorptive diarrhea with weight loss. Electron microscopic examination of tissue sections may be useful in identifying fine structures of a parasite (Fig. 50–5).

Medications, including antibiotics, antacids, antidiarrheal compounds, and certain enema and laxative preparations, as well as contrast material for radiographic studies can interfere with identification of an organism by altering morphologic features or causing a temporary disappearance of parasites from stool specimens. Patients should not receive these compounds for 48 to 72 hours before stools are collected for testing. *G. lamblia* and *Cryptosporidium* antigens in feces can be detected by use of one of several rapid and sensitive diagnostic tests.[148,220] *E. histolytica* can be diagnosed by microscopic examination of fresh stool specimens or bowel wall scrapings for cysts or trophozoites (see Fig. 50–2). A concentration technique may be helpful in demonstrating amebic cysts. Examination of several stool samples by an experienced technician may be necessary because excretion of cysts often is intermittent and making an interpretation is difficult. Confusion in differentiating amebic cysts from fecal leukocytes may occur. Microscopy can be used only as presumptive evidence of *E. histolytica* because the nonpathogen *E. dispar* is morphologically identical.[129] Several molecular techniques have been developed for detection and differentiation of *E. histolytica, E. dispar,* and *E. moshkovskii*.[142] Numerous serologic tests for amebiasis to detect different types and antibodies are available. Serologic test results for amebae almost always are positive in acute amebic dysentery and hepatic amebiasis. A liver scan may indicate the presence of a liver abscess.

Diagnosis of *Cryptosporidium, Isospora, Cyclospora*, and microsporidia is based on morphologic appearance and staining of stool or histologic examination of tissue sections.[159] Among the most widely used stains to visualize oocysts of *Cryptosporidium, Isospora,* and *Cyclospora* are standard acid-fast or modified acid-fast stains,

TABLE 50-9   Laboratory Evaluation of Patients with Presumed Bacterial Diarrhea

Organism	Tests
Aeromonas hydrophila	Screen colonies grown on MacConkey agar for positive oxidase test result
	Culture on modified blood agar
Bacillus cereus	Culture food ($>10^5$ organisms/g); demonstrate enterotoxin in food and stool by enzyme immunoassay
Campylobacter jejuni	Stool culture with special media incubated at 42° C with 5% O_2 and 10% CO_2
	Gram stain for "gull wing"–like organisms and fecal leukocytes; darkfield or phase contrast of stool for organisms with darting motility
	Nucleic acid probe
	Serology
Clostridium difficile	Culture feces anaerobically on cycloserine-cefoxitin-fructose agar
	Demonstrate toxins in stool by enzyme immunoassay or tissue culture cytotoxicity with neutralization with antitoxin
Clostridium perfringens	Culture food ($>10^5$ organisms/g) and feces; stools can be tested for enterotoxin
	Serotype organism
Escherichia coli	Standard stool culture for initial isolation
ETEC	
Stable toxin	Suckling mouse assay
	Gene probe hybridization assay
Labile toxin	Rabbit ileal loop
	Y-1 adrenal or Chinese hamster ovary cell assay
	Gene probe hybridization assay
	G_{M1} enzyme immunoassay
EPEC	Serogroup, gene probe assay
	Small bowel biopsy for routine microscopy and electron microscopy
EIEC	Gene probe assay
	Biologic assays for invasiveness (Serény or HeLa cell)
STEC	MacConkey sorbitol agar for O157:H7
	Gene probe or polymerase chain reaction to detect toxin gene sequences
	Serotyping
	Toxin enzyme immunoassay
	Free cytotoxin in stool by enzyme immunoassay or tissue culture
	Serologic responses to verotoxins or lipopolysaccharide of *E. coli* O157
EAEC	HEp-2 adherence assay, DNA probes
Listeria monocytogenes	Culture on blood agar
Plesiomonas shigelloides	Culture
Salmonella species	Standard stool culture; blood, bone marrow, and urine cultures if disseminated
	Serotype
Shigella species	Examine stool for fecal leukocytes
	Standard stool culture
Staphylococcus aureus	Culture food and skin lesions of food handlers
	Phage type
	Demonstrate enterotoxin in food, stool, and vomitus
Vibrio cholerae	Culture feces on thiosulfate–citrate–bile salt agar
	Serotype
Vibrio parahaemolyticus	Culture feces on thiosulfate–citrate–bile salt agar
	Test for Kanagawa reaction (beta-hemolysis on Wagatsuma agar), which is a marker for pathogenicity
Yersinia enterocolitica	Standard stool culture with cold enrichment; blood culture if disseminated
	Serology
	Lack of rhamnose fermentation by toxin-producing strains
	Suckling mouse assay for stable toxin

EAEC, enteroaggregative E. coli; STEC, Shiga toxin–producing E. coli; EIEC, enteroinvasive E. coli; EPEC, enteropathogenic E. coli; ETEC, enterotoxigenic E. coli.

which are based on the use of reagents that enhance the penetration of fuchsin into the organism without the need for heating (modified Kinyoun acid-fast stain). In a modified acid-fast stain, *Cryptosporidium* oocysts, which are 4 to 6 μm with four crescentic sporozoites, stain red and can be differentiated readily from yeasts that stain green.[172] Enzyme immunoassays[148,211] and fluorescent monoclonal antibody–based assays[149,345] for detection of *Cryptosporidium* antigen in stool specimens are available. In a study of seven microscopy-based *Cryptosporidium* oocyst detection methods, false-positive results were detected by acid-fast and auramine-rhodamine stains but not by monoclonal antibody–based methods.[23] Oocysts of *I. belli* often are visualized by wet-mount preparations because of their size, which is 20 to 30 μm with four sporozoites in two sporocysts. *Cyclospora* oocysts are 8 to 10 μm in diameter and are nonrefractile spherical organisms containing two sporozoites in two sporocysts that are seen easily on wet-mount preparations and are variably acid fast.

Microsporidia are difficult to differentiate from bacteria and debris because of the small size of the spores, which measure 1 to 2 μm. For detection, formalin-fixed stool or duodenal fluid can be stained with a calcofluor stain, a modified trichrome stain, or a fluorescent stain.[96,425] Gram, acid-fast, periodic acid–Schiff, and Giemsa stains also have been used to stain the organism.[367] A nonspecific fluorescence method or enzyme immunoassay may enhance speed and sensitivity. Small bowel biopsy may be more sensitive than is stool examination for establishing the diagnosis of intestinal microsporidiosis.[35] Spores are gram positive, and parts of the internal structure are positive for acid-fast or periodic acid–Schiff stains. After preliminary identification by these stains has been achieved, further examination by electron microscopy is needed to classify adequately the microsporidia into an appropriate genus. Routine histopathologic studies can provide presumptive identification in infected biopsy tissue; diagnostic confirmation requires electron microscopy. Reliable serologic

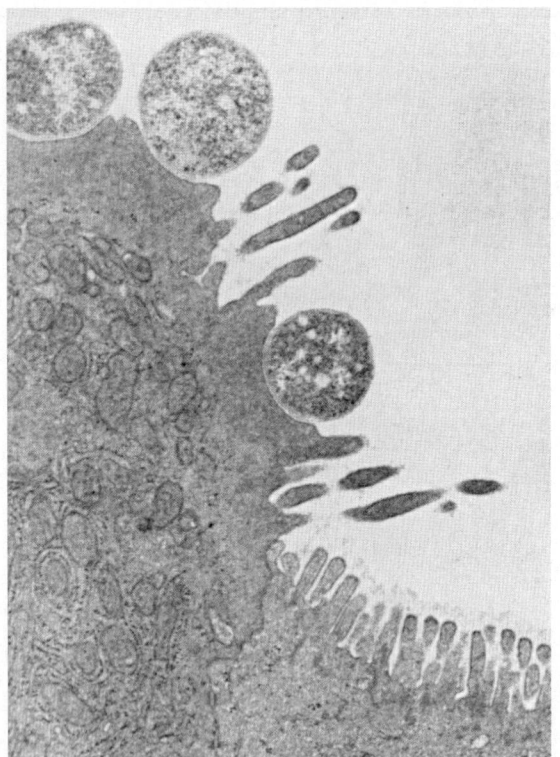

Figure 50–5 Electron micrograph of three *Escherichia coli* organisms adherent to enterocytes that have lost their microvilli and formed pedestals on which the bacteria lie (×25,000). *(Courtesy of Dr. R. J. Rothbaum.)*

tests are not available. Sensitive PCR assays are being evaluated for *E. bieneusi* and *E. intestinalis*.[89,133]

DIAGNOSTIC STOOL CULTURES

Obtaining of stool cultures cannot be justified in all patients with acute diarrhea.[178] Patients with mild, self-limited illness do not need to have stool specimens cultured. When culture is indicated, the specimen should be inoculated onto culture plate media adequate to isolate *E. coli*, *Shigella*, *Salmonella*, and *C. jejuni*. Fecal specimens can be transported to the laboratory in a non-nutrient holding medium, such as Cary-Blair, when culture cannot be performed immediately. This medium prevents drying or overgrowth of specific organisms.

E. coli grown in a hospital microbiology laboratory usually is considered to be normal flora. Proving pathogenicity is difficult because gene probe and PCR assays generally are available only in reference or research laboratories.[279,280] All stool specimens should be evaluated with sorbitol MacConkey medium for *E. coli* O157:H7.[47] *Shigella* organisms are identified in the standard evaluation of stool cultures. However, volunteer studies have shown that these organisms are not always isolated in culture from patients ill with shigellosis.

Salmonella organisms are isolated routinely by clinical microbiology laboratories. Speciation is important in salmonellosis because *S.* ser. *choleraesuis* and *S.* ser. *typhi* cause more severe disease than do other *Salmonella* spp. *S.* ser. *enteritidis* is more variable in severity. Serotyping of *S.* ser. *enteritidis* usually is not helpful in the individual case, although serotyping is crucial in evaluation of an outbreak. Because so many *Salmonella* serotypes exist, isolation of an unusual serotype can be of use in the investigation of a food-borne epidemic or identification of a potential

reptile source of infection. As with *Shigella*, isolation of a *Salmonella* spp., even without demonstration of virulence properties, is considered adequate to make an etiologic diagnosis. Serologic studies are of no value in the individual patient.

Some bacterial enteropathogens require modified laboratory procedures for identification.[178] If these agents are suspected, the laboratory should be notified so that appropriate culture methods can be used. *Listeria* is cultured on blood agar plates rather than on the usual enteric media.[410] *Y. enterocolitica* can be isolated from routine media, but a differential selective medium, such as cefsulodin–triclosan (Irgasan)–novobiocin agar, is more effective.[45] If routine enteric media are inoculated, recovery of organisms is optimized by plating them onto MacConkey agar, followed by incubation at 25° C for 48 hours. Cold-enrichment techniques may increase the yield of the organism from contaminated specimens, such as feces. Stool cultures positive for *Y. enterocolitica* only after prolonged cold enrichment may represent environmental strains of low virulence, unrelated to human disease. Biotyping and serotyping for O3, O8, and O9 are helpful in determining the clinical relevance of such isolates.

V. cholerae strains can be isolated from stool with use of thiosulfate–citrate–bile salt–sucrose agar, which is the most convenient and frequently used selective medium. This medium is suitable for most enteropathogenic *Vibrio* spp., except *V. hollisae*. Placement of the specimen into an enrichment broth, such as alkaline peptone water with 1 percent sodium chloride (pH 8.5) for 5 hours before placement on thiosulfate–citrate–bile salt–sucrose agar enhances the isolation of vibrios. Serotyping is necessary to classify organisms into those that cause typical epidemic cholera (i.e., O1 and O139 serotypes) and those that cause less severe disease (i.e., non-O1, or nonagglutinating vibrios).[209]

V. parahaemolyticus, like other vibrios, can be cultured on thiosulfate–citrate–bile salt–sucrose agar. Strains associated with diarrhea are Kanagawa-positive on Wagatsuma agar (i.e., show hemodigestion resembling beta-hemolysis), which is a marker for pathogenicity. *V. parahaemolyticus* can be serotyped on the basis of the O and K antigens.[87]

A. hydrophila can be overlooked easily on standard stool cultures. A specialized blood agar has been suggested for isolation.[16] Oxidase testing of organisms that resemble *E. coli* can select organisms as possible *Aeromonas* spp.[16] If oxidase-positive colonies are found, they can be evaluated biochemically to determine species.

C. difficile can be isolated by anaerobic stool culture on agar containing cycloserine, cefoxitin, and fructose. For establishing a definitive diagnosis, demonstration of the presence of cytotoxin in stool specimens and neutralization with antitoxin or by use of enzyme immunoassay or PCR-based assays are necessary.[14,324,355]

C. perfringens is isolated commonly from feces of well people. Diagnosis of *C. perfringens* food poisoning requires isolation of the organisms from epidemiologically implicated food in a significant quantity (more than 10^5 organisms/g) or demonstration of 10^6 organisms/g of stool from two or more ill people or demonstration of enterotoxin in stools of two or more ill people.[245]

S. aureus may be isolated from food and may not be the cause of illness because not all strains of *Staphylococcus* produce enterotoxin. Conversely, the absence of *S. aureus* from food that has been reheated just before being eaten does not exclude staphylococcal food poisoning because heating may destroy the organism without inactivating the toxin. Confirmation as a cause of foodborne disease requires isolation of the same phage type *S. aureus* from stools or vomitus of two or more ill persons or detection of enterotoxin in epidemiologically implicated food or isolation of 10^5 organisms/g from epidemiologically implicated food, provided the specimen is properly handled.[245]

B. cereus can be diagnosed by demonstration of greater than 10^5 organisms/g in the incriminated food or isolation of the organism from stool of two or more ill people and not from stool of control patients.[245]

SEROTYPING AND TOXIN DETECTION

Certain serotypes have been associated with ETEC, EIEC, EPEC, and STEC. Studies of somatic *E. coli* antigens are not helpful in establishing the diagnosis of ETEC because more than 50 different serogroups of *E. coli* have been shown to produce ST enterotoxins, HL enterotoxins, or both. Diagnosis of the various pathotypes of diarrheogenic *E. coli* is by assays that identify phenotype directly as well as with genotypic assays. Bacteria initially attach to epithelial cells that respond by forming cuplike pedestals composed of cytoskeletal protein and can be seen on electron micrographic examination in patients infected with EPEC (see Fig. 50–5). Identical lesions can be induced by human STEC strains.

VIRUS DETECTION

Rotavirus has been identified by examination of stool specimens for 70-nm particles by electron microscopy (see Fig. 50–1). Commercially available enzyme immunoassay and latex agglutination kits are available to detect rotavirus antigen in stool specimens. Assay procedures using monoclonal antibodies have improved the sensitivity and specificity to greater than 95 percent.[93,219] Other diagnostic methods less suitable for routine use include gel electrophoresis, PCR, and viral culture. Non–group A rotaviruses are not detected by the commercially available assays.

After the Norwalk virus was cloned and sequenced in 1990,[199] two major types of assays for diagnosing human noroviruses were developed. One type detects the viral antigens or antibodies against the antigens by recombinant enzyme immunoassays, and the other detects the viral RNA by reverse transcriptase–PCR.[269] The report of an in vitro cell culture infectivity assay for human norovirus may improve diagnostic abilities as well as understanding of the pathogenesis of norovirus.[388]

Diagnosis of enteric adenovirus can be established by immune electron microscopy of stool specimens, enzyme immunoassay of stool specimens, or propagation in a line of human embryonic kidney cells transformed by adenovirus type 5 (293 cells).[226] Restriction enzyme analysis is the definitive method for classifying individual enteric adenovirus isolates. Commercially available assays for detection of enteric adenovirus are available.[412]

Astroviruses grow well in human embryo kidney cells in the presence of trypsin. Electron microscopy, immune electron microscopy, immunofluorescence on cell culture, enzyme immunoassay, and PCR can be used as detection methods.[157]

PROCTOSIGMOIDOSCOPY

When symptoms of colitis are severe or the cause of an inflammatory enteritis syndrome remains obscure after laboratory evaluation, proctoscopic examination may help establish the diagnosis. Table 50–10 shows the usual proctoscopic findings in the various enteric syndromes that are characterized by fever, abdominal pain, and diarrhea with mucus and blood. Inflammatory bowel disease enters the differential diagnosis when symptoms of inflammatory enteritis become chronic. Proctitis with or without diarrhea may be related to milk allergy in infants, child abuse, or sexual practices. The etiology of proctitis includes all of these causes as well as *Neisseria gonorrhoeae*, herpes simplex virus, lymphogranuloma venereum, and *Chlamydia trachomatis*.

TREATMENT

Enteric infections generally are self-limited conditions, but nonspecific therapy can provide relief for some patients, and specific therapy may shorten the duration of the illness and eradicate fecal shedding of the organism. In caring for patients with diarrhea and dehydration, the major therapeutic considerations include fluid and electrolyte therapy, dietary manipulation, nonspecific therapy with antidiarrheal compounds, and specific therapy with antimicrobial agents. Increasing numbers of isolates resistant to antimicrobial agents and the risk for worsened illness (e.g., hemolytic-uremic syndrome occurring with Shiga toxin–producing *E. coli*) complicate antimicrobial and antimotility therapy.

TABLE 50–10 Proctoscopic Findings of Persistent Inflammatory Colitis

Organism or Disease	Gross Findings	Microscopic Findings
Shigella species	Diffuse erythema with loss of vascular pattern, mucopurulence, mild friability, occasional aphthoid ulcers	Edema, capillary congestion, focal hemorrhages, crypt hyperplasia, goblet cell depletion, mononuclear and polymorphonuclear leukocyte infiltrate, loss of epithelial cells with microulcerations
Salmonella species	Hyperemic, friable mucosa with petechiae and ulcerations; occasional pseudomembranous changes	Edema, inflammation, microabscesses, ulcerations
Campylobacter jejuni	Diffuse exudative edema	Inflammatory infiltrate with polymorphonuclear leukocytes, eosinophils, mononuclear cells, degeneration, loss of mucus, crypt abscesses, ulcerations
Clostridium difficile	Pseudomembranous colitis with 1- to 5-mm white-yellow nodules or plaques, minimal friability, sometimes nonspecific colitis	Fibrin, mucus, necrotic epithelial cells, leukocytes adherent to the underlying inflamed tissues
Clostridium perfringens	Rarely pseudomembranous colitis	Findings similar to those produced by *C. difficile*
Entamoeba histolytica	Discrete ulcers (millimeters to centimeters in diameter) with undermined edges amid normal mucosa	Trophozoites in flask-shaped ulcers that extend into submucosa, inflammatory cells near periphery but not near trophozoites; wet mount shows motile ameba containing erythrocytes
Ulcerative colitis	Friability, inflammatory polyps on heaped-up granulation tissue, deep linear ulcers	Mucosal ulceration extending to lamina propria, diffuse inflammation, vascular engagement, microabscesses in crypts
Crohn colitis	Hyperemic mucosa with linear ulcers	Inflammation involving all layers of bowel, with lymphocytes, histiocytes, and plasma cells forming granulomas

FLUID AND ELECTROLYTE THERAPY

Patients who develop diarrhea lose fluid and electrolytes through the GI tract by several mechanisms: vomiting, loss of fecal fluid caused by the infecting enteropathogen, and fecal water loss in excess of sodium caused by the intraluminal osmotic effect of unabsorbed nutrients.[179] The composition and amount of lost fluid depend on the rate of stool loss and the causative agent. The higher the rate of stool loss, the greater the sodium loss, probably as a result of rapid passage of intestinal contents through the colon, where sodium-potassium exchange occurs. Stools from patients with cholera or ETEC infection contain sodium in a concentration of 80 to 120 mEq/L, whereas stools from patients with rotavirus infection have sodium concentrations of less than 50 mEq/L.[357] In secretory diarrheal disorders, loss of fluid generally is derived from the small intestine, and colonic reabsorption is overwhelmed. In viral gastroenteritis, small bowel absorptive capacity primarily is impaired, and in dysenteric or invasive diarrhea, reabsorptive capacity of the large intestine is reduced. If vomiting also is a manifestation, this loss is compounded. Continued loss of fluid or electrolytes may lead to dehydration, with potentially severe sequelae. Children, especially infants, are more susceptible to dehydration because they have greater basal fluid and electrolyte requirements per kilogram and because they depend on others to meet these needs.

Important factors to be considered in evaluating patients with diarrhea and possible dehydration include an estimation of deficiency, ongoing daily requirements, continued losses and their replacement, and correction of the underlying cause.[18,179] The clinical signs and symptoms that may help in estimating deficiencies and determining the severity of dehydration include thirst, dryness of the mucous membranes, decrease in urinary output, tachycardia, loss of skin elasticity and turgor, and mottling and coolness of the skin.[18,66] These signs may be misleading in patients who are malnourished or in patients with hypertonic dehydration.

Fluids should not be withheld in treatment of any patient with diarrheal disease. Oral therapy should consist of rapid rehydration with replacement of ongoing losses during the first 6 to 12 hours of therapy with a glucose-electrolyte solution,[18,66,78,357] followed by early initiation of a modified diet.[66,250] If fluid and electrolyte deficits are significant, priority should be given to rehydration as rapidly as possible with oral electrolyte solutions. Ondansetron, an antiemetic, as a single dose reduced vomiting and facilitated oral rehydration in a study of children in an emergency department in the United States.[144]

Intravenous therapy is required only if the patient is in shock, is obtunded, or has ileus; otherwise, fluid and electrolyte therapy should be administered orally. Once the patient is rehydrated, an orally administered maintenance solution containing approximately 50 mEq/L of sodium should be used. Patients with mild diarrhea without clinical dehydration (<3% weight loss) can be managed at home by supplementing their diets with oral electrolyte solutions containing glucose. The glucose in these solutions is necessary to promote intestinal absorption of sodium and water in the small intestine.[370]

Commercial preparations of ready-to-feed glucose-electrolyte solutions are available in the United States and should be used in preference to homemade solutions. The sodium and potassium contents of various commercially available preparations are outlined in Table 50–11. Gatorade and other sports drinks do not supply the quantity of electrolytes necessary to replace those lost with the continued stool losses of severe diarrhea, and they are high in carbohydrate content. High concentrations of sugar are not tolerated well because high osmotic activity may exacerbate diarrhea. The carbohydrate concentration should not exceed the sodium concentration by more than 2:1. If it does, the excess carbohydrate produces osmotic retention of water in the intestine, with subsequent loss in stool.[18] The preparation of glucose and salt solutions at home is not recommended because errors in preparing the solutions may result in hypertonic dehydration in infants.[234] The use of rice-based oral rehydration solutions that contain glucose polymers and amino acids has been shown to increase the absorption of salt, water, and glucose from the intestine and may be more beneficial than are glucose-based oral rehydration solutions.[358,375] In a randomized, controlled trial in an emergency department in the United States, oral rehydration was as effective as intravenous rehydration of moderately dehydrated children.[384]

Other fluids that may be consumed at home include decarbonated soda beverages, fruit juices, and Jell-O. All contain inadequate amounts of sodium and potassium and excessive carbohydrate concentrations, which may exceed the absorptive capacity of the intestine[370] and, therefore, should not be used if rehydration requires more than one or two feedings. Kool-Aid and tea are not recommended because they are low in both sodium and potassium and thus have little advantage over sugar and water. Soon after the child has begun drinking a fluid and electrolyte solution, feeding should be restarted.[18,52,66]

DIETARY MANIPULATION

Of all common childhood illnesses, diarrhea has the most significant adverse nutritional effect. Restoration of feeding is important to reduce the nutritional defects caused by diarrhea.[18,66] However, optimal conditions have not been defined in nutritional management of different diarrheal states.[52] Once rehydration is complete, food may be reintroduced while the oral electrolyte solution is continued to replace ongoing losses from stools and for maintenance. Breast-feeding in infants should be resumed as soon as possible, preferably immediately after rehydration. Some

TABLE 50–11 Content of Representative Solutions Used for Oral Rehydration

Solution	Sodium (mmol/L)	Potassium (mmol/L)	Carbohydrate (mmol/L)	Osmolarity (mOsm/L)
Rehydration				
World Health Organization solution*	90	20	111	310
Reduced osmolar ORS (WHO/UNICEF)	75	20	75	245
Rehydralyte (Ross)	75	20	140	301
Maintenance or Prevention				
Infalyte (Mead Johnson)	50	25	70	200
Naturalyte (Unlimited Beverage)	45	20	140	265
Pedialyte (Ross)	45	20	140	250
Pediatric electrolyte (NutraMax)	45	20	140	250

*Packets of oral rehydration salts are available in the United States from Cera Products (410-997-2334) and Jianas Brothers (816-421-2880).

infants experience temporary lactose intolerance after having diarrheal illness,[29] although most young children with acute diarrhea can be managed successfully with continued feeding of undiluted nonhuman milk.[18,53,250] Routine dilution of milk and routine use of lactose-free milk formula are not necessary, especially when oral rehydration therapy and early feeding are part of the approach to the clinical management of acute diarrhea.

In some children and infants, the carbohydrate fraction of milk may exacerbate diarrhea because of disaccharidase deficiency acquired as a result of diarrhea.[29] Development of lactase deficiency during a diarrheal illness may require some alteration in diet. In children with moderate or severe acute diarrhea, reduction or elimination of lactose from the diet early in the illness may be necessary to minimize the effects of lactose intolerance. Relative lactose tolerance has been shown to persist for 2 to 6 weeks after some episodes of diarrhea. Other disaccharidases may be reduced during infection, influencing the absorption of other sugars. Soy-based, lactose-free formulas can be used safely during the acute phase of diarrheal illness in infants.[358] If diarrhea persists for more than 3 weeks, conditions that should be considered include not only disaccharidase deficiency but also celiac disease, cystic fibrosis, parasitic disease, allergic gastroenteropathy, bacterial overgrowth syndrome, congenital diarrhea disorders, EPEC or EAEC disease, and chronic nonspecific diarrhea.[41,240]

NONSPECIFIC THERAPY WITH ANTIDIARRHEAL COMPOUNDS

Many compounds are available for symptomatic treatment of patients with diarrhea. These substances are prescribed by physicians, administered by parents, or taken by patients who are eager to relieve the symptoms. Their purpose is to decrease the volume of diarrhea by increasing absorption of water and electrolytes, to decrease intestinal secretion, or to decrease intestinal motility. These over-the-counter and prescription preparations act on the GI tract by one or more of these mechanisms. Table 50–12 lists some commercially available antidiarrheal agents and their mechanisms of action, major value, and toxicity. Most of these

compounds are not approved for children younger than 2 to 3 years old.

Drugs that alter intestinal motility can be classified into antimuscarinics and synthetic or natural opium alkaloids.[18,110,321] These compounds usually have a rapid onset of action. They decrease the volume of stool output and relieve abdominal cramps and pain, probably by producing segmental contractions of the intestine, which retard movement of intestinal contents responsible for diarrhea and restrict the intestinal distention that normally causes abdominal pain. Drugs that affect intestinal motility may worsen the symptoms of *Shigella*, STEC, or other invasive and cytotoxin-producing bacteria by inhibiting intestinal transit and allowing the enteropathogen to be in contact with the intestinal mucosa for a longer time.[110,437] These agents may accelerate development of AAC.[287] Drugs that have central opiate–like effects can lead to overdose; fatalities in children have occurred.[152,153,321,344] Two to four doses of these compounds during a 24-hour period may be used in adolescents or adults to treat severe cramps, but prolonged therapy is not advised, and use in children is not recommended. The combination of TMP-SMX plus loperamide and the use of loperamide alone were effective in treating adults with traveler's diarrhea[54,127] and resulted in the shortest mean duration of diarrhea compared with that in patients taking placebo or TMP-SMX alone. In infants, loperamide can cause ileus, emesis, and drowsiness.[273] The practice parameter of the American Academy of Pediatrics does not recommend this class of compounds for treatment of diarrhea in children.[18]

Numerous chemically inert agents are used internally as adsorbents to bind toxins and water to reduce the number and to improve consistency of bowel movements. When these substances are given by mouth, they can adsorb not only bacteria and toxins but also drugs, nutrients, and enzymes. The only agents currently used widely are compounds containing activated attapulgite, which have been shown to be effective in animals by reducing diarrhea and producing formed stools,[139,329] but studies in humans are lacking. Disadvantages include nonspecific changes in adsorption of nutrients, enzymes, and antibiotics, particularly if the absorbent is used for a prolonged time.

TABLE 50–12   Antidiarrheal Compounds Used as Nonspecific Therapy for Patients with Acute Diarrhea

Mechanism of Action	Generic Name	Trade Name	Value	Comments
Alteration of intestinal motility	Loperamide	Imodium advanced, Imodium A-D, Maalox Antidiarrheal, Pepto Diarrhea Control	Decreases diarrhea, rapid onset of action	Numerous side effects and contraindications Not recommended or licensed for use in infants and young children May potentiate *Shigella*, *Salmonella*, or STEC infections or accelerate the course of antimicrobial-associated colitis
	Difenoxin and atropine	Motofen*		
	Diphenoxylate and atropine	Lomotil*		
	Tincture of opium	Paregoric*		
Alteration of secretion	Bismuth subsalicylate	Pepto-Bismol	Decreases diarrhea and cramps of travelers	Potential for salicylate or bismuth overdose, darkens stool
	Octreotide	Sandostatin*	Decreases diarrhea in patients with vasoactive intestinal peptide–secreting and metastatic carcinoid tumors	Used for relief of refractory AIDS-associated diarrhea; not licensed by the Food and Drug Administration for this condition
	Racecadotril	Not available	Decreases diarrhea	Decreases intestinal hypersecretion, enkephalinase inhibitor
Adsorption of toxins and water	Attapulgite	Diasorb, Donnagel, Kaopectate, Rheaban	Increases form of stool	Safe, minimally effective, decreases absorption of nutrients and drugs, causes abdominal fullness
Alteration of intestinal microflora	Probiotics (*Lactobacillus*, *Bifidobacterium*)	Pro-Bionate, Superdophilus	Value unproven	Safe, contraindicated in those with lactose tolerance

*Requires a prescription.
STEC, Shiga toxin–producing *Escherichia coli*.

Probiotics are live, nonpathogenic microorganisms that have been studied for prevention and treatment of a variety of disorders including diarrhea, irritable bowel syndrome, and inflammatory bowel disease. When given orally, these organisms recolonize the intestine with saccharolytic flora and alter the intestinal pH as a way of deterring potential pathogens.[17,318] Ingestion of probiotics results in an increased production of short-chain fatty acids and a decrease in pH in the intestine, which may inhibit the growth of *Salmonella* and *Shigella*. Feeding of selected microorganisms, including *Bifidobacterium bifidum*, *Saccharomyces boulardii*, *Lactobacillus acidophilus*, and *Streptococcus thermophilus*, to children and adults has been shown to be effective in prevention against and treatment of intestinal disease. Several meta-analyses have shown moderate clinical benefit of probiotics in treatment and prevention of diarrheal disease in children.[205,360,391,392] There is a need to better define and standardize the optimal probiotic for prevention and treatment of diarrheal disease caused by specific enteropathogens.[318]

Indomethacin, aspirin, chlorpromazine, and imidazole decrease intestinal secretion of fluid and electrolytes. Indomethacin has been shown to be effective in treating radiation-induced diarrhea, and chlorpromazine is effective in managing diarrhea caused by *V. cholerae*; however, the usefulness of these compounds in patients with various forms of acute infectious diarrhea is unknown. Laboratory studies showed that bismuth subsalicylate (Pepto-Bismol) inhibited intestinal secretion caused by *E. coli* and cholera enterotoxins,[126] reduced diarrhea in adult students who became ill in Mexico,[116] and prevented diarrhea among U.S. students traveling to Mexico.[113] Studies supporting its use in children are limited.[382,383] Potential problems with this compound relate to the absorption of salicylate[135,316] and bismuth.[262] Octreotide (Sandostatin) is a long-acting synthetic somatostatin analogue with pharmacologic actions mimicking those of the natural hormone somatostatin. Octreotide has been used in patients with AIDS who have severe refractory secretory diarrhea.[57]

Racecadotril (acetorphan) is an enkephalinase inhibitor that decreases intestinal hypersecretion but not motility in animals and humans by preventing breakdown of endogenous enkephalins in the GI tract. Racecadotril has been shown to decrease 48-hour stool output, median duration of diarrhea, and intake of oral rehydration solution in children with watery diarrhea.[354] The mechanisms and development of effective antisecretory drugs for diarrheal disease have been reviewed.[132] The potential immunomodulatory mechanisms involved in the interrelationships between micronutrients, including zinc and vitamin A, and infectious diseases, including diarrhea, have been reviewed.[7,189,396,419]

SPECIFIC THERAPY WITH ANTIMICROBIAL AGENTS

Antimicrobial therapy is administered to selected patients with gastroenteritis to abbreviate the duration of the clinical course and to decrease excretion of the causative organisms. A stool culture specimen should be obtained when antibiotic treatment is anticipated, and antibiotic susceptibility testing of any suspected pathogen should be performed to ensure optimal therapy. Changing susceptibility patterns renders the initial selection of an antimicrobial agent difficult. Antimicrobial agents should not be used routinely or liberally for gastroenteritis of unknown cause.

Shigella

Several antimicrobial agents have been used successfully in eradicating clinical symptoms and fecal shedding of *Shigella*, but a high prevalence of antimicrobial resistance in the United States limits treatment options.[374] Of the *Shigella* isolates reported in the National Antimicrobial Resistance Monitoring System (NARMS)

of the CDC in 2003, 88 percent were *S. sonnei* and 10 percent were *S. flexneri*. Among the 495 shigella isolates, 91 percent were resistant to one or more antimicrobial agents and 23 percent to five or more antimicrobial agents. Resistance to ampicillin occurred in 79 percent of isolates, to TMP-SMX in 38 percent, and to tetracycline in 29 percent. None of the isolates was resistant to ceftriaxone, imipenem, gentamicin, or ciprofloxacin. Susceptibility testing against azithromycin was not performed. Table 50–13 outlines suggested antimicrobial therapy for children and adults who are presumed to have shigellosis or from whom *Shigella* organisms are isolated from stool.

The history of resistance among *Shigella* strains has shown progressive acquisition of multiresistance, first to sulfonamides, shortly after their commercial availability; then to tetracycline, chloramphenicol, and streptomycin less than 10 years after they were introduced; and subsequently to ampicillin, kanamycin, and TMP-SMX.[308,333,394] In children with known ampicillin-susceptible or TMP-SMX–susceptible strains, either drug can be given, but neither should be used as empiric therapy because of increasing resistance. Amoxicillin is not as effective as is ampicillin in the treatment of shigellosis and should not be used.[283] Parenterally and orally administered, extended-spectrum cephalosporins have been used successfully in the treatment of children with shigellosis.[25,122,414] Two-day[122] and 5-day[414] courses of ceftriaxone were effective in eradicating *Shigella* from stool and reducing the duration of diarrhea, but a single parenteral dose of ceftriaxone produced only a moderate reduction in diarrhea and failed to eradicate *Shigella* strains from stools.[207] Cefixime and ceftibuten, orally administered extended-spectrum cephalosporins, have shown good in vitro activity against various enteric pathogens and promising clinical efficacy in patients with shigellosis; cefixime, however, no longer is manufactured in the United States.[25,325]

Ciprofloxacin, norfloxacin, and enoxacin have been used successfully to treat adults and children with shigellosis[217,251,369] and appear to be safe in children.[162] In a study evaluating dosing of ciprofloxacin in adults, 5 days of therapy were effective for patients infected with *S. dysenteriae* type 1. For other *Shigella* spp., a single 1-g dose was sufficient. Ciprofloxacin is approved by the FDA for treatment of GI tract infections caused by *S. sonnei* and *S. flexneri*. In a randomized, double-blind study of 120 children aged 2 to 15 years with shigellosis, ciprofloxacin and pivmecillinam given for 5 days were successful in providing a clinical cure and eradicating the organism from stool.[251] Ciprofloxacin was not associated with development of arthropathy in children in this study. A comparative study of a 5-day course of either azithromycin or ciprofloxacin in adults with shigellosis showed compa-

TABLE 50–13   Antimicrobial Therapy for Patients with Shigellosis

Strain Susceptibility	Antimicrobial Agent
Strain of unknown susceptibility	Ceftriaxone *or* azithromycin *or* ciprofloxacin* *or* ofloxacin*
Trimethoprim-sulfamethoxazole (TMP-SMX)–susceptible strains	TMP-SMX
Ampicillin-susceptible strain	Ampicillin
Suspected or proven multidrug-resistant strain	Ciprofloxacin* *or* ofloxacin*

*Not approved for patients younger than 18 years.

rable clinical and bacteriologic responses.[217] Patients who are transient asymptomatic carriers may be managed without antimicrobial therapy if they understand and employ excellent standards of personal hygiene. Treatment of these patients, however, reduces fecal shedding of the organism and prevents spread of infection.

Salmonella

Table 50–14 shows antimicrobial therapy for patients with various clinical manifestations of *Salmonella* infection.[260] The type of syndrome produced by *Salmonella* influences the selection and duration of antimicrobial therapy. Antibiotics should not be used in the treatment of patients who are nontyphoid *Salmonella* carriers or in most patients with mild gastroenteritis. Antimicrobial therapy may, on occasion, convert intestinal carriage into systemic disease with bacteremia,[337] prolong excretion of *Salmonella*,[24] produce a bacteriologic or symptomatic relapse,[24] or encourage development or selection of resistant strains. Antimicrobial agents should be considered for patients with enterocolitis if the disease appears to be evolving into one of the systemic syndromes and for patients with a condition that impairs host resistance to infection, including neonates, young infants, and patients with hemoglobinopathies including sickle-cell anemia, AIDS, leukemia, lymphoma, immunosuppression, congenital heart disease, valvular heart disease, prostheses, and uremia.[163] Antibiotic treatment of *Salmonella* infection should be given to all patients with typhoid fever, bacteremia caused by nontyphoidal strains, and dissemination with localized suppuration.

Selection of antimicrobial agents for therapy is complicated by the emergence of *Salmonella* strains that are resistant to multiple antibiotics[2,427] and by increased risk of acquiring *Salmonella* infection associated with prior antimicrobial exposure.[298] Rates of antibiotic resistance among certain serotypes have been increasing, with a substantial proportion of serotypes of Typhimurium and Newport isolates being resistant to multiple drugs.[58] In 2003, 23 percent of non-*typhi Salmonella* isolates tested by NARMS were resistant to one or more antimicrobial agents and 11 percent were resistant to five or more agents.[58] Only 2 percent of isolates were resistant to TMP-SMX, 0.4 percent to ceftriaxone, and 0.2 percent to ciprofloxacin. Azithromycin was not tested.

Several outbreaks of multiresistant *Salmonella* infection in the United States have been traced to animal sources.[91,151,158,266] Resistant strains of *Salmonella* are common findings in retail ground meats, possibly because of use of antibiotics in animals used for food.[432] Human isolates of *Salmonella* should have susceptibility testing performed to guide therapy. Recommended antimicrobial agents include ampicillin, chloramphenicol, TMP-SMX, ceftriaxone, cefotaxime, ceftazidime, and a fluoroquinolone, which is approved only for people older than 17 years.[260,381] Ciprofloxacin, ofloxacin, and azithromycin are active in vitro against *Salmonella*, including *S.* ser. *typhi*, and have been used clinically with success.[27,237,378,418]

Because of the high rate of *S.* ser. *typhi* transmission together with widespread indiscriminate use of antimicrobial agents in some areas of the world, an increase in resistance patterns to ampicillin, chloramphenicol, and TMP-SMX has occurred.[58,342] Of the *Salmonella typhi* isolates reported by NARMS, 26 percent were resistant to one or more antimicrobial agents. One isolate was resistant to ceftriaxone and ciprofloxacin.[58] Because of this high rate of resistance in *S.* ser. *typhi* strains imported by travelers, empiric treatment of *S.* ser. *typhi* should be provided with ceftriaxone or a fluoroquinolone if the patient is older than 17 years. Ampicillin, chloramphenicol, and TMP-SMX should be reserved for patients in whom susceptibility testing of the causative organism has shown susceptibility. Development of resistance of *S.* ser. *typhi* to ceftriaxone and fluoroquinolones needs to be monitored. In areas of the world where *S.* ser. *typhi* strains with reduced susceptibility to fluoroquinolones have been reported, azithromycin was effective for treatment of people with enteric fever,[77,145,155] as was cefixime.[261,306] In a prospective, randomized study of children and adults with confirmed typhoid fever, ceftriaxone administered for 5 days was as effective and safe as a 2- to 3-week course of chloramphenicol,[195] but in another study, short-course therapy failed.[40]

Corticosteroids can be beneficial in treating patients with typhoid fever in whom prompt relief of manifestations of toxemia might be lifesaving,[83] but corticosteroids may increase the relapse rate.[182]

Antibiotics listed in Table 50–14 can be used for treatment of *Salmonella* infections. Patients with defective host defense mechanisms, such as people with AIDS, should be treated with ampicillin or an expanded-spectrum cephalosporin.[380] Ciprofloxacin has been reported to be effective in treating acute diarrhea caused by *Salmonella*,[118,127,128] recurrent *Salmonella* sepsis,[81] and brain abscesses in a neonate.[430] Duration of therapy is influenced by the site of infection and by the host. Patients with bacteremia without a localized infection should be treated for 14 days, whereas those with localized infection, such as osteomyelitis or endocarditis, or patients with AIDS and bacteremia should receive at least 4 to 6 weeks of therapy.[40] In most cases, chronic carriage of *S.* ser. *typhi* is associated with gallbladder disease. The presence of cholelithiasis may significantly affect the efficacy of therapy. When gallbladder disease is present, the failure rate of ampicillin is approximately 75 percent.[204] In patients without gallbladder disease, ampicillin with probenecid or amoxicillin administered for 6 weeks is the treatment of choice for chronic enteric carriers.[305] Ciprofloxacin[137] has been reported to be successful in eradicating *S.* ser. *typhi* in adult chronic carriers. Resistance of clinical isolates and failure of treatment with ciprofloxacin have been noted in patients infected with *S.* ser. *typhi*.[320]

TABLE 50–14   Antimicrobial Therapy for Patients with *Salmonella* Infections

Clinical Manifestation	Antimicrobial Agent
Acute gastroenteritis*	None
Bacteremia or enteric fever†	Ceftriaxone *or* cefotaxime *or* fluoroquinolone† *or* ampicillin‡ *or* chloramphenicol‡ *or* trimethoprim-sulfamethoxazole‡ (TMP-SMX)
Dissemination with localized suppuration (osteomyelitis)† or bacteremia in patients with AIDS	Same as for bacteremia
Meningitis or ampicillin-chloramphenicol–resistant and TMP-SMX–resistant organisms	Cefotaxime or ceftriaxone

*Patients with hyperpyrexia and systemic signs or symptoms should be treated empirically until bacteremia is excluded. Although of unproven efficacy, antimicrobial therapy for children in the first 3 months of life also is recommended by most authorities; a 7- to 10-day course of therapy probably is sufficient.

†Ciprofloxacin or ofloxacin can be used to treat resistant organisms in patients 18 years of age and older. Both are available for intravenous as well as oral use. Neither is recommended for pregnant women. Azithromycin has been used with success in developing countries.

‡Can be used if the organism is susceptible.

Two typhoid fever vaccines for children older than 2 years, adolescents, and adults are available commercially in the United States for specific situations.[75] A *S. typhi* Vi conjugate vaccine has been shown to be safe, immunogenic, and 90 percent effective in children 2 to 5 years of age,[238] but this vaccine is not available commercially.

Campylobacter

Campylobacter jejuni isolates generally are susceptible to a wide variety of antimicrobial agents, including erythromycin, quinolones, furazolidone, aminoglycosides, tetracycline, chloramphenicol, imipenem, and clindamycin, whereas penicillin, ampicillin, cephalosporins, and TMP-SMX are relatively inactive. Isolation of *Campylobacter* from stool does not imply the need for antimicrobial therapy. In a meta-analysis of eight randomized, controlled trials of antimicrobial therapy versus placebo, antimicrobial therapy shortened the duration of intestinal symptoms by 1.32 days.[402] The decision concerning therapy should be individualized, but therapy should be considered in patients with high temperatures, bloody diarrhea, and severe diarrhea and in immunocompromised hosts. In patients with *Campylobacter* enteritis, erythromycin or azithromycin is the agent of choice when a decision has been made to initiate therapy.[260] Data from NARMS from 1977 to 2003 showed that less than 2 percent of the isolates were resistant to erythromycin and azithromycin.[58,165] In these and other studies, a higher frequency of erythromycin resistance was noted in hog isolates, most of which were *C. coli*.[147,198,285] Strains of *C. jejuni* and *C. coli* that show high-level resistance to erythromycin also appear to be resistant to clarithromycin and azithromycin.[397]

Ciprofloxacin has been licensed by the FDA for treatment of *C. jejuni* enteritis in patients older than 17 years. Development of resistance to ciprofloxacin in *Campylobacter* spp. has been reported.[58,165,347] Data from NARMS show that the rate of *C. jejuni/coli* isolates resistant to ciprofloxacin was 13 percent in 1997 and 18 percent in 2003.[58,165] These high rates of resistance have been related in part to introduction of fluoroquinolones in animal feed.[284,377] In double-blind, placebo-controlled trials of erythromycin for treatment of patients with enteritis caused by *C. jejuni*, erythromycin was shown to eradicate *C. jejuni* promptly from feces but not to alter the clinical course when begun 4 days or more after the onset of symptoms.[20] Studies in which therapy was started early showed that *C. jejuni* was eliminated rapidly from stools, but studies gave conflicting results with regard to resolution of clinical illness.[353,433] The treatment of choice for patients with septicemia caused by *C. jejuni* or *C. fetus* infection is gentamicin or imipenem.[260]

Other Bacterial Agents

Antimicrobial agents have been employed frequently in attempts to treat infantile gastroenteritis caused by EPEC and as a means of controlling the spread of EPEC strains in hospital nurseries (Table 50–15). Although no definitive studies support the effectiveness of these drugs, they may be useful in certain situations, particularly when life-threatening infection occurs or when epidemic spread of the strains continues, despite the use of strict handwashing and appropriate isolation. Agents used in the treatment of EPEC diarrhea include TMP-SMX, but strains may be resistant. If systemic infection is suspected, parenteral therapy should be started and modified according to antimicrobial susceptibility of the organism isolated.

Diarrhea caused by ETEC usually is limited, but studies in adults have shown that antimicrobial agents such as TMP-SMX and ciprofloxacin are effective treatments. The treatment in patients with diarrhea caused by EIEC is similar to that in patients with shigellosis (see Table 50–13). Travelers infected with EAEC

TABLE 50–15 Antimicrobial Therapy for Bacterial Pathogens Causing Gastroenteritis

Organism	Antibiotic Therapy
Campylobacter jejuni	
Gastroenteritis	None, or if colitis is present, erythromycin or azithromycin or ciprofloxacin
Sepsis	Aminoglycoside
Clostridium difficile (antimicrobial-associated colitis)	Metronidazole or vancomycin
Escherichia coli	
Enteropathogenic	None or TMP-SMX or fluoroquinolone*
Enterotoxigenic	TMP-SMX or fluoroquinolone* or cefixime
Enteroinvasive	Same as for shigellosis (see Table 50–13)
STEC	None
Vibrio cholerae	Doxycycline or tetracycline or TMP-SMX
Vibrio parahaemolyticus	None
Yersinia enterocolitica	
Gastroenteritis	Probably none
Sepsis	TMP-SMX or an aminoglycoside or cefotaxime or ceftizoxime or ciprofloxacin*

Approved only for patients 18 years of age or older.
STEC, Shiga toxin–producing E. coli; TMP-SMX, trimethoprim-sulfamethoxazole.

have shown response to ciprofloxacin.[156] Antimicrobial therapy of infants and children with hemorrhagic colitis caused by STEC has been reported to increase development of hemolytic-uremic syndrome,[437] but other studies have not supported this observation for STEC[348] or for *S. dysenteriae* type 1.[38]

Antimicrobial agents decrease the duration of diarrhea associated with cholera by eradicating the vibrios from the GI tract[420] and thus reducing the volume of fluid loss. Doxycycline is the drug of choice in most instances for O1 and O139 infections, including those in children, in whom the benefits of a 1- to 2-day course outweigh the risk for dental staining.[259,261] TMP-SMX can be used in children younger than 8 years for *V. cholerae* O1, but O139 strains often are resistant. Ampicillin probably is the safest agent for use during pregnancy. Other effective antimicrobial agents are the fluoroquinolones and azithromycin. Single-dose azithromycin has been effective in both children[218] and adults.[350] Single-dose ciprofloxacin has been successful in treatment of adults,[216,349] but resistance was reported in a study from Bangladesh.[350] Diarrhea caused by *V. parahaemolyticus* is self-limited, so antimicrobial therapy shortens neither the clinical course nor the duration of excretion.[87] Antimicrobial therapy has not been proved efficacious in the treatment of uncomplicated enterocolitis caused by *Y. enterocolitica*.[45] Patients with *Y. enterocolitica*-induced septicemia or extraintestinal focal infection or compromised hosts with enterocolitis should receive TMP-SMX, a fluoroquinolone if they are older than 17 years, an aminoglycoside, cefotaxime, or cefotaxime. Table 50–15 outlines the antimicrobial therapy of these bacterial pathogens.

Protozoal Agents

Several drugs have been shown to be effective in the treatment of patients with giardiasis (Table 50–16).[90,150,259,340] Metronidazole may be better tolerated than is quinacrine, is not approved for the treatment of patients with giardiasis in the United States, and is carcinogenic in animals. Quinacrine hydrochloride may produce a yellow discoloration of the skin that disappears after

TABLE 50-16   Antimicrobial Therapy for Patients with Giardiasis

Antimicrobial Agent	Comments
Furazolidone (Furoxone)	Nausea, vomiting, disulfiram-like reaction with alcohol, mild hemolysis in glucose-6-phosphate dehydrogenase–deficient people, hypoglycemia, allergic reactions
Metronidazole (Flagyl)*	Metallic taste, nausea, headache, dry mouth, mutagenic in bacteria, carcinogenic in animals, disulfiram-like reaction with alcohol
Quinacrine HCl	Dizziness, headache, vomiting, diarrhea, yellow-orange skin color; not available commercially but can be obtained†
Nitazoxanide	Abdominal pain, vomiting, and headache uniformly reported; data minimal for children younger than 12 months or older than 11 years and for patients with immune deficiencies
Paromomycin*	Not highly effective, proposed for use in pregnancy
Albendazole*	Anorexia, constipation; clinical trials have shown mixed results
Tinidazole	Given as one dose

*Not a U.S. Food and Drug Administration–licensed indication.
†Medical Center Pharmacy (203-688-6816) or Panorama Compounding Pharmacy (800-247-9767).

TABLE 50-17   Antimicrobial Therapy for Patients with Amebiasis

Asymptomatic amebic cyst	Iodoquinol (Yodoxin) or paromomycin (Humatin) or diloxanide furoate*
Mild to moderate intestinal disease	Metronidazole (Flagyl) followed by iodoquinol or paromomycin
Severe intestinal disease, liver abscess, or other extraintestinal disease	Metronidazole followed by iodoquinol or paromomycin

*Available in the United States from Panorama Compounding Pharmacy (800-247-9767) or Medical Center Pharmacy (203-688-6816).

the drug is stopped. Quinacrine is not available commercially but as a service can be compounded (see Table 50–16). Furazolidone is the only one of these three compounds available in liquid form; like quinacrine, it is less expensive than metronidazole. Furazolidone can be used in children if compliance is a problem with quinacrine and metronidazole, both of which have an objectionable taste. Clinical trials using albendazole to treat people with giardiasis have produced mixed results.[150] Treatment of children with albendazole for 5 days,[166] but not 3 days,[166,299] has been effective. Toxicity of albendazole is low, and this compound is effective against many helminths, rendering it useful for treatment when multiple intestinal parasites are identified or suspected. Nitazoxanide has been licensed by the FDA for treatment of children with diarrhea caused by *Giardia* or *Cryptosporidium*. Tinidazole, a nitroimidazole drug similar to metronidazole, is given as a single dose. Paromomycin is not absorbed and is not highly effective but has been proposed for use during pregnancy.[228]

In a review of comparative drug trials for the treatment of giardiasis, Davidson[90] reported that metronidazole cured 92 percent of 219 patients and furazolidone cured 84 percent of 150 patients. Approximately 7 percent of the metronidazole-treated patients and 10 percent of the furazolidone-treated patients had side effects that were serious enough to report. The drugs available in a liquid preparation are furazolidone and nitazoxanide.

In treatment of patients with amebiasis, iodoquinol and paromomycin are the recommended luminal amebicide drugs that are available in the United States.[259] Paromomycin may be used during pregnancy. Diloxanide furoate is an alternative, but it is not available commercially in the United States. These drugs are effective against both cysts and trophozoites in the lumen of the gut, but they are ineffective against tissue forms of the disease. Invasive amebiasis of the intestine, liver, or other organs necessitates the additional use of tissue amebicides, such as metronidazole or tinidazole. Liver abscess or other extraintestinal forms of disease should be treated with metronidazole or tinidazole in the dose recommended for intestinal disease. Table 50–17 lists the recommended drugs for the treatment of children and adults with various forms of amebiasis.

Patients with intestinal strongyloidiasis should receive ivermectin for 1 to 2 days or thiabendazole every 12 hours for four doses. Immunosuppressed patients with disseminated disease may require continued therapy for 2 to 3 weeks, but the mortality rate is high despite administration of therapy. A thorough examination should be performed before immunosuppressive therapy is given to a patient with a past history of infection with *S. stercoralis*.

Therapeutic agents generally have not proved consistently beneficial for treatment of patients with cryptosporidiosis, and only one drug (nitazoxanide) is approved by the FDA for this purpose.[1,143] Infection generally is self-limited in immunocompetent patients, and therapy usually is not warranted.[1,176] In patients with persistent disease, an underlying immunodeficiency should be considered. Spiramycin has been used but is ineffective.[435] Paromomycin may be effective in rapid resolution of chronic diarrhea.[138,421,431] In a prospective, randomized, double-blind, placebo-controlled trial in the treatment of adults with AIDS and symptomatic cryptosporidiosis,[176] paromomycin was not effective. Azithromycin has been shown to be effective in treatment of two children with cancer and four children with HIV infection who had severe diarrhea caused by *Cryptosporidium*.[177,413] Combination therapy with paromomycin and azithromycin has been effective in some patients with AIDS and chronic cryptosporidiosis.[379] In a prospective, randomized, double-blind, placebo-controlled study of 50 children and 50 adults, treatment with nitazoxanide reduced the duration of diarrhea and oocyst shedding.[339] A meta-analysis of immunocompromised people treated with nitazoxanide or paromomycin showed no evidence of effectiveness.[1] Evidence of cyst reduction was not significant for HIV-seropositive people. Nitazoxanide showed a significantly higher rate of achieving parasite clearance.[1] Nitazoxanide is licensed for treatment of children with diarrhea caused by cryptosporidiosis and giardiasis. The best approach for prevention of cryptosporidiosis in HIV-infected patients is maintenance of the immune system function by use of HAART because chronic cryptosporidiosis occurs only in severely immunocompromised individuals.

Hyperimmune bovine colostrum has been used with some success in a child with agammaglobulinemia[408] and in a patient with AIDS.[409] Immune bovine colostrum has been shown to neutralize *C. parvum* sporozoites and partially to protect mice against oral challenge with *C. parvum* oocysts,[304] and oral bovine transfer factor has been used for treatment of cryptosporidiosis.[242] Nonspecific therapy with octreotide may control the severe diarrhea that occurs in patients with AIDS but has no effect on the infection[57] and is not approved by the FDA.

For isosporiasis, TMP-SMX is effective and is the drug of choice.[259] In immunosuppressed patients, TMP-SMX, at a dose of 160 mg TMP and 800 mg SMX four times a day for 10 days, followed by the same dose twice a day for 3 weeks, is recommended for adults. In immunosuppressed children, TMP 5 mg/

kg with SMX 25 mg/kg four times a day for 10 days, followed by the same dose twice a day for 3 weeks, should be used. Ciprofloxacin can be used when TMP-SMX cannot be tolerated, although it is slightly less effective. Other drugs, including pyrimethamine-sulfadoxine (Fansidar), metronidazole, and furazolidone, have been reported to be successful for treating patients with isosporiasis.[296,428] Pyrimethamine has been an effective alternative in patients allergic to sulfa drugs.[296] Problems in the treatment of isosporiasis have been encountered in patients with AIDS, in whom a high incidence of recurrence has been reported after treatment has been stopped. Continuation of therapy indefinitely with either pyrimethamine-sulfadoxine or TMP-SMX in adults has been shown to be effective in preventing recurrence of disease.[296]

On the basis of in vitro studies, several drugs have been used to treat microsporidial infections in humans, but successful treatment with any of them in humans is limited. Therapy with antiparasitic drugs, diet alteration, and antidiarrheal medications often fails to relieve diarrhea and malabsorption associated with microsporidiosis, although octreotide may provide symptomatic relief,[57] and diet modification to include medium-chain triglyceride–based diets has produced clinical improvement.[423] E. intestinalis is susceptible to albendazole,[82,212,335] which has been reported to stop diarrhea and weight loss as well as to promote weight gain in patients infected with E. intestinalis,[104,267,406] although improvement has not been uniform. Infections caused by E. bieneusi are more difficult to treat, but oral fumagillin has been effective.[268] The use of HAART may lead to microbiologic and clinical response in HIV-infected patients with diarrhea due to microsporidia.

Patients with HIV and Cyclospora infection respond to TMP-SMX, but relapses are common occurrences.[247,259,417] As few as 7 days of treatment may be adequate in immunocompetent children. HIV-infected patients may need higher doses and long-term maintenance. Although ciprofloxacin is not as effective as is TMP-SMX, it is acceptable for patients who cannot tolerate TMP-SMX.[417]

Patients infected with S. stercoralis should be treated with ivermectin or, alternatively, thiabendazole.[260] In disseminated strongyloidiasis, ivermectin or thiabendazole therapy should be continued for at least 5 days. In immunocompromised patients and patients with Strongyloides hyperinfection, longer duration of therapy may be necessary[233]; however, the mortality rate is high despite therapy. A thorough examination should be performed before immunosuppressive therapy is given to a patient with a history of infection with S. stercoralis.

The clinical significance of B. hominis remains unclear, few studies have considered the treatment of large numbers of patients, and case-control studies are lacking.[388] Use of metronidazole or iodoquinol in the same dose as for mild to moderate intestinal disease from E. histolytica has been reported to be effective in uncontrolled studies,[388] and they are the recommended drugs of choice. TMP-SMX or paromomycin may be the most appropriate second-choice drug.[259] Treatment should be provided with caution, only after a thorough clinical review of other possible causes of symptoms has been performed.

REFERENCES

1. Abubakar, I., Aliyu, S. H., Arumugam, C., et al.: Treatment of cryptosporidiosis in immunocompromised individuals: Systematic review and meta-analysis. Brit. J. Clin. Pharmacol. 63:387-393, 2007.
2. Ackers, M.-L., Puhr, N. D., and Tauxe, R. V.: Laboratory-based surveillance of Salmonella serotype typhi infections in the United States. Antimicrobial resistance on the rise. J. A. M. A. 283:2668-2673, 2000.
3. Adachi, J. A., Jiang, Z. D., Mathewson, J. J., et al.: Enteroaggregative Escherichia coli as a major etiologic agent in traveler's diarrhea in 3 regions of the world. Clin. Infect. Dis. 32:1706-1709, 2001.
4. Adachi, J. A., Ostrosky-Zeichner, L., DuPont, H. L., et al.: Empirical antimicrobial therapy for traveler's diarrhea. Clin. Infect. Dis. 31:1079-1083, 2000.
5. Adachi, J. A., Ericsson, C. D., Jiang, Z. D., et al.: Azithromycin found to be comparable to levofloxacin for the treatment of US travelers with acute diarrhea acquired in Mexico. Clin. Infect. Dis. 37:1165-1171, 2003.
6. Adamkiewicz, T. V., Berkovitch, M., Krishnan, C., et al.: Infection due to Yersinia enterocolitica in a series of patients with beta-thalassemia: Incidence and predisposing factors. Clin. Infect. Dis. 27:1362-1366, 1998.
7. Aggarwal, R., Sentz, J., and Miller, M. A.: Role of zinc administration in prevention of childhood diarrhea and respiratory illnesses: A meta-analysis. Pediatrics 119:1120-1130, 2007.
8. Ahmed, L., El Rooby, A., Kassem, M. I., et al.: Ultrasonography in the diagnosis and management of 52 patients with amebic liver abscess in Cairo. Rev. Infect. Dis. 12:330, 1990.
9. Aho, K., Ahvonen, P., Alkio, P., et al.: HLA-27 in reactive arthritis following infection. Ann. Rheum. Dis. 34(Suppl.):29-30, 1975.
10. Akihara, S., Phan, T. G., Nguyen, T. A., et al.: Existence of multiple outbreaks of viral gastroenteritis among infants in a day care center in Japan. Arch. Virol. 150:2061-2075, 2005.
11. Albert, M. J., Ansaruzzaman, M., Talukder, K. A., et al.: Prevalence of enterotoxin genes in Aeromonas spp. isolated from children with diarrhea, healthy controls, and the environment. J. Clin. Microbiol. 38:3785-3790, 2000.
12. Albert, M. J., Faruque, A. S., Faruque, S. M., et al.: Case-control study of enteropathogens associated with childhood diarrhea in Dhaka, Bangladesh. J. Clin. Microbiol. 37:3458-3464, 1999.
13. Aldeen, W. E., Whisenant, J., Hale, D., et al.: Comparison of pooled formalin-preserved fecal specimens with three individual samples for detection of intestinal parasites. J. Clin. Microbiol. 31:144-145, 1993.
14. Alfa, M. J., Kabani, A., Lyerly, D., et al.: Characterization of a toxin A–negative, toxin B–positive strain of Clostridium difficile responsible for a nosocomial outbreak of Clostridium difficile–associated diarrhea. J. Clin. Microbiol. 38:2706-2714, 2000.
15. Allos, B. M.: Campylobacter jejuni infections: Update on emerging issues and trends. Clin. Infect. Dis. 32:1201-1206, 2001.
16. Altwegg, M., and Geiss, H. K.: Aeromonas as a human pathogen. C. R. C. Crit. Rev. Microbiol. 16:253, 1989.
17. Alvarez-Olmos, M. I., and Oberhelman, R. A.: Probiotic agents and infectious diseases: A modern perspective on a traditional therapy. Clin. Infect. Dis. 32:1567-1576, 2001.
18. American Academy of Pediatrics, Subcommittee on Acute Gastroenteritis: Practice parameter: The management of acute gastroenteritis in young children. Pediatrics 97:424-436, 1996.
19. American Academy of Pediatrics: Prevention of rotavirus disease: Guidelines for use of rotavirus vaccine. Pediatrics 119:171-182, 2007.
20. Anders, B. J., Paisley, J. W., Lauer, B. A., et al.: Double-blind placebo controlled trial of erythromycin for treatment of Campylobacter enteritis. Lancet 1:131-132, 1982.
21. Angulo, F. J., and Swerdlow, D. L.: Bacterial enteric infections in persons infected with human immunodeficiency virus. Clin. Infect. Dis. 21(Suppl. 1):S84-S93, 1995.
22. Arbo, A., and Santas, J. I.: Diarrheal disease in the immunocompromised host. Pediatr. Infect. Dis. J. 6:894-906, 1987.
23. Arrowood, M. J., and Sterling, C. R.: Comparison of conventional staining methods and monoclonal antibody–based methods for Cryptosporidium oocyst detection. J. Clin. Microbiol. 27:1490, 1989.
24. Aserkoff, B., and Bennett, J. V.: Effect of antibiotic therapy in acute salmonellosis on the fecal excretion of salmonellae. N. Engl. J. Med. 281:636-640, 1969.
25. Ashkenazi, S., Amir, J., Waisman, Y., et al.: A randomized, double-blind study comparing cefixime and TMP/SMX in the treatment of childhood shigellosis. J. Pediatr. 123:817-821, 1993.
26. Asmuth, D. M., DeGirolami, P. C., Federman, M., et al.: Clinical features of microsporidiosis in patients with AIDS. Clin. Infect. Dis. 18:819-825, 1994.
27. Asperilla, M. O., Smego, R. A., Jr., and Scott, L. K.: Quinolone antibiotics in the treatment of Salmonella infections. Rev. Infect. Dis. 12:873, 1990.
28. Aureli, P., Fiorucci, G. C., Caroli, D., et al.: An outbreak of febrile gastroenteritis associated with corn contaminated by Listeria monocytogenes. N. Engl. J. Med. 342:1236-1241, 2000.
29. Avery, G. B., Villavicencio, O., Lilly, J. R., et al.: Intractable diarrhea in early infancy. Pediatrics 41:712-722, 1968.
30. Bartlett, A. V., Reves, R. R., and Pickering, L. K.: Rotavirus in infant-toddler day care centers: Epidemiology relevant to disease control strategies. J. Pediatr. 113:435, 1988.
31. Bartlett, J. G.: Narrative review: The new epidemic of Clostridium difficile–associated enteric disease. Ann. Intern. Med. 145:758-764, 2006.
32. Bartlett, J. G., Tedesco, F. J., Shull, S., et al.: Symptomatic relapse after oral vancomycin therapy of antibiotic-associated pseudomembranous colitis. Gastroenterology 78:431-434, 1980.
33. Bartlett, J. G.: Clostridium difficile: History of its role as an enteric pathogen and the current state of knowledge about the organism. Clin. Infect. Dis. 18(Suppl. 4):S265-S272, 1994.
34. Beards, G. M., Green, J. G., Hall, C., et al.: An enveloped virus in stools of children and adults with gastroenteritis that resembles the Breda virus of calves. Lancet 1:1050, 1984.

35. Beauvais, B., Sarfati, C., Molina, J. M., et al.: Comparative evaluation of five diagnostic methods for demonstrating microsporidia in stool and intestinal biopsy specimens. Ann. Trop. Med. Parasitol. 87:99-102, 1993.

36. Benator, D. A., French, A. L., Beaudet, L. M., et al.: Isospora belli infection associated with acalculous cholecystitis in a patient with AIDS. Ann. Intern. Med. 121:663-664, 1994.

37. Benhamou, Y., Caumes, E., Gerosa, Y., et al.: AIDS-related cholangiopathy: Critical analysis of a prospective series of 26 patients. Dig. Dis. Sci. 38:1113-1118, 1993.

38. Bennish, M. L., Khan, W. A., Begum, M., et al.: Low risk of hemolytic uremic syndrome after early effective antimicrobial therapy for Shigella dysenteriae type 1 infection in Bangladesh. Clin. Infect. Dis. 42:356-362, 2006.

39. Bhan, M. K., Raj, P., Levine, M. M., et al.: Enteroaggregative E. coli associated with persistent diarrhea in a cohort of rural children in India. J. Infect. Dis. 159:1061, 1989.

40. Bhutta, A. A., Khan, I. A., and Shadmani, M.: Failure of short-course ceftriaxone chemotherapy for multidrug-resistant typhoid fever in children: A randomized controlled trial in Pakistan. Antimicrob. Agents Chemother. 44:450-452, 2000.

41. Binder, H. J.: Causes of chronic diarrhea. N. Engl. J. Med. 355:236-239, 2006.

42. Bishop, R. F., Davidson, G. P., Holmes, I. H., et al.: Virus particles in epithelial cells of duodenal mucosa from children with acute nonbacterial gastroenteritis. Lancet 2:1281-1283, 1973.

43. Blanton, L. H., Adams, S. M., Beard, R. S., et al.: Molecular and epidemiologic trends of caliciviruses associated with outbreaks of acute gastroenteritis in the United States, 2000-2004. J. Infect. Dis. 193:413-421, 2006.

44. Blossom, D. B., and McDonald, L. C.: The challenges posed by reemerging Clostridium difficile infection. Clin. Infect. Dis. 45:222-227, 2007.

45. Bottone, E. J.: Yersinia enterocolitica: The charisma continues. Clin. Microbiol. Rev. 10:257-276, 1997.

46. Bourke, B., Jones, N., and Sherman, P.: Helicobacter pylori infection and peptic ulcer disease in children. Pediatr. Infect. Dis. J. 15:1-13, 1996.

47. Boyle, T. G., Pemberton, A. G., Wells, J. G., et al.: Screening for Escherichia coli O157:H7: A nationwide survey of clinical laboratories. J. Clin. Microbiol. 33:3275-3277, 1995.

48. Braden, C. R.: Salmonella enterica serotype enteritidis and eggs: A national epidemic in the United States. Clin. Infect. Dis. 43:512-517, 2006.

49. Branda, J. A., Lin, T.-Y., Rosenberg, E. S., et al.: A rational approach to the stool ova and parasite examination. Clin. Infect. Dis 42:972-978, 2006.

50. Brandt, C. D., Kim, H. W., Rodriguez, W. J., et al.: Adenoviruses and pediatric gastroenteritis. J. Infect. Dis. 151:437-443, 1985.

51. Brenner, F. W., Villar, R. G., Angulo, F. J., et al.: Salmonella nomenclature. J. Clin. Microbiol. 38:2465-2467, 2000.

52. Brown, K. H., and McClean, W. C.: Nutritional management of acute diarrhea: An appraisal of the alternatives. Pediatrics 73:119-125, 1984.

53. Brown, K. H., Peerson, J. M., and Fontaine, O.: Use of nonhuman milks in the dietary management of young children with acute diarrhea: A meta-analysis of clinical trials. Pediatrics 93:17-27, 1994.

54. Caeiro, J. P., DuPont, H. L., Albrecht, H., et al.: Oral rehydration therapy plus loperamide versus loperamide alone in the treatment of traveler's diarrhea. Clin. Infect. Dis. 28:1286-1289, 1999.

55. Calva, J. J., Ruiz-Palacios, G. M., Lopez-Vidal, A. B., et al.: Cohort study of intestinal infection with Campylobacter in Mexican children. Lancet 1:503, 1988.

56. Carr, A., Marriott, D., Field, A., et al.: Treatment of HIV-1–associated microsporidiosis and cryptosporidiosis with combination antiretroviral therapy. Lancet 351:256-261, 1998.

57. Cello, J. P., Grendell, J. H., Basuk, P., et al.: Effect of octreotide on refractory AIDS-associated diarrhea: A prospective, multicenter trial. Ann. Intern. Med. 115:705-710, 1991.

58. Centers for Disease Control and Prevention: National Antimicrobial Resistance Monitoring System (NARMS): Enteric Bacteria. Human Isolates Final Report, 2003. Available at: www.cdc.gov/NARMS. Accessed August 2007.

59. Centers for Disease Control and Prevention: 1993 Revised classification system for HIV infection and expanded surveillance case definition for AIDS among adolescents and adults. M. M. W. R. Morb. Mortal. Wkly. Rep. 41(RR-17):1-19, 1992.

60. Centers for Disease Control and Prevention: Bacillus cereus food poisoning associated with fried rice at two child care centers: Virginia, 1993. M. M. W. R. Morb. Mortal. Wkly. Rep. 43:177-178, 1994.

61. Centers for Disease Control and Prevention: Cryptosporidiosis outbreaks associated with recreational water use—five states, 2006. M. M. W. R. Morb. Mortal. Wkly. Rep. 56:729-732, 2007.

62. Centers for Disease Control and Prevention: Diagnosis and management of foodborne illnesses: A primer for physicians. M. M. W. R. Morb. Mortal. Wkly. Rep. 50(RR-02):1-69, 2001.

63. Centers for Disease Control and Prevention: Giardiasis surveillance. United States, 1998-2002. M. M. W. R. Morb. Mortal. Wkly. Rep. 54(SS-1):9-16, 2005.

64. Centers for Disease Control and Prevention: Guidelines for preventing opportunistic infections among HIV-infected persons. M. M. W. R. Morb. Mortal. Wkly. Rep. 51:1-46, 2002.

65. Centers for Disease Control and Prevention: Laboratory-confirmed non-O157 shiga toxin–producing Escherichia coli—Connecticut, 2000-2005. M. M. W. R. Morb. Mortal. Wkly. Rep. 56:29-31, 2007.

66. Centers for Disease Control and Prevention: Managing acute gastroenteritis among children: Oral rehydration, maintenance, and nutritional therapy. M. M. W. R. Morb. Mortal. Wkly. Rep. 52(RR-16):1-16, 2003.

67. Centers for Disease Control and Prevention: Multistate outbreak of Listeriosis—United States, 2000. M. M. W. R. Morb. Mortal. Wkly. Rep. 49:1129-1130, 2000.

68. Centers for Disease Control and Prevention: Multistate outbreak of Salmonella serotype Tennessee infections associated with peanut butter—United States, 2006-2007. M. M. W. R. Morb. Mortal. Wkly. Rep. 56:521-524, 2007.

69. Centers for Disease Control and Prevention: Outbreak of gastroenteritis associated with Noroviruses on cruise ships—United States, 2002. M. M. W. R. Morb. Mortal. Wkly. Rep. 51:1112-1115, 2002.

70. Centers for Disease Control and Prevention: Preliminary FoodNet data on the incidence of infection with pathogens transmitted commonly through food—10 states, 2006. M. M. W. R. Morb. Mortal. Wkly. Rep. 56:336-339, 2007. Available at: www.cdc.gov/foodnet.

71. Centers for Disease Control and Prevention: Prevention of rotavirus gastroenteritis among infants and children: Recommendations of the Advisory Committee on Immunization Practices (ACIP). M. M. W. R. Morb. Mortal. Wkly. Rep. 55(RR-12):1-13, 2006.

72. Centers for Disease Control and Prevention: Responding to fecal accidents in disinfected swimming venues. M. M. W. R. Morb. Mortal. Wkly. Rep. 50:416-417, 2001.

73. Centers for Disease Control and Prevention: Summary of notifiable diseases, United States, 2005. M. M. W. R. Morb. Mortal. Wkly. Rep. 54:1-92, 2007.

74. Centers for Disease Control and Prevention: Two cases of toxigenic Vibrio cholera O1 infection after Hurricanes Katrina and Rita—Louisana, October 2005. M. M. W. R. Morb. Mortal. Wkly. Rep. 55:31-32, 2006.

75. Centers for Disease Control and Prevention: Typhoid immunization. M. M. W. R. Morb. Mortal. Wkly. Rep. 43:1-7, 1994.

76. Cerquetti, M., Luzzi, I., Caprioli, A., et al.: Role of Clostridium difficile in childhood diarrhea. Pediatr. Infect. Dis. J. 14:598-603, 1995.

77. Chinh, N. T., Parry, C. M., Ly, N. T., et al.: A randomized controlled comparison of azithromycin and ofloxacin for treatment of multidrug-resistant or nalidixic acid–resistant enteric fever. Antimicrob. Agents Chemother. 44:1855-1859, 2000.

78. CHOICE Study Group: Multicenter, randomized, double-blind clinical trial to evaluate the efficacy and safety of a reduced osmolarity oral rehydration salts solution in children with acute watery diarrhea. Pediatrics 107:613-618, 2001.

79. Clark, D. P.: New insights into human cryptosporidiosis. Clin. Microbiol. Rev. 12:554-563, 1999.

80. Cleary, T. G., Guerrant, R. L., and Pickering, L. K.: Microorganisms responsible for neonatal diarrhea. In Remington, J. S., Klein, J. O. (eds.): Infectious Diseases of the Fetus and Newborn Infant. 5th ed. Philadelphia, W. B. Saunders, 2000, pp. 1249-132.

81. Connolly, M. J., Snow, M. H., and Ingham, H. R.: Ciprofloxacin treatment of recurrent Salmonella septicaemia in a patient with acquired immune deficiency syndrome. J. Antimicrob. Chemother. 18:647, 1986.

82. Conteas, C. N., Berlin, O. G., Ash, L. R., and Pruthi, J. S.: Therapy for human gastrointestinal microsporidiosis. Am. J. Trop. Med. Hyg. 63:121-127, 2000.

83. Cooles, P.: Adjuvant steroids and relapse of typhoid fever. J. Trop. Med. Hyg. 89:229, 1986.

84. Cotte, L., Rabodonirina, M., Chapuis, F., et al.: Waterborne outbreak of intestinal microsporidiosis in persons with and without human immunodeficiency virus infection. J. Infect. Dis. 180:2003-2008, 1999.

85. Czeczulin, J. R., Balepur, S., Hicks, S., et al.: Aggregative adherence fimbria II, a second fimbrial antigen mediating aggregative adherence in enteroaggregative Escherichia coli. Infect. Immun. 65:4135-4145, 1997.

86. Dalton, C. B., Austin, C. C., Sobel, J., et al.: An outbreak of gastroenteritis and fever due to Listeria monocytogenes in milk. N. Engl. J. Med. 336:100-105, 1997.

87. Daniels, N. A., MacKinnon, L., Bishop, R., et al.: Vibrio parahaemolyticus infections in the United States, 1973-1998. J. Infect. Dis. 181:161-166, 2000.

88. Dansinger, M. L., Johnson, S., Jansen, P. C., et al.: Protein-losing enteropathy is associated with Clostridium difficile diarrhea but not with asymptomatic colonization: A prospective case-control study. Clin. Infect. Dis. 22:932-937, 1996.

89. DaSilva, A. J., Schwartz, D. A., Visvesvara, G. S., et al.: Sensitive PCR diagnosis of infections by Enterocytozoon bieneusi (microsporidia) using primers based on the region coding for small-subunit rRNA. J. Clin. Microbiol. 34:986-987, 1996.

90. Davidson, R. A.: Issues in clinical parasitology: The treatment of giardiasis. Am. J. Gastroenterol. 79:256-261, 1984.

91. Davis, M. A., Hancock, D. D., Besser, T. E., et al.: Changes in antimicrobial resistance among Salmonella enterica serovar typhimurium isolates from humans and cattle in the northwestern United States, 1982-1997. Emerg. Infect. Dis. 5:802-806, 1999.

92. DeHovitz, J. A., Pape, J. W., Boncy, M., et al.: Clinical manifestations and therapy of Isospora belli infection in patients with the acquired immunodeficiency syndrome. N. Engl. J. Med. 315:87, 1986.

93. Dennehy, P. H., Gauntlett, D. R., and Tente, W.: Comparison of nine commercial immunoassays for the detection of rotavirus in fecal samples. J. Clin. Microbiol. 26:1630, 1988.

94. Dennehy, P. H., Nelson, S. M., Spangenberger, S., et al.: A prospective case-control study of the role of astrovirus in acute diarrhea among hospitalized young children. J. Infect. Dis. 184:10-15, 2001.

95. DeVinney, R., Knoechel, D. G., and Finlay, B. B.: Enteropathogenic *Escherichia coli*: Cellular harassment. Curr. Opin. Microbiol. 2:83-88, 1999.

96. Didier, E. S., Orenstein, J. M., Aldras, A., et al.: Comparison of three staining methods for detecting microsporidia in fluids. J. Clin. Microbiol. 33:3138-3145, 1995.

97. Dierick, K., Van Coillie, E., Swiecicka, I., et al.: Fatal family outbreak of *Bacillus cereus*–associated food poisoning. J. Clin. Microbiol. 43:4277-4279, 2005.

98. Dietrich, D. T., Lew, E. A., Kotler, D. P., et al.: Treatment with albendazole for intestinal disease due to *Enterocytozoon bieneusi* in patients with AIDS. J. Infect. Dis. 169:178-183, 1994.

99. Dobell, C.: A revision of the coccidia parasitic in man. Parasitology 11:147, 1919.

100. Donnenberg, M. D., and Kaper, J. B.: Enteropathogenic *Escherichia coli*. Infect. Immun. 60:3953-3961, 1992.

101. Donnenberg, M. S., Giron, J. A., Nataro, J. P., et al.: A plasmid-encoded type IV fimbrial gene of enteropathogenic *Escherichia coli* associated with localized adherence. Mol. Microbiol. 6:3427-3437, 1992.

102. Donnenberg, M. S., Yu, J., and Kaper, J. B.: A second chromosomal gene necessary for intimate attachment of enteropathogenic *E. coli* to epithelial cells. J. Bacteriol. 175:4670-4680, 1993.

103. Donta, S. T., and Myers, M. G.: *Clostridium difficile* toxin in asymptomatic neonates. J. Pediatr. 100:431-434, 1982.

104. Dore, G. J., Marriott, D. J., Hing, M. C., et al.: Disseminated microsporidiosis due to *Septata intestinalis* in nine patients infected with the human immunodeficiency virus: Response to therapy with albendazole. Clin. Infect. Dis. 21:70-76, 1995.

105. Drobniewski, F. A.: *Bacillus cereus* and related species. Clin. Microbiol. Rev. 6:324-338, 1993.

106. DuPont, H. L.: Azithromycin for the self-treatment of traveler's diarrhea. Clin. Infect. Dis. 44:347-349, 2007.

107. DuPont, H. L., Jiang, Z. D., Belkind-Gerson, J., et al.: Treatment of travelers' diarrhea: Randomized trial comparing rifaximin, rifaximin plus loperamide, and loperamide alone. Clin. Gastroenterol. Hepatol. 5:451-456, 2007.

108. DuPont, H. L., Jiang, Z. D., Okhuysen, P. C., et al.: A randomized, double-blind, placebo-controlled trial of rifaximin to prevent travelers' diarrhea. Ann. Intern. Med. 42:805-812, 2005.

109. Dupont, H. L., and Capsuto, E. G.: Persistent diarrhea in travelers. Clin. Infect. Dis. 22:124-128, 1996.

110. DuPont, H. L., and Hornick, R. B.: Adverse effects of lomotil therapy in shigellosis. J. A. M. A. 226:1525-1528, 1973.

111. DuPont, H. L., and the Practice Parameters Committee of the American College of Gastroenterology: Guidelines on acute diarrhea in adults. Am. J. Gastroenterol. 92:1962-1975, 1997.

112. Dupont, H. L., Chappell, C. L., Sterling, C. R., et al.: The infectivity of *Cryptosporidium parvum* in healthy volunteers. N. Engl. J. Med. 332:855-859, 1995.

113. DuPont, H. L., Evans, D. G., Sullivan, P., et al.: Prevention of travelers' diarrhea (emporiatric enteritis) by prophylactic administration of bismuth subsalicylate. J. A. M. A. 243:237-241, 1980.

114. DuPont, H. L., Jiang, Z.-D., Ericsson, D. D., et al.: Rifaximin versus ciprofloxacin for the treatment of traveler's diarrhea: A randomized double-blind clinical trial. Clin. Infect. Dis. 33:1807-1815, 2001.

115. DuPont, H. L., Olarte, J., Evans, D. G., et al.: Comparative susceptibility of Latin American and United States students to enteric pathogens. N. Engl. J. Med. 295:1520-1521, 1976.

116. DuPont, H. L., Sullivan, P., Pickering, L. K., et al.: Symptomatic treatment of diarrhea with bismuth subsalicylate among students attending a Mexican university. Gastroenterology 73:715-718, 1977.

117. DuPont, H. L.: Therapy for and prevention of traveler's diarrhea. Clin. Infect. Dis. 45:S78-S84, 2007.

118. Dutta, P., Rasaily, R., Saha, M. R., et al.: Ciprofloxacin for treatment of severe typhoid fever in children. Antimicrob. Agents Chemother. 37:1197-1199, 1993.

119. Dworkin, M. S., Shoemaker, P. C., Goldoft, M. J., et al.: Reactive arthritis and Reiter's syndrome following an outbreak of gastroenteritis caused by *Salmonella enteritidis*. Clin. Infect. Dis. 33:1010-1014, 2001.

120. Dziuban, E. J., Liang, J. L., Craun, G. F., et al.: Surveillance for waterborne disease and outbreaks associated with recreational water—United States, 2003-2004. M. M. W. R. Surveill. Summ. 55(SS-12):1-30, 2006.

121. Eastaugh, J., and Shepherd, S.: Infectious and toxic syndromes from fish and shellfish consumption: A review. Arch. Intern. Med. 149:1735, 1989.

122. Eidlitz-Marcus, T., Cohen, Y. H., Nussinovitch, M., et al.: Comparative efficacy of two- and five-day courses of ceftriaxone for treatment of severe shigellosis in children. J. Pediatr. 123:822-824, 1993.

123. Eisenberg, M. S., Gaarslev, K., Brown, W., et al.: Staphylococcal food poisoning aboard a commercial aircraft. Lancet 2:595-599, 1975.

124. Enslava, C., Navarro-Garcia, F., Czeczulin, J. R., et al.: Pet, an autotransporter enterotoxin from enteroaggregative *Escherichia coli*. Infect. Immun. 66:3155-3163, 1998.

125. Ericsson, C., DuPont, H., Okhuysen, P., et al.: Loperamide plus azithromycin more effectively treats travelers' diarrhea in Mexico than azithromycin alone. J. Travel Med. 14:312-319, 2007.

126. Ericsson, C. D., DuPont, H. L., Evans, D. G., et al.: Bismuth subsalicylate inhibits activity of crude toxins of *Escherichia coli* and *Vibrio cholerae*. J. Infect. Dis. 136:693-696, 1977.

127. Ericsson, C. D., DuPont, H. L., Mathewson, J. J., et al.: Treatment of travelers' diarrhea with sulfamethoxazole and trimethoprim and loperamide. J. A. M. A. 263:257, 1990.

128. Ericsson, C. D., Pickering, L. K., Sullivan, P., et al.: The role of location of food consumption in the prevention of travelers' diarrhea in Mexico. Gastroenterology 79:812-816, 1980.

129. Espinosa-Cantellano, M., and Martinez-Palomo, A.: Pathogenesis of intestinal amebiasis: From molecules to disease. Clin. Microbiol. Rev. 13:318-331, 2000.

130. Estes, M. K., and Cohen, J.: Rotavirus gene structure and function. Microbiol. Rev. 53:410, 1989.

131. Fang, G. D., Lima, A. A., Martins, C. V., et al.: Etiology and epidemiology of persistent diarrhea in northeastern Brazil: A hospital-based, prospective case-control study. J. Pediatr. Gastroenterol. Nutr. 21:137-144, 1995.

132. Farthing, M. J.: Antisecretory drugs for diarrheal disease. Dig. Dis. 24:47-58, 2006.

133. Fedorko, D. P., Nelson, N. A., and Cartwright, C. P.: Identification of microsporidia in stool specimens by using PCR and restriction endonucleases. J. Clin. Microbiol. 33:1739-1741, 1995.

134. Feldman, R. J., Kallich, M., and Weinstein, M. P.: Bacteremia due to *Clostridium difficile*: Case report and review of extraintestinal *C. difficile* infections. Clin. Infect. Dis. 20:1560-1562, 1995.

135. Feldman, S., Chen, S. L., Pickering, L. K., et al.: Salicylate absorption from a bismuth subsalicylate antidiarrheal preparation. Clin. Pharmacol. Ther. 29:788-792, 1981.

136. Feng, X., and Jiang, X.: Library screen for inhibitors targeting norovirus binding to histo-blood group antigen receptors. Antimicrob. Agents Chemother. 51:324-331, 2007.

137. Ferreccio, C., Morriss, G., Valdivieso, C., et al.: Efficacy of ciprofloxacin in the treatment of chronic typhoid carriers. J. Infect. Dis. 157:1235, 1988.

138. Fichtenbaum, C. J., Ritchie, D. J., and Powderly, W. G.: Use of paromomycin for treatment of cryptosporidiosis in AIDS. Clin. Infect. Dis. 16:298-300, 1993.

139. Fioramonti, J., Droy-Lefaix, M. T., and Bueno, L.: Changes in gastrointestinal motility induced by cholera toxin and experimental osmotic diarrhoea in dogs: Effects of treatment with an argillaceous compound. Digestion 36:230, 1987.

140. Fischer, T. K., Viboud, C., Parashar, U., et al.: Hospitalizations and deaths from diarrhea and rotavirus among children <5 years of age in the United States, 1993-2003. J. Infect. Dis. 195:1117-1125, 2007.

141. Flanigan, T., Whalen, C., and Turner, J.: *Cryptosporidium* infection and CD4 counts. Ann. Intern. Med. 116:840-842, 1992.

142. Fotedar, R., Stark, D., Beebe, N., et al.: Laboratory diagnostic techniques for *Entamoeba* species. Clin. Microbiol. Rev. 20:511-532, 2007.

143. Fox, L., M., Ocfemia, M. C., Hunt, D. C., et al.: Emergency survey methods in acute cryptosporidiosis outbreak. Emerg. Infect. Dis. 11:729-731, 2005.

144. Freedman, S. B., Adler, M., Seshadri, R., et al.: Oral ondansetron for gastroenteritis in a pediatric emergency department. N. Engl. J. Med. 354:1698-1705, 2006.

145. Frenck, R. W., Jr., Nakhla, I., Sultan, Y., et al.: Azithromycin versus ceftriaxone for the treatment of uncomplicated typhoid fever in children. Clin. Infect. Dis. 31:1134-1138, 2000.

146. Furness, B. W., Beach, M. J., and Roberts, J. M.: Giardiasis surveillance—United States, 1992-1997. M. M. W. R. Morb. Mortal. Wkly. Rep. 49(SS-7):1-13, 2000.

147. Gallay, A., Prouzet-Mauléon, V., Kempf, I., et al.: *Campylobacter* antimicrobial drug resistance among humans, broiler chickens, and pigs, France. Emerg. Infect. Dis. 13:259-266, 2007.

148. Garcia, L. S., and Shimizu, R. Y.: Evaluation of nine immunoassay kits (enzyme immunoassay and direct fluorescence) for detection for *Giardia lamblia* and *Cryptosporidium parvum* in human fecal specimens. J. Clin. Microbiol. 35:1526-1529, 1997.

149. Garcia, L. S., Brewer, T. C., and Bruckner, D. A.: Incidence of *Cryptosporidium* in all patients submitting stool specimens for ova and parasites examination: Monoclonal antibody IFA method. Diagn. Microbiol. Infect. Dis. 11:25, 1988.

150. Gardner, T. B., and Hill, D. R.: Treatment of giardiasis. Clin. Microbiol. Rev. 14:114-128, 2001.

151. Gebreyes, W. A., Davies, P. R., Morrow, W. E. M., et al.: Antimicrobial resistance of *Salmonella* isolates from swine. J. Clin. Microbiol. 38:4633-4636, 2000.

152. Genta, R. M.: Global prevalence of strongyloidiasis: Critical review with epidemiologic insights into the prevention of disseminated disease. Rev. Infect. Dis. 11:755, 1989.

153. Ginsburg, C. M.: Lomotil (diphenoxylate and atropine) intoxication. Am. J. Dis. Child. 125:241, 1973.

154. Girard, D. E., and Keefe, E. B.: *Isospora* and travelers' diarrhea. Ann. Intern. Med. *106*:908, 1987.
155. Girgis, N. I., Butler, T., Frenck, R. W., et al.: Azithromycin versus cipro-floxacin for treatment of uncomplicated typhoid fever in a randomized trial in Egypt that included patients with multidrug resistance. Antimicrob. Agents Chemother. *43*:1441-1444, 1999.
156. Glandt, M., Adachi, J. A., Mathewson, J. J., et al.: Enteroaggregative *Escherichia coli* as a cause of traveler's diarrhea: Clinical response to ciprofloxacin. Clin. Infect. Dis. *29*:335-338, 1999.
157. Glass, R. I., Noel, J., Mitchell, D., et al.: The changing epidemiology of astro-virus-associated gastroenteritis. Arch. Virol. *12*(Suppl.):287-300, 1996.
158. Glynn, M. K., Bopp, D., Dewitt, W., et al.: Emergence of multidrug-resistant *Salmonella enterica* serotype typhimurium DT104 infections in the United States. N. Engl. J. Med. *338*:1333-1338, 1998.
159. Goodgame, R. W.: Understanding intestinal spore-forming protozoa: Cryptosporidia, microsporidia, isospora, and cyclospora. Ann. Intern. Med. *124*:429-441, 1996.
160. Gorbach, S. L., Carpenter, C. C. J., Grayson, R., et al.: Travelers' diarrhea: Consensus conference. J. A. M. A. *253*:2700-2704, 1985.
161. Gottlieb, S. L., Newbern, E. C., Griffin, P. M., et al.: Multistate outbreak of listeriosis linked to turkey deli meat and subsequent changes in US regulatory policy. Clin. Infect. Dis. *42*:29-36, 2006.
162. Green, S. D. R.: Ten years of pediatric experience with ciprofloxacin. Infect. Dis. Clin. Pract. 7(Suppl. 3):S175-S183, 1998.
163. Guerrant, R. L., Van Gilder, T., Steiner, T. S., et al.: Practice guidelines for the management of infectious diarrhea. Clin. Infect. Dis. *32*:331-350, 2001.
164. Guerrero, M. L., Noel, J. S., Mitchell, D. K., et al.: A prospective study of astrovirus diarrhea of infancy in Mexico City. Pediatr. Infect. Dis. J. *17*:723-727, 1998.
165. Gupta, A., Nelson, J. M., Barrett, T. J., et al.: Antimicrobial resistance among *Campylobacter* strains, United States, 1997-2001. Emerg. Infect. Dis. *10*:1102-1109, 2004.
166. Hall, A., and Nahar, Q.: Albendazole as a treatment for infections with *Giardia duodenalis* in children in Bangladesh. Trans. R. Soc. Trop. Med. Hyg. *87*:84-86, 1993.
167. Hanrahan, J. P., and Gordon, M. A.: Mushroom poisoning: Case reports and a review of therapy. J. A. M. A. *251*:1057-1061, 1984.
168. Hart, C. A., Baxby, D., and Blundell, N.: Gastroenteritis due to *Cryptosporidium*: A prospective survey in a children's hospital. J. Infect. *9*:264, 1984.
169. Hecht, D. W., Galang, M. A., Sambol, S. P., et al.: In vitro activities of 15 antimicrobial agents against 110 toxigenic *Clostridium difficile* clinical isolates collected from 1983 to 2004. Antimicrob. Agents Chemother. *51*:2716-2719, 2007.
170. Henderson, A. E., Gillespie, G. W., Kaplan, P., et al.: The human *Isospora*. Am. J. Hyg. *78*:302, 1963.
171. Hennessy, T. W., Hedberg, C. W., Slutsker, L., et al.: A national outbreak of *Salmonella enteritidis* infections from ice cream. N. Engl. J. Med. *334*:1281-1286, 1996.
172. Henricksen, S. A., and Pohlenz, J. F. L.: Staining of cryptosporidia by a modi-fied Ziehl-Neelsen technique. Acta Vet. Scand. *22*:594, 1981.
173. Herrington, D. A., Tzipori, S., Robins-Browne, R. M., et al.: In vitro and in vivo pathogenicity of *Plesiomonas shigelloides*. Infect. Immun. *55*:979, 1987.
174. Herwaldt, B. L., de Arroyave, K. R., Roberts, J. M., et al.: A multiyear prospec-tive study of the risk factors for and incidence of diarrheal illness in a cohort of Peace Corps volunteers in Guatemala. Ann. Intern. Med. *132*:982-988, 2000.
175. Herwaldt, B. L.: *Cyclospora cayetanensis*: A review, focusing on the outbreaks of cyclosporiasis in the 1990s. Clin. Infect. Dis. *31*:1040-1057, 2000.
176. Hewitt, R. G., Yiannoutsos, C. T., Higgs, E. S., et al.: Paromomycin: No more effective than placebo for treatment of cryptosporidiosis in patients with advanced human immunodeficiency virus infection. Clin. Infect. Dis. *31*:1084-1092, 2000.
177. Hicks, P., Zwiener, J., Squires, J., et al.: Azithromycin therapy for *Cryptosporidium parvum* infection in four children infected with human immu-nodeficiency virus. J. Pediatr. *129*:297-300, 1996.
178. Hines, J., and Nachamkin, I.: Effective use of the clinical microbiology laboratory for diagnosing diarrheal diseases. Clin. Infect. Dis. *23*:1292-1301, 1996.
179. Hirschhorn, N.: Treatment of acute diarrhea in children: Historical and physi-ological perspective. J. Clin. Nutr. *33*:637-663, 1980.
180. Hlady, W. G., and Klontz, K. C.: The epidemiology of *Vibrio* infections in Florida, 1981-1993. J. Infect. Dis. *173*:1176-1183, 1996.
181. Hlavsa, M. C., Watson, J. C., and Beach, M. J.: Cryptosporidiosis surveil-lance—United States 1999-2002. M. M. W. R. Morb. Mortal. Wkly. Rep. *54*(SS-1):1-8, 2005.
182. Hoffman, S. L., Punjabi, N. H., Kumala, S., et al.: Reduction of mortality in chloramphenicol-treated severe typhoid fever by high-dose dexamethasone. N. Engl. J. Med. *310*:82, 1984.
183. Hoge, C. W., Shlim, D. R., Echeverria, P., et al.: Epidemiology of diarrhea among expatriate residents living in a highly endemic environment. J. A. M. A. *275*:533-538, 1996.
184. Högenauer, C., Hammer, H. F., Krejs, G. J., et al.: Mechanisms and management of antibiotic-associated diarrhea. Clin. Infect. Dis. *27*:702-710, 1998.
185. Hohmann, E. L.: Nontyphoidal salmonellosis. Clin. Infect. Dis. *32*:263-269, 2001.
186. Holmberg, S. D., and Blake, P. A.: Staphylococcal food poisoning in the United States: New facts and old misconceptions. J. A. M. A. *251*:487-489, 1984.
187. Holmberg, S. D., Wachsmuth, I. K., Hickman-Brenner, F. W., et al.: *Plesiomonas* enteric infections in the United States. Ann. Intern. Med. *105*:690, 1986.
188. Holmes, S. J., Morrow, A. L., and Pickering, L. K.: Child care practices: Effects of social changes on epidemiology of infectious diseases and antibiotic resistance. Epidemiol. Rev. *18*:10-28, 1996.
189. Hoque, K. M., and Binder, H. J.: Zinc in the treatment of acute diarrhea: Current status and assessment. Gastroenterology *130*:2201-2205, 2006.
190. Hovius, S. E. R., and Rietra, P. J.: *Salmonella* colitis clinically presenting as pseudomembranous colitis. Neth. J. Surg. *34*:81-82, 1982.
191. Huang, D. B., Nataro, J. P., DuPont, H. L., et al.: Enteroaggregative *Escherichia coli* is a cause of acute diarrheal illness: A meta-analysis. Clin. Infect. Dis. *43*:556-563, 2006.
192. Hubert, B., Loo, V. G., Bourgault, A. M., et al.: A portrait of the geographic dissemination of the *Clostridium difficile* North American pulsed-field type 1 strain and the epidemiology of C. *difficile*–associated disease in Québec. Clin. Infect. Dis. *44*:238-244, 2007.
193. Hughes, J. M., Boyce, J. M., Aleem, A. R., et al.: *Vibrio parahaemolyticus* enterocolitis in Bangladesh: Report of an outbreak. Am. J. Trop. Med. Hyg. *27*:106-112, 1978.
194. Huicho, L., Campos, M., Rivera, J., et al.: Fecal screening tests in the approach to acute infectious diarrhea: A scientific overview. Pediatr. Infect. Dis. J. *15*:486-494, 1996.
195. Islam, A., Butler, T., Kabir, I., et al.: Treatment of typhoid fever with ceftri-axone for 5 days or chloramphenicol for 14 days: A randomized clinical trial. Antimicrob. Agents Chemother. *37*:1572-1575, 1993.
196. Janda, J. M., and Abbott, S. L.: Evolving concepts regarding the genus *Aeromonas*: An expanding panorama of species, disease presentations, and unanswered questions. Clin. Infect. Dis. *27*:332-344, 1998.
197. Janda, J. M., Powers, C., Bryant, R. G., et al.: Current perspectives on the epidemiology and pathogenesis of clinically significant *Vibrio* spp. Clin. Microbiol. Rev. *1*:245, 1988.
198. Jensen, L. B., and Aarestrup, F. M.: Macrolide resistance in *Campylobacter coli* of animal origin in Denmark. Antimicrob. Agents Chemother. *45*:371-372, 2001.
199. Jiang, X., Graham, D. Y., Wang, K., et al.: Norwalk virus genome cloning and characterization. Science *250*:1580-1583, 1991.
200. Jiang, X., Matson, D. O., Velazquez, F. R., et al.: A study of Norwalk-related viruses in Mexican children. J. Med. Virol. *47*:309-316, 1995.
201. Jiang, X., Turf, E., Hu, J., et al.: Outbreaks of gastroenteritis in elderly nursing homes and retirement facilities associated with human caliciviruses. J. Med. Virol. *50*:335-341, 1996.
202. Jimenez, S. G., Heine, R. G., Ward, P. B., et al.: *Campylobacter upsaliensis* gastroenteritis in childhood. Pediatr. Infect. Dis. J. *18*:988-992, 1999.
203. Johnson, S., Henderson, W., Crewe-Brown, H., et al.: Effect of human immu-nodeficiency virus infection on episodes of diarrhea among children in South Africa. Pediatr. Infect. Dis. J. *19*:972-979, 2000.
204. Johnson, W. D., Jr., Hook, E. W., Lindsey, E., et al.: Treatment of chronic typhoid carriers with ampicillin. Antimicrob. Agents Chemother. *3*:439-440, 1973.
205. Johnston, B. C., Supina, A. L., and Vohra, S.: Probiotics for pediatric antibi-otic-associated diarrhea: A meta-analysis of randomized placebo-controlled trials. C. M. A. J. *175*:377-383, 2006.
206. Jones, T. F., Buckingham, S. C., Bobb, C. A., et al.: From pig to paci-fier: Chitterling-associated yersiniosis outbreak among black infants. Emerg. Infect. Dis. *9*:1007-1009, 2003.
207. Kabir, I., Butler, T., and Khanam, A.: Comparative efficacies of single intrave-nous doses of ceftriaxone and ampicillin for shigellosis in a placebo-controlled trial. Antimicrob. Agents Chemother. *29*:645, 1986.
208. Kain, K. C., and Kelly, M. T.: Clinical features, epidemiology, and treatment of *Plesiomonas shigelloides* diarrhea. J. Clin. Microbiol. *27*:998, 1989.
209. Kaper, J. B., Morris, J. G., Jr., and Levine, M. M.: Cholera. Clin. Microbiol. Rev. *8*:48-86, 1995.
210. Karmali, M. A.: Infection by verocytotoxin-producing *Escherichia coli*. Clin. Microbiol. Rev. *2*:15, 1989.
211. Katanik, M. T., Schneider, S. K., Rosenblatt, J. E., et al.: Evaluation of ColorPAC *Giardia/Cryptosporidium* rapid assay and ProSpecT *Giardia/ Cryptosporidium* microplate assay for detection of *Giardia* and *Cryptosporidium* in fecal specimens. J. Clin. Microbiol. *39*:4523-4525, 2001.
212. Katiyar, S. K., and Edlind, T. D.: In vitro susceptibilities of the AIDS-associated microsporidian *Encephalitozoon intestinalis* to albendazole, its sulfox-ide metabolite, and 12 additional benzimidazole derivates. Antimicrob. Agents Chemother. *41*:2729-2732, 1997.
213. Keiser, P. B., and Nutman, T. B.: *Strongyloides stercoralis* in the immunocom-promised population. Clin. Microbiol. Rev. *17*:208-217, 2004.
214. Kelber, M., and Ament, M. E.: *Shigella dysenteriae* I: A forgotten cause of pseudomembranous colitis. J. Pediatr. *89*:595, 1976.
215. Keusch, G. T., and Bennish, M. L.: Shigellosis: Recent progress, persisting problems and research issues. Pediatr. Infect. Dis. *8*:713, 1989.
216. Khan, W. A., Bennish, M. L., Seas, C., et al.: Randomised controlled compari-son of single-dose ciprofloxacin and doxycycline for cholera caused by *Vibrio cholera* 01 and 0139. Lancet *348*:296-300, 1996.

217. Khan, W. A., Seas, C., Dhar, U., et al.: Treatment of shigellosis: V. Comparison of azithromycin and ciprofloxacin. Ann. Intern. Med. *126*:697-703, 1997.

218. Khan, W. A., Saha, D., and Rahman, A.: Comparison of a single-dose azithromycin and 12-dose, 3-day erythromycin for childhood cholera: A randomized, double-blind trial. Lancet *360*:1722-1727, 2002.

219. Knisley, C. V., Bednarz-Prashad, A. J., and Pickering, L. K.: Detection of rotavirus in stool specimens with monoclonal and polyclonal antibody-based assay systems. J. Clin. Microbiol. *23*:897-900, 1986.

220. Knisley, C. V., Englekirk, P. G., Pickering, L. K., et al.: Rapid detection of *Giardia* antigen in stool using enzyme immunoassays. Am. J. Clin. Pathol. *91*:704, 1989.

221. Koo, D., Maloney, K., and Tauxe, R.: Epidemiology of diarrheal disease outbreaks on cruise ships, 1986 through 1993. J. A. M. A. *275*:545-547, 1996.

222. Koopmans, M. P. G., Goosen, E. S. M., Lima, A. A. M., et al.: Association of torovirus with acute and persistent diarrhea in children. Pediatr. Infect. Dis. J. *16*:504-507, 1997.

223. Kotler, D. P., and Orenstein, J. M.: Clinical syndromes associated with microsporidiosis. Adv. Parasitol. *40*:321-349, 1998.

224. Kotler, D. P., Francisco, A., Clayton, F., et al.: Small intestinal injury and parasitic diseases in AIDS. Ann. Intern. Med. *113*:444, 1990.

225. Kotler, D. P.: Characterization of intestinal disease associated with human immunodeficiency virus infection and response to antiretroviral therapy. J. Infect. Dis. *179*(Suppl.):454-456, 1999.

226. Kotloff, K. L., Losonsky, G. A., Morris, J. G., et al.: Enteric adenovirus infection and childhood diarrhea: An epidemiologic study in three clinical settings. Pediatrics *84*:219, 1989.

227. Kourtis, A. P, Bansel, P., Posner, S. F., et al.: Trends in hospitalizations of HIV-infected children and adolescents in the United States: Analysis of data from the 1994-2003 Nationwide Inpatient Sample. Pediatrics *120*:e236-243, 2007.

228. Kreutner, A. K., Del Bene, V. E., and Amstey, M. S.: Giardiasis in pregnancy. Am. J. Obstet. Gynecol. *140*:895-901, 1981.

229. Kuritsky, J. N., Osterholm, M. T., Greenberg, H. B., et al.: Norwalk gastroenteritis: A community outbreak associated with bakery product consumption. Ann. Intern. Med. *201*:519-521, 1984.

230. Lagrotteria, D., Holmes, S., Smieja, M., et al.: Prospective, randomized inpatient study of oral metronidazole versus oral metronidazole and rifampin for treatment of primary episode of *Clostridium difficile*–associated diarrhea. Clin. Infect. Dis. *43*:547-552, 2006.

231. Lawson, A. J., Logan, J. M. J., O'Neil, G. L., et al.: Large-scale survey of *Campylobacter* species in human gastroenteritis by PCR and PCR–enzyme-linked immunosorbent assay. J. Clin. Microbiol. *37*:3860-3864, 1999.

232. Lee, L. A., Gerber, A. R., Lonsway, D. R., et al.: *Yersinia enterocolitica* O:3 infections in infants and children, associated with the household preparation of chitterlings. N. Engl. J. Med. *322*:984, 1990.

233. Lessnau, K. D., Can, S., and Talavera, W.: Disseminated *Strongyloides stercoralis* in human immunodeficiency virus–infected patients: Treatment failure and a review of the literature. Chest *104*:119-122, 1993.

234. Levine, M. M., Hughes, T. P., Black, R. E., et al.: Variability of sodium and sucrose levels of simple sugar/salt oral rehydration solutions prepared under optimal and field conditions. J. Pediatr. *97*:324-327, 1980.

235. Levine, W. C., Bennett, R. W., Choi, Y., et al.: Staphylococcal food poisoning caused by imported canned mushrooms. J. Infect. Dis. *173*:1263-1267, 1996.

236. Liang, J. L., Dziuban, E. J., Craun, G. F., et al.: Surveillance for waterborne disease and outbreaks associated with drinking water and water not intended for drinking—United States, 2003-2004. M. M. W. R. Surveill. Summ. *55*(SS-12):31-65, 2006.

237. Limson, B. M., and Littana, R. T.: Ciprofloxacin vs. co-trimoxazole in *Salmonella* enteric fever. Infection *17*:105, 1989.

238. Lin, F. Y. C., Ho, V. A., Khiem, H. B., et al.: The efficacy of a *Salmonella typhi* Vi conjugate vaccine in two- to five-year-old children. N. Engl. J. Med. *344*:1263-1269, 2001.

239. Lindsay, D. S., Dubey, J. P., and Blagburn, B. L.: Biology of *Isospora* spp. from humans, non-human primates, and domestic animals. Clin. Microbiol. Rev. *10*:19-34, 1997.

240. Lo, C. W., and Walker, W. A.: Chronic protracted diarrhea of infancy: A nutritional disease. Pediatrics *72*:786-800, 1983.

241. Loo, V. G., Poirier, L., Miller, M. A., et al.: A predominantly clonal multi-institutional outbreak of *Clostridium difficile*–associated diarrhea with high morbidity and mortality. N. Engl. J. Med. *353*:2442-2449, 2005.

242. Louie, E., Barkowsky, W., and Klesius, P. H.: Treatment of cryptosporidiosis with oral bovine transfer factor. Clin. Immunol. Immunopathol. *44*:329, 1987.

243. Lowry, P. W., Pavia, A. T., McFarland, L. M., et al.: Cholera in Louisiana: Widening spectrum of seafood vehicles. Arch. Intern. Med. *149*:2079, 1989.

244. Luby, S., Jones, J., Dowda, H., et al.: A large outbreak of gastroenteritis caused by diarrheal toxin-producing *Bacillus cereus*. J. Infect. Dis. *167*:1452-1455, 1993.

245. Lynch, M., Painter, J., Woodruff, R., et al.: Surveillance for foodborne-disease outbreaks—United States, 1998-2002. M. M. W. R. Surveill. Summ. *55*(SS-10):1-42, 2006.

246. MacKenzie, W. R., Hoxie, N. J., Proctor, M. E., et al.: A massive outbreak in Milwaukee of *Cryptosporidium* infection transmitted through the public water supply. N. Engl. J. Med. *331*:161-167, 1994.

247. Madico, G., McDonald, J., Gilman, R. H., et al.: Epidemiology and treatment of *Cyclospora cayetanensis* infection in Peruvian children. Clin. Infect. Dis. *24*:977-981, 1997.

248. Manabe, Y. C., Clark, D. P., Moore, R. D., et al.: Cryptosporidiosis in patients with AIDS: Correlates of disease and survival. Clin. Infect. Dis. *27*:536-542, 1998.

249. Manabe, Y. C., Vinetz, J. M., Moore, R. D., et. al.: *Clostridium difficile* colitis: An efficient clinical approach to diagnosis. Ann. Intern. Med. *123*:835-840, 1995.

250. Margolis, P. A., Litteer, T., Hare, N., et al.: Effects of unrestricted diet on mild infantile diarrhea. Am. J. Dis. Child. *144*:162, 1990.

251. Maslanka, S. E., Kerr, J. G., Williams, G., et al.: Molecular subtyping of *Clostridium perfringens* by pulsed-field gel electrophoresis to facilitate foodborne-disease outbreak investigations. J. Clin. Microbiol. *37*:2209-2214, 1999.

252. Mathewson, J. J., Johnson, P. C., DuPont, H. L., et al.: Pathogenicity of enteroadherent *Escherichia coli* in adult volunteers. J. Infect. Dis. *154*:524-527, 1986.

253. Mathis, A., Weber, R., and Deplazes, P.: Zoonotic potential of the microsporidia. Clin. Microb. Rev. *18*:423-445, 2005.

254. Matson, D. O., Estes, M. K., Burns, J. W., et al.: Serotype variation of human group A rotaviruses in two regions of the United States. J. Infect. Dis. *162*:605, 1990.

255. McDonald, L. C., Killgore, G. E., Thompson, A., et al.: An epidemic, toxin gene–variant strain of *Clostridium difficile*. N. Engl. J. Med. *353*:2433-2441, 2005.

256. McFarland, L. V.: Meta-analysis of probiotics for the prevention of antibiotic associated diarrhea and the treatment of *Clostridium difficile* disease. Am. J. Gastroenterol. *101*:812-822, 2006.

257. McFarland, L. V., Surawicz, C. M., and Stamm, W. E.: Risk factors for *Clostridium difficile* carriage and *C. difficile*–associated diarrhea in a cohort of hospitalized patients. J. Infect. Dis. *162*:678, 1990.

258. McLauglin, J. B., DePaola, A., Bopp, C. A., et al.: Outbreak of *Vibrio parahaemolyticus* gastroenteritis associated with Alaskan oysters. N. Engl. J. Med. *353*:1463-1470, 2005.

259. Medical Letter: Drugs for parasitic infections. *In* Pickering, L. K. (ed.): 2006 Red Book: Report of the Committee on Infectious Diseases. 27th ed. Elk Grove, IL, American Academy of Pediatrics, 2006, pp. 790-820.

260. Medical Letter: Treatment guidelines: Choice of antibacterial drugs. Med. Lett. *5*:33-50, 2007.

261. Memon, I. A., Billoo, A. G., and Memon, H. I.: Cefixime: An oral option for the treatment of multidrug-resistant enteric fever in children. South. Med. J. *90*:1204-1207, 1997.

262. Mendelowitz, P. C., Hoffman, R. S., and Weber, S.: Bismuth absorption and myoclonic encephalopathy during bismuth subsalicylate therapy. Ann. Intern. Med. *112*:140, 1990.

263. Mitchell, D. K., Monroe, S. S., Jiang, X., et al.: Virologic features of an astrovirus diarrhea outbreak in a day care center revealed by reverse transcriptase–polymerase chain reaction. J. Infect. Dis. *172*:1437-1444, 1995.

264. Mitchell, D. K., Snyder, J., and Pickering, L. K.: Gastrointestinal infections. *In* Pizzo, P. A., and Wilfert, C. M. (eds.): Pediatric AIDS: The Role of HIV Infections in Infants, Children, and Adolescents. 3rd ed. Baltimore, Williams & Wilkins, 1999, pp. 267-291.

265. Mitchell, D. K., Van, R., Mason, E. H., et al.: Prospective study of toxigenic *Clostridium difficile* in children given amoxicillin/clavulanate for otitis media. Pediatr. Infect. Dis. J. *15*:514-519, 1996.

266. Molbak, K., Baggesen, D. L., Aarestrup, F. M., et al.: An outbreak of multi-drug-resistant, quinolone-resistant *Salmonella enterica* serotype typhimurium DT 104. N. Engl. J. Med. *341*:1420-1425, 1999.

267. Molina, J.-M., Chastang, C., Goguel, J., et al.: Albendazole for treatment and prophylaxis of microsporidiosis due to *Encephalitozoon intestinalis* in patients with AIDS: A randomized double-blind controlled trial. J. Infect. Dis. *177*:1373-1377, 1998.

268. Molina, J. M., Tourneur, M., Sarfati, C., et al.: Fumagillin treatment of intestinal microsporidiosisn. N. Engl. J. Med. *346*:1963-1969, 2002.

269. Moreno-Espinosa, S., Farkas, T., and Jiang, X.: Human caliciviruses and pediatric gastroenteritis. Semin. Pediatr. Infect. Dis. *15*:237-245, 2004.

270. Morgan, D. R., Johnson, P. C., DuPont, H. L., et al.: Lack of correlation between known virulence properties of *Aeromonas hydrophila* and enteropathogenicity for humans. Infect. Immun. *50*:62, 1985.

271. Morris, J. G.: Cholera and other types of vibriosis: A story of human pandemics and oysters on the half shell. Clin. Infect. Dis. *37*:272-280, 2003.

272. Morse, D. L., Guzewich, J. J., Hanrahan, J. P., et al.: Widespread outbreaks of clam- and oyster-associated gastroenteritis: Role of Norwalk virus. N. Engl. J. Med. *314*:678-681, 1986.

273. Motala, C., Hill, I. D., Mann, M. D., et al.: Effect of loperamide on stool output and duration of acute infectious diarrhea in infants. J. Pediatr. *117*:467, 1990.

274. Murphy, T. V., Gargiullo, P. M., Massoudi, M. S., et al.: Intussusception among infants given an oral rotavirus vaccine. N. Engl. J. Med. *344*:564, 2001.

275. Murrell, T. G. C., Egerton, J. R., Rampling, A., et al.: The ecology and epidemiology of the pig-bel syndrome in man in New Guinea. J. Hyg. *64*:375-396, 1966.

276. Musher, D. M., Aslam, S., Logan, N., et al.: Relatively poor outcome after treatment of *Clostridium difficile* colitis with metronidazole. Clin. Infect. Dis. *40*:1586-1590, 2005.

277. Musher, D. M., Logan, N., Hamill, R. J., et al.: Nitazoxanide for the treatment of *Clostridium difficile* colitis. Clin. Infect. Dis. *43*:421-427, 2006.

278. Nachamkin, I., Allos, B. M., and Ho, T.: *Campylobacter* species and Guillain-Barré syndrome. Clin. Microbiol. Rev. *11*:555-567, 1998.

279. Nataro, J. P., and Kaper, J. B.: Diarrheagenic *Escherichia coli*. Microbiol. Rev. *11*:142-201, 1998.

280. Nataro, J. P., Mai, V., Johnson, J., et al.: Diarrheagenic *Escherichia coli* infection in Baltimore, Maryland, and New Haven, Connecticut. Clin. Infect. Dis. *43*:402-407, 2006.

281. National Association of State Public Health Veterinarians, Inc. (NASPHV): Compendium of measures to prevent disease associated with animals in public settings, 2007. M. M. W. R. Morb. Mortal. Wkly. Rep. *56*(RR-5):1-19, 2007. Available at: www.cdc.gov/mmwr/preview/

282. Navarro-Garcia, F., Canizalez-Roman, A., Luna J., et al.: Plasmid-encoded toxin of enteroaggregative *Escherichia coli* is internalized by epithelial cells. Infect. Immun. *69*:1053-1060, 2001.

283. Nelson, J. D., and Haltalin, K. C.: Amoxicillin less effective than ampicillin against *Shigella* in vitro and in vivo: Relationship of efficacy to activity in serum. J. Infect. Dis. *129*(Suppl.):222-227, 1974.

284. Nelson, J. M., Chiller, T. M. Powers, J. H., et al.: Fluoroquinolone-resistant *Campylobacter* species and the withdrawal of fluoroquinolones from use in poultry: A public health success story. Clin. Infect. Dis *44*:977-990, 2007.

285. Nesheim, S. R., Kapogiannis, B. G., Soe, M. M., et al.: Trends in opportunistic infections in the pre– and post–highly active antiretroviral therapy eras among HIV-infected children in the Perinatal AIDS Collaborative Transmission Study, 1986-2004. Pediatrics *120*:100-109, 2007.

286. Nilsson, M., Svenungsson, B., Hedlund, K. O., et al.: Incidence and genetic diversity of group C rotavirus among adults. J. Infect. Dis. *182*:678-684, 2000.

287. Novak, E., Lee, J. G., Seckman, C. E., et al.: Unfavorable effect of atropine-diphenoxylate (Lomotil) therapy in lincomycin-caused diarrhea. J. A. M. A. *235*:1451, 1976.

288. O'Connor, D., Hynes, P., and Cormican, M.: Evaluation of methods of detection of toxins in specimens of feces submitted for diagnosis of *Clostridium difficile*-associated diarrhea. J. Clin. Microbiol. *39*:2846-2849, 2001.

289. O'Ryan, M., Matson, D. O., Estes, M. K., et al.: Molecular epidemiology of rotaviruses in children attending day care centers in Houston. J. Infect. Dis. *162*:810, 1990.

290. Okhuysen, P. C.: Traveler's diarrhea due to intestinal protozoa. Clin. Infect. Dis. *33*:110-114, 2001.

291. Ooi, S. T., and Lorger B.: Gastroenteritis due to *Listeria monocytogenes*. Clin. Infect. Dis. *40*:1327-1332, 2005.

292. Ooi, W. W., Zimmerman, S. K., and Needham, C. A.: *Cyclospora* species as a gastrointestinal pathogen in immunocompetent hosts. J. Clin. Microbiol. *33*:1267-1269, 1995.

293. Ortega, Y. R., Sterling, C. R., Gilman R. H., et al.: *Cyclospora* species: A new protozoan pathogen of humans. N. Engl. J. Med. *328*:1308-1312, 1993.

294. Osterholm, M. T., MacDonald, K. L., White, K. E., et al.: An outbreak of brainerdiasis: An outbreak of a newly recognized chronic diarrhea syndrome associated with raw milk consumption. J. A. M. A. *256*:484-490, 1986.

295. Pape, J. W., and Johnson, W. D., Jr.: *Isospora belli* infection. Prog. Clin. Parasitol. *2*:119-127, 1991.

296. Pape, J. W., Verdier, R., Johnson, W. D., et al.: Treatment and prophylaxis of *Isospora belli* infection in patients with the acquired immunodeficiency syndrome. N. Engl. J. Med. *320*:1044, 1989.

297. Parsonnet, J., Trock, S. C., Bopp, C. A., et al.: Chronic diarrhea associated with drinking untreated water. Ann. Intern. Med. *110*:985, 1989.

298. Pavia, A. T., Shipman, L. D., Wells, J. G., et al.: Epidemiologic evidence that prior antimicrobial exposure decreases resistance to infection by antimicrobial-sensitive *Salmonella*. J. Infect. Dis. *161*:255, 1990.

299. Pengsaa, K., Sirivichayakul, C., Pojjaroen-anant, C., et al.: Albendazole treatment of *Giardia intestinalis* infections in school children. Southeast Asian J. Trop. Med. Public Health *30*:78-83, 1999.

300. Pépin, J., Alary, M.-E., Valiquette, L., et al.: Increasing risk of relapse after treatment of *Clostridium difficile* colitis in Quebec, Canada. Clin. Infect. Dis. *40*:1591-1597, 2005.

301. Pépin J., Routhier S., Gagnon S., et al.: Management and outcomes of a first recurrence of *Clostridium difficile*–associated disease in Quebec, Canada. Clin. Infect. Dis. *42*:758-764, 2006.

302. Pépin, J., Saheb, N., Coulombe, M.-A., et al.: Emergence of fluoroquinolones as the predominant risk factor for *Clostridium difficile*–associated diarrhea: A cohort study during an epidemic in Quebec. Clin. Infect. Dis. *41*:1254-1260, 2005.

303. Perl, T. M., Bedard, L., Kosatsky, T., et al.: An outbreak of toxic encephalopathy caused by eating mussels contaminated with domoic acid. N. Engl. J. Med. *322*:1775, 1990.

304. Perryman, L. E., Riggs, M. W., Mason, P. H., et al.: Kinetics of *Cryptosporidium parvum* sporozoite neutralization by monoclonal antibodies, immune bovine serum, and immune bovine colostrum. Infect. Immun. *58*:157, 1990.

305. Phillips, W. E.: Treatment of chronic carriers with ampicillin. J. A. M. A. *217*:913-915, 1971.

306. Phuong, C. X. T., Kneen, R., Anh, N. T., et al.: A comparative study of ofloxacin and cefixime for treatment of typhoid fever in childen. Pediatr. Infect. Dis. J. *18*:245-248, 1999.

307. Pichler, H. E. T., Divide, G., Stickler, K., et al.: Clinical efficacy of ciprofloxacin compared with placebo in bacterial diarrhea. Am. J. Med. *82*(Suppl. 4a):329-332, 1987.

308. Pickering, L. K.: Antimicrobial resistance among enteric pathogens. *In* Pollard, A. J., and Finn, A., (eds.): Hot Topics in Infection and Immunity in Children. New York, Springer, 2008.

309. Pickering, L. K., and Engelkirk, P. G.: *Giardia lamblia*. Pediatr. Clin. North Am. *35*:565, 1988.

310. Pickering, L. K., and Morrow, A. L.: Factors in human milk that protect against diarrhea disease. Infection *21*:355-357, 1993.

311. Pickering, L. K., Bartlett, A. V., Reves, R. R., et al.: Asymptomatic excretion of rotavirus before and after rotavirus diarrhea in children in day care centers. J. Pediatr. *112*:361, 1988.

312. Pickering, L. K., DuPont, H. L., Evans, D. G., et al.: Isolation of enteric pathogens in asymptomatic students from the United States and Latin America. J. Infect. Dis. *135*:1003-1005, 1977.

313. Pickering, L. K., DuPont, H. L., Olarte, J., et al.: Fecal leukocytes in enteric infections. Am. J. Clin. Pathol. *68*:562-565, 1977.

314. Pickering, L. K., Evans, D. G., DuPont, H. L., et al.: Diarrhea caused by *Shigella*, rotavirus, and *Giardia* in day care centers: Prospective study. J. Pediatr. *99*:51-56, 1981.

315. Pickering, L. K., Evans, D. G., Munoz, O., et al.: Prospective evaluation of enteropathogens in children with diarrhea in Houston and Mexico. J. Pediatr. *93*:383-388, 1978.

316. Pickering, L. K., Feldman, S., Ericsson, C. D., et al.: Absorption of salicylate and bismuth from a bismuth subsalicylate containing compound (Pepto-Bismol). J. Pediatr. *99*:654-656, 1981.

317. Pickering, L. K., Obrig, T. G., and Stapleton, F. B.: Hemolytic uremic syndrome and enterohemorrhagic *Escherichia coli*. Pediatr. Infect. Dis. J. *13*:459-475, 1994.

318. Pickering, L. K.: Biotherapeutic agents and disease in infants. *In* Newburg, D. S. (ed.): Bioactive Substances in Human Milk. New York, Plenum, 2001, pp. 365-373.

319. Pickering, L. K., Marano, N., Bocchini, J. A., and Angulo, F. J.: Exposure to nontraditional pets at home and to animals in public settings: Risks to children: Prepared for the Committee on Infectious Diseases, American Academy of Pediatrics. Pediatrics *122*:876, 2008.

320. Piddock, L. J. V., Griggs, D. J., Hall, M. C., et al.: Ciprofloxacin resistance in clinical isolates of *Salmonella typhimurium* obtained from two patients. Antimicrob. Agents Chemother. *37*:662-666, 1993.

321. Pitman, F. E.: Adverse effects of Lomotil. Gastroenterology *67*:408-410, 1974.

322. Pol, S., Romana, C. A., Richard, S., et al.: Microsporidia infection in patients with the human immunodeficiency virus and unexplained cholangitis. N. Engl. J. Med. *328*:95-99, 1993.

323. Pollard, D. R., Johnson, W. M., Lior, H., et al.: Rapid and specific detection of verotoxin genes in *Escherichia coli* by the polymerase chain reaction. J. Clin. Microbiol. *28*:540, 1990.

324. Pothoulakis, C.: Effects of *Clostridium difficile* toxins on epithelial cell barrier. Ann. N. Y. Acad. Sci. *915*:347-356, 2000.

325. Prado, D., Lopez, E., Liu, H., et al.: Ceftibuten and trimethoprim/sulfamethoxazole for treatment of *Shigella* and enteroinvasive *Escherichia coli* disease. Pediatr. Infect. Dis. J. *11*:644-647, 1992.

326. Proctor, M. E., Hamacher, M., Tortorello, M. L., et al.: Multistate outbreak of *Salmonella* serovar Muenchen infections associated with alfalfa sprouts grown from seeds pretreated with calcium hypochlorite. J. Clin. Microbiol. *39*:3461-3465, 2001.

327. Puthanakit, T., Aurpibul, L., Oberdorfer, P.: Hospitalization and mortality among HIV-infected children after receiving highly active antiretroviral therapy. Clin. Infect. Dis. *44*:599-604, 2007.

328. Qadri, F., Das, S. K., Faruque, A. S. G., et al.: Prevalence of toxin types and colonization factors in enterotoxigenic *Escherichia coli* isolated during a 1-year period from diarrheal patients in Bangladesh. J. Clin. Microbiol. *38*:27-31, 2000.

329. Rateau, J. G., Morgant, G., Droy-Priot, M. T., et al.: A histological, enzymatic and water-electrolyte study of the action of smectite, a mucoprotective clay, on experimental infectious diarrhoea in the rabbit. Curr. Med. Res. Opin. *8*:233, 1982.

330. Reid, J. A., White, D. G., Caul, E. O., et al.: Role of infected food handler in hotel outbreak of Norwalk-like viral gastroenteritis: Implications for control. Lancet *2*:321, 1988.

331. Rendtorff, R. C.: The experimental transmission of human intestinal protozoan parasites. II. *Giardia lamblia* cysts given in capsules. Am. J. Hyg. *59*:209-220, 1954.

332. Rennels, M. B.: The rotavirus vaccine story: A clinical investigator's view. Pediatrics *106*:123-125, 2000.

333. Replogle, M. L., Flemming, D. W., and Cieslak, P. R.: Emergence of antimicrobial-resistant shigellosis in Oregon. Clin. Infect. Dis. *30*:515-519, 2000.

334. Rich, C., Favre-Bronte, S., and Sapena, F.: Characterization of enteroaggregative *Escherichia coli* isolates. F. E. M. S. Microbiol. Lett. *173*:55-61, 1999.

335. Ridoux, O., and Drancourt, M.: In vitro susceptibilities of the microsporidia *Encephalitozoon cuniculi, Encephalitozoon bellem*, and *Encephalitozoon intestinalis*

to albendazole and its sulfoxide and sulfone metabolites. Antimicrob. Agents Chemother. *42*:3301-3303, 1998.

336. Rosenthal, P., and Liebman, W. M.: Comparative study of stool examination, duodenal aspiration and pediatric Entero-test for giardiasis in children. J. Pediatr. *96*:278-279, 1980.

337. Rosenthal, S. L.: Exacerbation of *Salmonella enteritis* due to ampicillin. N. Engl. J. Med. *280*:147-148, 1969.

338. Rossignol, J., Abu-Zekry, M., and Hussein, A.: Effect of nitazoxanide for treatment of severe rotavirus diarrhoea: Randomised double-blind placebo-controlled trial. Lancet *368*:124-129, 2006.

339. Rossignol, J., Ayoub, A., and Ayers, M. S.: Treatment of diarrhea caused by *Cryptosporidium parvum*: A prospective randomized double-blind, placebo-controlled study of nitazoxanide. J. Infect. Dis. *184*:103-106, 2001.

340. Rossignol, J., Ayoub, A., and Ayers, M. S.: Treatment of diarrhea caused by *Giardia intestinalis* and *Entamoeba histolytica* or *E. dispar*: A randomized double-blind, placebo-controlled study of nitazoxanide. J. Infect. Dis. *184*:381-384, 2001.

341. Rossignol, J., and El-Gohary, Y. M.: Nitazoxanide in the treatment of viral gastroenteritis: A randomized double-blind placebo-controlled clinical trial. Aliment. Pharmacol. Ther. *24*:1423-1430, 2006.

342. Rowe, B., Ward, L. R., and Threlfall, E. J.: Multidrug-resistant *Salmonella typhi*: A worldwide epidemic. Clin. Infect. Dis. *24*(Suppl. 1):S106-S109, 1997.

343. Ruiz-Palacios, G. M., Guerrero, L. M., Bautista-Márquez, A., et al.: Dose response and efficacy of a live, attenuated human rotavirus vaccine in Mexican infants. Pediatrics *120*:e253-e261, 2007.

344. Rumack, B. H., and Temple, A. R.: Lomotil poisoning. Pediatrics *53*:495, 1974.

345. Rusmak, J., Hadfield, T. L., Rhodes, M., et al.: Detection of *Cryptosporidium* oocysts in human fecal specimens by an indirect immunofluorescence assay with monoclonal antibodies. J. Clin. Microbiol. *27*:1135, 1989.

346. Ryder, R. W., Wells, J. G., and Gangarosa, E. J.: A study of travelers' diarrhea in foreign visitors to the United States. J. Infect. Dis. *136*:605-607, 1977.

347. Saenz, Y., Zarazaga, M., Lantero, M., et al.: Antibiotic resistance in *Campylobacter* strains isolated from animals, foods, and humans in Spain in 1997-1998. Antimicrob. Agents Chemother. *44*:267-271, 2000.

348. Safdar, N., Said, A., Gangnon, R. E., et al.: Risk of hemolytic uremic syndrome after antibiotic treatment of *Escherichia coli* O157:H7 enteritis. J. A. M. A. *288*:996-1001, 2002.

349. Saha, D., Kahn, W. A., Karim, M. M., et al.: Single-dose ciprofloxacin versus 12-dose erythromycin for childhood cholera: A randomised controlled trial. Lancet *366*:1085-1093, 2005.

350. Saha, D., Karim, M. M., Kahn, W. A., et al.: Single-dose azithromycin for the treatment of cholera in adults. N. Engl. J. Med. *354*:2452-2462, 2006.

351. Salam, M. A., Dhar, U., Khan, W. A., et al.: Randomised comparison of ciprofloxacin suspension and pivmecillinam for childhood shigellosis. Lancet *353*:522-527, 1998.

352. Salamina, G., Dalle Donne, E., Niccolini, A., et al.: A foodborne outbreak of gastroenteritis involving *Listeria monocytogenes*. Epidemiol. Infect. *117*:429-436, 1996.

353. Salazar-Lindo, E., Sack, B., Chea-Woo, E., et al.: Early treatment with erythromycin of *Campylobacter jejuni* associated dysentery in children. J. Pediatr. *109*:355, 1986.

354. Salazar-Lindo, E., Santisteban-Ponce, J., Chea-Woo, E., et al.: Racecadotril in the treatment of acute watery diarrhea in children. N. Engl. J. Med. *343*:463-467, 2000.

355. Sambol, J. S. P., Merrigan, M. M., Lyerly, D., et al.: Toxin gene analysis of a variant strain of *Clostridium difficile* that causes human clinical disease. Infect. Immun. *68*:5480-5487, 2000.

356. Sanchez, T. H., Brooks, J. T., Sullivan, P. S., et al.: Bacterial diarrhea in persons with HIV infection, United States, 1992-2002. Clin. Infect. Dis. *41*:1621-1627, 2005.

357. Santosham, M., and Greenough, W. B., III: Oral rehydration therapy: Global prospective. J. Pediatr. *118*:44-51, 1991.

358. Santosham, M., Foster, S., Reid, R., et al.: Role of soy-based, lactose-free formula during treatment of acute diarrhea. Pediatrics *76*:292-298, 1985.

359. Savarino, S. J., Fasano, A., Watson, J., et al.: Enteroaggregative *Escherichia coli* heat-stable enterotoxin 1 represents another subfamily of *E. coli* heat-stable toxin. Proc. Natl. Acad. Sci. U. S. A. *90*:3093-3097, 1993.

360. Sazawal, S., Hiremath, G., Dhingra, U., et al.: Efficacy of probiotics in prevention of acute diarrhoea: A meta-analysis of masked, randomised, placebo-controlled trials. Lancet Infect. Dis. *6*:374-382, 2006.

361. Scaletsky, I. C., Pedroso, M. D., Morais, M. B., et al.: Association of patterns of *Escherichia coli* adherence to Hep-2 cells with acute and persistent diarrhea. Arch. Gastroenterol. *36*:54-60, 1999.

362. Scallan, E.: Activities, achievements, and lesson learned during the first 10 years of the Foodborne Diseases Active Surveillance Network: 1996-2006. Clin. Infect. Dis. *44*:718-725, 2007.

363. Schantz, P. M.: The dangers of eating raw fish. N. Engl. J. Med. *320*:1143, 1989.

364. Schultsz, C., van den Ende, J., Cobelens, F., et al.: Diarrheagenic *Escherichia coli* and acute and persistent diarrhea in returned travelers. J. Clin. Microbiol. *38*:3550-3554, 2000.

365. Sears, C. L., and Kaper, J. B.: Enteric bacterial toxins: Mechanisms of action and linkage to intestinal secretion. Microbiol. Rev. *60*:167-215, 1996.

366. Sen, A., Kobayashi, N., Das, S., et al.: The evolution of human group B rotaviruses. Lancet *357*:198-199, 2001.

367. Shadduck, J. A., and Greeley, E.: *Microsporidia* and human infections. Clin. Microbiol. Rev. *2*:158, 1989.

368. Shane, A. L., Crump, J. A., Tucker, N. A., et al.: Sharing *Shigella*: Risk factors of a multi-community outbreak of shigellosis. Arch. Pediatr. Adolesc. Med. *157*:601-603, 2003.

369. Shanks, G. D., Smoak, B. L., Aleman, G. M., et al.: Single dose azithromycin or three-day course of ciprofloxacin as therapy for epidemic dysentery in Kenya. Clin. Infect. Dis. *29*:942-943, 1999.

370. Shedl, H. P., and Clifton, J. A.: Solute and water absorption by the human small intestine. Nature *199*:1264-1267, 1963.

371. Sheikh, R. A., Prindiville, T. P., Yenamandra, S., et al.: Microsporidial AIDS cholangiopathy due to *Encephalitozoon intestinalis*: Case report and review. Am. J. Gastroenterol. *95*:2364-2371, 2000.

372. Shinozaki, T., Araki, K., Ushijima, H., et al.: Antibody response to enteric adenovirus types 40 and 41 in sera from people in various age groups. J. Clin. Microbiol. *25*:1679, 1987.

373. Siddiqui, A. A., and Berk, S. L.: Diagnosis of *Strongyloides stercoralis* infection. Clin. Infect. Dis. *33*:1040-1047, 2001.

374. Sivapalasingam, S., Nelson, J. M., Joyce, K., et al.: High prevalence of antimicrobial resistance among *Shigella* isolates in the United States tested by the National Antimicrobial Resistance Monitoring System from 1999 to 2002. Antimicrob. Agents Chemother. *50*:49-54, 2006.

375. Sloven, D. G., Jirapinyo, P., and Lebenthal, E.: Hydrolysis and absorption of glucose polymers from rice compared with corn in chronic diarrhea in infancy. J. Pediatr. *116*:876, 1990.

376. Smith, H. R., Cheasty, T., and Rowe, B.: Enteroaggregative *Escherichia coli* and outbreaks of gastroenteritis in U.K. Lancet *350*:814-815, 1997.

377. Smith, K. E., Besser, J. M., Hedberg, C. W., et al.: Quinolone-resistant *Campylobacter jejuni* infections in Minnesota, 1992-1998. N. Engl. J. Med. *340*:1525-1532, 1999.

378. Smith, M. D., Duong, N. M., Hoa, N. T. T., et al.: Comparison of ofloxacin and ceftriaxone for short-course treatment of enteric fever. Antimicrob. Agents Chemother. *38*:1716-1720, 1994.

379. Smith, N. H., Cron, S., Valdez, L. M., et al.: Combination drug therapy for cryptosporidiosis in AIDS. J. Infect. Dis. *178*:900-903, 1998.

380. Smith, P. D., Macher, A. M., Bookman, M. A., et al.: *Salmonella typhimurium* enteritis and bacteremia in the acquired immunodeficiency syndrome. Ann. Intern. Med. *102*:207, 1985.

381. Soe, G. B., and Overturf, G. D.: Treatment of typhoid fever and other systemic salmonelloses with cefotaxime, ceftriaxone, cefoperazone, and other newer cephalosporins. Rev. Infect. Dis. *9*:719, 1987.

382. Soriano-Brücher, H. E., Avendaño, P., O'Ryan, M., et al.: Use of bismuth subsalicylate in acute diarrhea in children. Rev. Infect. Dis. *12*:S51, 1990.

383. Soriano-Brücher, H., Avendaño, P., O'Ryan, M., et al.: Bismuth subsalicylate in the treatment of acute diarrhea in children: A clinical study. Pediatrics *87*:18-27, 1991.

384. Spandorfer, P. R., Alessandrini, E. A., Jofee, M. D., et al.: Oral versus intravenous rehydration of moderately dehydrated children: A randomized, controlled trial. Pediatrics *115*:295-301, 2005.

385. Speelman, P., Kabir, I., and Islam, M.: Distribution and spread of colonic lesions in shigellosis: A colonoscopic study. J. Infect. Dis. *150*:899-903, 1984.

386. Steinberg, E. B., Greene, K. D., Bopp, C. A., et al.: Cholera in the United States, 1995-2000: Trends at the end of the twentieth century. J. Infect. Dis. *184*:799-802, 2001.

387. Steinmuller, N., Demma, L., Bender, J. B., et al.: Outbreaks of enteric disease associated with animal contact: Not just a foodborne problem anymore. Clin. Infect. Dis. *43*:1596-1602, 2006.

388. Stenzel, D. J., and Boreham, P. F. L.: *Blastomycosis hominis* revisited. Clin. Microbiol. Rev. *9*:563-584, 1996.

389. Straub, T. M., Höner zu Bentrup, K., Orosz-Coghlan, P. O., et al.: In vitro cell culture infectivity assay for human noroviruses. Emerg. Infect. Dis. *13*:396-402, 2007.

390. Szajewska, H., and Mrukowics, J.: Meta-analysis: Non-pathogenic yeast *Saccharomyces boulardii* in the prevention of antibiotic-associated diarrhoea. Aliment. Pharmacol. Ther. *22*:356-372, 2005.

391. Szajewska, H., Skorka, A., and Dylag, M.: Meta-analysis: *Saccharomyces boulardii* for treating acute diarrhoea in children. Aliment. Pharmacol. Ther. *25*:257-264, 2007.

392. Szajewska, H., Skorka, A., Ruszczyski, M., et al.: Meta-analysis: Lactobacillus GG for treating acute diarrhoea in children. Aliment. Pharmacol. Ther. *25*:871-881, 2007.

393. Tam, C. C., Rodrigues L. C., Petersen, I., et al.: Incidence of Guillain-Barré syndrome among patients with *Campylobacter* infection: A general practice research database study. J. Infect. Dis. *194*:95-97, 2006.

394. Tauxe, R. V., Puhr, N. D., Wells, J. G., et al.: Antimicrobial resistance of *Shigella* isolates in the U.S.A.: The importance of international travel. J. Infect. Dis. *162*:1107, 1990.

395. Tauxe, R. V.: Food safety and irradiation: Protecting the public from foodborne infections. Emerg. Infect. Dis. *7*(Suppl. 3):516-521, 2001.

396. Taylor, C. E., and Higgs, E. S.: A workshop on micronutrients and infectious diseases. Cellular and molecular immunomodulatory mechanisms. J. Infect. Dis. *182*(Suppl.):S1-S143, 2000.

397. Taylor, D. E., and Chang, N.: In vitro susceptibilities of *Campylobacter jejuni* and *Campylobacter coli* to azithromycin and erythromycin. Antimicrob. Agents Chemother. *35*:1917-1918, 1991.

398. Taylor, W. R., Schell, W. L., Wells, J. G., et al.: A foodborne outbreak of enterotoxigenic *Escherichia coli* diarrhea. N. Engl. J. Med. *306*:1093-1095, 1982.

399. Teasley, D. G., Gerding, D. N., Olson, M. M., et al.: Prospective randomized trial of metronidazole versus vancomycin for *Clostridium difficile*–associated diarrhea and colitis. Lancet *2*:1043-1046, 1983.

400. Teitelbaum, J. S., Zatorre, R. J., Carpenter, S., et al.: Neurologic sequelae of domoic acid intoxication due to the ingestion of contaminated mussels. N. Engl. J. Med. *322*:1781, 1990.

401. Telzak, E. E., Budnick, L. D., Greenberg, M. S. Z., et al.: A nosocomial outbreak of *Salmonella enteritis* infection due to the consumption of raw eggs. N. Engl. J. Med. *323*:394, 1990.

402. Ternhag, A., Asikainen, T., Giesecke J., et al.: A meta-analysis on the effects of antibiotic treatment on duration of symptoms caused by infection with *Campylobacter* species. Clin. Infect. Dis. *44*:696-700, 2007.

403. Thomas, M. R., Litin, S. C., Osmon, D. R., et al.: Lack of effect of *Lactobacillus* GG on antibiotic-associated diarrhea: A randomized placebo-controlled trial. Mayo Clin. Proc. *76*:883-889, 2001.

404. Tippen, P. S., Meyer, A., Blank, E. C., et al.: Aquarium-associated *Plesiomonas shigelloides* infection: Missouri. M. M. W. R. Morb. Mortal. Wkly. Rep. *38*:617, 1989.

405. Tjoa, W. S., DuPont, H. L., Sullivan, P., et al.: Location of food consumption and travelers' diarrhea. Am. J. Epidemiol. *106*:61-66, 1977.

406. Tremoulet A. H., Avila-Aguero, M. L. Paris, M. M., et al.: Albendazole therapy for *Microsporidium* diarrhea in immunocompetent Costa Rican children. Pediatr. Infect. Dis. J. *23*:915-918, 2004.

407. Turcios, R. M., Widdowson, M. A., Sulka, A. C., et al.: Reevaluation of epidemiological criteria for identifying outbreaks of acute gastroenteritis due to norovirus: United States, 1998-2000. Clin. Infect. Dis. *42*:964-969, 2006.

408. Tzipori, S., Roberton, D., and Chapman, C.: Remission of cryptosporidiosis in an immunodeficient child with hyperimmune bovine colostrum. B. M. J. *293*:1276, 1986.

409. Ungar, B. L., Ward, D. S., Fayer, R., et al.: Cessation of *Cryptosporidium*-associated diarrhea in an acquired immunodeficiency syndrome patient after treatment with hyperimmune bovine colostrum. Gastroenterology *98*:486, 1990.

410. Valazquez-Boland, J. A., Kuhn, M., Berche, P., et al.: *Listeria* pathogenesis and molecular virulence determinants. Clin. Microbiol. Rev. *14*:584-640, 2001.

411. Van Doorn, L. J., Verschuuren-van Haperen, A., Burnens, A., et al.: Rapid identification of thermotolerant *Campylobacter jejuni, Campylobacter coli, Campylobacter lari,* and *Campylobacter upsaliensis* from various geographic locations by a GTPase-based PCR–reverse hybridization assay. J Clin Microbiol. *37*:1790-1796, 1999.

412. Van, R., Wun, C. C., O'Ryan, M. L., et al.: Outbreaks of human enteric adenovirus types 40 and 41 in Houston day care centers. J. Pediatr. *120*:516-521, 1992.

413. Vargas, S. L., Shenep, J. L., Flynn, P. M., et al.: Azithromycin for treatment of severe *Cryptosporidium* diarrhea in children with cancer. J. Pediatr. *123*:154-156, 1993.

414. Varsano, I., Eidlitz-Marcus, T., Nassinovitch, M., et al.: Comparative efficacy of ceftriaxone and ampicillin for treatment of severe shigellosis in children. J. Pediatr. *118*:627-632, 1991.

415. Velazquez, F. R., Calva, J. J., Guerrero, M. L., et al.: Cohort study of rotavirus serotype patterns in symptomatic and asymptomatic infections in Mexican children. Pediatr. Infect. Dis. J. *12*:56-61, 1993.

416. Velazquez, F. R., Matson, D. O., Calva, J. J., et al.: Natural protection conferred by rotavirus infections: Implications for vaccine strategies. N. Engl. J. Med. *335*:1022-1028, 1996.

417. Verdier, R. I., Fitzgerald, D. W., Johnson, W. D., Jr., et al.: Trimethoprim-sulfamethoxazole compared with ciprofloxacin for treatment and prophylaxis of *Isospora belli* and *Cyclospora cayetanensis* infection in HIV-infected patients. A randomized, controlled trial. Ann. Intern. Med. *132*:885-888, 2000.

418. Vinh, H., Wain, J., Hanh, V. T. N., et al.: Two or three days of ofloxacin treatment for uncomplicated multidrug-resistant typhoid fever in children. Antimicrob. Agents Chemother. *40*:958-961, 1996.

419. Walker, C. L. F., and Black, R. E.: Micronutrients and diarrheal disease. Clin. Infect. Dis. *45*:S73-S77, 2007.

420. Wallace, C. K., Anderson, P. N., Brown, T. C., et al.: Optimal antibiotic therapy in cholera. Bull. World Health Organ. *39*:239-245, 1968.

421. Wallace, M. R., Nguyen, M.-T., and Newton, J. A., Jr.: Use of paromomycin for the treatment of cryptosporidiosis in patients with AIDS. Clin. Infect. Dis. *17*:1070-1071, 1993.

422. Walter, J. E., Briggs, J., Lourdes, G. M., et al.: Molecular characterization of a novel recombinant strain of human astrovirus associated with gastroenteritis in children. Arch. Virol. *146*:235, 2001.

423. Wanke, C. A., Plesko, D., DeGirolami, P. C., et al.: A medium chain triglyceride–based diet in patients with HIV and chronic diarrhea reduces diarrhea and malabsorption: A prospective, controlled trial. Nutrition *12*:766-771, 1996.

424. Warny M., Pepin J., Fang A., et al.: Toxin production by an emerging strain of *Clostridium difficile* associated with outbreaks of severe disease in North America and Europe. Lancet *366*:1079-1084, 2005.

425. Weber, R., Bryan, R. T., Owen, R. L., et al.: Improved light-microscopical detection of microsporidia spores in stool and duodenal aspirates. N. Engl. J. Med. *326*:161-166, 1992.

426. Weber, R., Bryan, R. T., Schwartz, D. A., et al.: Human microsporidial infections. Clin. Microbiol. Rev. *7*:426-461, 1994.

427. Wedel, S., Bender, J., Leano, F., et al.: Antimicrobial-drug susceptibility of human and animal *Salmonella* typhimurium, Minnesota, 1997-2003. Emerg. Infect. Dis. *11*:1899-1906, 2005.

428. Weiss, L. M., Perlman, D. C., Sherman, J., et al.: *Isospora belli* infection: Treatment with pyrimethamine. Ann. Intern. Med. *109*:474, 1988.

429. Wenisch, C., Parschalk, B., Masenhundl, M., et al.: Comparison of vancomycin, teicoplanin, metronidazole, and fusidic acid for the treatment of *Clostridium difficile*–associated diarrhea. Clin. Infect. Dis. *22*:813-818, 1996.

430. Wessalowski, R., Thomas, L., Kivit, J., et al.: Multiple brain abscesses caused by *Salmonella enteritis* in a neonate: Successful treatment with ciprofloxacin. Pediatr. Infect. Dis. J. *12*:683-688, 1993.

431. White, A. C., Chappell, C. L., Hayat, C. S., et al.: Paromomycin for cryptosporidiosis in AIDS: A prospective, double-blind trial. J. Infect. Dis. *170*:19-24, 1994.

432. White, D. G., Zhoa, S., Sudler, R., et al.: The isolation of antibiotic-resistant *Salmonella* from retail ground meats. N. Engl. J. Med. *345*:1147-1154, 2001.

433. Williams, D., Schorling, J., Barrett, L. J., et al.: Early treatment of *jejuni* enteritis. Antimicrob. Agents Chemother. *33*:248, 1989.

434. Willson, R., Harrington, R., and Stewart, B.: Human immunodeficiency virus 1–associated necrotizing cholangitis caused by infection with *Septata intestinalis*. Gastroenterology *108*:247-251, 1995.

435. Wittenberg, D. F., Miller, N. M., and Vanden Ende, J.: Spiramycin is not effective in treating *Cryptosporidium* diarrhea in infants: Results of a double-blind randomized trial. J. Infect. Dis. *159*:131, 1989.

436. Wittner, M., Turner, J. W., Jacquette, G., et al.: Eustrongylidiasis: A parasitic infection acquired by eating sushi. N. Engl. J. Med. *320*:1124, 1989.

437. Wong, C. S., Jelacic, S., Habeeb, R. L., et al.: The risk of the hemolytic uremic syndrome after antibody treatment of *Escherichia coli* O157:H7 infections. N. Engl. J. Med. *342*:1930-1936, 2000.

438. Yang, S., Leff, M. G., McTague, D., et al.: Multistate surveillance for food handling, preparation and consumption behaviors associated with foodborne diseases: 1995 and 1996 BRFSS food-safety questions. M. M. W. R. CDC Surveill. Sum. *47*(SS-4):33-57, 1998.

439. Yolken, R. H., Bishop, C. A., Townsend, T. R., et al.: Infectious gastroenteritis in bone-marrow transplant recipients. N. Engl. J. Med. *306*:1009-1012, 1982.

440. Yolken, R., Leister, F., Dubovi, E., et al.: Infantile gastroenteritis associated with excretion of pestivirus antigens. Lancet *1*:517, 1989.

441. Zar, F. A., Bakkanagari, S. R., Moorthi, K., et al.: A comparison of vancomycin and metronidazole for the treatment of *Clostridium difficile*–associated diarrhea, stratified by disease severity. Clin. Infect. Dis. *45*:302-307, 2007.

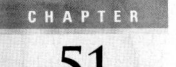

ANTIBIOTIC-ASSOCIATED COLITIS

George D. Ferry ☉ James Versalovic

Clostridium difficile colonization and infection accounts for 10 to 25 percent of antibiotic-associated diarrhea and is the major cause of antibiotic-associated pseudomembranous colitis.[8] Diarrhea and colitis develop when antibiotics, especially those with a broad spectrum of activity, disturb the bowel microbiota and allow overgrowth of *C. difficile*. Production of toxins then leads to inflammation and secretion of fluids from the colon, resulting in watery diarrhea. If inflammation progresses and pseudomembranous colitis develops, the diarrhea becomes bloody. Colitis induced by *C. difficile* has been reported without prior use of antibiotics, but it is an uncommon occurrence.

HISTORY

Pseudomembranous colitis was recognized as early as 1893[38] and derives its name from the numerous plaquelike lesions in the colon. The plaques are membranes of epithelial debris containing fibrin, mucus, and polymorphonuclear leukocytes overlying necrotic glands.[96] Not until the early 1950s was an association with antibiotics suggested. The organism that initially received the most attention as a possible cause was *Staphylococcus aureus*.[103] Stool cultures frequently were positive for *S. aureus* after antibiotic use, and autopsies showed enterocolitis with ulcers and pseudomembranes in both the small and the large bowel. The association with *C. difficile*, a gram-positive anaerobic bacillus, was shown in 1977 and 1978 with the reports of production of toxins related to pseudomembranous changes in the colon.[9,10,61] *C. difficile* can colonize the intestine without causing diarrhea and was identified as part of the normal microbiota of infants and newborns in 1935.[47] Early studies suggested that *Clostridium sordellii* might be related to pseudomembranous colitis, but subsequent investigation has shown that *C. sordellii* antitoxin neutralizes *C. difficile* cytotoxicity but is not a cause of colitis.[10]

ETIOLOGY AND PATHOGENESIS

C. difficile can be cultured in 7.6 percent of healthy adults,[34,51] but in hospitalized patients, the incidence of colonization and positive cultures reaches 20 percent or more.[74] *C. difficile*–associated diarrhea appears to have significantly increased in incidence in the United States, especially among the elderly,[70] and outbreaks with a more virulent and a more antibiotic resistant strain have been reported in the United States and Canada.[87] The specific *C. difficile* isolates responsible for some of these outbreaks have been characterized as restriction endonuclease analysis group BI, with an increased production of toxins A and B and also positive for the binary toxin CDT, a possible virulence factor.[4,67,71,72]

C. difficile spores are viable for long periods, up to 5 months,[54] and can be cultured from flooring, toilets, and bedding as well as from the stool and hands of carriers (Table 51–1).[34,54] Numerous studies have shown that neonates frequently are colonized with *C. difficile*.[47,49,117] In a London study, 2 to 52 percent of infants in three postnatal wards had positive cultures, but none developed diarrhea or colitis, and no evidence was found that infants were colonized from their mothers.[60] The rate of colonization appears to be related to the length of time infants are hospitalized.[100] In those older than 1 year, colonization decreases significantly.[46] Not only is *C. difficile* a common contaminant in hospitals,[34,54] but person-to-person transmission among children in daycare centers also has been reported.[53] A hospital outbreak of *C. difficile* in children 18 months to 18 years was reported from a pediatric orthopedic ward.[37]

Infection with *C. difficile* occurs commonly and accounts for 10 to 25 percent of cases of uncomplicated antibiotic-associated diarrhea.[8,109] Most infections cause watery diarrhea, but 5 to 10 percent progress to pseudomembranous colitis.[8,55] Pseudomembranous colitis can occur sporadically or in epidemics.[85,91] In daycare centers, the incidence of *C. difficile* infection not related to antibiotics may be as high as 50 percent.[8,53] Community-acquired diarrhea caused by *C. difficile* studied in a health maintenance organization population identified 51 cases, with an incidence of 7.7 cases per 100,000 person-years.[48] Half of these cases occurred after antibiotic use. Increased age and exposure to more than one antibiotic within a 42-day period increased the risk. *C. difficile* diarrhea was an uncommon occurrence in patients younger than 20 years. Risk factors included inflammatory bowel disease, infection with human immunodeficiency virus, and chronic treatment with antibiotics. In a report of 200 Canadian children with *C. difficile*–associated diarrhea, underlying factors

TABLE 51–1 Distribution of *Clostridium difficile* Isolates Taken from the Environment of Two Pediatric Units

	No. Positive/No. Sampled (%)	
Sites Cultured	**Pediatric Ward (case associated)**	**Newborn Intensive Care Unit (control)**
Surfaces		
Bedpan hoppers	0/25	0/15
Chart covers	1/30 (3.3)	0/20
Cribs (occupied)	2/45 (4.4)	1/20 (5)
Dust mops, dust pans on cleaning carts	2/6 (33.3)	0/4
Floors		
Bathroom	4/40 (10)	NA
Clean storage room	2/30 (6.7)	0/20
Patient's room	6/50 (12)	1/30 (3.3)
Soiled room	2/30 (6.7)	0/20
Hospital garments	0/20	0/11
Linens, blankets (clean)	0/20	0/8
Linens, blankets (in use)	5/50 (10)	3/37 (8.1)
Medical devices (e.g., stethoscopes)	0/25	0/20
Mobiles, toys	1/20 (5)	0/12
Scales	8/40 (20)	1/30 (3.3)
Washbasins, sinks, tubs	4/40 (10)	1/30 (3.3)
Air (30 cu. ft. per sample)	0/7	0/2
Total	37/478 (7.7)*	7/279 (2.5)*

*$p < .005$.

From Kim, K.-H., Fekety, R., Batts, D. H., et al.: Isolation of Clostridium difficile from the environment and contacts of patients with antibiotic-associated colitis. J. Infect. Dis. 143:44-50, 1981.

such as chemotherapy, Crohn disease, transplantation, immunodeficiency, and Hirschsprung disease were found in 19 percent of patients.[79] A history of antibiotic exposure in the previous 2 months was present in 74.5 and 55.5 percent of children who had been hospitalized. Elemental diets have been reported to increase the growth of *C. difficile*,[50] and both community- and hospital-acquired *C. difficile*–associated diarrhea are associated with the use of proton pump inhibitors.[26,27]

Virulence may differ among strains of *C. difficile*; some are highly toxigenic, and others have low virulence.[57] This difference may be related to S-layer proteins covering the surface of *C. difficile* serotypes known to cause disease.[94] Production of toxins by the organism and clinical illness are absent in 25 percent of patients with positive cultures.[35] Most toxigenic strains produce both toxin A and toxin B. Toxin B initially was thought to be a cytotoxin with little clinical effect[68,93]; however, more recent studies have shown that it has a significant effect once tissue damage has already occurred.[94] Toxin A produces necrosis and increased cell permeability, and both toxins lead to the production of tumor necrosis factor–α and other cytokines.[94] The increased permeability is responsible for the watery diarrhea.

Studies on the epithelial cell barrier have shown two additional pathways of cell injury.[86,92] *C. difficile* toxins disaggregate actin microfilaments in colonocytes, leading to cell destruction and opening of tight junctions. Toxin A also has a significant chemotactic effect on neutrophils, leading to local inflammation and release of inflammatory mediators.[93] Figure 51–1 illustrates these pathways. In experimental models, injection of toxin A into rabbit ileal loops results in increased fluid secretion, inflammation and necrosis of epithelial cells, and release of prostaglandin E_2 and leukotriene B_4 into the lumen.[113] Another mechanism for diarrhea may relate to decreased anaerobic microbiota and, subsequently, a decreased digestion of carbohydrates, leading to a decreased production of lactic acid and short-chain fatty acids and disturbed function of the colonic mucosa.[12]

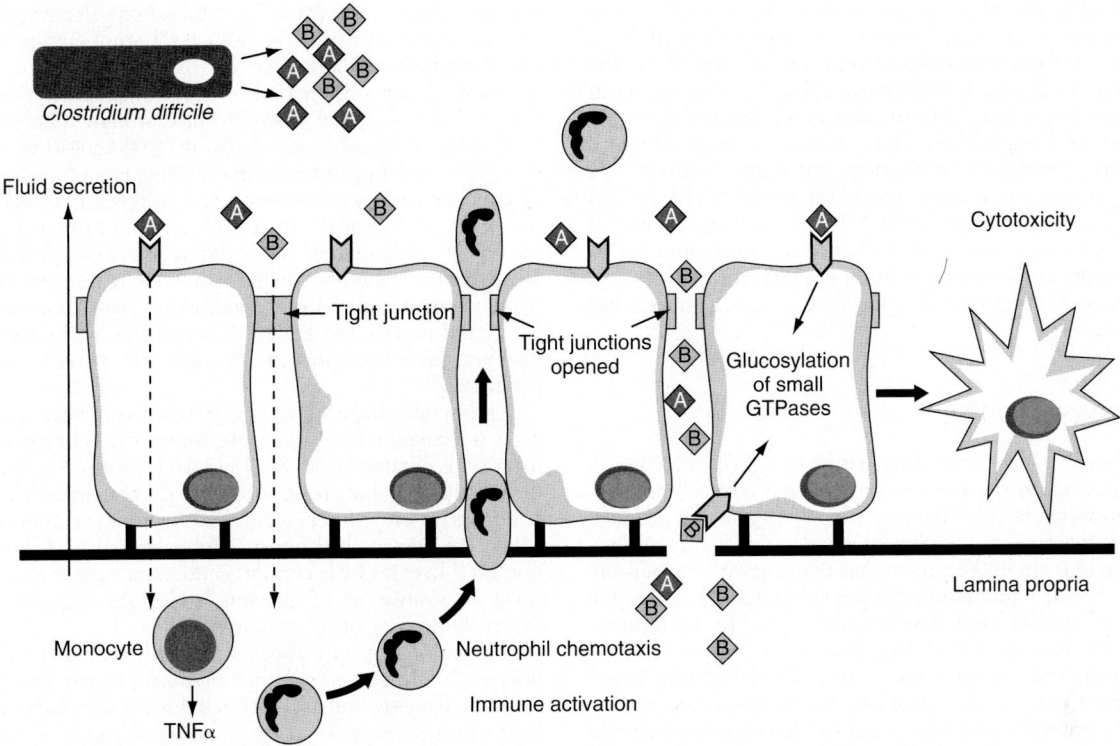

Figure 51–1 Actions of *Clostridium difficile* toxins A and B on intestinal epithelium. *(Courtesy of Ian R. Poxton, Professor of Microbial Infection and Immunity, Medical Microbiology, University of Edinburgh Medical School.)*

Serum antibodies to *C. difficile* toxins A and B occur commonly, being found in 60 to 70 percent of patients older than 3 years.[116] In adults, specific serum IgA and IgG antibodies to toxin A have been detected in 57 to 60 percent of patients.[52] Antibodies also have been found in colonic mucosa and duodenal aspirates in 10 percent of patients. Binding of toxin A was inhibited significantly by colonic aspirates with high-IgA antitoxin-A antibody. These antibodies appear to persist throughout life, and they may have a protective role against recurrence.[58]

Protection against diarrhea and pseudomembranous colitis in newborns may be due to a lack of the intestinal receptor for toxin A[30] or prematurity of the toxin receptor. A study by Enad and colleagues[32] showed that 87 infants colonized with toxin A–positive *C. difficile* had more days of diarrhea than did those who were toxin negative. Although breast milk contains antibody against *C. difficile*, whether it influences disease activity is unclear.[118] *C. difficile* has been suggested to be a causative agent in rare cases of necrotizing enterocolitis, but this suggestion remains controversial.[16,32]

In the normal host, many bacteria, especially lactobacilli, *Bacteroides*, enterococci, and *Escherichia coli*, inhibit growth of *C. difficile*.[99] Treatment with any antibiotic can result in overgrowth of *C. difficile* and lead to pseudomembranous colitis. Oral antibiotics are associated with colitis more often than are parenteral antibiotics, and broad-spectrum antibiotics are responsible for most cases. Multiple antibiotics, including clindamycin, ampicillin, cephalosporin, penicillin, chloramphenicol, gentamicin, trimethoprim-sulfamethoxazole, and rifampicin, have been implicated in antibiotic-associated diarrhea in children.[1,83,111] Fluoroquinolone administration was the most prominent risk factor for *C. difficile*–associated diarrhea (n = 5619 patients) during an epidemic in eastern Canada caused by a hypervirulent strain.[89] Proton pump inhibitors were not associated with disease in this study. Cefixime also has been associated with pediatric pseudomembranous colitis.[45] Long-term antibiotic treatment of acne has been complicated rarely by diarrhea or colitis.[33]

C. difficile infection has been reported in pediatric patients during chemotherapy.[31] The spectrum of illness has been mild to fulminant colitis, just as in antibiotic-associated disease. *C. difficile* also has occurred as an outbreak with associated diarrhea in patients with acquired immunodeficiency syndrome who were admitted to the same hospital ward.[5] In a study in 2005 of 75 pediatric outpatients presenting with diarrhea, positive bacterial isolates were found in 48 percent of patients, and eight children were positive for *C. difficile* toxin.[25]

CLINICAL MANIFESTATIONS

The spectrum of clinical signs and symptoms related to *C. difficile* infection ranges from the asymptomatic carrier state to a fulminant colitis and toxic megacolon.[112] Most patients have watery diarrhea, but 10 to 15 percent have bloody stools.[55] Diarrhea most often begins 3 to 21 days after the use of antibiotics. Most children with diarrhea have a self-limited illness with watery stools, fever, and abdominal pain.[105,111] Patients with pseudomembranous colitis present with cramping abdominal pain and fever, and watery, green, foul stools progress to bloody diarrhea.[29] Colitis often is a mild, self-limited illness once antibiotics are stopped, but it may be severe and require intensive antibiotic and supportive therapy.

Fulminant colitis is an uncommon occurrence but can lead to perforation and colectomy and a high mortality rate (35%).[56] Toxic megacolon, or toxic dilatation of the small bowel, may develop without preceding diarrhea. In these critically ill patients, colitis may lead to perforation and peritonitis. In a series of 201 surgical patients, toxic megacolon developed in five, and four of the five died.[95] Confirmation of the diagnosis may depend on finding the typical pseudomembranous ulcers on colonoscopy. Response to treatment generally is rapid; symptoms clear in 50 percent of patients within 6 to 14 days and in 100 percent by 1 month.

The role of *C. difficile* infection in inflammatory bowel disease has been controversial. Some studies have shown no significant association,[77] whereas others have implicated *C. difficile* in the relapse of Crohn disease and ulcerative colitis.[18,59] The organism has been found in 8 percent of patients in remission,[28] the same as in the general population. The presence of toxin seems to correlate with the degree of bleeding and disease activity.[44] In studies of 59 and 54 patients, toxin was found in 19 and 16 percent of individuals, respectively.[76,114] The majority, 64 and 90 percent of patients, respectively, had received antibiotics previously. These patients responded promptly to treatment with targeted antibiotics, suggesting that the flare of colitis was related to *C. difficile.*

LABORATORY STUDIES

The established standard for diagnosis of *C. difficile* infection is detection of enterotoxins A or B by immunoassays or cell culture–based cytotoxicity tests.[120] Because not all organisms produce toxin, a causative role for *C. difficile* in diarrhea and colitis is based on detection of toxin in the stool rather than a positive anaerobic culture.[42,62] Fresh, liquid stools are the specimens of choice for toxin testing,[24] and all specimens should be tested for both toxins A and B.[69] Production of *C. difficile* toxin can be diagnosed by a variety of techniques. Immunoassays, including laboratory-based enzyme-linked immunosorbent assays and point-of-care immunocard tests, are most commonly used for detection of toxigenic *C. difficile.* Although published sensitivities of these assays exceed 80 percent,[2,35] the reality is that most immunoassays have lower sensitivities when they are used in routine clinical practice. Repeated immunoassay testing usually is recommended when initial testing is negative for *C. difficile* toxin A or toxin B. An alternative and effective approach is the combination of *C. difficile* common antigen testing with toxin detection.[120] This two-pronged approach uses immunoassays to detect a species-specific antigen, glutamate dehydrogenase (GDH or *C. difficile* common antigen), and both enterotoxins A and B. GDH is found in both toxigenic and nontoxigenic strains. Commercial GDH tests are more sensitive than is direct toxin detection, and GDH-positive stools are evaluated subsequently by toxin A or B testing. This approach may detect stools positive for *C. difficile* that may be missed entirely by toxin screening. An enzyme immunosorbent assay test kit combining detection of toxin A and GDH has a negative predictive value for infection with *C. difficile* of 99.6 percent.[24]

Cell culture–based cytotoxicity assays were used widely before the introduction of commercial immunoassays and continue to be a useful approach for detection of *C. difficile* directly in stool specimens. Cell culture testing is tedious and time-consuming for the laboratory, but it may have superior sensitivity for toxin detection if technical expertise is available.[24,35] Fecal material is diluted, and cytopathic effects are evaluated with human fibroblast cell lines to assess the presence of toxin (primarily toxin B). Molecular methods show promise as next-generation methods for direct *C. difficile* enterotoxin gene detection. Polymerase chain reaction amplification, including real-time polymerase chain reaction methods, has demonstrated the ability to detect toxin A (*tcdA*) and toxin B (*tcdB*) genes (DNA) directly in human stool specimens. Published molecular studies described excellent concordance with toxin immunoassays[11,115] while enabling antigen-negative specimens to be detected.[63] Latex agglutination for *C. difficile* antigen is less sensitive than is culture and not as specific as the toxin assay.[42,90] Anaerobic culture of *C. difficile* from human stool specimens, although infrequently practiced in the United States today, may be coupled effectively with immunoassay-based or molecular detection of *C. difficile*

enterotoxins. *C. difficile* can be cultured on selective media, such as cycloserine-cefoxitin-fructose agar.[41] Stool culture alone does not determine the presence of toxigenic *C. difficile*, and this approach requires the tedious practice of anaerobic bacteriology for a test that frequently is performed at high volumes.[42]

Peripheral blood leukocytosis of 15,000 cells/mL or more is a common finding in hospitalized patients and may occur with diarrhea or with systemic symptoms of fever and toxicity before the onset of diarrhea.[20] In the appropriate setting, leukocytosis may be an early marker of *C. difficile* infection, with as many as 58 percent of patients being positive for toxins and responding to metronidazole.[119] Stool examination may show evidence of blood and mucus, but fecal leukocytes lack utility for screening because they are present in only 50 percent or less of patients.[35,98]

Endoscopic diagnosis of *C. difficile* is useful when urgent diagnosis is needed before laboratory confirmation of a positive assay for toxin is obtained (Fig. 51–2). Flexible sigmoidoscopy is a rapid diagnostic tool, but in one study of 29 patients with a positive toxin assay, only 55 percent had typical pseudomembranous colitis, 14 percent had nonspecific colitis, and 31 percent were normal.[13] In cases with a typical endoscopic appearance, *C. difficile* toxin is positive in 95 percent.[40] Flexible sigmoidoscopy will detect 90 percent of patients with colitis.[109]

The colon typically appears red with raised, circular, yellow plaques.[40,108] These pseudomembranous plaques vary from 2 to 5 mm in diameter and are scattered throughout the involved area. In the earliest stage, 1- to 2-mm ulcers may be seen but may not have an obvious membrane. Biopsy specimens of these small lesions show the same endothelial degeneration and pseudomembrane as larger lesions do.

Plain radiography of the abdomen in patients with colitis may show a variety of abnormalities, including colonic ileus, small bowel ileus, ascites, and nodular haustral thickening.[17] Colonic findings on computed tomography of the abdomen in adult patients show segmental wall thickening, but this finding is nonspecific.[3] Abdominal ultrasonography also has been used to diagnose cases of *C. difficile* infection.[97] In severely ill patients with pseudo-membranous colitis, leukocyte scintigraphy has demonstrated a constant and diffuse pattern of intense radiotracer.[84] Although not specific, this test may be useful whenever endoscopy cannot be performed.

The presence of *C. difficile* toxin A or toxin B may establish the etiology of diarrhea and colitis; the absence of toxin may not be conclusive. If symptoms are suggestive of antibiotic-associated diarrhea or colitis, studies of stools should be repeated several times before this diagnosis is ruled out.[73]

DIFFERENTIAL DIAGNOSIS

Bloody diarrhea occurring after recent use of antibiotics should suggest the possibility of pseudomembranous colitis. Stool specimens should be obtained for *C. difficile* toxins A and B, along with routine cultures for *Salmonella, Shigella, Campylobacter,* and enterohemorrhagic *E. coli.* Routine parasitologic testing for *Giardia lamblia* and *Cryptosporidium parvum* by ova and parasite examination or stool immunoassays should be performed. Enteric viruses such as rotaviruses may be an important consideration, especially in children, and may be evaluated with stool antigen immunoassays. The possibility of inflammatory bowel disease, either ulcerative colitis or Crohn disease of the colon, always should be considered, especially if treatment fails to resolve the colitis. A hemorrhagic colitis related to penicillin has been described, but no pseudomembranes were seen on colonoscopy, and studies for *C. difficile* yielded negative results.[80]

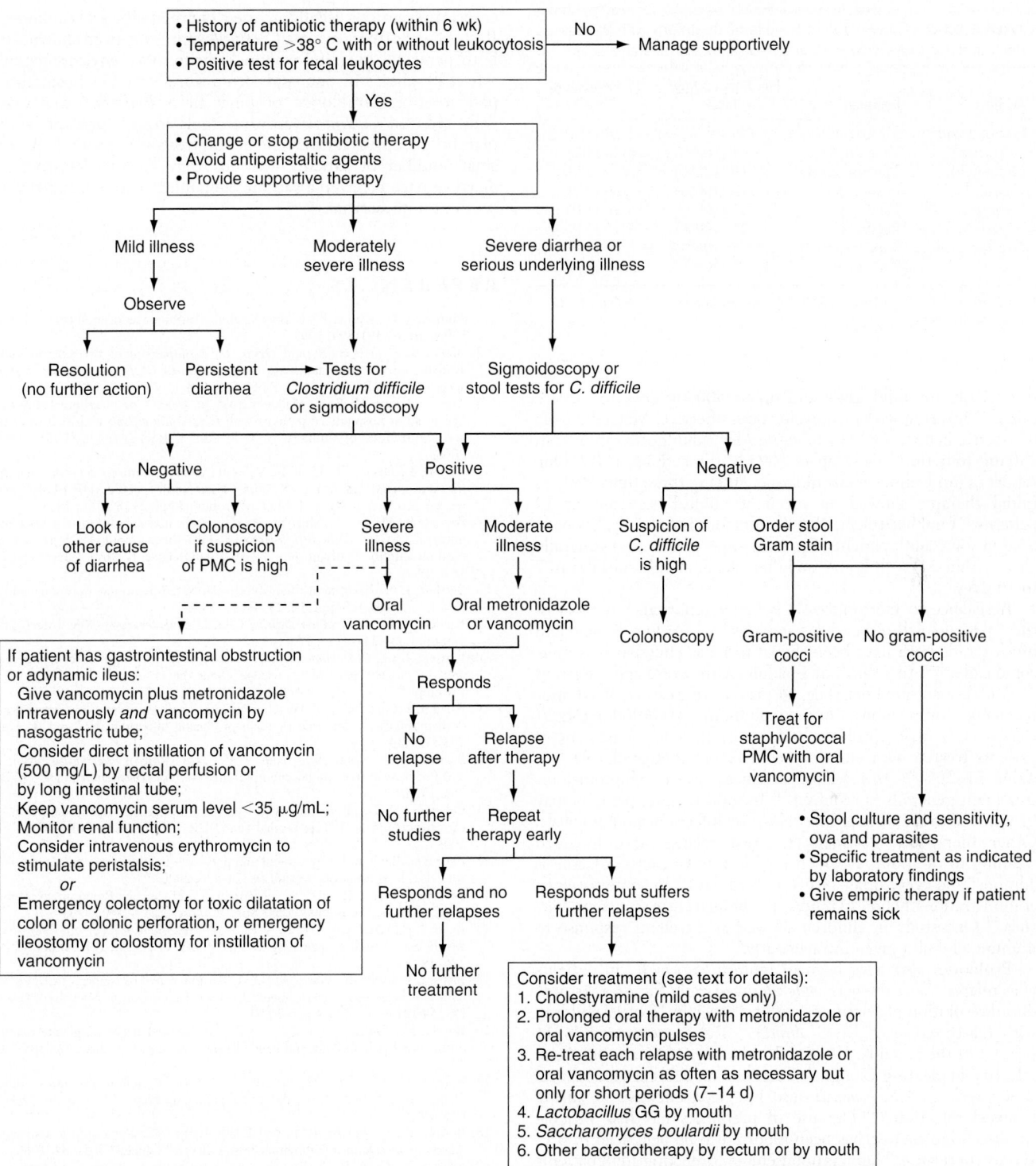

Figure 51–2 Algorithm for management of antibiotic-associated diarrhea and colitis. PMC, pseudomembranous colitis. *(From Fekety, R., and Shah, A. B.: Diagnosis and treatment of Clostridium difficile colitis. J. A. M. A. 269:72, 1993.)*

TREATMENT

In mild cases, discontinuation of antibiotics and implementation of supportive measures alone may lead to gradual resolution of symptoms.[19,108] In a study of 250 hospitalized children aged 5 to 12 years who developed diarrhea while receiving antibiotics, 45 (18%) children had stools positive for toxins A and B.[43] Although bloody diarrhea was a frequent occurrence in these patients, 68.9

percent of cases resolved with discontinuation of antibiotics. Antiperistaltic agents should be avoided because they may cause retention of toxins and complications.[23] Vancomycin has been the accepted treatment of choice for pseudomembranous colitis, but both vancomycin and metronidazole clear 80 to 100 percent of infections (Table 51–2), and metronidazole is considerably less expensive.[6,7,123] The effective oral dose of vancomycin is 40 to 50 mg/kg/day for 7 to 10 days. The adult dose is 125 mg four

TABLE 51-2   Comparison of Results of Treatment with Various Regimens for *Clostridium difficile*–Associated Diarrhea and Colitis

Author	Regimen	No. Responding/ Total	No. Relapsing/ Total
Gerding and Brazier[42]	Metronidazole	37/39 (95%)	2/39 (5%)
	Vancomycin	45/45 (100%)	6/45 (13%)
Greenfield et al.[44]	Metronidazole	19/19 (100%)	6/19 (32%)
	Fusidic acid	20/20 (100%)	5/20 (25%)
George et al.[41]	Vancomycin	21/21 (100%)	6/18 (33%)
	Bacitracin	21/21 (100%)	5/12 (42%)
Gremse et al.[45]	Vancomycin	15/15 (100%)	3/15 (20%)
	Bacitracin	12/15 (80%)	5/15 (33%)

From Bartlett, J. G.: Clostridium difficile: Clinical considerations. Rev. Infect. Dis. 12: S243-S251, 1990.

times daily for mild cases and up to 500 mg/dose for severe cases.[7,36] Intravenous vancomycin is not effective. Metronidazole is effective in doses of 20 to 40 mg/kg/day; adult doses range from 250 mg four times daily up to 500 mg three times a day. One report of intravenous metronidazole, 500 mg three times daily as initial therapy, showed an excellent clinical response in 10 patients.[39] Oral bacitracin, 25,000 units four times daily, has been used in some adult patients. Systemic signs of infection generally clear within 24 to 48 hours, and diarrhea gradually subsides in 7 to 10 days.

Resistance to metronidazole is being reported, but most of these patients will respond to vancomycin.[15,78,81] Fusidic acid and nitazoxanide both have been shown to be as effective as is metronidazole.[82,121] In a series of 14 adults with severe and recurrent *C. difficile*–associated diarrhea, 64 percent of cases resolved after receiving intravenous immunoglobulin (150-400 mg/kg).[75] Relapse is a major problem and occurs in 5 to 33 percent of patients treated with either vancomycin or metronidazole (see Table 51-2).[106,107] If a relapse produces severe symptoms, retreatment generally is required.[107] In mild relapse, patients may be watched to see whether they clear the infection spontaneously. Other therapeutic regimens to treat relapse have included weaning to the point at which vancomycin or metronidazole is administered every other or every third day.[110] In some patients, administration of cholestyramine has helped clear recurrent diarrhea.[35] One study in children showed an excellent response to immune globulin given intravenously.[64]

Probiotics also have been of interest, especially in patients who relapse. *Saccharomyces boulardii* given daily for 2 weeks produced resolution of symptoms within 1 week in 18 of 19 children with diarrhea caused by *C. difficile*.[21] Relapse occurred in 11 percent of the patients. *Lactobacillus rhamnosus* GG also has been effective in clearing *C. difficile* diarrhea.[14] A combination of oral vancomycin and *S. boulardii* also has been effective in curing relapsed infection.[104] The use of prebiotics has had variable results. Oligofructose has been reported to be beneficial in prevention of relapse,[65] but it is not useful in protecting adult patients while they are receiving antibiotics.[66]

Response to treatment is poor with ileus, toxic megacolon, or colonic perforation. In these cases, instillation of vancomycin by clamped nasogastric tube or direct colonic instillation can be tried.[101] The colonic vancomycin dose for adults is 2000 mg initially, followed by 100 mg every 6 hours.[88]

PREVENTION

To date, no effective means have been implemented to prevent the spread of and colonization with *C. difficile* or to prevent antibiotic-related pseudomembranous colitis. Private rooms and enteric precautions usually are used, but their efficacy is unknown. Bactericidal activity against *C. difficile* spores has been shown with both peracetyl ions and acidified nitrite, both environmentally safe materials.[122] In one study from Turkey of 151 hospitalized patients given antibiotics, prophylactic *S. boulardii* given twice daily reduced *C. difficile*–positive stools from 9 percent in the placebo group to 1.4 percent in the treatment group.[22] A very small number of patients with recurrent *C. difficile*–associated diarrhea have received a vaccine containing toxoid A and B with resolution of diarrhea.[102]

REFERENCES

1. Ahmad, S. H., Kumar, P., Fakhir, S., et al.: Antibiotic associated colitis. Indian J. Pediatr. *60*:591-594, 1993.
2. Altaie, S. S., Meyer, P., and Dryja, D.: Comparison of two commercially available enzyme immunoassays for detection of *Clostridium difficile* in stool specimens. J. Clin. Microbiol. *32*:51-53, 1994.
3. Ash, L., Baker, M. E., O'Malley, C. M., Jr., et al.: Colonic abnormalities on CT in adult hospitalized patients with *Clostridium difficile* colitis: Prevalence and significance of findings. A. J. R. Am. J. Roentgenol. *185*:1393-1400, 2006.
4. Barbut, F., Decre, D., Lalande, V., et al.: Clinical features of *Clostridium difficile*–associated diarrhea due to binary toxin (actin-specific ADP-ribosyltransferase)–producing strains. J. Med. Microbiol. *54*(pt. 2):181-185, 2005.
5. Barbut, F., Mario, N., Meyohas, M. C., et al.: Investigation of a nosocomial outbreak of *Clostridium difficile*–associated diarrhoea among AIDS patients by random amplified polymorphic DNA (RAPD) assay. J. Hosp. Infect. *26*:181-189, 1994.
6. Bartlett, J. G.: Treatment of antibiotic-associated pseudomembranous colitis. Rev. Infect. Dis. *6*(Suppl. 1):S235-S241, 1984.
7. Bartlett, J. G.: *Clostridium difficile*: Clinical considerations. Rev. Infect. Dis. *12*(Suppl. 2):S243-S251, 1990.
8. Bartlett, J. G.: *Clostridium difficile*: History of its role as an enteric pathogen and the current state of knowledge about the organism. Clin. Infect. Dis. *18*(Suppl. 4):S265-S272, 1994.
9. Bartlett, J. G., Chang, T. W., Gurwith, M., et al.: Antibiotic-associated pseudomembranous colitis due to toxin-producing clostridia. N. Engl. J. Med. *298*:531-534, 1978.
10. Bartlett, J. G., Moon, N., Chang, T. W., et al.: Role of *Clostridium difficile* in antibiotic-associated pseudomembranous colitis. Gastroenterology *75*:778-782, 1978.
11. Belanger, S. D., Boissinot, M., Clairoux, N., et al.: Rapid detection of *Clostridium difficile* in feces by real-time PCR. J. Clin. Microbiol. *41*:730-734, 2003.
12. Bergogne-Berezin, E.: Treatment and prevention of antibiotic associated diarrhea. Int. J. Antimicrob. Agents *16*:521-526, 2000.
13. Bergstein, J. M., Kramer, A., Wittman, D. H., et al.: Pseudomembranous colitis: How useful is endoscopy? Surg. Endosc. *4*:217-219, 1990.
14. Biller, J. A., Katz, A. J., Flores, A. F., et al.: Treatment of recurrent *Clostridium difficile* colitis with *Lactobacillus* GG. J. Pediatr. Gastroenterol. Nutr. *21*:224-226, 1995.
15. Bishara, J., Bloch, Y., Garty, M., et al.: Antimicrobial resistance of *Clostridium difficile* isolates in a tertiary medical center, Israel. Diagn. Microbiol. Infect. Dis. *54*:141-144, 2006. Epub 2006.
16. Boccia, D., Stolfi, I., Lana, S., et al.: Nosocomial necrotising enterocolitis outbreaks: Epidemiology and control measures. Eur. J. Pediatr. *160*:385-391, 2001.
17. Boland, G. W., Lee, M. J., Cats, A., et al.: Pseudomembranous colitis: Diagnostic sensitivity of the abdominal plain radiograph. Clin. Radiol. *49*:473-475, 1994.
18. Bolton, R. P., Sherriff, R. J., and Read, A. E.: *Clostridium difficile* associated diarrhoea: A role in inflammatory bowel disease? Lancet *1*:383-384, 1980.
19. Bricker, E., Garg, R., Nelson, R., et al.: Antibiotic treatment for *Clostridium difficile*–associated diarrhea in adults. Cochrane Database Syst. Rev. *25*:CD004610, 2005.
20. Bulusu, M., Narayan, S., Shetler, K., et al.: Leukocytosis as a harbinger and surrogate marker of *Clostridium difficile* infection in hospitalized patients with diarrhea. Am. J. Gastroenterol. *95*:3137-3141, 2000.
21. Buts, J. P., Corthier, G., and Delmee, M.: *Saccharomyces boulardii* for *Clostridium difficile*–associated enteropathies in infants. J. Pediatr. Gastroenterol. Nutr. *16*:419-425, 1993.
22. Can, M., Besirbellioglu, B. A., Avci, I. Y., et al.: Prophylactic *Saccharomyces boulardii* in the prevention of antibiotic-associated diarrhea: A prospective study. Med. Sci. Monit. *12*:P119-P122, 2006. Epub 2006.
23. Church, J. M., and Fazio, V. W.: A role for colonic stasis in the pathogenesis of disease related to *Clostridium difficile*. Dis. Colon Rectum *29*:804-809, 1986.
24. Delmee, M.: Laboratory diagnosis of *Clostridium difficile* disease. Clin. Microbiol. Infect. 7:411-416, 2001.

25. Denno, D. M., Stapp, J. R., Boster, D. R., et al.: Etiology of diarrhea in pediatric outpatient settings. Pediatr. Infect. Dis. J. *24*:142-148, 2005.

26. Dial, S., Alrasadi, K., Manoukian, C., et al.: Risk of *Clostridium difficile* diarrhea among hospital inpatients prescribed proton pump inhibitors: Cohort and case-control studies. C. M. A. J. *6*:171:33-38, 2004.

27. Dial, S., Delaney, J. A., and Barkun, A. N.: Use of gastric acid–suppressive agents and the risk of community acquired *Clostridium difficile*–associated disease. J. A. M. A. *294*:2989-2995, 2005.

28. Dorman, S. A., Liggoria, E., Winn, W. C., Jr., et al.: Isolation of *Clostridium difficile* from patients with inactive Crohn's disease. Gastroenterology *82*:1348-1351, 1982.

29. Drapkin, M. S., Worthington, M. G., Chang, T. W., et al.: *Clostridium difficile* colitis mimicking acute peritonitis. Arch. Surg. *120*:1321-1322, 1985.

30. Eglow, R., Pothoulakis, C., Israel, E., et al.: Age-related increase in receptor binding for *Clostridium difficile* toxin A (TxA) in rabbit intestine. Gastroenterology *96*:A136, 1989.

31. El-Mahallawy, H. A., El-Din, N. H., Salah, F., et al.: Epidemiologic profile of symptomatic gastroenteritis in pediatric oncology patients receiving chemotherapy. Pediatr. Blood Cancer *42*:338-342, 2004.

32. Enad, D., Meislich, D., Brodsky, N. L., et al.: Is *Clostridium difficile* a pathogen in the newborn intensive care unit? A prospective evaluation. J. Perinatol. *17*:355-359, 1997.

33. Facklam, D. P., Gardner, J. S., Neidert, G. L., et al.: An epidemiologic postmarketing surveillance study of prescription acne medications. Am. J. Public Health *80*:50-53, 1990.

34. Fekety, R., Kim, K. H., Brown, D., et al.: Epidemiology of antibiotic-associated colitis; isolation of *Clostridium difficile* from the hospital environment. Am. J. Med. *70*:906-908, 1981.

35. Fekety, R., and Shah, A. B.: Diagnosis and treatment of *Clostridium difficile* colitis. J. A. M. A. *269*:71-75, 1993.

36. Fekety, R., Silva, J., Kauffman, C., et al.: Treatment of antibiotic-associated *Clostridium difficile* colitis with oral vancomycin: Comparison of two dosage regimens. Am. J. Med. *86*:15-19, 1989.

37. Ferroni, A., Merckx, J., Ancelle, T., et al.: Nosocomial outbreak of *Clostridium difficile* diarrhea in a pediatric service. Eur. J. Clin. Microbiol. Infect. Dis. *16*:928-931, 1997.

38. Finney, J. M. T.: Gastroenterostomy for cicatrizing ulcer of the pylorus. Bull. Johns Hopkins Hosp. *4*:53, 1893.

39. Friedenberg, F., Fernandez, A., Kaul, V., et al.: Intravenous metronidazole for the treatment of *Clostridium difficile* colitis. Dis. Colon Rectum *44*:1176-1180, 2001.

40. Gebhard, R. L., Gerding, D. N., Olson, M. M., et al.: Clinical and endoscopic findings in patients early in the course of *Clostridium difficile*–associated pseudomembranous colitis. Am. J. Med. *78*:45-48, 1985.

41. George, W. L., Sutter, V. L., Citron, D., et al.: Selective and differential medium for isolation of *Clostridium difficile*. J. Clin. Microbiol. *9*:214-219, 1979.

42. Gerding, D. N., and Brazier, J. S.: Optimal methods for identifying *Clostridium difficile* infections. Clin. Infect. Dis. *16*(Suppl. 4):S439-S442, 1994.

43. Gogate, A., De, A., Nanivadekar, R., et al.: Diagnostic role of stool culture and toxin detection in antibiotic associated diarrhea due to *Clostridium difficile* in children. Indian J. Med. Res. *122*:518-524, 2005.

44. Greenfield, C., Aguilar Ramirez, J. R., Pounder, R. E., et al.: *Clostridium difficile* and inflammatory bowel disease. Gut *24*:713-717, 1983.

45. Gremse, D. A., Dean, P. C., and Farquhar, D. S.: Cefixime and antibiotic-associated colitis. Pediatr. Infect. Dis. J. *13*:331-333, 1994.

46. Hafiz, S., and Oakley, C. L.: *Clostridium difficile*: Isolation and characteristics. J. Med. Microbiol. *9*:129-136, 1976.

47. Hall, I. C., and O'Toole, E.: Intestinal flora in newborn infants. Am. J. Dis. Child. *49*:390, 1935.

48. Hirschhorn, L. R., Trnka, Y., Onderdonk, A., et al.: Epidemiology of community-acquired *Clostridium difficile*–associated diarrhea. J. Infect. Dis. *169*:127-133, 1994.

49. Holst, E., Helin, I., and Mardh, P. A.: Recovery of *Clostridium difficile* from children. Scand. J. Infect. Dis. *13*:41-45, 1981.

50. Iizuka, M., Itou, H., Konno, S., et al.: Elemental diet modulates the growth of *Clostridium difficile* in the gut flora. Aliment. Pharmacol. Ther. *20*(Suppl. 1):151-157, 2005.

51. Kato, H., Kita, H., Karasawa, T., et al.: Colonisation and transmission of *Clostridium difficile* in healthy individuals examined by PCR ribotyping and pulsed-field gel electrophoresis. J. Med. Microbiol. *50*:720-727, 2001.

52. Kelly, C. P., Pothoulakis, C., Orellana, J., et al.: Human colonic aspirates containing immunoglobulin A antibody to *Clostridium difficile* toxin A inhibit toxin A–receptor binding. Gastroenterology *102*:35-40, 1992.

53. Kim, K., DuPont, H. L., and Pickering, L. K.: Outbreaks of diarrhea associated with *Clostridium difficile* and its toxin in day-care centers: Evidence of person-to-person spread. J. Pediatr. *102*:376-382, 1983.

54. Kim, K. H., Fekety, R., Batts, D. H., et al.: Isolation of *Clostridium difficile* from the environment and contacts of patients with antibiotic-associated colitis. J. Infect. Dis. *143*:42-50, 1981.

55. Knoop, F. C., Owens, M., and Crocker, I. C.: *Clostridium difficile*: Clinical disease and diagnosis. Clin. Microbiol. Rev. *6*:251-265, 1993.

56. Koss, K., Clark, M. A., Sanders, D. S., et al.: The outcome of surgery in fulminant *Clostridium difficile* colitis. Colorectal Dis. *8*:149-154, 2006.

57. Kuijper, E. J., Oudbier, J. H., Stuifbergen, W. N., et al.: Application of whole-cell DNA restriction endonuclease profiles to the epidemiology of *Clostridium difficile*–induced diarrhea. J. Clin. Microbiol. *25*:751-753, 1987.

58. Kyne, L., Warny, M., Qamar, A., et al.: Association between antibody response to toxin A and protection against recurrent *Clostridium difficile* diarrhoea. Lancet *357*:189-193, 2001.

59. LaMont, J. T., and Trnka, Y. M.: Therapeutic implications of *Clostridium difficile* toxin during relapse of chronic inflammatory bowel disease. Lancet *1*:381-383, 1980.

60. Larson, H. E., Barclay, F. E., Honour, P., et al.: Epidemiology of *Clostridium difficile* in infants. J. Infect. Dis. *146*:727-733, 1982.

61. Larson, H. E., and Price, A. B.: Pseudomembranous colitis: Presence of clostridial toxin. Lancet *2*:1312-1314, 1977.

62. Lashner, B. A., Todorczuk, J., Sahm, D. F., et al.: *Clostridium difficile* culture-positive toxin-negative diarrhea. Am. J. Gastroenterol. *81*:940-943, 1986.

63. Lemee, L., Dhalluin, A., Testelin, S., et al.: Multiplex PCR targeting tpi (triose phosphate isomerase), tcdA (Toxin A), and tcdB (Toxin B) genes for toxigenic culture of *Clostridium difficile*. J. Clin. Microbiol. *42*:5710-5714, 2004.

64. Leung, D. Y., Kelly, C. P., Boguniewicz, M., et al.: Treatment with intravenously administered gamma globulin of chronic relapsing colitis induced by *Clostridium difficile* toxin. J. Pediatr. *118*(pt. 1):633-637, 1991.

65. Lewis, S., Burmeister, S., and Brazier, J.: Effect of the prebiotic oligofructose on relapse of *Clostridium difficile*–associated diarrhea: A randomized, controlled study. Clin. Gastroenterol. Hepatol. *3*:442-448, 2005.

66. Lewis, S., Burmeister, S., Cohen, S., et al.: Failure of dietary oligofructose to prevent antibiotic-associated diarrhoea. Ailment. Pharmacol. Ther. *21*:469-477, 2005.

67. Loo, V. G., Poirier, L., Miller, M. A., et al.: A predominantly clonal multi-institutional breakout of *Clostridium difficile*–associated diarrhea with high morbidity and mortality. N. Engl. J. Med. *353*:2442-2449, 2005. Epub 2005.

68. Lyerly, D. M., Krivan, H. C., and Wilkins, T. D.: *Clostridium difficile*: Its disease and toxins. Clin. Microbiol. Rev. *1*:1-18, 1988.

69. Markowitz, J. E., Brown, K. A., Mamula, P., et al.: Failure of single-toxin assays to detect *Clostridium difficile* infection in pediatric inflammatory bowel disease. Am. J. Gastroenterol. *96*:2688-2690, 2001.

70. McDonald, L. C., Owings, M., and Jernigan, D. B.: *Clostridium difficile* infection in patients discharged from US shortstay hospitals, 1996-2003. Emerg. Infect. Dis. *12*:409-415, 2006.

71. McDonald, L. C., Kilgore, G. E., Thompson, A., et al.: An epidemic, toxin gene–variant strain of *Clostridium difficile*. N. Engl. J. Med. *353*:2433-2441, 2006.

72. McEllistrem, M. C., Carman, R. J., Gerding, D. N., et al.: A hospital outbreak of *Clostridium difficile* disease associated with isolates carrying binary toxin genes. Clin. Infect. Dis. *40*:265-272, 2005. Epub 2004.

73. McFarland, L. V., Brandmarker, S. A., and Guandalini, S.: Pediatric *Clostridium difficile*: A phantom menace or clinical reality? J. Pediatr. Gastroenterol. Nutr. *31*:220-231, 2000.

74. McFarland, L. V., Mulligan, M. E., Kwok, R. Y., et al.: Nosocomial acquisition of *Clostridium difficile* infection. N. Engl. J. Med. *320*:204-210, 1989.

75. McPherson, S., Rees, C. J., Ellis, R., et al.: Intravenous immunoglobulin for the treatment of severe, refractory, and recurrent *Clostridium difficile* diarrhea. Dis. Colon Rectum *49*:640-645, 2006.

76. Meyer, A. M., Ramzan, N. N., Loftus, E. V., Jr., et al.: The diagnostic yield of stool pathogen studies during relapses of inflammatory bowel disease. J. Clin. Gastroenterol. *38*:772-775, 2004.

77. Meyers, S., Mayer, L., Bottone, E., et al.: Occurrence of *Clostridium difficile* toxin during the course of inflammatory bowel disease. Gastroenterology *80*:697-700, 1981.

78. Modena, S., Gollamudi, S., and Friedenberg, F.: Continuation of antibiotics is associated with failure of metronidazole for *Clostridium difficile*–associated diarrhea. J. Clin. Gastroenterol. *40*:49-54, 2006.

79. Morinville, V., and McDonald, J.: *Clostridium difficile*–associated diarrhea in 200 Canadian children. Can. J. Gastroenterol. *19*:497-501, 2005.

80. Moulis, H., and Vender, R. J.: Antibiotic-associated hemorrhagic colitis. J. Clin. Gastroenterol. *18*:227-231, 1994.

81. Musher, D. M., Aslam, S., Logan, N., et al.: Relatively poor outcome after treatment of *Clostridium difficile* colitis with metronidazole. Clin. Infect. Dis. *40*:1586-1590, 2005. Epub 2005.

82. Musher, D. M., Logan, N., Hamill, R. J., et al.: Nitazoxanide for the treatment of *Clostridium difficile* colitis. Clin. Infect. Dis. *43*:421-427, 2006. Epub 2006.

83. Nakajima, A., Yajima, S., Shirakura, T., et al.: Rifampicin-associated pseudomembranous colitis. J. Gastroenterol. *35*:299-303, 2000.

84. Nathan, M. A., Seabold, J. E., Brown, B. P., et al.: Colonic localization of labeled leukocytes in critically ill patients. Scintigraphic detection of pseudomembranous colitis. Clin. Nucl. Med. *20*:99-106, 1995.

85. Nolan, N. P., Kelly, C. P., Humphreys, J. F., et al.: An epidemic of pseudomembranous colitis: Importance of person to person spread. Gut *28*:1467-1473, 1987.

86. Nusrat, A., Eichel-Streiber, C., Turner, J. R., et al.: *Clostridium difficile* toxins disrupt epithelial barrier function by altering membrane microdomain localization of tight junction proteins. Infect. Immun. *69*:1329-1336, 2001.

87. Oldfield, E. C.: *Clostridium difficile*–associated diarrhea: Resurgence with a vengeance. Rev. Gastroenterol. Disord. *6*:79-96, 2006.

88. Pasic, M., Jost, R., Carrel, T., et al.: Intracolonic vancomycin for pseudomembranous colitis. N. Engl. J. Med. *329*:583, 1993.
89. Pepin, J., Saheb, N., Coulombe, M. A., et al.: Emergence of fluoroquinolones as the predominant risk factor for *Clostridium difficile*–associated diarrhea: A cohort study during an epidemic in Quebec. Clin. Infect. Dis. *41*:1254-1260, 2005.
90. Peterson, L. R., and Kelly, P. J.: The role of the clinical microbiology laboratory in the management of *Clostridium difficile*–associated diarrhea. Infect. Dis. Clin. North Am. 7:277-293, 1993.
91. Pierce, P. F., Jr., Wilson, R., Silva, J., Jr., et al.: Antibiotic-associated pseudomembranous colitis: An epidemiologic investigation of a cluster of cases. J. Infect. Dis. *145*:269-274, 1982.
92. Pothoulakis, C.: Effects of *Clostridium difficile* toxins on epithelial cell barrier. Ann. N. Y. Acad. Sci. *915*:347-356, 2000.
93. Pothoulakis, C., Sullivan, R., Melnick, D. A., et al.: *Clostridium difficile* toxin A stimulates intracellular calcium release and chemotactic response in human granulocytes. J. Clin. Invest. *81*:1741-1745, 1988.
94. Poxton, I. R., McCoubrey, J., and Blair, G.: The pathogenicity of *Clostridium difficile*. Clin. Microbiol. Infect. 7:421-427, 2001.
95. Prendergast, T. M., Marini, C. P., D'Angelo, A. J., et al.: Surgical patients with pseudomembranous colitis: Factors affecting prognosis. Surgery *116*:768-774, 1994.
96. Price, A. B., and Davies, D. R.: Pseudomembranous colitis. J. Clin. Pathol. *30*:1-12, 1977.
97. Razzaq, R., and Sukumar, S.A.: Ultrasound diagnosis of clinically undetected *Clostridium difficile* toxin colitis. Clin. Radiol. *61*:446-452, 2006.
98. Reddymasu, S., Sheth, A., and Banks, D. E.: Is fecal leukocyte test a good predictor of *Clostridium difficile* associated with diarrhea? Ann. J. Clin. Microbiol. Antimicrob. 5:9, 2005.
99. Rolfe, R. D., Helebian, S., and Finegold, S. M.: Bacterial interference between *Clostridium difficile* and normal fecal flora. J. Infect. Dis. *143*:470-475, 1981.
100. Sheretz, R. J., and Sarubbi, F. A.: The prevalence of *Clostridium difficile* and toxin in a nursery population: A comparison with patients with necrotizing enterocolitis and an asymptomatic group. J. Pediatr. *100*:435-439, 1982.
101. Shetler, K., Nieuwenhuis, R., Wren, S. M., et al.: Decompressive colonoscopy with intracolonic vancomycin administration for the treatment of severe pseudomembranous colitis. Surg. Endosc. *15*:653-659, 2001.
102. Sougioultzis, S., Kyne, L., Drudy, D., et al.: *Clostridium difficile* toxoid vaccine in recurrent *C. difficile*–associated diarrhea. Gastroenterology *128*:764-770, 2005.
103. Speare, G. S.: *Staphylococcus* pseudomembranous enterocolitis, a complication of antibiotic therapy. Am. J. Surg. *88*:523-534, 1954.
104. Surawicz, C. M., McFarland, L. V., Greenberg, R. N., et al.: The search for a better treatment for recurrent *Clostridium difficile* disease: Use of high-dose vancomycin combined with *Saccharomyces boulardii*. Clin. Infect. Dis. *31*:1012-1017, 2000.
105. Sutphen, J. L., Grand, R. J., Flores, A., et al.: Chronic diarrhea associated with *Clostridium difficile* in children. Am. J. Dis. Child. *137*:275-278, 1983.
106. Teasley, D. G., Gerding, D. N., Olson, M. M., et al.: Prospective randomised trial of metronidazole versus vancomycin for *Clostridium difficile*–associated diarrhoea and colitis. Lancet 2:1043-1046, 1983.
107. Tedesco, F. J.: Pseudomembranous colitis: Pathogenesis and therapy. Med. Clin. North Am. *66*:655-664, 1982.
108. Tedesco, F. J., Barton, R. W., and Alpers, D. H.: Clindamycin-associated colitis: A prospective study. Ann. Intern. Med. *81*:429-433, 1974.
109. Tedesco, F. J., Corless, J. K., and Brownstein, R. E.: Rectal sparing in antibiotic-associated pseudomembranous colitis: A prospective study. Gastroenterology *83*:1259-1260, 1982.
110. Tedesco, F. J., Gordon, D., and Fortson, W. C.: Approach to patients with multiple relapses of antibiotic-associated pseudomembranous colitis. Am. J. Gastroenterol. *80*:867-868, 1985.
111. Thompson, C. M., Jr., Gilligan, P. H., Fisher, M. C., et al.: *Clostridium difficile* cytotoxin in a pediatric population. Am. J. Dis. Child. *137*:271-274, 1983.
112. Triadafilopoulos, G., and Hallstone, A. E.: Acute abdomen as the first presentation of pseudomembranous colitis. Gastroenterology *101*:685-691, 1991.
113. Triadafilopoulos, G., Pothoulakis, C., Weiss, R., et al.: Comparative study of *Clostridium difficile* toxin A and cholera toxin in rabbit ileum. Gastroenterology *97*:1186-1192, 1989.
114. Trnka, Y. M., and LaMont, J. T.: Association of *Clostridium difficile* toxin with symptomatic relapse of chronic inflammatory bowel disease. Gastroenterology *80*:693-696, 1981.
115. van den Berg, R. J., Bruijnesteijn van Coppenraet, L. S., Gerritsen, H. J., et al.: Prospective multicenter evaluation of a new immunoassay and real-time PCR for rapid diagnosis of *Clostridium difficile*–associated diarrhea in hospitalized patients. J. Clin. Microbiol. *43*:5338-5340, 2005.
116. Viscidi, R., Laughon, B. E., Yolken, R., et al.: Serum antibody response to toxins A and B of *Clostridium difficile*. J. Infect. Dis. *148*:93-100, 1983.
117. Viscidi, R., Willey, S., and Bartlett, J. G.: Isolation rates and toxigenic potential of *Clostridium difficile* isolates from various patient populations. Gastroenterology *81*:5-9, 1981.
118. Wada, N., Nishida, N., Iwaki, S., et al.: Neutralizing activity against *Clostridium difficile* toxin in the supernatants of cultured colostral cells. Infect. Immun. *29*:545-550, 1980.
119. Wanahita, A., Goldsmith, E. A., Marino, B. J., et al.: *Clostridium difficile* infection in patients with unexplained leukocytosis. Am. J. Med. *115*:543-546, 2003.
120. Wilkins, T. D., and Lyerly, D. M.: *Clostridium difficile* testing: After 20 years, still challenging. J. Clin. Microbiol. *41*:531-534, 2003.
121. Wult, M., and Odenholt, I.: A double-blind randomized controlled trial of fusidic acid and metronidazole for treatment of an initial episode of *Clostridium difficile*–associated diarrhea. Antimicrob. Chemother. *54*:211-216, 2004. Epub 2004.
122. Wult, M., Odenholt, I., and Walder, M.: Activity of three disinfectants and acidified nitrite against *Clostridium difficile* spores. Infect. Control Hosp. Epidemiol. *24*:765-768, 2003.
123. Young, G. P., Ward, P. B., Bayley, N., et al.: Antibiotic-associated colitis due to *Clostridium difficile*: Double-blind comparison of vancomycin with bacitracin. Gastroenterology *89*:1038-1045, 1985.

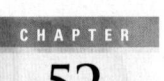

CHAPTER

52 | WHIPPLE DISEASE

Roberto A. Guerrero ❖ Mark A. Gilger

Whipple disease is a rare, systemic bacterial infection that can be potentially fatal without therapy. In its most common form, Whipple disease affects white, middle-aged men, causing diarrhea, weight loss, abdominal pain, arthralgias, and fever. Although it is extraordinarily rare in children, its recognition may be crucial. Simple treatment with appropriate antibiotics may be curative and lifesaving.[28] Despite successful cultivation of the bacterium *Tropheryma whipplei* (formerly *Tropheryma whippelii*) in 2000,[56] little progress has been made in the development of improved diagnostic tests.

HISTORY

Whipple disease was described in 1907 by George Hoyt Whipple,[77] at that time an Instructor in Pathology at The Johns Hopkins University.[6] Whipple's description probably was not the

first; Allchin and Webb apparently described a patient with "Whipple disease" in 1895.[48]

In Whipple's account, a 37-year-old medical missionary was admitted to the Johns Hopkins Hospital with low-grade fever, steatorrhea, and an abdominal mass. The patient had a 5-year history of sporadic migratory polyarthritis. These attacks of arthritis were associated with a gradual loss of weight and strength. His skin was pigmented with a brownish hue. Laboratory evaluation found severe anemia and an enormous number of fatty acid crystals in the stool. Explorative laparotomy revealed large, firm mesenteric lymph nodes, and a diagnosis of either Hodgkin disease or tuberculosis was made. The patient died 1 week later, and autopsy revealed marked fatty deposition within intestinal mucosa and the mesenteric and retroperitoneal lymph nodes. Other findings included polyserositis (peritonitis, pleuritis, and pericarditis) and endocarditis. Histologic examination revealed infiltration of the lamina propria of the small intestine by large, foamy mononuclear cells that did not stain for fat. Fatty acids and triglycerides were found in dilated lymph channels. Silver stains of the mesenteric lymph nodes showed "great numbers of rod-shaped organisms" that resembled the tubercle bacillus. Whipple suggested that these bacillus-like organisms in the nodes could be the cause.

Whipple[77] reported "a hitherto undescribed disease characterized anatomically by deposits of fat and fatty acids in the intestinal and mesenteric lymphatic tissues." He concluded that the patient had "an obscure disease of fat metabolism," and proposed the term *intestinal lipodystrophy*.[18] Whipple recognized the most important features of this disease except for the involvement of the central nervous system (CNS). In 1949, Black-Schaffer showed that macrophages within the intestinal mucosa of patients with Whipple disease are stained intensely by the periodic acid–Schiff method,[35] proving that the macrophages contained glycoprotein or mucopolysaccharide, not fat, as Whipple had suggested.

In 1992, Relman and colleagues[59] identified a gram-positive bacillus in association with Whipple disease by use of polymerase chain reaction (PCR). They reported a unique 1321-base pair, 16S ribosomal RNA sequence amplified by PCR on intestinal and lymph node tissue from five unrelated patients with Whipple disease. They suggested that the responsible bacillus is a member of the actinomycetes. Relman and colleagues[59] concluded that the phylogenetic relationships of the Whipple disease bacillus, the features of the illness, and its distinct morphologic characteristics provided sufficient grounds to propose a new genus and species name, *Tropheryma whippelii* (from the Greek *trophe*, or "nourishment"; *eryma*, or "barrier," because of the malabsorption it causes; and *whippelii*, in honor of Whipple).

EPIDEMIOLOGY

Whipple disease characteristically occurs in white middle-aged men. Its true incidence and prevalence are unknown because fewer than 1000 cases have been reported worldwide. It is an extremely rare disease in children,[1,2,4,10,34,73] with fewer than 10 cases reported. The youngest patient was a newborn,[15] and the oldest was 83 years old.[42] The peak age at presentation is 40 to 49 years.[24] In a literature review of 114 patients,[42] 88 percent were men and 12 percent were women. Most of these patients were white. Most patients reported as having Whipple disease are from continental Europe or the United States.[13] In an extensive review of 741 cases, Dobbins[20] found that most academic centers in the United States had records of three or four unreported cases. He estimated that for every published report, at least two or three unpublished cases exist, and approximately 1500 to 2000 individuals probably have had Whipple disease.[18]

ETIOLOGY AND PATHOGENESIS

Whipple disease is caused by an organism known as Whipple bacillus or *T. whipplei*.[24,42,56,77] Despite Whipple's account of "great numbers of rod-shaped organisms,"[77] culture of the organism was unsuccessful until more recently. In 2000, Raoult and associates[56] reported that the bacterium *T. whipplei* had been cultured successfully from an aortic valve vegetation in a patient with prolonged endocarditis. The bacteria were isolated after inoculation in a human fibroblast cell line (HEL). Analysis by PCR confirmed that the 16S ribosomal RNA gene of the cultured bacterium was identical to the *T. whipplei* sequence. Subcultures of the bacterium also were obtained, and high-titer polyclonal antibodies against *T. whipplei* were produced. Such antibodies potentially may allow serologic diagnosis to become a reality.

T. whipplei may be a member of the actinomycetes,[59] which are gram-positive bacteria with DNA rich in guanine and cytosine.[78] The genus consists of actinomycetes, streptomycetes, and the nocardioforms.[14] *T. whipplei* seems to be related most closely to the four actinobacteria *Dermatophilus congolensis*, *Arthrobacter globiformis*, *Terrabacter tumescens*, and *Micrococcus luteus*.[59] Using so-called bootstrap analysis, some researchers have argued that the Whipple bacillus is only 67 percent associated with actinobacteria, far from the level needed for scientific conclusion.[67] The Whipple bacillus may represent another, separate, fourth line of descent with the actinomycetes. Amplification, cloning, and sequencing of a 620-base pair fragment of *T. whipplei* heat shock protein led to the conclusion that *T. whipplei* is a member of the actinobacteria.[49]

Scant support exists for a primary humoral immunodeficiency in Whipple disease,[27] but stronger evidence exists for a distinct defect in the cell-mediated immune function. Dobbins[19] reviewed data of 30 patients with HLA-A and HLA-B locus typing and 47 patients with HLA-B27 typing. He found an increased incidence of patients who were positive for HLA-B27 (28%), even with absence of concomitant sacroiliitis. Other reports have failed to confirm the increased association with the HLA-B27 antigen.[3] Marth and associates[44] studied 27 patients with Whipple disease. They found a significantly reduced number of cells expressing the complement receptor 3 L-chain (CD11B), a reduced proliferation to phytohemagglutinin and to sheep red blood cells, and a hypoergic skin reaction. These findings indicated a defect of cell-mediated immunity.

In patients with active disease, the number of CD8[+] cells is increased, which results in a reduced CD4/CD8 ratio. Such defects of cellular immunity seem to persist in patients for several years, despite complete remission of the disease. Schoeden and associates[65] were able to culture *T. whipplei* in mononuclear phagocytes deactivated with interleukin-4 (IL-4), IL-10, and dexamethasone. IL-4 was found to be the crucial deactivating signal that rendered monocytes permissive for intracellular multiplication of *T. whipplei*. IL-4 is an immunoregulatory cytokine. Schoeden and associates[65] suggested that host factors, such as an imbalance in the T-helper 1 and T-helper 2 immune response, may contribute to the pathogenesis of Whipple disease.

Desnues and colleagues[17] reported a specific gene expression pattern associated with replication of *T. whipplei* in macrophages. *T. whipplei* organisms are killed by monocytes. The addition of exogenous IL-16 enabled *T. whipplei* to replicate in monocytes and increased bacterial replication in macrophages. *T. whipplei* replication in macrophages was completely prevented after blocking IL-16 activity with the use of anti-IL-16 antibodies. Untreated patients with Whipple disease were noted to have significantly higher circulating IL-16 than that of control subjects and patients treated for Whipple disease. They concluded that response of monocytes and macrophages to IL-16 likely is crucial for replication of *T. whipplei* to occur, in patients with Whipple disease.

Oral acquisition of the Whipple bacillus seems most likely,[24] emphasizing greater involvement of the duodenum and proximal jejunum than the more distal small intestine. Only three reports of siblings with this disease exist; contagious spread of Whipple disease seems unlikely.[32] *T. whipplei* has been identified free in the small intestine next to the glycocalyx of the enterocyte's microvilli, in epithelial cells, and in the lamina propria.[24] Even in patients with extraintestinal Whipple disease, the organism usually is identified in the small bowel.[24] The bacillus seems to spread through the lymphatics and through the systemic circulation[24,36,50] and then can involve several extraintestinal organs.

T. whipplei can be seen faintly by light microscopy. The bacilli are seen best by transmission electron microscopy, which reveals a rod-shaped organism 0.2 μm wide and 1.5 to 2.5 μm long (Fig. 52–1). The ultrastructure of the wall of *T. whipplei* is similar to that of other gram-positive bacteria, with the exception of an

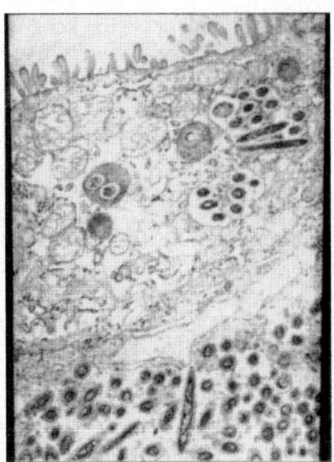

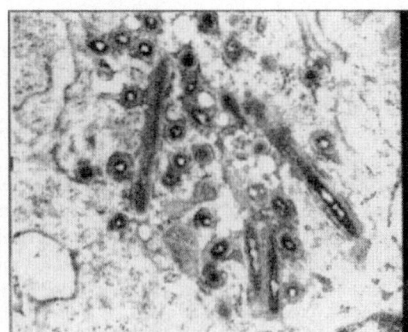

Figure 52–3 Electron micrograph illustrating numerous rod-shaped bacilliform bodies within the cytoplasm of a macrophage. (Magnification ×13,750.) *(From Tyor, M. P.: Whipple's disease: The Duke connection. N. C. Med. J. 55:237-240, 1994.)*

Figure 52–1 Electron micrograph of the invasion of enterocytes by Whipple bacilli. There are numerous bacilli within the lamina propria. (Magnification ×25,000.) *(From Tyor, M. P.: Whipple's disease: The Duke connection. N. C. Med. J. 55:237-240, 1994.)*

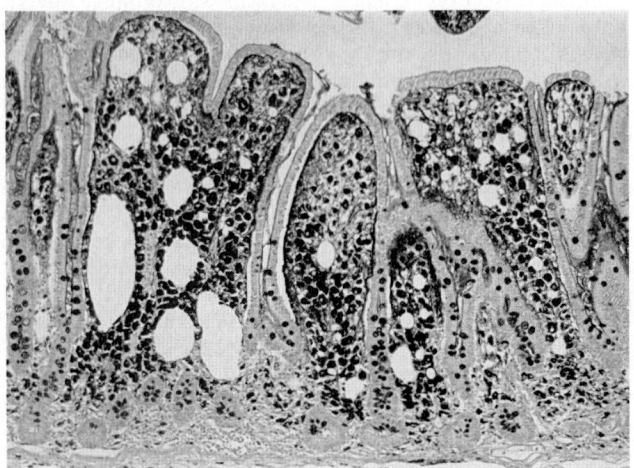

Figure 52–2 Light microscopic photograph of intestinal mucosa from the proximal jejunum of a patient with untreated Whipple disease. The villi appear blunted and swollen with periodic acid–Schiff-positive macrophages stuffed in the lamina propria. *(Courtesy of Kenneth P. Batts, M. D., Mayo Clinic, Rochester, MN; Jeffrey Craver, M. D., DePaul Health Center, Bridgeton, MO; and Milton J. Finegold, M. D., Baylor College of Medicine, Houston, TX.)*

additional surface membrane. This membrane is different from the outer membrane of gram-negative bacteria because it is thinner, has a symmetric profile, and has no periodic acid–Schiff-positive components.[67] After the bacillus has been ingested by the macrophage, the degenerative process that occurs leads to the accumulation of bacterial remnants that are resistant to degradation. The polysaccharide-containing portion of the bacillus wall correlates with these remnants, and its progressive accumulation leads to the typical intramacrophagic inclusions. These inclusions are periodic acid–Schiff-positive and one of the key features in the histologic diagnosis of Whipple disease.[67]

Biopsy specimens from the small intestine in patients with Whipple disease usually show characteristic changes. The intestinal villi are preserved,[24] but distortion of the architecture occurs.[27] A clubbed appearance of the intestinal villi[42] usually is present caused by the accumulation of foamy macrophages in the lamina propria.[24] The enterocytes may appear normal,[21,42] or they may show flattening and vacuolization and occasionally appear cuboidal (Fig. 52–2).[21,42] Lipid accumulation, with large fat drop-

lets within the lamina propria and smaller droplets within and between the absorptive cells, occurs commonly.[42] In some instances, prominent, dilated lacteals are present.[24] Ectors and associates[21] reported reduced and absent lactase and major histocompatibility complex class II (HLA-DR) expression. Lactase and major histocompatibility complex class II expression normalized within 3 to 6 months of starting antibiotic therapy.

The characteristic feature of Whipple disease is the presence of periodic acid–Schiff-positive, diastase-resistant macrophages.[32] These findings are not pathognomonic, however, because intestinal periodic acid–Schiff-positive macrophages can be found in other conditions,[24] such as histiocytosis, melanosis coli, and *Mycobacterium avium-intracellulare* infection, and even within macrophages in healthy individuals. The macrophages in Whipple disease do not stain with Ziehl-Neelsen.[21,32] A sickle-shaped appearance of the periodic acid–Schiff-positive granules often is present in the macrophages of patients with Whipple disease.[42]

Sieracki and Fine[66] observed systemic involvement in the autopsies of five patients with Whipple disease. The sickle-shaped, periodic acid–Schiff-positive macrophages were thought to be specific for Whipple disease, showing involvement of the entire gastrointestinal tract and the pancreas; diffuse involvement of the retroperitoneum and lymph nodes, the adrenals, the liver with sickle-form particles in Kupffer cells and in histiocytes, the brain, the heart, and the visceral pleura of the lungs; and minimal involvement of the genitourinary tract, skeletal muscles, and bone marrow. James and associates[36] examined the vessels of the gastrointestinal system and found abundant bacilli in the arteries of the small intestinal serosa and liver. They noted focal degeneration and fibrosis in the tunica media with arteritis and intimal proliferation. Rickman and coworkers[60] reported a case that confirmed the presence of *T. whipplei* in the vitreous of the eye.

T. whipplei produces a predominantly histiocytic inflammatory reaction, with infiltration by macrophages.[23] Noncaseating, epithelioid cell, sarcoid-like granulomata are located preferentially in peripheral lymph nodes and the liver.[16,23] These granulomata occasionally can be seen in different tissues, including three reports of granulomata in the intestinal tract.[23] Mesenteric lymph nodes often are strikingly enlarged.[13]

Electron microscopy can be useful, often revealing the presence of the rod-shaped bacterium (see Fig. 52–1).[28] Electron microscopy also shows intestinal macrophages containing bacteria with signs of lysis.[67] Silva and associates[67] described steps of a degradative process of the bacillus that starts with disorganization of the surface membrane and the thick outer wall. With the loss of intracellular material, bacterial ghosts composed of the three inner layers of the envelope are present. The two electron-dense layers of the cytoplasmic membrane become disorganized and solubilized, leaving the inner dense layer of the cell wall as the final bacterial remnant (Fig. 52–3).

CLINICAL MANIFESTATIONS

Whipple disease is viewed best as a multisystem illness. It usually manifests with arthralgias and then progresses to involve the gastrointestinal tract.[5] Malabsorption is the key feature of clinical disease, but no specific signs or symptoms for Whipple disease are known. Table 52–1 lists the major symptoms and signs of Whipple disease. In children, failure to thrive, malnutrition, and chronic diarrhea appear most frequently. Abdominal distention, abdominal pain, and generalized lymphadenopathy may be found.[2] Response to antibiotic treatment may be dramatic, with rapid weight gain and resolution of symptoms.[4]

GASTROINTESTINAL TRACT

One of the most common symptoms is weight loss, which is found in 65 to 100 percent of patients.[13,22,24,28,42] Weight loss may be the only symptom.[10] Diarrhea is reported in 60 to 85 percent of patients.[13,24,28,42] The diarrhea usually is watery or fatty in nature.[42] Several mechanisms have been proposed to explain the malabsorption and steatorrhea in Whipple disease.[24] Direct infection and secondary enterocyte dysfunction may prevent the esterification of fatty acids to triglycerides and inhibit the uptake of carbohydrates and amino acids. Blockage of transport of triglyceride-rich chylomicrons into lacteals may result from the deposition of foamy macrophages in the lamina propria. Lymphatic obstruction may occur by involvement of the mesenteric lymph nodes. Malabsorption and diarrhea tend to resolve within a few days after initiation of antibiotic treatment, whereas the lacteal dilation and periodic acid–Schiff-positive macrophages can remain for months to years. Occult gastrointestinal bleeding frequently is found, but melena and gross gastrointestinal bleeding are rare. Hematemesis was reported more recently.[11] Endoscopy revealed diffuse hemorrhagic duodenitis with bleeding on contact.

Abdominal pain is experienced by 60 percent of patients.[13,24,28,42] The pain is nonspecific, is generally epigastric, and may be worse after meals.[42] Abdominal pain and anorexia may lead to reduced calorie intake and further weight loss.[24] Abdominal distention occurs commonly and may be secondary to intra-abdominal lymphadenopathy or to thickening of loops of diseased intestine.[24,42] Ascites occasionally is seen and may be chylous, secondary to lymphatic obstruction.[10,28]

JOINTS

Arthralgia, the most frequent nongastrointestinal symptom in Whipple disease,[24,42] is present in 65 percent of adult cases.[42] Arthralgia may precede manifestation of gastrointestinal symptoms by many years or decades[24,39] and occurs less frequently in children. Generally, joint symptoms continue unchanged with the onset of gastrointestinal symptoms.[24] Acute migratory arthralgia or arthritis may last days or weeks[28,32,42] and may persist as the disease progresses. The involved joints, in decreasing order of frequency, are knees, ankles, hips, fingers, wrists, elbows, hands, and spine.[24] Examination may reveal joint pain, swelling, limited range of motion, and warmth.[63] Fever sometimes is present.[24] Spondylitis, with or without sacroiliitis, may develop.[4] Permanent joint destruction and deformity are uncommon occurrences, but can be severe.[24,63] Arthrocentesis may reveal an inflammatory arthritis, with cell counts of 6000 to 75,000, often with a polymorphonuclear leukocyte predominance.[24] Synovial biopsy may show periodic acid–Schiff-positive macrophages.[24]

CENTRAL NERVOUS SYSTEM

Whipple disease can be confined to the brain[61] but usually is accompanied by other manifestations.[28] CNS and neurologic manifestations, such as headache, diplopia, meningoencephalitis, depression, confusion, and personality changes, are uncommon manifestations[13,24,42] but may be significant.[13,24,27,42,51,53] Table 52–2 lists the spectrum of potential CNS involvement.

TABLE 52–1   Major Symptoms and Signs in Whipple Disease

Symptoms	Cases (%)
Weight loss	65-100
Chronic diarrhea	60-85
Arthralgia	65-80
Abdominal pain	60
Fever	10-55
Central nervous system–related complaints	10-40
Signs	
Malnutrition	90-95
Hypotension	70
Lymphadenopathy	55
Hyperpigmentation	45-55
Abdominal tenderness	50
Edema	30
Abdominal mass	20
Hepatomegaly	1-14
Splenomegaly	5-10
Ascites	8

Data from references 10, 23, 24, 35, 38.

TABLE 52–2   Central Nervous System Symptoms and Signs of Whipple Disease

Ataxia
Confusion
Convulsions
Dementia
Depression
Diplopia
Dizziness
Facial pain
Headache
Hearing loss
Hemiparesis
Hyperphagia
Hyperreflexia (± Babinski sign)
Incoordination
Lethargy, coma
Loss of vibratory and position sense
Meningoencephalitis
Mental and personality changes
Motor weakness
Muscle jerks and twitches
Muscle rigidity
Numbness
Nystagmus
Ophthalmoplegia
Papilledema
Polydipsia
Ptosis
Pupillary abnormalities
Sensory loss
Sleep disorders
Slurred speech
Stiff neck
Tinnitus
Visual difficulties (diplopia, blurring)

EYE

Indirect involvement of the CNS and direct involvement of the eye can produce visual problems.[24] Ophthalmoplegia and diplopia can occur with involvement of cranial nerves III, IV, and VI.[24] Reduced visual acuity and papilledema can occur with compromise of the optic nerve.[24] Numerous ophthalmologic findings, including vasculitis, vitritis, optic atrophy, uveitis, chorioretinitis, vitreous opacities, glaucoma, keratitis, retinal hemorrhages, disk edema, and lacrimal duct obstruction, have been reported.[24,75,76] Rickman and associates[60] reported a case of ocular disease without marked CNS or gastrointestinal disease.

SKIN

Hyperpigmentation of the skin in sun-exposed areas occurs in roughly half of cases.[27,42] The mechanism of hyperpigmentation is uncertain but is not related to adrenal insufficiency.[24] Subcutaneous nodules may be found and can reveal periodic acid–Schiff-positive macrophages and bacilli on electron microscopy.[31]

HEART

The heart frequently is involved in Whipple disease. Endocarditis, myocarditis, pericarditis, pancarditis, and coronary arteritis have been found.[24,46,74] A blood culture–negative endocarditis may be caused by Whipple disease.[24] Chronic aortic regurgitation is the most common clinical finding of endocardial involvement.[24] Pericarditis with polyserositis (pleuritis, peritonitis) has been found.[26] The abnormalities on electrocardiogram are nonspecific but include first-degree atrioventricular block, left ventricular hypertrophy, sinus tachycardia, left bundle branch block, intraventricular conduction delay, old inferior wall infarct, and short PR interval.[27] Sossai and associates[69] reported a case of regression of a right bundle branch block after treatment with antibiotics, but the block spontaneously recurred 2 years later.

SKELETAL MUSCLE

Skeletal muscle may be involved, diagnosed by electromyography or muscle biopsy.[71] Proximal muscle weakness occurs most commonly. Muscle biopsy reveals a nonspecific myopathy.

LYMPH NODES AND SPLEEN

Whipple disease may involve any lymph node in the body.[24] Mesenteric lymph nodes frequently are involved, and splenomegaly is found in 5 to 10 percent of cases.[42]

PULMONARY

Cough, pleuritic chest pain, and dyspnea have been reported.[72] Pleural involvement may appear as a pleural rub. Pleural adhesions and granulomata have been reported at autopsy.[4,72] Chest radiography often reveals pleural thickening, parenchymal shadowing, and elevation of the diaphragm.[72] Lung function tests may show decreased lung volumes.[72]

KIDNEY

Renal involvement in Whipple disease is rare.[24] Granulomata have been found, however, as has focal glomerulonephritis.[38]

HEMATOLOGIC

Anemia occurs commonly and usually is of a hypochromic, microcytic variety.[24,27,28] Macrocytic anemia caused by malabsorption of folate also may be seen. Leukocytosis, thrombocytosis,[52] and bone marrow involvement may be found.[57] Low serum iron concentration and an elevated erythrocyte sedimentation rate frequently are seen.[27] A single case of extraintestinal lymphoma in association with Whipple disease found at autopsy has been reported.[30]

DIAGNOSIS

Despite the successful culture of the organism in 2000,[56] no specific diagnostic tests have been developed. Anemia and low albumin probably are most common, being found in approximately 90 percent of patients. Low serum iron and folate concentrations are seen in approximately 30 percent of cases. Hypokalemia, hypocalcemia, low cholesterol and carotene, prolonged prothrombin time, and increased transaminases are less common findings. Elevated fecal fat is found in more than 90 percent of cases. The D-xylose malabsorption test result frequently is abnormal.

Barium x-ray studies of the small bowel may show marked thickening of the mucosal folds and separation of bowel loops, suggesting a malabsorptive disease. These findings usually resolve completely with successful antibiotic therapy. For CNS Whipple disease, characteristic abnormalities seen on computed tomography scans of the brain include atrophy, focal gray matter lesions, hydrocephalus, and white matter alterations.[73]

A key feature in the histologic diagnosis of Whipple disease is the accumulation of periodic acid–Schiff-positive, diastase-resistant macrophages in the lamina propria of the small intestine.[4,27,43] These findings are not pathognomonic, and infection with *Mycobacterium avium-intracellulare* must be excluded.[43] *T. whipplei* does not stain acid-fast,[43] whereas mycobacteria are identified readily. Small bowel involvement by *M. avium* complex can have endoscopic, histologic, and radiographic findings similar to those of Whipple disease.[55] Periodic acid–Schiff-positive macrophages occasionally can be seen in the mucosa of the large bowel and rectum in unrelated diseases, such as histiocytosis, and in benign conditions, such as melanosis coli and pneumatosis intestinalis.[43] Electron microscopy can confirm the diagnosis by visualization of the characteristic bacillus.[28,67]

Endoscopy of the small bowel may be helpful because characteristic lesions may be seen, and biopsy specimens can be obtained. No clear data suggest where the intestinal specimens should be taken[43] because intestinal involvement usually is patchy. Random biopsy samples of the small bowel are suggested, beginning at the ligament of Treitz.[47] Endoscopic findings include yellow-white plaques and an erythematous, erosive, friable mucosa.[29]

PCR amplification may be used to detect and identify bacterial pathogens. To set up a PCR, the only prerequisite information is the nucleotide sequences flanking each end of the target.[58] PCR has become an important method for establishing the diagnosis of Whipple disease. It may be especially helpful if the histopathologic examination findings are normal or in patients with unusual extraintestinal involvement. Specific identification of *T. whipplei* can be achieved by amplification of the 1321-base pair bacterial, 16S ribosomal RNA gene isolated from infected tissue.[59] Muller and associates[50] applied this PCR technique to show *T. whipplei* in peripheral blood mononuclear cells and cells derived from pleural effusion in a patient with Whipple disease. PCR techniques have been used to detect *T. whipplei* in erythrocytes,[41] cerebrospinal fluid,[6] and resected heart valves with infective endocarditis.[10,12,50]

Sloan and colleagues[68] reported in 2005 another real-time PCR method using a 213-base pair target sequence of the heat shock protein (hsp65) gene of *T. whipplei*. The sensitivity, specificity, and positive and negative values of this LightCycler real-time PCR were compared with the conventional 16S rRNA gene sequence PCR assay and were 98 percent (sensitivity), 99 percent (specificity), 94 percent (positive), and 100 percent (negative). The completion time of the LightCycler assay was approximately 5 hours, which was significantly less than the 2 to 3 days required for the traditional PCR assay.[68]

The diagnostic utility of PCR in Whipple disease is clear, but it cannot be taken as the sole basis for diagnosis. Ehrbar and associates[23] studied the specificity of PCR for *T. whipplei*. They performed elective gastroscopy on patients without known Whipple disease. PCR analysis was positive in 4.8 percent of duodenal biopsy specimens and 11.4 percent of gastric juice samples. Compared with the gold standard of histology and clinical signs, the specificity of PCR for *T. whipplei* was 95.2 percent for duodenal biopsy specimens and 88.6 percent for gastric juice. These findings suggest that *T. whipplei* or a closely related bacterium may be present in some people without known Whipple disease. Street and colleagues[70] detected *T. whipplei* DNA by PCR in the saliva of 35 percent of 40 healthy adults tested, which suggests that this organism can be an oral commensal.

TREATMENT

Antibiotics are the mainstay of therapy for Whipple disease.[13] In vitro antibiotic susceptibility testing using real-time PCR has identified penicillin, doxycycline, macrolides, ketolides, rifampin, aminoglycosides, teicoplanin, chloramphenicol, and trimethoprim-sulfamethoxazole (TMP-SMX) with activity.[7,8,45] Current antibiotic treatment strategies are empiric, based only on the accumulated anecdotal experience, although controlled trials are under way. Generally, response to antibiotics is good and often dramatic. Symptoms such as diarrhea quickly resolve, and weight gain is rapid. Several antibiotics that have been tried alone or in combination include chloramphenicol, penicillin, streptomycin, ampicillin, TMP-SMX, erythromycin, and doxycycline.[13,24,25,28] Keinath and associates[37] analyzed the antibiotic response rate of 88 patients with documented Whipple disease. Thirty-one patients experienced relapse, with a mean time to relapse of 4.2 years after initial diagnosis. CNS relapse occurred in 13 of 88, and all CNS and cardiac relapses were late (Table 52–3). In addition to diagnosis, PCR may prove useful in the monitoring of response to antibiotic therapy.[33,54]

All patients with Whipple disease should receive antibiotics that penetrate the blood-brain barrier.[37,62] Tetracycline and penicillin do not penetrate the blood-brain barrier well, unless the meninges are inflamed.[62] The preferred treatment in adults and children is TMP-SMX given orally twice a day for 1 year.[62] If the small bowel is involved, repeated small bowel biopsy is suggested at least 6 months to 1 year after treatment to document the disappearance of the bacillus. For patients who do not tolerate TMP-SMX, penicillin or ampicillin is recommended. Levy and associates[40] described a case of acquired resistance to TMP-SMX that responded to oral penicillin. Feurle and Marth[25] noted that TMP-SMX was more efficacious than tetracycline in inducing clinical remission of Whipple disease. They observed the development of aqueductal stenosis with hydrocephalus in a patient receiving TMP-SMX treatment, however, and indicated that even TMP-SMX is no safeguard against cerebral recurrence.

CNS relapse has a poor prognosis.[9,24,25,28,37] Feurle and Marth[25] suggested an experimental therapy for CNS recurrence with a highly active bactericidal compound, such as a third-generation cephalosporin, a quinolone, or intrathecal antibiotic therapy, that readily crosses the blood-brain barrier. In adult patients, Keinath and associates[37] recommended treatment with parenteral penicillin (1.2 million U daily) plus streptomycin (1 g daily) for 10 to 14 days, followed by TMP-SMX (1 double-strength tablet twice daily) for 1 year. Because of the extreme rarity of the occurrence of Whipple disease in children, prudent management dictates long-term surveillance after resolution of symptoms.

Because Whipple disease is a malabsorptive disorder, the patient's nutritional needs must be assessed carefully. Specific attention must be paid to replacement of any vitamin or mineral deficiencies. Iron, folate, vitamin D, and calcium typically are given until the steatorrhea resolves.

CONCLUSION

Whipple disease, despite its rarity, warrants diagnostic consideration in any child with failure to thrive, malnutrition, and chronic diarrhea. Such findings, especially with CNS manifestations or arthralgias, should raise the specter of Whipple disease. Diagnosis of Whipple disease can be made by histology, PCR, and clinical signs. PCR should not be the sole basis of diagnosis because *T. whipplei* DNA has been detected in samples from healthy individuals without Whipple disease.[64,70] Simple antibiotic treatment with oral TMP-SMX can result in dramatic resolution of symptoms, whereas failure to consider this rare disease can lead to catastrophic events.

TABLE 52–3   Treatment of Whipple Disease: Initial Antibiotic Regimen and Relapse

Antibiotics	No. Patients	Total No. Relapses	CNS Relapses
TCN* alone	49	21	9†
PCN + STM + TCN*	15	2	0
PCN/PCN*	8	3	2
PCN + STM	5	2	0
TMP-SMX*	3	0	0
Other	8	3	2
Totals	*88*	*31*	*13*

Oral therapy.
†*Includes two patients treated with TCN only in whom CNS relapse was the second relapse.*
CNS, central nervous system; PCN, penicillin; STM, streptomycin; TCN, tetracycline; TMP-SMX, trimethoprim-sulfamethoxazole.
Data from Keinath, R. D., Merrell, D. E., Vlietstra, R., et al.: Antibiotic treatment and relapse in Whipple's disease: Long-term follow-up of 88 patients. Gastroenterology 88:1867-1873, 1985.

REFERENCES

1. Ament, M. E.: Malabsorption syndromes in infancy and childhood. J. Pediatr. *81*:867-884, 1972.
2. Aust, C. H., and Smith, E. B.: Whipple's disease in a 3-month-old infant. Am. J. Clin. Pathol. *37*:66-74, 1962.
3. Bai, J. C., Mota, A. H., Maurino, E., et al.: Class I and class II HLA antigens in a homogeneous Argentinian population with Whipple's disease: Lack of association with HLA-B27. Am. J. Gastroenterol. *86*:992-994, 1991.
4. Barakat, A. Y., Bitar, J., and Nassar, V. H.: Whipple's disease in a seven-year-old child: Report of a case. Am. J. Proctol. *24*:312-315, 1973.
5. Bayless, T. M., and Knox, D. L.: Whipple's disease: A multisystemic infection. N. Engl. J. Med. *300*:920, 1979.
6. Birch, C. A.: Whipple's disease: George Hoyt Whipple (born 1878). Practitioner *212*(1270 Spec. No.):581-582, 1974.
7. Boulos, A., Rolain, J. M., Mallett, M. N., and Raoult, D.: Molecular evaluation of antibiotic susceptibility of *Tropheryma whipplei* in axenic medium. J. Antimicrob. Chemother. *55*:178, 2005.
8. Boulos, A., Rolain, J. M. and Raoult, D.: Antibiotic susceptibility of *Tropheryma whipplei* in MRC5 cells. Antimicrob. Agents Chemother. *48*:7477, 2004.

9. Brandle, M., Ammann, P., Spinas, G., et al.: Relapsing Whipple's disease presenting with hypopituitarism. Clin. Endocrinol. 50:399-403, 1999.
10. Bruni, R., and Massimo, L.: Descrizione un rarissimo caso di mallatia de Whipple nel eta pediatrica. Minerva Pediatr. 11:935-943, 1959.
11. Carney, P. W., Murugasu, A., and Duggan, A. E.: Whipple's disease: A rare cause of haematemesis and melaena. Eur. J. Gastroenterol. Hepatol. 17:779, 2005.
12. Celard, M., De Gevigney, G., Mosnier, S., et al.: Polymerase chain reaction analysis for the diagnosis of Tropheryma whippelii infective endocarditis in two patients with no previous evidence of Whipple's disease. Clin. Infect. Dis. 29:1348-1349, 1999.
13. Comer, G. M., Brandt, L. J., and Abissi, C. J.: Whipple's disease: A review. Am. J. Gastroenterol. 78:107-114, 1983.
14. Couper, R.: Whipple's disease: The bacillus unmasked. J. Pediatr. Gastroenterol. Nutr. 17:339-344, 1993.
15. DePra, M., Casagrande, A., and Guarino, M.: Whipple's disease: Apropos of a case demonstrating the existence of the congenital form. Minerva Pediatr. 26:1723-1743, 1974.
16. Desmet, V. J., and Geboes, K.: Review article: Liver lesions in inflammatory bowel disorders. J. Pathol. 151:247-255, 1987.
17. Desnues, B., Raoult, D., and Mege, J. L.: IL-16 is critical for Tropheryma whipplei replication in Whipples's disease. J. Immunol. 175:4575-4582, 2005.
18. Dobbins, W. O., III: Whipple's disease: An historical perspective. Q. J. M. 56:523-531, 1985.
19. Dobbins, W. O., III: HLA antigens in Whipple's disease. Arthritis Rheum. 30:102-105, 1987.
20. Dobbins, W. O., III: Whipple's disease. Mayo Clin. Proc. 63:623-624, 1988.
21. Ectors, N. L., Geboes, K. J., DeVos, R. M., et al.: Whipple's disease: A histological, immunocytochemical and electron microscopic study of the small intestinal epithelium. J. Pathol. 172:73-79, 1994.
22. Ectors, N., Geboes, K., Wynants, P., et al.: Granulomatous gastritis and Whipple's disease. Am. J. Gastroenterol. 87:509-515, 1992.
23. Ehrbar, H., Bauerfeind, P., Dutly, F., et al.: PCR-positive tests for Tropheryma whippelii in patients without Whipple's disease. Lancet 353:2214, 1999.
24. Feldman, M.: Southern Internal Medicine Conference: Whipple's disease. Am. J. Med. Sci. 291:56-67, 1986.
25. Feurle, G. E., and Marth, T.: An evaluation of antimicrobial treatment for Whipple's disease: Tetracycline versus trimethoprim-sulfamethoxazole. Dig. Dis. Sci. 39:1642-1648, 1995.
26. Finch, W.: Arthritis and the gut. Postgrad. Med. 86:229-235, 1989.
27. Flemin, J. L., Wiesner, R. H., and Shorter, R. G.: Whipple's disease: Clinical, biochemical and histopathologic features and assessment of treatment in 29 patients. Mayo Clin. Proc. 63:539-551, 1988.
28. Gaist, D., and Ladefoged, K.: Whipple's disease. Scand. J. Gastroenterol. 29:97-101, 1994.
29. Geboes, K., Ectors, N., Heidbuchel, H., et al.: Whipple's disease: Endoscopic aspects before and after therapy. Gastrointest. Endosc. 36:247-252, 1990.
30. Gillen, C. D., Coddington, R., Montieth, P. G., et al.: Extraintestinal lymphoma in association with Whipple's disease. Gut 34:1627-1629, 1993.
31. Good, A. E., Beals, T. F., Simmons, J. L., et al.: A subcutaneous nodule with Whipple's disease: Key to early diagnosis? Arthritis Rheum. 23:856-859, 1980.
32. Gran, J. T., and Husby, G.: Joint manifestations in gastrointestinal diseases. Dig. Dis. 10:295-312, 1992.
33. Gras, E., Matias, O., Guiu, X., et al.: PCR analysis in the pathological diagnosis of Whipple's disease: Emphasis on the extraintestinal involvement or atypical morphological features. J. Pathol. 188:318-321, 1999.
34. Hamilton, J. R.: Whipple disease. In Behrman, R. E., Vaughn, V., and Nelson, W. E. (eds.): Textbook of Pediatrics. Philadelphia, W. B. Saunders, 1983, p. 935.
35. Harvey, A. M.: Teacher and distinguished pupil: William Henry Welch and George Hoyt Whipple. Johns Hopkins Med. J. 135:178-190, 1974.
36. James, T. N., Bulkley, B. H., and Kent, S. P.: Case report: Vascular lesions of the gastrointestinal system in Whipple's disease. Am. J. Med. Sci. 288:125-129, 1984.
37. Keinath, R. D., Merrell, D. E., Vlietstra, R., et al.: Antibiotic treatment and relapse in Whipple's disease: Long-term follow-up of 88 patients. Gastroenterology 88:1867-1873, 1985.
38. Krauz, R. F.: Whipple's disease with cardiac and renal abnormalities. Arch. Intern. Med. 123:701-706, 1969.
39. Leirisalo-Repo, M.: Enteropathic arthritis, Whipple's disease, juvenile spondyloarthropathy and uveitis. Curr. Opin. Rheumatol. 6:385-390, 1994.
40. Levy, M., Poyart, C., Lamarque, D., et al.: Whipple's disease: Acquired resistance to trimethoprim-sulfamethoxazole. Am. J. Gastroenterol. 95:2390-2391, 2000.
41. Lowsky, R., Archer, G. L., Fyles, G., et al.: Brief report: Diagnosis of Whipple's disease by molecular analysis of peripheral blood. N. Engl. J. Med. 331:1343-1346, 1994.
42. Maizel, H., Ruffin, J. M., and Dobbins, W. O., III: Whipple's disease: A review of 19 patients from one hospital and a review of the literature since 1950. Medicine (Baltimore) 49:175-205, 1970.
43. Marbet, V. A., Stalder, G. A., and Gyr, K. E.: Whipple's disease: A multisystemic disease with changing presentation. Dig. Dis. 4:119-128, 1986.
44. Marth, T., Roux, M., VonHerbay, A., et al.: Persistent reduction of complement receptor 3 L-chain expressing mononuclear blood cells and transient

inhibitory serum factors in Whipple's disease. Clin. Immunol. Immunopathol. 72:217-226, 1994.
45. Masselot, F., Boulos, A., Maurin, M., et al.: Molecular evaluation of antibiotic susceptibility: Tropheryma whipplei paradigm. Antimicrob. Agents Chemother. 47:1658, 2003.
46. McAllister, H. A., and Fenoglio, J. J.: Cardiac involvement in Whipple's disease. Circulation 52:152-156, 1975.
47. Moorthy, S., Nolley, G., and Hermos, J. A.: Whipple's disease with minimal intestinal involvement. Gut 18:152-155, 1977.
48. Morgan, A. D.: The first recorded case of Whipple's disease. Gut 2:370-372, 1961.
49. Morgenegg, S., Dutly, F., and Altwegg, M.: Cloning and sequencing of a part of the heat shock protein 65 gene (hsp 65) of Tropheryma whippelii and its use for detection in clinical specimens by PDR. J. Clin. Microbiol. 38:2248-2253, 2000.
50. Muller, C., Stain, C., and Burghuber, O.: Tropheryma whippelii in peripheral blood mononuclear cells and cells of pleural effusion. Lancet 341:701, 1993.
51. Naegeli, B., Bannwart, F., and Bertel, O.: An uncommon cause of recurrent strokes: Tropheryma whippelii endocarditis. Stroke 31:2002-2003, 2000.
52. Nuzum, C. T., Sandler, R. S., and Paulk, H. T.: Thrombocytosis in Whipple's disease. Gastroenterology 80:1465-1467, 1981.
53. Ojeda, E., Redondo, J., Lapaza, J., et al.: Enfermedad de Whipple: Manifestaciones neurologicas y revision de los casos publicados en la literature nacional. Rev. Clin. Esp. 183:1465-1467, 1981.
54. Petrides, P., Muller-Hocker, J., Fredricks, D., et al.: PCR analysis of T. whippelii DNA in a case of Whipple's disease: Effect of antibiotics and correlation with histology. Am. J. Gastroenterol. 93:1579-1582, 1998.
55. Poorman, J. C., and Katon, R. M.: Small bowel involvement by Mycobacterium avium complex in a patient with AIDS: Endoscopic, histologic and radiographic similarities to Whipple's disease. N. Engl. J. Med. 342:620-625, 2000.
56. Raoult, D., Birg, M. L., Scola, B. L., et al.: Cultivation of the bacillus of Whipple's disease. N. Engl. J. Med. 342:620-625, 2000.
57. Rausing, A.: Bone marrow biopsy in diagnosis of Whipple's disease. Acta Med. Scand. 193:5-8, 1973.
58. Relman, D. A.: Whipple's disease: A disorder associated with a visible but uncultured bacillus. J. Infect. Dis. 168:1-8, 1993.
59. Relman, D. A., Schmidt, T. M., MacDermott, R. P., et al.: Identification of the uncultured bacillus of Whipple's disease. N. Engl. J. Med. 327:293-300, 1992.
60. Rickman, L. S., Freeman, W. R., Green, W. R., et al.: Brief report: Uveitis caused by Tropheryma whippelii (Whipple's bacillus). N. Engl. J. Med. 332:363-366, 1995.
61. Romanul, F. C. A., Radvany, J., and Rosales, R. K.: Whipple's disease confined to the brain: A case studied clinically and pathologically. J. Neurol. Neurosurg. Psychiatry 40:901-909, 1977.
62. Ryser, R. J., Locksley, R. M., Eng, S. C., et al.: Reversal of dementia associated with Whipple's disease by trimethoprim-sulfamethoxazole, drugs that penetrate the blood-brain barrier. Gastroenterology 86:745-752, 1984.
63. Scheib, J. S., and Quinet, R. J.: Whipple's disease with axial and peripheral joint destruction. South. Med. J. 83:684-687, 1990.
64. Schneemann, M., Schoedon, G.: Whipples's DNA is not Whipple's disease. J. Clin. Microbiol. 43:5414, 2005.
65. Schoeden, G., Goldenberger, D., Forrer, R., et al.: Deactivation of macrophages with interleukin-4 is the key to the isolation of Tropheryma whippelii. J. Infect. Dis. 176:672-677, 1997.
66. Sieracki, J. C., and Fine, G.: Whipple's disease: Observations on systemic involvement, II: Gross and histologic observations. Arch. Pathol. 67:81-93, 1959.
67. Silva, M. T., Macedo, P. M., and Moura Nunes, J. F.: Ultrastructure of bacilli and the bacillary origin of the macrophagic inclusions in Whipple's disease. J. Gen. Microbiol. 131:1001-1013, 1985.
68. Sloan, L. M., Rosenblatt, J. E., and Cockerill, F. J., III: Detection of Tropheryma whipplei DNA in clinical specimens by LightCycler Real-Time PCR. J. Clin. Microbiol. 43:3516-3518, 2005.
69. Sossai, P., DeBoni, M., and Cielo, R.: The heart and Whipple's disease. Int. J. Cardiol. 23:275-276, 1989
70. Street, S., Donoghue, H. D., and Neild, G. H.: Tropheryma whippelii DNA in saliva of healthy people. Lancet 354:1178-1179, 1999.
71. Swash, M., Schwartz, M. S., Vandenberg, M. J., et al.: Myopathy in Whipple's disease. Gut 18:800-804, 1977.
72. Symmons, D. P. N., Shepard, A. N., Boardman, P. L., et al.: Pulmonary manifestations of Whipple's disease. Q. J. M. 56:497-504, 1985.
73. Tan, T., Vogel, H., Tharp, B. R., et al.: Presumed central nervous system Whipple's disease in a child: Case report. Clin. Infect. Dis. 20:883-889, 1995.
74. Tyor, M. P.: Whipple's disease: The Duke connection. N. C. Med. J. 55:237-240, 1994.
75. Vine, A. K.: Retinal vasculitis. Semin. Neurol. 14:354-360, 1994.
76. von Weizsacker, F., and Blum, H. E.: Impact of molecular biology in gastroenterology. Digestion 54:125-129, 1993.
77. Whipple, G. H.: A hitherto undescribed disease characterized anatomically by deposits of fat and fatty acids in the intestinal mesenteric lymphatic tissues. Johns Hopkins Hosp. Bull. 18:382-391, 1907.
78. Woese, C. R.: Bacterial evolution. Microbiol. Rev. 51:221-271, 1987.

LIVER DISEASES

HEPATITIS

53
Gail J. Demmler-Harrison

Hepatitis, or inflammation of the liver, may be caused by a variety of infectious agents. Some agents, such as hepatitis A, B, C, D, and E viruses, are primarily hepatotropic and produce disease almost exclusively in the liver, whereas other agents, such as cytomegalovirus (CMV), Epstein-Barr virus (EBV), adenovirus, and the hemorrhagic fever viruses, produce hepatitis as part of a systemic or disseminated illness. With many infectious agents, hepatitis may be subclinical or silent, with very few, if any, signs or symptoms manifested in the patient. Symptomatic or clinical hepatitis may be acute or chronic at initial evaluation, and it may be associated with mild to severe or even fulminant or fatal disease.[64] Children of all ages, from neonates to young adults, both immunocompetent and immunocompromised, may contract infectious hepatitis, and the age and immune status of the host, as well as the history of exposure, may provide clues to identification of the most likely etiologic agent. Noninfectious causes such as autoimmune, genetic, and metabolic disorders, as well as exposure to toxins and idiosyncratic or hypersensitivity reactions to medications or drugs, also are important causes of hepatitis in children. Hepatic steatosis associated with childhood obesity and type 2 diabetes is a growing public health concern for our youth. Severe hypoxia also may damage the liver.

A general approach to an infant or child with hepatitis or hepatic dysfunction, from the perspective of an infectious disease specialist, is presented in this chapter. Detailed information regarding the diagnosis and management of each particular pathogen can be found in the respective chapters in the section of this textbook dedicated to infections with specific microorganisms.

HISTORY

Originally described by Hippocrates in the second century BCE, hepatitis has an ancient historical perspective. The earliest descriptions of outbreaks of hepatitis in the ancient world most likely involved hepatitis A virus (HAV), and it was known as *epidemic jaundice* and *catarrhal jaundice*, or *acute yellow atrophy of the liver* if the disease was severe or fulminant.[21] The earliest recorded outbreak in the United States occurred in Norfolk, Virginia, in 1812.[10] During wartimes, outbreaks of "camp jaundice" or "field jaundice" occurred and probably were caused by HAV, yellow fever, or leptospirosis. Not until 1973 was the cause of "infectious hepatitis" determined to be a 27-nm, nonenveloped viral particle, originally designated enterovirus 72 and now known as HAV.[39] Infection with hepatitis B virus (HBV) has a relatively more recent history. It probably was described originally in the late 1880s in an epidemiologic study published by Luerman in 1885 in Germany, where an outbreak of hepatitis in shipyard and warehouse workers who received smallpox vaccine contaminated with human material was associated with a prolonged form of hepatitis.[74] Other outbreaks of "serum hepatitis" associated with percutaneous therapies, such as gold used for rheumatoid arthritis or contaminated vaccines that were stabilized with

human serum have been described.[1,13,58] In the early 1970s, the complete HBV infectious particle identified in serum was called the *Dane particle*, and a specific serologic marker, originally called the *Australian (Au) antigen* because it was discovered first in the blood of an Australian aborigine and later designated hepatitis B surface antigen (HBsAg), also was characterized and subsequently used to diagnose serum hepatitis caused by HBV.[15,73,109] Not long thereafter, in the mid-1970s, parenterally transmitted "non-A, non-B hepatitis" was described and subsequently identified in 1989 as hepatitis C virus (HCV).[19,59,110,128] The 1970s also marked the discovery of hepatitis delta virus (HDV), a "defective helper virus" that replicates only in the presence of HBV and is associated with chronic or fulminant hepatitis.[114,115] In the 1990s, another enterically transmitted non-A, non-B hepatitis virus was found to be associated with outbreaks of infectious hepatitis in developing parts of the world.[11,52] It was characterized originally as a calicivirus-like particle and subsequently named hepatitis E virus (HEV).[113] No doubt, as our medical knowledge evolves, even more viruses and other infectious agents associated with hepatitis will be discovered and named.

CLINICAL MANIFESTATIONS AND EVALUATION

PATIENT HISTORY

The clinical approach to evaluating and managing a child with hepatitis includes careful attention to the age when first seen; evolution of the initial signs and symptoms; history of exposure to potential pathogens, toxins, or medications; the presence of underlying conditions; and a family history of liver or metabolic disorders. Initial symptoms in older children with acute hepatitis are nonspecific and may include fever, vomiting, poor feeding, anorexia or aversion to specific foods, indigestion, change in taste and smell, lethargy and malaise, mild weight loss, dark urine, pale stool, or jaundice, often with pruritus. Abdominal pain also is a common complaint, and it usually is mild, dull, or aching in quality; located in the right upper quadrant; and unaffected by meals, body position, or bowel movements. Often, an antecedent viral syndrome or "flulike" illness is noted 7 to 14 days before the onset of hepatitis. Rarely, a "serum sickness–like syndrome" may occur at the onset of the illness, before jaundice occurs, and is characterized by fever, rash, and arthritis. In contrast, neonates rarely have signs and symptoms from infection with the hepatotropic viruses and are more likely to have clinical disease with agents that cause congenital or perinatal infection, such as CMV, herpes simplex virus (HSV), rubella virus, parvovirus B19, or *Treponema pallidum*, especially if extrahepatic signs such as splenomegaly, skin lesions, microcephaly, or hearing loss are present. Newborns and young infants may become seriously ill with disseminated HSV, enteroviruses, or adenoviruses and show signs of acute, massive hepatocellular necrosis. A history of administration of blood products at any age suggests hepatitis B, C, or D or CMV, whereas previous attendance at summer camp or an institutional environment suggests HAV. A history of administration of antimicrobials such as the antifungal azoles, antibiotics, or isoniazid or medications such as acetaminophen suggests drug-induced hepatitis.[133] Exposure of older children to feral kittens is suggestive of infection with *Bartonella henselae* or *Toxoplasma gondii*. Children receiving cancer chemotherapy may have drug-induced hepatitis, and those who have experienced prolonged neutropenia may have fungal disease of the liver. Children with fulminant hepatitis are critically ill and initially may have persistent fever, protracted nausea and vomiting, severe abdominal pain, worsening jaundice, fluid retention with ascites, impaired clotting, and encephalopathy with seizures or coma. Patients with chronic hepatitis, on the other hand, often are clinically asymptomatic unless complications such as cirrhosis, chronic liver failure, or primary hepatocellular carcinoma develop.

PHYSICAL FINDINGS

Physical examination of a child with hepatitis should focus on the abdomen and liver, but it also should include a careful evaluation for extrahepatic manifestations of systemic disease. Tender hepatomegaly, with or without ascites, scleral icterus, and jaundiced skin, often is noted on physical examination of patients with acute hepatitis. Percussion or tapping over the right lower part of the thorax may produce right upper quadrant pain. Fever may or may not be present. Extrahepatic physical findings associated with the hepatotropic viruses, especially HAV, HBV, and HCV, include systemic vasculitis with rash or urticaria, polyarthralgia, and polyarthritis, similar to serum sickness or polyarteritis nodosa. A generalized papular rash, called *infantile papular acrodermatitis* (also known as *Gianotti disease* or *Gianotti-Crosti syndrome*), may accompany HBV infection, especially in young children. Rarely, a patient with acute viral hepatitis may exhibit the Raynaud phenomenon, bullous lesions, or erythema nodosa. Skin excoriations may be present if the jaundice-associated pruritus is severe, and older children and adolescents may have vascular spiders or exacerbation of acne. A child who also has conjunctivitis, pneumonitis, and a maculopapular rash may have a disseminated adenoviral disease. Generalized lymphadenopathy accompanied by pharyngitis and splenomegaly, in contrast, suggests systemic infection with CMV or EBV. Idiosyncratic reactions involving the liver may occur at any time; however, drug-related hypersensitivity hepatitis occurs 1 to 5 weeks after exposure to the agent and usually is accompanied by rash and fever on examination and evidence of nephritis, eosinophilia, and neutropenia. Neonates with acute fulminant hepatitis from disseminated infection with HSV, enteroviruses, or adenoviruses will have fever or hypothermia, respiratory distress, coagulopathy, and a sepsis-like syndrome. Physical examination of a child with fulminant hepatitis and liver failure may actually reveal a small liver or one that is shrinking in size and a child who is confused or has had personality changes. As hepatic failure ensues, the patient may be deeply jaundiced and encephalopathic or comatose, with hyperreflexia, decerebrate posturing, involuntary movements, and asterixis. A distinctive sweetish smell (also called *fetor hepaticus*) from the patient also may be appreciated by an astute observer. Physical examination of a child with chronic hepatitis, on the other hand, may be normal or reveal minimal enlargement of the liver. If the child is obese, fatty infiltration of the liver should be considered as a cause of liver inflammation and dysfunction.

LABORATORY DIAGNOSIS

Laboratory evaluation of a child with acute hepatitis should include a complete blood count and differential, urinalysis, tests of hepatic function, and specific serologic tests, cultures, or detection assays for specific pathogens of interest according to the patient's history or physical findings. In patients with severe or fulminant hepatitis or hepatic failure, serum albumin, electrolyte, and glucose levels also should be determined, in addition to performing a coagulopathy panel with fibrinogen, as well as determination of blood ammonia if encephalopathy is present. In many forms of viral hepatitis, the white blood cell count may be low, usually between 3000 and 4000/mm³. Atypical lymphocytes also may be seen. Eosinophilia suggests a drug hypersensitivity reaction. If significant leukocytosis is present, sepsis or fulminant hepatitis should be considered. Urinalysis may reveal dark urine and the presence of urobilinogen. In a neonate with jaundice or hepatic dysfunction, an infectious agent such as a gram-negative enteric organism (*Escherichia coli*, for example) may be identified in urine or blood, or evidence of viral infection may be detected in blood, cerebrospinal fluid (CSF), or body secretions. Hematuria with casts or other signs of nephritis in an older child may signify an autoimmune disorder or a drug-induced process as the cause of the hepatitis. Liver enzymes, especially aspartate aminotransferase and alanine aminotransferase, will be elevated in all patients with acute hepatitis, and frequently they are elevated before the onset of clinical symptoms occurs. Most forms of acute hepatitis will be accompanied by elevations of 500 IU/mL or greater. A neonate, however, with transaminase levels higher than 1000 IU/mL is likely to have a potentially life-threatening infection with HSV, enteroviruses, or adenoviruses. Similarly, older children with fulminant hepatitis or hepatic necrosis may have significantly elevated transaminase levels, which gradually fall to less than 500 IU/mL as the disease progresses. Prothrombin levels usually are normal in cases of uncomplicated acute viral hepatitis, but if they become prolonged, severe liver necrosis or fulminant hepatitis should be considered. Levels of alkaline phosphatase and gamma-glutamyltranspeptidase will be elevated in patients with acute hepatitis as well. Serum bilirubin, both conjugated and unconjugated, may be elevated, but it is rarely higher than 4 mg/dL unless fulminant hepatitis with hepatic failure is present. Exceptions to this rule include patients with underlying hemolytic states such as glucose-6-dehydrogenase deficiency or sickle-cell disease; such patients may exhibit marked jaundice and high indirect hyperbilirubinemia, even if the viral hepatitis otherwise is mild. Serum albumin often is normal in acute hepatitis, but it may be low in chronic hepatitis. Some patients will have low levels of nonspecific autoantibodies, such as an elevated homogeneous pattern of antinuclear antibodies, decreased complement levels, or false-positive VDRL (Venereal Disease Research Laboratory) test reactions. The erythrocyte sedimentation rate usually is normal or slightly increased in acute viral hepatitis.

Laboratory investigation to determine the specific etiology of the patient's hepatitis includes detection of HBsAg and anti–hepatitis B core antigen (HBcAg; IgM) in serum, anti-HAV (IgM) in serum and HAV RNA in saliva and serum by polymerase chain reaction (PCR), anti-HCV and HCV in serum by PCR, and anti-HDV antibody (especially if the hepatitis is fulminant) and anti-HEV antibody (if the travel history suggests exposure).[3] Many of the non-hepatitis viruses may be identified by serologic tests that detect virus-specific IgM antibody or by fourfold rises in viral-specific IgG antibody. However, isolation of the specific viral agent in cell culture or detection of viral nucleic acid by PCR in blood, CSF, body fluids such as saliva or stool, or liver tissue provides the most convincing evidence. Bacterial pathogens may be detected by culture or, for agents associated with granulomatous hepatitis, such as *Brucella* and *Mycobacterium*, by culture, serology, or appropriate skin tests. Non-infectious causes such as autoimmune hepatitis may be identified by persistent hypergammaglobulinemia and the presence of autoantibodies, such as positive lupus erythematosus cell tests and anti–liver-kidney-microsome antibodies (anti-LKM). Metabolic diseases may cause hepatic dysfunction that may mimic acute hepatitis. Laboratory tests that may help differentiate these diseases include sweat chloride or genetic screening for cystic fibrosis, α_1-antitrypsin levels, serum amino acids, and urine-reducing substances and organic acids for metabolic diseases. Serum ceruloplasmin and urine copper levels may help establish the laboratory diagnosis of Wilson disease. Acute hepatotoxicity from overdose of acetaminophen may be predicted from elevated acetaminophen levels. Anatomic causes of hepatic dysfunction, such as biliary atresia in infants and hepatic tumors or steatosis in older children, usually require diagnostic imaging such as ultrasound or liver biopsy for diagnosis.

INFECTIOUS CAUSES

VIRUSES

Hepatitis Viruses

Five hepatotropic viruses are known to cause infectious viral hepatitis in children: hepatitis A, B, C, D, and E. (Table 53–1).

HEPATITIS A VIRUS. HAV is a member of the *Picornaviridae* family and formerly was known as enterovirus 72.[78] A small, nonenveloped RNA virus with icosahedral symmetry (Fig. 53–1), HAV is transmitted by the fecal-oral route, and transplacental transmission has been documented on rare occasion.[27,44] It is transmitted most commonly among young and school-aged children receiving care in group settings such as daycare, summer camp, schools, and institutions.[60] The incubation period generally is 30 days but ranges from 15 to 50 days. HAV infection in young children often is asymptomatic, and usually outbreaks in children are recognized first when symptoms occur in adult caretakers. Older children are more likely to have the classic symptoms of nausea, malaise, jaundice, and tender hepatomegaly. Rarely, HAV causes fulminant hepatitis. Acute infection with HAV is diagnosed serologically by detecting the presence of HAV IgM antibody in serum. No licensed, specific antiviral treatment is available. However, prevention may be accomplished by passive immunization with immune globulin or active immunization with licensed inactivated HAV vaccines.

HEPATITIS B VIRUS. HBV, also known as *Dane particle* and *hepadnavirus type 1*, is a member of the *Hepadnaviridae* family and is a DNA virus that is a 42-nm, nonenveloped spherical particle (Fig. 53–2).[78] It is transmitted through close contact with blood or blood-contaminated secretions, objects, or products.[44] It also has been transmitted by organ transplantation, intravenous drug use, and sexual contact. The incubation period is prolonged, usually 90 days, with ranges of 45 to 160 days reported. Neonates may acquire HBV vertically from mothers who are actively infected with HBV, especially if the mothers also are positive for hepatitis B e antigen (HBeAg). Whereas newborns rarely are symptomatic, children and adults may have mild to moderate symptoms of acute hepatitis or progress to fulminant or fatal disease. HBV also is a common cause of chronic hepatitis in children. Chronic hepatitis will develop in approximately 10 percent of older children and adults infected with HBV; the figure rises to approximately 30 percent if the infection occurs during infancy or early childhood and reaches a striking 90 to 95 percent in infants born to infected mothers who are HBeAg-positive. Acute hepatitis B is diagnosed serologically by the presence of HBsAg or IgM antibody to HBcAg. HBV DNA also may be detected and quantified in serum by PCR during acute hepatitis. Individuals with HBeAg in their serum are highly infectious. Diagnosis of chronic hepatitis B requires a combination of

TABLE 53-1 Causes of Hepatitis in Children

Infectious
Viral
Primary hepatotropic
 Hepatitis A virus
 Hepatitis B virus
 Hepatitis C virus
 Hepatitis D virus
 Hepatitis E virus
DNA viruses
 Adenovirus
 Cytomegalovirus
 Epstein-Barr virus
 Erythrovirus (human parvovirus B-19)
 Herpes B virus
 Herpes simplex viruses 1 and 2
 Human herpesviruses 6, 7, and 8
 Varicella-zoster virus
RNA viruses
 Enteroviruses
 Hemorrhagic fever viruses
 Human immunodeficiency virus
 Measles virus
 Rubella virus
 Syncytial giant-cell hepatitis

Bacterial
Atypical mycobacteria
Bacille Calmette-Guérin (BCG)
Bacillus cereus toxin
Bartonella henselae and *Bartonella quintana*
Brucella species
Listeria monocytogenes
Mycobacterium tuberculosis
Sepsis syndrome with cholestatic jaundice
Urinary tract infection in neonates
Spirochetes
 Leptospira species
 Treponema pallidum
Rickettsiae
 Coxiella burnetii
Parasites
 Ascaris lumbricoides
 Entamoeba histolytica
 Plasmodium species
 Toxoplasma gondii

Fungal
Aspergillus species
Candida species
Cryptococcus neoformans
Histoplasma capsulatum

Non-infectious
Anoxic liver damage
Autoimmune hepatitis
Biliary atresia
Drugs and toxins
Hemophagocytic syndrome
Histiocytosis
Kawasaki disease
Lymphoma
Metabolic and genetic disorders
Obesity with hepatic steatosis (fatty infiltration)
Reye syndrome
Sarcoidosis
Sickle-cell crisis
Toxic shock syndrome
Tumors

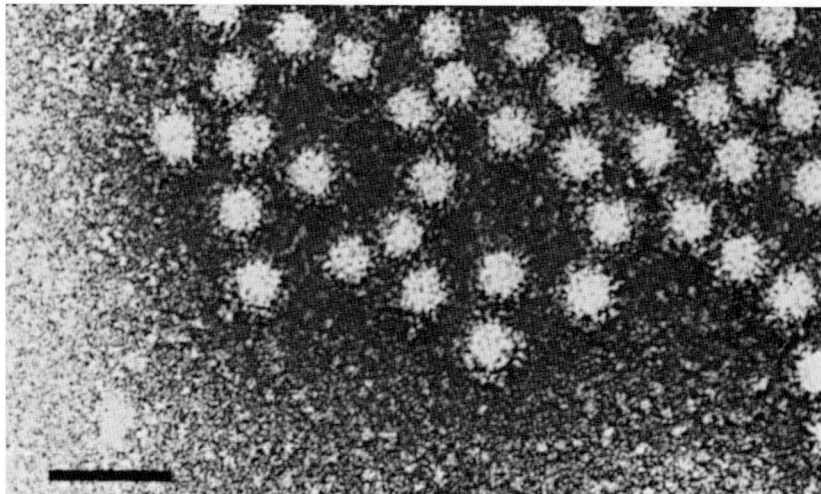

Figure 53–1 Twenty-seven-nanometer hepatitis A virus (HAV) isolated from the stool filtrate of a patient with acute HAV infection. The HAV particles are aggregated by convalescent serum containing anti-HAV antibodies. The *line* represents 100 nm. (*Courtesy of Dr. Jules Dienstag, taken at the Laboratory of Infectious Diseases, National Institute of Allergy and Infectious Diseases, National Institutes of Health, Department of Health, Education, and Welfare, Bethesda, MD.*)

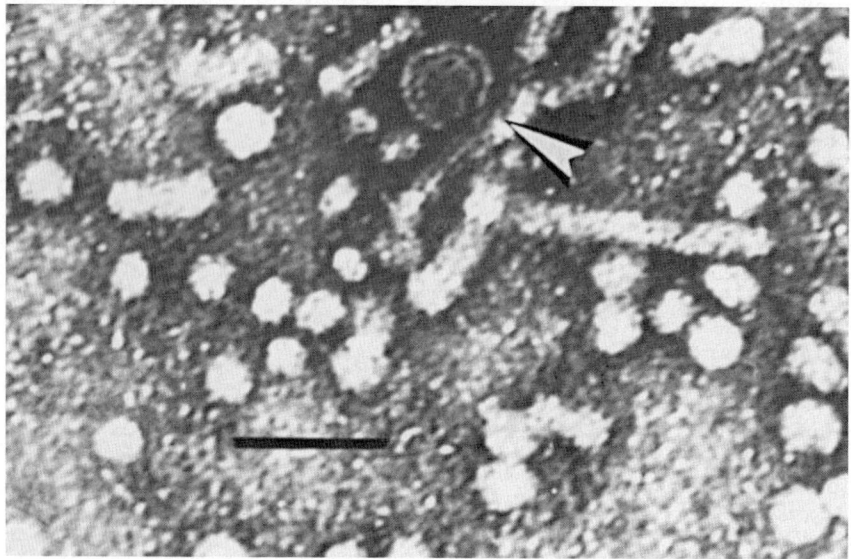

Figure 53–2 Electron micrograph of hepatitis B virus particles. Most particles are 20 to 25 nm in diameter and consist of both spheres and tubules. A larger, 42-nm Dane particle also is present (*arrowhead*). Hepatitis B surface antigen determinants are present on the surface of all three forms.

persistent clinical symptoms and laboratory abnormalities, persistence of specific serologic markers such as HBsAg over a period of at least 6 months, and histopathologic characteristics on liver biopsy. Primary hepatocellular carcinoma also is a long-term complication of infection with HBV. Successful resolution of infection with HBV is marked serologically by the presence of antibody to HBsAg. No licensed specific antiviral therapy is available for acute hepatitis caused by HBV; however, lamivudine and interferon-α may be helpful in treating chronic hepatitis. Famciclovir also has documented activity against HBV and has been used clinically in certain patients. Liver transplantation has been attempted in patients with end-stage HBV-associated cirrhosis, with variable results. Prevention is achieved by passive immunization with hepatitis B immune globulin (HBIG) and active immunization with licensed recombinant vaccines.[57]

HEPATITIS C VIRUS. HCV is a member of the *Flaviviridae* family. It is a small RNA virus with multiple genotypes that appear to have a variable effect on the development of clinical disease and response to antiviral therapy. It is transmitted most commonly to children and adolescents who have been exposed to blood products, clotting factor concentrates before 1987, hemodialysis, organ transplantation, intravenous drug use,

cocaine snorting, or tattoos and piercing procedures performed at parlors that do not practice sterile technique. Perinatal transmission from an HCV-seropositive mother to her infant also occurs at an estimated risk of 5 percent, especially if the mother is HCV RNA–positive at delivery.[92,97] Infection with HCV usually does not cause acute hepatitis; however, chronic hepatitis develops in more than 50 percent of children infected with HCV.[24] In adults, cirrhosis, end-stage liver failure, and hepatocellular carcinoma also may develop. Infection with HCV is diagnosed serologically by detecting the presence of HCV IgG antibody and by detecting and quantifying HCV RNA by PCR.[69] Treatment with ribavirin plus interferon may be beneficial in some patients. Liver transplantation may be performed in patients with end-stage liver disease. Currently, no biologic products or vaccines are licensed for prevention of infection with HCV.

HEPATITIS D VIRUS. HDV, also known as the *delta agent, delta virus, helper virus,* and *defective virus,* is a small, 37-nm RNA virus that requires the presence of HBV, especially HBsAg, to replicate.[107] HDV can co-infect a patient simultaneously or subsequent to infection with HBV. Like HBV, HDV is acquired by exposure to blood products or clotting factors, intravenous drug use, or sexual contact. It also may be transmitted by liver transplantation, and vertical transmission has been reported. Infection with HDV occurs more commonly in Europe, South America, Africa, and the Middle East and appears to be less common in the United States. The incubation period after superinfection occurs is 1 to 2 months, but it is similar to that for HBV (90 days) if co-infection occurs simultaneously. Co-infection with HDV is associated with more severe disease or progression to fulminant hepatitis in HBV-infected patients.[107] Laboratory diagnosis includes detection of antibody to HDV (anti-HDV) by commercial assays and reference laboratories that can detect IgM-specific HDV antibody, HDV antigen, and RNA by PCR. No specific antiviral therapy is available for HDV. Because HDV cannot be transmitted to or infect humans without HBV, prevention of HBV infection by vaccination prevents the acquisition of HDV infection. HDV co-infection of individuals already infected with HBV, however, cannot be prevented by any licensed biologic product or vaccine.

HEPATITIS E VIRUS. HEV is a small RNA virus that is transmitted by the fecal-oral route.[11,113] HEV infection in U.S. residents is a rare occurrence, but it may be a common cause of acute, self-limited viral hepatitis in developing countries and has been linked to outbreaks associated with contaminated water supplies.[52,101,108] The incubation period is unknown. HEV appears to cause a mild to moderate, acute hepatitis, especially in adults, and may have a high case-fatality in pregnant women. Similar to HAV, HEV does not appear to cause chronic hepatitis. Laboratory diagnosis is established by detection of IgG and IgM antibody to HEV in serum or detection of HEV RNA by PCR in serum or feces performed in reference laboratories or the Centers for Disease Control and Prevention (CDC). No antiviral agent is licensed for HEV, and prevention by immunoprophylaxis is not available. However, the results of clinical trials evaluating the efficacy of a new HEV vaccine may be available soon.

Herpesviruses

Herpesviruses are large DNA viruses with icosahedral symmetry and a glycoprotein envelope, and they share the biologic properties of latency and reactivation. Infections with this family of viruses, the *Herpesviridae*, may be primary or recurrent. All the human herpesviruses (HHVs) and one of the primate herpesviruses (herpes B virus) can cause acute hepatitis during the course of a systemic illness, but primary hepatitis with these viral agents is an unusual event.[42]

HERPES SIMPLEX VIRUS. HSV-1 and HSV-2 most often cause mucocutaneous vesicles or ulcers, and dissemination usually occurs during periods of relative immune compromise, such as pregnancy, the neonatal period, malnutrition, congenital or acquired immunodeficiency syndromes, or organ transplantation. Transient, subclinical hepatitis may occur during acute mucocutaneous HSV disease, but fulminant hepatitis with hepatic necrosis rarely has been documented in a normal host.[38,45,65,83] A special exception to this observation is HSV-associated primary hepatic necrosis and disseminated HSV disease in pregnant women.[45] Most cases occur during the late second or early third trimester, and most, but not all, cases are associated with primary infection with HSV-2.[132,134] Obvious skin lesions may not be present. This disease is associated with high mortality rates in both the mother and infant. Neonates, both term and preterm, are at risk for the development of neonatal HSV hepatitis as part of a disseminated HSV disease that includes viral sepsis–like syndrome, coagulopathy, pneumonitis with respiratory distress, and meningoencephalitis.[62] Skin lesions often are absent in this form of HSV disease. Neonatal HSV hepatitis develops most often in the child's first 2 weeks of life, and transaminase levels may be more than a thousand times higher than normal. Recipients of solid organ,

bone marrow, and stem cell transplants may have HSV infection with dissemination within the first 3 weeks after undergoing transplantation, most often as a result of reactivation.[43] Patients with hepatitis secondary to HSV infection may be shedding HSV from a mucocutaneous source or may be viremic, but some may require liver biopsy for confirmation. Acyclovir therapy is recommended for HSV-associated hepatitis, and post-transplant prophylaxis is very effective in preventing post-transplant HSV disease.[132] At least one neonate with HSV-induced fulminant hepatic failure successfully treated by liver transplantation combined with acyclovir therapy has been reported.[31]

VARICELLA-ZOSTER VIRUS. Varicella-zoster virus also causes mucocutaneous vesicles in both immunocompetent and immunocompromised hosts. Primary infection is known as *varicella* (also chickenpox) and is associated with primary and secondary viremias that often seed the visceral organs. Approximately a fourth of healthy children experiencing varicella will have silent hepatitis with transaminase levels at least twice normal.[41,91,105] Fulminant hepatitis with varicella occurs rarely, however, and generally is seen in immunocompromised hosts.[5,89,102,124] Patients have severe abdominal pain with little nausea or vomiting, skin lesions may or may not be present, and transaminases levels may be more than a thousand times higher than normal.[88,119,121] Zoster in a normal host is not associated with fulminant hepatitis, but immunocompromised hosts may experience disseminated zoster with hepatitis and hepatic necrosis.[40] The diagnosis often is based on clinical findings, but viral culture of cutaneous lesions, if present, or blood and liver biopsy also may help establish the diagnosis. Treatment with acyclovir is recommended. Varicella may be prevented or attenuated by passive immunization with varicella-zoster immune globulin (VZIG) or immune globulin intravenous (IGIV) or by active immunization with a licensed live virus vaccine.[17,25]

CYTOMEGALOVIRUS. CMV infection usually is asymptomatic or "silent." However, CMV in a normal host may cause gastroenteritis, pneumonitis, or a mononucleosis-like syndrome that consists of fever, lymphadenopathy, and atypical lymphocytosis. Hepatitis occurs as part of these syndromes but often is silent or mild and rarely is accompanied by jaundice.[67,82] Granulomatous hepatitis also may be associated with CMV.[28] Infants born congenitally infected with CMV frequently have hepatosplenomegaly, elevated transaminase levels, and direct hyperbilirubinemia.[29,129] The hepatitis that newborns and infants experience is self-limited and generally resolves within the first few months of life. If hepatitis with cholestasis persists, other diseases such as extrahepatic biliary atresia should be considered. Solid organ and marrow transplant recipients and patients with acquired immunodeficiency syndrome (AIDS) and other immunodeficiency states may experience persistent fever, malaise, leukopenia, and hepatitis caused by primary or recurrent infection with CMV. Severe liver disease can occur in transplant recipients and may be associated with graft-versus-host disease or graft rejection.[35,36] CMV-associated hepatitis may be diagnosed clinically and supported by virologic evidence of positive cultures, CMV viremia (or a viremia surrogate marker such as CMV antigenemia or CMV DNAemia), or demonstration of involvement of the end-organ by liver biopsy.[34,94] Treatment with ganciclovir, valganciclovir, foscarnet, or cidofovir appears to be beneficial in immunocompromised hosts, and prophylaxis or preemptive therapy with antiviral agents or CMV hyperimmune globulin may prevent the development of severe CMV disease in transplant recipients.[34,37,46]

EPSTEIN-BARR VIRUS. EBV infection also usually is asymptomatic or "silent," but it may cause a mononucleosis-like syndrome with mild hepatitis. However, in rare patients with a genetic X-linked predisposition, a severe, often fatal lymphoproliferative syndrome with prominent liver involvement may develop. Transplant recipients also may be susceptible to posttransplant lymphoproliferative disease (PTLPD), in which the liver may be involved.[8,22,116] In addition, patients with tumors associated with EBV, such as lymphoma, may have hepatic involvement. The diagnosis of mononucleosis usually is clinical and supported by a positive heterophile or "Monospot" test or by specific EBV serologic tests such as detection of IgM antibody to viral capsid antigen (VCA).[12] The immune response to EBV in immunocompromised hosts may be unusual, and the diagnosis of PTLPD generally is suspected by an increase in EBV DNA genome copies in peripheral blood, generalized adenopathy, or the presence of histopathologic features on biopsy. Treatment involves a reduction in immunosuppression, administration of rituximab (anti-CD20 monoclonal antibody), or adoptive immunotherapy.[26,51,99,120] Antiviral therapy with acyclovir also may be administered, but its effectiveness is controversial.

HUMAN HERPESVIRUSES 6, 7, AND 8. These viruses may involve the liver, especially in immunocompromised patients.[42] Hepatitis associated with HHV-6 may occur in solid organ transplant recipients. In recipients of liver transplants, infection with HHV-6, mostly reactivation, also has been associated with acute rejection, portal lymphocyte infiltration, and impaired function of the grafted liver. However, because HHV-6 is ubiquitous and commonly can be detected in blood and tissue, the role that the virus is playing in the liver disease observed in these patients is not entirely clear.[100] Normal hosts experiencing primary HHV-6 infection may have silent hepatitis with mild elevation of aminotransferase levels. Rarely, severe disseminated disease with fulminant hepatitis has been linked to HHV-6 and HHV-7.[2,9,54,79] HHV-8 (also known as *Kaposi sarcoma virus*) causes a complex neoplasm involving the skin, mucous membranes, and internal organs, most often in patients with severely compromised immune systems. It rarely is seen in children but has been reported in human immunodeficiency virus (HIV)-infected children with advanced AIDS. Recipients of solid organ transplants may be infected with HHV-8. The liver is a common site of visceral disease caused by HHV-8, which most often is associated with tumors rather than hepatitis.[23] Diagnosing infection with HHV-6, HHV-7, or HHV-8 is difficult because of the ubiquity of these viruses and their viral DNA in humans, but the diagnosis is supported by serologic evidence and by detection of viral DNA in blood, in secretions, or more specifically, in tissue.[100] No licensed specific antiviral therapy is available, but these viruses may be inhibited by ganciclovir, foscarnet, and cidofovir. Response also may be noted after withdrawal or reduction of immunosuppression, and with HHV-8, chemotherapy may be indicated.

HERPES B VIRUS. Also known as *herpesvirus simiae* or *cercopithecine herpesvirus 1*, herpes B virus is an alpha-herpesvirus of monkeys that causes severe disease in humans.[131] It can be transmitted from Asian monkeys, such as rhesus and cynomolgus monkeys, to humans through bites or contact with mucous membrane secretions from infected monkeys. The human disease associated with herpes B virus involves skin vesicles at the portal of entry, regional lymphadenitis, and hemorrhagic encephalitis. The virus also may disseminate to the liver and lungs and produce hemorrhagic necrosis, with a high mortality rate. The diagnosis is made by isolation of virus, and the virus is inhibited by acyclovir and ganciclovir.

Adenoviruses

Adenoviruses are small DNA viruses that are members of the viral family *Adenoviridae*. They usually are respiratory or enteric pathogens, but they also can cause disseminated disease with

hepatitis and hepatic necrosis in both immunocompetent and immunocompromised hosts and neonates.[56,81,96] Patients often have fever, malaise or lethargy, conjunctivitis, pharyngitis, cough, respiratory distress, vomiting and diarrhea, and a viral sepsis–like syndrome. Hepatitis is marked by hepatomegaly and by elevated aminotransferases and bilirubin. A specific viral diagnosis is made by isolation of adenovirus or detection of adenoviral DNA by PCR from respiratory secretions, blood, stool, or tissue. Adenovirus serotype 5 generally is associated with severe hepatitis, followed in frequency by types 1 and 2.[90] Viral surveillance cultures, blood DNA PCR testing, and virus serotyping and genotyping in immunocompromised patients, such as bone marrow and stem cell transplant recipients and liver transplant recipients at high risk for acquiring severe or fatal adenovirus-associated disease, may allow early intervention before severe, disseminated disease develops.[18,50,81] No licensed antiviral therapy is available, but the virus is inhibited to some extent by antiviral agents such as ribavirin and ganciclovir, and case reports suggest a potential clinical benefit in some patients with severe adenoviral hepatitis treated with cidofovir, an antiviral agent with broad-spectrum activity against many DNA viruses.[16,72]

Erythrovirus—Human Parvovirus B-19

Erythroviruses (i.e., human parvovirus B19) are small DNA viruses. They are members of the family *Parvoviridae* and are responsible for a variety of illnesses, including fifth disease (i.e., erythema infectiosum), arthritis, and anemia. Liver involvement, often severe, may be seen in intrauterine infection with hydrops fetalis.[4,80] Fulminant liver failure with massive hepatic necrosis associated with erythrovirus also has been reported in patients with aplastic anemia.[68] Persistent infection is seen in immunocompromised hosts. Parvovirus infection can be diagnosed by detection of virus-specific IgM antibodies or detection of viral DNA in blood, serum/plasma, bone marrow, secretions, urine, or tissue. No specific antiviral therapy is available, but immunocompromised patients with chronic infection may benefit from receiving IGIV. Severe fetal hydrops usually requires in utero and neonatal blood transfusions for anemia.

Enteroviruses

Enteroviruses are small RNA viruses and members of the *Picornaviridae* family, along with polioviruses and rhinoviruses. The non-polio enteroviruses usually are associated with mild respiratory or gastrointestinal illnesses, myocarditis, or aseptic meningitis, most often occurring in late summer or early fall. Significant hepatitis with hepatic necrosis, however, can occur, especially in neonates with disseminated disease. It often is accompanied by hepatomegaly, thrombocytopenia, viral sepsis syndrome, elevated aminotransferases, and elevated serum bilirubin.[84-86] Although any serotype can cause severe liver disease, echovirus 11 is associated most commonly with severe hepatitis or hepatitic necrosis, especially in neonates.[84] Coxsackie B and echoviruses 9 and 30 also are associated with fatal disease. Enteroviruses may be transmitted to neonates perinatally from the mother or through contact with ill family members. Nosocomial nursery outbreaks with enteroviruses also have been reported.[85] The diagnosis is established by isolation of the virus or detection of viral RNA by PCR in throat, stool, urine, blood, CSF, or tissue samples. Treatment is supportive; however, case reports suggest that IGIV, the investigational drug pleconaril, and even liver transplantation may have some clinical benefit in severely ill neonates.[6,20,63,112]

Measles Virus

Measles virus is an RNA virus that is a member of the *Paramyxoviridae* family, along with parainfluenza viruses, respiratory syncytial virus, metapneumovirus, and mumps virus. Of all the paramyxoviruses, measles virus is associated most often with hepatitis. Approximately 10 to 20 percent of children with measles will have subclinical hepatitis, and severe disease of the liver, lungs, and brain may occur in immunocompromised patients.[47,93,122] Rare reports of severe giant-cell hepatitis, often leading to liver failure, have implicated paramyxoviruses of undetermined type.[106] Measles and other paramyxoviruses may be identified by detection of virus-specific IgM antibody in serum and by isolation of virus in secretions, blood, or tissue. No specific antiviral therapy is licensed for measles virus; however, ribavirin, a broad-spectrum antiviral agent, may have some activity against the virus. Prevention is achieved by vaccination with the live measles vaccine or by postexposure administration of immunoglobulin or IGIV.

Rubella Virus

Rubella virus is a member of the *Togaviridae* family of RNA viruses. Clinical disease associated with infection by rubella virus generally is mild, but as many as 10 percent of children with rubella may have subclinical hepatitis with transient elevation of aminotransferase levels.[126] Congenital rubella syndrome caused by intrauterine infection with rubella virus is, however, associated with significant liver involvement, with hepatomegaly and jaundice being noted at birth.[33,87,125] Congenital rubella syndrome also is associated with intrauterine growth retardation, cataracts, congenital heart disease, thrombocytopenia, purpura, and hearing loss.[66] Because isolating the virus is difficult technically, the diagnosis of rubella most often is made serologically by detection of virus-specific IgM antibody. No specific antiviral therapy is available. Rubella can be prevented, however, by vaccination with the live rubella virus vaccine.

Hemorrhagic Fever Viruses

The hemorrhagic fever viruses are a diverse group of RNA viruses from a variety of different virus families. They include arenaviruses such as Lassa fever virus, bunyaviruses such as hantavirus, filoviruses such as Marburg and Ebola, and flaviviruses such as yellow fever virus and dengue. Hemorrhagic fever is characterized by fever, malaise or lethargy, headache, retro-orbital pain, myalgia, conjunctivitis, rash, and intravascular coagulation with hemorrhage. Liver involvement with hepatitis is a very common event, and elevation of aminotransferase levels to 500 IU/mL occurs in almost every patient, with a thousand times the normal range seen in patients who are severely ill.[32] Jaundice is a significant component of yellow fever.[61] The diagnosis is established by serologic means or by detection of the viral agent with electron microscopy or PCR techniques, which in most cases should be attempted only in biosafety level IV reference laboratories. Treatment of most hemorrhagic fevers is supportive; however, intravenous ribavirin reduces the mortality rate associated with Lassa fever and also may be of benefit to patients with hemorrhagic fever caused by other arenaviruses.[74,77]

BACTERIA

Nonviral acute hepatitis can be caused by bacterial illnesses (see Table 53–1).[95] Sepsis with gram-positive organisms, especially pneumococci, or with gram-negative organisms, particularly gram-negative enteric bacteria, can produce hepatic dysfunction, primarily from the cholestatic effects induced by bacterial endotoxins.[95,137] In this form of hepatic dysfunction, the patient will appear jaundiced with mild hepatomegaly, and conjugated bilirubin levels will be elevated out of proportion to the modest elevation in aminotransferase or alkaline phosphatase levels.

Neonates also may have jaundice secondary to urinary tract infection with gram-negative enteric organisms. The diagnosis is made by isolating the offending bacteria from blood, urine, or other usually sterile site. Treatment involves specific antimicrobial therapy.

Other bacterial diseases may cause chronic or granulomatous hepatitis, including actinomycosis, brucellosis, listeriosis, nocardiosis, bartonellosis (cat-scratch disease), and tuberculosis.[7,98] Diseases caused by atypical mycobacteria, especially *Mycobacterium avium-intracellulare* complex (MAC complex) or *Mycobacterium mucogenicum*, may be seen, particularly in patients with congenital or acquired immunodeficiency states.[48] Rarely, disseminated disease with hepatitis may occur as a complication of vaccination with bacille Calmette-Guérin (BCG) in children or, in adults, as a complication of bladder irrigation for bladder carcinoma.[7,49,71] A diagnosis of hepatitis caused by these unusual or indolent bacterial pathogens usually is accomplished by isolating the organism from blood or the affected organ. The diagnosis may be supported by positive skin test results in the case of tuberculosis or atypical mycobacterial disease, serologically by elevated titers to *Bartonella quintana* or *Bartonella henselae*, and by positive imaging studies that show hepatic microabscesses, as in the case of hepatic involvement with cat-scratch disease. Antimicrobial therapy is guided by the susceptibility of the offending pathogen.

Bacterial toxins, such as the emetic toxin of *Bacillus cereus*, also have been linked to fulminant hepatic failure in some patients.[75]

Spirochetes

Acute infection with *T. pallidum*, the agent of primary or early secondary syphilis in adolescents or adults, may cause acute or granulomatous hepatitis with serum aminotransferase levels up to 5 to 10 times normal.[70] Jaundice rarely develops, but a chancre of primary disease or a rash of secondary disease often is present. Congenital syphilis also is associated commonly with hepatosplenomegaly in the newborn, along with elevated aminotransferase and bilirubin levels. Other clinical manifestations of congenital syphilis include petechiae or purpura, thrombocytopenia, osteitis, and meningitis. Laboratory diagnosis is confirmed by reactive VDRL and positive fluorescent treponemal antibody tests. Treatment with penicillin is recommended.

Leptospirosis, or infection with the pathogenic bacterium *Leptospira interrogans*, can cause acute hepatitis.[55] Leptospirosis usually is an abrupt, anicteric, flulike illness, but approximately 10 percent of patients will have an icteric or septicemic syndrome with a biphasic clinical course. Patients with the icteric or severe form will exhibit jaundice, hepatomegaly, and characteristic conjunctival injection. Usually, levels of serum bilirubin are elevated out of proportion to the more modest elevations in serum aminotransferases, suggesting a defect in excretion of bilirubin rather than direct hepatic necrosis as the pathogenesis of the jaundice. Meningitis, renal failure, and even liver failure may occur in some patients. The diagnosis should be considered in older children and adolescents with a history of exposure to wild and domestic mammals, especially dogs, rats, and livestock, which may excrete *Leptospira* organisms in their urine, or with a history of exposure to contaminated water in ditches, lakes, or streams. The diagnosis is established by isolating the organisms on special media during the acute phase of illness. Serologic and PCR tests also are available in reference laboratories. Treatment with penicillin or doxycycline is recommended.

Rickettsiae

The rickettsial organism *Coxiella burnetii* causes Q fever, both the acute and chronic forms, in which hepatitis is a prominent feature along with persistent fever, malaise, weight loss, and pneumonitis.[14] Clinical jaundice is a rare finding, and most often the hepatitis is subclinical. A history of exposure to mammals or birds suggests the diagnosis, which can be confirmed serologically by reference clinical laboratories. Treatment with antibiotics, usually doxycycline, is recommended.

PARASITES AND FUNGI

A variety of parasites may invade the liver and occasionally cause hepatic dysfunction or disease.[95,135] Such parasites include *Plasmodium* spp. (malaria), *Entamoeba histolytica* (liver abscess), *Toxoplasma gondii* (toxoplasmosis), and *Toxocara canis* (visceral larval migrans). *Ascaris lumbricoides* (roundworms) may invade the common bile duct and cause acute obstructive jaundice.

Fungi also may invade the liver, usually with only minimal elevation of aminotransferase levels and rarely causing jaundice or elevated levels of bilirubin. Patients with a compromised immune system may have hepatic abscesses with *Candida* spp. or abscesses or necrotic lesions with *Aspergillus* spp., as well as other unusual fungal species. Both immunocompromised and normal hosts may have liver involvement with *Histoplasma capsulatum* or *Cryptococcus neoformans*.[95]

NONINFECTIOUS CAUSES

An important noninfectious cause of acute hepatitis is drug-related hepatitis (see Table 53–1).[133,136] It can range in severity from mild, with subclinical elevation of aminotransferase levels, to severe, with fulminant hepatic failure.[64] A careful history of ingestion of prescription or over-the-counter medications, as well as exposure to toxins or herbal remedies, should be elicited. Although almost any drug can cause acute hepatitis, the most common agents associated with hepatitis in children include acetylsalicylic acid (i.e., aspirin), acetaminophen, isoniazid, rifampin, phenytoin, valproic acid, phenobarbital, β-lactam antibiotics (e.g., oxacillin, nafcillin, and third-generation cephalosporins), sulfa drugs, and antifungal agents such as ketoconazole and fluconazole. The anesthetic drug halothane also can cause acute hepatitis with jaundice.[111] Gold and other metals used to treat arthritis have been associated with hepatitis as well. Carbon tetrachloride is a direct hepatic toxin. The *Amanita* mushroom, if ingested, causes severe liver injury. In addition, chronic hepatitis can develop in children, especially premature infants, who receive prolonged total parenteral nutrition.

Anoxic liver injury also can resemble acute viral hepatitis. It occurs in critically ill children after a period of hypotension, heart failure, or cardiopulmonary arrest. A history of such an inciting event supports the diagnosis. Anoxic liver injury is characterized by an abrupt onset of markedly elevated levels of aminotransferases, often hundreds of times higher than normal, without jaundice, and rapid recovery of enzyme levels to normal or nearly normal after the event has resolved.

Other diseases such as Kawasaki syndrome and toxic shock syndrome, which have been linked to or associated with infectious pathogens, may have hepatitis as part of their manifestation. Similarly, Reye syndrome, characterized by hepatomegaly with fatty infiltration of the liver and often fatal encephalopathy, may occur after a viral syndrome such as varicella or influenza.

Metabolic and genetic disorders may be manifested as hepatitis, especially in infants. Such disorders include cystic fibrosis, α_1-antitrypsin deficiency, galactosemia, glycogen storage disease, urea cycle deficiencies, organic acidemias, tyrosinemia, and lipid storage diseases such as Gaucher and Niemann-Pick disease.[105,127] Of note, cystic fibrosis in neonates may be associated with cholestatic jaundice in the absence of pulmonary disease.[123] Disorders of metal metabolism, such as Wilson disease, may cause acute,

chronic, or even fulminant hepatitis in older children.[104,117] In addition, patients with congenital disorders of bilirubin metabolism, such as Gilbert disease, may become jaundiced without significant elevation of aminotransferase levels, especially during an intercurrent viral illness. Sickle-cell crisis also may be manifested as hepatitis.[118]

Tumors of the liver and infiltrative diseases such as lymphoma, histiocytosis, and hemophagocytic syndrome may have hepatitis or hepatic failure as part of the initial manifestation.[53] Another multisystem disorder that may produce chronic granulomatous hepatitis is sarcoidosis.[30]

Anatomic causes of hepatic dysfunction in infants include extrahepatic biliary atresia, which usually develops in the first 2 months of life.[76,129]

Autoimmune hepatitis or other autoimmune disorders with liver involvement also may cause acute or chronic hepatitis, especially in older children and adolescents.[130] In autoimmune hepatitis, hypergammaglobulinemia and autoantibodies usually are present, as are other symptoms such as rash, arthritis, inflammatory bowel disease, thyroiditis, malaise, and persistent fever. Autoimmune hepatitis may respond to steroids or other immunosuppressive agents.

Hepatic steatosis (fatty infiltration) recently has been documented to occur in obese children, especially if they also have type 2 diabetes. These children may have enlarged or tender livers on examination, elevated transaminase levels in serum, abnormal imaging studies showing fatty infiltrates of the liver, and liver biopsies that show inflammation, fibrosis, and even cirrhosis in some cases. Treatment currently includes diet and lifestyle changes with weight loss and exercise.

REFERENCES

1. Aach, R. D., Lander, J. J., Sherman, L. A., et al.: Transfusion-transmitted viruses: Interim analysis of hepatitis among transfused and non-transfused patients. *In* Vyas, G. N., Cohen, S. N., and Schmid, R. (eds.): Viral Hepatitis. Philadelphia, Franklin Institute Press, 1978, p. 383.
2. Akashi, K., Eizuru, Y., Sumiyoshi, Y., et al.: Brief report: Severe infectious mononucleosis–like syndrome and primary human herpesvirus 6 infection in an adult. N. Engl. J. Med. 329:168-171, 1993.
3. Amado, L. A., Villar, L. M., dePaula, V. S., and Gaspar, A. M.: Comparison between serum and saliva for the detection of hepatitis A virus RNA. J. Virol. Methods 148:74-80, 2008.
4. Anand, A., Gray, E., Brown, T., et al.: Human parvovirus infection in pregnancy and hydrops fetalis. N. Engl. J. Med. 316:183-186, 1987.
5. Anderson, D. R., Schwartz, J., Hunter, N. J., et al.: Varicella hepatitis: A fatal case in a previously healthy, immunocompetent adult. Report of a case, autopsy, and review of the literature. Arch. Intern. Med. 154:2101-2106, 1994.
6. Aradottir, E., Alonoso, E. M., and Shulman, S. T.: Severe neonatal enteroviral hepatitis treated with pleconaril. Pediatr. Infect. Dis. J. 20:457-459, 2001.
7. Arisoy, E. S., Correa, A. G., Wagner, M. L., et al.: Hepatosplenic cat-scratch disease in children: Selected clinical features and treatment. Clin. Infect. Dis. 28:778-784, 1999.
8. Armes, J. E., Angus, P., Southey, M. D., et al.: Lymphoproliferative disease of donor origin arising in patients after orthotopic liver transplantation. Cancer 74:2436-2441, 1994.
9. Asano, Y., Yoshikawa, T., Suga, S., et al.: Fatal fulminant hepatitis in an infant with human herpesvirus-6 infection. Lancet 335:862-863, 1990.
10. Bachmann, L.: Infectious hepatitis in Europe. *In* Rodenwalt, E. (ed.): World Atlas of Epidemic Diseases. Part I. Hamburg, Germany, Falk-Verlag, 1952, p. 67.
11. Balayan, M. S., Andjaparidze, A. G., Savinskaya, S. S., et al.: Evidence for a virus in non-A/non-B hepatitis transmitted via the fecal oral route. Intervirology 20:23-26, 1983.
12. Basson, V., and Sharp, A. A.: Monospot: A differential slide test for infectious mononucleosis. J. Clin. Pathol. 225:324-325, 1969.
13. Beeson, P. B., Chesney, G., McFarlan, A. M., et al.: Hepatitis following injection of mumps convalescent plasma. Lancet 1:814-816, 1944.
14. Bernstein, M., Edmondson, H. A., and Barhour, B. H.: The liver lesion in Q fever: Clinical and pathologic features. Arch. Intern. Med. 116:491-500, 1965.
15. Blumberg, B. S., Stunick, A. I., and London, W. T.: Hepatitis and leukemia: Their relation to Australia antigen. Bull. N. Y. Acad. Med. 44:1566-1586, 1968.

16. Carter, B. A., Karpen, S. J., Quiros-Tejeira, R. E., et. al.: Intravenous cidofovir therapy for disseminated adenovirus in a pediatric liver transplant recipient. Transplantation 74:1050-1052, 2002.

17. Centers for Disease Control and Prevention: Prevention of varicella: Recommendations of the Advisory Committee on Immunization Practices (ACIP). M. M. W. R. Recomm. Rep. 45(RR-11):1-36, 1996.

18. Chakrabarti, S., Mauther, V., Osman, H., et al.: Adenovirus infections following allogeneic stem cell transplantation: Incidence and outcome in relation to graft manipulation, immunosuppression, and immune recovery. Blood 100:1619-1627, 2002.

19. Choo, Q.-L., Kuo, G., Weiner, A. J., et al.: Isolation of cDNA clone derived from a blood-borne non-A, non-B viral hepatitis genome. Science 244:359-362, 1989.

20. Chuang, E., Maller, E., Hoffman, M., et al.: Successful treatment of fulminant echovirus 11 infection in a neonate by orthotopic liver transplantation. J. Pediatr. Gastroenterol. Nutr. 17:211-214, 1993.

21. Cockayne, E. A.: Catarrhal jaundice sporadic and epidemic, and its relation to acute yellow atrophy of the liver. Q. W. J. Med. 6:1-5, 1912.

22. Cohen, J.: Epstein-Barr virus lymphoproliferative disease with acquired immunodeficiency. Medicine (Baltimore) 70:137-159, 1991.

23. Colina, F., Lopez-Rios, F., Lumbreras, C., et al.: Kaposi's sarcoma developing in a liver graft. Transplantation 61:1779-1781, 1996.

24. Committee on Infectious Diseases, American Academy of Pediatrics: Hepatitis C virus infection. Pediatrics 101:481-485, 1998.

25. Committee on Infectious Diseases, American Academy of Pediatrics: Varicella-zoster infections. In Pickering, L. K. (ed.): 2006 Red Book: Report of the Committee on Infectious Diseases. 27th ed. Elk Grove Village, IL, American Academy of Pediatrics, 2006, p. 711.

26. Cook, R. C., Connors, J. M., Gascoyne, R. D., et al.: Treatment of post-transplant lymphoproliferative disease with rituximab monoclonal antibody after lung transplantation. Lancet 354:1698-1699, 1999.

27. Cuthbert, J. A.: Hepatitis A: Old and new. Clin. Microbiol. Rev. 14:38-58, 2001.

28. de la Serna-Higuera, C., Gonzalez-Garcia, M., Milicua, J. M., and Munoz, V.: Cytomegalovirus granulomatous hepatitis in an immunocompetent patient. Gastroenterol. Hepatol. 22:230-231, 1999.

29. Demmler, G. J.: Summary of a Workshop on Surveillance for Congenital Cytomegalovirus Disease. Rev. Infect. Dis. 13:315-329, 1991.

30. Devaney, K., Goodman, Z. D., Epstein, M. S., et al.: Hepatic sarcoidosis: Clinicopathologic features in 100 patients. Am. J. Surg. Pathol. 17:1273-1280, 1993.

31. Egawa, H., Inomata, Y., Nakayama, S., et al.: Fulminant hepatic failure secondary to herpes simplex virus infection in a neonate: A case report of successful treatment with liver transplantation and perioperative acyclovir. Liver Transpl. Surg. 4:513-515, 1998.

32. Elisaf, M., Stafanaki, S., Reparti, M., et al.: Liver involvement in hemorrhagic fever with renal syndrome. J. Clin. Gastroenterol. 17:33-37, 1993.

33. Esterly, J., Slusser, R., and Ruebner, B.: Hepatic lesions in the congenital rubella syndrome. J. Pediatr. 71:676-685, 1967.

34. Evans, P. C., Soin, A., Wreghitt, T. G., et al.: Qualitative and semiquantitative polymerase chain reaction testing for cytomegalovirus DNA in serum allows prediction of CMV related disease in liver transplant recipients. J. Clin. Pathol. 51:914-921, 1998.

35. Falagas, M. E., Paya, C., Ruthazer, R., et al.: Significance of cytomegalovirus for long-term survival after orthotopic liver transplantation: A prospective derivation and validation cohort analysis. Transplantation. 66:1020-1028, 1998.

36. Falagas, M. E., Snydman, D. R., Griffith, J., et al.: Effect of cytomegalovirus infection status on first-year mortality rates among orthotopic liver transplant recipients. The Boston Center for Liver Transplantation CMVIG Study Group. Ann. Intern. Med. 126:275-279, 1997.

37. Falagas, M. E., Snydman, D. R., Ruthazer, R., et al.: Cytomegalovirus immune globulin (CMVIG) prophylaxis is associated with increased survival after orthotopic liver transplantation. The Boston Center for Liver Transplantation CMVIG Study Group. Clin. Transplant. 11:432-437, 1997.

38. Farr, R. W., Short, S., and Weissman, D.: Fulminant hepatitis during herpes simplex virus infection in apparently immunocompetent adults: Report of two cases and review of the literature. Clin. Infect. Dis. 24:1191-1194, 1997.

39. Feinstone, S. M., Kapikian, A. Z., and Purcell, R. H.: Hepatitis A: Detection by immune electron microscopy of a virus-like antigen associated with the acute illness. Science 182:1026-1028, 1973.

40. Feldman, S., Chaudary, S., Ossi, M., et al.: A viremic phase for herpes zoster in children with cancer. J. Pediatr. 91:597-600, 1977.

41. Feldman, S., Crout, J. D., and Andrew, M. E.: Incidence and natural history of chemically defined varicella-zoster virus hepatitis in children and adolescents. Scand. J. Infect. Dis. 29:33-36, 1997.

42. Fingeroth, J. D.: Herpesvirus infections of the liver. Infect. Dis. Clin. North Am. 14:1-34, 2000.

43. Fishman, J. A., and Rubin, R. H.: Infections in organ-transplant recipients. N. Engl. J. Med. 338:1741-1751, 1998.

44. Fishman, L. N., Jonas, M. M., and Lavine, J. E.: Update on viral hepatitis in children. Pediatr. Clin. North Am. 43:57-74, 1996.

45. Flewett, T. H., Parker, R. G., and Philip, W. M.: Acute hepatitis due to herpes simplex virus in an adult. J. Clin. Pathol. 22:60-66, 1969.

46. Gane, E., Saliba, F., Valdecasa, G. J., et al.: Randomized trial of efficacy and safety of oral ganciclovir in the prevention of cytomegalovirus disease in liver-transplant recipients. The Oral Ganciclovir International Transplantation Study Group. Lancet 350:1729-1733, 1997.

47. Gavish, D., Kleinman, Y., Morag, A., et al.: Hepatitis and jaundice associated with measles in young adults. Arch. Intern. Med. 143:674-677, 1983.

48. Goldblatt, M. R., and Ribes, J. A.: Mycobacterium mucogenicum isolated from a patient with granulomatous hepatitis. Arch. Pathol. Lab. Med. 126:73-75, 2002.

49. Gottke, M. U., Wong, P., Muhn, C., et al.: Hepatitis in disseminated bacillus Calmette-Guérin infection. Can. J. Gastroenterol. 14:333-336, 2000.

50. Gray, G. C., McCarthy T., Lebeck, M. G., et. al.: Genotype prevalence and risk factors for severe clinical adenovirus infections, United States, 2004-2006. Clin. Infect. Dis. 45:1120-1131, 2007.

51. Grillo-Lopez, A. J., White, C. A., Varns, C., et al.: Overview of the clinical development of rituximab: First monoclonal antibody approved for the treatment of lymphoma. Semin. Oncol. 26:66-73, 1999.

52. Gust, E. D., and Purcell, R. H.: Waterborne non-A, non-B hepatitis. J. Infect. Dis. 156:630-636, 1987.

53. Harrison, H. B., Middleton, H. M., Crosby, J. H., et al.: Fulminant hepatic failure: An unusual presentation of metastatic liver disease. Gastroenterology 80:820-825, 1981.

54. Hashida, T., Komura, E., Yoshida, M., et al.: Hepatitis in association with human herpes virus 7 infection. Pediatrics 96:783-785, 1995.

55. Heath, C. W., Jr., Alexander, A. D., and Galton, M. M.: Leptospirosis in the United States: Analysis of 483 cases in man 1949-1961. N. Engl. J. Med. 273:857-867, 1965.

56. Hierholzer, J. C.: Adenoviruses in the immunocompromised host. Clin. Microbiol. Rev. 5:262-274, 1992.

57. Hilleman, M. R.: Overview of the pathogenesis, prophylaxis, and therapeutics of viral hepatitis B, with focus on reduction to practical applications. Vaccine 19:1837-1848, 2001.

58. Hillis, W. D.: An outbreak of infectious hepatitis among chimpanzee handlers at a United States Air Force base. Am. J. Hyg. 73:316-320, 1961.

59. Hollinger, F. B., Gitnick, G. L., Aach, R. D., et al.: Non-A, non-B hepatitis transmission in chimpanzees: A project of the transfusion-transmitted viruses study group. Intervirology 10:60-68, 1978.

60. Hurwitz, E. S., Deseda, C. C., Shapiro, C. N., et al.: Hepatitis infections in the day-care setting. Pediatrics 94(Suppl.):1023-1024, 1994.

61. Ishak, K., Walker, D., Coetzer, J., et al.: Viral hemorrhagic fevers with hepatic involvement: Pathologic aspects with clinical correlations. Prog. Liver Dis. 7:495-515, 1982.

62. Jacobs, R. F.: Neonatal herpes simplex virus infections. Semin. Perinatol. 22:64-71, 1998.

63. Johnston, J., and Overall, J.: Intravenous immune globulin in disseminated neonatal echovirus 11 infection. Pediatr. Infect. Dis. J. 8:254-256, 1989.

64. Katelaris, P. H., and Jones, D. B.: Fulminant hepatic failure. Med. Clin. North Am. 73:955-970, 1989.

65. Kaufman, B., Gandhi, S. A., Louie, E., et al.: Herpes simplex virus hepatitis: Case report and review. Clin. Infect. Dis. 24:334-338, 1997.

66. Korones, S., Ainger, L., Monif, G., et al.: Congenital rubella syndrome: Study of 22 infants. Am. J. Dis. Child. 110:434-440, 1965.

67. Lamb, S. G., and Stern, H.: Cytomegalovirus mononucleosis with jaundice as a presenting sign. Lancet 2:1003-1006, 1966.

68. Langnas, A., Markin, R., Cattral, J., et al.: Parvovirus B19 as a possible causative agent of fulminant liver failure and associated aplastic anemia. Hepatology 22:1661-1665, 1995.

69. Lauer, G. M., and Walker, B. D.: Hepatitis C infection. N. Engl. J. Med. 345:41-52, 2001.

70. Lee, R. V., Thornton, G. F., and Conn, H. O.: Liver disease associated with secondary syphilis. N. Engl. J. Med. 284:1423-1430, 1971.

71. Leebeek, F. W. G., Ouwendijk, R. J. T., Kolk, A. H. U., et al.: Granulomatous hepatitis caused by bacillus Calmette-Guérin (BCG) infection after bladder instillation. Gut 38:616-618, 1996.

72. Legrand, F., Berrebi, D., Houhou, N., et al.: Early diagnosis of adenovirus infection and treatment with cidofovir after bone marrow transplantation in children. Bone Marrow Transplant. 27:621-626, 2001.

73. London, W. T., Sutnick, A. I., Blumberg, B. S., et al.: Australian antigen and acute viral hepatitis. Ann. Intern. Med. 70:55-59, 1969.

74. Luerman, A.: Eine Icterusepidemie. Berl. Klin. Wochenschr. 22:20-25, 1885.

75. Mahler, H., Pasi, A., Kramer, J. M., et al.: Fulminant liver failure in association with the emetic toxin of Bacillus cereus. N. Engl. J. Med. 33:1142-1148, 1997.

76. Manolaki, B., Larcher, V. F., Mowar, A. P., et al.: The prelaparotomy diagnosis of extra-hepatic biliary atresia. Arch. Dis. Child. 58:591-594, 1983.

77. McCormick, J. B., King, I. T., Webb, P. A., et al.: Lassa fever: Effective therapy with ribavirin. N. Engl. J. Med. 314:20-26, 1986.

78. Melnick, J. L.: Classification of hepatitis A as enterovirus 72 and of hepatitis B virus as hepadnavirus, type 1. Intervirology 18:105-110, 1982.

79. Mendel, I., de Matteis, M., Bertin, C., et al.: Fulminant hepatitis in neonates with human herpesvirus 6 infection. Pediatr. Infect. Dis. J. 14:993-997, 1995.

80. Metzman, R., Anand, A., DeGiulio, P., et al.: Hepatic disease associated with intrauterine parvovirus B19 infection in a newborn premature infant. J. Pediatr. Gastroenterol. Nutr. 9:112-114, 1989.

81. Michaels, M. G., Green, M., Wald, E. R., et al.: Adenovirus infection in pediatric liver transplant recipients. J. Infect. Dis. 165:170-174, 1992.

82. Miguelez, M., Gonzalez, A., and Perez, F.: Severe cytomegalovirus hepatitis in a pregnant woman treated with ganciclovir. Scand. J. Infect. Dis. 30:304-305, 1998.
83. Minuk, G. Y., and Nicolle, L. E.: Genital herpes and hepatitis in healthy young adults. J. Med. Virol. 19:269-272, 1986.
84. Modlin, J.: Fatal echovirus 11 disease in premature neonates. Pediatrics 66:775-779, 1980.
85. Modlin, J.: Perinatal echovirus infection: Insights from a literature review of 61 cases of serious infection and 16 outbreaks in nurseries. Rev. Infect. Dis. 8:918-926, 1986.
86. Modlin, J.: Perinatal echovirus and group B Coxsackie virus infections. Clin. Perinatol. 15:233-245, 1988.
87. Monif, G., Asofsky, R., and Sever, J.: Hepatic dysfunction in the congenital rubella syndrome. B. M. J. 1:1086-1088, 1966.
88. Morgan, E. R., and Smalley, L. A.: Varicella in immunocompromised children: Incidence of abdominal pain and organ involvement. Am. J. Dis. Child. 137:883-885, 1983.
89. Morishita, K., Kodo, H., Asano, S., et al.: Fulminant varicella hepatitis following bone marrow transplantation. J. A. M. A. 253:511-515, 1985.
90. Munoz, F., Piedra, P., and Demmler, G. J.: Disseminated adenovirus disease in immunocompromised and immunocompetent children. Clin. Infect. Dis. 27:1194-1200, 1998.
91. Myers, M. G.: Hepatic cellular injury during varicella. Arch. Dis. Child. 57:317-319, 1982.
92. Narkewicz, M. R., Cabrera, R., and Gonzalez-Peralta, R. P.: The "C" of viral hepatitis in children. Semin. Liver Dis. 27:295-311, 2007.
93. Nickell, M., Cannady, P., and Schwitzer, G.: Subclinical hepatitis in rubeola infections in young adults. Ann. Intern. Med. 90:354-355, 1979.
94. Niubo, J., Perez, J. L., Martinez-Lacasa, J. T., et al.: Associations of quantitative cytomegalovirus antigenemia with symptomatic infection in solid organ transplant recipients. Diagn. Microbiol. Infect. Dis. 24:19-24, 1996.
95. Novak, D. A., and Doloson, D. J.: Bacterial, parasitic, and fungal infections of the liver. In Suchy, F. J. (ed.): Liver Disease in Children. St. Louis, C. V. Mosby, 1994, pp. 550-568.
96. Odio, C., McCracken, G. H., Jr., Nelson, J. D., Jr., and Nelson, J. D.: Disseminated adenovirus infection: A case report and review of the literature. Pediatr. Infect. Dis. 3:46-49, 1984.
97. Ohto, H., Terazawa, S., Saski, N., et al.: Transmission of hepatitis C virus from mothers to infants. N. Engl. J. Med. 330:744-750, 1994.
98. Oliva, A., Duarte, B., Jonasson, O., and Nadimpalli, V.: The nodular form of local hepatic tuberculosis: A review. J. Clin. Gastroenterol. 12:166-173, 1990.
99. O'Reilly, R. J., Small, T. N., Papadopoulos, E., et al.: Biology and adoptive cell therapy of Epstein-Barr virus–associated lymphoproliferative disorders in recipients of marrow allografts. Immunol. Rev. 157:195-216, 1997.
100. Ozaki, Y., Tajiri, H., Tanaka-Taya, K., et al.: Frequent detection of the human herpesvirus 6–specific genomes in the livers of children with various liver diseases. J. Clin. Microbiol. 39:2173-2177, 2001.
101. Panda, S. K., Thakral, D., and Rehman, S.: Hepatitis E virus. Rev. Med. Virol. 17:151-180, 2007.
102. Patti, M. E., Selvaggi, K. J., and Kroboth, F. J.: Varicella hepatitis in the immunocompromised adult: A case report and review of the literature. Am. J. Med. 88:77-80, 1990.
103. Perlmutter, D. H.: Alpha-1-antitrypsin deficiency. Semin. Liver Dis. 18:217-225, 1998.
104. Perman, J. A., Werlin, S. L., Grand, R. J., et al.: Laboratory measures of copper metabolism in the differentiation of chronic active hepatitis and Wilson disease in children. J. Pediatr. 94:564-568, 1979.
105. Pitel, P. A., McCormick, K. L., Fitzgerald, T., et al.: Subclinical hepatic changes in varicella infection. Pediatrics 65:631-633, 1980.
106. Phillips, M. J., Blendis, L. M., Poucell, S., et al.: Syncytial giant-cell hepatitis: Sporadic hepatitis with distinctive pathologic features, a severe clinical course, and paramyxoviral features. N. Engl. J. Med. 324:455-460, 1991.
107. Polish, L. B., Gallagher, M., Fields, H. A., et al.: Delta hepatitis: Molecular biology and clinical and epidemiologic features. Clin. Microbiol. Rev. 6:211-229, 1993.
108. Purcell, R. H., and Emerson, S. U.: Hepatitis E: An emerging awareness of an old disease. J Hepatol. 48:494-503, 2008.
109. Prince, A. M.: An antigen detected in blood during the incubation period of serum hepatitis. Proc. Natl. Acad. Sci. U. S. A. 60:814-821, 1968.
110. Prince, A. M., Brotman, B., Grady, G. F., et al.: Long-incubation, post-transfusion hepatitis without serological evidence of exposure to hepatitis B virus. Lancet 2:241-246, 1974.
111. Ray, D. C., and Drummond, G. B.: Halothane hepatitis. Br. J. Anaesth. 67:84-99, 1991.
112. Rentz, A. C., Libbey J. E., Fujinami, R. S., et. al.: Investigation of treatment failure in neonatal echovirus 7 infection. Pediatr. Infect. Dis. J. 25:259-262, 2006.
113. Reyes, G. R., Purdy, M. A., Kim, J. P., et al.: Isolation of cDNA from the virus responsible for enterically transmitted non-A, non-B hepatitis. Science 247:1335-1339, 1990.
114. Rizzetto, M.: The delta agent. Hepatology 3:729-735, 1983.
115. Rizzetto, M., Canese, M. G., Avico, S., et al.: Immunofluorescence detection of a new antigen/antibody system (delta/anti-delta) associated with hepatitis B virus in liver and serum of HBsAg carriers. Gut 18:977-1003, 1977.
116. Robinson, J. E., Brown, N., Andiman, W., et al.: Diffuse polyclonal B-cell lymphoma during primary infection with Epstein-Barr virus. N. Engl. J. Med. 302:1293-1297, 1980.
117. Roche-Sicot, J., and Benhamou, J. P.: Acute intravascular hemolysis and acute liver failure associated with a first manifestation of Wilson's disease. Ann. Intern. Med. 86:301-310, 1977.
118. Rosenblate, H. J., Eisenstein, R., and Holmes, A. W.: The liver in sickle cell anemia. Arch. Pathol. Lab. 90:235-240, 1970.
119. Rowland, P., Wald, E. R., Mirro, J. R., Jr., et al.: Progressive varicella presenting with pain and minimal skin involvement in children with acute lymphoblastic leukemia. J. Clin. Oncol. 13:1697-1703, 1995.
120. Savoldo, B., Goss, J. A., Hammer, M. M., et. al.: Treatment of solid organ transplant recipients with autologous Epstein Barr virus–specific cytotoxic T lymphocytes (CTLs). Blood 108:2942-2949, 2006.
121. Schiller, G. J., Nimer, S. D., Gajewski, J. L., et al.: Abdominal presentation of varicella-zoster infection in recipients of allogeneic bone marrow transplantation. Bone Marrow Transplant. 7:489-491, 1991.
122. Shalev-Zimels, H., Weizman, Z., Lotan, C., et al.: Extent of measles hepatitis in various ages. Hepatology 8:1138-1139, 1988.
123. Sokol, R. J., and Durie, P. R.: Recommendations for management of liver and biliary tract disease in cystic fibrosis. J. Pediatr. Gastroenterol. Nutr. 28:511-513, 1999.
124. Soriano, V., Bru, F., and Gonzalez-Laoz, J.: Fatal varicella hepatitis in a patient with AIDS. J. Infect. 25:107-109, 1992.
125. Strauss, L., and Bernstein, J.: Neonatal hepatitis in congenital rubella. Arch. Pathol. 86:317-327, 1968.
126. Sugaya, N., Nirasawa, M., Mitamura, K., et al.: Hepatitis in acquired rubella infection in children. Am. J. Dis. Child. 142:817-818, 1988.
127. Svegar, T.: The natural history of liver disease in alpha-1-antitrypsin deficient children. Acta Pediatr. 77:847-851, 1995.
128. Tabor, E., Gerety, R. J., Drucker, J. A., et al.: Transmission of non-A, non-B hepatitis from man to chimpanzees. Lancet 1:463-466, 1978.
129. Tarr, P. I., Haas, J. E., and Christie, D. L.: Biliary atresia, cytomegalovirus, and age at referral. Pediatrics 97:828-831, 1996.
130. Van den Berg, A. P.: Autoimmune hepatitis: Pathogenesis, diagnosis, and treatment. Scand. J. Gastroenterol. Suppl. 225:66-69, 1998.
131. Whitley, R. J.: Cercopithecine herpes virus 1 (B virus). In Fields, B. N., Knipe, D. M., and Howley, P. M. (eds.): Fields Virology. 3rd ed. Philadelphia, Lippincott, Williams & Wilkins, 1999, pp. 2623-2630.
132. Whitley, R. J., and Kimberlin, D. W.: Treatment of viral infections during pregnancy and the neonatal period. Clin. Perinatol. 24:267-283, 1997.
133. Wu, S. S., Chao, C. S., Vargas, J. H., et. al.: Isoniazid-related hepatic failure in children: A survey of liver transplantation centers. Transplantation 27:173-179, 2007.
134. Young, E. J., Chafizadek, E., Oliveira, V. L., et al.: Disseminated herpesvirus infection during pregnancy. Clin. Infect. Dis. 22:51-58, 1996.
135. Zimmerman, H. J.: The differential diagnosis of jaundice. Med. Clin. North Am. 52:1417-1450, 1968.
136. Zimmerman, H. J.: Hepatotoxicity: The Adverse Effects of Drugs and Other Chemicals on the Liver. New York, Appleton-Century-Crofts, 1978.
137. Zimmerman, H. J., Fang, M., Utili, R., et al.: Clinical conference: Jaundice due to bacterial infection. Gastroenterology 77:362-373, 1979.

CHAPTER 54

CHOLANGITIS AND CHOLECYSTITIS

Valérie A. McLin ✪ Jason S. Soden ✪ Saul J. Karpen

CHOLANGITIS

The term *cholangitis* refers to any inflammation of the extrahepatic or intrahepatic biliary system. Clinically, it is seen most often as a consequence of infection in the setting of biliary tract disease or obstruction. The diagnosis of cholangitis implies microbial colonization of the biliary tract, increased biliary pressure, and systemic signs of infection, although all of these findings are not present in all patients. Generally, the etiology and treatment of infectious cholangitis are similar in adults and children. One specific pediatric population—children with biliary atresia and a hepatic portoenterostomy (HPE)—is particularly susceptible to cholangitis and its sequelae. This population and other patient groups at high risk of developing infectious cholangitis, such as patients with immunodeficiency states, congenital or acquired bile duct abnormalities, or liver transplants, are highlighted in this chapter. Biliary tract obstruction secondary to gallstone disease is discussed in the section on cholecystitis.

ETIOLOGY AND PATHOGENESIS

The central mechanisms leading to biliary tract infection are biliary colonization and stasis. Bile typically is sterile, implying that bactibilia develops either hematogenously via the portal venous system or directly via ascending infection from the gut lumen.[27]

Much is unknown regarding the route of bacterial infection of the biliary tree. Bacterial ascent may occur from the duodenum, most commonly in the presence of abnormal function of the sphincter of Oddi. In addition, bacterial invasion may occur hematogenously via increased gut translocation across the intestine into the portal circulation.[205] Earlier research indicates that infection of bile likely occurs via direct hematogenous spread of bacteria from portal venous flow across the gallbladder wall.[43] Although this mechanism has not been firmly established, the consensus is that transient episodes of bactibilia combined with biliary obstruction may lead to higher concentrations of bacteria in the biliary tract. As biliary pressure increases, bacteria likely migrate from the bile ducts into lymphatic and blood vessels, resulting in bacteremia and clinical signs and symptoms of cholangitis.[27]

In adults, cholangitis typically occurs in the presence of biliary tract obstruction secondary to impaction of gallstones in the common bile duct, leading to bile stasis and secondary infection. In approximately 85 percent of cases of cholangitis in adults, evidence of a common bile duct stone is present.[14] In adults with documented gallstones in the common bile duct (choledocholithiasis), the incidence of positive bile cultures is 30 to 90 percent.[119] Other potential causes of biliary obstruction in adults, possibly leading to a more chronic or recurrent presentation, include neoplasm of the biliary tree or head of the pancreas, other intrinsic or extrinsic strictures, parasitic disease, inflammatory conditions (e.g., primary biliary cirrhosis, primary sclerosing cholangitis [PSC]), and congenital bile duct anomalies. More recently, with improved imaging modalities and a better understanding of the pathogenesis of biliary lithiasis, it has become accepted that biliary sludge or microcalculi may be at the root of nonobstructive cholangitis and recurrent biliary infections.

In children, acute cholangitis occurs most frequently in patients with biliary atresia who have undergone HPE surgery.

The HPE, also known as a *Kasai operation*, provides a permissive setup for cholangitis: poor bile flow combined with damaged intrahepatic bile ducts and obligate bacterial colonization with enteric flora in the intestinal conduit.[79,80,103,116,176] In this setting, cholangitis is thought to arise from reflux of jejunal flora through the HPE (Roux-en-Y loop), directly contiguous with the hepatic porta. Cholangitis tends to occur more frequently within 1 year after surgery, usually in patients with evidence of good biliary flow. Decreased biliary and duodenal motility generally are accepted as being associated with a higher incidence of cholangitis,[47,207] but most predictors and exacerbants for the development of cholangitis remain unknown.

Microbiologic evidence of biliary tract infection ideally should involve at least 10^5 organisms per milliliter of bile.[43] Gram-negative rods, primarily *Escherichia coli* and *Klebsiella pneumonia*, are found in infected bile, but *Enterococcus* and *Enterobacter* spp. also often are encountered. Many cases of cholangitis are polymicrobial, lending support for use of broad-spectrum antibiotic treatment regimens. *E. coli* is the organism most commonly isolated, accounting for 20 to 68 percent of infections. Table 54–1 summarizes the frequencies of specific organisms found in adult and pediatric studies.[79,98,141] Anaerobes, such as *Bacteroides fragilis* and *Clostridium perfringens*, also may play a significant role and have been identified in 40 percent of biliary tract infections.[20] Specifically, the latter organism has been implicated in acute emphysematous cholecystitis. Despite these findings in bile, many patients with cholangitis have negative blood cultures, requiring clinicians to have a low index of suspicion for cholangitis in selected circumstances and patient populations.

In addition to bacterial infection, other pathogens—viral, fungal, and parasitic—have been reported in cases of pediatric cholangitis, particularly in immunodeficient patients (primarily patients with human immunodeficiency virus [HIV]; see later) and patients with environmental exposure to parasites in endemic settings. Cholangitis has been reported with viral disease; although most commonly associated with hepatocellular disease, hepatotropic viruses, primarily cytomegalovirus (CMV), hepatitis C, and hepatitis B, have been associated with pathologic findings of bile duct injury with apparent clinical significance.[24,67,110] Depending on the clinical setting and age of the patient, CMV can have a markedly varied presentation, ranging from bile duct paucity seen in congenital CMV infection to hepatomegaly and jaundice in infants and children with primary CMV infection. The role of CMV hepatitis and cholangitis is significant in immunocompromised patients and solid organ transplant recipients (see later).

Fungal cholangitis, specifically with *Cryptococcus neoformans* or *Candida albicans*, has been reported in immunocompromised and immunocompetent patients, although more commonly in the former than the latter population.[33] Although *Cryptosporidium* spp. typically are known to cause cholangitis in the immunocompromised host, one case of a child without a documented immunodeficiency has been reported.[65]

TABLE 54–1   Bacterial Pathogens Isolated from Bile Cultures in Cholangitis*

Organism	Hitch, 1978[80] (n = 283)	Keighley, 1975[99] (n = 231)	Lewis, 1987[114] (n = 23)	Boey, 1980[15] (n = 99)
Escherichia coli	230	65	15	46
Klebsiella	193	20	17	28
Enterococcus	179	22	6	14
Pseudomonas	150	1	—	17
Proteus	44	13	—	8
Bacteroides	28	—	2	—
Clostridium	—	11	9	—
Other species	23	—	10	23

*Pediatric and adult data used.[15,79,98,114]

The biliary tree also is susceptible to parasitic infections in normal hosts. Nematodes—*Ascaris* and, rarely, *Strongyloides*—commonly cause biliary disease in endemic regions. Migrating *Ascaris* larvae may cause either a direct inflammatory response if they pass through the biliary system or a secondary pyogenic cholangitis secondary to obstruction via the worms themselves or eggs. Liver flukes, such as *Clonorchis* (now *Opisthorchis*) *sinensis*, *Opisthorchis viverrini*, and *Opisthorchis felineus*, also may pass through the biliary system through their life cycle. Of these trematodes, *Clonorchis* is found frequently in cases of recurrent pyogenic cholangitis in Asian children.[148] Similar to the worms, the migration of the flukes (*Fasciola hepatica*) through the biliary tree may induce primary inflammation and, later, a secondary bacterial infection. Echinococcal cholangitis has been described in the setting of obstruction secondary to cyst formation from infection with either *Echinococcus granulosus* or *Echinococcus multilocularis*.[27,70,101] A thorough travel history should be obtained in all children presenting with new-onset cholangitis, in particular in patients in whom the most common causes are ruled out rapidly.

Finally, several cases of *Mycobacterium tuberculosis* cholangitis mimicking cholangiocarcinoma in immunocompromised and immunocompetent hosts have been reported in the adult literature.[12,50,104,155,163,219]

CLINICAL PRESENTATION

The classic presentation of cholangitis first described by Charcot in 1877 and known commonly as the *Charcot triad* is reported in 70 percent of patients with cholangitis (Table 54–2). It combines the clinical findings of fever, right upper quadrant pain, and jaundice.[94] The Reynold pentad adds septic shock and altered mental status to the Charcot triad.[115] Studies in children show that fever is the most common presenting symptom, occurring in 100 percent of 105 patients with cholangitis after undergoing HPE.[47] In addition, either acholic stools or an increase in serum bilirubin concentration occurs in 68 percent of patients. Older children and teenagers with cholangitis typically report abdominal pain that may or may not be associated with meals or localize to the right upper quadrant. Patients may report new-onset pruritus as a consequence of retained biliary constituents.

The findings of cholangitis may be markedly attenuated in infants and immunocompromised patients, suggesting that a low index of suspicion be employed in the evaluation of these children at risk. The presentation of cholangitis in an infant with biliary atresia, status post Kasai portoenterostomy, may be as varied as lethargy, increasing jaundice, abdominal tenderness, or fever alone. Finally, patients with ongoing hemolysis (e.g., patients with hemoglobin SS disease) are at high risk for developing cholecystitis and cholangitis from bilirubin stones, yet the symptoms may readily overlap with other causes of abdominal pain.

DIAGNOSTIC EVALUATION

Physical examination may reveal a varied range of toxic appearances, with vital signs suggesting serious systemic infection in more advanced cases (fever, tachycardia, hypotension). Physical examination typically reveals icteric sclera and a distended abdomen, with tenderness localized to the mid or right upper quadrant. Palpation of the liver edge may reveal tenderness. Laboratory studies may reveal an elevated erythrocyte sedimentation rate (81%), leukocytosis or leukopenia (56%), and increased serum levels of conjugated bilirubin.[47] Laboratory evaluations in children should include a standard complete blood count with differential and liver panel (alanine aminotransferase, aspartate aminotransferase, alkaline phosphatase, gamma-glutamyltransferase, and fractionated bilirubin [unconjugated and conjugated]). The differential diagnosis of fever, abdominal pain, and jaundice also should include sepsis and hepatitis. No single laboratory test or combination of tests can establish a diagnosis of cholangitis.

Attempts at identifying a microbiologic agent should be made, and blood cultures should be drawn before antimicrobial therapy is initiated. Most cases are polymicrobial, with a predominance of gut-derived organisms (see Table 54–1). Blood cultures may be positive in 50 percent of pediatric patients with cholangitis, as reported by Ecoffey and colleagues,[47] but this typically is not the case in routine pediatric practice. Other investigators have reported identification of organisms in blood in approximately 10 to 25 percent of patients, which is in keeping with our experience.[227] In patients with a history of hepatobiliary surgery, aerobic and anaerobic cultures should be considered, and in virtually all cases of young children with abdominal pain and jaundice, a urine culture should be considered.

A role for direct testing of hepatic tissue by percutaneous biopsy is controversial, but occasionally this testing may have a place in the setting of negative blood cultures. When used along with blood cultures, hepatic cultures have been shown to increase the diagnostic yield of identifying a microbiologic organism to 75 percent of patients, whereas histologic confirmation of cholangitis may be the only firm evidence of biliary tract infection in some cases.[47]

In practice, liver biopsy rarely is done, and patients are treated empirically. In cases of gallstone-associated biliary tract obstruction with cholangitis that requires endoscopic or surgical decompression, bile should be obtained and cultured at the time of the procedure. In an adult study, 22 of 23 patients with gallstone-associated cholangitis were found to have positive bile cultures.[114]

The initial and principal radiologic evaluation for suspected cholangitis is transabdominal ultrasound, with the primary goal being to search for evidence of biliary tract obstruction, usually associated with dilation of the common bile duct or intrahepatic ducts. Ultrasound examination may reveal anatomic biliary tract abnormalities (choledochal cyst), intrahepatic cysts, and hepatic or other intra-abdominal masses. Other noninvasive imaging modalities include computed tomography (CT) and magnetic resonance cholangiopancreatography (MRCP), which provide increasingly detailed images of the intrahepatic and extrahepatic biliary anatomy.[137,172]

Taken together, these noninvasive imaging techniques should be able to detect the presence of biliary tract obstruction and some congenital anatomic anomalies, although even experienced ultrasonographers still may miss small stones and sludge, especially in the common bile duct. It is important to recognize the technical limitations of the methodology and the possible presence of undetected stones or sludge in the gallbladder or common bile duct (choledocholithiasis) as a cause of biliary tract dilation. Ultrasound misses 40 percent of biliary tract stones.[191] Finally, ultrasound is only 51 to 85 percent sensitive in identifying biliary tract obstruction, which improves to approximately 90 percent with CT, and 95 to 99 percent with endoscopic retrograde cholangiopancreatography (ERCP).[164]

Newer modalities, including endoscopic ultrasound, laparoscopic ultrasound, and helical CT cholangiography, may improve detection in certain patient populations. The 2002 National

TABLE 54–2 Charcot Triad and Reynold Pentad	
Charcot Triad	**Reynold Pentad**
Fever	Fever
Right upper quadrant pain	Right upper quadrant pain
Jaundice	Jaundice
	Septic shock
	Altered mental status

Institutes of Health State-of-the-Science Consensus conference regarded endoscopic ultrasound, MRCP, and ERCP to have comparable sensitivity and specificity in detecting common bile duct stones.[146] In the hands of an experienced echoendoscopist, endoscopic ultrasound has been shown in adults to be the procedure of choice to identify small stones and sludge in the common bile duct. This method may prove useful in children as well, and may prevent the unnecessary use of ERCP and the risk of its associated complications.[54,173,191]

After HPE has been performed, imaging may be able to identify lakes of retained bile (bilomas), which may be a source of infection, in a patient with biliary atresia. Because of the inherent risks associated with invasive procedures in these infants, percutaneous drainage of bilomas for culture or other purposes rarely is performed. Similarly, ERCP is not indicated for patients with biliary atresia after HPE, for anatomic reasons.

Nuclear medicine (hepatobiliary iminodiacetic acid [HIDA]) scans have a limited role in the evaluation of cholangitis. HIDA scans may be most helpful in determining if a patient has a complete obstruction of the common bile duct, or if an isolated obstruction of the cystic duct (cholecystitis; see later) is present. Because most pediatric cases of cholangitis occur in patients with biliary atresia after HPE, involvement of the cystic duct rarely is a concern.

Invasive imaging has a role, especially when it may be coupled with therapeutic decompression of an obstructed, and potentially infected, biliary tree. ERCP has proved to be extremely useful in the evaluation and management of biliary tract obstruction and should be considered in the management of a child with evidence of an obstructed common bile duct (see later).[3,26,121,194,195,200,211,237] The role of ERCP in infants and small children is limited by the lack of experience of most pediatric gastroenterologists and should be considered in tertiary care centers that have the requisite expertise. ERCP is the most direct means of obtaining bile for microbial and chemical analysis and provides detailed imaging of the biliary tree.

Practically, ERCP may detect (and remove) small stones and sludge that are missed by ultrasound, CT, or MRCP. ERCP is helpful in establishing the differential diagnosis of biliary tract diseases, such as PSC, which may manifest in a fashion similar to that of infectious cholangitis but may have a characteristic radiographic appearance. In the future, as the use of endoscopic ultrasound in pediatrics increases, ERCP may be reserved for those patients in whom stones or sludge have been found by endoscopic ultrasound or in patients with a high pretest probablility of having choledocholithiasis (e.g., patients with sickle-cell conditions).[54,191] One more recent study showed that 34 percent of pediatric patients undergoing ERCP had a normal study.[89] Limiting the indications for ERCP could prevent complications such as pancreatitis and iatrogenic ascending cholangitis. Any child with a first episode of cholangitis warrants a detailed investigation of a possible underlying biliary tract anatomic abnormality.

DIFFERENTIAL DIAGNOSIS

The differential diagnosis for an acutely ill child with fever and clinical evidence of hyperbilirubinemia is broad; a thorough work-up must include consideration of infectious and noninfectious etiologies (Table 54-3). A thorough investigation for hepatic and biliary tract pathology with blood and radiologic studies must be initiated to evaluate for stones or other obstructive processes that may cause symptoms characteristic of the Charcot triad.

Acute viral hepatitis may manifest in numerous ways but often begins with nonspecific signs: fever, headache, anorexia, and jaundice. Laboratory studies typically reveal a greater elevation of serum aminotransferase levels (alanine aminotransferase and aspartate aminotransferase) than the biliary tract enzymes

TABLE 54-3 Differential Diagnosis of Fever, Abdominal Pain, and Jaundice

Cholangitis
Cholecystitis
Cholelithiasis
Sepsis
Hepatitis
Choledochal cyst
Pancreatitis
Urinary tract infection
Leptospirosis and other systemic infections with hepatic involvement
Spontaneous perforation of common bile duct
Biliary cyst
Appendicitis

alkaline phosphatase and gamma-glutamyltransferase. In a child with no other evidence of biliary tract obstruction, screening assays for hepatitis infection are warranted.

Pyogenic liver abscesses and amebic abscesses tend to manifest with fever, abdominal pain, hepatomegaly, and focal right upper quadrant tenderness.[148] Laboratory findings vary. CT is considered to be the most sensitive technique for evaluation of these diagnoses.[137] Numerous bacterial, parasitic, and spirochetal infections also should be considered in the differential diagnosis, including, but not limited to, typhoid fever, brucellosis, leptospirosis, borreliosis, amebiasis, and malaria. It is beyond the scope of this chapter to expand on the systemic infections associated with hepatic involvement.[154] Recurrent pyogenic cholangitis is another consideration, although it is rare in the Western Hemisphere and even more so in the pediatric population.[182]

Jaundice may occur with sepsis of any etiology, more commonly in a critically ill infant or child. Clinical evaluation may show a predominantly direct (conjugated) hyperbilirubinemia usually accompanied by a modest elevation of gamma-glutamyltransferase, although serum transaminase levels may not be elevated. These findings are caused by a hepatocellular cholestasis, owing to humoral mediators of sepsis (i.e., endotoxin and proinflammatory cytokines), but they can be exacerbated by biliary sludging that accompanies septicemia. Although sepsis-associated cholestasis historically was linked primarily to gram-negative sepsis, it can be seen in all forms of infection. In some cases, radiologic work-up or biopsy is warranted to rule out ductal obstruction or biliary tract pathology. Jaundice may occur as the sole presentation of sepsis in infants and children, however.[45] Evolving research into sepsis-induced cholestasis points to a complex, multifactorial etiopathogenesis.[30,59,138,215]

Drug-induced cholestasis tends to occur acutely with the onset of jaundice, pruritus, and other symptoms that may mimic cholangitis. It rarely is associated with fever, however. Among the main classes of drugs commonly used in pediatric practice that may lead to significant hepatotoxicity are antimicrobials (mainly trimethoprim-sulfamethoxazole [TMP-SMX], amoxicillin/clavulanate, clindamycin, minocycline, nitrofurantoin, erythromycin, cephalosporins, isoniazid, rifampicin, fluconazole), anticonvulsants (phenytoin, carbamazepine, valproate, felbamate), nonsteroidal anti-inflammatory drugs (aspirin, ibuprofen), antihypertensive agents (propranolol, diltiazem),[21,34] and herbal remedies such as kava kava. Although rarely used in pediatric patients, statins also lead to significant hepatotoxicity.[125] If the offending agent is identified in time, removing it typically leads to rapid improvement. Ceftriaxone warrants special mention because it has been linked directly to cholangitis and cholecystitis, possibly as a result of its biliary concentration and precipitation, leading to sludge and stones.[102,145]

Other systemic illnesses may occur with fever and evidence of biliary tract pathology, and their presentations may overlap with presentations of infectious cholangitis. PSC is defined as a chronic inflammation of the intrahepatic or extrahepatic ducts leading to a range of biliary tract pathologies, from dilation to obliteration and periductular fibrosis. PSC is seen most commonly in patients with inflammatory bowel disease and affects adolescent boys with inflammatory bowel disease more commonly than girls. Symptoms include systemic findings, such as fatigue, malaise, and weight loss, and evidence of cholangitis, including fever. PSC must be suspected in a jaundiced patient with inflammatory bowel disease or in an adolescent boy presenting for the first time with jaundice. Diagnosis is established best by ERCP or magnetic resonance cholangiography showing irregular narrowing and stricture of the hepatic and common bile ducts and the intrahepatic ducts.[124,169] Patients with PSC are at risk of developing intrahepatic and common bile duct strictures, with subsequent obstruction, sludge or stone formation, cholangitis, and ultimately cholangiocarcinoma.[112]

TREATMENT

Therapeutic goals in the treatment of cholangitis should include general support of the patient, early initiation of appropriate antibiotic therapy, and, in cases of obstruction by stones or stricture, decompression of biliary obstruction via ERCP or surgery. Consulting pediatric surgeons early in the course of evaluating a patient with suspected cholangitis generally is helpful. The importance of decompression and drainage of the bile tract in the face of systemic infection secondary to cholangitis cannot be overemphasized. Other potential etiologies of obstruction, such as choledochal cysts, ultimately require surgical consultation and repair.

Initial and conservative management should include appropriate inpatient monitoring, cessation of oral intake with intravenous fluid support, parenteral antibiotic therapy, and supportive management as warranted by the child's clinical status. Because blood cultures tend to have a low diagnostic yield in cholangitis, antibiotics should be selected empirically, and selection should not rely on culture results.

Selection of a drug or combination of drugs should be based on appropriate coverage of suspected or documented organisms (based on sensitivities) and ability to achieve adequate serum and tissue concentrations. Currently, no single antibiotic or combination is recognized universally as being the definitive therapy for cholangitis in children. Typically, antibiotic therapy is initiated before obtaining culture results. In the past, the goal was to achieve sufficient biliary concentrations, although adequate serum levels are probably a satisfactory surrogate.[43,115] Parenteral antibiotics are indicated in almost all cases of children with suspected biliary tract sepsis. Primary antibiotics should cover gram-negative enteric organisms—E. coli, Klebsiella, and Enterococcus. In the case of a child with clinical sepsis, it is reasonable to add coverage for anaerobic species, particularly Bacteroides.[20]

Previously, a combination of ampicillin or penicillin with an aminoglycoside was considered appropriate therapy. Studies in adults suggest, however, that the use of some antipseudomonal penicillins, such as mezlocillin, is more effective alone than is the ampicillin-gentamicin combination.[61] The general recommendation for treatment of a pediatric patient with suspected cholangitis is a semisynthetic penicillin (e.g., piperacillin or mezlocillin) or a third-generation cephalosporin (e.g., cefoperazone) in combination with an aminoglycoside for adequate coverage of Pseudomonas spp.[107,227] The addition of metronidazole helps to cover anaerobic gut flora.

Rothenberg and colleagues[176] reported a 62.7 percent success rate after treatment with imipenem-cilastatin or third-generation cephalosporins with or without aminoglycosides and a 58.2 percent success rate using semisynthetic penicillins with amino-

glycosides. A prospective trial involving 131 adults with biliary tract infections showed a "cure" in 85 percent of patients treated with ampicillin and tobramycin after a surgical procedure.[141] Although it is limited, a 1987 report of three patients suggests favorable results can be achieved using ciprofloxacin in pediatric patients with cholangitis after they have undergone a Kasai procedure.[84] TMP-SMX, which achieves a high biliary:serum concentration, has been used successfully in similar clinical settings.[80]

As mentioned previously, ceftriaxone probably should be avoided because it has been associated with biliary sludging and cholecystitis.[90] Currently, certain centers have reported the use of broad-spectrum antibiotics, such as meropenem, to cover optimally the enteric organisms most frequently associated with bacterial cholangitis.[201] Meropenem and other broad-spectrum β-lactam antibiotics with a β-lactamase inhibitor may be a good choice because many cholangitis episodes are polymicrobial.[221]

In clinical practice, the choice of antibiotic therapy often is empiric despite attempts to isolate a pathogenic organism. Antibiotic efficacy is determined by clinical and laboratory parameters, such as defervescence and improvement in biliary excretion. Antibiotic resistance is encountered more often in patients with repeated episodes of cholangitis.[47] The duration of antibiotic treatment varies, but a shorter course may result in recurrence.[176] The recommended course of therapy is 14 to 21 days, with longer duration recommended in special cases, such as recurrent or refractory cholangitis, and in the case of intrahepatic abscesses or hepatic surgery. Although oral antibiotic therapy generally has no place in the treatment of cholangitis in children, oral ciprofloxacin has been used in some adult populations.[227]

Ultimately, cholangitis or the risk thereof will not resolve in the presence of ongoing biliary obstruction. Although antibiotic therapy may treat septicemia, timely establishment of biliary drainage is imperative.[48] In 25 percent of adults with cholangitis, medical therapy is insufficient, and decompression via ERCP (or laparotomy) is indicated.[48,98,180] ERCP and percutaneous transhepatic cholangiography generally are recommended as first-line approaches because they pose a lower risk than does open surgical intervention.[157] These procedures can be diagnostic in the case of biliary obstruction and therapeutic, with sphincterotomy or stent placement.

Treatment of parasitic cholangitis should include appropriate treatment of biliary parasites based on regional sensitivities in addition to antibiotic coverage of secondary bacterial infections. Endoscopic or surgical intervention may be required to remove worms or cysts from the biliary tree.[35]

COMPLICATIONS OF CHOLANGITIS

Regardless of the patient's age at the time of presentation, cholangitis can be life-threatening. Other morbidities associated with cholangitis include pancreatitis. Because pediatric patients who present with cholangitis typically have underlying biliary or liver pathology, cholangitis may precipitate a rapid exacerbation of the underlying disease. In diseases such as biliary atresia, cholangitis may hasten the patient's course toward requiring organ replacement.

SPECIFIC POPULATIONS AND CHOLANGITIS

CHOLANGITIS AND BILIARY ATRESIA

In pediatrics, cholangitis is encountered most frequently in the setting of a patient with biliary atresia who has undergone a Kasai procedure. In 1959, Kasai and Suzuki[96] first reported relief of biliary obstruction in children with biliary atresia by HPE. The procedure, a Roux-en-Y hepatic portoenterostomy, is considered to be standard first-line surgical therapy for infants with biliary atresia, and it is associated with the highest success rates and long-term survival when performed early, usually by 60 days of life. Without this procedure, 90 percent of patients with biliary atresia die before reaching age 3 years, at an average age of 19 months.[95,199]

Cholangitis remains the most frequent complication of the Kasai procedure, occurring in 40 to 60 percent of patients.[152] A subgroup of patients with the pathologic finding of cystic dilation of the intrahepatic bile ducts seems to have the highest risk of developing postoperative cholangitis.[81] The development of cholangitis has been associated with a worsening in long-term prognosis of children with biliary atresia.[85] Complications of cholangitis are severe, ranging from inflammation and scarring, to alterations in biliary flow, and, eventually to biliary cirrhosis. Repeated bouts of cholangitis are associated with worsening liver function, impaired growth, and need for early transplantation. For this reason, early detection, appropriate management, and prompt intervention and treatment of cholangitis are important in this population.

Most cases of post–Kasai procedure cholangitis occur within 1 year postoperatively. In a 1976 review of 49 cases of children who underwent the procedure, 31 achieved good bile flow restoration. Of these, 20 subsequently developed cholangitis, 15 occurring within the first postoperative month and 3 within the second month.[149] Likewise, in a study of 105 cases of cholangitis developing in 101 children after they underwent hepatic portoenterostomies, Ecoffey and colleagues[47] showed that 63 percent of the cases occurred within 3 months after surgery, and 93 percent occurred within 1 year. Rarely, late cholangitis may occur; this has been reported to occur several years after HPE.[66]

The generally accepted mechanism for development of cholangitis after a Kasai procedure is ascending bacterial colonization. This theory is reinforced by reports of a higher incidence of cholangitis developing in patients with good or partial bile flow after the Kasai procedure (78%) than in patients with no obvious bile flow (13%).[47] A 1978 study of 19 patients concluded that all bilioenteric conduits after the procedure were colonized within 1 month, correlating with the high incidence of symptomatic infection at this early stage.[80] The retrograde bacterial colonization may be enhanced by overall changes in intestinal motility after the Roux-en-Y loop.[207] Over time, the intestinal conduit from hepatic porta to jejunum seems to "mature," and the number of episodes of cholangitis diminishes. How this adaptation happens is unknown. Late episodes of cholangitis, occurring 1 to 2 years after a Kasai procedure, likely are related to mechanical obstruction, such as adhesions, and warrant investigation.[116]

Gram-negative enteric organisms constitute most organisms causing ascending cholangitis after HPE. *E. coli* has been found in 50 percent of the first and second cholangitis episodes and in decreasing frequency in subsequent episodes.[47] Anaerobes also are common findings and should be considered when selecting antibiotic treatment.[20] Refractory or recurrent cases occurring after surgery may warrant consideration of fungal disease, principally *Candida*.[33] Attempts to isolate an organism generally are made, but blood cultures typically have a low yield.[176] Bile cultures tend to reflect the multiple enteric organisms that colonize the conduit, but may not specify the true pathogens. Percutaneous liver biopsy has been used successfully to obtain cultures, but it rarely is used for this indication in pediatric patients.[150]

In the intraoperative and postoperative management of children with biliary atresia, attempts have been made to prevent the incidence of cholangitis. Various modifications in the surgical configuration of the intestinal conduit have been suggested to reduce enteric reflux. Initial studies have documented a reduced incidence of ascending cholangitis in the presence of a surgically placed antireflux valve. Despite the reduction of intestinal reflux

in these cases, cholangitis continues to occur.[18] Cases of refractory cholangitis may require surgical intervention, especially if obstruction of the conduit or porta hepatis is suspected. The absolute indications for reoperation after HPE are unclear, however.

The role of corticosteroids in improving biliary drainage is controversial and has not been the subject of rigorous controlled trials. Perioperative steroid pulses, typically a 3- to 5-day course of intravenous methylprednisolone, have been shown, however, to be clinically beneficial by decreasing temperature, increasing bile flow, and improving liver function tests.[142,176] A multicenter, randomized, double-blind, placebo-controlled study sponsored by National Institutes of Health has been under way in 10 centers in the United States, to assess the safety and efficacy of using corticosteroids after the Kasai procedure (http://clinicaltrials.gov/ct2/show/NCT00294684?term=basitrank=3). The forthcoming results of this study should yield definitive information regarding the postoperative management of these children. The incidence of cholangitis in the treated and untreated arms is one of the outcomes.

In addition, some centers advocate the use of prophylactic antibiotics, typically TMP-SMX. The benefits of this practice are not well established, however.[32] In adults with recurrent cholangitis secondary to fixed obstruction, as in the case of malignancy, TMP-SMX and ciprofloxacin have been shown to be helpful in preventing episodes.[220] In our practice, TMP-SMX is used as a first-line agent. In selected patients with recurrent episodes of cholangitis on TMP-SMX and a functional HPE, we have used oral ciprofloxacin successfully.

In patients with post–Kasai procedure biliary atresia, each episode of cholangitis is associated with a 1 percent mortality risk. Some studies suggest that no significant clinical difference exists in overall survival rates between patients who have undergone the Kasai procedure and have or have not had cholangitis.[151] Previous studies suggest, however, an 88 percent mortality rate among patients who develop cholangitis within 1 month after undergoing the Kasai procedure, and 16 percent in patients who develop it more than 1 month later. More recent studies suggest that the occurrence of cholangitis is related to early postoperative mortality, and the number of repeated episodes is inversely related to survival.[231] Practically, because cholangitis can be life-threatening, patients with recurrent episodes frequently are considered for liver transplantation.

CHOLANGITIS AFTER LIVER TRANSPLANTATION

Infection remains the most common reason for morbidity and mortality after pediatric liver transplantation, accounting for 20 to 30 percent of postoperative deaths.[178,202,204] Bacterial infection that develops after transplantation tends to occur within the first 2 months postoperatively and generally is of either respiratory tract or intra-abdominal origin. Among patients with severe bacterial infections of intra-abdominal origin, cholangitis and biliary tract infections commonly develop. Gram-negative aerobic bacteria are encountered most commonly in this setting.[183] One adult study showed that 18 percent of 284 patients receiving liver transplantation had confirmed episodes of cholangitis.[222] Pediatric data suggest that the rate of cholangitis after liver transplantation for biliary atresia is 5 to 11 percent.

Biliary tract disease frequently occurs after the post–liver transplantation complication of hepatic artery thrombosis.[122,130] This complication was prevalent in the early days of pediatric liver transplantation. Although it remains a concern, the incidence has decreased owing to the use of microsurgical techniques. Hepatic artery thrombosis eventually leads to damage of the bile duct because the biliary blood supply is exclusively arterial, whereas the hepatic parenchyma is vascularized by the portal vein and the hepatic artery. Biliary injury leads to altered biliary anatomy and drainage, increasing the risk of development of infection in these patients. Although most pediatric liver transplant recipients have a Roux-en-Y biliary-enteric anastomosis from the donor bile duct to the recipient bowel, ascending cholangitis is rare in this population.

Cholangitis that develops after liver transplantation may manifest with fever, jaundice, elevated liver enzymes, and bacteremia. The variable nature of an immunocompromised patient's response to infection renders the reliability of each of these signs and symptoms suspect, however. Distinguishing these symptoms from the presentation of post-transplant rejection or infection (e.g., with CMV or Epstein-Barr virus) is important. For this reason, liver biopsy often is a necessary part of the evaluation of a post-transplant patient with fever and elevated liver tests.

CHOLANGITIS IN IMMUNOCOMPROMISED PATIENTS

Although biliary disease related to acquired immunodeficiency syndrome (AIDS) may be considered the most common cholangiopathy of immunocompromised hosts, it is not the most frequent one in pediatric practice. Cholangitis also may occur in children with non-AIDS immunodeficiency. Sclerosing cholangitis has been reported in cases of primary immunodeficiency, including familial T-cell deficiency, IgA/IgG deficiency, and X-linked hyper-IgM syndrome.[69,113] Patients with sclerosing cholangitis often present with superimposed bacterial cholangitis because of poor biliary drainage. Hepatobiliary infection also has been reported in children with leukemia.[58,105,189,197]

AIDS-related cholangitis is a well-known complication of AIDS. It tends to occur late in the course of the illness and is more common in adults than in children. With the decline in the number of new AIDS cases in the United States, especially in pediatric patients, this diagnosis has become rare. In 1989, Cello[29] described four distinct patterns of disease in AIDS-related cholangitis as seen on cholangiography—papillary stenosis, sclerosing cholangitis, combined papillary stenosis and sclerosing cholangitis, and long extrahepatic bile duct strictures. The pathogenesis of these changes is unknown and may be related to biliary inflammation secondary to immunodeficiency, infiltration of the mucosa by HIV itself, or opportunistic infection by known gut culprits in AIDS infection.

Opportunistic agents most commonly responsible are CMV, *Cryptosporidium*, *Microsporida*, and, uncommonly, *Mycobacterium avium-intracellulare* and *Isospora*.[144,235] One report of unexplained cholangitis in a small cohort of HIV-positive men identified *Enterocytozoon bieneusi* in the bile of all of the patients.[159] Although AIDS cholangiopathy is extremely rare in children, these pathogens can be found in pediatric patients with primary immunodeficiencies and associated PSC, and with secondary immunosuppression after undergoing solid organ transplantation.[1,40,132,170,228]

Clinical presentation is similar to that in non-HIV patients, with the exception of jaundice, which tends to be less common. In a series of 45 adults with AIDS-related cholangitis, abdominal pain was reported as the most common presenting symptom, occurring in 64 percent of patients, followed by diarrhea (22%), fever (20%), and jaundice (7%). A 1997 review reported that 90 percent of adults present with right upper quadrant or epigastric pain. Twenty percent of patients were asymptomatic and identified by routine blood work alone.[44] Cholangitis has been reported as the initial presentation of HIV infection in a few patients.[17,140]

Diagnostic steps include noninvasive imaging with sonography and CT, and ERCP. Abdominal ultrasound is abnormal in 75 percent of patients and typically shows dilation or wall thickening of the common bile duct. These findings, along with liver function studies, may be suggestive of the disease even in

children.[177] ERCP can show further characteristic changes in the biliary tract and has the added advantage of obtaining specimens for biopsy and culture and the possibility of therapeutic intervention.[232] Although AIDS-related cholangitis typically is not directly associated with mortality, most patients with AIDS-related cholangitis die within 1 year of being diagnosed because cholangitis usually occurs in patients with end-stage disease.[120] Therapy generally is symptomatic and should include coverage of bacterial cholangitis, which often is associated because of impaired biliary drainage.

CHOLANGITIS IN ASSOCIATION WITH CONGENITAL ANATOMIC ABNORMALITIES: CHOLEDOCHAL CYSTS AND CAROLI DISEASE

Choledochal cysts occur in 1 in 15,000 births in Western nations and 1 in 1000 live births in Japan.[148] Typically, presenting signs suggest cholestasis and may include jaundice, dark urine, and acholic stools, or patients may present with abdominal masses with or without jaundice. If diagnosed late or untreated, choledochal cysts may result in severe complications secondary to biliary tract obstruction, including cholangitis and pancreatitis. One series of 36 Indian patients reported 13 patients, more frequently children than infants, who presented with cholangitis.[158] Cholangitis is more likely to be the presenting sign for choledochal cyst in adult patients.[31]

Treatment of cholangitis associated with choledochal cysts involves supportive treatment of the patient, including appropriate antibiotic treatment. In the past, cyst-enteric drainage procedures were used as temporizing treatments, and this type of repair was associated with high rates of complications, including recurrent bouts of cholangitis, stones, and cholangiocarcinoma in the remnant duct.[168] The current surgical goal is complete surgical excision; compared with internal drainage procedures, this approach is associated with lower rates of postoperative cholangitis and mortality.[181] Five types of choledochal cysts have been identified, with solitary extrahepatic cysts (type I) being encountered most frequently. After this type of cyst has been excised, reconstruction of the biliary tract may involve a Roux-en-Y choledochojejunostomy or hepatojejunostomy.

Patients who undergo this surgery also are at risk for developing postoperative ascending cholangitis, with an incidence of 8 to 19 percent.[52,185] Although recurrent cholangitis may lead to chronic liver disease in the long-term, antibiotic prophylaxis is not recommended routinely.[92]

Caroli disease describes congenital dilation of the intrahepatic and extrahepatic biliary tree characterized by pure ductal ectasia.[37,38] More commonly, dilation of the intrahepatic ducts is attributed to ductal plate malformation in association with congenital hepatic fibrosis. The association of ductal ectasia with congenital hepatic fibrosis is more common than without and is termed *Caroli syndrome*. Both of these diseases may manifest with clinical signs of liver disease or renal disease secondary to the associated condition of autosomal recessive polycystic kidney disease, or both.[93,118,153] Dilation of the intrahepatic bile ducts results in biliary obstruction and places the patient at increased risk for development of intrahepatic stones and cholangitis, which significantly increases morbidity and mortality rates in Caroli disease and congenital hepatic fibrosis. Diagnosis is suspected in the case of recurrent cholangitis or portal hypertension of unknown etiology, and can be confirmed by ultrasound, cholangiography,[49] or MRCP.

Portosystemic shunting is considered the treatment of choice because this condition typically does not progress to liver failure. Suspicion of cholangitis, whether owing to signs of infection or sepsis or laboratory results suggesting inflammation, should be confirmed via a diagnostic liver biopsy for culture. Treatment of cholangitis in the setting of Caroli disease may be difficult.

Recurrent episodes may occur even after administration of intensive intravenous antibiotic therapy.[224] In some cases, drainage procedures may be used for refractory or recurrent infections. Orthotopic liver transplantation is the treatment of choice in recurrent, life-threatening episodes of cholangitis.[76,224]

Typically, patients with Caroli disease or Caroli syndrome present with cholangitis because the biliary malformation communicates with the extrahepatic biliary tree. Rarely, patients are seen with hepatic cysts associated with autosomal dominant polycystic kidney disease. These lesions are noncommunicating lesions and as such are not prone to infection. In the absence of a history of cholangitis, it is advisable that these rare patients not undergo invasive procedures of the biliary tree because of the risk of microbial seeding and subsequent suppurative cholangitis.[5,100,234]

CHOLANGITIS AFTER ENDOSCOPIC AND OTHER BILIARY PROCEDURES

Although at this point, experience in the use of ERCP in pediatric patients is limited, it is growing, and cholangitis is a known complication of this procedure in adults. In a series of 50 pediatric patients, low-grade fever, abdominal pain, nausea, and vomiting were reported as the most common complaints after undergoing ERCP; one patient was treated for mild cholangitis.[211] Another group reported three cases of sepsis in adults caused by multiresistant *Pseudomonas aeruginosa* after ERCP, ascribed to nosocomial transmission from the endoscope despite negative surveillance cultures.[41] In adults, and rarely in children, biliary stents are used to alleviate a common bile duct obstruction, most frequently malignant.

The major complication of these stents is obstruction and subsequent upstream infection. Clinicians have looked at ways to prolong stent patency. A meta-analysis of randomized or quasi-randomized studies examining the role of antibiotics or ursodeoxycholic acid to maintain stent patency showed no conclusive evidence in favor of either one in the prevention of stent occlusion. In certain children and adolescents with a history of recalcitrant cholangitis, percutaneous transhepatic biliary drainage is used by experienced centers to decompress the biliary tree upstream of the stricture or to dilate the stricture. This procedure is used primarily in patients with PSC and in transplant patients with biliary stenoses secondary to ischemia or rejection.[10,36,56,62,74,209] These patients also benefit from oral antibiotic prophylaxis, frequently ciprofloxacin for its excellent biliary penetration.

CHOLECYSTITIS

Gallstones are the prime initiating factor in cholecystitis. Gallstone disease is a common entity in adults, with more than 700,000 cholecystectomies performed each year in the United States among approximately 20 million adults with gallstones.[109] In children, gallstones and gallstone-related complications occur much less frequently than in adults. In certain pediatric populations, such as patients with hemolytic conditions, gallstone and gallbladder diseases are more common, however, and need to be considered in appropriate clinical settings.[192] In addition, because gallstones are associated with obesity, an increase in pediatric-onset cholelithiasis may occur soon owing to the epidemic in childhood obesity.[193]

The term *cholelithiasis* refers to the presence of gallstones, which may occur silently or in association with clinical symptoms. Biliary colic occurs in the setting of obstruction of either the cystic duct or the common bile duct secondary to gallstones and is associated with characteristic episodic, postprandial right upper quadrant pain. Acute cholecystitis involves inflammation of the gallbladder and can be seen with cholelithiasis (calculous) or in the absence of gallstones (acalculous). In adults, acute cholecystitis almost always is associated with gallstones—90 percent of adult cases occur secondary to gallstones. In contrast, 30 to 50 percent of pediatric cases are acalculous.[216] Acalculous cholecystitis is discussed separately at the end of this section.

ETIOLOGY AND PATHOGENESIS

Gallstones generally are classified as either pigment stones or cholesterol stones. Pigment stones can be divided further into either black or brown pigment stones. Black pigment stones occur in the face of a superabundance of unconjugated bilirubin in the bile and are seen most commonly in hemolytic disease, leading to increased biliary concentration of bilirubin and to calcium-bilirubinate stones. Brown pigment stones are less common and are associated with biliary infection or parasitic infestation, or with the presence of a foreign body (e.g., retained suture material) or biliary obstruction. Cholesterol stones are the end result of biliary cholesterol supersaturation secondary to an imbalance in the cholesterol : phospholipid : bile salt equilibrium or other precipitating factors.[42] These stones tend to occur in the face of either elevated cholesterol production or decreased bile salt pool.

In pediatric practice, pigment stones are seen more frequently than are cholesterol stones, in direct contrast to adult populations, in which cholesterol stones are more prevalent. Friesen and Roberts[55] described 693 pediatric cases of gallstone disease, of which 72 percent involved pigmented stones. The greatest experience with pigmented gallstones in children is in children with hemolytic diseases, primarily sickle-cell anemia and thalassemia, but also in patients with hereditary spherocytosis and other red cell membrane defects, pyruvate kinase deficiency, glucose-6-phosphate dehydrogenase deficiency, and autoimmune hemolytic anemia.[77,167,190] The prevalence of pigment gallstones in hemolytic disease increases with age. In children younger than 10 years old, the frequency is 12 to 14 percent; the frequency increases to 36 to 42 percent in individuals 10 to 20 years old.[16,188]

Total parenteral nutrition predisposes children to develop biliary tract disease, and in particular gallstone formation.[165] This condition occurs more commonly in premature neonates, especially neonates with enteral diseases, in which prolonged fasting, sepsis, immaturity of the enterohepatic circulation of bile acids, small bowel bacterial overgrowth, and prolonged duration of total parenteral nutrition contribute to biliary stasis and increased prevalence of gallstones and sludge.[6,99,106,187,208,226] The occurrence of gallstones secondary to total parenteral nutrition does not lead to increased prevalence of complications, however, because many of these gallstones are clinically silent.

Cholesterol stones are found most frequently in adults and have an increased prevalence in women from puberty to menopause and in obese patients.[184] Some of these characteristics may translate to pediatrics as well. Although boys and girls exhibit an equal incidence in gallstones at young ages, the incidence in girls increases significantly after puberty, and female predominance of gallstone disease continues through menopause.[147] Related risk factors for the presence of cholesterol stones in children and adolescents include obesity, pregnancy, and the use of oral contraceptives. In addition, conditions that are associated with decreased ileal bile salt resorption predispose to stone formation. This association includes patients who have undergone ileal resection or bypass and patients with Crohn disease.[174]

Gallstones are found in 28 percent of adults with cystic fibrosis at the time of autopsy.[196] The presence of gallstones in children with cystic fibrosis is well documented, but the pathogenesis likely is multifactorial.

TABLE 54-4 Patient Populations Predisposed to Gallstone Formation

Pigment Stones	Cholesterol Stones
Hemolytic disorders	Pregnancy
Total parenteral nutrition	Obesity
Biliary tract anomalies (e.g. Caroli disease)	Rapid weight loss
Parasitic disease (*Ascaris lubricoides*)*	Malabsorption (e.g., Crohn disease, ileal resection)
Ceftriaxone use	Genetic predisposition (e.g., *ABCB4* homozygosity)
Solid organ transplantation (heart, lung, kidney)	Cystic fibrosis and other cholestatic liver diseases

Brown pigment stones.

Finally, children with chronic liver disease, and in particular cholestasis, are at increased risk for gallstone formation, owing to a deficit of biliary excretion.[229] Table 54-4 summarizes the pediatric patient populations at risk for development of gallstones.[57]

The genetics of biliary stone formation has been the focus of intense research. The consensus is that biliary stone formation, affecting the gallbladder and the common bile duct, is the product of genetic predisposition and environmental risk factors. In adults, a distinction is made between the "common" polygenic predisposition to gallstones and the rarer oligogenic predisposition. Briefly, the first, polygenic group refers to patients with evidence of increased risk of developing biliary stone formation, probably associated with numerous factors, including lithogenic (*LITH*) genes. The oligogenic group refers to a small group of patients with known mutations in genes involved in bile synthesis and export.[72,229] The clearest examples to date are defects in the *ABCB4* transporter in humans[175] and the *Mdr2* homozygous null mutant in mice.[108] Both conditions lead to an increased propensity toward cholelithiasis and choledocholithiasis; however, whether these subjects have a profile of biliary tract infections different from that of the polygenic group is unknown.

The most likely cause of calculous cholecystitis is gallstone obstruction of the cystic duct, which leads to increased intraluminal pressure with gallbladder distention, mucosal damage, and release of inflammatory mediators. The end result is acute inflammation of the gallbladder. Any bacterial infection probably is a secondary occurrence to biliary obstruction.[109]

CLINICAL PRESENTATION

Acute cholecystitis typically manifests with abdominal pain and vomiting. Pain may be localized to the right upper quadrant; however, in pediatric patients, this making distinction can be difficult, and it may be difficult to differentiate from other causes of acute abdominal pain in children. As in the model of appendicitis, initial pain with obstruction of the cystic duct tends to be visceral pain that may be epigastric and poorly localized. With gallbladder inflammation, the pain becomes parietal—more localized to the right upper quadrant and associated with some peritoneal signs, such as pain with movement. With regard to the duration of pain, cholecystitis should produce pain that is more long-standing than uncomplicated biliary colic. Although obstruction of the cystic duct is associated with the acute onset of pain followed by resolution within 3 to 6 hours, true gallbladder inflammation may produce a more persistent pain, lasting 6 to 12 hours or longer.

The presence of jaundice with right upper quadrant pain and emesis in a patient without hemolysis or increasing jaundice in hemolytic patients warrants a thorough investigation for the possible presence of choledocholithiasis and cholecystitis. Fever, although classically described in the presentation of cholecystitis, is not universally present. In a retrospective study of 198 adults who presented to an emergency center with acute cholecystitis, 59 percent were afebrile.[71] Physical examination may show a tender right upper quadrant. The examiner should try to elicit Murphy's sign, for which tenderness on palpation of the right upper quadrant worsens with palpation of the liver edge or gallbladder and may be most apparent with deep inspiration. The patient may exhibit voluntary guarding or peritoneal signs. A palpable mass, representing the inflamed gallbladder with adjacent omentum, may be present.

EVALUATION

Laboratory evaluation may show leukocytosis, although this finding is not universally present in adults or children with cholecystitis.[71,165] Bilirubin levels may be elevated, especially in the setting of hemolysis. A conjugated hyperbilirubinemia should cause one to be concerned about choledocholithiasis, or sepsis-associated cholestasis. Transaminases and amylase and lipase are ordered frequently on initial evaluation to investigate for other causes of epigastric or right upper quadrant pain with vomiting or fever or both, such as pancreatitis and viral hepatitis. As in the evaluation of cholangitis, early consultation with a pediatric surgeon is appropriate.

Abdominal ultrasound is the test of choice in establishing the diagnosis of cholecystitis. Findings on ultrasound include a thickened or irregular, hyperreflexive gallbladder wall with or without the presence of gallstones. Experienced sonographers may be able to elicit tenderness over the gallbladder, the "sonographic Murphy sign." Ultrasound is useful for detecting gallstone disease, showing 90 percent in some cases, although in other studies, ultrasound has a markedly lower sensitivity to detected common duct stones.[54] Without suspicion of gallbladder inflammation, however, the finding of gallstones alone by sonogram does not indicate cholecystitis. Other false-positive studies may occur with the finding of thickened gallbladder walls in patients with hypoalbuminemia, renal failure, or heart failure.[156] The inability to visualize the gallbladder by ultrasound may indicate the finding of a diseased, chronically obstructed gallbladder.[68]

Hepatobiliary scintigraphy (HIDA scan) can be useful in confirming the diagnosis of acute cholecystitis. The study employs a technetium-labeled iminodiacetic acid agent that is excreted into the bile ducts. Subsequent images are taken, which in a normal study should fill the gallbladder, extrahepatic ducts, and duodenum. In the case of cystic duct obstruction, a positive study fails to show the gallbladder filling. The sensitivity and specificity of this study are high, with results approaching 90 to 100 percent and 90 to 95 percent.[143,166] The test may be augmented by attempts to stimulate gallbladder contraction using a cholecystokinin analogue. Plain abdominal radiographs and oral cholecystography are infrequently used in the current clinical environment.

ACALCULOUS CHOLECYSTITIS

Acalculous cholecystitis is a rare but important cause of cholecystitis in pediatric patients. Generally, acalculous gallbladder disease in children occurs in various clinical settings, ranging from congenital gallbladder abnormalities, to idiopathic gallbladder distention without inflammation (acute hydrops of the gallbladder), to acute or chronic cholecystitis. The exact pathogenesis of acute acalculous cholecystitis is unclear; however, stagnation of the bile may be an important factor, as suggested by several predisposing clinical conditions that lead to bile stasis. In addi-

TABLE 54–5   Conditions Associated with Acalculous Gallbladder Disease

Biliary tract anomaly (e.g., choledochal cyst)
Bone marrow transplant
Burns
Chemotherapy in oncology patients
Critical illness in ICU patients
Crohn disease, Kawasaki disease, systemic lupus erythematosus
Infectious agents (atypical microbes)
Postoperative state (e.g., cardiac surgery)
Sepsis
Sludge
Systemic inflammatory states
Total parenteral nutrition
Traumatic spinal cord injury

ICU, intensive care unit.

tion, sphincter of Oddi spasm or dysfunction, as occurs after administration of opiates, could lead to retrograde reflux of inflammatory enzymes or infectious agents. Alternatively, changes in the gallbladder vascular supply may weaken the gallbladder mucosa and allow biliary components to damage the gallbladder wall.[64] Acalculous cholecystitis has been associated with many infectious and noninfectious clinical scenarios. Bacterial, viral, and parasitic agents have been implicated in the setting of acalculous cholecystitis. Frequently, gallstone or biliary microlithiasis missed by standard diagnostic evaluations may lead the clinician to the presumptive diagnosis of acalculous cholecystitis. One adult study revealed that 33 of 35 patients with abdominal pain and a negative transabdominal sonogram had gallbladder sludge and stones, and 21 of those patients also had common bile duct involvement.[136]

Reports of true acalculous disease have been described with systemic infection from *Salmonella* spp., *Mycoplasma pneumoniae*, *Leptospira interrogans*, *Brucella* spp., Rocky Mountain spotted fever, group A streptococci, group B streptococci, and *Staphylococcus aureus*.[8,9,39,78,82,131,198,212,230] Examination and culture of cholecystectomy specimens from patients with acalculous cholecystitis have revealed positive cultures for *Helicobacter* spp. and *Campylobacter jejuni*.* Associations with viral disease include CMV, mumps virus, Epstein-Barr virus, and hepatitis A virus.[2,11,12,13,19,28,60,161] Acalculous cholecystitis has been associated with *Plasmodium falciparum* infections (malaria).[46,126,179,186,233] In immunosuppressed hosts, acalculous cholecystitis also has been described in fungal infections with *Candida* or *Aspergillus*, or parasitic infections with *Giardia* and *Cryptosporidium*.[144]

Noninfectious systemic diseases associated with acalculous cholecystitis or hydrops include neoplastic disease (i.e., leukemia), Henoch-Schönlein purpura, lupus erythematosus, and Kawasaki disease.[25,83,129] Table 54–5 lists several conditions with which acalculous cholecystitis has been reported.[86,88,171,203,213,214]

Clinical presentation is similar to that of patients with calculous disease, with right upper quadrant pain, nausea, vomiting, anorexia, and fever being the most common symptoms. Leukocytosis, jaundice, or a palpable right upper quadrant mass also may be present.[216] The most common setting for acalculous disease is in critically ill or chronically ill patients with concurrent acute or chronic symptoms. A high degree of clinical suspicion is crucial in making the diagnosis in these populations because often the findings suggestive of cholecystitis are obscured by the patient's systemic disease. The most common sonographic finding is a thickened gallbladder wall and a possible sonographic Murphy sign. Gallbladder distention, sludge, or pericholecystic

*See references 7, 22, 23, 53, 97, 111, 117, 128, 133, 134, 210, 223.

fluid also may be found on transabdominal ultrasound.[87] In addition to ultrasound, the HIDA scan is an important tool in the evaluation of acalculous cholecystitis. Failure to visualize the gallbladder on scintigraphy and a low ejection fraction in response to a cholecystokinin analogue are suggestive of acalculous disease.[127,143,162,236]

MANAGEMENT

Management strategies of gallstone disease in children vary, contingent on individual clinical scenarios. Silent gallstones, which are asymptomatic and often detected incidentally by ultrasound, can be followed conservatively and sonographically without emergent or elective surgery. Although conservative management of adults with asymptomatic stones is described in multiple reports, no such guidelines exist for children. Patients with hemolytic disease in whom gallstones are detected should be considered for early cholecystectomy, although this plan is controversial.[4,73,91,135,225] In patients with sickle-cell anemia, the benefit of timely surgery may outweigh the morbidity of associated abdominal pain crises and the overall morbidity and mortality of surgery in these patients, which increases with age.

In acute calculous cholecystitis, surgery is the mainstay of therapy. Patients should be admitted to the hospital for monitoring, intravenous hydration, and pain control. Antibiotic therapy often is initiated, even without clinical evidence of sepsis or perforation. The choice of antibiotics is similar to that for cholangitis and typically covers gut luminal flora (e.g., a synthetic penicillin plus an aminoglycoside with or without the addition of mezlocillin).[75,227] Surgical treatment may be limited to cholecystotomy, especially in chronically ill children with a high risk of developing complications. Generally, early cholecystectomy should be performed in patients with acute cholecystitis secondary to gallstone disease. Laparoscopic procedures are becoming more widely used in experienced pediatric surgical centers and are associated with positive outcomes in children and adults.

Optimal management of acalculous cholecystitis has not been investigated fully, primarily because of the lack of a diagnostic standard and varied patient population base. This situation leads to an individualized approach that typically starts conservatively with observation but may involve removing oral feeds and placing the patient on intravenous hydration and antibiotics, or it leads to more invasive management with cholecystectomy or biliary manometrics via ERCP.[63,87] Attempts should be made to diagnose and treat any underlying condition in the patient. A more recent treatment protocol supports the close monitoring of these patients with frequent examinations, ultrasonography, and blood tests to determine if the need for cholecystectomy or ERCP seems likely. If ultrasound shows improved findings, conservative management is continued with close follow-up. If biliary dyskinesia is suspected secondary to sphincter of Oddi dysfunction, ERCP offers a diagnostic and therapeutic option at experienced centers.[51,160,218]

COMPLICATIONS

Acute cholecystitis may lead to complications, even if it is recognized in a timely fashion. An inflamed, obstructed gallbladder may wall off to form an intraluminal abscess or empyema. Perforation of the gallbladder is the most frequent complication. A localized perforation may develop into a pericholecystic abscess that is palpable as a tender right upper quadrant mass on examination. Free perforation with peritonitis is associated with a 30 percent mortality rate, but it is found in only a few patients, estimated at 1 to 2 percent of adult patients.[109] In each of these situations, prompt surgical intervention and intravenous hydration and antibiotic therapy are crucial in management.

Aside from gallbladder inflammation, complications of gallstone disease may include pancreatitis and choledocholithiasis. Gallstone pancreatitis was a frequent complication of gallstone disease in a series of 50 pediatric patients.[165] Choledocholithiasis with ascending cholangitis, a well-known complication of gallstones, is a rare cause of cholangitis in pediatric patients. Secondary common bile duct stones, usually originating from the gallbladder, can be found in patients with acute cholecystitis by ultrasound, ERCP, MRCP, or intraoperative cholangiography. The possible presence of choledocholithiasis should be considered in any patient with known gallstone disease who presents with increasing jaundice, fever, and right upper quadrant pain, and requires urgent clinical investigation and decompression, typically via ERCP.[206]

BILIARY TRACT INFECTIONS AFTER CARDIOTHORACIC SURGERY

In adults, the association between cardiothoracic surgery and biliary complications is well known and covered extensively in the literature.[123,139,217] These complications frequently manifest as cholangitis or cholecystitis, commonly with stone or sludge formation. The high incidence of biliary complications that develop after cardiothoracic surgery is ascribed to prolonged fasting, metabolic disturbances, vagotomy, and hypoperfusion. The last, in particular, is thought to predispose the biliary tree, which is exquisitely reliant on adequate arterial perfusion, to development of focal ischemia and secondary strictures. In pediatrics, although it is commonly accepted by clinicians as a frequent association, no studies have been published. The clinical implications of the adult studies and unpublished pediatric observations is that patients may present after cardiothoracic surgery with acute biliary disease warranting aggressive empiric management occasionally in immunosuppressed hosts who have undergone thoracic organ transplantation.

Infections of the intrahepatic and extrahepatic biliary tree in children differ from infections in adults by the nature of the populations they affect. First, patients with biliary atresia and portoenterostomy are subject to ascending cholangitis and the risk of developing sepsis and rapidly progressive liver disease. Second, children with hemoglobinopathies are prone to developing cholecystitis because of their increased incidence of cholelithiasis. In these two groups and in other pediatric patients, the same principles of management apply: Biliary obstruction must be sought and alleviated when possible, and aggressive parenteral antimicrobial therapy must be initiated promptly because of the risk of developing sepsis and worsening liver disease.

REFERENCES

1. Abdo, A., Klassen, J., Urbanski, S., et al.: Reversible sclerosing cholangitis secondary to cryptosporidiosis in a renal transplant patient. J. Hepatol. 38:688, 2003.
2. Adolph, M. D., Bass, S. N., Lee, S. K., et al.: Cytomegaloviral acalculous cholecystitis in acquired immunodeficiency syndrome patients. Am. Surg. 59:679, 1993.
3. Allendorph, M., Werlin, S. L., Geenen, J. E., et al.: Endoscopic retrograde cholangiopancreatography in children. J. Pediatr. 110:206, 1987.
4. Al-Mulhim, A. S., Al-Mulhim, F. M., and Al-Suwaiygh, A. A.: The role of laparoscopic cholecystectomy in the management of acute cholecystitis in patients with sickle cell disease. Am. J. Surg. 183:668, 2002.
5. Ananthakrishnan, A. N., and Saeian, K.: Caroli's disease: Identification and treatment strategy. Curr. Gastroenterol. Rep. 9:151, 2007.
6. Angelico, M., and Della Guardia, P.: Review article: Hepatobiliary complications associated with total parenteral nutrition. Aliment. Pharmacol. Ther. 14(Suppl. 2):54, 2000.
7. Apostolov, E., Al-Soud, W. A., Nilsson, I., et al.: *Helicobacter pylori* and other *Helicobacter* species in gallbladder and liver of patients with chronic cholecystitis detected by immunological and molecular methods. Scand. J. Gastroenterol. 40:96, 2005.
8. Ashley, D., Vade, A., and Challapalli, M.: Brucellosis with acute acalculous cholecystitis. Pediatr. Infect. Dis. J. 19:1112, 2000.
9. Ayite, A., Etey, K., Tchatagba, K., et al.: [Acute acalculous cholecystitis of typhoid origin: A report of 5 cases]. Tunis Med. 74:257, 1996.
10. Barrioz, T., Ingrand, P., Besson, I., et al.: Randomised trial of prevention of biliary stent occlusion by ursodeoxycholic acid plus norfloxacin. Lancet 344:581, 1994.
11. Basar, O., Kisacik, B., Bozdogan, E., et al.: An unusual cause of acalculous cholecystitis during pregnancy: Hepatitis A virus. Dig. Dis. Sci. 50:1532, 2005.
12. Behera, A., Kochhar, R., Dhavan, S., et al.: Isolated common bile duct tuberculosis mimicking malignant obstruction. Am. J. Gastroenterol. 92:2122, 1997.
13. Bigio, E. H., and Haque, A. K.: Disseminated cytomegalovirus infection presenting with acalculous cholecystitis and acute pancreatitis. Arch. Pathol. Lab. Med. 113:1287, 1989.
14. Billhartz, L. E.: Gallstone disease and its complications. In Feldman, M., and Scharschmidt, B. F. (eds,): Sleisenger and Fordtran's Gastrointestinal and Liver Disease: Pathophysiology, Diagnosis, Management. 6th ed., Vol. 1. Philadelphia, W. B. Saunders, 1998.
15. Boey, J. H., and Way, L. W.: Acute cholangitis. Ann. Surg. 191:264, 1980.
16. Bond, L. R., Hatty, S. R., Horn, M. E., et al.: Gall stones in sickle cell disease in the United Kingdom. B. M. J. (Clin. Res. Ed.) 295:234, 1987.
17. Bouche, H., Housset, C., Dumont, J. L., et al.: AIDS-related cholangitis: Diagnostic features and course in 15 patients. J. Hepatol. 17:34, 1993.
18. Bowles, B. J., Abdul-Ghani, A., Zhang, J., et al.: Fifteen years' experience with an antirefluxing biliary drainage valve. J. Pediatr. Surg. 34:1711, 1999.
19. Brent, A. J., Hull, R., Jeffery, K. J., et al.: Acute cholecystitis complicating mumps. Clin. Infect. Dis. 42:302, 2006.
20. Brook, I., and Altman, R. P.: The significance of anaerobic bacteria in biliary tract infection after hepatic portoenterostomy for biliary atresia. Surgery 95:281, 1984.
21. Brown, S. J., and Desmond, P. V.: Hepatotoxicity of antimicrobial agents. Semin. Liver Dis. 22:157, 2002.
22. Bulajic, M., Maisonneuve, P., Schneider-Brachert, W., et al.: *Helicobacter pylori* and the risk of benign and malignant biliary tract disease. Cancer 95:1946, 2002.
23. Bulajic, M., Stimec, B., Milicevic, M., et al.: Modalities of testing *Helicobacter pylori* in patients with nonmalignant bile duct diseases. World J. Gastroenterol. 8:301, 2002.
24. Burgart, L. J.: Cholangitis in viral disease. Mayo Clin. Proc. 73:479, 1998.
25. Buyukasik, Y., Kosar, A., Demiroglu, H., et al.: Acalculous acute cholecystitis in leukemia. J. Clin. Gastroenterol. 27:146, 1998.
26. Cappell, M. S.: Endoscopic retrograde cholangiopancreatography with endoscopic sphincterotomy for symptomatic choledocholithiasis after recent myocardial infarction. Am. J. Gastroenterol. 91:1827, 1996.
27. Carpenter, H. A.: Bacterial and parasitic cholangitis. Mayo Clin. Proc. 73:473, 1998.
28. Casha, P., Rifflet, H., Renou, C., et al.: [Acalculous acute cholecystitis and viral hepatitis A]. Gastroenterol. Clin. Biol. 24:591, 2000.
29. Cello, J. P.: Acquired immunodeficiency syndrome cholangiopathy: Spectrum of disease. Am. J. Med. 86:539, 1989.
30. Chand, N., and Sanyal, A. J.: Sepsis-induced cholestasis. Hepatology 45:230, 2007.
31. Chaudhary, A., Dhar, P., Sachdev, A., et al.: Choledochal cysts—differences in children and adults. Br. J. Surg. 83:186, 1996.
32. Chaudhary, S., and Turner, R. B.: Trimethoprim-sulfamethoxazole for cholangitis following hepatic portoenterostomy for biliary atresia. J. Pediatr. 99:656, 1981.
33. Chen, C. C., Chang, P. Y., and Chen, C. L.: Refractory cholangitis after Kasai's operation caused by candidiasis: A case report. J. Pediatr. Surg. 21:736, 1986.
34. Chitturi, S., and George, J.: Hepatotoxicity of commonly used drugs: Nonsteroidal anti-inflammatory drugs, antihypertensives, antidiabetic agents, anticonvulsants, lipid-lowering agents, psychotropic drugs. Semin. Liver Dis. 22:169, 2002.
35. Chung, R. T., and Sheffer, E. C.: Case 28-2001: A 44-year-old woman with chills, fever, jaundice, and hepatic abscesses. N. Engl. J. Med. 345:817, 2001.
36. De Ledinghen, V., Person, B., Legoux, J. L., et al.: Prevention of biliary stent occlusion by ursodeoxycholic acid plus norfloxacin: A multicenter randomized trial. Dig. Dis. Sci. 45:145, 2000.
37. Desmet, V. J.: Congenital diseases of intrahepatic bile ducts: Variations on the theme "ductal plate malformation." Hepatology 16:1069, 1992.
38. Desmet, V. J.: Ludwig symposium on biliary disorders, part I: Pathogenesis of ductal plate abnormalities. Mayo Clin. Proc. 73:80, 1998.
39. Dickinson, S. J., Corley, G., and Santulli, T. V.: Acute cholecystitis as a sequel of scarlet fever. Am. J. Dis. Child. 121:331, 1971.
40. Dimicoli, S., Bensoussan, D., Latger-Cannard, V., et al.: Complete recovery from *Cryptosporidium parvum* infection with gastroenteritis and sclerosing cholangitis after successful bone marrow transplantation in two brothers with X-linked hyper-IgM syndrome. Bone Marrow Transplant. 32:733, 2003.

41. Doherty, D. E., Falko, J. M., Lefkovitz, N., et al.: *Pseudomonas aeruginosa* sepsis following retrograde cholangiopancreatography (ERCP). Dig. Dis. Sci. 27:169, 1982.

42. Donovan, J. M.: Physical and metabolic factors in gallstone pathogenesis. Gastroenterol. Clin. North Am. 28:75, 1999.

43. Dooley, J. S., Hamilton-Miller, J. M., Brumfitt, W., et al.: Antibiotics in the treatment of biliary infection. Gut 25:988, 1984.

44. Ducreux, M., Buffet, C., Lamy, P., et al.: Diagnosis and prognosis of AIDS-related cholangitis. AIDS 9:875, 1995.

45. Dunham, E. C.: Septicemia in the newborn. Am. J. Dis. Child. 45:229, 1933.

46. Dylewski, J. S., and Al-Azragi, T.: Acalculous cholecystitis associated with *Plasmodium falciparum* infection. Clin. Infect. Dis. 29:947, 1999.

47. Ecoffey, C., Rothman, E., Bernard, O., et al.: Bacterial cholangitis after surgery for biliary atresia. J. Pediatr. 111:824, 1987.

48. Elsakr, R., Johnson, D. A., Younes, Z., et al.: Antimicrobial treatment of intra-abdominal infections. Dig. Dis. 16:47, 1998.

49. Fagundes-Neto, U., Schettini, S. T., Wehba, J., et al.: Caroli's disease in childhood: Report of two new cases. J. Pediatr. Gastroenterol. Nutr. 2:708, 1983.

50. Fan, S. T., Ng, I. O., Choi, T. K., et al.: Tuberculosis of the bile duct: A rare cause of biliary stricture. Am. J. Gastroenterol. 84:413, 1989.

51. Fogel, E. L., Eversman, D., Jamidar, P., et al.: Sphincter of Oddi dysfunction: Pancreaticobiliary sphincterotomy with pancreatic stent placement has a lower rate of pancreatitis than biliary sphincterotomy alone. Endoscopy 34:280, 2002.

52. Fonkalsrud, E. W.: Choledochal cysts. Surg. Clin. North Am. 53:1275, 1973.

53. Fox, J. G., Dewhirst, F. E., Shen, Z., et al.: Hepatic *Helicobacter* species identified in bile and gallbladder tissue from Chileans with chronic cholecystitis. Gastroenterology 114:755, 1998.

54. Freitas, M. L., Bell, R. L., and Duffy, A. J.: Choledocholithiasis: Evolving standards for diagnosis and management. World J. Gastroenterol. 12:3162, 2006.

55. Friesen, C. A., and Roberts, C. C.: Cholelithiasis: Clinical characteristics in children: Case analysis and literature review. Clin. Pediatr. (Philadelphia) 28:294, 1989.

56. Galandi, D., Schwarzer, G., Bassler, D., et al.: Ursodeoxycholic acid and/or antibiotics for prevention of biliary stent occlusion. Cochrane Database Syst. Rev. CD003043, 2002.

57. Ganschow, R.: Cholelithiasis in pediatric organ transplantation: Detection and management. Pediatr. Transplant. 6:91, 2002.

58. Garcia-Ruiz, J. C., Hernandez, I., Munoz, F., et al.: Cholangitis due to *Aspergillus fumigatus* in a patient with acute leukemia. Clin. Infect. Dis. 26:228, 1998.

59. Geier, A., Fickert, P., and Trauner, M.: Mechanisms of disease: Mechanisms and clinical implications of cholestasis in sepsis. Nat. Clin. Pract. Gastroenterol. Hepatol. 3:574, 2006.

60. Gerain, J., Sculier, J. P., Malengreaux, A., et al.: Causes of deaths in an oncologic intensive care unit: A clinical and pathological study of 34 autopsies. Eur. J. Cancer 26:377, 1990.

61. Gerecht, W. B., Henry, N. K., Hoffman, W. W., et al.: Prospective randomized comparison of mezlocillin therapy alone with combined ampicillin and gentamicin therapy for patients with cholangitis. Arch. Intern. Med. 149:1279, 1989.

62. Ghosh, S., and Palmer, K. R.: Prevention of biliary stent occlusion using cyclical antibiotics and ursodeoxycholic acid. Gut 35:1757, 1994.

63. Glenn, F.: Acute acalculous cholecystitis. Ann. Surg. 189:458, 1979.

64. Glenn, F., and Becker, C. G.: Acute acalculous cholecystitis: An increasing entity. Ann. Surg. 195:131, 1982.

65. Goddard, E. A., Mouton, S. C., Westwood, A. T., et al.: Cryptosporidiosis of the gastrointestinal tract associated with sclerosing cholangitis in the absence of documented immunodeficiency: *Cryptosporidium parvum* and sclerosing cholangitis in an immunocompetent child. J. Pediatr. Gastroenterol. Nutr. 31:317, 2000.

66. Gottrand, F., Bernard, O., Hadchouel, M., et al.: Late cholangitis after successful surgical repair of biliary atresia. Am. J. Dis. Child. 145:213, 1991.

67. Grant, A., Sargent, C., Weller, I. V., et al.: Disseminated cytomegalovirus infection. Genitourin. Med. 68:75, 1992.

68. Greenberg, M., Kangarloo, H., Cochran, S. T., et al.: The ultrasonographic diagnosis of cholecystitis and cholelithiasis in children. Radiology 137:745, 1980.

69. Gremse, D. A., Bucuvalas, J. C., and Bongiovanni, G. L.: Papillary stenosis and sclerosing cholangitis in an immunodeficient child. Gastroenterology 96:1600, 1989.

70. Greulich, T., and Kohler, B.: [Obstructive jaundice caused by spontaneous rupture of an *Echinococcus granulosus* cyst into the bile duct system]. Z. Gastroenterol. 38:301, 2000.

71. Gruber, P. J., Silverman, R. A., Gottesfeld, S., et al.: Presence of fever and leukocytosis in acute cholecystitis. Ann. Emerg. Med. 28:273, 1996.

72. Grunhage, F., and Lammert, F.: Gallstone disease: Pathogenesis of gallstones: A genetic perspective. Best Pract. Res. Clin. Gastroenterol. 20:997, 2006.

73. Haberkern, C. M., Neumayr, L. D., Orringer, E. P., et al.: Cholecystectomy in sickle cell anemia patients: Perioperative outcome of 364 cases from the National Preoperative Transfusion Study. Preoperative Transfusion in Sickle Cell Disease Study Group. Blood 89:1533, 1997.

74. Halm, U., Schiefke, Fleig, W. E., et al.: Ofloxacin and ursodeoxycholic acid versus ursodeoxycholic acid alone to prevent occlusion of biliary stents: A prospective, randomized trial. Endoscopy 33:491, 2001.

75. Hanau, L. H., and Steigbigel, N. H.: Acute (ascending) cholangitis. Infect. Dis. Clin. North Am. 14:521, 2000.

76. Harjai, M. M., and Bal, R. K.: Caroli syndrome. Pediatr. Surg. Int. 16:431, 2000.

77. Heubi, J., Lewis, L. G., and Pohl, J.: Diseases of the gallbladder in infancy, childhood, and adolescence. *In* Suchy, F. J., Sokol, R. J., and Balistreri, W. F. (eds.): Liver Disease in Children. 2nd ed., Vol. 1. Philadelphia, Lippincott Williams & Williams, 2001.

78. Hirata, K., Torigoe, T., Fukuda, M., et al.: [A case of acute acalculous cholecystitis due to *Salmonella*]. Nippon Shokakibyo Gakkai Zasshi 93:137, 1996.

79. Hitch, D. C., and Lilly, J. R.: Identification, quantification, and significance of bacterial growth within the biliary tract after Kasai's operation. J. Pediatr. Surg. 13:563, 1978.

80. Hitch, D. C., Lilly, J. R., Reller, L. B., et al.: Biliary flora and antimicrobial concentrations after Kasai's operation. J. Pediatr. Surg. 14:648, 1979.

81. Honna, T., Tsuchida, Y., Kawarasaki, H., et al.: Further experience with the antireflux valve to prevent ascending cholangitis in biliary atresia. J. Pediatr. Surg. 32:1450, 1997.

82. Horii, Y., Sugimoto, T., Sakamoto, I., et al.: Acute acalculous cholecystitis complicating *Mycoplasma pneumoniae* infection. Clin. Pediatr. (Philadelphia) 31:376, 1992.

83. Hou, J. W., Chang, M. H., Wu, M. H., et al.: Kawasaki disease complicated by gallbladder hydrops mimicking acute abdomen: A report of three cases. Zhonghua Min Guo Xiao Er Ke Yi Xue Hui Za Zhi 30:52, 1989.

84. Houwen, R. H., Bijleveld, C. M., de Vries-Hospers, H. G.: Ciprofloxacin for cholangitis after hepatic portoenterostomy. Lancet 1:1367, 1987.

85. Houwen, R. H., Zwierstra, R. P., Severijnen, R. S., et al.: Prognosis of extrahepatic biliary atresia. Arch. Dis. Child. 64:214, 1989.

86. Hyams, J. S., Baker, E., Schwartz, A. N., et al.: Acalculous cholecystitis in Crohn's disease. J. Adolesc. Health Care 10:151, 1989.

87. Imamoglu, M., Sarihan, H., Sari, A., et al.: Acute acalculous cholecystitis in children: Diagnosis and treatment. J. Pediatr. Surg. 37:36, 2002.

88. Imhof, M., Raunest, J., Ohmann, C., et al.: Acute acalculous cholecystitis complicating trauma: A prospective sonographic study. World. J. Surg. 16:1160, 1992.

89. Issa, H., Al-Haddad, A., and Al-Salem, A. H.: Diagnostic and therapeutic ERCP in the pediatric age group. Pediatr. Surg. Int. 23:111, 2007.

90. Jacobs, R. F.: Ceftriaxone-associated cholecystitis. Pediatr. Infect. Dis. J. 7:434, 1988.

91. Johna, S., Shaul, D., Taylor, E. W., et al.: Laparoscopic management of gallbladder disease in children and adolescents. 1:241, 1997.

92. Joseph, V. T.: Surgical techniques and long-term results in the treatment of choledochal cyst. J. Pediatr. Surg. 25:782, 1990.

93. Jung, G., Benz-Bohm, G., Kugel, H., et al.: MR cholangiography in children with autosomal recessive polycystic kidney disease. Pediatr. Radiol. 29:463, 1999.

94. Kanter, M. A., and Geelhoed, G. W.: Biliary antibiotics: Clinical utility in biliary surgery. South. Med. J. 80:1007, 1987.

95. Karrer, F. M., Lilly, J. R., Stewart, B. A., et al.: Biliary atresia registry, 1976 to 1989. J. Pediatr. Surg. 25:1076, 1990.

96. Kasai, and Suzuki: A new operation for "non correctable" biliary atresia: Hepatic porto-enterostomy. Shujyutsu 13:733, 1959.

97. Kawaguchi, M., Saito, T., Ohno, H., et al.: Bacteria closely resembling *Helicobacter pylori* detected immunohistologically and genetically in resected gallbladder mucosa. J. Gastroenterol. 31:294, 1996.

98. Keighley, M. R., Drysdale, R. B., Quoraishi, A. H., et al.: Antibiotic treatment of biliary sepsis. Surg. Clin. North Am. 55:1379, 1975.

99. Kelly, D. A.: Liver complications of pediatric parenteral nutrition—epidemiology. Nutrition 14:153, 1998.

100. Kerkar, N., Norton, K., and Suchy, F. J.: The hepatic fibrocystic diseases. Clin. Liver Dis. 10:55, 2006.

101. Khuroo, M. S.: Ascariasis. Gastroenterol. Clin. North Am. 25:553, 1996.

102. Ko, C. W., Sekijima, J. H., and Lee, S. P.: Biliary sludge. Ann. Intern. Med. 130:301, 1999.

103. Kobayashi, A., Utsunomiya, T., Obe, Y., et al.: Ascending cholangitis after successful surgical repair of biliary atresia. Arch. Dis. Child. 48:697, 1973.

104. Kok, K. Y., and Yapp, S. K.: Tuberculosis of the bile duct: A rare cause of obstructive jaundice. J. Clin. Gastroenterol. 29:161, 1999.

105. Kosloske, A. M.: Acute abdomen due to acute cholangitis in a leukemic child. Pediatrics 56:469, 1975.

106. Kubota, A., Yonekura, T., Hoki, M., et al.: Total parenteral nutrition-associated intrahepatic cholestasis in infants: 25 years' experience. J. Pediatr. Surg. 35:1049, 2000.

107. Kuhls, T. L., and Jackson, M. A.: Diagnosis and treatment of the febrile child following hepatic portoenterostomy. Pediatr. Infect. Dis. 4:487, 1985.

108. Lammert, F., Wang, D. Q., Hillebrandt, S., et al.: Spontaneous cholecysto- and hepatolithiasis in Mdr2-/- mice: A model for low phospholipid-associated cholelithiasis. Hepatology 39:117, 2004.

109. Lee, S., and Ko, C.: Gallstones. *In* Yamada, T. (ed.): Textbook of Gastroenterology. 3rd ed., Vol. 2. Philadelphia, Lippincott Williams & Wilkins, 1999.

110. Lefkowitch, J. H.: Pathology of AIDS-related liver disease. Dig. Dis. *12*:321, 1994.
111. Leong, R. W., and Sung, J. J.: Review article: *Helicobacter* species and hepatobiliary diseases. Aliment. Pharmacol. Ther. *16*:1037, 2002.
112. Levy, C., and Lindor, K. D.: Primary sclerosing cholangitis: Epidemiology, natural history, and prognosis. Semin. Liver Dis. *26*:22, 2006.
113. Levy, J., Espanol-Boren, T., Thomas, C., et al.: Clinical spectrum of X-linked hyper-IgM syndrome. J. Pediatr. *131*:47, 1997.
114. Lewis, R. T., Goodall, R. G., Marien, B., et al.: Biliary bacteria, antibiotic use, and wound infection in surgery of the gallbladder and common bile duct. Arch. Surg. *122*:44, 1987.
115. Lillemoe, K. D.: Surgical treatment of biliary tract infections. Am. Surg. *66*:138, 2000.
116. Lilly, J. R., and Hitch, D. C.: Postoperative ascending cholangitis following portoenterostomy for biliary atresia: Measures for control. World J. Surg. *2*:581, 1978.
117. Lin, T. T., Yeh, C. T., Wu, C. S., et al.: Detection and partial sequence analysis of *Helicobacter pylori* DNA in the bile samples. Dig. Dis. Sci. *40*:2214, 1995.
118. Lipschitz, B., Berdon, W. E., Defelice, A. R., et al.: Association of congenital hepatic fibrosis with autosomal dominant polycystic kidney disease: Report of a family with review of literature. Pediatr. Radiol. *23*:131, 1993.
119. Lipsett, P. A., and Pitt, H. A.: Acute cholangitis. Surg. Clin. North Am. *70*:1297, 1990.
120. Liu, K. J., Atten, M. J., and Donahue, P. E.: Cholestasis in patients with acquired immunodeficiency syndrome: A surgeon's perspective. Am. Surg. *63*:519, 1997.
121. Livingston, E. H.: Endoscopic biliary drainage for acute cholangitis. N. Engl. J. Med. *327*:1176, 1992.
122. Lopez-Santamaria, M., Martinez, L., Hierro, L., et al.: Late biliary complications in pediatric liver transplantation. J. Pediatr. Surg. *34*:316, 1999.
123. Lord, R. V., Ho, S., Coleman, M. J., et al.: Cholecystectomy in cardiothoracic organ transplant recipients. Arch. Surg. *133*:73, 1998.
124. MacCarty, R. L., LaRusso, N. F., Wiesner, R. H., et al.: Primary sclerosing cholangitis: Findings on cholangiography and pancreatography. Radiology *149*:39, 1983.
125. Maddrey, W. C.: Role of antibiotics in the management of hepatic encephalopathy. Rev. Gastroenterol. Disord. *5*(Suppl. 1):S3, 2005.
126. Maggi, P., Coppola, S. L., Lamargese, V., et al.: Acute acalculous cholecystitis associated with co-infection by *Plasmodium falciparum* and *Plasmodium vivax*. J. Infect. *44*:136, 2002.
127. Mariat, G., Mahul, P., Prevt, N., et al.: Contribution of ultrasonography and cholescintigraphy to the diagnosis of acute acalculous cholecystitis in intensive care unit patients. Intensive Care Med. *26*:1658, 2000.
128. Matsukura, N., Yokomuro, S., Yamada, S., et al.: Association between *Helicobacter bilis* in bile and biliary tract malignancies: *H. bilis* in bile from Japanese and Thai patients with benign and malignant diseases in the biliary tract. Jpn. J. Cancer Res. *93*:842, 2002.
129. McCrindle, B. W., Wood, R. A., and Nussbaum, A. R.: Henoch-Schonlein syndrome: Unusual manifestations with hydrops of the gallbladder. Clin. Pediatr. (Philadelphia) *27*:254, 1988.
130. McDiarmid, S. V.: Management of the pediatric liver transplant patient. Liver Transpl. *7*:S77, 2001.
131. McKiernan, J., O'Brien, D. J., and Dundon, S.: Leptospirosis and acalculous cholecystitis. Irish Med. J. *69*:71, 1976.
132. McLauchlin, J., Amar, C. F., Pedraza-Diaz, S., et al.: Polymerase chain reaction-based diagnosis of infection with *Cryptosporidium* in children with primary immunodeficiencies. Pediatr. Infect. Dis. J. *22*:329, 2003.
133. Mertens, A., and De Smet, M.: *Campylobacter* cholecystitis. Lancet *1*:1092, 1979.
134. Metz, D. C.: *Helicobacter* colonization of the biliary tree: Commensal, pathogen, or spurious finding? Am. J. Gastroenterol. *93*:1996, 1998.
135. Miltenburg, D. M., Schaffer, R., 3rd, Breslin, T., et al.: Changing indications for pediatric cholecystectomy. Pediatrics *105*:1250, 2000.
136. Mirbagheri, S. A., Mohamadnejad, M., Nasiri, J., et al.: Prospective evaluation of endoscopic ultrasonography in the diagnosis of biliary microlithiasis in patients with normal transabdominal ultrasonography. J. Gastrointest. Surg. *9*:961, 2005.
137. Mortele, K. J., McTavish, J., and Ros, P. R.: Current techniques of computed tomography: Helical CT, multidetector CT, and 3D reconstruction. Clin. Liver Dis. *6*:29, 2002.
138. Moseley, R. H.: Sepsis and cholestasis. Clin. Liver Dis. *3*:465, 1999.
139. Mueller, X. M., Tevaearai, H. T., Stumpe, F., et al.: Extramediastinal surgical problems in heart transplant recipients. J. Am. Coll. Surg. *189*:380, 1999.
140. Mukhopadhyay, S., Monga, A., Rana, S. S., et al.: AIDS cholangiopathy as initial presentation of HIV infection. Trop. Gastroenterol. *22*:29, 2001.
141. Muller, E. L., Pitt, H. A., Thompson, J. E., Jr., et al.: Antibiotics in infections of the biliary tract. Surg. Gynecol. Obstet. *165*:285, 1987.
142. Muraji, T., and Higashimoto, Y.: The improved outlook for biliary atresia with corticosteroid therapy. J. Pediatr. Surg. *32*:1103, 1997.
143. Nadel, H. R.: Hepatobiliary scintigraphy in children. Semin. Nucl. Med. *26*:25, 1996.
144. Nash, J. A., and Cohen, S. A.: Gallbladder and biliary tract disease in AIDS. Gastroenterol. Clin. North Am. *26*:323, 1997.
145. Navarro, V. J., and Senior, J. R.: Drug-related hepatotoxicity. N. Engl. J. Med. *354*:731, 2006.
146. NIH state-of-the-science statement on endoscopic retrograde cholangiopancreatography (ERCP) for diagnosis and therapy. NIH Consens. State Sci. Statements *19*:1, 2002.
147. Nilsson, S.: Gallbladder disease and sex hormones: A statistical study. Acta Chir. Scand. *132*:275, 1966.
148. Novak: Bacterial, parasitic, and fungal infections of the liver. *In* Suchy, F. J., and Balistreri, W. F. (eds.): Liver Disease in Children. Philadelphia, Lippincott Williams & Wilkins, 2001.
149. Odievre, M., Valayer, J., Razemon-Pinta, M., et al.: Hepatic porto-enterostomy or cholecystostomy in the treatment of extrahepatic biliary atresia: A study of 49 cases. J. Pediatr. *88*:774, 1976.
150. Odom, F. C., Oliver, B. B., Kline, M., et al.: Gallbladder disease in patients 20 years of age and under. South. Med. J. *69*:1299, 1976.
151. Oh, M., Hobeldin, M., Chen, T., et al.: The Kasai procedure in the treatment of biliary atresia. J. Pediatr. Surg. *30*:1077, 1995.
152. Ohi, R.: Surgery for biliary atresia. Liver *21*:175, 2001.
153. Onuchic, L. F., Furu, L., Nagasawa, Y., et al.: PKHD1, the polycystic kidney and hepatic disease 1 gene, encodes a novel large protein containing multiple immunoglobulin-like plexin-transcription-factor domains and parallel beta-helix 1 repeats. Am. J. Hum. Genet. *70*:1305, 2002.
154. Pashankar, D. S., Schreiber, R. A.: Postnatal infections of the liver: Bacterial, parasitic, and other infections. *In* Walker, W. A., et al. (eds.): Pediatric Gastrointestinal Disease: Pathophysiology, Disease, and Management. Vol. 2. 4th ed. Hamilton, Ontario, B. C. Decker, 2004, pp. 1179-1190.
155. Patino, C., Fontes, B., Poggetti, R. S., et al.: Bile duct-duodenal fistula caused by AIDS/HIV-associated tuberculosis. Rev. Hosp. Clin. Fac. Med. Sao Paulo *58*:223, 2003.
156. Patriquin, H. B., DiPietro, M., Barber, F. E., et al.: Sonography of thickened gallbladder wall: Causes in children. A. J. R. Am. J. Roentgenol. *141*:57, 1983.
157. Pessa, M. E., Hawkins, I. F., and Vogel, S. B.: The treatment of acute cholangitis: Percutaneous transhepatic biliary drainage before definitive therapy. Ann. Surg. *205*:389, 1987.
158. Poddar, U., Thapa, B. R., Chhabra, M., et al.: Choledochal cysts in infants and children. Indian Pediatr. *35*:613, 1998.
159. Pol, S., Romana, C. A., Richard, S., et al.: Microsporidia infection in patients with the human immunodeficiency virus and unexplained cholangitis. N. Engl. J. Med. *328*:95, 1993.
160. Ponchon, T., and Pilleul, F.: Diagnostic ERCP. Endoscopy *34*:29, 2002.
161. Prassouli, A., Panagiotou, J., Vakaki, M., et al.: Acute acalculous cholecystitis as the initial presentation of primary Epstein-Barr virus infection. J. Pediatr. Surg. *42*:E11, 2007.
162. Prevot, N., Mariat, G., Mahul, P., et al.: Contribution of cholescintigraphy to the early diagnosis of acute acalculous cholecystitis in intensive-care-unit patients. Eur. J. Nucl. Med. *26*:1317, 1999.
163. Ratanarapee, S., and Pausawasdi, A.: Tuberculosis of the common bile duct. Hepatobiliary Surg. *3*:205, 1991.
164. Reddy, S. I., and Grace, N. D.: Liver imaging: A hepatologist's perspective. Clin. Liver Dis. *6*:297, 2002.
165. Reif, S., Sloven, D. G., and Lebenthal, E.: Gallstones in children: Characterization by age, etiology, and outcome. Am. J. Dis. Child. *145*:105, 1991.
166. Rescorla, F. J.: Cholelithiasis, cholecystitis, and common bile duct stones. Curr. Opin. Pediatr. *9*:276, 1997.
167. Rescorla, F. J., and Grosfeld, J. L.: Cholecystitis and cholelithiasis in children. Semin. Pediatr. Surg. *1*:98, 1992.
168. Rha, S. Y., Stovroff, M. C., Glick, P. L., et al.: Choledochal cysts: A ten year experience. Am. Surg. *62*:30, 1996.
169. Roberts, E. A.: Primary sclerosing cholangitis in children. J. Gastroenterol. Hepatol. *14*:588, 1999.
170. Rodrigues, F., Davies, E. G., Harrison, P., et al.: Liver disease in children with primary immunodeficiencies. J. Pediatr. *145*:333, 2004.
171. Romero Ganuza, F. J., La Banda, G., Montalvo, R., et al.: Acute acalculous cholecystitis in patients with acute traumatic spinal cord injury. Spinal Cord *35*:124, 1997.
172. Ros, P. R., and Mortele, K. J.: Hepatic imaging: An overview. Clin. Liver Dis. *6*:1, 2002.
173. Roseau, G., Palazzo, L., Dumontier, I., et al.: Endoscopic ultrasonography in the evaluation of pediatric digestive diseases: Preliminary results. Endoscopy *30*:477, 1998.
174. Roslyn, J. J., Pitt, H. A., Mann, L. L., et al.: Gallbladder disease in patients on long-term parenteral nutrition. Gastroenterology *84*:148, 1983.
175. Rosmorduc, O., Hermelin, B., Boelle, P. Y., et al.: ABCB4 gene mutation-associated cholelithiasis in adults. Gastroenterology *125*:452, 2003.
176. Rothenberg, S. S., Schroter, G. P., Karrer, F. M., et al.: Cholangitis after the Kasai operation for biliary atresia. J. Pediatr. Surg. *24*:729, 1989.
177. Rusin, J. A., Sivit, C. J., Rakusan, T. A., et al.: AIDS-related cholangitis in children: Sonographic findings. A. J. R. Am. J. Roentgenol. *159*:626, 1992.
178. Ryckman, F. C., Alonso, M. H., Bucuvalas, J. C., et al.: Long-term survival after liver transplantation. J. Pediatr. Surg. *34*:845, 1999.
179. Saha, A., Batra, P., Vilhekar, K. Y., et al.: Acute acalculous cholecystitis in a child with *Plasmodium falciparum* malaria. Ann. Trop. Paediatr. *25*:141, 2005.
180. Saharia, P. C., and Cameron, J. L.: Clinical management of acute cholangitis. Surg. Gynecol. Obstet. *142*:369, 1976.

181. Saing, H., Han, H., Chan, K. L., et al.: Early and late results of excision of choledochal cysts. J. Pediatr. Surg. 32:1563, 1997.
182. Saing, H., Tam, P. K., Choi, T. K., et al.: Childhood recurrent pyogenic cholangitis. J. Pediatr. Surg. 23:424, 1988.
183. Saint-Vil, D., Luks, F. I., Lebel, P., et al.: Infectious complications of pediatric liver transplantation. J. Pediatr. Surg. 26:908, 1991.
184. Sama, C., Labate, A. M., Taroni, F., et al.: Epidemiology and natural history of gallstone disease. Semin. Liver Dis. 10:149, 1990.
185. Samuel, M., and Spitz, L.: Choledochal cyst: Varied clinical presentations and long-term results of surgery. Eur. J. Pediatr. Surg. 6:78, 1996.
186. Sanchez, R., Portilla, J., Boix, V., et al.: Acalculous cholecystitis associated with *Plasmodium falciparum* malaria. Clin. Infect. Dis. 31:622, 2000.
187. Sandhu, I. S., Jarvis, C., and Everson, G. T.: Total parenteral nutrition and cholestasis. Clin. Liver Dis. 3:489, 1999.
188. Sarnaik, S., Slovis, T. L., Corbett, D. P., et al.: Incidence of cholelithiasis in sickle cell anemia using the ultrasonic gray-scale technique. J. Pediatr. 96:1005, 1980.
189. Scott, A. J.: Bacteria and disease of the biliary tract. Gut 12:487, 1971.
190. Senaati, S., Gumruk, F. U., Delbakhsh, P., et al.: Gallbladder pathology in pediatric beta-thalassemic patients: A prospective ultrasonographic study. Pediatr. Radiol. 23:357, 1993.
191. Sgouros, S. N., and Bergele, C.: Endoscopic ultrasonography versus other diagnostic modalities in the diagnosis of choledocholithiasis. Dig. Dis. Sci. 51:2280, 2006.
192. Shafer, A. D., Ashley, J. V., Goodwin, C. D., et al.: A new look at the multifactoral etiology of gallbladder disease in children. Am. Surg. 49:314, 1983.
193. Shaffer, E. A.: Gallstone disease: Epidemiology of gallbladder stone disease. Best Pract. Res. Clin. Gastroenterol. 20:981, 2006.
194. Shah, S. K., Mutignani, M., and Costamagna, G.: Therapeutic biliary endoscopy. Endoscopy 34:43, 2002.
195. Sharma, A. K., Wakhlu, A., and Sharma, S. S.: The role of endoscopic retrograde cholangiopancreatography in the management of choledochal cysts in children. J. Pediatr. Surg. 30:65, 1995.
196. Shen, G. K., Tsen, A. C., Hunter, G. C., et al.: Surgical treatment of symptomatic biliary stones in patients with cystic fibrosis. Am. Surg. 61:814, 1995.
197. Sindermann, J., Foerster, E., and Kienast, J.: Severe hepatobiliary complication in a patient with acute promyelocytic leukemia treated with all-trans retinoic acid. Acta Oncol. 35:499, 1996.
198. Singh, U. K., and Suman, S.: *Salmonella* cholecystitis in a neonate. Ann. Trop. Paediatr. 19:211, 1999.
199. Hays, D. M., and Snyder, W. H.: Lifespan in untreated biliary atresia. Surgery 54:373, 1963.
200. Soetikno, R. M., Montes, H., and Carr-Locke, D. L.: Endoscopic management of choledocholithiasis. J. Clin. Gastroenterol. 27:296, 1998.
201. Sokol, R. J., Mack, C., Narkewicz, M. R., et al.: Pathogenesis and outcome of biliary atresia: Current concepts. J. Pediatr. Gastroenterol. Nutr. 37:4, 2003.
202. SPLIT: Studies in Pediatric Liver Transplantation 2006 Annual Report, 2006.
203. Still, J., Scheirer, R., and Law, E.: Acute cholecystectomy performed through cultured epithelial autografts in a patient with burn injuries: A case report. J. Burn Care Rehabil. 17:429, 1996.
204. Sudan, D. L., Shaw, B. W., Jr., and Langnas, A. N.: Causes of late mortality in pediatric liver transplant recipients. Ann. Surg. 227:289, 1998.
205. Sung, J. Y., Shaffer, E. A., Olson, M. E., et al.: Bacterial invasion of the biliary system by way of the portal-venous system. Hepatology 14:313, 1991.
206. Tagge, E. P., Tarnasky, P. R., Chandler, J., et al.: Multidisciplinary approach to the treatment of pediatric pancreaticobiliary disorders. J. Pediatr. Surg. 32:158, 1997.
207. Takano, K., Iwafuchi, M., Uchiyama, M., et al.: Studies on intestinal motility and mechanism of cholangitis after biliary reconstruction. J. Pediatr. Surg. 24:1225, 1989.
208. Takiff, H., and Fonkalsrud, E. W.: Gallbladder disease in childhood. Am. J. Dis. Child. 138:565, 1984.
209. Tarnasky, P. R., and Cotton, P. B.: Randomized trial of prevention of biliary stent occlusion by ursodeoxycholic acid plus norfloxacin. Gastrointest. Endosc. 42:103, 1995.
210. Taziaux, P., Wahlen, C., and Drion, S.: [An unusual cause of non-lithiasic acute cholecystitis: *Campylobacter jejuni*]. J. Chir. (Paris) 128:554, 1991.
211. Teng, R., Yokohata, K., Utsunomiya, N., et al.: Endoscopic retrograde cholangiopancreatography in infants and children. J. Gastroenterol. 35:39, 2000.
212. Thambidorai, C. R., Shyamala, J., Sarala, R., et al.: Acute acalculous cholecystitis associated with enteric fever in children. Pediatr. Infect. Dis. J. 14:812, 1995.
213. Thurston, W. A., Kelly, E. N., and Silver, M. M.: Acute acalculous cholecystitis in a premature infant treated with parenteral nutrition. Can. Med. Assoc. J. 135:332, 1986.
214. Toursarkissian, B., Kearney, P. A., Holley, D. T., et al.: Biliary sludging in critically ill trauma patients. South. Med. J. 88:420, 1995.
215. Trauner, M., Fickert, P., and Stauber, R. E.: Inflammation-induced cholestasis. J. Gastroenterol. Hepatol. 14:946, 1999.
216. Tsakayannis, D. E., Kozakewich, H. P., and Lillehei, C. W.: Acalculous cholecystitis in children. J. Pediatr. Surg. 31:127, 1996.
217. Tsiotos, G. G., Mullany, C. J., Zietlow, S., et al.: Abdominal complications following cardiac surgery. Am. J. Surg. 167:553, 1994.
218. Tzovaras, G., and Rowlands, B. J.: Diagnosis and treatment of sphincter of Oddi dysfunction. Br. J. Surg. 85:588, 1998.
219. Valeja, R., Pal, S., Mann, M. S., et al.: Isolated common bile duct tuberculosis. Indian J. Gastroenterol. 18:125, 1999.
220. van den Hazel, S. J., Speelman, P., Tytgat, G. N., et al.: Successful treatment of recurrent cholangitis with antibiotic maintenance therapy. Eur. J. Clin. Microbiol. Infect. Dis. 13:662, 1994.
221. van Erpecum, K. J.: Gallstone disease: Complications of bile-duct stones: Acute cholangitis and pancreatitis. Best Pract. Res. Clin. Gastroenterol. 20:1139, 2006.
222. Wade, J. J., Rolando, N., Hayllar, K., et al.: Bacterial and fungal infections after liver transplantation: An analysis of 284 patients. Hepatology 21:1328, 1995.
223. Wadstrom, T., and Ljungh, A. A.: Chronic *Helicobacter* infection of the human liver and bile are common and may trigger autoimmune disease. Curr. Gastroenterol. Rep. 4:349, 2002.
224. Waechter, F. L., Sampaio, J. A., Pinto, R. D., et al.: The role of liver transplantation in patients with Caroli's disease. Hepatogastroenterology 48:672, 2001.
225. Walker, T. M., Hambleton, I. R., and Serjeant, G. R.: Gallstones in sickle cell disease: Observations from The Jamaican Cohort study. J. Pediatr. 136:80, 2000.
226. Wesdorp, I., Bosman, D., de Graaff, A., et al.: Clinical presentations and predisposing factors of cholelithiasis and sludge in children. J. Pediatr. Gastroenterol. Nutr. 31:411, 2000.
227. Westphal, J. F., and Brogard, J. M.: Biliary tract infections: A guide to drug treatment. Drugs 57:81, 1999.
228. Winkelstein, J. A., Marino, M. C., Ochs, H., et al.: The X-linked hyper-IgM syndrome: Clinical and immunologic features of 79 patients. Medicine (Baltimore) 82:373, 2003.
229. Wittenburg, H., and Lammert, F.: Genetic predisposition to gallbladder stones. Semin. Liver Dis. 27:109, 2007.
230. Wong, M. L., Kaplan, S., Dunkle, L. M., et al.: Leptospirosis: A childhood disease. J. Pediatr. 90:532, 1977.
231. Wu, E. T., Chen, H. L., Ni, Y. H., et al.: Bacterial cholangitis in patients with biliary atresia: Impact on short-term outcome. Pediatr. Surg. Int. 17:390, 2001.
232. Yabut, B., Werlin, S. L., Havens, P., et al.: Endoscopic retrograde cholangiopancreatography in children with HIV infection. J. Pediatr. Gastroenterol. Nutr. 23:624, 1996.
233. Yombi, J. C., Meuris, C. M., Van Gompel, A. M., et al.: Acalculous cholecystitis in a patient with *Plasmodium falciparum* infection: A case report and literature review. J. Travel Med. 13:178, 2006.
234. Yonem, O., and Bayraktar, Y.: Clinical characteristics of Caroli's syndrome. World J. Gastroenterol. 13:1934, 2007.
235. Yusuf, T. E., and Baron, T. H.: AIDS cholangiopathy. Curr. Treat. Options Gastroenterol. 7:111, 2004.
236. Ziessman, H. A.: Cholecystokinin cholescintigraphy: Clinical indications and proper methodology. Radiol. Clin. North Am. 39:997, 2001.
237. Zimmon, D. S.: The management of common duct stones. Adv. Intern. Med. 31:379, 1986.

CHAPTER 55

PYOGENIC LIVER ABSCESS

Sheldon L. Kaplan

Pyogenic liver abscesses are encountered infrequently in healthy children and generally have been reported more commonly in the compromised pediatric host. The rarity of liver abscesses may be explained partly by the rich blood supply, unique architecture, and extensive reticuloendothelial system of the liver, all of which present an effective barrier against bacterial invasion.

The precise incidence of pyogenic liver abscesses in children is unknown. Adult patients with hepatic abscesses constitute approximately 8 to 20 cases per 100,000 admissions; a 0.29 to 0.57 percent incidence of liver abscesses has been found in autopsies of adult patients.[11,48] In an early large series of liver abscesses in children, Dehner and Kissane[10] reported a 0.38 percent incidence at autopsy in patients younger than 15 years old; 11 of 27 (41%) patients were younger than 2 years, and 18 of 27 (67%) patients were younger than 6 years. In a review of admissions to Milwaukee Children's Hospital, Chusid[9] found five children (four of whom were <6 months old) with at least one hepatic abscess, and estimated an incidence of 3 cases for every 100,000 admissions. Pineiro-Carrero and Andres[43] estimated an incidence of approximately 25 cases per 100,000 admissions in their pediatric population (11 patients >14 years old). Pyogenic liver abscess in children is encountered more frequently in developing countries compared with developed countries.

PATHOGENESIS

Bacteria can establish an inflammatory focus in the liver by four major routes. Direct extension from contiguous structures is the most common mode in adults and precedes up to 60 percent of hepatic abscesses in adults.[7,24,44,48] Biliary tract infection (cholangitis, cholecystitis), pancreatitis, and penetrating gastric or duodenal ulcer are examples of diseases associated with liver abscesses caused by extension from a contiguous focus of infection. In a review of this problem at St. Louis Children's Hospital, 3 of 27 children (11%) were considered to have a liver abscess secondary to inflammation of contiguous organs.[10] Although biliary tract disease occurs infrequently in children, ascending cholangitis is a particularly frequent complication of the hepatic portoenterostomy procedure for congenital biliary atresia and may lead to infections of the liver in such patients.[14] Liver abscesses also may develop as a complication of liver transplantation, especially if technical problems related to vascular supply or biliary drainage develop.[30]

The portal system is the second most common route by which bacteria may reach the liver in adults; 6 to 27 percent of liver abscesses in adults derive from this source.[24,32,48] In newborns, solitary liver abscesses, especially abscesses caused by gram-negative organisms, have complicated the use of umbilical vein catheterization or have been secondary to omphalitis.[6] Prematurity and necrotizing enterocolitis also are important predisposing conditions.[13]

Portal vein inflammation and bacteremia can be associated with infections within the abdominal cavity. Appendicitis, diverticulitis, perirectal abscesses, regional enteritis, ulcerative colitis, and omphalitis are possible sources of portal vein sepsis.[10] A pyogenic liver abscess may be an unusual complication of an ingested foreign body, with subsequent development of portal venous bacteremia.[38] Since antibiotics have been available, portal vein inflammation and pyelophlebitis have become less common sources of hepatic infection in children.

Systemic bacteremia with hematogenous spread of bacteria to the liver through the hepatic artery seems to be the most common source of liver abscess in children, but it is implicated in less than 20 percent of adult patients. In the St. Louis series, the systemic hematogenous route was responsible for 21 of 27 (78%) cases of liver abscesses.[10] In five of the patients examined before 1940, the bacteremia was associated with infection that would be considered manageable today (pneumonia, cellulitis, and osteomyelitis). Seven of 13 patients encountered after 1940 had bacteremia associated with leukemia. Anaerobic bacteremia associated with retropharyngeal or peritonsillar abscesses presumably has preceded development of anaerobic liver abscesses in several children.[8] Likewise, liver abscesses in neonates may be preceded by a systemic bacteremia without evidence of portal or biliary tract involvement.[35]

Liver abscesses occur more frequently in compromised pediatric hosts than in healthy children. Johnston and Baehner[25] reported that hepatic or perihepatic abscesses were present in 41 of 92 (45%) patients with chronic granulomatous disease. In a registry of 368 patients with chronic granulomatous disease from the United States, a liver abscess occurred in 27 percent of patients.[57] Over the course of 10 years, 15 children were diagnosed with pyogenic liver abscess in a large referral center for pediatric liver disease in the United Kingdom.[36] Three children (20%) had chronic granulomatous disease. In addition to functional disorders of phagocytes, chronic neutropenia predisposes to the development of liver abscesses.[42] Wintch and colleagues[58] noted that 5 of 10 children with hepatic abscesses in their institution had an underlying defect in host defense. Primary hemochromatosis predisposes to multiple liver abscesses caused by *Yersinia enterocolitica* in particular.[54] Pyogenic liver abscesses also are associated with Papillon-Lefévre syndrome, a rare autosomal recessive disease characterized by palmoplantar keratoderma and periodontitis.[1]

Penetrating and nonpenetrating trauma to the liver may lead to liver abscesses, presumably caused by bacterial proliferation within small collections of blood and bile that result from the trauma. Hepatic abscess may be a rare complication of ventriculoperitoneal shunts after penetration of a peritoneal catheter into the liver.[39] This mode of infection has been reported in seven children.[22] Liver abscess also is a complication of percutaneous liver biopsy.[16]

Unexplained or cryptogenic hepatic abscesses are encountered in most series and accounted for 40 to 50 percent of cases in many series.[24] Lee and Block[33] have proposed that these cryptogenic liver abscesses "originate from anaerobic bacterial invasion of hepatic infarcts." This theory is supported by reports that describe pyogenic liver abscesses as a complication of hepatic infarction in patients with sickle-cell anemia.[50] Normal gastrointestinal bacterial flora were isolated from 9 of 11 patients with liver abscesses at the Mayo Clinic. This finding suggested to Lazarchick and associates[32] that unrecognized intra-abdominal collections of pus were responsible. Although the reasons are unclear, diabetes mellitus also predisposes to the development of liver abscesses.[21,44] Nematode infection with larvae migrating through the liver is thought to be another predisposing factor for the development of pyogenic abscesses in children. The larvae induce liver granulomata that trap bacteria, leading to formation of an abscess.[41] In one study from Brazil, positive serology for *Toxocara canis* was significantly more frequent for patients with pyogenic liver abscess (10 of 16) than for the 32 age-matched controls (4 of 32).[46]

Biliary tract disease generally predisposes to the development of multiple liver abscesses. In contrast, blunt trauma to the liver or portal system inflammation most commonly predisposes to a single abscess. In neonates, liver abscesses may be solitary or multiple because of systemic bacteria.[35,37] Solitary abscesses are the most common findings in the right lobe of the liver.[32]

Hepatic and splenic abscesses caused by *Candida* spp. are well described in patients with cancer.[52] Multiple abscesses are typical findings. These organs presumably are infected hematogenously, usually when the host is neutropenic.

MICROBIOLOGY

Gram-negative organisms have been the predominant isolates from liver abscesses in adults. *Escherichia coli, Klebsiella, Aerobacter, Pseudomonas,* and *Proteus* spp. have been implicated most frequently. *Klebsiella* spp. were the most common organism isolated from children with pyogenic liver abscess in Taiwan.[53] *Klebsiella* spp. also predominated in adult Asian patients in a report from New York.[45] Anaerobic organisms also are important; anaerobic organisms were recovered from 45 percent of patients with liver abscesses in the UCLA series.[49]

In contrast to the adult experience, Dehner and Kissane[10] reported that 33 percent of liver abscesses in children were caused by *Staphylococcus aureus*, whereas gram-negative organisms were found in only 32 percent. Two or more organisms were recovered from liver abscesses in 52 percent of children. In a review of 96 children (no neonates) with pyogenic liver abscesses, *S. aureus*, gram-negative enterics, and anaerobes were the organisms isolated most commonly, in that order.[28] *S. aureus* is the most common isolate that causes pyogenic liver abscess in patients with chronic granulomatous disease. In neonates, gram-negative enterics are isolated most commonly. Anaerobes, particularly *Fusobacterium necrophorum*, have been isolated from liver abscesses in children without underlying disease.[15] Human rotavirus–like particles were identified in the material aspirated from a liver abscess, but they were considered a secondary phenomenon and not the primary etiology of the liver abscess.[19] Fungi, particularly *Candida albicans*, have been associated with liver abscesses in children with leukemia and neutropenia who have received parenteral hyperalimentation.[3] Liver or splenic abscesses also may be an unusual complication of brucellosis.[55]

CLINICAL MANIFESTATIONS

The clinical manifestations of pyogenic liver abscesses are nonspecific. A high index of suspicion and an awareness of this illness are necessary to establish the diagnosis. A history of preceding abdominal surgery or trauma is helpful when present, as is the knowledge that the hosts response to infection is compromised.

Fever, nausea, vomiting, anorexia, weakness, and malaise are prominent symptoms that may last several weeks. Abdominal or pleuritic pain, weight loss, and diarrhea are less common manifestations. A history of abdominal pain and fever of unknown origin in an otherwise healthy child suggests the diagnosis of pyogenic liver abscess.[27] In contrast, fever often is not observed in neonates.[13] Patients with a macroscopic or single abscess frequently experience a subacute to chronic course. In contrast, patients with multiple abscesses generally experience a more acute febrile illness.

Hepatomegaly occurs in 40 to 80 percent of patients; abdominal tenderness occurs less frequently. Right upper quadrant tenderness or even a mass may be subtle and not appreciated, unless the physician specifically and carefully examines this region. Other physical findings include jaundice (generally associated with biliary tract disease and not liver abscesses), abdominal distention, and evidence of pleuropulmonary involvement (i.e., elevated or fixed hemidiaphragm, rales, and pleural effusion).

DIAGNOSIS

Routine laboratory studies are of little help in attempting to establish a diagnosis. Anemia, leukocytosis, and an elevation in C-reactive protein are common findings. Liver function tests generally reflect underlying disease of the liver itself and usually are not caused by the abscess. When abscesses occur secondary to biliary tract obstruction, alkaline phosphatase and bilirubin concentrations generally are elevated. Transaminase concentrations usually are normal to mildly elevated in most cases. A rapidly enlarging, tender liver in a patient with normal transaminase concentrations should alert the clinician to the possibility of liver abscess. Lazarchick and colleagues[32] found that the serum albumin concentration was the most important test with regard to prognosis; 14 of 16 patients with a serum albumin level of less than 2 g/dL died.

Blood cultures are positive more commonly in patients with multiple abscesses than in patients with solitary abscesses. Overall, however, blood cultures usually are sterile in children with pyogenic liver abscess.

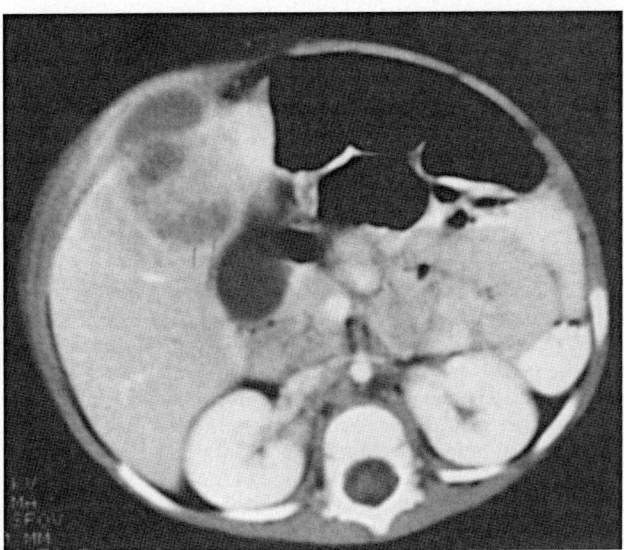

Figure 55–1 Abdominal computed tomography scan showing a 4-cm × 5-cm encapsulated, septate, circular mass within the liver. A low-density soft tissue mass is noted in the abdominal wall from apparent extension from the intrahepatic mass.

More than 50 percent of adult patients have abnormalities on chest radiography. Atelectasis, pulmonary infiltrates, pleural effusion, and elevated or fixed right hemidiaphragm are the most common findings.

Computed tomography (CT) currently provides the most accurate information concerning the size, location, and number of abscesses within the liver parenchyma (Fig. 55–1).[26,31,43] Lesions measuring 1 cm in diameter can be detected by CT. Multiple small abscesses may appear in clusters in a pattern suggesting early coalescence of the abscesses.[23] Liver abscesses appear as areas of low attenuation. The "target" lesions of hepatic candidiasis are not visualized by CT when the patient is neutropenic, and scans may need to be repeated before these characteristic lesions are observed.[52] Structures contiguous with the liver also are shown by CT; this information is important when a surgical approach to drainage is being planned.

Magnetic resonance imaging does not have any major advantages over CT for detecting or characterizing liver abscess but may show characteristic features to distinguish an abscess from other focal liver lesions in selected patients.[2,34] Ultrasonography also is a sensitive technique for detecting liver abscesses, and because it is noninvasive and does not require exposure to radiation, it is recommended for initial evaluation.[29,31] Hepatic angiography defines the vascular anatomy in the area of the liver abscess further and may provide information necessary for surgical management in selected cases. Nuclear medicine techniques rarely are indicated as a diagnostic method if liver abscess is suspected.

TREATMENT

Numerous reports have documented that patients with undiagnosed and untreated liver abscesses generally die and that surgical drainage of the solitary pyogenic liver abscess is the key to successful treatment. The choice of extraserous or transperitoneal open drainage or percutaneous closed aspiration depends on the location and size of the abscess and the experience and preference of the surgeon.[18,24,40,48]

Numerous groups have described percutaneous catheter drainage of liver abscesses in adults.[4,5,17,29] A catheter is placed into the cavity under CT or ultrasound guidance; material is aspirated, and when an abscess is documented, a draining catheter is placed. The cavity can be irrigated with saline initially. Criteria for the selection of patients for percutaneous drainage have been established.[17] Generally, percutaneous drainage is not indicated for patients with multiple large abscesses or multiloculated abscesses.[24] The optimal route of percutaneous aspiration is directly into the abscess cavity and does not involve any uninfected organs or space. Drainage may proceed for 2 weeks or more, or until drainage from the cavity is decreased, the patient is afebrile and improving, and radiography shows that the cavity is becoming smaller.[20] Surgical backup is mandatory when this drainage technique is used because spillage of abscess material into the peritoneal cavity, hemorrhage, and other complications may occur. Percutaneous drainage of liver abscesses in children has been performed successfully, and this technique should be considered an alternative approach to surgical drainage of such abscesses, especially in the right lobe of the liver.[12,43]

Appropriate antibiotic therapy initially is based on knowledge of the organisms most commonly involved, Gram stain of the purulent material, and culture and susceptibility to antibiotics of the organisms that are recovered. If a hematogenous source of infection is suspected or the host has an immunodeficiency disease, *S. aureus* and streptococci are more likely. Biliary tract disease and blunt trauma are associated more frequently with gram-negative aerobic and anaerobic organisms. A logical antibiotic combination for the initial therapy of children with liver abscesses includes a penicillinase-resistant penicillin, such as nafcillin, plus an aminoglycoside. Vancomycin or clindamycin is selected if strains of *S. aureus* resistant to methicillin are present in the community.

The optimal duration and route of administration of antibiotics for a child with a solitary pyogenic liver abscess that has been drained have not been determined. Generally, 2 to 4 weeks of antibiotic therapy administered parenterally, followed by an appropriate oral antibiotic to complete a minimum 4-week total course, should be adequate. Penicillin, ticarcillin-clavulanate, piperacillin-tazobactam, clindamycin, cefoxitin, or metronidazole is administered for anaerobic isolates, depending on susceptibility. Meropenem is useful for polymicrobial infections, including infections caused by gram-negative aerobic and anaerobic rods.

Multiple liver abscesses are more difficult to treat because achieving complete surgical drainage usually is impossible. Prolonged antibiotic therapy plus treatment of any underlying illnesses is the keystone to effective management. Duration of treatment can be modified, depending on the evidence for resolution of the abscesses as determined by repeated ultrasound examination or CT.

Fungal liver abscesses are difficult to document by culture of the abscess material; histologic evidence of a fungal infection of the liver must be sought.[3] Amphotericin B, with or without flucytosine, is administered in the treatment of fungal liver abscesses.[52] In a neutropenic rabbit model, combination therapy with amphotericin and flucytosine was superior to amphotericin B alone in clearing disseminated candidiasis.[51] The optimal duration of therapy is unknown, but prolonged therapy, guided by repeated CT scans and biopsies, should be provided until the lesions have resolved.[52] Liposomal preparations of amphotericin B or other antifungal agents, such as caspofungin, may be beneficial for selected children with hepatosplenic candidiasis who are intolerant of or failing treatment with traditional amphotericin B.[56]

COMPLICATIONS AND PROGNOSIS

Complications of hepatic abscesses vary and are relatively common. Twenty-eight percent of the patients described by

Rubin and associates[48] and 44 percent of the patients studied by Pitt and Zuidema[44] had one or more complications. Possible complications include pleural and pulmonary inflammation, peritonitis, subphrenic or subhepatic abscesses, and hemobilia.[10,48]

Polymicrobial bacteremia, hypoalbuminemia, multiple liver abscesses, or the presence of any complication is associated with increased mortality rates in patients with liver abscesses. Overall mortality rates depend largely on underlying pathologic processes and are difficult to interpret. Mortality figures from more recent reports range from 2.5 to 11 percent in adults.[24,45] In children, the prognosis for pyogenic liver abscess is excellent, generally with a low chance of mortality.[36] An increased awareness and suspicion of liver abscesses, in conjunction with ultrasound or CT of the liver, substantially reduces the mortality rate of this disease.

REFERENCES

1. Almuneef, M., Khenaizan, S. A., Ajaji. S. A., and Al-Anazi, A.: Pyogenic liver abscess and Papillon-Lefévre Syndrome: Not a rare association. Pediatrics 111: e85-e88, 2003.
2. Balci, N. C., Semelka, R. C., Noone, T. C., et al.: Pyogenic hepatic abscesses: MRI findings on T1- and T2-weighted and serial gadolinium-enhanced gradient-echo images. J. Magn. Reson. Imaging 9:285-290, 1999.
3. Bartley, D. L., Hughes, W. T., Parvey, L. S., et al.: Computed tomography of hepatic and splenic fungal abscesses in leukemic children. Pediatr. Infect. Dis. 1:317-321, 1982.
4. Berger, L. A., and Osborne, D. R.: Treatment of pyogenic liver abscesses by percutaneous needle aspiration. Lancet 1:132-134, 1982.
5. Bernardino, M. E., Berkman, W. A., Plemmons, M., et al.: Percutaneous drainage of multiseptated hepatic abscess. J. Comput. Assist. Tomogr. 8:38-41, 1984.
6. Brans, Y. M., Ceballos, R., and Cassady, G.: Umbilical catheters and hepatic abscesses. Pediatrics 53:264-265, 1974.
7. Branum, G. D., Tyson, G. S., Branum, M. A., et al.: Hepatic abscess: Changes in etiology, diagnosis, and management. Ann. Surg. 212:655, 1990.
8. Brook, I., and Fraizer, E. H.: Role of anaerobic bacteria in liver abscesses in children. Pediatr. Infect. Dis. J. 12:743, 1993.
9. Chusid, M. J.: Pyogenic hepatic abscess in infancy and childhood. Pediatrics 62:554-559, 1978.
10. Dehner, L. P., and Kissane, J. M.: Pyogenic hepatic abscesses in infancy and childhood. J. Pediatr. 74:763-773, 1969.
11. de la Maza, L. M., Faramary, N., and Berman, L. D.: The changing etiology of liver abscess. J. A. M. A. 227:161-163, 1974.
12. Diament, M. J., Stanley, P., Kangarloo, H., et al.: Percutaneous aspiration and catheter drainage of abscesses. J. Pediatr. 108:204-208, 1986.
13. Doerr, C. A., Demmler, G. J., Garcia-Pratts, J. A., et al.: Solitary pyogenic liver abscess in neonates: Report of three cases and review of the literature. Pediatr. Infect. Dis. J. 13:64, 1994.
14. Ecoffey, C., Rothman, E., Bernard, O., et al.: Bacterial cholangitis after surgery for biliary atresia. J. Pediatr. 111:824-829, 1987.
15. Embree, J. E., Williams, T., and Law, B. J.: Hepatic abscesses in a child caused by *Fusobacterium necrophorum*. Pediatr. Infect. Dis. 7:359-360, 1988.
16. Garcia-Arias, M. B., Rodriguez-Galindo, C., Hoffer, F. A., and Wang, W. C.: Pyogenic hepatic abscess after percutaneous liver biopsy in a patient with sickle cell disease. J. Pediatr. Hematol. Oncol. 27:103-105, 2005.
17. Gerzof, S. G., Robbins, A. H., Johnson, W. C., et al.: Percutaneous catheter drainage of abdominal abscesses: A five-year experience. N. Engl. J. Med. 305:353-357, 1981.
18. Goldsmith, H. S., and Chen, W. F.: Management of a pyogenic abscess of the liver. Surg. Clin. North Am. 53:711-715, 1973.
19. Grunow, J. E., Dunton, S. F., and Waner, J. L.: Human rotavirus-like particles in a hepatic abscess. J. Pediatr. 106:73-76, 1985.
20. Hoffer, F. A., Fellows, K. E., Wyly, J. B., et al.: Therapeutic catheter procedures in pediatrics. Pediatr. Clin. North Am. 32:1461, 1985.
21. Holt, J. M., and Spry, C. J. F.: Solitary pyogenic liver abscess in patients with diabetes mellitus. Lancet 2:198-200, 1966.
22. Huang, L.-T., Chen, C.-C., Shih, T.-Y., et al.: Pyogenic liver abscess complicating a ventriculoperitoneal shunt. Pediatr. Surg. Int. 13:6-7, 1998.
23. Jeffrey, R. B., Jr., Tolentino, C. S., Chang, F. C., et al.: CT of small pyogenic hepatic abscesses: The cluster sign. A. J. R. Am. J. Roentgenol. 151:487-489, 1988.
24. Johannsen, E. C., Sifri, C. D., and Madoff, L. C.: Pyogenic liver abscesses. Infect. Dis. Clin. N. Am. 14:547-563, 2000.
25. Johnston, R. B., and Baehner, R. L.: Chronic granulomatous disease: Correlation between pathogenesis and clinical findings. Pediatrics 48:730-739, 1971.
26. Kandel, G., and Marcon, N. E.: Pyogenic liver abscess: New concepts of an old disease. Am. J. Gastroenterol. 79:65-71, 1984.

27. Kaplan, S. L., and Feigin, R. D.: Pyogenic liver abscess in normal children with fever of unknown origin. Pediatrics *58*:614-616, 1976.
28. Kays, D. W.: Pediatric liver cysts and abscesses. Semin. Pediatr. Surg. *1*:107, 1992.
29. Kuligowska, E., Connors, S. K., and Shapiro, J. H.: Liver abscess: Sonography in diagnosis and treatment. A. J. R. Am. J. Roentgenol. *138*:253-257, 1982.
30. Kusne, S., Dummer, J. S., Singh, N., et al.: Infections after liver transplantation: An analysis of 101 consecutive cases. Medicine (Baltimore) *67*:132-143, 1988.
31. Laurin, S., and Kaude, J. V.: Diagnosis of liver-spleen abscesses in children: With emphasis on ultrasound for the initial and follow-up examinations. Pediatr. Radiol. *14*:198-204, 1984.
32. Lazarchick, J., DeSouza, E., Silvia, N. A., et al.: Pyogenic liver abscess. Mayo Clin. Proc. *48*:349-355, 1973.
33. Lee, J. F., and Block, G. E.: The changing clinical pattern of hepatic abscesses. Arch. Surg. *104*:456-470, 1972.
34. Mendez, R. J., Schiebler, M. L., Outwater, E. K., et al.: Hepatic abscesses: MR imaging findings. Radiology *190*:431, 1994.
35. Moss, T. J., and Pysher, T. J.: Hepatic abscess in neonates. Am. J. Dis. Child. *135*:726-728, 1981.
36. Muorah, M., Hinds, R., Verma, A., et al.: Liver abscesses in children: A single center experience in the developed world. J. Pediatr. Gastroenterol. Nutr. *42*:201-206, 2006.
37. Murphy, F. M., and Baker, C. J.: Solitary hepatic abscess: A delayed complication of neonatal bacteremia. Pediatr. Infect. Dis. 7:414-416, 1988.
38. Noel, G. J., and Karasic, R. B.: Liver abscess following ingestion of a foreign body. Pediatr. Infect. Dis. *3*:342-344, 1984.
39. Paone, R. F., and Mercer, L. C.: Hepatic abscess caused by a ventriculoperitoneal shunt. Pediatr. Infect. Dis. J. *10*:338, 1991.
40. Patterson, H. C.: Open aspiration in solitary liver abscess. Am. J. Surg. *119*:326-329, 1970.
41. Pereira, F. E., Musso, C., and Castelo, J. S.: Pathology of pyogenic liver abscess in children. Pediatr. Dev. Pathol. *2*:537-543, 1999.
42. Pincus, S. H., Boxer, L. A., and Stossel, T. P.: Chronic neutropenia in childhood: Analysis of 16 cases and a review of the literature. Am. J. Med. *61*:849-861, 1976.
43. Pineiro-Carrero, V. M., and Andres, J. M.: Morbidity and mortality in children with pyogenic liver abscess. Am. J. Dis. Child. *143*:1424-1427, 1989.
44. Pitt, H. A., and Zuidema, G. D.: Factors influencing mortality in the treatment of pyogenic hepatic abscess. Surg. Gynecol. Obstet. *140*:228-234, 1975.
45. Rahimian, J., Wilson, T., Oram, V., and Holzman R. S.: Pyogenic liver abscess: Recent trends in etiology and mortality. Clin. Infect. Dis. *39*:1654-1659, 2004.
46. Rayes, A. A., Teixeira, D., Serufo, J. C., et al.: Human toxocariasis and pyogenic liver abscess: A possible association. Am. J. Gastroenterol. *96*:563-566, 2001.
47. Rogers, C. A., Isenberg, J. N., Leonard, A. S., et al.: Ascending cholangitis diagnosed by percutaneous hepatic aspiration. J. Pediatr. *88*:83-86, 1976.
48. Rubin, R. H., Swartz, M. N., and Malt, R.: Hepatic abscess: Changes in clinical, bacteriologic and therapeutic aspects. Am. J. Med. 57:601-610, 1974.
49. Sabbaj, J.: Anaerobes in liver abscess. Rev. Infect. Dis. *6*:S152-S156, 1984.
50. Shulman, S. T., and Beem, M. O.: A unique presentation of sickle cell disease: Pyogenic hepatic abscess. Pediatrics 47:1019-1022, 1971.
51. Thaler, M., Bacher, J., O'Leary, T., et al.: Evaluation of single-drug combination antifungal therapy in an experimental model of candidiasis in rabbits with prolonged neutropenia. J. Infect. Dis. *158*:80-88, 1988.
52. Thaler, M., Pastakia, B., Shawker, T. H., et al.: Hepatic candidiasis in cancer patients: The evolving picture of the syndrome. Ann. Intern. Med. *108*:88-100, 1988.
53. Tsai, C. C., Chung, J. H., Ko, S. F., et al.: Liver abscess in children: A single institutional experience in southern Taiwan. Acta Paediatr. Taiwan *44*:282-286, 2003.
54. Vadillo, M., Corbella, X., and Pac, V.: Multiple liver abscesses due to *Yersinia enterocolitica* discloses primary hemochromatosis: Three case reports and review. Clin. Infect. Dis. *18*:938-941, 1994.
55. Vallejo, J. G., Stevens, A. M., Dutton, R. V., et al.: Hepatosplenic abscesses due to *Brucella melitensis*: Report of a case involving a child and review of the literature. Clin. Infect. Dis. *22*:485-489, 1996.
56. Walsh, T. J., Whitcomb, P., Piscitelli, S., et al.: Safety, tolerance, and pharmacokinetics of amphotericin B lipid complex in children with hepatosplenic candidiasis. Antimicrob. Agents Chemother. *41*:1944-1948, 1997.
57. Winkestein, J. A., Marino, M. C., Johnston, R. B., et al.: Chronic granulomatous disease: Report on a national registry of 368 patients. Medicine (Baltimore) *79*:155-169, 2000.
58. Wintch, R. W., Reines, H. D., and Rambo, W. M.: Liver abscess: A changing entity. Am. J. Surg. *48*:11-15, 1982.

CHAPTER 56

REYE SYNDROME

Eugene S. Hurwitz

A syndrome involving the acute onset of encephalopathy associated with fatty metamorphosis of the liver and occurring primarily in children was described first by Reye and colleagues[8] in Australia and by Johnson and associates[7] in the United States. The similarities of these two descriptions in separate countries led to the common designation of this clinicopathologic entity as *Reye-Johnson* or *Reye syndrome*. Reye syndrome occurs most frequently after a viral illness and is characterized by the onset of severe vomiting followed by the development of encephalopathy and hepatic dysfunction. The recognition in the early 1980s that the syndrome is associated with the ingestion of aspirin during the antecedent viral illness led to public awareness of this association, a decline in aspirin use for such illnesses in children, and a dramatic decline in the occurrence of this disease in the United States.[1]

EPIDEMIOLOGY

In the United States, national surveillance for Reye syndrome was conducted first during the 1973 to 1974 nationwide outbreak of influenza B and influenza A (H1N1). Such surveillance led to the recognition of outbreaks of Reye syndrome regionally and nationally that were associated with outbreaks of influenza in these and subsequent years.[2] During the first 5 years of surveillance, 250 to 550 cases were reported nationally—an underestimate because it was based on voluntary reporting.[9] Population-based studies conducted in several geographic locations showed that the average annual incidence of the syndrome

was one or two cases per 100,000 children younger than 18 years old. Adults rarely were affected. Case-fatality rates reported through national surveillance, initially 40 percent, declined to 20 to 30 percent in later years when the syndrome was prevalent, although this rate undoubtedly was an overestimate because of the tendency to report more severe and fatal cases through this system.

Between 1980 and 1982, four case-control studies reported an association between Reye syndrome and the ingestion of aspirin during an antecedent respiratory or chickenpox illness.[3,11,12] The results of these studies subsequently were confirmed in the Public Health Service Pilot and Main Studies of Reye Syndrome and Medications.[4,5] In these studies, more than 90 percent of patients with Reye syndrome compared with 40 to 70 percent of controls had received aspirin for the antecedent respiratory or chickenpox illness; reported odds ratios were 11.5 to 40. After these studies were reported, publicity and recommendations from various expert panels, including recommendations issued by the Food and Drug Administration in 1985, led to a decline in the use of aspirin and a decline in the incidence of Reye syndrome, particularly in the age group that had been affected most—children 5 to 15 years old.[1]

CLINICAL ILLNESS AND LABORATORY FINDINGS

Reye syndrome is described classically as an illness characterized by the abrupt onset of severe vomiting and progressive encephalopathy in a child who is just recovering from a viral illness, the most common of which are influenza and chickenpox. The onset of these symptoms typically occurs within several days after the onset of the viral illness and commonly during a period when the child seems to be recovering from this illness. In association with severe—often projectile—vomiting, which occurs for a transient period, are progressive encephalopathic changes that may follow stages from delirium through confusion, agitation, and lethargy to coma if untreated.

The definition used by the Centers for Disease Control and Prevention (CDC) and widely adopted for clinical purposes includes (1) evidence of acute encephalopathy manifested by alterations in consciousness and documented, when available, by cerebrospinal fluid with less than 9×10^6/L leukocytes or by biopsy or autopsy evidence of cerebral edema without perivascular or meningeal inflammation in histologic sections of the brain; (2) evidence of liver involvement, including either biopsy or autopsy findings of fatty metamorphosis of the liver if available or, in the absence of such specimens, elevations in liver enzymes (alanine aminotransaminase, aspartate aminotransaminase, or serum ammonia) that typically are more than three times normal levels; and (3) no other more reasonable explanation for the cerebral or hepatic abnormalities. The last requirement emphasizes that Reye syndrome is a diagnosis of exclusion, and that every effort should be undertaken to identify other possible causes for the clinical and laboratory abnormalities.

Liver biopsy or autopsy findings are considered characteristic and include panlobular microvesicular fat and mitochondrial abnormalities on electron microscopic examination showing peroxisome swelling and enlarged pleomorphic mitochondria with loss of dense granules. Additional findings include normal bilirubin levels and absence of jaundice. Most patients also have hypoglycemia and a prolonged prothrombin time. The typically elevated cerebrospinal fluid pressure in patients leads to progressive stages of coma.

Staging criteria for Reye syndrome have been used to define the level of encephalopathy. Patients have been reported with liver involvement, but without evidence of encephalopathy. These patients have been described as having stage 0 encephalopathy and, although they do not meet the Centers for Disease Control and Prevention criteria for Reye syndrome, are considered to have mild disease. Patients with stage I encephalopathy are difficult to arouse and lethargic, whereas patients with stage II are delirious and combative with some movement. Patients with higher stages of encephalopathy (III to V) cannot be aroused and have progressively deeper stages of coma. These patients have a poor prognosis, with a mortality rate approaching 50 percent for patients admitted with stage III or greater and 90 percent for patients admitted with stage V.

Exclusion of other diseases that may resemble Reye syndrome, such as salicylate toxicity, is essential in patients with symptoms resembling this entity. Intensive laboratory investigations should be undertaken to exclude such disorders. In young children, particularly children younger than 3 years of age, inherited metabolic disorders frequently may mimic Reye syndrome and must be excluded. Such metabolic disorders include disorders of fatty acid oxidation, urea cycle disorders, carnitine transport defects, and organic acidemias. Laboratory studies must be performed for the younger age group to exclude these disorders before a diagnosis of Reye syndrome is made, particularly because some of these disorders can be treated effectively. With the declining incidence of Reye syndrome in the typical age group (5 to 15 years) after virtual elimination of the use of aspirin in children, an increasing number of patients with features of Reye syndrome are in this younger age group and ultimately are found, after careful evaluation, to have one of the many metabolic disorders that mimic this syndrome.

TREATMENT AND PREVENTION

The mainstay of treatment of Reye syndrome is early recognition of disease and supportive care focusing on various measures to control intracranial pressure and electrolyte and other abnormalities. Patients should have glucose levels monitored, and early infusion of glucose is considered by many physicians to improve outcome. Comatose patients should be transferred to tertiary care centers that have experience in caring for such patients and can monitor and treat elevated intracranial pressure. When such measures were undertaken before the decline in incidence of this disease, they were associated with improved outcome and decreased mortality. Other therapeutic measures that have been used include efforts to reduce ammonia levels, such as exchange transfusions, peritoneal dialysis, and total-body washout via cardiopulmonary bypass. With advances in supportive care, the mortality rate declined to 10 to 20 percent in later years before Reye syndrome became extremely rare.

Since the association between Reye syndrome and aspirin has been recognized, aspirin no longer is recommended or used for the treatment of febrile illnesses in children. Alternative antipyretics, including nonsteroidal anti-inflammatory drugs and acetaminophen (Tylenol), have replaced aspirin as the primary therapy for such illnesses. These medications have not been associated with an increased risk for development of Reye syndrome. Children with some disorders, including juvenile rheumatoid arthritis and Kawasaki disease, continue to be given aspirin to treat these disorders. Efforts to reduce the risk of development of Reye syndrome in these children have included influenza vaccination annually and vaccination against chickenpox. Careful monitoring of these children also is necessary to ensure early recognition and treatment of Reye syndrome should it occur.

REFERENCES

1. Belay, E. D., Bresee, J. S., Holman, R. C., et al.: Reye's syndrome in the United States from 1981 through 1997. N. Engl. J. Med. 340:1377-1382, 1999.
2. Corey, L., Rubin, R. J., Hattwick, M. A., et al.: Nationwide outbreak of Reye's syndrome: Its epidemiologic relationship to influenza B. Am. J. Med. 61:615-625, 1976.
3. Halpin, T. J., Holtzhauer, F. J., Campbell, R. J., et al.: Reye's syndrome and medication use. J. A. M. A. 248:687-691, 1982.
4. Hurwitz, E. S., Barrett, M. J., Bregman, D., et al.: Public Health Service study on Reye's syndrome and medications: Report of the pilot phase. N. Engl. J. Med. 313:849-857, 1985.
5. Hurwitz, E. S., Barrett, M. J., Bregman, D., et al.: Public Health Service study of Reye's syndrome and medications: Report of the main study. [Erratum, J. A. M. A. 257:3366, 1987.] J. A. M. A. 257:1905-1911, 1987.
6. Hurwitz, E. S., Nelson, D. B., Davis, C., et al.: National surveillance for Reye syndrome: A five-year review. Pediatrics 70:895-900, 1982.
7. Johnson, G. M., Scurletis, T. D., and Carroll, N. B.: A study of sixteen fatal cases of encephalitis-like disease in North Carolina children. N. C. Med. J. 24:464-473, 1963.
8. Reye, R. D. K., Morgan, G., and Baral, J.: Encephalopathy and fatty degeneration of the viscera: A disease entity in childhood. Lancet 2:749-752, 1963.
9. Reye syndrome surveillance—United States, 1987 and 1988. M. M. W. R. Morb. Mortal. Wkly. Rep. 38:325-327, 1989.
10. Rowe, P. C., Valle, D., and Brusilow, S. W.: Inborn errors of metabolism in children referred with Reye's syndrome: A changing pattern. J. A. M. A. 260:3167-3170, 1988.
11. Starko, K. M., Ray, C. G., Dominguez, L. B., et al.: Reye's syndrome and salicylate use. Pediatrics 66:859-864, 1980.
12. Waldman, R. J., Hall, W. N., McGee, H., and Van Amburg, G.: Aspirin as a risk factor in Reye's syndrome. J. A. M. A. 247:3089-3094, 1982.

OTHER INTRA-ABDOMINAL INFECTIONS

APPENDICITIS AND PELVIC ABSCESS

Thomas L. Kuhls

The ability to diagnose appendicitis accurately in a child is one of the most fundamental skills that a pediatric surgeon has to master, although establishing the diagnosis often is difficult in young patients. The surgeon ultimately is responsible for deciding whether a child is taken to the operating room for an appendectomy; however, a primary care physician often is the first person to evaluate a patient who complains of abdominal pain. Pediatricians with expertise in infectious diseases frequently are involved in the care of children who present with subtle or atypical manifestations of appendicitis; have unusual microorganisms recovered from their appendices; or have complications as a result of appendiceal rupture, such as the development of wound infections, sepsis, peritonitis, intra-abdominal abscesses, and pelvic abscesses.

HISTORY

In the 16th century, physicians began describing patients with clinical manifestations suggestive of perforated appendicitis. Until the late 1800s, the inflammatory process was called *typhlitis* or *perityphlitis* because the illness was thought to originate from the cecum. In 1886, Fitz[52] recognized that the source of the inflammation was the appendix and suggested that a laparotomy be performed early in the course of the illness. Shortly afterward, McBurney[114] reported that in patients with appendicitis, tenderness was greatest 2 inches from the anterior iliac spine on a line drawn to the umbilicus. Despite intensive research and refinement of understanding of appendicitis during the 20th century, the rates of removing nondiseased appendices or finding already perforated appendices at laparotomy remained at approximately 20 percent until more recently when ultrasound and computed tomography (CT) examinations have been used routinely in children with suspected appendicitis, resulting in a possible decrease in misdiagnosis of the disease.

Despite the continued difficulties in diagnosing appendicitis, the mortality rate from appendicitis has decreased greatly since Fitz reported a 40 percent operative mortality rate. In 1936, Bancroft and Skoluda[16] reported a mortality rate of 8 percent and a complication rate of 11 percent for appendicitis, most likely because of the availability of general anesthesia and better aseptic surgical techniques. The second major improvement in outcome occurred in the 1940s, when sulfonamides and banked blood became widely available.[112] In the 1970s, anaerobes such as *Bacteroides fragilis* were found to cause postoperative infections frequently in patients with appendicitis, and treating these microorganisms was found to reduce further the rate of postoperative complications.[99] Currently, death from appendicitis is a rare occurrence in the United States.

EPIDEMIOLOGY

Reported incidences of acute appendicitis vary widely, depending on where the studies were performed and what methodologies were used. The consensus is that the number of cases of acute appendicitis has been decreasing during the past few decades.[86,115] Investigators have estimated that more than 70,000 children are diagnosed with appendicitis each year in the United States.[71] In 1997, appendicitis-related hospitalizations accounted for 0.6 percent of all hospitalizations in the United States, resulting in approximately 1 million hospital days and $3 billion in hospital charges.[40] Although appendicitis occurs in all age groups, the highest incidence occurs during the second decade of life.[3,107] Appendicitis is an uncommon event in children younger than 5 years of age and occurs extremely rarely in infants younger than 6 months. Researchers have suggested that patients with acquired immunodeficiency syndrome (AIDS) have a higher incidence of appendicitis than the normal population.[95]

Numerous studies have shown that the peak rates of appendicitis occur during the summer months, whereas the lowest rates occur during the winter months.[3,107] A study from Italy found a higher rate of pediatric appendicitis in winter, whereas appendicitis in adults was observed more frequently during the summer.[56] The reasons for these seasonal patterns are unknown, but changes in diet and exposure to allergens have been suggested as explanations.[107] Also, enteric infections occur most frequently during the summer and may play a role in increasing the incidence of appendicitis in summer.

Most studies show a modest increase in incidence of appendicitis in males compared with females.[3,107] An estimated lifetime risk for developing appendicitis is 8.6 percent for males and 6.7 percent for females.[3] In a study of acute appendicitis in California, the rate of appendicitis in whites was twice that of blacks and Asians.[107] More recently, Hispanics were shown to have the highest rate of appendicitis-related hospitalizations in the United States.[40] Whether the reported racial differences are due to errors of measurement, sociodemographic factors, environmental factors, factors related to body constitution, or genetic factors is unknown. Children with appendicitis more frequently have a history of having family members who previously have had appendicitis, suggesting that genetic background plays a role in the susceptibility to appendicitis.[18] Decreased dietary fiber and ingestion of refined carbohydrates also have been suggested to increase the risk for developing appendicitis.

The rates of perforation with appendicitis are significantly higher in Asian, Hispanic, and black children compared with non-Hispanic white children.[64,78,145,179] Similarly, children without health insurance or Medicaid have rates of perforation higher than those of children with private health insurance.[145,178]

Researchers have suggested that the pediatric rupture rate is a good candidate for inclusion in the National Healthcare Disparities Report.[78] Already, studies at local institutions have found no differences in perforation rates based on socioeconomic status, showing improved access to early medical care in their communities.[133,171]

PATHOPHYSIOLOGY

The initial event in the development of most cases of appendicitis is thought to be obstruction of the appendiceal lumen.[174] Microorganisms rarely invade the appendiceal mucosa and initiate the inflammatory process. Appendiceal obstruction can be caused by inspissated feces (fecalith), hypertrophied lymphoid tissue that develops during a systemic viral infection or bacterial enterocolitis, parasitic infestation, appendiceal wall hemorrhage associated with anaphylactic purpura, inspissated barium, or ingested seeds. Continued production of mucus by the appendiceal mucosa distal to the obstruction causes the appendix to distend. Vascular congestion and ischemia occur as the increased intraluminal pressure of the appendix becomes greater than the venous pressure, and edema develops as lymphatic flow becomes obstructed.

Stasis of intestinal flow and intestinal ischemia allow the microorganisms in the appendix to invade the tissues, enhancing the already developing inflammatory response. Bacteria may translocate across the appendiceal wall and reach the peritoneal cavity.[17] If the process is severe and arteriolar blood flow to the appendix is obstructed, transmural infarction occurs and the appendix ruptures. Microorganisms are liberated into the peritoneal cavity, causing generalized peritonitis and formation of an abscess. Animal studies have suggested that synergism occurring between enteric aerobes, such as *Escherichia coli*, and anaerobes, such as *B. fragilis*, is important in the development of intra-abdominal and pelvic abscesses after perforation.[62] An association between the development of an abscess after appendiceal perforation and the presence of *Streptococcus milleri* also apparently exists.[69]

As the appendix distends in the early stages of appendicitis, the visceral afferent autonomic nerves that enter the spinal cord at T8 to T10 are stimulated, referring the pain to the epigastric and periumbilical areas of the abdomen.[174] When the inflammatory response reaches the serosal surface of the appendix, the parietal peritoneum is stimulated, and the pain intensifies in the right lower quadrant. If perforation occurs, the peritoneal inflammatory response causes more generalized abdominal tenderness.

Although appendiceal obstruction may play an important role in the early stages of most cases of appendicitis, not all obstructed appendices become inflamed. Ten percent of normal appendices removed during abdominal surgical procedures contain inspissated fecal material. Also, children may develop recurrent, crampy abdominal pain, possibly from intermittent appendiceal obstruction.

The classic description of the pathophysiology of appendicitis does not explain easily many epidemiologic features of this disease, including its higher incidence in males and in certain races. The amount and reactivity of the lymphoid tissue in the wall of the appendix have been suggested to be key determinants to the development of appendicitis. The amount of lymphoid tissue in the appendix is greatest during adolescence, when the disease process is most prevalent, and the amount most likely is controlled genetically.

In a case-control study from Italy, prolonged breast-feeding during infancy was associated with a decreased risk for developing acute appendicitis later in life.[144] The investigators hypothesized that breast-feeding may have decreased the amount of stimulation to intestinal lymphocytes by microbial and food antigens early in life, so that appendiceal lymphoid tissues were less reactive to antigenic challenge during adolescence and adulthood. Appendicitis may be observed less frequently during infancy and the newborn period because the appendix is more funnel-shaped, the diet is primarily liquid, recumbent posture is maintained for prolonged periods, and gastrointestinal and respiratory infections develop less frequently during this time.[101]

CLINICAL MANIFESTATIONS

In school-aged children and adolescents with appendicitis, the median duration of symptoms before hospital admission is 24 to 28 hours.[151] Pain in the right iliac fossa is the most common sign of appendicitis, occurring in 88 to 99 percent of patients.[151,156] Pain shifts from the periumbilical area to the right lower quadrant of the abdomen in approximately two thirds of children with appendicitis. In three fourths of children, the pain worsens during movement. The characteristics of the abdominal pain do not always predict accurately which children have appendicitis. Of children found to have mesenteric adenitis at laparotomy, 25 percent report a shift in abdominal pain to the right iliac fossa and 33 percent experience worsening of pain during movement.[151]

Nausea and vomiting are found in 86 to 96 percent of children with appendicitis.[151,156] Vomiting usually occurs after the onset of abdominal pain but may precede pain in nearly 20 percent of cases. If only nausea or vomiting is present, it is less likely the child has appendicitis.[151] Anorexia occurs less commonly in children than in adults, occurring in 47 to 91 percent of cases of appendicitis. Because 50 percent of children found to have normal appendices at surgery complain of anorexia, differentiating appendicitis from other causes of right iliac fossa pain is not always helpful. Similarly, complaints of diarrhea (9-16%), constipation (5-28%), and dysuria (7%) occasionally can be elicited from children with appendicitis.[151,160] Fever may be helpful as a clinical sign of appendicitis if it is present (>37.5° C in 68-96% of cases), but absence of fever does not exclude the possibility of acute appendicitis. Very high temperatures (>39° C) suggest that perforation already has occurred or that another intra-abdominal process is present.[174] Rarely, children present with erythema and tenderness of the scrotum as the only manifestation of acute appendicitis.[216]

During the physical examination, the child frequently lies quietly on the examination table with the right hip flexed. Tenderness in the right iliac fossa is the most sensitive sign of appendicitis, occurring in 93 to 100 percent of cases of appendicitis.[151,156] The psoas muscle may become irritated from the inflamed appendix, causing the child to feel increased pain when the right hip is flexed actively. Likewise, if the obturator internus muscle is involved, pain is elicited when the flexed thigh is rotated internally.[174] Guarding is found in 80 to 91 percent of cases of appendicitis compared with 50 percent of cases of mesenteric adenitis and 8 percent of cases of nonspecific abdominal pain.[151] Similarly, rebound tenderness is found in 56 to 83 percent of cases of appendicitis, 33 percent of cases of acute mesenteric adenitis, and 1 percent of cases of nonspecific abdominal pain.[151]

The development of diffuse abdominal tenderness and the absence of bowel sounds usually indicate perforation. Extremely hyperactive bowel sounds suggest that the patient may not have appendicitis. Occasionally, a mass can be palpated in the right lower quadrant of the abdomen in children with appendicitis who are relaxed or well sedated. Rectal tenderness is present more commonly in children with appendicitis (44-68%) than in children with other causes of abdominal pain (12%); however, findings during the rectal examination seldom alter the clinical decision of the surgeon.[151]

In preschool-aged children, the diagnosis of appendicitis is more difficult to establish because of the inability of young children to express their symptoms and because they often do not cooperate during the physical examination.[210,211] Young children with appendicitis often are seen early in the course of their symptoms and are prescribed antibiotics, antihistamines, or antipyretics. By the time one realizes that the child has appendicitis, the appendix usually is perforated (50-90%).[210,211] In contrast to older children, in preschool-aged children vomiting is the initial symptom of appendicitis most frequently observed, and abdominal pain may be absent or may never localize in the right iliac fossa.[151] Sleep disturbances, irritability, restlessness, and crying are common manifestations of appendicitis in this age group. A preschool-aged child is more likely to have a palpable inflammatory mass at presentation.[174]

During the newborn period, appendicitis is an extremely rare occurrence.[101,164] Symptoms of neonatal appendicitis include abdominal distention; vomiting; irritability; diarrhea; erythema, edema, or cellulitis of the abdominal wall; gastrointestinal hemorrhage; abdominal rigidity; lethargy; and jaundice. Usually, the symptoms of neonatal appendicitis are indistinguishable from the symptoms of necrotizing enterocolitis. Underlying conditions, such as total colonic Hirschsprung disease, meconium plugs, or hernias, may predispose a newborn to developing this condition.

In children who are undergoing chemotherapy for leukemia, acute appendicitis may manifest with only vague abdominal pain, abdominal distention, lack of abdominal guarding, fever, dehydration, diarrhea, or unusual symptoms such as gastrointestinal bleeding.[8] Symptoms of appendicitis in immunocompromised patients may be identical to the symptoms of typhlitis.

The differential diagnosis of acute abdominal pain in children is extensive. Table 57–1 outlines conditions that can manifest with symptoms suggestive of acute appendicitis.

DIAGNOSIS

The diagnosis of acute appendicitis should be established without laboratory studies when a child complains of abdominal tenderness in the right lower quadrant that initially started in the periumbilical area, develops nausea and vomiting, and has rebound tenderness in the right lower quadrant with guarding during an abdominal examination.[21,174] The child should be taken to the operating room for an appendectomy as soon as possible before perforation occurs.[92] One third of children do not have all of the classic clinical manifestations of appendicitis, however; great emphasis has been placed on using various laboratory tests to help clinicians diagnose the disease accurately. Similarly, patients who have received prior oral antibiotics may have milder symptoms and signs of classic appendicitis, necessitating further diagnostic studies.[49]

For decades, physicians have valued peripheral blood leukocyte counts, neutrophil counts, C-reactive protein concentrations, and erythrocyte sedimentation rates to help them distinguish appendicitis from other causes of abdominal pain. When properly evaluated, these tests have been found, however, to be too insensitive to use as reliable tools for diagnosing appendicitis.[46,77,140,159] Normal results do not rule out the possibility that the child has appendicitis, although these tests help to confirm a physician's suspicions when results are positive. These nonspecific tests usually have elevated findings, however, during advanced disease, such as when perforation occurs.[5,136,142] Certain groups of patients commonly have normal leukocyte counts despite having acute appendicitis. Black patients with acute appendicitis frequently do not develop leukocytosis.[100,106] Patients with AIDS who develop appendicitis also frequently do not have elevated white blood cell counts.[24,124]

TABLE 57–1   Differential Diagnosis of Acute Appendicitis in Children

Cecal and Colonic Diseases
Constipation
Crohn disease
Infectious colitis (bacterial, parasitic)
Intestinal obstruction
Necrotizing enterocolitis (newborns)
Typhlitis (leukemia patients)

Small Intestinal Diseases
Duodenal ulcers (acute and perforated)
Gastroenteritis (including mesenteric adenitis)
Intestinal duplication
Intestinal obstruction
Intussusception
Meckel diverticulitis
Volvulus

Hepatobiliary and Pancreatic Diseases
Cholecystitis
Hepatitis
Hydrops of the gallbladder
Pancreatitis

Other Diseases
Omental torsion
Pneumonia
Psoas abscess
Spontaneous peritonitis

Reproductive Tract Diseases
Intrauterine and ectopic pregnancy
Ovarian torsion
Ovarian cysts
Pelvic inflammatory disease
Testicular torsion

Urinary Tract Diseases
Hydronephrosis
Pyelonephritis
Urachal abscess
Urolithiasis
Wilms tumor

Systemic Illnesses
Anaphylactoid purpura
Cytomegalovirus infection (in patients with AIDS)
Diabetic ketoacidosis
Kawasaki disease
Lymphoma (Burkitt)
Porphyria
Rocky Mountain spotted fever
Sickle-cell disease
Tuberculosis

AIDS, acquired immunodeficiency syndrome.

Routine radiographic studies for the diagnosis of appendicitis in children no longer are suggested. A chest radiograph often was obtained because right lower lobe pneumonia can cause severe abdominal pain in children. Radiographs of the abdomen are neither sensitive nor specific enough for diagnosing childhood appendicitis. Abnormalities described in association with acute appendicitis include an abnormal bowel gas pattern, a mass, a fecalith, and obliteration of normal fat planes in the right lower quadrant. Gas in the appendiceal lumen is thought to be diagnostic of acute appendicitis, but it may occur rarely in its absence. Most children do not have radiographic findings of appendicitis, or findings are nonspecific.

Graded compression ultrasonography has become the diagnostic procedure of choice in some institutions when evaluating a patient with possible appendicitis.[57,58] A transducer is used to apply gradual pressure to the abdomen. The technician must ensure that all gas and fluid contents from the loops of bowel are expressed for the examination to be adequate. A noncompressible, enlarged (>6 mm in diameter in adolescents) appendix or a fecalith is the major criterion used for diagnosing appendicitis by ultrasonography. Interruption in the continuity of the echogenic submucosa suggests necrosis of the appendiceal wall and impending perforation. An echogenic periappendiceal mass indicates inflammation of the mesenteric or omental fat. Loculated or generalized fluid collections suggest that perforation already has occurred.

Pooled studies of graded compression ultrasonography have shown that the procedure is 88 percent sensitive and 94 percent specific in diagnosing acute appendicitis in children.[44] False-positive ultrasound results occur in obese patients who have noncompressible appendices because of overlying fat and in children who have inflamed appendices caused by Crohn disease, ulcerative colitis, or adjacent salpingitis. False-negative results occur if retrocecally located appendices are not visualized properly; if the cecum is filled with gas or feces and is not compressed adequately; or if perforation has occurred, allowing the appendix to be compressible. In one study, a noncompressible appendix was identified in only 38 percent of pediatric patients with perforated appendicitis, rendering the other ultrasound findings of appendicitis important in diagnosing the disease.[146] The examination should be directed to diagnose other causes of abdominal pain that can mimic appendicitis when a normal appendix is found during the ultrasound evaluation.

The advantages of using ultrasonography over CT are that it is inexpensive, safe, and widely available. It is especially useful in adolescent girls with abdominal pain because gynecologic causes of the pain can be evaluated easily at the time of appendiceal examination.

Most North American pediatric surgeons prefer CT over ultrasonography as the diagnostic procedure of choice for appendicitis.[122] High-resolution CT has higher sensitivity (94%) and similar specificity (95%) than ultrasonography in diagnosing appendicitis, and it is less operator dependent.[44] Intravenous contrast agents and high-resolution, thin-section scanning techniques must be used to visualize the appendix adequately. An enlarged appendix with a circumferentially and symmetrically thickened bowel wall is the most common CT finding in appendicitis. Periappendiceal inflammatory reaction or fluid collections may be identified. If the appendix is not well visualized, the presence of a fecalith, along with pericecal inflammatory changes, strongly suggests appendicitis. Fecaliths can be visualized in normal appendices by CT, however, and are of no clinical significance unless other inflammatory changes are present.

In recent years, helical CT scanning techniques that are focused only to the right lower quadrant using rectal or no contrast material have been shown to be accurate in diagnosing appendicitis in children.[50,105] By using a focused approach, CT scans may be completed within 5 minutes. Because of the high accuracy rates of CT in diagnosing appendicitis, some physicians have suggested that all children with suspected disease should have a focused CT scan.[141] In most community hospitals and medical centers, waiting for results of a CT scan may delay a surgical consultation and increase the rate of perforation before surgery.[98] Also, CT scanning is expensive and uses significant amounts of ionizing radiation in children, who have greater radiosensitivity of organs and tissues than adults do.

Whether the increasing use of ultrasound and CT scans to diagnose appendicitis in children has decreased the misdiagnosis of the disease and subsequent negative appendectomy rate in hospitals is unclear.[53,82,84,110,111,218] In a single study, the misdiagnosis rate was lower in hospitals that perform frequent pediatric appendectomies.[178] Most children with appendicitis have surgery in nonchildren's hospitals, however.[37] Radiolabeled autologous leukocyte scans also have been used to diagnose appendicitis in children; however, this modality should be reserved for atypical presentations of disease when localizing signs are not present.[72]

MICROBIOLOGY

Numerous microorganisms have been implicated as a cause of acute appendicitis; considerable debate has ensued as to whether simply isolating an organism from the appendiceal lumen is sufficient proof to define causation (Table 57–2).[2]

BACTERIA

In most cases of appendicitis, bacteria do not seem to be involved directly in the initial stages of the inflammatory process. Microorganisms that normally inhabit the appendix are liberated into the peritoneal cavity when appendiceal perforation occurs or when translocation through the inflamed tissues is present, and polymicrobial infections develop as a complication of the disease process.[19,195] In a study of 30 adolescents and adults with nonperforated and perforated appendicitis, 223 different anaerobes and 82 aerobes were recovered from cultures of the appendiceal tissues, peritoneal fluid, and contents of abscesses.[19] An average of 10 different organisms were isolated per specimen collected.

In most microbiologic studies of appendiceal tissues and peritoneal fluid specimens from patients with appendicitis, *B. fragilis* is the strict anaerobe isolated most frequently, occurring in more than 70 percent of patients.[19,153] Other anaerobes that are isolated frequently include *Bacteroides* spp., *Bilophila wadsworthia*, *Peptostreptococcus* spp., *Fusobacterium* spp., and *Clostridium* spp.[201,213] A gram-negative anaerobic rod that develops a pigment in culture and is bile resistant also has been identified frequently.[152,153] Other anaerobes, such as *Turicibacter sanguinis*, continue to be newly described in patients with appendicitis.[23]

E. coli are the aerobic or facultative anaerobic bacteria isolated most frequently from children with appendicitis. *E. coli* are found in more than 75 percent of patients.[19,153] Researchers have suggested that certain *E. coli* strains with type 1C fimbriae may contribute to the development of appendiceal inflammation.[167] Enterohemorrhagic *E. coli* O157:H7 and O111:H have been isolated infrequently from the stools and peritoneal fluid of children with appendicitis.[199,205]

Viridans streptococci of the *S. milleri* group, including *Streptococcus anginosus*, can be found in more than 60 percent of cultures from children with appendicitis.[79,153] Group D streptococci are isolated in approximately 20 to 30 percent of patients with appendicitis, whereas *Pseudomonas* spp. are isolated slightly less frequently.[153] Other aerobes or facultative anaerobes that can be isolated from appendiceal tissues, abscesses, or blood include *Citrobacter* spp.; *Klebsiella* spp.; *Enterobacter* spp.; *Proteus* spp.; *Morganella morganii*; *Providencia rettgeri*; *Eikenella corrodens*; groups C, F, and G beta-hemolytic streptococci; and staphylococci.[45,70,81,148,153,195]

Rarely, encapsulated organisms, such as *Streptococcus pneumoniae*, *Haemophilus influenzae*, and *Haemophilus segnis*, have been isolated from appendiceal tissues or peritoneal fluid of young children with appendicitis, and often these organisms have been isolated in pure culture.[13,117,127] Very rarely, organisms such as *Pasteurella multocida*, *Streptococcus pyogenes*, and *Actinomyces* spp. have been cultured from patients with appendicitis.[149,162,169,198] *Shigella*, *Salmonella*, *Campylobacter*, and *Yersinia* spp. also have been isolated occasionally from appendiceal tissues or peritoneal fluid of patients with nonperforated and perforated appendicitis; whether they played a role in the pathogenesis of disease is

TABLE 57–2   Microorganisms Associated with Acute Appendicitis in Children

Anaerobes
Bacteroides spp.
Bilophilia wadsworthia
Clostridium spp.
Fusobacterium spp.
Peptostreptococcus spp.
Pigmented bile–resistant, gram-negative rod
Turicibacter sanguinis

Enteric Aerobes and Facultative Anaerobes
Campylobacter spp.
Citrobacter spp.
Enterobacter spp.
Enterococcus spp.
Escherichia coli
Klebsiella spp.
Morganella morganii
Proteus spp.
Providencia rettgeri
Salmonella spp.
Shigella spp.
Streptococcus milleri group
Yersinia spp.

Other Bacteria
Actinomyces spp.
Atypical mycobacteria (in patients with AIDS)
Brucella melitensis
Chromobacterium violaceum
Corynebacterium appendicis
Eikenella corrodens
Haemophilus spp.
Human monocytic ehrlichiosis
Kluyvera ascorbata
Pasteurella multocida
Pseudomonas spp.
Staphylococcus spp.
Streptococcus pneumoniae
Streptococcus pyogenes

Parasites
Angiostrongylus costaricensis
Anisakis spp.
Ascaris lumbricoides
Balantidium coli
Cryptosporidium parvum
Entamoeba histolytica
Enterobius vermicularis
Schistosoma spp.
Strongyloides stercoralis
Taenia spp.
Trichuris trichiura

Viruses
Adenoviruses
Coxsackieviruses B
Cytomegalovirus
Epstein-Barr virus
Measles

Fungi
Candida albicans
Histoplasma capsulatum
Mucor spp.

Rarely, *Kluyvera ascorbata*, *Arcobacter butzleri*, and *Chromobacterium violaceum* have been isolated from patients with appendicitis, as have newly described aerobes and facultative anaerobes, such as *Corynebacterium appendicis*.[31,33,97,215]

Rarely, isolated primary tuberculosis can occur in children.[66,147] The progression of disease usually is rapid. The clinician should be suspicious when caseating granulomas are observed in histopathologic sections of the appendix.

Adults and children with appendicitis usually are not bacteremic at the time they are diagnosed, especially if the appendix is not perforated. Occasionally, *Klebsiella pneumoniae*, *E. coli*, *B. fragilis*, and *B. wadsworthia* are isolated from the blood of patients with nonperforated appendicitis.[22,138,161] In a review of 1000 children and adults with appendicitis, 10 percent of patients with perforation had positive blood cultures, whereas none of the patients without perforation had bacteremia.[100] A higher rate of bacteremia may occur when laparoscopic surgery is done because of the air that is forced into the peritoneum, although the clinical significance of the induced bacteremia is unknown.[132]

In immunocompromised patients who develop appendicitis, the microorganisms that are isolated from appendiceal tissues or peritoneal cultures usually are identical to the microorganisms found in immunocompetent patients.[124] In adults infected with human immunodeficiency virus, appendicitis has been caused by cytomegalovirus infection and neoplastic obstruction of the base of the appendix by Kaposi sarcoma.[34,129] Patients with AIDS who have gastrointestinal *Mycobacterium avium* complex or *Mycobacterium tuberculosis* infections may develop symptoms that mimic appendicitis.[41,204] Atypical mycobacteria have been isolated from an appendiceal abscess from a child with AIDS.[48]

PARASITES

Roundworms, such as *Ascaris lumbricoides*, plausibly may obstruct the appendiceal lumen occasionally and initiate the cascade of inflammatory events leading to perforated appendicitis.[108,134] Parasites such as *Enterobius vermicularis* can be identified in the lumen of 1 to 12 percent of surgically removed appendices obtained from patients living in highly endemic areas.[10,38] Pinworms have been found more frequently, however, in appendices with no evidence of appendiceal inflammation in some studies, suggesting that pinworms probably are a part of the normal appendiceal flora and do not play a role in the pathogenesis of appendicitis.[38,163,217] Whether some parasites may cause abdominal pain that mimics the symptoms of appendicitis necessitating surgical intervention is unclear.

Scattered reports from mostly developing nations describe other worms, including *Taenia* spp., *Anisakis* spp., *Trichuris trichiura*, *Strongyloides stercoralis*, *Schistosoma* spp., and *Angiostrongylus costaricensis*, that have been identified in the lumina of appendices from patients with appendicitis.[11,55,65,91,165] Similarly, protozoa such as *Balantidium coli*, *Entamoeba histolytica*, and *Cryptosporidium parvum* have been found in inflamed appendices of immunocompromised and immunocompetent patients, but whether they play a role in the pathogenesis of disease is unknown.[27,43,67,150]

VIRUSES

The role that viruses play in causing appendicitis also has been debated. One suggestion is that a systemic viral infection may induce hypertrophied lymphoid aggregates that obstruct the appendiceal lumen. In the 1960s, elevated levels of antibodies against coxsackieviruses B and adenoviruses were found in the sera of some children with appendicitis.[196] A later study could not confirm this finding, however.[120] Six adolescents with infectious mononucleosis have developed appendicitis, and cytomegalovirus

unknown.[20,29,88,96,118] Much more commonly, these organisms cause enterocolitis or mesenteric adenitis, with symptoms mimicking those of appendicitis.[203]

In recent years, appendicitis has occurred during systemic infections caused by *Brucella melitensis* and *Ehrlichia chaffeensis*.[7,173]

has been observed occasionally in immunodeficient and otherwise healthy patients' inflamed appendices.[85,104,129,194] Other children have had histologic evidence of measles virus or adenovirus infection.[137,155] Because of the rarity of documented simultaneous viral infections and appendicitis, whether these viruses play a major role in the pathogenesis of acute appendicitis is doubtful.

FUNGI

Rarely, *Candida albicans* is isolated from inflamed appendices or abscess cultures, but its role in the pathogenesis of disease is unknown. Perforation of the appendix from intestinal mucormycosis has occurred in granulocytopenic patients and premature newborns.[130,193] Also, appendicitis has been described in individuals with histoplasmosis.[94]

TREATMENT

NONPERFORATED APPENDICITIS

In previously healthy children with signs of acute appendicitis and no clinical evidence of perforation, nasogastric suctioning should be established and imbalances in fluid and electrolyte concentrations should be corrected quickly. The child should be taken to the operating room as soon as possible for exploratory laparotomy and appendectomy. Many teaching hospitals now perform appendectomies only during day and evening hours, because of limitations on resident work hours and decreased services available at night.[122] No differences have been noted to date in perforation rates, lengths of stay, or complication rates in children who are diagnosed with appendicitis at night and given analgesics until a scheduled morning surgery.[1,191,214] Morphine can be used to reduce the severity of abdominal pain in children with appendicitis until the child is taken to the operating room and does not impede establishing the diagnosis in children under observation for suggestive symptoms and signs of appendiceal disease.[63]

Prophylactic antibiotics given perioperatively decrease the rate of postoperative wound infection, even in noncomplicated cases of childhood appendicitis.[4,175] No consensus exists concerning the appropriate antimicrobial agent or agents that should be used or the appropriate duration of treatment required after surgery to reduce the complication rate. Although some surgeons continue the antibiotics after surgery, prospective, randomized studies show that a single perioperative dose of appropriate antibiotic with antimicrobial activity against *E. coli* and enteric anaerobes is as effective as continuing the antibiotic for 1 to 5 days after surgery.[125,197]

Few data support the routine intraoperative collection of peritoneal fluid or appendiceal cultures in children with nonperforated appendicitis, although 5 to 20 percent of cultures grow enteric aerobes, anaerobes, or both.[32,60] Immunocompromised patients should undergo intraoperative cultures, including cultures for mycobacteria and cytomegalovirus.

Interest in performing laparoscopic appendectomies in children with nonperforated and perforated appendicitis has been increasing.[30,122,143] Advantages of the procedure are a reduction in wound infection, reduction in scarring, shorter hospital stay, and earlier return to normal activity, although the procedure must be done by a surgeon experienced in laparoscopic techniques.[14] The mean total cost of a laparoscopic appendectomy is similar to that of the more commonly performed open appendectomy, and more recent studies in pediatric patients have determined that no differences exist in postoperative pain, time to self-ambulation, and risk of developing a postoperative abscess.[175] In the future, the

use of smaller laparoscopic instruments may improve the speed of recovery of children.[121]

PERFORATED APPENDICITIS

Most surgeons advocate early intervention when perforation has occurred to prevent severe complications, such as fistula formation, abscess rupture, and death, despite the high chance of developing postoperative complications.[122] If a laparotomy is done, debate ensues as to whether the wound should be closed primarily and whether transperitoneal drains should be placed at the time of surgery. Surgeons increasingly are performing primary closures without placing drains in children.[47,116,122] A randomized prospective trial of appendiceal drains in children with perforated appendicitis showed no benefit in using drains compared with primary wound closure.[188] Laparoscopic surgery has been used for perforated appendicitis; nonetheless, caution, good surgical judgment, and a low threshold for conversion to an open procedure are advised.[102]

During the surgical procedure, most surgeons irrigate the peritoneal cavity with copious amounts of saline or antibiotics to reduce the quantity of bacteria in the abdomen.[122] To obtain sterile cultures of the lavage fluid, 6 L of lavage fluid per m² surface area of the child is required.[135] It is unclear whether the lavage fluid or the addition of antibiotics to the lavage fluid decreases the rate of postoperative complications in children with perforated appendicitis who are receiving systemic antibiotics.[113]

Controversy remains as to whether immediate appendectomy should be done in a child in whom a palpable mass is associated with the appendicitis or evidence of appendiceal rupture with or without abscess formation exists at the time of presentation.[174,207] Greater than 70 percent of children with palpable masses respond to conservative, nonoperative management consisting of administration of intravenous fluids and antibiotics.[174] If the child does not improve, or a walled-off abscess develops, drainage of the area and appendectomy should be done. If the child responds to conservative management, an interval appendectomy should be done 6 to 8 weeks after resolution of the symptoms. Proponents of initial conservative management consider that the complication rate after interval appendectomy is significantly lower than when a procedure is done during the acute stage of disease.

Antimicrobial agents should be administered routinely to children when perforation or appendiceal abscess is suspected or discovered during surgery. Antibiotics active against aerobes and anaerobes that normally inhabit the intestinal tract have been effective in treating children with perforated appendicitis. Treatment failures occur most commonly when *B. fragilis* or *Pseudomonas* spp. are isolated from intraoperative cultures and antimicrobial agents without activity against these organisms are used.[73] Controversy continues regarding the value of obtaining routine intraoperative peritoneal cultures in cases of perforated appendicitis, although most studies show that culture results seldom change the clinical management of patients.[32,60,87,90,182]

The antimicrobial combination of ampicillin, gentamicin, and clindamycin has been the gold standard of therapy since the 1970s. The importance of including ampicillin in the regimen for adequate enterococcal coverage continues to be controversial. Animal studies and clinical trials using antibiotics with poor enterococcal activity have shown that ampicillin probably is not required in the treatment of perforated appendicitis.[62] Because of the increasing problem of ampicillin resistance in enterococci, ampicillin probably should be reserved for the rare child with enterococcal bacteremia or with persistent intra-abdominal infection in which enterococci have been isolated. Some medical centers use metronidazole instead of clindamycin because of its broader activity against enteric anaerobes, whereas other institutions substitute cefotaxime or ceftriaxone for gentamicin.[170,186]

Efforts have been made to determine whether single antibiotics are effective in treating perforated appendicitis. The only agents that have been shown to be effective in treating children with perforated appendicitis are cefoxitin, imipenem-cilastatin, ticarcillin-clavulanate, piperacillin-tazobactam, ampicillin-sulbactam, meropenem, and ertapenem.[51,109,126,176,177,192,200,212] In a few medical centers, nearly 50 percent of *B. fragilis* isolates are resistant to cefoxitin, raising the question as to whether cefoxitin should be used routinely as a single agent in these institutions.[54] Generally, the convenience of monotherapy does not outweigh the potential development of resistance to these broad-spectrum agents and their associated increased costs.[87] They may be useful in the treatment of appendicitis in children with renal disease or hearing loss when avoiding the use of gentamicin is prudent.

Most patients with perforated appendicitis are treated with intravenous antibiotics for 5 to 10 days; however, limiting the duration of antibiotic use to 3 days does not lead to higher rates of wound infections or intra-abdominal abscesses.[122,180] Efforts have been made to shorten the hospital stay of children with perforated appendicitis. Some institutions have set criteria for hospital discharge and discontinuation of antibiotics, such as absence of fever for 24 hours, ability to eat well, and less than 3 percent band forms on the white blood cell differential.[74] Many surgeons switch to oral antibiotics at home after 3 to 5 days of intravenous antibiotics in the hospital, although the benefit of adding prolonged oral antibiotics to a short course of intravenous antibiotics has not been shown.[157,190] Providing home single intravenous antimicrobial therapy also can reduce costs and hasten hospital discharge in selected children with perforated appendicitis.[51,87,185]

PROGNOSIS AND EARLY COMPLICATIONS

Currently in the United States, the risk of dying as a result of appendicitis is very low. The estimated mortality rate for non-perforated and perforated appendicitis in California during the 1980s was 0.02 percent.[106] In smaller series of children and adults reported in the 1990s, the mortality rate was 0 percent.[112] It has been stated that the risk of death from appendicitis should be the risk of death from general anesthesia.[112] The mortality rate seems to be higher, however, in the rare newborn or premature infant who develops appendicitis. Also, factors contributing to the death of children rarely may include delay in establishing the diagnosis, inadequate fluid replacement, immunodeficiency, and postoperative vascular or infectious complications.

The most predictive factor of postoperative morbidity occurring from appendicitis is perforation.[154] Age, obesity, duration of the surgical procedure, and nutritional status also are risk factors for the development of complications. Wound infection rates in children who receive perioperative antibiotics should be less than 7 percent; infections generally are caused by the same organisms that are isolated in cultures obtained during appendectomy.[175,197] Occasionally, children develop peritonitis, intra-abdominal abscesses, psoas abscesses, fistulas, pyelophlebitis of the portal vein, scrotal abscesses, or pneumoperitoneum during treatment of appendicitis.[15,68,75,158,216] CT scans can be used successfully to detect postoperative abscesses in the first week after surgery.[9] If complications occur, another surgical procedure often is performed, and antibiotic treatment is prolonged. Abscesses may be treated successfully with antibiotics alone and without surgical drainage in stable patients after appendectomy.[42] The next section focuses on pelvic abscess as an early complication of appendicitis because the topic is not discussed elsewhere in this textbook.

PELVIC ABSCESS

The pelvic area is a common site for development of abscesses because it is the most dependent portion of the peritoneal cavity. Pelvic abscesses most commonly occur in children who have had intestinal perforations after appendicitis, have had penetrating abdominal or retroperitoneal injury, or have undergone an abdominal surgical procedure. Occasionally, adolescents with pelvic inflammatory disease or Crohn disease develop a pelvic abscess.[61]

In children with perforated appendicitis, a coexisting pelvic abscess often is diagnosed at the time of laparotomy. In patients who recently have had penetrating trauma to the abdomen, have had pelvic inflammatory disease, or have undergone gastrointestinal surgery, a pelvic abscess should be suspected when they have continued fever or complain of abdominal pain despite receiving adequate treatment of the initial disease process. Symptoms may not develop until days to months after therapy is ended. No characteristic physical findings are associated with a pelvic abscess, although abdominal palpation or rectal examination may elicit tenderness, or signs of intestinal obstruction may be present.

If a pelvic abscess is suspected, contrast-enhanced CT evaluation of the pelvis should be completed. The bladder should be filled before the procedure so that it can displace bowel loops from the pelvis, act as an anatomic marker, and act as a standard of fluidity against which an abscess cavity can be compared. Walled-off fluid collections in the pelvis can be identified, and sometimes the rectum, sigmoid colon, or bladder is compressed because of mass effect from the abscess cavity. Because most pelvic abscesses develop as complications of intestinal or pelvic infections, enteric aerobes and anaerobes are the organisms most commonly isolated from the abscess cavity. Yeasts only rarely cause pelvic abscesses.[202,209] An *Actinomyces*-related pelvic abscess developed in an adult who had an intrauterine device.[139] Rarely, tuberculous abscesses can develop as a complication of genital tuberculosis.[208]

When a pelvic abscess is identified, antibiotics covering intestinal aerobes and anaerobes, such as clindamycin and gentamicin, should be started, and the abscess contents should be drained. In most situations, reaching the abscess cavity by an anterior approach is difficult. Considerable interest has developed in using CT or ultrasonography to guide percutaneous drainage of pelvic abscesses by transgluteal, transrectal, transparacoccygeal, or transvaginal approaches.[28,59,80,103,131] Although placement of a transgluteal catheter is easiest, the sciatic nerve and gluteal vessels must be avoided. Also, an increased risk for development of a wound infection may occur because microorganisms may track along the outside of the catheter to the skin. Many surgeons prefer the transrectal approach because it often is the most direct route to the abscess. Transvaginal drainage has been used with good results in young women, however. Most often, drainage catheters can be removed after 7 to 10 days of treatment.

Abscesses also may develop within the muscles of the pelvic girdle, including the psoas and internal obturator muscles.[25,168,181,183,184,187] Similar to true pelvic abscesses, they usually cause fever and occasionally abdominal complaints in children. Most children begin to limp, refuse to walk, or complain of pain in the buttocks, thigh, or groin. Often, a suppurative hip infection is suspected initially. A pelvic muscle abscess usually is diagnosed by CT or magnetic resonance imaging. Labeled leukocyte scans sometimes are useful in localizing the infection to within the pelvis, especially when the child has no symptoms other than fever or refusing to walk.

Pelvic muscle abscesses can develop as a complication of Crohn disease or appendicitis; however, they often develop after an episode of bacteremia.[166] *Staphylococcus aureus* is the most common cause of a primary pelvic muscle abscess.[25,168,181,183] *S. pneumoniae*, *H. influenzae* type b, *E. coli*, *Enterococcus faecalis*,

S. milleri group, *Yersinia enterocolitica*, *Salmonella* spp., *Proteus mirabilis*, and *Actinomyces* spp. also have been reported to cause hematogenously acquired abscesses.[25,26,35,39,76,83,89,172] Bacteremia secondary to intravenous drug abuse or the presence of central lines occasionally predisposes patients to developing this type of infection.[93,206] Rarely, tuberculous psoas abscesses have been reported, often as a complication of vertebral osteomyelitis.[189]

Pelvic muscle abscesses usually are drained by a percutaneous or surgical approach, and antibiotic therapy is based on Gram stain and culture results. Successful therapy with antibiotics alone has been reported.[184] Duration of treatment is individualized and depends on the child's response and the drainage techniques that were used.

LATE COMPLICATIONS

Most children who have undergone appendectomy or drainage of a pelvic abscess do not have late complications. Occasionally, patients develop signs of bowel obstruction from peritoneal adhesions later. Some studies have suggested that the future risk for infertility is greater in women who have perforated appendices or pelvic abscesses, presumably because of adhesion formation that impairs the migration of ova in the reproductive tract.[123] Although some retrospective studies have suggested that patients with appendectomies have a higher rate of developing malignancies later in life, prospective and controlled studies have failed to show this association.[36,119] Patients who have had appendicitis have been reported to be three times more likely to develop right inguinal hernias than individuals who have not had the appendix removed.[12] It has been suggested that women have a higher long-term risk of developing Crohn disease if they had nonperforated appendicitis earlier in life, whereas patients with previous perforated appendicitis have a more severe course of inflammatory bowel disease.[6]

REFERENCES

1. Abou-Nukta, F., Bakhos, C., Arroyo, K., et al.: Effects of delaying appendectomy for acute appendicitis for 12 to 24 hours. Arch. Surg. *141*:504-507, 2006.
2. Addiss, D. G., and Juranek, D. D.: Lack of evidence for a causal association between parasitic infections and acute appendicitis. J. Infect. Dis. *164*:1036-1037, 1991.
3. Addiss, D. G., Shaffer, N., Fowler, B. S., et al.: The epidemiology of appendicitis and appendectomy in the United States. Am. J. Epidemiol. *132*:910-925, 1990.
4. Andersen, B. R., Kallehave, F. L., and Andersen, H. K.: Antibiotics versus placebo for prevention of postoperative infection after appendicectomy. Cochrane Database Syst. Rev. *3*:CD001439, 2005.
5. Andersson, R. E. B.: Meta-analysis of the clinical and laboratory diagnosis of appendicitis. Br. J. Surg. *91*:28-37, 2004.
6. Andersson, R. E., Olaison, G., Tysk, T., et al.: Appendectomy is followed by increased risk of Crohn's disease. Gastroenterology *124*:40-46, 2003.
7. Andriopoulos, P., Tsironi, M., and Asimakopoulos, G.: Acute abdomen due to *Brucella melitensis*. Scand. J. Infect. Dis. *35*:204-205, 2003.
8. Angel, C. A., Rao, B. N., Wrenn, E., et al.: Acute appendicitis in children with leukemia and other malignancies: Still a diagnostic dilemma. J. Pediatr. Surg. *27*:476-479, 1992.
9. Antevil, J. L., Egan, J. C., Woodbury, R. O., et al.: Abdominal computed tomography for postoperative abscess: Is it useful during the first week? J. Gastrointest. Surg. *10*:901-905, 2006.
10. Arca, M. J., Gates, R. L., Groner, J. I., et al.: Clinical manifestations of appendiceal pinworms in children: An institutional experience and a review of the literature. Pediatr. Surg. Int. *20*:372-375, 2004.
11. Arenal Vera, J. J., Marcos Rodriquez, J. L., Borrego Pintado, M. H., et al.: Anisakiasis as a cause of acute appendicitis and rheumatologic picture: The first case in medical literature. Rev. Esp. Enferm. Dig. *79*:355-358, 1991.
12. Arnbjornsson, E.: Development of right inguinal hernia after appendectomy. Am. J. Surg. *143*:174-175, 1982.
13. Astagneau, P., Goldstein, F. W., Francoual, S., et al.: Appendicitis due to both *Streptococcus pneumoniae* and *Haemophilus influenzae*. Eur. J. Clin. Microbiol. Infect. Dis. *11*:559-560, 1992.

14. Aziz, O., Athanasiou, T., Tekkis, P. P., et al.: Laparoscopic versus open appendectomy in children—a meta-analysis. Ann. Surg. *243*:17-27, 2006.
15. Babcock, D. S.: Ultrasound diagnosis of portal vein thrombosis as a complication of appendicitis. A. J. R. Am. J. Roentgenol. *133*:317-319, 1979.
16. Bancroft, F. W., and Skoluda, E. R.: Appendicitis: A study of 596 cases. N. Y. State J. Med. *36*:507-509, 1936.
17. Baron, E. J., Bennion, R., Thompson, J., et al.: Microbiological comparison between acute and complicated appendicitis. Clin. Infect. Dis. *14*:227-231, 1992.
18. Basta, M., Morton, N. E., Mulvihill, J. J., et al.: Inheritance of acute appendicitis: Familial aggregation and evidence of polygenic transmission. Am. J. Hum. Genet. *46*:377-382, 1990.
19. Bennion, R. S., Baron, E. J., Thompson, J. E., et al.: The bacteriology of gangrenous and perforated appendicitis revisited. Ann. Surg. *211*:165-171, 1990.
20. Bennion, R. S., Thompson, J. E., Gil, J., et al.: The role of *Yersinia enterocolitica* in appendicitis in the southwestern United States. Am. Surg. *57*:766-768, 1991.
21. Bergeron, E.: Clinical judgment remains of great value in the diagnosis of acute appendicitis. Can. J. Surg. *49*:96-100, 2006.
22. Bernard, D., Verschraegen, G., Claeys, G., et al.: *Bilophila wadsworthii* bacteremia in a patient with gangrenous appendicitis. Clin. Infect. Dis. *18*:1023-1024, 1994.
23. Bosshard, P. P., Zbinden, R., and Altwegg, M.: *Turicibacter sanguinis* gen. nov., sp. nov., a novel anaerobic, gram-positive bacterium. Int. J. Syst. Evol. Microbiol. *52*:1263-1266, 2002.
24. Bova, R., and Meagher, A.: Appendicitis in HIV-positive patients. Aust. N. Z. J. Surg. *68*:337-339, 1998.
25. Bresee, J. S., and Edwards, M. S.: Psoas abscess in children. Pediatr. Infect. Dis. J. *9*:201-206, 1990.
26. Brooks, D. J., Cant, A. J., Lambert, H. P., et al.: Recurrent *Salmonella* septicaemia with aortitis, osteomyelitis and psoas abscess. J. Infect. *7*:156-158, 1983.
27. Buch, K., Nguyen, S., Divino, C. M., et al.: Cryptosporidiosis presenting as acute appendicitis: A case report. Am. Surgeon *71*:537-538, 2005.
28. Cahill, A. M., Baskin, K. M., Kaye, R. D., et al.: Transgluteal approach for draining pelvic fluid collections in pediatric patients. Radiology *234*:893-898, 2005.
29. Campbell, L. K., Havens, J. M., Scott, M. A., et al.: Molecular detection of *Campylobacter jejuni* in archival cases of acute appendicitis. Mod. Pathol. *19*:1042-1046, 2006.
30. Canty, T. G., Sr., Collins, D., Losasso, B., et al.: Laparoscopic appendectomy for simple and perforated appendicitis in children: The procedure of choice? J. Pediatr. Surg. *35*:1582-1585, 2000.
31. Carter, J. E., and Evans, T. N.: Clinically significant *Kluyvera* infections—a report of seven cases. Am. J. Clin. Pathol. *123*:334-338, 2005.
32. Celik, A., Ergun, O., Ozcan, C., et al.: Is it justified to obtain routine peritoneal fluid cultures during appendectomy in children? Pediatr. Surg. Int. *19*:632-634, 2003.
33. Chen, C.-H., Lin, L.-C., Liu, C.-E., et al.: *Chromobacterium violaceum* bacteremia: A case report. J. Microbiol. Immunol. Infect. *36*:141-144, 2003.
34. Chetty, R., Slavin, J. L., and Miller, R. A.: Kaposi's sarcoma presenting as acute appendicitis in an HIV-1 positive patient. Histopathology *23*:590-591, 1993.
35. Coakham, H. B., and Ashby, E. C.: Actinomycosis in recurrent psoas abscess. Proc. R. Soc. Med. *65*:880, 1972.
36. Cope, J. U., Askling, J., Gridley, G., et al.: Appendectomy during childhood and adolescence and the subsequent risk of cancer in Sweden. Pediatrics *111*:1343-1350, 2003.
37. Cosper, G. H., Hamann, M. S., Stiles, A., et al.: Hospital characteristics affect outcomes for common pediatric surgical conditions. Am. Surgeon *72*:739-745, 2006.
38. Dahlstrom, J. E., and Macarthur, E. B.: *Enterobius vermicularis*: A possible cause of symptoms resembling appendicitis. Aust. N. Z. J. Surg. *64*:92-94, 1994.
39. Davies, D., King, S. M., Parekh, R. S., et al.: Psoas abscess caused by *Haemophilus influenzae*, type b. Pediatr. Infect. Dis. J. *10*:411-412, 1991.
40. Davies, G. M., Dasbach, E. J., and Teutsch, S.: The burden of appendicitis-related hospitalizations in the United States in 1997. Surg. Infect. *5*:160-165, 2004.
41. Dezfuli, M. G., Oo, M. M., Jones, B. E., et al.: Tuberculosis mimicking acute appendicitis in patients with human immunodeficiency virus infection. Clin. Infect. Dis. *18*:650-651, 1994.
42. Dobremez, E., Lavrand, F., Lefevre, Y., et al.: Treatment of post-appendectomy intra-abdominal deep abscesses. Eur. J. Pediatr. Surg. *13*:393-397, 2003.
43. Dodd, L. G.: *Balantidium coli* infestation as a cause of acute appendicitis. J. Infect. Dis. *163*:1392, 1991.
44. Doria, A. S., Moineddin, R., Kellenberger, C. J., et al.: US or CT for diagnosis of appendicitis in children and adults? A meta-analysis. Radiology *241*:83-94, 2006.
45. Dougherty, S. H., Saltzstein, E. C., Peacock, J. B., et al.: Perforated or gangrenous appendicitis treated with aminoglycosides. Arch. Surg. *124*:1280-1283, 1989.
46. Dueholm, S., Bagi, P., and Bud, M.: Laboratory aid in the diagnosis of acute appendicitis: A blinded, prospective trial concerning diagnostic value of

leukocyte count, neutrophil differential count, and C-reactive protein. Dis. Colon Rectum *32*:855-859, 1989.

47. Emil, S., Laberge, J.-M., Mikhail, P., et al.: Appendicitis in children: A ten-year update of therapeutic recommendations. J. Pediatr. Surg. *38*:236-242, 2003.

48. Enami, M. A., Frayha, H. H., and Halim, M. A.: An appendiceal abscess due to *Mycobacterium kansasii* in a child with AIDS. Clin. Infect. Dis. *27*:891-892, 1998.

49. England, R. J., and Crabbe, D. C. G.: Delayed diagnosis of appendicitis in children treated with antibiotics. Pediatr. Surg. Int. *22*:541-545, 2006.

50. Fefferman, N. R., Roche, K. J., Pinkney, L. P., et al.: Suspected appendicitis in children: Focused CT technique for evaluation. Radiology *220*:691-695, 2001.

51. Fishman, S. J., Pelosi, L., Klavon, S. L., et al.: Perforated appendicitis: Prospective outcome analysis for 150 children. J. Pediatr. Surg. *35*:923-926, 2000.

52. Fitz, R. H.: Perforating inflammation of the vermiform appendix, with special reference to its early diagnosis and treatment. Am. J. Med. Sci. *92*:321-346, 1886.

53. Flum, D. R., Morris, A., Koepsell, T., et al.: Has misdiagnosis of appendicitis decreased over time? A population-based analysis. J. A. M. A. *286*:1748-1753, 2001.

54. Fraulin, F. O. G., and Thurston, O. G.: Value of cultures of tissue samples taken at operation for lower intestinal perforation. Can. J. Surg. *36*:261-265, 1993.

55. Gabbi, C., Bertolotti, M., Iori, R., et al.: Acute abdomen associated with schistosomiasis of the appendix. Dig. Dis. Sci. *51*:215-217, 2006.

56. Gallerani, M., Boari, B., Anania, G., et al.: Seasonal variation in onset of acute appendicitis. Clin. Ter. *157*:123-127, 2006.

57. Garcia Pena, B. M., Cook, E. F., and Mandl, K. D.: Selective imaging strategies for the diagnosis of appendicitis in children. Pediatrics *113*:24-28, 2004.

58. Garcia Pena, B. M., Taylor, G. A., Fishman, S. J., et al.: Effect of an imaging protocol on clinical outcomes among pediatric patients with appendicitis. Pediatrics *110*:1088-1093, 2002.

59. Gervais, D. A., Brown, S. D., Connolly, S. A., et al.: Percutaneous imaging-guided abdominal and pelvic abscess drainage in children. RadioGraphics *24*:737-754, 2004.

60. Gladman, M. A., Knowles, C. H., Gladman, L. J., et al.: Intra-operative culture in appendicitis: Traditional practice challenged. Ann. R. Coll. Surg. Engl. *86*:196-201, 2004.

61. Golfieri, R., Cappelli, A., Giampalma, E., et al.: CT-guided percutaneous pelvic abscess drainage in Crohn's disease. Tech. Coloproctol. *10*:99-105, 2006.

62. Gorbach, S. L.: Intra-abdominal infections. Clin. Infect. Dis. *17*:961-967, 1993.

63. Green, R., Bulloch, B., Kabani, A., et al.: Early analgesia for children with acute abdominal pain. Pediatrics *116*:978-983, 2005.

64. Guagliardo, M. F., Teach, S. J., Huang, Z. J., et al.: Racial and ethnic disparities in pediatric appendicitis rupture rate. Acad. Emerg. Med. *10*:1218-1227, 2003.

65. Gupta, S. C., Gupta, A. K., Keswani, N. K., et al.: Pathology of tropical appendicitis. J. Clin. Pathol. *42*:1169-1172, 1989.

66. Gupta, S., Kaushik, R., Kaur, A., et al.: Tubercular appendicitis—a case report. World J. Emerg. Surg. *1*:22, 2006.

67. Guzman-Valdivia, G.: Acute amebic appendicitis. World J. Surg. *30*:1038-1042, 2006.

68. Haas, G. P., Shumaker, B. P., and Haas, P. A.: Appendicovesical fistula. Urology *24*:604-609, 1984.

69. Hardwick, R. H., Taylor, A., Thompson, M. H., et al.: Association between *Streptococcus milleri* and abscess formation after appendicitis. Ann. R. Coll. Surg. Engl. *82*:24-26, 2000.

70. Hasan, R. A., and Abuhammour, W.: Beta-hemolytic group F streptococcal bacteremia in children. Pediatr. Infect. Dis. J. *23*:468-470, 2004.

71. HCUPnet, Healthcare Cost and Utilization Project. Rockville, MD, Agency for Healthcare Research and Quality. Available at: http://www.ahrq.gov/data/hcup/hcupnet.htm. 2002.

72. Henneman, P. L., Marcus, C. S., Inkelis, S. H., et al.: Evaluation of children with possible appendicitis using technetium 99m leukocyte scan. Pediatrics *85*:838-843, 1990.

73. Heseltine, P. N. R., Yellin, A. E., Appleman, M. D., et al.: Perforated and gangrenous appendicitis: An analysis of antibiotic failures. J. Infect. Dis. *148*:322-329, 1983.

74. Hoelzer, D. J., Zabel, D. D., and Zern, J. T.: Determining duration of antibiotic use in children with complicated appendicitis. Pediatr. Infect. Dis. J. *18*:979-982, 1999.

75. Hoffer, F. A., Ablow, R. C., Gryboski, J. D., et al.: Primary appendicitis with an appendico-tuboovarian fistula. A. J. R. Am. J. Roentgenol. *138*:742-743, 1982.

76. Humphreys, H., Keane, C. T., Marron, P., et al.: Infective sacroiliac arthritis and psoas abscess caused by *Streptococcus milleri*. J. Infect. *19*:77-78, 1989.

77. Hyman, P., and Westring, D. W.: Leukocytosis in acute appendicitis: Observed racial difference. J. A. M. A. *229*:1630-1632, 1974.

78. Jablonski, K. A., and Guagliardo, M. F.: Pediatric appendicitis rupture rate: A national indicator of disparities in healthcare access. Population Health Met. *3*:4, 2005.

79. Jackson, D. S., Welch, D. F., Pickett, D. A., et al.: Suppurative infections in children caused by non-beta-hemolytic members of the *Streptococcus milleri* group. Pediatr. Infect. Dis. J. *14*:80-82, 1995.

80. Jaffe, T. A., Nelson, R. C., DeLong, D. M., et al.: Practice patterns in percutaneous image-guided intraabdominal abscess drainage: Survey of academic and private practice centers. Radiology *233*:750-756, 2004.

81. Jakobsen, J., Andersen, J. C., and Klausen, I. C.: Beta-haemolytic streptococci in acute appendicitis. Acta Chir. Scand. *154*:301-303, 1988.

82. Jones, K., Pena, A. A., Dunn, E. L., et al.: Are negative appendectomies still acceptable? Am. J. Surg. *188*:748-754, 2004.

83. Kahn, F. W., Glasser, J. E., and Agger, W. A.: Psoas muscle abscess due to *Yersinia enterocolitica*. Am. J. Med. *76*:947-949, 1984.

84. Kaiser, S., Mesas-Burgos, C., Soderman, E., et al.: Appendicitis in children—impact of US and CT on the negative appendectomy rate. Eur. J. Pediatr. Surg. *14*:260-264, 2004.

85. Kanafani, Z. A., Sharara, A. I., Shabb, N. S., et al.: Cytomegalovirus appendicitis following acute Epstein-Barr virus infection in an immunocompetent patient. Scand. J. Dis. *36*:505-507, 2004.

86. Kang, J. Y., Hoare, J., Majeed, A., et al.: Decline in admission rates for acute appendicitis in England. Br. J. Surg. *90*:1586-1592, 2003.

87. Kaplan, S.: Antibiotic usage in appendicitis in children. Pediatr. Infect. Dis. J. *17*:1047-1048, 1998.

88. Kazlow, P. G., Freed, J., Rosh, J. R., et al.: *Salmonella typhimurium* appendicitis. J. Pediatr. Gastroenterol. Nutr. *13*:101-103, 1991.

89. Knobel, B., Sommer, I., and Schwartz, G.: Primary psoas abscess three years after ipsilateral nephrectomy. Infection *13*:27-28, 1985.

90. Kokoska, E. R., Silen, M. L., Tracy, T. F., et al.: The impact of intraoperative culture on treatment and outcome in children with perforated appendicitis. J. Pediatr. Surg. *34*:749-753, 1999.

91. Komenaka, I. K., Wu, G. C. H., Lazar, E. L., et al.: *Strongyloides* appendicitis: Unusual etiology in two siblings with chronic abdominal pain. J. Pediatr. Surg. *38*:E37, 2003.

92. Kosloske, A. M., Love, C. L., Rohrer, J. E., et al.: The diagnosis of appendicitis in children: Outcomes of a strategy based on pediatric surgical evaluation. Pediatrics *113*:29-34, 2004.

93. Kwok, T., and Coles, J.: Psoas abscess as a complication of subclavian venous catheterization. Postgrad. Med. J. *66*:771-772, 1990.

94. Lamps, L. W., Molina, C. P., Haggitt, R. C., et al.: The pathologic spectrum of gastrointestinal and hepatic histoplasmosis. Am. J. Clin. Pathol. *113*:64-72, 2000.

95. LaRaja, R. D., Rothenberg, R. E., Odom, J. W., et al.: The incidence of intra-abdominal surgery in acquired immunodeficiency syndrome: A statistical review of 904 patients. Surgery *105*:175-179, 1989.

96. Lau, S. K. P., Woo, P. C. Y., Chan, C. Y. F., et al.: Typhoid fever associated with acute appendicitis caused by an H1-j strain of *Salmonella enterica* serotype Typhi. J. Clin. Microbiol. *43*:1470-1472, 2005.

97. Lau, S. K. P., Woo, P. C. Y., Teng, J. L. L., et al.: Identification by 16S ribosomal RNA gene sequencing of *Arcobacter butzleri* bacteraemia in a patient with acute gangrenous appendicitis. J. Clin. Pathol. Mol. Pathol. *55*:182-185, 2002.

98. Lee, S. L., Walsh, A. J., and Ho, H. S.: Computed tomography and ultrasonography do not improve and may delay the diagnosis and treatment of acute appendicitis. Arch. Surg. *136*:556-562, 2001.

99. Leigh, D. A., Simmons, K., and Normal, E.: Bacterial flora of the appendix fossa in appendicitis and postoperative wound infection. J. Clin. Pathol. *27*:997-1000, 1974.

100. Lewis, F., Holcroft, J., Boey, J., et al.: Appendicitis in critical review of diagnosis and treatment in 1000 cases. Arch. Surg. *110*:677-684, 1975.

101. Lin, Y. L., and Lee, C. H.: Appendicitis in infancy. Pediatr. Surg. Int. *19*:1-3, 2003.

102. Lintula, H., Kokki, H., Vanamo, K., et al.: Laparoscopy in children with complicated appendicitis. J. Pediatr. Surg. *37*:1317-1320, 2002.

103. Longo, J. M., Bilbao, J. I., deVilla, V. H., et al.: CT-guided paracoccygeal drainage of pelvic abscesses. J. Comput. Assist. Tomogr. *17*:909-914, 1993.

104. Lopez-Navidad, A., Domingo, P., and Cada Falch, G.: Acute appendicitis complicating infectious mononucleosis: Case report and review. Rev. Infect. Dis. *12*:297-302, 1990.

105. Lowe, L. H., Penney, M. W., Stein, S. M., et al.: Unenhanced limited CT of the abdomen in the diagnosis of appendicitis in children: Comparison with sonography. A. J. R. Am. J. Roentgenol. *176*:31-35, 2001.

106. Luckmann, R.: Incidence and case fatality rates for acute appendicitis in California: A population-based study of the effects of age. Am. J. Epidemiol. *129*:905-918, 1989.

107. Luckmann, R., and Davis, P.: The epidemiology of acute appendicitis in California: Racial, gender, and seasonal variation. Epidemiology *2*:323-330, 1991.

108. Malde, H. M., and Chadha, D.: Roundworm obstruction: Sonographic diagnosis. Abdom. Imag. *18*:274-276, 1993.

109. Maltezou, H. C., Nikolaidis, P., Lebesii, E., et al.: Piperacillin/tazobactam versus cefotaxime plus metronidazole for treatment of children with intra-abdominal infections requiring surgery. Eur. J. Clin. Microbiol. Infect. Dis. *20*:643-646, 2001.

110. Martin, A. E., Vollman, D., Adler, B., et al.: CT scans may not reduce the negative appendectomy rate in children. J. Pediatr. Surg. *39*:886-890, 2004.

111. Mathis, R. D., Chiumento, A. B., Yeh, B., et al.: An outcome study of the use of computed tomography for the diagnosis of appendicitis in a community-based emergency department. South. Med. J. *98*:1169-1172, 2005.

112. Maxwell, J. M., and Ragland, J. J.: Appendicitis: Improvements in diagnosis and treatment. Am. Surg. *57*:282-285, 1991.

113. McAllister, T. A., Fyfe, A. H., Young, D. G., et al.: Cefotaxime lavage in children undergoing appendicectomy. Drugs *35*(Suppl. 2):127-132, 1988.

114. McBurney, C.: Experience with early operative interference in cases of disease of the vermiform appendix. N. Y. State Med. J. *50*:676, 1889.

115. McCahy, P.: Continuing fall in the incidence of acute appendicitis. Ann. R. Coll. Surg. Engl. *76*:282-283, 1994.

116. Meier, D. E., Guzzetta, P. C., Barber, R. G., et al.: Perforated appendicitis in children: Is there a best treatment? J. Pediatr. Surg. *38*:1520-1524, 2003.

117. Miron, D., Dashkovsky, I., Zuker, M., et al.: Primary *Streptococcus pneumoniae* appendicitis in a child: Case report and review. Pediatr. Infect. Dis. J. *22*:282-284, 2003.

118. Miron, D., Sochotnick, I., Yardeni, D., et al.: Surgical complications of shigellosis in children. Pediatr. Infect. Dis. J. *19*:898-900, 2000.

119. Moertel, C. G., Nobrega, F. T., Elveback, L. R., et al.: A prospective study of appendectomy and predisposition to cancer. Surg. Gynecol. Obstet. *138*:549-553, 1974.

120. Morrison, J. D.: *Yersinia* and viruses in acute non-specific abdominal pain and appendicitis. Br. J. Surg. *68*:284-286, 1981.

121. Mostafa, G., Matthews, B. D., Sing, R. F., et al.: Mini-laparoscopic versus laparoscopic approach to appendectomy. B. M. C. Surg. *1*:1-4, 2001.

122. Muehlstedt, S. G., Pham, T. Q., and Schmeling, D. J.: The management of pediatric appendicitis: A survey of North American pediatric surgeons. J. Pediatr. Surg. *39*:875-879, 2004.

123. Mueller, B. A., Daling, J. R., Moore, D. E., et al.: Appendectomy and the risk of tubal infertility. N. Engl. J. Med. *315*:1506-1508, 1986.

124. Mueller, G. P., and Williams, R. A.: Surgical infections in AIDS patients. Am. J. Surg. *169*(Suppl. 5A):34S-38S, 1995.

125. Mui, L. M., Ng, C. S. H., Wong, S. K. H., et al.: Optimum duration of prophylactic antibiotics in acute non-perforated appendicitis. Aust. N. Z. J. Surg. *75*:425-428, 2005.

126. Nadler, E. P., Reblock, K. K., Ford, H. R., et al.: Monotherapy versus multidrug therapy for the treatment of perforated appendicitis in children. Surg. Infect. *4*:327-333, 2003.

127. Namnyak, S. S., Martin, D. H., Ferguson, J. D. M., et al.: *Haemophilus segnis* appendicitis. J. Infect. *23*:339-341, 1991.

128. Natesha, R., Barnwell, S., Weaver, W., et al.: Is there evidence for a racial difference in the misdiagnosis in patients explored for appendicitis? J. Natl. Med. Assoc. *81*:269-271, 1989.

129. Neumayer, L. A., Makar, R., Ampel, N. M., et al.: Cytomegalovirus appendicitis in a patient with human immunodeficiency virus infection. Arch. Surg. *128*:467-468, 1993.

130. Nichol, P. F., Corliss, R. F., Rajpal, S., et al.: Perforation of the appendix from intestinal mucormycosis in a neonate. J. Pediatr. Surg. *39*:1133-1135, 2004.

131. Nielsen, M. B., and Torp-Pedersen, S.: Sonographically guided transrectal or transvaginal one-step catheter placement in deep pelvic and perirectal abscesses. A. J. R. Am. J. Roentgenol. *183*:1035-1036, 2004.

132. Nordentoft, T., Bringstrup, F. A., Bremmelgaard, A., et al.: Effect of laparoscopy on bacteremia in acute appendicitis: A randomized controlled study. Surg. Laparosc. Endosc. Percutan. Tech. *10*:302-304, 2000.

133. Nwomeh, B. C., Chisolm, D. J., Caniano, D. A., et al.: Racial and socioeconomic disparity in perforated appendicitis among children: Where is the problem? Pediatrics *117*:870-875, 2006.

134. Ochoa, B.: Surgical complications of ascariasis. World J. Surg. *15*:222-227, 1991.

135. Ohno, Y., Furui, J., and Kanematsu, T.: Treatment strategy when using intraoperative peritoneal lavage for perforated appendicitis in children: A preliminary report. Pediatr. Surg. Int. *20*:534-537, 2004.

136. Okamoto, T., Sano, K., and Ogasahara, K.: Receiver-operating characteristic analysis of leukocyte counts and serum C-reactive protein levels in children with advanced appendicitis. Surg. Today *36*:515-518, 2006.

137. Paik, S.-Y., Oh, J.-T., Choi, Y.-J., et al.: Measles-related appendicitis. Arch. Pathol. Lab. Med. *126*:82-84, 2002.

138. Park, J.: *Escherichia coli* septicemia associated with acute appendicitis. South. Med. J. *84*:667-668, 1991.

139. Pearlman, M., Frantz, A. C., Floyd, W. S., et al.: Abdominal wall *Actinomyces* abscess associated with an intrauterine device. J. Reprod. Med. *36*:398-402, 1991.

140. Peltola, H., Ahlqvist, J., Rapola, J., et al.: C-reactive protein compared with white blood cell count and erythrocyte sedimentation rate in the diagnosis of acute appendicitis in children. Acta Chir. Scand. *152*:55-58, 1986.

141. Pena, B. M. G., Taylor, G. A., Lund, D. P., et al.: Effect of computed tomography on patient management and costs in children with suspected appendicitis. Pediatrics *104*:440-446, 1999.

142. Peng, Y.-S., Lee, H.-C., Yeung, C.-Y., et al.: Clinical criteria for diagnosing perforated appendix in pediatric patients. Pediatr. Emerg. Care *22*:475-479, 2006.

143. Phillips, S., Walton, J. M., Chin, I., et al.: Ten-year experience with pediatric laparoscopic appendectomy—are we getting better? J. Pediatr. Surg. *40*:842-845, 2005.

144. Pisacane, A., de Luca, U., Impagliazzo, N., et al.: Breast feeding and acute appendicitis. B. M. J. *310*:836-837, 1995.

145. Ponsky, T. A., Huang, Z. J., Kittle, K., et al.: Hospital- and patient-level characteristics and the risk of appendiceal rupture and negative appendectomy in children. J. A. M. A. *292*:1977-1982, 2004.

146. Quillin, S. P., Siegel, M. J., and Coffin, C. M.: Acute appendicitis in children: Value of sonography in detecting perforation. A. J. R. Am. J. Roentgenol. *159*:1265-1268, 1992.

147. Rabenandrasana, H. A., Ahmad, A., Samison, L. H., et al.: Child primary tubercular appendicitis. Pediatr. Int. *46*:374-376, 2004.

148. Raffensperger, J.: *Eikenella corrodens* infections in children. J. Pediatr. Surg. *21*:644-646, 1986.

149. Raffi, F., David, A., Mouzard, A., et al.: *Pasteurella multocida* appendiceal peritonitis: Report of three cases and review of the literature. Pediatr. Infect. Dis. *5*:695-698, 1986.

150. Ramsden, K., and Freeth, M.: Cryptosporidial infection presenting as an acute appendicitis. Histopathology *14*:209-211, 1989.

151. Rasmussen, O., and Hoffmann, J.: Assessment of the reliability of the symptoms and signs of acute appendicitis. J. R. Coll. Surg. Edinb. *36*:372-377, 1991.

152. Rautio, M., Lonnroth, M., Saxen, H., et al.: Characteristics of an unusual anaerobic pigmented gram-negative rod isolated from normal and inflamed appendices. Clin. Infect. Dis. *25*(Suppl. 2):S107-S110, 1997.

153. Rautio, M., Saxen, H., Siitonen, A., et al.: Bacteriology of histopathologically defined appendicitis in children. Pediatr. Infect. Dis. J. *19*:1078-1083, 2000.

154. Reid, R. I., Dobbs, B. R., and Frizelle, F. A.: Risk factors for post-appendicectomy intra-abdominal abscess. Aust. N. Z. J. Surg. *69*:373-374, 1999.

155. Reif, R. M.: Viral appendicitis. Hum. Pathol. *12*:193-196, 1981.

156. Reynolds, S. L., and Jaffe, D. M.: Diagnosing abdominal pain in a pediatric emergency department. Pediatr. Emerg. Care *8*:126-128, 1992.

157. Rice, H. E., Brown, R. L., Gollin, G., et al.: Results of a pilot trial comparing prolonged intravenous antibiotics with sequential intravenous/oral antibiotics for children with perforated appendicitis. Arch. Surg. *136*:1391-1395, 2001.

158. Robertson, F. M., Olsen, S. B., Jackson, M. R., et al.: Inguinal-scrotal suppuration following treatment of perforated appendicitis. J. Pediatr. Surg. *28*:267-268, 1993.

159. Rodriguez-Sanjuan, J. C., Martin-Parra, J. I., Seco, I., et al.: C-reactive protein and leukocyte count in the diagnosis of acute appendicitis in children. Dis. Colon Rectum *42*:1325-1329, 1999.

160. Rothrock, S. G., Skeoch, G., Rush, J. J., et al.: Clinical features of misdiagnosed appendicitis in children. Ann. Emerg. Med. *20*:45-50, 1991.

161. Ruff, M. E., Friedland, I. R., and Hickey, S. M.: *Escherichia coli* septicemia in nonperforated appendicitis. Arch. Pediatr. Adolesc. Med. *148*:853-855, 1994.

162. Sabbe, L. J. M., Van De Merwe, D., Schouls, L., et al.: Clinical spectrum of infections due to the newly described *Actinomyces* species *A. turicensis*, *A. radingae*, and *A. europaeus*. J. Clin. Microbiol. *37*:8-13, 1999.

163. Sah, S. P., and Bhadani, P. P.: *Enterobius vermicularis* causing symptoms of appendicitis in Nepal. Trop. Doctor *36*:160-162, 2006.

164. Sakellaris, G., Tilemis, S., and Charissis, G.: Acute appendicitis in preschool-age children. Eur. J. Pediatr. *164*:80-83, 2005.

165. Sartorelli, A. C., da Silva, M. G., Rodrigues, M. A. M., et al.: Appendiceal taeniasis presenting like acute appendicitis. Parasitol. Res. *97*:171-172, 2005.

166. Sauer, C., and Gutgesell, M.: Ballet dancer with hip and groin pain: Crohn disease and psoas abscess. Clin. Pediatr. *44*:731-733, 2005.

167. Saxen, H., Tarkka, E., Hannikainen, P., et al.: *Escherichia coli* and appendicitis: Phenotypic characteristics of *E. coli* isolates from inflamed and noninflamed appendices. Clin. Infect. Dis. *23*:1038-1042, 1996.

168. Scharschmidt, T. J., Weiner, S. D., and Myers, J. P.: Bacterial pyomyositis. Curr. Infect. Dis. Rep. *6*:393-396, 2004.

169. Schmidt, P., Koltai, J. L., and Weltzien, A.: Actinomycosis of the appendix in childhood. Pediatr. Surg. Int. *15*:63-65, 1999.

170. Schropp, K. P., Kaplan, S., Golladay, E. S., et al.: A randomized clinical trial of ampicillin, gentamicin and clindamycin versus cefotaxime and clindamycin in children with ruptured appendicitis. Surgery *172*:351-356, 1991.

171. Schweitzer, J., Fairman, N., Schreyer, K., et al.: Appendicitis, 2002: Relationship between payors and outcome. Am. Surgeon *69*:902-908, 2003.

172. Scott, B. D., and Schmidt, J. H.: Pneumococcal meningitis due to psoas abscess. South. Med. J. *82*:1310-1311, 1989.

173. Sehdev, A. E. S., Sehdev, P. S., Jacobs, R., et al.: Human monocytic ehrlichiosis presenting as acute appendicitis during pregnancy. Clin. Infect. Dis. *35*: E99-E102, 2002.

174. Silen, M. L., and Tracy, T. F.: The right lower quadrant "revisited." Pediatr. Clin. North Am. *40*:1201-1211, 1993.

175. Simpson, J., and Speake, W.: Appendicitis. Clin. Evid. *14*:529-535, 2005.

176. Sirinek, K. R., and Levine, B. A.: Antimicrobial management of surgically treated gangrenous or perforated appendicitis: Comparison of cefoxitin and clindamycin-gentamicin. Clin. Ther. *9*:420-428, 1987.

177. Sirinek, K. R., and Levine, B. A.: A randomized trial of ticarcillin and clavulanate versus gentamicin and clindamycin in patients with complicated appendicitis. Surg. Gynecol. Obstet. *172*:30-35, 1991.

178. Smink, D. S., Finkelstein, J. A., Kleinman, K., et al.: The effect of hospital volume of pediatric appendectomies on the misdiagnosis of appendicitis in children. Pediatrics *113*:18-23, 2004.

179. Smink, D. S., Fishman, S. J., Kleinman, K., et al.: Effects of race, insurance status, and hospital volume on perforated appendicitis in children. Pediatrics *115*:920-925, 2005.
180. Snelling, C. M. H., Poenaru, D., and Drover, J. W.: Minimum postoperative antibiotic duration in advanced appendicitis in children: A review. Pediatr. Surg. Int. *20*:838-845, 2004.
181. Snook, M. E., and LiPuma, J. J.: Pelvic muscle abscess: An unusual cause of gait disturbance in young children. Clin. Pediatr. *32*:298-299, 1993.
182. Soffer, D., Zait, S., Klausner, J., et al.: Peritoneal cultures and antibiotic treatment in patients with perforated appendicitis. Eur. J. Surg. *167*:214-216, 2001.
183. Song, K. S., and Lee, S. M.: Periplevic infections mimicking septic arthritis of the hip in children: Treatment with needle aspiration. J. Pediatr. Orthop. B. *21*:354-356, 2003.
184. Souid, A. K., Sadowitz, P. D., Weiner, L., et al.: Obturator internus muscle abscess: A case report and review of the literature. Am. J. Dis. Child. *147*:1278-1279, 1993.
185. Stovroff, M. C., Totten, M., and Glick, P. L.: PIC lines save money and hasten discharge in the care of children with ruptured appendicitis. J. Pediatr. Surg. *29*:245-247, 1994.
186. St. Peter, S. D., Little, D. C., Calkins, C. M., et al.: A simple and more cost-effective antibiotic regimen for perforated appendicitis. J. Pediatr. Surg. *41*:1020-1024, 2006.
187. Street, J., Lenehan, B., Mulcahy, D., et al.: Pelvic girdle sepsis in childhood an illustrative case of the difficulty in diagnosis. Acta Orthop. Belg. *71*:361-365, 2005.
188. Tander, B., Pektas, O., and Bulut, M.: The utility of peritoneal drains in children with uncomplicated perforated appendicitis. Pediatr. Surg. Int. *19*:548-550, 2003.
189. Tanomkiat, W., and Buranapanitkit, B.: Percutaneous drainage of large tuberculous iliopsoas abscess via a subinguinal approach: A report of two cases. J. Orthop. Sci. *9*:157-161, 2004.
190. Taylor, E., Berjis, A., Bosch, T., et al.: The efficacy of postoperative oral antibiotics in appendicitis: A randomized prospective double-blinded study. Am. Surgeon *70*:858-862, 2004.
191. Taylor, M., Emil, S., Nguyen, N., et al.: Emergent vs urgent appendectomy in children: A study of outcomes. J. Pediatr. Surg. *40*:1912-1915, 2005.
192. Teppler, H., Meibohm, A. R., and Woods, G. L.: Management of complicated appendicitis and comparison of outcome with other primary sites of intra-abdominal infection: Results of a trial comparing ertapenem and piperacillin-tazobactam. J. Chemother. *16*:62-69, 2004.
193. ter Borg, P., Kuijper, E. J., and van der Lelie, H.: Fatal mucormycosis presenting as an appendiceal mass with metastatic spread to the liver during chemotherapy-induced granulocytopenia. Scand. J. Infect. Dis. *22*:499-501, 1990.
194. Terry, N. E., and Fowler, C. L.: Cytomegalovirus enterocolitis complicated by perforated appendicitis in a premature infant. J. Pediatr. Surg. *41*:1476-1478, 2006.
195. Thadepalli, H., Mandal, A. K., Chuah, S. K., et al.: Bacteriology of the appendix and the ileum in health and in appendicitis. Am. Surg. *57*:317-322, 1991.
196. Tobe, I.: Inapparent virus infection as a trigger of appendicitis. Lancet *1*:1343-1346, 1965.
197. Tsang, T. M., Tam, P. K. H., and Saing, H.: Antibiotic prophylaxis in acute non-perforated appendicitis in children: Single dose of metronidazole and gentamicin. J. R. Coll. Surg. Edinb. *37*:110-112, 1992.
198. Tufariello, J. M., Kaleya, R. N., and Klein, R. S.: Group A streptococcal appendicitis in a patient with AIDS. Diagn. Microbiol. Infect. Dis. *38*:171-172, 2000.
199. Uchimura, M., Tsuruoka, Y., Hukuda, T., et al.: Isolation of vero toxin-producing *Escherichia coli* (enterohemorrhagic *E. coli*) 0111:H– from 2 cases diagnosed as appendicitis. Kansenshogaku Zasshi *65*:905-908, 1991.
200. Uhari, M., Seppanen, J., and Heikkinen, E.: Imipenem-cilastatin vs. tobramycin and metronidazole for appendicitis-related infections. Pediatr. Infect. Dis. J. *11*:445-450, 1992.
201. Urban, E., Hortobagyi, A., Szentpali, K., et al.: Two intriguing *Bilophila wadsworthia* cases from Hungary. J. Med. Microbiol. *53*:1167-1169, 2004.
202. Urizar, R. E., Lepow, M., Neumann, M., et al.: Fungal peritonitis with splenic-pelvic abscess in a patient on continuous ambulatory peritoneal dialysis. Perit. Dial. Int. *13*:162-163, 1993.
203. Van Noyen, R., Selderslaghs, R., Bekaert, J., et al.: Causative role of *Yersinia* and other enteric pathogens in the appendicular syndrome. Eur. J. Clin. Microbiol. Infect. Dis. *10*:735-741, 1991.
204. Visvanathan, K., Jones, P. D., and Truskett, P.: Abdominal mycobacterial infection mimicking acute appendicitis in an AIDS patient. Aust. N. Z. J. Surg. *63*:558-560, 1993.
205. Volinsky, J. B., Karrer, F. M., and Todd, J. K.: Hemolytic-uremic syndrome caused by *Escherichia coli* 0157:H7 after perforated appendix. Pediatr. Infect. Dis. J. *17*:846-847, 1998.
206. Walsh, T. R., Reilly, J. R., Hanley, E., et al.: Changing etiology of iliopsoas abscess. Am. J. Surg. *163*:413-416, 1992.
207. Weber, T. R., Keller, M. A., Bower, R. J., et al.: Is delayed operative treatment worth the trouble with perforated appendicitis is children? Am. J. Surg. *186*:685-689, 2003.
208. Wehner, J. H., De Bruyne, K., Kagawa, F. T., et al.: Pulmonary tuberculosis, amenorrhea, and a pelvic mass. West. J. Med. *161*:515-518, 1994.
209. Wiesenfeld, H. C., Berg, S. R., and Sweet, R. L.: *Torulopsis glabrata* pelvic abscess and fungemia. Obstet. Gynecol. *83*:887-889, 1994.
210. Williams, N., and Kapila, L.: Acute appendicitis in the preschool child. Arch. Dis. Child. *66*:1270-1272, 1991.
211. Williams, N., and Kapila, L.: Acute appendicitis in the under 5-year-old. J. R. Coll. Surg. Edinb. *39*:168-170, 1994.
212. Wilson, S. E.: Results of a randomized, multicenter trial of meropenem versus clindamycin/tobramycin for the treatment of intra-abdominal infections. Clin. Infect. Dis. *24*(Suppl. 2):S197-S206, 1997.
213. Woo, P. C. Y., Lau, S. K. P., Woo, G. K. S., et al.: Bacteremia due to *Clostridium hathewayi* in a patient with acute appendicitis. J. Clin. Microbiol. *42*:5947-5949, 2004.
214. Yardeni, D., Hirschl, R. B., Drongowski, R. A., et al.: Delayed versus immediate surgery in acute appendicitis: Do we need to operate during the night? J. Pediatr. Surg. *39*:464-469, 2004.
215. Yassin, A. F., Steiner, U., and Ludwig, W.: *Corynebacterium appendicis* sp. nov. Int. J. Syst. Evol. Microbiol. *52*:1165-1169, 2002.
216. Yasumoto, R., Kawano, M., Kawanishi, H., et al.: Left acute scrotum associated with appendicitis. Int. J. Urol. *5*:108-110, 1998.
217. Yildirim, S., Nursal, T. Z., Tarim, A., et al.: A rare cause of acute appendicitis: Parasitic infection. Scand. J. Infect. Dis. *37*:757-759, 2005.
218. York, D., Smith, A., Phillips, J. D., et al.: The influence of advanced radiographic imaging on the treatment of pediatric appendicitis. J. Pediatr. Surg. *40*:1908-1911, 2005.

PANCREATITIS

Thomas L. Kuhls

Pancreatitis previously was thought to be an uncommon cause of abdominal pain in children and a disease primarily of adults. Because of better recognition of symptoms in children and the more frequent use of medications that cause pancreatic inflammation, acute pancreatitis currently is being diagnosed more frequently in institutions specializing in pediatric care.[90,169]

Compared with causes of acute pancreatitis in adults—primarily alcoholism, cholelithiasis, and trauma—causes of childhood pancreatitis are more diverse. Microorganisms account for a significant proportion of cases of pancreatitis in children. In addition, antimicrobial agents have been associated with severe and occasionally fatal episodes of pancreatitis, and bacterial infections may complicate the natural history of acute and chronic pancreatitis. Pediatricians who care for children with pancreatitis must

have expertise in the diagnosis and treatment of infectious diseases.

CLINICAL MANIFESTATIONS

More than 80 percent of children with acute pancreatitis complain of abdominal pain.[16,169] Only 30 percent of pediatric patients have epigastric pain as usually described by adults, however.[165] In children, other sites of focal tenderness or diffuse pain include the right upper quadrant of the abdomen, the periumbilical area, the entire abdomen, and, less commonly, the right lower quadrant of the abdomen. The onset of pain usually is rapid and increases to a maximal intensity in a few hours, but occasionally the onset may be slow and gradual. Most often, the pain is sharp and excruciating in nature. Only one third of children complain of pain that radiates to other areas, including the back, lower part of the abdomen, upper abdominal quadrants, and anterior chest wall. In school-aged children, the pain often intensifies after meals.

Two thirds of children with acute pancreatitis have vomiting.[16] Children younger than 5 years old occasionally experience vomiting without abdominal tenderness.[176] Fever is present in only 30 percent of children with pancreatitis, but temperatures greater than 38.5° C are observed occasionally.[165]

On physical examination, children classically are found lying quietly on their sides with their knees flexed. They usually have epigastric tenderness to palpation and decreased or absent bowel sounds. Abdominal distention is found in 30 percent of children with pancreatitis and occurs more commonly in preschool-aged children.[165,176] Occasionally, rebound tenderness, guarding of the epigastrium, jaundice, an abdominal mass, or ascites is detected. Rarely, ecchymoses of the flanks (Turner sign) or the umbilical area (Cullen sign) can be identified, but usually only when life-threatening hemorrhagic pancreatitis is present. In severe pancreatitis, children may present with evidence of shock and multiorgan failure.

Chronic pancreatitis occurs when irreversible damage in the pancreatic architecture causes abnormalities in the function of the pancreas.[91] Children with chronic pancreatitis often have lengthy or recurrent bouts of abdominal pain and vomiting.

LABORATORY DIAGNOSIS

The most common useful laboratory test for the clinical diagnosis of pancreatitis in children is measurement of serum amylase, but the level correlates poorly with the severity of the disease.[58] In most studies of childhood pancreatitis, the diagnosis is confirmed when the serum amylase is greater than three times the normal level for the particular laboratory completing the test. The serum concentration increases quickly within hours after symptoms develop. High serum amylase concentrations can be observed, however, in numerous other illnesses, including acute cholecystitis, intestinal obstruction, perforated abdominal organs, appendicitis, salpingitis, ruptured ectopic pregnancy, and salivary gland disease. The serum amylase concentration can return to normal in 24 to 72 hours after the onset of symptoms, and the diagnosis of pancreatitis can be missed. In this situation, the urine amylase concentration can remain elevated for at least 1 week.

Serum amylase concentrations occasionally are not elevated during the course of pancreatitis in children.[133] In a series of children with pancreatitis, 83 percent of patients had elevated serum amylase levels.[169] In addition, marked hyperlipidemia may interfere with the laboratory measurement of amylase.[17] Serum lipase is useful in these situations; high serum concentrations often are not detected until 24 hours after the beginning of the illness. Because lipase is produced only in the pancreas and intestinal cells, measurement of the serum concentration helps distinguish children with high serum amylase concentrations of pancreatic as opposed to salivary origin. Measurement of serum trypsinogen may be the most sensitive and specific way of detecting acute pancreatitis, but it is unavailable in most clinical laboratories.[165]

Laboratory findings in children with severe acute pancreatitis may include leukocytosis with increased immature polymorphonuclear leukocytes, an elevated erythrocyte sedimentation rate, and elevated C-reactive protein level. In children with fulminate hemorrhagic pancreatitis, anemia develops quickly. Other associated findings include hyperglycemia, hypertriglyceridemia, hypoalbuminemia, and hypocalcemia. A new scoring system for children with pancreatitis has shown that severe pancreatitis is more likely when the child who presents is younger than 7 years of age, weighs less than 23 kg, has a total white blood cell count greater than 18,500 cells/mm³, has an admission lactate dehydrogenase greater than 2000 U/L, has a 48-hour calcium level less than 8.3 mg/dL, has a 48-hour albumin level less than 2.6 g/dL, has a 48-hour fluid sequestration greater than 75 mL/kg/48 hr, or has a 48-hour increase in blood urea nitrogen greater than 5 mg/dL.[32] Elevated transaminases and alkaline phosphatase generally are observed only when the episode of pancreatitis is caused by biliary obstruction, such as in gallstone-related disease.

The radiographic features of childhood pancreatitis also are nonspecific. Radiographs of the abdomen may show localized ileus of the jejunum in the midepigastric or left upper quadrant region adjacent to the pancreas (sentinel loop), a distended transverse colon without visualization of the descending colon because of adjacent pancreatic inflammation (colon cutoff sign), duodenal distention with air-fluid levels, or loss of the left psoas shadow.[63] Occasionally, chest radiography reveals an elevated left hemidiaphragm or pleural effusion.

In recent years, the ability to diagnose pancreatitis in children has been improved greatly by ultrasonography.[169] The echodensity of the pancreas normally is equal to or greater than that of the left lobe of the liver. During acute pancreatitis, edema causes the gland to enlarge and become less dense than the liver. These two findings can aid in establishing the diagnosis of pancreatitis, and complications such as abscesses and pseudocysts can be identified. Also, ultrasonography may delineate dilations of the pancreatic ducts caused by obstruction or ductal stones. Visualization of the pancreas by ultrasonography may be obscured because of overlying bowel gas. In such cases, computed tomography (CT) is useful to detect pancreatic size and density.

CT of the pancreas should be performed in complicated cases of pancreatitis after a few days of treatment to determine the severity of disease and extent of pancreatic necrosis. It is especially useful when surgery is being considered for drainage of abscesses and pseudocysts.

Endoscopic retrograde cholangiopancreatography (ERCP) is being used increasingly in children with pancreatitis to exclude or treat gallstones, pseudocysts, strictures, or *Ascaris* infection.[126,131] In recent years, magnetic resonance cholangiopancreatography has been used as a noninvasive technique for evaluating children with chronic pancreatitis.[11,99]

NONINFECTIOUS ETIOLOGIES

An etiology for pancreatitis in children can be determined now in more than 90 percent of cases if diagnostic evaluation is thorough, especially in children younger than 6 years of age.[90,176] The frequency of each specific cause depends on the patient population of the particular medical center. At Children's Hospital of Michigan, 33 percent of children with pancreatitis have biliary tract–related disease because of the large patient population with sickle-cell anemia.[176] At Yale–New Haven Hospital, drug-related pancreatitis accounts for 30 percent of the total cases of childhood pancreatitis because of the frequent use of immunosuppressive and cancer chemotherapeutic agents in this hospital.[63] Table 58–1 outlines the most common noninfectious causes of pancreatitis in children.

TRAUMA

In many older series of patients, trauma is the leading cause of acute pancreatitis in children. Because the highly vascular pancreas is immobilized by the stomach, duodenum, and vertebrae, it is susceptible to blunt and penetrating trauma. The less developed abdominal wall musculature in pediatric patients may

TABLE 58–1 Noninfectious Causes of Childhood Pancreatitis

Trauma
Blunt
Brain injury
Penetrating
Postoperative

Drugs
Antimicrobials—pentamidine, antimonials, sulfonamides,
 tetracycline, macrolides, metronidazole, dapsone, nitrofurantoin,
 isoniazid, ceftriaxone, gatifloxacin, nucleoside analogue reverse
 transcriptase inhibitors, interferon-α, liposomal amphotericin B
Atypical antipsychotics
Diuretics—thiazides, furosemide
Ethyl alcohol
Growth hormone
Immunosuppressives—azathioprine, steroids, asparaginase,
 mercaptopurine, tacrolimus
Metformin
Nonsteroidal anti-inflammatory drugs
Propofol
Proton pump inhibitors
Statins
Sulfasalazine
Valproic acid

Obstructive Diseases
Anatomic abnormalities
Cholelithiasis

Genetic and Metabolic Diseases
Aminoacidurias
Cystic fibrosis
Diabetes mellitus
Glycogen storage disease type I
Hyperlipoproteinemia types I, IV, V
Hyperparathyroidism
Recurrent hereditary pancreatitis

Vasculitic and Autoimmune Diseases
Crohn disease
Henoch-Schönlein purpura
Kawasaki syndrome
Systemic lupus erythematosus

Miscellaneous
Anticholinesterase insecticide intoxication
Chronic fibrosing pancreatitis
Lymphoma
Orthotopic liver transplantation
Reye syndrome
Scorpion stings
Tropical chronic pancreatitis

enhance their susceptibility to pancreatic injury after episodes of blunt trauma. Child abuse has been recognized increasingly as a cause of trauma-related pancreatitis. Postoperative pancreatitis occurs most commonly after abdominal or cardiac surgery.[43] Pancreatitis also may be associated with traumatic brain injury in children.[159]

MEDICATIONS

Medications used in pediatric practice increasingly are causing episodes of pancreatitis in children. In most recent pediatric studies, the anticonvulsant valproic acid is the most common medication associated with the development of pancreatitis.[169] The risk of developing pancreatitis does not depend on the serum level of valproic acid, and it is not related to the length of therapy.[142,168] Azathioprine, steroids, mercaptopurine, and aspar-

aginase have been associated with cases of childhood pancreatitis, and other immunosuppressive agents most likely play a role in post-transplantation pancreatitis.[80,135,143,167,171] Acute pancreatitis has been associated rarely with the use of diuretics, including hydrochlorothiazide and furosemide[96]; growth hormone[33,97]; sulfasalazine[49]; atypical antipsychotics[56,82]; statins[73]; propofol[20]; nonsteroidal anti-inflammatory agents, including ibuprofen[92,93]; metformin[46]; and proton pump inhibitors.[174] Alcohol consumption is an uncommon cause of pancreatitis in younger children; however, it can cause illness occasionally in adolescents.

Physicians with expertise in the management of infectious diseases are becoming more aware of drug-induced pancreatitis because many antimicrobial agents can cause pancreatic inflammation. Pentamidine isethionate is used in the treatment of *Pneumocystis carinii* pneumonia, African trypanosomiasis, and leishmaniasis. It may cause hypoglycemia because of toxicity to pancreatic islet cells and is associated with severe and occasionally fatal episodes of pancreatitis.[104,177] In children and adults, aerosolized pentamidine prophylaxis for *P. carinii* pneumonia also has been associated with severe cases of pancreatitis in patients with acquired immunodeficiency syndrome (AIDS).[59,104] Similarly, pentavalent antimonials, such as sodium stibogluconate and meglumine antimonate, used for the treatment of visceral leishmaniasis can induce pancreatic inflammation.[86,173]

Sulfonamides, including trimethoprim-sulfamethoxazole, have been implicated occasionally as a cause of acute pancreatitis in adults.[6,162] Symptoms have recurred when patients have been re-exposed to the medication. The abdominal pain often is accompanied by a hypersensitivity-type rash. Tetracycline-induced pancreatitis has been described in children with and without overt liver disease.[42,154] In addition, clarithromycin,[51,136] erythromycin,[149] rifampin,[125] roxithromycin,[129] dapsone,[31] nitrofurantoin,[112] isoniazid,[71] and metronidazole[116] have been added to the list of agents that can cause pancreatitis in previously healthy individuals when given in routine doses or when high amounts are consumed. Although uncommonly used in children, quinolone antibiotics, such as gatifloxacin, have been associated with hepatotoxicity and acute pancreatitis.[29] An adolescent who was receiving ceftriaxone also developed pancreatitis secondary to obstruction of the biliary tract from gallstones.[100]

Pancreatitis has been a major dose-limiting toxic effect of the human immunodeficiency virus (HIV)–inhibiting nucleoside analogue reverse transcriptase inhibitor class of medications, especially dideoxyinosine, in adult and pediatric patients.[21,22] Most episodes of pancreatitis occur when the dose is 360 mg/m²/day or more, and usually the pancreatic inflammation resolves when the medication is discontinued. Concomitant administration of pentamidine or another nucleoside analogue reverse transcriptase inhibitor, such as ribavirin, used in the treatment of hepatitis C infection with dideoxyinosine may increase the risk of developing pancreatitis.[108] In pediatric patients with AIDS, serum amylase concentrations often are elevated in patients without pancreatic symptoms, whereas children with pancreatitis can have normal serum amylase concentrations. The serum lipase concentration is useful in evaluating HIV-infected children for possible pancreatic inflammation.[22,104] Increased liver transaminase or lipase concentrations before the administration of dideoxyinosine may be helpful in predicting the children in whom pancreatitis would develop.[22] In all children with symptoms consistent with pancreatitis, dideoxyinosine should be withheld pending the results of a lipase assay, and it should be discontinued if the concentration is elevated. Similarly, dideoxyinosine should be discontinued for 1 week after treatment with pentamidine for *P. carinii* pneumonia.[47]

Interferon-α, which is used in the treatment of chronic hepatitis and malignancies, also has been associated with the development of pancreatitis.[26] Liposomal amphotericin B treatment rarely causes pancreatic toxicity.[147]

OBSTRUCTIVE DISEASES

Obstruction of the common bile duct, pancreatic duct, or sphincter of Oddi may cause pancreatitis.[7] Gallstones or congenital anatomic malformations, including an annular pancreas, pancreas divisum, choledochal cysts, and intrapancreatic duplication cysts, can cause pancreatitis by obstructing normal pancreatic flow. Pancreatitis observed in children with sickle-cell anemia may be caused by obstruction from stones, biliary sludge, or pancreatic microvascular occlusion and ischemia during crises.[3]

GENETIC AND METABOLIC DISEASES

Metabolic diseases often are associated with chronic recurrent episodes of pancreatitis. Such diseases include hyperlipoproteinemias, cystic fibrosis, diabetes mellitus, hyperparathyroidism, aminoacidurias, and glycogen storage disease type I.[54,63,75,160] Recurrent hereditary pancreatitis usually occurs in an autosomal dominant pattern, with onset occurring between infancy and adolescence.[76] It has been linked to chromosome 7q35. The mutation allows trypsinogen to become activated to trypsin within the pancreas. Other children and adults with chronic pancreatitis have been shown to have mutations in the cystic fibrosis transmembrane regulator (CFTR) gene similar to individuals with cystic fibrosis,[26] or to have a mutation causing a deficiency of trypsin-specific inhibitor that inactivates low levels of trypsin within acinar cells.[76]

VASCULITIC AND AUTOIMMUNE DISEASES

Pancreatitis also can occur in syndromes in which vasculitis is a major component of the disease process. It has been associated with common pediatric disorders, including Kawasaki syndrome, Henoch-Schönlein purpura, and systemic lupus erythematosus.[28,124,128,146] Increasing data suggest that numerous children with idiopathic chronic pancreatitis may have inflammation from an autoimmune process.[110] Pancreatitis has been a presenting manifestation of Crohn disease.[84]

MISCELLANEOUS CAUSES

Although no longer common, Reye syndrome has been associated with acute pancreatitis.[50] The venom of the scorpions *Tityus trinitatus*, *Tityus asthenes*, and *Leiurus quinquestriatus* can cause pancreatitis in patients who have been stung; however, these species do not live naturally in the United States.[15,121,144] The gastrointestinal symptoms observed in children with anticholinesterase insecticide poisoning may be caused by pancreatitis.[166] Also, tropical chronic pancreatitis seen in developing countries most likely is related to malnutrition and dietary intake of toxins, such as those from the tuber cassava.[14] Rarely, primary pancreatic lymphoma may manifest in children as acute pancreatitis.[41] Chronic fibrosing pancreatitis in which the pathogenesis of the disease process remains unsolved occurs only rarely in the United States.[57]

Although a much less common occurrence than in adults, acute pancreatitis after orthotopic liver transplantation is severe in children and often results in death.[152,153] The cause of pancreatitis in liver transplant recipients most likely is multifactorial but probably involves traumatic injury, biliary obstruction, and immunosuppressive therapy.

INFECTIOUS ETIOLOGIES

Infections caused by various microorganisms have been shown by culture, histologic examination, or elevation of antibody titer during the course of acute pancreatitis in humans (Table 58–2). A true causal relationship usually is not shown, however. Although not all of the following infectious agents have been shown to be associated with childhood pancreatitis, they must be considered as possible etiologic agents because adults with infectious pancreatitis have been described. Compared with previous decades, infectious agents are being encountered less as a cause of acute pancreatitis, most likely because of mumps vaccination.

VIRAL INFECTIONS

Group B coxsackieviruses and mumps virus are the best documented causes of pancreatitis in children. Group B coxsackieviruses usually cause pancreatitis along with other clinical manifestations, including aseptic meningitis, mild diarrhea, rash, and myocarditis.[23,67] They rarely have caused death in young

TABLE 58–2 Microorganisms Associated with Episodes of Acute Pancreatitis

Viruses
Adenoviruses
Cytomegalovirus
Epstein-Barr virus
Group B coxsackieviruses
Hepatitis A virus
Hepatitis B virus
Hepatitis E virus
Herpes simplex viruses
Human immunodeficiency virus
Measles virus
Mumps virus
Parainfluenza viruses
Rotavirus
Rubella virus
Varicella-zoster virus

Parasites
Ascaris lumbricoides
Clonorchis sinensis
Cryptosporidium parvum
Echinococcus granulosus
Fasciola hepatica
Plasmodium falciparum
Taenia saginata
Toxoplasma gondii
Wuchereria bancrofti

Mycoplasmas and Bacteria
Brucella melitensis
Campylobacter jejuni
Escherichia coli
Legionella spp.
Leptospira spp.
Moraxella catarrhalis
Mycobacterium tuberculosis
Mycoplasma pneumoniae
Salmonella spp.
Yersinia spp.

Fungi
Aspergillus spp.
Candida spp.
Cryptococcus neoformans

infants with myocarditis and pancreatitis.[36] How commonly these enteroviruses cause pancreatic inflammation is unknown. In one epidemiologic study, 31 percent of patients with aseptic meningitis during an epidemic of group B coxsackievirus infection had increased serum amylase concentrations.[111] Numerous studies have shown coxsackievirus-induced damage to pancreatic acinar cells in mouse models of infection.[65] Coxsackievirus B strains have been isolated from pancreatic biopsy samples of patients with chronic pancreatitis.[140]

Usually, mumps pancreatitis occurs in the presence of parotitis; however, abdominal pain and vomiting may occur for days before salivary swelling develops.[164] Rarely, mumps virus can cause pancreatitis without other common clinical manifestations.[109] Because more than 80 percent of children with mumps parotitis have elevated serum amylase concentrations, ultrasonography and serum lipase concentrations should be obtained to aid in establishing the diagnosis of pancreatitis.[55] An estimated 15 percent of children with mumps virus infection have abdominal tenderness and vomiting suggestive of pancreatitis.[63] In only a single report has the pancreatitis been hemorrhagic and severe.[44] Occasionally, chronic or recurring pancreatitis develops after mumps infection.[172]

Researchers previously thought that acute pancreatitis occurred in cases of viral hepatitis only when fulminate liver disease developed. Increasingly, children with mild hepatitis A infection and pancreatitis are being described, however.[2,105] In addition, a 16-year-old patient with acute hepatitis A infection died as a result of severe pancreatitis with multiorgan failure.[79] Individuals with acute hepatitis and pancreatitis also have been found to have hepatitis E viral infection.[69,105] Hepatitis B viral antigens have been detected in the pancreatic glandular cells of patients with severe acute hemorrhagic pancreatitis.[138] The role of hepatitis B virus in the pathogenesis of pancreatic inflammation in these patients is unknown; however, a young adult developed three episodes of acute pancreatitis during acute exacerbations of chronic hepatitis B infection that resolved after lamivudine therapy was given.[27]

Human herpesviruses are uncommon causes of childhood pancreatitis in immunocompetent patients. Occasionally, pancreatitis develops in children and adolescents with infectious mononucleosis.[83,107] Acute pancreatitis and occasionally pseudocyst formation also have been reported in previously healthy individuals with varicella infection.[95,155] In addition, adults have developed pancreatitis during a period in which seroconversion to cytomegalovirus was documented, or when antigens were identified in biopsy specimens obtained during ERCP.[78,119]

Viral pancreatitis also occurs in immunocompromised patients. Cytomegalovirus has been identified in pancreatic specimens from autopsies of patients who had AIDS, transplant recipients, and patients who had undergone cancer chemotherapy.[68,72] The symptoms of pancreatitis have resolved in a few patients with AIDS treated with ganciclovir or foscarnet.[30] Adenovirus has caused hemorrhagic pancreatitis and death in a child who received a bone marrow transplant, whereas an infant with disseminated adenoviral infection and pancreatitis survived with cidofovir therapy.[25,115] Varicella-zoster and herpes simplex viruses have caused pancreatitis and death in patients with various immunodeficient conditions.[45,139] A disseminated parainfluenza virus infection in an infant with severe combined immunodeficiency was associated temporally with the development of pancreatitis; however, no attempt was made to culture the virus from postmortem pancreatic tissue.[48]

Whether HIV directly causes pancreatitis is unclear. Laboratory-diagnosed episodes of pancreatitis in adults and children with AIDS do occur, but whether the pancreatic inflammation is caused by HIV or an unrecognized opportunistic pathogen is unknown.[175] HIV-infected children frequently have elevated

amylase and lipase levels with no correlation to antiviral therapy.[24] Also, increasing numbers of adults with primary manifestations of HIV infection have presented with acute pancreatitis, suggesting a role of HIV in the pathogenesis of the disease.[157]

Interstitial pancreatitis occurs commonly in children with congenital rubella syndrome.[106] In addition, severe pancreatitis has been identified in immunocompetent and immunocompromised patients with fatal measles virus infection.[161] An adolescent has been described with measles encephalitis and pancreatitis that responded to steroids.[148] One case of an adolescent with rotavirus gastroenteritis in whom pancreatitis developed has been reported.[35]

PARASITE INFESTATIONS AND INFECTIONS

Ascaris lumbricoides can migrate in the intestines to the ampulla of Vater and subsequently to the pancreatic duct or common bile duct. Obstruction of the biliary or pancreatic duct can cause acute pancreatitis.[1,11] Ascariasis is diagnosed when adult roundworms are identified in the duodenum by radiographs of the upper gastrointestinal tract (Fig. 58–1), or more commonly by ultrasonography or ERCP. Often, a history of seeing worms in the feces can be elicited. The flukes *Clonorchis sinensis* and *Fasciola hepatica* and the cestode *Taenia saginata* also can migrate to the pancreatic and biliary drainage systems and cause pancreatitis.[40,89,141] Rarely, hepatic hydatid cysts caused by *Echinococcus* can obstruct biliary drainage and cause pancreatic inflammation.[122] *Wuchereria bancrofti* occasionally has been found to cause chronic pancreatitis.[70] Parasitic infestations should be considered as a cause of pancreatitis, particularly in immigrant children and patients who have traveled to developing nations.

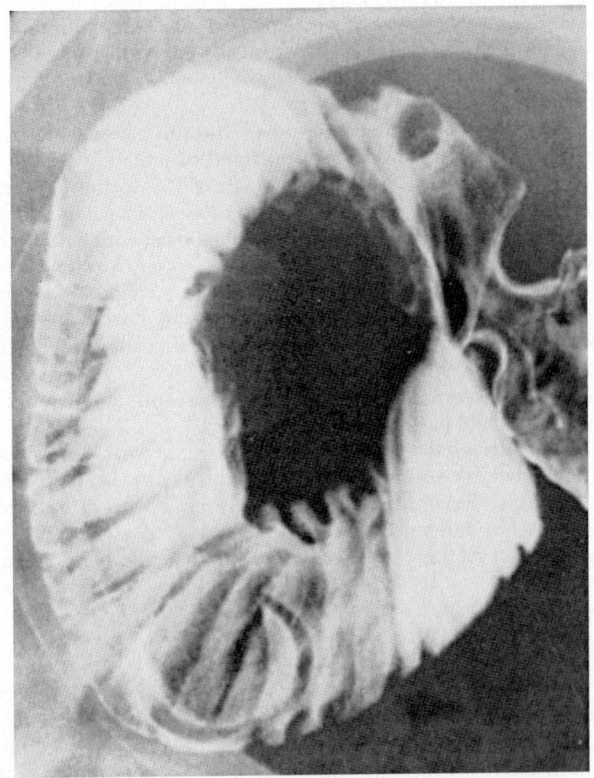

Figure 58–1 An ascaris close to the ampulla of Vater, the body and tail lying in the second and third parts of the duodenum. The patient is a 9-year-old girl with acute pancreatitis.

The protozoan *Cryptosporidium parvum* has been identified in the bile of a patient with AIDS with elevated serum amylase and right upper quadrant abdominal pain.[52] ERCP showed biliary and pancreatic ductal disease, but no other opportunistic pathogens were isolated. Cryptosporidia also have been observed in the interlobular pancreatic ducts of experimentally infected immunocompromised mice.[158] Whether cryptosporidial infection causes pancreatitis in immunocompetent patients is unknown; however, a previously healthy adolescent developed pancreatitis after having cryptosporidial diarrhea.[60] *Toxoplasma gondii* cysts have been found in the postmortem pancreatic tissue of patients with AIDS.[4,64] Rarely, pancreatitis occurs during acute episodes of falciparum malaria.[74] Other systemic manifestations of malaria that often are present include high fever, hepatitis, intestinal malabsorption, encephalitis, and pulmonary insufficiency.

MYCOPLASMAL AND BACTERIAL INFECTIONS

In older children and adults, moderately severe symptoms of pancreatitis have occurred just before or during the course of atypical pneumonia.[5,62] In these cases, most patients have had cold agglutinins in their sera, and all have had significant changes in *Mycoplasma pneumoniae* antibody titer. Some controversy has ensued over whether *M. pneumoniae* can cause acute pancreatitis without evidence of pneumonia. Although complement-fixing IgM antibodies against *M. pneumoniae* often increase significantly during the course of acute pancreatitis, researchers have argued that pancreatic cellular antigenic components similar to *Mycoplasma* lipid antigens are exposed during the disease process and that the antibodies elicited cross-react in *Mycoplasma* serologic assays.[88]

Along with *M. pneumoniae* infection, legionnaires' disease must be considered when acute pancreatitis develops along with pneumonia.[103,170] Miliary tuberculosis also can cause symptoms of pancreatitis.[132] Occasionally, pancreatitis may be the only manifestation of tuberculosis and usually is diagnosed by fine-needle aspiration of the pancreas.[58,113]

Common pyogenic bacteria usually do not cause acute pancreatitis. Secondary invasion of inflamed pancreatic tissue does occur. Some evidence exists that circulating endotoxin from *Escherichia coli* can cause extrahepatic cholestasis and pancreatitis.[37] Acute pancreatitis also has been seen in children with hemolytic-uremic syndrome.[130,134] Pancreatitis can occur during acute episodes of enteritis. *Salmonella typhimurium*, *Salmonella typhi*, *Campylobacter jejuni*, *Yersinia enterocolitica*, and *Yersinia pseudotuberculosis* all have been reported to cause clinically evident and laboratory-confirmed cases of pancreatitis.[10,34,137,145] A single case of *Moraxella catarrhalis* causing severe pancreatitis and death in a 4-year-old child has been reported.[118]

Pancreatitis has been reported in children with leptospirosis.[81,117] *Brucella melitensis* also has been added to the list of uncommon causes of acute pancreatitis.[123] *Helicobacter pylori* has been suggested to influence the clinical course of pancreatitis in humans, but data are still lacking to imply a role in pancreatic pathology.[98]

FUNGAL INFECTIONS

Fungal infections have not been reported to cause acute pancreatitis in immunocompetent patients. *Aspergillus* has caused fatal hemorrhagic pancreatitis, however, in an adult patient with cancer who was undergoing chemotherapy.[53] *Candida* spp. and *Cryptococcus neoformans* have been isolated from the pancreatic tissue of patients with AIDS, but whether they cause clinical symptoms of pancreatitis is unknown.[175]

PATHOGENESIS

Enzymes for polysaccharides, fats, and proteins are produced and stored in pancreatic acinar cells. They exist intracellularly in an inactive precursor form. After cholecystokinin stimulation, the proenzymes are released into the pancreatic ducts and flow into the duodenum. The enzymes normally do not become enzymatically active until they reach the intestinal lumen.

When trypsinogen is activated prematurely to trypsin within the pancreatic acinar cells, autodigestion occurs within the pancreas.[17] The mechanisms that activate trypsinogen and other proteolytic enzymes during specific pathologic processes have not been well elucidated. Drug-induced and infectious causes of pancreatitis are thought to be caused by direct toxic effects on acinar cells. Gallstones, *Ascaris* infection, and congenital abnormalities are thought to damage acinar cells by obstructing pancreatic flow. Traumatic pancreatitis probably occurs as a result of direct injury to the glandular cells, whereas vasculitis may cause changes in pancreatic blood flow, causing ischemia.

Autodigestion of the pancreas causes edema of pancreatic tissue, and microcirculation may be compromised, leading to ischemia, hemorrhage, or necrosis. An inflammatory response develops, which may be mild, as occurs commonly in episodes of infectious pancreatitis, or may be more severe with hemorrhagic necrosis. Major mediators of the intense immune response include tumor necrosis factor, interleukin-1, interleukin-6, interleukin-8, and platelet activation factor.[94] If an imbalance of the proinflammatory response occurs within the pancreas, a systemic inflammatory response including shock may occur, leading to high morbidity and mortality. Also, sepsis may occur because of extensive necrotic tissue within the pancreas and translocation of microorganisms from the intestines.

TREATMENT

Despite increasing recognition of cases of childhood pancreatitis, no major pharmacologic advances have been made in the treatment of the disease since the mid-1970s. Animal data have shown that medications such as glucagon, aprotinin, gabexate mesilate, 5-fluorouracil, octreotide, and somatostatin may be useful in the treatment of pancreatitis; however, trials in adults have not substantiated their efficacy.[38] The continuing main objectives of treatment are to relieve abdominal pain and treat aggressively systemic manifestations, such as shock, electrolyte abnormalities, and anemia. Meperidine continues to be the medication most commonly used for controlling pain.

In the past, children were kept in the fasted state and nasogastric suction was applied to decrease duodenal acid–stimulated secretin release. Feeding with carbohydrate solutions was not restarted until all symptoms had resolved. More recent studies in adults have shown, however, that feeding with a low-fat elemental diet decreases the complication rate of patients with acute pancreatitis and now is considered the treatment of choice over total parenteral nutrition.[101,151] A study has shown that patients with severe pancreatitis can be fed by slow infusion by the nasogastric route without worsening of pain or changes of nutritional status compared with being fed by a nasojejunal tube.[85] Intravenous fluids and colloids are used during the acute episode to maintain intravascular volume. During the entire course of acute pancreatitis, the hematologic and biochemical parameters of the child must be monitored closely.

If the episode of pancreatitis is drug-induced, use of the medication should be curtailed immediately. Often, the symptoms recur if the medication is restarted. Pancreatitis caused by *M. pneumoniae* or bacteria should be treated with proper antimicrobials. Obstructions to pancreatic flow (e.g., gallstones, roundworms, congenital abnormalities) may have to be excised or altered either by surgery or by endoscopy.[18,77,126]

COMPLICATIONS

During an acute episode of pancreatitis, the systemic inflammatory response syndrome may develop, leading to renal, hematologic, central nervous system, pulmonary, and cardiovascular complications. In 12 percent of children with pancreatitis, an inflammatory mass develops in the first weeks after the onset of illness; however, these masses more commonly occur after trauma.[163] Continued or increasing abdominal pain, nausea, or vomiting often accompanies the development of a phlegmon, abscess, or pseudocyst. An inflammatory phlegmon usually develops into a thin-walled pseudocyst of the lesser sac but may become secondarily infected and induce the formation of an abscess. Patients in whom an inflammatory mass develops must be monitored closely with frequent physical examinations and serial CT scans. In children with pseudocysts, acute abdominal pain accompanied by hypotension often signifies bleeding into the pseudocyst or rupture of the pseudocyst into the peritoneum. Slowly leaking pseudocysts may cause pancreatic ascites. Pseudocysts are resected surgically, drained externally, or drained by endoscopy when complications occur.[9] Approximately 33 percent of pseudocysts resolve spontaneously within 6 weeks.[127]

The development of fever and leukocytosis during pancreatitis should suggest the presence of an infected pseudocyst, pancreatic abscess, or sepsis. In adults, infectious complications account for 80 percent of deaths associated with acute pancreatitis.[19] Isolates from pancreatic abscesses have yielded intestinal flora, including anaerobes, in more than 90 percent of cases, but *Candida* spp. are being isolated more frequently in many medical centers.[8,39] Rarely, *Streptococcus pneumoniae* can be isolated from infected pancreatic tissues of adults with chronic pancreatitis.[150] Carbapenems, such as imipenem and meropenem, are used commonly to treat adult patients with suppurative complications of pancreatitis because these antibiotics penetrate well into pancreatic tissues and have activity against intestinal flora.

Even with early diagnosis and proper antibiotics and surgical intervention, the death rate from pancreatic abscesses is 22 to 57 percent in adults.[63,66] Performing percutaneous catheter drainage under CT guidance may reduce the mortality rate associated with treating pancreatic abscesses.[13] Rarely, fistulas from pseudocysts or abscesses to other abdominal organs may develop.[61]

The role of prophylactic antibiotics in preventing the suppurative complications of acute pancreatitis remains controversial despite 3 decades of debate.[120] Prophylactic antibiotics should be considered only when pancreatic necrosis is significant; however, antimicrobial trials have yielded conflicting results in adults.[87] A more recent meta-analysis on the subject concluded that prophylactic antibiotics do not prevent pancreatic necrosis from being infected and do not prevent death.[102] Infections, when they do occur after the administration of prophylactic antimicrobials, often are caused by multiresistant bacteria or by fungi.

Osteolytic lesions resembling osteomyelitis may develop weeks to months after an acute episode of pancreatitis.[114] Elevated systemic levels of lipase activity possibly may cause intramedullary fat necrosis in the bone. Usually, the lesions are asymptomatic and resolve spontaneously without therapy.

REFERENCES

1. Agarwal, A., Chowdhury, V., Srivastava, N., et al.: Pancreatic duct ascariasis: Sonographic diagnosis—a case report. Trop. Gastroenterol. 26:197-198, 2005.
2. Agarwal, K. S., Puliyel, J. M., Mathew, A., et al.: Acute pancreatitis with cholestatic hepatitis: An unusual manifestation of hepatitis A. Ann. Trop. Paediatr. 19:391-394, 1999.
3. Ahmed, S., Siddiqui, A. K., Siddiqui, R. K., et al.: Acute pancreatitis during sickle cell vaso-occlusive painful crisis. Am. J. Hematol. 73:190-193, 2003.
4. Ahuja, S. K., Ahuja, S. S., Thelmo, W., et al.: Necrotizing pancreatitis and multisystem organ failure associated with toxoplasmosis in a patient with AIDS. Clin. Infect. Dis. 16:432-434, 1993.
5. Al-Abassi, A.: Acute pancreatitis associated with *Mycoplasma pneumoniae*: A case report of missed diagnosis. Med. Princ. Pract. 11:112-115, 2002.
6. Alberti-Flor, J. J., Hernandez, M. E., Ferrer, J. P., et al.: Fulminant liver failure and pancreatitis associated with the use of sulfamethoxazole-trimethoprim. Am. J. Gastroenterol. 84:1577-1579, 1989.
7. Albu, E., Buiumsohn, A., Lopez, R., et al.: Gallstone pancreatitis in adolescents. J. Pediatr. Surg. 22:960-962, 1987.
8. Aloia, T., Solomkin, J., Fink, A. S., et al.: *Candida* in pancreatic infection: A clinical experience. Am. Surg. 60:793-796, 1994.
9. Al-Shanafey, S., Shun, A., and Williams, S.: Endoscopic drainage of pancreatic pseudocysts in children. J. Pediatr. Surg. 39:1062-1065, 2004.
10. Andrén-Sandberg, A., and Höjer, H.: Necrotizing acute pancreatitis induced by *Salmonella* infection. Int. J. Pancreatol. 15:229-230, 1994.
11. Arcement, C. M., Meza, M. P., Arumanla, S., et al.: MRCP in the evaluation of pancreaticobiliary disease in children. Pediatr. Radiol. 31:92-97, 2001.
12. Baldwin, M., Eisenman, R. E., Prelipp, A. M., et al.: *Ascaris lumbricoides* resulting in acute cholecystitis and pancreatitis in the Midwest. Am. J. Gastroenterol. 88:2119-2121, 1993.
13. Baril, N. B., Ralls, P. W., Wren, S. M., et al.: Does an infected peripancreatic fluid collection or abscess mandate operation? Ann. Surg. 23:361-367, 2000.
14. Barman, K. K., Premalatha, G., and Mohan, V.: Tropical chronic pancreatitis. Postgrad. Med. J. 79:606-615, 2003.
15. Bartholomew, C.: Acute scorpion pancreatitis in Trinidad. B. M. J. 1:666-668, 1970.
16. Benifla, M., and Weizman, Z.: Acute pancreatitis in childhood. J. Clin. Gastroenterol. 37:169-172, 2003.
17. Blake, R. L.: Acute pancreatitis. Prim. Care 15:187-199, 1988.
18. Bonnard, A., Seguier-Lipszyc, E., Liguory, C., et al.: Laparoscopic approach as primary treatment of common bile duct stones in children. J. Pediatr. Surg. 40:1459-1463, 2005.
19. Buggy, B. P., and Nostrant, T. T.: Lethal pancreatitis. Am. J. Gastroenterol. 78:810-814, 1983.
20. Bustamante, S. E., and Appachi, E.: Acute pancreatitis after anesthesia with propofol in a child with glycogen storage disease type 1A. Pediatr. Anesth. 16:680-683, 2006.
21. Butler, K. M., Husson, R. N., Balis, F. M., et al.: Dideoxyinosine in children with symptomatic human immunodeficiency virus infection. N. Engl. J. Med. 324:137-144, 1991.
22. Butler, K. M., Venzon, D., Henry, N., et al.: Pancreatitis in human immunodeficiency virus–infected children receiving dideoxyinosine. Pediatrics 91:747-751, 1993.
23. Capner, P., Lendrum, R., Jeffries, D. J., et al.: Viral antibody studies in pancreatic disease. Gut 16:866-870, 1975.
24. Carroccio, A., Fontana, M., Spagnuolo, M. I., et al.: Serum pancreatic enzymes in human immunodeficiency virus–infected children. Scand. J. Gastroenterol. 33:998-1001, 1998.
25. Carter, B. A., Karpen, S. J., Quiros-Tejeira, R. E., et al.: Intravenous cidofovir therapy for disseminated adenovirus in a pediatric liver transplant recipient. Pediatr. Infect. Dis. J. 74:1050-1052, 2002.
26. Cecchi, E., Forte, P., Cini, E., et al.: Pancreatitis induced by pegylated interferon alfa-2b in a patient affected by chronic hepatitis C. Emerg. Med. Austral. 16:473-475, 2004.
27. Chen, C., Changchien, C., Lu, S., et al.: Lamivudine treatment for recurrent pancreatitis associated with reactivation of chronic B hepatitis. Dig. Dis. Sci. 47:564-567, 2002.
28. Cheung, K. M., Mok, F., Lam, P., et al.: Pancreatitis associated with Henoch-Schönlein purpura. J. Paediatr. Child. Health. 37:311-313, 2001.
29. Cheung, O., Chopra, K., Yu, T., et al.: Gatifloxacin-induced hepatotoxicity and acute pancreatitis. Ann. Intern. Med. 140:73-74, 2004.
30. Colebunders, R., Van den Abbeele, K., Fleerackers, Y., et al.: Two AIDS patients with life-threatening pancreatitis successfully treated, one with ganciclovir, the other with foscarnet. Acta Clin. Belg. 49:229-232, 1994.
31. Corp, C. C., and Ghishan, F. K.: The sulfone syndrome complicated by pancreatitis and pleural effusion in an adolescent receiving dapsone for treatment of acne vulgaris. J. Pediatr. Gastroenterol. Nutr. 26:103-105, 1998.
32. DeBanto, J. R., Goday, P. S., Pedroso, M. R. A., et al.: Acute pancreatitis in children. Am. J. Gastroenterol. 97:1726-1731, 2002.
33. de Beaufort, C., Beck, P., Seligmann, R., et al.: Acute pancreatitis after growth hormone treatment: Disease or treatment linked? Eur. J. Pediatr. 165:652-653, 2006.
34. de Bois, M. H. W., Schoemaker, M. C., van der Werf, S. D. J., et al.: Pancreatitis associated with *Campylobacter jejuni* infections: Diagnosis by ultrasonography. B. M. J. 298:1004, 1989.
35. De La Rubia, L., Herrera, M. I., Cebrero, M., et al.: Acute pancreatitis associated with rotavirus infection. Pancreas 12:98-99, 1996.

36. Dettmeyer, R. B., Padosch, S. A., and Madea, B.: Lethal enterovirus-induced myocarditis and pancreatitis in a 4-month-old boy. Forensic Sci. Int. *156*:51-54, 2006.
37. Dev, G., Sikka, M., Sehgal, S., et al.: *Escherichia coli* infection producing pancreatitis and extrahepatic cholestasis. Indian Pediatr. *24*:249-253, 1987.
38. De Waele, J. J., and Hoste, E.: Current pharmacotherapeutic recommendations for acute pancreatitis. Exp. Opin. Pharmacother. *7*:1017-1025, 2006.
39. De Waele, J. J., Vogelaers, D., and Colardyn, F.: Fungal infections in patients with severe acute pancreatitis and the use of prophylactic therapy. Clin. Infect. Dis. *37*:208-213, 2003.
40. Echenique-Elizondo, M., Amondarain, J., and Liron de Robles, C.: Fascioliasis: An exceptional cause of acute pancreatitis. J. Pancreas *6*:36-39, 2005.
41. Eisenhuber, E., Schoefl, R., Wiesbauer, P., et al.: Primary pancreatic lymphoma presenting as acute pancreatitis in a child. Med. Pediatr. Oncol. *37*:53-54, 2001.
42. Elmore, M. F., and Rogge, J. D.: Tetracycline-induced pancreatitis. Gastroenterology *81*:1134-1136, 1981.
43. Feiner, H.: Pancreatitis after cardiac surgery: A morphologic study. Am. J. Surg. *131*:684-688, 1976.
44. Feldstein, J. D., Johnson, F. R., Kallick, C. A., et al.: Acute hemorrhagic pancreatitis and pseudocyst due to mumps. Ann. Surg. *180*:85-88, 1974.
45. Fernàndez, R. A., Varona, T. L., Jaquotot, J. M. K., et al.: Pancreatitis aguda asociada a infeccin por virus de la varicela-zoster en un paciente con sindrome de immunodeficiencia adquirida. Med. Clin. (Barcelona) *98*:339-341, 1992.
46. Fimognari, F. L., Corsonello, A., Pastorell, R., et al.: Metformin-induced pancreatitis. Diabetes Care *29*:1183, 2006.
47. Foisy, M. M., Slayter, K. L., Hewitt, R. G., et al.: Pancreatitis during intravenous pentamidine therapy in an AIDS patient with prior exposure to didanosine. Ann. Pharmacother. *28*:1025-1028, 1994.
48. Frank, J. A., Warren, R. W., Tucker, J. A., et al.: Disseminated parainfluenza infection in a child with severe combined immunodeficiency. Am. J. Dis. Child. *137*:1172-1174, 1983.
49. Garau, P., Orenstein, S. R., Neigut, D. A., et al.: Pancreatitis associated with olsalazine and sulfasalazine in children with ulcerative colitis. J. Pediatr. Gastroenterol. Nutr. *18*:481-485, 1994.
50. Glassman, M., Tahan, S., Hillemeier, C., et al.: Pancreatitis in patients with Reye's syndrome. J. Clin. Gastroenterol. *3*:165-169, 1981.
51. Gonzalez Carro, P., Perez Roldan, F., Legaz Huidobro, M. L., et al.: Acute pancreatitis and modified-release clarithromycin. Ann. Pharmacother. *38*:508-509, 2004.
52. Gross, T. L., Wheat, J., Bartlett, M., et al.: AIDS and multiple system involvement with *Cryptosporidium*. Am. J. Gastroenterol. *81*:456-458, 1986.
53. Guice, K. S., Lynch, M., and Weatherbee, L.: Invasive aspergillosis: An unusual cause of hemorrhagic pancreatitis. Am. J. Gastroenterol. *82*:563-565, 1987.
54. Haddad, N. G., Croffie, J. M., and Eugster, E. A.: Pancreatic enzyme elevations in children with diabetic ketoacidosis. J. Pediatr. *145*:122-124, 2004.
55. Haddock, G., Coupar, G., Youngson, G. G., et al.: Acute pancreatitis in children: A 15-year review. J. Pediatr. Surg. *29*:719-722, 1994.
56. Hanft, A., and Bourgeois, J.: Risperidone and pancreatitis. J. Am. Acad. Child Adolesc. Psychiatry *43*:1458-1459, 2004.
57. Harb, R., and Naon, H.: Idiopathic fibrosing pancreatitis in a 3-year-old girl: A case report and review of the literature. J. Pediatr. Surg. *40*:1335-1340, 2005.
58. Hari, S., Seith, A., Srivastava, D. N., et al.: Isolated tuberculosis of the pancreas diagnosed with needle aspiration: A case report and review of the literature. Trop. Gastroenterol. *26*:141-143, 2005.
59. Hart, C. C.: Aerosolized pentamidine and pancreatitis. Ann. Intern. Med. *111*:691, 1989.
60. Hawkins, S. P., Thomas, R. P., and Teasdale, C.: Acute pancreatitis: A new finding in *Cryptosporidium* enteritis. B. M. J. *294*:483-484, 1987.
61. Henderson, J. M., and MacDonald, J. A. E.: Fistula formation complicating pancreatic abscess. Br. J. Surg. *63*:233-234, 1976.
62. Herbaut, C., Tielemans, C., Burette, A., et al.: *Mycoplasma pneumoniae* infection and acute pancreatitis. Acta Clin. Belg. *38*:186-188, 1983.
63. Hillemeier, C., and Gryboski, J. D.: Acute pancreatitis in infants and children. Yale J. Biol. Med. *57*:149-159, 1984.
64. Hofman, P., Michiels, J.-F., Mondain, V., et al.: Pancréatite aiguë toxoplasmique. Gastroenterol. Clin. Biol. *18*:895-897, 1994.
65. Huber, S., and Ramsingh, A. I.: Coxsackievirus-induced pancreatitis. Viral Immunol. *17*:358-369, 2004.
66. Hurley, J. E., and Vargish, T.: Early diagnosis and outcome of pancreatic abscesses in pancreatitis. Am. Surg. *53*:29-33, 1987.
67. Imrie, C. W., Ferguson, J. C., and Sommerville, R. G.: Coxsackie and mumps virus infection in a prospective study of acute pancreatitis. Gut *18*:53-56, 1977.
68. Iwasaki, T., Tashiro, A., Satodate, R., et al.: Acute pancreatitis with cytomegalovirus infection. Acta Pathol. Jpn. *37*:1661-1668, 1987.
69. Jaroszewicz, J., Flisiak, R., Kalinowska, A., et al.: Acute hepatitis E complicated by acute pancreatitis. Pancreas *30*:382-384, 2005.
70. Jesudason, S. R. B., Mathai, V., Muthusami, J. C., et al.: *Wuchereria bancrofti* induced pancreatitis. Trop. Gastroenterol. *13*:115-118, 1992.
71. Jin, C.-F., and Sable, R.: Isoniazid-induced acute hepatitis and acute pancreatitis in a patient during chemoprophylaxis. J. Clin. Gastroenterol. *35*:100-101, 2002.
72. Joe, L., Ansher, A. F., and Gordin, F. M.: Severe pancreatitis in an AIDS patient in association with cytomegalovirus infection. South. Med. J. *82*:1444-1445, 1989.
73. Johnson, J. L., and Loomis, I. B.: A case of simvastatin-associated pancreatitis and review of statin-associated pancreatitis. Pharmacotherapy *26*:414-422, 2006.
74. Johnson, R. C., DeFord, J. W., and Carlton, P. K.: Pancreatitis complicating falciparum malaria. Postgrad. Med. *61*:181-183, 1977.
75. Kahler, S. G., Sherwood, W. G., Woolf, D., et al.: Pancreatitis in patients with organic acidemias. J. Pediatr. *124*:239-243, 1994.
76. Kandula, L., Whitcomb, D. C., and Lowe, M. E.: Genetic issues in pediatric pancreatitis. Curr. Gastroenterol. Rep. *8*:246-251, 2006.
77. Kawahara, H., Takahashi, T., and Okada, A.: Characteristics of duodenal duplications causing pancreatitis in children and adolescents: A case report and review of the literature. J. Pediatr. Gastroenterol. Nutr. *35*:372-376, 2002.
78. Keidar, S., Porath, E. B., Naftali, V., et al.: Acute pancreatitis associated with rising cytomegalovirus titer. Isr. J. Med. Sci. *23*:296-297, 1987.
79. Khanna, S., and Vij, J. C.: Severe acute pancreatitis due to hepatitis A virus infection in a patient of acute viral hepatitis. Trop. Gastroenterol. *24*:25-26, 2003.
80. Kirschner, B. S.: Safety of azathioprine and 6-mercaptopurine in pediatric patients with inflammatory bowel disease. Gastroenterology *115*:813-821, 1998.
81. Kishor, K. K., Rao, P. V., and Shastry, B. A.: Pancreatitis in Weil's disease. Trop. Doctor *32*:230-231, 2002.
82. Koller, E. A., Cross, J. T., Doraiswamy, P. M., et al.: Pancreatitis associated with atypical antipsychotics: From the Food and Drug Administration's MedWatch surveillance system and published reports. Pharmacotherapy *23*:1123-1130, 2003.
83. Koutras, A.: Epstein-Barr virus infection with pancreatitis, hepatitis, and proctitis. Pediatr. Infect. Dis. *2*:312-313, 1983.
84. Kugathasan, S., Halabi, I., Telega, G., et al.: Pancreatitis as a presenting manifestation of pediatric Crohn's disease: A report of three cases. J. Pediatr. Gastroenterol. Nutr. *35*:96-98, 2002.
85. Kumar, A., Singh, N., Prakash, S., et al.: Early enteral nutrition in severe acute pancreatitis: A prospective randomized controlled trial comparing nasojejunal and nasogastric routes. J. Clin. Gastroenterol. *40*:431-434, 2006.
86. Kuyucu, N., Kara, C., Bakirtac, A., et al.: Successful treatment of visceral leishmaniasis with allopurinol plus ketoconazole in an infant who developed pancreatitis caused by meglumine antimonate. Pediatr. Infect. Dis. J. *20*:455-457, 2001.
87. Lankisch, P. G., and Lerch, M. M.: The role of antibiotic prophylaxis in the treatment of acute pancreatitis. J. Clin. Gastroenterol. *40*:149-155, 2006.
88. Leinikki, P. O., Panzar, P., and Tykka, H.: Immunoglobulin M antibody response against *Mycoplasma pneumoniae* lipid antigen in patients with acute pancreatitis. J. Clin. Microbiol. *8*:113-118, 1978.
89. Liu, Y.-M., Bair, M.-J., Chang, W.-H., et al.: Acute pancreatitis caused by tapeworm in the biliary tract. Am. J. Trop. Med. Hyg. *73*:377-380, 2005.
90. Lopez, M. J.: The changing incidence of acute pancreatitis in children: A single-institution perspective. J. Pediatr. *140*:622-624, 2002.
91. Lowe, M. E.: Pancreatitis in children. Curr. Gastroenterol. Rep. *6*:240-246, 2004.
92. Magill, P., Ridgway, P. F., Conlon, K. C., et al.: A case of probable ibuprofen-induced acute pancreatitis. J. Pancreas *7*:311-314, 2006.
93. Mahjoub, W., Jarboui, S., Moussa, M. B., et al.: Indomethacin-induced pancreatitis: A second case report. J. Pancreas *7*:321-323, 2006.
94. Makhija, R., and Kingsnorth, A. N.: Cytokine storm in acute pancreatitis. J Hepatobil. Pancreat. Surg. *9*:401-410, 2002.
95. Malhi, N. S., Dutta, U., and Sathyanarayana, G.: Acute pancreatitis: Presenting manifestation of varicella infection. Trop. Gastroenterol. *25*:82-83, 2004.
96. Mallory, A., and Kern, F.: Drug-induced pancreatitis: A critical review. Gastroenterology *78*:813-820, 1980.
97. Malozowski, S., Hung, W., Scott, D. C., et al.: Acute pancreatitis associated with growth hormone therapy for short stature. N. Engl. J. Med. *332*:401-402, 1995.
98. Manes, G., Balzano, A., and Vaira, D.: *Helicobacter pylori* and pancreatic disease. J. Pancreas *4*:111-116, 2003.
99. Manfredi, R., Lucidi, V., Gui, B., et al.: Idiopathic chronic pancreatitis in children: MR cholangiopancreatography after secretin administration. Radiology *224*:675-682, 2002.
100. Maranan, M. C., Gerber, S. I., and Miller, G. G.: Gallstone pancreatitis caused by ceftriaxone. Pediatr. Infect. Dis. *17*:662-663, 1998.
101. Marik, P. E., and Zaloga, G. P.: Meta-analysis of parenteral nutrition versus enteral nutrition in patients with acute pancreatitis. B. M. J. *328*:1407-1410, 2004.
102. Mazaki, T., Ishii, Y., and Takayama, T.: Meta-analysis of prophylactic antibiotic use in acute necrotizing pancreatitis. Br. J. Surg. *93*:674-684, 2006.
103. Michel, O., Naeije, N., Csoma, M., et al.: Acute pancreatitis in Legionnaires' disease. Eur. J. Respir. Dis. *66*:62-64, 1985.
104. Miller, T. L., Winter, H. S., Luginbuhl, L. M., et al.: Pancreatitis in pediatric human immunodeficiency virus infection. J. Pediatr. *120*:223-227, 1992.
105. Mishra, A., Saigal, S., Gupta, R., et al.: Acute pancreatitis associated with viral hepatitis: A report of six cases with review of literature. Am. J. Gastroenterol. *94*:2292-2295, 1999.

106. Monif, G. R. G.: Rubella virus and the pancreas. Med. Chir. Dig. 3:195-197, 1974.
107. Mor, R., Pitlik, S., Dux, S., et al.: Parotitis and pancreatitis complicating infectious mononucleosis. Isr. J. Med. Sci. 18:709-710, 1982.
108. Moreno, A., Quereda, C., Moreno, L., et al.: High rate of didanosine-related mitochondrial toxicity in HIV/HCV-coinfected patients receiving ribavirin. Antiviral Ther. 9:133-138, 2004.
109. Naficy, K., Nategh, R., and Ghadimi, H.: Mumps pancreatitis without parotitis. B. M. J. 1:529-533, 1973.
110. Nahon Uzan, K., Levy, P., and O'Toole, D.: Is idiopathic chronic pancreatitis an autoimmune disease? Clin. Gastroenterol. Hepatol. 3:903-909, 2005.
111. Nakao, T., Nitta, T., Miura, R., et al.: Clinical and epidemiological studies on an outbreak of aseptic meningitis caused by Coxsackie B5 and A9 viruses in Aomori in 1961. Tohoku J. Exp. Med. 83:94-102, 1964.
112. Nelis, G. F.: Nitrofurantoin-induced pancreatitis: Report of a case. Gastroenterology 84:1032-1034, 1983.
113. Netherland, N. A., Chen, V. K., and Eloubeidi, M. A.: Intra-abdominal tuberculosis presenting with acute pancreatitis. Dig. Dis. Sci. 51:247-251, 2006.
114. Neuer, F. S., Roberts, F. F., and McCarthy, V.: Osteolytic lesions following traumatic pancreatitis. Am. J. Dis. Child. 131:738-740, 1977.
115. Niemann, T. H., Trigg, M. E., Winick, N., et al.: Disseminated adenoviral infection presenting as acute pancreatitis. Hum. Pathol. 24:1145-1148, 1993.
116. Nigwekar, S. U., and Casey, K. J.: Metronidazole induced pancreatitis: A case report and review of literature. J. Pancreas 5:516-519, 2004.
117. O'Brien, M. M., Vincent, J. M., Person, D. A., et al.: Leptospirosis and pancreatitis: A report of ten cases. Pediatr. Infect. Dis. J. 17:436-438, 1998.
118. Ohkusu, K., Nakamura, A., Horie, H., et al.: Fatal sepsis associated with acute pancreatitis caused by Moraxella catarrhalis in a child. Pediatr. Infect. Dis. J. 20:914-915, 2001.
119. Oku, T., Maeda, M., Waga, E., et al.: Cytomegalovirus cholangitis and pancreatitis in an immunocompetent patient. J. Gastroenterol. 40:987-992, 2005.
120. Oldfield, E. C.: Antibiotic prophylaxis in severe acute pancreatitis: The never-ending controversy. Rev. Gastoenterol. Disord. 5:183-194, 2005.
121. Otero, R., Navio, E., Cespedes, F. A., et al.: Scorpion envenoming in two regions of Colombia: Clinical, epidemiological and therapeutic aspects. Trans. R. Soc. Trop. Med. Hyg. 98:742-750, 2004.
122. Ozmen, M. M., Moran, M., Karakahya, M., et al.: Recurrent acute pancreatitis due to a hydatid cyst of the pancreatic head: A case report and review of the literature. J. Pancreas 6:354-358, 2005.
123. Papaioannides, D., Korantzopoulos, P., Sinapidis, D., et al.: Acute pancreatitis associated with brucellosis. J. Pancreas 7:62-65, 2006.
124. Penalva, J. C., Martinez, J., Pascual, S., et al.: Chronic pancreatitis associated with systemic lupus erythematosus in a young girl. Pancreas 27:275-277, 2003.
125. Perry, W., Jenkins, M. V., and Stamp, T. C. B.: Lysosomal enzymes and pancreatitis during rifampicin therapy. Lancet 1:492, 1979.
126. Poddar, U., Thapa, B. R., Bhasin, D. K., et al.: Endoscopic retrograde cholangiopancreatography in the management of pancreaticobiliary disorders in children. J. Gastroenterol. Hepatol. 16:927-931, 2001.
127. Pollak, E. W., Michas, C. A., and Wolfman, E. F.: Pancreatic pseudocyst: Management in 54 patients. Am. J. Surg. 135:199-201, 1978.
128. Ramanan, A. V., Thimmarayappa, A. D., and Baildam, E. M.: Acute lethal pancreatitis in childhood systemic lupus erythematosus. Rheumatology 41:467-469, 2002.
129. Renkes, P., Petitpain, N., Cosserat, F., et al.: Can roxithromycin and beta-methasone induce acute pancreatitis? A case report. J. Pancreas 4:184-186, 2003.
130. Robitaille, P., Gonthier, M., Grignon, A., et al.: Pancreatic injury in the hemolytic-uremic syndrome. Pediatr. Nephrol. 11:631-632, 1997.
131. Rocca, R., Castellino, F., Daperno, M., et al.: Therapeutic ERCP in paediatric patients. Dig. Liver Dis. 37:357-362, 2005.
132. Rushing, J. L., Hanna, C. J., and Selecky, P. A.: Pancreatitis as the presenting manifestation of miliary tuberculosis. West. J. Med. 129:432-436, 1978.
133. Ruzena, S.: Normal serum amylase in acute pancreatitis. Dig. Dis. Sci. 34:960-961, 1989.
134. Sass, D. A., Chopra, K. B., and Regueiro, M. D.: Pancreatitis and E. coli 0157:H7 colitis without hemolytic uremic syndrome. Dig. Dis. Sci. 48:415-416, 2003.
135. Sastry, J., Young, S., and Shaw, P. J.: Acute pancreatitis due to tacrolimus in a case of allogeneic bone marrow transplantation. Bone Marrow Transplant. 33:867-868, 2004.
136. Schouwenberg, B. J. J. W., and Deinum, J.: Acute pancreatitis after a course of clarithromycin. Neth. J. Med. 61:266-267, 2003.
137. Schulz, T. B.: Association of pancreas infection and yersiniosis. Acta Med. Scand. 205:255-256, 1979.
138. Shimoda, T., Shikata, T., Karasawa, T., et al.: Light microscopic localization of hepatitis B virus antigens in the human pancreas: Possibility of multiplication of hepatitis B virus in the human pancreas. Gastroenterology 81:998-1005, 1981.
139. Shintaku, M., Umehara, Y., Iwaisako, K., et al.: Herpes simplex pancreatitis. Arch. Pathol. Lab. Med. 127:231-234, 2003.
140. Shirobokov, V. P., Zhurba, T. B., and Zemlyansky, V. V.: Properties of the Coxsackie viruses isolated from pancreatic tissue of patients with chronic pancreatitis. Mikrobiol. Z. 50:78-81, 1988.
141. Shugar, R. A., and Ryan, J. J.: Clonorchis sinensis and pancreatitis. Am. J. Gastroenterol. 65:400-403, 1975.
142. Sinclair, D. B., Berg, M., and Breault, R.: Valproic acid-induced pancreatitis in childhood epilepsy: Case series and review. J. Child. Neurol. 19:498-502, 2004.
143. Sindhi, R., Webber, S., Venkataramanan, R., et al.: Sirolimus for rescue and primary immunosuppression in transplanted children receiving tacrolimus. Transplantation 72:851-855, 2001.
144. Sofer, S., Shalev, H., Weizman, Z., et al.: Acute pancreatitis in children following envenomation by the yellow scorpion Leiurus quinquestriatus. Toxicon 29:125-128, 1991.
145. Stauffer, W., Mantey, K., and Kamat, D.: Multiple extraintestinal manifestations of typhoid fever. Infection 30:113, 2002.
146. Stoler, J., Biller, J. A., and Grand, R. J.: Pancreatitis in Kawasaki disease. Am. J. Dis. Child. 141:306-308, 1987.
147. Stuecklin-Utsch, A., Hasan, C., Bode, U., et al.: Pancreatic toxicity after liposomal amphotericin B. Mycoses 45:170-173, 2002.
148. Takebayashi, K., Aso, Y., Wakabayashi, S., et al.: Measles encephalitis and acute pancreatitis in a young adult. Am. J. Med. Sci. 327:299-303, 2004.
149. Tenenbein, M. S., and Tenenbein, M.: Acute pancreatitis due to erythromycin overdose. Pediatr. Emerg. Care 21:675-676, 2005.
150. Thege, M. K., Pulay, I., Balla, E., et al.: Streptococcus pneumoniae as an etiologic agent in infectious complications of pancreatic disease. Microb. Drug Resist. 8:73-76, 2002.
151. Thomson, A.: Enteral versus parenteral nutritional support in acute pancreatitis: A clinical review. J. Gastroenterol. Hepatol. 21:22-25, 2006.
152. Tissieres, P., Durand, P., Chardot, C., et al.: Acute pancreatitis after orthotopic liver transplantation in children. Liver Transplant. Surg. 3:430-432, 1997.
153. Tissieres, P., Simon, L., Debray, D., et al.: Acute pancreatitis after orthotopic liver transplantation in children: Incidence, contributing factors, and outcome. J. Pediatr. Gastroenterol. Nutr. 26:315-320, 1998.
154. Torosis, J., and Vender, R.: Tetracycline-induced pancreatitis. J. Clin. Gastroenterol. 9:580-581, 1987.
155. Torre, J. A. C., Martin, J. J. D., Garcia, C. B., et al.: Varicella infection as a cause of acute pancreatitis in an immunocompetent child. Pediatr. Infect. Dis. J. 19:1218-1219, 2000.
156. Truninger, K., Malik, N., Ammann, R. W., et al.: Mutations of the cystic fibrosis gene in patients with chronic pancreatitis. Am. J. Gastroenterol. 96:2657-2661, 2001.
157. Tyner, R., and Turett, G.: Primary human immunodeficiency virus infection presenting as acute pancreatitis. South. Med. J. 97:393-394, 2004.
158. Ungar, B. L. P., Burris, J. A., Quinn, C. A., et al.: New mouse models for chronic Cryptosporidium infection in immunodeficient hosts. Infect. Immun. 58:961-969, 1990.
159. Urban, M., Splaingard, M., and Werlin, S. L.: Pancreatitis associated with remote traumatic brain injury in children. Childs Nerv. Syst. 10:388-391, 1994.
160. van Walraven, L. A., de Klerk, J. B. C., and Postema, R. R.: Severe acute necrotizing pancreatitis associated with lipoprotein lipase deficiency in childhood. J. Pediatr. Surg. 38:1407-1408, 2003.
161. Vargas, P. A., Bernardi, F. D. C., Alves, V. A. F., et al.: Uncommon histopathological findings in fatal measles infection: Pancreatitis, sialoadenitis and thyroiditis. Histopathology 37:141-146, 2000.
162. Versleijen, M. W. J., Naber, A. H. J., Riksen, N. P., et al.: Recurrent pancreatitis after trimethoprim-sulfamethoxazole rechallenge. Neth. J. Med. 63:275-277, 2005.
163. Warner, R. L., Othersen, H. B., and Smith, C. D.: Traumatic pancreatitis and pseudocyst in children: Current management. J. Trauma. 29:597-601, 1989.
164. Warren, W. R.: Serum amylase and lipase in mumps. Am. J. Med. Sci. 230:161-168, 1955.
165. Weizman, Z., and Durie, P. R.: Acute pancreatitis in childhood. J. Pediatr. 113:24-29, 1988.
166. Weizman, Z., and Sofer, S.: Acute pancreatitis in children with anticholinesterase insecticide intoxication. Pediatrics 90:204-206, 1992.
167. Werlin, S. L., Casper, J., Antonson, D., et al.: Pancreatitis associated with bone marrow transplantation in children. Bone Marrow Transplant. 10:65-69, 1992.
168. Werlin, S. L., and Fish, D. L.: The spectrum of valproic acid-associated pancreatitis. Pediatrics 118:1660-1663, 2006.
169. Werlin, S. L., Kugathasan, S., and Frautschy, B. C.: Pancreatitis in children. J. Pediatr. Gastroenterol. Nutr. 37:591-595, 2003.
170. Westblom, T. U., and Hamory, B. H.: Acute pancreatitis caused by Legionella pneumophila. South. Med. J. 81:1200-1201, 1988.
171. Willert, J. R., Dahl, G. V., and Marina, N. M.: Recurrent mercaptopurine-induced acute pancreatitis: A rare complication of chemotherapy for acute lymphoblastic leukemia in children. Med. Pediatr. Oncol. 38:73-74, 2002.
172. Wood, C. B., Bradbrook, R. A., and Blumgart, L. H.: Chronic pancreatitis in childhood associated with mumps virus infection. Br. J. Clin. Pract. 28:67-69, 1974.
173. Wortmann, G., Miller, R. S., Oster, C., et al.: A randomized, double-blind study of the efficacy of a 10- or 20-day course of sodium stibogluconate for the treatment of cutaneous leishmaniasis in United States military personnel. Clin. Infect. Dis. 35:261-267, 2002.

174. Youssef, S. S., Iskandar, S. B., Scruggs, J., et al.: Acute pancreatitis associated with omeprazole. Int. J. Clin. Pharmacol. Ther. *43*:558-561, 2005.
175. Zazzo, J. F., Pichon, F., and Regnier, B.: HIV and the pancreas. Lancet *2*:1212-1213, 1987.
176. Ziegler, D. W., Long, J. A., Philippart, A. I., et al.: Pancreatitis in childhood: Experience with 49 patients. Ann. Surg. *207*:257-261, 1988.
177. Zuger, A., Wolf, B. Z., El-Sadr, W., et al.: Pentamidine-associated fatal acute pancreatitis. J. A. M. A. *256*:2383-2385, 1986.

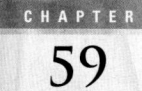

CHAPTER 59

PERITONITIS AND INTRA-ABDOMINAL ABSCESS

Judith R. Campbell ✦ John S. Bradley

Intra-abdominal infection can be a life-threatening condition that occurs spontaneously or as a result of intra-abdominal disease, injury, or surgery. Given the compartmental anatomy and physiology of the abdominal cavity, intra-abdominal infection frequently is categorized as peritonitis, intraperitoneal abscess, retroperitoneal abscess, and visceral abscess.[3] This chapter reviews peritonitis and intra-abdominal abscess; liver abscess and retroperitoneal abscess are reviewed in Chapters 55 (liver abscess) and 60 (retroperitoneal abscess).

PERITONITIS

ANATOMY

Knowledge of the anatomic relationships within the abdomen is important for understanding the source and routes of spread of infection. The peritoneal cavity extends from the undersurface of the diaphragm to the pelvis. In males, it is a closed space, whereas in females, the ends of the fallopian tubes penetrate into the peritoneal cavity. The transverse mesocolon and greater omentum separate the upper and lower peritoneal cavity. Peritoneal reflections divide the intraperitoneal space further into several compartments: the lesser sac, the paracolic gutters, and the subhepatic and subphrenic spaces (Fig. 59–1). The most dependent area of the peritoneal cavity is the pelvis. Exudate can extend to any of the recesses within the peritoneal cavity distant from the original source, however, and cause diffuse inflammation.[3] When inflamed, the anterior parietal peritoneum, which is supplied by somatic afferent nerves, gives the sensation of localized pain. Stimulation of the visceral peritoneum causes dull, poorly localized pain.

PATHOGENESIS

Peritonitis is defined as inflammation of the serosal lining of the abdominal cavity or the peritoneum and may be caused by any chemical or infectious agent that irritates the peritoneal surfaces. Noninfectious peritonitis is caused by extravasation of irritants, such as gastric juice, bile, urine, blood, pancreatic secretions, or the contents of a ruptured cyst, into the peritoneal cavity. Although chemical peritonitis generally is aseptic, it may be an important antecedent event to the development of infectious peritonitis.

After peritoneal contamination by bacteria has occurred, the first mechanism of host defense is lymphatic clearance. In experimental peritonitis, this clearance is so efficient that peritonitis and abscess formation occur only if adjuvant substances, such as hemoglobin or necrotic tissue, are present.[23,24,46] In the first hours after bacterial contamination occurs, local resident macrophages are the predominant phagocytic cells. The macrophages then are cleared by the lymphatic system. After bacterial proliferation

occurs, polymorphonuclear leukocytes become more numerous in the peritoneal cavity, and inflammation ensues. These peritoneal defense mechanisms also have adverse effects. Fibrin is deposited, which potentially entraps bacteria into a sequestered environment. An increase in splanchnic blood flow causes exudation of fluid into the peritoneal space, further impairing host defenses by diluting important peritoneal opsonins.[23,24] These host responses serve as a means of containing infection, but they also may contribute to the formation of abscesses.

Infectious peritonitis is subdivided into primary and secondary peritonitis based on the pathophysiology of the infection. Peritonitis that is associated with peritoneal dialysis or the presence of a ventriculoperitoneal shunt is a unique form of peritonitis that also is reviewed in this chapter. The microbial etiologies of peritonitis vary with the underlying cause and are summarized in Table 59–1.

PRIMARY PERITONITIS

Primary, or spontaneous, bacterial peritonitis is a rare infection defined as bacterial peritonitis in the absence of intra-abdominal findings, such as intestinal perforation. The incidence of spontaneous peritonitis in children is unknown; however, in the early 20th century, 8 to 10 percent of abdominal emergencies requiring surgical intervention were due to spontaneous peritonitis.[17,70] Freij and colleagues[29] conducted a 22-year review of children with primary peritonitis in Dallas, Texas. Primary peritonitis was diagnosed in 7 previously healthy children compared with 1840 cases of appendicitis during the same period. Currently, 1 to 2 percent of abdominal emergencies requiring surgical intervention are due to primary peritonitis.[37,40]

Now that this condition frequently is recognized clinically with the assistance of computed tomography (CT), the diagnosis often is made without exploratory laparotomy. The peak incidence of spontaneous peritonitis in children occurs when they are 5 to 9 years of age. In children, the most common predisposing factor is nephrotic syndrome, but this form of peritonitis also occurs in children with postnecrotic cirrhosis.[3,17,31,37,41,45,70,71] Spontaneous peritonitis rarely develops in previously healthy individuals without underlying conditions.[32,47]

The exact pathophysiologic mechanism for primary peritonitis is unknown; however, hematogenous inoculation is thought to be the most likely mechanism because the same organism frequently is recovered from cultures of blood and peritoneal fluid.[17,31,37] Alternative mechanisms include peritoneal seeding via the lymphatics, transmural migration through edematous bowel, and ascending infection from the female genitourinary tract.[31,37] In certain cases, impaired host defenses allow proliferation of bacteria that invade the peritoneal cavity, but a few children with primary peritonitis have no apparent impaired defense. Ascitic fluid from patients with nephrotic syndrome or cirrhosis contains lower levels of complement and immunoglobulin than does

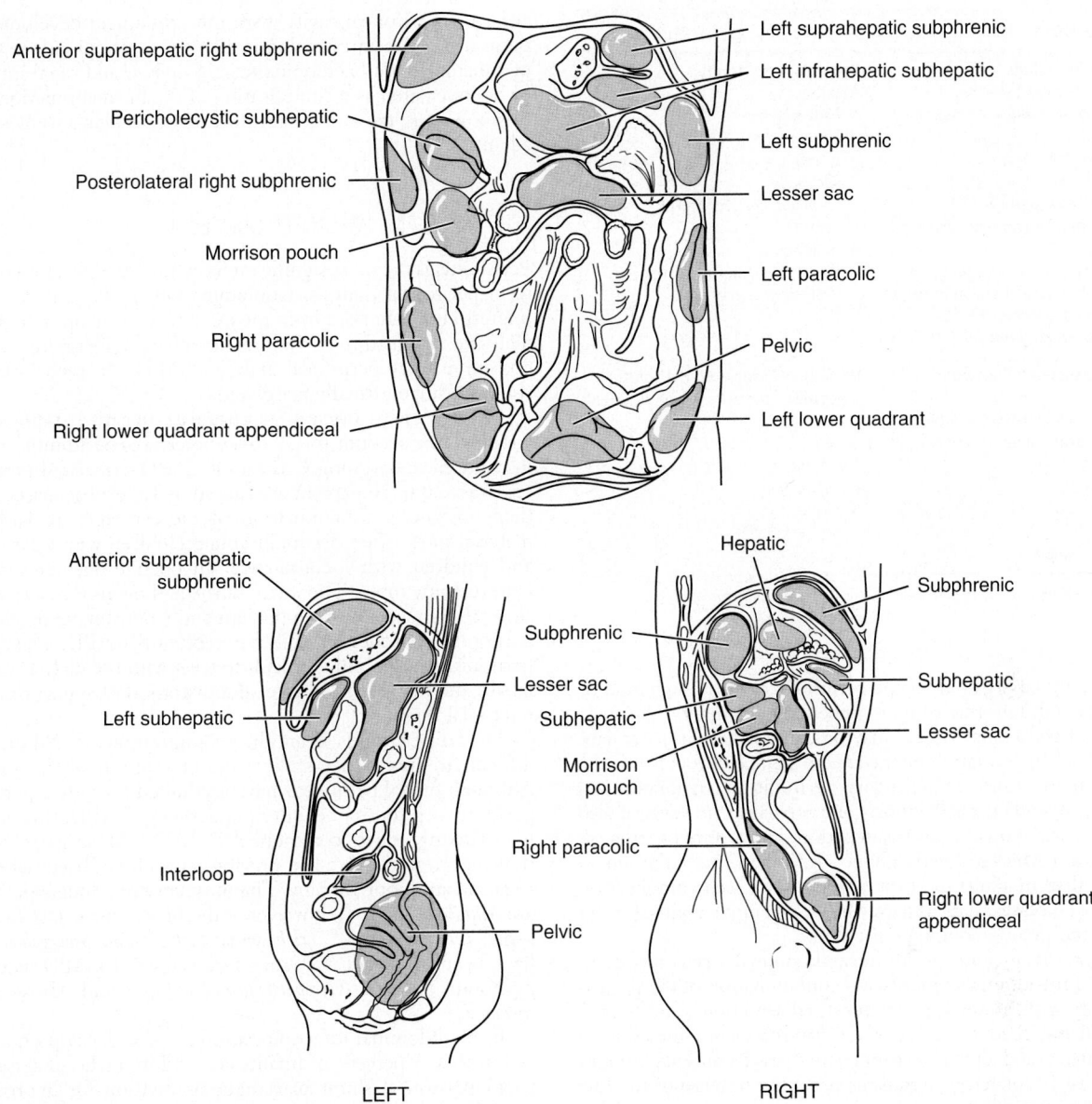

Figure 59–1 Anterior and sagittal views of the peritoneal cavity. (*From Altemeier, W. A., Culbertson, W. R., and Fullen, W. D.: Intra-abdominal sepsis. Adv. Surg. 5:281-333, 1971.*)

peritoneal fluid from a healthy host.[17,70] Deficiency of these important opsonins diminishes the natural clearance of organisms from the peritoneal cavity. Proliferation of organisms triggers the influx of phagocytes, release of inflammatory mediators, and localized or diffuse peritoneal irritation that gives rise to symptoms of abdominal pain and fever.

Since the pre-antibiotic era, researchers have recognized that primary peritonitis frequently is caused by *Streptococcus pneumoniae*,[31] *Streptococcus pyogenes*,[32] and *Staphylococcus aureus*.[17] Rarely, primary peritonitis in prepubescent girls is caused by extension of upper genital tract *S. pneumoniae* infection.[37,66] Since the 1960s, the bacteriology of primary peritonitis has shifted to include an increased proportion of infections caused by gram-negative enteric organisms, such as *Escherichia coli* and *Klebsiella* spp.[17,37,41,71] In some instances, primary *E. coli* peritonitis may occur concurrently with bacteremic urinary tract infection.

Tuberculous peritonitis may be caused by *Mycobacterium tuberculosis* or *Mycobacterium bovis*. It may occur as a complication of primary mycobacteremia or be caused by reactivation of latent intra-abdominal infection within lymphoid tissue, but only rarely does it seem to occur as a function of the ingestion of swallowed organisms from a pulmonary primary focus.[35,65,75] Peritoneal infection with *M. bovis*, which is clinically similar to *M. tuberculosis* peritonitis, is acquired from unpasteurized dairy products and has been reported in children living along the border between the United States and Mexico. These organisms may cause peritonitis from either mycobacteremia or erosion of organisms through the mesenteric lymph nodes or bowel wall into the peritoneal cavity.[20] *Salmonella* spp. rarely cause primary peritonitis and have been reported primarily in patients with underlying conditions.[47]

SECONDARY PERITONITIS

Secondary peritonitis, the most common form of peritonitis, arises as a complication of intra-abdominal injury or disease when microorganisms, secretions, and the particulate material of an

TABLE 59-1 Most Commonly Identified Etiologic Agents

Primary Peritonitis	Secondary Peritonitis
Escherichia coli (25-40%)	Aerobes
Haemophilus influenzae type b	*Enterobacter*
Klebsiella	*Enterococcus*
Mycobacterium bovis	*E. coli*
Mycobacterium tuberculosis	*Klebsiella*
Neisseria meningitidis	*Pseudomonas aeruginosa*
Other enteric gram-negative	*Serratia*
bacilli	Anaerobes
Other streptococci (alpha-	*Bacteroides fragilis* group
hemolytic and beta-hemolytic)	*Peptostreptococcus*
Staphylococcus aureus (2-4%)	
Streptococcus pneumoniae (30-50%)	
CAPD-Associated Peritonitis	**VP Shunt–Associated Peritonitis**
Candida	Coagulase-negative staphylococci
Coagulase-negative staphylococci	*Enterobacter*
Enteric gram-negative bacilli	*E. coli*
Mycobacterium	*Klebsiella*
Other fungi	*Pseudomonas*
Pseudomonas	*S. aureus*
S. aureus	
Stenotrophomonas	

CAPD, continuous ambulatory peritoneal dialysis; VP, ventriculoperitoneal.

intra-abdominal organ enter the peritoneal cavity. Congenital or acquired conditions that result in ischemia, inflammation, or perforation of abdominal viscera may be complicated by secondary peritonitis.[46] In premature infants, necrotizing enterocolitis is the most common cause of secondary peritonitis.[51] In infants and children, appendicitis is the most common cause; however, it also may occur with volvulus, intussusception, incarcerated hernia, or rupture of a Meckel diverticulum.[51] Although less common in children than in adults, peritonitis also occurs as a complication of mucosal diseases, such as peptic ulcer, ulcerative colitis, Crohn disease, and pseudomembranous colitis.[51]

Rupture of or injury to an intra-abdominal viscus results in spillage of the luminal contents and contamination of the peritoneal cavity with bacteria, gastrointestinal secretions, and debris. Chemical and infectious sources of inflammation are introduced. The stomach and upper gastrointestinal tract contents contain only 10^3 to 10^4 or fewer organisms per gram because of the low pH of gastric secretions. Gram-negative aerobic organisms colonize the upper gastrointestinal tract. In contrast, the colonic contents have predominantly anaerobes, with 10^{11} anaerobes and 10^8 aerobes per gram.[11,37,64]

Secondary peritonitis usually is a polymicrobial infection, with 5 to 10 different bacterial species of anaerobes and facultative gram-negative bacilli. Synergy among the various bacterial species enhances bacterial proliferation.[11] Members of the *Bacteroides fragilis* group and *Peptostreptococcus* spp. are the anaerobic organisms reported most commonly in secondary peritonitis. Of the aerobic organisms, *E. coli*, *Klebsiella* spp., *Pseudomonas aeruginosa*, and *Enterococcus* spp. are isolated most often. More recently, *P. aeruginosa* has been noted to be present in 20 to 30 percent of children with complicated ruptured appendicitis.[8,38] When secondary peritonitis occurs in patients with a history of prolonged hospitalization, underlying chronic conditions, or recent antibiotic therapy, the etiology may include nosocomial pathogens that have colonized the gastrointestinal tract, such as *P. aeruginosa*, *Enterobacter* spp., *Acinetobacter* spp., or other antibiotic-resistant organisms.

Focal suppurative infection may be present within an intra-abdominal or retroperitoneal solid organ or within intra-abdominal lymphoid tissue. Organisms spread from this purulent focus through the capsule of the organ or lymphoid tissue and enter the peritoneal cavity, with the subsequent development of peritonitis. The intra-abdominal organ or lymphoid tissue may be inoculated via bacteremia (e.g., *S. aureus* and renal infection) or be inoculated as a complication of the normal function of the organ (e.g., *E. coli* and renal infection or *Yersinia* and mesenteric adenitis).[13,36,42]

PERITONITIS AND IMPLANTED DEVICES

Peritonitis is the most significant infectious complication of long-term peritoneal dialysis. Contamination of the dialysis tubing, migration of skin flora from the exit site, or contamination of the dialysate may lead to peritonitis in patients undergoing continuous ambulatory peritoneal dialysis (CAPD). In each instance, a single pathogen usually is isolated.

Gram-positive organisms, coagulase-negative staphylococci, and *S. aureus* account for 30 to 45 percent of peritonitis episodes in children undergoing CAPD. Of CAPD-associated peritonitis episodes, 20 to 30 percent are caused by Enterobacteriaceae.[26] In these instances, contamination of the catheter site with fecal material most often occurs in young children who wear diapers and children with incontinence, an open urogenital sinus, or nephrostomy tubes. The water-borne pathogens *Pseudomonas* and *Acinetobacter* account for 6 percent and 4 percent, respectively, of peritonitis episodes in children receiving CAPD. *Pseudomonas* peritonitis is especially difficult to treat with the dialysis catheter in situ and may recur despite administration of appropriate antimicrobial therapy.[26]

Fungal peritonitis is another complication of CAPD that is difficult to treat successfully without removal of the catheter. Although fungal pathogens have accounted for only 2 percent of peritonitis episodes in children undergoing CAPD, this problem is occurring more commonly.[15,25,26,48,56,76] Most patients with fungal peritonitis have had previous episodes of bacterial peritonitis and antibiotic therapy. The most common fungal pathogens are *Candida* spp.[25,26]; however, rare fungi, such as *Curvularia* spp.,[15] *Fusarium* spp.,[26] *Trichosporon asahii*,[48] and *Aspergillus* spp.,[26] have been reported.[56,76] Other rare causes of CAPD-associated peritonitis include *Mycobacterium fortuitum* and *Mycobacterium chelonae*.[77]

Intra-abdominal infectious complications develop on average in less than 5 percent of infants and children who undergo ventriculoperitoneal shunt placement or revision for hydrocephalus.[43,55,68] Peritonitis, peritoneal pseudocyst, or perforation of the bowel by the abdominal catheter rarely occurs in children with such shunts.[5,30,33,60,61,63,67,72] Cerebrospinal fluid (CSF) in the peritoneal cavity may be seeded during transient bacteremia or a febrile illness or after abdominal trauma. In addition, peritonitis may develop as a complication of infection within the ventricles being drained[68] as organisms descend into the peritoneal cavity via the distal tubing.

A peritoneal pseudocyst containing CSF is the most common manifestation of peritoneal inflammation in patients with ventriculoperitoneal shunts. These patients often have a history of symptoms compatible with a shunt infection before the formation of a pseudocyst and may have signs of peritoneal inflammation and a palpable abdominal mass. The microbial etiology of ventriculoperitoneal shunt–associated peritonitis varies and reflects the pathogenesis of infection. Infections occurring within months of surgery often are caused by skin flora, *Staphylococcus epidermidis*, other coagulase-negative staphylococci, and *S. aureus*.[30,60] The microbiology of late shunt-associated peritonitis is similar to that of spontaneous bacterial peritonitis and may include gram-negative enteric organisms and gram-positive cocci.[60] Peritonitis caused by colonic flora also rarely has been associated with bowel perforation by the distal end of the ventriculoperitoneal shunt.[33,60,67]

CLINICAL MANIFESTATIONS

The initial signs and symptoms of primary bacterial peritonitis include nausea, vomiting, diarrhea, and diffuse abdominal pain.[37,40,41] These signs and symptoms are similar to those of secondary peritonitis caused by a ruptured appendix.

Rupture of the appendix is the most common cause of secondary peritonitis in children; the initial symptoms of anorexia, vomiting, and localized abdominal pain frequently precede the signs and symptoms of diffuse peritoneal inflammation. In primary and secondary peritonitis, patients typically lie very still because any movement exacerbates the abdominal pain. Physical findings include fever, tachycardia, abdominal distention, hypoactive bowel sounds, abdominal tenderness, rebound tenderness, abdominal wall rigidity, and tenderness on rectal or vaginal examination. Peritoneal inflammation is associated with an increase in splanchnic blood flow, capillary permeability, and a shift of fluid into the peritoneal space, which may lead to intravascular hypovolemia and shock, in addition to systemic absorption of endotoxin and bacteria.[46]

Fever and abdominal pain in any child undergoing peritoneal dialysis should be evaluated carefully. Turbid dialysate fluid raises the suspicion of CAPD-associated peritonitis. Similarly, symptomatic children with ventriculoperitoneal shunts should be evaluated for shunt-associated peritonitis.[61,68,80] In a retrospective report of 19 children with ventriculoperitoneal shunts and peritonitis, Reynolds and associates[61] noted that fever and abdominal pain were the most common symptoms in 14 of their patients. Stamos and colleagues[68] found that fever, lethargy, nausea, and vomiting were the most frequently reported symptoms in a review of 23 children with gram-negative infection of ventriculoperitoneal shunts.

Primary tuberculous peritonitis usually is gradual in onset and associated with weight loss, malaise, and nightsweats.[35,37,65] The degree of tenderness is less than that present with acute pyogenic peritonitis and may be nonexistent. Palpation of the abdomen may reveal an extensive, irregular collection of masses, often described as "doughy," caused by widespread granulomatous inflammation.[37]

DIAGNOSIS

Laboratory findings in a child with peritonitis often are nonspecific. The white blood cell count usually is elevated (16,000 to ≥25,000 cells/mm³), with a predominance of polymorphonuclear leukocytes and an increase in immature forms.[37] The hematocrit may be elevated because of dehydration and hemoconcentration. Mild pyuria is noted occasionally because of irritation of the urinary bladder or ureters.

Diagnostic imaging studies can be useful in evaluating intra-abdominal infections. Upright and lateral decubitus radiographs of the abdomen may show distended adynamic loops of bowel suggestive of ileus and obliteration of the peritoneal fat lines and psoas shadows. Free intraperitoneal air below the diaphragm indicates a ruptured viscus. The presence of a fecalith or right lower quadrant mass may be consistent with appendicitis. Abdominal ultrasound and CT may reveal an underlying cause of the peritonitis.[47,51]

Analysis of peritoneal fluid aspirate or lavage material may be helpful in differentiating primary from secondary peritonitis. Free air, blood, or bile indicates peritonitis secondary to intestinal perforation. In peritonitis, the leukocyte count in peritoneal fluid usually is greater than 250 to 300 white blood cells/mm³ and sometimes 3000 to 5000 white blood cells/mm³, with granulocytes predominating in 80 percent of cases.[37,45,70] A total protein content greater than 1 g/dL, a glucose level less than 50 mg/dL, or an elevated lactate dehydrogenase concentration (>25 mg/dL) is consistent with secondary peritonitis.[17,31,37,70]

If a Gram stain of peritoneal fluid shows only gram-positive cocci, primary peritonitis is most likely. The presence of gram-negative bacilli is consistent with primary or secondary peritonitis, but the presence of many different organisms on Gram stain is diagnostic of secondary peritonitis. Bacteremia occurs in 75 percent of patients with primary peritonitis. Specimens of peritoneal fluid and blood should be sent for culture.[37] Similarly, secondary peritonitis also can be associated with bacteremia, suggesting the need for obtaining cultures of blood in addition to peritoneal fluid. Specimens of peritoneal fluid should be processed to optimize the recovery of aerobic and anaerobic organisms, and the use of specific transport tubes or an airless, capped syringe is required.[11,37] The wide variety of pathogens isolated from intra-abdominal infections along with the variable antibiotic susceptibility of these pathogens supports taking an aggressive approach to obtaining samples for microbiologic evaluation.

A child undergoing CAPD who is suspected of having peritonitis should have dialysate sent for cell count, Gram stain, and culture for bacterial, mycobacterial, and fungal pathogens. If a child with a ventriculoperitoneal shunt is suspected of having peritonitis, CSF from the proximal portion of the shunt should be sent for culture, cell count, and determination of glucose and protein levels in addition to Gram stain and culture of peritoneal fluid.[30] Abdominal imaging by ultrasound or CT is useful in identifying a peritoneal pseudocyst and the location of distal tubing.

DIFFERENTIAL DIAGNOSIS

Other infectious diseases that may mimic primary or secondary bacterial peritonitis include mesenteric adenitis, gastroenteritis, hepatitis, streptococcal pharyngitis, lower lobe pneumonia, pyelonephritis, and pelvic inflammatory disease. Noninfectious diseases to be considered in the differential diagnosis are pancreatitis, diabetic ketoacidosis, Henoch-Schönlein purpura, ovarian torsion, sickle-cell pain crisis, and lead poisoning.[51]

TREATMENT

Optimal management of peritonitis involves prompt and aggressive physiologic support, surgical consultation, and antimicrobial therapy. Correction of fluid and electrolyte imbalances and hemodynamic stabilization should be initiated as soon as the diagnosis of peritonitis is suspected. Spontaneous bacterial peritonitis usually is managed medically, unless the diagnosis is uncertain, in which case exploratory laparotomy or laparoscopy is performed. Before resistant strains of S. pneumoniae emerged, primary peritonitis in children was treated with aqueous penicillin G.[17,31] Given the increased prevalence of S. pneumoniae with reduced susceptibility to penicillin, third-generation cephalosporins such as cefotaxime or ceftriaxone are recommended until susceptibility results are available.[45,71] If primary peritonitis is caused by gram-negative organisms, appropriate empiric therapy includes cefotaxime or ceftriaxone, with or without an aminoglycoside, a carbapenem, ticarcillin-clavulanate, or piperacillin-tazobactam, pending completion of culture and susceptibility testing.

Patients with secondary peritonitis may require either immediate surgery to control the source of contamination and to remove necrotic tissue, blood, and intestinal contents from the peritoneal cavity or a drainage procedure if a limited number of large abscesses can be shown.[43,47,52,79] In cases of phlegmon, or extensive inflammatory edema, surgery usually is not performed acutely because of the child's unstable metabolic state and friable intra-abdominal tissues. Surgery is delayed for several hours or weeks to allow the inflammation to resolve. Surgery also may be postponed indefinitely.[6,14,74]

Empiric antimicrobial therapy for secondary peritonitis should have activity against anaerobes, especially the *B. fragilis* group, and enteric gram-negative aerobes.[7] Although controversial, some regimens also include an antibiotic effective against enterococci. The gold standard for antimicrobial therapy historically has been clindamycin or metronidazole, gentamicin, and ampicillin.[7,11,27,43,46,52,62] Alternative efficacious regimens, as single or combination therapy, include aztreonam, cefotaxime, cefoxitin, imipenem-cilastatin, meropenem, piperacillin-tazobactam, and ticarcillin-clavulanate.[7,43,46,52,79] Rates of resistance to cefoxitin and clindamycin among the *B. fragilis* group have increased and are reported to be 49 percent; in some institutions, alternative regimens are used routinely.[2,46]

Other studies have examined the use of a single broad-spectrum antibiotic, which allows a portion of the therapy to be delivered less expensively on an outpatient basis. Fishman and coworkers[27] prospectively evaluated the clinical outcomes of 150 children with perforated appendicitis treated postoperatively with a 10-day course of piperacillin-tazobactam. They compared the outcome with that of historical controls treated with a 10-day course of ampicillin, gentamicin, and clindamycin. Rates of postoperative infectious complications were similar in both groups. Bradley and colleagues[8] prospectively identified 87 children with complicated appendicitis in five pediatric centers, also comparing costs and outcomes with historical controls. Although inpatient treatment courses were reduced by an average of 42 percent in meropenem-treated children, outcome measures were equivalent to those of historical controls.

Table 59-2 summarizes randomized trials of monotherapy versus combination therapy for ruptured appendicitis in children. Although no differences in outcome were observed, the potential of emerging resistance to broad-spectrum agents versus the convenience of monotherapy must be considered and balanced against the possible decreased risk of developing nosocomial infection among children who can receive a substantial component of parenteral therapy in the home.[38]

Empiric antibiotic treatment of CAPD-associated peritonitis should be effective against gram-positive and gram-negative organisms until culture results are available. Intraperitoneal antibiotics, with or without concomitant intravenous antibiotics, achieve adequate serum and dialysate concentrations. Vancomycin is used for empiric therapy for gram-positive infections, but if staphylococcal organisms are susceptible to β-lactam agents, treatment with cefazolin is effective.[26] Aminoglycosides (gentamicin or tobramycin) or cephalosporins are used for gram-negative infections; however, because most intraperitoneal antibiotics are absorbed into the systemic circulation, serum ami-

noglycoside or vancomycin concentrations should be monitored for possible toxicity. Therapy for fungal peritonitis usually is intravenous amphotericin B, although successful use of fluconazole or intraperitoneal amphotericin B has been reported.[26,56] Indications for removal of a dialysis catheter include persistent infection with *S. aureus* or *Pseudomonas*, tunnel infection, or fungal peritonitis.[26]

Treatment of peritonitis associated with ventriculoperitoneal shunts usually requires externalization of the distal end of the catheter in addition to institution of antibiotic therapy.[30] Empiric antibiotic therapy should include an antistaphylococcal agent active against coagulase-positive and coagulase-negative staphylococci. Coagulase-negative staphylococci are a common cause of ventriculoperitoneal shunt infection; vancomycin should be administered pending culture and susceptibility results. If Gram stain of ventricular CSF or peritoneal fluid reveals gram-negative organisms, cefotaxime, ceftriaxone, ceftazidime, or meropenem should be added.[5,61]

The duration of antibiotic therapy for peritonitis should be dictated by the clinical course of the patient because no single regimen or treatment course is accepted universally.[37] Indicators of sufficient therapy include resolution of fever and abdominal pain and return of the leukocyte and differential counts to normal.[37,52,69] Primary peritonitis caused by streptococci is treated successfully with a 10- to 14-day course of antibiotics.[17,37] Primary peritonitis with gram-negative organisms may require 10 days to 3 weeks of antibiotic treatment.[17] The duration of therapy for secondary peritonitis after adequate surgery usually is 5 to 10 days, but it depends on the clinical response to therapy.[37,52,69] Short-course therapy for 5 days has been shown to be efficacious in some patients,[37,52] but longer courses are required if fever persists, or abdominal signs and symptoms are present. Standard therapy for tuberculous peritonitis consists of a minimum of two antituberculous drugs. As with other forms of extrapulmonary tuberculosis in children, empiric therapy with isoniazid, rifampin, and pyrazinamide is advised pending culture and susceptibility results. Although *M. bovis* is resistant to pyrazinamide, most strains are susceptible to isoniazid and rifampin and to ethambutol.

COMPLICATIONS

Acute complications associated with peritonitis include septic shock, adult respiratory distress syndrome, septic thrombophlebitis of the portal vein, acute renal failure, and multiorgan system failure.[46] Postoperative complications include wound infection, adhesions, bowel obstruction, formation of a fistula, and formation of an intra-abdominal or retroperitoneal abscess.

Recurrent peritonitis (tertiary peritonitis) is an entity described as occurring late in the course of therapy for secondary peritoni-

TABLE 59-2   Monotherapy versus Combination Therapy for Ruptured Appendicitis in Children

Study	Monotherapy (A)	Combination Therapy (B)	No. Patients A	B	Complications* A (%)	B (%)
Meller et al.[49]	Cefoxitin	Clindamycin/gentamicin	29	27	1 (3)	4 (15)
Dougherty et al.[22]	Ticarcillin-clavulanate	Clindamycin/gentamicin ± ampicillin	79	45	14 (18)	5 (11)
Uhari et al.[73]	Imipenem-cilastatin	Metronidazole/tobramycin	9	10	2 (22)	1 (10)
Collins et al.[19]	Ampicillin-sulbactam ± aminoglycoside	Ampicillin/clindamycin ± aminoglycoside	75	39	2 (1)	1 (3)
Fishman et al.,[27] Lund and Murphy[43]	Pipercillin-tazobactam	Ampicillin/gentamicin/clindamycin	150	373	14 (9)	24 (6)
Bradley et al.[8]	Meropenem	Cefotaxime ± amikacin or tobramycin, clindamycin or metronidazole	22	13	2 (9)	1 (8)

Wound infections, intra-abdominal abscess, or rehospitalization.
Modified from Kaplan, S. L.: Antibiotic usage in appendicitis in children. Pediatr. Infect. Dis. J. 17:1047-1048, 1998.

tis.[37,44,79] Patients with this condition continue to have symptoms despite receiving appropriate antimicrobial therapy, and peritoneal fluid reveals persistent inflammation. Bacterial cultures often are negative or may yield an organism of low virulence. Multiorgan system failure and a poor outcome frequently are associated with tertiary peritonitis. The mechanism of ongoing peritoneal inflammation is unknown; however, some investigators have proposed that immunoregulatory dysfunction and poor nutrition are contributing factors.

INTRA-ABDOMINAL ABSCESS

Intra-abdominal abscesses often are categorized as intraperitoneal, visceral, or retroperitoneal (see Chapter 60).[4,10] In children, intraperitoneal abscesses are most common. The most common underlying conditions associated with an intra-abdominal abscess in children are appendicitis and trauma.[10,51] Reviews of gangrenous or perforated appendicitis in children indicate that 2 to 20 percent of cases are complicated by the formation of an abscess.[52,62]

Two basic mechanisms exist for the development of an intraperitoneal abscess. In the first mechanism, diffuse peritonitis may cause loculations of purulent material to form in the areas anatomically most dependent—typically the pelvic, subphrenic, and paracolic regions (see Fig. 59–1). The second mode of formation of an abscess involves a localized focus related to contiguous disease or injury in which host defenses and the inflammatory response prevent diffuse spread and peritonitis.[4] The microbiology of intraperitoneal abscesses is polymicrobial and reflects that of the intestinal flora. In a review of intra-abdominal abscess in 36 children, Brook[10,11] noted that the predominant organisms were the *B. fragilis* group, *Peptostreptococcus*, *E. coli*, and other Enterobacteriaceae.

The most common sites of visceral abscess in children are the liver (see Chapter 55), pancreas, and spleen. Underlying conditions that may lead to the development of a pancreatic abscess include pancreatic injury, pancreatitis, and biliary obstruction. Pancreatitis or surgical or accidental injury to the pancreas causes the release of pancreatic enzymes and focal necrosis.[28] Reflux of contaminated bile into the pancreatic duct is hypothesized to be the mechanism by which enteric organisms gain access to the injured pancreas and proliferate. A pancreatic abscess usually is a polymicrobial infection caused by aerobic (*E. coli*, *Klebsiella pneumoniae*, group D streptococci) or anaerobic (peptostreptococci, *B. fragilis* group) organisms that inhabit the gastrointestinal tract. Rare instances of *S. aureus* pancreatic abscess occur as a result of bacteremia.[12,13]

Splenic abscesses are unusual findings in infants and children. Before the 1970s, most reports involved solitary pyogenic abscesses. Since then, the number of reports of multiple splenic abscesses has increased.[16,39,58] Splenic abscess usually is associated with one of five underlying conditions: endocarditis, injury, hemoglobinopathy, immunodeficiency, or adjacent infection. Given the filtering function of the spleen, an abscess can form as a result of any metastatic hematogenous infection, such as endocarditis. Although rare, splenic abscess can be a delayed complication of the nonoperative management of splenic injuries. Splenic infarcts associated with hemoglobinopathies such as sickle-cell disease may become secondarily infected and form an abscess.[16] Immunodeficiency, such as malignancy or acquired immunodeficiency syndrome, is another significant risk factor for the development of multiple splenic abscesses.[39,53,58]

Rarely, infection or disease in a contiguous focus may extend to the spleen. In a review of 56 children with splenic abscesses, 7 (12.5%) were cryptogenic with no apparent cause.[39] In most instances, a single pathogen is isolated, with *S. aureus*, streptococci, *E. coli*, and *Salmonella* spp. being the most common. Fungi, most often *Candida* spp., have been isolated from splenic abscesses primarily in immunocompromised hosts.[39,53,58]

CLINICAL MANIFESTATIONS

The typical clinical features of an intra-abdominal abscess include fever, abdominal pain, and tenderness over the involved area. Subphrenic abscesses also may be manifested as referred pain or pulmonary or pleuritic symptoms. Pancreatic abscess may be associated with a palpable epigastric mass and elevated serum lipase and amylase.[12] Splenomegaly or a splenic mass may be noted in approximately half of patients with splenic abscesses.[39] In postoperative patients, persistence of abdominal symptoms or fever warrants evaluation for an intraperitoneal abscess.[3] Leukocytosis (20,000 to 50,000 cells/mm³) frequently is present in children with an intra-abdominal abscess.[3,37]

DIAGNOSIS

Imaging studies are helpful in diagnosing an intra-abdominal abscess. Plain radiographs are useful as an initial procedure and may show an extraintestinal air-fluid level, right lower quadrant mass, or localized ileus.[1] Chest radiographs should be obtained because subphrenic abscesses often are associated with a pleural effusion. In a series of 27 children with splenic abscesses, chest radiographs were abnormal in 20 cases, with the most common findings being left pleural effusion and an elevated left hemidiaphragm.[39] Ultrasonography is a useful noninvasive technique that can detect abdominal and pelvic abscesses. The quality of the images depends on the examiner, however. In addition, conditions such as ileus, postoperative drains, or dressings may hinder ultrasound detection of an abscess.[1,47,50] CT is the most sensitive tool for detecting an intra-abdominal abscess, and it provides good anatomic resolution. Disadvantages of CT are the radiation and, if used, exposure to intravenous, oral, or rectal contrast material.[1,47,50]

Although more recent experience with the use of magnetic resonance imaging for detecting an intraperitoneal abscess has been described in the literature,[54] this modality should be considered in children only when an abscess may not be detected more easily by other methods or in patients who should not have exposure to radiation.[54] Gallium scanning is a sensitive technique for diagnosing an abscess, but it is nonspecific, particularly in the abdomen.[1]

TREATMENT

Management of an intra-abdominal abscess includes physiologic and nutritional support, antimicrobial therapy, and drainage. After blood cultures have been obtained, empiric antibiotic therapy should be instituted with agents effective against anaerobes, Enterobacteriaceae, and other enteric flora as discussed earlier for peritonitis. Antibiotic therapy usually is begun before surgery is done to minimize any complications of bacteremia during the procedure. Abscess material should be obtained for culture of aerobic, anaerobic, fungal, and mycobacterial pathogens. Effective surgical management depends on accurate localization of the abscess, discrimination between single and multiple abscesses, and early and adequate drainage.[3,4,46] Traditional therapy for intraperitoneal abscesses has relied on open surgical drainage, although drainage of intraperitoneal abscesses percutaneously under ultrasound or CT guidance now is used often.[1,18,21,46,50,59]

In instances of multiple intraperitoneal abscesses or if the source of peritoneal contamination has not been controlled, laparotomy is indicated.[46] Pancreatic abscesses require intensive surgical and medical therapy. Antimicrobial therapy for mixed aerobic and anaerobic infection is suggested,[12] but splenectomy remains the definitive treatment of bacterial splenic abscesses. In selected patients, percutaneous drainage or splenotomy has the advantage of preserving splenic function, however.[39,53,58] Multiple small splenic abscesses and fungal lesions generally are treated medically.[39] Antibiotic therapy for a pyogenic splenic abscess should be guided by the pathogens associated with the child's underlying condition. Therapy should include antibiotics effective against *S. aureus*, streptococci, and gram-negative enteric bacilli. Specific therapy should be revised after culture and susceptibility results are available.

COMPLICATIONS

Intraperitoneal and visceral abscesses, if not adequately drained, may be associated with significant complications, including ongoing spread of the infectious process and, for splenic or pancreatic abscesses, a high mortality rate. Fistula formation, adhesions, and bowel obstruction may be late complications of intra-abdominal infection.

REFERENCES

1. Afshani, E.: Computed tomography of abdominal abscesses in children. Radiol. Clin. North Am. *19*:515-526, 1981.
2. Aldridge, K. E., Ashcraft, D., Cambre, K., et al.: Multicenter survey of the changing in vitro antimicrobial susceptibilities of clinical isolates of *Bacteroides fragilis* group, *Prevotella*, *Fusobacterium*, *Porphyromonas*, and *Peptostreptococcus* species. Antimicrob. Agents Chemother. *45*:1238-1243, 2001.
3. Altemeier, W. A., Culbertson, W. R., and Fuller, W. D.: Intra-abdominal sepsis. Adv. Surg. *5*:281-333, 1971.
4. Altemeier, W. A., Culbertson, W. R., Fuller, W. D., et al.: Intra-abdominal abscesses. Am. J. Surg. *125*:70-79, 1973.
5. Baird, C., O'Connor, D., and Pittman, T.: Late shunt infections. Pediatr. Neurosurg. *31*:269-273, 1999.
6. Blakely, M. L., Spurbeck, W. W., and Lobe, T. E.: Current status of laparoscopic appendectomy in children. Semin. Pediatr. Surg. *7*:225-227, 1998.
7. Bohnen, J. M., Solomkin, J. S., Dellinger, E. P., et al.: Guidelines for clinical care: Anti-infective agents for intra-abdominal infection. A Surgical Infection Society policy statement. Arch. Surg. *127*:83-89, 1992.
8. Bradley, J. S., Behrendt, C. E., Arrieta, A. C., et al.: Convalescent phase outpatient parenteral antiinfective therapy for children with complicated appendicitis. Pediatr. Infect. Dis. J. *20*:19-24, 2001.
9. Bradley, J. S., Faulkner, K. L., and Klugman, K. P.: Efficacy, safety and tolerability of meropenem as empiric antibiotic therapy in hospitalized pediatric patients. Pediatr. Infect. Dis. J. *15*:749-757, 1996.
10. Brook, I.: Intra-abdominal abscess in children: A 13 year experience. Hosp. Pract. *25*:20-23, 1990.
11. Brook, I.: Intra-abdominal infections in children: Pathogenesis, diagnosis and management. Drugs *46*:53-62, 1993.
12. Brook, I., and Frazier, E. H.: Microbiological analysis of pancreatic abscess. Clin. Infect. Dis. *22*:384-385, 1996.
13. Brook, I., and Frazier, E. H.: Aerobic and anaerobic microbiology of retroperitoneal abscesses. Clin. Infect. Dis. *26*:938-941, 1998.
14. Bufo, A. J., Shah, R. S., Li, M. H., et al.: Interval appendectomy for perforated appendicitis in children. J. Laparoendosc. Adv. Surg. Tech. A *8*:209-214, 1998.
15. Canon, H. L., Buckingham, S. C., Wyatt, R. J., et al.: Fungal peritonitis caused by *Curvularia* species in a child undergoing peritoneal dialysis. Pediatr. Nephrol. *16*:35-37, 2001.
16. Chun, C. H., Raff, M. J., Contreras, L., et al.: Splenic abscess. Medicine (Baltimore) *59*:50-65, 1980.
17. Clark, J. H., Fitzgerald, J. F., and Kleiman, M. B.: Spontaneous bacterial peritonitis. J. Pediatr. *104*:495-500, 1984.
18. Clark, R. A., and Towbin, R.: Abscess drainage with CT and ultrasound guidance. Radiol. Clin. North Am. *21*:445-459, 1983.
19. Collins, M. D., Dajani, A. S., Kim, K. S., et al.: Comparison of ampicillin/sulbactam plus aminoglycoside vs. ampicillin plus clindamycin plus aminoglycoside in the treatment of intraabdominal infections in children. Pediatr. Infect. Dis. J. *17*(Suppl.):15-18, 1998.

20. Dankner, W. M., and Davis, C. E.: *Mycobacterium bovis* as a significant cause of tuberculosis in children residing along the United States-Mexico border in the Baja California region. Pediatrics *105*:E79, 2000.
21. Diament, M. J., Stanley, P., Kangarloo, H., and Donaldson, J. S.: Percutaneous aspiration and catheter drainage of abscesses. J. Pediatr. *108*:204-208, 1986.
22. Dougherty, S. H., Sirinek, K. R., Schauer, P. R., et al.: Ticarcillin/clavulanate compared with clindamycin/gentamicin (with or without ampicillin) for the treatment of intra-abdominal infections in pediatric and adult patients. Am. Surg. *61*:297-303, 1995.
23. Dunn, D. L., Barke, R. A., Ahrenholz, D. H., et al.: The adjuvant effect of peritoneal fluid in experimental peritonitis: Mechanism and clinical implications. Ann. Surg. *199*:37-43, 1984.
24. Dunn, D. L., Barke, R. A., Knight, N. B., et al.: Role of resident macrophages, peripheral neutrophils, and translymphatic absorption in bacterial clearance from the peritoneal cavity. Infect. Immun. *49*:257-264, 1985.
25. Enriquez, J. L., Kalia, A., and Travis, L. B.: Fungal peritonitis in children on peritoneal dialysis. J. Pediatr. *117*:830-832, 1990.
26. Feinstein, E. I., Chesney, R. W., and Zelikovic, I.: Peritonitis in childhood renal disease. Am. J. Nephrol. *8*:147-165, 1988.
27. Fishman, S. J., Pelosi, L., Klavon, S. L., et al.: Perforated appendicitis: Prospective outcome analysis for 150 children. J. Pediatr. Surg. *35*:923-926, 2000.
28. Ford, E. G., Hardin, W. D., Mahour, G. H., et al.: Pseudocysts of the pancreas in children. Am. Surg. *56*:384-387, 1990.
29. Freij, B. J., Votteler, T. P., and McCracken, G. H.: Primary peritonitis in previously healthy children. Am. J. Dis. Child. *138*:1058-1061, 1984.
30. Gaskill, S. J., and Marlin, A. E.: Spontaneous bacterial peritonitis in patients with ventriculoperitoneal shunts. Pediatr. Neurosurg. *26*:115-119, 1997.
31. Gorensek, M. J., Lebel, M. H., and Nelson, J. D.: Peritonitis in children with nephrotic syndrome. Pediatrics *81*:849-856, 1988.
32. Graham, J. C., Moss, P. J., and McKendrick, M. W.: Primary group A streptococcal peritonitis. Scand. J. Infect. Dis. *27*:171-172, 1995.
33. Grosfeld, J. L., Cooney, D. R., Smith, J., et al.: Intra-abdominal complications following ventriculoperitoneal shunt procedures. Pediatrics *54*:791-796, 1974.
34. Gurkan, F., Ozates, M., Bosnak, M., et al.: Tuberculous peritonitis in 11 children: Clinical features and diagnostic approach. Pediatr. Int. *41*:510-513, 1999.
35. Jakubowski, A., Elwood, R. K., and Enarson, D. A.: Clinical features of abdominal tuberculosis. J. Infect. Dis. *158*:687-692, 1988.
36. Jelloul, L., Fremond, B., Dyon, J. F., et al.: Mesenteric adenitis caused by *Yersinia pseudotuberculosis* presenting as an abdominal mass. Eur. J. Pediatr. Surg. *7*:180-283, 1997.
37. Johnson, C. C., Baldessarre, J., and Levison, M. E.: Peritonitis: Update on pathophysiology, clinical manifestations, and management. Clin. Infect. Dis. *24*:1035-1047, 1997.
38. Kaplan, S. L.: Antibiotic usage in appendicitis in children. Pediatr. Infect. Dis. J. *17*:1047-1048, 1998.
39. Keidl, C. M., and Chusid, M. J.: Splenic abscesses in childhood. Pediatr. Infect. Dis. J. *8*:368-373, 1989.
40. Kimber, C. P., and Hutson, J. M.: Primary peritonitis in children. Aust. N. Z. J. Surg. *66*:169-170, 1996.
41. Krensky, A. M., Ingelfinger, J. R., and Grupe, W. E.: Peritonitis in childhood nephrotic syndrome. Am. J. Dis. Child. *136*:732-736, 1982.
42. Lamps, L. W., Madhusukhan, K. T., Greenson, J. K., et al.: The role of *Yersinia enterocolitica* and *Yersinia pseudotuberculosis* in granulomatous appendicitis: A histologic and molecular study. Am. J. Surg. Pathol. *25*:508-515, 2001.
43. Lund, D. P., and Murphy, E. U.: Management of perforated appendicitis in children: A decade of aggressive treatment. J. Pediatr. Surg. *29*:1130-1134, 1994.
44. Malangoni, M. A.: Evaluation and management of tertiary peritonitis. Am. Surg. *66*:157-161, 2000.
45. Markenson, D. S., Levine, D., and Schacht, R.: Primary peritonitis as a presenting feature of nephrotic syndrome: A case report and review of the literature. Pediatr. Emerg. Care *15*:407-409, 1999.
46. McClean, K. L., Sheehan, G. J., and Harding, G. K. M.: Intraabdominal infection: A review. Clin. Infect. Dis. *19*:100-116, 1994.
47. McConkey, S. J., McCarthy, N. D., and Keane, C. T.: Primary peritonitis due to nonenteric salmonellae. Clin. Infect. Dis. *29*:211-212, 1999.
48. Melez, K. A., Cherry, J., Sanchez, C., et al.: Successful outpatient treatment of *Trichosporon beigelii* peritonitis with oral fluconazole. Pediatr. Infect. Dis. J. *14*:1110-1113, 1995.
49. Meller, J. L., Reyes, H. M., Loeff, D. S., et al.: One drug versus two-drug antibiotic therapy in pediatric perforated appendicitis: A prospective randomized study. Surgery *110*:764-768, 1991.
50. Montgomery, R. S., and Wilson, S. E.: Intraabdominal abscesses: Image-guided diagnosis and therapy. Clin. Infect. Dis. *23*:28-36, 1996.
51. Neblett, W. W., Pietsch, J. B., and Holcomb, G. W., Jr.: Acute abdominal conditions in children and adolescents. Surg. Clin. North Am. *68*:415-430, 1988.
52. Neilson, I. R., Laberge, J. M., Nguyen, L. T., et al.: Appendicitis in children: Current therapeutic recommendations. J. Pediatr. Surg. *25*:1113-1116, 1990.
53. Nelken, N., Ignatius, J., Skinner, M., et al.: Changing clinical spectrum of splenic abscess: A multicenter study and review of the literature. Am. J. Surg. *154*:27-34, 1987.

54. Noone, T. C., Semelka, R. C., Worawattanakul, S., et al.: Intraperitoneal abscesses: Diagnostic accuracy of and appearances at MR imaging. Radiology 208:525-528, 1998.
55. Odio, C., McCracken, G. H., and Nelson, J. D.: CSF shunt infections in pediatrics: A seven-year experience. Am. J. Dis. Child. 138:1103-1108, 1984.
56. Oh, S. H., Conley, S. B., Rose, G. M., et al.: Fungal peritonitis in children undergoing peritoneal dialysis. Pediatr. Infect. Dis. J. 4:62-66, 1985.
57. Olika, D., Yamini, D., Udani, V. M., et al.: Nonoperative management of perforated appendicitis without periappendiceal mass. Am. J. Surg. 179:177-181, 2000.
58. Phillips, G. S., Radosevich, M. D., and Lipsett, P. A.: Splenic abscess: Another look at an old disease. Arch. Surg. 132:1331-1336, 1997.
59. Ramakrishnan, M. R., and Sarathy, T. K. P.: Percutaneous drainage of splenic abscess: Case report and review of literature. Pediatrics 79:1029-1031, 1987.
60. Rekate, H. L., Yonas, H., White, R. J., et al.: The acute abdomen in patients with ventriculoperitoneal shunts. Surg. Neurol. 11:442-445, 1979.
61. Reynolds, M., Sherman, J. O., and Mclone, D. G.: Ventriculoperitoneal shunt infection masquerading as an acute surgical abdomen. J. Pediatr. Surg. 18:951-955, 1983.
62. Schwartz, M. Z., Tapper, D., and Solenberger, R. I.: Management of perforated appendicitis in children: The controversy continues. Ann. Surg. 197:407-411, 1983.
63. Sells, C. J., and Loeser, J. D.: Peritonitis following perforation of the bowel: A rare complication of a ventriculoperitoneal shunt. J. Pediatr. 83:823-824, 1973.
64. Simon, G. L., and Gorbach, S. L.: Intestinal flora in health and disease. Gastroenterology 86:174-193, 1984.
65. Sioson, P. B., Stechenberg, B. W., Courtney, R., et al.: Tuberculous peritonitis in a three-year-old boy: Case report and review of the literature. Pediatr. Infect. Dis. J. 11:409-411, 1992.
66. Sirotnak, A. P., Eppes, S. C., and Klein, J. D.: Tuboovarian abscess and peritonitis caused by Streptococcus pneumoniae serotype 1 in young girls. Clin. Infect. Dis. 22:993-996, 1996.
67. Snow, R. B., Lavyne, M. H., and Fraser, R. A. R.: Colonic perforation by ventriculoperitoneal shunts. Surg. Neurol. 25:173-177, 1986.
68. Stamos, J. K., Kaufman, B. A., and Yogev, R.: Ventriculoperitoneal shunt infections with gram-negative bacteria. Neurosurgery 33:858-862, 1993.
69. Stone, H. H., Bourneuf, A. A., and Stinson, L. D.: Reliability of criteria for predicting persistent or recurrent sepsis. Arch. Surg. 120:17-20, 1985.
70. Such, J., and Runyon, B. A.: Spontaneous bacterial peritonitis. Clin. Infect. Dis. 27:669-676, 1998.
71. Tain, Y. L., Lin, G. J., and Cher, T. W.: Microbiological spectrum of septicemia and peritonitis in nephrotic children. Pediatr. Nephrol. 13:835-837, 1999.
72. Tchirkow, G., and Verhagen, A. D.: Bacterial peritonitis in patients with ventriculoperitoneal shunt. J. Pediatr. Surg. 14:182-184, 1979.
73. Uhari, M., Seppanen, J., and Heikkinen, E.: Imipenem-cilastatin vs. tobramycin and metronidazole for appendicitis-related infections. Pediatr. Infect. Dis. J. 11:445-450, 1992.
74. Vargas, H. I., Averbook, A., and Stamos, M. J.: Appendiceal mass: Conservative therapy followed by interval laparoscopic appendectomy. Am. Surg. 60:753-758, 1994.
75. Veeragandham, R. S., Lynch, F. P., Canty, T. G., et al.: Abdominal tuberculosis in children: Review of 26 cases. J. Pediatr. Surg. 31:170-176, 1996.
76. Warady, B. A., Bashir, M., and Donaldson, L. A.: Fungal peritonitis in children receiving peritoneal dialysis: A report of the NAPRTCS. Kidney Int. 58:384-389, 2000.
77. White, R., Abreo, K., Flanagan, R., et al.: Nontuberculous mycobacterial infections in continuous ambulatory peritoneal dialysis patients. Am. J. Kidney Dis. 22:581-587, 1993.
78. Wilfert, C. M., and Katz, S. L.: Etiology of bacterial sepsis in nephrotic children 1963-1967. Pediatrics 42:840-843, 1968.
79. Wittmann, D. H., Schein, M., and Condon, R. E.: Management of secondary peritonitis. Ann. Surg. 224:10-18, 1996.
80. Younger, J. J., Simmons, J. C. H., and Barrett, F. F.: Occult distal ventriculoperitoneal shunt infections. Pediatr. Infect. Dis. J. 4:557-558, 1985.

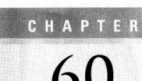

RETROPERITONEAL INFECTIONS

CHAPTER 60

Alice Pong ☯ **John S. Bradley**

Retroperitoneal infections consist primarily of suppurative bacterial infections that originate within the retroperitoneal structures or as an extension from another primary site. In children, these infections are much less common than are intra-abdominal infections; however, they can lead to significant morbidity if missed. Establishing a diagnosis can be difficult because symptoms often are indolent and poorly localized.

The retroperitoneal structures are separated from the intra-abdominal organs by the posterior peritoneal fascia (Fig. 60–1). Structures posterior to this fascia layer, in the anterior retroperitoneal space, include the duodenum, pancreas, and parts of the colon. The kidneys and ureters are encased further by the renal fascia. The iliopsoas and psoas muscles lie at the posterior aspect of the retroperitoneal space and are separated from the other retroperitoneal structures by the transversalis fascia. Pelvic structures, including the bladder, uterus, and rectum, that lie inferior to the pelvic peritoneum constitute the pelvic portion of the retroperitoneal space. The fascial layers limit the spread of retroperitoneal infections. However, the deep location can be difficult to assess by physical examination.

ETIOLOGY AND PATHOGENESIS

Retroperitoneal infections in children arise in numerous anatomic structures. Brook[6] reviewed cases of retroperitoneal infections from five U.S. hospitals from 1974 to 1994. Of 41 children identified, 21 had infections in the anterior retroperitoneal space related to the pancreas (4) and intestines (13), 6 had perinephric abscesses, 7 had iliopsoas abscesses, and 7 had pelvic retroperitoneal abscesses (Fig. 60–2).

Primary infection of the retroperitoneal space can be hematogenous in origin or complicate an ascending urinary tract infection. Secondary infections occur as a direct extension from gastrointestinal perforations, such as ruptured appendices or those related to Crohn disease.[6,19,20] Greenstein and associates[19] reported retroperitoneal abscesses in 12 of 231 patients with Crohn disease. Retroperitoneal infections also can develop secondary to primary infections of the vertebral spine, pelvic bones, and sacroiliac joint.[21,33,36] Suppurative iliac or retroperitoneal lymph nodes are another source of retroperitoneal infections. Prior surgery has been reported as a predisposing factor in perinephric abscesses[7,16] and in vascular grafts in adults.[8] Pancreatic abscesses are seen more frequently in adult patients and are associated with underlying biliary tract disease, alcoholism, surgery, and trauma.[9]

Infections of the perinephric retroperitoneal space include those involving the kidney and adrenal glands. Perinephric abscesses can result from bacteremic inoculation of renal tissue or as a consequence of an ascending urinary tract infection. Nephronia (i.e., focal renal cellulitis) is thought to be an intermediate stage of renal infection between pyelonephritis and renal abscess, resulting from an ascending infection of the urinary tract.[31] Adrenal abscesses are reported more frequently in neonates than in older children and are thought to be related to adrenal hemorrhages that become secondarily infected.[28]

Iliopsoas abscesses may be a consequence of hematogenous seeding of the muscle, with trauma as a predisposing factor (see Fig. 60–2).[20,32] Although primary infection occurs most commonly,[5] the iliopsoas muscle extends from the ribs and lumbar vertebrae to its insertion on the femur and is exposed to the risk of extension of infection from numerous adjacent structures.

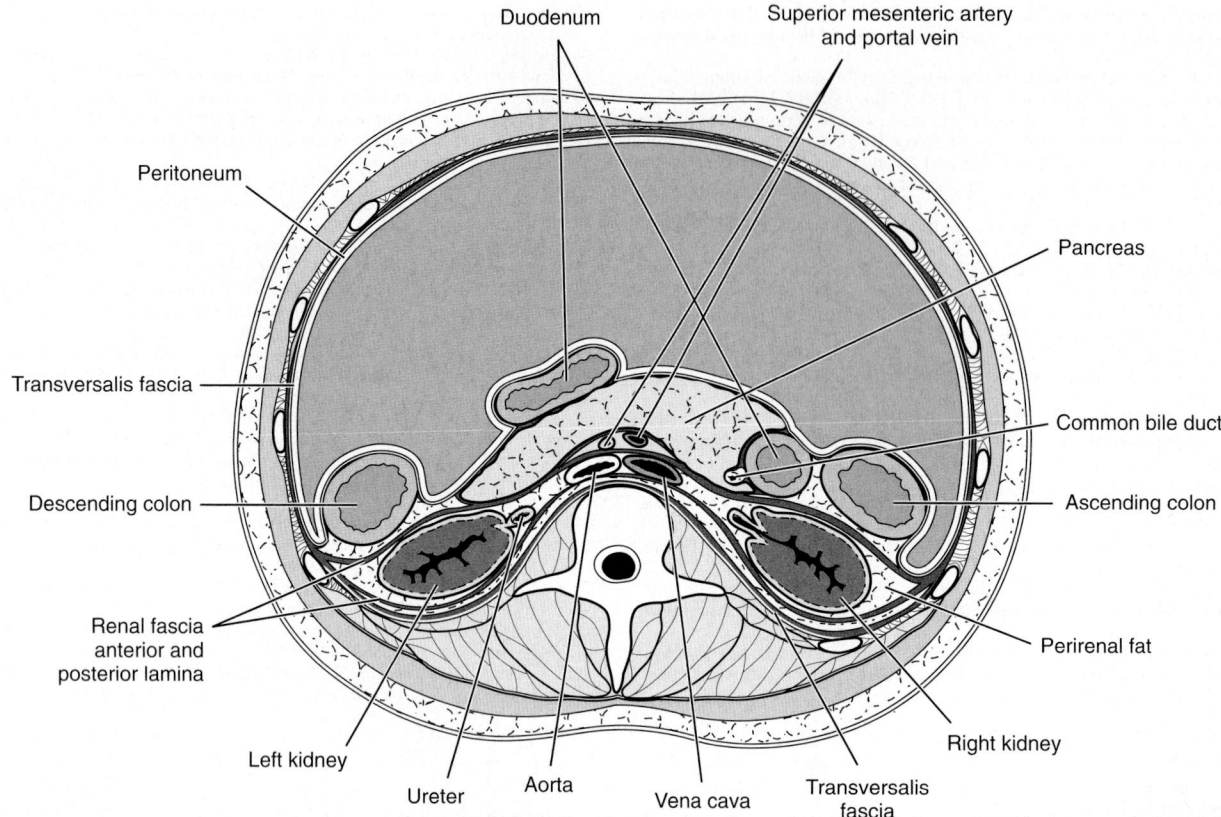

Figure 60–1 A cross section of abdomen at L2 shows the structures within the retroperitoneal space. *(From Altemeier, W. A., and Alexander, J. W.: Retroperitoneal abscess. Arch. Surg. 83:515, 1961, with permission.)*

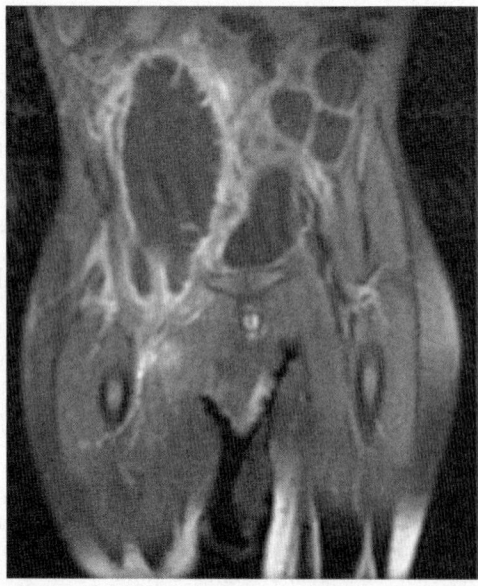

Figure 60–2 Large iliopsoas abscess seen on magnetic resonance imaging. Coronal view with contrast enhancement.

Psoas abscesses have developed as a consequence of vertebral infections, intestinal perforations, and genitourinary sources and as an extension of primary pelvic osteomyelitis.[20,22,31,33] Neonatal iliopsoas abs-cesses also have been reported and present with symptoms similar to those of a septic hip.[14,17,30]

Complications of retroperitoneal abscesses include both rupture into the intraperitoneal space and extension of the infec-tion along fascial planes to adjacent muscles that extend from origins in the pelvis and trunk to insertion sites on the femur. Rupture into the thoracic cavity also has been reported.[1] Other reported complications include pneumonia, recurrent abscess, renal failure, and venous and arterial thrombosis.[12]

MICROBIOLOGY

The microbiology of retroperitoneal infections is determined by the source of the infection and the retroperitoneal compart-ment involved. Most primary infections thought to result from bacteremia are caused by *Staphylococcus aureus*. Secondary infection related to the gastrointestinal tract is caused by mixed bowel flora including *Escherichia coli*, other gram-negative enteric bacteria, *Pseudomonas* spp., and gastrointestinal anaerobes, particularly *Bacteroides fragilis* and *Peptostreptococcus*.[6] Most infections in the anterior retroperitoneal space are associ-ated with a gastrointestinal source and may be polymicrobial.[4] *Actinomyces* infections, although seen more commonly in the cervicofacial area, also can present as retroperitoneal infections.[3,25]

Ascending infections from the urinary tract usually are caused by *E. coli*. However, perinephric abscesses also are reported as a complication of renal infection caused by *S. aureus*, group B streptococcus, and *Salmonella*.[16,38,39]

S. aureus is the leading pathogen isolated in iliopsoas abscesses unless the infection is secondary to erosion of a primary gastro-intestinal focus. In that situation, gram-negative enteric bacteria and anaerobes are more likely to be the causative agents.[5,32] Ret-roperitoneal necrotizing fasciitis from group A streptococcus also has been reported.[13]

Tuberculosis caused by *Mycobacterium tuberculosis* or *Mycobacterium bovis* may involve the retroperitoneal space as an extension of vertebral tuberculous osteomyelitis.[1,15,22] Abdominal tuberculosis usually is manifested as an intraperitoneal infection but can produce retroperitoneal adenopathy.

CLINICAL PRESENTATION

Children with retroperitoneal infections present clinically in a variety of ways, ranging from nonspecific fever to overwhelming sepsis. The most common clinical symptoms associated with retroperitoneal infections include fever and pain in the hip, back, and abdomen.[12,26] Psoas abscesses often are manifested with the child's limping or refusing to walk.[5] Neonates with a retroperitoneal abscess may present with an abdominal mass.[34] Symptoms often are vague, and pain is not well localized. Patients often have been evaluated previously for fevers and have been treated with antibiotics before a diagnosis has been made.[5,24,33] A delay in establishing the diagnosis is not uncommon.

DIFFERENTIAL DIAGNOSIS

Retroperitoneal infections can be confused with a variety of other infections. Limp and fever caused by pyogenic arthritis of the hip and infection of the sacroiliac joint and pelvic bones occur more commonly than do retroperitoneal infections. Abdominal pain and fever are seen more frequently in patients with intra-abdominal infections, including appendicitis and intra-abdominal abscesses. Trauma and malignant disease are more frequent causes of retroperitoneal masses compared with infectious causes and should be considered.

SPECIFIC DIAGNOSIS

Laboratory tests often are nonspecific and of minimal benefit. Sedimentation rates and leukocyte counts often are elevated.[5,6,32,33] Pyuria often is absent in children with perinephric and renal abscesses, and the urine culture may be negative.[7,16,37,38] However, in patients with nephronia, pyuria and positive urine cultures are more likely.[24,31] Blood cultures may be helpful in identifying a bacterial pathogen. Brook[6] reported that 40 percent of blood cultures were positive for the same organism isolated from abscesses in children with retroperitoneal infections who had blood culture specimens collected. For children with psoas abscesses, Santaella and colleagues[32] reported that 71 percent of blood cultures were positive.

Imaging studies are the most useful diagnostic tools. Ultrasonography can be used to diagnose perinephric infections[7,37] and has been used to diagnose abscesses of the iliopsoas muscle.[20] Computed tomography (CT) with contrast enhancement appears to be the most helpful[11,12,32] because of superior delineation of organ involvement and the extent of infection as well as wide availability and rapid imaging times compared with magnetic resonance imaging (MRI). CT also can provide clues about the primary focus of the infection, thereby helping guide empiric antibiotic therapy. Abscess fluid is seen on CT as areas of low attenuation, often with an enhancing rim.[11,23,38] Percutaneous drainage and biopsy of the lesions also may be accomplished with CT. Although alternative diagnoses also can be evaluated with CT,[35] hematomas and certain tumors may not be distinguished easily radiographically from infection. These noninfectious entities may be identified better by MRI. Another advantage of MRI over CT is superior visualization of bone and inflamed muscle tissue, although calcifications may not be as well identified.[29]

TREATMENT

Percutaneous or open surgical drainage should be considered for all retroperitoneal infections for both diagnostic and treatment purposes. Culture of the aspirated fluid for aerobic and anaerobic bacteria, mycobacteria, and fungi is vital to selection of appropriate antimicrobial therapy. Reports of percutaneous drainage of perinephric abscesses and iliopsoas abscesses are increasing in number.[5,22] These procedures usually are performed with ultrasound or CT guidance. Treatment of patients with antibiotics alone without surgical drainage may not be effective, particularly in cases involving larger abscesses.[1,11]

Initial antimicrobial therapy for retroperitoneal infections should be directed by the presumed source of the infection, with definitive therapy guided by microbiologic culture results. Infections related to gastrointestinal perforation should include coverage directed primarily against enteric gram-negative bacteria and gastrointestinal anaerobes such as β-lactamase–producing *B. fragilis*. Coverage for *Pseudomonas* and *Enterococcus* spp. also should be considered. Historically, antibiotic combinations such as ampicillin for enterococcus, metronidazole or clindamycin for anaerobes, and a third-generation cephalosporin or aminoglycoside for gram-negative bacteria have been used. However, carbapenems such as meropenem, imipenem, and ertapenem as single agents may be more cost effective, particularly if any outpatient antibiotic therapy is being considered. The β-lactam and β-lactamase inhibitor combinations (e.g., ticarcillin-clavulanate, piperacillin-tazobactam), with or without an aminoglycoside, also are likely to be effective.

Infections of renal origin, usually caused by *E. coli* or other gram-negative enteric organisms, can be treated with extended-spectrum cephalosporins such as ceftriaxone or, if abscesses have been drained successfully, with aminoglycosides such as gentamicin and tobramycin. The activity of aminoglycosides may be compromised by the acidic environment of abscess cavities and may lead to clinical failures despite in vitro susceptibility of the organism.[10] Increasingly, resistance to ampicillin is seen in *E. coli*,[2,4] rendering it unreliable for empiric use in severe urinary tract infections. *Pseudomonas* is not an uncommon pathogen in children with recurrent infections caused by anatomic genitourinary abnormalities.[2] *Pseudomonas* spp. usually are resistant to ceftriaxone; extended-spectrum cephalosporins, such as ceftazidime and cefepime, or carbapenems may be needed. Urine culture and susceptibility results help focus the choice of an antibiotic to the narrowest spectrum agent required.

Psoas abscesses and primary perinephric abscesses caused by *S. aureus* should be treated with an antistaphylococcal agent such as nafcillin (or oxacillin or methicillin) or a first-generation cephalosporin such as cefazolin. The prevalence of community-acquired methicillin-resistant *S. aureus* (CA-MRSA) has increased significantly as a soft tissue pathogen, particularly in children.[18,27] Vancomycin or clindamycin should be considered as empiric therapy for serious infections in areas with high rates of CA-MRSA (>5% of all invasive *S. aureus* infections) until culture results are available. These agents also may be effective in treating the patient who is unable to tolerate penicillin or cephalosporin antibiotics.

Infections originating in the vertebrae usually are caused by *S. aureus* or may result from tuberculosis. Empiric antistaphylococcal therapy can be started, but culture and histologic examination of tissue are needed to direct appropriate therapy. For the child with risk factors for acquiring tuberculosis, a positive tuberculin skin test result, and a negative Gram stain result, empiric therapy with three or four antituberculous antibiotics should be considered. A chest radiograph should be obtained to look for evidence of pulmonary tuberculosis.

After adequate drainage is achieved, the duration of antimicrobial therapy depends on several factors, including the organism, the site and extent of infection, and the clinical improvement. Most drained retroperitoneal bacterial abscesses of renal or muscle origin are treated for 2 to 3 weeks with initial parenteral and follow-up oral antibiotics. Infections involving bone may require 6 to 8 weeks or longer, depending on how quickly the infection responds to treatment. Radiographic studies, erythrocyte sedimentation rate, and C-reactive protein measurements can be helpful to monitor recovery. Tuberculous infections are treated for 6 to 12 months, depending on the presence of bone involvement. *Actinomyces* infection can be difficult to treat because of lack of susceptibility to many antibiotics and the need for prolonged courses of antibiotic therapy, preferentially with penicillin.

PROGNOSIS

Historically, retroperitoneal abscesses are reported to have high morbidity and mortality rates. However, with modern imaging techniques enabling physicians to make more timely diagnoses, the overall prognosis is good, and most children with no underlying disease recover without sequelae.

REFERENCES

1. Altemeier, W. A., and Alexander, J. W.: Retroperitoneal abscess. Arch. Surg. *83*:512-524, 1961.
2. Ashkenazi, S., Even-Tov, S., Samra, Z., et al.: Uropathogens of various childhood populations and their antibiotic susceptibility. Pediatr. Infect. Dis. J. *10*:742-746, 1991.
3. Benammar, S., Helardot, P. F., Sapin, E., et al.: Childhood actinomycosis: Report of two cases. Eur. J. Pediatr. Surg. *5*:180-183, 1995.
4. Bonadio, W. A., Smith, D. S., Madagame, E., et al.: *Escherichia coli* bacteremia in children. Am. J. Dis. Child. *145*:671-674, 1991.
5. Bresee, J. S., and Edwards, M. S.: Psoas abscess in children. Pediatr. Infect. Dis. J. *9*:201-206, 1990.
6. Brook, I: Microbiology of retroperitoneal abscesses in children. J. Med. Microbiol. *48*:697-700, 1999.
7. Brook, I.: The role of anaerobic bacteria in perinephric and renal abscesses in children. Pediatrics *93*:261-264, 1994.
8. Brook, I., and Frazier, E. H.: Aerobic and anaerobic microbiology of retroperitoneal abscesses. Clin. Infect. Dis. *26*:938-941, 1998.
9. Brook, I., and Frazier, E. H.: Microbiological analysis of pancreatic abscess. Clin. Infect. Dis. *22*:384-385, 1996.
10. Bryant, R. E., Fox, K., Oh, G., and Morthland, V. H.: β-Lactam enhancement of aminoglycoside activity under conditions of reduced pH and oxygen tension that may exist in infected tissues. J. Infect. Dis. *165*:676-682, 1992.
11. Chen, W. C., Huang, J. K., Chen, K. K., et al.: Retroperitoneal abscesses. Chin. Med. J. *46*:208-212, 1990.
12. Crepps, J. T., Welch, J. P., and Orlando, R., III: Management and outcome of retroperitoneal abscesses. Ann. Surg. *205*:276-281, 1987.
13. Devin, B., McCarthy, A., Mehran, R., and Auger, C.: Necrotizing fasciitis of the retroperitoneum: An unusual presentation of group A *Streptococcus* infection. Can. J. Surg. *41*:156-160, 1998.
14. Dib, M., Bedu, A., Garel, C., et al.: Ilio-psoas abscess in neonates: Treatment by ultrasound-guided percutaneous drainage. Pediatr. Radiol. *30*:677-680, 2000.
15. Dinc, H., Onder, C., Turhan, A. U., et al.: Percutaneous catheter drainage of tuberculous and nontuberculous psoas abscesses. Eur. J. Radiol. *23*:130-134, 1996.
16. Edelstein, H., and McCabe, R. E.: Perinephric abscess in pediatric patients: Report of six cases and review of the literature. Pediatr. Infect. Dis. J. *8*:167-170, 1989.
17. Feo, C. F., Dessanti, A., Franco, B., et al.: Retroperitoneal abscess and omphalitis in young infants. Acta Paediatr. *92*:122-125, 2003.
18. Frank, A. L., Marcinak, J. F., Mangat, D., et al.: Community-acquired and clindamycin susceptible methicillin-resistant *Staphylococcus aureus* in children. Pediatr. Infect. Dis. J. *18*:993-1000, 1999.
19. Greenstein, A. J., Dreiling, D. A., and Aufses, A. H., Jr.: Crohn's disease of the colon. Am. J. Gastroenterol. *64*:306-318, 1975.
20. Hoffer, F. A., Shamberger, R. C., and Teele, R. L.: Ilio-psoas abscess: Diagnosis and management. Pediatr. Radiol. *17*:23-27, 1987.
21. Holliday, P. O., III, Davis, C. H., Jr., and Shaffner, L. S: Intervertebral disc space infection in a child presenting as a psoas abscess: Case report. Neurosurgery 7:395-397, 1980.
22. Kang, M., Gupta, S., Gulati, M., and Suri, S.: Ilio-psoas abscess in the paediatric population: Treatment by US-guided percutaneous drainage. Pediatr. Radiol. *28*:478-481, 1998.
23. Kuhns, L. R.: Computed tomography of the retroperitoneum in children. Radiol. Clin. North Am. *19*:495-501, 1981.
24. Kline, M. W., Kaplan, S. L., and Baker, C. J.: Acute focal bacterial nephritis: Diverse clinical presentations in pediatric patients. Pediatr. Infect. Dis. J. 7:346-349, 1988.
25. Latawiec-Mazurkiewicz, I., Juszkiewicz, P., Pacanowski, J., et al.: Tumour-like inflammatory abdominal conditions in children. Eur. J. Pediatr. Surg. *15*:38-43, 2005.
26. March, A. W., Riley, L. H., and Robinson, R. A.: Retroperitoneal abscess and septic arthritis of the hip in children. J. Bone Joint Surg. Am. *54*:67-74, 1972.
27. Martinez-Aguilar, G., Avalos-Mishaan, A., Hulten, K., et al.: Community-acquired, methicillin-resistant and methicillin-susceptible *Staphylococcus aureus* musculoskeletal infections in children. Pediatr. Infect. Dis. J. *23*:701-706, 2004.
28. Mondor, C., Gauthier, M., Garel, L., et al.: Nonsurgical management of neonatal adrenal abscess. J. Pediatr. Surg. *23*:1048-1050, 1988.
29. Negus, S., and Sidhu, P. S.: MRI of retroperitoneal collections: A comparison with CT. Br. J. Radiol. 73:907-912, 2000.
30. Okada, Y., Yamataka, A., Ogasawara, Y., et al.: Ilio-psoas abscess caused by methicillin-resistant *Staphylococcus aureus* (MRSA): A rare but potentially dangerous condition in neonates. Pediatr. Surg. Int. *20*:73-74, 2004.
31. Rathore, M. H., Barton, L. L., and Luisiri, A.: Acute lobar nephronia: A review. Pediatrics 87:728-734, 1991.
32. Santaella, R. O., Fishman, E. K., and Lipsett, P. A.: Primary vs secondary iliopsoas abscess. Arch. Surg. *130*:1309-1313, 1995.
33. Schwaitzberg, S. D., Pokorny, W. J., Thurston, R. S., et al.: Psoas abscess in children. J. Pediatr. Surg. *20*:339-342, 1985.
34. Sedaghatian, M. R., Barkhordar, J., and Gerami, S.: Retroperitoneal abscess presenting as an abdominal mass in neonate. J. Pediatr. Surg. *13*:544-545, 1978.
35. Siegel, M. J., Balfe, D. M., McClennan, B. L., and Levitt, R. G.: Clinical utility of CT in pediatric retroperitoneal disease: 5 years' experience. A. J. R. Am. J. Roentgenol. *138*:1011-1017, 1982.
36. Simons, G. W., Sty, J. R., and Starshak, R. J.: Retroperitoneal and retrofascial abscesses. J. Bone Joint Surg. Am. *65*:1041-1058, 1983.
37. Vachvanichsanong, P., Dissaneewate, P., Patrapinyokul, S., et al.: Renal abscess in healthy children: Report of three cases. Pediatr. Nephrol. *6*:273-275, 1992.
38. Wippermann, C. F., Schofer, O., Beetz, R., et al.: Renal abscess in childhood: Diagnostic and therapeutic progress. Pediatr. Infect. Dis. J. *10*:446-450, 1991.
39. Woods, C. R., and Edwards, M. S.: Renal abscess caused by group B *Streptococcus*. Clin. Infect. Dis. *18*:662-663, 1994.

MUSCULOSKELETAL INFECTIONS

OSTEOMYELITIS

Paul Krogstad

The term *osteomyelitis* denotes inflammation of bone and marrow but generally implies the presence of infection. Osteomyelitis is considered acute if diagnosed within 2 weeks of the onset of symptoms, or subacute if symptoms have been present for more than 2 weeks at the time of presentation. Although bacteria are the most common cause, fungi, parasites, and other microorganisms also may cause osteomyelitis.[108] Acute osteomyelitis may evolve into a chronic process, especially if not treated adequately, leading to extensive necrosis of bone.

The incidence of osteomyelitis in normal children has been examined in several populations. Estimates have varied from 1 in 20,000 adolescent girls in New Zealand to 1 in 1000 Australian Aboriginals.[26,45,82] Boys seem to be at greater risk and contract the disease 1.2 to 3.7 times more often than do girls.[82,158,189] Osteomyelitis occurs most often in the first 2 decades of life. Approximately 25 percent of children with osteomyelitis are younger than 2 years old, and 50 percent are younger than 5 years old.[83,121,154,214] The incidence is increased in patients with sickle-cell disease and in some other immunocompromised patients (see the section on special populations).

Microorganisms can be introduced into bone in three ways: (1) by direct inoculation, usually traumatic, but also during surgery; (2) by local invasion from a contiguous focus of infection; and (3) by hematogenous delivery. In children, osteomyelitis generally is of hematogenous origin. Regardless of the route of infection, the common denominator is microscopic bone death. The goal of treatment is to arrest the infection and limit the extent of the injury to bone.

USUAL MICROBIAL ETIOLOGY

Although cultures frequently fail to identify bacterial pathogens in osteomyelitis, most microbiologically confirmed infections are caused by single organisms.[5,154,162] Gram-positive bacteria are responsible for most cases of osteomyelitis in children. *Staphylococcus aureus* is incriminated in 89 percent of cases of osteomyelitis in immunocompetent children.[83,171,207,211] Group A streptococci are next in frequency (Table 61–1). Historically, *Streptococcus pneumoniae* has been a frequent cause of osteomyelitis, but protein conjugate vaccines are likely to diminish markedly the incidence of pneumococcal osteomyelitis. In contrast, *Kingella kingae*, a fastidious gram-negative organism, is being identified increasingly in children as a cause of osteoarticular infection, including osteomyelitis, diskitis, and septic arthritis, and may explain many cases of culture-negative osteoarticular disease.[46,88,134,215,228] Even in more affluent countries, *Salmonella* spp. frequently are a cause of osteomyelitis in immunocompetent patients. *Salmonella* spp. are the most common organism found in cases of osteomyelitis in patients with sickle-cell disease (discussed later). (The microbiologic peculiarities of osteomyelitis in other immunocompromised patients and special populations are discussed in later sections.)

Other aerobic gram-negative bacteria are less common causes of osteomyelitis. Before the development of protein conjugate vaccines, *Haemophilus influenzae* was reported consistently in pediatric case series and caused approximately 5 to 8 percent of cases.[121,154,171,211] As with other invasive *H. influenzae* infections, osteomyelitis caused by this organism usually occurs in children 3 months to 6 years of age.[62,71,89,199] With the advent of effective immunization, cases of *H. influenzae* osteomyelitis are noticeably absent from more recent case series.[5,83,114] Osteomyelitis caused by other gram-negative organisms is an uncommon finding but generally occurs in neonates and young infants. Hematogenous osteomyelitis caused by *Pseudomonas aeruginosa* has been associated with injection of illicit drugs.[102,128,223]

Four distinct clinical entities of infection caused by anaerobic bacteria are recognized: (1) bacteremic seeding of previously normal bones in children and young adults; (2) superinfection of a fracture site already infected with *S. aureus*; (3) indolent (months to years after surgery) infection of a prosthetic device; and (4) contiguous chronic infection,[201] which most often occurs in the skull and the extremities. *Bacteroides* spp. are found most commonly and are associated with paranasal, sinus, or mastoid infection. In most cases, a foul odor is noted when the bone is incised or the focus is opened; trauma often has been an inciting influence.[129]

As noted previously, most cases of osteomyelitis in children develop after an episode of bacteremia and are caused by a single organism. Polymicrobial infections generally reflect the spread of infection from contiguous infectious foci and most often occur in the skull, face, hands, or feet. Distal extremities compromised by vascular insufficiency or immobilized because of peripheral neuropathy also are sites of polymicrobial osteomyelitis (including paraplegia caused by spina bifida). Osteomyelitis caused by fungi and atypical bacterial pathogens occasionally occurs in children and is discussed in greater detail later.

HEMATOGENOUS OSTEOMYELITIS

PATHOGENESIS

In long tubular bones, hematogenous osteomyelitis generally begins in the metaphysis, the broad cancellous end of the bone shaft adjacent to the epiphyseal growth plate. The cartilaginous epiphyseal growth plate (the physis) is nourished by diffusion of nutrients from a narrow plexus of capillaries fed by the metaphyseal branches of the nutrient artery; these capillaries drain into a large sinusoidal plexus that ultimately joins the large sinusoidal veins in the bone marrow (Fig. 61–1).[100] Trauma or emboli lead to occlusion of the slow-flowing sinusoidal vessels, establishing a nidus for infection. Blood-borne bacteria can seed the poorly perfused area and proliferate.[40,111,209]

The high frequency of *S. aureus* in osteomyelitis may reflect specific pathogenic properties of the organism. It has the ability

TABLE 61-1   Etiology of Acute Hematogenous Osteomyelitis in Children: Number of Bacteriologically Confirmed Cases

Organisms	Nelson[154] (n = 296) (%)	LaMont et al.[121] (n = 90) (%)	Unkila-Kallio et al.[211] (n = 44) (%)	Roine et al.[171] (n = 38) (%)	Goegens et al.[83] (n = 45) (%)
Gram-Positive Bacteria					
Staphylococcus aureus	67	70	89	89	85
Coagulase-negative staphylococci	3	1			
Streptococcus pneumoniae	2	5	2		4
Other streptococci	12	16	2	1	8
Gram-Negative Bacteria					
Haemophilus influenzae	4	8	7	8	0
Pseudomonas aeruginosa	3				
Salmonella spp.	2				
Escherichia coli	<1				
Kingella kingae	<1				
Mixed or unusual organisms	4				

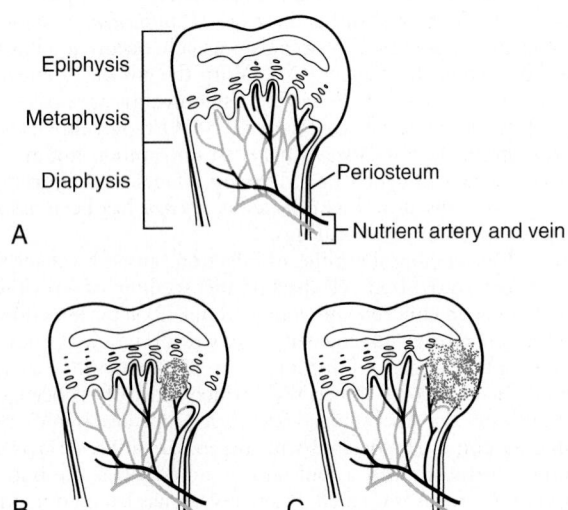

Epiphysis

Metaphysis

Diaphysis

A

Periosteum

Nutrient artery and vein

B

C

Figure 61-1 A, The sluggish blood flow in the sinusoidal venous connections located at the metaphyseal-epiphyseal junction predisposes to the development of traumatic thrombosis and infarction. **B,** Bacteremic seeding of the avascular area initiates the infection, which spreads through the Volkmann canals and the haversian systems and causes septic thrombosis. **C,** Infection tends to spread laterally through the cortex and elevates or ruptures through the periosteum.

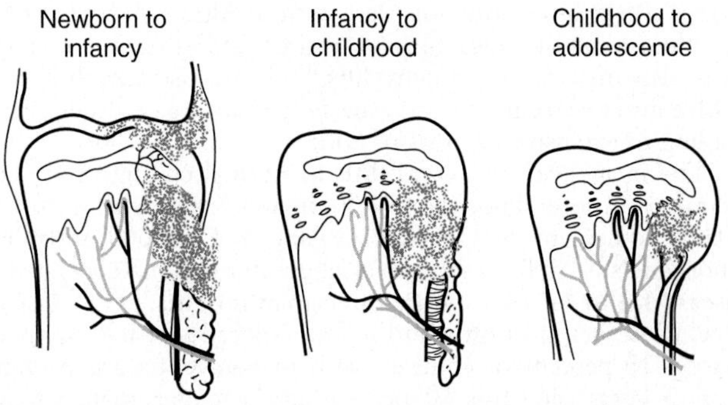

Newborn to infancy   Infancy to childhood   Childhood to adolescence

Figure 61-2 In young infants and neonates, particularly in the hip where the epiphyseal growth plate is traversed by nutrient vessels terminating in the distal ossification center, septic thrombophlebitis of the nutrient vessels can lead to growth discrepancies. With the capsule of the joint extending to the metaphysis, rupture of the infection through the cortex leads to the development of septic arthritis. Because of the thin cortex and loose periosteum, the osteomyelitis may come to medical attention as a deep soft tissue abscess. In older infants and young children, the thicker cortex and denser periosteum are a greater barrier to infection. Local tenderness from subperiosteal edema or abscess is the rule. In late childhood and adolescence, the lesion is extremely well localized and rarely penetrates the bony cortex. In this age group, invasive procedures, such as windowing or drilling, are necessary to obtain infected material.

to adhere to type I collagen of bone fibrils.[32] When *S. aureus* binds to collagen, bacterial replication gives rise to microcolonies surrounded by a glycocalyx.[94] Continued injury, elicited by *S. aureus* exoproducts and the host cellular inflammatory response to the injury, causes the accumulation of exudate under pressure. The pressure compresses blood vessels of bone and produces focal bone necrosis. The low ratio of surface area to mass, combined with the blood vessel anatomy described earlier, interferes with reabsorption of necrotic cortical bone[40,111] and the effectiveness of host defense mechanisms.

Since the late 1990s, community-acquired methicillin-resistant *S. aureus* (CA-MRSA) isolates have become a common cause of musculoskeletal infections in the United States and other countries. As described further later, most of these CA-MRSA isolates carry genes encoding the Panton-Valentine leukocidin (pvl).[22] Pvl-positive CA-MRSA has been associated frequently with sepsis, venous thrombosis, and polyostotic disease, suggesting that this or other factors contribute to the development and severity of hematogenous osteomyelitis.[26a,140] The very early stages of osteomyelitis may be aborted by administration of

appropriate chemotherapy. In the absence of therapy, necrosis of cortical bone and marrow continues. The exudate under pressure is forced through the haversian systems and Volkmann canals and into the cortex (see Fig. 61-1).

SIGNS AND SYMPTOMS

The bacteremic phase of hematogenous osteomyelitis may be entirely subclinical and associated only with malaise and low-grade fever, or it may be characterized by severe constitutional symptoms with a temperature of 40° C. The subsequent clinical manifestations of osteomyelitis are not related to the severity of initial constitutional signs of infection but are influenced by the age of the child and the etiologic agent (Fig. 61-2).

In newborns, the thin cortex and loosely attached periosteum are poor barriers to the spread of infection. Consequently, the purulence rapidly ruptures through both of these structures into the contiguous muscle bed. With progression of the infection, the purulent material often dissects the muscle bundles, with the swollen, discolored limb taking the appearance of a sausage. In addition, nutrient metaphyseal capillaries perforate the epiphyseal growth plate in newborns, and the capsule of the diarthrodial joints frequently extends to or is slightly distal to the epiphyseal plate. These anatomic characteristics permit an infection arising in the metaphysis to involve the epiphysis and to extend into the adjacent joint cavity.

In older infants, the cortex (see Fig. 61–2) is thicker and the periosteum is slightly more dense. Consequently, the infection spreads less often to the soft tissues of the extremity. Subperiosteal abscess and contiguous edema readily develop, however. The nutrient metaphyseal capillaries in older infants are atrophic, which, although more recently disputed,[159] is thought to decrease the risk of spread of infection into the adjacent joint space. The subperiosteal purulence almost always is at the metaphysis, the area in which the cortex is the thinnest.[91]

In children and adolescents (4-16 years old), the metaphyseal cortex is considerably thicker, with a dense, fibrous periosteum. The pathogenesis of the infection is the same in this age group, but the infection rarely ruptures and spreads to the outer cortical lamellae. As a result, the signs and symptoms of osteomyelitis in these older children and adolescents usually are more focal.

A newborn with osteomyelitis usually is irritable and displays evidence of pain when the affected extremity is touched or moved. Pseudoparalysis may occur, and if the disease remains untreated, massive swelling of the extremity may be seen. Obtaining a plain radiograph is invaluable in this age group; most of these patients have changes consistent with osteomyelitis on the initial radiograph.[118,147,220] In infants and young children, pain usually is present, as is a limp because osteomyelitis occurs more commonly in the lower extremities. The child refuses to use the affected extremity and displays variable constitutional symptoms.

In older children and adolescents, less restriction of function of the extremity is found compared with infants and young children. The point tenderness is circumscribed more sharply and may be found only as a small area of discomfort at rest. This disease most often affects the lower extremities and produces a mild limp. Most commonly, tubular bones are involved, but osteomyelitis occurs throughout the skeleton (Table 61–2). The hallmark of the disease is the focal nature of symptoms; point tenderness and well-localized pain suggest the diagnosis. Percussion of the long bone away from the area of point tenderness often elicits pain at the site of osteomyelitis in older children and adolescents.

The clinical features of osteomyelitis are influenced by the organisms involved. Osteomyelitis caused by CA-MRSA seems to be more complex and severe than are infections caused by methicillin-susceptible *S. aureus* (MSSA). Life-threatening infections caused by CA-MRSA have been reported in adolescents, and polyostotic disease is more common (15% in one more recent series compared with 2% in a large series that preceded the emergence of CA-MRSA).[22,154] Myositis, pyomyositis, intraosseous and subperiosteal abscesses, and septic thrombophlebitis also seem to occur more frequently with CA-MRSA than with MSSA.[5,86,87,140] In contrast, osteoarticular infections caused by *Kingella* spp. generally have an indolent course, with limb pain often present for longer than a week before initial medical evaluation is made.[134,227] Osteomyelitis caused by *H. influenzae* seems to occur primarily in the upper extremities.[61,62,89,199]

Culture-negative osteomyelitis generally is mild. In one series comparing 45 culture-positive patients with 40 patients with culture-negative osteomyelitis, symptoms were of longer duration, and overlying skin changes were seen less frequently in patients with negative disease. Treatment with β-lactams generally was successful and associated with skeletal sequelae in only one case.[69] Whether these features of culture-negative osteomyelitis suggest a more effective host defense or infection by a less virulent and more fastidious pathogen, such as *K. kingae*, which has been identified in culture-negative disease, is unclear.[215]

TABLE 61–2   Site of Involvement in Acute Hematogenous Osteomyelitis*

Bone Type	%
Tubular	
Femur	25
Tibia	24
Humerus	13
Phalanges	5
Fibula	4
Radius	4
Ulna	2
Metatarsal	2
Clavicle	0.5
Metacarpal	0.5
Cuboidal	
Calcaneus	5
Talus	0.8
Carpals	0.5
Cuneiform	0.5
Cuboid	0.3
Irregular	
Ischium	4
Ilium	2
Vertebra	2
Pubis	0.8
Sacrum	0.8
Flat	
Skull	1
Rib	0.5
Sternum	0.5
Scapula	0.5
Maxilla	0.3
Mandible	0.3

*The bone classification is according to Jaffe.[108]
Data from Nelson, J. D.: Acute osteomyelitis in children. Infect. Dis. Clin. North. Am. 4:513-522, 1990.

DIFFERENTIAL DIAGNOSIS

Osteomyelitis can be confused with many other conditions associated with fever, pain, and tenderness in an extremity, including fractures, rheumatic fever, septicemia, septic arthritis, cellulitis, Ewing sarcoma, leukemia, reflex neurovascular dystrophy, thrombophlebitis, bone infarction secondary to sickle-cell or Gaucher disease, and toxic synovitis.

DIAGNOSIS

The diagnosis of osteomyelitis generally is suspected based on typical findings, such as fever, focal skeletal pain, warmth, and swelling, and a limp or refusal to use an extremity. The diagnosis is confirmed by an organism shown by culture or Gram stain in an aspirate of bone, or by histopathologic analysis of surgical specimens. In an otherwise healthy individual, the diagnosis is probable when a patient has fever, leukocytosis, elevated acute-phase reactants (elevated C-reactive protein [CRP] or erythrocyte sedimentation rate [ESR]), or a positive blood culture plus one or more of the following: abnormal imaging studies (plain radiograph, magnetic resonance imaging [MRI], or computed tomography [CT]), scintigraphy, or physical findings consistent with osteomyelitis.

Microbiology

The cornerstone of the diagnosis of osteomyelitis is isolation of bacteria or other microbes from bone or from anatomic structures contiguous to bone. Overall, such cultures (bone, subperiosteal exudate, or joint fluid) provide a bacteriologic diagnosis in 66 to 76 percent of cases. Blood cultures yield an organism in about half of cases (36-74% of patients in three series).[154,207,212,215]

In neonates, needle aspiration of soft tissue or incision and drainage of bone may yield the offending organism. In infants and young children, subperiosteal needle aspiration can be done if the point tenderness is localized. In older children and adolescents, noninvasive culturing of the bone is less rewarding. In this age group, windowing or drilling to drain pus from the bone yields valuable material for culture but is controversial; some orthopedic surgeons consider the risk of causing epiphyseal damage and subsequent length discrepancy secondary to the procedure too great. Consequently, blood cultures and imaging methods often represent the extent of the diagnostic evaluation. Nonetheless, it is important to attempt to obtain bacterial cultures early in the evaluation of suspected osteomyelitis because decisions about the type and duration of antimicrobial therapy are greatly facilitated by knowing the susceptibility profile of the etiologic agent.

Radiology

PLAIN RADIOGRAPHS

Conventional radiographs are crucial in establishing the diagnosis of pediatric osteomyelitis and always should be obtained.[26a,39,96]

Because bone density must decrease 50 percent to be detected by radiographs,[8] changes in the less ossified bones of neonates are detected more readily than are changes in older children. In contrast, Waldvogel and Papageorgiou[216] found in adults that plain radiographs were of no diagnostic value in 23 percent and were misleading in an additional 16 percent.

Radiographic changes occur in three stages.[34] The first stage, which occurs approximately 3 days after the onset of symptoms, is the formation of a small area of localized, deep soft tissue swelling, usually in the region of the metaphysis (Fig. 61–3). When diagnosis of osteomyelitis is sought early, examination of the radiograph should be directed to the soft tissue rather than the bone. During the second stage, which occurs 3 to 7 days after the onset of symptoms, swelling of the muscles with obliteration of the interposed translucent fat planes can be noted. It is caused by continued spread of edema fluid and can progress, particularly in neonates and young infants, to superficial soft tissue edema; the skin may acquire an orange-peel texture.

Radiographic evidence of bone destruction usually is not detected until 10 to 21 days after the onset of symptoms. The first changes detected include subperiosteal bone resorption, areas of bone destruction, and periosteal new bone formation. The variability depends on the specific bone involved; generally, long tubular bones tend to show bony changes 2 to 3 weeks earlier than membranous or irregular bones.

MAGNETIC RESONANCE IMAGING

MRI is becoming the imaging modality of choice when additional imaging is needed.[39] The major advantages of MRI are that it accurately delineates subperiosteal or soft tissue collections of pus that might require surgical drainage without using ionizing

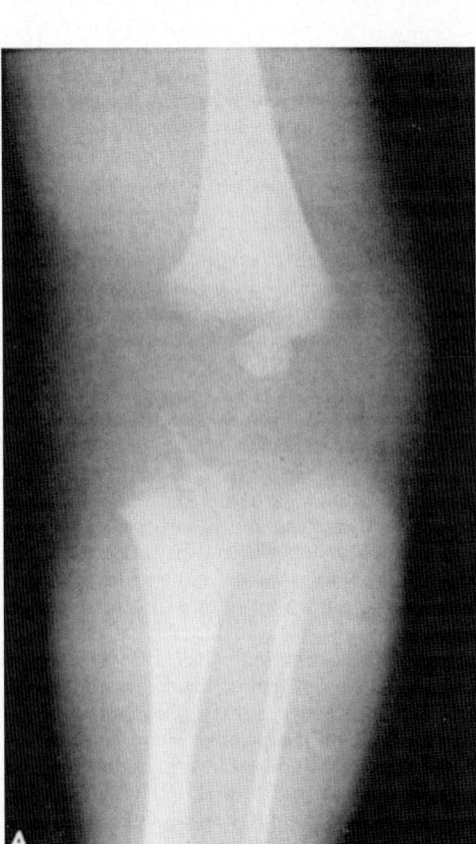
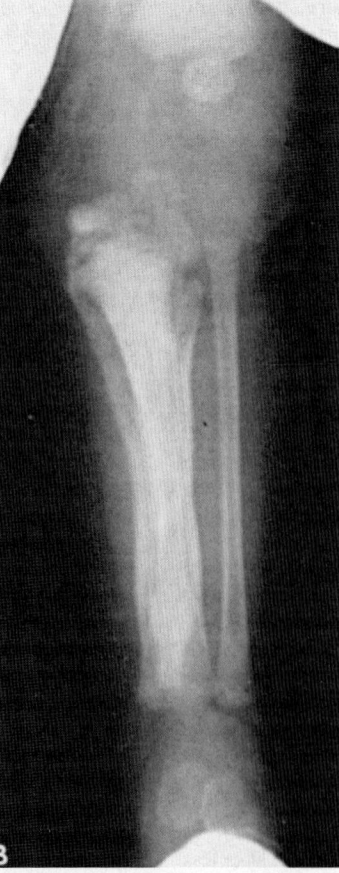

Figure 61–3 A, The left knee of an infant shows diffuse soft tissue swelling around the proximal ends of the tibia and fibula. **B,** Six weeks later, the subcutaneous fat lines between the muscles and the skin can be seen, as can an involucrum involving almost all of the tibia.

radiation, and it can identify sinus tracts for removal (Fig. 61–4).[26a,68,164,197] MRI often provides more specific anatomic information than CT or plain radiography.

In acute osteomyelitis, bone marrow edema caused by the accumulation of purulent material leads to decreased signal on T1-weighted images. On T2-weighted images of the same area, increased signal is seen. With commonly used sequences, the sensitivity of MRI for the detection of acute osteomyelitis may approach 100 percent.[141] Fat-suppression sequences, including short-tau inversion recovery, decrease the signal from fat. Inversion recovery sequences allow more sensitive detection of bone marrow edema. MRI may have a particular advantage in establishing the diagnosis of spinal osteomyelitis because a clear distinction can be made between the vertebral body and the adjacent disk. Loss of this border is one of the first abnormalities detected by MRI in spinal osteomyelitis.

The need for sedation in most infants and children and the cost of MRI are the major disadvantages that continue to limit its use. In addition, infarction and other processes can alter the appearance of bone marrow and lower the specificity of MRI and must be considered in the interpretation of the imaging study.

RADIONUCLIDE IMAGING

Radionuclide scanning has been used for decades in the evaluation of suspected osteomyelitis. Despite the fact that bone scanning involves exposure to ionizing radiation, it continues to be used widely because of its ready availability and utility in detecting multifocal disease.[56] Bone imaging employing technetium 99m (Tc 99m) diphosphonate scintigraphy is used most frequently. After being injected, the phosphate adduct is adsorbed to the surface of the hydroxyapatite crystal in bone, and Tc 99m becomes concentrated in the cement line located at the junction of osteoid and mineralized bone.[204]

Most institutions perform a three-phase bone scan for evaluation of infection. Shortly after injection (2-5 seconds), a nuclear angiogram (flow phase) of the area of suspected osteomyelitis is obtained. The second phase (the blood pool phase) consists of a single image obtained 5 to 10 minutes after injection. The third image is obtained 2 to 4 hours after injection. In this later phase, specificity of the diphosphonate compounds for the bone is revealed. Anything increasing local blood flow to the area, particularly if accompanied by inflammation, results in increased general uptake in the first two phases, but osteomyelitis results in focal uptake in the third phase, with the intensity of the signal detected reflecting the level of osteoblastic activity.[36,48,50,56,80,119,180]

Acute osteomyelitis in children is often diagnosed by a Tc 99m scan and treated successfully before bone changes are detected by plain radiographs (see Fig. 61–4).[206] With sensitivity reported to be as high as 95 percent, bone scanning has until recently been a reliable tool in establishing the diagnosis of osteomyelitis.[34] Unfortunately, in one recent report, bone scintigraphy detected only osteomyelitis caused by community acquired-MRSA cases in 53 percent (26/49) of children.[26a] This apparent lack of sensitivity for CA-MRSA may reflect the acuity of disease caused by this pathogen, as changes in radionuclide scans are more characteristic when patients have had an illness of longer duration.[182]

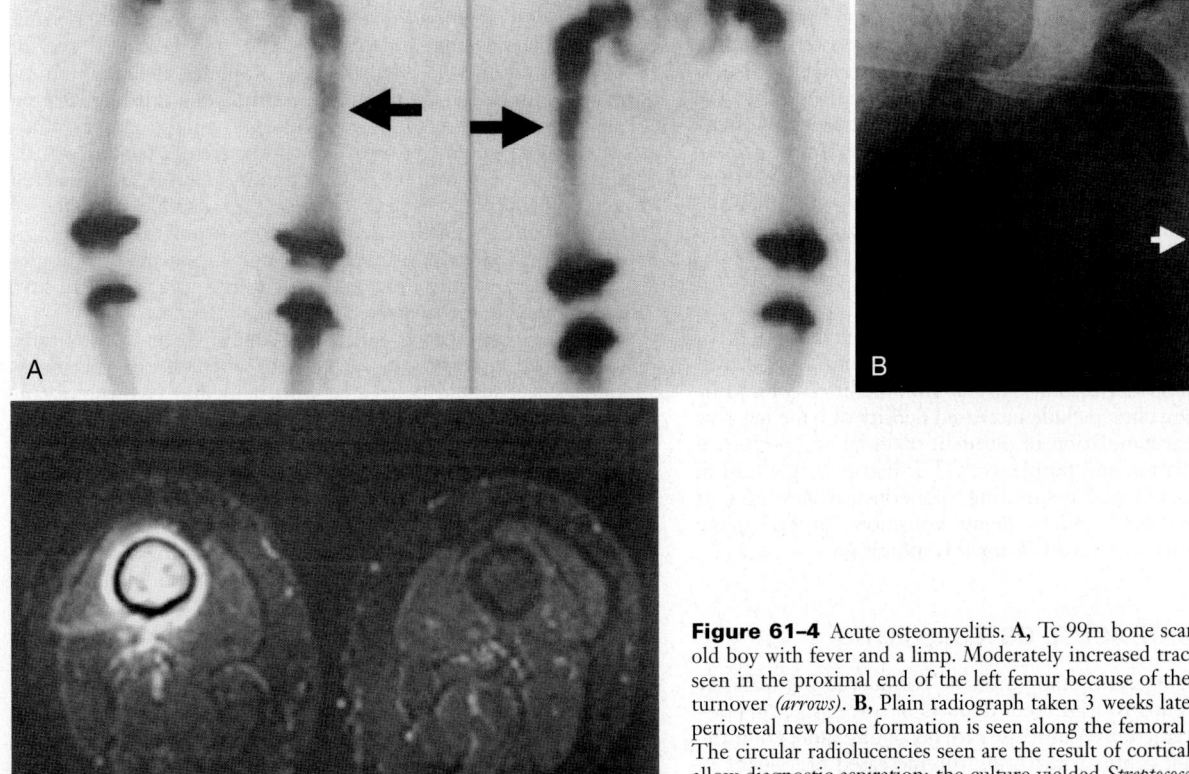

Figure 61–4 Acute osteomyelitis. **A,** Tc 99m bone scan of a 2-year-old boy with fever and a limp. Moderately increased tracer activity is seen in the proximal end of the left femur because of the increased bone turnover *(arrows)*. **B,** Plain radiograph taken 3 weeks later. Unilamellar periosteal new bone formation is seen along the femoral shaft *(arrows)*. The circular radiolucencies seen are the result of cortical drilling to allow diagnostic aspiration; the culture yielded *Streptococcus pyogenes*. **C,** Axial T2-weighted magnetic reasonance image of the thigh from a different patient shows abnormally high signal intensity throughout the marrow cavity. The band of high signal surrounding the cortex represents periostitis. *(Courtesy of Dr. Leanne Seeger.)*

In addition, bone scans that use Tc 99m may be nondiagnostic in neonates.[6,71] Destruction of cortical bone occurs, and periosteal new bone formation often is present on plain-film radiographs of bones with normal Tc 99m uptake. The false-negative result of bone scans probably is due to the paucity of mineralization in neonates' bones. Ischemia of bone, probably caused by infarction, also has been noted on the initial bone scan.[147] Overall, the sensitivity of bone scans in neonates is uncertain, but may be only 30 percent.[71]

Older infants with osteomyelitis and a nondiagnostic Tc 99m bone scan also have been described.[17,95] In such instances, a gallium 67 (Ga 67) scan may be valuable. Ga 67 is a transition metal that, similar to iron, is bound to plasma proteins; the unbound portion (10-25%) is excreted in urine. It localizes in inflammatory foci because of increased capillary permeability (leaking plasma proteins), in vivo leukocyte labeling, binding to lactoferrin in the lesion, and perhaps direct bacterial uptake. Because of the slower elimination of gallium from blood, its uptake in an inflammatory focus depends less on blood flow. Delayed elimination often results in poor contrast of bone to soft tissue, however, and delays making a reliable interpretation for 24 to 72 hours after injection.[101] In one study, 15 of 16 cases of osteomyelitis with a nondiagnostic Tc 99m scan had changes on Ga 67 scan typical of osteomyelitis.[188] Combined evaluation with Ga 67 imaging and Tc 99m bone scanning may lead to greater diagnostic certainty when the studies are not conclusively diagnostic.[185,226] Despite these successes, Ga 67 scans are seldom employed because MRI, repeating plain radiographs, and clinical improvement during therapy usually are sufficient to resolve initial diagnostic uncertainties.

Numerous studies have been conducted to examine the utility of indium 111–labeled leukocyte scans for the diagnosis of osteomyelitis. This method involves removing leukocytes and injecting them back into the patient after in vitro labeling. It has a sensitivity of approximately 86 percent.[177] The sensitivity seems to be best for the detection of lesions in long bones. False-positive scans can result from a variety of processes, including fracture and infarction. Enthusiasm for this modality also is limited by the higher organ absorption of the radiation dose.[73] Numerous other scintigraphic methods for the detection of osteomyelitis, including Tc 99m hexamethylpropyleneamine oxime–labeled leukocytes and monoclonal antibodies, have been examined. At present, these alternative methods do not offer any advantage over MRI and older radionuclide imaging approaches.

COMPUTED TOMOGRAPHY

CT is used occasionally in the diagnosis and management of osteomyelitis because it provides excellent definition of cortical bone and high spatial resolution. CT abnormalities commonly found in osteomyelitis include increased density of bone marrow caused by the accumulation of purulent material and periosteal new bone formation and purulence. CT is particularly useful in detecting sequestra and delineating subperiosteal abscesses. It previously has been used to define infections of the spine; however, MRI has replaced CT for this indication.

TREATMENT OF ACUTE OSTEOMYELITIS

The need for surgical therapy must be considered immediately when osteomyelitis is diagnosed. Reports of soft tissue, subperiosteal, and intramedullary abscesses are becoming more common in the early 21st century, mirroring the increased prevalence of skin, soft tissue, and musculoskeletal infections caused by CA-MRSA.[5,112,140] MRI, ultrasound, and CT imaging may prove useful in assessing these purulent foci.[26a] Drainage of these sites by surgical or interventional radiology techniques also provides the opportunity to obtain cultures to confirm a microbiologic diagnosis. Sequestra, if present at presentation, should be removed. If contiguous infectious foci are present, they should be débrided adequately and treated with effective antimicrobial therapy. Immobilization of the affected extremity or splinting may afford relief from pain and sometimes is used to prevent the development of pathologic fractures when extensive bone involvement is detected by plain radiography.

Although the choice of antimicrobial agents used often is modified during a course of therapy, the therapy initially chosen always should have potent activity against S. aureus and group A streptococci because these pathogens represent the primary causes of osteomyelitis. Acute bacterial hematogenous osteomyelitis should be treated initially with parenteral anti-infective agents, in view of the high mortality rate in S. aureus osteomyelitis seen in the pre-antibiotic era and more recent reports of fulminant disease with CA-MRSA.[86,87,91,140] The choice of initial therapy has become more complex with the marked increase in prevalence of CA-MRSA in the United States and other countries.

In areas where most (≥90%) S. aureus isolates remain methicillin-susceptible, initial therapy may consist of a penicillinase-resistant, semisynthetic penicillin, such as nafcillin or oxacillin, administered parenterally in a dosage of 150 to 200 mg/kg/day in four divided doses.[90,105,171] Cefuroxime, a second-generation cephalosporin, also has been used for empiric therapy, with good results.[154] In areas where CA-MRSA is common, either vancomycin or clindamycin (if >90% of CA-MRSA isolates are susceptible) should be included in the initial empiric therapy for CA-MRSA.[112,139] Currently, most isolates of CA-MRSA remain susceptible to clindamycin, but clinical laboratories should screen for inducible macrolide-lincosamide-streptogramin resistance using the D-test or similar methodology.[5,112,127]

Although protein conjugate vaccines have rendered invasive H. influenzae infections rare occurrences in the United Sates, antimicrobial coverage for this possibility may be considered for younger children who have not yet completed their immunization series. In these circumstances, addition of a third-generation cephalosporin (ceftriaxone or cefotaxime) to the empiric anti-staphylococcal agent (vancomycin, clindamycin, oxacillin, or nafcillin) might be warranted. Other agents may be administered when epidemiologic factors suggest the possible presence of other pathogens: third-generation cephalosporins or chloramphenical for Salmonella osteomyelitis, ceftazidime and aminoglycosides for P. aeruginosa or for enteric gram-negative organisms, and clindamycin for suspected anaerobic infections.[63,170]

When an organism is isolated or identified by other means, antimicrobial therapy can be chosen with greater specificity. Staphylococci should be treated with penicillin G if the organisms are susceptible to this antibiotic. In most cases, staphylococci must be treated with a penicillinase-resistant penicillin (oxacillin or nafcillin), clindamycin, or vancomycin. Ceftriaxone also has proved successful in the treatment of most cases of MSSA. Oxazolidinone (linezolid) and streptogramin (quinupristin-dalfopristin) drugs have been used successfully for the treatment of osteomyelitis in some adults with MRSA and MSSA[54] and for the treatment of vancomycin-resistant enterococci. They may prove useful in cases of pediatric osteomyelitis caused by S. aureus with decreased susceptibility to vancomycin, but experience with these agents is still limited.

Trimethoprim-sulfamethoxazole and the lipophilic tetracyclines (minocycline and doxycycline) have been used successfully in the treatment of osteomyelitis in children and adults and are readily absorbed by the oral route. Experience with these agents in treating CA-MRSA infections in which pneumonia and bacteremia seem to be common is limited, however, and the potential for dental staining should be considered with the tetracyclines. Daptomycin, a bactericidal lipopeptide antimicrobial agent, has excellent activity against CA-MRSA, but pediatric pharmacokinetic data and clinical experience also are limited. Daptomycin seems to have poor activity in lung tissue. Reports of pneumonia and sepsis in association with osteomyelitis add to concerns about the utility of daptomycin for the treatment of osteomyelitis.[86,87,112]

Osteomyelitis caused by *S. pneumoniae* strains with decreased susceptibility to penicillin have been managed successfully with a variety of agents, including ceftriaxone, vancomycin, and clindamycin.[74] β-Lactam antibiotics, including oxacillin, nafcillin, and cephalosporins, have been used successfully in the treatment of *K. kingae* infection.[46,88,227,228]

Decades of experience and clinical investigation have led to wide acceptance of sequential use of the intravenous and oral routes of administration of antibiotics to treat pediatric osteomyelitis, which previously was controversial. Completing treatment with oral therapy avoids the cost, pain, inconvenience, and well-known complications of long-term administration of intravenous antibiotics. Central venous catheters have not obviated these concerns. To the contrary, local skin infections, bacteremia, and malfunctions of the catheters seem to be common occurrences, especially among young children.[175]

Oral therapy is most likely to succeed, and oral therapy is an acceptable option when the following criteria are met: An organism has been identified, the patient has the ability to swallow and retain an appropriate medication, the laboratory is able to monitor the degree of antibiotic absorption, and the patient has a clear clinical response to intravenously administered antibiotics.[154,156] In most series in which oral therapy has been evaluated,[29,52,154,203,217] treatment was continued with intravenous antibiotics until the patient was afebrile, until local signs and symptoms of infection were reduced considerably, and until the patient was maintaining caloric and fluid balances by the oral route. In severe or complicated cases, an advisable approach is to delay switching to the oral route until the peripheral leukocyte count has normalized, and the ESR has decreased by 20 percent or more, or until a marked decrease in the concentration of CRP has occurred.[171,212] A review of case series employing sequential therapy affirmed these recommendations and found no evidence that a fixed period of intravenous therapy is beneficial or essential. A transition to oral therapy within 7 days of diagnosis seemed to be equal in outcome to therapy with a fixed initial period of parenteral therapy.[126]

When oral therapy is begun, most antibiotics administered orally for osteomyelitis must be given in doses higher than the doses used for the treatment of other infections.[8,155,203] Specific antibiotics and the recommended starting doses are listed in Table 61-3. Dosages of β-lactams often can be increased to 200 mg/kg/day without having serious adverse side effects. Diarrhea, an infrequent complication of high-dose, oral β-lactam

therapy, can be mitigated by a reduction in dose and the administration of probenecid (40 mg/kg/day every 6 hours; maximal dose 2 g/day).[29,154,203] Clindamycin readily achieves high bone levels and does not require higher dose therapy when given orally.[113,139]

The assumption implicit in successful oral therapy is that the antibiotic reaches an effective concentration at the focus of infection. Compliance with the prescribed dose and frequency and absorption into the bloodstream are necessary to fulfill this assumption. Patient (or parent) education and a continuing time commitment by a physician or nurse are essential to maintaining the compliance required for successful treatment. Although eschewed by some physicians,[137,158] therapeutic drug monitoring is recommended by some specialists to show that adequate absorption of orally administered antibiotics is occurring.[155] Rare patients have inadequate serum levels despite receiving high oral dosages.[203] If bacteria have been isolated from the patient, a peak serum bactericidal titer of 1:8 or greater is sought.[165,203]

A disadvantage of assessing serum bactericidal activity is the difficulty of performing the test when other antibiotics are present in the serum sample. Nafcillin administered intravenously would interfere with evaluating the bioactivity of dicloxacillin. Chemical assays of a specific agent circumvent this problem. Dicloxacillin can be administered orally and the dose adjusted based on dicloxacillin measurements before the intravenous administration of another β-lactam has been discontinued. This procedure avoids several days of inadequate therapy should the dosage of the oral agent need to be adjusted.

In most cases, clinical improvement is evident within 3 to 7 days of the initiation of appropriate therapy. To help show that effective therapy is under way, it is helpful to monitor acute-phase reactants. Although CRP and ESR typically increase during the first 3 days of therapy, CRP then begins to decrease rapidly, and typically returns to normal in 7 to 10 days. CRP returns to normal levels in blood more rapidly in children with an uneventful clinical course than in children who ultimately require repeated surgical drainage.[171] A slow decline in serum CRP to normal levels has been associated with more extensive radiographic changes or persistent symptoms 1 to 2 months after discharge from the hospital. Similar to CRP, ESR generally increases during the first several days but declines in the weeks that follow.[212] Failure of ESR to decrease during the second week of treatment may indicate a need for surgical drainage or the development of chronic osteomyelitis.[196]

The outcome of acute osteomyelitis depends heavily on the duration of therapy. In one early report of 45 cases of osteomyelitis, four treatment failures occurred; all had been treated for 10 days or less.[97] Likewise, Dich and colleagues[52] noted a 19 percent failure rate in 37 patients treated for 3 weeks or less; the rate was 2 percent in 48 patients treated for 21 to 50 days. Blockey and Watson[21] provided similar data. The minimal duration of therapy for hematogenous osteomyelitis to minimize the risk of recurrence seems to be more than 3 weeks. A conservative but individualized approach is to administer antibiotics until ESR and CRP are within the normal range, which usually requires 4 to 6 weeks of treatment.[112,154-156,196]

SPECIAL MANIFESTATIONS OF HEMATOGENOUS OSTEOMYELITIS

EPIPHYSEAL OSTEOMYELITIS

Rarely, hematogenous osteomyelitis may arise in the epiphyses of the tubular bones of young children.[78,133,208] Although the pathogenesis is unclear, it may involve delivery of microorganisms to the epiphyses by transphyseal vessels. After the child

TABLE 61-3 Initial Antibiotic Doses for Oral Treatment of Osteomyelitis

Drug	Dose (mg/kg/day)	Interval between Doses (hr)
Amoxicillin	100	6
Cephalexin	150	6
Chloramphenicol	75	8
Clindamycin	40	8
Cloxacillin	125	6
Dicloxacillin	100	6
Penicillin V	125	4

Data from references 29, 76, 154, 203.

reaches 15 to 18 months of age, these vessels are lost, and the physis acts as a physical barrier to the spread of infection from the metaphysis. The vascular anatomy of the epiphysis is very similar to that of the metaphysis, however, and in some cases infection may occur when bacteria are delivered to venous sinusoids by terminal branches of the epiphyseal arteries.

Hematogenous epiphyseal osteomyelitis may be acute or subacute. In the acute manifestation, septic arthritis initially may be diagnosed when joint swelling occurs, and abnormal fluids are removed by diagnostic aspiration. In cases with a more indolent course, pain, limp, or other symptoms prompt an evaluation for the possibility of an osteoarticular infection. The correct diagnosis typically is established when a radionuclide bone scan or plain radiographs taken weeks later show evidence of increased bone turnover or the lytic changes characteristic of osteomyelitis. Administration of appropriate therapy for epiphyseal osteomyelitis has been followed by complete recovery without apparent sequelae 2 to 6 years after diagnosis.

INVOLVEMENT OF NONTUBULAR BONES

Less than 20 percent of all cases of osteomyelitis involve nontubular bones. Infection of the calcaneus seems to be the most common.[154] In patients with hematogenous infection, destruction occurs just under the epiphyseal line in the metaphysis posteriorly and medially, where the blood supply is greatest. It is present in all patients, in addition to destruction of the adjacent epiphysis, particularly in its middle to superior portion. Periosteal new bone formation occurs very late, with 3 to 4 months required for reossification. Osteomyelitis in the other cuboidal bones rarely occurs.

Almost equal in frequency to infection of the calcaneus is infection of the bones of the pelvis.[154] Of the bones of the pelvis, the ischium is involved most commonly. The next most frequently involved bone is the ilium, followed by the sacroiliac joint. The pubis is involved in only 20 percent of cases of pelvic osteomyelitis.[99,152] Pelvic osteomyelitis causes an increase in the ESR in nearly all patients, and two thirds have a peripheral leukocyte count greater than 10,000 cells/mm^3.[152] The most common organism causing pelvic osteomyelitis is *S. aureus*, which is isolated from either blood or an aspirate from the bone lesions in approximately 80 percent of cases.

Establishing the diagnosis of pelvic osteomyelitis often is difficult. Most patients are judged to have disease in the hip at the time that medical attention is sought. Most often, patients with pelvic osteomyelitis have hip pain and a gait abnormality but allow their hips to be put through a passive range of motion. Point tenderness at the site of the lesion can be elicited in approximately 50 percent of these patients. Sacroiliitis frequently is difficult to identify by clinical examination. Pressing down on the pelvis, which stresses the sacroiliac joint, produces local pain. Tenderness in the buttocks or the sciatic notch, if present, is an invaluable diagnostic finding.[1,38,55,148,221] Pelvic osteomyelitis can mimic appendicitis and urinary tract infection[221]; it occurs more frequently in individuals with inflammatory bowel disease. In most patients, plain films of the pelvis are not rewarding, whereas Tc 99m bone scans indicate the diagnosis in approximately 90 percent of cases.[135,152] CT may reveal infection not evident by bone scanning. MRI also is likely to identify pelvic osteomyelitis.[210]

Antibiotic therapy alone is adequate in most cases of pelvic osteomyelitis. Surgery is indicated only when a lack of response to antimicrobial therapy occurs. Osteomyelitis in the pelvic bones has a uniformly good prognosis; chronic infection and sequelae are rare events.

Hematogenous osteomyelitis of the flat bones occurs rarely. It has been described in the skull, ribs, sternum, and scapula.[83,149,154,211]

SPINAL OSTEOMYELITIS

Spinal osteomyelitis can involve either the intervertebral disk or the vertebral bodies per se. Conceptualizing these infections as different entities is worthwhile because of the different pathophysiology and prognosis.[65]

DISKITIS

The intervertebral disk consists of three components: the paired cartilaginous articulation, the fibrous ring (annulus fibrosus), and the nucleus pulposus.[23,65] The axial vessels that parallel the fetal notochord are atrophied by birth, with the avascular, mucilaginous nucleus pulposus remaining. The disk has two arterial supplies: periosteal vessels and vessels descending from the central portion of the vertebral body.[42,64] The vessel from the central portion of the adjacent vertebra begins to atrophy in the first year and is obliterated completely by the time the child is 10 years old. This condition leaves only the capillary network in the annulus fibrosus, which is derived from the terminal radial ramifications of the periosteal vessels. If loss of this vascular supply is precipitous, idiopathic disk necrosis ensues, usually manifested as asymptomatic calcification.[178,194,200] If bacteremia occurs during loss of the blood supply, however, infection of an intervertebral disk may occur.

Infection of an intervertebral disk has no sex preponderance, and most children are younger than 5 years old.[65,184] It occurs almost exclusively in the lumbar region (the L4 and L5 disks are involved most frequently, followed by L3 and L4). The disease comes to medical attention with the patient's refusal to walk. Backache and a progressive limp may be present. Nonambulatory infants often become irritable and refuse to sit. On examination, the most striking feature is percussion tenderness over the contiguous spine; hip pain and stiffness with loss of lordosis of the lower part of the back are observed. Occasionally, compression of the spine produces pain at the infected disk. The mean duration of symptoms before diagnosis is established ranges from 1 day to 18 months. Most patients have had symptoms for several weeks.

Lesions in higher locations (T8 to L1) can mimic gastrointestinal disease with abdominal pain, ileus, and vomiting, but the most important entities in the differential diagnosis are vertebral osteomyelitis and spinal or paraspinal tumors. Most patients have a history of a recent upper respiratory infection.[116,122,169,174,187] Fever generally is absent or low-grade. Peripheral leukocytosis is present in one third of patients, and virtually all have an increased ESR. A few patients undergoing biopsy have cultures that grow microorganisms. Most commonly, *S. aureus* is recovered, along with rare isolates of pneumococci and gram-negative organisms, including *K. kingae*. Evaluation for suspected diskitis usually involves careful elicitation of the history and physical examination, a complete blood count, determination of the ESR, a blood culture, and plain lateral radiographs of the lumbosacral spine.[65]

Typical plain radiographic findings are shown in Figure 61–5. The first finding is narrowing of the disk space, usually not detectable until 2 to 4 weeks after the onset of symptoms. Frequently, this narrowing is overlooked if loss of the normal progressive (from cephalad to caudad) increase in disk width is not appreciated. It is followed by destruction of the adjacent cartilaginous vertebral end-plates and, subsequently, by herniation of the disk into the vertebral body. Rarely, compression or wedging of the vertebral body is noted. In older children, anterior spontaneous fusion is a common finding. In all individuals, reactive bone proliferation is a rare finding, as are paravertebral soft tissue masses.

Because of overlap of this syndrome with noninfectious disk necrosis, investigators in the earlier literature advocated treating

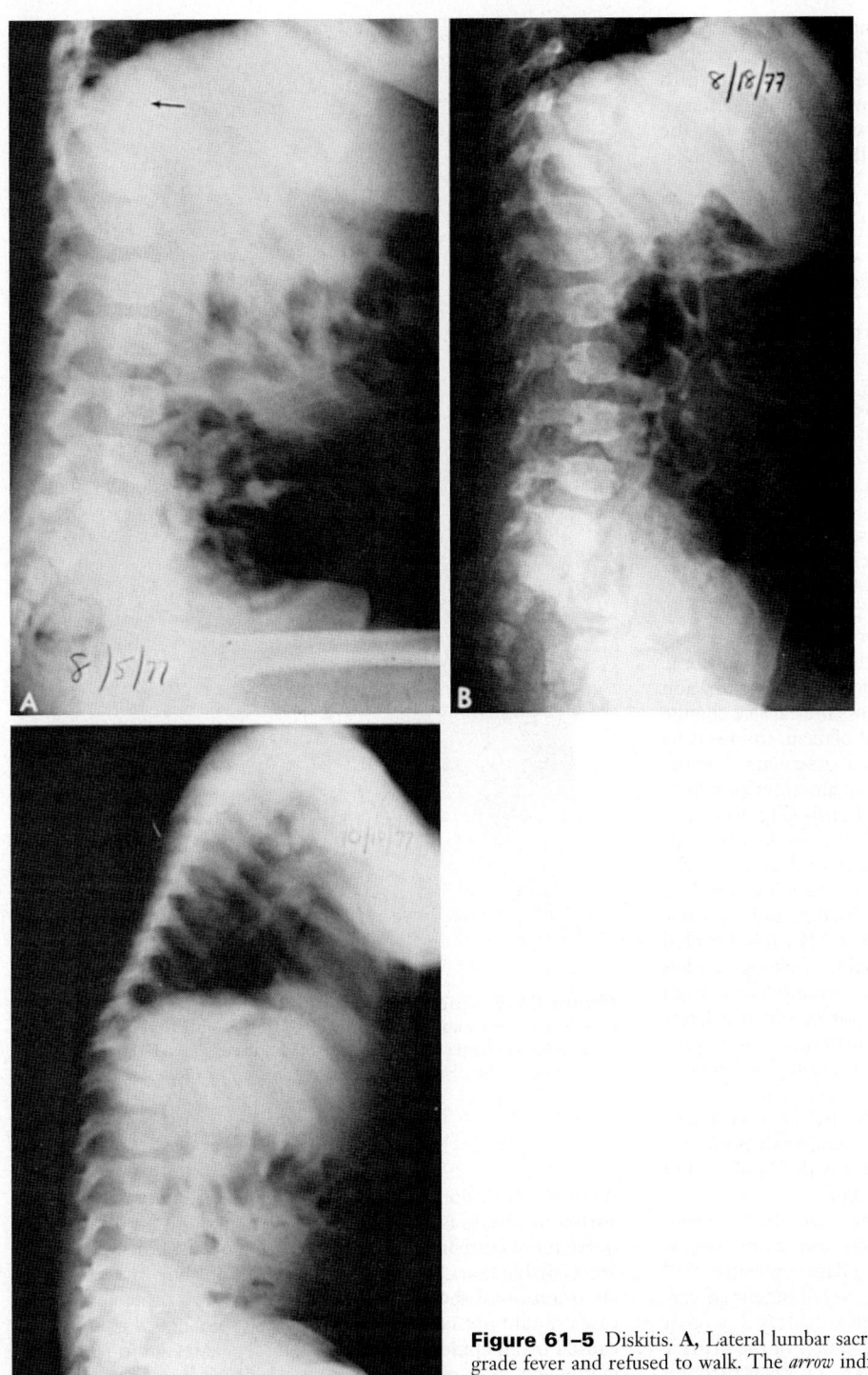

Figure 61–5 Diskitis. **A,** Lateral lumbar sacral spine of a 13-month-old child who had low-grade fever and refused to walk. The *arrow* indicates the narrow disk space. **B,** Follow-up examination 2 weeks later shows almost complete collapse of the intervertebral body. **C,** Two months later, destruction of the contiguous vertebra with marked kyphosis was apparent. *(Courtesy of Dr. Joel Blumhagen.)*

this disease solely by bed rest. In view of the low yield and generally favorable prognosis of diskitis, biopsy or aspiration for culture generally is unnecessary. Although controversial, oral antistaphylococcal therapy often is administered for a prolonged period (5-6 months).[65] Other physicians have suggested giving 5 to 7 days of intravenous antistaphylococcal therapy, followed by 7 to 14 days of a similar oral agent.[44] Very young children generally do well, and the disk space is preserved; spontaneous spinal fusion occurs commonly in older individuals.

VERTEBRAL OSTEOMYELITIS

The intervertebral disk loses its vascular supply with age, a process usually completed by 30 years of age. As a result, bacteremic pyogenic infections of the spine occur most often in the vertebral bodies. The venous drainage of the vertebral bodies is composed of three different freely communicating, but valveless, systems. Intraosseous vertebral veins drain the center of each body and form a large channel that exits through the nutrient foramen. They anastomose with the anterior and posterior internal plexus (between the dura mater and the vertebral body). The internal venous plexus has anastomotic connections with the external venous plexus through the vertebral ligaments. The external venous plexus communicates freely with the segmental veins on the ventral surface of the body wall (Batson plexus).

Reversal of blood flow or thrombosis in the sluggishly flowing vertebral veins is thought to be the first event in the development of vertebral osteomyelitis. Because of the vascular communication, osteomyelitis usually involves two adjacent vertebral bodies, with the interposed disk initially skipped. The same process of septic thrombophlebitis involving the internal venous plexus can produce an epidural abscess (with cord compression) and infarction of the vertebral body. Spread along the external venous plexus can lead to a paraspinous mass. In the thoracic area, it may produce mediastinitis,[47] and in the cervical area, a retropharyngeal abscess can occur. The lumbar area is involved much more frequently than is the thoracic area, which is involved more frequently than is the cervical region.[2,110,193]

Children with vertebral osteomyelitis usually are older than 8 years of age and seek medical attention because of constant back pain. They may appear toxic and have a low-grade fever (>39° C) after an indolent course (2 weeks to several months).[65] Percussion of the spinal dorsal process frequently elicits exquisite tenderness. Usually, the paraspinous muscles around the involved vertebrae are in spasm, with rigidity of the area. Radiographic examination of a patient with vertebral osteomyelitis shows the earliest change to be localized rarefaction of one vertebral plateau, followed by involvement of adjacent vertebrae. Marked destruction of the bone, usually anteriorly, is followed by abundant anterior osteophytic reactions with bridging and bone sclerosis (Fig. 61–6).

Obtaining an MRI study is useful in establishing the diagnosis of vertebral osteomyelitis[146] because the vertebral disk and the vertebral body are clearly discernible. Most cases of vertebral osteomyelitis begin at the margin between the disk and the anterior part of the vertebral body. In some cases, MRI has detected evidence of osteomyelitis when radionuclide imaging studies were normal.[205] Distinguishing pyogenic osteomyelitis from tuberculous lesions radiologically is impossible, but the latter usually are characterized by less bone destruction, less bone proliferation, and less sclerosis. The osteophytic bridging between adjacent vertebrae is extremely rare in spinal tuberculosis.

Tc 99m and Ga 67 are taken up by the lesion in vertebral osteomyelitis. A possible advantage of scanning with both isotopes is identification of paraspinous abscess with Ga 67,[176] but MRI probably would accomplish the same goal.

Most cases of vertebral osteomyelitis are caused by *S. aureus*. Organisms causing urinary tract infection can cause osteomyelitis, presumably by local spread through Batson plexus.[27,98,124] Urinary tract infection rarely precedes the development of vertebral osteomyelitis, however, and only approximately 2 percent of all cases can be shown to be related to infection of the urinary tract.[77] The best method of establishing the diagnosis is through examination of bone biopsy specimens and cultures.[153] *P. aeruginosa* also has been recognized as a pathogen in vertebral osteomyelitis. All patients were intravenous drug abusers, and the organisms presumably were inoculated along with the illicit drug. Young heroin addicts have been found to have *P. aeruginosa* infection in their intervertebral disks.[28,181] In areas of the world where brucellosis is endemic, spinal osteomyelitis caused by *Brucella* spp. needs to be considered.[130] Fungal pathogens causing vertebral osteomyelitis include *Coccidioides immitis* in endemic areas and *Candida* spp. (often in immunocompromised patients).[144] *Bartonella henselae* also has been found to cause vertebral osteomyelitis.[65]

Therapy for spinal osteomyelitis includes immobilization. Whether immobilization should be accomplished by simple bed

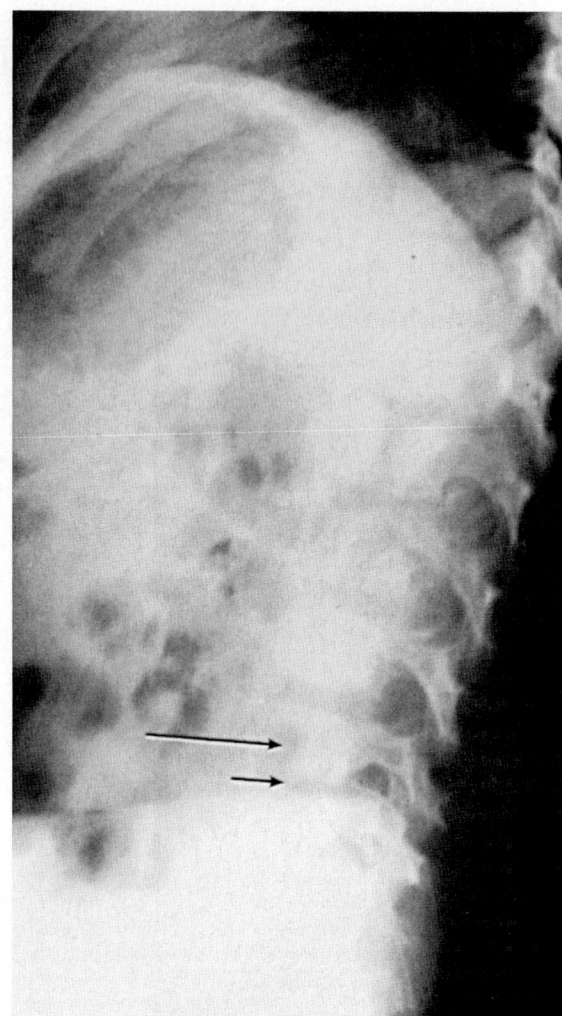

Figure 61–6 Vertebral osteomyelitis. The *large arrow* indicates the lytic lesion with some anterior sclerosis in the lumbar vertebra. The *small arrow* indicates involvement of the adjacent lower vertebra and narrowing of the disk space. *(Courtesy of Dr. Joel Blumhagen.)*

rest or with a body cast is controversial. Administration of an antibiotic always is indicated. The average duration of treatment of bacterial vertebral osteomyelitis is 2 months; however, no data are available that can be used for determining the most appropriate duration of therapy. The need for surgical drainage in some cases should not be overlooked because spinal cord compression caused by an epidural or subdural abscess can lead to permanent paraplegia. A paraspinal mass may rupture into the abdominal cavity or erode the aorta; both events are catastrophic complications.[72] The optimal therapy for fungal infection of the vertebra is unclear.

BRODIE ABSCESS

Osteomyelitis occasionally is indolent in presentation. Perhaps the best defined example is subacute osteomyelitis with the development of an intraosseous abscess (Brodie abscess).[191] These patients most often are adolescents with complaints of long bone pain and tenderness. A bony defect with sclerotic margins is detected by plain radiography in most patients. A distinctive "target" lesion has been described in MRI studies of

Brodie abscesses.[138] Concentric layers are seen and reflect a central abscess cavity surrounded by an inner ring of granulation tissue, an outer ring of fibrotic reaction, and a peripheral rim of endosteal reaction that is hypointense on T1-weighted images.

ESR usually is normal. Treatment consists of surgical drainage and curettage followed by antimicrobial therapy, as for other forms of hematogenous osteomyelitis. A variety of organisms, including *H. influenzae*, have been isolated from these lesions,[120] but *S. aureus* and other gram-positive cocci are the pathogens usually involved. The prognosis generally is good, although deformities occur in some cases.

HEMATOGENOUS OSTEOMYELITIS IN SPECIAL POPULATIONS

OSTEOMYELITIS IN NEWBORNS

Infection of the bones of newborns has distinct physiologic and clinical features that warrant emphasis.[7,49,226] Although it is rare, neonatal osteomyelitis may occur in newborns with certain risk factors, such as prematurity, skin infections, and complicated delivery.[72,118] As indicated earlier, the epiphyseal-metaphyseal junction frequently is within the joint capsule, and blood vessels that penetrate the epiphysis are common findings, particularly in the hip, shoulder, and knee of the newborn.

In newborns, osteomyelitis in the long tubular bones frequently (50-70% of cases) is accompanied by contiguous septic arthritis. Fever is present in one third to one half of the newborns; of these, half have a septic or toxic appearance. Half of infants have multiple bones involved. Antecedent infections are present in half of the cases and usually are nosocomial; infections of heel puncture sites, arterial cannulas, lungs, and cut-down sites and cephalhematoma have been described.[7] *S. aureus* is the etiologic agent in more than 90 percent of cases; gram-negative bacilli cause a few cases. Osteomyelitis often is identified when a search is instituted for the source or focus of bacteremia.[226] As noted earlier, plain radiographs often reveal evidence of osteomyelitis at the time of diagnosis, whereas bone scanning may be negative. Bone scanning may be useful, however, in excluding the diagnosis of osteomyelitis; in one study, the negative predictive value was estimated at 82 percent.[226]

Although staphylococci seem to be the most common cause of osteomyelitis in infants, group B streptococci have been found consistently.[58] Infants with group B streptococcal osteomyelitis generally are older (2-4 weeks old), have no recognized preceding infection, and have only a single bone involved, often the right tibia or humerus.[7]

Osteomyelitis in the skull, an uncommon disease, can occur in neonates. Frequently, it is associated with a cephalhematoma, with or without loss of skin integrity,[123] but it can be caused by fetal monitoring without a cephalhematoma.[142] Numerous bacteria have been isolated from such lesions; as one might expect, most of these bacteria have been present as vaginal flora. Radiographic changes (i.e., bony erosion) are a late finding, but CT of the skull seems to assist in establishing the diagnosis. Infection of a cephalhematoma should be considered if it is enlarging, if it is inflamed, or if laboratory evidence of infection is present, such as an increased CRP concentration or leukocyte count. In most cases, the lesion is drained and treated with an antibiotic appropriate for the infecting organism.

In older descriptions of neonatal osteomyelitis, sequelae were common findings. In more recent series,[118,224] approximately three fourths of all cases have had good outcomes, even when the hip has been involved. When seen, sequelae include avascular necrosis of the femoral head, bony deformities, and shortening of the involved limb.[161]

OSTEOMYELITIS IN LONG-TERM HEMODIALYSIS PATIENTS

Patients undergoing long-term hemodialysis, with multiple invasions of the vascular compartment, seem to be at greater risk for development of hematogenous osteomyelitis.[125] Their indwelling intravenous cannulas can be colonized with coagulase-negative staphylococci or *S. aureus*, and osteomyelitis may develop. The thoracic spine and ribs are the bones most commonly involved; other tubular and cuboidal bones that have been traumatized also can become infected.

OSTEOMYELITIS IN CHILDREN WITH HEMOGLOBINOPATHIES

After pneumonia, osteomyelitis is the most common serious infection in children with sickle-cell disease.[11] Children at risk are children with hemoglobin SS, hemoglobin S-Thal, or hemoglobin SO-Arab and certain children with hemoglobin SC disease.[93,186] The clinical manifestations of osteomyelitis are similar to those of other children with osteomyelitis, but there is a propensity for simultaneous involvement of multiple sites, a tendency toward recurrence, and a greater frequency in children 18 to 48 months of age.

As noted earlier, the microbiology of osteomyelitis in children with sickle-cell disease is complex and dominated by *Salmonella* spp.[11,31] Seventy percent of all lesions or blood cultures in children with hemoglobinopathy and presumptive osteomyelitis yield *Salmonella* microorganisms; 10 percent contain *S. aureus*; and aerobic gram-negative rods, including *Shigella sonnei*,[173] *Escherichia coli*,[92] *Serratia* spp.,[70] and *Arizona hinshawii*,[103] are isolated in 7 percent. Although *Salmonella* osteomyelitis occurs in less than 1 percent of normal patients with *Salmonella* bacteremia,[222] the frequency of *Salmonella* osteomyelitis in sickle-cell disease is several hundred times that occurring in the general population, with an incidence estimated at 0.36 percent per annum.[11,53,163]

Many factors probably contribute to the greater incidence of osteomyelitis in patients with sickle-cell hemoglobinopathy. Injuries to the intestinal mucosa from local thrombosis during a thrombotic crisis may facilitate the entrance of *Salmonella* and other enteric organisms into the bloodstream.[31,222] When infection of the bloodstream occurs, the splenic dysfunction in these patients may allow a prolonged period or greater magnitude of bacteremia. Evidence of impaired production of opsonic antibodies also exists. Whether bacteria lodge in infarcted bone, or whether a different pathogenesis exists is unclear. Infarction occurs in the capital femoral epiphysis, hands, feet, and vertebrae, whereas osteomyelitis involves the metaphyseal-diaphyseal junction of long tubular bones.[60,163]

Infants with hand and foot syndrome are not distinguished easily from infants with osteomyelitis of the phalanges of the hands or tarsal bones of the feet.[16,41,219] The changes caused by osteomyelitis that are seen on plain radiographs are more severe than the changes expected in uncomplicated sickle-cell disease. The most common radiographic findings are a longitudinal intracortical diaphyseal fissure and overabundant periosteal new bone formation. The cortical fissures are thought to represent a layer of purulent exudate in and between the periosteal new bone and dead bone.[53]

Radionuclide scans also are used frequently to help differentiate osteomyelitis from bone infarction. In theory, bone infarction should have decreased uptake of Tc 99m in the early "blood pool" phase of the scan; increased uptake would be found only as the lesion healed.[115] In one series with 34 sites of infarction, increased Tc 99m uptake occurred in 10, normal uptake occurred in 9, and decreased uptake surrounded by zones of increased concentration occurred in the remaining 15 sites.[81] Ga 67 or bone marrow scans of lesions with Tc 99m sulfur colloid also may be valuable in differentiating infarction from infection; increased uptake of the radionuclide is seen more frequently with infection than with infarction.[166] Acute infarction and osteomyelitis cannot always be differentiated by MRI, perhaps because of pre-existing abnormalities in bone marrow. MRI may be useful, however, for presurgical evaluation. Ultrasound imaging also has been used to distinguish osteomyelitis and sickle-cell crisis and, if confirmed, may prove to be a useful adjunct to other imaging modalities.[23]

Generally, patients with bony infarcts have had dactylitis as an infant and multiple episodes; their temperature usually is less than 39° C. Children with hemoglobinopathy and osteomyelitis may lack this history and have a modest leukocytosis of immature granulocytes.[105] If fever, leukocytosis, and local symptoms persist despite provision of hydration and other supportive measures, needle aspiration of the area must be considered. Identification of an infectious pathogen is particularly important because of the large number of possible organisms involved.

OSTEOMYELITIS IN PATIENTS WITH HUMAN IMMUNODEFICIENCY VIRUS INFECTION

Although recurrent invasive bacterial infections often complicate human immunodeficiency virus (HIV) infection in children and adults, few reports of osteomyelitis in these patients exist.[104,143,190] Many of the existing reports involve patients with recent intravenous drug use, which probably acted as a predisposing factor. *S. aureus* was recovered most commonly, although *E. coli, Salmonella enteritidis, Cryptococcus neoformans, Mycobacterium kansasii, Histoplasma capsulatum*, and other organisms also were seen in individual cases. To date, no evidence supports the view that the initial signs and symptoms or treatment needed for recovery from osteomyelitis is affected by co-infection with HIV.

OSTEOMYELITIS IN PATIENTS AFTER CLOSED FRACTURES

Acute hematogenous osteomyelitis sometimes develop after closed fractures of tubular bones occur.[33,218] The diagnosis generally is not recognized until fluctuation is apparent at the fracture site. A clue to diagnosis is that after the initial post-fracture pain has subsided, the pain of osteomyelitis occurs. It begins 1 to 6 weeks after the injury occurs. The pain differs from that associated with the fracture by being progressive, and it is not relieved by immobilization. When the cast is removed, local erythema and warmth are apparent and are increased when these findings would seem to be resolving if they were secondary to the fracture. Patients are febrile and may be thought to have another focus of infection before osteomyelitis is discovered. Anaerobic superinfection of staphylococcal osteomyelitis at the fracture site has been recognized.[201] Adequate débridement, administration of appropriate antibiotics, and external fixation have been used in such cases. The outcome varies, however.

OSTEOMYELITIS IN PATIENTS WITH CHRONIC GRANULOMATOUS DISEASE

The phagocytes of patients with chronic granulomatous disease fail to kill intracellular organisms, and infections with catalase-positive bacteria or fungi are frequent complications. Although staphylococci are a common cause of cutaneous infection in chronic granulomatous disease, osteomyelitis is caused most often by *Serratia* and *Aspergillus* spp. Osteomyelitis is attributed less often to staphylococci, *Pseudomonas, Burkholderia, Nocardia*, and other bacterial and fungal species.[225]

NONHEMATOGENOUS OSTEOMYELITIS

Nonhematogenous infections of the bone arise either through inoculation or from a contiguous focus of infection.

PUNCTURE WOUND OSTEOMYELITIS

Inoculation osteomyelitis most often involves either the patella or the bones of the foot. Soft tissue infections occur after puncture wounds of the foot approximately 15 percent of the time, and osteomyelitis occurs in 1.5 percent of these injuries.[67] Osteomyelitis of the foot that develops after children sustain puncture wounds should be termed *osteochondritis* because it commonly includes infection of the articular cartilage in the metatarsals. Most patients are aged 9 to 18 years. After the initial pain of the puncture wound subsides (in 24-48 hours), the signs of osteochondritis appear after another 48 to 72 hours. Typically, joint tenderness and localized swelling, erythema, and pain over the entrance of the puncture wound are present. Fever is an infrequent finding, and the patient seldom has any other constitutional symptoms. No peripheral leukocytosis is noted, and ESR is increased minimally.

Although the offending organism most commonly is *P. aeruginosa* (90% of the time), staphylococci, streptococci, *Stenotrophomonas maltophilia*,[9] and *Serratia marcescens*[151] also have been isolated.[25,67,106,107,109] In some series,[107] 20 percent of the cases involved infection with *P. aeruginosa* and *S. aureus*. The predominance of *Pseudomonas* can be explained partially on the basis of the mechanism of injury. *Pseudomonas* is not found commonly in surveys of the microbial flora of the skin of the feet,[85,145,198] but often it is found by culture of the sponge liner from children's sneakers.[66] In addition, many patients in whom *P. aeruginosa* osteochondritis develops have received prophylactic treatment with oral antibiotics that have activity against gram-positive bacteria. A semisynthetic penicillinase-resistant penicillin and an aminoglycoside or ceftazidime often are used as initial therapy.[106,107]

Surgical débridement of necrotic cartilage is a key element of treatment because foreign material frequently is found embedded in the soft tissue; débridement also provides the opportunity to identify organisms resistant to the initial antibiotic agents. The local signs and symptoms of infection usually resolve 4 to 5 days after adequate débridement is performed, and the patient is able to bear weight on the foot. In contrast, antibiotic therapy alone after diagnostic aspiration may need to be continued 6 to 8 weeks before weight bearing is possible. Long-term follow-up of *P. aeruginosa* osteochondritis indicates that many patients have asymptomatic radiographic abnormalities.[13] Radiographic abnormalities are found more commonly in patients in whom an adjacent joint was involved initially.[13]

Osteomyelitis also has been described repeatedly after puncture wounds occur from stepping on wooden toothpicks. In these cases, *Eikenella corrodens*, a member of the human oral flora, has been found with other organisms. Surgical débridement to remove toothpick fragments and drain local abscesses is essential.[168]

Osteomyelitis of the patella is a disease of children aged 5 to 15 years old, the time in life during which the patella is vascularized. By adulthood, the vessels are almost completely atrophied. In almost all cases, the diagnosis shows the cause to be by inoculation, such as kneeling on a needle. The most common etiologic agent is *S. aureus*; signs of osteomyelitis appear 1 week after the puncture occurs. No constitutional symptoms occur, but extension of the leg produces pain over the anterior aspect of the patella. The diagnosis is made by isolating the organism from the patella. Radiographic confirmation of the diagnosis often requires 2 to 3 weeks. Because the bone lacks periosteum, no periosteal elevation is present, but rarefaction and sclerosis may be seen on the profile view or on tomograms. Treatment of this disease is similar to that for other forms of osteomyelitis.

OSTEOMYELITIS CAUSED BY SPREAD OF INFECTION FROM A CONTIGUOUS FOCUS

In children, osteomyelitis related to an infected contiguous focus is a rare finding. Almost all cases of osteomyelitis from a contiguous source in childhood are nosocomial or are caused by an infected burn wound. The probability of postoperative osteomyelitis developing is a function of the surgeon's experience, the technique, the length of time that the wound was open, and whether prophylactic antibiotics were administered.[192] The interval between the precipitating event and pain and the appearance of persistent sinus drainage or ulceration is 2 to 4 weeks. The peripheral white blood cell count often is normal, as is ESR. More than half of cases are caused by multiple organisms. When small draining sinuses are present, correlation between sinus culture and bone biopsy findings is good. With large open areas, organisms obtained by culture of the wound may not be important etiologically, and obtaining a bone biopsy specimen is necessary for making a definitive bacteriologic diagnosis. Staphylococci and streptococci predominate; however, nosocomial gram-negative organisms often are seen.

ORTHOPEDIC FIXATOR DEVICES

Infection involving the wires or pins used for orthopedic stabilization represents a diagnostic and therapeutic challenge. Osteomyelitis is suspected when evidence of inflammation or infection is noted near these materials, but it seldom can be proved.[20] Plain radiographs are essential because they may reveal bone destruction at the site of entry of fixation pins. No controlled studies of treatment are available. Soft tissue débridement and removal of necrotic bone should be done as soon as possible, but fixation devices generally are left in place.[10,160] Prolonged therapy usually is given, guided by the susceptibility pattern of any organisms recovered from local cultures.[160]

UNUSUAL MICROBIAL CAUSES OF OSTEOMYELITIS

ACTINOMYCES

More than half of all actinomycotic infections involve the facial or cervical area. The most common site of actinomycotic bone infection is the jaw, with the mandible being involved more frequently than the maxilla. Local signs and symptoms of fever and discharge from a sinus indicate the presence of the disease. Radiographically, periosteal elevation is followed by lytic changes. Often, several "eggshell" areas of new bone are present.

Forty percent of all actinomycotic infections occur in the vertebral bodies. In this illness, the infection almost always is associated with a focus elsewhere; the condition comes to medical attention because of mild pain, tenderness, and some stiffness. It can be distinguished from tuberculosis radiographically by the diffuse honeycombing of the vertebral bodies and the periosteal reaction; large lytic lesions usually are absent. Although no controlled trials of therapy have been done, long-term (>3 months) penicillin G therapy is indicated at doses of 150,000 U/kg body weight per day (i.e., approximately 100 mg/kg/day). Extensive débridement may be needed and has been linked to successful short-term treatment of mandibular actinomycosis.[12]

BRUCELLA

Although an uncommon cause of osteomyelitis in developed countries, *Brucella* spp. are a well-known cause of skeletal infections, most often following the consumption of unpasteurized milk products. *Brucella* spp. can produce abscesses in the vertebral bodies or long bones, although they are not striking features of the disease. The disease often is subacute in presentation, and malaise, headaches, night sweats, and minimally tender cervical adenopathy with hepatosplenomegaly are common initial findings.

FUNGI

Osteomyelitis may be caused by numerous endemic and opportunistic fungal agents, including *C. immitis*, cryptococci, *Candida* spp., *Blastomyces* spp., and *Aspergillus* spp. Coccidioidomycosis may be characterized by cough, chest pain, night sweats, and anorexia, and it often is associated with erythema nodosum or erythema multiforme. This disease commonly is found in the southwestern United States. Extrapulmonary involvement is suggested by persistent high temperature and toxicity. *C. immitis* occurs primarily in cancellous bone (e.g., vertebral bodies, distal tubular bones, and the skull).[167] These lesions are not radiographically distinct from the lesions seen in osteomyelitis from other causes.[183] Débridement of bone lesions often is needed initially, and years of therapy are required. Oral triazole agents generally are recommended.[74]

Blastomycosis may mimic coccidioidomycosis, but the pulmonary involvement is much more varied, and fusion of the vertebral bodies rarely occurs. A propensity for the development of verrucous, reddened, weeping skin lesions has been noted, and prostate involvement may be seen. Bone involvement occurs frequently, with the skull and vertebral bodies being infected most often. Distinguishing it from other forms of osteomyelitis is impossible by radiographic examination.

Aspergillus osteomyelitis is being recognized with increasing frequency.[35] Most commonly, it is a disease of immunosuppressed patients, with *Aspergillus* pneumonia seen initially followed by disseminated disease. Bone disease occurring by hematogenous spread has developed, however, in normal individuals and after injectable drug use.[43,172] *Aspergillus* osteomyelitis developing after trauma also has been reported.

Other fungi are causes of osteomyelitis. The medical literature contains dozens of reports of osteomyelitis caused by *C. neoformans*, generally in immunocompromised patients and in the setting of disseminated or pulmonary infection. The few reports in pediatric patients generally have involved immunocompromised adolescents. In adolescents and adults, usually only one bone is involved. The lesions generally are slowly destructive, very discrete lesions occurring primarily in the long tubular bones without marginal sclerosis. This radiologic reaction is confused most commonly with tumor and, occasionally, with tuberculosis. Infection of the ribs and skull also has been reported. Although experience with this disease is limited, débridement of the lesions and medical therapy seem to be highly effective.[14,30,37,84,131,132] Cases of *Rhizopus* osteomyelitis have been reported intermittently and apparently are hematogenous in origin.[57]

CHRONIC OSTEOMYELITIS

Chronic osteomyelitis often is the result of bone infection that develops after a surgical procedure or major trauma.[209] Inadequate treatment of acute hematogenous osteomyelitis also can lead to the development of chronic osteomyelitis. The diagnosis of chronic osteomyelitis usually is straightforward; patients generally have a painful, nonfunctional extremity and may have chronically draining sinuses. Cultures of the purulent exudate or necrotic bone usually reveal *S. aureus*. Gram-negative bacteria, including *H. influenzae*,[120] may be isolated from an intraosseous abscess. Plain radiographs, CT, and MRI all play roles in medical and surgical management by revealing details of the bony and soft tissue involvement, including the formation of abscesses[164] and sequestra (Fig. 61–7).

Treatment of chronic osteomyelitis involves the removal of devitalized bone, management of soft tissue disease, and long-term administration of appropriate antibiotics. Few controlled trials comparing different modes of therapy have been performed. Antimicrobial regimens for chronic staphylococcal osteomyelitis that have been studied include oral cloxacillin plus probenecid for 6 to 12 months; 9 of 19 patients apparently were treated successfully.[15] In another study, the outcome of a 6-week course of nafcillin was compared with that of nafcillin and oral rifampin. No statistically significant differences were observed with the addition of rifampin, but most (10 of 17) of the patients showed no evidence of disease activity 2 years after the cessation of treatment with antibiotics.[157]

The high failure rate in these and other studies has led to investigation of a variety of adjunctive measures to improve the outcome of chronic osteomyelitis. Local irrigation with antibiotic solutions, with[136] and without[3] added detergents, has been examined. The use of surgically implanted polymethyl methacrylate beads impregnated with an antibiotic (usually gentamicin) has been compared with conventional antibiotic therapy and with therapy with both.[19] No differences were seen among the three groups in a preliminary analysis. Hyperbaric oxygen also has been suggested as an aid to therapy, but no comparative studies have been done.[150]

Because perpetuation of chronic infection seems to be caused by the presence of avascular bone and tissue, advances such as laser Doppler flowmetry ultimately may improve the outcome of this disease.[195] Surgical approaches to close open wounds after débridement and improve blood flow with mobilized tissue flaps also seem to bring about prolonged remission in some patients.[4] Meticulous surgical technique is essential to avoid thermal injury and to retain the vascular supply to compromised areas.[202] Complications of chronic osteomyelitis include secondary amyloidosis and local sarcomatosis or carcinomatous changes at the site of infection. The high likelihood of a poor outcome in chronic osteomyelitis must be kept in mind during treatment of acute hematogenous osteomyelitis. Failure to comply with a regimen of oral therapy may result in chronic infection.[196]

CHRONIC RECURRENT MULTIFOCAL OSTEOMYELITIS

Giedion and coworkers[79] first described chronic recurrent multifocal osteomyelitis, an illness characterized by multiple chronic focal, inflammatory lesions in bone with periodic exacerbation and remission, moderate bone pain, and sterile lesions.[213] Initially, this disease is difficult to distinguish from pyogenic osteomyelitis; the only difference seems to be the apparent absence of an infecting agent. Repeated biopsy of lesions that prove to be sterile usually leads to the diagnosis. It occurs more commonly in girls younger than 10 years of age.

At initial evaluation, slightly more than 50 percent of patients have fever, and virtually all have an increased ESR (or increased CRP). The lesions occur primarily in the distal femoral, distal tibial, and proximal tibial regions. Virtually all tubular bones can be involved.[179] Patients may have 1 to 18 lesions at a time; biopsy specimens show a nonspecific chronic inflammatory process. Occasionally, a predominance of plasma cells is present, which erroneously leads to this disease being termed *plasma-cell osteomyelitis*. In the first reported cases, the lesions were symmetric. This feature has not been present consistently, however, as more cases have been described. Many of the cases are in children of northern European origin.[18,117]

Approximately 20 percent of patients have a pustular eruption of the palms and soles at the same time that they come to medical attention with bone lesions; this condition is termed *pustulosis palmaris et plantaris*. Some patients also may have Sweet syndrome, in which painful, indurated, cutaneous plaques are accompanied by fever and leukocytosis. Sweet syndrome and pustulosis palmaris et plantaris may be variations of the same illness. Sweet syndrome and congenital dyserythropoietic anemia also have been associated with chronic recurrent multifocal osteomyelitis.[59]

The long-term outlook in children with this disease generally is good, although numerous relapses may occur.[18] Glucocorti-

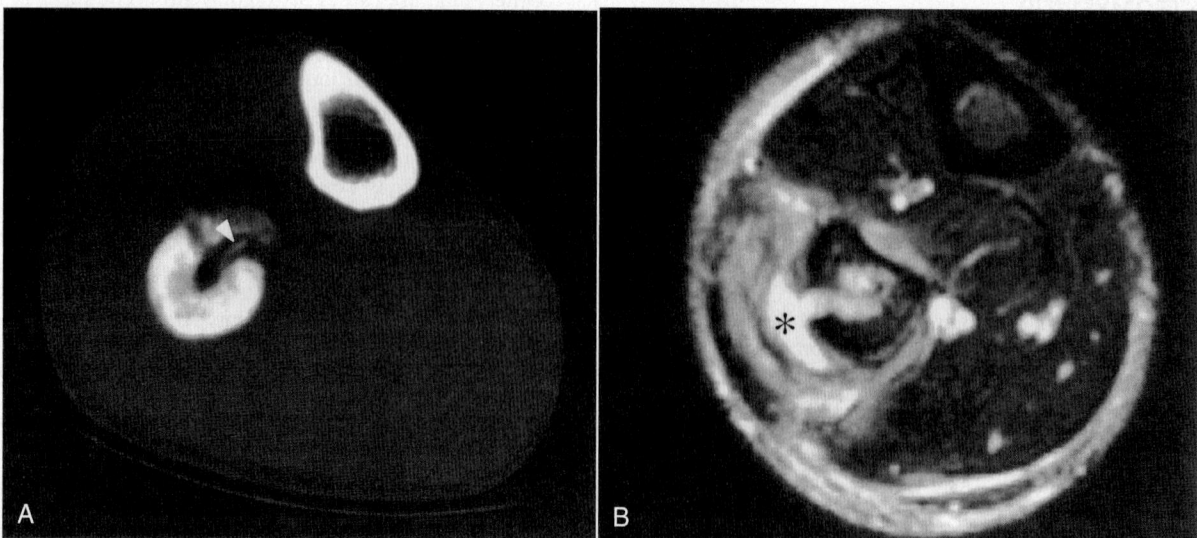

Figure 61–7 Chronic osteomyelitis. **A,** Computed tomography reveals thickening of the fibular cortex and a sinus tract that contains a sequestrum *(arrowhead)*. **B,** T2-weighted axial magnetic resonance imaging from a different level shows a lateral sinus tract through the cortex communicating with a soft tissue abscess *(asterisk)*. Edema is surrounding the entire fibula. *(Courtesy of Dr. Leanne Seeger.)*

coids and nonsteroidal anti-inflammatory drugs have been administered to children with this disease and afford transient relief. Patients usually have a recurrence of symptoms and lesions, however, when these agents are discontinued. Treatment with interferon-γ and tumor necrosis factor–α blocking agents also has been reported to be helpful.[51,75]

REFERENCES

1. Ailsby, R., and Staheli, L.: Pyogenic infections of the sacroiliac joint in children. Clin. Orthop. *100*:96-100, 1974.
2. Ambrose, G. B., Alpert, M., and Neer, C. S.: Vertebral osteomyelitis: A diagnostic problem. J. A. M. A. *197*:619-622, 1966.
3. Anderson, L. D., and Horn, L. G.: Irrigation-suction technic in the treatment of acute hematogenous osteomyelitis, chronic osteomyelitis, and acute and chronic joint infections. South. Med. J. *63*:745-754, 1970.
4. Anthony, J. P., and Mathes, S. J.: Update on chronic osteomyelitis. Clin. Plast. Surg. *18*:515-523, 1991.
5. Arnold, S. R., Elias, D., Buckingham, S. C., et al.: Changing patterns of acute hematogenous osteomyelitis and septic arthritis: Emergence of community-associated methicillin-resistant *Staphylococcus aureus*. J. Pediatr. Orthop. *26*:703-708, 2006.
6. Ash, J. M., and Gilday, D. L.: The futility of bone scanning in neonatal osteomyelitis: Concise communication. J. Nucl. Med. *21*:417-420, 1980.
7. Asmar, B. I.: Osteomyelitis in the neonate. Infect. Dis. Clin. N. Am. *6*:117-132, 1992.
8. Babaiantz, L.: Les osteopathies atrophiques. J. Radiol. Radiother. Nucl. Med. *19*:333, 1948.
9. Baltimore, R. S., and Jenson, H. B.: Puncture wound osteochondritis of the foot caused by *Pseudomonas maltophilia*. Pediatr. Infect. Dis. J. *9*:143-144, 1990.
10. Barret, J. P., Desai, M. H., and Herndon, D. N.: Osteomyelitis in burn patients requiring skeletal fixation. Burns *26*:487-489, 2000.
11. Barrett-Connor, E.: Bacterial infection and sickle cell anemia: An analysis of 250 infections in 166 patients and a review of the literature. Medicine (Baltimore) *50*:97-112, 1971.
12. Bartkowski, S. B., et al.: Actinomycotic osteomyelitis of the mandible: Review of 15 cases. J. Craniomaxillofac. Surg. *26*:63-67, 1998.
13. Barton, L. L., et al.: Long-term radiologic outcome of *Pseudomonas* osteomyelitis of the foot. Pediatrics *9*:476-478, 1980.
14. Behrman, R. E., Masci, J. R., and Nicholas, P.: Cryptococcal skeletal infections: Case report and review. Rev. Infect. Dis. *12*:181-190, 1990.
15. Bell, S. M.: Further observations on the value of oral penicillins in chronic staphylococcal osteomyelitis. Med. J. Aust. *2*:591-593, 1976.
16. Bennett, O. M.: *Salmonella* osteomyelitis and the hand-foot syndrome in sickle cell disease. J. Pediatr. Orthop. *12*:534-538, 1992.
17. Berkowitz, I. D., and Wenzel, W.: 'Normal' technetium bone scans in patients with acute osteomyelitis. Am. J. Dis. Child. *134*:828-830, 1980.
18. Bjorksten, B., et al.: Chronic recurrent multifocal osteomyelitis and pustulosis palmoplantaris. J. Pediatr. *93*:227-231, 1978.
19. Blaha, J. D., et al.: Comparison of the clinical efficacy and tolerance of gentamicin PMMA beads on surgical wound versus combined and systemic therapy for osteomyelitis. Clin. Orthop. *295*:8-12, 1993.
20. Blasier, R. D., Aronson, J., and Tursky, E. A.: External fixation of pediatric femur fractures. J. Pediatr. Orthop. *17*:342-346, 1997.
21. Blockey, N. J., and Watson, J. T.: Acute osteomyelitis in children. J. Bone Joint Surg. *52*:77-87, 1970.
22. Bocchini, C. E., Hulten, K. G., Mason, E. O., Jr., et al.: Panton-Valentine leukocidin genes are associated with enhanced inflammatory response and local disease in acute hematogenous *Staphylococcus aureus* osteomyelitis in children. Pediatrics *117*:433-440, 2006.
23. Booz, M. M., et al.: The value of ultrasound and aspiration in differentiating vaso-occlusive crisis and osteomyelitis in sickle cell disease patients. Clin. Radiol. *54*:636-639, 1999.
24. Bradley, J. S., et al.: Pediatric pneumococcal bone and joint infections. The Pediatric Multicenter Pneumococcal Surveillance Study Group (PMPSSG). Pediatrics *102*:1376-1382, 1998.
25. Brand, R. A., and Black, H.: *Pseudomonas* osteomyelitis following puncture wounds in children. J. Bone Joint Surg. Am. *56*:1637-1642, 1974.
26. Bremnet, A., and Neligan, G.: Pyogenic osteitis. *In* Gairdners, D. (ed): Recent Advances in Pediatrics. London, T. A. Churchill Ltd., 1958.
26a. Browne, L. P., Mason, E. O., Kaplan, S. L., et al.: Optimal imaging strategy for community-acquired *Staphylococcus aureus* musculoskeletal infections in children. Pediatr. Radiol. *38*:841-847, 2008.
27. Bruno, M. S., and Neligan, G.: Embolic osteomyelitis of the spine as a complication of infection of the urinary tract. Am. J. Med. *19*:865-878, 1958.
28. Bryan, V., Franks, L., and Torres, H.: *Pseudomonas aeruginosa* cervical diskitis with chondro-osteomyelitis in an intravenous drug abuser. Surg. Neurol. *1*:142-144, 1973.
29. Bryson, Y. J., et al.: High-dose oral dicloxacillin treatment of acute staphylococcal osteomyelitis in children. J. Pediatr. *94*:673-675, 1979.
30. Burch, K. H., et al.: *Cryptococcus neoformans* as a cause of lytic bone lesions. J. A. M. A. *231*:1057-1059, 1975.
31. Burnett, M. W., Bass, J. W., and Cook, B. A.: Etiology of osteomyelitis complicating sickle cell disease. Pediatrics *101*:296-297, 1998.
32. Buxton, T. B., et al.: Binding of a *Staphylococcus aureus* bone pathogen to type I collagen. Microb. Pathog. *8*:441-448, 1990.
33. Canale, S. T., et al.: Acute osteomyelitis following closed fractures: Report of three cases. J. Bone Joint Surg. Am. *57*:415-418, 1975.
34. Capitanio, M. A., and Kirkpatrick, J. A.: Early roentgen observations in acute osteomyelitis. Am. J. Roentgenol. Radium Ther. Nucl. Med. *108*:488-496, 1970.
35. Casscells, S. W.: *Aspergillus* osteomyelitis of the tibia: A case report. J. Bone Joint Surg. Am. *60*:994-995, 1978.
36. Charkes, N. D.: Skeletal blood flow: Implications for bone-scan interpretation. J. Nucl. Med. *21*:91-98, 1980.
37. Ching, N., et al.: Enlarging parietal mass with lytic skull lesion. Pediatr. Infect. Dis. J. *23*:589, 595-596, 2004.
38. Chung, S. M., and Borns, P.: Acute osteomyelitis adjacent to the sacroiliac joint in children: Report of two cases. J. Bone Joint Surg. Am. *55*:630-634, 1973.
39. Chung, T.: Magnetic resonance imaging in acute osteomyelitis in children. Pediatr. Infect. Dis. J. *21*:869-870, 2002.
40. Collin, D. H.: Pathology of Bone. London, Butterworths, 1966.
41. Constant, E., Green, R. L., and Wagner, D. K.: *Salmonella* osteomyelitis of both hands and the hand-foot syndrome. Arch. Surg. *102*:148-151, 1971.
42. Conventry, M. B., Ghormley, R. K., and Kernohan, J.: Intervertebral disc: Its microscopic anatomy and pathology. J. Bone Joint Surg. Am. *27*:105-112, 1945.
43. Corrall, C. J., et al.: *Aspergillus* osteomyelitis in an immunocompetent adolescent: A case report and review of the literature. Pediatrics *70*:455-461, 1982.
44. Cushing, A. H.: Diskitis in children. Clin. Infect. Dis. *17*:1-6, 1993.
45. Dahl, L. B., et al.: Acute osteomyelitis in children: A population-based retrospective study 1965 to 1994. Scand. J. Infect. Dis. *30*:573-577, 1998.
46. de Groot, R., et al.: Bone and joint infections caused by *Kingella kingae*: Six cases and review of the literature. Rev. Infect. Dis. *10*:998-1004, 1988.
47. Delorimier, A. A., Haskin, D., and Massie, F.: Mediastinal mass caused by vertebral osteomyelitis. Am. J. Dis. Child. *111*:639-643, 1966.
48. Demopulos, G. A., Bleck, E. E., and McDougall, I. R.: Role of radionuclide imaging in the diagnosis of acute osteomyelitis. J. Pediatr. Orthop. *8*:558-565, 1988.
49. Deshpande, P. G., et al.: Neonatal osteomyelitis and septic arthritis. Indian Pediatr. *27*:453-457, 1990.
50. Deutsch, S. D., Gandsman, E. J., and Spraragen, S. C.: Quantitative regional blood-flow analysis and its clinical application during routine bone-scanning. J. Bone Joint Surg. Am. *63*:295-305, 1981.
51. Deutschmann, A., Mache, C. J., Budo, K., et al.: Successful treatment of chronic recurrent multifocal osteomyelitis with tumor necrosis factor-alpha blockage. Pediatrics *116*:1231-1233, 2005.
52. Dich, V. Q., Nelson, J. D., and Haltalin, K. C.: Osteomyelitis in infants and children: A review of 163 cases. Am. J. Dis. Child. *129*:1273-1278, 1975.
53. Diggs, L. W.: Bone and joint lesions in sickle-cell disease. Clin. Orthop. *52*:119-143, 1967.
54. Drew, R. H., et al.: Treatment of methicillin-resistant *Staphylococcus aureus* infections with quinupristin-dalfopristin in patients intolerant of or failing prior therapy. For the Synercid Emergency-Use Study Group. J. Antimicrob. Chemother. *46*:775-784, 2000.
55. Dunn, E. J., et al.: Pyogenic infections of the sacro-iliac joint. Clin. Orthop. *118*:113-117, 1976.
56. Duszynski, D. O., et al.: Early radionuclide diagnosis of acute osteomyelitis. Radiology *117*:337-340, 1975.
57. Echols, R. M., et al.: Rhizopus osteomyelitis: A case report and review. Am. J. Med. *66*:141-145, 1979.
58. Edwards, M. S., et al.: An etiologic shift in infantile osteomyelitis: The emergence of the group B streptococcus. J. Pediatr. *93*:578-583, 1978.
59. Edwards, T. C., et al.: Sweet's syndrome with multifocal sterile osteomyelitis. Am. J. Dis. Child. *140*:817-818, 1986.
60. Epps, C. H., Jr., and Bryant, D. D.: Osteomyelitis in patients who have sickle-cell disease: Diagnosis and management. J. Bone Joint Surg. Am. *73*:1281-1294, 1991.
61. Farr, H.: Acute hematogenous osteomyelitis due to type B *Haemophilus* osteomyelitis and arthritis. Lancet *1*:517-518, 1966.
62. Farrand, R. J., Johnstone, J. M., and McCabe, A. F.: *Haemophilus* osteomyelitis and arthritis. B. M. J. *2*:334-336, 1968.
63. Feigin, R. D., et al.: Clindamycin treatment of osteomyelitis and septic arthritis in children. Pediatrics *55*:213-223, 1975.
64. Ferguson, W. R.: Some observations on circulation in fetal and infant spine. J. Bone Joint Surg. Am. *32*:640-648, 1950.
65. Fernandez, M., Carrol, C. L., and Baker, C. J.: Discitis and vertebral osteomyelitis in children: An 18-year review. Pediatrics *105*:1299-1304, 2000.
66. Fisher, M. C., Goldsmith, J. F., and Gilligan, P. H.: Sneakers as a source of *Pseudomonas aeruginosa* in children with osteomyelitis following puncture wounds. J. Pediatr. *106*:607-609, 1985.
67. Fitzgerald, R. H., Jr., and Cowan, J. D.: Puncture wounds of the foot. Orthop. Clin. North Am. *6*:965-972, 1975.

68. Fletcher, B. D., Scoles, P. V., and Nelson, A. D.: Osteomyelitis in children: Detection by magnetic resonance. Work in progress. Radiology 150:57-60, 1984.
69. Floyed, R. L., and Steele, R. W.: Culture-negative osteomyelitis. Pediatr. Infect. Dis. J. 22:731-736, 2003.
70. Fonk, J., and Coonrod, J. D.: Serratia osteomyelitis in sickle cell disease. J. A. M. A. 217:80-81, 1970.
71. Fox, L., and Sprunt, K.: Neonatal osteomyelitis. Pediatrics 62:535-542, 1978.
72. Freehafer, A. A., Furey, J. G., and Pierce, D. S.: Pyogenic osteomyelitis of the spine resulting in spinal paralysis. J. Bone Joint Surg. Am. 44:710-716, 1962.
73. Gainey, M. A., et al.: Indium-111-labeled white blood cells: Dosimetry in children. J. Nucl. Med. 29:689-694, 1988.
74. Galgiani, J. N., et al.: Practice guideline for the treatment of coccidioidomycosis. Infectious Diseases Society of America. Clin. Infect. Dis. 30:658-661, 2000.
75. Gallagher, K. T., et al.: Treatment of chronic recurrent multifocal osteomyelitis with interferon gamma. J. Pediatr. 131:470-472, 1997.
76. Geddes, A. M., et al.: The Treatment of Pediatric Infections with Clindamycin. Baltimore, University Park Press, 1972.
77. Genster, H. G., and Anderson, J. J. F.: Spinal osteomyelitis complicating urinary tract infection. J. Urol. 107:109-111, 1971.
78. Gibson, W. K., Bartosh, R., and Timperlake, R.: Acute hematogenous epiphyseal osteomyelitis. Orthopedics 14:705-707, 1991.
79. Giedion, A., et al.: [Subacute and chronic "symmetrical" osteomyelitis]. Ann. Radiol. (Paris) 15:329-342, 1972.
80. Gilday, D. L., Paul, D. J., and Paterson, J.: Diagnosis of osteomyelitis in children by combined blood pool and bone imaging. Radiology 117:331-335, 1975.
81. Gilfand, M. J., and Harche, H. T.: Skeletal imaging in sickle cell disease. J. Nucl. Med. 19:698-709, 1978.
82. Gillespie, W. J.: Epidemiology in bone and joint infection. Infect. Dis. Clin. N. Am. 4:361-376, 1990.
83. Goergens, E. D., McEvoy, A., Watson, M., et al.: Acute osteomyelitis and septic arthritis in children. J. Paediatr. Child Health 41:59-62, 2005.
84. Goldshteyn, N., Zanchi, A., Cooke, K., and Aqha, R.: Cryptococcal osteomyelitis of the humeral head initially diagnosed as avascular necrosis. South. Med. J. 99:1140-1141, 2006.
85. Goldstein, E. J., et al.: Source of Pseudomonas in osteomyelitis of heels. J. Clin. Microbiol. 12:711-713, 1980.
86. Gonzalez, B. E., Hulten, K. G., Bishop, M. K., et al.: Pulmonary manifestations in children with invasive community-acquired Staphylococcus aureus infection. Clin. Infect. Dis. 41:583-590, 2005.
87. Gonzalez, B. E., Teruya, J., Mahoney, D. H., Jr., et al.: Venous thrombosis associated with staphylococcal osteomyelitis in children. Pediatrics 117:1673-1679, 2006.
88. Goutzmanis, J. J., Gonis, G., and Gilbert, G. L.: Kingella kingae infection in children: Ten cases and a review of the literature. Pediatr. Infect. Dis. J. 10:677-683, 1991.
89. Granoff, D. M., Sargent, E., and Jolivette, D.: Haemophilus influenzae type b osteomyelitis. Am. J. Dis. Child. 132:488-490, 1976.
90. Green, J. H.: Cloxacillin in treatment of acute osteomyelitis. B. M. J. 2:414-416, 1967.
91. Green, W. T.: Osteomyelitis of infants: A disease different from osteomyelitis of older children. Arch. Surg. 32:462-493, 1936.
92. Greenburg, L. W., and Haynes, R. E.: Escherichia coli osteomyelitis in an infant with sickle cell disease. Clin. Pediatr. (Philadelphia) 9:436-438, 1990.
93. Griesemer, D. A., Winkelstein, J. A., and Luddy, R.: Pneumococcal meningitis in patients with a major sickle hemoglobinopathy. J. Pediatr. 92:82-84, 1978.
94. Gristina, A. G., et al.: Adherent bacterial colonization in the pathogenesis of osteomyelitis. Science 228:990-993, 1985.
95. Handmaker, H., and Giammona, S. T.: Improved early diagnosis of acute inflammatory skeletal-articular diseases in children: A two-radiopharmaceutical approach. Pediatrics 73:661-669, 1984.
96. Harcke, H. T.: Role of imaging in musculoskeletal infections in children. J. Pediatr. Orthop. 15:141-143, 1995.
97. Harris, N. H.: Some problems in the diagnosis and treatment of acute osteomyelitis. J. Bone Joint Surg Am. 42:535-542, 1960.
98. Henson, N. H.: Some problems in the diagnosis and treatment of acute osteomyelitis. Surg. Gynecol. Obstet. 102:207-214, 1956.
99. Highland, T. R., and LaMont, R. L.: Osteomyelitis of the pelvis in children. Pediatrics 73:661-669, 1984.
100. Hobo, T.: Zur Pathogenese der Vitalfarbungalehre. Acta Sch. Med. Univ. Kioto 4:1-29, 1921.
101. Hoffer, P.: Gallium and infection. J. Nucl. Med. 21:484-488, 1980.
102. Holzman, R. S., and Bishko, F.: Osteomyelitis in heroin addicts. Ann. Intern. Med. 75:693-696, 1971.
103. Hruby, M. A., Honig, G. R., Lolekha, S., Gotoff, S. P.: Arizoni hinshawii osteomyelitis in sickle cell anemia. Am. J. Dis. Child. 125:867-868, 1973.
104. Hughes, R. A., et al.: Septic bone, joint and muscle lesions associated with human immunodeficiency virus infection. Br. J. Rheumatol. 31:381-388, 1992.
105. Jackson, M. A., and Nelson, J. D.: Etiology and medical management of acute suppurative bone and joint infections in pediatric patients. J. Pediatr. Orthop. 2:313-323, 1982.
106. Jacobs, R. F., et al.: Management of Pseudomonas osteochondritis complicating puncture wounds of the foot. Pediatrics 69:432-435, 1982.
107. Jacobs, R. F., McCarthy, R. E., and Elser, J. M.: Pseudomonas osteochondritis complicating puncture wounds of the foot in children: A 10-year evaluation. J. Infect. Dis. 160:657-661, 1989.
108. Jaffe, H. L.: Degenerative and Inflammatory Diseases of the Bones and Joints. Philadelphia, Lea & Febiger, 1972.
109. Johanson, P. H.: Pseudomonas infections of the foot following puncture wounds. J. A. M. A. 204:262-264, 1968.
110. Jordan, M. C., and Kirby, W. M.: Pyogenic vertebral osteomyelitis: Treatment with antimicrobial agents and bed rest. Arch. Intern. Med. 128:405-410, 1971.
111. Kahn, D. S., and Pritzker, K. P.: The pathophysiology of bone infection. Clin. Orthop. 96:12-19, 1973.
112. Kaplan, S. L.: Osteomyelitis in children. Infect. Dis. Clin. N. Am. 19:787-797, vii, 2005.
113. Kaplan, S. L., Mason, E. O., Jr., and Feigin, R. D.: Clindamycin versus nafcillin or methicillin in the treatment of Staphylococcus aureus osteomyelitis in children. South. Med. J. 75:138-142, 1982.
114. Karwowska, A., Davies, H. D., and Jadavji, T.: Epidemiology and outcome of osteomyelitis in the era of sequential intravenous-oral therapy. Pediatr. Infect. Dis. J. 17:1021-1026, 1998.
115. Keeley, K., and Buchanan, G. R.: Acute infarction of long bones in children with sickle cell anemia. J. Pediatr. 101:170-175, 1982.
116. Kemp, H., Jackson, J., and Jeremia, J.: Pyogenic infections occurring primarily in intervertebral discs. J. Bone Joint Surg. Am. 55:698-714, 1963.
117. King, S. M., et al.: Chronic recurrent multifocal osteomyelitis: A noninfectious inflammatory process. Pediatr. Infect. Dis. J. 6:907-911, 1987.
118. Knudsen, C. J., and Hoffman, E. B.: Neonatal osteomyelitis. J. Bone Joint Surg. Br. 72:846-851, 1990.
119. Kozin, F., et al.: Computed tomography in the diagnosis of sacroiliitis. Am. J. Dis. Child. 134:828-830, 1980.
120. Kurlandsky, L. E., Quinn, P. H., and Sills, E. M.: Haemophilus influenzae as a cause of Brodie's abscess in an infant. Johns Hopkins Med. J. 144:15-17, 1979.
121. LaMont, R. L., et al.: Acute hematogenous osteomyelitis in children. J. Pediatr. Orthop. 7:579-583, 1987.
122. Lascari, A. D., Graham, M. H., and MacQueen, J. C.: Intervertebral disk infection in children. J. Pediatr. 70:751-757, 1967.
123. Lee, P. Y.: Infected cephalhaematoma and neonatal osteomyelitis. J. Infect. 21:191-193, 1990.
124. Leigh, T. F., Kelly, R. P., and Weens, H. S.: Spinal osteomyelitis associated with urinary tract infections. Radiology 65:334-342, 1955.
125. Leonard, A., et al.: Osteomyelitis in hemodialysis patients. Ann. Intern. Med. 78:651-658, 1973.
126. Le Saux, O., Beck, K., Sachsinger, C., et al.: Evidence for a founder effect for pseudoxanthoma elasticum in the Afrikaner population of South Africa. Hum. Genet. 111:331-338, 2002.
127. Lewis, J. S., 2nd, and Jorgensen, J. H.: Inducible clindamycin resistance in staphylococci: Should clinicians and microbiologists be concerned? Clin. Infect. Dis. 40:280-285, 2005.
128. Lewis, R., Gorbach, S., and Altner, P.: Spinal Pseudomonas chondroosteomyelitis in heroin users. N. Engl. J. Med. 286:1303, 1972.
129. Lewis, R. P., Sutter, V. L., and Finegold, S. M.: Bone infections involving anaerobic bacteria. Medicine (Baltimore) 57:279-305, 1978.
130. Lifeso, R. M., Harder, E., and McCorkell, S. J.: Spinal brucellosis. J. Bone Joint Surg. Br. 67:345-351, 1985.
131. Littman, M. L., and Walter, J. E.: Cryptococcosis: Current status. Am. J. Med. 45:922-932, 1968.
132. Liu, P. Y.: Cryptococcal osteomyelitis: Case report and review. Diagn. Microbiol. Infect. Dis. 30:33-35, 1998.
133. Longjohn, D. B., Zionts, L. E., and Stott, N. S.: Acute hematogenous osteomyelitis of the epiphysis. Clin. Orthop. 316:227-234, 1995.
134. Lundy, D. W., and Kehl, D. K.: Increasing prevalence of Kingella kingae in osteoarticular infections in young children. J. Pediatr. Orthop. 18:262-267, 1998.
135. Majeed, H. A., Kalaawi, M., Mohanty, D., et al.: Congenital dyserythropoietic anemia and chronic recurrent multifocal osteomyelitis in three related children and the association with Sweet syndrome in two siblings. J. Pediatr. 115:730-734, 1989.
136. Makin, M., Geller, R., Jacobs, J., Sacks, T.: Non-toxic detergent irrigation of chronic infections: An experimental evaluation. Clin. Orthop. 320-324, 1973.
137. Marshall, G. S., Mudido, P., Rabalais, G. P., et al.: Organism isolation and serum bactericidal titers in oral antibiotic therapy for pediatric osteomyelitis. South. Med. J. 89:68-70, 1996.
138. Martí-Bonmati, L., Aparisi, F., Poyatos, C., Vilar, J.: Brodie abscess: MR imaging appearance in 10 patients. J. Magn. Reson. Imaging 3:543-546, 1993.
139. Martinez-Aguilar, G., et al.: Clindamycin treatment of invasive infections caused by community-acquired, methicillin-resistant and methicillin-susceptible Staphylococcus aureus in children. Pediatr. Infect. Dis. J. 22:593-598, 2003.
140. Martinez-Aguilar, G., Avalos-Mishaan, A., Hulten, K., et al.: Community-acquired, methicillin-resistant and methicillin-susceptible Staphylococcus aureus musculoskeletal infections in children. Pediatr. Infect. Dis. J. 23:701-706, 2004.

141. Mazur, J. M., et al.: Usefulness of magnetic resonance imaging for the diagnosis of acute musculoskeletal infections in children. J. Pediatr. Orthop. 15:144-147, 1995.

142. McGregor, J. A., and McFarren, T.: Neonatal cranial osteomyelitis: A complication of fetal monitoring. Obstet. Gynecol. 73:490-492, 1989.

143. Medina, F., et al.: Salmonella pyomyositis in patients with the human immunodeficiency virus. Br. J. Rheumatol. 34:568-571, 1995.

144. Miller, D. J., and Mejicano, G. C.: Vertebral osteomyelitis due to Candida species: Case report and literature review. Clin. Infect. Dis. 33:523-530, 2001.

145. Miller, E. H., and Semian, D. W.: Gram-negative osteomyelitis following puncture wounds of the foot. Medicine (Baltimore) 57:279-205, 1978.

146. Modic, M. T., et al.: Vertebral osteomyelitis: Assessment using MR. Radiology 157:157-166, 1985.

147. Mok, P. M., Reilly, B. J., and Ash, J. M.: Osteomyelitis in the neonate: Clinical aspects and the role of radiography and scintigraphy in diagnosis and management. Radiology 145:677-682, 1982.

148. Morgan, A., and Yates, A. K.: The diagnosis of acute osteomyelitis of the pelvis. Postgrad. Med. J. 42:74-78, 1966.

149. Morrey, B. F., Bianco, A. J., and Rhodes, K. H.: Hematogenous osteomyelitis at uncommon sites in children. Mayo Clin. Proc. 53:707-713, 1978.

150. Morrey, B. F., Dunn, J. M., Heimbach, R. D., and Davis, J.: Hyperbaric oxygen and chronic osteomyelitis. Clin. Orthop. 121-127, 1979.

151. Murray, M. M., Welch, D. F., and Kuhls, T. L.: Serratia osteochondritis after puncture wounds of the foot. Pediatr. Infect. Dis. J. 9:523-525, 1990.

152. Mustafa, M. M., et al.: Acute hematogenous pelvic osteomyelitis in infants and children. Pediatr. Infect. Dis. J. 9:416-421, 1990.

153. Nagal, D. A., Albright, J. A., and Keggi, K. J.: Closer look at spinal lesions: Open biopsy of vertebral lesions. J. A. M. A. 191:975-978, 1965.

154. Nelson, J. D.: Acute osteomyelitis in children. Infect. Dis. Clin. N. Am. 4:513-522, 1990.

155. Nelson, J. D.: Toward simple but safe management of osteomyelitis. Pediatrics 99:883-884, 1997.

156. Nelson, J. D., Bucholz, R. W., Kusmiesz, H., Shelton, S.: Benefits and risks of sequential parenteral-oral cephalosporin therapy for suppurative bone and joint infections. J. Pediatr. Orthop. 2:255-262, 1982.

157. Norden, C. W., et al.: Chronic osteomyelitis caused by Staphylococcus aureus: Controlled clinical trial of nafcillin therapy and nafcillin-rifampin therapy. South. Med. J. 79:947-951, 1986.

158. Peltola, H., Unkila-Kallio, L., and Kallio, M. J.: Simplified treatment of acute staphylococcal osteomyelitis of childhood. The Finnish Study Group. Pediatrics 99:846-850, 1997.

159. Perlman, M. H., et al.: The incidence of joint involvement with adjacent osteomyelitis in pediatric patients. J. Pediatr. Orthop. 20:40-43, 2000.

160. Perry, J. W., et al.: Wound infections following spinal fusion with posterior segmental spinal instrumentation. Clin. Infect. Dis. 24:558-561, 1997.

161. Peters, W., Irving, J., and Letts, M.: Long-term effects of neonatal bone and joint infection on adjacent growth plates. J. Pediatr. Orthop. 12:806-810, 1992.

162. Pichichero, M. E., and Friesen, H. A.: Polymicrobial osteomyelitis: Report of three cases and review of the literature. Rev. Infect. Dis. 4:86-96, 1982.

163. Piehl, F. C., Davis, R. J., and Prugh, S. I.: Osteomyelitis in sickle cell disease. J. Pediatr. Orthop. 13:225-227, 1993.

164. Poyhia, T., and Azouz, E. M.: MR imaging evaluation of subacute and chronic bone abscesses in children. Pediatr. Radiol. 30:763-768, 2000.

165. Prober, C. G., and Yeager, A. S.: Use of the serum bactericidal titer to assess the adequacy of oral antibiotic therapy in the treatment of acute hematogenous osteomyelitis. J. Pediatr. 95:131-135, 1979.

166. Rao, S., et al.: Scintigraphic differentiation of bone infarction from osteomyelitis in children with sickle cell disease. J. Pediatr. 107:685-688, 1985.

167. Rhangos, W. C., and Chick, E. W.: Mycotic infections of bone. South. Med. J. 57:664-674, 1964.

168. Robinson, L. G., and Kourtis, A. P.: Tale of a toothpick: Eikenella corrodens osteomyelitis. Infection 28:332-333, 2000.

169. Rocco, H. D., and Eyring, E. J.: Intervertebral disk infections in children. Am. J. Dis. Child. 123:448-451, 1972.

170. Rodriguez, W., Ross, S., Kahn, W., McKay, D., et al.: Clindamycin in the treatment of osteomyelitis in children: A report of 29 cases. Am. J. Dis. Child. 131:1088-1093, 1977.

171. Roine, I., et al.: Serial serum C-reactive protein to monitor recovery from acute hematogenous osteomyelitis in children. Pediatr. Infect. Dis. J. 14:40-44, 1995.

172. Roselle, G. A., and Baird, I. M.: Aspergillus flavipes group osteomyelitis. Arch. Intern. Med. 139:590-592, 1995.

173. Rubin, H. M., Eardley, W., and Nichols, B. L.: Shigella sonnei osteomyelitis and sickle-cell anemia. Am. J. Dis. Child. 116:83-87, 1968.

174. Rubin, R. C., Jacobs, G. B., Cooper, P. R., and Wille, R. L.: Disc space infections in children. Childs Brain 3:180-190, 1977.

175. Ruebner, R., et al.: Complications of central venous catheters used for the treatment of acute hematogenous osteomyelitis. Pediatrics 117:1210-1215, 2006.

176. Sapico, F. L., and Montgomerie, J. Z.: Pyogenic vertebral osteomyelitis: Report of nine cases and review of the literature. Rev. Infect. Dis. 1:754-776, 1979.

177. Schauwecker, D. S.: Osteomyelitis: Diagnosis with In-111-labeled leukocytes. Radiology 171:141-146, 1989.

178. Schechter, L. S., Smith, A., and Pearl, M.: Intervertebral disk calcification in childhood. Am. J. Dis. Child. 123:608-611, 1972.

179. Schultz, C., et al.: Chronic recurrent multifocal osteomyelitis in children. Pediatr. Infect. Dis. J. 18:1008-1013, 1999.

180. Scoles, P. V., Hilty, M. D., and Sfakianakis, G. N.: Bone scan patterns in acute osteomyelitis. Clin. Orthop. 153:210-217, 1980.

181. Selby, R. C., and Pillay, K. V.: Osteomyelitis and disc infection secondary to Pseudomonas aeruginosa in heroin addiction: Case report. J. Neurosurg. 37:463-466, 1972.

182. Sfakianakis, G. N., Scoles, P., Welch, M., et al.: Evolution of bone imaging findings in osteomyelitis. J. Nucl. Med. 199:706, 1978.

183. Smith, C. E., and Beard, R. R.: Varieties of coccidioidal infection in relation to epidemiology and control of the disease. Am. J. Public Health 36:1394-1402, 1946.

184. Smith, R. F., and Taylor, T. K.: Inflammatory lesions of intervertebral discs in children. J. Bone Joint Surg. Am. 49:1508-1520, 1967.

185. Sorsdahl, O. A., et al.: Quantitative bone gallium scintigraphy in osteomyelitis. Skeletal Radiol. 22:239-242, 1993.

186. Specht, E. E.: Hemoglobinopathic Salmonella osteomyelitis: Orthopedic aspects. Clin. Orthop. 79:110-118, 1971.

187. Spiegel, P. G., Kengla, K. W., Isaacson, A. S., and Wilson, J. C., Jr.: Intervertebral disc-space inflammation in children. J. Bone Joint Surg. Am. 54:284-296, 1972.

188. Staab, E. V., and McCartney, W. H.: Role of gallium 67 in inflammatory disease. Semin. Nucl. Med. 8:219-234, 1978.

189. Starr, C. L.: Acute hematogenous osteomyelitis. Arch. Surg. 4:567-587, 1922.

190. Steinbach, L. S., Tehran Zaden, J., Fleckenstein, J. L., et al.: Human immunodeficiency virus infection: Musculoskeletal manifestations. Radiology 186:833-838, 1993.

191. Stephens, M. M., and MacAuley, P.: Brodie's abscess: A long-term review. Clin. Orthop. 234:211-216, 1988.

192. Stevens, J.: Post-operative orthopedic infections. J. Bone Joint Surg. Am. 46:96, 1964.

193. Stone, D. B., and Bonfiglio, M.: Pyogenic vertebral osteomyelitis: A diagnostic pitfall for the internists. Arch. Intern. Med. 112:491-500, 1963.

194. Swick, H. M.: Calcification of intervertebral discs in childhood. J. Pediatr. 86:364-369, 1975.

195. Swiontkowski, M. F.: Surgical approaches in osteomyelitis: Use of laser Doppler flowmetry to determine nonviable bone. Infect. Dis. Clin. N. Am. 4:501-512, 1990.

196. Syrogiannopoulos, G. A., and Nelson, J. D.: Duration of antimicrobial therapy for acute suppurative osteoarticular infections. Lancet 1:37-40, 1988.

197. Tang, J. S., Gold, R. H., Bassett, L. W., and Seeger, L. L.: Musculoskeletal infection of the extremities: Evaluation with MR imaging. Radiology 166:205-209, 1988.

198. Taplin, D.: Environmental influences on the microbiology of the skin. Arch. Environ. Health 11:546, 1968.

199. Taylor, J. C., and Fallon, R. J.: Osteomyelitis due to Hemophilus influenzae. Lancet 1:715, 1964.

200. Taylor, J. R.: Growth of human intervertebral discs and vertebral bodies. J. Anat. 120:49-68, 1975.

201. Templeton, W. C., 3rd, Wawrukiewicz, A., Melo, J. C., et al.: Anaerobic osteomyelitis of long bones. Rev. Infect. Dis. 5:692-712, 1983.

202. Tetsworth, K., and Cierny, G.: Osteomyelitis débridement techniques. Clin. Orthop. 360:87-96, 1999.

203. Tetzlaff, T. R., McCracken, G. H., Jr., and Nelson, J. D.: Oral antibiotic therapy for skeletal infections of children, II: Therapy of osteomyelitis and suppurative arthritis. J. Pediatr. 92:485-490, 1978.

204. Tilden, R. L., Jackson, J., Jr., Enneking, W. F., et al.: 99m Tc-polyphosphate: Histological localization in human femurs by autoradiography. J. Nucl. Med. 14:576-578, 1973.

205. Torda, A. J., Gottlieb, T., and Bradbury, R.: Pyogenic vertebral osteomyelitis: Analysis of 20 cases and review. Clin. Infect. Dis. 20:320-328, 1995.

206. Treves, S., Khettry, J., Broker, F. H., et al.: Osteomyelitis: Early scintigraphic detection in children. Pediatrics 57:173-186, 1976.

207. Tröbs, R., Möritz, R., Bühligen, U., et al.: Changing pattern of osteomyelitis in infants and children. Pediatr. Surg. Int. 15:363-372, 1999.

208. Trueta, J.: The three types of acute hematogenous osteomyelitis. J. Bone Joint Surg. Am. 41:671-680, 1959.

209. Tsukayama, D. T.: Pathophysiology of posttraumatic osteomyelitis. Clin. Orthop. 360:22-29, 1999.

210. Unger, E., Moldofsky, P., Gatenby, R., et al.: Diagnosis of osteomyelitis by MR imaging. A. J. R. Am. J. Roentgenol. 150:605-610, 1988.

211. Unkila-Kallio, L., Kallio, M. J., and Peltola, H.: Acute haematogenous osteomyelitis in children in Finland. Finnish Study Group. Ann. Med. 25:545-549, 1993.

212. Unkila-Kallio, L., Kallio, M. J., Peltola, H., and Eskola, J.: Serum C-reactive protein, erythrocyte sedimentation rate, and white blood cell count in acute hematogenous osteomyelitis of children. Pediatrics 93:59-62, 1994.

213. Van Howe, R. S., Starshak, R. J., and Chusid, M. J.: Chronic, recurrent multifocal osteomyelitis: Case report and review of the literature. Clin Pediatr (Philadelphia) 28:54-59, 1989.

214. Vaughan, P. A., Newman, N. M., and Rosman, M. A.: Acute hematogenous osteomyelitis in children. J. Pediatr. Orthop. 7:652-655, 1987.

215. Verdier, I., Gayet-Ageron, A., Ploton, C., Taylor, P., et al.: Contribution of a broad range polymerase chain reaction to the diagnosis of osteoarticular infections caused by *Kingella kingae*: Description of twenty-four recent pediatric diagnoses. Pediatr. Infect. Dis. J. *24*:692-696, 2005.
216. Waldvogel, F. A., and Papageorgiou, P. S.: Osteomyelitis: The past decade. N. Engl. J. Med. *303*:360-370, 1980.
217. Walker, S. H.: Staphylococcal osteomyelitis in children: Success with cephaloridine-cephalexin therapy. Clin Pediatr (Philadelphia) *12*:98-100, 1973.
218. Watson, F. M., and Whitesides, T. E., Jr.: Acute hematogenous osteomyelitis complicating closed fractures. Clin. Orthop. 296-302, 1976.
219. Watson, R. J., Burko, H., Megas H., and Robinson, M.: The hand-foot syndrome in sickle cell disease in young children. Pediatrics *31*:505-509, 1963.
220. Weissberg, E. D., Smith, A. L., and Smith, D. H.: Clinical features of neonatal osteomyelitis. Pediatrics *53*:505-510, 1974.
221. Weld, P. W.: Osteomyelitis of the ileum, masquerading as acute appendicitis. J. A. M. A. *173*:634-636, 1960.
222. Widen, A. L., and Cardon, L.: *Salmonella typhimurium* osteomyelitis with sickle cell-hemoglobin C disease: A review and case report. Ann. Intern. Med. *54*:510-521, 1961.
223. Wiesseman, G. J., Wood, V. E., Kroll, L. L., and Linda, L.: *Pseudomonas* vertebral osteomyelitis in heroin addicts: Report of five cases. J. Bone Joint Surg. Am. *55*:1416-1424, 1973.
224. Williamson, J. B., Galasko, C. S., and Robinson, M. J.: Outcome after acute osteomyelitis in preterm infants. Arch. Dis. Child. *65*:1060-1062, 1990.
225. Winkelstein, J. A., Marino, M. C., Johnston, R. B., Jr., et al.: Chronic granulomatous disease: Report on a national registry of 368 patients. Medicine (Baltimore) *79*:155-169, 2000.
226. Wong, M., Isaacs, D., Howman-Giles, R., and Uren, R.: Clinical and diagnostic features of osteomyelitis occurring in the first three months of life. Pediatr. Infect. Dis. J. *14*:1047-1053, 1995.
227. Yagupsky, P.: *Kingella kingae*: From medical rarity to an emerging paediatric pathogen. Lancet Infect. Dis. *4*:358-367, 2004.
228. Yagupsky, P., Howard, C. B., Einhorn, M., and Dagan, R.: *Kingella kingae* osteomyelitis of the calcaneus in young children. Pediatr. Infect. Dis. J. *12*:540-541, 1993.

CHAPTER 62

SEPTIC ARTHRITIS

Paul Krogstad

This chapter addresses acute infection of the joints caused by bacteria, fungi, and viruses. Bacterial infections occur most frequently. The terms *septic arthritis, acute suppurative pyarthrosis,* and *infectious arthritis* are used interchangeably with regard to bacterial infections; they refer to the presence of organisms in the joint space.

EPIDEMIOLOGY

Septic arthritis occurs most frequently in childhood. The overall incidence of septic arthritis in children has been estimated as 5.5 to 12 cases per 100,000 individuals.[32] Describing the age distribution of septic arthritis is difficult because of the varying age intervals selected by authors of different studies. In a review from the pre-antibiotic era, half of the patients were younger than 20 years old.[45] In a later study, performed after antibiotics became available for systemic use, 31 of 66 patients (47%) were younger than 20 years old.[6] Males are affected more often than are females by ratios of 1.2 to 2.1, and most cases occur in children younger than 10 years old.[10,34,55,59,77,91]

PATHOPHYSIOLOGY

Synovial joints, also termed *diarthrodial joints,* are freely movable articulations containing synovia. Synovia is a transparent viscous fluid that lubricates the joint and nourishes the avascular articular cartilage. The synovium, a connective tissue layer interposed between the fibrous joint capsule and the fluid-filled synovial cavity, is responsible for formation of the joint fluid. The synovium contains a prominent capillary supply embedded in a connective tissue network containing at least two types of cells. One morphologic type (type A) seems to be related to mononuclear phagocytes; fibroblast-like type B cells seem to be responsible for the synthesis of hyaluronic acid. Joint fluid (synovia) is formed by filtration through the capillary network (i.e., the net balance of back-diffusion into the capillary bed and diffusion into the joint space). Diarthrodial joints normally contain small amounts of fluid (e.g., 0.5 to 3 mL in the knee),[81] with glucose and electrolyte concentrations equal to those in plasma. An oxygen partial pressure of 60 to 70 mm Hg, an albumin concentration of 10 to 20 g/L, and an IgG content of 500 mg/L are typical.[22,24,30,81]

Diffusion from the joint space is increased by any mechanism that increases pressure (distention with injected solution, active or passive motion, or external massage). Particulate material is removed from the joint space by synovial membrane macrophages and free monocytes (the latter usually are present in concentrations of $<60 \times 10^6$/L).[75] The viscosity of joint fluid is due to hyaluronic acid; enzymatic depolymerization produces a viscosity approximately equivalent to that of water. With the loss of hyaluronidase from the synovia, the articular cartilage, with continued use, becomes eroded and sclerotic.[9] The vasculature of the synovial membrane is innervated, which has two consequences: Joint pain is localized poorly because it results from stretching of the fibrous joint capsule, and inflammation within the joint cavity elicits an axon reflex leading to vasodilation and warmth over an infected joint. Lymphatic channels drain to the regional lymph nodes and are present in all the joint tissues except cartilage.

Microorganisms can enter the joint space by hematogenous spread, direct inoculation, or extension of a contiguous focus of infection. The synovial membrane has been shown to have highly effective blood flow, approximately equal to that of the brain (if one assumes that 1 g of synovial membrane is in an adult knee joint). Numerous bacteria in blood potentially are delivered to the synovial membrane during transient bacteremia. A history of trauma often is cited as a predisposing factor for development of bacterial arthritis, but the significance of such a history is unclear in view of the great frequency of minor trauma in childhood.

Upper respiratory tract infections frequently precede the development of septic arthritis caused by *Haemophilus influenzae* and *Kingella kingae* and oral ulcers with *Kingella* infections. Similar to traumatic injuries, they are presumed to increase the likelihood of bacteremia occurring.[10,90] Septic arthritis also may develop after joint surgery and joint injections. Gram-negative organisms are the most frequent pathogens when septic arthritis occurs after surgery or instrumentation of the urinary or intestinal tract. *Salmonella* septic arthritis may develop during the course of *Salmonella* bacteremia in a normal host, but it occurs with increased frequency in patients with sickle-cell disease and related hemoglobinopathies. Although septic arthritis occurs in children and adults infected with human immunodeficiency virus (HIV),[58] as yet no data have substantiated that HIV increases the incidence of musculoskeletal infections in children. Septic arthritis has been described during varicella, presumably caused by bacteremia resulting from infection of skin lesions. It must be differentiated from the apparent ability of varicella-zoster virus to cause joint inflammation on its own.[61,74] Arthritis also occurs during acute infection with other viruses (e.g., variola, Epstein-Barr virus, *Erythrovirus* [parvovirus B19], mumps, measles, and enteroviruses).

Inoculation arthritis occurs after invasion of the joint by a contaminated object. In one series, 5 of 35 cases of septic arthritis were caused by such a mechanism. A predilection for the knee exists; four of five cases cited in this study were secondary to kneeling on sewing needles.[77]

Aside from joint involvement during osteomyelitis, contiguous extension of an infection into the joint space rarely occurs. In one series, 10 of 77 patients with septic arthritis had disease originating from a contiguous focus.[18] None involved the joints of the foot, and eight occurred before the availability of many antibiotics (1951). This high frequency of septic arthritis caused by spread of infection from a contiguous focus has not been seen in more recent studies.

ETIOLOGY

Staphylococcus aureus is the most common agent causing septic arthritis, and infection with community-acquired methicillin-resistant *S. aureus* (MRSA) is now commonly reported.[3,57] Streptococci (especially group A beta-hemolytic organisms and pneumococci) have been responsible for most other gram-positive infections (Table 62–1). *H. influenzae* type b historically has been an important cause of septic arthritis in children younger than 2 years, but now is seen only rarely in areas with widespread immunization.[13,41,55] Arthritis caused by *Streptococcus pneumoniae* also generally occurs in children younger than 2 years old and may diminish in frequency with broader use of protein conjugate vaccines. *K. kingae* has been recognized increasingly as a cause of septic arthritis,[23,39,55,91] perhaps because of improvements in laboratory methods.[92] In one series from Israel, *Kingella* was the most common bacterial isolate (48% of cases), and *S. aureus* was not found.[91] In a few cases, septic arthritis is seen with acute *Neisseria meningitidis* infection. In newborns and sexually active adolescents with suspected septic arthritis, *Neisseria gonorrhoeae* should be considered.[35,51,53]

Salmonella spp. cause approximately 1 percent of the total cases of septic arthritis. Beyond the newborn period, infections with other enteric gram-negative bacteria are rare occurrences in pediatric septic arthritis and often are associated with inoculation, instrumentation, or an immunocompromised state.[35] Infections with *Serratia, Aeromonas, Enterobacter, Bacteroides,* and *Campylobacter* generally occur in patients with malignancy who are immunosuppressed.[1,6,19,35,56,63,67] *Pseudomonas aeruginosa* infections are associated with arthritis in infants, with infection of puncture wounds, or with injectable drug use.[59,63,83] Other rare bacterial causes of septic arthritis include *Propionibacterium acnes,*[93] *Corynebacterium pyogenes,*[67] and *Pasteurella multocida.*[38] *Streptobacillus moniliformis* infection of joints may become evident 2 to 3 days after a rat bite occurs; a macular rash commonly is present at initial evaluation. Discussion of Lyme arthritis is beyond the scope of this chapter, but intermittent, inflammatory arthritis is seen in many patients after *Borrelia burgdorferi* is transmitted by a tick bite.[49,80] *Brucella,* mycobacteria (*Mycobacterium tuberculosis* and atypical species), and *Nocardia asteroides* may cause a chronic monarticular arthritis with a granulomatous reaction.

DIAGNOSIS

CLINICAL FINDINGS

Almost all patients have fever and constitutional symptoms within the first few days of acquiring infection with the most common bacterial pathogens.[31] Table 62–2 presents the frequency of specific joint involvement in hematogenous septic arthritis of childhood. Lower extremity (knee, hip, and ankle) infections consistently account for approximately 80 percent of all cases.[34,45,59,63,77] Focal findings in the joint involved almost always are present.

In infants, in whom the hip is one of the most frequent joints involved, swelling, tenderness, and heat may be absent. Most commonly, the infant lies with the involved leg abducted and externally rotated. Often, dislocation occurs.[65] When the capsule of the joint can be examined, swelling is noted; effusion was present in 22 of 24 cases in one series.[87] Because pain fibers are located in the capsule, any maneuver that increases intracapsular pressure also produces pain. In the hip, this pain can be elicited by compression of the head of the femur into the acetabulum. A portal of entry almost never is apparent, and bilateral hip joint infection occurs in a few cases.[69] Pyogenic sacroiliitis often is accompanied by tenderness detected by pressure applied over the sacrum during a digital rectal examination and by pain experienced during simultaneous flexion, abduction, and external rotation at the hip.[2]

Gonococcal arthritis in newborns has nonspecific prodromal symptoms, including poor feeding, irritability, and fever. The

TABLE 62–1   Bacterial Etiology of Septic Arthritis in Children

Year of Report	Gram-Positive Bacteria				Gram-Negative Bacteria							Total Cases
	Staphylococcus aureus	Streptococci	*Streptococcus pneumoniae*	CNS	*Haemophilus influenzae*	*Kingella kingae*	*Neisseria meningitidis*	*Salmonella*	Non-*Salmonella* Enterobacteriaceae	*Neisseria gonorrhoeae*	Other	
1941[45]	50	45	2	10	0	0	0	0	0	14	0	121
1958[77]	18	8	5	2	3	0	0	2	0	0	1	38*
1972[63]	40	20	8	5	37	0	4	2	7	13	11	146*
1975[59]	37	10	0	5	14	0	0	0	2	0	7	75
1987[10]	40	8	5	0	20	0	4	0	2	2	9	90
1995[91]	0	2	3	0	8	19	1	1	4	2	5	40
1999[55]	10	5	2	2	1	3	3	0	4	2	1	33
Total	195	98	25	24	83	22	12	3	18	31	34	543
Percentage of all isolates	36	18	5	4	15	4	2	1	3	6	6	

Two isolates in one case each.
CNS, coagulase-negative staphylococci.

TABLE 62-2   Joints Involved in Septic Arthritis of Children

Reference	Knee	Hip	Ankle	Wrist	Elbow	Shoulder	Small Diarthrodial Joints
Heberling[45]	40	50	13	3	8	9	2
Watkins et al.[88]	8	13	2	6	9	2	3
Samilson et al.[77]	8	19	2	0	6	3	0
Nelson[63]	103	48	38	12	35	10	4
Gillespie[31]	37	41	13	2	3	3	0
Yagupsky et al.[91]	16	6	13	1	2	3	1
Goergens et al.[34]	15	15	4	2	4	1	3
Total	227	192	85	26	67	31	13
Percentage of all cases	35	30	13	4	10	5	2

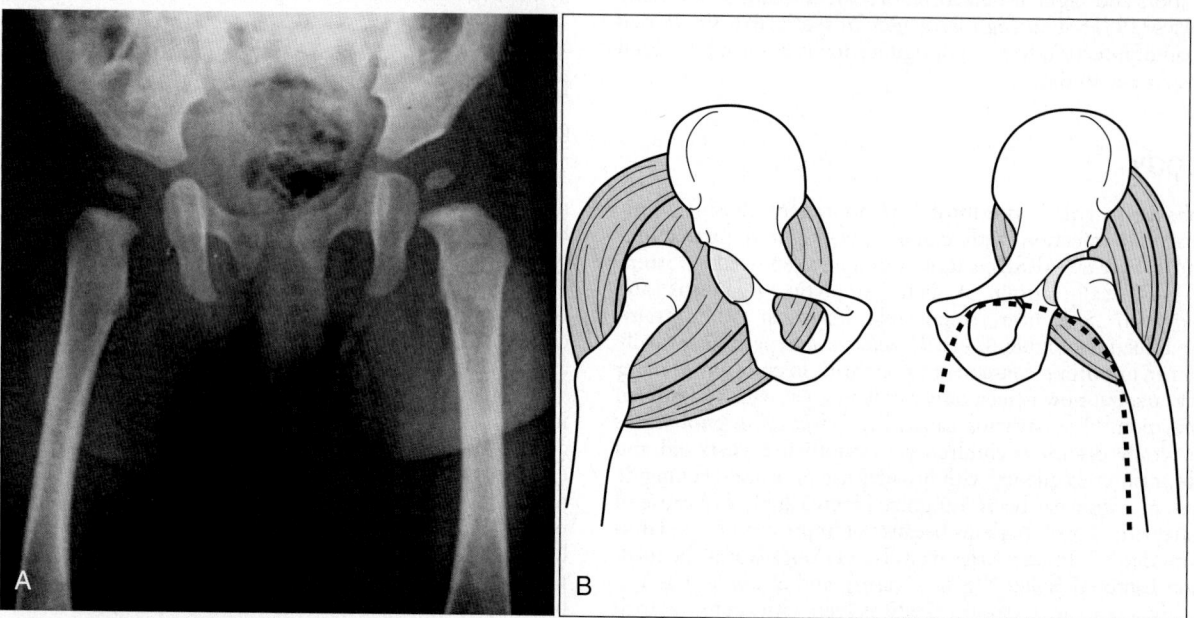

Figure 62–1 A and **B,** The obturator sign in the hip is one of the oldest signs of septic arthritis. Another consistent finding is obliteration or lateral displacement of the gluteal fat lines and loss of continuity of the Shenton line. These findings are illustrated radiographically **(A)** and schematically **(B).**

portal of entry is unknown, and the joints below the hip usually are involved (knee, ankle, and metatarsal). During adolescence, gonococcal arthritis occurs as a manifestation of sepsis with fever, chills, rash, and multiple small joint involvement, often with tenosynovitis.[29] The illness frequently follows the onset of menses by a few days.

RADIOLOGIC FINDINGS

Findings on plain-film radiographs are due to capsular swelling. In the joints readily accessible to physical examination, radiographs add little to the diagnostic evaluation, but when septic arthritis of the hip is suspected in a child, they are a valuable adjunct and may identify other causes of hip pain, such as Legg-Calvé-Perthes disease, slipped capital femoral epiphysis, and fracture. Films of the hip should be made with the child in the frog-leg position and with the legs extended at the knee and slightly internally rotated. The early signs of septic arthritis are caused by swelling of the capsule, which displaces the fat lines. One of the oldest signs is the obturator sign: As the tendon of the obturator internus passes over the capsule of the hip joint, the margins of this muscle are displaced medially into the pelvis (Fig. 62–1).[46] With continued swelling of the hip joint capsule, the femoral head is displaced laterally and upward.[20]

One of the most consistent findings is obliteration or lateral displacement of the gluteal fat lines (see Fig. 62–1).[89] Coincident with filling of the capsule with exudate, the femoral portion of the Shenton line is raised, and its arc is widened.[89] If a technetium bone scan is performed, increased uptake on either side of the joint is seen during the "blood pool" phase of the scan.[86] Ultrasound evaluation has proved useful in evaluation of septic arthritis of the hip.[48,94] In a series of 96 patients, none of the 40 patients with normal ultrasound findings had septic arthritis.[94] Bacterial infections causing pyogenic sacroiliitis may be particularly difficult to diagnose. Bone scans and computed tomography may be negative initially. Magnetic resonance imaging seems to be the diagnostic radiologic method of choice.[2,27]

LABORATORY EVALUATION

Diagnostic evaluation for suspected septic arthritis generally includes determination of the erythrocyte sedimentation rate or C-reactive protein, and the peripheral blood leukocyte count and differential. These may be only mildly elevated in cases of proven infection, however.[26,94] Blood for culture always should be obtained because blood cultures sometimes may yield the pathogen when joint fluid cultures do not.[52]

Joint fluid should be collected in a heparinized syringe so that the large clot that usually forms in fluid obtained from patients with septic arthritis or juvenile rheumatoid arthritis does not preclude enumeration of leukocytes. A cell and differential count should be performed on aspirated joint fluid, and it must be Gram-stained and cultured. Identification of organisms in joint fluid is the primary criterion for diagnosis of septic arthritis. Careful examination of a Gram-stained smear of joint fluid aspirates must be emphasized because joint fluid exerts a bacteriostatic effect on microorganisms and organisms that can be seen but may not grow in culture. Approximately 35 percent of joint aspirates are sterile in patients with other clinical and laboratory findings of a septic joint, including positive blood cultures.[10,63] Joint fluid should be cultured aerobically and under anaerobic conditions. The use of cell lysis culture bottles may enhance the recovery of *K. kingae* and other organisms.[92] *N. gonorrhoeae* is a highly fastidious organism, and oropharyngeal, rectal, and urogenital cultures or detection of gonococcal DNA in urine may be needed to confirm the diagnosis of gonococcal arthritis. Polymerase chain reaction analysis of joint fluid is likely to become a useful adjunct to the diagnosis of culture-negative disease, although it remains investigational.[60,84]

The median synovial fluid leukocyte count in bacterial arthritis in one study was 60.5×10^9 cells/L.[79] In this and other surveys,[75] polymorphonuclear leukocytes accounted for 75 to 90 percent of the white blood cells. Cell density generally is lower in fluid obtained from patients with acute rheumatic fever, juvenile rheumatoid arthritis, and other inflammatory causes of arthritis (Table 62–3).[8,75,79] The glucose concentration often is decreased in septic arthritis, but it may be normal.[79,87] It also may be depressed in rheumatoid arthritis and other conditions. A joint fluid leukocyte density of 5 to 8×10^9 cells/L has been found in joint fluid from patients ultimately proved to have septic arthritis.[75] Minimally turbid fluid with a seemingly low number of cells still should be processed for bacterial culture and Gram stain. Examination of the fluid for uric acid and other types of crystals should be considered in certain children (e.g., children with hyperuricemia).

DIFFERENTIAL DIAGNOSIS

Although bacterial infections are the most common cause of septic arthritis, other microorganisms, including viruses (varicella-zoster, *Erythrovirus* [parvovirus B19], rubella, chikungunya and other togaviruses, variola, vaccinia, certain enteroviruses, others), mycobacteria, and fungi (*Coccidioides immitis*, *Sporothrix schenckii*, *Blastomyces dermatitidis*, *Candida* spp.), may be involved. The differential diagnosis includes obturator internus muscle abscess,[85] epiphyseal osteomyelitis, traumatic arthritis, bacterial endocarditis, villonodular synovitis, leukemia, deep cellulitis, serum sickness, ulcerative colitis, granulomatous colitis, Schönlein-Henoch purpura, traumatic arthritis, fracture, Legg-Calvé-Perthes disease, slipped femoral capital epiphysis, and metabolic diseases affecting joints (e.g., ochronosis in adults with alkaptonuria).

Toxic (or transient) synovitis (also referred to as *irritable hip* and *reactive synovitis*) frequently is seen in children and has milder

presenting features than bacterial infections of the hip. The combination of fever, elevated white blood cell count, erythrocyte sedimentation rate (>40 mm/hr), C-reactive protein, and inability to bear weight permits septic arthritis to be distinguished from transient synovitis with high accuracy; greater than 90 percent sensitivity for the detection of septic arthritis has been reported when all of these factors are present.[15,26,52,94] Septic (suppurative) bursitis, although rare in childhood, can be difficult to distinguish from septic arthritis. Children with septic bursitis frequently have a history of recent trauma and fever along with limitation of joint movement.[44,71] Careful physical examination and aspiration of bursal fluid allow the entities to be differentiated.

TREATMENT

ANTIBIOTIC THERAPY

Antibiotic treatment of septic arthritis should target the most common pathogens. In children beyond the neonatal period, *S. aureus* and other gram-positive organisms currently predominate.[13,55,63] Although the risk of acquiring invasive *H. influenzae* infection is low in areas with effective immunization, rare cases continue to be reported. Children younger than 2 years who have not been immunized against *H. influenzae* type b should be treated initially with a regimen that contains an antistaphylococcal agent, such as nafcillin, vancomycin, or clindamycin, and an agent active against this agent (e.g., cefotaxime). Cefuroxime, which is active against *S. aureus* (and other gram-positive pathogens) and *H. influenzae*, is a useful alternative. As with osteomyelitis, vancomycin or clindamycin should be used as the empiric antistaphylococcal agent in areas where community-acquired MRSA is a concern.[3,57] Some authorities advocate that this be done when community-acquired MRSA represents more than 10 percent of *S. aureus* in a geographic area.[50] At present, no regimen is preferred for the treatment of penicillin-nonsusceptible *S. pneumoniae*, but ceftriaxone, cefotaxime, and clindamycin have been used successfully.[14] If β-lactam resistance continues to increase in *S. pneumoniae* and *S. aureus*, other regimens that target highly resistant gram-positive organisms may be needed. Ceftriaxone and cefotaxime are appropriate for the treatment of gonococcal infection.

All antibiotics that have been studied penetrate into joint fluid readily; soon after administration, at the time of peak serum levels, the joint fluid concentration averages 30 percent of the serum value.[5,7,62,73] The efflux of antibiotic from joint fluid back to serum is slow, however. Immediately before the next systemic dose is administered, joint fluid antibiotic concentrations frequently exceed the concentrations present in serum. Antibiotics, whether administered orally or parenterally, can achieve efficacious concentrations in joint fluid.

Injecting antibiotics into the joint space usually is unnecessary because of their excellent penetration. Many antibiotics (e.g., cephalothin) are capable of evoking an intense inflammatory reaction, much as they do if they are infiltrated beneath the skin. Tetzlaff and associates[82] have shown that septic arthritis can be treated for 1 week (or less) parenterally, with the balance of the

---

TABLE 62–3 Joint Fluid Findings in Childhood Arthritides

Diagnosis	Spontaneous Clotting	Mucin Clot	Leukocytes/mL	% Polymorphonuclear Leukocytes	Glucose as Percentage of Blood Value
Septic arthritis	Rapid formation of large clot	Curdled milk	73,000	90	30
Rheumatic fever	Small to absent	Tightrope	18,000	60	75
Juvenile rheumatoid arthritis	Large clot	Small, friable masses	15,000	60	75

From Ropes, M.: Joint fluid findings in disease. Bull. Rheum. Dis. 7(Suppl.):21, 1957.

drug given orally. These investigators caution that the drug dosage should be adjusted for each patient to ensure a peak serum bactericidal titer of at least 1:8, and that the patient should remain hospitalized so that compliance can be ensured. These investigators considered the minimal duration of therapy to be 3 weeks.

The adequacy of antibiotic therapy can be assessed by serial joint fluid examinations, leukocyte density, and culture results.[87] The time required for resolution of joint symptoms and the time for the synovia to become sterile are proportional to the duration of symptoms before the initiation of appropriate antibiotic therapy.[47] In one study, some patients still had cultures yielding bacteria after undergoing 1 week of therapy. In these patients, cellular density ranged from 25 to 253×10^9 cells/L (mean 109×10^9 cells/L) at the beginning of therapy; 92 percent of the cells were polymorphonuclear leukocytes. By the end of 2 weeks of therapy, all cultures were sterile, and leukocyte density ranged from 4.9 to 23×10^9 cells/L (mean of 12.3×10^9 cells/L).[87] Similar studies of the rate of resolution of indicators of inflammation in joint fluid have suggested that after receiving 9 days of treatment, patients who ultimately recovered completely had a density of 5×10^9 cells/L; however, in patients with recrudescent infection or a poor outcome, the density was 6×10^{10} cells/L.[35]

When an effusion reaccumulates, one should remove it by arthrocentesis, not only to make the patient more comfortable, but also to permit serial assessment of therapy. Generally, disease caused by *S. aureus* and Enterobacteriaceae requires longer treatment than disease caused by *H. influenzae* or meningococci. Radiographs should be obtained during therapy to seek bone changes indicating that osteomyelitis may have been present. Osteomyelitis may require surgical intervention or more prolonged antibiotic therapy.

SURGICAL TREATMENT

In infants, septic arthritis in the hips or shoulders is a surgical emergency; these joints should be drained as soon as the diagnosis is apparent to prevent bony destruction.[69] In a study in adults, the outcome of septic arthritis was better in patients treated by repeated needle aspiration than in patients treated by surgical drainage.[36,37] Eighty percent of the patients treated by needle aspiration were thought to have a good outcome versus 47 percent treated by surgical drainage. All wrist joint infections in this series were treated only by needle aspiration; in treatment of septic arthritis of the knee, however, the outcome was almost equivalent. Similar findings have been reported by others.[11] The investigators suggested that surgical drainage should be performed in any joint whenever the presence of large amounts of fibrin, tissue debris, or loculation prevents adequate drainage by needle aspiration.

PROGNOSIS

Sequelae, including hip dislocation, are more likely to develop in infants and patients with symptoms of longer duration.[87,88] In one study, seven of eight patients in whom "permanent" hip dislocation developed had symptoms for 7 or more days before receiving treatment.[88] Similarly, all patients with spontaneous ankylosis had symptoms longer than 7 days.[88] Comparable data were obtained by Samilson and colleagues.[77] Eight of 10 patients with pathologic dislocation of the hip had symptoms for longer than 7 days.

A detailed analysis of factors affecting satisfactory outcomes in hematogenous septic arthritis of childhood showed no significant difference in the joint when arthrotomy, with or without irrigation, was compared with repeated aspiration.[59] Likewise, the specific antibiotic used had no effect on outcome as long as it was

effective against the infecting organism. The literature does suggest that septic arthritis caused by Enterobacteriaceae is associated with more frequent sequelae than when caused by other pathogens.[37,64] *S. aureus* is more likely to cause sequelae than *H. influenzae*.[10] A single randomized, placebo-controlled study has examined the impact of a brief course of dexamethasone on the outcome of bacteriologically confirmed cases of septic arthritis of hematogenous origin in children. Children younger than 3 months were excluded from participation, and *H. influenzae* was responsible for 13 percent of cases among the 100 evaluable patients. After 1 year of follow-up, limping, joint pain, and restriction of movement were found in 26 percent of patients who received a placebo, but in only 1 of 50 patients treated with dexamethasone. If confirmed, this anti-inflammatory therapy may prove useful to limit the sequelae of septic arthritis.[70]

SPECIAL PROBLEMS

NEONATAL SEPTIC ARTHRITIS

Neonatal septic arthritis is a problem that warrants special attention because of its subtle signs and symptoms,[21] its potential for catastrophic consequences of untreated disease,[68] and the unusual organisms occasionally seen. Any newborn who has swelling in the region of the thigh and the buttock and holds that leg flexed with slight abduction and external rotation at the hip should be suspected to have femoral-acetabular septic arthritis. It can occur 1 to 28 days after femoral venipuncture (in most newborns, 5 to 9 days) and should not be confused with femoral vein thrombosis.[4,17]

In most newborns, no toxemia, fever, or leukocytosis is present. More than one joint may be involved when initially evaluated. The progression of disease in newborns can be so indolent that the hip spontaneously drains along the obturator internus, and the condition is manifested as a lower abdominal mass just above the inguinal canal.[28] Problems in recognizing the disease in newborns undoubtedly contribute to the poor outcome. In one series, the delay from onset to diagnosis was an average of 1 week; only two of the nine infants in this series had a normal hip examination at follow-up.[68]

In most series, the causative agents are staphylococci and streptococci,[4,12,17,21,68] but gram-negative organisms often are found. More importantly, arthritis caused by *Candida albicans* has been described,[23] and the gonococcus should not be forgotten. In gonococcal arthritis, the symptoms, which usually become apparent in infants 1 to 5 weeks of age, generally are polyarthritic (more than one joint involved).[33] As previously noted, other symptoms of neonatal gonococcal arthritis are no different from symptoms caused by other pathogens.

Initial antibiotic therapy for neonatal septic arthritis should be directed toward *S. aureus* and the nosocomial gram-negative bacteria that are prevalent in the nursery. Antibiotic therapy can be altered when the susceptibility of the causative bacterium is known. As noted earlier, the usual duration of therapy is 3 to 4 weeks, and radiography should be performed toward the end of treatment. Oral therapy has been used successfully to complete treatment of septic arthritis in newborns,[72] but absorption of antibiotics in this age range is unpredictable.[78] Consequently, either intravenous therapy or measurement of serum bactericidal activity should be used to verify absorption.[82]

FUNGAL ARTHRITIS

Fungal arthritis is rare in children, but may be seen with pathogens of endemic mycoses, such as *Histoplasma capsulatum*, *C. immitis*, and *B. dermatitidis*, and with opportunistic fungal pathogens (e.g., *Candida* spp., *Cryptococcus neoformans*).[55,63] These pathogens usually manifest after an indolent course. The recommended medical treatment generally is that required for other systemic infections caused by these organisms.

JOINT INFECTIONS DURING RHEUMATOID ARTHRITIS

Joint infections that develop during a case of rheumatoid arthritis seem to occur more frequently in adults with rheumatoid arthritis than in children. In one series, only 2 of 17 patients were younger than 10 years.[6] The notable features are that the hips generally are not involved, and infection of multiple joints (17 of 44 patients had more than one joint involved) frequently occurs. Because of the preexisting joint disease, the diagnosis often is delayed, and the outcome usually is poor. Septic arthritis should be considered if an unusual worsening of one joint occurs during a flare-up of rheumatoid arthritis.

REACTIVE ARTHRITIS

After infections with *Shigella* spp.,[16,66] *Chlamydia trachomatis*, *Salmonella* spp.,[43] and *Yersinia* spp., a reactive arthritis can occur.[54] This postinfectious joint inflammation seems to develop with greater frequency in individuals who express the histocompatibility antigen HLA-B*27, perhaps as a result of molecular similarities between bacterial antigens and the human protein. In addition, during the initial infection, bacterial antigens apparently may be deposited in the synovium and may persist for a long time and lead to pathogenic inflammation.[40,54] Generally, the onset of joint symptoms occurs a few days to several weeks after a transient and often mild episode of diarrhea. The arthritis may mimic rheumatic fever and is characterized by daily low-grade fever and an increased erythrocyte sedimentation rate. Reactive arthritis generally can be distinguished from septic arthritis by analysis of synovial fluid; infectious arthritis usually is associated with high white blood cell fluid numbers.[8] Resolution of joint symptoms in reactive cases takes 7 to 10 days.

Reactive arthritis also may occur after acute infections with *N. meningitidis*[42] and *H. influenzae*.[76] Symptoms and signs of joint inflammation often appear 1 week or more after the acute septic episode and resolve without sequelae.

REFERENCES

1. Ament, M. E., and Gaal, S. A.: Bacteroides arthritis. Am. J. Dis. Child. *114*:427-428, 1967.
2. Aprin, H., and Turen, C.: Pyogenic sacroiliitis in children. Clin. Orthop. *287*:98-106, 1993.
3. Arnold, S. R., et al.: Changing patterns of acute hematogenous osteomyelitis and septic arthritis: Emergence of community-associated methicillin-resistant *Staphylococcus aureus*. J. Pediatr. Orthop. *26*:703-708, 2006.
4. Asnes, R. S., and Arendar, G. M.: Septic arthritis of the hip: A complication of femoral venipuncture. Pediatrics *38*:837-841, 1966.
5. Baciocco, E. A., and Iles, R. L.: Ampicillin and kanamycin concentrations in joint fluid. Clin. Pharmacol. Ther. *12*:858-863, 1971.
6. Baitch, A.: Recent observations of acute suppurative arthritis. Clin. Orthop. *22*:157-166, 1962.
7. Balboni, V., Shapiro, I. M., and Kydd, D. M.: The penetration of penicillin into joint fluid following intramuscular administration. Am. J. Med. Sci. *210*:588-591, 1945.
8. Baldassare, A. R., Chang, F., and Zuckner, J.: Markedly raised synovial fluid leucocyte counts not associated with infectious arthritis in children. Ann. Rheum. Dis. *37*:404-409, 1978.
9. Barnett, C., Davies, D. V., and MacConcill, M. A.: Synovial Joints. Springfield, IL, Charles C. Thomas, 1961.
10. Barton, L. L., Dunkle, L. M., and Habib, F. H.: Septic arthritis in childhood: A 13-year review. Am. J. Dis. Child. *141*:898-900, 1987.
11. Betz, R. R., Cooperman, D. R., Wopperer, J. M., et al.: Late sequelae of septic arthritis of the hip in infancy and childhood. J. Pediatr. Orthop. *10*:365-372, 1990.
12. Bodganovitich, A.: Neonatal arthritis due to *Proteus vulgaris*. Arch. Dis. Child. *23*:65-66, 1948.
13. Bowerman, S. G., Green, N. E., and Mencio, G. A.: Decline of bone and joint infections attributable to *Haemophilus influenzae* type b. Clin. Orthop. *341*:128-133, 1997.
14. Bradley, J. S., et al.: Pediatric pneumococcal bone and joint infections. The Pediatric Multicenter Pneumococcal Surveillance Study Group (PMPSSG). Pediatrics *102*:1376-1382, 1998.
15. Caird, M. S., et al.: Factors distinguishing septic arthritis from transient synovitis of the hip in children: A prospective study. J. Bone Joint Surg. Am. *88*:1251-1257, 2006.
16. Calin, A., and Fries, J. F.: An "experimental" epidemic of Reiter's syndrome revisited: Follow-up evidence on genetic and environmental factors. Ann. Intern. Med. *84*:564-566, 1976.
17. Chacha, P. B.: Suppurative arthritis of the hip joint in infancy: A persistent diagnostic problem and possible complication of femoral venipuncture. J. Bone Joint Surg. Am. *53*:538-544, 1971.
18. Chartier, Y., Martin, W. J., and Kelly, P. J.: [Bacterial arthritis: Experiences in the treatment of 77 patients]. Ann. Intern. Med. *50*:1462-1474, 1959.
19. Chmel, H., and Armstrong, D.: Acute arthritis caused by *Aeromonas hydrophila*: Clinical and therapeutic aspects. Arthritis Rheum. *19*:169-172, 1976.
20. Chont, L.: Roentgen sign of early suppurative arthritis of the hip in infancy. Radiology *38*:708-714, 1942.
21. Chung, S. M., and Pollis, R. E.: Diagnostic pitfalls in septic arthritis of the hip in infants and children. Clin. Pediatr. (Philadelphia) *14*:758-761, 1975.
22. Curtiss, P. H., Jr.: The pathophysiology of joint infections. Clin. Orthop. *96*:129-135, 1973.
23. Dan, M.: Septic arthritis in young infants: Clinical and microbiologic correlations and therapeutic implications. Rev. Infect. Dis. *6*:147-155, 1984.
24. Daniel, D., Akeson, W., Amiel, D., et al.: Lavage of septic joints in rabbits: Effects of chondrolysis. J. Bone Joint Surg. Am. *58*:393-395, 1976.
25. de Groot, R., Glover, D., Clausen, C., et al.: Bone and joint infections caused by *Kingella kingae*: Six cases and review of the literature. Rev. Infect. Dis. *10*:998-1004, 1988.
26. Del Beccaro, M. A., Champoux, A. N., Bockers, T., et al.: Septic arthritis versus transient synovitis of the hip: The value of screening laboratory tests. Ann. Emerg. Med. *21*:1418-1422, 1992.
27. Doita, M., Yoshiya, S., Nabeshima, Y., et al.: Acute pyogenic sacroiliitis without predisposing conditions. Spine *28*:E384-E399, 2003.
28. Freiberg, J. A., and Perlman, R.: Pelvic abscesses associated with acute purulent infection of the hip joint. J. Bone Joint Surg. Am. *18*:417-427, 1936.
29. Garcia-Kutzbach, A., and Masi, A. T.: Acute infectious agent arthritis (IAA): A detailed comparison of proved gonococcal and other blood-borne bacterial arthritis. J. Rheumatol. *1*:93-101, 1974.
30. Gardner, E. D.: Physiology of joints. J. Bone Joint Surg. Am. *45*:152-159, 1963.
31. Gillespie, R.: Septic arthritis of childhood. Clin. Orthop. *96*:152-159, 1973.
32. Gillespie, W. J.: Epidemiology in bone and joint infection. Infect. Dis. Clin. North Am. *4*:361-376, 1990.
33. Glaser, S., Boxerbaum, B., and Kennell, J. H.: Gonococcal arthritis in the newborn: Report of a case and review of the literature. Am. J. Dis. Child. *112*:185-188, 1966.
34. Goergens, E. D., McEvoy, A., Watson, M., et al.: Acute osteomyelitis and septic arthritis in children. J. Paediatr. Child Health *41*:59-62, 2005.
35. Goldenberg, D. L., Brandt, K. D., Cathcart, E. S., et al.: Acute arthritis caused by gram-negative bacilli: A clinical characterization. Medicine (Baltimore) *53*:197-208, 1974.
36. Goldenberg, D. L., Brandt, K. D., Cohen, A. S., et al.: Treatment of septic arthritis: Comparison of needle aspiration and surgery as initial modes of joint drainage. Arthritis Rheum. *18*:83-90, 1975.
37. Goldenberg, D. L., and Cohen, A. S.: Acute infectious arthritis: A review of patients with nongonococcal joint infections (with emphasis on therapy and prognosis). Am. J. Med. *60*:369-377, 1976.
38. Gomez-Reino, J. J., Shah, M., Gorevic, P., et al.: *Pasteurella multocida* arthritis: Case report. J. Bone Joint Surg. Am. *62*:1212-1213, 1980.
39. Goutzmanis, J. J., Gonis, G., and Gilbert, G. L.: *Kingella kingae* infection in children: Ten cases and a review of the literature. Pediatr. Infect. Dis. J. *10*:677-683, 1991.
40. Granfors, K., Jalkanen, S., von Essen R., et al.: *Yersinia* antigens in synovial-fluid cells from patients with reactive arthritis. N. Engl. J. Med. *320*:216-221, 1989.
41. Granoff, D. M., Sargent, E., and Jolivette, D.: *Haemophilus influenzae* type b osteomyelitis. Am. J. Dis. Child. *132*:488-490, 1978.
42. Greenwood, B. M., Whittle, H. C., and Bryceson, A. D.: Allergic complications of meningococcal disease, II: Immunological investigations. B. M. J. *2*:737-740, 1973.
43. Hakansson, U., Eitrem, R., Löw, B., et al.: HLA-B27 and reactive arthritis in an outbreak of salmonellosis. Tissue Antigens *6*:366-367, 1975.
44. Harwell, J. I., and Fisher, D.: Pediatric septic bursitis: Case report of retrocalcaneal infection and review of the literature. Clin. Infect. Dis. *32*:E102-E104, 2001.
45. Heberling, J. A.: A review of two hundred and one cases of suppurative arthritis. J. Bone Joint Surg. *23*:917-921, 1941.
46. Hefke, H. W., and Turner, V. C.: The obturator sign as the earliest roentgenographic sign in the diagnosis of septic arthritis and tuberculosis of the hip. J. Bone Joint Surg. *24*:857-869, 1942.
47. Ho, G., Jr., and Su, E. Y.: Therapy for septic arthritis. J. A. M. A. *247*:797-800, 1982.
48. Jamillo, D., Treves, S. T., Kasser, J. R., et al.: Osteomyelitis and septic arthritis in children: Appropriate use of imaging to guide treatment. A. J. R. Am. J. Roentgenol. *165*:339-403, 1995.
49. Kalishm, R.: Lyme disease. Rheum. Dis. Clin. North Am. *19*:399-426, 1993.

50. Kaplan, S. L.: Osteomyelitis in children. Infect. Dis. Clin. North Am. *19*:787-797, vii, 2005.
51. Kleiman, M. B., and Lamb, G. A.: Gonococcal arthritis in a newborn infant. Pediatrics *52*:285-287, 1973.
52. Kocher, M. S., Zurakowski, D., and Kasser, J. R.: Differentiating between septic arthritis and transient synovitis of the hip in children: An evidence-based clinical prediction algorithm. J. Bone Joint Surg. Am. *81*:1662-1670, 1999.
53. Kohen, D. P.: Neonatal gonococcal arthritis: Three cases and review of the literature. Pediatrics *53*:436-440, 1974.
54. Koopman, W. J.: Host factors in the pathogenesis of arthritis triggered by infectious organisms: Overview. Rheum. Dis. Clin. North Am. *19*:279-292, 1993.
55. Luhmann, J. D., and Luhmann, S. J.: Etiology of septic arthritis in children: An update for the 1990s. Pediatr. Emerg. Care *15*:40-42, 1999.
56. Martin, C. M., Merrill, R. H., and Barrett, O., Jr.: Arthritis due to *Serratia*. J. Bone Joint Surg. *52*:1450-1452, 1970.
57. Martinez-Aguilar, G., Hammerman, W. A., Mason, E. O., Jr., et al.: Clindamycin treatment of invasive infections caused by community-acquired, methicillin-resistant and methicillin-susceptible *Staphylococcus aureus* in children. Pediatr. Infect. Dis. J. *22*:593-598, 2003.
58. Merchan, E. C., Magallon, M., Manso, F., et al.: Septic arthritis in HIV positive haemophiliacs: Four cases and a literature review. Int. Orthop. *16*:302-306, 1992.
59. Morrey, B. F., Bianco, A. J., Jr., and Rhodes, K. H.: Septic arthritis in children. Orthop. Clin. North Am. *6*:923-934, 1975.
60. Moumile, K., Merckx, J., Glorion, C., et al.: Osteoarticular infections caused by *Kingella kingae* in children: Contribution of polymerase chain reaction to the microbiologic diagnosis. Pediatr. Infect. Dis. J. *22*:837-839, 2003.
61. Mulhern, L. M., Friday, G. A., and Perri, J. A.: Arthritis complicating varicella infection. Pediatrics *48*:827-829, 1971.
62. Nelson, J. D.: Antibiotic concentrations in septic joint effusions. N. Engl. J. Med. *284*:349-353, 1971.
63. Nelson, J. D.: The bacterial etiology and antibiotic management of septic arthritis in infants and children. Pediatrics *50*:437-440, 1972.
64. Newman, J. H.: Review of septic arthritis throughout the antibiotic era. Ann. Rheum. Dis. *35*:198-205, 1976.
65. Nicholson, J.: Pyogenic arthritis with pathologic dislocation of the hip in infants. J. A. M. A. *141*, 1949.
66. Noer, H. R.: An "experimental" epidemic of Reiter's syndrome. J. A. M. A. *198*:693-698, 1966.
67. Norenberg, D. D., Bigley, D. V., Virata, R. L., et al.: *Corynebacterium pyogenes* septic arthritis with plasma cell synovial infiltrate and monoclonal gammopathy. Arch. Intern. Med. *138*:810-811, 1978.
68. Obletz, B. E.: Acute suppurative arthritis of the hip in the neonatal period. J. Bone Joint Surg. Am. *42*:23-30, 1960.
69. Obletz, B. E.: Suppurative arthritis of the hip joint in infants. Clin. Orthop. *22*:27-33, 1962.
70. Odio, C. M., Ramirez, T., Arias, G., et al.: Double blind, randomized, placebo-controlled study of dexamethasone therapy for hematogenous septic arthritis in children. Pediatr. Infect. Dis. J. *22*:883-888, 2003.
71. Paisley, J. W.: Septic bursitis in childhood. J. Pediatr. Orthop. *2*:57-61, 1982.
72. Perkins, M. D., Edwards, K. M., Heller, R. M., et al.: Neonatal group B streptococcal osteomyelitis and suppurative arthritis: Outpatient therapy. Clin. Pediatr. (Philadelphia) *28*:229-230, 1989.
73. Plott, M. A., and Roth, H.: Penetration of clindamycin into synovial fluid. Clin. Pharmacol. Ther. *11*:577-580, 1970.
74. Priest, J. R., Urick, J. J., Groth, K. E., et al.: Varicella arthritis documented by isolation of virus from joint fluid. J. Pediatr. *93*:990-992, 1978.
75. Ropes, M.: Joint fluid findings in disease. Bull. Rheum. Dis. 7(Suppl.):21, 1957.
76. Rush, P. J., Shore, A., Inman, R., et al.: Arthritis associated with *Haemophilus influenzae* meningitis: Septic or reactive? J. Pediatr. *109*:412-415, 1986.
77. Samilson, R. L., Bersani, F. A., and Watkins, M. B.: Acute suppurative arthritis in infants and children: The importance of early diagnosis and surgical drainage. Pediatrics *21*:798-804, 1958.
78. Schwartz, G. J., Hegyi, T., and Spitzer, A.: Subtherapeutic dicloxacillin levels in a neonate: Possible mechanisms. J. Pediatr. *89*:310-312, 1976.
79. Shmerling, R. H., Delbanco, T. L., Tosteson, A. N., et al.: Synovial fluid tests: What should be ordered? J. A. M. A. *264*:1009-1014, 1990.
80. Steere, A. C.: Lyme disease. N. Engl. J. Med. *345*:115-125, 2001.
81. Stravino, V. D.: The synovial system. Am. J. Phys. Med. *51*:312-320, 1972.
82. Tetzlaff, T. R., McCracken, G. H., Jr., and Nelson, J. D.: Oral antibiotic therapy for skeletal infections of children, II: Therapy of osteomyelitis and suppurative arthritis. J. Pediatr. *92*:485-490, 1978.
83. Tindel, J. R., and Crowder, J. G.: Septic arthritis due to *Pseudomonas aeruginosa*. J. A. M. A. *218*:559-561, 1971.
84. Verdier, I., Gayet-Ageron, A., Ploton, C., et al.: Contribution of a broad range polymerase chain reaction to the diagnosis of osteoarticular infections caused by *Kingella kingae*: Description of twenty-four recent pediatric diagnoses. Pediatr. Infect. Dis. J. *24*:692-696, 2005.
85. Viani, R. M., Bromberg, K., and Bradley, J. S.: Obturator internus muscle abscess in children: Report of seven cases and review. Clin. Infect. Dis. *28*:117-122, 1999.
86. Volberg, F. M., Sumner, T. E., Abramson, J. S., et al.: Unreliability of radiographic diagnosis of septic hip in children. Pediatrics *74*:118-120, 1984.
87. Ward, J., Cohen, A. S., and Bauer, W.: The diagnosis and therapy of acute suppurative arthritis. Arthritis Rheum. *3*:522-535, 1960.
88. Watkins, M. B., Samilson, R. L., and Winter, D. M.: Acute suppurative arthritis. J. Bone Joint Surg. *28*:1313-1320, 1956.
89. White, H.: Roentgen findings of acute infectious disease of the hip in infants and children. Clin. Orthop. *22*:34-42, 1962.
90. Yagupsky, P.: *Kingella kingae*: From medical rarity to an emerging paediatric pathogen. Lancet Infect. Dis. *4*:358-367, 2004.
91. Yagupsky, P., Bar-Ziv, Y., Howard, C. B., et al.: Epidemiology, etiology, and clinical features of septic arthritis in children younger than 24 months. Arch. Pediatr. Adolesc. *149*:537-540, 1995.
92. Yagupsky, P., and Press, J.: Use of the isolator 1.5 microbial tube for culture of synovial fluid from patients with septic arthritis. J. Clin. Microbiol. *35*:2410-2412, 1997.
93. Yocum, R. C., McArthur, J., Petty, B. G., et al.: Septic arthritis caused by *Propionibacterium acnes*. J. A. M. A. *248*:1740-1741, 1982.
94. Zawin, J. K., Hoffer, F. A., Rand, F. F., et al.: Joint effusion in children with an irritable hip: US diagnosis and aspiration. Radiology *187*:459-463, 1993.

BACTERIAL MYOSITIS AND PYOMYOSITIS

CHAPTER 63

Charles Grose

Myositis is not a common manifestation of bacterial infection, but when it occurs, the consequences to the patient may be severe or even fatal. *Staphylococcus aureus* and group A streptococci are the most likely causative organisms. Myositis also has been associated with several other infectious agents, including viruses, fungi, and parasites. These pathogens are listed in Table 63–1; they are discussed briefly herein and more thoroughly in the chapters on the specific microorganisms. This chapter focuses on two forms of pyogenic myositis, designated as *acute bacterial myositis* and *tropical pyomyositis*. The former is caused primarily by group A streptococci and the latter by *S. aureus*. Tropical (or staphylococcal) pyomyositis is the more common of the two bacterial diseases and should be considered a distinct nosologic entity.

TABLE 63–1 Infectious Causes of Myositis

Bacterial
Tropical pyomyositis
Acute bacterial myositis

Viral
Influenza myositis
Coxsackievirus myositis

Fungal
Disseminated candidiasis

Parasitic
Trichinosis
Cysticercosis
Toxoplasmosis

PYOMYOSITIS

The pathologic entity termed *spontaneous acute myositis* was recognized by Virchow in the mid-19th century, but the first clinical description of suppurative myositis generally is attributed to the Japanese surgeon Scriba.[20] In 1904, another Japanese surgeon, Miyake,[17] extensively reviewed the subject of skeletal muscle abscesses and added 33 more cases. As the British and French expanded their colonial empires at the turn of the 20th century, the disease was recognized with increasing frequency in the native populations and in the soldiers who lived in the tropical areas of Asia and Africa.[26] It acquired the name by which it now is known widely—*tropical pyomyositis.*[9,10]

The suitability of this designation was confirmed by an epidemiologic study in East Africa, which discovered that the disease was found commonly only in regions with a truly tropical climate (i.e., a fairly constant high temperature and high relative humidity) at an altitude below 4000 ft.[15] Pyomyositis has been described, however, in children from geographic regions of the United States as diverse as New England,[9] northern California,[2] Iowa,[16] and Texas.[11,19,21] Numerous reported cases within the continental United States have occurred in and around San Antonio, Texas.[5] In a 10-year chart review, 1 or 2 cases of pyomyositis per 4000 pediatric admissions occurred annually. In contrast, a review of consultations of pediatric infectious diseases at the University of Iowa Hospital disclosed fewer cases of pyomyositis among children younger than 16 years old.[7] Pyomyositis seems to occur more commonly in children who live in the southernmost regions of the United States (e.g., Texas) than in children who live in the northern regions (e.g., Iowa).

PATHOPHYSIOLOGY

The etiologic agent of the skeletal muscle abscesses in more than 90 percent of cases is *S. aureus.* Phage typing of many isolates in different countries has not identified a particular staphylococcal strain that is more likely to cause pyomyositis.[11] The second most common bacteriologic isolate is *Streptococcus,* including group A and nonhemolytic strains. Whether more virulent streptococcal infections are occurring at the beginning of the 21st century is an issue that remains unresolved.

Miyake[17] studied extensively the experimental conditions under which staphylococci cause muscle abscesses. When healthy rabbits were given boluses of staphylococci intravenously, they occasionally developed small abscesses in the kidney, liver, or spleen but never in the skeletal muscles. When specific muscles were damaged by mechanical pinching or electric current 24 or 48 hours before the intravenous injection of bacteria was administered, small abscesses developed within 2 to 28 days at some of

the injured sites in nearly half of the animals. Abscesses were not found in healthy muscle tissue.

The role of trauma was supported further by a study of pyomyositis in the British Army.[3] After physicians found this disease to be a common problem in Gurkha army recruits, they investigated 32 cases and made several observations: Two thirds of the men recalled having experienced trauma at the affected site, the incidence of abscesses increased as the severity of physical training increased, and the abscesses occurred three times more commonly on the dominant (right) side of the body. In an analysis of 78 cases in Uganda, abscesses also were found more commonly on the right side of the body.[15]

From experimental evidence and clinical observations, two conditions commonly are found when pyomyositis occurs: muscle injury and bacteremia, usually staphylococcal. A reported case is illustrative.[11] A 12-year-old girl caught her left foot in the wheel of a moving bicycle and tumbled to the ground. One week later, she developed a furuncle of the foot, and within the next 2 weeks, she developed painful lumps in muscles of the thigh, shoulder, and chest wall (which had been injured during the original accident). Cultures from the furuncle and blood and from the incised muscle abscesses grew *S. aureus.* All isolates were identified as phage type 94. The initial episode of trauma resulted in a staphylococcal skin lesion and, presumably, a bacteremia that seeded sites of previously bruised muscle.

Seven children with pyomyositis are described in Table 63–2. An analysis of all seven cases illustrates the association of pyomyositis with trauma. The sources of muscle trauma have ranged from bicycle accidents to strenuous aerobic exercises. These cases also may explain the predilection of the disease to occur in warmer climates; concomitant skin infections and muscle trauma are more likely to occur in a climate in which children can play or work outside wearing fewer clothes for most of the year.

In tropical countries, pyomyositis is said to occur in individuals who are malnourished and who have multiple parasitic infections. This association has not been confirmed, however, in children with pyomyositis seen in the United States or Australia.[5,7,13] The children have not been malnourished or vitamin-deficient, and they have not had parasitic infestation or marked eosinophilia. Extensive immunologic evaluations also have been normal; the tests included quantitative immunoglobulins, enumeration of T-lymphocyte subpopulations, total hemolytic complement levels, and leukocyte function as tested by reduction of nitroblue tetrazolium.

CLINICAL PRESENTATION

Pyomyositis often is considered a disease of adolescents and young adults, even though it occurs in individuals of all ages, including infants and young children.[2,6,13] Boys are affected more

TABLE 63–2 Pyomyositis and Trauma

Case*	Sex	Age (yr)	Source of Trauma	Circumstances of Trauma	Extent of Disease
1	F	12	Bicycle accident	Thrown from bicycle onto street after foot was caught in the wheel	Right deltoid/right chest wall/left thigh/right groin
2	M	3	Fall while running	Fell while running on street	Left calf/right scapula/right buttock
3	M	11	Hay bale accident	Struck in abdomen by bale of hay thrown from a hay baler	Abdominal wall musculature
4	M	6	Blunt trauma to abdomen	Struck in abdomen during mock fistfight with sibling	Abdominal wall musculature
5	F	17	Aerobic exercises	Injured while instructing others in aerobic exercises	Left thigh
6	M	7	Bicycle accident	Fell from fast-moving bicycle onto street	Left calf
7	F	13	Volleyball accident	Fell several times diving for volleyball during training exercises	Left iliopsoas

*Cases 1 and 2 from reference 11, cases 3 and 4 from reference 5, cases 5 and 6 from reference 7, and case 7 from reference 16.

often than are girls. As more girls enter competitive sporting activities, however, pyomyositis is being reported in female athletes.[16] Most children with pyomyositis have a solitary lesion, but multiple lesions are common findings. The most common site of abscess formation is the thigh, followed by the calf, buttock, arm, scapula, and chest wall. The muscle lesions are firm or "woody" to palpation, with a well-defined border. The sign of fluctuation may be difficult to elicit. Erythema and warmth often are not apparent because of the deep location of the masses, although diffuse tenderness usually occurs. When a muscle in an extremity is involved, the entire limb may be swollen. Occasionally, pyomyositis also can occur in muscles of the pelvis, in which case pain may be transferred to the hip.[14,19]

In case reports with a clinical history, children with pyomyositis often had similar presenting complaints.[7,11] Many had incurred a recent accidental injury (often involving a leg) that usually was not considered serious. After a few days, the children developed low-grade fever (38.3° C to 39° C), muscle pain, and, occasionally, an impaired gait. These symptoms persisted a few days to a few weeks until a mass appeared. When first examined, many of the patients were considered to have only a contusion or a hematoma; occasionally, a child was diagnosed as having a rhabdomyosarcoma. Although the disease usually occurs in individuals who are otherwise healthy, pyomyositis has been reported in patients with malignancy. Pyomyositis also may develop in children with acquired immunodeficiency syndrome or other immunodeficiency.[13] The pathophysiology of pyogenic muscle abscess may not be the same, however, in immunodeficient individuals with increased susceptibility to bacterial infection. Most children with pyomyositis have no definable immunologic abnormalities.

An unusual clinical presentation is acute abdominal pain. Beck and Grose[5] described two children with pyomyositis whose initial complaints were confined to the abdominal wall. One patient, a 6-year-old child, had been struck in the abdomen in a mock fist-fight with an older sibling. One week later, he developed a low-grade fever and began to walk with a stoop; after another week, his mother detected a "knot" in his right mid-abdominal wall. The second case involved the 11-year-old son of a rancher; the boy was struck in the abdomen by a bale of hay tossed from a hay baler. When he subsequently developed symptoms of abdominal pain, the diagnosis of appendicitis was entertained. When a mass later became palpable in his abdominal wall, rhabdomyosarcoma was suspected. A correct diagnosis was made after the use of scintigraphy and sonography, as described later.[5] A review from Nigeria found muscle abscesses in the anterior abdominal wall to be common.[2]

DIAGNOSIS

The diagnosis of pyomyositis should be considered in any child with fever and muscle pain, especially if a recent history of trauma exists. When a child has visible masses at commonly involved sites, such as the thigh, the diagnosis of pyomyositis can be made by needle aspiration of a mass. If a febrile child complains of myalgia in an extremity but has no palpable masses, the differential diagnosis must include more common inflammatory and infectious conditions of the bone or joint. A definitive diagnosis usually depends on one or more radiologic procedures. Plain films may show a soft tissue swelling or even a widened fascial plane suggestive of a mass lesion. A combination of plain radiography and radionuclide (technetium 99m phosphate) bone scintigraphy often can exclude osteomyelitis and pyoarthritis. If the diagnosis still is in question, scanning with gallium or indium can localize a muscle abscess precisely and can visualize other intramuscular abscesses too small to palpate (Fig. 63–1). Alternatively, ultrasonography can detect muscle abscesses and may be prefer-

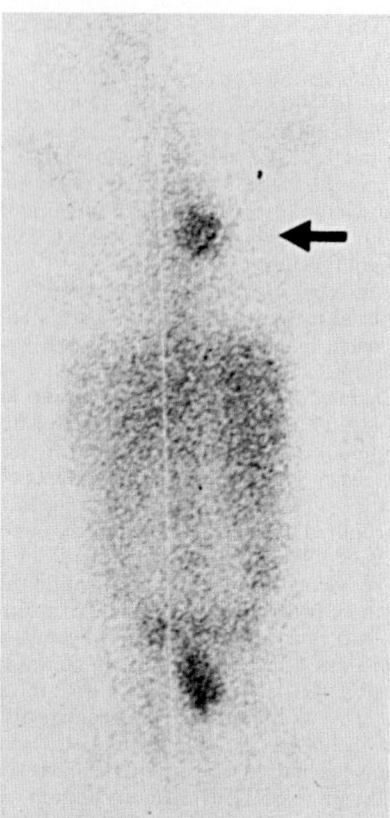

Figure 63–1 Scintigram of a patient with pyomyositis. Posterior gallium 67 citrate scan shows abnormally high uptake over the right scapula (*arrow*), where an abscess cavity was located within the muscle. Increased radioactivity also is observed in the bladder, which is a normal finding.

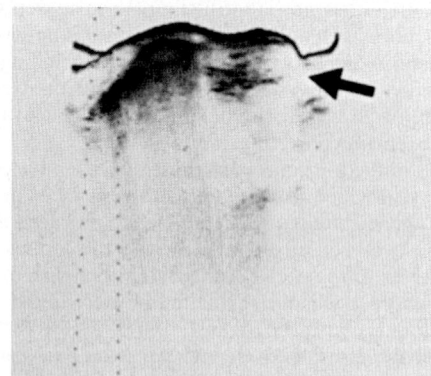

Figure 63–2 Sonogram of the abdominal wall of a patient with pyomyositis. The transverse view of the abdomen shows an abscess cavity in the right belly of the rectus abdominis muscle (*arrow*).

able as an initial procedure because it avoids the radiation exposure from computed tomography (CT) or scintigrams (Fig. 63–2).[27]

Magnetic resonance imaging (MRI) is very helpful in delineating the extent of a muscle abscess. In many cases, the abscess is much larger than suspected by physical symptoms and signs. The MRI scans of an illustrative case are presented in Figure 63–3. The patient was a 17-year-old girl with a swollen left lower thigh. She worked part-time as an attendant in an athletic club, where she participated in some of the vigorous exercise programs. Radiographs of the knee were normal, whereas a technetium

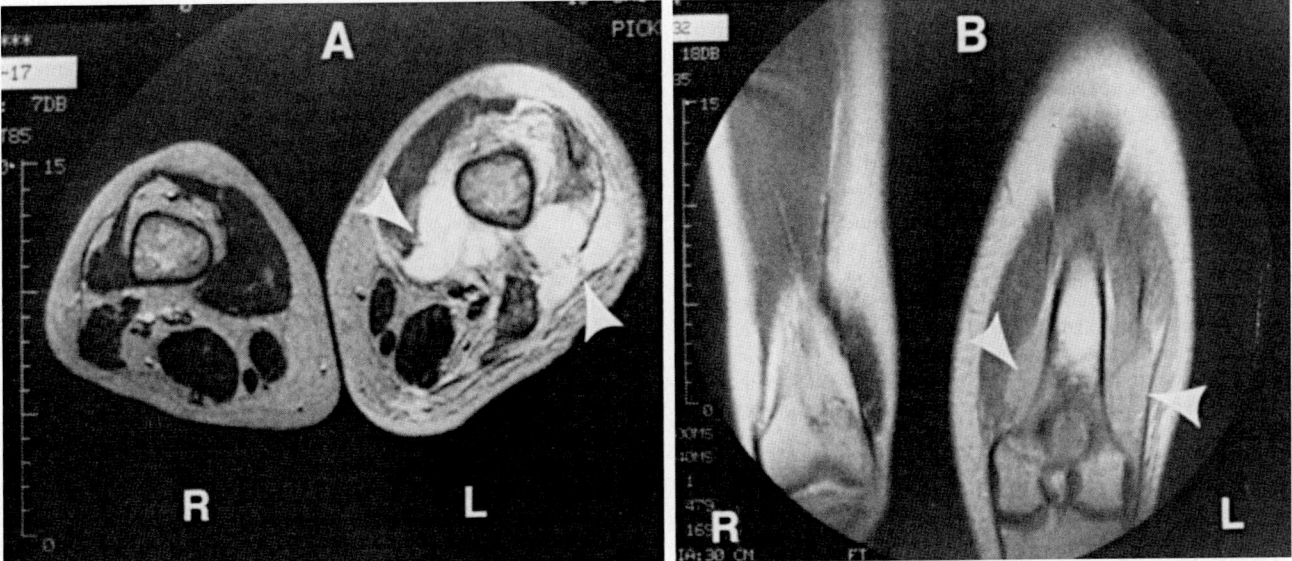

Figure 63–3 Magnetic resonance imaging of the thighs of a patient with pyomyositis. **A,** Axial images of the right (*R*) and left (*L*) thighs. **B,** Coronal images around the distal femoral shafts and femoral condyles. The scans show several well-defined areas of extremely high intensity in the muscle bundles and fascial planes from the middle to distal left femur (*arrows*). The high signal intensity suggests a fluid collection (e.g., an abscess), rather than a neoplastic process. Edema of the subcutaneous tissues also is evident in the lateral aspect of the swollen left thigh. There are no abnormal signals within the bone.

bone scan showed slightly increased radionuclide uptake in the soft tissues around the distal left femur. MRI of the left and right thighs showed a large fluid collection extending from the middle to distal left femur. Surgical exploration identified extensive abscess formation around the posterior aspect of the femur; the culture grew *S. aureus.* The affected muscle groups included the vastus medialis, vastus intermedius, vastus lateralis, and biceps femoris. The bone was not involved. For the reasons described, MRI has become the preferred procedure for establishing the diagnosis of pyomyositis.[14,22,27]

TREATMENT

Because pyomyositis is an abscess of skeletal muscle, the treatment is surgical incision and drainage.[2] Several physicians have seen that smaller lesions resolve spontaneously, even before the antibiotic era. An important role for systemic antibiotics is to prevent the formation of further muscle abscesses, especially in a patient with proven bacteremia. Because *S. aureus* is the most likely agent, a semisynthetic penicillinase-resistant penicillin is the preferred antibiotic in communities with little or no methicillin-resistant *S. aureus* (MRSA). Usually, nafcillin or oxacillin is administered intravenously every 6 hours at a total daily dosage of 150 to 200 mg/kg. When pyomyositis occurs in a patient with penicillin hypersensitivity, clindamycin, 40 mg/kg/day, divided every 8 hours, can be substituted because of its excellent coverage of gram-positive cocci. Parenteral therapy is continued until clinical improvement is evident, usually within a few days after surgical drainage. Thereafter, the antibiotics can be given orally at a reduced dosage for an additional 2 to 3 weeks. A penicillin derivative (dicloxacillin, 25 mg/kg/day, or cefadroxil, 30 mg/kg/day) or clindamycin, 20 to 30 mg/kg/day, is acceptable.

In many communities, MRSA is now a common agent. In a clinical analysis of 182 patients with pyomyositis from Texas Children's Hospital in Houston, Texas,[19] more than 50 percent of the isolated *S. aureus* strains were MRSA. In these communities, initial antibiotic management must include either intravenous clindamycin or vancomycin, 40 mg/kg/day, divided every 6 hours. Clindamycin can be continued as an oral antibiotic. For MRSA

isolates resistant to clindamycin, treatment with intravenous vancomycin can be followed by administration of oral linezolid, 30 mg/kg/day, divided every 8 hours, for children younger than 12 years; for children 12 years and older, 20 mg/kg/day, divided every 12 hours, is given. Therapy of MRSA infection may require a longer duration, from 3 to 4 weeks. Before discontinuing antibiotics, the patient should have documented normal levels of C-reactive protein and erythrocyte sedimentation rate.

ACUTE BACTERIAL MYOSITIS

Far less common than tropical pyomyositis is acute bacterial myositis, usually caused by group A streptococci. In this condition, the bacterial infection often is not confined to distinct abscesses within the muscle, but instead it extends diffusely through one or more muscle groups. As with pyomyositis, the disease occurs more commonly in males than in females and usually is associated with prior physical exertion and perhaps minor trauma. In contrast to pyomyositis, most published cases of acute bacterial myositis have occurred in adults and not in children.[4] The disease has been divided by Svane[25] into the following four main types:

1. A malignant form with septicemia and a uniformly fatal outcome
2. An acute form with a more protracted clinical course and other foci of suppuration, such as the bones, joints, or viscera
3. A subacute form with a better clinical prognosis
4. A benign type associated with more distinct muscle abscesses

The benign type of acute bacterial myositis by the Svane classification is the same disease process as described in the preceding section on pyomyositis.

CLINICAL PRESENTATION

The main clinical difference between the acute myositis syndrome and the pyomyositis syndrome is the virulence of the former disease, especially the malignant type. A case in a San Antonio, Texas, native is illustrative. The patient was a 23-year-old jackhammer operator who was admitted because of high fever, malaise, and pains in his arms. On examination, both upper extremities were tender to palpation, and faint erythema was visible over the same areas. He soon became incoherent, and his general condition quickly deteriorated. Death followed within 24 hours. Blood cultures drawn before death grew group A streptococci, and cultures of the biceps muscles obtained at autopsy grew the same organism. This case is similar to others described in the literature.[4,25] The patient worked as a jackhammer operator, who presumably would incur considerable minor trauma to the muscles of the upper arms and shoulders. Two reported cases of streptococcal myositis in children involved the left thigh and the left paravertebral muscles.[18] The first child developed septic shock and required intensive care for 27 days before a definitive diagnosis was made by CT.

A case of generalized myositis with staphylococcal septicemia has been described in a 15-year-old boy.[1] The patient presented with signs of fever and very diffuse muscle swelling and tenderness. All muscle groups of the extremities appeared to be inflamed and markedly tender; the creatine phosphokinase enzyme levels were markedly elevated. Culture of a muscle biopsy specimen grew *S. aureus*, as did previously drawn blood cultures. The patient experienced a stormy hospital course with severe hypotension and shock syndrome, requiring treatment with intravenous fluids, corticosteroids, dopamine, heparin, and assisted ventilation. He also received a total of 4 weeks of antistaphylococcal antibiotic therapy.

DIAGNOSIS

Blood cultures are positive most often in patients with the most significant clinical symptoms. Cultures of muscle biopsy specimens may yield a profuse growth of bacteria. Rarely, myositis has occurred as a delayed complication of chickenpox, often together with fasciitis.[12,17,23] In this situation, bacteremia may not be documented because the bacterial process usually is the result of contiguous spread from a secondarily infected pock lesion. These streptococcal complications of chickenpox often occur in an extremity, which may become swollen and painful. Under these circumstances, MRI can be an extremely valuable diagnostic tool to gauge the depth and extent of inflammation.[27]

TREATMENT AND THE EAGLE EFFECT

The treatment of acute streptococcal or staphylococcal myositis of the malignant type is a medical emergency. As soon as the diagnosis is suspected, bacteriologic cultures should be obtained, and intravenous therapy should be initiated with a high-dose semisynthetic penicillin (e.g., nafcillin, 50 mg/kg every 6 hours) and vancomycin. If the cultures yield group A streptococci rather than *Staphylococcus*, the antibiotic can be switched to penicillin G at an equivalent high dosage. Surgical consultation is required to evaluate the need for débridement and drainage. Obtaining MRI scans may be advisable to document the extent of the disease and the response to antibiotic therapy. In severe cases of bacterial myositis, the total duration of hospitalization can exceed 4 weeks.[1,18]

The apparent resurgence of serious streptococcal infection has led to an increased interest in what has been called the *Harry Eagle effect*, named after the scientist who first described the failure of penicillin to eradicate group A streptococcal infection in a mouse model.[8] Eagle inoculated mice intramuscularly with group A streptococci and observed a markedly retarded bactericidal action of penicillin on organisms in the older abscesses, even

though the bacteria remained highly sensitive to the antibiotic. Even massive doses of penicillin 10,000 times greater than the minimum inhibitory concentration were not effective at eradicating the bacteria. Subsequent studies by other investigators confirmed the existence of the Eagle effect and disclosed that clindamycin showed superior efficacy to penicillin in treatment of streptococcal myositis in the mouse model.[24] In an editorial comment, Stevens[23] observed that penicillin most likely fails to kill stationary-phase streptococci in muscle infections, an explanation for the Eagle effect. He suggested that streptococcal myositis or fasciitis be treated with intravenous clindamycin, 40 mg/kg/day, if the condition fails to respond to penicillin therapy.

MISCELLANEOUS CAUSES OF MYOSITIS

Viral infection occasionally leads to myositis (see Table 63–1). The most common example undoubtedly is myositis associated with influenza virus infection in children. Typically, school-aged children are affected. Muscle groups of the legs often are involved, associated with a marked elevation of serum creatine phosphokinase. Clinical symptoms generally last 2 to 4 days. Another, far less common myositis is caused by coxsackievirus B infection. This disease is called *epidemic pleurodynia* because the myositis frequently involves the chest and upper abdomen. The enteroviral infection is known as *Bornholm disease*, named after the Danish island where it was first described.

Fungal infection (e.g., *Candida albicans*) can cause myositis. Candidal myositis is uncommon, however, and usually occurs in patients who are severely immunocompromised. Frequently, other sites also are involved by the disseminated fungal infection in addition to muscle.

Parasitic infection can cause myositis. The best known is trichinosis, caused by ingestion of the encysted larvae of *Trichinella spiralis*. The larvae typically are found in products containing pork and wild game, such as bear meat. The first signs of illness are fever and abdominal pain. Later, muscle pain is noted in the neck and chest. Eventually, calcifications form in the involved muscles. Treatment of the acute disease with mebendazole or albendazole may be beneficial. Another parasite more common in Central and South America is *Taenia solium*. Ingestion of eggs of this pork tapeworm leads to cysticercosis, with calcified densities in skeletal muscle. Finally, toxoplasmosis infection can lead to symptoms of myositis. During acute infection, *Toxoplasma gondii* can encyst in the skeletal muscle and lead to an inflammatory myopathy closely resembling dermatomyositis.

REFERENCES

1. Adamski, G. B., Garin, E. H., Ballinger, W. E., et al.: Generalized non-suppurative myositis with staphylococcal septicemia. J. Pediatr. *96*:694-697, 1980.
2. Ameh, E. A.: Pyomyositis in children: Analysis of 31 cases. Ann. Trop. Paediatr. *19*:263-265, 1999.
3. Ashken, M. H., and Cotton, R. E.: Tropical skeletal muscle abscesses (pyomyositis tropicans). Br. J. Surg. *50*:846-852, 1963.
4. Barrett, A. M., and Gresham, G. A.: Acute streptococcal myositis. Lancet *1*:347-351, 1958.
5. Beck, W., and Grose, C.: Pyomyositis presenting as acute abdominal pain. Pediatr. Infect. Dis. *3*:445-448, 1984.
6. Chacha, P. B.: Muscle abscesses in children. Clin. Orthop. *70*:174-180, 1970.
7. Diamandakis, V., and Grose, C.: Bad consequences of bicycle accidents. Pediatr. Infect. Dis. J. *13*:422-425, 1994.
8. Eagle, H.: Experimental approach to the problem of treatment failure with penicillin, I: Group A streptococcal infection in mice. Am. J. Med. *13*:389-399, 1952.
9. Echeverria, P., and Vaughn, M. C.: Tropical pyomyositis: A diagnostic problem in temperate climates. Am. J. Dis. Child. *129*:856-857, 1975.
10. Goldberg, J. S., London, W. L., and Nagel, D. M. Tropical pyomyositis: A case report and review. Pediatrics *63*:298-300, 1979.

11. Grose, C.: Staphylococcal pyomyositis in south Texas. J. Pediatr. *93*:457-458, 1978.
12. Grose, C.: Varicella-zoster virus infections: Chickenpox, shingles, and varicella vaccine. *In* Glaser, R., and Jones, J. F. (eds.): Herpesvirus Infections. New York, Marcel Dekker, 1994, pp. 117-185.
13. Gubbay, A. J., and Issacs, D.: Pyomyositis in children. Pediatr. Infect. Dis. J. *19*:1009-1012, 2000.
14. Karmazyn, B., Kleiman, M. B., Buckwalter, K., et al. Acute pyomyositis of the pelvis: The spectrum of clinical presentations and MR findings. Pediatr. Radiol. *36*: 338-343, 2006.
15. Marcus, R. T., and Foster, W. D.: Observations on the clinical features, etiology and geographic distribution of pyomyositis in East Africa. East Afr. Med. J. *45*:167-176, 1968.
16. Meehan, J., Grose, C., Soper, R. T., and Kimura, K. Pyomyositis in an adolescent female athlete. J. Pediatr. Surg. *30*:127-128, 1995.
17. Miyake, H.: Beitrage zur kenntnis der sogenannten myositis infectiosa. Mitt. Grenageb. Med. Chir. *13*:155-198, 1904.
18. Moore, D. L., Delage, G., Labelle, H., et al.: Peracute streptococcal pyomyositis: Report of two cases and review of the literature. J. Pediatr. Orthop. *6*:232-235, 1986.
19. Pannaraj, P. S., Hulten, K. G., Gonzalez, B. E., et al.: Infective pyomyositis and myositis in children in the era of community acquired methicillin resistant *Staphylococcus aureus*. Clin. Infect. Dis. *43*:953-960, 2006.
20. Scriba, J.: Beitrag zur aetiologie der myositis acuta. Dtsch. Z. Chir. *22*:497-502, 1885.
21. Sirinavin, S., and McCracken, G. H.: Primary suppurative myositis in children. Am. J. Dis. Child. *133*:263-265, 1979.
22. Solar, R., Rodriguez, E., Aguiler, C., and Fernandez, R.: Magnetic resonance imaging of pyomyositis in 43 cases. Eur. J. Radiol. *35*:59-64, 2000.
23. Stevens, D. L.: Editorial response: Varicella gangrenosa with toxic shock-like syndrome. Clin. Infect. Dis. *20*:1061-1062, 1995.
24. Stevens, D. L., Gibbons, A. E., Bergstrom, R., and Winn, V.: The Eagle effect revisited: Efficacy of clindamycin, erythromycin, and penicillin in the treatment of streptococcal myositis. J. Infect. Dis. *158*:23-28, 1988.
25. Svane, S.: Peracute spontaneous streptococcal myositis. Acta Chir. Scand. *137*:155-163, 1971.
26. Traquair, R. N.: Pyomyositis. J. Trop. Med. Hyg. *50*:81-89, 1947.
27. Trusen, A., Beissert, M., Schultz, G., and Darge, K.: Ultrasound and MRI features of pyomyositis in children. Eur. Radiol. *13*:1050-1055, 2003.

SKIN INFECTIONS

CHAPTER

64

CUTANEOUS MANIFESTATIONS OF SYSTEMIC INFECTIONS

James D. Cherry

Many illnesses caused by infectious agents have associated cutaneous manifestations. In some cases, the exanthem may be the hallmark of the disease; in others, it may be only a vague indicator of a more significant underlying process. When an exanthem occurs, it often offers important clues to the etiology of a patient's illness. Although most exanthematous illnesses in children are benign, their differential diagnosis is critical because the early manifestations of potentially fatal bacterial and rickettsial diseases frequently have cutaneous findings.

HISTORY

Exanthematous manifestations of infectious illnesses have been important since medical antiquity. Major epidemics of both measles and smallpox occurred in the Roman Empire and in China at the beginning of the Christian era.[25,130] Scarlet fever was recognized as a distinct entity in the 17th century, and chickenpox and rubella were identified in the 18th and 19th centuries, respectively.[49]

In the writings of the early 20th century, maculopapular exanthematous illnesses of children frequently were referred to by number. Scarlet fever and measles historically were the first two classic maculopapular exanthems of childhood. Which one had the honor of being the "first disease" is unknown today. The "third disease" was rubella, which was recognized by the beginning of the 20th century as a distinct entity.[68,70,87,157,178–180] In 1900, Dukes[68] described an exanthematous illness with the characteristics of both rubella and scarlet fever, which he suggested was a "fourth disease." The general opinion today is that his disease was not a distinct entity. Shaw[180] suggested that Dukes' cases had mild atypical scarlet fever, and Powell[157] raised the possibility that the illness resulted from epidermolytic toxin–producing staphylococci. Most probably, rubella and scarlet fever both were epidemic in the student population under Dr. Dukes' care; combined infections led to the confusion.

Erythema infectiosum (see Chapter 164) commonly is referred to as the *fifth disease*, and roseola infantum (see Chapter 65) qualifies as the *sixth disease*.[179]

During the last 55 years, interest in exanthematous diseases has been renewed because a large number of previously unknown viruses and other infectious agents that cause cutaneous manifestations have been discovered. In addition, the pattern of disease caused by classic exanthem-producing agents has changed; smallpox has been eradicated, the epidemiology of measles and rubella has been altered by immunization, and ecologic changes have resulted in differences in viral and bacterially induced rashes.

ETIOLOGIC AGENTS

Many different types of viruses, chlamydiae, rickettsiae, mycoplasmas, bacteria, fungi, and protozoan and metazoan agents cause illnesses with associated cutaneous manifestations. Although this chapter is devoted to systemic infectious diseases with cutaneous manifestations, the demarcation between exanthematous disease of systemic and local origin is not always readily apparent. For example, the recurrent cold sore caused by herpes simplex virus (HSV) infection frequently is considered a local problem, although its nature and pathogenesis involve central virus latency and host systemic immune functions. Similarly, superficial fungal diseases and other local infections, such as warts, may be quite dependent on more general immunologic functions of the host. The exanthems of enteroviral infections frequently are confused with those caused by insect bites and allergic problems.

Table 64–1 presents viruses that have cutaneous manifestations in humans. Erythema infectiosum is caused by human parvovirus B19.[7,205] This virus also is an important cause of the papular-purpuric gloves and socks syndrome that is an uncommon occurrence and mainly affects young adults.[3,6,50,85,91,184,185] Human parvovirus B19 also has been associated with a vesiculopustular exanthem, erythema multiforme, and other petechial and purpuric rashes. In one study, an erythematous maculopapular rash was noted in 9 percent of children with human bocavirus infections.[8] Adenovirus types 1, 2, 3, 4, 7, and 7a have been isolated from children and young adults with exanthem.[49,110,208,209] The overall clinical expression rate of exanthem in adenovirus infection rarely has been studied. Fukumi and associates[79] noted that rash occurred in 2 percent of adenoviral infections; Hope-Simpson and Higgins[98] indicated a rate of approximately 8 percent.

Eight species in the *Herpesvirus* genus have cutaneous manifestations associated with infection, but clinical expression rates vary greatly. Nearly all primary varicella infections are associated with exanthem, whereas exanthem with acquired cytomegalovirus infection is a rare manifestation.[19,22,49,166,190,208] The incidence of exanthem in Epstein-Barr virus infection varies from 3 percent to nearly 100 percent, depending on whether concomitant ampicillin is administered.[16,28,95,104,111,146,159,197,198] Although firm data are lacking, probably less than 10 percent of primary infections with HSV type 1 are associated with cutaneous manifestations. Erythema multiforme occasionally occurs with recurrent HSV infections.[36,76,107,144] Human herpesvirus–6 (HHV-6) is a major cause of roseola infantum.[11,205,217] HHV-7 also is a cause of roseola infantum[10]; in addition, some evidence suggests that this virus may play a role in pityriasis rosea.[66] HHV-8 infection is necessary

Text continued on p. 762

TABLE 64-1   Clinical Characteristics of Viral Infections with Cutaneous Manifestations

Virus	Disease or Syndrome	Incubation Period (days)	Main Season	Clinical Characteristics	Exanthem Lesions	Exanthem Distribution	Usual Duration (days)
Human parvovirus B19 (see Figs. 64–6 to 64–8)	Erythema infectiosum; gloves and socks syndrome	7–17	Winter and spring	Biphasic illness with mild prodromal period with headache and malaise for 2–3 days, then 7-day symptom-free period, followed by typical exanthema	Three-stage exanthema: initially, rash on cheeks (slapped-cheek appearance) and then erythematous maculopapular rash on trunk and limbs; finally, rash develops a reticular pattern	Starts on face More prominent on extensor surfaces of extremities	7–21
Human bocavirus			Fall, winter, and spring	Fever, cough, coryza, respiratory distress (bronchitis, bronchiolitis, pneumonia)	Erythematous maculopapular	Mainly face, chest, and trunk	
Human papillomaviruses	Warts		Nonseasonal	Local cutaneous disease	Papular or nodular isolated lesions	Most common on extremities	100+
Adenovirus types 1, 2, 3, 4, 7, and 7a		6–9	Winter and spring	Fever and signs and symptoms of respiratory illness Occasionally, rash occurs after defervescence (roseola-like)	Most commonly erythematous, maculopapular, and discrete (rubelliform), but occasionally confluent (morbilliform) Rarely, erythema multiforme and Stevens-Johnson syndrome	Usually starts on face and spreads downward to trunk and extremities	3–5
Herpes simplex types 1 and 2 (see Fig. 64–5)	Cold sores, genital herpes, neonatal herpes, or other	2–12	Nonseasonal	Primary disease associated with fever and systemic symptoms Recurrent disease caused by exogenous and endogenous infections	Singular or grouped vesicular lesions varying in size from 2 to 10 mm, frequently on a mildly erythematous base Occasionally, erythema multiforme, Stevens-Johnson syndrome, and erythema nodosum	Lesions in primary infection with type 1 virus are mainly in and around the mouth Recurrent type 1 lesions usually perioral Primary and recurrent type 2 lesions usually on genitals	7–14
Human herpesvirus-6 (HHV-6)	Roseola infantum		Nonseasonal	Fever 3–5 days in duration, rapid defervescence, and then the appearance of rash	Erythematous macular or maculopapular	Most prominent on neck and trunk Face and extremities may be affected	1–2
Human herpesvirus-7 (HHV-7)	Roseola infantum		Nonseasonal	Fever 3–5 days in duration, rapid defervescence, and then the appearance of rash	Erythematous macular or maculopapular	Most prominent on neck and trunk Face and extremities may be affected	1–2
Human herpesvirus-8 (HHV-8)	Kaposi sarcoma	Months to years	Nonseasonal	Asymptomatic infection Most commonly noted in AIDS patients but occurs in other immunodeficiency states	Purple to blue nodular, raised lesions	Any epidermal or mucosal surface	Months to years
Varicella-zoster (see Fig. 64-4)	Chickenpox (varicella)	12–20	Late fall, winter, and spring	Malaise and fever of 5–6 days duration	Basic lesion is vesicular, but lesions go through stages: macules, papules, vesicles, and crusts Lesions occur in crops	Lesions more profuse on trunk than on extremities Proximal end of extremities more involved than distal end	8–10
	Herpes zoster		Nonseasonal	Endogenous infection Pain and paresthesia with dermatome distribution	Basic lesion is vesicular, but lesions go through stages: macules, papules, vesicles, and crusts	Lesions localized to area of skin innervated by a single sensory ganglion	10–28

Virus	Disease	Incubation (days)	Season	Associated findings	Skin lesions	Distribution	Duration (days)
Epstein-Barr	Infectious mononucleosis	28–49	Nonseasonal	Fever, pharyngitis, and lymphadenopathy; Exanthem occurs in 3–13% of cases; If ampicillin is administered, then exanthema in 50% of cases	Most commonly erythematous, macular, maculopapular, and discrete (rubelliform); In association with ampicillin administration, the rash may be more vivid; Erythema multiforme and urticaria may occur	Mainly on trunk and proximal end of extremities	2–7
Cytomegalovirus	Cytomegalovirus mononucleosis		Nonseasonal	Acquired: mild febrile illness with lymphadenopathy; Congenital: disseminated disease	Erythematous, maculopapular, and discrete; Vesicular or petechial in congenital infection	Located mainly on trunk and proximal end of extremities	2–7
Vaccinia	Roseola vaccinatum, eczema vaccinatum, vaccination "take," or disseminated vaccinia		Nonseasonal	Illness caused by direct exposure via vaccination or exposure to a vaccinee	Vaccination and eczema vaccinatum lesions go through stages: papule, vesicle, pustule, and scab; Roseola vaccinatum: erythematous maculopapular lesions; Occasionally erythema multiforme; Disseminated vaccinia: papular or vesicular lesions	Lesions in roseola vaccinatum, eczema vaccinatum, and disseminated vaccinia are generalized	7–14
Variola	Smallpox	8–17	Seasonal by geographic area	Abrupt onset of high fever, headache, and muscle and joint pain; Rash appears 2–4 days after onset	Basic lesion is vesicular, but lesions go through stages: macules, papules, vesicles, pustules, and crusts	Most prominent on exposed body surfaces; Starts on extremities and face; Spreads centripetally	12–20
Monkeypox				Similar to mild smallpox; Exposure to monkeys; No human-to-human spread	Similar to mild smallpox	Similar to mild smallpox	
Orf	Ecthyma contagiosum	4–7	Spring	Disease of sheep acquired by humans	Initially erythematous papule; Becomes umbilicated, nodular, and then vesicular; Occasionally erythema multiforme	Solitary lesion, usually on hands	30–40
Molluscum contagiosum	Molluscum contagiosum			Local cutaneous disease	Umbilicated nodular lesions: singular or clusters	Most common on face, inner aspect of thigh, breasts, and genitalia	100+
Paravaccinia	Milker's nodules	4–7		Human infection acquired from infected calves	Nodular lesion; Occasionally erythema multiforme; Umbilicated vesicular lesion	Solitary lesion, usually on hands	30–40
Tanapox				A virus of monkeys; Human infection associated with fever and regional lymphadenopathy		Upper part of body; Solitary lesion	35–56
Coxsackieviruses A2, A4, A5, A7, A9, A10, and A16; coxsackieviruses B1-B5; echoviruses 1-7, 9, 11-14, 16-19, 22, 24, 25, 30, and 33; enterovirus 71 (see Figs. 64–9 to 64–16)		4–7	Summer and fall	Fever and mild to moderate pharyngitis; Occasionally, herpangina, meningitis, and other manifestations of systemic viral infection; Exanthem occurs in 5–50% of infections, depending on virus type; Rash may occur during fever or after defervescence; hand, foot, and mouth syndrome	Most commonly erythematous, maculopapular, and discrete; May have macular, petechial, vesicular, and urticarial components; Rarely erythema multiforme	Usually starts on face and spreads downward to trunk and extremities; May have peripheral distribution (hand, foot, and mouth syndrome)	3–7

TABLE 64–1 Clinical Characteristics of Viral Infections with Cutaneous Manifestations—cont'd

Virus	Disease or Syndrome	Incubation Period (days)	Main Season	Clinical Characteristics	Exanthem Lesions	Exanthem Distribution	Usual Duration (days)
Rhinoviruses (many types)		2-4	Fall, winter, and spring	Mild fever and signs and symptoms of respiratory illness Exanthem occurs in about 5% of cases	Erythematous or maculopapular and discrete	Starts on face and spreads downward to trunk and extremities	1-4
Foot and mouth		3-4		Direct animal contact Fever, sore mouth, and lymphadenopathy Vesicles and ulcers within the mouth	Vesicular lesions	Hands and feet	3-6
Colorado tick fever		3-5	Summer	Fever, chills, eye pain, myalgia, and headache Diphasic course Rash in only about 10% of cases	Occasionally maculopapular but usually petechial	Maculopapular rash is generalized Petechial rash most prominent on arms, legs, and trunk	2-7
Reovirus 2 and 3		4-7	Summer	Fever, mild pharyngitis, and cervical adenopathy	Erythematous or maculopapular Discrete or confluent Occasionally vesicular	Starts on face and spreads downward to trunk and extremities	3-9
Rotavirus	Gianotti-Crosti syndrome; infantile acute hemorrhagic edema	2-4	Fall, winter, and spring	Gastroenteritis	Petechial and morbilliform	Generalized	7-14
Chikungunya, o'nyong-nyong, Ross River, Sindbis			During periods of arthropod prevalence	Fever, headache, eye pain, and marked myalgia, arthralgia, and arthritis Geographically localized diseases	Rubelliform and morbilliform Frequently vesicular and petechial	Starts on face and spreads downward to trunk and extremities	
Rubella (see Fig. 64-3)	Rubella (German measles)	15-21	Winter and spring	Mild symptoms with onset 1-5 days before rash Fever usually <38.5° C (101.5° F) Headache, malaise, and suboccipital and postauricular lymphadenopathy	Erythematous, maculopapular, and discrete	Starts on face and spreads downward to trunk and extremities	4-7
West Nile				Sudden onset of fever, chills, and drowsiness Rash may appear during or after fever Geographically localized disease	Erythematous, macular, and maculopapular	Starts on trunk and spreads to extremities	3-6
Dengue and Kunjin		7	During periods of specific arthropod prevalence	Sudden onset of high fever, then severe headache, myalgia, arthralgia, abdominal pain, and marked diaphoresis Fever lasts 5-6 days and ends by crisis Rash appears within 48 hours of onset of fever Geographically localized diseases	Initially, macular, flushed appearance, then erythematous, maculopapular rash May be scarlatiniform Frequently becomes petechial and purpuric Small vesicles occur in Kunjin virus infection	Initial macular rash is more prominent centrally Maculopapular rash may start on hands and feel and spread to trunk	3-10
Influenza A and B		2-5	Fall, winter, and spring	Fever, cough, headache, and muscle aches and pains Usually in young children Rash an occasional occurrence	Erythematous, maculopapular, and discrete (rubelliform) Rarely erythema multiforme	Starts on face and trunk and spreads to extremities	1-3
Respiratory syncytial		2-5	Fall, winter, and spring	Fever, coryza, and respiratory distress (bronchitis, bronchiolitis, or pneumonia) Usually in children <2 years	Erythematous, maculopapular, and discrete (rubelliform)	Starts on face and trunk and spreads to extremities	1-3
Human metapneumovirus			Fall, winter, and spring	Fever, coryza, and respiratory distress (bronchitis, bronchiolitis, or pneumonia)	Erythematous, maculopapular		

Virus	Disease	Incubation period (days)	Seasonal occurrence	Signs and symptoms	Rash characteristics	Distribution	Duration (days)
Parainfluenza 1-3		2-5	Fall, winter, and spring	Fever, coryza, nasopharyngitis, croup, and bronchitis; Usually in young children	Erythematous, maculopapular, and discrete (rubelliform)	Starts on face and trunk and spreads to extremities	1-3
Mumps		14-21	Fall, winter, and spring	Fever, headache, and salivary gland swelling	Erythematous, maculopapular, and discrete; also, urticaria and vesicles; rarely, erythema multiforme	Most prominent on trunk	2-5
Measles (see Figs. 64-1 and 64-2)		8-12	Winter and spring	Onset with fever, cough, coryza, and conjunctivitis; About 2 days after onset, appearance of enanthem (Koplik spots); and 2 days later, onset of exanthem	Erythematous, maculopapular, and confluent; Develops a brownish appearance, and fine desquamation occurs	Starts behind ears and on forehead; Spreads downward over body; Confluence most prominent on face, trunk, and proximal end of extremities	5-7
Lassa	Lassa fever		Nonseasonal	Sudden onset of fever, chills, headache, and sore throat; Progresses to pneumonia and renal failure	Macular and sometimes petechial	Localized or general	
Hepatitis B	Papular acrodermatitis of childhood	50-180		Geographically localized outbreaks; Insidious onset with arthralgia, arthritis, and rash occurring before jaundice	Maculopapular, macular, or urticarial; In young children, papular (Gianotti-Crosti syndrome or papular acrodermatitis of childhood); Rarely, erythema multiforme	Generalized	4-10
Hepatitis C	Mixed cryoglobulinemia (not reported in children)	7-14	Nonseasonal	Acute hepatitis followed by chronic infection; Skin findings occur late in disease	Palpable purpura	Mostly buttocks, lower extremities	Variable
Marburg	Hemorrhagic fever	5-7	Occurs in outbreaks	Headache, conjunctivitis, photophobia, myalgia, vomiting, diarrhea, and fever (biphasic); Exposure to vervet monkeys	Initially erythematous macular, then discrete maculopapular, and finally confluent maculopapular; Exfoliation occurs; Occasionally purpura	Generalized	2-14
Ebola	Hemorrhagic fever	5-10	Occurs in outbreaks	Febrile illness that progresses to hemorrhage, shock, and coma	Maculopapular rash that appears toward end of first week of illness	Lateral sides of trunk, groin, and axillae; Can become generalized but spares the face	14-60
Hantavirus	Hemorrhagic fever with renal syndrome (nephropathia epidemica)	14-60	Spring and summer outbreaks	Febrile illness with hemorrhagic and renal manifestations	Flushing and petechial rash	Face (flushing), skin folds (petechiae)	14-28
HIV			Nonseasonal	Fever, pharyngitis, myalgia, arthralgias, adenopathy, and rash	Macular	Mainly chest and abdomen	7
Human T-lymphotropic virus	Infective dermatitis		Nonseasonal	Acute onset of eczema	Severe exudative eczema with a crusting, generalized, fine papular rash	Scalp, eyelid margins, perinasal skin, retroauricular areas, axillae, and groin	Months to years

Data from references 1, 2, 4, 6, 7-12, 16, 19, 22, 26, 36, 39, 42, 44, 46, 48-50, 52, 57, 58, 60, 62, 63, 65, 76-79, 85, 91, 95, 97, 98, 102, 104, 106, 111, 114, 116, 117, 120, 121, 126, 135, 137-141, 144, 150, 152, 158, 164, 166, 167, 169-171, 174, 175, 184, 185, 189, 193, 197, 198, 202, 205, 207-209, 216, 217.

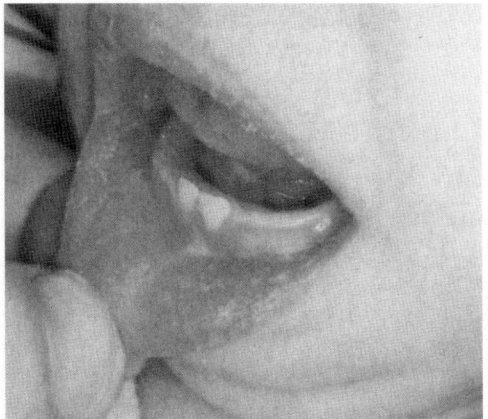

Figure 64–1 Koplik spots with involvement of the buccal and lower labial mucosa. (See companion Expert Consult web site for color version.)

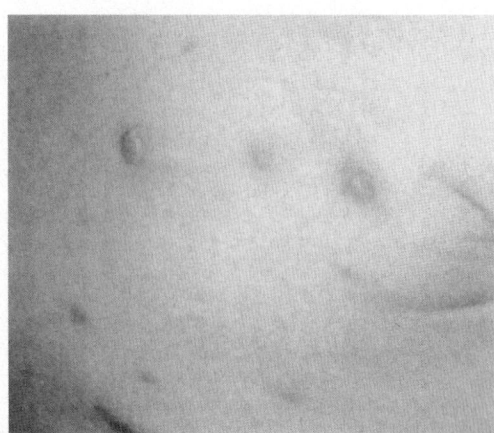

Figure 64–4 Chickenpox exanthem. Typical lesions in all stages: vesicles, papulovesicles, and papules. (See companion Expert Consult web site for color version.) *(From Cherry, J. D.: Newer viral exanthems. Adv. Pediatr. 16:233-286, 1969.)*

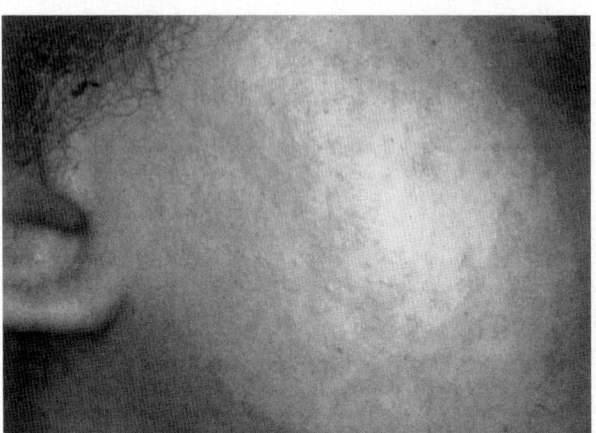

Figure 64–2 Measles exanthem. Note the generalized erythematous confluent base supporting small papular and microvesicular lesions. (See companion Expert Consult web site for color version.)

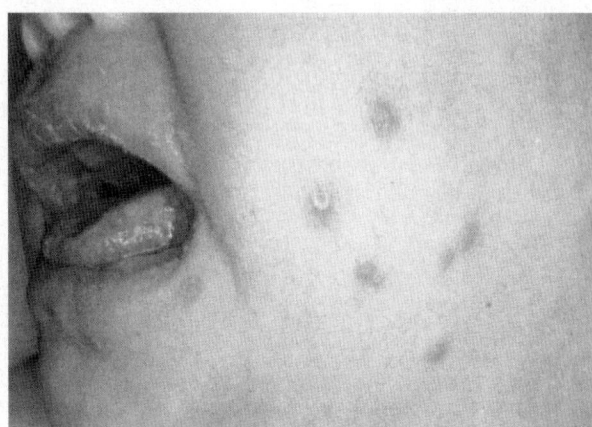

Figure 64–5 Primary herpes simplex virus infection in an infant. Note the severe stomatitis and papulovesicular and vesicular lesions under the lower lip and on the cheek. (See companion Expert Consult web site for color version.)

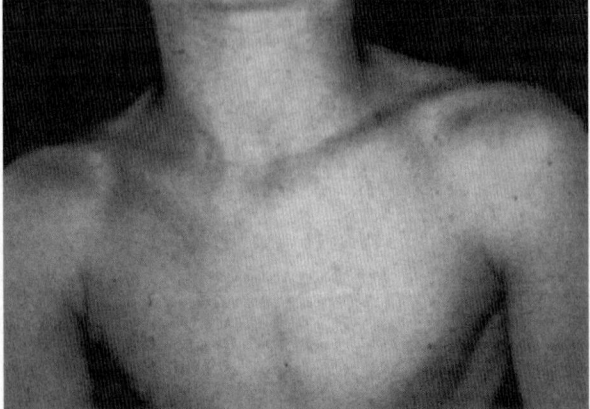

Figure 64–3 Rubella exanthem. The rash is erythematous, maculopapular, and discrete. (See companion Expert Consult web site for color version.) *(From Cherry, J. D.: Newer viral exanthems. Adv. Pediatr. 16:233-286, 1969.)*

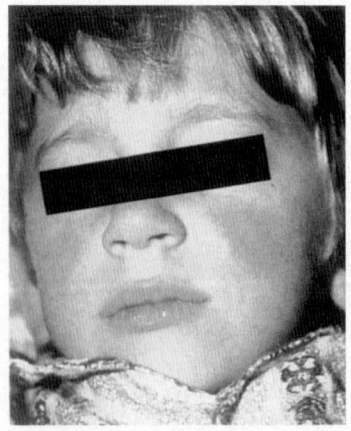

Figure 64–6 Slapped-cheek appearance with a relative circumoral maculopapular rash in erythema infectiosum. (See companion Expert Consult web site for color version.)

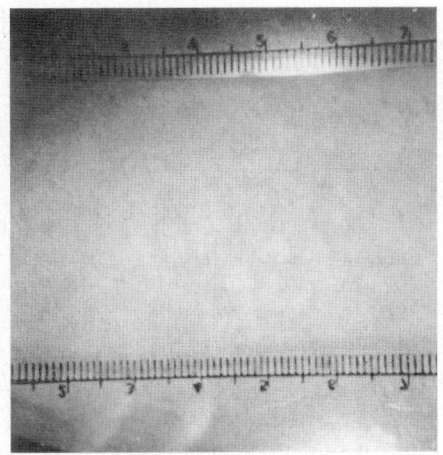

Figure 64–7 Rash with a lacelike, or reticular, pattern in erythema infectiosum. (See companion Expert Consult web site for color version.)

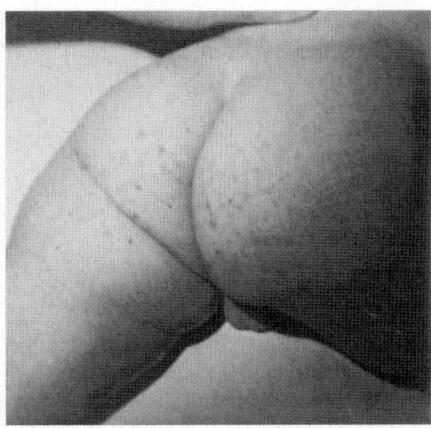

Figure 64–10 Erythematous maculopapular lesions on the buttocks as part of the hand, foot, and mouth syndrome caused by coxsackievirus A16. (See companion Expert Consult web site for color version.) *(From Cherry, J. D., and Jahn, C. L.: Hand, foot, and mouth syndrome: Report of six cases due to coxsackievirus, group A, type 16. Pediatrics 37:637, 1966. Copyright American Academy of Pediatrics 1966.)*

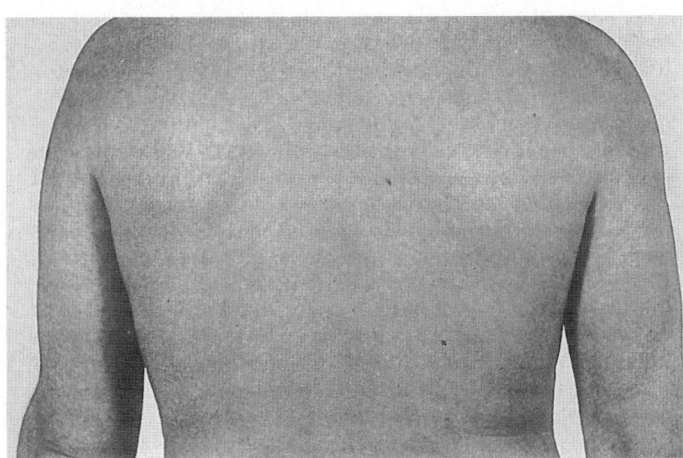

Figure 64–8 Confluent exanthem in a patient with human parvovirus infection. (See companion Expert Consult web site for color version.)

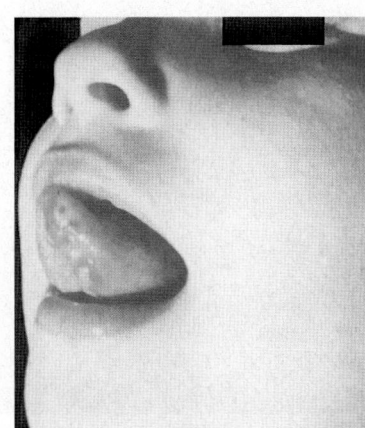

Figure 64–11 Two large ulcerative lesions on the underside of the tongue in a patient with hand, foot, and mouth syndrome caused by coxsackievirus A16. (See companion Expert Consult web site for color version.)

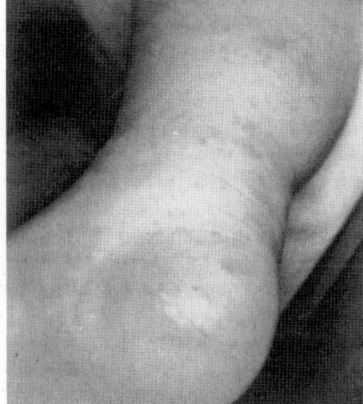

Figure 64–9 Vesicular and maculopapular lesions on the foot and lower part of the leg as part of the hand, foot, and mouth syndrome caused by coxsackievirus A16. (See companion Expert Consult web site for color version.) *(From Cherry, J. D., and Jahn, C. L.: Hand, foot, and mouth syndrome: Report of six cases due to coxsackievirus, group A, type 16. Pediatrics 37:637, 1966. Copyright American Academy of Pediatrics 1966.)*

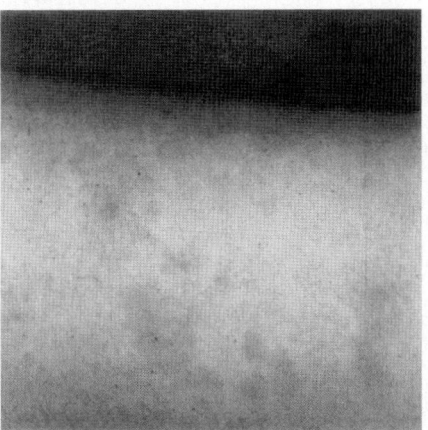

Figure 64–12 Papular-urticarial lesions in coxsackievirus A9 infection. (See companion Expert Consult web site for color version.) *(From Cherry, J. D.: Newer viral exanthems. Adv. Pediatr. 16:233-286, 1969.)*

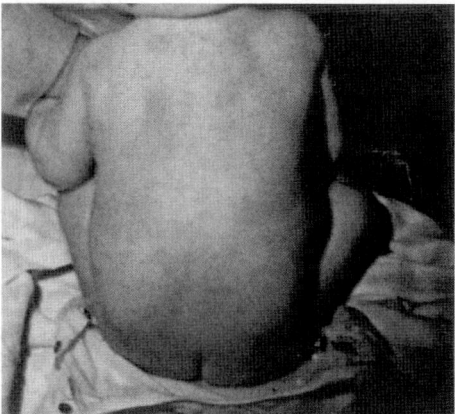

Figure 64–13 Erythematous, discrete, maculopapular, and petechial rash of echovirus 9 infection. (See companion Expert Consult web site for color version.) *(From Cherry, J. D.: Newer viral exanthems. Adv. Pediatr. 16:233-286, 1969.)*

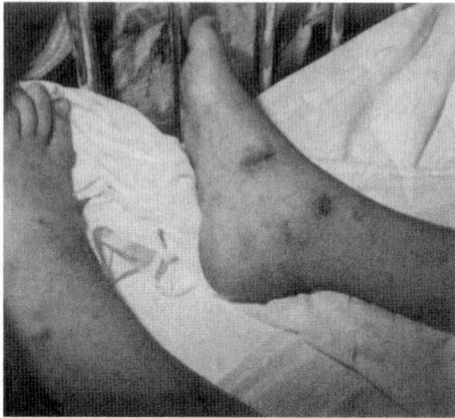

Figure 64–14 Petechial and purpuric rash in a child with coxsackievirus A9 infection. (See companion Expert Consult web site for color version.)

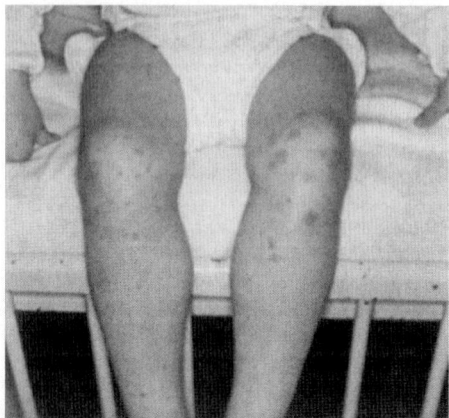

Figure 64–15 Erythematous, papular, papulovesicular, and petechial lesions suggestive of anaphylactic purpura in a child with coxsackievirus A4 infection. (See companion Expert Consult web site for color version.)

Figure 64–16 Acute urticaria in a child with hand, foot, and mouth syndrome caused by coxsackievirus A16 infection. (See companion Expert Consult web site for color version.)

for the development of Kaposi sarcoma in patients with acquired immunodeficiency syndrome (AIDS) and other immunodeficiency states.[102,114,135]

At present, human illnesses with cutaneous manifestations caused by poxviruses rarely occur. Because smallpox as a disease has ceased to exist, the use of vaccinia virus for immunization has decreased dramatically. However, the terrorist events of 2001 raised concern about the possible use of smallpox virus as a terrorist weapon. Because of this potential danger, smallpox vaccines are being produced and used again. With the increased use of these vaccines, cutaneous complications of vaccinia virus infection can be expected. Monkeypox, orf, and paravaccinia (milker's nodules) continue to occur as isolated events in exposed individuals.[170,208,209] Human infection with tanapox virus is a geographically related illness occurring in limited areas of Kenya.

In the present era, enteroviruses are the leading cause of infection-related exanthematous diseases.[51,55,109,208,209] Thirty-seven types have been associated with rash illnesses. The clinical expression rate varies greatly among the different types; it is as high as 50 percent in children with coxsackievirus A16 and echovirus 9 infections. Only approximately 15 percent of individuals infected with echovirus 4 have exanthem, and rash is a rare occurrence in echovirus 6 infection. Hope-Simpson and Higgins[98] noted exanthem in approximately 5 percent of patients with rhinoviral respiratory illness.

A young adult research worker had an influenza-like illness and a hand, foot, and mouth syndrome–like rash caused by infection with a calicivirus (San Miguel sea lion virus serotype 5) of oceanic origin.[183]

Two percent of patients with Colorado tick fever encephalitis have exanthem.[51] Although infection with reoviruses occurs commonly, exanthem has been noted on only nine occasions.[51,121] A morbilliform rash has been observed in one adult with a rotavirus infection, and a 4-year-old boy was noted to have a petechial rash in association with a rotaviral illness.[60,167] Di Lernia and Ricci[63] described three cases of Gianotti-Crosti syndrome and one child with infantile acute hemorrhagic edema associated with rotavirus infections.

Of the *Togaviridae* family of viruses, rubella virus is the most important as a worldwide cause of exanthematous disease. Several alphaviruses also frequently cause exanthems.[108,141,208,209] Each of these viruses has a marked geographic distribution. Similarly, flaviviruses also have exanthem as part of their clinical expression, and they too have specific geographic boundaries.[208,209] In the New York City area outbreak of West Nile virus infection in 1999, 19 percent of patients had exanthem.[138] The rash was erythematous macular, papular, or morbilliform.

Exanthem generally is not considered to be a manifestation of influenza virus infection, but Hope-Simpson and Higgins[98] noted exanthem in approximately 8 percent of patients from whom influenza B virus was isolated and in 1 or 2 percent of those infected with influenza A virus. Measles virus is the most notable of the *Paramyxoviridae* family with an associated exanthem. However, exanthem occurs rather frequently in young children infected with parainfluenza virus types 1, 2, and 3 and also in those with respiratory syncytial virus (RSV) illnesses.[81,93,94,199,202] Hope-Simpson and Higgins[98] noted a 15 percent incidence of rash in RSV infection and an approximately 15 percent incidence in parainfluenza virus infection. Rash, which was not described further, was observed in four children with respiratory illnesses caused by human metapneumovirus infections.[158] Exanthem also has been noted on rare occasion with mumps virus infection.[49]

Lassa fever virus, Marburg virus, Ebola virus, and hepatitis B virus all have been associated with exanthem on occasion.[42,46,62,75,152,208] Hepatitis B virus is the main cause of papular acrodermatitis (Gianotti-Crosti syndrome) in children.[46,171,175] Chronic hepatitis C virus infection occasionally causes systemic vasculitis and cryoglobulinemia in adults, with purpuric lesions concentrated on the lower extremities.[2,97] Other cutaneous manifestations of chronic hepatitis C virus infection include urticaria, erythema nodosum, lichen planus, and nodular prurigo.[106,216]

Hantaviruses cause two major syndromes throughout the world: hemorrhagic fever with renal syndrome and hantavirus pulmonary syndrome.[4,39,150,174] Exanthem (facial flushing and petechial lesions in skin folds) occurs in approximately 30 percent of patients with hemorrhagic fever with renal syndrome, but rash is not reported in the hantavirus pulmonary syndrome. A macular rash has been noted in association with acute infection with human immunodeficiency virus type 1 (HIV-1).[137,139,140,189] Several reports have associated human T-lymphotropic virus type 1 (HTLV-1) with an atypical form of eczema called infective dermatitis. This exanthem has an acute onset and is somewhat recalcitrant to treatment.[116,117,126]

Chlamydiae, rickettsiae, and mycoplasmas associated with cutaneous manifestations are listed in Table 64–2. Of the chlamydiae, only *Chlamydia psittaci* has been associated with exanthem. In contrast, all rickettsiae that infect humans, with the exception of *Coxiella burnetii*, usually display some cutaneous manifestations as part of their systemic disease.[31,69,84,115,122,143,147,173] Approximately 4 to 7 percent of adults with Q fever have exanthem.[40,187] Of the mycoplasmas that infect humans, only *Mycoplasma pneumoniae* is associated with exanthem.[13,51,53] In epidemics, exanthem occurs in approximately 15 percent of persons with respiratory illness.

In Table 64–3, bacterial agents for which cutaneous manifestations are part of the clinical illness are presented (see Chapter 66). The clinical expression of exanthem varies tremendously among the different etiologic agents, as do the conditions associated with a specific infection. For example, infection with phage group 2 staphylococci usually results in cutaneous disease in young infants, whereas the same organisms rarely cause illness in adults. Symptomatic infection with *Streptococcus pneumoniae* is associated with cutaneous manifestations only occasionally; on the other hand, similar systemic disease with *Neisseria meningitidis* virtually always is associated with the characteristic petechial exanthem. Of the other bacterial agents listed in Table 64–3, exanthem is most important in the following: *Neisseria gonorrhoeae*, *Salmonella typhi*, *Streptobacillus moniliformis*, *Spirillum minus*, *Pseudomonas aeruginosa*, and *Treponema pallidum*.

Fungal, protozoan, and metazoan agents associated with cutaneous manifestations in humans are listed in Tables 64–4, 64–5, and 64–6, respectively. These agents and their diseases, discussed more completely in other chapters, are included here for completeness of the differential diagnosis.

EPIDEMIOLOGY

Tables 64–1 through 64–6 clearly show that exanthematous disease has many possible etiologic agents; hence, no unified epidemiology exists. Epidemiologic events related to specific agents are considered in the appropriate sections throughout this text. Each agent with exanthem as a clinical manifestation has a unique epidemiologic pattern that, if understood, distinguishes it from many of the other agents that cause otherwise identical clinical illnesses. In the evaluation of all patients with rash, exposure, season, and incubation period are important aspects of the diagnostic process.

PATHOPHYSIOLOGY AND PATHOLOGY OF EXANTHEMS

Even though the skin can respond in only a limited number of ways, what is obvious from the extensive number of etiologic agents is that multiple pathogenic mechanisms must occur. In many sections of this book, the pathology and pathophysiology of specific agents are presented in detail. An overview is presented here.

Small vessel vasculitis (leukocytoclastic vasculitis) is a leading event in most exanthematous illnesses caused by infectious agents.[186] The cutaneous manifestations of systemic diseases can be separated into three broad categories. The first category involves dissemination of infectious agents by blood (viremia, bacteremia, and so on), which results in secondary infection at the cutaneous site. The clinical cutaneous findings in this type of infection can be the direct result of infectious agents in the epidermis, dermis, or dermal capillary endothelium or can be the result of an immune response between the organism and antibody or cellular factors in the cutaneous location. The possible events in the skin with this type of infection are presented in Table 64–7. Chickenpox, many enteroviral infections, and meningococcemia are examples of diseases in which infectious agents have reached the skin through the blood and are causing the cutaneous findings without the additional contribution of host immune factors. In illnesses such as measles, rubella, and gonococcemia, the timing, histologic picture, and difficulty of direct recovery of the agent by culture suggest both a direct effect and an immune-mediated response.

The second category of pathogenesis relates to the dissemination of known specific toxins of infectious agents. The infection is in a localized area of the body, but the toxin liberated by the infectious agents reaches the skin by blood-borne dissemination. Three examples of toxin-mediated exanthematous disease are streptococcal scarlet fever, staphylococcal scalded skin syndrome, and toxic shock syndrome.

The third category of pathogenesis in systemic disease with exanthem is poorly understood but appears to have an immunologic basis. Most important in this category are the clinical pictures of erythema multiforme, erythema multiforme exudativum (Stevens-Johnson syndrome), and erythema nodosum. In erythema multiforme associated with *M. pneumoniae* and HSV infection, the respective organisms have been isolated or identified at the skin site. In most instances, however, neither antigen localization nor disseminated toxin has been identified.

Important clinical aspects of exanthematous diseases are the distribution and progression of the lesions, yet little is known of the cause of these aspects. Differences in skin thickness, vascularity, proliferation rate, temperature, and metabolic activity are important in animal diseases with cutaneous manifestations.[51,75,124,134,154] In humans, similar factors must be important but obviously affect the various etiologic agents differently (e.g., the more central exanthem of chickenpox versus that of the hand, foot, and mouth syndrome of coxsackievirus A16 infection).

Text continued on p. 770

TABLE 64-2   Clinical Characteristics of Chlamydial, Rickettsial, and Mycoplasmal Infections with Cutaneous Manifestations

Agent	Disease or Syndrome	Incubation Period (days)	Main Season	Clinical Characteristics	Exanthem		Usual Duration (days)
					Lesions	Distribution	
Chlamydia psittaci	Psittacosis	7-14	Nonseasonal	Fever, chills, headache, and cough; Respiratory distress	Erythematous macules; Occasionally erythema multiforme or erythema nodosum	Mainly on trunk	2-7
Rickettsia akari	Rickettsialpox	7-14	Nonseasonal	Fever, chills, headache, backache, and malaise 4-7 days after onset of primary lesion at site of mite bite; Geographically localized disease	Initial lesion at site of mite bite is papular and then vesicular, and finally an eschar forms; Two days after onset of fever, erythematous maculopapular discrete rash occurs; Lesions progress to small vesicles and later to scabs	Most prominent on trunk and proximal end of extremities	7-10
Rickettsia typhi	Endemic, murine typhus	7-14	Nonseasonal	Fever and headache; Rash appears on 4th-7th day; Geographically localized disease	Initially discrete macules and then erythematous maculopapular; May become purpuric	Initially upper part of trunk and axilla; Progresses to entire body except face, palms, and soles	7-21
Rickettsia prowazekii	Epidemic typhus	10-14	Nonseasonal	Sudden onset of fever, chills, headache, and myalgias; Rash appears on 4th-7th day; Geographically localized disease	Initially discrete macules and then progresses to maculopapular and petechial lesions; Sometimes purpuric	Appears first on trunk and spreads to extremities; Spares palms and soles	7-14
Rickettsia tsutsugamushi	Scrub typhus	7-21	Nonseasonal	Sudden onset of chills, fever, and headache	Local lesion at site of chigger bite is present at onset of symptoms; characterized by vesicle, ulcer, and eschar; Maculopapular rash occurs 5-8 days after onset of fever	Maculopapular rash first occurs on trunk and then becomes generalized	7-14
Rickettsia rickettsii	Rocky Mountain spotted fever	3-12	Summer	Abrupt onset of fever, chills, and headache; Rash appears 2-4 days after onset	Early maculopapular, then petechial, and sometimes purpuric	Rash starts on distal end of extremities; Rarely involves the trunk	7-14
Other tick-borne rickettsiae R. sibirica (North Asian tick-borne rickettsiosis) R. australis (Queensland tick typhus) R. conorii (Boutonneuse fever) R. africae (African tick fever)			Tick seasons	Similar to mild Rocky Mountain spotted fever	Similar to Rocky Mountain spotted fever; eschar at site of tick bite	Similar to Rocky Mountain spotted fever	7-14
Coxiella burnetii	Q fever	20-40	Nonseasonal	Acute febrile illness with chills, headache, and myalgia	Fine discrete macular rash occurring during febrile illness; Transient urticarial rash also noted	Mainly on trunk	2-7
Ehrlichia species	Ehrlichiosis	14-28	Tick seasons	Similar to Rocky Mountain spotted fever, but rash usually not on palms and soles	Similar to endemic typhus	Similar to endemic typhus	7-14
Mycoplasma pneumoniae		21	All seasons	Gradual onset of fever, malaise, headache, and cough	Maculopapular rash occurs in 5-15% of cases; Vesicular and bullous lesions common (Stevens-Johnson syndrome); more common in males; Papular, petechial, and urticarial lesions also noted; Erythema multiforme common	Rash most prominent on trunk and proximal end of extremities	7-14

Data from references 13, 14, 18, 31, 35, 40, 51, 53, 69, 84, 92, 115, 122, 129, 136, 143, 147, 160, 173, 187, 210, 215.

TABLE 64–3   Bacteria Associated with Cutaneous Manifestations

Agent	Disease or Syndrome	Clinical Characteristics	Exanthem	
			Lesions	Distribution
Gram-positive cocci				
Staphylococcus aureus, exfoliative toxin-producing, mainly phage group 2 (see Figs. 64–17 and 64–18)	Bullous impetigo	Usually occurs in neonates May be epidemic	Rapid progression from vesicles to bullous lesions	Most common in diaper area
	Scalded skin syndrome Toxic epidermal necrolysis (Ritter disease in infants <4 months; Lyell syndrome in older children)	Usually occurs in infants and children 1 month–5 years of age Mucopurulent nasal and eye discharge Fever	Scarlatiniform eruption with exfoliation Nikolsky sign present Crusty appearance around eyes and under nose	Generalized Most marked on trunk
	Staphylococcal scarlet fever or staphylococcal scarlatiniform eruption	Fever and staphylococcal infection in throat, but no evidence of pharyngitis	Scarlet fever–like rash with desquamation Pastia lines present	Generalized
Staphylococcus aureus, non–exfoliative toxin-producing	Septicemic disease	Severe septicemia with osteomyelitis, arthritis, endocarditis, or pneumonia	Diffuse, erythematous, confluent, and macular rash (flush) With endocarditis, may have petechiae and splinter hemorrhages, Osler nodes, Janeway spots	Trunk and proximal end of extremities
Staphylococcus aureus, toxin-l (TSST-1)–producing	Toxic shock syndrome	Fever, intense myalgias, vomiting, and diarrhea Mental confusion and hypotension	Erythematous, deep red (sunburn-like) rash Desquamation occurs	Generalized
Staphylococcus aureus, non–exfoliative toxin-producing	Folliculitis, furuncles, or carbuncles	See primary skin infections, Chapter 66		
Streptococcus pyogenes	Scarlet fever	Fever, pharyngitis, and cervical lymphadenitis Rash onset within 2 days of first symptoms Incubation period 3-4 days	Diffuse erythematous and fine maculopapular (looks and feels like red sandpaper) Rash darker in skin folds (Pastia lines) Desquamation occurs	Circumoral pallor Generalized rash, with trunk and proximal end of extremities being most involved
	Erysipelas	Fever, headache, and vomiting Localized infection	Circumscribed area that is raised and erythematous Advancing edge is irregular	Anywhere
	Impetigo	Localized superficial pyoderma See primary skin infections, Chapter 66	Discrete and coalescent lesions of a vesicular nature Quickly becomes more pustular and then crusts over with a yellowish brown appearance	Forearms, legs, and face
	Septicemia	Fever and systemic foci of infection	Petechiae	Diffuse
	Miscellaneous skin manifestations of *S. pyogenes* infections		Erythema multiforme, erythema nodosum, and erythema marginatum	
Streptococcus pneumoniae	Septicemia	Fever	Petechiae	Diffuse
Enterococcal and viridans group streptococci	Endocarditis	Endocarditis	Petechiae, splinter hemorrhages, Osler nodes, and Janeway spots	
Gram-negative cocci				
Neisseria gonorrhoeae	Gonococcemia	Fever and polyarthralgias	Papular, petechial purpuric, pustular, or necrotic lesions	Most common on extremities Extensor surfaces over joints
Neisseria meningitidis	Meningococcemia	Fever and pharyngitis Sudden onset of rash	Characteristic rash is petechial or purpuric Early lesions may be erythematous maculopapular, or urticarial	Generalized
Moraxella catarrhalis	Bacteremia	Fever and pharyngitis	Maculopapular and petechial	Generalized

TABLE 64–3   Bacteria Associated with Cutaneous Manifestations—cont'd

Agent	Disease or Syndrome	Clinical Characteristics	Exanthem Lesions	Exanthem Distribution
Gram-positive bacilli				
Bacillus anthracis	Anthrax	Fever, headache, malaise, and joint pain	Initially, macular, pruritic lesion; Later, a papule forms and then vesiculation; Vesicles last 2-6 days, and then eschar forms	Usually, single lesion initially at point of exposure, secondary lesions in area develop later
Listeria monocytogenes	Listeriosis	Neonatal meningitis with hepatosplenomegaly	Maculopapular, discrete lesions; Pustules	Trunk and legs
Erysipelothrix rhusiopathiae	Crab or fishnet dermatitis	Fever and local pain	Erysipeloid lesion (violet or red)	Hands
Corynebacterium diphtheriae	Cutaneous diphtheria	Secondary infection in cutaneous wounds	Impetigo or ecthyma-like; Rarely, erythema multiforme	Exposed surfaces
Arcanobacterium hemolyticum	Scarlet fever–like illness	Fever and pharyngitis	Scarlet fever–like rash; Occasionally, rubelliform	Generalized rash with peripheral predominance
Enteric gram-negative bacilli				
Salmonella typhi	Typhoid fever	Malaise, headache, and marked fever; Rash onset 10 days after onset of fever	Rose spots, 2- to 4-mm macular lesions	Discrete lesions on abdomen
Other *Salmonella* species	Septicemic salmonellosis	Similar to mild typhoid fever	Similar to typhoid fever	Similar to typhoid fever
Shigella sonnei	Shigellosis	Diarrhea	Urticaria	Diffuse
Campylobacter species	Gastroenteritis		Skin pustules and erythema nodosum	Lower part of legs
Other gram-negative bacilli				
Francisella tularensis	Tularemia	Chills, fever, headache, and localized lymphadenopathy	Initial papule that later ulcerates	Site of inoculation
Haemophilus ducreyi	Chancroid	Local pain and tenderness	Pustular lesions that ulcerate	External genitalia
Haemophilus influenzae	Septicemia	Fever	Petechiae; Reddish purple cellulitis	Diffuse; Cellulitis mainly on cheeks and extremities
Streptobacillus moniliformis	Rat-bite fever	Fever, chills, malaise, headache, and polyarthritis	Erythematous, maculopapular rash that may become petechial	Most prominent on extremities, including palms and soles
Yersinia pestis	Septicemic plague	Sudden onset of fever	Initial generalized erythema followed by petechiae and purpura	Generalized
Yersinia pseudotuberculosis		Mesenteric lymphadenitis	Erythema nodosum and scarlatiniform eruption	Lower part of legs and generalized
Yersinia enterocolitica	Yersiniosis	Enterocolitis	Erythema nodosum and urticaria	Lower part of legs and generalized
Bartonella bacilliformis	Bartonellosis, Carrión disease, or Oroya fever	Initially intermittent fever, malaise, and myalgias; 30-60 days after initial fever, exanthem appears	Erythematous maculopapular; Later recurrent nodules	Face and extensor surface of extremities
Bartonella quintana	Trench fever	Usually mild fever, headache, chills, and tibial bone pain	Macular rash	Mainly on trunk
Calymmatobacterium granulomatis	Granuloma inguinale	See *Calymmatobacterium granulomatis*, Chapter 141	Nodular, ulcerovegetative, hypertrophic, or cicatricial lesions	Genitals
Pseudomonas aeruginosa	Ecthyma gangrenosa	Septicemia (usually in immunocompromised patients)	Initially vesicular and then hemorrhagic; Become ulcerated with central black necrotic eschar	Anywhere
	Pseudomonas folliculitis (health spa dermatitis)	Headache, malaise, and fatigue	Papular and pustular	Generalized
Burkholderia mallei	Glanders, melioidosis	Fever, malaise, chills, arthralgia, and muscle pains	Nodule or ulcer at site of inoculation and then widespread papules, bullae, and pustules	Generalized
Brucella species	Brucellosis	Acute or subacute febrile illness; Exanthem in 8% of cases	Erythematous and maculopapular; Occasionally vesicles	Generalized
Legionella pneumophila	Legionnaires' disease	Severe pneumonia	Maculopapular	Anterior of trunk

TABLE 64–3   Bacteria Associated with Cutaneous Manifestations—cont'd

Agent	Disease or Syndrome	Clinical Characteristics	Exanthem Lesions	Exanthem Distribution
Bartonella henselae	Cat-scratch fever	Subacute regional lymphadenitis	Erythematous maculopapular, morbilliform, petechial, erythema nodosum, erythema multiforme, and erythema marginatum May be pruritic	Generalized
Acid-fast bacilli				
Mycobacterium tuberculosis	Lupus vulgaris	Usually associated with other manifestations of tuberculosis	Reddish brown nodular or scaling lesions	Mainly on face and neck
	Papulonecrotic tuberculids	Associated with disseminated tuberculosis	Initially vesicular Become pustules, umbilical, and ulcerated and then form scabs and leave scars	Single or multiple lesions anywhere
Atypical mycobacteria			Granulomatous and ulcerative lesions at site of superficial injury	Usually on hands
Mycobacterium leprae	Erythema nodosum leprosum	General findings of lepromatous leprosy	Erythematous nodular lesions	Disseminated Most prominent on face and extremities
Spirochetes				
Treponema pallidum	Primary syphilis Secondary syphilis	Chancre	Large ulcers with indurated edges Erythematous maculopapules that frequently are scaly (psoriasiform)	Genitals Generalized, including palms and soles
Treponema pertenue	Yaws		Papular lesions at sites of inoculations Lesions ulcerate, leaving a wart-like appearance	Anywhere
Borrelia burgdorferi	Lyme disease (erythema chronicum migrans)	Skin, cardiac, neurologic, and joint abnormalities	Expanding erythematous, annular lesions	Thighs, buttocks, or axillae
Treponema carateum	Pinta		Initially, erythematous, papular lesions; increase in size during 1-month period and become scaly	Exposed surfaces of body
Spirillum minus	Rat-bite fever	Fever and chills	Discrete, macular rash	Trunk and extremities, including palms and soles
Leptospira species	Leptospirosis	Fever, conjunctivitis, and anorexia Rash rarely noted	Erythematous maculopapular rash	Mainly on trunk
Borrelia species	Relapsing fever	Relapsing fever, headache, myalgia, and photophobia	Morbilliform and petechial Erythema multiforme	Generalized

Data from references 5, 17, 21, 24, 29, 30, 32-34, 37, 38, 41, 54, 59, 64, 67, 69, 71, 74, 86, 88, 90, 99, 100, 101, 103, 105, 112, 113, 118, 119, 123, 125, 128, 132, 142, 145, 149, 151, 153, 155, 156, 161, 162, 168, 172, 177, 188, 190-192, 194-196, 201, 204, 206, 211, 213, 214, 218.

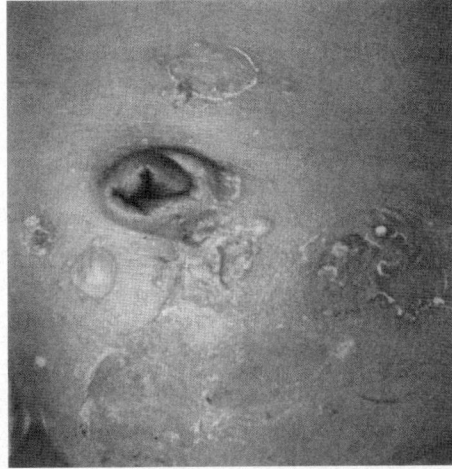

Figure 64–17 Bullous impetigo in a newborn infant caused by exfoliative toxin–producing *Staphylococcus aureus*. (See companion Expert Consult web site for color version.)

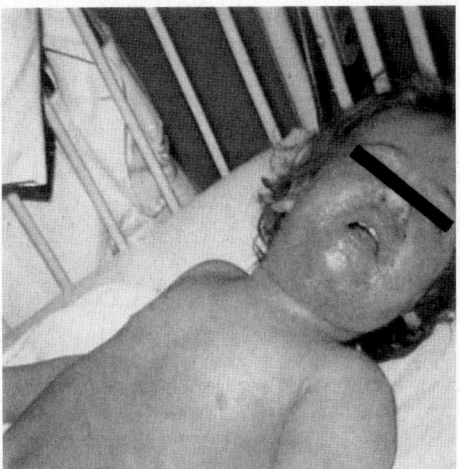

Figure 64–18 Scalded skin syndrome caused by exfoliative toxin–producing *Staphylococcus aureus*. (See companion Expert Consult web site for color version.)

TABLE 64–4 Fungi Associated with Cutaneous Manifestations

Agent	Disease or Syndrome	Clinical Characteristics	Exanthem Lesions	Distribution
Dermatophytic fungi	Tinea capitis, tinea cruris, tinea pedis, or tinea circinata		Localized, brownish, maculopapular lesions that are scaly Erythema nodosum	
Candida albicans	Congenital cutaneous candidiasis	Congenital infection	Discrete vesicular lesions	Generalized
	Chronic mucocutaneous candidiasis	Immunodeficiency disease	Confluent, erythematous, and exudative lesions	Generalized, including scalp
	Acquired candidiasis		Confluent, fiery red lesions	Most common in diaper area
Candida spp.	Systemic candidiasis	Severe opportunistic infection	Erythematous nodular lesions	Generalized
Histoplasma capsulatum	Histoplasmosis	Primary respiratory infection	Erythema nodosum, erythema multiforme, and erythematous maculopapular	
Cryptococcus neoformans	Cryptococcosis	Primary respiratory infection	Erythema nodosum and acneiform eruptions	
Coccidioides immitis	Coccidioidomycosis	Primary respiratory infection	Initially, erythematous, maculopapular rash Later, erythema multiforme and erythema nodosum	Generalized maculopapular rash
Sporotrichum schenckii	Sporotrichosis	Cutaneous inoculation	Nodular lesions that ulcerate	Usually, hands, arms, and legs
Blastomyces dermatitidis	Blastomycosis	Primary respiratory infection	Nodular lesions that ulcerate Erythema nodosum	
Scedosporium spp.	No specific syndrome	Severe opportunistic infection	Nodular or necrotic skin lesions	Generalized
Fusarium spp.	No specific syndrome	Severe opportunistic infection	Nodular skin lesions, abscesses	Generalized
Aspergillus spp.	No specific syndrome	Severe opportunistic infection	Nodular and purpuric lesions	Generalized

Data from references 14, 15, 23, 27, 43, 69, 73, 80, 82, 127, 131, 163, 182, 203, 212.

TABLE 64–5 Cutaneous Manifestations of Protozoan and Helminthic Infections

Agent	Disease or Syndrome	Cutaneous Manifestations
Plasmodium spp.	Malaria	Occasionally generalized urticaria in chronic infection
Toxoplasma gondii	Acquired toxoplasmosis	Occasionally generalized erythematous, maculopapular rash
	Congenital toxoplasmosis	Generalized petechial rash
Giardia lamblia	Giardiasis	Rarely urticaria
Entamoeba histolytica	Amebiasis	Rarely urticaria
Leishmania tropica	Oriental sore	Red nodular lesion that ulcerates; lasts 2-3 months
Leishmania braziliensis and *mexicana*	American cutaneous leishmaniasis	Erythematous papular lesion that vesiculates and ulcerates
Trypanosoma gambiense	African trypanosomiasis	Red nodular lesion at site of bite, followed by generalized, pruritic, erythema multiforme–like rash
Trypanosoma cruzi	American trypanosomiasis or Chagas disease	Nodular lesion at site of bite; generalized recurrent erythematous, maculopapular rash
Trichomonas vaginalis	Vulvovaginalis	Rarely urticaria and erythema multiforme
Ascaris lumbricoides	Roundworm infestation	Erythema nodosum
Enterobius vermicularis	Pinworm infestation	Rarely urticaria
Necator americanus	Hookworm disease	Papules and papulovesicles on exposed surfaces (feet); generalized urticaria
Trichinella spiralis	Trichinosis	Urticaria common; also, generalized maculopapular rash may occur; petechiae frequently develop
Strongyloides stercoralis	Strongyloidiasis; also, creeping eruption (cutaneous larva migrans)	Erythematous, maculopapular lesions on feet; creeping eruption
Ancylostoma braziliense	Creeping eruption (cutaneous larva migrans)	Creeping eruption
Dermatobia hominis	Cutaneous myiasis	Creeping eruption, subacute draining lesions
Schistosoma haematobium, mansoni, and *japonicum*	Schistosomiasis	Pruritic papular eruption where exposed; generalized urticaria and granulomatous lesions
Trichobilharzia ocellata, physellae, and *stagnicolae*	Swimmer's itch or collector's itch	Initial erythema and urticaria followed by papules and vesiculation; pruritic
Wuchereria bancrofti	Filariasis	Localized erythema urticaria and erythema nodosum
Onchocerca volvulus	Onchocerciasis	Chronic, papular, scaly rash
Echinococcus granulosus and *multilocularis*	Echinococcosis	Frequent urticaria

Data from references 14, 20, 43, 56, 69, 72, 83, 89, 133.

TABLE 64-6   Cutaneous Manifestations of Arthropod Bites and Stings

Agent	Disease or Syndrome	Cutaneous Manifestations
Spiders		
Loxosceles rectus	Recluse spider bite or brown spider bite	Erythema followed by blister and necrosis
Ticks	Tick bite	Initial pruritus at site; becomes ulcerated and granulomatous
Mites		
Sarcoptes scabiei	Scabies	Pruritic burrows in body creases and generalized; become erythematous and then papular urticaria
Trombicula irritans	Chigger bite	Marked pruritus and then papular urticaria
Other mites: food, grain, murine, and fowl		Marked pruritus and then papular urticaria
Lice		
Pediculus humanus	Body lice or pediculosis	Erythematous, maculopapular, pruritic lesions; sometimes urticaria
Phthirus pubis	Crabs	Pruritus and erythema under pubic hair
Bedbugs and kissing bugs		
Cimex lectularius	Bedbug bite	Pruritic papular urticaria
Triatoma sanguisuga	Kissing bug bite	Papular urticaria; occasionally hemorrhagic nodular lesions
Gypsy moth caterpillar		
Lymantria dispar	Gypsy moth rash	Pruritic blotchy erythema and maculopapular
Moths		
Hylesia alinda	Moth-associated dermatitis	Erythema and pruritus; feeling of warmth in area of rash; may have vesicular lesions
Ants		
Solenopsis saevissima	Fire ant bite	Painful papular urticarial lesions that become pustular and then nodular
Fleas		
Pulex irritans (human flea) and fleas of many animals	Flea bite	Papular urticaria
Flies and mosquitoes	Fly and mosquito bite	Papular, nodular, and urticarial lesions in sensitive persons

Data from references 45, 47, 61, 69, 96, 148, 165, 176, 181.

TABLE 64-7   Aspects of Pathogenesis in Exanthems Associated with Blood-borne Dissemination of the Infectious Agent

Anatomic Location	Spread of Agent		Histology	Clinical Expressions	Pathophysiology
Blood	Free in plasma	Associated with leukocytes			
	→ Infection ←		Damage to vessel, endothelial swelling, perivascular edema, cellular infiltration, hemorrhage	Macule, papule, petechia	Direct effect of agent or immune reaction with pathologic consequences
Dermal capillary endothelium					
	To dermis through breaks in basement membrane (secondary to trauma)	To dermis by diapedesis			
		Contiguous spread			
Dermis	Infection		Edema, cellular infiltration, hemorrhage, microscopic visualization of organism	Papule, urticaria, purpura, vesicle	Direct effect of agent or immune reaction with pathologic consequences; histamine release
	Contiguous spread				
Epidermis	Infection		Cytopathic effects (inclusions, ballooning, vacuolation, necrosis, nuclear disruption), microscopic visualization of organism	Papule, vesicle, ulcer	Direct effect of agent

Modified from Cherry, J. D.: Newer viral exanthems. Adv. Pediatr. 16:233-286, 1969.

CLINICAL MANIFESTATIONS

The clinical findings in exanthematous diseases resulting from systemic infections are varied and depend on the inciting pathogens. By examination of skin alone, differentiating an exanthematous disease resulting from systemic infection (e.g., coxsackievirus A9, rubella virus infection) from primary cutaneous diseases of infectious and noninfectious origin (insect bites, acne, and contact with poison ivy) frequently is difficult. In Tables 64–1 through 64–6, the clinical characteristics of viral, chlamydial, rickettsial, bacterial, fungal, parasitic, and arthropod-induced illnesses with primary or secondary cutaneous manifestations are presented. In Tables 64–8 through 64–17, etiologic agents and clinical manifestations are presented on the basis of the more pronounced cutaneous manifestations or syndrome associations. The clinician must keep in mind that other aspects of an illness (e.g., exposure, season, incubation period, geographic location, patient age, associated signs and symptoms) may be more important in determining the underlying etiologic agent. Clinical manifestations of specific exanthematous diseases are presented in greater detail in other chapters of this book.

ERYTHEMATOUS MACULAR EXANTHEMS

When all infectious diseases with exanthems are taken into consideration, the occurrence of illnesses in which the lesions are just macular is rare. However, many important, severe diseases have a transitory erythematous macular rash early in their course, and recognition of this fact can be lifesaving. Infectious agents associated with illnesses in which macular exanthems have been observed are presented in Table 64–8.

The most common rash in infectious mononucleosis is erythematous and maculopapular, but rarely (most often in association with the administration of ampicillin) the exanthem is generalized, confluent, fiery red, and macular. Blotchy or diffuse

TABLE 64–8   Infectious Agents Associated with Illness in Which a Macular Exanthem Has Been Observed

Infectious Agent	Illness
Human herpesvirus–6, –7	Roseola infantum
Epstein-Barr virus	Infectious mononucleosis
Coxsackieviruses Bl, B2, B5	—
Echoviruses 2, 4, 5, 14, 17-19, 30	—
Enterovirus 71	—
Dengue virus	Dengue fever
Lassa virus	Lassa fever
Marburg virus	Marburg fever
Parvovirus	Erythema infectiosum
HIV-1	Manifestation of acute infection
Hantavirus	Hemorrhagic fever with renal syndrome
Chlamydia psittaci	Psittacosis
Rickettsia typhi	Murine typhus
Rickettsia prowazekii	Epidemic typhus
Rickettsia quintana	Trench fever
Coxiella burnetii	Q fever
Mycoplasma pneumoniae	—
Staphylococcus aureus	Septicemia and toxic shock syndrome
Streptococcus pyogenes	Scarlatina and septicemia
Bacillus anthracis	Anthrax
Salmonella typhi	Typhoid fever
Salmonella species	Septicemic salmonellosis
Spirillum minus	Rat-bite fever
Leptospira species	Leptospirosis
Yersinia pestis	Plague

erythematous macular rashes have been caused specifically by 12 different enterovirus types. Most of these descriptions involve neonates, other very young infants, and adults; children in the peak ages for enteroviral exanthematous diseases do not seem to have solely macular lesions. In neonates, enteroviral disease with a blotchy macular rash in association with fever and lethargy usually is confused with bacterial sepsis.

Patients with dengue, Lassa, and Marburg viral infections frequently have a macular, flushed appearance before other cutaneous manifestations develop. Similarly, in both murine and epidemic typhus, the initial skin manifestations are macular but progress rapidly to more pronounced findings.

Bacterial septicemia with both common and exotic organisms is associated frequently with a generalized flush. In staphylococcal disease, the rash is particularly apparent in endocarditis and osteomyelitis. The most famous disease with a macular rash is typhoid fever. Rose spots occur most commonly on the abdomen, but they also are seen on the chest and back. They are erythematous, macular lesions 2 to 4 mm in size. Lesions likewise have been noted in leptospirosis and psittacosis. In addition, rose spots are seen occasionally in septicemic illnesses caused by other *Salmonella* spp.

The slapped-cheek appearance in erythema infectiosum (Fig. 64–6) is caused by an erythematous macular flush of the cheeks. The full-blown rash in streptococcal scarlet fever is maculopapular, but frequently in mild cases and in those altered by antibiotic therapy, the exanthem is only macular in character (scarlatina).

ERYTHEMATOUS MACULOPAPULAR EXANTHEMS

An erythematous maculopapular rash is the most common cutaneous manifestation of systemic infection (Figs. 64–2, 64–8, 64–10, and 64–13). It also is an exceedingly common occurrence in allergic conditions. However, all too frequently, the rash of an infectious illness is ascribed to an allergic reaction to an administered drug rather than correctly to the disease process. The converse—an allergic rash illness that is attributed mistakenly to an infectious agent—rarely occurs. Infectious agents associated with illnesses in which maculopapular exanthems occur are presented in Table 64–9.

Both by the number of possible etiologic agents and by total infections, viruses account for the vast majority of illnesses with maculopapular eruptions. Although the distribution and progression of rashes are important aspects relating to the differential diagnosis, the single most important point is whether the lesions are discrete (rubelliform) or confluent (morbilliform). Adenoviruses are not uncommon causes of erythematous maculopapular eruptions. In most instances, signs and symptoms of upper respiratory infection are present. Most commonly, the lesions are discrete, but occasionally, a confluent morbilliform rash is present. A roseola infantum picture—occurrence of rash after the fever falls by crisis—frequently occurs. As a rule, the exanthem in adenoviral infections starts on the head and spreads to the trunk and extremities.

Enteroviruses account for the greatest number of erythematous maculopapular rash illnesses; 36 different serologic types have been implicated. The enteroviral types most commonly associated with maculopapular exanthems are coxsackieviruses A9 and B5 and echoviruses 4, 9, and 16. Echovirus 9 has been the most frequent cause of enteroviral exanthem for the last 35 years (Fig. 64–13). Although morbilliform rashes do occur, the more usual cutaneous manifestation is one suggestive of rubella. The exanthem usually starts on the head and upper part of the trunk and spreads to the extremities.

Although they are not common manifestations of respiratory viruses (rhinoviruses, influenza A and B viruses, RSV, and para-

TABLE 64–9   Infectious Agents Associated with Illnesses in Which Maculopapular Exanthems Occur

Infectious Agent	Illness	Character of Rash	
		Discrete	**Confluent**
Parvovirus	Erythema infectiosum	+++	+
Human bocavirus		++++	
Adenoviruses 1, 2, 3, 4, 7, 7a		+++	+
Human herpesvirus–6	Roseola infantum	+++	+
Epstein-Barr virus	Infectious mononucleosis	+++	+
Cytomegalovirus		++++	
Vaccinia virus	Roseola vaccinatum	+++	+
Coxsackieviruses A2, A4, A5, A7, A9, A10, A16		+++	+
Coxsackieviruses B1-B5		+++	+
Echoviruses 1-7, 9, 11, 13, 14, 16-19, 22, 25, 30, 33		+++	+
Enterovirus 71		++++	
Rhinoviruses (many types)		++++	
Colorado tick fever virus	Colorado tick fever	++++	
Reoviruses 2, 3		++	++
Rotavirus	Gianotti-Crosti syndrome; infantile acute hemorrhagic edema	++++	
Alphaviruses: chikungunya, Sindbis, o'nyong-nyong fever, Ross River		++	++
Rubella virus	Rubella (German measles)	+++	+
Flavivirus: dengue, Kunjin, West Nile	Dengue, Kunjin fever	++	++
Influenza viruses A, B		++++	
Respiratory syncytial virus		++++	
Parainfluenza viruses 1-4		++++	
Mumps virus	Mumps	++++	
Measles virus	Measles	+	+++
Hepatitis B virus		++++	
Marburg virus	Marburg fever	++	++
Ebola virus	Ebola hemorrhagic fever	+++	+
Rickettsia akari	Rickettsialpox	++++	
Rickettsia typhi	Murine typhus	+++	+
Rickettsia prowazekii	Epidemic typhus	+++	+
Rickettsia tsutsugamushi	Scrub typhus	+++	+
Rickettsia rickettsi	Rocky Mountain spotted fever		++++
Ehrlichia species	Ehrlichiosis	+++	+
Mycoplasma pneumoniae		+++	+
Staphylococcus aureus (exfoliative toxin producing)	Staphylococcal scarlet fever		++++
Streptococcus pyogenes	Scarlet fever		++++
Arcanobacterium hemolyticum		++	++
Neisseria meningitidis	Meningococcemia	++++	
Moraxella catarrhalis		++++	
Listeria monocytogenes	Listeriosis	++++	
Streptobacillus moniliformis	Rat-bite fever	+++	+
Yersinia pseudotuberculosis			++++
Bartonella bacilliformis	Bartonellosis	++++	
Brucella species	Brucellosis	++++	
Legionella pneumophila	Legionnaires' disease	++++	
Bartonella henselae	Cat-scratch fever	+++	+
Treponema pallidum	Secondary syphilis	+++	+
Leptospira species	Leptospirosis	++++	
Borrelia species	Relapsing fever		++++
Coccidioides immitis	Coccidioidomycosis	+++	+
Toxoplasma gondii	Toxoplasmosis	++++	
Strongyloides stercoralis	Strongyloidiasis	++++	

influenza viruses types 1 through 4), exanthems probably occur more often than is generally realized. Because children infected with these agents frequently are given antibiotics, confusion often occurs between an allergic and an infectious etiology. With all the respiratory viruses, the signs and symptoms of respiratory illness (cough, coryza, croup, bronchiolitis, and so on) are prominent. The exanthems virtually are always discrete and rubelliform in character.

In dengue, the exanthem goes through several stages. Initially, it is macular, then erythematous maculopapular, and finally hemorrhagic. Similarly, the exanthems in the rickettsial diseases go through stages that vary in relation to the specific agent (see Table 64–2). In Rocky Mountain spotted fever, the rash starts on the distal ends of extremities. Although the hallmark of meningococcemia is a petechial or purpuric rash, in the initial stages, the exanthem may be erythematous and maculopapular. In addition, maculopapular eruptions are observed in chronic meningococcemia. The most notable cutaneous lesion in coccidioidomycosis is erythema nodosum, but a rubelliform rash early in infection is not an unusual manifestation.

VESICULAR EXANTHEMS

The three main categories of vesicular exanthems are single or localized lesions, generalized lesions in greatest concentration on

TABLE 64–10 Infectious Agents Associated with Illnesses in Which Vesicular Exanthems Occur

Infectious Agent	Illness
Human parvovirus B19	
Herpes simplex virus types 1 and 2	Cold sores, genital herpes, or neonatal herpes
Varicella-zoster virus	Chickenpox (varicella) or herpes zoster
Vaccinia virus	Disseminated vaccinia or eczema vaccinatum
Variola virus	Smallpox
Monkeypox virus	
Orf virus	Ecthyma contagiosum
Tanapox virus	
Coxsackieviruses A4, A5, A8, A10, A16	
Coxsackieviruses Bl-B3	
Echoviruses 6, 9,11, 17	
Enterovirus 71	
Reovirus 2	
Calicivirus of oceanic origin	
Alphaviruses: chikungunya, o'nyong-nyong fever, Ross River, Sindbis	
Kunjin virus	
Mumps virus	Mumps
Measles virus	Atypical measles
Rickettsia akari	Rickettsialpox
Rickettsia tsutsugamushi	
Mycoplasma pneumoniae	
Streptococcus pyogenes	Impetigo
Pseudomonas aeruginosa	
Brucella species	Brucellosis
Bacillus anthracis	Anthrax
Mycobacterium tuberculosis	Papulonecrotic tuberculids
Candida albicans	Congenital cutaneous candidiasis
Leishmania braziliensis	American cutaneous leishmaniasis
Necator americanus	Hookworm disease

TABLE 64–11 Infectious Agents Associated with Illness in Which Petechial and Purpuric Exanthems Occur

Infectious Agent	Illness
Human parvovirus B19	Glove and socks syndrome
Varicella-zoster virus	Hemorrhagic chickenpox
Cytomegalovirus	Congenital cytomegalovirus infection
Variola virus	Hemorrhagic smallpox
Coxsackieviruses A4, A9	
Coxsackieviruses B2-B4	
Echoviruses 4, 7, 9	
Colorado tick fever virus	Colorado tick fever
Rotavirus	
Alphaviruses: chikungunya, o'nyong-nyong fever, Ross River, Sindbis	
Rubella virus	Rubella (German measles) or congenital rubella
Respiratory syncytial virus	
Measles virus	Hemorrhagic (black measles) or atypical measles
Lassa virus	Lassa fever
Marburg virus	
Hepatitis C virus	Mixed cryoglobulinemia
Hantavirus	Hemorrhagic fever with renal syndrome
Rickettsia typhi	Murine typhus
Rickettsia prowazekii	Epidemic typhus
Rickettsia rickettsii and other tick-borne rickettsiae	Rocky Mountain spotted fever
Ehrlichia species	Ehrlichiosis
Mycoplasma pneumoniae	
Streptococcus pyogenes	Scarlet fever or septicemia
Streptococcus pneumoniae	Pneumococcal septicemia
Enterococcal and viridans group streptococci	Endocarditis
Neisseria gonorrhoeae	Gonococcemia
Neisseria meningitidis	Meningococcemia
Moraxella catarrhalis	
Haemophilus influenzae	*H. influenzae* septicemia
Pseudomonas aeruginosa	Ecthyma gangrenosa
Streptobacillus moniliformis	
Yersinia pestis	Septicemic plague (black death)
Bartonella henselae	Cat-scratch fever
Treponema pallidum	Congenital syphilis
Borrelia species	Relapsing fever
Toxoplasma gondii	Congenital toxoplasmosis
Trichinella spiralis	Trichinosis

the trunk and head, and generalized lesions with the greatest concentration on the extremities (Figs. 64–4, 64–5, and 64–9). Infectious agents associated with illnesses in which vesicular rashes develop are presented in Table 64–10. The exanthem in primary or recurrent HSV infection is localized, as it is in recurrent endogenous varicella-zoster infection (herpes zoster), ecthyma contagiosum, tanapox, scrub typhus, anthrax, and papulonecrotic tuberculids (Fig. 64–5).

The vesicular exanthematous disease that occurs most commonly in children today is chickenpox (Fig. 65–4). It should be a readily recognizable disease, but is all too frequently confused with enteroviral infections or insect bites and allergic conditions. Chickenpox has a long incubation period (16 days) and is associated with mild fever and an exanthem that starts on the head and upper part of the trunk and spreads to the extremities. The rash always is more prominent on the trunk than on the extremities. At any time during the first few days of the rash, lesions in all stages (macules, papules, and vesicles) can be seen. Individual lesions in chickenpox form scabs that persist for approximately 7 days.

In contrast to that of chickenpox, the exanthem in enteroviral infections frequently is peripheral in distribution, and the lesions generally heal without scabs. The incubation period (5 days) is much shorter than that of chickenpox. The hand, foot, and mouth syndrome is a common manifestation of enteroviral vesicular rash illnesses (Figs. 64–9 to 64–11). The most frequent etiologic agent in the hand, foot, and mouth syndrome is coxsackievirus A16, but

the syndrome also has been attributed to coxsackieviruses A5, A9, A10, B1, and B3 and enterovirus 71.

Enteroviral infections with vesicular exanthems in which the hand, foot, and mouth distribution is not present quite frequently are diagnosed erroneously as insect bites or poison ivy.

PETECHIAL AND PURPURIC EXANTHEMS

A large number of infectious agents are associated with petechial and purpuric skin manifestations (Figs. 64–14 and 64–15). They are listed in Table 64–11. Infectious diseases with hemorrhagic rash can be fulminant fatal events or relatively benign illnesses. On a worldwide basis, meningococcemia is perhaps the most important and feared, although it is not the most prevalent of the petechial and purpuric exanthematous diseases. The relatively sudden onset of fever and a petechial rash must be considered and treated as meningococcemia unless another etiology can be established with absolute certainty. The most important of the differential diagnostic problems is exanthem caused by enteroviral infection. Many different entero-virus illnesses have a sudden onset with accompanying fever and petechial rash. In addition, the situation frequently is complicated further by the occurrence of meningitis. The most important enterovirus in its ability to mimic meningococcemia is echovirus 9.

Purpuric and petechial lesions in infectious illnesses can result from a direct or indirect (immunologic) effect of the infectious agent at the cutaneous site or from the occurrence of thrombocytopenia. Thrombocytopenia is noted most commonly in acquired rubella virus infections.

URTICARIAL EXANTHEMS

The occurrence of urticaria all too frequently leads the physician to suspect an allergic or dermatologic condition (Figs. 64–12 and 64–16).[199,200] However, what has become quite evident in recent years is that when urticaria develops in association with an acute febrile illness, the cutaneous reaction is a direct effect of an infectious agent, and its mediation does not require an allergic response. Listed in Table 64–12 are infectious agents associated with urticarial exanthems.

Papular urticaria occurs very commonly in children in the summer and fall and most frequently is the result of insect bites (see Table 64–6). However, virtually identical lesions occur in infections with coxsackievirus A as well as with other enteroviruses (Fig. 64–12). The main point for differentiation is that fever regularly develops in the virus-induced exanthems but is not a characteristic associated with insect bites.

Early in the course of meningococcemia, the exanthem can be urticarial, so an illness of sudden onset with fever and this cutaneous manifestation never should be taken lightly.

TABLE 64–12 Infectious Agents Associated with Illness in Which Urticarial Exanthems Occur

Infectious Agent	Illness
Epstein-Barr virus	Infectious mononucleosis
Coxsackieviruses A9, A16, B4, B5	
Echovirus 11	
Mumps virus	Mumps
Hepatitis B virus	
Hepatitis C virus	
Mycoplasma pneumoniae	
Neisseria meningitidis	Meningococcemia
Shigella sonnei	Shigellosis
Yersinia enterocolitica	Yersiniosis
Borrelia burgdorferi	Lyme disease
Plasmodium species	Malaria
Coxiella burnetii	Q fever
Giardia lamblia	Giardiasis
Entamoeba histolytica	Amebiasis
Trichomonas vaginalis	Vulvovaginalis
Enterobius vermicularis	Pinworm infestation
Necator americanus	Hookworm disease
Trichinella spiralis	Trichinosis
Schistosoma species	Schistosomiasis
Trichobilharzia species	Swimmer's itch or collector's itch
Wuchereria bancrofti	Filariasis
Echinococcus species	Echinococcosis
Sarcoptes scabiei	Scabies
Trombicula irritans	Chigger bites
Other mites	Mite bites
Pediculus humanus	Pediculosis
Bedbugs, kissing bugs, ants, fleas, flies, and mosquitoes	Bites and stings

PAPULAR, NODULAR, AND ULCERATIVE LESIONS

In many instances, the lesions in this category occur as single events at the site of primary inoculation. Specific illnesses and etiologic agents are listed in Table 64–13.

DISTINCTIVE CLINICAL FEATURES OR SYNDROMES

(Figs. 64–19 to 64–24)

Erythema Multiforme

Erythema multiforme is a self-limited skin eruption that is erythematous and characterized by distinctive target or iris lesions or both. Small vesicles and urticarial areas also may develop. On occasion, the disease is severe and associated with mucosal involvement and genital lesions. In this latter illness—the Stevens-Johnson syndrome, bullous erythema multiforme, erythema multiforme exudativum major—severe ulcerative, oral, and genital lesions occur; generalized exanthems become bullous, and

TABLE 64–13 Infectious Agents Associated with Papular, Nodular, and Ulcerative Lesions

Agent	Illness
Wart virus	Warts (P and N)
Orf virus	Ecthyma contagiosum (N)
Molluscum contagiosum virus	Molluscum contagiosum (P and N)
Hepatitis B virus	Gianotti-Crosti syndrome (P)
Paravaccinia virus	Milker's nodules (N)
Francisella tularensis	Tularemia (U)
Haemophilus ducreyi	Chancroid (U)
Bartonella bacilliformis	Bartonellosis (N)
Calymmatobacterium granulomatis	Granuloma inguinale (N and U)
Pseudomonas aeruginosa	Ecthyma gangrenosa (U)
	Pseudomonas folliculitis (P)
Burkholderia mallei	Glanders (N and U)
Mycobacterium tuberculosis	Lupus vulgaris (N)
	Papulonecrotic tuberculids (U)
Atypical mycobacteria	(U)
Mycobacterium leprae	(N)
Treponema pallidum	Chancre (U)
Treponema pertenue	Yaws (P and U)
Sporotrichum schenckii	Sporotrichosis (U)
Blastomyces dermatitidis	Blastomycosis (N and U)
Fusarium species	Opportunistic infection (N)
Scedosporium species	Opportunistic infection (N)
Candida albicans	Systemic candidiasis (N)
Leishmania tropica	Oriental sore (N and U)
Leishmania braziliensis and mexicana	American cutaneous leishmaniasis (P and U)
Trypanosoma species	Trypanosomiasis (N)
Necator americanus	Hookworm disease (P)
Schistosoma species	Schistosomiasis (P)
Trichobilharzia species	Swimmer's itch or collector's itch (P)
Onchocerca volvulus	Onchocerciasis (P)
Loxosceles reclusa	Recluse spider bites (U)
Ticks	Tick bites (U)
Sarcoptes scabiei	Scabies (P)
Trombicula irritans	Chigger bites (P)
Other mites	Mite bites (P)
Cimex lectularius	Bedbug bites (P)
Triatoma sanguisuga	Kissing bug bites (P and N)
Solenopsis saevissima	Fire ant bites (P and N)
Fleas	Flea bites (P)
Flies and mosquitoes	Fly and mosquito bites (P)

N, nodular; P, papular U, ulcerative.

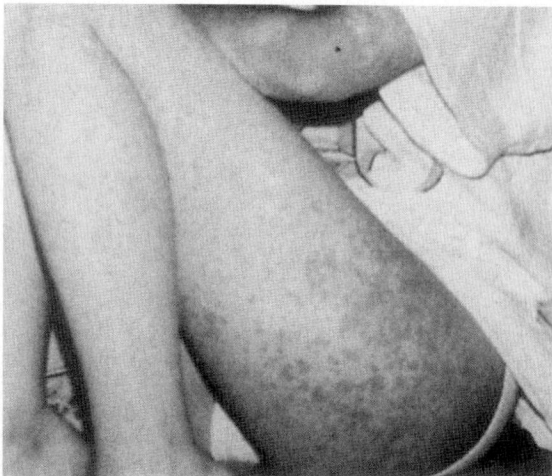

Figure 64–19 An erythematous maculopapular discrete and confluent rash on the thigh and arm of a 16-year-old girl with pharyngitis and *Arcanobacterium haemolyticum* isolated from her throat. (See companion Expert Consult web site for color version.) *(From Mackenzie, A., Fuite, L. A., Chan, F. T. H., et al.: Incidence and pathogenicity of Arcanobacterium haemolyticum during a 2-year study in Ottawa. Clin. Infect. Dis. 21:177-181, 1995.)*

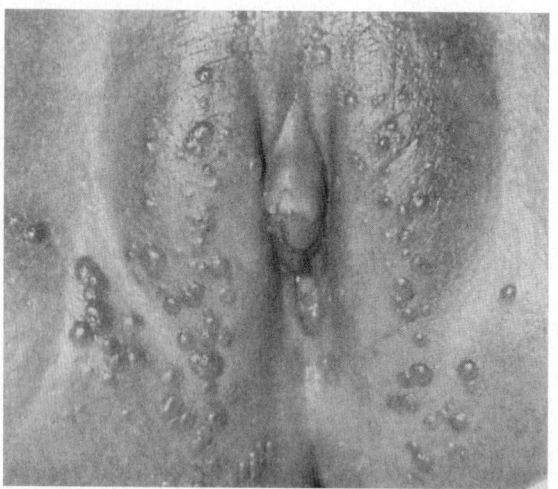

Figure 64–20 Numerous flat-topped and dome-shaped, slightly erythematous papules over the skin of the perineum of a young girl with bowenoid papulosis. (See companion Expert Consult web site for color version.)

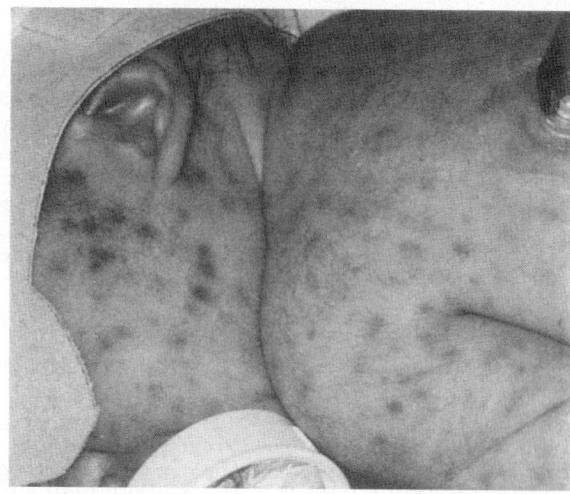

Figure 64–21 Numerous isolated purple papules of dermal erythropoiesis overlying the icteric skin of a neonate with congenital cytomegalovirus infection. (See companion Expert Consult web site for color version.)

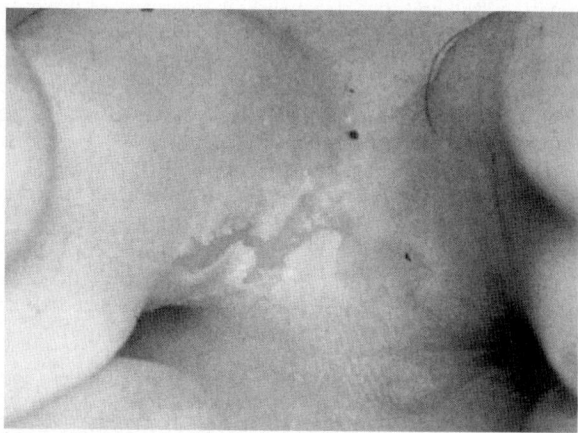

Figure 64–22 Tinea pedis. Peeling, macerations, and fissuring in the fourth interdigital space of the foot are characteristic of dermatophytic infections. (See companion Expert Consult web site for color version.)

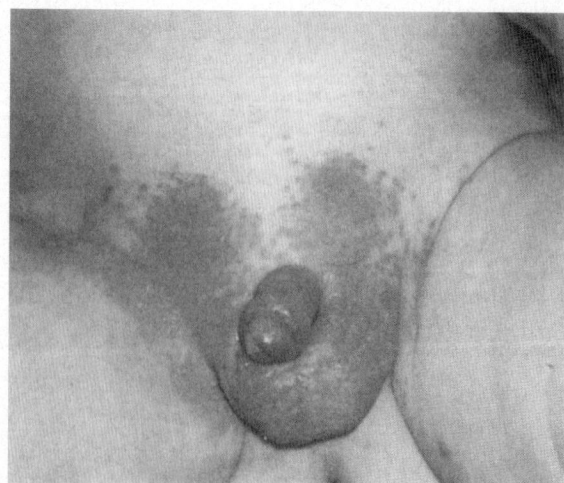

Figure 64–23 Clinical photograph of an infant with *Candida* diaper dermatitis. Confluent and discrete erythematous papules and plaques involving the scrotum, penis, and suprapubic and inguinal area are evident. (See companion Expert Consult web site for color version.)

conjunctivitis is present. The illness is associated with fever and general distress.

Although the pathogenesis of erythema multiforme is unknown, what is clear is that multiple factors, including infectious agents, are responsible for its occurrence. Infectious agents associated with erythema multiforme are listed in Table 64–14. The single most important infectious cause of erythema multiforme and Stevens-Johnson syndrome is *M. pneumoniae*. When *M. pneumoniae* is the instigating agent, the patient nearly always has concomitant pneumonia.

HSV frequently has been recovered from the throats of persons with erythema multiforme, but the cause-and-effect relationship in many cases must be questioned. However, in a recent study, HSV DNA was found in the skin lesions of 11 of 31 patients with erythema multiforme.[58]

TABLE 64–14 Infectious Agents Associated with Erythema Multiforme

Agent	Illness
Human parvovirus B19	Erythema infectiosum
Adenovirus 7	Respiratory infection
Herpes simplex virus type 1	Perioral or respiratory infection
Epstein-Barr virus	Infectious mononucleosis
Varicella virus	Chickenpox
Coxsackieviruses A10, A16, B5	Enterovirus syndrome
Echovirus 6	Enterovirus syndrome
Poliomyelitis virus	Poliomyelitis
Vaccinia virus	Smallpox vaccination
Variola virus	Smallpox
Orf virus	Ecthyma contagiosum
Paravaccinia virus	Milker's nodules
Influenza A virus	Influenza
Mumps	Mumps
Hepatitis B virus	Serum hepatitis
Chlamydia psittaci	Psittacosis
Chlamydia trachomatis	Lymphogranuloma venereum
Mycoplasma pneumoniae	Respiratory symptoms
Staphylococcus aureus	Septicemia
Streptococcus pyogenes	Respiratory symptoms
Neisseria gonorrhoeae	Gonorrhea
Corynebacterium diphtheriae	Diphtheria
Pseudomonas aeruginosa	Septicemia
Salmonella species	Gastroenteritis
Francisella tularensis	Tularemia
Yersinia species	Gastrointestinal symptoms
Vibrio parahaemolyticus	Gastroenteritis
Treponema pallidum	Syphilis
Bartonella henselae	Cat-scratch fever
Mycobacterium tuberculosis	Tuberculosis
Mycobacterium leprae	Leprosy
Coccidioides immitis	Coccidioidomycosis
Histoplasma capsulatum	Histoplasmosis
Trichomonas vaginalis	Vulvovaginalis

TABLE 64–15 Infectious Agents Associated with Erythema Nodosum

Agent	Illness
Herpes simplex virus	Perioral or respiratory infection
Epstein-Barr virus	Infectious mononucleosis
Chlamydia psittaci	Psittacosis
Chlamydia trachomatis	Lymphogranuloma venereum
Streptococcus pyogenes	Respiratory infection
Neisseria meningitidis	Meningococcemia
Corynebacterium diphtheriae	Diphtheria
Campylobacter species	Gastroenteritis
Haemophilus ducreyi	Chancroid
Salmonella species	Salmonellosis
Yersinia species	Gastrointestinal symptoms
Brucella species	Brucellosis
Treponema pallidum	Syphilis
Bartonella henselae	Cat-scratch fever
Mycobacterium tuberculosis	Tuberculosis
Mycobacterium leprae	Leprosy
Trichophyton species	Kerion of scalp
Histoplasma capsulatum	Histoplasmosis
Cryptococcus neoformans	Cryptococcosis
Coccidioides immitis	Coccidioidomycosis
Blastomyces dermatitidis	Blastomycosis
Ascaris lumbricoides	Roundworm infestation
Wuchereria bancrofti	Filariasis

Erythema nodosum occurs less commonly today than it did 4 decades ago, and the frequency of specific associated infectious agents also is different. In the past, streptococcal and mycobacterial infections were the agents most commonly related. Now, the exanthem most often is associated with respiratory infection with *Histoplasma capsulatum*, *Cryptococcus neoformans*, and *Coccidioides immitis*. Infectious agents associated with erythema nodosum are listed in Table 64–15.

Hand, Foot, and Mouth Syndrome

The hand, foot, and mouth syndrome is a clearly recognizable viral illness characterized by vesicular lesions in the anterior of the mouth and on the hands and feet in association with fever. Although several enteroviruses (coxsackieviruses A5, A9, A10, A16, B1, and B3 and enterovirus 71) have been implicated, as have HSV and foot and mouth disease virus, most of these cases are caused by coxsackievirus A16.

Roseola-like Illness

Roseola infantum is a classic pediatric illness characterized by fever of 3 to 5 days' duration, rapid defervescence, and then the appearance of an erythematous macular or maculopapular rash that persists for 1 to 2 days. Roseola is an age-related response to infection with many viruses. Recent studies suggest that a leading cause of roseola infantum is primary infection with HHV-6. The following other viruses have been noted in association with roseola: adenoviruses 1, 2, 3, and 14; coxsackieviruses A6, A9, B1, B2, B4, and B5; echoviruses 9, 11, 16, 25, 27, and 30; parainfluenza virus type 1; and measles vaccine virus.

Rocky Mountain Spotted Fever–like Illness

Rocky Mountain spotted fever is a clinical illness characterized by fever and a petechial rash located mainly on the distal ends of extremities. The illness is caused by *Rickettsia rickettsii* and is prevalent in many areas of North America; the infectious agent is transmitted to humans by ticks. In other areas of the world,

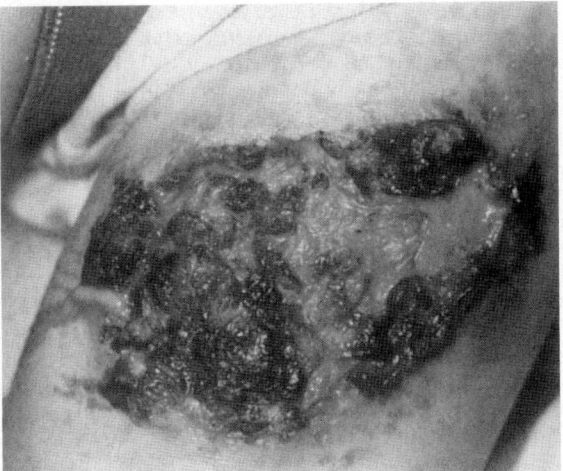

Figure 64–24 An extensive crusted erosion on the left thigh of a child with a cryptococcal skin infection. (See companion Expert Consult web site for color version.)

Erythema Nodosum

Erythema nodosum most commonly occurs on the anterior aspect of the lower part of the legs but may be seen anywhere on the body. The lesions are raised, erythematous, and painful to touch. Their usual size is approximately 2 to 4 cm, with a duration of 2 to 6 weeks.

other tick-borne rickettsiae (*Rickettsia sibirica, Rickettsia australis, Rickettsia conorii*) produce similar human illness. Infection with *Ehrlichia canis* also can cause an illness similar to Rocky Mountain spotted fever.

The most important illness confused with Rocky Mountain spotted fever is atypical measles (see Chapter 192). This illness, which has both the constitutional symptoms of Rocky Mountain spotted fever and a rash most prominent on the extremities, occurs almost exclusively after exposure to measles virus in some persons previously immunized with inactivated (killed) measles vaccine.

Rat-bite fever caused by *S. moniliformis* also has been misdiagnosed as Rocky Mountain spotted fever.[156]

Exanthem and Meningitis

Aseptic and also bacterial meningitis frequently are characterized by both exanthem and symptoms and signs of neurologic involvement. Infectious agents associated with exanthem and meningitis are presented in Table 64–16. Of most importance in this category is the differential diagnosis of enteroviral syndromes and meningococcemia.

Exanthem and Pulmonary Involvement

Infectious agents associated with exanthem and pulmonary involvement are listed in Table 64–17. In patients older than 5 years old, the leading cause of exanthem and pneumonia is *M. pneumoniae* infection. In younger children, adenoviruses are the most important etiologic agents. With the exception of enteroviral infections, which are more likely to involve young children, most of the illnesses listed in Table 64–17 occur in older children and young adults.

Gianotti-Crosti Syndrome (Papular Acrodermatitis)

Gianotti-Crosti syndrome is a distinct clinical entity characterized by a papular (lichenoid) exanthem, generalized lymphadenopathy, hepatomegaly, and acute anicteric hepatitis.[46,170,173] In most instances, this illness has been associated with hepatitis B virus infection. The syndrome also has been noted in association with Epstein-Barr virus, cytomegalovirus, coxsackievirus B virus, and RSV infections.[65,111,171,193]

Cutaneous Manifestations Associated with Infections in Immunocompromised Patients

All infectious agents that cause exanthems in immunologically normal children can cause infections in immunocompromised children. However, the clinical manifestations may be different. For example, measles virus infection in a child who is T-cell-deficient may be associated with a severe, progressive pneumonia but not the typical rash. Other viral exanthems that are self-limited in normal children, such as varicella, may be progressive and develop into hemorrhagic skin lesions with disseminated organ involvement in children with T-cell-deficiency.

Of particular concern are bacterial and fungal infections, which are rarely a problem in normal children but are rapidly fatal in granulocytopenic children. These patients have characteristic skin lesions resulting from disseminated infections. Of importance are ecthyma gangrenosa resulting from *Pseudomonas aeruginosa* septicemia and the nodular and purpuric lesions of disseminated fungal infections caused by *Aspergillus, Candida,* and other less common agents.

DIAGNOSIS

DIFFERENTIAL DIAGNOSIS

The diagnosis of infectious exanthems frequently is considered an impossible task by many physicians. Other physicians glibly call the first maculopapular exanthem of childhood "roseola" and the first vesicular rash "chickenpox" without consideration of more appropriate choices. The hallmark of diagnosis in exanthematous disease is careful elicitation of historic data. Differential diagnosis requires the consideration of noninfectious etiologies as well as different infectious agents. Listed in Table 64–18 are the major considerations in the diagnosis of diseases with cutaneous manifestations.

A history of exposure is most important in making a differential diagnosis. For example, was the patient exposed to poison ivy, insects, or a person ill with a specific disease? In infectious illnesses with high clinical expression rates (measles, chickenpox, rubella), proper questioning usually reveals a contact case or at least other cases in the community. On the other hand, in ill-

TABLE 64–16 Infectious Agents Associated with Exanthem and Meningitis

Agent	Illness
Herpes simplex virus type 2	Recurrent genital herpes
Coxsackieviruses A2, A9, B1, B4, B5	Enterovirus syndrome
Echoviruses 4, 6, 9, 11, 14, 17, 25, 33	Enterovirus syndrome
Colorado tick fever virus	Colorado tick fever
Reovirus 2	Respiratory infection
West Nile virus	Meningoencephalitis
Neisseria meningitidis	Meningococcemia
Borrelia burgdorferi	Lyme disease
Listeria monocytogenes	Listeriosis
Toxoplasma gondii	Toxoplasmosis

TABLE 64–17 Infectious Agents Associated with Exanthem and Pulmonary Involvement

Agent	Illness
Adenoviruses 7,7a	Respiratory infection
Herpes simplex virus type 1	Respiratory infection
Varicella-zoster virus	Chickenpox pneumonia
Epstein-Barr virus	Infectious mononucleosis
Coxsackievirus A9	Enterovirus syndrome
Echovirus 11	Enterovirus syndrome
Reovirus 3	Respiratory infection
Measles virus	Measles pneumonia and atypical measles
Chlamydia psittaci	Psittacosis
Mycoplasma pneumoniae	*M. pneumoniae* pneumonia
Neisseria meningitidis	Meningococcal pneumonia
Mycobacterium tuberculosis	Tuberculosis
Histoplasma capsulatum	Histoplasmosis
Cryptococcus neoformans	Cryptococcosis
Coccidioides immitis	Coccidioidomycosis

TABLE 64–18 Important Aspects in the Diagnosis of Exanthematous Illness

Exposure	Types of Rash
Season	Distribution of rash
Incubation period	Progression of rash
Age	Exanthem
Previous exanthems	Other associated symptoms
Relationship of rash to fever	Laboratory tests
Adenopathy	

From Cherry, J. D.: Newer viral exanthems. Adv. Pediatr. 16:233-286, 1969.

nesses with low rates of clinical expression of exanthem, such as adenoviral and some enteroviral infections, the source may not be apparent.

Consideration of the seasonal occurrence of different infectious agents, as well as insects, is particularly useful in making a differential diagnosis. In temperate climates, enteroviral and arthropod-mediated diseases occur in the summer and fall. Exanthems with measles, varicella-zoster, and rubella viruses occur most often in the winter and spring. The diagnosis of rubella is important because of fetal consequences. All too frequently, rubella is overdiagnosed and underdiagnosed, both of which can be avoided if its seasonal prevalence is understood.

The incubation period is important in separating the exanthem caused by rubella, varicella-zoster, or measles viruses from rash illnesses caused by enteroviruses or common respiratory viruses. The former have long incubation periods, whereas in the others, the period from exposure to the onset of illness is less than 1 week. Age can be useful. Today in the United States, measles and rubella often are illnesses of adolescents and young adults. Enteroviral exanthem frequency is related inversely to age.

Questioning to obtain a pertinent history of previous exanthems can give useful information if it is done with care. For example, if patients are asked whether they had rubella, the answer is quite unreliable. However, if the past illness is documented by year, season, and symptoms, accurate information often is obtained. The relationship of rash to fever is most significant in the diagnosis of roseola. The presence or absence of fever is important in separating exanthems of infectious and noninfectious etiology. Frequently, insect bites are diagnosed as chickenpox by parents and physicians as well. Chickenpox rarely occurs without fever.

The type and distribution of exanthem obviously are important. They virtually are diagnostic in hand, foot, and mouth syndrome, Rocky Mountain spotted fever, and atypical measles. Enanthem can lead to a specific diagnosis (Koplik spots in measles [Fig. 64–1]) or a category diagnosis (herpangina in enteroviral infections). Other characteristics, such as those listed in Tables 64–8 through 64–17, obviously are useful in delineating a specific illness.

SPECIFIC DIAGNOSIS

As with other infectious diseases, establishing specific diagnosis depends on the acquisition of proper cultures, serologic tests, and microscopic study of secretions or histologic or cytologic preparations. These techniques are discussed in other chapters of this book.

Vesicular lesions always should be scraped for cytologic study or direct antigen identification (varicella, herpes simplex), and, frequently, petechial lesions should be scraped and stained in a search for infectious agents (meningococci). The etiology of viral infections can be established by isolation of virus, direct antigen detection, or serologic methods. In most instances, a virus recovered from the throat indicates acute infection and is the probable cause of a particular illness. Serologic study without culture is useful in diagnosing rickettsial diseases, some viral infections, and a few illnesses of bacterial origin. Serologic study without virus isolation generally is not useful in diagnosing enteroviral illnesses.

TREATMENT, PROGNOSIS, AND PREVENTION

The treatment, prognosis, and prevention of exanthematous diseases are presented in appropriate chapters throughout this text.

REFERENCES

1. Africk, J. A., and Halprin, K. M.: Infectious mononucleosis presenting as urticaria. J. A. M. A. 209:1524-1525, 1969.
2. Agnello, V., and Abel, G.: Localization of hepatitis C virus in cutaneous vasculitic lesions in patients with type II cryoglobulinemia. Arthritis Rheum. 40:2007-2015, 1997.
3. Aguilar-Bernier, M., Bassas-Vila, J., Torne-Gutierrez, J. I., et al.: Presence of perineuritis in a case of papular purpuric gloves and socks syndrome associated with mononeuritis multiplex attributable to B19 parvovirus. J. Am. Acad. Dermatol. 54:896-899, 2006.
4. Ahlm, C., Settergren, B., Gothfors, L., et al.: Nephropathia epidemica (hemorrhagic fever with renal syndrome) in children: Clinical characteristics. Pediatr. Infect. Dis. J. 13:45-49, 1994.
5. Ahvonen, P.: Human yersiniosis in Finland. II. Clinical features. Ann. Clin. Res. 4:39-48, 1972.
6. Alfadley, A., Aljubran, A., Hainau, B., et al.: Papular-purpuric "gloves and socks" syndrome in a mother and daughter. J. Am. Acad. Dermatol. 48:941-944, 2003.
7. Anderson, M. J., Lewis, E., Kidd, I. M., et al.: An outbreak of erythema infectiosum associated with human parvovirus infection. J. Hyg. (Lond.) 93:85-93, 1984.
8. Arnold, J. C., Singh, K. K., Spector, S. A., et al.: Human bocavirus: Prevalence and clinical spectrum at a children's hospital. Clin. Infect. Dis. 43:283-288, 2006.
9. Arkwright, J. A.: Foot-and-mouth disease in man. Lancet 1:1191-1192, 1928.
10. Asano, Y., Suga, S., Yoshikawa, T., et al.: Clinical features and viral excretion in an infant with primary human herpesvirus 7 infection. Pediatrics 95:187-190, 1995.
11. Asano, Y., Yoshikawa, T., Suga, S., et al.: Viremia and neutralizing antibody response in infants with exanthem subitum. J. Pediatr. 114:535-539, 1989.
12. Athreya, B. H., and Coriell, L. L.: Erythema multiforme exudativum major: A review and report of four cases. Clin. Pediatr. (Phila.) 3:68-74, 1964.
13. Azimi, P. H., Chase, P. A., and Petru, A. M.: Mycoplasmas: Their role in pediatric disease. Curr. Probl. Pediatr. 14:7-46, 1984.
14. Baer, R. L.: Erythema multiforme—1976. Am. J. Med. Sci. 271:119-120, 1976.
15. Baley, J. E., Kliegman, R. M., and Fanaroff, A. A.: Disseminated fungal infections in very low-birth weight infants: Clinical manifestations and epidemiology. Pediatrics 83:144-152, 1984.
16. Balfour, H. H., Jr., Forte, F. A., Simpson, R. B., et al.: Penicillin-related exanthems in infectious mononucleosis identical to those associated with ampicillin. Clin. Pediatr. (Phila.) 11:417-421, 1972.
17. Baron, J., and Shapiro, E. D.: Unsuspected bacteremia caused by *Branhamella catarrhalis*. Pediatr. Infect. Dis. 4:100-101, 1985.
18. Barrett, P. K. M., and Greenberg, M. J.: Outbreak of ornithosis. B. M. J. 2:206-207, 1966.
19. Baumgartner, J. D., Glauser, M. P., Burgo-Black, A. L., et al.: Severe cytomegalovirus infection in multiply transfused, splenectomised, trauma patients. Lancet 2:63-66, 1982.
20. Beall, G. N.: Urticaria: A review of laboratory and clinical observations. Medicine (Baltimore) 43:131-151, 1964.
21. Benoit, F. L.: Chronic meningococcemia: Case report and review of the literature. Am. J. Med. 35:103-112, 1963.
22. Berant, M., Naveh, Y., and Weissman, I.: Papular acrodermatitis with cytomegalovirus hepatitis. Arch. Dis. Child. 58:1024-1025, 1983.
23. Berenguer, J., Rodriguez-Tudela, J. L., Richard, C., et al.: Deep infections caused by *Scedosporium prolificans*. Medicine (Baltimore) 76:256-265, 1997.
24. Berger, B. W.: Erythema chronicum migrans of Lyme disease. Arch. Dermatol. 120:1017-1021, 1984.
25. Black, F. L.: Measles. In Evans, A. S. (ed.): Viral Infections of Humans: Epidemiology and Control. New York, Plenum, 1976, pp. 297-316.
26. Blatt, J., Kastner, O., and Hodes, D. S.: Cutaneous vesicles in congenital cytomegalovirus infection. J. Pediatr. 92:509, 1978.
27. Bodey, G. P., and Fainstein, V.: Systemic candidiasis. In Bodey, G. P., and Fainstein, V. (eds.): Candidiasis. New York, Raven Press, 1985, pp. 135-168.
28. Boughton, C. R.: Glandular fever: A study of hospital series in Sydney. Med. J. Aust. 2:529-535, 1970.
29. Bowmer, E. J., McKiel, J. A., Cockcroft, W. H., et al.: *Listeria monocytogenes* infections in Canada. Can. Med. Assoc. J. 109:125-135, 1973.
30. Bowmer, M. I., Leggat, I., and Barrowman, J. A.: Disseminated gonococcal infection. Can. Med. Assoc. J. 126:1188-1190, 1982.
31. Bradford, W. D., and Hawkins, H. K.: Rocky Mountain spotted fever in childhood. Am. J. Dis. Child. 131:1228-1232, 1977.
32. Breese, B. B.: Streptococcal pharyngitis and scarlet fever. Am. J. Dis. Child. 132:612-616, 1978.
33. Breese, B. B.: Pharyngitis and scarlet fever. In Breese, B. B., and Hall, C. B. (eds.): Beta Hemolytic Streptococcal Diseases. Boston, Houghton Mifflin, 1978, pp. 65-78.
34. Breese, B. B.: Streptococcal skin infections. In Breese, B. B., and Hall, C. B. (eds.): Beta Hemolytic Streptococcal Diseases. Boston, Houghton Mifflin, 1978, pp. 176-211.
35. Brettman, L. R., Lewin, S., Holzman, R. S., et al.: Rickettsialpox: Report of an outbreak and a contemporary review. Medicine (Baltimore) 60:363-372, 1981.

36. Brody, I.: Topical treatment of recurrent herpes simplex and post-herpetic erythema multiforme with low concentrations of zinc sulphate solution. Br. J. Dermatol. *104*:191-194, 1981.

37. Browne, S. G.: Mycobacterial diseases: Leprosy. *In* Fitzpatrick, T. B., Eisen, A. Z., Wolff, K., et al. (eds.): Dermatology in General Medicine. New York, McGraw-Hill, 1979, pp. 1492-1505.

38. Bruhn, F. W.: Lyme disease. Am. J. Dis. Child. *138*:467-470, 1984.

39. Bruno, P., Harrison Hassell, L., Brown, J., et al.: The protean manifestations of hemorrhagic fever with renal syndrome: A retrospective review of 26 cases from Korea. Ann. Intern. Med. *113*:385-391, 1990.

40. Buckley, B.: Q fever epidemic in Victorian general practice. Med. J. Aust. *1*:593-595, 1980.

41. Burnett, J. W.: Uncommon bacterial infections of the skin. Arch. Dermatol. *86*:597-607, 1962.

42. Bwaka, M. A., Bonnet, M. J., Calain, P., et al.: Ebola hemorrhagic fever in Kitwit, Democratic Republic of the Congo: Clinical observations of 103 patients. J. Infect. Dis. *179*(Suppl.):1-7, 1999.

43. Caputo, R. V., and Solomon, L. M.: Vascular reactive diseases. *In* Solomon, L. M., Esterly, N. B., and Loeffel, E. D. (eds.): Adolescent Dermatology. Philadelphia, W. B. Saunders, 1978, pp. 404-432.

44. Carlstrom, G., Alden, J., Belfrage, S., et al.: Acquired cytomegalovirus infection. B. M. J. *2*:521-525, 1968.

45. Carslaw, R. W.: Skin infestation. Practitioner *216*:154-158, 1976.

46. Castellano, A., Schweitzer, R., Tong, M. J., et al.: Papular acrodermatitis of childhood and hepatitis B infection. Arch. Dermatol. *114*:1530-1532, 1978.

47. Centers for Disease Control and Prevention: Moth-associated dermatitis—Cozumel, Mexico. M. M. W. R. Morb. Mortal. Wkly. Rep. *39*(13):219-220, 1990.

48. Chanarin, I., and Walford, D. M.: Thrombocytopenic purpura in cytomegalovirus mononucleosis. Lancet *2*:238-239, 1973.

49. Cherry, J. D.: Newer viral exanthems. Adv. Pediatr. *16*:233-286, 1969.

50. Cherry, J. D.: Parvovirus infections in children and adults. Adv. Pediatr. *46*:245-269, 1999.

51. Cherry, J. D., Hurwitz, E. S., and Welliver, R. C.: *Mycoplasma pneumoniae* infections and exanthems. J. Pediatr. *87*:369-373, 1975.

52. Cherry, J. D., and Jahn, C. L.: Exanthem and enanthem associated with mumps virus infection. Arch. Environ. Health *12*:518-521, 1966.

53. Cherry, J. D., and Welliver, R. C.: *Mycoplasma pneumoniae* infections of adults and children. West. J. Med. *125*:47-55, 1976.

54. Chesney, P. J., Davis, J. P., Purdy, W. K., et al.: Clinical manifestations of toxic shock syndrome. J. A. M. A. *246*:741-748, 1981.

55. Chonmaitree, T., Menegus, M. A., and Powell, K. R.: The clinical relevance of "CSF viral culture": A two-year experience with aseptic meningitis in Rochester, New York. J. A. M. A. *247*:1843-1847, 1982.

56. Clark, R. F.: Localized urticaria due to *Enterobius vermicularis*. Arch. Dermatol. *84*:1026, 1961.

57. Cowdrey, S. C., and Reynolds, J. S.: Acute urticaria in infectious mononucleosis. Ann. Allergy *27*:182-187, 1969.

58. Darragh, T. M., Egbert, B. M., Berger, T. G., et al.: Identification of herpes simplex virus DNA in lesions of erythema multiforme by the polymerase chain reaction. J. Am. Acad. Dermatol. *24*:23-36, 1991.

59. Daye, S., McHenry, J. A., and Roscelli, J. D.: Pruritic rash associated with cat scratch disease. Pediatrics *81*:559-561, 1988.

60. Delage, G., McLaughlin, B., and Berthiaume, L.: A clinical study of rotavirus gastroenteritis. J. Pediatr. *93*:455-457, 1978.

61. Derbes, V. J.: Arthropod bites and stings. *In* Fitzpatrick, T. B., Eisen, A. Z., Wolff, K., et al. (eds.): Dermatology in General Medicine. New York, McGraw-Hill, 1979, pp. 1656-1668.

62. Dienstag, J. L., Rhodes, A. R., Bhan, A. K., et al.: Urticaria associated with acute viral hepatitis type B: Studies of pathogenesis. Ann. Intern. Med. *88*:34-40, 1978.

63. Di Lernia, V., and Ricci, C.: Skin manifestations with *Rotavirus* infections. Int. J. Dermatol. *45*:759-761, 2006.

64. Dooley, J. R.: Haemotropic bacteria in man. Lancet *2*:1237-1239, 1980.

65. Draelos, Z. K., Hansen, R. C., and James, W. D.: Gianotti-Crosti syndrome associated with infections other than hepatitis B. J. A. M. A. *256*:2386-2388, 1986.

66. Drago, F., Ranieri, E., Malaguti, F., et al.: Human herpesvirus 7 in pityriasis rosea. Lancet *349*:1367-1368, 1997.

67. Dryer, R. F., Goellner, P. G., and Carney, A. S.: Lyme arthritis in Wisconsin. J. A. M. A. *241*:498-499, 1979.

68. Dukes, C.: On the confusion of two different diseases under the name of rubella (rose-rash). Lancet *2*:89-94, 1900.

69. Duncan, W. C.: Cutaneous manifestations of infectious diseases. *In* Hoeprich, P. D. (ed.): Infectious Diseases: A Modern Treatise of Infectious Processes. Hagerstown, MD, Harper & Row, 1977, pp. 68-74.

70. Editor's Reply: First, second, third, fourth and fifth diseases. Am. J. Dis. Child. *108*:440-441, 1964.

71. Ellis, M. E., Pope, J., Mokashi, A., et al.: *Campylobacter* colitis associated with erythema nodosum. B. M. J. *285*:937, 1982.

72. Farah, F. S.: Protozoan and helminth infections. *In* Fitzpatrick, T. B., Eisen, A. Z., Wolff, K., et al. (eds.): Dermatology in General Medicine. New York, McGraw-Hill, 1979, pp. 1635-1656.

73. Fass, R. J., and Saslaw, S.: Earth day histoplasmosis: A new type of urban pollution. Arch. Intern. Med. *128*:588-590, 1971.

74. Fell, H. W. K., Nagington, J., Naylor, G. R. E., et al.: *Corynebacterium haemolyticum* infections in Cambridgeshire. J. Hyg. (Lond.) *79*:269-275, 1977.

75. Fenner, F.: The clinical features and pathogenesis of mouse-pox (infectious ectromelia of mice). J. Pathol. Bacteriol. *60*:529-552, 1948.

76. Fiumara, N. J., and Solomon, J.: Recurrent herpes simplex virus infections and erythema multiforme: A report of three patients. Sex. Transm. Dis. *10*:144-146, 1983.

77. Flaum, A.: Foot-and-mouth disease in man. Acta Pathol. Microbiol. Scand. *16*:197-213, 1939.

78. Formenty, P., Hatz, C., Le Guenno, B., et al.: Human infection due to Ebola virus, subtype Cote d'Ivoire: Clinical biologic presentation. J. Infect. Dis. *179*(Suppl.):48-53, 1999.

79. Fukumi, H., Nishikawa, F., Kokubu, Y., et al.: Isolation of adenovirus from an exanthematous infection resembling roseola infantum. Jpn. J. Med. Sci. Biol. *10*:87-91, 1957.

80. Game, M. A., Owen, W. C., and Mitchell, D. K.: Cutaneous manifestations of disseminated fungal infection in an immunocompromised child. J. Pediatr. *133*:466, 1998.

81. Gardner, S. D.: The isolation of parainfluenza 4 subtypes A and B in England and serological studies of their prevalence. J. Hyg. (Camb.) *67*:545-550, 1969.

82. Goodwin, R. A., Loyd, J. E., and Des Prez, R. M.: Histoplasmosis in normal hosts. Medicine (Baltimore) *60*:231-266, 1981.

83. Gordon, P. M., Hepburn, N. C., Williams, A. E., et al.: Cutaneous myiasis due to *Dermatobia hominis*: A report of six cases. Br. J. Dermatol. *132*:811-814, 1995.

84. Griffith, G. L., and Luce, E. A.: Massive skin necrosis in Rocky Mountain spotted fever. South. Med. J. *71*:1337-1340, 1978.

85. Grilli, R., Izquierdo, M. J., Farina, M. C., et al.: Papular-purpuric "gloves and socks" syndrome: Polymerase chain reaction demonstration of parvovirus B19 DNA in cutaneous lesions and sera. J. Am. Acad. Dermatol. *41*:793-796, 1999.

86. Gustafson, T. L., Band, J. D., Hutcheson, R. H., Jr., et al.: *Pseudomonas folliculitis*: An outbreak and review. Rev. Infect. Dis. *5*:1-8, 1983.

87. Hall, C. B.: The exanthematous family tree: Diseases one, two, three and five? Am. J. Dis. Child. *131*:816, 1977.

88. Halliday, H. L., and Hirata, T.: Perinatal listeriosis: A review of twelve patients. Am. J. Obstet. Gynecol. *133*:405-410, 1979.

89. Hamrick, H. J., and Moore, G. W.: Giardiasis causing urticaria in a child. Am. J. Dis. Child. *137*:761-763, 1983.

90. Hannuksela, M., and Ahvonen, P.: Skin manifestations in human yersiniosis. Ann. Clin. Res. *7*:368-373, 1975.

91. Harel, L., Straussberg, I., Zeharia, A., et al.: Papular purpuric rash due to parvovirus B19 with distribution on the distal extremities and the face. Clin. Infect. Dis. *35*:1558-1561, 2002.

92. Harrison, D. L.: A case of human ornithosis presenting as an obscure febrile illness associated with macular rash. Practitioner *190*:245-246, 1963.

93. Herrmann, E. C., Jr., and Hable, K. A.: Experiences in laboratory diagnosis of parainfluenza viruses in routine medical practice. Mayo Clin. Proc. *45*:177-188, 1970.

94. Hilleman, M. R., Hamparian, V. V., Ketler, A., et al.: Acute respiratory illnesses among children and adults: Field study of contemporary importance of several viruses and appraisal of the literature. J. A. M. A. *180*:445-453, 1962.

95. Hoagland, R. J.: The clinical manifestations of infectious mononucleosis: A report of two hundred cases. Am. J. Med. Sci. *240*:55-62, 1960.

96. Honig, P. J.: Bites and parasites. Pediatr. Clin. North Am. *30*:563-581, 1983.

97. Hoofnagle, J. H.: Hepatitis C: The clinical spectrum of disease. Hepatology *26*(Suppl.):15-20, 1997.

98. Hope-Simpson, R. E., and Higgins, P. G.: A respiratory virus study in Great Britain: Review and evaluation. Prog. Med. Virol. *11*:354-407, 1969.

99. Horton, J. M., and Blaser, M. J.: The spectrum of relapsing fever in the Rocky Mountains. Arch. Intern. Med. *145*:871-875, 1985.

100. Humphrey, T., Sanders, S., and Stadius, M.: Leptospirosis mimicking MLNS. J. Pediatr. *91*:853-854, 1977.

101. Jacobs, R. F., Hsi, S., Wilson, C. B., et al.: Apparent meningococcemia: Clinical features of disease due to *Haemophilus influenzae* and *Neisseria meningitidis*. Pediatrics *72*:469-472, 1983.

102. Jaffe, H. W., and Pellett, P. E.: Human herpesvirus 8 and Kaposi's sarcoma—some answers, more questions. N. Engl. J. Med. *340*:1912-1913, 1999.

103. Johnson, R. A.: Atypical mycobacteria. *In* Fitzpatrick, T. B., Eisen, A. Z., Wolff, K., et al. (eds.): Dermatology in General Medicine. New York, McGraw-Hill, 1979, pp. 1505-1508.

104. Joncas, J., Chiasson, J. P., Turcotte, J., et al.: Studies on infectious mononucleosis. III. Clinical data, serologic and epidemiologic findings. Can. Med. Assoc. J. *98*:848-854, 1968.

105. Kalis, P., LeFrock, J. L., Smith, W., et al.: Listeriosis. Am. J. Med. Sci. *271*:159-169, 1976.

106. Kanazawa, K., Yaoita, H., Tsuda, F., et al.: Hepatitis C virus infection in patients with urticaria. J. Am. Acad. Dermatol. *35*:195-198, 1996.

107. Kazmierowski, J. A., Peizner, D. S., and Wuepper, K. D.: Herpes simplex antigen in immune complexes of patients with erythema multiforme: Presence following recurrent herpes simplex infection. J. A. M. A. *247*:2547-2550, 1982.

108. Kennedy, A. C., Fleming, J., and Solomon, L.: Chikungunya viral arthropathy: A clinical description. J. Rheumatol. *7*:231-236, 1980.

109. Kennett, M. L., Birch, C. J., Lewis, F. A., et al.: Enterovirus type 71 infection in Melbourne. Bull. World Health Organ. *51*:609-615, 1974.

110. Kiernan, J. P., Schanzlin, D. J., and Leveille, A. S.: Stevens-Johnson syndrome associated with adenovirus conjunctivitis. Am. J. Ophthalmol. *92*:543-545, 1981.

111. Konno, M., Kikuta, H., Ishikawa, N., et al.: A possible association between hepatitis B antigen-negative infantile papular acrodermatitis and Epstein-Barr virus infection. J. Pediatr. *101*:222-224, 1982.

112. Krause, V. W., Embree, J. E., MacDonald, S. W., et al.: Congenital listeriosis causing early neonatal death. Can. Med. Assoc. J. *127*:36-38, 1982.

113. Krober, M. S., Bass, J. W., and Barcia, P. J.: Scarlatiniform rash and pleural effusion in a patient with *Yersinia pseudotuberculosis* infection. J. Pediatr. *102*:879-881, 1983.

114. Kusenbach, G., Rubben, A., Schneider, E. M., et al.: Herpes virus (KSHV) associated Kaposi sarcoma in a 3-year-old child with non–HIV-induced immunodeficiency. Eur. J. Pediatr. *156*:440-443, 1997.

115. Lackman, D. B.: A review of information on rickettsialpox in the United States. Clin. Pediatr. (Phila.) *2*:296-301, 1963.

116. La Grenade, L., Hanchard, B., Feltcher, V., et al.: Infective dermatitis of Jamaican children: A marker for HTLV-I infection. Lancet *336*:1345-1347, 1990.

117. La Grenade, L., Hanchard, B., Feltcher, V., et al.: Clinical, pathologic, and immunologic features of human T-lymphotropic virus type I–associated infective dermatitis in children. Arch. Dermatol. *134*:439-444, 1998.

118. Lambie, J. A., and Gustafson, A. A.: Contagious ecthyma in man: Report of two cases with laboratory studies. Lancet *87*:400-402, 1967.

119. Le, C. T.: Tick-borne relapsing fever in children. Pediatrics *66*:963-966, 1980.

120. Leavell, U. W., Jr., McNamara, M. J., Meulling, R. J., et al.: Ecthyma contagiosum (orf). South. Med. J. *58*:239-243, 1965.

121. Lerner, A. M., Cherry, J. D., Klein, J. O., et al.: Infections with reoviruses. N. Engl. J. Med. *267*:947-952, 1962.

122. Linnemann, C. C., Jr., and Janson, P. J.: The clinical presentations of Rocky Mountain spotted fever: Comments on recognition and management based on a study of 63 patients. Clin. Pediatr. (Phila.) *17*:673-679, 1978.

123. Litt, I. F., Edberg, S. C., and Finberg, L.: Gonorrhea in children and adolescents: A current review. J. Pediatr. *85*:595-607, 1974.

124. Liu, C., and Coffin, D. L.: Studies on canine distemper infection by means of fluorescein-labeled antibody. I. The pathogenesis, pathology, and diagnosis of the disease in experimentally infected ferrets. Virology *3*:115-131, 1957.

125. Maki, M., Vesikari, T., Rantala, I., et al.: *Yersinia* in children. Arch. Dis. Child. *55*:861-865, 1980.

126. Maloney, E. M., Hisada, M., Palmer, P., et al.: Human T cell lymphotropic virus type I–associated infective dermatitis in Jamaica: A case report of clinical and biologic correlates. Pediatr. Infect. Dis. J. *19*:560-565, 2000.

127. Martinez-Roig, A., Llorens-Terol, J., and Torres, J. M.: Erythema nodosum and kerion of the scalp. Am. J. Dis. Child. *136*:440-442, 1982.

128. Mast, W. E., and Burrows, W. M.: Erythema chronicum migrans in the United States. J. A. M. A. *236*:859-860, 1976.

129. McDade, J. E.: Ehrlichiosis: A disease of animals and humans. J. Infect. Dis. *161*:609-617, 1990.

130. McNeill, W. H.: Plagues and Peoples. Garden City, New York, Anchor Press–Doubleday, 1976, pp. 105, 119.

131. Medeiros, A. A., Marty, S. D., Tosh, F. E., et al.: Erythema nodosum and erythema multiforme as clinical manifestations of histoplasmosis in a community outbreak. N. Engl. J. Med. *274*:415-420, 1966.

132. Melish, M. E., and Glasgow, L. A.: Staphylococcal scalded skin syndrome: The expanded clinical syndrome. J. Pediatr. *78*:958-967, 1971.

133. Milder, J. E., Walzer, P. D., Kilgore, G., et al.: Clinical features of *Strongyloides stercoralis* infection in an endemic area of the United States. Gastroenterology *80*:1481-1488, 1981.

134. Mims, C. A.: Pathogenesis of rashes in virus diseases. Bacteriol. Rev. *30*:739-760, 1966.

135. Moore, P. S.: The emergence of Kaposi's sarcoma–associated herpesvirus (human herpesvirus 8). N. Engl. J. Med. *343*:1411-1413, 2000.

136. Moraga, F. A., Martinez-Roig, A., Alonso, J. L., et al.: Boutonneuse fever. Arch. Dis. Child. *57*:149-151, 1982.

137. Myskowski, P., and Ahkami, R.: Dermatologic complications of HIV infection. Med. Clin. North Am. *80*:P1415-P1435, 1996.

138. Nash, D., Mostashari, F., Fine, A., et al.: The outbreak of West Nile virus infection in the New York City area in 1999. N. Engl. J. Med. *344*:1807-1814, 2001.

139. Needlestick transmission of HTLV-III from a patient infected in Africa. Lancet *2*:1376-1377, 1984.

140. Neisson-Vernant, C., Arfi, S., Mathez, D., et al.: Needlestick HIV seroconversion in a nurse. Lancet *2*:814, 1986.

141. Niklasson, B., Espmark, A., LeDuc, J. W., et al.: Association of a Sindbis-like virus with Ockelbo disease in Sweden. Am. J. Trop. Med. Hyg. *33*:1212-1217, 1984.

142. Nussbaum, M., Scalettar, H., and Shenker, I. R.: Gonococcal arthritis-dermatitis (GADS) as a complication of gonococcemia in adolescents. Clin. Pediatr. (Phila.) *14*:1037-1040, 1975.

143. Older, J. J.: The epidemiology of murine typhus in Texas, 1969. J. A. M. A. *214*:2011-2017, 1970.

144. Orton, P. W., Huff, J. C., Tonnesen, M. G., et al.: Detection of a herpes simplex viral antigen in skin lesions of erythema multiforme. Ann. Intern. Med. *101*:48-50, 1984.

145. Patamasucon, P., Schaad, U. B., and Nelson, J. D.: Melioidosis. J. Pediatr. *100*:175-182, 1982.

146. Patel, B. M.: Skin rash with infectious mononucleosis and ampicillin. Pediatrics *40*:910-911, 1967.

147. Paterson, P. Y., and Taylor, W.: Rickettsialpox. Bull. N. Y. Acad. Med. *42*:579-587, 1966.

148. Perlman, F.: Arthropod sensitivity. *In* Criep, L. H. (ed.): Dermatologic Allergy. Philadelphia, W. B. Saunders, 1967, pp. 222-244.

149. Peter, G.: Leptospirosis: A zoonosis of protean manifestations. Pediatr. Infect. Dis. *1*:282-288, 1982.

150. Pether, J. V. S., and Lloyd, G.: The clinical spectrum of human hantavirus infection in Somerset, UK. Epidemiol. Infect. *111*:171-175, 1993.

151. Pfister, L. E., Gallagher, M. V., Potterfield, T. G., et al.: *Neisseria catarrhalis*: Bacteremia with meningitis. J. A. M. A. *193*:399-401, 1965.

152. Pittsley, R. A., Shearn, M. A., and Kaufman, L.: Acute hepatitis B simulating dermatomyositis. J. A. M. A. *239*:959, 1978.

153. Place, E. H., and Sutton, L. E.: Erythema arthriticum epidemicum (Haverhill fever). Arch. Intern. Med. *54*:659-684, 1934.

154. Platt, H.: The susceptibility of the skin and epidermoid mucous membranes to virus infection in man and other animals. J. Pathol. Bacteriol. *76*:479-497, 1948.

155. Pollowitz, J. A.: Acute urticaria associated with shigellosis: A case report. Ann. Allergy *45*:302-303, 1980.

156. Portnoy, B. L., Satterwhite, T. K., and Dyckman, J. D.: Rat bite fever misdiagnosed as Rocky Mountain spotted fever. J. South. Med. Assoc. *72*:607-609, 1979.

157. Powell, K. R.: Filatow-Dukes' disease: Epidermolytic toxin-producing staphylococci as the etiologic agent of the fourth childhood exanthem. Am. J. Dis. Child. *133*:88-90, 1979.

158. Principi, N., Bosis, S., and Esposito, S.: Human metapneumovirus in paediatric patients. Clin. Microbiol. Infect. *12*:301-308, 2006.

159. Pullen, H., Wright, N., and Murdoch, J. M.: Hypersensitivity reactions to antibacterial drugs in infectious mononucleosis. Lancet *2*:1176-1178, 1967.

160. Raoult, D., Fournier, P. E., Fenollar, F., et al.: *Rickettsia africae*, a tick-borne pathogen in travelers to sub-Saharan Africa. N. Engl. J. Med. *344*:1504-1510, 2001.

161. Rasmussen, J. E., and Graves, W. H.: *Pseudomonas aeruginosa*, hot tubs, and skin infections. Am. J. Dis. Child. *136*:553-554, 1982.

162. Resnick, S. D.: Toxic shock syndrome: Recent developments in pathogenesis. J. Pediatr. *1*:321-328, 1990.

163. Richter, H. S.: Coccidioidomycosis: A report of 300 new cases. G. P. *39*:89-92, 1969.

164. Robbins, F. C.: Measles: Clinical features. Am. J. Dis. Child. *103*:266-273, 1962.

165. Rook, A.: Papular urticaria. Pediatr. Clin. North Am. *8*:817-833, 1961.

166. Rustgi, V. K., Sacher, R. A., O'Brien, P., et al.: Fatal disseminated cytomegalovirus infection in an apparently normal adult. Arch. Intern. Med. *143*:372-373, 1983.

167. Ruzicka, T., Rosendahl, C., and Braun-Falco, O.: A probable case of rotavirus exanthem. Arch. Dermatol. *121*:253-254, 1985.

168. Saari, T. N., and Triplett, D. A.: *Yersinia pseudotuberculosis* mesenteric adenitis. J. Pediatr. *85*:656-659, 1974.

169. Sabin, A. B.: Research on dengue during World War II. Am. J. Trop. Med. *1*:30-50, 1952.

170. Sanchez, R. L., Hebert, A., Lucia, H., et al.: Orf: A case report with histologic, electron microscopic, and immunoperoxidase studies. Arch. Pathol. Lab. Med. *109*:166-170, 1985.

171. San Joaquin, V. H., and Marks, M. I.: Gianotti disease or Gianotti-Crosti syndrome? J. Pediatr. *101*:216-217, 1982.

172. Saslaw, S.: Chronic meningococcemia: Report of a case. N. Engl. J. Med. *266*:605-607, 1962.

173. Schaffner, W.: The rickettsioses. *In* Fitzpatrick, T. B., Eisen, A. Z., Wolff, K., et al. (eds.): Dermatology in General Medicine. New York, McGraw-Hill, 1979, pp. 1563-1570.

174. Schmaljohn, C., and Hjelle, B.: Hantaviruses: A global disease problem. Emerg. Infect. Dis. *3*:95-104, 1997.

175. Schneider, J. A., Poley, J. R., Millunchick, E. W., et al.: Papular acrodermatitis (Gianotti-Crosti syndrome) in a child with anicteric hepatitis B, virus subtype adw. J. Pediatr. *101*:219-222, 1982.

176. Shama, S. K., Etkind, P. H., Odell, T. M., et al.: Gypsy-moth-caterpillar dermatitis. N. Engl. J. Med. *306*:1300-1301, 1982.

177. Shanson, D. C., Gazzard, B. G., Midgley, J., et al.: *Streptobacillus moniliformis* isolated from blood in four cases of Haverhill fever: First outbreak in Britain. Lancet *2*:92-94, 1983.

178. Shapiro, L.: The numbered diseases: First through sixth. J. A. M. A. *194*:210, 1965.

179. Shapiro, L.: On the numbered exanthemata. Clin. Pediatr. (Phila.) *6*:611-612, 1967.

180. Shaw, E. B.: Fifth disease. Am. J. Dis. Child. *131*:816, 1977.

181. Shelley, E. D., Shelley, W. B., Pula, J. F., et al.: The diagnostic challenge of nonburrowing mite bites: *Cheyletiella yasguri*. J. A. M. A. *251*:2690-2691, 1984.

182. Siewers, C. M. F., and Cramblett, H. G.: Cryptococcosis (torulosis) in children: A report of four cases. Pediatrics 34:393-400, 1964.
183. Smith, A. W., Berry, E. S., Skilling, D. E., et al.: In vitro isolation and characterization of a calicivirus causing a vesicular disease of the hands and feet. Clin. Infect. Dis. 26:434-439, 1998.
184. Smith, P. T., Landry, M. L., Carey, H., et al.: Papular-purpuric gloves and socks syndrome associated with acute parvovirus B19 infection: Case report and review. Clin. Infect. Dis. 27:164-168, 1998.
185. Smith, S. B., Libow, L. F., Elston, D., M., et al.: Gloves and socks syndrome: Early and late histopathologic features. J. Am. Acad. Dermatol. 47:749-754, 2002.
186. Somer, T., and Finegold, S. M.: Vasculitides associated with infections, immunization, and antimicrobial drugs. Clin. Infect. Dis. 20:1010-1036, 1995.
187. Spelman, D. W.: Q fever: A study of 111 consecutive cases. Med. J. Aust. 1:547-553, 1982.
188. Steere, A. C., Broderick, T. F., and Malawista, S. E.: Erythema chronicum migrans and Lyme arthritis: Epidemiologic evidence for a tick vector. Am. J. Epidemiol. 108:312-321, 1978.
189. Stricof, R. L., and Morse, D. L.: HTLV-III/LAV seroconversion following a deep intramuscular needlestick injury. N. Engl. J. Med. 314:1115, 1986.
190. Strong, W. B.: Petechiae and streptococcal pharyngitis. Am. J. Dis. Child. 117:156-160, 1969.
191. Swartz, M. N., and Weinberg, A. N.: Infections due to gram-positive bacteria. In Fitzpatrick, T. B., Eisen, A. Z., Wolff, K., et al. (eds.): Dermatology in General Medicine. New York, McGraw-Hill, 1979, pp. 1426-1445.
192. Swartz, M. N., and Weinberg, A. N.: Miscellaneous bacterial infections with cutaneous manifestations. In Fitzpatrick, T. B., Eisen, A. Z., Wolff, K., et al. (eds.): Dermatology in General Medicine. New York, McGraw-Hill, 1979, pp. 1459-1473.
193. Taieb, A., Plantin, P., DuPasquier, P., et al.: Gianotti-Crosti syndrome: A study of 26 cases. Br. J. Dermatol. 115:49-59, 1986.
194. Taylor, P. R., Weinstein, W. M., and Bryner, J. H.: *Campylobacter* fetus infection in human subjects: Association with raw milk. Am. J. Med. 66:779-783, 1979.
195. Tertti, R., Granfors, K., Lehtonen, O. P., et al.: An outbreak of *Yersinia pseudotuberculosis* infection. J. Infect. Dis. 149:245-250, 1984.
196. Thomas, P., Moore, M., Bell, E., et al.: *Pseudomonas* dermatitis associated with a swimming pool. J. A. M. A. 253:1156-1159, 1985.
197. Timar, L., Budai, J., Gero, A., et al.: Rare complications and unusual syndromes associated with Epstein-Barr virus. Pediatr. Infect. Dis. 4:212-213, 1985.
198. Timar, L., Budai, J., and Koller, M.: A prospective study on infectious mononucleosis in childhood—symptoms, serology, Epstein-Barr virus specific leukocyte migration inhibition. Infection 10:139-143, 1982.
199. Toth, M., Barna, M., and Voltay, B.: Aetiology of acute respiratory diseases in infants and children. Acta Paediatr. Hung. 6:367-374, 1966.
200. Tudor, R. B.: Urticaria in childhood. Lancet 82:273-274, 1962.
201. Turner, T. W., and Wilkinson, D. S.: *Pasteurella pseudotuberculosis* as a cause of erythema nodosum. Br. J. Dermatol. 81:823-826, 1969.
202. Unger, A., Tapia, L., Minnich, L. L., et al.: Atypical neonatal respiratory syncytial virus infection. J. Pediatr. 100:762-764, 1982.
203. Utz, J. P., and Shadomy, H. J.: Deep fungus infections. In Fitzpatrick, T. B., Eisen, A. Z., Wolff, K., et al. (eds.): Dermatology in General Medicine. New York, McGraw-Hill, 1979, pp. 1533-1563.
204. Van Arsdall, J. A., Wunderlich, H. F., Melo, J. C., et al.: The protean manifestations of legionnaires disease. J. Infect. Dis. 7:51-62, 1983.
205. Ware, R.: Human parvovirus infection. J. Pediatr. 114:343-348, 1989.
206. Weinberg, A. N., and Swartz, M. N.: Gram-negative coccal and bacillary infections. In Fitzpatrick, T. B., Eisen, A. Z., Wolff, K., et al. (eds.): Dermatology in General Medicine. New York, McGraw-Hill, 1979, pp. 1445-1459.
207. Weller, T. H.: The cytomegaloviruses: Ubiquitous agents with protean clinical manifestations. I and II. N. Engl. J. Med. 285:203-214, 267-274, 1971.
208. Wenner, H. A.: Virus diseases associated with cutaneous eruptions. Prog. Med. Virol. 16:269-336, 1973.
209. Wenner, H. A., and Lou, T. Y.: Virus diseases associated with cutaneous eruptions. Prog. Med. Virol. 5:219-294, 1963.
210. Whiteford, S. F., Taylor, J. P., and Dumler, J. S.: Clinical, laboratory, and epidemiology features of murine typhus in 97 Texas children. Arch. Pediatr. Adolesc. Med. 155:396-400, 2001.
211. Wiesenthal, A. M., and Todd, J. K.: Toxic shock syndrome in children aged 10 years or less. Pediatrics 74:112-117, 1984.
212. Winn, W. A., Levine, H. B., Broderick, J. E., et al.: A localized epidemic of coccidioidal infection: Primary coccidioidomycosis occurring in a group of ten children infected in a backyard playground in the San Joaquin Valley of California. N. Engl. J. Med. 268:867-870, 1963.
213. Wolff, K.: Mycobacterial diseases: Tuberculosis. In Fitzpatrick, T. B., Eisen, A. Z., Wolff, K., et al. (eds.): Dermatology in General Medicine. New York, McGraw-Hill, 1979, pp. 1473-1492.
214. Wong, M. L., Kaplan, S., Dunkle, L. M., et al.: Leptospirosis: A childhood disease. J. Pediatr. 90:532-537, 1977.
215. Woodward, T. E.: Rocky mountain spotted fever: Epidemiological and early clinical signs are keys to treatment and reduced mortality. J. Infect. Dis. 150:465-468, 1984.
216. Yamamoto, T., and Yokoyama, A.: Hepatitis C virus infection and nodular prurigo. Br. J. Dermatol. 135:489-504, 1996.
217. Yamanishi, K., Shiraki, K., Kondo T., et al.: Identification of human herpesvirus-6 as a causal agent for exanthem subitum. Lancet 1:1065-1067, 1988.
218. Young, E. J.: Human brucellosis. Rev. Infect. Dis. 5:821-842, 1983.

CHAPTER
65

ROSEOLA INFANTUM (EXANTHEM SUBITUM)

James D. Cherry

Roseola infantum (i.e., exanthem subitum, pseudorubella, exanthem criticum, sixth disease, or 3-day fever) is a common, acute illness of young children characterized by a fever of 3 to 5 days' duration, rapid defervescence, and then the appearance of an erythematous macular or maculopapular rash that persists for 1 to 2 days.

HISTORY

Zahorsky[80] generally is given credit for the original description of roseola infantum. In his writings, he pointed out, however, that the syndrome was described in earlier pediatric and dermatology texts.[81-83] Altschuler[1] observed that a British dermatologist, Willan, presented a description of the illness in his 1809 book *On Cutaneous Diseases*. The descriptions in the older literature did not separate the syndrome from the known exanthematous diseases (i.e., measles, rubella, and scarlet fever), an omission that Zahorsky corrected.

In 1921, Veeder and Hempelmann[75] described the syndrome further and noted that leukopenia and relative lymphocytosis occurred. These investigators objected to the name *roseola infantum*, which in the past had been used to describe a large group of diseases with indefinite causes. They suggested the term *exanthem subitum* because it was "descriptive of the most striking clinical symptom, namely, the sudden, unexpected appearance of the eruption on the fourth day." Currently, the term *roseola* is used most commonly to describe the syndrome.

From 1920 through 1940, many excellent clinical descriptions of the syndrome were published.* From 1940 through 1988, articles relating to roseola were concerned with unusual manifestations and complications[8,11-13,22,32,46,48,49,53,56,63] and attempts to recover an etiologic agent.[26,30,40,45,64] In 1988, Yamanishi and associates[78] identified human herpesvirus–6 (HHV-6) in the blood of infants with roseola, and since then, the association between this virus and the disease has been confirmed on many occasions.† HHV-7 also has been found to be the cause of many cases of roseola.[3,14,31,68,71,72,74]

---

*See references 6, 7, 10, 17, 18, 20, 24, 25, 36, 83, 84.
†See references 2-5, 9, 19, 21, 27, 28, 33-35, 39, 41-44, 54, 58, 60, 66-69, 76, 85.

EPIDEMIOLOGY

In his original article, Zahorsky[80] reported that roseola occurred most commonly in the fall. In his second article, he observed a year-round incidence[81]; in 1925, he pointed out that most cases occurred in the spring, summer, and fall.[82] Breese[10] noted that the greatest number of cases occurred in the summer and early fall. In contrast, 55 percent of Clemens' cases occurred in February, March, and April; 16 percent were seen in October.[17] In a review of 243 cases during a 10-year period, Juretic[38] observed that the peak month was May. Juretic also reviewed the seasonal incidence in 10 other studies and found only minor variations by month. Prevalence was greatest in March, April, and October and least in December. One epidemic of roseola in a maternity hospital occurred in the summer,[36] another epidemic in an infants' home occurred in the fall,[6] and a hospital outbreak occurred in the winter.[18]

Roseola predominantly is an illness of young children. It occurs rarely in infants younger than 3 months old or children older than 4 years. In a review of 1462 cases, the peak age range prevalence was 7 to 13 months of age; 55 percent of the cases occurred within the first year of life, and 90 percent occurred within the first 2 years of life.[38] Occasionally, cases have been seen in older children, adolescents, and young adults and in neonates and other infants younger than 6 months.[25,36]

Although Faber and Dickey[20] found twice as many girls as boys with the syndrome, the sex ratio in most large studies has been equal.[7,10,17,25,45] Although three epidemics have been reported, and cases frequently occur in groups by season, most cases occur sporadically without known exposure. The syndrome, when seen sporadically, generally is considered to be noncontagious, but secondary cases have been reported occasionally.[6,10,18,36] The incubation period range in epidemics is 5 to 15 days.[6,10,18]

The attack rate of roseola has not been well studied. Berenberg and associates[7] stated that roseola is the exanthem most commonly encountered in children younger than 2 years old. Breese[10] found that 16 percent of a group of infants he followed for the first 12 months of life had definite roseola. He estimated that 30 percent of children would have clinical roseola. Juretic[38] looked at the frequency of roseola in 6735 children; the yearly attack rate during a 10-year period ranged from 1 to 10 percent, with a mean of 3.3 percent.

ETIOLOGY

In 1941, Breese[10] reported vigorous attempts to isolate a filterable virus from three children with pre-eruptive roseola. These studies included extensive animal inoculations, but no viral agents were uncovered. In 1950, Kempe and associates[40] reported the passage of the illness to a 6-month-old susceptible infant by the intravenous injection of serum from an 18-month-old child with pre-eruptive roseola. Febrile illnesses without exanthem also were produced in monkeys with serum and throat washings from a child with the syndrome. In similar experiments, Hellström and Vahlquist[30] produced the syndrome in three children aged 6 to 9 days after the intramuscular administration of blood from typical roseola cases.

In electron microscopic studies, Reagan and associates[61] observed uniform virus-like particles (100-110 nm) in the blood of an 18-month-old child with the syndrome. Febrile illness was produced in two monkeys after concentrated virus-containing material was inoculated.

Since the advent of modern diagnostic virology in the early 1950s, numerous viral agents have been recovered from children with roseola. In 1951, Neva and associates[52] studied an epidemic exanthematous illness (i.e., Boston exanthem) caused by echovirus 16, in which many of the illnesses were characteristic of roseola. In 1954, Neva[50] observed additional cases of roseola-like illness associated with echovirus 16 infection. In 1974, Hall and colleagues[27] reported four additional echovirus 16 infections with clinical manifestations of roseola. The reporting of roseola in Rochester, New York, nearly doubled during the time of echovirus 16 activity in the area. Roseola-like illnesses that also have been associated with these enteroviruses are caused by coxsackievirus A6, A9, B1, B2, B4, and B5 and echovirus 9, 11, 25, 27, and 30.[15,16,27,66,77] Outbreaks of roseola that occur in the summer and fall probably are caused by enteroviral infections.

In addition to enteroviruses, adenovirus types 1, 2, 3, and 14 and parainfluenza type 1 virus have been recovered from children with roseola.[23,37,51,77] Saitoh and associates[64] detected rotavirus capsomeres in fecal specimens of nine children with roseola. In contrast to these findings, Gurwith and colleagues[26] studied fecal specimens from five children with roseola, and in none were viral particles identified. One of 13 children in this study did develop antibody to rotavirus around the time of illness, however. In addition to the occurrence of roseola associated with numerous natural viral infections, its pattern (i.e., fever and then rash with defervescence) was observed frequently in recipients of Edmonton B measles vaccine.[15]

In 1988, Yamanishi and associates[78] isolated HHV-6 from four infants with roseola, and all four had significant titer increases for this virus. Shortly after this finding was reported, several other investigators noted similar findings.[2,4,19,33,42,69,73] The implication from these studies, as suggested by the various investigators, is that HHV-6 is the cause of roseola. This viewpoint overlooks or ignores the past experience in which other viral agents have been associated with the clinical syndrome. Subsequent studies indicate that HHV-6 is a major cause of roseola and the cause of acute febrile illness without exanthem in infants.* Since 1993, HHV-7 has been accepted as an additional causative agent in roseola.[3,14,31,68,71,76]

In a study of 1653 infants and young children with acute febrile illnesses, Hall and colleagues[27] found that 160 (9.7%) had primary HHV-6 infections; 27 (17%) of the children who were infected with HHV-6 had roseola. Zerr and associates[85] identified 80 children with primary HHV-6 infections, and of these, 30 percent had roseola. In the same population-based study, 3 of 80 (4%) children without primary HHV-6 infection also had roseola. In a study of clinical roseola, Okada and associates[54] found that 81 percent had serologic evidence of HHV-6 infection, and that 8 percent had an echovirus-18 infection. In a study of roseola in Italy, Braito and Uberti[9] found serologic evidence of HHV-6 infection in only 30 percent of the cases. In 33 percent of the remaining cases, they attributed the illnesses to another infectious agent. In 1994, Hidaka and associates[31] estimated that 73.5 percent, 10.2 percent, and 16.3 percent of their roseola cases were caused by HHV-6, HHV-7, and other viruses. HHV-6 seems to be the major cause of roseola.

PATHOPHYSIOLOGY

The pathophysiology of roseola is unknown. Watson[77] suggested that roseola is not an infection caused by one particular pathogen, but is the result of an immunizing reaction against many different viruses. He also suggested that the rash is caused by the neutralization of virus in the skin at the end of the period of viremia.

Because viremia is common in HHV-6, HHV-7, enteroviral, and adenoviral infections, a reasonable conclusion is that the rash in roseola is related to an immunologic event resulting from the virus that is localized in the skin. Why the pattern of fever and then rash with defervescence is so clearly age-dependent is

---

*See references 5, 9, 27, 34, 41, 44, 54, 58, 60, 67, 76, 85.

unknown. Most of the viruses that in the past have been associated with roseola cause other exanthematous manifestations in older patients.[15]

CLINICAL PRESENTATION

The basic clinical pattern of roseola is a febrile period of 3 to 5 days, defervescence, and the appearance of a rash that persists for 1 to 2 days. Because the syndrome is caused by many different viruses, the illness apparently may be associated with numerous other symptoms and signs. The major manifestations have been reviewed elsewhere.[7,10,17,25,38,81]

Illness usually occurs with the apparent abrupt onset of fever. Slight irritability and malaise occur frequently, but more commonly, the child's temperature is taken because a parent notices that the child feels warm. The temperature usually is in the range of 38.9°C to 40.6°C (102°F to 105°F). Despite the high fever, the child usually is active, alert, and generally unphased. The fever is constant or intermittent, with its greatest degree occurring in the early evening. Restlessness and irritability occur with higher temperatures. The usual duration of fever is 3 to 5 days, but it has persisted for 9 days. The temperature most often returns to normal by crisis, but in some cases, temperature "lysis" occurs over the course of 24 to 36 hours.

Mild cough and coryza are seen frequently in cases occurring in the winter and spring. Headache and abdominal pain are reported in older children, mainly in the summer and fall. Vomiting and diarrhea occur infrequently.

On initial physical examination during the febrile period, most children appear to be happy, alert, and playful. With high temperatures, some children are irritable; occasionally, a child appears to be sick, which suggests more serious illness, such as meningitis or septicemia. Examination within the oral cavity frequently reveals one or more abnormalities. Mild inflammation of the pharynx and tonsils occurs most commonly. Occasionally, small exudative follicular lesions are noted on the tonsils. In other cases, small ulcerative lesions on the soft palate, uvula, and tonsillar pillars are observed. Usually, the lesions on the soft palate consist of only erythematous macules and maculopapules, presumably because of lymphoid hyperplasia.

Mild injection of the tympanic membranes occurs commonly. Enlargement of the suboccipital, posterior cervical, and post-auricular lymph nodes is a common finding, but the degree is not remarkable.

Berliner[8] noticed that children with roseola had palpebral edema. He suggested that the "heavy eyelids" or "droopy" or "sleepy" appearance resulting from this edema was diagnostic of the syndrome before the appearance of the rash. Bulging of the anterior fontanelle also has been observed in roseola.[56]

Appearance of the rash in roseola usually coincides with the subsidence of fever, but it may occur after an afebrile interlude of several hours to 2 days. When defervescence occurs by lysis, onset of the exanthem can occur before the temperature has returned entirely to normal. By definition, it is incorrect, however, to call an illness roseola if the fever and rash are truly concomitant.

Zahorsky[80,81] originally described the rash as morbilliform, but his use of morbilliform was not the same as ours is today (i.e., measles-like, erythematous, maculopapular with confluence). The rash is erythematous and macular or maculopapular, and the lesions are discrete. The lesions are 2 to 5 mm in diameter, and they blanch on pressure. Frequently, individual lesions are surrounded by a whitish ring. The rash is most prominent on the neck and trunk, but the proximal extremities and the face also may be affected. Although they have been reported,[17,24] pruritus and desquamation usually do not occur. The rash usually persists for 24 to 48 hours. In occasional cases, well-documented rashes

have been observed to appear and resolve within 2 to 4 hours. Yoshida and associates[79] described a 7-month-old boy with HHV-6 infection and typical roseola initially. On the ninth day of illness, vesicular lesions appeared on the face and limbs, however. These lesions persisted for 12 days.

Except for the white blood cell count, routine laboratory studies are of little use in roseola. The total white blood cell count usually is low. Early in the febrile period, high counts occasionally are found, however. The total count reaches its nadir by the third to sixth day of illness, and then gradually returns to normal over the ensuing 7 to 10 days. During the same time frame, the percentage of lymphocytes increases from a normal value of about 50 percent to 60 to 80 percent on days 3 to 10, and then returns to normal over the next 7 days. Frequently, extreme counts in the range of 3000 cells/mm^3 with 90 percent lymphocytes are found, which raises the consideration of a granulocytic defect.

CLINICAL COMPLICATIONS

The most important complications of roseola are convulsions and other neurologic symptoms.* The incidence of convulsions has varied widely among reports. Juretic[38] did not find one instance of convulsions in the 243 cases in his study. Breese[10] did not report convulsions in any of 100 roseola attacks that he studied. In contrast, Greenthal[25] noted convulsions in 6 percent of his cases, and Faber and Dickey[20] found seizures in 8 of 26 cases of roseola. Möller[48] observed that 8 percent of children admitted to the hospital because of febrile convulsions eventually were diagnosed with roseola infantum.

Möller[48] also reported cerebrospinal fluid evaluations in 29 cases of roseola and febrile convulsions. In six instances, the pressure was elevated; in two, there were 5 white blood cells/mm^3; and in another instance, there were 9 white blood cells/mm^3. In most other cerebrospinal fluid examinations, the findings have been normal, but mild pleocytosis with mononuclear cells has been identified occasionally.[7,32] A surprising number of cases of encephalitis associated with roseola have been reported,[13,22,32,35] and residua have been common. Hemiplegia has occurred after illness,[13,22,59,62] and permanent paresis and mental retardation have occurred in some affected patients. The syndrome of inappropriate secretion of antidiuretic hormone has been reported in roseola associated with HHV-6 infection.[55,65] Facial nerve palsy and Guillain-Barré syndrome also have been noted after HHV-6 induced roseola.[47,57]

Thrombocytopenic purpura was noted in one report in five children with roseola; all of these patients recovered.[53] In a more recent study, Hashimoto and colleagues[29] noted five children with thrombocytopenia during the acute phase of roseola caused by HHV-6 infection. Their data suggested that the thrombocytopenia was due to bone marrow suppression, rather than immune-mediated peripheral consumption. A 14-month-old girl developed a generalized eruptive histiocytoma with rapid progression and then resolution after roseola.[70]

DIAGNOSIS

Although detecting leukopenia with relative lymphocytosis is fortuitous, the only necessity in establishing the diagnosis of roseola is to document the fever, defervescence, and exanthem pattern. Frequently, the first exanthematous illness that a child has is called roseola, regardless of whether the exanthem and the fever are concomitant, or the child has no febrile period at all.

*See references 2, 7, 11-13, 20, 22, 25, 32, 35, 43, 48, 59, 62, 63.

The only problem in the differential diagnosis occurs when a febrile child is receiving antibiotics and a rash follows defervescence. This event occurs frequently, and the child usually is labeled allergic to the antibiotic, rather than suspected of having roseola. In most instances of drug allergy, the exanthem lasts longer than roseola does, and in allergic cases, pruritus and fever may accompany the rash.

TREATMENT AND PROGNOSIS

No specific treatment for roseola exists. When fever is a problem, it may be treated with acetaminophen. Acetaminophen can alter the temperature curve, possibly obscuring the correct diagnosis. Febrile seizures and other neurologic complications should be treated vigorously.

In most cases, the outlook is excellent. When encephalitis occurs, the prognosis must be guarded. Because roseola is the result of infection with multiple different viruses, no practical way to prevent it exists.

REFERENCES

1. Altschuler, E. L.: Oldest description of roseola and implications for the antiquity of human herpesvirus 6. Pediatr. Infect. Dis. 19:903, 2000.
2. Asano, Y., Nakashima, T., Yoshikawa, T., et al.: Severity of human herpesvirus-6 viremia and clinical findings in infants with exanthem subitum. J. Pediatr. 118:891-895, 1991.
3. Asano, Y., Suga, S., Yoshikawa, T., et al.: Clinical features and viral excretion in an infant with primary human herpesvirus 7 infection. Pediatrics 95:187-190, 1995.
4. Asano, Y., Yoshikawa, T., Suga, S., et al.: Viremia and neutralizing antibody response in infants with exanthem subitum. J. Pediatr. 114:535-539, 1989.
5. Asano, Y., Yoshikawa, T., Suga, S., et al.: Clinical features of infants with primary human herpesvirus 6 infection (exanthem subitum, roseola infantum). Pediatrics 93:104-108, 1994.
6. Barenberg, L. H., and Greenspan, L.: Exanthema subitum (roseola infantum). Am. J. Dis. Child. 58:983-993, 1939.
7. Berenberg, W., Wright, S., and Janeway, C. A.: Roseola infantum (exanthem subitum). N. Engl. J. Med. 241:253-259, 1949.
8. Berliner, B. C.: A physical sign useful in diagnosis of roseola infantum before the rash. Pediatrics 25:1034, 1960.
9. Braito, A., and Uberti, M.: Roseola infantum and its correlation with HHV6. Eur. J. Pediatr. 153:209, 1994.
10. Breese, B. B., Jr.: Roseola infantum (exanthem subitum). N. Y. State J. Med. 41:1854-1859, 1941.
11. Broberger, A. O.: Exanthema subitum och feberkramper. Nord. Med. 59:523-525, 1958.
12. Brunner, V. N.: 172 Fälle von exanthema subitum aus praxis und klinik. Helv. Paediatr. Acta 14:408-425, 1959.
13. Burnstine, R. C., and Paine, R. S.: Residual encephalopathy following roseola infantum. Am. J. Dis. Child. 98:144-152, 1959.
14. Caserta, M. T., Hall, C. B., Schnabel, K., et al.: Primary human herpesvirus 7 infection: A comparison of human herpesvirus 7 and human herpesvirus 6 infections in children. J. Pediatr. 133:386-389, 1998.
15. Cherry, J. D.: Newer viral exanthems. Adv. Pediatr. 16:233, 1969.
16. Cherry, J. D., Lerner, A. M., Klein, J. O., et al.: Coxsackie B5 infections with exanthems. Pediatrics 31:455-462, 1963.
17. Clemens, H. H.: Exanthem subitum (roseola infantum): Report of eighty cases. J. Pediatr. 26:66-77, 1945.
18. Cushing, H. B.: An epidemic of roseola infantum. Can. Med. Assoc. J. 17:905-906, 1927.
19. Enders, G., Biber, M., Meyer, G., et al.: Prevalence of antibodies to human herpesvirus 6 in different age groups, in children with exanthema subitum, other acute exanthematous childhood diseases, Kawasaki syndrome, and acute infections with other herpesviruses and HIV. Infection 18:12-15, 1990.
20. Faber, H. K., and Dickey, L. B.: The symptomatology of exanthem subitum. Arch. Pediatr. 44:491-496, 1927.
21. Fox, J. D., Ward, P., Briggs, M., et al.: Production of IgM antibody to HHV6 in reactivation and primary infection. Epidemiol. Infect. 104:289-296, 1990.
22. Friedman, J. H., Golomb, J., and Aronson, L.: Hemiplegia associated with roseola infantum (exanthem subitum). N. Y. State J. Med. 50:1749-1750, 1950.
23. Fukumi, H., Nishikawa, F., Kokubu, Y., et al.: Isolation of adenovirus from an exanthematous infection resembling roseola infantum. Jpn. J. Med. Sci. Biol. 10:87-91, 1957.
24. Greenthal, R. M.: An unusual exanthem occurring in infants. Am. J. Dis. Child. 23:63-65, 1922.
25. Greenthal, R. M.: Roseola infantum (exanthem subitum). Wisc. Med. J. 40:25-27, 1941.
26. Gurwith, M., Gurwith, D., Wenman, W., et al.: Exanthem subitum not associated with rotavirus. N. Engl. J. Med. 305:174-175, 1981.
27. Hall, C. B., Cherry, J. D., Hatch, M. H., et al.: The return of Boston exanthem: Echovirus 16 infections in 1974. Am. J. Dis. Child. 131:323-326, 1977.
28. Hall, C. B., Long, C. E., Schnabel, K. C., et al.: Human herpesvirus-6 infection in children: A prospective study of complications and reactivation. N. Engl. J. Med. 331:432-438, 1994.
29. Hashimoto, H., Maruyama, H., Fujimoto, K., et al.: Hematologic findings associated with thrombocytopenia during the acute phase of exanthem subitum confirmed by primary human herpesvirus-6 infection. J. Pediatr. Hematol. Oncol. 24:211-214, 2002.
30. Hellström, B., and Vahlquist, B.: Experimental inoculation of roseola infantum. Acta Paediatr. 40:189-197, 1951.
31. Hidaka, Y., Okada, K., Kusuhara, K., et al.: Exanthem subitum and human herpesvirus 7 infection. Pediatr. Infect. Dis. 13:1010-1011, 1994.
32. Holliday, P. B., Jr.: Pre-eruptive neurological complications of the common contagious diseases: Rubella, rubeola, roseola, and varicella. J. Pediatr. 36:185-198, 1950.
33. Huang, L. M., Lee, C. Y., Chen, J. Y., et al.: Primary human herpesvirus 6 infections in children: A prospective serologic study. J. Infect. Dis. 165:1163-1164, 1992.
34. Irving, W. L., Chang, J., Raymond, D. R., et al.: Roseola infantum and other syndromes associated with acute HHV6 infection. Arch. Dis. Child. 65:1297-1300, 1990.
35. Ishiguro, N., Yamada, S., Takahashi, T., et al.: Meningoencephalitis associated with HHV-6-related exanthem subitum. Acta Paediatr. Scand. 79:987-989, 1990.
36. James, U., and Freier, A.: Roseola infantum: An outbreak in a maternity hospital. Arch. Dis. Child. 23-24:54-58, 1948-1949.
37. Jansson, E., Wager, O., Forssell, P., et al.: An exanthema subitumlike rash in patients with adenovirus infection. Ann. Paediatr. Fenn. 7:3-11, 1961.
38. Juretic, M.: Exanthema subitum: A review of 243 cases. Helv. Paediatr. Acta 18:80-95, 1963.
39. Kawaguchi, S., Suga, S., Kozawa, T., et al.: Primary human herpesvirus-6 infection (exanthem subitum) in the newborn. Pediatrics 90:628-630, 1992.
40. Kempe, C. H., Shaw, E. B., Jackson, J. R., et al.: Studies on the etiology of exanthema subitum (roseola infantum). J. Pediatr. 37:561-568, 1950.
41. Knowles, W., and Gardner, S.: High prevalence of antibody to human herpesvirus 6 and seroconversion associated with rash in 2 infants. Lancet 2:912-913, 1988.
42. Kodo, S., Kondo, K., Kondo, T., et al.: Detection of human herpesvirus 6 DNA in throat swabs by polymerase chain reaction. J. Med. Virol. 32:139-142, 1990.
43. Kondo, K., Nagafuji, H., Hata, A., et al.: Association of human herpesvirus 6 infection of the central nervous system with recurrence of febrile convulsions. J. Infect. Dis. 167:1197-1200, 1993.
44. Kusuhara, K., Ueda, K., Okada, K., et al.: Do second attacks of exanthema subitum result from human herpesvirus-6 reactivation or reinfection? Pediatr. Infect. Dis. J. 10:468-469, 1991.
45. Letchner, A.: Roseola infantum: A review of fifty cases. Lancet 2:1163-1165, 1955.
46. McEnery, J. T.: Postoccipital lymphadenopathy as a diagnostic sign in roseola infantum (exanthem subitum). Clin. Pediatr. 9:512-514, 1970.
47. Miyake, F., Yoshikawa, T., Suzuki, K., et al.: Guillain-Barré syndrome after exanthem subitum. Pediatr. Infect. Dis. J. 21:569-570, 2002.
48. Möller, K. L.: Exanthema subitum and febrile convulsions. Acta Paediatr. 45:534-540, 1956.
49. Moore, W. F., Jr.: Roseola infantum. Hawaii Med. J. 22:431-434, 1963.
50. Neva, F. A.: A second outbreak of Boston exanthem disease in Pittsburgh during 1954. N. Engl. J. Med. 254:838, 1956.
51. Neva, F. A., and Enders, J. F.: Isolation of a cytopathogenic agent from an infant with a disease in certain respects resembling roseola infantum. J. Immunol. 72:315-321, 1954.
52. Neva, F. A., Feemster, R. F., and Gorback, I. J.: Clinical and epidemiological features of an unusual epidemic exanthem. J. A. M. A. 155:544, 1954.
53. Nishimura, K., and Igarashi, M.: Thrombocytopenic purpura associated with exanthem subitum. Pediatrics 60:260, 1977.
54. Okada, K., Ueda, K., Kusuhara, K., et al.: Exanthema subitum and human herpesvirus 6 infection: Clinical observations in fifty-seven cases. Pediatr. Infect. Dis. 12:204-208, 1993.
55. Okafuji, T., Uchiyama, H., Okabe, N., et al.: Syndrome of inappropriate secretion of antidiuretic hormone associated with exanthem subitum. Pediatr. Infect. Dis. 16:532-533, 1997.
56. Oski, F. A.: Roseola infantum: Another case of bulging fontanel. Am. J. Dis. Child. 101:376-378, 1961.
57. Pitkäranta, A., Lahdenne, P., and Piiparinen, H.: Facial nerve palsy after human herpesvirus 6 infection. Pediatr. Infect. Dis. J. 23:688-659, 2004.
58. Portolani, M., Cermelli, C., Moroni, A., et al.: Human herpesvirus-6 infections in infants admitted to hospital. J. Med. Virol. 39:146-151, 1993.
59. Posson, D. D.: Exanthem subitum (roseola infantum) complicated by prolonged convulsions and hemiplegia. J. Pediatr. 35:235-236, 1949.
60. Pruksananonda, P., Hall, C. B., Insel, R. A., et al.: Primary human herpesvirus 6 infection in young children. N. Engl. J. Med. 326:1445-1450, 1992.

61. Reagan, R. L., Chang, S. C., Moolten, S. E., et al.: Electron microscopic studies of the roseola infantum (exanthem subitum) virus. Tex. Rep. Biol. Med. *13*:929-933, 1955.
62. Rosenblum, J.: Roseola infantum (exanthem subitum) complicated by hemiplegia. Am. J. Dis. Child. *69*:234-236, 1945.
63. Rothman, P. E., and Naiditch, M. J.: Nervous complications of exanthem subitum. Calif. Med. J. *88*:39-44, 1958.
64. Saitoh, Y., Matsuno, S., and Mukoyama, A.: Exanthem subitum and rotavirus. N. Engl. J. Med. *304*:845, 1981.
65. Shimura, N., Kim, H., Sugimoto, H.. et al.: Syndrome of inappropriate secretion of antidiuretic hormone as a complication of human herpesvirus-6 infection. Pediatr. Int. *46*:497-498, 2004.
66. St. Geme, J. W., Jr., Prince, J. T., Scherer, W. F., et al.: A clinical study of an exanthem due to ECHO virus type 9. J. Pediatr. *54*:459-467, 1959.
67. Suga, S., Yazaki, T., Kajita, Y., et al.: Detection of human herpesvirus 6 DNAs in samples from several body sites of patients with exanthem subitum and their mothers by polymerase chain reaction assay. J. Med. Virol. *46*:52-55, 1995.
68. Suga, S., Yoshikawa, T., Nagai, T., et al.: Clinical features and virological findings in children with primary human herpesvirus 7 infection. Pediatrics *99*:e4, 1997.
69. Takahashi, K., Sonoda, S., Kawakami, K., et al.: Human herpesvirus 6 and exanthem subitum. Lancet *1*:1463, 1988.
70. Tamiya, H., Tsuruta, D., Takeda, E., et al.: Generalized eruptive histiocytoma with rapid progression and resolution following exanthema subitum. Clin. Exp. Dermatol. *30*:294-307, 2005.
71. Tanaka, K., Kondo, T., Torigoe, S., et al.: Human herpesvirus 7: Another causal agent for roseola (exanthem subitum). J. Pediatr. *125*:1-5, 1994.

72. Torigoe, S., Kumamoto, T., Koide, W., et al.: Clinical manifestations associated with human herpesvirus 7 infection. Arch. Dis. Child. *72*:518-519, 1995.
73. Ueda, K., Kusuhara, K., Hirose, M., et al.: Exanthem subitum and antibody to human herpesvirus-6. J. Infect. Dis. *159*:750-752, 1989.
74. Ueda, K., Kusuhara, K., Okada, K.: Primary human herpesvirus 7 infection and exanthem subitum. Pediatr. Infect. Dis. J. *13*:167-168, 1994.
75. Veeder, B. S., and Hempelmann, T. C.: A febrile exanthem occurring in childhood (exanthem subitum). J. A. M. A. 77:1787-1789, 1921.
76. Ward, K. N.: The natural history and laboratory diagnosis of human herpesviruses-6 and -7 infections in the immunocompetent. J. Clin. Virol. *32*:183-193, 2005.
77. Watson, G. I.: The roseolar reaction. B. M. J. *4*:719-720, 1974.
78. Yamanishi, K., Okuno, T., Shiraki, K., et al.: Identification of human herpesvirus-6 as a causal agent for exanthem subitum. Lancet *1*:1065-1067, 1988.
79. Yoshida, M., Fukui, K., Orita, T., et al.: Exanthem subitum (roseola infantum) with vesicular lesions. Br. J. Dermatol. *132*:614-616, 1995.
80. Zahorsky, J.: Roseola infantilis. Pediatrics 22:60-64, 1910.
81. Zahorsky, J.: Roseola infantum. J. A. M. A. *61*:1446-1450, 1913.
82. Zahorsky, J.: Roseola infantum: The rose rash of infants. Arch. Pediatr. *42*:610-613, 1925.
83. Zahorsky, J.: Roseola infantum: A critical survey of some recent literature. Arch. Pediatr. 57:405-409, 1940.
84. Zahorsky, J.: Roseola infantum, a critical survey of recent literature. Arch. Pediatr. *64*:579-583, 1947.
85. Zerr, D. M., Meier, A. S., Selke, S. S., et al.: A population-based study of primary human herpesvirus 6 infection. N. Engl. J. Med. *352*:768-776, 2005.

CHAPTER 66

BACTERIAL SKIN INFECTIONS

Mary Anne Jackson

NORMAL SKIN

ANATOMY

The epidermal skin layer provides the primary barrier to invasion by microorganisms and an interface between the body and the environment. Hair follicles, sebaceous glands, nails, and sweat glands are considered epidermal appendages and as such may be involved in skin infection. A dermal layer composed of collagen and elastic fibers gives skin its elasticity; however, other cell elements that are present, including mast cells, blood and lymph vessels, and cutaneous nerves, may be involved in the inflammatory process in response to infection. The subcutaneous fat layer is just beneath the dermis and contributes primarily to thermal stability, but it also may be involved when infection extends beyond the epidermal-dermal layer.

FLORA

Colonization is defined as the presence of a microorganism on the skin without either clinical signs or symptoms of infection at the time of isolation. Normal bacterial skin colonization is divided into resident and transient flora. Resident flora predominates and includes typical nonpathogens, such as *Staphylococcus epidermidis* and *Propionibacterium acnes*, in addition to other anaerobic diphtheroids and micrococci. Transient flora include pathogenic organisms, such as *Staphylococcus aureus*, streptococci, gram-negative enterics, and *Candida albicans*; these pathogens usually are present in smaller numbers than the resident flora and may be removed by skin cleansing. Acutely or chronically damaged skin, contact with animate and inanimate environmental sources, and exposure to antimicrobial agents or indwelling devices can modify the skin flora and predispose to infection by resident or acquired transient flora.[80,90]

CUTANEOUS INFECTION AND DERMATOLOGIC MANIFESTATIONS OF SYSTEMIC DISEASE

Dermatologic manifestations of infection can occur when the skin is infected primarily or as a secondary phenomenon. Prompt diagnosis and treatment of certain systemic or disseminated diseases may be accomplished when the secondary dermatologic manifestations are recognized. Empiric treatment of systemic diseases such as endocarditis (septic emboli) or septicemia caused by bacterial pathogens, such as *Neisseria meningitidis* or *Pseudomonas aeruginosa*, is possible when the dermatologic manifestations (purpura fulminans, ecthyma gangrenosum) are noted. Generalized viral infections may be heralded by pathognomonic skin findings, such as occur in varicella or measles. Alternatively, skin manifestations may be mediated by toxin (staphylococcal scalded skin syndrome or toxic shock syndrome [TSS]) or by immunologic mechanisms (gonococcemia).

The list of bacterial infectious agents associated with skin infections is extensive (Table 66–1). This chapter focuses on the bacterial skin infections most frequently encountered by practicing clinicians.

IMPETIGO

NONBULLOUS OR SIMPLE SUPERFICIAL IMPETIGO

The bacterial skin infection most commonly encountered in children is nonbullous impetigo, which accounts for more than 70 percent of impetigo cases in children. This superficial infection is seen predominantly in summer, with insect bites, cutaneous injuries, and primary dermatitis serving as the portal of entry.[46,61]

TABLE 66–1 Bacterial Infectious Agents Associated with Cutaneous Manifestations

Anthrax	*Bacillus anthracis*
Blistering dactylitis	*Streptococcus pyogenes*
	Streptococcus agalactiae
	Staphylococcus aureus
Cellulitis	*S. pyogenes*
	Staphylococcus aureus
	Haemophilus influenzae type b
	Streptococcus pneumoniae
Chancroid	*Haemophilus ducreyi*
Diphtheria	*Corynebacterium diphtheriae*
Ecthyma gangrenosum	*Pseudomonas aeruginosa*
Erysipelas	*S. pyogenes*
	S. agalactiae; group C, G streptococci
	S. pneumoniae
Erysipeloid	*Erysipelothrix rhusiopathiae*
Folliculitis	*S. aureus*
	Coagulase-negative staphylococci
	Klebsiella spp.
	Enterobacter spp.
	Escherichia coli
	P. aeruginosa
	Proteus spp.
Erythrasma	*Corynebacterium minutissimum*
Furunculosis	*S. aureus*
Hidradenitis suppurativa	*S. aureus*
	Streptococcus milleri
	E. coli
	Anaerobic streptococci
Granuloma inguinale	*Calymmatobacterium granulomatis*
Impetigo	
Simple superficial	*S. aureus*
	S. pyogenes
Bullous	*S. aureus*
Lymphogranuloma venereum	*Chlamydia trachomatis*
Melioidosis	*Burkholderia pseudomallei*
Necrotizing fasciitis	*S. pyogenes*
	Polymicrobial
Nocardiosis	*Nocardia brasiliensis*
	Nocardia asteroides
Paronychia	Polymicrobial
Perianal dermatitis	*S. pyogenes*
Pitted keratolysis	Coryneform bacteria
Syphilis	*Treponema pallidum*

Entries in bold are discussed in the text.

Nonbullous impetigo, sometimes called *thick crusted impetigo*, is characterized by the appearance of erythematous maculopapules that rapidly evolve from a vesicular to a pustular stage. Centrally crusted plaques range in size from a few millimeters to 1 cm and are surrounded by a distinct margin of erythema. The honey-colored crust is a classic feature, and removal of the crust results in the reaccumulation of fresh exudate. Regional lymphadenopathy can occur and often is the reason that the patient seeks medical attention. Spread to exposed areas, usually the face, neck, and limbs, occurs frequently. This form of pyoderma often is associated with a 2- to 3-week delay in establishing the diagnosis because the lesions are slow to progress, only mildly tender at the site of the lesion, and generally not associated with systemic signs or symptoms.

Nonbullous impetigo classically has been associated with infection caused by group A beta-hemolytic streptococci (GABHS). More recent data underscore the importance of *S. aureus*, however, which now accounts for most cases of nonbullous impetigo in the United States.[6,50]

Primarily a disease of children, nonbullous impetigo is spread within families and by close physical contact. It is prevalent during warm, humid seasons and is seen year-round in tropical regions. Endemic disease occurs in the southeastern United States and Hawaii.

Epidemics of streptococcal impetigo have been associated with postinfectious glomerulonephritis, and streptococcal strains, including types 2, 31, 49, 53, 55, 56, 57, and 60, have been implicated in such outbreaks.[12,67] Studies published in the 1950s and 1960s from the Red Lake Indian Reservation in Minnesota first confirmed the association of impetigo in school-aged children with a postinfectious nephritis that occurred 18 to 21 days after the onset of impetigo and implicated the so-called Red Lake strain, M-type 49.[5] Further studies in this population performed in the early 1970s found that GABHS was isolated from normal skin in 23 of 31 high-risk children a mean of 10 days before the development of impetigo.[34] Local trauma and other environmental factors seemed to explain the predilection of exposed skin to streptococcal infection, especially the skin of the legs, where 62 percent of the total lesions were noted. Secondary acquisition of streptococcal isolates in other family members occurred a mean of 5 days after the primary case, a time frame that was noted to be significantly shorter than that of secondary respiratory acquisition.[52] Rheumatic fever does not occur as a postinfectious sequela of streptococcal skin infection.

Cutaneous botryomycosis, an indolent infection reminiscent of crusted impetigo, usually is caused by *S. aureus*. Characterized by plaquelike lesions with superficial pustules and crusts, this entity has a predilection for patients with altered immune function.[23] Histologic examination may suggest the diagnosis of actinomycosis if a granulomatous lesion with granules resembling those seen with *Actinomyces* is noted. Successful treatment can be accomplished after the bacterial pathogen has been identified.

BULLOUS IMPETIGO

Bullous impetigo is diagnosed when the primary lesion begins as small vesicles and later appears as flaccid, painless bullae, generally measuring greater than 1 cm (see Fig. 64–17). Initially filled with clear fluid, the lesions eventually may exhibit a purulent fluid level. Rupture of the thin bullae usually reveals a moist, erythematous base that dries to a shiny lacquer-like appearance, sometimes described as a varnished finish (Fig. 66–1). Systemic toxicity is not seen except in neonates, in whom disseminated disease may occur.

In contrast to thick, crusted impetigo, in virtually all cases of bullous impetigo, staphylococci are isolated in pure culture from aspirated bulla fluid. Other bullous dermatitides of childhood, such as pemphigus or Stevens-Johnson syndrome, may be excluded by isolation of the organism. Occasionally, biopsy is done in cases in which extensive bullae or an atypical clinical appearance is noted. Confirmation of a cleavage plane high in the epidermis with gram-positive organisms and polymorphonuclear leukocytes present is a definitive diagnosis of bullous staphylococcal disease.

Infection generally is caused by phage group II strains, particularly phage type 71, but also 3A, 3C, and 55, which are noted to elaborate epidermolytic toxins A and B. Pathologically, these toxins act by disrupting the intercellular attachment of epidermal cells of the stratum granulosum. The toxin is thought to function as a protease in separating the upper layers of the epidermis of adult and infant human skin. Production of antibody to epidermolytic toxin occurs with age; however, it does not protect against the development of new bullous lesions during the localized impetiginous stage of this staphylococcal disease.

Epidemiologically, large outbreaks of bullous impetigo have been traced most notably to hospital nurseries, where identification of infected infants always occurs within the first month of life but after the infant has been sent home. A more severe, generalized form of the epidermolytic toxin-mediated disease (Ritter disease) may be seen in a few infants during one of these out-

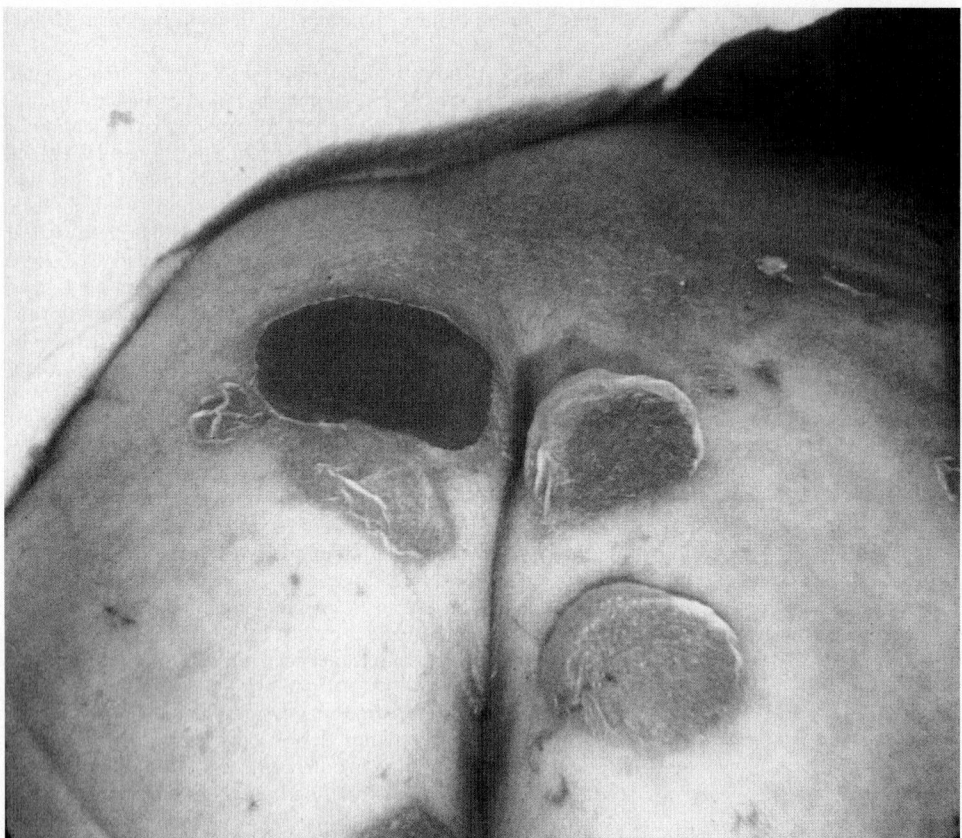

Figure 66–1 Flaccid bullae and shiny lacquer base of staphylococcal impetigo.

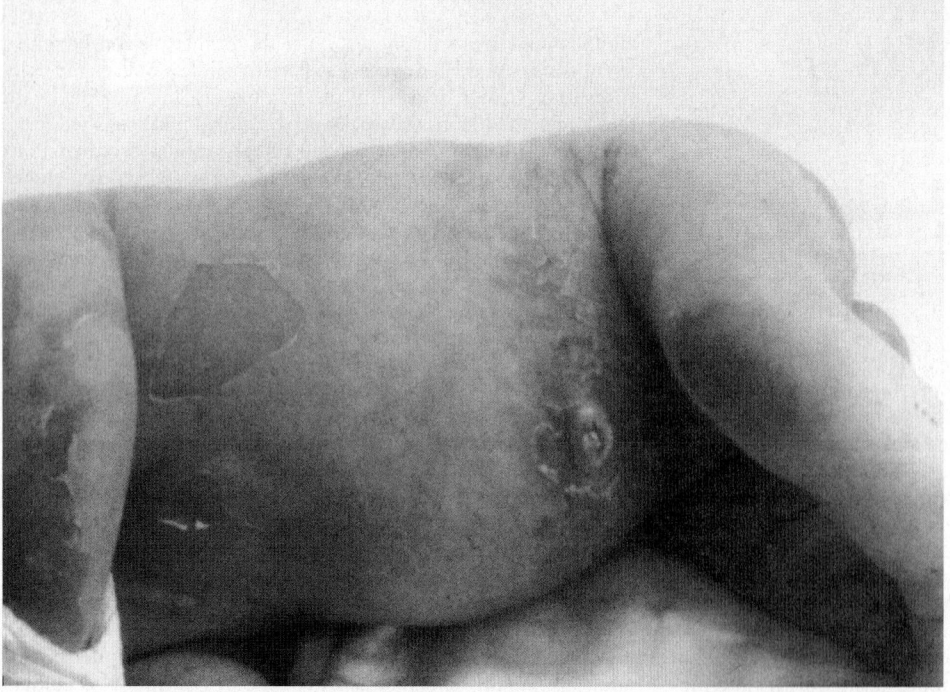

Figure 66–2 Typical appearance of a neonate with Ritter disease.

breaks, underscoring the importance of infection control surveillance practices in recognizing such an outbreak (Fig. 66–2).

TREATMENT OF IMPETIGO

Topical mupirocin may be used in cases of nonbullous impetigo in which adequate coverage of the affected sites can be ensured.[18,33,99] In other cases, systemic treatment with an oral antistaphylococcal antimicrobial agent, such as cephalexin, should be employed.[38,39,45,109] As in other staphylococcal diseases, an increase in community-acquired, methicillin-resistant *S. aureus* (MRSA) cases has been noted in the last decade.[62,63,72,124] In cases for which traditional antistaphylococcal agents are unsuccessful or in patients with recurrent disease, culture should be done to identify the bacterial strain and susceptibility pattern. Currently, most community-acquired MRSA isolates are susceptible to clindamycin.[17,24]

PERIANAL STREPTOCOCCAL DERMATITIS

Formerly called *perianal cellulitis*, perianal streptococcal dermatitis, a commonly recognized superficial skin infection, is characterized by the presence of marked, well-demarcated, perirectal erythema with associated swelling, pruritus, and tenderness but an absence of systemic symptoms or progressive disease. Approximately half of patients complain of significant rectal pain on defecation, and a third note blood in their stools.[4,29,70,98]

Heavy growth of GABHS is seen on perianal culture, and in one study, isolation of a specific T-type streptococcus (T 28) raised the question of whether certain streptococcal strains have tropism for the perineal region.[104] Asymptomatic patients were evaluated in two studies, and only sparse growth of GABHS was noted in 6 percent of cases.

Perianal streptococcal dermatitis is treated with oral penicillin agents. Topical mupirocin also has been used successfully. Recurrences are noted commonly, however. In one large series of patients, one third had recurrent disease.[87] Intrafamilial spread of disease frequently occurs and may provide a vector for recurrence. For patients with recurrent or persistent disease, clindamycin or a β-lactam agent plus rifampin may be used, and identification and treatment of other affected family members may be necessary.

BLISTERING DISTAL DACTYLITIS

Most commonly identified in school-aged children, blistering distal dactylitis is a distinctive superficial skin infection classically associated with GABHS.[13] Bullae 2 cm in diameter develop over the anterior fat pad of the distal phalanges, sometimes extending to involve the nail folds. Involvement of the proximal phalanges or the palms occasionally is noted. Frankly pustular lesions may occur, but the lesions themselves usually are asymptomatic or only mildly tender. A thin purulent exudate generally is apparent on incision and drainage.[71]

The diagnosis is confirmed by recovery of the etiologic agent on culture, most commonly GABHS, although group B streptococci and *S. aureus* also have been noted.[58] Concurrent recovery of GABHS in the pharynx has been reported in a few cases. Treatment includes a 10-day course of an oral β-lactam agent, usually penicillin or amoxicillin, in addition to incision and drainage of any tense bullae.

ERYSIPELAS

The superficial cellulitis erysipelas, referred to as *St. Anthony's fire* in the Middle Ages, is characterized by the appearance of a bright erythematous plaque with a distinct, elevated border that sharply demarcates affected from unaffected skin. The lesion most often involves the face or lower extremity, although extensive involvement of the trunk has been noted. The involved skin is warm and tender and may have a peau d'orange appearance. Large tension bullae may be seen in the erythematous zone.[65] The patient generally appears toxic and is highly febrile, and rapid extension of the affected skin may occur over the course of hours.[31,66,136]

Histopathologic findings include intense edema with vascular dilation of the dermis and uppermost subcutaneous tissue. Involvement of lymphatic channels and tissue spaces with polymorphonuclear leukocytes is a typical finding.

Surgical wounds, the umbilicus of the neonate, or any break in the skin may serve as the portal of entry; however, the initial lesion may be inapparent. Localized edema, such as occurs from a renal or lymphatic source, is a predisposing factor, and antecedent respiratory infection often is reported. An increased risk for development of erysipelas has been noted in patients with hypogammaglobulinemia, certain malignancies such as lymphoma, or lymphedema complicating radiation therapy.

The diagnosis generally is recognized on clinical grounds, and GABHS traditionally has been isolated by aspiration of the advancing margin of the lesion. A few case reports have identified other streptococci (including group B, C, and G), *Moraxella* spp., *Haemophilus influenzae*, and *Streptococcus pneumoniae* as etiologic agents.[15,30,42,88,102,123,137] A combination of intravenous penicillin and clindamycin should be used until the results of culture are available. Erysipelas has a classic clinical appearance, and appropriate diagnosis and therapy result in a prompt clinical response in most cases. Penicillin prophylaxis may be considered for patients with recurrent erysipelas, particularly patients with underlying risk factors.[16,40]

ECTHYMA

Ecthyma gangrenosa is a deep-seated infectious process that manifests as a necrotic ulcer covered by a black eschar. Usually, the initial lesion, a vesicopustule, sits on an erythematous base; it eventually erodes through the epidermis to the dermis, where it forms a crusted ulcer with heaped-up borders and then becomes frankly necrotic.[64]

This process rarely occurs in an otherwise healthy child, and if it does, an immunodeficiency work-up should ensue. *Chromobacterium violaceum* has been reported to cause ecthyma and similarly should result in an immunologic evaluation focusing on neutrophil defects, including disorders such as chronic granulomatous disease.[22]

Ecthyma can occur as a primary cutaneous infection in an immunocompetent host, and other etiologic agents that have been confirmed include *S. aureus*, *Aeromonas hydrophila*, and GABHS.[48,57,73,84,96,105,134] A similar-appearing lesion is seen with cutaneous anthrax; however, extensive nonpitting edema of the surrounding soft tissues is an important clue to this diagnosis. Ecthymatous-like lesions have been seen in patients with herpes simplex infection.[85] Additionally, human orf infections result in ulcerative skin lesions that appear similar to lesions of ecthyma; the clue to establishing the diagnosis is contact with an infected animal, usually sheep or goats, or a contaminated fomite.[26]

When an ecthymatous lesion is noted in a febrile neutropenic host, it generally signals disseminated infection. *P. aeruginosa* is the etiologic pathogen identified most commonly in such cases, but other gram-negative pathogens and fungi, including *Enterobacter*, *Escherichia coli*, *Morganella*, *Pseudomonas cepacia*, *Serratia marcescens*, *Stenotrophomonas maltophilia*, *Aspergillus*, *Mucor*, *Fusarium*, and *C. albicans*, have been implicated in ecthyma gangrenosum in compromised hosts.[36,51,53,97,107,112,117,122] Ecthyma has been seen as the heralding manifestation of acute lymphoblastic leukemia in children.[111] Empiric antimicrobial therapy for ecthyma gangrenosum in a neutropenic host should include intravenous therapy with an anti-*Pseudomonas* agent plus an aminoglycoside. Biopsy of the lesion may provide more specific etiologic information and allow for confirmation of antimicrobial susceptibility.

FOLLICULITIS, FURUNCULOSIS, AND CARBUNCLES

Folliculitis, furunculosis, and carbuncles represent a group of infections characterized by their origin in the hair follicles and the formation of abscesses. Virtually always caused by *S. aureus*, these infections were seen commonly in the 1950s in disease that often involved multiple family members. Outbreaks among athletes likewise have been reported.[130]

By definition, these infections involve sites where body hair is present, including the axilla, breast area, perineum, neck, and extremities. Lesions of folliculitis represent abscesses of a single hair follicle with limited surrounding tissue involvement. When deeper inflammatory nodules are associated with tissue edema, furunculosis is diagnosed. When several interconnecting furuncles are present, the lesion is referred to as a carbuncle. Generally, older children and adolescents are predisposed to the development of follicular infections, and individuals with diabetes mellitus, abnormal neutrophil chemotaxis, and impaired circulation may have recurrent disease.

Although *S. aureus* nearly always is the cause of folliculitis as in the past, outbreaks of so-called hot tub folliculitis have been described and almost always are caused by *P. aeruginosa*; rarely, other gram-negative organisms have been reported.[27,28] Folliculitis in an immunocompromised host often is caused by unusual fungal pathogens.[3,115,127] Although typically associated with hot tubs and whirlpools, a large outbreak of *Pseudomonas* folliculitis reported in 1984 involved 117 individuals after swimming in an indoor pool. An incubation period of 24 to 30 hours could be ascertained, and a typical follicular, pustular eruption was noted. The mean duration of the folliculitis, 15 days, is consistent with other reports, but some patients continued to complain of rash for weeks, and recurrent pustules appearing months later have been reported in other studies.[56]

A more recent report has identified four cases of *Mycobacterium fortuitum* complex furunculosis that developed after pedicures, suggesting this pathogen may be added to the differential diagnosis in such cases when a patient presents with nonhealing furuncles on the lower legs, especially when bacterial cultures have been negative, or the disease is unresponsive to antistaphylococcal therapy (including MRSA).[114] Early recognition and institution of appropriate therapy are essential, and the history of pedicures may be a clue to establishing the diagnosis. Cutaneous myiasis has been reported to manifest as a chronic boil or furuncle, but the diagnosis should be considered only in such cases in which an appropriate travel history is elicited.[32]

Recognition of the typical skin lesion usually is sufficient to establish the diagnosis. Unless the patient has a history of exposure to a hot tub or whirlpool, or recently has had a pedicure, a regimen of antistaphylococcal therapy should be sufficient. In the era of MRSA infection, local susceptibility profiles should be used to confirm appropriate therapy. Isolated boils resolve with drainage alone. Systemic therapy may be considered in cases in which lesions are large or multiple. Trimethoprim-sulfamethoxazole is a good choice for a nontoxic patient older than 2 months. Clindamycin is a good choice for most locales, although resistance may be increasing.[82,91] Because MRSA now accounts for 75 percent of cases in which children present with skin and soft tissue infection, treatment should be individualized, based on type of presentation, patient age, and underlying disease.[81] Systemic agents should be used for 7 to 10 days in patients who are toxic, who have extensive disease, or who have associated cellulitis. Large lesions, specifically larger than 5 cm, should be incised and drained, and culture should be done in all cases to confirm susceptibility testing. In some patients, hematogenous metastatic spread may occur, and a search for foci in the heart, bones, joints, deep tissues, or brain should be done in patients with significant systemic toxicity.

For patients in whom recurrent disease develops, chronic dermatoses, such as eczema, should be identified, and in obese adolescents, the diagnosis of diabetes mellitus should be considered.[7] The patient should be cautioned to refrain from sharing washcloths or towels, and skin trauma and use of irritants such as deodorants should be avoided.

The utility of decolonizing regimens with topical agents, such as mupirocin (nares and perianal area) and chlorhexidine or bleach baths (skin), may be considered in certain cases. *S. aureus* colonization of the nares, rectum, or skin can be detected by culture of these areas, but confirmation of carriage is likely necessary only in specific cases for which decolonization is desirable. The indications for and benefit of decolonization vary depending on host factors, underlying disease, and circumstances related to the health care setting.[126] Outbreaks of MRSA colonization/infection require a multifaceted approach, including attention given to handwashing, cohorting, barrier measures, and decolonization strategies. Examples of special circumstances include the following: (1) patients who are immunosuppressed and colonized, and at risk for development of systemic infections; (2) patients who are more likely to spread the organisms, owing to behavior (e.g., mentally retarded patients); or (3) patients who have repeated infections caused by the MRSA strain that they carry.

Most children with recurrent furunculosis are otherwise healthy, and no specific immunologic evaluation is necessary; however, cases of recurrent furunculosis in patients with hyper-IgE syndrome and common variable immunodeficiency have been reported, and an association with mannose-binding lectin deficiency was confirmed in a family.[78,83,125] Rarely, children with white blood cell defects may have recurrent staphylococcal skin abscesses, and tests of white blood cell function may be considered in specific patients. Data suggest that vitamin C may be beneficial in cases of recurrent folliculitis.[93,94]

HIDRADENITIS SUPPURATIVA

Hidradenitis suppurativa, a chronic, debilitating condition, is a disorder of the apocrine glands that involves primarily skin in the axilla and anogenital region, although scalp, umbilical, and breast involvement has been reported. Seen mainly in adolescents, this androgen-dependent condition is manifested by the development of multiple painful nodules and the formation of deep abscesses in the skin in areas where apocrine glands are present. The formation of fistulas, ulcers, and contracted scars may complicate the course, and recurrent relapses may be noted. Infection usually is polymicrobial, and pathogens to consider include *S. aureus*, gram-negative enterics, and anaerobes. Drainage of abscesses and institution of systemic antimicrobial therapy may be necessary. When fistulas associated with anogenital disease develop, adjacent structures, including the urethra, bladder, and rectum, may be involved. Surgery usually is required for cure. Carbon dioxide laser treatment in some cases may be beneficial.[89]

CELLULITIS

The diagnosis of cellulitis is made when the subcutaneous tissues and dermis are involved in a clinical process manifested as localized edema, erythema, warmth, and tenderness of the tissues. The leading edge of the involved site may be notable, but it is not raised and well demarcated as in erysipelas.

Infection usually is caused by coagulase-positive staphylococci and GABHS; however, infection also is caused by group B streptococci (neonates) and *S. pneumoniae*, and, in the past, *H. influenzae* type b (Hib) cellulitis was described.[131] Streptococcal and staphylococcal cellulitis can involve patients of any age and any site, although the extremity is noted most often. Frequently, the patient has a history of antecedent trauma at the site of involvement, but the injury may not have appeared significant. Some researchers advocate culture of the cellulitic site, but in practice, it rarely is performed. Blood cultures are valuable in individuals

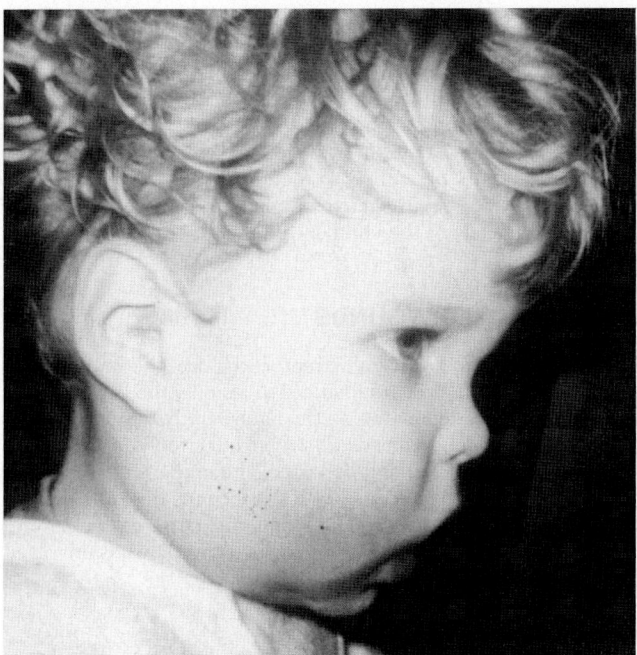

Figure 66–3 Buccal involvement in an infant with invasive *Haemophilus influenzae* type b disease.

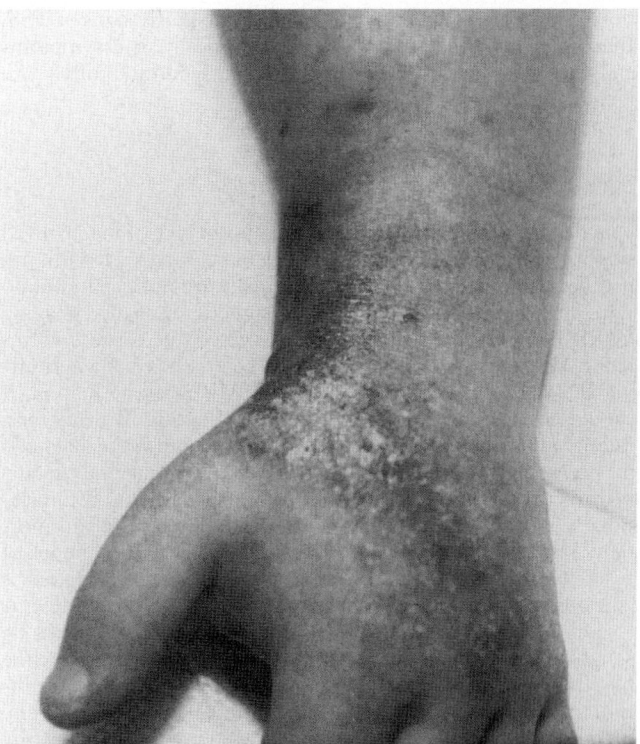

Figure 66–4 Necrotizing fasciitis in a toddler with varicella.

with disease caused by group B streptococci, *S. pneumoniae*, and Hib.[75]

Group B streptococcal cellulitis occurs in neonates and generally is seen as part of invasive, late-onset disease. Unilateral involvement of the face or submandibular sites occurs most commonly, but inguinal, scrotal, and prepatellar involvement has been described.[10,69] When cellulitis occurs in an infant younger than 3 months old, group B streptococcal bacteremia should be suspected, even in the absence of other signs of systemic infection.

Pneumococcal soft tissue infections are common findings.[110] Patients with connective tissue disorders, such as systemic lupus erythematosus, seem especially prone, although these infections can occur in healthy infants and children. Sites of involvement include the head, neck, leg, and torso.

Hib cellulitis often involves the face of infants (Fig. 66–3). A violaceous hue of the cellulitic area, which some researchers thought to be pathognomonic, might be observed. This process nearly always was the result of hematogenous seeding by Hib, and meningitis occurred in 15 to 20 percent of such patients.[68,129,140] As has been the case with other forms of Hib disease, almost complete eradication has been achieved in the last decade with the use of conjugate vaccine.

Treatment of simple cellulitis in patients with a clear-cut area of preceding trauma should include an agent that is active against *S. aureus* and GABHS, and in most locales, clindamycin remains a good choice for therapy, although resistance for *S. aureus* (10-15%) and GABHS (2-3%) is noted. The aforementioned caveats for treating staphylococcal skin infections should be followed. In infants with buccal or periorbital involvement or in infants with soft tissue involvement but without a clear-cut focus of infection, a third-generation cephalosporin, such as cefotaxime or ceftriaxone, should be included with clindamycin. Vancomycin always should be included in cases of a patient who is toxic and when metastatic suppurative disease is suspected.

NECROTIZING FASCIITIS

Necrotizing fasciitis is a rapidly progressive bacterial infection of the soft tissues associated with a fulminant course and a high mortality rate. This infection spreads rapidly in the plane between the subcutaneous tissue and superficial muscle fascia and causes widespread necrosis. Prompt and aggressive medical and surgical management is necessary to ensure a good outcome.

In children, necrotizing fasciitis usually is caused by GABHS; traumatic lesions involving the skin, including varicella, burns, or eczema, may predispose to this aggressive process.[19,47,55,59,76,108,119,120,142] An association has been noted among varicella, ibuprofen use, and invasive GABHS infection, although no data convincingly link this triad to necrotizing infection.[54,92,143] Patients with congenital or acquired immunodeficiencies are at greater risk for the development of necrotizing fasciitis, and in neonates, omphalitis and circumcision are predisposing conditions.

CLINICAL MANIFESTATIONS

The child generally has a high fever and is fussy. In infants, the irritability may be profound and may not appear to be localized to an involved site, unless the clinician is meticulous in conducting the examination. An extremity most commonly is involved, and older infants and children often refuse to bear weight or move the affected extremity. Swelling of soft tissue usually is noted, but the erythema may be subtle. The hallmark tip-off on examination is the finding of intense pain on manipulation of the involved site that is out of proportion to the cutaneous signs. Skin changes that occur during the subsequent 24 to 48 hours include blistering with bleb formation, and a dusky appearance of the involved site is noted as vessels are thrombosed, and cutaneous ischemia develops. Skin necrosis is a late sign and indicates a poor prognosis (Fig. 66–4).[79,135]

Recognition of the manifestations of TSS is crucial because mortality rates of 60 percent have been reported in patients with associated fasciitis. Multisystem complaints, including vomiting, diarrhea, and severe myalgia, are present when GABHS fasciitis is associated with streptococcal TSS. Tachycardia out of proportion to fever and altered mental status may be early signs of TSS. Renal and hepatic dysfunctions occur typically, and symptoms and signs of adult respiratory distress syndrome often are identified.

DIAGNOSIS

The diagnosis cannot be based on the appearance of the involved site because none of the early findings of necrotizing fasciitis are pathognomonic. Plain radiographs usually are normal and of no value in establishing the diagnosis. Magnetic resonance imaging (MRI) is the preferred technique to detect soft tissue involvement. MRI permits visualization of the soft tissue edema infiltrating the fascial planes.[21,113,144] Although MRI may be helpful, it should not delay performing surgical intervention. Waiting for a radiographic procedure to be performed to confirm the diagnosis may serve only to delay implementing definitive surgical therapy and to increase the risk for development of systemic complications, contributing further to the increased morbidity and mortality rates. In the typical clinical scenario in which the index of suspicion for necrotizing fasciitis is high, surgical exploration is appropriate, even in the presence of "normal" MRI findings.

Laboratory manifestations of streptococcal TSS should be sought in any pediatric patient with fasciitis. Typically, the white blood cell count is normal; however, most patients have a significant increase in band forms (>50%) noted on the peripheral blood smear. Thrombocytopenia and evidence of coagulopathy are found commonly, and marked hypoalbuminemia with hypocalcemia is a typical finding. Laboratory findings associated with renal failure, myocardial dysfunction, and adult respiratory distress syndrome may develop during the first 48 to 72 hours.

A microbiologic diagnosis can be made by isolating bacteria from blood, tissue, or wound culture. In some cases, a polymicrobial etiology has been noted, particularly in patients with so-called Fournier gangrene or necrotizing fasciitis of the perineum.[49,74] In these cases, *S. aureus*, GABHS, and one or more anaerobes, including *Peptostreptococcus*, *Prevotella*, *Bacteroides fragilis*, and *Porphyromonas*, have been implicated in infection.[20] Fasciitis caused by *P. aeruginosa* or *Clostridium septicum* has been seen in neutropenic patients. In the last decade, GABHS has been reported widely as a single pathogen and is the etiologic agent in most cases of pediatric fasciitis. As in other cases of invasive disease caused by GABHS, virulence is related to certain structural characteristics of the organism and to its ability to produce biologically active substances, some of which facilitate invasion and spread of the pathogen.

TREATMENT

Surgical débridement of necrotic tissue is the key to managing necrotizing fasciitis, and increased mortality rates have been observed when débridement is delayed more than 24 hours.[106] Mandatory return to the operating room for examination and repeat débridement should occur during the following 24 to 48 hours. Careful management of fluids, attention to pain control, anticipation and management of multisystem organ failure, and administration of appropriate parenteral antimicrobial therapy should be initiated promptly. The use of intravenous immunoglobulin may be considered in cases of TSS-associated fasciitis.[25]

Appropriate therapy includes intravenous penicillin, 150,000 U/kg/day divided into four to six doses; clindamycin, 40 mg/kg/day divided into four doses; and vancomycin, 40 mg/kg/day divided into three to four doses. The use of additional coverage with agents active against *P. aeruginosa* and gram-negative enterics should be considered in neutropenic patients.

Response to therapy is assessed by careful serial examination. Control of pain is crucial in such patients, while keeping in mind that persistent, severe pain suggests ongoing tissue necrosis and may signal the need for further surgical intervention. Careful attention to nutritional support should be maintained throughout the child's hospital stay. Physical therapy is necessary for most patients, especially patients who require amputation, skin grafting, or extensive reconstructive surgery, and providing for the psychosocial needs of the child and the family is imperative.

CONTAMINATED WOUNDS

Although staphylococci and streptococci are the most likely causes of infection after traumatic skin lesions, the list of causes may be extensive, depending on the nature of the injury. Specific pathogens should be considered when infections develop after human or animal bites, soil or water contamination, or various types of injury. Management of such infections depends on recognizing infection patterns and obtaining cultures for careful identification of the specific organism or organisms involved (Table 66–2).

HUMAN BITES

Two types of human bites are described: occlusional and clenched fist (see also Chapter 259). Occlusional bites are related most commonly to child abuse, although in a pediatric patient, a biting toddler may be the culprit. Accidental bites may occur during sporting activities and generally involve the face of a teammate. Clenched-fist injuries are associated with the most prevalent and severe infections that occur after human bites. Rapidly progressive infection may follow despite the patient's receiving early medical attention.[11] When clenched-fist injuries are associated with bite wounds, laceration and puncture wounds commonly occur along the dorsal aspect of the third metacarpophalangeal joint, and bone, joint capsule, or tendon structures may be involved.

Polymicrobial infection is the usual finding, and in such cases, broad-spectrum empiric antimicrobial coverage should be initiated promptly, after adequate drainage has been performed.[118] In a multicenter study of infected human bites, the median number of isolates per wound was four, and aerobes and anaerobes were

TABLE 66–2   Infections Associated with Animal Bites

Nature of Injury	Pathogens Involved
Human bites	Staphylococci
	Anaerobic and aerobic streptococci
	Eikenella corrodens
Animal bites	
Dog/cat	*Pasteurella* species
	Staphylococcus aureus
	Streptococci
	Anaerobes
	Capnocytophaga canimorsus, Capnocytophaga cynodegmi
	Moraxella species
	Corynebacterium species
	Neisseria species
Reptile	Enteric gram-negatives
	Anaerobes
Horse and sheep	*Actinobacillus* species, *Pasteurella* species
Pig	*Flavobacterium* species, *Actinobacillus* species, *Pasteurella aerogenes*
Rat	*Streptobacillus moniliformis, S. aureus*

identified. The common pathogens were *Streptococcus anginosus*, *S. aureus*, *Eikenella corrodens*, *Fusobacterium nucleatum*, and *Prevotella melaninogenica*. *Candida* spp. were noted less commonly.[132] Many strains of *Prevotella* and *S. aureus* are β-lactamase producers, and *E. corrodens* is intrinsically resistant to clindamycin and cephalosporins. Ampicillin with clavulanate given orally (simple infections) or ampicillin-sulbactam given intravenously for more complicated infections may be used as a single agent. Unusual pathogens rarely occur. A report of a human bite infection caused by *Mycobacterium ulcerans* is noted; this pathogen is emerging rapidly in West African countries.[35] Antimicrobial prophylaxis should be considered for patients with human bites to the hands, feet, and skin overlying joints and for patients with bites that penetrate deeper than the epidermal layer.[116]

ANIMAL BITES

Animal bite wounds occur commonly, with more than 4 million reported annually in the United States (see also Chapter 260). Children account for more than half of patients who go to emergency departments for care of bite wounds.[2] Although one survey has revealed that rodents and lagomorphs are the biting animals most commonly reported, wounds related to these bites seldom are associated with infection. By contrast, cats and dogs together account for approximately 40 percent of bites, and their bites are associated more frequently with morbidity. The etiology of animal bite infections often is related to the species of animal involved (see Table 66–2).[41,44,77,95]

Approximately 1000 emergency department visits related to dog bites occur each day, at a cost of more than $100 million/yr.[128] The incidence of infection related to dog bites has been estimated at 3 to 17 percent.[9,37] Cat bites are most likely to become infected, probably because of the puncture-like nature of the injury. One study suggests that half of cat bites result in infection, prompting recommendations for prophylaxis of such bites, especially if they involve the face or hands. In the presence of infection, exploration plus débridement of devitalized tissue is necessary, and purulent collections should be drained.

Although *Pasteurella multocida* is implicated most frequently, numerous other pathogens, including *S. aureus*, *Capnocytophaga canimorsus*, and other aerobic and anaerobic bacteria, are associated with dog and cat bites. Depending on the depth of the wound's penetration, underlying structures such as bones, joints, and tendons may be involved in such infections.[60] The wound itself may not appear significant, particularly in the case of puncture wounds, but several clinical features should influence treatment decisions. The presence of tissue edema and point tenderness on palpation over the site should signal that deeper structures may be involved. Soft tissue imaging may be necessary, and appropriate drainage or débridement of involved sites should be pursued.

As with human bites, oral amoxicillin-clavulanate may be used for prophylaxis or treatment of simple infections. Indications for prophylaxis of bite wounds include bites associated with a crush or puncture injury and bites involving the face, hands, feet, and genitalia. Wounds in immunocompromised, especially asplenic, individuals should be considered for prophylaxis. Intravenous ampicillin-sulbactam or ticarcillin-clavulanate can be used for more serious infections. For individuals who have a history of anaphylaxis with penicillin or cephalosporins, a combination of clindamycin plus trimethoprim-sulfamethoxazole or ciprofloxacin can be used.[113,115] Antimicrobial therapy may be modified further depending on the biting animal and suspected pathogen (see Table 66–2).[14]

Appropriate prophylaxis against tetanus should be considered for all bites. Hepatitis B can be transmitted by human bites, and appropriate management should be ensured for susceptible

patients. Rabies vaccine should be administered after bat, skunk, or raccoon bites; public health information should be accessed to decide whether rabies vaccine is indicated for other animal bites.

SOIL-CONTAMINATED AND WATER-CONTAMINATED WOUNDS

Four factors that must be considered in the acute care of contaminated wounds include the (1) mechanism of injury, (2) the length of time that transpires from injury to treatment, (3) the type of pathogens that occur in the environment, and (4) the presence of underlying disease in the host.[43] When a traumatic wound becomes infected, a polymicrobial etiology is typical, and common pathogens such as *S. aureus*, gram-negative enterics, and anaerobes characteristically are involved.[1] Unusual and rare organisms, such as nontuberculous mycobacteria, *Nocardia*, *Actinomyces*, fungi including *Aspergillus* spp., and unusual gram-negative organisms, occasionally may be encountered (Table 66–3).[86,100,101,103,138] *A. hydrophila* has been implicated in infections associated with injuries contaminated by fresh water and may produce rapidly progressive wound infection with fascia, tendon, muscle, bone, or joint involvement.[121]

Managing wounds contaminated by soil or water is difficult, especially if the mechanism of injury is a catastrophic event with complex bone and soft tissue injuries. In the acute setting of such an event, complete exploration and thorough débridement with copious irrigation are performed primarily, and signs of infection generally are not present. Days later, the clinician often is faced with the dilemma of a patient who is receiving antimicrobial prophylaxis with broad-spectrum agents and in whom new signs or symptoms develop acutely. Separating infectious from noninfectious complications often is difficult; however, the onset of fever in such a patient, especially in the setting of an open fracture or dural tear, should prompt further evaluation. Careful serial examination of the site of injury is necessary, and more extensive evaluation generally is indicated. Such assessment may include radiographic imaging and specific evaluation of body fluids with appropriate cultures. Because open fractures are associated with an increased risk for development of infection, the utility of antibiotic-impregnated implants, which are biodegradable and osteoconductive, may prove beneficial in such cases.[133,139]

Infections associated with foreign bodies such as wood generally cannot be cured until the foreign body is identified and removed.[141] Puncture wounds should be explored carefully, and

TABLE 66–3 Infections Associated with Soil-Contaminated or Water-Contaminated Wounds

Soil-Contaminated Wounds
Staphylococcus aureus
Group A beta-hemolytic streptococci
Many gram-negative enterics
Enterobacter cancerogenus
Anaerobes
Nocardia asteroides, *Nocardia otitidis-caviarum*
Mycobacterium fortuitum, *Mycobacterium abscessus*
Actinomyces
Aspergillus species
Enterococcus species

Water-Contaminated Wounds
Aeromonas hydrophila
Pseudomonas species
Many gram-negative enterics
Edwardsiella tarda (catfish injury)
Mycobacterium marinum

further débridement of necrotic tissue or drainage of involved sites such as joints may be necessary.[8]

Treatment of simple wound infections associated with soil or water contamination should include an agent such as ciprofloxacin, although deeper tissue infection may develop after a seemingly innocuous injury, and tissue débridement may be necessary. Determining the appropriate therapy for a patient with infection involving extensive soft tissue injury and open fractures is problematic. Administration of an empiric regimen with an agent such as piperacillin-tazobactam, imipenem, or a fluoroquinolone plus vancomycin may be reasonable after evaluation and appropriate culturing have been done.

REFERENCES

1. Abbott, S. L., and Janda, J. M.: *Enterobacter cancerogenus* ("*Enterobacter taylorae*") infections associated with severe trauma or crush injuries. Am. J. Clin. Pathol. *107*:359-361, 1997.
2. Aghabian, R. V., and Conte, J. E., Jr.: Mammalian bite wounds. Ann. Emerg. Med. *9*:79-83, 1980.
3. Alves, E. V., Martins, J. E., Ribeiro, E. B., et al.: *Pityrosporum folliculitis*: Renal transplantation case report. J. Dermatol. *27*:49-51, 2000.
4. Amren, D. P., Anderson, A. S., and Wannamaker, L. W.: Perianal cellulitis associated with group A streptococci. Am. J. Dis. Child. *112*:546-552, 1966.
5. Anthony, B. F., Perlman, L. V., and Wannamaker, L. W.: Skin infections and acute nephritis in American Indian children. Pediatrics *39*:263-279, 1967.
6. Aranow, H., and Wood, W. B.: Staphylococcal infections simulating scarlet fever. J. A. M. A. *119*:1491-1495, 1942.
7. Aroni, K., Aivaliotis, M., and Davaris, P.: Disseminated and recurrent infundibular folliculitis (D. R. I. F.): Report of a case successfully treated with isotretinoin. J. Dermatol. *25*:51-53, 1998.
8. Ashford, R. U., Sargeant, P. D., and Lum, G. D.: Septic arthritis of the knee caused by *Edwardsiella tarda* after a catfish puncture wound. Med. J. Aust. *168*:443-444, 1998.
9. Avner, J. R., and Baker, M. D.: Dog bites in urban children. Pediatrics *88*:55-57, 1991.
10. Baker, C. J.: Group B streptococcal cellulitis-adenitis in infants. Am. J. Dis. Child. *136*:631-633, 1982.
11. Baker, M. D., and Moore, S. E.: Human bites in children: A six-year experience. Am. J. Dis. Child. *141*:1285-1290, 1987.
12. Baraff, L. J., Fine, R. N., and Knutson, D. W.: Poststreptococcal acute glomerulonephritis: Fact and controversy. Ann. Intern. Med. *91*:76-86, 1979.
13. Barnett, B. O., and Frieden, I. J.: Streptococcal skin diseases in children. Semin. Dermatol. *11*:3-10, 1992.
14. Benaoudia, F., Escande, F., and Simonet, M.: Infection due to *Actinobacillus lignieresii* after a horse bite. Eur. J. Clin. Microbiol. Infect. Dis. *13*:439-440, 1994.
15. Binnick, A. N., Klein, R. B., and Baughman, R. D.: Recurrent erysipelas caused by group B streptococcus organisms. Arch. Dermatol. *116*:798-799, 1980.
16. Bitnun, S.: Prophylactic antibiotics in recurrent erysipelas. Lancet *1*:345, 1985.
17. Bratcher, D.: Methicillin-resistant *Staphylococcus aureus* in the community. Pediatr. Infect. Dis. J. *20*:1167-1168, 2001.
18. Britton, J. W., Fajardo, J. E., and Krafte-Jacobs, B.: Clinical and laboratory observations: Comparison of mupirocin and erythromycin in the treatment of impetigo. J. Pediatr. *117*:827-829, 1990.
19. Brogan, T. V., Nizet, V., Waldhausen, J. H., et al.: Group A streptococcal necrotizing fasciitis complicating primary varicella: A series of fourteen patients. Pediatr. Infect. Dis. J. *14*:588-594, 1995.
20. Brook, I., and Frazier, E. H.: Clinical and microbiological features of necrotizing fasciitis. J. Clin. Microbiol. *33*:2382-2387, 1995.
21. Brothers, T. E., Tagge, D. U., Stutley, J. E., et al.: Magnetic resonance imaging differentiates between necrotizing and non-necrotizing fasciitis of the lower extremity. J. Am. Coll. Surg. *187*:416-421, 1998.
22. Brown, K. L., Stein, A., and Morrell, D. S.: *Ecthyma gangrenosum* and septic shock syndrome secondary to *Chromobacterium violaceum*. J. Am. Acad. Dermatol. *54*(Suppl.):S224-S228, 2006.
23. Buescher, E. S., Hebert, A., and Rapini, R. P.: Staphylococcal botryomycosis in a patient with the hyperimmunoglobulin E-recurrent infection syndrome. Pediatr. Infect. Dis. J. *7*:431-433, 1988.
24. Bukharie, H. A., Abdelhadi, M. S., Saeed, I. A., et al.: Emergence of methicillin-resistant *Staphylococcus aureus* as a community pathogen. Diagn. Microbiol. Infect. Dis. *40*:1-4, 2001.
25. Cawley, M. J., Briggs, M., Haith, L. R., et al.: Intravenous immunoglobulin as adjunctive treatment for streptococcal toxic shock syndrome associated with necrotizing fasciitis: Case report and review. Pharmacotherapy *19*:1094-1098, 1999.
26. Centers for Disease Control and Prevention: Orf virus infection in humans—New York, Illinois, California, and Tennessee, 2004-2005. M. M. W. R. Morb. Mortal. Wkly. Rep. *55*:65-68, 2006.
27. Chandrasekar, P. H., Rolston, K. V. I., Kannangara, W., et al.: Hot tub-associated dermatitis due to *Pseudomonas aeruginosa*: Case report and review of the literature. Arch. Dermatol. *120*:1337-1340, 1984.
28. Chastain, M. A.: A cycle: Recurrent gram-negative folliculitis with *Citrobacter diversus* (koseri) following eradication of recurrent staphylococcal pyoderma. Arch. Dermatol. *136*:803, 2000.
29. Combs, J. T.: Perianal streptococcal disease. Clin. Pediatr. (Philadelphia) *39*:500, 2000.
30. Cox, N. H., Knowles, M. A., and Porteus, I. D.: Pre-septal cellulitis and facial erysipelas due to *Moraxella* species. Clin. Exp. Dermatol. *19*:321-323, 1994.
31. Crickx, B., Chevron, F., Sigal-Nahum, M., et al.: Erysipelas: Epidemiological, clinical and therapeutic data (111 cases). Ann. Dermatol. Venereol. *118*:545-546, 1991.
32. Dada-Adegbola, H. O., and Oluwatoba, O. A.: Cutaneous myiasis presenting as chronic furunculosis—case report. West Afr. J. Med. *24*:346-347, 2005.
33. Dagan, R., and Bar-David, Y.: Double-blind study comparing erythromycin and mupirocin for treatment of impetigo in children: Implications of a high prevalence of erythromycin-resistant *Staphylococcus aureus* strains. Antimicrob. Agents Chemother. *36*:287-290, 1992.
34. Dajani, A. S., Ferrieri, P., and Wannamaker, L. W.: Natural history of impetigo, II: Etiologic agents and bacterial interactions. J. Clin. Invest. *51*:2863-2871, 1972.
35. Debacker, M., Zinsou, C., Aguiar, J., et al.: First case of *Mycobacterium ulcerans* disease (Buruli ulcer) following a human bite. Clin. Infect. Dis. *36*:e67-e68, 2003.
36. Del Pozo, J., Garcia-Silva, J., Almagro, M., et al.: Ecthyma gangrenosum-like eruption associated with *Morganella morganii* infection. Br. J. Dermatol. *139*:520-521, 1998.
37. de Melker, H. E., and de Melker, R. A.: Dog bites: Publications on risk factors, infections, antibiotics, and primary wound closure. Ned. Tijdschr. Geneeskd. *140*:709-713, 1996.
38. Demidovich, C. W., Wittler, R. R., Ruff, M. E., et al.: Impetigo: Current etiology and comparison of penicillin, erythromycin, and cephalexin therapies. Am. J. Dis. Child. *144*:1313-1315, 1990.
39. Dillon, H. C.: The treatment of streptococcal skin infections. J. Pediatr. *76*:676-684, 1970.
40. Duvanel, T., Merot, Y., Harms, M., et al.: Prophylactic antibiotics in erysipelas. Lancet *1*:1401, 1985.
41. Ejlertsen, T., Gahrn-Hansen, B., Sogaard, P., et al.: *Pasteurella aerogenes* isolated from ulcers or wounds in humans with occupational exposure to pigs: A report of 7 Danish cases. Scand. J. Infect. Dis. *28*:567-570, 1996.
42. Eriksson, B. K.: Anal colonization of group G beta-hemolytic streptococci in relapsing erysipelas of the lower extremity. Clin. Infect. Dis. *29*:1319-1320, 1999.
43. Eron, L. J.: Targeting lurking pathogens in acute traumatic and chronic wounds. J. Emerg. Med. *17*:189-195, 1999.
44. Escande, F., Bailly, A., Bone, S., et al.: *Actinobacillus suis* infection after a pig bite. Lancet *348*:888, 1996.
45. Esterly, N. B., and Markowitz, M.: The treatment of pyoderma in children. J. A. M. A. *212*:1667-1670, 1970.
46. Esterly, N. B., Nelson, D. B., and Dunne, W. M., Jr.: Impetigo. Am. J. Dis. Child. *145*:125-126, 1991.
47. Falcone, P. A., Pricolo, V. E., and Edstrom, L. E.: Necrotizing fasciitis as a complication of chickenpox. Clin. Pediatr. (Philadelphia) *27*:339-343, 1988.
48. Farber, S., and Vawter, G. F.: Clinical pathological conference: The Children's Hospital Medical Center, Boston, Mass. J. Pediatr. *69*:485-489, 1966.
49. Farrell, L. D., Karl, S. R., Davis, P. K., et al.: Postoperative necrotizing fasciitis in children. Pediatrics *82*:874-879, 1988.
50. Feldman, C. A.: Staphylococcal scarlet fever. N. Engl. J. Med. *267*:877-878, 1962.
51. Fergie, J. E., Patrick, C. C., and Lott, L.: *Pseudomonas aeruginosa* cellulitis and ecthyma gangrenosum in immunocompromised children. Pediatr. Infect. Dis. J. *10*:496-500, 1991.
52. Ferrieri, P., Dajani, A. S., Wannamaker, L. W., et al.: Natural history of impetigo, I: Site sequence of acquisition and familial patterns of spread of cutaneous streptococci. J. Clin. Invest. *51*:2851-2862, 1972.
53. Fine, J. D., Miller, J. A., Harrist, T. J., et al.: Cutaneous lesions in disseminated candidiasis mimicking ecthyma gangrenosum. Am. J. Med. *70*:1133-1135, 1981.
54. Forbes, N., and Rankin, A. P.: Necrotizing fasciitis and non-steroidal anti-inflammatory drugs: A case series and review of the literature. N. Z. Med. J. *114*:3-6, 2001.
55. Ford, L. M., and Waksman, J.: Necrotizing fasciitis during primary varicella. Pediatrics *103*:783-790, 1999.
56. Fox, A. B., and Hambrick, G. W.: Recreationally associated *Pseudomonas aeruginosa* folliculitis. Arch. Dermatol. *120*:1304-1307, 1984.
57. Francis, Y. F., Richman, S., Hussain, S., et al.: *Aeromonas hydrophila* infection: Ecthyma gangrenosum with aplastic anemia. N. Y. State J. Med. *82*:1461-1464, 1982.
58. Frieden, I. J.: Blistering dactylitis caused by group B streptococci. Pediatr. Dermatol. *6*:300-302, 1989.

59. Givner, L. B., Abramson, J. S., and Wasilauskas, B.: Apparent increase in the incidence of invasive group A beta-hemolytic streptococcal disease in children. J. Pediatr. *118*:341-346, 1991.

60. Goldstein, E. J.: Current concepts on animal bites: Bacteriology and therapy. Curr. Clin. Top. Infect. Dis. *19*:99-111, 1999.

61. Gonzalez, A., Schachner, L. A., Cleary, T., et al.: Pyoderma in childhood. Adv. Dermatol. *4*:127-141, 1989.

62. Gorak, E. J., Yamada, S. M., and Brown, J. D.: Community-acquired methicillin-resistant *Staphylococcus aureus* in hospitalized adults and children without known risk factors. Clin. Infect. Dis. *29*:797-800, 1999.

63. Gosbell, I. B., Mercer, J. L., Neville, S. A., et al.: Non-multiresistant and multiresistant methicillin resistant *Staphylococcus aureus* in community-acquired infections. Med. J. Aust. *174*:627-630, 2001.

64. Greene, S. L., Su, W. P., and Muller, S. A.: Ecthyma gangrenosum: Report of clinical, histopathologic, and bacteriologic aspects of eight cases. J. Am. Acad. Dermatol. *11*:781-787, 1984.

65. Guberman, D., Gilead, L. T., Zlotogorski, A., et al.: *Bullous erysipelas*: A retrospective study of 26 patients. J. Am. Acad. Dermatol. *41*:733-737, 1999.

66. Gucluer, H., Ergun, T., and Demircay, Z.: Ecthyma gangrenosum. Int. J. Dermatol. *38*:299-302, 1999.

67. Hall, W. D., Blumberg, R. W., and Moody, M. D.: Studies in children with impetigo: Bacteriology, serology, and incidence of glomerulonephritis. Am. J. Dis. Child. *125*:800-806, 1973.

68. Halperin, S. A.: *Haemophilus influenzae* type b and its role in diseases of the head and neck. J. Otolaryngol. *19*:169-174, 1990.

69. Hauger, S. B.: Facial cellulitis: An early indicator of group B streptococcal bacteremia. Pediatrics *67*:376-377, 1981.

70. Hayden, G. F.: Skin diseases encountered in a pediatric clinic: A one-year prospective study. Am. J. Dis. Child. *139*:36-38, 1985.

71. Hays, G. C., and Mullard, J. E.: Blistering distal dactylitis: A clinically recognizable streptococcal infection. Pediatrics *56*:129-131, 1975.

72. Herold, B. C., Immergluck, L. C., Maranan, M. C., et al.: Community-acquired methicillin-resistant *Staphylococcus aureus* in children with no identified predisposing risk. J. A. M. A. *279*:593-598, 1998.

73. Hewitt, W. D., and Farrar, W. E.: Bacteremia and ecthyma caused by *Streptococcus pyogenes* in a patient with acquired immunodeficiency syndrome. Am. J. Med. Sci. *295*:52-54, 1988.

74. Hirn, M., and Niinikoski, J.: Management of perineal necrotizing fasciitis (Fournier's gangrene). Ann. Chir. Gynaecol. *78*:277-281, 1989.

75. Ho, P. W., Pien, F. D., and Hamburg, D.: Value of cultures in patients with acute cellulitis. South. Med. J. *72*:1402-1403, 1979.

76. Hoeger, P. H., Lenz, W., Boutonnier, A., et al.: Staphylococcal skin colonization in children with atopic dermatitis: Prevalence, persistence, and transmission of toxigenic and nontoxigenic strains. J. Infect. Dis. *165*:1064-1068, 1992.

77. Hsieh, S., and Babl, F. E.: *Serratia marcescens* cellulitis following an iguana bite. Clin. Infect. Dis. *28*:1181-1182, 1999.

78. Hsu, C. T., Lin, Y. T., Yang, Y. H., and Chiang, B. L.: The hyperimmunoglobulin E syndrome. J Microbiol. Immunol. Infect. *37*:121-123, 2004.

79. Jackson, M. A., Colombo, J., and Boldrey, A.: *Streptococcal fasciitis* with toxic shock syndrome in the pediatric patient. Orthop. Nurs. *22*:4-8, 2003.

80. Jarvis, W. R.: The epidemiology of colonization. Infect. Control Hosp. Epidemiol. *17*:47-52, 1996.

81. Kaplan, S. L.: Community-acquired methicillin-resistant *Staphylococcus aureus* infection in children. Semin. Pediatr. Infect. Dis. *17*:113-119, 2006.

82. Kaplan, S. L., Hulten, K. G., Gonzalez, B. E., et al.: Three-year surveillance of community-acquired *Staphylococcus aureus* infections in children. Clin. Infect. Dis. *40*:1785-1791, 2005.

83. Kars, M., van Dijk, H., Salimans, M. M., et al.: Association of furunculosis and familial deficiency of mannose-binding lectin. Eur. J. Clin. Invest. *35*:531-534, 2005.

84. Kelly, C., Taplin, D., and Allen, A. M.: Streptococcal ecthyma: Treatment with benzathine penicillin G. Arch. Dermatol. *103*:306-310, 1971.

85. Kimyai-Asadi, A., Tausk, F. A., and Nousari, H. C.: Ecthyma secondary to herpes simplex virus infection. Clin. Infect. Dis. *29*:454-455, 1999.

86. Kocher, M. S., Coombs, C. J., and Upton, J., 3rd: Actinomycetoma of the phalanx in an immunocompromised patient: A case report. J. Hand Surg. [Am.] *21*:515-517, 1996.

87. Kokx, N. P., Comstock, J. A., and Facklam, R. R.: Streptococcal perianal disease in children. Pediatrics *80*:659-663, 1987.

88. Lacroix, J., Cau, D., Pascal, C., et al.: A case of erysipelas caused by *Haemophilus influenzae*. Union Med. Can. *112*:272, 1983.

89. Lapins, J., Sartorius, K., and Emtestam, L.: Scanner-assisted carbon dioxide laser surgery: A retrospective follow-up study of patients with hidradenitis suppurativa. J. Am. Acad. Dermatol. *47*:280-285, 2002.

90. Larson, E. L., Hughes, C. A., Pyrek, J. D., et al.: Changes in bacterial flora associated with skin damage on hands of health care personnel. Am. J. Infect. Control *26*:513-521, 1998.

91. Le, J., and Lieberman, J. M.: Management of community-associated methicillin-resistant *Staphylococcus aureus* infections in children. Pharmacotherapy *26*:1758-1770, 2006.

92. Lesko, S. M., O'Brien, K. L., Schwartz, B., et al.: Invasive group A streptococcal infection and nonsteroidal antiinflammatory drug use among children with primary varicella. Pediatrics *107*:1108-1115, 2001.

93. Levy, R., and Schlaeffer, F.: Successful treatment of a patient with recurrent furunculosis by vitamin C: Improvement of clinical course and of impaired neutrophil functions. Int. J. Dermatol. *32*:832-834, 1993.

94. Levy, R., Shriker, O., Porath, A., et al.: Vitamin C for the treatment of recurrent furunculosis in patients with impaired neutrophil functions. J. Infect. Dis. *173*:1502-1505, 1996.

95. Lion, C., Conroy, M. C., Dupuy, M. L., et al.: Pasteurella "SP" group infection after a guinea pig bite. Lancet *346*:901-902, 1995.

96. Loebl, E. C., Marvin, J. A., Curreri, P. W., et al.: Survival with ecthyma gangrenosum, a previously fatal complication of burns. J. Trauma *14*:370-377, 1974.

97. Mandell, I. N., Feiner, H. D., Price, N. M., et al.: *Pseudomonas cepacia* endocarditis and ecthyma gangrenosum. Arch. Dermatol. *113*:199-202, 1977.

98. Marks, V. J., and Maksimak, M.: Perianal streptococcal cellulitis. J. Am. Acad. Dermatol. *18*:587-588, 1988.

99. McLinn, S.: A bacteriologically controlled, randomized study comparing the efficacy of 2% mupirocin ointment (Bactroban) with oral erythromycin in the treatment of patients with impetigo. J. Am. Acad. Dermatol. *22*:883-885, 1990.

100. Meredith, F. T., and Sexton, D. J.: *Mycobacterium abscessus* osteomyelitis following a plantar puncture wound. Clin. Infect. Dis. *23*:651-653, 1996.

101. Mereghetti, L., van der Mee-Marquet, N., Dubost, A. F., et al.: *Nocardia otitidis-caviarum* infection of a traumatic skin wound. Eur. J. Clin. Microbiol. Infect. Dis. *16*:383-384, 1997.

102. Milstein, P., and Gleckman, R.: Pneumococcal erysipelas: A unique case in an adult. Am. J. Med. *59*:293-296, 1975.

103. Miron, D., El, A. L., Zuker, M., et al.: *Mycobacterium fortuitum* osteomyelitis of the cuboid after nail puncture wound. Pediatr. Infect. Dis. J. *19*:483-485, 2000.

104. Mogielnicki, N. P., Schwartzman, J. D., and Elliott, J. A.: Perineal group A streptococcal disease in a pediatric practice. Pediatrics *106*:276-281, 2000.

105. Moyer, C. D., Sykes, P. A., and Rayner, J. M.: *Aeromonas hydrophila* septicaemia producing ecthyma gangrenosum in a child with leukaemia. Scand. J. Infect. Dis. *9*:151-153, 1977.

106. Murphy, J. J., Granger, R., Blair, G. K., et al.: Necrotizing fasciitis in childhood. J. Pediatr. Surg. *30*:1131-1134, 1995.

107. Murphy, O., Marsh, P. J., Gray, J., et al.: Ecthyma gangrenosum occurring at sites of iatrogenic trauma in pediatric oncology patients. Med. Pediatr. Oncol. *27*:62-63, 1996.

108. O'Brien, K., Schwartz, B., Lesko, S. M., et al.: Necrotizing fasciitis during primary varicella. Pediatrics *103*:783-790, 1999.

109. Ohana, N., Keness, J., Verner, E., et al.: Skin-isolated, community-acquired *Staphylococcus aureus*: In vitro resistance to methicillin and erythromycin. J. Am. Acad. Dermatol. *21*:544-546, 1989.

110. Patel, M., Ahrens, J. C., Moyer, D. V., et al.: Pneumococcal soft-tissue infections: A problem deserving more recognition. Clin. Infect. Dis. *19*:149-151, 1994.

111. Pouryousefi, A., Foland, J., Michie, C., et al.: Ecthyma gangrenosum as a very early herald of acute lymphoblastic leukaemia. J. Paediatr. Child Health *35*:505-506, 1999.

112. Rabinowitz, R., and Lewin, E. B.: Gangrene of the genitalia in children with *Pseudomonas* sepsis. J. Urol. *124*:431-432, 1980.

113. Rahmouni, A., Chosidow, O., Mathieu, D., et al.: MR imaging in acute infectious cellulitis. Radiology *192*:493-496, 1994.

114. Redbord, K. P., Shearer, D. A., Gloster, H., et al.: Atypical *Mycobacterium furunculosis* occurring after pedicures. J. Am. Acad. Dermatol. *54*:520-524, 2006.

115. Rhie, S., Turcios, R., Buckley, H., et al.: Clinical features and treatment of *Malassezia folliculitis* with fluconazole in orthotopic heart transplant recipients. J. Heart Lung Transplant. *19*:215-219, 2000.

116. Rittner, A. V., Fitzpatrick, K., and Corfield, A.: Best evidence topic report: Are antibiotic indicated following human bites? Emerg. Med. J. *22*:654, 2005.

117. Rodot, S., Lacour, J. P., van Elslande, L., et al.: Ecthyma gangrenosum caused by *Klebsiella pneumoniae*. Int. J. Dermatol. *34*:216-217, 1995.

118. Rolle, U.: *Haemophilus influenzae* cellulitis after bite injuries in children. J. Pediatr. Surg. *31*:1408-1409, 2000.

119. Roujeau, J. C.: Necrotizing fasciitis: Clinical criteria and risk factors. Ann. Dermatol. Venereol. *128*:376-381, 2001.

120. Schwarz, G., Sagy, M., and Barzilay, Z.: Multifocal necrotizing fasciitis in varicella. Pediatr. Emerg. Care *5*:31-33, 1989.

121. Semel, J. D., and Trenholme, G.: *Aeromonas hydrophila* water-associated traumatic wound infections: A review. J. Trauma *30*:324-327, 1990.

122. Sevinsky, L. D., Viecens, C., Ballesteros, D. O., et al.: Ecthyma gangrenosum: A cutaneous manifestation of *Pseudomonas aeruginosa* sepsis. J. Am. Acad. Dermatol. *29*:104-106, 1993.

123. Shama, S., and Calandra, G. B.: Atypical erysipelas caused by group G streptococci in a patient with cured Hodgkin's disease. Arch. Dermatol. *118*:934-936, 1982.

124. Shopsin, B., Mathema, B., Martinez, J., et al.: Prevalence of methicillin-resistant and methicillin-susceptible *Staphylococcus aureus* in the community. J. Infect. Dis. *182*:359-362, 2000.

125. Sidwell, R. U., Ibrahim, M. A., and Bunker, C. B.: A case of common variable immunodeficiency presenting with furunculosis. Br. J. Dermatol. *147*:364-367, 2002.

126. Simor, A. E., Phillips, E., McGeer, A., et al.: Randomized controlled trial of chlorhexidine gluconate for washing, intranasal mupirocin, and rifampin and doxycycline versus no treatment for the eradication of methicillin-resistant *Staphylococcus aureus* colonization. Clin. Infect. Dis. *44*:178-185, 2007.

127. Smith, K. J., Neafie, R., Yeager, J., et al.: Micrococcus folliculitis in HIV-1 disease. Br. J. Dermatol. *141*:558-561, 1999.

128. Smith, P. F., Meadowcroft, A. M., and May, D. B.: Treating mammalian bite wounds. J. Clin. Pharm. Ther. *25*:85-99, 2000.

129. Sokol, R. J., and Bowden, R. A.: An erysipelas-like scalp cellulitis due to *Haemophilus influenzae* type b. J. Pediatr. *96*:60-61, 1980.

130. Sosin, D. M., Gunn, R. A., Ford, W. L., et al.: An outbreak of furunculosis among high school athletes. Am. J. Sports Med. *17*:828-832, 1989.

131. Stone, L., Codére, F., and Ma, S. A.: Streptococcal lid necrosis in previously healthy children. Can. J. Ophthalmol. *26*:386-390, 1991.

132. Talan, D. A., Abrahamian, F. M., Moran, G. J., et al.: Clinical presentation and bacteriologic analysis of infected human bites in patients presenting to emergency departments. Clin. Infect. Dis. *37*:1481-1489, 2003.

133. Thomas, D. B., Brooks, D. E., Bice, T. G., et al.: Tobramycin-impregnated calcium sulphate prevents infection in contaminated wounds. Clin. Orthop. *441*:366-371, 2005.

134. Turnbull, D., and Parry, M. F.: Ecthyma-like skin lesions caused by *Staphylococcus aureus*. Arch. Intern. Med. *141*:689, 1981.

135. Umbert, I. J., Winkelmann, R. K., Oliver, G. F., et al.: Necrotizing fasciitis: A clinical, microbiologic, and histopathologic study of 14 patients. J. Am. Acad. Dermatol. *20*:774-781, 1989.

136. Vaillant, L.: Diagnostic criteria for erysipelas. Ann. Dermatol. Venereol. *128*:326-333, 2001.

137. Varghese, R., Melo, J. C., Chun, C. H., et al.: Erysipelas-like syndrome caused by *Streptococcus pneumoniae*. South. Med. J. *72*:757-758, 1979.

138. Wenger, P. N., Brown, J. M., McNeil, M. M., et al.: *Nocardia farcinica* sternotomy site infections in patients following open heart surgery. J. Infect. Dis. *178*:1539-1543, 1998.

139. Wenke, J. C., Owens, B. D., Svoboda, S. J., and Brooks, D. E.: Effectiveness of commercially-available antibiotic-impregnated implants. J. Bone Joint Surg. Br. *88*:1102-1104, 2006.

140. Wilfert, C. M.: Epidemiology of *Haemophilus influenzae* type b infections. Pediatrics *85*:631-635, 1990.

141. Zentner, J., Hassler, W., and Petersen, D.: A wooden foreign body penetrating the superior orbital fissure. Neurochirurgia *34*:188-190, 1991.

142. Zerr, D. M., Alexander, E. R., Duchin, J. S., et al.: A case-control study of necrotizing fasciitis during primary varicella. Pediatrics *105*:1372-1373, 2000.

143. Zerr, D. M., and Rubens, C. E.: NSAIDs and necrotizing fasciitis. Pediatr. Infect. Dis. J. *18*:724-725, 1999.

144. Zittergruen, M., and Grose, C.: Magnetic resonance imaging for early diagnosis of necrotizing fasciitis. Pediatr. Emerg. Care *9*:26-28, 1993.

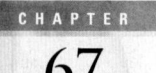

CHAPTER 67

VIRAL AND FUNGAL SKIN INFECTIONS

Meena R. Julapalli ✣ Moise L. Levy

VIRAL INFECTIONS

Cutaneous manifestations of viral infections are common. Exanthems often accompany acute viral infections. The Dukes numbering system of six exanthems is well known to clinicians but is now primarily of historic interest only (Table 67–1). With rare exceptions, skin manifestations that mimic the "typical" features of the six exanthems are seen with multiple infectious agents. Other infections result in lesions such as warts or molluscum contagiosum. This chapter focuses on the common viral illnesses that manifest with cutaneous manifestations. More detailed information on each of these illnesses can be found in the chapters devoted to specific viral agents.

Viruses can invade the skin indirectly as a result of viremia or directly, as with warts or molluscum. Other mechanisms of producing exanthems include interactions between the infecting agent and humoral or cell-mediated factors or a systemic immune response in the absence of viral antigen in the skin.[78]

The type of exanthem encountered depends on the virus, the pathophysiologic mechanisms involved, the location of the eruption, and local and systemic immune factors. A single virus may manifest with a variety of cutaneous reactions within the same host. Clinicians caring for a patient with an exanthem usually are faced with a challenge to determine its cause. Most viral exanthems are benign and self-limited, but understanding the exact cause can be important when evaluating immunocompromised patients or in the setting of a fetus. Similarly, distinguishing a viral exanthem from skin eruptions caused by other infectious agents or drugs is important.

Generally, children presenting with fever and a rash cannot be diagnosed accurately by the presentation of the eruption.[53] The distribution and character of exanthems, such as the often characteristic reticulated erythema after "slapped cheek" exanthem typical of parvovirus B19 infections, are helpful; however, the virus can manifest with several other cutaneous findings.[20,81,86] Typical hand, foot, and mouth syndrome is caused by coxsackievirus, although it has been related more recently to enterovirus 71.[25] The concurrent administration of antibiotics in the setting of Epstein-Barr virus infection is important to know, as is the possible relationship between human herpesvirus infection and certain drugs resulting in drug rash with eosinophilia and systemic symptoms.[35]

Laboratory studies, in addition to specific viral cultures, polymerase chain reaction, and serologies, may be helpful in distinguishing between viral and bacterial diseases or drug eruptions. Coagulation studies may help clarify whether a purpuric eruption is caused by a primary coagulopathy or a viral process. Other laboratory tests, such as streptococcal screens or throat cultures or both, serum antibody titers, viral cultures, and antigen detection methods, are required for evaluating exanthems, depending on the state of the patient being evaluated.

TABLE 67–1 Dukes Classification of Exanthems

First disease*	Measles
Second disease	Scarlet fever
Third disease	Rubella
Fourth disease†	Dukes disease
Fifth disease	Erythema infectiosum
Sixth disease	Roseola infantum

*It is not known definitively if measles or scarlet fever was the first disease.
†This disorder had characteristics of many infections and today is not believed to represent a distinct entity.
Data from Cherry, J. D.: Cutaneous manifestations of systemic disease. In Feigin, R. D., and Cherry, J. D. (eds.): Textbook of Pediatric Infectious Diseases. 3rd ed. Philadelphia, W. B. Saunders, 1992, pp. 755-782; Frieden, I. J., and Penneys, N. S.: Viral infections. In Schachner, L. A., and Hansen, R. C. (eds.): Pediatric Dermatology. New York, Churchill Livingstone, 1988, pp. 1371-1413; Hurwitz, S.: Clinical Pediatric Dermatology. 2nd ed. Philadelphia, W. B. Saunders, 1993, pp. 318-371.

WARTS

Although most warts are easily recognized by practitioners and manifest with nothing more than local discomfort or embarrassment for school-aged children, some carry more ominous associations. Human papillomaviruses (HPV), which are DNA viruses, cause this infection. Approximately 120 different serotypes exist, and subclinical infections have been documented.[75] The common wart, or verruca vulgaris, is caused by infection with HPV type 2 or 4. Infection is transmitted by direct contact, and some site specificity exists for each HPV type. Some HPV types, such as 11 and 16, have documented associations with malignancy.[75,124] A vaccine directed against HPV types 6, 11, 16, and 18 has been released in an attempt to address this problem.[24,47] Immunocompromised patients, such as renal transplant recipients, can have persistence of a variety of HPV types, although not always the types having a malignant risk.[9] In healthy hosts, warts can resolve spontaneously within 2 years in most patients.[6] Persistence of infection can be a source of great concern, however, leading to consultation regarding treatment options.

No specific treatments are available for warts. Most treatments are physically destructive in nature, although some incite local immune responses. When discussing treatment options with patients or families, being frank about the lack of predictably useful therapies is important. One of the only therapies subjected to appropriately controlled trials is salicylic acid, which has shown efficacy in approximately 65 percent of the patients so managed. Office therapies using liquid nitrogen, acids such as trichloroacetic acid, or cantharidin have been used with variable success. Over-the-counter cryotherapy units typically do not freeze the lesions as quickly or as thoroughly as does liquid nitrogen. Laser such as carbon dioxide or erbium:YAG lasers are classic destructive lasers. Pulsed-dye lasers also have been useful for some patients through selective destruction of the vasculature. Multiple other modalities, such as duct tape, first suggested in 1978 and more recently by several authors, and antivirals such as cidofovir have been used. The goal of management of this infection must be tailored to the patient and the nature of the lesions.

The finding of condyloma in a young child always raises concern for sexual abuse. When a condyloma is seen in children younger than 2 to 3 years of age, vertical transmission is well recognized to be a means of transmission.[75,124] Caretakers known to have warts also are obvious transmitters of viruses causing such lesions. In these children or in the case of older children, obtaining a careful history regarding the child's behavior and caretakers and examining the child thoroughly for any signs of physical abuse always are important.

MOLLUSCUM CONTAGIOSUM

Molluscum contagiosum represents a common viral infection of the skin (and sometimes mucous membranes) of children and adolescents. It is caused by a poxvirus and has not been grown in culture. The virus replicates within the cytoplasm[38] and is represented by four viral types based on DNA analysis: MCV-1 to MCV-4.[73] MCV-1 accounts for more than 90 percent of infections in the United States.[38,73] The subtypes do not show site specificity. MCV-2 was reported to be seen most commonly in patients infected with human immunodeficiency virus (HIV).[40,73]

EPIDEMIOLOGY

The disease is seen with increasing frequency in sexually active and immunodeficient individuals. Infection occurs at any age, with the highest frequency seen in patients younger than 5 to 10 years old.[17,38] The infection is two to three times more common in school-aged and sexually active males than in females. Transmission is via close contact. Spread is reported to occur via fomites. The incidence of disease is highest in warm climates and in areas of overcrowding.

CLINICAL MANIFESTATIONS

The incubation period for molluscum contagiosum is 2 to 7 weeks, but it has been reported to occur at 1 week of age. Typical lesions are 1 to 5 mm in size, dome-shaped, skin-colored or pink papules with a distinctive central umbilication (Fig. 67–1). Giant lesions 1 to 2 cm can be seen. According to an epidemiologic survey conducted at three pediatric dermatology centers, fewer than 15 lesions usually are seen.[38] In children, molluscum contagiosum is seen most frequently on the face, neck, trunk, and extremities but may be seen on any part of the body, including the mucous membranes.[17,38,72] Periocular lesions may lead to secondary keratoconjunctivitis or trachoma. In some cases, molluscum contagiosum is a sexually transmitted disease, raising the issue of sexual abuse when infection is seen in the genital area. The most common etiology of genital molluscum contagiosum is autoinoculation; however, if the lesions occur solely in the genital area, or a question exists about the patient's social situation, the possibility of abuse should be explored.

Atypical lesions of molluscum contagiosum are seen more commonly, particularly with the improved survival rates of patients with acquired immunodeficiency syndrome (AIDS) and other immunocompromised states. The incidence of molluscum contagiosum in HIV infection is 5 to 18 percent. With improved antiretroviral therapies, molluscum contagiosum has decreased in this population.[21,38]

Molluscum contagiosum lesions in immunocompromised patients often are large, are situated more deeply in the epider-

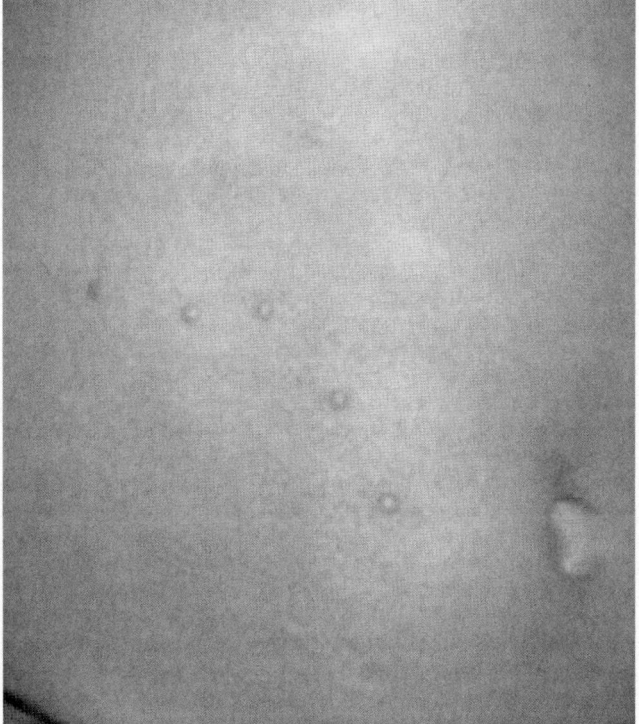

Figure 67–1 Grouped dome-shaped papules of molluscum contagiosum on the skin of the abdomen. (See companion Expert Consult web site for color version.)

mis, and may number in the hundreds. HIV-positive adults usually have molluscum contagiosum on the face, neck, and trunk. In a study of immunocompromised children, molluscum contagiosum was not considered to be common or severe, however. This study included only six patients, and two were disease-free and thought to be immunocompetent at the time of onset of the infection. This and other studies suggest that the presence and degree of cellular immunodeficiency are important in the presentation of molluscum contagiosum.

Patients with atopic dermatitis may be predisposed to develop more severe molluscum contagiosum infection. Available information is insufficient to know if this development is related to the dermatitis itself with its well-described barrier dysfunction or to the use of corticosteroids or other topical agents. The term *molluscum dermatitis* is used to describe an eczematous eruption, more commonly seen in patients with atopic dermatitis, which may occur around molluscum contagiosum lesions and is thought to represent a delayed-type hypersensitivity reaction to viral antigens in the dermis.

Molluscum contagiosum infections in healthy individuals usually resolve spontaneously over the course of several months to 3 to 5 years. For this reason, limited infections can be observed expectantly. More diffuse infections or infections that show continued extension can be considered for treatment. No definitive treatments are available for molluscum contagiosum. Most treatments, similar to those used for warts, are destructive in nature. Immune enhancement for these infections has been tried, but its utility has not been proven. Multiple treatments have been used, although utility is uncertain in all but curettage.

PARVOVIRUS B19 INFECTIONS

The most well-known infection caused by parvovirus B19 is erythema infectiosum or fifth disease.[86] The infection also is termed *slapped cheek disease* because of its initial skin manifestation of bilateral facial erythema (Fig. 67–2). Other manifestations include a papular purpuric glove-and-socks eruption and an eruption with pustules in a bathing-trunk distribution.

The virus is a single-stranded DNA virus that infects erythroid cells. The infection is spread via the respiratory route, with an incubation period of approximately 2 weeks. Most patients are asymptomatic. Serologic assays for IgG and IgM antibodies are used for confirmation of infection. The exanthem of fifth disease coincides with the presence of IgM antibodies. Viral DNA has been found in infected tissues.

Children with fifth disease or erythema infectiosum generally are not ill-appearing. Mild complaints of myalgias or low-grade fevers may be reported. As in adults, arthritis may be seen in older children and adolescents. Outbreaks often spread through schools

or families. Most patients present to their physicians with a typical-appearing reticulated blanching erythema. The slapped cheek appearance characteristic of the disorder may be missed or elicited only on questioning.

The papular, purpuric glove-and-socks syndrome is another condition caused by infection with parvovirus B19.[62] When patients present with the eruption, they are infectious based on the finding of viral DNA. The eruption shows a curious distribution of the hands and feet with clear "cutoff" at the wrists and ankles. Changes in oral skin and mucous membrane may be seen, in addition to mild systemic complaints.

Diagnosis of erythema infectiosum or papular purpuric glove-and-socks syndrome is confirmed by serologic testing for antibodies or polymerase chain reaction. A report of loop-mediated isothermal amplification has shown its utility for rapid diagnosis of such infections and has compared favorably with polymerase chain reaction.[134]

GIANOTTI-CROSTI SYNDROME (PAPULAR ACRODERMATITIS OF CHILDHOOD)

Gianotti-Crosti syndrome (papular acrodermatitis of childhood) is a viral exanthem first reported in 1955 by Gianotti,[50] who described a group of children who presented with predominately acrally located, skin-colored or slightly erythematous, lichenoid papules (Fig. 67–3).[120] The flexures usually were spared. Involvement of the buttocks or trunk was seen in some cases. No involvement of mucous membranes occurred. Patients generally were healthy. The initial reports showed prior infection with hepatitis B. The eruption lasted 2 weeks to 2 months.

Since the initial report, similar cases have been associated with other infections, such as Epstein-Barr virus, coxsackievirus, echovirus, other viruses, and streptococcal disease.[85] Most cases are thought to be viral in origin and often caused by Epstein-Barr virus. Topical therapies do not hasten resolution of the exanthem.

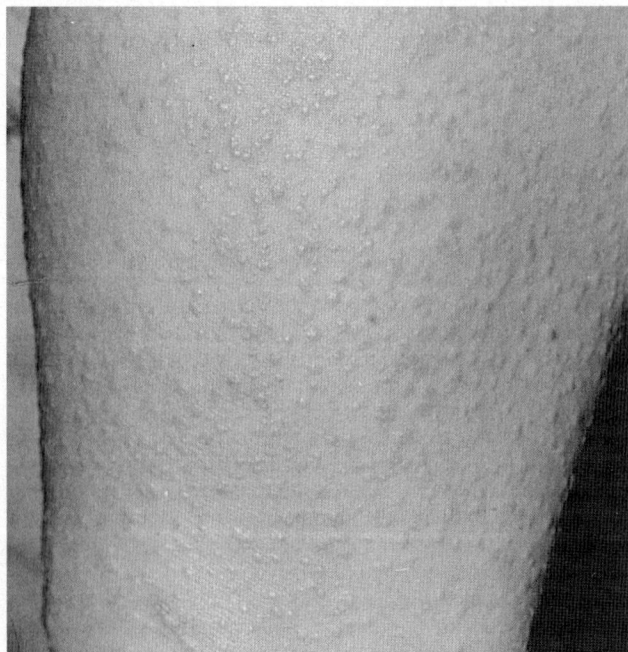

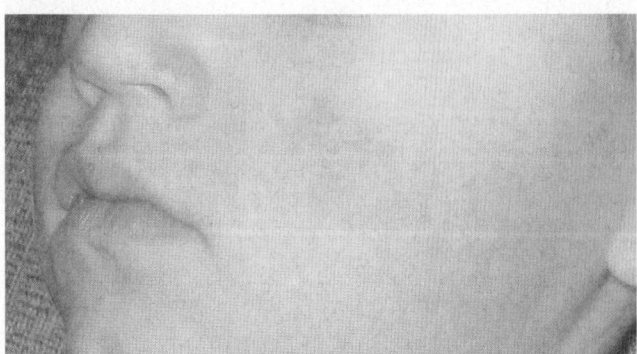

Figure 67–2 Reticulated erythema on the face of a child with erythema infectiosum. (See companion Expert Consult web site for color version.)

Figure 67–3 Diffusely distributed, isolated, monomorphous skin-colored papules on the thigh of a child typical of Gianotti-Crosti syndrome.

ASYMMETRIC PERIFLEXURAL VIRAL EXANTHEM

Some children have been described with discrete or grouped lichenoid papules or urticarial papules beginning around flexures or the torso (Fig. 67–4).[49] The eruption generalizes over several days and can appear as a more diffuse case of the papular acrodermatitis of childhood. The condition also has been described as the unilateral laterothoracic viral exanthem and seems to be associated with the same infectious agents as described in papular acrodermatitis of childhood.[15] The evolution of this condition is similar to that in the papular acrodermatitis of childhood.

HAND, FOOT, AND MOUTH SYNDROME

Patients presenting with a distinctive eruption of sausage-shaped vesicles on the palms and soles with oral mucosal erosions after a mild viral gastroenteritis represent the classic case of hand, foot, and mouth syndrome. Patients may have erythematous papules found on the skin of the buttocks as well. Cases tend to cluster within homes, daycare centers, or schools. Most cases resolve spontaneously without sequelae over the course of 2 to 3 weeks. Hand, foot, and mouth syndrome traditionally is attributed to infection with coxsackievirus A16; however, more recent data suggest enterovirus 71 as a predominant cause as well.

A more recent publication followed a large outbreak of hand, foot, and mouth syndrome (and herpangina) in Taiwan.[25] As with known epidemiologic data, most cases occurred in younger children (93%, <4 years old; 75%, <1 year old). Enterovirus 71 and coxsackievirus A16 were the viruses predominantly recovered. Enterovirus 71 was seen in 66 percent of these patients. The authors emphasized the potential for mortality from this virus, particularly as a result of pulmonary edema or hemorrhage, although encephalitis also was seen. Enterovirus 71 was seen primarily in inpatients, whereas coxsackievirus A16 was recovered from outpatients.

HERPES SIMPLEX VIRUS

Herpes simplex virus (HSV) types 1 and 2 are members of the herpesvirus family, which includes varicella-zoster virus, Epstein-Barr virus, cytomegalovirus, and human herpesvirus. HSV-1 and HSV-2 infections may be asymptomatic or associated with classic and unusual clinical manifestations. Although a predilection exists for involvement of the oral mucosa for HSV-1 and the genitalia for HSV-2, either can infect any site. These infections occur worldwide and are transmitted by direct contact. Asymptomatic carrier states exist and are known to be the source of infection in patients. Immunity to HSV-1 generally is acquired during childhood, whereas HSV-2 immunity usually is seen after adolescence.

The virus replicates within the epidermis and travels to regional nerve ganglia. The incubation period ranges from 2 to 20 days. Recurrences, which occur in the same site as the original infection, usually are less severe than is the primary infection. In immunocompetent patients, the infection usually remains localized.

CLINICAL MANIFESTATIONS

Children most often present with oral or perioral disease, such as gingivostomatitis or herpes labialis.[124] Painful vesicles and discrete "punched-out" erosions can be seen on the lips, anterior surface of the tongue, or hard palate. Herpes pharyngitis can be seen in older children and can be caused by HSV-2 infection. Feeding problems and foul-smelling breath can occur in these settings. Grouped vesicles on an erythematous base are a common cutaneous finding (Fig. 67–5).

Disease manifestations can last 10 to 14 days. Herpes gladiatorum is caused by transmission of HSV by direct contact. The name derives from exposure and infection between wrestlers, although the infection also can occur in the setting of close contact between participants of other sports. Eczema herpeticum occurs when cutaneous HSV infection spreads over the skin of individuals with an abnormal skin barrier, such as in atopic dermatitis. Infections can be localized or very diffuse and can be associated with systemic involvement. Herpetic whitlow manifests as painful deep-seated vesicles or pustules on the tips of fingers (Fig. 67–6). This infection results from direct contact with active lesions of HSV. A common presentation is in an infant or

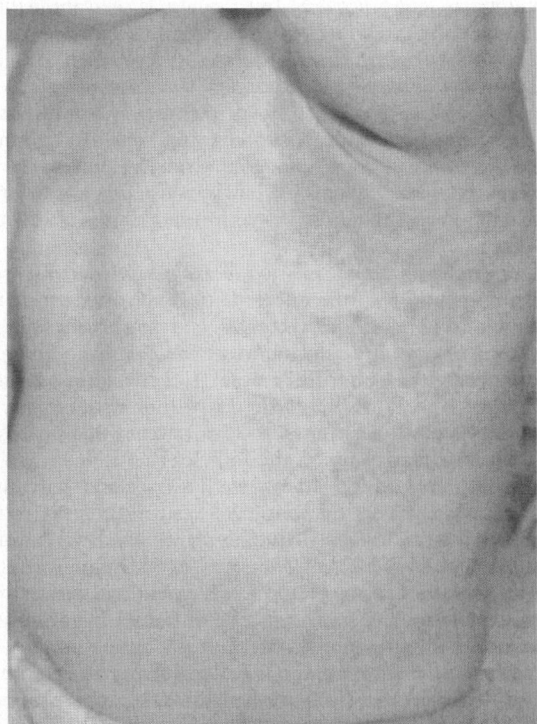

Figure 67–4 Lichenoid papules involving the lateral trunk typical of the unilateral periflexural viral exanthem. (See companion Expert Consult web site for color version.)

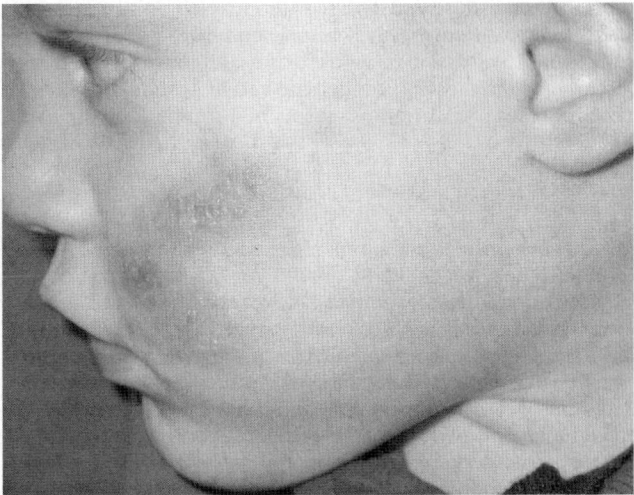

Figure 67–5 Tense vesicles overlying erythematous plaque caused by herpes simplex virus. (See companion Expert Consult web site for color version.)

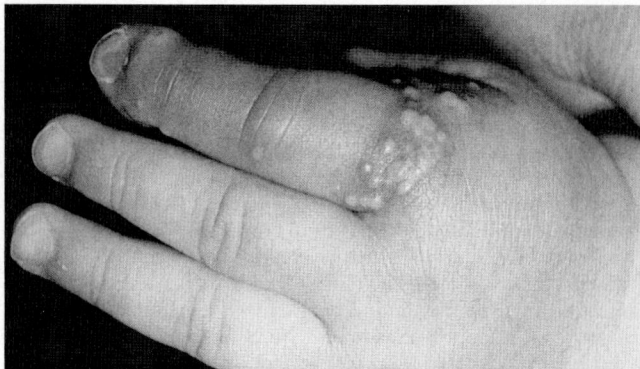

Figure 67–6 Photograph of the left hand of a young child shows grouped tense vesicles typical of a herpetic whitlow.

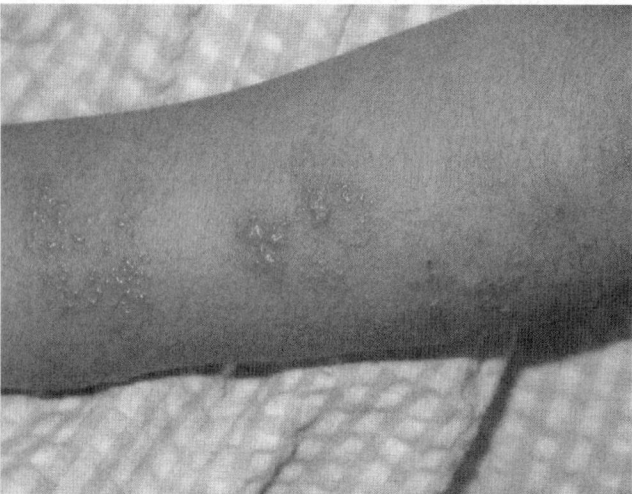

Figure 67–7 Linear array of vesicles caused by herpes zoster. (See companion Expert Consult web site for color version.)

young child who has manipulated a lesion of herpes labialis on a parent. Lastly, HSV infection is perhaps the most common cause of recurrent erythema multiforme.[129] Clinicians should keep this association in mind.

Localized disease and disease without systemic symptoms can be treated symptomatically. Local wound care is appropriate, as indicated. Acyclovir or valacyclovir is useful for cases when antiviral therapy is chosen. Prophylactic antivirals should be considered for cases of recurrent erythema multiforme.

VARICELLA-ZOSTER VIRUS

Chickenpox is the most common presentation of varicella-zoster virus infection in childhood. After a 2-week incubation period, vesicles on erythematous bases ("dewdrops on rose petals") are seen on the head and neck and spread rapidly to the trunk. Involvement of mucous membranes occurs frequently. Lesions are seen in all stages. Constitutional symptoms also may be seen. Unless bacterial infection occurs, scarring seldom occurs. An uncommon and perhaps under-recognized presentation of varicella is photolocalized disease. Several cases of varicella presenting in a photodistributed fashion (i.e., over sun-exposed skin) have been reported.[126]

Shingles or herpes zoster occurs after primary infection with varicella-zoster virus or receipt of vaccination (Fig. 67–7).[112,125]

Healthy children who have had a case of chickenpox before reaching 6 to 12 months of age are at risk for developing shingles.[74] Immunocompromised children are at risk for acquiring this infection as well. Ramsay Hunt syndrome is caused by infection of the geniculate ganglion in this setting.[124]

Most cases of chickenpox do not require antiviral therapy. Management of systemic symptoms and local skin care are needed. Antivirals are needed when treating neonates or immunocompromised patients or normal patients with severe skin disease. There is considerable anecdotal experience using corticosteroids and antivirals for the management of Ramsay Hunt syndrome.

FUNGAL INFECTIONS

Superficial fungal infections, which include dermatophytes, yeast, or dematiaceous fungi, are encountered frequently in general pediatric practice. Particularly in an immunocompromised patient, fungal infections also may involve deeper cutaneous structures and other organ systems. This section focuses on the skin manifestations, diagnosis, and treatment of pediatric fungal infections.

SUPERFICIAL FUNGAL INFECTIONS

DERMATOPHYTE INFECTIONS

Dermatophytes invade and grow in hair, nails, and the outer layer of the skin known as the *stratum corneum*. These lesions vary in appearance based on the site of infection and are named accordingly.

Tinea Capitis

Also known as *scalp ringworm*, tinea capitis is seen frequently in prepubertal children. The causative organisms vary according to country; in North America, tinea capitis is caused largely by *Trichophyton tonsurans* and less often by *Microsporum canis*.[101,121,128] *M. canis*, a zoophilic dermatophyte common to suburban and rural areas, can be transmitted to children who handle infected animals such as cats, dogs, and certain rodents; however, it does not spread between humans.[121] Thick, white patches of broken hair that fluoresce under Wood lamp examination characterize these lesions.

Human-to-human transmission of *T. tonsurans* occurs through the shedding of spores from infected skin scales and hair on items such as clothing, bed linen, combs, and hairbrushes. Lesions caused by *T. tonsurans* do not fluoresce under a Wood lamp and vary in appearance from diffuse scaling of the scalp to circumscribed areas of scaling and erythema with or without hair loss, and, in dark-haired individuals, to scaly patches of hair loss that may leave small dark hairs in the follicles (black-dot ringworm) (Fig. 67–8). Tinea capitis lesions may be associated with suboccipital or posterior cervical lymphadenopathy and may produce more inflammatory lesions, including scaly, pustular areas of hair loss and formation of a kerion—a boggy, erythematous mass with follicular pustules that may lead to permanent hair loss and scarring if left untreated (Fig. 67–9).[28,101,128] Another hypersensitivity response to the dermatophyte infection is a dermatophytid or id reaction, which involves papulovesicular inflammatory eruptions adjacent to or distant from the site of the primary infection (Fig. 67–10).[12]

Tinea capitis must be distinguished from alopecia areata, which consists of patches of total hair loss without scalp changes, and trichotillomania, which may be associated with excoriations,

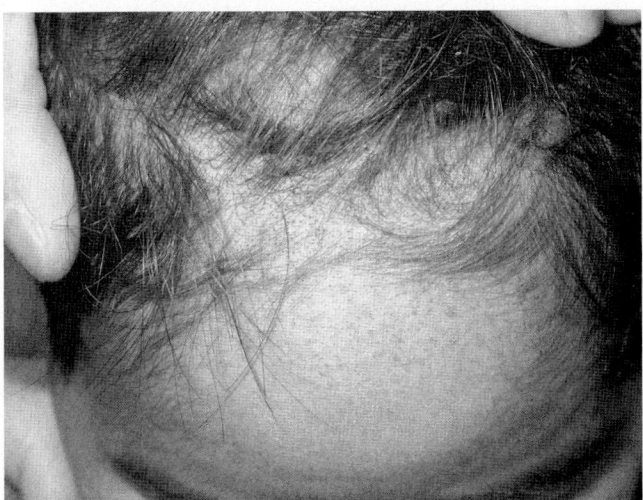

Figure 67–8 Nonscarring alopecia associated with tinea capitis. (See companion Expert Consult web site for color version.)

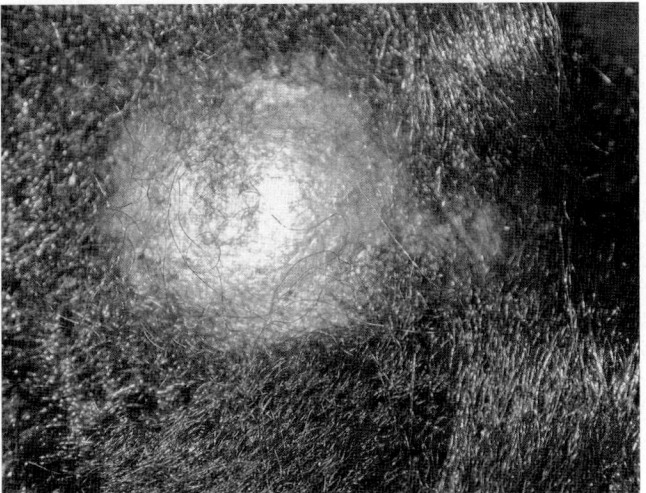

Figure 67–9 Indurated tumor on the scalp typical of kerion. (See companion Expert Consult web site for color version.)

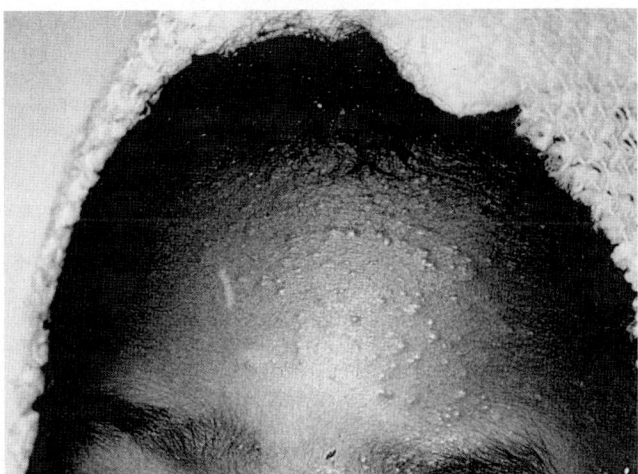

Figure 67–10 Multiple skin-colored papules and pustules on the forehead typical of an id reaction to tinea capitis.

varying lengths of broken hairs, and ill-defined patterns of hair loss. Differential diagnosis also includes traction alopecia, seborrheic dermatitis, psoriasis, and pityriasis amiantacea. In addition, inflammatory lesions of tinea capitis may be confused with bacterial pyodermas of the scalp.[28,121,128]

Tinea Corporis

Tinea corporis refers to dermatophyte infection of the trunk or extremities. Lesions appear as erythematous patches or plaques with well-demarcated, annular borders that may be scaly, pustular, or vesicular.[28,121,128] The application of potent topical corticosteroids may obscure these characteristic borders, resulting in a manifestation termed *tinea incognito*.[121] The differential diagnosis includes seborrheic, atopic, and contact dermatitides; psoriasis; and granuloma annulare.[28,128]

Tinea Faciei

Dermatophyte infections of the face in children are characterized by erythematous, scaly plaques that may be unilateral or occur in a "butterfly" distribution, mimicking cutaneous findings of systemic lupus erythematosus and other collagen vascular diseases (Fig. 67–11). As with tinea corporis, differential diagnosis includes seborrheic, atopic, and contact dermatitides.[28,128]

Tinea Pedis

Tinea pedis, which occurs more commonly in adolescents than in prepubertal children, characterizes dermatophyte infection involving the feet. Findings vary and may be vesicles or erosions over the instep of the feet, fissuring between the toes with surrounding erythema and scaling, or diffuse scaling of the soles in a "moccasin-like" distribution. Differential diagnosis includes juvenile plantar dermatosis, dyshidrotic eczema, atopic dermatitis, contact dermatitis, granuloma annulare, scabies, psoriasis, and erythrasma.[28,121,128]

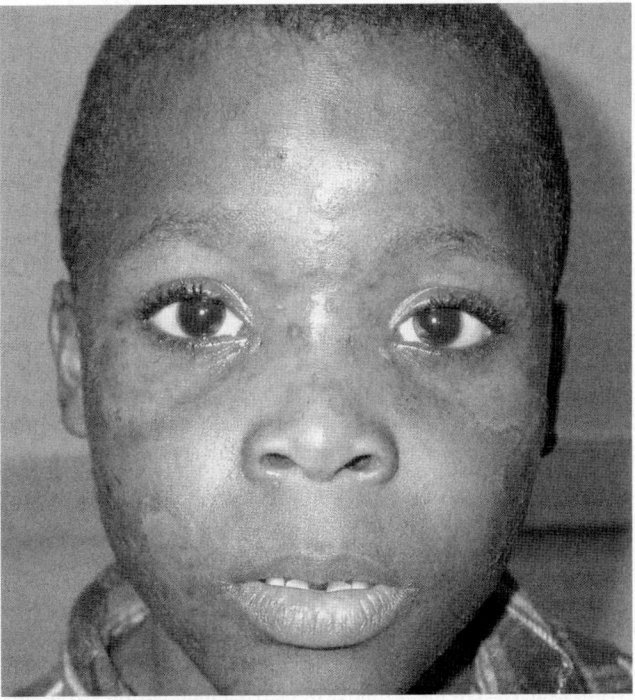

Figure 67–11 Diffuse scaling plaques on the face caused by tinea faciei. (See companion Expert Consult web site for color version.)

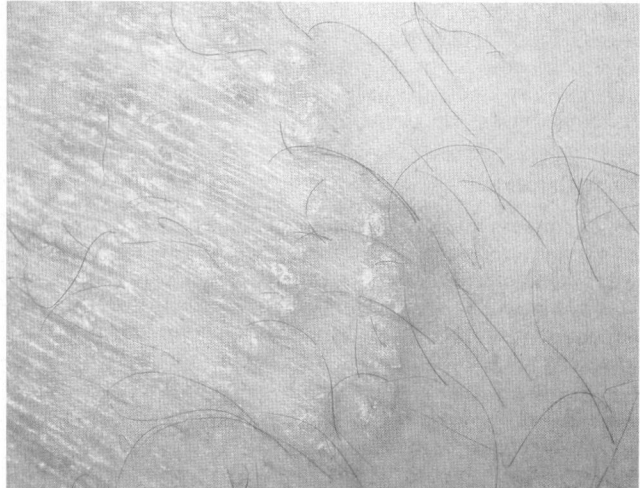

Figure 67–12 Annular scaling plaque on the upper inner thigh caused by tinea cruris. (See companion Expert Consult web site for color version.)

Tinea Cruris

Also predominately seen in adolescents, particularly boys, tinea cruris often occurs in association with tinea pedis and is transmitted through indirect or direct contact with infected skin scales or hair. Risk factors include obesity, friction, moisture, and tight clothing. The characteristic lesions are usually symmetric, well-demarcated, erythematous, scaly eruptions in the inguinal and inner thigh area with potential spread to the buttocks and perianal region. These lesions also may have a raised papular or pustular edge and often are very pruritic, leading to lichenification in chronic disease (Fig. 67–12). The differential diagnosis includes seborrheic dermatitis, *Candida* intertrigo, flexural psoriasis, irritant dermatitis, contact dermatitis, and erythrasma.[28,121,128]

Tinea Unguium

The term *onychomycosis* refers to fungal invasion of the nail plate, which is termed *tinea unguium* when the infection is caused by dermatophytes. The lower incidence of tinea unguium in children compared with adults may be due to faster nail growth, decreased likelihood of nail trauma, and less exposure to tinea pedis, which often is seen concurrently with onychomycosis.[63,106] Clinical findings of infection include superficial white patches on the surface of the nail plate, white spots under the nail, and yellowing and thickening of the nail plate that usually extends from the distal to the proximal end (Figs. 67–13 and 67–14). The differential diagnosis includes psoriasis, lichen planus, hereditary onychodystrophy, and acquired trachyonychia, all of which may be distinguished from tinea unguium by their diffuse nail involvement as opposed to the more limited disease of a dermatophyte infection. Tinea unguium also may mimic *Candida* infection of the nails, but the latter disease differs in that it tends to spread distally from the proximal nail plate.[28,57,63,101,106,128]

DIAGNOSIS

Light microscopy examination with potassium hydroxide should show spores in infected scalp hairs of tinea capitis and branching hyphae in affected nail samples or skin scrapings from advancing margins of lesions on the body (see Fig. 67–14). Fungal culture on Sabouraud dextrose agar treated with chloramphenicol and

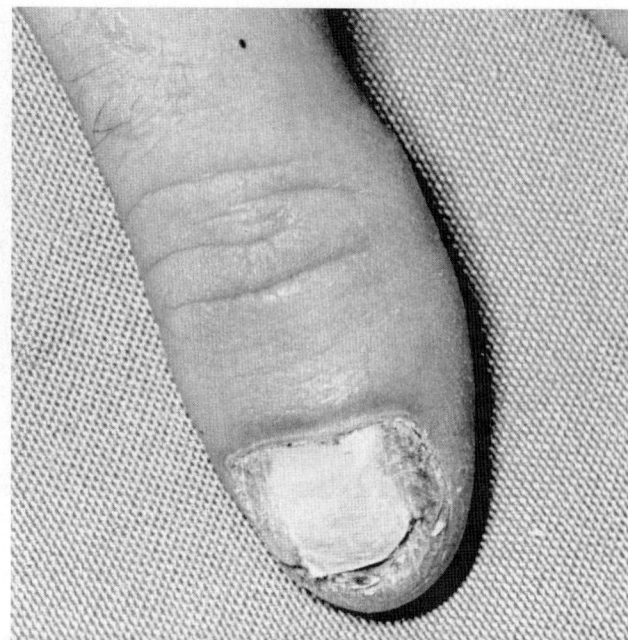

Figure 67–13 Clinical photograph illustrating onychodystrophy and subungual hyperkeratosis involving the left thumb of a child with onychomycosis.

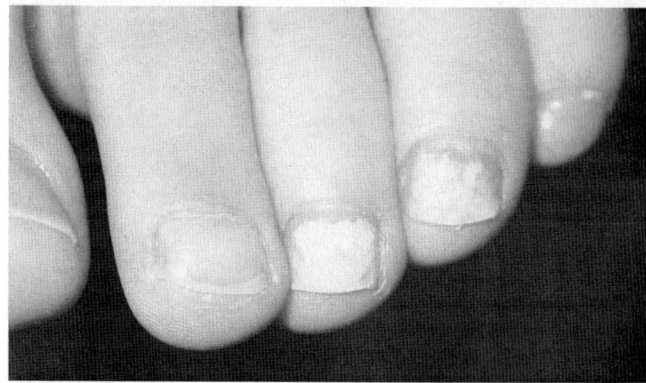

Figure 67–14 White superficial plaques typical of superficial white onychomycosis. (See companion Expert Consult web site for color version.)

cycloheximide provides a growth medium selective for dermatophytes and may aid in differentiating various species. Rarely, biopsy may be required for definitive diagnosis.[28,101,121,128]

TREATMENT

Localized lesions of tinea corporis, faciei, pedis, and cruris generally respond to a 2- to 4-week course of topical antifungals, such as clotrimazole, tolnaftate, ciclopirox olamine, amorolfine, or terbinafine.[101] Severe or refractory disease may require oral antifungal medications. Recurrence of tinea pedis can be prevented by avoiding occlusive footwear and keeping the feet clean and dry.[121]

Griseofulvin is the only oral antifungal medication that is approved by the U.S. Food and Drug Administration (FDA) for use in children. Many agents, including terbinafine, itraconazole, and fluconazole, have been used successfully as off-label alternatives, however, despite limited data regarding their safety and efficacy in children.

Griseofulvin remains the gold standard for the treatment of tinea capitis in the United States. The approved dose of micro-sized griseofulvin is 11 mg/kg/day for 6 to 8 weeks; however, 20 to 25 mg/kg/day often is required to achieve an adequate response.[114] A 2- to 4-week course of terbinafine also has been shown to be as effective as is griseofulvin, particularly in the treatment of tinea capitis caused by *Trichophyton* spp.[42,45,54,115] For *Microsporum* infections, higher doses or longer duration of therapy with terbinafine may be required.[42,45,54,76,115] Studies have shown that a fluconazole regimen of 6 mg/kg/day for 3 to 6 weeks has a cure rate comparable to that of griseofulvin.[43,54,114] Continuous or pulse itraconazole therapy of 5 mg/kg/day has been noted to result in significant improvement and even cure in *Trichophyton* and *Microsporum* tinea capitis by 6 weeks; however, infection with *Microsporum* may require a longer duration of treatment with itraconazole compared with effective courses for *Trichophyton* infection.[51,54,55] In addition, concomitant topical therapy with selenium sulfide 1 to 2.5 percent shampoo in affected individuals and household contacts reduces the number of viable spores and prevents the spread of infection.[52,105,121]

At present, no antifungal agent is approved by the FDA for treatment of onychomycosis in children, and data are limited regarding efficacy of topical and oral antifungal agents. Topical agents have poor penetration into the nail plate, usually leading to an inadequate response rate. Treating concurrent tinea pedis infections with topical therapy may help prevent recurrences of tinea unguium, however. Although griseofulvin is the drug of choice for treating other dermatophyte infections, it is not recommended for the treatment of onychomycosis because of the lengthy course (≤18 months), inadequate response, and high recurrence rate.

Terbinafine (3 to 6 mg/kg/day for 6 to 12 weeks), continuous or pulse itraconazole therapy (5 mg/kg/day for 3 months), and fluconazole (3 to 6 mg/kg once a week for 12 to 26 weeks) have been reported as safe, effective, and well-tolerated alternatives.[57,59,93,115] Because of their keratinophilic and lipophilic natures, these agents accumulate in the stratum corneum and persist at high concentrations in the nails for months, allowing for shorter courses of therapy.[55,57,59,63,115] Terbinafine may be crushed and taken with or without food. Optimal bioavailability with itraconazole capsules occurs when taken with fatty foods, whereas itraconazole solution should be taken on an empty stomach and may be associated with a higher incidence of gastrointestinal side effects than capsules. Studies regarding use of fluconazole for treatment of onychomycosis in children are limited, but successful therapy has been reported at a pulsed dose of 3 to 6 mg/kg once a week for 3 months.[57,59,115]

CANDIDA

The most common cause of fungal infection in healthy and immunocompromised children is *Candida*, and *Candida albicans* accounts for most cases. These yeast forms have a predilection for moist, warm areas of the body such as mucosal surfaces and intertriginous regions and often colonize these areas, becoming part of the normal flora. Disease is caused by overgrowth and infiltration into the epidermis. Superficial infections may be seen in healthy individuals and individuals with predisposing risk factors, such as prematurity; low birth weight; diabetes mellitus; antibiotic, corticosteroid, or oral contraceptive therapy; and other immunocompromised states. These individuals also are more likely to develop systemic candidiasis.[46,101,128]

Thrush is characterized by superficial, sometimes tender, white plaques on oral mucosa that reveal denuded, erythematous bases when scraped off (Fig. 67–15). These manifestations must be distinguished from other oral cavity lesions, such as aphthous stomatitis, epidermolysis bullosa, herpes simplex, hairy leukoplakia,

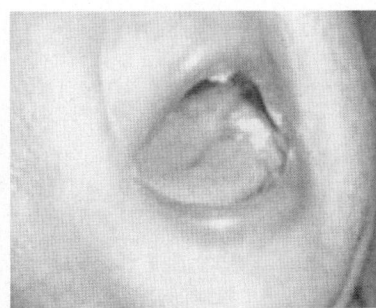

Figure 67–15 White patches on buccal mucosa caused by *Candida albicans*. (See companion Expert Consult web site for color version.)

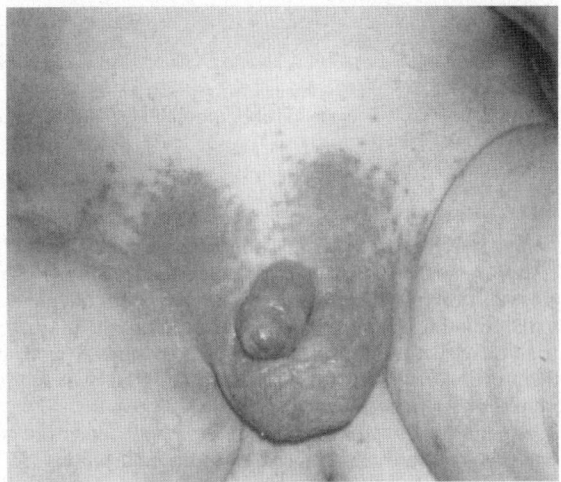

Figure 67–16 Clinical photograph of an infant with *Candida* diaper dermatitis. Confluent and discrete erythematous papules and plaque involving the scrotum, penis, and superpubic and inguinal area.

lichen planus, geographic tongue, erythema multiforme, and burns.[128] Use of pacifiers in infants may increase the risk of development of thrush and colonization of the organism.[11] Oropharyngeal candidiasis may spread to the esophagus in immunocompromised individuals and lead to difficulty with feeding.

Diaper candidiasis appears as beefy, erythematous plaques that involve the inguinal creases and perianal region and often are associated with satellite (or surrounding) erythematous papules, plaques, or pustules (Fig. 67–16). These lesions may cause discomfort when the infant urinates onto affected skin. Superinfection with *Candida* should be suspected when irritant diaper dermatitis fails to improve within several days. Other lesions that may be confused with diaper candidiasis include psoriasis, Langerhans cell histiocytosis, and seborrheic dermatitis.[128]

Thumb-sucking or other trauma near nail beds may lead to nontender, erythematous swelling at the base of the nails termed *paronychia* (Fig. 67–17). Some cases are complicated by *Candida* infection. Differential diagnosis of these lesions includes psoriasis, bacterial infection, lichen planus, and pachyonychia congenita. *Candida* also may produce onychomycosis, but its distribution usually involves the proximal nail plate, in contrast to dermatophytosis of the nails, which more commonly affects the distal nail plate.[128]

Adolescent girls may present with vulvovaginal candidiasis, which is characterized by thick, white discharge and white plaques on irritated, erythematous vaginal mucosa. These lesions may cause vaginal itching and dysuria.[128]

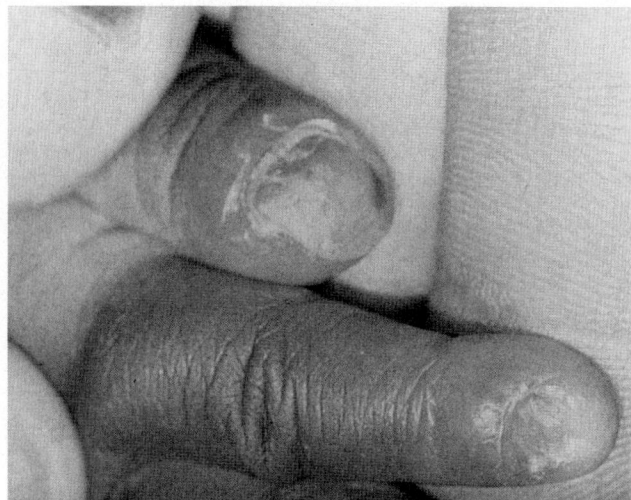

Figure 67–17 Onychodystrophy involving the thumb and index finger, with erythema and edema of the paronychium. These features are typical of *Candida* paronychia.

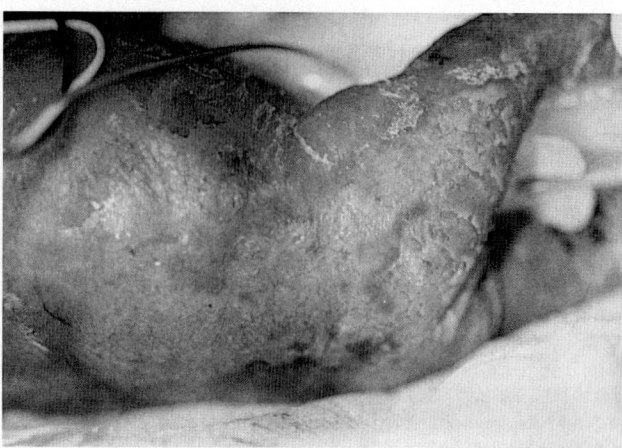

Figure 67–18 Dense crusting overlying the flank and buttocks of a neonate with *Candida* dermatitis. *(From Rowen, J. L., Atkins, J. T., Levy, M. L., et al.: Invasive fungal dermatitis in the 1000-gram neonate. Pediatrics 95:682-687, 1995.)*

Diagnosis of localized *Candida* infection usually is made clinically. Microscopic examination of potassium hydroxide–prepared scrapings of skin and mucosal lesions reveals pseudohyphae and elongated budding yeast forms. Positive cultures of infected material on Sabouraud dextrose agar or cornmeal agar may signify infection or benign colonization. Biopsy rarely is required for establishing a definitive diagnosis.

Treatment of localized *Candida* infection depends on good hygiene practices and maintenance of a dry environment in the susceptible area. Localized infections usually respond well to topical antifungal therapy. Nystatin solution is the first-line agent used for thrush, but oral fluconazole or itraconazole and intravenous amphotericin B may be required to treat recurrent, refractory, or extensive disease, especially in immunocompromised children.[65] Nystatin or imidazole creams in conjunction with frequent diaper changes, barrier creams, and sometimes low-strength topical steroids are the recommended treatment for diaper candidiasis. Paronychia also is susceptible to nystatin and imidazole creams but may require oral therapy. Vulvovaginal candidiasis often can be treated successfully with topical azole medications, but oral azoles are recommended for refractory or recurrent cases. Adolescents can be treated with a single, 150-mg dose of oral fluconazole.[22,65]

Congenital candidiasis, a rare form of infection acquired in utero as a result of *Candida* chorioamnionitis, can manifest in full-term and premature neonates within the first few days of life as a diffuse, erythematous, papular eruption that progresses to formation of vesicles and pustules, and subsequently crusting and desquamation. Palms and soles also may be affected. Term infants with congenital candidiasis rarely develop systemic manifestations, and the infection usually resolves spontaneously or with topical antifungal agents, such as nystatin, imidazoles, or allylamines. Premature, very-low-birth-weight neonates are at risk for developing ecchymosis and necrosis of the skin with dissemination of the *Candida* infection, requiring treatment with systemic antifungal medication. Congenital candidiasis in these premature infants may manifest as sepsis or pneumonia without cutaneous findings as well.[2,101,119]

Differential diagnosis of congenital candidiasis includes epidermolysis bullosa and infection with *Listeria monocytogenes*, *Staphylococcus*, herpesvirus, and syphilis.[36] Early diagnosis is established by histologic examination of the placenta and umbilical cord, which shows the characteristic pseudohyphae and spores

and white microabscesses.[2,36] Microscopic examination and culture of the skin lesions can confirm the diagnosis.

Systemic candidiasis, in which *Candida* spp. can be isolated from the blood, urine, or cerebrospinal fluid, is seen more commonly in immunocompromised individuals, who often present with skin manifestations that include desquamation, abscesses at indwelling catheter sites, and progressive diaper candidiasis. Systemic candidiasis may be associated with signs of sepsis, such as hemodynamic and temperature instability, and respiratory changes.[65,128]

Invasive fungal dermatitis is a rare manifestation of *Candida* infection in premature, very-low-birth-weight infants. *Aspergillus*, *Trichosporon*, and *Curvularia* spp. also have been implicated in this type of infection, but *Candida* is the most common etiologic agent. Besides low birth weight and prematurity, additional risk factors for acquisition of invasive fungal dermatitis include hyperglycemia, steroid use, and vaginal birth. In contrast to congenital candidiasis, invasive fungal dermatitis usually does not manifest until after several days of life. Skin findings include erythematous, macerated plaques and crusted erosions that can spread rapidly over the body and may lead to development of systemic fungemia, with a high mortality rate (Fig. 67–18). Biopsy of these lesions shows invasion through the stratum corneum into the epidermis with occasional extension into the dermis.[107] Survival depends on prompt initiation of systemic antifungal medications.[94,119]

Treatment of disseminated *Candida* infection requires removal of infected indwelling catheters in addition to administration of systemic antifungal therapy. Intravenous amphotericin B is the drug of choice for treating disseminated disease and sometimes is administered in combination with 5-fluorocytosine for synergism. Other options include systemic itraconazole and fluconazole; however, some *Candida* spp. have shown resistance to fluconazole.[2,101,119] Azoles also have been used as prophylaxis for systemic fungal infections in neutropenic patients with hematologic malignancies and bone marrow transplant recipients,[30,66,90] but this practice, especially in preterm neonates, is controversial because of the potential for resistance.[19,23] Newer antifungal agents, such as voriconazole, posaconazole, and caspofungin, have been reported to be effective treatments, particularly in resistant candidemia.[5,85,88,91,114,118] Avoidance of prolonged antibiotic and steroid administration may aid in clearance of *Candida* infection.[65,128]

MALASSEZIA

Malassezia spp., most notably *Malassezia furfur,* are lipophilic yeast forms that are found more readily in humid, tropical environments and are part of the normal skin flora in humans. Colonization begins in the neonatal period and increases with age.[10] *Malassezia* is the organism thought to be responsible for neonatal cephalic pustulosis and tinea (or pityriasis) versicolor in older children, adolescents, and young adults. Invasion of the organism through indwelling catheters, particularly catheters being used for intralipid infusion, in premature, very-low-birth-weight infants also may lead to sepsis and death.[7,103,119] *Malassezia* also has been implicated in the pathogenesis of seborrheic dermatitis, atopic dermatitis, and psoriasis, although this implication is controversial.[7,28,56,84,92,110,123]

Neonatal cephalic pustulosis is a self-limited disease characterized by scattered, erythematous papules and pustules in a head-and-neck distribution (Fig. 67–19). Follicular accentuation and comedones are not observed. Diagnosis usually is made clinically, but may be confirmed by microscopic findings.[10,101,119]

Tinea versicolor is characterized by macules with fine scales that are distributed on the upper body and neck. The macules may appear hypopigmented in dark-skinned individuals or tan or dark brown in lighter skinned individuals (Fig. 67–20). Differential diagnosis includes vitiligo, pityriasis alba, pityriasis rosea, postinflammatory hypopigmentation, melasma, seborrheic dermatitis, contact dermatitis, and tinea corporis. Lesions of tinea versicolor are fluorescent yellow to orange under Wood lamp. Microscopic examination of potassium hydroxide–prepared scrapings of the lesions shows a "spaghetti and meatball" appearance owing to the presence of short, curved hyphae and round spores. Biopsy of the lesions, which usually is unnecessary, reveals the characteristic hyphae and spores invading the stratum corneum.

The recommended treatment is application of 2.5 percent selenium sulfide or ketaconazole shampoo. Other topical agents, such as ciclopirox, terbinafine solutions, sodium hypochlorite, and other azoles, also may be effective. Short 1- to 5-day courses of oral itraconazole, fluconazole, and ketoconazole in single daily doses have been suggested as effective treatments; however, these agents are not approved by the FDA for treating tinea versicolor in children because of their limited safety and efficacy profiles.[12,41,100] It is important to advise patients that skin discolorations may take months to resolve and that recurrences are very common and may require retreatment.[28,100,101,119,128] *Malassezia* sepsis responds well to removal of indwelling catheters and rarely requires systemic antifungal therapy.[119]

CHROMOBLASTOMYCOSIS

Fonsecaea pedrosoi, and less commonly *Cladophialophora carrionii* and *Phialophora verrucosa,* are found in tropical climates and are organisms responsible for causing chromoblastomycosis, a chronic granulomatous disease affecting skin and subcutaneous tissue. Infection is acquired through traumatic inoculation into the skin. Cutaneous manifestations are described as pink papules that progressively enlarge to become tender, pruritic, hyperkeratotic nodules or verrucous plaques (Fig. 67–21). Scratching may lead to secondary infection or result in autoinoculation of the organism to other areas of the body. Infection may lead to scarring of lymphatic vessels causing obstruction and lymphedema.[16,97,102,107]

Differential diagnosis includes tuberculosis, sporotrichosis, blastomycosis, leishmaniasis, and squamous cell carcinomas. Potassium hydroxide smears of skin scrapings reveal characteristic dark brown, round, sclerotic bodies with horizontal or vertical septa and thick, pigmented hyphae. Sclerotic bodies also are identified easily on hematoxylin and eosin stain. In addition, biopsy of the chromoblastomycosis lesions shows granulomatous inflammation with macrophages and neutrophils and a hyperkeratotic, hyperplastic epidermis with microabscesses.[16,102,107]

Treatment of localized lesions involves surgical excision, cryotherapy, or heat therapy. Chemotherapy with 5-fluorocytosine

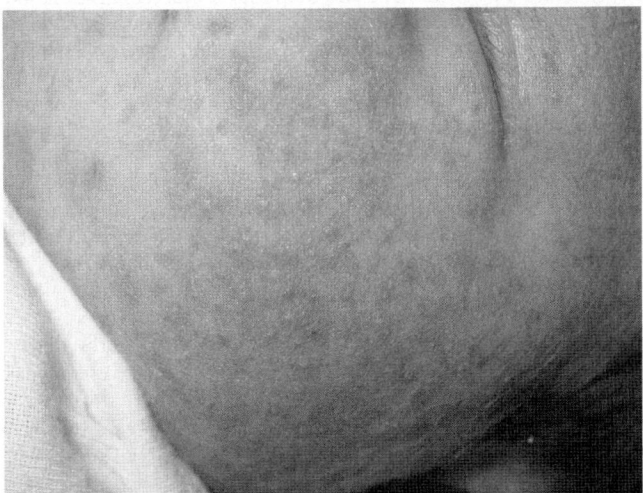

Figure 67–19 Pustules and papules on the face and scalp owing to neonatal cephalic pustulosis. (See companion Expert Consult web site for color version.)

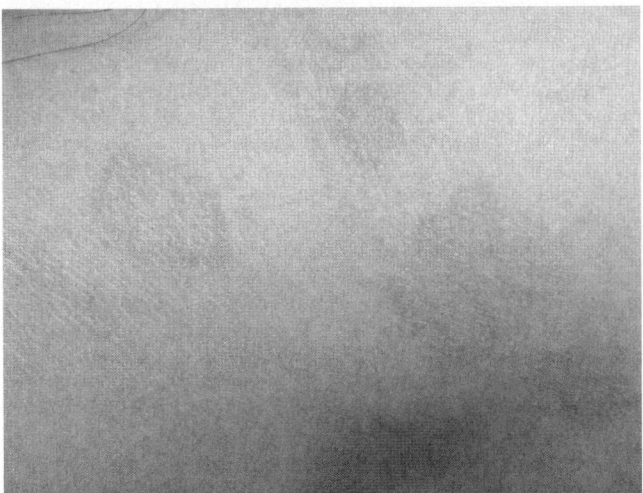

Figure 67–20 Well-circumscribed annular scaling plaques on the neck typical of tinea versicolor. (See companion Expert Consult web site for color version.)

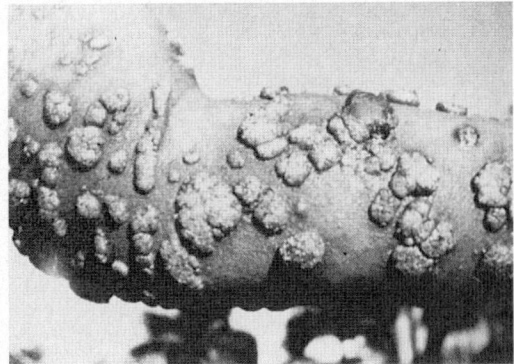

Figure 67–21 Chromoblastomycosis. The warty-like growth of epidermis and dermis is a result of traumatic implantation of the etiologic agent and subsequent autoinoculation from scratching. The agent was *Fonsecaea pedrosoi.*

and antifungal agents such as azoles, amphotericin B, and terbinafine has been used with some success in more widespread disease.[16,107,116]

TINEA NIGRA

Tinea nigra, caused by the organism *Phaeoannellomyces werneckii*, is a superficial fungal infection seen primarily in children and adolescents.[28,80,95] The organism is found in soil, wood, sewage, salted dried fish, and vegetation, mainly in beach environments of Central and South America, Africa, Asia, and, less frequently, in the United States and Europe. Transmission occurs by direct contact.[80,95,96]

Tinea nigra usually is characterized by an asymptomatic, well-demarcated, single brown to black macule or patch primarily on the palm, but may involve other areas of the body as well (Fig. 67–22). Lesions grow slowly and usually are nonscaly.[28,95] Tinea nigra lesions may mimic melanoma, lentigines, junctional nevi, and the hyperpigmented patches of Addison disease.[28,95,96] Under microscopic examination, potassium hydroxide–prepared scrapings of the lesion show yellow to light brown, branched, septate hyphae (Fig. 67–23).[28,96] Diagnosis is confirmed further by

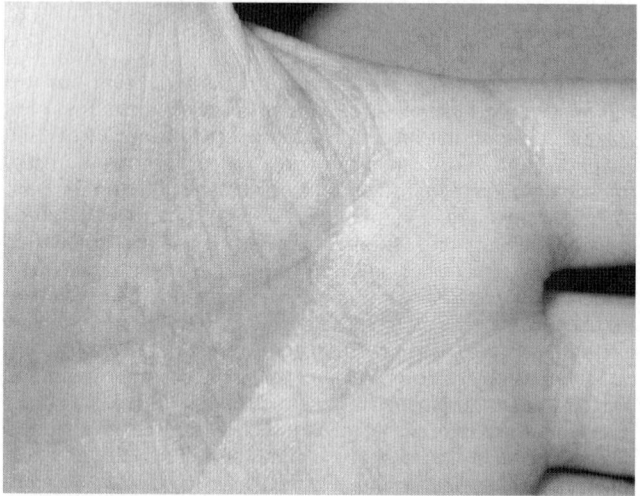

Figure 67–22 Brown patch on the palm of the hand caused by tinea nigra palmaris. (See companion Expert Consult web site for color version.)

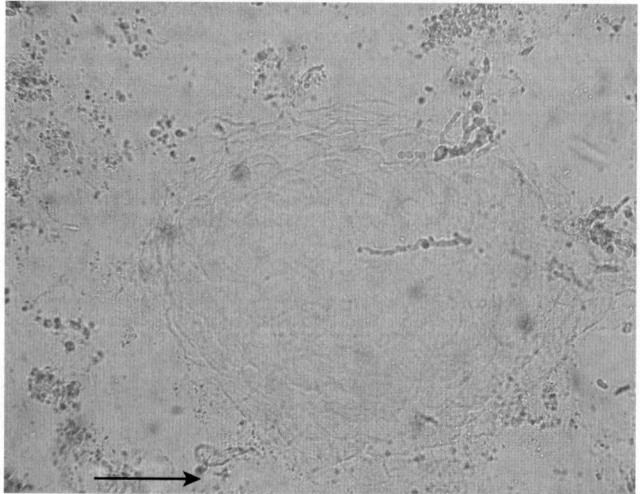

Figure 67–23 Septate hyphae seen by potassium hydroxide examination of scale from the patient in Figure 67–22. (See companion Expert Consult web site for color version.)

culture, which grows oval to spindle-shaped, moist, shiny, black colonies on Sabouraud agar.[95]

Tinea nigra has been treated successfully with keratolytic ointments or solutions, which include salicylic acid and benzoic acid and azole and allylamine creams.[28,95,96] Scraping the lesion with a scalpel also can remove the discoloration.[96]

TRICHOSPORONOSIS

Trichosporon spp., which are found in soil, vegetation, animal feces, and stagnant or fresh water, have a worldwide distribution with a predilection for tropical climates. They also may colonize human skin and digestive, respiratory, and urinary tracts. In immunocompetent individuals, *Trichosporon* organisms produce superficial fungal infections of the hair shaft termed *white piedra* and, less commonly, are one of the causes of onychomycosis. Systemic disease, termed *trichosporonosis*, may develop in immunocompromised patients, particularly neutropenic patients with hematologic malignancies, and in premature, very-low-birth-weight infants with colonization of indwelling catheters.[68,101]

White piedra is described as soft white, tan, or reddish-green nodules encircling the hair shaft that may be associated with scalp hyperkeratosis, brittle hair, and alopecia. These concretions do not fluoresce under Wood lamp examination. Differential diagnosis includes tinea capitis, pediculosis, black piedra, monilethrix, trichomycosis axillaris or pubis, and trichorrhexis nodosa.[70,135] Skin manifestations of disseminated infection include desquamation and serous drainage, purpuric papules or nodules with central ulceration or necrosis, and white plaques.[101,109]

Fungal blood culture reveals germ tube–negative and urease-positive yeast. Potassium hydroxide mounts of affected hair show hyaline septate hyphae, pseudohyphae, rectangular arthroconidia, and spherical blastoconidia that circumscribe the hair shaft.[70,107,109] Culture on Sabouraud dextrose agar shows cream-colored colonies that become wrinkled in a few weeks.[69] Biopsy specimen of skin lesions shows perivascular inflammation with budding yeast cells.[99]

White piedra is a difficult disease to treat because of the high recurrence rate. Although the American Academy of Dermatology Guidelines Committee recommends shaving affected hair to eradicate white piedra,[39] cosmetic and social considerations render this approach an unfavorable option for most patients. Topical antifungal agents that have been tried with varying degrees of success include ciclopirox olamine, imidazoles, chlorhexidine solution, 2.5 percent sulfide shampoo, zinc pyrithione, Castellani paint, mercury bichloride solution, 5 percent sulfur ointment, 5 percent ammoniated mercury ointment, and amphotericin B lotion. Although topical treatments may clear hair shaft concretions, they are not as effective at preventing recurrence. Because of their ability to bind keratin and their excretion in sebum, oral antifungal agents such as itraconazole may achieve higher concentrations in hair follicles and lead to greater success in eliminating colonized *Trichosporon* organisms and preventing relapse.[69,70]

Disseminated trichosporonosis is associated with high morbidity and mortality rates. It has been treated with varying degrees of success using amphotericin B with or without 5-fluorocytosine and the newer azole drugs, such as voriconazole.[4,68]

DEEP FUNGAL INFECTIONS

ASPERGILLOSIS

Aspergillosis, an opportunistic fungal infection caused by *Aspergillus* spp., affects primarily immunocompromised hosts, such as premature infants and children undergoing chemotherapy for

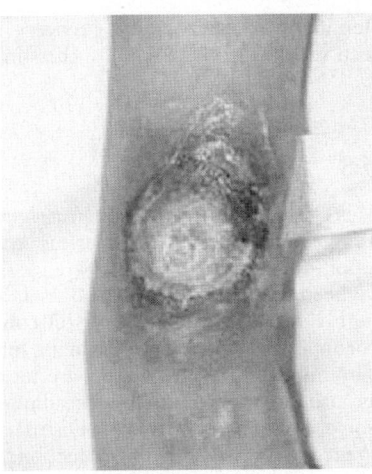

Figure 67–24 Eschar overlying eroded skin on a child with invasive aspergillosis. (See companion Expert Consult web site for color version.)

leukemia. It is acquired most commonly by inhalation of spores into the respiratory tract, with subsequent hematogenous spread to other organ systems including the skin. Cutaneous manifestations of aspergillosis may represent disseminated disease or, less commonly, infection limited to the skin. Premature infants have been reported to develop primary cutaneous aspergillosis at sites of skin trauma caused by adhesive tape, monitor leads, or placement of an intravenous catheter. Lesions appear as erythematous papules, pustules, nodules, or plaques that progressively enlarge and develop necrosis with formation of eschar (Fig. 67–24).[3,14,99,101,119] Differential diagnosis includes ecthyma gangrenosum, cutaneous candidiasis, mucormycosis, vasculitis, and pyoderma gangrenosum.[99,101]

Culture and histopathologic examination, revealing granulomatous inflammation with branched septate hyphae, of the skin biopsy specimen confirms the diagnosis.[14,99,101,119] Treatment of cutaneous aspergillosis includes surgical débridement or excision and administration of systemic antifungals.[101,119] Although amphotericin B remains the drug of choice, itraconazole and newer azoles such as voriconazole and other antifungal agents, including lipid-associated amphotericin B preparations and echinocandins such as caspofungin, also seem to be effective in individuals who cannot tolerate or are refractory to amphotericin B.[44,77,98,111,114] Data regarding safety and efficacy of these alternative therapies in children are limited.

BLASTOMYCOSIS

Blastomyces dermatitidis, a dimorphic fungus that causes North American blastomycosis, is found in the soil in the midwestern United States near the Ohio and Mississippi River valleys and the Great Lakes region, Canada, Central and South America, and tropical areas of Asia and Africa. Human disease is acquired through inhalation of spores, causing lung disease, and, rarely, through direct inoculation into the skin, which may cause primary cutaneous blastomycosis. Infection of the skin usually is due to hematogenous spread from a primary pulmonary focus, however.[13,48,99,113,125,136]

Cutaneous lesions are seen more frequently on sun-exposed areas and may begin as papules or pustules that progressively enlarge; become verrucous or ulcerative; and develop elevated, crusted borders. The central regions may heal, leaving an atrophic, hypopigmented scar, whereas the advancing borders remain active. Subcutaneous nodules with surface pustules and abscess formation may be seen as well. Erythema nodosum has

been described as a reactive skin manifestation of pulmonary blastomycosis.[13,48,99,113,136]

Biopsy specimens show noncaseating granulomas with giant cells and microabscesses, and potassium hydroxide smears of purulent material obtained from lesions or biopsy specimens may reveal broad-based budding yeast forms with thick cell walls. Culture on Sabouraud dextrose agar confirms the diagnosis.[13,48,99,113,136]

Amphotericin B is the recommended treatment for blastomycosis with central nervous system involvement and disease in immunocompromised individuals or individuals with severe, disseminated disease. For mild to moderate blastomycosis, itraconazole, sometimes after a course of amphotericin B, is preferred.[13,48,99,113,136] Research on the development of a vaccine against *B. dermatitidis* for immunocompromised individuals in endemic areas or individuals with high exposure is in progress.[34,133]

COCCIDIOIDOMYCOSIS

Coccidioides immitis is a dimorphic fungus endemic to the southwestern United States, Mexico, and Central and South America. Transmission occurs through inhalation of spores from the soil, and the primary site of infection usually is in the lung.[29,99,117] Shortly after the onset of symptoms, primary pulmonary disease may be associated with reactive skin lesions, which do not contain viable organisms. These findings include a generalized, erythematous exanthem, erythema multiforme, Sweet syndrome, or interstitial granulomatous dermatitis.[29,37,99]

Erythema nodosum may be seen 1 to 3 weeks after the onset of infection. The exanthem, which may last several weeks, varies from macular, papular, morbilliform, to urticarial. The exanthem and erythema multiforme lesions may be associated with involvement of the oral cavity, pruritus, target-like lesions, and desquamation of the palms. Sweet syndrome, or acute febrile neutrophilic dermatosis, is characterized by abrupt onset of fever; leukocytosis; and tender, erythematous, well-demarcated papules or plaques. These lesions result from dense, neutrophilic infiltration of the dermis and respond well to topical corticosteroids. Interstitial granulomatous dermatitis, which may persist for 2 months, is a reactive eruption of indurated papules, nodules, and plaques that are caused by interstitial dermal infiltration with macrophages, neutrophils, eosinophils, and leukocytoclastic debris. Erythema nodosum manifests as painful, erythematous, subcutaneous nodules usually found on the lower extremities.[37]

Coccidioidomycosis may spread hematogenously to the skin, a common site of disseminated disease, and produce abscesses, sinus tracts, and granulomatous verrucous nodules or plaques. In contrast to the reactive skin manifestations, these lesions show the characteristic organism under microscopic examination. In extremely rare cases, traumatic inoculation into the skin may result in primary cutaneous coccidioidomycosis characterized by painless, ulcerated, and indurated nodules or plaques associated with regional lymphadenitis. Affected lymph nodes also may ulcerate.[37,99]

Histopathologic examination of infected cerebrospinal fluid and pleural fluid, bronchoalveolar lavage, and biopsy specimens of skin lesions may reveal large spherules containing endospores. Spherules may be seen on culture as well, but specimens should be handled using appropriate safety precautions because the organism may convert to active form during growth on culture plates. Serum antibody titers may be helpful for confirming the disease.[29,37,99,117]

Because uncomplicated primary coccidioidomycosis is self-limited in most patients, administration of antifungal treatment is unnecessary. Individuals with severe or disseminated disease or individuals with risk factors such as immunosuppression should receive treatment. Amphotericin B is the recommended treatment for severe or progressive disease; otherwise, oral azole antifungals, such as itraconazole and fluconazole, are used most often for initial therapy of nonmeningeal coccidioidomycosis.[29,37,82,99,117] Oral fluconazole with or without administration of intrathecal amphotericin B is recommended for central nervous system involvement.[29,82,117] Additionally, surgical excision of localized infection with or without administration of antifungal therapy may be considered. Immunocompromised patients and patients with meningeal disease may require lifelong suppressive antifungal therapy with an azole to prevent recurrence.[29,37,117] The development of a vaccine against coccidioidomycosis is in progress.[31]

CRYPTOCOCCOSIS

Cryptococcus neoformans, the causative species of cryptococcosis, is an encapsulated yeast found worldwide in soil, fruits, and avian stool. Cryptococcosis affects primarily immunocompromised adults, particularly patients with AIDS, but it also may be seen in children. Infection usually is acquired through inhalation but rarely may spread through direct inoculation. Cutaneous findings, which often mimic other skin diseases, such as molluscum contagiosum and Kaposi sarcoma, vary as papules, nodules, vesicles, purpuric plaques, cellulitis, ulcers, abscesses, and sinus tracts.[27,32,64,99]

Diagnosis of these polymorphic lesions as a manifestation of cryptococcosis is established by visualizing the characteristic encapsulated yeast cells in culture on Sabouraud dextrose agar and on histopathologic examination of a skin sample stained with methenamine silver, periodic acid–Schiff, or mucicarmine. Another diagnostic method includes identification of the organism on smears of infected material prepared with potassium hydroxide and India ink.[27,32,64,99] Although a few cases of isolated cutaneous cryptococcosis have been reported, involvement of the skin usually reflects disseminated disease. Patients whose skin lesions show *C. neoformans* should undergo further evaluation for systemic disease and for cell-mediated immunodeficiencies.[27,32]

Although studies in children are limited, current treatment recommendations for cryptococcosis include a 6- to 12-week course of oral fluconazole or itraconazole for mild to moderate disease in immunocompetent individuals and intravenous amphotericin B in combination with oral fluconazole or flucytosine for more severe disease.[32,64,82,99] Immunocompromised patients continue on lifelong maintenance antifungal therapy because of the high rate of recurrence.[32,82]

FUSARIOSIS

Fusarium spp. are ubiquitous saprophytic fungi that affect primarily immunocompromised hosts, particularly neutropenic patients with hematologic malignancies. Fusariosis may produce localized infection of the nails, cornea, or skin and disseminated disease through hematogenous spread. Rarely, skin disease may result from traumatic inoculation. Lesions are seen most often on the extremities and manifest as tender, erythematous macules or plaques that develop central necrosis, form an eschar, and may become hemorrhagic.[79,87,99,107]

Because the mortality rate of disseminated *Fusarium* infection in neutropenic patients is 80 percent,[79,107] promptly establishing the diagnosis through biopsy and culture is important. Culture of tissue specimens reveals sickle-shaped macroconidia. On microscopic examination, *Fusarium* spp. appear as branched, septate hyphae with a perivascular distribution. Fungal blood cultures also may aid in establishing the diagnosis.[79,87,99,107]

Prognosis of *Fusarium* infection is poor, and treatment options are limited. Combination antifungal therapy with amphotericin

B lipid complex and voriconazole and recovery of neutrophil counts have been reported to have some success in resolving the disease.[72,79,87,107,114]

HISTOPLASMOSIS

Histoplasmosis is caused by the organism *Histoplasma capsulatum*, a dimorphic fungus endemic to the Americas, particularly the Ohio, Mississippi, Missouri, and St. Lawrence River valleys. Cases also have been reported in Africa and Asia. The disease is acquired through inhalation of spores in soil contaminated by bird and bat droppings, producing a primary lung infection.[1] Most cases in immunocompetent patients are localized pulmonary infections, producing an influenza-like illness with symptoms that resolve within a few weeks. Disease also may be produced by reactivation of a latent infection.[82] Patients at extremes of age and patients who are immunocompromised, especially patients with AIDS and low CD4 lymphocyte counts, are at risk for developing progressive, disseminated disease.[1,58,60,82,122]

Involvement of the skin, causing chancriform lesions associated with regional lymphadenopathy, rarely has been described as a consequence of direct inoculation. These lesions typically resolve spontaneously in several months. Acute or chronic pulmonary histoplasmosis may produce reactive skin changes, such as erythema nodosum, erythema multiforme, and exfoliative dermatitis. Cutaneous manifestations through hematogenous spread in disseminated histoplasmosis include papules, nodules, ulcerative, or granulomatous lesions often involving oral mucosa. These lesions may progress to thick, verrucous vegetations that cause obstruction of the affected regions.[71,99]

Differential diagnosis includes tuberculosis, *Pneumocystis carinii* pneumonia, and other fungal infections caused by dimorphic fungi.[99] Biopsy specimens of skin lesions show granulomatous inflammation with macrophages, histiocytes, and giant cells and round, narrow-necked, budding yeast cells within phagocytes. Culture of involved tissue, bone marrow, blood, or sputum specimens provides the definitive diagnosis, but *H. capsulatum* may take several weeks to months for growth on culture media to occur. *Histoplasma* antigen may be detected in urine samples of individuals with disseminated histoplasmosis; however, this test is inconsistent in patients with localized infections.[1,99,104,108]

Self-limited disease in immunocompetent individuals does not require treatment. Amphotericin B remains the drug of choice for severe, disseminated histoplasmosis, whereas azole drugs can be effective for treating less advanced disease.[1,130] Itraconazole also is used for lifelong suppressive therapy in immunocompromised patients.[60,82]

MUCORMYCOSIS

Mucormycosis is an opportunistic fungal infection that affects primarily immunosuppressed hosts. Common risk factors include prematurity, diabetes mellitus, malignancies, neutropenia, burns, or malnutrition. Transmission may result from inhalation of spores or, in the case of primary skin disease, from direct inoculation through contaminated occlusive dressings or at sites of invasive procedures, trauma, or burns. Cutaneous manifestations may occur alone or in conjunction with disseminated disease. Mucormycosis has a tendency to invade vascular tissues, leading to inflammation, thrombosis, necrosis, and septic emboli. Infection may spread hematogenously to the skin, causing cellulitis with erythematous papules and pustules that progressively enlarge and develop necrosis with formation of eschar (Fig. 67–25).[89,99,101,132]

Differential diagnosis includes pyoderma gangrenosum, bacterial cellulitis, and necrotizing fasciitis. Tissue biopsy examina-

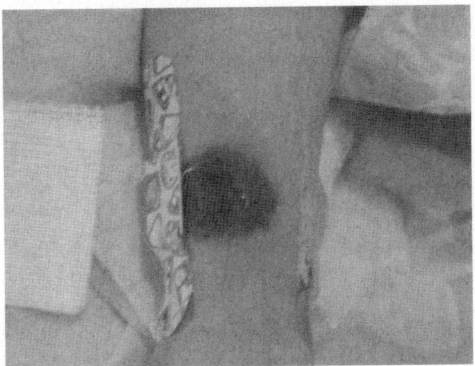

Figure 67–25 Purpura and ulceration in a patient with mucormycosis. (See companion Expert Consult web site for color version.)

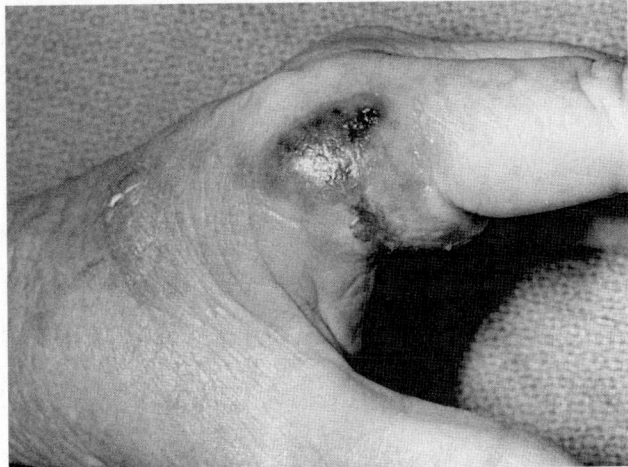

Figure 67–26 Two erythematous nodules on the dorsum of the left hand of a patient with sporotrichosis.

tion of mucormycosis lesions shows characteristic nonseptate hyphae with right angle branches, vascular invasion, necrosis, and inflammatory infiltrate. Administration of intravenous amphotericin B in addition to surgical débridement and wide excision of the skin disease is the recommended treatment.[89,99,101,132]

SPOROTRICHOSIS

Sporothrix schenckii, the organism responsible for sporotrichosis, is found in soil and plants worldwide with a predilection for tropical climates. Sporotrichosis usually is transmitted through inoculation at sites of trauma; however, pulmonary disease may be acquired through inhalation of spores. Infection with *S. schenckii* may produce four forms of disease, with lymphocutaneous being the most common and fixed cutaneous, disseminated skin, and extracutaneous disease being less common.[33,61,83,99,131] Children and individuals with prior exposure to the fungus may present more often with localized skin manifestations.[18] Characteristic lesions include erythematous papules, nodules, and scaly, verrucous plaques that progressively enlarge and ulcerate (Fig. 67–26). Regional lymphadenopathy and spread along the lymphatic drainage may soon follow. Scarring is a common occurrence. Although bone and joints are the most frequent sites of extracutaneous infection, hematogenous spread to almost every other organ system has been described. Disseminated disease should raise the suspicion of immunodeficiency in the affected individual.[33,61,83,99,131]

Definitive diagnosis is made by culture of wound material on Sabouraud agar. Itraconazole is the drug of choice for treating skin disease, whereas intravenous amphotericin B is the recommended treatment for severe, disseminated disease. Saturated solution of potassium iodide at 1 to 2 drops per the child's year of age administered three times daily also has been used as an effective treatment for uncomplicated cutaneous sporotrichosis in pediatric patients.[18,67]

REFERENCES

1. Adderson, E. E.: Histoplasmosis in a pediatric oncology center. J. Pediatr. *144*:100-106, 2004.
2. Aldana-Valenzuela, C., Morales-Marquec, M., Castellanos-Martinez, J., et al.: Congenital candidiasis: A rare and unpredictable disease. J. Perinatol. *25*:680-682, 2005.
3. Andresen, J., Nygaard, E. A., and Stordal, K.: Primary cutaneous aspergillosis (PCA)—a case report. Acta Paediatr. *94*:761-762, 2005.
4. Antachopoulos, C., Papakonstantinou, E., Dotis, J., et al.: Fungemia due to *Trichosporon asahii* in a neutropenic child refractory to amphotericin B: Clearance with voriconazole. J. Pediatr. Hematol. Oncol. *27*:283-285, 2005.
5. Antachopoulos, C., and Walsh, T. J.: New agents for invasive mycoses in children. Curr. Opin. Pediatr. *17*:78-87, 2005.
6. Armour, K., and Orchard, D.: Treatment of palmoplantar warts with a diphencyprone and salicylic acid ointment. Australas. J. Dermatol. *47*:182-185, 2006.
7. Ashbee, H. R., and Evans, E. G.: Immunology of diseases associated with *Malassezia* species. Clin. Microbiol. Rev. *15*:21-57, 2002.
8. Bayrou, O., Pecquet, C., Flahault, A., et al.: Head and neck atopic dermatitis and *Malassezia-furfur*-specific IgE antibodies. Dermatology *211*:107-113, 2005.
9. Berkhout, R. J. M., Bouwes Bavinck, J. N., and ter Schegget, J.: Persistence of human papillomavirus DNA in benign and (pre)malignant skin lesions from renal transplant recipients. J. Clin. Microbiol. *38*:2087-2096, 2000.
10. Bernier, V., Weill, F. X., Hirigoyen, V., et al.: Skin colonizations by *Malassezia* species in neonates: A prospective study and relationship with neonatal cephalic pustulosis. Arch. Dermatol. *138*:215-218, 2002.
11. Bessa, C. F., Santos, P. J., Aguiar, M. C., and do Carmo, M. A.: Prevalence of oral mucosal alterations in children from 0 to 12 years old. J. Oral Pathol. Med. *33*:17-22, 2004.
12. Bhogal, C. S., Singal, A., and Baruah, M. C.: Comparative efficacy of ketoconazole and fluconazole in the treatment of pityriasis versicolor: A one year follow-up study. J. Dermatol. *28*:535-539, 2001.
13. Blastomycosis. *In* Pickering, L. K., Baker, C. J., Long, S. S., et al. (eds.): Red Book: 2006 Report of the Committee on Infectious Diseases. 27th ed. Elk Grove Village, IL, American Academy of Pediatrics, 2006, pp. 232-233.
14. Blum, M. D., and Wiedermann, B. L.: Aspergillus Infections. *In* Feigin, R. D., Cherry, J. D., and Demmler, G. J., et al. (eds.): Textbook of Pediatric Infectious Diseases. 5th ed. Philadelphia, W. B. Saunders, 2004, pp. 2550-2560.
15. Bodemer, C., and de Prost, Y.: Unilateral laterothoracic exanthem in children: A new disease? J. Am. Acad. Dermatol. *27*:693-696, 1992.
16. Bonifaz, A., Carrasco-Gerard, E., and Saul, A.: Chromoblastomycosis: Clinical and mycologic experience of 51 cases. Mycoses *44*:1-7, 2001.
17. Braue, A., Ross, F., Varigos, G., et al.: Epidemiology and impact of childhood molluscum contagiosum: A case series and critical review of the literature. Pediatr. Dermatol. *22*:287-294, 2005.
18. Burch, J. M., Morelli, J. G., and Weston, W. L.: Unsuspected sporotrichosis in childhood. Pediatr. Infect. Dis. J. *20*:442-445, 2001.
19. Burwell, L. A., Kaufman, D., Blakely, J., et al.: Antifungal prophylaxis to prevent neonatal candidiasis: A survey of perinatal physician practices. Pediatrics *118*:1019-1026, 2006.
20. Butler, G. J., Mendelsohn, S., and Franks, A.: Parvovirus B19 infection presenting as 'bathing trunk' erythema with pustules. Austral. J. Dermatol. *47*:286-288, 2006.
21. Calista, D., Boschini, A., and Landi, G.: Resolution of disseminated molluscum contagiosum with highly active anti-retroviral therapy (HAART) in patients with AIDS. Eur. J. Dermatol. *9*:211-213, 1999.
22. Candidiasis. *In* Pickering, L. K., Baker, C. J., Long, S. S., et al. (eds.): Red Book: 2006 Report of the Committee on Infectious Diseases. 27th ed. Elk Grove Village, IL, American Academy of Pediatrics, 2006, pp. 242-246.
23. Chapman, R. L.: Prevention and treatment of *Candida* infections in neonates. Semin. Perinatol. *31*:39-46, 2007.
24. Charo, R. A.: Politics, parent, and prophylaxis—mandating HPV vaccination in the United States. N. Engl. J. Med. *356*:1905-1908, 2007.
25. Chen, K. T., Chang, H. L., Wang, S. T., et al.: Epidemiologic features of hand-foot-mouth disease and herpangina caused by enterovirus 71 in Taiwan, 1998-2005. Pediatrics *120*:e244-e252, 2007.
26. Choong, K. Y., and Roberts, L. J.: Molluscum contagiosum, swimming and bathing: A clinical analysis. Austral. J. Dermatol. *40*:89-92, 1999.

27. Christianson, J. C., Engber, W., and Andes, D.: Primary cutaneous crypto-coccosis in immunocompetent and immunocompromised hosts. Med. Mycol. *41*:177-188, 2003.

28. Clayton, Y. M.: Superficial fungal infections. *In* Harper, J., Oranje, A., and Prose, N. (eds.): Textbook of Pediatric Dermatology. Oxford, Blackwell Sciences, 2000, pp. 447-472.

29. Coccidioidomycosis. *In* Pickering, L. K., Baker, C. J., Long, S. S., et al. (eds.): Red Book: 2006 Report of the Committee on Infectious Diseases. 27th ed. Elk Grove Village, IL, American Academy of Pediatrics, 2006, pp. 265-267.

30. Cornely, O. A., Maertens, J., Winston, D. J., et al.: Posaconazole vs. flucon-azole or itraconazole prophylaxis in patients with neutropenia. N. Engl. J. Med. *356*:348-359, 2007.

31. Cox, R. A., and Magee, D. M.: Coccidioidomycosis: Host response and vac-cine development. Clin. Microbiol. Rev. *17*:804-839, 2004.

32. Cryptococcosis. *In* Pickering, L. K., Baker, C. J., Long, S. S., et al. (eds.): Red Book: 2006 Report of the Committee on Infectious Diseases. 27th ed. Elk Grove Village, IL, American Academy of Pediatrics, 2006, pp. 269-270.

33. da Rosa, A. C., Scrofernecker, M. L., Vettorato, R., et al.: Epidemiology of sporotrichosis: A study of 304 cases in Brazil. J. Am. Acad. Dermatol. *52*:451-459, 2005.

34. Deepe, G. S., Jr., Wuthrich, M., and Klein, B. S.: Progress in vaccination for histoplasmosis and blastomycosis: Coping with cellular immunity. Med. Mycol. *43*:381-389, 2005.

35. Descamps, V., Valance, A., Edlinger, C., et al.: Association of human herpes-virus 6 infection with drug reaction with eosinophilia and systemic symptoms. Arch. Dermatol. *137*:301-304, 2001.

36. Diana, A., Epiney, M., Ecoffey, M., et al.: White dots on the placenta and red dots on the baby: Congenital cutaneous candidiasis—a rare disease of the neonate. Acta Paediatr. *93*:996-999, 2004.

37. DiCaudo, D. J.: Coccidioidomycosis: A review and update. J. Am. Acad. Dermatol. *55*:929-942, 2006.

38. Dohil, M. A., Lin, P., Lee, J., et al.: The epidemiology of molluscum conta-giosum in children. J. Am. Acad. Dermatol. *54*:47-54, 2006.

39. Drake, L. A., Dinehart, S. M., Farmer, E. R., et al.: Guidelines of care for superficial mycotic infections of the skin: Piedra-guidelines/outcomes com-mittee. J. Am. Acad. Dermatol. *34*:122-124, 1996.

40. Epstein, W. L.: Molluscum contagiosum. Semin. Dermatol. *11*:184-189, 1992.

41. Farschian, M., Yaghoobi, R., and Samadi, K.: Fluconazole versus ketoconazole in the treatment of tinea versicolor. J. Dermatol. Treat. *13*:73-76, 2002.

42. Fleece, D., Gaughan, J. P., and Aronoff, S. C.: Griseofulvin versus terbinafine in the treatment of tinea capitis. Pediatrics *114*:1312-1315, 2004.

43. Foster, K. W., Friedlander, S. F., Panzer, H., et al.: A randomized controlled trial assessing the efficacy of fluconazole in the treatment of pediatric tinea capitis. J. Am. Acad. Dermatol. *53*:798-809, 2005.

44. Frankenbusch, K., Eifinger, F., Kribs, A., et al.: Severe primary cutaneous aspergillosis refractory to amphotericin B and the successful treatment with systemic voriconazole in two premature infants with extremely low birth weight. J. Perinatol. *26*:511-514, 2006.

45. Friedlander, S. F., Aly, R., Krafchik, B., et al.: Tinea Capitis Study Group. Terbinafine in the treatment of *Trichophyton* tinea capitis: A randomized, double-blind, parallel-group, duration-finding study. Pediatrics *109*:602-607, 2002.

46. Fukushima, C., Matsuse, H., Tomari, S., et al.: Oral candidiasis associated with inhaled corticosteroid use: Comparison of fluticasone and beclometha-sone. Ann. Allergy Asthma Immunol. *90*:646-651, 2003.

47. Future II Study Group. Quadrivalent vaccine against human papillomavirus to prevent hight-grade cervical lesions. N. Engl. J. Med. *356*:1915-1927, 2007.

48. Garvey, K., Hinshaw, M., and Vanness, E.: Chronic disseminated cutaneous blastomycosis in an 11-year old, with a brief review of the literature. Pediatr. Dermatol. *23*:541-545, 2006.

49. Gelmetti, C., and Caputo, R.: Asymmetric periflexural exanthem of childhood: Who are you? J. Eur. Acad. Dermatol. Venereol. *15*:293-294, 2001.

50. Gianotti, F.: Papular acrodermatitis of childhood: An Australia antigen dis-ease. Arch. Dis. Child. *48*:794-799, 1973.

51. Ginter-Hanselmayer, G., Smolle, J., and Gupta, A.: Itraconazole in the treat-ment of tinea capitis caused by *Microsporum canis*: Experience in a large cohort. Pediatr. Dermatol. *21*:499-502, 2004.

52. Givens, T. G., Murray, M. M., and Baker, R. C.: Comparison of 1% and 2.5% selenium sulfide in the treatment of tinea capitis. Arch. Pediatr. Adolesc. Med. *149*:808-811, 1995.

53. Goodyear, H. M., Laidler, P. W., Price, E. H., et al.: Acute infectious erythe-mas in children: A clinicopathological study. Br. J. Dermatol. *124*:433-438, 1991.

54. Gupta, A. K., Adam, P., Dlova, N., et al.: Therapeutic options for the treat-ment of tinea capitis caused by *Trichophyton* species: Griseofulvin versus the new oral antifungal agents, terbinafine, itraconazole, and fluconazole. Pediatr. Dermatol. *18*:433-438, 2001.

55. Gupta, A. K., Cooper, E. A., and Ginter, G.: Efficacy and safety of itracon-azole use in children. Dermatol. Clin. *21*:521-535, 2003.

56. Gupta, A. K., Madzia, S. E., and Batra, R.: Etiology and management of sebor-rheic dermatitis. Dermatology *208*:89-93, 2004.

57. Gupta, A. K., and Skinner, A. R.: Onychomycosis in children: A brief overview with treatment strategies. Pediatr. Dermatol. *21*:74-79, 2004.

58. Hajjeh, R. A., Pappas, P. G., Henderson, H. D., et al.: National Institute of Allergy and Infectious Diseases Mycoses Study Group. Multicenter case-control study of risk factors for histoplasmosis in human immunodeficiency virus-infected people. Clin. Infect. Dis. *32*:1215-1220, 2002.

59. Heikkilä, H., and Stubb, S.: Onychomycosis in children: Treatment results of forty-seven patients. Acta Derm. Venereol. *82*:484-485, 2002.

60. Histoplasmosis. *In* Pickering, L. K., Baker, C. J., Long, S. S., et al. (eds.): Red Book: 2006 Report of the Committee on Infectious Diseases. 27th ed. Elk Grove Village, IL, American Academy of Pediatrics, 2006, pp. 371-374.

61. Horii, K. A., Jackson, M. A., and Sharma, V.: Localized cutaneous sporotri-chosis in a child. Arch. Dermatol. *142*:1369-1370, 2006.

62. Hsieh, M. Y., and Huang, P. H.: The juvenile variant of papular-purpuric gloves and socks syndrome and its association with viral infections. Br. J. Dermatol. *151*:201-206, 2004.

63. Huang, P. H., and Paller, A. S.: Itraconazole pulse therapy for dermatophyte onychomycosis in children. Arch. Pediatr. Adolesc. Med. *154*:614-618, 2000.

64. Hughes, W. T.: Cryptococcosis. *In* Feigin, R. D., Cherry, J. D., and Demmler, G. J., et al. (eds.): Textbook of Pediatric Infectious Diseases. 5th ed. Philadelphia, W. B. Saunders, 2004, pp. 2602-2607.

65. Hughes, W. T., and Flynn, P. M.: Candidiasis. *In* Feigin, R. D., Cherry, J. D., and Demmler, G. J., et al. (eds.): Textbook of Pediatric Infectious Diseases. 5th ed. Philadelphia, W. B. Saunders, 2004, pp. 2550-2560.

66. Ito, Y., Ohyashiki, K., Yoshida, I., et al.: The prophylactic effect of itra-conazole capsules and fluconazole capsules for systemic fungal infections in patients with acute myeloid leukemia and myelodysplastic syndromes: A Japanese multicenter randomized, controlled study. Int. J. Hematol. *85*:121-127, 2007.

67. Kauffman, C. A., Hajjeh, R., and Chapman, S. W.: Practice guidelines for the management of patients with sporotrichosis. Clin. Infect. Dis. *30*:684-687, 2000.

68. Kendirli, T., Ciftci, E., Ince, E., et al.: Successful treatment of *Trichosporon mucoides* infection with lipid complex amphotericin B and 5-fluorocytosine. Mycoses *49*:251-253, 2006.

69. Khandpur, S., and Reddy, B. S.: Itraconazole therapy for white piedra affecting scalp hair. J. Am. Acad. Dermatol. *47*:415-418, 2002.

70. Kiken, D. A., Sekaran, A., Antaya, R. J., et al.: White piedra in children. J. Am. Acad. Dermatol. *55*:956-961, 2006.

71. Kleiman, M. B.: Histoplasmosis. *In* Feigin, R. D., Cherry, J. D., and Demmler, G. J., et al. (eds.): Textbook of Pediatric Infectious Diseases. 5th ed. Philadelphia, W. B. Saunders, 2004, pp. 2607-2629.

72. Kontoyiannis, D. P., Bodey, G. P., Hanna, H., et al.: Outcome determinants of fusariosis in a tertiary care cancer center: The impact of neutrophil recov-ery. Leuk. Lymphoma *45*:139-141, 2004.

73. Laxmisha, C., Thappa, D. M., and Jaisankar, T. J.: Clinical profile of mollus-cum contagiosum in children versus adults. Dermatol. Online J. *9*:1-9, 2003.

74. Leung, A. K. C., Robson, W. L. M., and Leong, A. G.: Herpes zoster in child-hood. J. Pediatr. Child Health Care *20*:300-303, 2006.

75. Lipke, M. M.: A armamentarium of wart treatments. Clin. Med. Res. *4*:273-293, 2006.

76. Lipozencic, J., Skerlev, M., Orofino-Costa, R., et al.: Tinea Capitis Study Group. A randomized, double-blind, parallel-group, duration-finding study of oral terbinafine and open-label, high-dose griseofulvin in children with tinea capitis due to *Microsporum* species. Br. J. Dermatol. *146*:816-823, 2002.

77. Maertens, J., Raad, I., Petrikkos, G., et al.: Caspofungin Salvage Aspergillosis Study Group. Efficacy and safety of caspofungin for treatment of invasive aspergillosis in patients refractory to or intolerant of conventional antifungal therapy. Clin. Infect. Dis. *39*:1563-1571, 2004.

78. Mancini, A. J., and Bodemer, C.: Viral Infections. *In* Schachner, L. S., and Hansen, R. C. (eds.): Pediatric Dermatology. 3rd ed. St. Louis, Mosby, 2003, pp. 1059-1092.

79. Mays, S. R., Bogle, M. A., and Bodey, G. P.: Cutaneous fungal infections in the oncology patient: recognition and management. Am. J. Clin. Dermatol. *7*:31-43, 2006.

80. McKinlay, J. R., Barrett, T. L., and Ross, E. V.: Picture of the month. Tinea nigra. Arch. Pediatr. Adolesc. Med. *153*:305-306, 1999.

81. McNeely, M., Friedman, J., and Pope, E.: Generalized petechial eruption induced by parvovirus B19 infection. J. Am. Acad. Dermatol. *52*:S109-S113, 2005.

82. Mofenson, L. M., Oleske, J., Serchuck, L., et al.: Treating opportunistic infec-tions among HIV-exposed and infected children: Recommendations from CDC, the National Institutes of Health, and the Infectious Diseases Society of America. M. M. W. R. Morb. Mortal. Wkyl. Rep. Recomm. Rep. *53*:1-92, 2004.

83. Morris-Jones, R.: Sporotrichosis. Clin. Exp. Dermatol. *27*:427-431, 2002.

84. Nakabayashi, A., Sei, Y., and Guillot, J.: Identification of *Malassezia* species isolated from patients with seborrhoeic dermatitis, atopic dermatitis, pityriasis versicolor and normal subjects. Med. Mycol. *38*:337-341, 2000.

85. Natarajan, G., Lulic-Botica, M., Rongkavilit, C., et al.: Experience with caspofungin in the treatment of persistent fungemia in neonates. J. Perinatol. *25*:770-777, 2005.

86. Nelson, J. S. B., and Stone, M. S.: Update on selected viral exanthems. Curr. Opin. Pediatr. *12*:359-364, 2000.

87. Nucci, M., Anaissie, E. J., Queiroz-Telles, F., et al.: Outcome predictors of 84 patients with hematologic malignancies and *Fusarium* infection. Cancer *98*:315-319, 2003.

88. Odio, C. M., Araya, R., Pinto, L. E., et al.: Caspofungin therapy of neonates with invasive candidiasis. Pediatr. Infect. Dis. J. 23:1093-1097, 2004.

89. Oh, D., and Notrica, D.: Primary cutaneous mucormycosis in infants and neonates: Case report and review of the literature. J. Pediatr. Surg. 37:1607-1611, 2002.

90. Oren, I., Rowe, J. M., Sprecher, H., et al.: A prospective randomized trial of itraconazole vs fluconazole for the prevention of fungal infections in patients with acute leukemia and hematopoietic stem cell transplant recipients. Bone Marrow Transplant. 38:127-134, 2006.

91. Pannaraj, P. S., Walsh, T. J., and Baker, C. J.: Advances in antifungal therapy. Pediatr. Infect. Dis. J. 24:921-922, 2005.

92. Parry, M. E., and Sharpe, G. R.: Seborrhoeic dermatitis is not caused by an altered immune response to *Malassezia* yeast. Br. J. Dermatol. 139:254-263, 1998.

93. Partap, R., Kaur, I., Chakrabarti, A., et al.: Single-dose fluconazole versus itraconazole in pityriasis versicolor. Dermatology 208:55-59, 2004.

94. Passeron, T., Desruelles, F., Gari-Toussaint, M., et al.: Invasive fungal dermatitis in a 770 gram neonate. Pediatr. Dermatol. 21:260-261, 2004.

95. Pegas, J. R., Criado, P. R., Lucena, S. K., et al.: Tinea nigra: Report of two cases in infants. Pediatr. Dermatol. 20:315-317, 2003.

96. Perez, C., Colella, M. T., Olaizola, C., et al.: Tinea nigra: Report of twelve cases in Venezuela. Mycopathologia 160:235-238, 2005.

97. Perez-Blanco, M., Hernandez Valles, R., Garcia-Humbria, L., et al.: Chromoblastomycosis in children and adolescents in the endemic area of the Falcon State, Venezuela. Med. Mycol. 44:467-471, 2006.

98. Perfect, J. R., Marr, K. A., Walsh, T. J., et al.: Voriconazole treatment for less-common, emerging, or refractory fungal infections. Clin. Infect. Dis. 36:1122-1131, 2003.

99. Pierini, A. M.: Deep mycoses and opportunistic infections. *In* Harper, J., Oranje, A., and Prose, N. (eds.): Textbook of Pediatric Dermatology. Oxford, Blackwell Sciences, 2000, pp. 473-496.

100. Pityriasis versicolor. *In* Pickering, L. K., Baker, C. J., Long, S. S., et al. (eds.): Red Book: 2006 Report of the Committee on Infectious Diseases. 27th ed. Elk Grove Village, IL, American Academy of Pediatrics, 2006, pp. 522-523.

101. Pong, A. L., and McCuaig, C. C.: Fungal infections, infestations, and parasitic infections in neonates. *In* Eichenfeld, L. F, Frieden, I. J., and Esterly, N. B. (eds.): Textbook of Neonatal Dermatology. Philadelphia, W. B. Saunders, 2001, pp. 223-240.

102. Pradhan, S. V., Talwar, O. P., Ghosh, A., et al.: Chromoblastomycosis in Nepal: A study of 13 cases. Indian J. Dermatol. Venereol. Leprol. 73:176-178, 2007.

103. Prohic, A., and Ozegovic, L.: *Malassezia* species isolated from lesional and non-lesional skin in patients with pityriasis versicolor. Mycoses 50:58-63, 2007.

104. Ramdial, P. K., Mosam, A., Dlova, N. C., et al.: Disseminated cutaneous histoplasmosis in patients infected with human immunodeficiency virus. J. Cutan. Pathol. 29:215-225, 2002.

105. Roberts, B. J., and Friedlander, S. F.: Tinea capitis: A treatment update. Pediatr. Ann. 34:191-200, 2005.

106. Romano, C., Papini, M., Ghilardi, A., et al.: Onychomycosis in children: A survey of 46 cases. Mycoses 48:430-437, 2005.

107. Rowen, J. L.: Miscellaneous mycoses. *In* Feigin, R. D., Cherry, J. D., and Demmler, G. J., et al. (eds.): Textbook of Pediatric Infectious Diseases. 5th ed. Philadelphia, W. B. Saunders, 2004, pp. 2640-2653.

108. Saidinejad, M., Burns, M. M., and Harper, M. B.: Disseminated histoplasmosis in a nonendemic area. Pediatr. Infect. Dis. J. 23:781-782, 2004.

109. Salazar, G. E., and Campbell, J. R. Trichosporonosis, an unusual fungal infection in neonates. Pediatr. Infect. Dis. J. 21:161-165, 2002.

110. Sandstrom Falk, M. H., Tengvall Linder, M., Johansson, C., et al.: The prevalence of *Malassezia* yeasts in patients with atopic dermatitis, seborrhoeic dermatitis and healthy controls. Acta Derm. Venereol. 85:17-23, 2005.

111. Santos, R. P., Sanchez, P. J., Mejias, A., et al.: Successful medical treatment of cutaneous aspergillosis in a premature infant using liposomal amphotericin B, voriconazole and micafungin. Pediatr. Infect. Dis. J. 26:364-366, 2007.

112. Sauerbrei, A., Uebe, B., and Wutzler, P.: Molecular diagnosis of zoster post varicella vaccination. J. Clin. Virol. 27:190-199, 2003.

113. Schutze, G. E.: Blastomycosis. *In* Feigin, R. D., Cherry, J. D., and Demmler, G. J., et al. (eds.): Textbook of Pediatric Infectious Diseases. 5th ed. Philadelphia, W. B. Saunders, 2004, pp. 2560-2568.

114. Scott, L. J., and Simpson, D.: Voriconazole: A review of its use in the management of invasive fungal infections. Drugs 67:269-298, 2007.

115. Sethi, A., and Antaya, R.: Systemic antifungal therapy for cutaneous infections in children. Pediatr. Infect. Dis. J. 25:643-644, 2006.

116. Sharma, N. L., Sharma, R. C., Grover, P. S., et al.: Chromoblastomycosis in India. Int. J. Dermatol. 38:846-851, 1999.

117. Shehab, Z. M.: Coccidioidomycosis. *In* Feigin, R. D., Cherry, J. D., and Demmler, G. J., et al. (eds.): Textbook of Pediatric Infectious Diseases. 5th ed. Philadelphia, W. B. Saunders, 2004, pp. 2580-2591.

118. Smith, P. B., Steinbach, W. J., Cotten, C. M., et al.: Caspofungin for the treatment of azole resistant candidemia in a premature infant. J. Perinatol. 27:127-129, 2007.

119. Smolinski, K. N., Shah, S. S., Honig, P. J., et al.: Neonatal cutaneous fungal infections. Curr. Opin. Pediatr. 17:486-493, 2005.

120. Taieb, A., Plantin, P., Du Pasquier, P., et al.: Gianotti-Crosti syndrome: A study of 26 cases. Br. J. Dermatol. 115:49-59, 1986.

121. Tinea capitis, tinea corporis, tinea cruris, tinea pedis and tinea unguium. *In* Pickering, L. K., Baker, C. J., Long, S. S., et al. (eds.): Red Book: 2006 Report of the Committee on Infectious Diseases. 27th ed. Elk Grove Village, IL, American Academy of Pediatrics, 2006, pp. 654-660.

122. Tobon, A. M., Agudelo, C. A., Rosero, D. S., et al.: Disseminated histoplasmosis: A comparative study between patients with acquired immunodeficiency syndrome and non-human immunodeficiency virus-infected individuals. Am. J. Trop. Med. Hyg. 73:576-582, 2005.

123. Tollesson, A., Frithz, A., and Stenlund, K.: *Malassezia furfur* in infantile seborrheic dermatitis. Pediatr. Dermatol. 14:423-425, 1997.

124. Trizna, Z.: Viral diseases of the skin. Pediatr. Drugs 4:9-19, 2002.

125. Uebe, B., Sauerbrei, A., Burdach, S., et al.: Herpes zoster by reactivated vaccine varicella zoster virus in a healthy child. Eur. J. Pediatr. 161:442-444, 2002.

126. Varella, T. C., and Machado, M. C.: Photolocalized varicella. Acta Derm. Venereol. 84:494-495, 2004.

127. Walsh, C. M., Morris, S. K., Brophy, J. C., et al.: Disseminated blastomycosis in an infant. Pediatr. Infect. Dis. J. 25:656-658, 2006.

128. Weston, W. L., Lane, A. T., and Morelli, J. G.: Fungal and yeast infections of the skin. *In*: Color Textbook of Pediatric Dermatology. 3rd ed. St. Louis, Mosby, 2002, pp. 63-76.

129. Weston, W. L., and Morelli, J. G.: Herpes simplex virus-associated erythema multiforme in prepubertal children. Arch. Pediatr. Adolesc. Med. 151:1014-1016, 1997.

130. Wheat, L. J., Sarosi, G. A., McKinsey, D., et al.: Practice guidelines for the management of patients with histoplasmosis. Clin. Infect. Dis. 30:688-695, 2000.

131. Wiedermann, B. L.: Sporotrichosis. *In* Feigin, R. D., Cherry, J. D., and Demmler, G. J., et al. (eds.): Textbook of Pediatric Infectious Diseases. 5th ed. Philadelphia, W. B. Saunders, 2004, pp. 2629-2633.

132. Wiedermann, B. L.: Zygomycosis. *In* Feigin, R. D., Cherry, J. D., and Demmler, G. J., et al. (eds.): Textbook of Pediatric Infectious Diseases. 5th ed. Philadelphia, W. B. Saunders, 2004, pp. 2633-2640.

133. Wuthrich, M., Filutowicz, H. I., and Klein, B. S.: Mutation of the WI-1 gene yields an attenuated *Blastomyces dermatitidis* strain that induces host resistance. J. Clin. Invest. 106:1381-1389, 2000.

134. Yamada, Y., Itoh, M., and Yoshida, M.: Sensitive and rapid diagnosis of human parvovirus B19 infection by loop-mediated isothermal amplification. Br. J. Dermatol. 155:50-55, 2006.

135. Youker, S. R., Andreozzi, R. J., Appelbaum, P. C., et al.: White piedra: Further evidence of a synergistic infection. J. Am. Acad. Dermatol. 49:746-749, 2003.

136. Zampogna, J. C., Hoy, M. J., and Ramos-Caro, F. A.: Primary cutaneous North American blastomycosis in an immunosuppressed child. Pediatr. Dermatol. 20:128-130, 2003.

OCULAR INFECTIONS

CHAPTER
68

OCULAR INFECTIOUS DISEASES

Kimberly G. Yen ☉ **Madhuri C. Chilakapati** ☉ **David K. Coats** ☉
Aaron M. Miller ☉ **Evelyn A. Paysse** ☉ **Paul G. Steinkuller**

The eye may be affected by a wide spectrum of infections and infestations manifested as primary disease or as part of a larger systemic process. Many infections are vision-threatening, whereas others have important implications affecting the generalized disease process. Findings in the eye, for example, can aid in narrowing the differential diagnosis in some cases of systemic disease, such as congenital viral infections. A helpful approach to delineating the ophthalmic manifestations of infectious diseases is to use an anatomic scheme that considers the primary site of involvement. This chapter proceeds systematically from infections involving the eyelids and ocular surface to those involving intraocular structures and concludes with a discussion of infections involving deeper tissues in the orbit. Some overlap and duplication are unavoidable because disease involvement that truly is isolated to a single anatomic component of the eye or orbit is an unusual occurrence. Most infectious processes involving the eye can be diagnosed accurately with a careful history and detailed ophthalmic examination. Simple tools such as a penlight and a direct ophthalmoscope facilitate establishing a diagnosis in many instances. In some cases, however, special ophthalmologic testing such as slit-lamp examination, indirect ophthalmoscopy, ocular ultrasound, and even biopsy or culture (or both) is required.

INFECTIONS OF THE EYELIDS

Despite being only 2 mm thick, the anatomy of the eyelids is complex and elegant. The eyelids are composed of dense connective tissue, hair follicles, sweat and sebaceous glands, smooth and striated muscles, sensory and motor nerves, and vascular elements. The skin covering the eyelids is the thinnest of the entire body. The internal surface of the eyelid, the part adjacent to the eye, is covered by the palpebral conjunctiva. Bulbar conjunctiva covers the surface of the globe itself. Sebaceous glands, known as the glands of Zeis, are associated with hair follicles. Meibomian glands, located within the tarsal plates of the eyelids, also are sebaceous and drain at the posterior aspect of the lid margin.

Infection of the eyelids may be generalized or focal. Involvement of the skin by an infectious agent is referred to as *dermatoblepharitis*. *Staphylococcus aureus* and *Staphylococcus epidermidis* infections predominate. The exception is angular blepharitis, characterized by inflammation in the lateral canthal region, which frequently is caused by *Moraxella* spp. Impetigo or erysipelas of the eyelids may be caused by *Streptococcus pyogenes*. A variety of infestations, including *Demodex folliculorum*, *Sarcoptes scabiei* (scabies), *Pediculus capitis*, and the pubic louse *Phthirus pubis*, may involve the eyelids.

Though more commonly found in adults, infection of the lid margin does occur in children. Infections of the anterior lid margin most frequently encountered include bacterial blepharitis, molluscum contagiosum, and parasitic diseases. Infections of the posterior lid margin include those associated with chronic meibomian gland dysfunction. Herpes simplex virus (HSV) and herpes zoster virus may involve the lid and lid margin and are discussed elsewhere in this chapter.

ANTERIOR EYELID INFECTION

Staphylococcal Blepharitis

Staphylococcal eyelid infection may be an acute or chronic condition. Typically, the chronic form of the disease is manifested as crusting of the lid margins, especially on awakening. Thickening of the lid margin, seen most easily on slit-lamp examination, is a frequent manifestation. Mild, chronic conjunctival infection often occurs as a spillover phenomenon caused by local reaction to materials secreted by the infecting organism. A child with staphylococcal blepharitis may be completely asymptomatic or may complain of ocular discomfort, burning, a foreign body sensation, or any combination of these symptoms. Lid hygiene usually is all that is required to treat the condition and can be accomplished through eyelid scrubs, with attention given to the lid margin. Tap water can be used, or in refractory cases, the eyelids and lid margins can be cleansed once or twice daily with a 50 : 50 mixture of baby shampoo and warm water. This mixture is applied gently with a clean washcloth. Lid hygiene is effective in decreasing the concentration of local bacterial flora and reducing or eliminating symptoms from chronic staphylococcal infection. A 2- to 4-week course of erythromycin or bacitracin ophthalmic ointment applied twice daily may hasten resolution and reduce exacerbation and recurrence. Because ophthalmologic ointments can produce temporary blurred vision, they often are used only at night before sleeping.

Molluscum Contagiosum Infection

Molluscum contagiosum is caused by a member of the family *Poxviridae*. Infection of the eyelid may be unilateral or bilateral. Infection may be transmitted by skin-to-skin contact, through fomites, or by auto-inoculation. Widespread development of lesions can occur as a result of auto-inoculation. Epidemics in people who live in closed communities have been reported.[160] Eyelid manifestations typically include an isolated nodule or nodules with mild surrounding inflammation (Fig. 68–1). The nodules vary in size but generally are 1 to 3 mm in diameter. Older lesions frequently become umbilicated and develop a white or waxy-appearing core. Mild conjunctival injection frequently accompanies lesions on or near the margin of the eyelid. The associated conjunctivitis occasionally can be severe and chronic. In chronic cases, corneal epithelial disease may develop.

Molluscum infection is considered to be self-limited, with most lesions resolving spontaneously within a few months.

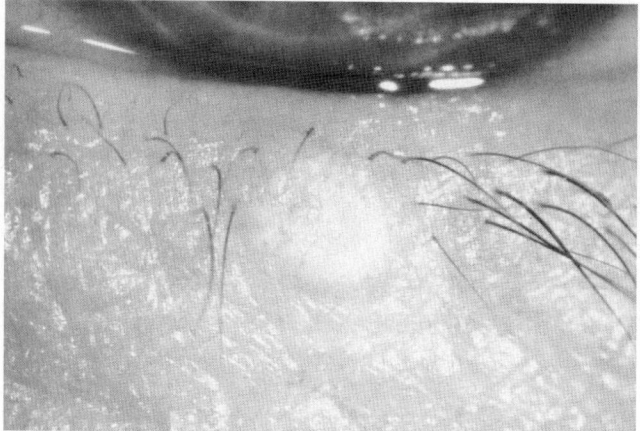

Figure 68–1 *Molluscum contagiosum* typically is manifested as an isolated nodule or nodules approximately 1 to 3 mm in diameter. Older lesions often become umbilicated and develop a white or waxy-appearing core. (See companion Expert Consult web site for color version.)

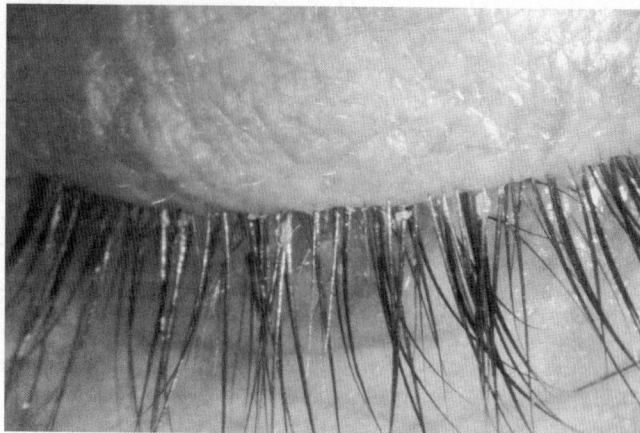

Figure 68–2 Slit-lamp photo of *Phthirus pubis* infestation demonstrating adult lice firmly adherent to the eyelashes and egg cases (i.e., nits) attached to the proximal ends of the hair shafts. (See companion Expert Consult web site for color version.)

However, the infection can be recalcitrant and problematic, especially in immunocompromised patients.[226,234] The presence of recalcitrant or atypical molluscum contagiosum lesions involving the eye have been reported in patients infected with human immunodeficiency virus (HIV).[144,188] Despite the self-limited nature of the disease in immunocompetent individuals, treatment often is advocated to prevent auto-inoculation, which may prolong the course of the disease. Treatment also may be offered to provide symptomatic relief. Mechanical treatments such as cryotherapy, expression or curettage of the central core, excision, and cautery have been effective.[46] Medical treatments that have been effective against molluscum infection remote from the eye include 1 percent imiquimod cream[202] and podophyllotoxin.[203] These agents are not recommended for the treatment of periocular lesions, however, because of the possibility of injury to the eye.

PARASITIC EYELID DISEASE

Phthirus pubis Infestation

The crab louse *Phthirus pubis* is a tiny insect well adapted to living in coarse, widely spaced hair. Infestation most commonly involves pubic, axillary, and body hair. The organism is transmitted by direct person-to-person contact and possibly by fomites.[192] Infestation of the eyelid often is a marker for sexually transmitted diseases, especially in adult patients.[192] Affected patients typically have unilateral, chronic blepharoconjunctivitis, but some patients may be asymptomatic. Although unmagnified ocular examination may reveal signs of the disease, diagnosis is facilitated by slit-lamp examination, which offers a magnified view of the eyelid margins and eyelashes (Fig. 68–2). Slit-lamp examination reveals adult lice firmly adherent to the eyelashes and egg cases (i.e., nits) attached to the proximal ends of the hair shafts. Reddish brown flecks of louse excreta frequently are found at the base of the lashes.[44]

Treatment can be facilitated by simple mechanical removal of the lice and associated nits under magnification offered by the slit lamp or other devices. Medical treatment often is preferred for young children because of their inability to tolerate mechanical removal. The organisms can be smothered by the application of a bland ointment such as petrolatum jelly applied four times each day to the eyelids. Physostigmine ointment administered twice a day frequently is used by ophthalmologists to treat eye lesions.[44] The agent inhibits nerve transmission in the insect and

thus is directly toxic to the insect. It should be used with caution in infants and small children. If physostigmine comes into contact with the eye, it has several significant side effects, the most bothersome of which is stimulation of accommodation, which can produce blurred vision that may last for several hours. Medical treatment should be continued for as long as 2 weeks to ensure eradication of lice that emerge from nits during the normal life cycle of the organism.[44]

Patients also should undergo a general physical examination to assess for involvement of other body regions. Lindane shampoo scrubs of the scalp, pubic hair, and body are recommended if infestation is found in these areas. Clothing and bed linen should be laundered, and family members should be examined and treated as necessary. Follow-up at 4 to 6 weeks after treatment is recommended to detect re-infestation.

Demodex Infection

Demodex folliculorum and *Demodex brevis* are mites that frequently infest hair follicles in humans, including the hair follicles of the eyelids.[70] The organisms historically have been considered nonpathogenic parasites,[118] although they have been postulated to cause increased hordeola formation as a result of obstruction of sebaceous glands in the eyelids. *Demodex* is found commonly in patients with rosacea, although a causal relationship is difficult to establish.[172] Rosacea-like eruptions also have been attributed to *Demodex*, and one pathologic report demonstrated a granulomatous dermal inflammation associated with *Demodex* infection.[164] *Demodex* is found more commonly on eyelashes with cylindrical dandruff (Fig. 68–3).[80] Treatment with topical pilocarpine gel was shown in one study to alleviate the ocular itching associated with *Demodex* infection.[79] Because of the frequency of infestation and the paucity of definitive disease caused by the organism, treatment often is considered unnecessary.

POSTERIOR EYELID INFECTION

Hordeolum

A hordeolum (i.e., stye) is an infection of the sebaceous glands in the eyelids. When the glands of Zeis are involved, the term *external hordeolum* is used. The lesion typically points to the skin surface. When the meibomian glands are involved, the term *internal hordeolum* is used. An internal hordeolum may point toward the skin or toward the palpebral conjunctiva. *S. aureus*

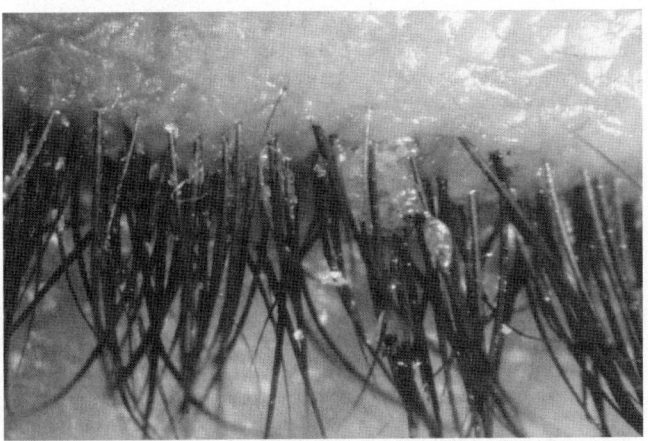

Figure 68–3 *Demodex folliculorum* and *Demodex brevis* are mites that can infect the hair follicles of the eyelids and are found more commonly on eyelashes with cylindrical dandruff. (See companion Expert Consult web site for color version.)

is the most common causal agent of internal and external hordeola.

Patients with disease of the lid margin, such as those with chronic blepharitis, seborrhea, or rosacea, are prone to recurrent hordeola, especially during the first decade of life. Hordeola are manifested as erythematous, elevated, tender nodules. Nodules typically are 5 to 10 mm in diameter and usually are solitary, although they may be multiple or bilateral. Patients with a history of recurrent hordeola may have them in various stages of evolution or resolution.

The lesions usually are self-limited and typically resolve within 5 to 7 days with spontaneous drainage of the abscess. Warm compresses may hasten resolution and improve comfort. Parents should be advised to place a clean washcloth soaked in warm tap water on the involved eyelid for 10 to 15 minutes several times each day. Parents should be advised to ensure that the water is not hot enough to result in a burn. For significant coexisting blepharitis, a topical antibiotic such as erythromycin ointment may prove useful by reducing the normal bacterial skin flora of the eyelid and decreasing the risk of recurrence. Systemic antibiotics rarely are indicated for acute hordeola. Children with frequent recurrences, however, may benefit from a short course of systemic antibiotics such as erythromycin (younger than 12 years) or tetracycline (older than 12 years). These agents further decrease the bacterial flora on the eyelid and may reduce the risk of recurrence even more. Lid hygiene efforts, as described for the treatment of staphylococcal blepharitis, should be instituted and maintained for children with recurrent hordeola. Surgical drainage of a hordeolum usually is unnecessary.

Chalazion

Cytologically, a chalazion may represent either a mixed-cell granulomatous inflammation or a suppurating granuloma.[57] The lesion occurs in a meibomian gland as a result of a foreign body reaction to secretions produced by the gland that have been extruded into surrounding tissue. A chalazion may develop after resolution of an internal hordeolum, in which case it is preceded by an acute stage, or it may develop primarily, without a preceding acute inflammatory phase. A typical chalazion appears as a round, nontender nodule within the substance of the eyelid. Multiple and bilateral chalazia may occur in susceptible patients. Recurrent lesions are not uncommon findings. They are typically 2 to 10 mm in diameter.

Spontaneous resolution of smaller chalazia can be anticipated after a period of observation without treatment, sometimes as long as several months. Larger lesions, particularly those greater than 10 mm in diameter, frequently do not resolve without specific treatment. In patients with an acute or chronic inflammatory component, application of warm compresses may be beneficial. Surgical intervention may be warranted to treat medium to large chalazia that are cosmetically objectionable, produce astigmatism by pressing on the cornea, result in mechanical ptosis, or cause other symptoms. The most common surgical treatment offered is incision and curettage through an internal incision on the palpebral conjunctival surface. Surgery is highly effective. It can be performed in the office, but general anesthesia is required for most young children. Because of the need for general anesthesia, we typically recommend deferring surgical treatment until several months has elapsed without spontaneous resolution. Earlier intervention may be recommended if the chalazion is particularly large, if pigmentary changes have developed in the overlying skin, or if astigmatism or ptosis is present in a young child at risk for the development of amblyopia.

Chalazia can be treated by intralesional steroid injection, surgical incision,[58] or both.[72] Dhaliwal and Bhatia[58] reported that incision plus curettage was the procedure of choice for lesions that have been present for 8.5 months or longer and for lesions 11.4 mm or larger in size, based on the results of a prospective study. The major potential drawback of intralesional steroid injection is the risk of complications developing with an otherwise relatively benign condition. Rarely, steroid injection can result in sterile abscess formation or eyelid necrosis. Intralesional injections are done best with a chalazion clamp in place to protect the underlying globe from accidental needle trauma during injection. This device places a metal plate between the chalazion and the eye.

DACRYOADENITIS

Dacryoadenitis is an uncommon ophthalmic condition. Even in a busy ophthalmology practice, dacryoadenitis was diagnosed in approximately 1 in every 10,000 patient visits.[176] The clinical manifestation is variable. Localized tenderness and swelling of the temporal aspect of the upper eyelid usually occur and often produce an S-shaped deformity of the lid margin. Pain is frequently a predominant feature. Associated signs and symptoms include fever, follicular conjunctivitis, mucopurulent discharge, limited extraocular movement, and proptosis.[176] Keratoconjunctivitis sicca has been reported as a consequence of Epstein-Barr virus (EBV)-associated dacryoadenitis in a child.[139]

Before the era of widespread immunization, mumps was a leading cause of dacryoadenitis. Bacteria such as staphylococci, streptococci, and gonococci also have been implicated. Exceedingly rare organisms such as *Brucella* are involved occasionally in bacterial cases.[13] EBV has been implicated as the etiologic agent in a large proportion of nonsuppurative cases. Marked regional lymphadenopathy may be a distinguishing feature of EBV dacryoadenitis.[176]

Appropriate laboratory evaluation includes Gram stain and culture of mucopurulent discharge from the eye. Neuroimaging is indicated when the patient has severe inflammation, proptosis, limitation of extraocular movement, or other orbital signs to rule out a more generalized orbital process. The condition easily can be confused clinically with orbital cellulitis when signs and symptoms are severe. Biopsy of the lacrimal gland may be required to confirm the diagnosis in patients not responding to standard medical treatment or when atypical features are identified on clinical examination or radiographic studies. Blood cultures are indicated for patients with signs of systemic toxicity.

Intravenous nafcillin or vancomycin is a reasonable initial antibiotic choice for severe dacryoadenitis caused by gram-positive organisms. Oral anti-staphylococcal agents may be used for less severe cases. For gram-negative cases, ceftazidime or other similar agents should be considered. For suppurative cases without Gram-stain guidance, intravenous nafcillin or vancomycin should be considered as initial therapy for severe cases and oral anti-staphylococcal agents for less acute cases.

Therapy in the form of warm compresses and oral analgesics is indicated for nonsuppurative dacryoadenitis. Serum testing for evidence of EBV infection should be considered in patients with regional lymphadenopathy.[176] Noninfectious causes of dacryoadenitis include sarcoidosis, Sjögren syndrome, leukemia, lymphoma, eosinophilic granuloma, and orbital pseudotumor. Noninfectious cases of dacryoadenitis sometimes can be difficult to distinguish from infectious cases. Lacrimal gland biopsy and neuroimaging usually are necessary to establish a diagnosis in noninfectious cases.[129] Intralesional steroid injection has been shown to be effective in the management of acute idiopathic dacryoadenitis; it results in marked improvement of symptoms within 7 days of treatment in most cases.[145]

DACRYOCYSTITIS

Dacryocystitis may result from congenital or acquired lacrimal outflow obstruction. Simple membranous nasolacrimal duct obstruction occurs in as many as 6 percent of the newborn population, and intermittent, mild, self-limited bacterial infection is a commonly associated feature. More severe infection of the lacrimal sac results in dacryocystitis. This condition is manifested as acute erythema, pain, and swelling in the medial canthal region. The swelling typically is located below the medial canthal tendon. Marked epiphora generally is present, and a mucopurulent discharge frequently can be expressed through the lacrimal punctum if the proximal aspect of the lacrimal drainage system is not obstructed. If the infection has resulted in or from obstruction proximal and distal to the lacrimal sac, the overlying skin may become tense as the nasolacrimal sac distends in response to the infectious process. Formation of a fistula to the overlying skin may occur as a result of dacryocystitis, and surgical excision of the fistula tract often is needed after the acute process has resolved. Dacryocystitis is a particularly common finding in neonates with a dacryocele, with dacryocystitis developing in as many as 60 percent of affected neonates.[163]

Aerobic and anaerobic bacteria and fungi may produce dacryocystitis.[29,30] In one study, S. epidermidis and Pseudomonas spp. were the aerobic organisms identified most frequently, and Peptostreptococcus spp. and Propionibacterium spp. were the anaerobes isolated most frequently. Less common agents include Escherichia coli, Pseudomonas spp., Haemophilus influenzae, Pasteurella multocida, and various anaerobes. Laboratory investigation should include aerobic and anaerobic culture of mucopurulent discharge from the lacrimal sac. Mild massage of the lacrimal sac may be used to facilitate expression of material for Gram stain and culture. A sepsis work-up should be considered for children who are acutely ill and for young infants.

Intravenous nafcillin, vancomycin, or both are good initial therapeutic choices for serious gram-positive infections. Mild cases in older children can be treated with oral antibiotics. Intravenous ceftazidime is a reasonable initial antibiotic choice for gram-negative dacryocystitis. Oral ciprofloxacin is useful for less severe cases in adult patients, although the drug is not approved for use in children. Intravenous nafcillin or vancomycin typically provides good initial empiric therapy in patients when Gram stain guidance is not available.

Ophthalmologic consultation should be requested in all cases of acute dacryocystitis. Decompression of the lacrimal sac by aspiration, incision and drainage, or probing the proximal lacrimal drainage system may be needed to hasten resolution. Probing of the distal lacrimal system often is deferred until the acute infection has subsided, although probing during the acute infection has been reported to be a safe and effective adjunct to treatment.[167] Mucopurulent material obtained during surgical decompression should be sent for appropriate culture.

PRESEPTAL (PERIORBITAL) CELLULITIS

The term *preseptal cellulitis* refers to an infectious process in the eyelids that is isolated to regions anterior to the orbital septum. The orbital septum is a thin layer of fascia that extends vertically from the periosteum of the orbital rim to the tarsal plate within the eyelids. Though penetrated by nerves and vascular structures, the septum provides a barrier that slows the spread of infectious agents into deeper orbital and retro-orbital structures.[198] Typical signs and symptoms of preseptal cellulitis include erythema and edema of the eyelids. Distinctively absent are signs of deeper orbital involvement such as restricted ocular motility, pain with eye movement, and proptosis. Preseptal cellulitis may occur after trauma or be caused by spread of infection from adjacent structures, such as skin and the upper respiratory system.[224]

Post-traumatic Preseptal Cellulitis

Post-traumatic preseptal cellulitis occurs after puncture wounds on the lids, face, or scalp. It also may occur after blunt trauma with no obvious entry wound. The etiologic agents most commonly identified are S. aureus and S. pyogenes, and polymicrobial infections can occur. Other bacterial causes include non–spore-forming anaerobes such as Peptococcus, Peptostreptococcus, and Bacteroides. Infection by aerobic gram-negative bacilli is an uncommon finding.[10] P. multocida is a common organism that produces post-traumatic preseptal cellulitis after dog and cat bites.[124,127] Cellulitis secondary to methicillin-resistant S. aureus (MRSA) is a common cause of community-acquired cellulitis in some locations.

Clinical signs and symptoms are determined in large part by the severity of the injury, the interval since injury, and the infecting organisms. The involved lids are edematous, erythematous, and typically quite tender. Fluctuation of subcutaneous tissue may be seen if an abscess has developed. Swelling of the uninvolved contralateral eyelids may occur as a result of lymphedema. As with any form of isolated preseptal cellulitis, vision is unaffected, and proptosis and eye movement disturbances are absent. On rare occasion, eyelid edema may be sufficiently severe to preclude adequate evaluation of the eye. Neuroimaging is required in such cases to assess the globe and rule out involvement of structures posterior to the orbital septum. Ophthalmologic consultation is critical in cases of severe post-traumatic preseptal cellulitis because of the potential for concurrent globe injury.

Laboratory analysis includes Gram stain and aerobic and anaerobic culture of mucopurulent material to aid in therapeutic decisions. Amoxicillin-clavulanate or a related agent is the drug of choice for treating post-traumatic cellulitis caused by a dog bite because of the high prevalence of P. multocida. Tetanus prophylaxis should be guided by standard recommendations. Surgical drainage of large abscesses may be required if a rapid response to antimicrobial therapy does not occur.

Nontraumatic Preseptal Cellulitis

The clinical features of nonsuppurative, nontraumatic preseptal cellulitis depend to a large degree on the causative agent. Erythema and swelling of the involved eyelids are typical and often are accompanied by pain. Signs of orbital infection, such as altered vision, proptosis, and eye movement abnormalities, are absent.

Before the advent of *H. influenzae* type b (Hib) vaccine, this organismly frequently was a cause of nonsuppurative preseptal cellulitis in children. Hib is seen infrequently as a cause of preseptal cellulitis today.[62] It was a particularly dangerous agent because of a high risk of spread to the central nervous system (CNS), which occurred in as many as 2 to 3 percent of patients. Though rare today, Hib infections still may be encountered. Like many infecting organisms, Hib gains access to subcutaneous tissue through infected nasal passages.

Streptococcus pneumoniae is now the most common bacterial cause of preseptal cellulitis in the pediatric age group.[62] It occurs in association with upper respiratory tract infection, although constitutional symptoms usually are less pronounced than those associated with Hib infection. A variety of other bacterial agents may cause preseptal cellulitis, but they are seen less commonly. Preseptal cellulitis occasionally has been reported to be due to a variety of other organisms, including *Trichophyton* (ringworm),[218] tuberculosis,[170] and anthrax.[35]

Adenovirus is another particularly common cause of preseptal cellulitis in children. Adenovirus is an important consideration in the differential diagnosis of childhood preseptal cellulitis because, despite being self-limited, the condition can occasionally mimic bacterial infection and prompt unnecessary treatment with antibiotics. Adenovirus can be recognized by its characteristic copious discharge, which may be serous. Swelling of the lid may be prominent, but erythema usually is minimal. Preauricular lymphadenopathy often occurs in older children, and marked conjunctival hyperemia with or without chemosis and subconjunctival hemorrhage may be present. Photophobia also may be noticed in cases of concurrent punctate keratopathy. A history of recent contact with other infected individuals frequently is noted and should be sought. Care should be taken to avoid spreading infection to family members, medical personnel, and others.

Hospital admission should be considered for children younger than 1 year of age with bacterial preseptal cellulitis. Hospitalization also is important for children with signs of systemic toxicity and those with inadequate *H. influenzae* immunization. A sepsis work-up is indicated for children with signs of systemic toxicity and for extremely young children. Ophthalmologic consultation is recommended if orbital involvement is suspected or if clinical examination is inconclusive. Computed tomography (CT) usually is unnecessary for isolated preseptal cellulitis. Cultures of blood obtained from patients with preseptal cellulitis generally are negative but are more likely to be positive in children younger than 2 years. Culture of conjunctival discharge is done often but rarely has significant diagnostic benefit.

A severity index for scoring preseptal cellulitis in children has been reported to help guide treatment decisions.[221] Antibacterial treatment should include intravenous agents for infants and those with signs of serious systemic infection. Intravenous cefuroxime or a combination of nafcillin plus cefotaxime or ceftriaxone frequently is recommended for empiric therapy. Outpatient treatment with intramuscular or oral antibiotics is reasonable for older, less acutely ill children. Intracranial infection has been associated with preseptal cellulitis in pediatric patients. Intracranial involvement should be suspected in any patient 7 years or older with preseptal or orbital cellulitis associated with an orbital subperiosteal abscess, Pott puffy tumor, concurrent sinusitis, complaints of headache, and persistent fever despite intravenous antibiotics.[175]

Systemic antibiotics should be continued for 7 to 10 days. Patients in whom intravenous antibiotics are started initially can switch to an oral antibiotic after they have been afebrile for at least 24 hours and otherwise have improved clinically, unless the possibility of development of sepsis or meningitis remains a concern.

ORBITAL CELLULITIS

Bacterial infection of orbital structures posterior to the orbital septum is the most frequent cause of acute orbital inflammation. Orbital cellulitis occurs more commonly in children and more frequently during cold weather, when sinusitis is more prevalent.

Initial signs and symptoms can vary from mild inflammation to severe and fulminant orbital disease. Cardinal signs and symptoms of infectious orbital cellulitis include proptosis, limited eye movement (including total ophthalmoplegia), pain with eye movement, and an abnormal pupillary response. Decreased vision or even blindness can occur as the most serious ophthalmic complication.[183] Death can result from intracranial extension of the infection if appropriate treatment is not initiated. Elevated intraocular pressure and chemosis of the conjunctiva are common ancillary signs. Preseptal cellulitis often coexists with orbital cellulitis but is not a prerequisite.

Most cases of orbital cellulitis are caused by spread of infection from an adjacent infected sinus.[40,151] Ethmoid sinusitis is the most common predisposing factor. Rare cases are due to penetrating orbital trauma or skin infection involving the face, with spread of organisms into the orbit. Orbital cellulitis may occur infrequently after orbital, ocular, or periocular surgery.[161,230] Orbital cellulitis and cavernous sinus thrombosis have been reported to occur after dental infections and dental surgery.[32]

Comprehensive evaluation of a patient with confirmed or suspected orbital cellulitis includes ophthalmologic and systemic examination. Assessment of visual acuity in both eyes is important for excluding vision loss and establishing a baseline to aid in monitoring progression of the disease or the effects of therapy. Evaluation of optic nerve dysfunction by examining the pupils for an afferent pupillary defect (APD) is important before pupillary dilation is performed to assess the retina. Careful evaluation of extraocular movement should be performed in all extreme positions of gaze to identify restriction of ocular duction and elicit pain on eye movement. The presence or absence of proptosis can be assessed clinically by viewing the eyes from above (bird's-eye view) or below (worm's-eye view) and by comparing their relative positions within the orbits. In severe cases of orbital cellulitis, funduscopic examination may reveal dilation of the retinal venules and signs of compressive optic neuropathy such as optic disk edema. Central retinal artery occlusion has been reported occasionally.[112] Systemic evaluation includes determination of temperature, which usually is in the range of 39° C to 40° C (102° F to 104° F). Sinus examination, a screening neurologic examination, and evaluation for signs and symptoms of sepsis and meningitis should be performed.

In any case of clinically definite or suspected orbital cellulitis, CT of the orbit and brain is indicated. CT can establish or confirm the diagnosis of orbital cellulitis and provides critical information needed to manage the patient. Imaging of the brain is important because orbital cellulitis can evolve into a brain abscess, meningitis, or cavernous sinus thrombosis. However, when a clinical response to treatment is noted, improvement in CT findings frequently is delayed. Therefore, recurrent CT scanning of a child with clinically improving findings is not indicated absolutely unless new signs or symptoms of concern develop.

Microbiologic studies often are acutely unhelpful for the routine patient with orbital cellulitis. Nonetheless, baseline studies remain important because critical information sometimes is acquired. Blood cultures should be obtained at a minimum, and a lumbar puncture with culture of cerebrospinal fluid (CSF) should be considered in infants and those with signs of CNS infection. Culture of the ocular, nasal, and nasopharyngeal mucous membranes is of limited value and can be omitted. However, if surgical drainage is performed, cultures of any material removed should be obtained.

Optimal management of a child with orbital cellulitis requires a multidisciplinary approach. In addition to evaluation and management by an experienced pediatrician, ophthalmologic and otolaryngologic consultation should be obtained. Neurosurgical consultation is required when involvement of the CNS is diagnosed or suspected. In atypical cases and those not responding to treatment, consultation with an infectious disease specialist is warranted.

The most common offending etiologic bacteria are *S. aureus*, *Streptococcus* spp., and *Haemophilus* spp. (other than *H. influenzae*). *S. pneumoniae* also is implicated frequently, and a variety of less common organisms have been reported. *H. influenzae* orbital cellulitis rarely has occurred since widespread use of the Hib vaccine was implemented.[3,62] Fungal infection of the orbit occasionally is encountered, typically in immunocompromised individuals.[137]

The differential diagnosis of orbital inflammation in children includes a broad range of noninfectious conditions, including cavernous sinus thrombosis, idiopathic inflammatory orbital pseudotumor, Wegener granulomatosis, sarcoidosis, leukemic infiltration, lymphoma, rhabdomyosarcoma, necrotic retinoblastoma, metastatic carcinoma, and histiocytosis X. Thyroid ophthalmopathy also can be manifested as an acute orbital inflammatory process, although usually its onset is slow and insidious.

Treatment of all patients with orbital cellulitis requires hospitalization and initiation of intravenous antibiotics as soon as possible after material has been obtained for culture. Infection with penicillin-resistant organisms is an increasingly common occurrence and must be considered during treatment.[37,181] Appropriate initial antibiotic therapy may include nafcillin, metronidazole, and cefotaxime as combination therapy. Given the increasing incidence of MRSA, initial treatment with vancomycin or clindamycin should be considered.[148,181] Other antimicrobial agents may be useful, and local susceptibility patterns should guide the choice of initial antimicrobial therapy. Antibiotic coverage should be modified according to the clinical course and culture results. If the patient fails to respond to antibiotic treatment within 24 to 48 hours, consultation with an infectious disease specialist and a repeat CT scan to look for the development of an orbital abscess should be considered (Fig. 68–4). The mean hospital stay for uncomplicated cases of orbital cellulitis is 10 to 14 days, and oral antibiotics should be prescribed for 7 to 10 days after discharge. A nasal decongestant commonly is prescribed at the time that the diagnosis is established to aid in opening the sinus ostia, promoting drainage of the infected sinus, and speeding resolution. Nasal decongestants should be continued for 7 to 10 days after initiation.

Although treatment of orbital cellulitis with steroids remains controversial, their use in the treatment of acute and chronic sinusitis has become increasingly common. Studies have shown that steroids can reduce levels of inflammatory cytokines in the sinonasal mucosa of individuals with sinusitis.[34,223] In a recent study on the use of steroids in children with orbital cellulitis, Yen and Yen[232] reported no adverse effects of this adjunct treatment with systemic antibiotics. Prospective studies on the use of steroids in orbital cellulitis have been proposed to determine whether they have any clinical benefit.

Children with orbital cellulitis require diligent follow-up while in the hospital. Vision should be assessed at the bedside daily; results may be more accurate if a single examiner routinely assesses vision for a given patient. Pupillary examination for an APD should be performed at each examination. Development of an APD indicates compromise of the optic nerve, warrants escalation of treatment, and usually requires urgent surgical intervention. Reduction of vision, development of an APD, onset of CNS signs, or worsening of systemic status should prompt emergency repeat neuroimaging of the brain and orbit, with further inter-

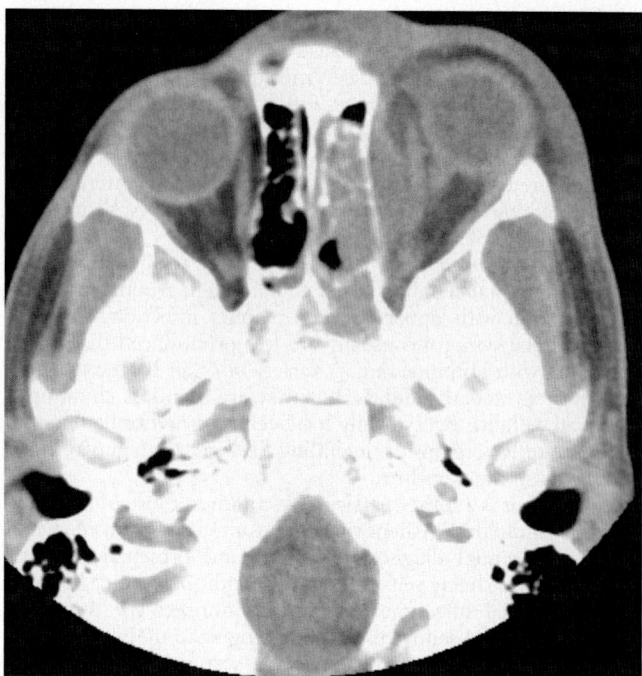

Figure 68–4 Failure of response of orbital cellulitis to antibiotic treatment may be a sign of development of a subperiosteal orbital abscess (seen here in the right medial orbit).

vention as dictated by results of the scan. The close anatomic relationship of the orbit to the brain, with the orbital venous system freely anastomosing with the facial venous plexus and cranial venous sinus system through a series of valveless veins, seriously increases the potential for spread of infection to contiguous structures, including the brain.

Acute surgical intervention to decompress the orbit or drain an orbital or subperiosteal abscess is indicated if vision loss or an APD is identified at any point during treatment. Immediate neurosurgical consideration is indicated if CNS involvement is documented. Most patients without evidence of vision loss, optic nerve dysfunction, or CNS involvement can be managed successfully medically. The surgical adage that all abscesses should be subjected to incision and drainage does not apply to abscesses associated with orbital cellulitis. Most subperiosteal abscesses located in the medial orbit can be managed successfully with medical therapy alone.[89,180] Formation of an abscess within the substance of the orbit (as opposed to a subperiosteal abscess) seldom occurs. Guidelines for surgical drainage are similar to those for subperiosteal abscess,[180] although such abscesses are more likely to require surgical intervention because of treatment failure or spread of infection to contiguous structures.[89] Provided that clinical improvement continues, no worrisome signs or symptoms of CNS involvement develop, and the patient's overall clinical status does not worsen, repeat neuroimaging of patients with an orbital abscess is unnecessary. Short-term resolution of an orbital abscess often is not obvious on CT. The radiographic appearance of the abscess typically remains unchanged on early follow-up scans, although it may no longer contain viable organisms.

Sinus drainage by an otolaryngologist frequently is required to hasten resolution. Formation of an abscess is not a prerequisite for surgical intervention, and orbital cellulitis without abscess formation may progress to the point of requiring surgery. Despite prompt and appropriate treatment, serious complications such as permanent vision loss and brain abscess can occur.[97,175,183] Most patients, however, can be treated effectively with no permanent sequelae.

Orbital cellulitis caused by fungal infection has a course and prognosis markedly different from those of bacterial orbital cellulitis, particularly cellulitis caused by mucormycosis and aspergillosis. Fungal orbital cellulitis typically occurs in patients who are immunocompromised or patients with metabolic acidosis, such as those with poorly controlled diabetes. Orbital cellulitis may be manifested as a subacute or chronic process. Orbital apex syndrome is considered to be the most severe form, with loss of function of all cranial nerves traversing the orbital apex into the orbit (i.e., cranial nerves II, III, IV, V, and VI). A black eschar-like lesion may form in the oropharynx or nasopharynx.

Aspergillus orbital infections (most commonly caused by *A. flavus, A. fumigatus,* or *A. oryzae*) are rare findings in children and may take a slow, chronic course over a period of months or years. No clear predisposing factors exist, but it has a predilection for humid climates and most cases occur in otherwise healthy individuals. Signs and symptoms of orbital infection caused by *Aspergillus* spp. include loss of vision, constant dull pain, decreased or absent ocular motility, and proptosis with firm resistance to retropulsion. Palate and nasopharyngeal lesions occur but are rare. Biopsy is required for establishing the diagnosis.[88]

Effective treatment of orbital fungal infection requires correction of systemic and metabolic disturbances and administration of intravenous antifungal agents such as amphotericin B. Though still considered experimental, posaconazole has been shown to be effective as an alternative treatment in those who fail to respond to or cannot tolerate treatment with amphotericin B.[182] Surgical débridement of the orbit or adjacent infected sinuses frequently is required. Treatment often is unsuccessful, and fatalities are not uncommon, particularly with mucormycosis.

The larva of *Echinococcus granulosus* can produce a hydatid cyst in the orbit. The dog is the definitive host animal, although the organism also may live in the intestines of sheep, goats, cattle, pigs, and other animals. The disease is endemic in the Middle East, Africa, and Asia. Humans become infected by eating contaminated food, typically meat, and infection may occur in any age group. Affected patients have noninflammatory proptosis, decreased ocular motility, and dull orbital pain. Surgical excision is required for treatment. The cyst may be injected with hypertonic saline to kill the parasite, followed by excision.[86]

CONJUNCTIVAL INFECTIONS

The conjunctiva is the mucous membrane covering the inner surfaces of the eyelids and the anterior surface of the sclera. The mucous membrane lining the inner surface of the eyelids is called the *palpebral conjunctiva*, and that covering the globe is called the *bulbar conjunctiva*. The conjunctiva contains numerous small glands that produce most of the aqueous and mucous components of tears that are responsible for producing a smooth, uniform tear film over the cornea. The conjunctiva may be infected by a wide variety of bacterial and viral agents, as well as by noninfectious allergic and toxic agents.

Patients with conjunctivitis may complain of burning, itching, or a foreign body sensation. Significant itching usually signifies an allergic or viral cause. The conjunctival injection (erythema) in eyes with infectious conjunctivitis is located away from the cornea. Conjunctival injection concentrated adjacent to the cornea (i.e., limbal or ciliary flush) suggests keratitis (i.e., inflammation of the cornea), iritis (inflammation of the iris), or iridocyclitis (i.e., inflammation of the iris and ciliary body). When the eye is severely infected, however, such a differentiating pattern may not be discernible. Conjunctivitis usually is accompanied by a discharge that has some important diagnostic properties. Purulence suggests a bacterial cause, a mucoid discharge is seen most often with viral infections, and a serous discharge usually is seen with viral or allergic causes. Patients with isolated conjunctivitis do not have any significant alteration in vision. Conjunctivitis with poor vision warrants search for another diagnosis.[83,135]

BACTERIAL CONJUNCTIVITIS

Bacterial conjunctivitis is a common form of infectious conjunctivitis in children. It is characterized by a purulent discharge and can be unilateral or bilateral. It is useful clinically to divide bacterial conjunctivitis into mild and severe forms because treatment approaches are different.

Mild Bacterial Conjunctivitis

The agents most commonly causing mild bacterial conjunctivitis in children aged 5 years or older are *S. pneumoniae* and *Moraxella* spp.[83] *H. influenzae* was a prominent causative agent before the availability of Hib vaccine. *S. aureus* conjunctivitis is seen most frequently after trauma or surgical manipulation. Conjunctival stains and cultures usually are not necessary because the disease is self-limited or responds rapidly to topical antibiotics.

Many appropriate topical antimicrobial agents for treatment of bacterial conjunctivitis are readily available and include topical moxifloxacin, gatifloxacin, ciprofloxacin, ofloxacin, norfloxacin, tobramycin, gentamicin, erythromycin, sulfacetamide, and combination antibiotics. Aminoglycoside-containing compounds such as neomycin occasionally can cause a dramatic allergic blepharoconjunctivitis that can be worse than the original problem. The choice of using either drops or ointment is best left to the person who will be instilling the medication because neither has any proven therapeutic advantage. With the emergence of multidrug-resistant organisms in many parts of the country, the choice of antibiotic should be modified accordingly. Newer agents, such as the fourth-generation fluoroquinolones (moxifloxacin and gatifloxacin), have many advantages over older drugs, including broad-spectrum coverage, ease of dosing, and pH neutrality. A typical regimen for treatment of mild conjunctivitis is 1 drop or a 0.25-inch bead of ointment placed into the inferior conjunctival fornix three to six times daily for 5 to 7 days, depending on the actual medication. Persistent infection should prompt a return to the physician for reconsideration of the diagnosis. Mild bacterial conjunctivitis generally resolves spontaneously in 7 to 14 days without treatment.[82,83]

Severe Bacterial Conjunctivitis

Severe bacterial conjunctivitis, characterized by pronounced conjunctival infection and copious purulent discharge, usually is caused by *Neisseria gonorrhoeae, Neisseria meningitidis, S. aureus, S. pneumoniae,* and, in children younger than 5 years, *H. influenzae.* A hyperpurulent state in which the copious purulent discharge reaccumulates in a matter of minutes is characteristic of infection with *N. gonorrhoeae.*[96,194]

Severe conjunctivitis demands a comprehensive microbiologic evaluation consisting of stains and cultures. Samples from both eyes should be cultured separately, even if only one eye is involved, to allow the uninvolved eye to serve as a useful control.[205] Gram stains of conjunctival scrapings should be done at the time of culture. A useful culture technique includes the use of a cotton or calcium alginate swab (Calgiswab, Spectrum, Houston) gently rubbed against the palpebral conjunctiva of the lower lid and inoculated onto blood and chocolate agar. If *N. gonorrhoeae* is suspected, culture for chlamydia also is indicated because concurrent infection with both organisms is a common occurrence.

Treatment of severe bacterial conjunctivitis is based initially on results of the stains and later modified according to culture and sensitivities. If *Neisseria* is strongly suspected, the patient should be treated as though the disease is present, even if the laboratory results are not confirmatory. Ocular *N. gonorrhoeae* infection is a vision- and life-threatening disease. This organism can penetrate the intact cornea and cause microbial keratitis, corneal perforation, and endophthalmitis, in addition to conjunctivitis. *N. gonorrhoeae* conjunctivitis should be considered in three patient groups: neonates after passage through an infected birth canal, sexually active individuals, and victims of suspected sexual abuse. Pediatric infection with *N. gonorrhoeae* requires hospital admission and administration of a systemic antibiotic. Because of the prevalence of penicillin-resistant strains, a broad-spectrum (third-generation) cephalosporin, such as ceftriaxone, is the most appropriate choice of antibiotic.[92] Adjunctive treatment of *N. gonorrhoeae* conjunctivitis with topical moxifloxacin and simple saline irrigation for 5 days can be helpful, but topical agents should never be used as an isolated treatment.[96] Moxifloxacin is a particularly good antibiotic choice because it is effective against chlamydia as well.

Conjunctivitis caused by gram-positive cocci can be treated with topical moxifloxacin, gatifloxacin, ciprofloxacin, or erythromycin. Systemic nafcillin, a second- or third-generation cephalosporin, or both can be added as needed for more extensive infections. Gram-negative bacterial conjunctivitis can be treated with topical erythromycin ointment or an aminoglycoside drip such as gentamicin or tobramycin. Systemic antibiotics can be added if needed.[205]

VIRAL CONJUNCTIVITIS

Adenoviral Conjunctivitis

Viruses are another common cause of infectious conjunctivitis in children. Many pediatric cases of viral conjunctivitis are caused by adenovirus. Serotypes 1, 2, 3, 4, 7, and 10 produce an acute form of conjunctivitis with prominent conjunctival follicles. Serotypes 3 and 7 also may cause pharyngoconjunctival fever. This entity is characterized by conjunctivitis, fever, and pharyngitis.[21] Serotypes 8, 19, and 37 primarily cause epidemic keratoconjunctivitis.[205] The keratitis is characterized by a combination of a punctate epithelial keratitis and an immune response that results in subepithelial infiltrates. Photophobia is a prominent feature, and vision may be decreased markedly with this entity. Epidemic keratoconjunctivitis commonly is associated with pharyngitis and rhinitis, which may precede or coexist with the conjunctivitis.

Adenoviral conjunctivitis is highly contagious. It is transmitted easily from an infected individual to others at home or school. The incubation period is 5 to 10 days but may be as long as 21 days. The virus is shed from the infected conjunctiva for 7 to 12 days after the onset of infection. Frequently, a prodromal upper respiratory infection consisting of fever, pharyngitis, or otitis media occurs.[205] Ocular signs and symptoms include photophobia (with corneal involvement), foreign body sensation, epiphora, bulbar and palpebral conjunctival injection and chemosis (edema), and subconjunctival hemorrhage.[100] Formation of grayish pink friable membranes on the palpebral conjunctiva is a hallmark of the disease and may result in bleeding when removed. Preauricular lymphadenopathy is a common feature in older children and adults. Keratitis may be prolonged, with mild to moderate reduction of vision lasting weeks to months.[100,136]

The diagnosis of adenoviral conjunctivitis usually is clinical. Rarely is laboratory confirmation necessary. Viral cultures are possible when indicated, and a rapid enzyme immunoassay test is available.[228] Treatment of adenoviral conjunctivitis is supportive, aimed at decreasing symptoms. Cool compresses and acetaminophen are helpful, and removal of conjunctival membranes with a cotton swab may relieve the foreign-body sensation. A small

amount of bleeding often occurs after removal of these membranes, and the membranes can recur after several days. If corneal subepithelial infiltrates cause significant discomfort or an unacceptable decrease in vision, treatment with a short course of topical steroids may provide symptomatic relief and speed resolution. The use of steroid preparations requires careful monitoring,[135,205] and they should be prescribed only by an ophthalmologist.

The clinician should wear gloves when examining patients with suspected adenovirus infection. Careful handwashing is essential after direct contact. Instruments or equipment used in examining an infected patient should be cleaned with 10 percent sodium hypochlorite solution or other solutions known to eradicate adenovirus. Mini-epidemics have originated in physicians' offices.[113] At home, families should exercise caution and separate the towels and bed clothes of the patient from those of others in the household. Children of school age should be kept home for approximately 7 days or longer to reduce the risk of transmitting the infection to classmates.[205]

Herpes Simplex Virus Conjunctivitis and Complex Forms

HSV conjunctivitis may occur as a primary or as a secondary infection. Ocular infection usually is caused by HSV-1, except in newborns, in whom HSV-2 predominates.[42] Typical initial signs of HSV conjunctivitis include a serous discharge, scant conjunctival follicle formation on the inferior palpebral conjunctiva, and preauricular lymphadenopathy. Eighty percent of cases are unilateral. Eyelid vesicles often occur in primary infections. Bulbar conjunctival ulceration is an unusual occurrence, but when present, it is virtually pathognomonic of primary HSV-1 infection. Keratitis occurs in as many as 50 percent of primary cases and is characterized by mild epithelial irregularities. Dendrites can occur in primary infections. Reactivated HSV keratitis has the characteristic dendritic pattern of epithelial disease. Lid vesicles usually do not develop in reactivated HSV infection.[117]

Primary HSV dermatoblepharitis is seen most commonly in children younger than 6 years old, but it may occur at any age. The initial episode may be associated with an upper respiratory infection, and recurrences are common. Clinical signs include an eyelid vesicular reaction, mild follicular conjunctivitis, preauricular lymphadenopathy, and, occasionally, atypical epithelial keratitis. Secondary bacterial infection can occur. Systemic acyclovir is a safe and effective treatment, although the disease itself typically is self-limited and does not require treatment.[117]

The diagnosis of HSV keratoconjunctivitis usually is made on the basis of the clinical appearance alone. Antigen detection tests or viral cultures can be used when the diagnosis is in question.[113] Viral cultures, when necessary, require special handling.[205] In primary HSV infection, after the skin surface has been swabbed with an alcohol sponge, a tuberculin syringe with a 30-gauge needle is used to aspirate fluid from an intact vesicle. If no vesicles are present, a Dacron swab is wiped on the palpebral conjunctiva of the lower lid. In either case, the viral transport medium is inoculated and taken to the laboratory for special handling.

Treatment of HSV conjunctivitis alone (in the absence of corneal epithelial disease) is somewhat controversial. Oral acyclovir may be used for severe cases of primary HSV infection.[189,201] Three topical antiviral agents are available: iododeoxyuridine, vidarabine, and trifluridine.

When epithelial HSV keratitis is reactivated and the typical dendritic (branched) epithelial lesions are seen, the cornea usually is hypoesthetic. Iritis commonly is associated with HSV keratitis and is characterized by miosis, photophobia, ocular pain, and a foreign-body sensation. Vision may be decreased if the epithelial disease involves the visual axis.[205] Epithelial HSV may be atypical, more severe, or more complicated in patients receiving topical steroids and in immunocompromised patients.

Treatment with topical trifluridine or vidarabine is indicated in all cases of HSV keratitis. Topical steroid is effective in decreasing corneal scarring caused by HSV stromal keratitis. When using a topical steroid, coverage with a topical antiviral agent such as vidarabine always should be included to reduce the risk for recurrent active viral proliferation during the course of steroid treatment. Oral acyclovir is not effective for treating active HSV keratitis, but it may be useful in treating HSV uveitis.[201] Ancillary treatments include cycloplegic eyedrops to dilate the pupil and pain medications.

Though not helpful in treating acute epithelial disease, chronic suppression with oral acyclovir is effective in reducing the number of recurrences of HSV epithelial and stromal keratitis, especially in patients with stromal keratitis.[201,205] Interferon also significantly adds to the efficacy of topical antiviral therapy, but the adverse side effects of interferon must be weighed against its potential benefits.[201]

External Ocular Infections with Varicella-Zoster Virus

Childhood varicella infection (chickenpox) commonly is accompanied by conjunctivitis. Vesicles, ulcers, or both occur occasionally on the bulbar or palpebral conjunctiva. Conjunctivitis associated with varicella infection does not result in permanent visual sequelae. Corneal involvement rarely occurs and typically heals without sequelae. Occasionally, it may result in stromal scarring and produce irregular astigmatism and reduced vision.

After primary varicella infection occurs, the virus may persist in latent form in the trigeminal nerve ganglia. Herpes zoster ophthalmicus occurs when the ophthalmic division of the trigeminal nerve is affected by reactivation of the virus. The condition occurs more commonly in immunocompromised patients, and recurrences occur infrequently except in these patients.

The diagnosis of herpes zoster ophthalmicus almost always is made on the basis of the characteristic clinical feature of a painful, tender vesicular eruption in the V1 dermatome. Ocular involvement may include keratitis and uveitis. Corneal epithelial lesions may appear dendritiform, with or without subepithelial infiltrates. Uveitis may occur with or without associated keratitis. Usually it is mild, but occasionally it may be severe, with the formation of a hypopyon or hyphema. Immunofluorescence testing of vesicular base scrapings or viral cultures may be helpful if the manifestation is atypical or the diagnosis is in doubt.[125]

Treatment of herpes zoster ophthalmicus involves the administration of oral or intravenous acyclovir. Treatment is most effective when initiated within 72 hours of the appearance of vesicles. Keratitis and uveitis do not respond to topical antiviral therapy.[201] Sometimes topical steroids can be helpful in treating varicella keratitis and uveitis, but such treatment should be administered under the direction of an ophthalmologist.[135]

Chlamydial Conjunctivitis and Trachoma

Chlamydia spp. can cause conjunctivitis and trachoma. *Chlamydia psittaci* rarely causes ocular disease in humans. *Chlamydia trachomatis*, however, has numerous serotypes that affect the eye. Serotypes A, B, Ba, and C cause trachoma, and serotypes B, C, D, Da, D–, E, F, G, H, I, Ia, J, and K cause inclusion conjunctivitis, including neonatal inclusion conjunctivitis. Neonatal chlamydial conjunctivitis is discussed in the section "Neonatal Conjunctivitis."

Inclusion conjunctivitis in older children and adults is manifested as subacute or chronic inflammation of the conjunctiva. The condition may be unilateral or bilateral. A mucopurulent discharge typically occurs, as do follicles on the bulbar and peri-limbal conjunctiva. Preauricular lymphadenopathy is a common

finding. Punctate epithelial keratitis with subepithelial infiltrates and a superior micropannus (i.e., vascular growth on the cornea) may develop.[52]

The differential diagnosis of inclusion conjunctivitis is sizable and includes viral and bacterial conjunctivitis, molluscum contagiosum, and toxic keratoconjunctivitis from chronic administration of topical agents. Laboratory testing may be necessary to confirm the diagnosis. Giemsa staining of conjunctival scrapings may demonstrate the classic intracytoplasmic inclusions. A fluorescent antibody detection test or enzyme immunoassay is used to make a rapid diagnosis.[205] Rarely are chlamydial cultures needed except when the diagnosis remains in doubt.

Treatment consists of oral erythromycin or doxycycline if systemic infection is suspected. Topical erythromycin or tetracycline alone four times each day for 7 days is effective treatment of infection limited to the conjunctiva.[52,205] Moxifloxacin recently has been shown to be effective against chlamydia as well but is not yet the recommended treatment of choice.

Trachoma remains a leading cause of blindness worldwide, ranking second or third, depending on the region studied. It is a disease of impoverished populations that is exacerbated by inadequate supplies of water and by poor hygiene. Trachoma seldom is seen in developed countries. In the United States, it is encountered on Native American reservations in the Southwest and in individuals arriving in endemic areas of the United States. Eye-seeking flies play an important role in transmission of *Chlamydia* from one person to another.[205]

Trachoma causes blindness by producing chronic inflammation of the palpebral conjunctiva of the upper eyelid with secondary scar formation. Contracture of the palpebral conjunctiva scar causes entropion of the eyelid and trichiasis. Eventually, this situation leads to corneal opacification and vision loss.[204,205] Less commonly, the cornea may be infected directly. The complete course of the disease from initial infection to blindness generally takes decades.

The diagnosis of trachoma usually is made on the basis of clinical findings alone. The disease passes through characteristic stages, from simple inflammation to scarring, entropion, and trichiasis. Multiple stages may coexist in various parts of the eyelids. The World Health Organization classifies the stages of trachoma as follows: TF, trachomatous follicular response; TI, diffuse trachomatous conjunctival inflammation; TS, trachomatous scarring of the palpebral conjunctiva; TT, trachomatous trichiasis; and TO, trachomatous corneal opacification. In the pediatric population, physicians usually encounter only stages TI and TF.[214] The scars on the palpebral conjunctiva, referred to as *Arlt lines*, are linear and multidirectional. Slit-lamp examination may reveal a superior limbal micropannus and Herbert pits (i.e., hollowed-out areas in the superior limbus), which represent sites of resolved follicles.

Treatment of trachoma consists of topical tetracycline or erythromycin ointment instilled twice daily for 2 months and, more importantly, improved sanitation and hygiene to prevent recurrence.[205] Trachoma can be self-limited if hygiene alone is improved.[204] In patients who do not respond promptly to topical treatment or in those with severe disease, systemic antimicrobial agents should be instituted. For those older than 8 years, doxycycline should be administered orally daily for 40 days. Erythromycin can be substituted in younger children or in patients intolerant of doxycycline.

NEONATAL CONJUNCTIVITIS

Neonatal conjunctivitis, or ophthalmia neonatorum, is a common vision-threatening disorder throughout the world, although it has been relegated to a position of secondary importance in the industrialized world, where screening and prophylactic measures are widespread. It remains a significant cause of childhood ocular morbidity in developing countries.

Dilute topical silver nitrate solution instilled just after birth for prophylaxis against ophthalmia neonatorum was the first treatment used. It was responsible for reducing the prevalence of gonococcal ophthalmia neonatorum from 10 to 0.17 percent of live births in Europe.[205] A mild, self-limited chemical conjunctivitis is associated with the use of silver nitrate,[154] but it lasts 2 to 4 days and resolves with no treatment. Topical erythromycin largely has replaced silver nitrate in developed countries because it is effective without producing a chemical conjunctivitis.[94] In the developing world, regional conflicts, political instability, and burgeoning refugee populations often result in underuse of these simple prophylactic measures.[78,94]

Causes of neonatal conjunctivitis are highly variable among populations. In areas that use silver nitrate drops for prophylaxis, chemical conjunctivitis is the most common cause of neonatal conjunctivitis.[154] Infectious conjunctivitis occurs in 0.5 to 6.0 percent of live births in the United States. The leading infection is *C. trachomatis*.[15,99,185,205] Neonatal infection is caused by ocular exposure to contaminated maternal discharge during normal birth, although it may occur in infants born by cesarean section, especially if the membranes rupture prematurely. Other important infectious agents that may cause ophthalmia neonatorum are *N. gonorrhoeae* and *S. aureus*.[77,194] Bacteria that normally reside in the vaginal or gastrointestinal tract occasionally are implicated in ophthalmia neonatorum. Such bacteria include *Streptococcus* spp., *Haemophilus* spp., *Pseudomonas aeruginosa*, *Moraxella* spp., *Moraxella catarrhalis*, *N. meningitidis*, *E. coli*, and *Enterobacter cloacae*.[185,200]

Viruses occasionally produce neonatal conjunctivitis. Rarely, HSV may cause keratoconjunctivitis.[78] It is associated with distinctive vesicular skin changes and systemic signs, and the diagnosis seldom is in doubt.[9] Life-threatening HSV meningoencephalitis is a serious potential complication of HSV ophthalmia neonatorum.[152] Other viruses occasionally implicated include adenovirus, coxsackievirus A9, cytomegalovirus (CMV), and echovirus.[199]

Certain clinical features may help establish the specific etiologic diagnosis in cases of ophthalmia neonatorum (Table 68–1), but considerable overlap in findings exists, and physicians cannot rely on the history and physical examination alone to make a definitive diagnosis. Even when all appropriate investigative modalities are used, the cause may remain unknown in some cases.

Variations in the time of onset after birth, severity of inflammation, and character of the ocular discharge are common, and none is considered pathognomonic of a specific infectious process, but general considerations are worth reviewing.[185] Silver nitrate conjunctivitis typically begins during the first 48 hours of life and produces a watery discharge with mild inflammation. It is self-limited and resolves within 48 to 72 hours of its appearance.[154] *C. trachomatis* conjunctivitis generally begins 1 to 21 days after birth and usually is apparent by day 7. A moderately copious

mucopurulent discharge may be present but can be variable.[99,149] *S. aureus* conjunctivitis also begins during the first 3 weeks of life and can produce a moderately profuse mucopurulent discharge. Many other bacterial agents produce an overlapping clinical picture. Conjunctivitis caused by *N. gonorrhoeae* ordinarily begins somewhat earlier, usually by the third day of life, but it may appear as late as 3 weeks after birth. The hallmark is a copious, hyperpurulent discharge that can reaccumulate in a matter of minutes after it is removed. *N. gonorrhoeae* can penetrate an initially intact cornea and result in perforation of the eye and endophthalmitis.[96,187,199] Conjunctivitis caused by gastrointestinal flora often begins within a few days of birth and can produce a copious purulent discharge.

Viral neonatal conjunctivitis is a rare occurrence. HSV infection may begin during the first 3 weeks of life and usually produces a serous or serosanguineous discharge.[78,152] Other viruses have highly variable characteristics, but a serous discharge is a common finding.

The differential diagnosis of neonatal conjunctivitis includes congenital glaucoma, dacryostenosis with or without dacryocystitis, keratitis, and uveitis. Dacryostenosis is manifested as epiphora and a watery or purulent discharge. Occasionally, conjunctivitis may develop. Because epiphora caused by congenital dacryostenosis ordinarily is not seen until the second or third week of life, it rarely is a serious consideration. Newborns with congenital glaucoma often are photophobic and irritable.[222] They may exhibit increased tearing, conjunctival injection, and corneal edema. Both keratitis and uveitis most often are accompanied by photophobia and pain. The discharge with keratitis can vary but with bacterial causes is purulent. The discharge with uveitis, if present, is watery.

Laboratory testing is important in establishing a specific diagnosis and should include Gram and Giemsa stains, a chlamydial immunoassay, and cultures for aerobic and anaerobic bacteria. Cotton-tipped swabs should be used to obtain material for culture from the conjunctival fornices. Viral and chlamydial cultures and immunoassays can be considered but usually are unnecessary.[14,207] Gonococcal immunoassay and HSV immunochemical tests are available but not in widespread use.

The initial treatment of neonatal conjunctivitis depends on the suspected infectious agent. Broad-spectrum treatment should be considered if the diagnostic possibilities cannot be narrowed. Silver nitrate–induced conjunctivitis is self-limited and does not require treatment. *C. trachomatis* conjunctivitis is treated with tetracycline (1%) or erythromycin (0.5%) ointment four times daily for 3 weeks and with systemic erythromycin for 2 to 3 weeks to prevent or to treat chlamydial pneumonia. Sulfonamides can be used to treat chlamydial conjunctivitis if erythromycin is not tolerated. Topical antibiotics alone are insufficient for the treatment of neonatal *Chlamydia* infection.[87,95,99] Staphylococcal conjunctivitis can be treated with erythromycin ointment or a variety of other topical antimicrobial agents every 4 to 6 hours for 3 to 7 days. Appropriate systemic antibiotic treatment should be considered if the infection is particularly severe.[205]

N. gonorrhoeae infection requires systemic treatment in all cases. Aqueous penicillin G can be considered if resistant strains are unlikely. However, one dose of intramuscular ceftriaxone is the treatment of choice in the United States because it is effective against all *N. gonorrhoeae* strains.[92,171] Eyes should be irrigated with saline every hour until the discharge clears and then in reduced frequency as necessary to reduce the risk for development of corneal infection. This interval usually is 24 to 48 hours after the initiation of systemic treatment. Penicillin G drops are recommended by some ophthalmologists, but such drops do not appear to improve the overall prognosis or speed of recovery.

HSV neonatal conjunctivitis is treated with systemic acyclovir in appropriate doses for as long as 3 weeks.[78] Treatment should be instituted on an emergency basis because of the potential for

TABLE 68–1 Clinical Characteristics of Neonatal Conjunctivitis Caused by Various Agents

Agent	Day of Life at Onset	Discharge
Silver nitrate	1 (0-2)	Serous
Chlamydia trachomatis	7 (1-21)	Mucopurulent
Staphylococcus aureus	5 (1-21)	Mucopurulent
Neisseria gonorrhoeae	3 (0-21)	Purulent
Other bacteria	7 (1-21)	Mucopurulent
Herpes simplex virus	5 (0-21)	Serosanguineous
Other viruses	Not established	Probably serous

development of serious permanent neurologic sequelae and death if treatment is delayed. Topical ophthalmic vidarabine or trifluridine also should be applied to the eyes four times daily for 2 to 3 weeks.

Prevention of ophthalmia neonatorum is simple and requires only instillation of an antibiotic or antiseptic agent within the first hour after birth. Silver nitrate drops (1%), erythromycin ointment (0.5%), and tetracycline ointment (1%) have been effective treatment against *N. gonorrhoeae* and *C. trachomatis*.[95,205] A 5 percent solution of povidone-iodine also has been effective and economical in prophylaxis against a variety of agents, including gonococcal neonatal conjunctivitis. It may be particularly useful in developing countries.[110] As with other sexually transmitted diseases, neonatal conjunctivitis caused by *N. gonorrhoeae*, *C. trachomatis*, or HSV should be addressed according to standard public health policies, with reporting, investigation, and case identification as required by local law.

KERATITIS: CORNEAL INFECTION

The cornea, with its overlying tear film, is the major refracting component of the human eye. Keratitis means inflammation of the cornea. Any irregularity of the corneal surface or an opacity involving the central visual axis of the cornea may impair vision.

The cornea is composed of five distinct layers: epithelium, Bowman membrane, stroma, Descemet membrane, and endothelium. The epithelium is several layers thick and, when healthy, can regenerate without scarring after an insult. The Bowman membrane lies beneath the epithelium. It does not regenerate and, when injured, heals with a scar. The stroma, approximately 0.5 mm in thickness, is the thickest part of the cornea. It is composed of regularly arranged collagen fibrils embedded in a matrix of mucoproteins and glycoproteins. The arrangement of the fibrils is more regular in the posterior aspect of the stroma. Like the Bowman membrane, the stroma heals with scarring. The Descemet membrane is the basement membrane of the corneal endothelium. It can regenerate after an insult and does not opacify. The innermost layer, the endothelium, is derived from neuroectoderm. It consists of a single layer of cells that do not have significant regenerative capacity. The cornea is an avascular structure that is kept clear by virtue of the regular arrangement of collagen fibers in the stroma and by the pumping action of the endothelium, which keeps the stroma relatively dehydrated. The cornea will become edematous and opacify if the endothelium is significantly damaged or diseased.

The external corneal surface is protected from injury and exposure by the eyelids. Reflex tearing in response to mechanical irritation provides further protection. The blink response to threat and the antimicrobial properties of the normal tear film further protect the cornea from injury and infection.

Keratitis is a potentially vision-threatening condition that refers to inflammatory reactions and infectious processes of the cornea. Persons with keratitis usually have erythema of the perilimbal bulbar conjunctiva and eye pain. Additional complaints may include decreased vision and photophobia. The diagnosis of keratitis depends on the presence of a corneal epithelial or stromal infiltrate. The infiltrate can be extremely difficult to see in uncooperative infants and young children. Ideally, the patient is examined with a slit lamp; sometimes sedation is required for adequate examination of uncooperative children. Stains and cultures often are required to establish the diagnosis, and an ophthalmologist should be consulted promptly. Rarely, biopsy of the cornea is needed to obtain material for culture, and corneal transplantation is required occasionally to halt progression of an infection or to treat corneal perforation. Etiologic diagnosis is based on clinical findings and examination of stains and cultures.

ISOLATED EPITHELIAL KERATITIS

Keratitis can be classified further according to the layer of cornea involved. Most infections involve the epithelium or stroma. Isolated epithelial keratitis usually is caused by one of several viruses: HSV, varicella-zoster virus (VZV), adenovirus, EBV, and measles virus (rubeola). The first three organisms are discussed in an earlier section.

EBV causes HSV-like dendritic corneal epithelial lesions. Stromal disease also may occur. The lesions are self-limited and do not respond to antiviral therapy.[136] When measles involves the cornea, it usually does so in the context of transient epithelial infiltrates, which resolve without permanent sequelae.[117] In malnourished children with vitamin A deficiency, however, measles represents a serious threat to life and vision. Deep corneal ulcers may develop during the first few days of measles infection. Rapid progression culminating in corneal perforation and ultimate loss of the eye may occur.[20,75] Whether the ulcers are caused by direct measles virus infection, by the keratomalacia of vitamin A deficiency, or by some combination of these factors has been debated for some time. Measles immunization programs and vitamin A administration programs can reduce the prevalence of childhood blindness in developing nations significantly.

STROMAL KERATITIS

Syphilis and unique parasitic and viral infections can cause a nonsuppurative keratitis isolated to the corneal stroma. Congenital syphilis produces interstitial (stromal) keratitis in children, although the condition usually does not become apparent until late in the first decade of life. An indolent, peripheral corneal haze develops and slowly progresses centrally. Ghost vessels devoid of blood flow are seen in the corneal stroma on slit-lamp examination.[206] The condition is manifested as a bilateral inactive stromal process[190] in 80 percent of cases and is accompanied by iritis, iridocyclitis, or scleritis at some point in the course of the disease. When ocular syphilis is diagnosed, systemic infection is present by definition. The systemic disease should be treated according to accepted guidelines.

BACTERIAL KERATITIS

Bacterial keratitis (i.e., corneal ulcer) most often occurs after trauma that disrupts the normal integrity of the corneal epithelium. The trauma can be mild and occult, such as that caused by lens wear. *S. aureus*, *S. pneumoniae*, *P. aeruginosa*, and *Moraxella* spp. are the most common bacterial causes of severe necrotizing bacterial keratitis.[8,127,217] Other organisms, such as *S. epidermidis*, *Actinomyces* spp., viridans streptococci, and a variety of others, have been implicated in less severe cases.

Accurate identification of the offending organism facilitates treatment. A specimen is obtained by scraping the edge of the ulcer with a sterile platinum spatula. Smears should be fixed in 70 percent methanol, not by heat, and Gram stain for bacteria and acridine orange stain for fungi and *Acanthamoeba* are recommended. The yield of culture-positive cases is higher in laboratories skilled in handling corneal cultures. Material for culture should be inoculated onto fresh media such as blood and chocolate agar (aerobes and facultative anaerobes), Sabouraud agar (fungi), and thioglycolate broth (anaerobic bacteria). Thayer-Martin agar should be plated if *N. gonorrhoeae* is suspected. Initial treatment is based on the resulting stains (Table 68–2) and modified pending cultures (Table 68–3).[17,126]

Medical treatment of bacterial keratitis includes fourth-generation fluoroquinolones, fortified topical antibiotics, and, occasionally, subconjunctival antibiotic injection (see Table

TABLE 68–2   Treatment of Keratitis Based on Smear Morphology

Organism	Antibiotic	
	Ocular	Systemic*
Gram-positive cocci, gram-positive bacilli	Cefazolin[†]	Nafcillin, IV
Gram-positive filaments	Amikacin[‡]	Trimethoprim-sulfamethoxazole, IV
Gram-negative cocci	Ceftriaxone[†] or ciprofloxacin[‡,§]	Ceftriaxone, IV or IM
Gram-negative bacilli	Tobramycin[†]	Tobramycin, IV
Acid-fast bacilli	Amikacin[‡]	
Hyphal fragments	Natamycin,[‡] fluconazole[¶]	Fluconazole, PO
Yeasts	Amphotericin B,[‡] fluconazole[¶]	Fluconazole, PO
Cysts, trophozoites	Polyhexamethylene, biguanide,[‡] paromomycin,[‡] and propamidine isethionate[†]	Itraconazole, PO

*Standard age-appropriate milligram-per-kilogram dosages.
[†]Topical and periocular use only.
[‡]Topical use only.
[§]Use in children 12 years or older.
[¶]Periocular use only.
IM, intramuscularly; IV, intravenously; PO, orally.

TABLE 68–3   Treatment Based on Identification of Organisms

Organism	Antibiotic	
	Ocular	Systemic
Micrococcus, Staphylococcus (penicillin-resistant)	Cefazolin*	Nafcillin, IV
Micrococcus, Staphylococcus (methicillin-resistant)	Vancomycin*	Vancomycin, IV
Streptococcus	Penicillin G*	Penicillin G, IV
Enterococcus	Vancomycin* and gentamicin*	Vancomycin, IV, and gentamicin, IV
Anaerobic gram-positive coccus	Penicillin G*	Penicillin G, IV
Corynebacterium species	Penicillin G*	Penicillin G, IV
Mycobacterium fortuitum-chelonae	Amikacin[†]	Amikacin, IV,* or clarithromycin, PO
Nocardia	Amikacin[†]	Trimethoprim-sulfamethoxazole, IV
Neisseria gonorrhoeae	Ceftriaxone*	Ceftriaxone, IV or IM
Pseudomonas species	Ceftazidime,* Tobramycin*	Ceftazidime, IV or IM
Other aerobic, gram-negative bacilli	Ceftazidime* Tobramycin*	Ceftazidime, IV or IM
Filamentous fungi	Natamycin[†] Fluconazole[‡]	Fluconazole, PO
Candida species	Amphotericin B[†] Fluconazole[‡]	Fluconazole, PO
Acanthamoeba	Polyhexamethylene biguanide,[†] paromomycin,[†] and propamidine isethionate[†]	Itraconazole, PO

*Topical and periocular use.
[†]Topical use only.
[‡]Periocular use only.
IM, intramuscularly; IV, intravenously.

68–2).[38,156,205] Antibiotics are administered as often as every 15 to 30 minutes initially. Systemic antibiotics are required only for gonococcal, chlamydial, and onchocercal keratitis, as well as for actual or threatened perforation of the cornea, extension of infection to the sclera, or worsening of the process during topical or periocular treatment (or both). Topical steroids are useful if the resulting inflammation threatens to destroy the mechanical or optical integrity of the cornea, but steroids never are used as isolated treatment.[205]

FUNGAL KERATITIS

The most common causes of fungal keratitis include *Candida*, *Aspergillus*, and *Fusarium*. Mycotic keratitis associated with the filamentous fungi *Aspergillus* and *Fusarium* is thought to occur with trauma, whereas keratitis caused by *Candida* is associated more commonly with a preexisting ocular (e.g., dry eye) or systemic

(e.g., diabetes mellitus, immunosuppression) condition.[210] Fungal keratitis tends to be relatively indolent in comparison to bacterial keratitis. Typically, white stromal infiltrates with irregular and indistinct borders are detected. Satellite lesions, or those independent of the main lesion, may be evident. Mild concurrent iritis is a common finding. Severe iritis with hypopyon can occur but is an infrequent manifestation of fungal corneal disease.[157] Acridine orange stain is recommended, and culture on a Sabouraud agar plate is indicated. Hyphal fungi are treated with topical natamycin, topical fluconazole, systemic fluconazole, or some combination of these medications. Yeasts are treated with topical or systemic amphotericin B, fluconazole, or both agents.[76]

PROTOZOAN KERATITIS

Protozoan keratitis is a particularly serious vision-threatening process. It usually is caused by *Acanthamoeba* and occurs more frequently in wearers of soft contact lenses. Use of homemade saline solution is a significant risk factor and should be discouraged.[31] Amebae are ubiquitous organisms in soil, water, and air. They have been identified in hot tubs and in the feces of domestic animals.[134] People living in rural areas may be at special risk. *Acanthamoeba* keratitis also has been reported in children without a history of contact lens use or trauma.[53]

Acanthamoeba corneal ulcers are pleomorphic.[109] Older lesions may exhibit a ringlike infiltrate around a central ulcer. Iritis or iridocyclitis may be intense, and severe pain is a hallmark of the disease. Acridine orange and calcofluor white stains aid in establishing an early diagnosis of the condition. Tandem scanning confocal microscopy of corneal specimens may increase diagnostic accuracy, and the organism may grow on blood and chocolate agar.[31,131,133,138,166]

Treatment of *Acanthamoeba* keratitis is complex and suboptimal. Topical application of polyhexamethylene biguanide (0.02%),[123] chlorhexidine (0.02%), paromomycin (0.1%), or propamidine isethionate (Brolene) drops may be effective. Oral itraconazole (Sporanox) has been used successfully in adults.[127,131,138] Cycloplegic agents are recommended to improve the patient's comfort, and pain medications often are required. Corneal transplantation is needed if the infection progresses despite treatment, if perforation occurs, or if significant corneal opacification remains after the disease is eradicated.

Onchocerca volvulus is a filarial parasite that causes river blindness (i.e., onchocerciasis). The disease is endemic in sub-Saharan West Africa and in areas of Central and South America. The organism is transmitted by the bite of a blackfly of the family Simuliidae.[179] Larvae migrate to subcutaneous tissue and pass through several molts to become adult worms, which encapsulate in nodules and produce microfilariae that pass into blood, skin, and other organs, including the eyes. The conjunctiva, cornea, aqueous humor, vitreous, retina, uveal tract, sclera, and optic nerve all may be infested. Corneal involvement can lead to vision loss caused by corneal opacification, but most severe vision loss is caused by choroidal, retinal, and optic nerve disease.[93] Although children often are infected, blindness usually does not occur until they reach the third or fourth decade of life.[213,220]

Current treatment of onchocercal infection is administration of ivermectin every 6 to 12 months to all individuals living in endemic areas. Ivermectin kills the microfilariae but not the adult worms, which remain until their death.[209] The adult worm may live 10 or more years. Because of the long life span, ivermectin should be taken every 6 months for at least 10 years to treat microfilariae as they develop.

Microsporidia are intracellular protozoa that represent a new emerging ocular pathogen. Interest in the organism has increased in the last decade because of its association with HIV and acquired immunodeficiency syndrome (AIDS). The ocular manifestation corresponds to both the immune status of the patient and the genus of microsporidia involved.[115] Typically, keratoconjunctivitis occurs in immunocompromised individuals, and stromal keratitis is seen in immunocompetent individuals. Keratoconjunctivitis is manifested as bilateral conjunctival inflammation and epithelial keratopathy, which may lead to decreased vision. Stromal keratitis is manifested as an insidious diskiform keratitis with uveitis similar to that seen in HSV stromal keratitis and may require penetrating keratoplasty because of perforation or scarring.

Potassium hydroxide plus calcofluor white and acid-fast stains are thought to be the most efficient means of establishing the diagnosis of microsporidial keratitis.[114] Transmission electron microscopy provides specificity in identification of the genus and possibly the species, but it may lack sensitivity and is laborious.[115] Knowledge of the genus and species may help guide management. Albendazole, fumagillin, itraconazole, metronidazole, and topical propamidine isethionate have been used as therapeutic agents.[43,115]

INFECTIONS PRIMARILY INVOLVING THE UVEA

The uveal tract is the vascular middle coat of the eye. It is situated between the sclera and the retina. Its major function is to provide nourishment for intraocular tissues, including the retina, lens, and cornea. The uveal tract is composed of the iris, ciliary body, and choroid.

Uveitis is a nonspecific term for inflammation of the uvea. If the inflammatory process primarily affects the iris, it is called *iritis*. If the ciliary body is involved, the process is called *cyclitis*. If these two structures together are involved, the process is called *iridocyclitis* (i.e., anterior uveitis). The term *intermediate uveitis* (i.e., pars planitis) applies to inflammation in the region of the ciliary body and peripheral retina. The term *posterior uveitis* usually applies to combined inflammation of the retina and choroids, also called *chorioretinitis*. If the choroid alone is involved, it is called *choroiditis*; inflammation of the retina alone is called *retinitis*. Because of the thinness and close apposition of these two tissue layers, inflammation in one layer frequently "spills over" into the other. The vitreous body occupies the central area of the eye behind the lens. It is composed of water, mucopolysaccharides, and collagen. Though transparent in a normal, healthy eye, the vitreous is subject to inflammation or vitritis, usually as a result of inflammation in adjacent retinal tissue or in the pars plana.

Causes of uveitis are numerous but can be categorized into two main groups: infectious and noninfectious. Infectious causes are discussed in this chapter. Uveitis in any area of the eye may result in pain, conjunctival or episcleral hyperemia, photophobia, lacrimation, and decreased vision, although these symptoms vary relative to the site and the aggressiveness of the inflammation.

With slit-lamp examination, the hallmark of anterior uveitis is the finding of hazy, proteinaceous aqueous humor, called *flare*, and the presence of leukocytes in the anterior chamber. The cell and flare components are graded independently on a 1+ to 4+ scale. If present in sufficiently great numbers, leukocytes can precipitate in the anterior chamber (with location dependent on gravity) and form a mass called a *hypopyon*. The cells can aggregate on the back of the cornea and create fine, medium, and large lesions known as *keratic precipitates*. The conjunctiva usually is injected or hyperemic. With chronic inflammation, the border of the pupil often adheres to the anterior surface of the lens. Such adhesions are called *posterior synechiae* and may cause the pupil to have an irregular shape and size, as well as poor reactivity to light. Chronic or recurrent anterior segment inflammation may lead to the formation of a cataract. Iris nodules or atrophy may develop with long-standing inflammation. Anterior vitreous cells may occur as a spillover phenomenon in the setting of a prolonged or vigorous anterior chamber reaction. Although inflammatory effects on the ciliary body generally compromise its production of aqueous humor and thereby reduce intraocular pressure, cellular and proteinaceous debris can occlude aqueous humor outflow channels and lead to elevated intraocular pressure.

Inflammation primarily involving the posterior segment of the eye usually leads to decreased vision, which may be the symptom for which treatment initially is sought. Pain may be minimal or absent. Inflammatory lesions of the retina and choroid also may lead to the development of cellular debris in the vitreous and cause the patient to perceive "floaters." Initially, the borders of the retinal or choroidal inflammatory foci often are indistinct and cream-colored. In the healing phase, the borders of these lesions increasingly become distinct, and a defined, partially pigmented scar results. Inflammatory perivascular sheathing of the retinal vessels may occur as well. Involvement of the macula with edema or exudates may result from inflammation of the posterior segment, and long-standing edema may evolve into a cystic configuration and cause loss of central visual acuity. The optic nerve may exhibit an inflammatory response; if the optic disk is so involved, the response is called *papillitis*. Inflammatory debris also may be found in the vitreous.[4,159,233]

Under normal circumstances, the amount of immune traffic within the eye, especially in the anterior chamber, is held to a minimum by a group of immunomodulatory pathways that together form anterior chamber–associated immune deviation (ACAID). Chief among these deviations is active suppression of delayed hypersensitivity; distinctive ocular antigen-presenting cells migrate to the spleen, where they generate an immune response deficient in CD4+ cells but high in CD8+ cells. These regulatory T cells return to the eye to suppress the CD4+ populace, thereby minimizing the arm of inflammation most likely to impair visual clarity.[74,200]

EPIDEMIOLOGY

In the United States, most uveitis cases have noninfectious causes. Large samples demonstrate a predominance of anterior rather than posterior uveitis. The most common category of anterior uveitis is idiopathic; the most common infectious cause of anterior uveitis is herpetic kerato-uveitis (simplex and zoster). Posterior uveitis is caused most frequently by *Toxoplasma gondii*. In developing nations, infectious uveitis plays a larger role. In West Africa, *T. gondii* probably accounts for most cases of intraocular inflammation.[177,178]

VIRAL UVEITIS

Herpes Simplex Virus

Most of the uveal inflammation associated with HSV (typically iridocyclitis) results from the corneal disease. Occasionally, a patient will have iritis as an isolated finding, but most patients with ocular HSV demonstrate conjunctivitis, keratitis, chorioretinitis, or retinal vasculitis. The iritis may require treatment with topical steroids and topical antivirals as prophylaxis against the development of corneal epithelial disease.[216,233]

Varicella-Zoster Virus

Occasionally, varicella infection (i.e., chickenpox) may be associated with a transient iritis that requires no treatment. Though rare, cases of unifocal choroiditis causing visual loss but responsive to acyclovir in children with primary varicella have been reported.[146]

Herpes zoster virus may cause iridocyclitis during the acute stage of the disease; the anterior chamber reaction can persist or recur long after resolution of the cutaneous component of the condition. Herpes zoster always should be considered in the differential diagnosis of chronic unilateral iridocyclitis. Topical steroids are indicated for iritis, with the addition of oral or intravenous acyclovir for severe cases. Segmental iris atrophy is a characteristic sequela of herpes zoster uveitis. Glaucoma, hyphema, retinitis, vasculitis, and extraocular muscle palsy occasionally occur in patients with herpes zoster ophthalmicus. In a profoundly immunosuppressed patient, VZV can cause a devastating retinitis known as *progressive outer retinal necrosis*.[125]

VZV and HSV-2 have been implicated as causes of acute retinal necrosis syndrome. Patients in whom this syndrome is diagnosed range from 13 to 71 years of age, with an average age of 43 years. The syndrome typically occurs in healthy patients. The virus causes a triad of acute vitritis, retinal vasculitis, and peripheral necrotizing retinitis and is bilateral in 33 percent of patients. Treatment consists of intravenous acyclovir. Prophylactic laser photocoagulation may prevent retinal detachment. The visual prognosis is guarded.[22,125]

Epstein-Barr Virus

Ocular EBV involvement has been reported primarily in patients with infectious mononucleosis. Follicular conjunctivitis may be diagnosed in 2 to 40 percent of patients. Corneal stromal inflammation, iritis, episcleritis, optic neuritis, and chorioretinitis occur less commonly. Systemic corticosteroids and acyclovir may be useful in treating sight-threatening complications of chronic intraocular inflammation from EBV infection.[135] Postinfectious uveitis also has been described and is discussed later.

Enteroviruses

Coxsackievirus A24 and enterovirus 70 may cause a painful follicular conjunctivitis called acute hemorrhagic conjunctivitis. Rarely, chorioretinitis may be diagnosed. Treatment of these infections primarily is supportive.[159]

Rubella Virus

Rubella virus can cause congenital and acquired infections. Ocular manifestations of acquired rubella include conjunctivitis in 70 percent of patients, superficial keratitis, and iritis. Rarely, retinitis has been reported.

Congenital rubella syndrome can be manifested as cataracts, glaucoma, microphthalmos, and retinitis. Cataracts occur in 15 percent of patients and glaucoma in 10 percent. Retinal examination reveals a "salt-and-pepper fundus" caused by the alternating pattern of hypopigmentation and hyperpigmentation of the retinal pigment epithelium. The prognosis for patients with retinitis alone usually is good, with vision between 20/20 and 20/40. Glaucoma resulting from rubella commonly requires surgery, as do the cataracts. Iritis is reported less commonly.[23,135]

Mumps Virus

Ocular manifestations of mumps virus includes dacryoadenitis, conjunctivitis, iritis, optic neuritis, and keratitis. Retinitis also has been reported. The prognosis for visual recovery from the retinitis is good, and sequelae of the iritis are rare occurrences.[76,135]

Measles Virus

Measles virus can cause congenital and acquired infections. In congenital infections, a "salt-and-pepper" retinopathy and cataract formation may occur, similar to that found in rubella. Ocular manifestations in acquired measles include conjunctivitis and, much less commonly, retinitis, retinal vasculitis, and optic nerve edema.[12,159]

Subacute Sclerosing Panencephalitis

Between 30 and 75 percent of patients with subacute sclerosing panencephalitis (SSPE or Dawson inclusion body encephalitis) have ocular findings. SSPE is caused by a variant of the measles virus; it differs from the wild-type virus by alteration or absence of viral M protein. Optic nerve edema, inflammation, and subsequent optic atrophy have been reported. Macular retinitis is a common finding, and the contiguous non-neural tissues (vitreous and choroid) almost never are involved. The visual prognosis of survivors is poor.[155,159]

Creutzfeldt-Jakob Disease

The most common ocular manifestation of Creutzfeldt-Jakob disease is cortical blindness. Optic atrophy may result from degeneration of the neurons of the optic nerve.[159]

Human Immunodeficiency Virus and Acquired Immunodeficiency Syndrome

As many as 75 percent of patients with advanced AIDS have ocular findings. Cotton-wool spots occur in more than 50 percent of patients and are bilateral in more than 80 percent. Cotton-wool patches represent focal infarctions of the neural layer of the retina and are the most common ocular finding in patients with AIDS. They generally produce no symptoms and do not decrease vision. These spots are white and fluffy and occur most commonly in the macular portion of the retina. They resolve in 4 to 6 weeks with no residual scars. Occasionally, flame-shaped hemorrhages are detected as well. The retina and choroid in these patients may become infected with HSV, CMV, VZV, syphilis, tuberculosis, ocular histoplasmosis, *Candida*, toxoplasmosis and *Pneumocystis*, although in the highly active antiretroviral therapy (HAART) era, the incidence of CMV retinitis has declined and its advance in existing cases has been slowed or halted. Symptomatic anterior uveitis in the absence of the aforementioned pathogens occurs rarely in patients with AIDS and may be caused by HIV itself.[111]

Cytomegalovirus Infection

CMV infections may occur in preterm neonates and immunosuppressed patients, especially those with AIDS. In neonates with symptoms of CMV infection (i.e., low birth weight, microcephaly, jaundice, thrombocytopenia, hepatosplenomegaly, or petechial rash), congenital CMV infection[18] (i.e., prenatal transmission) may be manifested in the fundus as chorioretinal scars (21%) and optic atrophy (7%).[41]

CMV retinitis develops in approximately 30 percent of adult patients with AIDS, usually those with $CD4^+$ counts less than $50/mm^3$.[63] In the pediatric AIDS population, $CD4^+$ counts of less than $20/mm^3$ may be required for appearance of the retinitis.[64] The disease is less common in pediatric patients with AIDS. Patients with CMV retinitis have no external ocular signs but may complain of loss of vision. Children may not complain of such loss, and the problem may become apparent only after bilateral severe vision loss has occurred.[64] The retinal lesions of CMV typically are yellow-white and often are associated with hemorrhage. The retinitis generally follows a perivascular distribution. The retina becomes necrotic and eventually atrophies, with a gliotic scar. CMV optic neuritis also may develop. Treatment consists of intravenous or intravitreal ganciclovir, intravenous or intravitreal cidofovir, or intravenous foscarnet[64,233] and can often be discontinued when the $CD4^+$ count rises above $100/mm^3$.[212]

Parvovirus Infection

Bilateral panuveitis has been reported to be associated with parvovirus B19 infection.[130]

Human T-Cell Lymphotrophic Virus Infection

Human T-cell lymphotrophic virus (HTLV) is endemic in several regions of the globe: Japan, the Caribbean islands, and parts of central Africa. It probably is responsible for several cases of self-limited, occasionally recurrent uveitis in these regions.[153]

Lymphocytic Choriomeningitis Virus Infection

Lymphocytic choriomeningitis virus (LCMV) is an arenavirus endemic in mice; it is reported in hamsters as well and occasionally is transmitted to humans by direct contact with the rodent or through aerosolization of its feces or urine. Postnatal exposure results in asymptomatic seroconversion or aseptic meningitis, but intrauterine infection can have devastating consequences. Spontaneous abortion, congenital hydrocephalus, psychomotor retardation, and chorioretinitis have been documented. Diffuse chorioretinal scarring identified postnatally may bode a grim visual prognosis. LCMV may be an underdiagnosed cause of unexplained congenital chorioretinitis. The diagnosis is confirmed by elevated LCMV antibody titers. A survey of severely retarded, visually disabled children revealed immunologic evidence pointing to LCMV as the cause of the visual loss in approximately half of those surveyed.[140,143]

BACTERIAL UVEITIS

Syphilis

Syphilis (*Treponema pallidum*) should be considered as a possible cause in all cases of intraocular inflammation. Any patient with confirmed syphilitic uveitis should undergo a lumbar puncture to rule out asymptomatic neurosyphilis.

Ocular manifestations of congenital syphilis include interstitial keratitis, a mottled "salt-and-pepper" fundus, and chorioretinal scarring. Acute interstitial keratitis occurs as a late manifestation of congenital syphilis (5-25 years of age) and is thought to be a hypersensitivity response to treponemal antigen in the cornea. Patients complain of pain and photophobia and have a diffusely opaque cornea and anterior uveitis. Blood vessels invade the inflamed cornea and eventually are obliterated, with ghost vessels left in the corneal stroma. Glaucoma may occur. A unilateral manifestation of interstitial keratitis suggests postnatally acquired lues.

Secondary syphilis may involve any layer of the eye. Episcleritis, scleritis, iridocyclitis (acute, chronic, or recurrent), iris capillary dilation (i.e., iris roseata), vascular papules of the iris (i.e., iris papulosa), inflammatory nodules (i.e., iris nodosa), choroiditis, chorioretinitis, and retinal vasculitis all have been reported, as have optic neuritis and subsequent atrophy.

Tertiary syphilis may have associated gummata of the iris and an Argyll Robertson pupil (i.e., miotic, irregularly shaped pupil with loss of response to light but preservation of the near response). Intraocular inflammation seldom occurs at this stage.

Ocular inflammation secondary to syphilis should be treated as neurosyphilis. With the appropriate doses of penicillin G, the inflammation typically resolves rapidly. Occasionally, topical regional steroids are required to control local inflammation. Treatment of ocular syphilis may lead, at least initially, to a vigorous local and systemic self-limited, febrile response, presumably caused by liberation of spirochetal antigens or toxins. Topical oral corticosteroids may be required to quell this response, which is also known as a *Jarisch-Herxheimer reaction*.[4,132,159]

Lyme Disease

A mild follicular conjunctivitis occurs in 11 percent of patients with stage 1 Lyme disease, caused by *Borrelia burgdorferi*. During the second and third stages, neuro-ophthalmic manifestations, including cranial neuropathy (most often cranial nerves III, IV, VI, and VII), optic neuritis, bilateral keratitis, bilateral iridocyclitis, diffuse choroiditis, vasculitis, intermediate uveitis, and Parinaud oculoglandular syndrome, may be seen. The most frequent manifestation of late Lyme disease is arthritis. Ocular inflammation occurs in approximately 4 percent of children with Lyme arthritis.[108] Early, localized Lyme disease may be treated with doxycycline (8 years and older) or amoxicillin. More advanced or persistent disease is treated best with intravenous ceftriaxone.[6] Antibiotic treatment early in the course of the disease carries a better prognosis than does therapy initiated at later stages.[19]

Leptospirosis

Leptospirosis may cause an anterior uveitis that occurs months after the acute infection. Leptospirosis is identified as an important cause of epidemic panuveitis in southern India; the most common posterior segment manifestations in this group are vasculitis and vitritis.[39]

Tuberculosis

Any structure of the eye may be affected by tuberculosis. Allergic and infectious processes have been implicated as important causes of tuberculous uveitis. Anterior uveitis with or without keratitis has been attributed to tuberculosis. Choroiditis, optic neuritis, and orbital infections have been detected in cases of miliary tuberculosis. The most frequent manifestations of ocular tuberculosis are choroidal nodules and scars; anterior uveitis is an uncommon occurrence.[26] Treatment should be undertaken with the appropriate antituberculous medications. Corticosteroids often are necessary in conjunction with antimicrobial therapy.

Leprosy

Because *Mycobacterium leprae*, the cause of leprosy, grows best at lower temperatures, corneal infections predominate. Corneal involvement is associated with prominence of the corneal nerves, interstitial keratitis, and corneal hypoesthesia, but corneal opacities are often peripheral and not visually significant.[49] Uveal involvement in leprosy frequently is silent and accounts for a large number of the ocular complications from the disease.[48,49]

Brucella Infection

Ocular manifestations of *Brucella* infection are rare but include iritis, focal nodular choroiditis, and panophthalmitis.[159]

Cat-Scratch Disease

Bartonella henselae is a gram-negative rod transmitted to humans by the bite or scratch of an infected animal, often a young cat or kitten. Regional lymphadenopathy is the predominant nonocular finding. A striking stellate neuroretinitis characterized by swelling of the optic nerves and lipid deposition in the retina is the most easily identifiable complication of ocular infection. Other manifestations include intermediate uveitis, optic disk swelling, multifocal choroiditis, and serous macular detachment. The discrete foci of multifocal choroiditis are the most common findings in the posterior segment. The role of antibiotics in this condition is debated.[119,195]

FUNGAL UVEITIS

Histoplasmosis

The diagnosis of presumed ocular histoplasmosis syndrome is based on the clinical picture of disseminated punched-out retinal "histo spots," atrophic retinal changes around the optic nerve, and a clear vitreous.[168] Later in the course of the disease, subretinal hemorrhage and retinal detachment may occur. Ocular histoplasmosis often is bilateral and can result in legal blindness from the loss of macular vision. Presumed ocular histoplasmosis syndrome may occur after an episode of benign systemic histoplasmosis during childhood. Active inflammation and vitreous cells usually are not seen in this syndrome, although case series have documented active chorioretinal inflammation as new-onset lesions and as reactivation of previously quiescent lesions.[36,116] The hallmark histoplasmosis spots appear as white, punched-out, well-demarcated chorioretinal scars and represent healed fungal lesions. Generally, they first appear during adolescence, do not reduce vision, and do not require treatment. Macular disease, which may reduce vision, does not develop until after the patient reaches the second decade of life. Subretinal neovascularization may develop at the site of a macular histoplasmosis spot, with fluid, blood, and lipid accumulating in the subretinal space. This process plus local scarring can result in a marked reduction in central vision.

Macular neovascularization may be treated suitably with laser photocoagulation in an attempt to salvage the remaining central vision. Antifungal drugs may play a role in the unusual setting of demonstrated active histoplasmosis choroiditis.[184]

Candidiasis

Candida spp., including *C. albicans*, are fungi with yeast and filamentous forms. Candidiasis is encountered in immunocompromised patients and in situations involving indwelling catheters, intravenous therapy, chronic antibiotic use, poorly controlled diabetes, and intravenous drug abuse. Candidal chorioretinitis can develop in approximately 9 percent of patients with blood cultures positive for the fungus,[60] although more recent studies have demonstrated that ocular involvement (either chorioretinitis or endophthalmitis) in children is a rare occurrence.[61]

In the eye, *Candida* infection usually begins in the choroid and eventually causes multifocal white chorioretinal lesions. If the fungus proliferates unchecked, it may break through the retina into the vitreous and produce the classic, white, snowball-like "fungus ball." Candidal infection that progresses to endophthalmitis is exceedingly rare if appropriate intravenous antifungals are started promptly on notice of a positive blood culture.

Intravenous amphotericin B is the drug of choice. Other antifungal agents such as fluconazole, flucytosine, and miconazole also may be effective, but none is dramatically so. Surgical treatment of intraocular *Candida* disease is discussed in the section on endophthalmitis.

Aspergillosis

Aspergillus spp. can infect the choroid, retina, and vitreous of immunocompromised individuals. One group of investigators found a high rate (7%) of these unusual infections on reviewing records of deceased liver transplant recipients.[107]

Coccidioidomycosis

Coccidioides spp. have yeast and filamentous forms. Ocular disease consists of a multifocal chorioretinitis that develops during the course of systemic coccidioidomycosis. The lesions initially appear similar to those seen in histoplasmosis; in severe cases, endophthalmitis results, and vitrectomy may need to be performed. In less severe cases, the lesions may respond to intravenous amphotericin B. Occasionally, an isolated granulomatous iridocyclitis may develop.[147]

Cryptococcosis

Cryptococcus neoformans is a yeast-like fungus that can cause multifocal chorioretinitis and endophthalmitis. Most patients with cryptococcosis are severely immunocompromised; many have AIDS. The CNS and eye are involved commonly, and elevated intracranial pressure may cause papilledema and sixth cranial nerve palsy. Intravenous amphotericin B in combination with oral flucytosine is the treatment regimen of choice.[6,120]

Sporotrichosis

The dimorphic fungus *Sporothrix schenckii* is encountered commonly in rotting vegetable matter, wood, and soil. The fungus gains access to the host by traumatic implantation or inhalation. It has been reported to be responsible for anterior uveitis in the setting of a suggestive lesion on a finger of the dominant hand, with presumed hand-to-eye transmission.[219]

PROTOZOAL UVEITIS

Leishmaniasis

Ocular leishmaniasis has been described. Manifestations include conjunctivitis, blepharitis, and anterior uveitis. This trio of findings responds to systemic treatment with sodium stibogluconate.[68]

HELMINTHIC UVEITIS

Toxocariasis

Toxocara canis causes visceral larva migrans, which is not associated with ocular disease. In the retina, larvae get trapped in small capillaries and burrow into surrounding tissue; the dead larvae incite an intense eosinophilic abscess. Ocular toxocariasis has three classic clinical manifestations, almost always involving one eye only. One form occurs in children 2 to 9 years of age and causes an indolent endophthalmitis and leukokoria (i.e., white pupil). Tractional retinal detachment may occur. The eye typically shows little or no external evidence of inflammation, and the patient experiences no pain.

A second form appears in children between 4 and 14 years of age. These patients have reduced vision but little or no external inflammation and no pain. The reduced vision may cause strabismus, which may be the first sign. An inflammatory granuloma is seen in the macula.

The third form of ocular toxocariasis occurs in patients between 6 and 40 years of age but may not be recognized until years later. Patients with this form of toxocariasis have good vision, but a peripheral retinal granuloma is seen on routine eye examination. Vision may be affected if a traction band from the granuloma distorts the macula.

Inactive *Toxocara* granulomata do not respond to medication. When active intraocular inflammation exists in such a magnitude that it poses a further threat to vision, administration of periocular or systemic steroids may be necessary. Anthelmintic agents eradicate migrating larvae, but their effect on "residing" larvae is questionable. When giving antihelmintics, one should combine them with a short course of corticosteroids because death of the larvae may incite vigorous inflammation. Cryotherapy and laser therapy may be useful when the *Toxocara* granuloma is located away from the macula and optic nerve. Vitrectomy may be helpful if significant traction on the retina occurs. Antihelmintic drugs should not be administered after the patient has undergone posterior segment surgery. Visual prognosis is poor if the macula is involved.[159,186,191,229]

Onchocerciasis

Onchocerciasis often causes a severe choroiditis with an overlying retinitis. The various ocular manifestations of infestation with *O. volvulus* are discussed in the section on keratitis.

Loiasis

The *Loa loa* worm can migrate through the tissues of the eye and cause conjunctivitis, iridocyclitis, vitritis, and chorioretinitis. The disease is transmitted by the bite of a mango fly. Vascular obstruction with intraretinal hemorrhage and retinal exudation may occur as well. Medical treatment with diethylcarbamazine can kill the adult worms and microfilariae. Adult worms also can be removed from the eye surgically.[159]

Cysticercosis

The tapeworm *Taenia solium* causes cysticercosis. When the larva gains access to the eye, cysts form in the vitreous or subretinal space in 13 to 46 percent of patients. The living worm may be seen undulating in these spaces. With death of the organism, severe panuveitis can occur. Orbital and subconjunctival involvement occurs less commonly. Surgical removal of the intraocular cysts may prevent the severe inflammation that occurs on death of the worm. Praziquantel can kill the organism, but the ensuing increase in inflammation may be dramatic.[159]

UVEITIS CAUSED BY INSECT-INDUCED DISEASE

Ophthalmomyiasis is the ocular disorder caused by infestation with fly larvae, most commonly the larval form of the sheep botfly *Oestrus ovis*. Maggots may be seen in the conjunctival fornix (cul-de-sac) or inside the eye. Internal ophthalmomyiasis can be diagnosed by noting a motile larva in the anterior chamber, vitreous, or subretinal space. The maggot may leave trails ("railroad tracks") behind throughout the retina. A mild inflammatory response in the anterior chamber (e.g., iritis, iridocyclitis) or vitreous may occur. Treatment is surgical removal of the larva. Corticosteroids may be used to treat the accompanying intraocular inflammation.[65,159]

POSTINFECTIOUS UVEITIS

Increasingly, attention is being given to the role of bacterial and viral systemic illness in the eventual development of sterile intraocular inflammation. This type of uveitis is thought to be caused by an autoimmune response that occurs between sensitized lymphocytes and host tissues that bear some antigenic similarity to the recently cleared pathogen. Disruption of the ACAID is probably a prerequisite for the development of these postinfectious syndromes. Several reports exist of nongranulomatous anterior uveitis occurring weeks or months after streptococcal infection. These uveitides may be associated with other poststreptococcal findings (e.g., arthritis, glomerulonephritis) or may be the sole manifestation. Treatment with cycloplegics and topical corticosteroids is sufficient for the ocular manifestations.[16,215,231]

Uveitis, predominantly of the anterior type, has been reported to occur after illnesses caused by gram-negative enteric bacteria such as *Klebsiella*, *Salmonella*, and *Yersinia*. These gram-negative–induced uveitides are much more likely to occur in the setting of HLA-B27 positivity. The ocular findings often parallel the development of arthritis, thus suggesting that parallel immunologic processes are occurring in both these mesenchymal cavities (i.e., the joint space and the anterior chamber). An association between recent EBV infection and acute tubulointerstitial nephritis and anterior uveitis has been described, with onset of the renal and ocular inflammation occurring several months after the characteristic acute EBV infection.[90]

INFECTIONS INVOLVING PRIMARILY THE RETINA

EYE MANIFESTATIONS OF INTRAUTERINE INFECTIONS (TORCHS COMPLEX)

The TORCHS complex is a group of congenital and perinatal infections that may cause severe systemic and ophthalmic abnormalities. The effect of infection with one of the TORCHS organisms—*T. gondii*, others (LCMV, EBV), rubella virus, CMV, herpesvirus, and syphilis—may be evident at birth or be manifest later in childhood or adulthood. Congenital EBV infection (infectious mononucleosis) has been reported to be associated, possibly, with congenital cataracts.[85] All these infections commonly cause either mild or no clinically evident disease in the mother.[141] The diagnosis cannot always be established on clinical grounds alone, and neonatal and maternal serologic tests must be performed to confirm the clinical suspicion.

Toxoplasmosis

T. gondii is an obligate intracellular parasite that has an affinity for the CNS and retina. The parasite has three forms: tachyzoite, bradyzoite, and sporozoite or oocyst. Human infection may be congenital or acquired. Acquired infection results from the ingestion of undercooked meat contaminated with oocysts or from exposure to the feces of an infected cat, the definitive host. The oocysts release tachyzoites, which multiply intracellularly and result in cell death. In adults, primary acquired infection usually is asymptomatic. The immune response then transforms the tachyzoite into a bradyzoite, which encysts and remains dormant in tissues for years. These cysts have the propensity to rupture sometime later and cause an inflammatory response resulting in recurrent infection.

Congenital infection is transmitted through the transplacental route. In the United States, the reported incidence of congenital toxoplasmosis is one case per 1000 to 10,000 births.[9,47] Seventy percent of the obstetric population is negative for antibodies and, therefore, at risk for infection and transplacental transmission to the fetus.[141] Congenital infection is most severe when acquired in the first trimester and can result in chorioretinitis, intracranial calcifications, microcephaly, mental retardation, and deafness.[47,71,73] Symptomatic neonates with disseminated disease have hepatosplenomegaly, lymphadenopathy, jaundice, fever, anemia, pneumonitis, and a poor prognosis. Other ocular manifestations include cataracts, strabismus, microcornea, vitritis, retinal detachment, optic atrophy, microphthalmos, nystagmus, and ptosis.[141] In a prospective study, 15 percent of infected newborns had chorioretinal scars, indicative of infection in utero; 4 percent had active chorioretinitis; and, in 10 percent, retinal lesions developed by the time that the children were 1 to 2 years of age. Long-term follow-up studies have found that chorioretinal lesions develop in 82 to 85 percent of children with subclinical *Toxoplasma* infection, some with severe visual loss. Infants with asymptomatic toxoplasmosis should undergo regular ophthalmologic examination because retinal involvement can occur later in childhood or adulthood.[27,71,121] Some researchers have suggested that all neonates with toxoplasmosis should receive drug therapy, even if they are asymptomatic.[71]

Toxoplasmosis is the leading cause of acquired necrotizing retinitis and, in many cases, represents reactivation of congenitally acquired infection. Clinically, an area of active retinochoroiditis is adjacent to the border of a chorioretinal scar.[73,174] Associated choroiditis and vitritis may be present. Primary acquired ocular toxoplasmosis manifested as retinochoroiditis is well-documented also, and reports suggest that this route of infection may be more common than originally thought.[27,105]

Recurrent ocular disease with postnatally acquired toxoplasmosis has been reported.[25]

T. gondii causes a focal necrotizing retinitis with secondary choroiditis and vitritis. Patients may have floaters, blurred vision, and photophobia. Those with macular involvement can suffer significant visual loss. After the inflammation has resolved, a flat, pigmented chorioretinal scar develops. Visual loss depends on the location of the retinal lesion, with peripheral lesions resulting in little or no visual disturbance and macular lesions capable of producing profound visual loss.

Toxoplasma retinochoroiditis is an emerging problem in patients with AIDS and may be the initial manifestation of this syndrome.[225] The clinical appearance often is atypical.[193] Chronic suppressive therapy is necessary because infection recurs with discontinuation of treatment. A combination of pyrimethamine and clindamycin has been reported to be most effective as prophylaxis.[225]

The diagnosis of *Toxoplasma* retinochoroiditis usually is presumptive and is based on clinical appearance and serologic testing. Several serologic tests are available. The standard serologic diagnosis is based on the presence of anti-*Toxoplasma* IgM in any sample or demonstration of a significant rise in antibody titer in paired sera taken 4 to 6 weeks apart. However, in reactivated congenital infections, which many cases are, *Toxoplasma* IgM results are not positive. The antibody tests most commonly used are indirect immunofluorescent assay (IFA) and enzyme-linked immunosorbent assay (ELISA) for IgM and IgA.[85] False-positive results can occur with both tests in the presence of rheumatoid factor. If clinical infection is suspected and the initial testing results are negative, repeat testing or an alternative testing technique should be considered.

Standard treatment of *Toxoplasma* retinochoroiditis is triple therapy with sulfadiazine (100 to 200 mg/kg/day in four divided doses [maximum, 1.5 g]), pyrimethamine (2 mg/kg/day for 3 days, then 1 mg/kg/day [maximum, 25 mg/day]), and leucovorin (folinic acid) (10 to 25 mg given orally daily for 6 weeks). Folinic acid prevents the leukopenia and thrombocytopenia that may result from pyrimethamine therapy. Weekly complete blood counts and platelet counts are required to monitor toxicity from therapy. Alternative therapy with clindamycin (40 mg/kg/day in four divided doses [maximum, 2.4 g] for 6 weeks) rather than sulfadiazine also has been effective.[208] This therapy is less toxic than is triple therapy and, therefore, is better tolerated. In patients with severe intraocular inflammation, systemic corticosteroids can be used with concurrent antimicrobial therapy.

Preventive measures are twofold: first, avoidance of raw meat and cat feces during pregnancy, especially during the first trimester, and second, treatment of a mother known to have contracted the disease during pregnancy with spiramycin because it has no known teratogenic effects.[45,55,56] In utero pyrimethamine and sulfadiazine treatment of a fetus known to be infected may be effective.[45,47,102]

Lymphocytic Choriomeningitis Infection

LCMV, an arenavirus discovered in 1933, was recognized as a cause of intrauterine infection in 1955 (also see the earlier section "Viral Uveitis").[142] The common house mouse *Mus musculus* is the natural host and reservoir of the virus, but laboratory mice and pet hamsters also may be infected.[7,101] LCMV may be transmitted to humans by airborne means, rodent bites, or food contaminated by rodent urine, feces, or saliva; the fetus may be infected by transplacental transmission.[85] The diagnosis may be confirmed by LCMV titers.

Systemic manifestations, often devastating, include hydrocephaly, microcephaly, periventricular calcifications, neonatal meningitis, hepatosplenomegaly, cerebral palsy, mental retardation, and seizures.[85] Ocular findings include chorioretinitis, optic atrophy, nystagmus, microphthalmos, strabismus, and cataracts[142]; the chorioretinitis may mimic congenital toxoplasmosis.[28] The most common ocular findings are peripheral chorioretinal scars, although macular involvement is a common occurrence as well. At present there is no effective treatment. Prevention involves avoidance of mice and hamsters by pregnant women.[85,142]

Rubella Infection

The rubella virion is an RNA virus of the family *Togaviridae* that causes a febrile exanthem. Before the advent of rubella vaccine in 1969, rubella, or "German measles," epidemics occurred every 6 to 9 years. The last major outbreak in the United States took place in 1964.[11] With preschool immunization programs, most primary cases now reported occur in individuals between 15 and 24 years of age. Transmission occurs by inhalation of aerosolized droplets in the nasopharynx. Primary infection in adults results in a mild febrile illness associated with lymphadenopathy and a rash. The proportion of susceptible nonimmunized women of child-bearing age ranges from 10 to 25 percent. Fetal infection occurs transplacentally, and the likelihood of transmission from mother to fetus is highest (90%) in the first trimester; transmission at this stage can produce severe fetal damage and result in spontaneous abortion, stillbirth, or multiple congenital anomalies.

The classic congenital rubella syndrome, first described by Sir Norman McAlister in Australia in 1949,[142] is characterized by cardiac defects, ocular abnormalities, and hearing deficits. The incidence of ocular and cardiac defects is higher with exposure early in the first trimester; hearing deficits appear to be associated with exposure late in the first trimester. Givens and associates[84] reported that 88 percent had multiorgan involvement. Hearing loss is the most frequent nonocular manifestation.[142] The most common cardiac defects are patent ductus arteriosus, pulmonary artery stenosis, and pulmonary valve stenosis. Other features include microcephaly, thrombocytopenia, hepatosplenomegaly, and mental retardation.

Ocular involvement occurs in approximately 50 percent of infected infants.[81] Pigmentary retinopathy (i.e., "salt-and-pepper" retinopathy) affects 22 percent of infected infants. The retina has a mottled appearance, most frequently observed in the posterior pole; the optic nerve and vessels usually are normal unless the patient also has glaucoma.

Nuclear cataracts, which affect between 15 and 27 percent of patients, are the second most frequent ocular complication. Glaucoma is seen in approximately 10 percent of eyes; the combination of cataracts and glaucoma is an uncommon finding. Microphthalmos (which occurs in 10-63% of affected individuals), iris atrophy, and iritis also have been reported.[23] Live virus may persist for years in the lens, so appropriate precautions must be taken during cataract surgery to prevent transmission.[85]

The retinopathy associated with rubella usually is asymptomatic and does not necessitate treatment. In some cases, it can be complicated by subretinal neovascularization, which may require laser or macular surgery. Cataracts cause most visual morbidity. Visual rehabilitation depends on early cataract extraction to prevent deprivation amblyopia, correction of aphakia with spectacles or contact lenses, and careful follow-up. Glaucoma in infants and children can be temporized with topical medications, but most cases require glaucoma surgery.

Congenital rubella has long-term consequences for all organs involved. In nearly two thirds of infants with no manifestations at birth, hearing loss or psychomotor deficits subsequently develop. From an ophthalmic standpoint, individuals with congenital rubella need continued follow-up.[84]

Cytomegalovirus Infection

CMV is an enveloped DNA virus of the family *Herpesviridae*. An estimated 80 percent of adults are infected by the time that they reach 40 years of age.[196] In immunocompetent adults, infection is asymptomatic or can cause a mononucleosis syndrome. Individuals can shed virus in saliva, urine, and other body fluids for months to years after initial infection. Transmission occurs through exposure to body fluids, sexual contact, blood transfusion, or organ transplantation, or it can occur transplacentally. Primary infection acquired in the birth canal is not likely to result in serious disease.

Congenital CMV is the most common congenital infection in humans[197] and can result from exposure to the virus in utero or in the birth canal. In utero infection produces more serious disease. CMV infection occurs in 1 percent of all live births, and only 5 to 10 percent of infants with congenital CMV infection are symptomatic. Maternal infection may be primary or recurrent, but primary infection carries the greatest risk (30-40%) for transmission of symptomatic CMV disease to the newborn.[196] Blood transfusions from CMV antibody–positive donors also can result in severe CMV infection in the newborn. Systemic manifestations include intrauterine growth retardation (IUGR), thrombocytopenic purpura, microcephaly with periventricular calcifications, hepatosplenomegaly, pneumonia, and sensorineural deafness.[54]

In symptomatic congenital CMV infection, the retina is the primary site of ocular involvement. Cytomegalic inclusion bodies are seen in all layers of the retina. Patchy white areas of necrotic retina with hemorrhage and vascular sheathing are seen in the peripheral portion of the retina, although the posterior pole can be affected as well.[128] Nonhemorrhagic retinitis also may be seen, and most affected infants do not have active retinitis at birth, although scars may be visible as evidence of previous disease.[41] Resolution of the retinitis results in an atrophic scar with areas of hyperpigmentation. If retinitis involves the retinal periphery, vision may be normal. However, visual loss may occur if the posterior pole is involved or if optic atrophy or retinal detachment occurs. CMV retinopathy develops in 5 to 30 percent of infants with clinically apparent disease.[66] Microphthalmos, optic nerve hypoplasia, optic atrophy, optic nerve colobomata, anophthalmia, corneal opacities, and anterior segment dysgenesis also have been associated with congenital CMV infection.[103] In addition, cyclopia and anophthalmia have been reported.[33]

The diagnosis of CMV retinitis is based on the clinical appearance and the constellation of systemic symptoms and signs. Recovery of the virus from urine, maternal cervical secretions, saliva, or aqueous humor can confirm the diagnosis. Complement fixation can identify IgM antibodies to CMV that do not cross-react with other herpesviruses. Immunofluorescence techniques are more sensitive but less specific than is complement fixation.[128]

Treatment of neonatal or pediatric CMV retinitis is based on the results of treatment of adults with CMV retinitis. Ganciclovir has been shown to stabilize and prevent spread of the disease in infants. Maintenance therapy is not required, but continued follow-up is necessary to detect recurrence. Granulocytopenia and thrombocytopenia can result. Retinal detachment requires vitrectomy, membrane peel, and silicone oil to tamponade the detached retina.[104]

Herpes Simplex Virus Infection

HSV is a double-stranded enveloped DNA virus. Both subtypes, HSV-1 and HSV-2, can cause a vesicular skin eruption. HSV-1 typically is isolated from oral-facial infections; HSV-2 usually is isolated from genital infections. After primary infection occurs, HSV can maintain latency in neuronal ganglion cells and reactivate. Transmission occurs by exposure to infected body fluids such as saliva, and the risk of transmission is higher when the individual is symptomatic.[152]

Maternal-fetal transmission occurs through infected genital secretions in the birth canal (HSV-2) or exposure to infected individuals with oral-facial herpetic disease (HSV-1) in the postnatal period. In mothers with active genital disease, the risk of transmission to the neonate is 50 percent with vaginal delivery. Most series report that between 70 and 80 percent of neonatal HSV infection is caused by HSV-2. Neonatal HSV infection is life-threatening, and the mortality rate without treatment is 80 percent.[227] The diagnosis is suspected by the clinical findings: lethargy, respiratory distress, anorexia, vomiting, cyanosis, low birth weight, IUGR, microcephaly, seizures, intracranial calcifications, pneumonia, hepatosplenomegaly, and skin vesicles. The virus may be isolated from skin vesicles or from nasal or conjunctival secretions, CSF, or blood. The mortality rate of untreated neonatal HSV is 49 percent.[85]

Ocular sequelae develop in less than 1 percent of immunocompetent adults with HSV infection. In contrast, 17 to 40 percent of infected neonates have ocular disease.[135,196] Thirteen percent of neonates with HSV have eye involvement. Ocular involvement can range from mild conjunctivitis to severe bilateral necrotizing retinitis and may be unilateral or bilateral. Conjunctivitis is the most common manifestation. Conjunctivitis, keratitis, and, occasionally, retinitis develop 2 to 14 days after birth. HSV retinitis causes punctate, white-yellow lesions in the periphery and the posterior pole accompanied by choroiditis, vascular sheathing, hemorrhage, and vitritis. Chorioretinal atrophic scars with variable amounts of pigmentation around the border result after resolution of acute infection.[106,173] Visual prognosis depends on the severity of disease, macular scarring, optic atrophy, or CNS involvement of the visual pathways. Severe chorioretinitis and cortical blindness are the usual sequelae of HSV infection acquired through transplantation, a rare mode of transmission.

El Azazi and colleagues[67] examined children with serologically proven HSV infection 1 to 15 years after neonatal exposure and found a higher prevalence of chorioretinal scars than noted in previous reports (28% versus 4%). This finding suggests that HSV remains dormant in the retina and reactivates later in childhood or adulthood. Chorioretinitis, cataracts, optic atrophy, and microphthalmos have been reported.[91] Acute retinal necrosis from reactivation of HSV-2 has occurred as well.[211]

Ocular HSV infection can be seen in conjunction with a vesicular rash or disseminated disease. The differential diagnosis of ophthalmic complications from HSV includes infection with any of the TORCHS organisms. Identification of neonatal IgM antibody to HSV confirms the diagnosis of in utero infection. Demonstration of intranuclear inclusions and multinucleated giant cells in skin, conjunctiva, and oral and genital lesions may be diagnostic.

The drug of choice to treat neonatal HSV infection is intravenous acyclovir, 30 to 60 mg/kg/day.[165] Conjunctival and corneal disease also can be treated by débridement and topical antivirals such as vidarabine. In neonatal HSV infection, systemic acyclovir should be given regardless of topical treatment. Early diagnosis and treatment can reduce ocular morbidity.

Varicella-Zoster Virus Infection

VZV is a DNA virus of the family *Herpesviridae*; enveloped virions are the infectious agents. Primary infection results in chickenpox, a highly communicable febrile illness with a vesicular rash that appears after 48 to 72 hours of incubation. VZV can remain dormant in sensory ganglion neurons and reactivate as herpes zoster, a painful rash in the dermatomal distribution of the sensory ganglion.

Congenital varicella syndrome is considered a rare entity. One prospective series reported a 24 percent incidence of congenital

varicella with serologic or clinical confirmation of maternal infection during pregnancy. Mortality rates can be high if maternal infection develops 5 days before delivery to 2 days after delivery. Systemic complications of VZV infection include cranial nerve palsy, hemiparesis, cicatricial skin lesions, IUGR, developmental delay, seizures, neurogenic bladder, and learning difficulty.[122,162]

Ocular abnormalities in children with congenital VZV infection include chorioretinitis, cataracts, Horner syndrome, optic atrophy and optic nerve hypoplasia, retinal coloboma, and microphthalmos. The chorioretinal scars of VZV infection have a deeply pigmented center with depigmented borders or a gliotic white center with hyperpigmented edges. The neurotropic nature of VZV infection may explain the association of Horner syndrome. Ocular involvement can be unilateral or bilateral. VZV chorioretinitis affects the macula, periphery, or both.

Serologic testing for IgG and IgM antibodies to VZV, a history of maternal infection during pregnancy, and the constellation of systemic findings help establish the diagnosis. Because active infection may occur early in pregnancy, the neonate may have IgG but no detectable IgM antibodies to VZV by the time of delivery. The persistence of elevated IgG antibodies beyond 6 months, when passive immunity through maternal antibodies has waned, without evidence of primary VZV infection postnatally is a helpful indication of infection in utero.

Syphilis

Syphilis is caused by the spirochete *T. pallidum*. Acquired syphilis is a sexually transmitted chronic disease and has three stages of infection. Primary infection is characterized by painless, indurated chancres of the skin or mucous membranes at the site of inoculation. The secondary stage appears as a maculopapular rash, classically involving the palms and soles. Generalized lymphadenopathy, fever, malaise, sore throat, headache, and arthralgias can accompany the rash. Hypertrophic lesions (i.e., condyloma lata) occur in moist mucous membranes. Approximately a third of untreated cases progress to the tertiary stage, which occurs after a variable latent period that may have occasional recurrences of secondary syphilis. Transmission to the fetus can occur with any stage of maternal syphilis.[206]

Pigmentary retinopathy is the most common early ocular manifestation of congenital syphilis. Diffuse mottling in the periphery (i.e., salt-and-pepper retinopathy) is indicative of chorioretinitis in utero. Pigment clumping in the periphery usually has no effect on vision, but macular involvement can cause decreased vision. Retinal changes can appear later in adulthood, thus suggesting that inflammatory changes caused by congenital infection can occur after birth. Salt-and-pepper retinopathy is evidence of previous inflammation, and no treatment is required. Interstitial keratitis (see the section "Stromal Keratitis") is the hallmark of congenital syphilis and occurs in 75 percent of these patients.[206] It usually is not detected until late in the first decade of life. Other reported ocular manifestations include optic neuritis and iritis.

Testing the serum by nontreponemal and treponemal methods confirms the diagnosis of congenital infection. The American Academy of Pediatrics recommends physical examination, quantitative nontreponemal serologic testing, a CSF Venereal Disease Research Laboratory (VDRL) test, long bone radiographs, and antitreponemal IgM testing, as specified by the Centers for Disease Control and Prevention (CDC). The CDC states that congenital syphilis is presumptively diagnosed with a positive VDRL and at least one of the following: physical examination evidence of congenital syphilis, characteristic radiographic long bone findings, VDRL + CSF, an otherwise unexplained elevated CSF protein or cell count, quantitative nontreponemal serologic titer four times greater than the mother's, or a positive FTA-

ABS-19s-IgM test.[5] Treatment is with intravenous penicillin G for 10 to 14 days.[6,132]

ENDOPHTHALMITIS

Endophthalmitis is an infection within the eye that may arise endogenously during septicemia or exogenously from accidental or surgical trauma.[144,153] Sixty-two percent of cases occur after intraocular surgery, 20 percent after penetrating trauma, and 10 percent after glaucoma surgery; 8 percent result from metastatic infection.[60,169] The patient usually has severe ocular pain and visual loss at initial evaluation. Rarely, patients may be asymptomatic. Signs of endophthalmitis include conjunctival injection, vitritis, uveitis, hypopyon, and intraocular membrane formation.

Endophthalmitis is an ophthalmic emergency and necessitates immediate evaluation of aqueous and vitreous cultures and institution of intravitreal antibiotic therapy. Any significant delay in recognition and treatment of endophthalmitis can result in permanent vision loss.

Postsurgical endophthalmitis occurs in 0.086 percent of cataract operations.[2] The source of postsurgical infection may be from the eyelids, conjunctiva, contaminated instruments and irrigating solutions, or contamination by operating room personnel. The routine use of subconjunctival antibiotics after intraocular surgery does not prevent all cases of postoperative endophthalmitis. Vitreous loss, which may occur occasionally as a complication of cataract surgery, increases the risk of infection developing. Patients who have undergone glaucoma filtering surgery are particularly prone to endophthalmitis, primarily because sclerostomy is performed routinely as part of this procedure and the only remaining protection that the eye has from infective organisms is a thin layer of conjunctiva overlying the sclerostomy. Local antimetabolites, often used in conjunction with glaucoma filtering procedures, predispose the conjunctiva to bleb leaks that allow direct access of microorganisms to the eye.

Endogenous (metastatic) endophthalmitis should be suspected when ocular inflammation occurs in a septicemic patient, particularly if the patient is immunocompromised or has an underlying systemic illness such as diabetes or leukemia.[24,150,158]

Post-traumatic endophthalmitis should be considered in any patient with a history of injury and visual loss. A history of a high-velocity projectile presents great concern for a penetrating injury, and apparently minor accidental ocular trauma may result in perforation of the globe with or without a retained foreign body. The likelihood of post-traumatic endophthalmitis occurring increases directly with the extent of the injury and the degree of intraocular contamination.

After the diagnosis is suspected, immediate referral to an ophthalmologist is necessary. Once the patient has been examined, a vitreous and aqueous aspirate is obtained under general anesthesia and material is evaluated with Gram and Giemsa stains. Staining with calcofluor white or acridine orange is performed if fungal infection is a concern. The material is cultured on blood and chocolate agar, thioglycolate broth, and Sabouraud agar. Vancomycin (1 mg) to cover gram-positive organisms and ceftazidime (2.25 mg) to cover gram-negative organisms are injected into the vitreous cavity. If fungal infection is suspected, intravitreal amphotericin B is given. Occasionally, the ophthalmologist uses intravitreal dexamethasone to control associated, intense intraocular inflammation. Gram stain results often are inconsistent with cultures.

The role of vitrectomy in postoperative endophthalmitis has been addressed in the Endophthalmitis Vitrectomy Study (EVS).[69] In eyes with better than light perception vision at initial evaluation, outcome measurements were equal between the vitrectomy group and the vitreous tap or biopsy group. In eyes with light perception–only vision, the EVS found that patients who underwent immediate pars plana vitrectomy did significantly better than those who underwent vitreous tap or biopsy alone.

The most common infectious agents in endophthalmitis are *S. epidermidis*, *Bacillus* spp., *Streptococcus* spp., *S. aureus*, and various fungi. *Bacillus cereus* is isolated in 30 to 40 percent of cases and can cause severe ocular morbidity.[1,50,51,59,98] *S. epidermidis* is the predominant organism in postoperative cases, and *Streptococcus* spp. with filtering blebs and *B. cereus* are the organisms associated most frequently with penetrating trauma. Approximately 65 percent of cases are culture-positive.

Fungal endophthalmitis has become a relatively common form of endophthalmitis in childhood because of the prolonged hospital care required for severely ill immunocompromised children. The most common organism is *C. albicans*. Children with a central line catheter or receiving prolonged intravenous therapy of any type are particularly prone to infection. In patients with *Candida* endophthalmitis, the vitreous may be hazy, and small, white "snowball" localizations of infected material may appear in the vitreous or on the surface of the retina. Daily careful observation may be required during intravenous amphotericin B therapy. If the endophthalmitis clears, no ocular surgical intervention is indicated. If the infection is not adequately controlled with intravenous therapy, vitrectomy with injection of intravitreal amphotericin may be required.

REFERENCES

1. Alfaro, D. V., Roth, D., and Liggett, P. E.: Posttraumatic endophthalmitis. Causative organisms, treatment, and prevention. Retina 14:206-211, 1994.
2. Allen, H. F., and Mangiaracine, A. B.: Bacterial endophthalmitis after cataract extraction. II. Incidence in 36,000 consecutive operations with special reference to preoperative topical antibiotics. Arch. Ophthalmol. 91:3-7, 1974.
3. Ambati, B. K., Ambati, J., Azar, N., et al.: Periorbital and orbital cellulitis before and after the advent of Haemophilus influenzae type B vaccination. Ophthalmology 107:1450-1453, 2000.
4. American Academy of Ophthalmology: Basic and Clinical Science Course. Section 9: Intraocular Inflammation and Uveitis. San Francisco, American Academy of Ophthalmology, 1995, pp. 57-61.
5. American Academy of Ophthalmology, Section 6: Pediatric ophthalmology and strabismus, In Liesegang, T. J. (ed.): Basic and Clinical Science Course 2006-2006. San Francisco, American Academy of Ophthalmology, 2005, pp. 203-209.
6. American Academy of Pediatrics: 1997 Red Book: Report of the Committee on Infectious Diseases. 24th ed. Elk Grove Village, IL, American Academy of Pediatrics, 1997.
7. Armstrong, D., Fortner, J. G., Rowe, W. P., and Parker, J. C.: Meningitis due to lymphocytic choriomeningitis virus endemic in a hamster colony. J. A. M. A. 209:265-267, 1969.
8. Asbell, P., and Stenson, S.: Ulcerative keratitis, survey of 30 years' laboratory experience. Arch. Ophthalmol. 100:77-80, 1982.
9. Bale, J. F., Jr., and Murph, J. R.: Congenital infections and the nervous system. Pediatr. Clin. North Am. 39:669-690, 1992.
10. Barkin, R. M., Todd, J. K., and Amer, J.: Periorbital cellulitis in children. Pediatrics 62:390-392, 1978.
11. Bart, K. J., Orenstein, W. A., Preblud, S. R., et al.: Elimination of rubella and congenital rubella from the United States. Pediatr. Infect. Dis. 4:14-21, 1985.
12. Bedrossian, R. H.: Neuroretinitis following measles. J. Pediatr. 46:329-331, 1955.
13. Bekir, N. A., Gungor, K., and Namiduru, M.: Brucella melitensis dacryoadenitis: A case report. Eur. J. Ophthalmol. 10:259-261, 2000.
14. Bell, T. A., Kuo, C. C., Stamm, W. E., et al.: Direct fluorescent monoclonal antibody stain for rapid detection of infant Chlamydia trachomatis infections. Pediatrics 74:224-228, 1984.
15. BenEzra, D.: Ocular Inflammation: Basic and Clinical Concepts. London, Martin Dunitz, 1999, pp. 427-444.
16. Benjamin, A., Tufail, A., and Holland, G. N.: Uveitis as the only clinical manifestation of poststreptococcal syndrome. Am. J. Ophthalmol. 123:259-260, 1997.
17. Benson, W. H., and Lanier, J. D.: Current diagnosis and treatment of corneal ulcers. Curr. Opin. Ophthalmol. 9:45-49, 1998.
18. Berenberg, W., and Nankervis, G.: Long-term follow-up cytomegalic inclusion disease of infancy. Pediatrics 46:403, 1970.
19. Bertuch, A. W., Rocco, E., and Schwartz, E. G: Lyme disease: Ocular manifestations. Ann. Ophthalmol. 20:376-378, 1988.

20. Bhaskaram, P., Mathur, R., Rao, V., et al.: Pathogenesis of corneal lesions in measles. Hum. Nutr. Clin. Nutr. *40*:197-204, 1986.

21. Birenbaum, E., Linder, N., Varsano, N., et al.: Adenovirus type 8 conjunctivitis outbreak in a neonatal intensive care unit. Arch. Dis. Child. *68*:610-611, 1993.

22. Blumenkranz, M., Clarkson, J., Culbertson, W. W., et al.: Visual results and complications after retinal reattachment in the acute retinal necrosis syndrome: The influence of operative technique. Retina *9*:170-174, 1989.

23. Boniuk, M. M., and Zimmerman, L. E.: Ocular pathology in the rubella syndrome. Arch. Ophthalmol. *77*:455-473, 1967.

24. Borne, M. J., Shields, J. A., Shields, C. L., et al.: Bilateral viral endophthalmitis as the presenting sign of severe combined immunodeficiency. Arch. Ophthalmol. *112*:1280-1281, 1994.

25. Bosch-Driessen, E. H., and Rothova, A.: Recurrent ocular disease in postnatally acquired toxoplasmosis. Am. J. Ophthalmol. *128*:421-425, 1999.

26. Bouza, E., Merino, P., Sanchez-Carrillo, C., et al.: Ocular tuberculosis: A prospective study in a general hospital. Medicine (Baltimore) *76*:53-61, 1997.

27. Brézin, A. P., Kasner, L., Thulliez, P., et al.: Ocular toxoplasmosis in the fetus. Immunohistochemistry analysis and DNA amplification. Retina *14*:19-26, 1994.

28. Brézin, A. P., Thullilez, P., Cisneros, B., et al.: Lymphocytic choriomeningitis virus chorioretinitis mimicking ocular toxoplasmosis in two otherwise normal children. Am. J. Ophthalmol. *130*:245-247, 2000.

29. Brook, I.: Dacryocystitis caused by anaerobic bacteria in the newborn. Pediatr. Infect. Dis. J. *17*:172-173, 1998.

30. Brook, I., and Frazier, E. H.: Aerobic and anaerobic microbiology of dacryocystitis. Am. J. Ophthalmol. *125*:552-554, 1998.

31. Buck, S. L., Rosenthal, R. A., and Schlech, B. A.: Methods used to evaluate the effectiveness of contact lens care solutions and other compounds against *Acanthamoeba*: A review of the literature. C. L. A. O. J. *26*:72-84, 2000.

32. Bullock, J. D., and Fleishman, J. A.: Orbital cellulitis following dental extraction. Trans. Am. Ophthalmol. Soc. *82*:111-133, 1984.

33. Byrne, P. J., Silver, M. M., Gilbert, J. M., et al.: Cyclopia and congenital cytomegalovirus infection. Am. J. Med. Genet. *28*:61-65, 1987.

34. Cable, B. B., Wassmuth, Z., Mann, E. A., et al.: The effect of corticosteroids in the treatment of experimental sinusitis. Am. J. Rhinol. *14*:217-222, 2000.

35. Caca, I., Cakmak, S. S., Unlü, K., et al.: Cutaneous anthrax on eyelids. Jpn. J. Ophthalmol. *48*:268-271, 2004.

36. Callanan, D., Fish, G. E., and Anand, R.: Reactivation of inflammatory lesions in ocular histoplasmosis. Arch. Ophthalmol. *116*:470-484, 1998.

37. Chang, C. H., Lai, Y. H., Wang, H. Z., et al.: Antibiotic treatment of orbital cellulitis: An analysis of pathogenic bacteria and bacterial susceptibility. J. Ocul. Pharmacol. Ther. *16*:75-79, 2000.

38. Charukamnoetkanok, P., and Pineda, R., 2nd.: Controversies in management of bacterial keratitis. Int. Ophthalmol. Clin. *45*:199-210, 2005.

39. Chu, K. M., Rathinam, R., Namperumalsamy, P., et al.: Identification of *Leptospira* species in the pathogenesis of uveitis and determination of clinical ocular characteristics in south India. J. Infect. Dis. *177*:1314-1321, 1998.

40. Clary, R., Weber, A. L., Eavey, R., and Oot, R. F.: Orbital cellulitis with abscess formation caused by sinusitis. Ann. Otol. Rhinol. Laryngol. *97*:211-212, 1988.

41. Coats, D. K., Demmler, G. J., Paysse, E. A., et al.: Ophthalmologic findings in children with congenital cytomegalovirus infection. J. A. A. P. O. S. *4*:110-116, 2000.

42. Corey, L.: Herpes simplex viruses. *In* Braunwald, E., Isselbacher, K. J., Petersdorf, R. G., et al. (eds.): Harrison's Principles of Internal Medicine. 14th ed. New York, McGraw-Hill, 1998, pp. 1080-1086.

43. Costa, S. F., and Weiss, L. M.: Drug treatment of microsporidiosis. Drug Resist. Update *3*:384-399, 2000.

44. Couch, J. M., Green, W. R., Hirst, L. W., and de la Cruz, Z. C.: Diagnosing and treating *Phthirus pubis* palpebrarum. Surv. Ophthalmol. *26*:219-225, 1982.

45. Couvreur, J., Thulliez, P., Daffos, F., et al.: In utero treatment of toxoplasmic fetopathy with the combination pyrimethamine-sulfadiazine. Fetal Diagn. Ther. *8*:45-50, 1993.

46. Credo, B. V., and Dyment, P. G.: Molluscum contagiosum. Adolesc. Med. *7*:57-62, 1996.

47. Daffos, F., Forestier, F., Capella-Pavlovsky, M., et al.: Prenatal management of 746 pregnancies at risk for congenital toxoplasmosis. N. Engl. J. Med. *318*:271-275, 1988.

48. Daniel, E., Ebenezer, G. J., and Job, C. K.: Pathology of iris in leprosy. Br. J. Ophthalmol. *81*:490-492, 1997.

49. Daniel, E., Ffytche, T. J., Kempen, J. H., et al.: Incidence of ocular morbidity among multibacillary leprosy patients during a 2 year course of multidrug therapy. Br. J. Ophthalmol. *90*:568-573, 2006.

50. Davey, R. T., Jr., and Tauber, W. B.: Posttraumatic endophthalmitis: The emerging role of *Bacillus cereus* infection. Rev. Infect. Dis. *9*:110-123, 1987.

51. David, D. B., Kirkby, G. R., and Noble, B. A.: *Bacillus cereus* endophthalmitis. Br. J. Ophthalmol. *78*:577-580, 1994.

52. Dawson, D. R., and Sheppard, J. D.: Follicular conjunctivitis. *In* Tasman, W., and Jaeger, E. A. (eds.): Duane's Clinical Ophthalmology. Philadelphia, J. B. Lippincott, 1990, pp. 16-18.

53. Demirci, G., Ay, G. M., Karabas, L. V., et al.: *Acanthamoeba* keratitis in a 5-year-old boy without a history of contact lens usage. Cornea *25*:356-358, 2006.

54. Demmler, G. J.: Congenital cytomegalovirus infection and disease. Adv. Pediatr. Infect. Dis. *11*:135-162, 1996.

55. Desmonts, G., and Couvreur, J.: Congenital toxoplasmosis. A prospective study of 378 pregnancies. N. Engl. J. Med. *290*:1110-1116, 1974.

56. Desmonts, G., and Couvreur, J.: [Congenital toxoplasmosis. Prospective study of the outcome of pregnancy in 542 women with toxoplasmosis acquired during pregnancy.] Ann. Pediatr. (Paris) *31*:805-809, 1984.

57. Dhaliwal, U., Arora, V. K., Singh, N., and Bhatia, A.: Cytopathology of chalazia. Diagn. Cytopathol. *31*:118-122, 2004.

58. Dhaliwal, U., and Bhatia, A.: A rationale for therapeutic decision-making in chalazia. Orbit *24*:227-230, 2005.

59. Diamond, J. G.: Intraocular management of endophthalmitis. A systematic approach. Arch. Ophthalmol. *99*:96-99, 1981.

60. Donahue, S. P., Greven, C. M., Zuravleff, J. J., et al.: Intraocular candidiasis in patients with candidemia. Clinical implications derived from a prospective multicenter study. Ophthalmology *101*:1302-1309, 1994.

61. Donahue, S. P., Hein, E., and Sinatra, R. B.: Ocular involvement in children with candidemia. Am. J. Ophthalmol. *135*:886-887, 2003.

62. Donahue, S. P., and Schwartz, G.: Preseptal and orbital cellulitis in childhood. A changing microbiologic spectrum. Ophthalmology *105*:1902-1905; discussion 1905-1906, 1998.

63. Drew, W. L.: Cytomegalovirus infection in patients with AIDS. J. Infect. Dis. *158*:449-456, 1988.

64. Du, L. T., Coats, D. K., Paysse, E. A., et al.: Incidence of presumed cytomegalovirus retinitis in HIV-infected pediatric patients. J. A. A. P. O. S. *3*:245-249, 1999.

65. Edwards, K. M., Meredith, T. A., Hager, W. S., et al.: Ophthalmomyiasis interna causing visual loss. Am. J. Ophthalmol. *97*:605-610, 1984.

66. Eichenwald, H. F., and Shinefield, H. R.: Viral infections of the fetus and of the premature and newborn infant. Adv. Pediatr. *12*:249-305, 1962.

67. el Azazi, M., Malm, G., and Forsgren, M.: Late ophthalmologic manifestations of neonatal herpes simplex virus infection. Am. J. Ophthalmol. *109*:1-7, 1990.

68. El Hassan, A. M., Khalil, E. A., el Sheikh, E. A., et al.: Post kala-azar ocular leishmaniasis. Trans. R. Soc. Trop. Med. Hyg. *92*:177-179, 1998.

69. Endophthalmitis Vitrectomy Study Group: Results of the Endophthalmitis Vitrectomy Study. A randomized trial of immediate vitrectomy and of intravenous antibiotics for the treatment of postoperative bacterial endophthalmitis. Endophthalmitis Vitrectomy Study Group. Arch. Ophthalmol. *113*:1479-1496, 1995.

70. English, F. P., and Nutting, W. B.: Demodicosis of ophthalmic concern. Am. J. Ophthalmol. *91*:362-372, 1981.

71. Engstrom, R. E., Jr., Holland, G. N., Nussenblatt, R. B., Jabs, D. A.: Current practices in the management of ocular toxoplasmosis. Am. J. Ophthalmol. *111*:601-610, 1991.

72. Epstein, G. A., and Putterman, A. M.: Combined excision and drainage with intralesional corticosteroid injection in the treatment of chronic chalazia. Arch. Ophthalmol. *106*:514-516, 1988.

73. Fair, J. R.: Clinical eye findings in congenital toxoplasmosis. Surv. Ophthalmol. *6*:923-935, 1961.

74. Feltkamp, T. E. W., and Ringrose, J. H.: Acute anterior uveitis and spondyloarthropathies. Curr. Opin. Rheumatol. *10*:314-318, 1998.

75. Foster, A., and Sommer, A.: Corneal ulceration, measles, and childhood blindness in Tanzania. Br. J. Ophthalmol. *71*:331-343, 1987.

76. Foster, C. S.: Fungal keratitis. Infect. Dis. Clin. North Am. *6*:851-857, 1992.

77. Fox, K. R., and Golomb, H. S.: Staphylococcal ophthalmia neonatorum and the staphylococcal scalded skin syndrome. Am. J. Ophthalmol. *88*:1052-1055, 1979.

78. Friendly, D. S.: Ophthalmia neonatorum. Pediatr. Clin. North Am. *30*:1033-1042, 1983.

79. Fulk, G. W., Murphy, B., and Robins, M. D.: Pilocarpine gel for the treatment of demodicosis—a case series. Optom. Vis. Sci. *73*:742-745, 1996.

80. Gao, Y. Y., Di Pascuale, M. A., Li, W., et al.: High prevalence of *Demodex* in eyelashes with cylindrical dandruff. Invest. Ophthalmol. Vis. Sci. *46*:3089-3094, 2005.

81. Geltzer, A. I., Guber, D., and Sears, M. L.: Ocular manifestations of the 1964-65 rubella epidemic. Am. J. Ophthalmol. *63*:221-229, 1967.

82. Gigliotti, F., Hendley, J. O., Morgan, J., et al.: Efficacy of topical antibiotic therapy in acute conjunctivitis in children. J. Pediatr. *104*:623-626, 1984.

83. Gigliotti, F., Williams, W. T., Hayden, F. G., et al.: Etiology of acute conjunctivitis in children. J. Pediatr. *98*:531-536, 1981.

84. Givens, K. T., Lee, D. A., Jones, T., and Ilstrup, D. M..: Congenital rubella syndrome: Ophthalmic manifestations and associated systemic disorders. Br. J. Ophthalmol. *77*:358-363, 1993.

85. Goldberg, G. N., Fulginiti, V. A., Ray, C. G., et al.: In utero Epstein-Barr virus (infectious mononucleosis) infection. J. A. M. A. *246*:1579-1581, 1981.

86. Gomez Morales, A., Croxatto, J. O., Crovetto, L., and Ebner, R.: Hydatid cysts of the orbit. A review of 35 cases. Ophthalmology *95*:1027-1032, 1988.

87. Goscienski, P. J.: Inclusion conjunctivitis in the newborn infant. J. Pediatr. *77*:19-26, 1970.

88. Green, W. R., Font, R. L., and Zimmerman, L. E.: Aspergillosis of the orbit. Report of ten cases and review of the literature. Arch. Ophthalmol. *82*:302-313, 1969.

89. Greenberg, M. F., and Pollard, Z. F.: Medical treatment of pediatric subperiosteal orbital abscess secondary to sinusitis. J. A. A. P. O. S. *2*:351-355, 1998.

90. Grefer, J., Santer, R., Ankermann, T., et al.: Tubulointerstitial nephritis and uveitis in association with Epstein-Barr virus infection. Pediatr. Nephrol. *13*:336-339, 1999.

91. Hagler, W. S., Walters, P. V., and Nahmias, A. J.: Ocular involvement in neonatal herpes simplex virus infection. Arch. Ophthalmol. *82*:169-176, 1969.

92. Haimovici, R., and Roussel, T. J.: Treatment of gonococcal conjunctivitis with single-dose intramuscular ceftriaxone. Am. J. Ophthalmol. *107*:511-514, 1989.

93. Hall, L. R., and Pearlman, E.: Pathogenesis of onchocercal keratitis. Clin. Microbiol. Rev. *12*:445-453, 1999.

94. Hammerschlag, M. R.: Neonatal conjunctivitis. Pediatr. Ann. *22*:346-351, 1993.

95. Hammerschlag, M. R., Chandler, J. W., Alexander, E. R., et al.: Erythromycin ointment for ocular prophylaxis of neonatal chlamydial infection. J. A. M. A. *244*:2291-2293, 1980.

96. Hansen, T., Burns, R. P., and Allen, A.: Gonorrheal conjunctivitis: An old disease returned. J. A. M. A. *195*:1156, 1966.

97. Hartstein, M. E., Steinvurzel, M. D., and Cohen, C. P.: Intracranial abscess as a complication of subperiosteal abscess of the orbit. Ophthal. Plast. Reconstr. Surg. *17*:398-403, 2001.

98. Hemady, R., Zaltas, M., Paton, B., et al.: *Bacillus*-induced endophthalmitis: New series of 10 cases and review of the literature. Br. J. Ophthalmol. *74*:26-29, 1990.

99. Hess, D. L.: *Chlamydia* in the neonate. Neonatal Netw. *12*:9-12, 1993.

100. Hierholzer, J. C. H., and Hatch, M.: Acute hemorrhagic conjunctivitis. *In* Darnell R. W. (ed.): Viral Diseases of the Eye. Philadelphia, Lea & Febiger, 1985, pp. 165-196.

101. Hirsch, M. S., Moellering, R. C., Jr., Pope, H. G., and Poskanzer, D. C..: Lymphocytic-choriomeningitis-virus infection traced to a pet hamster. N. Engl. J. Med. *291*:610-612, 1974.

102. Hohlfeld, P., Daffos, F., Thulliez, P. L., et al.: Fetal toxoplasmosis: Outcome of pregnancy and infant follow-up after in utero treatment. J. Pediatr. *115*:765-769, 1989.

103. Holland, G. N.: Infectious diseases. *In* Isenberg S. (ed.): The Eye in Infancy. Chicago, Year Book, 1989.

104. Holland, G. N.: An update on AIDS-related cytomegalovirus retinitis. *In* Focal Points: Clinical Modules for Ophthalmologists. San Francisco, American Academy of Ophthalmology, 1991, module 5.

105. Holland, G. N.: Reconsidering the pathogenesis of ocular toxoplasmosis. Am. J. Ophthalmol. *128*:502-505, 1999.

106. Honda, Y., Nakazawa, Y., and Chihara, E.: Necrotizing chorioretinitis induced by herpes simplex virus infection in the neonate. Metab. Pediatr. Syst. Ophthalmol. *7*:147-152, 1983.

107. Hunt, K. E., and Glasgow, B. J.: *Aspergillus* endophthalmitis: An unrecognized endemic disease in orthotopic liver transplantation. Ophthalmology *103*:757-767, 1996.

108. Huppertz, H.-I., Munchmeier, D., Lieb, W.: Ocular manifestations in children and adolescents with Lyme arthritis. Br. J. Ophthalmol. *83*:1149-1152, 1999.

109. Illingworth, C. D., and Cook, S. D.: *Acanthamoeba* keratitis. Surv. Ophthalmol. *42*:493-508, 1998.

110. Isenberg, S. J., Apt, L., and Wood, M.: A controlled trial of povidone-iodine as prophylaxis against ophthalmia neonatorum. N. Engl. J. Med. *332*:562-566, 1995.

111. Jabs, D. A., Green, W. R., Fox, R., et al.: Ocular manifestations of AIDS. Ophthalmology *96*:1092-1099, 1989.

112. Jarrett, W. H., 2nd, and Gutman, F. A.: Ocular complications of infection in the paranasal sinuses. Arch. Ophthalmol. *81*:683-688, 1969.

113. Jones, D. B.: Viral and chlamydial conjunctivitis. *In* Symposium on Medical and Surgical Diseases of the Cornea: Transactions of the New Orleans Academy of Ophthalmology. St. Louis, C. V. Mosby, 1980, pp. 497-523.

114. Joseph, J., Murthy, S., Garg, P., and Sharma, S.: Use of different stains for microscopic evaluation of corneal scrapings for diagnosis of microsporidial keratitis. J. Clin. Microbiol. *44*:583-585, 2006.

115. Joseph, J., Vemuganti, G. K., and Sharma, S.: Microsporidia: Emerging ocular pathogens. Indian J. Med. Microbiol. *23*:80-91, 2005.

116. Katz, B. J., Scott, W. E., and Folk, J. C.: Acute histoplasmosis choroiditis in 2 immunocompetent brothers. Arch. Ophthalmol. *115*:1470-1472, 1997.

117. Kaufman, H. E.: Treatment of viral diseases of the cornea and external eye. Prog. Retin. Eye Res. *19*:69-85, 1998.

118. Kemal, M., Sümer, Z., Toker, M. I., et al.: The prevalence of *Demodex folliculorum* in blepharitis patients and the normal population. Ophthalmic Epidemiol. *12*:287-290, 2005.

119. Kerkhoff, F. T., Ossewaarde, J. M., de Loos, W. S., et al.: Presumed ocular bartonellosis. Br. J. Ophthalmol. *83*:270-275, 1999.

120. Kestelyn, P., Taelman, H., Bogaerts, J., et al.: Ophthalmic manifestations of infections with *Cryptococcus neoformans* in patients with the acquired immunodeficiency syndrome. Am. J. Ophthalmol. *116*:721-727, 1993.

121. Koppe, J. G., Kloosterman, G. J., de Roever-Bonnet, H., et al.: Toxoplasmosis and pregnancy, with a long-term follow-up of children. Eur. J. Obstet. Gynecol. Reprod. Biol. *4*:101-110, 1974.

122. Laforet, E. G., and Lynch, C. L., Jr.: Multiple congenital defects following maternal varicella. Report of a case. N. Engl. J. Med. *236*:534-537, 1947.

123. Larkin, D. F. P., Kilvington, S., and Dart, J. K. G.: Treatment of *Acanthamoeba* keratitis with polyhexamethylene biguanide. Ophthalmology *99*:185-191, 1992.

124. Lewis, K. T., and Stiles, M.: Management of cat and dog bites. Am. Fam. Physician *52*:479-485, 489-490, 1995.

125. Liesegang, T. J.: Diagnosis and therapy of herpes zoster ophthalmicus. Ophthalmology *98*:1216-1229, 1991.

126. Liesegang, T. J.: Bacterial keratitis. Infect. Dis. Clin. North Am. *6*:815-829, 1992.

127. Liesegang, T. J., and Forster, R. K.: Spectrum of microbial keratitis in South Florida. Am. J. Ophthalmol. *90*:38-47, 1980.

128. Lonn, L. I.: Neonatal cytomegalic inclusion disease chorioretinitis. Arch. Ophthalmol. *88*:434-438, 1972.

129. Mafee, M. F., Edward, D. P., Koeller, K. K., and Dorodi, S..: Lacrimal gland tumors and simulating lesions. Clinicopathologic and MR imaging features. Radiol. Clin. North Am. *37*:219-239, xii, 1999.

130. Maini, R., and Edelsten, C.: Uveitis associated with parvovirus infection. Br. J. Ophthalmol. *83*:1403-1404, 1999.

131. Mannis, M. J., Tamaru, R., Roth, A. M., et al.: *Acanthamoeba* sclerokeratitis: Determining diagnostic criteria. Arch. Ophthalmol. *104*:1313-1317, 1986.

132. Margo, C. E., and Hamed, L. M.: Ocular syphilis. Surv. Ophthalmol. *37*:203-220, 1992.

133. Marines, H. M., Osato, M. S., and Font, R. L.: The value of calcofluor white in the diagnosis of mycotic and acanthamoeba infections of the eye and ocular adnexa. Ophthalmology *94*:23-26, 1987.

134. Mathers, W. D., Sutphin, J. E., Folberg, R., et al.: Outbreak of keratitis presumed to be caused by *Acanthamoeba*. Am. J. Ophthalmol. *121*:129-142, 1996.

135. Matoba, A. Y.: Ocular viral infections. Pediatr. Infect. Dis. *3*:358-368, 1984.

136. Matoba, A. Y.: Ocular disease associated with Epstein-Barr virus infection. Surv. Ophthalmol. *35*:145-150, 1990.

137. McCarty, M. L., et al.: Manifestations of fungal cellulitis of the orbit in children with neutropenia and fever. Ophthal. Plast. Reconstr. Surg. *20*:217-223, 2004.

138. McCulley, J. P., Alizadeh, H., and Niederkorn, J. Y.: The diagnosis and management of *Acanthamoeba* keratitis. C. L. A. O. J. *26*:47-51, 2000.

139. Merayo-Lloves, J., Baltatzis, S., and Foster, C. S.: Epstein-Barr virus dacryoadenitis resulting in keratoconjunctivitis sicca in a child. Am. J. Ophthalmol. *132*:922-923, 2001.

140. Mets, M. B.: Childhood blindness and visual loss: An assessment at two institutions including a "new" cause. Am. Ophthalmol. Soc. *97*:653-696, 1999.

141. Mets, M. B.: Eye manifestations of intrauterine infections. Ophthalmol. Clin. North Am. *14*:521-531, 2001.

142. Mets, M. B., Barton, L. L., Khan, A. S., and Ksiazek, T. G.: Lymphocytic choriomeningitis virus: An underdiagnosed cause of congenital chorioretinitis. Am. J. Ophthalmol. *130*:209-215, 2000.

143. Mets, M. B., Bechtel, R. T., Haught, K. A., et al.: Lymphocytic choriomeningitis virus: A new addition to the TORCH evaluation. Arch. Ophthalmol. *115*:680-681, 1997.

144. Meyer, D.: Eye signs that alert the clinician to a diagnosis of AIDS. S. A. D. J. *60*:386-387, 2005.

145. Mohammad, A. N.: Intralesional steroid injection for management of acute idiopathic dacryoadenitis: A preliminary result. Ophthal. Plast. Reconstr. Surg. *21*:138-141, 2005.

146. Moinfar, N., Wagner, D. G., Chrousos, G. A., et. al.: Paediatric varicella choroiditis. Br. J. Ophthalmol. *82*:1092-1093, 1998.

147. Moorthy, R. S., Rao, N. A., Sidikaro, Y., and Foos, R. Y.: Coccidioidomycosis iridocyclitis. Ophthalmology *101*:1923-1928, 1994.

148. Moran, G. J., Krishnadasan, A., Gorwitz, R. J., et al.: Methicillin-resistant *S. aureus* infections among patients in the emergency department. N. Engl. J. Med. *355*:666-674, 2006.

149. Mordhorst, C. H., and Dawson, C.: Sequelae of neonatal inclusion conjunctivitis and associated disease in parents. Am. J. Ophthalmol. *71*:861-867, 1971.

150. Nagelberg, H. P., Petashnick, D. E., To, K. W., and Woodcome, H. A., Jr.: Group B streptococcal metastatic endophthalmitis. Am. J. Ophthalmol. *117*:498-500, 1994.

151. Nageswaran, S., Woods, C. R., Benjamin, D. K., Jr., et al.: Orbital cellulitis in children. Pediatr. Infect. Dis. J. *25*:695-699, 2006.

152. Nahmias, A. J., Visintine, A. M., Caldwell, D. R., and Wilson, L. A.: Eye infections with herpes simplex viruses in neonates. Surv. Ophthalmol. *21*:100-105, 1976.

153. Nakao, K., Ohba, N., Nakagawa, M., et al.: Clinical course of HTLV-1–associated uveitis. Jpn. J. Ophthalmol. *43*:404-409, 1999.

154. Nishida, H., and Risemberg, H. M.: Silver nitrate ophthalmic solution and chemical conjunctivitis. Pediatrics *56*:368-373, 1975.

155. Obenour, L. C.: Subacute sclerosing panencephalitis. Int. Ophthalmol. Clin. *12*:215-223, 1972.

156. O'Brien, T. P.: Management of bacterial keratitis: Beyond exorcism towards consideration of organism and host factors. Eye *17*:957-974, 2003.

157. O'Day, D. M., and Head, W. S.: Advances in the management of keratomycosis and *Acanthamoeba* keratitis. Cornea *19*:681-687, 2000.

158. Okada, A. A., Johnson, R. P., Liles, W. C., et al.: Endogenous bacterial endophthalmitis. Report of a ten-year retrospective study. Ophthalmology *101*:832-838, 1994.

159. Opremcak, E. M.: Uveitis: A Clinical Manual for Ocular Inflammation. New York, Springer-Verlag, 1994, pp. 1-183.
160. Oren, B., and Wende, S. O.: An outbreak of molluscum contagiosum in a kibbutz. Infection 19:159-161, 1991.
161. Palamar, M., Uretmen, O., and Kose, S.: Orbital cellulitis after strabismus surgery. J. A. A. P. O. S. 9:602-603, 2005.
162. Paryani, S. G., and Arvin, A. M.: Intrauterine infection with varicella-zoster virus after maternal varicella. N. Engl. J. Med. 314:1542-1546, 1986.
163. Paysse, E. A., Coats, D. K., Bernstein, J. M., et al.: Management and complications of congenital dacryocele with concurrent intranasal mucocele. J. A. A. P. O. S. 4:46-53, 2000.
164. Pena, G. P., and Andrade Filho, J. S.: Is Demodex really non-pathogenic? Rev. Inst. Med. Trop. Sao Paulo 42:171-173, 2000.
165. Pepose, J., Holland, G., and Wilhelmus, K.: Ocular Infection and Immunology. St. Louis, C. V. Mosby, 1996.
166. Pfister, D. R., Cameron, J. D., Krachmer, J. H., et al.: Confocal microscopy findings of Acanthamoeba keratitis. Am. J. Ophthalmol. 121:119-128, 1996.
167. Pollard, Z. F.: Treatment of acute dacryocystitis in neonates. J. Pediatr. Ophthalmol. Strabismus 28:341-343, 1991.
168. Prasad, A. G., and Van Gelder, R. N.: Presumed ocular histoplasmosis syndrome. Curr. Opin. Ophthalmol. 16:364-368, 2005.
169. Puliafito, C. A., Baker, A. S., Haaf, J., and Foster, C. S.: Infectious endophthalmitis. Review of 36 cases. Ophthalmology 89:921-929, 1982.
170. Raina, U. K., Jain, S., Monga, S., et al.: Tubercular preseptal cellulitis in children: A presenting feature of underlying systemic tuberculosis. Ophthalmology 111:291-296, 2004.
171. Raucher, H. S., Newton, M. J., and Stern, R. H.: Ophthalmia neonatorum caused by penicillinase-producing Neisseria gonorrhoeae. J. Pediatr. 100:925-926, 1982.
172. Rebora, A.: The management of rosacea. Am. J. Clin. Dermatol. 3:489-496, 2002.
173. Reersted, P., and Hansen, B.: Chorioretinitis of the newborn with herpes simplex virus type 1. Report of a case. Acta. Ophthalmol. (Copenh.) 57:1096-1100, 1979.
174. Remington, J. S., and Desmote, G.: Toxoplasmosis. In Remington, J. S., and Klein J. O. (eds.): Infectious Diseases of the Fetus and Newborn. 3rd ed. Philadelphia, W. B. Saunders, 1990, pp. 89-105.
175. Reynolds, D. J., Kodsi, S. R., Rubin, S. E., and Rodgers, I. R.: Intracranial infection associated with preseptal and orbital cellulitis in the pediatric patient. J. A. A. P. O. S. 7:413-417, 2003.
176. Rhem, M. N., Wilhelmus, K. R., and Jones, D. B.: Epstein-Barr virus dacryoadenitis. Am. J. Ophthalmol. 129:372-375, 2000.
177. Rodriguez, A., Calonge, M., Petroza-Sers, M., et al.: Referral patterns of uveitis in a tertiary eye care center. Arch. Ophthalmol. 114:593-599, 1996.
178. Ronday, M. J., Stilma, J. S., Barbe, R. F., et al.: Aetiology of uveitis in Sierra Leone, West Africa. Br. J. Ophthalmol. 80:956-961, 1996.
179. Rowe, S. G., and Durand, M.: Blackflies and white water: Onchocerciasis and the eye. Int. Ophthalmol. Clin. 38:231-240, 1998.
180. Rubin, S. E., Rubin, L. G., Zito, J., et al.: Medical management of orbital subperiosteal abscess in children. J. Pediatr. Ophthalmol. Strabismus 26:21-27, 1989.
181. Rutar, T., Chambers, H. F., Crawford, J. B., et al.: Ophthalmic manifestations of infections caused by the USA300 clone of community-associated methicillin-resistant Staphylococcus aureus. Ophthalmology 113:1455-1462, 2006.
182. Rutar, T., and Cockerham, K. P.: Periorbital zygomycosis (mucormycosis) treated with posaconazole. Am. J. Ophthalmol. 142:187-188, 2006.
183. Rutar, T., Zwick, O. M., Cockerham, K. P., and Horton, J. C.: Bilateral blindness from orbital cellulitis caused by community-acquired methicillin-resistant Staphylococcus aureus. Am. J. Ophthalmol. 140:740-742, 2005.
184. Ryan, S. J., Jr.: De novo subretinal neovascularization in the histoplasmosis syndrome. Arch. Ophthalmol. 94:321-327, 1976.
185. Sandstrom, K. I., Bell, T. A., Chandler, J. W., et al. Diagnosis of neonatal purulent conjunctivitis caused by Chlamydia trachomatis and other organisms. In Marah, P. A., Holmes, K. K., Oriel, J. D., et al. (eds.): Chlamydial Infections. Amsterdam, Elsevier, 1982, pp. 217-220.
186. Schantz, P. M., and Glickman, L. T.: Toxocara visceral larva migrans. N. Engl. J. Med. 298:436-439, 1978.
187. Schneider, G.: Silver nitrate prophylaxis. Can. Med. Assoc. J. 131:193-196, 1984.
188. Schulz, D., Sarra, G. M., Koerner, U. B., and Garweg, J. G.: Evolution of HIV-1–related conjunctival molluscum contagiosum under HAART: Report of a bilaterally manifesting case and literature review. Graefes Arch. Clin. Exp. Ophthalmol. 242:951-955, 2004.
189. Schwab, I. R.: Oral acyclovir in the management of herpes simplex ocular infections. Ophthalmology 95:423-430, 1988.
190. Schwartz, G. S., Harrison, A. R., and Holland, E. J.: Etiology of immune stromal (interstitial) keratitis. Cornea 17:278-281, 1998.
191. Shields, J. A.: Ocular toxocariasis: A review. Surv. Ophthalmol. 28:361-381, 1984.
192. Skinner, C. J., Viswalingam, N. D., and Goh, B. T.: Phthirus pubis infestation of the eyelids: A marker for sexually transmitted diseases. Int. J. S. T. D. A. I. D. S. 6:451-452, 1995.
193. Smith, R. E.: Toxoplasmic retinochoroiditis as an emerging problem in AIDS patients. Am. J. Ophthalmol. 106:738-739, 1988.
194. Snowe, R. J., and Wilfert, C. M.: Epidemic reappearance of gonococcal ophthalmia neonatorum. Pediatrics 51:110-114, 1973.
195. Solley, W. A., Martin, D. F., Newman, N. J., et al.: Cat scratch disease: Posterior segment manifestations. Ophthalmology 106:1546-1553, 1999.
196. Stagno, S.: Cytomegalovirus. In Remington, J. S., and Klein J. O. (eds.): Infectious Diseases of the Fetus and Newborn Infant. 3rd ed. Philadelphia, W. B. Saunders, 1990.
197. Stagno, S., and Whitley, R. J.: Herpesvirus infections of pregnancy. Part I: Cytomegalovirus and Epstein-Barr virus infections. N. Engl. J. Med. 313:1270-1274, 1985.
198. Steinkuller, P. G., and Jones, D. B.: Microbial preseptal and orbital cellulitis. In Duane, T. D. (ed.): Clinical Ophthalmology. Hagerstown, MD, Harper & Row, 1997, p. 8.
199. Stenson, S., Newman, R., and Fedukowicz, H.: Conjunctivitis in the newborn: Observations on incidence, cause, and prophylaxis. Ann. Ophthalmol. 13:329-334, 1981.
200. Streilein, J. W.: Anterior chamber associated immune deviation: The privilege of immunity in the eye. Surv. Ophthalmol. 35:67-73, 1990.
201. Sudesh, S., and Laibson, P. R.: The impact of the herpetic eye disease studies on the management of herpes simplex virus ocular infections. Curr. Opin. Ophthalmol. 10:230-233, 1999.
202. Syed, T. A., Goswami, J., Ahmadpour, O. A., and Ahmad, S. A.: Treatment of molluscum contagiosum in males with an analog of imiquimod 1% in cream: A placebo-controlled, double-blind study. J. Dermatol. 25:309-313, 1998.
203. Syed, T. A., Lundin, S., and Ahmad, M.: Topical 0.3% and 0.5% podophyllotoxin cream for self-treatment of molluscum contagiosum in males. A placebo-controlled, double-blind study. Dermatology 189:65-68, 1994.
204. Tabbara, K. F.: Trachoma: Have we advanced in the last 20 years? Int. Ophthalmol. Clin. 30:23-27, 1990.
205. Tabbara, K. F., and Hyndiuk, R. A. (eds.): Infections of the Eye. 2nd ed. Boston, Little, Brown, 1996, pp. 323-347, 361-385, 423-431, 433-478, 603-606.
206. Taber, L. H.: Syphilis. In Kaplan, S. L. (ed.): Current Therapy in Pediatric Infectious Disease. St. Louis, C. V. Mosby, 1993, pp. 243-245.
207. Talley, A. R., Garcia-Ferrer, F., Laycock, K. A., et al.: Comparative diagnosis of neonatal chlamydial conjunctivitis by polymerase chain reaction and McCoy cell culture. Am. J. Ophthalmol. 117:50-57, 1994.
208. Tate, G. W., Jr., and Martin, R. G.: Clindamycin in the treatment of human ocular toxoplasmosis. Can. J. Ophthalmol. 12:188-195, 1977.
209. Taylor, H. R., and Dax, E. M.: Ocular onchocerciasis. In Tabbara, K. F., and Hyndiuk, R. A. (eds.): Infections of the Eye. Boston, Little, Brown, 1996, pp. 673-683.
210. Thomas, P. A.: Fungal infections of the cornea. Eye 17:852-862, 2003.
211. Thompson, W. S., Culbertson, W. W., Smiddy, W. E., et al.: Acute retinal necrosis caused by reactivation of herpes simplex virus type 2. Am. J. Ophthalmol. 118:205-211, 1994.
212. Thorne, J. E., Jabs, D. A., Kempen, J. H., et al.: Incidence of and risk factors for visual acuity loss among patients with AIDS and cytomegalovirus retinitis in the era of highly active antiretroviral therapy. Ophthalmology 113:1432-1440, 2006.
213. Thylefors, B.: Onchocerciasis: An overview. Int. Ophthalmol. Clin. 30:21-22, 1990.
214. Thylefors, B., Dawson, C. R., Jones, B. R., et al.: A simple system for the assessment of trachoma and its complications. Bull. World Health Organ. 65:477-483, 1987.
215. Ur Rehman, S., Anand, S., Reddy, A., et al.: Poststreptococcal syndrome uveitis: A descriptive case series and literature review. Ophthalmology 113:701-706, 2006.
216. Van der Lelij, A., Ooijman, F. M., Kijlstra, A., and Rothova, A.: Anterior uveitis with sectoral iris atrophy in the absence of keratitis. Ophthalmology 107:1164-1170, 2000.
217. Varaprasathan, G., Miller, K., Lietman, T., et al.: Trends in the etiology of infectious corneal ulcers at the F. I. Proctor Foundation. Cornea 23:360-364, 2004.
218. Velazquez, A. J., Goldstein, M. H., and Driebe, W. T.: Preseptal cellulitis caused by Trichophyton (ringworm). Cornea 21:312-314, 2002.
219. Vieira-Dias, D., Sena, C. M., Orefice, F., et al.: Ocular and concomitant cutaneous sporotrichosis. Mycoses 40:197-201, 1997.
220. von Noorden, G. K., and Buck, A. A.: Ocular onchocerciasis: An ophthalmological and epidemiological study in an African village. Arch. Ophthalmol. 80:26-34, 1968.
221. Vu, B. L., Dick, P. T., Levin, A. V., and Pirie, J.: Development of a clinical severity score for preseptal cellulitis in children. Pediatr. Emerg. Care 19:302-307, 2003.
222. Wagner, R. S.: Glaucoma in children. Pediatr. Clin. North Am. 40:855-867, 1993.
223. Wallwork, B., Coman, W., Feron, F., et al.: Clarithromycin and prednisolone inhibit cytokine production in chronic rhinosinusitis. Laryngoscope 112:1827-1830, 2002.
224. Weiss, A., Friendly, D., Eglin, K., et al.: Bacterial periorbital and orbital cellulitis in childhood. Ophthalmology 90:195-203, 1983.
225. Weiss, A., Margo, C. E., Ledford, D. K., et al.: Toxoplasmic retinochoroiditis as an initial manifestation of the acquired immune deficiency syndrome. Am. J. Ophthalmol. 101:248-249, 1986.

226. Wheaton, A. F., Timothy, N. H., Dossett, J. H., and Manders, E. K.: The surgical treatment of molluscum contagiosum in a pediatric AIDS patient. Ann. Plast. Surg. *44*:651-655, 2000.
227. Whitley, R. J.: Herpes simplex virus infections. *In* Remington, J. S., and Klein J. O. (eds.): Infectious Diseases of the Fetus and Newborn Infant. 3rd ed. Philadelphia, W.B. Saunders, 1990.
228. Wiley, L., Springer, D., Kowalski, R. P., et al.: Rapid diagnostic test for ocular adenovirus. Ophthalmology *95*:431-433, 1988.
229. Wilkinson, C. P., and Welch, R. B.: Intraocular *Toxocara*. Am. J. Ophthalmol. *71*:921-930, 1971.
230. Wilson, M. E., and Paul, T. O.: Orbital cellulitis following strabismus surgery. Ophthalmic Surg. *18*:92-94, 1987.
231. Wirostko, W. J., Connor, T. B., and Wagner, P. F.: Recurrent poststreptococcal uveitis. Arch. Ophthalmol. *117*:1649-1650, 1999.
232. Yen, M. T., and Yen, K. G.: Effect of corticosteroids in the acute management of pediatric orbital cellulitis with subperiosteal abscess. Ophthal. Plast. Reconstr. Surg. *21*:363-366; discussion 366-367, 2005.
233. Yoser, S. L., Forster, D. J., and Rao, N. A.: Systemic viral infections and their retinal and choroidal manifestations. Surv. Ophthalmol. *37*:313-352, 1993.
234. Yoshinaga, I. G., Conrado, L. A., Schainberg, S. C., and Grinblat, M.: Recalcitrant molluscum contagiosum in a patient with AIDS: Combined treatment with CO(2) laser, trichloroacetic acid, and pulsed dye laser. Lasers Surg. Med. *27*:291-294, 2000.

CHAPTER
69

BACTEREMIA AND SEPTIC SHOCK
Sheldon L. Kaplan ☼ Jesus G. Vallejo

One of the most serious and potentially life-threatening infectious diseases in childhood is a bacteremic illness. Bacteremia may be caused by a wide variety of gram-positive or gram-negative microorganisms, and it may or may not be associated with a specific focus of infection, such as pneumonia or meningitis. Some bacteremias are transient and self-limited; they are not discussed in this chapter.

The incidence of bacteremia in children has been studied in hospital and ambulatory settings. In otherwise normal children, beyond the newborn age group, *Streptococcus pneumoniae*, *Escherichia coli*, *Staphylococcus aureus*, group A streptococcus, *Salmonella* spp., and *Neisseria meningitidis* are the most common microorganisms causing bacteremia.[99,234] Children with underlying illnesses that depress the host response to infection may develop bacteremia caused by these same microorganisms; however, in this population of children, especially when hospitalized, Enterobacteriaceae, *S. aureus*, coagulase-negative staphylococci, and fungi are the most important organisms commonly isolated from blood cultures.[6,170] Indwelling vascular lines, urinary catheters, endotracheal tubes, and other foreign material further predispose already compromised children to nosocomial infections. The incidence of diagnosed septicemia has increased over the years, partly owing to improved medical technology and the greater numbers of individuals with immunocompromising conditions who previously would not have survived.[160]

Gray and colleagues[91] reported that the incidence of bloodstream infections in a pediatric intensive care unit (ICU) during a 3-year period was 39 cases per 1000 admissions. Of the episodes, 64 percent were acquired in the ICU and 20.6 percent were community-acquired infections. Gram-positive and gram-negative organisms accounted for 62 percent and 31 percent of the isolates. Yeasts were isolated in 5.6 percent of episodes. Children with acquired immunodeficiency syndrome or severe immunosuppression caused by human immunodeficiency virus infection also are at increased risk for developing bacteremias caused by gram-negative bacilli, especially *Pseudomonas aeruginosa*.[189]

Using a seven-state hospital discharge database, Watson and associates[234] estimated that the U.S. age-adjusted and sex-adjusted annual incidence of severe sepsis was 0.56 cases per 1000 children, or more than 42,000 cases per year. The highest age-specific incidence occurred in infants (5.16 cases per 1000), with the incidence declining to 0.20 cases per 1000 for children 10 to 14 years old. Half of the children had underlying comorbidity, with neuromuscular, cardiovascular, and respiratory disorders being the most common.

One potential consequence of bacteremia is septic shock, a state characterized by inadequate tissue perfusion that is associated frequently with endotoxemia. Although most children with septic shock have infections caused by gram-negative enteric bacteria, *P. aeruginosa*, or *N. meningitidis*, organisms with endotoxin or lipopolysaccharide (LPS) within cell walls, septic shock also is associated with disease caused by gram-positive bacteria (especially *S. aureus*, *Streptococcus pyogenes*, and viridans streptococci), viruses, rickettsiae, and fungi. New clones of community-acquired methicillin-resistant *S. aureus* (MRSA) in particular have been associated with severe sepsis and septic shock in young children and adolescents.[87] In adults, the frequency of septic shock continues to increase as the population ages, new technology including more complicated surgery and immunosuppressive agents is developed, and antibiotic resistance grows.[194]

Dupont and Spink[64] reviewed the cases of 172 children, 30 days to 16 years of age, who were hospitalized at the University of Minnesota Medical Center with gram-negative bacteremia. Shock occurred in 25 percent of the children, and 98 percent of children with shock died. In meningococcal infections, 11 to 40 percent of children develop hypotension.[56,116,228] During a 10-month study period, Naqvi and colleagues[157] reported that shock occurred in 5 of 39 (13%) episodes of gram-negative bacillary sepsis, with three deaths. Jacobs and associates[107] reviewed the admissions of previously normal children to a pediatric ICU in a large children's hospital for a 30-month period. Hypotension or evidence of peripheral hypoperfusion occurred in 143 children with confirmed bacterial sepsis, mostly *Haemophilus influenzae* type b (Hib), or apparent meningococcemia. Among 1058 consecutive admissions of 916 children to a pediatric ICU in Canada from July 1, 1991, to July 31, 1992, 25 episodes (2%) of septic shock occurred.[178] During a 12-month period, 140 episodes of septicemia (135 bacterial and 5 fungal) were documented in 100 pediatric hematology-oncology patients.[5] Septic shock occurred in 19 percent.

The organisms and case-fatality rates in the study by Watson and colleagues[234] are outlined in Table 69–1. *N. meningitidis* and fungi were associated with the highest mortality rates. Early-onset group B streptococcal infections in neonates and overwhelming *S. pneumoniae* infections in children with splenic dysfunction or asplenia are associated with shock in a high percentage of cases. *S. aureus* or group A streptococcus may cause hypotension in a child with or without other manifestations of toxic shock syndrome.[202]

Advances in understanding of the pathogenesis and pathophysiology of septic shock with respect to the host response to infection have required that more precise clinical definitions of sepsis and expanded syndromes be developed. Much of the impetus for this effort is related to the ability to identify more readily patients with infections who may benefit from administration of newer (expensive) adjunctive measures. An American College of Chest Physicians and Society of Critical Care Medicine Consensus Conference in 1991 developed new terminology to define sepsis and its sequelae.[28] This terminology has been modified for use in children by an international consensus panel of 20 experts in sepsis and clinical research (Table 69–2).[84]

TABLE 69–1   Occurrence and Case-Fatality Rates of Selected Pathogens among Children with Severe Sepsis Based on Age*

Organism	<1 Year (N = 4643)		1-10 Years (N = 2724)		11-19 Years (N = 2308)	
	Cases (%)	Case-Fatality (%)	Cases (%)	Case-Fatality (%)	Cases (%)	Case-Fatality (%)
Neisseria meningitidis	0.3	20	8	10.4	2.3	15.1
Haemophilus influenzae	1.6	4.2	2.4	1.6	1.9	6.8
Pseudomonas	3.6	14.6	7.7	12.4	6.9	9.4
Staphylococcus aureus	2.3	5.7	2.9	0	3.5	3.8
Group A streptococcus	0.3	0	0.7	5	0.2	0
Group B streptococcus	3.1	7.6	0.1	50	0.8	5.6
Fungus	10	10.8	13.3	16.8	10.4	11.6

*Represents data from a seven-state hospital discharge database in 1995.
Modified from Watson, R. S., Carcillo, J. A., Linde-Zwirble, W. T., et al.: The epidemiology of severe sepsis in children in the United States. Am. J. Respir. Care Med. 167:695-701, 2003.

TABLE 69–2   Consensus Definitions of Systemic Inflammatory Response Syndrome (SIRS), Infection, Sepsis, Severe Sepsis, and Septic Shock

SIRS

The presence of ≥2 of the following 4 criteria, one of which must be abnormal temperature or white blood cell count:
Core temperature (rectal, bladder, oral, or central catheter probe) >38.5°C or <36°C
Tachycardia defined as >2 standard deviations above normal for age in the absence of external factors or drugs; *or* otherwise unexplained persistent elevation of a 0.5- to 4-hr time period; *or* for children <1 yr old, bradycardia defined as a mean heart rate <10th percentile for age in the absence of external factors or drugs or otherwise unexplained persistent depression over a 0.5-hr period
Mean respiratory rate >2 standard deviations for age *or* mechanical ventilation for an acute process not related to an underlying neuromuscular disease or to general anesthesia
Peripheral white blood cell count elevated or depressed for age unrelated to medications or >10% immature neutrophils

Infection

A suspected or proven (by culture, tissue stain, polymerase chain reaction assay) infection caused by any pathogen *or* a clinical syndrome associated with a high probability of infection
Sepsis
SIRS in the presence of or caused by suspected or proven infection
Severe Sepsis
Sepsis plus 1 of the following: cardiovascular organ dysfunction, acute respiratory distress syndrome *or* ≥2 other organ dysfunction as defined in the consensus statement
Septic Shock
Sepsis and cardiovascular organ dysfunction as defined in the consensus statement

Modified from Goldstein, B., Giroir, B., Randoph, A.; and the Members of the International Consensus Conference on Pediatric Sepsis: International pediatric sepsis conference: Definitions for sepsis and organ dysfunction in pediatrics. Pediatr. Crit. Care Med. 6:2-8, 2005.

PATHOPHYSIOLOGY

The pathophysiology of bacteremia is highly variable and depends on the specific microorganism isolated, the immune status of the host, and other factors such as the locations of indwelling catheters. Highly encapsulated organisms, such as *S. pneumoniae*, *N. meningitidis*, and Hib, normally may reside in the nasopharynx and, for reasons that are poorly understood, are capable of invading beyond mucosal barriers into the bloodstream. A preceding viral upper respiratory tract infection may play some role in alterations in local host defense mechanisms that result in bacteremia.[117,143]

Using human columnar nasopharyngeal tissue in organ cultures, Stephens and colleagues[208] showed that *N. meningitidis*

organisms were ingested by the columnar cells, then found within phagocytic vacuoles, and later observed within subepithelial tissues, suggesting that the meningococci had penetrated the epithelial layer. In this same model, Hib organisms attach to nonciliated columnar epithelial cells and subsequently are found in the intercellular spaces in association with a preceding disruption of the tight junctions of epithelial cells.[66] After passing the mucosal barriers, Hib may enter the bloodstream directly through pharyngeal blood vessels.[192] Pneumococci adhere to specific ligands on respiratory cells. The inflammatory mediators generated during viral infections up-regulate platelet-activating factor receptor on respiratory cells to which the pneumococci adhere more avidly and subsequently invade.[223] Pili or adhesins of gram-negative enteric organisms seem to be important in attachment and adherence of these microorganisms to specific receptors expressed on epithelial surfaces. Pili also have been shown to be important in the pathogenesis of some gram-positive infections, such as *S. pyogenes*, group B streptococcus, and *S. pneumoniae*.[18,152]

The placement of an endotracheal tube unmasks a greater number of these receptors, presumably through increased protease activity of secretions and decreased cell-bound fibronectin, and leads to colonization of the upper respiratory tract with gram-negative organisms, which are ubiquitous in the environment of an ICU.[244] Altered host defense mechanisms allow these organisms to move beyond epithelial surfaces and cause bacteremia.

The gastrointestinal and genitourinary tracts are major sources of gram-negative organisms responsible for bacteremia. These organisms first may cause localized abscesses or peritonitis if intestinal perforation occurs, or they may translocate the intestinal mucosa, particularly when the mucosa is affected by antineoplastic agents. Viridans streptococci can cause bacteremia in a neutropenic patient with severe mucositis that develops after the patient undergoes chemotherapy.[204] Microorganisms within the bladder may ascend the genitourinary tract and presumably enter the bloodstream through the kidneys. *S. aureus* and *S. pyogenes* are common inhabitants of the skin and skin structures. Any skin wound or foreign matter within the skin tissue renders the skin more susceptible to bacterial invasion. Staphylococci have a unique capability of adhering to solid surfaces, such as catheters, which may be an important prerequisite to colonization and subsequent catheter-related bacteremia.[173]

The pathophysiology of septic shock is very complex. Septic shock associated with gram-negative organisms has been studied most extensively, especially with respect to endotoxin or bacterial LPS, which has multiple biologic effects. Bacterial LPS has three basic components, as follows:

1. Terminal side chains consist of repeating oligosaccharides that differ from strain to strain and are responsible for the antigenic specificity of the O antigens.

2. A core LPS also consists of oligosaccharides but has less diversity in structure among strains than do the terminal side chains.

3. Lipid A is very similar among the different strains and is responsible for most of the biologic activity of endotoxin.

Endotoxin shock has been the subject of intensive animal research, and much of what is known about the pathogenesis of endotoxin shock has been derived from animal models. Although septic shock in humans is not simulated precisely in these animal models because the animals do not have underlying host defense defects, much of what has been learned about endotoxin shock in animals has been corroborated in the human host.

ENDOTOXIN SHOCK IN ANIMALS

Most animal models of endotoxin shock employ infusions of live gram-negative bacteria, usually *Escherichia coli*, or purified endotoxin, after which observations are made. The effects of purified endotoxin depend partly on the species of animal being studied. The effects of endotoxin in animal models are summarized in Table 69–3.

Numerous mediators induced by endotoxin play pivotal roles in the pathogenesis of endotoxin shock. Tumor necrosis factor (TNF) or cachectin, a polypeptide hormone, is a key cytokine mediating septic shock.[219] The tissue injury induced by TNF largely is a result of other mediators that are induced by TNF, including interleukin-1β (IL-1β), IL-6, eicosanoids, and platelet-activating factor.[62,103,217,220] TNF is synthesized by a wide variety of cells (including monocytes/macrophages, natural killer cells, microglial cells, hepatic Kupffer cells) after stimulation by LPS, C5a, viruses, and enterotoxins, among other agents. TNF initiates a cascade of events that leads to endothelial cell injury, an

enhanced inflammatory response, and, ultimately, the characteristic findings of endotoxic shock.

Nitric oxide (i.e., endothelium-derived relaxing factor) is the final pathway by which endogenous vasodilators stimulated by endotoxin result in hypotension from altered control of microcirculation. LPS through the release of cytokines induces a form of the enzyme nitric oxide synthase II, which leads to increased production of nitric oxide.[150] Inhibitors of nitric oxide synthase, such as N^G-monomethyl-l-arginine, can reverse or prevent hypotension in animals challenged with LPS.[142]

The pathophysiology of septic shock caused by gram-positive bacteria is similar to that described for gram-negative organisms.[206] Cell wall components, such as peptidoglycan and teichoic acid, promote proinflammatory activity, but are less potent than endotoxin.

ENDOTOXIN SHOCK IN HUMANS

The pathophysiology of septic shock is highly complex and is related predominantly to actions of endogenous mediators released as part of the systemic inflammatory response to an infection. The cascade of events is intertwining, with production of one cytokine stimulating the synthesis of others; synergistic, in that the activities of certain cytokines act in concert; and sometimes antagonistic, with the production of other molecules to inhibit or compete with various cytokines. This complicated response to an infectious stimulus has been studied best for LPS, but a similar series of events occurs in response to gram-positive infections. Although the best understood system is the one that recognizes bacterial LPS, others exist for sensing the presence of bacterial peptidoglycan, DNA, lipopeptides, flagella, viral double-stranded RNA, and other conserved microbial molecules.

The first host protein involved in the recognition of LPS is LPS-binding protein. LPS-binding protein is an acute-phase protein; its role is to bring LPS to the cell surface by binding to LPS and forming a ternary complex with the LPS receptor molecule, CD14.[235,245] Formation of the complex between LPS and CD14 facilitates the transfer of LPS to the LPS receptor complex, which is composed of toll-like receptor 4 (TLR4) and MD2. Studies over the course of several years led to the discovery of the TLR4/MD2 receptor complex as the signaling entity for LPS (Fig. 69–1).[23,24] MD2 is a secreted glycoprotein that functions as an indispensable extracellular adapter molecule for LPS-initiated signaling events, perhaps by aiding in ligand recognition. The resulting signal promotes mononuclear phagocytes to produce reactive oxygen molecules, cytokines, and arachidonic acid metabolites, including prostaglandin and leukotrienes. A counterregulatory protein is a bactericidal, permeability-increasing protein that is stored in the granules of polymorphonuclear leukocytes and inhibits the effects of LPS.[77]

TNF is largely responsible for the biologic effects, including fever, shock, myocardial suppression, capillary leak (i.e., endothelial damage), coagulation alterations, and metabolic changes,[39,40,144,177,218] of LPS in humans. In children, including neonates, the role of cytokines in sepsis caused by a variety of organisms, but especially *N. meningitidis*, is well-documented.[34,56,81,213,228] LPS and TNF each can induce the synthesis of other proinflammatory cytokines, such as IL-1β and IL-6.[63] IL-6 levels in plasma correlate with mortality. IL-8 plasma concentrations also are increased after infusion of LPS or IL-1β.[63,93]

The anti-inflammatory cytokine IL-10 is produced after LPS is injected and inhibits the production of TNF, IL-1β, and IL-6.[138] Naturally occurring inhibitors of TNF or IL-1β are present in serum samples of patients with the sepsis syndrome.[59,60,83] IL-1 receptor antagonist (IL-1a) binds competitively to the IL-1

TABLE 69–3   Endotoxin Shock in Animal Models

Effects	Mediators
Cardiovascular Effects	
Decreased peripheral vascular resistance[158]	Histamine, bradykinin,[145] serotonin, complement activation, prostaglandins, anaphylatoxins
Decreased cardiac output[8,13,180]	
Depressed myocardial function[140]	
Decreased systemic blood pressure[48]	
Metabolic Effects[180]	
Hyperglycemia[54]	Hypoinsulinemia
Hypoglycemia[70]	
Increased adrenocorticotropic hormone, growth hormone, and antidiuretic hormone[241]	
Decreased calcium[213]	
Increased triglycerides[97]	
Decreased iron, transferrin, and zinc	
Pulmonary Effects	
Congestive atelectasis[29]	Polymorphonuclear leukocytes
Increased capillary permeability[32,101]	Polymorphonuclear leukocytes
Vasoconstriction	Thromboxane, prostacyclin
Bronchoconstriction[23]	Leukotrienes
Central Nervous System Effects	
Decreased regional and total cerebral blood flow[158]	
Increased cerebral oxygen consumption[179]	

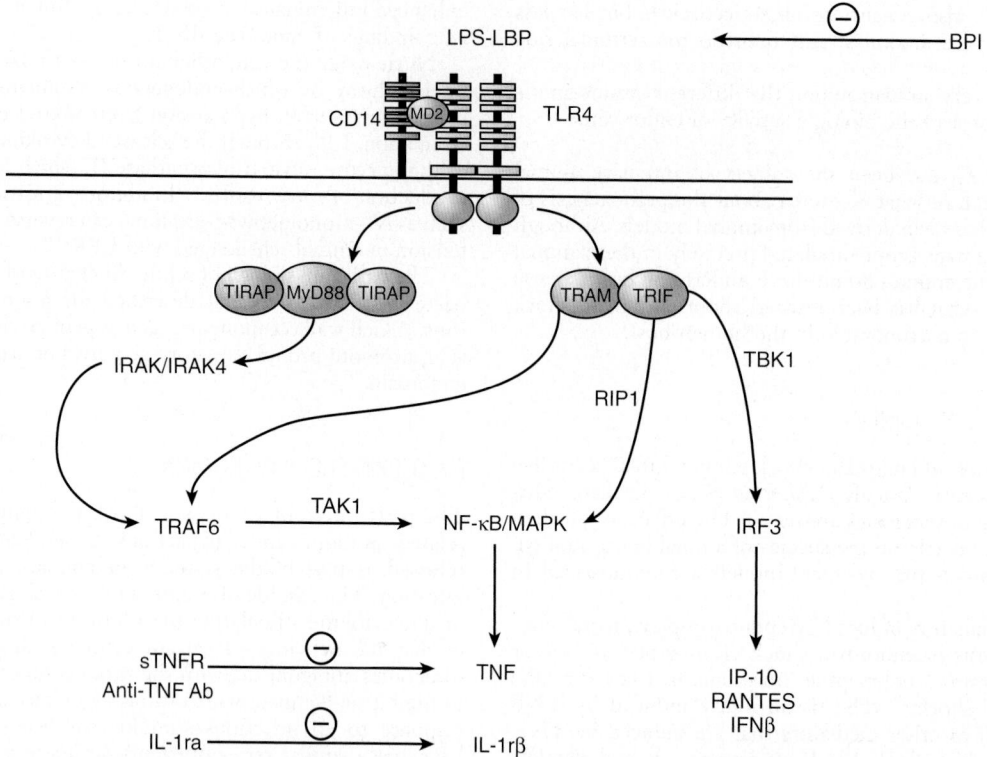

Figure 69–1 Activation of the cytokine network by lipopolysaccharide (LPS). Circulating lipopolysaccharide-binding protein (LBP) recognizes LPS in the plasma and brings it to CD14. This aids the loading of LPS onto the LPS receptor complex, which is composed of dimerized toll-like receptor 4 (TLR4) receptors and two molecules of the extracellular adapter MD-2. Signals activated by TLR4 can be subdivided into signals dependent on MyD88 (and Mal), which occur early (represented by the events illustrated on the left-hand side of the diagram), and signals independent of MyD88, which occur later and use the adapters TRIF and TRAM (depicted on the right). IL-1ra, interleukin-1 receptor antagonist; sTNFr, soluble tumor necrosis factor receptor.

receptor to block the action of IL-1. Soluble TNF receptors bind to circulating TNF, which prevents its proinflammatory actions (see Fig. 69-1).

In humans, gram-negative bacteremia is followed by a decrease in systemic vascular resistance and mean blood pressure and an increase in cardiac output.[24,237] Decreased systemic vascular resistance may be accompanied by activation of the complement and kinin systems.[145] After this early phase, the blood pressure decreases further without change in the central venous pressure. Certain patients, especially children, are able to maintain their cardiac output and cardiac index, and this ability may be associated with increased rates of survival. When peripheral resistance is measured within 12 to 24 hours of the onset of shock, its decrease is significant in patients who survive compared with patients who die.[162] In contrast, cardiac output is reduced significantly in other patients; this decrease is associated with increased concentration of blood lactate, decreased arterial blood pH, and decreased rates of survival.

Depression of myocardial function has been shown in adult and pediatric patients in septic shock.[69] These patients have a reduced ejection fraction, left ventricular dilation, and significantly altered ventricular performance in response to infusion of volume.[164] This depression of myocardial function is transient in survivors, however, reverting to normal within 1 to 4 days.[167] Parker and colleagues[168] found that patients who did not survive septic shock did not have left ventricular dilation or reduction in the ejection fraction. When the systemic vascular resistance index was averaged over the course of time, nonsurvivors had a significantly ($p < 0.05$) lower index than that of survivors of septic shock. This study included three children who were 9 to 17 years of age. Abraham and associates[1] sequentially monitored hemodynamic

and oxygen transport measurements in 33 patients with septic shock. In the 24-hour period before the onset of hypotension, the survivors showed significantly greater cardiac index, left cardiac work index, oxygen delivery, and oxygen consumption than the nonsurvivors.

A circulating myocardial depressant factor in patients with septic shock was proposed more than 50 years ago, but myocardial dysfunction was not quantitatively linked to a serum factor until the late 1980s.[140,169,181] Kumar and colleagues[121] later reported that the myocardial depressant activity of sera obtained from patients with septic shock could be eliminated by the immunoprecipitation of TNF and IL-1β. Several investigators also have shown that TNF and IL-1β synergistically depress myocardial function in vitro, and that this effect can be abolished by an inhibitor of nitric oxide.[38,166] Germane to this discussion is the observation that LPS-induced biosynthesis of TNF mRNA and protein is not strictly confined to peripheral mononuclear cells but also may occur within many different tissue compartments. Experimental studies have shown that the cardiac compartment can be a significant source of TNF during septic shock. Kapadia and colleagues[111] showed that administration of LPS leads to intramyocardial production of TNF mRNA and protein in vivo.

These observations raise the possibility that the myocardial depression occurring in sepsis may develop directly in response to the compartmentalized production of TNF and other cytokines within the heart, as opposed to systemic production of these mediators by circulating mononuclear cells. TLR4 is expressed in the heart, and investigators have suggested that it is involved in signaling the cytokine production induced by LPS within the heart.[20]

In children, the most comprehensive investigation of myocardial dysfunction has been in meningococcal septic shock. Thiru and coworkers[214] measured serum concentrations of the cardiac muscle–specific protein cardiac troponin I, which is released from injured cardiac myocytes, in 101 children with meningococcal septicemia. Minimum left ventricular ejection fraction was inversely related to peak cardiac troponin I levels. The degree of myocardial dysfunction, as determined by inotrope measurement, was related directly to peak cardiac troponin I concentrations. Their results suggested that myocardial cell death might contribute, at least in part, to the cardiac dysfunction associated with meningococcal septic shock.

Hematologic changes, such as leukocytosis, leukopenia, and thrombocytopenia, have been observed in human volunteers after receiving an infusion of endotoxin. Thrombocytopenia commonly occurs in association with sepsis of any cause.[50] Septic shock is one of the most common causes of disseminated intravascular coagulation in children. Hageman factor (i.e., factor XII), which initiates the coagulation cascade, can be activated directly by LPS or through endothelial damage induced by bacteria.[134] In septic shock, concentrations of Hageman factor, prekallikrein, high-molecular-weight kininogen, and factor VII are decreased partly as a result of consumption.[53,110] Similarly, levels of inactivators of clotting factors, such as C1 esterase inhibitor, α_2-macroglobulin, and antithrombin III, also are diminished. Corrigan and Jordan[53] diagnosed disseminated intravascular coagulation in 24 of 26 children with septic shock and found that improvement in coagulation parameters seemed to be related most to restoration of blood pressure. Gram-negative bacteremia may be associated with a coagulopathy that is not disseminated intravascular coagulation but is characterized by prolongation of the prothrombin and partial thromboplastin times caused by a reduction in the vitamin K–dependent coagulation factors.[52]

LPS or cell wall components of gram-positive organisms, through cytokine production, activate blood coagulation predominantly through the extrinsic pathway. The procoagulant state is enhanced further by decreased protein C activity, which is an important inhibitor of coagulation factors Va and VIIIa. The fibrinolytic system also is altered by endotoxemia and is mediated by plasminogen activator inhibitor 1–induced suppression. The coagulopathy associated with septic shock is characterized by a procoagulant state and inhibition of fibrinolysis.[125,130] Protein C has anti-inflammatory properties. The antithrombotic, profibrinolytic, and anti-inflammatory actions of activated protein C counteract the effects of cytokine activation, but a deficiency of protein C may be acquired during severe sepsis. Low levels of protein C have been associated with increased morbidity and mortality rates in patients with severe sepsis and septic shock.[73] For meningococcal disease in particular, dysfunction of the protein C activation pathway is a key factor in the development of the thrombosis associated with purpura fulminans. Downregulation of the endothelial thrombomodulin–endothelial protein C receptor pathway seems to be the mechanism for impaired activation of protein C during severe meningococcal sepsis.[67]

LPS can activate the complement cascade by the classic or the alternate pathway. Significantly depressed concentrations of C3 occur in patients with bacteremia and hypotension compared with normal individuals or with patients with uncomplicated bacteremia, and C3 is activated primarily by the alternate pathway.[68,110,136] In patients with bacteremia and hypotension, C1, C4, and C2 levels were not depressed significantly from values found in normal controls or in normotensive patients with bacteremia. In contrast, C3, C5, C6, C9, properdin, and factor B levels were decreased significantly ($p < 0.05$) in bacteremic patients with shock. In children with meningococcal disease, Tubbs[222] found a mean C3 concentration (as a percentage of

normal values) of 132 ± 21 percent for survivors versus 91 ± 21 percent for nonsurvivors. The C3 levels did not correlate with endotoxin levels in sera.

Many metabolic alterations have been documented in the human host during endotoxin shock. Hyperglycemia followed by hypoglycemia can complicate the shock state induced by sepsis.[70,146] Whole-body use of glucose is increased during sepsis, which probably is cytokine-mediated.[147] Glycolysis and gluconeogenesis are increased, but insulin resistance occurs in skeletal muscle. Children with underlying liver disease or with reduced glycogen stores are most likely to develop hypoglycemia during septic shock. Lactic acidosis develops as a result of poor tissue perfusion and cellular hypoxia. Lactic acid concentrations are increased in nonsurvivors and patients with poor or low-flow cardiac output during sepsis.

In clinical studies, Clowes and associates[47] identified a subgroup of patients with low-flow septic shock in whom concentrations of serum insulin were lower than concentrations in a control population. In children with meningococcal sepsis, van Waardenburg and colleagues[225] found higher blood glucose concentrations and significantly lower insulin levels on day 2 or 3 of hospitalization in children with shock compared with children without shock. Levels of plasma insulin and soluble TNF receptor 75 were inversely correlated in these children. Their findings were consistent with the inflammatory response inhibiting insulin secretion.

Hypocalcemia and decreased serum ionized calcium concentrations occur frequently during bacterial sepsis. In one study, 12 (20%) of 60 critically ill adults with bacterial sepsis had hypocalcemia.[247] The mortality rate in the hypocalcemic patients was 50 percent compared with 30 percent in the patients who were normocalcemic. Cardenas-Rivero and associates[42] studied calcium homeostasis in 145 children admitted to an ICU. Of eight children with confirmed sepsis or meningitis (or both) not caused by Hib, seven had hypocalcemia, and six of seven had ionized hypocalcemia. Five of the six children with ionized hypocalcemia had inappropriately normal concentrations of parathyroid hormone, which suggests that transient hypoparathyroidism occurs in some children with sepsis. Hypocalcemia also occurs commonly in patients with toxic shock syndrome.[240] In women with toxic shock syndrome and hypocalcemia, serum concentrations of calcitonin are elevated by unknown mechanisms.[45] Hypocalcemia and elevated calcitonin concentrations also have been documented in children with fulminant meningococcemia.[131]

Procalcitonin levels are elevated in several conditions associated with systemic inflammatory response syndrome, including sepsis, and have been proposed as adjunctive laboratory tests for the early detection of, and indicators for prognosis of, meningococcal disease.[43,96,122] These changes in calcium levels are especially critical because the level of ionized calcium and cardiac output in septic shock can be correlated.[243] Other metabolic changes may occur during septic shock in humans, as follows:

1. Increased concentrations of cortisol and growth hormone (including in neonates[215])[229]
2. Depression of triiodothyronine and thyroxine levels related to poor nutrition[186]
3. Elevations in total concentrations of amino acid in plasma and the preferential use of branched-chain amino acids as an energy source for skeletal muscle[147]
4. Muscle proteolysis, possibly induced by one or more circulating agents in the plasma of patients with serious infections[46]
5. Elevations in concentrations of plasma thromboxane, which are observed in nonsurvivors of septic shock[183]
6. Elevations in concentrations of triglycerides and free fatty acid during gram-negative bacteremia[78,118]

Liver dysfunction is an important aspect of endotoxin shock in adults. Banks and colleagues[16] found that clinical jaundice was apparent in 63 percent of their patients with septic shock, that it was found more commonly in nonsurvivors than in survivors, and that the degree of biochemical liver abnormalities was related to the duration of shock. Postmortem findings included focal liver necrosis, Kupffer cell hyperplasia, portal tract inflammation, venous congestion, and intrahepatic cholestasis.

Adult respiratory distress syndrome (ARDS), or shock lung, is a major complication of septic shock in children.[104,175] The lungs of children with ARDS have characteristic changes consisting of increased lung weight reflecting congestion and atelectasis, alveoli lined with hyaline membranes, microthrombi, hemorrhage, and interstitial edema.[104] Increased capillary permeability and intrapulmonary shunts have been documented in patients with ARDS.[4,55] C5a, a potent chemotactic factor, causes aggregation of polymorphonuclear neutrophils, is elevated in the sera of patients who ultimately develop ARDS, and is found in increased concentrations in bronchoalveolar lavage fluid obtained from patients with ARDS.[94,187] Leukocyte aggregates are thought to be trapped in lung tissue and may cause damage to the endothelium of the pulmonary microvasculature through the release of oxygen radicals, lysosomal enzymes, and products of arachidonic acid metabolism. Although neutrophils play a critical role in the pathogenesis of ARDS, other factors also are important, considering that ARDS can develop in patients who are neutropenic.[163,238] Thromboxane, platelet-activating factor, fibrin, and other substances contribute to the lung injury in ARDS.[190]

The effects of endotoxin shock on the central nervous system have not been studied carefully in humans.[90] The encephalopathy associated with sepsis seems to be caused partly by altered phenylalanine metabolism; concentrations of phenylalanine and its metabolite, phenylacetic acid, are increased in the sera and cerebrospinal fluid of septic adults who are stuporous or comatose.[148]

Endotoxin has been implicated in the pathogenesis of acute renal failure associated with sepsis. Wardle[231,232] showed that 12 of 16 patients with acute tubular necrosis had endotoxemia. Renal arterial blood flow and renal vascular resistance are decreased significantly in baboons 2 to 4 hours after infusion of endotoxin. Inadequate perfusion pressure was associated with renal ischemia and negligible urine output in these animals shortly after administration of endotoxin.[197] Pathologic examination of the kidneys revealed focal necrosis of the proximal tubular epithelium, eosinophilic casts within proximal and distal tubules, and microthrombi in the glomerular capillaries. Endothelin, a potent vasoconstrictor peptide produced by endothelial cells, is elevated in concentration in the plasma of patients with septic shock. Because endothelin contributes to the regulation of regional blood flow, elevated levels suggest that it may relate to renal vasoconstriction and dysfunction.[227]

Endotoxin can be measured in the plasma of patients with gram-negative bacteremia. The presence of circulating endotoxin does not mean that bacteremia is present or ever has occurred because endotoxin presumably may be "absorbed or leak" into the circulation from the gastrointestinal tract.[126,211,221] Endotoxemia may be a valid indicator, however, of impending gram-negative septicemia in febrile patients.[61] Preformed antibody to LPS or lipid A is associated with protection against shock and death caused by gram-negative bacteremia in adults. McCartney and colleagues[138] detected endotoxin in the blood (after chloroform extraction) of patients with gram-negative septic shock; all 18 patients with persistently positive endotoxin assays died. In contrast, nine patients who initially had endotoxemia but subsequently had negative assays survived. Other studies confirm the association between endotoxemia and outcome.[123] Evidence exists that human endotoxin is cleared from the circulation by the liver

and can be detoxified by neutrophil enzymes (i.e., acyloxacyl hydrolases).[135,153]

The sequence of events in the evolution of endotoxin shock has been outlined by several investigators.[159] Bacteria, endotoxin, or other bacterial products stimulate the production of TNF and other cytokines, which in concert with endotoxin set off a whole series of events. Potent mediators, including C3a, C5a, eicosanoids, platelet-activating factor, histamine, and myocardial depressant substance, are released. Potent vasodilators cause peripheral vasodilation, and decreased systemic peripheral resistance leads to pooling of blood and decreased venous return to the heart. Mean blood pressure may be low, or it may be normal if cardiac output increases sufficiently to compensate for these alterations despite depression of ventricular function. The central venous pressure, which partially depends on myocardial performance, may be low or in the normal range.

If intravascular volume is increased by the administration of sufficient fluids, shock may be prevented or corrected. Continued hypotension and diminished perfusion pressure may lead, however, to cellular hypoxia and increased production of lactic acid from pyruvate. The microcirculation is altered by local tissue acidosis. Capillary beds become congested, and intravascular fluid may leak into the interstitial spaces. Increased secretion of catecholamine leads to arteriolar and venular constriction and increased peripheral resistance. Pooling of blood is enhanced, which leads to a further diminution in venous return and a reduction of cardiac output. Oliguria, coagulation abnormalities, and additional metabolic alterations indicate multiple organ system failure and presage the death of the patient.

CLINICAL PRESENTATION AND DIAGNOSIS

The signs and symptoms of bacteremia vary, greatly depending on the age and underlying disease of the patient, the duration of illness, and the specific microorganisms. Young, otherwise healthy children aged 3 months to 3 years may present with fever and evidence of an upper or lower respiratory tract infection or no focus of infection and yet have unsuspected bacteremia. Most studies indicated that the risk of developing bacteremia increases as the body temperature increases and that after the temperature exceeds 41°C, almost 25 percent of these children may be bacteremic.[19] In a previously healthy child, the persistence of irritability and the inability to console the child despite optimal environmental conditions have been proposed as key points in the physical examination that should alert the clinician to the possibility of a serious infection, such as bacteremia or meningitis.[137,203]

Underlying illnesses with splenic dysfunction place a child at increased risk for acquisition of infections caused by encapsulated organisms, whereas children with leukemia or other immunosuppressive diseases or children in the ICU are more likely to be infected with gram-negative bacilli or S. aureus. A history of diarrhea may suggest Salmonella spp. as a possible cause of illness. Preceding skin infections or wounds are important clues to infection caused by S. aureus or group A streptococcus. An indwelling vascular catheter may precipitate overlying erythema in a patient with evidence of phlebitis proximally. Gram-positive cocci and gram-negative bacilli can be associated with catheter-related sepsis.[199] Toxic shock syndrome should be considered in a hypotensive girl or woman with a recent menstrual period and history of tampon use, although toxic shock also is associated with S. aureus sepsis in males and nonmenstruating females.[87,202] Evidence of osteomyelitis, with or without venous thrombosis, is a very common finding in staphylococcal sepsis.[88] Intra-abdominal sources of infection increase the likelihood of developing anaerobic bacteremia.

Petechiae may be associated with many microorganisms, especially invasive disease caused by *N. meningitidis*.[161] Purpura is an ominous finding and frequently is associated with overwhelming infection caused by *N. meningitidis*, *S. pneumoniae*, and Hib. *P. aeruginosa* is associated specifically with erythema gangrenosum. Almost half of children presenting with erythroderma (diffuse erythema) either had shock at presentation or developed shock in one study.[37] Other skin and soft tissue manifestations of gram-negative sepsis include bullous lesions, cellulitis, fasciitis, thrombophlebitis, and symmetrical peripheral gangrene with disseminated intravascular coagulation.[154] Signs of meningeal irritation or increased intracranial pressure are important because they may modify the approach to management of fluids in a child in shock.

The onset of bacteremia may be heralded by chills, fever, nausea, vomiting, diarrhea, rashes, and petechiae. Initially, the skin feels warm and appears flushed. A change or impairment in mental status may be the first clue to the presence of shock. Hyperventilation also may develop before the onset of clinical shock occurs, which can alert the physician to impending circulatory insufficiency.[25] In time, cold, clammy extremities; a weak pulse; tachycardia; tachypnea; hypotension; and oliguria may occur. The skin over the extremities, the tip of the nose, and the earlobes especially are prone to cyanosis. Auscultation of the lungs may reveal rales, indicating pneumonia or pulmonary edema. Abnormal distention or tenderness to palpation and guarding may be evidence of peritonitis. Costovertebral angle tenderness suggests acute pyelonephritis as a source of bacteremias.

The physician must distinguish among the following three main types of shock in children:

1. *Hypovolemic shock*, such as occurs with blood loss, fluid and electrolyte loss, adrenal insufficiency, or other causes
2. *Cardiogenic shock*, which is associated with drug intoxication, cardiac surgery, arrhythmias, and pericardial tamponade, among other causes
3. *Distributive shock*, which indicates abnormal distribution of blood flow leading to inadequate tissue perfusion (e.g., septic shock, anaphylaxis)

The laboratory evaluation of a child with bacteremia, septic shock, or both conditions should provide information concerning the cause and the data required for optimal supportive management. Several studies showed that a total white blood cell (WBC) count exceeding 15,000 cells/mm^3 in a 3- to 36-month-old child with a temperature greater than 39°C to 40°C and without a focus of infection is an indication that the child is at increased risk for having bacteremia, especially pneumococcal bacteremia.[17] Since the introduction of the pneumococcal conjugate vaccine, pneumococcal bacteremia in this scenario has been greatly reduced.[99,196,210] An erythrocyte sedimentation rate greater than 30 mm/hr and C-reactive protein levels also have been suggested as useful screening tools for detecting serious bacterial infections. A low peripheral WBC count also may suggest septicemia and commonly is observed during episodes of overwhelming bacteremic illnesses.

Procalcitonin levels are elevated in bacteremic children and are related to the severity of illness, such as organ failure and even mortality.[96,122] Commercial kits for the rapid measurement of concentrations of procalcitonin are available in some countries. Hemoglobin and hematocrit results should help differentiate between septic and hemorrhagic shock. Examination of the peripheral smear may disclose evidence of splenic dysfunction (i.e., Howell-Jolly bodies) or fragmented red blood cells, as seen in disseminated intravascular coagulation. Thrombocytopenia, prolongation of prothrombin time and partial prothrombin time, and the presence of fibrin split products are consistent with disseminated intravascular coagulation.[42]

Hyponatremia is a common finding. Concentrations of serum bicarbonate may be depressed, which may signify a state of metabolic acidosis. Elevated lactic acid concentrations result from inadequate tissue perfusion, and in some reports have been significantly greater in nonsurvivors or patients with low-flow states than in survivors or patients with high-flow shock.[47] In pediatric studies, serial lactate levels showing normalization are associated with recovery.[30] Hyperglycemia or hypoglycemia may be encountered. In one study, serum glucose levels greater than 178 mg/dL were associated with a greater risk of death caused by septic shock.[31] Transaminase levels may be elevated and presumably reflect cellular injury. Serum calcium concentrations (preferably ionized calcium levels) should be checked periodically because hypocalcemia may interfere with optimal myocardial function.

A chest radiograph may reveal a pulmonary source of infection or show a secondary pulmonary manifestation of an invasive infection such as pneumonia or septic emboli in children with staphylococcal sepsis.[86] Arterial blood gases obtained early in endotoxin shock usually reveal hypocapnia and normal to elevated pH.[25,26] At this point, the patient has a mixed metabolic acidosis and respiratory alkalosis. If the shock state progresses, the metabolic acidosis becomes so severe that respiratory compensation is ineffective, and the patient becomes acidotic. In some patients, respiratory acidosis accompanies metabolic acidosis. In either case, decompensated metabolic acidosis in a patient with septic shock is associated with a grave prognosis. A major consequence of ARDS is hypoxemia. For patients with ARDS, the chest radiograph characteristically shows bilateral and diffuse hazy infiltrates; opacification of all lung fields usually is seen during the late phases of ARDS.

Concentrations of blood urea nitrogen and serum creatinine may be elevated. Jones and Weil[109] found that the ratio of urine to plasma osmolality was the most valuable indicator of renal impairment in adult patients with shock. When this ratio was greater than 1.5, the likelihood of developing progressive renal failure was remote. A urine osmolality value greater than 400 mOsm/kg also indicated adequate renal function. Many WBCs or WBC casts in the urine may suggest the genitourinary tract as the source of bacteremia. If one or more gram-negative rods are seen on the Gram stain of unspun urine, more than 10^5 colony-forming units/mL of bacteria are likely to be present.

Isolating the organism responsible for bacteremia or septic shock is important for documenting the infection and for providing optimal antimicrobial therapy. With instruments that continuously monitor growth in the blood culture bottles, growth can be detected sooner than if the bottles are inspected just once or twice daily. Before the use of the pneumococcal conjugate vaccine became routine, many authorities recommended that a blood culture be obtained in a 3- to 36-month-old child with temperature greater than 39°C to 40°C and a total WBC count greater than or equal to 15,000 cells/mm^3 and without a specific focus of infection. In this way, instances of "unsuspected" or "outpatient" bacteremia could be identified. In an outpatient setting, almost 90 percent of blood cultures growing true pathogens were positive within 24 hours of incubation using a continuously monitored system.[141] This approach is now less useful in the era of administration of pneumococcal conjugate vaccine to young infants.

In an infant who has received three or more doses of the conjugate pneumococcal vaccine, the likelihood of developing invasive pneumococcal infection is reduced approximately 90 percent. The proportion of children with high fever without localizing findings and a WBC count of 15,000/mm^3 or greater who might have occult pneumococcal bacteremia may be less than 1 percent, a level that no longer justifies this approach. Most organisms isolated from blood cultures in these patients are now more likely to be a contaminant than a true pathogen. Currently, the approach to a febrile child without a source has changed in many emergency departments such that more selective criteria for obtaining blood cultures are being developed.

When appropriate, cerebrospinal fluid, urine, and other pertinent sites should be cultured before initiating antibiotic therapy, if possible. When an intra-abdominal source of infection is likely, blood and other cultures should be processed anaerobically. Gram stain or acridine orange stain of a buffy coat smear of peripheral blood may reveal evidence of the causative microorganism, especially in an overwhelming infection.[119] Gram stain of material obtained from petechial or purpuric lesions may show gram-negative diplococci suggestive of meningococcus. Polymerase chain reaction for detecting *N. meningitidis* is available in selected laboratories and may be the only method by which infection is documented when cultures are sterile. Bacterial polysaccharide antigens can be detected rapidly in many body fluids by latex agglutination tests. Rapid diagnostic procedures for evaluating outpatients with suspected bacteremia are unreliable. Pneumococcal antigenuria is not detected readily when bacteremia occurs without a specific focus of infection. The value of assays for detecting circulating endotoxin is unclear.

TREATMENT

The initial selection of antibiotics for administration to a child with suspected bacteremia is based on the clinical situation (Table 69–4). If untreated initially, children with occult bacteremia are at risk of developing serious complications, such as meningitis or pneumonia.[133,155] Empiric antibiotic therapy for children who are selected carefully and followed seems reasonable.[17] Two prospective studies of empiric administration of penicillin or amoxicillin in this situation reached different conclusions, however.[44,108] Ceftriaxone has been compared with amoxicillin or amoxicillin-clavulanate in two large studies involving children 3 to 36 months old. Ceftriaxone was marginally superior at best to the oral agents with regard to efficacy.[19,74]

In children who have not received more than two doses of the pneumococcal conjugate vaccine, one approach may be to obtain a blood culture from children aged 3 to 36 months with a temperature of 39°C or greater who have no focal findings and whose peripheral WBC count is greater than or equal to 15,000/mm³. In such patients, the decision to administer antibiotics expectantly may be based on several factors, especially the ability of the parents to observe the child and communicate this information back to the physician in a timely manner.

TABLE 69–4   Empiric Antibiotic Regimens for Septic Shock in Infants and Children under Selected Clinical Circumstances

Circumstances	Antibiotics
Normal Child	
Skin findings suggesting meningococcemia or preceding skin trauma or varicella	Cefotaxime or ceftriaxone + vancomycin ± nafcillin
Urinary tract source	Cefotaxime or ceftriaxone + aminoglycoside
Intra-abdominal source	Clindamycin + gentamicin + ampicillin or piperacillin or piperacillin-tazobactam
Immunocompromised Child	
Malignancy or immunodeficiency or neutropenia or central line	Vancomycin + aminoglycoside + ticarcillin-clavulanate piperacillin-tazobactam or ceftazidime
Asplenia or splenic dysfunction	Vancomycin + cefotaxime or ceftriaxone

Ceftriaxone given parenterally, an oral agent such as amoxicillin and amoxicillin-clavulanate, or other oral antibiotics can be administered. If treatment is initiated, a properly collected urine specimen for urinalysis or urine culture also should be obtained so that a urinary tract infection would not be treated inadvertently. Occult bacteremia caused by *S. pneumoniae* intermediate or resistant to penicillin or intermediate to ceftriaxone in an otherwise normal child should resolve with any of the options noted earlier.[115] This approach probably is less useful in an infant or child who has received three or more doses of the conjugate pneumococcal vaccine.

Children who subsequently are determined to have *S. pneumoniae* bacteremia and who have been treated with antibiotics expectantly need to be re-evaluated as soon as the results of the blood cultures are known. If the child appears well and has been afebrile for at least 24 hours and if the parents can observe the child carefully and are able to communicate frequently with the physician, outpatient management can be continued. For children who were not treated initially, who remain febrile, and who are called back to be re-evaluated for a positive blood culture, a parenteral dose of antibiotics is recommended.[15] Close contact with the parents and patient is mandatory no matter how these children are managed initially. Hospitalization for intravenous antibiotics is indicated if the child appears "toxic" or has other signs suggesting a serious infection.

For children with suspected bacteremia who are ill and require admission to the hospital, antibiotics are selected to cover the most serious organisms causing that infection. In normal children aged 3 months or older, a combination of nafcillin (150 to 200 mg/kg/day) or another semisynthetic antistaphylococcal penicillin plus cefotaxime (150 to 200 mg/kg/day) or ceftriaxone (75 to 100 mg/kg/day) covers most of the likely pathogens (e.g., *S. pneumoniae, S. aureus, S. pyogenes, N. meningitidis*, Hib). In areas of the United States where community-acquired MRSA is a problem, an agent effective against MRSA should be included in the initial empiric regimen.[98,113] Vancomycin (45 to 60 mg/kg/day) is the gold standard for treating infections caused by MRSA. Whether adding an aminoglycoside or rifampin to vancomycin is beneficial is unclear. For most community-acquired MRSA isolates, clindamycin (40 mg/kg/day in four divided doses) also is an effective antibiotic. Some experts recommend adding clindamycin to vancomycin or nafcillin theoretically to reduce toxin production. This reduction occurs in vitro, but no clinical data indicate that this approach leads to a decrease in the incidence of morbidity or mortality.[209]

Treatment of bacteremia associated with a genitourinary or gastrointestinal source requires antibiotics to which gram-negative enterics are susceptible. In such cases, initial therapy could consist of an aminoglycoside with an additional antibiotic active against anaerobes, such as clindamycin, metronidazole, ticarcillin-clavulanate, or piperacillin-tazobactam, for a gastrointestinal focus of infection. Extended-spectrum cephalosporins, such as cefotaxime or ceftriaxone, are possible alternative drugs for treating serious gram-negative enteric infections.[112] Optimal management of intra-abdominal or other abscesses usually requires surgical drainage, which should be undertaken as soon as the child's condition allows.

Immunosuppressed children or children with serious illnesses in the ICU require a different initial approach to suspected bacteremia. Gram-negative enterics, *P. aeruginosa, S. aureus*, and coagulase-negative staphylococcus are likely to be isolated from these patients.[6] Empiric therapy of nosocomial infection is based on the current antibiotic susceptibility pattern within the hospital.[216] *E. coli, Klebsiella* spp., and *Enterobacter* spp. are among the most common organisms causing bacteremia in patients in the pediatric ICU.[185] *E. coli* and *Klebsiella* spp. frequently produce β-lactamases that lead to resistance to ticarcillin or piperacillin. Generally, a combination of an antistaphylococcal semisynthetic penicillin or vancomycin (if a central line is present) or, if MRSA is a relatively common nosocomial pathogen, an aminoglycoside and an extended-spectrum penicillin (e.g., ticarcillin-clavulanate, piperacillin-tazobactam) is administered initially until a specific pathogen is isolated.[105] Broad-spectrum penicillins and aminoglycosides frequently exhibit synergy in vitro against gram-negative organisms, especially against *P. aeruginosa*.[124,198] In critically ill patients, a synergistic combination of antibiotics may be beneficial for treating bacteremia caused by *P. aeruginosa* or *Klebsiella* spp., although this subject remains controversial.[100,120]

After a specific organism is identified and antibiotic susceptibilities are known, the most appropriate agent is selected. If *E. coli* or *Klebsiella* spp. are isolated, these organisms can produce extended-spectrum β-lactamases, and the isolates should be tested for this possibility.[172] An extended-spectrum, β-lactamase–producing organism may seem susceptible to the extended-spectrum cephalosporins with minimal inhibitory concentrations of 2 to 8 μg/mL, but treatment failures may occur. If an extended-spectrum, β-lactamase–producing organism is identified, treatment with an extended-spectrum cephalosporin (e.g., cefotaxime, ceftriaxone, ceftazidime) is not recommended.[171] In this case, a carbapenem, such as imipenem-cilastatin or meropenem, is suggested.[171]

Enterobacter spp. may hyperproduce β-lactamase enzymes or be induced to hyperproduce these enzymes and are resistant or can become resistant to the extended-spectrum cephalosporins.[174] In many institutions, more than 30 percent of *Enterobacter cloacae* isolates are resistant to ceftazidime.[35] Cefepime may be more active than is ceftazidime or cefotaxime against *Enterobacter* spp. and other Amp C, β-lactamase enzyme–producing, gram-negative bacilli.[195] A carbapenem with an aminoglycoside is the treatment regimen recommended for treating infections caused by *Enterobacter* spp. resistant to ceftazidime.

In these patients, rapidly achieving therapeutic aminoglycoside levels in the plasma is important.[151] Serum concentrations of the aminoglycoside should be measured within 24 hours of initiation of therapy to ensure that therapeutic concentrations have been reached.

Antibiotics should be administered as soon as the diagnosis of septic shock is suspected. The selection of antibiotics is the same as that for bacteremia. If *S. aureus* is suspected among the potential causes of septic shock, antibiotic therapy is complicated by two factors: MRSA may make up more than 50 percent of community-acquired isolates[114] and nafcillin or oxacillin is superior to vancomycin for the treatment of serious infections caused by MRSA.[89] Nafcillin or oxacillin plus an aminoglycoside may be synergistic against staphylococci, but adding an aminoglycoside increases the risk for nephrotoxicity to develop. Some authorities include nafcillin or oxacillin plus vancomycin plus gentamicin in the initial empiric therapy of patients with life-threatening infections possibly caused by *S. aureus*.[9]

The management of septic shock is directed toward three main objectives: (1) control of the infectious process, (2) restoration of adequate tissue perfusion, and (3) maintenance of efficient respiratory function. Details of management have been the subject of numerous reports.[36,41,194] The reader is referred to these reviews for expert detailed guidance in the fluid management, use of vasoactive agents, and respiratory treatments in children with septic shock.

The benefits of therapy with high doses of corticosteroids in the treatment of endotoxin shock remain unproved. Extensive experimental data document the salutary hemodynamic, metabolic, microcirculatory, and cellular effect of steroids in laboratory models of endotoxin shock.[102] High-dose steroids were never found to be efficacious, however, in randomized controlled trials conducted in adults with severe sepsis or septic shock.[30,205,213]

On the basis of these studies, the routine use of high-dose corticosteroids in patients with severe sepsis or septic shock is not recommended. Later, results of small studies enrolling adults suggested that lower stress doses of hydrocortisone might be beneficial in managing patients with septic shock.[27,33] In one of these trials, placebo was compared with a 100-mg loading dose of hydrocortisone followed by a continuous infusion of 0.18 mg/kg/hr with a reduction of the infusion after shock had been reversed. Twenty patients were randomly assigned to each treatment arm. Infusion of stress doses of hydrocortisone reduced the time to discontinuing the vasopressor therapy and was associated with a trend toward earlier resolution of sepsis-induced organ dysfunction. Overall reversal of shock and mortality rates was unchanged, however. The role of low-dose hydrocortisone in children with septic shock remains controversial.[12,224] Randomized studies are needed to clarify the role of stress doses of hydrocortisone in children with septic shock.

Every effort should be made to ensure an adequate airway, which may require periodic suctioning if the patient is unable to clear pooled secretions. Humidified oxygen in concentrations required to maintain an adequate partial pressure of oxygen should be provided early. The method of oxygen administration (e.g., mask, ventilator) depends on the clinical state of the patient. Intubation and assisted ventilation are indicated if the child shows evidence of impending respiratory failure.

ARDS, usually appearing within 2 days after the onset of shock, may complicate the respiratory and fluid management.[104] Pulmonary edema, atelectasis, decreased pulmonary compliance, and ventilation-perfusion abnormalities are some factors that can lead to inadequate oxygenation. Administration of excessive fluids may contribute to ARDS. The central venous pressure may remain normal, despite the presence of pulmonary edema. Positive end-expiratory pressure, oxygen, and careful attention to cardiovascular parameters are the mainstays of therapy for ARDS.[104,175,191] Steroids are not beneficial after ARDS has been diagnosed.

The general supportive care of a child with septic shock includes attention to nutritional and metabolic requirements.[182] Administration of fluids containing 10 percent glucose may be necessary to prevent development of hypoglycemia. Parenteral alimentation may be the only means by which to provide nutrition, although the optimal amount and composition of elemental nutrients for children with septic shock are unknown. Hypocalcemia should be corrected. Platelet transfusions or fresh-frozen plasma may be necessary to correct coagulopathies. Continuous venovenous hemofiltration with or without dialysis may be instituted for complications of renal failure, such as fluid overload with pulmonary edema or hyperkalemia. It is not surprising that children who have acute renal failure complicating severe septic shock have a significantly higher mortality rate than that of children without acute renal failure.[176]

INVESTIGATIVE THERAPIES

Based on the evolving understanding of the pathophysiology of septic shock, many large, randomized, double-blind, multicenter trials have been conducted to assess the efficacy of agents that neutralize or counteract toxins or cytokines that are important in the evolution of septic shock. These immunomodulating strategies have been used on the basis of experimental data from animal studies. The conditions seen in experimental animal models of sepsis do not reflect the pathophysiologic situation seen in patients with severe sepsis or septic shock, however, which has led to many negative clinical trials (Table 69–5).

Antibody to Lipopolysaccharide

Endotoxemia frequently can be documented in patients with gram-negative sepsis. Endotoxin is released when bacteria are

TABLE 69-5 Clinical Trials of Sepsis Medications in Adults

Trial	Agent Studied	Total Patients (no.)	28-Day Mortality (%)	
			Medications	Controls
CHESS	HA-1A human monoclonal antibody[139]	1578	41	37
INTERSEPT	Anti-TNF[49]	564	37.3	39.5
	Steroids[30]	1267	39	35
	IL1-RA[72]	893	31	35
	Soluble TNF receptor[71]	141	40	38
COMPASS	Platelet-activating factor acetylhydrolase[165]	1425	25	24
KyberSept	Antithrombin III[233]	2314	38.9	38.7
OPTIMIST	Tissue factor pathway inhibitor[3]	1754	34.2	33.9
PROWESS	Activated protein C[22]	1690	24.7	30.8
ADDRESS	Activated protein C[2]	2613	17	18.5

TNF, tumor necrosis factor.

killed by bactericidal antibiotics.[200,201] This release may help explain why some patients develop shock after parenteral antibiotics are administered. Because endotoxin is responsible directly or through mediators for many of the adverse effects of gram-negative bacteremia, attempts to neutralize endotoxin have been undertaken. One problem with this approach is that only patients with septic shock caused by endotoxin-producing organisms may benefit from this treatment, and distinguishing a gram-positive from a gram-negative infection is impossible on patient presentation.

Neither E-5[29,92,95] (XMMEN-OEJ; XOMA Corp., Berkeley, CA), a murine monoclonal antibody, nor HA-1A[139,248] (Centoxin; Centocor, Malvern, PA), a different human monoclonal antibody against lipid A, were found to be efficacious in randomized, multicenter trials of gram-negative sepsis in adults. Children were not included in either study, although the pharmacokinetics and safety of HA-1A were established in children.[188] In the one study performed, HA-1A did not reduce the mortality rate in children with meningococcal disease.[57]

Other Potential Adjunctive Therapies

Antibody to TNF, soluble TNF receptors, antiplatelet activating factor, recombinant IL-1 receptor antagonist, antibradykinin, nitric oxide synthase inhibitor, and other therapies have undergone evaluation in large clinical trials of adjunctive therapy for adults with sepsis syndrome. None has proved beneficial.[4,14,72] Some combination of therapies may provide significant benefit in humans with gram-negative septic shock, as has been shown in animals.[193] Using recombinant soluble CD14 is another approach for blocking the action of endotoxin.[97]

Recombinant bactericidal/permeability-increasing protein (rBPI$_{23}$), a human-derived recombinant protein that expresses the amino-terminal half of the whole bactericidal, permeability-increasing protein molecule, has been studied in children with severe meningococcal sepsis.[149] Preliminary evaluation of rBPI$_{23}$ in 26 children with severe meningococcal sepsis in an open-label phase I/II trial was associated with fewer cases of mortality than in historical control patients.[82] A subsequent large, multicenter, randomized, double-blind trial in which 395 children were enrolled was conducted in 22 centers throughout the United States and the United Kingdom.[127] Mortality rates (7.4%) were not diminished significantly in the rBPI$_{23}$ group because the mortality rate in the control group was only 9.9 percent, a rate much less than anticipated. Children receiving rBPI$_{23}$ did have fewer amputations and a better functional outcome than did children receiving placebo. rBPI$_{23}$ is not being developed further.

Based on the complex interaction of the inflammatory and procoagulation responses of the host to infection as outlined in the pathophysiology section, recombinant human activated

protein C (drotrecogin alfa activated [rhAPC]) was evaluated for adjunctive treatment of severe sepsis in patients 18 years old and older. In a multicenter, double-blind, placebo-controlled study conducted in several countries, placebo or rhAPC was infused at a rate of 24 µg/kg/hr for 96 hours to patients with severe sepsis.[22] Selected demographic and clinical characteristics of the patients showed that the patients were matched well. The mortality rate at 28 days was 30.8 percent for the 840 patients in the placebo group and 24.7 percent for the patients receiving rhAPC ($p = 0.005$). The relative risk of mortality was reduced in the rhAPC group by 19.4 percent (95% confidence interval 6.6 to 30.5). The major difference in serious adverse effects was for serious bleeding, which occurred in 3.5 percent and 2 percent of the rhAPC and placebo patients. Recombinant human activated protein C has been approved for use in adults by the U.S. Food and Drug Administration.

Protein C concentrate has been administered to several children with fulminant meningococcemia and thought to be associated with enhanced survival and decreased amputations.[7,239] These findings supported the continued evaluation of rhAPC in the adjunctive treatment of septic shock in children. Phase I and II studies evaluated the pharmacokinetics and safety of rhAPC in children with severe sepsis.[129] An infusion rate of 24 µg/kg/hr resulted in mean serum concentrations of 67 ng/mL in 43 infants and children. (The mean concentration found in adults was 52 ng/mL.) rhAPC did not accumulate during a 96-hour infusion. The estimated half-life was 0.91 hours, and plasma clearance was 0.49 L/hr/kg. In 2005, however, the Food and Drug Administration and the manufacturer announced the discontinuation of a randomized, placebo-controlled trial of rhAPC in pediatric patients with severe sepsis (information available online at www.fda.gov/medwatch/SAFETY/2005/safety05.htm#Xigris2). An interim analysis showed that rhAPC was highly unlikely to show a benefit over placebo in the primary end-point (time to complete organ failure resolution over 14 days). rhAPC was associated with a significantly higher risk for central nervous system bleeding. The risk for intracranial hemorrhage was particularly elevated in patients younger than 60 days. The use of rhAPC is not indicated for use in pediatric severe sepsis.[156]

Intravenous immunoglobulin is recommended for adjunctive therapy for patients with toxic shock syndrome caused by either group A streptococcus or *S. aureus* that is not responding to aggressive therapy after several hours or after appropriate drainage of focal infections.[10] The value of intravenous immunoglobulin in the treatment of septic shock caused by *S. aureus* infection but not associated with toxic shock syndrome has not been established.[80] Tefibazumab is a monoclonal antibody directed against clumping factor A, an adhesin on the surface of *S. aureus*, that is being investigated to determine if it improves the outcome of adults with *S. aureus* bacteremia.[236]

Polymyxin B is an antibiotic that can neutralize endotoxin possibly through a detergent-like action. In experimental models, polymyxin B moderates some of the cardiovascular, metabolic, and lethal consequences of *E. coli* sepsis in rabbits and overwhelming Hib disease in infant rats.[75,230] Clinical studies of polymyxin B have not been conducted in humans with sepsis or septic shock.

Pentoxifylline is a phosphodiesterase inhibitor that has anti-inflammatory properties, including the ability to suppress endotoxin-induced mononuclear cell production of TNF. Pentoxifylline decreases endotoxin or TNF-induced lung injury and increases survival in animals infected with *E. coli* or infused with endotoxin.[128] In a study of human volunteers, a 500-mg dose of pentoxifylline infused 30 minutes before a 100-ng injection of endotoxin from *Salmonella abortus equi* blunted the TNF response but did not affect IL-6 serum levels after administration of endotoxin.[246] Clinical effects, such as fever, myalgia, and headache, were not affected by pentoxifylline. In one small study of 51 patients, a continuous infusion of pentoxifylline was associated with improvement in organ dysfunction scores, Pao_2/Fio_2 ratio, and the pressure-adjusted heart rate compared with placebo-treated patients.[207] Larger clinical studies of pentoxifylline or similar agents are warranted for the adjunctive treatment of sepsis and septic shock.

Plasmapheresis, exchange transfusions, and extracorporeal membrane oxygenation are heroic measures that seem to be beneficial in selected patients not responding to standard management.[21,58,79] These procedures may be considered for such patients when, in the opinion of experienced clinicians, their use is justified and they are the last hope for a successful outcome.[76]

PROGNOSIS

The morbidity and mortality rates for septic shock in children vary with age, the presence or absence of underlying diseases, and the specific microorganisms responsible for the septicemic state. Dupont and Spink[64] reported a 98 percent mortality rate in their series of children with septic shock and gram-negative bacteremia. Jacobs and colleagues[107] reported a 9.8 percent case-fatality rate for otherwise normal children with septic shock. In the pediatric HA-1A study, the overall mortality rate for severe sepsis or septic shock was 31 percent.[188] The overall mortality rate for children with meningococcal infection was 8 percent in a 10-center surveillance study.[116] For the seven-state sepsis cohort, the overall mortality rate was approximately 10 percent.[234] Much progress has been made in the treatment of sepsis and septic shock since the report of Dupont and Spink was published.[64] As with many infections, prevention is more desirable than is treatment. Careful attention given to sterile techniques for insertion and maintenance of intravascular or other lines and other procedures is crucial and may prevent some episodes of bacteremia and septic shock.

REFERENCES

1. Abraham, E., Bland, R. D., Cobo, J. C., et al.: Sequential cardiorespiratory patterns associated with outcome in septic shock. Chest *85*:75-80, 1984.
2. Abraham, E., Laterre, P. F., Garg, R., et al.: Drotrecogin alfa (activated) for adults with severe sepsis and a low risk of death. N. Engl. J. Med. *353*:1332-1341, 2005.
3. Abraham, E., Reinhart, K., Opal, S., et al.: Efficacy and safety of tifacogin (recombinant tissue factor pathway inhibitor) in severe sepsis. J. A. M. A. *290*:238-247, 2003.
4. Abraham, E., Wunderink, R., Silverman, H., et al.: Efficacy and safety of monoclonal antibody to human tumor necrosis factor α in patients with sepsis syndrome: A randomized, controlled, double-blind, multicenter clinical trial. J. A. M. A. *273*:934-941, 1995.
5. Adem, P. V., Montgomery, C. P., Husain, A. N., et al.: *Staphylococcus aureus* sepsis and the Waterhouse-Friderichsen syndrome in children. N. Engl. J. Med. *353*:1245-1251, 2005.

6. Albano, E. A., and Pizzo, P. A.: Infectious complications in childhood acute leukemias. Pediatr. Clin. North Am. *35*:873-901, 1988.
7. Alberio, L., Lämmle, B., and Esmon, C. T.: Protein C replacement in severe meningococcemia: Rationale and clinical experience. Clin. Infect. Dis. *32*:1338-1346, 2001.
8. Aledo, A., Heller, G., Gardner, S., et al.: Septicemia and septic shock in pediatric patients: 140 consecutive cases on a pediatric hematology-oncology service. J. Pediatr. Hematol. Oncol. *20*:215-221, 1998.
9. American Academy of Pediatrics: Staphylococcal infections. *In* Pickering, L. K., Baker C. J., Long, S. S., and McMillan, J. (eds.): 2006 Red Book: Report of the Committee on Infectious Diseases. 25th ed. Elk Grove Village, IL, American Academy of Pediatrics, 2006, pp. 598-610.
10. American Academy of Pediatrics: Toxic shock syndrome. *In* Pickering, L. K., Baker, C. J., Long, S. S., and McMillan, J. A. (eds.): 2006 Red Book: Report of the Committee on Infectious Diseases. 25th ed. Elk Grove Village, IL, American Academy of Pediatrics, 2006, pp. 650-655.
11. Anderson, R. R., Holliday, R. L., Driedger, A. A., et al.: Documentation of pulmonary capillary permeability in the adult respiratory distress syndrome accompanying human sepsis. Am. Rev. Respir. Dis. *119*:869-877, 1979.
12. Aneja, R., and Carcillo, J. A.: What is the rationale for hydrocortisone treatment in children with infection-related adrenal insufficiency and septic shock? Arch. Dis. Child. *92*:165-169, 2007.
13. Archer, L. T., Benjamin, B. A., Beller-Todd, B. K., et al.: Does LD$_{100}$ *E. coli* shock cause myocardial failure? Cir. Shock *9*:7-16, 1982.
14. Astiz, M. E., and Rackow, E. C.: Septic shock. Lancet *351*:1501-1505, 1998.
15. Bachur, R., and Harper, M. B.: Reevaluation of outpatients with *Streptococcus pneumoniae* bacteremia. Pediatrics *105*:502-509, 2000.
16. Banks, J. G., Foulis, A. K., Ledingham, I. M., et al.: Liver function in septic shock. J. Clin. Pathol. *35*:1249-1252, 1982.
17. Baraff, L. J., Bass, J. W., Fleisher, G. R., et al.: Practice guideline for the management of infants and children 0 to 36 months of age with fever without source. Pediatrics *92*:1-12, 1993.
18. Barocchi, M. A., Ries, J., Zogaj, X., et al.: A pneumococcal pilus influences virulence and host inflammatory responses. Proc. Natl. Acad. Sci. U. S. A. *103*:2857-2862, 2006.
19. Bass, J. W., Steele, R. W., Wittler, R. R., et al.: Antimicrobial treatment of occult bacteremia: A multicenter cooperative study. Pediatr. Infect. Dis. J. *12*:466-471, 1993.
20. Baumgarten, G., Knuefermann, P., Nozaki, N., et al.: In vivo expression of proinflammatory mediators in the adult heart after endotoxin administration: The role of toll-like receptor-4. J. Infect. Dis. *183*:1617-1624, 2001.
21. Beca, J., and Butt, W.: Extracorporeal membrane oxygenation for refractory septic shock in children. Pediatrics *93*:726-729, 1994.
22. Bernard, G. R., Vincent, J. L., Laterre, P. F., et al.: Efficacy and safety of recombinant human activated protein C for severe sepsis. N. Engl. J. Med. *344*:699-709, 2001.
23. Beutler, B., and Poltorak, A.: Sepsis and evolution of the innate immune response. Crit. Care Med. *29*(Suppl. 1):S2-S6, 2001.
24. Blain, C. M., Anderson, T. O., Pietras, R. J., et al.: Immediate hemodynamic effects of gram-negative vs. gram-positive bacteremia in man. Arch. Intern. Med. *126*:260-265, 1970.
25. Blair, E.: Hypocapnea and gram-negative bacteremic shock. Am. Surg. J. *119*:433-438, 1970.
26. Blair, E.: Acid-base balance in bacteremic shock. Arch. Intern. Med. *127*:731-739, 1971.
27. Bollaert, P. E., Charpentier, C., Levy, S., et al.: Reversal of late septic shock with supraphysiologic doses of hydrocortisone. Crit. Care Med. *26*:645-650, 1998.
28. Bone, R. C., Balk, R. A., Cerra, F. B., et al.: Definitions for sepsis and organ failure and guidelines for the use of innovative therapies in sepsis. Chest *101*:1644-1655, 1992.
29. Bone, R. C., Balk, R. A., Fein, A. M., et al.: A second large controlled clinical study of E5, a monoclonal antibody to endotoxin: Results of a prospective, multicenter, randomized, controlled trial: The E5 sepsis study group. Crit. Care Med. *23*:994-1006, 1995.
30. Bone, R. C., Fisher, C. J., Jr., Clemmer, T. P., et al.: A controlled clinical trial of high dose methylprednisolone in the treatment of severe sepsis and septic shock. N. Engl. J. Med. *317*:653-658, 1987.
31. Branco, R. G., Garcia, P. C. R., Piva, J. P., et al.: Glucose level and risk of mortality in pediatric septic shock. Pediatr. Crit. Care Med. *6*:470-472, 2005.
32. Brigham, K. L., and Meyrick, B.: Endotoxin and lung injury. Am. Rev. Respir. Dis. *133*:913-927, 1986.
33. Briegel, J., Forst, H., Haller, M., et al.: Stress doses of hydrocortisone reverses hyperdynamic septic shock: A prospective, randomized, double-blind, single-center study. Crit. Care Med. *27*:723-732, 1999.
34. Buck, C., Bundschu, J., Gallati, H., et al.: Interleukin-6: A sensitive parameter for early diagnosis of neonatal bacterial infection. Pediatrics *93*:54-58, 1994.
35. Burwen, D. R., Banerjee, S. N., Gaynes, R. P., and the National Nosocomial Infections Surveillance System: Ceftazidime resistance among selected nosocomial gram-negative bacilli in the U.S. J. Infect. Dis. *170*:1622-1625, 1994.
36. Butt, W.: Septic shock. Pediatr. Clin. North Am. *48*:601-625, 2001.
37. Byer, R. L., and Bachur, R. G.: Clinical deterioration among patients with fever and erythroderma. Pediatrics *118*:2450-2460, 2006.

38. Cain, B. S., Meldrum, D. R., Dinarello, C. A., et al.: Tumor necrosis factor-α and interleukin-1β synergistically depress human myocardial function. Crit. Care Med. 27:1309-1318, 1999.

39. Calandra, T., Baumgartner, J. D., Grau, G. E., et al.: Prognostic values of tumor necrosis factor/cachectin, interleukin-1, interferon-alpha, and interferon-gamma in the serum of patients with septic shock. J. Infect. Dis. 161:982-987, 1990.

40. Cannon, J. G., Tompkins, R. G., Gelfand, J. A., et al.: Circulating interleukin-1 and tumor necrosis factor in septic shock and experimental endotoxin fever. J. Infect. Dis. 161:79-84, 1990.

41. Carcillo, R. A., Fields, A. I.; and the Task Force Committee Members: Clinical practice parameters for hemodynamic support of pediatric and neonatal patients in septic shock. Crit. Care Med. 30:1365-1378, 2002.

42. Cardenas-Rivero, N., Chernow, B., Stoiko, M. A., et al.: Hypocalcemia in critically ill children. J. Pediatr. 114:946-951, 1989.

43. Carrol, E. D., Newland, P., Thomson, A. P., and Hart, C. A.: Prognostic value of procalcitonin in children with meningococcal sepsis. Crit. Care Med. 33:224-225, 2005.

44. Carroll, W. L., Farrell, M. K., Singer, J. L., et al.: Treatment of occult bacteremia: A prospective randomized clinical trial. Pediatrics 72:608-612, 1983.

45. Chesney, R. W., McCarron, D. M., Haddad, J. G., et al.: Pathogenic mechanisms of the hypocalcemia of the staphylococcal toxic-shock syndrome. J. Lab. Clin. Med. 101:576-585, 1983.

46. Clowes, G. H. A., George, B. C., Villee, C. A., et al.: Muscle proteolysis induced by a circulating peptide in patients with sepsis or trauma. N. Engl. J. Med. 308:545-552, 1983.

47. Clowes, G. H. A., O'Donnell, T. F., Ryan, V. T., et al.: Energy metabolism in sepsis: Treatment based on different patterns in shock and high output stage. Ann. Surg. 179:684-696, 1974.

48. Coalson, J. J., Archer, L. T., Hall, N. K., et al.: Prolonged shock in the monkey following live E. coli organism infusion. Circ. Shock 6:343-355, 1979.

49. Cohen, J., and Carlet, J.: INTERSEPT: An international, multicenter, placebo-controlled trial of monoclonal antibody to human tumor necrosis factor-alpha in patients with sepsis. Crit. Care Med. 24:1431-1440, 1996.

50. Corrigan, J. J.: Thrombocytopenia: A laboratory sign of septicemia in infants and children. J. Pediatr. 85:219-221, 1974.

51. Corrigan, J. J.: Disseminated intravascular coagulopathy. Pediatrics 64:37-45, 1979.

52. Corrigan, J. J.: Vitamin K-dependent coagulation factors in gram-negative septicemia. Am. J. Dis. Child. 138:240-242, 1984.

53. Corrigan, J. J., and Jordan, C. M.: Heparin therapy in septicemia with disseminated intravascular coagulation. N. Engl. J. Med. 283:778-782, 1970.

54. Cryer, P. E., Coran, A. G., Soda, J., et al.: Lethal Escherichia coli septicemia in the baboon: Alpha-adrenergic inhibition in insulin secretion and its relationship to the duration of survival. J. Lab. Clin. Med. 79:622-638, 1972.

55. Dantzsker, D. R., Brook, C. J., Hebart, P., et al.: Ventilation-perfusion distributions in the adult respiratory distress syndrome. Am. Rev. Respir. Dis. 120:1039-1052, 1979.

56. DeBont, E. S. J. M., Raan, M. J., Samson, G., et al.: Tumor necrosis factor-α, interleukin-1β, and interleukin-6 plasma levels in neonatal sepsis. Pediatr. Res. 33:330-383, 1993.

57. Derkx, B., Wittes, J., McCloskey, R.; and the European Pediatric Meningococcal Septic Shock Trial Study Group: Randomized placebo-controlled trial of HA-1A, a human monoclonal antibody to endotoxin in children with meningococcal septic shock. Clin. Infect. Dis. 28:770-777, 1999.

58. Deuren, M., Santman, F. W., Dalen, R., et al.: Plasma and whole blood exchange in meningococcal sepsis. Clin. Infect. Dis. 15:424-430, 1992.

59. Deuren, M., Ven-Jongekrijg, J., Bartelink, A. K. M., et al.: Correlation between proinflammatory cytokines and antiinflammatory mediators and severity of disease in meningococcal infections. J. Infect. Dis. 172:433-439, 1995.

60. Deuren, M., Ven-Jongekrijg, J., Demacker, P. N. M., et al.: Differential expression of proinflammatory cytokines and their inhibitors during the course of meningococcal infections. J. Infect. Dis. 169:157-161, 1994.

61. Deventer, S. J. H. V., Bulter, H. R., Cate, J. W. T., et al.: Endotoxaemia: An early predictor of septicaemia in febrile patients. Lancet 1:605-609, 1988.

62. Dinarello, C. A.: Interleukin-1 and its biologically related cytokines. Adv. Immunol. 44:153-203, 1989.

63. Dinarello, C. A., and Wolff, S. M.: The role of interleukin-1 in disease. N. Engl. J. Med. 328:106-113, 1993.

64. Dupont, H. L., and Spink, W. W.: Infections due to gram-negative organisms: An analysis of 860 patients with bacteremia at the University of Minnesota Medical Center, 1958-1966. Medicine (Baltimore) 48:307-332, 1969.

65. Edwards, M. S., and Baker, C. J.: Complications and sequelae of meningococcal infections in children. J. Pediatr. 99:540-545, 1981.

66. Farley, M. M., Stephens, D. S., Mulks, M. H., et al.: Pathogenesis of IgA1 protease producing and non producing Haemophilus influenzae in human nasopharyngeal organ cultures. J. Infect. Dis. 154:752-759, 1986.

67. Faust, S. N., Levin, M., Harrison, O. B., et al.: Dysfunction of endothelial protein C activation in severe meningococcal sepsis. N. Engl. J. Med. 345:408-416, 2001.

68. Fearson, D. T., Ruddy, S., Schur, P. H., et al.: Activation of the properdin pathway of complement in patients with gram-negative bacteremia. N. Engl. J. Med. 292:937-940, 1975.

69. Feltes, T. F., Pignatelli, R., Kleinert, S., and Mariscalco, M.: Quantitated left ventricular systolic mechanics in children with septic shock utilizing noninvasive wall-stress analysis. Crit. Care Med. 22:1647-1648, 1994.

70. Filkins, J. P., and Cornell, R. P.: Depression of hepatic gluconeogenesis and the hypoglycemia of endotoxin shock. Am. J. Physiol. 227:778-781, 1974.

71. Fisher, C. J., Agosti, J. M., Opal, S. M., et al.: Treatment of septic shock with the tumor necrosis factor receptor:Fc fusion protein. N. Engl. J. Med. 334:1697-1702, 1996.

72. Fisher, C. J., Dhainaut, J.-F. A., Opal, S. M., et al.: Recombinant human interleukin 1 receptor antagonist in the treatment of patients with sepsis syndrome: Results from a randomized, double-blind, placebo-controlled trial. J. A. M. A. 271:1836-1843, 1995.

73. Fisher, C. J., Jr., and Yan, S. B.: Protein C levels as a prognostic indicator of outcome in sepsis and related diseases. Crit. Care Med. 28:S49-S56, 2000.

74. Fleisher, G. R., Rosenberg, N., Vinci, R., et al.: Intramuscular versus oral antibiotic therapy for the prevention of meningitis and other bacterial sequelae in young, febrile children at risk for occult bacteremia. J. Pediatr. 124:504-512, 1994.

75. Flynn, P. M., Shenep, J. L., Stokes, D. C., et al.: Polymyxin B moderates acidosis and hypotension in established experimental gram-negative septicemia. J. Infect. Dis. 156:706-712, 1987.

76. Fortenberry, J. P., and Paden, M. L.: Extracorporeal therapies in the treatment of sepsis: Experience and promise. Semin. Pediatr. Infect. Dis. 17:72-79, 2006.

77. Froon, A. H. M., Dentener, M. A., Greve, J. W. M., et al.: Lipopolysaccharide toxicity-regulating proteins in bacteremia. J. Infect. Dis. 171:1250-1257, 1995.

78. Gallin, J. I., Kaye, D., and O'Leary, W. M.: Serum lipids in infections. N. Engl. J. Med. 281:1081-1086, 1969.

79. Garlund, B., Sjölin, J., Nilsson, A., et al.: Plasmapheresis in the treatment of primary septic shock in humans. Scand. J. Infect. Dis. 25:757-761, 1993.

80. Gauduchon, V., Cozon, G., Vandenesch, F., et al.: Neutralization of Staphylococcus aureus Panton Valentine leukocidin by intravenous immunoglobulin in vitro. Clin. Infect. Dis. 189:346-353, 2004.

81. Girardin, E., Grau, G. E., Dayer, J. M., et al.: Tumor necrosis factor and interleukin-1 in the serum of children with severe infectious purpura. N. Engl. J. Med. 319:397-400, 1988.

82. Giroir, B. P., Quint, P. A., Barton, P., et al.: Preliminary evaluation of recombinant amino-terminal bactericidal/permeability-increasing protein in children with severe meningococcal sepsis. Lancet 350:1439-1443, 1997.

83. Goldie, A. S., Fearon, K. C. H., Ross, J. A., et al.: Natural cytokine antagonists and endogenous antiendotoxin core antibodies in sepsis syndrome. J. A. M. A. 274:172-177, 1995.

84. Goldstein, B., Giroir, B., Randoph, A.; and the Members of the International Consensus Conference on Pediatric Sepsis: International pediatric sepsis conference: Definitions for sepsis and organ dysfunction in pediatrics. Pediatr. Crit. Care Med. 6:2-8, 2005.

85. Goldstein, S. L., Currier, H., Graf, J. M., et al.: Outcome in children receiving continuous venovenous hemofiltration. Pediatrics 107:1309-1312, 2001.

86. Gonzalez, B. E., Hulten, K. G., Dishop, M. E., et al.: Pulmonary manifestations in children with invasive community-acquired Staphylococcus aureus infection. Clin. Infect. Dis. 41:583-590, 2005.

87. Gonzalez, B. E., Martinez-Aguilar, G., Hulten, K. G., et al.: Severe staphylococcal sepsis in adolescents in the era of community-acquired methicillin-resistant Staphylococcus aureus. Pediatrics 115:642-648, 2005.

88. Gonzalez, B. E., Teruya, J., Mahoney, D. J., Jr., et al.: Venous thrombosis associated with staphylococcal osteomyelitis in children. Pediatrics 117:1673-1679, 2006.

89. Gonzalez, C., Rubio, M., Romero-Vivas, J., et al.: Bacteremic pneumonia due to Staphylococcus aureus: A comparison of disease caused by methicillin-resistant and methicillin-susceptible organisms. Clin. Infect. Dis. 29:1171-1177, 1999.

90. Graham, D. L., Behan, P. O., and More, I. A. R.: Brain damage complicating septic shock: acute hemorrhagic leukoencephalitis as a complication of the generalized Schwartzman reaction. J. Neurol. Neurosurg. Psychiatry 42:19-28, 1979.

91. Gray, J., Gossain, S., and Morris, K.: Three-year survey of bacteremias and fungemia in a pediatric intensive care unit. Pediatr. Infect. Dis. J. 20:416-421, 2001.

92. Greenman, R. L., Schein, R. M., Martin, M. A., et al.: A controlled clinical trial of E5 murine monoclonal IgM antibody to endotoxin in the treatment of gram-negative sepsis. J. A. M. A. 266:1097-1102, 1991.

93. Hack, C. E., Hart, M., Strack, R. J. M., et al.: Interleukin-8 in sepsis: Relation to shock and inflammatory mediators. Infect. Immun. 60:2835-2842, 1992.

94. Hammerschmidt, D. E., Weaver, L. J., Hudson, L. D., et al.: Association of complement activation and elevated plasma-C5a with adult respiratory distress syndrome: Pathophysiologic relevance and possible prognostic value. Lancet 1:947-949, 1980.

95. Harkonen, S., Scannon, P., Mischak, R. P., et al.: Phase I study of a murine monoclonal antilipid A antibody in bacteremic and nonbacteremic patients. Antimicrob. Agents Chemother. 32:710-716, 1988.

96. Hatherill, M., Tibby, S. M., Turner, C., et al.: Procalcitonin and cytokine levels: Relationship to organ failure and mortality in pediatric septic shock. Crit. Care Med. 28:2591-2594, 2000.

97. Haziot, A., Rong, G. W., Lin, X.-Y., et al.: Recombinant soluble CD14 prevents mortality in mice treated with endotoxin (lipopolysaccharide). J. Immunol. 154:6529-6532, 1995.

98. Herold, B. C., Immergluck, L. C., Maranan, M. C., et al: Community-acquired methicillin-resistant Staphylococcus aureus in children with no identified predisposing risks. J. A. M. A. 279:593-598, 1998.

99. Herz, A. M., Greenhow, T. L., Alcantara, J., et. al.: Changing epidemiology of outpatient bacteremia in 3- to 36-month old children after the introduction of the heptavalent-conjugated pneumococcal vaccine. Pediatr. Infect. Dis. J. 25:293-300, 2006.

100. Hilf, M., Yu, V. L., Sharp, J., et al.: Antibiotic therapy for Pseudomonas aeruginosa bacteremia: Outcome correlations in a prospective study of 200 patients. Am. J. Med. 87:540-546, 1989.

101. Hill, S. L., Eblings, V. B., and Lewis, F. R.: Changes in lung water and capillary permeability following sepsis and fluid overload. J. Surg. Res. 28:140-150, 1980.

102. Hinshaw, L. B., Beller-Todd, B. K., Archer, L. T., et al.: Effectiveness of steroid/antibiotic treatment in primates administered LD₁₀₀ Escherichia coli. Ann. Surg. 194:51-56, 1981.

103. Hinshaw, L. B., Tekamp-Olson, P., Chang, A. C. K., et al.: Survival of primates in LD₁₀₀ septic shock following therapy with antibody to tumor necrosis factor (TNF). Circ. Shock 30:279-292, 1990.

104. Holbrook, P. R., Taylor, G., Pollack, M. M., et al.: Adult respiratory distress syndrome in children. Pediatr. Clin. North Am. 27:677-685, 1980.

105. Hughes, W. T., Armstrong, D., Bodey, G. P., et al.: 2002 Guidelines for the use of antimicrobial agents in neutropenic patients with cancer. Clin. Infect. Dis. 34:730-751, 2002.

106. Ingalls, R. R., Heine, H., Lien, E., et al.: Lipopolysacchaide recognition, CD14, and lipopolysaccharide receptors. Infect. Dis. Clin. North Am. 13:341-353, 1999.

107. Jacobs, R. F., Sowell, M. K., Moss, M. M., et al.: Septic shock in children: Bacterial etiologies and temporal relationships. Pediatr. Infect. Dis. J. 9:196-200, 1990.

108. Jaffe, D. M., Tanz, R. R., Davis, A. T., et al.: Antibiotic administration to treat possible occult bacteremia in febrile children. N. Engl. J. Med. 317:1175-1180, 1987.

109. Jones, L. W., and Weil, M. H.: Water, creatinine and sodium excretion following circulatory shock with renal failure. Am. J. Med. 51:314-318, 1971.

110. Kalter, E. S., Daha, M. R., Cate, J. W. T., et al.: Activation and inhibition of Hageman factor-dependent pathways and the complement system in uncomplicated bacteremia or bacterial shock. J. Infect. Dis. 151:1019-1027, 1985.

111. Kapadia, S., Torre-Amione, G., Birdsall, H. H., et al.: Tumor necrosis factor-α gene and protein expression in adult feline myocardium after endotoxin administration. J. Clin. Invest. 96:1042-1052, 1995.

112. Kaplan, S. L.: Serious pediatric infections. Am. J. Med. 88(Suppl. 4A):18S-24S, 1990.

113. Kaplan, S. L.: Implications of methicillin-resistant Staphylococcus aureus as a community-acquired pathogen in pediatric patients. Infect. Dis. Clin. North Am. 19:747-757, 2005.

114. Kaplan, S. L., Hulten, K. G., Gonzalez, B. E., et al.: Three-year surveillance of community-acquired Staphylococcus aureus infections in children. Clin. Infect. Dis. 40:1785-1791, 2005.

115. Kaplan, S. L., Mason, E. O., Jr., Barson, W. J., et al.: Outcome of invasive infections outside the central nervous system caused by Streptococcus pneumoniae isolates nonsusceptible to ceftriaxone in children treated with beta-lactam antibiotics. Pediatr. Infect. Dis. J. 20:392-396, 2001.

116. Kaplan, S. L., Schutze, G. E., Leake, J. A. D., et al.: Multicenter surveillance of invasive meningococcal infections in children. Pediatrics 118:e979-e984, 2006.

117. Kaplan, S. L., Taber, L. H., Frank, A. L., et al.: Nasopharyngeal viral isolates in children with Haemophilus influenzae type b meningitis. J. Pediatr. 99:591-593, 1981.

118. Kaufmann, R. L., Matson, C. F., and Beisel, W. R.: Hypertriglyceridemia produced by endotoxin: Role of impaired triglyceride disposal mechanisms. J. Infect. Dis. 133:548-555, 1976.

119. Kleiman, M. B., Reynolds, J. K., Schreiner, R. L., et al.: Rapid diagnosis of neonatal bacteremia with acridine orange-stained buffy coat smears. J. Pediatr. 105:419-421, 1984.

120. Korvick, J. A., Bryan, C. S., Farber, B., et al.: Prospective observational study of Klebsiella bacteremia in 230 patients: Outcome for antibiotic combinations versus monotherapy. Antimicrob. Agents Chemother. 36:2639-2644, 1992.

121. Kumar, A., Thota, V., Dee, L., et al.: Tumor necrosis factor α and interleukin 1β are responsible for in vitro myocardial cell depression induced by human septic shock serum. J. Exp. Med. 183:949-958, 1996.

122. Lacour, A. G., Gervaix, A., Zamora, S. A., et al.: Procalcitonin, IL-6, IL-8, IL receptor antagonist and C-reactive protein as identificators of serious bacterial infections in children with fever without localizing signs. Eur. J. Pediatr. 160:95-100, 2001.

123. Langevelde, P. V., Joop, K., Loon, J. V., et al.: Endotoxin, cytokines, and procalcitonin in febrile patients admitted to the hospital: Identification of subjects at high risk of mortality. Clin. Infect. Dis. 31:1343-1348, 2000.

124. Lau, W. K., Young, L. S., Black, R. E., et al.: Comparative efficacy and toxicity of amikacin/carbenicillin versus gentamicin/carbenicillin in leukopenic patients: A randomized prospective trial. Am. J. Med. 62:959-966, 1977.

125. Levi, M., ten Cate, H., Poll, T., et al.: Pathogenesis of disseminated intravascular coagulation in sepsis. J. A. M. A. 270:975-979, 1993.

126. Levin, J., Poore, T. E., Young, N. S., et al.: Gram-negative sepsis: Detection of endotoxemia with the Limulus test. Ann. Intern. Med. 76:1-7, 1972.

127. Levin, M., Quint, P. A., Goldstein, B., et al.: Recombinant bactericidal/permeability-increasing protein (rBPI₂₃) as adjunctive treatment for children with severe meningococcal sepsis: A randomized trial. Lancet 356:961-967, 2000.

128. Lilly, C. M., Sandhu, J. S., Ishizaka, A., et al.: Pentoxifylline prevents tumor necrosis factor-induced lung injury. Am. Rev. Respir. Dis. 139:1361-1368, 1989.

129. Lilly Research Laboratories: Briefing document for XIGRIS for the treatment of severe sepsis. FDA Anti-Infective Drugs Advisory Committee, September 12, 2001. Available at www.fda.gov/ohrms/dockets/ac/01/briefing/3787b1_01_Sponsor.pdf.

130. Lorente, J. A., Garcia-Frade, L. J., Landin, L., et al.: Time course of hemostatic abnormalities in sepsis and its relation to outcome. Chest 103:1536-1542, 1993.

131. Mallet, E., Lanse, X., Devaux, A. M., et al.: Hypercalcitoninaemia in fulminant meningococcaemia in children. Lancet 1:294, 1983.

132. Marchant, A., Devière, J., Byl, B., et al.: Interleukin-10 production during septicemia. Lancet 343:707-708, 1994.

133. Marshall, R., Teele, D. W., and Klein, J. O.: Unsuspected bacteremia due to Haemophilus influenzae: Outcome in children not initially admitted to hospital. J. Pediatr. 95:690-695, 1979.

134. Mason, J. W., Kleeberg, V., Dolan, P., et al.: Plasma kallikrein and Hageman factor in gram-negative bacteremia. Ann. Intern. Med. 73:545-551, 1970.

135. Matuschak, G. M., and Rinaldo, J. E.: Organ interactions in the adult respiratory distress syndrome during sepsis: Role of the liver in host defense. Chest 94:400-406, 1988.

136. McCabe, M. R.: Serum complement levels in bacteremia due to gram-negative organisms. N. Engl. J. Med. 288:21-23, 1973.

137. McCarthy, P. L.: Controversies in pediatrics: What tests are indicated for the child under 2 with fever? Pediatr. Rev. 1:51-56, 1979.

138. McCartney, A. C., Banks, J. G., Clements, G. B., et al.: Endotoxemia in septic shock: Clinical and post-mortem correlations. Intensive Care Med. 9:117-122, 1983.

139. McCloskey, R. V., Straube, R. C., Sanders, C., et al.: Treatment of septic shock with human monoclonal antibody HA-1A: A randomized, double-blind, placebo-controlled trial. Ann. Intern. Med. 121:1-5, 1994.

140. McConn, R., Greineder, J. K., Wasserman, F., et al.: Is there a humoral factor that depresses ventricular function in sepsis? Circ. Shock 1(Suppl.):9-27, 1979.

141. McGowan, K. L., Foster, J. A., and Coffin, S. E.: Outpatient pediatric blood cultures: Time to positivity. Pediatrics 106:251-255, 2000.

142. Meyer, J., Traber, L. D., Nelson, S., et al.: Reversal of hyperdynamic response to continuous endotoxin administration by inhibition of NO synthesis. J. Appl. Physiol. 73:324-328, 1992.

143. Michaels, R. H., Myerowitz, R. L., and Klaw, R.: Potentiation of experimental meningitis due to Haemophilus influenzae by influenza A virus. J. Infect. Dis. 135:641-645, 1977.

144. Michie, H. R., Manoque, K. R., Spriggs, D. R., et al.: Detection of circulating tumor necrosis factor after endotoxin administration. N. Engl. J. Med. 318:1481-1486, 1988.

145. Miller, R. L., Reichgott, M. J., and Melmon, K. L.: Biochemical mechanisms of generation of bradykinin by endotoxin. J. Infect. Dis. 128(Suppl.):144-156, 1973.

146. Miller, S. I., Wallace, R. J., Musher, D. M., et al.: Hypoglycemia as a manifestation of sepsis. Am. J. Med. 68:649-654, 1980.

147. Mizock, B.: Metabolic derangements in sepsis and septic shock. Crit. Care Clin. 16:319-336, 2000.

148. Mizock, B. A., Sabelli, H. C., Dubin, A., et al.: Septic encephalopathy: Evidence for altered phenylalanine metabolism and comparison with hepatic encephalopathy. Arch. Intern. Med. 150:443-449, 1990.

149. Möhlen, M. A. M., Kimmings, A. N., Wedel, N. I., et al.: Inhibition of endotoxin-induced cytokine release and neutrophil activation in humans by use of recombinant bactericidal/permeability-increasing protein. J. Infect. Dis. 172:144-151, 1995.

150. Moncada, S., and Higgs, A.: The l-arginine-nitric oxide pathway. N. Engl. J. Med. 329:2002-2012, 1993.

151. Moore, R. D., Smith, C. R., and Lietman, P. S.: The association of aminoglycoside plasma levels with mortality in patients with gram-negative bacteremia. J. Infect. Dis. 199:443-448, 1984.

152. Mora, M., Bensi, G., Capo, S., et al.: Group A streptococcus produces pilus-like structures containing protective antigens and Lancefield T antigens. Proc. Natl. Acad. Sci. U. S. A. 102:15641-15646, 2005.

153. Munford, R. S., and Hall, C.: Detoxification of bacterial lipopolysaccharides (endotoxins) by a human neutrophil enzyme. Science 234:203-205, 1986.

154. Musher, D. M.: Cutaneous and soft-tissue manifestations of sepsis due to gram-negative enteric bacilli. Rev. Infect. Dis. 2:854-866, 1980.

155. Myers, M. G., Wright, P. F., Smith, A. L., et al.: Complications of occult pneumococcal bacteremia in children. J. Pediatr. 84:656-660, 1974.

156. Nadel, S., Goldstein, B., Williams, M. D., et al.: Drotrecogin alfa (activated) in children with severe sepsis: A multicentre phase III randomized controlled trial. Lancet 369:836-843, 2007.

157. Naqvi, S. H., Chundu, K. R., and Friedman, A. D.: Shock in children with gram-negative bacillary sepsis and *Haemophilus influenzae* type b sepsis. Pediatr. Infect. Dis. *5*:512-515, 1986.

158. Natanson, C., Fink, M. P., Ballantyne, H. K., et al.: Gram-negative bacteremia produces both severe systolic and diastolic cardiac dysfunction in a canine model that simulates human septic shock. J. Clin. Invest. *78*:259-270, 1986.

159. Natanson, C., Hoffman, W. D., Suffredini, A. F., et al.: Selected treatment strategies for septic shock based on proposed mechanisms of pathogenesis. Ann. Intern. Med. *120*:771-783, 1994.

160. National Center for Health Statistics: Increase in national hospital discharge survey rates for septicemia: United States, 1979-1987. M. M. W. R. Morb. Mortal. Wkly. Rep. *39*:31-34, 1990.

161. Nguyen, Q. V., Nguyen, E. A., and Weiner, L. B.: Incidence of invasive bacterial disease in children with fever and petechiae. Pediatrics *74*:77-80, 1984.

162. Nishijima, J., Weil, M. H., Subin, H., et al.: Hemodynamic and metabolic studies on shock associated with gram-negative bacteremia. Medicine (Baltimore) *52*:287-294, 1973.

163. Ognibene, F. P., Martin, S. E., Parker, M. M., et al.: Adult respiratory distress syndrome in patients with severe neutropenia. N. Engl. J. Med. *315*:547-551, 1986.

164. Ognibene, F. P., Parker, M. M., Natanson, C., et al.: Depressed left ventricular performance: Response to volume infusion in patients with sepsis and septic shock. Chest *93*:903-910, 1988.

165. Opal, S., Laterre, P. F., Abraham, E., et al.: Recombinant human platelet-activating factor acetylhydrolase for treatment of severe sepsis: Results of a phase III, multicenter, randomized, double-blind, placebo-controlled, clinical trial. Crit. Care Med. *32*:332-341, 2004.

166. Panas, D., Khadour, F. H., Szabo, C., and Schulz, R.: Proinflammatory cytokines depress cardiac efficiency by a nitric oxide-dependent mechanism. Am. J. Physiol. *275*:H1016-H1023, 1998.

167. Parker, M. M., and Parillo, J. E.: Septic shock: Hemodynamics and pathogenesis. J. A. M. A. *250*:3324-3327,1983.

168. Parker, M. M., Shelhamer, J. H., Bacharach, S. L., et al.: Profound but reversible myocardial depression in patients with septic shock. Ann. Intern. Med. *100*:483-490, 1984.

169. Parrillo, J. E., Burch, C., Shelhamer, J. H., et al.: A circulating myocardial depressant substance in humans with septic shock: Septic shock patients with a reduced ejection fraction have a circulating factor that depresses in vitro myocardial cell performance. J. Clin. Invest. *76*:1539-1553, 1985.

170. Patrick, C. C.: Coagulase-negative staphylococci: Pathogens with increasing clinical significance. J. Pediatr. *116*:497-507, 1990.

171. Patterson, D. L., Ko, W.-C., Gottberg, A. V., et al.: Outcome of cephalosporin treatment for serious infections due to apparently susceptible organisms producing extended-spectrum β-lactamases: Implications for the clinical laboratory. J. Clin. Microbiol. *39*:2206-2212, 2001.

172. Patterson, D. L., and Yu, V. L.: Editorial response: Extended-spectrum β-lactamases: A call for improved detection and control. Clin. Infect. Dis. *29*:1419-1422, 1999.

173. Peters, G., Locci, R., and Pulverer, G.: Adherence and growth of coagulase-negative staphylococci on surfaces of intravenous catheters. J. Infect. Dis. *146*:479-482, 1982.

174. Pfaller, M. A., Jones, R. N., Marshall, S. A., et al.: Inducible Amp C β-lactamase producing gram-negative bacilli from bloodstream infections: Frequency, antimicrobial susceptibility, and molecular epidemiology in a national surveillance program (SCOPE). Diagn. Microbiol. Infect. Dis. *28*:211-219, 1997.

175. Pfenniger, J., Gerber, A., Tschappeler, H., et al.: Adult respiratory distress syndrome in children. J. Pediatr. *101*:352-357, 1982.

176. Plotz, F. B., Hulst, H. E., Twisk, J. W., et al.: Effect of acute renal failure on outcome in children with severe septic shock. Pediatr. Nephrol. *20*:1177-1181, 2005.

177. Poll, T. V. D., Büller, H. R., Cate, H. T., et al.: Activation of coagulation after administration of tumor necrosis factor to normal subjects. N. Engl. J. Med. *322*:1622-1627, 1990.

178. Proulx, F., Fayon, M., Farrell, C. A., et al.: Epidemiology of sepsis and multiple organ dysfunction syndrome in children. Chest *109*:1033-1037, 1996.

179. Raymond, R. M., and Emerson, T. E.: Cerebral metabolism during endotoxin shock in the dog. Circ. Shock *5*:407-414, 1978.

180. Reichgott, M. L., Melmon, K. L., Forsyth, R. P., et al.: Cardiovascular and metabolic effects of whole or fractionated gram-negative bacterial endotoxin in the unanesthetized rhesus monkey. Circ. Res. *33*:346-352, 1973.

181. Reilly, J. M., Cunnion, R. E., Burch-Whitman, C., et al.: A circulating myocardial depressant substance is associated with cardiac dysfunction and peripheral hypoperfusion (lactic acidemia) in patients with septic shock. Chest *95*:1072-1080, 1989.

182. Reimer, S. L., Michener, W. M., and Steiger, E.: Nutritional support of the critically ill child. Pediatr. Clin. North Am. *27*:647-660, 1980.

183. Reines, H. D., Cook, J. A., Halushka, P. V., et al.: Plasma thromboxane concentrations are raised in patients dying with septic shock. Lancet *11*:174-175, 1982.

184. Rey, C., Los Arcos, M., Concha, A., et al.: Procalcitonin and C-reactive protein as markers of systemic inflammatory response syndrome severity in critically ill children. Intensive Care Med. *33*:477-484, 2007.

185. Richards, M. J., Edwards, J. R., Culver, D. H., et al.: Nosocomial infections in the pediatric intensive care units in the United States. Pediatrics *103*:e39, 1999.

186. Richmond, D. A., Molitch, M. E., and O'Donnell, T. F.: Altered thyroid hormone levels in bacterial sepsis: The role of nutritional adequacy. Metabolism *29*:936-942, 1980.

187. Robbins, R. A., Russ, W. D., Rasmussen, J. K., et al.: Activation of the complement system in the adult respiratory distress syndrome. Am. Rev. Respir. Dis. *135*:651-658, 1987.

188. Romano, M. J., Kearns, G. L., Kaplan, S. L., et al.: Single-dose pharmacokinetics and safety of HA-1A, a human IgM anti-lipid-A monoclonal antibody, in pediatric patients with sepsis syndrome. J. Pediatr. *122*:974-981, 1993.

189. Rongkavilit, C., Rodriguez, Z. M., Gomez-Marin, O., et al.: Gram-negative bacillary bacteremia in human immunodeficiency virus type 1-infected children. Pediatr. Infect. Dis. J. *19*:122-128, 1998.

190. Royall, J. P., and Levin, D. L.: Adult respiratory distress syndrome in pediatric patients, I: clinical aspects, pathophysiology, pathology, and mechanisms of lung injury. J. Pediatr. *112*:169-180, 1988.

191. Royall, J. P., and Levin, D. L.: Adult respiratory distress syndrome in pediatric patients, II: Management. J. Pediatr. *112*:335-347, 1988.

192. Rubin, L. G., and Moxon, E. R.: Pathogenesis of bloodstream invasion with *Haemophilus influenzae* type b. Infect. Immun. *41*:280-284, 1983.

193. Russell, D. A., Tucker, K. K., Chinookoswong, N., et al.: Combined inhibition of interleukin-1 and tumor necrosis factor in rodent endotoxemia: Improved survival and organ function. J. Infect. Dis. *171*:1528-1538, 1995.

194. Russell, J. A.: Management of sepsis. N. Engl. J. Med. *355*:1699-1713, 2006.

195. Sanders, C. C.: Cefepime: The next generation? Clin. Infect. Dis. *17*:369-379, 1993.

196. Sard, B., Bailey, M. C., and Vinci, R.: An analysis of pediatric blood cultures in the postpneumococcal conjugate vaccine era in a community hospital emergency department. Pediatr. Emerg. Care *22*:295-300, 2006.

197. Schmyer, J. P., Reynolds, D. G., and Swan, K. G.: Renal blood flow during endotoxin shock in the subhuman primate. Surg. Gynecol. Obstet. *137*:3-6, 1973.

198. Shales, D. M., and Bass, S. N.: Combination antimicrobial therapy. Pediatr. Clin. North Am. *30*:121-134, 1983.

199. Shapiro, E. D., Wald, E. R., Nelson, K. A., et al.: Broviac catheter-related bacteremia in oncology patients. Am. J. Dis. Child. *136*:679-681, 1982.

200. Shenep, J. L., Barton, R. P., and Mogan, K. A.: Role of antibiotic class in the rate of liberation of endotoxin during therapy for experimental gram-negative bacterial sepsis. J. Infect. Dis. *151*:1012-1018, 1985.

201. Shenep, J. L., Flynn, P. M., Barrett, F. F., et al.: Serial quantitation of endotoxemia and bacteremia during therapy for gram-negative bacterial sepsis. J. Infect. Dis. *157*:565-568, 1988.

202. Shulman, S. T., and Ayoub, E. M.: Severe staphylococcal sepsis in adolescents. Pediatrics *58*:59-66, 1976.

203. Smith, A. L.: Commentary: The febrile infant. Pediatr. Rev. *1*:35-36, 1979.

204. Sotiropoulos, S. V., Jackson, M. A., Woods, G. M., et al.: Alpha-streptococcal septicemia in leukemic children treated with continuous or large dosage intermittent cytosine arabinoside. Pediatr. Infect. Dis. J. *8*:755-758, 1989.

205. Sprung, C. L., Caralis, P. V., Marcial, E. H., et al.: The effects of high-dose corticosteroids in patients with septic shock: A prospective, controlled study. N. Engl. J. Med. *311*:1137-1143, 1984.

206. Sriskandan, S., Cohen, J.: Gram-positive sepsis: Mechanisms and differences from gram-negative sepsis. Infect. Dis. Clin. North Am. *13*:392-412, 1999.

207. Staubach, K. H., Schroder, L., Stuber, F., et al.: Effect of pentoxifylline in severe sepsis: Results of a randomized, double-blind, placebo-controlled study. Arch. Surg. *133*:94-100, 1998.

208. Stephens, D. S., Hoffman, L. H., and McGee, Z. A.: Interaction of *Neisseria meningitidis* with human nasopharyngeal mucosa: Attachment and entry into columnar epithelial cells. J. Infect. Dis. *148*:369-376, 1983.

209. Stevens, D. L., Ma, Y., Salmi, D. B., McIndoo, E., et al.: Impact of antibiotics on expression of virulence-associated exotoxin genes in methicillin-sensitive and methicillin-resistant *Staphylococcus aureus*. J. Infect. Dis. *195*:202-211, 2007.

210. Stoll, M. L., and Rubin, L. G.: Incidence of occult bacteremia among highly febrile children in the era of the pneumococcal conjugate vaccine: A study from a Children's Hospital Emergency Department and Urgent Care Center. Arch. Pediatr. Adolesc. Med. *158*:671-675, 2004.

211. Stumacher, R. J., Kovnat, M. J., and McCabe, W. R.: Limitations of the usefulness of the Limulus assay for endotoxin. N. Engl. J. Med. *288*:1261-1264, 1973.

212. Suffredini, A. F., Fromm, R. E., Parker, M. M., et al.: The cardiovascular response of normal humans to the administration of endotoxin. N. Engl. J. Med. *321*:280-287, 1989.

213. Sullivan, J. S., Kilpatrick, L., Costarino, A. T., et al.: Correlation of plasma cytokine elevations with mortality rate in children with sepsis. J. Pediatr. *120*:510-515, 1992.

214. Thiru, Y., Pathan, N., Bignall, S., et al.: A myocardial cytotoxic process is involved in the cardiac dysfunction of meningococcal septic shock. Crit. Care Med. *28*:2979-2983, 2000.

215. Togari, H., Sugiyama, S., Ogino, T., et al.: Interactions of endotoxin with cortisol and acute phase proteins in septic shock neonates. Acta Paediatr. Scand. *75*:69-74, 1986.

216. Toltzis, P., and Blumer, J. L.: Antibiotic-resistant gram-negative bacteria in the critical care setting. Pediatr. Clin. North Am. *42*:687-702, 1995.
217. Tracey, K. J., Beutler, B., Lowry, S. F., et al.: Shock and tissue injury induced by recombinant human cachectin. Science *234*:470-474, 1986.
218. Tracey, K. J., and Cerami, A.: Tumor necrosis factor: An updated review of its biology. Crit. Care Med. *21*:S415-S422, 1993.
219. Tracey, K. J., Lowry, S. F., and Cerami, A.: Cachectin: A hormone that triggers acute shock and chronic cachexia. J. Infect. Dis. *157*:413-420, 1988.
220. Tracey, K. J., Vlassara, H., and Cerami, A.: Cachectin/tumor necrosis factor. Lancet *1*:1122-1126, 1989.
221. Triger, D. R., Boyer, T. D., and Levin, J.: Portal and systemic bacteremia and endotoxaemia in liver disease. Gut *19*:935-939, 1978.
222. Tubbs, H. R.: Endotoxin in meningococcal infections. Arch. Dis. Child. *55*:808-819, 1980.
223. Tuomanen, E. I.: The biology of pneumococcal infections. Pediatr. Res. *42*:253-258, 1997.
224. van Schaik, S. M.: Do pediatric patients with septic shock benefit for steroid therapy? A critical appraisal of "Low-dose hydrocortisone improves shock reversal and reduces cytokine levels in early hyperdynamic septic shock" by Oppert et al. (Crit. Care Med. *33*:2457-2464, 2005). Pediatr. Crit. Care Med. *8*:174-176, 2007.
225. van Waardenburg, D. A., Jansen, T. C., Vos, G. D., and Buurman, W. A.: Hyperglycemia in children with meningococcal sepsis and septic shock: The relation between plasma levels of insulin and inflammatory mediators. J. Clin. Endocrinol. Metab. *91*:3916-3921, 2006.
226. Veterans Administration Systemic Sepsis Cooperative Study Group: Effect of high-dose glucocorticoid therapy on mortality in patients with clinical signs of systemic sepsis. N. Engl. J. Med. *317*:659-665, 1987.
227. Voerman, H. J., Stehouwer, C. D. A., Kamp, G. J., et al.: Plasma endothelin levels are increased during septic shock. Crit. Care Med. *20*:1097-1101, 1992.
228. Waage, A., Brandtzaeg, P., Halstensen, A., et al.: The complex pattern of cytokines in serum from patients with meningococcal septic shock: Association between interleukin 6, interleukin 1, and fatal outcome. J. Exp. Med. *169*:333-338, 1989.
229. Wajchenberg, B., Leme, C. E., Tambascia, M., et al.: The adrenal response to exogenous adrenocorticotrophin in patients with infections due to *Neisseria meningitidis*. J. Infect. Dis. *138*:387-391, 1978.
230. Walterspiel, J. W., Kaplan, S. L., and Mason, E. O., Jr.: Protective effect of subinhibitory polymyxin B alone and in combination with ampicillin for overwhelming *Haemophilus influenzae* type b infection in the infant rat: Evidence for in vivo and in vitro release of free endotoxin after ampicillin treatment. Pediatr. Res. *20*:237-241, 1986.
231. Wardle, E. N.: Endotoxin and acute renal failure. Nephron *14*:321-332, 1975.
232. Wardle, E. N.: Acute renal failure in the 1980's: The importance of septic shock and of endotoxaemia. Nephron *30*:193-200, 1982.
233. Warren, B. L., Eid, A., Singer, P., Pillay, S. S., et al.: High-dose antithrombin III in severe sepsis: A randomized controlled trial. J. A. M. A. *286*:1869-1878, 2000.
234. Watson, R. S., Carcillo, J. A., Linde-Zwirble, W. T., et al.: The epidemiology of severe sepsis in children in the United States. Am. J. Respir. Care Med. *167*:695-701, 2003.
235. Watson, R. W. G., Redmond, H. P., and Bouchier-Hayes, D.: Role of endotoxin in mononuclear phagocyte-mediated inflammatory responses. J. Leukoc. Biol. *56*:95-103, 1994.
236. Weems, J. J., Jr., Steinberg, J. P., Filler, S., et al.: Phase II, randomized, double-blind, multicenter study comparing the safety and pharmacokinetics of tefibazumab to placebo for treatment of *Staphylococcus aureus* bacteremia. Antimicrob. Agents Chemother. *50*:2751-2755, 2006.
237. Weil, M. H., and Nishijima, H.: Cardiac output in bacterial shock. Am. J. Med. *64*:920-922, 1978.
238. Weiland, J. E., Davis, W. B., Holter, J. F., et al.: Lung neutrophils in the adult respiratory distress syndrome: Clinical and pathophysiologic significance. Am. Rev. Respir. Dis. *133*:218-225, 1986.
239. White, B., Livingston, W., Murphy, C., et al.: An open-label study of the role of adjuvant hemostatic support with protein C replacement therapy in purpura fulminans-associated meningococcemia. Blood *96*:3719-3724, 2000.
240. Wiesenthal, A. M., and Todd, J. K.: Toxic shock syndrome in children aged 10 years or less. Pediatrics *74*:112-117, 1984.
241. Wilson, M. D., Brackett, D. J., Hinshaw, L. B., et al.: Vasopressin release during sepsis and septic shock in baboons and dogs. Surg. Gynecol. Obstet. *153*:869-872, 1981.
242. Wong, V. K., Hitchcock, W., and Mason, W. H.: Meningococcal infections in children: A review of 100 cases. Pediatr. Infect. Dis. J. *8*:224-227, 1989.
243. Woo, P., Carpenter, M. A., and Trunkey, D.: Ionized calcium: The effect of septic shock in the human. J. Surg. Res. *26*:605-610, 1979.
244. Woods, D. E., Strauss, D. C., Johanson, W. G., Jr., et al.: Role of salivary protease activity in adherence of gram-negative bacilli to mammalian buccal epithelial cells in vivo. J. Clin. Invest. *68*:1435-1440, 1981.
245. Wright, S. D., Ramos, R. A., Tobias, P. S., et al.: CD14, a receptor for complexes of lipopolysaccharide (LPS) and LPS binding protein. Science *249*:1431-1433, 1990.
246. Zabel, P., Schönharting, M. M., Wolter, D. T., et al.: Oxpentifylline in endotoxaemia. Lancet *2*:1474-1477, 1989.
247. Zaloga, G. P., and Chernow, B.: The multifactorial basis for hypocalcemia during sepsis: Studies of the parathyroid hormone-vitamin D axis. Ann. Intern. Med. *107*:36-41, 1987.
248. Ziegler, E., Fisher, C., Sprung, C., et al.: Treatment of gram-negative bacteremia and septic shock with HA-1A human monoclonal antibody against endotoxin. N. Engl. J. Med. *324*:429-436, 1991.

CHAPTER 70

FEVER WITHOUT SOURCE AND FEVER OF UNKNOWN ORIGIN

Debra L. Palazzi ✿ Ralph D. Feigin

Petersdorf and Beeson[76] in 1961 proposed that the term *fever of unknown origin* (FUO) be reserved for persons with an illness persisting for 3 or more weeks and accompanied by temperatures higher than 38.4° C (101.2° F) on at least several occasions. They further specified that the cause of the fever should remain undetermined after at least 1 week of investigation in the hospital. Although this definition was arbitrary, it was useful at that time, when many of the diagnostic tests now in routine use were unknown. The purpose of their precise definition was to explore the cause of fever in this select group of adult patients and to permit comparison of data from different investigations. This exacting definition probably never was applied rigorously in pediatric practice. In children, the term FUO should be reserved for fever of at least 8 days' duration and for which no diagnosis is apparent after the initial work-up in the hospital or as an outpatient.

Many investigators prefer using the term *fever without source* (FWS) for fever of recent onset with no adequate explanation

determined by the history or physical examination. The distinction between FUO and FWS is of more than academic interest for several reasons. First, although overlap exists, the differential diagnoses of these clinical conditions are distinct, and the most frequent causes of one are different from the most frequent causes of the other. Second, a child with fever of recent onset generally warrants more immediate evaluation than does a child with FUO. The latter usually does not occur as an emergency and requires timely, but not urgent, diagnostic or therapeutic intervention. Third, although expectant antibiotic treatment of children with FUO generally is not indicated, expectant treatment of infants with FWS is recommended in most cases.

FEVER WITHOUT SOURCE

A convenient definition of FWS *is the occurrence of fever for 1 week or less in a child in whom a careful history and physical examination fail to reveal a probable cause of the fever.* An estimated 14 to 40 percent of children with fever have no localizing signs or symptoms.[7,12] Stein[89] found that the peak incidence occurs during the second year of life. On the basis of a review of private pediatric practices in upstate New York, Hoekelman and colleagues[43] predicted that every 4 to 5 days a practicing pediatrician would see one child between 1 and 24 months of age with FWS.

Most children with fever of recent onset have acute infectious diseases, the majority of which are self-limited.[100] A few of these patients have serious acute infectious diseases, including meningitis and bacteremia, and a very few have acute noninfectious diseases or chronic disorders. For example, an occasional patient with FWS is discovered to have a disorder such as heat illness, drug poisoning, Kawasaki disease, malignancy, or connective tissue disease. However, these disorders occur infrequently. A physician faced with a child with FWS should consider the possibility of a noninfectious cause or the onset of a chronic disease, but unless a clinical clue suggests one of these entities, investigation in this direction is not warranted.

Many children with FWS are in the prodromal stages of an acute infectious illness, and evidence of a specific infection, such as pharyngitis, otitis media, or pneumonia, develops within hours to days of first being evaluated by a physician. Fever can precede the appearance of specific signs and symptoms by as long as 3 days, as in measles, Rocky Mountain spotted fever, and leptospirosis. In some infections, such as roseola, viral hepatitis, infectious mononucleosis, typhus, and typhoid fever, the interval between the onset of fever and the appearance of specific findings often is more than 3 days.

OCCULT BACTEREMIA

One major concern regarding a young child with FWS is the possibility that the child has occult bacteremia. The patient does not appear ill, is judged clinically well enough to be managed as an outpatient, and does not have an infection commonly associated with bacteremia such as pneumonia, but the blood culture yields pathogenic bacteria such as *Streptococcus pneumoniae, Neisseria meningitidis, Haemophilus influenzae, Escherichia coli, Salmonella,* or *Staphylococcus aureus.* Before introduction of the pneumococcal conjugate vaccine, the incidence of occult bacteremia in children with FWS was approximately 3 to 5 percent.[14,25,60,70,93,100] More recent data report an incidence of 0.2 to 3 percent, although this figure can vary depending on vaccine coverage rates in the population studied.[2,3,42,74,85,91] Few prospective, large studies have been performed to further investigate the impact of the pneumococcal conjugate vaccine on the incidence of occult bacteremia in children.[79] Historically, occult bacteremia has been found to occur more commonly in children with FWS than in febrile children of the same age with infections such as pharyngitis, otitis media, or upper respiratory tract infection. In the 1970s, investigators[60] reported the incidence of bacteremia in febrile children without an obvious source of infection to be 9.9 percent, as opposed to 3.3 percent in children with otitis media, upper respiratory tract infection, or a flu-like syndrome. During the same era, Teele and colleagues[93] found a 3.9 percent incidence of bacteremia in children with FWS and a 1.5 percent incidence in comparably febrile children with otitis media or pharyngitis.

The risk of occult bacteremia developing in a child with FWS is age-related, with most cases occurring in children younger than 24 months old. Numerous studies have demonstrated a higher risk for bacteremia or other serious bacterial infections (SBIs) in febrile infants younger than 3 months old.[58,60,84,93] In a group of children with clinically unsuspected meningococcemia, all 12 patients who initially looked well enough to be treated as outpatients were younger than 24 months of age.[31] Bonadio and colleagues[20] found the incidence of positive bacterial cultures to be 12 percent in febrile infants younger than 4 weeks and 6 percent in those between 4 and 8 weeks of age.

The risk of having occult bacteremia and other SBIs increases with the severity of fever. In a prospective study of bacteremia in children seen in the outpatient department, McCarthy and colleagues[61] identified a small, but statistically significant, difference in the incidence of bacteremia between children with temperatures of 40° C (104° F) or higher and those with temperatures of 40.5° C (104.9° F) or higher. In a prospective study in which blood was obtained for culture from all febrile children younger than 2 years old seen in a walk-in clinic, no positive blood cultures were found in 44 children with FWS and rectal temperatures lower than 38.9° C (102° F), whereas five (3.9%) positive blood cultures were found in 129 children with FWS and rectal temperatures of 38.9° C (102° F) or higher.[93] Other studies have reported similar findings.[14,58,85] Several series of children with fevers of 41° C (105.8° F) or higher found a relatively high prevalence of bacteremia and other SBIs, especially meningitis and pneumonia.[19,58,81] However, even in this group of children with very high fever, most of those older than 2 or 3 months of age who looked well did not have an SBI.

The white blood cell (WBC) count has been studied extensively as a potential tool in the diagnosis of occult bacteremia. On the basis of a study of hospitalized children, Todd[94] reported that the absolute number of polymorphonuclear leukocytes and the absolute number of nonsegmented polymorphonuclear leukocytes were more sensitive than was the total WBC count, the percentage of polymorphonuclear leukocytes, or the percentage of nonsegmented polymorphonuclear leukocytes. However, whether information based on hospitalized children—presumably all of whom had serious localized infections or looked ill enough to warrant hospitalization—can be applied to children with FWS who look well enough to be treated on an ambulatory basis is questionable.

Considerable debate continues over the usefulness of the WBC count in febrile children evaluated in the outpatient setting. McCarthy and associates[61] concluded that a WBC count of 15,000/mm³ or greater was helpful in identifying patients at greatest risk for the development of bacteremia. Dershewitz[32] found a direct relationship between the total leukocyte count and the prevalence of bacteremia and stated that "knowledge of the count was a helpful but limited predictor of patients with positive blood cultures." Other investigators reported that the incidence of bacteremia increased with an increased WBC count[85] and that bacteremia most commonly occurred in patients with counts of 20,000/mm³ or higher.[66]

Other studies have examined the utility of the WBC count specifically in children with FWS who look well enough to be treated on an outpatient basis. One such study found a sensitivity of 1.0 and a positive predictive value of 0.11 for a total WBC count of 15,000/mm³.[93] Using a WBC count of 20,000/mm³ would have decreased the sensitivity to 0.4 while increasing the positive predictive value to only 0.13. In another series, the sensitivity for a WBC count of 15,000/mm³ was 0.87, with a specificity of 0.73.[14] Kline and coworkers[50] found that a WBC count of 15,000/mm³ was more sensitive for *S. pneumoniae* bacteremia than for *H. influenzae* bacteremia. Although a total WBC count of 15,000/mm³ does not accurately predict which child is or is not bacteremic, it is helpful in dividing the population of children with FWS into high- and low-risk groups.

Some investigators have found the erythrocyte sedimentation rate to be no more useful than the WBC count in predicting bacteremia in ambulatory febrile patients.[61] Others have reported that the serum concentration of C-reactive protein (CRP) may be more accurate than is the complete blood count or erythrocyte sedimentation rate in distinguishing bacterial from viral infections.[59,75] However, recent studies reported conflicting data regarding the utility of the CRP test in screening children aged 3 to 36 months old for occult bacteremia.[44,82] An elevated serum procalcitonin level has been found by some investigators to be at least as sensitive and specific as is CRP in predicting SBI in children with fever and no localizing signs.[51,80]

Other hematologic findings that suggest bacteremia include thrombocytopenia,[29] Döhle inclusion bodies, toxic granulations, and vacuolization of neutrophils. In one study, peripheral blood smears of children younger than 24 months old with acute febrile illnesses were reviewed the following day by a single investigator to determine whether vacuolization and toxic granulations were present; when both abnormalities were present, the positive predictive value for bacteremia was 0.76.[53] The presence of these findings should be considered when estimating the risk for bacteremia.[1,29,69]

Several studies have examined the response to acetaminophen and found no difference in the rate of reduction of temperature or improvement in clinical appearance between bacteremic and nonbacteremic children.[9,95,102] Mazur and associates,[57] however, found that febrile children aged 2 months to 6 years old who did not respond to a dose of acetaminophen by a reduction in temperature of at least 0.8°C in 2 hours had a statistically significant increased risk of developing occult bacteremia in comparison to those who did respond.

The most important aspects of assessment of a febrile child are a careful history and physical examination. Laboratory data are secondary and should be ordered on the basis of the clinical assessment. By definition, a child with FWS has no localizing signs to explain the fever or indicate a site of infection. Many physicians suggest that a general impression can indicate whether the child has occult bacteremia. Some physicians have suggested that careful clinical judgment, based on extensive experience, can identify most, if not all, children with serious illnesses.[18] McCarthy and colleagues,[62-64] in a series of carefully designed studies, elucidated the variables of history and observation that were most useful in assessing febrile children. They found that observation of the variable *playfulness* had the strongest correlation with overall assessment.[63] However, they observed that even an experienced attending pediatrician could identify only 57 percent of seriously ill children by initial impression before performing a full physical examination. Dershewitz[32] found that private pediatricians were no more accurate than were pediatric residents in identifying children with occult bacteremia and that in the private office, pediatricians were no better at predicting bacteremia in familiar patients than in first-time patients.

In a study of 292 consecutive febrile children seen in an emergency department, Waskerwitz and Berkelhammer[97] identified a subgroup of patients who had no localizing signs and who looked so well that they were predicted not to have bacteremia. The physicians were assisted in their assessment by a functional scale that gave 0 to 2 points for the child's eating, drinking, sleeping, and play activities, with a best possible score of 8. The group of patients who had functional scores of 5 or greater, with no localized infection and predicted clinically not to have bacteremia, were free of bacteremia, whereas 14 of 202 patients with functional scores of 4 or less were bacteremic. In this study, the physicians were not able to identify which patients had bacteremia and which did not; rather, they were able to identify one subgroup at high risk for having bacteremia and another at very low risk. Teach and Fleisher[92] found that although Yale Observation Scale scores were higher in patients with bacteremia than in those without, the difference was not clinically useful in detecting bacteremia in well-looking febrile children without a discernible focus of infection. The clinician's overall assessment of the degree of illness of the child appears to be a valuable, but not infallible, tool in estimating the risk of occult bacteremia in children with FWS.

CLINICAL MANAGEMENT OF FEVER WITHOUT SOURCE

As many as 3 percent of children with FWS are bacteremic. Numerous studies (all performed before institution of the routine use of *H. influenzae* vaccine) have shown that if these children were not treated with antibiotics at the time of the initial clinical encounter, 5 to 10 percent would return with bacterial meningitis, 10 percent with localized bacterial infection, and another 30 percent with continued fever and persistent bacteremia.[14,21,43,56,60,61,66,93] In all of these retrospective studies, patients treated initially with antibiotics fared better than those not treated initially, although the decision regarding treatment always was at the discretion of the physician and was not randomized.

In a prospective, randomized investigation, Carroll and associates[25] studied 96 children between the ages of 6 and 24 months who had FWS and a temperature higher than 40°C (104°F). Of 10 patients who were bacteremic, 5 were treated initially with antibiotics on an outpatient basis and 5 were not treated. The difference in outcome between the two groups was statistically significant in favor of the treatment group; four of the five treated patients were improved clinically, as opposed to none of the five untreated patients. Bacterial meningitis did not develop in any of the treated patients, whereas it did develop in two of the five untreated patients. In a prospective, randomized, placebo-controlled study of empiric treatment with amoxicillin in children at risk for developing occult bacteremia, Jaffee and colleagues[46] showed no difference existed between treatment and nontreatment groups. However, the power of this study was low, and a true difference in outcome easily could have been missed.[5] The dosage of amoxicillin used was 125 mg three times daily for children who weighed 10 kg or less and 250 mg three times daily for those weighing more than 10 kg, so some children may have received as little as 37.5 mg/kg/day. Although this dosage is close to the usual recommended dosage of 40 mg/kg/day for infections such as otitis media, Baron and coworkers[15] suggested that considerably higher doses might be required to treat occult bacteremia. In a retrospective study of a private pediatric practice, these investigators found that no complications developed in 11 infants with FWS and bacteremia who initially received 150 mg/kg/day or more of amoxicillin (*p* = 0.03). In contrast, in 5 of 12 such infants not treated or treated with less than 100 mg/kg/day of amoxicillin, complications did develop. A study of the outcome of outpatient management of febrile children who proved to have pneumococcal bacteremia found that those not treated with antibiotics and those still febrile on re-evaluation were most likely to have persistent bacteremia.[6]

One should not be dogmatic about the management of children with FWS. One reasonable approach, based on a careful history, thorough physical examination, and overall clinical impression, is to classify these children as being at low or high risk for the development of occult bacteremia and other SBIs. For the low-risk group, no laboratory investigation is required routinely. For the high-risk group, a complete blood count and blood culture should be obtained. Lumbar puncture, chest radiography, urinalysis, and urine culture are considered on an individual basis. If the patient appears ill, admission to the hospital may be justified, even if all test results are negative. When high-risk children look well enough to be sent home, they are reasonable candidates for expectant antibiotic therapy, pending the outcome of blood culture. For patients clinically considered to be at moderate risk (not clearly high or low risk), the physician has the option of obtaining a WBC count and using the results to decide whether to draw blood for culture and prescribe antibiotics expectantly.

Table 70–1 lists risk factors for the development of occult bacteremia. Current information is not sufficient to warrant the use of scoring systems except as part of investigational series. In the final analysis, the clinician's judgment, taking into account all

TABLE 70–1   Risk Factors for Occult Bacteremia

Factor	High Risk	Low Risk
Age	≤24 mo	>36 mo
Magnitude of fever	≥40°C (104°F)	≤39.4°C (103°F)
White blood cell count	≥15,000/mm³	<15,000/mm³
Peripheral blood smear	Toxic granulation or vacuolization of polymorphonuclear leukocytes, thrombocytopenia	Unremarkable
Underlying chronic disorder	Sickle-cell disease, immunodeficiency, malnutrition	None
History of contact with bacterial disease	Contact with *Neisseria meningitidis* or *Haemophilus influenzae*	None
Clinical appearance	Appears ill, "toxic," or unhappy; inconsolable; irritable or lethargic; not eating or drinking enough	Looks well, playful, eating normally, not irritable

available clinical and laboratory data about each patient, is the guide to selecting which children require a diagnostic work-up and expectant therapy with antibiotics.

If the physician elects to prescribe antibiotics while awaiting the results of blood culture, such antibiotic therapy should provide adequate coverage for *S. pneumoniae*, *N. meningitidis*, and *H. influenzae*, although the frequency of *H. influenzae* has decreased dramatically with current immunization practice. A single injection of 50 to 75 mg/kg of ceftriaxone given while awaiting the results of blood culture has been successful in resolving fever, clearing bacteremia, and preventing meningitis and was found to be superior to oral regimens in several series.[13,16,38] Children with a positive blood culture should be recalled for re-evaluation, even if they are afebrile.

Because *S. pneumoniae* is a dominant cause of occult bacteremia, routine use of pneumococcal vaccine is expected to diminish the occurrence of occult bacteremia significantly. Children who have been immunized against both *H. influenzae* and *S. pneumoniae* should be considered to be at relatively low risk for the development of occult bacteremia and may require less work-up, unless they appear ill or have a very high fever.

Infants younger than 90 days old pose a special problem because they have an increased risk for developing SBI, clinical evaluation is more difficult, and a broader spectrum of invading organisms (e.g., group B *Streptococcus*, *E. coli*, *Listeria monocytogenes*) exists. Baker and coworkers[8] showed the safety of managing selected low-risk infants (i.e., normal WBC count, urinalysis, lumbar puncture, and chest roentgenogram and, if diarrhea was present, negative smear for fecal leukocytes) 30 to 90 days of age on an outpatient basis without antibiotics. Jaskiewicz and coworkers[48] found the Rochester criteria (WBC count of 5000 to 15,000/mm³, band count <1500/mm³, spun urine specimen <10 WBCs/high-power field, stool specimen [if diarrhea] <5 WBCs/high-power field) to have a 98.9 percent negative predictive value in well-appearing, previously healthy infants younger than 90 days old with no focal infections. One reasonable practice guideline for managing infants with FWS is to hospitalize and treat all who appear toxic and all younger than 28 days. Those between 28 and 90 days of age can be managed as outpatients if they look well and the blood count, urinalysis, and cerebrospinal fluid analysis are within normal limits.[10,11]

FEVER OF UNKNOWN ORIGIN

The exact definition of FUO is a subject of considerable disagreement, and series in the pediatric literature differ in their criteria for inclusion. Brewis[22] defined FUO in children as a temperature of 38.3°C (101°F) or higher for 5 to 7 consecutive days without localizing signs or symptoms. In sharp contrast, McClung[65] and Lohr and Hendley[54] considered children with fever for at least 3 weeks on an outpatient basis or 1 week in the hospital to have FUO. Pizzo and associates,[78] however, required only that the fever be present for 2 weeks, with no distinction made between outpatient or in-hospital status. A reasonable working definition of FUO for clinical purposes is the presence of fever for 8 or more days in a child for whom a careful and thorough history and physical examination and preliminary laboratory data fail to reveal a probable cause of the fever.

Most cases of FUO in children are caused by relatively common diseases. In four series of FUO totaling 418 children, only 5 patients would be considered to have rare disorders (i.e., Behçet syndrome, ichthyosis, variant of "blue diaper" syndrome, diencephalic seizure disorder, and "possible chronic lead and/or arsenic intoxication").[22,54,65,78] The adage that FUO is more likely to be caused by an unusual manifestation of a common disorder than by a common manifestation of a rare disorder certainly is true in pediatrics. The three most common discernible causes of FUO in children, in order of decreasing frequency, are infectious diseases, connective tissue diseases, and neoplasms. In approximately 10 to 20 percent of cases, a definitive diagnosis never is established.

In the United States, the systemic infectious diseases diagnosed most frequently in children with FUO include tuberculosis, brucellosis, tularemia, salmonellosis, and infections caused by rickettsia, spirochetes (e.g., leptospirosis), Epstein-Barr virus, cytomegalic inclusion virus, human immunodeficiency virus, hepatitis viruses, and other viruses. The most common causes of localized infection are upper respiratory tract infections (e.g., sinusitis, otitis, tonsillitis), urinary tract infection, osteomyelitis, and occult abscesses, including hepatic and pelvic abscesses.

The connective tissue disease most commonly manifested as FUO in children is juvenile rheumatoid arthritis, which accounts for more than 90 percent of connective tissue diseases in most series, followed by systemic lupus erythematosus and then by undefined vasculitis.[54,65,68,78] Frequently, a definitive diagnosis of juvenile rheumatoid arthritis can be made only after an extended period of observation because physical examination may yield no findings and the results of specific serologic studies generally are normal or negative.

Malignancy is a less frequent cause of FUO in children than in adults and usually is the third-largest group, after infectious diseases and connective tissue diseases. Malignancy accounted for 7 percent of FUO cases in the series reported by Pizzo and associates[78] and for 13 percent in the Lohr and Hendley[54] series. Leukemia and lymphoma are responsible for most cases of cancer manifested as FUO in children. Other tumors less commonly reported as causing FUO include neuroblastoma, hepatoma, sarcoma, and atrial myxoma.

Although the prognosis for children with FUO is better than that for adults and even though most children with FUO have treatable or self-limited disease, the overall prognosis is far from benign. Mortality rates were 9 percent in the series reported by Pizzo and associates[78] and 6 percent in Lohr and Hendley's series.[54] The prognosis for children in whom a definitive diagnosis is not established during the initial hospitalization is mixed. In most cases, the fever eventually resolves.[36] In some patients, a specific diagnosis is established, whereas other patients continue to have fever without a definitive diagnosis. McClung[65] described 11 such patients, most of whom appeared to do well despite having recurrent episodes of fever.

DIAGNOSTIC APPROACH TO A CHILD WITH FEVER OF UNKNOWN ORIGIN

A child with FUO is admitted to the hospital for more than simply laboratory investigation. Hospitalization provides an opportunity to observe the child, repeat the history and physical examination, analyze all available data, and investigate every potential diagnostic lead. In the Lohr and Hendley[54] series of 54 children with FUO, an incomplete history delayed establishing the diagnosis in 9 cases, and physical findings that were ignored delayed rendering the diagnosis in 4 cases. In McClung's report[65] of 99 pediatric cases of FUO, errors in the history or physical examination obscured the correct diagnosis for at least 10 patients. Failure to use existing laboratory data correctly is another common factor preventing early determination of the diagnosis in children with FUO.[54,78]

Clinical Evaluation

The first and most important step in the diagnostic work-up of a child with FUO is obtaining a complete and detailed history and conducting a physical examination. The clinical evaluation must be thorough and careful, and it must be repeated frequently. Often, a patient or parent eventually recalls information that was omitted or forgotten when the initial history was obtained. Physical findings change, and abnormalities not originally present can appear subsequently. Lohr and Hendley[54] noted that in more than 25 percent of children admitted to the hospital with FUO, significant physical findings developed that were not present at the time of admission.

A detailed history should be obtained regarding contact with infected or otherwise ill persons and any exposure to animals, including pets and wild animals. The number of children with zoonotic infections is increasing each year. Immunization of domestic animals such as the dog against leptospirosis can prevent canine disease, but it does not prevent carriage, excretion, and transmission of this infection. A history of travel extending back to birth must be elicited. Re-emergence of histoplasmosis, coccidioidomycosis, blastomycosis, or malaria years after visiting or living in an endemic area can occur. Inquiring about prophylactic immunizations, precautions taken against the ingestion of contaminated food or water, and malarial prophylaxis is important. Questioning should include the possibility that rocks, soil, or artifacts from geographically distant regions may have been brought into the home, as well as the possibility that contact with persons who have visited distant countries has occurred. Even contact with insects can be important. Tick bites can be a clue to Rocky Mountain spotted fever or tick-borne relapsing fever. North American mosquitoes and some ticks carry a variety of arboviruses.

The physician should determine whether the patient has eaten game meat, raw meat, or raw shellfish. A history of pica should be sought routinely. Ingestion of dirt can suggest a diagnosis of visceral larva migrans, toxoplasmosis, or other infectious diseases. A detailed history regarding all medications, including topical agents and nonprescription items, must be elicited carefully. Any history of surgical procedures should be explored.

Questions designed to determine the genetic or ethnic background of the patient can reveal information that specifically suggests or largely excludes diagnoses such as nephrogenic diabetes insipidus (found in Ulster Scots), familial Mediterranean fever (found in Armenians, Arabs, and Sephardic Jews), familial dysautonomia (found in Jews), and Kikuchi-Fujimoto disease, a benign and self-limited histiocytic necrotizing lymphadenitis (found mostly in young Asian females and characterized by fever, lymphadenopathy, and malaise).

The history should be exacting regarding the duration, height, and pattern of the fever, as well as the circumstances under which temperature elevation occurs, whether the child appears ill or any signs or symptoms develop, and how well the fever responds to antipyretic drugs. A history of "fever" occurring only after exercise or late in the afternoon can indicate parental concern about normal variations in body temperature. A history of high fever occurring in the absence of malaise or other generalized signs can be a clue to factitious fever. The physician also should obtain a careful history regarding how well the fever has been documented. Has a thermometer been used, by whom, and in whose presence? A history of sweating and heat intolerance can indicate hyperthyroidism, whereas a history of heat intolerance with the absence of sweating can be a clue to ectodermal dysplasia.

Several investigators have found that neither the pattern of fever nor its duration was useful in pointing to or establishing a diagnosis in children with FUO.[54,78] However, occasionally the character of the fever can be helpful. *Intermittent fever* is characterized by a return of temperature to normal at least once daily. If the peak of fever is high and the rate of defervescence quick, this pattern often is referred to as *hectic* or *spiking*. Intermittent fevers suggest pyogenic infections but also occur with tuberculosis, lymphoma, and juvenile rheumatoid arthritis. In *remittent fever*, the temperature fluctuates but does not return to normal. A *sustained fever* pattern is characterized by persistent fever with little or no fluctuation and can occur in typhoid fever or typhus. Antipyretic agents can make a remittent or sustained fever appear intermittent. *Relapsing fever* refers to a pattern in which the patient is afebrile for 1 or more days between episodes of fever and can be seen with malaria, rat-bite fever, infection with *Borrelia*, and lymphoma. Recurrent episodes of fever of more than a year's duration can suggest metabolic defects, central nervous system abnormalities in temperature control, and immunodeficient states.

The general activity and appearance of the patient should be observed, vital signs checked, and growth parameters measured. Weight loss is an important, though nonspecific, finding. Impairment of linear growth or short stature can be a clue to inflammatory bowel disease, an intracranial lesion involving the pituitary gland, or a long-standing chronic disease. Examining the patient during an episode of fever to observe the presence or absence of sweating, the effect of the fever on the heart and respiratory rate, the presence or absence of malaise or other symptoms, and the appearance of "toxicity" is helpful. The rash of juvenile rheumatoid arthritis characteristically is evanescent and may be present only during periods of temperature elevation.

Some special aspects of the physical examination merit mention. Hypohidrosis, anomalous dentition, and sparse hair, particularly involving the eyebrows and eyelashes, suggest anhidrotic ectodermal dysplasia. Palpebral conjunctivitis can be a clue to the presence of infectious mononucleosis, Newcastle disease, or lupus erythematosus, whereas predominantly bulbar conjunctivitis can suggest leptospirosis or Kawasaki disease. Phlyctenular conjunctivitis can signal tuberculosis.

Absence of the pupillary constrictor response can be caused by a deficiency of the constrictor sphincter muscle of the eye. This muscle, derived from ectoderm rather than mesoderm, develops embryologically at the same time that hypothalamic structures and function are undergoing differentiation. Absence of this muscle can suggest that the elevation in temperature is the result of hypothalamic or autonomic dysfunction. Careful funduscopic examination can disclose evidence of miliary tuberculosis, vasculitis, or toxoplasmosis. Lack of tears, absence of corneal reflexes, and a smooth tongue with absence of the fungiform papillae suggest familial dysautonomia.

Purulent or persistent nasal discharge can be a sign of sinusitis. The physician should palpate for tenderness over the sinuses.

Hyperemia of the pharynx, even in the absence of exudate or specific symptoms, can be a clue to the diagnosis of infectious mononucleosis, cytomegalic inclusion disease, toxoplasmosis, tularemia, or leptospirosis. Gingival hypertrophy or inflammation and loosening or loss of teeth can indicate leukemia or Langerhans cell histiocytosis.

The bones and muscles should be palpated carefully. Tenderness over a bone can be found in cases of osteomyelitis or marrow invasion by neoplastic disease. Muscle tenderness can be associated with trichinosis, dermatomyositis, polyarteritis, or various arboviral infections.

The search for skin lesions and rash must be careful, extensive, and repeated. Petechiae can indicate endocarditis or other sources of bacteremia but also can occur with viral and rickettsial infections. A seborrheic rash can be a sign of histiocytosis.

A careful rectal examination is imperative for patients of all ages and can reveal pararectal tenderness or a mass indicative of a pelvic abscess or tumor. A test for occult blood should be performed on any stool found on the examining finger. Examination of the external genitalia should be completed on patients of all ages, and sexually active adolescent females should undergo a pelvic examination.

Laboratory Evaluation

The extent of laboratory investigation depends on the age of the patient, duration of the fever, and history and physical examination findings. Laboratory studies should be directed, as much as possible, toward the most likely diagnostic possibilities. The tempo of the diagnostic evaluation should be adjusted to the severity of the illness. In a critically ill child, speedy evaluation is important. If the patient is less severely ill, however, the evaluation can proceed more slowly; sometimes the fever can disappear without apparent explanation before a definitive diagnosis can be established and any invasive diagnostic procedures have been undertaken.

A complete blood count and careful examination of the peripheral smear are indicated for all patients. Anemia, thrombocytosis, and thrombocytopenia should be noted. Although mild or moderate changes in the total WBC or differential count usually are of no help, in some series, children with more than 10,000 polymorphonuclear leukocytes or 500 nonsegmented neutrophils/mm³ were found to have a greater likelihood of having SBI.[89,94] Atypical lymphocytes generally indicate viral infection, whereas bizarre or immature forms can suggest leukemia. Although the erythrocyte sedimentation rate is of no specific diagnostic value, it is a general indicator of inflammation and can help in ruling out factitious fever, determining the need for further evaluation, and monitoring the progress of the disease process.

Blood should be obtained from all patients for aerobic and anaerobic culture. In select cases, media appropriate for the isolation of *Francisella* organisms, *Leptospira*, and *Spirillum* also should be used.

Urine analysis and culture should be completed for all patients. In one series of FUO in children, failure to perform urinalysis and failure to investigate pyuria adequately were the most common laboratory errors.[65] Radiographic study of the urinary tract, however, should be performed only when indicated.

All patients should undergo radiographic examination of the chest. Diagnostic imaging of the nasal sinuses, mastoids, and gastrointestinal tract is performed initially only for specific indications but should be done eventually in all children whose fever persists without explanation for a long period. Persistent fever and elevation of the erythrocyte sedimentation rate, with or without anemia, abdominal complaints, anorexia, and weight loss, are sufficient indications for radiographic study to rule out inflammatory bowel disease.

All patients should have an intradermal tuberculin skin test. Control skin tests with antigens such as *Candida* are of limited value because the anergy may be specific for tuberculosis rather

than universal for all skin-testing materials.[55,67,71,72] A positive control test result and negative tuberculin test result do not rule out tuberculosis.

Bone marrow examination is most useful in diagnosing cancer (especially leukemia), histiocytic disorders, and hemophagocytic disease. It is less useful in determining infection. Hayani and associates[41] reviewed the results of 414 bone marrow examinations for FUO in children. In only one case was an organism (*Salmonella* group D) recovered from the marrow that also was not recovered from blood or another source. Noninfectious causes of FUO were found in 8 percent of specimens: malignancy (6.7%), hemophagocytic syndrome (HPS, 0.7%), histiocytosis (0.5%), and hypoplastic anemia (0.2%). In most of these cases, the diagnosis had been suspected clinically before the bone marrow was examined.

All patients should undergo a serum test for human immunodeficiency virus infection. Other appropriate serologic tests can help establish a diagnosis of cat-scratch disease, brucellosis, tularemia, Epstein-Barr virus infection, cytomegalic inclusion virus infection, other viral infections, toxoplasmosis, and certain fungal infections.

Hepatic enzymes and serum chemistry, including electrolytes, urea nitrogen, and creatinine, should be determined in all patients. Serum antinuclear antibody should be measured in those older than 5 years. Serum hepatitis antigens, electrocardiography, electroencephalography, echocardiography, and stool culture and examination for ova and parasites generally should be performed in selected cases. Other tests to be considered for individual patients include ophthalmologic examination by slit lamp, radiographic bone survey, technetium bone scan, liver-spleen scan, and abdominal imaging by ultrasonography or computed tomography.[24,77] Computed tomographic scanning, gallium scanning, and indium 111 scanning[37] can detect inflammatory lesions and tumors. Such scanning procedures offer a relatively noninvasive technique for screening patients with FUO for a variety of disorders. Although Steele and associates[88] found that radionucleotide scans seldom led to unsuspected diagnoses in children and suggested that they not be used indiscriminately, gallium scanning has been helpful in diagnosing adult patients with FUO,[40] and it may be a reasonable test for selected children. Lymph node biopsy, liver biopsy, and exploratory laparoscopy are reserved for patients with evidence of involvement of these organs.

In general, antibiotics or other medications should not be administered empirically as a diagnostic measure in children with FUO. Exceptions include the use of nonsteroidal agents in children with presumed juvenile rheumatoid arthritis and the use of antituberculous drugs in critically ill children thought to have disseminated tuberculosis. Empiric trials of broad-spectrum antibiotics generally do more to obscure than illuminate the etiology of FUO and can mask or delay establishing the diagnosis of infections such as meningitis, parameningeal infection, endocarditis, or osteomyelitis.

Examples of disorders that can be manifested as FUO in children are listed in Table 70–2. A few of these disorders are discussed briefly in the following sections.

INFECTIOUS CAUSES OF FEVER OF UNKNOWN ORIGIN

Infectious causes of FUO can be divided into systemic and localized. Immunodeficient states may be considered under the general classification of infections.

Generalized Infections

BRUCELLOSIS

The manifestation of this disease as FUO is explained by the nonspecific symptoms that it engenders and by the chronicity of

TABLE 70-2 Causes of Fever of Unknown Origin in Children

Infectious Diseases
Bacterial
Bacterial endocarditis
Brucellosis
Cat-scratch disease
Leptospirosis
Liver abscess
Mastoiditis (chronic)
Osteomyelitis
Pelvic abscess
Perinephric abscess
Pyelonephritis
Salmonellosis
Sinusitis
Subdiaphragmatic abscess
Tuberculosis
Tularemia

Viral
Cytomegalovirus
Epstein-Barr virus (infectious mononucleosis)
Hepatitis viruses

Chlamydial
Lymphogranuloma venereum
Psittacosis

Rickettsial
Q fever
Rocky Mountain spotted fever

Fungal
Blastomycosis (nonpulmonary)
Histoplasmosis (disseminated)

Parasitic
Malaria
Toxoplasmosis
Visceral larva migrans

Unclassified
Sarcoidosis

Collagen Vascular Diseases
Juvenile rheumatoid arthritis
Polyarteritis nodosa
Systemic lupus erythematosus

Malignancies
Hodgkin disease
Leukemia/lymphoma
Neuroblastoma

Miscellaneous
Central diabetes insipidus
Drug fever
Ectodermal dysplasia
Factitious fever
Familial dysautonomia
Granulomatous colitis
Hemophagocytic syndrome
Infantile cortical hyperostosis
Kikuchi-Fujimoto disease
Nephrogenic diabetes insipidus
Pancreatitis
Periodic fever
Serum sickness
Thyrotoxicosis
Ulcerative colitis

untreated infection. Many physicians, particularly in urban areas, tend to ignore the possibility of this disease and neglect to inquire about a history of exposure to animals or animal products, especially the consumption of unpasteurized goat's milk cheese (see Chapter 139).

CAT-SCRATCH DISEASE

During recent years, many children with FUO have proved to be infected with *Bartonella henselae*. Cat-scratch disease is one of the most common causes of FUO in patients seen at the infectious disease service at Texas Children's Hospital in Houston.[4] Most of the children with this manifestation of cat-scratch disease have hepatosplenic involvement. Jacobs and Schutze[45] reported that *B. henselae* infection was the cause of 4.8 percent of all cases of FUO at the Arkansas Children's Hospital and 10.9 percent of the cases of FUO caused by infection. *B. henselae* infection is best diagnosed by serologic evaluation (i.e., immunofluorescence assay that detects serum antibody to *B. henselae*). Biopsy of lesions (e.g., lymph nodes, liver, bone marrow) may allow visualization of bacilli with the Warthin-Starry silver stain; however, this finding is not specific for *B. henselae*. Management of patients with cat-scratch disease is primarily symptomatic because the disease usually is self-limited. Antimicrobial therapy can be helpful in acutely or severely ill patients, especially those with hepatosplenic disease. Several oral antimicrobial regimens (rifampin, trimethoprim-sulfamethoxazole, azithromycin) and parenteral gentamicin have been used successfully for the treatment of this disease. In particular, rifampin at a dose of 20 mg/kg/day in two divided doses for 14 days has been particularly efficacious.[4] However, the optimal duration of therapy is not known.

LEPTOSPIROSIS

Leptospirosis is caused by a single family of organisms composed of multiple serotypes; it is one of the most widespread zoonoses in the world. Transmission of infection from animal to human can occur by direct contact with the blood, tissue, organs, or urine of infected animals or indirectly by exposure to an environment that has been contaminated by leptospires. The organism also can be acquired from soil or from fresh water after ingestion. Reports indicate that leptospirosis is not a rare disease, that many infections are not associated with occupational exposure, and that urban and suburban cases are becoming more prevalent.[26] Clinical manifestations of leptospirosis usually are not specific. A variety of laboratory aids are available, but specimens must be collected and handled properly. In some cases, establishing a definitive diagnosis may be impossible; negative cultures or failure to demonstrate a rise in antibody titer does not exclude the possibility that the patient has active infection because the organism may not be present in the specimens that have been cultured, the antibody titer may have peaked before an acute-phase specimen was collected, and antibiotic therapy may suppress the development of positive titers or delay their appearance (see Chapter 154).

TOXOPLASMOSIS

Toxoplasmosis should be considered in any child with persistent fever. Cervical or supraclavicular adenopathy is present in most cases, but occasionally fever is the only manifestation. The diagnosis is established by demonstration of a rising serologic titer; antibody to *Toxoplasma gondii* is so prevalent that demonstration of a high titer alone is not diagnostic of acute infection. Demonstration of *Toxoplasma* in tissue sections or body fluid is highly suggestive, although the organism can persist in tissue for years. Isolation of the parasite is not absolutely diagnostic of recent infection (see Chapter 235).

MALARIA

Malaria also should be considered in children with FUO. In addition to fever, splenomegaly usually is present. A history of travel to endemic areas should be sought, although malaria has occurred in patients who never traveled outside the United States. Disease can occur even in persons who have taken antimalarial drugs when they visited the endemic region. A hiatus of several months can occur between the development of infection and the onset of symptoms. The infection can be transmitted from a person who has visited an endemic area to one who has not when an appropriate mosquito vector is present. Malaria also can be acquired by blood transfusion or by the use of needles and syringes contaminated by the parasite. Demonstration of malarial organisms on appropriately stained thin or thick smears of blood is diagnostic (see Chapter 231).

SALMONELLOSIS

Salmonella organisms are contaminants in many food products. In view of the nonspecific signs and symptoms with which salmonellosis can occur, its association with FUO in children is not surprising. Repetitive blood and stool cultures are most helpful in establishing a diagnosis (see Chapter 121).

TUBERCULOSIS

Tuberculosis is an important cause of FUO in children, as well as in adults. Nonpulmonary tuberculosis is manifested as FUO more frequently than pulmonary tuberculosis is, which usually is evident on routine chest radiographs. FUO occurs most commonly with disseminated tuberculosis or infection of the liver, peritoneum, pericardium, or genitourinary tract. Active disseminated tuberculosis has been well documented in children with negative results on chest radiography and tuberculin skin tests.[72,90] A high index of suspicion and a careful history of possible contacts can be the best diagnostic tools. Funduscopic examination can reveal choroid tubercles. Liver and bone marrow frequently are involved in children with miliary tuberculosis; liver biopsy specimens and bone marrow aspirates should be obtained and processed for morphologic evaluation and culture. If the chest radiograph yields abnormal results, cultures of gastric aspirates, sputum, or both should be obtained. Because nontuberculous mycobacteria (i.e., atypical organisms) are present in the gastric contents of normal individuals, demonstration of acid-fast organisms on smears of gastric secretion does not indicate disease necessarily. Rarely, a patient with tuberculous pericarditis has fever, weight loss, and weakness but no precordial pain or other specific cardiac complaints. Disseminated infection with atypical mycobacteria generally is seen in patients infected with human immunodeficiency virus (see Chapter 107).

TULAREMIA

Generally, failure to consider tularemia in children with FUO may be attributed to a lack of appreciation of the many sources of infection and the various routes of inoculation. The organism can be acquired from contact with a variety of animal species, as well as from ticks, mosquitoes, lice, fleas, flies, and contaminated water. The organism can penetrate mucous membranes and broken or unbroken skin, or it can be inhaled or swallowed. Patients and parents should be questioned about animal contact and the ingestion of rabbit or squirrel meat (see Chapter 144).

VIRAL INFECTIONS

Infection by most viruses produces an illness that is relatively brief. Exceptions to this rule include infections by cytomegalovirus, Epstein-Barr virus, hepatitis viruses, and certain arboviruses. In all of these diseases, symptoms are extremely variable and signs and symptoms frequently are nonspecific. The diagnosis can be established by appropriate cultures and serologic studies (see Section 17 and Chapter 264).

IMMUNODEFICIENCY

A variety of congenital and acquired immunodeficiency states can be manifested as FUO. Patients with immunoglobulin deficiencies (e.g., Bruton agammaglobulinemia) may have a long history of recurrent fever, with or without evident infection, whereas patients with abnormalities in lymphocyte function are more likely to have prolonged fever caused by persistent viral or parasitic infection.

Localized Infections

BACTERIAL ENDOCARDITIS

Infective endocarditis is an infrequent cause of FUO in children. Acute bacterial endocarditis tends to be fulminant in nature, but the subacute form begins insidiously, generally at the site of a preexisting cardiac lesion. Subacute bacterial endocarditis is a rare occurrence in infants and increases in frequency with advancing age. The organisms most commonly encountered are viridans streptococci, enterococci, *S. aureus*, and *Staphylococcus epidermidis*. The absence of a cardiac murmur does not exclude the possibility of endocarditis, especially when the infection is limited to the right side of the heart. Endocarditis also can occur in the absence of positive blood cultures, particularly in association with the following factors: use of antibiotics for an undefined febrile illness, right-sided cardiac lesions, prolonged duration of disease, infection by unusual organisms such as *Brucella* or *Coxiella burnetii*, and inadequate culture methods for the detection of infection with anaerobic organisms. Frequently associated laboratory findings include anemia, leukocytosis, and an elevated erythrocyte sedimentation rate. Several blood cultures (aerobic and anaerobic) should be obtained before starting antibiotics. Echocardiography and gallium scanning can reveal vegetations, but negative results do not rule out endocarditis (see Chapter 32).

BONE AND JOINT INFECTIONS

Infections of bones and joints usually can be diagnosed clinically but occasionally are manifested as FUO. This manifestation occurs commonly in young children who cannot explain where they hurt and is more likely to occur with osteomyelitis than with septic arthritis. Infection of the pelvic bones is implicated most often in this regard. Radioisotopic bone scan and magnetic resonance imaging are more sensitive than are plain radiographs of the bones (see Chapters 61 and 62).

INTRA-ABDOMINAL ABSCESSES

Subphrenic, perinephric, and pelvic abscesses may be manifested as FUO. A history of previous intra-abdominal disease or abdominal surgery or a history of vague abdominal complaints should heighten suspicion of an intra-abdominal collection of pus. The organisms involved most commonly are *S. aureus*, streptococci, *E. coli*, and anaerobic flora. Fever may be the only sign of a pelvic, perinephric, or psoas abscess. Urinalysis generally yields normal results, but the mass can be demonstrated by ultrasound examination, gallium scan, or computed tomography.

LIVER ABSCESS AND OTHER HEPATIC INFECTIONS

Pyogenic liver abscesses are encountered most frequently in immunocompromised pediatric patients but can be seen in otherwise normal children.[49] In some patients, persistent fever is the only finding. Blood cultures usually are sterile, and serum levels of liver enzymes generally are close to or within normal limits. Many patients have hepatomegaly and right upper quadrant abdominal tenderness. The diagnosis can be established by examination of the liver by ultrasonography, radioisotope scanning, computed tomography, or magnetic resonance imaging; a body gallium scan also can yield positive results. Bacterial hepatitis and bacterial cholangitis can occur in the absence of jaundice and other specific signs of liver dysfunction.[98,101] Granulomatous hepatitis is not a specific disease but rather a syndrome characterized by granuloma formation within the liver. A specific cause cannot be determined in every case. Although most reported cases have been in adults,[86] pediatric cases do occur, particularly with Epstein-Barr virus infection and with cat-scratch disease. The diagnosis can be made by ultrasound or other diagnostic imaging (see Chapter 55).

UPPER RESPIRATORY TRACT INFECTIONS

Frequently, infections of the upper respiratory tract and related organs are manifested as FUO.[54,65,78] Although obvious signs or symptoms would be expected, the complaints often appear trivial and may be ignored. Reported cases of FUO have occurred in children with mastoiditis, sinusitis, chronic or recurrent otitis media, chronic or recurrent pharyngitis, tonsillitis, peritonsillar abscess, and nonspecific upper respiratory tract infection. A parapharyngeal inflammatory pseudotumor manifested as FUO has been reported in a 3-year-old girl in whom anemia and weight loss also developed. The cause never was discerned, but the symptoms resolved after surgical removal of the inflammatory mass.[27]

A syndrome of periodic fever has been associated with recurrent aphthous stomatitis, pharyngitis, and cervical adenitis. Symptoms recur at 4- to 6-week intervals, generally beginning abruptly and resolving spontaneously in 4 to 5 days. The cause of this syndrome remains unknown.[35]

NONINFECTIOUS CAUSES OF FEVER OF UNKNOWN ORIGIN

Central Nervous System Dysfunction

Children with severe brain damage can have dysfunctional thermoregulation, and body temperature in some of these patients can remain elevated for months. Cases of otherwise neurologically normal children who have had fever as a result of central dysfunction also have been reported. Berger[17] discussed a 16-year-old child with recurrent episodes of fever that were thought to represent a form of epilepsy but disappeared when treatment with phenytoin was begun. Wolff and associates[99] reported a 14-year-old child with cyclic episodes of fever, nausea, vomiting, and emotional disturbance caused by a central nervous system lesion.

Diabetes Insipidus

Central and nephrogenic diabetes insipidus can cause FUO in infants and young children. Polyuria and polydipsia may not be appreciated during infancy. Hyperthermia, weight loss, and peripheral vascular collapse can ensue. Signs of dehydration or an increased serum concentration of sodium suggests the diagnosis. The diagnosis is established by simultaneous measurements of urine and serum electrolytes and osmolality during periods of normal hydration and after carefully controlled periods of water deprivation. Serum levels of antidiuretic hormone also can be measured by radioimmunoassay.

Drug Fever

Nearly any medication can be associated with an allergic reaction, including fever. The offending agent may be a prescribed drug, an over-the-counter preparation, or a street drug such as amphetamine or PCP (1-[1-phenylcyclohexyl]piperidine, phencyclidine). Atropine, whether taken systemically or used topically in the form of eyedrops, can cause elevation of temperature. Phenothiazines and anticholinergic drugs can inhibit sweating and impair regulation of temperature. Epinephrine and related compounds can affect thermoregulatory control mechanisms and produce fever. Drug fever can be low-grade or high and spiking. Fever can be continuous or intermittent. Discontinuation of the drug generally is followed by disappearance of the fever within 48 hours, but it sometimes persists for as long as a month as a result of slow excretion of the offending agent.

Factitious Fever

A parent or patient may report the presence of fever that does not exist. The reading of the thermometer can be increased by immersing the bulb in hot liquid or by rinsing the mouth with hot liquid immediately before inserting the thermometer. Clues to factitious fever include absence of tachycardia, malaise, or discomfort despite a markedly elevated temperature; apparent rapid defervescence unaccompanied by diaphoresis; failure of the temperature curve to follow the normal diurnal variation of body temperature; hyperpyrexia; and normal temperature reading when the temperature is obtained rectally by someone who remains in attendance during the procedure. The presence of fever also can be confirmed or excluded by measuring the temperature of a freshly voided urine specimen. The current use of electronic thermometers in most hospitals decreases the possibility of factitious fever in that setting because the nurse or aide usually brings in the thermometer and stays in attendance during the relatively brief period of insertion. In more unusual cases, the patient or parent can induce fever by the injection of infective or foreign materials.

Familial Dysautonomia

Familial dysautonomia (Riley-Day syndrome), an autosomal recessive disorder, is characterized by autonomic and peripheral sensory nerve dysfunction. Eighty percent of patients are children of Jewish parentage, particularly Ashkenazi Jews. Defective regulation of temperature can result in hypothermia or hyperthermia.[30]

A careful history and physical examination can reveal the following: poorly coordinated swallowing movements that lead to recurrent aspiration and pneumonia; recurrent episodes of vomiting; excessive salivation; excessive or diminished sweating; diminished formation of tears; periods of hypotension, hypertension, or both; and erythema or blanching of the skin. The fungiform papillae of the tongue are absent or diminished in number, and the sensation of taste is deficient.[87] Self-mutilation or multiple sites of skin trauma can reflect diminished or absent pain sensation peripherally. Deep tendon reflexes are diminished; corneal reflexes are impaired; and mental deficiency, dysarthria, and emotional lability are common findings.

Excretion of vanillylmandelic acid in urine can be diminished, and excretion of homovanillic acid can be increased. Administration of histamine intradermally can produce a wheal but no flare or pain at the site of injection. Placement of methacholine (2.5%) into the conjunctival sac produces pupillary constriction in children with familial dysautonomia but no response in a normal child. Intravenous infusion of norepinephrine is followed by an exaggerated pressor response, and the hypotensive response to infusion of methacholine is increased.

Hemophagocytic Syndrome

HPS is characterized by prolonged fever, hepatosplenomegaly, cytopenia, and hemophagocytosis in the bone marrow, liver, spleen, or lymph nodes.[47,73] It is a life-threatening and unusual disorder in which uncontrolled proliferation of activated lymphocytes and histiocytes results in unregulated hypersecretion of inflammatory cytokines. HPS can be primarily a familial disease or can be manifested as a reactive process triggered by infection, malignancy, immunologic disease, or drugs.

The diagnosis of HPS is suggested by fever, hepatosplenomegaly, cytopenia in at least two cell lines, hypertriglyceridemia or hypofibrinogenemia, and an elevated ferritin level. Because HPS can be manifested initially as FUO and progress to masquerade as overwhelming sepsis, a high index of suspicion is required for establishing the diagnosis. Further investigation should include evaluation of bone marrow, cerebrospinal fluid, or lymph nodes for the presence of hemophagocytosis. Therapy should include treatment of the underlying infection or trigger, if one exists, in addition to appropriate immune modulation therapies. A substantial proportion of HPS cases progress rapidly to death despite administration of appropriate chemotherapy.[47,73]

Inflammatory Bowel Disease

Fever is a prominent feature in many children with inflammatory bowel disease.[28,52,96] A greater percentage of children than adults with regional enteritis have fever. Appropriate contrast-enhanced radiographic studies of the intestines should be undertaken in children with prolonged FUO, even in the absence of findings specifically referable to the gastrointestinal tract, especially if the erythrocyte sedimentation rate is elevated and if the patient has anemia, weight loss, failure of linear growth, or a positive stool guaiac test.

Ulcerative colitis can be manifested as FUO, though less commonly than with regional enteritis. In patients with ulcerative colitis, symptoms referable to the gastrointestinal tract generally are present at the time that the patient is febrile.

Infantile Cortical Hyperostosis

The cause of infantile cortical hyperostosis (i.e., Caffey disease) is unknown. The decreased incidence in recent years suggests an infectious, possibly a viral, cause. Spontaneous hyperplasia of subperiosteal bone begins during infancy and is associated with swelling of the overlying tissues. The skull, mandible, clavicles, scapula, and ribs are affected most frequently, but in some children the long bones and even the metatarsal bones can be involved. Most patients have persistent fever, sometimes as high as 40°C (104°F). Tenderness over the affected regions, irritability, elevated erythrocyte sedimentation rate, and leukocytosis are common findings. The diagnosis is established by the clinical picture in conjunction with radiographically demonstrated periosteal involvement.

Juvenile Rheumatoid Arthritis

Juvenile rheumatoid arthritis is a chronic inflammatory disorder that usually is manifested as one of three distinct syndromes: the systemic form, characterized by high, spiking temperatures (generally once or twice each day), evanescent rash, and lymphadenopathy; a polyarticular form; and a monarticular or pauciarticular form. Fever is associated with all three manifestations but occurs most commonly in the systemic form, in which case it is present in nearly 100 percent of patients. This form also is the one most likely to be manifested as FUO.[23] Arthritis may not develop for months to years after onset of the fever. The diagnosis often needs to be made by exclusion because serologic tests generally are negative.

Periodic Fevers

Familial Mediterranean fever is characterized by episodic fever and abdominal pain.[34] This disease, found in persons of Mediterranean ancestry, is inherited as an autosomal recessive trait. The pattern of recurrent fever, however, is irregular, with varying periods of normality between episodes of fever.

Reimann[83] called attention to a group of patients with recurrent episodes of fever at regular intervals, usually 7 to 21 days. Some of the patients had leukopenia and abdominal or thoracic pain. Reasons for the fever and its periodicity remain unknown. Patients with cyclic neutropenia frequently have fever during acute episodes, but not all the patients reported by Reimann had neutropenia. Cases of children with periodic fever and hyperimmunoglobulinemia D, with or without chills, cervical lymphadenopathy, and occasionally abdominal pain, have been reported,[33,39] primarily from Europe. The cause of the syndrome remains unknown.

REFERENCES

1. Adams, K. C., Dixon, J. H., and Eichner, E. R.: Clinical usefulness of polymorphonuclear leukocyte vacuolization in predicting septicemia in febrile children. Pediatrics 62:67-70, 1978.
2. Alpern, E. R., Alessandrini, E. A., Bell, L. M., et al.: Occult bacteremia from a pediatric emergency department: Current prevalence, time to detection and outcome. Pediatrics 106:505-511, 2000.
3. Alpern, E. R, Alessandrini, E. A., McGowan, K. L., et al.: Serotype prevalence of occult pneumococcal bacteremia. Pediatrics 108:e23, 2001.
4. Arisoy, E. S., Correa, A. G., Wagner, M. L., and Kaplan, S. L.: Hepatosplenic cat-scratch disease in children: Selected clinical features and treatment. Clin. Infect. Dis. 28:778-784, 1999.
5. Ayus, C. J., Krothapalli, R. K., and Arieff, A. I.: Occult bacteremia in febrile children. N. Engl. J. Med. 318:1338-1339, 1988.
6. Bachur, R., and Harper, M.: Reevaluation of outpatients with Streptococcus pneumoniae bacteremia. Pediatrics 105:502-509, 2000.
7. Baker, M. D., Bell, L. M., and Avner, J. R.: Outpatient management without antibiotics of fever in selected infants. N. Engl. J. Med. 329:1437-1441, 1993.
8. Baker, M. D., Bell, L. M., and Avner, J. R.: The efficacy of routine outpatient management without antibiotics of fever in selected infants. Pediatrics 103:627-631, 1999.
9. Baker, R. C., Tiller, T., Bausher, J. C., et al.: Severity of disease correlated with fever reduction in febrile infants. Pediatrics 83:1016-1019, 1989.
10. Baraff, L. J.: Management of fever without source in infants and children. Ann. Emerg. Med. 36:602-614, 2000.
11. Baraff, L. J., Bass, J. W., Fleisher, G. R., et al.: Practice guidelines for the management of infants and children 0 to 36 months of age with fever without source. Pediatrics 92:1-12, 1993.
12. Baraff, L. J., and Lee, S. I.: Fever without source: Management of children 3 to 36 months of age. Pediatr. Infect. Dis. J. 11:146-151, 1992.
13. Baraff, L. J., Oslund, S., and Prather, M.: Effect of antibiotic therapy and etiologic microorganism on the risk of bacterial meningitis in children with occult bacteremia. Pediatrics 92:140-143, 1993.
14. Baron, M. A., and Fink, H. D.: Bacteremia in private pediatric practice. Pediatrics 66:171-175, 1980.
15. Baron, M. A., Fink, H. D., and Cicchetti, D. V.: Blood cultures in private pediatric practice: An eleven-year experience. Pediatr. Infect. Dis. 8:2-7, 1989.
16. Bass, J. W., Steel, R. W., Wittler, R. R., et al.: Antimicrobial treatment of occult bacteremia: A multicenter cooperative study. Pediatr. Infect. Dis. J. 12:466-473, 1993.
17. Berger, H.: Fever: An unusual manifestation of epilepsy. Postgrad. Med. 40:479-481, 1966.
18. Bloom, H. R.: Must we teach clinical judgment? Pediatrics 67:745-746, 1981.
19. Bonadio, W. A.: Systemic bacterial infections in children with fever greater than 41°C. Pediatr. Infect. Dis. J. 8:120-121; 1989.
20. Bonadio, W. A., Webster, H., Wolfe, A., and Gorecki, D.: Correlating infectious outcome with clinical parameters of 1130 consecutive febrile infants aged zero to eight weeks. Pediatr. Emerg. Care 9:84-86, 1993.
21. Bratton, L., Teele, D. W., and Klein, J. O.: Outcome of unsuspected pneumococcemia in children not initially admitted to the hospital. J. Pediatr. 90:703-706, 1977.
22. Brewis, E. C.: Undiagnosed fever. Br. Med. J. 1:107-110, 1965.
23. Calabro, J. J., and Marchesano, J. M.: Juvenile rheumatoid arthritis. N. Engl. J. Med. 277:746-749, 1967.
24. Carey, B. M., Williams, C. E., and Arthur, R. J.: Ultrasound demonstration of pericardial empyema in an infant with pyrexia of undetermined origin. Pediatr. Radiol. 18:349-350, 1988.
25. Carroll, W. L., Farrell, M. K., Singer, J. I., et al.: Treatment of occult bacteremia: A prospective randomized clinical trial. Pediatrics 72:608-611, 1983.
26. Centers for Disease Control and Prevention: Annual Survey of Leptospirosis for 1972. Atlanta, Centers for Disease Control and Prevention, 1974.

27. Chan, Y. F., Ma, L. T., Yeung, L. T., et al.: Parapharyngeal inflammatory pseudotumor presenting as fever of unknown origin in a 3-year-old girl. Pediatr. Pathol. 8:195-203, 1988.

28. Chron, B. B., and Yarnis, H.: Continuous fever of intestinal origin. Ann. Intern. Med. 26:858-862, 1947.

29. Corrigan, J. J.: Thrombocytopenia: Laboratory sign of septicemia in infants and children. J. Pediatr. 85:219-223, 1974.

30. Dancis, J., and Smith, A. A.: Familial dysautonomia. N. Engl. J. Med. 274:207-209, 1966.

31. Dashefsky, B., Teele, D. W., and Klein, J. O.: Unsuspected meningococcemia. J. Pediatr. 102:69-72, 1983.

32. Dershewitz, R. A.: A comparative study of the prevalence, outcome and prediction of bacteremia in children. J. Pediatr. 103:352-358, 1983.

33. Drenth, J. P. H., Haagsma, C. J., and van Der Meer, J. W. H.: Hyperimmunoglobulinemia D and periodic fever syndrome. Medicine (Baltimore) 73:133-144, 1994.

34. Ehrenfeld, E. N., Eliakin, M., and Rachmilewitz, M.: Recurrent polyserositis (familial Mediterranean fever, periodic disease): A report of 55 cases. Am. J. Med. 31:107-123, 1961.

35. Feder, H. M. J., and Bialecki, C. A.: Periodic fever associated with aphthous stomatitis, pharyngitis and cervical adenitis. Pediatr. Infect. Dis. 8:186-189, 1989.

36. Feigin, R. D., and Shearer, W. T.: Fever of unknown origin in children. Curr. Probl. Pediatr. 6:2-57, 1976.

37. Fineman, D. S., Palestno, C. J., Kim, C. K., et al.: Detection of abnormalities in febrile AIDS patients with In-111–labelled leukocyte and Ga-67 scintigraphy. Radiology 170:677-680, 1989.

38. Fleishner, G. R., Rosenberg, N., Vinci, R., et al.: Intramuscular versus oral antibiotic therapy for the prevention of meningitis and other bacterial sequelae in young febrile children at risk for occult bacteremia. J. Pediatr. 124:504-512, 1994.

39. Gross, C., Schnetzer, J. R., Ferrante, A., and Vladutiu, A. O.: Children with hyperimmunoglobulinemia D and periodic fever syndrome. Pediatr. Infect. Dis. J. 15:72-77, 1996.

40. Habibian, M. R., Staab, E. V., and Matthews, H. A.: Gallium citrate Ga 67 scans in febrile patients. J. A. M. A. 233:1073-1076, 1975.

41. Hayani, A., Mahoney, D. H., and Fernback, D. J.: Role of bone marrow examination in the child with prolonged fever. J. Pediatr. 116:919-920, 1990.

42. Herz, A. M., Greenhow, T. L., Alcantara, J., et al.: Changing epidemiology of outpatient bacteremia in 3- to 30-month-old children after the introduction of the heptavalent-conjugated pneumococcal vaccine. Pediatr. Infect. Dis. J. 25:293-300, 2006.

43. Hoekelman, R., Lewin, E. B., and Shapira, M. D., et al.: Potential bacteremia in pediatric practice. Am. J. Dis. Child. 133:1017-1019, 1979.

44. Isaacman, D. J., and Burke, D. L.: Utility of the serum C-reactive protein for detection of occult bacterial infection in children. Arch. Pediatr. Adolesc. Med. 156:905-909, 2002.

45. Jacobs, R. F., and Schutze, G. E.: *Bartonella henselae* as a cause of prolonged fever and fever of unknown origin in children. Clin. Infect. Dis. 26:80-84, 1988.

46. Jaffee, D. M., Tanz, R. R., Davis, T., et al.: Antibiotic administration to treat possible occult bacteremia in febrile children. N. Engl. J. Med. 317:1175-1180, 1987.

47. Janka, G. E.: Familial and acquired hemophagocytic lymphohistiocytosis. Eur. J. Pediatr. 166:95-109, 2007.

48. Jaskiewicz, J. A., McCarthy, C. A., Richardson, A. C., et al.: Febrile infants at low risk for serious bacterial infection—an appraisal of the Rochester criteria and implications of management. Pediatrics 94:390-396, 1994.

49. Kaplan, S. L., and Feigin, R. D.: Pyogenic liver abscess in normal children with fever of unknown origin. Pediatrics 58:614-616, 1976.

50. Kline, M. W., Smith, E. O., Kaplan, S. L., et al.: Effects of causative organism and presence or absence of meningitis on white blood cell counts in children with bacteremia. J. Emerg. Med. 6:33-35, 1988.

51. Lacour, A. G., Gervaix, A., Zamora, S. A., et al.: Procalcitonin, IL-6, IL-8, IL-1 receptor antagonist and C-reactive protein as identificators of serious bacterial infections in children with fever without localising signs. Eur. J. Pediatr. 160:95-100, 2001.

52. Lee, F. I., and Davies, D. M.: Crohn's disease presenting as pyrexia of unknown origin. Lancet 1:1205-1206, 1961.

53. Liu, C., Lehan, C., Speer, M. E., et al.: Early detection of bacteremia in an outpatient clinic. Pediatrics 75:827-831, 1985.

54. Lohr, J. A., and Hendley, J. O.: Prolonged fever of unknown origin: Record of experience with 54 childhood patients. Clin. Pediatr. (Phila.) 16:768-773, 1977.

55. Margolis, M. T.: Specific anergy in tuberculosis. N. Engl. J. Med. 309:1388, 1983.

56. Marshall, R., Teele, D. W., and Klein, J. O.: Unsuspected bacteremia due to *Haemophilus influenzae*: Outcome in children not initially admitted to hospital. J. Pediatr. 95:690-695, 1979.

57. Mazur, L. J., Jones, T., and Kozinetz, C. A.: Temperature response to acetaminophen and risk of occult bacteremia: A case control study. J. Pediatr. 115:888-891, 1989.

58. McCarthy, P. L., and Dolan, T. F.: Hyperpyrexia in children: Eight-year emergency room experience. Am. J. Dis. Child. 130:849-851, 1976.

59. McCarthy, P. L., Frank, A. L., Ablow, R. C., et al.: Value of the C-reactive protein test in the differentiation of bacterial and viral pneumonia. J. Pediatr. 92:454-459, 1978.

60. McCarthy, P. L., Grundy, G. W., Spiesel, S. Z., et al.: Bacteremia in children: An outpatient review. Pediatrics 57:861-868, 1976.

61. McCarthy, P. L., Jekel, J. F., and Dolan, T. F.: Temperature greater than or equal to 40°C in children less than 24 months of age: A prospective study. Pediatrics 59:663-668, 1977.

62. McCarthy, P. L., Jekel, J. F., Stashwick, C. A., et al.: History and observation variables in assessing febrile children. Pediatrics 65:1090-1095, 1980.

63. McCarthy, P. L., Jekel, J. F., Stashwick, C. A., et al.: Further definition of history and observation variables in assessing febrile children. Pediatrics 67:687-693, 1981.

64. McCarthy, P. L., Sharpe, M. R., Spiesel, S. Z., et al.: Observation scales to identify serious illness in febrile children. Pediatrics 70:802-809, 1982.

65. McClung, H. J.: Prolonged fever of unknown origin in childhood. Am. J. Dis. Child. 124:544-550, 1972.

66. McGowan, J. E., Bratton, L., Klein, J. O., et al.: Bacteremia in febrile children seen in a walk-in pediatric clinic. N. Engl. J. Med. 288:1309-1312, 1973.

67. McMurray, D. N., and Echeverri, A.: Cell-mediated immunity in anergic patients with pulmonary tuberculosis. Am. Rev. Respir. Dis. 118:827-834, 1978.

68. Miller, M. L., Szer, I., Yogev, R., and Bernstein, B.: Fever of unknown origin. Pediatr. Clin. North Am. 42:999-1011, 1995.

69. Morens, D. W.: WBC and differential: Value in predicting bacterial disease in children. Am. J. Dis. Child. 133:25-27, 1979.

70. Murray, D. L., Zonana, J., Seidel, J. S., et al.: Relative importance of bacteremia and viremia in the course of acute fevers of unknown origin in outpatient children. Pediatrics 68:157-160, 1981.

71. Nash, D. R., and Douglas, J. E.: Anergy in active pulmonary tuberculosis: A comparison between positive and negative reactors and an evaluation of 5 TU and 250 TU skin test doses. Chest 77:32-37, 1980.

72. Ostrow, J. H.: Tuberculin negative tuberculosis. Am. Rev. Respir. Dis. 107:882-883, 1973.

73. Palazzi, D. L., McClain, K. L., and Kaplan, S. L. Hemophagocytic syndrome in children: An important diagnostic consideration in fever of unknown origin. Clin. Infect. Dis. 36:306-312, 2003.

74. Pantell, R. H., Newman, T. B., Bernzweig, J., et al.: Management and outcomes of care of fever in early infancy. J. A. M. A. 291:1203-1212, 2004.

75. Peltola, H.: C-reactive protein in rapid differentiation of acute epiglottitis from spasmodic croup and acute laryngotracheitis: Preliminary report. J. Pediatr. 102:713-715, 1983.

76. Petersdorf, R. G., and Beeson, P. B.: Fever of unexplained origin: Report on 100 cases. Medicine (Baltimore) 40:1-30, 1961.

77. Picus, D., Siegel, M. J., and Balfe, D. M.: Abdominal computed tomography in children with unexplained prolonged fever. J. Comput. Assist. Tomogr. 8:851-856, 1984.

78. Pizzo, P. A., Lovejoy, F. H., and Smith, D. H.: Prolonged fever in children: Review of 100 cases. Pediatrics 55:468-473, 1975.

79. Poehling, K. A., Talbot, T. R., Griffin, M. R., et al.: Invasive pneumococcal disease among infants before and after introduction of pneumococcal conjugate vaccine. J. A. M. A. 295:1668-1674, 2006.

80. Prat, C., Dominguez, J., Rodrigo, C., et al.: Use of quantitative and semiquantitative procalcitonin measurements to identify children with sepsis and meningitis. Eur. J. Clin. Microbiol. Infect. Dis. 23:136-138, 2004.

81. Press, S.: Association of hyperpyrexia with serious disease in children. Clin. Pediatr. (Phila.) 33:19-25, 1994.

82. Pulliam, P. N., Attia, M. W., and Cronan, K. M.: C-reactive protein in febrile children 1 to 36 months of age with clinically undetectable serious bacterial infection. Pediatrics 108:1275-1279, 2001.

83. Reimann, H. A.: Periodic disease, periodic fever, periodic abdominalgia, cyclic neutropenia, intermittent arthralgia, angioneurotic edema, anaphylactoid purpura and periodic paralysis. J. A. M. A. 141:175-183, 1949.

84. Roberts, K. B., and Borzy, M. S.: Fever in the first eight weeks of life. Johns Hopkins Med. J. 141:9-13, 1977.

85. Sard, B., Bailey, M. C., and Vinci, R.: An analysis of pediatric blood cultures in the postpneumococcal conjugate vaccine era in a community hospital emergency department. Pediatr. Emerg. Care 22:295-300, 2006.

86. Simon, H. B., and Wolff, S. M.: Granulomatous hepatitis and prolonged fever of unknown origin: A study of 13 patients. Medicine (Baltimore) 52:1-21, 1973.

87. Smith, A. A., Farbman, A., and Dancis, J.: Tongue in familial dysautonomia. Am. J. Dis. Child. 110:152-153, 1965.

88. Steele, R. W., Jones S. M., Lowe, B. A., et al.: Usefulness of scanning procedures for diagnosis of fever of unknown origin in children. J. Pediatr. 119:526-530, 1991.

89. Stein, R. C.: The white blood cell count in fevers of unknown origin. Am. J. Dis. Child. 124:60-63, 1972.

90. Steiner, P., and Portugulea, C.: Tuberculous meningitis in children. Am. Rev. Respir. Dis. 107:22-29, 1973.

91. Stoll, M. J., and Rubin L. G.: Incidence of occult bacteremia among highly febrile young children in the era of the pneumococcal conjugate vaccine. Arch. Pediatr. Adolesc. Med. 158:671-675, 2004.

92. Teach, S. J., and Fleisher, G. R.: Efficacy of an observation scale in detecting bacteremia in febrile children three to thirty six months of age, treated as outpatients. J. Pediatr. 126:877-881, 1995.

93. Teele, D. W., Pelton, S. I., Grant, M. J., et al.: Bacteremia in febrile children under 2 years of age: Results of cultures of blood of 600 consecutive febrile children in a "walk-in" clinic. J. Pediatr. 87:227-230, 1975.

94. Todd, J. K.: Childhood infections: Diagnostic value of peripheral white blood cell and differential cell counts. Am. J. Dis. Child. 127:810-816, 1974.

95. Torrey, S. B., Henretig, F., Fleisher, G., et al.: Temperature response to antipyretic therapy in children. Am. J. Emerg. Med. 3:190-192, 1985.

96. Walker, S. H.: Periodic fever in juvenile regional enteritis. J. Pediatr. 60:561-565, 1962.

97. Waskerwitz, S., and Berkelhammer, J. E.: Outpatient bacteremia: Clinical findings in children under two years with initial temperatures of 39.5°C or higher. J. Pediatr. 99:231-233, 1981.

98. Weinstein, L.: Bacterial hepatitis: A case report on an unrecognized cause of fever of unknown origin. N. Engl. J. Med. 299:1052-1054, 1978.

99. Wolff, S. M., Ward, S. B., and Landy, M.: A syndrome of periodic hypothalamic discharge. Am. J. Med. 36:956-966, 1964.

100. Wright, P. F., Thompson, J., McKee, K. T., Jr., et al.: Patterns of illness in the highly febrile young child: Epidemiologic, clinical and laboratory correlates. Pediatrics 67:694-700, 1981.

101. Wyllie, R., and Fitzgerald, J. F.: Bacterial cholangitis in a 10-week-old infant with fever of undetermined origin. Pediatrics 65:164-167, 1980.

102. Yamamoto, L. T., Wigder, H. N., Fligner, D. J., et al.: Relationship of bacteremia to antipyretic therapy in febrile children. Pediatr. Emerg. Care. 3:223-226, 1987.

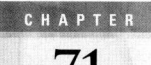

CHAPTER 71

TOXIC SHOCK SYNDROME

Jeffrey Suen ⊛ P. Joan Chesney ⊛ Jeffrey P. Davis

Much has been learned about the pathogenesis and pathophysiology of toxic shock syndrome (TSS) since its initial description in 1978 by Dr. James K. Todd and colleagues.[305] The clinical illness is defined by the criteria listed in the case definition formulated for epidemiologic studies (Table 71–1). Though often confused with septic shock, TSS has unique clinical manifestations not generally noted in septic shock, including diffuse erythroderma,

delayed desquamation of the palms and soles, conjunctival and pharyngeal hyperemia, muscle injury, rapidly accelerated renal failure, and gastrointestinal symptoms. The capillary leak syndrome, or rapid and massive loss of fluid from capillaries into the interstitial space, loss of peripheral vascular resistance, and subsequent multisystem end-organ failure further characterize this entity. The histopathologic findings are minimal and nonspecific, with extensive interstitial edema of all tissues and minimal perivascular mononuclear cellular infiltrates. TSS can recur after both menstrual and nonmenstrual cases. The highest recurrence rate of 65 percent was reported in a subset of untreated women with menstrual TSS who continued to use tampons during menses.

When first described, TSS had unique geographic, age, sex, and racial characteristics. It was associated with menses, particularly tampon use, as well as with a phenotypically distinctive type of *Staphylococcus aureus*. In 1994, at least 42 percent of reported cases of TSS were nonmenstrual. *S. aureus* exotoxins now are recognized to be "superantigens," and the endogenous mediators produced by these exotoxins appear to mediate manifestations of the disease.

TSS toxin I (TSST-I) and the staphylococcal enterotoxins are extremely potent stimuli of the in vitro macrophage production of interleukin-1 (IL-1) and tumor necrosis factor-α (TNF-α) and the T-lymphocyte production of IL-2, lymphotoxin (TNF-β), and interferon-γ. These staphylococcal exotoxins are functionally bivalent mitogens that highly selectively bind to major histocompatibility complex (MHC) class II receptors on antigen-processing cells and to selected V_β elements of the T-cell receptor (TCR) specific for each toxin. They now are known as superantigens. Besides *S. aureus*, other bacteria, particularly *Streptococcus pyogenes*, also can produce exotoxins that function as superantigens and produce a toxic shock–like syndrome.

TABLE 71–1   Clinical Case Definition of Toxic Shock Syndrome

Clinical Findings

Fever: Temperature ≥38.9°C

Rash: Diffuse macular erythroderma

Desquamation: 1-2 wk after onset of illness, particularly on palms, soles, fingers, and toes

Hypotension: Systolic blood pressure ≤90 mm Hg for adults; <5th percentile by age for children <16 yr old; orthostatic drop in diastolic blood pressure ≥15 mm Hg from lying to sitting; orthostatic syncope or orthostatic dizziness

Involvement of three or more of the following organ systems:

  Gastrointestinal: Vomiting or diarrhea at onset of illness

  Muscular: Severe myalgia or creatinine phosphokinase level greater than twice the upper limit of normal for the laboratory

  Mucous membrane: Vaginal, oropharyngeal, or conjunctival hyperemia

  Renal: BUN or serum creatinine greater than twice the upper limit of normal or ≥5 white blood cells per high-power field in the absence of a urinary tract infection

  Hepatic: Total bilirubin, AST, or ALT greater than twice the upper limit of normal for the laboratory

  Hematologic: platelets <100,000/mm³

  Central nervous system: disorientation or alterations in consciousness without focal neurologic signs when fever and hypotension are absent

Negative results on the following tests, if obtained:

  Blood, throat, or cerebrospinal fluid cultures; blood culture may be positive for *Staphylococcus aureus*

  Serologic tests for Rocky Mountain spotted fever, leptospirosis, or measles

Case Classification

Probable: A case with 5 of the 6 clinical findings described above

Confirmed: A case with all 6 of the clinical findings described above, including desquamation, unless the patient dies before desquamation could occur

ALT, alanine transaminase; AST, aspartate transaminase; BUN, blood urea nitrogen.
From Wharton, M., Chorba, T. L., Vogt, R. L., et al.: Case definitions for public health surveillance. M. M. W. R. Recomm. Rep. 39(RR-13): 1-43, 1990.

HISTORY

Illnesses resembling TSS and associated with *S. aureus* have been reported since 1927,[7,95,108,293,325] but the initial description of the illness as a disease of children was published in 1978.[305] A Kawasaki-like syndrome described in adults subsequently was recognized to be TSS.[201] The first 12 cases of TSS identified in Wisconsin and Minnesota between July 1979 and January 1980 were reported by state epidemiologists to the Centers for Disease Control and Prevention (CDC) in January 1980.[75,277,315] All 12 cases had occurred in women, and a possible association with menses was noted. The probable recurrent nature of the illness also was reported.[75,315] In May 1980, the CDC reported findings of the first 55 nationally reported cases,[315] 95 percent of which occurred in women. Of 40 patients for whom a menstrual history was obtained, 38 (95%) had onset during menstruation. Thirteen patients had experienced recurrent episodes of TSS.

By June 1980, case-control studies statistically linking the occurrence of menstrual TSS with tampons had been completed by the Wisconsin Division of Health[75] and the CDC,[277] and similar trends had been noted by the Utah Department of Health.[162] In September 1980, the CDC reported that although TSS had been associated with many tampon brands, women using one particular brand of tampon, Rely (Procter & Gamble), were at greatest risk. This brand was withdrawn immediately and voluntarily from the market by the manufacturer.[24,120,264] Subsequent frequent updates by the CDC documented a decrease in reported cases.[316,317,320]

Microbiologic studies have established that most patients with menses-associated TSS (menstrual TSS) have evidence of vaginal or cervical colonization with *S. aureus*.[22] These strains of *S. aureus* made a characteristic toxin initially called *staphylococcal enterotoxin F*[23] and *pyrogenic exotoxin C*[270] and now known as *TSST-I*.

EPIDEMIOLOGY

SURVEILLANCE AND INCIDENCE

Statewide surveillance for cases of TSS began in Wisconsin[77] and Minnesota[229] in January 1980, in Utah in February 1980,[175] and in other states after the national communications about TSS in spring 1980. In 1982, TSS became a nationally notifiable disease. Between 1983 and 1994, the CDC received reports of 4192 cases of TSS through the National Electronic Telecommunications System for Surveillance (NETSS).[296] The National Center for Infectious Diseases at the CDC maintains a database of TSS cases, including those reported before 1983. In addition, in January 1981, the National Center for Health Statistics recommended use of the International Classification of Diseases (ICD) code 040.89 for TSS, and a study involving reviews of records in 97 percent of Wisconsin general hospitals demonstrated that by 1983 the sensitivity and specificity of using this code in this review of discharge coding was 85 and 95 percent, respectively.[137] Since 1983, a continued downward trend in passively reported cases has been noted (Fig. 71-1).[330]

Of 2509 confirmed cases reported to the CDC through April 1984, 95 percent occurred in females.[249] Among the 2295 women with known menstrual histories, 89 percent had an onset of TSS associated with menstruation. Of 1716 menses-associated cases for which information related to tampon use was available, 99 percent occurred in tampon users and 1 percent in women using napkins or minipads.

The results of an active surveillance study conducted by the CDC in 1986 and 1987 in five states and Los Angeles County confirmed the trends previously noted in the CDC passive surveillance system.[127] The incidence of menstrual TSS was found to be 1 case per 100,000 women aged 15 to 44 years. This rate is a substantial reduction from the reported rates of 2.4 to 12.3 cases per 100,000 women of menstruating age in 1980.[75,175,229,241] Only 55 percent of the cases detected in the 1986-1987 study occurred in women, and 45 percent of all cases were menstrually associated.[38,127] The nationally reported TSS-related mortality rate for menstrual cases decreased from 5.5 percent in 1979 and 1980 to 2.8 percent in 1981 to 1986, then to 1.8 percent in 1987 to 1996 (chi-square for linear trend, $p = 0.0001$).[133]

The striking reduction in the incidence of menstrual TSS was attributed to a decrease in tampon absorbency, changes in com-

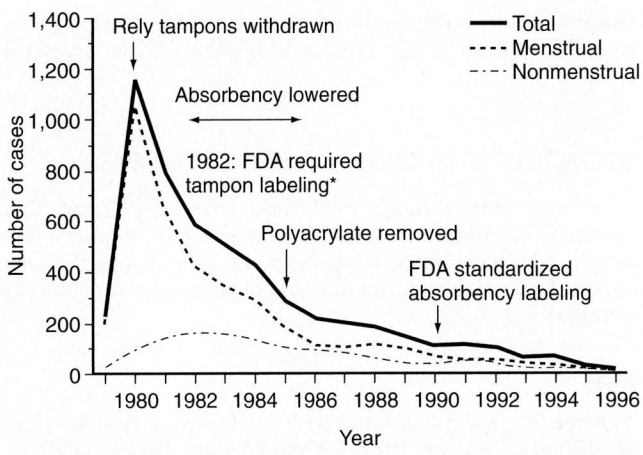

*FDA, Food and Drug Administration, including definite and probable toxic shock syndrome cases

Figure 71-1 Menstrual and nonmenstrual toxic shock syndrome cases reported to the Centers for Disease Control and Prevention by year, 1979 to 1996. (*From Hajjeh, R. A., Reingold, A., Weil, A., et al.: Toxic-shock syndrome in the United States: Surveillance update, 1979-1996. Emerg. Infect. Dis. 5:807-810, 1999.*)

position of tampons and patterns of use, and the impact of publicity on early recognition of symptoms.[77,78,111,228,248,274] Since the 1980s, there has been a paucity of active surveillance data on TSS. Passive reporting during 2000 to 2003 in Minneapolis–St. Paul, Minnesota, suggested an increasing incidence of menstrual TSS cases from 0.8 per 100,000 to 3.4 per 100,000 women of menstrual age.[271] Subsequently, a medical record search for illnesses during 2000 to 2003 that had TSS-based, ICD-9 discharge codes (040.82 or 040.89) and a 20 percent random sample of five other shock or sepsis codes with review of cases was conducted in 25 Minneapolis–St. Paul metropolitan area hospitals. The incidence was not calculated, but the number of menstrual TSS cases ($n = 23$) was similar to the number of nonmenstrual cases ($n = 21$), and the gradual increase in total cases from 2000 ($n = 9$) to 2003 ($n = 13$) was not significant. Cases associated with methicillin-resistant *S. aureus* (MRSA) and new sites of staphylococcal infection (lung, urinary tract) were noted.[86]

In 1986 and 1987, the incidence of nonmenstrual TSS in women (0.25 case per 100,000 women) and TSS in men (0.16 case per 100,000 men) had changed little since 1980. However, with the declining trend in menstrual TSS, nonmenstrual TSS has accounted for a greater proportion of overall TSS cases. In 1994, only 192 cases of TSS were reported to the CDC through the NETSS (0.1 case per 100,000 population). Among confirmed cases, 42 percent were nonmenstrual.[296] The proportion of nonmenstrual cases reported after surgical procedures increased from 14 percent during 1979 to 1986 to 27 percent during 1987 to 1996.[133] Overall, no significant change in the case-fatality ratio for nonmenstrual cases has occurred: 8.5 percent for 1979 and 1980, 5.3 percent for 1981 to 1986, and 6 percent for 1987 to 1996.[38,133]

Although cases in the United States have been reported in all 50 states and the District of Columbia, significant differences in incidence were noted among the states through 1983.[249] Through mid-1983, the five states of Wisconsin, Minnesota, Colorado, Utah, and California accounted for 44 percent of the total reported cases but represented only 16 percent of the U.S. population.[309] Although intensified surveillance may have been a factor, regional differences in the degree of immunity to TSS-associated *S. aureus* toxins and in the distribution of toxin-producing organisms may have been important factors.[322]

Geographic differences in the occurrence of TSS continued even with the increase in the relative proportion of nonmenstrual cases.[38]

RISK FACTORS FOR MENSTRUAL TOXIC SHOCK SYNDROME

From early 1980 through 1990, most reported cases of TSS occurred in previously healthy, young white menstruating women who were using tampons at the time of onset of the illness. The explanation for this combination of risk factors is complex.

Age

The median age of patients with confirmed menstrual TSS (median age: 21 years, 1979 to 1980; 20 years, 1981 to 1986; 25 years, 1987 to 1996) has varied little since 1980.[127,133,249] Roughly a third of cases occur in adolescents 15 to 19 years of age[249] (Fig. 71–2). The mean age of patients with nonmenstrual TSS (27 years through 1982, 30 years in 1986) is significantly higher than that for menses-associated cases.[127,250] The precise reason for the increased incidence of TSS in adolescent girls is not known, but a lower prevalence of antibody to TSST-I may increase susceptibility in this age group.[324]

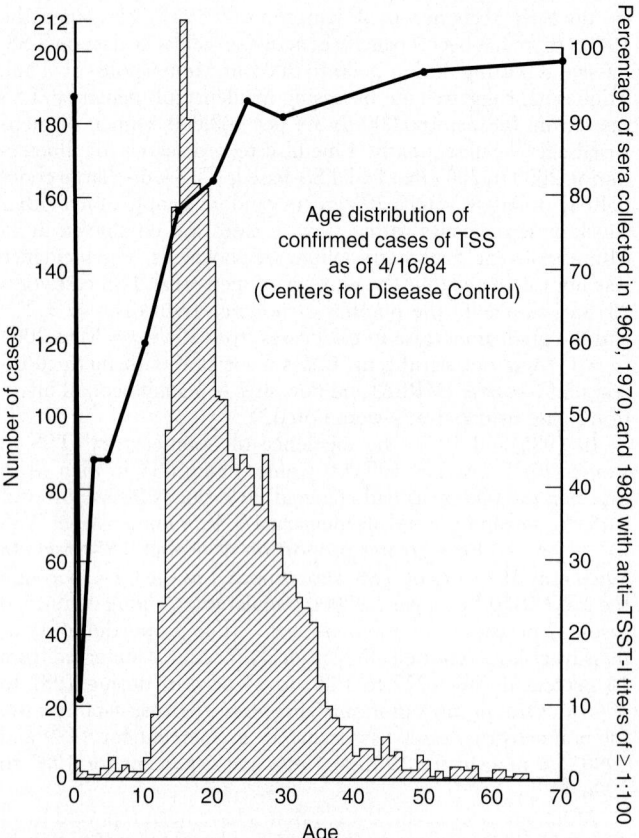

Figure 71–2 Age distribution of patients with confirmed toxic shock syndrome (TSS) reported to the Centers for Disease Control and Prevention before April 16, 1984. The age-specific prevalence of antibodies to toxic shock syndrome toxin I (TSST-I) in a normal population in Wisconsin in the years 1960, 1970, and 1980 is indicated by the *solid connected line*. (*Data from Vergeront, J. M., Stolz, S. J., Crass, B. A., et al.: Prevalence of serum antibody to staphylococcal enterotoxin F among Wisconsin residents: Implications for toxic shock syndrome. J. Infect. Dis. 148:692-698, 1983.*)

Race

A striking race-ethnicity distribution is present for menstrual TSS; 97 percent of such cases have occurred in whites, who make up 83 percent of the U.S. population. This distribution is not as striking for nonmenstrual TSS in that 87 percent of nonmenstrual cases have occurred in whites. The reasons for racial differences are not clear and only partially explained by differences in menses-related practices.[111,249,250] Racial differences in antibody to TSST-I may explain to some degree the differences in the distribution of cases.[322]

Menstruation and Tampon Use

The initial observations in 1980 that a high proportion of patients with TSS had an onset during menses is well documented now. The use of tampons as a significant risk factor for the development of TSS was established clearly in six case-control studies conducted in 1980[75,138,162,227,264,277] and one conducted in 1987.[127] Even though these studies varied in design and methodologic technique, all demonstrated that in at least 97 percent of affected individuals, use of tampons during menstrual periods was associated with disease onset. Although 76 to 89 percent of matched control individuals used tampons during temporally comparable menstrual periods, the use of tampons was associated with menstrual TSS in each of these studies, with odds ratios ranging from 11 to 18.[38]

Despite the fact that TSS has occurred and continues to occur with the use of all brands of tampons, the second CDC case-control study demonstrated a greater relative risk for menstrual TSS with the use of one tampon brand, Rely.[120,264] The Tri-State (Minnesota, Wisconsin, and Iowa) TSS Study established that tampons of increasing absorbency were associated with an increasing relative risk for the development of menstrual TSS and that the risk of development of menstrual TSS associated with Rely tampons was greater than that predicted by absorbency alone.[227]

Reasons listed earlier for the striking reduction in incidence of menstrual TSS may be the decrease in absorbency of tampons and changes in composition of tampons.[248] In 1980, products very high in absorbency were used by 42 percent of tampon users.[229] By 1983, this proportion had decreased to 18 percent and, by 1986, to 1 percent.[248] Overall, the absorbency of available tampon brand styles, as measured by the Syngina test,[217] ranged from 10.3 to 20.5 g in 1980 to less than 6 to 15 g in 1990, indicative of an industry-wide decrease in tampon absorbency. The composition of tampons also has changed since 1980. Tampons currently available are composed of cotton or cotton and rayon combinations. In 1980, additives included polyacrylate, polyester foam, cross-linked carboxymethylcellulose, and several surfactants, including Pluronic L-92.[267] Whether these additives enhanced the risk for development of TSS independently or in combination with their increasing absorbency is unclear.[24,227,264]

Two subsequent case-control studies conducted by the CDC and involving patients with an onset of TSS in 1983 and 1984 (CDC III) and 1986 and 1987 (CDC IV) confirmed the Tri-State TSS Study results of a linearly increasing risk for TSS related to increasing tampon absorbency; for each 1-g increase in absorbency, the risk for TSS increased by 34 to 37 percent.[24,116] In addition, the Tri-State TSS Study and the CDC III study both suggested that the effects of absorbency and chemical composition of tampons on TSS risk were independent.[24,38,227]

Continuous use of tampons was associated with a greater risk for the development of TSS than noncontinuous use was in one case-control study[277]; however, this finding was not confirmed in a subsequent investigation.[227] No association between TSS and the frequency of changing tampons has been demonstrated.

As a result of these studies demonstrating the importance of tampons in menses-associated TSS, as well as the voluntary withdrawal of Rely, several other changes in the manufacture, labeling, and distribution of tampons have occurred. After a request by the Food and Drug Administration (FDA) in November 1980 that tampon manufacturers place warnings on tampon packages, on June 22, 1982, an FDA regulation required that information on TSS and tampon-associated risks appear on tampon packages.[90] In April 1985, two additional tampon manufacturers withdrew their superabsorbent tampons containing polyacrylate from the market on the basis of an in vitro study[208] and a judicial decision.[222] In 1990, the FDA published the in vitro rating system to be used by manufacturers to inform the public about tampon absorbency.[182,217,301]

RISK FACTORS FOR NONMENSTRUAL TOXIC SHOCK SYNDROME

Before 1986, less than 20 percent of confirmed cases of TSS reported to the CDC were nonmenstrual. In the 1986 and 1987 multistate active surveillance study (CDC IV), 54 percent of cases were found to be nonmenstrual.[127] Although the mean age of nonmenstrual cases is higher than that of menstrual cases and the ratio of males to females with nonmenstrual TSS is closer to that in the general population, the clinical findings and complications of nonmenstrual TSS are the same as those occurring in menstrual TSS. The number of confirmed cases of TSS reported in children younger than 10 years of age is surprisingly low, particularly in light of their demonstrated low antibody titers to TSST-I and the increased prevalence of nasal colonization (10%) with TSST-I–positive strains.[38,153,324,334]

Data on risk factors (Table 71–2) were obtained for 559 nonmenstrual TSS cases reported to the CDC through 1986.[38] Associated infections or procedures included nonsurgical cutaneous and subcutaneous infections, 22 percent; childbirth or abortion, 15 percent; infections after a wide variety of surgical procedures, 15 percent; vaginal infections occurring at times other than during menses, 6 percent; vaginal contraceptive sponge use, 5 percent[73]; diaphragm use, 6 percent; and other or unknown sources of infection, 31 percent. The proportion of all nonmenstrual cases reported after surgical procedures increased from 14 percent during 1979 to 1986 to 27 percent during 1987 to 1996. The proportion of female nonmenstrual case patients using barrier contraceptives was significantly less in 1987 to 1996 (6%) than in 1979 to 1986 (14%).[133]

In 1994, nonmenstrual cases accounted for at least 42 percent of all cases of TSS reported to the CDC through the passive surveillance system.[296] The three risk factors necessary for the acquisition of nonmenstrual disease include colonization (or acquisition) of a toxin-producing strain of *S. aureus*, absence of protective antitoxin antibody, and an infected site. TSS has been reported in association with *S. aureus* infections of almost every type, including primary staphylococcal infections and those occurring after surgery, infections associated with disruption of skin or a mucous membrane, and infections occurring after placement of a foreign body[22] (see Table 71–2). Numerous patients with TSS have been reported for whom no obvious focus of infection was found.[38,250] Trauma or surgery in areas of the body frequently colonized with *S. aureus* (nose, skin, vagina) places individuals at enhanced risk for infection and subsequent TSS.

HOST RISK FACTORS: GENERAL

Colonization with Exotoxin-Producing *Staphylococcus aureus*

For TSS to develop, an individual must be colonized with or acquire a strain of *S. aureus* that produces TSST-I or one of the

TABLE 71–2 Risk Factors for Nonmenstrual Toxic Shock Syndrome

I. Colonization with toxin-producing *Staphylococcus aureus*
II. Absence of protective antitoxin antibody
III. Infected site
  A. Primary *S. aureus* infection
    Carbuncle
    Cellulitis
    Dental abscess
    Empyema
    Endocarditis
    Folliculitis
    Mastitis
    Osteomyelitis
    Peritonitis
    Peritonsillar abscess
    Pneumonia
    Pyarthrosis
    Pyomyositis
    Sinusitis
    Tracheitis
  B. After surgery: wound infection
    Abdominal
    Breast
    Cesarean section
    Dermatologic
    Ear, nose, and throat
    Genitourinary
    Neurosurgery
    Orthopedic
  C. Skin or mucous membrane disruption
    Burns (chemical, scald, etc.)
    Dermatitis
    Influenza
    Pharyngitis
    Postpartum (vaginal delivery)
    Superficial/penetrating trauma (insect bite, needle-stick)
    Viral infection
    Varicella
  D. After surgical or nonsurgical foreign body placement
    Augmentation mammoplasty
    Catheters
    Diaphragm
    Sponge (contraceptive)
    Surgical prostheses/stents/packing material/sutures
  E. No obvious focus of infection (vaginal or pharyngeal colonization)

staphylococcal enterotoxins. Evidence that staphylococcal enterotoxin B (SEB) alone and, uncommonly, staphylococcal enterotoxin A (SEA) or staphylococcal enterotoxin C (SEC) alone, as well as TSST-I, may be responsible for the manifestations of TSS is compelling. Although many genotypically different strains of *S. aureus* possess the *tst*H gene, one clone has been isolated from 88 percent of menstrual cases and 54 percent of nonmenstrual cases.[214] Colonization with this clone, particularly in menstruating women, clearly provides a significant risk factor. Future work may identify other clones with unique adherence properties to other mucosal or skin sites.

Absence of Protective Antibody Levels

A necessary factor for the development of TSS is the absence of protective antibody levels for the toxin (TSST-I or enterotoxin) produced by the isolate associated with TSS. Thus, more than 90 percent of women with menstrual TSS associated with TSST-I–positive strains have antibody titers of 1:10 or lower, whereas a titer of 1:100 or higher is considered protective.[22] Because most adults acquire these antibodies without the development of disease, absent antibody levels may be the result of lack of exposure to a toxin-producing organism or a lacunar inability to respond to the toxin. The failure of most patients, menstrual and nonmenstrual, to form antibody during convalescence may reflect this lacunar nonrecognition of staphylococcal protein antigen, or it may be a reflection of the superantigenic nature of these proteins and failure of the toxin proteins to be presented to the TCR as conventional antigens. In mice and one patient with TSS, in vivo TSST-I–induced proliferation was followed by hyporesponsiveness of TSST-I–responsive $V_\beta 2^+$ T cells.[181]

Interruption of a Mucosal or Skin Surface

Primary deep-tissue staphylococcal infections (e.g., osteomyelitis, pyarthrosis, pyomyositis,[4] endocarditis,[242,331] renal carbuncles, bacteremia) rarely are associated with TSS. Most nonmenstrual cases occur in patients with an altered skin or mucosal surface. Examples of skin disruption associated with TSS include burns, insect bites, needle-sticks, surgical incisions, and varicella. Cases of disruption of mucous membranes can be divided into those associated with respiratory and those associated with genital mucosae. Damage to respiratory mucosa may occur after nasal or other surgery, particularly with placement of stents or packing, in association with a viral respiratory infection such as influenza, or as a result of primary sinusitis, tracheitis, or a parapharyngeal abscess. Heavy colonization of the pharynx also has been associated with TSS. The vaginal mucosa may be damaged in numerous ways, including during placement of tampons or barrier contraceptives,[105,275,313] postpartum,[22,233] or after genital surgery or genital mucosal damage.[106,231,257] Heavy colonization of the vagina without any other apparent risk factor likewise has been associated with TSS.[250] These mucosal infections may provide the right conditions for production of TSST-I, including an aerobic environment, high carbon dioxide concentration, neutral pH, high protein and low glucose concentrations, and low to normal magnesium concentration.[296]

Presence of a Foreign Body

Tampons create an aerobic environment in the vagina, which normally is anaerobic. Tampons of three different types have been shown in humans to change the partial pressure of oxygen of the vaginal wall from an anaerobic environment to that of atmospheric air throughout the 90-minute interval after insertion.[326] Because oxygen is required for the production of TSST-I, researchers have suggested that tampons with enhanced absorbency allow the introduction of increasing concentrations of oxygen to enhance production of toxin.

Several alternative explanations for the role of tampons have been proposed. Tampons may remove vaginal substrates that normally inhibit the growth of *S. aureus*.[22] Another suggested role for tampons is that of inducing cervicovaginal ulceration. Such ulcers have been suggested to enhance bacterial growth or toxin absorption and expose submucosal fibronectin for binding of *S. aureus*.[68,70,329] Tampons can induce chronic cervicovaginal ulcers after long-term continuous use or superficial micro-ulcerations after a brief insertion in otherwise healthy women. However, vaginal ulcerations of the type typically seen in TSS have been found during postmortem examination in women who had never used tampons. This finding suggests that vaginal ulceration, such as that seen in the esophagus and bladder in TSS, may be induced by TSST-I.[174]

Investigations to determine whether individual tampon components can induce or amplify the production of TSST-I in vitro have provided conflicting data, in part because no consensus exists on how best to test tampons and their components to determine their potential to increase risk for the development of

TSS. In one setting, although bacterial growth was unaffected, production of TSST-I varied from undetectable levels to 300 μg/mL, depending on the particular brand and style of tampon studied.[22] Other investigators have found that most tampons tested were inhibitory to both bacterial growth and production of TSST-I and that none consistently increased the production of TSST-I.[22]

Two studies clearly demonstrated enhanced production of TSST-I in vitro by the Rely tampon, which is composed of cross-linked carboxymethylcellulose and polyester foam.[238,268] The polyacrylate rayon included in two tampons now removed from the market increased the production of TSST-I under certain conditions,[208] as did the surfactant Pluronic L-92 used in at least one tampon.[268] Neither cotton nor rayon amplifies the production of TSST-I in vitro, nor do cotton tampons adsorb TSST-I or prevent its production.[238,268] Thus, cotton tampons cannot be claimed to be safer than cotton/rayon combinations, although this contention has been disputed.[303] The role of magnesium in controlling the production of TSST-I in the presence of tampons is unclear.[208]

Implanted foreign material such as sutures, central venous lines, and metallic or polymeric implants have been documented repeatedly to enhance the risk of acquiring bacterial infection.[22,155] These infections are characterized by limited spread beyond the tissues in immediate contact with the implants, poor response to antibiotics, and poor healing without removal of the foreign material. Two important differences between TSS and other *S. aureus* infections related to foreign material are the added ability of the organism to produce a toxin that readily disseminates and the limited ability of these strains to produce inflammation.[107] Researchers have suggested that the increased number of surgically associated TSS cases may be related to the number of implanted materials.[133]

The enhanced risk of acquiring infection by *S. aureus* in the presence of foreign material has been defined experimentally in animals. Rats remained asymptomatic after the subcutaneous injection of more than 1×10^6 colony-forming units of *S. aureus*, whereas 3×10^2 colony-forming units invariably led to infection in the presence of a suture. In addition, the ability of sutured tissue to resist infection varies with the kind of material implanted, particularly its physical or chemical configuration. For example, bacterial adherence is eightfold higher for braided sutures of silk, silicone-heated blue polyester, and absorbable polyglycolic acid than for monofilament nylon.[155]

In addition to sutures, other foreign materials associated with TSS-related wound infection are Teflon splints, gauze packing, and mammary implants.[22]

OTHER POTENTIAL HOST RISK FACTORS

Other factors have been examined in an attempt to identify individuals who may be at increased risk for the development of TSS.[80] Some of these factors have included HLA typing,[22] neutrophil function,[140] adherence of *S. aureus* to vaginal epithelial cells,[20] alteration of the cervicovaginal flora,[22] hormonal factors, and personal hygiene practices.[80] Of all these factors, those of potential importance included cervicovaginal flora and hormonal factors.

Vaginal co-colonization with *S. aureus* and one of the Enterobacteriaceae has been postulated to enhance the risk of development of TSS.[55] Prospective examination of 495 healthy women revealed a 7 percent vaginal colonization rate for *S. aureus* TSST-I–positive strains. Women who were colonized with toxin-producing *S. aureus* also were colonized with *Escherichia coli* or other Enterobacteriaceae statistically significantly more often than were women colonized with non–toxin-producing or no *S. aureus*. *E. coli* isolation rates were 54 percent in women with

TSST-I–positive isolates, 15 percent in women with TSST-I–negative isolates, and 11 percent in women with no *S. aureus*. Co-isolation of *E. coli* was the only identified factor associated with vaginal carriage of TSST-I–positive *S. aureus*. Additionally, among the 14 patients with TSS monitored in this study, 9 had *E. coli* as well as TSST-I–positive *S. aureus* co-isolated during the acute TSS episode. The significance of these observations and their relationship to postulated roles for endotoxin in TSS are not clear.

The results of early case-control studies suggested that oral contraceptive steroids may have an effect on vaginal *S. aureus* organisms that may produce or release TSS-associated toxins[75,227] and that this effect was protective. However, one case-control study found no protective effect or enhanced risk associated with oral contraceptive use.[127] Hormonal control is known to be responsible for numerous cyclic changes in vaginal pH and flora, but the role of hormonal factors in the pathogenesis of TSS has not been examined well.

HISTOPATHOLOGY

The histopathologic findings on postmortem examination support the concept that TSS is a toxin-mediated disease.[1,28,36,174,230,333] Striking histopathologic similarities exist between patients with TSS and those with "scarlet fever" reported in 1936.[36] Typically, a total absence of tissue invasion by bacteria and minimal evidence of an inflammatory reaction in most organs are noted. Findings thought to be due to a direct effect of the toxin or mediators (or both) and unrelated to hypoperfusion have included subepidermal ulcerations in the cervix, vagina, esophagus, and bladder; depletion of lymphocytes in lymph nodes; a subepidermal cleavage plane in the skin; and mild inflammatory changes in the kidney, liver, heart, and muscle.

Cervicovaginal ulcerations are the only characteristic lesions noted in the genital tract of patients with fatal menstrual TSS, and such ulcers have been found in a patient with menstrual TSS who had never used tampons.[174,233] The ulcerations are superficial. Capillary vasodilation and thrombosis with inflammation of the mucosa are present, but no deep-tissue bacterial invasion is seen. The layer of vacuolization and separation in the ulcers occurs beneath the basal layer. The same type of ulcer also has been found in the bladder and esophagus, which suggests that these ulcerations may be caused by the toxins or mediators and not by the use of tampons.

Although the myocardium was described as normal in one postmortem series of TSS, in another series of eight fatal cases, all patients had evidence of focal round-cell infiltration with variable degrees of congestion, edema, and hemorrhage.[174,230] Myxoid degeneration was found in all heart valves from four patients in one series. Sections of skeletal muscle have demonstrated only congestion, edema, focal hemorrhage or fiber necrosis, and a mild acute inflammatory infiltrate.

Varying degrees of triaditis or periportal lymphocytic inflammation have been the most consistent findings in the liver; centrilobular congestion with necrosis and mild cellular degeneration also has been described.[150] In the kidney, toxin-mediated mononuclear interstitial nephritis may result from perivasculitis of the adventitia of the renal venules, lesions that probably precede the development of hypotension-induced acute tubular necrosis. The most characteristic findings in the spleen and lymph nodes have been lymphocyte depletion; inactive hypocellular, hypoplastic lymphoid follicles with edema; marked histiocytosis in the interfollicular areas; and hemophagocytosis.

Perivascular lymphocytic infiltrates and bullae that separate at the basement membrane are characteristic of the early skin changes in TSS.[8,10,140] No evidence of vasculitis has been reported.

CLINICAL SPECTRUM

ACUTE PHASE: MODERATE TO SEVERE DISEASE*

Multisystem end-organ damage secondary to loss of peripheral vascular resistance, loss of intravascular volume as a result of endothelial damage and the capillary leak syndrome, and interstitial edema constitute the most important mediator-induced changes of TSS. Prolonged hypotension, interstitial edema, and vascular congestion additionally may result in ischemic organ damage.

The onset of illness in patients with moderate to severe disease is abrupt, with symptoms and signs including fever, chills, malaise, headache, sore throat, myalgia, muscle tenderness, fatigue, vomiting, diarrhea, abdominal pain, and orthostatic dizziness or syncope (Figs. 71–3 and 71–4).

During the first 24 to 48 hours, diffuse erythroderma, severe watery diarrhea (often with incontinence), decreased urine output, cyanosis, and edema of the extremities may be noted. Some patients may have purpura fulminans.[168] Cerebral ischemia and edema rapidly result in somnolence, confusion, irritability, agitation, and occasionally hallucinations, even in individuals without hypotension. Patients with TSS have had signs and symptoms of encephalopathy, cerebral infarction, meningismus,[15,27,135,179,283] and the cauda equina syndrome.[8]

During initial physical examination of a moderately to severely ill patient, fever, tachycardia, tachypnea, a low or unobtainable blood pressure, erythroderma (generally not seen in patients with severe hypotension or in those without T cells)[159] (see Fig. 71–4A), and muscle tenderness are noted in conjunction with peripheral cyanosis and edema, conjunctival hyperemia, subconjunctival hemorrhages (see Fig. 71–4B), beefy red edematous mucous membranes, somnolence, disorientation, and agitation. In menstrual TSS, edema and erythema of the inner aspect of the thighs and the perineum may be noted in conjunction with normal findings on uterine and adnexal examination. In nonmenstrual cases, vaginitis or another focus of infection will be present. In most postoperative cases, the surgical wound is not inflamed. If erythroderma is present, it will be most intense surrounding the infected focus.

Surgical wounds and some abscesses colonized or infected with *S. aureus* and responsible for postoperative or nonmenstrual TSS may have minimal or no signs of inflammation.[6,17,93,250] The production of TNF-α by macrophages in response to TSST-I inhibits neutrophil mobilization in vitro,[107] which may provide an explanation for the absence of signs of inflammation. The incubation period for postoperative or postpartum TSS may be as short as 12 to 48 hours. Relatively few cases have been associated with deep-tissue infection.[22]

Laboratory Changes

Abnormalities in clinical laboratory tests will reflect the endogenous cytokine release, shock, and organ failure associated with TSS. Leukocytosis may not be present, but the total proportion of mature and immature neutrophils generally exceeds 90 percent. The proportion of immature neutrophils usually is 25 to 50 percent of the total number of neutrophils and is associated with a profound and absolute lymphopenia. Thrombocytopenia and anemia are present during the first few days and frequently are accompanied by prolonged prothrombin and partial thromboplastin times. Disseminated intravascular coagulation may be present. Sterile pyuria and cerebrospinal fluid pleocytosis are indicative of generalized involvement of the mucous membranes and serosal surfaces. Elevated blood urea nitrogen and creatinine

*See references 47, 56, 76, 114, 116, 139, 192, 277, 305, 311.

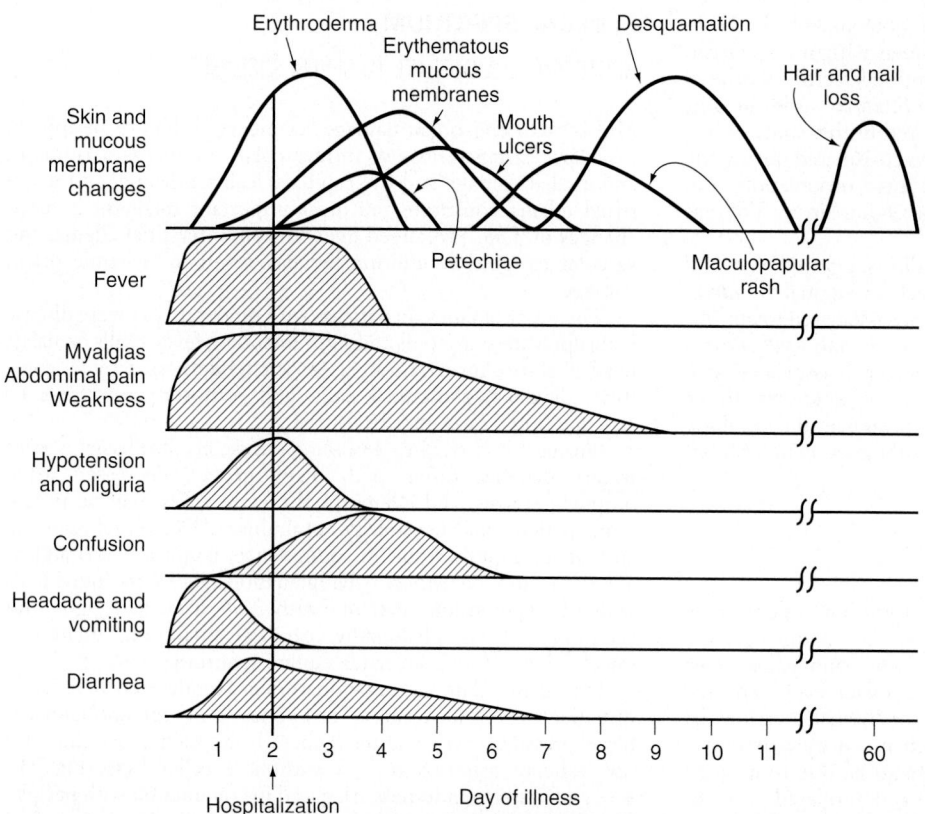

Figure 71–3 Composite drawing of the major systemic skin and mucous membrane manifestations of toxic shock syndrome. *(From Chesney, P. J., Davis, J. P., Purdy, W. K., et al.: The clinical manifestations of toxic shock syndrome. J. A. M. A. 246:741-748, 1981. Copyright 1981, American Medical Association.)*

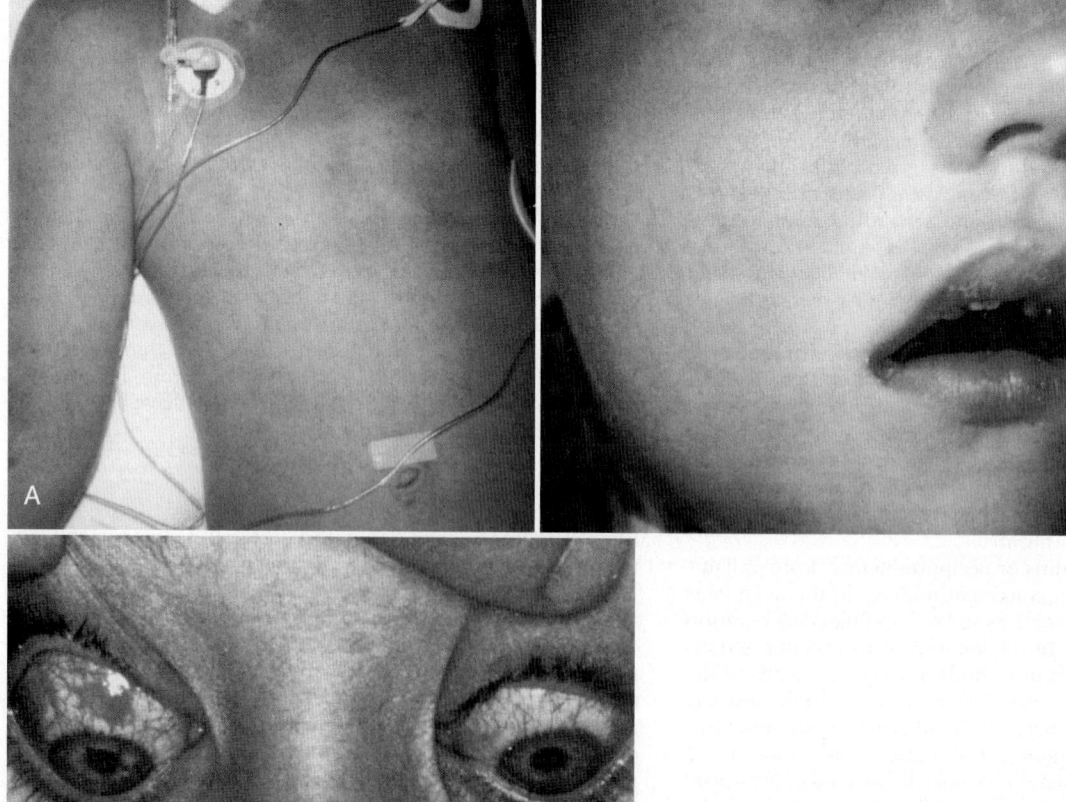

Figure 71–4 Skin and mucous membrane manifestations present at the onset of toxic shock syndrome (TSS). **A,** Diffuse erythroderma in a 7-year-old child with nonmenstrual TSS associated with osteomyelitis of the fibula. **B,** Bulbar conjunctival infection and subconjunctival hemorrhage in a 24-year-old woman with nonmenstrual TSS. *(B, from Bach, M. C.: Dermatologic signs in toxic shock syndrome: Clues to diagnosis. J. Am. Acad. Dermatol. 8:343-347, 1983.)*

TABLE 71–3 Therapeutic Principles for Management of Toxic Shock Syndrome

1. Identify the focus of infection: débride and irrigate extensively and remove any foreign material
2. Isolate the organism for antimicrobial susceptibility studies
3. Administer parenteral antimicrobial therapy
   Stop enzyme/toxin production with a protein synthesis inhibitor (e.g., clindamycin, erythromycin, gentamicin)
   and
   Eradicate the organism with a bacterial cell wall inhibitor (e.g., β-lactamase–resistant antistaphylococcal antimicrobial agent)
   Consider intravenous immunoglobulin to provide antitoxin antibodies for a subset of patients, including those with the following:
   • Disease refractory to initial fluid replacement and several hours of vasopressor support
   • A focus of infection that cannot be drained
   • Persistent oliguria despite massive fluid replacement and in the presence of pulmonary edema
   Consider additional measures, such as the following:
   • Methylprednisolone to suppress cytokine production and the inflammatory response
   • Fluid therapy to maintain adequate venous return and cardiac filling pressure and to prevent end-organ damage
4. Anticipate the management of multisystem organ failure

levels reflect kidney damage,[50] abnormalities in tests of liver function reflect liver damage and acute cholestasis,[130,150] and the profound hypocalcemia may reflect both hypoproteinemia and high serum levels of a calcitonin-like material.[51,286] Muscle involvement is noted by an elevated creatine phosphokinase level, and the hypophosphatemia that occurs despite impaired renal function is unexplained.[14,51,319] Most of these test results will return to normal within 7 to 10 days of disease onset. *S. aureus* will be cultured from the cervix or vagina in more than 85 percent of patients with menstrual TSS and from the focus of infection in patients with nonmenstrual TSS. Positive blood culture results are rare findings.[69] Antibody to TSST-I or to the staphylococcal enterotoxins will be absent at the onset of disease in more than 85 percent of patients.[23,33,66,259,281,332]

Treatment

The four general principles of treatment of TSS (Table 71-3) are (1) identification and drainage of the focus of toxin production, (2) identification and susceptibility testing of the organism, (3) administration of antimicrobial therapy to block synthesis of the toxin and to kill *S. aureus*, and (4) management of the systemic multiorgan actions of the toxins or mediators.*

LOCATION AND DRAINAGE OF THE INFECTED SITE

The focus of infection should be identified rapidly, any foreign bodies should be removed, and the site should be drained or irrigated completely, even if it does not appear to be inflamed. Performing this procedure is of utmost importance because perpetuation of even a small, undrained focus of infection may result in serious clinical consequences. If TSS occurs in the immediate postoperative period, the wound should be assumed to be the source of infection, regardless of its benign appearance.

IDENTIFICATION AND SUSCEPTIBILITY TESTING OF THE ORGANISM

The incidence of community-acquired MRSA infections has increased dramatically in incidence during the past 10 years.[129]

*See references 47, 56, 75, 76, 114, 116, 139, 192, 264, 289, 311.

These MRSA strains differ from the long-standing hospital-acquired MRSA strains in that they are acquired in the community by well individuals with no risk factors and are not multiresistant. Most strains are susceptible to clindamycin. Because MRSA strains are fully capable of producing TSST-I,[89,272] community-acquired menstrual and nonmenstrual cases of TSS may be caused by either community or multiresistant hospital-acquired strains of MRSA.[96] To date, vancomycin-resistant strains of *S. aureus* are rare findings.[143,288] Thus, every effort should be made to obtain the organism for susceptibility testing.

ADMINISTRATION OF ANTIMICROBIAL AGENTS

Administration of antistaphylococcal antibiotics is indicated to eradicate organisms and prevent recurrence.[75,76] The infection may be a superficial or deep-tissue infection and may be associated with *S. aureus* bacteremia or bacteriuria. Antistaphylococcal antimicrobial agents should be administered intravenously at maximal doses for age and should be initiated as soon as possible.

Once the patient is stable, no longer vomiting or having diarrhea, and able to take food by mouth, high doses of an oral antimicrobial agent to which the organism is susceptible can be given to complete a total course of 10 to 14 days.

Subinhibitory concentrations of the protein synthesis inhibitors clindamycin, lincomycin, erythromycin, clarithromycin, kanamycin, gentamicin, tetracycline, and linezolid have been shown to suppress TSST-I production in vitro.[88,237,269,291] In one study, clindamycin concentrations $^{1}/_{64}$ the minimal inhibitory concentration (MIC) were effective in totally blocking TSST-I production.[237] In a mouse model of myositis caused by *S. pyogenes*, another superantigen-producing organism, clindamycin and erythromycin were more efficacious than penicillin.[97,289,292]

Data suggest that subinhibitory concentrations of β-lactam antibiotics actually may *increase* TSST-I production by *S. aureus*. At a concentration of half the MIC, nafcillin can *increase* toxin production 10-fold more than do control conditions.[5] A similar effect has been described for nafcillin and the staphylococcal alpha-toxin.[163] The effect is not seen with vancomycin, another cell-wall-active drug, thus suggesting specificity beyond merely a cell wall effect. Co-administration of a protein synthesis inhibitor with a β-lactam antibiotic blocks the effect.[5]

The choice of initial empiric antimicrobial therapy has become more complex as a result of an increase in the number of community-acquired MRSA infections and the spread of multiresistant MRSA strains in hospitals.[161] The severity of TSS warrants initiating maximally effective therapy. Once the results of susceptibility testing of the organism are available, therapy can be adjusted appropriately. In the past, the most effective initial empiric therapy was a combination of a β-lactamase–resistant penicillin and clindamycin. If there is concern for MRSA strains causing TSS, consideration should be given to initiating therapy with vancomycin and clindamycin. This situation clearly is difficult because most patients with TSS have a degree of renal failure. In addition, if the organism is susceptible to methicillin, the β-lactamase–resistant penicillins generally are more efficacious than is vancomycin. As an option to vancomycin, linezolid has been used successfully for the treatment of staphylococcal TSS.[291] An infectious disease consultation should be considered to help in the management of these patients.

MANAGEMENT OF SYSTEMIC MULTIORGAN ACTIONS OF THE TOXINS OR MEDIATORS

Intravenous Immunoglobulin

Not surprisingly, given the high prevalence of antibodies to TSST-I in adults,[324] high levels of antibody to TSST-I are present in IVIG preparations.[46,52,196,233,300] In animal models of TSS, human IVIG given at the time of inoculation of TSST-I–positive *S. aureus* prevented the development of TSS. When IVIG was administered 8 hours later, it decreased the mortality rate from 90 percent in control rabbits to 16 percent. When IVIG was given 29 hours after administration of TSST-I, the increase in survival rates in the IVIG-treated animals still was significant. No adverse reactions were noted in the treated animals, and no evidence was found of disease mediated by the formation of antigen-antibody complexes.[196,197,199,200] Monoclonal antibodies to TSST-I can prevent the development of manifestations of TSS in the rabbit model completely.[34,235,276]

High concentrations of antibodies to TSST-I and the staphylococcal enterotoxins (SEA; SEB; SEC types 1, 2, and 3; SED; and SEE) have been demonstrated in pooled IVIG.[46,52,233,300] These antibodies may inhibit the binding of toxins to MHC class II antigen-processing cells or interfere with presentation of toxin by these cells to the TCR. As a result, production of TNF-α and TNF-β is inhibited by these antibodies in vitro in an apparent toxin-specific manner.[300] Down-regulation of the production of lymphokine induced by streptococcal pyrogenic exotoxin A by IVIG also has been demonstrated in vitro.[215,281]

The results of these in vitro studies have supported the use of IVIG for both streptococcal and staphylococcal TSS.[253] Anecdotal case reports have indicated a beneficial effect on both streptococcal[16,215,338] and staphylococcal[2,52,61,221,233] TSS in humans. The efficacy of IVIG as adjunctive therapy for streptococcal TSS was evaluated in a multicenter, randomized, double-blind, placebo-controlled trial.[72] Although the trial was prematurely terminated because of slow patient recruitment, results from 21 enrolled patients (10 IVIG recipients and 11 placebo recipients) showed 3.6-fold higher mortality in the placebo group. Even though statistical significance was not reached, the trial provides support for IVIG as adjunctive therapy for streptococcal TSS.

Because IVIG is expensive and most patients respond rapidly once standard therapeutic measures are initiated, some authors would reserve IVIG for patients with an inaccessible focus of infection or for those who continue to deteriorate after receiving fluid and vasopressor support for several hours (see Table 71–3). The dose most often used has been 400 mg/kg given as a single dose over the course of several hours. This dose results in a serum antibody titer of greater than 1:100, much higher than that appearing to provide immunity to TSST-I.[233] Some studies have used IVIG doses of up to 2 g/kg.[72] Because early administration of IVIG possibly could blunt the immune response to TSST-I or other toxins and increase the possibility of a recurrent episode, the potential risks and benefits of this form of therapy must be considered for each patient.

The role of endotoxin in the pathogenesis of TSS is unclear. The failure of polymyxin B and anti-J5 antiserum to alter the course of TSST-I–positive TSS in a rabbit model suggests that endotoxin may not be an important mediator of TSS in humans.[198]

Early and sporadic case reports of TSS have suggested therapeutic benefit with naloxone,[59] calcium,[233] and exchange transfusion in severely ill patients unresponsive to the usual forms of therapy.

Corticosteroids

Short courses of methylprednisolone or dexamethasone, if given early in the course of the disease, have been associated with a reduction in the duration of fever and the severity of illness but no reduction in mortality rates.[307] In vitro, dexamethasone has been shown to down-regulate TSST-I–induced cytokine production.[167] Because no controlled prospective study has demonstrated efficacy, the use of steroids probably should be restricted to hypotensive patients unresponsive to fluid resuscitation, antimicrobial agents, and intravenous immunoglobulin (IVIG).

Fluid Replacement

The most important aspect of the nonspecific treatment of symptomatic patients is fluid replacement.[304] Intravascular volume and cardiac filling pressure must be restored rapidly to achieve adequate tissue perfusion. Because of the ongoing capillary leakage, this fluid replacement may far exceed the estimated fluid requirements based on calculated maintenance and fluid deficit volumes. Some adults have required vasopressors and as much as 12 L of fluid during the first 24 hours to stabilize the circulating blood pressure. Pleural, pericardial, and peritoneal effusions and interstitial edema inevitably occur as a result of the continued vascular capillary fluid leak. Close monitoring in an intensive care unit will facilitate determining when the correct intravascular volume has been achieved, as well as detecting and appropriately monitoring and treating myocardial dysfunction, hemodynamic derangements, pulmonary edema, adult respiratory distress syndrome, acute renal failure, encephalopathy, and disseminated intravascular coagulation.

SUBACUTE PHASE: AFTER TREATMENT IS INITIATED

Once treatment is initiated, response usually is rapid. Temperature returns to normal within 48 hours. The hemodynamic changes are observed initially as tachycardia, decreased systemic vascular resistance, decreased central venous pressure, hypovolemia, normal pulmonary artery wedge pressure, and an increased cardiac index.[13,41,67,114,117] Once aggressive fluid therapy has been initiated, myocardial edema and potential failure, along with pulmonary and cerebral edema in the face of renal failure, become the most critical management issues. The reasons for myocardial failure are unclear but probably are related to perivascular inflammation of the coronary vessels, edema, and postulated myocardial depressant factors.[174,230] TSST-I has been shown to inhibit systolic function in isolated rabbit atria, though at higher than usual circulating concentrations.[224] Arrhythmias may result from myocardial damage or electrolyte abnormalities.[193,255] Endomyocardial biopsy in one patient with severe global hypokinesis of the left ventricle revealed no substantial inflammatory infiltrate but a mild to moderate number of T cells scattered diffusely throughout the biopsy specimen.[67]

During the decompensated stage of myocardial dysfunction, the cardiac index falls and pulmonary wedge pressure increases, with both left atrial and ventricular and diastolic diameters being at the upper limits of normal.[114] Reversible electrocardiographic findings include sinus tachycardia, diffuse loss of voltage, flattened T waves, and diffuse nonspecific ST-T wave changes. If fatal arrhythmia does not occur during the decompensated stage, the toxic cardiomyopathy is reversible and rarely results in permanent changes. This process is similar to "stunned myocardium," a transient, postischemic myocardial dysfunctional state.[67]

Pulmonary edema and adult respiratory distress syndrome occur commonly in patients with severe disease when massive fluid replacement is necessary and the capillary leak syndrome continues in the lungs. Pulmonary edema appears rapidly once fluid replacement is initiated and often necessitates intubation and respirator management for several days.[304]

Forms of TSS-associated acute renal failure include prerenal azotemia and both nonoliguric and oliguric renal failure.[50] The type of renal failure manifested may be dependent on the degree of intravascular volume depletion. Unless severe acute tubular necrosis necessitates temporary hemodialysis, repletion of intravascular volume usually results in rapid restoration of renal function and, ultimately, diuresis. Permanent renal damage is an extremely rare event.[46]

The gastrointestinal, musculoskeletal, and hepatic changes resolve rapidly. Sequelae associated with these changes are rare, except for prolonged muscle weakness.[46,79] Joint manifestations generally are self-limited.[22,119]

Management of fluids, electrolytes, and metabolic acidosis in patients with TSS is complex. Although tetany is a rare occurrence, this common severe hypocalcemia may be life-threatening and should be corrected.[51,235,286] Most patients require potassium replacement and management of metabolic acidosis. The use of colloid for fluid replacement and removal of the toxin stimulus for capillary leak syndrome ultimately correct the hypoproteinemia.

The typical dermatologic manifestations follow a predictable sequence (see Fig. 71–3). A dandruff-like flaky desquamation begins on the trunk and extremities 5 to 7 days after the onset of symptoms. From days 10 to 12 and for as long as a month, the characteristic full-thickness desquamation of the fingers, toes, palms, and soles takes place (Fig. 71–5). A variety of atypical dermatologic manifestations, including petechiae and subepidermal bullae, have been described.[10,101,146]

Early in the acute phase, many patients exhibit desquamation of the mucous membranes, which is particularly painful when the oral mucous membranes are involved.[47] In addition, a small number of patients will have reactivated herpes simplex virus type 1 or 2 lesions with the acute illness.[47] A late-onset pruritic maculopapular rash with edema and low-grade fever probably unrelated to antimicrobial therapy occurs in more than 50 percent of menses-associated cases within 7 to 14 days of disease onset.[47,84] The cause of this late-onset rash is unknown.

Telogen effluvium, a common sequela, is a nonspecific response to severe trauma, sepsis, or stress that results in disturbed metabolism and keratinization of the hair follicles and nails. The hair follicles appear to transform prematurely from the growth, or anlagen, phase to the telogen, or resting, phase. Hair and nail loss occurs 4 to 16 weeks after onset of the illness, with restoration taking place in 5 to 6 months.[22,26,47]

The hematologic system seldom is involved with major complications in TSS. Although disseminated intravascular coagulation may be present, gastrointestinal, uterine, or cerebral bleeding rarely occurs. Thrombocytopenia may be present initially in patients with disseminated intravascular coagulation; thrombocytosis is characteristic of the recovery phase. Mild to moderate normocytic, normochromic anemia, which probably is dilutional and a result of suppressed red blood cell synthesis, develops in virtually all moderately to severely ill patients with TSS and resolves during convalescence.[47,49] Hypoferrinemia occurs commonly.[49]

The relatively common toxic or ischemic encephalopathy, rarely complicated by seizures, resolves slowly during the first 4 to 5 days of hospitalization.

Outcome and Sequelae

Death associated with TSS usually takes place within the first few days of hospitalization, but it may occur as late as 15 days after admission. Fatalities have been attributed to refractory cardiac arrhythmias, cardiomyopathy, irreversible respiratory failure, and, rarely, bleeding caused by coagulation defects.[174,230] The duration of circulation of toxins and mediators and the associated hypotension may be the best predictors of the severity of the end-organ damage.

After being discharged, more patients experience prolonged fatigue, muscle weakness, and pain.[46] Sequelae attributed to TSS that appear to be related to a prolonged period of hypotension have included chronic renal failure, gangrene, and telogen effluvium.[79,158,202,258,262] Other sequelae, such as neuropsychological abnormalities, prolonged myalgia and weakness, carpal tunnel syndrome, chronic dermatitis, Raynaud syndrome, new allergies, and recurrences, are explained less easily. Abnormalities such as impaired memory and poorly sustained concentration have been found in patients who did not require any therapy other than intravenous fluids to restore their blood pressure.[258] In one center, patients with nonmenstrual TSS had more serious short- and long-term neuropsychological complications than did patients with menstrual TSS.[158] Sequelae related primarily to the neuromuscular system have resulted in speculation that the TSS-associated toxin may have a direct effect on nerve or muscle tissue. In one patient with TSS, cauda equina syndrome with partial paralysis developed after lumbar laminectomy and staphylococcal meningitis, thus suggesting a neurotoxic effect of the intrathecally produced SEC.[8]

One study compared the sequelae and other long-term effects in 183 (174 menstrual cases) women with TSS and 366 control women hospitalized for appendicitis and appendectomy and matched for age, race, and duration of follow-up.[79] Each subject completed two comprehensive phone interviews. When compared with controls, women with TSS were significantly more likely to report sequelae involving fatigue, the integument (hair loss and nail changes), mental and cognitive skills (problems with concentration, reading difficulty, and memory loss), emotions (menses attitude and emotional changes), and multiple organ

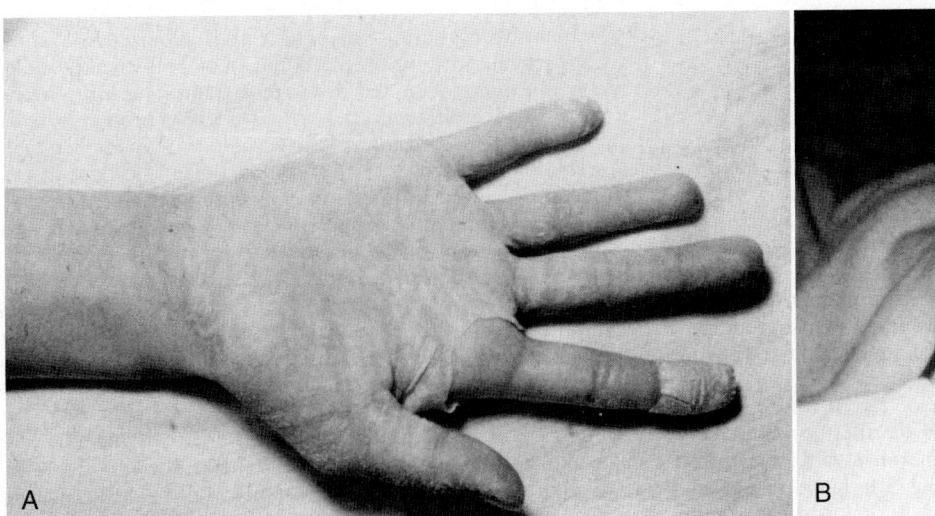
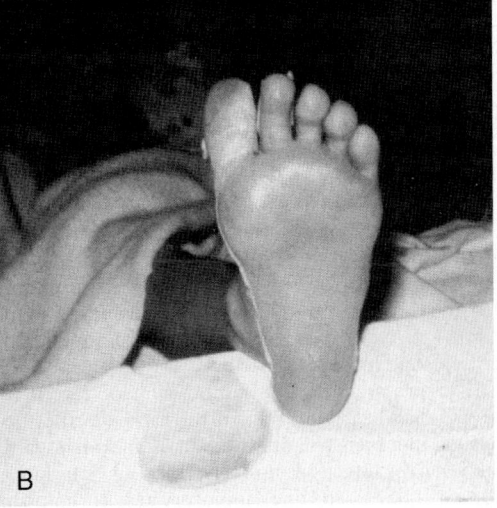

Figure 71–5 Universal full-thickness desquamation of the hands (**A**) and feet (**B**) first noted 7 to 14 days after disease onset and persisting for up to 30 days.

systems (conditions involving the joint, cardiac, muscle, and genitourinary systems). In addition, women with TSS were significantly more likely than controls to report persistence of symptoms. Fertility patterns and pregnancy outcomes were similar in controls and women with TSS, both before and after the index illness.[79]

Recurrences

One of the most puzzling aspects of the pathophysiology of TSS is the high rate of recurrence in patients with inadequately treated menstrual or nonmenstrual disease.[6,47,75,76,191,294] A small number of patients with menstrual disease and repeated tampon exposure have experienced as many as 6 to 12 recurrences. Recurrences associated with menstrual disease have no predictable pattern. In most patients the first episode is the most severe. However, asymptomatic menses may occur between symptomatic episodes, and the most severe episode may occur after one or more milder episodes.[76] The use of antistaphylococcal antimicrobial therapy to which the organism is susceptible in doses recommended for serious infections for 10 to 14 days and discontinuation of tampon use can be expected to reduce the rate of recurrence significantly.[76] Recurrences after nonmenstrual TSS are well described and usually are associated with inadequate initial therapy.[6,158,233] Cisplatin administration resulting in significant hypomagnesemia precipitated several recurrent episodes of TSS in an immunocompromised adult.[25]

The absent or delayed antibody response to TSST-I found in both menstrual and nonmenstrual TSS patients probably accounts for the continued susceptibility to TSS and for the high recurrence rate.[22,33,181,259,281,294,332] The fact that superantigenic toxins are not processed by antigen-processing cells and T lymphocytes as conventional antigens may provide an explanation for the poor convalescent antibody response to these antigens.[166]

Culture-negative, menses-associated, recurrent episodes of TSS continue to occur in a small number of patients despite discontinuation of tampon use and administration of appropriate antimicrobial therapy during the acute episode.[76] Administration of an oral β-lactamase–resistant antistaphylococcal antimicrobial agent during menses has been tried in an attempt to prevent these recurrences but is not always successful. In recurrent cases resistant to this form of prophylaxis, consideration could be given to the untested and empiric use of rifampin, clindamycin, erythromycin, or IVIG (if the patient has no antibody to TSST-I) or to the use of an oral contraceptive.[191]

ATYPICAL MANIFESTATIONS

Mild Disease

Recognition of mild episodes of TSS is particularly important in patients with menstrual TSS because repeated use of tampons and the risk for recurrence are episodic.[48,85,310] Patients with mild or severe menstrual TSS typically do not form antibody to TSST-I during convalescence[22,33,259,281,332] and, without appropriate therapy, may have one or more recurrences. Such recurrences may be mild or severe.[75,76,192] Patients with nonmenstrual TSS also do not form antibodies in convalescence. A mild episode may be recognized only in retrospect, after desquamation or a recurrent episode (or both) develop.[233]

The presence of any combination of fever, headache, sore throat, diarrhea, vomiting, orthostatic dizziness, syncope, and myalgia in a menstruating woman or an individual with a potential S. aureus infection, no matter how trivial, should raise suspicion of TSS. A specific laboratory test to confirm the clinical diagnosis is not available. A bacterial culture positive for S. aureus may be helpful but is not diagnostic of menstrual cases because

S. aureus may be cultured from the cervix or vagina in as many as 33 percent of menstruating women.[186,239]

Other laboratory data usually do not reflect multisystem involvement in mild disease, and assays for TSST-I in body fluids are investigational.[195,323] Diagnostic support for the theory that the patient's signs and symptoms represent mild TSS often depends on the constellation of findings present, including subsequent typical desquamation of the palms, soles, toes, or fingers; demonstration that S. aureus isolates from the site of infection produce TSST-I or an enterotoxin; absence of antibody to TSST-I or enterotoxins in acute-phase serum; and recurrent disease, if it develops.

Nonmenstrual Disease

The incidence of postoperative cases of TSS after all types of surgery has been estimated to be 3 per 100,000 population.[131] For ear, nose, and throat surgery, the incidence is higher (16.5/100,000 population).[152] A striking feature of most postoperative cases with rapid onset is the absence of any signs of wound infection.[17,131,246,260] The mean time from surgery to the onset of symptoms is 2 to 4 days.[17] Nosocomial acquisition of TSST-I–positive organisms rarely has been documented for postoperative cases.[9,169,212] A wide variety of types of surgery have been associated with TSS.[22,43,211,223,252,278,282]

Burn wounds provide a particularly rich environment for growth of S. aureus and the production of toxins.* In burn centers, TSS occurs predominantly in young children with small burns.[98] In one large pediatric burn center, S. aureus normally was not cultured from any site on admission.[52] However, it was acquired within a few days of admission and became the most common wound pathogen. Of all wound isolates of S. aureus, just 16 percent produced TSST-I. Only 50 percent of the children had antibodies to TSST-I on admission, which reflects the low prevalence of antibodies in this population.[324] Of blood products administered, 76 percent had antibodies to TSST-I, and seroconversion occurred in children receiving these products. A toxic shock–like syndrome developed in 13 percent (7/53) of children, only one of whom had TSST-I–producing S. aureus isolated from the wound. SEA and SEB were produced by isolates from three patients. In burn patients, issues regarding the use of prophylactic antibiotics and occlusive dressings and enhancement of TSST-I production by topical antimicrobial agents are unsettled.[99] The mortality rate associated with TSS in children with burns may be as high as 57 percent.[122] Skin disrupted in any way, including disruption by varicella or a tattoo, also may be a focus for TSS.[22,37,65]

Patients whose anterior nares have been colonized by S. aureus are at particular risk for the development of TSS when the respiratory mucosa is disrupted by surgery, trauma, or a respiratory infection such as influenza.[22,63,180,312,314] TSS has been reported in association with sinusitis,[22,109] pharyngitis,[22,263] parapharyngeal abscesses,[263] tracheitis,[22,71,92,125,218] pneumonia,[22,74] rubeola,[297] and submandibular space abscesses. TSS occurring after ear, nose, and throat surgery has been associated with the use of nasal splints and packing materials and in part may be the result of interruption of the ciliary blanket.[3,22,121,207,339]

After orthopedic procedures or in association with bone and joint infections, the clinical manifestation of TSS may be confusing as a result of the intense and generalized myalgias associated with TSS, which may be misinterpreted as postoperative musculoskeletal symptoms. The wounds usually appear to be benign.[22,206,240,302,318] Infected abrasions under casts may be focal sites of TSST-I production.[285]

In one center, when cases of nonmenstrual TSS were compared with menstrual cases, patients with nonmenstrual disease

---

*See references 11, 52, 60, 98, 122, 124, 128, 142, 183, 188, 328.

were found to have a delayed onset of symptoms after the precipitating event, more frequent central nervous system manifestations, less frequent musculoskeletal involvement (myalgia and arthralgia), and a higher degree of anemia.[158] Recurrences occurred in both groups in untreated patients, and mortality rates were not different. Clinical differences between the two categories are suggested to be related to differences in the types of toxins produced. TSST-I was produced with comparable frequency in both groups. SEA was produced less often by nonmenstrual isolates, and menstrual isolates more often produced both TSST-I and SEA. SEB was produced more frequently by nonmenstrual isolates.

Several patients with TSS have been reported to be simultaneously infected with *S. aureus* and *S. pyogenes*.[100] Determining which infection primarily was responsible for the manifestations or whether an amplified effect of exotoxins from both organisms was present was not possible.

Recalcitrant Erythematous Desquamating Disorder

An atypical, subacute variant of TSS has been described in patients with acquired immunodeficiency syndrome (AIDS) and labeled recalcitrant erythematous desquamating disorder. *S. aureus* strains producing TSST-I, SEA, or SEB have been isolated from patients with AIDS and prolonged erythema, extensive cutaneous desquamation, hypotension, tachycardia, and multiple and variable organ involvement.[61,91,164] The illness is recalcitrant, prolonged, and characterized by multiple recurrences. In one patient, elevated levels of TNF and IL-6 were found during severe episodes. When antitoxin antibodies have been measured during recurrence, they have been undetectable. Two patients responded well to IVIG.[61,164] Patients with the combined cellular and humoral immunodeficiencies of AIDS may be at particular risk for the development of severe, frequent, and prolonged recurrent episodes of TSS.[61,91,112,164,284] TSST-I and the enterotoxins may activate human immunodeficiency virus type 1 (HIV-1) gene expression in vivo, as has been observed in vitro.[123]

Neonatal Toxic Shock Syndrome–like Exanthematous Disease

A toxic shock–like illness related to MRSA producing TSST-I, neonatal toxic shock syndrome–like exanthematous disease (NTED), was described initially in neonates in Japan[299] and subsequently recognized in France.[321] These infants are seen in the first week of life with the combination of a generalized erythematous macular rash, thrombocytopenia, elevated acute-phase reactants, and fever. Patients are colonized with MRSA belonging to a single clonal type that produces TSST-I and SEC.[147] Although no focus of infection is present and no exotoxins are detectable in serum, analysis of T cells shows selective expansion of V$_\beta$2-positive T cells during the acute phase as a result of selective activation of TSST-I–reactive T cells.[298,299] Maternal IgG antibody to TSST-I plays a protective role in preventing NTED.[298] Although complications occur in premature neonates, term infants typically recover within 5 days without active treatment. The limited disease in comparison to TSS has been attributed to the minute amount of exotoxin from colonized sites and to the high susceptibility to induction of anergy in the immature T cells of neonates.[298,299]

Streptococcal and Other Toxic Shock Syndromes

An increase in the incidence and severity of invasive *S. pyogenes* infections was recognized in the 1980s. Manifestations of severe disease have included septicemia with or without a focus of infection; severe, painful cellulitis; necrotizing fasciitis; and in some cases, streptococcal TSS with or without a focus of infection. Streptococcal TSS is similar to staphylococcal TSS in that it appears to be mediated by superantigenic toxins and results in endothelial damage, hypotension, and multisystem organ involvement. In 1993, the Working Group on Severe Streptococcal Infections proposed a consensus definition for streptococcal TSS with clinical criteria, including isolation of group A streptococci from a normally sterile site, hypotension, and two or more of the following: renal impairment, coagulopathy, liver dysfunction, adult respiratory distress syndrome, erythematous macular rash, and soft tissue necrosis.[336]

Streptococcal toxic shock–like syndrome differs from staphylococcal TSS in numerous respects, including a slower onset over the course of several days; usual absence of vomiting, profuse diarrhea, and conjunctival infection; frequent absence of erythroderma or the presence of only a sandpaper-like rash; severe generalized hyperesthesia; extreme pain at the site of skin involvement; and a mortality rate of 40 to 50 percent.[62,290] Both cell-associated and soluble streptococcal virulence factors, including M protein and pyrogenic exotoxins A and B, have been implicated as superantigens mediating the systemic effects of streptococcal TSS.[39,103,141]

Clostridium sordellii has been reported to cause a toxic shock–like syndrome after medical abortion with mifepristone and intravaginal misoprostol.[58,113,279]

UNIQUE MANIFESTATIONS

Work with superantigens suggests that the pathophysiologic events observed in TSS are the result of release of endogenous mediators after monocyte and T-cell activation by TSST-I or the staphylococcal enterotoxins.

The physiologic changes induced by this dysregulation of the immune system are striking in their rapidity of onset and progression and the involvement of almost all body tissues and organs. The consequent functional disorders of many organs appear to be the result of extensive endothelial damage and loss of peripheral vascular resistance. The generalized decrease in vasomotor tone results in pooling of blood in the peripheral vasculature, vascular congestion, and probably relaxation of the microcirculation. Rapid, nonhydrostatic leakage of fluid from the intravascular to the interstitial space, or "second spacing," does occur and is manifested as extensive generalized anasarca-like, nonpitting edema. The universal hypoproteinemia and hypoalbuminemia in patients with TSS suggest that the fluid leaking from the vasculature is high in protein.

Unique clinical manifestations include profuse vomiting and diarrhea, often associated with incontinence; generalized erythroderma; intense erythema of the mucous membranes, including conjunctival injection and subconjunctival hemorrhages; absence of inflammation in surgical wounds and other focal sites of infection; absence of bacteremia; severe hypocalcemia and hypophosphatemia; rapidly accelerated renal dysfunction; universal desquamation of the palms, soles, fingers, and toes; and risk for recurrent disease and long-term cognitive sequelae.

DIAGNOSIS

Application of the case definition for a single episode[330] or recurrent episodes[76] to the patient's illness is currently the only way to confirm the diagnosis (see Table 71–1). Aggressive attempts to find the focus of *S. aureus* replication that always should be undertaken include culture of the cervix and vagina in patients with menses-associated illness and culture of other potentially infected sites that may not appear to be infected obviously in patients with nonmenstrual illness. *S. aureus* isolates could be examined, when possible, for their ability to produce TSST-I, although such testing seldom is indicated. This test is of limited usefulness for nonmenstrual cases because TSST-I is produced by only 40 to 60 percent of *S. aureus* isolates from such patients.[126] Isolates from these patients could be examined for the presence of the other enterotoxins. Acute and convalescent sera can be tested for the presence of antibodies to TSST-I and the other enterotoxins.[144] Elevated levels of anti–TSST-I in the acute-phase serum of a patient with menstrual-associated TSS would be highly unusual.

In most instances, toxin detection tests are of value only for research or for the rare patient with chronic recurrent or otherwise puzzling disease. Genes for TSST-I and the enterotoxins have been detected in *S. aureus* strains by polymerase chain reaction[19,157,178,194,219,273] and hybridization techniques.[156,216,226] A noncompetitive enzyme-linked immunosorbent assay allows quantitation of TSST-I in clinical samples.[195,209] Reversed passive latex agglutination has been used in hospital laboratories to detect TSST-I and in research laboratories to detect enterotoxins.[83,104] Research laboratories also have developed techniques for detecting the selective expansion of V$_\beta$2-positive T cells as evidence of host response to superantigenic toxins.[54,187]

DIFFERENTIAL DIAGNOSIS

The differential diagnosis of TSS includes clinical entities in which a rapid onset of fever, erythroderma-like rash, hypotension, and multisystem involvement are observed[42,110,210,233,241,243] (Table 71–4).

PREVENTION AND PROPHYLAXIS

To decrease the risk of development of menstrual TSS, in 1982 the Institute of Medicine Committee on TSS recommended that

women, particularly adolescents, minimize their use of high-absorbency tampons.[244] The committee also recommended that women who have had TSS not use tampons because of the increased risk of recurrence and that postpartum women be informed that the use of tampons might increase their risk for the development of TSS.

Although the frequency of changing tampons during a menstrual period has not been associated with risk for the development of TSS, the use of an individual tampon for no more than 12 hours at a time might decrease the risk for menstrual TSS. Women using intravaginal contraceptive devices also should be informed of the potential increase in risk for development of TSS.[275]

Although postoperative TSS is a rare event, it generally occurs in healthy people. As a result of the unexpected and potentially severe consequences of TSS, issues regarding surgical antimicrobial prophylaxis for prevention have been raised. Perioperative systemic antistaphylococcal antibiotics did not prevent TSS in four patients[35,260] and do not eradicate nasal carriage of *S. aureus*.[154] TSS with onset after 48 hours of amoxicillin therapy was reported in two patients after they underwent endonasal sinus surgery.[2] Topical bacitracin ointment on nasal packing does not prevent the development of TSS.[35,87,152,154]

Most authors contend that the rare risk of development of postoperative TSS is comparable to the risk of having a severe antimicrobial reaction and that perioperative antimicrobial prophylaxis is not indicated for clean procedures of short duration.[131,246] Effort should be intensified to recognize postoperative cases early; to open, explore extensively, and irrigate wounds; and to provide immediate antimicrobial and supportive therapy for suspected TSS.

CHARACTERISTICS OF TOXIC SHOCK SYNDROME–ASSOCIATED *STAPHYLOCOCCUS AUREUS* ISOLATES

The ability to produce TSST-I, a previously uncharacterized protein, is the single most distinguishing characteristic of TSS-associated *S. aureus* strains. More than 90 percent of *S. aureus* isolates from patients with menstrual TSS[23,270] and 40 to 60 percent of isolates from patients with nonmenstrual disease[126] produce TSST-I as compared with less than 20 percent of non-TSS strains.

S. aureus strains isolated from patients with TSS are phenotypically different from other strains of *S. aureus*.[22,306] They produce less beta-hemolysis on sheep blood agar and less frequently harbor plasmids than control strains do. An increase in protease production and proteolytic activity by TSS-associated strains has been noted.[306] Next to TSST-I production, production of protease is the most characteristic marker for these strains.

Unlike non-TSS *S. aureus* strains, most TSST-I–positive strains of *S. aureus* require tryptophan for growth and production.[57] In one study, 91 percent of 27 TSST-I–positive vaginal *S. aureus* isolates were tryptophan auxotrophs as compared with 6 percent of 32 TSST-I–negative vaginal *S. aureus* isolates. Eight of 22 TSST-I–producing tryptophan auxotrophs were blocked at the tryptophan synthetase B locus, thus suggesting that the TSST-I gene cluster may have been inserted into this locus and disrupted its function.

Additional differences between TSS and non-TSS strains of *S. aureus* include the resistance of TSS strains to cadmium, arsenate, and penicillin, characteristics that usually are plasmid mediated but, in TSS strains, are chromosomally mediated. As such, these traits must be the result of heterologous insertions. These characteristics are not co-transferred with and therefore presum-

TABLE 71–4   Differential Diagnosis of Toxic Shock Syndrome Based on Clinical Manifestations

Diagnosis	Fever	Exanthem	Shock
Severe invasive *Streptococcus pyogenes* infection	+	+	+
Meningococcemia	+	+	+
Rocky Mountain spotted fever	+	+	±
Ehrlichiosis	+	+	±
Kawasaki disease	+	+	−
Staphylococcal scalded skin syndrome	+	+	−
Toxic epidermal necrolysis	+	+	−
Viral syndromes	+	+	−
Leptospirosis	+	+	−
Systemic lupus erythematosus	+	+	−
Erythema multiforme	+	+	−
Septic shock	+	−	+
Hantavirus pulmonary syndrome	+	−	+
Salmonella infections	+	−	±
Gastroenteritis	+	−	−
Urinary tract infection	+	−	−
Drug reactions			
Phenytoin (Dilantin)	+	+	±
Cocaine	+	+	±
Pseudoephedrine	+	+	±
Inhalational mercury	+	+	±
Quinidine	+	+	−
Sulfonamides	+	+	−
β-Lactam antibiotics	+	+	−
Quinolones	+	+	−

ably not closely linked to the gene segment responsible for TSST-I production.[22,306] TSST-I production is unrelated to methicillin susceptibility or resistance.[272]

ROLE OF STAPHYLOCOCCAL EXOTOXIN TSST-I AND THE ENTEROTOXINS IN TOXIC SHOCK SYNDROME

ROLE OF TSST-I

TSST-I appears to be an important toxin in TSS. Factors supporting this statement include (1) the observation that more than 90 percent of isolates from patients with TSS produce TSST-I, (2) the absence of acute-phase antibody to TSST-I in more than 90 percent of patients with menstrual TSS, (3) the increase in anti–TSST-I antibody during recovery in nonmenstrual cases, (4) absent or low levels of antibody in patients with recurrent menstrual TSS, (5) comparable illness inducible with TSST-I in in vivo animal models, and (6) neutralization of IL-1 stimulation and response to TSST-I by antibody to TSST-I.

Most convincing are experiments in which the ability to cause TSS followed bacteriophage-mediated transfer of the TSST-I–positive chromosomal segment into a recipient *S. aureus* strain without the segment.[82,233] Experiments demonstrating the effectiveness of monoclonal antibodies to TSST-I in reversing the effects of TSST-I provide additional strong support.[171]

ROLE OF ENTEROTOXINS

Because 40 to 60 percent of nonmenstrual TSS *S. aureus* isolates and 5 to 10 percent of menstrual TSS isolates do not produce TSST-I, a role for other staphylococcal exotoxins, including the enterotoxins, has been proposed.[22,66,177,190,234,266,337] Patients with nonmenstrual disease infected with TSST-I–negative strains may have a higher mortality rate.[126] Significant increases in the titer of antibody to the staphylococcal enterotoxins during convalescence strongly suggest a role for these proteins in the pathogenesis of TSS.[12]

In rabbit models, the morbidity and mortality occurring after the injection of TSST-I–negative TSS isolates were comparable to those occurring after infection with TSST-I–positive strains and significantly greater than after inoculation with TSST-I–negative non-TSS isolates.[126] Administration of staphylococcal enterotoxins to animals results in many of the manifestations characteristic of TSS.[21,102]

When large numbers of isolates from patients with TSS have been examined, production of TSST-I alone is the toxin pattern identified most commonly.[22,66,184] Other patterns identified include production of TSST-I in combination with one or more of the identified enterotoxins, production of enterotoxins *only* (one or more), and nonproduction of TSST-I and enterotoxins. Of the TSS strains producing TSST-I, 60.6 percent also produce an enterotoxin.[66,184] SEA is co-expressed with TSST-I frequently, particularly in menstrual isolates. A clone producing both TSST-I and SEA is associated with 88 percent of menstrual TSS cases and may account for as many as 54 percent of isolates from nonmenstrual TSS cases.[44] Seroconversion to SEA occurs more commonly in TSS than in non-TSS *S. aureus* infection, thus further suggesting a role for SEA. TSST-I and SEA have a common MHC class II binding domain and share overlapping domains critical for superantigenic and lethal activities. A monoclonal antibody to TSST-I inhibits these SEA-induced activities.[172]

The third most common pattern of toxin production by TSS isolates is that of TSST-I plus SEC. These isolates have been associated with both menstrual and nonmenstrual cases and par-

ticularly with severe respiratory tract TSS-associated infections.[66] NTED also has been associated with MRSA isolates exhibiting a clonal pattern with TSST-1 and SEC production.[147]

The fourth most common pattern of toxin production is that of SEB alone. In one study, strains producing SEB alone accounted for 38 percent of all nonmenstrual TSS isolates.[177,266] This prevalence is significantly higher than that for isolates from non-TSS *S. aureus* infections (15%) or asymptomatic carriers (13%). SEB never is co-expressed with TSST-I. Even though all TSST-I–positive isolates contain the SEB genetic determinant, none produces SEB. SEB is produced only by isolates that have the SEB gene and no TSST-I gene. Given that production of both toxins is mutually exclusive and both genes are located close together on the chromosome, researchers have suggested that the TSST-I genetic determinant may have a preferred site of insertion within the SEB genetic element. Because the TSST-I gene is associated with a variable genetic element and such mobile genetic elements are known to be capable of gene disruption, the gene possibly was inserted within the SEB gene or in a position that interferes with its transcription.[83]

A TSS isolate producing TSST-I along with two other enterotoxins is the fifth most common combination, and an isolate producing no known toxins is the sixth. The identification of new enterotoxins[251,295] capable of producing TSS-like disease in rabbits may account for isolates previously identified as producing no toxins. Isolates producing a non-SEB enterotoxin alone are the least common.

PREVALENCE OF EXOTOXIN-PRODUCING *STAPHYLOCOCCUS AUREUS* STRAINS AND ANTIBODY TO THE EXOTOXINS

PREVALENCE OF EXOTOXIN-PRODUCING ORGANISMS

TSST-I–positive strains of *S. aureus* have been present since at least 1957, and antibody to TSST-I was as prevalent in the general population in 1960 as it was in 1999.[236,324] Thus, the increase in incidence of TSS from 1980 to 1985 is assumed to have been the result of newly introduced cofactors rather than an increase in the prevalence of TSST-I–positive organisms.

At any given time, *S. aureus* is present in 20 to 40 percent of cultures from the anterior nasal vestibule of adults and in as many as 33 percent of nasal cultures from children.[151] A study of 3012 menstruating women between 13 and 40 years of age in North America from 1998 to 1999 showed that 26 percent were colonized with *S. aureus* in at least one of three body sites (nose, vagina, or anus) and 9 percent were colonized vaginally.[236] In women, the prevalence of *S. aureus* in vaginal cultures is higher during menses than at midcycle.[186,225] Vaginal carriage rates vary from 7 percent in premenarcheal and nonmenstruating women to 33 percent in menstruating women.[236,239] TSST-I–positive *S. aureus* is present in 1 to 5 percent of vaginal cultures in women, 7 percent of nasal cultures in hospitalized patients, and 18 percent of nasal cultures in children. In prospective studies of *S. aureus* isolates from healthy individuals and from specimens received for other purposes, 14 to 39 percent of all isolates produced TSST-I and 7 to 14 percent produced SEB.[85,233,236] Overall, between 1 and 7 percent of healthy individuals at any given time are colonized at a mucosal site with TSST-I–positive *S. aureus*.

Of 60 *S. aureus* isolates from blood cultures of patients who did not have TSS, 28 percent produced TSST-I.[46] Presumably, these patients had circulating antibody to TSST-I that prevented the development of TSS despite *S. aureus* infection. Adults and children with persistent nasal carriage of a TSST-I–positive strain have high levels of antibody to TSST-I.[236,254]

Evidence suggests that a single clone of *S. aureus* causes most cases of TSS.[44,214] Multilocus enzyme electrophoresis has demonstrated that the TSST-I gene *tst*H is distributed widely over the whole spectrum of *S. aureus* genotypes. Of 315 *S. aureus* strains collected from around the world, 88 percent of menstrual TSS strains and 53 percent of nonmenstrual strains were indistinguishable by multilocus enzyme electrophoresis. The same clone also was found in 28 percent of vaginal isolates from asymptomatic women. This remarkable phenomenon may reflect the unique ability of this clone to colonize the urogenital epithelium or the unique capability of this clone to cause disease. Although TSS strains are similar in gene content, indicative of a common ancestor, their considerable heterogeneity indicates that the common ancestor was not recent in evolutionary time.[118] Thus, the TSS outbreak was the result of a change in the host environment and not geographic dissemination of a new "hypervirulent" strain.[118]

Even though TSST-I–positive strains may cluster within families, living units, and hospital settings, the occurrence of TSS clusters is a rare event.[169,212] Probable TSS has developed within 24 hours in a husband and wife[115] and in two mother-daughter pairs. Nosocomial acquisition and transmission of TSST-I–positive organisms have been described.[9,169,212]

PREVALENCE OF ANTIBODY TO EXOTOXINS

The prevalence of antibody to TSST-I in 689 Wisconsin residents was found to be 47 percent at 1 year of age, 58 percent at 5 years, 70 percent at 10 years, 88 percent at 20 years, and 96 percent for ages 30 to 50 during the years 1960 to 1983 (see Fig. 71–2).[315] The presence of transplacentally acquired antibody in more than 90 percent of infants also was demonstrated.[324] A study of 3012 menstruating women between 13 and 40 years of age across North America in 1998 and 1999 found similar results, with 85 percent overall and 81 percent of subjects aged 13 to 18 years having positive antibody to TSST-1.[236] Among carriers of toxigenic *S. aureus*, a significantly lower percentage of black women (89%) than white or Hispanic women (98% and 100%, respectively) had positive antibody titers. Mucosal colonization with TSST-I–positive *S. aureus* strains is assumed to result in antibody formation.[254] Coworkers of a nurse in whom recurrent TSS developed were demonstrated to be colonized by TSST-I–positive strains and to form antibody to TSST-I, but not to acquire TSS during a period of several months.[9] Subclinical and mild, unrecognized disease[48] may result in the formation of antibodies as well.

Acquisition of antibodies to the enterotoxins also is age related. By the time that children reach the age of 10 years, the proportion with antibody titers of 1:100 or higher is 15 percent for SEA, 65 percent for SEB, 30 percent for SEC, 5 percent for SED, and 20 percent for SEE. By 22 years of age, the numbers increase to 55 percent for SEA, 77 percent for SEB, and 98 percent for SEC.[22]

Former studies suggested that the prevalence of antibody varies from one area of the country to another. During 1982, of 1017 serum samples obtained from U.S. Air Force recruits between the ages of 17 and 26 years, 35 percent from the Mountain and Pacific states were serosusceptible to TSST-I versus 3 percent from the south Atlantic states and 5 percent from the east south central states. Because low titers appear to indicate susceptibility, the findings in this study suggest that differences in the incidence of TSS among states and regions were explained in part by differences in host susceptibility.[322] However, the 2005 multicenter study of 3012 women from Ohio, New Jersey, Florida, Arizona, and Manitoba, Canada, found no significant regional differences in rates of *S. aureus* colonization or prevalence of antibody.[236]

Sera randomly selected from 87 control women were seronegative more frequently for antibody to TSST-I (24%) than were those from 66 control men (9%), which led to the suggestion that women may be more susceptible than men to TSS.[259] Patients in whom TSS develops have significantly lower levels of antibody to SEB and SEC, as well as to TSST-I, than the general population does.[22,66]

As noted in the discussion on recurrence, acute-phase sera of patients with TSS uniformly demonstrate absent or low levels of antibody to TSST-I. The antibody response to TSST-I is absent or delayed in both menstrual and nonmenstrual TSS.[233,294]

PHYSICOCHEMICAL AND BIOLOGIC CHARACTERISTICS OF TSST-I

PHYSICOCHEMICAL PROPERTIES

The mature secreted TSST-I protein is a single polypeptide chain with a molecular weight of 22,000 daltons and an isoelectric point of 7.2. It is resistant to proteolytic digestion by trypsin but is hydrolyzed by pepsin at pH 4.5. In sterile solution at neutral pH, it is stable for months. When lyophilized, it is a white powder that easily dissolves in distilled water. No loss of serologic activity of the lyophilized powder occurs for at least a year. TSST-I can be heated to 100°C for longer than an hour without loss of biologic activity.[29]

Purification of TSST-I has yielded diffraction-quality crystals that have led to an understanding of its three-dimensional structure.[29] The molecule is folded into two closely associated domains that create two major grooves, the front and backside grooves. The backside groove is larger and more exposed to the external environment. The crystal structures of all the protein superantigens have striking similarity in the two-domain conformational architecture, even though the primary protein segments are different.[189]

REGULATION OF PRODUCTION

S. aureus is highly adaptable and able to live and grow in extremes of temperature, pH, and oxygen concentration. TSST-I production, however, is controlled tightly. TSST-I is not produced in unfavorable conditions, including an anaerobic environment, pH values lower than 6.0 and greater than 8.0, concentrations of clindamycin below the MIC of the organism, glucose concentrations greater than 3 percent, and temperatures lower than 37°C or greater than 40°C.[22,29,335] Conditions and factors that enhance production of TSST-I include uniform aeration of medium through shaking or a roller apparatus, complex medium containing animal protein and low glucose concentrations, a neutral pH, incubation in 5 percent carbon dioxide (under some in vitro conditions), and temperatures of 37°C to 40°C. The role of magnesium is unclear.[88] Twice as much toxin is produced at 40°C as at 37°C. The addition of blood to media does not increase production of TSST-I reliably. Depending on in vitro growth conditions, most strains of TSST-I–negative *S. aureus* produce 3 μg/mL of TSST-I, but some may produce up to 30 μg/mL.

Under optimal in vitro growth conditions, TSST-I production lags behind but parallels bacterial growth. Like other *S. aureus* exotoxins, TSST-I is made primarily during the postexponential phase of growth, when nutrients are scarce and cell density is great.[85] Levels of TSST-I remain stable throughout the stationary phase, even after the organisms begin to die. Under less than optimal conditions, synchronous production of TSST-I and growth of *S. aureus* do not occur. For example, bacterial growth may be reduced only twofold in an anaerobic environment, whereas TSST-I production is inhibited. Likewise, clindamycin at concentrations below the MIC for the organism will inhibit the production of toxins without altering growth.[269]

Most strains of *S. aureus* do not have the genes for TSST-I or the enterotoxins. TSST-I thus is not necessary for bacterial homeostasis, and its production is a variable genetic trait.

The gene *tst*H is encoded by a transposon-like mobile genetic element.[57,83,148,170] The chromosomal fragment with the structural gene for production of TSST-I is a 10.6-kilobase (kb) unit that has been cloned in *E. coli. tst*H has been sequenced and encodes a 234–amino acid protein that is converted by the removal of a signal peptide of 40 amino acids to the mature exotoxin of 194 amino acids.[29,85,170] *tst*H has been inserted in the chromosome to disrupt both the tryptophan synthetase B and SEB genes, thereby preventing the production of both proteins.[57,83]

Production of TSST-I and other post–exponential-phase virulence factors is regulated by three separate genetic loci: the accessory gene regulator (*agr*), the staphylococcal accessory regulator (*sar*), and the extracellular protein regulator (*xpr*).[12,29,85] All three regulators affect gene expression primarily at the level of transcription. During the late log phase of bacterial growth, they activate the expression of TSST-I, alpha- and gamma-hemolysins, serine protease, and nuclease and down-regulate the expression of cell wall–associated proteins, fibronectin-binding protein, protein A, and coagulase. Beta-hemolysin, SEB, SEC, and exfoliative toxin A are regulated less tightly by *agr* than TSST-I is. SEA appears to be independent of *agr* in some strains. This complex regulation of exoprotein synthesis probably is the result of a complex interaction between environmental factors and gene products.[29,85] These regulatory functions explain why the production of TSST-I is stimulated under some conditions without SEA or SEC stimulation.[335]

Glyceryl monolaurate is a mild surfactant and emulsifier commonly used in the food and cosmetic industries. It is capable of inhibiting the production of staphylococcal and streptococcal exotoxins at concentrations subinhibitory to growth.[40,245,267] As a lipophilic compound, the mechanism of action appears to be insertion into the cell membrane with resulting interruption of signal transduction. Other surfactants used in the tampon industry have been found to both inhibit and enhance[268] the production of TSST-I in vitro.

KINETICS OF DISTRIBUTION

Detecting TSST-I in body fluids is difficult. In humans, nanogram quantities have been detected by radioimmunoassay in the breast milk of a woman with TSS,[149,323] in serum early during illness in two of four patients,[195] in urine, and in vaginal washings in a small number of patients.[195] By means of the rabbit subcutaneous Wiffle ball abscess model, TSST-I can be detected first in abscess fluid 4 hours after *S. aureus* has been inoculated into the Wiffle ball and in urine 48 hours after inoculation.[195]

For further examination of in vivo target tissues for TSST-I activity, purified TSST-I radiolabeled with iodine 139 has been injected intravenously into rabbits. Measurement of plasma clearance demonstrated a half-life of 1.5 hours. Within 15 minutes of injection, TSST-I was concentrated fourfold in blood cells in comparison to plasma. Toxin persisted in the cellular compartment, and plasma concentrations fell. After 3 hours, most of the radiolabel was found in the spleen.

TSST-I, SEA, and SEB can cross epithelial membranes intact in a fully functional form.[134] In a cellular model of the blood-brain barrier, TSST-1 showed slow bidirectional movement consistent with restricted paracellular diffusion.[18]

CELLULAR INTERACTIONS

TSST-I has been shown to inhibit systolic function in isolated rabbit atria.[224] It also can bind directly to human and porcine endothelial cells and is cytotoxic to porcine endothelial cells because it permits leakage across endothelial cell monolayers.[173,176] However, concentrations of TSST-I needed to induce these and other diverse cytotoxic changes in vitro are higher than the usual tissue and serum levels. Interactions of TSST-I and the enterotoxins with T lymphocytes and antigen-processing cells are described in the next section.

BIOLOGIC FUNCTIONS

Animal Models

Much information regarding pathogenesis has been obtained from both the subcutaneous Wiffle ball and the vaginal tampon rabbit models and a primate model.[81] Rabbits, primates, and other species have been examined for sensitivity to TSST-I or TSS-associated strains of *S. aureus*.[232] Rabbits and baboons exhibit clinical and laboratory changes most consistent with the human syndrome, including pyrogenicity and lethality.* The signs and symptoms observed in these animals after the intravenous injection of purified TSST-I include skin erythema, conjunctivitis, diarrhea, lethargy, tachypnea, respiratory distress, central nervous system changes, and increased capillary permeability, as demonstrated by the skin bluing technique. A variety of laboratory abnormalities consistent with those described in human TSS have been reported for these models.

Immunoregulatory Activities

The absence of in vitro cytotoxicity of TSST-I[22,232] despite potent in vivo biologic effects has suggested an important role for endogenous mediators in TSS. The ability of SEB to induce dramatic T-cell proliferation was recognized a decade ago.[160,166,185] Subsequent work has shown it to be a feature of other bacterial exotoxins, including TSST-I, the staphylococcal enterotoxins, the streptococcal pyrogenic exotoxins A and C, a new streptococcal superantigen, and a streptococcal M surface protein.[166] Since the late 1980s, activation of T cells by these bacterial components or products has become an area of intense interest. The term *superantigen* was coined in 1989 to describe antigens that at concentrations lower than those of conventional antigens (picomolar concentrations) can stimulate proliferation of a large percentage of T cells bearing a TCR beta-chain variable (V_β) sequence or sequences specific for each superantigen. Such activation and proliferation of T cells result in profound alterations in immune system homeostasis by inducing the release of large quantities of monokines (IL-1, TNF-α) and lymphokines (IL-2, TNF-β).[166,280,341]

T cells are activated to produce lymphokines as a result of TCR-antigen binding and activation of signal transduction.[45,94,287] Antigens can bind to the TCR in one of two forms: as conventional antigens or as superantigens. Conventional antigens enter antigen-processing cells by endocytosis. They are broken into small peptides in the lysosomal compartments of the antigen-processing cell and targeted to small vesicles, where they form complexes with one of the allele-restricted MHC class II molecules (HLA-DQ, HLA-DP, and HLA-DR).[280] The complex then is transported to the cell surface, where it is bound in the groove on the heavy chain formed by the alpha and beta chains of the class II molecule. Certain amino acids in residues at critical points

---

*See references 31, 32, 81, 82, 196, 198, 200, 234, 247, 270, 276.

in the peptide's sequence anchor the peptides in the groove, and this interaction is moderately specific for each different allelic form of the MHC molecule.[280] This complex of peptide and MHC molecule of the same allelic type as the T cell is recognized by the TCR.

The TCR is composed of both alpha and beta glycoprotein chains, each of which is composed of variable (V) and joining (J) segments. The beta chain has an additional diversity (D) segment. As many as 50 V_β and 32 V_α segments are present on human T cells. The $V_{\alpha\beta\alpha\beta\beta}$ segments each are encoded by different genes that undergo gene rearrangement to give more than 10,000 possible combinations to recognize conventional antigenic peptides presented by antigen-processing cells.[16,280] Conventional antigens presented as peptides must be recognized by a specific combination of these elements. Thus, one peptide will activate only 1 in 10^4 to 10^6 T cells, and only CD4+ T cells respond to conventional antigens.

In contrast, superantigens are presented to T lymphocytes in a very different fashion. They bind first as intact proteins (small fragments are inactive) to most allelic forms of MHC class II molecules in an unrestricted fashion at a site outside the peptide-binding groove. They then react with the TCR only through the V_β element or elements specific for that molecule and will react with all T cells carrying that V_β element.[145] Because only 25 to 50 major families of V_β genes exist in humans, each superantigen can interact with 5 to 20 percent of resting T cells, depending on the frequency of T cells expressing that V_β family in each individual's repertoire. Both CD4+ and CD8+ T cells are activated. Features unique to the presentation of superantigens to the TCR V_β receptor thus include the requirement for initial binding of superantigen to the MHC class II molecule (even if unrestricted and not self) outside the antigen-presenting groove and the requirement for an intact superantigen protein.

Once the T cell has recognized the superantigen,[132] both antigen-processing cell and T-cell activation by signal transduction[45] results in release of cytokine by the antigen-processing cell (IL-1, TNF-α) and the lymphocyte (IL-2, TNF-β). In mice and possibly also in humans, the initial T-cell activation occurs in lymph nodes.[205] Within hours of T-cell activation by superantigens, cytokines are detected in vitro and in serum in vivo.

TSST-I binds only to the $V_\beta 2$ element.[256] In humans with TSS caused by TSST-I–secreting *S. aureus*, within 10 to 14 days 30 to 70 percent of the circulating T-cell population will be T cells bearing the $V_\beta 2$ element.[53,54,187] The number of circulating $V_\beta 2$ T cells does not return to normal for several months. In contrast, patients with TSS caused by *S. pyogenes* have a consistent pattern of depletion of certain V_β T-cell types after T-cell activation.[166,220,327] In mice, such depletion is thought to be the result of programmed cell death (apoptosis).[203,204]

Thus, activation of T cells by superantigens may result in massive cytokine release with subsequent selected V_β T-cell expansion, T-cell deletion, or apoptosis, depending on the superantigen and species. The fact that superantigens bind only to selected and specific V_β elements distinguishes them from the nondiscriminating mitogens.

Activation of monocytes and lymphocytes by superantigens involves signal transduction. Activation of both src protein tyrosine kinases and protein kinase C occurs in a manner common to that of other immunoglobulin supergene family members. MHC class II cells also are expressed on beta, endothelial, and dendritic cells. In some instances, superantigens may activate these cells uniquely.

Convincing evidence from the mouse model supports a central role for T-lymphocyte activation in superantigen-mediated disease. Mice that have received cyclosporine to block T-cell activation and lymphokine production or mice with severe combined immunodeficiency disease are protected against SEB-induced lethal shock. Repopulation with T cells results in susceptibility to SEB. The same mice are not protected against endotoxin-induced shock because lipopolysaccharide activates only monocytes.[203-205]

Mononuclear production of IL-1 and TNF-α is central to the shock induced by endotoxin. Production of these two cytokines in addition to production of the lymphokines IL-2, IFN-α, and TNF-β may explain the enhanced severity of superantigen-associated TSS.[30,132,166] These powerful effects on the immune system may account for the tenacity of shock in otherwise healthy individuals. If more than one superantigen is produced by an organism (e.g., TSST-I plus one or more enterotoxins), different V_β specificities would result in an even greater number of T cells being activated, with the potential for development of disease with enhanced severity and mortality.

Once superantigens have resulted in monokine and lymphokine release, the subsequent pathophysiologic events appear to be related to the many and complex interactions of these cytokines,[30,136,340] with the ultimate result being profound endothelial damage. TNF-α and TNF-β and the complex interaction of cytokines, leukotrienes, prostaglandins, adhesion molecules, nitric oxide, platelet-activating factor, complement components, neutrophils, platelets, and endothelium-derived factors appear to be responsible for the extensive endothelial damage and resulting capillary fluid leakage and the decrease in peripheral vascular resistance.[30,136,261,340] In a different setting of antineoplastic therapy, high doses of IL-2 and lymphokine-activated killer cells induce the capillary leak syndrome, which is characterized by rapid weight gain, anasarca, pulmonary edema, hypoalbuminemia, and multiple organ dysfunction in humans.[64,165]

Endotoxin Enhancement

A striking property of TSST-I is its marked ability to enhance the susceptibility of some animals to lethal endotoxic shock.[29,265,270] Intravenous administration of TSST-I to rabbits at less than $1/2$ the median lethal dose (LD$_{50}$) followed 2 hours later by endotoxin at less than $1/500$ the LD$_{50}$ results in 50 to 100 percent mortality, a 10,000-fold enhancement. In vitro, endotoxin enhances IL-1 production by TSST-I–stimulated monocytes.[20] Whether enhanced endotoxin susceptibility plays any role in human disease is not clear.[55]

STRUCTURE-FUNCTION RELATIONSHIPS

Effort to understand the molecular actions of TSST-I has focused on separating regions that interact with the TCR from those required for lethality.[29,31,32,213] Through the use of TSST-I variants (TSST-ovine and TSST-bovine) and TSST-I molecules with single–amino acid mutations, the areas responsible for binding of TSST-I to both the TCR and the macrophage class II MHC molecule have been defined.[29] In animal models, lethality, induction of fever, and endotoxin susceptibility do not depend on T-cell proliferation as measured by superantigenic activity but must involve interaction of toxin with other host-cell receptors in the body.[29]

Most secreted bacterial superantigens are small, compact globular proteins of 20 to 30 kd.[29] They are protease-, heat-, and acid-resistant and share immunologic, biologic, and functional properties. However, they do not share sequence homology. Although they do not share obvious structural features that would predict their superantigen properties, they may share a common conformational structure.[166] The secreted exotoxins can be divided into two groups based on their amino acid sequence homology. In group 1, SEA, SED, and SEE share 54 to 90 percent homology. In group 2, streptococcal pyrogenic exotoxin A, SEB, and SEC-1, SEC-2, and SEC-3 share 46 to 68 percent homology. In group 3, TSST-I, the exfoliative toxins, and streptococcal pyrogenic exotoxin show no significant homology to each other or to any of the members of group 1 or 2. However, all the secreted superantigens may share a three-dimensional conformation that allows them to interact simultaneously with two different receptors on two different cell types.[29,166]

The structure and binding sites of SEB to the MHC class II molecule have been determined by crystallographic conformation. Two different MHC class II binding sites for SEB exist. The amino-terminal domain forms most of the contact, but residues at the carboxy-terminal domain also contact the MHC class II molecule, as well as the TCR. Although TSST-I is very similar to SEB on the basis of their crystallographic structure, the two proteins do not compete with each other for the same MHC class II HLA-DR sites. Likewise, SEA and SEE have greater than 90 percent amino acid sequence homology but quite distinct patterns of V_β specificity. TSST-I and the exfoliative toxins A and B are unrelated structurally but have the same $V_\beta2$ specificity.[166,185]

REFERENCES

1. Abdul-Karim, F. W., Lederman, M. M., Carter, J. R., et al.: Toxic shock syndrome: Clinicopathologic findings in a fatal case. Hum. Pathol. 12:16-22, 1981.
2. Abram, A. C., Bellian, K. T., Giles, W. J., et al.: Toxic shock syndrome after functional endonasal sinus surgery: An all or none phenomenon? Laryngoscope 104:927-931, 1994.
3. Allen, S. T., Liland, J. B., Nichols, C. G., et al.: Toxic shock syndrome associated with use of latex nasal packing. Arch. Intern. Med. 150:2587-2588, 1990.
4. Alsoub, H.: Toxic shock syndrome associated with pyomyositis. Postgrad. Med. J. 70:309-312, 1994.
5. Andrews, M. M., Giacobbe, K. D., and Parsonnet, J.: Induction of toxic shock syndrome toxin-1 (TSST-1) and beta-lactamase by subinhibitory concentrations of beta-lactam antibiotics. Abstract N-IN-0011. Presented at Biomedicine '96, May 3-6, 1996, Washington, DC.
6. Andrews, M. M., Parent, E. M., Barry, M., and Parsonnet, J.: Recurrent nonmenstrual toxic shock syndrome: Clinical manifestations, diagnosis, and treatment. Clin. Infect. Dis. 32:1470-1479, 2001.
7. Aranow, H., Jr., and Wood, W. B., Jr.: Staphylococcic infection simulating scarlet fever. J. A. M. A. 119:1491-1495, 1942.
8. Arend, S. M., Steenmeyer, A. V., Mosmans, P. C. M., et al.: Postoperative cauda syndrome caused by *Staphylococcus aureus*. Infection 21:248-250, 1993.
9. Arnow, P. M., Chou, T., Weil, D., et al.: Spread of a toxic-shock syndrome–associated strain of *Staphylococcus aureus* and measurement of antibodies to staphylococcal enterotoxin F. J. Infect. Dis. 149:103-107, 1984.
10. Bach, M. C.: Dermatologic signs in toxic shock syndrome: Clues to diagnosis. J. Am. Acad. Dermatol. 8:343-347, 1983.
11. Bacha, E. A., Sheridan, R. L., Donohue, G. A., et al.: Staphylococcal toxic shock syndrome in a paediatric burn unit. Burns 20:499-502, 1994.
12. Balaban, N., and Novick, R. P.: Autocrine regulation of toxin synthesis by *Staphylococcus aureus*. Proc. Natl. Acad. Sci. U. S. A. 92:1619-1623, 1995.
13. Bannister, B., and Platts, A. J.: Some cardiological findings in toxic shock syndrome. J. Infect. 3:293-294, 1981.
14. Baracos, V., Rodemann, P., Dinarello, C. A., et al.: Stimulation of muscle protein degradation and prostaglandin E₂ release by leucocytic pyrogen (interleukin-1). N. Engl. J. Med. 308:553-558, 1983.
15. Barrett, J. A., and Graham, D. R.: TSS presenting as encephalopathy. J. Infect. 12:276, 1986.
16. Barry, W., Hudgins, L., Donta, S. T., et al.: Intravenous immunoglobulin therapy for toxic-shock syndrome. J. A. M. A. 267:3315-3317, 1992.
17. Bartlett, P., Reingold, A. L., Graham, D. R., et al.: Toxic shock syndrome associated with surgical wound infections. J. A. M. A. 247:1448-1450, 1982.
18. Batisson, M., Strazielle, N., Hejmadi, M., et al.: Toxic shock syndrome toxin-1 challenges the neuroprotective functions of the choroidal epithelium and induces neurotoxicity. J. Infect. Dis. 194:341-349, 2006.
19. Becker, K., Roth, R., and Peters, G.: Rapid and specific detection of toxigenic *Staphylococcus aureus*: Use of two multiplex PCR enzyme immunoassays for amplification and hybridization of staphylococcal enterotoxin genes, exfoliative toxin genes, and toxic shock syndrome toxin 1 gene. J. Clin. Microbiol. 36:2548-2553, 1998.
20. Beezhold, D. H., Best, G. K., Bonventre, P. F., et al.: Endotoxin enhancement of TSST-1–induced secretion of interleukin-1 by murine macrophages. Rev. Infect. Dis. 11(Suppl.):289-293, 1989.
21. Beisel, W. R.: Pathophysiology of staphylococcal enterotoxin, type B, (SEB) toxemia after the intravenous administration to monkeys. Toxicon 10:433, 1972.
22. Bergdoll, M. S., and Chesney, P. J.: Toxic-Shock Syndrome. Boca Raton, FL, CRC Press, 1991.
23. Bergdoll, M. S., Crass, B. A., Reiser, R. F., et al.: A new staphylococcal enterotoxin, enterotoxin F, associated with toxic-shock syndrome *Staphylococcus aureus* isolates. Lancet 1:1017-1021, 1981.
24. Berkley, S. F., Hightower, A. W., Broome, C. W., et al.: The relationship of tampon characteristics to menstrual toxic-shock syndrome. J. A. M. A. 258:917-920, 1987.
25. Berman, A. C., and Boly, L. R.: Cisplatin therapy–associated recurrent toxic shock syndrome. West. J. Med. 155:415-416, 1991.
26. Bernstein, G. M., Crollick, J. S., and Hassett, J. M., Jr.: Post febrile telogen effluvium in critically ill patients. Crit. Care Med. 16:98-99, 1988.
27. Black, D. A., and Maw, D. S.: Toxic shock syndrome presenting as cerebral infarct. Corres. J. Neurol. Neurosurg. Psychiatry 47:568, 1984.
28. Blair, J. D., Livingston, D. G., and Vongsnichakul, R.: Tampon-related toxic-shock syndrome: Histopathologic and clinical findings in a fatal case. Am. J. Clin. Pathol. 78:372-376, 1982.
29. Bohach, G. A., Dinges, M. M., Mitchell, D. T., et al.: Staphylococcal exotoxins. In Leung, D. Y. M., Huber, B. T., and Schlievert, P. M. (eds.): Superantigens: Molecular Biology, Immunology and Relevance to Human Disease. New York, Marcel Dekker, 1997.
30. Bone, R. C.: The pathogenesis of sepsis. Ann. Intern. Med. 115:457-469, 1991.
31. Bonventre, P. F., Heeg, H., Cullen, C., et al.: Toxicity of recombinant toxic shock syndrome toxin 1 and mutant toxins produced by *Staphylococcus aureus* in a rabbit infection model of toxic shock syndrome. Infect. Immun. 61:793-799, 1993.
32. Bonventre, P. F., Heeg, H., Edwards, C. K., III, et al.: A mutation at histidine residue 135 of toxic shock syndrome toxin yields an immunogenic protein with minimal toxicity. Infect. Immun. 63:509-515, 1995.
33. Bonventre, P. F., Linnemann, C., Weckback, L. S., et al.: Antibody responses to toxic-shock-syndrome (TSS) toxin by patients with TSS and by healthy staphylococcal carriers. J. Infect. Dis. 150:662-666, 1984.
34. Bonventre, P. F., Thompson, M. R., Adinolfi, L. E., et al.: Neutralization of TSST-1 by monoclonal antibodies in vitro and in vivo. Infect. Immun. 50:135, 1987.
35. Breda, S. D., Jacobs, J. B., Lebowitz, A. S., et al.: Toxic shock syndrome in nasal surgery: A physiochemical and microbiologic evaluation of Merocel and NuGauze nasal packing. Laryngoscope 97:1388, 1987.
36. Brody, H., and Smith, L. W.: The visceral pathology in scarlet fever and related *Streptococcus* infections. Am. J. Pathol. 12:373, 1936.
37. Brook, M. G., and Bannister, B. A.: Staphylococcal enterotoxins in scarlet fever complicating chicken pox. Postgrad. Med. J. 67:1013-1014, 1991.
38. Broome, C. V.: Epidemiology of TSS in the United States: Overview. Rev. Infect. Dis. 11(Suppl.):14-21, 1989.
39. Brown, E. J.: The molecular basis of streptococcal toxic shock syndrome. N. Engl. J. Med. 350:2093-2094, 2004.
40. Brown-Skrobot, S. K., Irving, M. M., and Wojnarowicz, L.: Tampon additives and toxic shock syndrome toxin-1 (TSST-1) production. Abstract B18. Presented at the 91st General Meeting of the American Society of Microbiology, 1991, Chicago, p. 28.
41. Burns, J. R., and Menpace, F. J.: Acute reversible cardiomyopathy complicating toxic shock syndrome. Arch. Intern. Med. 142:1032-1034, 1982.
42. Cavanah, D. K., and Ballas, Z. K.: Pseudoephedrine reaction presenting as recurrent toxic shock syndrome. Ann. Intern. Med. 119:302-303, 1993.
43. Cederna, J. P.: Toxic shock syndrome after transverse rectus abdominis musculocutaneous flap breast reconstruction. Ann. Plast. Surg. 34:73-75, 1995.
44. Chang, A. H., Musser, J. M., and Chow, A. W.: A single clone which produces both TSST-1 and SEA causes the majority of menstrual toxic shock syndrome. Abstract. Clin. Res. 39:36, 1991.
45. Chatila, T., and Geha, R. S.: Signal transduction by microbial superantigens via MHC class II molecules. Immunol. Rev. 131:43-59, 1993.
46. Chesney, P. J., Crass, B. A., Polyak, M. B., et al.: Toxic-shock syndrome: Management and long-term sequelae. Ann. Intern. Med. 96:847-851, 1982.
47. Chesney, P. J., Davis, J. P., Purdy, W. K., et al.: The clinical manifestations of toxic shock syndrome. J. A. M. A. 246:741-748, 1981.
48. Chesney, P. J., Slama, S. L., Hawkins, R. L., et al.: Outpatient diagnosis and management of toxic-shock syndrome. N. Engl. J. Med. 304:1426, 1981.
49. Chesney, P. J., and Zimmerman, J. J.: Hypoferrinemia in toxic-shock syndrome (TSS). Abstract. Pediatr. Res. 20:306, 1986.
50. Chesney, R. W., Chesney, P. J., Davis, J. P., et al.: Renal manifestations of the staphylococcal toxic-shock syndrome. Am. J. Med. 71:583-588, 1981.
51. Chesney, R. W., McCarren, D. M., Haddad, J. G., et al.: Pathogenic mechanisms of the hypocalcemia of the staphylococcal toxic-shock syndrome. J. Lab. Clin. Med. 101:576-585, 1983.
52. Childs, C., Edwards-Jones, V., Healthcote, D. M., et al.: Patterns of *Staphylococcal aureus* colonization, toxin production, immunity and illness in burned children. Burns 20:514-521, 1994.
53. Choi, Y., Kotzin, B., Herron, L., et al.: Interaction of *Staphylococcus aureus* toxin "superantigens" with human T cells. Proc. Natl. Acad. Sci. U. S. A. 86:8941-8945, 1989.
54. Choi, Y., Lafferty, J. A., Clements, J. R., et al.: Selective expansion of T cells expressing V beta 2 in toxic-shock syndrome. J. Exp. Med. 172:981-984, 1990.

55. Chow, A.: Microbiology of toxic shock syndrome: Overview. Rev. Infect. Dis. 1:55-60, 1989.
56. Chow, A. W., Wong, C. K., MacFarlane, A. M., et al.: Toxic shock syndrome: Clinical and laboratory findings in 30 patients. Can. Med. Assoc. J. 130:425-430, 1984.
57. Chu, M. C., Kreiswirth, B. N., Pattee, P. A., et al.: Association of toxic shock toxin-1 determinant with a heterologous insertion at multiple loci in the Staphylococcus aureus chromosome. Infect. Immun. 56:2702-2708, 1988.
58. Clostridium sordellii toxic shock syndrome after medical abortion with mifepristone and intravaginal misoprostol—United States and Canada, 2001-2005. M. M. W. R. Morb. Mortal. Wkly. Rep. 54(20):724, 2005.
59. Cohen, K. R., Emmons, K. M., and Goldstein, M. F.: Naloxone treatment of toxic shock syndrome. Arch. Intern. Med. 143:1072, 1983.
60. Cole, R. P., and Shakespeare, P. G.: Toxic-shock syndrome in scalded children. Burns 16:221-224, 1990.
61. Cone, L. A., Woodward, D. R., Byrd, R. G., et al.: A recalcitrant, erythematous, desquamating disorder associated with toxin-producing staphylococci in patients with AIDS. J. Infect. Dis. 165:638-643, 1992.
62. Cone, L. A., Woodard, D. R., Schlievert, P. M., et al.: Clinical and bacteriologic observations of a toxic-shock–like syndrome due to Streptococcus pyogenes. N. Engl. J. Med. 317:146-149, 1987.
63. Conway, E. E., Jr., Haber, R. S., Gumprecht, J., et al.: Toxic shock syndrome following influenza A in a child. Crit. Care Med. 19:123-125, 1991.
64. Cotran, R. S., Proba, J. S., Gimbrone, M. A., et al.: Endothelial activation during IL-2 immunotherapy: A possible mechanism for the vascular leak syndrome. J. Immunol. 139:1883, 1987.
65. Cowan, R. K., and Martens, M. G.: Toxic shock syndrome mimicking pelvic inflammatory disease presumably resulting from tattoo. South. Med. J. 86:1427-1431, 1993.
66. Crass, B. A., and Bergdoll, M. S.: Toxin involvement in toxic shock syndrome. J. Infect. Dis. 153:918-926, 1986.
67. Crews, J. R., Harrison, J. K, Corey, G. R., et al.: Stunned myocardium in the toxic shock syndrome. Ann. Intern. Med. 117:912-913, 1992.
68. Crowder, W. E., and Shannon, F. C.: Colposcopic diagnosis of vaginal ulcerations in toxic-shock syndrome. Obstet. Gynecol. 61:505-535, 1983.
69. Crowther, M. A., and Ralph, E. D.: Menstrual toxic shock syndrome complicated by persistent bacteremia: Case report and review. Clin. Infect. Dis. 16:288-289, 1993.
70. Danielson, R. W.: Vaginal ulcers caused by tampons. Am. J. Obstet. Gynecol. 146:547-549, 1983.
71. Dann, E. J., Weinberger, M., Gillis, S., et al.: Bacterial laryngotracheitis associated with toxic-shock syndrome in an adult. Clin. Infect. Dis. 18:437-439, 1994.
72. Darenberg, J., Ihendyane, N., Sjolin, J., et al.: Intravenous immunoglobulin G therapy in streptococcal toxic shock syndrome: A European randomized, double-blind, placebo-controlled trial. Clin. Infect. Dis. 37:333-340, 2003.
73. Dart, R. C., and Levitt, M. A.: Toxic-shock syndrome associated with the use of the vaginal contraceptive sponge. J. A. M. A. 253:1877, 1985.
74. Davidson, A. C., Creach, M., and Cameron, I. R.: Staphylococcal pneumonia, pneumatoceles, and the toxic shock syndrome. Thorax 45:639-640, 1990.
75. Davis, J. P., Chesney, P. J., Wand, P. J., et al.: Toxic shock syndrome: Epidemiologic features, recurrences, risk factors and prevention. N. Engl. J. Med. 303:1429-1435, 1980.
76. Davis, J. P., Osterholm, M. T., Helms, C. M., et al.: Tristate toxic-shock syndrome study. II. Clinical and laboratory findings. J. Infect. Dis. 145:441-448, 1982.
77. Davis, J. P., and Vergeront, J. M.: The effect of publicity on the reporting of toxic-shock syndrome in Wisconsin. J. Infect. Dis. 145:449-457, 1982.
78. Davis, J. P., and Vergeront, J. M.: A review of toxic shock syndrome surveillance in Wisconsin: The effect of media publicity and laboratory services on reporting of illness. Ann. Intern. Med. 96:883-886, 1982.
79. Davis, J. P., Vergeront, J. V., Amsterdam, L. E., et al.: Long-term effects of TSS in women: Sequelae, subsequent pregnancy, menstrual history, and long-term trends in catamenial product use. Rev. Infect. Dis. 11(Suppl.):50, 1989.
80. Davis, J. P., Vergeront, J. M., and Chesney, P. J.: Possible host-defense mechanisms in toxic shock syndrome. Ann. Intern. Med. 96:986-991, 1982.
81. de Azavedo, J. C. S.: Animal models for toxic-shock syndrome: Overview. Rev. Infect. Dis. 11(Suppl.):205-209, 1989.
82. de Azavedo, J. C. S., Foster, T. J., Hartigan, J., et al.: Expression of the cloned toxic shock syndrome toxin 1 gene (tst) in vivo with a rabbit uterine model. Infect. Immun. 50:304-309, 1985.
83. De Boer, M. L., and Chow, A. W.: Toxic shock syndrome toxin 1–producing Staphylococcus aureus isolates contain the staphylococcal enterotoxin B genetic element but do not express staphylococcal enterotoxin B. J. Infect. Dis. 170:818-827, 1994.
84. Deetz, T. R., Reves, R., and Septimus, E.: Secondary rash in toxic shock syndrome. N. Engl. J. Med. 304:174, 1981.
85. Deresiewicz, R. L.: Staphylococcal toxic shock syndrome. In Leung, D. Y. M., Huber, B. T., and Schlievert P. M. (eds.): Superantigens: Molecular Biology, Immunology and Relevance to Human Disease. New York, Marcel Dekker, 1997.
86. DeVries, A., Leshser, L., and Lynfield, R.: Staphylococcal toxic shock syndrome, Minnesota, 2000-2003. Abstract 379. Presented at 44th Annual Meeting of the Infectious Diseases Society of America, San Francisco, October 2006, p. 118.
87. deVries, N., and Vander Baan, S.: Toxic shock syndrome after nasal surgery: Is prevention possible? A case report and review of literature. Rhinology 27:125-128, 1989.
88. Dickgiesser, N., and Wallach, U.: Toxic shock syndrome toxin-1 (TSST-1): Influence of its production by subinhibitory antibiotic concentrations. Infection 15:351-353, 1987.
89. Diep, B. A., Carleton, H. A., Chang, R. F., et al.: Roles of 34 virulence genes in the evolution of hospital- and community-associated strains of methicillin-resistant Staphylococcus aureus. J. Infect. Dis. 193:1495-1503, 2006.
90. Donawa, M. E., Schmid, G. R., and Osterholm, M. T.: Toxic shock syndrome: Chronology of state and federal epidemiologic studies and regulatory decision-making. Public Health Rep. 99:342-350, 1984.
91. Dondorp, A. M., Veenstra, J., vanderPoll, T., et al.: Activation of the cytokine network in a patient with AIDS and the recalcitrant erythematous desquamating disorder. Clin. Infect. Dis. 18:942-945, 1994.
92. Donnelly, B. W., McMillan, J. A., and Weiner, L. B.: Bacterial tracheitis: Report of eight new cases and a review. Rev. Infect. Dis. 12:729-735, 1990.
93. Dornan, K. J., Thompson, D. M., Conn, A. R., et al.: Toxic shock syndrome in the postoperative patient. Surg. Gynecol. Obstet. 154:65-68, 1982.
94. Driessen, C., Hirv, K., Kirchner, H., et al.: Zinc regulates cytokine induction by superantigens and lipopolysaccharide. Immunology 84:272-277, 1995.
95. Dunnet, U. B., and Schallibaum, E. M.: Scarlet fever–like illness due to staphylococcal infection. Lancet 2:1227-1229, 1960.
96. Durand, G., Bes, M., Meugnier, H., et al.: Detection of new methicillin-resistant Staphylococcus aureus clones containing the toxic shock syndrome toxin 1 gene responsible for hospital- and community-acquired infections in France. J. Clin. Microbiol. 44:847-853, 2006.
97. Eagle, H.: Experimental approach to the problem of treatment failure with penicillin. I. Group A streptococcal infection in mice. Am. J. Med. 13:389-399, 1952.
98. Edwards-Jones, V., Dawson, M. M., and Childs, C.: A survey into toxic shock syndrome (TSS) in UK burn units. Burns 26:323-333, 2000.
99. Edwards-Jones, V., and Foster, H. A.: The effect of topical antimicrobial agents on the production of toxic shock syndrome toxin-1. J. Med. Microbiol. 41:408-413, 1994.
100. Ejlertsen, T., and Porsborg, P. A.: Toxic-shock syndrome related to simultaneous Staphylococcus aureus epiglottic abscess and group A streptococcal pharyngitis with bacteremia. A. P. M. I. S. 102:956-959, 1994.
101. Elbaum, D. J., Wood, C., Abuabara, F., et al.: Bullae in a patient with toxic shock syndrome. J. Am. Acad. Dermatol. 10:267-272, 1984.
102. Elsberry, D. D., Rhoda, D. A., and Beisel, W. R.: Hemodynamics of staphylococcal B enterotoxemia and other types of shock in monkeys. J. Appl. Physiol. 27:164, 1969.
103. Eriksson, B., Anderson, J., Bergholm, A. M., et al.: Invasive group A streptococcal infections: T1M1 isolates expressing pyrogenic exotoxins A and B in combination with selective lack of toxin-neutralizing antibodies are associated with increased risk of streptococcal toxic shock syndrome. J. Infect. Dis. 180:410-418, 1999.
104. Espersen, F., Baek, L., Kjaeldgaard, P., et al.: Detection of staphylococcal toxic shock syndrome toxin 1 by a latex agglutination kit. Scand. J. Infect. Dis. 20:449-450, 1988.
105. Faich, G., Pearson, K., and Fleming, D., et al.: Toxic-shock syndrome and the vaginal contraceptive sponge. J. A. M. A. 255:216-218, 1986.
106. Farley, D. E., Katz, V. L., and Dotters, D. J.: Toxic shock syndrome associated with vulvar necrotizing fasciitis. Obstet. Gynecol. 82:660-662, 1993.
107. Fast, D. J., Schlievert, P. M., and Nelson, R. D.: Nonpurulent response to toxic shock syndrome toxin-1–producing Staphylococcus aureus. J. Immunol. 140:949-953, 1988.
108. Feldman, C. A.: Staphylococcal scarlet fever. N. Engl. J. Med. 267:877-888, 1962.
109. Ferguson, M. A., and Todd, J. K.: Toxic-shock syndrome associated with Staphylococcus aureus sinusitis in children. J. Infect. Dis. 161:953-955, 1990.
110. Fichtenbaum, C. J., Peterson, L. R., and Weil, G. J.: Ehrlichiosis presenting as a life-threatening illness with features of the toxic shock syndrome. Am. J. Med. 95:351-357, 1993.
111. Finkelstein, J. W., and von Eye, A.: Sanitary product use by white, black and Mexican American women. Public Health Rep. 105:491, 1990.
112. Finkelstein, S., and Hyland, R. H.: Toxic shock syndrome as the AIDS defining diagnosis. Chest 104:950-951, 1993.
113. Fischer M., Bhatnagar J., Guarner J., et al.: Fatal toxic shock syndrome associated with Clostridium sordellii after medical abortion. N. Engl. J. Med. 353:2352-2360, 2005.
114. Fisher, C. J., Jr., Horowitz, Z., and Albertson, T. E.: Cardiorespiratory failure in toxic shock syndrome: Effect of dobutamine. Crit. Care Med. 13:160-165, 1985.
115. Fisher, C. J., Jr., Horowitz, B. Z., and Nolan, S. M.: The clinical spectrum of toxic shock syndrome. West. J. Med. 15:175-182, 1981.
116. Fisher, R. F., Goodpasture, H. C., Peterie, J. D., et al.: Toxic shock syndrome in menstruating women. Ann. Intern. Med. 94:156-163, 1981.
117. Fitz, J. D., Weeks, K. D., and Duff, P.: Left ventricular dysfunction in a patient with toxic shock syndrome. Am. J. Obstet. Gynecol. 146:467-468, 1983.
118. Fitzgerald, J. R., Sturdevant, D. E., Mackie, S. M., et al.: Evolutionary genomics of Staphylococcus aureus: Insights into the origin of methicillin-resistant

strains and the toxic shock syndrome epidemic. Proc. Natl. Acad. Sci. U. S. A. *98*:8821-8826, 2001.
119. Foley-Nolan, D., Coughlan, R. J., and Sugrue, D.: Toxic shock syndrome associated arthropathy. *Staphylococcus aureus*: A further triggering event in reactive arthritis? Ann. Rheum. Dis. *48*:331, 1989.
120. Follow-up on toxic-shock syndrome—United States. M. M. W. R. Morb. Mortal. Wkly. Rep. *29*:441-445, 1980.
121. Fornadley, J. A., Gomez, P. J., Crane, R. T., et al.: Toxic shock syndrome following submandibular gland excision. Head Neck *12*:66-68, 1990.
122. Frame, J. D., Eve, M. D., Hackett, M. E., et al.: The toxic shock syndrome in burned children. Burns *11*:234-241, 1985.
123. Fuleihan, R., Trede, N., Chatila, T., et al.: Superantigens activate HIV-1 gene expression in monocytic cells. Clin. Immunol. Immunopathol. *72*:357-361, 1994.
124. Galea, P., and Goel, K. M.: Toxic shock syndrome (TSS) in children. Scott. Med. J. *32*:28-29, 1987.
125. Gallagher, P. G., and Myer, C. M.: An approach to the diagnosis and treatment of membranous laryngotracheobronchitis in infants and children. Pediatr. Emerg. Care 7:337-342, 1991.
126. Garbe, P. L., Arko, R. J., and Reingold, A. L., et al.: *Staphylococcus aureus* isolates from patients with non-menstrual toxic shock syndrome: Evidence for additional toxins. J. A. M. A. *253*:2538-2542, 1985.
127. Gaventa, S., Reingold, A. L., Hightower, A. W., et al.: Active surveillance for TSS in the United States. Rev. Infect. Dis. *11*(Suppl.):28-34, 1989.
128. Glazowski, M. J., Ostergaard, G. Z., Arpi, M., et al.: Toxic shock syndrome: A case of a child with burns. Ugeskr. Laeger *154*:868-869, 1992.
129. Gosbell, I. B.: Epidemiology, clinical features and management of infections due to community methicillin-resistant *Staphylococcus aureus* (cMRSA). Intern. Med. J. *35*(Suppl. 2):S120-S135, 2005.
130. Gourley, G. R., Chesney, P. J., Davis, J. P., et al.: Acute cholestasis in patients with toxic-shock syndrome. Gastroenterology *81*:928-931, 1981.
131. Graham, D. R., O'Brien, M., Hayes, J. M., et al.: Postoperative toxic shock syndrome. Clin. Infect. Dis. *20*:895-899, 1995.
132. Hackett, S. P., and Stevens, D. L.: Superantigens associated with staphylococcal and streptococcal toxic shock syndrome are potent inducers of tumor necrosis factor β synthesis. J. Infect. Dis. *168*:232-235, 1993.
133. Hajjeh, R. A., Reingold, A., Weil, A., et al.: Toxic shock syndrome in the United States: Surveillance update, 1979-1996. Emerg. Infect. Dis. *5*:807-810, 1999.
134. Hamad, A. R. A., Marrach, P., and Kappler, J. W.: Transcytosis of staphylococcal superantigen toxins. J. Exp. Med. *185*:1447-1454, 1997.
135. Hanafiah, S. R., and Chong, S. K. F.: Toxic shock syndrome presenting as an acute encephalopathy and diarrhoea. J. R. Soc. Med. *84*:48-49, 1991.
136. Hauschildt, S., Bessler, W. G., and Scheipers, P.: Engagement of major histocompatibility complex class II molecules leads to nitrite production in bone marrow–derived macrophages. Eur. J. Immunol. *23*:2988-2992, 1993.
137. Hayward, J., Vergeront, J. M., Stolz-LaVerriere, S. J., et al.: A hospital discharge code review of toxic shock syndrome in Wisconsin. Am. J. Epidemiol. *123*:876-883, 1986.
138. Helgerson, S. D., and Foster, L. R.: Toxic shock syndrome in Oregon: Epidemiologic findings. Ann. Intern. Med. *96*:909-911, 1982.
139. Helms, C. M., Lengeling, R. W., Pinsky, R. L., et al.: Toxic shock syndrome: A retrospective study of 25 cases from Iowa. Am. J. Med. Sci. *282*:50-60, 1981.
140. Hensler, T., Koller, M., Geoffroy, C., et al.: *Staphylococcus aureus* toxic shock syndrome toxin 1 and *Streptococcus pyogenes* erythrogenic toxin A modulate inflammatory mediator release from human neutrophils. Infect. Immun. *61*:1055-1061, 1993.
141. Herwald, H., Cramer, H., Morgelin, M, et al.: M protein, a classical bacterial virulence determinant, forms complexes with fibrinogen that induce vascular leakage. Cell *116*:367-379, 2004.
142. Heywood, A. J., and al-Essa, S.: Toxic shock syndrome in child with only 2% burn. Lancet *335*:867, 1990.
143. Hiramatsu, K.: Vancomycin-resistant *Staphylococcus aureus*: A new model of antibiotic resistance. Lancet Infect. Dis. *1*:147-155, 2001.
144. Hirose-Kumagai, A., Whipple, F. H., Ikejima, T., et al.: A comparison of neutralizing and antigen-binding assays for human antibodies against toxic-shock-syndrome 1. J. Infect. Dis. *150*:788, 1984.
145. Hurley, J. M., Shimonkevitz, R., Hanagan, A., et al.: Identification of class II major histocompatibility complex and T cell receptor binding sites in the superantigen toxic shock syndrome toxin 1. J. Exp. Med. *181*:2229, 1995.
146. Hurwitz, R. M., and Ackerman, A. B.: Cutaneous pathology of the toxic shock syndrome. Am. J. Dermatopathol. 7:563, 1985.
147. Kikuchi, K., Takahashi, N., Piao, C., et al.: Molecular epidemiology of MRSA strains causing neonatal TSS-like exanthematous disease in neonatal and perinatal wards. J. Clin. Microbiol. *41*:3001-3006, 2003.
148. Iandolo, J. J.: Genetic analysis of extracellular toxins of *Staphylococcus aureus*. Annu. Rev. Microbiol. *43*:375-402, 1989.
149. Ikejima, T., and Dinarello, C. A.: Distribution of radiolabeled toxic shock syndrome toxin: Implications for the pathogenesis of interleukin-1–mediated toxic shock syndrome. J. Leukoc. Biol. *37*:714, 1985.
150. Ishak, K. G., and Rogers, W. A.: Cryptogenic acute cholangitis: Association with toxic shock syndrome. Am. J. Clin. Pathol. 76:619-626, 1981.
151. Jacobson, J. A., Kasworm, E. M., and Bolte, R. G., et al.: Prevalence of nasal carriage of toxigenic *Staphylococcus aureus* and antibody to TSST-1 in Utah children. Rev. Infect. Dis. *11*(Suppl.):324-325, 1989.
152. Jacobson, J. A., Kasworm, E., and Daly, J. A.: Risk of developing TSS associated with TSST-1 following nongenital staphylococcal infection. Rev. Infect. Dis. *11*(Suppl.):8-13, 1989.
153. Jacobson, J. A., Kasworm, E. M., Reiser, R. F., et al.: Low incidence of toxic shock syndrome in children with staphylococcal infection. Am. J. Med. Sci. *294*:403-407, 1987.
154. Jacobson, J. A., Stevens, M. H., and Kasworm, E. M.: Evaluation of single-dose cefazol in prophylaxis for toxic-shock syndrome. Arch. Otolaryngol. Head Neck Surg. *114*:326-327, 1988.
155. James, R. C., and MacLeod, C. J.: Induction of staphylococcal infections in mice with small inocula introduced on sutures. Br. J. Exp. Pathol. *42*:266, 1961.
156. Jaulhac, B., Bes, M., Bornstein, N., et al.: Synthetic DNA probes for detection of genes for enterotoxins A, B, C, D, E and for TSST-1 in staphylococcal strains. J. Appl. Bacteriol. *72*:386-392, 1992.
157. Johnson, W. M., Tyler, S. D., Ewan, E. P., et al.: Detection of genes for enterotoxins, exfoliative toxins, and toxic shock syndrome toxin 1 in *Staphylococcus aureus* by the polymerase chain reaction. J. Clin. Microbiol. *29*:426-430, 1991.
158. Kain, K. C., Schulzer, M., and Chow, A. W.: Clinical spectrum of nonmenstrual toxic shock syndrome (TSS): Comparison with menstrual TSS by multivariate discriminant analyses. Clin. Infect. Dis. *16*:100-106, 1993.
159. Kamel, N. S., Banks, M. C., Dosik, A., et al.: Lack of mucocutaneous signs of toxic shock syndrome when T cells are absent: S. aureus shock in immunodeficient adults with multiple myeloma. Clin. Exp. Immunol. *128*:131-139, 2002.
160. Kappler, J., Kotzin, B., Herron, L., et al.: Vβ-specific stimulation of human T-cells by staphylococcal toxins. Science *244*:811-813, 1989.
161. Kato, K., and Tanaka, T.: MRSA infection and toxic shock syndrome in burn patients. Jpn. J. Clin. Med. *50*:1104-1111, 1992.
162. Kehrberg, M. W., Latham, R. H., Haslam, B. T., et al.: Risk factors for staphylococcal toxic-shock syndrome. Am. J. Epidemiol. *114*:873-879, 1981.
163. Kernodle, D. S., McGraw, P. A., Barg, N. L., et al.: Growth of *Staphylococcus aureus* with nafcillin in vitro induces α-toxin production and increases the lethal activity of sterile broth filtrates in a murine model. J. Infect. Dis. *172*:410-419, 1995.
164. Kline, M. W., and Dunkle, L. M.: Toxic shock syndrome and the acquired immunodeficiency syndrome. Pediatr. Infect. Dis. J. 7:736-738, 1988.
165. Kotasek, D., Vercelloti, G. M., Ochoa, A. C., et al.: Mechanism of cultured endothelial injury induced by lymphokine activated killer cells. Cancer Res. *48*:5528, 1988.
166. Kotb, M.: Bacterial pyrogenic exotoxins as superantigens. Clin. Microbiol. Rev. 8:411-426, 1995.
167. Krakauer, T.: Inhibition of toxic shock syndrome toxin-1–induced cytokine production and T cell activation by interleukin-10, interleukin-4 and dexamethasone. J. Infect. Dis. *172*:988-992, 1995.
168. Kravitz, G. R., Dries, D. J., Peterson, M. L., et al.: Purpura fulminans due to *Staphylococcus aureus*. Clin. Infect. Dis. *40*:941-947, 2005.
169. Kreiswirth, B. N., Kravitz, G. R., Schlievert, P. M., et al.: Nosocomial transmission of a strain of *Staphylococcus aureus* causing toxic shock syndrome. Ann. Intern. Med. *105*:704, 1986.
170. Kreiswirth, B. N., Projan, S. J., Schlievert, P. M., et al.: Toxic shock syndrome toxin 1 is encoded by a variable genetic element. Rev. Infect. Dis. *11*(Suppl.):83-88, 1989.
171. Ku, W. W. S., and Chow, A. W.: Monoclonal antibodies (MAb5 and MAb4) protect against the lethal effect of toxic shock syndrome toxin-1 in the D-galactosamine sensitized mouse mode. Abstract. J. Invest. Med. *110*:68, 1996.
172. Kum, W. W., and Chow, A. W.: Inhibition of staphylococcal enterotoxin A–induced superantigenic and lethal activities by a monoclonal antibody to toxic shock syndrome toxin-1. J. Infect. Dis. *183*:1739-1748, 2001.
173. Kushnaryov, V. M., MacDonald, H. S., Reiser, R. F., et al.: Reaction of TSST-1 with endothelium of human umbilical cord vein. Rev. Infect. Dis. *11*(Suppl.):282-287, 1989.
174. Larkin, S. M., Williams, D. N., Osterholm, M. T., et al.: Toxic shock syndrome: Clinical, laboratory, and pathologic findings in nine fatal cases. Ann. Intern. Med. *96*:858-864, 1982.
175. Latham, R. H., Kehrberg, M. W., Jacobson, J. A., et al.: Toxic shock syndrome in Utah: A case-control and surveillance study. Ann. Intern. Med. *96*:906-908, 1982.
176. Lee, P. K., Vercellotti, G. M., Deringer, J. R., et al.: Effects of staphylococcal toxic shock syndrome toxin 1 on aortic endothelial cells. J. Infect. Dis. *164*:711-719, 1991.
177. Lee, V. T. P., Chang, A. H., and Chow, A. W.: Detection of staphylococcal enterotoxin B among toxic-shock syndrome (TSS) and non-TSS associated *Staphylococcus aureus* isolates. J. Infect. Dis. *166*:911-915, 1992.
178. Lovseth, A., Loncarevic, S., Berdal, K. G., et al.: Modified multiplex PCR method for detection of pyrogenic exotoxin genes in staphylococcal isolates. J. Clin. Microbiol. *42*:3869-3872, 2004.
179. Lund, L., Nielsen, D., and Anderson, E. S.: Meningismus as the main symptom in toxic shock syndrome. Acta Obstet. Gynecol. Scand. 67:395, 1988.
180. MacDonald, K. L., Osterholm, M. T., Hedberg, C. W., et al.: Toxic shock syndrome: A newly recognized complication of influenza and influenza like illness. J. A. M. A. *257*:1053-1058, 1987.

181. Malknecht, U., Hunter, M., Hoffmann, M. K., et al.: The toxic shock syndrome toxin-1 induces anergy in human T cells in vivo. Hum. Immunol. *45*:42-45, 1996.

182. Marlowe, D. E., Weigle, R. M., and Stauffenberg, R. S.: Measurement of Tampon Absorbency: Evaluation of Tampon Brands. Rockville, MD, FDA Bureau of Biologics, 1981.

183. Marodi, L., Kaposzta, R., Rozgonyi, F., et al.: Staphylococcal enterotoxin A involvement in the illness of a 20-month-old burn patient. Pediatr. Infect. Dis. J. *14*:632-634, 1995.

184. Marples, R. R., and Wienecke, A. A.: Enterotoxins and toxic-shock syndrome-1 in non-enteric staphylococcal disease. Epidemiol. Infect. *110*:477-488, 1993.

185. Marrack, P., and Kappler, J.: The staphylococcal enterotoxins and their relatives. Science *248*:705-711, 1990.

186. Martin, R. R., Buttram, V., Besch, P., et al.: Nasal and vaginal *Staphylococcus aureus* in young women: Quantitative studies. Ann. Intern. Med. *96*:951-953, 1982.

187. Matsuda, Y., Kato, H., Yamada, R., et al.: Early and definitive diagnosis of toxic shock syndrome by detection of marked expansion of T-cell-receptor V$_\beta$2-positive T cells. Emerg. Infect. Dis. *9*:387-389, 2003.

188. McAllister, R. M., Mercer, N. S., Morgan, B. D., et al.: Early diagnosis of staphylococcal toxemia in burned children. Burns *19*:22-25, 1993.

189. McCormick, J. K., Yarwood, J. M., and Schlievert, P. M.: Toxic shock syndrome and bacterial superantigens: An update. Annu. Rev. Microbiol. *55*:77-104, 2001.

190. McGann, V. G., Rollins, J. B., and Mason, D. W.: Evaluation of resistance to staphylococcal enterotoxin B: Naturally acquired antibodies of man and monkey. J. Infect. Dis. *124*:206-213, 1971.

191. McIvor, M. E., and Levin, M. L.: Treatment of recurrent toxic shock syndrome with oral contraceptive agents. Md. Med. J. *31*:56-57, 1982.

192. McKenna, U. G., Meadows, J. A., III, Brewer, N. S., et al.: Toxic shock syndrome, a newly recognized disease entity: Report of 11 cases. Mayo Clin. Proc. *55*:663-672, 1980.

193. McMahon, W. S., Patrenos, M. E., McConnell, M. E., et al.: Complete heart block in toxic shock syndrome. Am. J. Dis. Child. *144*:748, 1990.

194. Mehrotra, M., Wang, G., Johnson, W. M., et al.: Multiplex PCR for detection of genes for *Staphylococcus aureus* enterotoxins, exfoliative toxins, toxic shock syndrome toxin 1, and methicillin resistance. J. Clin. Microbiol. *38*:1032-1035, 2000.

195. Melish, M. E., Chen, F. S., and Murata, M. S.: Quantitative detection of toxic shock marker protein in human and experimental toxic shock syndrome. Abstract. Clin. Res. *31*:122, 1983.

196. Melish, M. E., Frogner, K. S., Hirata, S. A., et al.: Use of IVGG for therapy in the rabbit model of TSS. Abstract. Clin. Res. *35*:220, 1987.

197. Melish, M. E., Murata, S., Fukunaga, C., et al.: Corticosteroid and immunoglobulin therapy in toxic shock syndrome (TSS). Abstract. Clin. Res. *36*:781, 1988.

198. Melish, M. E., Murata, S., Fukunaga, C., et al.: Endotoxin is not an essential mediator in TSS. Rev. Infect. Dis. *11*(Suppl.):219-228, 1989.

199. Melish, M. E., Murata, S., Fukunaga, C., et al.: Vaginal tampon model for toxic shock syndrome. Rev. Infect. Dis. *11*(Suppl.):238-246, 1989.

200. Melish, M. E., Murata, S., Fukunaga, C., et al.: Corticosteroid and immunoglobulin therapy in TSS. Rev. Infect. Dis. *11*(Suppl.):332-333, 1989.

201. Michels, T. C.: Mucocutaneous lymph node syndrome in adults: Differentiation from toxic shock syndrome. Am. J. Med. *80*:724, 1986.

202. Michie, C. A., Davis, T., and MacAllister, M.: The sequelae of toxic shock syndrome. Abstract. Pediatr. Res. *39*:179, 1996.

203. Miethke, T., Duschek, K., Wahl, C., et al.: Pathogenesis of the toxic shock syndrome: T-cell–mediated lethal shock caused by the superantigen TSST-1. Eur. J. Immunol. *23*:1494-1500, 1993.

204. Miethke, T., Wahl, I. C., Heeg, K., et al.: T-cell–mediated lethal shock triggered in mice by the superantigen staphylococcal enterotoxin B: Critical role of tumor necrosis factor. J. Exp. Med. *175*:91-98, 1992.

205. Miethke, T., Wahl, C., Regele, D., et al.: *Staphylococcus aureus* mediated shock: A cytokine release syndrome. Immunobiology *189*:270-284, 1993.

206. Miller, S. D.: Postoperative toxic shock syndrome after lumbar laminectomy in a male patient. Spine *19*:1182-1185, 1994.

207. Miller, W., and Stankiewicz, J. A.: Delayed toxic shock syndrome in sinus surgery. Otolaryngol. Head Neck Surg. *111*:121-123, 1994.

208. Mills, J. T., Parsonnet, J., Hickman, R. K., et al.: Control of production of toxic-shock syndrome toxin-1 (TSST-1) by magnesium ion. J. Infect. Dis. *151*:1158-1161, 1985.

209. Miwa, K., Fukuyama, M., Kunitomo, T., et al.: Rapid assay for detection of toxic shock syndrome toxin 1 from human sera. J. Clin. Microbiol. *32*:539-542, 1994.

210. Mohan, S. B., Tamilarasan, A., and Buhl, M.: Inhalational mercury poisoning masquerading as toxic shock syndrome. Anaesth. Intensive Care *22*:305-306, 1994.

211. Mohsenipour, M., Deusch, E., Twerdy, K., et al.: Toxic shock syndrome in transsphenoidal neurosurgery. Acta Neurochir. *128*:169-170, 1994.

212. Moyer, M. A., Edwards, L. D., and Bergdoll, M. S.: Nosocomial toxic shock syndrome in two patients after knee surgery. Am. J. Infect. Control *11*:83-87, 1983.

213. Murray, D. L., Earhart, C. A., Mitchell, D. T., et al.: Localization of biologically important regions on toxic shock syndrome toxin-1. Infect. Immun. *64*:371-374, 1996.

214. Musser, J. M., Schlievert, P. M., Chow, A. W., et al.: A single clone of *Staphylococcus aureus* causes the majority of cases of toxic-shock syndrome. Proc. Natl. Acad. Sci. U. S. A. *87*:225-229, 1990.

215. Nadal, D., Lauener, R. P., Braegger, C. P., et al.: T-cell activation and cytokine release in streptococcal toxic shock–like syndrome. J. Pediatr. *122*:727-729, 1993.

216. Neill, R. J., Fanning, G. R., Delahoz, F., et al.: Oligonucleotide probes for detection and differentiation of *Staphylococcus aureus* strains containing genes for enterotoxins A, B, and C and toxic shock syndrome toxin 1. J. Clin. Microbiol. *28*:1514-1518, 1990.

217. Nightingale, S. L.: New requirements for tampon labeling. Am. Fam. Physician *41*:999, 1990.

218. Nijssen-Jordan, C., Donaldson, J. D., and Halperin, S. A.: Bacterial tracheitis associated with respiratory syncytial virus infection and toxic-shock syndrome. Can. Med. Assoc. J. *142*:233-234, 1990.

219. Nishi, J., Yoshinaga, M., Miyanohara, H., et al.: An epidemiologic survey of methicillin-resistant *Staphylococcus aureus* by combined use of mec-HVR genotyping and toxin genotyping in a university hospital in Japan. Infect. Control Hosp. Epidemiol. *23*:506-510, 2002.

220. Norrby-Teglund, A., Pauksens, K., Holm, S. E., et al.: Relation between low capacity of human sera to inhibit streptococcal mitogens and serious manifestation of disease. J. Infect. Dis. *170*:585-591, 1994.

221. Ogawa, M., Ueda, S., Anzai, N., et al.: Toxic shock syndrome after staphylococcal pneumonia treated with intravenous immunoglobulin. Vox Sang. *68*:59-60, 1995.

222. O'Gilvie vs. International Playtex, No. 83-1845, Vol. 37 (DC Kansas March 21, 1985, post-trial motions and court findings).

223. Olesen, L. L., Ejlertsen, T., and Nielsen, J.: Toxic shock syndrome following insertion of breast prostheses. Br. J. Surg. *78*:585-586, 1991.

224. Olson, R. D., Stevens, D. L., and Melish, M. E.: Direct effects of purified staphylococcal TSST-1 on myocardial function of isolated rabbit atria. Rev. Infect. Dis. *11*(Suppl.):313-315, 1989.

225. Onderdonk, A. B., Delaney, M. L., Zamarchi, G. R., et al.: Normal vaginal microflora during use of various forms of catamenial protection. Rev. Infect. Dis. *11*(Suppl.):61-67, 1989.

226. Orden, J. A., Goyache, J., Hernandez, F. J., et al.: Detection of staphylococcal enterotoxin and toxic shock syndrome toxin-1 (TSST-1) by immunoblot combined with a semiautomated electrophoresis system. J. Immunol. Methods *144*:197-202, 1991.

227. Osterholm, M. T., Davis, J. P., Gibson, R. W., et al.: Tri-state toxic-shock syndrome study. I. Epidemiologic findings. J. Infect. Dis. *145*:431-440, 1982.

228. Osterholm, M. T., Davis, J. P., Gibson, R. W., et al.: Toxic shock syndrome: Relation to catamenial products, personal health and hygiene, and sexual practices. Ann. Intern. Med. *96*:954-958, 1982.

229. Osterholm, M. T., and Forfang, J. C.: Toxic-shock syndrome in Minnesota: Results of an active-passive surveillance system. J. Infect. Dis. *145*:458-464, 1982.

230. Paris, A. L., Herwaldt, L. A., Blum, D., et al.: Pathologic findings in twelve fatal cases of toxic-shock syndrome. Ann. Intern. Med. *96*:852-857, 1982.

231. Parkin, D. E.: Fatal toxic shock syndrome following endometrial resection. Br. J. Obstet. Gynaecol. *102*:163-164, 1995.

232. Parsonnet, J.: Mediators in the pathogenesis of TSS: Overview. Rev. Infect. Dis. *11*(Suppl.):263-269, 1989.

233. Parsonnet, J.: Nonmenstrual toxic shock syndrome: New insights into diagnosis, pathogenesis and treatment. Curr. Clin. Top. Infect. Dis. *16*:1-20, 1996.

234. Parsonnet, J., Gillis, Z. A., and Pier, G. B.: Induction of interleukin-1 by strains of *Staphylococcus aureus* from patients with non-menstrual toxic shock syndrome. J. Infect. Dis. *154*:55-63, 1986.

235. Parsonnet, J., Gillis, Z. A., Thompson, M. R., et al.: Effects of monoclonal antibody on biologic function of TSST-1 in vitro and in vivo. Rev. Infect. Dis. *11*(Suppl.):318-319, 1989.

236. Parsonnet, J., Hansmann, M. A., Delaney, M. L., et al.: Prevalence of toxic shock syndrome toxin 1–producing *Staphylococcus aureus* and the presence of antibodies to this superantigen in menstruating women. J. Clin. Microbiol. *43*:4628-4634, 2005.

237. Parsonnet, J., Modern, P. A., and Giacobbe, K.: Effect of subinhibitory concentrations of antibiotics on production of toxic shock syndrome toxin-1 (TSST-1). Abstract 29. Presented at the 32nd Annual Meeting of the Infectious Diseases Society of America, 1994, Washington, DC.

238. Parsonnet, J., Modern, P. A., and Giacobbe, K. D.: Effect of tampon composition on production of toxic shock syndrome toxin-1 by *Staphylococcus aureus* in vitro. J. Infect. Dis. *173*:98-103, 1996.

239. Parsonnet, J., Tosteson, A., Modern, P., et al.: Antibody to toxic shock syndrome toxin-1 (TSST-1) and vaginal colonization by TSST-1 producing *S. aureus* among adolescent women. Abstract 1327. Presented at the 33rd Interscience Conference on Antimicrobial Agents and Chemotherapy, American Society for Microbiology, 1993, Washington, DC.

240. Paterson, M. P., Hoffman, E. B., and Roux, P.: Severe disseminated staphylococcal disease associated with osteitis and septic arthritis. J. Bone Joint Surg. Br. *72*:94-97, 1990.

241. Petitti, D. B., Reingold, A., and Chin, J.: The incidence of toxic shock syndrome in northern California: 1972 through 1983. J. A. M. A. *255*:368-372, 1986.
242. Pokriefka, R., Rabah, M., Saravolatz, L., et al.: Toxic shock syndrome in an injection drug user with *Staphylococcus aureus* endocarditis. Infect. Med. *11*:34-36, 48-49, 1994.
243. Potter, T., DiGregorio, F., Stiff, M., et al.: Dilantin hypersensitivity syndrome imitating staphylococcal toxic shock. Arch. Dermatol. *130*:856-858, 1994.
244. Prevention and Recognition of TSS: Institute of Medicine: Toxic Shock Syndrome: Assessment of Current Information and Future Research Needs. Washington, DC, National Academy Press, 1982, pp. 85-86.
245. Projan, S. J., Brown-Skrobot, S., and Schlievert, P. M.: Glycerol monolaurate inhibits the production of beta-lactamase, toxic shock toxin-1, and other staphylococcal exoproteins by interfering with signal transduction. J. Bacteriol. *176*:4204-4209, 1994.
246. Raab, M. G., O'Brien, M., Hayes, J. M., et al.: Postoperative toxic shock syndrome. Am. J. Orthop. *24*:130-136, 1995.
247. Rasheed, J. K., Arko, R. J., Feeley, J. C., et al.: Acquired ability of *Staphylococcus aureus* to produce toxic shock–associated protein and resulting illness in a rabbit model. Infect. Immun. *47*:598-604, 1985.
248. Reduced incidence of menstrual toxic-shock syndrome—United States, 1980-1990. M. M. W. R. Morb. Mortal. Wkly. Rep. *39*(25):421-423, 1990.
249. Reingold, A. L.: Epidemiology of toxic-shock syndrome, United States, 1960-1984. M. M. W. R. C. D. C. Surveill. Summ. *33*(3):19SS-22SS, 1984.
250. Reingold, A. L., Hargrett, N. T., Dan, B. B., et al.: Nonmenstrual toxic shock syndrome: A review of 130 cases. Ann. Intern. Med. *96*:871-874, 1982.
251. Ren, K., Bannan, J. D., Pancholi, V., et al.: Characterization and biological properties of a new staphylococcal exotoxin. J. Exp. Med. *180*:1675-1683, 1994.
252. Rhee, C. A., Smith, R. J., and Jackson, I. T.: Toxic shock syndrome associated with suction-assisted lipectomy. Aesthetic Plast. Surg. *18*:161-163, 1994.
253. Rich, R. R.: Intravenous IgG: Supertherapy for superantigens. J. Clin. Invest. *91*:378, 1993.
254. Ritz, H. L., Kirkland, J. J., Bond, G. G., et al.: Association of high levels of serum antibody to staphylococcal toxic shock antigen with nasal carriage of toxic shock antigen–producing strains of *Staphylococcus aureus*. Infect. Immun. *43*:954-958, 1984.
255. Rolston, R. D., Yabek, S. M., Florman, A. L., et al.: Severe cardiac conduction abnormalities associated with atypical toxic-shock syndrome. J. Pediatr. *117*:89, 1990.
256. Romagne, F., Besnardeau, L., and Malissen, B.: A versatile method to produce antibodies to human T cell receptor V beta segments: Frequency determination of human V beta 2+ T cells that react with toxic-shock syndrome toxin-1. Eur. J. Immunol. *22*:2749-2752, 1992.
257. Rose, P. G., and Wilson, G.: Advanced cervical carcinoma presenting with toxic shock syndrome. Gynecol. Oncol. *52*:264-266, 1994.
258. Rosene, K. A., Copass, M. K., Kastner, L. S., et al.: Persistent neuropsychological sequelae of toxic shock syndrome. Ann. Intern. Med. *96*:865-870, 1982.
259. Rosten, P. M., Bartlett, K. H., and Chow, A. W.: Serologic responses to toxic shock syndrome (TSS) toxin-1 in menstrual and nonmenstrual TSS. Clin. Invest. Med. *11*:187-192, 1988.
260. Rovner, R. A., Baird, R. A., and Malerich, M. M.: Fatal toxic-shock syndrome as a complication of orthopedic surgery. J. Bone Joint Surg. Am. *66*:952-954, 1984.
261. Royall, J. A., Berkow, R. L., Beckman, J. S., et al.: Tumor necrosis factor and interleukin 1α increase vascular endothelial cell permeability. Am. J. Physiol. *257*:L399-L410, 1989.
262. Sahs, A. L., Helms, C. M., and DuBois, C.: Carpal tunnel syndrome: Complication of toxic shock syndrome. Arch. Neurol. *40*:414-415, 1983.
263. Sales, J. H., Kennedy, K. S., Galantich, P. T., et al.: Toxic shock syndrome associated with pharyngitis and submandibular space abscess. Ann. Otol. Rhinol. Laryngol. *100*:540-543, 1991.
264. Schlech, W. F., III, Shands, K. N., Reingold, A. L., et al.: Risk factors for development of toxic shock syndrome: Association with a tampon brand. J. A. M. A. *7*:835-839, 1982.
265. Schlievert, P. M.: Enhancement of host susceptibility to lethal endotoxin shock by staphylococcal pyrogenic exotoxin type C. Infect. Immun. *36*:123-128, 1982.
266. Schlievert, P. M.: Staphylococcal enterotoxin B and toxic-shock syndrome toxin-1 are significantly associated with non-menstrual TSS. Lancet *1*:1149, 1986.
267. Schlievert, P. M.: Comparison of cotton and cotton/rayon tampons for effect on production of toxic shock syndrome toxin. J. Infect. Dis. *172*:1112-1114, 1995.
268. Schlievert, P. M., Deringer, J. R., Kim, M. H., et al.: Effect of glycerol monolaurate on bacterial growth and toxin production. Antimicrob. Agents Chemother. *36*:626-632, 1992.
269. Schlievert, P. M., and Kelly, J. A.: Clindamycin-induced suppression of toxic-shock syndrome–associated exotoxin production. J. Infect. Dis. *149*:471, 1984.
270. Schlievert, P. M., Shands, K. N., Dan, B. B., et al.: Identification and characterization of exotoxin from *Staphylococcus aureus* associated with toxic shock syndrome. J. Infect. Dis. *143*:509-516, 1981.
271. Schlievert, P. M., Tripp, T. J., Peterson, M. L.: Reemergence of staphylococcal toxic shock syndrome in Minneapolis–St. Paul, Minnesota, during the 2000-2003 surveillance period. J. Clin. Microbiol. *42*:2875-2876, 2004.
272. Schmitz, F. J., Mackenzie, C. R., Geisel, R., et al.: Enterotoxin and toxic shock syndrome toxin-1 production of methicillin resistant and methicillin sensitive *Staphylococcus aureus* strains. Eur. J. Epidemiol. *13*:699-708, 1997.
273. Schmitz, F. J., Steiert, M., Hofmann, B., et al.: Development of a multiplex-PCR for direct detection of the genes for enterotoxin B and C, and toxic shock syndrome toxin-1 in *Staphylococcus aureus* isolates. J. Med. Microbiol. *47*:335-340, 1998.
274. Schuchat, A., and Broome, C. V.: Toxic shock syndrome and tampons. Epidemiol. Rev. *13*:99-112, 1991.
275. Schwartz, B., Gaventa, S., Broome, C. V., et al.: Nonmenstrual TSS associated with barrier contraceptives: Report of a case-control study. Rev. Infect. Dis. *11*(Suppl.):43-48, 1989.
276. Scott, D. F., Best, G. K., Kling, J. M., et al.: Passive protection of rabbits infected with TSS associated strains of *Staphylococcus aureus* by monoclonal antibody to TSST-1. Rev. Infect. Dis. *11*(Suppl.):214-217, 1989.
277. Shands, K. N., Schmid, G. P., Dan, B. B., et al.: Toxic-shock syndrome in menstruating women: Association with tampon use and *Staphylococcus aureus* and clinical features in 52 cases. N. Engl. J. Med. *303*:1436-1442, 1980.
278. Shlasko, E., Harris, M. T., Benjamin, E., et al.: Toxic shock syndrome after pilonidal cystectomy: Report of a case. Dis. Colon Rectum *34*:502-505, 1991.
279. Sinave, C., Le Templier, G., Blouin, D., et al.: Toxic shock syndrome due to *Clostridium sordellii*: A dramatic postpartum and postabortion disease. Clin. Infect. Dis. *35*:1441-1443, 2002.
280. Sissons, J. G.: Superantigens and infectious disease. Lancet *341*:1627-1629, 1993.
281. Skansen-Saphir, U., Andersson, J., Bjork, L., et al.: Lymphokine production induced by streptococcal pyrogenic exotoxin A is selectively down regulated by pooled human IgG. Eur. J. Immunol. *24*:916-922, 1994.
282. Slingluff, C. L., Jr., Burns, W. W., and Cooperberg, C.: Toxic shock syndrome after inguinal hernia repair: Report of a case with patient survival. Am. Surg. *56*:610-612, 1990.
283. Smith, D. B., and Gulinson, J.: Fatal cerebral edema complicating toxic shock syndrome. Neurosurgery *22*:598-599, 1988.
284. Sparano, J., and Ferranti, E.: The acquired immunodeficiency syndrome and non-menstrual toxic shock syndrome. Ann. Intern. Med. *105*:300-301, 1986.
285. Spearman, P. W., and Barson, W. J.: Toxic shock syndrome occurring in children with abrasive injuries beneath casts. J. Pediatr. Orthop. *12*:169-172, 1992.
286. Sperber, S. J., Blevins, D. D., and Francis, J. B.: Hypercalcitonemia, hypocalcemia, and toxic-shock syndrome. Rev. Infect. Dis. *12*:736-739, 1990.
287. Spertini, F., Spits, H., and Geha, R. S.: Staphylococcal exotoxins deliver activation signals to human T-cell clones via major histocompatibility complex class II molecules. Proc. Natl. Acad. Sci. U. S. A. *88*:7533-7537, 1991.
288. *Staphylococcus aureus* resistant to vancomycin—United States, 2002. M. M. W. R. Morb. Mortal. Wkly. Rep. *51*(26):565-567, 2002.
289. Stevens, D. L., Gibbons, A. E., Bergstrom, R., et al.: The eagle effect revisited: Efficacy of clindamycin, erythromycin, and penicillin in the treatment of streptococcal myositis. J. Infect. Dis. *158*:23-28, 1988.
290. Stevens, D. L., Tanner, M. H., Winship, J., et al.: Severe group A streptococcal infections associated with a toxic shock–like syndrome and scarlet fever toxin A. N. Engl. J. Med. *321*:1-7, 1989.
291. Stevens, D. L., Wallace, R. J., Hamilton, S. M., et al.: Successful treatment of staphylococcal toxic shock syndrome with linezolid: A case report and in vitro evaluation of the production of toxic shock syndrome toxin type 1 in the presence of antibiotics. Clin. Infect. Dis. *42*:729-730, 2006.
292. Stevens, D. L., Yan, S., and Bryant, A. E.: Penicillin-binding protein expression at different growth stages determines penicillin efficacy in vitro and in vivo: An explanation for the inoculum effect. J. Infect. Dis. *167*:1401-1405, 1993.
293. Stevens, F. A.: The occurrence of *Staphylococcus aureus* infection with a scarlatiniform rash. J. A. M. A. *18*:1957-1958, 1927.
294. Stolz, S. J., Davis, J. P., Vergeront, J. M., et al.: Development of serum antibody to toxic shock toxin among individuals with toxic shock syndrome in Wisconsin. J. Infect. Dis. *151*:883-889, 1985.
295. Su, Y. C., and Wong, A. C.: Identification and purification of a new staphylococcal enterotoxin, H. Appl. Environ. Microbiol. *61*:1438-1443, 1995.
296. Summary of notifiable diseases, United States, 1994. M. M. W. R. Morb. Mortal. Wkly. Rep. *43*(53):1-80, 1994.
297. Swift, J. D., Barruga, M. C., Perkin, R. M., et al.: Respiratory failure complicating rubeola. Chest *104*:1786-1787, 1993.
298. Takahashi, N., Kato, H., Imanishi, K., et al.: Immunopathophysiological aspects of an emerging neonatal infectious disease induced by a bacterial superantigen. J. Clin. Invest. *106*:1409-1415, 2000.
299. Takahashi, N., Nishida, H., Kato, H., et al.: Exanthematous disease induced by toxic shock syndrome toxin I in the early neonatal period. Lancet *351*:1614-1619, 1998.
300. Takei, S., Arora, Y. K., and Walker, S. M.: Intravenous immunoglobulin contains specific antibodies inhibitory to activation of T cells by staphylococcal toxin superantigens. J. Clin. Invest. *91*:602-607, 1993.
301. Tampon packages carry TSS information. F. D. A. Drug Bull. *3*(3):19-20, 1982.

302. Thompson, T. D., and Friedman, A. L.: Simultaneous occurrence of *Staphylococcus aureus*–associated septic arthritis and toxic shock syndrome. Clin. Pediatr. (Phila.) *33*:243-245, 1994.
303. Tierno, P. M., Jr., and Hanna, B. A.: Propensity of tampons and barrier contraceptives to amplify *Staphylococcus aureus* toxic shock syndrome toxin-1. Infect. Dis. Obstet. Gynecol. *2*:140-145, 1994.
304. Todd, J. K.: Therapy of toxic shock syndrome. Drugs *39*:856-861, 1990.
305. Todd, J. K., Fishaut, M., and Kapral, F., et al.: Toxic-shock syndrome associated with phage-group-1 staphylococci. Lancet *2*:1116-1118, 1978.
306. Todd, J. K., Franco-Buff, A., Lawellin, D. W., et al.: Phenotypic distinctiveness of *Staphylococcus aureus* strains associated with toxic shock syndrome. Infect. Immun. *45*:339-344, 1984.
307. Todd, J. K., Ressman, M., Caston, S. A., et al.: Corticosteroid therapy for patients with toxic shock syndrome. J. A. M. A. *252*:3399-3402, 1984.
308. Todd, J. K., Todd, B. H., Franco-Buff, A., et al.: Influence of focal growth conditions on the pathogenesis of toxic shock syndrome. J. Infect. Dis. *155*:673-681, 1987.
309. Todd, J. K., Weisenthal, A. M., Ressman, M., et al.: Toxic shock syndrome. II. Estimated occurrence in Colorado as influenced by case ascertainment methods. Am. J. Epidemiol. *22*:857-867, 1985.
310. Tofte, R. W., and Williams, D. N.: Toxic shock syndrome: Evidence of a broad clinical spectrum. J. A. M. A. *246*:2163-2167, 1981.
311. Tofte, R. W., and Williams, D. N.: Clinical and laboratory manifestations of toxic shock syndrome. Ann. Intern. Med. *96*:843-847, 1982.
312. Tolan, R. W., Jr.: Toxic shock syndrome complicating influenza A in a child: Case report and review. Clin. Infect. Dis. *17*:43-45, 1993.
313. Toxic-shock syndrome and the vaginal contraceptive sponge. M. M. W. R. Morb. Mortal. Wkly. Rep. *33*(4):43-44, 49, 1984.
314. Toxic shock syndrome following influenza—Oregon, United States; update on influenza activity—United States. M. M. W. R. Morb. Mortal. Wkly. Rep. *36*(5):64-65, 1987.
315. Toxic-shock syndrome—United States. M. M. W. R. Morb. Mortal. Wkly. Rep. *29*:229-230, 1980.
316. Toxic-shock syndrome—United States, 1970-1980. M. M. W. R. Morb. Mortal. Wkly. Rep. *30*(3):25-28, 33, 1981.
317. Toxic-shock syndrome, United States, 1970-1982. M. M. W. R. Morb. Mortal. Wkly. Rep. *31*(16):201-204, 1982.
318. Tracey, K. J., Lowry, S. F., Beutler, B., et al.: Cachectin/tumor necrosis factor mediates changes of skeletal muscle plasma membrane potential. J. Exp. Med. *164*:1368-1373, 1986.
319. Turker, R., Lubicky, J. P., and Vogel, L. C.: Toxic shock syndrome in patients with external fixators. J. Pediatr. Orthop. *12*:658-662, 1992.
320. Update: Toxic shock syndrome—United States. M. M. W. R. Morb. Mortal. Wkly. Rep. *32*(30):398-400, 1983.
321. Van der Mee-Marquet, N., Lina, G., Quentin, R., et al.: Staphylococcal exanthematous disease in a newborn due to a virulent methicillin-resistant *Staphylococcus aureus* strain containing the TSST-1 gene in Europe: An alert for neonatologists. J. Clin. Microbiol. *41*:4883-4884, 2003.
322. Vergeront, J. M., Blouse, L. E., Crass, B. A., et al.: Regional differences in the prevalence of serum antibody to toxic-shock toxin (anti-TST). Abstract 610.

Presented at the 24th Interscience Conference on Antimicrobial Agents and Chemotherapy, 1984, Atlanta, p. 193.
323. Vergeront, J. M., Evenson, M. L., Crass, B. A., et al.: Recovery of staphylococcal enterotoxin F from the breast milk of a woman with toxic-shock syndrome. J. Infect. Dis. *146*:456-459, 1982.
324. Vergeront, J. M., Stolz, S. J., Crass, B. A., et al.: Prevalence of serum antibody to staphylococcal enterotoxin F among Wisconsin residents: Implications for toxic shock syndrome. J. Infect. Dis. *148*:692-698, 1983.
325. Vic-Dupont, M. P., Duval, P., and Kamaliv, S. R.: Scarlatiniform staphylococcal diseases. Soc. Med. Hop. Paris *116*:51, 1965.
326. Wagner, G., Bohr, L., Wagner, P., et al.: Tampon-induced changes in vaginal oxygen and carbon dioxide tensions. Am. J. Obstet. Gynecol. *148*:147-150, 1984.
327. Watanabe-Ohnishi, R., Low, D. E., McGeer, A., et al.: Selective depletion of V_β-bearing T cells in patients with severe invasive group A streptococcal infections and streptococcal toxic shock syndrome. J. Infect. Dis. *171*:74-84, 1995.
328. Weinzweig, J., Gottlich, L. J., and Krizek, T. J.: Toxic shock syndrome associated with the use of Biobrane in a scald burn victim. Burns *20*:180-181, 1994.
329. Weissberg, S. M., and Dodson, M. G.: Recurrent vaginal and cervical ulcers associated with tampon use. J. A. M. A. *250*:1430-1431, 1983.
330. Wharton, M., Chorba, T. L., Vogt, R. L., et al.: Case definitions for public health surveillance. M. M. W. R. Recomm. Rep. *39*(RR-13):1-43, 1990.
331. Whitby, M., Fraser, S., Gemmell, C. G., et al.: Toxic shock syndrome and endocarditis. B. M. J. *286*:1613, 1983.
332. Whiting, J. L., Rosten, P. M., and Chow, A. W.: Determination by Western blot (immunoblot) of seroconversions to toxic shock syndrome (TSS) toxin 1 and enterotoxin A, B, or C during infection with TSS- and non–TSS-associated *Staphylococcus aureus*. Infect. Immun. *57*:231-234, 1989.
333. Wick, M. R., Bahn, R. C., and McKenna, U. G.: Toxic shock syndrome: A fatal case with autopsy findings. Mayo Clin. Proc. *57*:583-589, 1982.
334. Wiesenthal, A. M., and Todd, J. K.: Toxic shock syndrome in children aged 10 years or less. Pediatrics *74*:112-117, 1984.
335. Wong, A. C. L., and Bergdoll, M. S.: Effect of environmental conditions on production of toxic shock syndrome toxin 1 by *Staphylococcus aureus*. Infect. Immun. *58*:1026-1029, 1990.
336. Working Group on Severe Streptococcal Infections: Defining the group A streptococcal toxic shock syndrome: Rationale and consensus definition. The Working Group on Severe Streptococcal Infections. J. A. M. A. *269*:390-391, 1993.
337. Yagoob, M., McClelland, P., Murray, A. E., et al.: Staphylococcal enterotoxins A and C causing toxic shock syndrome. J. Infect. *20*:176-178, 1990.
338. Yong, J. M.: Necrotising fasciitis. Lancet *343*:1427, 1994.
339. Younis, R. T., Gross, C. W., and Lazar, R. H.: Toxic shock syndrome following functional endonasal sinus surgery: A case report. Head Neck *13*:247-248, 1991.
340. Zembowicz, A., and Vane, J. R.: Induction of nitric oxide synthase activity by toxic shock syndrome toxin 1 in a macrophage-monocyte cell line. Proc. Natl. Acad. Sci. U. S. A. *89*:2051-2055, 1992.
341. Zumla, A.: Superantigens, T cells and microbes. Clin. Infect. Dis. *15*:313-320, 1992.

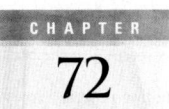

ACUTE RESPIRATORY DISTRESS SYNDROME IN CHILDREN

CHAPTER 72

Christopher M. Oermann ⬥ **Peter W. Hiatt**

Ashbaugh and associates[11] first used the term *adult respiratory distress syndrome* in a case series that they reported in 1967. In it, they described a clinical syndrome of diverse etiology that was characterized by the development of fulminant respiratory failure associated with rapidly progressive bilateral pulmonary infiltrates in the absence of cardiac failure. Although the mortality rate in their patients was 67 percent, four individuals treated with continuous positive airway pressure and high positive end-expiratory pressure (PEEP) survived. Postmortem examination of the lungs from nonsurvivors revealed significant pulmonary edema and hyaline membrane formation. They assumed that the presence of hyaline membranes and the favorable response to positive pressure indicated an acquired surfactant deficiency. The term *adult respiratory distress syndrome* was used as an analogy to neonatal respiratory distress syndrome (hyaline membrane disease)

caused by insufficient surfactant production and is now referred to as *acute respiratory distress syndrome* (ARDS).

ARDS now is recognized as a relatively common sequela of a variety of local or systemic diseases that result in damage to the vascular endothelium, alveolar epithelium, and alveolar-capillary membrane. Compromise of these structures leads to the final common pathway of ARDS: pulmonary vascular leak, noncardiogenic pulmonary edema, and respiratory failure. The clinical syndrome consists of tachypnea, dyspnea, and marked hypoxemia caused by edema and reduced total lung compliance. Radiographs demonstrate diffuse bilateral opacities. Although considerable research has been conducted in an attempt to identify factors predisposing individuals to ARDS and even more in therapeutic trials, ARDS remains poorly understood and therapy is primarily supportive. Even though mortality rates in adults and children have decreased during the past 20 years, ARDS remains a life-threatening disease.[77,102,123]

ARDS initially was described in adults, but it has been recognized as a leading cause of mortality in pediatric patients in critical care units. More than 500 cases have been reported in children ranging in age from 2 weeks to 17 years.* The true incidence of pediatric ARDS is unknown but has been estimated to be between 8.5 and 10.4 cases per 100 pediatric intensive care unit (ICU) admissions.[107] The prevalence rate of ARDS in pediatric patients in ICUs has been reported to be 0.6 to 7.2 percent.[23,27] A recent population-based study of pediatric ARDS in Germany reported a prevalence of 5.5×10^{-5} cases per year and an incidence of 3.4×10^{-5} cases per year.[18] As in adults, ARDS in children can result from a variety of injuries that all lead to increased vascular permeability, pulmonary edema, and clinical respiratory failure. Also as in adults, ARDS develops in most children as a result of sepsis, pneumonia, and aspiration.[30,33,44,91,141] Advances in supportive therapy for ARDS have improved outcomes in adults, and the results of several adult clinical trials have been extrapolated for use in children. The overall mortality rates have decreased in both adults and children during the past decade, with recent pediatric studies reporting mortality rates of 22 to 31 percent.[30,33,35,44,141]

DEFINITION

Defining ARDS has been the source of much confusion and, at times, heated debate. Initially, ARDS signified a disease of adults, but the reporting of numerous cases in children prompted the use of *acute* rather than *adult* respiratory distress syndrome. Although both terms occasionally appear, *acute respiratory distress syndrome* currently is the preferred designation. Early attempts at defining ARDS resulted in the use of criteria proposed by the National Heart, Lung, and Blood Institute (NHLBI) that included (1) acute and rapidly progressing pulmonary disease of a noncardiac nature; (2) progressive, diffuse, bilateral pulmonary infiltrates on chest radiographs; and (3) hypoxemia, defined as a ratio of arterial oxygen tension to the fractional concentration of inspired oxygen (Pao_2/Fio_2) of less than 150 without PEEP or less than 200 with PEEP. Continued interest in the systematic study of ARDS from epidemiologic and therapeutic standpoints, combined with continued difficulty in comparing data because of differences in definition, led to the formation of an international discussion group. The European-American Consensus Committee on ARDS then published a unifying definition of ARDS that included (1) impaired oxygenation with a Pao_2/Fio_2 ratio less than 200, regardless of PEEP; (2) bilateral densities demonstrated on chest radiographs; and (3) pulmonary artery wedge pressure less than 18 mm Hg with no evidence of left atrial hypertension.[15] Although this definition of ARDS in pediatric populations is widely accepted, recent evaluation suggests that the Pao_2/Fio_2 ratio used may need to be modified in children.[103]

PATHOPHYSIOLOGY

The pathophysiologic abnormalities associated with ARDS, though studied extensively since the syndrome was originally described in 1967, remain incompletely understood. A host of seemingly unrelated systemic diseases and local insults to the respiratory tract have been reported to result in ARDS. Despite efforts to elucidate the precise chain of events that lead from these initial triggers to massive cellular injury and rapidly pro-

gressive respiratory failure, much of the process remains a mystery. Nonetheless, certain cellular and biochemical markers, as well as physiologic characteristics associated with ARDS, have been identified. In addition, the histologic findings seen in ARDS follow a characteristic pattern that has been well described. These pathophysiologic events and findings generally correlate with the clinical findings seen in ARDS.

As mentioned earlier, a wide variety of apparently unrelated disorders and injuries have been associated with the development of ARDS[22,26,33,35,70,91,107,135] and include a broad spectrum of infections (bacterial, viral, and other), inhalation/aspiration injuries, sepsis syndromes, trauma, drug reactions and metabolic disorders, transfusion and stem cell transplantation reactions, and malignancies, among other causes (Tables 72–1 and 72–2). Although the mechanism or mechanisms of injury that unite this group are unknown, underlying damage to the vascular endothelium, alveolar epithelium, or alveolar-capillary membrane (or any combination of such damage) clearly must be present. Several hypotheses have been proposed and are summarized in review articles.[105,111] These hypotheses include activation of the complement cascade, excessive neutrophil and macrophage activity, surfactant dysfunction, and others. A more recent review of ARDS summarizes the importance of disruption of the alveolar-capillary barrier and its constituents—the microvascular endothelium and the alveolar epithelium.[145]

Complement activation occurs after trauma, pancreatic damage, endothelial damage, exposure to endotoxin, and other systemic and respiratory injuries.[99] By-products of complement activation then cause recruitment and activation of neutrophils, which in turn escalate the inflammatory cycle and damage the

TABLE 72–1   Noninfectious Conditions Associated with Acute Respiratory Distress Syndrome

Direct Injury to the Lung	Secondary Injury to the Lung
Inhalation	Anaphylaxis
NO_2	Shock—any cause
Cl_2	Sepsis
SO_2	Trauma
NH_3	Multiple trauma
Phosgene	Fractures
Smoke	Burns
Oxygen toxicity	Head trauma
Aspiration	Blood disorders
Foreign body	Diffuse intravascular coagulation
Gastric fluid (especially	Massive blood transfusion
with a pH < 2.5)	Drug overdose
Near drowning (fresh or	Heroin
salt water)	Methadone
Hydrocarbons	Barbiturates
Emboli	Ethchlorvynol
Air	Salicylates
Fat	Propoxyphene
Amniotic fluid	Deferoxamine
Pulmonary contusion	Metabolic disorders
Radiation pneumonitis	Diabetic ketoacidosis
Asphyxiation/strangulation	Uremia
	Pancreatitis
	Increased intracranial pressure
	Cardiopulmonary bypass
	Hemodialysis
	Cardioversion
	Paraquat ingestion
	Malignancy/lymphoproliferative disorder

From Royall, J. A., and Levin, D. L.: Adult respiratory distress syndrome in pediatric patients. I. Clinical aspects, pathophysiology, pathology, and mechanisms of lung injury. J. Pediatr. 112:169-180, 1988.

---

*See references 13, 27, 33, 35, 53, 59, 70, 84, 90, 107, 109, 111, 112, 136.

TABLE 72–2 Infectious Conditions Associated with Acute Respiratory Distress Syndrome in Children

Author	Year	No. of Patients	Mortality	Viral Isolates	Bacterial Isolates	Fungal	Other
Lyrene and Troug[70]	1981	15	9/15 (60%)	0	*Enterococcus*	0	0
Pfenninger et al.[91]	1982	20	8/20 (40%)	0	Intra-abdominal process, 7/20, NS	0	0
Nussbaum[79]	1983	7	2/7 (29%)	0	*Haemophilus influenzae* type b	0	0
Katz et al.[59]	1984	23	8/23 (35%)	2/23, NS	*Pneumococcus*	0	0
Tamburro et al.[128]	1991	37	19/37 (51%)	Adenovirus, cytomegalovirus, varicella	*Staphylococcus aureus*	0	0
DeBruin et al.*[35]	1992	100	72/100 (72%)	HIV, cytomegalovirus, respiratory syncytial virus	Septic shock syndrome, 64/100, NS; *Bordetella pertussis*	5/100, NS	*Pneumocystis carinii*, 14/100
Davis et al.[33]	1993	60	37/60 (62%)	Respiratory syncytial virus, influenza virus, cytomegalovirus, varicella	Sepsis syndrome, 22/60, NS	4/60, NS	0

*Children with malignancy, compromised immunity, or both.
HIV, human immunodeficiency virus; NS, organism not specified.

pulmonary parenchyma through the release of oxygen radicals, proteolytic enzymes, and eicosanoids. A strong association has been demonstrated between complement activation and the development of ARDS.[50] However, other investigators have reported that complement activation is nonspecific in predicting the development of ARDS.[40,64,83,150] Additional evidence suggests that the combination of circulating endotoxin and complement activation is potentially more important in the development of ARDS than is complement activation alone.[82] Complement activation further stimulates an inflammatory cascade involving tumor necrosis factor-α (TNF-α), interleukin-1β (IL-1β), IL-6, IL-8, and other mediators.[14] Additional studies suggest possible roles for other proinflammatory elements, as well as genetic influences related to the inflammatory response.[31,48,89]

Significant, though again not conclusive, evidence suggests a key role for neutrophils in the genesis of ARDS.[14,129] Once activated, neutrophils can damage the lung parenchyma by the release of proteolytic enzymes, generation of toxic oxygen radicals, and initiation of arachidonic acid metabolism. Numerous studies have indicated potential roles for superoxide radicals in the development of ARDS or the presence of elevated concentrations of peroxide in the breath of ARDS patients.[54,124,125] Patients with ARDS similarly have elevated concentrations of elastase and collagenase and increased leukotriene B4 in bronchoalveolar lavage fluid, findings consistent with neutrophil degranulation.[124,127] Although neutrophils are capable of causing widespread parenchymal lung damage, are characteristically found in ARDS, and probably play some role in the pathogenesis or propagation of ARDS (or both), the occurrence of ARDS in severely neutropenic individuals suggests that they are not essential or singly responsible for its development.[80,115]

Alveolar macrophages may play a critical role in the pathogenesis of ARDS. They are found in abundance in normal airways, and when stimulated by endotoxin or endogenous proinflammatory cytokines, alveolar macrophages synthesize and release TNF and IL-1.[111] Both products promote neutrophil chemotaxis, degranulation, and release of oxygen metabolites, thereby creating a cycle of inflammation within the pulmonary parenchyma. Administration of TNF to animals in experimental models produces pulmonary edema, decreased pulmonary compliance, increased cellularity, and increased lung water, the primary physiologic markers of ARDS.[121,138,139] Conversely, anti-TNF antibody offered protection from ARDS in a baboon septicemia model.[140]

In his review article, Royall[105] also discusses putative roles for oxygen radicals, platelet-derived eicosanoids, proteolytic enzymes, fibrin and its degradation products, and other processes that may be involved in the pathogenesis of ARDS. Likewise, secondary injuries, such as acquired surfactant deficiency, oxygen toxicity, and barotrauma, are thought to contribute to the pulmonary damage. As noted in the same article, a single mediator or mechanism probably is not responsible for all the findings seen in ARDS, and simultaneous activity on several fronts most likely occurs.

The physiologic hallmark of ARDS is damage to the capillary endothelium and alveolar epithelial barriers, leading to disruption of the alveolar-capillary membrane, increased permeability, and noncardiogenic pulmonary edema.[107] Increasing fluid within the alveoli and interstitial spaces leads to decreased total lung compliance, decreased functional residual capacity, increased airway resistance, and increased dead space. The resultant ventilation-perfusion mismatch creates the large intrapulmonary shunt responsible for the profound hypoxemia seen clinically.[63] Additional physiologic derangements seen in ARDS include alterations in peripheral oxygen delivery and consumption, pulmonary hypertension with right ventricular compromise, and end-organ damage (liver, kidney, intestine, bone marrow).[23,111,148]

The histologic findings seen at postmortem examination of patients dying as a result of ARDS are very consistent and have been well described.[12,60,95,137] Historically, three interrelated and overlapping phases are described. They correlate well with clinical progression of the syndrome and include the exudative, proliferative, and fibrotic phases.[14] The early exudative phase typically is recognized from 12 to 96 hours after the onset of respiratory failure.[107,111,137] It is characterized by increased fluid in the alveoli and interstitium and hemorrhagic alveolitis. Grossly, the lungs are rigid, dusky, red-blue, and very heavy.[137] The alveolar fluid is protein-rich, often hemorrhagic, and associated with hyaline membranes.[95] A combined neutrophilic and monocytic infiltrate is observed in the pulmonary capillaries, interstitium, and alveoli (Fig. 72–1A). Although capillaries also contain fibrin plugs and microthrombi, endothelial cells show only subtle abnormalities when compared with the alveolar surfaces, which undergo degeneration and sloughing.[107]

The proliferative phase occurs 3 to 10 days after the onset of ARDS and is characterized by organization of the alveolar and interstitial exudates acquired during the exudative phase.[137] Gross examination reveals the lungs to be solid, pale gray, and slippery because of the generation of connective tissue. The proliferation of type II cuboidal epithelial cells occurs as early as 3 days after onset, with fibrosis visible by 10 days. Type II pneumocytes are metabolically active and responsible for the production of surfactant, and they evolve into the type I epithelial cells that line the alveolar spaces (see Fig. 72–1B). Within the alveolar walls, fibro-

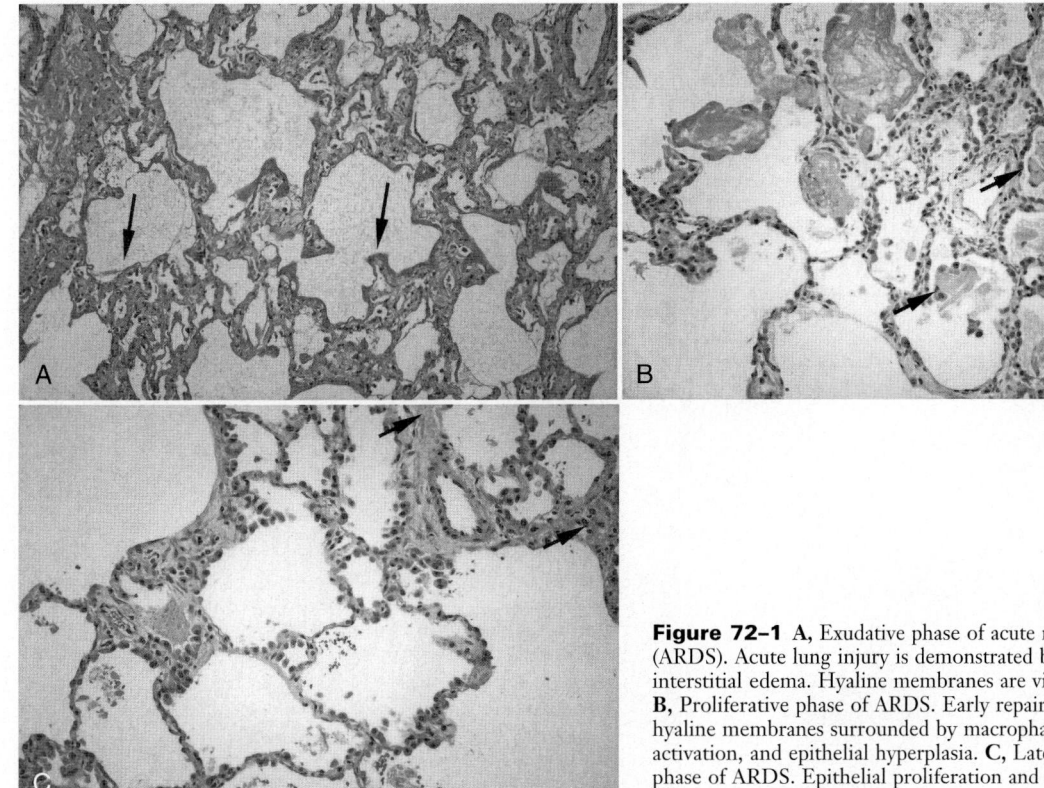

Figure 72–1 A, Exudative phase of acute respiratory distress syndrome (ARDS). Acute lung injury is demonstrated by diffuse alveolar and interstitial edema. Hyaline membranes are visible within the alveoli (*arrows*). **B,** Proliferative phase of ARDS. Early repair is evident, with residual hyaline membranes surrounded by macrophages (*arrows*), early fibroblast activation, and epithelial hyperplasia. **C,** Late proliferative to early fibrotic phase of ARDS. Epithelial proliferation and hyperplasia persist with increasing evidence of fibroblast activation (*arrows*).

blasts and myofibroblasts also proliferate and migrate through the basement membrane into the alveolar space. In addition, early resolution of the hyaline membranes and pulmonary edema begins. This phase is considered to be reparative in nature.

Phase III, the fibrotic stage, begins to develop 7 to 10 days after the onset of respiratory failure and is characterized by progressive fibrosis that distorts the primary acinar architecture of the lung. The lungs appear pale and spongy with a cobblestone surface. Cellularity is reduced, alveolar fluid organizes, and fibrosis develops in and around the terminal respiratory units (see Fig. 72–1C). Airspaces are irregularly enlarged and separated by thick bands of collagenous connective tissue. Extensive fibrosis appears to be related to irreversible respiratory failure.[12]

CLINICAL MANIFESTATIONS

The clinical features of ARDS are a reflection of the pathophysiologic changes previously discussed and generally follow a typical course regardless of the initiating event or injury. The syndrome progresses through four stages: the acute injury, a latent period, acute respiratory failure, and a period of severe physiologic derangement.[105,107,111] During the period of acute injury, the physical, laboratory, and radiographic findings associated with the causative disease or injury generally overshadow those associated with ARDS itself. Disorders associated with primary lung injury (e.g., aspiration pneumonitis or inhalation injury) may demonstrate significant physical or radiographic findings, whereas individuals with trauma or sepsis syndromes may have entirely normal auscultative or radiographic examinations of the chest.

The latent period is said to occur from 6 to 48 hours after the onset of ARDS and is characterized by cardiopulmonary stabilization or even improvement in the patient's condition. Subtle physical examination findings (mild tachypnea), radiographic findings (fine reticular infiltrates), and laboratory abnormalities (increased $Paco_2$, increased pulmonary vascular resistance, decreased tissue oxygen delivery, increased serum von Willebrand factor antigen) may suggest the development of ARDS during this phase.[1,108,114]

The diagnosis of ARDS generally is made during the period of acute respiratory failure and is based on appropriate clinical and laboratory findings supportive of the diagnosis combined with a preexisting condition known to be associated with ARDS. The physical examination is remarkable for tachypnea, tachycardia, dyspnea, and cyanosis. The chest is quiet generally, but fine crackles may be present. Hypoxemia refractory to supplemental oxygen therapy is one of the hallmarks of the syndrome. Chest radiographs demonstrate diffuse, bilateral infiltrates suggestive of both interstitial fluid and alveolar filling or atelectasis (Fig. 72–2). Computed tomography may be helpful in characterizing the nature of the pulmonary infiltrates or even distinguishing the cause of the ARDS.[38] Respiratory failure and profound hypoxemia require intubation. The hypoxemia often worsens rapidly despite assisted ventilation, and many patients progress to the phase of severe physiologic abnormalities. During this stage, hypoxemia and hypercapnia refractory to high levels of ventilatory support often denote an irreversible pulmonary process. Multiorgan system failure frequently ensues at this point. The clinical course thereafter depends on the severity and character of the initial illness and the development of complications such as sepsis, disseminated intravascular coagulation, and pulmonary air leak syndromes.

TREATMENT

Although tremendous energy and resources have been invested in research aimed at defining the mechanism of lung injury in

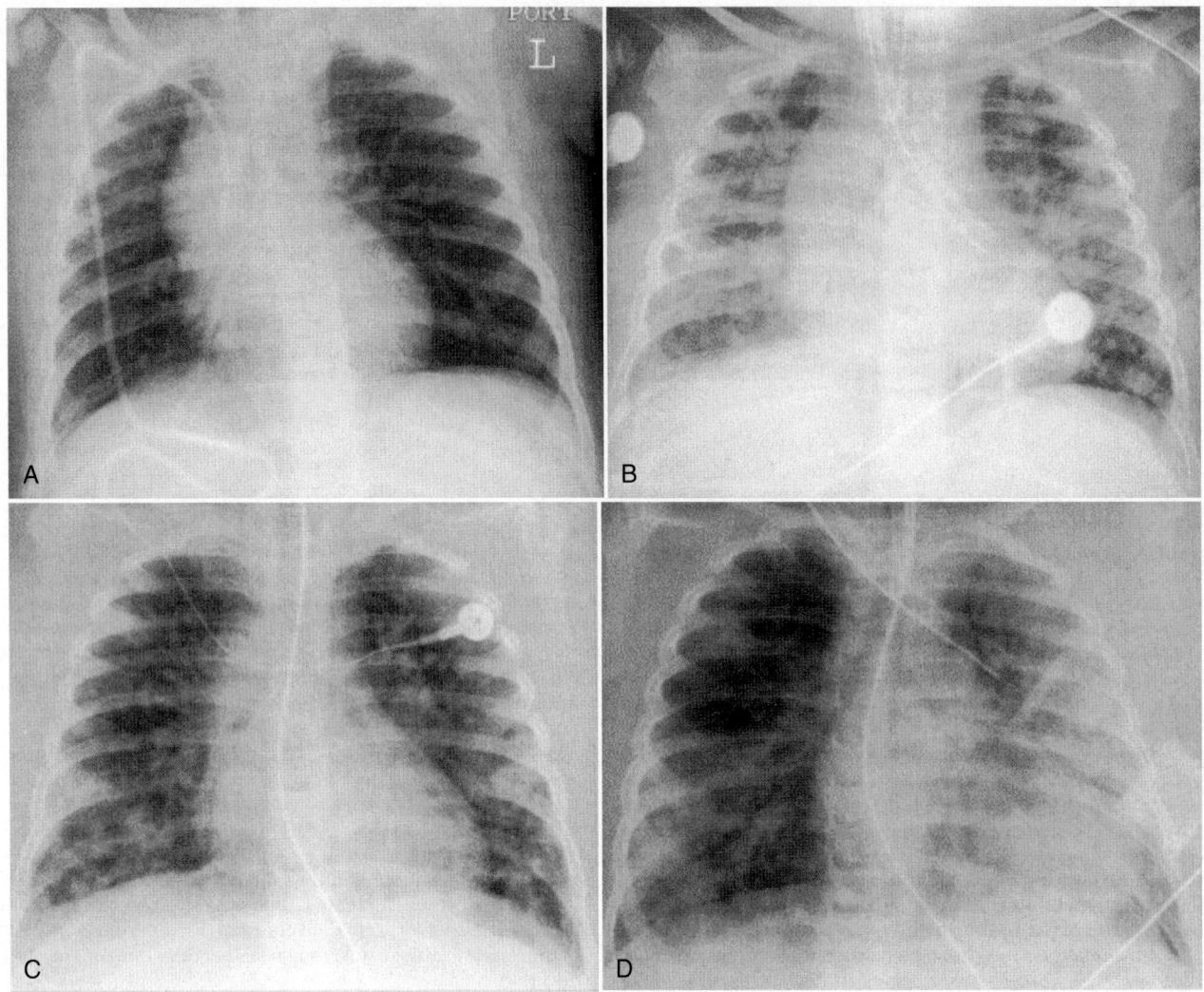

Figure 72–2 Chest radiographs of a 4-year-old child with central line sepsis and acute respiratory distress syndrome. Note the diffuse bilateral infiltrates suggestive of alveolar filling, interstitial fluid, and atelectasis. The time from **A** to **B** was 24 hours, but the intervals from **B** to **C** and from **C** to **D** were several days.

ARDS, a definitive answer and, thus, definitive therapeutic interventions have remained elusive. For this reason, management of ARDS historically has been primarily supportive. The traditional goals of therapy have been to treat the underlying or predisposing condition, maintain adequate end-organ oxygenation through the use of oxygen and supportive ventilation, and minimize complications of therapy or acute/chronic illness (oxygen toxicity, barotrauma, nosocomial infections, negative nitrogen balance, and multisystem organ dysfunction).[106,111] Only in the past decade have significant advances been made in improving supportive care and have attempts been made to treat some of the underlying pathologies encountered in ARDS.

Both Sarnaik and Lieh-Lai[111] and Royall[105] have stressed the importance of adequate monitoring of patients with ARDS. Invasive and noninvasive monitoring modalities allow the physician to assess pulmonary mechanics, the adequacy of peripheral oxygen delivery and consumption, cardiac function, and other critical physiologic parameters. Pulse oximetry, arterial catheters, and central venous pressure monitors are suggested as a minimum, with the use of pulmonary artery catheters as indicated by the patient's clinical status.

Positive-pressure ventilation is a major component of care for patients with ARDS. Several randomized trials have evaluated the usefulness of low–tidal volume ventilation as a method to improve survival and decrease complications. Experimental animal data suggested that high–tidal volume ventilation was associated with inflammation and increased release of inflammatory mediators from the lung into the systemic circulation (e.g., TNF-α, IL-6) when compared with low–tidal volume ventilation strategies.[62,142] Initial human trials with relatively small sample sizes yielded conflicting results.[5,20,21,122] A large multicenter trial sponsored by the NHLBI's ARDS Network (ARMA) enrolled 861 patients at ten sites to compare a ventilatory protocol consisting of tidal volumes of less than 6 mL/kg with conventional ventilation using higher tidal volumes. Plateau pressures were maintained at less than that of 30 cm H_2O.[132] The study reported that the group undergoing low–tidal volume ventilation had a lower rate of mortality than that of controls (31% versus 40%), more mean days free of mechanical ventilation, and more days free of nonpulmonary organ failure. Thus, high tidal volumes and high plateau pressures were associated with worse outcomes in patients treated for ARDS and should be avoided if possible in these patients. Other treatment parameters outlined in the publication suggest maintaining pH between 7.3 to 7.45 by changing the respiratory rate and adjusting the fraction of inspired oxygen and PEEP to achieve adequate oxygenation (Pao_2, 55 to 80 mm Hg, or Spo_2, 88%-95%).

High-frequency oscillation is a mode of ventilation that delivers small tidal volumes and has been proposed as a better method of ventilation for ARDS. Two randomized trials in adults and one in children demonstrated improved oxygenation in patients receiving high-frequency ventilation, but mortality rates were not significantly different from those of patients undergoing conventional ventilation.[10,19,37] These studies had considerably fewer patients than did the ARMA trial. Pediatric case series suggest that this mode of ventilation is safe and can be used as rescue therapy; however, large randomized trials in pediatrics are needed.[9,55,94] The role of high-frequency oscillation versus low–tidal volume ventilation in the routine treatment of ARDS remains to be determined and will require further investigation.

The historical approach to the respiratory management of ARDS has focused on the use of oxygen and PEEP. PEEP is a critical component of mechanical ventilation in the treatment of patients with ARDS. Hypoxemia is profound in patients with ARDS and is refractory to supplemental oxygen given by face mask. The vast majority of patients require intubation and supportive mechanical ventilation. Once the patient is intubated, high concentrations of supplemental oxygen and high levels of PEEP often are needed. PEEP improves pulmonary function in ARDS by reducing ventilation-perfusion mismatch and decreasing intrapulmonary shunting,[32,113] which is accomplished by increasing functional residual capacity by enlarging open alveoli and recruiting atelectatic airspaces. PEEP additionally reduces the repetitive expansion and collapse of terminal airways and redistributes alveolar fluid. The improved lung compliance and decreased ventilation-perfusion mismatch may allow a reduction in F_{IO_2}, thereby decreasing the potential for oxygen toxicity and possibly protecting the lung.[87,151]

Although PEEP is used to treat patients with ARDS, the optimal values have not been established. Several randomized trials have not demonstrated a significant change in mortality rates with increased levels of PEEP.[132,134,144] To determine the effect of high PEEP in the treatment of ARDS, the NHLBI sponsored a multicenter randomized trial comparing patients randomized to high PEEP (12-24 cm H_2O) with a comparable group randomized to low PEEP (5-24 cm H_2O).[134] No significant differences were observed between the two groups in mortality rates, yet the high-PEEP group had improved oxygenation. All patients in the trial were ventilated with low tidal volumes. Mean days of mechanical ventilation and the duration of nonpulmonary organ failure were comparable in both groups. Thus, PEEP should be used to maintain adequate oxygenation, yet the optimal pressure will vary, depending on the severity of the patient's disease.

PEEP significantly improves ventilation-perfusion mismatch, but it can affect cardiac output. Decreased venous return to the heart and a shift in the interventricular cardiac septum can occur with high pressure. These complications are treated by a reduction in left ventricular afterload. PEEP should be used to maximize oxygen delivery at the lowest pressure that achieves this goal. Additional methods of improving mechanical ventilation are prone positioning, inverse-ratio ventilation, partial liquid ventilation, and noninvasive ventilation. Randomized controlled trials of prone positioning have demonstrated that improved oxygenation is achieved with a change in positioning; however, mortality rates in these trials did not significantly decrease with its use.[28,46,49,71,98] For selected patients with an F_{IO_2} requirement of greater than 0.6 or refractory hypoxemia, use of the prone position may be helpful. Because extubation is a potential complication with repositioning, prone positioning should be used with caution at centers unfamiliar with this technique. Studies using perfluorocarbons for partial liquid ventilation have not shown improved outcomes over standard methods of ventilation.[52,56] Noninvasive positive-pressure ventilation is useful in selected

patients with acute lung injury, such as pediatric cancer,[92] but it will not provide sufficient ventilatory support for the majority of patients with ARDS.

Many of the predisposing conditions associated with ARDS result in cardiovascular instability. Cardiovascular function should be monitored and maintained with additional therapies (e.g., inotropic agents, fluids) as needed. Patients seen in the early stages of septic shock often require vigorous fluid resuscitation to maintain adequate tissue perfusion.[101] Once the patient has been stabilized for a minimum of 12 hours, a conservative fluid strategy to maintain cardiovascular function and keep the patient's fluid balance stable with no net gain should be considered. A large randomized trial by the Acute Respiratory Distress Network reported more ventilator-free days and ICU-free days with a conservative fluid treatment approach than with a liberal fluid strategy; however, no significant differences were observed in mortality rates.[4] Furthermore, the need for renal dialysis and the prevalence of shock were not significantly different between the conservative and liberal fluid management groups. Patients in shock still should receive fluid resuscitation as needed and would not be candidates for the conservative fluid management strategy. Colloid or crystalloid is used for volume resuscitation.[24,152] A recent large randomized trial reported the equivalence of saline resuscitation and albumin volume resuscitation[43]; however, albumin with furosemide may be useful in patients with hypoproteinemia.[6] Once patients are hemodynamically stable, fluids are restricted to decrease vascular leak and subsequent pulmonary edema. Patients frequently are given diuretics to reduce fluid in the interstitium and alveoli. Positive inotropic support with dopamine or dobutamine may be required.

The overall goal of cardiopulmonary management of ARDS is to maintain good cardiac output and optimize oxygen delivery to the periphery. Other important aspects of the supportive care required for management of ARDS include maintenance of adequate nutrition, avoidance or treatment of complications related to therapy (barotrauma and oxygen toxicity) or prolonged illness (infection), and support of other organ systems.[106] Poor nutrition is a common problem in critically ill children and results in inadequate tissue repair, multiple organ system dysfunction, respiratory muscle weakness, and immune deficiency.[93,120] Hence, nutritional support is of paramount importance in ARDS and must be maintained.[97] The related issues of oxygen toxicity and barotrauma are considered later. Infection is both a common precipitating event in ARDS and an important factor in its course and outcome.[106] Infections typically take the form of bacteremia/sepsis or nosocomial pneumonia. Organisms frequently isolated from the lower respiratory tract are *Klebsiella* and *Pseudomonas*; however, *Escherichia coli*, *Candida albicans*, and *Staphylococcus epidermidis* are not uncommon isolates.[111] A high index of suspicion and a low threshold for initiating therapy should be maintained. Finally, prevention, detection, and treatment of multisystem organ dysfunction or its complications are critical in the overall management of children with ARDS.

As suggested earlier, many of the innovations in the supportive care of ARDS have come in the arena of ventilatory support. Pressure-limited ventilation with a reversed inspiratory-to-expiratory ratio, permissive hypercapnia, high-frequency ventilation (positive pressure, jet, and oscillating), prone positioning, and extracorporeal membrane oxygenation have been reported.* Patients unresponsive to conventional mechanical ventilation may benefit, in terms of improved oxygenation, from any of these methods. Additionally, patients may benefit from lower F_{IO_2} and peak airway pressure to decrease the potential oxygen toxicity and barotrauma. Although many of these newer forms of ventilation

*See references 5, 10, 47, 51, 57, 61, 65, 67, 84, 85.

show promise for children with ARDS, none has been demonstrated conclusively to be superior to another, and all will require more research and clinical experience. At present, many of them are considered "rescue therapy."

Numerous pharmacologic agents have been used for the treatment of ARDS during the past decade. Therapeutic trials with corticosteroids, vasodilators, and prostaglandin E_1 have been reported.[7,16,29,106,149] Improved outcomes have been achieved with short-course corticosteroid therapy for early-phase ARDS and moderate-dose therapy for prolonged ARDS, yet a 7-year multicenter trial did not find a change in mortality rates with moderate-dose methylprednisolone for 14 days in patients with persistent ARDS.[6,25,43,45,72,100,101,133,152] In addition, starting corticosteroid therapy more than 2 weeks after the onset of ARDS was associated with increased mortality rates at 60 and 180 days.[133] Few data exist on the benefits of steroid therapy in pediatrics. Therefore, the role of corticosteroid therapy in the routine treatment of ARDS remains unresolved at the present time. Small trials with a host of other agents have failed to identify universally effective therapies.[61,75] Among the many pharmacologic agents studied, corticosteroid therapy, exogenous surfactant, and inhaled nitric oxide (NO) have been evaluated in large, multicenter trials.

The relative or acquired surfactant deficiency seen in ARDS renders surfactant replacement therapy an attractive area of investigation. In 1993, Lewis and Jobe[66] presented a comprehensive review of the rationale behind surfactant use in ARDS. Theoretically, replacement of endogenous surfactant by exogenous material would increase total lung compliance, decrease atelectasis, and improve pulmonary mechanics, thereby leading to decreased ventilation-perfusion mismatch, improved oxygenation, and less potential oxygen toxicity and barotrauma. The results of several trials have been reported in recent years and appear to offer some hope of improving outcomes in children with ARDS.[41,68,73,117,126,154] Early phase I and II trials in adults were encouraging, but larger randomized trials with synthetic surfactant[8] and natural and recombinant surfactant[118,119] have not demonstrated improvement in the mortality rate. In contrast, a recent randomized trial in children reported a decrease in the mortality rate and improved oxygenation.[153] The randomized trial enrolled 153 infants, children, and adolescents with acute lung injury. Although the mortality rate was greater in the placebo group, no significant differences were observed in the number of ventilator-free days or the duration of respiratory failure. Problems with surfactant therapy include difficulty with delivery and inactivation by lung fluid proteins. As the aforementioned references suggest, solutions to these and other issues related to surfactant therapy for ARDS are being sought aggressively, and researchers hope that surfactant will prove to be a valuable therapy in the future.

Another area of active research for the treatment of ARDS is the use of inhaled NO. NO has been shown to be a potent vasodilator and has been used in numerous settings for infants and children with a variety of cardiopulmonary diseases.[3,58] Numerous clinical trials have suggested a potential role for NO in the treatment of ARDS.[2,34,36,59,76,78,81] However, several randomized trials have not reported a reduction in mortality rates with its use. Improved oxygenation is observed on initiation of therapy, but it often is transient, with the effect lasting just a few days.[36,69,76,104,130,143] NO should be considered rescue therapy pending further investigation.[116,131] Some authors have questioned its use altogether.[74,86] Additional study is required to answer questions regarding the best use of NO therapy for ARDS. Other pharmacologic agents being investigated for the treatment of ARDS include beta-agonists,[88] granulocyte-macrophage colony-stimulating factor (GM-CSF),[96] and activated protein C.[17,110,146,147]

PROGNOSIS

Despite the huge investments of time, money, energy, and talent that have gone into research on the basic pathophysiologic mechanisms involved in the development of ARDS and equal amounts into potential therapies, many questions remain unanswered. Mortality rates have decreased during the past decade since this disease first was described in children. Mortality rates have decreased from 40 to 70 percent (see Table 72–2) to 20 to 31 percent.[30,44,141] New supportive and therapeutic interventions have improved the care of children with ARDS. Most children who survive ARDS eventually have normal radiographic results, and pulmonary function improves gradually with only a mild reduction in forced vital capacity.[42] Long-term physiologic abnormalities show a strong correlation with the severity of the acute illness and the degree of support required in the acute phase of ARDS. The search for innovative therapies to decrease the acuity of illness during the acute phase of the disease and reduce the incidence of iatrogenic complications holds some hope for the future.

REFERENCES

1. Aberle, D. R., and Brown, K.: Radiologic considerations in the adult respiratory distress syndrome. Clin. Chest Med. 11:737-754, 1990.
2. Abman, S. H., Griebel, J. L., Parker, D. K., et al.: Acute effects of inhaled nitric oxide in children with severe hypoxemic respiratory failure. J. Pediatr. 124:881-888, 1994.
3. Abman, S. H., and Kinsella, J. P.: Inhaled nitric oxide therapy for pulmonary disease in pediatrics. Curr. Opin. Pediatr. 10:236-242, 1998.
4. Acute Respiratory Distress Syndrome Network: Comparison of two fluid-management strategies in acute lung injury. N. Engl. J. Med. 354:2564-2575, 2006.
5. Amato, M. B., Barbas, C. S., Medeiros, D. M., et al.: Effect of a protective-ventilation strategy on mortality in the acute respiratory distress syndrome. N. Engl. J. Med. 338:347-354, 1998.
6. American Thoracic Society: Evidence-based colloid use in the critically ill: American Thoracic Society consensus statement. Am. J. Respir. Crit. Care Med. 170:1247-1259, 2004.
7. Annest, S. J., Rhodes, G. R., Stratton, H. H., et al.: Increased intrapulmonary shunt following infusion of nitroglycerine or nitroprusside in patients with posttraumatic respiratory distress. Surg. Forum 30:22-24, 1979.
8. Anzueto, A., Baughman, R. P., Guntupalli, K. K., et al.: Aerosolized surfactant in adults with sepsis-induced acute respiratory distress syndrome: Exosurf Acute Respiratory Distress Syndrome Sepsis Study Group. N. Engl. J. Med. 334:1417-1421, 1996.
9. Arnold, J. H., Anas, N. G., Luckett, P., et al.: High frequency oscillatory ventilation in pediatric respiratory failure: A multicenter experience. Crit. Care Med. 28:3912-3919, 2000.
10. Arnold, J. H., Hanson, J. H., Toro-Figuero, L. O., et al.: Prospective, randomized comparison of high-frequency oscillatory ventilation and conventional mechanical ventilation in pediatric respiratory failure. Crit. Care Med. 22:1530-1539, 1994.
11. Ashbaugh, D. G., Bigelow, D. B., Petty, T. L., et al.: Acute respiratory distress in adults. Lancet 2:319-323, 1967.
12. Bachofen, M., and Weibel, E. R.: Structural alterations of lung parenchyma in the adult respiratory distress syndrome. Clin. Chest Med. 3:35-56, 1982.
13. Beaufils, F., Mercier, J. C., Farnoux, C., et al.: Acute respiratory distress syndrome in children. Curr. Opin. Pediatr. 9:207-212, 1997.
14. Bellingan, G. J.: The pulmonary physician in critical care—6: The pathogenesis of ALI/ARDS. Thorax 57:540-546, 2002.
15. Bernard, G. R., Artigas, A., Brigham, K. L., et al.: The American-European Consensus Conference on ARDS. Definitions, mechanisms, relevant outcomes, and clinical trial coordination. Am. J. Respir. Crit. Care Med. 149:818-824, 1994.
16. Bernard, G. R., Luce, J. M., Sprung, C. L., et al.: High-dose corticosteroids in patients with the adult respiratory distress syndrome. N. Engl. J. Med. 317:1565-1570, 1987.
17. Bernard, G. R., Vincent, J. L., Laterre, P. F., et al.: Efficacy and safety of recombinant human activated protein C for severe sepsis. N. Engl. J. Med. 344:699-709, 2001.
18. Bindl, L., Dresbach, K., Lentze, M. J.: Incidence of acute respiratory distress syndrome in German children and adolescents: A population-based study. Crit. Care Med. 33:209-312, 2005.
19. Bollen, C. W., van Well, G. T., Sherry, T., et al.: High frequency oscillatory ventilation compared with conventional mechanical ventilation in adult

respiratory distress syndrome: A randomized controlled trial. Crit. Care *9*: R430-R439, 2005.

20. Brochard, L., Roudot-Thoraval, F., Roupie, E., et al.: Tidal volume reduction for prevention of ventilator-induced lung injury in acute respiratory distress syndrome. Am. J. Respir. Crit. Care Med. *158*:1831-1838, 1998.

21. Brower, R. G., Shanholtz, C. B., Fessler, H. E., et al.: Prospective, randomized, controlled clinical trial comparing traditional versus reduced tidal volume ventilation in acute respiratory distress syndrome patients. Crit. Care Med. *27*:1492-1498, 1999.

22. Church, G. D., Price, C., Sanchez, R., and Looney, M. R.: Transfusion-related acute lung injury in the paediatric patient: Two case reports and a review of the literature. Transfus. Med. *16*:343-348, 2006.

23. Clarke, C., Edwards, J. D., Nightingale, P., et al.: Persistence of supply dependency of oxygen uptake at high levels of delivery in adult respiratory distress syndrome. Crit. Care Med. *19*:497-502, 1991.

24. Cochrane Injuries Group Albumin Reviewers: Human albumin administration in critically ill patients: Systematic review of randomised controlled trials. B. M. J. *317*:235-240, 1998.

25. Cook, D.: Is albumin safe? N. Engl. J. Med. *350*:2294-2296, 2004.

26. Cooke, K. R.: Acute lung injury after allogeneic stem cell transplantation: From the clinic, to the bench and back again. Pediatr. Transplant. *9*(Suppl. 7):25-36, 2005.

27. Costil, J., Cloup, M., Leclerc, F., et al.: Acute respiratory distress syndrome (ARDS) in children: Multicenter Collaborative Study of the French Group of Pediatric Intensive Care. Pediatr. Pulmonol. Suppl. *11*:106-107, 1995.

28. Curley, M. A., Hibberd, P. L., Fineman, L. D., et al.: Effect of prone positioning on clinical outcomes in children with acute lung injury: A randomized controlled trial. J. A. M. A. *294*:229-237, 2005.

29. Dahlem, P., van Aalderen, W. M., deNeef, M., et al.: Randomized controlled trial of aerosolized prostacyclin therapy in children with acute lung injury. Crit. Care Med. *32*:1055-1060, 2004.

30. Dahlem, P., van Aalderen, W. M., Hamaker, M. E., et al.: Incidence and short term outcome of acute lung injury in mechanically ventilated children. Eur. Respir. J. *22*:980-985, 2003.

31. Dal-Pizzol, F., Di Leone, L. P., Ritter, C., et al.: Gastrin-releasing peptide receptor antagonist effects on an animal model of sepsis. Am. J. Respir. Crit. Care Med. *173*:84-90, 2006.

32. Dantzker, D. R.: Gas exchange in the adult respiratory distress syndrome. Clin. Chest Med. *3*:57-67, 1982.

33. Davis, S. L., Furman, D. P., and Costarino, A. T.: ARDS in children: Associated disease, clinical course, and predictors of death. J. Pediatr. *123*:35-45, 1993.

34. Day, R. W., Allen, E. M., and Witte, M. K.: A randomised, controlled study of the 1-hour and 24-hour effects of inhaled nitric oxide therapy in children with acute hypoxemic respiratory failure. Chest *112*:1324-1331, 1997.

35. DeBruin, W., Notterman, D., Magid, M., et al.: Acute hypoxemic respiratory failure in infants and children: Clinical and pathologic characteristics. Crit. Care Med. *20*:1223-1234, 1992.

36. Dellinger, R. P., Zimmerman, J. L., Taylor, R. W., et al.: Effects of inhaled nitric oxide in patients with acute respiratory distress syndrome: Results of a randomized phase II trial. Inhaled Nitric Oxide in ARDS Study Group. Crit. Care Med. *26*:15-23, 1998.

37. Derdak, S., Mehta, S., Stewart, T. E., et al.: High-frequency oscillatory ventilation for acute respiratory distress syndrome in adults: A randomized, controlled trial. Am. J. Respir. Crit. Care Med. *166*:801-808, 2002.

38. Desai, S. R., and Hansell, D. M.: Lung imaging in the adult respiratory distress syndrome: Current practice and new insights. Intensive Care Med. *23*:7-15, 1997.

39. Dobyns, E. L., Cornfield, D. N., Anas, N. G., et al.: Multicenter randomized controlled trial of the effects of inhaled nitric oxide therapy on gas exchange in children with acute hypoxemic respiratory failure. J. Pediatr. *134*:406-412, 1999.

40. Duchateau, J., Haas, M., Schreyen, H., et al.: Complement activation in patients at risk of developing the adult respiratory distress syndrome. Am. Rev. Respir. Dis. *130*:1058-1064, 1984.

41. Evans, D. A., Wilmott, R. W., and Whitsett, J. A.: Surfactant replacement therapy for adult respiratory distress syndrome in children. Pediatr. Pulmonol. *21*:328-336, 1996.

42. Fanconi, S., Kraemer, R., Weber, J., et al.: Long-term sequelae in children surviving adult respiratory distress syndrome. J. Pediatr. *106*:218-222, 1985.

43. Finfer, S., Bellomo, R., Boyce, N., et al.: A comparison of albumin and saline for fluid resuscitation in the intensive care unit. N. Engl. J. Med. *350*:2247-2256, 2004.

44. Flori, H. R., Glidden, D. V., Rutherford, G. W., et al.: Pediatric acute lung injury: Prospective evaluation of risk factors associated with mortality. Am. J. Respir. Crit. Care Med. *171*:995-1001, 2005.

45. Freire, A. X., Bridges, L., Umpierrez, G. E., et al.: Admission hyperglycemia and other risk factors as predictors of hospital mortality in a medical ICU population. Chest *128*:3109-3116, 2005.

46. Gattinoni, L., Tognoni, G., Pesenti, A., et al.: Effect of prone positioning on the survival of patients with acute respiratory failure. N. Engl. J. Med. *345*:568-573, 2001.

47. Gauger, P. G., Pranikoff, T., Schreiner, R. J., et al.: Initial experience with partial liquid ventilation in pediatric patients with the acute respiratory distress syndrome. Crit. Care Med. *24*:16-22, 1996.

48. Gong, M. N.: Genetic epidemiology of acute respiratory distress syndrome: Implications for future prevention and treatment. Clin. Chest Med. *27*:705-724, 2006.

49. Guerin, C., Gaillard, S., Lemasson, S., et al.: Effects of systematic prone positioning in hypoxemic acute respiratory failure: A randomized controlled trial. J. A. M. A. *292*:2379-2387, 2004.

50. Hammerschmidt, D. E., Weaver, L. J., Hudson, L. D., et al.: Association of complement activation and elevated plasma-C5a with adult respiratory distress syndrome. Lancet *1*:947-949, 1980.

51. Hickling, K. G., Walsh, J., Henderson, S., et al.: Low mortality rate in adult respiratory distress syndrome using low-volume, pressure limited ventilation with permissive hypercapnia: A prospective study. Crit. Care Med. *22*:1568-1578, 1994.

52. Hirschl, R. B., Croce, M., Gore, D., et al.: Prospective, randomized, controlled pilot study of partial liquid ventilation in adult acute respiratory distress syndrome. Am. J. Respir. Crit. Care Med. *165*:781-787, 2002.

53. Holbrook, P. R., Taylor, G., Pollack, M. M., et al.: Adult respiratory distress syndrome in children. Pediatr. Clin. North Am. *27*:677-685, 1980.

54. Holman, R. G., and Maier, R. V.: Superoxide production by neutrophils in a model of adult respiratory distress syndrome. Arch. Surg. *123*:1491-1495, 1988.

55. Jaballah, N. B., Khaldi, A., Mnif, K., et al.: High-frequency oscillatory ventilation in pediatric patients with acute respiratory failure. Pediatr. Crit. Care Med. *7*:362-367, 2006.

56. Kacmarek, R. M., Wiedemann, H. P., Lavin, P. T., et al.: Partial liquid ventilation in adult patients with acute respiratory distress syndrome. Am. J. Respir. Crit. Care Med. *173*:882-889, 2006.

57. Kallas, H. J.: Non-conventional respiratory support modalities applicable in the older child. High frequency ventilation and liquid ventilation. Crit. Care Clin. *14*:655-683, 1998.

58. Kass, L. J., and Apkon, M: Inhaled nitric oxide in the treatment of hypoxemic respiratory failure. Curr. Opin. Pediatr. *10*:284-290, 1998.

59. Katz, R., Pollack, M., and Spady, D.: Cardiopulmonary abnormalities in severe acute respiratory failure. J. Pediatr. *104*:357-364, 1984.

60. Katzenstein, A. L., Bloor, C. M., and Leibow, A. A.: Diffuse alveolar damage—the role of oxygen, shock, and related factors. Am. J. Pathol. *85*:209-228, 1976.

61. Kollef, M. H.: Rescue therapy for the acute respiratory distress syndrome (ARDS). Chest *111*:845-846, 1997.

62. Kolobow, T., Moretti, M. P., Fumagalli, R., et al.: Severe impairment in lung function induced by high peak airway pressure during mechanical ventilation: An experimental study. Am. Rev. Respir. Dis. *135*:312-315, 1987.

63. Lamy, M., Fallat, R. J., Koeniger, E., et al.: Pathologic features and mechanisms of hypoxemia in adult respiratory distress syndrome. Am. Rev. Respir. Dis. *114*:267-284, 1976.

64. Langlois, P. F., and Gawryl, M. S.: Complement activation occurs through both classical and alternative pathways prior to onset and resolution of adult respiratory distress syndrome. Clin. Immunol. Immunopathol. *47*:152-163, 1988.

65. Lewandowski, K.: Extracorporeal membrane oxygenation for severe acute respiratory failure. Crit. Care *4*:156-168, 2000.

66. Lewis, J. F., and Jobe, A. H.: Surfactant and the adult respiratory distress syndrome. Am. Rev. Respir. Dis. *147*:218-233, 1993.

67. Linden, V., Palmer, K., Reinhard, J., et al.: High survival in adult patients with acute respiratory distress syndrome treated by extracorporeal membrane oxygenation, minimal sedation, and pressure supported ventilation. Intensive Care Med. *26*:1630-1637, 2000.

68. Lopez-Herce, J., de Lucas, N., Carrillo, A., et al.: Surfactant treatment for acute respiratory distress syndrome. Arch. Dis. Child. *80*:248-252, 1999.

69. Lundin, S., Mang, H., Smithies, M., et al.: Inhalation of nitric oxide in acute lung injury: Results of a European multicentre study: The European Study Group of Inhaled Nitric Oxide. Intensive Care Med. *25*:911-919, 1999.

70. Lyrene, R. K., and Troug, W. E.: Adult respiratory distress syndrome in a pediatric intensive care unit: Predisposing conditions, clinical course, and outcome. Pediatrics *67*:790-795, 1981.

71. Mancebo, J., Fernandez, R., Blanch, L., et al.: A multicenter trial of prolonged prone ventilation in severe acute respiratory distress syndrome. Am. J. Respir. Crit. Care Med. *173*:1233-1239, 2006.

72. Mangialardi, R. J., Martin, G. S., Bernard, G. R., et al.: Hypoproteinemia predicts acute respiratory distress syndrome development, weight gain, and death in patients with sepsis: Ibuprofen in Sepsis Study Group. Crit. Care Med. *28*:3137-3145, 2000.

73. Marraro, G. A., Luchetti, M., Galassini, E. M., et al.: Natural surfactant supplementation in ARDS in paediatric age. Minerva Anestesiol. *65*(Suppl.):92-97, 1999.

74. Matthay, M. A., Pittet, J. F., and Jayr, C.: Just say NO to inhaled nitric oxide for the acute respiratory distress syndrome. Crit. Care Med. *26*:1-2, 1998.

75. McIntyre, R. C., Jr., Pulido, E. J., Bensard, D. D., et al.: Thirty years of clinical trials in acute respiratory distress syndrome. Crit. Care Med. *28*:3314-3331, 2000.

76. Michael, J. R., Barton, R. G., Saffle, J. R., et al.: Inhaled nitric oxide versus conventional therapy: Effect on oxygenation in ARDS. Am. J. Respir. Crit. Care Med. 157:1372-1380, 1998.

77. Milberg, J. A., Davis, D. R., Steinberg, K. P., et al.: Improved survival of patients with acute respiratory distress syndrome (ARDS): 1983-1993. J. A. M. A. 273:306-309, 1995.

78. Nakagawa, T. A., Morris, A., Gomez, R. J., et al.: Dose response to inhaled nitric oxide in pediatric patients with pulmonary hypertension and acute respiratory distress syndrome. J. Pediatr. 131:63-69, 1997.

79. Nussbaum, E.: Adult type respiratory distress syndrome in children. Clin. Pediatr. (Phila.) 22:401-406, 1983.

80. Ognibene, F. P., Martin, S. E., Parker, M. M., et al.: Adult respiratory distress syndrome in patients with severe neutropenia. N. Engl. J. Med. 315:547-551, 1986.

81. Okamato, K., Hamaguchi, M., Kukuta, K., et al.: Efficacy of inhaled nitric oxide in children with ARDS. Chest 114:827-833, 1998.

82. Parsons, P. E., and Giclas, P. C.: The terminal complement complex (sC5b-9) is not specifically associated with the development of the adult respiratory distress syndrome. Am. Rev. Respir. Dis. 141:98-103, 1990.

83. Parsons, P. E., Worthen, G. S., Moore, E. E., et al.: The association of circulating endotoxin with the development of the adult respiratory distress syndrome. Am. Rev. Respir. Dis. 140:294-301, 1989.

84. Paulson, T. E., Spear, R. M., and Peterson, B. M.: New concepts in the treatment of children with acute respiratory distress syndrome. J. Pediatr. 127:163-175, 1995.

85. Paulson, T. E., Spear, R. M., Silva, P. D., et al.: High-frequency pressure-control ventilation with high positive end-expiratory pressure in children with acute respiratory distress syndrome. J. Pediatr. 129:566-573, 1996.

86. Payen, D. M.: Is nitric oxide inhalation a "cosmetic" therapy in acute respiratory distress syndrome? Am. J. Respir. Crit. Care Med. 157:1361-1362, 1998.

87. Pepe, P. E., Hudson, L. D., and Carrico, C. J.: Early application of positive end-expiratory pressure in patients at risk for the adult respiratory-distress syndrome. N. Engl. J. Med. 311:281-286, 1984.

88. Perkins, G. D., McAuley, D. F., Thickett, D. R., et al.: The β-Agonist Lung Injury Trial (BALTI): A randomized placebo-controlled clinical trial. Am. J. Respir. Crit. Care Med. 173:281-287, 2006.

89. Perkins, G. D., Roberts, J., McAuley, D. F., et al.: Regulation of vascular endothelial growth factor bioactivity in patients with acute lung injury. Thorax 60:153-158, 2005.

90. Pfenninger, J.: Acute respiratory distress syndrome (ARDS) in neonates and children. Paediatr. Anaesth. 6:173-181, 1996.

91. Pfenninger, J., Gerber, A., Tschäppeler, H., et al.: Adult respiratory distress syndrome in children. J. Pediatr. 101:352-357, 1982.

92. Piastra, M., Antonelli, M., Chiaretti, A., et al.: Treatment of acute respiratory failure by helmet-delivered non-invasive pressure support ventilation in children with acute leukemia: A pilot study. Intensive Care Med. 30:472-476, 2004.

93. Pingleton, S. K., and Harmon, G. S.: Nutritional management in acute respiratory failure. J. A. M. A. 257:3094-3099, 1987.

94. Playfor, S. D.: The role of high-frequency oscillatory ventilation in paediatric intensive care. Crit. Care 9:249-250; 2005.

95. Pratt, P. C., Vollmer, R. T., Shelburne, J. D., et al.: Pulmonary morphology in a multihospital collaborative extracorporeal membrane oxygenation project. I. Light microscopy. Am. J. Pathol. 95:191-214, 1979.

96. Presneill, J. J., Harris, T., Stewart, A. G., et al.: A randomized phase II trial of granulocyte-macrophage colony-stimulating factor therapy in severe sepsis with respiratory dysfunction. Am. J. Respir. Crit. Care Med. 166:138-143, 2002.

97. Reimer, S. L., Michener, W. M., and Steiger, E.: Nutritional support of the critically ill child. Pediatr. Clin. North Am. 27:647-660, 1980.

98. Relvas, M. S., Silver, P. C., and Sagy, M.: Prone positioning of pediatric patients with ARDS results in improvement in oxygenation if maintained >12 h daily. Chest 124:269-274, 2003.

99. Rinaldo, J. E., and Christman, J. W.: Mechanisms and mediators of the adult respiratory distress syndrome. Clin. Chest Med. 11:621-632, 1990.

100. Rivers, E. P.: Fluid-management strategies in acute lung injury: Liberal, conservative, or both? N. Engl. J. Med. 354:2564-2575, 2006.

101. Rivers, E., Nguyen, B., Havstad, S., et al.: Early goal-directed therapy in the treatment of severe sepsis and septic shock. N. Engl. J. Med. 345:1368-1377, 2001.

102. Rocco, T. R., Jr., Reinert, S. E., Cioffi, W., et al.: A 9-year, single-institution, retrospective review of death rate and prognostic factors in adult respiratory distress syndrome. Ann. Surg. 233:414-422, 2001.

103. Rodriguez Martinez, C. E., Guzman, M. C., Castillo, J. M., et al.: Evaluation of clinical criteria for the acute respiratory distress syndrome in pediatric patients. Pediatr. Crit. Care Med. 7:335-339, 2006.

104. Rossaint, R., Falke, K. J., Lopez, F., et al.: Inhaled nitric oxide for the adult respiratory distress syndrome. N. Engl. J. Med. 328:399-405, 1993.

105. Royall, J. A.: Adult respiratory distress syndrome in children. Semin. Respir. Med. 11:223-234, 1990.

106. Royall, J. A., and Levin, D. L.: Adult respiratory distress syndrome in pediatric patients. 1. Clinical aspects, pathophysiology, pathology, and mechanisms of lung injury. J. Pediatr. 112:169-180, 1988.

107. Royall, J., and Levin, D. L.: Adult respiratory distress syndrome in pediatric patients. II. Management. J. Pediatr. 112:335-347, 1988.

108. Rubin, D. B., Wiener-Kronish, J. P., Murray, J. F., et al.: Elevated von Willebrand factor antigen is an early plasma predictor of acute lung injury in nonpulmonary sepsis syndrome. J. Clin. Invest. 86:474-480, 1990.

109. Sachdeva, R. C., and Guntupalli, K. K.: Acute respiratory distress syndrome. Crit. Care Clin. 13:503-521, 1997.

110. Sapru, A., Wiemels, J. L., Witte, J. S., et al.: Acute lung injury and the coagulation pathway: Potential role of gene polymorphisms in the protein C and fibrinolytic pathways. Intensive Care Med. 32:1293-1303, 2006.

111. Sarnaik, A. P., and Lieh-Lai, M.: Adult respiratory distress syndrome in children. Pediatr. Clin. North Am. 41:337-363, 1994.

112. Scannell, G., Waxman, K., and Tominagam G. T.: Respiratory distress in traumatized and burned children. J. Pediatr. Surg. 30:612-614, 1995.

113. Shapiro, B. A., Cane, R. D., and Harrison, R. A.: Positive end-expiratory pressure therapy in adults with special reference to acute lung injury: A review of the literature and suggested clinical correlations. Crit. Care Med. 12:127-141, 1984.

114. Shoemaker, W. C., Appel, P., Czerm, L. S., et al.: Pathogenesis of respiratory failure (ARDS) after hemorrhage and trauma: I. Cardiorespiratory patterns preceding the development of ARDS. Crit. Care Med. 8:504-512, 1980.

115. Sivan, Y., Mor, C., al-Jundi, S., et al.: Adult respiratory distress syndrome in severely neutropenic children. Pediatr. Pulmonol. 8:104-108, 1990.

116. Sokol, J., Jacobs, S. E., Bohn, D.: Inhaled nitric oxide for acute hypoxemic respiratory failure in children and adults. Cochrane Database Syst. Rev. 1: CD002787, 2003.

117. Spragg, R. G.: Surfactant replacement therapy. Clin. Chest Med. 21:531-541, 2000.

118. Spragg, R. G., Lewis, J. F., Walmrath, H. D., et al.: Effect of recombinant surfactant protein C–based surfactant on the acute respiratory distress syndrome. N. Engl. J. Med. 351:884-892, 2004.

119. Spragg, R. G., Lewis, J. F., Wurst, W., et al.: Treatment of acute respiratory distress syndrome with recombinant surfactant protein C surfactant. Am. J. Respir. Crit. Care Med. 167:1562-1566, 2003.

120. Steffee, W. P.: Malnutrition in hospitalized patients. J. A. M. A. 244:2630-2635, 1980.

121. Stephens, K. E., Ishizaka, A., Larrick, J. W., et al.: Tumor necrosis factor causes increased pulmonary permeability and edema: Comparison to septic acute lung injury. Am. Rev. Respir. Dis. 137:1364, 1988.

122. Stewart, T. E., Meade, M. O., Cook, D. J., et al.: Evaluation of a ventilation strategy to prevent barotrauma in patients at high risk for acute respiratory distress syndrome: Pressure- and Volume-Limited Ventilation Strategy Group. N. Engl. J. Med. 338:355-361, 1998.

123. Suchyta, M. R., Clemmer, T. P., Elliot, C. G., et al.: The adult respiratory distress syndrome. A report of survival and modifying factors. Chest 101:1074-1079, 1992.

124. Swank, D. W., and Moore, S. B.: Roles of the neutrophil and other mediators in adult respiratory distress syndrome. Mayo Clin. Proc. 64:1118-1132, 1989.

125. Sznajder, J. I., Fraiman, A., Hall, J. B., et al.: Increased hydrogen peroxide in the expired breath of patients with acute hypoxemic respiratory failure. Chest 96:606-612, 1989.

126. Taeusch, H. W.: Treatment of acute (adult) respiratory distress syndrome. The holy grail of surfactant therapy. Biol. Neonate 77(Suppl.):2-8, 2000.

127. Tamakuma, S., Ogawa, M., Aikawa, N., et al.: Relationship between neutrophil elastase and acute lung injury in humans. Pulm. Pharmacol. Ther. 17:271-279, 2004.

128. Tamburro, R. F., Bugnitz, M. C., and Stidham, G. L.: Alveolar-arterial oxygen gradient as a predictor of outcome in patients with non-neonatal pediatric respiratory failure. J. Pediatr. 119:935-938, 1991.

129. Tate, R. M., and Repine, J. E.: Neutrophils and the adult respiratory distress syndrome. Am. Rev. Respir. Dis. 128:552-559, 1983.

130. Taylor, R. W., Zimmerman, J. L., Dellinger, R. P., et al.: Low-dose inhaled nitric oxide in patients with acute lung injury: A randomized controlled trial. J. A. M. A. 291:1603-1609, 2004.

131. Thammasitboon, S., Thammasitboon, S.: A critical appraisal of a systemic review: Sokol J, Jacob SE, Bohn D: Inhaled nitric oxide for acute hypoxemia respiratory failure in children and adults. Cochrane Database Syst Rev 1: CD002787, 2003, Pediatr. Crit. Care Med. 6:340-343, 2005.

132. The Acute Respiratory Distress Syndrome Network: Ventilation with lower tidal volumes as compared with traditional tidal volumes for acute lung injury and the acute respiratory distress syndrome. N. Engl. J. Med. 342:1301-1308, 2000.

133. The Acute Respiratory Distress Syndrome Network: Efficacy and safety of corticosteroids for persistent acute respiratory distress syndrome. N. Engl. J. Med. 354:1671-1684, 2006.

134. The National Heart Lung and Blood Institute ARDS Clinical Trials Network: Higher versus lower positive end-expiratory pressures in patients with the acute respiratory distress syndrome. N. Engl. J. Med. 351:327-336, 2004.

135. Timmons, O.: Infection in pediatric acute respiratory distress syndrome. Semin. Pediatr. Infect. Dis. 17:65-71, 2006.

136. Timmons, O. D., Dean, J. M., and Vernon, D. D.: Mortality rates and prognostic variables in children with adult respiratory distress syndrome. J. Pediatr. 119:896-899, 1991.

137. Tomashefski, J. F., Jr.: Pulmonary pathology of the adult respiratory distress syndrome. Clin. Chest Med. *11*:593-619, 1990.

138. Tracey, K. J., Beutler, B., Lowry, S. F., et al.: Shock and tissue injury induced by recombinant human cachectin. Science *234*:470-474, 1986.

139. Tracey, K. J., Fong, Y., Hessem, D. G., et al.: Anti-cachectin/TNF monoclonal antibodies prevent septic shock during lethal bacteraemia. Nature *330*:662-664, 1987.

140. Tracey, K. J., Lowry, S. F., Fahey, T. J., III, et al.: Cachectin/tumor necrosis factor induces lethal shock and stress hormone responses in the dog. Surg. Gynecol. Obstet. *164*:415, 1987.

141. Trachsel, D., McCrindle, B. W., Nakagawa, S., et al: Oxygenation index predicts outcome in children with acute hypoxemic respiratory failure. Am. J. Respir. Crit. Care Med. *172*:206-211, 2005.

142. Tremblay, L., Valenza, F., Ribeiro, S. P., et al.: Injurious ventilatory strategies increase cytokines and c-fos m-RNA expression in an isolated rat lung model. J. Clin. Invest. *99*:944-952, 1997.

143. Troncy, E., Collet, J. P., Shapiro, S., et al.: Inhaled nitric oxide in acute respiratory distress syndrome: A pilot randomized controlled study. Am. J. Respir. Crit. Care Med. *157*:1483-1488, 1998.

144. Villar, J., Kacmarek, R. M., Perez-Mendez, L., et al.: A high positive end-expiratory pressure, low tidal volume ventilatory strategy improves outcome in persistent acute respiratory distress syndrome: A randomized, controlled trial. Crit. Care Med. *34*:1311-1318, 2006.

145. Ware, L. B.: Pathophysiology of acute lung injury and the acute respiratory distress syndrome. Semin. Respir. Crit. Care Med. *27*:337-349, 2006.

146. Ware, L. B., Camerer, E., Welty-Wolf, K. E., et al.: Bench to bedside: Targeting coagulation and fibrinolysis in acute lung injury. Am. J. Physiol. Lung Cell. Mol. Physiol. *291*:L307-L311, 2006.

147. Ware, L. B., Fang, X., Matthay, M. A.: Protein C and thrombomodulin in human acute lung injury. Am. J. Physiol. Lung Cell. Mol. Physiol. *285*:L514-L521, 2003.

148. Weg, J. G.: Oxygen transport in adult respiratory distress syndrome and other acute circulatory problems: Relationship of oxygen delivery and oxygen consumption. Crit. Care Med. *19*:650-657, 1991.

149. Weigelt, J. A., Norcross, J. F., Borman, K. R., et al.: Early steroid therapy for respiratory failure. Arch. Surg. *120*:536-540, 1985.

150. Weinberg, P. F., Matthay, M. A., Webster, R. O., et al.: Biologically active products of complement and acute lung injury in patients with the sepsis syndrome. Am. Rev. Respir. Dis. *130*:791-796, 1984.

151. Weisman, I. M., Rinaldo, J. E., Rogers, R. M.: Current concepts: Positive end-expiratory pressure in adult respiratory failure. N. Engl. J. Med. *307*:1381-1384, 1982.

152. Wilkes, M. M., Navickis, R. J.: Patient survival after human albumin administration: A meta-analysis of randomized, controlled trials. Ann. Intern. Med. *135*:149-164, 2001.

153. Willson, D. F., Thomas, N. J., Markovitz, B. P., et al.: Effect of exogenous surfactant (calfactant) in pediatric acute lung injury: A randomized controlled trial. J. A. M. A. *293*:470-476, 2005.

154. Wiswell, T. E., Smith, R. M., Katz, L. B., et al.: Bronchopulmonary segmental lavage with Surfaxin (KL(4)-surfactant) for acute respiratory distress syndrome. Am. J. Respir. Crit. Care Med. *160*:1188-1195, 1999.

INFECTIONS OF THE FETUS AND NEWBORN

VIRAL INFECTIONS OF THE FETUS AND NEONATE

Pablo J. Sánchez ✪ Gail J. Demmler-Harrison

GENERAL ASPECTS OF VIRAL INFECTIONS OF THE FETUS AND NEWBORN

The fetus and newborn infant are highly susceptible to many different viruses that in most instances cause little or no disease in older age groups. However, relatively few of the hundreds of viruses to which humans constantly are exposed are ever transmitted to the fetus or cause infection in newborn infants. Nonetheless, viral infections are an important cause of neonatal morbidity and mortality. The cumulative frequency of viral infections in the fetus or newborn infant may be as high as 6 to 8 percent of all live births, whereas systemic bacterial disease occurs in only 1 to 2 percent of neonates.[188,229]

Contributing to the frequency of viral infections in this age group is that the infection can be acquired at several different periods during intrauterine and neonatal life: in utero (congenital infection), at the time of birth (natal infection), or after birth but during the neonatal period (postnatal infection). In addition, numerous different outcomes of infection are possible. Congenital infections can result in resorption of the embryo; abortion; stillbirth; congenital malformation; prematurity; intrauterine growth restriction; acute disease apparent in utero, at birth, or shortly thereafter; asymptomatic infection in the neonatal period, but a persistent postnatal infection with neurologic sequelae later in life; or a normal infant with no apparent sequelae. Natal or postnatal infections can cause acute systemic illness leading to death, persistent infection with late sequelae, self-limited disease with no discernible damage, or asymptomatic infection.[188,229]

Recent developments in the fields of diagnostic virology, epidemiology, and viral immunology have expanded our knowledge tremendously and modified our understanding of fetal and neonatal viral infections and their contribution to disease, not only in the neonatal period but also later in life.[188,229] In addition, the development of rubella vaccine and antiviral drugs effective against a few of the agents offers hope for prevention or control of these infections. This chapter provides the physician with an approach to diagnosis and management of, as well as prognostic information about, viral infections that occur in the fetus and newborn infant. Human immunodeficiency virus (HIV), an important perinatal viral pathogen, is covered in another chapter.

PATHOGENESIS

Congenital Viral Infections

Congenital viral infections are secondary to exposure of the fetus during maternal viral infection. Evidence from both humans and experimental animals indicates that most fetal infections are preceded by a systemic viral infection in the mother, with hematogenous spread of the virus to the placenta and subsequently to the fetus (Fig. 73–1). Ascending infection through amniotic membranes also may occur while the fetus is still in utero. Viral infections that occur in the mother during pregnancy and that are limited to the respiratory or gastrointestinal tract may not pose a risk to the fetus but later may be transmitted perinatally to the newborn infant. Even if viremia does occur in the mother, maternal host defense mechanisms and the placenta appear to provide a protective barrier for the fetus. With most viruses known to cause fetal infection—cytomegalovirus (CMV), rubella virus, herpes simplex virus (HSV), varicella-zoster virus (VZV), and vaccinia virus–placental involvement by the virus also has been documented.[74,550] Viruses may reach the fetal circulation by (1) replication through the layers of the placenta, (2) production of virus-induced vascular lesions in the placenta resulting in abnormal communications between the maternal and fetal circulation, or (3) diapedesis of virus-infected maternal leukocytes through the layers of the placenta to the fetal circulation.[74,475,635] Damage to the fetus also may occur in the absence of actual fetal viral infection as a result of severe systemic illness in the mother or alteration of placental function (e.g., abortion or stillbirth in maternal measles, influenza). Viruses demonstrated to have caused congenital infection are listed in Table 73–1. Proof of congenital infection usually consists of the presence of infection or disease caused by the virus or demonstration of the pathogen in the fetus before birth or in the neonate at birth or shortly thereafter.

The effect that congenital infection with various viruses can have on the fetus is shown in Table 73–2.[581-583] Abortion or stillbirth usually occurs when the mother is infected very early in gestation (e.g., rubella) or when the systemic illness in the mother is severe (e.g., measles, influenza). The reasons that premature birth occurs in congenital viral infection are not well understood. Infants with congenital viral infection who are small for gestational age have intrauterine growth restriction, usually the result of decreased numbers of cells in organs.[444,445]

Developmental malformations result from infection of the fetus with the virus (see Table 73–2). Rubella virus is the classic known teratogen; that is, it causes disturbances in organogenesis. VZV has been shown to cause limb hypoplasia and developmental malformations of the eye.[243] Other viruses that result in congenital defects, such as CMV and HSV, cause inflammatory, destructive lesions of already developed organs. Type B coxsackieviruses have been associated with a variety of congenital malformations of the heart,[93-95] and mumps has been linked to endocardial fibroelastosis,[595] but these associations require further substantiation before a causative role can be assigned.

In Table 73–2, congenital disease refers to any manifestation of illness present at birth or shortly thereafter that is secondary to transplacental infection with the virus. Some of the viruses that result in congenital disease cause a chronic persistent infection (CMV, rubella, and hepatitis B virus [HBV]), whereas others cause acute, self-limited, or fatal infection (echovirus, coxsackie-

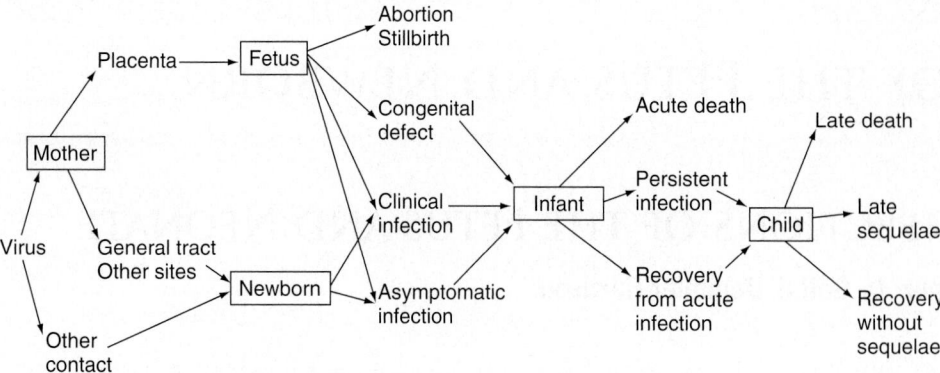

Figure 73–1 Pathogenesis of viral infections in the fetus and newborn.

TABLE 73–1   Period of Transmission of Selected Viruses to the Fetus or Newborn Infant

Viruses	Congenital	Natal	Postnatal
Adenovirus	+	+	+
Cytomegalovirus	++	++	++
Echoviruses	+	+	+
Epstein-Barr	+	–	–
Hepatitis A	–	++	+
Hepatitis B	+	++	+
Hepatitis C	+	++	–
Herpes simplex	+	++	+
Herpesvirus-6	+	–	+
Human immunodeficiency virus	+	++	+
Human parvovirus B19	+	–	–
Influenza	(+)	–	–
Lymphocytic choriomeningitis virus	++	–	–
Measles	+	–	–
Mumps	+	–	–
Parechovirus	–	–	+
Polioviruses	+	–	–
Rubella	++	–	–
Smallpox	+	–	–
St. Louis encephalitis virus	(+)	–	(+)
Type B coxsackieviruses	+	+	+
Vaccinia	+	–	–
Varicella-zoster	++	–	+
West Nile virus	+	–	+
Western equine encephalitis	+	–	–

++, major demonstrated route; +, minor demonstrated route; (+), suggested route, few supporting data; –, route not demonstrated.

virus B, poliovirus, measles, vaccinia, smallpox, western equine encephalitis, and human parvovirus B19). HSV and VZV can cause chronic persistent intrauterine infection, as well as acute transplacental infection at the time of delivery. Because HSV has a relatively short incubation period, ascending amniotic infection with HSV, in association with premature rupture of membranes and maternal genital herpes infection, may cause acute disease that is evident at birth or shortly thereafter. Other viruses, including adenoviruses, Epstein-Barr virus, and respiratory syncytial virus (RSV), also have been detected in the amniotic fluid of both normal fetuses and fetuses with structural abnormalities; however, the direct role these viruses play in fetal infection and disease is not currently known.[418]

Viruses and Congenital Malformation

The role of viruses as etiologic agents in congenital malformations merits special mention. After the recognition by Gregg[198,250]

in 1941 that congenital cataracts and other defects occurred in the offspring of mothers with German measles, the concept of an infectious origin for congenital malformations was established firmly. Major malformations occur in 2 to 3 percent of all live births. Although great strides have been made in the diagnosis and management of these defects, their etiologic basis remains largely undefined. Approximately 10 percent are caused by environmental agents such as infections, drugs, or radiation. Another 10 percent have genetic origin and result from familial inheritance or demonstrable chromosomal abnormalities.[475] The remaining 80 percent are of unknown etiology. Most congenital defects may not be caused by environmental or genetic factors acting individually but rather in concert with one another. A genetically predisposed fetus is exposed to the appropriate environmental factor at a particular stage during organogenesis, which then leads to the development of malformations. Because control of the genetic factors contributing to fetal malformation is unlikely to be developed to the point of practical application in the near future, efforts to identify environmental factors that are amenable to control appear warranted.

For several reasons, viruses have been considered to be likely contributors to the 80 percent of malformations that are of unknown etiology. First, the precedent is established that rubella virus and VZV infections during pregnancy do cause congenital defects. Second, most women are expected to have one or more viral infections at some time during pregnancy,[570] so the potential exposure rate is high. Third, a viral infection could be unrecognized in the mother yet produce significant disease in the fetus, which could lead to the occurrence of a "congenital defect of unknown etiology." Fourth, viruses are known to multiply readily in rapidly dividing immature cells, with resultant cell destruction or altered cell function.[426] In the case of more destructive viruses (e.g., measles, vaccinia), fetal death with abortion or stillbirth may occur, whereas with less cytolytic agents (e.g., rubella, CMV), the fetus may survive but defects are produced. Finally, experimental animals provide numerous examples of infection with a virus resulting in little or no disease in the pregnant mother, yet the fetuses are aborted or the newborn offspring are deformed.[208] Therefore, physicians caring for newborn infants should not only be familiar with the patterns of congenital defects currently known to be caused by viruses (CMV, rubella, HSV, and VZV) but also be aware that additional viruses may be added to the list of causative agents in the future.

Natal Viral Infections

Natal viral infections are the result of exposure of the newborn to virus replicating in the genital tract (CMV, HSV, HBV) or to fecal virus contaminating genital secretions (enteroviruses) (see Fig. 73–1 and Table 73–1). Because the incubation periods of HSV and enteroviruses are short, acute postnatal disease may appear in the neonate within 5 to 7 days after natal infection with

TABLE 73-2   Effect of Specific Viruses on the Fetus and Newborn Infant

	Abortion, Stillbirth	Prematurity	Small for Gestational Age	Developmental Malformations	Congenital Disease	Acute Postnatal Disease	Persistent Postnatal Infection
Adenovirus	(+)	–	–	–	(+)	+	–
Cytomegalovirus	+	+	+	+	+(C)	+	+
Echoviruses	–	–	–	–	+(A)	+	–
Epstein-Barr	–	–	+	+	+(C)	–	+
Hepatitis B	–	+	–	–	+(C)	+	+
Herpes simplex	+	+	+	+	+(C,A)	+	+
Influenza	+	–	–	–	–	(+)	–
Lymphocytic choriomeningitis virus	(+)	–	–	+	+(A)	(+)	–
Measles	+	+	–	–	+(A)	–	–
Mumps	+	–	–	(+)	–	–	–
Parechoviruses	(+)	–	–	–	+(A)	+	–
Parvovirus B19	+	–	–	–	+(C,A)	+	+
Polioviruses	+	+	–	–	+(A)	–	–
Rubella	+	+	+	+	+(C)	–	+
Smallpox	+	+	–	–	+(A)	–	–
St. Louis encephalitis	(+)	–	–	(+)	(+)	+	–
Type B coxsackieviruses	+	–	–	(+)	+(A)	+	–
Vaccinia	+	+	–	–	+(A)	–	–
Varicella-zoster	–	+	+	+	+(C,A)	+	+
West Nile	(+)	–	–	(+)	(+)	+	–
Western equine encephalitis	–	–	–	–	+(A)	–	–

+, effect established; –, effect not established; (+), effect suggested, but not proved; (A), acute fatal or self-limited infection; (C), chronic persistent infection.

these agents occurs (see Table 73–2). In contrast, the incubation periods of CMV and HBV are long, and clinically apparent disease, if it occurs, may not be observed for several weeks or even months after birth (see Table 73–2). Persistent postnatal infection can occur after natal infection with CMV, HSV, and HBV.

Postnatal Viral Infections

The source of exposure for postnatal infections of a newborn infant often is the mother, but other sources have been observed and include personnel or other infants in the nursery or newborn intensive care unit and family members (see Fig. 73–1). Neonatal infections, as well as hospital-associated outbreaks of enterovirus[34,526] and parechovirus,[429,654] RSV,[260] rotavirus, adenovirus, rhinovirus, parainfluenza virus, and influenza virus infection, have occurred in nurseries. In addition, health-care-associated HSV infections have occurred in neonates (see Table 73–1).[262,321,487,542,650] Although the maternal respiratory and gastrointestinal tracts are the most common sites from which virus can be transmitted to the neonate postnatally, other viruses, including HIV, human T-cell leukemia virus types 1 and 2 (HTLV I and II), CMV,[277] West Nile virus, rubella virus, hepatitis C virus (HCV), and HBV,[381] have been recovered from breast milk. HSV and VZV lesions on the breast of a mother also may be a source of transmission of virus for the breast-feeding neonate, even though these viruses probably are not present in the breast milk. Finally, HIV, CMV,[697] and HBV[201] have been transmitted to newborn infants by blood transfusion.[199,692] Although most postnatal infections are acute, self-limited processes, severe disease and fatalities have been reported, especially in preterm infants infected with enteroviruses, adenoviruses, or RSV, and persistent postnatal infection may occur with CMV and HBV (see Table 73–2).

EPIDEMIOLOGY

Factors Influencing the Frequency of Infection

Many factors can influence the frequency of infections in the fetus and newborn infant (Table 73–3). Because the mother is the

TABLE 73-3   Factors Influencing Frequency and Severity of Viral Infections in the Fetus and Newborn Infant

	Time of Fetal or Neonatal Infection		
Factors	Congenital	Natal	Postnatal
Absence of vaccine	++	–	–
Geographic location	++	++	++
Gestational age of fetus	++	+	+
Maternal age	++	+	++
Method of case identification	++	++	++
Presence of epidemic in community	++	+	++
Primary infection in mother	++	++	++
Season of year	++	+	++
Sexual promiscuity	+	++	–
Socioeconomic status	++	++	++

++, major influence; +, minor influence; –, little or no influence.

source of the virus causing fetal and neonatal infection in most instances, factors influencing the frequency of maternal infection are of major importance. Except for CMV infection, most congenital infections of the fetus occur after primary viral infection has occurred in the mother. Congenital CMV infection may occur as frequently in mothers known to be seropositive before conception as in seronegative mothers.[603] Congenital rubella, on the other hand, occurs only rarely in immune mothers.[532] Transplacental HBV infection occurs much more often in mothers with acute, primary, symptomatic infection, whereas natal infection is the primary route of transmission in chronic carrier mothers.[470,559] Fetal parvovirus B19 infection and perinatal enteroviral and adenovirus infections acquired from the mother almost always are the result of primary maternal infection. In contrast, natal infections with CMV, HBV, and HSV may result from primary or persistent or recurrent infections in the mother.

The time during pregnancy when the mother is infected (the gestational age of the fetus) is a major factor influencing both the frequency of transmission and the severity of congenital rubella.

One hundred percent of infants who have congenital rubella infection during the first 11 weeks of pregnancy have malformations associated with congenital rubella syndrome, 30 percent who have congenital infection from 12 to 20 weeks have malformations, and no malformations develop with infections occurring after 20 weeks.[442] A similar phenomenon occurs with congenital parvovirus B19, CMV, and VZV infections.[282,488,598] In contrast, transplacental HBV and HSV infections appear to develop more frequently when the acute, symptomatic maternal infection occurs in the third trimester rather than the first or second.[704] With viruses such as polio, measles, vaccinia, and smallpox, early-gestation maternal disease results in abortion or stillbirth, whereas late-gestation infection results in congenital disease with acute symptoms in the early neonatal period (see Table 73–2).

Several social and environmental factors may influence the likelihood of development of maternal infection and thereby affect the frequency of infection in the fetus and neonate. The development of rubella vaccine and its licensure in 1969 reduced the incidence of congenital rubella syndrome significantly.[54,473] The successful eradication of smallpox worldwide and discontinuation of the need for smallpox vaccine (vaccinia virus) have eliminated fetal infection with these viruses. Although measles and mumps vaccines have reduced significantly the frequency of occurrence of these diseases in children, whether waning immunity in women of child-bearing age who were vaccinated as infants will predispose to reinfection in pregnant women and subsequent fetal or neonatal disease remains unclear. The presence of epidemics in the community, such as those caused by rubella or enteroviruses, certainly can influence the frequency of maternal and, therefore, congenital, natal, and postnatal infections. The incidence of infection with some viruses (e.g., rubella, primary VZV, enteroviruses, measles, mumps, influenza) clearly is higher during certain months of the year, so the season can influence maternal and neonatal infection rates. In contrast, other viruses causing congenital or natal infection, such as CMV, HBV, or HSV, do not occur in an epidemic or seasonal fashion. Geographic location also can be influential, probably because of differences in the ethnic (and, therefore, genetic) origin of populations in different locations. Rates of chronic carriage of hepatitis B surface antigen (HBsAg) in mothers and the frequency of congenital and natal HBV infection in neonates are much higher in Taiwanese than in U.S. residents.[704] The incidence of numerous maternal viral infections is known to be higher in populations with a lower socioeconomic status, thereby influencing the frequency of congenital, natal, and postnatal infections. Other social factors such as drug abuse, which is associated with higher rates of HBV infection, also can affect the frequency of congenital and natal infections. Because CMV, HBV, and HSV all have been shown to be transmitted venereally, sexual promiscuity in the mother can influence the frequency of these infections in the neonate.

Case identification is a major factor that can have some bearing on the frequency of recognized infection in the neonate. Because most neonates with congenital CMV, rubella virus, or HBV infection are asymptomatic, the use of clinical case-finding methods alone significantly underestimates the true frequency of these infections. Epidemiologic observations (e.g., rubella or enterovirus epidemic in the community), clinical or laboratory information about the mother (e.g., viral illness with a rash or the presence of HBsAg in serum), or screening tests in the newborn (e.g., elevated quantitative IgM in umbilical cord blood) often have been used to select a group of neonates at high risk of contracting congenital infection. The performance of additional laboratory tests in these high-risk neonates to identify potential specific causative agents often has led to the demonstration of infection rates much higher than previously suspected.

Frequency of Infection in the Mother and Neonate

Table 73–4 shows the approximate frequency of the most common viral infections in the mother during pregnancy and in the newborn infant. Although the figures have been obtained by a variety of laboratory methods and some are based on a relatively small or nonrepresentative population sample, they do provide an estimate of the relative frequency of the infections. In many studies, prospective screening of mothers for viral infection during pregnancy or screening of infants for elevated cord blood serum immunoglobulin M (IgM) levels was done to select a population of neonates at high risk of acquiring congenital infection for more detailed virologic investigation.

CMV clearly is the most common cause of viral infection, both in the mother and in the neonate.[105] Surveys in the United States indicate that 30 to 110 per 1000 women excrete virus in urine during pregnancy and that 60 per 1000 are excreters at the time of delivery.[225,284,341,435,452,528] Isolation from cervical swabs is even more common: 80 to 120 per 1000 women during pregnancy and 110 to 130 per 1000 at delivery.[130,341,435,528] Most maternal CMV infections occurring during pregnancy are recurrent rather than primary.[600] Extrapolation from data obtained at the same institution[528,600,605] suggests that two thirds to three quarters of CMV shedding in the cervix or urine during pregnancy is the result of recurrent rather than primary CMV infection in the mother. The frequency of primary CMV infection occurring during pregnancy averages 20 to 25 per 1000 (range, 10 to 40), with higher rates occurring in populations with a larger percentage of susceptible persons (seronegative at the beginning of pregnancy).[251,598] Several factors are known to be associated with increased rates of recurrent urine or cervical shedding: (1) sampling on several occasions rather than a single time; (2) collection of specimens during the third rather than the first trimester because shedding rates are known to increase as gestation progresses; (3) Asian, black, or Native American versus white populations; (4) younger maternal age; (5) lower socioeconomic status; (6) a greater number of lifetime sexual partners; and (7) a history of sexually transmitted diseases.[130,341,452,606] An even more important source for transmission of CMV to the neonate may be breast milk. Postpartum shedding from colostrum or breast milk, the cervix, urine, or saliva was demonstrated in 130 to 280 per 1000 unselected women, and breast milk was the most common site by far.[202,598,605,607]

Congenital CMV infection has been documented in 6 to 24 per 1000 live births, as determined by isolation of virus from the urine of the neonate within the first few days of life.[73,178,530,603] In contrast to rubella, congenital infection with CMV occurs in mothers with either primary or recurrent infections during pregnancy.[603] Congenital CMV infection rates are significantly higher

TABLE 73–4 Approximate Frequency of Infections in the Mother during Pregnancy and in the Newborn Infant

Viruses	Mother (No./1000 Pregnancies)	Neonate (No./1000 Live Births)
Cytomegalovirus		
During pregnancy, congenital	30-120	6-24
At delivery, natal	80-130	20-60
After delivery, postnatal	130-280	140-210
Rubella		
1964 epidemic	20-40	3-7
Interepidemic prevaccine	0.1-2.0	0.1-0.7
Postvaccine	0.15-0.3	0.03
Hepatitis B	1-160	0-61
Enteroviruses	90-600	2-38
Herpes simplex	1-7	0.1-0.6

in lower socioeconomic groups (1.6%) than in middle to upper ones (0.6%).[600] However, among low-income mothers, the status of immunity to CMV is high (82%), and most congenital infections (81%) are associated with recurrent CMV infection during pregnancy. In contrast, seroimmunity to CMV in middle- to upper-income women is lower (55%), and the frequency of congenital infection associated with recurrent maternal CMV also is lower (47%). Although the rate of total congenital CMV infection is lower in mid- to high-income mothers, the proportion of infants born after primary CMV infection is acquired during pregnancy is higher (53% versus 19%). Pooled data from several studies indicate that 30 to 40 percent (range, 20-52%) of mothers with primary CMV infection during pregnancy deliver congenitally infected infants.[12,13,251,364,598,600] Congenitally infected babies born to mothers with primary rather than recurrent CMV infection during pregnancy have a greater frequency of symptoms of CMV disease at birth, higher levels of IgM in cord serum, higher titers of virus in urine, and a greater likelihood of having neurologic sequelae at follow-up.[11,12,598,600] The time during gestation when maternal primary CMV infection occurs does not appear to influence the rate of fetal infection, but fetal damage seems to occur more frequently and to be more severe after the acquisition of maternal infection during the first half than during the second half of pregnancy.[11,251,509,598]

The frequency of natal and postnatal acquisition of CMV by newborn infants is far greater than that of congenital infection. Natally acquired CMV infection occurs at an incidence of 20 per 1000 live births.[528,604] Because approximately one half the infants born to mothers known to be cervical excreters at the time of delivery acquire natal infection[528] and because as many as 130 per 1000 mothers from a low socioeconomic group are excreting CMV at this time, the actual rate of natally acquired CMV infection may be as high as 60 per 1000 live births. A more frequent source for infection of the neonate with CMV is postnatal consumption of virus-infected colostrum or breast milk. In two studies, 58 to 69 percent of infants of nursing mothers who excreted CMV in milk acquired infection.[202,605] Shedding of virus occurred most frequently between 2 and 12 weeks postpartum, and the onset of infant viruria usually occurred when the infants were between 1 and 6 months of age. The aforementioned rates of postnatal infection would project to between 140 and 210 infections per 1000 live births in the United States. These rates, of course, would be affected by all the factors mentioned earlier that influence maternal CMV infection rates, as well as the frequency and duration of breast-feeding.

Yet another source for transmission of CMV to neonates is blood transfusion in infants in neonatal intensive care units. Risk factors include birth weight less than 1250 g, a CMV-seronegative mother, hospitalization for a period longer than 4 weeks, receipt of multiple blood transfusions or a total volume of more than 50 mL, and receipt of blood from a CMV-seropositive donor.[10,50,228,697] The infection rate in high-risk infants may be high: 24 to 31 percent. Morbidity and mortality rates with these infections also are high: clinical disease developed in 88 percent of 34 reported cases, and 24 percent died (CMV was thought to be causal or contributory).

In summary, several factors contribute to the high rates of fetal and neonatal CMV infection: (1) virus can be transmitted from both immune mothers (recurrent infection) and nonimmune mothers (primary infection); (2) virus may be shed or carried in many different sites in the mother's blood (for transplacental infection), urine, cervix, breast milk, and saliva; (3) infection may occur at different times—congenitally, natally, and postnatally; and (4) infection may come from sources other than the mother (e.g., hospital-acquired infection from blood transfusion).

The use of rubella vaccine has modified the epidemiologic patterns of this disease in the United States.[54,184,473] Vaccination has eliminated endemic rubella in the United States. Rates of maternal and congenital rubella during the 1964 epidemic were many times higher than in interepidemic periods. Nonetheless, a comparison of the incidence during the 1964 epidemic with the rates during prevaccine interepidemic periods and what may be happening currently provides useful information. The frequency of serologically proven clinical rubella among 30,000 pregnant women in the Collaborative Perinatal Research Study was approximately 1 per 1000 during the interepidemic years before vaccine licensure but rose to 22 per 1000 during the epidemic. The total figure for rubella during pregnancy is likely to be at least two times higher because as many as one half to two thirds of maternal rubella infections are subclinical or not diagnosed as rubella.[568] An incidence of congenital rubella of 0.7 per 1000 live births was demonstrated during the interepidemic period in a study screening cord blood sera for the presence of rubella-specific IgM antibody.[15] During the 1964 epidemic, an estimated 20,000 babies were born with congenital rubella syndrome in the United States among approximately 4 million live births, an incidence of 5 per 1000 live births.[454] During 1980 to 1982, an average of 11 cases of confirmed congenital rubella syndrome were reported to the Centers for Disease Control and Prevention (CDC) each year.[473] Correcting for under-reporting and missed cases yielded an annual estimate of 110 cases.[473] With an annual national birth rate of 3.5 million per year, this figure projects to 0.03 cases of congenital rubella syndrome per 1000 live births currently in the United States. Assuming a 10 to 20 percent rate of congenital rubella infection during pregnancy, the current estimate is thought to be 0.15 to 0.3 cases of maternal rubella per 1000 pregnancies. Importantly, however, a resurgence in acquired and congenital rubella, particularly in unvaccinated women in correctional institutions and unimmunized communities,[116,412] emphasizes the need for continued surveillance for rubella disease and proper use of the vaccine.

HBV infection during pregnancy may result in acute clinical disease in the mother or, more commonly, may result in an asymptomatic chronic carrier state.[560] The frequency of HBsAg in the serum of pregnant women varies highly and is influenced by geographic location, ethnic origin, socioeconomic status, and other social factors such as illicit drug use and sexual promiscuity. An incidence of 1 to 160 per 1000 pregnancies has been reported in several series.* Infection with HBV in the neonate is even more variable, for several reasons. First, transmission of the virus to the fetus or neonate may occur by several routes: (1) transplacental; (2) natal, from the genital tract; (3) postnatal, by intrafamilial spread through unknown mechanisms; and (4) postnatal, by blood transfusion. Second, infants born to mothers with hepatitis B may follow one of these courses: (1) serum from the infant remains negative for HBsAg, and hepatitis B never develops; (2) umbilical cord blood is positive for HBsAg, but the antigenemia clears and no disease is evident, presumably representing transplacental transmission of antigen only or insufficient virus to cause true infection in the neonate; (3) umbilical cord blood is HBsAg-positive, and clinical or subclinical infection develops with or without persistent hepatitis B antigenemia; or (4) cord blood is antigen-negative, but infection occurs, sometimes not until several months after birth, and persistent antigenemia may or may not develop. Third, because exposed infants may follow one of several courses and because HBV infection may be demonstrable at various times after birth, serial blood specimens must be obtained for evaluation of the true frequency of neonatal infection. Serial blood specimens are difficult to obtain in this age group, and published reports may have based their estimates of infection on one or two blood specimens per infant. Fourth, transplacental infection occurs much more commonly in mothers

---

*See references 31, 66, 183, 200, 347, 381, 469, 486, 560, 615, 687.

with acute, symptomatic hepatitis, particularly during the second or third trimester of pregnancy, than it does in mothers who are chronic carriers.[560] Finally, even in these mothers, true differences in the rates of transplacental transmission occur: Asians have a much higher incidence than whites do,[704] and mothers who are hepatitis B e antigen (HBeAg)-positive are much more likely to transmit infection than are mothers who have anti-HBe antibody or lack e-antigen markers.[469] Therefore, the incidence of HBV infection in the neonate varies from 0 to 61 per 1000 live births in different reports.*

Data from several studies indicate that perinatal enteroviral infections occur much more frequently than previously realized.[106,307,318,429,436,536,93-95,353,567] Serologic surveys indicate a surprisingly high rate of seroconversion to at least one enterovirus during pregnancy (first serum at the time of enrollment for obstetric care, second serum at delivery): 90 to 600 per 1000 pregnancies.[93-95,353,567] Several factors complicate arriving at an interpretation of the data concerning the frequency of occurrence of maternal enteroviral infections. First, only 2 to 13 of the almost 70 nonpolio enterovirus serotypes were used for antibody testing, thereby resulting in an underestimate of the true frequency for all enteroviruses. Second, the data are reported as the total number of enteroviral infections for a group of pregnant women rather than the percentage of pregnancies complicated by at least one enteroviral infection. Use of these data for calculating the number of pregnancies per 1000 complicated by enteroviral infection would result in an overestimation because more than 25 percent of women may have more than one enteroviral infection during the 9 months of pregnancy.[93]

Data concerning the actual frequency of neonatal enteroviral and parechoviral infection also are difficult to summarize because of differences in the study designs used in the various published results. Modlin and associates[432] reported four echovirus 11 infections among 158 consecutive neonates who had stool samples taken when they were 3 days and 2 weeks of age during the 3-week period of an outbreak of echovirus 11 in Boston. Assuming that live births are distributed evenly throughout the year and that no additional cases of enteroviral infection occurred during the remainder of the year, this incidence translates into two enteroviral infections per 1000 live births. These calculations probably underestimate the true frequency markedly because only echovirus 11 was sought in the diagnostic virology laboratory evaluation of these 158 infants, and, obviously, enteroviral infections occur for more than a 3-week period of the year. A prospective study of all enteroviral infections acquired during the patient's first month of life in Rochester, New York, during the peak enterovirus season (June to October) demonstrated 75 (12.8%) nonpolio enteroviral infections in 586 infants.[307] Fourteen (18.7%) of these 75 infected infants were hospitalized for "suspected sepsis." By using the estimated number of live births per year in the Rochester area and assuming that no additional cases of neonatal enteroviral infection occurred during the remaining 7 months of the year, the authors projected a rate of seven neonatal enteroviral infections serious enough to require hospitalization per 1000 live births. If one considered the total 75 enteroviral infections (14 hospitalized and 61 not hospitalized), the rate would be 38 per 1000 live births. A survey by Kaplan and associates[318] of 77 cases of coxsackievirus B infection occurring during the first 3 months of life in infants hospitalized at the Nassau County Medical Center between 1970 and 1979 yielded an estimated rate of 0.5 per 1000 live births. Because group B coxsackieviruses account for only 45 percent of all enteroviral infections during early infancy[351] and because only 18 to 19 percent of all enterovirus-infected infants may require hos-

pitalization,[307] the actual rate for all enteroviral infections may be 6 per 1000 live births. Despite the variation in estimates, enteroviral infections are clearly a frequent cause of maternal and neonatal infection. Parechovirus infections are being diagnosed and described in the medical literature with increased frequency, but current knowledge of the epidemiology of this infection in neonates is still evolving.[654] The infected genital tract of the mother is the source of virus for most neonatal HSV infections. However, other sources, such as nongenital sites in the mother, family members, and even other infants or caretakers in the nursery, have been implicated. Both genital and neonatal herpes have increased in frequency in recent years.[67,623] Current estimates are that culture-positive genital herpes may occur at a rate of one to seven per 1000[75,77,97-102] during pregnancy and at a rate of one to four per 1000 at the time of delivery.[97,101,450,513,632] However, culture is not the most sensitive method to detect genital HSV-2 infection. Seroprevalence studies have demonstrated HSV-2–specific antibody in 32 percent of women in private obstetric practices,[362] and polymerase chain reaction (PCR) detected HSV DNA in 9 percent of asymptomatic women in labor.[149] Higher rates are associated with lower socioeconomic status, increased numbers of sexual partners, and occurrence of other sexually transmitted diseases. Rates of neonatal herpes have been estimated at 0.1 to 0.6 per 1000 live births.[97,623,669] The greatest risk of acquiring neonatal infection occurs when the mother has an initial genital infection at the time of vaginal delivery.

The frequency of infection with the other viruses listed in Tables 73–1 and 73–2 is so low that numeric estimates per 1000 pregnancies or live births cannot be made.

APPROACH TO DIAGNOSIS

Fetal viral infection may be suspected if the mother is exposed to or experiences an infection with a virus known to transmit to the fetus; or abnormalities detected on routine fetal ultrasound may suggest fetal infection. Fetal abnormalities detected during prenatal evaluation that may be caused by in utero virus infection include intrauterine growth retardation, microcephaly, cerebral ventriculomegaly or hydrocephalus, cataracts, hepatosplenomegaly, hepatic or intracranial calcifications, echogenic bowel, fetal ascites, cardiomegaly, congestive heart failure, fetal hydrops, or poly- or oligohydramnios.[173] Intrauterine cardiac abnormalities, myocarditis, and heart failure may be associated with HIV, parvovirus B19, mumps virus, or adenovirus, and cardiac structural defects may be associated with rubella virus. Limb deformities or dysplasias, especially if they are associated with eye or central nervous system (CNS) abnormalities, may be caused by intrauterine VZV or HSV infection. Consultation with a maternal-fetal medicine specialist is recommended if fetal viral infection is suspected because intervention strategies are now available for many of these infections, which may lessen the morbidity and mortality rates associated with viral infections in the fetus.[1,173,461]

The usual set of circumstances leading one to consider the diagnosis of viral infection in a newborn infant is the presence of clinical or laboratory features in the neonate that suggest this possibility (Table 73–5). Icterus, petechiae, or hepatosplenomegaly at the time of birth or shortly thereafter in a small-for-gestational-age infant suggests a chronic in utero viral infection. On the other hand, acute viral infection in a neonate with suspected sepsis may be present when cultures of blood, spinal fluid, and urine fail to yield a bacterial or fungal agent.

Evaluation of the Mother

Once the suspicion of a viral infection in a newborn infant has been raised, one should proceed with an evaluation of the mother for features that might add further evidence to this possibility.

---

*See references 31, 66, 183, 200, 347, 381, 469, 486, 560, 576, 615, 687.

TABLE 73–5 Common Manifestations of Viral Infections in the Newborn Infant

Asymptomatic Infection
Chronic Infection (Early Gestation to Midgestation Congenital)
General Characteristics
Manifestations present at birth or shortly thereafter
Presence of congenital defects
Specific Features

General	Small for gestational age
Central nervous system	Microcephaly, seizures, cerebral calcification, hypertonia or hypotonia, cerebrospinal fluid pleocytosis, encephalitis, hydrocephalus, hearing loss
Skin	Icterus, petechiae, purpura, vesicles, hypopigmentation
Eye	Chorioretinitis, cataracts, glaucoma, microphthalmos, optic atrophy
Heart	Patent ductus arteriosus, pulmonary artery stenosis
Abdomen	Hepatosplenomegaly, hepatitis
Lung	Pneumonitis
Musculoskeletal	Bone lesions, limb hypoplasia

Acute Infection (Late Gestation Congenital, Natal, or Postnatal)
General Characteristics
Manifestations usually appear several days to weeks after birth
Absence of congenital defects
Specific Features

General	Hyperthermia or hypothermia, irritability, lethargy, jitters, poor feeding, vomiting
Central nervous system	Seizures, hypertonia or hypotonia, full fontanelle, meningitis, encephalitis, hearing loss
Skin	Icterus, petechiae, purpura, vesicles, maculopapular rash
Eye	Conjunctivitis, keratitis
Heart	Myocarditis
Abdomen	Hepatosplenomegaly, hepatitis
Lung	Pneumonitis, respiratory distress, cyanosis

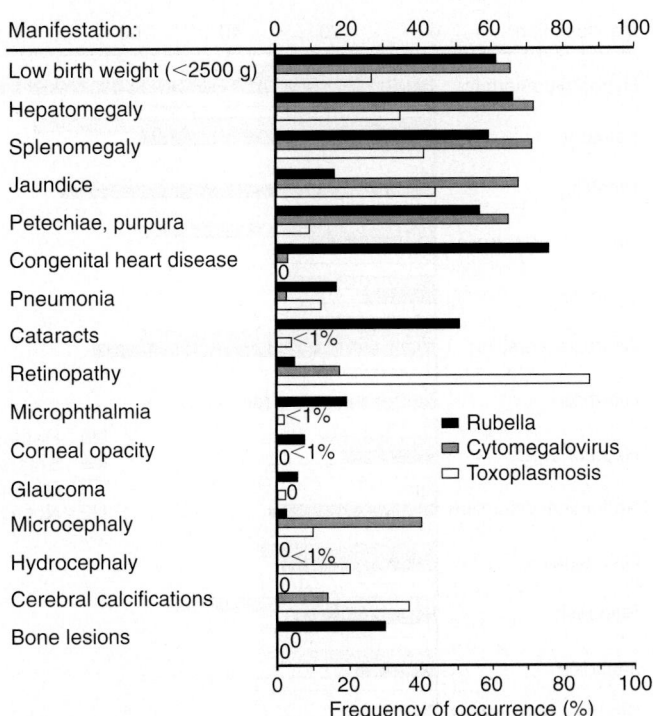

Figure 73–2 Manifestations of symptomatic congenital rubella virus and cytomegalovirus infections and toxoplamosis.

For example, the occurrence of maternal viral illness with an associated maculopapular rash suggests rubella or enterovirus infection in the neonate, whereas ulcerative genital lesions suggest HSV and heterophile-negative infectious mononucleosis is suggestive of CMV. Maternal rash with arthralgias may be caused by parvovirus B19. One should note, however, that most maternal viral infections that lead to fetal or neonatal infection (almost all cases of CMV and HBV infection[612,687] and one half to two thirds of rubella virus and HSV infections[450,568,669,675]) are asymptomatic in the mother. Therefore, the absence of a history of viral infection in the mother certainly does not rule out the possibility of a viral infection in her neonate.

Specimens from the mother for isolation or detection of the viral agent usually are not available. However, the presence of HBsAg- or CMV-specific IgM antibody in maternal serum or isolation of CMV or HSV from the genital tract or an enterovirus from the stool at the time of delivery certainly should lead one to consider these agents in her newborn infant. Serologic documentation of a specific viral illness in the mother during pregnancy requires serum specimens that bracket the illness. Unfortunately, these specimens rarely are available when the pediatrician is considering the possibility of a congenital or neonatal viral illness. Routine IgG antibody determinations on a single specimen obtained from the mother after the birth of a neonate with suspected congenital viral infection are not likely to yield useful information, except if the mother lacks IgG antibody to the pathogen in question. Such a finding in the face of a symptomatic infant would rule out that organism as the cause of the infant's disease. Although the presence of specific IgM antibody against CMV,[253,269,608] rubella virus,[246] parvovirus B19, or HSV[447] in a single maternal serum specimen is highly suggestive of recent infection, IgM tests are known to produce false-positive results and need to be interpreted accordingly. On the other hand, if the maternal viral infection occurs near the time of delivery (e.g., enterovirus meningitis, coxsackievirus B pleurodynia, initial genital herpes), acute and convalescent serum specimens may be obtained from the mother that do demonstrate the diagnostic fourfold or greater rise in antibody titer against a specific agent. Documentation of a particular causative agent in the mother does not constitute proof that the same agent is causing disease in the neonate, but it certainly does provide strong suggestive evidence. Definitive proof, therefore, must come from studies in the newborn infant.

Clinical Features in the Neonate

Certain clinical manifestations of viral disease in the neonate may provide helpful clues to the specific etiologic agent. However, most viral infections are asymptomatic in neonates: more than 95 percent of CMV, two thirds of rubella virus, and most HBV infections. In contrast, less than 1 percent of HSV infections in the neonate are subclinical. To complicate the effort to pinpoint the diagnosis further, the clinical and laboratory manifestations of symptomatic disease caused by numerous agents often have similar patterns (see Table 73–5; Figs. 73–2 and 73–3). However, infants whose congenital viral infections were incurred in early gestation to midgestation have manifestations of disease at birth or shortly thereafter, whereas infants with late-gestation congenital infections or natal or postnatal infections usually do not

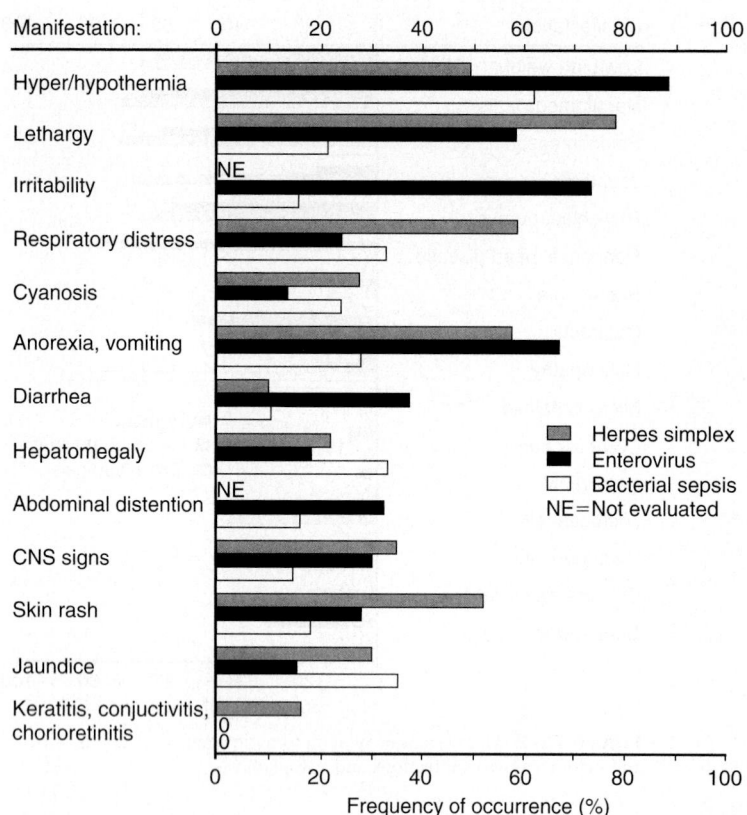

exhibit signs and symptoms for several days to several weeks after birth (see Table 73–5). In addition, newborn infants who acquire congenital infections in early gestation to midgestation exhibit congenital defects and intrauterine growth retardation, whereas neonates who acquire viral infections near the time of birth have acute disease resembling bacterial sepsis or the viral syndrome typically seen in older children (e.g., enterovirus exanthem, chickenpox) (see Table 73–5). Because the viral agents that commonly cause chronic intrauterine infections are different from those that result in acute neonatal diseases (see Tables 73–1 to 73–3), recognition of these two different patterns helps define a specific etiologic agent.

The most common manifestations of congenital CMV and rubella infection in symptomatic newborn infants are shown in Figure 73–2. Also shown in this figure are the features observed in infants with congenital toxoplasmosis because this infection is important to consider in the differential diagnosis. (Infection with *Toxoplasma gondii* is covered in another chapter.) Note that many nonspecific manifestations, such as low birth weight caused by intrauterine growth retardation, hepatomegaly, splenomegaly, jaundice, and petechiae/purpura, occur with a similar frequency in the three infections. However, certain specific findings may be helpful in the differential diagnosis. The presence of cataracts, congenital heart disease, bone lesions, or microphthalmos is highly suggestive of rubella, whereas chorioretinitis, cerebral calcifications, and hydrocephaly are findings against this diagnosis. In congenital CMV infection, microcephaly, cerebral calcifications, and sensorineural hearing loss are relatively common findings, but congenital heart disease, eye abnormalities, and bone lesions rarely occur. Chorioretinitis, cerebral calcifications, or hydrocephaly should suggest toxoplasmosis or lymphocytic chorriomeningitis virus (LCMV). The cerebral calcifications in CMV infection tend to be periventricular, whereas those in toxoplasmosis are scattered through the parietal lobes of the cerebrum. An important note is that some manifestations may not be

evident for several months after birth: congenital heart disease, chorioretinitis, microcephaly, hydrocephaly, and cerebral calcifications.

The most frequent findings in the common acute viral infections of the neonate—HSV and enterovirus infections—are shown in Figure 73–3. Because the features in infants with these two kinds of viral infection resemble those associated with bacterial sepsis, the manifestations in neonates with septicemia also are presented. Again, the more common nonspecific features, such as fever or hypothermia, respiratory distress, cyanosis, anorexia or vomiting, and hepatomegaly, occur at a relatively similar frequency in the three infections.[106,107] Lethargy, irritability, and CNS signs are found more commonly with HSV and enterovirus infections, probably because encephalitis and meningitis, respectively, occur more frequently with these two infections. Features that suggest a diagnosis of HSV infection are a vesicular rash and keratitis or conjunctivitis, whereas enterovirus infection usually is associated with diarrhea and abdominal distention. The rash in enterovirus infection usually is erythematous and maculopapular, but petechiae can occur with overwhelming infection. The skin lesions in bacterial sepsis generally are pustules, abscesses, cellulitis, or purpura.

DIFFERENTIAL DIAGNOSIS

The differential diagnosis in a fetus or newborn infant with a suspected viral infection is extensive. In the fetus, noninfectious and genetic etiologies may cause signs and symptoms similar to congenital virus syndromes. Many of the neonatal manifestations shown in Figures 73–2 and 73–3, such as lethargy, irritability, respiratory distress, cyanosis, and anorexia, can be caused by the most common diseases occurring in sick newborn infants—hyaline membrane disease, prematurity, intraventricular hemorrhage, metabolic disturbances, and bacterial sepsis.[106,107,674] Infants with low birth weight caused by intrauterine growth restriction (small for gestational age) may have congenital malformations, chromosomal abnormalities, placental insufficiency, and inborn errors of metabolism. Hepatosplenomegaly usually is caused by one of the infectious diseases of the neonate. In infants with jaundice, ABO and Rh hemolytic disease and physiologic jaundice should be considered. Noninfectious causes of petechiae/purpura include idiopathic or drug-induced (including transplacental passage) thrombocytopenia, erythroblastosis fetalis, and disseminated intravascular coagulation.

Little firm evidence indicates that infectious agents other than rubella can cause congenital heart disease. However, in utero mumps, adenovirus, CMV, and parvovirus B19 may produce myocarditis and congestive heart failure. Diffuse pulmonary infiltrates early in the neonatal period most commonly are caused by hyaline membrane disease, but in older neonates one should consider bronchopulmonary dysplasia and chlamydial infection. Causes of cataracts other than congenital rubella, HSV, and VZV infection include congenital galactosemia and the oculocerebrorenal (Lowe) syndrome. Chorioretinitis or retinopathy usually is caused by infection with *Taxoplasma gondii* or with viruses such as HSV, CMV, rubella, or LCMV. Microcephaly also can be caused by infection with HSV or VZV; noninfectious causes include Down syndrome, perinatal anoxia, phenylketonuria, and maternal irradiation. Hydrocephalus generally is caused by a congenital malformation of the ventricular aqueductal or subarachnoid space system. In a neonate with manifestations of an acute infection, major diagnostic considerations include serious bacterial infections such as sepsis, meningitis, urinary tract infection, or pneumonia. However, neonatal viral infections also are common causes of fever and sepsis syndrome in the neonate.[92,106-108,236,654,654a] After appropriate samples for bacterial and viral cultures have been obtained from the neonate, systemic antibiotics should be administered until a bacterial infection has been ruled out. Because of the frequency of neonatal HSV disease and its severe morbidity and mortality if untreated, and because results of recent studies have shown viral testing and antiviral treatment to be cost-effective as well as life-saving, some experts recommend administering intravenous acyclovir as well to selected neonates who present with fever or sepsis syndrome and appear to be at high risk for having neonatal HSV infection.[106-108]

LABORATORY DIAGNOSIS

Because the clinical manifestations in the various neonatal viral infections frequently overlap, establishing a specific etiologic diagnosis usually depends on the laboratory. General laboratory tests may show abnormalities suggestive of viral infection. For example, the peripheral white blood cell count may show neutropenia or lymphocytosis, with thrombocytopenia, and liver function tests may be elevated. The approach to the specific laboratory diagnosis of viral infection in a newborn infant is outlined in Table 73–6. Details of the various methods for each virus are covered in the respective chapters for these agents; only general comments relevant to the diagnosis of infection in the fetus or neonate are presented here.

Historically, histopathologic methods were used to attempt to establish a diagnosis of viral infection. For example, examination of stained cells from urine for CMV inclusions or examination of cells scraped from the base of a vesicle or from the conjunctiva for multinucleated giant cells with intranuclear inclusions characteristic of HSV or VZV (Tzanck-stained smear) were performed previously, but they are rarely performed currently. In addition, tissue obtained by biopsy or at postmortem examination may reveal intranuclear inclusions and multinucleated giant cells characteristic of the herpesviruses. Electron microscopy may reveal viral particles in vesicle fluid or tissue. Except for the pro-

TABLE 73–6 Laboratory Diagnosis of Viral Infection in the Newborn Infant

Procedure	Details, Comments
Routine histopathologic methods	Urine cells stained for inclusions
	Scraping of vesicle base or conjunctiva for multinucleated giant cells
	Examination of biopsy or autopsy tissue
Isolation of detection of infectious agents	Isolation of infectious agent in cell culture or animals
	Detection of viral particles by electron microscopy
	Detection of viral antigen by immunologic methods
	Detection of viral nucleic acid by DNA probes, often after amplification by PCR
IgG antiviral antibody	Persistence of antibody in serum of infant beyond age of normal decline in maternal transplacental antibody—usually 4-6 mo
	Variety of methods available (CF, neut, HI, IHA, IFA, ELISA, etc.)—sensitivity of method varies according to specific virus
IgM-specific antiviral antibody	IgM not normally passed transplacentally, presence in cord blood or neonatal serum diagnostic
	IgM-specific antibodies not always present in neonate
	False-positive and false-negative results
Quantitative IgM level	Not a specific diagnostic test, suggests intrauterine infection

CF, complement fixation; ELISA, enzyme-linked immunosorbent assay; HI, hemagglutination inhibition; IFA, immunofluorescent assay; IHA, indirect hemagglutination; neut, neutralization; PCR, polymerase chain reaction. Modified from Hanshaw, J. R., Dudgeon, J. A., and Marshall, W. C.: Viral Disease of the Fetus and Newborn. 2nd ed. Philadelphia, W. B. Saunders, 1985.

pensity to involve certain organs (e.g., rubella virus, the heart; HBV, the liver), the pathologic changes induced by viruses other than the herpes group rarely are sufficiently specific to enable one to make an etiologic diagnosis. Even for the herpesviruses, the routine histopathologic methods are only one half to two thirds as sensitive as is isolation of the virus.

The most direct, definitive, and preferred method of establishing the diagnosis is isolation of the agent from an appropriate site in the fetus or neonate. Prenatal diagnosis of fetal viral infection may be established by testing amniotic fluid for viral culture and PCR and fetal blood sample or viral-specific IgM and PCR.[310,628] The following sites generally are used in neonates: urine, saliva, and blood for CMV; throat, cataracts, and occasionally spinal fluid or urine for rubella; skin vesicles, buffy coat or whole blood, cerebrospinal fluid (CSF), conjunctivae, throat, stool, and urine for HSV; throat, stool, urine, CSF, or serum/buffy coat for enteroviruses; and skin vesicles for VZV. In addition, isolation of virus can be attempted from biopsy or autopsy specimens. Recovery of a virus from internal body fluids (buffy coat, CSF, urine), vesicle fluid, or tissue from organs is strong evidence of an etiologic association. Electron-microscopic examination of vesicle fluid can demonstrate typical herpesvirus particles in both HSV and VZV infection but cannot distinguish between the two. Immunofluorescence and immunoperoxidase methods are available for many of the viruses and can demonstrate and type viral antigen in cells scraped from lesions or in biopsy material. HBsAg is demonstrable in serum by radioimmunoassay or enzyme-linked immunosorbent assay (ELISA).

Methods for amplifying a particular segment of a viral genome, using methods such as traditional and real-time PCR, are now available in many hospital laboratories and most reference laboratories. Most commonly, testing for CMV, HBV, HSV, VZV, parvovirus B19, adenovirus, and the enteroviruses and parechoviruses is performed in neonates.[479] However, almost any viral pathogen may now be detected using molecular techniques. In general, PCR and other molecular amplification methods are more rapid and sensitive than is virus isolation and are quite specific and may become the diagnostic test of choice for many viral infections. Molecular diagnostic tests also may be performed on any body fluid, but most commonly on blood and CSF. In addition, molecular methods also have been applied recently to diagnose congenital viral infections retrospectively from archived dried blood spots and used prospectively to develop newborn screening programs.[51,659]

Though not as sensitive, immediate, or direct as is isolation or detection of the viral agent using molecular methods, serologic studies are a readily available and traditional means for laboratory diagnosis of viral infection in a fetus or newborn infant. They should be used only when isolation or detection of the organism is not possible. The "TORCH" screen for antibodies (*Toxoplasma*, other, rubella, cytomegalovirus, and herpes simplex) was developed for this purpose. However, proper interpretation of serologic tests in newborn infants requires an understanding of the kinetics of the humoral immune response in the fetus and newborn infant, as well as an appreciation of the transplacental passage of antibodies from mother to fetus. Figure 73–4 illustrates the pattern of immunoglobulin concentrations in the serum of the fetus and newborn infant, as well as older infants and children. Maternal IgG, which contains antibody against viruses to which the mother has been exposed, passes transplacentally, beginning at midgestation. Peak levels are reached in fetal serum at the time of birth (umbilical cord blood); they decline to undetectable levels by the time that the infant reaches 6 to 12 months of age. However, the use of more sensitive assays for IgG antibody detection, such as immunoblotting, has demonstrated that maternal IgG antibody may persist for as long as 15 to 18 months.

In contrast, maternal IgM antibody normally is not passed transplacentally. Because the fetus is in a "protected" environment and usually does not receive an antigenic challenge in utero, fetal immunoglobulin levels remain low and do not begin to rise until after birth, when exposure to a variety of antigens occurs. However, the fetus is capable of mounting a humoral immune response when exposed to an antigen (a virus) in utero. Elevated levels of fetal immunoglobulins, therefore, can be detected at birth in umbilical cord blood. Because maternal IgG is present

in such high concentration in cord blood serum, assays for IgM are performed. A fetus challenged in utero with a virus can have specific IgM antibodies against the viral agent, as well as elevated levels of the total IgM fraction. Often, a fetus with detectable virus-specific IgM will have severe in utero disease caused by the virus. Typically, three approaches can be used to make a serologic diagnosis of viral infection in a newborn infant: (1) assay of maternal serum and serum specimens from the infant at birth and at 5 to 6 months of age for antiviral antibody (predominantly IgG activity), (2) assay of neonatal serum for IgM antibody against a specific viral agent, and (3) assay of neonatal serum for quantitative IgM levels, a nonspecific indication of antigenic challenge in utero.

For purposes of illustration, the rubella hemagglutination-inhibition titers of two mother/infant pairs are shown in Table 73–7. Both mothers were exposed to someone with a rubella-like rash during pregnancy. The first mother was susceptible; subclinical rubella developed, and she delivered an infant with congenital rubella, whereas the second mother was immune and delivered an uninfected normal infant. The serum specimen obtained from the first mother at the time of exposure showed no detectable hemagglutination-inhibition titer, whereas the serum at delivery and 6 months postpartum showed high titers indicative of acute rubella virus infection during pregnancy. Serum specimens from her infant at birth and at 6 months of age demonstrated rubella virus hemagglutination-inhibition antibodies at approximately the same level, thus indicating the persistence of antibody formed by the infant and substantiating the occurrence of congenital infection. In the second mother, the rubella hemagglutination-inhibition titers remained unchanged in all three specimens. Her infant had evidence of transplacental maternal antibody in serum obtained at birth but no detectable antibody at 6 months of age. Similar results could be expected from serologic studies with the other viral agents listed in Tables 73–1 and 73–2, not only for congenital infections but also for natal and postnatal infections in which primary viral infection occurred in the mother. Even with natal infections in immune mothers and postnatal infections from nonmaternal sources, the serologic responses in the neonate would be similar to those shown in Table 73–7.

The presence of IgM antibodies in maternal, fetal, or neonatal serum against a specific virus usually is considered to be diagnostic of acute or recent infection with that agent. However, both false-positive and false-negative results can occur. False-positive findings can result from cross-reaction between viruses, espe-

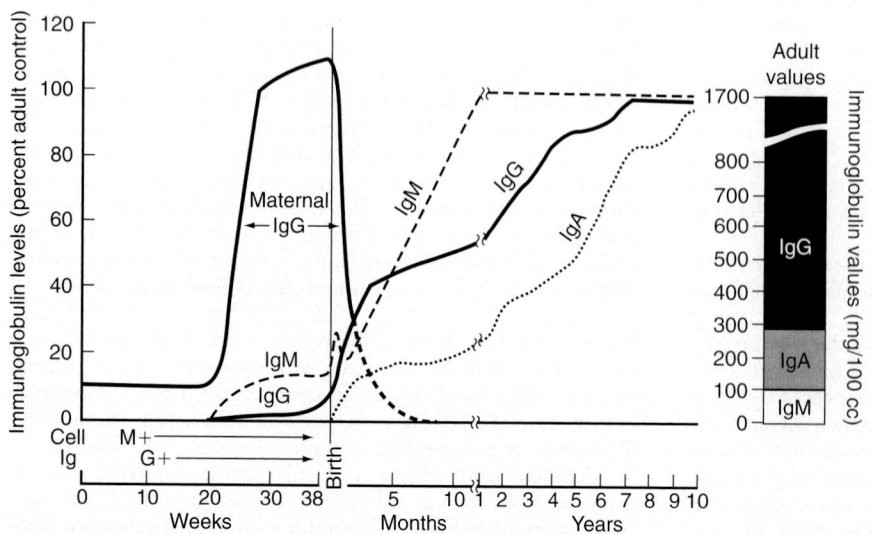

Figure 73–4 Kinetics of fetal and neonatal immunoglobulins. (*From Alford, C. A.: Immunoglobulin determinations in the diagnosis of fetal children. Pediatr. Clin. North Am. 18:99–113, 1971.*)

TABLE 73–7 Mother and Infant Serologic Response in Congenital Rubella

Serum Specimens	Rubella Hemagglutination-Inhibition Antibody Titers			
	Mother A	Infant A	Mother B	Infant B
At exposure	<8	–	128	–
At birth	1024	1024	128	256
6 mo postpartum	1024	2048	250	<8
Comment	Congenital rubella		Passive transfer of antibody; no congenital rubella	

cially the herpesviruses,[458] and the presence of rheumatoid factor (IgM antibody that binds to the Fc portion of IgG) in serum.[129] False-negative results can occur because of a poor or delayed humoral immune response in the fetus/neonate. For example, CMV IgM antibody was present in the serum of only 70 percent of congenitally infected infants, as demonstrated by isolation of virus from urine in the first few days of life.[608]

Determination of a quantitative IgM level in cord-blood serum often has been recommended as a screening test for congenital viral infection. Values above 20 mg/dL are considered to be abnormal, but the normal values in local laboratories should be used as a guide.[18] Unfortunately, contamination of cord-blood serum samples by maternal blood may occur in one half to two thirds of specimens.[15,425] Contamination is determined by demonstrating that the concentration of cord-blood serum IgA, which also is not passed transplacentally, is higher than the IgM level. If one excludes contaminated specimens, the incidence of congenital infection in infants with an elevated IgM level is many times higher than that in infants with normal levels. However, at least 50 percent of infants with a proven congenital infection, particularly those with asymptomatic infection, have a normal IgM level. In two thirds of infants with elevated IgM, infection with a specific etiologic agent could not be diagnosed.[15,18] Therefore, high rates of both false-positive and false-negative results occur. Finally, an elevated IgM level does not enable a specific etiologic diagnosis; it merely provides strong evidence for an intrauterine infection of some type.

The similarities in the clinical signs and physical findings associated with congenital and perinatal infection have led to the recommendation that for establishing appropriate diagnoses of these infections, submission of maternal and neonatal serum specimens for the "TORCH" screen or, in selected instances, a single neonatal specimen for specific IgM antibodies is best. The use of a "TORCH" battery of serologic tests, however, no longer can be recommended routinely because of poor diagnostic return; these tests are difficult to interpret because of transplacental passage of maternal IgG antibodies, and IgM assays may result in false-positive findings.[1] Instead, the laboratory test or tests that should be performed must be dictated by which congenital infection or infections one is trying to diagnose or rule out. As seen in Table 73–6, the variety of tests that are available for establishing the diagnosis of any of the multitude of different potential congenital pathogens renders a "TORCH" assay, and by inference the term "TORCH" itself, obsolete by current standards. Finally, if a congenital infection is suspected in the delivery room, the placenta should be sent for histopathologic studies.

CYTOMEGALOVIRUS

CMV is a ubiquitous agent that usually causes asymptomatic infection in a normal infant, child, or adult. CMV is the most common congenital infection in humans. Overall, the birth prevalence for congenital CMV infection has been estimated at 0.64 percent, with ranges between 0.4 and 1.2 percent reported. Con-

genital CMV infection occurs after both maternal primary and recurrent infections during pregnancy. It remains a worldwide public health problem for which interventions are critically necessary.[105,323,535] However, patients with immature or impaired host defenses, such as a fetus, newborn infant, or immunosuppressed patient, may exhibit a variety of clinical manifestations during the acute infection and have a greater potential for developing long-term neurologic sequelae.[17,178,228,267,451]

MICROBIOLOGY AND EPIDEMIOLOGY

CMV is a member of the herpesvirus group, which includes HSV, VZV, and Epstein-Barr virus, as well as human herpesvirus 6 (HHV6), HHV7, and HHV8. Several different genotypes or genetic strains of CMV differ, and an individual can have more than one CMV genotype or strain infection.[17,178,228] Different genotypes are associated with congenital CMV infection and disease; gB3 genotype appears to predominate in some studies, but no clear association between genotype and pathogenesis has been identified.[47,691]

Human CMV is limited to the human host and grows only in human cells in tissue culture. Its distribution is worldwide, and no predilection for either sex or a particular season of the year exists.* Studies of antibody prevalence and virus isolation have indicated two peak ages for acquisition of infection: (1) infancy and early childhood and (2) early adulthood (in the sexually active).[228,699] Infection rates are higher and exposure to the virus occurs earlier in life in developing countries, lower socioeconomic groups in industrial nations, and Asian populations.[228] The major source of infection of young infants is the mother, whereas transmission in the daycare setting is an important source for older infants and toddlers.[490,599] Approximately 50 percent of susceptible children between the ages of 1 to 3 years who are in group daycare acquire CMV, mostly by transfer of virus present in saliva on hands and toys. Within 3 to 7 months of their child's acquiring CMV infection in the daycare center, as many as 33 percent of the seronegative mothers become infected.[7] Transmission of CMV from a child in daycare to his mother and her fetus has been confirmed. Thus, CMV infection in young children in daycare has become an important source of maternal and fetal infection.[323,491] In young adults, intimate interpersonal contact appears to be necessary for transmission and an infected sexual partner also may be the source of infection for a pregnant woman and her fetus.

The usual sites for isolation of virus are the urine, cervix, and saliva,[228] but CMV also has been recovered from amniotic fluid,[171] semen,[375,376] breast milk,[202,277] feces,[159] and autopsy and biopsy tissue. Excretion of virus in urine, saliva, or the cervix may be prolonged after primary infection, particularly with congenital disease.[17,178,603,606] Intermittent, recurring shedding also may occur in a significant proportion of seropositive young adults.[528,604,606] Despite this prevalence of virus excretion, CMV seems to be of low communicability.[228] Beyond the neonatal period,

---

*See references 17, 52, 105, 170, 178, 228, 302, 305, 323, 535, 660.

infection appears to require prolonged or intimate contact and presumably is transmitted through contact with oropharyngeal or genital secretions.[105] Researchers have assumed that CMV may be transmitted sexually because of the frequency of isolation of virus from genital secretions and because the prevalence of antibody is higher in sexually active populations.[17,178] Finally, transmission of CMV by blood transfusion has been documented, particularly in the event of multiple seropositive blood donors.[10,228]

Prenatal transmission of CMV to the fetus presumably is associated with maternal viremia and transplacental passage of the virus, perhaps within virus-infected leukocytes.[17,178] An important observation is that congenital CMV infection occurs in the infants of mothers known to be immune to CMV, thus indicating that transplacental transmission is possible despite circulating antibody in maternal serum.[600,603] In addition, mothers have delivered more than one congenitally infected infant in successive pregnancies.[603,604] Analysis of CMV isolates obtained from the same mothers on repeated occasions are antigenically and genetically identical, whereas strains from different mothers are not.[297] In addition, strains obtained from pairs of mothers and their congenitally infected infant pairs, as well as congenitally infected siblings, usually, but not always, are identical. These results suggest that most CMV transmission from immune mothers to their fetuses or newborns is the result of reactivated latent infection. Recently, however, Boppana and colleagues[82] have documented that acquisition of a new strain of CMV by pregnant immune women can lead to symptomatic congenital CMV infection in their offspring. Fetal CMV infection also may occur in HIV-infected pregnant women.[194,443,558] Symptomatic congenital CMV infection has been documented in a preterm infant who died of disseminated CMV infection and was born to an HIV-infected, CMV-immune mother with acquired immunodeficiency syndrome (AIDS).[558] Among HIV-infected, CMV-immune women without advanced HIV disease, the rate of congenital CMV infection in their infants was similar to that of a comparison group of infants born to CMV-immune, HIV-uninfected mothers.[354,443] In another study, among a cohort of infants born to HIV-infected mothers, infants who were infected with HIV were significantly more likely to have congenital CMV infection than were non–HIV-infected infants, 21 versus 4 percent, respectively.[194] Importantly, HIV-infected infants who are co-infected with CMV appear to have greater immunosuppression and progression of disease than do those infected with HIV alone.[194,354,459]

Natal transmission of CMV results from exposure of the neonate to infected genital secretions at the time of delivery.[17,528,529] If the mother is excreting virus at the time of delivery, 40 to 50 percent of exposed infants become infected.[528] The level of maternal antibody did not influence the frequency or time of onset of infection in the neonate. The usual incubation period for natal infection is 5 to 6 weeks.[529]

The importance of breast milk and blood transfusion as sources for postnatal acquisition of CMV was mentioned earlier in the section "Frequency of Infection in the Mother and Neonate." Although nosocomial transmission of CMV from baby to baby via fomites or health care workers' hands in the neonatal intensive care unit has been documented,[593] it rarely occurs.[8,219]

PATHOGENESIS AND PATHOLOGY

Congenital infection results from transplacental transmission during maternal viremia.[17] However, CMV placentitis may occur without transplacental transmission of virus.[278] If transplacental transmission occurs, the virus spreads through the fetus by the hematogenous route.[400,550] The severity of congenital disease in the neonate usually, but not always, correlates with intrauterine

infection at an earlier gestational age.[598] With the exception of blood transfusion-associated infection, natal and postnatal infection with CMV usually is acquired secondary to challenge of the nasopharynx or oropharynx of the infant with virus from infected maternal genital secretions or breast milk.[17,178] Replication of virus in the neonate occurs in the mucosa of the respiratory or gastrointestinal tract, with subsequent viremic spread to target organs. With blood transfusion-associated infection, virus is inoculated directly into the bloodstream. The major target organs are the CNS, eyes, lungs, liver, and kidneys.[17] Of interest is that overt disease in the neonate appears to be associated more commonly with the hematogenous route of inoculation: transplacental infection or infection secondary to blood transfusion.

CMV appears to have a particular affinity for epithelial cells, for ependymal cells lining the ventricles of the brain, and for the organ of Corti and neurons of the eighth nerve.[602] The characteristic pathologic features of CMV infection are cytolysis, focal necrosis and an inflammatory response, the formation of enlarged cells with intranuclear inclusions (cytomegalic cells), and the production of multinucleated giant cells. Healing results in fibrosis and often calcifications, which cause structural damage to the fetal developing organs. Damage may continue after birth because of persistent postnatal viral replication.[17] Replication of CMV in the epithelial cells of blood vessels may result in vascular damage and secondary structural defects. The intrauterine growth restriction associated with symptomatic congenital infection appears to be the result of a reduction in the numbers of cells in various organs rather than a diminution in cell size.[444] Abnormalities resulting from faulty organogenesis secondary to CMV infection are limited primarily to the brain and include microcephaly, optic atrophy, aplasia of various parts of the brain, and microphthalmos.[265] Although a variety of congenital malformations outside the CNS have been observed in infants with congenital CMV infection, they probably are coincidental rather than true teratogenic effects of the virus.[265] Such malformations include a variety of heart lesions, clubfoot deformities, indirect inguinal hernias, high arched palate, dental defects, and hypospadias.[17,265] Other than inguinal hernia in male infants and tooth enamel defects, the extraneural defects in infants with congenital CMV infection have been infrequent, sporadic, and diverse occurrences.

The fetus is capable of mounting a humoral immune response to CMV, as evidenced by the presence of elevated IgM levels and specific CMV IgM antibody in cord serum.[17,530,608] Excessive production of IgM and IgG in the presence of virus replication during the early postnatal course of congenital CMV has resulted in the formation of circulating immune complexes and rheumatoid factor, thereby providing a potential risk for tissue damage to occur by immune complexes.[609] The factors contributing to prolonged replication and excretion of CMV in involved infants are not understood fully, but it does not appear to be a matter of immunologic tolerance because infants do produce specific antibody against CMV.[17]

However, abnormalities in other aspects of the immune response of congenitally infected infants, including decreased lymphocyte blastogenesis and production of immune interferon in response to CMV antigen,[527,613] a decreased percentage of T cells in peripheral blood,[548] and a diminished interferon response in leukocytes challenged with Newcastle disease virus in vitro, have been observed.[210] The degree of suppression of these responses appears to correlate with the presence and amount of virus excretion and the severity of the disease.[529,613] Further investigations are necessary to determine the contribution of these immunologic aberrations to the pathogenesis of congenital CMV infection. The clinical relevance of these immunologic impairments is uncertain. Infants with congenital CMV infection do not have a higher incidence or severity of bacterial infections, although three fatal cases of overwhelming sepsis secondary to

Staphylococcus epidermidis have been described in CMV-infected, low-birth-weight infants.[365] Recently, *Pneumocystis carinii* pneumonia was reported in a 4-month-old infant who had congenital CMV infection; this infant was not infected with HIV but was severely malnourished.[386]

CLINICAL MANIFESTATIONS

From 90 to 95 percent of neonates with congenital CMV infection are asymptomatic in the neonatal period. Babies born to mothers with primary CMV infection during pregnancy are much more likely to be symptomatic as neonates than are newborns of mothers with recurrent infection.[11,17,23,178,510,600] The clinical manifestations present in those with overt disease in the neonatal period are shown in Figure 73–2. These features may occur singly or in combination. The constellation of findings seen in infants with multiorgan disease that primarily affects the reticuloendothelial system and CNS historically has been referred to as *cytomegalic inclusion disease*, a term that rarely, if ever, is used today.

Typical clinical features of symptomatic congenital CMV disease include small size for gestational age, hepatomegaly, splenomegaly, jaundice, petechiae or purpura, pneumonia, microcephaly, chorioretinitis, and cerebral calcifications.[589] The enlargement of the liver and spleen is caused by mild hepatitis, a reticuloendothelial response to chronic infection, and extramedullary hematopoiesis. Hepatitis is associated with direct- and indirect-reacting hyperbilirubinemia and mild elevation of liver enzymes. Liver biopsy specimens have revealed local infiltration and necrosis, multinucleated giant cells, large inclusion-bearing cells, cholangitis, fatty metamorphosis, interstitial fibrosis, and bile stasis.[17,178] Although hepatomegaly and mild alteration in liver function test results may persist for several months after birth, severe chronic liver disease with cirrhosis rarely occurs. Splenomegaly is a common event and may be the only abnormality present at birth. Petechiae and purpura are the result of thrombocytopenia, which usually resolves within a few weeks or months but may persist through the first year of life. Thrombocytopenia may be the only manifestation of CMV infection. "Blueberry muffin spots" are discrete, well-circumscribed lesions often mistaken for purpura; they represent dermal erythropoiesis in the more severely affected infants. A diffuse interstitial pneumonitis occurs in less than 1 percent of newborns with symptomatic disease. Congenital CMV infection also has been associated with defective enamelization of the deciduous teeth.[601]

Involvement of the CNS by CMV results in the most severe sequelae of the disease. CMV infection of the brain causes encephalitis and periependymitis, with resultant ventriculomegaly, gliosis, and calcification. The cerebral calcifications typically are periventricular, a pattern that may be distinguished from the more diffuse pattern observed in congenital toxoplasmosis. In addition, linear calcifications along the lenticulostriate vessels within the basal ganglia and thalamus have been associated with CMV infection. Intracranial calcifications are best visualized by unenhanced computed tomography (CT) scan of the brain; however, cranial ultrasound and brain magnetic resonance imaging (MRI) also have been applied to discern abnormalities.[128] As many as 70 percent of symptomatic infants have neurologic findings, with the most common being microcephaly. Microcephaly may not be present at birth but may become apparent when the child is 1 year of age or older, a period in which differences in growth rates between the brain and somatic tissues are observed. When associated with cerebral calcifications and chorioretinitis, microcephaly carries a high probability of developmental disabilities.[465] On occasion, microcephaly is associated with obstruction of the fourth ventricle, with subsequent development of hydrocephalus. As many as 37 percent of congenitally

infected infants with neuroradiologic abnormalities will develop seizures.[623]

The most common ocular abnormalities are chorioretinitis, strabismus, and optic atrophy.[145] Central vision loss may occur in neonates with severe CNS involvement.[145] Although microphthalmos, cataracts, and other eye abnormalities have been observed in congenitally infected infants, they are rare occurrences and most likely are not caused by CMV, but rather represent a coincidental finding with another etiology.[145,265] Permanent vision loss may occur as long-term sequela.

Deafness is the most common sequela of congenital CMV infection. Sensorineural hearing loss occurs in approximately 50 to 75 percent of symptomatic infants and 7 to 15 percent of those with asymptomatic congenital infection. Hearing loss associated with symptomatic infection usually is severe and bilateral, whereas the hearing loss in asymptomatically infected infants usually is unilateral. Both forms of hearing loss are progressive.[230,678] Approximately 20 percent of infants with congenital CMV have late-onset hearing loss that will not manifest until after the child reaches 1 year of age.

Most naturally acquired natal and postnatal CMV infections in full-term newborn infants are asymptomatic and not associated with late neurologic sequelae such as hearing loss and psychomotor retardation. Most of these infections result from reactivation of latent maternal CMV, and infants are born with transplacentally acquired maternal IgG antibody that ameliorates the disease. However, mostly pneumonitis, but also hepatosplenomegaly and lymphadenopathy, has been noted in some infants.[366,597,670,698] Severe disease manifested also by neutropenia and thrombocytopenia has been reported predominantly in preterm infants and is associated with the development of chronic lung disease.[698] In addition, exacerbation of congenital CMV infection has been documented in premature infants receiving corticosteroid therapy for chronic lung disease of prematurity.[648] Similarly, postnatal acquisition of CMV through breast-feeding nearly always is an asymptomatic infection in full-term infants because of the presence of maternal antibodies. CMV infection acquired through breast milk by premature infants with a birth weight of 1000 g or less has been associated with a sepsis-like illness consisting of apnea and bradycardia, hepatosplenomegaly, a distended bowel, pallor, thrombocytopenia, and elevated liver function test results.[263,656]

Transfusion-acquired CMV infection is an important clinical syndrome associated with multiple blood transfusions from seropositive donors to very-low-birth-weight infants in neonatal intensive care units.[10,50,692,697] Eighty-eight percent of babies had hepatosplenomegaly, a "septic" appearance, deterioration in respiratory status, a peculiar gray pallor, and atypical lymphocytosis approximately 4 to 12 weeks after receiving transfusions.[10,50,697] The illness lasted 2 to 3 weeks in most infants, although 24 percent died.

DIAGNOSIS AND DIFFERENTIAL DIAGNOSIS

Primary CMV infection occurring during pregnancy is documented by demonstration of IgG seroconversion with sera obtained before or during early pregnancy and at delivery. Detection of anti-CMV IgM in a single specimen is considered a presumptive primary infection.[12,13,253,364,452,509,608] Caution, however, must be exercised when analyzing the results of CMV IgM tests. Even with the best commercially available assays, at least 5 percent of positive serum IgM tests represent false-positive results. On the other hand, a negative CMV IgG antibody test in the mother of an infant in whom the diagnosis of CMV infection is in question would exclude congenital transmission as a possible source of CMV. CMV avidity tests can be helpful in distinguishing recent primary infections from past recurrent

CMV infections in CMV-seropositive women. The prenatal diagnosis of congenital CMV infection can be accomplished by amniocentesis, with detection of CMV in amniotic fluid by culture and PCR. Fetal blood sampling for CMV IgM determination, complete blood count (CBC) with platelet count, and serial fetal ultrasound examinations can help identify fetuses at high risk for developing disease and sequelae.[41,213,388]

Because the signs and symptoms of symptomatic CMV infection in newborns so often overlap with those in other diseases during this period of life, establishing a definitive diagnosis requires the use of laboratory tests. Isolation of virus from urine or saliva collected within the first 21 days of life is considered proof of congenital infection and is the most sensitive and recommended means of diagnosis.[17,178] The usual specimens for isolation of CMV are urine and saliva,[48] but virus may be recovered from CSF, buffy coat, nasopharynx, tears, and biopsy and postmortem tissue.[465] Congenitally infected infants are known to excrete virus for several years after birth. Isolation of virus in an infant beyond 3 weeks of age does not, by itself, differentiate between natal or postnatal infection and congenital infection, unless negative cultures have been obtained previously. Detection of CMV DNA by PCR in urine, saliva, blood,[235,311] or CSF also may confirm congenital infection, although the sensitivity and specificity of PCR performed on urine may be less than those for viral culture.[179,455] On the other hand, PCR is preferred for detection of CMV in CSF and blood because CMV culture usually is negative.[203,365,643] The presence of CMV DNA by PCR in the CSF of congenitally infected infants has correlated with abnormal neurologic outcome.[643] Similarly, the finding of a positive serum or whole blood CMV PCR in infants with congenital CMV infection has been associated with the development of hearing loss.[86] Quantitative CMV PCR assays also may be used to follow antiviral therapy.

Serologic tests, such as "TORCH" titers performed for specific antibody determination in neonates, rarely are helpful and are not recommended for establishing a diagnosis of congenital infection. If serologic tests that predominantly measure IgG are used, serial serum specimens from birth are required to differentiate congenital from natal or postnatal infection. One observes maintenance of a stable antibody titer during the first 6 months of life in infants with a congenital infection. In contrast, with natal and postnatal infection, a drop in antibody titer occurs during the first 2 to 3 months of life as maternal passive antibody declines, followed by a rise by the time the infant reaches 5 to 6 months of age.[529,607] If the infant is not evaluated until several months of age and serum specimens from earlier life are not available, determining whether the infection is congenital, natal, or postnatal in origin may not be possible.

Detection of CMV antigenemia in blood can be achieved by means of a commercial assay that uses monoclonal antibodies to pp65, a tegument protein of the virus that is present in infected polymorphonuclear leukocytes.[190] Its major use may be for evaluation of a symptomatic infant who has natally or postnatally acquired CMV infection, for which making a differentiation between congenital and acquired CMV infection is difficult at best and the finding of a positive urine CMV culture may be only incidental. The assay is quantitative, so it also may be used to follow antiviral treatment.

Examination for inclusion-bearing cells in urine carries historical significance, but this test yields positive results in only 20 to 50 percent of known virus-positive cases, and it is rarely, if ever, used today.[17,178] Typical intranuclear inclusions also may be seen in biopsy tissue or in megakaryocytes of bone marrow aspirates,[17,178] but virus may be isolated from tissue when these pathologic findings are absent.

The major diseases to consider in the differential diagnosis include congenital syphilis, congenital rubella, congenital toxoplasmosis, erythroblastosis fetalis, disseminated HSV infection, LCMV, neonatal sepsis, and enterovirus infection. Congenital syphilis is suggested by the presence of osteochondritis and periostitis on radiographs of the long bones in an infant born to a mother with reactive serologic tests for syphilis. Darkfield examination of spirochete-laden nasal secretions in infants with rhinitis confirms the diagnosis. The presence of congenital heart disease and cataracts suggests rubella, and chorioretinitis, hydrocephalus, and intracranial calcifications suggest toxoplasmosis, but a definitive diagnosis depends on the laboratory findings. In uncomplicated erythroblastosis, the direct bilirubin and liver function study results remain normal. Vesicular skin lesions suggest HSV or VZV infection. Positive blood cultures confirm the diagnosis of neonatal sepsis. Congenital CMV infection seldom is complicated by bacterial sepsis in a newborn. Neonatal enterovirus infections are seasonal; associated with maternal symptoms of enteroviral disease; and characterized by aseptic meningitis, hepatitis, myocarditis, or gastroenteritis. Biliary atresia, as well as noninfectious and genetic and metabolic disorders, also may mimic congenital CMV disease.

TREATMENT

Although treatment with idoxuridine,[148] floxuridine,[223] 5-fluorodeoxyuridine,[506] cytosine arabinoside,[357,405,506] adenine arabinoside,[58,138] interferon inducers,[506] human interferon,[38,211] and acyclovir[505] has been tried in infants with congenital CMV infection, the only effect was a transient alteration in viral excretion. Unfortunately, little or no effect on the clinical course of the disease was achieved with these early antiviral compounds. Foscarnet, cidofovir, ganciclovir, and valganciclovir are currently licensed for treatment of life- and sight-threatening CMV infections. Of these antivirals, only ganciclovir has been subjected to clinical trials that evaluated the pharmacokinetics and efficacy in treatment of newborns with virologically proven CMV disease.* Neither standard nor CMV hyperimmune intravenous immunoglobulin is recommended for the treatment of congenital CMV infection. However, in nonrandomized studies, maternal administration for in utero fetal treatment with CMV hyperimmune globulin has shown possible benefit in preventing transmission to the fetus and in ameliorating fetal disease.[440,462] Also, the extremely premature infant who develops CMV disease postnatally, after maternal IgG levels have declined and after administration of only CMV-seronegative blood products, may be devoid of virus-specific CMV antibody and, therefore, if CMV IgG levels are nil or negative, may possibly benefit from administration of IGIV or CMV hyperimmune globulin. However, there are no clinical trials published that evaluate the supportive role of immune globulin in the treatment of CMV disease in these special infants.

Clinical studies and experience support the use of ganciclovir in selected neonates. A phase II study of intravenous ganciclovir (4 or 6 mg/kg per dose every 12 hours for 6 weeks) in 47 neonates with congenital CMV infection involving the CNS found that the preferred dose was 12 mg/kg/day.[671] Adverse effects of ganciclovir included neutropenia in 16 (34%) infants, increases in aspartate aminotransferase in 6 (13%), and direct hyperbilirubinemia in 3 (6%). Hearing was improved or stabilized in 16 percent of infants at 6 months or longer of follow-up, thus suggesting efficacy.

Furthermore, a phase III, multicenter randomized study of ganciclovir therapy for infants with congenital CMV infection involving the CNS was performed by the Collaborative Antiviral Study Group (CASG) from 1991 to 1999.[335] This study evaluated

*See references 25, 180, 286, 330, 335, 411, 420, 421, 460, 462, 555, 590, 629, 646, 648.

the safety and efficacy of intravenous ganciclovir (6 mg/kg per dose every 12 hours for 6 weeks) versus no therapy in 100 enrolled CMV-infected neonates with neurologic involvement (≥32 weeks of gestation, birth weight ≥1200 g). Among 47 evaluable infants who completed all protocol follow-up evaluations, those who received ganciclovir were significantly more likely to have either improved or normal hearing at 6 months than were untreated infants, and none of the ganciclovir-treated infants had worse hearing. At 1 year or longer, those who received ganciclovir also were significantly less likely to have worse hearing than were those in the untreated group. Other beneficial effects of ganciclovir therapy included a significant decrease in the median time to normalization of alanine transaminase, as well as improved weight gain and head circumference after 6 weeks of therapy, but no change in mortality rates. Neutropenia developed in 63 percent of ganciclovir recipients, reversible with adjustment or discontinuation of medication. In addition, neurodevelopmental assessments in neonates at 6 to 12 months of age showed that treated neonates had fewer milestone delays and improved growth in head circumference compared with untreated neonates, suggesting another potential benefit of ganciclovir therapy.[335]

Currently, offering ganciclovir therapy to CMV-infected neonates with CNS disease seems reasonable because 90 to 95 percent of these infants will have significant neurologic and sensory sequelae. The decision to treat should be individualized and carefully considered.[25] Because 6 weeks of therapy may not be sufficient for optimal benefit, a phase I/II pharmacokinetic evaluation of oral valganciclovir in neonates with CMV infection of the CNS has been published recently, with the hope that studies evaluating the effects of long-term oral suppressive therapy will be soon conducted.[330,335] Ganciclovir also may be beneficial in treating critically ill neonates, especially preterm infants, with life-threatening CMV disease manifested by viral sepsis syndrome, persistent thrombocytopenia, recurrent or progressive sight threatening retinitis, persistent or severe pneumonitis, persistent hepatitis, or encephalitis.[179]

PROGNOSIS

The major long-term sequelae of neonatal CMV infection are neurodevelopmental, motor, and sensory disabilities.[231,269,367,530,541,602] The most guarded prognosis occurs in neonates born to mothers with primary CMV infection during pregnancy; in infants with symptoms at birth, particularly those of the CNS; in infants with the triad of microcephaly, intracranial calcifications, and chorioretinitis; and in neonates who have elevated quantitative IgM or in whom CMV-specific IgM is present.[17,81,178,231,252,367,465,466,678] The duration of CMV urinary excretion has not been associated with abnormalities in growth or neurodevelopmental deficits.[465] Overall, 25 percent of infants born to mothers with primary CMV infection during pregnancy will have at least one sequela, versus 8 percent of those born to mothers with recurrent infection.[231] Of symptomatic, congenitally infected neonates, approximately 8 percent die in the neonatal period.[82,589] Six percent of symptomatic infants die after the neonatal period, and death often is caused by progressive liver disease, failure to thrive, seizures, or intercurrent illnesses. Death beyond infancy is a result of malnutrition, aspiration pneumonia, or overwhelming infection. Of survivors with symptomatic congenital CMV disease, as many as 90 percent have some evidence of CNS abnormality, such as microcephaly, impaired intellect or development, neuromuscular disorders (seizures, cerebral palsy, spasticity, hemiparesis), sensorineural hearing loss, and ocular abnormalities (usually chorioretinitis).[147,231,492,596,679] Neurologic sequelae of congenital CMV disease, especially sensorineural hearing loss, may progress after the first year of life.[80]

For this reason, the recommendation is that CMV-infected newborns have close audiologic and neurodevelopmental follow-up through childhood and adolescence. Cochlear transplantation performed in children as young as 11 months of age, accompanied by intensive speech language therapy, has been used successfully in infants who have profound bilateral hearing loss from congenital CMV disease.

Ninety to 95 percent of infants with congenital CMV infection are asymptomatic in the neonatal period. As many as 25 percent of these infants will have abnormal brain CT scans. Several long-term follow-up studies have indicated that as many as 15 percent will have progressive hearing loss, and at least 10 percent of these infants may have neurodevelopmental and auditory processing differences and disabilities, possibly caused by CMV. The following abnormalities were noted in infected infants when compared with matched control children: IQ less than 90 (32 vs. 16%), significant hearing loss (23 vs. 9%), predicted school failure (36 vs. 14%), and microcephaly (15 vs. 5%).[268,530] Auditory imperception problems also have been associated with congenital CMV infection in children with normal hearing. In addition, approximately 2 percent of infants with asymptomatic congenital infection may have silent, unrecognized chorioretinitis.[145]

As many as one third of neonates who acquire CMV natally from maternal cervical secretions may have acute disease associated with the onset of viruria, regardless of birth weight.[366,698] However, birth weight and age of onset of viral excretion appear to influence the development of neurologic sequelae significantly. Full-term neonates with natally acquired CMV do not have significantly altered behavioral, neurologic, audiologic, speech, and language examinations on long-term follow-up when compared with uninfected controls.[367] In contrast, infants with birth weight less than 2000 g and onset of CMV excretion before they reach 8 weeks of age have associated severe cardiopulmonary disease during the neonatal intensive care unit stay (perhaps because of CMV worsening the pulmonary disease) and a significantly greater percentage of severe handicaps on long-term follow-up than do matched controls.[489] The relationships among low birth weight, early onset of CMV excretion, lower levels of transplacental antibody, and more severe cardiopulmonary disease and their contribution to neurologic sequelae require further evaluation, but natal acquisition of CMV appears to contribute to the development of sequelae in selected situations. CMV disease acquired from blood transfusion in very-low-birth-weight infants also may contribute to neurologic sequelae.[10,17,697]

Infants with congenital CMV infection have many special needs. These infants and children require physical, occupational, and speech therapy, as well as audiologic follow-up to assess their need for hearing aids and cochlear implantation. Ophthalmologic follow-up also is necessary because strabismus, optic atrophy, and, rarely, late onset chorioretinitis may develop and affect visual acuity. Failure to thrive secondary to swallowing dysfunction, such as microaspiration and gastroesophageal reflux, often is present in the more severely affected infants, which renders the need for gastrostomy tube feeding essential for survival. This decision often becomes an ethical issue, as is establishment of resuscitation orders. Severely affected children also may have sleep disorders that may require the use of nighttime sedatives. In less severely affected children, school function must be assessed carefully. Finally, all these issues bring stress to the family unit, and the need for family support cannot be overemphasized.

PREVENTION

Routine serologic screening of pregnant women currently is not recommended routinely by all experts because no prophylactic or therapeutic interventions, such as vaccines or antivirals, are available during pregnancy. However, many experts recommend that women of child-bearing years be aware of their CMV serostatus and also be aware of the most likely sources of CMV infection.[105] In addition, physicians caring for women who may become or are pregnant should counsel them about hygienic precautions that may reduce the risk of acquiring CMV infection during pregnancy, and educational materials are available to assist in counseling (*www.cdc.gov/cmv* or *www.bcm.edu/pedi/infect/cmv*). During pregnancy, meticulous adherence to standard precautions, especially handwashing after exposure to urine or saliva from young infants and toddlers and avoidance of kissing and sharing utensils with toddlers and young children who are likely to be shedding CMV, currently may be the most effective means of preventing transmission of CMV infection to susceptible pregnant women.[25,105,124,308] CMV often is transmitted within the family settings and in daycare centers caring for infants, toddlers, and young children. The rate of transmission of CMV in the hospital setting appears to be low[181,228] because prolonged or intimate contact seems to be necessary for spread to occur.[17,181,228,693] For this reason and because of the ubiquity of the virus, pregnant women are not excluded routinely from caring for patients infected with CMV.[25] Adherence to universal, standard precautions for all patients is adequate to prevent CMV transmission to patients and health care workers.[181]

Blood transfusion–associated CMV infection in low-birth-weight infants in neonatal intensive care units virtually has been eliminated by the use of CMV-seronegative blood donors,[6,88,374,385] frozen deglycerolized red cells,[88,631] removal of the buffy coat by saline washing,[179] and filtration to remove white blood cells. Pasteurization of breast milk effectively kills CMV, although freezing at −20°C significantly reduces but does not eliminate infectivity. If donor breast milk is provided to premature infants or full-term infants born to nonimmune mothers, only that from a seronegative mother should be used.

Passive immunoprophylaxis with CMV hyperimmune globulin has been reported in uncontrolled studies to reduce transmission of CMV and morbidity in the fetus of women experiencing primary CMV infection while pregnant.[462] Randomized, controlled, multicenter trials should be performed, however, to determine if this approach can be beneficial enough to be routinely recommended.

Several vaccine candidates, including two live-attenuated CMV vaccines (AD-169 and Towne strains), have been evaluated in phase I and II clinical trials, and chimeric vaccines combining Towne and Toledo strains have been evaluated.[79,17,90,178] Currently, subunit vaccines using CMV glycoprotein gB, a principal target of the neutralizing antibody response, attached to an adjuvant, is a promising vaccine candidate that has been shown to be safe and immunogenic in phase I trials and currently awaits phase II and III trials. Development of a safe and effective CMV vaccine that can prevent severe congenital CMV disease remains a top priority and is a realistic and attainable goal.[36a,325,551]

RUBELLA

Rubella usually is a mild, often subclinical disease involving school-aged children and young adults. However, rubella virus also can cross the placenta, infect the fetus, and cause fetal death or congenital malformations. Since the original observations were made by the Australian ophthalmologist Norman McAlister were Gregg,[198,250] in which maternal rubella was associated with the birth of offspring with defects of the eye and heart, rubella has been the prototype for congenital viral infection.

MICROBIOLOGY AND EPIDEMIOLOGY

Rubella virus, an enveloped RNA virus in the family *Togaviridae*, has only a single antigenic type but has several newly characterized genotypes.[152,310,518] Genotyping is now used to track the molecular epidemiology of rubella strains associated with outbreaks.[310,518,628] Rubella virus grows in tissue culture from a variety of animal species, but commonly, a viral interference assay with African green monkey kidney cells is used for isolation in the diagnostic virology laboratory.[134] Several serologic tests, including complement fixation, hemagglutination inhibition, immunofluorescence, radioimmunoassay, and enzyme immunoassay (EIA), are available.[134,281] Although hemagglutination inhibition[619] has been the gold standard, many diagnostic virology laboratories now use more sensitive and practical methods such as ELISA, latex agglutination, or fluorescent assay kits.[134] In addition, traditional and real-time PCR assays can now detect and genotype rubella virus RNA in clinical samples.[310,518]

Rubella is worldwide in distribution. Human beings are the only host, and transmission occurs from person to person.[152,681] In the era before rubella vaccine was available, epidemics occurred at 6- to 9-year intervals, and pandemics occurred every 10 to 20 years.[681] Since the vaccine was licensed in 1969, this epidemic pattern has been interrupted; the last major outbreak in the United States was in 1964.[54,473] The peak seasonal incidence is in the spring.[681] In the prevaccine era, the peak age incidence was between 5 and 14 years of age,[681] but in the mid-1970s, the peak age was 15 to 19 years.[473] Currently, no peak age exists. Approximately 5 to 25 percent of women of child-bearing age lack rubella antibody and are susceptible to primary infection.[54,116] The attack rate for rubella in susceptible populations with prolonged intimate exposure is high—95 to 100 percent.[152,681] The frequency of transmission after brief exposure, however, is low.[152,681] The frequency of subclinical infections is much higher in adults than in children, although some serologically diagnosed infections in adults actually may be reinfections rather than primary disease.[293,294,566]

The incubation period for acquired rubella ranges from 14 to 23 days but usually is 16 to 18 days.[566] Virus may be isolated from the throat from 1 week before until 2 weeks after the onset of rash. Rubella virus infection may be subclinical in one third to a half of children and in half to two thirds of adults.[293,566] Rubella hemagglutination-inhibition antibody is detectable in serum within 2 to 3 days after the onset of rash, with peak titers being reached in 3 to 4 weeks.[134] Complement-fixation antibody rises more slowly, with peak titers noted at 4 to 6 weeks after the rash appears. Primary rubella virus infection is associated with an initial response in IgM-specific antibody, followed by an increase in IgG antibody. Reinfection with rubella virus is known to occur, and rates are higher in vaccine-immune than in naturally immune subjects.[293] The vast majority of congenital rubella virus infections occur after primary infection, but a few cases have been reported after reinfection.[131,206,532] If no evidence of rubella-specific IgM can be found in mothers with subclinical reinfection during pregnancy, the fetus is unlikely to be at risk.

PATHOGENESIS AND PATHOLOGY

Transplacental infection of the fetus with rubella virus occurs secondary to maternal viremia during the course of primary infection.[14,16,249] Fetal infection appears to result from embolization of pieces of necrotic placental vascular endothelium.[414] However, involvement of the placenta with rubella virus does not always result in fetal infection, particularly after the first trimester.[16] After maternal immunity, the next most critical factor determining the frequency of fetal infection and the severity of disease in neonates is the time during gestation that rubella virus infection occurs. Studies of the frequency of fetal infection and congenital defects according to gestational age at the time of maternal infection have used more sensitive methods to detect maternal and neonatal infection and long-term follow-up to detect abnormalities that were not apparent during infancy.[422] These studies indicated higher fetal infection rates than previously realized: 90 percent during the first 11 weeks, 50 percent during weeks 11 to 20, 37 percent from 20 to 35 weeks, and 100 percent during the last month. The congenital defect rate was 100 percent for the first 11 weeks, 30 percent during weeks 11 to 20, and none thereafter. Neonatal purpura and cataracts or glaucoma are observed when maternal rubella occurs during the first 2 months of gestation; congenital heart disease, during the first 3 months; deafness and neurologic deficit, during the first 4 months; and retinopathy, during the first 5 months.[422,646]

Excretion of rubella virus from the throat of congenitally infected infants may continue for several months after birth; approximately 10 to 20 percent of infected infants shed virus in nasopharyngeal secretions at 6 months of age. A small number will continue to shed virus for 1 year or more, and the virus has been recovered from tissues up to several years later.[16,154] Persistence of viral replication after birth may result in continuing damage to involved tissues, especially in the CNS and the eye and lens. In fact, hearing loss and neurologic deficits may appear long after birth in children previously considered well, or the clinical severity of these sequelae actually may worsen as the child's condition is being monitored.[136,154,185]

Rubella virus is a proven teratogenic viral agent that may cause congenital malformations.[475] Knowledge of the mechanisms by which rubella virus causes deformities may lead to a basic understanding of the pathogenesis of these malformations. Rubella virus is noncytolytic in certain tissues in that it does not destroy the cells in which it replicates. This characteristic, if manifested in the fetus, would tend to allow survival but result in disordered function of cells, tissues, and organs. On the other hand, selective cell destruction also may occur in fetal tissues.

In studies of the pathology of therapeutically aborted, rubella-infected fetuses, scattered foci of necrotic cellular damage without inflammatory infiltrates were noted in the endothelial cells of blood vessels and in myocardial cells.[635] Rubella-induced defects could result in defective formation or function of developing tissues by direct cellular destruction or by hypoxic damage secondary to blood vessel obliteration. For example, alteration of the elastic or muscle fibers in the ductus arteriosus could result in failure of postnatal ductus closure. Studies of tissue obtained from infants with rubella syndrome and maintained in culture showed that the cells were infected with rubella virus persistently and had a decreased growth rate and shortened survival time.[521] Naeye and Blanc[445] noted that the growth retardation of infants with rubella syndrome was the result of decreased numbers of cells in organs. This impaired cellular growth, if it occurred during a crucial phase in cardiac development, for example, could result in such cardiac anomalies as septal defects.

Increased numbers of chromosome breaks have been noted in leukocyte cultures of children with congenital rubella.[467] Chromosomal injury possibly results in cell loss during rapid organ development and is, in part, responsible for the congenital anomalies. Persistence of virus possibly results in continuing cell destruction or immunopathologic damage to tissues. In addition, two studies have demonstrated circulating rubella antigen-antibody complexes in 10 infants with congenital rubella and late-onset manifestations such as interstitial pneumonia, hepatosplenomegaly, rash, lymphocytic meningitis, and rapid neurologic deterioration.[78,630] IgG levels were low and IgM levels were elevated, with a diminished number of T cells and an increased proportion of B cells. Delayed maturation of the

immune response in congenital rubella was postulated to predispose possibly to persistent antigenemia complexed with IgM and deposition of circulating immune complexes in tissues. Finally, antibodies against thyroid microsomes or thyroglobulin were found in a much larger percentage of children with congenital rubella syndrome than in control subjects.[142] A significant number of the patients with congenital rubella and thyroid antibodies also had thyroid dysfunction. These observations suggest that autoimmunity, induced in some way by persistent infection with rubella virus, plays a role in the late-onset endocrine dysfunction that occurs in children and young adults with congenital rubella syndrome.

Specific pathologic lesions in infants with congenital rubella depend on the gestational age at the time of infection and the particular organs involved. One common finding is necrosis of vascular endothelium, which may be accompanied by damage to organs secondary to vascular obstruction.[416,635] Diffuse intimal changes have been observed in the pulmonary and systemic arteries, as well as the ductus arteriosus.[416] Focal inflammation and necrosis have been seen in the myocardium[352] and structures of the inner ear.

The fetus is capable of an immune response to rubella virus: specific IgM and, occasionally, IgA have been observed in fetal and cord-blood specimens. In fact, hypergammaglobulinemia may be observed during early life in some infants with congenital rubella.[264] On the other hand, hypogammaglobulinemia has been noted in a few infants.[264,504] In 10 to 20 percent of infants with congenital rubella, hemagglutination-inhibition antibody declines to undetectable levels when they reach 1 to 4 years of age.[154,270] Several of these infants failed to respond to immunization with rubella vaccine.[151] In fact, infants with congenital rubella have been reinfected with rubella virus later in life.[414] Several defects in cell-mediated immunity, including diminished responsiveness of peripheral blood leukocytes to phytohemagglutinin and diminished lymphocyte transformation, interferon production, and synthesis of leukocyte migration inhibitory factor in response to challenge with rubella virus antigen, have been observed in infants with congenital rubella.[104,472] Normal responses were observed in healthy, seropositive children and adults. Researchers have presumed, but have not proved, that these abnormalities in cell-mediated immunity play a role in persistent viral excretion in congenitally infected infants.

CLINICAL MANIFESTATIONS

Although the typical clinical features of rubella may occur in pregnant women, as many as one half to two thirds of these infections are subclinical.[568] Typical features that might occur in symptomatic postpubertal women include fever, rash, posterior auricular and postoccipital adenopathy, and arthralgia or arthritis.

As many as two thirds of infants with proven congenital rubella may be asymptomatic in the neonatal period.[549] However, evidence of long-term sequelae was noted in almost three quarters of such infants within the first 5 years of life.[549] The clinical manifestations of congenital rubella syndrome vary highly, not only with regard to specific features but also in relation to the age during which the specific feature occurs. The collected features may be divided into three broad categories: (1) transient—those that are present in the neonatal period and clear after a few months, such as thrombocytopenia and hepatitis; (2) permanent—major malformations that persist and may even worsen as the child grows older, such as congenital heart lesions, cataracts, or hearing loss; and (3) developmental—aspects that do not emerge until childhood or young adulthood, such as behavioral disorders or endocrine dysfunction.[151,569] This categorization of abnormal features may be useful in determining the prognosis and management of these children.

The manifestations of congenital rubella that are symptomatic in the neonatal period, compiled from several series,[153,292,351,392,540] are illustrated in Figure 73–2. The low birth weight of infants with rubella syndrome results from intrauterine growth restriction; even when born prematurely, the infant often is small for gestational age. The frequency of purpura in most series ranges from 15 to 50 percent. Thrombocytopenia almost always was present in association with the purpura and usually resolved spontaneously in the first month of life. Neonatal thrombocytopenic purpura is a poor prognostic sign because it generally occurs in severely affected infants with multiple manifestations. Thirty-five percent of 58 patients with purpura in one series[153] died during the first year, in contrast to a mortality rate of only 13 percent during the first 18 months for patients from the entire series. Although the thrombocytopenia frequently was profound, death rarely was caused by hemorrhage.

Direct involvement of the liver by rubella virus results in neonatal hepatitis, as evidenced by hepatomegaly, predominantly direct-reacting hyperbilirubinemia, and elevation of liver enzymes.[217] Pathology studies usually demonstrate hepatocellular disease with necrosis, giant-cell formation, bile stasis, and fibrosis, but extrahepatic biliary obstruction also has been demonstrated.[620]

Congenital heart disease occurs frequently and generally is detectable in the neonatal period, although specific lesions may not be defined until later in life. The most common lesions in 87 catheterized patients with congenital rubella were patent ductus arteriosus in 78 percent, right pulmonary artery stenosis in 70 percent, left pulmonary artery stenosis in 56 percent, valvular pulmonic stenosis in 40 percent, mild aortic valvular stenosis in 14 percent, aberrant subclavian artery in 11 percent, and ventricular septal defect in 10 percent.[154] Evidence of active myocardial disease has been noted in some infants.[352]

Interstitial pneumonia with cough, tachypnea, and breathlessness as the major manifestation of congenital rubella has been reported.[498] Most patients with pneumonitis died in the first year of life as a result of their pulmonary disease. Cardiac abnormalities also were present but were thought not to be significant either clinically or from autopsy findings. Microscopic studies revealed acute to subacute chronic interstitial pneumonitis. Rubella virus was isolated from all of the four lung specimens cultured.

Although cataracts are the most characteristic ocular lesion in rubella syndrome, they may not be visualized until after the neonatal period. Worldwide, vision loss from cataracts associated with congenital rubella syndrome remains a global public health problem.[518,650] Retinopathy is described as widespread, with mottled or blotchy, black pigmentary deposits of variable size and location: the "salt and pepper" retinitis.[358] Retinal function usually is not affected adversely. The frequency of retinopathy in the combined data from six series of children monitored for several years was 36 percent.

Bone lesions are another finding in congenital rubella in the neonatal period. Radiographic studies reveal small linear areas of radiolucency and increased bone density in the longitudinal axis of the metaphyseal area of the long bones of the lower and upper extremities.[540] This abnormality results from disturbances in deposition and calcification of osteoid and usually resolves by the time the child is 2 to 3 months of age.

Involvement of the CNS frequently is evident in symptomatic infants. Lethargy, irritability, disturbances in tone, and a bulging fontanelle are common findings. One or more seizures developed in 27 of 100 infants in one series.[185,186] However, they usually occurred after the neonatal period. In most infants with CNS involvement, CSF protein is elevated, but increased cell counts are seen less frequently. Rubella virus may be isolated from the CSF; in one series, 25 percent of 99 CSF specimens obtained during the first 3 months of life from patients with CNS symptoms were positive.[185,186] The extent of impairment at 18 months of age was not readily predictable on the basis of clinical symptoms or isolation of virus in the first few weeks of life. However, severe involvement was found more frequently in infants with seizures and high levels of CSF protein in the first few months of life.[185,186] An important emphasis is the chronic nature of congenital rubella infection, and one should note that although most infants may be asymptomatic in the neonatal period, evidence of disease was seen on follow-up examination in up to 70 percent.

DIAGNOSIS AND DIFFERENTIAL DIAGNOSIS

Because many maternal rubella cases are subclinical and other diseases may mimic symptomatic rubella, establishing a definitive diagnosis in the mother depends on the laboratory. Although rubella virus may be isolated from the throat during the acute phase of the illness, such culture frequently is not a practical means of establishing the diagnosis. The tissue culture cells required for isolation of rubella virus are not always available in routine virology laboratories. Widely used serologic tests include hemagglutination inhibition, ELISA, and fluorescent assay.[127,134] Susceptible individuals lack IgG antibody. Detectable antibody is present in the blood within a few days after onset of the rash, and peak titers are reached within 2 to 3 weeks. If serum specimens are not available until some time after the onset of illness, complement-fixation antibody titers may be useful because peak titers are not reached for 4 to 6 weeks after the rash is manifested. If only a single specimen is available, rubella-specific IgM antibody may be demonstrable by ELISA or immunofluorescence methods, peak 3 to 6 weeks after infection occurs, and persist for several months.[134,281] If maternal rubella infection is diagnosed, then prenatal diagnosis of congenital rubella infection can be made through amniocentesis to obtain amniotic fluid for viral rubella culture and rubella virus RNA detection by PCR and by fetal blood sampling for rubella IgM determination. Laboratory tests ideally should be combined with serial fetal ultrasound evaluations to determine the extent of fetal involvement if the fetus is identified as being infected with rubella.[308,627] Detection of viral RNA by PCR on chorionic villi samples obtained very early in gestation also has been used for prenatal diagnosis.

The most characteristic clinical features of congenital rubella are congenital heart disease, cataracts, microphthalmos, corneal opacity, glaucoma, and radiolucent bone lesions. In infants with these classic features, the clinical diagnosis correlates with laboratory confirmation of congenital rubella 80 percent of the time. However, many of the features, such as low birth weight, hepatosplenomegaly, icterus, and petechiae/purpura, overlap with those found in other infectious diseases of the newborn, and definitive diagnosis requires laboratory confirmation. The diagnosis of congenital rubella is confirmed by isolation of virus from the throat or urine; in addition, virus has been recovered from cataracts, conjunctivae, CSF, feces, bone marrow, and circulating leukocytes. The lens is an excellent site for recovery of virus, especially because cataracts are removed from these infants within the first few weeks of life. The diagnosis of congenital rubella also can be made by serologic means. Because rubella IgG antibody is passed transplacentally, serum levels determined early in the neonatal period mimic those of the mother. Stable or rising serum concentrations of rubella-specific IgG antibody in the serum of infants during their first 4 to 6 months of life can be considered diagnostic of congenital rubella when the clinical picture is compatible. The presence of specific IgM antibody in a single serum specimen obtained from an infant early in life also can be diagnostic, but false-positive test results have been reported. Whenever possible, isolation of virus should be performed for definitive diagnosis. PCR performed on nasopharyngeal secretions ultimately may aid in establishing the diagnosis.[176,658]

The finding during pregnancy that a mother is immune to rubella is not sufficient to exclude the diagnosis because reinfection may have occurred or maternal infection may have developed before the screen was performed. If the diagnosis of congenital rubella is suspected clinically when the mother is thought to be immune, the infant should be screened with rubella-specific IgM ELISA and viral culture or PCR of appropriate clinical specimens. The diagnosis of congenital rubella infection can be eliminated if the mother is nonimmune when the infant manifests clinical signs of possible congenital infection.

The principal diseases to consider in the differential diagnosis include congenital CMV infection, congenital toxoplasmosis, erythroblastosis fetalis, disseminated herpes simplex, neonatal sepsis and congenital syphilis. Infants with congenital CMV infection more commonly have chorioretinitis and microcephaly, whereas congenital heart disease and eye malformations are unusual findings. Infants with symptomatic congenital toxoplasmosis have chorioretinitis, hydrocephaly, and cerebral calcifications but not congenital heart disease, cataracts, or glaucoma. In uncomplicated erythroblastosis, the direct bilirubin and liver function studies remain normal. Disseminated herpes simplex should be differentiated on the basis of the characteristic vesicular skin lesions or the presence of keratoconjunctivitis. Positive blood cultures identify neonatal sepsis. The bone lesions in congenital syphilis are associated with periosteal new bone formation; rhinitis and lesions of the skin and mucous membranes also are seen. Because of overlapping clinical features, however, definitive diagnosis requires laboratory confirmation.

TREATMENT

No specific antiviral therapy exists for congenital rubella. Although amantadine hydrochloride inhibits rubella virus in vitro, treatment with this drug was not shown to alter the clinical or virologic course of the disease.[504] Sensorineural hearing loss associated with congenital rubella syndrome now may be treated with cochlear implantation combined with speech language therapy, and vision loss associated with cataracts can be restored with ophthalmologic surgical procedures that remove the opaque lens and replace it.[317,518,651]

PROGNOSIS

The most common long-term sequelae of congenital rubella are listed in Table 73–8. Deafness is the most frequent finding and

TABLE 73–8 Frequency of Defects in Children with Congenital Rubella

Defect	Percentage of Cases
Deafness	67
Congenital heart disease	48
Psychomotor retardation	45
Retinopathy	39
Cataracts	29
Neonatal purpura	23
No defect	19
Deaths	16
Glaucoma	3

Data from 376 children studied in the New York Rubella Birth Defect Project. Modified from Cooper, L. Z., Ziring, P. R., Ockerse, A. B., et al.: Rubella: Clinical manifestations and management. Am. J. Dis. Child. 118:18-29, 1969.

may not be apparent for several months to several years after birth. In 15 to 20 percent of children, it may be the only abnormality detectable.[154] Approximately one half of the children may have absent or hyporeactive responses to tests of vestibular function.[424] The hearing loss may be profound and, thus, a major contributor to speech impairment and learning disability. Cochlear implantation and speech language therapy, however, may restore hearing, improve receptive and expressive language abilities, and improve communication skills and school performance.[317] In approximately 50 percent of children with mental retardation, the deficiency is moderate to severe. Although retinopathy is present in a significant proportion of infants, it does not appear to interfere with vision. Cataracts, of course, certainly can interfere with the development of vision, and they should be removed surgically in the first few weeks of life. Most fatalities from congenital rubella occur in the first year of life and are associated with severe congenital heart disease and general debility from multiple defects.[154]

Long-term follow-up evaluation of children with congenital rubella syndrome is available.[136,185,186,414,569] Among 205 children examined at 8 to 9 years of age, 26 percent had severe mental retardation, 18 percent had reactive behavior disorder, 12 percent showed behavior disorder with neurologic damage, and 6 percent displayed autism. Of 29 children with neurologic manifestations of congenital rubella between birth and 18 months of age but with normal intelligence, 93 percent had hearing loss when examined at 9 to 12 years of age; 61 percent, poor balance; 54 percent, muscular weakness; 52 percent, learning deficits; 48 percent, behavioral disturbance; and 41 percent, deficits in tactile perception. Head circumference appears to correlate poorly with intellectual function in patients with congenital rubella.[398] Diabetes mellitus has been observed in 15 to 20 percent of adults with congenital rubella.[415] Onset usually occurs in the second or third decade of life. Other late manifestations[569] of congenital rubella syndrome include hyperIgM syndrome,[481] autoimmune disorders such as chronic lymphocytic thyroiditis,[706] thymic hypoplasia,[238] abnormal dermatoglyphics,[154] chromosomal abnormalities,[33] pancreatic insufficiency,[191] and progressive panencephalitis.[642,663] As one might expect, the severity of long-term sequelae appears to correlate with the number of defects observed in early life.[136,154]

PREVENTION

Active immunization with live, attenuated rubella virus vaccine is the most effective means of preventing congenital rubella syndrome.[539] It has led to the elimination of endemic rubella in the United States and progress toward elimination in Europe and other parts of the world.[117,377,503] The development and use of rubella vaccine in the United States clearly have reduced the frequency of congenital rubella.[54,285,473] Since 2001, fewer than 25 reported cases of congenital rubella syndrome have occurred each year, and genotype analysis showed all cases that have occurred originated in parts of the world other than the United States. However, outbreaks of rubella and congenital rubella syndrome have occurred in the United States, especially in South Texas near the Mexico border. In addition, Hispanic populations and foreign-born individuals from countries that do not have rubella vaccination programs appear to be the highest risk for rubella outbreaks.[377,705] The target population in the United States has been preschool- and school-aged children, whereas in Great Britain, selective vaccination of 11- to 14-year-olds and women immediately after delivery has been the goal. The strategy used in the United States is more effective in decreasing the incidence of congenital rubella syndrome. More recently, immunization programs in the United States have emphasized the need to vaccinate susceptible women of child-bearing age.[54,285,473] Moreover, routine prenatal screening for rubella immunity should be performed, and all nonimmune women should be vaccinated during the immediate postpartum period and before being discharged. Breast-feeding is not a contraindication to postpartum immunization. Although the vaccine virus may be transmitted in breast milk, the infection in the neonate is asymptomatic. Immunization with rubella vaccine, however, is contraindicated during pregnancy, and physicians recommend that a woman not conceive during the 3-month period after being immunized.[97,368] Data collected by the CDC from more than 500 pregnancies show that vaccine viruses can cross the placenta and infect the fetus but do not produce the defects associated with congenital rubella syndrome. The rate of isolation of vaccine virus from the products of conception is only 3 percent for the currently used RA 27/3 vaccine. Studies of fetal risk associated with inadvertent administration of rubella vaccine during pregnancy have confirmed rubella vaccine safety in pregnant women and their fetuses.[43] Thus, inadvertent administration of rubella vaccine during the first trimester of pregnancy is not an indication for termination of pregnancy.

Continuing concerns with regard to rubella include reinfection with wild rubella virus in vaccine-immune subjects,[293] failure of rubella herd immunity during an epidemic,[340] arthralgia and arthritis as side effects of the vaccine in children and particularly postpubertal women even though the risk of developing chronic arthropathy is not increased,[328,662] waning immunity that is more profound after immunization than after natural infection,[54,285,473] and, more recently, outbreaks of rubella among unvaccinated pregnant women in custodial institutions, immigration camps in border states, or selected communities, including Hispanic populations and groups of foreign-born individuals from countries with no rubella vaccine program.[16,114,412]

Although administration of gamma-globulin to women during pregnancy may reduce the frequency of symptomatic disease in the mother, it appears to have little effect on the frequency or severity of fetal and neonatal disease.[91,406] Infants with congenital rubella syndrome are considered to be contagious and are maintained with contact precautions until they are at least 1 year of age, unless repeated nasopharyngeal and urine cultures performed after they reach 3 months of age are negative for rubella virus. Health care workers are required to report all suspected and confirmed cases of congenital rubella to their local health department. Therefore, physicians who serve populations at high risk for rubella should be aware of the signs and symptoms of rubella and congenital rubella syndrome so that they may recognize the disease if it occurs in their patients.

MEASLES AND MUMPS

Measles during pregnancy may have severe complications, including maternal pneumonitis, hepatitis, and hemorrhagic sepsis syndrome. On rare instances, maternal measles during pregnancy may be fatal. The adverse fetal effects include spontaneous abortion or premature delivery, and neonates may be born with congenital measles syndrome.[39,136,204]

Mumps rarely if ever causes severe illness in pregnancy. However, mumps RNA has been detected in the myocardium of fetuses and neonates with myocarditis and endocardial fibroelastosis, providing molecular evidence for the long suspected role of mumps virus in these disease processes.[457]

HEPATITIS

Since the late 1970s, a veritable explosion of information concerning infection with hepatitis A virus (HAV), HBV,

HCV, hepatitis D virus (HDV), and hepatitis E virus (HEV) has occurred.* HAV has been grown in cell cultures, and two purified viral glycoprotein vaccines have been licensed and recommended for use in high-risk individuals aged 2 years and older.[143,289,383,384] HBV and HCV are discussed later. HDV is a defective virus that infects only persons with acute or chronic HBV infection.[507] The major cause of enterically transmitted non-A, non-B (NANB) hepatitis, a problem confined largely to developing countries,[652] has been shown to be HEV, an RNA virus of the family *Calicivirus*.[355,634] Epidemic NANB hepatitis occurs more frequently during pregnancy and can result in fulminant hepatic failure in these women.

HAV and HDV rarely cause infection of the fetus and newborn.[614,704] Natal transmission of hepatitis A to the newborn can occur if the mother has jaundice or had acute hepatitis within the 2 weeks before and 1 week after delivery. Although most infants are asymptomatic, researchers have recommended that exposed infants receive 0.02 mL/kg of immunoglobulin intramuscularly as soon as possible after delivery. The infant should be maintained with contact precautions for 6 weeks, or for 1 week after the onset of symptoms. Preterm infants may excrete HAV antigen and RNA for several months after acquiring acute infection. Nosocomial transmission of hepatitis A within nurseries has been documented. A report from India indicated a relatively high rate of vertical transmission among eight women with third-trimester HEV infection[326]; more investigations are necessary to determine the true significance of maternal HEV infection for the fetus and newborn infant in the United States. The following section focuses on HBV and HCV.

MICROBIOLOGY AND EPIDEMIOLOGY

HBV, a double-stranded DNA virus with a DNA polymerase, is the prototype member of the family Hepadnaviridae.[296,346] Sero-epidemiologic investigation of HBV infection has been enhanced by the identification and development of three major antigen systems, antibody systems, or both: surface antigen (HBsAg and anti-HBs), core antigen (total anti-HBc and IgM anti-HBc), and e antigen (HBeAg and anti-HBe).[296,346] Tests for HBsAg are used widely for establishing the diagnosis of acute or chronic infection with HBV. Anti-HBc is a marker of continuing viral replication in the liver, IgM anti-HBc is present during acute but not chronic HBV infection, and HBeAg is a more specific indicator of infectivity than HBsAg is.[120,288,296,346,572]

HBV accounts for 40 to 50 percent of all cases of hepatitis in the United States and 10 percent of those associated with blood transfusion.[120,572] Between 5 and 10 percent of patients infected with HBV become chronic carriers, and many of them have benign chronic persistent hepatitis or the more serious chronic active hepatitis.[296,346,396,572] A strong association has been noted, particularly in Asian males, between chronic carriage of HBsAg and death from cirrhosis or primary hepatocellular carcinoma.[24,62,409] The age at which HBV infection occurs has a significant effect on the occurrence of clinically overt hepatitis and the development of a chronic carrier state.[241] The vast majority of neonates who acquire HBV from their mothers have subclinical infection, but 60 to 95 percent of infected infants become chronic carriers, particularly when the mother is HBeAg-positive.[60,61,66,183,242,469,614,618,686]

In the United States, the frequency of HBsAg in the general population is 0.2 to 0.9 percent.[115] The highest prevalence of HBV antigenemia in the United States is in Asian immigrants/refugees (13%), Alaskan Natives/Pacific Islanders (5-15%), clients in institutions for the developmentally disabled (10-20%), users of illicit parenteral drugs (7%), sexually active homosexual

---

*See references 109, 111, 120, 164, 248, 291, 296, 346, 356, 361, 507, 572, 617, 649.

men (6%), household contacts of HBV chronic carriers (3-6%), and patients in hemodialysis units (3-10%).[115] Only 10 to 15 percent of persons reactive for HBsAg have a history of contracting hepatitis. In chronic carriers of HBsAg, antigen has been detected in saliva, feces, urine, wound exudates, vaginal secretions, breast milk, amniotic fluid, and semen.[296,346,572] The prevalence of anti-HBs in the general population is approximately 11 percent; this frequency increases with advancing age and is related inversely to socioeconomic status.[115]

Among children and adults, HBV is transmitted by the parenteral route (blood transfusion, needle-sticks), but infection by nonparenteral routes also occurs.[59,63,572,637] Hepatitis B is not transmitted by the fecal-oral route. In the United States, transmission by blood and blood products now is a rare event because of routine screening of blood donors and viral inactivation of certain blood products.

Clustering of HBV infections in families is known to occur; family members of a known antigen-positive index case have a 10-fold higher prevalence of HBsAg or anti-HBs than do control families of the same ethnic background.[627] Although this clustering within families initially was considered to have a genetic basis,[627] "vertical" transmission of HBV infection from the mother to the infant may be a source.[183,242,469] However, person-to-person spread clearly occurs, but the exact mechanism is not known.[59,637,704] It has been seen in household settings from child to child but not in daycare centers.

Moreover, transmission of HBV has occurred in children born to HBsAg-negative mothers who immigrated to the United States from countries where HBV infection is endemic.[59,637,704] The incubation period for the onset of HBV antigenemia after parenteral inoculation is 2 weeks to 2 months, depending on the dose of virus received. In nonparenteral exposure, the incubation period for antigenemia is 2 to 3 months. The onset of elevated liver enzymes and clinical symptoms follows the onset of antigenemia by 2 weeks to 2 months.[346]

In the fetus and neonate, transmission by the following routes has been suggested: transplacental, either during pregnancy or at the time of delivery secondary to placental leaks; natal, by exposure to HBsAg in amniotic fluid, cervical and vaginal secretions, or maternal blood; and postnatal, by contact with household members who are infected or are chronic carriers or, rarely, by transfusion of blood or blood products. Ninety-five percent of infections occur at the time of delivery, whereas only 5 percent occur in utero. The fetus or newborn infant, therefore, can be infected by hematogenous (transplacental, blood transfusion) or nonparenteral (contamination of the oropharynx or breaks in the skin) routes. Differences in the time of exposure (congenital, natal, postnatal) and in the route of viral inoculation (parenteral, nonparenteral) may account for the wide variation in time of onset of antigenemia in the neonate after birth. The usual age at onset of antigenemia in neonates born to chronic carrier mothers is 2 to 5 months,[31,183,200,381,470,576,615] which is consistent with exposure at the time of birth. Infections secondary to blood transfusion in the neonatal period also are associated with the onset of antigenemia at younger than 2 months of age.[201] Infants with an onset of antigenemia at younger than 2 months of age presumably were exposed to HBV in utero.[200,242,381,470,559,576] In general, infants of mothers with acute hepatitis near the time of birth have antigenemia at an earlier age (1-2 months), thus suggesting transplacental transmission of HBV.[242,559] Infants with an onset of antigenemia after they reach 6 months of age can be assumed to have had postnatal exposure,[559] but the exact source of virus in these infants is unclear.

In summary, evidence is good that infection with HBV can occur transplacentally, at the time of birth, and postnatally by blood transfusion or contamination of the oropharynx with infected secretions.[614] Several studies indicate that transmission by breast milk is a rare occurrence.[65,183,687] Further substantiation

for the mother as the primary source of virus for the neonate comes from observations that the HBV serotype almost always is the same in infants and their carrier mothers.[242,470,615]

From 0.1 to 15.6 percent of pregnant women are asymptomatic chronic carriers of HBsAg. The lowest rates occur in the United States and in northern European populations,[183,200,588,687] and the highest rates occur in Chinese populations, regardless of geographic location.[31,66,185,381,615] Intermediate rates are observed in Japanese,[469,576] African,[183,687] South Asian,[183,687] and Mediterranean populations.[486] Rates of transmission of HBsAg from infected mothers to neonates vary highly and are influenced by the sensitivity of the HBsAg assay system used in the study, whether neonatal serum is examined for anti-HBs as well as for HBsAg, the frequency of bleeding and length of follow-up of infants, and the e antigen/antibody status of the mother. In general, HBsAg in a cord-blood specimen is not a reliable indicator of neonatal infection because of the possibility of contamination with antigen-positive maternal blood or vaginal secretions and because of the possibility of transient noninfectious antigenemia from the mother.[183,381,485,687] Demonstration of HBsAg in the serum of the infant during the first several months of life can be considered diagnostic of infection with HBV in the absence of immunization with hepatitis B vaccine. HBsAg may be detected for up to 1 week after the administration of a dose of vaccine. Most infants demonstrate antigenemia by the time they are 6 months of age, with peak acquisition occurring at 3 to 4 months of age.[31,242,381,576]

Factors known to be associated with higher rates of HBV transmission to neonates include the presence of HBeAg and the absence of anti-HBe in maternal serum—attack rates of 80 to 95 percent;[66,183,206,381,469,485,687] an Asian racial origin, particularly Chinese—attack rates of 40 to 70 percent;[31,183,381,576,615] maternal acute hepatitis in the third trimester of pregnancy or the immediate postpartum period—attack rates of 60 to 70 percent;[242,559,560] a higher titer of HBsAg in maternal serum—attack rates parallel the titer;[66,381,615] and the presence of antigenemia in older siblings.[31,469,615] Factors *not* related to transmission include the presence or absence of breast-feeding,[65,183,687] the particular HBV subtype in the mother,[242,470,615] the presence or absence of HBsAg in amniotic fluid,[381] and the presence or absence of anti-HBc in cord blood.[183,200,242] Data conflict regarding the significance of HBsAg in cord blood. Some studies have found no relationship between its presence or absence and subsequent infection of the neonate, whereas others have found a correlation. The reasons for this difference are not understood.[183,381,485,615,687]

From 75 to 100 percent of infants in whom HBsAg develops in serum within the first several months of life have persistent or chronic antigenemia.[31,183,242,469,470,576,615] In some infants, anti-HBs may develop after transient carriage of HBsAg, and in a few (usually those born to asymptomatic carrier mothers), anti-HBs may develop without the infant ever having detectable antigen.[485,576]

Transmission of HBV to infants in successive pregnancies of the same mother has been documented,[192,199] and such transmission has, on occasion, been associated with the development of fatal hepatitis.

PATHOGENESIS AND PATHOLOGY

HBV transmitted to the neonate by the hematogenous route probably seeds the liver directly, whereas nonparenteral exposure requires replication at the portal of entry before spread to the liver through the bloodstream occurs. Electron-microscopic studies of liver biopsy specimens from chronic carrier infants indicate that replication of HBV appears to occur in the nuclei of hepatocytes and that 50 to 100 percent of cells are involved.[197,559] Histopathologic examination demonstrates a diffuse hydropic appearance of the liver cells, with effacement of the normal cord pattern and the creation of a "cobblestone appearance" in the liver lobule.[559] Only small foci of hepatocytolysis surrounded by macrophages and lymphocytes are present. Infants with symptomatic acute hepatitis have more widespread hepatic necrosis with surrounding inflammatory infiltrates, including giant cells.[199,319] In fulminant disease, massive necrosis with little or no inflammatory response is present.[199,319] In some infants with symptomatic hepatitis, the disease may progress to chronic persistent hepatitis, chronic active hepatitis, cirrhosis, or hepatocellular carcinoma.[184,201,319,399,636,647,690]

CLINICAL MANIFESTATIONS

Although clinically typical acute hepatitis may occur in mothers of infants in whom HBV infection develops, most are asymptomatic chronic carriers of HBsAg. Therefore, routine screening of serum for antigen in all pregnant women is necessary for the identification of infants at risk for development of HBV infection. Maternal HBV infection has not been associated with abortion, stillbirth, congenital malformations, or intrauterine growth retardation.[183,201,576] However, prematurity has been observed, particularly when the mother has acute hepatitis during pregnancy.[559]

A fetus or newborn infant exposed to HBV may follow one of several courses: (1) asymptomatic transient hepatitis B antigenemia, followed by the production of anti-Hbs[200,485]; (2) asymptomatic persistent antigenemia, variably associated with mild and fluctuating elevations in liver enzymes[31,200,242,576,599]; (3) symptomatic hepatitis with recovery and clearance of the antigen[201,222]; (4) symptomatic hepatitis that becomes chronically persistent or chronically active with continued presence of hepatitis B antigenemia[199,201,319,690]; (5) acute fulminant hepatitis with death[201,222]; and (6) asymptomatic neonatal/infant infection with progression to cirrhosis or liver cancer.[84,636,647] Most infants with HBsAg in their serum become asymptomatic chronic carriers. However, liver function studies may be abnormal in some of these infants, and liver biopsy specimens usually show evidence of mild, unresolved hepatitis.[183,201,242,559,576] The long-term significance of these persistent abnormalities in asymptomatic chronic carrier infants is unknown. The factors that determine which pattern of HBV infection occurs in a given newborn infant and the mechanisms responsible for chronic carriage of HBsAg in many infants are not understood.

The source of virus for 29 infants with symptomatic HBV infection in the first few months of life was blood transfusion in 15 (52%), a chronic carrier mother in 9 (31%), and unknown in 5 (17%).[201] The type of clinical disease in these infants was acute, self-limited hepatitis in 16 (55%), severe or fulminant hepatitis in 9 (31%), chronic persistent hepatitis in 2 (7%), chronic active hepatitis in one, and an asymptomatic chronic carrier state in 1. Most patients with fulminant hepatitis died.

DIAGNOSIS AND DIFFERENTIAL DIAGNOSIS

HBV infection in an infant generally is diagnosed by the demonstration of HBsAg in serum. If positive, infants also should be tested for HBeAg and anti-HBc IgM. In addition, PCR is available for detecting HBV DNA in blood. The major diseases to be considered in the differential diagnosis include biliary atresia and acute hepatitis caused by other viruses—HAV, CMV, rubella virus, enteroviruses, adenoviruses, and HSV.

TREATMENT

Treatment with human interferon has resulted in the termination or transient cessation of hepatitis B antigenemia in chronic hepatitis of adults,[249,291,497] but experience in neonates and children is limited.[320,370,453] Lamivudine also is licensed for the treatment of chronic infection in adults. Treatment of established disease in infants with hepatitis B immunoglobulin (HBIG) has not altered the course of illness.[199,222] Therefore, treatment of neonatal HBV infection primarily is supportive.

PROGNOSIS

The long-term outcome of asymptomatic infants with persistent antigenemia is guarded because chronic active and progressive hepatitis occur, as do death from cirrhosis, liver failure, and hepatocellular carcinoma. Death from fulminant HBV infection in neonates or young infants is a rare event but has occurred, particularly in successive children born to the same chronic carrier mother.[192,222]

PREVENTION

Remarkable advances have occurred in the prophylaxis of neonates born to mothers with HBV infection. Initial studies in infants born to HBeAg-positive, chronic carrier mothers demonstrated that administration of HBIG significantly reduced the development of a chronic carrier state.[61,64,192,309,347,523] The most successful regimens were those that began as soon as possible after birth and used multiple doses of HBIG. Anti-HBs developed in most infants who were protected against becoming chronic carriers, thus indicating that passive/active immunization had occurred. However, protection against persistent antigenemia was only 50 to 75 percent effective. Twenty to 30 percent of infants became infected during the second and third years after the protective effects of their passive immunoglobulin subsided.[61,64] This finding suggests that the risk of developing infection continues beyond the time of birth and that active immunization would be necessary to provide long-term protection.

Hepatitis B vaccine (Heptavax B; licensed but no longer produced in the United States) then was demonstrated to be both safe and effective in inducing protective levels of anti-HBs in 95 percent or more of infants receiving three doses of the vaccine.[53,382] Because passive/active immunization (HBIG plus three doses of HBV vaccine) in adults was shown to be safe and as effective in inducing long-term protective titers of anti-HBs as was a dosage of three doses of vaccine alone[702] this regimen was tried in infants. Several investigations have demonstrated 85 to 96 percent efficacy in preventing chronic antigenemia with the combined HBIG/vaccine regimen.[60,396,618,685] Persistent antibody against HBsAg developed in virtually all protected infants. Vaccine failures were thought to occur in babies who already were infected with HBV in utero and, hence, could not be protected by the HBIG/vaccine regimen initiated at birth. Subsequent studies using recombinant DNA vaccines (Recombivax HB, Engerix-B) showed them to be safe and highly immunogenic in neonates (>95%), with an efficacy of 90 to 95 percent.[508,616]

The concentration of HBsAg protein differs in the two vaccines; the pediatric formulation of Recombivax HB contains 10 μg/mL, whereas Engerix-B has 20 mg/mL. The two vaccines are interchangeable, and neither one contains thimerosal.

Because most chronic carrier mothers are asymptomatic, serologic screening during pregnancy would be required to identify neonates needing prophylaxis beginning at birth. Initial recommendations suggested screening during pregnancy in populations with high-risk factors: (1) Asian, Alaskan, or Pacific Island descent; (2) birth in Haiti, sub-Saharan Africa, Eastern Europe, the Middle East, the Caribbean, or Central or South America; (3) acute or chronic liver disease; (4) work or treatment in a dialysis unit; (5)

work or residence in an institution for the mentally retarded; (6) rejection as a blood donor; (7) blood transfusion on repeated occasions; (8) frequent occupational exposures to blood in medical or dental settings; (9) household contact with an HBV carrier or hemodialysis patient; (10) multiple episodes of sexually transmitted disease; or (11) percutaneous use of illicit drugs.[111,115,591] Because routine prenatal history to screen for these risk factors will miss one half to two thirds of asymptomatic chronic carrier mothers,[613,363] the current recommendation is to screen *all* pregnant women for HBsAg early in pregnancy.[35,36,112,119,617] Testing should be repeated late in pregnancy for women who are negative initially and at high risk for acquiring HBV infection or who have had clinical hepatitis since the screening was performed.[123]

Perinatal transmission is prevented in more than 90 percent of cases by the intramuscular administration of 0.5 mL of HBIG and hepatitis B vaccine to both term and preterm infants of HBsAg-positive mothers as soon as possible but within 12 hours of delivery.[115] HBIG efficacy decreases markedly if treatment is delayed beyond 48 hours. HBV vaccine is administered intramuscularly at a separate site at birth (preferably) or within 7 days, and in infants with a birth weight of 2 kg or more, administration is repeated at 1 to 2 months and 6 months after administration of the first dose. In infants with a birth weight less than 2 kg, the initial dose of hepatitis B vaccine does not count toward completion of the hepatitis B vaccine series, and administration of three additional doses of hepatitis B vaccine should commence when the infant is 1 month of age.[122] By the chronologic age of 1 month, all premature infants, regardless of initial birth weight or gestational age, are likely to respond as adequately as do older and larger infants.[329,365,397,494] Testing for HBsAg and anti-HBs is recommended at 1 to 3 months after completion of the vaccine series. The presence of anti-HBs along with the absence of HBsAg indicates successful prophylaxis and immunization. An HBsAg-positive result indicates failure of prophylaxis or in utero infection. Infants who are negative for anti-HBs and HBsAg should receive three additional doses of vaccine at a 0-, 1-, and 6-month schedule, followed by retesting for anti-HBs 1 month after the third dose. Alternatively, additional doses of vaccine (one to three) can be administered and the infant tested for anti-HBs 1 month after each dose has been administered to determine whether subsequent doses are necessary. Household members and sexual contacts of HBsAg-positive mothers should be screened, and if no evidence of previous HBV infection is noted, they also should be immunized.

Infants delivered by HBsAg-positive women are bathed as soon as possible after delivery to remove all maternal blood and secretions. Intramuscular injections should be delayed until bathing is completed; if such bathing is not possible, meticulous cleaning of the site with alcohol is necessary. These infants require standard precautions. Infants who have received both active and passive prophylaxis may be breast-fed.

In 1991, the Advisory Committee on Immunization Practices of the CDC[119] and, in 1992, the Committee on Infectious Diseases of the American Academy of Pediatrics[146] recommended the universal use of hepatitis B vaccine in all infants as the optimal strategy for prevention of HBV infection.[617] Current recommendations continue to support these opinions.[27] For infants with a birth weight of 2 kg or greater and born to mothers whose HBsAG status is negative, the first dose of HBV vaccine should be administered at or soon after birth, the second dose at 1 month or more after the first dose, and the third dose at 6 to 18 months of age. The minimal interval between the second and third doses is 2 months, and the third dose should not be given before 6 months. For infants who receive their first dose after they have reached 2 months of age, the minimal interval between the first and third doses is 4 months. An alternative schedule of the three doses administered at 2, 4, and 6 to 18 months of age concur-

rently with other routine vaccines may be used for HBsAg-negative infants not vaccinated at birth.

Seroconversion rates in premature infants who have a birth weight of less than 2 kg and are vaccinated shortly after birth are lower than those in larger preterm infants and full-term infants vaccinated at birth.[380] For this reason, for premature infants weighing less than 2 kg at birth and born to HBsAg-negative mothers, initiation of the vaccination series is delayed until they are 1 month of age.[122] The schedule for follow-up doses is the same as for other infants.

Infants with a birth weight of 2 kg or more and born to mothers whose HBsAg status is unknown should receive the first dose of vaccine within 12 hours of birth. Blood should be drawn from the mother at delivery to determine her HBsAg status. If it is positive, HBIG should be given as soon as possible, but no later than when the infant is 1 week of age. If the infant's birth weight is less than 2 kg, HBIG in addition to vaccine should be given within 12 hours of birth. This initial vaccine dose should not be counted as part of the three-dose schedule. The subsequent vaccine schedule is based on the mother's HBsAg status. If it remains unknown, the infant should be treated as though the mother were HBsAg-positive.

Because the rate of perinatal transmission is greatest in mothers who are HBeAg-positive or those who are negative for both HBeAg and anti-HBe, some researchers have suggested administering prophylaxis to neonates born only to this group of mothers.[534,577] However, the occurrence of several cases of hepatitis in babies born to mothers with anti-HBe[174,585] and the demonstration that measurements such as HBV DNA polymerase or HBV DNA by PCR may be more accurate indicators of infectivity than are measurements of HBe antigen or antibody[280,637] indicate that prophylaxis should be given to neonates of all chronic carrier mothers, regardless of their e antigen/antibody status.[27] Because the combined HBIG/vaccine regimen results in effective and long-term protection, breast-feeding is allowed and encouraged in chronic carrier mothers. These significant developments in prophylaxis against perinatal transmission of hepatitis B should reduce the frequency of chronic carriers strikingly and thereby decrease the number of cases of chronic active or progressive hepatitis and death from cirrhosis, liver failure, and hepatocellular carcinoma.

HEPATITIS C VIRUS INFECTION

The remarkable molecular biology effort to isolate and clone the gene of HCV[141] and to express a major nonstructural protein[368] led to the demonstration that HCV is the predominant cause of NANB hepatitis and a major contributor to chronic hepatitis in developed countries.[21-23,121,164,649] Rates of HCV seroprevalence are highest (60-90%) in those with repeated exposure to blood or blood products (e.g., injection drug users, hemophilia patients), intermediate (20%) in those with repeated or inapparent percutaneous exposure (e.g., hemodialysis patients), lower (1-10%) in those with high-risk sexual behavior or household contacts of infected persons, and lowest (0.5-1%) in blood donors.[22,164,649] Overall, an estimated 1.8 percent of the population, including pregnant women, in the United States is infected with HCV.[28]

Among studies of infants born to anti-HCV-positive women, an average of 5 percent (range, 0-25%) of infants were persistently positive for second-generation assay anti-HCV antibody or HCV RNA during a follow-up period of at least 10 months.* The risk of vertical transmission is correlated with higher concentrations of plasma HCV RNA[390,468]; with HIV-1 co-infection, especially in those with advanced stages of AIDS; with the specific genotype of HCV; and, possibly, with the vaginal route of deliv-

*See references 373, 390, 402, 464, 468, 524, 538, 633, 664, 665, 703.

ery. HCV RNA has been detected in the breast milk of infected women, but transmission by breast milk has not been documented, and HCV infection is not a contraindication to breast-feeding.[391]

HCV infection can be diagnosed by antibody titers and molecular methods to detect and quantitate viral RNA. Antigen-detection tests and IgM assays are not available. Antibody titers in infants are confounded by maternal transplacental antibody; this effect presumably is gone by the time that the infant reaches 18 months of age.[27] Antibody testing involves a screening EIA, with repeat positive results confirmed by a recombinant immunoblot assay (RIBA), analogous to what is done for the serologic diagnosis of HIV infection. The second-generation EIA (EIA-2) and RIBA are 95 percent sensitive and 97 percent specific.[254] Infants born to HCV antibody-positive mothers should be screened for anti-HCV with the EIA-2 after they are 18 months of age. RIBA may be used as a supplemental test for specificity; both the EIA-2 and RIBA measure IgG antibody to recombinant HCV antigens. Detection of HCV RNA in infant blood is also available commercially and should be performed when the infant is between 1 and 2 months of age.[29,254] Infants who are infected perinatally should be referred to a hepatologist and have annual screening of liver enzymes, even if they remain asymptomatic.

Controlled trials of interferon therapy in children with chronic hepatitis C are limited.[144] Long-term prognosis for HCV infection in infants and children is not clear, but 85 percent of adults become chronically infected, and HCV is known to be associated with cirrhosis and hepatocellular carcinoma.[22,164,649]

The development of a successful vaccine for hepatitis C must overcome several obstacles, including multiple genotypes of the virus, lack of cross-protective immunity among the genotypes, lack of long-term protection with the same genotype, and lack of successful cultivation of the virus in cell culture.[22,164] In February 1994, the Advisory Committee on Immunization Practices reviewed the available data and concluded that no support was found for the use of immunoglobulin for postexposure prophylaxis. This recommendation is still the current opinion of experts.[28] Immunoglobulin is not protective because blood from anti-HCV-positive donors is excluded from the pool used for preparation and no neutralizing antibody for HCV has been identified as yet. Routine screening of all pregnant women and their newborns for HCV infection cannot be recommended at this time, but screening should be considered in those with known risk factors. For example, infants who received 1 U or more of blood or blood products before 1992 or who received Gammagard/Polygam (Baxter Healthcare Corporation, Glendale, CA) in 1993 or 1994 were screened with liver transaminase tests and for anti-HCV antibody.

HERPES SIMPLEX

HSV, the etiologic agent of cold sores, keratitis, encephalitis, and genital ulcers in older children and adults, causes serious disease in neonates, with high mortality rates and severe neurologic sequelae.

MICROBIOLOGY AND EPIDEMIOLOGY

The two types of HSV, type 1 and type 2, may be distinguished by antigenic, biochemical, molecular, and biologic differences.[156,667] HSV-1 (the "oral strain") usually causes mouth lesions, eye infections, and endemic encephalitis, whereas HSV-2 (the "genital strain") usually is associated with sexually transmitted genital infections.[156,667] However, 8 to 50 percent of genital herpes disease is now caused by HSV-1.[476] Most neonatal disease is caused by HSV-2, but HSV-1 neonatal disease appears in recent studies to be increasing in certain populations.[98]

Antiviral collaborative studies indicate that 4 percent of neonatal herpes cases are acquired in utero, 86 percent natally, and 10 percent postnatally. Three quarters of natal/postnatal cases of neonatal herpes are caused by HSV-2, and the remainder are caused by HSV-1 strains.[480] Virtually all neonatal HSV-2 infections probably are acquired from mothers having an active genital herpes infection at the time of delivery.[477,623,675,695] The majority of neonates with HSV appear to acquire the infection by contact with infected genital secretions at or during delivery from an asymptomatic mother who acquired her first episode of genital herpes infection in the third trimester or near the time of delivery.[96,97,100,102] Because 60 to 80 percent of these mothers have no signs or symptoms of genital herpes at the time of labor and delivery and have a negative past history of genital herpes or sexual contact with a partner who had a genital vesicular rash, some experts recommend routine serologic screening of pregnant women and their partners to identify potential at-risk mothers.[96-98,404,668,674] In a study of 140 pregnant women with cytologically diagnosed genital herpes, only 36 percent had clinically recognized herpetic lesions.[450] Twenty-one percent had nonspecific abnormal findings, and 43 percent were asymptomatic. In addition, 20 to 40 percent of nonpregnant women from whose genital secretions HSV is isolated are asymptomatic.[306,680] Use of more sensitive techniques, such as PCR, detects genital HSV shedding in asymptomatic women even more frequently.[149]

Neonates with HSV-1 infection can acquire the virus from several sources: maternal genital, oral, or breast lesions[97,98,196,389,622,695]; oral herpes in the father or other family members[193,623,695]; or health care–associated transmission from other infected babies or health care workers.[262,393] Although HSV-1 cold sores and asymptomatic oral shedding may be common findings in nursery personnel,[275,276] transmission to a neonate from this source appears to be rare.[414,533,650]

Because most fetal and neonatal HSV infections are transmitted from the mother, a summary of several aspects of herpes infection during pregnancy is appropriate. Fulminant or disseminated primary HSV disease may occur in pregnancy, but whether it develops more often than in nonpregnant women is not clear. A review[495] of seven such cases revealed (1) infection during the third trimester in all; (2) four beginning as a genital HSV infection and three as oral disease; (3) hepatitis in six, encephalitis in two, and pancreatitis in two; (4) maternal death in three (43%)—two from hepatitis and one from encephalitis; and (5) three instances of fetal death—each secondary to severe maternal systemic illness rather than direct infection with HSV. Evidence of visceral disease in a pregnant woman with either genital or oral HSV infection is an indication for providing systemic antiviral therapy.[369]

An increased rate of spontaneous abortion occurs in women with primary genital herpes during early pregnancy, regardless of socioeconomic status.[100,271,274,450,480] Premature delivery does not occur more commonly in prospectively monitored women with recurrent genital herpes,[274,480,657,682] but most reports of neonatal herpes cases find a greater preponderance of premature infants than in the general population.[480,668,675,695] This finding, however, may reflect a higher susceptibility of premature infants to HSV infection secondary to a lack of transplacentally acquired IgG neutralizing antibodies rather than being a cause of the prematurity. Recurrent genital herpes in middle-class pregnant women is no more severe or frequent than in nonpregnant ones,[271,657,682] but older studies demonstrated more frequent and longer episodes in women of lower socioeconomic groups.[450,456] Between 74 and 88 percent of middle-class pregnant women with a history of genital herpes had at least one clinical recurrence during an observed pregnancy.[271,657,682] A mean of 2.7 to 3.0 episodes occurred during gestation, and HSV was isolated from lesions in 56 to 75 percent of the recurrences and in 0.6 to 12 percent of concomitant cervical cultures obtained during the recurrence. Asymptomatic shedding of HSV from the cervix, either between clinical recurrences or in a history-positive woman with no episodes during the observed pregnancy, was detected in 0.5 to 2.3 percent of the cultures obtained. Importantly, the presence of HSV shedding during the latter weeks of pregnancy was not predictive of shedding at the time of delivery.[37,682]

The number of cases of neonatal herpes occurring in the United States each year is far less than one would expect from the probable number of pregnancies complicated by genital herpes. Of the 3.5 million annual pregnancies, 7000 to 200,000 of these women have genital herpes at some time during the pregnancy and 3500 to 14,000 have positive HSV cultures at the time of delivery.[75,255,274,632,657,673,682] The actual number of cases of neonatal herpes per year in Seattle and Atlanta (0.1 and 0.3 per 1000 live births, respectively) would project to a national estimate of 350 to 1050 per year in the United States.[623] Because asymptomatic HSV infection of the neonate rarely occurs, subclinical cases or missed diagnoses probably do not account for the differences between the estimated number of maternal and neonatal infections. More likely, neonatal infection rates in the babies of mothers with genital herpes are far lower than currently assumed, possibly because of the preventive measures used. The estimated infection rates quoted most often currently are: (1) a 33 to 50 percent rate for infants vaginally delivered by mothers with primary genital herpes, (2) a 3 to 5 percent rate for infants vaginally delivered by mothers with recurrent lesions, and (3) less than 3 percent for those delivered by mothers with recurrent asymptomatic shedding at the time of delivery.[75,97,155,480,682] In the early 1970s, Nahmias and associates[450] reported the following neonatal infection rates in babies born to mothers with genital herpes during pregnancy: (1) 33 percent in mothers with primary disease after the 32nd week of gestation, (2) 3 percent in mothers with recurrent episodes after 32 weeks, and (3) 42 percent in mothers with virus-positive lesions at the time of delivery (primary versus recurrent episodes not specified). More recent studies have determined a significant risk of neonatal herpes occurring in babies born to mothers with asymptomatic shedding at the time of vaginal delivery: 33 percent with subclinical first episodes[97] and 0 to 3 percent with recurrent shedding.[97,106-108,481,511] Accurate knowledge of the actual neonatal infection risk is important for making decisions about management (e.g., cesarean section, prophylactic antiviral therapy). However, because researchers have estimated that as many as 75 percent of neonates with HSV disease are born to mothers with no history or clinical findings suggestive of active HSV infection during pregnancy, labor, or delivery, not all neonatal HSV disease is preventable by management decisions made on the basis of current knowledge of known risk factors.[26,101,106-108]

Several factors influence the risk of acquiring neonatal herpes and the severity of neonatal disease once the infection develops. The greater risk of transmitting neonatal infection by mothers with primary, as opposed to recurrent, vesicular or ulcerative lesions at the time of delivery is well established. Also, a woman with virus-positive recurrent lesions at the time of delivery is likely to be a greater risk than is a woman who is asymptomatic and shedding virus identified by HSV surveillance cultures. Other aspects of the anatomic site and the severity of maternal genital herpes also may be associated with a greater risk of development of neonatal disease: (1) cervical as opposed to vulvar or buttock skin involvement—resulting in more virus being shed into vaginal secretions; (2) multiple as opposed to single vesicles or ulcers—again, more virus from multiple lesions; (3) higher titer of virus in vaginal secretions—cultures positive sooner or more intensely positive in the diagnostic virology laboratory; and (4) longer duration of fetal exposure to infected vaginal secretions because of prolonged rupture of membranes, or fetal scalp monitors.[155,478,480]

Investigations by Yeager and associates[695,696] indicate that no anti-HSV antibody or a low titer of such antibody in maternal and neonatal serum is associated with a greater risk of acquisition of neonatal infection and more serious disease and that high-titer antibody is associated with a lower risk. Studies of HSV antibody titers in neonates enrolled in the CASG trial do not show an association between antibody titer and outcome of disease.[676] More investigations are required, therefore, to determine the potential protective role of maternal transplacental anti-HSV antibody.

Premature infants have accounted for 40 to 50 percent of cases of neonatal herpes,[668,676] in contrast to the usual prematurity rates of 6 to 18 percent reported in the general maternal population. Whether the increased frequency of prematurity among neonates with herpes indicates a greater propensity of mothers with genital herpes to deliver prematurely or a greater susceptibility of premature infants to HSV infection is not known. Premature infants appear more likely to have a fatal outcome.[108,668,669]

Instrumentation of the neonate, particularly scalp electrodes for fetal monitoring, is known to increase the risk of acquiring neonatal HSV infection.[205,321,487] Mortality rates appear to be higher in neonates with HSV-2 than in those with HSV-1 infection, probably because of the greater proportion of HSV-2–infected babies with dissemination.[669] In neonatal herpes survivors, neurologic damage occurs much more frequently in infants with HSV-2 than in those with HSV-1 infection.[157,669] Finally, the body sites of involvement in the neonate clearly influence outcome. Babies with disseminated infection (liver, lungs, adrenals), with or without CNS involvement, have the highest mortality rates (70-80%); those with encephalitis have only intermediate rates (30-40%); and those with infection limited to the skin, eye, or mouth have the lowest rates (0%).[676] Babies delivered in a high-risk situation might be given anticipatory antiviral chemotherapy after appropriate cultures have been obtained, whereas those in low-risk situations might be cultured and observed closely for evidence of neonatal herpes.[480,481]

PATHOGENESIS AND PATHOLOGY

As mentioned previously, HSV may be transmitted to the neonate in utero either by a transplacental (congenital infection) or ascending route, at the time of birth (natal infection), or after birth (postnatal infection). Congenital infection probably results from transplacental transmission of virus secondary to leukocyte-associated viremia in a mother with genital herpes, but no direct evidence supports this hypothesis. HSV-2 viremia has been documented in two women with primary genital herpes.[160] A report of 13 neonates with intrauterine HSV infection indicated that primary genital herpes was present during pregnancy in four mothers, recurrent disease was present in one, and no history of genital herpes was elicited in the remaining eight.[301] In the fetus, HSV appears to be transmitted directly from the placenta through the bloodstream to target organs. Because of the known tropism of HSV for the CNS, one is not surprised that most infants with congenital infection have evidence of brain involvement at birth.[301] Intrauterine infection also may occur by an ascending route from an infected maternal genital tract, and such transmission is supported by the development of clinical signs of HSV infection in the first 5 days of life.

The natal infection presumably is acquired secondary to aspiration of infected vaginal secretions into the nares, oropharyngeal cavity, conjunctivae, and upper respiratory tract of the infant. Other portals of entry for natal infection include the scalp, skin, and umbilical cord.[480,668] In postnatal HSV infection, no evidence supports the genital tract as a source of virus. Most postnatally acquired infections appear to result from contact with saliva from persons with oral herpes or with virus carried on the hands of

TABLE 73-9 Congenital Herpes Simplex Virus Infection: Features in 30 Cases*

Feature	Number	Percentage
Culture-positive vesicles or bullae	28/30	93
HSV-2	24/27	89
Low birth weight	22/26	85
Microcephaly, seizures, diffuse brain damage, intracranial calcification	20/30	67
Chorioretinitis, microphthalmos	17/30	57
Small for gestational age	9/25	36

Other features: retinal dysplasia, scars on skin or digits, cataracts, pneumonitis, hepatomegaly.
Features present at birth or shortly thereafter.
From Hutto, C., Arvin, A., Jacob, R., et al.: Intrauterine herpes simplex virus infections. *J. Pediatr.* 110:97-101, 1987.

personnel.[389,668,695] After natal or postnatal acquisition of HSV occurs, initial replication of the virus occurs at the portal of entry, with subsequent viremic dissemination to viscera. Involvement of the CNS occurs either from hematogenous spread to the brain in infants with disseminated disease, which results in multiple areas of cortical hemorrhagic necrosis, or from retrograde axonal transport of the virus to the CNS from superficial replication in the skin, eye, or mouth.[324,451,668]

CLINICAL MANIFESTATIONS

The clinical features of genital herpes in women have been discussed in detail elsewhere.[99,155,256,449,476] Women with initial or primary infections may have multiple, small, painful, and tender vesicles and ulcers involving the cervix, vagina, vulva, and skin of the perineal region. In addition, patients may complain of inguinal or pelvic pain that is caused by associated lymphadenopathy. Systemic symptoms consisting of fever, malaise, and myalgia usually are present. The total duration of pain is 10 days to 2 weeks, whereas the total duration of lesions may be 2 to 3 weeks. Peak lesion virus titers, from 10^4 to 10^5 plaque-forming units per milliliter, occur during the first week of illness.[99] The total duration of viral shedding lasts from 10 to 14 days.[99,155] Lesions on dry skin progress through the well-defined vesicle, ulcer, crust, and healed stages described for herpes simplex labialis.[594] On moist mucous membranes, vesicles quickly rupture to form shallow ulcers that persist for days and gradually heal from the periphery.[99]

Recurrent genital herpes in women usually is milder and of shorter duration than is primary infection, the vesicles and ulcers are more circumscribed and fewer in number, and the disease appears to be limited largely to the external genitals.[99] Peak virus titers occur during the first few days and are lower, 10^3 to 10^4 plaque-forming units per milliliter. The total duration of pain is 5 to 9 days, duration of vesicles and ulcers is 8 to 11 days, and the duration of viral shedding is 5 to 8 days.[99,155] Women with both primary or initial and recurrent genital herpes may be asymptomatic.[97]

The clinical spectrum in infants with congenital HSV infection is different from that observed in babies with natal or postnatal disease. The most prominent features summarized from 30 cases of congenital infection reported in the literature are shown in Table 73-9.* A vesicular rash, bullae, or cutaneous scars present at birth or within a few days of birth were noted in almost all infants. In some cases, the extent and severity of these lesions resulted in an initial diagnosis of epidermolysis bullosa. At least

*See references 195, 227, 290, 301, 348, 378, 427, 434, 571, 580, 592, 621.

one case report of limb hypoplasia, similar to congenital varicella syndrome, has been shown to be caused by HSV-2.[312] Two thirds of infants demonstrate extensive involvement of the CNS at birth, either clinically or from autopsy findings: diffuse brain damage, microcephaly, or intracranial calcifications. In some infants, eye findings, including chorioretinitis, microphthalmos, retinal scars and retinal dysplasia, and cataracts, have been noted.[401]

As indicated in Figure 73-3, infants with natal or postnatal herpes commonly have a clinical picture resembling that of bacterial sepsis: alterations in temperature, lethargy, respiratory distress, anorexia or vomiting, and cyanosis.[106-108,266,674,675] The three general patterns of infection are categorized by the extent of disease: (1) disseminated infection with or without CNS involvement, present in 25 percent of cases; (2) infection localized to the CNS in 30 percent of cases; and (3) infection localized to the skin, eye, or mouth in 45 percent of cases.[106-108,334]

The frequency of disseminated disease has decreased after a high of 51 percent reported in the years 1973 to 1981; this decrease probably represents earlier diagnosis and treatment of localized infection before dissemination occurs.[672] The disseminated form of infection in the earlier years of recognition presented in infants between 9 and 11 days of age and usually involved the liver, where it caused fulminant hepatitis with disseminated intravascular coagulation, and the adrenal glands, and it most closely resembled the picture of bacterial sepsis.[279,640] Current reports show disseminated neonatal HSV may present as early as the first week of life, without cutaneous or localizing signs, similar to bacterial sepsis, and confirm that HSV remains an important cause of neonatal morbidity and mortality.[106-108,644] A disseminated infection can affect multiple organs, including the brain, larynx, trachea, lungs, esophagus, stomach, lower gastrointestinal tract, spleen, kidneys, pancreas, and heart. Pneumonia occurs in 37 percent of infants. Markedly elevated transaminase levels, direct hyperbilirubinemia, coagulopathy, and thrombocytopenia are common findings. Approximately 60 to 75 percent of infants with disseminated disease have hematogenously acquired CNS involvement, as manifested by irritability, a bulging fontanelle, localized or generalized seizures, flaccid or spastic paralysis, opisthotonos, decerebrate rigidity, or coma. Importantly, 39 percent of infants with disseminated disease do not have skin vesicles at initial evaluation, and vesicles do not develop during the acute HSV disease; only 56 percent initially have fever, and many are hypothermic on presentation.[106,107,334]

CNS disease from retrograde axonal transmission of virus presents later than does disseminated disease, usually when the infant is 11 to 17 days old but occasionally when the infant is as old as 4 to 6 weeks of age. Typically, these infants have focal seizures that subsequently generalize. Examination of CSF demonstrates mononuclear pleocytosis with a predominance of lymphocytes, a moderately low glucose concentration, and elevated protein levels. A normal cell count, glucose, and protein concentration, however, may be found on the initial lumbar puncture, if performed early in the disease process.[106,107,664] An elevated red blood cell count secondary to hemorrhagic brain involvement may be present but by itself is an unreliable sign. Fever is present at initial evaluation in only 44 percent of infants with HSV encephalitis, and 32 percent of infants do not have skin vesicles either initially or during the course of their illness.

Localized skin, eye, or mouth disease usually presents within the infant's first 7 to 10 days of life. Approximately 83 percent of these neonates have skin lesions: usually single vesicles, occasionally vesicle clusters, and rarely a zoster-like rash.[442] As many as 46 to 80 percent of neonates with skin lesions have 1 to 12 recurrences during the first 6 to 12 months of life.[295,337,669] Approximately 13 to 25 percent of infants have eye involvement; disease is limited to only the eye in one third of these cases. Common manifestations include conjunctivitis, keratitis, and chorioretinitis.[258,448] As many as 83 percent of infants are afebrile initially.[106,107] One third of all infants have evidence of herpetic mouth lesions, but involvement of this site alone rarely occurs.

DIAGNOSIS AND DIFFERENTIAL DIAGNOSIS

Up to 80 percent of infants have classic features that would suggest herpes simplex, such as skin vesicles, mouth ulcers, or keratoconjunctivitis. One half of the remaining 15 to 20 percent have either (1) focal or diffuse encephalitis or (2) a sepsis syndrome with pneumonitis, hepatitis, encephalitis, and frequently, disseminated intravascular coagulopathy.[106,107,480] A clinical picture of encephalitis certainly should suggest HSV infection; the combination of pneumonitis, hepatitis, and encephalitis seldom is seen in bacterial sepsis/meningitis and should alert the clinician that a neonatal viral infection is more likely. As many as 32 percent of all HSV-infected neonates do not have vesicular skin lesions that would prompt clinical suspicion and a more rapid diagnosis. Kimberlin and colleagues[334] with the CASG compared the clinical characteristics of neonates with HSV disease in two multicenter studies that they conducted, one from 1981 to 1988 and the other from 1989 to 1997. They found that no progress has been made in decreasing the time interval between the onset of HSV symptoms and the initiation of antiviral therapy; the mean time between the earliest manifestation of an HSV symptom and initiation of acyclovir therapy was between 5 and 7 days. Recent studies have shown neonatal HSV disease presents more commonly than previously appreciated and appears similar in incidence to bacterial meningitis.[106-108] Although acyclovir should not be part of routine antibiotic therapy for all neonates with presumed sepsis, intravenous acyclovir should be provided promptly, similar to the paradigm of bacterial sepsis, pending results of viral studies, if the diagnosis of neonatal HSV is in the differential diagnosis.

The most definitive means of establishing a diagnosis of HSV infection in a neonate is isolation or identification of the virus in clinical or autopsy specimens. Samples for isolation of virus in cell culture should be obtained prior to initiating antiviral therapy and may be obtained from the skin vesicles, nares, throat, nasopharynx, conjunctivae, stool, urine, peripheral blood buffy coat, CSF, brain tissue, and liver biopsy and autopsy material.[187] HSV has been isolated from CSF in up to 25 to 40 percent of cases of encephalitis. HSV also has been isolated from duodenal aspirates of infants with hepatitis. Ideally, specimens should be processed immediately or frozen at −70°C if testing cannot be performed until later. However, HSV is stable for 2 to 3 days at 4°C in commercial viral transport media or media containing trypticase soy broth or brain-heart infusion broth.[694] In cell culture, the typical HSV cytopathic effect often is evident within 1 to 2 days after inoculation. Studies using centrifugation of the specimen onto a cell monolayer at the bottom of a shell vial, followed by staining for HSV antigen the next day, yielded 99 percent sensitivity and 100 percent specificity.[479] Typing of HSV should be performed because recent evidence suggests that neurologic outcomes may be worse with neonatal infection caused by HSV-2 than with infection caused by HSV-1. Moreover, typing might help establish the mode of transmission and provide information useful for future counseling regarding preventive measures.

Direct immunofluorescence assays (DFAs) or immunoperoxidase techniques are available to demonstrate HSV-1 or HSV-2 antigens in cells scraped from the base of vesicles or the conjunctivae or in biopsy or autopsy material.[321,554] Scraping from the base of a vesicle reveals intranuclear inclusions and multinucleated giant cells by the Tzanck test or Wright stain in 60 to 70 percent of cases. Detection of specific HSV antigen from skin and mucocutaneous ulcers by immunofluorescence is preferred

and can be accomplished in 70 to 80 percent of cases. Direct detection of HSV antigen by commercial EIA has variable reliability compared with that of traditional cell culture and DFA.[653]

The diagnosis of HSV encephalitis has been improved greatly by the development of PCR for detection of HSV DNA in CSF.[332,333,372,644] PCR has supplanted the need for biopsy testing of brain tissue for HSV diagnostic purposes. It has a sensitivity of 48 to 98 percent and a specificity of 94 to 100 percent. HSV DNA can be detected by PCR in most culture-positive CSF even after 1 week of acyclovir therapy. HSV DNA detection by PCR on infant serum and whole blood is a useful method to document HSV viremia and disseminated HSV infection.[106-108,333,610] Other tests that aid in the detection of CNS abnormalities and help establish CNS involvement with HSV include electroencephalography, enhanced brain CT, and MRI. The characteristic electroencephalographic abnormality is a periodic slow and sharp wave discharge; more commonly, multiple independent foci of periodic activity are present. CT scanning may be normal early in the course of the disease, with characteristic abnormalities appearing 3 to 5 days later. The findings most frequently observed in the acute phase are (1) patchy areas of low attenuation with brain edema in both cerebral hemispheres or (2) hemorrhage or calcification in the thalamus, insular cortex, and periventricular white matter and along the corticomedullary junction. Late findings include multicystic encephalomalacia and ventriculomegaly as a result of brain atrophy and destruction. MRI is sensitive in detecting early abnormalities in the periventricular white matter and in defining the extent of parenchymal lesions.

In most circumstances, serologic assays are not useful for establishing the diagnosis of maternal or neonatal herpes during the acute phase of the disease.[187] Antibody assays may be used for documenting initial or primary genital herpes infection in the mother, as well as for determining whether the mother has a past history of HSV-2 infection. New serologic assays are available that reliably detect serum HSV-2 IgG antibodies.[123] The persistent lack of HSV-2 antibody on repeated samples taken over time in a mother whose infant has clinical evidence of possible HSV infection would render HSV-2 unlikely. However, the possibility of the infection being caused by HSV-1 remains. Immunofluorescent techniques to quantify HSV-specific IgM antibodies have been developed, but these antibodies usually are not detected in serum for 2 or more weeks after onset of the infection in neonates.[447]

The major diseases to be considered in the differential diagnosis of neonatal HSV include bacterial sepsis and meningitis, adenovirus and enterovirus infection, and, to a lesser extent, congenital infection with CMV, rubella virus, and VZV. Inquiry about illness in the mother and other epidemiologic features may be helpful. For example, mothers of neonates with HSV infection may (but often do not) have a history of having had genital lesions or sexual contact with someone who has genital herpes. Infants with sepsis usually have associated factors known to predispose to bacterial infection, such as maternal peripartum infection, premature rupture of membranes, and procedures performed in the intensive care unit or nursery. Enterovirus infection of infants tends to occur in the summer and fall and is associated with signs and symptoms of enterovirus disease in the mother. Adenoviruses, however, occur year-round and may have slight increase in frequency during winter/spring months. Varicella in the neonate usually presents with a history of maternal varicella near the time of delivery or close contact with a caretaker with varicella.

TREATMENT

Studies conducted by the CASG of the National Institute of Allergy and Infectious Diseases (NIAID) have shown that antivi-

TABLE 73–10 Neonatal Herpes: Antiviral Therapy

Outcome	Total (%)	Skin, Eyes, Mouth (%)	Encephalitis (%)	Disseminated (%)
Mortality				
ACV, Ara-A*	17	0	14	54
Historical controls†	49	7	37	76
Developmental Normal				
ACV, Ara-A*	67	94	36	59
Historical controls†	26	73	19	54

*Data from Whitley, R., Arvin, A., Prober, C., et al.: A controlled trial comparing vidarabine with acyclovir in neonatal herpes simplex virus infection. N. Engl. J. Med. 324:444-449, 1991.
†Data from Nahmias, A. J., Keyserling, H. L, and Kerrick, G. M.: Herpes simplex. In Remington, J. S., and Klein, J. O. (eds.): Infectious Diseases of the Fetus and Newborn Infant. 2nd ed. Phidelphia, W. B. Saunders, 1983, pp. 636-678.
ACV, acyclovir; Ara-A, vidarabine (adenine arabinoside).

ral therapy for neonatal HSV disease significantly improves mortality rates and long-term outcomes of infected neonates. Vidarabine was the first commercially available drug for the treatment of neonatal HSV disease.[139] Placebo-controlled trials demonstrated that adenine arabinoside (vidarabine, ara-A) at doses of 15 or 30 mg/kg/day given as a 12-hour infusion significantly reduced the mortality rate from 62 percent in historic cases and placebo controls to 35 percent in treated cases and increased the percentage of normal survivors from 19 to 43 percent.[676] Results were best in infants with disseminated infection and disease localized to the CNS, with the mortality rate being reduced from 70 to 40 percent and the percentage of normal survivors increased from 10 to 30 percent. No difference was found between the 15-mg and the 30-mg dose in side effects, but the higher dose appeared to inhibit more effectively the progression of disease from skin-eye-mouth involvement to disseminated or CNS disease.[674] None of the 49 treated patients had significant adverse clinical reactions or laboratory abnormalities attributable to the drug. On the negative side, 21 percent of infants progressed to more serious disease while receiving therapy, and serious neurologic sequelae developed in 27 percent of the total. Fifteen percent of babies with disseminated or CNS disease continued to excrete HSV in the throat after 10 days of therapy.

The results of a vidarabine-acyclovir comparison trial in the treatment of neonatal herpes did not show any difference in efficacy and safety between the two drugs.[668] When the results with vidarabine and vidarabine-acyclovir were combined, the mortality rate was reduced from 49 percent in untreated historical controls to 17 percent in treated patients (Table 73–10). Normal survivors increased from 26 to 67 percent. Although the results in the total group of patients were encouraging, the outcome in the group of patients with disseminated disease was not: a mortality rate of 54 percent in treated patients versus 76 percent in untreated historical controls and normal development in 59 percent of treated survivors versus 54 percent of controls (see Table 73–10). Factors that predicted mortality and their relative risk were as follows: disseminated disease, 33; CNS disease, 5.8; semicoma or coma, 5.2; disseminated intravascular coagulation, 3.8; prematurity, 3.7; and pneumonitis, 3.6.[669] Factors significantly associated with neurologic sequelae in survivors and their relative risk in these studies were as follows: skin-eye-mouth disease with three or more recurrent skin lesions after completion of acute therapy, 21; skin-eye-mouth disease caused by HSV-2, 14; HSV-2 infection, regardless of disease category, 4.9; CNS disease, 4.4; and seizures, 3.0. In infants with HSV disease limited to the skin, eye, or mouth, neonates with HSV-1 infection were all normal developmentally at 1 year of age as compared with 86 percent of those with HSV-2 infection. Among the latter infants, those with impaired neurologic outcome were significantly more

likely to have had three or more skin recurrences in the first 6 months of life.

Because of greater ease of administration, intravenous acyclovir has supplanted vidarabine as the drug of choice for the treatment of neonatal HSV infection. Vidarabine no longer is available commercially. Because mortality and morbidity in neonates with HSV infection remained high using standard (30 mg/kg/day) dosing of acyclovir for 10 days, the CASG evaluated intermediate-dose (45 mg/kg/day) and high-dose (60 mg/kg/day) intravenous acyclovir for 21 days in 79 neonates with neonatal HSV infection.[335] Data were compared with those of a previous CASG study in which all infants received standard doses of acyclovir (30 mg/kg/day) for 10 days. Overall, after stratification for disease category, the survival rate for patients treated with high-dose acyclovir was significantly higher than that for patients treated with the standard dose. Specifically, in neonates who received high-dose acyclovir, those with disseminated disease but not encephalitis had a significantly higher survival rate. The mortality rate at 24 months for patients with disseminated disease who received 21 days of high-dose acyclovir was 31 percent, compared with 57 percent for patients who received an intermediate dose for 21 days and 61 percent for those who received the standard dose for 10 days in the earlier CASG trial. For encephalitis, the mortality rate of infants at 24 months was 6 percent with high-dose acyclovir, 20 percent with the intermediate dose, and 19 percent with the standard dose. In addition, recipients of high-dose acyclovir had less morbidity than did historical control infants who received the standard dose of acyclovir. Patients treated with high-dose acyclovir were 6.6 times as likely to have normal development at 12 months of age. Among infants with encephalitis, however, 31 percent of high-dose acyclovir recipients were developing normally at 12 months as compared with 29 percent of patients treated with the standard dose. With respect to toxicity in the high-dose acyclovir recipients, 21 percent had a transient neutropenia that resolved either during continuation of high-dose acyclovir or after its cessation. Nephrotoxicity occurred in four (6%) infants who had disseminated disease. Because acyclovir is eliminated by the kidneys, the dose should be adjusted for renal disease.[216] High-dose acyclovir did not impede the development of an adequate antibody response to HSV in infected infants.

These studies have led to the current recommendation for the use of intravenous acyclovir at a dose of 60 mg/kg/day for 21 days to treat neonatal CNS and disseminated HSV disease and for 14 days for skin-eye-mouth disease.[26,331] In addition, infants with ocular involvement should receive a topical ophthalmic drug (1-2% trifluridine, 1% idoxuridine, or 3% vidarabine). Consultation with an ophthalmologist is also recommended to assist in the management of ocular HSV in the neonate. All patients with HSV CNS infection should have a repeat lumbar puncture performed at the completion of acyclovir therapy to determine resolution of abnormal CSF parameters and to document whether the CSF specimen is HSV culture and PCR-negative. A positive CSF HSV PCR at this time is an indication for continuing intravenous acyclovir therapy and for performing repeat neuroimaging studies to evaluate the extent of CNS damage. Repeat samples of blood and CSF should be obtained weekly until HSV studies are negative and provide a guideline for duration of antiviral therapy.

Concern has been raised that some infants may have progressive neurologic injury after acquiring neonatal herpes encephalitis.[257] In addition, infants who have three or more skin recurrences with HSV-2 in the first 6 months of life have been shown to be at increased risk for having neurodevelopmental abnormalities at follow-up, whether as a consequence of previously undetected CNS infection or because of CNS dissemination during skin reactivation.[669] Suppression of HSV skin reactivation by the administration of acyclovir (300 mg/m^2 per dose given orally three times daily) for 6 months is recommended by some experts for selected patients. The infant's blood counts should be monitored while receiving oral acyclovir long term because Kimberlin and coworkers[336] documented suppressive therapy resulted in neutropenia in 50 percent of treated infants and emergence of an acyclovir-resistant HSV isolate in one infant. Acyclovir suppression should be considered after the initial recurrence of skin lesions in the first 2 to 3 months of age or after a recurrent episode of HSV encephalitis. Acyclovir suppression also has been used after development of HSV eye infection in which reactivation might imperil vision.

General supportive measures, such as maintenance of fluid and electrolyte balance, correction of hypoglycemia, management of disseminated intravascular coagulation and shock, control of seizures with anticonvulsants, mechanical support of the respiratory system, nutritional support, and antimicrobial therapy for complicating bacterial infections, also are critical in improving the outcome for neonates with HSV infection.

PROGNOSIS

As indicated in Table 73–10, the overall mortality rate from untreated neonatal HSV infection is 49 percent, and only 26 percent of survivors develop normally. The most guarded prognosis is natal infection that is disseminated, with pneumonitis, or presents as encephalitis localized to the CNS. Between 50 and 60 percent of infants with HSV infection limited to the skin, eye, and mouth who do not receive antiviral therapy progress to having CNS or disseminated disease. As shown in Table 73–10, neurologic sequelae develop in an appreciable proportion of survivors. All infants with neonatal herpes, therefore, require antiviral chemotherapy, regardless of the type or severity of disease at initial evaluation.

The major sequelae in infants surviving neonatal herpes involve the CNS. Diffuse brain damage, seizures, microcephaly, spasticity, paralysis, growth retardation, and chorioretinitis with visual loss all have been observed.[676] Serial CT or MRI of the head may be useful in these infants and can provide prognostic information.[674] Physical therapy and developmental interventions will help optimize the infant's abilities. Most infants with skin involvement have recurrent lesions, which can be managed with oral suppression therapy.

PREVENTION

The major approaches to the prevention of neonatal herpes involve interruption of transmission from sites of HSV infection and disease at the time of delivery and postnatally from a variety of potential sources. Because in utero transplacental congenital

infection occurs so infrequently[668] and predicting the occurrence of congenital infection during pregnancy is not possible,[301] no standard recommendations for prophylaxis are available.

Cesarean delivery within 4 hours of rupture of fetal membranes in a mother with active genital herpes at the time of delivery is recommended to reduce the risk of natal infection. Because serial vaginal cultures taken during the latter stages of pregnancy have failed to predict shedding at the time of delivery,[37,71,682] such monitoring is not recommended. Cesarean delivery is recommended only for women with active vesicular or ulcerative lesions at the time of delivery.[45,244,274,485,511,561] Cesarean delivery is not always 100 percent protective, even if the membranes are intact.[274,480,511,561] Between 1.2 and 3 percent and, in one study, up to 33 percent of neonates with HSV infection are delivered by cesarean delivery.[102,673] The cost-effectiveness of performing a cesarean delivery in women with recurrent lesions at delivery has been questioned by some experts, but it remains the current recommendation in the United States.[519] Multiple clinical trials have shown that administration of prophylactic acyclovir and valacyclovir beginning at 36 weeks gestation reduces the risk of clinically apparent HSV genital vesicles and ulcers at delivery, reduces the risk of HSV viral shedding at delivery, and also reduces the incidence of cesarean delivery.[286,562,573,574,673] However, although the hope is that the risk of HSV disease in the neonate also would be reduced, in none of these studies was sufficient power or evidence available to determine the effect of peripartum prophylaxis on the incidence of neonatal HSV. No adverse effects have been seen in infants exposed to maternal acyclovir during pregnancy. Because fetal scalp electrode monitor, forceps, and maneuvers that might cause a break in the infant's skin during delivery appear to increase the risk for acquisition of neonatal HSV, they should be used only with clear indication and a careful assessment of the risk-to-benefit ratio.

The results of antenatal genital HSV cultures from pregnant women with a history of genital herpes do not predict the infant's risk of exposure to HSV at delivery. Because 60 to 80 percent of mothers of babies with neonatal herpes are asymptomatic or have unrecognized infection, the optimal approach may be to perform a screening test to identify women shedding or likely to shed HSV at the time of delivery. Although HSV rapid antigen-detection tests continue to be developed commercially,[479] their sensitivity in *asymptomatic* women still is only 60 to 75 percent. Screening of pregnant women for non–type-specific HSV antibody would be confounded by the presence of HSV-1 antibody, which is present in 60 to 80 percent of the population.[476] The presence of HSV-1 antibody probably represents oral herpes, which poses little risk to the neonate. Although type-specific antibody assays are available to identify pregnant women infected with HSV-2,[123,313] such an approach would miss women with genital HSV-1 infection[155,511] or those with asymptomatic primary HSV-2 infection near the time of delivery before antibody is detectable.[97,511] Its use has been recommended in identifying discordant couples, that is, women with no history of having genital HSV infection but whose sexual partner has had previous infection, so barrier precautions may be used before delivery to decrease the chance of development of a maternal primary infection that poses a greater risk to her infant.[123] Culturing the genital tract of women at the time of vaginal delivery would identify infants exposed to HSV and allow anticipatory management.[478,485,511] However, because genital HSV infection rates are only 0.1 to 0.4 percent,[97,450,513] this approach likely would not be practical or cost-effective for *all* women. Culturing of *selected* women at delivery could focus on (1) positive or partner-discordant HSV-2 serologic tests, (2) those women with a history of genital herpes in themselves or their sexual partners, (3) those women with a history of another sexually transmitted disease or multiple sexual partners, and (4) mothers with a history of maternal fever in labor. However, routine or selective serologic screening, although recommended by some experts, is not currently a standard recommendation, and further investigation is required to determine whether screening of pregnant women to prevent neonatal herpes is beneficial, practical, and cost-effective.[26,106-108,169]

No studies have been conducted on the optimal management of asymptomatic infants exposed to maternal HSV infection at delivery, although some guidelines on obtaining viral cultures and prophylactic or anticipatory antiviral therapy are available.[26,478-480,511,561] In general, appropriate cultures for HSV should be performed for all infants born to mothers with active genital HSV infection at delivery. In asymptomatic infants, cultures of the conjunctiva, throat, rectum, and possibly urine should be done at 24 to 36 hours of age. Cultures obtained at birth may indicate only contaminating virus, whereas those obtained 1 to 2 days after birth probably represent HSV newly replicating in the mucous membranes. If the infant is delivered by cesarean section within 4 hours of rupture of membranes, no prophylactic antiviral therapy is indicated. If the infant is born vaginally or by cesarean section performed more than 4 hours after rupture of membranes, further management is dependent on the presence of other risk factors. If the mother has primary infection at delivery, a situation in which the neonatal infection rate may be as high as 30 to 50 percent, intravenous acyclovir (60 mg/kg/day) should be initiated. If the mother has recurrent infection, in which the risk of neonatal disease occurring after vaginal delivery is probably less than 3 percent, acyclovir may be withheld pending the results of culture or the development of clinical illness in the neonate that could be caused by HSV. Situations that increase the risk of neonatal transmission despite maternal recurrent disease include prematurity, the use of a scalp electrode monitor, or skin lacerations; prophylactic acyclovir should be considered in these instances if the infant has been delivered vaginally or by cesarean section more than 4 hours after rupture of membranes. In all instances, acyclovir can be discontinued when HSV cultures are negative at 48 to 72 hours and the infant has remained well. All infants should be monitored closely for any clinical evidence of HSV infection. Any positive culture or the occurrence of signs or symptoms suggesting HSV infection in the neonate suggests that a full virologic evaluation, including blood and CSF analysis for HSV by PCR, should be performed and antiviral therapy initiated. Antiviral therapy also should be administered to neonates with positive HSV cultures of mucosal sites, and these neonates should not be assessed as being merely colonized, as all require intravenous acyclovir therapy.[26] The duration of therapy, however, probably can be shortened to 7 or 10 days if no other site of infection is found and the infant remains asymptomatic. Breast-feeding is contraindicated only if the mother has a vesicular lesion on her breast. Physicians also have recommended that circumcision be delayed for 1 month in infants at highest risk of transmission.

Prevention of postnatally acquired neonatal infection needs to take into account the potential sources of HSV: (1) maternal oral herpes or breast lesions; (2) household member, such as father or sibling, or other close contact, such as grandparent or caretaker, with oral herpes or herpetic gingivostomatitis; and (3) health care–associated transmission from other infected babies or health care workers.[193,262,393,622,623,695] Transmission to the neonate from family members with oral herpes lesions can be interrupted by education, avoidance of kissing and nuzzling of the neonate if they have oral herpes ulcers, and avoidance of touching the neonate if they have a herpetic skin lesion or whitlow, as well as common sense personal hygiene, including handwashing. Health care–associated transmission can be reduced by contact isolation and hospital infection control measures, as well as universal precautions and good handwashing techniques.[327,339] Personnel with herpetic whitlow should not have direct patient care responsibili-

ties until the lesion has healed. Infants with HSV infection should be placed in contact isolation for the duration of the illness.[26] The median duration of viral shedding from skin vesicles and mucosal sites in infants receiving acyclovir is approximately 5 to 8 days.[335] Asymptomatic but high-risk infants born to mothers with herpes at delivery also should be in contact isolation; alternatively, they may room-in with the mother in a private room.

ENTEROVIRUS AND PARECHOVIRUS

The enteroviruses and parechoviruses are small RNA viruses that are members of the virus family Picornaviridae. The enteroviruses currently include the polioviruses types 1, 2, and 3; the coxsackieviruses A and B; and the echoviruses. Currently, there are four known parechoviruses: PeV1 (formerly enterovirus 22), PeV2 (formerly enterovirus 23), PeV3, and PeV4.[654] Enteroviruses are common infections in neonates, children, and adults. Coxsackievirus and echovirus infections are fairly common events in young infants and, as with other viral agents, often result in more severe disease in neonates. Neonatal poliomyelitis, however, is a rare occurrence in the United States and is not covered in this section. All four known parechoviruses have caused disease in neonates.[76,654]

MICROBIOLOGY AND EPIDEMIOLOGY

Twenty-three types of type A coxsackieviruses, six types of type B coxsackieviruses, 30 types of echoviruses, three types of polioviruses, five types of other enteroviruses (68 to 72), and four types or parechoviruses are currently recognized.[76,413,653] Most strains grow in tissue culture, but some, particularly type A coxsackieviruses, require inoculation in suckling mice. Because no common or group antigens for the enteroviruses exist, separate antibody titration must be performed for each virus. Therefore, to make a laboratory diagnosis of enteroviral infection by serologic means alone is not recommended. However, antibody titers can be performed after a specific enterovirus has been isolated from the patient or when a concurrent epidemic with a known virus occurs in the community. Detection of enterovirus and parechovirus RNA by reverse transcriptase (RT)-PCR is now a common method of establishing a diagnosis.[158]

The attack rate for enteroviral infections is highest during infancy and early childhood.[109,165-167,359,403,429,436,684] In addition, severe disease occurs much more commonly in neonates than in older children or adults.[429,684] Sixty to 70 percent of neonates infected with enterovirus are males, whereas one study has shown females may predominate in parechovirus infections.[318,371,427,436,517,654] Enteroviruses are worldwide in distribution, and in temperate climates, infections occur predominantly during the summer and fall months, with peaks in July, August, and September.[109,307,413] Parechovirus infection also occurs during summer and fall months.[654] The incubation period for enteroviral infections in children and adults usually is 5 to 8 days, with a range of 2 to 12 days.[543,660] Of the cases reported to the CDC from 1970 to 1979, echoviruses accounted for 57 percent; type B coxsackieviruses, 25 percent; polioviruses, 9 percent; type A coxsackieviruses, 8 percent; and enterovirus types 68 to 71, 0.1 percent.[109] In infants younger than 2 months of age, echoviruses accounted for 51 percent of infections; type B coxsackieviruses, 45 percent; and type A coxsackieviruses, 4 percent.[394,436] In any given year in the United States, usually an epidemic occurs that is caused by a few enterovirus types: echovirus 11 and coxsackieviruses B2 and B4 in 1979, echoviruses 9 and 4 in 1978, echovirus 6 in 1977, coxsackievirus B4 in 1976, and echovirus 9 in 1975.[109]

Outbreaks of enteroviral disease have occurred in normal nurseries and in neonatal intensive care units.*

Acute enteroviral and parechoviral infections may be acquired congenitally, natally, or postnatally.[135,536] However, confusion concerning the incubation period and source of virus for neonatal infection often has ensued. Late-gestation congenital infection is presumed to occur in infants with an onset of illness at birth or within the first few days of life, when their mothers had symptoms of enteroviral disease just before or immediately after delivery.[5,107,133,172,371,429,499] Further evidence of congenital infection is the observation that viremia with echoviruses and coxsackieviruses is known to occur in pregnant women,[135] and virus has been isolated from the placenta of infants with an onset of disease early in life.[89,429] Infants with an onset of enteroviral disease between 3 and 8 to 10 days of age probably acquired the infection from their mothers at the time of birth (natal infection), whereas those with illness appearing after this time probably acquired it postnatally. At least one case of congenital parechovirus infection has been documented in a neonate who presented at 1 day of age.[654] The source of enterovirus for most cases in nurseries appears to be the mother because the age of the infants at the time that the first symptoms appear is usually less than 10 days.[5,107,133,172,371,429,499] However, in some cases and outbreaks, the infection clearly appears to be associated with health care, presumably through spread of virus from other infected neonates by the hands of personnel or from infected personnel themselves.[161,407,429]

Some investigations indicate that enteroviral infections acquired in the community are a common cause of hospitalization for a febrile illness in young infants.[107,165-167,307,359] Enteroviral infections were estimated to account for 20,000 to 40,000 hospitalizations per year in young infants in the United States. Viruses appear more frequently than do bacteria as a cause of fever in the neonate.[107] One study of 182 infants younger than 3 months of age and hospitalized for fever over the course of a year showed viral pathogens were isolated in 41 percent and bacteria in only 15 percent.[359] Enteroviruses accounted for 85 percent of the viral isolates. Among a cohort of 586 newborns prospectively monitored during the enteroviral season in Rochester, New York, 24 (4%) were hospitalized during the first month of life.[307] Two thirds of these 24 were infected with enteroviruses. Risk factors associated with development of infection and more severe enteroviral disease included a particular serotype of virus (e.g., echovirus 22, presumably a more virulent strain); lower socioeconomic status, probably with associated crowding and an increased rate of transmission; bottle feeding (absence of passive antibody in breast milk); and absence of antibody in cord serum.[166,307,429,432]

Evidence suggests that coxsackieviral infections in early pregnancy may cause congenital malformations in the fetus. Brown and colleagues[94,95] demonstrated a significant association between serologic evidence of coxsackievirus A9, B2, B3, or B4 infection in mothers during pregnancy and the birth of infants with anomalies of the cardiovascular, urogenital, and digestive systems. However, specific viral isolation and antibody studies were not performed on the involved infants, and no seasonal distribution was noted in their births. In addition, the observations of Brown and colleagues[94,95] have not been confirmed by others.[207,353,502] The association between maternal infection with coxsackieviruses and congenital malformations, therefore, remains suggestive but not proven. Moreover, no conclusive evidence supports any relationship between maternal infection with type B coxsackieviruses and congenital CNS malformations.[207] More studies are necessary to determine whether or not parechoviral infections are associated with congenital malformations.

PATHOGENESIS AND PATHOLOGY

Our knowledge of the pathogenesis of congenital enteroviral and parechoviral infections is incomplete because they are rare events. However, studies in gravid mice support the transplacental passage of enteroviruses with resultant fetal infection.[2,311,365,484] By inference from these studies and our understanding of congenital CMV and rubella virus infections, transplacental transmission secondary to maternal viremia probably occurs. Virus then is transmitted through fetal blood to target organs, principally the CNS, liver, heart, lungs, kidneys, and adrenal glands. In congenital infections that are fatal in the early neonatal period, type B coxsackieviruses involve primarily the heart, CNS, liver, and lungs,[239,318,371,684] and echoviruses involve the liver, adrenals, kidneys, CNS, and lungs.[133,299,259,360,428,429,499] Histopathologic findings have consisted of focal myocardial necrosis with type B coxsackieviruses[239,684]; massive hepatic necrosis with echoviruses[299,360,429,499]; and evidence of disseminated intravascular coagulation and adrenal, pulmonary, and renal hemorrhage with both virus groups.[133,239,299,360,371,429,499,684,684] Of interest is that the onset of illness in most neonates with fatal coxsackievirus B and echovirus infection occurred at birth or within the first few days of life, suggesting that transplacental infections carry a worse prognosis.[5,133,299,360,371,429,499] In addition, lack of transplacental transfer of maternal antibody before delivery could play a role.[426,427] Only a few isolated cases of congenital coxsackievirus A infection have been reported.[135]

Natal infection is secondary to aspiration and swallowing of enterovirus-contaminated vaginal secretions at the time of birth. Postnatal acquisition is the result of fecal-oropharyngeal spread of the virus on the hands of the mother, other family members, or hospital personnel.[135,429] Pathogenesis of natal and postnatal infection is similar to that observed in older infants and children. Because most infants with postnatal infection survive, the pathologic features are not well characterized.

CLINICAL MANIFESTATIONS

The clinical features in 134 neonates and very young infants with echoviral and coxsackieviral infections are shown in Figure 73–3. The most common findings, hyperthermia or hypothermia, anorexia or vomiting, and lethargy, are relatively nonspecific findings and are encountered with similar frequency in neonates with other viral infections or bacterial sepsis. Features that appear to be characteristic of enteroviral infection include signs and symptoms of aseptic meningitis and meningoencephalitis (irritability, CNS signs, including seizures); gastroenteritis (anorexia, vomiting, diarrhea, abdominal distention); and an erythematous, maculopapular exanthem. In addition, neonates may manifest a mild, nonspecific febrile illness, a severe sepsis-like disease, respiratory illness, hepatitis that may be fulminant with resultant hepatic necrosis and death, and cardiovascular manifestations secondary to myocarditis. Enteroviral DNA also has been detected by PCR in the respiratory tract of infants with sudden death.[245]

Infants with more serious disease may have a biphasic course that begins as a mild illness with slight elevation of temperature, coryza, anorexia, and diarrhea. After an apparent recovery period lasting 1 to 5 days, infants may have more severe symptoms of aseptic meningitis; myocarditis (tachycardia, tachypnea, respiratory distress, and cyanosis); hepatitis with elevated transaminases; or disseminated infection (abdominal distention, hepatomegaly, petechial rash, disseminated intravascular coagulation).

Milder forms of disease, such as pneumonitis, undifferentiated febrile illness, exanthematous illness, or gastroenteritis lasting only a few days, also occur.[303,371] In a survey of 338 infants younger than 2 months of age with enteroviral infections reported to the

---

*See references 42, 89, 132, 161, 221, 379, 403, 429, 473, 536, 626.

TABLE 73-11 Characteristics Associated with Parechovirus and Enteroviral Infection in Neonates

Seasonal occurrence—summer and fall
Presence of known epidemic in the community
History of maternal viral illness near the time of delivery
Absence of factors predisposing to bacterial sepsis
Nursery outbreak of infectious illness with negative bacterial cultures
Development of culture-negative sepsis or aseptic meningitis in the neonate
Development of myocarditis, hepatitis, or erythematous maculopapular exanthem in the neonate

CDC, 74 percent had severe disease, and 26 percent had mild disease.[436] Five (1%) of these infants died, all in the group with severe disease. Asymptomatic infections in neonates have been detected during outbreaks in nurseries or when routine virologic surveillance was being performed in a nursery.[89] An outbreak of neonatal herpangina caused by coxsackievirus A5 was observed in Thailand.[132] Parechoviruses in neonates also may cause both mild and serious illnesses that cannot be differentiated clinically from enteroviruses and that include fever, seizures, rash, irritability, apnea, tachypnea, diarrhea, meningoencephalitis, hepatitis, and acute myocarditis.[653]

DIAGNOSIS AND DIFFERENTIAL DIAGNOSIS

The major epidemiologic and clinical features that suggest a diagnosis of enteroviral or parechoviral infection in a neonate are listed in Table 73–11. Because the signs and symptoms in neonates with enteroviral and parechoviral disease often mimic those of bacterial sepsis and meningitis, antibiotic therapy generally should be initiated until a bacterial etiology is ruled out. In addition to sepsis and meningitis, the major diseases to be considered in the differential diagnosis include HSV infection, adenovirus, and, to a lesser extent, congenital infection with CMV and rubella virus. HSV infection is nonseasonal, endemic, and may be associated with genital ulcerative lesions in the mother. Symptomatic congenital CMV and rubella infections are associated with intrauterine growth retardation and a chronic rather than an acute infectious clinical picture in the infant.

The most direct means of establishing a diagnosis of enteroviral infection in neonates is isolation of the virus in tissue culture or suckling mice.[479] Virus may be recovered from throat swab, stool, CSF, serum or buffy coat, and biopsy and autopsy tissue. Ideally, specimens should be processed immediately, but enteroviruses may remain stable at 4°C for several days if testing cannot be performed until later. Isolation of virus from CSF, blood, or tissue can be considered diagnostic. A throat, urine, or stool isolate also can be considered etiologic in most neonatal illnesses. RT-PCR performed for detection of enterovirus or parechovirus RNA in CSF or blood samples is more sensitive and rapid than is isolation of virus[526] and is the preferred method for diagnosing meningitis or disseminated infection caused by these viruses in most circumstances.[547,552] Because of genetic differences, parechoviruses cannot be identified by primers used in enterovirus RT-PCR assays. Therefore, RT-PCR for both types of these viruses should be performed for optimal diagnostic sensitivity.[158,654]

TREATMENT

No licensed and effective antiviral chemotherapy exists for enteroviruses. Pleconaril administered orally on a compassionate basis to neonates with severe disseminated enteroviral disease has resulted in clinical recovery.[34,322,537] In adults, pleconaril has decreased the duration of clinical symptomatology in aseptic meningitis significantly and has resulted in cessation of viral shedding in immunocompromised individuals. Case reports and series on administration of pleconaril to neonates with enterovirus infection are published.[34,525,531] Clinical trials evaluating the benefits of pleconaril in neonatal enteroviral sepsis syndrome with liver or cardiac involvement are in progress through the NIAID CASG. Intravenous immunoglobulin often is recommended, especially if myocarditis is present, because it may improve survival.[4,168,261,314]

PROGNOSIS

The outcome is influenced by several factors: the enterovirus serotype causing the infection, the route of transmission of virus to the neonate, the age at acquisition of the infection, prematurity, and severity of the disease in the neonate. Mortality rates are highest for coxsackievirus B infections, intermediate for echovirus infections, and lowest for coxsackievirus A infections.[135,239,318,371] Most of the neonatal deaths caused by enteroviruses reported in recent years have occurred in infants whose onset of disease was at or within a few days of birth and who, therefore, had congenital disease.[133,299,365,371] Infection and mortality rates both appear to be higher for premature infants.[89,429] Death is most likely to occur in infants with acute myocarditis, encephalitis, or severe hepatitis.[135,429] Neurologic sequelae have been observed to occur after meningoencephalitis in the neonatal period,[135,565,677] although most infants who survive enteroviral meningitis appear to have an excellent long-term prognosis.[70] Long-term cardiac sequelae also do not appear to complicate most neonatal enteroviral myocarditis.[239] Long-term follow-up studies of neonates infected with parechovirus have not been performed.

PREVENTION

Polio vaccine has reduced maternal and neonatal poliomyelitis to an extremely rare occurrence, but poliovirus infections still occur in underdeveloped countries without polio vaccination programs. No prospects exist for vaccines for the echoviruses or coxsackieviruses or parechoviruses at this time. With the appearance of a case of enteroviral or parechoviral disease in a newborn nursery or intensive care unit, initiation of vigorous infection control measures involving contact precautions, including such measures for suspected cases and renewed emphasis on handwashing and exclusion of personnel with symptoms of enteroviral disease, is indicated. Of emphasis is that infection control measures applied in the nursery do not prevent congenital or natal transmission of virus from the mother to the infant. The continued appearance of cases in neonates younger than 8 to 10 days of age may reflect a persistent epidemic among pregnant women rather than a failure of nursery infection control measures and spread within the nursery.[626]

VARICELLA-ZOSTER VIRUS

VZV causes both varicella ("chickenpox"), the result of primary infection with the virus, and zoster, caused by reactivation of latent virus.[240,243,476] VZV infection of a pregnant woman results in three separate and distinct syndromes that become apparent in neonates and infants: (1) congenital varicella syndrome with congenital defects secondary to intrauterine VZV infection, (2) neonatal varicella, and (3) zoster in infants.[212,214,240,243,493] Transmission to the fetus occurs as a consequence of maternal viremia and may result in congenital varicella syndrome, fetal hydrops, or fetal death.[240,243,273] Transmission to the neonate occurs through exposure to virus-infected secretions or lesions present in the mother or close contact and may result in neonatal varicella.

MATERNAL VARICELLA

Knowledge of several features of chickenpox in the mother is necessary to understand the pathogenesis of VZV infection in the fetus and neonate. Because antibody to VZV is present in approximately 90 percent of women of child-bearing age,[243] varicella occurring during pregnancy is a relatively uncommon event. Pregnant women with varicella may develop severe disease, with severe constitutional symptoms, and potentially fatal pneumonia.[272] Maternal chickenpox has been reported to occur in only 0.7 per 1000 pregnancies.[570] The incubation period for chickenpox (from exposure to the onset of rash) usually is between 14 and 16 days, with a range of 10 to 21 days.[240,243]

CONGENITAL VARICELLA SYNDROME

In several large prospective studies, no increase in anomalies was apparent in the offspring of women who had varicella during pregnancy.[87,581-583] However, a prospective study[410] of 43 pregnancies complicated by varicella indicated that (1) 21 percent of the women experienced appreciable morbidity, (2) 24 percent of 33 infants tested had clinical or immunologic evidence of intrauterine VZV infection, and (3) congenital varicella syndrome occurred in 9 percent of 11 women with first-trimester varicella. Pooling of results from several prospective studies indicates an approximate 2 percent risk of fetal malformations caused by maternal varicella during the first 20 weeks of pregnancy.[214,419,493] Of the reported cases of congenital varicella syndrome, 93 percent have occurred after maternal chickenpox and only 7 percent after maternal zoster. Seven percent of reported cases occurred after maternal varicella was acquired at less than the 20th week, with the latest being at 28 weeks of gestation.[19] In another recent prospective multicenter study of 347 pregnant women with varicella, the incidence of congenital varicella syndrome was 0.4 percent, with fetal death and fetal hydrops also observed.[273] One case of congenital varicella syndrome occurring after maternal varicella developed in the third trimester of pregnancy has been reported.[350]

The abnormalities present in 77 infants with congenital varicella syndrome are summarized in Table 73-12. The defects apparently are the result of VZV replication in and destruction of developing fetal ectodermal tissue: skin, peripheral nerves, cervical and lumbosacral spinal cord, brain, and eye.[41,44,233,463,482,545] Diagnosis of the syndrome usually is clinical: a history of varicella in the mother and recognition of the characteristic findings in the fetus or neonate. Prenatal diagnosis may be established by amniocentesis with demonstration of VZV in amniotic fluid by culture or PCR and by cordocentesis and demonstration of VZV-specific IgM in a fetal blood sample. Prenatal ultrasound and fetal MRI imaging may detect abnormalities and document the extent of involvement.[417,655] Virus has not been isolated from these infants, and serologic studies often have been inconclusive.[232,243] However, detection of varicella-zoster DNA by PCR has been used to confirm the syndrome in some cases.[438,461,514,544] Infants with varicella embryopathy do not require isolation. Severely affected neonates may die in infancy.[232,243] However, some children may survive and enjoy productive lives.[556] Children with congenital varicella syndrome also may experience apparent reactivation disease, involving skin and, rarely, brain or other organs.[85,545] Universal vaccination against varicella may decrease the importance of this virus in congenital and neonatal disease.

TABLE 73-12   Abnormalities in 77 Infants with Congenital Varicella Syndrome

Features	Percentage
Skin scars*	61
Eye abnormalities	56
Chorioretinitis	27
Horner syndrome/anisocoria	16
Microphthalmos	19
Cataract	19
Nystagmus	13
Abnormal limb[†]	47
Hypoplasia	36
Equinovarus	14
Abnormal/absent digits	10
Cortical atrophy/mental retardation	40
Prematurity, low birth weight	36
Early death	26
Dysphagia/aspiration	19
Gastrointestinal tract abnormalities	12
Urinary tract abnormalities	10

*Cicatricial in 37 (79%).
[†]Eleven of 28 (39%) with a hypoplastic limb had mental retardation or early death.
Data from Gershon, A. A.: Chickenpox, measles and mumps. In Remington, J. S., and Klein, J. O. (eds.): Infectious Diseases of the Fetus and Newborn Infant. Philadelphia, W. B. Saunders, 2001, p. 698.

TABLE 73-13   Congenital Varicella Syndrome: Outcome in Relation to Rash Onset in Mother and Neonate

Day of Rash Onset	Neonatal Cases	Neonatal Deaths	
		Number	Percentage
Mother, antepartum			
5 or more	23	0	0
0 to 4	13	4	31
Neonate, after delivery			
0 to 4	22	0	0
5 to 10	19	4	21

Modified from Gershon, A. A.: Chickenpox, measles and mumps. In Remington, J. S., and Klein, J. O. (eds.): Infectious Diseases of the Fetus and Newborn Infant. Philadelphia, W. B. Saunders, 1990, pp. 395-445, as modified from Meyers, J. D.: Congenital varicella in term infants: Risk reconsidered. J. Infect. Dis. 729:215-217, 1974, with permission from the University of Chicago.

NEONATAL VARICELLA

Neonatal varicella refers to the onset of varicella ("chickenpox") within the first 28 days of life.[546] The incubation period, defined as the interval between the onset of rash in the mother and onset in the fetus or neonate, usually is 9 to 15 days, with a range between 1 and 16 days. Neonatal varicella occurs when a pregnant woman experiences varicella during the last 1 to 2 weeks of pregnancy or within the first few days postpartum. The attack rate is approximately 25 to 50 percent. As indicated in Table 73-13, the timing of the onset of disease in the mother and the neonate is a critical factor influencing the outcome in the infant. If disease onset occurs in the mother 5 or more days before delivery or in the neonate during the first 4 days of life, the infection is mild. In contrast, if disease onset in the mother is within 4 days before delivery or in the neonate between 5 and 10 days of age, the infection usually is disseminated and fulminant, and approximately one third of the infants die.[243,423] Other investigations have found that the risk period of the onset of maternal rash extends from 7 days before to 16 days after delivery.[28,512] The generally accepted explanation for this observation is that when illness in the mother occurs more than 5 days before delivery or when illness in the baby occurs during the first 4 days of life, maternal antibody has time to pass transplacentally and provide passive protection for the infant. However, passive protection does not have time to occur when illness in the mother occurs within 4 days of delivery. Presumably, the immune responses of the neonate are insufficient to retard the growth and dissemination of VZV after intravenous inoculation via the placenta, and disseminated disease results.

The milder form of neonatal varicella resembles the disease in normal, older children, whereas the disseminated variety is similar to that seen in immunosuppressed, leukemic children. In the latter, diffuse pneumonia, severe hepatitis, and meningoencephalitis are the most common clinical manifestations. The diagnosis usually can be established clinically from the characteristic appearance of skin vesicles, and VZV antigen can be demonstrated by immunofluorescence testing of vesicular fluid. Less commonly, VZV may be isolated from vesicular fluid by tissue culture during the first 3 days of the rash, but VZV is difficult to isolate in commercial virology laboratories.[479] VZV DNA can be demonstrated in vesicular fluid by PCR.[300] The major disease to consider in the differential diagnosis is disseminated neonatal HSV infection. With HSV infection, a history of maternal genital herpes may be elicited; characteristic keratoconjunctivitis, mouth lesions, or both may be present in the infant, and growth of the virus in cell culture is markedly different.[476,479] Immunofluorescence testing of vesicular lesions with commercially available specific monoclonal antibodies will rapidly differentiate the two.

Varicella-zoster immunoglobulin (Vari-ZIG) should be administered as soon as possible after birth to a neonate born to a mother with an onset of chickenpox rash between 5 days before delivery and 2 days after delivery.[512] If Vari-ZIG is not available, some experts recommend IGIV, intravenous acyclovir, or both in combination, as an effective alternative.[297] Breakthrough varicella has occurred in neonates properly treated with Var-ZIG, however.[46] Therefore, these infants still must be considered potentially infective and isolated with airborne precautions in a negative-pressure room for 16 days after maternal onset of rash because the incubation period with in utero exposure is decreased. If the newborn is exposed to maternal varicella at delivery, airborne precautions are extended until 21 days after exposure (28 days when Vari-ZIG is given) if hospitalization is required. Exposed infants do not need to be separated from their mothers; on the contrary, rooming-in may be a preferable alternative. If breakthrough neonatal varicella occurs despite Vari-ZIG immunoprophylaxis and the neonatal varicella appears to be becoming severe (extensive skin lesions, high fever and toxicity, hepatitis, pneumonitis), treatment with intravenous acyclovir at 1500 mg/m²/day or 45 mg/kg/day divided every 8 hours should be administered.[575]

Infants born to mothers with zoster do not require Vari-ZIG immunoprophylaxis because they already have high levels of transplacentally acquired maternal VZV IgG antibody. No special precautions are indicated except that the maternal lesions should be covered and good handwashing when handling the infant must be stressed.

ZOSTER IN INFANCY AND CHILDHOOD

Epidemiologic and serologic evidence indicates zoster is a reactivated infection with VZV.[240,476] Persons with zoster, therefore, have had a previous episode of chickenpox. The vast majority of zoster occurs in older adult patients. The occurrence of zoster in infants and children is somewhat of a paradox because many of these patients have a negative history of having had chickenpox.[103,243,408] However, with several of these cases of childhood

zoster, particularly those occurring in infants and young children, the mother had a history of chickenpox during pregnancy.[103,214,240,390] The presumption is that fetal VZV infection occurred, with recovery and no evidence of disease in the neonate at birth. In a few other instances, an infant born to a VZV-immune mother may be exposed to chickenpox or zoster during early life at a time when maternal transplacental antibody still would be present. This passive antibody could provide protection against chickenpox and modify the disease to a subclinical or mild form that was not recognized.[224] Both situations could result in a patient with (1) an unrecognized episode of varicella and (2) the occurrence of zoster as the first overt manifestation of VZV infection.

The major disease in the differential diagnosis of neonatal varicella is HSV infection. Patients with neonatal herpes may have a clinical picture resembling that of zoster,[442] and laboratory evaluation is required to differentiate the two diseases.

HUMAN PARVOVIRUS B19 (*ERYTHROVIRUS*)

Human parvovirus B19 (*Erythrovirus*) is a small, single-stranded DNA virus with two viral capsid proteins, VP1 and VP2.[175] It is the cause of erythema infectiosum, or fifth disease, a mild exanthematous illness in school-aged children.[32] Parvovirus B19 infection in pregnant women is associated with spontaneous abortion, stillbirth, and nonimmune hydrops fetalis secondary to transplacental passage of the virus.[30,338,342,345,578,638,648,661,685] A summary of 22 published case reports of parvovirus fetal infection revealed that (1) only half the mothers had parvovirus-like clinical illness 4 to 13 weeks before fetal death; (2) all fetuses had hydrops fetalis and probable myocarditis; and (3) 19 died in utero at 16 to 26 weeks, and the remaining 3 died within 24 hours of delivery.[26] Laboratory evidence of parvovirus infection includes (1) maternal parvovirus IgM antibody, (2) elevated maternal alpha-fetoprotein, and (3) the presence of parvovirus DNA in amniotic fluid.[32,638,639] Maternal blood also may contain high titers of parvovirus DNA that is detectable by PCR assays. Persistent parvovirus B19 DNA-emia often occurs, and supplementary measurement of VP1 IgG avidity and VP2 IgG epitope-type specificity may be helpful in timing the infection in some cases.[214]

Hydrops fetalis occurs from replication of parvovirus in the fetal bone marrow and resultant profound fetal anemia, with myocarditis playing a potential secondary role.[32,174] Fortunately, not all pregnancies complicated by parvovirus infection result in fetal infection, and hydrops does not develop in all infected fetuses. A British study of 186 pregnant women who had parvovirus IgM antibody and were monitored to term demonstrated that fetal loss occurred in 16 percent (no data on fetal loss rates in a control population) and that 43 percent of 14 fetal tissues tested showed parvovirus DNA.[112,514] Extrapolation from these figures yielded a maximal parvovirus-associated adverse fetal outcome of 7 percent in pregnancies with laboratory-proven parvovirus infection. Extrapolation to the community level yielded the following estimates of fetal death in a pregnant woman exposed to active parvovirus infection: 1.8 percent with home exposure and 1.1 percent or less with school exposure.[112,514] Figures used in this estimate are 7 percent fetal death rate with documented maternal infection cited earlier. Furthermore, only approximately 50 percent of women of child-bearing age are seronegative and, therefore, susceptible, and infection rates after exposure to parvovirus infection are 50 percent in the home and 30 percent with a *widespread* school outbreak. More recent studies have indicated a total fetal infection rate of 25 to 50 percent, but an adverse fetal outcome rate of less than 1 to 2 percent.[247,343,-345,648] Overall, after an acute parvovirus B19 infection during pregnancy, the vertical transmission rate is approximately 30 to 50 percent, the risk of fetal death is between 2 and 6 percent, and most infected newborns are asymptomatic. In addition, maternal parvovirus B19 infection during pregnancy has not been associated with congenital anomalies. CNS abnormalities, however, have been reported in a few infants with in utero infection.[150] Abnormalities consisted of cerebral atrophy, ventricular enlargement, basal ganglia and periventricular calcifications, and diffuse cortical dysplasia, with hypotonia and later development of cerebral palsy and developmental delay. These findings could be secondary to parvovirus infection of the fetal brain; alternatively, they could be a result of the profound anemia that can occur in the fetus.

Fetal infection is diagnosed best by demonstration of parvovirus B19 DNA in amniotic fluid or determination of parvovirus B19 IgM antibody and DNA levels in fetal blood obtained by cordocentesis. Presence and severity of fetal anemia and thrombocytopenia also can be determined and corrected by intrauterine fetal transfusions into the fetal vein.[162,552] Mild or asymptomatic fetal infections may be managed conservatively with weekly fetal ultrasound examinations because some cases resolve without fetal interventions.[316] Fetal hydrops is readily detectable and monitored by antenatal ultrasound.[661]

In the neonate, detection of virus in blood and CSF can document parvovirus B19 infection. Assays for detection of human parvovirus B19 IgG and IgM antibodies are available commercially. Many infected newborns lack specific parvovirus IgM antibody at birth but will demonstrate persistence of parvovirus B19 IgG antibody beyond infancy, thus documenting infection.

No specific therapy is available. Intravenous immunoglobulin therapy has suppressed or controlled parvovirus-associated chronic anemia in immunosuppressed patients,[233] although no evidence indicates that it would be beneficial in pregnant women with parvovirus infection. Intrauterine transfusions have been used in cases of fetal hydrops associated with severe anemia, although some cases of hydrops resolve spontaneously.

Recent studies on the long-term neurodevelopmental outcome of infants after fetal transfusions for non-immune hydrops associated with parvovirus B19 infection show normal or near normal development in most survivors, supporting the use of intrauterine transfusions for correction of severe anemia and hydrops associated with this intrauterine infection.[177,445] Because some infants have experienced neurodevelopmental disabilities, some experts suggest that parvovirus B19 possibly may invade the fetal and neonatal CNS and produce neurodevelopmental sequelae. However, further studies are necessary to investigate this hypothesis.

Prevention consists largely of the rational use of infection control measures, including handwashing and disposal of used facial tissues. To isolate or quarantine otherwise normal children who have the rash of erythema infectiosum makes no sense because viral shedding has ceased by the time that the rash appears.[32] On the other hand, hemoglobinopathy patients with parvovirus-induced aplastic crisis or immunosuppressed patients with parvovirus-associated chronic anemia are highly infectious,[69] so droplet precautions should be instituted.

LYMPHOCYTIC CHORIOMENINGITIS VIRUS

LCMV is an RNA virus and a member of the Arenaviridae family. It causes a chronic infection with virus excretion in rodents, but it also may infect humans worldwide, especially in Europe, Africa, and the Americas. LCMV most commonly causes a nonspecific febrile illness, aseptic meningitis, or encephalitis. In adults, it also has been associated with nonbacterial orchitis, parotitis, and sudden-onset deafness. On rare occasion, congenital infection and disease have been documented.[55] The incidence of congenital infection with this virus, however, has not been studied systemati-

cally, and some experts suggest that it may be under-recognized as a pathogen of the fetus and newborn.[55,79,417,689,700] Congenital infection with LCMV appears to be a common cause of ocular abnormalities such as chorioretinitis, chorioretinal scars, and optic atrophy. Rarely, microphthalmos and cataracts have been observed. Other neurologic abnormalities noted at birth include microcephaly, hydrocephalus, abnormal corpus callosum, cerebellar hypoplasia, porencephalic cysts, and periventricular calcifications. Sequelae such as cognitive delays, major motor disabilities, ataxia, seizures, and vision loss have been seen in these infants. In contrast to other congenital viral infections, signs such as hydrops, hepatosplenomegaly, skin lesions, thrombocytopenia, and hearing loss are uncommon findings in children born with congenital LCMV infection.

The diagnosis of congenital LCMV infection should be suspected in an infant who appears to have a congenital viral infection or congenital toxoplasmosis, but the routine laboratory evaluation for the usual "TORCH" agents does not identify one of these infections. Supporting evidence for congenital LCMV infection includes a mother with prenatal exposure to wild, pet, or laboratory rodents such as mice, hamsters, or gerbils. The laboratory diagnosis of LCMV most commonly is established serologically, and detection of LCMV-specific IgG and IgM antibodies in serum or CSF supports the diagnosis. Detection of the virus by culture or RT-PCR–based methods is also available in reference laboratories. The virus also has been isolated from the CSF of an infant with congenital LCMV.[555] Currently, management is supportive because antiviral therapy has not been evaluated in clinical trials. Prevention of congenital LCMV infection includes minimizing exposure of pregnant women to rodents in the home and workplace.

ADENOVIRUSES

Adenoviruses are DNA viruses and common respiratory and gastrointestinal pathogens of children and adults. Fetal infection with adenovirus has been diagnosed by detection of viral DNA by PCR in amniotic fluid and has been associated with intrauterine myocarditis, fetal tachyarrhythmia, and non-immune hydrops fetalis.[56,140,520,641] Echogenic liver lesions and CNS anomalies also have been described in association with detection of adenovirus DNA in amniotic fluid and fetal tissues. Postnatal adenovirus infections in both term and preterm neonates also occur and may cause keratoconjunctivitis, as well as severe multisystem disease involving the liver, lungs, and brain.[1,72,500] Fatalities are most often associated with prematurity and pneumonitis.[1,92,218,474,625] The virus is transmitted easily in the health care setting and by ophthalmologic instruments, and it can cause outbreaks in neonatal intensive and special care units.[218,226,500]

Diagnosis is established by isolation of adenovirus from blood, CSF, conjunctival swabs, stool or urine specimens, and oropharyngeal or respiratory secretions. Tissue obtained by biopsy or autopsy also may reveal adenoviruses by culture or adenovirus particles by electron microscopy.[474] Histopathology may show smudge cells in lung tissue, and virus-specific immunohistochemical staining may reveal adenovirus antigens in tissue. Direct detection of adenovirus antigen in clinical specimens using rapid immunochromatographic assays or direct immunofluorescence assays can support the diagnosis.[497] Detection and quantification of viral DNA using PCR assays also can provide laboratory diagnosis.[641] Treatment is primarily supportive, and neonates with severe necrotizing pneumonitis may require mechanical ventilation or extracorporeal membrane oxygenation. The antivirals cidofovir and ribavirin have activity against adenoviruses and both have been used to treat severe disseminated adenovirus disease. Neonates with suspected or proven adenovirus infection should be isolated and all ophthalmologic instruments thoroughly disinfected to prevent health care–associated transmission of the virus.[72,226]

RESPIRATORY VIRUSES—RESPIRATORY SYNCYTIAL VIRUS, INFLUENZA VIRUSES, PARAINFLUENZA VIRUSES, CORONAVIRUSES, HUMAN METAPNEUMOVIRUS

The RNA viruses; influenza A and B viruses (Orthomyxoviridae family), as well as RSV; the parainfluenza viruses types 1, 2, 3, and 4 (Paramyxoviridae family); coronaviruses; and human metapneumovirus are common seasonal winter respiratory pathogens in children and adults. These viruses also may infect neonates, who present with upper or lower respiratory signs and symptoms, or sepsis syndrome. These viruses also may cause health care–associated outbreaks in special care units with cases of serious, even fatal, pneumonia in this special age group.[236,237,315,432,441,583,587,701] Coronavirus, RSV, and influenza A virus appear most frequently, followed by influenza B virus and parainfluenza virus type 3. Neonatal infections with human metapneumovirus and parainfluenza viruses 1, 2, and 4 are less well documented. An outbreak of parainfluenza virus type 3 in an intermediate care nursery was associated with upper respiratory symptoms (nasal discharge and cough), as well as lower respiratory illness, including pneumonia and oxygen requirement. No ventilatory support or fatalities, however, occurred. The outbreak was contained with institution of barrier isolation, reinforcement of hand washing, and temporary closure of the special care unit.[432] Influenza A virus also has been associated with an outbreak in a neonatal intensive care unit.[439] Rapid diagnostic techniques helped identify infected infants, and reinforcement of infection control measures limited the outbreak. Amantadine resistance also was documented in influenza virus isolated from one treated neonate. Term and preterm neonates, especially those infants with chronic lung disease or congenital heart disease, may experience severe or fatal disease with community or health care–acquired RSV infection.[584] More recently, coronaviruses and human metapneumoviruses have been identified as causes of acute illness in neonates, especially premature infants.[236,237,587] Outbreaks of coronavirus infection in neonatal intensive care units also have been documented. Symptoms and signs in infected neonates at presentation included fever, bradycardia, apnea, hypoxemia, and abdominal distension, and chest radiographics showed diffuse pneumonitis.[587] Respiratory viral pathogens should be considered in the differential diagnosis of neonates with fever, apnea, bradycardia, sepsis syndrome, or pneumonitis in whom bacterial and fungal cultures are negative. Rapid diagnostic techniques that detect viral antigens by immunochromatographic assays that provide results within minutes, DFAs that provide same-day diagnosis, and viral culture and viral RNA detection using PCR-based methods are now routinely available and should be used for laboratory diagnosis and confirmation of viral respiratory pathogens in high-risk neonates. Antiviral therapy may be considered in selected neonates with severe respiratory viral disease. The long-term impact on pulmonary function in neonates, both term and preterm, infected with any of these viral pathogens requires further study and investigation.

ARBOVIRUSES

West Nile virus, a single-stranded RNA flavivirus, has caused severe disease in pregnant women. West Nile virus infection in pregnancy has been associated with spontaneous abortion, as well as congenital and neonatal infection.[645] Transmission of West Nile virus appears to occur in less than 5 percent of neonates born to women with West Nile virus infection during pregnancy. Most of these neonatal infections appear asymptomatic. However, congenital abnormalities, including chorioretinitis and CNS abnormalities, have been described in neonates with laboratory evidence of congenital in utero infection with West Nile virus. Possible perinatal transmission of West Nile virus to a neonate through breast milk also has been reported. Neonates with West Nile virus infection may present with fever and encephalitis and may have severe or even fatal illness.[125,126] Neonatal infection with St. Louis encephalitis virus also has been documented in a 19-day-old neonate who presented with fever and seizures.[688] If arbovirus infection, especially West Nile virus infection, is documented during pregnancy, the fetus should be assessed with ultrasound imaging. Fetal infection may be documented by presence of virus-specific IgM in fetal blood obtained by cordocentesis. At delivery, the umbilical cord and placenta may be examined for evidence of virus infection. The infant should be followed for evidence of neurodevelopmental and sensory disabilities, and repeat serologic testing with virus specific IgG and IgM should be performed at 6 months of age, to confirm whether or not infection had occurred. No specific antiviral therapies are available at this time, and studies on the long-term neurodevelopmental outcome of these infants are necessary.

REFERENCES

1. Abdel-Fattah, S., Bhat, A., Illanes, S., et al.: TORCH test for fetal medicine indications: Only CMV is necessary in the United Kingdom. Prenat. Diagn. 25:1028, 2005.
2. Abzug, M.: Maternal factors affecting the integrity of the late gestation placental barrier to murine enterovirus infection. J. Infect. Dis. 176:41, 1997.
3. Abzug, M., Beam, A., Byorkos E, et al.: Viral pneumonia in the first month. Pediatr. Infect. Dis. J. 9:881, 1990.
4. Abzug, M., Keyerling, H., Lee, M. L., et al.: Neonatal enterovirus infection: Virology, serology, and effects of intravenous immune globulin. Clin. Infect. Dis. 20:1201, 1995.
5. Abzug, M., Levin, M., and Rotbart, H.: Profile of enterovirus disease in the first two weeks of life. Pediatr. Infect. Dis. J. 12:820, 1993.
6. Adler, S.: Transfusion-associated cytomegalovirus infections. Rev. Infect. Dis. 5:977, 1983.
7. Adler, S.: Molecular epidemiology of cytomegalovirus: Viral transmission among children attending a day care center, their parents, and caretakers. J. Pediatr. 112:366, 1988.
8. Adler, S., Baggett, J., Wilson, M., et al.: Molecular epidemiology of cytomegalovirus in a nursery: Lack of evidence for nosocomial transmission. J. Pediatr. 108:117, 1986.
9. Adler, S., Hempfling, S., Starr, S., et al.: Safety and immunogenicity of the Towne strain cytomegalovirus vaccine. Pediatr. Infect. Dis. J. 17:200, 1998.
10. Adler, S., Tattamangalam, C., Lawrence, L., et al.: Cytomegalovirus infections in neonates acquired by blood transfusions. Pediatr. Infect. Dis. 2:114, 1983.
11. Ahlfors, K., Forsgren, M., Ivarsson, S., et al.: Congenital cytomegalovirus infection: On the relation between type and time of maternal infection and infant's symptoms. Scand. J. Infect. Dis. 15:129, 1983.
12. Ahlfors, K., Ivarsson, S., Harris, S., et al.: Congenital cytomegalovirus infection and disease in Sweden and the relative importance of primary and secondary maternal infections. Scand. J. Infect. Dis. 16:129, 1984.
13. Ahlfors, K., Ivarsson, S., Johnsson, T., et al.: Primary and secondary maternal cytomegalovirus infections and their relation to congenital infection. Acta Paediatr. 71:109, 1982.
14. Alestig, K., Bartsch, F., Nilsson, L., et al.: Studies of amniotic fluid in women infected with rubella. J. Infect. Dis. 129:79, 1974.
15. Alford, C. Jr., Foft, J., Blankenship, W., et al: Subclinical central nervous system disease of neonates: A prospective study of infants born with increased levels of IgM. J. Pediatr. 75:1167, 1969.
16. Alford, C., Jr., Neva, F., and Weller, T.: Virologic and serologic studies on human products of conception after maternal rubella. N. Engl. J. Med. 271:1275, 1964.
17. Alford, C., Stagno, S, Pass, R, et al.: Congenital and perinatal cytomegalovirus infections. Rev. Infect. Dis. 12:745, 1990.
18. Alford, C., Jr., Stagno, S., and Reynolds, D.: Diagnosis of chronic perinatal infections. Am. J. Dis. Child. 129:455, 1975.
19. Alkalay, A., Pomerance, J., and Rimoin, D.: Fetal varicella syndrome. J. Pediatr. 111:322, 1987.
20. Alpert, S., Ferguson, J., Noel, L., et al.: Intrauterine West Nile virus: Ocular and systemic findings. A. J. Ophthalmol. 136:733, 2003.

21. Alter, H. J., Purcell, R. H., Shih, J. W., et al.: Detection of antibody to hepatitis C virus in prospectively followed transfusion recipients with acute and chronic non-A, non-B hepatitis. N. Engl. J. Med. *321*:1492-1500, 1989.

22. Alter, M: The detection, transmission, and outcome of hepatitis C virus infection. Infect. Agents. Dis. *2*:155, 1993.

23. Alter, M., Hadler, S., Judson, F., et al.: Risk factors for acute non-A, non-B hepatitis in the United States and association with hepatitis C virus infection. J.A.M.A. *264*:2231, 1990.

24. Alward, W., McMahon, B., Hall, D., et al.: The long-term serological course of asymptomatic hepatitis B virus carriers and the development of primary hepatocellular carcinoma. J. Infect. Dis. *151*:604, 1985.

25. American Academy of Pediatrics: Cytomegalovirus. *In* Pickering, L. K. (ed.): 2006 Red Book: Report of the Committee on Infectious Diseases. 27th ed. Elk Grove Village, IL, American Academy of Pediatrics, 2006, pp. 227-230.

26. American Academy of Pediatrics: Herpes simplex. *In* Pickering, L. K. (ed.): 2006 Red Book: Report of the Committee on Infectious Diseases. 27th ed. Elk Grove Village, IL, American Academy of Pediatrics, 2006, pp. 309-318.

27. American Academy of Pediatrics: Hepatitis B. *In* Pickering, L. K. (ed.): 2006 Red Book: Report of the Committee on Infectious Diseases. 27th ed. Elk Grove Village, IL, American Academy of Pediatrics, 2006, pp. 341-354.

28. American Academy of Pediatrics: Hepatitis C. *In* Pickering, L. K. (ed.): 2006 Red Book: Report of the Committee on Infectious Diseases. 27th ed. Elk Grove Village, IL, American Academy of Pediatrics, 2006, pp. 355-361.

29. American Academy of Pediatrics: Varicella-zoster virus. *In* Pickering, L. K. (ed.): 2006 Red Book: Report of the Committee on Infectious Diseases. 27th ed. Elk Grove Village, IL, American Academy of Pediatrics, 2006, pp. 711-725.

30. Anand, A., Gray, E., Brown, T., et al: Human parvovirus infection in pregnancy and hydrops fetalis. N. Engl. J. Med. *316*:183, 1987.

31. Anderson, K., Stevens, C., Tsuei, J., et al: Hepatitis B antigen in infants born to mothers with chronic hepatitis B antigenemia in Taiwan. Am. J. Dis. Child. *129*:1389, 1975.

32. Anderson, L.: Human parvoviruses. J. Infect. Dis. *161*:603, 1990.

33. Ansari, B., and Mason, M.: Chromosomal abnormality in congenital rubella. Pediatrics *59*:13, 1977.

34. Aradottir, E., Alonso, and E., Shulman, S.: Severe neonatal enteroviral hepatitis treated with pleconaril. Pediatr. Infect. Dis. J. *20*:457, 2001.

35. Arevalo, J.: Hepatitis B in pregnancy. West. J. Med. *150*:668, 1989.

36. Arevalo, J., and Washington, A.: Cost-effectiveness of prenatal screening and immunization for hepatitis B virus. J. A. M. A. *259*:365, 1988.

36a. Arvin, A., Fest, P., Myers, M., et al.: Vaccine development to prevent CMV disease: Report from the National Vaccine Advisory Committee. Clin. Infect. Dis. *39*:233, 2004.

37. Arvin, A., Hensleigh, P., Prober, C., et al.: Failure of antepartum maternal cultures to predict the infant's risk of exposure to herpes simplex virus at delivery. N. Engl. J. Med. *315*:796, 1986.

38. Arvin, A., Yeager, A., and Merigan, T.: Effect of leukocyte interferon on urinary excretion of cytomegalovirus by infants. J. Infect. Dis. *133*(Suppl.):A205, 1976.

39. Atmar, R., Englund, J., and Hammill, H.: Complications of measles during pregnancy. Clin. Infect. Dis. *14*:217, 1992.

40. Avram, M., Gobel, V., and Stpehr, A.: Case records of the Massachusetts General Hospital—Case 30-2007. A newborn girl with skin lesions. N. Engl. J. Med. *257*:1327, 2007.

41. Azam, A., Vial, Y., Fawer, C., et al.: Prenatal diagnosis of congenital cytomegalovirus infection. Obstet. Gynecol. *97*:443, 2001.

42. Bacon, C., and Sims, D.: Echovirus 19 infection in infants under six months. Arch. Dis. Child. *51*:631, 1976.

44. Bai, P., and John, T.: Congenital skin ulcers following varicella in late pregnancy. J. Pediatr. *94*:65, 1979.

45. Baker, D.: Herpes and pregnancy: New management. Clin. Obstet. Gynecol. *33*:253, 1990.

46. Bakshi, S., Miller, T., Kaplan, M., et al.: Failure of varicella-zoster immunoglobulin in modification of severe congenital varicella. Pediatr. Infect. Dis. *5*:699, 1986.

47. Bale, J., Murph, J., Demmler, G., et al.: Intrauterine cytomegalovirus infection and glycoprotein B genotypes. J. Infect. Dis. *182*:933, 2000.

48. Balkarek, K., Warren, W., Smith, R., et al.: Neonatal screening for congenital cytomegalovirus infection by detection of virus in saliva. J. Infect. Dis. *167*:1433, 1993.

50. Ballard, R., Drew, W., Hufnagle, K., et al.: Acquired cytomegalovirus infection in preterm infants. Am. J. Dis. Child. *133*:482, 1979.

51. Barbi, M., Binda, S., Caroppo, S., et al.: Neonatal screening for congenital cytomegalovirus infection and hearing loss. J. Clin. Virol. *35*:206, 2006.

52. Barbi, M., Binda, S., Caroppo, S., et al.: Multicity Italian study of congenital cytomegalovirus infection. Pediatr. Infect. Dis. J. *25*:156, 2006.

53. Barin, F., Goudeau, A., Denis, F., et al.: Immune response in neonates to hepatitis B vaccine. Lancet *1*:251, 1982.

54. Bart, K., Orenstein, W., Preblud, S., et al.: Elimination of rubella and congenital rubella from the United States. Pediatr. Infect. Dis. *4*:14, 1985.

55. Barton, L., and Mets, M.: Congenital lymphocytic choriomeningitis virus infection: Decade of rediscovery. Clin. Infect. Dis. *33*:370, 2001.

56. Baschat, A., Towbin, J., Bowles, N., et al.: Prevalence of viral DNA in amniotic fluid of low-risk pregnancies in the second trimester. J. Matern. Fetal. Neonatal. Med. 13:381, 2003.

57. Baschat, A., Towbin, J., Bowles, N., et al.: Is adenovirus a fetal pathogen? Obstet. Gynecol. 189:758, 2003.

58. Baublis, J., Whitley, R., Ch'ien, L., et al.: Treatment of cytomegalovirus infection in infants and adults. *In* Pavan-Langston, D., and Buchanan, R. A. (eds.): Adenine Arabinoside: An Antiviral Agent. New York, Raven Press, 1975, pp. 247-260.

59. Beasley, R., and Hwang, L.-Y.: Postnatal infectivity of hepatitis B surface antigen-carrier mothers. J. Infect. Dis. *147*:185, 1983.

60. Beasley, R., Hwang, L.-Y., Lee, G., et al.: Prevention of perinatally transmitted hepatitis B virus infections with hepatitis B immune globulin and hepatitis B vaccine. Lancet 2:1099, 1983.

61. Beasley, R., Hwang, L.-Y., Lin, C.-C., et al.: Hepatitis B immune globulin (HBIG) efficacy in the interruption of perinatal transmission of hepatitis B virus carrier state. Lancet 2:388, 1981.

62. Beasley, R., Hwang, L.-Y., Lin, C.-C., et al.: Hepatocellular carcinoma and hepatitis B virus: A prospective study of 22,707 men in Taiwan. Lancet 2:1129, 1981.

63. Beasley, R. P., Hwang, L.-Y., Lin, C.-C., et al.: Incidence of hepatitis B virus infections in preschool children in Taiwan. J. Infect. Dis. *146*:198, 1982.

64. Beasley, R., Hwang, L.-Y., Stevens, C. E., et al.: Efficacy of hepatitis B immune globulin for prevention of perinatal transmission of the hepatitis B virus carrier state: Final report of a randomized double-blind, placebo-controlled trial. Hepatology *3*:135, 1983.

65. Beasley, R., Shiao, I.-S., Stevens, C., et al.: Evidence against breast-feeding as a mechanism for vertical transmission of hepatitis B. Lancet 2:740, 1975.

66. Beasley, R., Trepo, C., Stevens, C., et al.: The e antigen and vertical transmission of hepatitis B surface antigen. Am. J. Epidemiol. *105*:94, 1977.

67. Becker, T. M., Blount, J., and Guinan, M. E.: Genital herpes infections in private practice in the United States, 1966 to 1981. J. A. M. A. *253*:1601, 1985.

68. Behrman, R. E.: The high-risk infant. *In* Vaughan, V. C., III, McKay, R., Jr., and Behrman, R. (eds.): Nelson Textbook of Pediatrics. Philadelphia, W. B. Saunders, 1979, pp. 398-414.

69. Bell, L., Naides, S., Stoffman, P., et al: Human parvovirus B19 infection among hospital staff members after contact with infected patients. N. Engl. J. Med. *321*:485, 1989.

70. Bergman, I., Painter, M., Wald, E., et al.: Outcome in children with enteroviral meningitis during the first year of life. J. Pediatr. *110*:705, 1987.

71. Binkin, N., Koplan, J., and Cates, W., Jr.: Preventing neonatal herpes: The value of weekly viral cultures in pregnant women with recurrent genital herpes. J. A. M. A. *251*:2816, 1984.

72. Birenbaum, E., Linder, N., Varsano, N., et al.: Adenovirus type 8 conjunctivitis outbreak in a neonatal intensive care unit. Arch. Dis. Child. *68*:610, 1993.

73. Birnbaum, G., Lynch, J., Margileth, A., et al.: Cytomegalovirus infections in newborn infants. J. Pediatr. *75*:789, 1969.

74. Blanc, W.: Pathology of the placenta and cord in some viral infections. *In* Hanshaw, J., and Dudgeon, J. (eds.): Viral Diseases of the Fetus and Newborn. Philadelphia, W. B. Saunders, 1978, pp. 237-258.

75. Boehm, F., Estes, W., Wright, P., et al.: Management of genital herpes simplex virus infection occurring during pregnancy. Am. J. Obstet. Gynecol. *141*:735, 1981.

76. Bolvin, G., Abed, Y., Boucher, F.: Human parechovirus 3 and neonatal infections. Emerg. Infect. Dis. *11*:103, 2005.

77. Bolognese, R., Corson, S., Fuccillo, D., et al.: Herpesvirus hominis type II infections in asymptomatic pregnant women. Obstet. Gynecol. 48:507, 1976.

78. Boner, A., Wilmott, R., Dinwiddie, R., et al.: Desquamative interstitial pneumonia and antigen-antibody complexes in two infants with congenital rubella. Pediatrics 72:835, 1983.

79. Bonthius, D., Wright, R., Tseng, B., et al.: Congenital cytomegalovirus infection: Specifics of disease. Ann. Neurol. *62*:347, 2007.

80. Boppana, S., Amos, C., Britt, W., et al.: Late onset and reactivation of chorioretinitis in children with congenital cytomegalovirus infection. Pediatr. Infect. Dis. J. *13*:1139, 1994.

81. Boppana, S., Fowler, K. B., Vaid, Y., et al.: Neuroradiographic findings in the newborn period and long-term outcome in children with symptomatic congenital cytomegalovirus infection. Pediatrics 99:409, 1997.

82. Boppana, S., Pass, R., Britt, W., et al.: Symptomatic congenital cytomegalovirus infection: Neonatal morbidity and mortality. Pediatr. Infect. Dis. J. *11*:93, 1992.

83. Boppana, S., Rivera, L., Fowler, K., et al.: Intrauterine transmission of cytomegalovirus to infants of women with preconceptional immunity. N. Engl. J. Med. *344*:1366, 2001.

84. Bortolotti, F., Caizia, R., Cadrobbi, P., et al.: Liver cirrhosis associated with chronic hepatitis B virus infection in childhood. J. Pediatr. *108*:224, 1986.

85. Boussault, P., Boralevi, F., Labke, L., et al.: Chronic varicella-zoster skin infection complicating the central nervous system. Pediatr. Dermatol. *24*:429, 2007.

86. Bradford, R., Cloud, G., Lakeman, F., et al.: Detection of cytomegalovirus (CMV) DNA by polymerase chain reaction is associated with hearing loss in newborns with symptomatic congenital CMV infection involving the central nervous system. J. Infect. Dis. *191*:227, 2005.

87. Bradford-Hill, A., Doll, R., Galloway, T., et al.: Virus diseases in pregnancy and congenital defects. Br. J. Prev. Soc. Med. *12*:1, 1958.

88. Brady, M., Milam, J., Anderson, D., et al.: Use of deglycerolized red blood cells to prevent posttransfusion infection with cytomegalovirus in neonates. J. Infect. Dis. *150*:334, 1984.

89. Brightman, V., Scott, T., Westphal, M., et al.: An outbreak of Coxsackie B-5 virus infection in a newborn nursery. J. Pediatr. *69*:179, 1966.

90. Britt, W. J.: Vaccines against human cytomegalovirus: Time to test. Trends Microbiol. *4*:34, 1996.

91. Brody, J., Sever. J., and Schiff, G.: Prevention of rubella by gamma globulin during an epidemic in Barrow, Alaska, in 1964. N. Engl. J. Med. *272*:127, 1965.

92. Brown, M., Rossier, E., Carpenter, B., et al.: Fatal adenovirus type 35 infection in neonates. Pediatr. Infect. Dis. J. 10:955, 1991.

93. Brown, G.: Maternal virus infection and congenital anomalies. Arch. Environ. Health *21*:362, 1970.

94. Brown, G., and Evans, T. N.: Serologic evidence of coxsackievirus etiology of congenital heart disease. J. A. M. A. *199*:183, 1967.

95. Brown, G., and Karunas, R.: Relationship of congenital anomalies and maternal infection with selected enteroviruses. Am. J. Epidemiol. *95*:207, 1972.

96. Brown, Z.: Herpes simplex virus-2 specific serology should be offered routinely to antenatal patients. Rev. Med. Virol. 10:141, 2000.

97. Brown, Z., Benedetti, J., Ashley, R., et al.: Neonatal herpes simplex virus infection in relation to asymptomatic maternal infection at the time of labor. N. Engl. J. Med. *324*:1247, 1991.

98. Brown, E., Gardella, C., Maim, G., et al.: Effect of maternal HSV serostatus and HSV type on risk of neonatal herpes. Acta Obstet. Gynecol. Scand. *86*:523, 2007.

99. Brown, Z., Kern, E., Spruance, S., et al.: Clinical and virologic course of herpes simplex genitalis. West. J. Med. *130*:414, 1979.

100. Brown, Z., Selke, S., Zeh, J., et al.: The acquisition of HSV during pregnancy. N. Engl. J. Med. *337*:509, 1997.

101. Brown, Z., Vontver, L., Benedetti, J., et al.: Effects on infants of a first episode of genital herpes during pregnancy. N. Engl. J. Med. *317*:1246, 1987.

102. Brown, Z., Wald, A., Morrow, R., et al.: Effect of serologic status and Cesarean delivery on the rates of HSV from mother to infant. J. A. M. A. *289*:203, 2003.

103. Brunell, P., Miller, L., and Lovejoy, F.: Zoster in children. Am. J. Dis. Child. *115*:432, 1968.

104. Buimovici-Klein, E., Lang, P., Ziring, P., et al.: Impaired cell-mediated immune response in patients with congenital rubella: Correlation with gestational age at time of infection. Pediatrics *64*:620, 1979.

105. Cannon, M., and Davis, K.: Washing our hands of the congenital CMV disease epidemic. BMC Public Health *5*:70, 2005.

106. Caviness, A. C., Demmler, G., Almenderez, Y., et al.: The prevalence of neonatal herpes simplex virus infection compared to serious bacterial illness in hospitalized neonates. J. Pediatr., *153*:164-169, 2008.

107. Caviness, A. C., Demmler, G., Selwyn, B.: Clinical and laboratory features of neonatal herpes simplex virus infection: A case-control study. Pediatr. Infect. Dis. J 27:1, 2008.

108. Caviness, A. C., Demmler, G., Swint, M., et. al.: Cost-effectiveness analysis of herpes simplex virus testing and treatment strategies in febrile neonates. Arch. Pediatr. Adolesc. Med. *162*:1, 2008.

109. Centers for Disease Control and Prevention: Immune globulins for protection against viral hepatitis. M. M. W. R. Morb. Mortal. Wkly. Rep. *30*:423428, 433-435, 1981.

110. Centers for Disease Control and Prevention: Enterovirus surveillance report, 1970-1979. Issued November 1981.

111. Centers for Disease Control and Prevention: Recommendations for protection against viral hepatitis. M. M. W. R. Morb. Mortal. *34*:313-324, 329-335, 1985.

112. Centers for Disease Control and Prevention: Prevention of perinatal transmission of hepatitis B virus: Prenatal screening of all pregnant women for hepatitis B surface antigen. M. M. W. R. Wkly. Rep. *37*:341-346, 351, 1988.

113. Centers for Disease Control and Prevention: Risks associated with human parvovirus B19 infection. M. M. W. R. Morb. Mortal. Wkly. Rep. *38*:81-88, 93-97, 1989.

114. Centers for Disease Control and Prevention: Rubella vaccination during pregnancy: United States, 1971-1988. M. M. W. R. Morb. Mortal. Wkly. Rep. *38*:289-293, 1989.

115. Centers for Disease Control and Prevention: Protection against viral hepatitis. Recommendations of the Immunization Practices Advisory Committee (ACIP). M. M. W. R. Recomm. Rep. *39*:1-26, 1990.

116. Centers for Disease Control and Prevention: Increase in rubella and congenital rubella syndrome-United States, 1988-1990. M. M. W. R. Morb. Mortal. Wkly. Rep. *40*:93-99, 1991.

117. Centers for Disease Control and Prevention: Elimination of rubella and congenital rubella syndrome—United States, 1969-2004. M. M. W. R. Morb. Mortal. Wkly. Rep. *54*:279, 2005.

118. Centers for Disease Control and Prevention: Progress towards elimination of measles and prevention of congenital rubella infection—European results 1990-2004. M. M. W. R. Morb. Mortal. Wkly. Rep. *54*:175, 2005.

119. Centers for Disease Control and Prevention: Hepatitis B virus: A comprehensive strategy for eliminating transmission in the United States through universal childhood vaccination. Recommendations of the Immunization Practices Advisory Committee (ACIP). M. M. W. R. Recomm. Rep. *40*:1-25, 1991.

120. Centers for Disease Control and Prevention: Hepatitis Surveillance Report No. 55, 1994, pp. 1-34.

121. Centers for Disease Control and Prevention: Recommendations for prevention and control of hepatitis C virus (HCV) infection and HCV-related chronic disease. M. M. W. R. Recomm. Rep. *47*:1-39, 1998.

122. Centers for Disease Control and Prevention: General recommendations on immunization. Recommendations of the Advisory Committee on Immunization Practices (ACIP) and the American Academy of Family Physicians (AAFP). M. M. W. R. Recomm. Rep. *51*:1-35, 2002.

123. Centers for Disease Control and Prevention: Sexually transmitted diseases treatment guidelines 2002. M. M. W. R. Recomm. Rep. *51*:1-78, 2002.

124. Centers for Disease Control and Prevention: Knowledge and practices of obstetricians and gynecologists regarding cytomegalovirus during pregnancy—United States, 2007. M. M. W. R. Morb. Mort. Wkly. Rep. *57*:65, 2008.

125. Centers for Disease Control and Prevention: Interim guidelines for the evaluation of infants born to mothers infected with West Nile virus during pregnancy. M. M. W. R. Morb. Mort. Wkly. Rep. *53*:154, 2004.

126. Centers for Disease Control and Prevention: Intrauterine West Nile virus infection—New York, 2002. J. A. M. A. *289*:295, 2003.

127. Chairez, R., Cesario, A., Barrett, J., et al.: Evaluation of CMV antibody EIA: An enzyme immunoassay for detection of antibodies to cytomegalovirus. Diagn. Microbiol. Infect. Dis. *3*:403, 1985.

128. Chamnanvanakij, S., Rogers, C., Luppino, C., et al.: Linear hyperechogenicity within the basal ganglia and thalamus of preterm infants. Pediatr. Neurol. *23*:129, 2000.

129. Champsaur, H., Fattal-German, M., and Arranhado, R.: Sensitivity and specificity of viral immunoglobulin M determination by indirect enzyme-linked immunosorbent assay. J. Clin. Microbiol. *26*:328, 1988.

130. Chandler, S., Alexander, E., and Holmes, K.: Epidemiology of cytomegaloviral infection in a heterogeneous population of pregnant women. J. Infect. Dis. *2*:249, 1985.

131. Chang, T: Rubella reinfection and intrauterine involvement. J. Pediatr. *84*:617, 1974.

132. Chawareewong, S., Kiangsiri, S., Lokaphadhana, K., et al.: Neonatal herpangina caused by coxsackie A-5 virus. J. Pediatr. *93*:492, 1978.

133. Cheeseman, S., Hirsch, M., Keller, E., et al.: Fatal neonatal pneumonia caused by echovirus type 9. Am. J. Dis. Child. *131*:1169, 1977.

134. Chernesky, M., and Mahony, J.: Rubella virus. *In* Murray, P., Barron, E., Pfaller, M., et al. (eds.): Manual of Clinical Microbiology. Washington, DC, American Society of Microbiology, 1995, pp. 968-973.

135. Cherry, J.: Enteroviruses. *In* Remington, J., and Klein, J. (eds.): Infectious Diseases of the Fetus and Newborn Infant. 5th ed. Philadelphia, W. B. Saunders, 2001, pp. 477-518.

136. Chess, S., Fernandez, P., and Korn, S.: Behavioral consequences of congenital rubella. J. Pediatr. *93*:699, 1978.

137. Chiba, M., Saito, M., Suzuki, N., et al.: Measles infection in pregnancy. J. Infect. Dis. *47*:407, 2003.

138. Ch'ien, L., Cannon, N., Whitley, R., et al.: Effect of adenine arabinoside on cytomegalovirus infections. J. Infect. Dis. *130*:32, 1974.

139. Ch'ien, L., Whitley, R., Nahmias, A., et al.: Antiviral chemotherapy and neonatal herpes simplex virus infection: A pilot study—Experience with adenine arabinoside (ARA-A). Pediatrics *55*:678, 1975.

140. Chiou, C., Soong, W., Hwang, B., et al.: Congenital adenoviral infection. Pediatr. Infect. Dis. J. 13:664, 1994.

141. Choo, Q.-L., Kuo, G., Weiner, A., et al.: Isolation of a cDNA clone derived from a blood-borne non-A, non-B viral hepatitis genome. Science *244*:359, 1989.

142. Clarke, W., Shaver, K., Bright, G., et al.: Autoimmunity in congenital rubella syndrome. J. Pediatr. *104*:370, 1984.

143. Clemens, R., Safary, A., Hepburn, A., et al.: Clinical experience with an inactivated hepatitis A vaccine. J. Infect. Dis. *171*(Suppl. 1):44, 1995.

144. Clemente, M., Congia, M., Lai, M., et al.: Effect of iron overload on the response to recombinant interferon-alfa treatment in transfusion dependent patients with thalassemia major and chronic hepatitis C. J. Pediatr. *125*:123, 1994.

145. Coats, D., Demmler, G., Payssee, E., et al.: Ophthalmologic findings in children with congenital cytomegalovirus infection. J. AAPOS *4*:110, 2000.

146. Committee on Infectious Diseases: Universal hepatitis B immunization. Pediatrics *89*:795, 1992.

147. Conboy, T., Pass, R., Stagno, S., et al.: Early clinical manifestations and intellectual outcome in children with symptomatic congenital cytomegalovirus infection. J. Pediatr. *111*:343, 1987.

148. Conchie, A., Barton, B., and Tobin, J.: Congenital cytomegalovirus infection treated with idoxuridine. B.M.J. *4*:162, 1968.

149. Cone, R., Hobson, A., Brown, Z., et al.: Frequent detection of genital herpes simplex virus DNA by polymerase chain reaction among pregnant women. J. A. M. A. *272*:792, 1994.

150. Conry, J., Török, T., and Andrews, P.: Perinatal encephalopathy secondary to in utero human parvovirus B-19 (HPV) infection. Abstract 736S. Neurology *43*(Suppl):346, 1993.

151. Cooper, L.: The history and medical consequences of rubella. Rev. Infect. Dis. *7*(Suppl. 1):2, 1985.

152. Cooper, L., and Alford, C., Jr.: Rubella. *In* Remington J and Klein J (eds.): Infections of the Fetus and Newborn Infant. 5th ed. Philadelphia, W. B. Saunders, 2001, pp. 347-388.

153. Cooper, L., Green, R., Krugman, S., et al.: Neonatal thrombocytopenic purpura and other manifestations of rubella contracted in utero. Am. J. Dis. Child. *110*:416, 1965.

154. Cooper, L., Ziring, P., Ockerse, A., et al.: Rubella: Clinical manifestations and management. Am. J. Dis. Child. *118*:18, 1969.

155. Corey, L., Adams, H. G., Brown, Z. A., et al.: Genital herpes simplex virus infections: Clinical manifestations, course, and complications. Ann. Intern. Med. 98:958-972, 1983.

156. Corey, L., and Spear, P.: Infections of herpes simplex viruses. N. Engl. J. Med. 314:686, 1986.

157. Corey, L., Whitley, R., Stone, E., et al.: Difference between herpes simplex virus type 1 and type 2 neonatal encephalitis in neurological outcome. Lancet 1:1, 1988.

158. Corless, C., Guiver, M., Borrow, R., et al.: Development and evaluation of a real-time RT-PCR for the detection of enterovirus and parechovirus RNA in CSF and throat swabs. J. Med. Virol. 67:555, 2003.

159. Cox, F., and Hughes, W.: Fecal excretion of cytomegalovirus in disseminated cytomegalic inclusion disease. J. Infect. Dis. 129:732, 1974.

160. Craig, C., and Nahmias, A.: Different patterns of neurologic involvement with herpes simplex virus types 1 and 2: Isolation of herpes simplex virus type 2 from the buffy coat of two adults with meningitis. J. Infect. Dis. 127:365, 1973.

161. Cramblett, H., Haynes, R., Azimi, P., et al.: Nosocomial infection with echovirus type 11 in handicapped and premature infants. Pediatrics 51:603, 1973.

162. Crane, J.: Parvovirus B19 infection in pregnancy. J. Obstet. Gynaecol. Can. 24:727, 2002.

163. Cruz, A., Frentzen, B., and Behnke, M.: Hepatitis B: A case for prenatal screening of all patients. Am. J. Obstet. Gynecol. 156:1180, 1987.

164. Cuthbert, J.: Hepatitis C: Progress and problems. Clin. Microbiol. Rev. 7:505, 1994.

165. Dagan, R., Hall, C., Powell, K., et al: Epidemiology and laboratory diagnosis of infection with viral and bacterial pathogens in infants hospitalized for suspected sepsis. J. Pediatr. 115:351, 1989.

166. Dagan, R., Jenista, J., and Menegus, M.: Clinical, epidemiological, and laboratory aspects of enterovirus infection in young infants. In de la Maza L. M., and Peterson, E. (eds.): Medical Virology IV. Hillsdale, NJ, L. Erlbaum Associates, 1985, pp. 123-151.

167. Dagan, R., Jenista, J., Prather, S., et al.: Viremia in hospitalized children with enterovirus infections. J. Pediatr. 106:397, 1985.

168. Dagan, R., Prather, S., Powell, K., et al.: Neutralizing antibodies to non-polio enteroviruses in human immune serum globulin. Pediatr. Infect. Dis. 2:454, 1983.

169. Daling, J., and Wolf, M.: The role of decision and cost analyses in the treatment of pregnant women with recurrent genital herpes. J. A. M. A. 251:2828, 1984.

170. Das, S., Ramachandran, V., Arora, R.: Cyotmegalovirus and rubella infection in children and pregnant mothers in a hospital based study. J. Commun. Dis. 39:113, 2007.

171. Davis, L., Tweed, G., Chin, T., et al.: Intrauterine diagnosis of cytomegalovirus infection: Viral recovery from amniocentesis fluid. Am. J. Obstet. Gynecol. 109:1217, 1971.

172. De Backer, S., Samule, K., Carton, D., et al.: Neonatal Coxsackie B3 sepsis. Acta Paediatr. Belg. 29:55, 1976.

173. Degani S: Sonographic findings in fetal viral infection: A systematic review. Obstet. Gynecol. Surv. 61:329, 2006.

174. Delaplane, D., Yogev, R., Crussi, F., et al.: Fatal hepatitis B in early infancy: The importance of identifying HBsAg-positive pregnant women and providing immunoprophylaxis to their newborns. Pediatrics 72:176-180, 1983.

175. DeHaan, T., Oepkes, D., Beersman, M., et al.: Aetiology, diagnosis, and treatment of hydrops fetalis. Curr. Perinat. Rev. I:63, 2005.

176. Del Mar Mosquera, M., de Ory, F., Moreno, M., and Echevarria, J.: Simultaneous detection of measles virus, rubella virus, and parvovirus B19 by using multiplex PCR. J. Clin. Microbiol. 40:111, 2002.

177. Dembinski, J., Haverkamp, F., Maara, H., et al.: Neurodevelopmental outcome after intrauterine red cell transfusion for parvovirus B19 induced fetal hydrops. B.J.O.G. 109:1232, 2002.

178. Demmler, G.: Summary of a workshop on surveillance for congenital cytomegalovirus disease. Rev. Infect. Dis. 13:315, 1991.

179. Demmler, G., Buffone G., Schimbor C., et al: Detection of cytomegalovirus in urine from newborns by using polymerase chain reaction DNA amplification. J. Infect. Dis. 158:1177, 1988.

180. Demmler, G.: Congenital cytomegalovirus infection treatment. Pediatr. Infect. Dis. J. 22:1005, 2003.

181. Demmler, G., Yow, M., Spector, S., et al.: Nosocomial cytomegalovirus infection within two hospitals caring for infants and children. J. Infect. Dis. 156:9:1987.

182. Demmler, G., Brady, M., Bijou, H., et al.: Post-transfusion cytomegalovirus infection in neonates: Role of saline-washed RBCs. J. Pediatr. 108:762, 1986.

183. Derso, A., Boxall, E. H., Tarlow, M. J., et al.: Transmission of HBsAg from mother to infant in four ethnic groups. B. M. J. 1:949-952, 1978.

184. Desmond, M.: Social upheaval and technological Progress. In Desmond, M.: Newborn medicine and society: European background and American practitioners 1750-1975. Austin, TX, Eakin Press, 1998, pp. 206-207.

185. Desmond, M., Fisher, E., Vorderman, A., et al.: The longitudinal course of congenital rubella encephalitis in nonretarded children. J. Pediatr. 93:584, 1978.

186. Desmond, M., Wilson, G., and Melnick, J.: Congenital rubella encephalitis. J. Pediatr. 71:311, 1967.

187. Diamond, C., Mohan, K., Hobson, A., et al.: Viremia in neonatal herpes simplex virus infections. Pediatr. Infect. Dis. J. 18:487, 1999.

188. Dickinson, J., and Gonik, B.: Teratogenic viral infections. Clin. Obstet. Gynecol. 33:242, 1990.

189. Distefano, A., Alonso, A., Martin, F., et al.: Human cytomegalovirus: Detection of congenital and perinatal infection in Argentina. B. M. C. Pediatr. 23:11, 2004.

190. Dodt, K., Jacobsen, P., Hofmann, B., et al.: Development of cytomegalovirus (CMV) disease may be predicted in HIV-infected patients by CMV polymerase chain reaction and the antigenemia test. A I D S 11:F21, 1997.

191. Donowitz, L., and Gryboski, J.: Pancreatic insufficiency and the congenital rubella syndrome. J. Pediatr. 87:241, 1975.

192. Dosik, H., and Jhaveri, R.: Prevention of neonatal hepatitis B infection by high-dose hepatitis B immune globulin. N. Engl. J. Med. 298:602, 1978.

193. Douglas, J., Schmidt, O., and Corey, L.: Acquisition of neonatal HSV-1 infection from a paternal source contact. J. Pediatr. 103:908, 1983.

194. Doyle, M., Atkins, J., and Rivera-Matos, I. R.: Congenital cytomegalovirus infection in infants infected with human immunodeficiency virus type 1. Pediatr. Infect. Dis. J. 15:1102, 1996.

195. Dublin, A., and Merten, D.: Computed tomography in the evaluation of herpes simplex encephalitis. Radiology 125:133, 1977.

196. Dunkle, L., Schmidt, R., and O'Connor, D.: Neonatal herpes simplex infection possibly acquired via maternal breast milk. Pediatrics 63:250, 1979.

197. Dunn, A., Peters, R., Schweitzer, I., et al.: Virus-like particles in livers of infants with vertically transmitted hepatitis. Arch. Pathol. 94:258, 1972.

198. Dunn, P. M.: Perinatal lessons from the past: Sir Norman Gregg, ChM, MC, of Sydney (1892-1966) and rubella embryopathy. Arch. Dis. Child. Fetal Neonatal. Ed. 92: F513-F514, 2007.

199. Dupuy, J., Frommel, D., and Alagille, D.: Severe viral hepatitis type B in infancy. Lancet 1:191, 1975.

200. Dupuy, J., Giraud, P., Dupuy, C., et al.: Hepatitis B in children. II. Study of children born to chronic HBsAg carrier mothers. J. Pediatr. 92:200, 1978.

201. Dupuy, J. M., Kostewicz, E., and Alagille, D.: Hepatitis B in children. I. Analysis of 80 cases of acute and chronic hepatitis B. J. Pediatr. 92:17-20, 1978.

202. Dworsky, M., Yow, M., Stagno, S., et al.: Cytomegalovirus infection of breast milk and transmission in infancy. Pediatrics 72:295, 1983.

203. Dzierzahowska, D., Augustynowicz, F., Gyzl, A., et al.: Application of polymerase chain reaction (PCR) for the detection of DNA-HCMV in cerebrospinal fluid of neonates and infants with cytomegalovirus infection. Neurol. Neurochir. Pol. 31:447, 1997.

204. Eberhart-Phillips, J. E., Frederick, P., Baron, R., et al.: Measles in pregnancy: A descriptive study of 58 cases. Obstet. Gynecol. 82:797, 1993.

205. Echeverria, P., Miller, G., Campbell, A., et al.: Scalp vesicles within the first week of life: A clue to early diagnosis of herpes neonatorum. J. Pediatr. 83:1062, 1973.

206. Eilard, T., and Strannegard, Ö.: Rubella reinfection in pregnancy followed by transmission to the fetus. J. Infect. Dis. 129:594, 1974.

207. Elizan, T. S., Ajero-Froehlich, L., Fabiyi, A., et al.: Viral infection in pregnancy and congenital CNS malformations in man. Arch. Neurol. 20:115-119, 1969.

208. Elizan, T., and Fabiyi, A.: Congenital and neonatal anomalies linked with viral infections in experimental animals. Am. J. Obstet. Gynecol. 106:147, 1970.

209. Emanuel, D., Cunningham, I., Jules-Elysee, K., et al.: Cytomegalovirus pneumonia after bone marrow transplantation successfully treated with the combination of ganciclovir and high-dose intravenous immune globulin. Ann. Intern. Med. 109:777, 1988.

210. Emodi, G., and Just, M.: Impaired interferon response of children with congenital cytomegalovirus disease. Acta. Paediatr. 63:183-187, 1974.

211. Emodi, G., O'Reilly, R., Müller, A., et al.: Effect of human exogenous leukocyte interferon in cytomegalovirus infections. J. Infect. Dis. 133(Suppl.):A199, 1976.

212. Enders, G: Varicella-zoster virus infection in pregnancy. Prog. Med. Virol. 29:166, 1984.

213. Enders, G., Bader, U., Lindemann, L., et al.: Prenatal diagnosis of congenital cytomegalovirus infection in 189 pregnancies with known outcome. Prenatal. Diagn. 21:362, 2001.

214. Enders, G., Miller, E., and Cradock-Watson, J.: Consequences of varicella and herpes zoster in pregnancy: Prospective study of 1379 cases. Lancet 343:1547, 1994.

215. Enders, M., Weidner, A., Rosenthal, T., et al.: Improved diagnosis of gestation parvovirus B19 infection at the time of nonimmune hydrops. J. Infect. Dis. 197:58, 2008.

216. Englund, J., Courtney, F., and Balfour, H.: Acyclovir therapy in neonates. J. Pediatr. 119:129, 1991.

217. Esterly, J., Slusser, R., and Ruebner, B.: Hepatic lesions in the congenital rubella syndrome. J. Pediatr. 71:676, 1967.

218. Faden, H., Wynn, R., Campagna, L., et al.: Outbreak of adenovirus type 30 in a neonatal intensive care unit. J. Pediatr. 146:523, 2005.

219. Faix, R.: Survival of cytomegalovirus on environmental surfaces. J. Pediatr. 106:649, 1986.

220. Farmer, K., MacArthur, B., and Clay, M.: A follow-up study of 15 cases of neonatal meningoencephalitis due to coxsackievirus B5. J. Pediatr. 87:568, 1975.

221. Faulkner, R., and van Rooyen, C.: Echovirus type 17 in the neonate. Can. Med. Assoc. J. 108:878, 1973.

222. Fawaz, K., Grady, G., Kaplan, M., et al.: Repetitive maternal-fetal transmission of fatal hepatitis B. N. Engl. J. Med. 293:1357, 1975.
223. Feigin, R., Shackleford, P., Haymond, M., et al.: Floxuridine treatment of congenital cytomegalovirus inclusion disease. Pediatrics 48:318, 1971.
224. Feldman, G: Herpes zoster neonatorum. Arch. Dis. Child. 27:126, 1952.
225. Feldman, R. A.: Cytomegalovirus infection during pregnancy. Am. J. Dis. Child. 117:517, 1969.
226. Finn, A., Andy, E., Talbot, G.: An epidemic of adenovirus 7a in a neonatal nursery: Course, morbidity, and management. Infect. Control. Hosp. Epidem. 9:398, 1988.
227. Florman, A., Gershon, A., Blackett, P., et al.: Intrauterine infection with herpes simplex virus. J. A. M. A. 225:129, 1973.
228. Forbes, B.: Acquisition of cytomegalovirus infection: An update. Clin. Microbiol. Rev. 2:204, 1989.
229. Forbes, B.: Perinatal viral infections. Clin. Microbiol. News 14:169, 1992.
230. Fowler, K., McCollister, F., Dahle, A., et al.: Progressive and fluctuating sensorineural hearing loss in children with asymptomatic congenital cytomegalovirus infection. J. Pediatr. 130:624, 1997.
231. Fowler, K., Stagno, S., and Pass, R., et al.: The outcome of congenital cytomegalovirus infection in relation to maternal antibody status. N. Engl. J. Med. 326:667, 1992.
232. Frey, H. M., Bailkin, G., and Gershon, A. A.: Congenital varicella: Case report of a serologically proved long-term survivor. Pediatrics 59:110-112, 1977.
233. Frickhofen, N., Abkowitz, J., Safford, M., et al.: Persistent B19 parvovirus infection in patients infected with human immunodeficiency virus type-1 (HIV-1): A treatable cause of anemia in AIDS. Ann. Intern. Med. 113:926, 1990.
234. Fujita. H., Yoshii. A., Maeda. J., et al.: Genitourinary anomaly and congenital varicella syndrome: case report and review. Pediatr. Nephrol. 19:554, 2004.
235. Funato, T., Satou, N., Abukawa, D., et al.: Quantitative evaluation of cytomegalovirus DNA in infantile hepatitis. J. Viral. Hepat. 8:217, 2001.
236. Gagneur, A., Sizum, J., Vallet, S., et al.: Coronavirus—nosocomial viral respiratory infection in a neonatal and paediatric intensive care unit: A prospective study. J. Hosp. Infect. 51:59, 2002.
237. Gagneur, A., Vallet, S., Talbot, P., et al.: Outbreaks of human coronavirus in a paediatric and neonatal intensive care unit. Eur. J. Pediatr. Mar 12, 2008, Epub ahead of print.
238. Garcia, A., Olinto, F., and Fortes, T.: Thymic hypoplasia due to congenital rubella. Arch Dis Child 49:181, 1974.
239. Gear, J., and Measroch, V.: Coxsackievirus infections of the newborn. Prog. Med. Virol. 15:42, 1973.
240. Gelb, L.: Varicella-zoster virus. In Fields, B., and Knipe, D. (eds.): Virology. New York, Raven Press, 1990, pp. 2011-2054.
241. Gerety, R., Hoofnagle, J., Markenson, J., et al.: Exposure to hepatitis B virus and development of the chronic HBAg carrier state in children. J. Pediatr. 84:661, 1974.
242. Gerety, R., and Schweitzer, I.: Viral hepatitis type B during pregnancy, the neonatal period, and infancy. J. Pediatr. 90:368, 1977.
243. Gershon, A.: Chickenpox, measles and mumps. In Remington, J., and Klein, J. (eds.): Infectious Diseases of the Fetus and Newborn Infant. 5th ed. Philadelphia, W. B. Saunders, 2001, pp. 683-732.
244. Gibbs, R., Amstey, M., Sweet, R., et al.: Management of genital herpes infection in pregnancy. Obstet. Gynecol. 71:779, 1988.
245. Grangeot-Keros, L., Broyer, M., Briand, E., et al.: Enterovirus in sudden unexpected deaths in infants. Pediatr. Infect. Dis. 15:123, 1996.
246. Grangeot-Keros, L., Pillot, J., Daffos, F., et al.: Prenatal and postnatal production of IgM and IgA antibodies to rubella virus studied by antibody capture immunoassay. J. Infect. Dis. 158:138, 1988.
247. Gratacos, E., Torres, P.-J., Vidal, J., et al.: The incidence of human parvovirus B19 infection during pregnancy and its impact on perinatal outcome. J. Infect. Dis. 171:1360, 1995.
248. Greenberg, D.: Pediatric experience with recombinant hepatitis B vaccines and relevant safety and immunogenicity studies. Pediatr. Infect. Dis. J. 12:438, 1993.
249. Greenberg, H., Pollard, R., Lutwick, L., et al.: Effect of human leukocyte interferon on hepatitis B virus infection in patients with chronic active hepatitis. N. Engl. J. Med. 295:517, 1976.
250. Gregg, N.: Congenital cataract following German measles in the mother. Trans. Ophthalmol. Soc. Aust. 3:35, 1941.
251. Griffiths, P., and Baboonian, C.: A prospective study of primary cytomegalovirus infection during pregnancy: Final report. Br. J. Obstet. Gynaecol. 91:307, 1984.
252. Griffiths, P., Stagno, S., Pass, R., et al.: Congenital cytomegalovirus infection: Diagnostic and prognostic significance of the detection of specific immunoglobulin M antibodies in cord serum. Pediatrics 69:544, 1982.
253. Griffiths, P., Stagno, S., Pass, R., et al.: Infection with cytomegalovirus during pregnancy: Specific IgM antibodies as a marker of recent primary infection. J. Infect. Dis. 145:647, 1982.
254. Gross, J., Jr., and Persing, D.: Hepatitis C: Advances in diagnosis. Mayo. Clin. Proc. 70:296, 1995.
255. Grossman, J., III: Herpes simplex virus (HSV) infections. Clin. Obstet. Gynecol. 25:555, 1982.
256. Gupta, R., Warren, T., Wald, A.: Genital herpes. Lancet 370:2127, 2007.
257. Gutman, L., Wilfert, C., and Eppes, S.: Herpes simplex virus encephalitis in children: Analysis of cerebrospinal fluid and progressive neurodevelopmental deterioration. J. Infect. Dis. 154:415, 1986.
258. Hagler, W. S., Walters, P. V., and Nahmias, A. J.: Ocular involvement in neonatal herpes simplex virus infection. Arch. Ophthalmol. 82:169-176, 1969.
259. Halfon, N., and Spector, S.: Fatal echovirus type 11 infections. Am. J. Dis. Child. 135:1017, 1981.
260. Hall, C., Douglas, R., Jr., Gelman, J., et al.: Nosocomial respiratory syncytial virus infections. N. Engl. J. Med. 293:1343, 1975.
261. Hammond, J., Lukes, H., Wells, B., et al.: Maternal and neonatal neutralizing antibody titers to selected enteroviruses. Pediatr. Infect. Dis. J. 4:32, 1985.
262. Hammerberg, O., Watts, J., Chernesky, M., et al.: An outbreak of herpes simplex virus type I in an intensive care nursery. Pediatr. Infect. Dis. 2:290, 1983.
263. Hamprecht, K., Maschmann, J., Vochem, M., et al.: Epidemiology of transmission of cytomegalovirus from mother to preterm infant by breastfeeding. Lancet 357:513, 2001.
264. Hancock, M., Huntley, C., and Sever, J.: Congenital rubella syndrome with immunoglobulin disorder. J. Pediatr. 72:636, 1968.
265. Hanshaw, J.: Developmental abnormalities associated with congenital cytomegalovirus infection. Adv. Teratol. 4:64, 1970.
266. Hanshaw, J.: Herpesvirus hominis infections in the fetus and the newborn. Am. J. Dis. Child. 126:546, 1973.
267. Hanshaw, J.: Congenital cytomegalovirus infection. Pediatr. Ann. 23:124, 1994.
268. Hanshaw, J., Scheiner, A., Moxley, A., et al: School failure and deafness after "silent" congenital cytomegalovirus infection. N. Engl. J. Med. 295:468, 1976.
269. Hanshaw, J., Steinfeld, H., and White, C.: Fluorescent-antibody test for cytomegalovirus macroglobulin. N. Engl. J. Med. 279:566, 1968.
270. Hardy, J. B., Sever, J. L., and Gilkeson, M. R.: Declining antibody titers in children with congenital rubella. J. Pediatr. 75:213-220, 1969.
271. Harger, J.: Indications for antepartum HSV screening cultures. Infect. Surg. 8:24, 1989.
272. Harger, J, Ernest, J., Thurnau, G., et al.: Risk factors and outcome of varicella zoster virus pneumonia in pregnant women. J. Infect. Dis. 185:422, 2002.
273. Harger, J., Ernest, J., Turnau, G., et al.: Frequency of congenital varicella syndrome in a prospective cohort of 347 pregnant women. Obstet. Gynecol. 100:260, 2002.
274. Harger, J., Pazin, G., Armstrong, J., et al: Characteristics and management of pregnancy in women with genital herpes simplex virus infection. Am. J. Obstet. Gynecol. 145:784, 1983.
275. Hatherley, L., Hayes, K., Hennessy, E., Jack, I.: Herpesvirus in an obstetric hospital. I. Herpetic eruptions. Med. J. Aust. 2:205, 1980.
276. Hatherley, L., Hayes, K., and Jack, I.: Herpesvirus in an obstetric hospital. II. Asymptomatic virus excretion in staff members. Med. J. Aust. 2:273, 1980.
277. Hayes, K., Danks, D., Gibas, H., et al.: Cytomegalovirus in human milk. N. Engl. J. Med. 287:177, 1972.
278. Hayes, K., and Gibas, H.: Placental cytomegalovirus infection without fetal involvement following primary infection in pregnancy. J. Pediatr. 79:401, 1971.
279. Haynes, R., Azimi, P., and Cramblett, H.: Fatal herpesvirus hominis (herpes simplex virus) infections in children: Clinical, pathologic, and virologic characteristics. J. A. M. A. 206:312, 1968.
280. Heijtink, R., Boender, P., Schalm, S., et al.: Hepatitis B virus DNA in serum of pregnant women with HBsAg and HBeAg or antibodies to HBe. J. Infect. Dis. 150:462, 1984.
281. Herrmann, K.: Available rubella serologic tests. Rev. Infect. Dis. 7(Suppl 1):108, 1985.
282. Higa, K., Dan, K., and Manabe, H.: Varicella-zoster virus infections during pregnancy: Hypothesis concerning the mechanisms of congenital malformations. Obstet. Gynecol. 69:214, 1987.
283. Hinckley, A., O'Leary, D., Hayes, E.: Transmission of West Nile virus through human breast milk is thought to be rare. Pediatrics 119:e666, 2007.
284. Hildebrandt, R., Sever, J., Margileth, A., et al.: Cytomegalovirus in the normal pregnant woman. Am. J. Obstet. Gynecol. 98:1125, 1967.
285. Hinman, A.: Prevention of congenital rubella infection: Symposium summary. Pediatrics 75:1162, 1985.
286. Hocker, J., Cook, L., Adams, G., et al.: Ganciclovir therapy of congenital cytomegalovirus pneumonia. Pediatr. Infect. Dis. J. 9:743, 1990.
287. Hollier, L., and Werdel, J.: Third trimester antiviral prophylaxis for prevention of maternal genital herpes simplex virus recurrence and neonatal infection. Cochrane Database System Rev CD004949, Jan 23, 2008.
288. Hollinger, F.: Serologic evaluation of viral hepatitis. Hosp. Pract. 22:101, 1987.
289. Holzer, B., and Egger, M.: Hepatitis A vaccine. Curr. Opin. Infect. Dis. 8:186, 1995.
290. Honig, P., and Brown, D.: Congenital herpes simplex virus infection initially resembling epidermolysis bullosa. J. Pediatr. 101:958, 1982.
291. Hoofnagle, J.: Therapy of acute and chronic viral hepatitis. Adv. Intern. Med. 39:241, 1994.
292. Horstmann, D., Banatvala, J., Riordan, J., et al.: Maternal rubella and the rubella syndrome in infants: Epidemiologic, clinical, and virologic observations. Am. J. Dis. Child. 110:408, 1965.

293. Horstmann, D., Liebhaber, H., Le Bouvier, G. L., et al.: Rubella: Reinfection of vaccinated and naturally immune persons exposed in an epidemic. N. Engl. J. Med. 283:771, 1970.

294. Horstmann, D., Pajot, T., and Liebhaber, H.: Epidemiology of rubella: Subclinical infection and occurrence of reinfection. Am. J. Dis. Child. 118:133, 1969.

295. Hovig, D., Hodgman, J., Mathies, A., Jr., et al.: Herpesvirus hominis (simplex) infection: With recurrences during infancy. Am. J. Dis. Child. 115:438, 1968.

296. Hsu, H., Feinstone, S., and Hoofnagle, J.: Acute viral hepatitis. In Mandell, G., Bennett, J., and Dolin, R. (eds): Principles and Practice of Infectious Diseases. 4th ed. New York, Churchill Livingstone, 1995, pp. 1136-1153.

297. Huang, E.-S., Alford, C,, Reynolds, D. W., et al.: Molecular epidemiology of cytomegalovirus infections in women and their infants. N. Engl. J. Med. 303:958, 1980.

298. Huang, Y., Lin, T., Lin, Y., et al.: Prophylaxis of intravenous immunoglobulin and acyclovir in perinatal varicella. Eur. J. Pediatr. 160:91, 2001.

299. Hughes, J. R., Wilfert, C. M., Moore, M., et al.: Echovirus 14 infection associated with fatal neonatal hepatic necrosis. Am. J. Dis. Child. 123:61-67, 1972.

300. Hughes, P., LaRusso, P., Pearce, J., et al.: Transmission of varicella-zoster virus from a vaccinee with underlying leukemia, demonstrated by polymerase chain reaction. J. Pediatr. 124:932, 1994.

301. Hutto, C., Arvin, A., Jacob, R., et al.: Intrauterine herpes simplex virus infections. J. Pediatr. 110:97, 1987.

302. Istas, A., Demmler, G., Dobbins, J., et al.: Surveillance for congenital cytomegalovirus disease: A report from the National Congenital Cytomegalovirus Disease Registry. Clin. Infect. Dis. 20:665, 1995.

303. Jahn, C. L., and Cherry, J. D.: Mild neonatal illness associated with heavy enterovirus infection. N. Engl. J. Med. 274:394, 1966.

304. Jamieson, D., Kourtis, A., Bell, M., et al.: Lymphocytic choriomeningitis virus: An emerging obstetrical pathogen? Am. J. Obstet. Gynecol. 194:1532, 2006.

305. Ivarsson, S., Jonsson, K., and Jonsson, B.: Birth characteristics and growth pattern in children with congenital CMV infection. J. Pediatr. Endocr. Metab. 16:1233, 2003.

306. Jeansson, S., and Molin, L.: On the occurrence of genital herpes simplex virus infection: Clinical and virological findings and relation to gonorrhoea. Acta Dermatol. Venereol. (Stockh.) 54:479, 1974.

307. Jenista, J., Powell, K., and Menegus, M.: Epidemiology of neonatal enterovirus infection. J. Pediatr. 104:685, 1984.

308. Jeaon, J., Victor, M., Adler, S., et al.: Knowledge and awareness of congenital CMV among women. Infect. Dis. Obstet. Gynecol. 2006:80383, 2006.

309. Jhaveri, R., Rosenfeld, W., Salazar, J., et al.: High titer multiple dose therapy with HBIG in newborn infants of HBsAg positive mothers. J. Pediatr. 97:305, 1980.

310. Jin, L., and Thomas, B.: Application of molecular and serological assays to case-based investigation of rubella and congenital rubella syndrome. J. Med. Virol. 79:1017, 2007.

311. Johansson, P., Jonsson, M., Ahlfors, K., et al.: Retrospective diagnosis of congenital cytomegalovirus infection performed by polymerase chain reaction in blood stored on filter paper. Scand. J. Infect. Dis. 29:465, 1997.

312. Johansson, A., Rassart, A., Blum, D., et al.: Lower-limb hypoplasia due to intrauterine infection with HSV-2: Possible confusion with intrauterine varicella zoster virus syndrome. Clin. Infect. Dis. 38:e57, 2004.

313. Johnson, R., Nahmias, A., Magder, L., et al.: A seroepidemiologic survey of the prevalence of herpes simplex virus type 2 infection in the United States. N. Engl. J. Med. 321:7, 1989.

314. Johnston, J., and Overall, J., Jr.: Intravaneous immunoglobulin in disseminated neonatal echovirus 11 infection. Pediatr. Infect. Dis. J. 8:254, 1989.

315. Joshi, W., Escobar, M., Stewart, L., et al.: Fatral influenza A2 virus pneumonia in a newborn infant. Am. J. Dis. Child. 126:839, 1973.

316. Kallasam, C., Brennard, J., and Cameron, A.: Congenital parvovirus B19 infection: Experience of a recent epidemic. Fetal. Diagn. Ther. 16:18, 2001.

317. Kanchanelarp, C., Cheewaruangroi, W., Thaurin, C., et al.: Indication and surgical consideration of coclear implants at Ramathibodi Hospital. J. Med. Assoc. Thai. 89:1171, 2006.

318. Kaplan, M., Klein, S., McPhee, J., et al.: Group B coxsackie infections in infants younger than three months of age: A serious childhood illness. Rev. Infect. Dis. 5:1019, 1983.

319. Kattamis, C., Demetrios, D., and Matsaniotis, N.: Australia antigen and neonatal hepatitis syndrome. Pediatrics 54:157, 1974.

320. Kay, M., Wyllie, R., Deimler, C., et al.: Alpha interferon therapy in children with chronic active hepatitis B and delta virus infection. J. Pediatr. 123:1001, 1993.

321. Kaye, E., and Dooling, E.: Neonatal herpes simplex meningoencephalitis associated with fetal monitor scalp electrodes. Neurology 31:1045, 1981.

322. Kearns, G., Bradley, J., Jacobs, R., et al.: Single dose pharmacokinetics of pleconaril in neonates. Pediatr. Infect. Dis. J. 19:833, 2000.

323. Kenneson, A., and Cannon, M.: Review and metaanalysis of the epidemiology of congenital cytomegalovirus infection. Rev. Med. Virol. 17:253, 2007.

324. Kern, E., Overall, J., Jr., and Glasgow, L.: Herpesvirus hominis infection in newborn mice. I. An experimental model and therapy with iododeoxyuridine. J. Infect. Dis. 128:290, 1973.

325. Khanna, R., and Diamond, D.: HCMV vaccine: Time to look for alternative options. Trends. Mol. Med. 12:26, 2006.

326. Khuroo, M., Kamili, S., and Jameel, S.: Vertical transmission of hepatitis E virus. Lancet 345:1025, 1995.

327. Kibrick, S.: Herpes simplex infection at term: What to do with mother, newborn, and nursery personnel. J. A. M. A. 243:157, 1980.

328. Kilroy, A., Schaffner, W., Fleet, W., Jr., et al: Two syndromes following rubella immunization: Clinical observations and epidemiological studies. J. A. M. A. 214:2287, 1980.

329. Kim, S., Chung, E., Hodinka, R., et al.: Immunogenicity of hepatitis B vaccine in preterm infants. Pediatrics 99:534, 1997.

330. Kimberlin, D., Acosta, E., Sanchez, P., et al.: Pharmacokinetic and pharmacodynamic assessment of oral valganciclovir in the treatment of symptomatic congenital CMV disease. J. Infect. Dis. 197:836-845, 2008.

331. Kimberlin, D.: Herpes simplex virus infection in the newborn. Semin. Perinatol. 31:19, 2007.

332. Kimberlin, D., Lakeman, F., Arvin, A., et al.: Application of the polymerase chain reaction to the diagnosis and management of neonatal herpes simplex virus disease. J. Infect. Dis. 174:1162, 1996.

333. Kimberlin, D., Lin, C.-Y., Jacobs, R., et al.: Natural history of neonatal herpes simplex virus infections in the acyclovir era. Pediatrics 108:223, 2001.

334. Kimberlin, D., Lin, C.-Y., Jacobs, R., et al.: Safety and efficacy of high-dose intravenous acyclovir in the management of neonatal herpes simplex virus infections. Pediatrics 108:230, 2001.

335. Kimberlin, D., Lin, C.-Y., Sanchez, P. J., et al.: Effect of ganciclovir therapy on hearing in symptomatic congenital cytomegalovirus disease involving the central nervous system: A randomized controlled trial. J Pediatr 143:16, 2003.

336. Kimberlin, D., Powell, D., Gruber, W., et al.: Administration of oral acyclovir suppressive therapy after neonatal herpes simplex virus disease limited to the skin, eyes, and mouth: Results of a phase I/II trial. Pediatr. Infect. Dis. J. 15:247, 1996.

337. Kimura, H., Futamara, M., Kito, H., et al.: Detection of viral DNA in neonatal herpes simplex virus infections: Frequent and prolonged presence in serum and cerebrospinal fluid. J. Infect. Dis. 164:289, 1991.

338. Kinney, J., Anderson, L., Farrar, J., et al.: Risk of adverse outcomes of pregnancy after human parvovirus B19 infection. J. Infect. Dis. 157:663, 1988.

339. Kleiman, M., Schreiner, R., Eitzen, H., et al.: Oral herpesvirus infection in nursery personnel: Infection control policy. Pediatrics 70:609, 1982.

340. Klock, L., and Rachelefsky, G.: Failure of rubella herd immunity during an epidemic. N. Engl. J. Med. 288:69, 1973.

341. Knox, G., Pass, R., Reynolds, D., et al.: Comparative prevalence of subclinical cytomegalovirus and herpes simplex virus infections in the genital and urinary tracts of low-income, urban women. J. Infect. Dis. 140:419, 1979.

342. Koch, W., and Adler, S.: Human parvovirus B19 infections in women of childbearing age and within families. Pediatr. Infect. Dis. J. 8:83, 1989.

343. Koch, W., and Adler, S.: Detection of human parvovirus B19 DNA by using the polymerase chain reaction. J. Clin. Microbiol. 28:65, 1990.

344. Koch, W., Adler, S., and Harger, J.: Intrauterine parvovirus B19 infection may cause an asymptomatic or recurrent postnatal infection. Pediatr. Infect. Dis. J. 12:747, 1993.

345. Koch, W., Harger, J., Barnstein, B., and Adler, S.: Serologic and virologic evidence for frequent intrauterine transmission of human parvovirus B19 with a primary maternal infection during pregnancy. Pediatr. Infect. Dis. J. 17:489, 1998.

346. Koff, R.: Hepatitis B today: Clinical and diagnostic overview. Pediatr. Infect. Dis. J. 12:428, 1993.

347. Kohler, P., Dubois, R., Merrill D, et al: Prevention of chronic neonatal hepatitis B virus infection with antibody to the hepatitis B surface antigen. N. Engl. J. Med. 291:1378, 1974.

348. Komorous, J., Wheeler, C., Briggaman, R., et al.: Intrauterine herpes simplex infections. Arch. Dermatol. 113:918, 1977.

349. Kono, R., Hayakawa, Y., Hibi, M., et al.: Experimental vertical transmission of rubella virus in rabbits. Lancet 1:343, 1969.

350. Koren, G.: Congenital varicella syndrome in the third trimester. Lancet 366:1591, 2005.

351. Korones, S., Ainger, L., Monif, G., et al.: Congenital rubella syndrome: New clinical aspects with recovery of virus from affected infants. J. Pediatr. 67:166, 1965.

352. Korones, S., Ainger, L., Monif, G., et al.: Congenital rubella syndrome: Study of 22 infants. Myocardial damage and other new clinical aspects. Am. J. Dis. Child. 110:434, 1965.

353. Koskimies, O., Lapinleimu, K., and Saxen, L.: Infections and other maternal factors as risk indicators for congenital malformations: A case-control study with paired serum samples. Pediatrics 61:832, 1978.

354. Kovacs, A., Schluchter, M., Easley, K., et al.: Cytomegalovirus infection and HIV-1 disease progression in infants born to HIV-1-infected women. N. Engl. J. Med. 341:77, 1999.

355. Krawczynski, K., and Bradley, D.: Enterically transmitted non-A, non-B hepatitis: Identification of virus-associated antigen in experimentally infected cynomolgus macaques. J. Infect. Dis. 159:1042, 1989.

356. Krawitt, E.: Chronic hepatitis. In Mandell. G., Bennett, J., and Dolin, R. (eds): Principals and Practice of Infectious Diseases. 4th ed. New York, Churchill Livingstone, 1995, pp. 1153-1159.

357. Kraybill, E., Sever, J., Avery, G., et al.: Experimental use of cytosine arabinoside in congenital cytomegalovirus infection. J. Pediatr. 80:485, 1972.

358. Krill, A.: The retinal disease of rubella. Arch. Ophthalmol. 77:445, 1967.

359. Krober, M., Bass, J., Powell, J., et al.: Bacterial and viral pathogens causing fever in infants less than 3 months old. Am. J. Dis. Child. 139:889, 1985.

360. Krous, H., Dietzman, D., and Ray, C.: Fatal infections with echovirus types 6 and 11 in early infancy. Am. J. Dis. Child. *126*:842, 1973.

361. Krugman, S: Viral hepatitis: A, B, C, D and E infection. Pediatr. Rev. *13*:203, 1992.

362. Kulhanjian, J., Soroush, V., Au, D., et al.: Identification of women at unsuspected risk of primary infection with herpes simplex virus during pregnancy. N. Engl. J. Med. *326*:916, 1992.

363. Kumar, M., Dawson, N., McCullough, A., et al.: Should all pregnant women be screened for hepatitis B? Ann. Intern. Med. *107*:273, 1987.

364. Kumar, M., Gold, E., Jacobs, I., et al.: Primary cytomegalovirus infection in adolescent pregnancy. Pediatrics *74*:493, 1984.

365. Kumar, M., Jensen, H., and Dahms, B.: Fatal *Staphylococcal epidermidis* infections in very low-birth-weight infants with cytomegalovirus infection. Pediatrics 76:110, 1985.

366. Kumar, M., Nankervis, G., Cooper, A., et al.: Postnatally acquired cytomegalovirus infections in infants of CMV-excreting mothers. J. Pediatr. *104*:669, 1984.

367. Kumar, M., Nankervis, G., Jacobs, I., et al.: Congenital and postnatally acquired cytomegalovirus infections: Long-term follow-up. J. Pediatr. *104*:674, 1984.

368. Kuo, G., Choo, Q.-L., Alter, H. J., et al.: An assay for circulating antibodies to a major etiologic virus of human non-A, non-B hepatitis. Science *244*:362, 1989.

369. Lagrew, D., Jr., Furlow, T., Harger, W., et al.: Disseminated herpes simplex virus infection in pregnancy: Successful treatment with acyclovir. J. A. M. A. *252*:2058, 1984.

370. Lai, C.-L., Lin, H.-J., Yeoh, E.-K., et al.: Placebo-controlled trial of recombinant α₂-interferon in Chinese HBsAg-carrier children. Lancet *2*:877, 1987.

371. Lake, A., Lauer, B., Clark, J., et al.: Enterovirus infections in neonates. J. Pediatr. *89*:787, 1976.

372. Lakeman, F., and Whitley, R.: Collaborative Antiviral Study Group: Diagnosis of herpes simplex encephalitis: Application of polymerase chain reaction to cerebrospinal fluid from brain-biopsied patients and correlation with disease. National Institute of Allergy and Infectious Diseases. J. Infect. Dis. *171*:857, 1995.

373. Lam, J., McOmish, F., Burns, S., et al.: Infrequent vertical transmission of hepatitis C virus. J. Infect. Dis. *167*:572, 1993.

374. Lamberson, H., Jr., McMillan, J., Weiner, L., et al.: Prevention of transfusion-associated cytomegalovirus (CMV) infection in neonates by screening blood donors for IgM to CMV. J. Infect. Dis. *157*:820, 1988.

375. Lang, D., and Kummer, J.: Cytomegalovirus in semen: Observations in selected populations. J. Infect. Dis. *132*:472, 1975.

376. Lang, D., Kummer, J., and Hartley, D. P.: Cytomegalovirus in semen: Persistence and demonstration in extracellular fluids. N. Engl. J. Med. *291*:121, 1974.

377. Lanzieri, T., Pinto, D., and Prevots, D.: Impact of rubella vaccination strategy on the occurrence of congenital rubella syndrome. J. Pediatr. (Rio J.) *83*:415, 2007.

378. Lapinleimu, K., Cantell, K., Koskimies, O., et al.: Association between maternal herpesvirus infections and congenital malformations. Lancet *1*:1127, 1974.

379. Lapinleimu, K., and Hakulinen, A.: A hospital outbreak caused by echovirus type 11 among newborn infants. Ann. Clin. Res. *4*:183, 1972.

380. Lau, Y., Tam, A., Ng, K., et al.: Response of preterm infants to hepatitis B vaccine. J. Pediatr. *121*:962, 1992.

381. Lee, A., Ip, H., and Wong, V.: Mechanisms of maternal-fetal transmission of hepatitis B virus. J. Infect. Dis. *138*:668, 1978.

382. Lee, G., Hwang, L., Beasley, R., et al.: Immunogenicity of hepatitis B virus vaccine in healthy Chinese neonates. J. Infect. Dis. *148*:526, 1983.

383. Lemon, S.: Type A viral hepatitis: New developments in an old disease. N. Engl. J. Med. *313*:1059, 1985.

384. Lemon, S.: Inactivated hepatitis A vaccines. J. A. M. A. *271*:1363, 1994.

385. Lentz, E., Dock, N., McMahon, C., et al.: Detection of antibody to cytomegalovirus-induced early antigens and comparison with four serologic assays and presence of viruria in blood donors. J. Clin. Microbiol. *26*:133, 1988.

386. Leung, T., Ng, P., Fok, T., et al.: *Pneumocystis carinii* pneumonia in an immunocompetent infant with congenital cytomegalovirus infection. Infection 28:184, 2000.

387. Lewkonia, I., and Jackson, A.: Infantile herpes zoster after intra-uterine exposure to varicella. B. M. J. *3*:149, 1973.

388. Liesanard, C., Donner, C., Brancart, F., et al.: Prenatal diagnosis of congenital CMV infection: Prospective study of 237 pregnancies at risk. Obstet. Gynecol. *95*:881, 2000.

389. Light, I. J.: Postnatal acquisition of herpes simplex by the newborn infant: A review of the literature. Pediatrics *63*:480, 1979.

390. Lin, H.-H., Kao, J.-H., Hsu, H.-Y., et al.: Possible role of high titered maternal viremia in perinatal transmission of hepatitis C virus. J. Infect. Dis. *169*:638, 1994.

391. Lin, H.-H., Kao, J.-H., Hsu, H.-Y., et al.: Absence of infection in breast-fed infants born to hepatitis C virus-infected mothers. J. Pediatr. *126*:589, 1995.

392. Lindquist, J., Plotkin, S., Shaw, L., et al.: Congenital rubella syndrome as a systemic infection: Studies of affected infants born in Philadelphia, U. S. A. B. M. J. 2:1401, 1965.

393. Linnemann, C., Jr., Light, I., Buchman, T., et al.: Transmission of herpes simplex virus type 1 in a nursery for the newborn identification of viral isolates by D.N.A. "fingerprinting." Lancet *1*:964, 1978.

394. Linnemann, C., Jr., Steichen, J., Sherman, W., et al.: Febrile illness in early infancy associated with ECHO virus infection. J. Pediatr. *84*:49, 1974.

395. Lo, K.-J., Tong, M., Chien, M.-C., et al.: The natural course of hepatitis B surface antigen-positive chronic active hepatitis in Taiwan. J. Infect. Dis. *146*:205, 1982.

396. Lo, K., Tsai, Y.-T., Lee, S.-D., et al.: Immunoprophylaxis of infection with hepatitis B virus in infants born to hepatitis B surface antigen-positive carrier mothers. J. Infect. Dis. *152*:817, 1985.

397. Losonsky, G., Wasserman, S., Stephens, I., et al.: Hepatitis B vaccination of premature infants: A reassessment of current recommendations for delayed immunization. Pediatrics *103*:e14, 1999.

398. Macfarlane, D., Boyd, R., Dodrill, C., et al.: Intrauterine rubella, head size, and intellect. Pediatrics 55:797, 1975.

399. Maggiore, G., De Giacomo, C., Marzani, D., et al.: Chronic viral hepatitis B in infancy. J. Pediatr. *103*:749, 1983.

400. Majdji, E., Genbacer, O., Chang, H., et al.: Developmental regulation of hCMV receptors in cytotrophoblasts correlates with distinct replication sites in the placenta. J. Virol. *81*:4701, 2007.

401. Malik, A., Hildebrand, G., Sekhri, R., et al.: Bilateral macular scars following intrauterine HSV2 infection. J. AAPOS *12*:305-306, 2008.

402. Manzini, P., Saracco, G., Cerchier, A., et al.: Human immunodeficiency virus infection as risk factor for mother-to-child hepatitis C virus transmission: Persistence of anti-hepatitis C virus in children is associated with mother's anti-hepatitis C virus immunoblotting pattern. Hepatology *21*:328, 1995.

403. Marier, R., Rodriguez, W., Chloupek, R., et al.: Coxsackievirus B5 infection and aseptic meningitis in neonates and children. Am. J. Dis. Child. *129*:321, 1975.

404. Mark, K., Kim, H., Wald, A., et al.: Targeted prenatal HSV testing: Can we identify women at risk for transmission to the neonate? Am. J. Obstet. Gynecol. *194*:408, 2006.

405. McCracken, G., Jr., and Luby, J.: Cytosine arabinoside in the treatment of congenital cytomegalic inclusion disease. J. Pediatr. *80*:488, 1972.

406. McDonald, J., and Peckham, C.: Gammaglobulin in prevention of rubella and congenital defect: A study of 30,000 pregnancies. B. M. J. 3:633, 1967.

407. McDonald, L., St. Geme, J., Jr., and Arnold, B.: Nosocomial infection with echovirus type 31 in a neonatal intensive care unit. Pediatrics *47*:995, 1971.

408. McKendrick, G., and Raychoudhury, S.: Herpes zoster in childhood. Scand. J. Infect. Dis. *4*:23, 1972.

409. McMahon, B., Alberts, S., Wainwright, R., et al.: Hepatitis B-related sequelae: Prospective study in 1400 hepatitis B surface antigen-positive Alaska native carriers. Arch. Intern. Med. *150*:1051, 1990.

410. McMahon, B., Alward, W., Hall, D., et al.: Acute hepatitis B virus infection: Relation of age to the clinical expression of disease and subsequent development of the carrier state. J. Infect. Dis. *151*:599, 1985.

411. Meine-Jansen, C., Toet, M., Rademaker, C., et al.: Treatment of symptomatic congenital CMV infection with valganciclovir. J. Perinat. Med. *33*:364, 2005.

412. Mellinger, A., Cragan, J., Atkinson, W., et al.: High incidence of congenital rubella syndrome after a rubella outbreak. Pediatr. Infect. Dis. J. *14*:573, 1995.

413. Melnick, J.: Enteroviruses: Polioviruses, coxsackieviruses, echoviruses, and newer enteroviruses. In Fields, B., and Knipe, D. (eds): Virology. 2nd ed. New York, Raven Press, 1990, pp. 549-605.

414. Menser, M., Dods, L., and Harley, J.: A twenty-five year follow-up of congenital rubella. Lancet *2*:1347, 1967.

415. Menser, M., Forrest, J., and Bransby, R.: Rubella infection and diabetes mellitus. Lancet *1*:57, 1978.

416. Menser, M., and Reye, R.: The pathology of congenital rubella: A review written by request. Pathology 6:215, 1974.

417. Meyberg-Solomayer, G., Felim, T., Muller-Harsen, I., et al.: Prenatal ultrasound diagnosis, followup and outcome of congenital varicella syndrome. Fetal. Diagn. Ther. *21*:296, 2006.

418. Mets, M., Barton, I., Khan, A., et al.: Lymphocytic choriomeningitis virus: An underdiagnosed cause of congenital chorioretinitis. Am. J. Ophthal. *130*:209, 2000.

419. Meyers, J.: Congenital varicella in term infants: Risk reconsidered. J. Infect. Dis. *129*:215, 1974.

420. Michaels, M., Greenberg, D., Sabo, D., et al.: Treatment of children with congenital CMV infection with ganciclovir. Pediatr. Infect. Dis. J. *22*:504, 2003.

421. Michaels, M: Treatment of congenital CMV: Where are we now? Expert Rev. Anti. Infect. Ther. *5*:441, 2007.

422. Miller, E., Cradock-Watson, J., and Pollock, T.: Consequences of confirmed maternal rubella at successive stages of pregnancy. Lancet *2*:781, 1982.

423. Miller, E., Cradock-Watson, J., and Ridehalgh, M.: Outcome in newborn babies given anti-varicella-zoster immunoglobulin after perinatal maternal infection with varicella-zoster virus. Lancet *2*:371, 1989.

424. Miller, M., Rabinowitz, M., Frost, J., and Seager, G.: Audiological problems associated with maternal rubella. Laryngoscope *79*:417, 1969.

425. Miller, M., Sunshine, P., and Remington, J.: Quantitation of cord serum IgM and IgA as a screening procedure to detect congenital infection: Results of 5006 infants. J. Pediatr. 75:1287, 1969.

426. Mims, C.: Pathogenesis of viral infections of the fetus. Prog. Med. Virol. *10*:194, 1968.

427. Mitchell, J., and McCall, F.: Transplacental infection by herpes simplex virus. Am. J. Dis. Child. *106*:207, 1963.

428. Modlin, J.: Fatal echovirus 11 disease in premature neonates. Pediatrics *66*:775, 1980.

429. Modlin, J.: Perinatal echovirus infection: Insights from a literature review of 61 cases of serious infection and 16 outbreaks in nurseries. Rev. Infect. Dis. *8*:918, 1986.

430. Modlin, J., and Crumpacker, C.: Coxsackievirus B infection in pregnant mice and transplacental infection of the fetus. Infect. Immunol. *37*:222, 1982.

431. Modlin, J., Herrmann, K., Brandling-Bennett, A., et al.: Risk of congenital abnormality after inadvertent rubella vaccination of pregnant women. N. Engl. J. Med. *294*:972, 1976.

432. Modlin, J., Polk, B., Horton, P., et al.: Perinatal echovirus infection: Risk of transmission during a community outbreak. N. Engl. J. Med. *305*:368, 1981.

433. Moisuk, S., Robson, D., Klass, L., et al.: Outbreak of parainfluenza virus type 3 in an intermediate care neonatal nursery. Pediatr. Infect. Dis. J. *17*:49, 1998.

434. Montgomery, J., Flanders, R., and Yow, M.: Congenital anomalies and herpes-virus infection. Am. J. Dis. Child. *126*:364, 1973.

435. Montgomery, R., Youngblood, L., and Medearis, D., Jr.: Recovery of cytomegalovirus from the cervix in pregnancy. Pediatrics *49*:524, 1972.

436. Morens, D.: Enteroviral disease in early infancy. J. Pediatr. *92*:374, 1978.

437. Moseley, R., Corey, L., Benjamin, D., et al.: Comparison of viral isolation, direct immunofluorescence, and indirect immunoperoxidase techniques for detection of genital herpes simplex virus infection. J. Clin. Microbiol. *13*:913, 1981.

438. Mouly, F., Mirlesse, V., Meritet, J., et al.: Prenatal diagnosis of fetal varicella-zoster virus infection with polymerase chain reaction of amniotic fluid in 107 cases. Am. J. Obstet. Gynecol. *177*:894, 1997.

439. Muller, A., Eis-Hubinger, A., Brandhorst, G., et al.: Oral valganciclovir for symptomatic congenital cytomegalovirus infection in an extremely low birth weight infant. J. Perinatol. *28*:74, 2008.

440. Moxley, K., and Knudtson, E.: Resolution of hydrops secondary to CMV after maternal and fetal treatment with hCMV hyperimmune globulin. Obstet. Gynecol. *111*:524, 2008.

441. Munoz, F., Campbell, J., Atmar, R., et al.: Influenza A virus outbreak in a neonatal intensive care unit. Pediatr. Infect. Dis. J. *18*:811, 1999.

442. Music, S. T., Fine, E. M., and Togo, Y.: Zoster-like disease in the newborn due to herpes-simplex virus. N. Engl. J. Med. *284*:24-26, 1971.

443. Mussi-Pinhata, M., Yamamoto, A., Figueiredo, L., et al.: Congenital and perinatal cytomegalovirus infection in infants born to mothers infected with human immunodeficiency virus. J. Pediatr. *132*:285, 1998.

444. Naeye, R. L.: Cytomegalic inclusion disease: The fetal disorder. Am. J. Clin. Pathol. *47*:738-744, 1967.

445. Naeye, R., and Blanc, W.: Pathogenesis of congenital rubella. J. A. M. A. *194*:1277, 1965.

446. Nagel, H., deHaan, T., Vandenbussche, F., et al.: Long term outcome after fetal transfusion for hydrops associated with parvovirus B19 infection. Obstet. Gynecol. *109*:42, 2007.

447. Nahmias, A., Dowdle, W., Josey, W., et al.: Newborn infection with herpes-virus hominis types 1 and 2. J. Pediatr. *75*:1194, 1969.

448. Nahmias, A., and Hagler, W.: Ocular manifestations of herpes simplex in the newborn (neonatal ocular herpes). Int. Ophthalmol. Clin. *12*:191, 1972.

449. Nahmias, A., Josey, W., and Naib, Z.: Significance of herpes simplex virus infection during pregnancy. Clin. Obstet. Gynecol. *15*:929, 1972.

450. Nahmias, A., Josey, W., Naib, Z., et al.: Perinatal risk associated with maternal genital herpes simplex virus infection. Am. J. Obstet. Gynecol. *110*:825, 1971.

451. Nankervis, G.: Cytomegaloviral infections: Epidemiology, therapy, and prevention. Pediatr. Rev. 7:169, 1985.

452. Nankervis, G., Kumar, M., Cox, F., et al.: A prospective study of maternal cytomegalovirus infection and its effect on the fetus. Am. J. Obstet. Gynecol. *149*:435, 1984.

453. Narkiewicz, M., Smith, D., Silverman, A., et al.: Clearance of chronic hepatitis B virus infection in young children after alpha interferon treatment. J. Pediatr. *127*:815, 1995.

454. National Communicable Disease Center: Rubella Surveillance, June 1969.

455. Nelson, C., Istas, A., Wilkerson, M., and Demmler, G.: PCR detection of cytomegalovirus DNA in serum as a diagnostic test for congenital cytomegalovirus infection. J. Clin. Microbiol. *33*:3317, 1995.

456. Ng, A., Reagan, J., and Yen, S.: Herpes genitalis. Obstet. Gynecol. *36*:645, 1970.

457. Ni, J., Bowles, N., Kim, Y., et al.: Viral infection of the myocardium in endocardial fibroelastosis: Molecular evidence for the role orf mumps virus as etiologic agent. Circulation *95*:133, 1997.

458. Nielsen, C., Hansen, K., Andersen, H., et al.: An enzyme labeled nuclear antigen immunoassay for detection of cytomegalovirus IgM antibodies in human serum: Specific and nonspecific reaction. J. Med. Virol. 7:111, 1987.

459. Nigro, G., Krzysztofiak, A., Gattinara, G., et al.: Rapid progression of HIV disease in children with cytomegalovirus DNAemia. AIDS *10*:1127, 1996.

460. Nigro, G., Scholz, H., and Bartmann, U: Ganciclovir therapy for symptomatic congenital cytomegalovirus infection in infants: A two-regimen experience. J. Pediatr. *124*:318, 1994.

461. Nigro, G., Adler, S., LaTorre, R., et al.: Passive immunization during pregnancy for congenital cytomegalovirus infection. N. Engl. J. Med. *353*:1350, 2005.

462. Nigro, G., Sali, E., Anceschi, M., et al.: Foscarnet therapy for congenital cytomegalovirus liver fibrosis following perinatal ascites. J. Matern. Fetal. Neo. Med. *15*:325, 2004.

463. Nikkels, A., Delbecque, K., Pierard, G., et al.: Distribution of VZV DNA and gene products in tissue of a first trimester fetus. J. Infect. Dis. *191*:540, 2005.

464. Novati, R., Thiers, V., Monforte, A. D., et al.: Mother-to-child transmission of hepatitis C virus detected by nested polymerase chain reaction. J. Infect. Dis. *165*:720, 1992.

465. Noyola, D., Demmler, G., Williamson, W., et al.: Cytomegalovirus urinary excretion and long term outcome in children with congenital cytomegalovirus infection. Congenital CMV Longitudinal Study Group. Pediatr. Infect. Dis. J. *19*:505, 2000.

466. Noyola, D., Demmler, G., Nelson, C., et al.: Early predictors of neurodevelopmental outcome in symptomatic congenital cytomegalovirus infection. J. Pediatr. *138*:325, 2001.

467. Nusbacher, J., Hirschhorn, K., and Cooper, L.: Chromosomal abnormalities in congenital rubella. N. Engl. J. Med. *276*:1409, 1967.

468. Ohto, H., Terazawa, S., Sasaki, N., et al.: Transmission of hepatitis C virus from mothers to infants. N. Engl. J. Med. *330*:744, 1994.

469. Okada, K., Kamiyama, I., Inomata, M., et al.: e Antigen and anti-e in the serum of asymptomatic carrier mothers as indicators of positive and negative transmission of hepatitis B virus to their infants. N. Engl. J. Med. *294*:746, 1976.

470. Okada, K., Yamada, T., Miyakawa, Y., et al.: Hepatitis B surface antigen in the serum of infants after delivery from asymptomatic carrier mothers. J. Pediatr. *87*:360, 1975.

471. O'Learny, D., Kuhn, S., Knis, K., et al.: Birth outcomes following West Nile virus infection of pregnant women in the U.S. 2003-2004. Pediatrics *117*:e537, 2006.

472. Olson, G., Dent, P., Rawls, W., et al.: Abnormalities of in vitro lymphocyte responses during rubella virus infections. J. Exp. Med. *128*:47, 1968.

473. Orenstein, W., Bart, K., Hinman, A., et al.: The opportunity and obligation to eliminate rubella from the United States. J. A. M. A. *251*:1988, 1984.

474. Osamora, T., Mizuta, R., Yoshioka, H., et al.: Isolatin of adenovirus type 11 from the brain of a neonate with pneumonia and encephalitis. Eur. J. Pediatr. 152, 496, 1993.

475. Overall, J., Jr.: Intrauterine virus infections and congenital heart disease. Am. Heart. J. *84*:823, 1972.

476. Overall, J., Jr.: Dermatologic viral diseases. *In* Galasso, G., Merigan, T., and Buchanan, R. (eds.): Antiviral Agents and Viral Diseases of Man. 2nd ed. New York, Raven Press, 1984, pp. 247-312.

477. Overall, J., Jr.: Genital and perinatal herpes simplex virus infections. *In* de la Maza, L., and Peterson, E. (eds): Medical Virology. IV. Hillsdale, NJ, L. Erlbaum Associates, 1985, pp. 253-304.

478. Overall, J., Jr.: Empiric therapy with acyclovir for suspected neonatal herpes simplex infections. Pediatr. Infect. Dis. J. *8*:808, 1989.

479. Overall, J., Jr.: Diagnostic virology. *In* McClatchy, K. (ed.): Clinical Laboratory Medicine. Baltimore, Williams & Wilkins, 1994, pp. 1359-1385.

480. Overall, J., Jr.: Herpes simplex virus infection of the fetus and newborn. Pediatr. Ann. *23*:131, 1994.

481. Overall, J., Jr., Whitley, R., Yeager, A., et al.: Prophylactic or anticipatory antiviral therapy for newborns exposed to herpes simplex infection. Pediatr. Infect. Dis 3:193, 1984.

482. Palacin, P., Castilla, Y., Garzon, P., et al.: Congential rubella syndrome, hyper IgM syndrome and autoimmunity in an 18 year old girl. J. Paediatr. Child. Health *43*:716, 2007.

483. Palano, G., DiPietro, M., Scuderi, A., et al.: Microcephaly due to varicella infection: A case report. Minerva Pediatr. *57*:433, 2005.

484. Palmer, A., Rotbart, H., Tyson, R., et al.: Adverse effects of maternal enterovirus infection on the fetus and placenta. J. Infect. Dis. *176*:1437, 1997.

485. Papaevangelou, G., and Hoofnagle, J.: Transmission of hepatitis B virus infection by asymptomatic chronic HBsAg carrier mothers. Pediatrics *63*:602, 1979.

486. Papaevangelou, G., Hoofnagle, J., and Kremastinou, J.: Transplacental transmission of hepatitis-B virus by symptom-free chronic carrier mothers. Lancet 2:746, 1974.

487. Parvey, L., and Ch'ien, L.: Neonatal herpes simplex virus infection introduced by fetal-monitor scalp electrodes. Pediatrics *65*:1150, 1980.

488. Paryani, S., and Arvin, A.: Intrauterine infection with varicella-zoster virus after maternal varicella. N. Engl. J. Med. *314*:1542, 1986.

489. Paryani, S., Yeager, A., Hosford-Dunn, H., et al.: Sequelae of acquired cytomegalovirus infection in premature and sick term infants. J. Pediatr. *107*:451, 1985.

490. Pass, R., August, A., Dworsky, M., et al.: Cytomegalovirus infection in a daycare center. N. Engl. J. Med. *307*:477, 1982.

491. Pass, R., Little, E., Stagno, S., et al.: Young children as a probable source of maternal and congenital cytomegalovirus infection. N. Engl. J. Med. *316*:1366, 1987.

492. Pass, R., Stagno, S., Myers, G., et al.: Outcome of symptomatic congenital cytomegalovirus infection: Results of long-term longitudinal follow-up. Pediatrics *66*:758, 1980.

493. Pastuszak, A., Levy, M., Schick, B., et al.: Outcome after maternal varicella infection in the first 20 weeks of pregnancy. N. Engl. J. Med. *330*:901, 1994.

494. Patel, D., Butler, J., Feldman, S., et al.: Immunogenicity of hepatitis B vaccine in healthy very low birth weight infants. J. Pediatr. *131*:641, 1997.

495. Peacock, J., Jr., and Sarubbi, F.: Disseminated herpes simplex virus infection during pregnancy. Obstet. Gynecol. *61*(Suppl.):13, 1983.

496. Percivalle, E., Sarasini, A., Torsellini, M., et al.: A comparison of methods for detecting adenovirus type 8 keratoconjunctivitis during a nosocomial outbreak in a neonatal intensive care unit. J. Clin. Virol. *28*:257, 2003.

497. Perrillo, R., Schiff, E., Davis, G., et al.: A randomized, controlled trial of interferon alpha-2b alone and after prednisone withdrawal for the treatment of chronic hepatitis B. N. Engl. J. Med. *323*:295, 1990.

498. Phelan, P., and Campbell, P.: Pulmonary complications of rubella embryopathy. J. Pediatr. *75*:202, 1969.

499. Philip, A. G. S., and Larson, E. J.: Overwhelming neonatal infection with ECHO 19 virus. J. Pediatr. *82*:391-397, 1973.

500. Piedra, P., Kasel, J., Norton, H., et al.: Description of an adenovirus type 8 outbreak in hospitalized neonates born prematurely. Pediatr. Infect. Dis. J. *11*:460, 1992.

501. Pinto, A., Beck, R., and Jadaji, T.: Fatal neonatal pneumonia caused by adenovirus type 35. Report of one case and review of the literature. Arch. Pathol. Lab. Med. *116*:95, 1992.

502. Plager, H., Beebe, R., and Miller, J.: Coxsackie B-5 pericarditis in pregnancy. Arch. Intern. Med. *110*:735, 1962.

503. Plotkin, S.: The history of rubella and rubella vaccination leading to elimination. Clin. Infect. Dis. *43*:S164, 2006.

504. Plotkin, S., Klaus, R., and Whitely, J.: Hypogammaglobulinemia in an infant with congenital rubella syndrome: Failure of 1-adamantanamine to stop virus excretion. J. Pediatr. *69*:1085, 1966.

505. Plotkin, S., Starr, S., and Bryan, C.: In vitro and in vivo responses of cytomegalovirus to acyclovir. Am. J. Med. *73*:257, 1982.

506. Plotkin, S., and Stetler, H.: Treatment of congenital cytomegalic inclusion disease with antiviral agents. Antimicrob. Agents. Chemother. *9*:372, 1969.

507. Polish, L., Gallagher, M., Fields, H., et al.: Delta hepatitis: Molecular biology and clinical and epidemiologic features. Clin. Microbiol. Rev. *6*:211, 1993.

508. Poovorawan, Y., Sanpavat, S., Pongpunlert, W., et al.: Protective efficacy of a recombinant DNA hepatitis B vaccine in neonates of HBe antigen-positive mothers. J. A. M. A. *261*:3278, 1989.

509. Preece, P., Blount, J., Glover, J., et al.: The consequences of primary cytomegalovirus infection in pregnancy. Arch. Dis. Child. *58*:970, 1983.

510. Preece, P., Pearl, K., and Peckham, C.: Congenital cytomegalovirus infection. Arch. Dis. Child. *59*:1120, 1984.

511. Prober, C., Corey, L., Brown, Z., et al.: The management of pregnancies complicated by genital infection with herpes simplex virus. Clin. Infect. Dis. *15*:1031, 1992.

512. Prober, C., Gershon, A., Grose, C., et al.: Consensus: Varicella-zoster infections in pregnancy and the perinatal period. Pediatr. Infect. Dis. J. *9*:865, 1990.

513. Prober, C., Hensleigh, P., Boucher, F., et al.: Use of routine viral cultures at delivery to identify neonates exposed to herpes simplex virus. N. Engl. J. Med. *318*:887, 1988.

514. Public Health Laboratory Service Working Party on Fifth Disease: Prospective study of human parvovirus B19 infection in pregnancy. B. M. J. *300*:1166, 1990.

516. Puchhammer-Stockl, E., Kunz, C., Wagner, G., and Enders, G.: Detection of varicella-zoster virus (VZV) in fetal tissue by polymerase chain reaction. J. Perinat. Med. *22*:65, 1994.

517. Purdham, D., Purdham, P., Wood, B., et al.: Severe echo 19 virus infection in a neonatal unit. Arch. Dis. Child. *51*:634, 1976.

518. Rajasundari, T., Sundaresan, P., Vijayalakshmi, P., et al.: Laboratory confirmation of congenital rubella syndrome in infants: An eye hospital-based investigation. J. Med. Virol. *80*:536, 2008.

519. Randolph, A., Washington, A., and Prober, C.: Cesarean delivery for women presenting with genital herpes lesions: Efficacy, risks, and costs. J. A. M. A. *270*:77, 1993.

520. Ranucci-Weiss, D., Yerpairojkit, B., Bowles, N., et al.: Intrauterine adenoviral infection associated with fetal nonimmune hydrops. Prenat. Diagn. *18*:182, 1998.

521. Rawls, W., and Melnick, J.: Rubella virus carrier cultures derived from congenitally infected infants. J. Exp. Med. *123*:795, 1966.

522. Reddy, U., Baschat, A., Ziatnik, M., et al.: Detection of viral DNA in amniotic fluid: association with fetal malformation and pregnancy abnormalities. Fetal Diagn. Ther. *20*:203, 2005.

523. Reesink, H., Reerink-Brongers, E., Lafeber-Schut, B., et al.: Prevention of chronic HBsAg carrier state in infants of HBsAg-positive mothers by hepatitis B immunoglobulin. Lancet *2*:436, 1979.

524. Reinus, J., Leikin, E., Alter, H., et al.: Failure to detect vertical transmission of hepatitis C virus. Ann. Intern. Med. *117*:881, 1992.

525. Revello, M., Cerna, G.: Diagnosis and management of human CMV infection in the mother, fetus, and newborn infant. Clin. Microbiol. Rev. *15*:680, 2002.

526. Rentz, A., Libbey, J., Fujinami, R., et al.: Investigations of treatment failure in neonatal ECHO 7 infection. Pediatr. Infect. Dis. J. *25*:259, 2006.

527. Reynolds, D., Dean, P., Pass, R., et al.: Specific cell-mediated immunity in children with congenital and neonatal cytomegalovirus infection and their mothers. J. Infect. Dis. *140*:493, 1979.

528. Reynolds, D., Stagno, S., Hosty, T., et al.: Maternal cytomegalovirus excretion and perinatal infection. N. Engl. J. Med. *289*:1, 1973.

529. Reynolds, D., Stagno, S., Reynolds, R., et al.: Perinatal cytomegalovirus infection: Influence of placentally transferred maternal antibody. J. Infect. Dis. *137*:564, 1978.

530. Reynolds, D., Stagno, S., Stubbs, G., et al.: Inapparent congenital cytomegalovirus infection with elevated cord IgM levels. N. Engl. J. Med. *290*:291, 1974.

531. Rittichier, K., Bryan, P., Bassett, K., et al.: Diagnosis and outcomes of enterovirus infections in young infants. Pediatr. Infect. Dis. J. *24*:546, 2005.

532. Robinson, J., Lemay, M., and Vaudry, W. L.: Congenital rubella after anticipated maternal immunity: Two cases and a review of the literature. Pediatr. Infect. Dis. J. *13*:812, 1994.

533. Roizman, B., and Buchman, T.: The molecular epidemiology of herpes simplex viruses. Hosp. Pract. *14*:95, 1979.

534. Rosendahl, C., Kochen, M., Kretschmer, R., et al.: Avoidance of perinatal transmission of hepatitis B virus: Is passive immunisation always necessary? Lancet *1*:1127, 1983.

535. Ross, D., Dollard, S., Victor, M., et al.: The epidemiology and prevention of congenital CMV infection and disease: activities of the CDC. J. Womans Health *15*:224, 2006.

536. Rotbart, H.: Human Enterovirus Infections. Washington, DC, ASM Press, 1995.

537. Rotbart, H., and Webster, A.: Treatment of potentially life-threatening enterovirus infections with pleconaril. Clin. Infect. Dis. *32*:228, 2001.

538. Roudot-Thoraval, F., Pawlotsky, J.-M., Thiers, V., et al.: Lack of mother-to-infant transmission of hepatitis C virus in human immunodeficiency virus-seronegative women: A prospective study with hepatitis C virus RNA testing. Hepatology *17*:772, 1993.

539. Roysh, S., and Murphy, T.: Vaccine Preventable Diseases Table Working Group: Historical comparisons of morbidity and mortality for vaccine-preventable diseases in the U.S. J. A. M. A. *298*:2155, 2007.

540. Rudolph, A., Singleton, E., Rosenberg, H., et al.: Osseous manifestations of the congenital rubella syndrome. Am. J. Dis. Child. *110*:428, 1965.

541. Saigal, S., Lunyk, O., Larke, R., et al.: The outcome in children with congenital cytomegalovirus infection: A longitudinal follow-up study. Am. J. Dis. Child. *136*:896, 1982.

542. Sakaoka, H., Saheki, Y., Uzuki, K., et al.: Two outbreaks of herpes simplex virus type 1 nosocomial infection among newborns. J. Clin. Microbiol. *24*:36, 1986.

543. Sanford, J.: Coxsackievirus and echovirus infections. *In* Hoeprich, P. (ed.): Infectious Diseases. New York, Harper & Row, 1977, pp. 1107-1117.

544. Sauerbrai, A., Muller, D., Eichhorn, U., and Wutzler, P.: Detection of varicella-zoster virus in congenital varicella syndrome: A case report. Obstet. Gynecol. *88*:687, 1996.

545. Sauerbrai, A., Pawlak, J., Luger, C., et al.: Intracerebral varicella zoster virus reactivation in congenital varicella syndrome. Dev. Med. Child. Neurol. 45:837, 2003.

546. Sauerbrai, A., and Wutzler, P.: Neonatal varicella. J. Perinatol. 21:545, 2001.

547. Sawyer, M., Holland, D., Aintablian, N., et al.: Diagnosis of enteroviral central nervous system infection by polymerase chain reaction during a large community outbreak. Pediatr. Infect. Dis. J. *13*:177, 1994.

548. Schauf, V., Strelkauskas, A., and Deveikis, A.: Alteration of lymphocyte sub-populations with cytomegalovirus infection in infancy. Clin. Exp. Immunol. *26*:478, 1976.

549. Schiff, G., Sutherland, J., and Light, I.: Congenital rubella. *In* Thalhammer, O. (ed.): Prenatal Infections. Stuttgart, Germany, Georg Thieme Verlag, 1971, pp. 31-36.

550. Schleiss, M., Aranow, B., and Werger, S.: Cytomegalovirus infection of human syncytiotrophoblast cells strongly interferes with expression of genes involved in placental differentiation and tissue integrity. Pediatr. Res. *61*:565, 2007.

551. Schleiss, M.: Prospects for development and potential impact of a vaccine against congenital CMV infection. J. Pediatr. *151*:564, 2007.

552. Schlesinger, Y., Sawyer, M., and Storch, G.: Enteroviral meningitis in infancy: Potential role for polymerase chain reaction in patient management. Pediatrics *94*:157, 1994.

553. Schild, R., Bald, R., Plath, H., et al.: Intrauterine management of fetal parvovirus B19 infection. Ultrasound Obstet. Gynecol. *13*:161, 199.

554. Schmidt, N., Dennis, J., Devlin, V., et al.: Comparison of direct immunofluorescence and direct immunoperoxidase procedures for detection of herpes simplex virus antigen in lesion specimens. J. Clin. Microbiol. *18*:445, 1983.

555. Schulzke, S., and Buhner, C.: Valganciclovir for treatment of congenital cytomegalovirus infection. Eur. J. Pediatr. *165*:575, 2006.

556. Schulze, A., and Dietzsch, H.: The natural history of varicella embryopathy: A 25-year followup. J. Pediatr. 137:871, 2000.

557. Schulte, D., Corner, J., Erickson, B., et al.: Congenital lymphocytic choriomeningitis virus: An underdiagnosed cause of neonatal hydrocephalus. Pediatr. Infect. Dis. J. *25*:560, 2006.

558. Schwebke, K., Henry, K., Balfour, H., Jr., et al.: Congenital cytomegalovirus infection as a result of nonprimary cytomegalovirus disease in a mother with acquired immunodeficiency syndrome. J. Pediatr. *126*:293-295, 1995.

559. Schweitzer, I. L., Dunn, A. E. G., Peters, R., et al.: Viral hepatitis B in neonates and infants. Am. J. Med. *55*:762, 1973.
560. Schweitzer, I., Mosley, J., Ashcaval, M., et al.: Factors influencing neonatal infection by hepatitis B virus. Gastroenterology *65*:277, 1973.
561. Scott, L.: Perinatal herpes: Current status and obstetric management strategies. Pediatr. Infect. Dis. J. *14*:827, 1995.
562. Scott, L., Hollier, L., McIntire, D., et al.: Acyclovir suppression to prevent recurrent genital herpes at delivery. Infect. Dis. Obstet. Gynecol. *10*:71, 2002.
563. Scott, L., Sánchez, P., Jackson, G., et al.: Acyclovir suppression to prevent cesarean delivery after first-episode genital herpes. Obstet. Gynecol. *87*:69, 1996.
564. Seale, H., Macintyre, C., Dwyer, D., et al.: The changing epidemiology of severe CMV disease in Australia. Human Vaccin. *3*;239, 2007.
565. Sells, C., Carpenter, R., and Ray, C.: Sequelae of central-nervous-system enterovirus infections. N. Engl. J. Med. *293*:1, 1975.
566. Sever, J., Brody, A., Schiff, G., et al.: Rubella epidemic on St. Paul Island in the Pribilofs, 1963. II. Clinical and laboratory findings for the intensive study population. J. A. M. A. *191*:624, 1965.
567. Sever, J., Huebner, R., Castellano, G., et al.: Serologic diagnosis "en masse" with multiple antigens. II. Am. Rev. Respir. Dis. *88*:342, 1963.
568. Sever, J., Nelson, K., and Gilkeson, M.: Rubella epidemic, 1964: Effect on 6000 pregnancies. I. Preliminary clinical and laboratory findings through the neonatal period: A report from the Collaborative Study on Cerebral Palsy. Am. J. Dis. Child. *110*:395, 1965.
569. Sever, J., South, M., and Shaver, K.: Delayed manifestations of congenital rubella. Rev. Infect. Dis. *7*:164, 1985.
570. Sever, J., and White, L.: Intrauterine viral infections. Annu. Rev. Med. *19*:471, 1968.
571. Shackelford, G., and Kirks, D.: Neonatal hepatic calcification secondary to transplacental infection. Radiology *122*:753, 1977.
572. Shapiro, C.: Epidemiology of hepatitis B. Pediatr. Infect. Dis. J. *12*:433, 1993.
573. Sheffield, J., Hill, J., Hollier, L., et al.: Valacyclovir prophylaxis to prevent recurrent herpes at delivery: A randomized clinical trial. Obstet. Gynecol. *108*:141, 2006.
574. Sheffield, J., Hollier, L., Hill, J., et al.: Acyclovir prophylaxis to prevent HSV recurrence at delivery: A systemic review. Obstet. Gynecol. *102*:1396, 2003.
575. Shepp, D., Dandliker, P., and Meyers, J.: Treatment of varicella-zoster virus infection in severely immunocompromised patients: A randomized comparison of acyclovir and vidarabine. N. Engl. J. Med. *314*:208, 1986.
576. Shiraki, K., Yoshihara, N., Kawana, T., et al.: Hepatitis B surface antigen and chronic hepatitis in infants born to asymptomatic carrier mothers. Am. J. Dis. Child. *131*:644, 1977.
577. Shiraki, K., Yoshihara, N., Sakurai, M., et al.: Acute hepatitis B in infants born to carrier mothers with the antibody to hepatitis B e antigen. J. Pediatr. *97*:768, 1980.
578. Shmoys, S., and Kaplan, C.: Parvovirus and pregnancy. Clin. Obstet. Gynecol. *33*:268, 1990.
579. Shyamala, G., Sowmya, P., Madhavan, H., et al.: Relative efficiency of PCR and ELISA in determination of viral etiology in congenital cataracts in infants. J. Postgrad. Med. *54*:17, 2008.
580. Sieber, O., Fulginiti, V., Brazie, J., et al.: In utero infection of the fetus by herpes simplex virus. J. Pediatr. *69*:30, 1966.
581. Siegel, M: Congenital malformations following chickenpox, measles, mumps, and hepatitis: Results of a cohort study. J. A. M. A. *226*:1521, 1973.
582. Siegel, M., and Fuerst, H.: Low birth weight and maternal virus diseases: A prospective study of rubella, measles, mumps, chickenpox, and hepatitis. J. A. M. A. *197*:680, 1966.
583. Siegel, M., Fuerst, H., and Peress, N.: Comparative fetal mortality in maternal virus diseases: A prospective study on rubella, measles, mumps, chickenpox, and hepatitis. N. Engl. J. Med. *274*:768, 1966.
584. Simon, A., Amann, R., Wilkesmann, A.: Eur. J. Pediatr. *166*:1273, 2007.
585. Sinatra, F., Shah, P., Weissman, J., et al.: Perinatal transmitted acute icteric hepatitis B in infants born to hepatitis B surface antigen-positive and anti-hepatitis B e-positive carrier mothers. Pediatrics *70*:557, 1982.
586. Singalavarija, S., Limpongsanvrte, W., Horpoapan, S., et al.: Neonatal varicella: Report of 26 cases. J. Med. Assoc. Thai. *82*:957, 1999.
587. Sizum, J., Soupre, D., Legrand, M., et al.: Neonatal nosocomial respiratory infection with coronaviruses: A prospective study in a neonatal intensive care unit. Acta. Pediatr. *84*:617, 1995.
588. Skinhoj, P., Sardemann, H., Cohn, J., et al.: Hepatitis-associated antigen (HAA) in pregnant women and their newborn infants. Am. J. Dis. Child. *123*:380, 1972.
589. Snider, M., Griesser, C., Noyola, D., et al.: 15 years of the Congenital CMV Disease Registry 1990-2005—targets for treatment and prevention revealed. Pediatric Academic Societies Annual Meeting, Honolulu, Hawaii, May 2-6, 2008.
590. Smets, K., DeCoen, K., Dhooge, I., et al.: Selecting neonates with congenital CMV infection for ganciclovir therapy. Eur. J. Pediatr. *165*:885, 2006.
591. Snydman, D.: Hepatitis in pregnancy. N. Engl. J. Med. *313*:1398, 1985.
592. South, M., Tompkins, W., Morris, C., et al.: Congenital malformation of the central nervous system associated with genital type (type 2) herpesvirus. J. Pediatr. *75*:13, 1969.
593. Spector, S.: Transmission of cytomegalovirus among infants in hospital documented by restriction-endonuclease-digestion analyses. Lancet *1*:378, 1983.
594. Spruance, S., Overall, J., Jr., Kern, E., et al.: The natural history of recurrent herpes simplex labialis: Implications for antiviral therapy. N. Engl. J. Med. *297*:69, 1977.
595. St. Geme, J., Jr., Noren, G., and Adams, P., Jr.: Proposed embryopathic relation between mumps virus and primary endocardial fibroelastosis. N. Engl. J. Med. *275*:339, 1966.
596. Stagno, S.: Cytomegalovirus. *In* Remington, J., and Klein, J. (eds.): Infectious Diseases of the Fetus and Newborn Infant. 5th ed. Philadelphia, W. B. Saunders, 2001, pp. 389-424.
597. Stagno, S., Brasfield, D., Brown, M. C. et al.: Infant pneumonitis associated with cytomegalovirus, *Chlamydia, Pneumocystis* and *Ureaplasma*—a prospective study. Pediatrics *68*:322, 1981.
598. Stagno, S., Pass, R., Cloud, G., et al.: Primary cytomegalovirus infection in pregnancy: Incidence, transmission to fetus, and clinical outcome. J. A. M. A. *256*:1904, 1986.
599. Stagno, S., Pass, R., Dworsky, M., et al.: Congenital and perinatal cytomegalovirus infections. Semin. Perinatol. 7:31, 1983.
600. Stagno, S., Pass, R., Dworsky, M., et al.: Congenital cytomegalovirus infection: The relative importance of primary and recurrent maternal infection. N. Engl. J. Med. *306*:945, 1982.
601. Stagno, S., Pass, R., Thomas, J., et al.: Defects of tooth structure in congenital cytomegalovirus infection. Pediatrics *69*:646, 1982.
602. Stagno, S., Reynolds, D., Amos, C., et al.: Auditory and visual defects resulting from symptomatic and subclinical congenital cytomegalovirus and *Toxoplasma* infections. Pediatrics *59*:669, 1977.
603. Stagno, S., Reynolds, D., Huang, E.-S., et al.: Congenital cytomegalovirus infection: Occurrence in an immune population. N. Engl. J. Med. *296*:1254, 1977.
604. Stagno, S., Reynolds, D., Lakeman, A., et al.: Congenital cytomegalovirus infection: Consecutive occurrence due to viruses with similar antigenic compositions. Pediatrics *52*:788, 1973.
605. Stagno, S., Reynolds, D., Pass, R., et al.: Breast milk and the risk of cytomegalovirus infection. N. Engl. J. Med. *302*:1073, 1980.
606. Stagno, S., Reynolds, D., Tsiantos, A., et al.: Cervical cytomegalovirus excretion in pregnant and nonpregnant women: Suppression in early gestation. J. Infect. Dis. *131*:522, 1975.
607. Stagno, S., Reynolds, D., Tsiantos, A., et al.: Comparative serial virologic and serologic studies of symptomatic and subclinical congenitally and natally acquired cytomegalovirus infections. J. Infect. Dis. *132*:568, 1975.
608. Stagno, S., Tinker, M., Elrod, C., et al.: Immunoglobulin M antibodies detected by enzyme-linked immunosorbent assay and radioimmunoassay in the diagnosis of cytomegalovirus infections in pregnant women and newborn infants. J. Clin. Microbiol. *21*:930, 1985.
609. Stagno, S., Volanakis, J., Reynolds, D., et al.: Immune complexes in congenital and natal cytomegalovirus infections of man. J. Clin. Invest. *60*:838, 1977.
610. Stanberry, L., Floyd-Reising, S., Connelly, B., et al.: Herpes simplex viremia: Report of eight pediatric cases and review of the literature. Clin. Infect. Dis. *18*:401, 1994.
611. Staras, S., Dollard, S., Radford, K., et al.: Seroprevalence of CMV infection in the U.S. 1988-1994. Clin. Infect. Dis. *43*:143, 2006.
612. Starr, J.: Cytomegalovirus infection in pregnancy. N. Engl. J. Med. *282*:50, 1970.
613. Starr, S., Tolpin, M., Friedman, H., et al.: Impaired cellular immunity to cytomegalovirus in congenitally infected children and their mothers. J. Infect. Dis. *140*:500, 1979.
614. Stevens, C.: In utero and perinatal transmission of hepatitis viruses. Pediatr. Ann. 23:152, 1994.
615. Stevens, C., Beasley, R., Tsui, J., et al.: Vertical transmission of hepatitis B antigen in Taiwan. N. Engl. J. Med. *292*:771, 1975.
616. Stevens, C., Taylor, P., Tong, M., et al.: Yeast-recombinant hepatitis B vaccine: Efficacy with hepatitis B immune globulin in prevention of perinatal hepatitis B transmission. J. A. M. A. *257*:2612, 1989.
617. Stevens, C., Toy, P., Taylor, P., et al.: Prospects for control of hepatitis B virus infection: Implications of childhood vaccination and long-term protection. Pediatrics *90*:170, 1992.
618. Stevens, C., Toy, P., Tong, M., et al.: Perinatal hepatitis B virus transmission in the United States: Prevention by passive-active immunization. J. A. M. A. *253*:1740, 1985.
619. Stewart, G., Parkman, P., Hopps, H., et al.: Rubella-virus hemagglutination-inhibition test. N. Engl. J. Med. *276*:554, 1967.
620. Strauss, J., and Bernstein, J.: Neonatal hepatitis in congenital rubella. Arch. Pathol. *86*:317, 1968.
621. Strawn, E., and Scrimenti, R.: Intrauterine herpes simplex infection. Am. J. Obstet. Gynecol. *115*:581, 1973.
622. Sullivan-Bolyai, J., Fife, K., Jacobs, R., et al.: Disseminated neonatal herpes simplex virus type 1 from a maternal breast lesion. Pediatrics *71*:455, 1983.
623. Sullivan-Bolyai, J., Hull, H., Wilson, C., et al.: Neonatal herpes simplex virus infection in King County, Washington: Increasing incidence and epidemiologic correlates. J. A. M. A. *250*:3059, 1983.
624. Suzuki, Y., Toribe, Y., Mogami, Y., et al.: Epilepsy in patients with congenital CMV infection. Brain. Dev. *30*:420-424, 2008.
625. Sun, C., Duara, S.: Fatal adenovirus pneumonia in two newborn infants, one cased caused by adenovirus type 30. Pediatr. Pathol. *4*:247, 1985.

626. Swender, P., Shott, R., and Williams, M.: A community and intensive care nursery outbreak of coxsackievirus B5 meningitis. Am. J. Dis. Child. *127*:42, 1974.

627. Szmuness, W., Harley, E., and Prince, A. M.: Intrafamilial spread of asymptomatic hepatitis B. Am. J. Med. Sci. *270*:292, 1975.

628. Tang, J., Aaron, S., Hesketh, L., et al.: Prenatal diagnosis of congenital rubella infection in the second trimester of pregnancy. Prenat. Diag. *23*:509, 2003.

629. Tanaka-Kitajima, N., Sugaya, N., Futatani, T., et al.: Ganciclovir therapy for congenital CMV infection in 6 infants. Pediatr. Infect. Dis. J. *24*:782, 2005.

630. Tardieu, M., Grospierre, B., Durandy, A., et al.: Circulating immune complexes containing rubella antigens in late-onset rubella syndrome. J. Pediatr. *97*:370, 1980.

631. Taylor, B., Jacobs, R., Baker, R., et al.: Frozen deglycerolyzed blood prevents transfusion-acquired cytomegalovirus infections in neonates. Pediatr. Infect. Dis. *5*:188, 1986.

632. Tejani, N., Klein, S., and Kaplan, M.: Subclinical herpes simplex genitalis infections in the perinatal period. Am. J. Obstet. Gynecol. *135*:547, 1979.

633. Thaler. M., Park, C.-K., Landers, D., et al.: Vertical transmission of hepatitis C virus. Lancet *338*:17, 1991.

634. Ticehurst, J.: Hepatitis E virus. *In* Murray, P., Baron, E., Pfaller, M., et al. (eds.): Manual of Clinical Microbiology. 6th ed. Washington, DC, ASM Press, 1995, pp. 1056-1067.

635. Tondury, G., and Smith, D.: Fetal rubella pathology. J. Pediatr. *68*:867, 1966.

636. Tong, M., and Govindarajan, S.: Primary hepatocellular carcinoma following perinatal transmission of hepatitis B. West. J. Med. *148*:205, 1988.

637. Tong, M., Thursby, M., Lin, J-H. et al.: Studies on the maternal-infant transmission of the hepatitis B virus and HBV infection within families. Prog. Med. Virol. *27*:137, 1981.

638. Torok, T.: Human parvovirus B19 infections in pregnancy. Pediatr. Infect. Dis. J. *9*:772, 1990.

639. Torok, T., Wang, Q.-Y., Gary, G., Jr., et al.: Prenatal diagnosis of intrauterine infection with parvovirus B19 by the polymerase chain reaction technique. J. Infect. Dis. *14*:149, 1992.

640. Torphy, D., Ray, C., McAlister, R., et al.: Herpes simplex virus infection in infants: A spectrum of disease. J. Pediatr. *76*:405, 1970.

641. Towbin, J., Griffin, L., Martin, A., et al.: Intrauterine adenoviral myocarditis presenting as nonimmune hydrops fetalis: Diagnosis by PCR. Pediatr. Infect. Dis. J. *13*:144, 1994.

642. Townsend, J., Baringer, J., Wolinsky, J., et al.: Progressive rubella panencephalitis: Late onset after congenital rubella. N. Engl. J. Med. *292*:990, 1975.

643. Troendle-Atkins, J., Demmler, G., Williamson, W., et al.: Polymerase chain reaction to detect cytomegalovirus DNA in the cerebrospinal fluid of neonates with congenital infection. J. Infect. Dis. *169*:1334, 1994.

644. Troendle-Atkins, J., Demmler, G., Buffone, G.: Rapid diagnosis of HSV encephalitis by using PCR. J. Pediatr. *123*:376, 1993.

645. Tsai, T.: Congenital arbovirus infections: Something new, something old. Pediatrics *117*:936, 2006.

646. Ueda, K., Nishida, Y., Oshima, K., et al.: Congenital rubella syndrome: Correlation of gestational age at time of maternal rubella with type of defect. J. Pediatr. *94*:763, 1979.

646. Vajro, P., Hadchouel, P., Hadchouel, M., et al.: Incidence of cirrhosis in children with chronic hepatitis. J. Pediatr. *117*:392, 1990.

647. Vallejo, J., Englund, J., Garcia-Prats, J., et al.: Ganciclovir treatment of steroid-associated cytomegalovirus disease in a congenitally-infected neonate. Pediatr. Infect. Dis. J. *13*:239, 1994.

648. Valeur-Jensen, A., Pedersen, C., Westergaard, T., et al.: Risk factors for parvovirus B19 infection in pregnancy. J. A. M. A. *281*:1099, 1999.

649. Van der Poel, C., Cuypers, H., and Reesink, H.: Hepatitis C virus 6 years on. Lancet *344*:1475, 1994.

650. Van Dyke, R., and Spector, S.: Transmission of herpes simplex virus type 1 to a newborn infant during endotracheal suctioning for meconium aspiration. Pediatr. Infect. Dis. *3*:153, 1984.

651. Vijayalokshmi, P., Rajasundai, T., Pragad, N., et al.: Prevalence of eye signs in congenital rubella syndrome in South India: A role for population screening. Br. J. Ophthal. *91*:1467, 2007.

652. Velazquez, O., Stetler, H., Avila, C., et al.: Epidemic transmission of enterically transmitted non-A, non-B hepatitis in Mexico, 1986-1987. J. A. M. A. *263*:3281, 1990.

653. Verano, L., and Michalski, F.: Herpes simplex virus antigen direct detection in standard virus transport medium by DuPont Herpchek enzyme-linked immunosorbent assay. J. Clin. Microbiol. *28*:2555, 1990.

654. Verboon-Maclolek, M., Krediet, T., Gerards, L., et al.: Severe neonatal parechovirus infection and similarity with enterovirus infection. Pediatr. Infect. Dis. J. *27*:241, 2008.

654a. Verboon-Maciolek, M., Krediet, T., Gerardis, L., et al.: Clinical and epidemiologic characteristics of viral infections in a neonatal intensive care unit during a 12-year period. Pediatr. Infect. Dis. J. *24*:901, 2005.

655. Verstraelen, H., Vanzieleghem, B., Defoort, P., et al.: Prenatal ultrasound and MRI in fetal varicella syndrome: Correlation with pathologic findings. Prenat. Diagn. *23*:705, 2003.

656. Vochem, M., Hamprecht, K., Jahn, G., et al.: Transmission of cytomegalovirus to preterm infants through breast milk. Pediatr. Infect. Dis. J. *17*:53, 1998.

657. Vontver, L., Hickok, D., Brown, Z., et al.: Recurrent genital herpes simplex virus infection in pregnancy: Infant outcome and frequency of asymptomatic recurrences. Am. J. Obstet. Gynecol. *143*:75, 1982.

658. Vyse, A., and Jin, L.: An RT-PCR assay using oral fluid samples to detect rubella virus genome for epidemiological surveillance. Mol. Cell. Probes *16*:93, 2002.

659. Walter, S., Atkinson, C., Sharland, M., et al.: Congenital CMV: Association between dried blood spot viral load and hearing loss. Arch. Dis. Child. Fetal Neonatal Ed. Nov 26, 2007, Epub ahead of publication.

660. Waner, J., Weller, T., and Kevy, S.: Patterns of cytomegaloviral complement-fixing antibody activity: A longitudinal study of blood donors. J. Infect. Dis. *127*:538, 1973.

661. Wattre, P., Deilde, A., Subtil, D., et al.: A clinical and epidemiological study of human parvovirus B19 infection in fetal hydrops using PCR Southern blot hybridization and chemiluminescence detection. J. Med. Virol. *54*:140, 1998.

662. Weibel, R. E., Stokes, J., Jr., Buynak, E., et al.: Rubella vaccination in adult females. N. Engl. J. Med. *280*:682, 1969.

663. Weil, M., Itabashi, H., Cremer, N., et al.: Chronic progressive panencephalitis due to rubella virus simulating subacute sclerosing panencephalitis. N. Engl. J. Med. *292*:994, 1975.

664. Weinstock, H., Bolan, G., Reingold, A., et al.: Hepatitis C virus infection among patients attending a clinic for sexually transmitted diseases. J. A. M. A. *269*:392, 1993.

665. Wejstal, R., Widell, A., Mansson, A.-S., et al.: Mother-to-infant transmission of hepatitis C virus. Ann. Intern. Med. *117*:887, 1992.

666. Wenner, H.: Viral meningitis. *In* Hoeprich, P. (ed.): Infectious Diseases. New York, Harper & Row, 1977, pp. 881-888.

667. Whitley, R.: Congenital CMV infection: Epidemiology and treatment. Adv. Exp. Med. Biol. *549*:155, 2004.

668. Whitley, R., Arvin, A., Prober, C., et al.: A controlled trial comparing vidarabine with acyclovir in neonatal herpes simplex virus infection. N. Engl. J. Med. *324*:444, 1991.

669. Whitley, R., Arvin, A., Prober, C., et al: Predictors of morbidity and mortality in neonates with herpes simplex virus infections. N. Engl. J. Med. *324*:450, 1991.

670. Whitley, R., Brasfield, D., Reynolds, D., et al.: Protracted pneumonitis in young infants associated with perinatally acquired cytomegaloviral infection. J. Pediatr. *89*:16, 1976.

671. Whitley, R., Cloud, G., Gruber, W., et al.: Ganciclovir treatment of symptomatic congenital cytomegalovirus infection: Results of a phase II study. J. Infect. Dis. *175*:1080, 1997.

672. Whitley, R., Corey, L., Arvin, A., et al.: Changing presentation of herpes simplex virus infection in neonates. J. Infect. Dis. *158*:109, 1988.

673. Whitley, R., Davis, E., Suppapanya, N.: Incidence of neonatal HSV infection in a managed care population. Sex. Trans. Dis. *34*:704, 2007.

674. Whitley, R., and Hutto, C.: Neonatal herpes simplex virus infections. Pediatr. Rev. 7:119, 1985.

675. Whitley, R., Nahmias, A., Visintine, A., et al.: The natural history of herpes simplex virus infection of mother and newborn. Pediatrics *66*:489, 1980.

676. Whitley, R. J., Yeager, A., Kartus, P., et al.: Neonatal herpes simplex virus infection: Follow-up evaluation of vidarabine therapy. Pediatrics *72*:778-785, 1983.

677. Wilfert, C., Thompson, R., Sunder, T., et al.: Longitudinal assessment of children with enteroviral meningitis during the first three months of life. Pediatrics *67*:811, 1981.

678. Williamson, W. D., Demmler, G., Percy, A., et al.: Progressive hearing loss in infants with asymptomatic congenital cytomegalovirus infection. Pediatrics *90*:862, 1992.

679. Williamson, W. D., Desmond, M., LaFevers, N., et al.: Symptomatic congenital cytomegalovirus: Disorders of language, learning, and hearing. Am. J. Dis. Child. *136*:896, 1982.

680. Willmott, F., and Mair, H.: Genital herpesvirus infection in women attending a venereal diseases clinic. Br. J. Vener. Dis. *54*:341, 1978.

681. Witte, J., Karchmer, A., Herrmann, K., et al.: Epidemiology of rubella. Am. J. Dis. Child. *118*:107, 1969.

682. Wittek, A., Yeager, A., Au, D., et al.: Asymptomatic shedding of herpes simplex virus from the cervix and lesion site during pregnancy: Correlation of antepartum shedding with shedding at delivery. Am. J. Dis. Child. *138*:439, 1984.

683. Woernle, C., Anderson, L., Tattersall, P., et al.: Human parvovirus B19 infection during pregnancy. J. Infect. Dis. *156*:17, 1987.

684. Wong, S., Tam, A, Ng, T., et al.: Fatal Coxsackie B1 virus infection in neonates. Pediatr. Infect. Dis. J. *8*:638, 1989.

685. Wong, V., Ip, H., Reesink, H., et al.: Prevention of the HBsAg carrier state in newborn infants of mothers who are chronic carriers of HBsAg and HBeAg by administration of hepatitis-B vaccine and hepatitis-B immunoglobulin. Lancet *1*:921, 1984.

686. Wong, V., Lee, A., and Ip, H.: Transmission of hepatitis B antigens from symptom free carrier mothers to the fetus and the infant. Br. J. Obstet. Gynaecol. *87*:958, 1980.

687. Woo, D., Cummins, M., Davies, P., et al.: Vertical transmission of hepatitis B surface antigen in carrier mothers in two west London hospitals. Arch. Dis. Child. *54*:670, 1979.

688. Wootton, S., Kaplan, S., Perotta, D., et al.: St. Louis encephalitis in early infancy. Pediatr. Infect. Dis. J. *23*:951, 2004.

689. Wright, R., Johnson, D., Neumann, M., et al.: Congenital lymphocytic choriomeningitis virus syndrome: A disease that mimics congenital toxoplasmosis and cytomegalovirus infection. Pediatrics 100:e9-e14, 1997.

690. Wright, R., Perkins, J., Bower, B., et al.: Cirrhosis associated with the Australia antigen in an infant who acquired hepatitis from her mother. B. M. J. 4:719, 1970.

691. Yan, H., Koyano, S., Inami, Y., et al.: Genetic variation in the gB, UL 144 and UL 149 genes of hCMV strains collected from congenital and postnatally infected Japanese children. Arch. Virol. 153:667, 2008.

692. Yeager, A.: Transfusion-acquired cytomegalovirus infection in newborn infants. Am. J. Dis. Child. 128:478, 1974.

693. Yeager, A.: Longitudinal, serological study of cytomegalovirus infections in nurses and in personnel without patient contact. J. Clin. Microbiol. 2:448, 1975.

694. Yeager, A.: Storage and transport of cultures for herpes simplex virus type 2. Am. J. Clin. Pathol. 72:977, 1979.

695. Yeager, A., and Arvin, A.: Reasons for the absence of a history of recurrent genital infections in mothers of neonates infected with herpes simplex virus. Pediatrics 73:188, 1984.

696. Yeager, A., Arvin, A., Urbani, L., et al.: Relationship of antibody to outcome in neonatal herpes simplex virus infections. Infect. Immun. 29:532, 1980.

697. Yeager, A., Grumet, F., Hafleigh, E., et al.: Prevention of transfusion-acquired cytomegalovirus infections in newborn infants. J. Pediatr. 98:281, 1981.

698. Yeager, A., Palumbo, P., Malachowski, N., et al.: Sequelae of maternally derived cytomegalovirus infections in premature infants. J. Pediatr. 102:918, 1983.

699. Yow, M., White, N., Taber, L., et al.: Acquisition of cytomegalovirus infection from birth to 10 years: A longitudinal serologic study. J. Pediatr. 110:37, 1987.

700. Yu, J., Culican, S., and Tychsen, L.: Aicardi-like chorioretinitis and maldevelopment of the corpus callosum in congenital lymphocytic choriomeningitis virus. J. AAPOS 10:58, 2006.

701. Yusuf, K., Soralsham, A., Fonseca, K.: Fatal influenza B virus pneumonia in a preterm neonate: Case report and review of the literature. J. Perinatol. 27:623, 2007.

702. Zachoval, R., Jilg, W., Lorbeer, B., et al.: Passive/active immunization against hepatitis. B. J. Infect. Dis. 150:112, 1984.

703. Zanetti, A., Tanzi, E., Paccagnini, S., et al.: Mother-to-infant transmission of hepatitis C virus. Lancet 345:289, 1995.

704. Zeldis, J., and Crumpacker, C.: Hepatitis. *In* Remington, J., and Klein, J. (eds): Infectious Diseases of the Fetus and Newborn Infant. 4th ed. Philadelphia, W. B. Saunders, 1995, pp. 805-834.

705. Zimmerman, L., and Reef, S.: Incidence of congenital rubella syndrome at a hospital serving predominantly Hispanic population, El Paso, Texas. Pediatrics 107:e40, 2001.

706. Ziring, P. R., Gallo, G., Finegold, M., et al.: Chronic lymphocytic thyroiditis: Identification of rubella virus antigen in the thyroid of a child with congenital rubella. J. Pediatr. 90:419, 1977.

CHAPTER 74

CHLAMYDIA TRACHOMATIS INFECTIONS IN THE NEONATE

Margaret R. Hammerschlag

HISTORY

At the beginning of the 20th century, before expectant mothers began being screened for sexually transmitted diseases (STDs), the term *ophthalmia neonatorum* was, for all practical purposes, synonymous with gonococcal conjunctivitis. As neonatal conjunctivitis came under control with silver nitrate prophylaxis, the importance of another form of ophthalmia neonatorum, *inclusion blennorrhea*, was noted. The relationship between maternal genital infection and conjunctivitis of the newborn associated with inclusion bodies within epithelial cells was established by Lindner, Halbstader, Von Prowazek, and others.[10,29] Respiratory infection in infants caused by *Chlamydia trachomatis* probably was reported first in 1941 by Botsztejn,[5] who described an entity that he called *pertussoid eosinophilic pneumonia*.

EPIDEMIOLOGY

C. trachomatis is the most common sexually transmitted pathogen in the United States.[6] The rate of cervical infection with *C. trachomatis* during pregnancy varies from 1 to 37 percent, with the highest rates occurring in women aged 25 years and younger.

C. trachomatis infection is acquired by the infant from the mother during parturition, as demonstrated in a number of well-controlled prospective studies conducted in the 1970s and 1980s of maternal-infant infection in which infection occurred only in infants born to infected mothers.[11,13,27] No convincing evidence demonstrates horizontal transmission from mother to infant, from other family members to the infant, or from infant to infant after delivery. Infection after cesarean delivery, usually associated with rupture of the membranes, or infection through intact membranes is a rare event but may occur.[3] The overall risk of an infant born to a mother with active chlamydial infection becoming infected at any anatomic site has been reported to be approximately 50 to 75 percent in various studies (Table 74–1).[11,13,27] Infants can be infected at more than one site, including the conjunctiva, nasopharynx, rectum, and vagina. The most frequent clinical manifestation of neonatal chlamydial infection, inclusion conjunctivitis, has been reported to occur in 15 to 37 percent of infants born to mothers with untreated cervical chlamydial infection.[11-13,27] The most frequent site of infection, however, is the nasopharynx, with 78 percent of infected infants having positive nasopharyngeal cultures in one study.[12] Approximately half of infants with inclusion conjunctivitis also will be infected in the nasopharynx. In only a minority of infants with nasopharyngeal

TABLE 74–1 Selected Studies of Perinatal Chlamydial Infection

	Prevalence of Maternal Genital Infection		Proportion of Infants with Chlamydial Infection Born to Infected Mothers				
Author, Year, City	Total	No. Infected (%)	Total	Conjunctivitis (%)	Pneumonia (%)	NP (%)	Rectum/Vagina (%)
Frommell et al., 1979, Denver[11]	340	30 (8.8)	67	39	11	6	NS
Schachter et al., 1986, San Francisco[27]	5531	262 (4.7)	131	17.6	16	11.5	14
Hammerschlag et al., 1989, Brooklyn[13]	4357	341 (7.8)	45	15	1	4	NS

NP, nasopharynx; NS, not studied.

infection does chlamydial pneumonia eventually develop; Hammerschlag and colleagues found that pneumonia subsequently developed in only 4 of 12 (33%) infants with isolated nasopharyngeal infection.[12] The overall risk of pneumonia developing in infants born to chlamydia-positive mothers has been reported to range from 1 to 22 percent.[11,13,27]

Data on the risk of acquiring rectal or vaginal infection are more limited. Bell and colleagues[4] demonstrated that perinatally acquired *C. trachomatis* infection may persist for months to years. Twenty-two infants born to women with culture-documented chlamydial infection were monitored, and positive cultures from the nasopharynx and oropharynx in the infants were detected as late as 28.5 months after birth. Rectal and vaginal infections were asymptomatic and persisted for at least 1 year, which can become an important confounding variable when young children are tested for the presence of *C. trachomatis* during evaluation for suspected sexual abuse.

CONJUNCTIVITIS

C. trachomatis was the most frequent identifiable infectious cause of neonatal conjunctivitis, and conjunctivitis was the major clinical manifestation of neonatal chlamydial infection in the United States in the 1990s.[11,13,27] The introduction of systematic screening and treatment of pregnant women has resulted in a dramatic decrease in the number of perinatal chlamydial infections. However, in countries in which pregnant women are not screened routinely, including many developing countries, *C. trachomatis* remains the most frequent cause of neonatal conjunctivitis.[10-12] The incubation period of *C. trachomatis* conjunctivitis is 5 to 14 days after delivery—or earlier if premature rupture of membranes has occurred. At least 50 percent of infants with chlamydial conjunctivitis also will have nasopharyngeal infection. The manifestation is extremely variable and ranges from mild conjunctivitis with scant mucoid discharge to severe conjunctivitis with copious purulent discharge, chemosis, and pseudomembrane formation. The conjunctiva can be very friable and may bleed when stroked with a swab. Eyelid erythema and edema frequently are present. A Gram-stained conjunctival smear initially may reveal a predominance of polymorphonuclear leukocytes. Chlamydial conjunctivitis needs to be differentiated from gonococcal ophthalmia in some infants, especially those born to mothers who did not receive any prenatal care, had gonorrhea during pregnancy, or abused drugs. An overlap in both incubation periods and clinical findings can occur. Bilateral infections are present in two thirds of cases. A follicular reaction is not seen because infants younger than 3 months old do not have the requisite lymphoid tissue present in the conjunctiva. Though an uncommon finding, chlamydial neonatal conjunctivitis has been noted to induce the long-term sequelae of corneal neovascularization and scarring. However, Hammerschlag and colleagues[12] did not detect micropannus at 1 year of age in seven infants who had culture-documented neonatal *C. trachomatis* conjunctivitis.

PNEUMONIA

As stated previously, approximately 70 percent of infected infants will have positive nasopharyngeal cultures, but the majority of these infections are asymptomatic. Chlamydial pneumonia develops in only approximately 30 percent of infants with nasopharyngeal infection.[12] In infants in whom pneumonia does develop, the manifestations and clinical findings are very characteristic.[1,17,30] The children usually are seen initially when they are between the ages of 4 and 12 weeks. A few cases have been reported in infants as young as 2 weeks of age, but no cases have been seen in infants older than 4 months. The infants frequently have a history of

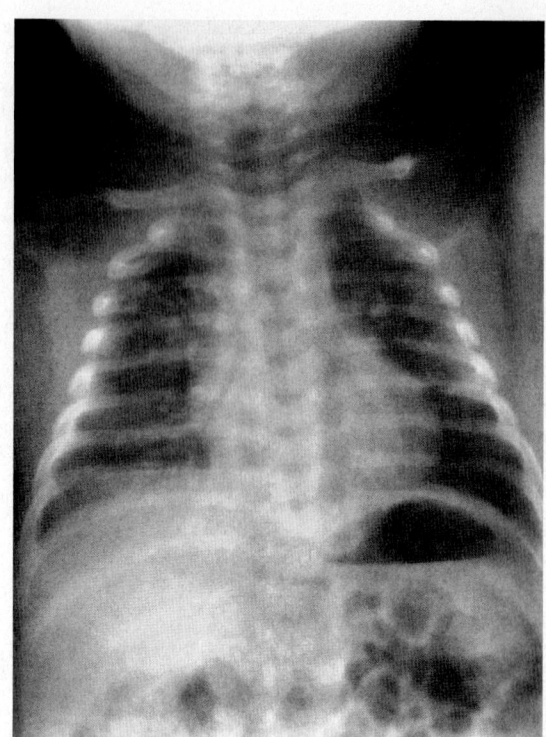

Figure 74–1 Anteroposterior chest radiograph of a severely ill 1-month-old male infant with chlamydial pneumonitis. Diffuse interstitial infiltrates and hyperaeration with a flattened diaphragm are prominent.

cough and congestion with an absence of fever. On physical examination, the infant is tachypneic, and rales are heard on auscultation of the chest; wheezing is a distinctly uncommon finding.[1,17,20] No specific radiographic findings except hyperinflation are found (Fig. 74–1). Significant laboratory findings include peripheral eosinophilia (>300 cells/cm^3) and elevated serum immunoglobulins. If cultures are performed, infants with *C. trachomatis* pneumonia may remain symptomatic and shed the organism from the nasopharynx for protracted periods.[4,12] Generally, infantile pneumonia caused by *C. trachomatis* appears to be self-limited. Most infants can be managed as outpatients, although a few cases of severe disease requiring hospitalization and assisted ventilation have been reported. *C. trachomatis* pneumonia in infants also appears to be associated with few sequelae, although data are limited. Rarely, infants with *C. trachomatis* pneumonia may have concomitant otitis media.[30]

DIAGNOSIS

The diagnosis of neonatal conjunctivitis cannot be made on clinical grounds alone. Significant overlap in both incubation period and clinical findings occurs with infections by other organisms, especially *Neisseria gonorrhoeae*. In a high-risk population, particularly infants born to women with no prenatal care, gonococcal ophthalmia must be considered seriously.[13] The incubation period for gonococcal conjunctivitis is usually 3 to 5 days, but it can be longer. The incubation period for chlamydial conjunctivitis is approximately 5 to 14 days. Most cases will be evident by the time that the infant is 2 weeks of age, which is after the infant leaves the hospital. Epidemiologic clues can help the physician decide whether gonococcal ophthalmia needs to be considered. Hammerschlag and colleagues[13] noted that seven of the eight infants with gonococcal conjunctivitis were born to mothers who had not received any prenatal care. Five of these women were abusers of crack cocaine. Another epidemiologic clue is a history of gonorrhea or other STD during pregnancy.

The clinical manifestation of *C. trachomatis* pneumonitis in infants is fairly characteristic, and one may be able to establish a clinical diagnosis with a degree of certainty.

LABORATORY DIAGNOSIS OF *C. TRACHOMATIS* INFECTION IN INFANTS

The "gold standard" for diagnosis of *C. trachomatis* infection in infants and children remains isolation of *C. trachomatis* by culture from the conjunctiva, nasopharynx, vagina, or rectum. *C. trachomatis* culture has been defined further by the Centers for Disease Control and Prevention (CDC) as isolation of the organism in tissue culture and confirmation by microscopic identification of the characteristic inclusions, preferably by staining with a fluorescein-conjugated, species-specific monoclonal antibody.[6] Enzyme immunoassays (EIAs) have been used by some commercial laboratories as a "screen" for culture confirmation; however, use of EIAs for confirmation of culture results has been associated with a significant number of false-positive results, especially with rectal and vaginal specimens.[7] The CDC has stated strongly that the use of EIAs for this indication is not acceptable.[7] Several nonculture tests, specifically EIAs and direct fluorescent antibody (DFA) tests, have been approved for the diagnosis of chlamydial conjunctivitis in infants. The only EIA and DFA tests still available in the United States are the Pathfinder Chlamydia DFA and EIA Microplate (Bio-Rad Laboratories). These tests appear to perform well with conjunctival specimens, and sensitivities of 90 percent or greater and specificities of 95 percent or greater in comparison to culture have been achieved.[15,24] Unfortunately, their performance with nasopharyngeal specimens has not been as good, with sensitivities ranging from 33 to higher than 90 percent.[15,24] The DNA probe Pace II (GenProbe, San Diego, CA), which is still used in many laboratories, does not have approval for any site in children, including the conjunctiva.

There are currently three Food and Drug Administration (FDA)-approved, commercially available nucleic acid amplification tests (NAATs) for the diagnosis of *C. trachomatis* infection: polymerase chain reaction (PCR) (Amplicor; Roche Molecular Diagnostics, Nutley, NJ), strand displacement amplification (SDA) (ProbeTec; Becton Dickson, Sparks, MD), and transcription-mediated amplification (TMA) (GenProbe). These assays currently have FDA approval for cervical swabs from women, urethral swabs from men, and urine from men and women. Preliminary data suggest that PCR is equivalent to culture for detection of *C. trachomatis* in the conjunctiva and nasopharynx of infants with conjunctivitis.[16] Hammerschlag and associates evaluated Amplicor for the detection of *C. trachomatis* in ocular and nasopharyngeal specimens from 75 infants with suspected chlamydial conjunctivitis.[16] Amplicor was equivalent to culture for eye specimens, with a sensitivity and specificity of 92.3 and 100 percent, respectively. The sensitivity and specificity for nasopharyngeal specimens were 100 and 97.2 percent, respectively. PCR also detected *C. trachomatis* in the urine of 12 of 12 mothers of culture-positive infants.

TREATMENT OF CHLAMYDIAL CONJUNCTIVITIS AND PNEUMONIA IN INFANTS

Oral erythromycin suspension (ethylsuccinate or stearate) (50 mg/kg/day for 14 days) is the therapy of choice for the treatment of chlamydial conjunctivitis and pneumonia in infants.[2,7] It provides better and faster resolution of the conjunctivitis, in addition to treating any concurrent nasopharyngeal infection, which prevents the development of pneumonia. Additional topical

therapy is not needed. The efficacy of this regimen has been reported to range from 80 to 90 percent; however, as many as 20 percent of infants may require another course of therapy.[7,12] Erythromycin given at the same dose for 2 weeks is the treatment of choice for pneumonia and does result in clinical improvement, as well as elimination of the organism from the respiratory tract.

Treatment with oral erythromycin has been associated with hypertrophic pyloric stenosis in infants younger than 6 weeks old who were given the drug for prophylaxis after nursery exposure to pertussis.[9,18] Erythromycin is a motilin receptor agonist. Data on the use of other macrolides, including azithromycin or clarithromycin, for the treatment of neonatal chlamydial infection are limited. No studies of clarithromycin have been published; only one small study evaluated azithromycin and found that a short course of azithromycin suspension (20 mg/kg/day orally, one dose daily for 3 days) was as effective as was 2 weeks of erythromycin for eradication of *C. trachomatis* from the conjunctivae and nasopharynx of infants with conjunctivitis.[14]

PREVENTION AND CONTROL STRATEGIES

Because *C. trachomatis* infections are transmitted vertically from mother to infant during delivery, several possible options for intervention exist. The results of several prospective studies of mother-to-infant transmission of *C. trachomatis* demonstrated that neonatal ocular prophylaxis with silver nitrate, erythromycin, and tetracycline ophthalmic ointment does not prevent the development of chlamydial conjunctivitis.[8,13,20] In 1989, Hammerschlag and colleagues[13] compared silver nitrate, erythromycin, and tetracycline as neonatal ocular prophylaxis in a large urban hospital in Brooklyn, New York. The prophylaxis preparations were given within 30 minutes of birth. Chlamydial conjunctivitis developed in 20 percent (15 of 76) of infants born to infected mothers who received silver nitrate drops, 14 percent (13 of 92) of those who received erythromycin, and 11 percent (7 of 62) of those who received tetracycline. There was no effect on the incidence of nasopharyngeal infection and pneumonia. A subsequent study from Taiwan compared silver nitrate, the two antibiotics, and no prophylaxis.[8] This study, in contrast to previous studies, did not specifically monitor infants born to women with culture-documented chlamydial infection but instead monitored all infants delivered during the period of the study—for 4 weeks or until conjunctivitis developed. Again, no difference occurred in the incidence of neonatal chlamydial conjunctivitis among the four groups. The incidence of chlamydial conjunctivitis in the tetracycline, erythromycin, silver nitrate, and no-prophylaxis groups was 1.3, 1.5, 1.7, and 1.6 percent, respectively. Diagnosis of *C. trachomatis* was by DFA rather than culture. No data were given on the prevalence of maternal infection with *C. trachomatis* or *N. gonorrhoeae*. Differences in the prevalence of maternal infection among the four groups could lead to different rates of *C. trachomatis* conjunctivitis in the infants that were unrelated to prophylaxis. Respiratory infection was not assessed. A similar study from a clinic in Kenya compared povidone-iodine, erythromycin ophthalmic ointment, and silver nitrate drops as neonatal ocular prophylaxis.[19] Povidone-iodine was selected because it has a broad antibacterial spectrum in vitro; it also is antiviral and very inexpensive in comparison to the other prophylaxis agents. As with the study from Taiwan, the pregnant women were not screened for *C. trachomatis* prenatally, and chlamydial conjunctivitis in the infants was diagnosed by DFA. Mothers were told to bring their infants back if conjunctivitis developed. Use of povidone-iodine appeared to result in a 50 percent reduction in *C. trachomatis* conjunctivitis in comparison to silver nitrate (5.5% versus 10.5% of infants) and an approximately 30 percent reduction in comparison to erythromycin

(7.4%). There was no difference in the proportions of infants in whom gonococcal ophthalmia developed. As a result of the structure of the study, one cannot be certain whether every infant in whom conjunctivitis developed returned to the clinic. Because the prevalence of chlamydial infection among the pregnant women in the population was unknown, the investigators did not know how many cases of chlamydial ophthalmia to expect. The CDC does not recommend the use of povidone-iodine because of subsequent data that suggest lower efficacy than antibiotics for prevention of gonococcal ophthalmia.[7] Silver nitrate drops no longer are manufactured in the United States. Another approach that has been considered is oral prophylaxis with erythromycin or azithromycin for infants born to mothers with untreated *C. trachomatis* infection.[25] However, several analyses have found this approach to be very expensive in comparison to watching and treating the infants when they become symptomatic. In addition, there is the issue of compliance, and no data exist on the efficacy of either oral erythromycin or azithromycin for prophylaxis.

The most effective method of control of perinatal *C. trachomatis* infection is screening and treatment of pregnant women. In the 1980s, McMillan and colleagues[22] and Schachter and coworkers[28] reported that treatment of pregnant women infected with *C. trachomatis* with erythromycin resulted in a dramatic decrease in chlamydial infection (conjunctivitis and nasopharyngeal infection) in their infants in comparison to infants born to untreated infected women. The introduction of NAATs for diagnosis and the use of well-tolerated antibiotic regimens, including amoxicillin and single-dose azithromycin, have increased the efficacy of prenatal screening and treatment. This approach has been validated by a dramatic decrease in perinatal chlamydial infection in the United States and persistence of these infections in countries in which screening and treatment of pregnant women are not standard practice, such as the Netherlands, India, and China.[21,23,26,31] Rours and colleagues[26] reported that from 1996 through 2001, *C. trachomatis* was responsible for 61 to 64 percent of cases of neonatal conjunctivitis seen in a large university-affiliated hospital in Rotterdam. Even though the rate of *C. trachomatis* infection among pregnant women in Rotterdam exceeded 5 percent, prenatal screening and treatment are not part of routine prenatal care in the Netherlands.

Reasons for failure of maternal treatment to prevent infantile chlamydial infection include poor compliance and reinfection from untreated or new sexual partners. Even with effective screening, some infected women will be missed, depending on the methods used. Additionally, some women do not seek prenatal care.

REFERENCES

1. Beem, M. O., and Saxon, E. M.: Respiratory-tract colonization and a distinctive pneumonia syndrome in infants infected with *Chlamydia trachomatis*. N. Engl. J. Med. *296*:306-310, 1977.
2. Beem, M. O., Saxon, E., and Tipple, M. A.: Treatment of chlamydia pneumonia of infancy. Pediatrics *63*:198-203, 1979.
3. Bell, T. A., Stamm, W. E., Kuo, C. C., et al.: Risk of perinatal transmission of *Chlamydia trachomatis* by mode of delivery. J. Infect. *29*:165, 1994.
4. Bell, T. A., Stamm, W. E., Wang, S. P., et al.: Chronic *Chlamydia trachomatis* infections in infants. J. A. M. A. *267*:400-402, 1992.
5. Botsztejn, A.: Die pertossoide eosinophile Pneumoniae des Sauglings. Ann. Paediatr. (Basel) *157*:28-46, 1941.
6. Centers for Disease Control and Prevention: Sexually Transmitted Disease Surveillance, 2004. Atlanta, U. S. Department of Health and Human Services, C. D. C., National Center for H. I. V. , S. T. D. , and T. B. Prevention, 2005.
7. Centers for Disease Control and Prevention: Sexually transmitted diseases treatment guidelines—2006. M. M. W. R. Recomm. Rep. *55*(RR-11):1-100, 2006.
8. Chen, J. Y.: Prophylaxis of ophthalmia neonatorum: Comparison of silver nitrate, tetracycline, erythromycin and no prophylaxis. Pediatr. Infect. Dis. J. *12*:1026-1030, 1992.
9. Copper, W. O., Griffin, M. R., Arbogast, P., et al.: Very early exposure to erythromycin and infantile hypertrophic pyloric stenosis. Arch. Pediatr. Adolesc. Med. *156*:64-50, 2002.
10. Darville, T.: *Chlamydia trachomatis* infections in neonates and young children. Semin. Pediatr. Infect. Dis. *16*:235-244, 2005.
11. Frommell, G. T., Rothenberg, R., Wang, S. P., et al.: Chlamydial infection of mothers and their infants. J. Pediatr. *95*:28-32, 1979.
12. Hammerschlag, M. R., Chandler, J. W., Alexander, E. R., et al.: Longitudinal studies of chlamydial infection in the first year of life. Pediatr. Infect. Dis. *1*:395-401, 1982.
13. Hammerschlag, M. R., Cummings, C. C., Roblin, P. M., et al.: Efficacy of neonatal ocular prophylaxis for the prevention of chlamydia and gonococcal conjunctivitis. N. Engl. J. Med. *320*:769-772, 1989.
14. Hammerschlag, M. R., Gelling, M., Roblin, P. M., et al.: Treatment of neonatal chlamydial conjunctivitis with azithromycin. Pediatr. Infect. Dis. J. *17*:1049-1050, 1998.
15. Hammerschlag, M. R., Roblin, P. M., Gelling, M., et al.: Comparison of two enzyme immunoassays to culture for the diagnosis of chlamydial conjunctivitis and respiratory infections in infants. J. Clin. Microbiol. *28*:1725-1727, 1990.
16. Hammerschlag, M. R., Roblin, P. M., Gelling, M., et al.: Use of polymerase chain reaction for the detection of *Chlamydia trachomatis* in ocular and nasopharyngeal specimens from infants with conjunctivitis. Pediatr. Infect. Dis. J. *16*:293-297, 1997.
17. Harrison, H. R., English, M. G., Lee, C. K., et al.: *Chlamydia trachomatis* infant pneumonitis: Comparison with matched controls and other infant pneumonitis. N. Engl. J. Med. *298*:702-708, 1978.
18. Honein, M. A., Paulozzi, L. J., Himelright, I. M., et al.: Infantile hypertrophic pyloric stenosis after pertussis prophylaxis with erythromycin: A case review and cohort study. Lancet *354*:2101-2105, 1999.
19. Isenberg, S. J., Apt, L., and Wood, M. A.: A controlled trial of povidone-iodine as prophylaxis against ophthalmia neonatorum. N. Engl. J. Med. *332*:562-566, 1995.
20. Laga, M., Plummer, F. A., Piot, P., et al.: Prophylaxis of gonococcal and chlamydial ophthalmia neonatorum: A comparison of silver nitrate and tetracycline. N. Engl. J. Med. *318*:653-1149, 1988.
21. Lawton, B., Rose, S., Bromhead, C., et al.: Rates of *Chlamydia trachomatis* testing and chlamydial infection in pregnant women. N. Z. Med. J. *117*:U889, 2004.
22. McMillan, J. A., Weiner, L. B., Lamberson, H. V., et al.: Efficacy of maternal screening and therapy in the prevention of chlamydia infection in the newborn. Infection *13*:263-266, 1985.
23. Mohile, M., Dorari, A. K., Satpathy, G., et al.: Microbiologic study of neonatal conjunctivitis with special reference to *Chlamydia trachomatis*. Indian J. Ophthalmol. *50*:295-299, 2002.
24. Roblin, P. M., Hammerschlag, M. R., Cummings, C. C., et al.: Comparison of two rapid microscopic methods and culture for detection of *Chlamydia trachomatis* in ocular and nasopharyngeal specimens from infants. J. Clin. Microbiol. *27*:968-670, 1989.
25. Rosenman, M. B., Mahon, B. E., Downs, S. M., et al.: Oral erythromycin prophylaxis vs. watchful waiting in caring for newborns exposed to *Chlamydia trachomatis*. Arch. Pediatr. Adolesc. Med. *157*:565-571, 2003.
26. Rours, G. I. J. G., Hammerschlag, M. R., de Faber, J. T. H. N., et al.: *Chlamydia trachomatis* as a cause of neonatal conjunctivitis in Dutch infants. Pediatrics *121*: e321-e326, 2008.
27. Schachter, J., Grossman, M.., Sweet, R. L., et al.: Prospective study of perinatal transmission of *Chlamydia trachomatis*. J. A. M. A. *255*:3374-3377, 1986.
28. Schachter, J., Sweet, R. L., Grossman, M., et al.: Experience with the routine use of erythromycin for chlamydia infections in pregnancy. N. Engl. J. Med. *314*:276-279, 1986.
29. Thygeson, P., and Stone, W.: Epidemiology of inclusion conjunctivitis. Arch. Ophthalmol. *27*:91-122, 1942.
30. Tipple, M. A., Beem, M. O., and Saxon, E. M.: Clinical characteristics of the afebrile pneumonia associated with *Chlamydia trachomatis* infection in infants less than 6 months of age. Pediatrics *63*:192-197, 1979.
31. Wu, S. X., Yang, J., and Liu, G.: A clinical study in China of neonatal conjunctivitis caused by *Chlamydia trachomatis*. Clin. Pediatr. (Phila.) *42*:83, 2003.

MYCOPLASMA AND *UREAPLASMA* INFECTIONS OF THE NEONATE

Vladana Milisavljevic ☉ James D. Cherry

Mycoplasmas are the smallest free-living microorganisms and are characterized by lack of a cell wall. *Mycoplasma hominis*, *Ureaplasma urealyticum*, and *Ureaplasma parvum* are the genital mycoplasmas with clinical significance in neonatal disease.[26,62,164] The two *Ureaplasma* spp. were described previously as the two biovars of *Ureaplasma urealyticum*. Biovar 1 is now *U. parvum*, and biovar 2 is *U. urealyticum*.[70,91,92]

EPIDEMIOLOGY

M. hominis and *Ureaplasma* spp. are sexually transmitted organisms that colonize the urogenital tract of women at rates of 20 to 50 percent and 40 to 80 percent, respectively.[18,105,149] Colonization rates are similar in pregnant and nonpregnant women. High rates of colonization have been associated with younger age, lower socioeconomic status, sexual activity with multiple partners, black ethnicity, and use of oral contraceptives.

In general, cervicovaginal colonization with *Ureaplasma* spp. and *M. hominis* during pregnancy is not predictive of adverse outcomes such as premature delivery, low-birth-weight infants, and spontaneous abortion.[29,49,164] High-density genital ureaplasmal colonization, though, has been associated with chorioamnionitis and preterm delivery.[4] Both *Ureaplasma* spp. and *M. hominis* appear to be capable of invading the upper genital tract in a subpopulation of women, as evidenced by their isolation from the endometrium,[95] placenta,[47,94] and amniotic fluid.[21,25,28,51,65,76,152,173,174] *Ureaplasma* spp. have been associated strongly with histologic chorioamnionitis, postpartum fever, and endometritis.[10-12,23,28,29,143] *M. hominis* is a recognized cause of pelvic inflammatory disease, postpartum septicemia, and endometritis,[26,46,84,106,111] and it has been associated with surgical wound infection after cesarean delivery.[100,127] The role of these organisms in causing spontaneous abortion and premature birth, however, remains controversial and currently unproven.[48,164]

TRANSMISSION

Vertical transmission of *Ureaplasma* ssp. and *M. hominis* from a colonized mother to her newborn occurs in utero or during delivery.[6,8,63,132,164] The relative frequency of occurrence at each time point is not fully known. Acquisition of mycoplasmas by newborns can occur at the time of delivery through contact with a colonized birth canal, but they also have been found on the mucosal surfaces of newborns delivered by cesarean section performed before the onset of labor and rupture of amniotic membranes.[135,147] In utero transmission occurs either transplacentally by the hematogenous route or via an ascending intrauterine infection from a colonized maternal genital tract. Mycoplasmas have been isolated from maternal blood at the time of delivery and from umbilical cord blood, amniotic fluid, endometrium, chorioamnion, placenta, and aborted fetal tissue. Specific IgM antibody responses have been detected in neonatal serum. Postpartum or nosocomial transmission probably occurs, but definitive proof is lacking. The idea was suggested by the finding of ureaplasmal colonization in infants at 3 to 4 weeks of age who were not previously shown to be colonized with *Ureaplasma* spp. while in a neonatal intensive care unit (NICU).[135]

The rate of vertical transmission of *Ureaplasma* spp. ranges from 0.9 to 55 percent in full-term infants and 8.5 to 58 percent in preterm infants, depending on the number and type of mucosal surfaces sampled.[8,31,112,132,134,135,147] *M. hominis* has been isolated from the nasopharyngeal aspirates and gastric secretions of 30 to 42 percent[31,32] and 8 percent,[63] respectively, of infants born to colonized mothers. The rate of vertical transmission of *Ureaplasma* spp. is not affected by the method of delivery or the duration of time after rupture of membranes. Vertical transmission is increased significantly in the presence of chorioamnionitis and intraamniotic infection.[43,140] Colonization of newborn infants increases with decreasing gestational age and birth weight,[7] and it is highest in infants weighing less than 1000 g at birth.[135] Female newborns are more likely than are males to be colonized with *Ureaplasma* because the vagina is a common site of colonization.[52,134]

Colonization with *Ureaplasma* persists through early infancy; 68, 33, and 37 percent of full-term newborns colonized in the throat, eye, and vagina, respectively, are still colonized at 3 months of age.[147] However, most of them lose colonization by the time they reach 2 years of age.[52] Among preterm infants, 65 percent remain colonized at the time of discharge from the NICU or at 28 days of life.[135] Overall, the prevalence of ureaplasmal colonization varies from 2 to 86 percent among infants admitted to NICUs, and as many as 14 to 41 percent of infants have endotracheal aspirate cultures positive for *Ureaplasma* spp.[42,45,71,79,119,132]

CLINICAL MANIFESTATIONS

The roles of *Ureaplasma* spp. and *M. hominis* in neonatal disease continue to be investigated and defined. *M. hominis* and *Ureaplasma* spp. have been recovered from the lungs, brain, heart, and viscera of aborted fetuses and stillborn infants, with histologic findings of bronchopneumonia present in the lungs.[101,148] *Ureaplasma* spp. were isolated from blood in as many as 34 percent of infants younger than 34 weeks' gestational age.[117] Twenty-six percent of preterm infants had positive endotracheal aspirate cultures for *Ureaplasma* spp. in one study.[27] Genital mycoplasmas have been also isolated from the blood, urine, cerebrospinal fluid (CSF), and lung tissue of infants with clinical signs of infection. These organisms frequently colonize the mucosal surfaces of newborns,[88,134] and ascribing disease often is difficult. However, isolation from normally sterile body fluids in symptomatic infants has led to the recognition that these organisms are neonatal pathogens.

NEONATAL PNEUMONIA

Fatal neonatal pneumonia in a term infant was documented by isolation of *Ureaplasma* from lung tissue at autopsy, with demonstrated elevated serum IgG and IgM titers to the organism.[125] Afebrile pneumonitis was reported in infants younger than 3 months old.[144] Pneumonia and persistent pulmonary hypertension were documented in three infants from whom *Ureaplasma* spp. were isolated from blood, endotracheal aspirates, pleural fluid, or lung tissue (or any combination of these sites) at autopsy.[161] Cultrera and colleagues[40] reported finding an association between colonization of the lower respiratory tract by *Ureaplasma* spp., particularly by *U. parvum* in preterm newborns, and respiratory distress syndrome. The potential role of *Ureaplasma* in neonatal pneumonia[19,54,60,120] has been strengthened by the demonstration of histologic evidence of pneumonia in the lungs of newborn mice and premature baboons; ureaplasmal isolates were obtained from the pleural fluid, lung biopsy specimens, and lung tissue of these experimental pneumonia models.[26,129,167] Crouse and associates[35] demonstrated that pneumonia is produced in newborn mice, but significantly less often in mice older than 14 days, and is potentiated by oxygen therapy. *Ureaplasma* spp. have been shown to induce ciliostasis and mucosal lesions in human fetal tracheal organ cultures.[26] In addition, *Ureaplasma* can induce the production of alveolar macrophage proinflammatory cytokines in vitro,[96] and both *Ureaplasma* spp. and *M. hominis* stimulate the production of tumor necrosis factor-α (TNF-α) and inducible nitric oxide synthase from murine macrophages.[36] Viscardi and colleagues[157] developed the first juvenile mouse model of *Ureaplasma* pneumonia. Their data suggest that *Ureaplasma* alone may cause limited inflammation and minimal tissue injury in the early phase of infection but may promote a mild chronic inflammatory response in the later phase of infection (days 14 to 28), similar to the process that occurs in human newborns.[153] *M. hominis* also has been associated with pneumonia.[153]

CHRONIC LUNG DISEASE

Isolation of *Ureaplasma* spp. from endotracheal secretions, the nasopharynx, the throat, or gastric aspirates (or any combination of these sites) has been associated with chronic lung disease of prematurity. Development of chronic lung disease was described in low-birth-weight infants whose respiratory tracts were colonized with *Ureaplasma* spp. in the first week of life.*

The results from a meta-analysis performed by Wang and colleagues[172] involving 17 publications supported a significant association between ureaplasmal colonization and the subsequent development of chronic lung disease. Crouse and associates[37,38] noted that infants who weighed 1250 g or less at birth, had respiratory disease, and were colonized with *Ureaplasma* spp. in their tracheal secretions were more likely to have radiographic evidence of more severe pulmonary disease than were infants who were not colonized. These findings were not supported by studies of Cordero and colleagues,[33] who did not detect any specific radiographic abnormalities in 183 infants with a birth weight of 1250 g or less and who had endotracheal colonization with *Ureaplasma* spp., gram-negative cocci, or gram-negative bacilli. However, Ollikainen and associates[118] found that preterm infants colonized with *Ureaplasma* spp. had higher leukocyte counts on the first 2 days of life and that they required high-frequency oscillatory ventilation more often than did those not colonized. In addition, the isolation by Walsh and colleagues[168] of *Ureaplasma* spp. from the lungs of infants with chronic lung disease implies an invasive bacterial process as part of the pathogenesis of lung injury. In a retrospective study of 60 ventilated babies born at less than 30 weeks' gestation, 25 of whom were *Ureaplasma* culture–positive, Theilen and associates[151] found that the ventilated babies with *Ureaplasma* in their tracheal secretions had a different clinical and radiologic course than that of infants who were culture-negative. Specifically, they had less acute lung disease but an earlier onset of chronic lung disease.

In contrast to these studies, Heggie,[71] Da Silva,[42] and Couroucli[34] and their colleagues found no association between *Urea-*

plasma and the development of bronchopulmonary dysplasia (BPD). Bowman and colleagues[16] used erythromycin to treat extremely-low-birth-weight infants colonized with *Ureaplasma* and found no association between the initial colonization and the development of chronic lung disease. They also called attention to the fact that in the study by Heggie and coworkers,[71] a substantial proportion of the colonized infants were treated with erythromycin, which might explain the lack of an association between colonization and subsequent chronic lung disease. In 1997, Van Waarde and associates[155] noted that preterm infants who were at the highest risk for the development of chronic lung disease (i.e., those with the lowest gestational age and birth weight) also were the ones most likely to be colonized with *Ureaplasma* spp. Castro-Alcaraz and coworkers[30] found that a persistently positive colonization pattern, which accounted for 45 percent of the *Ureaplasma*-positive infants, was associated with a significantly increased risk for the development of chronic lung disease.

One theory suggests that *Ureaplasma* is not the primary cause of BPD but that it might be the cause of undetected pneumonia.[24] This pneumonia results in an increased requirement for supplemental oxygen, and BPD is the result of oxygen toxicity caused by the supplemental oxygen therapy. Viscardi and associates,[156] using the preterm baboon model, suggested that a prolonged proinflammatory response initiated by intrauterine *Ureaplasma* infection contributed to the early development of fibrosis and altered developmental signaling in the immature lung.

The possibility that ureaplasmal colonization of the respiratory tract induces an inflammatory response without direct pulmonary invasion and infection cannot be excluded.[66,98] It has been supported by the finding of elevated levels of TNF-α, interleukin-6 (IL-6), IL-8, and monocyte chemoattractant protein-1 (MCP-1) in the tracheal secretions of colonized infants,[14,26,67,102,146] as well as by elevated white blood cell counts and eosinophilia in infants whose respiratory tract is colonized by *Ureaplasma* spp.[114,118,121] The contribution of *U. urealyticum* and *U. parvum* was evaluated by Heggie and colleagues.[71] Both species colonized preterm infants with a birth weight of less than 1500 g; however, no association was seen between endotracheal colonization with either species and the development of chronic lung disease. In a study performed by Katz and colleagues,[83] *U. parvum* was detected more often than was *U. urealyticum*, but they found no significant difference or trend in the prevalence of either species between infants with or without BPD.

In a meta-analysis, Schelonka and colleagues[137] reviewed 36 articles in which cohorts of neonates were screened for the presence of *Ureaplasma* by culture with or without polymerase chain reaction (PCR) and monitored prospectively for the development of BPD. They concluded that colonization with *Ureaplasma* was associated with higher reported rates of BPD. However, the greatest reported effect was seen in the small studies, and, therefore, reporting bias may be partially responsible for the higher rates of BPD in colonized infants.

NEONATAL CENTRAL NERVOUS SYSTEM INFECTIONS

Both *Ureaplasma* spp. and *M. hominis* have been isolated from the CSF of both full-term and preterm infants.* The repeated isolation of these organisms from the CSF of predominantly preterm infants with suspected meningitis and their association with a CSF pleocytosis consisting of polymorphonuclear or mononuclear cells, hypoglycorrhachia, and elevated protein content support their role in causing neonatal meningitis. Waites and

---

*See references 2, 7, 8, 14, 22, 26, 55, 69, 75, 78, 81, 82, 93, 120, 122, 123, 133, 142, 168-170.

*See references 9, 56-58, 73, 74, 87, 103, 107, 109, 139, 141, 145, 154, 162, 165.

colleagues[165] noted hemiplegia, hydrocephalus, and developmental delay in survivors. Isolation of *Ureaplasma* spp. from the CSF of preterm infants also has been associated with severe intraventricular hemorrhage.[3,116,165] However, Likitnukul and associates[97] cultured the CSF and blood of 203 infants with suspected sepsis and failed to isolate *Ureaplasma* spp. Primarily in full-term infants, isolation of *Ureaplasma* spp. and *M. hominis* often has been associated with minimal if any CSF abnormalities, and these infants have done well without receiving specific antimicrobial therapy.[72,109,137,154,162] In such instances, the presence of these organisms remains of unclear clinical significance, and their role in producing disease is questionable.

SYSTEMIC INFECTIONS

Nonimmune hydrops fetalis was reported in a newborn at 32 weeks' gestation in whom *U. urealyticum* was isolated from bronchial secretions and lung and brain tissue at autopsy.[115] *M. hominis* has been associated with neonatal septicemia.[26,153]

OTHER INFECTIONS

Osteomyelitis of the femur was associated with isolation of *Ureaplasma* from the blood of a preterm infant.[59] *Ureaplasma* was recovered from a scalp abscess at the site of an internal fetal electrode monitor.[68] *M. hominis* infections have been noted in association with brain and scalp abscesses, ventriculitis, submandibular adenitis, abscesses of subcutaneous tissue, pericarditis, and conjuctivitis.[1,61,80,108,124,131] The clinical significance of isolation of genital mycoplasmas from urine obtained by suprapubic bladder aspiration in infants remains to be determined.[97] In such instances, analysis of urinary sediment has been normal.

DIAGNOSIS

Because of the frequent colonization of newborn infants with mycoplasmas, an etiologic role for these agents cannot be supported by detection of organisms on mucosal surfaces only. The diagnosis of mycoplasmal infection is made by isolating the organism from a normally sterile body fluid or suppurative focus. Genital mycoplasmas may be isolated on special broth and solid media that are available commercially. Shepard 10B broth and A8 agar have been used successfully for cultivation of both *Ureaplasma* spp. and *M. hominis*.[26] Cultures generally become positive within 2 to 5 days.

Cassell and colleagues[22,26] recommended that mucosal specimens be obtained with a Dacron or calcium alginate swab and be placed in a specific mycoplasmal transport medium such as Shepard 10B broth. Specimens should be refrigerated at 4°C until they are transported to the laboratory and be protected from drying. Alternatively, specimens in appropriate transport media can be frozen at −70°C because both *Ureaplasma* spp. and *M. hominis* are stable for long periods of time under these conditions. Specimens should be diluted serially in 10B broth to at least 10^{-3} (preferably to 10^{-5}) to overcome any potential inhibitory substances or metabolites, and an aliquot of the original sample and dilution should be plated directly onto A8 agar. Body fluids (e.g., blood, CSF, pleural fluid) should be inoculated into 10B broth in an approximate 1:10 ratio (usually 0.1 mL of fluid per 0.9 mL of 10B broth). Blood should be collected free of anticoagulants. Broth cultures and agar plates are incubated under 95 percent nitrogen and 5 percent carbon dioxide. The presence of mycoplasmal growth in 10B medium is indicated by a change in color from yellow to pink, which is caused by an alkaline shift in the media as a result of either the urease activity

of ureaplasmas or arginine hydrolysis by *M. hominis*. Growth of mycoplasmas in broth culture as indicated by a change in color should be confirmed by inoculation of a broth specimen onto A8 agar. Characteristic colonies of *Ureaplasma* spp. and *M. hominis* can be identified readily on A8 agar after 24 to 72 hours of incubation.

Serologic tests have been used to measure antibody to genital mycoplasmas. Such tests include the metabolic inhibition assay, enzyme-linked immunosorbent assay, mycoplasmacidal test, indirect hemagglutination, indirect immunofluorescence, and IgG and IgM immunoblotting.[26,44,53,126] Use of these tests for establishing the diagnosis of mycoplasmal infection in infants remains problematic and is not well established. None is available commercially, and, therefore, diagnosis of newborns relies on culture results.

PCR assays involving the urease gene, 16S RNA genes, and the multiple-banded antigen genes have been used to detect *Ureaplasma* spp. in neonatal clinical specimens.* On endotracheal secretions, Blanchard and associates[15] reported finding a sensitivity of 100 percent and a specificity of 99 percent in comparison to culture. PCR assays using 16S rRNA and ribosomal DNA targets are available for *M. hominis*.[5,64,99] Ultimately, PCR may aid in identifying colonized or infected infants more readily (results available in 1 day) and reliably, given the fastidious nature of these organisms and the scarcity of microbiology laboratories that routinely perform mycoplasmal culture.

TREATMENT

The decision to treat an infant for possible mycoplasmal infection should be based on the clinical picture and culture results. In general, isolation of mycoplasmas from a normally sterile site in an ill neonate is an indication for consideration of treatment. However, no large randomized clinical trials have determined the efficacy of treatment in neonates. Experience on which to base treatment decisions, the choice of drug, and the duration of therapy is very limited.[171]

In a preterm infant with clinical evidence of sepsis or central nervous system disease in whom routine bacterial and viral cultures are sterile and the infant is not responding to antibacterial or antiviral therapy, the presence of mycoplasmal disease should be suspected and appropriate samples obtained for culture of mycoplasmas. Isolation of mycoplasmas from endotracheal secretions is not diagnostic of pneumonia, and most of these infants do not require any antimycoplasmal therapy. However, if pneumonia is suspected and the infant's clinical condition is deteriorating, a trial of therapy may be indicated despite the unknown efficacy of treatment.

Mycoplasmas are not susceptible to the antimicrobial agents routinely used to treat neonatal infections.[17,159,160,163] Because they lack a cell wall, mycoplasmas are insensitive to penicillins, cephalosporins, polymyxins, sulfonamides, and vancomycin. Although they may have moderate sensitivity to the aminoglycosides, the minimal inhibitory concentrations (MICs) of these agents for genital mycoplasmas usually are too high for therapeutic use. The drugs of choice for the treatment of infection caused by *M. hominis* are chloramphenicol, clindamycin, doxycycline, and tetracycline; for the treatment of ureaplasmal infections, erythromycin or other macrolides, doxycycline, tetracycline, and chloramphenicol are recommended.[89,104,159,166] When possible, antibiotic susceptibility testing should be performed on all clinically significant isolates because of the occurrence of multidrug resistance.

M. hominis is resistant to erythromycin, but in *Ureaplasma* spp., high-level resistance to erythromycin (MIC ≥ 32 mg/mL)

---

*See references 5, 6, 15, 41, 98, 99, 110, 128, 138, 150.

is found very infrequently. Cardiac toxicity consisting of acute cardiorespiratory deterioration possibly secondary to cardiac arrhythmias has been reported in neonates treated with intravenous erythromycin lactobionate for presumed ureaplasmal pneumonia.[50] Ototoxicity has been seen in adults but not in neonates.[39] Oral erythromycin has been associated with hypertrophic pyloric stenosis in infants younger than 6 weeks.[77] Although the exact duration of therapy is not known, a 10- to 14-day course seems reasonable when clinical improvement and microbiologic eradication are observed during that period.

Azithromycin and clarithromycin are active in vitro against *Ureaplasma* spp. but not *M. hominis*,[90,130,158] but their use in neonates has not been evaluated thoroughly. When given orally to very-low-birth-weight infants colonized with *Ureaplasma* spp., serum levels of clarithromycin at a dose of 7.5 mg/kg every 12 hours were subtherapeutic.[136] For this reason, a dose of 15 mg/kg every 12 hours is recommended.

PREVENTION

Erythromycin administered between 26 and 35 weeks' gestation to pregnant women colonized with *Ureaplasma* spp. was not effective in reducing adverse outcomes such as preterm delivery, low birth weight, or premature rupture of membranes.[49] In the ORACLE I study,[85] in which the use of broad-spectrum antibiotics was evaluated in mothers with premature rupture of membranes, use of erythromycin was associated with prolongation of pregnancy, reduction in neonatal treatment with surfactant, decrease in oxygen dependence at 28 days of age and older, fewer major cerebral abnormalities on ultrasonography before discharge, and fewer positive blood cultures. The ORACLE II study, which consisted of 6295 women with spontaneous preterm labor, intact membranes, and no evidence of clinical infection, showed that none of the trial antibiotics was associated with a lower rate of the composite primary outcome events than occurred in placebo recipients.[86] Because erythromycin therapy does not eliminate *Ureaplasma* spp. from the lower genital tract, it most likely also does not prevent neonatal ureaplasmal colonization.[113] Its effect on prevention of neonatal disease has not been evaluated fully.[13] Administration of erythromycin to preterm infants whose mothers had *Ureaplasma* spp. in their lower genital tract reduced respiratory tract colonization but did not decrease the duration of supplemental oxygen therapy[82] or chronic lung disease.[16,98] Treating very-low-birth-weight infants who have respiratory tract colonization with *Ureaplasma* spp. to prevent chronic lung disease cannot be recommended at present.[20]

REFERENCES

1. Abdel-Haq, N., Asmar, B., and Brown, W.: *Mycoplasma hominis* scalp abscess in the newborn. Pediatr. Infect. Dis. J. 21:1171-1173, 2002.
2. Abele-Horn, M., Genzel-Boroviczeny, O., Uhlig, T., et al.: *Ureaplasma urealyticum* colonization and bronchopulmonary dysplasia: A comparative prospective multicentre study. Eur. J. Pediatr. 157:1004, 1998.
3. Abele-Horn, M., Peters, J., Genzel-Boroviczeny, O., et al.: Vaginal *Ureaplasma urealyticum* colonization: Influence on pregnancy outcome and neonatal morbidity. Infection 25:286, 1997.
4. Abele-Horn, M., Scholz, M., Wolff, C., et al.: High-density vaginal *Ureaplasma urealyticum* colonization as a risk factor for chorioamnionitis and preterm delivery. Acta Obstet. Gynecol. Scand. 79:973, 2000.
5. Abele-Horn, M., Wolff, C., Dressel, P., et al.: Polymerase chain reaction versus culture for detection of *Ureaplasma urealyticum* and *Mycoplasma hominis* in the urogenital tract of adults and the respiratory tract of newborns. Eur. J. Clin. Microbiol. Infect. Dis. 15:595, 1996.
6. Abele-Horn, M., Wolff, C., Dressel, P., et al.: Association of *Ureaplasma urealyticum* biovars with clinical outcome for neonates, obstetric patients, and gynecological patients with pelvic inflammatory disease. J. Clin. Microbiol. 35:1199, 1997.
7. Agarwal, P., Rajadurai, V. S., Pradeepkumar, V. K., and Tan, K. W.: *Ureaplasma urealyticum* and its association with chronic lung disease in Asian neonates. J. Paediatr. Child Health 36:487, 2000.

8. Alfa, M. J., Embree, J. E., Degagne, P., et al.: Transmission of *Ureaplasma urealyticum* from mothers to full and preterm infants. Pediatr. Infect. Dis. J. 14:341, 1995.
9. Alonso-Vega, C., Wauters, N., Vermeylen, D., et al.: A fatal case of *Mycoplasma hominis* meningoencephalitis in a full-term newborn. J. Clin. Microbiol. 35:286-287, 1997.
10. Andrews, W. W., Hauth J. C., Cliver, S. P., et al.: Randomized clinical trial of extended spectrum antibiotic prophylaxis with coverage for *Ureaplasma urealyticum* to reduce post-cesarean delivery endometritis. Obstet. Gynecol. 101:1183-1189, 2003.
11. Andrews, W., Shah, S., Goldenberg, R., et al.: Post-cesarean endometritis: Role of asymptomatic antenatal colonization of the chorioamnion with *Ureaplasma urealyticum*. Am. J. Obstet. Gynecol. 170:416, 1994.
12. Andrews, W. W., Shah, S. R., Goldenberg, R. L., et al.: Association of post-cesarean delivery endometritis with colonization of the chorioamnion by *Ureaplasma urealyticum*. Obstet. Gynecol. 85:509, 1995.
13. Antsaklis, A., Daskalakis, G., Michalas, S., et al.: Erythromycin treatment for subclinical *Ureaplasma urealyticum* infection in preterm labor. Fetal Diagn. Ther. 12:89, 1997.
14. Baier, R. J., Loggins, J., and Kruger, T. E.: Monocyte chemoattractant protein-1 and interleukin-8 are increased in bronchopulmonary dysplasia: Relation to isolation of *Ureaplasma urealyticum*. J. Invest. Med. 49:362, 2001.
15. Blanchard, A., Hentschel J., Duffy, L., et al.: Detection of *Ureaplasma urealyticum* by polymerase chain reaction in the urogenital tract of adults, in amniotic fluid, and in the respiratory tract of newborns. Clin. Infect. Dis. 17(Suppl. 1):148, 1993.
16. Bowman, E. D., Dharmalingam, A., Fan, W. Q., et al.: Impact of erythromycin on respiratory colonization of *Ureaplasma urealyticum* and the development of chronic lung disease in extremely low birth weight infants. Pediatr. Infect. Dis. J. 17:615, 1998.
17. Braun, P., Klein, J. O., and Rass, E. H.: Susceptibility of *Mycoplasma hominis* and T-strains to 14 antimicrobial agents. Appl. Microbiol. 19:62, 1970.
18. Braun, P., Klein, J. O., Lee, Y. H., et al.: Methodologic investigations and prevalence of genital mycoplasmas in pregnancy. J. Infect. Dis. 121:391, 1970.
19. Brus, F., van Waarde, W. M., Schoots, C., et al.: Fatal ureaplasmal pneumonia and sepsis in a newborn infant. Eur. J. Pediatr. 150:782, 1991.
20. Buhrer, C., Hoehn, T., and Hentschel, J.: Role of erythromycin for treatment of incipient chronic lung disease in preterm infants colonised with *Ureaplasma urealyticum*. Drugs 61:1893, 2001.
21. Caspi, E., Herczeg, E., Solomon, F., et al.: Amnionitis and T strain mycoplasmemia. Am. J. Obstet. Gynecol. 111:1102, 1971.
22. Cassell, G. H., Blanchard, A., Duffy, L., et al.: Mycoplasmas. In Howard B. J., Klaas, J., III, Rubin, S. J., et al. (eds.): Clinical and Pathogenic Microbiology. St. Louis, Mosby–Year Book, 1994, pp. 491-502.
23. Cassell, G. H., Clyde, W. A., Kenny, G. E., et al.: Ureaplasmas of humans with emphasis on maternal and neonatal infections. Pediatr. Infect. Dis. J. 6(Suppl.):221, 1986.
24. Cassell, G. H., Crouse, D. T., Waites, K. B., et al.: Does *Ureaplasma urealyticum* infection cause respiratory disease in newborns? Pediatr. Infect. Dis. J. 7:535-541, 1988.
25. Cassell, G. H., Davis, R. O., Waites, K. B., et al.: Isolation of *Mycoplasma hominis* and *Ureaplasma urealyticum* from amniotic fluid at 16-20 weeks gestation. Potential effect on pregnancy outcome. Sex. Transm. Dis. 10:294, 1983.
26. Cassell, G. H., Waites, K. B., and Crouse, D. T.: Mycoplasmal infections. In Remington, J. S., and Klein, J. O. (eds.): Infectious Diseases of the Fetus and Newborn Infant. 5th ed. Philadelphia, W. B. Saunders, 2001, pp. 733-767.
27. Cassell, G. H., Waites, K. B., Crouse, D. T., et al.: Association of *Ureaplasma urealyticum* infection of the lower respiratory tract with chronic lung disease and death in very low birthweight infants. Lancet 2:240, 1988.
28. Cassell, G. H., Waites, K. R., Gibbs, R. S., et al.: The role of *Ureaplasma urealyticum* in amnionitis. Pediatr. Infect. Dis. J. 5(Suppl.):247, 1986.
29. Cassell, G. H., Waites, K. B., Watson, H. L., et al.: *Ureaplasma urealyticum* intrauterine infection: Role in prematurity and disease in newborns. Clin. Microbiol. Rev. 6:69, 1993.
30. Castro-Alcaraz, S., Greenberg, E. M., Bateman, D. A., et al.: Patterns of colonization with *Ureaplasma urealyticum* during neonatal intensive care unit hospitalizations of very low birth weight infants and the development of chronic lung disease. Pediatrics 110:e45, 2002.
31. Chua, K. R., Ngeow, Y. F., Lim, C. T., et al.: Colonization and transmission of *Ureaplasma urealyticum* and *Mycoplasma hominis* from mothers to full and preterm babies by normal vaginal delivery. Med. J. Malaysia 54:242, 1999.
32. Chua, K. R., Ngeow, Y. F., Ng, K. B., et al.: *Ureaplasma urealyticum* and *Mycoplasma hominis* isolation from cervical secretions of pregnant women and nasopharyngeal secretions of their babies at delivery. Singapore Med. J. 39:300, 1998.
33. Cordero, L., Coley, R. D., Miller, R. L., et al.: Bacterial and *Ureaplasma* colonization of the airway: Radiologic findings in infants with bronchopulmonary dysplasia. J. Perinatol. 17:428, 1997.
34. Coroucli, X. I., Welty, S. E., Ramsay, P. L., et al.: Detection of microorganisms in the tracheal aspirates of preterm infants by polymerase chain reaction: Association of adenovirus infection with bronchopulmonary dysplasia. Pediatr. Res. 47:225-232, 2000.

35. Crouse, D. T., Cassell, G. H., Waites, K. R., et al.: Hyperoxia potentiates *Ureaplasma urealyticum* pneumonia in newborn mice. Infect. Immun. *58*:3487, 1990.

36. Crouse, D. T., English, R. K., Livingston, L., and Meals, E. A.: Genital mycoplasmas stimulate tumor necrosis factor-alpha and inducible nitric oxide synthase production from a murine macrophage cell line. Pediatr. Res. *44*:785, 1998.

37. Crouse, D. T., Odrezin, G. T., Cutter, G. R., et al.: Radiographic changes associated with tracheal isolation of *Ureaplasma urealyticum* from neonates. Clin. Infect. Dis. *17*(Suppl. 1):122-130, 1993.

38. Crouse, D. T., Odrezin, G. T., Cutter, G. R., et al.: Radiographic changes associated with tracheal isolation of *Ureaplasma urealyticum* in a neonatal intensive care population. J. Paediatr. Child Health *29*:295, 1993.

39. Crouse, D. T., Waites, K. R., Geerts, M. H., et al.: Parenteral erythromycin is not associated with hearing loss in preterm infants. Abstract. Clin. Res. *39*:832, 1991.

40. Cultrera, R., Seraceni, S., Germani, R., et al.: Molecular evidence of *Ureaplasma urealyticum* and *Ureaplasma parvum* colonization in preterm infants during respiratory distress syndrome. B. M. C. Infect. Dis. *6*:166, 2006.

41. Cunliffe, N. A., Fergusson, S., Davidson, F., et al.: Comparison of culture with the polymerase chain reaction for detection of *Ureaplasma urealyticum* in endotracheal aspirates of preterm infants. J. Med. Microbiol. *45*:27, 1996.

42. Da Silva, O., Gregson, D., and Hammerberg, O.: Role of *Ureaplasma urealyticum* and *Chlamydia trachomatis* in development of bronchopulmonary dysplasia in very low birth weight infants. Pediatr. Infect. Dis. J. *16*:364, 1997.

43. Dinsmoor, M. J., Ramamurthy, R. S., and Gibbs, R. S.: Transmission of genital mycoplasmas from mother to neonate in women with prolonged membrane rupture. Pediatr. Infect. Dis. J. *8*:483, 1989.

44. Dinsmoor, M. J., Ramaril Urthy, R. S., Cassell, G. H., et al.: Neonatal serologic response at term to the genital mycoplasmas. Pediatr. Infect. Dis. J. *8*:487, 1989.

45. Dyke, M. P., Grauaug, A., Kohan, R., et al.: *Ureaplasma urealyticum* in a neonatal intensive care population. J. Paediatr. Child Health *29*:295, 1993.

46. Edelin, K. C., and McCormack, W. M.: Infection with *Mycoplasma hominis* in postpartum fever. Lancet *2*:1217, 1980.

47. Embree, J. E., Krause, V. W., Embil, J. A., et al.: Placental infection with *Mycoplasma hominis* and *Ureaplasma urealyticum*: Clinical correlation. Obstet. Gynecol. *56*:475, 1980.

48. Eschenbach, D. A.: *Ureaplasma urealyticum* and premature birth. Clin. Infect. Dis. *17*(Suppl. 1):100, 1993.

49. Eschenbach, D. A., Nugent, R. P., Rao, A. V., et al.: A randomized placebo-controlled trial of erythromycin for the treatment of *Ureaplasma urealyticum* to prevent premature delivery. Am. J. Obstet. Gynecol. *164*:734, 1991.

50. Farrar, H. C., Walsh-Sukys, M. C., Pharmd, K. K., et al.: Cardiac toxicity associated with intravenous erythromycin lactobionate: Two case reports and a review of the literature. Pediatr. Infect. Dis. J. *12*:688, 1993.

51. Foulon, W., Naessens, A., Dewaele, M., et al.: Chronic *Ureaplasma urealyticum* amnionitis associated with abruptio placentae. Obstet. Gynecol. *68*:280, 1986.

52. Foy, H. M., Kenny, G. E., Levinsohn, E. M., et al.: Acquisition of mycoplasmata and T-strains during infancy. J. Infect. Dis. *121*:579, 1970.

53. Gallo, D., Dupuis, K. W., Schmidt, N. J., et al.: Broadly reactive immuno-fluorescence test for measurement of immunoglobulin M and G antibodies to *Ureaplasma urealyticum* in infant and adult sera. J. Clin. Microbiol. *17*:614, 1983.

54. Gannon, H.: *Ureaplasma urealyticum* and its role in neonatal lung disease. Neonat. Network *12*:13, 1993.

55. Garland, S. M., and Bowman, E. D.: Role of *Ureaplasma urealyticum* and *Chlamydia trachomatis* in lung disease in low birth weight infants. Pathology *28*:266, 1996.

56. Garland, S., and Murton, L. J.: Neonatal meningitis caused by *Ureaplasma urealyticum*. Pediatr. Infect. Dis. J. *6*:868, 1987.

57. Gewitz, M., Dinwiddle, R., Rees, L., et al.: *Mycoplasma hominis*: A cause of neonatal meningitis. Arch. Dis. Child. *54*:231, 1979.

58. Gilbert, G. L., Law, F., and Macinnes, S. J.: Chronic *Mycoplasma hominis* infection complicating severe intraventricular hemorrhage in a premature neonate. Pediatr. Infect. Dis. *5*:285, 1973.

59. Gjuric, G., Prislin-Muskic, M., Nikolic, E., et al.: *Ureaplasma urealyticum* osteomyelitis in a very low birth weight infant. J. Perinat. Med. *22*:79, 1994.

60. Gjuric, G., Prislin-Muskic, M., Zurga, B., et al.: *Ureaplasma urealyticum* infection in newborns: Three case reports. Eur. J. Pediatr. *152*:599, 1993.

61. Glaser, J. B., Engelbert, M., and Hammerschlag, M.: Scalp abscess associated with *Mycoplasma hominis* infection complicating intrapartum monitoring. Pediatr. Infect. Dis. J. *2*:468, 1983.

62. Glass, J. I., Lefkowitz, E. J., Glass, J. S., et al.: The complete sequence of the mucosal pathogen *Ureaplasma urealyticum*. Nature *407*:757, 2000.

63. Grattard, F., Soleiliac, B., de Barbeyrac, B., et al.: Epidemiologic and molecular investigations of genital mycoplasmas from women and neonates at delivery. Pediatr. Infect. Dis. J. *14*:853, 1995.

64. Grau, O., Kovacic, R., Griffais, R., et al.: Development of PCR-based assays for the detection of two human mollicute species, *Mycoplasma penetrans* and *M. hominis*. Mol. Cell Probes *8*:139-147, 1994.

65. Gray, D. J., Robinson, H. B., Malone, J., et al.: Adverse outcome in pregnancy following amniotic fluid isolation of *Ureaplasma urealyticum*. Prenat. Diagn. *12*:111, 1992.

66. Groneck, P., Goetze-Speer, B., and Speer, C. P.: Inflammatory bronchopulmonary response of preterm infants with microbial colonization of the airways at birth. Arch. Dis. Child. Fetal Neonatal Ed. *74*:F51, 1996.

67. Groneck, P. J., Schmale, V., Soditt, H., et al.: Bronchoalveolar inflammation following airway infection in preterm infants with chronic lung disease. Pediatr. Pulmonol. *31*:331-338, 2001.

68. Hamrick, H. J., and Mangum, M. E.: *Ureaplasma urealyticum* abscess at site of an internal fetal heart rate monitor. Pediatr. Infect. Dis. J. *12*:410, 1993.

69. Hannaford, K., Todd, D. A., Jeffery, H., et al.: Role of *Ureaplasma urealyticum* in lung disease of prematurity. Arch. Dis. Child. Fetal Neonatal Ed. *81*:F162, 1999.

70. Harasawa, R., and Kanamoto, Y.: Differentiation of two biovars of *Ureaplasma urealyticum* based on the 168-238 rRNA intergenic spacer region. J. Clin. Microbiol. *37*:4135, 1999.

71. Heggie, A. D., Bar-Shain, D., Boxerbaum, B., et al.: Identification and quantification of ureaplasmas colonizing the respiratory tract and assessment of their role in the development of chronic lung disease in preterm infants. Pediatr. Infect. Dis. J. *20*:854, 2001.

72. Heggie, A. D., Jacobs, M. R., Butler, V. T., et al.: Frequency and significance of isolation of *Ureaplasma urealyticum* and *Mycoplasma hominis* from cerebrospinal fluid and tracheal aspirate specimens from low birth weight infants. J. Pediatr. *124*:956, 1994.

73. Hentschel, J., Abele-Horn, M., and Peters, J.: *Ureaplasma urealyticum* in the cerebrospinal fluid of a premature infant. Acta Paediatr. *82*:690, 1993.

74. Hjelm, E., Jousell, E., Linglof, T., et al.: Meningitis in a newborn infant caused by *Mycoplasma hominis*. Acta Paediatr. Scand. *68*:415, 1980.

75. Horowitz, S., Landau, D., Shinwell, E. S., et al.: Respiratory tract colonization with *Ureaplasma urealyticum* and bronchopulmonary dysplasia in neonates in southern Israel. Pediatr. Infect. Dis. J. *11*:847, 1992.

76. Horowitz, S., Mazor, M., Romero, R., et al.: Infection of the amniotic cavity with *Ureaplasma urealyticum* in the midtrimester of pregnancy. J. Reprod. Med. *40*:375, 1995.

77. Hypertrophic pyloric stenosis in infants following pertussis prophylaxis with erythromycin—Knoxville, Tennessee, 1999. M. M. W. R Morb. Mortal. Wkly. Rep. *48*(49):1117, 1999.

78. Iles, R., Lyon, A., Ross, P., and McIntosh, N.: Infection with *Ureaplasma urealyticum* and *Mycoplasma hominis* and the development of chronic lung disease in preterm infants. Acta Paediatr. *85*:482, 1996.

79. Izraeli, S., Samra, Z., Sirota, L., et al.: Genital mycoplasmas in preterm infants: Prevalence and clinical significance. Eur. J. Pediatr. *150*:804, 1991.

80. Jones, D. M., and Tobin, B.: Neonatal eye infections due to *Mycoplasma hominis*. B. M. J. *2*:467, 1968.

81. Jonsson, R., Karell, A. C., Ringertz, S., et al.: Neonatal *Ureaplasma urealyticum* colonization and chronic lung disease. Acta Paediatr. *83*:927, 1994.

82. Jonsson, R., Rylander, M., and Faxelius, G.: *Ureaplasma urealyticum*, erythromycin and respiratory morbidity in high-risk preterm neonates. Acta Paediatr. *87*:1079, 1998.

83. Katz, B., Patel, P., Duffy, L., et al.: Characterization of ureaplasmas isolated from preterm infants with and without bronchopulmonary dysplasia. J. Clin. Microbiol. *43*:4852-4854, 2005.

84. Kelly, V. N., Garland, S. M., and Gilbert, G. L.: Isolation of genital mycoplasmas from the blood of neonates and women with pelvic infection using conventional SPS-free blood culture media. Pathology *19*:277, 1987.

85. Kenyon, S. L., Taylor, D. J., and Tarnow-Mordi, W.: Broad-spectrum antibiotics for preterm, prelabour rupture of fetal membranes: The ORACLE I randomised trial. ORACLE Collaborative Group. Lancet *357*:979-988, 2001.

86. Kenyon, S. L., Taylor, D. J., and Tarnow-Mordi, W.: Broad-spectrum antibiotics for spontaneous preterm labour: The ORACLE II randomised trial. ORACLE Collaborative Group. Lancet. *357*:989-994, 2001.

87. Kirk, N., and Kovar, I.: *Mycoplasma hominis* meningitis in a preterm infant. J. Infect. *15*:109, 1987.

88. Klein, J. O., Buckland, D. O., and Finland, M.: Colonization of newborn infants by mycoplasmas. N. Engl. J. Med. *20*:1025, 1969.

89. Knausz, M., Niederland, T., Dosa, E., and Rozgonyi, F.: Meningoencephalitis in a neonate caused by maternal *Mycoplasma hominis* treated successfully with chloramphenicol. J. Med. Microbiol. *51*:187, 2002.

90. Kober, M. R., and Mason, R. A.: Colonization of the female genital tract by resistant *Ureaplasma urealyticum* treated successfully with azithromycin. Clin. Infect. Dis. *27*:401, 1998.

91. Kong, F., James, G., Ma, Z., et al.: Phylogenetic analysis of *Ureaplasma urealyticum*—support for the establishment of a new species, *Ureaplasma parvum*. Int. J. Syst. Bacteriol. *49*:1879, 1999.

92. Kong, F., Ma, Z., James, G., et al.: Species identification and subtyping of *Ureaplasma parvum* and *Ureaplasma urealyticum* using PCR-based assays. J. Clin. Microbiol. *38*:1175, 2000.

93. Kotecha, S., Hodge, R., Schaber, J. A., et al.: Pulmonary *Ureaplasma urealyticum* is associated with the development of acute lung inflammation and chronic lung disease in preterm infants. Pediatr. Res. *55*:61-68, 2004.

94. Kundsin, R. B., Driscoll, S. G., Monson, R. R., et al.: Association of *Ureaplasma urealyticum* in the placenta with perinatal morbidity and mortality. N. Engl. J. Med. *310*:941, 1984.

95. Lamey, J. R, Fay, H. M., and Kenny, G. E.: Infection with *Mycoplasma hominis* and T-strains in the female genital tract. Obstet. Gynecol. *44*:703, 1974.

96. Li, Y. H., Brauner, A., Jonsson, B., et al.: *Ureaplasma urealyticum*–induced production of proinflammatory cytokines by macrophages. Pediatr. Res. *48*:114, 2000.

97. Likitnukul, S., Kusmiesz, H., Nelson, J. D., et al.: Role of genital mycoplasmas in young infants with suspected sepsis. J. Pediatr. *109*:971, 1986.

98. Lyon, A. J., McColm, J., Middlemist, L., et al.: Randomised trial of erythromycin on the development of chronic lung disease in preterm infants. Arch. Dis. Child. Fetal Neonatal Ed. *78*:F10, 1998.

99. Luki, N., Lebel, P., Boucher, M., et al.: Comparison of polymerase chain reaction assay with culture for detection of genital mycoplasmas in perinatal infections. Eur. J. Clin. Microbiol. Infect. Dis. *17*:255, 1998.

100. Maccato, M., Faro, S., and Summers, K. L.: Wound infections after cesarean section with *Mycoplasma hominis* and *Ureaplasma urealyticum*: A report of three cases. Diagn. Microbiol. Infect. Dis. *13*:363, 1990.

101. Madan, E., Meyer, M. P., and Amortegui, A. J.: Isolation of genital mycoplasmas and *Chlamydia trachomatis* in stillborn and neonatal autopsy material. Arch. Pathol. Lab. Med. *112*:749, 1988.

102. Manimtim, W. M., Hasday, J. D., Hester, L., et al.: *Ureaplasma urealyticum* modulates endotoxin-induced cytokine release by human monocytes derived from preterm and term newborns and adults. Infect. Immun. *69*:3906, 2001.

103. Mardh, P. A.: *Mycoplasma hominis* infection of the central nervous system in newborn infants. Sex. Transm. Dis. *10*:332, 1990.

104. Matlow, A., Th'ng, C., Kovach, D., et al.: Susceptibilities of neonatal respiratory isolates of *Ureaplasma urealyticum* to antimicrobial agents. Antimicrob. Agents Chemother. *42*:1290, 1998.

105. McCormack, W. M., Rosner, B., Alpert, S., et al.: Vaginal colonization with *Mycoplasma hominis* and *Ureaplasma urealyticum*. Sex. Transm. Dis. *134*:67, 1986.

106. McCormack, W. M., Rosner, B., Lee, Y. H., et al.: Isolation of genital mycoplasmas from blood obtained shortly after vaginal delivery. Lancet *1*:596, 1975.

107. McDonald, J. C.: *Mycoplasma hominis* meningitis in a premature infant. Pediatr. Infect. Dis. J. *7*:795, 1988.

108. Miller, T. C., Baman, S. I., and Albers, W. H.: Massive pericardial effusion due to *Mycoplasma hominis* in a newborn. Am. J. Dis. Child. *136*:271, 1982.

109. Neal, T. J., Roe, M. F., and Shaw, N. J.: Spontaneously resolving *Ureaplasma urealyticum* meningitis. Eur. J. Pediatr. *153*:342, 1994.

110. Nelson, S., Matlow, A., Johnson, G., et al.: Detection of *Ureaplasma urealyticum* in endotracheal tube aspirates from neonates by PCR. J. Clin. Microbiol. *36*:1236, 1998.

111. Neman-Simha, V., Renaudin, H., de Barbeyrac, B., et al.: Isolation of genital mycoplasmas from blood of febrile obstetrical-gynecologic patients and neonates. Scand. J. Infect. Dis. *24*:317, 1992.

112. Ogasawara, K. K., and Goodwin, T. M.: The efficacy of prophylactic erythromycin in preventing vertical transmission of *Ureaplasma urealyticum*. Am. J. Perinatol. *14*:233, 1997.

113. Ogasawara, K. K., and Goodwin, T. M.: Efficacy of azithromycin in reducing lower genital *Ureaplasma urealyticum* colonization in women at risk for preterm delivery. J. Matern. Fetal Med. *8*:12, 1999.

114. Ohlsson, A., Wang, E., and Vearncombe, M.: Leukocyte counts and colonization with *Ureaplasma urealyticum* in preterm neonates. Clin. Infect. Dis. *17*(Suppl. 1):144, 1993.

115. Ollikainen, J., Hiekkaniemi, H., Korppi, M., et al.: Hydrops fetalis associated with *Ureaplasma urealyticum*. Acta Paediatr. *81*:851, 1992.

116. Ollikainen, J., Hiekkaniemi, H., Korppi, M., et al.: *Ureaplasma urealyticum* cultured from brain tissue of preterm twins who die of intraventricular hemorrhage. Scand. J. Infect. Dis. *25*:528, 1993.

117. Ollikainen, J., Heikkaniemi, H., Korppi, M., et al.: *Ureaplasma urealyticum* infection associated with acute respiratory insufficiency and death in premature infants. J. Pediatr. *122*:756, 1993.

118. Ollikainen, J., Heiskanen-Kosma, T., Korppi, M., et al.: Clinical relevance of *Ureaplasma urealyticum* colonization in preterm infants. Acta Paediatr. *87*:1075, 1998.

119. Ollikainen, J., Korppi, M., Heiskanen-Kosma, T., and Heinonen, K: Chronic lung disease of the newborn is not associated with *Ureaplasma urealyticum*. Pediatr. Pulmonol. *32*:303, 2001.

120. Pacifico, L., Panero, A., Roggini, M., et al.: *Ureaplasma urealyticum* and pulmonary outcome in a neonatal intensive care population. Pediatr. Infect. Dis. J. *16*:579, 1997.

121. Panero, A., Pacifico, L., Rossi, N., et al.: *Ureaplasma urealyticum* as a cause of pneumonia in preterm infants: Analysis of the white cell response. Arch. Dis. Child. Fetal Neonatal Ed. *73*:F37-F40, 1995.

122. Payne, N. R., Steinberg, S., Stefan, H., et al.: New prospective studies of the association of *Ureaplasma urealyticum* colonization and chronic lung disease. Clin. Infect. Dis. *17*(Suppl. 1):117, 1993.

123. Perzigian, R. W., Adams, J. T., Weiner, G. M., et al.: *Ureaplasma urealyticum* and chronic lung disease in very low birth weight infants during the exogenous surfactant era. Pediatr. Infect. Dis. J. *17*:620, 1998.

124. Powell, D. A, Miller, K., and Clyde, W. A., Jr.: Submandibular adenitis in a newborn caused by *Mycoplasma hominis*. Pediatrics *63*:789, 1979.

125. Quinn, P. A., Gillian, J. E., Markestad, T., et al.: Intrauterine infection with *Ureaplasma urealyticum* as a cause of fatal neonatal pneumonia. Pediatr. Infect. Dis. J. *4*:538, 1985.

126. Quinn, P. A., Li, H. C., Th'ng, C., et al.: Serological response to *Ureaplasma urealyticum* in the neonate. Clin. Infect. Dis. *17*(Suppl. 1):136, 1993.

127. Roberts, S., Maccato, M., Faro, S., et al.: The microbiology of postcesarean wound morbidity. Obstet. Gynecol. *81*:383, 1993.

128. Robertson, J. A., Vekris, A., Bebear, C., et al.: Polymerase chain reaction using 16S rRNA gene sequences distinguishes the two biovars of *Ureaplasma urealyticum*. J. Clin. Microbiol. *31*:824-830, 1993.

129. Rudd, P. T., Cassell, G. H., Waites, K. R., et al.: Experimental production of *Ureaplasma urealyticum* pneumonia and demonstration of age-related susceptibility. Infect. Immun. *57*:918, 1989.

130. Rylander, M., and Hallander, H. O.: In vitro comparison of the activity of doxycycline, tetracycline, erythromycin and a new macrolide, CP 62993, against *Mycoplasma pneumoniae*, *Mycoplasma hominis* and *Ureaplasma urealyticum*. Scand. J. Infect. Dis. Suppl. *53*:12-17, 1988.

131. Sacker, I., and Brunnell, P. A.: Abscess in newborn infants caused by *Mycoplasma*. Pediatrics *46*:303, 1970.

132. Sanchez, P. J.: Perinatal transmission of *Ureaplasma urealyticum*: Current concepts based on review of the literature. Clin. Infect. Dis. *17*(Suppl. 1):107, 1993.

133. Sanchez, P. J., and Regan, J. A.: *Ureaplasma urealyticum* colonization and chronic lung disease in low birth weight infants. Pediatr. Infect. Dis. J. *78*:542, 1988.

134. Sanchez, P., and Regan, J. A.: Vertical transmission of *Ureaplasma urealyticum* in full term infants. Pediatr. Infect. Dis. J. *6*:825, 1988.

135. Sanchez, P. J., and Regan, J. A.: Vertical transmission of *Ureaplasma urealyticum* in preterm infants. Pediatr. Infect. Dis. J. *9*:398, 1990.

136. Sanchez, P. J., Zeray, F., Priest, C., et al.: Pharmacokinetic analysis of clarithromycin in very-low-birth-weight infants colonized with *Ureaplasma urealyticum*. Abstract 110. Poster presented at the 37th Interscience Conference on Antimicrobial Agents and Chemotherapy, September 28-October 1, 1997, Toronto.

137. Schelonka, R., Katz, B., Waites, K. B., et al.: Critical appraisal of the role of *Ureaplasma* in the development of bronchopulmonary dysplasia with metaanalytic techniques. Pediatr. Infect. Dis. *24*:1033-1039, 2005.

138. Scheurlen, W., Frauendienst, G., Schrod, L., et al.: Polymerase chain reaction-amplification of urease genes: Rapid screening for *Ureaplasma urealyticum* infection in endotracheal aspirates of ventilated newborns. Eur. J. Pediatr. *151*:740, 1992.

139. Shaw, N. J., Pratt, R. C., and Weindling, A. M.: *Ureaplasma* and *Mycoplasma* infections of the central nervous system in preterm infants. Lancet *23*:1530, 1989.

140. Shurin, P. A., Alpert, S., Rosner, B., et al.: Chorioamnionitis and colonization of the newborn infant with genital mycoplasmas. N. Engl. J. Med. *293*:5, 1975.

141. Siber, G. R., Alpert, S., Smith, D. L., et al.: Neonatal central nervous system infection due to *Mycoplasma hominis*. J. Pediatr. *90*:625, 1977.

142. Smyth, A. R., Shaw, N. J., Pratt, B. C., et al.: *Ureaplasma urealyticum* and chronic lung disease. Eur. J. Pediatr. *152*:931, 1993.

143. Sompolinsky, D., Solomon, F., Leiba, H., et al.: Puerperal sepsis due to T-strain *Mycoplasma*. Isr. J. Med. Sci. 7:745, 1971.

144. Stagno, S., Brasfield, D. M., Brown, M. B., et al.: Infant pneumonitis associated with cytomegalovirus, *Chlamydia*, *Pneumocystis*, and *Ureaplasma*: A prospective study. Pediatrics 68:322, 1981.

145. Stahelin-Massik, J., Levy, F., Friderich, P., et al.: Meningitis caused by *Ureaplasma urealyticum* in a full term neonate. Pediatr. Infect. Dis. J. *13*:419, 1994.

146. Stancombe, B. B., Walsh, W. F., Derdak, S., et al.: Induction of human neonatal pulmonary fibroblast cytokines by hyperoxia and *Ureaplasma urealyticum*. Clin. Infect. Dis. *17*(Suppl. 1):154, 1993.

147. Syrogiannopoulos, G. A., Kapatais-Zoumbox, K., Decavalas, G. D., et al.: *Ureaplasma urealyticum* colonization of full term infants: Perinatal acquisition and persistence during early infancy. Pediatr. Infect. Dis. J. *9*:236, 1990.

148. Tafari, N., Ross, S., Naeye, R. L., et al.: *Mycoplasma* "T" strains and perinatal death. Lancet *1*:108, 1976.

149. Taylor-Robinson, D., and McCormack, W. M.: The genital mycoplasmas. N. Engl. J. Med. *302*:1003, 1980.

150. Teng, L. J., Zheng, X., Glass, J. I., et al.: *Ureaplasma urealyticum* biovar specificity and diversity are encoded in multiple-banded antigen gene. J. Clin. Microbiol. *32*:1464-1469, 1994.

151. Theilen, U., Lyon A. J., Fitzgerald, T., et al.: Infection with *Ureaplasma urealyticum*: Is there a specific clinical and radiological course in the preterm infant? Arch. Dis. Child. Fetal Neonatal Ed. *89*:F163-F167, 2004.

152. Thomsen, A. C., Taylor-Robinson, D., Hanson, K. B., et al.: The infrequent occurrence of mycoplasmas in amniotic fluid from women with intact fetal membranes. Acta Obstet. Gynecol. Scand. *3*:425, 1983.

153. Unsworth, P. F., Taylor-Robinson, D., Sho, E. E., et al.: Neonatal mycoplasmemia: *Mycoplasma hominis* as a significant cause of disease? J. Infect. *10*:163, 1985.

154. Valencia, G. B., Banzon, F., Cummings, M., et al.: *Mycoplasma hominis* and *Ureaplasma urealyticum* in neonates with suspected infection. Pediatr. Infect. Dis. J. *12*:571, 1993.

155. Van Waarde, W. M., Brus, F., Okken, A., and Kimpen, J. L.: *Ureaplasma urealyticum* colonization, prematurity and bronchopulmonary dysplasia. Eur. Respir. J. *10*:886, 1997.

156. Viscardi, R. M., Atamas, S. P., Luzina, I. G., et al.: Antenatal *Ureaplasma urealyticum* respiratory tract infection stimulates proinflammatory, profibrotic responses in the preterm baboon lung. Pediatr. Res. *60*:141-146, 2006.

157. Viscardi, R. M., Kaplan, J., Lovchik, J. C., et al.: Characterization of a murine model of *Ureaplasma urealyticum* pneumonia. Infect. Immun. *70*:5721-5729, 2002.

158. Waites, K. B., Cassell, G. R., Canupp, K. C., et al.: In vitro susceptibilities of mycoplasmas and ureaplasmas to new macrolides and arylfluoroquinolones. Antimicrob. Agents Chemother. *32*:1500, 1988.

159. Waites, K. B., Crouse, D. T., and Cassell, G. R.: Antibiotic susceptibilities and therapeutic options for *Ureaplasma urealyticum* infections in neonates. Pediatr. Infect. Dis. J. *11*:23, 1992.

160. Waites, K. B., Crouse, D. T., and Cassell, G. R.: Therapeutic consideration for *Ureaplasma urealyticum* infections in neonates. Clin. Infect. Dis.. *17*(Suppl. 1):208, 1993.

161. Waites, K. B., Crouse, D. T., Phillips, J. G., et al.: *Ureaplasma* pneumonia and sepsis associated with persistent pulmonary hypertension of the newborn. Pediatrics *83*:84, 1991.

162. Waites, K. B., Duffy, L. B., Crouse, D. T., et al.: Mycoplasmal infection of cerebrospinal fluid in newborn infants from a community hospital population. Pediatr. Infect. Dis. J. *9*:241, 1990.

163. Waites, K. B., Figarola, T. A., Schmid, T., et al.: Comparison of agar versus broth dilution techniques for determining antibiotic susceptibilities of *Ureaplasma urealyticum*. Diagn. Microbiol. Infect. Dis. *14*:265, 1991.

164. Waites, K. B., Katz, B., and Schelonka, R. L.: Mycoplasmas and ureaplasmas as neonatal pathogens. Clin. Microbiol. Rev. *18*:757-789, 2005.

165. Waites, K. B., Rudd, P. T., Crouse, D. T., et al.: Chronic *Ureaplasma urealyticum* and *Mycoplasma hominis* infections of central nervous systems in preterm infants. Lancet *2*:17, 1988.

166. Waites, K. B., Sims, P. J., Crouse, D. T., et al.: Serum concentrations of erythromycin after intravenous infusion in preterm neonates treated for *Ureaplasma urealyticum* infection. Pediatr. Infect. Dis. J. *13*:287, 1994.

167. Walsh, W. F., Butler, J., Coalson, J., et al.: A primate model of *Ureaplasma urealyticum* infection in the premature infant with hyaline membrane disease. Clin. Infect. Dis. *17*(Suppl. 1):158, 1993.

168. Walsh, W. F., Stanley, S., Lally, K. P., et al.: *Ureaplasma urealyticum* demonstrated by open lung biopsy in newborns with chronic lung disease. Pediatr. Infect. Dis. J. *10*:823, 1991.

169. Wang, E. L., Cassell, G. R., Sanchez, P., et al.: *Ureaplasma urealyticum* and chronic lung disease of prematurity: Critical appraisal of the literature on causation. Clin. Infect. Dis. *17*(Suppl. 1):112, 1993.

170. Wang, E. E., Frayha, R., Watts, J., et al.: The role of *Ureaplasma urealyticum* and other pathogens in the development of chronic lung disease of prematurity. Pediatr. Infect. Dis. J. *7*:547, 1988.

171. Wang, E. E., Matlow, A. G., Ohlsson, A., and Nelson, S. C.: *Ureaplasma urealyticum* infections in the perinatal period. Clin. Perinatol. *24*:91, 1997.

172. Wang, E. E. L., Ohlsson, A., and Kellner, J. D.: Association of *Ureaplasma urealyticum* colonization with chronic lung disease of prematurity: Results of a metaanalysis. J. Pediatr. *127*:640, 1995.

173. Yonn, B. R., Romero, R., Kim, M., et al.: Clinical implications of detection of *Ureaplasma urealyticum* in the amniotic cavity with the polymerase chain reaction. Am. J. Obstet. Gynecol. *183*:1130, 2000.

174. Yoon, B. R., Romero, R., Park, J. S., et al.: Microbial invasion of the amniotic cavity with *Ureaplasma urealyticum* is associated with a robust host response in fetal, amniotic, and maternal compartments. Am. J. Obstet. Gynecol. *179*:1254, 1998.

CHAPTER 76

YEAST AND FUNGAL INFECTIONS OF THE FETUS AND NEONATE

Gail J. Demmler-Harrison

The improved survival of preterm infants since the early 1980s has resulted in the emergence of yeasts and fungi as significant neonatal pathogens.* *Candida albicans* remains the most frequently isolated pathogenic yeast overall, but other *Candida* spp., especially *Candida parapsilosis* and *Candida tropicalis*, and less common pathogenic yeasts, such as *Malassezia*, *Trichosporon*, *Rhodotorula*, and *Pichia/Hansenula*, have increased in frequency. The incidence of invasive fungal disease, often with fatal outcomes, caused by *Aspergillus* and Zygomycetes (*Mucor*, *Rhizopus*, *Rhizomucor*, and *Absidia*) also has increased in neonates, especially infants who were born premature or with an inherited metabolic disorder or primary immunodeficiency.[309]

Reports about premature neonates with serious or fatal infection with rare, darkly pigmented fungi, such as *Phialemonium obovatum*, also have emerged more recently, perhaps heralding an increasing trend for unusual fungal infections in this special age group.[138] In addition, the rare vertical transmission of the endemic pathogenic yeast and fungi *Cryptococcus*, *Coccidioides*, and *Blastomyces* continues to be documented, especially in neonates born to mothers infected with human immunodeficiency virus (HIV).[67] Prompt recognition of pathogenic yeast or invasive fungal disease in neonates and institution of aggressive management that includes appropriate antifungal therapy and, when required, surgical intervention, are important to minimize rates of morbidity and mortality from these serious, often fatal, infections.

NEONATAL CANDIDIASIS

Candida spp. account for approximately 9 percent of all nosocomial infections in the neonatal intensive care unit (NICU).

Candida spp. infect approximately 1 to 6 percent of infants with a birth weight less than 1500 g (very low birth weight [VLBW]) and 5 to 10 percent of infants with a birth weight less than 1000 g (extremely low birth weight [ELBW]).[177,292,295] The overall case-fatality rate is approximately 30 percent, with a range of 4 to 40 percent reported.[190,211,220,343,411] Neurodevelopmental disabilities also are more common findings in premature infants with invasive candidiasis.[98] In addition to excess mortality and disability rates, neonatal candidiasis is associated with increased length of hospitalizations and excess hospital costs.[343,411]

The species isolated most frequently is *C. albicans*,[27,28,37,41] which represents approximately 40 to 60 percent of isolates from neonates with systemic disease and is the most common *Candida* spp. associated with NICU outbreaks.[18,74,121,313] *Candida* spp. other than *C. albicans* have become increasingly more prevalent, however, and in some NICUs may be isolated more frequently than is *C. albicans*.[63,112,139,306] Among these organisms, *C. parapsilosis* is the most common,* followed by *C. tropicalis*;[124,303] both of them have caused outbreaks in NICUs. *Candida glabrata*,[26,112] *Candida guilliermondii*,[312,314,315] *Candida lusitaniae*,[316] and *Candida krusei*[133,304] also have caused invasive disease in neonates. Most recently, *Candida haemulonii*[193] has emerged as a neonatal pathogen and caused an outbreak in an NICU.[193] Manifestations of neonatal candidiasis range from commonly encountered benign oral and cutaneous candidiasis to systemic infection with candidemia to more severe and often fatal disseminated candidiasis.[27,28,31]

TRANSMISSION, PATHOGENESIS, AND RISK FACTORS

Candida transmitted to the fetus in utero by an ascending route from the colonized vagina of the mother results in

---

*See references 31, 37, 61, 149, 154, 161, 177, 332, 335, 341.

*See references 41, 85, 96, 113, 115, 166, 211, 218, 319, 373, 395, 405.

congenital candidiasis. Transplacental infection has not been described.[106,170,176,180,215,222] More frequently, vertical transmission to a newborn occurs during birth through the mother's colonized birth canal, which results in the development of oral candidiasis, or thrush, in an otherwise healthy infant.[10,27,65,76,306,382] *Candida* also may be acquired by the infant during breast-feeding if the mother's skin is colonized and from inadequate sterilization of feeding bottles and nipples.[113] Subsequent colonization of the gastrointestinal tract and the presence of *Candida* in stool lead to superficial cutaneous infection involving primarily the perineal area.[27]

Nosocomial transmission occurs and has resulted in nursery outbreaks. Even though *Candida* spp. have been detected on environmental surfaces and from the air samples of neonatal units, person-to-person transmission is the most important mode of transmission.[202,376,382] Horizontal transmission from health care worker to newborn with subsequent colonization of conjunctivae, mucosa, or skin and infant-to-infant transmission via the hands of health care workers have been documented in outbreak investigations that used molecular analysis of *Candida* isolates.* In addition, systemic candidiasis in ELBW infants has been linked to use of topical petrolatum ointment for skin care.[63]

Candidal colonization of the oropharynx of preterm neonates in NICUs is a common occurrence; it occurs in approximately 2.5 to 19 percent of infants in the first few days of life and increases with age and time in the NICU.[121,313] Subsequent colonization of the gastrointestinal tract and endotracheal tube in ventilated neonates seems to predispose them to development of invasive candidiasis.[27,310,314,315] Baley and colleagues[27] studied 146 infants with a birth weight less than 1500 g during an 11-month period. They performed fungal cultures of pharynx, rectum, and endotracheal aspirates within 24 hours of birth, and then weekly while the infants were in the NICU. The overall colonization rate was 27 percent; by 2 weeks of age, 85 percent of the infants were colonized with *Candida* spp. Mucocutaneous disease developed in 28 percent of the colonized infants, and systemic candidiasis was seen in 8 percent.

In high-risk neonates, gastrointestinal colonization also may lead to bloodstream dissemination, particularly if the integrity of the intestinal mucosal lining is disrupted by surgery, ischemia, or enterocolitis.[56,61,108,314,315] In addition, the immature skin of ELBW infants may predispose them to invasive candidal infection.[276,306] Gastrointestinal colonization with *Candida* occurs before the development of candidemia in most preterm infants.[314,315] In addition, Rowen and colleagues[310] showed that VLBW infants with endotracheal colonization by *Candida* had a sixfold increased risk for development of invasive disease.

The relationships among adhesion proteins, lymphocytes, and neutrophils may contribute to yeast pathogenicity in colonized neonates. The ability of *C. albicans* to invade oral and gastrointestinal mucosal tissues and enter the bloodstream may be a major determinant of virulence. In vitro studies of interaction of *C. albicans* with epithelial cells have shown that *C. albicans* invades mucosal tissues by promoting the proteolytic degradation of the junction adherin protein E-cadherin, allowing an increase in cell permeability.[129,160,379] Candidal dissemination in neonates is aided further by abnormal neonatal leukocyte function, as shown by an impaired ability of polymorphonuclear leukocytes to adhere to, ingest, and kill *Candida*, and a reduced capacity of lymphocytes to inhibit candidal growth.[331,357]

In addition, proteomic studies have begun decoding serologic responses to *Candida* cell wall proteins.[285,286] Antibodies made to *C. albicans* cell wall proteins, such as antiwall enolase antibodies, by survivors of systemic candidiasis may provide

the basis for novel diagnostic and prognostic indicators and may be candidates for possible future vaccine development. More recently, *Candida* antigens identified by proteomic approaches were shown in murine models to induce protective responses, providing the basis for possible future human clinical vaccine trials.[286]

Risk factors for neonates colonized with *Candida* to progress to systemic infection include prematurity; VLBW and ELBW; prolonged endotracheal intubation with mechanical ventilation; bronchopulmonary dysplasia; indwelling intravenous catheters; prolonged administration of third-generation cephalosporin antibiotics, hyperalimentation solutions, H_2 blockers, and steroids; lack of enteral feedings; abdominal surgery; skin care practices; and early neutropenia.* Several risk factors consistently have been associated with systemic candidiasis, the most common being prematurity and VLBW and ELBW, with attendant impairment of host defense mechanisms; indwelling intravenous catheters; and prolonged use of broad-spectrum antimicrobial therapy, in particular, third-generation cephalosporins, which suppress normal gastrointestinal flora.[314,327,334] Although aminophylline is able to inhibit the activity of human granulocytes in vitro, its use has not been associated clinically with systemic candidiasis in neonates. Studies by Hostetter[37,160] suggested the use of heparin may be another predisposing factor; this in vitro finding also has not been confirmed in the clinical setting, however.

CLINICAL MANIFESTATIONS

ORAL CANDIDIASIS

Oral candidiasis is the most common form of infection with *Candida* spp.[242] Lesions on the mucous membranes of the mouth and oropharynx usually appear on the 7th to 10th day of life as whitish gray plaques that can be scraped easily from the mucosa to expose an erythematous base. Persistent or recurrent infection may be caused by the continued use of bottle nipples and pacifiers that harbor *Candida* on their surface. Primary and acquired immunodeficiency states, including infection with HIV, should be considered if oral thrush fails to clear with appropriate therapy.

CUTANEOUS CANDIDIASIS

Cutaneous candidiasis typically is manifested by erythematous, vesiculopustular lesions found primarily on the skin of the perineum, axilla, and intertriginous areas.[346] The periumbilical area also can be involved.[242] Benign diaper dermatitis with so-called satellite lesions is a frequent occurrence in an otherwise healthy infant, and the peak incidence occurs at 3 to 4 months of age. In VLBW and ELBW premature infants, seemingly benign mucocutaneous lesions, including lesions in the perineum or diaper area, may progress rapidly to invasive dermatitis, producing cutaneous scales, crusting, erosions, ulcerations, or extensive maceration of skin, and result in a potentially lethal systemic candidiasis (Fig. 76–1).[31,72,159,276,306] Scattered, faint, erythematous maculopapular lesions of the skin may be an expression of a serious disseminated candidiasis.[31,306,309] Chronic mucocutaneous candidiasis may be diagnosed in an otherwise well-appearing infant, if *Candida* infections of the skin, mucous membranes, and nails persist or recur, despite administration of antifungal therapy. These neonates have a congenital defect in T-lymphocyte function specific to *Candida* spp.

---

*See references 18, 119, 124, 163, 165, 167, 218, 295, 303, 304, 373.

*See references 57, 63, 209, 220, 221, 226, 304, 309, 310, 314, 315, 327, 335, 389.

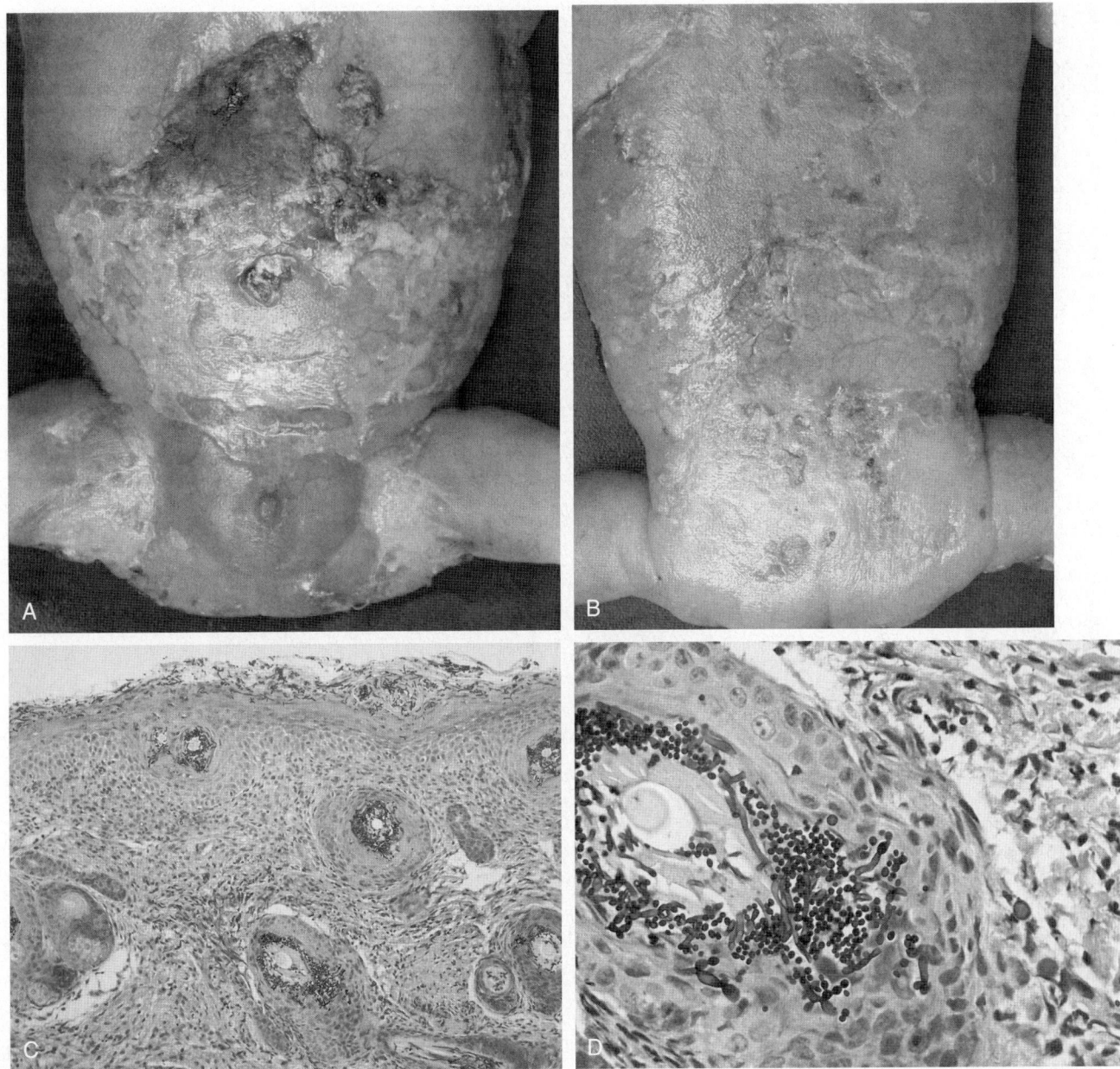

Figure 76–1 A-D, Invasive cutaneous candidiasis. A 3-week-old, former 24-2/7 weeks' gestation premature infant with fatal invasive candidiasis. The skin on the abdomen (**A**) and back (**B**) showed extensive cutaneous ulceration and exudates caused by *Candida* infection. Autopsy examination showed disseminated candidiasis with thromboemboli, infarction, and microabscesses involving the brain, lungs, and kidneys. Skin biopsy specimen showed numerous ovoid yeasts and pseudohyphae infiltrating the stratum corneum and within hair follicles (periodic acid–Schiff stain, 100× original magnification) (**C**) and infiltration of yeasts deep into the dermal connective tissue (periodic acid–Schiff stain, 400× original magnification) (**D**). (See companion Expert Consult web site for color version.) *(Courtesy of Dr. Megan K. Dishop, Department of Pathology, Baylor College of Medicine and Texas Children's Hospital, Houston, TX.)*

CONGENITAL CANDIDIASIS

Congenital candidiasis may cause fetal infection with onset of premature labor or intrauterine demise; it may be evident at birth, or it may appear within the first 24 to 48 hours of life.* Term and preterm neonates may be affected (Fig. 76–2).[348,349] Congenital candidiasis usually is caused by *C. albicans*, but other

Candida spp., including *C. tropicalis* and *C. glabrata*, also have been reported to cause congenital candidiasis.[230,260]

Congenital cutaneous candidiasis most often manifests as a widespread, mucocutaneous infection, with erythematous maculopapular or vesiculopustular rash.[349,399] Congenital pneumonia also may be a part of the disease, with or without the mucocutaneous or systemic signs.[66,120,185] Congenital systemic candidiasis may manifest as life-threatening, early-onset sepsis syndrome, especially in premature neonates (see Fig. 76–2) with septic shock or meningitis; it also may be accompanied by leukocytosis or neutropenia, or it may mimic congenital leukemia.[66,268] Twins

---

*See references 32, 59, 60, 66, 106, 170, 173, 176, 180, 203, 237, 305, 306, 328.

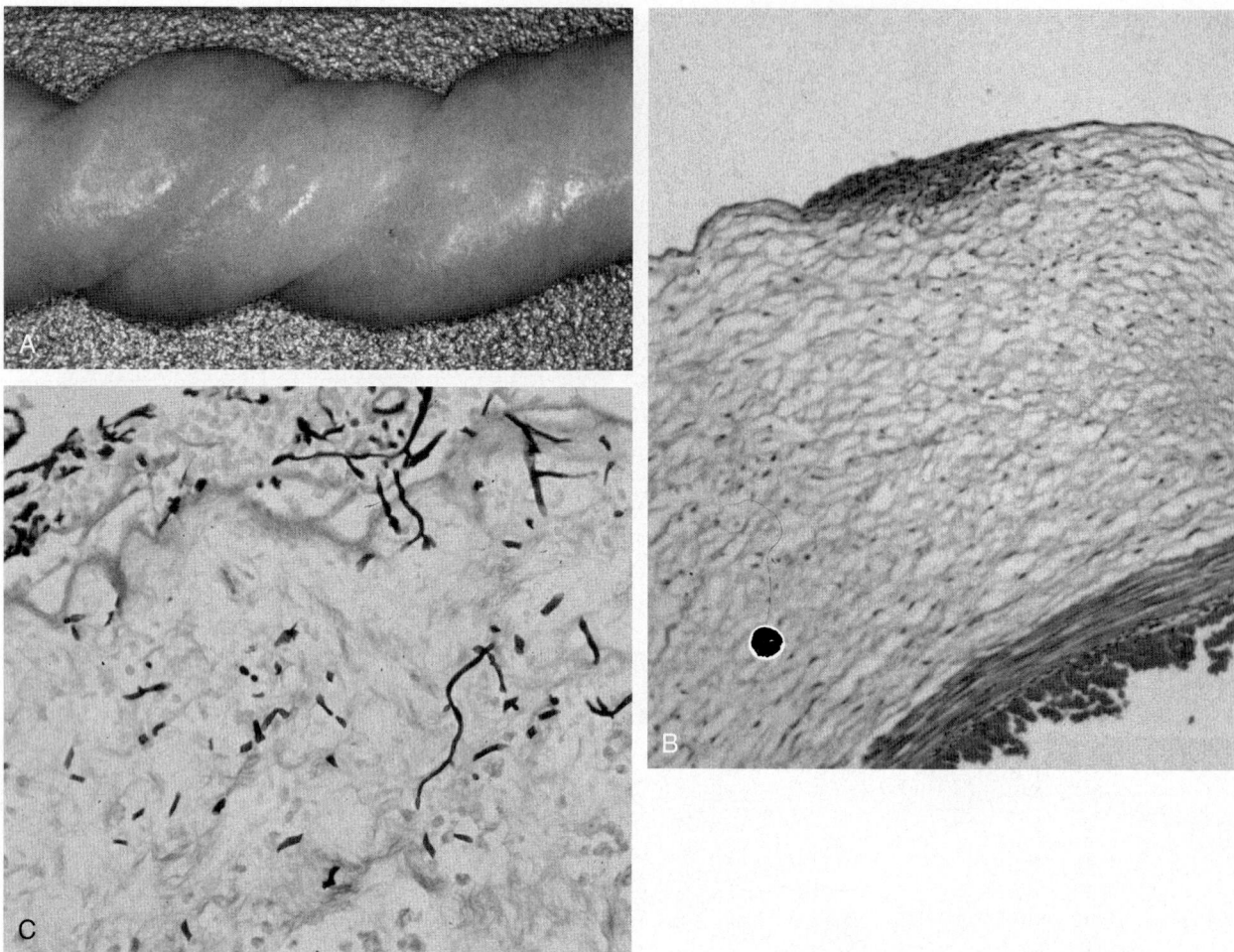

Figure 76–2 **A-C,** Umbilical cord funisitis in congenital candidiasis. **A,** Umbilical cord from a term infant born with congenital candidiasis (*C. albicans*). Gross examination showed cord edema with pinpoint yellow-white lesions on the surface. **B** and **C,** Umbilical cord from premature infant, born at 24 weeks' gestation with a birth weight of 610 g, to a mother with *Candida* vaginitis at the time of delivery. The infant presented at birth with septic shock associated with disseminated congenital candidiasis. Examination of the umbilical cord showed extensive funisitis with *Candida* microabscesses (hematoxylin and eosin stain, 40× original magnification) (**B**). Microscopic examination showed *Candida* funisitis with budding yeasts and invasive pseudohyphae (methenamine silver nitrate stain, 200× original magnification) (**C**). *(Courtesy of Dr. Edwina J. Popek, Department of Pathology, Baylor College of Medicine and Texas Children's Hospital, Houston, TX.)*

may be affected, sometimes with different *Candida* spp., manifestations, and outcomes for each twin.[203,326,350]

Prenatal diagnosis of intrauterine infection with *Candida* may be determined by amniocentesis.[49,237,305] A presumptive diagnosis in a neonate can be made by identifying budding yeast organisms on potassium hydroxide preparations or Gram-stained smears of the pustular or vesicular skin lesions, blood buffy coat, or gastric fluid aspirate.[294] Growth of *Candida* in culture provides confirmatory evidence. Term newborns with congenital candidiasis usually have infection limited to the skin, mucous membranes, lungs, or gastrointestinal tract; *Candida* rarely is isolated from blood or other sterile body sites. In contrast, premature neonates with congenital candidiasis often have more severe disease, with positive blood cultures and evidence of disseminated disease, including meningitis.[141,348,349] The umbilical cord from a fetus or newborn with congenital candidiasis may show *Candida* funisitis with yellow-white nodules and fungal microabscesses (see Fig. 76–2); the placenta also may have nodules and shows chorioamnionitis on histologic examination.[230,291,325]

Maternal risk factors include a history during pregnancy of *Candida* vaginitis, use of antibiotics, retained intrauterine contraceptive device, cervical cerclage, and prolonged rupture of fetal membranes, although none of these factors may be present in the history.[32,59,76,237,305,328] Poor prognostic factors for neonates include the presence of pneumonia or sepsis, prematurity, and early-onset neutropenia at presentation.[411]

SYSTEMIC CANDIDIASIS

Systemic candidiasis refers to the isolation of *Candida* or its histopathologic demonstration in a normally sterile body site. The most common forms of this clinical syndrome include (1) catheter-associated sepsis, in which *Candida* is isolated from the blood of infants who have central venous catheters, but no evidence of focal infection or disseminated disease; (2) disseminated candidiasis, in which *Candida* is isolated from the bloodstream in association with other foci of infection, such as skin or intestine, regardless of whether the infant has a central venous catheter[61]; and (3) focal disease of an organ or disseminated disease caused by *Candida* spp., without a positive blood culture. No significant differences in presentation of systemic candidiasis caused by different *Candida* spp. have been apparent.[41,43,112,116,163,165,166]

The clinical and laboratory signs of systemic candidiasis usually are nonspecific and resemble signs seen with bacterial sepsis.[37,41,43,220,221] Knowledge of prior colonization with *Candida* spp. or presence of cutaneous crusting or erosions, dermatitis, or skin maceration provides clinical clues that a sepsis syndrome in a premature neonate may be caused by invasive *Candida* spp. (see Fig. 76–1A and B).[31,61,276,306,309] Signs and symptoms most commonly reported in neonates with systemic candidiasis include respiratory deterioration (74%), apnea and bradycardia (60%), carbohydrate intolerance (56%), skin manifestations (53%),[28,31,37] abdominal distention (49%), temperature instability (35%), guaiac-positive stools (26%), and hypotension (21%).[61,85]

The frequency of end-organ involvement in neonates with systemic candidiasis is difficult to determine precisely. Based on several retrospective, single-center medical literature reviews and one meta-analysis report, the sites most frequently involved in systemic neonatal candidiasis include blood (60-80%), the central nervous system (CNS) (meningoencephalitis, 25-60%),[113,114,123,199] the lungs (pneumonia, 70%),[28,74,185,277] the kidneys (renal candidiasis, 60%),[28,41,107,126,197,272,283,289] the liver and spleen (19%),[42,163,263] and the eyes (endophthalmitis, 30%).[24,25,263] End-organ disease is accompanied most often by positive blood or urine cultures, especially if cultures are persistently positive for more than 5 days.[39,73,263] Not all neonates with end-organ disease with *Candida* spp. have positive blood or urine cultures, however.

The organ involved most frequently in systemic candidiasis seems to be the kidney.[28,39,107,126,197,263] *Candida* may be isolated from the urine of 73 percent of neonates with systemic candidiasis with positive blood cultures, but only 5 to 15 percent of such neonates have documented *Candida* pyelonephritis with renal infiltration, mycetoma, or renal abscess.[7,22,41,153,192,198,206,368] The kidney seems to be particularly vulnerable to the formation of renal cortical abscesses and obstructive masses, which usually occur at the ureteropelvic junction. A neonate with persistently positive urine or blood cultures, hypertension, renal insufficiency or acute renal failure, or oliguria or anuria should undergo ultrasound imaging to determine the presence of a bezoar-associated obstructive uropathy, which requires immediate attention.[22,44,229,289,381,403,404] Urinary catheters or nephrostomy tubes may become colonized with *Candida* and result in secondary infections that may range from asymptomatic to invasive disease with obstruction.[44,229]

CNS involvement occurs in 3 to 23 percent of neonates with systemic candidiasis; percentages of 54 to 64 percent have been reported in a few series.[39,77,79,118,171] In addition to causing meningitis, *Candida* may invade the brain tissue, through hematogenous dissemination, producing focal nodular encephalitis, with minimal inflammation of the meninges (Fig. 76–3). The diagnosis of candidal meningoencephalitis requires a high index of suspicion, followed by thoughtful and careful evaluation.[113,114,123,199]

Candida meningitis may occur in the absence of positive blood cultures; cerebrospinal fluid (CSF) pleocytosis may be minimal or absent, and elevated protein or hypoglycorrhachia is an inconsistent finding. Gram-stained smears of CSF rarely reveal budding yeast, even when CSF cultures are positive for *Candida*.[40,90,123,169] More recent reviews determined that meningitis with *Candida* isolated from the CSF occurred in 8 percent of ELBW infants, but only 37 to 52 percent had *Candida*-positive blood cultures.[40,90,169] CSF findings in neonates diagnosed with *Candida* meningitis also may vary. Of neonates with *Candida* meningitis, 43 percent may have normal CSF.[90] Fernandez and associates,[123] in a 10-year review of candidal meningitis in 23 infants in an NICU, reported that pleocytosis occurred in only 39 percent of infants, and hypoglycorrhachia occurred in 25 percent, despite a positive CSF culture for *Candida* in 74 percent of infants. The remaining neonates are diagnosed when a positive blood culture occurs with an abnormal, but culture-negative, CSF.[98,114,208,254] *Candida* also may colonize and infect external ventricular drains placed for management of hydrocephalus.

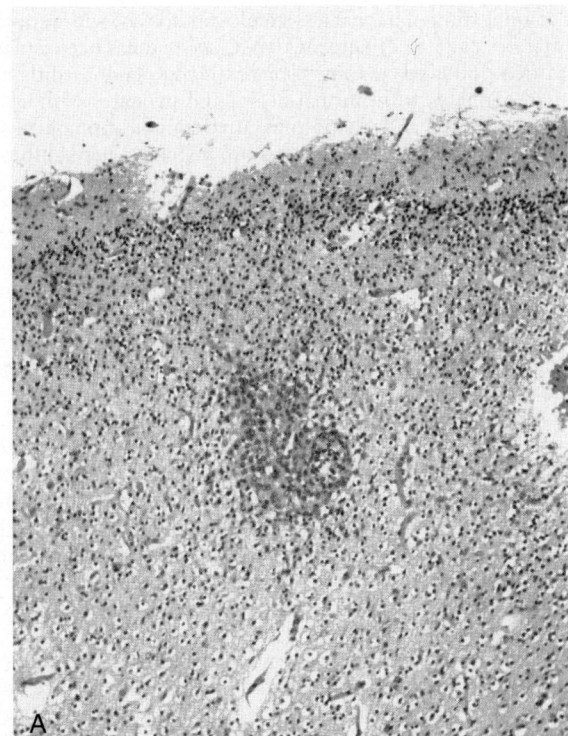

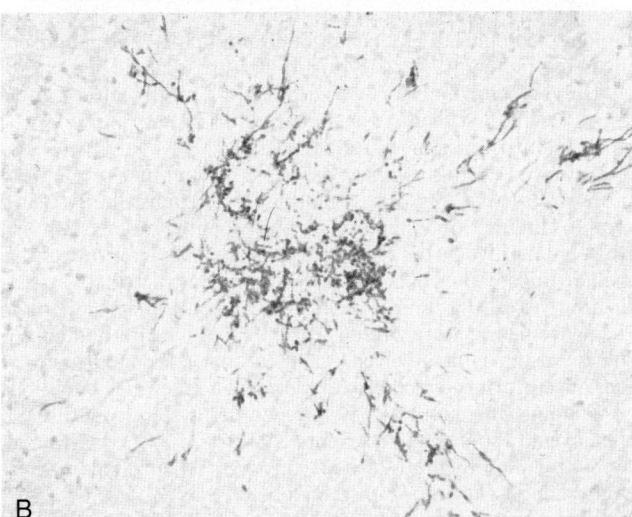

Figure 76–3 **A** and **B,** Invasive candidiasis (*C. albicans*) of the central nervous system. Autopsy examination of a premature infant born at 25 weeks' gestation who died at 1 month of age of disseminated invasive candidiasis. **A,** Central nervous system involvement, with brain microglial nodules, was seen at autopsy examination (hematoxylin and eosin stain, 40× original magnification). **B,** Brain microglial nodules contained *Candida* yeasts and invasive ribbon-like *Candida* pseudohyphae (Gomori methenamine silver stain, 100× original magnification). (*Courtesy of Dr. Edwina J. Popek, Department of Pathology, Baylor College of Medicine and Texas Children's Hospital, Houston, TX.*)

Ventriculitis, brain abscesses, and brain calcifications are unusual complications of *Candida* meningitis that can be diagnosed with brain imaging procedures.[58,141,181,197,198] Mortality or neurodevelopmental disabilities in survivors may occur in 73 percent of neonates with *Candida* meningitis.[40,98,208,254]

Endocarditis is estimated to occur in 5 to 15 percent of neonates with systemic candidiasis.* It is a serious and potentially

---

*See references 39, 117, 128, 174, 216, 217, 263, 264, 284, 317, 414.

fatal complication of neonatal systemic candidiasis, with reported fatality rates of 25 to 73 percent.[216,217] *C. albicans* has been isolated most often, followed by *C. parapsilosis. Candida* endocarditis may occur in neonates with normal hearts and neonates with structural heart disease, and as a postoperative complication of cardiac surgery.[236,246] *Candida* endocarditis in neonates may differ in presentation from *Candida* endocarditis in older children and adults.[115,233] It usually occurs in premature neonates with persistent candidemia associated with an indwelling vascular catheter. Most neonates with *Candida* endocarditis have structurally normal hearts, however, and not all reported cases in neonates have been associated with vascular devices.[104,151,246]

The presentation of *Candida* endocarditis in neonates may be acute and associated with an episode of persistent candidemia, or late onset, often discovered weeks or months after a presumably silent or resolved episode of candidemia.[39,96,179,212,246,301] Cardiac murmurs may be absent. Early literature reports consisted mostly of autopsy diagnoses; however, more recently, echocardiography has proved to be a valuable tool in establishing the diagnosis of *Candida* endocarditis.[236,246,256] Intracardiac vegetations on the mitral, tricuspid, and aortic valves, or the presence of a right atrial mass, in association with persistently positive blood cultures for *Candida*, strongly supports the diagnosis of endocarditis.

Eye disease may occur in 3 to 11 percent of neonates with systemic candidiasis; figures as high as 45 percent have been reported.[77,246,263] Candidal eye disease may complicate systemic candidiasis in term, near-term, and preterm infants.[24-26] More recent reports suggest, however, that the prevalence of ophthalmologic complications in hospitalized infants and children, including premature VLBW infants who are treated aggressively and survive candidemia, may be decreasing.[100,127] Eye disease may occur on the first day of systemic candidiasis but more often is associated with prolonged candidemia.[25,99,263]

Advanced eye disease may be visible on routine examination; however, establishing the diagnosis of endophthalmitis early requires indirect ophthalmoscopy by an ophthalmologist.[77,248,269] Most lesions involve the retina and choroids; characteristic lesions include unilateral or bilateral yellow-white fluffy, retinal, or free-floating vitreal opacities or balls, often accompanied by hemorrhage or inflammatory vitreous haze.[12,24,25,269] The iris and lens of the eye also may be involved.[330,367] Lens abscesses manifesting as lens opacities or cataracts also may occur, and they may be a nidus of ongoing infection poorly reached by systemic antifungal therapy and a source for recurrent disease.[87,103,254,330,367] Untreated, *Candida* endophthalmitis also may progress and produce corneal thinning and perforation of the globe.[240] Rarely, *Candida* endophthalmitis may mimic retinoblastoma.[336] In addition, VLBW infants who experience candidemia may have concomitant endophthalmitis and retinopathy of prematurity, or they may develop more severe retinopathy of prematurity (stage 3 or beyond) or retinal detachment and require laser therapy.[49,136,145,184,245,262] Premature, high-risk, VLBW infants with candidemia should be monitored closely for *Candida* eye disease and for progression of retinopathy of prematurity.[262]

Osteoarthritis is a rare manifestation of systemic candidiasis in neonates.[2,146,162,199,361,387,390,393] It may occur temporarily associated with persistent candidemia or as a late complication, weeks to months later, after apparent resolution of an episode of candidemia.[146,162,390] In addition to premature infants, newborns with underlying inherited disorders of metabolism also may be at increased risk. Clinical features of candidal osteoarthritis in neonates are similar to the features of osteoarthritis caused by bacterial pathogens and include warmth, pain, tenderness, and swelling of the extremity and diminished range of motion. Imaging may show swelling of soft tissue and joint and cortical bone erosion. Culture of aspirated joint fluid or biopsy of bone tissue positive for *Candida* spp. confirms the diagnosis.[387,393]

Intra-abdominal infections, including enteritis, necrotizing enterocolitis (NEC), and peritonitis, and intra-abdominal and hepatosplenic abscesses are estimated to occur in 8 percent of neonates with invasive systemic candidiasis (Fig. 76–4).[39] *Candida* peritonitis and sepsis may complicate surgical procedures performed on the intestine for congenital bowel atresias or bowel perforation associated with NEC.[26,56,99,182,243] Distinct from NEC is idiopathic spontaneous focal intestinal perforation (SFIP), which occurs rarely in VLBW infants and has been associated with systemic candidiasis in half of cases.[1,88,243,290,299,307] SFIP is approximately 12-fold less common than is NEC in preterm neonates and has a distinct combination of clinical and laboratory features that help distinguish it from NEC. Prognosis and management differ, so it is important to understand the difference between these two clinical entities.

Neonates with SFIP are more likely than are neonates with NEC to be smaller at birth, have lower Apgar scores, experience early hypotension or hypothermia, and require more intensive

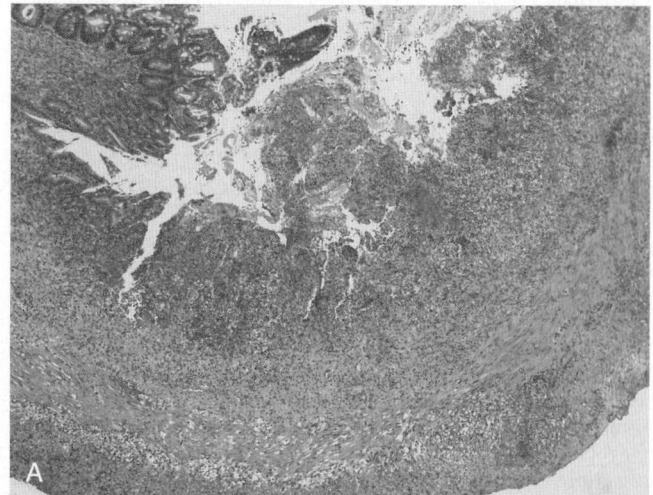

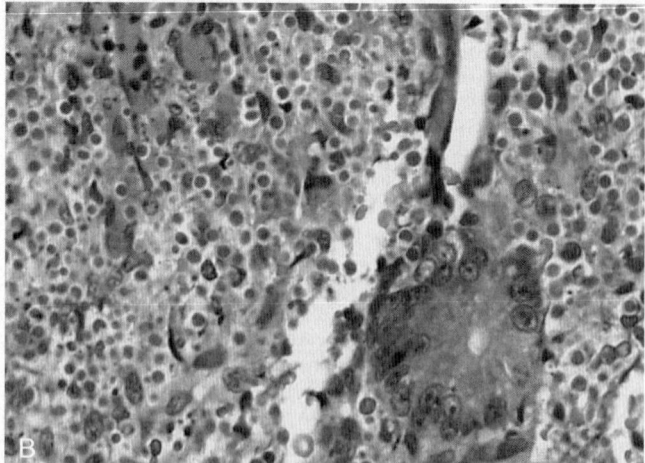

Figure 76–4 A and B, *Candida* infection complicating necrotizing enterocolitis. A 2-week-old extremely-low-birth-weight premature infant with invasive *Candida* infection associated with necrotizing enterocolitis with perforation. **A,** A large segment of resected bowel showed extensive mucosal erosion and hemorrhage with transmural inflammation (hematoxylin and eosin stain, 40× original magnification). **B,** Numerous yeast organisms infiltrated the eroded mucosa (hematoxylin and eosin stain, 400× original magnification). (See companion Expert Consult web site for color version.) *(Courtesy of Dr. Megan K. Dishop, Department of Pathology, Baylor College of Medicine and Texas Children's Hospital, Houston, TX.)*

neonatal resuscitation.[182,307] Neonates with SFIP present acutely in the second or third week of life (mean, 16.7 days of life), with distention and a bluish discolored abdomen. Radiographs in SFIP reveal a gasless abdomen without pneumatosis intestinalis or portal venous gas commonly associated with NEC. SFIP frequently is an easily resectable focal area of necrosis associated with a single perforation less than 1 cm in size, often located in the terminal ileum, but also may involve the colon or stomach. The remaining bowel may be covered with serosal exudate, but otherwise it appears normal. In contrast, NEC often involves large areas of transmural bowel necrosis that are difficult to resect completely in many patients; *Candida* and other organisms may be seen in multiple sections of resected bowel (see Fig. 76–3B). Histologic findings in SFIP show focal hemorrhagic necrosis, often with *Candida* invading the bowel wall at the site of perforation only, and otherwise healthy bowel. *Candida* spp. and *Staphylococcus epidermidis* or coagulase-negative staphylococci are the predominant pathogens isolated in SFIP, whereas Enterobacteriaceae predominate in peritonitis caused by NEC-associated perforations, with *Candida* spp. isolated in approximately 10 percent of cases of NEC.[1,88,182,243,248,290] A peritoneal culture should be obtained in all neonates with intestinal perforation, regardless of cause, because results of cultures determine the most appropriate antimicrobial therapy for bacteria and *Candida* spp.

Pulmonary candidiasis is seen frequently in congenital candidiasis.[66,185] VLBW infants with endotracheal colonization with *Candida* spp. have an increased risk for development of systemic candidiasis.[132,310] Acquired pulmonary candidiasis with pneumonia may occur in 8 to 10 percent of ventilated premature neonates and must be differentiated clinically and radiographically from asymptomatic *Candida* colonization and pneumonia caused by other pathogens.[132,185,226,277,306,309]

DIAGNOSIS

Congenital or acquired cutaneous candidiasis may be diagnosed by the presence of budding yeast organisms in scrapings of skin lesions, and the species involved is established by culture. Invasive dermatitis caused by *Candida* can be differentiated from benign cutaneous dermatitis by skin biopsy. Histopathologic evidence of organisms beyond the stratum corneum is evidence of more serious invasive dermatitis that leads to potentially fatal systemic candidiasis (see Fig. 76–1C and D).[306,309]

The diagnosis of systemic candidiasis in a fetus or neonate is established by isolation of *Candida* spp. in culture from a normally sterile body fluid, such as amniotic fluid, urine, blood, or CSF, or from an involved site, such as joint or bone. Culture of *Candida* spp. from abscesses and intraoperative tissue specimens also establishes the diagnosis of invasive *Candida* disease. The presence of characteristic yeast or fungal elements in tissue specimens from the placenta, the umbilical cord, or the neonate provides supportive evidence for invasive *Candida* disease, but isolation of the organism from the tissue is required to establish the diagnosis. Methods of detection of *Candida* in blood or CSF by polymerase chain reaction amplification of *C. albicans* DNA or 18S rRNA and detection of *Candida* antigens, such as mannan, in blood or CSF have been developed by a variety of different laboratories; however, they have not been evaluated in neonates and should not replace culture as the definitive test to establish the diagnosis.[285,286,365,366,378] A high index of suspicion is the key to establishing an early and accurate diagnosis, which improves outcome. Systemic candidiasis has been diagnosed first in 20 to 50 percent of infants at autopsy, and a mean delay of 11 days has been reported between the onset of symptomatic disease and the initiation of antifungal therapy.[28]

The diagnosis often is made when a routine blood culture from an infant evaluated for possible bacterial sepsis yields a *Candida* organism. In as little as 4 hours, but usually within 48 to 72 hours, *Candida* grows in routine blood cultures processed in the automated systems used by most clinical laboratories. Yeast also may be detected in smears of blood or buffy coats in high-risk neonates.[287,294] In the evaluation of an infant for possible candidemia, blood for culture should be obtained from a peripheral vein or artery and through all intravascular catheters in place at the time.[311] In addition, at least one blood culture should be obtained after removal of a colonized catheter to determine if candidemia persists after the catheter is removed.

Culture of CSF should be performed if candidemia is documented, even if CSF indices are normal. A CSF specimen that grows *Candida* in a high-risk neonate should not be dismissed as a culture contaminant.

Urine obtained by suprapubic bladder aspiration, often facilitated by ultrasound guidance, is an excellent source for recovery of *Candida*.[283] If the urine grows *Candida*, renal or systemic infection is suggested. Bag specimens of urine are unreliable for establishing the diagnosis because of the high rate of perineal candidal colonization in infants. Catheterized urine specimens, although preferable to specimens obtained by bag, may be contaminated from contact with perineum and penis. Urine obtained from an indwelling urinary catheter may represent colonization of the catheter; a repeat specimen obtained using sterile technique, at least 24 hours after removal of the catheter, is recommended. Fungal culture of urine may yield candidal growth in a premature neonate with disseminated candidiasis, even when other body fluids, such as blood and CSF, do not. Microscopic analysis of urine, Gram-stained smear of urine, or potassium hydroxide preparation of freshly obtained urine may show evidence of yeast or fungi, providing evidence for a presumptive diagnosis and early initiation of antifungal therapy.

In addition to cultures of blood, CSF, and urine, cultures of all involved sites, such as joints, bones, and abscesses, should be performed. The peritoneal fluid from infants with NEC or SFIP who require surgical intervention should be stained and cultured, and resected bowel should be sent for histopathologic examination and culture. Endotracheal cultures positive for *Candida* spp. may represent colonization in an infant at risk for having invasive disease; however, if positive respiratory cultures for *Candida* are associated with pneumonia and respiratory deterioration, invasive pulmonary candidiasis may be present.[132,310]

In addition to culture and histopathology, routine laboratory evaluations may support the diagnosis of systemic or invasive candidiasis.[61] Persistent thrombocytopenia is a frequent early finding in infants with systemic candidiasis. Additional laboratory tests, such as a complete blood cell count, liver function tests, and determination of serum glucose, blood urea nitrogen, and creatinine, may be helpful in assessing the degree of systemic involvement.

Infants whose urine, blood, or CSF cultures yield *Candida*, especially if persistently positive, should have further evaluation done to detect any evidence of dissemination that would influence the prognosis and duration of antifungal therapy.[61,73,254,311] Ultrasound or enhanced computed tomography evaluation of the abdomen, kidneys, and bladder should be done to assess for possible liver or splenic abscesses and evidence of renal infiltration or obstructive lesions.[39,72,197,198,201] Cranial ultrasound may be a useful screen for CNS pathology, such as hydrocephalus. Infants with a positive CSF culture or who are otherwise suspected to have CNS involvement should undergo enhanced computed tomography or magnetic resonance imaging of the brain to detect abscesses, nodules, infarction, or parenchymal calcified granulomata.[141,181] Careful ophthalmologic examination also is recommended, especially if candidemia is persistent, to detect endophthalmitis or lens abscesses. Infants with persistent candidemia, structural or postoperative heart disease, or new-onset heart murmur should have an echocardiogram done for possible valvular endocarditis or intracardiac mass.[317]

TREATMENT

MANAGEMENT STRATEGIES

Oral candidiasis or thrush in an otherwise healthy infant is treated with oral nystatin suspension or gentian violet. Superficial cutaneous candidiasis in an otherwise healthy neonate is treated with topical nystatin cream or powder. When the diaper area is extensively involved, oral nystatin therapy may be administered as well in an attempt to eliminate the yeast from the gastrointestinal tract. Cutaneous candidiasis that persists or evolves into invasive candidiasis requires systemic antifungal therapy, usually with amphotericin B or fluconazole.

Congenital candidiasis usually requires only topical antifungal therapy in an otherwise healthy newborn; neonates who have pulmonary involvement or who are preterm should receive systemic antifungal therapy because they are at greater risk for dissemination and a poor outcome.[61,66] In these instances, amphotericin B or fluconazole may be used for approximately 10 to 25 days, until clinical signs and symptoms have resolved.

Candidemia is now a common cause of late-onset sepsis in VLBW and ELBW neonates.[255,279] Because it is associated with significant morbidity and mortality rates, and potential risk factors for candidemia among high-risk neonates have been identified, some experts suggest that empiric antifungal therapy with amphotericin B or fluconazole should be administered along with antibiotics at the time that a blood culture is obtained for suspected sepsis in VLBW, extremely premature neonates with gestational ages of less than 28 weeks, especially if they have thrombocytopenia or a history of exposure to third-generation cephalosporin or carbapenem in the previous week.[38,63,220,221,335]

Although many antifungal medications are available, data from well-designed, randomized clinical trials in neonates, especially premature neonates, are insufficient to favor a recommendation of one antifungal agent or combination of agents for invasive or systemic candidiasis.* Most information published is derived from analyses of case series and retrospective reviews.[86,101,253] Published studies on pharmacokinetic profiles, studies evaluating optimal dose or duration of therapy, and studies with safety and toxicity data on neonates are difficult to find.[†] Recommendations for treatment are based on published experience in adults and older children and opinions of experts in neonatal medicine and pediatric infectious diseases. It is hoped that new data specific to neonates and premature neonates will emerge.

Most experts agree that evaluation for disseminated disease and prompt systemic antifungal therapy, usually with amphotericin B or fluconazole, is indicated if even a single blood culture from a neonate is positive for *Candida* spp.[72,311] Consensus seems to be lacking, however, on which antifungal compound or combination is preferred for treatment of complications such as meningitis, and for how long treatment should be administered.[72,79,123,169,178,253] The most appropriate management for an individual neonate should consider the *Candida* spp. prevalent in the nursery, the *Candida* spp. isolated from the patient, and the usual or known antifungal susceptibility patterns; the site of infection; the availability of pharmacokinetic, efficacy, and safety data; and the ability of the host to metabolize and eliminate the medication.[122,132,140,253,380,410,413]

Isolation of *Candida* from blood obtained through a vascular catheter means the device is colonized with the organism and must be removed promptly to eradicate the infection and reduce the risk of morbidity and mortality.[94,111,352] *Candida* is difficult to eradicate from catheters, and persistence of positive blood cultures from blood obtained through the catheter increases the rates of complications and mortality associated with candidemia.[73,111] In addition to removal of the catheter, systemic antifungal therapy should be administered for 10 to 14 days. If the peripheral blood culture also is positive for *Candida* spp., dissemination via the bloodstream may have occurred, and most experts recommend duration of antifungal therapy to be at least 25 to 30 days.[61,62,311]

Isolation of *Candida* spp. from urine obtained from an indwelling catheter suggests possible colonization of the catheter, requiring removal of the catheter if the infection is to be eradicated. Isolation of *Candida* spp. from a urine specimen obtained by sterile technique denotes invasive renal or systemic disease and requires further evaluation and systemic antifungal therapy. In some patients, medical therapy alone may eradicate the *Candida* infection, even if partial obstruction is present.[7,22,368] Some neonates may require an urgent surgical or endoscopic procedure, however, to relieve the obstruction and restore renal function.[44,51,153,229,289,381,403] Duration of antifungal therapy required for cure may range from 25 to 42 days or longer and should be guided by microbiologic cure and resolution of lesions by imaging studies.[51]

Treatment of meningoencephalitis caused by *Candida* spp. in a neonate usually requires systemic therapy for at least 30 days; longer courses of treatment may be required if ventriculitis or brain abscesses or nodules are present.[79,80,123,169,316] Repeat CSF examination and culture before discontinuing antifungal therapy is recommended to document sterilization and improved CSF parameters of white cells, glucose, and protein.[90] If *Candida* ventriculitis is associated with an indwelling ventricular drain or shunt, prompt removal of the device also is indicated. Repeat CSF examination and culture should be done every 24 to 48 hours until sterile, and treatment should be continued when, and for sometime after, the drain or shunt is replaced.

Treatment of endocarditis or septic thrombophlebitis caused by *Candida* spp. requires prolonged antifungal treatment, at least 30 days and usually 42 to 60 days, depending on clearance of candidemia, clinical progress, and resolution of intracardiac vegetations or lesions as documented by echocardiography.[115,128,233,263] Consultation with a cardiologist or cardiovascular surgeon is recommended.[96,104,246] If septic thrombophlebitis with vascular abscess is present, or an enlarging valvular mass obstructs blood flow, surgical intervention may be considered.[104,115,151,216,241] Reports of resolution of endocarditis with medical therapy alone suggest, however, that it may be a valid option to consider, especially for neonates who are hemodynamically stable, with right-sided, nonvalvular lesions.[115,117,128,151,183,212,317,414]

Treatment of eye disease, such as endophthalmitis, requires systemic antifungal therapy for 25 to 42 days, and consultation with an ophthalmologist is recommended to assess the extent of disease, presence or progression of comorbid retinopathy of prematurity, and response to therapy.[100,136,223,263,356] If an abscess of the lens is present, surgical drainage or lensectomy may be necessary.[25,87,103,330,356,367] Long-term follow-up of neonates with *Candida* endophthalmitis suggests that early medical therapy results in cure for most neonates who survive systemic candidiasis and that invasive procedures usually performed in adults with *Candida* eye disease, such as vitreous taps or intravitreal injections of medications, are unnecessary in most neonates.[12,25,127,136] Neonates with invasive candidiasis should be observed closely, however, for progression of retinopathy of prematurity.[49,145]

Renal disease caused by invasive *Candida* spp. usually responds to systemic antifungal therapy, the duration of which usually is

*See references 8, 29, 52, 62, 68, 86, 101, 102, 131, 140, 145, 172, 253, 265, 274, 321, 354, 410, 413.
†See references 30, 53, 78, 148, 157, 158, 255, 275, 320, 344, 347, 353, 363, 397.

at least 25 days.[7,41,44,153,263] Longer duration of therapy may be required to eradicate renal mycetomas, abscesses, or masses ("fungal balls"). If obstructive uropathy is present, urologic consultation is recommended to determine if nephrostomy or other diverting procedure is indicated to relieve the obstruction temporarily.*

Treatment of osteoarthritis caused by *Candida* spp. usually requires prolonged duration of systemic antifungal therapy (≥42 days).[361,387,393] Aspiration or surgical drainage by an orthopedic surgeon may be necessary if there is an infected joint or bone abscess.[2,146,162,199]

Peritonitis associated with NEC or SFIP usually requires at least 25 days of systemic antifungal therapy, but longer duration may be required if intra-abdominal abscesses develop.[39,88] Surgical management of SFIP also differs from that of NEC; simple surgical procedures, such as suturing or resection with primary anastomosis, may be all that is required for treatment of SFIP, whereas NEC may require extensive bowel resection.†

Duration of systemic antifungal treatment for pulmonary candidiasis is not well established. Treatment should be guided by clinical and radiographic improvement; however, 25 days is likely to be adequate for most patients.[39,132,310]

ANTIFUNGAL AGENTS

The choice of antifungal agents available to treat neonatal candidiasis has expanded beyond the traditional polyene antibiotics, nystatin and amphotericin B deoxycholate, and the pyrimidine analogue 5-flucytosine (5-FC). Lipid formulations of amphotericin B are safe and effective when administered to neonates.[3,51,68] The first antifungal azoles administered to neonates were imidazoles (miconazole and ketoconazole) with unpredictable absorption and toxicities.[83,359,369] First-generation triazoles (fluconazole and itraconazole), available now for almost 2 decades, seem to be effective and safe when administered to most neonates.[44,47,54,375] Rare reports of fetal malformations associated with fluconazole administered prenatally to pregnant women are of potential concern.[5] Newer compounds, including second-generation triazoles (posaconazole, ravuconazole, and voriconazole) and echinocandins (caspofungin, micafungin, and anidulafungin), have emerged as potentially valuable agents to treat resistant yeast and fungal infections in neonates.[8,72,150,158,253,337]

Amphotericin B

Amphotericin B deoxycholate, a polyene macrolide antibiotic, remains the drug of choice for most neonates with systemic candidiasis caused by susceptible *Candida* spp.‡ *Candida* spp. most commonly isolated, including *C. albicans*, usually are susceptible to amphotericin B; however, more recent reports suggest the incidence of amphotericin B resistance may be 20 to 25 percent in *C. albicans* and *C. parapsilosis* isolated from pediatric patients, including neonates.[18,405,410] In addition, resistance is a common finding in *C. lusitaniae* and *C. haemulonii*. Also, the compound seems to be less active in vitro against some species, including *C. parapsilosis*, *C. tropicalis*, and *C. guilliermondii*.[384]

The limited pharmacokinetic data available suggest neonates exhibit considerable interindividual variability in metabolism of the drug, and this variation is speculated to be due partly to genomic factors that affect drug metabolism.[8,353] The usual recommended dose is 1 mg/kg/day infused over the course of 2 to 4 hours; however, dosage ranges of 0.5 to 1.5 mg/kg/day have

been used, depending on the diagnosis and organism isolated. Administration of a small initial test dose, slow escalation of doses, and premedication to prevent infusion-related reactions are unnecessary in neonates. The duration of therapy varies with the severity and type of *Candida* infection. For uncomplicated, catheter-associated candidemia in which prompt removal of the intravascular device results in rapid clinical and laboratory improvement, a cumulative dose of 7 to 10 mg/kg usually is sufficient.[62] For disseminated infection, cumulative doses of at least 25 mg/kg often are necessary.[62,311] For meningitis, a 30-mg/kg cumulative dose often is preferred,[79] whereas for endocarditis and osteoarthritis, cumulative doses of 40 to 50 mg/kg have been administered in some cases.[317]

Intrathecal amphotericin B deoxycholate has been used to treat refractory candidal meningitis, but it rarely is needed. The initial intrathecal dose is 0.01 mg, which is increased gradually over 5 to 7 days to 0.1 mg given every other or every third day.

Adverse effects of amphotericin B deoxycholate include nephrotoxicity in 15 percent of neonates, manifested by azotemia, hypokalemia, and hypomagnesemia, often with an elevated serum creatinine concentration and oliguria.[62,78,156,353] Hypokalemia occurs frequently and reflects tubular injury resulting in increased urinary excretion of potassium.[156] Nephrotoxicity may be minimized by avoiding concomitant use of other potentially nephrotoxic drugs during administration of amphotericin B. Animal and adult studies also have suggested higher sodium intake may prevent renal compromise during amphotericin B therapy. More recently, a study of the effects of fluid and electrolyte management on amphotericin B–induced nephrotoxicity in VLBW neonates suggested nephrotoxicity occurred more frequently in neonates with hyponatremia and suggested hydration and higher sodium intake may provide some protection against amphotericin B–induced nephrotoxicity in VLBW neonates.[156]

Hepatic enzyme abnormalities, hyperbilirubinemia,[172,267] anemia, and thrombocytopenia[69] also have been reported, but rarely occur in neonates. Similarly, neonates do not experience the fever, rigors, shaking, chills, or vomiting that are common infusion-related events in older children and adults.

Lipid preparations of amphotericin B, such as liposomal amphotericin B (L-AmB; AmBisome), amphotericin B lipid complex (ABLC; Abelcet), and amphotericin B colloidal dispersion (ABCD; Amphocil, Amphotec), in usual daily doses of 3 to 5 mg/kg (range 2.5 to 7.5 mg/kg), have been used safely and successfully in neonates with invasive candidiasis of many forms caused by a variety of *Candida* spp.* More recent pharmacokinetic and clinical information support their use in neonates, but optimal dosage with standardized duration of therapy has not been established in randomized controlled trials.[86,200,321]

Some reports suggest lipid preparations may eradicate *Candida* infection more rapidly than does amphotericin B deoxycholate when used as first-line therapy for some forms of invasive candidiasis and may benefit neonates who do not respond clinically and microbiologically to amphotericin B deoxycholate therapy.[179,183,200] Although experience with lipid formulations has increased dramatically in recent years, superior efficacy or safety for neonatal candidiasis has not been proven. In addition, lipid formulations are more costly than is amphotericin B deoxycholate, so they are not recommended universally for routine or first-line treatment in neonates.[134,142,152,171,206,386,402] In most centers, lipid preparations are reserved for clinical or microbiologic failure, or when toxicity, primarily renal, occurs during the course of conventional amphotericin B deoxycholate therapy.

Of the lipid preparations, liposomal amphotericin B may have improved CNS penetration; however, some preparations may not penetrate the kidney well.[142] Because these preparations prefer-

---

*See references 22, 44, 107, 126, 198, 207, 229, 272, 277, 289, 381.
†See references 1, 34, 56, 88, 175, 182, 243, 248, 290, 299, 301.
‡See references 8, 29, 30, 37, 52, 61, 62, 86, 123, 131, 354, 413.

*See references 3, 8, 52, 68, 86, 134, 152, 171, 172, 178, 179, 183, 200, 206, 321, 394, 413.

entially accumulate in organs of the reticuloendothelial system, they may be more useful for the treatment of hepatic or splenic candidal abscesses.[386] Toxicities associated with lipid preparations of amphotericin B are similar to the toxicities seen with amphotericin B deoxycholate and include hypokalemia, hypomagnesemia, renal insufficiency, and hepatic dysfunction; however, occurrence of toxicities may be less frequent or less severe than those of amphotericin B deoxycholate.[68,172,179,394]

5-Flucytosine

The compound 5-FC is a synthetic pyrimidine analogue that is administered orally in a dose of 50 to 150 mg/kg/day divided every 6 hours, in combination with amphotericin B formulations, when meningitis is present.[79,80,311] Some experts also consider using 5-FC if endophthalmitis, endocarditis, persistent candidemia, or osteoarthritis is present, whereas others prefer to use amphotericin B alone and monitor for clinical and microbiologic response.[61,62] Most *Candida* spp. are highly susceptible to 5-FC, and synergy of 5-FC with amphotericin B has been documented.[249] It also is well absorbed from the gastrointestinal tract and diffuses well into the CSF and eye.[53,80]

The dose of 5-FC should be decreased if renal insufficiency is present or suspected, and all neonates should have serum levels monitored frequently to ensure they have adequate levels and to avoid development of toxicity. Recommended therapeutic serum levels range from 25 to 100 mg/L. Some centers recommend steady-state serum levels of 40 to 60 mg/L, whereas others prefer predose and 2-hour postdose serum therapeutic ranges of 30 to 40 mg/L and 70 to 80 mg/L.[275,347] Levels greater than 100 mg/L are associated with toxicity and should be avoided. More recent studies on 5-FC therapeutic monitoring in pediatric patients, including neonates, have shown that the standard recommended daily dose of 100 mg/kg is associated with significantly higher serum concentrations in neonates, prompting recommendations for adjusted dosage schedules in this special age group.[275,336]

Approximately 4 to 8 percent of *C. albicans* isolates, and as many as 22 percent of non-*albicans* isolates, mostly *C. tropicalis* and *C. krusei*, are resistant to 5-FC.[366] The drug should never be used alone to treat candidiasis because resistance is likely to emerge even in susceptible *Candida* spp. if 5-FC is used as monotherapy. Side effects can be significant and include renal toxicity, hepatotoxicity, bone marrow suppression, gastrointestinal intolerance, and hemorrhagic enterocolitis.[53,186,317] These effects usually are associated with elevated serum levels greater than 100 μg/mL; nonetheless, it is prudent to monitor blood counts and liver and renal function tests in all neonates who receive 5-FC. Because of the potential for development of significant toxicity, the need for oral administration in premature neonates who may be unable to tolerate enteral feeds and recommended monitoring of drug levels, and the need for successful clinical experience with amphotericin B monotherapy, routine use of 5-FC requires thoughtful consideration.[62]

Triazoles (Fluconazole, Itraconazole, Voriconazole)

Fluconazole is a first-generation triazole antifungal agent with excellent antifungal activity against most isolates of *C. albicans*.[380] *C. krusei* and the more recently recognized *C. haemulonii* seem to be inherently resistant to fluconazole, and some strains of *C. glabrata*, *C. tropicalis*, *C. parapsilosis*, and *C. guilliermondii* may have reduced susceptibility.[164,193,311,380] Fluconazole resistance also has been detected more recently in *C. parapsilosis*, *C. albicans*, and *C. tropicalis* isolates from neonates.[50,139,319,380,410]

Fluconazole seems to be a safe and effective agent for treatment of neonatal systemic candidiasis and may be first-line therapy in some centers for uncomplicated, catheter-associated candidemia in neonates.* Breakthrough candidemia has been described, however, in neonates receiving fluconazole therapy.[204,246] Because it has excellent penetration of CSF, fluconazole also has been used occasionally to treat neonates with candidal meningitis.[169] Adverse effects associated with use of fluconazole in neonates are minimal and include elevated liver enzymes and skin rashes. Usual recommended doses for term neonates are 3 to 6 mg/kg/day for mucocutaneous disease and up to 6 to 12 mg/kg/day every 24 hours for systemic disease. In premature neonates, the dose interval should be adjusted to every 48 to 72 hours, depending on gestational and chronologic postnatal age. Duration of therapy should be at least 28 days for systemic candidiasis; shorter durations may be acceptable for isolated catheter colonization or mild, noninvasive mucocutaneous candidiasis.

Itraconazole, an oral first-generation triazole with activity against most *Candida* spp. except *C. krusei* is not approved for use in children or neonates. Nonetheless, it has been used rarely to treat systemic candidiasis in neonates.[47,375] Because it does not cross the blood-brain barrier well, itraconazole should not be used to treat neonates in whom *Candida* meningitis is suspected or proven. Clinical experience seems to be limited; similar to fluconazole, emergence of itraconazole resistance has been documented in *C. albicans* and *C. tropicalis* strains isolated from neonates.[140]

The second-generation triazole, voriconazole, has expanded antifungal activity that includes not only *Candida* spp., but also *Cryptococcus neoformans*, *Aspergillus*, *Fusarium*, and *Trichosporon beigelii*. Voriconazole displays nonlinear pharmacokinetics in adults, but it seems to have linear pharmacokinetics in children and neonates.[354] Higher doses in smaller patients may be needed to avoid treatment failures. Experience in neonates is very limited, and the drug is not approved for use in this age group. Nonetheless, isolated case reports of use of the drug in difficult cases appear in the literature. In one case report, the addition of intravenous voriconazole administered in the pediatric dose of 6 mg/kg/dose every 12 hours resulted in subtherapeutic levels; however, 6 mg/kg every 8 hours achieved acceptable serum concentrations and eliminated disseminated fluconazole-resistant *C. albicans* infection in a neonate with persistent infection while receiving liposomal amphotericin B alone.[255] In addition, voriconazole has been administered successfully to neonates with vertically transmitted cryptococcal meningitis and invasive dermatitis caused by *Aspergillus* spp.[130,189,318,333]

Currently, no data on neonates are available on the use of posaconazole, ravuconazole, isavuconazole, or albaconazole, which are antifungal azoles currently in preclinical and clinical development stages.[274]

Echinocandins (Caspofungin, Micafungin)

The echinocandins include caspofungin, micafungin, anidulafungin, and aminocandin and have activity against most *Candida* spp., including *C. krusei*.[64,239,282] Clinical trials showed caspofungin to be comparable to amphotericin B for treatment of candidemia in adult patients.[281] Caspofungin is not approved for use in children, however, and the appropriate dose and safety of this drug have not been established in neonates. Limited published experience using caspofungin to treat neonates with persistent candidemia or progressive invasive candidiasis caused by *C. albicans* or other *Candida* spp., resistant or unresponsive to amphotericin B or fluconazole, suggests that caspofungin may be a safe and effective alternative in selected neonates, alone or when added to amphotericin B.[55,150,224,257,265,334,405]

Caspofungin penetrates the kidneys well, and good levels are achieved in urine. It does not penetrate into CSF or the eye well,

---

*See references 54, 101, 102, 122, 169, 300, 311, 320, 324, 384, 397.

however, and it should not be used to treat neonates in whom *Candida* meningitis or endophthalmitis is suspected or proven.[137] It also may be less effective for *Candida* endocarditis. Available pharmacokinetic data suggest that caspofungin also requires higher doses in children and neonates, calculated using body surface area rather than body weight (70 mg/m² first day, then 50 mg/m² once daily).[274]

Micafungin, the newest echinocandin, is not approved for use in this age group. It has been administered to preterm neonates, however, in phase I clinical trials, and case reports of micafungin administered in combination with voriconazole and amphotericin B to treat severe cutaneous aspergillosis in preterm infants have been published.[157,158,318] Limited pharmacokinetic and safety data suggest that VLBW preterm infants tolerate doses up to 3 mg/kg daily, but may require a larger dose (8 to 15 mg/kg) or more frequent dosing compared with older children and adults.[157,363] Neonatal rabbit models suggest that micafungin does not reliably penetrate the CSF; studies administering micafungin to treat human neonates with *Candida* meningitis are unavailable.[157] Currently, no data or published experiences are available on administration of anidulafungin or aminocandin to neonates with invasive candidiasis.

Immunomodulators

Because antibody to fungal proteins is associated with recovery from invasive candidiasis, immunoglobulin and other immunomodulators may be evaluated eventually for treatment or prevention of invasive *Candida* infections. Currently, preclinical assessments of recombinant antibodies (hsp90, Mycograb, Efungumab) show antifungal activity against *Candida* spp. and *C. neoformans*, and synergy with antifungal chemotherapy agents.[155,231,261] No clinical trials evaluating specific antibody preparations for treatment or prevention of invasive yeast or fungal disease in neonates have been performed.

PREVENTION

FLUCONAZOLE PROPHYLAXIS

The high frequency and significant morbidity and mortality rates associated with *Candida* infections in VLBW neonates have been the impetus behind animal models and clinical studies of preventive strategies using antifungal agents.[187,338,377] In early studies evaluating prophylactic regimens, oral nystatin reduced fungal colonization and disease in preterm infants with a birth weight of less than 1250 g, and it has been used to control a nursery outbreak of *Candida* infection.[92,337] Miconazole oral gel decreased rectal fungal colonization, a predisposing factor for the development of systemic candidiasis, compared with placebo in infants with a birth weight of less than 1750 g.[383] Several single-center and cohort studies and a large, multicenter, randomized, double-blind, placebo-controlled trial have shown that fluconazole prophylaxis reduces *Candida* colonization, invasive candidiasis, or mortality rates in high-risk, VLBW premature neonates.*

These published studies presented slightly different methods of selection criteria for neonates for prophylaxis (universal for all infants weighing <1000 or <1500 g versus risk-based selection), doses (3 to 6 mg/kg/day), dosage schedules (daily versus every other day versus twice weekly), routes of administration (intravenous only versus intravenous followed by oral versus oral alone), and duration of prophylaxis (4 weeks versus 6 weeks), and slightly different outcome measures. Fluconazole administration was not associated with significant toxicity in any of the studies. Despite these encouraging findings, however, not all centers have adopted

*See references 19, 46, 84, 187, 188, 194, 225, 234, 235, 273, 319.

or advocate universal prophylaxis for VLBW infants with birth weight of less than 1500 to 1000 g. Some centers prefer a risk-based strategy, selecting only VLBW neonates with an additional risk factor, such as *Candida* surface colonization, central venous catheter in place, endotracheal intubation, or recent administration of third-generation cephalosporin.[234] Some centers advocate twice-weekly, rather than daily, prophylaxis to reduce health care costs and to minimize neonates' exposure to antifungals, with the speculation that lower and less frequent dosing may delay or prevent emergence of resistant *Candida* spp.[188]

Most studies of fluconazole prophylaxis in neonates did not report changes in patterns of colonization or rates of invasive disease caused by *Candida* spp. other than *C. albicans*, or emergence of resistance to fluconazole.[188,225,228] These studies may not have had sufficient duration of exposure or power, however, to determine a difference during the study period.[228] More recent reports have documented emergence of *Candida* spp. other than *C. albicans* as predominant pathogens[193,273,319] and emergence of resistance to fluconazole in *C. albicans* and other *Candida* spp.[140,380,410] One center with more than 10 years of experience using fluconazole prophylaxis documented emergence of a resistant strain of *C. parapsilosis* that caused invasive candidiasis in neonates.[319]

Similar to well-documented emergence of bacteria that become resistant to frequently used antibiotics, the emergence of *Candida* spp. resistant to antifungal agents is becoming an important consideration in clinical management of invasive candidiasis.[319,410,411] In addition, emergence of invasive yeasts other than *Candida* spp. may occur. An outbreak of *Rhodotorula mucilaginosa*, a fluconazole-resistant yeast, occurred more recently in an NICU that routinely administered prophylactic fluconazole.[280,371]

OTHER PREVENTIVE STRATEGIES

Preventive strategies other than administration of antifungal agents to reduce *Candida* infections in neonates, are important approaches to investigate. Oral supplementation of breast milk feedings with the probiotic *Lactobacillus casei* subspecies *rhamnosus* was shown more recently to reduce significantly the incidence and intensity of enteric colonization with *Candida* spp. in VLBW neonates.[227] Bloodstream infections with *Candida* spp. occurred in neonates enrolled in previous studies evaluating intravenous immunoglobulin for prevention of nosocomial infections in VLBW neonates; however, no studies have evaluated immunoprophylaxis strategies designed specifically for prevention of nosocomial *Candida* infections in VLBW neonates.[391]

The role of patient cohorting or single-room isolation of neonates with *Candida* colonization or infection also was reviewed more recently.[72,247] Published evidence shows that transmission of *Candida* in the NICU occurs by direct or indirect contact, and cross-infection by health care workers has been documented.[18,63,163,165,167,247,303] Guidelines for isolation procedures are unavailable, most likely because currently available information neither supports nor refutes the use of isolation measures to reduce transmission of *Candida* infections in high-risk neonates.[247]

INVASIVE YEASTS OTHER THAN *CANDIDA*

Disseminated candidiasis is the most common fungal infection in neonates. The dimorphic fungi may infect pregnant women and rarely may be transmitted to the fetus or newborn. More recent reports have suggested that unusual yeasts are becoming important causes of invasive disease in neonates and NICU outbreaks, often with high morbidity and mortality rates.[346] It is important to be aware of emerging pathogenic yeasts because a timely diagnosis and effective management may improve neonatal morbidity and mortality from these often challenging and difficult infections.

CRYPTOCOCCUS

Congenital and perinatal infections with the encapsulated yeast, *C. neoformans*, have been reported.[67,110,189,339,342] Fetal demise may occur, especially in pregnant women with untreated or severe disease.[110] Neonates also may aspirate the organism during delivery and present with fever and respiratory symptoms; meningitis, gastrointestinal involvement, and disseminated disease also may occur.[189] Neonates and young infants who present with disseminated *C. neoformans* also may have a congenital immune disorder, such as severe combined immunodeficiency.[342] Systemic antifungal treatment with amphotericin B is preferred, used in combination with 5-FC. Although *C. neoformans* seems to be susceptible to triazole agents, experience using these compounds to treat neonates with cryptococcosis is limited.[333]

MALASSEZIA

Malassezia genus of yeasts includes seven species. The six lipophilic species are *Malassezia furfur, Malassezia globosa, Malassezia obtuse, Malassezia restricta, Malassezia slooffiae*, and *Malassezia sympodialis*, and one species, *Malassezia pachydermatis*, is not strictly lipophilic.[17] *Malassezia* spp. frequently colonize the skin of neonates.[16,20,346] By the time they are 1 week old, 5 percent of neonates have positive skin cultures for *Malassezia* spp.; by 2 weeks of age, 37 to 51 percent of VLBW premature neonates have positive skin cultures. By the time they reach 3 to 6 months of age, healthy newborns have been observed to have colonization rates of 48 to 91 percent, as have preterm neonates in the NICU.[16,20,36] *Malassezia* spp. can be introduced into the NICU on the hands of health care workers and be transmitted to neonates; it also seems to persist on environmental surfaces such as incubators.[70,82,396] The species most frequently associated with neonatal infections and NICU outbreaks include *M. furfur, M. pachydermatis, M. sympodialis*, and *M. globosa*.

Skin infections with *M. furfur* and *M. sympodialis* have been associated with nonfollicular pustulosis skin conditions, such as neonatal cephalic pustulosis and neonatal acne, in neonates.[20,45,259,293] Skin scrapings of the pustules may show neutrophilic cells and fungal or yeast organisms when examined under the microscope, and fungal culture confirms the organism.[20,293] Neonatal cephalic pustulosis usually is a benign, self-limited condition of the skin and responds to topical antifungal therapy. It must be differentiated, however, from more invasive forms of yeast and fungal diseases. Skin infections with *M. globosa* and, to a lesser extent, *M. sympodialis* are associated with pityriasis versicolor.[17]

Intravascular catheters may become colonized with *M. furfur* or *M. pachydermatis* and cause bloodstream infections, often with serious complications in VLBW preterm neonates.[93,392] Risks for development of invasive disease include previous treatment with broad-spectrum antibiotics and prolonged use of intravascular catheters and intravenous fat emulsions or lipid infusions.[82,396] Neonates may present with systemic signs of sepsis, pulmonary decompensation, and thrombocytopenia.[360] Complications of

catheter-associated bloodstream infections with *M. furfur* include peripheral thrombophlebitis, thromboembolism, catheter occlusion, adhesion of the vascular catheter to the vein wall, and endocarditis with intracardiac mass and thromboembolic phenomena.[21,95,191,195,323] Neonatal meningitis and urinary tract infections associated with *M. furfur* and *M. pachydermatis* also have been reported.[70]

Cultures of blood, catheter tip, urine, CSF, and involved tissue should be obtained. The organism also has been seen on peripheral blood smear.[48] Diagnosis may be elusive, however, because recovery of *Malassezia* spp. in routine cultures is rare; if the diagnosis is suspected, special fungal cultures on Sabouraud dextrose agar overlaid with sterile olive oil or media containing long-chain fatty acids may enhance recovery of lipophilic *Malassezia* spp. Treatment involves immediate removal of the catheter and discontinuation of lipid infusions. *Malassezia* spp. seem to be susceptible to most triazole agents and amphotericin B.[144,244] Administration of intravenous amphotericin B deoxycholate is recommended for treatment of neonates with invasive disease caused by *Malassezia* spp.

PICHIA

Pichia (Hansenula) anomala and *Pichia ohmeri* are emerging yeasts that may cause infection in preterm VLBW neonates and infants with severe combined immunodeficiency. In some NICUs, 17 percent of preterm neonates may be colonized, and single cases and NICU outbreaks associated with indwelling catheters, administration of total parenteral nutrition solutions, and abdominal surgery have been described.[13,23,219,256,278,338,364,401] Invasive diseases in preterm neonates include bloodstream infections, sepsis syndrome, abscesses, and meningitis with ventriculitis. Management includes removal of indwelling catheters and systemic antifungal therapy. Although *Pichia* spp. seem to be susceptible to amphotericin B and some antifungal triazoles, no standard treatment recommendations are available. Amphotericin B in combination with 5-FC usually has been administered as treatment for neonates with invasive *Pichia* spp. infections.[23,219,256,364,401]

TRICHOSPORON

Trichosporon spp. colonize the hair, skin, mucous membranes, and gastrointestinal tract. *T. beigelii* has caused invasive dermatitis, late-onset sepsis, pulmonary infiltrates, and urinary tract infections in VLBW preterm neonates with intravascular catheters.* It also may cause endophthalmitis and endocarditis. *Trichosporon asahii* infection in neonates has been reported more recently, suggesting that this species has emerged as a neonatal pathogen.[270,407]

Trichosporon spp. have been isolated from blood, urine, tracheal aspirates, skin lesions, and catheter tip cultures from neonates.[338] The organism may be identified preliminarily as a germ-tube negative yeast and be confused initially with *Candida* spp. Breakthrough *Trichosporon* infections in patients receiving antifungal agents for candidemia have been reported. The clinician may erroneously attribute persistently positive cultures to a resistant *Candida* spp. rather than *Trichosporon* spp.[35,298] *Trichosporon* spp. also share heat-stable antigens with *C. neoformans*, and produce false-positive cryptococcal antigen tests. A real-time polymerase chain reaction assay to detect *T. asahii* DNA in sera has been developed and may help facilitate rapid establishment of the diagnosis of this potentially fatal infection.[238]

---

*See references 15, 16, 20, 21, 36, 45, 70, 82, 95, 161, 191, 195, 259, 288, 293, 297, 323, 332, 360, 374, 396.

*See references 35, 125, 140, 147, 196, 270, 298, 338, 362, 385, 407, 408.

The organism has unpredictable susceptibility to antifungal agents, and there are no standardized recommendations for management of neonates with invasive *Trichosporon* infection. Most neonates have been treated with amphotericin B deoxycholate or liposomal amphotericin B.[338,407] The organism may be tolerant or resistant to amphotericin B, caspofungin, and posaconazole, and treatment failures with all of these agents may occur.[385] The organism seems to be susceptible to voriconazole, and isolated case reports of successful therapy in older patients using voriconazole, in combination with amphotericin B, have been published, but no published experience in neonates is available.[35,196,298]

RHODOTORULA

Rhodotorula spp. are another emerging opportunistic yeast that has caused catheter-associated bloodstream infections, endocarditis, peritonitis, meningitis, and endophthalmitis in immunocompromised patients and patients in intensive care units.[280,371] *R. mucilaginosa* and, less frequently, *Rhodotorula glutinis* have been documented to cause disease. *Rhodotorula* spp. usually are susceptible to amphotericin B, itraconazole, and voriconazole, but commonly are resistant to fluconazole. More recently, an outbreak of catheter-associated bloodstream infections with *R. mucilaginosa* in preterm neonates in an NICU administering routine fluconazole prophylaxis was reported.[280] Successful management of infected neonates included removal of the catheters and administration of systemic amphotericin B.

INVASIVE FUNGAL DISEASES

CONGENITAL AND PERINATAL TRANSMISSION

Fetal demise, congenital infection, and perinatal transmission associated with the endemic dimorphic fungi, *Coccidioides immitis* and *Blastomyces dermatitidis*, have been described.* Published case reports are very rare, however. Third-trimester acute infection with *C. immitis* seems to carry increased risk of developing severe illness for the mother and fetus. Perinatal transmission for both organisms likely occurs from neonatal aspiration of infected cervicovaginal secretions from a chronically infected maternal genitourinary tract. Cultures of urine, respiratory secretions, and lung tissue are most likely to yield the organisms. If coccidioidomycosis or blastomycosis is diagnosed in a neonate, treatment with systemic amphotericin B is recommended.

ACQUIRED INVASIVE FUNGAL DISEASE

Invasive fungal disease acquired by VLBW or ELBW premature neonates involves primarily the skin, lungs, or gastrointestinal tract. Because many of the invasive fungi that affect neonates also are angioinvasive, sepsis syndrome with hematogenous dissemination to lung, liver, spleen, CNS, and eye may occur rapidly.

ASPERGILLUS

Aspergillus spp. include *Aspergillus flavus, Aspergillus fumigatus, Aspergillus glaucus, Aspergillus nidulans, Aspergillus niger,* and *Aspergillus terreus. Aspergillus* spp. frequently are found in the environment and the hospital. Infection in neonates and outbreaks in NICUs have been associated with nearby construction

*See references 5, 75, 89, 210, 214, 232, 329, 370, 388, 398, 409.

or renovation.[9,11,143,271] Diseases associated with *Aspergillus* infection of the neonate include primary cutaneous aspergillosis or invasive dermatitis, pulmonary aspergillosis, and disseminated aspergillosis. Disseminated disease may involve the heart, liver, spleen, lungs, CNS, or eye.*

Neonatal aspergillosis usually manifests in the second week of life.[271,308,400] Risk factors include extreme prematurity and VLBW or ELBW, administration of steroids and broad-spectrum antibiotics, hyperglycemia, and trauma of the extremely vulnerable skin of the premature infant.[143,308] The delicate skin of VLBW infants can be macerated easily by adhesive tape, traumatized at the site of insertion of an indwelling intravascular catheter or by surgical procedures, or damaged by pressure sores, providing a portal of entry for the fungus. Invasive fungal dermatitis then occurs (Fig. 76–5). *Aspergillus* spp. also may gain entry through the lungs and cause invasive pulmonary aspergillosis.[143] Because the fungus has a predilection for invasion of blood vessels, it can disseminate quickly in the bloodstream and occlude vessels, causing thrombosis, infarction, and necrosis of tissue (see Fig. 76–5B and C).

Establishment of the diagnosis requires a high index of suspicion and documentation of the fungus by histopathologic examination and culture of the involved tissue or organ. Suspicious skin lesions may appear early as erythematous plaques, vesicles, scales, or persistent maceration; advanced disease may show dark, necrotic skin lesions; skin biopsy that shows invasion below the stratum corneum establishes the diagnosis of invasive fungal dermatitis (see Fig. 76–5A and B).[400] *Aspergillus* also may be recovered from tracheal aspirate cultures, ascites, and CSF.[135,143] No studies have evaluated the performance of galactomannan antigen tests for the early diagnosis of invasive aspergillosis in neonates.

Early diagnosis followed by prompt and aggressive treatment of a neonate with invasive aspergillosis is important to minimize the usually high morbidity and mortality rates associated with this disease. Traditional treatment has included prolonged, high-dose amphotericin B deoxycholate or lipid complex and surgical excision of accessible tissue, such as the skin and soft tissue, if local disease progresses despite administration of systemic antifungal therapy.[10,271,281] Treatment failures frequently occur.[130,135,143,149] More recently, case reports of premature neonates with primary cutaneous aspergillosis who were treated successfully with voriconazole alone or in combination with amphotericin B lipid complex and micafungin have been published.[130,318]

ZYGOMYCETES (ABSIDIA, RHIZOPUS, MUCOR, RHIZOMUCOR)

Zygomycosis, a term preferred now over mucormycosis, usually is caused by the following species of fungi: *Absidia* (*Absidia corymbifera*), *Rhizopus* (*Rhizopus arrhizus, Rhizopus microsporus*), *Mucor* (*Mucor amphibiorum, Mucor circinelloides, Mucor hiemalis, Mucor indicus, Mucor racemosus, Mucor ramsissimus*), or *Rhizomucor* (*Rhizomucor pusillus, Rhizomucor miehei, Rhizomucor variabilis*). Zygomycosis in a neonate usually manifests during the second and third weeks of life.[296,340,412] Health care–associated outbreaks have been linked to contaminated dressings, bandages, or armboards. Risk factors for acquisition of infection include VLBW, extreme prematurity, indwelling intravascular catheters, exposure to elastic bandages, adhesive dressings and tapes, and armboards or tongue depressors used to split extremities, and host factors such as congenital immunodeficiency or genetic disorders of metabolism that cause metabolic acidosis.[213,252,412]

The Zygomycetes are angiotrophic and aggressively invade blood vessels very early in the disease process (Fig. 76–6C). Invasion of blood vessels leads to thrombosis, infarction, and tissue

*See references 9, 11, 130, 135, 143, 149, 159, 271, 281, 308, 309, 318, 400.

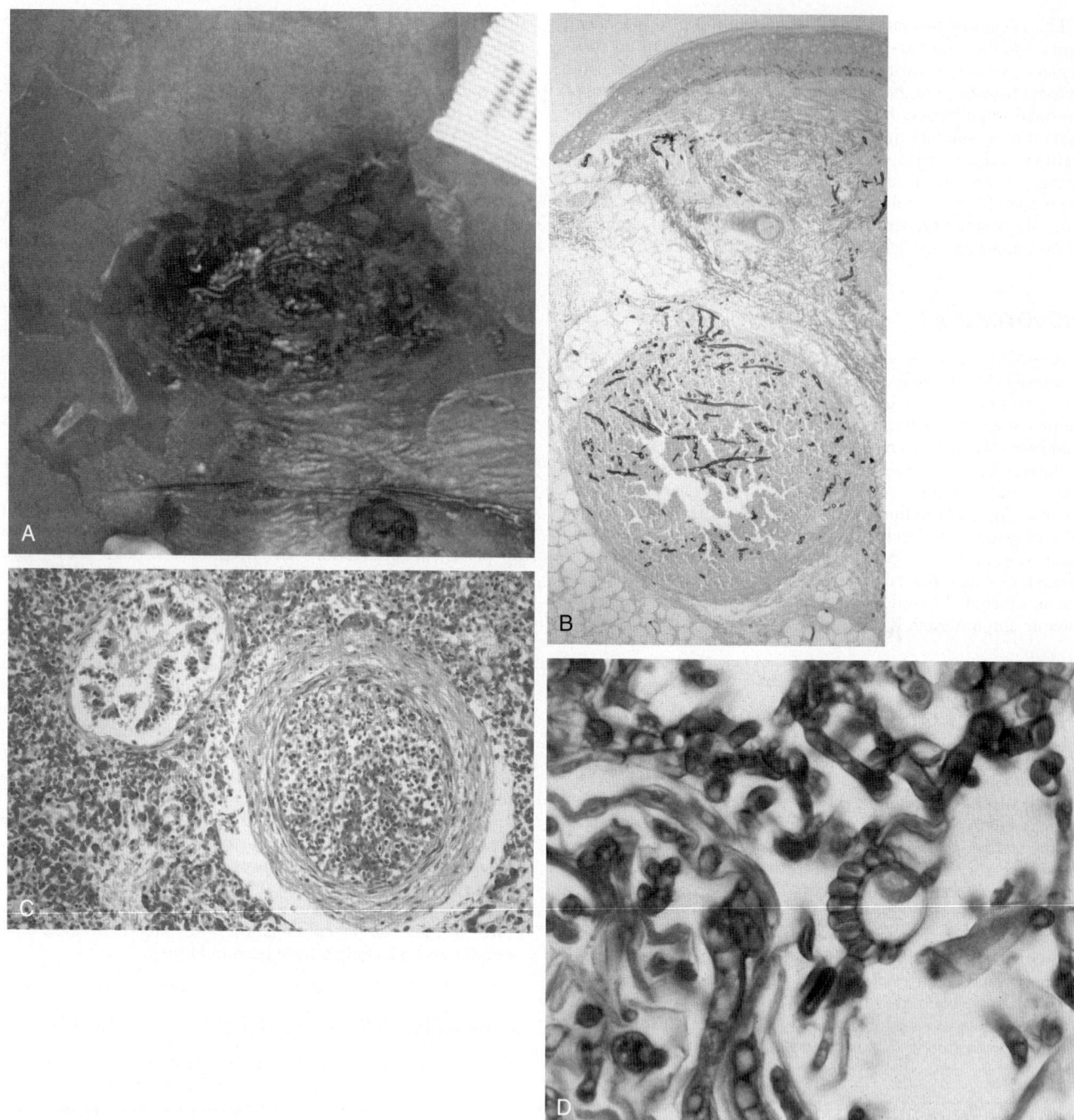

Figure 76–5 A-D, Invasive fungal dermatitis in a premature neonate caused by *Aspergillus flavus*. **A,** Fatal invasive fungal dermatitis with necrotizing fasciitis and disseminated fungal disease in a 23-day-old premature infant born at 26 weeks' gestation. **B-D,** Autopsy examination impressively showed angioinvasive nature of *A. flavus* with infected thrombus in skin (**B**) and lung (**C**) tissue. Uniformly broad, hyaline, septated, right angle branching hyphae with dramatic fungal fruiting body of *A. flavus* were seen in a lung lesion of this infant (**D**) (methenamine silver nitrate stain, 40×, 100×, and 400×, respectively, original magnification). *(Courtesy of Dr. Edwina J. Popek, Department of Pathology, Baylor College of Medicine and Texas Children's Hospital, Houston, TX.)*

necrosis; destruction of local tissue can be extensive, and the fungus may disseminate throughout the body and CNS. The most common presentation of invasive zygomycosis in neonates is primary cutaneous disease. Cutaneous zygomycosis usually begins at an area of minor skin trauma or at the site of intravenous catheter insertion that has come in contact with adhesive tape or bandages, first appearing as a cluster of necrotic vesicles or scales, which then rapidly progresses to extensive necrotizing cellulitis.[14,91,105,168,195,213,252,266,322] It usually involves the skin and

soft tissues of the upper extremities, but the lower extremities, abdominal wall, or face also may be presenting sites.

Gastrointestinal zygomycosis in a premature neonate often mimics NEC clinically, but without the characteristic radiographic bowel patterns; rarely, it has presented as Hirschsprung disease.[6,412] Intestinal perforation, of small or large bowel or appendix, with secondary peritonitis, may occur (see Fig. 76–6).[4,6,81,91,97,296,340] Rhinocerebral zygomycosis classically manifests in diabetics with ketoacidosis, but it also may affect neonates with

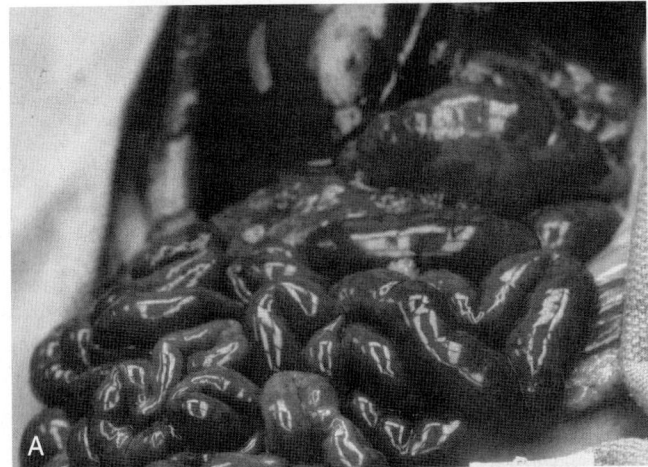

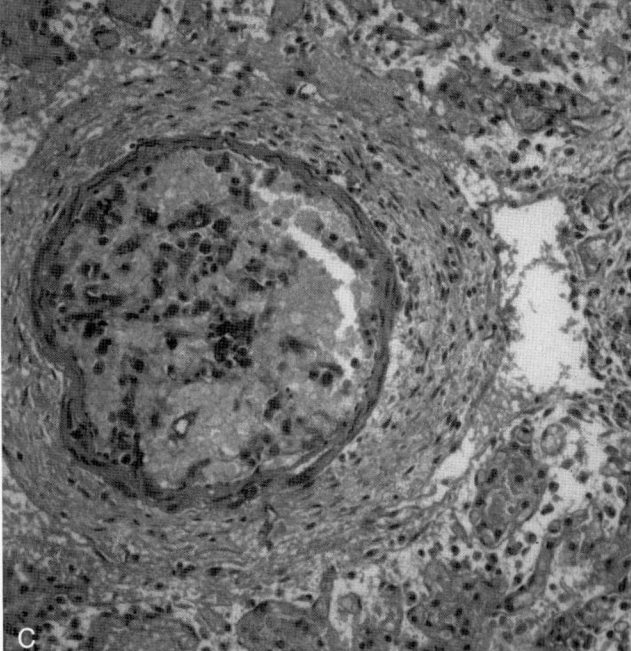

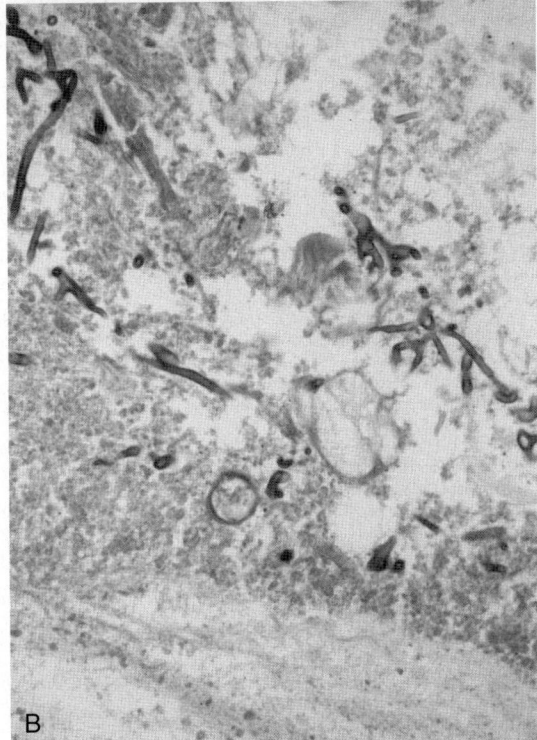

Figure 76–6 A-C, Invasive zygomycosis associated with necrotizing enterocolitis in a premature neonate. **A,** Intestinal bowel of an 11-day-old premature neonate born at 26 1/7 weeks' gestation, showing necrotizing enterocolitis associated with invasive zygomycosis (*Mucor* spp.). **B** and **C,** Angioinvasive nature of this pathogenic fungus was shown on autopsy examination by the presence of broad, thin-walled, nonseptated or sparsely septated, and irregular branching fungal hyphae (*Mucor* spp.) invading the intestine (**B**) and blood vessels (**C**) (methenamine silver nitrate stain, 100× original magnification). (*Courtesy of Dr. Edwina J. Popek, Department of Pathology, Baylor College of Medicine and Texas Children's Hospital, Houston, TX.*)

conditions associated with metabolic acidosis and premature infants. The fungus enters via the nasal passages and invades the sinus cavities and orbits, spreading to the CNS by fungal thrombosis of cavernous sinus and internal carotid artery.[413] Pulmonary zygomycosis also may occur, either as a primary pneumonia with consolidation and necrosis or secondary to vascular dissemination from a cutaneous or gastrointestinal source.[413] Disseminated zygomycosis is a fatal fungal sepsis syndrome, usually involving all major organ systems and the CNS.

Diagnosis is established by histopathologic examination of tissue, in which characteristic fungal elements invading the tissue and blood vessels can be seen. Fungal culture confirms the identification of the fungus. Successful management includes early diagnosis and aggressive surgical débridement and resection of involved tissues, to clear margins of resection.[252] Amputation or extensive skin grafts may be necessary in some patients.[205] Aggressive surgery is important because the fungus is resistant to most currently available antifungal agents, including the echinocandins

and first-generation and second-generation triazoles. The fungus may be inhibited by amphotericin B given in high doses (1.5 mg/kg/day of amphotericin B deoxycholate or ≥5 mg/kg of lipid formulations), which should be administered as soon as the diagnosis is suspected. The newest triazole compound, posaconazole, seems to have activity against zygomycetes, but experience in administering this new agent to neonates is unavailable.[302]

RARE AND UNUSUAL PATHOGENIC FUNGI

Other unusual pathogenic fungi that have been reported to cause invasive, and often fatal, disease in neonates include *Curvularia* (especially *Curvularia lunata*), which caused invasive fungal dermatitis in a premature infant, caused sternal wound infection complicating cardiac surgery in another neonate, and complicated disseminated neonatal herpes simplex infection in a third neonate (unpublished data) (Fig. 76–7).[309,406] *Phialemonium obova-*

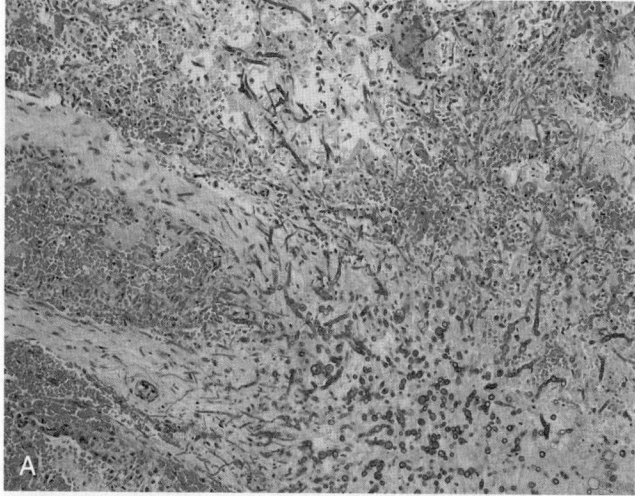

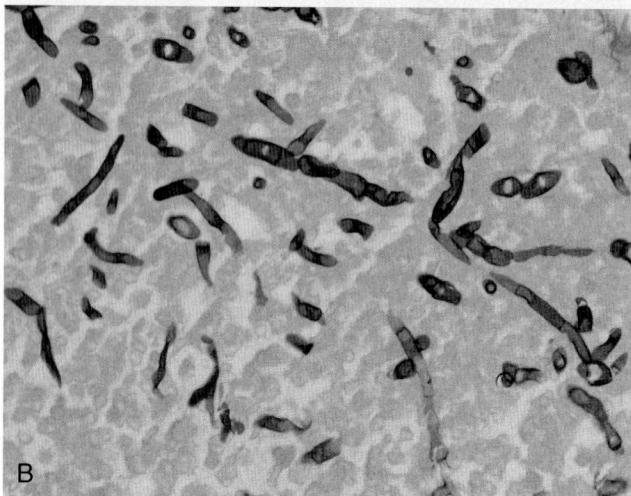

Figure 76–7 A and **B,** Disseminated *Curvularia* infection. Fatal invasive fungal infection with *Curvularia* in a 2-week-old term neonate with liver failure because of neonatal herpes simplex virus infection. **A,** The lungs showed angioinvasive fungal hyphae extending from the lumen of a thrombosed vessel into the adjacent alveolated lung parenchyma (hematoxylin and eosin stain, 100× original magnification). **B,** The fungal hyphae of *Curvularia* are narrow, frequently septated, with acute angle branching (methenamine silver nitrate stain, 400× original magnification). (See companion Expert Consult web site for color version.) *(Courtesy of Dr. Megan K. Dishop, Department of Pathology, Baylor College of Medicine and Texas Children's Hospital, Houston, TX.)*

tum reportedly has caused fatal endocarditis in a premature neonate.[138] *Bipolari spicifera* has caused invasive fungal dermatitis with dissemination in a preterm neonate.[250] Several cases of *Trichophyton* (*Trichophyton rubrum* and *Trichophyton violaceum*) causing localized scalp lesions, similar to tinea capitis, in neonates have been reported.[33,71,258,372]

REFERENCES

1. Adderson, E., Pappin, A., and Pavia, A.: Spontaneous intestinal perforation in premature infants: A distinct clinical entity associated with systemic candidiasis. J. Pediatr. Surg. *33*:1463, 1998.
2. Adler, S., Randall, J., and Plotkin, S.: Candidal osteomyelitis and arthritis in a neonate. Am. J. Dis. Child. *123*:595, 1972.
3. Adler-Shohet, F., Waskin, H., and Lieberman, J.: Amphotericin B lipid complex for neonatal invasive candidiasis. Arch. Dis. Child. Fetal Neonatal Ed. *84*: F131, 2001.
4. Agarwal, K., Sharma, M., Singh, S., et al.: Antemortem diagnosis of gastrointestinal mucormycosis in neonates: Report of two cases and review of the literature. Indian J. Pathol. Microbiol. *49*:430, 2006.
5. Aleck, K., and Bartley, D.: Multiple malformation syndrome following fluconazole use in pregnancy: Report of an additional patient. Am. J. Med. Genet. *72*:253, 1997.
6. Alexander, P., Alladi, A., Correa, M., et al.: Neonatal colonic mucormycosis—a tropical perspective. J. Trop. Pediatr. *51*:54, 2005.
7. Alkalay, A., Srugo, I., Blifeld, C., et al.: Noninvasive medical management of fungus ball uropathy in a premature infant. Am. J. Perinatol. *8*:330, 1991.
8. Almirante, B., and Rodriguez, D.: Antifungal agents in neonates: Issues and recommendations. Paediatr. Drugs *9*:311, 2007.
9. Amod, F., Coovadia, T., Pillay, T., et al.: Primary cutaneous aspergillosis in ventilated neonates. Pediatr. Infect. Dis. J. *19*:482, 2000.
10. Anderson, N., Sage, N., and Spaulding, E.: Oral moniliasis in newborn infants. Am. J. Dis. Child. *67*:450, 1944.
11. Andresen, J., Nygaard, E., and Stordal, K.: Primary cutaneous aspergillosis (PCA)—a case report. Acta Paediatr. *94*:761, 2005.
12. Annabie, W., Kachmer, M., DiMarco, M., et al.: *Pichia anomala* outbreak in a nursery: Exogenous source? Pediatr. Infect. Dis. J. *20*:843, 2001.
13. Aragao, P., Oshiro, I., Manrique, E., et al.: *Pichia anomala* outbreak in a nursery: Exogenous source? Pediatr. Infect. Dis. J. *20*:843, 2001.
14. Arisoy, A., Arisoy, E., Correa-Calderon, A., et al.: *Rhizopus* necrotizing cellulitis in a preterm infant: A case report and review of the literature. Pediatr. Infect. Dis. J. *12*:1029, 1993.
15. Aschner, J., Punsalang, A., Manisacalco, W., et al.: Percutaneous central venous catheter colonization with *Malassezia furfur*: Incidence and clinical significance. Pediatrics *80*:535, 1987.
16. Ashbee, H., Leck, A., Puntis, J., et al.: Skin colonization by *Malassezia* in neonates and infants. J. Infect. Control Hosp. Epidemiol. *23*:212, 2002.
17. Aspiroz, C., Ara, M., Varea, M., et al.: Isolation of *Malassezia globosa* and *M. sympodialis* from patients with pityriasis versicolor in Spain. Mycopathologia *154*:111, 2002.
18. Asticcioli, S., Nucleo, E., Perotti, G., et al.: *Candida albicans* in a neonatal intensive care unit: Antifungal susceptibility and genotype analysis. New Microbiol. *30*:303, 2007.
19. Austin, N., and Darlow, B.: Prophylactic oral antifungal agents to prevent systemic *Candida* infection in preterm infants. Cochrane Database Syst. Rev. *1*:CD003478, 2004.
20. Ayhan, M., Sancak, B., Karaduman, A., et al.: Colonization of neonate skin by *Malassezia* species: Relationship with neonatal cephalic pustulosis. J. Am. Acad. Dermatol. *57*:1012, 2007.
21. Azimi, P., Levernier, K., Lefrak, L., et al.: *Malassezia furfur*: A cause of occlusion of percutaneous central venous catheters in infants in the intensive care nursery. Pediatr. Infect. Dis. J. *7*:100, 1988.
22. Baetz-Greenwalt, B., Debaz, B., and Kumar, M.: Bladder fungus ball: A reversible cause of neonatal obstructive uropathy. Pediatrics *81*:826, 1988.
23. Bakir, M., Cerikcioglu, N., Tirtir, A., et al.: *Pichia anomala* fungaemia in immunocompromised children. Mycoses *47*:231, 2004.
24. Baley, J., Annable, W., and Kliegman, R.: *Candida* endophthalmitis in the premature infant. J. Pediatr. *98*:458, 1981.
25. Baley, J., and Ellis, F.: Neonatal candidiasis: Ophthalmologic infection. Semin. Perinatol. *27*:401, 2003.
26. Baley, J., Kliegman, R., Annabie, W., et al.: *Torulopsis glabrata* sepsis appearing as necrotizing enterocolits and endophthalmitis. Am. J. Dis. Child. *138*:965, 1984.
27. Baley, J., Kliegman, R., Boxerbaum, B., et al.: Fungal colonization in the very low birth weight infant. Pediatrics *78*:225, 1986.
28. Baley, J., Kliegman, R., and Fanaroff, A.: Disseminated fungal infections in very low birth weight infants: Clinical manifestations and epidemiology. Pediatrics *73*:144, 1984.
29. Baley, J., Kliegman, R., and Fanaroff, A.: Disseminated fungal infections in very low birth weight infants: Therapeutic toxicity. Pediatrics *73*:152, 1984.
30. Baley, J., Meyers, C., Kliegman, R., et al.: The pharmacokinetics, outcome and toxicity of amphotericin B and 5-fluorocytosine in neonates. J. Pediatr. *116*:791, 1990.
31. Baley, J., and Silverman, R.: Systemic candidiasis: Cutaneous manifestations in low birth weight infants. Pediatrics *82*:211, 1988.
32. Barth, T., Broscheit, J., Bussen, S., et al.: Maternal sepsis and intrauterine fetal death resulting from *Candida tropicalis* in a woman with a retained intrauterine contraceptive device. Acta Obstet. Gynecol. Scand. *81*:981, 2002.
33. Battin, M., and Wilson, E.: *Trichophyton rubrum* skin infection in two premature infants. J. Paediatr. Child Health *41*:377, 2005.
34. Bayer, A., Blumenkrantz, M., Montgamerie, J., et al.: *Candida* peritonitis: Report of 22 cases and review of the English literature. Am. J. Med. *61*:832, 1976.
35. Bayramoglu, G., Sonmez, M., Tosun, I., et al.: Breakthrough *Trichosporon asahii* fungemia in neutropenic patient with acute leukemia while receiving caspofungin. Infection *36*:68, 2008.
36. Bell, L., Alpert, G., Slight, P., et al.: *Malassezia furfur* skin colonization in infancy. Infect. Control Hosp. Epidemiol. *9*:151, 1988.
37. Bendel, C., and Hostetter, M.: Systemic candidiasis and other fungal infections in the newborn. Semin. Pediatr. Infect. Dis. *5*:35, 1994.

38. Benjamin, D., DeLong, E., Steinbach, W., et al.: Empirical therapy for neonatal candidemia in very low birth weight infants. Pediatrics *112*:543, 2003.

39. Benjamin, D., Poole, C., Steinbach, W., et al.: Neonatal candidemia and end-organ damage: A critical appraisal of the literature using meta-analytic techniques. Pediatrics *112*:634, 2003.

40. Benjamin, D., Stoll, B., Fanaroff, A., et al.: National Institute of Child Health and Human Development Neonatal Research Network. Pediatrics *117*:84, 2006.

41. Benjamin, D., Jr., Fisher, R., McKinney, R., et al.: Candidal mycetoma in a neonatal kidney. Pediatrics *104*:1126, 1999.

42. Benjamin, D., Jr., Garges, H., and Steinback, W.: *Candida* blood stream infection in neonates. Semin. Perinatol. 27:375, 2003.

43. Benjamin, D., Jr., Ross, K., McKinney, R., Jr., et al.: When to suspect fungal infection in neonates: A clinical comparison of *Candida parapsilosis* fungemia with coagulase-negative staphylococcal bacteremia. Pediatrics *106*:712, 2000.

44. Bergman, K., Meis, J., Horrevorts, A., et al.: Acute renal failure in a neonate due to pelviureteric candidal bezoars successfully treated with long-term systemic fluconazole. Acta Paediatr. *81*:709, 1992.

45. Bernier, V., Weill, F., Hirigoyen, V., et al.: Skin colonization by *Malassezia* species in neonates: A prospective study and relationship with neonatal cephalic pustulosis. Arch. Dermatol. *138*:215, 2002.

46. Bertini, G., Perugi, A., Dani, C., et al.: Fluconazole prophylaxis prevents against fungal colonization and invasive infection in very low birth weight infants. J. Pediatr. *147*:162, 2005.

47. Bhandari, V., Narang, A., Kumar, B., et al.: Itraconazole therapy for disseminated candidiasis in very low birth weight neonate. J. Pediatr. Child Health. *28*:323, 1992.

48. Bhargava, P., and Longhi, L.: Images in clinical medicine: Peripheral smear with *Malassezia furfur*. N. Engl. J. Med. *356*:e25, 2007.

49. Bharwani, S., and Dhanireddy, R.: Systemic fungal infection is associated with the development of retinopathy of prematurity in very low birth weight infants: A meta-review. J. Perinatol. *28*:61-66, 2008.

50. Bilgen, H., Ozek, E., Korten, V., et al.: Treatment of systemic neonatal candidiasis with fluconazole. Infection *23*:394-395, 1995.

51. Biyiki, N., Tugtepe, H., Akpinar, I., et al.: The longest use of liposomal amphotericin B and 5-fluorocytosine in neonatal renal candidiaisis. Pediatr. Nephrol. *19*:801, 2004.

52. Bliss, J., Wellington, M., and Gigliotti, F.: Antifungal pharmacotherapy for neonatal candidiasis. Semin. Perinatol. 27:365, 2003.

53. Block, E., and Bennett, J.: Pharmacological studies with 5-fluorocytosine. Antimicrob. Agents Chemother. *1*:476, 1972.

54. Bode, S., Pederson-Bjergaard, L., and Hjelt, K.: *Candida albicans* septicemia in a premature infant successfully treated with oral fluconazole. Scand. J. Infect. Dis. *24*:673, 1992.

55. Bolet, N., Cifti, E., Ince, E., et al.: Caspofungin treatment in two infants with persistent fungaemia due to *Candida lipolytica*. Scand. J. Infect. Dis. *38*:559, 2006.

56. Bond, S., Stewart, D., and Bendon, R.: Invasive *Candida* enteritis of the newborn. J. Pediatr. Surg. *35*:1496, 2000.

57. Botas, C., Kurlat, I., Young, S., et al.: Disseminated candidal infections and intravenous hydrocortisone in preterm infants. Pediatrics *95*:883, 1995.

58. Boxynski, M., Naglie, R., and Russell, E.: Real-time ultrasonographic surveillance in the detection of CNS involvement in systemic candidiasis. Pediatr. Radiol. *16*:235, 1986.

59. Bruner, J., Elliott, J., and Kilbride, H., et al.: *Candida* chorioamnionitis diagnosed by amniocentesis with subsequent fetal infection. Am. J. Perinatol. *3*:213, 1986.

60. Buchanan, R., Sworn, M., and Noble, A.: Abortion associated with intrauterine infection by *Candida albicans*: Case report. Br. J. Obstet. Gynaecol. *86*:741, 1979.

61. Butler, K., and Baker, C.: *Candida*: An increasingly important pathogen in the nursery. Pediatr. Clin. North Am. *35*:543, 1988.

62. Butler, K., Rench, M., and Baker, C.: Amphotericin B as a single agent in the treatment of systemic candidiasis in neonates. Pediatr. Infect. Dis. J. *9*:51, 1990.

63. Campbell, J., Zaccaria, E., and Baker, C.: Systemic candidiasis in extremely low birth weight infants receiving topical petrolatum ointment for skin care: A case-control study. Pediatrics *105*:1041, 2000.

64. Cappelletty, D., and Eiselstein-McKitrick, K.: The echinocandins. Pharmacotherapy 27:369, 2007.

65. Caramalac, D., da Silva, R., and de Batista, G.: *Candida* isolated from vaginal mucosa of mothers and oral mucosa of neonates: Occurrence and biotypes concordance. Pediatr. Infect. Dis. J. 26:553, 2007.

66. Carmo, K., Evans, N., and Isaacs, D.: Congenital candidiasis presenting as septic shock without rash. Arch. Dis. Child. *92*:627, 2007.

67. Castro, G., Cervi, M., and Martinez, R.: Vertical transmission of *Cryptococcus neoformans* from a mother coinfected with human immunodeficiency virus: Case report. Rev. So. Bras. Med. Trop. *39*:501, 2006.

68. Cetin, H., Yalez, M., and Akisu, M.: The efficacy of two different lipid-based amphotericin B in neonatal *Candida* septicemia. Pediatr. Int. *47*:676, 2005.

69. Chan, C., Tuazon, C., and Lessin, L.: Amphotericin-B-induced thrombocytopenia. Ann. Intern. Med. *96*:332, 1982.

70. Chang, H., Miller, H., Watkins, N., et al.: An epidemic of *Malassezia pachydermatis* in an intensive care nursery associated with colonization of health care workers' pet dogs. N. Engl. J. Med. *338*:706, 1998.

71. Chang, S., Kang, S., Choi, J., et al.: Tinea capitis due to *Trichophyton rubrum* in a neonate. Pediatr. Dermatol. *19*:356, 2002.

72. Chapman, R.: Prevention and treatment of *Candida* infections in neonates. Semin. Perinatol. *31*:39, 2007.

73. Chapman, R., and Faix, R.: Persistently positive cultures and outcome in invasive neonatal candidiasis. Pediatr. Infect. Dis. J. *19*:822, 2000.

74. Chapman, R., and Faix, R.: Invasive neonatal candidiasis an overview. Semin. Perinatol. *27*:352, 2003.

75. Charlton, V., Ramsdell, K., and Sehring, S.: Intrauterine transmission of coccidioidomycosis. Pediatr. Infect. Dis. J. *18*:516, 1999.

76. Chen, C., Weng, Y., Su, L., et al.: Molecular evidence of congenital candidiasis associated with maternal candidal vaginitis. Pediatr. Infect. Dis. J. *25*:655, 2006.

77. Chen, J.: Neonatal candidiasis associated with meningitis and endophthalmitis. Acta Paediatr. Jpn. *36*:261, 1994.

78. Cherry, J., Lloyd, C., Quilty, J., et al.: Amphotericin B therapy in children. J. Pediatr. *75*:1063, 1969.

79. Chesney, P., Justman, R., and Bogdanowicz, W.: *Candida* meningitis in newborn infants: A review and report of combined amphotericin B-flucytosine therapy. Johns Hopkins Med. J. *142*:155, 1976.

80. Chesney, P., Teets, K., Mulvihill, J., et al.: Successful treatment of *Candida* meningitis with amphotericin B and 5-fluorocytosine in combination. J. Pediatr. *89*:1017, 1976.

81. Chouldhury, M., Kahkashan, E., and Choudhury, S.: Neonatal gastrointestinal mucormycosis—a case report. Trop. Gastroenterol. *28*:81, 2007.

82. Chryssanthou, E., Broberger, U., and Petrini, B.: *Malassezia pachydermatis* fungaemia in a neonatal intensive care unit. Acta Paediatr. *90*:323, 2001.

83. Clarke, M., and Davies, D.: Neonatal systemic candidiasis treated with miconazole. B. M. J. *281*:354, 1980.

84. Clerihew, L., Austin, N., and McGuire, W.: Prophylactic systemic antifungal agents to prevent mortality and morbidity in very low birth weight infants. Cochrane Database Syst. Rev. *4*:CD003850, 2007.

85. Clerihew, L., Lamagni, T., Brocklehurst, P., et al.: *Candida parapsilosis* infection in very low birthweight infants. Arch. Dis. Child. Fetal Neonatal Ed *92*: F127, 2007.

86. Clerihew, L., and McGuire, W.: Systemic antifungal drugs for invasive fungal infection in preterm infants. Cochrane Database Syst. Rev. *1*:CD003953, 2004.

87. Clinch, T., Duker, J., Eagle, R., et al.: Infantile endogenous *Candida* endophthalmitis presenting as a cataract. Surv. Ophthalmol. *34*:107, 1989.

88. Coates, E., Karlowicz, M., Croitoru, D., et al.: Distinctive distribution of pathogens associated with peritonitis in neonates with focal intestinal perforation compared with necrotizing enterocolitis. Pediatrics *116*:e241, 2005.

89. Cohen, I.: Absence of congenital and teratogensis in three children born to mothers with blastomycosis and treated with amphotericin B during pregnancy. Pediatr. Infect. Dis. J. *6*:76, 1987.

90. Cohen-Wolkowiez, M., Smith, P., Mangum, B., et al.: Neonatal *Candida* meningitis: Significance of cerebrospinal fluid parameters and blood cultures. J. Perinatol. *27*:97, 2007.

91. Craig, N., Lueder, F., Pensler, J., et al.: Disseminated *Rhizopus* infection in a premature infant. Pediatr. Dermatol. *11*:346, 1994.

92. Damjanovic, V., Connolly, C., van Saene, F., et al.: Selective decontamination with nystatin for control of a *Candida* outbreak in a neonatal intensive care unit. J. Hosp. Infect. *24*:245, 1993.

93. Dankner, W., Spector, S., Fierer, J., et al.: *Malassezia* fungemia in neonates and adults: Complication of hyperalimentation. Rev. Infect. Dis. *9*:743, 1987.

94. Dato, V., and Dajani, A.: Candidemia in children with central venous catheters: Role of catheter removal and amphotericin B therapy. Pediatr. Infect. Dis. J. *9*:309, 1990.

95. Devlin, R.: Invasive fungal infections caused by *Candida* and *Malassezia* species in the neonatal intensive care unit. Adv. Neonatal Care *6*:68, 2006.

96. Divekar, A., Rebekya, I., and Soni, R.: Late onset *Candida parapsilosis* endocarditis after surviving nosocomial candidemia in an infant with structural heart disease. Pediatr. Infect. Dis. J. *23*:472, 2004.

97. Diven, S., Angel, C., Hawkins, H., et al.: Intestinal zygomycosis due to *Absidia corymbifera* mimicking necrotizing enterocolitis in a preterm infant. J. Perinatol. *24*:794, 2004.

98. Doctor, B., Newman, N., Minich, N., et al.: Clinical outcomes of neonatal meningitis in very-low-birth-weight infants. Clin. Pediatr. *40*:473, 2001.

99. Doi, O., Takada, Y., Yamauchi, Y., et al.: Systemic candidiasis with disseminated intravascular coagulation and candida endophthalmitis in a post-operative neonate. Aust. Paediatr. J. *25*:372, 1989.

100. Donahue, S., Hein, E., and Sinatra, R.: Ocular involvement in children with candidiasis. Am. J. Ophthalmol. *135*:886, 2003.

101. Driessen, M., Ellis, J., Cooper, P., et al.: Fluconazole vs. amphotericin B for the treatment of neonatal fungal septicemia: A prospective randomized trial. Pediatr. Infect. Dis. J. *15*:1107, 1996.

102. Driessen, M., Ellis, J., Muzai, F., et al.: The treatment of systemic candidiasis in neonates with oral fluconazole. Ann. Trop. Paediatr. *7*:263, 1997.

103. Drohan, L., Colby, C., Brindle, M., et al.: *Candida* (amphotericin-sensitive) lens abscess associated with decreasing arterial blood flow in a very low birth weight preterm infant. Pediatrics *110*:e65, 2002.

104. du Plessis, F., Helbing, W., and Bogers, A.: Excision of the tricuspid valve in a baby with *Candida* endocarditis. Cardiol. Young *17*:545, 2007.

105. du Plessis, P., Wentzel, L., Delport, S., et al.: Zygomycotic necrotizing cellulitis in a premature infants. Dermatology 195:179, 1997.

106. Dvorak, A., and Gavaller, B.: Congenital systemic candidiasis. N. Engl. J. Med. 10:540, 1966.

107. Eckstein, C., and Kass, E.: Anuria in a newborn secondary to bilateral uteropelvic fungus balls. J. Urol. 127:109, 1982.

108. Ekenna, O., and Sherertz, R.: Factors affecting colonization and dissemination of Candida albicans from the gastrointestinal tract of mice. Infect. Immun. 55:1558, 1987.

109. El-Masry, F., Neal, T., and Subhedar, N.: Risk factors for invasive fungal infection in neonates. Acta Paediatr. 91:198, 2002.

110. Ely, E., Peacock, J., Haponik, E., et al.: Cryptococcal pneumonia complicating pregnancy. Medicine 77:153, 1998.

111. Eppes, S., Troutman, J., and Gutman, L.: Outcome of treatment of candidemia in children whose central catheters were removed or retained. Pediatr. Infect. Dis. J. 8:99, 1989.

112. Fairchild, K., Tomkoria, S., Sharp, E., et al.: Neonatal Candida glabrata sepsis: Clinical and laboratory features compared with other Candida species. Pediatr. Infect. Dis. J. 21:39, 2002.

113. Faix, R.: Candida parapsilosis meningitis in premature infant. Pediatr. Infect. Dis. J. 2:462, 1983.

114. Faix, R.: Systemic Candida infections in infants in intensive care nurseries: High incidence of central nervous system involvement. J. Pediatr. 105:616-622, 1984.

115. Faix, R.: Nonsurgical treatment of candida endocarditis. J. Pediatr. 120:665, 1992.

116. Faix, R.: Invasive neonatal candidiasis: Comparison of albicans and parapsilosis. Pediatr. Infect. Dis. J. 11:88, 1992.

117. Faix, R., Feick, H., Frommelt, P., et al.: Successful medical treatment of Candida parapsilosis endocarditis in a premature infant. Am. J. Perinatol. 7:272, 1990.

118. Faix, R., and Chapman, R.: Central nervous system candidiasis in the high-risk neonate. Semin. Perinatol. 27:384, 2003.

119. Faix, R., Finkel, D., Anderson, R., et al.: Genotypic analysis of a cluster of systemic Candida albicans infections in a neonatal intensive care unit. Pediatr. Infect. Dis. J. 14:1063, 1995.

120. Faix, R., Naglie, R., and Bart, M., Jr.: Intrapleural inoculation of Candida in an infant with congenital cutaneous candidiasis. Am. J. Perinatol. 3:119, 1986.

121. Farmaki, E., Evdoridou, J., Pouliou, T., et al.: Fungal colonization in the neonatal intensive care unit: Risk factors, drug susceptibility, and association with invasive fungal infections. Am. J. Perinatol. 24:127, 2007.

122. Fasano, C., O'Keefe, J., and Gibbs, D.: Fluconazole treatment of neonates and infants with severe fungal infections not treatable with conventional agents. Eur. J. Clin. Microbiol. Infect. Dis. 13:351, 1994.

123. Fernandez, M., Moylett, E., Noyola, D., et al.: Candidal meningitis in neonates: A 10-year review. Clin. Infect. Dis. 31:458, 2000.

124. Finkelstein, R., Reinhertz, G., Hashman, N., et al.: Outbreak of Candida tropicalis fungemia in a neonateal intensive care unit. Infect. Control Hosp. Epidemiol. 14:587, 1993.

125. Fisher, D., Christy, C., Spafford, P., et al.: Neonatal Trichosporon beigelii infection: Report of a cluster of cases in a neonatal intensive care unit. Pediatr. Infect. Dis. J. 12:149, 1993.

126. Fisher, J., Chew, W., Shadomy, S., et al.: Urinary tract infections due to Candida albicans. Rev. Infect. Dis. 4:1107, 1982.

127. Fisher, R., Karlowicz, M., and Lall-Trail, J.: Very low prevalence of endophthalmitis in very low birthweight infants who survive candidemia. J. Perinatol. 25:208, 2005.

128. Foker, J., Bass, J., Thompson, T., et al.: Management of intracardiac fungal masses in premature infants. J. Thorac. Cardiovasc. Surg. 87:244, 1984.

129. Frank, C., and Hostetter, M.: Cleavage of E-cadherin: A mechanism for disruption of the intestinal epithelial barrier by Candida albicans. Transl. Res. 149:211, 2007.

130. Frankenbusch, K., Elfinger, F., Kribs, A., et al.: Severe primary cutaneous aspergilllosis refractory to amphotericin B and the successful treatment with systemic voriconazole in two premature infants with extremely low birth weight. J. Perinatol. 26:511, 2006.

131. Frattarelli, D., Reed, M., Giacoia, G., et al.: Antifungals in systemic neonatal candidiasis. Drugs 64:949, 2004.

132. Frezza, S., Maggio, L., DeCarolis, M., et al.: Risk factors for pulmonary candidiasis in preterm infants with a birth weight of less than 1250 g. Eur. J. Pediatr. 164:88, 2005.

133. Fridkin, S., Kaufman, D., and Edwards, J.: Changing incidence of Candida bloodstream infections among NICU patients in the United States: 1995-2004. Pediatrics 117:1680, 2005.

134. Friedlich, P., Steinberg, I., Fujitani, A., et al.: Renal tolerance with the use of intralipid-amphotericin B in low-birth-weight neonates. Am. J. Perinatol. 14:377, 1997.

135. Fuchs, H., vonBaum, H., Meth, M., et al.: CNS-manifestation of aspergillosis in an extremely low-birth-weight infant. Eur. J. Pediatr. 165:476, 2006.

136. Gago, L., Capone, A., and Trese, M.: Bilateral presumed endogenous Candida endophthalmitis and state 3 retinopathy of prematurity. Am. J. Ophthalmol. 135:747, 2002.

137. Gauthier, G., Nork, T., Prince, R., et al.: Subtherapeutic ocular penetration of caspofungin and associated treatment failure in Candida albicans endophthalmitis. Clin. Infect. Dis. 41:e27, 2005.

138. Gavin, P., Sutton, D., and Katz, B.: Fatal endocarditis in a neonate caused by the dematiaceous fungus Phlaemonium obovatum: Case report and review of the literature. J. Clin. Microbiol. 40:2207, 2002.

139. Giusiano, G., Mangiaterra, M., Rojas, F., et al.: Yeasts species distribution in neonatal intensive care units in northeast Argentina. Mycoses 47:300, 2004.

140. Giusiano, G., Mangiaterra, M., Rojas, F., et al.: Azole resistance in neonatal intensive care units in Argentina. J. Chemother. 17:347, 2005.

141. Goldsmith, L., Rubenstein, S., Wolfson, B., et al.: Cerebral calcifications in a neonate with candidiasis. Pediatr. Infect. Dis. J. 9:451, 1990.

142. Groll, A., Giri, N., Petraitis, V., et al.: Comparative efficacy and distribution of lipid formulations of amphotericin B in experimental Candida albicans infection of the central nervous system. J. Infect. Dis. 182:274, 2000.

143. Groll, A., Jaeger, G., Allendorf, A., et al.: Invasive pulmonary aspergillosis in a critically ill neonate: Case report and review of invasive aspergillosis during the first 3 months of life. Clin. Infect. Dis. 27:437, 1998.

144. Gupta, A., Kohli, Y., Li, A., et al.: In vitro susceptibility of the seven Malassezia species to ketoconazole, voriconazole, itraconazole, and terbinafine. Br. J. Dermatol. 142:758, 2000.

145. Haroon-Parupia, M., and Dhanireddy, R.: Association of postnatal dexamethasone use and fungal sepsis in the development of severe retinopathy of prematurity and progression to laser therapy in extremely low-birth-weight infants. J. Perinatol. 21:242, 2001.

146. Harris, M., Pereira, R., Myers, M., et al.: Candidal arthritis in infants previously treated for systemic candidiasis during the newborn period: Report of three cases. Pediatr. Emerg. Care 16:249, 2000.

147. Henwick, S., Henrickson, K., Storgion, S., et al.: Disseminated neonatal Trichosporon beigelii. Pediatr. Infect. Dis. J. 11:50, 1992.

148. Heresi, G., Gerstman, D., Reed, M., et al.: The pharmacokinetics and safety of micafungin, a novel echinocandin, in premature infants. Pediatr. Infect. Dis. J. 25:1110, 2006.

149. Herron, M., Vanderhooft, S., Byington, C., et al.: Aspergillosis in a 24-week newborn: A case report. J. Perinatol. 23:256, 2003.

150. Hesseling, M., Weindling, M., and Neal, T.: First reported use of caspofungin in an extremely low-birth-weight neonate. J. Matern. Fetal Neonatal Med. 14:212, 2003.

151. Heydarian, M., Werthammer, J., and Kelly, P.: Echocardiographic diagnosis of Candida mass of the right atrium in a premature infant. Am. Heart. J. 113:402, 1987.

152. Hiemenz, J., and Walsh, J.: Lipid formulations of amphotericin B: Recent progress and future directions. Clin. Infect. Dis. 22(Suppl.):133, 1996.

153. Hitchcock, R., Pallett, A., Hall, M., et al.: Urinary tract candidiasis in neonates and infants. Br. J. Urol. 76:252, 1995.

154. Ho, N.: Systemic candidiasis in premature infants. Aust. Pediatr. J. 20:127, 1984.

155. Hodgetts, S., Nooney, L., Al-Akeel, R., et al.: Efungumab and caspofungin: Preclinical data supporting synergy. J. Antimicrob. Chemother. 61:1132-1139, 2008.

156. Holler, B., Omar, S., Farid, M., et al.: Effects of fluid and electrolyte management on amphotericin B-induced nephrotoxicity among extremely low birth weight infants. Pediatrics 113:e608, 2004.

157. Hope, W., Mickiene, D., Petraitis, V., et al.: The pharmacokinetics and pharmacodynamics of micafungin in experimental hematogenous Candida meningoencephalitis: Implications for echinocandin therapy in neonates. J. Infect. Dis. 197:163, 2008.

158. Hope, W., Seibel, N., Schwartz, C., et al.: Population pharmacokinetics of micafungin in pediatric patients and implications for antifungal dosing. Antimicrob. Agents Chemother. 51:3714, 2007.

159. Horii, K., and Nopper, A.: Emerging cutaneous infections in the premature neonate. Adv. Dermatol. 23:177, 2007.

160. Hostetter, M.: Integrin-like proteins in Candida spp. and other microorganisms. Fungal Genet. Biol. 21:1212, 2001.

161. Hruszkewycz, V., Holtrop, P., and Batton, D.: Complications associated with central venous catheters inserted in critically ill neonates. Infect. Control Hosp. Epidemiol. 12:544, 1991.

162. Hsieh, W., and Leung, C.: Candidal arthritis after complete treatment of systemic candidiasis. J. Chin. Med. Assoc. 68:191, 2005.

163. Huang, S., Lin, T., Peng, H., et al.: Outbreak of Candida albicans fungaemia in a neonatal intensive care unit. Scand. J. Infect. Dis. 30:137, 1998.

164. Huang, Y., Kao, H., Lin, T.: Antifungal susceptibility testing and the correlation with clinical outcome in neonatal candidemia. Am. J. Perinatol. 18:141, 2001.

165. Huang, Y., Lin, T., Leu, H., et al.: Outbreak of Candida parapsilosis fungemia in neonatal intensive care units: Clinical implications and genotyping analysis. Infection 27:97, 1999.

166. Huang, Y., Lin, T., Lian, R., et al.: Candidemia in special care nurseries: Comparison of albicans and parapsilosis infection. J. Infect. 40:171, 2000.

167. Huang, Y., Su, L., Wu, T., et al.: Genotyping analysis of colonizing candidal isolates from very-low-birth-weight infants in a neonatal intensive care unit. J. Hosp. Infect. 58:200, 2004.

168. Hughes, C., Driver, S., and Alexander, K.: Successful treatment of abdominal wall Rhizopus necrotizing cellutis in a preterm infant. Pediatr. Infect. Dis. J. 14:336, 1995.

169. Huttova, M., Hartmanova, I., Kralinsky, K., et al.: Candida fungemia in neonates treated with fluconazole: Report of forty cases, including eight with meningitis. Pediatr. Infect. Dis. J. 17:1012, 1998.

170. Jahn, C., and Cherry, J.: Congenital cutaneous candidiasis. Pediatrics *33*:440, 1966.
171. Jarlov, J., Born, P., and Bruun, B.: *Candida albicans* meningitis in a 27 weeks premature infant treated with liposomal amphotericin B (AmBisome). Scand. J. Infect. Dis. *27*:419, 1995.
172. Jeon, G., Kee, S., Lee, J., et al.: A comparison of AmBisome to amphotericin B for treatment of systemic candidiasis in very low birth weight infants. Yonsei Med. J. *31*:619, 2007.
173. Jin, Y., Endo, A., Shimada, M., et al.: Congenital systemic candidiasis. Pediatr. Infect. Dis. J. *14*:818, 1995.
174. Johnson, D., Bass, J., Thompson, T., et al.: *Candida* septicemia and right atrial mass secondary to umbilical vein catheterization. Am. J. Dis. Child. *135*:275, 1981.
175. Johnson, D., Conroy, M., Foker, J., et al.: *Candida* peritonitis in the newborn infant. J. Pediatr. *97*:298, 1980.
176. Johnson, D., Thompson, T., and Ferrieri, P.: Congenital candidiasis. Am. J. Dis. Child. *135*:273, 1981.
177. Johnson, D., Thompson, T., Green, T., et al.: Systemic candidiasis in very low-birth-weight infants (<1500 grams). Pediatrics *73*:138, 1984.
178. Juster-Reicher, A., Flidel-Rimon, O., Amitay, M., et al.: High-dose liposomal amphotericin B in the therapy of systemic candidiasis in neonates. Eur. J. Clin. Microbiol. Infect. Dis. *22*:603, 2003.
179. Juster-Reicher, A., Leibovitz, E., Linder, N., et al.: Liposomal amphotericin B (AmBisome) in the treatment of neonatal candidiasis in very low birth weight infants. Infection *28*:233, 2000.
180. Kam, L., and Giaoia, G.: Congenital cutaneous candidiasis. Am. J. Dis. Child. *129*:1215, 1975.
181. Kamitsuka, M., Nugent, N., Conrad, P., et al.: *Candida albicans* brain abscesses in a premature infant treated with amphotericin B, flucytosine and fluconazole. Pediatr. Infect. Dis. J. *14*:329, 1995.
182. Kaplan, M., Eidelman, A., Dollberg, L., et al.: Necrotizing bowel disease with *Candida* peritonitis following severe neonatal hypothermia. Acta Paediatr. Scand. *79*:876, 1990.
183. Karatza, A., Dimitriou, G., Marangos, M., et al.: Successful resolution of cardiac myceteomas by combined liposomal amphotericin B with fluconazole treatment in premature neonates. Eur. J. Pediatr. *167*:1021-1023, 2008.
184. Karlowicz, M., Giannone, P., Pestian, J., et al.: Does candidemia predict threshold retinopathy of prematurity in extremely low birth weight (<1000 g) neonates? Pediatrics *105*:1036, 2000.
185. Kassner, E., Kauffman, S., Yoon, J., et al.: Pulmonary candidiasis in infants: Clinical, radiologic and pathologic features. A. J. R. Am. J. Roentgenol. *137*:707, 1981.
186. Kauffman, C., and Frame, P.: Bone marrow toxicity associated with 5-fluorocytosine therapy. Antimicrob. Agents Chemother. *11*:244, 1977.
187. Kaufman, D., Boyle, R., Hazen, K., et al.: Fluconazole prophylaxis against fungal colonization and infection in preterm infants. N. Engl. J. Med. *345*:1660, 2001.
188. Kaufman, D., Boyle, R., Hazen, K., et al.: Twice weekly fluconazole prophylaxis for prevention of invasive *Candida* infection in high-risk infants of <1000 grams birth weight. J. Pediatr. *147*:172, 2005.
189. Kaur, R., Mittal, N., Rawat, D., et al.: Cryptococcal meningitis in a neonate. Scand. J. Infect. Dis. *34*:542, 2002.
190. Keller, M., Sellers, B., Melish, M., et al.: Systemic candidiasis in infants. Am. J. Dis. Child. *131*:1260, 1977.
191. Kessler, A., Kourtis, A., and Simon, N.: Peripheral thromboembolism associated with *Malassezia furfur* sepsis. Pediatr. Infect. Dis. J. *21*:356, 2002.
192. Khan, M.: Anuria from *Candida* pyelonephritis and obstructing fungal balls. Urology *21*:421, 1983.
193. Khan, Z., Al-Sweih, N., Ahmad, S., et al.: Outbreak of fungemia among neonates caused by *Candida haemulonii* resistant to amphotericin B, itraconazole, and fluconazole. J. Clin. Microbiol. *45*:2025, 2007.
194. Kicklighter, S., Springer, S., Cox, T., et al.: Fluconazole for prophylaxis against candidal rectal colonization in the very low birth weight infant. Pediatrics *107*:293, 2001.
195. Kim, E., Cohen, R., Ramachandran, P., et al.: Adhesion of percutaneously inserted Silastic central venous lines to the vein wall associated with *Malassezia furfur* infectin. J. Parenter. Enteral Nutr. *17*:458, 1993.
196. Kim, Y., Kim, S., Kim, Y., et al.: Successful treatment of septic shock with purpura fuliminas caused by *Trichosporon asahii* in an immunocompetent patient. Ann. Clin. Lab. Sci. *37*:366, 2007.
197. Kintanar, C., Cramer, B., Reid, W., et al.: Neonatal candidiasis: Sonographic diagnosis. A. J. R. Am. J. Roentgenol. *147*:801, 1986.
198. Kirpekar, M., Abiri, M., Hilfer, C., et al.: Ultrasound in the diagnosis of systemic candidiasis (renal and cranial) in very low birth weight premature infants. Pediatr. Radiol. *16*:17, 1986.
199. Klein, J., Yamauchi, T., and Horlick, S.: Neonatal candidiasis, meningitis and arthritis: Observations and a review of the literature. J. Pediatr. *81*:31, 1972.
200. Knoppert, D., Salama, H., and Lee, S.: Eradication of severe neonatal systemic candidiasis with amphotericin B lipid complex. Ann. Pharmacother. *35*:1032, 2001.
201. Kossoff, E., Buescher, E., and Karlowicz, M.: Candidemia in a neonatal intensive care unit: Trends during fifteen years and clinical features of 111 cases. Pediatr. Infect. Dis. J. *17*:504, 1998.
202. Krajewska-Kulak, E., Lukaszuk, C., Tsokantaridis, C., et al.: Indoor air studies of fungi contamination at the Neonatal Department and Intensive Care Unit

and Palliative Care in Kavala Hospital in Greece. Adv. Med. Sci. *52*(Suppl. 1):11, 2007.
203. Krallis, N., Tzioras, S., Giapros, V., et al.: Congenital candidiasis caused by different *Candida* species in a dizygotic pregnancy. Pediatr. Infect. Dis. J. *25*:958, 2006.
204. Kremery, V., Huttova, M., Mateicka, F., et al.: Breakthrough fungaemia in neonates and infants caused by *Candida albicans* and *Candida parapsilosis* susceptible to fluconazole in vitro. J. Antimicrob. Chemother. *48*:521, 2001.
205. Kumar, V., Aggarwal, A., Taneja, A., et al.: Primary cutaneous mucormycosis in a premature neonate and its management by tumescent skin grafting. Br. J. Plast. Surg. *58*:852, 2005.
206. Lackner, H., Schwinger, W., Urban, C., et al.: Liposomal amphotericin-B (AmBisome) for treatment of disseminated fungal infections in two infants of very low birth weight. Pediatrics *89*:1259, 1992.
207. Laufer, J., Reichman, B., Graif, M., et al.: Anuria in a premature infant due to ureteropelvic fungal bezoars. Eur. J. Pediatr. *145*:125, 1986.
208. Lee, B., Cheung, P., Robinson, J., et al.: Comparative study of mortality and morbidity in premature infants (birth weight, <1,250 g) with candidemia or candidal meningitis. Clin. Infect. Dis. *27*:559, 1998.
209. Leibovitz, E., Iuster-Reicher, A., Amitai, M., et al.: Systemic candidal infections associated with the use of peripheral venous catheters in neonates: A 9-year experience. Clin. Infect. Dis. *14*:485, 1992.
210. Lemos, L., Soofi, M., and Amir, E.: Blastomycosis and pregnancy. Ann. Diagn. Pathol. *6*:211, 2002.
211. Levy, I., Rubin, L., Vasishtha, S., et al.: Emergence of *Candida parapsilosis* as the predominant species causing candidemia in children. Clin. Infect. Dis. *26*:1086, 1998.
212. Levy, I., Shalit, I., Birk, E., et al.: *Candida* endocarditis in neonates: Report of five cases and review of the literature. Mycoses *49*:43, 2006.
213. Linder, N., Keler, N., Huri, C., et al.: Primary cutaneous mucromycosis in a premature infant: Case report and review of the literature. Am. J. Perinatol. *15*:35, 1998.
214. Linsangan, L., and Ross, L.: *Coccidioides immitis* infection of the neonate: Two routes of infection. Pediatr. Infect. Dis. J. *18*:171, 1999.
215. Lopez, E., and Aterman, K.: Intra-uterine infection by *Candida*. Am. J. Dis. Child. *115*:663, 1968.
216. Luciani, G., Casali, G., Viscardi, F., et al.: Tricuspid valve repair in an infant with multiple obstructive *Candida* mycetomas. Ann. Thorac. Surg. *80*:2378, 2005.
217. Lundstrom, N., and Bjorkhem, G.: Mitral and tricuspid valve vegetations in infancy diagnosed by echocardiography. Acta Paediatr. Scand. *68*:345, 1979.
218. Lupetti, A., Tavanti, A., Davini, P., et al.: Horizontal transmission of *Candida parapsilosis* candidemia in a neonatal intensive care unit. J. Clin. Microbiol. *40*:236, 2002.
219. Ma, J., Chen, P., Chen, C., et al.: Neonatal fungemia caused by *Hansenula anomala*: A case report. J. Microbiol. Immunol. Infect. *33*:267, 2000.
220. Makhoul, I., Bental, Y., Weisbrod, M., et al.: Candidal versus bacterial late-onset sepsis in very low birthweight infants in Israel: A national survey. J. Hosp. Infect. *65*:237, 2007.
221. Makhoul, I., Kassis, I., Smolkin, T., et al.: Review of 49 neonates with acquired fungal sepsis: Further characterization. Pediatrics *107*:61, 2001.
222. Mamlok, R., Richardson, C., Mamlok, V., et al.: A case of intrauterine pulmonary candidiasis. Pediatr. Infect. Dis. J. *4*:692, 1985.
223. Manfredi, R., and Sabbatani, S.: Severe *Candida albicans* panophthalmitis treated with all available and potentially effective antifungal drugs: Fluconazole, liposomal amphotericin B, caspofungin, and voriconazole. Scand. J. Infect. Dis. *38*:950, 2006.
224. Manzar, S., Kamat, M., and Pyati, S.: Caspofungin for refractory candidemia in neonates. Pediatr. Infect. Dis. J. *25*:282, 2006.
225. Manzoni, P., Arisio, R., Mostert, M., et al.: Prophylactic fluconazole is effective in preventing fungal colonization and fungal systemic infections in preterm neonates: A single-center, 6-year, retrospective cohort study. Pediatrics *117*:e22, 2006.
226. Manzoni, P., Farina, D., Monetti, C., et al.: Early-onset neutropenia is a risk factor for *Candida* colonization in very-low-birth-weight neonates. Diagn. Microbiol. Infect. Dis. *57*:77, 2007.
227. Manzoni, P., Mostert, M., Leonessa, M., et al.: Oral supplementation with *Lactobacillus casei* subspecies *rhamnosus* prevents enteric colonization by *Candida* species in preterm neonates: A randomized study. Clin. Infect. Dis. *42*:1735, 2006.
228. Manzoni, P., Stolfi, I., Pugni, L., et al.: A multicenter, randomized trial of prophylactic fluconazole in preterm neonates. N. Engl. J. Med. *356*:2483, 2007.
229. Matsumoto, A., Dejter, W., Barth, K., et al.: Percutaneous nephrostomy drainage in the management of neonatal anuria secondary to renal candidiasis. J. Pediatr. Surg. *25*:1295, 1990.
230. Matsuzawa, S., Ohyama, M., Kawataki, M., et al.: Congenital *Candida glabrata* infection without specific nodules on the placenta and umbilical cord. Pediatr. Infect. Dis. J. *24*:744, 2005.
231. Matthews, R., Rigg, G., Hodgetts, S., et al.: Preclinical assessment of the efficacy of mycograb, a human recombinant antibody against fungal HSP90. Antimicrob. Agents Chemother. *47*:2208, 2003.
232. Maxson, S., Miller, S., Tryka, A., et al.: Perinatal blastomycosis: A review. Pediatr. Infect. Dis. J. *11*:760, 1992.
233. Mayayo, E., Moralejo, J., Camps, J., et al.: Fungal endocarditis in premature infants: Case report and review. Clin. Infect. Dis. *22*:366, 1996.

234. McCrossan, B., McHenry, E., O'Neill, F., et al.: Selective fluconazole prophylaxis in high-risk babies to reduce invasive fungal infection. Arch. Dis. Child. Fetal Neonatal Ed. *92*:F454, 2007.

235. McGuire, W., Clerihew, L., and Austin, N.: Prophylactic intravenous antifungal agents to prevent mortality and morbidity in very low birth weight infants. Cochrane Database Syst. Rev. *1*:CD003850, 2004.

236. Mecrow, I., and Ladusans, E.: Infective endocarditis in newborn infants with structurally normal hearts. Acta Paediatr. *83*:35, 1994.

237. Meizoso, T., Rivera, T., Fernandez-Acenero, M., et al.: Intrauterine candidiasis: Report of four cases. Arch. Gynecol. Obstet. *278*:173-176, 2008.

238. Mekha, N., Sugita, T., Ikeda, R., et al.: Real-time PCR assay to detect DNA in sera for the diagnosis of deep-seated trichosporonosis. Microbiol. Immunol. *51*:633, 2007.

239. Messer, S., Diekema, D., Boyken, L., et al.: Activities of micafungin against 315 invasive clinical isolates of fluconazole-resistant *Candida* spp. J. Clin. Microbiol. *44*:324, 2006.

240. Michelson, P., Rupp, R., and Efhimiadis, B.: Endogenous *Candida* endophthalmitis leading to bilateral corneal perforation. Am. J. Ophthalmol. *80*:800, 1975.

241. Millar, B., Jugo, J., and Moore, J.: Fungal endocarditis in neonates and children. Pediatr. Cardiol. *26*:517, 2005.

242. Miller, M. J.: Fungal infections. *In* Remington, J. S., and Klein, J. O. (eds.): Infectious Diseases of the Fetus and Newborn Infant. 5th ed. Philadelphia, W. B. Saunders, 2001, p. 813.

243. Mintz, A., and Applebaum, H.: Focal gastrointestinal perforations not associated with necrotizing enterocolitis in very low birth weight neonates. J. Pediatr. Surg. *28*:857, 1993.

244. Miranda, K., deAraujo, C., Costa, C., et al.: Antifungal activities of azole agents against the *Malassezia* species. Int. J. Antimicrob. Agents *29*:281, 2007.

245. Mittal, M., Dhanireddy, R., and Higgins, R.: *Candida* sepsis and association with retinopathy of prematurity. Pediatrics *101*:654, 1998.

246. Mogyorosy, G., Soos, G., and Nagy, A.: *Candida* endocarditis in a premature infant. J. Perinat. Med. *28*:407, 2000.

247. Mohan, P., Eddama, O., and Weisman, L.: Patient isolation measures for infants with *Candida* colonization or infection for preventing or reducing transmission of *Candida* in neonatal units. Cochrane Database Syst. Rev. *3*: CD006068, 2007.

248. Mollit, D., Tepas, J., and Talbert, J.: The microbiology of neonatal peritonitis. Arch. Surg. *123*:176, 1988.

249. Montgomery, J., Edwards, J., and Guze, L.: Synergism of amphotericin B and 5-fluorocytosine for *Candida* species. J. Infect. Dis. *132*:82, 1975.

250. Moore, M., Collins, G., Hawk, B., et al.: Disseminated *Bipolaris spicifera* in a neonate. J. Perinatol. *21*:399, 2001.

251. Mora-Duarte, J., Betts, R., Rotstein, C., et al.: Caspfungin Invasive Candidiasis Study Group. Comparison of caspofungin and amphotericin B for invasive candidiasis. N. Engl. J. Med. *347*:2020, 2002.

252. Morales-Aguirre, J., Aguero-Echeverria, W., Ornelas-Carsolio, M., et al.: Successful treatment of a primary cutaneous zygomycosis caused by *Absidia corymbifera* in a premature newborn. Pediatr. Infect. Dis. J. *23*:470, 2004.

253. Moreira, M.: Controversies about the management of invasive fungal infections in very low birth weight infants. J. Pediatr. (Rio J.) *81*:S52, 2005.

254. Moylett, E.: Neonatal *Candida* meningitis. Semin. Pediatr. Infect. Dis. *14*:115, 2003.

255. Muldrew, K., Maples, H., Stowe, C., et al.: Intravenous voriconazole therapy in a preterm infant. Pharmacotherapy *25*:893, 2995.

256. Murphy, N., Buchanan, C., Damjanovic, V., et al.: Infection and colonization of neonates by *Hansenula anomala*. Lancet *1*:291, 1986.

257. Natarajan, G., Lulic-Botica, M., Rongkailt, C., et al.: Experience with caspofungin in the treatment of persistent fungemia in neonates. J. Perinatol. *25*:770, 2005.

258. Ng, P., and Dear, P.: Phycomycotic abscesses in a preterm infant. Arch. Dis. Child. *64*:862, 1989.

259. Niamba, P., Weill, F., and Sarlangue, J.: Is common neonatal cephalic pustulosis (neonatal acne) triggered by *Malassezia sympodialis*? Arch. Dermatol. *134*:995, 1998.

260. Nichols, A., Khong, T., and Crowther, C.: *Candida tropicalis* chorioamnionitis. Am. J. Obstet. Gynecol. *172*:1045, 1995.

261. Nooney, L., Matthews, R., and Burnie, J.: Evaluation of Mycograb, amphotericin B, caspofungin, and fluconazole in combination against *Cryptococcus neoformans* by checkerboard and time-kill methodologies. Diagn. Microbiol. Infect. Dis. *51*:19, 2005.

262. Noyola, D., Bohra, L., Paysse, E., et al.: Association of candidemia and retinopathy of prematurity in very low birthweight infants. Ophthalmology *109*:80, 2002.

263. Noyola, D., Fernandez, M., Moylett, E., et al.: Ophthalmologic, visceral, and cardiac involvement in neonates with candidemia. Clin. Infect. Dis. *32*:1018, 2001.

264. O'Calligan, C., and McDougall, P.: Infective endocarditis in neonates. Arch. Dis. Child. *63*:53, 198.

265. Odio, C., Araya, R., Pinto, L., et al.: Caspofungin therapy of neonates with invasive candidiasis. Pediatr. Infect. Dis. J. *23*:1093, 2004.

266. Oh, D., and Notrica, D.: Primary cutaneous mucormycosis in infants and neonates: Case report and review of the literature. J. Pediatr. Surg. *37*:1607, 2002.

267. Olin, J., and Spooner, L.: Amphotericin B-associated hyperbilirubinemia: Case report and review of the literature. Pharmacotherapy *26*:1011, 2006.

268. Ozkiraz, S., Tarcan, A., Gokmen, Z., et al.: Invasive *Candida albicans* infection mimicking leukemia in a neonate. J. Matern. Fetal Neonatal Med. *20*:555, 2007.

269. Palmer, E.: Endogenous *Candida* endophthalmitis in infants. Am. J. Ophthalmol. *89*:388, 1980.

270. Panagopoulou, P., Evoridou, J., and Bibashi, E.: *Trichosporon asahii*: An unusual cause of invasive infection in neonates. Pediatr. Infect. Dis. J. *21*:169, 2002.

271. Papouili, M., Roilides, E., Bibashi, E., et al.: Primary cutaneous aspergillosis in neonates: Case report and review. Clin. Infect. Dis. *22*:1102, 1996.

272. Pappu, L., Purohit, D., Bradford, B., et al.: Primary renal candidiasis in two preterm neonates. Am. J. Dis. Child. *138*:923, 1984.

273. Parikh, T., Nanvati, R., Patankar, C., et al.: Fluconazole prophylaxis against fungal colonization and invasive fingal infection in very low birth weigt infants. Indian Pediatr. *44*:832, 2007.

274. Pasqualotto, A., and Denning, D.: New and emerging treatments for fungal diseases. Antimicrob. Chemother. *61*(Suppl. 1):119, 2008.

275. Pasqualotto, A., Howard, S., Moore, C., et al.: Flucytosine therapeutic monitoring: 15 years experience from the UK. J. Antimicrob. Chemother. *59*:791, 2007.

276. Passeron, T., Desruelles, R., Gari-Toussaint, M., et al.: Invasive fungal dermatitis in a 770 gm neonate. Pediatr. Dermatol. *21*:260, 2004.

277. Patriquin, H., Lebowitz, R., Perreault, G., et al.: Neonatal candidiasis: Renal and pulmonary manifestations. A. J. R. Am. J. Roentgenol. *135*:1205, 1980.

278. Paula, C., Krebs, V., Auler, M., et al.: Nosocomial infection in newborns by *Pichia anomala* in a Brazilian intensive care unit. Med. Mycol. *44*:479, 2006.

279. Perez-Gonzalez, L., Ruiz-Gonzalez, J., and Noyola, D.: Nosocomial bacteremia in children: A 15-year experience at a general hospital in Mexico. Infect. Control Hosp. Epidemiol. *28*:418, 2007.

280. Perniola, R., Faneschi, M., Manso, E., et al.: *Rhodotorula mucilaginosa* outbreak in neonatal intensive care unit: Microbiological features, clinical presentation, and analysis of related variables. Eur. J. Clin. Microbiol. Infect. Dis. *25*:193, 2006.

281. Perzigian, R., and Faix, R.: Primary cutaneous aspergillosis in a preterm infant. Am. J. Perinatol. *10*:269, 1993.

282. Pfaller, M., Boyken, L., and Hollis, R.: In vitro susceptibility of invasive isolates of *Candida* spp. to anidulafungin, caspofungin, and micafungin: six years of global surveillance. J. Clin. Microbiol. *46*:150, 2008.

283. Phillips, J., and Karlowicz, M.: Prevalence of *Candida* species in hospital-acquired urinary tract infections in a neonatal intensive care unit. Pediatr. Infect. Dis. J. *16*:190, 1997.

284. Picarelli, D., Surraco, J., Zuniga, C., et al.: Surgical management of active infective endocarditis in a premature neonate weighing 950 grams. J. Thorac. Cardiovasc. Surg. *119*:380, 2000.

285. Pitarch, A., Abian, J., Carrascal, M., et al.: Proteomics-based identification of novel *Candida albicans* antigens for diagnosis of systemic candidiasis in patients with underlying hematological malignancies. Proteomics *4*:3084, 2004.

286. Pitarch, A., Jimenez, A., Nombela, C., et al.: Decoding serological response to *Candida* cell wall immunome into novel diagnostic prognostic, and therapeutic candidates for systemic candidiasis by proteomic and bioinformatic analyses. Mol. Cell Proteom. *5*:79, 2006.

287. Portnoy, J., Wolf, P., Webb, M., et al.: *Candida* blastospores and pseudohyphae in blood smears. N. Engl. J. Med. *285*:1010, 1971.

288. Powell-Hayes, J., Currell, D., Miller, M., et al.: *Malassezia furfur* skin colonization of infants hospitalized in intensive care units. J. Pediatr. *111*:217, 1987.

289. Prat, O., Schurr, D., Pomeranz, A., et al.: Renal candidiasis in infancy—a case with fungus ball obstruction. Int. J. Pediatr. Nephrol. *5*:223, 1984.

290. Pumberger, W., Mayr, M., Kohlhauser, C., et al.: Spontaneous localized intestinal perforation in very-low-birth-weight infants: A distinct clinical entity different from necrotizing enterocolitis. J. Am. Coll. Surg. *195*:796, 2002.

291. Qureshi, F., Jacques, S., Bendon, R., et al.: *Candida* funisitis: A clinicopathologic study of 32 cases. Pediatr. Dev. Pathol. *1*:118, 1998.

292. Rangel-Fausto, M., Wiblin, T., Blumberg, H., et al.: National Epidemiology of Mycosis Survey (NEMIS): Variations in rates of bloodstream infections due to *Candida* species in 7 surgical intensive care units and 6 neonatal intensive care units. Clin. Infect. Dis. *29*:253, 1999.

293. Rapelanoro, R., Mortureaux, P., Couprie, B., et al.: Neonatal *Malassezia furfur* pustulosis. Arch. Dermatol. *133*:190, 1996.

294. Reddy, T., Chakrabart, A., Singh, M., et al.: Role of buffy coat examination in the diagnosis of neonatal candidiasis. Pediatr. Infect. Dis. J. *15*:718, 1996.

295. Reef, S., Lasker, B., Butcher, D., et al.: Nonperinatal nosocomial transmission of *Candida albicans* in a neonatal intensive care unit: Prospective study. J. Clin. Microbiol. *36*:1255, 1998.

296. Reimund, E., and Ramos, A.: Disseminated neonatal gastrointestinal mucormycosis: A case report and review of the literature. Pediatr. Pathol. *14*:385, 1994.

297. Richet, H., McNeil, M., Edwards, M., et al.: Cluster of *Malassezia furfur* pulmonary infections in infants in a neonatal intensive-care unit. J. Clin. Microbiol. *27*:1197, 1989.

298. Rieger, C., Geiger, S., Herold, T., et al.: Breakthrough infection of *Trichosporon asahii* during posaconazole treatment in a patient with acute myeloid leukaemia. Eur. J. Clin. Microbiol. Infect. Dis. *26*:843, 2007.

299. Robertson, N., Kuna, J., and Cox, P.: Spontaneous intestinal perforation and *Candida* peritonitis presenting as extensive necrotizing enterooclitis. Acta Paediatr. 92:258, 2003.

300. Robinson, L., Jain, L., and Kourtis, A.: Persistent candidemia in a premature infant treated with fluconazole. Pediatr. Infect. Dis. J. 18:735, 1999.

301. Rodriquez, D., Almirante, B., Park, B., et al.: Neonatal candidemia in neonatal intensive care units in Barcelona, Spain. Pediatr. Infect. Dis. J. 25:224, 2006.

302. Rogers, T.: Treatment of zygomycosis: current and new options. J. Antimicrob. Chemother. 61(Suppl.):35, 2008.

303. Roilides, E., Farmaki, E., Evdoridou, J., et al.: *Candida tropicalis* in a neonatal intensive care unit: Epidemiologic and molecular analysis of an outbreak of infection with an uncommon neonatal pathogen. J. Clin. Microbiol. 41:735-741, 2003.

304. Roilides, E., Farmaki, E., Evdoridou, J., et al.: Neonatal candidiasis: Analysis of epidemiology, drug susceptibility, and molecular typing of causative isolates. Eur. J. Clin. Microbiol. Infect. Dis. 23:745, 2007.

305. Roque, H., Abdeihak, Y., and Young, B.: Intra amniotic candidiasis: Case report and meta-analysis of 54 cases. J. Perinat. Med. 27:253, 1999.

306. Rowen, J.: Mucocutaneous candidiasis. Semin. Perinatol. 27:406, 2003.

307. Rowen, J., Atkins, J., Levy, M., et al.: Invasive fungal dermatitis in the 1000-gram neonate. Pediatrics 95:682, 1995.

308. Rowen, J., Correa, A., Sokol, D., et al.: Invasive aspergillosis in neonates: Report of five cases and review. Pediatr. Infect. Dis. J. 11:269, 1993.

309. Rowen, J., Ragouilliaux, C., Keeneu, S., et al.: Maternal factors in extremely low birth weight infants who develop spontaneous intestinal perforation. Pediatrics 120:e1458, 2007.

310. Rowen, J., Rench, M., Kozinetz, C., et al.: Endotracheal colonization with *Candida* enhances risk of systemic candidiasis in very low birth weight neonates. J. Pediatr. 124:789, 1994.

311. Rowen, J., and Tate, J. M.: Management of neonatal candidiasis. Neonatal Candidiasis Study Group. Pediatr. Infect. Dis. J. 17:1007, 1998.

312. Rowen, J., Tate, J., Nordoff, N., et al.: *Candida* isolates from neonates: Frequency of misidentification and reduced fluconazole susceptibility. J. Clin. Microbiol. 11:3735, 1999.

313. Ruiz-Diez, B., Martinez, V., Alvarez, M., et al.: Molecular tracking of *Candida albicans* in a neonatal care unit: Long-term colonization versus catheter-related infections. J. Clin. Microbiol. 35:3032, 1997.

314. Saiman, L., Ludington, E., Dawson, J. D., et al.: Risk factors for *Candida* species colonization of neonatal intensive care unit patients. Pediatr. Infect. Dis. J. 20:1119, 2001.

315. Saiman, L., Ludington, E., Pfaller, M., et al.: Risk factors for candidemia in neonatal intensive care unit patients. Pediatr. Infect. Dis. J. 19:319, 2000.

316. Sanchez, P., and Cooper, B. H.: *Candida lusitaniae*: Sepsis and meningitis in a neonate. Pediatr. Infect. Dis. J. 6:758, 1987.

317. Sanchez, P., Siegel, J., and Fishbein, J.: *Candida* endocarditis: Successful medical management in three preterm infants and review of the literature. Pediatr. Infect. Dis. J. 10:239, 1991.

318. Santos, R., Sanchez, P., Mejias, A., et al.: Successful medical treatment of cutaneous aspergillosis in a premature infants using amphotericin B, voriconazole, and micafungin. Pediatr. Infect. Dis. J. 26:364, 2007.

319. Sarvikivi, E., Lyytikainen, O., Soll, D., et al.: Emergence of fluconazole resistance in a *Candida parapsilosis* strain that caused infections in a neonatal intensive care unit. J. Clin. Microbiol. 43:2729, 2005.

320. Saxen, H., Hoppu, K., and Pohjavuori, M.: Pharmacokinetics of fluconazole in very low birth weight infants during the first two weeks of life. Clin. Pharmacol. Ther. 54:269, 1993.

321. Scarcella, A., Pasquariello, M., Giugliano, B., et al.: Liposomal amphotericin B treatment for neonatal fungal infections. Pediatr. Infect. Dis. J. 17:146, 1998.

322. Scheffler, E., Miller, G., and Classen, D.: Zygomycotic infection of the neonatal upper extremity. J. Pediatr. Surg. 38:816, 2003.

323. Schleman, K., Tullis, G., and Blum, R.: Intracardiac mass complicating *Malassezia furfur* fungemia. Chest 118:1828, 2000.

324. Schwarze, R., Penk, A., and Pittow, L.: Treatment of candidal infections with fluconazole in neonates and infants. Eur. J. Med. Res. 5:203, 2000.

325. Schwartz, D., and Reef, S.: *Candida albicans* placentitis and funisitis: Early diagnosis of congenital candidemia by histopathologic examination of umbilical cord vessels. Pediatr. Infect. Dis. J. 9:661, 1990.

326. Schwesinger, G.: Disseminated candidiasis in premature twins: Case report. Mycoses 42S:60, 1999.

327. Seelig, M.: The role of antibiotics in the pathogenesis of *Candida* infections. Am. J. Med. 40:887, 1966.

328. Segal, D., Gohar, J., Hulelhel, M., et al.: Fetal death associated with asymptomatic intrauterine *Candida albicans* infection and a retained intrauterine contraceptive device. Scand. J. Infect. Dis. 33:77, 2001.

329. Shafai, T.: Neonatal coccidioidomycosis in premature twins. Am. J. Dis. Child. 132:634, 1978.

330. Shah, G., Vander, J., and Eagle, R.: Intralenticular *Candida* species abscess in a premature infant. Am. J. Ophthalmol. 129:390, 2000.

331. Shareef, M., Myers, T., Mathews, H., et al.: Reduced capacity of neonatal lymphocytes to inhibit the growth of *Candida albicans*. Biol. Neonate 75:31, 1999.

332. Shattuck, K., Cochran, C., Zabransky, R., et al.: Colonization and infection associated with *Malassezia* and *Candida* species in a neonatal unit. J. Hosp. Infect. 34:123, 1996.

333. Shen, Y., Wang, J., and Lu, H.: Voriconazole in an infant with cryptococcal meningitis. Chin. Med. J. (Engl.) 121:286, 2008.

334. Sherertz, R., Gledhill, S., Hampton, K., et al.: Outbreak of *Candida* bloodstream infections associated with retrograde medication administration in a neonatal intensive care unit. J. Pediatr. 120:455, 1992.

335. Shetty, S., Harrison, L., Hajjeh, R., et al.: Determining risk factors for candidemia among newborn infants from population-based surveillance: Baltimore, Maryland, 1998-2000. Pediatr. Infect. Dis. J. 24:601, 2005.

336. Shields, J., Shields, C., Eagles, R., et al.: Endogenous endophthalmitis simulating retinoblastoma. The 1993 David and Mary Sesien Endowment Lecture. Retina 15:213, 1995.

337. Sims, M., Yoo, Y., You, H., et al.: Prophylactic oral nystatin and fungal infections in very-low-birth-weight infants. Am. J. Perinatol. 5:33, 1988.

338. Singh, K., Chakrabarti, A., Narang, A., et al.: Yeast colonization and fungaemia in preterm neonates in a tertiary care centre. Indian J. Med. Res. 110:169, 1999.

339. Sirinavin, S., Intusoma, U., and Tuntirungsee, S.: Mother-to-child transmission of *Cryptococcus neoformans*. Pediatr. Infect. Dis. J. Hum. Pathol. 23:278, 2004.

340. Siu, K., and Lee, W.: A rare cause of intestinal perforation in an extreme low birth weight infant—gastrointestinal mucormycosis: A case report. J. Perinatol. 24:319, 2004.

341. Smith, H., and Congdon, P.: Neonatal systemic candidiasis. Arch. Dis. Child. 60:365, 1985.

342. Smith, J., Nichols, M., Goldman, A., et al.: Disseminated *Cryptococcus* in an infant with severe combined immunodeficiency. Hum. Pathol. 13:500, 1982.

343. Smith, P., Morgan, J., Benjamin, J., et al.: Excess costs of hospital care associated with neonatal candidemia. Pediatr. Infect. Dis. J. 26:197, 2007.

344. Smith, P., Olson, J., Constable, D., et al.: Effect of dosing regimen on accumulation, retention and prophylactic efficacy of liposomal amphotericin B. J. Antimicrob. Chemother. 59:941, 2007.

345. Smith, P., Steinbach, W., Cotton, C., et al.: Caspofungin for the treatment of azole resistant candidemia in a premature infant. J. Perinatol. 27:127, 2007.

346. Smolinski, K., Shah, S., Honig, P., et al.: Neonatal cutaneous fungal infections. Curr. Opin. Pediatr. 17:486, 2005.

347. Soltani, M., Tobin, C., Bowker, K., et al.: Evidence of excessive concentrations of 5-flucytosine in children aged below 12 years: A 12-year review of serum concentrations from a UK clinical assay reference laboratory. Int. J. Antimicrob. Agents 28:574, 2006.

348. Sonnenschein, H., Clark, H., and Taschdjian, C.: Congenital cutaneous candidiasis in a premature infant. Am. J. Dis. Child. 99:81, 1960.

349. Sonnenschein, H., Taschdjian, C., and Clark, D.: Congenital cutaneous candidiasis in a premature infant. Am. J. Dis. Child. 107:260, 1964.

350. Sood, S., Majumdar, T., Chatterjee, A., et al.: Disseminated candidosis in premature twins. Mycoses 41:417, 1998.

351. Speer, M., Hittner, H., and Rudolph, A.: *Candida* endophthalmitis: A manifestation of candidiasis in the neonate. South. Med. J. 73:1407, 1980.

352. Stamos, J., and Rowley, A.: Candidemia in a pediatric population. Clin. Infect. Dis. J. 20:571, 1995.

353. Starke, J., Mason, E., Kramer, W., et al.: Pharmacokinetics of amphotericin B in infants and children. J. Infect. Dis. 155:766, 1987.

354. Steinbach, W., and Benjamin, D.: New antifungal agents under development in children and neonates. Curr. Opin. Infect. Dis. 18:484, 2005.

355. Stephenson, J.: Can a common medical practice transform *Candida* infections from benign to deadly? J. A. M. A. 286:2531, 2001.

356. Stern, J., Calvano, C., and Simon, J.: Recurrent endogenous candidal endophthalmitis in a premature infant. J. Am. Assoc. Pediatr. Ophthalmol. Strabismus 5:50, 2001.

357. Stoll, B., Gordon, T., Korones, S., et al.: Late-onset sepsis in very low birth weight neonates: A report from the National Institute of Child Health and Human Development Neonatal Research Network. J. Pediatr. 129:63, 1996.

358. Stopfkuchen, H., Benzing, F., Jungst, B., et al.: Echocardiographic diagnosis of *Candida* endocarditis of the tricuspid valve and of the right atrium in a young infant. Pediatr. Cardiol. 4:49, 1983.

359. Sung, J., Rajani, K., Chopra, D., et al.: Miconazole therapy for systemic candidiasis in conjoined (Siamese) twin and a premature newborn. Am. J. Surg. 138:688, 1979.

360. Surmont, I., Gavilanes, A., Vandepitte, J., et al.: *Malassezia furfur* fungaemia in infants receiving intravenous lipid emulsions: A rarity or just underestimated. Eur. J. Pediatr. 148:435, 1989.

361. Svirsky-Fein, S., Langer, L., Milbauer, B., et al.: Neonatal osteomyelitis caused by *Candida tropicalis*. J. Bone Joint Surg. Am. 61:455, 1979.

362. Sweet, D., and Reid, M.: Disseminated neonatal *Trichosporon beigelii* infection: Successful treatment with liposomal amphotericin B. J. Infect. 36:120, 1998.

363. Tabata, K., Katashima, M., Kawamura, A., et al.: Linear pharmacokinetics of micafungin and its active metabolites in Japanese pediatric patients with fungal infections. Biol. Pharm. Bull. 29:1706, 2006.

364. Taj-Aldeen, S., Doiphode, S., and Han, X.: *Kodamaea (Pichia) ohmeria* fungaemia in a premature neonate. J. Med. Microbiol. 55:237, 2006.

365. Thomas, D., Viudes, A., Monteagudo, C., et al.: Proteomics-based identification of novel *Candida albicans* antigens for diagnosis of systemic candidiasis in patients with underlying hematological malignancies. Proteomics 4:3084, 2004.

366. Tirodker, U., Nataro, J., Smith, S., et al.: Detection of fungemia by polymerase chain reaction in critically ill neonates and children. J. Perinatol. 23:117, 2003.

367. Todd Johnston, W., and Cogen, M.: Systemic candidiasis with cataract formation in a premature infant. J. Am. Assoc. Pediatr. Ophthalmol. Strabismus 4:386, 2000.

368. Triolo, V., Gari-Toussaint, M., Casagrande, F., et al.: Fluconazole therapy for Candida albicans urinary tract infections in infants. Pediatr. Nephrol. 17:550, 2002.

369. Tuck, S.: Neonatal systemic candidiasis treated with miconazole. Arch. Dis. Child. 55:903, 1980.

370. Tuthill, W.: Disseminated blastomycosis with intrauterine transmission. South. Med. J. 78:1526, 1985.

371. Tuon, F., de Almeida, G., and Costa, S.: Central venous catheter-associated fungemia due to Rhodotorula spp.—systematic review. Med. Mycol. 45:441, 2007.

372. Valari, M., Stefanaki, C., Karteri, G., et al.: Tinea capitis due to Trichophyton rubrum in a 3 month old infant. Mycoses 49:439, 2006.

373. van Asbeck, E., Huang, Y., Markham, A., et al.: Candida parapsilosis fungemia in neonates: Genotyping results suggest healthcare workers hands as source, and review of published studies. Mycopathologia 164:287, 2007.

374. van Belkum, A., Boekhout, T., and Bosboom, R.: Monitoring spread of Malassezia infections in a neonatal intensive care unit by PCR-mediated genetic typing. Clin. Microbiol. 32:2528, 1994.

375. van den Anker, J.: Treatment of neonatal Candida albicans septicemia with itraconazole. Pediatr. Infect. Dis. J. 11:684, 1992.

376. Vaudry, W., Tierney, A., and Wenman, W.: Investigation of a cluster of systemic Candida albicans infections in a neonatal intensive care unit. J. Infect. Dis. 158:1375, 1988.

377. Venkatesh, M., Pham, D., Fein-Kong, L., et al.: Neonatal coinfection model of coagulase-negative Staphylococcus (Staphylococcus epidermidis) and Candida albicans: Fluconazole prophylaxis enhances survival and growth. Antimicrob. Agents Chemother. 51:1240, 2007.

378. Verduyn-Lunel, F., Voss, A., Kuijper, E., et al.: Detection of the Candida antigen mannan in cerebrospinal fluid specimens from patients suspected of having Candida meningitis. J. Clin. Microbiol. 43:867, 2004.

379. Villar, C., Kashleva, H., Nobile, C., et al.: Mucosal tissue invasion by Candida albicans is associated with E-cadherin degradation, mediated by transcription factor Rim101p and protease Sap5p. Infect. Immun. 75:2126, 2007.

380. Vinod Kumar, C., and Neelagund, Y.: Incidence and antifungal susceptibility of Candida species in neonatal septicemia. J. Commun. Dis. 36:182, 2004.

381. Visser, D., Monnens, L., Feitz, W., et al.: Fungal bezoars as a cause of renal insufficiency in neonates and infants—recommended treatment strategy. Clin. Nephrol. 49:198, 1998.

382. Waggoner-Fountain, L., Walker, M., Hollis, J., et al.: Vertical and horizontal transmission of unique Candida species to premature newborns. Clin. Infect. Dis. 22:803, 1996.

383. Wainer, S., Cooper, P., Funk, E., et al.: Prophylactic miconazole oral gel for the prevention of neonatal fungal rectal colonization and systemic infection. Pediatr. Infect. Dis. J. 11:713, 1992.

384. Walsh, T., Gonzalez, C., Lyman, C., et al.: Invasive fungal infections in children: Recent advances in diagnosis and treatment. Adv. Pediatr. Infect. Dis. 11:187, 1996.

385. Walsh, T., Melcher, G., Rinaldi, M., et al.: Trichosporon beigelii, an emerging pathogen resistant to amphotericin B. J. Clin. Microbiol. 28:1616, 1990.

386. Walsh, T., Seibel, N., Arndt, C., et al.: Amphotericin B lipid complex in pediatric patients with invasive fungal infections. Pediatr. Infect. Dis. J. 18:702, 1999.

387. Ward, R., Sattler, F., and Dalton, A.: Assessment of antifungal therapy in an 800 gram infant with candidal arthritis and osteomyelitis. Pediatrics 72:234, 1983.

388. Watts, E., Gard, P., and Tuthill, W.: First reported case of intrauterine transmission of blastomycosis. Pediatr. Infect. Dis. J. 2:308-310, 1983.

389. Weese-Mayer, D. E., Fondriest, D., Brouillette, R. T., et al.: Risk factors associated with candidemia in the neonatal intensive care unit: A case-control study. Pediatr. Infect. Dis. J. 6:190, 1987.

390. Weigh, J.: Candida arthritis in a premature infant treated successfully with oral fluconazole for six months. Ann. Acad. Med. Singapore 29:253, 2000.

391. Weisman, L., Stoll, B., Kueser, T., et al.: Intravenous immune globulin prophylaxis for late-onset sepsis in premature neonates. J. Pediatr. 125:922, 1994.

392. Weiss, S., Schoch, P., and Cunha, B.: Malassezia furfur fungemia associated with central venous catheter lipid emulsion infusion. Heart Lung 20:87, 1991.

393. Weisse, M., Person, D., and Berkenbaugh, J.: Treatment of Candida arthritis with flucytosine and amphotericin B. J. Perinatol. 13:402, 1993.

394. Weitkamp, J., Poets, C., Sievers, R., et al.: Candida infection in very low birth-weight infants: Outcome and nephrotoxicity of treatment with liposomal amphotericin B (AmBisome). Infection 26:11, 1998.

395. Welbel, S., McNeil, M., Kuykendall, R., et al.: Candida parapsilosis bloodstream infections in neonatal intensive care unit patients: Epidemiologic and laboratory confirmation of a common source outbreak. Pediatr. Infect. Dis. J. 15:998, 1996.

396. Welbel, S., McNeil, M., Pramanik, A., et al.: Nosocomial Malassezia pachydermatis bloodstream infections in a neonatal intensive care unit. Pediatr. Infect. Dis. J. 13:104, 1994.

397. Wenzl, T., Schefels, J., Hörnchen, H., et al.: Pharmacokinetics of oral fluconazole in premature infants. Eur. J. Pediatr. 157:661, 1998.

398. Westley, C., and Haak, W.: Neonatal coccidioidomycosis in a southwestern Pima Indian. South. Med. J. 67:855, 1974.

399. Whyte, R., Hussain, Z., and deSa, D.: Antenatal infections with Candida species. Arch. Dis. Child. 57:528, 1982.

400. Woodruff, C., and Hebert, A.: Neonatal primary cutaneous aspergillosis: Case report and review of the literature. Pediatr. Dermatol. 19:439, 2002.

401. Wong, A., Ibrahim, H., Van Rostenberghe, H., et al.: Hansenula anomala infection in a neonate. J. Paediatr. Child Health 36:609, 2000.

402. Wong-Beringer, A., Jacobs, R. A., and Guglielmo, B. J.: Lipid formulations of amphotericin B: Clinical efficacy and toxicities. Clin. Infect. Dis. 27:603, 1998.

403. Wu, K., Chen, W., Chiang, L., et al.: Ureteropelvic fungal bezoar causing oliguric renal failure in a premature infant. Zhonghua. Min. Guo. Xiao. Er. Ke. Yi. Xue. Hui. Za. Zhi. 36:292, 1995.

404. Yadin, O., Gradus Ben-Ezer, D., Golan, A., et al.: Survival of a premature neonate with obstructive anuria due to Candida: The role of early sonographic diagnosis and antimycotic treatment. Eur. J. Pediatr. 147:653, 1988.

405. Yalaz, M., Akisu, M., Hillmioglu, S., et al.: Successful caspofungin treatment of multidrug resistant Candida parapsilosis septicaemia in an extremely low birth weight neonate. Mycoses 49:242, 2006.

406. Yau, Y., deNanassy, J., Summerbell, R., et al.: Fungal sternal wound infection due to Curvularia lunata in a neonate with congenital heart disease: Case report and review. Clin. Infect. Dis. 19:735, 1994.

407. Yildiran, A., Kucukoduk, S., Sanic, A., et al.: Disseminated Trichosporon asahii infection in a preterm. Am. J. Perinatol. 20:269, 2003.

408. Yoss, B., Sautter, R., and Brenker, H.: Trichosporon beiglii, a new neonatal pathogen. Am. J. Perinatol. 14:113, 1997.

409. Young, L., and Schutze, G.: Perinatal blastomycosis: The rest of the story. Pediatr. Infect. Dis. J. 14:83, 1995.

410. Zaoutis, T., Foraker, E., McGowan, K., et al.: Antifungal susceptibility of Candida spp. isolated from pediatric patients: A survey of 4 children's hospitals. Diagn. Microbiol. Infect. Dis. 52:295, 2005.

411. Zaoutis, T., Heydon, K., Localio, R., et al.: Outcomes attributable to neonatal candidiasis. Clin. Infect. Dis. 44:1187, 2007.

412. Zaoutis, T., Roilides, E., Chiou, C., et al.: Zygomycosis in children: A systematic review and analysis of reported cases. Pediatr. Infect. Dis. J. 26:723, 2007.

413. Zaoutis, T., and Walsh, T.: Antifungal therapy for neonatal candidiasis. Curr. Opin. Infect. Dis. 20:592, 2007.

414. Zenker, P., Rosenberg, E., Van Dyke, R., et al.: Successful medical treatment of presumed Candida endocarditis in critically ill infants. J. Pediatr. 119:472, 1991.

CHAPTER

77

CONGENITAL TOXOPLASMOSIS

James B. McAuley ⊙ Kenneth M. Boyer

Toxoplasma gondii is an obligate intracellular protozoan parasite (phylum Apicomplexa, class Sporozoasida, order Eucoccidiida).[126] The first report of human infection occurred in 1908.[18] In 1937, Wolf and Cowen[132] reported a case of congenital granulomatous encephalitis, which Sabin[103] later correctly attributed to T. gondii infection. Congenital toxoplasmosis results from placental infection that develops after primary maternal infection and subse-

quent hematogenous spread to the fetus.[95] Toxoplasma is ubiquitous in nature, with the cat family being the definitive host.[35,37]

The organism exists in three forms: (1) oocyst, which is excreted in cat feces and is infectious within 2 to 5 days after sporulation; (2) a proliferative stage called a tachyzoite; and (3) a tissue cystic stage called a bradyzoite. Mammals or birds ingest oocysts from contaminated plants and soil, or, if carnivorous, they may ingest bradyzoites. When ingested, *Toxoplasma* replicate asexually, and tissue cysts accumulate in the organs and skeletal muscle of these animals. Possible routes of infection for humans are direct ingestion of sporulated oocysts from soil, water, fruits, or vegetables that have been contaminated by cat feces, or ingestion of undercooked meat containing bradyzoites.[6,8,26,95] Humans also have become infected after undergoing organ transplantation, after receiving blood product transfusions, and after having laboratory accidents.[95]

The prevalence of antibody to *T. gondii* in women of childbearing age in the United States varies from approximately 3 to 30 percent, depending on the region of the country.[57,58,111] The lowest seroprevalence rates have been found in the Mountain states, where a dry climate does not favor survival of oocysts in the soil. The highest rates have been noted in the northeastern and southeastern states. In contrast, the seropositivity rate for women in Paris may be 70 percent. These widely disparate seroprevalence rates in different adult populations throughout the world are explained by differences in eating and sanitation practices and conditions that affect survival of oocysts in the environment.[58,95] More recent studies have documented a declining prevalence of infection in the United States.[57] This decline likely is related to decreased rates of contamination of commercial meats with *Toxoplasma* and increased educational efforts aimed at informing the public about avoiding acquisition of infection.[27,58]

The prevalence of congenital infection in the United States has been documented to be 0.08 per 1000 births (1 in 12,000 births) by IgM screening of blood specimens collected on filter paper from newborns in Massachusetts and New Hampshire.[49] This figure compares with a rate of 3 to 10 per 1000 live births in Paris and Vienna. In Massachusetts, a case-control study involving 14 years of newborn screening for congenital toxoplasmosis found that birth of the mother outside the United States, particularly in Cambodia and Laos, and the educational level and higher gravidity of the mother were strongly predictive of congenital infection.[55]

TRANSMISSION

Infection of the fetus occurs during maternal parasitemia, with subsequent infection of the placenta caused by tachyzoites.[36,95] Placental infection represents an important intermediary step between maternal and fetal infection. A delay of 16 weeks between placental infection and subsequent infection of the fetus has been noted and is termed the *prenatal incubation period*.[95] Fetal infection occurs as a consequence of maternal primary infection acquired during pregnancy.[36,83,95] Rare instances of transmission have been reported in women with primary infection shortly before conception.[40,122] Reactivation of latent *Toxoplasma* infection during pregnancy does not lead to fetal infection except rarely in immunocompromised women, such as women infected with human immunodeficiency virus (HIV).[80,87,95,134] In these instances, congenital infection has been documented, although the risk is very low.[30] Maternal re-infection leading to congenital toxoplasmosis also has been reported rarely.[40,95] Congenital toxoplasmosis has occurred in twins and triplets.[13,95] Despite these occasional case reports, most congenital infections are the result of primary maternal infection during pregnancy.

The overall fetal infection rate from untreated maternal infection during pregnancy is approximately 40 percent, although the rate depends on when in pregnancy the mother becomes infected (Table 77-1).[31,95,134] Although the actual rate of fetal infection increases as pregnancy advances, the severity of clinical manifestations is greatest when maternal infection is acquired during the first trimester.[31,95,134] Transmission during breast-feeding in humans has not been shown, although the organism has been detected in human milk.

TABLE 77-1 Vertical Transmission and Severity of Disease for *Toxoplasma gondii* by the Timing of Maternal Infection during Pregnancy

	Trimester of Maternal Infection		
	First	**Second**	**Third**
Overall transmission rate (%)	15	30	60
Proportion of infected children with specific disease severity			
Stillborn/perinatal death (%)	35	7	0
Subclinical (asymptomatic) (%)	18	67	90
Mild disease (%)	6	18	10
Severe disease (%)	41	8	0

CLINICAL MANIFESTATIONS

Acute maternal infection acquired early in pregnancy may lead to fulminant fetal infection and result in stillbirth, nonimmune fetal hydrops, preterm birth, and perinatal death.[1,5,49,95] Chronic *Toxoplasma* infection has been associated only rarely with sporadic abortion.[95] Most infants born with congenital *Toxoplasma* infection are asymptomatic in the neonatal period, with clinical signs and symptoms being present in only approximately 25 percent of infants.[2,55,63,73] Long-term follow-up of these asymptomatically infected infants reveals eye or neurologic disease, or both, in 80 to 90 percent by the time they reach adulthood.[20,31,49,55,116,124] The clinical manifestations of congenital toxoplasmosis in newborns generally are indistinguishable from the manifestations associated with other agents of congenital infection, such as cytomegalovirus and *Treponema pallidum*. The most characteristic clinical findings, frequently referred to as the *classic triad of congenital toxoplasmosis*, are chorioretinitis, intracranial calcifications, and hydrocephalus.[32,95] They are seen in approximately 86 percent (chorioretinitis), 37 percent (intracranial calcifications), and 20 percent (hydrocephalus) of symptomatic infants. These conditions often are accompanied by a combination of signs and symptoms including anemia (59%), jaundice (43%), splenomegaly (41%), seizures (41%), fever (40%), hepatomegaly (34%), lymphadenopathy (32%), microcephaly (9%), and eosinophilia (9%).[32,95]

Involvement of the central nervous system is a hallmark of congenital *Toxoplasma* infection.[12a,13,20,32,72,95,100,111] Hydrocephalus usually is obstructive and often requires ventriculoperitoneal shunting.[95,111] It may be the only manifestation of disease. Abnormalities in cerebrospinal fluid (CSF) occur in approximately 63 percent of infected infants; characteristically, they consist of lymphocytic pleocytosis and an elevated protein level.[32,72,95] The markedly high protein concentrations in ventricular fluid, often exceeding 1 g/dL, and hydrocephalus are explained by periaqueductal and periventricular vasculitis with necrosis, which are associated specifically with toxoplasmosis.[95] Inflammation and necrosis involving the hypothalamus have resulted in hypothermia and hyperthermia. When microcephaly is present, it indicates severe brain damage. Intracranial calcifications may be single or multiple but typically are generalized and located in the caudate nucleus, choroid plexus, meninges, and subependyma.[25,88,95] Periventricular calcifications similar to those associated with cytomegalovirus also have been described. They are visualized best by computed tomography (CT),[72] although ultrasonography has been shown to have excellent correlation with CT findings.[10] The calcifications may resolve with appropriate antimicrobial therapy.[88]

Neurologic sequelae from untreated congenital toxoplasmosis include mental retardation (87%), seizures (82%), spasticity and palsies (71%), and deafness (15%).[32,72,95,111] *Toxoplasma* has been detected in the inner ear and mastoid, with the associated inflammation resulting in deafness. An ascending flaccid paralysis with myelitis also has been reported.[95]

Chorioretinitis caused by *Toxoplasma* occurring at any age is likely to be a result of congenital infection, although acute acquired toxoplasmosis was reported to cause approximately 40 percent of childhood chorioretinitis in one study.[44,79,95] In infants, the most common manifestation is strabismus, whereas defects in visual acuity predominate in older children and adults. The characteristic lesion consists of a focal necrotizing retinitis that often is bilateral.[79] Organisms are present in the retina, and they have a predilection for the macula, with resultant loss of vision. Involvement of the optic nerve also may occur. Other complications include iridocyclitis and cataracts.[79]

Other manifestations of congenital toxoplasmosis include nonspecific maculopapular or petechial rash, myocarditis, pneumonitis, thrombocytopenia, nephrotic syndrome, and abnormalities in immunoglobulin production.[32,95] Bony abnormalities consisting of metaphyseal radiolucencies similar to those seen in congenital syphilis also have been reported. A variety of endocrine abnormalities, including hypothyroidism, diabetes insipidus,[72,95] precocious puberty, and growth hormone deficiency, may occur. All these abnormalities are related to the fact that the organism is capable of widespread dissemination throughout the brain and body, with involvement of virtually all organ systems.

DIAGNOSIS

The diagnosis of congenital toxoplasmosis can be established by isolating the organism from infected body fluids and tissues, such as the placenta, amniotic fluid, fetal blood obtained by cordocentesis, umbilical cord blood, infant blood, and CSF.[22,82,131] Such isolation involves inoculation of the specimen intraperitoneally into laboratory mice and requires approximately 4 to 6 weeks for confirmation. Testing is not widely available but can be done at the Toxoplasma Serology Laboratory, Palo Alto Medical Foundation (860 Bryant Street, Palo Alto, CA 94301; 415-326-8120).

Alternatively, a diagnosis can be established by histopathologic examination of the placenta in which tachyzoites are revealed. Polymerase chain reaction (PCR) has been used successfully to detect *Toxoplasma* DNA in amniotic fluid, placenta, CSF, and fetal and infant blood.[22,48,50,82,101,102,131] PCR performed on amniotic fluid obtained by amniocentesis is the preferred method of confirming in utero infection. A negative amniotic fluid PCR result does not always rule out congenital infection, however.[82,131] In addition, interlaboratory variability in performance of PCR assays has been documented.

The most practical and widely used method of establishing the diagnosis is by testing maternal and newborn blood for serologic evidence of *Toxoplasma* infection. Major problems associated with serologic diagnosis include determining the acuity of the maternal infection and differentiating endogenous from transplacentally acquired antibodies in neonatal/fetal infection. In addition, many commercially available immunoglobulin M (IgM) assays have been associated with significant false-positive and false-negative results.[125,131] Table 77–2 is a brief overview of strategies for establishing the serologic diagnosis in maternal and fetal/neonatal sera, including when to send sera for testing in a reference laboratory.

Tests are available that detect *T. gondii*–specific IgG, and they include the Sabin-Feldman dye test,[104] which is considered to be the gold standard but requires live organisms/tachyzoites; the indirect immunofluorescent antibody test; IgG enzyme-linked immunosorbent assay (ELISA); and direct agglutination.[2,82,93,131,133] An AC/HS differential agglutination test has been developed as a confirmatory test to differentiate acute and chronic maternal infection.[16,24,68] This test compares the IgG serologic titer obtained with the use of formalin-fixed tachyzoites (HS antigen) with the titer obtained with acetone-fixed (or methanol-fixed) tachyzoites (AC antigen). The latter preparation contains stage-specific *Toxoplasma* antigens that are recognized by IgG antibodies only during early infection. The enzyme-linked immunofiltration assay compares the immunologic profile of the mother's antibody response and that of her child at delivery and allows discrimination between

TABLE 77–2   Guidelines for Interpretation of Serologic Tests for Toxoplasmosis in Newborns

Newborn Serology		Interpretation
IgG	*IgM*	
Positive	Negative	For newborns, 25% have false-negative IgM (competition with high maternal IgG or failure to produce adequate IgM). Repeat testing on second specimen. Consider using alternative assay (IgM ELISA if IFA was used first, IgM IFA if ELISA was used first)
		If clinically high suspicion (documented acute maternal primary infection in pregnancy *or* compatible illness in infant), specimen should be sent to a reference laboratory for further testing. Clinical evaluation may be initiated (see below)
		Reference Laboratory: 0.5 mL serum to Toxoplasma Serology Laboratory, Palo Alto Medical Foundation, 860 Bryant Street, Palo Alto, CA 94301, 415-326-8120
Positive	Positive	IgM ELISA can be false-positive in the presence of rheumatoid factor, and IgM IFA can be false-positive in the setting of antinuclear antibodies. Further testing needed (IgM ISAGA, IgA EIA, IgE EIA/ISAGA, AC/HS antigen, placental PCR) in reference laboratory (see above)
		If high likelihood of infection (known maternal primary infection *or* child with clinically compatible illness), begin work-up while reference laboratory tests are pending
		Initial clinical evaluation of the infant should include ophthalmologic examination, auditory brain stem response to 20 dB of sound, serum alanine aminotransferase, total and direct bilirubin, complete blood count, CSF examination (cell count, glucose, protein, and total IgG), and brain CT for calcifications (more recent data suggest excellent agreement between CT and ultrasound, which can be obtained more quickly and without the need for sedation)
Positive	Equivocal	Repeat testing on second specimen. Consider using alternative assay (IgM ELISA if IFA was used first, IgM IFA if ELISA was used first). If clinically high suspicion (documented acute maternal primary infection in pregnancy *or* compatible illness in infant), specimen should be sent to a reference laboratory (see above)
Negative	Negative	Newborn IgG reflects maternal antibody, so no evidence of maternal infection. Newborn not infected
Negative	Positive	Newborn IgG reflects maternal antibody, so no evidence of maternal infection. Newborn not likely to be infected; consider false-positive IgM. Repeat assay on second specimen (IgG and IgM). Consider using alternative assay (IgM ELISA if IFA was used first, IgM IFA if ELISA was used first)

AC/HS, differential agglutination acetone-fixed/formalin-fixed tachyzoites; CSF, cerebrospinal fluid; CT, computed tomography; EIA, enzyme immunoassay; ELISA, enzyme-linked immunosorbent assay; IFA, immunofluorescent assay; Ig, immunoglobulin; ISAGA, immunosorbent agglutination assay; PCR, polymerase chain reaction.

IgG antibodies of maternal origin and IgG synthesized by the fetus; it has a reported sensitivity of 94 percent and a specificity of 99 percent. The IgG avidity test may be more widely available than is the AC/HS test, which requires working with tachyzoites, and allows timing of the infection from a single maternal specimen.[10,131]

After primary infection occurs, the avidity of IgG antibody for *T. gondii* antigen is low. Urea dissociates low-avidity antibodies, and by determining the percentage of antibodies that resist elution by 6 mol/L urea, one can differentiate infection acquired within the past 12 weeks from an older infection. This test is useful in the first 12 weeks of gestation because the presence of high-avidity antibodies excludes the acquisition of infection in the previous 3 months.

Tests that detect *T. gondii*–specific IgM include (1) the double-sandwich IgM ELISA, which has a sensitivity of 75 percent and a specificity of 100 percent[23,94]; (2) the IgM immunosorbent agglutination assay, which is the most sensitive test but should not be performed on umbilical cord blood because even small quantities of maternal IgM antibodies contaminating the specimen would result in a false-positive test result[84-86]; and (3) the IgM immunofluorescent antibody test, which is not recommended as a first screening test for IgM antibodies because of lower sensitivity than that of either the IgM ELISA or the IgM immunosorbent agglutination assay but may be useful in conjunction with the IgM ELISA.[2,7,23,131] Other tests that can help differentiate acute infection further include a *T. gondii*–specific IgA ELISA and IgA immunofiltration assay; a *T. gondii*–specific IgE immuno-filtration assay; and IgG, IgM, and IgA immunoblotting tests.[19,22,82,92,93,113,131]

Evaluation of a pregnant woman and fetus typically is prompted initially either by detection of seroconversion in the context of a screening program or by serologic evaluation in the context of an acute illness compatible with toxoplasmosis. If the initial IgG is negative, a follow-up test needs to be performed to exclude seroconversion. If the initial test on a pregnant woman reveals IgG antibody, an attempt needs to be made to determine if the primary infection occurred during gestation. An IgM antibody test should be ordered, but the clinician must be aware of the potential for false-positive and false-negative results.[82,125,131] The IgG avidity test can be helpful if the pregnancy is within the first 12 weeks, with a high avidity test virtually excluding infection within the past 12 weeks. If the IgM is determined to be truly positive, and the IgG avidity test does not allow the clinician to exclude acute infection during pregnancy, the clinician needs to move to more sophisticated testing through a reference laboratory (see earlier) because IgM may persist for 12 to 18 months after acute infection.

If recent maternal infection is documented, the fetus should be evaluated and therapy should be started in the mother (see treatment section). The fetus is evaluated by ultrasound, and amniotic fluid should be tested for specific *Toxoplasma* DNA by PCR. PCR has supplanted the need for cordocentesis, and a positive result confirms fetal infection.[95] Postnatally, serologic testing of paired maternal and infant sera should be performed at a reliable laboratory that includes assays for IgG, IgM, IgA, and IgE antibodies. Subinoculation of placental tissue, amniotic fluid, and umbilical cord blood into mice should be considered. If the results of these tests suggest the possible presence of infection, the newborn should be evaluated fully by a complete blood cell count and platelet determination, liver function tests, CSF evaluation (including tests for IgG and IgM antibodies and PCR),[7,72,95] ophthalmologic examination, and CT scan or ultrasound of the head.

The presence of neonatal IgM antibody in serum or CSF or a positive PCR in serum or CSF indicates congenital infection. In addition, at-risk infants should have serologic follow-up to detect increasing serum IgG titers during the first year of life or persistent IgG antibody beyond 12 to 15 months of age, which would be indicative of congenital infection.[7,72] Uninfected infants have a continuous decline in *Toxoplasma* IgG titer, with no detectable IgM or IgA antibodies.

Low IgG titers and an AC/HS differential agglutination test that indicates remote maternal infection do not require further evaluation of the mother or infant, unless the mother is infected with HIV. Because fetal infection has occurred during chronic *Toxoplasma* infection in HIV-infected pregnant women, infants of co-infected mothers should be evaluated serologically at birth for evidence of congenital infection. Whether HIV-infected pregnant women who have low CD4+ counts and who are seropositive for *Toxoplasma* antibody should receive empiric therapy to prevent fetal infection remains unclear. At present, available data are insufficient for routinely recommending such therapy.

TREATMENT

PREGNANT WOMEN

Treatment of an acutely infected woman during pregnancy with spiramycin may prevent transmission of the infection to the fetus.[14,33,127] A meta-analysis including 20 cohorts with 1721 infected mothers and 506 infected children suggested a reduction in transmission (odds ratio 0.48, 95% confidence interval 0.28 to 0.80) if therapy was started within 3 weeks of maternal seroconversion.[120] These results, considered along with the numerous women studied by individual investigators, strongly suggest that intrauterine treatment does reduce transmission of maternal infection to the fetus.[3,15,21,39,47,51] Contrary to the many individual studies, the meta-analysis failed to show that intrauterine treatment ameliorated the manifestations of congenital infection in the children who were born infected.

Spiramycin treatment of pregnant women with recently acquired primary infection should be instituted empirically while further testing is being done, in the hope of preventing spread of infection to the fetus. When fetal infection has occurred, however, maternal treatment with spiramycin does not seem to alter the evolution and severity of disease in the fetus, which is why evaluation of a potentially exposed fetus by PCR amplification of amniotic fluid permits informed decisions to be made concerning termination of pregnancy or treatment of the fetus in utero with pyrimethamine-sulfadiazine.

SEQUENTIAL FETAL AND POSTNATAL TREATMENT

Reports have described improved outcomes in patients treated in utero with continuing treatment during the first year of life compared with historical controls.[39,51] Pregnancies in which fetuses had obvious manifestations on ultrasound examination and most pregnancies with definite first-trimester infection were terminated, however.

Nonetheless, what is remarkable is that when this method of initiating aggressive treatment of fetuses in utero was applied, retinal disease was reported in only 3 of 50 such infants monitored until they reached 2 years of age. This finding contrasts with the presence of retinal or neurologic involvement in 50 percent of asymptomatic newborns detected by serologic screening in Massachusetts[49] and in 75 percent of children whose pediatricians referred them to our National Collaborative Treatment Trial for treatment in the perinatal period.[72] The outcome of pregnancies with infection acquired in the first trimester after in utero treatment also has been reported to be favorable in another study[5] in which only pregnancies in which the fetus had hydrocephalus were terminated.

TABLE 77–3   Treatment Guidelines for Congenital Toxoplasmosis

Condition	Medication	Dosage	Length of Therapy
Congenital infection	Pyrimethamine +	2 mg/kg/day for 2 days, then 1 mg/kg/day for 6 mo, then 3 times weekly (M-W-F) for 6 mo	1 year; monitor weekly complete blood counts and platelets
	Sulfadiazine +	100 mg/kg/day divided twice daily	
	Folinic acid +	5-10 mg 3 times weekly	Dose adjusted to maintain adequate complete blood count
	Prednisone	1 mg/kg/day divided twice daily	Until resolution of elevated CSF protein (<1 g/dL) or sight-threatening chorioretinitis resolves
Pregnant women—acute infection first 21 wk of gestation	Spiramycin—available on request from the Food and Drug Administration (301-827-2127)	1.5 g q12h without food	Until fetal infection documented or excluded (amniotic fluid PCR) at 21 wk gestation. If fetus infected, change to pyrimethamine + sulfadiazine + folinic acid until delivery
Pregnant women—fetal infection confirmed (amniotic fluid PCR positive)	Pyrimethamine +	100 mg/day divided twice daily for 2 days, then 50 mg/day	Until delivery
	Sulfadiazine +	100 mg/kg/day divided twice daily (maximum 3 g/day)	
	Folinic acid	5-20 mg/day	

CSF, cerebrospinal fluid; M-W-F, Monday, Wednesday, Friday; PCR, polymerase chain reaction.

CONGENITAL INFECTION

POSTNATAL TREATMENT

Data regarding the efficacy of postnatal treatment of infants with congenital *Toxoplasma* infection are becoming available.[45,46,49,72] The controlled National Collaborative Treatment Trial is in progress in Chicago.[72] This study seeks to define optimal therapeutic regimens. Physicians treating patients with congenital *Toxoplasma* infection who are younger than 2.5 months may wish to contact this multidisciplinary group regarding potential enrollment of their patients in that study (773-834-4152).

Outcomes to date from the National Collaborative Treatment Trial are substantially better for most, but not all, infants treated from the neonatal period for 12 months with pyrimethamine-sulfadiazine and leucovorin (Table 77–3) than for historical controls receiving no or short-course therapy.[72] Signs of active infection resolve within weeks of initiation of treatment. Overall, 18 of 66 (27%) children in the National Collaborative Treatment Trial have IQ results less than 70 compared to 86 of 101 (85%) in the reported literature.[32,72] No significant diminution in cognitive function occurs over the course of time, and most treated children are functioning well in regular school classrooms. No sensorineural hearing loss has been ascribable to congenital toxoplasmosis in treated children.[72,100,116] A subset of children with significant irreversible neurologic damage already present in the perinatal period have manifested profound developmental delay, motor impairment, and seizures. For the most part, these were children with hydrocephalus, high CSF protein, minimal improvement in brain CT scans after shunting, and often substantial delays in shunt placement or needed revision for shunt failure or other intercurrent medical problems.[116]

Although treatment during the first year of life arrests all signs of active disease, results in normal cognitive and motor outcome for most children and may result in resolution of seizures without recurrence for some treated children, the currently available drugs do not eradicate all cysts containing bradyzoites.[51] In most children, serologic titers of *T. gondii*–specific antibodies rebound 3 to 4 months after treatment is discontinued.[123] To date, new retinal lesions have occurred in 17 of 58 children in the National Collaborative Treatment Trial during 3 to 10 years of follow-up

after the 1-year course of treatment.[72] Infected children undergo retinal examination each month for 3 months after discontinuing treatment around their first birthday, then every 3 months until they are old enough to describe visual symptoms accurately, and then every 6 months. In addition, an ophthalmologic evaluation should be performed promptly for any acute visual signs or symptoms that may be related to recrudescence of congenital ocular toxoplasmosis.[79]

Toxoplasmosis and coexistent HIV infection in children is increasingly rare since the advent of highly active antiretroviral therapy for HIV. Most children reported with toxoplasmosis and HIV have had congenital toxoplasmosis and have been symptomatic. For such children, therapy with pyrimethamine-sulfadiazine plus folinic acid is recommended in the doses presented in Table 77–3.

Indications for corticosteroid therapy with prednisone (0.5 mg/kg twice a day) are a CSF protein concentration of 1 g/dL or greater or chorioretinitis that threatens vision. Prednisone is continued until these findings are resolved.

PREVENTION

Routine serologic screening of women during pregnancy has been an effective means of prevention in France and Austria, and it has been advocated in other areas where the incidence of congenital toxoplasmosis remains high.[15] Such strategies have been criticized regarding the cost-effectiveness and feasibility of such strategies and the lack of randomized controlled trials definitively proving benefit.[44,121] Although such studies would be helpful, they are unlikely to be performed, given the current cohort data supporting the interventions. Neonatal screening for IgM antibody also has been advocated so that asymptomatic infants can be detected and treated before neurologic symptoms develop.[45,46,49,61,69,98] This strategy does not detect approximately 25 percent of infected infants who lack anti-*Toxoplasma* IgM antibody, but it allows postnatal treatment, which seems to ameliorate symptoms. The focus of prevention should be on educating women of child-bearing age to avoid ingesting oocysts in cat feces, fruits, or vegetables and encysted bradyzoites in raw meat.[8,11,12,33]

Acknowledgments

The authors acknowledge the contribution of Pablo J. Sánchez, M.D., to this chapter in the previous edition of this text.

REFERENCES

1. Alford, C. A., Jr., Stagno, S., and Reynolds, D. W.: Congenital toxoplasmosis: Clinical, laboratory and therapeutic considerations, with special reference to subclinical disease. Bull. N. Y. Acad. Med. *50*:160, 1974.
2. Araujo, F. G., Barnett, E. V., Gentry, L. O., et al.: False positive anti-*Toxoplasma* fluorescent antibody tests in patients with antinuclear antibodies. Appl. Microbiol. *22*:270, 1971.
3. Aspock, H.: Prevention of congenital toxoplasmosis by serological surveillance during pregnancy: Current strategies and future perspectives. *In* Marget, W., Lang, W., and Gabler-Sandberger, E. (eds.): Parasitic Infections, Immunology, Mycotic Infections, General Topics. Vol. 3. Munich, Medizin Verlag, 1986, pp. 69-72.
4. Beach, P. G.: Prevalence of antibodies to *Toxoplasma gondii* in pregnant women in Oregon. J. Infect. Dis. *140*:780, 1979.
5. Berrebi, A., Kobuch, W. E., Bessieres, M. H., et al.: Termination of pregnancy for maternal toxoplasmosis. Lancet *344*:36-38, 1994.
6. Bowie, W. R., King, A. S., Werker, D. H., et al.: Outbreak of toxoplasmosis associated with municipal drinking water. Lancet *350*:173-177, 1997.
7. Boyer, K. M.: Diagnostic testing for congenital toxoplasmosis. Pediatr. Infect. Dis. J. *20*:59-60, 2001.
8. Boyer, K.M., Holfels, E., Roizen, N., et al.: Risk factors for *Toxoplasma gondii* infection in mothers of infants with congenital toxoplasmosis: Implications for prenatal management and screening. Am. J. Obstet. Gynecol. *192*:564-571, 2005.
9. Brezin, A. P., Kasner, L., Thulliez, P., et al.: Ocular toxoplasmosis in the fetus: Immunohistochemistry analysis and DNA amplification. Retina *14*:19-26, 1994.
10. Candolfi, E., Pastor, R., Huber, R., et al.: IgG avidity assay firms up the diagnosis of acute toxoplasmosis on the first serum sample in immunocompetent pregnant women. Diag. Microbiol. Infect. Dis. *58*:83-88, 2007.
11. Carter, A. O., Gelmon, S. B., Wells, G. A., et al.: The effectiveness of a prenatal education programme for the prevention of congenital toxoplasmosis. Epidemiol. Infect. *103*:539-545, 1989.
12. Centers for Disease Control and Prevention: Preventing congenital toxoplasmosis. M. M. W. R. Morb. Mortal. Wkly. Rep. *49*(RR-2):57-75, 2000.
12a. Conley, F. K., Jenkins, H. T., and Remington, J. S.: *Toxoplasma gondii* infection of the central nervous system. Hum. Pathol. *12*:690, 1981.
13. Couvreur, J., and Desmonts, G.: Congenital and maternal toxoplasmosis: A review of 300 congenital cases. Dev. Med. Child. Neurol. *4*:519-530, 1962.
14. Couvreur, J., Desmonts, G., and Thulliez, P.: Prophylaxis of congenital toxoplasmosis: Effect of spiramycin on placental infection. J. Antimicrob. Chemother. *22*:193-200, 1988.
15. Daffos, F., Forestier, F., Capella-Pavlovsky, M., et al.: Prenatal management of 746 pregnancies at risk for congenital toxoplasmosis. N. Engl. J. Med. *318*:271-275, 1988.
16. Dannemann, B. R., Vaughan, W. C., Thulliez, P., et al.: The differential agglutination test for diagnosis of recently acquired infection with *Toxoplasma gondii*. J. Clin. Microbiol. *28*:1928-1933, 1990.
17. Darde, M. L.: Genetic analysis of the diversity in *Toxoplasma gondii*. Ann. Ist. Super Sanita. *40*:57-63, 2004.
18. Darling, S. T.: Sarcosporidiosis: With report of a case in man. Proc. Canal Zone Med. Assoc. *1*:141, 1908.
19. Decoster, A., Darcy, F., Caron, A., et al.: IgA antibodies against P30 as markers of congenital and acute toxoplasmosis. Lancet *2*:1104, 1988.
20. Desmonts, G., and Couvreur, J.: Congenital toxoplasmosis: A prospective study of 378 pregnancies. N. Engl. J. Med. *290*:1110, 1974.
21. Desmonts, G., and Couvreur, J.: Congenital toxoplasmosis: A prospective study of the offspring of 54 women who acquired toxoplasmosis during pregnancy: Pathophysiology of congenital disease. *In* Thalhammer, O., Baumgarten, K., and Pollak, A. (eds.): Perinatal Medicine. Sixth European Congress, Vienna, 1978. Stuttgart, Georg Thieme, 1979, 51-60.
22. Desmonts, G., Daffos, F., Forestier, F., et al.: Prenatal diagnosis of congenital toxoplasmosis. Lancet *1*:500, 1985.
23. Desmonts, G., Naot, Y., and Remington, J. S.: Immunoglobulin M immunosorbent agglutination assay for diagnosis of infectious disease: Diagnosis of acute congenital and acquired *Toxoplasma* infections. J. Clin. Microbiol. *14*:486, 1981.
24. Desmonts, G., and Remington, J. S.: Direct agglutination test for diagnosis of *Toxoplasma* infection: Method for increasing sensitivity and specificity. J. Clin. Microbiol. *11*:562, 1980.
25. Diebler, C., Dussler, A., and Dulac, O.: Congenital toxoplasmosis: Clinical and neuroradiological evaluation of the cerebral lesions. Neuroradiology *27*:125-130, 1985.
26. Dubey, J. P.: Toxoplasmosis—a waterborne zoonosis. Vet. Parasitol. *126*:57-72, 2004.
27. Dubey, J. P., Hill, D. E., Jones, J. L., et al.: Prevalence of viable *Toxoplasma gondii* in beef, chicken, and pork from retail meat stores in the United States: Risk assessment to consumers. J. Parasitol. *91*:1082-1093, 2005.
28. Dubey, J. P., Miller, N. L., and Frenkel, J. K.: The *Toxoplasma gondii* oocyst from cat feces. J. Exp. Med. *132*:636-662, 1970.
29. Dubremetz, J. F.: Rhopteries are major players in *Toxoplasma gondii* invasion and host cell interaction. Cell. Microbiol. *9*:841-848, 2007.
30. Dunn, D., Newell, M. L., and Gilbert, R.: Low risk of congenital toxoplasmosis in children born to women infected with human immunodeficiency virus. Pediatr. Infect. Dis. J. *16*:84, 1997.
31. Dunn, D., Wallon, M., Peyron, F., et al.: Mother-to-child transmission of toxoplasmosis: Risk estimates for clinical counseling. Lancet *353*:1829, 1999.
32. Eichenwald, H. G.: A study of congenital toxoplasmosis. *In* Siim, J. C. (ed.): Human Toxoplasmosis. Copenhagen, Munksgaard, 1960, pp. 41-49.
33. Foulon, W., Naessens, A., and Ho-Yen, D.: Prevention of congenital toxoplasmosis. J. Perinat. Med. *28*:337-345, 2000.
34. Frenkel, J. K.: Toxoplasmosis. *In* Marcial-Rojas, R. A. (ed.): Pathology of Protozoal and Helminthic Diseases. Baltimore, Williams & Wilkins, 1971, pp. 254-290.
35. Frenkel, J. K.: Toxoplasmosis: A parasite life cycle, pathology, and immunology. *In* Hammond, D. M. (ed.): The Coccidian. Baltimore, University Park Press, 1973, pp. 343-410.
36. Frenkel, J. K.: Pathology and pathogenesis of congenital toxoplasmosis. Bull. N. Y. Acad. Med. *50*:182-191, 1974.
37. Frenkel, J., Dubey, J. P., and Miller, N. L.: *Toxoplasma gondii* in cats: Fecal stage identified as coccidian oocysts. Science *167*:893-896, 1970.
38. Frenkel, J. K., Weber, R. W., and Lunde, M. N.: Acute toxoplasmosis: Effective treatment with pyrimethamine, sulfadiazine, leucovorin calcium and yeast. J. A. M. A. *173*:1471-1476, 1960.
39. Galanakis, E., Manoura, A., Antoniou, M., et al.: Outcome of toxoplasmosis acquired during pregnancy following treatment in both pregnancy and early infancy. Fetal Diag. Ther. *22*:444-448, 2007.
40. Garcia, A. G. P.: Congenital toxoplasmosis in two successive sibs. Arch. Dis. Child. *43*:705-709, 1979.
41. Gazzinelli, R. T., Hayashi, S., Wysocka, M., et al.: Role of IL-12 in the initiation of cell-mediated immunity by *Toxoplasma gondii* and its regulation by IL-10 and nitric oxide. J. Eukaryot. Microbiol. *41*(Suppl.):9, 1994.
42. Gazzinelli, R. T., Oswald, I. P., James, S. L., et al.: IL-10 inhibits parasite killing and nitrogen oxide production by IFN-γ-activated macrophages: IL-10 prevents IFN-γ from inducing activity against *T. gondii* and increasing production of RNIs by murine macrophages. J. Immunol. *148*:1792-1796, 1992.
43. Gilbert, R., and Dezateux, C.: Newborn screening for congenital toxoplasmosis: Feasible, but benefits are not established. Arch. Dis. Child. *91*:629-631, 2006.
44. Gilbert, R., Tan, H. K., Cliffe, S., et al.: Symptomatic toxoplasma infection due to congenital and postnatally acquired infection. Arch. Dis. Child. *91*:495-498, 2006.
45. Gomez-Martin, J. E., Gonzalez, M. M., Montoya, M. T., et al.: A newborn screening programme for congenital toxoplamsosis in the setting of a country with less income. Arch. Dis. Child. *92*:88, 2007.
46. Gomez-Martin, J. E., and delaTorre, A.: Positive benefit of postnatal treatment in congenital toxoplasmosis. Arch. Dis. Child. *92*:88-89, 2007.
47. Gras, L., Wallon, M., Pollak, A., et al.: Association between prenatal treatment and clinical manifestations of congenital toxoplasmosis in infancy: A cohort study in 13 European centers. Acta Paediatr. *94*:1721-1731, 2005.
48. Grover, C. M., Thulliez, P., Remington, J. S., et al.: Rapid prenatal diagnosis of congenital *Toxoplasma* infection using polymerase chain reaction and amniotic fluid. J. Clin. Microbiol. *28*:2297, 1990.
49. Guerina, N. G., Hsu, H.-W., Meissner, H. C., et al.: Neonatal serologic screening and early treatment for congenital *Toxoplasma gondii* infection. N. Engl. J. Med. *33*:1858-1863, 1994.
50. Hohlfeld, P., Daffos, F., Costa, J. M., et al.: Prenatal diagnosis of congenital toxoplasmosis with a polymerase-chain reaction test on amniotic fluid. N. Engl. J. Med. *331*:695-699, 1994.
51. Hohlfeld, P., Daffos, F., Thulliez, P., et al.: Fetal toxoplasmosis: Outcome of pregnancy and infant follow-up after in utero treatment. J. Pediatr. *115*:765-769, 1989.
52. Holfels, E., McAuley, J., Mack, D., et al.: In vitro effects of artemisinin ether, cycloguanil hydrochloride (alone and in combination with sulfadiazine), quinine sulfate, mefloquine, primaquine phosphate, trifluoperazine hydrochloride, and verapamil on *Toxoplasma gondii*. Antimicrob. Agents Chemother. *38*:1392-1396, 1994.
53. Huskinson-Mark, J., Araujo, F. G., and Remington, J. S.: Evaluation of the effect of drugs on the cyst form of *Toxoplasma gondii*. J. Infect. Dis. *164*:170-177, 1991.
54. Hutchison, W. M., Dunachie, J. F., Siim, J. C., et al.: Coccidian-like nature of *Toxoplasma gondii*. B. M. J. *1*:142, 1970.
55. Jara, M., Hsu, H. W., Eaton, R. B., and Demaria, A., Jr.: Epidemiology of congenital toxoplasmosis identified by population-based newborn screening in Massachusetts. Pediatr. Infect. Dis. J. *20*:1132, 2001.
56. Johnson, A., McLeod, R., Cesbron-Delauw, M. F., et al.: Vaccine Development and Technology to Prevent Toxoplasmosis. Fontevraud, France, WHO Working Group, 1992, p. 1.

57. Jones, J. L., Kruszon-Moran, D., Sanders-Lewis, K., and Wilson, M.: *Toxoplasma gondii* infection in the United States, 1999-2004, decline from prior decade. Am. J. Trop. Med. Hyg. 77:405-410, 2007.

58. Jones, J. L., Kruszon-Moran, D., Wilson, M., et al.: *Toxoplasma gondii* infection in the United States: Seroprevalence and risk factors. Am. J. Epidemiol. 154:357-365, 2001.

59. Khan, A., Jordan, C., Muccioli, C., et al.: Genetic divergence of *Toxoplasma gondii* strains associated with ocular toxoplasmosis, Brazil. Emerg. Infect. Dis. 12:942-949, 2006.

60. Khan, I. A., Ely, K. H., and Kasper, L. H.: A purified parasite antigen (p30) mediates CD8+ T cell immunity against fatal *Toxoplasma gondii* infection in mice. J. Immunol. 147:3501-3506, 1991.

61. Kim, K.: Time to screen for congenital toxoplasmosis? Clin. Infect. Dis. 42:1395-1397, 2006.

62. Koppe, J. G., Kloosterman, G. J., de Roever-Bonnet, H., et al.: Toxoplasmosis and pregnancy, with a long-term follow-up of the children. Eur. J. Obstet. Gynaecol. Reprod. Biol. 413:101-110, 1974.

63. Koppe, J. G., Loewer-Sieger, D. H., and de Roever-Bonnet, H.: Results of 20-year follow-up of congenital toxoplasmosis. Lancet 1:254-256, 1986.

64. Lago, E. G., Baldisserotto, M., Hoefel Filho, J. R., et al.: Agreement between ultrasonography and computed tomography in detecting intracranial calcifications in congenital toxoplasmosis. Clin. Radiol. 62:1004-1011, 2007.

65. Luft, B. J., and Remington, J. S.: Acute *Toxoplasma* infection among family members of patients with acute lymphadenopathic toxoplasmosis. Arch. Intern. Med. 144:53, 1984.

66. Mack, D. G., Johnson, J. J., Roberts, F., et al.: Murine and human MHC class II genes determine susceptibility to toxoplasmosis. Int. J. Parasitol. 29:1351-1358, 1999.

67. Masur, H., Jones, T. C., Lempert, J. A., et al.: Outbreak of toxoplasmosis in a family and documentation of acquired retinochoroiditis. Am. J. Med. 64:396, 1978.

68. McCabe, R., Gibbons, D., Brooks, R. G., et al.: Agglutination test for diagnosis of toxoplasmosis in AIDS. Lancet 2:680, 1983.

69. McCabe, R. E., and Remington, J. S.: Toxoplasmosis: The time has come. N. Engl. J. Med. 318:313-315, 1988.

70. McGee, T., Wolters, C., Stein, L., et al.: Absence of sensorineural hearing abnormalities in treated infants with congenital toxoplasmosis. Otolaryngol. Head Neck Surg. 106:75-80, 1992.

71. McLeod, R., Beem, M. O., and Estes, R. G.: Lymphocyte anergy specific to *Toxoplasma gondii* antigens in a baby with congenital toxoplasmosis. J. Clin. Lab. Immunol. 17:149, 1985.

72. McLeod, R., Boyer, K. M., Karrison, T., et al.: Outcome of treatment for congenital toxoplasmosis, 1981-2004: The national collaborative Chicago-based, congenital toxoplasmosis study. Clin. Infect. Dis. 42:1383-1394, 2006.

73. McLeod, R., Boyer, K. M., Roizen, N., et al.: The child with congenital toxoplasmosis. Curr. Clin. Top. Infect. Dis. 20:189-208, 2000.

74. McLeod, R., Brown, C., and Mack, D.: Immunogenetics influence outcome of *Toxoplasma gondii* infection. J. Immunol. 142:3247-3255, 1989.

75. McLeod, R., Frenkel, J. K., Estes, R. G., et al.: Subcutaneous and intestinal vaccination with tachyzoites of *Toxoplasma gondii* and acquisition of immunity to peroral and congenital *Toxoplasma* challenge. J. Immunol. 140:1632-1637, 1988.

76. McLeod, R., and Mack, D.: A new micromethod to study the effects of antimicrobial agents of *Toxoplasma gondii*: Comparison of sulfadoxine and sulfadiazine individually and in combination with pyrimethamine and study of clindamycin, metronidazole, and cyclosporin A. Antimicrob. Agents Chemother. 26:26-30, 1984.

77. McLeod, R., Mack, D. G., Boyer, K. M., et al.: Phenotypes and functions of lymphocytes in congenital toxoplasmosis. J. Lab. Clin. Med. 116:623-635, 1990.

78. McLeod, R., Mack, D., Foss, R., et al.: Levels of pyrimethamine in sera and cerebrospinal and ventricular fluids from infants treated for congenital toxoplasmosis. Antimicrob. Agents Chemother. 36:1040-1048, 1992.

79. Mets, M. B., Holfels, E. M., Boyer, K. M., et al.: Eye manifestations of congenital toxoplasmosis. Am. J. Ophthalmol. 122:309-324, 1996.

80. Mitchell, C. D., Erlich, S. S., Mastrucci, M. T., et al.: Congenital toxoplasmosis occurring in three infants perinatally infected with the human immunodeficiency virus (HIV-1). Pediatr. Infect. Dis. J. 9:512, 1990.

81. Mitchell, W.: Neurological and developmental effects of HIV and AIDS in children and adolescents. Ment. Retard. Dev. Disabil. Res. Rev. 7:211-216, 2001.

82. Montoya, J. G.: Laboratory diagnosis of *Toxoplasma gondii* infection and toxoplasmosis. J. Infect. Dis. 185(Suppl.):73-82, 2002.

83. Montoya, J. G., and Liesenfeld, O.: Toxoplasmosis. Lancet 363:1965-1976, 2004.

84. Naot, Y., Barnett, E. V., and Remington, J. S.: Method for avoiding false positive results occurring in immunoglobulin M enzyme-linked immunosorbent assays due to presence of both rheumatoid factor and antinuclear antibodies. J. Clin. Microbiol. 14:73, 1981.

85. Naot, Y., Desmonts, G., and Remington, J. S.: IgM enzyme-linked immunosorbent assay test for the diagnosis of congenital *Toxoplasma* infection. J. Pediatr. 98:32, 1981.

86. Naot, Y., and Remington, J. S.: An enzyme-linked immunosorbent assay for detection of IgM antibodies to *Toxoplasma gondii*: Use for diagnosis of acute acquired toxoplasmosis. J. Infect. Dis. 142:757, 1981.

87. O'Donohoe, J. M., Brueton, M. J., and Holliman, R. E.: Concurrent congenital human immunodeficiency virus infection and toxoplasmosis. Pediatr. Infect. Dis. J. 10:627, 1991.

88. Patel, D. V., Hofels, E., Vogel, N., et al.: Resolution of intracerebral calcifications in children with treated congenital toxoplasmosis. Radiology 199:433-440, 1996.

89. Peyron, F., and Wallon, M.: Options for the pharmacotherapy of toxoplasmosis during pregnancy. Exp. Opin. Pharmacother. 2:1269, 2001.

90. Pfefferkorn, E. R., Nothnagel, R. F., and Borotz, S. E.: Parasiticidal effect of clindamycin on *Toxoplasma gondii* grown in cultured cells and selection of a drug-resistant mutant. Antimicrob. Agents Chemother. 36:1091-1096, 1992.

91. Pinkerton, H., and Weinman, D.: *Toxoplasma* infection in man. Arch. Pathol. 30:374, 1940.

92. Pinon, J. M., Chemla, C., Villena, I., et al.: Early neonatal diagnosis of congenital toxoplasmosis: Value of comparative enzyme linked immunofiltration assay immunological profiles and anti-*Toxoplasma gondii* immunoglobulin M (IgM) or IgA immunocapture and implications for postnatal therapeutic strategies. J. Clin. Microbiol. 34:579-583, 1996.

93. Pinon, J. M., Dumon, H., Chemla, C., et al.: Strategy for diagnosis of congenital toxoplasmosis: Evaluation of methods comparing mothers and newborns and standard methods for postnatal detection of immunoglobulin G, M, and A antibodies. J. Clin. Microbiol. 39:2267, 2001.

94. Remington, J., Eimstad, W., and Araujo, F.: Detection of immunoglobulin M antibodies with antigen-tagged latex particles in an immunosorbent assay. J. Clin. Microbiol. 17:939, 1983.

95. Remington, J. S., McLeod, R., Thulliez, P., et al.: Toxoplasmosis. *In* Remington, J. S., Klein, J. O., Wilson, C. B., et al. (eds.): Infectious Diseases of the Fetus and Newborn. 6th ed. Philadelphia, W. B. Saunders, 2006, pp. 947-1092.

96. Roberts, F., Mets, M. B., Ferguson, D. J. P., et al.: Histopathological features of ocular toxoplasmosis in the fetus and infant. Arch. Ophthalmol. 19:51-58, 2001.

97. Roberts, F., Roberts, C. W., Johnson, J. J., et al.: Evidence for the shikamate pathway in apicomplexan parasites. Nature 393:801-805, 1998.

98. Roberts, T., and Frenkel, J. K.: Estimating income losses and other preventable costs caused by congenital toxoplasmosis in people in the United States. J. A. M. A. 2:249-257, 1990.

99. Roizen, N., McLeod, R., Boyer, K. M., et al. Impact of visual impairment on measures of cognitive function for children with congenital toxoplasmosis: Implications for compensatory intervention strategies. Pediatrics 118:379-90, 2006.

100. Roizen, N., Swisher, C., Stein, M. A., et al.: Neurologic and developmental function in treated congenital toxoplasmosis. Pediatrics 95:11-20, 1995.

101. Romand, D. S., Chosson, M., Franck, J., et al.: Usefulness of quantitative polymerase chain reaction in amniotic fluid as early prognostic marker of fetal infection with *Toxoplasma gondii*. Am. J. Gynecol. 90:797-802, 2004.

102. Romand, D. S., Wallon, M., Franck, J., et al.: Prenatal diagnosis using polymerase chain reaction on amniotic fluid for congenital toxoplasmosis. Obstet. Gynecol. 97:296-300, 2001.

103. Sabin, A. B.: Toxoplasmic encephalitis in children. J. A. M. A. 116:801-807, 1941.

104. Sabin, A. B., and Feldman, H. A.: Dyes as microchemical indicators of a new immunity phenomenon affecting a protozoon parasite (*Toxoplasma*). Science 108:660, 1948.

105. Sacks, J. J., Roberto, R. R., and Brooks, N. F.: Toxoplasmosis infection associated with raw goat's milk. J. A. M. A. 248:1728, 1982.

106. Schoondermark-Van de Ven, E., Galama, J., Camps, W., et al.: Pharmacokinetic of spiramycin in the rhesus monkey: Transplacental passage and distribution in tissue in the fetus. Antimicrob. Agents Chemother. 38:1922-1929, 1994.

107. Schoondermark-Van de Ven, E., Melchers, W., Camps, W., et al.: Effectiveness of spiramycin for treatment of congenital *Toxoplasma gondii* infection in rhesus monkeys. Antimicrob. Agents Chemother. 38:1930-1936, 1994.

108. Shenep, J. L., Barenkamp, S. J., Brammeier, S. A., et al.: An outbreak of toxoplasmosis on an Illinois farm. Pediatr. Infect. Dis. 3:518, 1984.

109. Sher, A., Oswald, I. P., Hieny, S., et al.: *Toxoplasma gondii* induces a T-independent IFN-γ response in natural killer cells that requires both adherent accessory cells and tumor necrosis factor-α. J. Immunol. 150:3982-3989, 1993.

110. Sibley, L. D., Pfefferkorn, E. R., and Boothroyd, J. C.: Development of genetic systems for *Toxoplasma gondii*. Parasitol. Today 9:392-395, 1993.

111. Smith, K. L., Wilson, M., Hightower, A. L., et al.: Prevalence of *Toxoplasma gondii* antibodies in U.S. military recruits in 1989: Comparison with data published in 1965. Clin. Infect. Dis. 23:1182-1183, 1996.

112. Soheilian, M., Sadoughi, M. M., Ghajarnia, M., et al.: Prospective randomized trial of trimethoprim/sulfamethoxazole versus pyrimethamine and sulfadiazine in the treatment of ocular toxoplasmosis. Ophthalmology 112:1876-1882, 2005.

113. Stepick-Biek, P., Thulliez, P., Araujo, F. G., et al.: IgA antibodies for diagnosis of acute congenital and acquired toxoplasmosis. J. Infect. Dis. 162:270, 1990.

114. Stray-Pedersen, B.: Infants potentially at risk for congenital toxoplasmosis: A prospective study. Am. J. Dis. Child. 134:638, 1980.

115. Suzuki, Y., Orellana, M. A., Schreiber, R. D., et al.: Interferon-γ: The major mediator of resistance against *Toxoplasma gondii*. Science 240:516, 1988.

116. Swisher, C. N., Boyer, K., and McLeod, R.: Congenital toxoplasmosis. The Toxoplasmosis Study Group. Semin. Pediatr. Neurol. 1:4-25, 1994.

117. Tabbara, K., and O'Connor, R.: Treatment of ocular toxoplasmosis with clindamycin and sulfadiazine. Ophthalmology 87:129, 1980.
118. Tan, H. K., Schmidt, D., Stanford, M., et al.: Risk of visual impairment in children with congenital toxoplasmic retinochoroiditis. Am. J. Ophthalmol. 144:648-653, 2007.
119. Teutsch, S. M., Juranek, D. D., Sulzer, A., et al.: Epidemic toxoplasmosis associated with infected cats. N. Engl. J. Med. 300:695, 1979.
120. The SYROCOT Study Group, Theibaut, R., Leproust, S., Chene, G., and Gilbert, R. E.: Effectiveness of prenatal treatment for congenital toxoplasmosis: A meta-analysis of individual patients' data. Lancet 369:115-122, 2007.
121. Thiebaut, R., Leroy, V., Alioum, A., et al.: Biases in observational studies of the effect of prenatal treatment for congenital toxoplasmosis. Eur. J. Obstet. Gynaecol. Reprod. Biol. 124:3-9, 2005.
122. Vogel, N., Kirisits, M., Michael, E., et al.: Congenital toxoplasmosis transmitted from an immunologically competent mother infected before conception. Clin. Infect. Dis. 23:1055-1060, 1996.
123. Wallon, M., Cogan, G., Ecochard, R., et al.: Serological rebound in congenital toxoplasmosis: Long-term follow-up of 133 children. Eur. J. Pediatr. 160:534-540, 2001.
124. Wallon, M., Kodjikian, L., Binquet, C., et al.: Long-term ocular prognosis in 327 children with congenital toxoplasmosis. Pediatrics 113:1567-1572, 2004.
125. Walls, K. W., and Remington, J. S.: Evaluation of a commercial latex agglutination method for toxoplasmosis. Diagn. Microbiol. Infect. Dis. 1:265, 1983.
126. Weiss, L., and Kim, K. (eds.): Toxoplasma gondii, the Model Apicomplexan Parasite: Perspectives and Methodology. London, Elsevier Academic Press, 2007.

127. Wilson, C. B.: Treatment of congenital toxoplasmosis during pregnancy. J. Pediatr. 116:1003-1004, 1990.
128. Wilson, C. B., Desmonts, G., Couvreur, J., et al.: Lymphocyte transformation in the diagnosis of congenital Toxoplasma infection. N. Engl. J. Med. 302:785, 1980.
129. Wilson, C. B., and Remington, J. S.: What can be done to prevent congenital toxoplasmosis? Am. J. Obstet. Gynecol. 138:357, 1980.
130. Wilson, C. B., Remington, J. S., Stagno, S., et al.: Development of adverse sequelae in children born with subclinical congenital Toxoplasma infection. Pediatrics 66:767, 1980.
131. Wilson, M., Jones, J. L., McAuley, J. B.: Toxoplasma. In Murray, P. R., Baron, E. J., Jorgenson, J. H., et al. (eds.): Manual of Clinical Microbiology. 8th ed. Washington, D.C., ASM Press. 2006, pp. 1970-1980.
132. Wolf, A., and Cowen, D.: Granulomatous encephalomyelitis due to an Encephalitozoon (encephalitozoic encephalomyelitis): A new protozoan disease of man. Bull. Neurol. Inst. N. Y. 6:307, 1937.
133. Wong, S. Y., Hajdu, M. P., Ramirez, R., et al.: The role of specific immunoglobulin E in the diagnosis of acute Toxoplasma infection and toxoplasmosis. J. Clin. Microbiol. 31:2952-2959, 1993.
134. Wong, S. Y., and Remington, J. S.: Toxoplasmosis in pregnancy. Clin. Infect. Dis. 18:853-862, 1994.
135. Zufferey, J., Hohlfeld, P., Bille, J., et al.: Value of the comparative enzyme-linked immunofiltration assay for early neonatal diagnosis of congenital Toxoplasma infection. Pediatr. Infect. Dis. J. 18:971, 1999.

CHAPTER 78

PERINATAL BACTERIAL DISEASES

Dora Estripeaut ✿ Xavier Sáez-Llorens

In this chapter, we update relevant information on neonatal bacterial infections, with emphasis on epidemiology, pathogenesis, diagnosis, treatment, and prevention strategies. Aspects of the clinical manifestations, laboratory features, and management that are peculiar to the newborn infant are stressed. More complete descriptions of the bacterial pathogens, host-parasite relationships, and spectrum of diseases in older infants and children are presented elsewhere in the text.

ANTIBIOTIC DOSAGE SCHEDULES FOR NEONATES

Much has been written about the irrational use of antimicrobial agents in newborn infants. The "therapeutic misadventures" (i.e., the gray baby syndrome of chloramphenicol, kernicterus associated with sulfisoxazole, enamel hypoplasia after tetracycline therapy, and deafness from streptomycin and kanamycin) of past decades primarily resulted from lack of knowledge about pharmacologic concepts in neonates. Dosage recommendations for babies were calculated from simplified formulas that pared down the usual dosage for adults or from armchair reasoning based on information obtained from healthy men and women. In either case, the amount of antibiotic administered to neonates often was as subtherapeutic as it was toxic.

Physicians have come to realize that many of the physiologic and metabolic processes of the newborn constantly change during the first few days of life and that these alterations profoundly affect the pharmacokinetics of antibiotics. Since 1979, systematic investigations of these drugs have produced a clearer understanding of the factors influencing absorption, distribution, metabolism, and excretion of antimicrobials in newborn infants. As a result, the dosage and intervals of administration for the drugs most commonly used have been defined (Table 78–1).[312,420] These dosage schedules are offered as a guide to the safe and effective use of antibiotics in newborn infants. The suggested regimens must be modified in premature babies weighing less than 1200 g

at birth, in patients with reduced renal or hepatic function, and in infants with altered metabolic or physiologic states (e.g., congestive heart failure, shock, hypothyroidism, during exchange transfusions and extracorporeal membrane oxygenation), in whom the volume of drug distribution in the body may be affected profoundly. Under such circumstances, the most effective means of prescribing antibiotics is to monitor serum concentrations and adjust the dosage accordingly.

EPIDEMIOLOGY AND PATHOGENESIS

Throughout pregnancy and until the membranes rupture, the infant's environment usually is sterile. Not until delivery and the immediate neonatal period is the infant exposed to many microorganisms. The human birth canal is host to large numbers of aerobic and anaerobic bacteria, *Mycoplasma*, *Ureaplasma*, *Chlamydia*, fungi, yeast, and viruses. *Staphylococcus epidermidis*, lactobacilli, diphtheroids, and alpha-hemolytic streptococci are found in 50 to 100 percent of vaginal cultures of pregnant women and constitute the predominant aerobic flora.[40,276,485] Significant but less common isolates include *Gardnerella vaginalis*, *Proteus* and *Klebsiella* spp., and group B and D streptococci; miscellaneous organisms, such as *Citrobacter*, *Acinetobacter*, and the *Campylobacter* group, are identified even less commonly.

Certain microorganisms are associated with the occurrence of stillbirths. Among these bacterial agents are *Escherichia coli*, group B streptococci, *Ureaplasma urealyticum*, *Listeria monocytogenes*, and *Treponema pallidum*. In countries with a high prevalence of syphilis, as many as half of all stillbirths are caused by this bacterium.[186,187] In the United States, stillbirths occur in nearly 7 per 1000 of all births, and 10 to 25 percent of them appear to be caused by a maternal/fetal infection. In developing countries, the relative contribution of infection may be even greater.[186]

Obligate anaerobes are present in most vaginal cultures of normal, healthy women.[189] Commonly, multiple anaerobic and aerobic species are present in the same host. Approximately 85

TABLE 78-1   Antibiotic Dosage Schedules in Neonates

Antibiotics	Route	Individual Dose (mg/kg) and Frequency of Administration									
		Weight <1200 g		Weight 1200-2000 g				Weight >2000 g			
		Ages: 0-4 Weeks		0-7 Days		>7 Days		0-7 Days		>7 Days	
Amikacin	IV, IM	7.5	q12h	7.5	q12h	7.5	q8h	10	q12h	10	q8h
Ampicillin*	IV, IM	25	q12h	25	q12h	25	q8h	25	q8h	25	q6h
Cefazolin	IV, IM	20	q12h	20	q12h	20	q12h	20	q12h	20	q8h
Cefotaxime	IV, IM	50	q12h	50	q12h	50	q8h	50	q12h	50	q8h
Ceftazidime	IV, IM	50	q12h	50	q12h	50	q8h	50	q12h	50	q8h
Ceftriaxone‡	IV, IM	50	q24h	50	q24h	50	q24h	50	q24h	75	q24h
Cephalothin	IV	20	q12h	20	q12h	20	q8h	20	q8h	20	q6h
Ciprofloxacin†	IV	—	—	—	—	10-20	q24h	—	—	20-30	q12h
Clindamycin	IV, IM, PO	5	q12h	5	q12h	5	q8h	5	q8h	5	q6h
Erythromycin	PO	10	q12h	10	q12h	10	q8h	10	q12h	10	q8h
Gentamicin	IV, IM	2.5	q18h	2.5	q12h	2.5	q8h	2.5	q12h	2.5	q8h
Imipenem	IV, IM	—	—	20	q12h	20	q12h	20	q12h	20	q8h
Meropenem	IV, IM	—	—	20	q12h	20	q12h	20	q12h	20	q8h
Metronidazole	IV, PO	7.5	q48h	7.5	q24h	7.5	q12h	7.5	q12h	15	q12h
Mezlocillin	IV, IM	75	q12h	75	q12h	75	q8h	75	q12h	75	q8h
Nafcillin*	IV	25	q12h	25	q12h	25	q8h	25	q8h	37.5	q6h
Netilmicin	IV, IM	2.5	q18h	2.5	q12h	2.5	q8h	2.5	q12h	2.5	q8h
Oxacillin*	IV, IM	25	q12h	25	q12h	25	q8h	25	q8h	37.5	q6h
Penicillin G (U/kg)*	IV	25,000	q12h	25,000	q12h	25,000	q8h	25,000	q8h	25,000	q6h
Piperacillin	IV, IM	75	q12h	75	q12h	75	q8h	75	q8h	75	q6h
Piperacillin/tazobactam	IV	50	q12h	50	q12h	100	q8h	100	q12h	100	q8h
Ticarcillin	IV, IM	75	q12h	75	q12h	75	q8h	75	q8h	75	q6h
Tobramycin	IV, IM	2.5	q18h	2	q12h	2	q8h	2	q12h	2	q8h
Vancomycin	IV	15	q24h	10	q12h	10	q12h	10	q8h	10	q8h

For meningitis, double the recommended dosage.
†*Doses based on anecdotal clinical experience. Not recommended routinely for neonates.*
‡*Not recommended for premature and/or hyperbilirubinemic neonates.*

percent of women with genital colonization by anaerobes harbor *Bacteroides* spp., including *Bacteroides fragilis* in a third of cases. Anaerobic streptococci, *Peptostreptococcus* and *Peptococcus*, are found in approximately 40 percent of women, and *Clostridium* is present in 20 percent. Uncommon anaerobic isolates include *Veillonella*, *Bifidobacterium*, and *Eubacterium*. Vaginal cultures of pregnant women also yield mixed aerobic and anaerobic species, but the number of anaerobes decreases from early pregnancy to delivery.[276]

During the process of delivery, encounters with some of these bacteria initiate colonization of the infant's respiratory and gastrointestinal tracts. In most infants, the microbial flora is established without incident; however, disease caused by one of these organisms develops occasionally in an infant. Factors influencing conversion from colonization to disease are not understood well. Some women have asymptomatic bacterial vaginosis that has been associated with preterm labor and significant vaginal isolation of anaerobic flora.[193]

Worldwide, 1.6 million neonates die every year of infection. In the United States, the infant mortality rate is approximately 6.85 infant deaths per 1000 live births. Neonatal bacterial sepsis corresponds to the eighth leading cause of fatality.[31,233] The incidence of neonatal sepsis ranges from one to eight cases per 1000 live births, with the higher figures corresponding to developing countries. Low birth weight, male sex, and congenital malformation are important risk factors.[61] Extreme prematurity is the greatest risk factor for early-onset sepsis and is associated with an increased risk of having adverse outcomes, including respiratory distress syndrome, bronchopulmonary dysplasia, severe intraventricular hemorrhage, and periventricular leukomalacia.[477] Between 1962 and 1987, the overall incidence of neonatal sepsis in Panorama City, California, was 2.2 cases per 1000 live births; it was 18.6 for infants with birth weights less than 2500 g versus 1.2 for those with birth weights of 2500 g or greater.[263] In the

same study, the incidence of meningitis was 0.3 case per 1000 live births and 2.8 and 0.07 for those with birth weights less than and greater than 2500 g, respectively. The highest age-specific incidence of bacterial meningitis occurs during the first month of life.[262]

Socioeconomic factors appear to be important in determining whether infants are at risk for infection. Premature infants and infants with low birth weight are born more frequently to mothers of low socioeconomic class than to those of average or high socioeconomic class.

Although no noticeable sex predilection has been observed for infants with intrauterine infections, a male preponderance is reported in almost all studies. The greater susceptibility of male infants is more evident in cases of sepsis caused by gram-negative enteric bacilli. The reasons behind this male preponderance are unknown but may be related to sex-linked factors in host susceptibility.

The bacterial cause of neonatal sepsis and meningitis varies from one geographic area to another. Although bacterial causes of neonatal sepsis in Western European countries are similar to those in the United States, a different pattern has been identified in Latin America, Asia, and Africa.[36,115] In the latter sites, gram-negative rods are the most frequent pathogens, followed by *Staphylococcus aureus* (Table 78-2).[25,530] Poor sterility standards in preparing intravenous solutions and performing invasive procedures might contribute to these etiologic patterns.[296]

The bacterial pathogens that cause infection in the nursery are different from those encountered when the infant arrives home. In the nursery, besides organisms acquired vertically from mothers, staphylococci (coagulase-positive and coagulase-negative) and gram-negative bacilli constitute the predominant etiologic agents causing nosocomial disease. At home, the infant is exposed to a different environment and to members and pets of the household, which provides opportunity for infection to

TABLE 78-2 Neonatal Pathogens of Sepsis in Hospitals in Different Geographic Areas (1990 to 2004)

	Latin America, Caribbean (%)	Africa	South Asia
All gram-positive	533 (41.7)	606 (38.8)	1857 (31.0)
Staphylococcus aureus	178 (13.9)	224 (14.3)	1206 (20.2)
Coagulase-negative staphylococci	246 (19.2)	122 (7.8)	356 (5.9)
Group B streptococci	53 (4.1)	133 (8.5)	31 (0.5)
Group D streptococci	22 (1.7)	27 (1.7)	132 (2.2)
Listeria spp.	6 (0.5)	7 (0.4)	ND
All gram-negative	709 (55.4)	938 (60.0)	3793 (63.4)
Klebsiella spp	204 (15.9)	441 (28.2)	1450 (24.2)
Escherichia coli	116 (9.1)	155 (9.9)	984 (16.4)
Pseudomonas spp	92 (7.2)	51 (3.3)	576 (9.6)
Acinetobacter spp	26 (2.0)	4 (0.3)	251 (4.2)
Citrobacter spp	11 (1.3)	42 (2.7)	54 (0.9)

Modified from Zaidi, A. K., Huskins, W. C., Thaver, D., et al.: Hospital-acquired neonatal infections in developing countries. Lancet 365:1175-1188, 2005.

develop in the newborn and probably in the household from the newborn.

The current most common bacterial pathogens of the neonatal period in very-low-birth-weight (VLBW) infants (401 to 1500 g) are *E. coli*, group B *Streptococcus* (GBS), and coagulase-negative staphylococci.[409,477] These three organisms account for approximately 65 percent of all bacterial sepsis cases in this population.[477] The bacteria usually are acquired from the mother during the intrapartum period, after the onset of labor or rupture of membranes.[444] The acute septicemic form of group B streptococcal disease can be caused by any of the group B types (B_I to B_{VIII}), and the specific B type causing disease in the infant usually is found in the maternal vaginal tract.[21,22] The gastrointestinal tract is the natural reservoir for GBS and the probable source of vaginal colonization.[79,135,444]

Epidemiologic studies have shown that approximately 10 to 30 percent of pregnant women are colonized vaginally, rectally, or both with GBS, with the highest percentage occurring in developed countries.[79,135,275,400] After routine implementation of maternal cultures and antibiotic prophylaxis guidelines, the incidence of invasive group B streptococcal infection among pregnant women in the United States has decreased dramatically in the past decade.[307]

In a report from Panama,[334] only 5 percent of poor pregnant women seen in a public hospital were colonized by GBS, and approximately 2 percent of documented neonatal sepsis cases were caused by these organisms; in contrast, almost 20 percent of "septic" neonates born to mothers with better socioeconomic status and higher vaginal colonization (seen in a hospital that is only 5 miles away) had group B streptococcal disease.[418] Possibly, better hygienic practices contribute to eradication of many microorganisms from vaginal sites, thereby allowing GBS to colonize the vagina without interference by other microbes. Currently, a sepsis group B streptococcal etiology is relatively common in our country (personal communication).

Vertical transmission from mother to infant occurs in 40 to 70 percent of women colonized with this organism.[1,35,157,528] Infants born to heavily colonized women are more likely to harbor the organism, frequently at multiple sites, than are those born to lightly colonized women.[12,245,370] Some mothers of infants who are infected with GBS are at high risk for having babies in the future who are infected similarly. A low titer of serum antibodies to the type of infecting GBS and persistence of the organism in the mother have been demonstrated.[90]

Although intrapartum mother-to-infant transfer is the initial mode of acquisition of GBS by the newborn, it is not the sole

way in which the baby becomes colonized.[1,15,35,369] In a Houston nursery, infant colonization rates increased from 20 to 25 percent at 1 day of age to 60 to 65 percent at 3 to 5 days of age, without a concomitant increase in parturient colonization rates.[369] Nosocomial spread of organisms from the hands of nursery personnel to the infant probably explains the remarkable increase in colonization rates in this nursery. Analysis of the serotype distribution of GBS discloses no significant differences among parturients, 1-day-old infants, nursery personnel, and infants at hospital discharge.

The major sites of colonization in infants are the skin, nasopharynx, and rectum. GBS persists in the nasopharynx for weeks to months, whereas its cutaneous location usually is lost by the time that the infant reaches several weeks of age. For every 100 infants colonized with GBS, disease caused by this organism will develop in an estimated one or two infants.

Group B streptococcal meningitis is caused almost exclusively by the B_{III} organism.[22] These organisms may be acquired from nonmaternal sites. Clusters of three or four cases of group B streptococcal meningitis have occurred in nurseries during short intervals, thus suggesting nosocomial acquisition.[1,27,473]

E. coli is the other important agent implicated in neonatal bacterial disease, with an annual incidence of approximately 6.8 per 1000 live births, and it is the most common gram-negative bacterium causing meningitis during this period.[131,307,477] The *Escherichia* genus is antigenically complex, with at least 177 somatic (O), 103 capsular (K), and 53 flagellar (H) antigens.[56] The epidemiology of this agent in relation to newborn infection was defined more clearly with discovery of the association between the K1 capsular polysaccharide antigen and invasive disease.[403] Strains with K1 antigen are responsible for approximately 80 percent of neonatal meningitis cases caused by *E. coli* and 50 percent of sepsis cases.[20,335,430] K1 strains are associated with more severe disease than non-K1 strains are.[267,313]

Sepsis caused by *E. coli* is associated with greater morbidity and mortality rates than is early-onset group B streptococcal infection. This finding, however, may be confounded by the higher frequency of prematurity among the former infected group.[307]

The explanation for the association between *E. coli* K1 strains and neonatal meningitis is unknown. Animal studies have demonstrated that *E. coli* strains with K1 are highly virulent in mice and that this lethal effect can be prevented completely by pretreatment of mice with minute amounts of specific K1 antibody.[403] The proclivity of K1 strains for the meninges also has been demonstrated in infant rats, in which oral feeding of *E. coli* K1 strains resulted in septicemia and meningitis in approximately 20 percent of experimental animals.[182] Similar feeding experiments with *E. coli* K92 and K100 strains did not cause disease in this animal model. Recently, K1 strains have been categorized into two groups based on their profile for putative virulence factors, lipoproteins, proteases, and outer membrane proteins, which suggests that *E. coli* K1 may use different mechanisms to induce meningitis.[525]

Neonatal colonization with *E. coli* often results from maternal transmission during delivery.[430] Thus, vaginal colonization, observed in 3 to 20 percent of pregnant women, seems to be an important step in neonatal infection. Approximately half of all vaginal strains express the K1 antigen.[11,271] The *E. coli* strains responsible for invasive neonatal infections come from intestinal flora. Evidence suggests, however, that the vagina and amniotic fluid are two barriers that favor selection of a population of highly virulent *E. coli* strains. Most *E. coli* strains that cause neonatal meningitis and septicemia belong to the clone ECOR B2 group.[511]

The highest prevalence rates for rectal colonization with *E. coli* K1 strains are found in pregnant and nonpregnant women aged 16 to 31 years. Approximately 45 to 50 percent of this population have K1 organisms on rectal culture.[430] Studies of pediatric populations have disclosed colonization rates of 20 to 30 percent for newborns on the second day of life, 40 percent for infants 4 weeks to 1 year of age, and 35 percent for children 1 year to 16 years of age. As expected, the organism is dispersed widely among hospital personnel, who have rectal carriage rates of approximately 40 percent.

Vertical (mother-to-infant) and horizontal (nursery staff–to-infant, infant-to-infant) modes of transmission have been documented for *E. coli* K1 infections.[55,430] Approximately 50 to 70 percent of infants born to culture-positive women acquire *E. coli* K1 strains during the first 48 hours of life; in these instances of vertical transmission, serologic concordance exists for the O and H types of the *E. coli* cultured from the mother and baby.[11] Approximately 10 to 15 percent of infants colonized with K1 strains are born to K1-negative mothers. For this group of babies, *E. coli* is acquired at a later age (3-4 days), presumably from horizontal transmission. Vertical acquisition of K1 organisms has been documented in approximately three fourths of neonates with *E. coli* K1 meningitis. Based on a colonization rate of approximately 200 to 300 infants per 1000 live births and an attack rate of 1 per 1000 live births, the colonization-to-disease ratio for *E. coli* is approximately 200:1 to 300:1.

E. coli containing the K1 antigen was isolated from women throughout their pregnancy and at delivery, and 50 percent of the babies were colonized if their mothers were positive for this organism at the time of delivery.

E. coli infection is highly associated with preterm delivery at less than 34 weeks' gestation and with VLBW neonates and occurs more frequently in infants of women who are heavily colonized.[271] Infants with early-onset *E. coli* sepsis had a poor outcome, with high mortality rates and neurodevelopmental sequelae in 30 percent of survivors. Although amoxicillin resistance is a common finding, a low prevalence of gentamicin resistance exists in coliform isolates.[14] Ampicillin-resistant *E. coli* infections tend to be severe and fatal and appear to be seen more frequently when ampicillin instead of penicillin is used for maternal group B streptococcal prophylaxis.[450] Characterization and comparison of virulence genotypes and phylogenetic analysis will help in understanding the origins and spread of virulence factors within the population of *E. coli* neonatal meningitis isolates.[60,66]

Listeria is a ubiquitous soil organism, and although the animal reservoir for this organism is large, transfer from animals to humans is a rare event and occurs in high-risk persons, such as farmers and veterinarians.[365,399,439] *L. monocytogenes* appears to be a common transient colonizer of the human gastrointestinal tract but with little propensity to cause invasive infection unless host risk factors are present or the gut inoculum is large enough to overwhelm local gastrointestinal preventive barriers. Host factors that increase the risk for *Listeria* infection include pregnancy, acquired immunosuppression associated with organ transplantation, cytotoxic chemotherapy, hemochromatosis, diabetes mellitus, and renal failure.[192,425,439]

The annual incidence of listeriosis in infants younger than 1 year old varies between 1.0 and 11.9 per 100,000, and it is seen more commonly in males. Rates in women of child-bearing age (15-39 years) are between 0.1 and 1.1 per 100,000, with the higher numbers being observed in the Hispanic population.[278,372] Perinatal infection constituted 34 percent (470 of 1378) of cases of listeriosis.[175,461]

Epidemiologic information implicating food as a vehicle for transmission of listeriosis from animals to humans now appears to be established firmly. Food-borne outbreaks have been traced to cabbage, dairy products, and vegetables. Undercooked chicken and hot dogs appear to be frequent sources of infection, as are delicatessen meats and unpasteurized cheese products, especially soft cheese.[367,439] In an outbreak in Canada,[440] *Listeria*-contaminated sheep manure was used to fertilize locally grown cabbage that was stored for the winter in the cold, where the organism is known to survive for long periods. Clinical disease occurred in pregnant women who consumed the processed cabbage months after its original contamination. In 1985, the first well-documented outbreak of listeriosis in humans through contaminated milk products was reported.[163] The milk, which came from a group of farms where listeriosis in dairy cattle was known to have occurred, was well pasteurized, which indicated that pasteurization might not be sufficient to eradicate a large inoculum of *L. monocytogenes*. Linnan and associates[292] reported a large outbreak of perinatal listeriosis in southern California that appeared to be caused by Mexican-style cheese contaminated with raw milk. In a report from Costa Rica, a nosocomial outbreak of listeriosis was associated with the use of contaminated mineral oil for bathing neonates.[448] In 2000, a small outbreak of listeriosis in two previously healthy adults occurred in Ontario, Canada, and was associated with the intake of imitation crab meat. In 2002, 47 cases of human listeriosis were related to ripening solutions used in a cheese-making process.[173,367]

Several large prospective epidemiologic studies have demonstrated that few women are colonized with *Listeria* strains during pregnancy and that the organism is cultured infrequently from healthy premature and term infants or from stillborn fetuses.[229,518] These studies suggest that human carriage of this bacterium does not appear to be of the same magnitude as that for GBS and *E. coli* K1, but asymptomatic colonization with *Listeria* does occur. *Listeria* has been found occasionally in the genitourinary tracts of pregnant women, in the throats of children, and in the noses of men.[197] *L. monocytogenes* rectal carriage rates of 1 to 30 percent of all pregnant or nonpregnant women have been reported.[283] The *Listeria* colonization rate in fecal surveys in the community is approximately 2 to 10 percent.[295,446] A possible venereal nature of listerial colonization has been suggested.[196]

Since the 1980s, epidemic and endemic colonization and disease of the newborn infant with methicillin-resistant *S. aureus* (MRSA) have been reported with increasing frequency in the United States and Europe. Table 78–4 demonstrates the relative frequency of infections caused by *S. aureus* versus those caused by other common neonatal pathogens in nurseries at Parkland Memorial Hospital in Dallas, Texas.

Epidemics of disease caused by MRSA have been reported in the United States and several other countries. Risk factors associated with the development of MRSA infection include lengthy hospitalization, previous antibiotic administration, overcrowding and understaffing, and the presence of predisposing factors such as indwelling central venous catheters, cerebrospinal shunts, mechanical ventilation, and prematurity.[264]

Potential reservoirs of MRSA in the hospital environment include colonized or infected neonates, hospital personnel, and the hospital inanimate environment. MRSA is spread by contact and by air and may circulate among patients, staff, and visitors for several months during an outbreak in hospitals, long-term care facilities, and the community.[64,272,284,327] Although chronic nasal carriage of MRSA by hospital personnel has been implicated in several hospital outbreaks, it generally is an uncommon event and is not necessary for initiation or propagation of hospital outbreaks.[489] Limited data suggest that the hospital inanimate environment may become contaminated with MRSA, thereby possibly sustaining outbreaks of infection.[64,489] Colonized patients without clinical disease contribute substantially to the inpatient reservoir of MRSA. In recent years, an increase in the incidence of community-acquired MRSA infections has occurred in healthy patients without obvious risk factors.[92,224,237]

Coagulase-negative staphylococci also have been found increasingly to be important neonatal pathogens. They are the most common species of the normal flora on the skin, nasal mucosa, and umbilicus of the newborn. With sensitive culture techniques, rates of colonization of the nose, umbilicus, gastrointestinal tract, and cutaneous areas of the neonate with coagulase-negative staphylococci can be as high as 83 percent at 4 days of age.[463] The ubiquitous presence of the organisms and their tolerance to drying and temperature changes contribute to the increased presence of coagulase-negative staphylococci in neonates. Coagulase-negative staphylococci are the most common late-onset organisms isolated in neonatal intensive care units (48% of all infections and 68% of gram-positive infections).[80,239,477,478] In some neonatal intensive care units, disease caused by coagulase-negative staphylococci exceeds that of group B streptococci and *E. coli*.[387]

Prematurity, high rates of colonization, and aggressive treatment of newborn infants in intensive care units (e.g., placement of umbilical or central venous catheters, intravenous parenteral nutrition, and mechanical ventilation) account for coagulase-negative staphylococci becoming important invasive nosocomial pathogens.[478,482] Despite plausible evidence of an increasing prevalence of these organisms as neonatal pathogens, distinguishing between infection and contamination of blood cultures by them often is difficult.[80,208,478]

Most studies have shown that infections with coagulase-negative staphylococci are not associated with significant mortality rates or morbidity in infected infants.[239,251,320] Recently, however, an outbreak of coagulase-negative staphylococcal sepsis characterized by persistent bacteremia and severe thrombocytopenia was reported at the Children's and Women's Health Centre of British Columbia. Some experts suggest that this neonatal infection may not be as benign as has been perceived historically and recommend a large prospective evaluation.[256]

Group D streptococci are normal inhabitants of the gastrointestinal tract and can cause invasive disease. These bacteria are the third most frequent gram-positive organisms associated with late-onset sepsis.[103,422,478] Outbreaks of bacteremia and meningitis related to *Enterococcus faecium* were reported from neonatal intensive care units at the Medical College of Virginia and the Children's Hospital of Denver, Colorado.[119] These organisms have become resistant to ampicillin and vancomycin in many hospitals.[61] Disease caused by these multidrug-resistant enterococci often is difficult to treat. An outbreak of *E. faecium* resistant to vancomycin and teicoplanin was reported in South Korea, where all isolates are shown to have the vanA gene.[281]

Maternal, environmental, and host factors determine the infants in whom invasive bacterial infections will develop when exposed to a potentially pathogenic organism. The presence of any of the following factors can be associated with a 10-fold or greater increased risk for the development of systemic infection: premature onset of labor, prolonged rupture of fetal membranes, chorioamnionitis, and maternal fever. Twin pregnancy remains an independent risk factor for the acquisition of infection with GBS and other organisms after correction for low birth weight. The first-born twin is at a higher risk of contracting ascending intrauterine infection than the second-born is. Infection developed in 3 of 56 twin births, or 54 per 1000 live births, as compared with 7 infections in 603 single births, or 12 per 1000 live births.[371] The basis for the increased risk of acquisition of infection in twins includes the common features of virulent organisms, absence of protective antibody, and similar genetic heritage. Substance abuse by the mother (e.g., heroin) has been shown to alter T-cell activity significantly in the neonate, and such alterations persist through the first year of life.[121] Although numerous microorganisms have been documented to cause maternal bacteremia before delivery, infants born to mothers with bacteremia usually remain well. This phenomenon most likely is explained by a balance among the presence of maternal antibody, the virulence of the organism, and the effectiveness of the placenta in preventing transmission of the organism to the fetus.

Klebsiella pneumoniae is one of the most important neonatal pathogens in developing countries, with an incidence between 4.1 and 6.3 per 1000 live births and fatality rates of 18 to 68

percent. It is the second most frequent gram-negative organism associated with late-onset sepsis in developed nations.[478,530] Although *Klebsiella* strains are part of the normal gastrointestinal and vaginal flora, the resistant nature of the hospital isolates indicates their presence in contaminated environmental reservoirs.[102,296,349]

All arms of the defense system are relatively immature (i.e., lack of previous experience with microorganisms) in a healthy neonate and are impaired further by conditions such as prematurity, hypoxia, acidosis, jaundice, and metabolic derangements. Infants with galactosemia particularly are susceptible to the development of sepsis by gram-negative enteric bacilli.[287] *E. coli* is by far the organism most commonly encountered as a cause of sepsis and meningitis in these infants. The umbilical stump may serve as the portal of entry of microorganisms to the bloodstream. Closure of the umbilical vessels plus subsequent aseptic necrosis of the cord, which begins soon after birth, results in an ideal environment for microorganisms to multiply and invade deeper tissues, with resultant omphalitis. Complications of omphalitis include septic umbilical arteritis, suppurative thrombophlebitis of the umbilical or portal vein, peritonitis, liver abscess, endocarditis, superficial abscess, and necrotizing fasciitis.[10,299]

Of the various microbial virulence factors, the polysaccharide capsule has been studied most thoroughly. Bloodstream infections in infant rats and mice caused by *E. coli* K1 or any of the GBS serotypes can be prevented by pretreatment with type-specific capsular polysaccharide antibody. In infants, mortality and long-term sequelae were increased in cases of meningitis caused by *E. coli* K1 strains versus those caused by non-K1 strains.[217] K1 capsular polysaccharide has been detected in cerebrospinal fluid (CSF) by counterimmunoelectrophoresis in higher concentrations and for longer durations in patients who died or were impaired neurologically than in those who were normal survivors.[217] Concentrations and persistence of K1 capsular polysaccharide in the CSF of neonates with *E. coli* meningitis have been correlated with concentrations and persistence of endotoxin and interleukin-1β in CSF.[311] *E. coli* strains also have been found to resist phagocytosis by normal adult polymorphonuclear leukocytes, thereby resulting in delayed clearance of bacteria from the bloodstream. This delay allows the organism to multiply and achieve the concentration of 1000 colony-forming units per milliliter of blood or more, an inoculum that generally is considered essential for invasion of the meninges. The presence of K1 antigen alone, however, does not appear to account fully for an organism's virulence because nonpathogenic *E. coli* K12 strains that are transformed by plasmid containing the cloned K1 antigen gene do not become virulent on expression of the K1 antigen.[462]

E. coli causing neonatal meningitis usually belongs to the phylogenetic group B2 and to the main serotype O18:K1.[66,244,335] Virulence factors such as fimbrial adhesion S (sfaS), invasion IbeA (ibeA), and cytotoxic necrotizing factor (cnf1), in conjunction with the K1 antigen, facilitate penetration of the brain barrier. These extraintestinal pathogenicity genes of *E. coli* usually are clustered in chromosomal genomic structures known as pathogenicity islands.[66,235,258]

Detailed studies of type III GBS demonstrated that the quantity of sialic acid residues in the capsular polysaccharide and the spatial conformation of the antigenic molecule determine the antiphagocytic properties of this organism. A gene sequence that is specific for type III GBS has been identified and cloned. Strains with multiple copies of the gene sequence repeated within the chromosome have a lower lethal dose required to kill 50 percent of infected animals (LD_{50}) in the infant rat model of disease and are more resistant to opsonophagocytosis than are strains that do not contain the gene structure or have only one or two copies of that sequence.[413]

Studies in children and adults have demonstrated clearly that protection from disease caused by bacteria (i.e., *Haemophilus influenzae* type b, *Neisseria meningitidis*, and *Streptococcus pneumoniae*) possessing polysaccharide capsules is afforded by specific antibody directed against these structures.[331,441] Resistance to bloodstream clearance probably relates in part to relative resistance of the encapsulated organisms to complement. The capsule may protect the deep somatic antigen structures capable of activating the alternative complement pathway. Opsonization is essential for phagocytosis and intracellular killing of these organisms and depends primarily on anticapsular antibody. Studies indicate that levels of B_{III} antibody correlate with in vitro opsonic activity[13] and with in vivo protection in animals experimentally infected with GBS.[502] The lack of type-specific maternal opsonizing antibody is a significant risk factor for the development of systemic disease caused by GBS in the mother and infant.[27,222]

Most pregnant women colonized with group B_{III} organisms have increased concentrations of antibody in their circulation that pass transplacentally to the fetus. Both mother and baby in this instance are protected against disease by that specific B type. Conversely, infants born to mothers with undetectable concentrations of antibody are susceptible to invasion by the group B organisms. In one study, protective B_{III} antibody titers were detected in 73 percent of women whose newborns were well as compared with 17 percent of mothers whose newborn infants contracted group B streptococcal sepsis or meningitis.[26] The same study documented lower concentrations of B_{III} antibody in sick neonates than in healthy infants born to mothers with vaginal colonization. Other studies have shown that premature infants have lower concentrations of B_{Ia}, B_{II}, and B_{III} antibody than do term neonates.[74,107] This finding may explain in part the higher incidence and case-fatality rates of group B streptococcal disease observed in premature infants. Probably, a lack of K1 antibody in the sera of neonates predisposes them to *E. coli* K1 disease as well.[314] Mouse protection studies lend credence to this contention.[403]

Strong parallels exist between the host-parasite relationships found with GBS and with *E. coli*. Both organisms possess immunochemical structures as components of the surface polysaccharide capsule that appear to confer virulence. In both cases, neonatal immunity is mediated, at least in part, by maternally derived serum antibody. For both organisms, asymptomatic infection (i.e., colonization) occurs commonly and clinical disease rarely (i.e., colonization-to-disease ratios of 100:1 to 200:1). Questions concerning the precise role of the complement system in opsonization of these and other bacterial pathogens, the exact concentration of antibody that confers protection, and the feasibility of screening large populations for the absence of antibody need further investigation. The role of local immunity in determining invasion of these bacteria from their sites of colonization (i.e., respiratory and gastrointestinal tracts) needs clarification.

The meninges can be invaded directly from an adjacent infected site, such as skin lesions, meningomyelocele, or a skull fracture. Most cases of meningitis, however, result from bacteremia. After gaining access to the blood, bacteria probably enter the CSF space through the choroid plexus of the lateral ventricle and then spread to the subarachnoid space along normal paths of CSF flow. Because of the absence of antibody and complement in the subarachnoid space, bacteria multiply logarithmically, and as many as 10^8 colony-forming units/mL can be cultured from lumbar CSF. The larger the number of bacteria in CSF, the poorer the prognosis.

As a response to the interaction of bacteria or their cell wall components with central nervous system (CNS) tissues, the local production of inflammatory mediators, such as tumor necrosis factor and interleukin-1β, is an initial step in the cascade of events leading to inflammation and tissue destruction.[340,395,421] Experiments in animals demonstrated that interleukin-1β, tumor necro-

sis factor, and other mediators can act synergistically in altering the function of the cerebral capillary endothelium (i.e., blood-brain barrier) and in promoting attachment of leukocytes through the expression of adhesion receptors.[421,437] The net result is injury and increased permeability of the usually highly efficient blood-brain barrier that allows transendothelial passage of phagocytic cells and low-molecular-weight serum proteins, including complement. Despite this influx, the opsonic activity of CSF remains low; as a result, phagocytosis is inefficient, thereby allowing continued bacterial growth and meningeal inflammation.

Accumulation of inflammatory exudate and inflammation of the arachnoid villi can alter CSF flow, which coupled with loss of autoregulation of cerebral blood flow, can result in increased intracranial pressure. Hydrocephalus results from aqueductal obstruction by fibrinous debris or from reduced CSF outflow caused by inflammation of the arachnoid villi. The raised intracranial pressure, occlusion of blood vessels traversing the subarachnoid space, and edema of vascular endothelial cells can result in cerebral ischemia and possibly cerebral infarction. Anaerobic glycolysis by poorly perfused cerebral tissue results in increased CSF lactate concentrations and hypoglycorrhachia, which further potentiates swelling of glial and neuronal cells through failure of the adenosine triphosphate–dependent sodium pump; in turn, failure of the sodium pump results in accumulation of intracellular sodium. Inappropriate secretion of antidiuretic hormone also can contribute to cerebral edema.

SEPSIS NEONATORUM

Sepsis neonatorum is a bacterial disease of infants 30 days of age or younger. It involves primarily the bloodstream, although spread to the meninges or other organs occurs in a substantial portion of affected infants.[457] No obvious focus of infection of the bloodstream can be found in most cases. The presence of clinical and laboratory findings distinguishes this condition from the transient bacteremia observed in some healthy neonates. Terminology guidelines to classify infants and children with a systemic inflammatory response syndrome resulting from an infectious process are *sepsis*, *severe sepsis*, *septic shock*, and *multiple organ dysfunction syndrome*.[188,419,423]

Different opinions exist on the appropriate age for differentiating between early- and late-onset sepsis. Although the usual range is 2 to 7 days of age for the early-onset variety, more than 80 to 90 percent of infections in the first week of life have their onset in the infant's first 2 days of life.[476,478] Early-onset sepsis commonly is associated with vertical transmission and late-onset sepsis with the hospital environment or acquisition from human contact.

PREDISPOSING FACTORS

The skin is an important component of innate immunity. Preterm infants are particularly susceptible to the development of infections because the skin lacks the vernix (the naturally protective cutaneous biofilm[527]) and is developmentally immature, easily injured, and functionally compromised, thus becoming an additional risk factor for developing nosocomial sepsis.[116,126] This cutaneous barrier also is affected by malnutrition in developing countries.[125]

In a trial in Egypt consisting of topical application of sunflower seed oil to preterm infants, a substantial improvement in skin condition and a decrease in the risk for late-onset sepsis were observed. Nonetheless, a recent Cochrane review of four trials performed in developed countries using different emollient ointments with mineral oil found an increased risk for the development of coagulase-negative staphylococcal infection and fungal nosocomial infections, so further clinical studies are warranted before recommending this practice.[116]

Many prepartum and intrapartum obstetric complications are associated with an increased risk for the acquisition of infection in newborn infants. Among these complications are premature onset of labor, prolonged rupture of fetal membranes, uterine inertia with high forceps extraction, and maternal pyrexia.[49,315,363]

Group B streptococcal disease is associated more frequently than are other causes of sepsis with frequent vaginal examinations and intrapartum fever.[450] Preterm delivery is identified consistently as a strong risk factor for the development of group B streptococcal infection. A multicenter study found that approximately 80 percent of group B streptococcal disease occurred in infants born at 37 weeks or fewer and that only 40 percent of cases of early-onset, non–group B streptococcal disease occurred in term infants.[450]

Sophisticated equipment for respiratory and nutritional support combined with invasive techniques provides life support to ill infants. Arterial and venous umbilical catheters, central venous catheters, peripheral arterial and venous cannulas, indwelling urinary catheters, and tracheal intubation provide enormous opportunity for relatively nonvirulent pathogens to establish infection and invade the host.[3,33,78,114,217,242,269,480] The frequency of these infections varies, and they usually are sporadic. Recognizing these opportunistic infections may be difficult because of the severe underlying illnesses requiring intensive therapy and the frequent use of antimicrobial agents in these infants.

CLINICAL MANIFESTATIONS

The newborn infant responds to many varieties of noxious stimuli (e.g., infectious, metabolic, respiratory, traumatic) with a limited repertoire of stereotyped reactions. As a result, many of the manifestations of sepsis have their counterparts in hypoglycemia, hypocalcemia, hypoxemia, hemolytic blood disorders, drug reactions, and surgical events. Most infectious problems in infants cannot be differentiated from other neonatal disorders on the basis of the initial clinical manifestations. The major signs and symptoms of sepsis relate to disturbances in thermoregulation, respiration, and gastrointestinal function.[140,315,354,465]

Abnormalities in temperature regulation frequently are observed as initial complaints. They may take the form of hypothermia (in 40% of cases) or, less commonly, hyperthermia.[61,122,147,503] With the introduction of isolette care of premature infants to maintain an optimal thermic environment, thermoregulatory disturbances commonly become obvious when the nurse reports the need to make frequent changes in the isolette's thermostat to accommodate the infant's loss of regulatory control. Fever can result from a variety of noninfectious causes, such as dehydration, elevation in ambient temperature, and hematomas, or from central origins secondary to neonatal conditions such as anoxia, CNS hemorrhage, and kernicterus.

Another frequent condition seen is respiratory distress manifested as tachypnea, grunting respirations, cyanosis, intercostal and substernal retractions, and apnea. A heart rate persistently in excess of 160 beats per minute can be a sensitive indicator of early-onset neonatal sepsis.[195] Although these findings are indicative of early-onset group B streptococcal disease in particular, they have been associated with infection caused by all of the pathogens commonly encountered in the neonatal period.

Approximately a third of infants have gastrointestinal findings, including poor feeding, regurgitation, vomiting, weak sucking, abdominal distention, diarrhea, and, rarely, gallbladder distention.[376] Although in most cases conditions other than sepsis can explain these findings, bacterial disease always must be consid-

ered. In most patients, ruling out sepsis on clinical grounds alone is impossible. Appropriate laboratory studies and therapeutic intervention frequently are necessary in the assessment of these nonspecific clinical manifestations.

Only a small percentage of infants have cutaneous findings (except for jaundice). Such findings include cellulitis, impetiginous lesions, furunculosis, papular lesions (i.e., listeriosis), vascular lesions (i.e., *Pseudomonas*), and exfoliative dermatitis (i.e., phage group II staphylococcal disease). Jaundice develops in approximately a third of infants with sepsis and can occur in infants with urinary tract infection. Occasionally, jaundice is the only sign of infection and occurs in septic infants, regardless of the type of bacterial pathogen.

In utero infection is identified by the presence of bacteria in blood obtained at delivery. Signs of fetal distress may be the first indication of infection in the newborn. Schiano and associates[438] suggested fetal tachycardia in the second stage of labor as a sign of intrauterine infection. Pneumonia or sepsis occurred in 3 of 8 infants with fetal heartbeats more rapid than than 180 per minute, in 7 of 32 infants with a rate of 160 to 179 beats per minute, and in 1 of 167 infants with lower heart rates.

One report suggests that infants with documented sepsis or a sepsis-like illness have abnormal heart rate characteristics for as long as 24 hours preceding their clinical signs. These abnormalities included reduced baseline variability and short-lived decelerations in heart rate. If these findings are confirmed, monitoring of these parameters in neonates at risk for sepsis may lead to earlier suspicion of disease and initiation of more effective and prompt therapy.[200]

ETIOLOGY

Since the middle of the 20th century, a shift has occurred in the microorganisms responsible for neonatal septicemia and meningitis.[140,168,183,315,354] In the 1930s and 1940s, the predominant organism was the group A beta-hemolytic *Streptococcus*. It was replaced in the 1950s by the phage group I *S. aureus* and by coliform organisms. In the last cohort of VLBW infants, gram-negative organisms accounted for 60 percent of infections, with 44 percent caused by *E. coli* and group B beta-hemolytic streptococci accounting for approximately 10 to 11 percent of all infections (Table 78–3).[477] *S. epidermidis* has emerged as an important

TABLE 78–3 Distribution of Pathogens in Early-Onset Neonatal Sepsis in the United States (Neonatal Research Network) 1998 to 2000

Gram-Negative Organisms	
Escherichia coli	37 (44.0)
Haemophilus influenza	7 (8.3)
Citrobacter	2 (2.4)
Other	5 (6.0)
Gram-Positive Organisms	
Group B streptococci	9 (10.7)
Viridans streptococci	3 (3.6)
Other streptococci	4 (4.8)
Listeria monocytogenes	2 (2.4)
Coagulase-negative staphylococci	9 (10.7)
Other	4 (4.8)
Fungi	
Candida albicans	2 (2.4)
Total	84 (100)

Modified from Stoll, B. J., Hansen, N., Fanaroff, A. A., et al.: Changes in pathogens causing early-onset sepsis in very-low-birth-weight infants. N. Engl. J. Med. 347:240-247, 2002.

pathogen in neonates and is responsible for a large proportion of cases of sepsis in newborn intensive care facilities.[39,91,336] A study of VLBW neonates (401 to 1500 g) born between 1998 and 2000 at 15 neonatal centers that belong to the Neonatal Research Network of the National Institute of Child Health and Human Development (NICHD) found a rate of early-onset sepsis of 15.4 per 1000 live births in this group, not a significant decline from the 19.3 per 1000 live births reported between 1991 and 1992. The important differences were a reduction in group B streptococcal sepsis from 5.9 to 1.7 per 1000 live births of VLBW infants and an increase in *E. coli* sepsis from 3.2 to 6.8 when compared with a previous cohort from 1991 to 1993.[477] In a survey of high-risk nurseries participating in the National Nosocomial Infection Surveillance System of the Centers for Disease Control and Prevention (CDC) conducted from October 1986 through September 1994, the pathogen most commonly reported as the cause of nosocomial bacteremia was coagulase-negative staphylococci, which accounted for 51 percent of isolates.[174] The apparent increased incidence of *S. epidermidis* sepsis has been associated with increased survival of very small premature infants and the introduction of invasive procedures.[208] MRSA also has emerged as a nosocomial pathogen of major importance in some nurseries. Prevalence rates for a specific bacterial pathogen vary from nursery to nursery and may change abruptly in any one unit.[38,41,168,183,222] Knowledge of the bacteria most commonly isolated in a nursery or intensive care unit, as well as the antimicrobial susceptibility of these organisms, is invaluable in treating infants with suspected sepsis neonatorum.

In 2004, a total of 308 cases of neonatal group B streptococcal disease, including 146 (47%) early-onset cases and 162 (53%) late-onset cases, were reported to the Emerging Infections Program. Between 1993 (pre-prophylaxis era) and 2003, the absolute difference in the incidence of early-onset disease between blacks and whites had declined by 68 percent. However, racial disparities in the incidence of both early- and late-onset group B streptococcal disease persist. In 2004, rates of early-onset disease per 1000 live births for black infants were 0.73, followed by 0.26 for white infants and 0.15 for those of other races.[95]

During 1999 to 2001, the incidence of early-onset disease in the United States was 0.47 case per 1000 live births; it declined to 0.32 and 0.34 in 2003 and 2004, respectively. In Parkland Memorial Hospital in Dallas, Texas, the incidence of cases has been diminished with the use of obstetric and neonatal chemoprophylaxis since 1995 (Fig. 78–1). Between 1995 and 1999, with implementation of the chemoprophylaxis protocol, no deaths as a result of GBS were reported in Parkland Memorial Hospital, as opposed to 8 percent from 1986 to 1994.[500] During the period from 1996 to 2004, late-onset disease occurred in 0.35 per 1000 live births (range, 0.29 to 0.39 per 1000). The rate of late-onset disease surpassed that of early-onset disease for the first time in 2003, a trend that continued in 2004 (Fig. 78–2).[95]

The etiologic agents of neonatal sepsis and meningitis at Parkland Memorial Hospital in Dallas, Texas, for 1987 through 1999 are shown in Table 78–4.

Coliform bacteria, including *E. coli*, *Klebsiella* spp., and *Enterobacter* spp., were recovered more frequently in Panama and Mal-

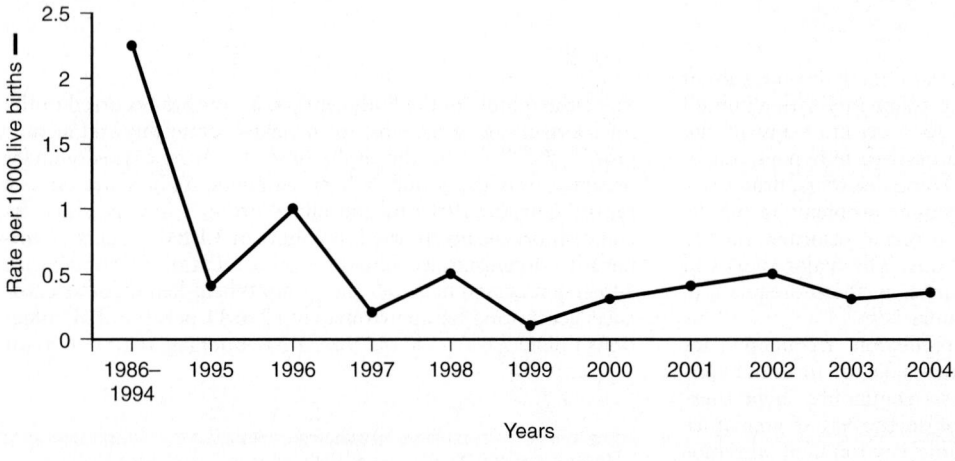

Figure 78–1 Cases of early-onset group B streptococcal infection by year at Parkland Memorial Hospital. *(From Parkland Memorial Hospital, Dallas, Texas [1986-2004]. Data provided by Pablo Sánchez, M.D. Combined obstetric and neonatal chemoprophylaxis was used routinely from 1995 to the present.)*

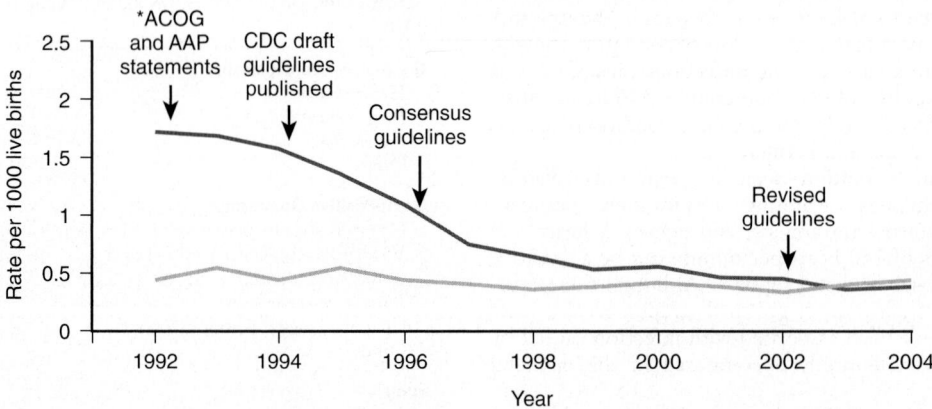

Figure 78–2 Early- and late-onset invasive group B streptococcal disease in infants per 1000 live births from 1992 to 2004, United States. AAP, American Academy of Pediatrics; ACOG, American College of Obstetricians and Gynecologist; CDC, Centers for Disease Control and Prevention. *(Adapted from Centers for Disease Control and Prevention. Early-onset and late-onset neonatal group B streptococcal disease—United States, 1996-2004. M. M. W. R. Morb. Mortal. Wkly. Rep. 54:1205-1208, 2005; and Schrag, S. J., Zywicki, S., Farley, M. M., et al.: Group B streptococcal disease in the era of intrapartum antibiotic prophylaxis. N. Engl. J. Med. 342:15-20, 2000.)*

TABLE 78–4 Main Etiologic Agents Isolated from the Blood and Cerebrospinal Fluid of Neonates with Suspected Sepsis According to Age at Onset and Time Period*

Etiologic Agents	1987-1994		1995-1999	
	Early Onset	Late Onset	Early Onset	Late Onset
Gram-positive bacteria	290	426	39	161
Streptococcus agalactiae	233	61	32	5
Enterococci	13	42	1	17
Other streptococci	25	12	2	1
Staphylococcus aureus	8	100	2	22
Coagulase-negative *Staphylococcus*	10	210	0	116
Listeria monocytogenes	1	0	2	0
Gram-negative bacteria	49	80	18	56
Escherichia coli	23	34	13	28
Klebsiella spp.	3	16	1	13
Enterobacter spp.	3	18	1	8
Pseudomonas spp.	1	4	0	2
Acinetobacter spp.	1	2	0	0
Others	18	6	3	5
Total live births	117,478		67,869	
Rate of infection with group B streptococci[†]				
Early onset (≤3 days)	2		0.5	
Late onset (>3 days)	0.5		0.1	

*Parkland Memorial Hospital, Dallas, Texas (1987 to 1999).
[†]Cases per 1000 live births.
Data provided by Sithembiso Velaphi, M.D. Intrapartum prophylaxis was used routinely in the 1995-1999 period.

lorca than in Dallas.[225] *S. aureus* was recovered relatively commonly in the three nurseries; a large percentage of the strains isolated in the United States were methicillin-resistant, which underscores the importance of these organisms in some neonatal units. Coagulase-negative staphylococci also were recovered frequently from infants with neonatal sepsis. Anaerobes were responsible for a small percentage of cases of septicemia. Because special techniques for isolation of these relatively fastidious organisms were not used, the actual contribution of these bacteria to the development of sepsis may have been underestimated considerably.

H. influenzae, *S. pneumoniae*, and *N. meningitidis* are occasional causes of neonatal sepsis. Viridans streptococci are being isolated with increased frequency and, in one series, were the major pathogens in neonates with streptococcal septicemia. From 1987 to 1989, viridans streptococci were recovered from the blood of 20 of 273 infants with neonatal sepsis in nurseries at Parkland Memorial Hospital in Dallas, Texas.

The changing distribution of etiologic agents over the course of time has been demonstrated in both developed and developing countries.[294,359,467] In nurseries in the United States, gram-negative enteric organisms were the isolates most frequently recovered 2 decades ago; gram-positive bacteria (mostly GBS and staphylococci) constitute the predominant pathogens today. In the largest public hospital of Panama during an 18-year period (1975 to 1992), the proportional incidence of gram-negative infections also declined with time, whereas that of gram-positive infections increased.[334]

SPECIFIC CLINICAL SYNDROMES

Group B Beta-Hemolytic Streptococcal Infection

Group B streptococcal infection may become evident in a variety of ways, ranging from asymptomatic bacteremia to septicemia, pneumonia, and meningitis. Skin infections, such as impetigo, cellulitis, erythema nodosum–like lesions, adenitis, breast abscess, and scalp abscesses, also may occur.[20,231,345] Group B streptococcal infection may be manifested initially as conjunctivitis, orbital cellulitis, otitis media, or ethmoiditis. These organisms are

responsible for an increasing proportion of suppurative arthritis and osteomyelitis cases during the newborn period and have been incriminated in unusual infections such as retropharyngeal cellulitis, pleural empyema, endocarditis, peritonitis, and adrenal abscess.[17,97,231,505,513]

Group B streptococcal colonization can be transient, chronic, or intermittent. Maternal intrapartum colonization is a major risk factor for early-onset disease in infants, and vertical transmission of this organism from mother to fetus occurs primarily after the onset of labor or rupture of membranes. However, colonization early in pregnancy is not predictive of neonatal sepsis.[401]

Culture screening of both the vagina and rectum for GBS late in gestation during prenatal care can detect women who are likely to be colonized at the time of delivery and thus are at higher risk for perinatal transmission of the organism.[72] Almost 21 percent of women are colonized vaginorectally with GBS, and the most frequent capsular serotypes are III and IA.[246]

The most important risk factors for the acquisition of group B streptococcal early-onset disease, in addition to colonization, include gestational age less than 37 weeks, prolonged rupture of membranes (≥18 hours), chorioamnionitis (intrapartum fever ≥38.0°C) , young maternal age, black race, Hispanic ethnicity, and low maternal levels of anticapsular antibody.[26,72,444,447,449,450,477] A multivariable analysis of a large multistate birth cohort in 1998 and 1999 found that intrapartum fever and a previous infant with GBS were associated with greater than a fivefold increase in risk.[444] Six or more vaginal examinations performed during delivery have been associated with a threefold risk for acquisition of group B streptococcal infection, and these factors were not associated with other organisms, probably because of differences in the route of transmission. GBS generally is acquired by vertical transmission, and non-GBS cases usually were seen after the first day of life and may be acquired during hospitalization or through contact.[450]

Universal administration of single-dose intramuscular penicillin to neonates at birth has been considered as an alternative strategy for prevention of early-onset group B streptococcal disease. Randomized trials have shown that this intervention alone[389,458,459] or in combination with a risk-based intrapartum prophylaxis approach can result in significant prevention of early-onset invasive group B streptococcal disease.[374,500]

Animals studies that explore GBS based on a conserved surface protein that is expressed by all GBS serotypes found that it induced a strong systemic and mucosal antibody response in mice. This finding raises hope that a protein vaccine that would be effective against all serotypes also may prevent maternal colonization with this pathogen and protect neonates against invasive disease.[236] Phase I and II trials of candidates for capsular polysaccharide–protein conjugate group B streptococcal vaccines have been conducted in healthy, nonpregnant adults, and phase I safety and immunogenicity trials were conducted in pregnant women and yielded promising results.[14,31,253]

After implementation of the American College of Obstetricians and Gynecologists and the American Academy of Pediatrics statements in 1992, the CDC chemoprophylaxis draft guidelines in 1994, and the official CDC guidelines in 1996 for prevention of group B streptococcal disease, a reduction in the prevalence of early-onset group B streptococcal sepsis has been documented, from 1.8 per 1000 live births in 1990[253,305,444,531] to 0.5 per 1000 live births in 1999 with an estimate of 4500 early-onset cases and 225 deaths being prevented per year. There was a plateau of tendencies during 1999 to 2002, but then the rates declined 34 percent in 2003 with an overall incidence of 0.32 (Fig. 78–2).[93,94,445] The efficacy of intrapartum prophylaxis adjusted for the presence of fever has been estimated to be 85 percent against early-onset group B streptococcal sepsis and 63 percent against early-onset sepsis attributable to other organisms.[450]

The previous guidelines for intrapartum antibiotic prophylaxis recommended a screen- and risk-based approach, and the modified 2002 guidelines recommend universal screening by vaginal and rectal GBS cultures for all pregnant women at 35 to 37 weeks of gestation.[253,444]

Intrapartum antibiotic prophylaxis is effective in preventing early-onset group B streptococcal sepsis, but the widespread use of antibiotics has led to concern about possible selection for other more virulent organisms and increased antibiotic resistance.[307,477]

Two clinically and epidemiologically distinct forms of illness have been described.[23,37,165,231] The early- or acute-onset form is seen in the first 3 days of life (usually within the first 6 to 12 hours) and is characterized by a high incidence of maternal complications. These infants usually are very ill within hours of delivery and exhibit unexplained apnea or tachypnea, respiratory distress, hypoxemia, and shock. Chest radiographs reveal a diffuse pulmonary infiltrate similar to that seen after aspiration or findings indistinguishable from those of hyaline membrane disease. One of the major diagnostic problems associated with the acute-onset syndrome is clinical differentiation of it from respiratory distress syndrome. Several features of early-onset group B streptococcal disease may be helpful in differentiating it from respiratory distress syndrome. Obstetric complications are encountered commonly in mothers of infants with group B streptococcal disease, whereas they seldom occur in mothers of infants with respiratory distress syndrome.[37,165] Evidence indicates that prenatal complications may protect the infant from respiratory distress syndrome because of increased corticosteroid secretion by the mother.

The proportion of infants with meningitis is higher in those with late-onset infections.[444] Intrauterine infection of the fetus results from ascending spread of GBS from the vagina of a colonized woman, who typically is asymptomatic. Fetal aspiration of infected amniotic fluid can lead to stillbirth, neonatal pneumonia, or sepsis. Infants also can become infected with GBS during passage through the birth canal, although the majority of infants who are exposed to the organism through this route become colonized on skin or mucous membranes but remain asymptomatic.[444]

When compared with infants who have respiratory distress syndrome, infants with streptococcal disease usually are sicker early in the course of illness, and apnea, shock, or both occur within 12 to 24 hours of the onset of infection. Infants with respiratory distress syndrome experience a more gradual evolution of events. In some infants with group B streptococcal disease, rapid progression to respiratory failure and death occurs within 12 hours. This situation is an unusual occurrence in infants with uncomplicated respiratory distress syndrome. The peak inspiratory pressures required to ventilate babies with streptococcal disease are said to be lower than those necessary for infants with respiratory distress syndrome.[2] In preterm infants, leukopenia with increased numbers of band forms occurs commonly in infected cases.[2,300]

The chest radiograph may be helpful in differentiating these two illnesses. Neonatal pneumonia is found in approximately 40 percent of infants with group B streptococcal disease. In the others, a diffuse reticulogranular pattern with air bronchograms is seen and cannot be distinguished from that observed in infants with respiratory distress syndrome. Hyaline membranes are seen pathologically in both illnesses.

The second major form of neonatal group B streptococcal disease is the late-onset syndrome. In contrast to the acute fulminant disease of the first day of life, the late-onset syndrome has an insidious onset after the infant reaches 5 to 7 days of age, although it occasionally may be fulminant.[23,238] The disease almost invariably involves the meninges. Most infants are initially seen in the second through fourth weeks of life, but documented cases have occurred at up to 12 weeks of age. A history of maternal obstetric complications usually is lacking, and the infant almost always has an unremarkable early neonatal history, although late-onset disease does occur occasionally in premature infants.[136] The case-fatality rate is low, on the order of 5 to 15 percent. Some cases of necrotizing fasciitis have been reported, with prematurity probably being the most important risk factor.[274]

GBS can be immunologically subclassified into nine different capsular serotypes (Ia, Ib, and II to VIII); Ia, II, III, and V uniformly are attributed as causes of early-onset disease, and the group B_{III} organism is responsible for approximately 90 percent of all late-onset cases[22,223] (irrespective of clinical manifestation) and cases of meningitis in infants (irrespective of the age at onset). This apparently virulent effect of type III strains, which account for two thirds of group B streptococcal infections in infants, appears to be restricted to young infants. In contrast, type II strains are predominant in isolates from adults with meningitis, but this serotype rarely is isolated from the CSF of infants with meningitis. All the capsular types, especially serotype III, are poorly immunogenic, which helps GBS avoid immune clearance by masking its surface proteins, and the capsular polysaccharide inhibits complement deposition and phagocytosis.[223,268]

The mode of acquisition of B_{III} is uncertain because this organism usually cannot be recovered from maternal sites at onset of the infant's illness. Horizontal transmission of the pathogen from nursery personnel, caregivers at home, and other individuals to the newborn has been proposed as the most reasonable mode of acquisition.[1,22,373]

The clinical features of illness are indistinguishable from those of other forms of purulent meningitis in this age group. An exception to the normal pattern of late-onset infection is the intensive care unit setting, where nosocomially acquired clusters of disease in low-birth-weight infants have been reported.[353,512] In such circumstances, the spectrum of clinical expression is similar to that of early-onset disease, although serotype III still predominates.[353]

The gastrointestinal tract serves as the natural reservoir for GBS and is the probable source of vaginal colonization. Vaginal colonization is an unusual occurrence in children but becomes a more common finding in older adolescents.[210]

Resistance among group B streptococci has been limited to certain agents, such as macrolides and clindamycin, but not to penicillin. Resistance to erythromycin and clindamycin occurs in as many as 25 and 15 percent of clinical isolates, respectively.[14,221,443]

The impact of intrapartum antibiotic prophylaxis on neonatal infections caused by organisms other than GBS is not clear inasmuch as different studies have shown a range of results, including an increase, no change, and a decrease in frequency.[104,239,317,450,477] The incidence of ampicillin-resistant *E. coli* strains seems to be increasing, but the role of intrapartum prophylaxis in this trend remains unclear. Although the incidence of *E. coli* sepsis increased in VLBW infants in one report (from 3.2 to 6.8 cases per 1000 births), the occurrence of other types of gram-negative sepsis declined in the same report (from 5.1 to 2.6 per 1000 births).[477]

OTHER STREPTOCOCCAL DISEASE

Group A beta-hemolytic streptococcal disease does not occur as frequently now as in previous decades. Disease caused by this organism varies from low-grade chronic omphalitis to fulminant septicemia and meningitis. Because of the explosive nature of this organism in nursery settings, constant surveillance for colonized infants and prompt recognition of illness are mandatory to avert a nursery outbreak of group A streptococcal disease.[178]

Necrotizing fasciitis caused by group A streptococci is a rare event that occurs in approximately 0.018 percent of hospitalized neonates, with a mortality rate of 18 percent but with a long-term morbidity rate of 91 percent.[201] Maternal carriage is considered an important risk factor for neonatal infection, with an approximate rate of 0.03 percent for vaginal and rectal carriage.[319,328]

Group D and G streptococci have been reported to cause an illness indistinguishable from early-onset group B streptococcal sepsis.[141,456] Viridans streptococci are the second most frequent gram-positive organisms in early-onset sepsis, and they usually cause a less severe illness with a lower incidence of respiratory distress, shock, and white blood cell (WBC) count abnormalities.[450,468,477] Dobson and Baker,[138] in a review of 56 neonates with enterococcal septicemia from a single hospital in Houston, Texas, from 1977 through 1986, described two distinct clinical syndromes. Infants older than 7 days were more premature, had lower birth weights, and, in most cases, had infections characterized by a nosocomial origin. When compared with early-onset disease (5 days of age or younger), which was manifested as mild illness with respiratory distress or diarrhea without focal infection, late-onset enterococcal sepsis was heralded by severe apnea, bradycardia, circulatory collapse, and increased ventilation requirements. Focal infections, such as meningitis, pneumonia, scalp abscess, and catheter-related illnesses, were common occurrences.

Staphylococcus Infection

In the mid-1950s, phage group I *S. aureus* was the most common bacterial agent causing serious bacterial disease in newborn infants. Its unique invasive properties caused disseminated disease, including mastitis, furunculosis, suppurative arthritis, osteomyelitis, septicemia, and meningitis, with widespread manifestations. Because bloodstream infection usually occurs after local invasion, the primary focus must be searched for carefully in all septic babies. Changes in the epidemiologic characteristics of the organism, coupled with intensified microbial surveillance and infection control measures, have reduced colonization and disease rates attributable to phage group I *Staphylococcus*.

Coagulase-positive staphylococcal disease in nurseries also has been caused by phage group II organisms.[316] These organisms

produce an exotoxin (i.e., exfoliatin) that results in intraepidermal cleavage through the granular cell layer because of disruption of desmosomes.[322] Clinical disease may take one of several forms, including bullous impetigo, toxic epidermal necrolysis (i.e., Ritter disease), and nonstreptococcal scarlatina. The initial finding in Ritter disease is intense, with painful erythema followed by the formation of bullae, which when ruptured leave a tender, weeping erythematous area. A characteristic desquamation of large epidermal sheets occurs approximately 3 to 5 days after onset of the disease. Fine desquamation is observed commonly in the perioral region. Bullous impetigo has been the disease associated most commonly with nursery outbreaks of group II staphylococcal infections.[6]

In premature infants, the risk of acquiring staphylococcal infection increases as a result of poorly developed host defense mechanisms; the presence of central venous, upper gastrointestinal tract, or endotracheal catheters; procedures causing interruption in skin integrity; prolonged total parenteral nutrition; and the use of steroids.[220] By the third day of life, *S. aureus* and coagulase-negative staphylococci colonize the nasopharyngeal compartment of nearly all infants with birth weights lower than 1750 g.[159]

In the 1980s, MRSA emerged as a nosocomial pathogen of considerable importance. MRSA demonstrates resistance to the penicillinase-resistant penicillin class of antibiotics, which includes methicillin, nafcillin, oxacillin, cloxacillin, and dicloxacillin. The mechanism of resistance involves, in part, alteration of penicillin-binding proteins in the periplasm of the bacterium, thereby resulting in a decrease in affinity for these antibiotics. The spectrum of clinical disease caused by MRSA is similar to that caused by methicillin-susceptible *S. aureus*, except that patients with MRSA bacteremia were reported to be less likely to have bone or joint infection.[479] Between 2000 and 2005, the incidence of MRSA infection in the Parkland nursery has varied between 0.12 to 0.45 per 1000 live births. There appears to be a more frequent colonization rate as well (P. Sanchez, personal communication, 2006).[426]

MRSA infection emerged in the late 1990s in healthy children and adults in the community setting. Community-acquired MRSA is associated more frequently with skin and soft tissue infections; however, some cases may progress to invasive infection and death.[169,246] In hospitalized neonates, different clinic characteristics, consisting of omphalitis, preseptal cellulites, otitis externa, pustulosis, mastitis, and bacteremia, can be present.[220]

Staphylococcal infections are a frequent and important cause of morbidity and mortality in nurseries.[19] Outbreaks of skin infections in neonates have been associated with colonized nurses.[54]

Coagulase-negative *Staphylococcus* is the most common organism associated with late-onset sepsis. However, determining which blood culture isolates represent an infection or contamination remains difficult.[330,478] Isolation of these organisms should be considered significant when they grow in aerobic and anaerobic blood culture bottles, when growth occurs within 72 hours, or when they are isolated from two or more sites or from the same site at different times.[39,336,352] *S. epidermidis* disease tends to occur as a late-onset infection (i.e., nosocomial acquisition) and is associated with the usual signs and symptoms of sepsis. WBC count abnormalities are found in approximately half of all infected infants. Major risk factors include prematurity, low birth weight, invasive procedures, central venous catheters, and total parenteral nutrition. Exposure to intravenous lipid emulsions was the major determinant of bacteremia caused by coagulase-negative staphylococci in VLBW infants in one case-control study.[167] These infections frequently are associated with colonization of central venous catheters and involvement of other sites, such as the CNS. Infected patients usually are not very ill and respond well to antimicrobial therapy, but frequently the central venous catheters must be removed to prevent further seeding of the bloodstream. The mortality rate is low and ranges from 0 to 15 percent in different series.[39,162,336,352] In a cohort of 1313 VLBW infants with late-onset sepsis (Neonatal Research Network), infants with sepsis attributable to coagulase-negative staphylococci were not more likely to die than were infants who were not infected, but the results can be misleading because of the difficulty of determining which patients have true infections.[478]

Escherichia coli Infection

E. coli strains are the most common gram-negative bacteria that cause septicemia in neonates. Unlike illnesses caused by GBS and *L. monocytogenes*, *E. coli* infections do not fit into distinct clinical syndromes of early- and late-onset disease. Approximately 40 percent of *E. coli* strains causing septicemia possess K1 capsular antigen.[430] The clinical features of *E. coli* sepsis generally are similar to those observed in infants with disease caused by other pathogens. Localized *E. coli* infections have included breast abscess, cellulitis, meningitis, pneumonia, lung abscess, empyema, osteomyelitis, septic arthritis, urinary tract infection, ascending cholangitis, and otitis media.

In recent reviews of early-onset sepsis, *E. coli* isolates have shown an increase in resistance to ampicillin, with figures of higher than 80 percent reported in developed and developing countries. Women with ampicillin-resistant *E. coli* infections were more likely to have received intrapartum ampicillin than were those with susceptible strains.[477,530]

Klebsiella pneumoniae Infection

K. pneumoniae is the major pathogen responsible for neonatal sepsis in many developing countries. The incidence of infections varies from 4.1 to 6.3 per 1000 live births, with a fatality rate of 16 to 68 percent. A substantial number of infections occur as early-onset disease. Although species of *Klebsiella* can be normal flora in gastrointestinal and vaginal sites, isolation of resistant strains is more likely related to hospital acquisition in heavily contaminated environmental reservoirs, particularly in developing countries.[58,145,349,530]

Listeria monocytogenes Infection

The pathogenesis and clinical spectrum of diseases caused by *L. monocytogenes* are similar to those caused by GBS. Because the most common foci for neonatal infection are the lung and gut, the fetus probably is infected by the mother swallowing contaminated liquor and through the transplacental route. Infants acquire the infection in two ways, from mothers who are colonized in the gastrointestinal tract after eating contaminated food, with occult sepsis developing and resulting in chorioamnionitis, or from mothers carrying *Listeria* in the gastrointestinal or perianal regions that contaminates the skin and respiratory tract of their babies during birth.[439] Chorioamnionitis diagnosed by transabdominal amniocentesis in pregnant women with intact fetal membranes has been reported,[378] thus favoring the blood-borne route of infection. Early gestational *Listeria* can be associated with abortion or stillbirth. Premature labor in mothers with *Listeria* infection is a common occurrence; in approximately 70 percent of cases, delivery occurs before 35 weeks' gestation.

Evidence of preceding maternal illness often is described in infants with early-onset disease. Symptoms in mothers can be vague (i.e., malaise and myalgia) or distinctive (i.e., fever and chills) and may alert the physician to a risk for *Listeria* infection. Blood cultures often (35%) are positive for *Listeria* in such mothers.

In neonates, two types of illness have been described. "Early-onset" listeriosis can develop after maternal sepsis, and chorioamnionitis can cause abortion, stillbirth, or premature delivery

of a severely infected infant. These patients can have pustular skin lesions (granulomatosis infantisepticum) and granulomatous hepatitis, findings often detected at autopsy. The associated mortality rate can reach up to 20 percent.[150,388] The pathogen is acquired transplacentally[499] or by aspiration at the time of vaginal delivery.[42] The infant frequently has hypothermia, is lethargic, and feeds poorly.[451] The organism can be found in the infant's blood, CSF, skin, and placenta; the primary clinical picture is severe sepsis with multiorgan involvement.

A characteristic rash consisting of small, salmon-colored papules scattered primarily on the trunk may be observed in some infants.

Listeria infection should be suspected in premature infants with early passage of meconium. Because meconium is an extremely unusual finding in premature infants younger than 32 weeks' gestational age, its presence should alert the physician to the possibility of *Listeria* infection. Chest radiographs show parenchymal infiltrates suggesting aspiration pneumonitis in most infants. A miliary type of bronchopneumonia also can be seen in some infants. No cases of acute-onset listeriosis mimicking the radiographic picture of hyaline membrane disease have been reported. *Listeria* serotypes Ia, Ib, and IVb produce the early-onset disease, whereas serotype IVb is the predominant type in late-onset meningitic disease.[7]

A delayed form of neonatal listeriosis (late-onset disease) occurs during the second through eighth weeks of life and involves the meninges in almost all cases.[318] Infected infants usually are the term products of an uncomplicated labor and delivery. The onset of symptoms and signs is relatively insidious, and they are indistinguishable from those observed with meningitis caused by other pathogens. Acute *Listeria* encephalitis, which usually is fatal within a few days, is a rare disease in humans. Other clinical forms of disease at this age include *Listeria*-induced colitis with associated diarrhea and sepsis but without meningitis. The bacteriology laboratory should be forewarned of the clinical suspicion of listerial meningitis because these microorganisms frequently are discarded as contaminants because of their tinctorial and morphologic similarities with diphtheroids. Overnight refrigeration of spinal fluid specimens frequently enhances growth of this organism.

The peripheral WBC count usually shows a brisk leukocytosis with a predominance of polymorphonuclear leukocytes in the differential count. A significant elevation in the number of monocytes to 7 to 21 percent of the total WBC count has been documented on admission laboratory evaluation of infected infants.[501] Likewise, a monocytosis of this magnitude can be demonstrated in most of the remaining infants on repetitive determination of the peripheral WBC count. In contrast, monocytes are not found typically in the spinal fluid of infants infected with *L. monocytogenes*. Polymorphonuclear leukocytes predominate in approximately 75 percent of cases, with a relative lymphocytosis detected in the remaining 25 percent. As with other pyogenic meningitides, hypoglycorrhachia and elevated protein concentrations are frequent findings. Examination of stained smears of spinal fluid has not been rewarding in more than 50 percent of cases, a reflection of the relatively low concentration of organisms in this fluid,[155] the atypical morphology, and the variable decoloration resulting from the Gram-staining procedure, which may result in organisms appearing as gram-negative rods or gram-positive cocci.

Pseudomonas aeruginosa Infection

Pseudomonas septicemia may be manifested as characteristic violaceous papular lesions in which central necrosis develops after several days (i.e., ecthyma gangrenosum). Noma (i.e., gangrenous lesions of the nose, lips, and mouth) has been associated with *P. aeruginosa* bacteremia. It is caused by a suppurative vasculitis, and deep-seated abscess formation is a common finding.[398] A neonate treated with broad-spectrum antimicrobial agents while in an environment potentially contaminated by "water bugs" (e.g., respirators, moist oxygen) particularly is prone to acquisition of disease caused by *Pseudomonas* spp. or other fastidious commensals. The organism usually is a cause of late-onset disease.[282,478] Stevens and colleagues,[475] however, reported nine cases of *Pseudomonas* sepsis, four of which developed in the infants' first 72 hours of life. The clinical and radiologic findings in these four infants were similar to those of hyaline membrane disease.

DIAGNOSIS

The diagnosis of sepsis neonatorum relies heavily on the clinical judgment and diagnostic acumen of the physician. Signs and symptoms may be vague and frequently misleading. Bacterial infection may masquerade as metabolic disease, respiratory distress, environmental stress, and other noninfectious conditions. A physician evaluating an infant with possible sepsis must be guided by a complete perinatal history to elicit factors that place the infant at high risk, by a thorough physical examination with attention to signs suggestive of infection, and by clinical experience. When infection is likely, a laboratory work-up is indicated. When infection is unlikely and not substantiated by the history, physical examination, and clinical judgment, investigating for an infectious process usually is unnecessary. If doubt exists, as frequently is the case, good practice is to proceed with a laboratory work-up.

Recovery of an organism from a meaningful site, such as blood, CSF, urine, abscesses, pleural and peritoneal spaces, joints, bones, and middle ear cavities, substantiates the clinical impression of systemic bacterial disease. Isolation of an organism from mucocutaneous sites, such as the skin, ear canal, nasopharynx, gastric aspirate, and rectum, usually does not reflect the microbiologic status of normally sterile body fluids or tissues.[159] A point of emphasis is that the colonization-to-disease ratio for the major neonatal pathogens is approximately 100:1 to 200:1. For every infant with documented systemic bacterial disease, 100 or more infants are colonized superficially with this organism but are free of systemic bacterial disease.

Several sites to sample blood for culture give reliable results: peripheral vein, umbilical artery, and capillary blood. The preferred site is the peripheral vein. Venipuncture should be performed after the skin has been prepared properly by cleansing with an iodine-containing solution.[146] A two-phase antisepsis procedure using 70 percent isopropyl alcohol followed by chlorhexidine or povidone-iodine has been shown to be superior to one using chlorhexidine or povidone-iodine alone in reducing skin colonization by *S. epidermidis*.[100] The theoretical minimal amount of blood needed for detecting bacteremia is a function of the number of organisms circulating at any given time. Infants with *E. coli* sepsis have 5 to more than 1000 colony-forming units per milliliter of blood.[133] Culturing as little as 0.2 mL of blood should be sufficient for detecting *E. coli* bacteremia in these patients. On the basis of experimental *E. coli* sepsis in rabbits, a cultured volume of blood of 0.2 mL is as sensitive as is 1 mL in detecting bacteremia at a threshold level of five organisms per milliliter of circulating blood.[160] To improve culture sensitivity, a prudent procedure is to obtain at least 0.5 to 1 mL of blood for culture in infants aged birth to 2 months. Optimal results are obtained when the cultured volume of blood is 5 to 10 percent of the total amount of liquid growth medium to be inoculated.

Bacterial growth is seen in most blood cultures within 48 hours. With the use of conventional culture techniques and subcultures at 4 and 14 hours, only 4 percent of cultures that had positive results required more than 48 hours of incubation.[383] With the use of radiometric technique, 98 percent of cultures

growing GBS and *E. coli* were identified within 24 hours.[412] We generally recommend obtaining one or two blood cultures before initiating antibiotic therapy. Urine and CSF should be obtained for examination and culture before starting therapy.

Many laboratory tests have been recommended for the evaluation of suspected bacterial disease in neonates. The WBC count is a simple, readily available test that can help in the early detection of sepsis.[46,300,301] Elevated total WBC counts, absolute neutrophils counts, and absolute band counts generally are not helpful singly as indicators of sepsis. Although neutropenia in neonates is caused by infection in most cases, it frequently is associated with other conditions, such as birth asphyxia and pregnancy-induced hypertension.[148]

The usefulness of abnormal WBC counts in the detection of sepsis is enhanced by measurement of the immature-to-total neutrophil ratio; a ratio of 0.2 or greater is a relatively sensitive indicator of neonatal sepsis.[108,379,380] Numerous studies that have evaluated the immature-to-total neutrophil ratio have shown that the ratio is too unreliable to achieve more than limited clinical usefulness. Sensitivities ranging from 90 to 60 percent or less have been reported.[52,53] Elevated ratios caused by a variety of perinatal conditions have been seen in 25 to 50 percent of noninfected, ill infants.[177,260] The ratio's greatest value is thought to be in its good negative predictive value; if the ratio is normal, the likelihood that infection is absent is very high.[177,260] An immature-to-total ratio of 0.8 or greater indicates depletion of bone marrow neutrophil reserves and is a poor prognostic indicator. A combination of all these laboratory findings (i.e., hematologic scoring system), rather than those of any test alone, increases the diagnostic specificity of a bacterial infection.[406] This scoring system is of limited value in late-onset, coagulase-negative staphylococcal infections.[128]

Determining the WBC count and immature-to-total ratio again 6 to 8 hours after the initial evaluation is important because studies in animals and human infants have demonstrated that the WBC count can be normal at the onset of group B streptococcal sepsis and abnormal 4 to 8 hours later. Morphologic changes in neutrophils, such as vacuolization and toxic granulation, suggest the presence of infection. The degree of these degenerative changes in the neutrophils of infected neonates provides no implication of the severity or potential outcome of the illness.[293] Identical morphologic findings can occur as artifacts in citrated blood samples stored for longer than 1 hour before smears are made.

A reduced platelet count associated with placental insufficiency is the most frequent cause of early-onset thrombocytopenia in neonates.[404] The presence of severe thrombocytopenia, or less than 50,000 cells/mL, within 72 hours of birth is an uncommon occurrence and more likely is related to perinatal asphyxia or early bacterial infection (e.g., group B streptococcal sepsis). Late-onset thrombocytopenia almost always is caused by bacterial sepsis or necrotizing enterocolitis. In these cases, platelets fall rapidly, with a nadir at 24 to 48 hours, to counts less than 50,000 cells/mL and tend to persist until the infection is controlled. Slow recovery of platelet counts over a period of 1 to 2 weeks is common.[98,337,404]

The erythrocyte sedimentation rate in infected patients generally is elevated above the normal range of 1 to 2 mm/hr at 12 hours of age to 17 to 20 mm/hr at 14 days of age.[4] Elevated rates usually are not observed until 24 to 48 hours after clinical signs of disease first occur. Other acute-phase reactants, such as C-reactive protein, haptoglobin, prealbumin, orosomucoid, and transferrin, may be useful in establishing the diagnosis of neonatal sepsis and in monitoring the course of the infection.[381] The most extensively studied of these acute-phase reactants is C-reactive protein. Concentrations of this protein increase significantly within a few hours of the onset of infection. In general, other perinatal events have little impact on neonatal C-reactive protein values.[442] C-reactive protein concentrations decrease rapidly in infected neonates who respond to therapy and, conversely, are elevated persistently in neonates whose infections fail to respond to therapy.[241,429] Reliance on a single C-reactive protein determination as an early indicator of neonatal bacterial infection is not recommended. Serial determinations are helpful, especially in combination with other hematologic tests, when making a decision to stop antimicrobial therapy safely.[65,382]

Fibronectin is a glycoprotein that has been identified on cell surfaces and in extracellular fluids. The concentration of fibronectin in fetal plasma increases with gestational age to values at term of approximately half those found in healthy adults. Plasma concentrations fall significantly during an episode of sepsis[177] but may decrease in noninfectious neonatal conditions such as perinatal asphyxia and respiratory distress syndrome.[526] More data are needed to determine the value of fibronectin concentrations as an indicator of bacterial sepsis.

Detection of interleukin-6 in plasma samples of newborns has been suggested as a reliable early indicator of sepsis.[83,203,218] Interleukin-6 is a pleiotropic cytokine involved in many aspects of the immune system. It is synthesized and released in response to inflammatory stimuli by monocytes, endothelial cells, and fibroblasts after production of tumor necrosis factor and interleukin-1. Interleukin-6 is the major inducer for the synthesis of hepatic proteins, including C-reactive protein, fibrinogen, and other acute-phase reactants. Its sensitivity in the diagnosis of sepsis and necrotizing enterocolitis appears to be high.[218] One study suggests that measuring serum concentration of platelet-activating factor can identify septic infants at risk for necrotizing enterocolitis.[392] An analysis of all studies published indicates that the main diagnostic importance of measuring interleukin-6 in neonates appears to relate to its very high negative predictive value. An initial interleukin-6 value below 20 pg/mL excludes the possible presence of sepsis in more than 90 percent of infants; if it is still below this value when repeated several hours later, its usefulness as a negative predictor of sepsis is even stronger.[158,252,297] More studies are needed, however, to evaluate the precise role of interleukin-6 measurement in guiding physicians to a better diagnostic approach to systemic neonatal infections.

Procalcitonin

Procalcitonin (PCT) has been proposed as a sensitive and specific marker of bacterial infection.[105,176] Several recent studies have found that an elevated serum PCT concentration can be useful in diagnosing antenatal and early-onset infection because of its high positive and negative predictive values. Infants with viral infection, bacterial colonization, and sterile inflammatory stress have normal or slightly raised concentrations.[176] Some studies suggest that this test will be useful in evaluating the severity of the infection and monitoring the clinical course.[105] However, very high serum concentrations have been detected in patients with respiratory distress syndrome, acute lung and inhalation injuries, hemodynamic failure, and severe trauma.[351] Administration of antibiotics during the prenatal, intranatal, and postnatal periods also may alter the relationship between PCT and infection. Although cutoff values usually differ among studies, a concentration of 2 ng/mL is considered reliable in distinguishing between viral and bacterial infection.[498] More extensive investigations are needed to determine whether PCT measurement, in a single or repeated sampling, would be of value in differentiating between bacterial infection and colonization and in reducing the number of patients treated unnecessarily with antibiotics.[248]

Other Diagnostic Tests

Detection of bacterial antigens in blood, urine, or CSF confirms the presence of systemic bacterial disease. Diagnostic techniques include countercurrent immunoelectrophoresis, latex particle agglutination, and coagglutination procedures. Countercurrent immunoelectrophoresis is specific but has low sensitivity and can be used to detect infections caused by E. coli K1 and GBS.[32,215] Latex particle agglutination and coagglutination tests are more sensitive than is countercurrent immunoelectrophoresis, but they have been associated with a small percentage of false-positive and false-negative reactions.[170,215] They can be used for the detection of disease caused by GBS, N. meningitidis, S. pneumoniae, and H. influenzae type b. The highest yield is achieved by testing concentrated heat-treated urine specimens and CSF. The sensitivity of this test is 90 to 98 percent, with an average false-positive rate of 2 to 6 percent. Perineal contamination may cause false-positive results in healthy colonized infants in the absence of invasive disease when the urine tested is obtained by bag collection.[427] The absence of antigen does not rule out infection. A positive result in the urine antigen test with negative results on blood culture can imply occult infection (e.g., osteomyelitis), partial treatment by intrapartum antibiotic therapy, or a false-positive result. The E. coli K1 antigen is identical immunologically to the N. meningitidis group B antigen and, therefore, can be detected by N. meningitidis group B kits. The usefulness of this test is much decreased, however, by its low sensitivity and the high contamination rate of urine collected by bag with E. coli from the gastrointestinal tract.

Direct examination of Gram- or methylene-stained blue buffy coat smears can help in the early detection of neonatal bacteremia if bacteria engulfed by neutrophils are visualized.[152] Some physicians consider only smears with intragranulocytic bacteria to be positive. Bacteria are seen more readily when acridine orange stain is used.[261] This technique requires a smaller volume of blood but cannot distinguish between gram-positive and gram-negative bacteria. Identification of bacteria on Gram-stained smears of tracheal secretions obtained in the first 12 hours of life from infants who require intubation is associated with bacteremia in approximately half of these cases.[452]

Endotoxin elaborated from gram-negative bacteria circulates in blood and is present in urine for considerable periods of time after these fluids have been sterilized. Detection of endotoxin by the Limulus amebocyte lysate assay may be helpful in the early identification of infected infants.[254,436] Endotoxin may be present in the blood of septic-appearing infants who have sterile blood cultures. Transient endotoxemia perhaps is responsible for "clinical sepsis" in these infants. The source of endotoxin may be the gram-negative bacterial flora of the bowel. Endotoxin possibly enters the circulation through injured and permeable gastrointestinal mucosa.

Several serologic tests for establishing the diagnosis of listeriosis have been described, but none has become an established routine method. Agglutination reactions, complement fixation, enzyme-linked immunosorbent assay, precipitin, indirect hemagglutination, and antigen fixation tests are available and may help occasionally. Caution is warranted, however, in attempts to use these tests for diagnostic purposes. Genetic studies have shown that an extracellular hemolysin, listeriolysin O, is essential for the intracellular multiplication of Listeria. Molecular tests, including DNA hybridization and polymerase chain reaction (PCR), also have been developed for rapid identification of Listeria spp. and for differentiating L. monocytogenes from other Listeria spp.[172]

In one study,[47] French investigators examined whether detection of specific anti-listeriolysin O could be used for the serodiagnosis of human listeriosis. Sera from 28 patients (13 were newborn) infected with L. monocytogenes and 101 controls were tested by dot-blot titration with purified listeriolysin O. Twenty-seven patients (96%) with Listeria infection produced specific anti-listeriolysin O, which was detected in low titer in 16 percent of healthy controls and in 12 percent of persons who had various bacterial, fungal, and viral infections. Anti-listeriolysin O could be detected soon after infection and persisted for at least several months. Although this test might be useful for epidemiologic surveys and serodiagnosis of listeriosis, more data are needed before it can be used routinely for the serodiagnosis of human listeriosis.

TREATMENT

After the diagnosis of sepsis is suspected or established and the appropriate samples have been obtained for culture, antibiotic therapy should be instituted. When the infant's condition prompts an evaluation for sepsis, initiation of empiric parenteral antibiotic treatment usually is prudent, despite the fact that only 5 to 10 percent of blood cultures are positive. For practical purposes, we have summarized the recommended empiric antimicrobial treatment of the various bacterial infections occurring during the neonatal period based on the published etiologic organisms identified; therapeutic alternatives also are provided (Table 78–5).

Infants with suspected sepsis should be treated with a combination that includes a penicillin and an aminoglycoside. The choice of antibiotics must be based on the infectious history of the nursery, the antimicrobial susceptibilities of bacteria recently isolated from sick and healthy neonates, the probable etiologic agent, CSF penetration of antibiotics, and the infant's hepatic and renal function. Factors that determine the probable infecting organism include patient age and birth weight; environment (home versus hospital); previous antibiotic therapy; perinatal or nosocomial exposure to pathogens (e.g., MRSA); presence of central lines, drains, or endotracheal tube; and identification of specific infections, such as meningitis, necrotizing enterocolitis, peritonitis, thrombophlebitis, pneumonia, and soft tissue infections.

For treating early-onset sepsis neonatorum, we recommend ampicillin and gentamicin. Ampicillin is effective in vitro and clinically against GBS, *Listeria*, *Proteus*, most enterococci, and 15 to 30 percent of current *E. coli* strains.[450,477] The aminoglycosides have broader antimicrobial activity against many Enterobacteriaceae, including most *E. coli*, *Klebsiella-Enterobacter*, and *Proteus* strains, and, with the exception of kanamycin, against *P. aeruginosa*. Although gentamicin frequently is used, the choice of aminoglycoside (e.g., amikacin, tobramycin, netilmicin) should be based on the antimicrobial susceptibility of nosocomial bacteria within individual nurseries. For infections caused by gentamicin-resistant coliforms, amikacin or third-generation cephalosporins such as cefotaxime and ceftazidime should be used.[232,249,435,496]

Cephalosporins are not active against *Listeria* or enterococci and should not be used without concomitant administration of ampicillin. Moreover, when used with ampicillin, cephalosporins do not offer the advantage of synergism that aminoglycosides do against strains of enterococci. Staphylococci, nosocomial gram-negative organisms, and fungi rarely are encountered in early-onset sepsis neonatorum, and empiric coverage for them generally is not required. When the epidemiologic experience of the nursery suggests *Pseudomonas*, an extended-spectrum penicillin (i.e., ticarcillin or piperacillin) or ceftazidime combined with an aminoglycoside should be administered (see Table 78–1 for dosages). Therapeutic drug monitoring is recommended when aminoglycosides are used, especially in low-birth-weight neonates, and adjustment of the dosage is essential for infants with impaired renal function. Recent interest has focused on evaluating the use of extended intervals for aminoglycoside administration in the neonatal period,[358] and guidelines for drug monitoring in these circumstances need to be evaluated carefully.

Because late-onset sepsis neonatorum is more heterogeneous in its epidemiology than is early-onset disease and may reflect maternal, family, community, or nosocomial sources for the infecting pathogen, the organisms involved cover a broad taxonomic spectrum. As a result, empiric antimicrobial regimens vary. In a previously healthy infant who already has been discharged from the hospital, ampicillin and an aminoglycoside or cefotaxime are recommended unless staphylococcal infection is highly suspected, in which case an antistaphylococcal agent (e.g., oxacillin, nafcillin) should replace ampicillin. Selection of empiric antibiotic regimens can be more difficult for a septic premature infant who has had a prolonged hospitalization, previous antibiotic therapy, possible prolonged tracheal intubation, and placement of a central or peripheral intravascular catheter.

In these patients, major pathogens include coagulase-negative and coagulase-positive staphylococci (including MRSA), amino-glycoside-resistant coliforms, highly resistant opportunistic organisms (e.g., *Pseudomonas*, *Serratia*), fungi, and possibly enterococci. As a result, empiric regimens in this situation should be individualized. Examples include ampicillin, amikacin, and clindamycin for suspected necrotizing enterocolitis, vancomycin and an aminoglycoside or cefotaxime for patients with indwelling central vascular lines, and nafcillin and an aminoglycoside for babies with skin infection. Avoiding empiric vancomycin therapy seems to be a reasonable approach for treating late-onset sepsis because coagulase-negative staphylococci are common contaminants of blood cultures and are associated with a very low frequency of fulminant infection. In institutions with a high

TABLE 78–5 Recommended Empiric Antimicrobial Treatment of Several Neonatal Bacterial Infections on the Basis of Probable Etiologic Microorganisms

Bacterial Infection	Recommendation	Alternatives	Observations
Sepsis			
Early onset (<5 days)	AMPI + GENTA	AMPI + CEFO	
Late onset	AMPI + GENTA	AMPI + CEFO	Readmission of the neonate at term
Nosocomial	VAN ± OXA/NAF + GENTA or AMIK	VAN + CEFTA	Consider AMPHO
Meningitis	AMPI + CEFO	AMPI + GENTA	
Otitis media	AMOX/CLAV	CEFUROXIME	Given orally unless systemic signs present
Urinary infection	AMPI + GENTA	AMPI + CEFO	
Osteoarticular infection	VAN ± OXA/NAF + CEFO	VAN + CEFO	Consider AMPHO
Cellulitis/fasciitis/funisitis/omphalitis	VAN ± OXA/NAF or CLIN + GENTA or AMIK	VAN + CEFTA	Surgery
Pneumonia			
Early onset (<5 days)	AMPI + GENTA	AMPI + CEFO	
Nosocomial	VAN ± OXA/NAF + GENTA or AMIK	VAN + CEFTA	Consider macrolide

AMIK, amikacin; AMOX/CLAV, amoxicillin/clavulanate; AMPHO, amphotericin B; AMPI, ampicillin; CEFO, cefotaxime; CEFTA, ceftazidime; GENTA, gentamicin; NAF, nafcillin; OXA, oxacillin; VAN, vancomycin.

prevalence of MRSA infection, vancomycin generally is used as initial therapy for suspected staphylococcal disease.[251] For infants who fail antimicrobial therapy or have superficial cultures positive for *Candida albicans*, empiric use of amphotericin should be considered. Ceftazidime and cefotaxime should not be used routinely in neonatal units because of the potential for emergence of resistant *Enterobacter* and *Serratia* spp.

After culture and susceptibility studies are available, changes in therapy may be necessary. Ampicillin alone is preferred for enterococcal and *Listeria* infections, whereas ampicillin or penicillin can be used for group B streptococcal disease. Infants infected with these organisms usually receive a combination of ampicillin and an aminoglycoside for the first 3 to 5 days, followed by ampicillin for the balance of 7 to 10 days. The minimal inhibitory concentration (MIC) and minimal bactericidal concentration of ampicillin or penicillin against streptococci and that of nafcillin or oxacillin against *S. aureus* should be considered for the purpose of detecting tolerant strains of these organisms.[259,408,416,460] Tolerant strains are inhibited but not killed by concentrations of these antibiotics, which usually can be achieved in body fluids and are treated best by the addition of an aminoglycoside to ampicillin or nafcillin. The clinical significance of tolerance is uncertain. For *S. epidermidis* infection, vancomycin is the drug of choice unless the isolate demonstrates in vitro susceptibility to nafcillin or oxacillin; most are resistant to these latter drugs. In selected neonates, the addition of rifampin to vancomycin therapy may be beneficial in clearing persistent bacteremia caused by coagulase-negative staphylococci.[484]

Central venous catheters or other foreign bodies frequently must be removed to eliminate the source of these organisms. If a gram-negative enteric isolate is susceptible to ampicillin and aminoglycosides, treatment with either antibiotic alone can be adequate, but we prefer treatment with both drugs for at least a portion of the treatment period. For *Pseudomonas* infections, combined therapy with ticarcillin, piperacillin, or ceftazidime and an aminoglycoside should be used for the duration of therapy. In certain circumstances, antibiotics not approved for infants (i.e., cefepime, imipenem or meropenem, ciprofloxacin) need to be used to treat an infection caused by a multidrug-resistant gram-negative isolate. A few anecdotal reports have been published suggesting successful outcomes of treated neonates.[68,255,270,341]

Although the third-generation cephalosporins have attractive features for the treatment of sepsis neonatorum, such as excellent in vitro activity against GBS and gram-negative enteric bacilli, provision of high serum and CSF concentrations, and no dose-related toxicity, we do not recommend their routine use in the nursery. Clinical studies suggest that they are comparable but not superior to ampicillin and gentamicin and that gram-negative enteric bacilli can become resistant rapidly when third-generation cephalosporins are used for presumptive treatment of neonatal sepsis.

In a 1989 survey of directors of programs in pediatric infectious disease in the United States and Canada, most physicians favored the traditional regimen of ampicillin and gentamicin for initial empiric treatment of sepsis and meningitis.[324] Use of a cephalosporin (cefotaxime in most cases) in conjunction with ampicillin was considered to be appropriate alternative therapy when meningitis was diagnosed. Antibiotics that have the potential to displace bilirubin from albumin-binding sites, such as ceftriaxone and sulfonamides, should be avoided in the newborn period.[338] Currently, no rationale exists for the routine use of chloramphenicol in newborn infants because of individual variations in pharmacokinetics in neonates that are associated with increased risk for the development of toxicity and that necessitate monitoring of the serum drug concentration, its bacteriostatic action against most gram-negative enteric pathogens in vitro, its antagonism with ampicillin against enteric gram-negative rods and GBS, and the availability of equally potent, safer β-lactam antibiotics.

The duration of antimicrobial therapy for neonatal sepsis usually is 7 to 10 days or approximately 5 to 7 days after the clinical signs and symptoms of infection have disappeared. Delayed clinical improvement or persistently positive blood cultures during therapy may indicate that inappropriate antibiotics have been selected or that occult sites of infection (e.g., endocarditis, abscesses, infected foreign bodies) exist.

Blood cultures in bacteremic neonates become positive in 96 percent of infants by 48 hours and in 98 percent by 72 hours.[383] For infants whose initial bacterial cultures are sterile after 48 to 72 hours of incubation, antimicrobial therapy can be discontinued. If no pathogen has been isolated but bacterial sepsis cannot be excluded, a negative C-reactive protein test at 72 hours can help support the decision to discontinue antibiotics.[470] Because postmortem blood cultures can be negative in infants with unequivocal evidence of sepsis (in 18% of patients in one study[469]), blood cultures from septic infants probably are sterile in some at the time of initial evaluation.

A good outcome depends critically on giving careful attention to fluid and electrolyte balance; correcting hypoxia, acidosis, hypoglycemia, and other metabolic abnormalities; and providing nutritional support. The use of fresh-frozen plasma and exchange transfusion as adjunctive therapy in severe neonatal sepsis has not been studied adequately, and no recommendations for their use can be made.[510] Infusion of intravenous immunoglobulin with functional activity against GBS to neonates produces a significant increase in GBS-specific immunoglobulin G that is sustained for several days.[161] Potential therapeutic benefits of intravenous immunoglobulin include enhanced chemotaxis and opsonophagocytosis and improved bactericidal activity of neonatal sera for these organisms. In animal models, a therapeutic effect is achieved only when immunoglobulins are given early in the course of disease.[397]

Experience with human immunoglobulin for intravenous use in septic neonates is limited, but such use appears to be safe. In a double-blind, placebo-controlled study, Weisman and colleagues[516] evaluated the effect of intravenous immunoglobulin (500 mg/kg) on the outcome of 31 premature infants with early-onset sepsis. During the first 7 days after therapy, 5 (29%) of 17 albumin-treated patients and none of 14 patients treated with intravenous immunoglobulin died ($p < .05$). The survival rate at 56 days of age, however, was not improved significantly. Very large doses of intravenous immunoglobulin may induce a blockade of the neutrophil receptors that are necessary for opsonophagocytosis of GBS. Additional studies are required to demonstrate efficacy, safety, and optimal dosage before immunoglobulin therapy can be recommended confidently.

The efficacy of granulocyte transfusions in reducing mortality from severe neonatal sepsis has been reported by several researchers.[88,109,277] Christensen and associates[109] conducted a randomized, prospective, controlled trial of granulocyte transfusions in 16 septic neonates with depleted bone marrow reserves. None of seven infants receiving the transfusions died, whereas only one of nine neonates survived among those not receiving granulocyte transfusions. Cairo and coworkers[88] evaluated the early administration of granulocyte transfusions to neonates with clinical sepsis. Of 23 infants in their study, only 3 had depleted neutrophil storage pools. These researchers also found that the survival rate was improved in neonates with sepsis who received these transfusions as compared with control neonates. Only infants with granulocyte-depleted storage pools are likely to benefit from receiving transfusions. Neither clinical severity nor the degree of neutropenia predicted neutrophil storage pool depletion in septic infants; bone marrow aspiration is required for determining the status of the granulocyte storage pool.[34]

Although these studies are encouraging, they involve a small number of patients, and larger, carefully designed studies are needed. Currently, this strategy is used sporadically in a few nurseries around the world. The granulocytes normally are obtained from healthy adult volunteers by leukapheresis and then irradiated for prevention of graft-versus-host disease. Approximately 0.5 to 1×10^9 granulocytes per kilogram of recipient body weight are transfused in 20 to 30 minutes.[510] These transfusions usually are tolerated well by neonates, but potential risks include blood group sensitization, graft-versus-host disease, transmission of cytomegalovirus and hepatitis viruses, and volume overload from hydroxyethyl starch.

A more practical and safer approach to reverse sepsis-associated neonatal neutropenia and potentially improve survival is the use of recombinant human granulocyte-macrophage colony-stimulating factor (rhGM-CSF). Several small studies have documented that subcutaneous administration of rhGM-CSF (5 to 10 µg/kg/day for 5 to 7 consecutive days) to septic infants with neutropenia significantly increases the number of various phagocytic cells and decreases mortality rates.[59,77,266,471] Large trials are needed to confirm these benefits before administration of hematopoietic factors can be recommended routinely.

Other nonconventional therapeutic approaches that are being evaluated include extracorporeal membrane oxygenation of neonates with early-onset GBS disease,[227] administration of colony-stimulating factors to neutropenic infants,[87] and immunomodulating strategies (e.g., anticytokine agents, steroids, pentoxifylline, nitric oxide inhibitors).[419] The precise role, if any, of these approaches for the management of newborns with systemic infection needs to be demonstrated in rigorous, carefully designed, double-blind clinical studies.

PREVENTION

Chemoprophylaxis

Studies on the prevention of neonatal infection have focused on those caused by GBS because of its greater prevalence and immunogenicity in comparison to other common neonatal pathogens. Methods proposed for the prevention of neonatal group B streptococcal disease are aimed either at decreasing the likelihood of exposure of the infant to GBS by the use of antibiotic chemoprophylaxis or at decreasing the susceptibility of the exposed infant through improved host defenses by passive or active immunoprophylaxis.

The efficacy of antepartum, intrapartum, or postpartum administration of ampicillin or penicillin has been evaluated in numerous studies. The results have established that selective intrapartum chemoprophylaxis can prevent colonization and disease caused by GBS in the first days of life and prevent postpartum maternal infection with this organism.

Many investigators have attempted to eradicate group B streptococcal colonization from pregnant women during the last trimester. In a prospective, randomized study of women known to be colonized with GBS, Hall and associates[207] demonstrated that treatment with ampicillin (500 mg four times daily for 1 week) briefly reduced maternal colonization, but no difference was found in maternal or infant colonization at the time of delivery. Reinfection from the untreated sexual partner or re-emergence of GBS from an undetectably low population of organisms remaining after antibiotic treatment probably explains failure of antepartum chemoprophylaxis. Gardner and associates[171] treated colonized women in the last trimester of pregnancy and their husbands simultaneously with oral penicillin for 12 to 14 days. Before therapy, 63 percent of husbands also were colonized with GBS in the genital tract, with concordance of isolated serotypes in 88 percent of colonized couples. Such treatment was found to have no effect on the colonization rate of the maternal genital tract at delivery. Other studies also

demonstrated that antibiotic therapy had little effect on carriage of GBS.

In contrast, Merenstein and associates[324] demonstrated that treatment of colonized pregnant women with 500 mg of penicillin four times daily at 38 weeks' gestation until delivery resulted in a significant reduction in maternal and infant colonization. Such an approach may eliminate colonization in infants delivered after 38 weeks' gestation; however, because 30 percent of infants with early-onset disease are preterm, the timing of such treatment is inappropriate. The bulk of evidence indicates that antepartum oral antibiotic prophylaxis generally is unacceptable for prevention of early-onset GBS disease.

Parenteral administration of antibiotics during labor has been examined in an attempt to overcome the potential shortcomings of antibiotic administration during pregnancy. In the first published study of intrapartum therapy, 34 women with group B streptococcal genital colonization early in the third trimester were treated at term with intravenously administered ampicillin (500 mg every 6 hours until delivery) at hospital admission.[529] This approach uniformly interrupted vertical transmission of the organism to the infants of treated mothers, which would be expected in approximately 50 percent of infants born to genitally colonized women. Easmon and colleagues[142] conducted a prospective, controlled trial of 87 colonized parturient patients based on vaginal and anorectal cultures obtained at 36 weeks' gestation. Intrapartum prophylaxis with benzylpenicillin during labor significantly reduced the rate of transmission of GBS from mothers to their babies from 45 percent (untreated controls) to 3 percent ($p < .001$). Allerdice and associates[9] prospectively identified 57 women with prenatal group B streptococcal colonization and treated them intrapartum with ampicillin. Seven percent of infants born to treated women were found to have group B streptococcal colonization, and none had invasive disease; 46 percent of infants born to untreated women were colonized, and 7 percent had invasive disease.

Intrapartum chemoprophylaxis given to women with proven GBS reliably prevents colonization of the newborn in the postpartum period. Universal prophylaxis of all pregnant women with group B streptococcal colonization, however, would result in a large number of pregnant women being treated unnecessarily and clearly is unacceptable. Realizing this limitation, researchers started to investigate the feasibility of providing selective, rather than universal, intrapartum chemoprophylaxis.

Boyer and Gotoff[73] were the first to document the efficacy of maternal chemoprophylaxis in high-risk parturients for the prevention of neonatal sepsis. Infants born to women with prenatal cultures positive for GBS and gestation of less than 37 weeks, rupture of amniotic membranes more than 12 hours before delivery, or both, were studied. Eighty women were randomized to receive ampicillin (2 g intravenously and then 1 g every 4 hours until delivery) or no therapy. Infants whose mothers had received ampicillin also were given ampicillin (50 mg/kg body weight every 12 hours intramuscularly for 4 days). Only 1 (2%) of 43 infants born to treated mothers was colonized as compared with 13 (35%) of 37 born to untreated mothers. Boyer and associates,[70,73] in a randomized controlled trial of selective intrapartum chemoprophylaxis using the same selection criteria, demonstrated the efficacy of this approach for prevention of neonatal sepsis and postpartum maternal febrile morbidity.[71] In none of the 85 infants born to mothers in the treatment group versus 5 (6%) of 79 infants born to mothers in the untreated control group did group B streptococcal bacteremia develop ($p = .024$). Additionally, in none of the parturient women did an intrapartum temperature higher than $37.5°C$ develop in the ampicillin-treated group as compared with four in the control group ($p < .01$). The investigators estimated that their approach had the potential to eliminate more than 50 percent of cases of early-onset group B streptococcal disease and 75 percent of associated deaths in the United States.

A prospective epidemiologic study of early-onset GBS disease for a 9-year period has provided additional data regarding risk factors for the development of early-onset disease.[70] In this study the relative risk of early-onset disease developing was 7.3 for infants whose birth weight was 2500 g or less (versus those weighing more than 2500 g), 7.2 for infants delivered more than 18 hours after rupture of membranes, and 4.0 for those born to women with intrapartum fever. Overall, 74 percent of the 61 infants had one of these perinatal risk factors at the time that the pregnant women were admitted to the hospital in labor. In Finland, Tupperainen and coworkers,[494] using a rapid latex agglutination test, selected patients solely on the basis of healthy intrapartum colonization. Early-onset group B streptococcal infection developed in 7 (12%) of 58 babies born to mothers who did not receive penicillin, whereas infection developed in only one (3%) of 36 infants whose mothers received penicillin. That infant had intrauterine pneumonia thought to be caused probably by GBS.

Morales and associates[333] selected patients in labor who had positive results on serial coagglutination tests performed on vaginal secretions obtained prenatally. Patients were stratified according to whether their test results were positive after 5 hours' preincubation, which indicated heavy colonization, or after 20 hours' preincubation, which indicated light colonization. None of the infants born to treated, highly colonized mothers was colonized at birth versus 35 percent of the control babies ($p <$ .001). In no infant in either group did invasive group B streptococcal disease develop. None of the infants born to treated, heavily colonized mothers was colonized at birth or had early-onset disease; in contrast, 80 percent of the control babies whose mothers were untreated was colonized ($p <$ .001), and early-onset group B strepococcal disease developed in three of these control infants ($p =$ .08). In another study by the same group,[332] only preterm patients who had premature rupture of membranes were studied, again with use of the results of a rapid coagglutination test on vaginal secretions obtained at the time of hospital admission. Treatment of 36 women with ampicillin resulted in no cases of chorioamnionitis or neonatal sepsis, whereas chorioamnionitis developed in 23 percent of untreated mothers and early-onset group B streptococcal sepsis developed in 27 percent of the babies.

Together, these studies establish the efficacy of selective chemoprophylaxis to prevent early-onset group B streptococcal disease in neonates and postpartum infections in their mothers. Despite endorsement of this approach by the American Academy of Pediatrics and the American College of Obstetricians and Gynecologists, many physicians involved in the management of mothers and their infants are not aware of or do not follow widely published guidelines to prevent acquisition of group B streptococcal disease.[240]

Chemoprophylaxis also has been targeted to neonates at birth. The observation in 1978 that early-onset group B streptococcal disease did not develop in infants born at Mount Sinai Hospital in New York who received intramuscular penicillin at birth for prevention of gonococcal ophthalmia prompted two prospective, randomized studies for evaluation of this regimen. Siegel and colleagues[458,459] studied preterm and term infants and demonstrated the efficacy of a single dose of penicillin administered at birth. The population in this study was characterized by group B streptococcal infection, mostly in term infants who acquired infection at the time of delivery, as evidenced by a delayed onset of symptoms. Because blood for culture was not obtained before penicillin was administered, whether some infections were suppressed inadvertently was unknown. The other investigation of chemoprophylaxis at birth was reported by Pyati and associates.[389] They studied only infants weighing 2000 g or less at birth

and found no beneficial effect of penicillin administered at birth. These infants were infected in utero, as determined by the presence of positive blood cultures at the time of delivery in 21 of 24 infants with group B streptococcal disease. Infection had been established before the administration of penicillin at delivery. The population in each of these studies had unique characteristics, and, therefore, the results may not be broadly applicable to all nurseries.

Intrapartum ampicillin prophylaxis coupled with a dose of penicillin to the neonate immediately after birth has been used for years at Parkland Memorial Hospital in Dallas, Texas.[500] This policy has resulted in an approximately 75 percent reduction of group B streptococcal infection rates in neonates (see Table 78–4) without altering the incidence of infections caused by other pathogens. A substantial decline in neonatal early-onset group B streptococcal sepsis related to routine intrapartum prophylaxis also has been documented by the CDC and other U.S. institutions.[44,298] In our Dallas, Texas, series, the incidence of late-onset group B streptococcal sepsis also has declined.

Three special circumstances merit chemoprophylaxis. The first is an asymptomatic twin of an infant with group B streptococcal disease. This twin has an approximately 25-fold increased risk for the development of invasive group B streptococcal disease.[143] Cultures of blood and CSF should be obtained from the twin, and close observation in the hospital with or without treatment is indicated until cultures have been sterile for 72 hours. The second situation is chemoprophylaxis for a pregnant woman who previously has delivered an infant with invasive group B streptococcal disease. Starting at the end of the second trimester, rectal and vaginal cultures are recommended on three occasions at regular intervals for isolation of GBS. If cultures are negative and delivery occurs at term in the absence of maternal risk factors for neonatal infection, prophylaxis can be withheld. If one or more cultures are positive or delivery occurs before 37 weeks' gestation, intrapartum ampicillin should be administered intravenously. The condition of the newborn infant should be assessed; clinical findings and maternal obstetric factors may warrant further laboratory evaluation and antimicrobial therapy. Initiation of chemoprophylaxis in all women colonized with GBS who have two or more risk factors for invasive infection of the neonate seems prudent.[24,179,390]

Several studies[158,286,323,486,493] have indicated that routine administration of prophylactic ampicillin during labor to women with risk factors for GBS-associated infections has facilitated the proliferation of resistant gram-negative bacteria in the vaginal and rectal maternal mucosa and resulted in an increased incidence of neonatal sepsis caused by these organisms, particularly by *E. coli*. Based on these findings, switching to exclusive use of intrapartum penicillin for prevention of early group B streptococcal sepsis in neonates seems reasonable.

Prevention of early sepsis caused by gram-negative bacilli is important in areas of the world where these organisms are prevalent. Unfortunately, no evidence-based medical guidelines on the epidemiology, risk factors, and prophylactic approaches exist for making a clear recommendation. Empiric administration of aminoglycosides during labor frequently is used in Latin American countries, but no published reports have shown its usefulness. We demonstrated that a single, 1-g parenteral injection of ceftriaxone given to high-risk Panamanian pregnant women (i.e., gestation of less than 37 weeks, prolonged rupture of membranes of more than 12 hours, or both) during labor is associated with decreased bacterial colonization and early-onset infection caused by gram-negative enteric bacilli and possibly by GBS.[417] Although this prophylactic strategy seems to be safe and attractive, analysis of cost-effectiveness and careful evaluation for the potential emergence of ceftriaxone-resistant organisms must be done before recommending it for routine use in selected mothers.

Immunoprophylaxis

Effective immunoprophylaxis would be preferable to chemoprophylaxis because of the limitations of antibiotic prophylaxis and because an immunologic approach is more likely to prevent early- and late-onset group B streptococcal disease in neonates and postpartum febrile morbidity in the pregnant woman. The underlying principle is that IgG antibody directed against the type-specific polysaccharide antigen critical to protection against invasive group B streptococcal disease would be provided by passive or active immunization. GBS type-specific polysaccharide vaccines have been developed and found to be associated with low rates of side effects.[28] However, the immune response was unsatisfactory in as many as 40 percent of nonimmune pregnant women who received type III polysaccharide vaccine. These nonresponders did not develop specific antibody, even after repeated vaccine challenge.[28] Response to vaccine possibly is determined genetically, and some of the women in whom antibodies do not respond to vaginal colonization by GBS may be the same women in whom the vaccine will fail. Pregnant women with the highest risk may not benefit from vaccination. Studies of conjugated GBS vaccines using capsular polysaccharide are in progress. Candidate vaccines are immunogenic in adult women, but immune responses are poor even after protein conjugation. Thus, these vaccines are going to be limited for administration to pregnant women. Their use in pregnancy, however, is associated with many medicolegal difficulties.[25,31,181,368]

Maternal immunizations with type III GBS conjugate vaccines have demonstrated 77 percent placental transport of antibodies and persistence of titers in infants up to the age of 2 months. Infant sera uniformly promoted opsonization of type III GBS strains and killing by neutrophils in vitro, thus suggesting that this approach might be an option for the prevention of early- and late-onset disease.[25,31] A recent analysis published by Sinha and coworkers[464] showed that maternal immunization strategies are superior to all other prophylactic strategies, with prevention of 61 to 67 percent of early-onset and 70 to 72 percent of late onset neonatal disease versus a global 55 percent rate of prevention with the current practice of culture-based chemoprophylaxis. Maternal immunization, however, does not prevent disease in neonates who are born before 32 weeks' gestation because not enough antibody would pass transplacentally.

Prevention of late-onset infection, as opposed to early-onset disease, in neonates by the administration of intravenous immunoglobulin to preterm babies has undergone intense clinical scrutiny.[29,30,153,515,517] Premature babies, particularly those born before 32 weeks' gestation, are relatively hypogammaglobulinemic at birth and become more so during the first several weeks of life. Because these same infants are at high risk for the development of infection beyond the first week of life (late onset), intravenous immunoglobulin infusion may provide opsonizing antibody to prevent late-onset infections. Three of the five early clinical trials that examined the efficacy of intravenous immunoglobulin in preventing infection in neonates demonstrated significant favorable responses.[106,112,206,472] Problems with these studies included small sample size, definition of infection, and lack of a blind design.

A well-controlled multicenter study demonstrated the efficacy of intravenous immunoglobulin infusion in reducing late-onset infection rates.[30] Study infants received intravenous immunoglobulin (500 mg/kg) or placebo at 3 to 7 days of age, 1 week later, and every 2 weeks for a total of five infusions or until hospital discharge. Infusions were tolerated well. Although no significant differences in mortality rates or reduction of infections in infants weighing more than 1500 g occurred, the incidence of bacterial infections was reduced significantly in infants weighing less than 1500 g at birth, and the duration of hospitalization was significantly shorter in recipients of intravenous immunoglobu-

lin. Most infections were bacterial in origin, and approximately 70 percent of them were caused by gram-positive organisms, primarily staphylococci. In contrast to the beneficial effect found in this study, two larger, multicenter, well-designed trials showed no significant differences in the rate of nosocomial infection or in the mortality rate between control and treated groups.[153,517] At this time, intravenous immunoglobulin cannot be recommended as routine prophylaxis for low-birth-weight infants. Investigations now are directed at evaluating the usefulness of pathogen-specific hyperimmunoglobulin for the prevention and treatment of sepsis caused by the most common etiologic agents.[515]

PURULENT MENINGITIS

As many as a fourth of neonates with bacterial sepsis have a simultaneous meningeal infection. The incidence of neonatal meningitis varies greatly among institutions in North America. Rates are approximately 0.2 to 0.4 case per 1000 live births but may be as high as 1 case per 1000 live births in some nurseries. In general, group B beta-hemolytic streptococci and E. coli strains account for two thirds of all cases of neonatal meningitis in North America. Gram-negative enteric bacilli predominate in many developing areas of the world (Table 78–6).

Information about the bacteria isolated from the CSF cultures of 257 neonates with meningitis treated at Children's Medical Center or Parkland Memorial Hospital in Dallas, Texas, from 1969 to 1989 is presented in Table 78–6. One hundred thirty-six (53%) of these 257 infants had disease caused by GBS. An additional 49 infants (19%) had meningitis caused by E. coli strains. L. monocytogenes added an additional 7 percent of cases. These three agents accounted for 79 percent of cases seen during the 20-year period. E. coli and Klebsiella-Enterobacter strains accounted for 77 percent of the gram-negative organisms causing meningitis. For an etiologic comparison, the distribution of meningeal pathogens in a developing setting[329] also is displayed in the same table.

PATHOLOGY

The pathologic findings are similar, regardless of the bacterial cause. Studies of the fulminant, early-onset form of group B streptococcal disease have shown primarily bronchopneumonia with or without hyaline membranes and usually no histologic

TABLE 78–6 Etiologic Agents of Neonatal Meningitis in Nurseries from a Developed and Developing Country

Organism	Isolation Rate in	
	Dallas (1969-1989) N = 257	Panama (1975-1992) N = 105
Gram-negative bacteria	88 (35%)	68 (64%)
Escherichia coli	19%	16%
Klebsiella species	8%	25%
Other gram-negative rods	4%	16%
Pseudomonas aeruginosa	2%	5%
Haemophilus influenzae	1%	1%
Neisseria meningitidis	1%	1%
Gram-positive bacteria	169 (65%)	37 (36%)
Group B *Streptococcus*	53%	5%
Coagulase-negative *Staphylococcus*	<1%	18%
Staphylococcus aureus	2%	10%
Listeria monocytogenes	7%	1%
Enterococci	2%	1%
Streptococcus pneumoniae	1%	<1%

evidence of meningeal involvement. The most consistent finding at necropsy of meningitis cases is a purulent exudate of the meninges and ependymal surfaces of the ventricles.[52] The inflammatory response of neonates is similar to that observed in adults with meningitis, with the exception that babies have a scarcity of plasma cells and lymphocytes during the subacute stage of meningeal reactions. Some patients also have perivascular inflammation. Hydrocephalus and a noninfectious encephalopathy can be demonstrated in approximately 50 percent of infants dying of meningitis.

Subdural effusions occur rarely in neonates. In contrast, effusions are observed commonly (i.e., by computed tomography or magnetic resonance imaging) in infants with meningitis who are aged 3 to 12 months. Various degrees of phlebitis and arteritis of intracranial vessels can be found in all infants. Thrombophlebitis with occlusion of veins may occur in the subependymal zone. K1 antigen has been demonstrated in the brain tissue of infants succumbing to *E. coli* K1 infection.[430] High concentrations of interleukin-1β have been detected in the brain and meningeal tissue of infants succumbing to meningitis.[34]

CLINICAL MANIFESTATIONS

The early signs and symptoms of neonatal meningitis frequently are indistinguishable from those of septicemia and other disorders occurring in the neonatal period. The most frequent signs are temperature instability, respiratory distress, irritability, lethargy, and poor feeding or vomiting. GBS occasionally has been reported to be manifested as hydrocephalus without other signs of infection. Signs suggestive of meningeal involvement, such as a stiff neck, bulging fontanelle, convulsions, and opisthotonos, are the exception in neonates with meningitis. The frequency of these findings as culled from the literature is 17 percent for a bulging fontanelle, 33 percent for opisthotonos, 23 percent for a stiff neck, and 12 percent for convulsions.[52,315,363] The sensitivity of these findings in distinguishing infection of the pia-arachnoid is poor. All newborns being evaluated for sepsis should undergo examination of CSF, especially if antimicrobial therapy is to be instituted.

DIAGNOSIS

Interpretation of CSF values in newborn infants may be difficult. During the first several days of life, the mean WBC count is 15 ± 30 cells/mm³ (95% confidence limit, 12 to 18 cells/mm³) in the CSF of healthy or high-risk uninfected babies.[362,431] Approximately 60 percent of these cells are polymorphonuclear leukocytes. During the first week of life, the cell count slowly diminishes in term infants and increases in premature infants. Cell counts in the range of 0 to 10 cells/mm³ (median, 4 cells/mm³) are observed in infants at approximately 2 to 4 weeks of age. The WBC count is uncertain when bleeding occurs after the lumbar puncture has been performed. The fixed relationship between the number of WBCs in CSF and peripheral blood has been disputed. A repeat lumbar puncture may need to be performed in 12 to 24 hours to resolve the ambiguity of the traumatic lumbar puncture.

The mean cerebrospinal protein concentration in the first month of life is 64 ± 24 mg/dL, although individual values can be as great as 170 mg/dL, especially in low-birth-weight, premature infants. The ratio of cerebrospinal glucose to blood glucose is 60 to 70 percent and can be greater than 100 percent in term and preterm infants.[431] The upper limits of normal for cellular and chemistry values are higher in uninfected VLBW infants.[67]

These data indicate that CSF values must be interpreted in relation to these normal findings if a diagnosis of neonatal meningitis is to be made early. Comparison of the results of initial

CSF evaluations obtained from newborns with proven bacterial meningitis with those from normal or high-risk infants revealed considerable overlap in the findings.[431] For example, approximately 30 percent of infants with group B streptococcal meningitis had normal spinal fluid leukocyte counts (<32 cells/mm³), whereas only 4 percent of neonates with meningitis caused by gram-negative organisms had normal counts.[432] The ratio of CSF to blood glucose was normal in 45 percent and 15 percent of patients with streptococcal and coliform meningitis, respectively. However, when the total CSF evaluation (including Gram-stained smears) was considered, less than 1 percent of babies with bacteriologically proven meningitis had totally normal CSF on initial lumbar tap. The likelihood of suppurative meningitis is diminished greatly but not impossible if evaluation of CSF discloses no abnormalities. In some patients in whom the diagnosis is obscured, a repeat CSF examination performed 4 to 6 hours after the initial tap (regardless of whether therapy has been instituted in the interim) may help establish the diagnosis. In premature infants with meningitis caused by *S. epidermidis*, the CSF analysis may be only mildly abnormal despite compatible clinical findings.[204]

Careful examination of the stained smears of CSF from every infant with suspected meningitis is important. Grossly clear fluid may contain few WBCs and many bacteria. The stained smears from approximately 20 percent of neonates with proven meningitis are interpreted as showing no bacteria. Because of the low concentrations of organisms, most Gram-stained smears of CSF from infants with *L. monocytogenes* meningitis do not reveal bacteria. The CSF findings in an infant with a brain abscess may include a pleocytosis of up to a few hundred cells, a predominance of mononuclear cells, and an elevated protein concentration. Bacteria may not be seen on a Gram-stained smear of CSF if meningitis is not present. Ventriculitis is diagnosed on the basis of an elevated WBC count (>100 cells/mm³), identification of an organism by culture, detection of antigen on a Gram-stained smear, increased intraventricular pressure, and dilated ventricles. A cranial computed tomogram with contrast material may show enhancement of the lining tissue of the ventricles.

Several techniques for establishing rapid diagnosis of bacterial meningitis have been described. The first, counterimmunoelectrophoresis, is used to detect bacterial capsular antigens in CSF and other body fluids. Depending on the source of antisera used in this method, meningitis can be diagnosed with counterimmunoelectrophoresis in almost all patients with *H. influenzae* type b and meningococcal groups B and C meningitis if spinal fluid, serum, and urine are tested.[154] Approximately 70 percent of infants with *E. coli* K1 meningitis have detectable K1 antigen in CSF, serum, or both.[301] Group B_III streptococcal antigen has been detected in the CSF, serum, and urine of approximately 90 percent of infected infants.[32] Quantitation of antigen is a helpful means of establishing the prognosis of infants with *E. coli* K1 and type III group B streptococcal meningitis.[32,313]

Latex particle agglutination and staphylococcal coagglutination tests have been developed for detection of bacterial antigens in body fluid. The latex particle agglutination method has been found useful in detecting antigen in the CSF of older infants and children with meningitis caused by *H. influenzae* type b; *N. meningitidis* groups A, B, and C; and *S. pneumoniae*.[350,519] This method is more sensitive than is counterimmunoelectrophoresis for measuring the capsular antigen of *H. influenzae*.[508] The staphylococcal coagglutination test has not been used extensively in pediatric patients, but the polyribose phosphate antigen of *H. influenzae* has been detected in body fluids by this method.[481] Both methods can be used for the detection of group B streptococcal infection.

The *Limulus* lysate test detects the presence of endotoxin, a soluble lipopolysaccharide constituent of the cell wall of gram-negative bacteria.[285] Endotoxin can be measured in the CSF of patients with meningitis caused by coliform bacteria, *H. influen-*

zae, and *N. meningitidis*.[304] Endotoxin has been detected in initial CSF specimens obtained from infants with meningitis caused by *E. coli* and other coliforms. Both counterimmunoelectrophoresis and the *Limulus* lysate technique require approximately 1 hour to run and can be performed in most hospital laboratories. If both methods are used, approximately 80 percent of neonates with coliform meningitis can be identified as having disease within an hour of the initial lumbar tap. However, these results are no better than those obtained from a carefully prepared and examined stained smear of CSF, in which bacteria can be identified in approximately 80 percent of patients with documented bacterial meningitis.[431]

TREATMENT

Selection of appropriate antibiotic therapy for meningitis is based in part on achievable CSF concentrations of these drugs in relation to the susceptibility of the pathogens causing disease. The highest concentrations of penicillin or ampicillin in CSF are at least 10 to 100 times greater than the susceptibilities (i.e., MICs) of GBS and *L. monocytogenes*. As a result, sufficient activity remains in CSF for at least 40 to 60 percent of the dosing interval, and most infants with meningitis caused by these two organisms respond promptly to ampicillin or penicillin therapy. CSF cultures usually are sterile within 24 to 36 hours of initiation of therapy. In contrast, concentrations of aminoglycosides (i.e., kanamycin, gentamicin, tobramycin, and amikacin) in CSF usually are equal to or several times greater than the MIC values for coliform organisms and *P. aeruginosa*. Because killing of bacteria by aminoglycosides is concentration-dependent and requires CSF drug concentrations at least fourfold to eightfold the minimal bactericidal concentration, cultures of CSF from infants with meningitis caused by these organisms often remain positive for 2 or 3 days or longer. Documenting bacteriologic cure in patients with meningitis is important because outcome is correlated with the time necessary to eradicate the bacterial pathogen.

Ampicillin and gentamicin or cefotaxime are recommended for initial empiric treatment of neonatal meningitis (for dosages, see Table 78–1). All infants should undergo repeat CSF examination and culture 24 to 36 hours after initiation of therapy. If organisms are observed on methylene blue– or Gram-stained smears of fluid, modification of the therapeutic regimen should be considered. For many years physicians have attempted to increase antibiotic concentrations in CSF by instilling drugs directly into the lumbar intrathecal space. The first Neonatal Meningitis Cooperative Study evaluated 117 prospectively enrolled, randomly treated infants to determine the role of intrathecal gentamicin therapy in the management of neonatal meningitis caused by coliform bacilli.[309] No statistically significant differences were seen in mortality rates, long-term morbidity, or days that CSF cultures remained positive in infants who received lumbar intrathecal gentamicin plus systemic therapy and those who were treated with systemic drugs only.

Data from the Neonatal Meningitis Cooperative Study and from adult neurosurgical patients with meningitis demonstrated that lumbar CSF concentrations of aminoglycoside drugs administered locally usually exceed the MIC values for coliform organisms by 10- to 50-fold.[309,393] However, lumbar instillation does not result consistently in diffusion of these drugs to the level of the cisterna or into ventricular fluid. In contrast, instillation of aminoglycosides into unobstructed ventricles results in rapid and uniform distribution of drug throughout the CSF space.

Data obtained from the second Neonatal Meningitis Cooperative Study demonstrated ventricular fluid gentamicin concentrations were 10 to 130 µg/mL at 1 to 6 hours after administration of a 2.5-mg intraventricular dose and were 1 to 24 µg/mL at 16 to 24 hours later.[308,310] Concentrations in lumbar CSF at comparable intervals after intraventricular administration were 8 to 85 µg/mL and 1.8 to 4.2 µg/mL, respectively. However, results of the intraventricular regimen were inferior to those obtained with systemic therapy alone. The mortality rate was significantly higher in infants who had meningitis and ventriculitis and received intraventricular gentamicin and systemic antibiotics (43%) than in those who were given systemic therapy only (12.5%). The duration of positive CSF cultures was 1 day shorter in those receiving intraventricular therapy. With the use of serial CSF samples from patients enrolled in this study, we demonstrated some years later that intraventricular gentamicin therapy, which resulted in higher gentamicin CSF concentrations, was associated with higher ventricular CSF endotoxin and interleukin-1β concentrations and greater CNS inflammation (i.e., higher CSF leukocyte count, higher protein concentration, and lower glucose concentration), most likely as a result of lysis of organisms.[339] This finding possibly could explain the poor outcomes in these patients versus infants who received parenteral antibiotic therapy only.[339]

On the basis of the findings from the second Neonatal Meningitis Cooperative Study, intraventricular therapy cannot be recommended for the routine management of neonatal meningitis caused by gram-negative enteric bacilli. A controlled study[316] found that ampicillin and moxalactam therapy (a broad-spectrum cephalosporin no longer available) for neonatal coliform meningitis was as effective as is a conventional regimen of ampicillin and amikacin. In that study, moxalactam achieved greater CSF and ventricular fluid concentrations, and bactericidal titers were considerably greater than those achieved with conventional therapy, but this increase did not translate into more rapid sterilization of the CSF, lower case-fatality rates, or improved neurologic outcome in survivors. Although no large controlled trials have evaluated the use of cefotaxime, clinical experience indicates that it can be used safely and effectively for the treatment of gram-negative meningitis in neonates. CSF examination and culture should be repeated 48 to 72 hours after initiation of therapy. If the results still are positive, computed tomography should be performed to rule out the possibility of subdural empyema, brain abscess, or ventriculitis. In all cases caused by *Citrobacter diversus*, cranial computed tomograms should be obtained early because of the frequent association with brain abscess. The duration of antibiotic therapy should be extended, depending on clinical evolution and resolution of the lesion based on repeated tomography. A neurosurgeon should be consulted early for needle aspiration or excision of the abscess. Aminoglycosides probably should not be used because of decreased activity in abscess cavities that have low pH and anaerobic conditions.

Third-generation cephalosporins possess attractive features, including lower MICs for gram-negative enteric bacilli than with aminoglycosides, good penetration into CSF in the presence of inflamed meninges, and a wide therapeutic index, for the treatment of bacterial meningitis in newborn infants. These agents are active against most streptococci but inactive against *L. monocytogenes* and enterococci. Only ceftazidime provides adequate activity against *P. aeruginosa*. Among these agents, cefotaxime is preferred for the treatment of neonatal meningitis because of extensive experience with this drug in the neonatal period and because it does not alter the bowel flora substantially. Cefotaxime can be used singly or in combination with an aminoglycoside. Ceftazidime has been shown to be effective in treating patients with *P. aeruginosa* meningitis. Because of high biliary excretion and marked alteration of the normal intestinal flora and because of potential concern for displacement of bilirubin, we do not recommend routine use of ceftriaxone during the neonatal period. A prospective study of neonatal bacterial meningitis conducted in England indicated that treatment with third-generation cephalosporins has been associated with a decrease in mortality rates from disease seen during the past decade, especially that related to gram-negative bacillary infection.[219]

For premature infants hospitalized in the nursery for pro-longed periods, staphylococci, enterococci, and gentamicin-resistant gram-negative organisms are potential pathogens; an alternative antimicrobial regimen should be considered for initial empiric treatment. A combination of nafcillin or oxacillin and amikacin or ceftazidime or cefotaxime could be used as initial empiric therapy. When MRSA or *S. epidermidis* is a potential cause of infection, vancomycin and amikacin or cefotaxime can be used initially. Imipenem, meropenem, cefepime, and cipro-floxacin have been used to treat neonatal meningitis caused by multiresistant gram-negative bacteria. Greater experience is required before they can be recommended for routine use. For neonatal meningitis caused by *Flavobacterium meningosepticum* isolates, combined use of parenteral vancomycin and rifampin has been suggested as the best therapeutic option.[137]

After the pathogen has been identified and susceptibility studies are available, the single drug or combination of drugs that is most effective should be used. In general, penicillin G or ampicillin is preferred for group B streptococcal meningitis, ampicillin for *L. monocytogenes* and enterococci, ampicillin plus an amino-glycoside or cefotaxime for coliforms, and ceftazidime or ticarcillin and an aminoglycoside for *Pseudomonas* infections. The duration of systemic therapy in neonatal meningitis depends on the causative agent and the time necessary to sterilize CSF cultures. As a rule, therapy is given for approximately 2 weeks after bacteriologic cure has been achieved. For meningitis caused by GBS or *Listeria*, approximately 2 weeks of therapy usually is satisfactory. Because delayed sterilization is a common occurrence in infants with gram-negative enteric disease, systemic therapy is given for a minimum of 3 weeks and in some babies for many additional weeks. Final judgment about when to discontinue therapy must be based on the clinical course of the illness and on CSF findings at the time that this decision is to be made.

Despite the beneficial effects of dexamethasone achieved in several prospective, randomized, double-blind studies for the treatment of infants and children with bacterial meningitis,[415] especially that caused by *H. influenzae*,[434] no such data are available for its use in newborns; the use of steroids in neonatal meningitis cannot be recommended. A prospective trial performed in Jordan found lack of effectiveness of dexamethasone for neonatal meningitis in terms of mortality and sequelae rates when compared with the nonsteroid group.[124] Because this study was small (not sufficient statistical power), not blinded, and without a placebo group, additional studies are required to determine whether dexamethasone has a beneficial effect in neonates with meningitis.

PROGNOSIS

Acute complications of bacterial meningitis include communicating and noncommunicating hydrocephalus, subdural effusions (approximately 1% of patients), deafness, and blindness. Ventriculitis occurs in approximately 70 percent of neonates with coliform meningitis and usually is detected at the time of initial diagnosis. Brain abscess is an infrequent complication, except in infants with *C. diversus* meningitis, in whom abscess develops approximately 70 percent of the time.[194,309,310,316] A 30 to 50 percent incidence in neurologic sequelae has been reported in surviving infants.[202] Although gross retardation and neurologic deficits may be obvious in some infants at discharge, most babies appear "well" at this time. Only after prolonged and careful follow-up do the perceptual difficulties, behavioral problems, and other subtle neurologic signs become apparent. Within 4 to 6 weeks of recovering from meningitis, hearing should be evaluated by evoked response audiometry.

Case-fatality rates in neonates with meningitis range from 15 to greater than 30 percent.[131,315,363] A mortality rate of 30 percent

was observed in 117 neonates with coliform meningitis enrolled in the first Neonatal Meningitis Cooperative Study.[309] In this project, term infants had a significantly lower rate (18%) than that observed in low-birth-weight (<2500 g) babies (45%) and in infants older than 30 days (48%). Poor outcome after gram-negative enteric meningitis is correlated directly with the presence of ventriculitis, the persistence of positive CSF cultures, the presence and persistence of elevated endotoxin and interleukin-1β concentrations in CSF, a CSF cell count of greater than 10,000/mm^3, and a CSF protein concentration higher than 500 mg/dL.[257] When meningitis is caused by *E. coli* K1, poor outcome is associated with persistence of large quantities of K1 capsular polysaccharide antigen in CSF.[311,313]

Long-term follow-up studies of babies with coliform meningitis enrolled in the Neonatal Meningitis Cooperative Study have revealed that approximately 65 percent of survivors were normal 3 to 7 years after illness. An additional 30 percent were classified as having mild to moderate neurologic sequelae. Many of these latter patients had only slightly abnormal neurologic or psychological evaluations and were considered normal on routine physical examination. About 5 to 10 percent of survivors had severe neurologic or mental impairment requiring custodial care. Approximately 15 to 20 percent of survivors of group B streptococcal meningitis have major sequelae, including spastic quadriplegia, profound mental retardation, hemiparesis, deafness, and blindness.[109] Hydrocephalus develops in 11 percent, and 13 percent have a seizure disorder. The survivors without major sequelae on physical examination, however, appear to function within normal limits and comparable to their siblings.

Edwards and associates[144] reported a 21 percent morbidity rate after group B streptococcal meningitis. Of the survivors, 29 percent had severe neurologic sequelae, 21 percent had minor deficits, and 50 percent were functioning normally. Factors at initial evaluation associated with death or severe disability included coma, decreased perfusion, CSF protein greater than 300 mg/dL, an absolute neutrophil count of less than 1000, and a total leukocyte count of less than 5000/mm^3. A report from Canada noted that duration of seizures longer than 72 hours, presence of coma, use of inotropes, and leukopenia were the most important predictors of an adverse outcome.[265] Our experience with gram-negative enteric bacillary meningitis in 98 identified neonates managed from 1969 through 1989 revealed a case-fatality rate of 17 percent; 61 percent of survivors had long-term sequelae that included seizure disorders, hydrocephalus, physical disability, developmental delay, and hearing loss.[497]

OTITIS MEDIA

Otitis media is diagnosed infrequently in neonates because of the paucity of clinical findings and the difficulty of examining an infant's tympanic membrane. The external canal is narrow and tortuous and often is filled with debris. Because a healthy baby's membrane may appear thickened and dull, mobility of the drum determined by pneumatoscopy should be used as the single most reliable indicator of middle ear abnormalities. The examiner must beware of mistaking movement of the distal interior canal wall for movement of the tympanic membrane. Movement of a normal membrane is seen best in the posterior portion. A reddish or reddish orange color of the tympanic membrane usually indicates infection, provided that the infant is not crying.

The exact incidence of disease is unknown, but a prospective study found that in 34 percent of 70 infants monitored from birth, the first episode of otitis media occurred before they reached 2 months of age.[302] Otitis media develops more commonly in premature than in term infants and occurs almost exclusively in bottle-fed babies. It is a frequent finding in neonates receiving intensive care, especially those with prolonged nasotracheal intubation.[53] The ears of 127 infants with birth weights of less than 2300 g were examined by Warren and Stool[509] three times weekly until discharge from the nursery; in only three patients (2%) did otitis media develop. In contrast, in a study of 125 premature infants in a neonatal intensive care unit, Berman and associates[53] found that 38 infants (30%) had middle ear fluid compatible with the diagnosis of otitis media; this finding was confirmed by tympanocentesis in 13 patients in whom the procedure was performed. Development of otitis media was correlated significantly with nasotracheal intubation for longer than 7 days.

Meconium staining of amniotic fluid and prolonged rupture of membranes are two other risk factors for the subsequent development of middle ear disease.[377] Neonates with cleft palate, Down syndrome, or maxillofacial anomalies are at high risk for the development of chronic middle ear disease. The onset of illness is insidious, and the most common manifestations are rhinorrhea, irritability, and failure to thrive. Fever higher than 38°C is a rare finding. The presence of lethargy, hypotonia, hypothermia, high fever, or jaundice suggests septic complications such as bacteremia or meningitis.

The cause of neonatal otitis media is similar to that observed in older infants and children. *S. pneumoniae*, *H. influenzae*, and *Moraxella catarrhalis* account for more than 50 percent of cases.[62,63,455,487] The important difference from disease in older patients is that 10 to 15 percent of neonates have disease caused by coliforms, GBS, or *S. aureus*. In a review of 137 medical records of infants younger than 2 months with acute otitis media who underwent tympanocentesis in the emergency room of Soroka University Medical Center between January 1995 and May 1999, 20 percent of *S. pneumoniae* isolates were not susceptible to penicillin, thus indicating that antibiotic resistance already may be present at an early age. Pathogens isolated from the middle ear fluid of these infants were *S. pneumoniae* in 46 percent of cases, *H. influenzae* in 34 percent, group A *Streptococcus* in 10 percent, enteric gram-negative bacilli in 7 percent, *M. catarrhalis* in 2 percent, and *Streptococcus faecalis* in 1 percent. Mixed infections were recorded in 20 patients.[495] We occasionally have encountered neonates with otitis media associated with septicemia and pneumonia or meningitis. GBS or coliform organisms were the causative agents in these cases.

The importance of establishing the diagnosis and cause of otitis media in neonates and using appropriate therapy cannot be overemphasized. When otologic examination demonstrates middle ear disease, the infant should be examined carefully for other sites of infection. If none is found, which is the usual case, the infant can be treated on an outpatient basis. Because a small percentage of these cases are caused by coliform bacilli or *S. aureus*, drugs that include those organisms in their spectrum of activity (i.e., second-generation cephalosporin or amoxicillin-clavulanate) are preferable to the aminopenicillins. The patient's condition should be re-evaluated 8 to 72 hours after therapy is initiated to determine whether clinical improvement has occurred and whether the middle ear infection is resolving. In patients demonstrating no improvement, tympanocentesis should be performed for examination of stained smears of middle ear fluid and for culture of the contents. Changes in therapy should be based on the findings of these examinations. If gram-negative organisms or staphylococci are observed, the infant probably is managed best in the hospital by means of parenteral therapy, with administration of an aminoglycoside if coliforms are suspected or an antistaphylococcal penicillin for *S. aureus*. If organisms are not observed in infants with unresolving disease, nafcillin and gentamicin or cefuroxime can be used until the results of culture and susceptibility studies are available. CSF examination should be performed before parenteral therapy is initiated.

All infants with otitis media should be monitored carefully for many months after illness. Misdiagnosis or improper therapy may

result in chronic middle ear disease and, occasionally, extension of infection to adjacent structures such as the mastoid or CNS. Infants in whom the first episode of otitis media develops before they reach 2 months of age may require 3 to 4 months to clear the effusions, and recurrent or chronic otitis media is reported to develop in a third of them.[302]

DIARRHEAL DISEASE

Although diarrheal disease during the neonatal period usually is brief and self-limited, it may cause significant morbidity in some infants and represents a potential danger to other infants in the nursery. The advent of modern sterilization practices and increased emphasis on hospital infection control measures has reduced the incidence of nosocomial diarrheal disease significantly.

Numerous factors, including underdevelopment of local and systemic immune responses; lack of fully developed aerobic and anaerobic enteric flora, which protects the gastrointestinal tract of older infants and children; a less effective gastric bactericidal barrier; less intestinal mucus; and less motility, contribute to increased susceptibility to neonatal enteric infections.[357] The infant may have been fed powdered formula that could have been mixed with contaminated water, or a critically ill newborn may have received a broad-spectrum antibiotic in intensive care, in which case highly resistant nosocomial flora pose a special risk.

The importance of breast-feeding in preventing diarrheal disease in infants cannot be overemphasized. The protective effects of breast-feeding have been confirmed in surveys of sporadic gastroenteritis, in community epidemics, and in outbreaks in newborn nurseries. Antibacterial and antiviral factors in breast milk, including lactoferrin, lysozyme, phagocytes, specific secretory immunoglobulins, and lymphocytes sensitive to organisms such as *E. coli*, *Salmonella*, *Shigella*, *Clostridium difficile* toxins A and B, and rotavirus, are well documented.[197,209,357,492] Breast-fed infants are less susceptible to diarrheal diseases than are bottle-fed infants.[205,357]

ETIOLOGY AND PATHOGENESIS

The most common cause of diarrhea in young infants is alteration of diet and feeding practices rather than specific bacterial or viral pathogens. Diarrhea can be a nonspecific symptom of sepsis or urinary tract infection in a newborn infant. Of the infectious causes, rotaviruses are important in infantile diarrheal disease.[326,415] They have been associated with nursery outbreaks of gastroenteritis and necrotizing enterocolitis.[111,410] Studies from France have shown that approximately a third of all neonates shed rotavirus in their stool; of these infants, only 29 percent have associated diarrhea.[101]

Transplacental transfer of rotaviral group-specific or type-specific maternal antibodies to neonates appears to have little effect on the incidence of infection or illness by rotaviruses.[135,136,355] The essential pathogenic feature of rotavirus infection is destruction of the absorptive cells lining the duodenum, jejunum, and possibly the ileum.[325] Lactase exists only in the brush borders of differentiated epithelial cells at these sites and has been suggested to act as a combined receptor and uncoating enzyme for the virus, which may explain why rotavirus infection occurs less commonly in infants of less than 32 weeks' gestation than in more mature infants.[89] In infants between 26 and 34 weeks' gestation, lactase activity is approximately 30 percent of that found in term infants.[280]

Enteropathogenic *E. coli* serotypes once were considered the most common bacterial agents responsible for diarrhea in young infants. Failure to demonstrate on rectal cultures specific serotypes of *E. coli* designated as enteropathogenic does not rule out coliform disease. Enterotoxigenic strains of *E. coli* possessing nonenteropathogenic serotypes have been identified in nursery outbreaks of diarrheal disease.[75,360] These organisms inhabit the small bowel, where they attach to but do not invade the intestinal mucosa. The enterotoxin produced by these organisms stimulates cyclic adenosine monophosphate, which inhibits sodium and chloride transport across the intestinal wall. As a result, these salts are lost into the lumen of the upper bowel, followed passively by water, which causes a net loss of stools containing high concentrations of electrolytes. *Vibrio cholerae*, some *E. coli* serotypes (almost exclusively nonenteropathogenic strains), *Vibrio parahaemolyticus*, *Aeromonas*, and possibly some *Campylobacter* and *Yersinia* strains are examples of bacteria that cause diarrhea by this mechanism.

The importance of recognizing this form of diarrheal disease was emphasized in a nursery outbreak in the southwestern United States. Severe, watery diarrhea was observed in 59 infants during a 9-month period; in the 7 percent of infants who died, death resulted from altered hepatic function and a hemorrhagic diathesis.[75] An O142/K86/H6 *E. coli* strain was responsible for the outbreak. Because this organism is not a classic enteropathogenic serotype, it was not identified as a pathogen, which thereby delayed establishing the definitive diagnosis and institution of proper infection control techniques. Only by special laboratory techniques was this *E. coli* strain shown to produce labile enterotoxin.

A second mechanism involved in the development of bacterial diarrhea is invasion of the intestinal mucosa. *Shigella* dysentery is the classic example of this disease. Colonic invasion with subsequent destruction of the mucosa causes an outpouring of polymorphonuclear cells and mucus. The resultant diarrhea usually is bloody and contains mucus and pus. *Salmonella* spp. also invade the intestinal mucosa, but destruction is not extensive. The epithelial lining is left intact, and the organisms reach the lamina propria, where an inflammatory response is elicited.[483] *Campylobacter*, *Yersinia*, *Aeromonas* spp., and *C. difficile* also can cause bloody diarrhea.

Although serotyping of *E. coli* to identify the traditional enteropathogenic strains no longer is available routinely, the epidemiologic evidence is strong enough to support a pathogenic role for these strains, even though the mechanism of pathogenicity is unknown. When an index case of diarrhea caused by enteropathogenic *E. coli* or other pathogens is recognized in a nursery, secondary cases are likely to occur. In any nursery infant with diarrhea, a potentially communicable disease should be suspected. For all infants in proximity to the index case, rectal swabs should be tested by culture or by fluorescent antibody technique, which is more sensitive in identifying asymptomatic carriers of enteropathogenic *E. coli*. Ill and healthy colonized infants should be segregated and treated with orally administered neomycin (100 mg/kg/day in three or four divided doses) or with colistin sulfate (15 mg/kg/day in three or four divided doses) for 5 days. Neomycin causes rapid disappearance of the organism and abbreviates the duration diarrhea, but approximately 20 percent of infants revert to an asymptomatic carrier state (J. D. Nelson, personal communication, 1990). Repeated surveillance of infants is necessary until the pathogenic strain has been eliminated from the nursery. A report from Yugoslavia identified a multiresistant strain of enteroaggregative *E. coli* (O4 serogroup) associated with an outbreak of transient, self-limited diarrhea in a neonatal nursery ward.[113]

Campylobacter, a curved, gram-negative bacterium, has been recognized increasingly as a common cause of enteritis. Of the 14 known species, *Campylobacter fetus* and *Campylobacter jejuni* cause human disease most frequently. *C. fetus* causes prenatal and neonatal infections that result in abortion, premature delivery, bacteremia, and meningitis. Infections caused by *C. fetus* appear to be the most common type of *Campylobacter* infection in the first 3 weeks of life and are associated with a high incidence of fetal and neonatal morbidity.[205] In contrast, the most common syndrome produced by a *Campylobacter* species is enteritis caused by *C. jejuni*. Unlike the serious neonatal disease caused by *C. fetus*, infections with *C. jejuni* usually result in mild gastroenteritis, although meningitis occurs rarely. Nursery outbreaks of gastroenteritis caused by *C. jejuni* have been documented definitively.[205]

Although some diarrheal episodes in neonates probably can be caused by *C. difficile*, the diagnostic criteria used in older children and adults are inadequate to establish a definitive diagnosis in this age group. *C. difficile* is a gram-positive anaerobic bacillus that produces an enterotoxin (i.e., toxin A) that causes fluid secretion and a cytotoxin that damages cells (i.e., toxin B).[85,288] *C. difficile* colonic overgrowth and toxin production can result from the selective pressure of antibiotic therapy. A wide variety of antibiotic, antifungal, and antituberculous agents have been associated with *C. difficile* colitis.[205] Although healthy children older than 1 year and healthy adults rarely carry the organisms, as many as two thirds of neonates can be demonstrated to have both *C. difficile* and its cytotoxins in their stool.[205] This high frequency of colonization and the presence of cytotoxin have led to skepticism about the pathogenic potential of this organism in neonates.

CLINICAL MANIFESTATIONS

Although the cause of diarrhea in infants and children may be suspected on clinical grounds, usually this is not possible in newborn infants. As a general rule, diarrhea caused by enteropathogenic strains of *E. coli* is insidious in onset, is associated with 7 to 10 green watery stools daily, and generally is without blood or mucus. These infants do not appear to be acutely ill. Complications rarely occur and primarily are related to dehydration and electrolyte disturbances. *Shigella* infection seldom occurs, usually is episodic in neonates, and generally does not spread within nurseries.[211] Shigellosis in a newborn may occur as a diarrheic or dysenteric syndrome or may be evidenced only by a septic- or toxic-appearing infant. Suppurative complications are rare events, but dehydration and electrolyte disturbances are common and need immediate and constant attention. *C. jejuni* infection typically involves the gastrointestinal tract and produces watery diarrhea or a dysentery-like illness with fever and bloody mucoid stools. Extraintestinal infections related to *C. jejuni*, other than bacteremia, are rare occurrences but include cholecystitis, urinary tract infection, and meningitis.[205] The clinical manifestations in neonates with *C. fetus* infection are similar to those caused by the common neonatal pathogens.[205] *C. jejuni* has been reported to cause bloody diarrhea in otherwise asymptomatic neonates.[84]

A useful procedure for differentiating enteroinvasive from enterotoxigenic diarrhea is examination of fecal material for polymorphonuclear cells. Feces from many patients with dysentery show significant numbers of polymorphonuclear leukocytes, whereas those from patients with enterotoxigenic disease usually show few neutrophils.

TREATMENT

The most important aspect of therapy for diarrheal disease of newborn infants is maintenance of hydration and electrolyte balance. As a rule, parenteral solutions containing appropriate electrolytes should be administered during the time of active diarrhea, and the infant should be examined and weighed frequently to ensure that proper rehydration has been achieved and to prevent the development of complications. Estimates of fluid loss from diarrhea and vomiting should be recorded carefully and used as a basis for replacement therapy.

Selection of appropriate antimicrobial therapy depends in part on the mechanism of diarrhea. In general, an orally administered, absorbable antibiotic such as ampicillin or trimethoprim-sulfamethoxazole is indicated for disease caused by invasive bacteria (e.g., shigellosis), whereas orally administered, nonabsorbable drugs such as neomycin and colistin sulfate are used for noninvasive organisms that produce enterotoxin (e.g., some *E. coli*).

Antimicrobial therapy for uncomplicated *Salmonella* gastroenteritis is controversial. We do not recommend antibiotics for most infants and children with uncomplicated *Salmonella* disease because such therapy does not shorten the course of illness and can be associated with an increased likelihood of prolonged asymptomatic excretion of the organism. However, neonates and infants younger than 3 or 4 months should be treated with a 7-day course of amoxicillin because of their propensity for the development of a protracted illness or bloodstream invasion with distant foci of infection.[130] Trimethoprim-sulfamethoxazole is a suitable alternative for ampicillin-resistant strains. The asymptomatic carrier state requires no therapy.

Ampicillin formerly was the antibiotic of choice for shigellosis, but in recent years significant resistance to this agent has been observed in many areas of the country. Some strains are susceptible to trimethoprim-sulfamethoxazole in a daily dosage of 10 mg of trimethoprim and 50 mg of sulfamethoxazole per kilogram per day in two divided doses. Sulfa drugs are contraindicated in newborns with jaundice. For multiresistant *Shigella* strains, some authorities recommend third-generation cephalosporins given parenterally (e.g., ceftriaxone) or orally (e.g., cefixime).

Erythromycin is the preferred drug for treating symptomatic *C. jejuni* enteritis. Frequently, if erythromycin therapy is initiated within the first 4 days of illness, excretion of the organism is reduced and symptoms resolve rapidly. An aminoglycoside is the drug of choice for treating *C. fetus* infections; chloramphenicol is an alternative.

Any infant with diarrhea must be isolated from other babies in the nursery. Surveillance of all infants in contact with the index case and institution of infection control measures are mandatory, as discussed earlier.

Probiotics (generally strains of *Bifidobacterium*, *Lactobacillus*, or *Saccharomyces*) have been used for the treatment of acute gastroenteritis with beneficial results. In murine experiments, however, administration of probiotic has shown the potential to causes sepsis in athymic mice, thus suggesting that the presence of immune deficiency in neonates may put them at risk for development of probiotic-induced sepsis. Accordingly, its use is not recommended at present.[76]

URINARY TRACT INFECTIONS

The incidence of bacteriuria in newborn infants ranges from 0.5 to 1 percent for term infants and is approximately 3 percent for premature infants.[348] Urinary tract infections occur more commonly in babies born to bacteriuric mothers and in boys during the neonatal period. The latter observation contrasts with the preponderance of infection in girls beyond the first months of life. The frequency of urinary tract infection and bacteremia is significantly higher in uncircumcised male neonates and young infants.[522] Circumcision reduces the frequency of urinary tract infection by approximately 90 percent. Bacterial colonization of both the prepuce and female perineum may occur because of the presence of maternal urinary tract infection. This prevalence was shown in a study in which 24 percent of infants were bacteriuric when delivered by mothers who had bacteriuria, whereas control infants whose mothers had not been bacteriuric had no bacteri-

uria. Clinical pyelonephritis occurred in 3 percent of these bacteriuric infants, but only 0.2 percent of 500 control infants of nonbacteriuric mothers had pyelonephritis.[375]

ETIOLOGY

E. coli is the most common etiologic agent of urinary tract infections and accounts for approximately 90 percent of acute infections and 70 to 80 percent of recurrent disease. Approximately 70 percent of *E. coli* strains belong to one of eight common somatic (O) antigen groups, similar to those found in older persons. Several capsular polysaccharide antigens (K1, K2, K12, and K13) are found more often in children with upper tract disease than in those with cystitis.[250,520] The association between K1 antigen and upper tract disease is found significantly more often in newborn and young infants than in older infants and children with *E. coli* urinary tract infection.[520] Fimbriated *E. coli* can attach to specific receptors or uroepithelial cells. Glycolipids of the P blood group constitute a specific receptor that is thought to be associated with pyelonephritis in patients who do not have reflux. When compared with asymptomatic bacteriuric infants, those with febrile urinary tract infections were found to have significantly increased inflammatory signs (e.g., C-reactive protein, microsedimentation rate) and attaching *E. coli*.[304] This finding suggests that bacterial properties determine not only the location of the urinary tract infection but also the severity of inflammation in individual patients.

Proteus, *Klebsiella*, and *Pseudomonas* spp. are encountered in patients with recurrent disease, particularly those receiving prolonged antimicrobial prophylaxis. Gram-positive bacteria, with the exception of enterococci, rarely are encountered as pathogens for the urinary tract. Only a few neonatal cases of renal abscess have been reported in the literature. *S. aureus* and coliforms were the predominant etiologic agents.[466]

CLINICAL MANIFESTATIONS

Most infants with significant bacteriuria are asymptomatic or have nonspecific signs and symptoms. The neonate may appear septic or may have decreased activity, feeding problems, and the other constitutional signs that are seen with infections of other organ systems. Jaundice, hepatomegaly, and thrombocytopenia may be observed in a few infants with urinary tract infection; these findings are associated with septicemia or cholestatic hepatitis in some babies.[50] Localizing signs suggesting urinary tract involvement are unusual findings. When present, they usually consist of a weak urinary stream on voiding or an abdominal tumor from bladder distention, hydronephrosis, or both.

DIAGNOSIS

The diagnosis of urinary tract infection is confirmed by examination and culture of urine. The results of these tests depend largely on the method of urine collection. Most pediatricians obtain urine with a sterile, plastic receptacle applied to the cleansed perineum. However, urine obtained by this method may have an elevated cell count because of recent circumcision, vaginal reflux of urine, or contamination from the perineum. Neonatal asphyxia also may increase the urine cell count. WBCs must be differentiated from round epithelial cells, which appear in the urine in significant numbers during the early days of life. Although pyuria commonly accompanies significant bacteriuria, cells can be few or absent. Direct microscopic examination of uncentrifuged, fresh urine is useful. If bacteria are seen readily in each high-power field, they generally number greater than 10^5 cells/mL.

Glitter cells are thought by many physicians to be diagnostic of urinary tract infection.

Quantitative urine cultures from infants with documented disease usually contain more than 100,000 colonies/mL of a single bacterial species. Any number of bacteria in a urine specimen obtained by percutaneous needle puncture of the bladder should be considered significant. This latter procedure is the single best source of urine for culture and is safe in most newborn infants.[343] The procedure should not be performed in infants who are dehydrated or have bleeding problems. Minor, transient hematuria is an uncommon occurrence, and serious problems from hemorrhage or perforation of the bowel have been rare events. If a "bagged urine specimen" contains fewer than 100,000 colonies/mL of a single species of bacteria or if the culture yields a mixed bacterial population, a repeat urine specimen should be obtained by suprapubic bladder aspiration or catheterization for culture.

Examination of the urinary sediment for antibody-coated bacteria has been found to be useful in differentiating upper tract disease from cystitis in adult patients.[247] Some reports have suggested, however, that this technique is not applicable to infants and children.[520] These studies have demonstrated false-positive and false-negative rates of approximately 30 percent. Because acute pyelonephritis is associated with enlargement of the kidneys secondary to edema and acute inflammatory infiltrate of the medulla and pelvis, ultrasound volume measurements of the kidneys provide a noninvasive method for identifying the probable site of urinary tract infection.[243] Fifteen of 18 children with upper urinary tract infection had increases in volume of 30 percent or greater in at least one kidney, whereas only 4 of 21 children with lower urinary tract infection had increases of greater than 30 percent ($p < .005$).

TREATMENT

Blood and urine should be obtained for culture from all newborn infants with suspected or proven urinary tract infection before antimicrobial therapy is initiated. Antibiotics initially are administered parenterally because sepsis is associated with urinary tract infection in 20 to 30 percent of infants[180] and absorption of antibiotics after oral administration is erratic in some babies. Therapy is initiated with an aminoglycoside and ampicillin to provide antibacterial coverage for the anticipated coliforms, enterococci, and GBS. If the patient has renal impairment, ampicillin and cefotaxime constitute an alternative empiric regimen. Because urine concentrations of these drugs exceed the MIC values of the urinary pathogens manyfold, the usual dosages may be reduced after septicemia has been ruled out.[312] Infants with renal or perirenal abscesses require percutaneous drainage under sonographic guidance or open surgical drainage if the former fails.

A repeat urine culture performed 48 to 72 hours after initiation of appropriate therapy should be sterile or show a substantial reduction in the bacterial count. Infants with persistent bacteriuria should be evaluated for the possibility of inappropriate therapy, obstruction, or perinephric abscess. In uncomplicated disease, therapy usually is continued for a period of 7 to 10 days. Approximately 1 week after discontinuance of therapy, a repeat urine culture is performed.

All infants with documented infection should undergo radiologic evaluation of the urinary tract. An intravenous pyelogram or renal sonograph is obtained during the course of therapy to rule out the possibility of gross congenital abnormalities of the urinary system. Renal sonography is preferred over intravenous pyelography in the acute phase of disease. Congenital malformations are unusual findings in the first week of life but may be present in a significant proportion of infants with urinary tract infections after this age. If obstruction is demonstrated, urologic procedures to ensure proper drainage are mandatory if therapy is to be successful. A voiding cystourethrogram or a radionuclide cystourethrogram should be obtained several weeks after therapy is discontinued. Radiologic abnormalities are found in approximately 45 percent of infants, especially in girls.[69,180]

Physicians have the responsibility of ascertaining that neonates with urinary tract infections do not have congenital abnormalities of the urinary system.[402] In these patients, recurrent urinary tract infections are common events, and physical growth may be retarded until definitive surgery has been performed. Every infant with urinary tract infection should undergo long-term follow-up studies for detection of recurrent infections, many of which are asymptomatic.

Infants found to have anatomic abnormalities (e.g., vesicoureteral reflux) must be protected from reinfection by prophylactic administration of trimethoprim-sulfamethoxazole or nitrofurantoin, and urine cultures or urinary nitrite tests should be performed soon thereafter for children. Although no absolute medical indication exists for routine circumcision of the newborn, cumulative data suggest that circumcision protects against urinary tract infections during early infancy.[523] When compared with the complications of urinary tract infections, short-term complications of circumcision are rare occurrences and mostly minor.[522]

SUPPURATIVE ARTHRITIS AND OSTEOMYELITIS

Osteomyelitis and suppurative arthritis rarely occur in the first 4 weeks of life. The incidence has not changed for many years and is estimated to be one to three cases of bone or joint infections per 1000 nursery admissions. A review of osteoarticular infections from Dallas, Texas, revealed 18 cases (3%) of neonatal arthritis and 18 cases (5%) of osteomyelitis out of 632 arthritis and 365 osteomyelitis cases in infants and children managed from 1959 to 1986.[343] Male infants are affected more often than female infants are (1.6:1), and the incidence is higher in premature than in term infants.

Bone and joint infections can be difficult to detect in neonates and young infants. Early establishment of the diagnosis and appropriate management are vital in preventing orthopedic abnormalities later in life.

ETIOLOGY AND PATHOGENESIS

The infecting organisms in osteomyelitis and septic arthritis vary, but the predominant ones are *S. aureus*, GBS, and gram-negative enteric organisms such as *Klebsiella*, *Proteus*, and *E. coli*. In a study of neonates in Dallas, Texas, *S. aureus* was the etiologic agent in 50 and 44 percent of cases of osteomyelitis and arthritis, respectively, whereas streptococci were responsible for 6 and 22 percent of such cases, respectively. GBS has become the single most common agent associated with arthritis in many areas of the United States.[164] Osteomyelitis and arthritis caused by gram-negative enteric bacilli have remained uncommon events despite the frequency of neonatal bacteremia caused by these organisms. Coliforms caused 11 percent of cases in Dallas and 5 percent in a children's hospital in Stockholm.[45] In Africa and Asia, rates as high as 45 percent have been described.[273] We reported that coliforms and *S. aureus* accounted for two thirds of isolates in neonates with osteoarticular infections in Panama.[424] Gonococcal arthritis and tenosynovitis were common occurrences in previous decades, but they are seen only occasionally today.[117] Other causative agents associated infrequently with newborn infection are *Salmonella*, *Pseudomonas*, *C. albicans*, and *U. urealyticum*.[123,385,386]

Osteomyelitis and arthritis have been reported in newborns after several invasive procedures, including heel puncture, femoral venipuncture, exchange transfusions, fetal monitoring with electrodes, serial lumbar puncture, and umbilical artery catheterization.[18,48,290,342,364,386,391] Osteomyelitis of cranial bones has complicated infected cephalohematomas. The use of peripheral and central intravascular catheters in neonates has been associated with the development of bacterial and fungal osteomyelitis.[148] Septic embolization from catheter tip thrombi, together with local hypoxia from partial occlusion of the vessel by the catheter, may explain this association.[164,291] A very strong correlation exists between the site of the catheter and localization of infection in the limb; for example, the knees and hips are involved in most cases associated with aortic catheters.[291] Usually, the origin is unknown and presumed to be hematogenous.

During the infant's first month of life, the epiphyseal plate is traversed by multiple small transepiphyseal vessels that provide direct communication between the articular space and the metaphysis of the long bones.[356] As a result, infection of the metaphysis (i.e., osteomyelitis) can spread across the growth plate and penetrate the epiphysis or enter the joint space. Because the perforating vessels disappear when the child is approximately 1 year of age, septic arthritis usually is not associated with osteomyelitis in older infants and children. The two exceptions to this rule are osteomyelitis of the proximal ends of the femur and humerus. The capsule of the hip and shoulder attaches below the proximal metaphysis of the femur and humerus, respectively. Infection of the epiphyseal cartilage may rupture through the periosteum, enter the joint space, and produce purulent arthritis. Because the capsular articulation of the hip and shoulder is permanent, osteomyelitis and septic arthritis may coexist, thus rendering the origin of infection difficult to establish.

The large vascular spaces and thin spongy structure of the metaphyseal cortex in infants permit early decompression of the primary abscess into the subperiosteal space. The abscess then dissects rapidly between the loosely attached periosteum. As pressure increases from the accumulating pus, a subcutaneous abscess can develop that may point and drain spontaneously through the skin and form a sinus tract. Free communication between the original site of osteomyelitis and the subperiosteal space prevents the necrosis and extensive spread of infection within bone that occurs frequently in older children and adults.

CLINICAL MANIFESTATIONS

Two distinct clinical syndromes that may be associated with osteomyelitis in the newborn period have been described.[132,199,490] The first is a benign form in which the earliest sign of bone and joint infection in newborns is failure to move an extremity spontaneously or apparent pain on movement without systemic evidence of infection. Swelling, erythema, and heat localized to the affected part are late findings. Multiple bones or joints can be involved, especially when disease is caused by *S. aureus*. The striking feature of this form is the satisfactory general condition of the infant despite the intensity of the local process. The fatality rate is exceedingly low, and healing is prompt. The second syndrome, a severe form, is characterized by systemic manifestations of sepsis; only later are multiple sites of bone and visceral involvement noted.

Two other clinical entities unique to the newborn are maxillary bone involvement and osteomyelitis caused by GBS. Maxillitis or osteomyelitis of the superior maxilla is an unusual form of bone infection in newborn infants.[289,290] More than 85 percent of all maxillary infections in infants take place in the first 3 months of life, with the peak incidence occurring in the second to fourth weeks.[303] Swelling of the cheek, associated with unilateral nasal discharge of pus, and swelling of the alveolar ridge of the maxilla should alert the physician to this entity. Initially,

dacryocystitis or orbital cellulitis may be suspected. The etiologic agent usually is *S. aureus*. Septicemia and death occur commonly in untreated cases.

Group B streptococcal osteomyelitis is manifested during the third and fourth weeks of life (i.e., late onset) and is caused predominantly by type III strains. It affects girls more often than boys, and the humerus is the most common site of involvement. In contrast to the fulminant onset and poor outcome that occur in some infants with late-onset meningitis, group B streptococcal bone and joint infection has an indolent nature and an almost uniformly good outcome. Occasionally, a diagnosis of Erb palsy may be entertained when inflammatory signs are minimal and diminished use of an arm is marked. Manipulations known to predispose neonates to bone and joint infections caused by other organisms have not been reported in infants with group B streptococcal arthritis or osteomyelitis.[299]

DIAGNOSIS

Conventional radiography remains the most useful means of establishing the diagnosis in patients with suspected suppurative arthritis; radiographs may be normal or show enlargement of the joint space. Later in the course of disease, subluxation and destruction of the joint are common findings. In early osteomyelitis, the normal radiographic water markings of tissues adjacent to the affected bone may be obliterated, an indication of deep-tissue inflammation and swelling. Lifting of the periosteum also may be observed, but cortical bone destruction seldom occurs before the second week of illness. A complete skeletal survey should be performed because of the frequent involvement of multiple sites.[164,329] In approximately 10 percent of patients, radiographic abnormalities are not seen during the course of disease. Although radionuclide bone scans are useful in establishing an early diagnosis of osteomyelitis in infants and children, they can be normal in newborn and young infants with confirmed infection. A report indicates a sensitivity of 90 percent for three-phase bone scintigraphy in the diagnosis of neonatal osteomyelitis.[5] Magnetic resonance imaging has been used successfully for establishing the diagnosis of osteomyelitis in the newborn period.

Blood should be obtained for culture from all infants with osteomyelitis or septic arthritis. In view of the varied etiologic bacteria, obtaining specimens of bone or a joint aspirate for culture is imperative, as is percutaneous needle aspiration of intra-articular pus in patients with suspected suppurative arthritis or aspiration of sequestrum in those with suspected osteomyelitis. If pus is obtained, the material should be Gram-stained and cultured.

TREATMENT

Selection of initial antimicrobial therapy is guided by preliminary identification of the pathogen from stained smears of material obtained by needle aspiration. If no microorganisms are seen, initiating treatment with two drugs, a penicillinase-resistant penicillin (e.g., nafcillin, oxacillin) and cefotaxime, is advisable. Vancomycin should be added if MRSA is a possibility. Use of an aminoglycoside with the antistaphylococcal penicillin does not provide adequate coverage for GBS. Definitive treatment is based on culture and susceptibility results. Direct instillation of an antibiotic into the joint space is unnecessary because most drugs penetrate the inflamed synovium and adequate concentrations are achieved in purulent material.[344] The same applies to treatment of osteomyelitis; direct instillation of antibiotics into acutely inflamed bone is unnecessary.[488]

Surgical removal of infected material is an integral part of treatment. Open drainage is essential for managing septic hip disease. The inflammation in osteomyelitis or septic arthritis can occupy the epiphyseal and metaphyseal sides of the growth plate and result in ischemia and necrosis of the plate and permanent orthopedic damage. For other joints, repeated daily evacuation of fluid with a needle and syringe usually is adequate. In patients with osteomyelitis, the subperiosteal space and the metaphysis should be drained if pus is obtained during diagnostic aspiration. If only a small amount of bloody material is obtained at aspiration, surgery does not need to be performed immediately, and the patient generally can be managed with antibiotic therapy alone as long as the local and systemic signs resolve. If improvement is unsatisfactory, repeat aspiration or open surgical drainage may need to be performed.

Antimicrobial treatment of neonatal musculoskeletal infections caused by staphylococci or coliform organisms is continued for a minimum of 3 to 6 weeks. Group B streptococcal infection is treated with penicillin G or ampicillin for at least 2 weeks. Ten days of therapy usually is adequate for treating gonococcal infection. Use of oral antibiotics as a substitute for parenteral therapy during the second and third weeks of treatment is unwise unless compliance can be ensured and serum bactericidal activity or the antibiotic concentration is satisfactory, which indicates adequate absorption of the orally administered drug. Parenteral antibiotic therapy can be administered at home if the infant can be assessed routinely by a physician.

As a general rule, systemic symptoms disappear within several days of initiation of therapy and adequate surgical drainage, although such local signs as heat, erythema, and swelling may persist for 4 to 7 days. Full range of motion may not return to the involved limb for several months. The erythrocyte sedimentation rate is a useful guide for determining the duration of therapy. The rate usually returns to within the normal range within 2 to 4 weeks; in contrast, C-reactive protein becomes normal sooner. As reported for older infants and children, serial determinations of C-reactive protein may be valuable in assessing the clinical course, but experience is inadequate to use this test in guiding the duration of antimicrobial therapy for neonatal osteoarticular infections.[407] Complete resolution of the radiographic changes may take several months.

Physical therapy to ensure full range of motion should be started as soon as the pain has abated. Assessing residual joint abnormalities and abnormal bone growth patterns in infants frequently is difficult until many months or years have passed. Maintaining good long-term follow-up after treatment has concluded is important.

CONJUNCTIVITIS AND ORBITAL CELLULITIS

Infections of the eye of the newborn can be caused by a variety of microorganisms, including *Neisseria gonorrhoeae*, *Chlamydia trachomatis*, *S. aureus*, and *P. aeruginosa*. From a review of more than 300 eye infections in newborns at Grady Memorial Hospital in Atlanta, Georgia,[16] researchers determined that 29 percent were caused by *Chlamydia*, 14 percent by gonococci, 10 percent by staphylococci, 2 percent by chemical reactions, and 1 percent by mixed gonococcal and chlamydial infections. The remaining 44 percent were of uncertain cause. A prospective, controlled study found that the major microbial causes of neonatal conjunctivitis were *Haemophilus* spp. in 17 percent, *S. aureus* in 17 percent, *C. trachomatis* in 14 percent, *S. pneumoniae* in 11 percent, and enterococci in 8 percent.[428] Other less frequently encountered organisms included *M. catarrhalis*, *Pasteurella multocida*, *N. meningitidis*, and herpes simplex virus.

The incidence of ophthalmia neonatorum has not paralleled the large increase in gonococcal disease rates among adolescent and young adults, almost certainly a result of universal neonatal prophylaxis with 1 percent silver nitrate solution, antibiotic ointment, or systemic penicillin G. Today, we rarely see the invasive,

destructive ophthalmitis described so vividly in the early literature.[151]

Numerous agents have been shown to be effective prophylactically against gonococci. The largest series was published by Greenberg and Vandow[198] and involved 250,000 infants treated with 1 percent silver nitrate. A failure rate of 6.6 per 100,000 infants treated with silver nitrate compared favorably with the rate of 22.5 per 100,000 in 86,000 infants who received no prophylaxis. Of the topical antimicrobial agents, tetracycline or erythromycin appears to be comparable in efficacy to silver nitrate and has the advantage of causing fewer cases of chemical conjunctivitis.[361] Penicillin applied topically or given intramuscularly also is effective, although the ointment no longer is available commercially. Bacitracin ointment is ineffective.[110,306] Ceftriaxone as a single dose of 50 mg/kg (for low-birth-weight infants, 25 to 50 mg/kg) can be useful for prophylaxis when the risk is high. Infants born to mothers with active gonorrhea should receive a single 125-mg dose of ceftriaxone intravenously or intramuscularly. Ceftriaxone should not be given to hyperbilirubinemic infants, especially premature ones.

A study by Hammerschlag and associates[211] showed that neonatal ocular prophylaxis with erythromycin or tetracycline ophthalmic ointment does not reduce the incidence of chlamydial conjunctivitis significantly in the offspring of mothers with *Chlamydia* infection when compared with silver nitrate. The investigators concluded that better management of maternal *Chlamydia* infection is required if the incidence of conjunctivitis caused by this organism is to be reduced. They suggested that a small but appreciable incidence of neonatal gonococcal ophthalmia could be prevented by performing better prenatal screening and treating maternal gonococcal infections.

DIAGNOSIS

Any infant with a conjunctival discharge should be evaluated carefully to determine the cause. Three tests should be performed: Gram and methylene blue stain of the exudate, culture of the exudate, and Giemsa stain and culture for *Chlamydia*, if available, of scrapings made from the lower palpebral conjunctiva after the exudate has been removed. The results of the stained smears determine the appropriate therapy. Direct detection of chlamydial antigens in eye scrapings now is possible by means of a commercially available enzyme-linked immunoassay (e.g., Chlamydiazyme). Limited experience in neonates suggests that it is a sensitive and specific test that can provide rapid and reliable results.[213]

DIFFERENTIAL DIAGNOSIS

Conjunctivitis occurring in the first days of life can be chemical or bacterial. Chemical irritants, such as silver nitrate, cause transient conjunctival hyperemia and a watery discharge that rarely turns purulent.

Gonococcal ophthalmia usually becomes apparent within the first 5 days of life and is characterized initially by a clear watery discharge. Conjunctival hyperemia and chemosis are associated with a copious discharge of thick, white purulent material. Both eyes generally are involved, though not necessarily to the same degree. Untreated gonococcal ophthalmia may extend to involve the cornea (i.e., keratitis) and the anterior chamber of the eye. Corneal perforation and blindness can result. Before adequate prophylactic measures were introduced, ophthalmia neonatorum was the most frequent cause of acquired blindness in the United States.

If gram-negative rods are seen in the stained exudate, the greatest concern is *P. aeruginosa* because of the virulent necrotizing endophthalmitis that can result. In this condition, a relatively mild conjunctivitis can progress to infection of the entire globe within 12 to 24 hours. Invasion of the cornea by small blood vessels (pannus) is characteristic of *Pseudomonas* conjunctivitis. Perforation of the cornea may occur, and blindness from corneal opacity occurs commonly. The ophthalmic disease occasionally can be followed by bacteremia and septic foci in other organs.[86] Prompt diagnosis and immediate institution of appropriate antimicrobial therapy are mandatory.[86]

Conjunctivitis during the second or third week of life can be caused by viral, bacterial, or chlamydial agents. Viral conjunctivitis frequently is associated with other symptoms of respiratory tract disease, such as rhinorrhea, cough, and rash, and several individuals in the family or nursery may have disease simultaneously. The discharge in viral conjunctivitis usually is watery or mucopurulent but rarely purulent. A hemorrhagic discharge can be seen with adenoviral infection. Preauricular adenopathy is a common finding. Staphylococci, streptococci, *Haemophilus*, and occasionally gonococci cause conjunctivitis in this age group. A smear of purulent material helps differentiate these bacterial agents. However, the presence of bacteria on a Gram-stained smear of exudate is not necessarily related etiologically to the conjunctivitis. The exudate may contain normal inhabitants of the skin and mucous membranes, such as staphylococci, diphtheroids, and *Neisseria* spp.

Chlamydial eye infection may begin on the first days of life but usually does not come to the attention of the physician until the second or third week. Conjunctivitis develops in approximately a third of infants exposed to *Chlamydia* during vaginal delivery.[127] Clinical manifestations of chlamydial infection (inclusion blennorrhea) vary from mild conjunctivitis to intense inflammation and swelling of the lids in conjunction with a copious purulent discharge.[190,411] Pseudomembrane formation and a diffuse "matte" injection of the tarsal conjunctiva are common findings. The cornea rarely is affected, and preauricular adenopathy is an unusual occurrence. In the early stages of disease, one eye may appear more swollen and infected than the other, but both eyes are involved almost invariably.

The diagnosis is established by scraping the tarsal conjunctiva and looking for typical cytoplasmic inclusions within epithelial cells (not in the exudate). Exudates are not sufficient for *Chlamydia* testing because specimens must contain epithelial cells that harbor the infecting organism. Newborns with conjunctivitis should have specimens obtained from both the conjunctiva and pharynx.[127]

Specially prepared tissue culture cells for *Chlamydia* are available in some centers, and immunoassays are available commercially for a rapid and specific diagnosis. The conjunctival material obtained is layered carefully onto a microscope slide and stained by the Giemsa method. Without treatment, the acute inflammation continues for several weeks and merges into a subacute phase of slight conjunctival infection with scant purulent material. Occasionally, chronicity develops; some cases persist for longer than a year. The PCR method is used comparably for detection of *C. trachomatis* in conjunctival and nasopharyngeal specimens from infants with conjunctivitis.[214]

TREATMENT

Initial therapy is based on the results of stained smears of exudate and epithelial cells. If gonococci are seen, parenteral penicillin or ceftriaxone therapy is administered. If staphylococci are detected, nafcillin or another penicillinase-resistant penicillin analogue is used. The necessity of using topical antibiotics in these two bacterial infections is dubious. In the presence of acute inflammation, ample antibiotic is present in eye secretions to inhibit bacteria.

Since the beginning of the 1980s, gonococci resistant to penicillin have appeared in the United States and other parts of the world.[139,396] These strains are susceptible to spectinomycin, erythromycin, and the new-generation cephalosporins (e.g., ceftriaxone, cefotaxime). Experience in treating gonococcal ophthalmia with these drugs is limited, as are pharmacologic data for spectinomycin in newborns. Infants with documented gonococcal infections at any site, including the eye, should be examined for disseminated gonococcal infection. This investigation should include a careful physical examination, especially of the joints, and evaluation of blood and CSF cultures. Term, nonhyperbilirubinemic infants with gonococcal ophthalmia should be treated for 4 to 7 days with ceftriaxone (50 mg/kg given intravenously or intramuscularly every 24 hours). Limited data suggest that uncomplicated gonococcal ophthalmia in infants can be cured with a single injection of ceftriaxone (50 mg/kg, up to 125 mg). If the gonococcal isolate is susceptible to penicillin, crystalline penicillin G can be given. The dose is 100,000 U/kg/day given in two doses (or four doses in infants older than 1 week). The eye should be irrigated with buffered saline solution until the eye discharge has cleared. In patients who do not respond satisfactorily, co-infection with *Chlamydia* should be considered. The mother and infant should be tested routinely for *Chlamydia* infection.

Pseudomonas eye infection always should be treated with parenteral therapy consisting of ticarcillin or ceftriaxone and gentamicin. Gentamicin ophthalmic drops are used for simple *Pseudomonas* conjunctivitis, and subtenon injections of gentamicin may be indicated for endophthalmitis.[185]

Orally administered erythromycin (50 mg/kg/day in four divided doses for 14 days) is superior to topically applied tetracycline or sodium sulfacetamide in the treatment of chlamydial conjunctivitis. Topical therapy suppresses chlamydial growth only, whereas erythromycin eradicates the organism in most patients. Topical and oral erythromycin regimens have comparable efficacy, but oral therapy has the advantage of eradicating nasopharyngeal carriage of *Chlamydia*.[373] Although infantile hypertropic pyloric stenosis has been associated with erythromycin administered orally to infants younger than 6 months old, erythromycin remains the antibiotic of choice for the treatment of *C. trachomatis* disease in infants.[228] Eight infants with documented chlamydial conjunctivitis were treated with azithromycin (20 mg/kg once daily for 3 days); failure to eradicate the organism occurred in three patients, but compliance was doubtful in these cases.[212] In infants who do not tolerate erythromycin, oral sulfisoxazole (150 mg/kg/day in four divided doses) can be used after the immediate newborn period. Most cases heal without residua, but if not treated, infection may persist and cause corneal and conjunctival scarring.[127,191] Approximately 25 percent of infants with gonococcal ophthalmia have concomitant infection with *Chlamydia* that requires therapy.

Patients with gonococcal ophthalmia should be segregated, and strict handwashing techniques should be used because the exudate is highly contagious.

CUTANEOUS AND GLANDULAR INFECTIONS

PUSTULAR AND VESICULAR LESIONS

Superficial pustular staphylococcal disease (i.e., impetigo neonatorum) is the most common skin infection of neonates. The lesions tend to concentrate in the periumbilical and diaper areas and rarely become invasive, except when extensive areas are involved or when monitoring devices, catheters, or other invasive devices are used in a gravely ill infant. The lesions respond to simple topical measures; systemic antibiotic treatment usually is not indicated unless extensive involvement of the skin occurs.

The organisms should be phage-typed (they usually belong to group I) so that if additional cases are encountered in the same nursery, the infected infants and their cohorts can be evaluated for the possibility of nosocomial staphylococcal disease. If these infections are caused by the same staphylococcal phage type, prompt measures should be instituted to determine the source and extent of infection to prevent further colonization and disease.

A second form of staphylococcal disease has been recognized with increased frequency in recent years. The disease takes one of several clinical forms, including bullous impetigo, the most common manifestation, and Ritter disease, the eponymic equivalent in newborns of toxic epidermal necrolysis of older infants.[321] These illnesses usually are caused by phage group II staphylococci, which produce an exotoxin (i.e., exfoliatin) that causes intraepidermal cleavage through the granular cell layer as a result of disruption of desmosomes.[322] The initial finding in Ritter disease is intense, painful erythema, not unlike a severe sunburn. During the next hours, bullus formation occurs, and when the bullae rupture, a tender, weeping, erythematous area is left. A characteristic desquamation of large epidermal sheets occurs approximately 3 to 5 days after onset of the illness. A finer desquamation commonly is seen periorally.

Bacteremic complications occur more commonly in neonates than in older infants with the scalded skin syndrome. Treatment consists of systemically administered, penicillinase-resistant penicillin because most phage group II staphylococci are resistant to penicillin. The cleavage plane in this syndrome is very superficial in the epidermis, so little risk for the development of superinfection exists. Steroids are contraindicated. Maceration may occur in intertriginous areas, which should be treated by local soaks with Burow solution.

CELLULITIS AND FASCIITIS

Group A streptococci are the usual cause of diffuse, well-demarcated cellulitis (or erysipelas), although we have seen the same diseases also caused by group B organisms. The involved skin usually is intensely red, hot, and moderately indurated. Occasionally, streptococci can be recovered from material aspirated from the lesion, but blood culture rarely is positive. Parenteral therapy is with penicillin G, and, although the borders continue to advance for the first 12 to 24 hours, stabilization of body temperature and improvement in general appearance of the infant give reassurance that the diagnosis and therapy are correct.

Necrotizing fasciitis is a virulent form of cellulitis that is a relatively rare event in newborns but has a case-fatality rate of up to 50 percent in this age group. Initially, it resembles uncomplicated cellulitis, but the baby rapidly becomes "toxic," the lesion advances progressively, and the central portion becomes discolored and anesthetic. The lesion has borders that generally are indistinct when compared with erysipelas, in which the borders are raised and palpated easily. The disease may be associated with surgical procedures, birth trauma, previous omphalitis, fetal monitoring, or cutaneous infection and has been reported after the infant has undergone circumcision. The abdominal wall is the usual site of involvement, but other areas such as the thorax, back, scalp, and extremities also can be involved.[234] Causative agents include several streptococci, *S. aureus*, *P. aeruginosa*, *E. coli*, and anaerobic bacteria.[394,514,521] In this condition, subcutaneous tissues, including muscle layers, are invaded, and the organism spreads along fascial planes. Extensive surgery involving resection of destroyed tissue is imperative in treating necrotizing fasciitis.[521] Blood and tissue cultures should be performed, and initial antibiotic therapy should consist of a penicillinase-resistant penicillin or clindamycin or vancomycin and an aminoglycoside, pending

results of these cultures. Hypocalcemia and hypoproteinemia may complicate the illness. If the infant survives the first days, extensive skin grafting generally is necessary. In a retrospective review, the overall mortality rate for 66 neonatal cases was 59 percent.[234] Having a high index of suspicion, performing prompt aggressive surgery, and providing appropriate antibiotics and optimal supportive care are the mainstays of management.[81,149,234] The role of adjuvant hyperbaric oxygen is controversial, and very limited information is available.

FUNISITIS AND OMPHALITIS

The umbilical cord may be colonized with numerous different potential bacterial pathogens, some of which may have significant epidemiologic importance. Hexachlorophene was used in many institutions in an attempt to reduce or eliminate the staphylococci that were responsible for nursery epidemics in the late 1950s and early 1960s. Although this antiseptic is effective in reducing staphylococcal colony counts, it is not effective in controlling nosocomial staphylococcal disease in nursery units. Widespread use of hexachlorophene occasionally has been associated with CNS spongiform degeneration, particularly in premature infants.[454] A single application of triple dye to the cord results in a significant reduction of all bacteria, particularly staphylococci, streptococci, and coliforms, but its use for care of the umbilical stump at home can delay the time until the cord separates.[99,347,384] Mupirocin ointment applied to the cord or the nasal mucosa also is effective in eradicating staphylococcal carriage.[226]

Group A streptococci may colonize the umbilical cord and be important as a focal point for epidemic streptococcal disease in a nursery. Unlike staphylococci, they tend to cause an inflammatory reaction.[134,347] Streptococcal funisitis (i.e., inflammation of the cord) is mild and is characterized by a wet, malodorous umbilical stump with minimal inflammation. Disseminated disease is an uncommon occurrence, but when present, it results from bloodstream invasion or direct extension to the peritoneal cavity by way of the umbilical vessels. Treatment consists of systemic penicillin G and topical therapy with antibiotic ointment or triple dye. Local therapy is provided for epidemiologic reasons to eliminate surface colonization. Identification of a single infant with group A streptococcal disease in a nursery necessitates immediate institution of infection control measures for identification and segregation of all colonized persons. When a nursery outbreak is suspected, specific M and T typing of the organism is useful in defining the source and spread of infection. A single injection of benzathine penicillin G is satisfactory for treatment of mild superficial infection or for elimination of the organism from colonized persons.[178,347]

Omphalitis, or infection of the umbilicus, has many causes and occurs more frequently in low-birth-weight infants and those with complicated deliveries. The incidence is estimated to be approximately 2 percent, and symptoms start at an average age of 3 days. Culture and susceptibility test results are necessary for the selection of an appropriate antibiotic. *S. aureus* is the most frequent pathogen isolated, followed by gram-negative rods.[433] Some of the complications secondary to omphalitis reported in the literature are spontaneous evisceration of the small bowel through the umbilical cicatrix, necrotizing fasciitis, small bowel obstruction, peritonitis, and superficial, retroperitoneal, or hepatic abscesses.[10,156,166]

BREAST ABSCESS

Breast abscesses are encountered most frequently during the second or third week of life and are more common findings in girls, particularly those older than 2 weeks.[414] The disease does not occur in premature infants, presumably because of underdevelopment of the mammary glands in these infants. Bilateral disease is a rare event, but a case caused by GBS has been reported.[345]

The major clinical finding is swelling of the affected breast with or without accompanying erythema and warmth. Systemic manifestations are uncommon occurrences, and only a fourth of patients have low-grade fever. The disease sometimes can progress rapidly and involve breast tissue and the entire subcutaneous tissue beyond the breast's anatomic area.[453] This condition is associated with considerable toxicity and systemic signs and symptoms. *S. aureus* is the major pathogen, but coliform bacteria and GBS have become more common causes in the past decade.[414,474] Mixed infection rarely occurs. In 36 infants with mastitis seen in Dallas, Texas, during a 16-year period, 32 cases were caused by *S. aureus*, 1 case by *E. coli*, 2 cases by *Salmonella* spp., and 1 case by both *S. aureus* and *E. coli*.

Breast abscess is diagnosed by examination of stained purulent material obtained from gentle manipulation of the nipple or by needle aspiration of the abscess. If gram-positive cocci are identified, nafcillin or another penicillinase-resistant penicillin is given. For gram-negative bacilli, an aminoglycoside or cefotaxime is appropriate. When no organisms are seen, nafcillin and an aminoglycoside or cefotaxime should be used initially until results of culture are available. Bacteremia is a rare finding in this condition.

If the patient has only mild cellulitis and no discernible fluctuance, antibiotic treatment alone may suffice. We have managed several patients with GBS mastitis successfully in this fashion. In most instances, however, surgical incision and drainage by a skilled surgeon are required. The duration of treatment depends on the rate of response. It generally is rapid, and we have found that healing is complete within 5 to 7 days in most instances. Long-term follow-up studies suggest that some girls will have diminished breast tissue on the affected side.[414]

SUPPURATIVE PAROTITIS

Suppurative parotitis of the newborn usually is easy to recognize, although occasionally it is confused with infection of a preauricular or superior anterior cervical lymph node. We have encountered one instance in which delay in initiating therapy was caused by attributing the swelling to trauma from obstetric forceps. Infection occurs more commonly in low-birth-weight infants than in term infants and boys. Dehydration predisposes to stasis of parotid secretions and subsequent infection. Bilateral infection is a rare event.

Although *S. aureus* accounts for most cases, disease may be caused by coliform bacteria, *Pseudomonas*, pneumococci, and group A streptococci.[129,279] The clinical manifestations include fever, anorexia, irritability, and failure to gain weight. Erythema, swelling, and tenderness over the involved gland may occur. The diagnosis can be confirmed by expressing pus through the parotid duct or by needle aspiration of a fluctuant area. Gram staining of this material helps identify the causative agent; however, one should recognize that material expressed from the duct may be contaminated by mouth microflora.

Selection of antimicrobial therapy should be based on interpretation of the Gram-stained smear of expressed pus. If gram-positive cocci are seen, nafcillin or another penicillinase-resistant penicillin should be used. Vancomycin should be added if MRSA is a possibility. Gram-negative organisms are treated best with an aminoglycoside, cefotaxime, or ceftazidime to cover both coliform bacteria and *Pseudomonas*. If no organisms are seen in the purulent material, a combination of nafcillin and gentamicin or

cefotaxime should be used until the results of culture are available. In most cases, antibiotic therapy alone suffices, and surgical incision and drainage are unnecessary. The gland should not be extirpated. Response to therapy generally is rapid. Most patients require only 7 to 10 days of therapy until healing is complete.

SCALP ABSCESS

Scalp abscesses usually are a complication of fetal monitoring with scalp electrodes.[82,504] The number of vaginal examinations, use of more than one electrode, and fetal scalp blood sampling are risk factors for the development of scalp abscesses. Pathogens incriminated include staphylococci, gonococci, and gram-negative enteric bacteria. A polymicrobial flora, including anaerobic organisms, frequently is isolated in scalp abscesses caused by electronic fetal monitoring electrodes. Incision and drainage of the infected site usually is sufficient. If an associated cellulitis occurs, antibiotics are administered and continued for 5 to 7 days.

LOWER RESPIRATORY TRACT INFECTIONS

Neonatal lower respiratory tract infections may be acquired congenitally or postnatally. Perinatal infection results from transplacental transfer of the agent (i.e., congenital infection) or from inhalation of infected amniotic fluid (usually associated with prolonged rupture of membranes) or infected vaginal secretions during delivery. Viruses, bacteria, *Chlamydia*, and spirochetes are the most common causative agents that produce perinatal pneumonia. Common viral agents include cytomegalovirus, rubella, and herpes simplex virus. Common bacterial agents are GBS, *L. monocytogenes*, and coliform bacilli. *Chlamydia* organisms have been implicated as the cause of a chronic interstitial pneumonitis of early infancy (i.e., eosinophilic pertussis-like pneumonia).[43] *Treponema pallidum* produces a severe, sometimes fatal pneumonitis, and mycoplasmas have caused a rare form of fatal congenital pneumonia. We also have seen in Panama in the last 4 years a few cases of congenital pneumonia caused by *Candida* spp. (unpublished observation).

Perinatal lower respiratory tract disease generally becomes apparent clinically in infants from birth to 7 days, occasionally up to 2 weeks of age. Of emphasis is that inhalation of amniotic fluid or maternal vaginal secretions usually is not associated with infection, nor is meconium inhalation, in which case the pneumonitis has a chemical cause. Only a small percentage of inhalation pneumonias are bacterial in origin; the pathogens most commonly encountered in such cases are GBS and coliform organisms. The clinical signs of inhalation pneumonia are caused by obstruction, chemical inflammation, or both.

The second category of pneumonia is acquired postnatally and usually beyond the first week of life. These diseases may be caused by viral or bacterial agents and most frequently are bronchopneumonic in type. Viral disease may be sporadic or occur as part of a nosocomial nursery outbreak. Respiratory syncytial virus is the most important pathogen of lower respiratory tract disease in young infants.[51] This agent causes particularly severe disease in infants with congenital heart disease. The parainfluenza viruses and adenoviruses also cause bronchiolitis and pneumonia during early infancy. An obliterating, necrotizing bronchiolitis may be caused by adenoviruses and result in radiographic hyperlucency of a segment or a lobe in later infancy and childhood.[184]

Documented nursery outbreaks of lower respiratory tract disease have been associated with respiratory syncytial virus, adenoviruses, echoviruses, influenza A and B viruses, and parainfluenza virus infections. During these outbreaks, many infants are colonized with the epidemic strains, but only a few have clinical disease.

Common bacterial pathogens causing postnatally acquired pneumonia are *S. aureus*, coliform bacilli, and *Pseudomonas*. These infections occur sporadically or epidemically and often are of nosocomial origin. They may be rapidly progressive, necrotic pneumonias that result in pyogenic complications (e.g., empyema, pulmonary abscesses) and metastatic disease in the bones or meninges.

CLINICAL MANIFESTATIONS

The early signs of respiratory disease in neonates and young infants frequently are nonspecific and include change in feeding status, listlessness or irritability, and poor color. More specific findings that may not be present at the onset of illness are tachypnea, dyspnea, cyanosis, alteration of temperature (i.e., hypothermia or fever), coughing, and grunting. Accentuation of the normal irregularity of breathing is a common finding in neonates.

The physical findings of pneumonia are variable. Flaring of the alae nasi, rapid respirations, and sternal and subcostal retractions are common findings. Coughing indicates lower respiratory tract involvement; brassy coughing is found frequently in viral disease. Dullness to percussion is difficult to demonstrate, but when present, it indicates consolidation or effusion. Breath sounds also may be diminished over the affected area. Crackles or wheezes usually can be heard on deep inspiration (or when the baby is crying) but may be absent early in disease. The clinician frequently is surprised by the meager clinical signs in the face of clearly demonstrable and sometimes extensive radiographic findings of pneumonitis.

DIAGNOSIS

The WBC count usually does not help differentiate viral from bacterial pneumonia. An exception is seen in premature infants with acute respiratory distress syndrome caused by GBS. In these patients, the WBC count often reveals leukopenia with an increased proportion of band forms.[308]

Cultures of blood and material from the trachea frequently help in defining the etiologic agent of neonatal pneumonia. Results of cultures of the ear canal, throat, and other external sites typically are unreliable in defining the cause of pneumonia; more often, they are misleading. Lung puncture should be considered for severely ill infants with consolidated pneumonia when the cause is unknown or for an infant who fails to respond to conventional antimicrobial therapy. Material obtained by needle aspiration is Gram-stained for direct visualization and cultured.

A chest radiograph should be obtained for all babies with suspected lower respiratory tract disease. Radiographic evidence of pneumonia may not exist in the absence of specific physical findings. Although the cause of neonatal pneumonia usually can be determined from a radiograph, certain radiologic patterns are associated with specific diseases. With acute-onset group B streptococcal disease, the radiograph may mimic one showing hyaline membrane disease. A consolidating bronchopneumonia with pneumatoceles, with or without empyema, suggests staphylococcal disease. When a lobar infiltrate is associated with expansion of the lobe, *K. pneumoniae* infection should be considered. A miliary type of bronchopneumonia in a septic neonate is characteristic of listeriosis.

SPECIFIC CLINICAL SYNDROMES

Staphylococcal Pneumonia

Primary staphylococcal pneumonia occurs quite frequently in young infants. Epidemics of staphylococcal disease caused by phage group I organisms are rare events today. In the epidemic setting, many infants are colonized with a virulent strain, but only a few have disease. Concomitant viral respiratory tract infections possibly play a role in promoting dissemination of staphylococci among infants and in converting colonization to disease, but such has not been established.

Staphylococci cause a confluent bronchopneumonia consisting of extensive areas of hemorrhagic necrosis and irregular areas of cavitation. The pleural surface usually is covered by a thick layer of fibrinopurulent exudate. Multiple, small abscesses are scattered throughout the affected lung. Rupture of a small subpleural abscess may result in pyopneumothorax. If erosion into a large bronchus occurs, a bronchopleural fistula results.

Most patients with staphylococcal pneumonia have radiographic evidence of bronchopneumonia early in the illness. The infiltrate may be patchy and limited in extent or dense and homogeneous and involve an entire lobe or hemithorax. Bilateral disease occurs in half of affected patients. Pleural effusion or empyema is detected in most infants. Pneumatoceles of various size are common findings. Although no radiographic picture can be considered absolutely diagnostic, progression over the course of a few hours from bronchopneumonia to empyema or pyopneumothorax, with or without pneumatoceles, strongly suggests staphylococcal disease.

Klebsiella pneumoniae Pneumonia

Primary *K. pneumoniae* infection is an unusual event in infants and young children. However, nursery epidemics of *Klebsiella* infection have been reported. During these epidemics, colonization rates are high, but most infants remain asymptomatic. Contaminated fomites are the primary source of nosocomial infection with this organism.

K. pneumoniae pneumonia may be difficult to distinguish clinically from pneumonia attributable to other causes. The disease may have a fulminant course characterized by copious, thick purulent secretions and the formation of pulmonary abscesses and cavitation. The case-fatality rate in sporadic cases is approximately 50 percent but is considerably lower during epidemics.

Pertussis

During 1994 to 2004, the reported pertussis rate per 100,000 inhabitants increased from 1.8 to 8.9. This is the highest figure since 1959. In 2004, 10 percent of the cases occurred in infants 6 months or younger; these infants were too young to have received the first three doses of diphtheria and tetanus toxoids and acellular pertussis (DTaP) vaccine. Adolescents and adults accounted for the majority (67%) of notified cases, which led to a recommendation by the CDC's Advisory Committee on Immunization Practices for the routine use of DTaP vaccine in adolescents aged 11 to 18 years.[96] Although infants formerly acquired disease from siblings, in the past years infection usually has been acquired from one or both parents whose illnesses have not been diagnosed correctly as pertussis. The reason for these epidemiologic changes most likely is better vaccination of schoolchildren. Because immunity starts to wane in adolescence, parents of young infants are susceptible to infection.[346] The infants of these women also are susceptible to the development of infection because of the lack of transplacental immunity.

The onset of disease generally is in the second to sixth weeks of life; the earliest onset reported was at 10 days of age. Most young infants do not have a characteristic whoop. Pertussis should be suspected when an infant has a paroxysmal cough with excessive mucus. Because apneic spells are common occurrences in these infants, as they also are in those with respiratory syncytial virus, *Chlamydia*, or influenza virus infection, all infants with pertussis are admitted to the hospital for management. Fluorescent antibody testing provides a means of making a rapid diagnosis, but false-negative and false-positive results are common occurrences. Cultures for *Bordetella* should be performed in all infants. PCR-based testing may become the most sensitive means of documenting *Bordetella pertussis* in the future. Mucus for examination is obtained from patients with a flexible nasopharyngeal wire swab or by nasopharyngeal washing or aspiration.

The greatest hazards to an infant with pertussis are asphyxia and secondary bacterial pneumonia. Supportive care is essential. Excessive mucus must be suctioned, and equipment for emergency airway intubation should be at hand. Administration of fluid therapy is necessary, and maintaining adequate nutritional intake may present the greatest challenge. Infants with pertussis should not be placed in mist tents. Mist therapy provides no substantial amelioration of paroxysmal coughing episodes, and it increases the risk for development of secondary infection with *P. aeruginosa* (or with other commensals).

Atelectasis caused by mucus plugs is a common complication of pertussis in small babies. After the infant has passed the stage of severe paroxysms, chest physiotherapy can be initiated. In almost all cases the atelectasis resolves within 2 to 3 weeks.

Chlamydial Pneumonia

Chlamydial pneumonia is manifested between the 4th and 11th weeks of life in most infants.[491] Infants typically are afebrile and tachypneic, and they have a characteristic staccato cough. Only half of the patients have a history of conjunctivitis. Otitis media occurs frequently.[127]

On chest auscultation, rales may be heard, but wheezes are uncommon findings. The chest radiograph reveals hyperexpanded lungs with bilateral interstitial infiltrates. Approximately half of the infants have peripheral eosinophilia (>400 cells/mm^3). A definitive diagnosis made by isolating the organism from the respiratory tract is not possible in many institutions. The role of immunologic techniques for identifying *Chlamydia* in throat swabs is yet to be determined. Serologic testing is available more readily. These infants usually respond to therapy with erythromycin. The clinical course and duration of nasopharyngeal shedding of *Chlamydia* are shortened by treatment with this antibiotic. If left untreated, these infants remain sick for several weeks but do not become acutely ill. Death from this infection seldom occurs.

TREATMENT

Initial antibiotic treatment of suspected bacterial pneumonia should consist of ampicillin or nafcillin and an aminoglycoside or cefotaxime. The most suitable combination of these drugs depends on the clinical features of the illness and the recent experience with bacterial diseases in the local nursery or community. For patients in whom the cause never is defined and staphylococcal disease cannot be ruled out, therapy with nafcillin or vancomycin and an aminoglycoside or cefotaxime is indicated. If the organism is identified, the single most effective drug should be used. Penicillin G or ampicillin is effective against GBS and penicillin-susceptible staphylococci, ampicillin against *Listeria*, and nafcillin or another suitable antistaphylococcal penicillin against penicillinase-producing *S. aureus*. Vancomycin should be used for disease caused by MRSA or coagulase-negative staphylococci. For pneumonia caused by gram-negative bacilli (e.g., *K. pneumoniae* and others), an aminoglycoside or a third-generation cephalosporin should be used. *Pseudomonas* pneumonia is treated best with ticarcillin or ceftazidime in combination with an aminoglycoside. Therapy is continued for 10 to 14 days for disease caused by GBS and *Listeria* and for a minimum of 3 weeks for pneumonia caused by staphylococci or gram-negative bacilli.

Nosocomial pneumonia is a relatively frequent condition of mechanically ventilated premature infants and can be caused by a vast array of microorganisms. Accordingly, treatment with an empiric regimen of broad-spectrum antibiotics is advised until microbial identification is made. Nonetheless, the physician should realize that isolation of bacteria from tracheal aspirates usually represents airway colonization and not necessarily the etiologic agents. For a reliable etiologic approach, a combination of clinical, radiographic, laboratory, and microbiologic findings is recommended. An important matter to recognize is that antimicrobial therapy commonly fails to eradicate microorganisms from the airway of ventilated infants despite clinical and radiographic resolution of pneumonia.[118]

Empyema is managed best by closed drainage and use of chest tubes with the largest possible caliber. Generally, placement of one tube high and anteriorly and a second tube low and posterolaterally is necessary to achieve optimal drainage. Pyopneumothorax is another indication for immediate insertion of a catheter into the pleural space. After the infant has improved clinically and the amount of drainage is minimal, the tubes should be removed. In general, they should not remain in the chest for more than 5 to 7 days. Instillation of antimicrobial agents or enzymes into the pleural space does not help control infection or promote drainage.

Pneumonia may be one manifestation of generalized congenital viral infection. Distinguishing these infections from congenital syphilis and bacterial pneumonia secondary to inhalation is important.

Most infants with inhalation pneumonia do not require antimicrobial therapy. Differentiating infants inhaling sterile fluid from those inhaling infected material frequently is difficult. If doubt exists, therapy with ampicillin and an aminoglycoside should be initiated and continued until the results of cultures are available.

Therapy for pertussis consists of erythromycin administered orally. Antibiotic therapy may lessen the symptoms of pertussis if administered early in the paroxysmal stage and is valuable for rendering the patient noncontagious. Hyperimmune serum probably is not beneficial.

Associations between bronchopulmonary dysplasia and respiratory colonization by *U. urealitycum*, *C. trachomatis*, *M. hominis*, and adenovirus have been shown in different studies.[57,120,216,506]

In a prospective cohort study, isolation of *U. urealyticum* from respiratory tract secretions was associated with radiographic evidence of pneumonia within 7 days of birth, precocious development of bronchopulmonary dysplasia, and a severe pulmonary outcome.[366] A few case reports have suggested that eradication of *Ureaplasma* with erythromycin contributes to faster resolution of symptoms or to a better outcome in neonates with this chronic disease.[8,230,507] Controlled studies are needed to verify these preliminary observations. No experience with the use of newer macrolides in neonates exists.

Recognition of the role of endogenous surfactant inactivation in the pathogenesis of bacterial pneumonia suggests that therapy with exogenous surfactant, in conjunction with antimicrobial drugs, could be beneficial for the management of affected infants. Large, prospective, placebo-controlled randomized trials are needed to explore the effect of surfactant therapy for neonatal bacterial pneumonia.[405]

REFERENCES

1. Aber, R. C., Allen, N., Howell, J. T., et al.: Nosocomial transmission of group B streptococci. Pediatrics 58:346, 1976.

2. Ablow, R. C., Driscoll, S. G., Effmann, E. L., et al.: A comparison of early-onset group B streptococcal neonatal infection and the respiratory-distress syndrome of the newborn. N. Engl. J. Med. 294:65, 1976.

3. Adams, J. M., Speer, M. E., and Rudolph, A. J.: Bacterial colonization of radial artery catheters. Pediatrics 65:94, 1980.

4. Adler, S. M., and Denton, R. L.: The erythrocyte sedimentation rate in the newborn period. J. Pediatr. 86:942, 1975.

5. Aigner, R. M., Fueger, G. F., and Ritter, G.: Results of three-phase bone scintigraphy and radiography in 20 cases of neonatal osteomyelitis. Nucl. Med. Commun. 17:20-28, 1996.

6. Albert, S., Baldwin, R., Czekajewski, S., et al.: Bullous impetigo due to group II *Staphylococcus aureus*: An epidemic in a normal newborn nursery. Am. J. Dis. Child. 120:10, 1970.

7. Albritton, W. L., Wiggins, G. L., and Feeley, J. C.: Neonatal listeriosis: Distribution of serotypes in relation to age at onset of disease. J. Pediatr. 88:481, 1976.

8. Alfa, M. J., Embree J. E., Degagne P., et al.: Transmission of *Ureaplasma urealyticum* from mothers to full and preterm infants. Pediatr. Infect. Dis. J. 14:341, 1995.

9. Allerdice, J. G., Baskett, T. F., Seshia, M. M. K., et al.: Perinatal group B streptococcal colonization and infection. Am. J. Obstet. Gynecol. 142:617, 1982.

10. Ameh, E. A., and Nmadu, P. T.: Major complications of omphalitis in neonates and infants. Pediatr. Surg. Int. 18:413-416, 2002.

11. Amstey, M. S., Lewin, E., and Colaice. J.: Vaginal colonization with invasive *Escherichia coli* during pregnancy. Am. J. Obstet. Gynecol. 137:534-535, 1980.

12. Ancona, R. J., Ferrieri, P., and Williams, P. P.: Maternal factors that enhance the acquisition of group B streptococci by newborn infants. J. Med. Microbiol. 13:273, 1980.

13. Anderson, D. C., Edwards, M. S., and Baker, C. J.: Luminol-enhanced chemiluminescence for evaluation of type III group B streptococcal opsonins in human sera. J. Infect. Dis. 141:370, 1980.

14. Andrews, J. I., Diekema, D. J., Hunter, S. K., et al.: Group B streptococci causing neonatal bloodstream infection: Antimicrobial susceptibility and serotyping results from SENTRY centers in the Western Hemisphere. Am. J. Obstet. Gynecol. 183:859-862, 2000.

15. Anthony, B. F., Okada, D. M., and Hobel, C. J.: Epidemiology of the group B *Streptococcus*: Maternal and nosocomial sources for infant acquisitions. J. Pediatr. 95:431, 1979.

16. Armstrong, J. H., Zacarias, F., and Rein, M. F.: Ophthalmia neonatorum: A chart review. Pediatrics 57:884, 1976.

17. Asmar, B. I.: Neonatal retropharyngeal cellulitis due to group B *Streptococcus*. Clin. Pediatr. (Phila.) 26:183, 1987.

18. Asnes, R. S., and Arendar, G. M.: Septic arthritis of the hip: A complication of femoral venipuncture. Pediatrics 38:837, 1966.

19. Auriti, C., Maccallini, A., Di Liso, G., et al.: Risk factors for nosocomial infections in a neonatal intensive-care unit. J. Hosp. Infect. 53:25-30, 2003.

20. Baker, C. J.: Group B streptococcal cellulitis-adenitis in infants. Am. J. Dis. Child. 136:631, 1982.

21. Baker, C. J., and Barrett, F. F.: Transmission of group B streptococci among parturient women and their neonates. J. Pediatr. 83:919, 1973.

22. Baker, C. J., and Barrett, F. F.: Group B streptococcal infections in infants: The importance of the various serotypes. J. A. M. A. 230:1158, 1974.

23. Baker, C. J., Barrett, F. F., Gordon, R. C., et al.: Suppurative meningitis due to streptococci of Lancefield group B: A study of 33 infants. J. Pediatr. 82:724, 1973.

24. Baker, C. J., and Edwards, M. S.: Group B streptococcal infections. *In* Remington, J. S., and Klein, J. O. (eds.): Infectious Diseases of the Fetus and Newborn Infants. 3rd ed. Philadelphia, W. B. Saunders, 1990, pp. 742-811.

25. Baker, C. J., and Edwards, M. S.. Group B streptococcal conjugate vaccines. Arch. Dis. Child. 88:375-378, 2003.

26. Baker, C. J., Edwards, M. S., and Kasper, D. L.: Role of antibody to native type III polysaccharide of group B *Streptococcus* in infant infection. Pediatrics 68:544, 1981.

27. Baker, C. J., and Kasper, D. L.: Correlation of maternal antibody deficiency with susceptibility to neonatal group B streptococcal infection. N. Engl. J. Med. 294:753, 1976.

28. Baker, C. J., and Kasper, D. L.: Group B streptococcal vaccines. Rev. Infect. Dis. 7:458, 1985.

29. Baker, C. J., Melish, M. E., Hall, R. T., et al.: Intravenous immune globulin for the prevention of nosocomial infection in low-birth-weight neonates. N. Engl. J. Med. 327:213, 1992.

30. Baker, C. J., and Neonatal IVIG Collaborative Study Group: Multicenter trial of intravenous immunoglobulin (IVIG) to present late-onset infection in preterm infants: Preliminary results. Abstract. Pediatr. Res. 25:275A, 1989.

31. Baker, C. J., Rench, M. A., and McInnes, P.: Immunization of pregnant women with group B streptococcal type III capsular polysaccharide–tetanus toxoid conjugate vaccine. Vaccine 21:3468-3472, 2003.

32. Baker, C. J., Webb, B. J., Jackson, C. V., et al.: Counter-current immunoelectrophoresis in the evaluation of infants with group B streptococcal disease. Pediatrics 65:1110, 1980.

33. Balagtas, R. C., Bell, C. E., Edwards, L. D., et al.: Risk of local and systemic infections associated with umbilical vein catheterization: A prospective study in 86 newborn patients. Pediatrics 48:359, 1971.

34. Baley, J. E., Stork, E. K., Warkentin, P. I., et al.: Buffy coat transfusions in neutropenic neonates with presumed sepsis: A prospective, randomized trial. Pediatrics 80:712, 1987.

35. Band, J. D., Clegg, H. W., II, Hayes, P. S., et al.: Transmission of group B streptococci: Traced by use of multiple epidemiologic markers. Am. J. Dis. Child. 135:355, 1981.

36. Barclay, N.: High frequency of *Salmonella* species as a cause of neonatal meningitis in Ibadan, Nigeria: A review of thirty-eight cases. Acta Paediatr. Scand. 60:540, 1971.

37. Barton, L. L., Feigin, R. D., and Lins, R.: Group B beta hemolytic streptococcal meningitis in infants. J. Pediatr. 82:719, 1973.

38. Battisti, O., Mitchison, R., and Davies, P. A.: Changing blood culture isolates in a referral neonatal intensive care unit. Arch. Dis. Child. 56:775, 1981.

39. Baumgart, S., Hall, S. E., Campos, J. M., et al.: Sepsis with coagulase-negative staphylococci in critically ill newborns. Am. J. Dis. Child. 137:461, 1983.

40. Beargie, R., Lynd, P., Tucker, E., et al.: Perinatal infection and vaginal flora. Am. J. Obstet. Gynecol. 122:31, 1975.

41. Beck-Sague, C. M., Azimi, P., Fonseca, S. N., et al.: Bloodstream infections in neonatal intensive care unit patients: Results of a multicenter study. Pediatr. Infect. Dis. J. 13:1110, 1994.

42. Becroft, D. M. O., Farmer, K., Seddon, R. J., et al.: Epidemic listeriosis in the newborn. Br. Med. J. 3:747, 1971.

43. Beem, M. O., and Saxon, E. M.: Respiratory-tract colonization and a distinctive pneumonia syndrome in infants with *Chlamydia trachomatis*. N. Engl. J. Med. 296:306, 1977.

44. Benitz, W. E., Gould, J. B., and Druzin, M. L.: Antimicrobial prevention of early-onset group B streptococcal sepsis: Estimates of risk reduction based on a critical literature review. Pediatrics 103:e78, 1999.

45. Bennet, R., Eriksson, M., and Zetterström, R.: Increasing incidence of neonatal septicemia: Causative organisms and predisposing risk factors. Acta Paediatr. Scand. 70:207, 1981.

46. Benuck, I., and David, R. J.: Sensitivity of published neutrophil indexes in identifying newborn infants with sepsis. J. Pediatr. 103:961, 1983.

47. Berche, P., Reich, K. A., Bonnichon, M., et al.: Detection of anti–listeriolysin O for serodiagnosis of human listeriosis. Lancet 335:624, 1990.

48. Bergman, J., Wald, E. R., Meyer, J. D., et al.: Epidural abscess and vertebral osteomyelitis following serial lumbar punctures. Pediatrics 72:476, 1983.

49. Bergqvist, G., Eriksson, M., and Zetterström, R.: Neonatal septicemia and perinatal risk factors. Acta Paediatr. Scand. 68:337, 1979.

50. Bergstrom, T., Larson, H., Lincoln, K., et al.: Studies of urinary tract infections in infancy and childhood. XII. Eighty consecutive patients with neonatal infection. J. Pediatr. 80:858, 1972.

51. Berkovich, S., and Taranko, L.: Acute respiratory illness in the premature nursery associated with respiratory syncytial virus infections. Pediatrics 34:753, 1964.

52. Berman, P. H., and Banker, B. Q.: Neonatal meningitis: A clinical and pathological study of 29 cases. Pediatrics 38:6, 1966.

53. Berman, S. A., Balkany, T. J., and Simmons, M. A.: Otitis media in the neonatal intensive care unit. Pediatrics 62:198, 1978.

54. Bertini, G., Nicoletti, P., Scopetti, F., et al.: *Staphylococcus aureus* epidemic in a neonatal nursery: A strategy of infection control. Eur. J. Pediatr. 165:530-535, 2006.

55. Bettelheim, K. A., and Lennox-King, S. M. J.: The acquisition of *Escherichia coli* by new-born babies. Infection 4:174, 1976.

56. Beutin, L., Kong, Q., Feng, L., et al.: Development of PCR assays targeting the genes involved in synthesis and assembly of the new *Escherichia coli* O 174 and O 177 O antigens. J. Clin. Microbiol. 43:5143-5149, 2005.

57. Bhandari, V., Hussain, N., Rosenkrantz, T., and Kresch, M.: Respiratory tract colonization with mycoplasma species increases the severity of bronchopulmonary dysplasia. J. Perinat. Med. 26:37-42, 1998.

58. Bhutta, Z. A., and Yusuf, K.: Early-onset neonatal sepsis in Pakistan: A case control study of risk factors in a birth cohort. Am. J. Perinatol. 14:577-581, 1997.

59. Bilgin, K., Yaramis, A., Haspolak, K., et al.: A randomized trial of granulocyte-macrophage colony-stimulating factor in neonates with sepsis and neutropenia. Pediatrics 107:36-41, 2001.

60. Bingen, E., Picard, B., Brahimi, N., et al.: Phylogenetic analysis of *Escherichia coli* strains causing neonatal meningitis suggests horizontal gene transfer from a predominant pool of highly virulent B2 group strains. J. Infect. Dis. 177:642-650, 1998.

61. Bizzarro, M. J., Raskind, C., Baltimore, R. S., and Gallagher, P. G.: Seventy-five years of neonatal sepsis at Yale: 1928-2003. Pediatrics 116:595-602, 2005.

62. Bland, R. D.: Otitis media in the first six weeks of life: Diagnosis, bacteriology, and management. Pediatrics 49:187, 1972.

63. Bluestone, C. D., and Klein, J. O.: Otitis Media in Infants and Children. Philadelphia, W. B. Saunders, 1988.

64. Blythe, D., Keenlyside, D., Dawson, S. J., and Galloway, A.: Environmental contamination due to methicillin-resistant *Staphylococcus aureus* (MRSA). J. Hosp. Infect. 38:67-69, 1998.

65. Bomela, H. N., Ballot, D. E., Cory, B. J., et al.: Use of C-reactive protein to guide duration of empiric antibiotic therapy in suspected early neonatal sepsis. Pediatr. Infect. Dis. J. 19:531-535, 2000.

66. Bonacorsi, S., Clermont, O., Houdouin, V., et al.: Molecular analysis and experimental virulence of French and North American *Escherichia coli* neonatal meningitis isolates: Identification of a new virulent clone. J. Infect. Dis. 187:1895-1906, 2003.

67. Bonadio, W. A., Stanco, L., Bruce, R., et al.: Reference values of normal cerebrospinal fluid composition in infants ages 0 to 8 weeks. Pediatr. Infect. Dis. J. 11:589, 1992.

68. Boswald, M., Dobig, C., Kandler, C., et al.: Pharmacokinetic and clinical evaluation of serious infections in premature and newborn infants under therapy with imipenem/cilastatin. Infection 27:299-304, 1999.

69. Bourchier, D., Abbott, G. D., and Maling, T. M. J.: Radiological abnormalities in infants with urinary tract infections. Arch. Dis. Child. 59:620, 1984.

70. Boyer, K. M., Gadzala, C. A., Burd, L. I., et al.: Selective intrapartum chemoprophylaxis of neonatal group B streptococcal early-onset disease. I. Epidemiologic rationale. J. Infect. Dis. 148:795, 1983.

71. Boyer, K. M., Gadzala, C. A., Kelly, P. D., et al.: Selective intrapartum chemoprophylaxis of neonatal group B streptococcal early-onset disease. III. Interruption of mother-to-infant transmission. J. Infect. Dis. 148:810, 1983.

72. Boyer, K. M., Gadzala, C. A., Kelly, P. D., et al.: Selective intrapartum chemoprophylaxis of neonatal group B streptococcal early-onset disease. II. Predictive value of prenatal cultures. J. Infect. Dis. 148:802-809, 1983.

73. Boyer, K. M., and Gotoff, S. P.: Prevention of early-onset neonatal group B streptococcal disease with selective intrapartum chemoprophylaxis. N. Engl. J. Med. 314:1665, 1986.

74. Boyer, K. M., Papierniak, C. K., Gadzala, C. A., et al.: Transplacental passage of IgG antibody to group B *Streptococcus* serotype Ia. J. Pediatr. 104:618, 1984.

75. Boyer, K. M., Petersen, N. J., Farzaneh, I., et al.: An outbreak of gastroenteritis due to *E. coli* 0142 in a neonatal nursery. J. Pediatr. 86:919, 1975.

76. Boyle, R. J., Robins-Browne, R. M., and Tang, M. L.: Probiotic use in clinical practice: What are the risks? Am. J. Clin. Nutr. 83:1256-1264; quiz 1446-1447, 2006.

77. Bracho, F., Goldman, S., and Cairo, M. S.: Potential use of granulocyte colony-stimulating factor and granulocyte-macrophage colony-stimulating factor in neonates. Curr. Opin. Hematol. 5:215-220, 1998.

78. Brans, Y. W., Ceballos, R., and Cassady, G.: Umbilical catheters and hepatic abscesses. Pediatrics 53:264, 1974.

79. Brimil, N., Barthell, E., Heindrichs, U., et al.: Epidemiology of *Streptococcus agalactiae* colonization in Germany. Int. J. Med. Microbiol. 296:39-44, 2006.

80. Brodie, S. B., Sands, K. E., Gray, J. E., et al.: Occurrence of nosocomial bloodstream infections in six neonatal intensive care units. Pediatr. Infect. Dis. J. 19:56-65, 2000.

81. Brook, I.: Microbiology of necrotizing fasciitis associated with omphalitis in the newborn infant. J. Perinatol. 18:28-30, 1998.

82. Brook, I., and Frazier, E. H.: Microbiology of scalp abscess in newborns. Pediatr. Infect. Dis. J. 11:766, 1992.

83. Buck, C., Bundschu, J., Gallati, H., et al.: Interleukin-6: A sensitive parameter for the early diagnosis of neonatal bacterial infection. Pediatrics 93:54, 1994.

84. Buck, G. E., Kelly, M. T., Pichanick, A. M., et al.: *Campylobacter jejuni* in newborns: A cause of asymptomatic bloody diarrhea. Am. J. Dis. Child. 136:744, 1982.

85. Burdon, D. W., Thompson, H., Candy, D. C. A., et al.: Enterotoxin(s) of *Clostridium difficile*. Lancet 2:258, 1981.

86. Burns, R. P., and Rhodes, D. H., Jr.: *Pseudomonas* eye infection as a cause of death in premature infants. Arch. Ophthalmol. 65:517, 1961.

87. Cairo, M. S.: Review of G-CSF and GM-CSF effects on neonatal neutrophil kinetics. Am. J. Pediatr. Hematol. Oncol. 11:238, 1989.

88. Cairo, M. S., Rucker, R., Bennetts, G. A., et al.: Improved survival of newborns receiving leukocyte transfusions for sepsis. Pediatrics 74:887, 1984.

89. Cameron, D. J. S., Bishop, R. F., Veenstra, A., et al.: Nonculturable viruses and neonatal diarrhea: Fifteen-month survey in a newborn special care nursery. J. Clin. Microbiol. 8:93, 1978.

90. Carstensen, H., Christensen, K. K., Grennert, I., et al.: Early-onset neonatal group B streptococcal septicemia in siblings. J. Infect. 17:201, 1988.

91. Centers for Disease Control and Prevention: Nosocomial infection surveillance, 1980-1982. M. M. W. R. C. D. C. Surveill. Summ. 32:1SS-16SS, 1983.

92. Centers for Disease Control and Prevention: Four pediatric deaths from community-acquired methicillin-resistant *Staphylococcus aureus*—Minnesota and North Dakota, 1997-1999. J. A. M. A. 282:1123-1125, 1999.

93. Centers for Disease Control and Prevention: Early-onset group B streptococcal disease, United States, 1998-1999. M. M. W. R. Morb. Mortal. Wkly. Rep. 49:793-796, 2000.

94. Centers for Disease Control and Prevention: Diminishing racial disparities in early-onset neonatal group B streptococcal disease—United States, 2000-2003. M. M. W. R. Morb. Mortal. Wkly. Rep. 53:502-505, 2004.

95. Centers for Disease Control and Prevention: Early-onset and late-onset neonatal group B streptococcal disease—United States, 1996-2004. M. M. W. R. Morb. Mortal. Wkly. Rep. 54:1205-1208, 2005.

96. Centers for Disease Control and Prevention: Preventing tetanus, diphtheria, and pertussis among adolescents: Use of tetanus toxoid, reduced diphtheria

toxoid and acellular pertussis vaccines—United States. M. M. W. R. Recomm. Rep 55(RR-3):1-34, 2006.

97. Chadwick, E. G., Shulman, S. T., and Yogev, R.: Peritonitis as a late manifestation of group B streptococcal disease in newborns. Pediatr. Infect. Dis. 2:142, 1983.

98. Chakravorty, S., Murray, N., and Roberts, I.: Neonatal thrombocytopenia. Early Hum. Dev. 81:35-41, 2005.

99. Chamnanvanakij, S., Decharachakul, K., Rasamimaree, P., and Vanprapar, N.: A randomized study of 3 umbilical cord care regimens at home in Thai neonates: Comparison of time to umbilical cord separation, parental satisfaction and bacterial colonization. J. Med. Assoc. Thai. 88:967-972, 2005.

100. Champagne, S., Fussell, S., and Scheifele, D.: Evaluation of skin antisepsis prior to blood culture in neonates. Infect. Control. 5:489, 1984.

101. Champsaur, H., Questiaux, E., Prevot, J., et al.: Rotavirus carriage, asymptomatic infection, and disease in the first two years of life. I. Virus shedding. J. Infect. Dis. 149:667, 1984.

102. Chandrashekar, M. R., Rathish, K. C., and Nagesha, C. N.: Reservoirs of nosocomial pathogens in neonatal intensive care unit. J. Indian Med. Assoc. 95:72-74, 77, 1997.

103. Chapman, R. L., and Faix, R. G.: Persistent bacteremia and outcome in late onset infection among infants in a neonatal intensive care unit. Pediatr. Infect. Dis. J. 22:17-21, 2003.

104. Chen, K. T., Tuomala, R. E., Cohen, A. P., et al.: No increase in rates of early-onset neonatal sepsis by non–group B *Streptococcus* or ampicillin-resistant organisms. Am. J. Obstet. Gynecol. 185:854-858, 2001.

105. Chiesa, C., Panero, A., Rossi, N., et al.: Reliability of procalcitonin concentrations for the diagnosis of sepsis in critically ill neonates. Clin. Infect. Dis. 26:664-672, 1998.

106. Chirico, G., Rondini, G., Plebani, A., et al.: Intravenous gammaglobulin therapy for prophylaxis of infection in high-risk neonates. J. Pediatr. 110:437, 1987.

107. Christensen, K. K., Christensen, P., Duc, G., et al.: Correlation between serum antibody-levels against group B streptococci and gestational age in newborns. Eur. J. Pediatr. 142:86, 1984.

108. Christensen, R. D., Bradley, P. P., and Rothstein, G.: The leukocyte left shift in clinical and experimental neonatal sepsis. J. Pediatr. 98:101, 1981.

109. Christensen, R. D., Rothstein, G., Anstall, H. B., et al.: Granulocyte transfusions in neonates with bacterial infection, neutropenia, and depletion of mature marrow neutrophils. Pediatrics 70:1, 1982.

110. Christian, J. R.: Comparison of ocular reactions with the use of silver nitrate and erythromycin ointment in ophthalmia neonatorum prophylaxis. J. Pediatr. 57:55, 1960.

111. Chrystie, I. L., Totterdell, B., Baker, M. J., et al.: Rotavirus infections in a maternity unit. Lancet 2:79, 1975.

112. Clapp, D. W., Kliegman, R. M., Baley, J. E., et al.: The use of intravenously administered immune globulin to prevent nosocomial sepsis in low birth weight infants: Report of a pilot study. J. Pediatr. 115:973, 1989.

113. Cobeljic, M., Miljkovic-Selimovic, B., Paunovic-Todosijevic, D., et al.: Enteroaggregative *Escherichia coli* associated with an outbreak of diarrhoea in a neonatal nursery ward. Epidemiol. Infect. 117:11-16, 1996.

114. Cochran, W. D., Davis, H. T., and Smith, C. A.: Advantages and complications of umbilical artery catheterization in the newborn. Pediatrics 42:769, 1968.

115. Collado, M., Kretschmer, R. R., Becker, I., et al.: Colonization of Mexican pregnant women with group B *Streptococcus*. J. Infect. Dis. 143:134, 1981.

116. Conner, J. M., Soll, R. F., Edwards, W. H.: Topical ointment for preventing infection in preterm infants. Cochrane Database Syst. Rev. 1:CD001150, 2004.

117. Cooperman, M. B.: *Gonococcus* arthritis in infancy: A clinical study of forty-four cases. Am. J. Dis. Child. 33:932, 1927.

118. Cordero, L., Sananes, M., and Ayers, L. W.: Failure of systemic antibiotics to eradicate gram-negative bacilli from the airway of mechanically ventilated very low-birth-weight infants. Am. J. Infect. Control. 28:286-290, 2000.

119. Coudron, P. E., Mayhall, C. G., Fracklam, R. R., et al.: *Streptococcus faecium* outbreak in a neonatal intensive care unit. J. Clin. Microbiol. 20:1044, 1984.

120. Couroucli, X. I., Welty, S. E., Ramsay, P. L., et al.: Detection of microorganisms in the tracheal aspirates of preterm infants by polymerase chain reaction: Association of adenovirus infection with bronchopulmonary dysplasia. Pediatr. Res. 47:225-232, 2000.

121. Culver, K. W., Ammann, A. J., Partridge, J. C., et al.: Lymphocyte abnormalities in infants born to drug-abusing mothers. J. Pediatr. 111:230, 1987.

122. Dagan, R., and Gorodischer, R.: Infections in hypothermic infants younger than 3 months old. Am. J. Dis. Child. 138:483, 1984.

123. Dan, M.: Septic arthritis in young infants: Clinical and microbiologic correlations and therapeutic implications. Rev. Infect. Dis. 6:147, 1984.

124. Daoud, A. S., Batieha, A., Al-Sheyyab, M., et al.: Lack of effectiveness of dexamethasone in neonatal bacterial meningitis. Eur. J. Pediatr. 158:230-233, 1999.

125. Darmstadt, G. L., Badrawi, N., Law, P. A., et al.: Topically applied sunflower seed oil prevents invasive bacterial infections in preterm infants in Egypt: A randomized, controlled clinical trial. Pediatr. Infect. Dis. J. 23:719-725, 2004.

126. Darmstadt, G. L., and Dinulos, J. G.: Neonatal skin care. Pediatr. Clin. North Am. 47:757-782, 2000.

127. Darville, T.: *Chlamydia trachomatis* infections in neonates and young children. Semin. Pediatr. Infect. Dis. *16*:235-244, 2005.

128. DaSilva, O., and Hammerberg, O.: Diagnostic value of leukocyte indices in late neonatal sepsis. Pediatr. Infect. Dis. J. *13*:409, 1994.

129. David, R. B., and O'Connell, E. J.: Suppurative parotitis in children. Am. J. Dis. Child. *119*:332, 1970.

130. Davis, R. C.: *Salmonella* sepsis in infancy. Am. J. Dis. Child. *135*:1096, 1981.

131. Dawson, K. G., Emerson, J. C., and Burns, J. L.: Fifteen years of experience with bacterial meningitis. Pediatr. Infect. Dis. J. *18*:816-822, 1999.

132. Dennison, W. M.: Haematogenous osteomyelitis of the newborn. Lancet *2*:474, 1955.

133. Dietzman, D. E., Fischer, G. W., and Schoenknecht, F. D.: Neonatal *Escherichia coli* septicemia: Bacterial counts in blood. J. Pediatr. *85*:128, 1974.

134. Dillon, H. C., Jr.: Group A type 12 streptococcal infection in a newborn nursery: Successfully treated neonatal meningitis. Am. J. Dis. Child. *112*:177, 1966.

135. Dillon, H. C., Jr., Gray, E., Pass, M. A., et al.: Anorectal and vaginal carriage of group B streptococci during pregnancy. J. Infect. Dis. *145*:794, 1982.

136. Dillon, H. C., Jr., Khane, S., and Gary, B. M.: Group B streptococcal carriage and disease: A 6-year prospective study. J. Pediatr. *110*:31, 1987.

137. Di Pentima, M. C., Mason, E. O., and Kaplan, S. L.: In vitro antibiotic synergy against *Flavobacterium meningosepticum*: Implications for therapeutic options. Clin. Infect. Dis. *26*:1169-1176, 1998.

138. Dobson, S. R. M., and Baker, C. J.: Enterococcal sepsis in neonates: Features by age at onset and occurrence of focal infection. Pediatrics *85*:165, 1990.

139. Doraiswamy, B., Hammerschlag, M. R., Pringle, G. F., et al.: Ophthalmia neonatorum caused by β-lactamase–producing *Neisseria gonorrhoeae*. J. A. M. A. *250*:790, 1983.

140. Dunham, E. C.: Septicemia in the new-born. Am. J. Dis. Child. *45*:229, 1933.

141. Dyson, A. E., and Read, S. E.: Group G streptococcal colonization and sepsis in neonates. J. Pediatr. *99*:944, 1981.

142. Easmon, C. S. F., Hastings, M. J. G., Deeley, J., et al.: The effect of intrapartum chemoprophylaxis on the vertical transmission of group B streptococci. Br. J. Obstet. Gynaecol. *90*:633, 1983.

143. Edwards, M. S., Jackson, C. V., and Baker, C. J.: Increased risk of group B streptococcal disease in twins. J. A. M. A. *245*:2044, 1981.

144. Edwards, M. S., Rench, M. A., Haffar, A. A. M., et al.: Long-term sequelae of group B streptococcal meningitis in infants. J. Pediatr. *106*:717, 1985.

145. Efird, M. M., Rojas, M. A., Lozano, J. M., et al.: Epidemiology of nosocomial infections in selected neonatal intensive care units in Colombia, South America. J. Perinatol. *25*:531-536, 2005.

146. Eitzman, D. V., and Smith, R. T.: The significance of blood cultures in the newborn period. Am. J. Dis. Child. *94*:601, 1957.

147. El-Radhi, A. S., Jawad, M. H., Mansor, N., et al.: Infection in neonatal hypothermia. Arch. Dis. Child. *58*:143, 1983.

148. Engle, W. D., and Rosenfeld, C. R.: Neutropenia in high-risk neonates. J. Pediatr. *105*:982, 1984.

149. Epps, C., and Brown, M.: Necrotizing fasciitis: A case study. Neonatal Netw. *16*:19-25, 1997.

150. Evans, J. R., Allen, A. C., Stinson, D. A., et al.: Perinatal listeriosis: Report of an outbreak. Pediatr. Infect. Dis. *4*:237-241, 1985.

151. Evanston, R. T., and Maunsell, H.: A Practical Treatise on the Management and Diseases of Children [first American edition from the first Irish edition in 1836]. Philadelphia, Haswell, Barrington, & Haswell, 1838, pp. 193-194.

152. Faden, H. S.: Early diagnosis of neonatal bacteremia by buffy-coat examination. J. Pediatr. *88*:1032, 1976.

153. Fanaroff, A. A., Korones, S. B., Wright, L. L., et al.: Controlled trial of intravenous immune-globulin to reduce nosocomial infections in very-low-birth-weight infants. N. Engl. J. Med. *330*:1107-1113, 1994.

154. Feigin, R. D., Wong, M., Shackelford, P. G., et al.: Countercurrent immunoelectrophoresis of urine as well as of CSF and blood for diagnosis of bacterial meningitis. J. Pediatr. *89*:773, 1976.

155. Feldman, W. E.: Relation of concentrations of bacteria and bacterial antigen in cerebrospinal fluid to prognosis in patients with bacterial meningitis. N. Engl. J. Med. *296*:433, 1977.

156. Feo, C. F., Dessanti, A., Franco, B., et al.: Retroperitoneal abscess and omphalitis in young infants. Acta Paediatr. *92*:122-125, 2003.

157. Ferrieri, P., Cleary, P. P., and Seeds, A. E.: Epidemiology of group-B streptococcal carriage in pregnant women and newborn infants. J. Med. Microbiol. *10*:103, 1977.

158. Figueroa-Damian, R., Arrendondo-García, J. L., and Mancilla-Ramírez, J.: Amniotic fluid interleukin-6 and the risk of early-onset sepsis among preterm infants. Arch. Med. Res. *30*:198-202, 1999.

159. Finelli, L., Livengood, J. R., and Saiman, L.: Surveillance of pharyngeal colonization: Detection and control of serious bacterial illness in low birth weight infants. Pediatr. Infect. Dis. J. *13*:854, 1994.

160. Fischer, G. W., Crumrine, M. H., and Jennings, P. B.: Experimental *Escherichia coli* sepsis in rabbits. J. Pediatr. *85*:117, 1974.

161. Fischer, G. W., Weisman, L. B., Hemming, V. G., et al.: Intravenous immunoglobulin in neonatal group B streptococcal disease: Pharmacokinetic and safety studies in monkeys and humans. Am. J. Med. *76*(Suppl. 3A):117, 1984.

162. Fleer, A., Senders, R. C., Visser, M. R., et al.: Septicemia due to coagulase-negative staphylococci in a neonatal intensive care unit: Clinical and bacteriological features and contaminated parenteral fluids as a source of sepsis. Pediatr. Infect. Dis. *2*:426, 1983.

163. Fleming, D. W., Cochi, S. L., MacDonald, K. L., et al.: Pasteurized milk as a vehicle of infection in an outbreak of listeriosis. N. Engl. J. Med. *312*:404, 1985.

164. Fox, L., and Sprunt, K.: Neonatal osteomyelitis. Pediatrics *62*:535, 1978.

165. Franciosi, R. A., Knostman, J. D., and Zimmerman, R. A.: Group B streptococcal neonatal and infant infections. J. Pediatr. *82*:707, 1973.

166. Fraser, N., Davies, B. W., and Cusack, J.: Neonatal omphalitis: A review of its serious complications. Acta Paediatr. *95*:519-522, 2006.

167. Freeman, J., Goldmann, D. A., Smith, N. E., et al.: Association of intravenous lipid emulsion and coagulase-negative staphylococcal bacteremia in neonatal intensive care units. N. Engl. J. Med. *323*:301-308, 1990.

168. Freedman, R. M., Ingram, D. L., Gross, I., et al.: A half century of neonatal sepsis at Yale: 1928 to 1978. Am. J. Dis. Child. *135*:140, 1981.

169. Fridkin, S. K., Hageman, J. C., Morrison, M., et al.: Methicillin-resistant *Staphylococcus aureus* disease in three communities. N. Engl. J. Med. *352*:1436-1444, 2005.

170. Friedman, C. A., Wender, D. F., and Rawson, J. E.: Rapid diagnosis of group B streptococcal infection utilizing a commercially available latex agglutination assay. Pediatrics *73*:27, 1984.

171. Gardner, S. E., Yow, M. D., Leeds, L. J., et al.: Failure of penicillin to eradicate group B streptococcal colonization in the pregnant woman: A couple study. Am. J. Obstet. Gynecol. *135*:1062, 1979.

172. Gasanov, U., Hughes, D., Hansbro, P. M.: Methods for the isolation and identification of *Listeria* spp. and *Listeria monocytogenes*: A review. F. E. M. S. Microbiol. Rev. *29*:851-875, 2005.

173. Gaulin, C., Ramsay, D., Ringuette, L., and Ismail, J.: First documented outbreak of *Listeria monocytogenes* in Quebec, 2002. Can. Commun. Dis. Rep. *29*:181-186, 2003.

174. Gaynes, R. P., Edwards, J. R., Jarvis, W. R., et al.: Nosocomial infections among neonates in high-risk nurseries in the United States. Pediatrics *98*:357-361, 1996.

175. Gellin, B. G., Broome, C. V., Bibb, W. F., et al.: The epidemiology of listeriosis in the United States—1986. Listeriosis Study Group. Am. J. Epidemiol. *133*:392-401, 1991.

176. Gendrel, D., Assicot, M., Raymond, J., et al.: Procalcitonin as a marker for the early diagnosis of neonatal infection. J. Pediatr. *128*:570-573, 1996.

177. Gerdes, J. S., and Polin, R. A.: Sepsis screen in neonates with evaluation of plasma fibronectin. Pediatr. Infect. Dis. J. *6*:443, 1987.

178. Gezon, H. M., Schaberg, M. J., and Klein, J. O.: Concurrent epidemics of *Staphylococcus aureus* and group A *Streptococcus* disease in a newborn nursery: Control with penicillin G and hexachlorophene bathing. Pediatrics *51*:383, 1973.

179. Gibbs, R. S., Hall, R. T., Yow, M. D., et al.: Consensus: Perinatal prophylaxis for group B streptococcal infection. Pediatr. Infect. Dis. J. *11*:179, 1992.

180. Ginsburg, C. M., and McCracken, G. H., Jr.: Urinary tract infections in young infants. Pediatrics *69*:409, 1982.

181. Glezen, W. P.: Maternal vaccines. Prim. Care *28*:791-806, vi-vii, 2001.

182. Glode, M. P., Sutton, A., Moxon, E. R., et al.: Pathogenesis of neonatal *Escherichia coli* meningitis: Induction of bacteremia and meningitis in infant rats fed *E. coli* K1. Infect. Immun. *16*:75, 1977.

183. Gluck, L., Wood, H. F., and Fousek, M. D.: Septicemia of the newborn. Pediatr. Clin. North Am. *13*:1131, 1966.

184. Gold, R., Wilt, J. C., Adhikari, P. K., et al.: Adenoviral pneumonia and its complications in infancy and childhood. J. Can. Assoc. Radiol. *20*:218, 1969.

185. Golden, B.: Subtenon injection of gentamicin for bacterial infections of the eye. J. Infect. Dis. *124*:S271, 1971.

186. Goldenberg, R. L., Culhane, J. F., Johnson, D. C.: Maternal infection and adverse fetal and neonatal outcomes. Clin. Perinatol. *32*:523-559, 2005.

187. Goldenberg, R. L., and Thompson, C.: The infectious origins of stillbirth. Am. J. Obstet. Gynecol. *189*:861-873, 2003.

188. Goldstein, B., Giroir, B., and Randolph, A.: International pediatric sepsis consensus conference: Definitions for sepsis and organ dysfunction in pediatrics. Pediatr. Crit. Care Med. *6*:2-8, 2005.

189. Gorbach, S. L., Menda, K. B., Thadepalli, H., et al.: Anaerobic microflora of the cervix in healthy women. Am. J. Obstet. Gynecol. *117*:1053, 1973.

190. Goscienski, P. J.: Inclusion conjunctivitis in the newborn infant. J. Pediatr. *77*:19, 1970.

191. Goscienski, P. J., and Sexton, R. R.: Follow-up studies in neonatal inclusion conjunctivitis. Am. J. Dis. Child. *124*:180, 1972.

192. Goulet, V., and Marchetti, P.: Listeriosis in 225 non-pregnant patients in 1992: Clinical aspects and outcome in relation to predisposing conditions. Scand. J. Infect. Dis. *28*:367-374, 1996.

193. Goyal, R., Sharma, P., Kaur, I., et al.: Bacterial vaginosis and vaginal anaerobes in preterm labour. J. Indian Med. Assoc. *102*:548-550, 553, 2004.

194. Graham, D. R., Anderson, R. L., Ariel, F. E., et al.: Epidemic nosocomial meningitis due to *Citrobacter diversus* in neonates. J. Infect. Dis. *144*:203, 1981.

195. Graves, G. R., and Rhodes, P. G.: Tachycardia as a sign of early onset neonatal sepsis. Pediatr. Infect. Dis. *3*:404, 1984.

196. Gray, M. L.: Genital listeriosis as a cause of repeated abortion. Lancet *2*:315, 1960.

197. Gray, M. L.: Epidemiological aspects of listeriosis. Am. J. Public Health. *53*:554, 1963.

198. Greenberg, M., and Vandow, J. E.: Ophthalmia neonatorum: Evaluation of different methods of prophylaxis in New York City. Am. J. Public Health 51:836, 1961.
199. Greengard, J.: Acute hematogenous osteomyelitis in infancy. Med. Clin. North Am. 30:135, 1946.
200. Griffin, M. P., and Moorman, J. R.: Toward the early diagnosis of neonatal sepsis and sepsis-like illness using novel heart rate analysis. Pediatrics 107:97-104, 2001.
201. Griffiths, A. N., Sudhahar, A. A., and Ashraf, M.: Neonatal necrotising fasciitis and late maternal pelvic abscess formation: A late complication of group A Streptococcus. J. Obstet. Gynaecol. 25:197-198, 2005.
202. Grimwood, K., Anderson, P., Anderson, V., et al.: Twelve year outcomes following bacterial meningitis: Further evidence for persisting effects. Arch. Dis. Child 83:111-116, 2000.
203. Groll, A. H., Meiser, A., Weise, M., et al.: Interleukin-6 as early mediator in neonatal sepsis. Pediatr. Infect. Dis. J. 11:496, 1992.
204. Gruskay, J., Harris, M. C., Costarino, A. T., et al.: Neonatal Staphylococcus epidermidis meningitis with unremarkable CSF examination results. Am. J. Dis. Child. 143:580, 1989.
205. Guerrant, R. L., Cleary, T. G., and Pickering, L. K.: Microorganisms responsible for neonatal diarrhea. In Remington, J. S., and Klein, J. O. (eds.): Infectious Diseases of the Fetus and Newborn Infant. 3rd ed. Philadelphia, W. B. Saunders, 1990, pp. 901-989.
206. Hague, K. N., Zaidi, M. H., Hazne, S. K., et al.: Intravenous immunoglobulin for prevention of sepsis in preterm and low birth weight infants. Pediatr. Infect. Dis. J. 5:622, 1986.
207. Hall, R. T., Barnes, W., Krishnan, et al.: Antibiotic treatment of parturient women colonized with group B streptococci. Am. J. Obstet. Gynecol. 124:630, 1976.
208. Hall, S. L.: Coagulase-negative staphylococcal infections in neonates. Pediatr. Infect. Dis. J. 10:57, 1991.
209. Haltalin, K. C.: Neonatal shigellosis: Report of 16 cases and review of the literature. Am. J. Dis. Child. 114:603, 1967.
210. Hammerschlag, M. R., Baker, C. J., Alpert, S., et al.: Colonization with group B streptococci in girls under 16 years of age. Pediatrics 60:473-476, 1977.
211. Hammerschlag, M. R., Cummings, C., Roblin, P. M., et al.: Efficacy of neonatal ocular prophylaxis for the prevention of Chlamydia and gonococcal conjunctivitis. N. Engl. J. Med. 320:769, 1989.
212. Hammerschlag, M. R., Gelling, M., Roblin, P. M., et al.: Treatment of neonatal chlamydial conjunctivitis with azithromycin. Pediatr. Infect. Dis. J. 17:1049-1050, 1998.
213. Hammerschlag, M. R., Herrmann, J. E., Cox, P., et al.: Prospective comparison of Chlamydiazyme to chlamydial cultures for the diagnosis of neonatal conjunctivitis. Presented at the 24th Interscience Conference on Antimicrobial Agents and Chemotherapy, October, 1984, Washington, D. C.
214. Hammerschlag, M. R., Roblin, P. M., Gelling, M., et al.: Use of polymerase chain reaction for the detection of Chlamydia trachomatis in ocular and nasopharyngeal specimens from infants with conjunctivitis. Pediatr. Infect. Dis. J. 16:293-297, 1997.
215. Hamoudi, A. C., Marcon, M. J., Cannon, H. J., et al.: Comparison of three major antigen detection methods for the diagnosis of group B streptococcal sepsis in neonates. Pediatr. Infect. Dis. 2:432, 1983.
216. Hannaford, K., Todd, D. A., Jeffery, H., et al.: Role of ureaplasma urealyticum in lung disease of prematurity. Arch. Dis. Child. Fetal Neonatal Ed. 81:F162-F167, 1999.
217. Harris, H., Wirtschafter, D., and Cassady, G.: Endotracheal intubation and its relationship to bacterial colonization and systemic infection of newborn infants. Pediatrics 58:816, 1976.
218. Harris, M. C., Costarino, A. T., Sullivan, J. S., et al.: Cytokine elevations in critically ill infants with sepsis and necrotizing enterocolitis. J. Pediatr. 124:105, 1994.
219. Harvey, D., Holt, D. E., and Bedford, H.: Bacterial meningitis in the newborn: A prospective study of mortality and morbidity. Semin. Perinatol. 23:218-225, 1999.
220. Healy, C. M., Hulten, K. G., Palazzi, D. L., et al.: Emergence of new strains of methicillin-resistant Staphylococcus aureus in a neonatal intensive care unit. Clin. Infect. Dis. 39:1460-1466, 2004.
221. Heelan, J. S., Hasenbein, M. E., and McAdam, A. J.: Resistance of group B Streptococcus to selected antibiotics, including erythromycin and clindamycin. J. Clin. Microbiol. 42:1263-1264, 2004.
222. Hemming, V. G., Hall, R. T., Rhodes, P. G., et al.: Assessment of group B streptococcal opsonins in human and rabbit serum by neutrophil chemiluminescence. J. Clin. Invest. 58:1379, 1976.
223. Herbert, M. A., Beveridge, C. J., and Saunders, N. J.: Bacterial virulence factors in neonatal sepsis: Group B Streptococcus. Curr. Opin. Infect. Dis. 17:225-229, 2004.
224. Herold, B. C., Immergluck, L. C., Maranan, M. C., et al.: Community-acquired methicillin-resistant Staphylococcus aureus in children with no identified predisposing risk. J. A. M. A. 279:593-598, 1998.
225. Hervás, J. A., Alomar, A., Salvá, F., et al.: Neonatal sepsis and meningitis in Mallorca, Spain, 1977-1991. Clin. Infect. Dis. 16:719, 1993.
226. Hitomi, S., Kubota, M., Nori, N., et al.: Control of a methicillin-resistant Staphylococcus aureus outbreak in a neonatal intensive care unit by unselective use of nasal mupirocin ointment. J. Hosp. Infect. 46:123-129, 2000.
227. Hocker, J. R., Simpson, P. M., Rabalais, G. P., et al.: Extracorporeal membrane oxygenation and early-onset group B streptococcal sepsis. Pediatrics 89:1, 1992.
228. Honein, M. A., Paulozzi, L. J., Himelright, I. M., et al.: Infantile hypertrophic pyloric stenosis after pertussis prophylaxis with erythromycin: A case review and cohort study. Lancet 354:2101-2105, 2000.
229. Hood, M.: Listeriosis as an infection of pregnancy manifested in the newborn. Pediatrics 27:390, 1961.
230. Horowitz, S., Landau, D., Shinwell, E. S., et al.: Respiratory tract colonization with Ureaplasma urealyticum and bronchopulmonary dysplasia in neonates in southern Israel. Pediatr. Infect. Dis. J. 11:847, 1992.
231. Howard, J. B., and McCracken, G. H., Jr.: The spectrum of group B streptococcal infections in infancy. Am. J. Dis. Child. 128:815, 1974.
232. Howard, J. B., and McCracken, G. H., Jr.: Reappraisal of kanamycin usage in neonates. J. Pediatr. 86:949, 1975.
233. Hoyert, D. L., Heron, M. P., Murphy, S. L., and Kung, H.-C.: Deaths: Final Data for 2003. National Vital Statistics Reports 54:1-120, 2006.
234. Hsieh, W. S., Yang, P. H., Chao, H. C., et al.: Neonatal necrotizing fasciitis: A report of three cases and review of the literature. Pediatrics 103:e53, 1999.
235. Huang, S. H., Chen, Y. H., Kong, G., et al.: A novel genetic island of meningitic Escherichia coli K1 containing the ibeA invasion gene (GimA): Functional annotation and carbon-source–regulated invasion of human brain microvascular endothelial cells. Funct. Integr. Genomics 1:312-322, 2001.
236. Hunter, S. K., and Andracki, M.: Univalent GBS vaccine utilizing C5A peptidase encapsulated within biodegradable polymeric microspheres. Presented at the 2004 Annual Scientific Meeting and Symposium of the Infectious Diseases Society for Obstetrics and Gynecology, August, 2004, San Diego, CA.
237. Hussain, F. M., Boyle-Vavra, S., Bethel, C. D., and Daum, R. S.: Current trends in community-acquired methicillin-resistant Staphylococcus aureus at a tertiary care pediatric facility. Pediatr. Infect. Dis. J. 19:1163-1166, 2000.
238. Isaacman, S. H., Heroman, W. M., and Lightsey, A. L.: Purpura fulminans following late-onset group B β-hemolytic streptococcal sepsis. Am. J. Dis. Child. 138:915, 1984.
239. Isaacs, D., and Royle, J. A.: Intrapartum antibiotics and early onset neonatal sepsis caused by group B Streptococcus and by other organisms in Australia. Australasian Study Group for Neonatal Infections. Pediatr. Infect. Dis. J. 18:524-528, 1999.
240. Jafari, H. S., Schuchat, A., Hildson, R., et al.: Barriers to prevention of perinatal group B streptococcal disease. Pediatr. Infect. Dis. J. 14:662, 1995.
241. Jincharadze, N., Abelashvili, D., McHedlishvili, M., and Kacharava, M.: Diagnostic value of C-reactive protein test at early-onset sepsis in preterm infants. Georgian Med. News 130:87-91, 2006.
242. Johns, A. W., Kitchen, W. H., and Leslie, D. W.: Complications of umbilical vessel catheters. Med. J. Aust. 2:810, 1972.
243. Johnson, C. E., DeBaz, B. P., Shurin, P. A., et al.: Renal ultrasound evaluation of urinary tract infection in children. Pediatrics 78:871, 1986.
244. Johnson, J. R., Oswald, E., O'Bryan, T. T., et al.: Phylogenetic distribution of virulence-associated genes among Escherichia coli isolates associated with neonatal bacterial meningitis in the Netherlands. J. Infect. Dis. 185:774-784, 2002.
245. Jones, D. E., Kanarek, K. S., and Lim, D. V.: Group B streptococcal colonization patterns in mothers and their infants. J. Clin. Microbiol. 20:438, 1984.
246. Jones, N., Oliver, K., Jones, Y., et al.: Carriage of group B Streptococcus in pregnant women from Oxford, UK. J. Clin. Pathol. 59:363-366, 2006.
247. Jones, S. R., Smith, J. W., and Sanford, J. P.: Localization of urinary-tract infections by detection of antibody-coated bacteria in urine sediment. N. Engl. J. Med. 290:591, 1974.
248. Joram, N., Boscher, C., Denizot, S., et al.: Umbilical cord blood procalcitonin and C reactive protein concentrations as markers for early diagnosis of very early onset neonatal infection. Arch. Dis. Child. Fetal Neonatal Ed. 91:F65-F66, 2006.
249. Kafetzis, D. A., Brater, D. C., Kapiki, A. N., et al.: Treatment of severe neonatal infections with cefotaxime: Efficacy and pharmacokinetics. J. Pediatr. 100:483, 1982.
250. Kaijser, B., Hanson, L. A., Jodal, U., et al.: Frequency of E. coli K antigens in urinary-tract infections in children. Lancet 1:663, 1977.
251. Karlowicz, M. G., Buescher, E. S., and Surka, A. E.: Fulminant late-onset sepsis in a neonatal intensive care unit, 1988-1997, and the impact of avoiding empiric vancomycin therapy. Pediatrics 106:1387-1390, 2000.
252. Kashlan, F., Smulian, J., Shen-Schwarz, S., et al.: Umbilical vein interleukin 6 and tumor necrosis factor alpha plasma concentrations in the very preterm infant. Pediatr. Infect. Dis. J. 19:238-243, 2000.
253. Kasper, D. L., Paoletti, L. C., Wessels, M. R., et al.: Immune response to type III group B streptococcal polysaccharide–tetanus toxoid conjugate vaccine. J. Clin. Invest. 98:2308-2314, 1996.
254. Kelsey, D. L., Lipscomb, A. P., and Mowles, J. M.: Limulus amoebocyte lysate endotoxin test: An aid to the diagnosis in the septic neonate? J. Infect. 4:69, 1982.
255. Khaneja, M., Naprawa, J., Kumar, A., et al.: Successful treatment of late-onset infection due to resistant Klebsiella pneumoniae in an extremely low birth weight infant using ciprofloxacin. J. Perinatol. 19:311-314, 1999.
256. Khashu, M., Osiovich, H., Henry, D., et al.: Persistent bacteremia and severe thrombocytopenia caused by coagulase-negative Staphylococcus in a neonatal intensive care unit. Pediatrics 117:340-348, 2006.

257. Klinger, G., Chin, C. N., Beyene, J., et al.: Predicting the outcome of neonatal bacterial meningitis. Pediatrics *106*:477-482, 2000.

258. Kim, K. S.: *Escherichia coli* translocation at the blood-brain barrier. Infect. Immun. *69*:5217-5222, 2001.

259. Kim, K. S., and Anthony, B. F.: Penicillin tolerance in group B streptococci isolated from infected neonates. J. Infect. Dis. *144*:411, 1981.

260. King, J. C., Berman, E. D., and Wright, P. F.: Evaluation of fever in infants less than 8 weeks old. South. Med. J. *80*:948, 1987.

261. Kleiman, M. B., Reynolds, J. K., Schreiner, R. L., et al.: Rapid diagnosis of neonatal bacteremia with acridine orange–stained buffy coat smears. J. Pediatr. *105*:419, 1984.

262. Klein, J. O., Feigin, R. D., and McCracken, G. H., Jr.: Report of the task force on diagnosis and management of meningitis. Pediatrics 78(Suppl.):959, 1986.

263. Klein, J. O., and Marcy, S. M.: Bacterial sepsis and meningitis. *In* Remington, J. S., and Klein, J. O. (eds.): Infectious Diseases of the Fetus and Newborn Infant. 3rd ed. Philadelphia, W. B. Saunders, 1990, p. 60.

264. Kline, M. W., and Mason, E. O., Jr.: Methicillin-resistant *Staphylococcus aureus*: Pediatric perspective. Pediatr. Clin. North Am. *35*:613, 1988.

265. Klinger, G., Chin, C. N., Beyene, J., et al.: Predicting the outcome of neonatal bacterial meningitis. Pediatrics *106*:477-482, 2000.

266. Kocherlakota, P., and La Gamma, E. F.: Preliminary reports: rhG-CSF may reduce the incidence of neonatal sepsis in prolonged preeclampsia-associated neutropenia. Pediatrics *102*:1107-1111, 1998.

267. Korhonen, T. K., Valtonen, M. V., Parkkinen, J., et al.: Serotypes, hemolysin production, and receptor recognition of *Escherichia coli* strains associated with neonatal sepsis and meningitis. Infect. Immun. *48*:486-491, 1985.

268. Koskiniemi, S., Sellin, M., and Norgren, M.: Identification of two genes, cpsX and cpsY, with putative regulatory function on capsule expression in group B streptococci. FEMS Immunol. Med. Microbiol. *21*:159-168, 1998.

269. Krauss, A. N., Albert, R. F., and Kannan, M. M.: Contamination of umbilical catheters in the newborn infant. J. Pediatr. *77*:965, 1970.

270. Krcmery, V., Filka, J., Uher, J. et al.: Ciprofloxacin in treatment of nosocomial meningitis in neonates and in infants: Report of 12 cases and review. Diagn. Microbiol. Infect. Dis. *35*:75-80, 1999.

271. Krohn, M. A., Thwin, S. S., Rabe, L. K., et al.: Vaginal colonization by *Escherichia coli* as a risk factor for very low birth weight delivery and other perinatal complications. J. Infect. Dis. *175*:606-610, 1997.

272. Kumari, D. N., Haji, T. C., Keer, V., et al.: Ventilation grilles as a potential source of methicillin-resistant *Staphylococcus aureus* causing an outbreak in an orthopaedic ward at a district general hospital. J. Hosp. Infect. *39*:127-133, 1998.

273. Kumari, S., Bhargava, S. K., Baijal, V. N., et al.: Neonatal osteomyelitis: A clinical and follow-up study. Indian Pediatr. *15*:393, 1978.

274. Lang, M. E., Vaudry, W., and Robinson, J. L.: Case report and literature review of late-onset group B streptococcal disease manifesting as necrotizing fasciitis in preterm infants: Is this a new syndrome? Clin. Infect. Dis. *37*:e132-e135, 2003.

275. Larcher, J. S., Capellino, F., De Giusto, R., et al.: [Group B streptococcus colonization during pregnancy and prevention of early onset of disease.] Medicina (B. Aires) *65*:201-206, 2005.

276. Larsen, B., and Galask, R. P.: Vaginal microbial flora: Practical and theoretic relevance. Obstet. Gynecol. *55*:100S, 1980.

277. Laurenti, F., Ferro, R., Isacchi, G., et al.: Polymorphonuclear leukocyte transfusion for the treatment of sepsis in the newborn infant. J. Pediatr. *98*:118, 1981.

278. Lay, J., Varma, J., Marcus, R., et al. Higher incidence of *Listeria* infections among Hispanics: FoodNet, 1996-2000. Presented at an International Conference on Emerging Infectious Diseases, March 2002, Atlanta.

279. Leake, D., and Leake, R.: Neonatal suppurative parotitis. Pediatrics *46*:203, 1970.

280. Lebenthal, E.: Lactose malabsorption and milk consumption in infants and children. Am. J. Dis. Child. *133*:21, 1979.

281. Lee, H. K., Lee, W. G., and Cho, S. R.: Clinical and molecular biological analysis of a nosocomial outbreak of vancomycin-resistant enterococci in a neonatal intensive care unit. Acta Paediatr. *88*:651-654, 1999.

282. Leigh, L., Stoll, B. J., Rahman M., et al.: *Pseudomonas aeruginosa* infection in very low birth weight infants: A case-control study. Pediatr. Infect. Dis. J. *14*:367, 1995.

283. Lennon, D., Lewis, B., Mantell, C., et al.: Epidemic perinatal listeriosis. Pediatr. Infect. Dis. *3*:30, 1984.

284. Lessing, M. P., Jordens, J. Z., and Bowler, I. C.: Molecular epidemiology of a multiple strain outbreak of methicillin-resistant *Staphylococcus aureus* amongst patients and staff. J. Hosp. Infect. *31*:253-260, 1995.

285. Levin, J., and Bang, F. B.: Clottable protein in *Limulus*: Its localization and kinetics of its coagulation by endotoxin. Thromb. Diath. Haemorrh. *19*:186, 1968.

286. Levine, E. M., Ghai, V., Barton, J. J., et al.: Intrapartum antibiotic prophylaxis increases the incidence of gram-negative neonatal sepsis. Infect. Dis. Obstet. Gynecol. 7:210-213, 1999.

287. Levy, H. L., Sepe, S. J., Shih, V. E., et al.: Sepsis due to *Escherichia coli* in neonates with galactosemia. N. Engl. J. Med. *297*:1403, 1977.

288. Libby, J. M., Donta, S. T., and Wilkins, T. D.: *Clostridium difficile* toxin A in infants. J. Infect. Dis. *148*:606, 1983.

289. Lieberman, H., and Brem, J.: Syndrome of acute osteomyelitis of the superior maxilla in early infancy. N. Engl. J. Med. *260*:318, 1959.

290. Lilien, L. D., Harris, V. J., Ramamurthy, R. S., et al.: Neonatal osteomyelitis of the calcaneus: Complication of heel puncture. J. Pediatr. *88*:478, 1976.

291. Lim, M. O., Gresham, E. L., Franken, E. A., Jr., et al.: Osteomyelitis as a complication of umbilical artery catheterization. Am. J. Dis. Child. *131*:142, 1977.

292. Linnan, M. J., Mascola, L., Lou, X. D., et al.: Epidemic listeriosis associated with Mexican-style cheese. N. Engl. J. Med. *319*:823, 1988.

293. Liu, C.-H., Lehan, C., Speer, M. E., et al.: Degenerative changes in neutrophils: An indicator of bacterial infection. Pediatrics 74:823, 1984.

294. MacFarlane, D. E.: Neonatal group B streptococcal septicemia in a developing country. Acta Pediatr. Scand. 76:470, 1987.

295. MacGowan, A. P., Marshall, R. J., MacKay, I. M., and Reeves, D. S.: *Listeria* faecal carriage by renal transplant recipients, haemodialysis patients and patients in general practice: Its relation to season, drug therapy, foreign travel, animal exposure and diet. Epidemiol. Infect. *106*:157-166, 1991.

296. Macias, A. E., Munoz, J. M., Galvan, A., et al.: Nosocomial bacteremia in neonates related to poor standards of care. Pediatr. Infect. Dis. J. *24*:713-716, 2005.

297. Magudumana, M. O., Ballot, D. E., Cooper, P. A., et al.: Serial interleukin 6 measurements in the early diagnosis of neonatal sepsis. J. Trop. Pediatr. *46*:267-271, 2000.

298. Main, E. K., and Slagle, T.: Prevention of early-onset invasive neonatal group B streptococcal disease in a private hospital setting: The superiority of culture-based protocols. Am. J. Obstet. Gynecol. *182*:1344-1354, 2000.

299. Manikoth, P., George, M., Vaishnav, A., and Sajwani, M. J.: Omphalitis. Lancet 364:1522, 2004.

300. Manroe, B. L., Rosenfeld, C. R., Weinberg, A. G., et al.: The differential leukocyte count in the assessment and outcome of early-onset neonatal group B streptococcal disease. J. Pediatr. *91*:632, 1977.

301. Manroe, B. L., Weinberg, A. G., Rosenfeld, C. R., et al.: The neonatal blood count in health and disease. I. Reference values for neutrophilic cells. J. Pediatr. *95*:89, 1979.

302. Marchant, C. D., Shurin, P. A., Turczyk, V. A., et al.: Course and outcome of otitis media in early infancy: A prospective study. J. Pediatr. *104*:826, 1984.

303. Marcy, S. M.: Bacterial infections of the bones and joints. *In* Remington, J. S., and Klein, J. O. (eds.): Infectious Diseases of the Fetus and Newborn Infant. 3rd ed. Philadelphia, W. B. Saunders, 1990, p. 674.

304. Marild, S., Wettergren, B., Hellstrom, M., et al.: Bacterial virulence and inflammatory response in infants with febrile urinary tract infection or screening bacteriuria. J. Pediatr. *112*:348, 1988.

305. Marodi, L., Kaposzta, R., and Nemes, E.: Survival of group B streptococcus type III in mononuclear phagocytes: Differential regulation of bacterial killing in cord macrophages by human recombinant gamma interferon and granulocyte-macrophage colony-stimulating factor. Infect. Immun. *68*:2167-2170, 2000.

306. Mathieu, P. L.: Comparison study: Silver nitrate and oxytetracycline in newborn eyes: A comparison of the incidence of conjunctivitis following the instillation of silver nitrate or oxytetracycline into the eyes of newborn infants. Am. J. Dis. Child. *95*:609, 1958.

307. Mayor-Lynn, K., Gonzalez-Quintero, V. H., O'Sullivan, M. J., et al.: Comparison of early-onset neonatal sepsis caused by *Escherichia coli* and group B *Streptococcus*. Am. J. Obstet. Gynecol. *192*:1437-1439, 2005.

308. McCracken, G. H., Jr.: Intraventricular treatment of neonatal meningitis due to gram-negative bacilli. J. Pediatr. *91*:1037, 1977.

309. McCracken, G. H., Jr., and Mize, S. G.: A controlled study of intrathecal antibiotic therapy in gram-negative enteric meningitis of infancy: Report of the Neonatal Cooperative Study Group. J. Pediatr. *89*:66, 1976.

310. McCracken, G. H., Jr., Mize, S. G., and Threlkeld, N.: Intraventricular gentamicin therapy in gram-negative bacillary meningitis of infancy: Report of the Second Neonatal Meningitis Cooperative Study Group. Lancet *1*:787, 1980.

311. McCracken, G. H., Jr., Mustafa, M. M., Ramilo, O., et al.: Cerebrospinal fluid interleukin-1 beta and tumor necrosis factor concentrations and outcome from neonatal gram-negative enteric bacillary meningitis. Pediatr. Infect. Dis. J. 8:155, 1989.

312. McCracken, G. H., Jr., and Nelson, J. D.: Antimicrobial Therapy for Newborns. 2nd ed. New York, Grune & Stratton, 1983.

313. McCracken, G. H., Jr., Sarff, L. D., Glode, M. P., et al.: Relation between *Escherichia coli* K1 capsular polysaccharide antigen and clinical outcome in neonatal meningitis. Lancet 2:246, 1974.

314. McCracken, G. H., Jr., Sarff, L. D., Robbins, J. B., et al.: Ontogeny of serum and secretory K1 antibodies. Presented at a meeting of the American Pediatric Society, April 1976, St. Louis.

315. McCracken, G. H., Jr., and Shinefield, H. R.: Changes in the pattern of neonatal septicemia and meningitis. Am. J. Dis. Child. *112*:33, 1966.

316. McCracken, G. H., Jr., Threlkeld, N., Mize, S., et al.: Moxalactam therapy for neonatal meningitis due to gram-negative enteric bacilli: A prospective controlled evaluation. J. A. M. A. *252*:1427, 1984.

317. McDuffie, R. S., Jr., McGregor, J. A., and Gibbs, R. S.: Adverse perinatal outcome and resistant Enterobacteriaceae after antibiotic usage for premature rupture of the membranes and group B streptococcus carriage. Obstet. Gynecol. *82*:487-489, 1993.

318. McLauchlin, J.: Human listeriosis in Britain, 1967-85, a summary of 722 cases. 1. Listeriosis during pregnancy and in the newborn. Epidemiol. Infect. *104*:181-189, 1990.

319. Mead, P. B., and Winn, W. C.: Vaginal-rectal colonization with group A streptococci in late pregnancy. Infect. Dis. Obstet. Gynecol. 8:217-219, 2000.

320. Mehr, S. S., Sadowsky, J. L., Doyle, L. W., and Carr, J.: Sepsis in neonatal intensive care in the late 1990s. J. Paediatr. Child Health 38:246-251, 2002.

321. Melish, M. E., and Glasgow, L. A.: Staphylococcal scalded skin syndrome: The expanded clinical syndrome. J. Pediatr. 78:958, 1971.

322. Melish, M. E., Glasgow, L. A., and Turner, M. D.: The staphylococcal scalded-skin syndrome: Isolation and partial characterization of the exfoliative toxin. J. Infect. Dis. 125:129, 1972.

323. Mercer, B. M., Carr, T. L., Beazley, D. D. et al.: Antibiotic use in pregnancy and drug-resistant infant sepsis. Am. J. Obstet. Gynecol. 181:16-21, 1999.

324. Merenstein, G. B., Todd, W. A., Brown, G., et al.: Group B beta-hemolytic Streptococcus: Randomized controlled treatment study at term. Obstet. Gynecol. 55:315, 1980.

325. Middelton, P. J.: Pathogenesis of rotaviral infection. J. Am. Vet. Med. Assoc. 173:544, 1978.

326. Middelton, P. J., Szymanski, M. T., and Petric, M.: Viruses associated with acute gastroenteritis in young children. Am. J. Dis. Child. 131:733, 1977.

327. Mitsuda, T., Arai, K., Ibe, M., et al.: The influence of methicillin-resistant Staphylococcus aureus (MRSA) carriers in a nursery and transmission of MRSA to their households. J. Hosp. Infect. 42:45-51, 1999.

328. Miyairi, I., Berlingieri, D., Protic, J., and Belko, J.: Neonatal invasive group A streptococcal disease: Case report and review of the literature. Pediatr. Infect. Dis. J. 23:161-165, 2004.

328. Mok, P. M., Reilly, B. J., and Ash, J. M.: Osteomyelitis in the neonate. Radiology. 145:677, 1982.

330. Molina-Cabrillana, J., Santana-Reyes, C., Hernandez, J., et al.: [Incidence of nosocomial infections at a neonatal intensive care unit: A six-year surveillance study.] Enferm. Infecc. Microbiol. Clin. 24:307-312, 2006.

331. Monto, A. S., Brandt, B. L., and Artenstein, M. S.: Response of children to Neisseria meningitidis polysaccharide vaccines. J. Infect. Dis. 127:394, 1973.

332. Morales, W. J., and Lim, D. V.: Reduction of group B streptococcal maternal and neonatal infections in preterm pregnancies with premature rupture of membranes through a rapid identification test. Am. J. Obstet. Gynecol. 157:13, 1987.

333. Morales, W. J., Lim, D. V., and Walsh, A. F.: Prevention of neonatal group B streptococcal sepsis by the use of rapid screening test and selective intrapartum chemoprophylaxis. Am. J. Obstet. Gynecol. 155:979, 1986.

334. Moreno, M. T., Vargas, S., Poveda, R., et al.: Neonatal sepsis and meningitis in a developing Latin American country. Pediatr. Infect. Dis. J. 13:516, 1994.

335. Mulder, C. J. J., van Alphen, L., and Zanen, H. C.: Neonatal meningitis caused by Escherichia coli in the Netherlands. J. Infect. Dis. 150:935, 1984.

336. Munson, D. P., Thompson, T. R., Johnson, D. E., et al.: Coagulase-negative staphylococcal septicemia: Experience in a newborn intensive care unit. J. Pediatr. 101:602, 1982.

337. Murray, N. A., Howarth, L. J., McCloy, M. P., et al.: Platelet transfusion in the management of severe thrombocytopenia in neonatal intensive care unit patients. Transfus. Med. 12:35-41, 2002.

338. Mustafa, M. M., and McCracken, G. H., Jr.: Antimicrobial agents in pediatrics. Infect. Dis. Clin. North Am. 3:491, 1989.

339. Mustafa, M. M., Mertsola, J., Ramilo, O., et al.: Increased endotoxin and interleukin-1 beta concentrations in cerebrospinal fluid of infants with coliform meningitis and ventriculitis associated with intraventricular gentamicin therapy. J. Infect. Dis. 160:891, 1989.

340. Mustafa, M. M., Ramilo, O., Olsen, K. D., et al.: Tumor necrosis factor in mediating experimental Haemophilus influenzae type b meningitis. J. Clin. Invest. 84:1253, 1989.

341. Nejjari, N., Benomar, S., and Lahbabi, M. S.: Nosocomial infections in neonatal and pediatric intensive care: The appeal of ciprofloxacin. Arch. Pediatr. 7:1268-1273, 2000.

342. Nelson, D. L., Hable, K. A., and Matsen, J. M.: Proteus mirabilis osteomyelitis in two neonates following needle puncture: Successful treatment with ampicillin. Am. J. Dis. Child. 125:109, 1973.

343. Nelson, J. D.: Duration of neomycin therapy for enteropathogenic Escherichia coli diarrheal disease: A comparative study of 113 cases. Pediatrics 48:248, 1971.

344. Nelson, J. D.: Antibiotic concentrations in septic joint effusions. N. Engl. J. Med. 284:349, 1971.

345. Nelson, J. D.: Bilateral breast abscess due to group B Streptococcus. Am. J. Dis. Child. 130:567, 1976.

346. Nelson, J. D.: The changing epidemiology of pertussis in young infants: The role of adults as reservoirs of infection. Am. J. Dis. Child. 132:371, 1978.

347. Nelson, J. D., Dillon, H. C., Jr., and Howard, J. B.: A prolonged nursery epidemic associated with a newly recognized type of group A Streptococcus. J. Pediatr. 89:792, 1976.

348. Nelson, J. D., and Peters, P. C.: Suprapubic aspiration of urine in premature and term infants. Pediatrics 36:132, 1965.

349. Newman, M. J.: Neonatal intensive care unit: Reservoirs of nosocomial pathogens. West Afr. J. Med. 21:310-312, 2002.

350. Newman, R. B., Stevens, R. W., and Gaafar, H. A.: Latex agglutination test for the diagnosis of Haemophilus influenzae meningitis. J. Lab. Clin. Med. 76:107, 1970.

351. Ng, P. C.: Diagnostic markers of infection in neonates. Arch. Dis. Child. Fetal Neonatal Ed. 89:F229-235, 2004.

352. Noel, G. J., and Edelson, P. J.: Staphylococcus epidermidis bacteremia in neonates: Further observations and the occurrence of focal infection. Pediatrics 74:832, 1984.

353. Noya, F. J. D., Rench, M. N., Metzger, T. A., et al.: Unusual occurrence of an epidemic of type Ib/c group B streptococcal sepsis in a neonatal intensive care unit. J. Infect. Dis. 115:1135, 1987.

354. Nyhan, W. L., and Fousek, M. D.: Septicemia of the newborn. Pediatrics 22:268, 1958.

355. Offit, P. A., and Clarke, H. F.: Protection against rotavirus-induced gastroenteritis in a murine model by passively acquired gastrointestinal but not circulatory antibodies. J. Virol. 54:58, 1985.

356. Ogden, J. A., and Lister, G.: The pathology of neonatal osteomyelitis. Pediatrics 55:474, 1975.

357. Ogra, P. L., and Fishaut, M.: Human breast milk. In Remington, J. S., and Klein, J. O. (eds.): Infectious Diseases of the Fetus and Newborn Infant. 3rd ed. Philadelphia, W. B. Saunders, 1990, pp. 68-88.

358. Ohler, K. H., Menke, J. A., and Fuller, L.: Use of higher dose extended interval aminoglycosides in a neonatal intensive care unit. Am. J. Perinatol. 17:285-290, 2000.

359. Ohlsson, A., Baily, T., and Takiedine, F.: Changing etiology and outcome of neonatal septicemia in Riyadh, Saudi Arabia. Acta Paediatr. Scand. 75:540, 1986.

360. Olarte, J., and Ramos-Alvares, M.: Epidemic diarrhea in premature infants: Etiologic significance of a newly recognized type of Escherichia coli (0142: K86[B]:H6). Am. J. Dis. Child. 109:436, 1965.

361. Oriel, J. D.: Ophthalmia neonatorum: Relative efficacy of current prophylactic practices and treatment. J. Antimicrob. Chemother. 14:209, 1984.

362. Otila, E.: Studies on the cerebrospinal fluid in premature infants. Acta Paediatr. 35(Suppl. 8):9, 1948.

363. Overall, J. C., Jr.: Neonatal bacterial meningitis: Analysis of predisposing factors and outcome compared with matched control subjects. J. Pediatr. 76:499, 1970.

364. Overturf, G. D., and Balfour, G.: Osteomyelitis and sepsis: Severe complications of fetal monitoring. Pediatrics 55:244, 1975.

365. Owen, C. R., Meis, A., Jackson, J. W., et al.: A case of primary cutaneous listeriosis. N. Engl. J. Med. 262:1026, 1960.

366. Pacifico, L., Panero, A., Roggini, M., et al.: Ureaplasma urealyticum and pulmonary outcome in a neonatal intensive care population. Pediatr. Infect. Dis. J. 16:579-586, 1997.

367. Pagotto, F., Ng, L. K., Clark, C., and Farber, J.: Canadian listeriosis reference service. Foodborne Pathog. Dis. 3:132-137, 2006.

368. Paoletti, L. C., and Kasper, D. L.: Conjugate vaccines against group B Streptococcus types IV and VII. J. Infect. Dis. 186:123-126, 2002.

369. Paredes, A., Wong, P., Mason, E. O., Jr., et al.: Nosocomial transmission of group B streptococci in a newborn nursery. Pediatrics 59:679, 1977.

370. Pass, M. A., Gray, B. M., Khare, S., et al.: Prospective studies of group B streptococcal infections in infants. J. Pediatr. 95:437, 1979.

371. Pass, M. A., Khare, S., and Dillon, H. C., Jr.: Twin pregnancies: Incidence of group B streptococcal colonization and disease. J. Pediatr. 97:635, 1980.

372. Pass, M., Samual, M., Karchmer, T., et al.: Trend in listeriosis in FoodNet Sites: 1996-1998. Presented at the 2nd International Conference on Emerging Infectious Diseases, July 2000, Atlanta.

373. Patamasucon, P., Rettig, P. J., Faust, K. L., et al.: Oral v topical erythromycin therapies for chlamydial conjunctivitis. Am. J. Dis. Child. 136:817, 1982.

374. Patel, D. M., Rhodes, P. G., LeBlanc, M. H., et al.: Role of postnatal penicillin prophylaxis in prevention of neonatal group B Streptococcus infection. Acta Paediatr. 88:874-879, 1999.

375. Patrick, M. J.: Influence of maternal renal infection on the fetus and infant. Arch. Dis. Child. 42:208, 1967.

376. Peevy, K. J., and Wiseman, H. J.: Gallbladder distension in septic neonates. Arch. Dis. Child. 57:75, 1982.

377. Pestalozza, G.: Otitis media in newborn infants. Int. J. Pediatr. Otorhinolaryngol. 8:109, 1984.

378. Petrilli, E. S., d'Ablaig, G., and Ledger, W. J.: Listeria monocytogenes chorioamnionitis: Diagnosis by transabdominal amniocentesis. Obstet. Gynecol. 55:5S, 1980.

379. Philip, A. G. S.: Decreased use of antibiotics using a neonatal sepsis screening technique. J. Pediatr. 98:795, 1981.

380. Philip, A. G. S.: Detection of neonatal sepsis of late onset. J. A. M. A. 247:489, 1982.

381. Philip, A. G. S.: Acute-phase proteins in neonatal infection. J. Pediatr. 105:940, 1984.

382. Philip, A. G., and Mills, P. C.: Use of C-reactive protein in minimizing antibiotic exposure: Experience with infants initially admitted to a well-baby nursery. Pediatrics 106:E4, 2000.

383. Pichichero, M. E., and Todd, J. K.: Detection of neonatal bacteremia. J. Pediatr. 94:958, 1979.

384. Pildes, R. S., Ramamurthy, R. S., and Vidyasagar, D.: Effect of triple dye on staphylococcal colonization in the newborn infant. J. Pediatr. 82:987, 1973.

385. Pinna, G. S., Skevaki, C. L., and Kafetzis, D.A.: The significance of Ureaplasma urealyticum as a pathogenic agent in the paediatric population. Curr. Opin. Infect. Dis. 19:283-289, 2006.

386. Pittard, W. B., III, Thullen, J. D., and Fanaroff, A. A.: Neonatal septic arthritis. J. Pediatr. 88:621, 1976.

387. Placezek, M. M., and Whitelaw, A.: Early and late septicemia. Arch. Dis. Child. 58:728, 1983.

388. Potel, J.: Zur granulomatosis infantiseptica. Zentral Bakteriol. Orig. 158:329-331, 1952.

389. Pyati, S. P., Pildes, R. S., Jacobs, N. M., et al.: Penicillin in infants weighing two kilograms or less with early-onset group B streptococcal disease. N. Engl. J. Med. 308:1383, 1983.

390. Pylipow, M., Gaddis, M., and Kinney, J. S.: Selective intrapartum prophylaxis for group B Streptococcus colonization: Management and outcome of newborns. Pediatrics 93:631, 1994.

391. Qureshi, M. E., and Puri, S. P.: Osteomyelitis after exchange transfusion. Br. Med. J. 2:28, 1971.

392. Rabinowitz, S. S., Dzakpasu, P., Piecuch, S., et al.: Platelet-activating factor in infants at risk for necrotizing enterocolitis. J. Pediatr. 138:81-86, 2001.

393. Rahal, J. J., Jr., Hyams, P. J., Simberkoff, M. S., et al.: Combined intrathecal and intramuscular gentamicin for gram-negative meningitis: Pharmacologic study of 21 patients. N. Engl. J. Med. 290:1394, 1974.

394. Ramamurthy, R. S., Srinivasan, G., and Jacobs, N. M.: Necrotizing fasciitis and necrotizing cellulitis due to group B Streptococcus. Am. J. Dis. Child. 131:1169, 1977.

395. Ramilo, O., Mertsola, J., Mustafa, M. M., et al.: Interleukin-1β appears to mediate CSF inflammation in rabbits. Abstract No. 708. Presented at the 29th Interscience Conference on Antimicrobial Agents and Chemotherapy, September, 1989, Houston.

396. Raucher, H. S., Newton, M. J., and Stern, R. H.: Ophthalmia neonatorum caused by penicillinase-producing Neisseria gonorrhoeae. J. Pediatr. 100:925, 1982.

397. Redd, H., Christensen, R. D., and Fisher, C. W.: Circulating and storage neutrophils in septic neonatal rats treated with immunoglobulin. J. Infect. Dis. 157:705, 1988.

398. Reed, R. K., Larter, W. E., Sieber, O. F., et al.: Peripheral nodular lesions in Pseudomonas sepsis: The importance of incision and drainage. J. Pediatr. 88:977, 1976.

399. Regan, E. J., Harrison, G. A., Butler, S., et al.: Primary cutaneous listeriosis in a veterinarian. Vet. Rec. 157:207, 2005.

400. Regan, J. A., Klebanoff, M. A., and Nugent, R.P.: The epidemiology of group B streptococcal colonization in pregnancy. Vaginal Infections and Prematurity Study Group. Obstet. Gynecol. 77:604-610, 1991.

401. Regan, J. A., Klebanoff, M. A., Nugent, R. P., et al.: Colonization with group B streptococci in pregnancy and adverse outcome. VIP Study Group. Am. J. Obstet. Gynecol. 174:1354-1360, 1996.

402. Reid, B. S., and Binder, T. M.: Radiographic evaluation of children with urinary tract infections. Radiol. Clin. North Am. 26:933, 1988.

403. Robbins, J. B., McCracken, G. H., Jr., Gotschlich, E. C., et al.: Escherichia coli K1 capsular polysaccharide associated with neonatal meningitis. N. Engl. J. Med. 290:1216, 1974.

404. Roberts, I. A., and Murray, N. A.: Neonatal thrombocytopenia. Curr. Hematol. Rep. 5:55-63, 2006.

405. Rodriguez, R. J., and Martin, R. J.: Exogenous surfactant therapy in newborns. Respir. Care Clin. North Am. 5:595-616, 1999.

406. Rodwell, R. L., Faims, K., Taylor, K., et al.: Hematologic scoring system in early diagnosis of sepsis in neutropenic newborns. Pediatr. Infect. Dis. J. 12:372, 1993.

407. Roine, I., Faingezicht, I., Arguedas, A., et al.: Serial serum C-reactive protein to monitor recovery from acute hematogenous osteomyelitis in children. Pediatr. Infect. Dis. J. 14:40, 1995.

408. Rolston, K. V. I., Chandrasekar, P. H., and LeFrock, J. L.: Antimicrobial tolerance in group C and group G streptococci. J. Antimicrob. Chemother. 13:389, 1984.

409. Ronnestad, A., Abrahamsen, T. G., Medbo, S., et al.: Septicemia in the first week of life in a Norwegian national cohort of extremely premature infants. Pediatrics 115:e262-e268, 2005.

410. Rotbart, H. A., Levin, M. J., Yolken, R. H., et al.: An outbreak of rotavirus-associated neonatal necrotizing enterocolitis. J. Pediatr. 103:454, 1983.

411. Rowe, D. S., Aicardi, E. Z., Dawson, C. R., et al.: Purulent ocular discharge in neonates: Significance of Chlamydia trachomatis. Pediatrics 63:628, 1979.

412. Rowley, A. H., and Wald, E. R.: Incubation period necessary to detect bacteremia in neonates. Pediatr. Infect. Dis. J. 5:590, 1986.

413. Rubens, C. E., Heggan, L., and Wessels, M.: A genetic marker for virulence of the type III group B streptococci. Abstract 1076. Pediatr. Res. 23:380A, 1988.

414. Rudoy, R. C., and Nelson, J. D.: Breast abscess during the neonatal period: A review. Am. J. Dis. Child. 129:1031, 1975.

415. Ryder, R. W., McGowan, J. E., Hatch, M. H., et al.: Reovirus-like agent as a cause of nosocomial diarrhea in infants. J. Pediatr. 90:698, 1977.

416. Sabath, L. D., Wheeler, N., Laverdiere, M., et al.: A new type of penicillin resistance of Staphylococcus aureus. Lancet 1:443, 1977.

417. Sáez-Llorens, X., Ah Chu, M. S., Castano, E., et al.: Intrapartum prophylaxis with ceftriaxone decreases rates of bacterial colonization and early-onset infection in newborns. Clin. Infect. Dis. 21:876, 1995.

418. Sáez-Llorens, X., Espino, R. T., Moreno, M. T., and Vargas, S.: Sepsis neonatal: Diferencias en la epidemiologia y microbiologia de dos unidades materno-infantiles metropolitanas (1975-1992). Bol. Soc. Panam. Pediatr. 24:26-33, 1995.

419. Sáez-Llorens, X., and McCracken, G. H.: Sepsis syndrome and septic shock in pediatrics: Current concepts on terminology, pathophysiology, and management. J. Pediatr. 123:497, 1993.

420. Sáez-Llorens, X., and McCracken, G. H.: Clinical pharmacology of antibacterial agents. In Remington, J. S., and Klein, J. O. (eds.): Infectious Diseases of the Fetus and Newborn Infant. 4th ed. Philadelphia, W. B. Saunders, 1995, pp. 1287-1336.

421. Sáez-Llorens, X., Ramilo, O., Mustafa, M., et al.: The molecular pathophysiology of bacterial meningitis: Current concepts and therapeutic implications. J. Pediatr. 116:671, 1990.

422. Sáez-Llorens, X., and Siegel, J. D.: Neonatal septicemia, meningitis, and pneumonia. In Gellis & Kagan's Current Pediatric Therapy. 14th ed. Philadelphia, W. B. Saunders, 1993, pp. 544-549.

423. Sáez-Llorens, X., Vargas, S., Guerra, F., et al.: Application of new sepsis definitions to evaluate outcome of pediatric patients with severe systemic infections. Pediatr. Infect. Dis. J. 14:557, 1995.

424. Sáez-Llorens, X., Velarde, J., and Cantón, C.: Pediatric osteomyelitis in a developing country. Clin. Infect. Dis. 19:323, 1994.

425. Safdar, A., Papadoupoulous, E. B., and Armstrong, D.: Listeriosis in recipients of allogeneic blood and marrow transplantation: Thirteen year review of disease characteristics, treatment outcomes and a new association with human cytomegalovirus infection. Bone Marrow Transplant. 29:913-916, 2002.

426. Sánchez P.: MRSA in Parkland Memorial Hospital nursery, Dallas, 2006. Personal communication.

427. Sánchez, P. J., Siegel, J. D., Cushion, N. B., et al.: Significance of a positive urine group B streptococcal latex agglutination test in neonates. J. Pediatr. 116:601, 1990.

428. Sandström, K. I., Bell, T. A., Chandler, J. W., et al.: Microbial causes of neonatal conjunctivitis. J. Pediatr. 105:706, 1984.

429. Sann, L., Bienvenu, F., Bienvenu, J., et al.: Evolution of serum prealbumin, C-reactive protein, and orosomucoid in neonates with bacterial infection. J. Pediatr. 105:977, 1984.

430. Sarff, L. D., McCracken, G. H., Jr., Schiffer, M. S., et al.: Epidemiology of Escherichia coli K1 in healthy and diseased newborns. Lancet 1:1099, 1975.

431. Sarff, L. D., Platt, L. H., and McCracken, G. H., Jr.: Cerebrospinal fluid evaluation in neonates: Comparison of high-risk infants with and without meningitis. J. Pediatr. 88:473, 1976.

432. Sarman, G., Moise, A. A., and Edwards, M. S.: Meningeal inflammation in neonatal gram-negative bacteremia. Pediatr. Infect. Dis. J. 14:701, 1995.

433. Sawardekar, K. P.: Changing spectrum of neonatal omphalitis. Pediatr. Infect. Dis. J. 23:22-26, 2004.

434. Schaad, U. B., Kaplan, S. L., and McCracken, G. H.: Steroid therapy for bacterial meningitis. Clin. Infect. Dis. 20:685, 1995.

435. Schaad, U. B., McCracken, G. H., Jr., Threlkeld, N., et al.: Clinical evaluation of a new broad-spectrum oxa-beta-lactam antibiotic, moxalactam, in neonates and infants. J. Pediatr. 98:129, 1981.

436. Scheifele, D. W., Melton, P., and Whitchelo, V.: Evaluation of the Limulus test for endotoxemia in neonates with suspected sepsis. J. Pediatr. 98:899, 1981.

437. Scheld, W. M., Quagliarello, V. J., and Wispelwey, B.: The potential role of host cytokines in Haemophilus influenzae lipopolysaccharide-induced blood-brain barrier permeability. Pediatr. Infect. Dis. J. 8:910, 1989.

438. Schiano, M. A., Hauth, J. C., and Gilstrap, L. C.: Second-stage fetal tachycardia and neonatal infection. Am. J. Obstet. Gynecol. 148:779, 1984.

439. Schlech, W. F., 3rd.: Foodborne listeriosis. Clin. Infect. Dis. 31:770-775, 2000.

440. Schlech, W. F., III, Lavigne, P. M., Bortolussi, R., et al.: Epidemic listeriosis: Evidence of transmission by food. N. Engl. J. Med. 308:203, 1983.

441. Schneerson, R., Rodrigues, L. P., Parke, J. C., Jr., et al.: Immunity to disease caused by Hemophilus influenzae type b. II. Specificity and some biologic characteristics of "natural," infection-acquired, and immunization-induced antibodies to the capsular polysaccharide of Hemophilus influenzae type b. J. Immunol. 107:1081, 1971.

442. Schouten-Van Meeteren, N. Y., Rietveld, A., Moolenaar, A. J., et al.: Influence of perinatal conditions on C-reactive protein production. J. Pediatr. 120:621, 1992.

443. Schrag, S., and Schuchat, A.: Prevention of neonatal sepsis. Clin. Perinatol. 32:601-615, 2005.

444. Schrag, S. J., Zell, E. R., Lynfield, R., et al.: A population-based comparison of strategies to prevent early-onset group B streptococcal disease in neonates. N. Engl. J. Med. 347:233-239, 2002.

445. Schrag, S. J., Zywicki, S., Farley, M. M., et al.: Group B streptococcal disease in the era of intrapartum antibiotic prophylaxis. N. Engl. J. Med. 342:15-20, 2000.

446. Schuchat, A., Deaver, K., Hayes, P. S., et al.: Gastrointestinal carriage of Listeria monocytogenes in household contacts of patients with listeriosis. J. Infect. Dis. 167:1261-1262, 1993.

447. Schuchat, A., Deaver-Robinson, K., Plikaytis, B. D., et al.: Multistate case-control study of maternal risk factors for neonatal group B streptococcal disease. The Active Surveillance Study Group. Pediatr. Infect. Dis. J. 13:623-629, 1994.

448. Schuchat, A., Lizano, C., Broome, C. V., et al.: Outbreak of neonatal listeriosis associated with mineral oil. Pediatr. Infect. Dis. J. 10:183, 1991.

449. Schuchat, A., Oxtoby, M., Cochi, S., et al.: Population-based risk factors for neonatal group B streptococcal disease: Results of a cohort study in metropolitan Atlanta. J. Infect. Dis. 162:672-677, 1990.

450. Schuchat, A., Zywicki, S. S., Dinsmoor, M. J., et al.: Risk factors and opportunities for prevention of early-onset neonatal sepsis: A multicenter case-control study. Pediatrics 105:21-26, 2000.

451. Seeliger, H. P. R.: Listeriosis. New York, Hafner, 1961.

452. Sherman, M. P., Chance, K. H., and Goetzman, B. W.: Gram's stains of tracheal secretions predict neonatal bacteremia. Am. J. Dis. Child. 138:848, 1984.

453. Shinefield, H. R.: Staphylococcal infections. In Remington, J. S., and Klein, J. O. (eds.): Infectious Diseases of the Fetus and Newborn Infant. 3rd ed. Philadelphia, W. B. Saunders, 1990, pp. 866-900.

454. Shuman, R. M., Leech, R. W., and Alvord, E. C., Jr.: Neurotoxicity of hexachlorophene in the human. I. A clinicopathologic study of 248 children. Pediatrics 54:689, 1974.

455. Shurin, P. A., Howie, V. M., Pelton, S. I., et al.: Bacterial etiology of otitis media during the first six weeks of life. J. Pediatr. 92:893, 1978.

456. Siegel, J. D., and McCracken, G. H., Jr.: Group D streptococcal infections. J. Pediatr. 93:542, 1978.

457. Siegel, J. D., and McCracken, G. H., Jr.: Sepsis neonatorum. N. Engl. J. Med. 304:642, 1981.

458. Siegel, J. D., McCracken, G. H., Jr., Threlkeld, N., et al.: Single-dose penicillin prophylaxis against neonatal group B streptococcal infection. N. Engl. J. Med. 303:769, 1980.

459. Siegel, J. D., McCracken, G. H., Jr., Threlkeld, N., et al.: Single-dose penicillin prophylaxis of neonatal group-B streptococcal disease: Conclusion of a 41 month controlled trial. Lancet 1:1426, 1982.

460. Siegel, J. D., Shannon, K. M., and DePasse, B. M.: Recurrent infection associated with penicillin-tolerant group B streptococci: A report of two cases. J. Pediatr. 99:920, 1981.

461. Siegman-Igra, Y., Levin, R., Weinberger, M., et al.: Listeria monocytogenes infection in Israel and review of cases worldwide. Emerg. Infect. Dis. 8:305-310, 2002.

462. Silver, R. P., Finn, C. W., Vann, W. F., et al.: Molecular cloning of the K1 capsular polysaccharide genes of E. coli. Nature 289:696, 1981.

463. Simpson, R. A., Spencer, A. F., Speller, D. C. E., et al.: Colonization by gentamicin-resistant Staphylococcus epidermidis in a special care baby unit. J. Hosp. Infect. 7:108, 1986.

464. Sinha, A., Lieu, T. A., Paoletti, L. C., et al.: The projected health benefits of maternal group B streptococcal vaccination in the era of chemoprophylaxis. Vaccine 23:3187-3195, 2005.

465. Smith, R. T., Platou, E. S., and Good, R. A.: Septicemia of the newborn: Current status of the problem. Pediatrics 17:549, 1956.

466. Sood, K., Mulvihill, D., and Daum, R. S.: Intrarenal abscess caused by Klebsiella pneumoniae in a neonate: Modern management and diagnosis. Am. J. Perinatol. 6:367, 1989.

467. Speer, C. P., Hauptmann, D., Stubbe, P., et al.: Neonatal septicemia and meningitis in Göttingen, West Germany. Pediatr. Infect. Dis. 4:36, 1985.

468. Spigelblatt, L., Saintonge, J., Chicoine, R., et al.: Changing pattern of neonatal streptococcal septicemia. Pediatr. Infect. Dis. 4:56, 1985.

469. Squire, E., Favara, B., and Todd, J.: Diagnosis of neonatal bacterial infection: Hematologic and pathologic findings in fatal and nonfatal cases. Pediatrics 64:60, 1979.

470. Squire, E. N., Jr., Reich, H. M., Merenstein, G. B., et al.: Criteria for the discontinuation of antibiotic therapy during presumptive treatment of suspected neonatal infection. Pediatr. Infect. Dis. 1:85, 1982.

471. Sreenan, C., and Osiovich, H.: Myeloid colony-stimulating factors: Use in the newborn. Arch. Pediatr. Adolesc. Med. 153:984-988, 1999.

472. Stabile, A., Miceli Sopo, S., Romanelli, V., et al.: Intravenous immunoglobulin for prophylaxis of neonatal sepsis in premature infants. Arch. Dis. Child. 63:441, 1988.

473. Steere, A. C., Aber, R. C., Warford, L. R., et al.: Possible nosocomial transmission of group B streptococci in a newborn nursery. J. Pediatr. 87:784, 1975.

474. Stetler, H., Martin, E., Plotkin, S., et al.: Neonatal mastitis due to Escherichia coli. J. Pediatr. 76:611, 1970.

475. Stevens, D. C., Kleiman, M. B., and Schreiner, R. L.: Early onset Pseudomonas sepsis of the neonate. Perinatol. Neonatol. 6:75, 1982.

476. Stoll, B. J., Gordon, T., Korones, S. B., et al.: Early-onset sepsis in very low birth weight neonates: A report from the National Institute of Child Health and Human Development Neonatal Research Network. J. Pediatr. 129:72-80, 1996.

477. Stoll, B. J., Hansen, N., Fanaroff, A. A., et al.: Changes in pathogens causing early-onset sepsis in very-low-birth-weight infants. N. Engl. J. Med. 347:240-247, 2002.

478. Stoll, B. J., Hansen, N., Fanaroff, A. A., et al.: Late-onset sepsis in very low birth weight neonates: The experience of the NICHD Neonatal Research Network. Pediatrics 110:285-291, 2002.

479. Storch, G. A., and Rajagopalan, L.: Methicillin-resistant Staphylococcus aureus bacteremia in children. Pediatr. Infect. Dis. J. 5:59, 1986.

480. Storm, W.: Transient bacteremia following endotracheal suctioning in ventilated newborns. Pediatrics 65:487, 1980.

481. Suksanong, M., and Dajani, A. S.: Detection of Haemophilus influenzae type b antigens in body fluids, using specific antibody-coated staphylococci. J. Clin. Microbiol. 5:81, 1977.

482. Sung, L., Ramotar, K., Samson, L. M., and Toye, B.: Bacteremia due to persistent strains of coagulase-negative staphylococci in a neonatal intensive-care unit. Infect. Control Hosp. Epidemiol. 20:349-351, 1999.

483. Szanton, V. L.: Epidemic salmonellosis: A 30-month study of 80 cases of Salmonella oranienburg infection. Pediatrics 20:794, 1957.

484. Tan, T. Q., Mason, E. O., Jr., Ou, C. N., and Kaplan, S. C.: Use of intravenous rifampin in neonates with persistent staphylococcal bacteremia. Antimicrob. Agents Chemother. 37:2401-2406, 1993.

485. Tashjian, J. H., Coulam, C. B., and Washington, J. A., II.: Vaginal flora in asymptomatic women. Mayo Clin. Proc. 51:557, 1976.

486. Terrone, D. A., Rinehart, B. K., Einstein, M. H., et al.: Neonatal sepsis and death caused by resistant Escherichia coli: Possible consequences of extended maternal ampicillin administration. Am. J. Obstet. Gynecol. 180:1345-1348, 1999.

487. Tetzlaff, T. R., Ashworth, C., and Nelson, J. D.: Otitis media in children less than 12 weeks of age. Pediatrics 59:827, 1977.

488. Tetzlaff, T. R., Howard, J. B., McCracken, G. H., Jr., et al.: Antibiotic concentrations in pus and bone of children with osteomyelitis. J. Pediatr. 92:135, 1978.

489. Thompson, R. L., Cabezudo, I., and Wenzel, R. P.: Epidemiology of nosocomial infections caused by methicillin-resistant Staphylococcus aureus. Ann. Intern. Med. 97:309, 1982.

490. Thomson, J., and Lewis, I. C.: Osteomyelitis in the newborn. Arch. Dis. Child. 25:273, 1950.

491. Tipple, M. A., Beem, M. O., and Saxon, E. M.: Clinical characteristics of the afebrile pneumonia associated with Chlamydia trachomatis infection in infants less than 6 months of age. Pediatrics 63:192, 1979.

492. Totterdell, B. M., Chrystie, I. L., and Banatvala, J. E.: Cord blood and breast milk antibodies in neonatal rotavirus infection. Br. Med. J. 1:828, 1980.

493. Towers, C. V., Carr, M. H., Padilla, G., et al.: Potential consequences of widespread antepartal use of ampicillin. Am. J. Obstet. Gynecol. 179:879-883, 1998.

494. Tupperainen, N., Osterlund, K., and Hallman, M.: Selective intrapartum penicillin prophylaxis of early onset group B streptococcal disease. Abstract. Pediatr. Res. 20:403A, 1986.

495. Turner, D., Leibovitz, E., Aran, A., et al.: Acute otitis media in infants younger than two months of age: Microbiology, clinical presentation and therapeutic approach. Pediatr. Infect. Dis. J. 21:669-674, 2002.

496. Umaña, M. A., Odio, C. M., Salas, J. L., et al.: Comparative evaluation of aztreonam/ampicillin versus amikacin/ampicillin in neonates with bacterial infections. Presented at the 27th Interscience Conference on Antimicrobial Agents and Chemotherapy, October, 1987, New York.

497. Unhanand, M., Mustafa, M. M., McCracken, G. H., et al.: Gram-negative enteric bacillary meningitis: A twenty-one-year experience. J. Pediatr. 122:15, 1993.

498. Van Rossum, A. M., Wulkan, R. W., and Oudesluys-Murphy, A. M.: Procalcitonin as an early marker of infection in neonates and children. Lancet Infect. Dis. 4:620-630, 2004.

499. Vawter, G. F.: Perinatal listeriosis. In Rosenberg, H. S., and Bernstein, J. (eds.): Perspectives in Pediatric Pathology. Vol. 6. New York, Masson Publishing, 1981, p. 153.

500. Velaphi, S., Siegel, J. D., Wendel, G. D., Jr., et al.: Early-onset group B streptococcal infection after a combined maternal and neonatal group B streptococcal chemoprophylaxis strategy. Pediatrics 111:541-547, 2003.

501. Visintine, A. M., Oleske, J. M., and Nahmias, A. J.: Listeria monocytogenes infection in infants and children. Am. J. Dis. Child. 131:393, 1977.

501. Vogel, L. C., Kretschmer, R. R., Boyer, K. M., et al.: Human immunity to group B streptococci measured by indirect immunofluorescence: Correlation with protection in chick embryos. J. Infect. Dis. 140:682, 1979.

503. Voora, S., Srinivasan, G., Lilien, L. D., et al.: Fever in full-term newborns in the first four days of life. Pediatrics 69:40, 1982.

504. Wagener, M. M., Rycheck, R. R., Yee, R. B., et al.: Septic dermatitis of the neonatal scalp and maternal endomyometritis with intrapartum internal fetal monitoring. Pediatrics 74:81, 1984.

505. Walker, K. M., and Coyer, W. F.: Suprarenal abscess due to group B Streptococcus. J. Pediatr. 94:970, 1979.

506. Walsh, W. F., Stanley, S., Lally, K. P., et al.: Ureaplasma urealyticum demonstrated by open lung biopsy in newborns with chronic lung disease. Pediatr. Infect. Dis. J. 10:823, 1991.

507. Wang, E. L., Cassell, G. H., Sánchez, P. J., et al.: Ureaplasma urealyticum and chronic lung disease of prematurity: Critical appraisal of the literature on causation. Clin. Infect. Dis. 17:S112, 1993.

508. Ward, J. I., Siber, G. R., Scheifele, D. W., et al.: Rapid diagnosis of Hemophilus influenzae type b infections by latex particle agglutination and counterimmunoelectrophoresis. J. Pediatr. 93:37, 1978.

509. Warren, W. S., and Stool, S. E.: Otitis media in low-birth weight infants. J. Pediatr. 79:740, 1971.

510. Wasserman, R. L.: Unconventional therapies for neonatal sepsis. Pediatr. Infect. Dis. 2:421, 1983.

511. Watt, S., Lanotte, P., Mereghetti, L., et al.: Escherichia coli strains from pregnant women and neonates: Intraspecies genetic distribution and prevalence of virulence factors. J. Clin. Microbiol. 41:1929-1935, 2003.

512. Weems, J. J., Jr., Jarvis, W. R., and Colman, G.: A cluster of late onset group B streptococcal infections in low birth weight premature infants: No evidence of horizontal transmission. Pediatr. Infect. Dis. J. 5:715, 1986.

513. Weinberg, A. G., and Laird, W. P.: Group B streptococcal endocarditis detected by echocardiography. J. Pediatr. *92*:335, 1978.

514. Weinberger, M., Haynes, R. E., and Morse, T. S.: Necrotizing fasciitis in a neonate. Am. J. Dis. Child. *123*:591, 1972.

515. Weissman, C. L. E., Anthony B. F., Hemming, V. G., et al.: Comparison of group B streptococcal hyperimmune globulin and standard intravenously administered immune globulin in neonates. J. Pediatr. *122*:929, 1993.

516. Weissman, C. L. E., Stoll, B. J., Kueser, T. J., et al.: Intravenous immune globulin therapy for early-onset sepsis in premature neonates. J. Pediatr. *121*:434, 1992.

517. Weissman, C. L. E., Stoll, B. J., Kueser, T. J., et al.: Intravenous immune globulin prophylaxis of late-onset sepsis in premature neonates. J. Pediatr. *125*:922, 1994.

518. Welshimer, H. J., and Winglewish, N. G.: Listeriosis: Summary of seven cases of *Listeria* meningitis. J. A. M. A. *171*:1319, 1959.

519. Whittle, H. C., Tugwell, P., Egler, L. J., et al.: Rapid bacteriological diagnosis of pyogenic meningitis by latex agglutination. Lancet *2*:619, 1974.

520. Wientzen, R. L., McCracken, G. H., Jr., Petruska, M. L., et al.: Localization and therapy of urinary tract infections of childhood. Pediatrics *63*:467, 1979.

521. Wilson, H. D., and Haltalin, K. C.: Acute necrotizing fasciitis in childhood: Report of 11 cases. Am. J. Dis. Child. *125*:591, 1973.

522. Wiswell, T. E., and Geschke, D. W.: Risk from circumcision during the first month of life compared with those for uncircumcised boys. Pediatrics *83*:1011, 1989.

523. Wiswell, T. E., and Roscelli, J. D.: Corroborative evidence for the decreased incidence of urinary tract infections in circumcised male infants. Pediatrics *78*:96, 1986.

524. Word, B. M., and Klein, J. O.: Therapy of bacterial sepsis and meningitis in infants and children: 1989 poll of directors of programs in pediatric infectious diseases. Pediatr. Infect. Dis. J. *8*:635, 1989.

525. Yao, Y., Xie, Y., and Kim, K. S.: Genomic comparison of *Escherichia coli* K1 strains isolated from the cerebrospinal fluid of patients with meningitis. Infect. Immun. *74*:2196-2206, 2006.

526. Yoder, M. C., Douglas, S. D., Gerdes, J., et al.: Plasma fibronectin in healthy newborn infants: Respiratory diseases syndrome and perinatal asphyxia. J. Pediatr. *102*:777, 1983.

527. Yoshio, H., Tollin, M., Gudmundsson, G. H., et al.: Antimicrobial polypeptides of human vernix caseosa and amniotic fluid: Implications for newborn innate defense. Pediatr. Res. *53*:211-216, 2003.

528. Yow, M. D., Leeds, L. J., Thompson, P. K., et al.: The natural history of group B streptococcal colonization in the pregnant woman and her offspring. I. Colonization studies. Am. J. Obstet. Gynecol. *137*:34, 1980.

529. Yow, M. D., Mason, E. O., Leeds, L. J., et al.: Ampicillin prevents intrapartum transmission of group B *Streptococcus*. J. A. M. A. *241*:1245, 1979.

530. Zaidi, A. K., Huskins, W. C., Thaver, D., et al.: Hospital-acquired neonatal infections in developing countries. Lancet *365*:1175-1188, 2005.

531. Zangwill, K. M., Schuchat, A., and Wenger, J. D.: Group B streptococcal disease in the United States, 1990: Report from a multistate active surveillance system. M. M. W. R. C. D. C. Surveill. Summ. *41*:25-32, 1992.

INFECTIONS OF THE COMPROMISED HOST

PRIMARY IMMUNODEFICIENCIES

Javier Chinen ✪ Mark W. Kline ✪ William T. Shearer

Primary immunodeficiencies include a broad range of congenital and hereditary disorders that manifest with a defect in the development or function of the immune system and, as a consequence, with increased susceptibility to infections and autoimmunity. Although the molecular defects are present from birth, clinical manifestations may not be evident until much later in life. Previously considered of rare occurrence, primary immunodeficiency disorders are estimated to occur in 1 in 10,000 live births, with a wide range of severity depending on the degree of compromise of the immune function, including mild presentation variants that are clinically subtle and difficult to diagnose. This rate is minimal and considered underestimated because it is based on hospital records and does not include two frequent conditions that usually manifest with only minor immunologic abnormalities: DiGeorge syndrome (1 in 3000 live births) and selective IgA deficiency (1 in 500 individuals).

In contrast to primary immunodeficiencies, secondary immunodeficiencies are acquired disorders, with immune dysfunction occurring as a result of exogenous factors or along with some other non-immune primary disease process. Causes of secondary immunodeficiency include infection (e.g., human immunodeficiency virus [HIV]), drugs (e.g., corticosteroids), malnutrition, and neoplastic or metabolic diseases (e.g., Hodgkin disease, diabetes mellitus). Secondary immunodeficiency disorders, such as those resulting from malnutrition or HIV infection, are diagnosed far more frequently than primary immunodeficiencies.

Pediatricians refer children for immunologic evaluation when they present with unusually frequent or severe infections or when they present with infections that are caused by uncommon organisms (Table 79–1). Most of these children are immunocompetent and may have risk factors for increased frequency of infections, such as allergic disorders, anatomic abnormalities, or other clinical conditions that secondarily produce increased susceptibility to development of infections, as discussed earlier. Some evaluated children have a known primary immunodeficiency and benefit from early diagnosis and management.

Understanding of primary immunodeficiencies has increased in recent years with the significant scientific progress that has been made, especially with the description of gene defects responsible for most of the observed immunodeficiency syndromes and leading to the restoration of immune function by gene therapy in two forms of severe combined immunodeficiency (SCID) (see later).

This chapter discusses the elements of the medical history and physical examination that can help to establish the diagnosis of a primary immunodeficiency, in addition to screening laboratory tests that are useful to assess clinically significant immune dysfunction. The most common primary antibody, cellular immunity, complement, and phagocyte deficiencies are described. Also, a few rare but distinctive conditions, including ataxia-telangiectasia and Wiskott-Aldrich Syndrome (WAS), are reviewed.

INITIAL EVALUATION FOR SUSPECTED IMMUNODEFICIENCY

MEDICAL HISTORY

A comprehensive medical history is the key element in identifying children who are likely to have an immunodeficiency. Children with immunodeficiencies often have a history of frequent and severe infections (e.g., pneumonia, meningitis, septicemia, osteomyelitis, abscess of soft tissue or an internal organ). Although infections occur commonly throughout childhood, epidemiologic studies have established a range for the average number of infections that a normal child may have per year. Otherwise healthy children younger than 5 years old average three to eight episodes of upper respiratory infection annually.[14,38] By 1 year of age, 62 percent of children have had at least one episode of acute otitis media, and 17 percent have had three or more episodes.[101] By 3 years of age, more than 80 percent of children have had at least one episode of acute otitis media, and 46 percent have had three or more episodes. Although these studies have not been repeated since routine anti–*Haemophilus influenzae* type b (Hib) and anti-pneumococcal vaccinations were introduced, the frequency of respiratory infections has not changed; however, the causal agents have been replaced by viral and other bacterial pathogens.

Approximately 2 percent of children 1 to 5 years old develop symptomatic urinary tract infection.[92] The incidence of gastroenteritis among children in the United States is approximately two to three episodes per child-year, with rates of five episodes per child-year among children attending daycare centers.[12,44] Occurrence of these infections during infancy or early childhood in normal children is the result of several factors, including immunologic immaturity or naiveté (lack of prior exposure to infectious agents); poor hygiene; mouthing behavior; allergic disease; and frequent exposure to ill contacts in the home, school, or daycare setting.

The courses of individual episodes of infection in an immunodeficient child may be unusually prolonged or associated with unexpected complications (e.g., lung abscess in a child with pneumonia or skull bone osteomyelitis as a complication of sinusitis). Generally, infections that develop over time at multiple body sites are more suggestive of immunodeficiency than are infections occurring at only one site (e.g., recurrent otitis media). In the latter circumstance, a mechanical or anatomic explanation for the infections (e.g., foreign body or occult tracheoesophageal fistula in a child with recurrent pneumonia, congenital fistulous tract to the middle ear in a child with recurrent bacterial meningitis) should be considered.

A history of recurrent infections of defined cause is more meaningful than a history of frequent, self-limited infections of presumed viral cause. Children with primary antibody deficien-

TABLE 79–1 When to Suspect an Immunodeficiency Disorder

Increased number of infections
Increased severity of infectious disease
Poor response to antibiotic therapy
Unusual organisms (opportunistic infections)
Failure to thrive
Poor wound healing
"Cold" *Staphylococcus* species infection (absence of pus)
Recurrent periodontitis
Low granulocyte or lymphocyte count

TABLE 79–2 Common Pathogens in Children with Primary Immunodeficiency

Immunodeficiency	Common Pathogens
Antibody deficiencies	*Streptococcus pneumoniae, Haemophilus influenzae, Staphylococcus aureus, Pseudomonas aeruginosa, Mycoplasma* species, *Salmonella* species, *Shigella* species, *Campylobacter* species, rotavirus, enteroviruses, *Giardia* species
Cellular and combined immunodeficiencies	Mycobacteria, *S. pneumoniae, P. aeruginosa, Candida* species, *Pneumocystis jiroveci,* herpesviruses, adenoviruses
Complement deficiencies	*S. pneumoniae, H. influenzae, Neisseria* species
Phagocyte deficiencies	*S. aureus, Nocardia* species, *P. aeruginosa, Serratia* species, enteric gram-negative bacilli, *Candida* species, *Aspergillus* species

cies typically experience infections caused by extracellular bacteria with polysaccharide capsules (e.g., *Streptococcus pneumoniae*, Hib). In contrast, children with primary cellular immunodeficiencies often have infections with unusual or opportunistic viruses, fungi, protozoa, and mycobacteria (Table 79–2). Because of the impairment of T-cell–dependent antibody responses, infections with common bacteria also may be observed. Children with primary deficiencies of complement components typically have recurrent neisserial infections, and children with phagocyte deficiencies may have infections with a variety of catalase-positive bacterial (e.g., *Staphylococcus aureus, Pseudomonas aeruginosa, Serratia marcescens*) and fungal (e.g., *Candida* spp., *Aspergillus* spp.) organisms. Severe infections with atypical mycobacteria often indicate a defect in interleukin-12 (IL-12)–mediated or interferon-γ–mediated responses.

In addition to the microbial cause of infections, several other items of historical information may help to define the risk for and possible nature of a primary immunodeficiency. Because young infants are afforded some protection by the presence of maternal IgG, children with primary antibody deficiencies generally have an initial period of relative well-being, with onset of infections occurring when they are 3 to 18 months of age. Children with severe T-cell, complement, or phagocyte deficiencies may have onset of infections in the first days or weeks of life.

Omphalitis and poor wound healing suggest phagocyte deficiency. Hypocalcemic seizures in the neonatal period and congenital heart disease may be clues to the presence of DiGeorge syndrome. Severe disease associated with administration of live vaccines (e.g., bacille Calmette-Guérin, measles, poliomyelitis, varicella) suggests an immune defect. The absence of potential causes for secondary immunodeficiency should be sought and shown.

Family history can offer important clues to the presence of a primary immunodeficiency. A family history of consanguinity or deaths from infection or from unexplained causes during infancy

TABLE 79–3 X-Linked Primary Immunodeficiency Disorders

X-linked agammaglobulinemia (Bruton disease)
Immunodeficiency with hyper-IgM (CD40 ligand deficiency)
X-linked ectodermal dysplasia with immunodeficiency (NEMO defect)
Immunodeficiency, polyendocrinopathy, enteropathy, X-linked (IPEX)
X-linked lymphoproliferative syndrome
Severe combined immunodeficiency (common gamma-chain deficiency)
Properdin deficiency
Wiskott-Aldrich syndrome
X-linked chronic granulomatous disease (most cases)

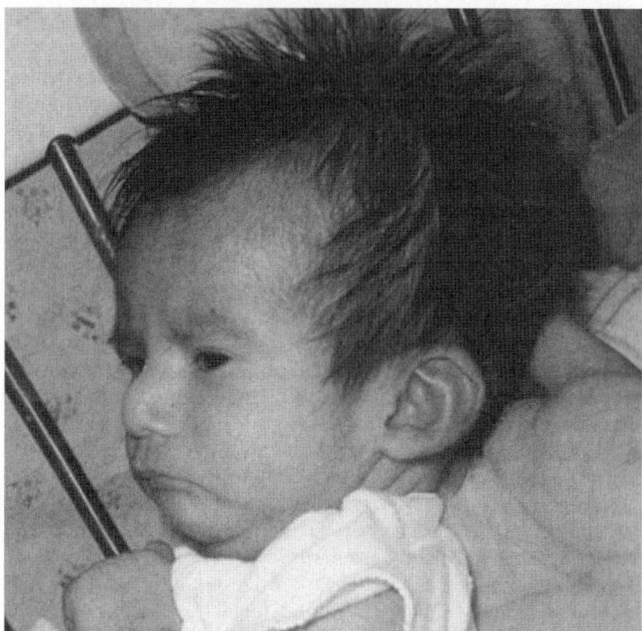

Figure 79–1 Typical facial appearance of a child with DiGeorge anomaly. Notice the microstomia, hypertelorism, upturned nose, and posteriorly rotated and small, low-set ears. (See companion Expert Consult web site for color version.)

or early childhood suggests a genetic defect. Many immunodeficiency syndromes have X-linked inheritance patterns (Table 79–3), which explains the male-to-female ratio of 5:1 among children with primary immunodeficiencies seen in the pediatrician's office.

PHYSICAL EXAMINATION

Except for patients with DiGeorge syndrome, who have distinctive dysmorphic features, or Omenn syndrome, which is characterized by severe rash during the newborn period, the physical examination in children with primary immunodeficiency may not be revealing, especially when patients are very young and have not been exposed to potential pathogens. Short stature is a feature of some of these congenital disorders (e.g., chronic granulomatous disease [CGD]), with wasting or failure to thrive likely being secondary to recurrent infections or other chronic conditions such as intestinal malabsorption. Oral candidiasis, omphalitis, and multiple skin abscesses may indicate an underlying immune disorder. A paucity of lymphoid tissues (e.g., tonsils, lymph nodes) suggests poor lymphocyte development.

Examples of helpful physical stigmata include the characteristic facial features (Fig. 79–1) and cardiac malformations in children with DiGeorge syndrome. Telangiectasia of the bulbar conjunctivae (Fig. 79–2), nasal bridge, ears, and flexor surfaces of the extremities, with or without ataxia, suggests ataxia telangiectasia. Chronic eczema is observed in hyper-IgE and Wiskott-Aldrich syndromes, and severe gingivitis and periodontitis with loss of alveolar bone and dentition can occur in children with LAD (Fig. 79–3).

LABORATORY TESTS

The initial evaluation for immunodeficiency can be done with commonly available, inexpensive laboratory tests to exclude most serious disorders (Table 79–4). This evaluation should be targeted to the type of immunodeficiency (e.g., antibody deficiency versus T-cell defect) suggested by the medical history and physical examination findings. Laboratory test results must be interpreted in the context of the child's age because average normal serum immunoglobulin levels, T-cell counts, and other immune parameters physiologically change with age.[37]

The initial evaluation for immunodeficiency includes a complete blood count and examination of the peripheral blood smear. Because 50 to 70 percent of circulating lymphocytes are T cells, children with severe cellular (e.g., complete DiGeorge syndrome) or combined (e.g., SCID) immunodeficiencies may have lymphopenia. Children with Wiskott-Aldrich syndrome have reduced numbers of platelets, which are small (decreased mean platelet volume), a characteristic that is unique for this syndrome and the related X-linked thrombocytopenia. Large neutrophil cytoplasmic granules are observed in children with Chédiak-Higashi syndrome.

A complete blood count also is useful in excluding congenital neutropenia. Children with LAD often have the opposite, with markedly increased neutrophil and total white blood cell counts. The presence of Howell-Jolly bodies, with or without thrombocytosis, suggests anatomic or functional asplenia. Other tests to rule out HIV infection, malnutrition, or metabolic disorders as causes of secondary immunodeficiency should be considered.

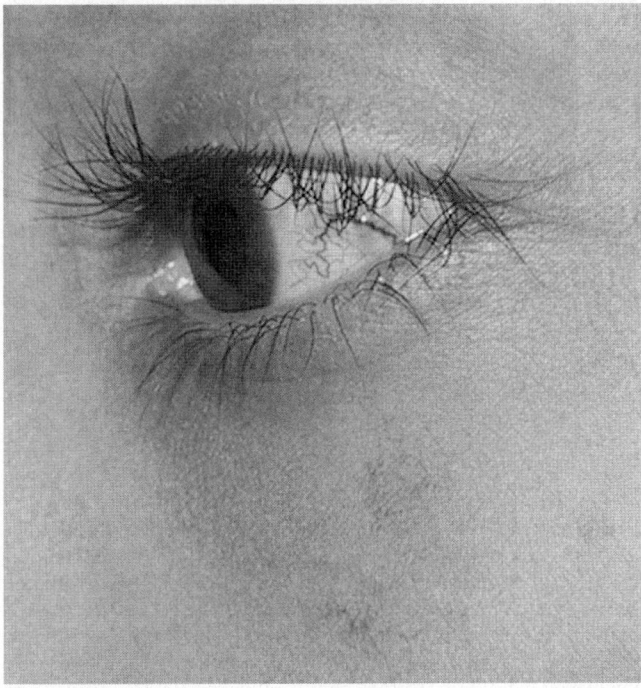

Figure 79–2 Telangiectases of the bulbar conjunctivae in a child with ataxia telangiectasia. (See companion Expert Consult web site for color version.)

TABLE 79–4 Screening Tests for Suspected Primary Immunodeficiency

Immunodeficiency	Screening Tests
All types	Complete blood cell count
	Peripheral blood smear, for percentage of leukocyte types
Antibody deficiency	Quantitative serum immunoglobulins, IgG, IgA, IgM
	Post-immunization antibody titers
	Isohemagglutinins
Cellular immunodeficiency	Delayed hypersensitivity skin tests
	Chest radiography or chest CT for thymus size
	Lymphocyte phenotyping for CD3, CD4, CD8, CD19
Complement deficiency	Total hemolytic complement (CH50) assay
Phagocyte deficiency	Nitroblue tetrazolium dye test
	Dihydrorhodamine (DHR)-1,2,3
	Neutrophil CD11a,b,c/CD18 expression

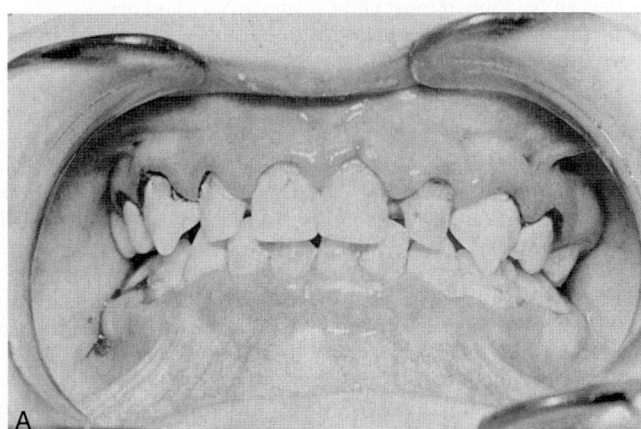

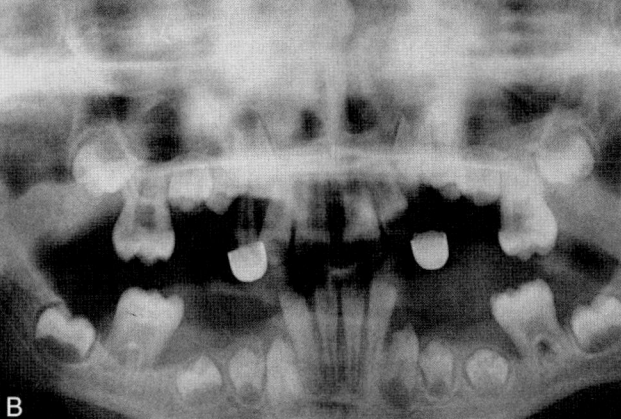

Figure 79–3 A, Chronic periodontitis in a boy with leukocyte adhesion deficiency. **B,** Radiograph of the same patient shows extensive alveolar bone loss. *(Courtesy of Dr. Bruce Carter, Texas Children's Hospital, Houston, TX.)*

Evaluation of Humoral Immunity

Screening evaluation of a child with suspected antibody deficiency should include quantitative measurement of serum immunoglobulins and functional assessment of specific antibody responses. Except for the rare deficiency of antibody response to specific antigens, children with primary antibody deficiencies have abnormalities of serum immunoglobulin concentrations. Measurement of serum IgG, IgA, and IgM concentrations identifies children with panhypogammaglobulinemia and children with deficiency of a particular immunoglobulin isotype, such as selective IgA deficiency. Because of marked age-related changes in serum immunoglobulin concentrations, use of age-appropriate normal values for assessment purposes is important.

Functional antibody production usually is evaluated by measuring antibody titers generated in response to immunization with vaccines, such as diphtheria and tetanus toxoids. Antibody responses to polysaccharide antigens do not require cooperation of T cells and are evaluated separately using the pneumococcal polysaccharide vaccine (Pneumovax 23; Merck & Co., West Point, PA) after the child reaches 24 months of age. Younger infants are thought to have a functional immaturity in the ability to respond to this class of antigens. Alternatively, because ABO blood group antigens are polysaccharides and cross-reacting environmental antigen epitopes are ubiquitous, production of anti-polysaccharide antibodies can be assessed by measuring serum isohemagglutinin titers, taking into consideration that children with blood type AB do not form isohemagglutinins. The conjugated pneumococcal (Prevnar; Wyeth-Ayerst, Philadelphia, PA) and Hib (several brand names) vaccines are not suitable for the assessment of anti-polysaccharide antibody responses because they are not pure polysaccharides. Patients vaccinated with the conjugated pneumococcal vaccine still can be evaluated for production of anti-polysaccharide antibodies because the pneumococcal polysaccharide vaccine contains serotype antigens against which the conjugated vaccine does not protect.

Measurement of serum IgG subclasses may be indicated for children with apparent abnormalities in functional antibody production. Further evaluation of children whose screening tests indicate significant quantitative and functional antibody abnormalities should include enumeration of T and B cells in the peripheral blood and in vitro studies of mitogen-induced or antigen-induced B-cell proliferation. The antibody response to neoantigens (e.g., bacterial phages) may be useful for the evaluation of patients receiving immunoglobulin therapy.

Evaluation of Cellular Immunity

The screening evaluation for cellular immunodeficiency starts with delayed hypersensitivity skin tests and, in young infants, posteroanterior and lateral chest radiographs for the assessment of the thymus size (Fig. 79–4). A chest computed tomography or ultrasound scan also may be helpful if available.

Delayed hypersensitivity skin tests are performed using vaccine or microbial antigens to which the child has had prior exposure. Commonly used antigens include tetanus toxoid and *Candida albicans*. Standard initial dilutions are 1:100 for both antigens, but a *C. albicans* dilution of 1:10 may be more appropriate for children aged 5 years or younger because they are less likely to have been exposed to this antigen. The diluted antigen is administered intradermally, and the skin reaction is read at 24 and 48 hours for the presence of wheal formation.

Delayed hypersensitivity skin test responses have low specificity because they depend on previous exposure to the antigen tested and often are absent in children younger than 2 years old. Enumeration of peripheral blood T cells, T-cell subset phenotyping (i.e., CD4+ or CD8+ lymphocyte counts), and mitogen-induced and antigen-induced lymphocyte proliferation studies

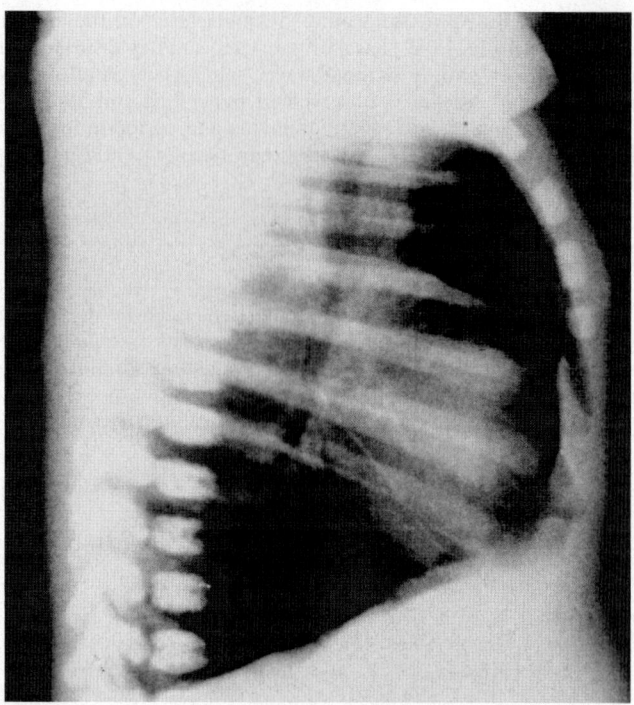

Figure 79–4 Lateral chest radiograph of an infant with severe combined immunodeficiency. Notice absence of the normal thymic shadow.

may be needed to make a reliable assessment of cellular immune function.[37]

Evaluation of the Complement System

Deficiencies of components of the classic complement pathway can be detected by performing the total serum hemolytic complement (CH_{50}) assay. This test measures the ability of proteins contained in the fresh patient serum to lyse antibody-coated sheep erythrocytes and reflects the activity of all numbered components of the classic complement pathway from C1 through C9. Complete deficiency of any of these components results in very low levels of CH_{50}. Often, mildly abnormal CH_{50} values are obtained because of inadequate sample handling. Single complement component levels and function should be investigated only when CH_{50} value is zero or near zero, taking into consideration that primary complement deficiencies are rare occurrences. Additionally, measuring the levels of complement components C3 and C4 can be done in most clinical laboratories and may be ordered when complement deficiency is suspected.

Evaluation of Phagocyte Function

A variety of assays are available for assessment of phagocyte function. The nitroblue tetrazolium (NBT) dye test uses the reduction of NBT to formazan by activated phagocytes to measure the oxidative metabolic responses that accompany phagocytosis. Children with CGD show reduced dye reduction (<10% of cells are formazan positive); carriers of X-linked CGD typically have 20 to 90 percent formazan-positive cells. The specificity and sensitivity of this test depend largely on the expertise of the performing laboratory. Flow cytometry is being used increasingly to detect production of hydrogen peroxide in phagocytes, using dihydrorhodamine (DHR)-1,2,3 as the fluorescent indicator, and has proven to be more reliable and sensitive.[50] More sophisticated tests, including assays of chemotaxis, phagocytosis, and bactericidal activity, may be done when the NBT and DHR test results

TABLE 79-5 Gene Defects in Primary Immunodeficiencies

Immunodeficiency	Gene Defect	Chromosome
Antibody Deficiency		
Agammaglobulinemia	Immunoglobulin heavy chain	14q23
	Bruton tyrosine kinase	Xq22
Hyper-IgM syndrome	Activation-induced deaminase	12p13
	CD40 ligand (CD154)	Xq26
Cellular Immunodeficiency		
DiGeorge syndrome	Unknown, TBX1?	22q11.2, 10p13
Severe combined immunodeficiency	RAG1, RAG2	11p13
	JAK3	19p13.1
	Adenosine deaminase	20q13.11
	Common gamma chain	Xq13.1
	IL-7 receptor	5p13
Ataxia telangiectasia	ATM, DNA kinase	11q22.3
Wiskott-Aldrich syndrome	WASP, cytoskeleton protein	Xp11.23
Phagocyte Deficiency		
Chronic granulomatous disease	gp67phox	1q25
	gp47phox	7q11.23
	gp22phox	16q24
	gp91phox	Xp21.1
LAD type I	CD18	21q22

Note: More than 120 gene defects have been shown to cause immunodeficiency syndromes. A more comprehensive list has been compiled by Notarangelo and associates[73] and Geha and colleagues.[41a]

are abnormal, or when high clinical suspicion of a phagocyte disorder exists.[51] Enumeration of CD11a,b,c+/CD18+ white blood cells is indicated when a diagnosis of LAD is suspected.

Genetic Testing

More than 120 gene defects responsible for immunodeficiency disorders have been identified (Table 79-5).[73] Currently, testing for these gene defects is available only in a few specialized laboratories, but testing should be pursued when a primary immunodeficiency with a known genetic defect is suspected. Genetic testing is strongly recommended for an affected patient who is ill, for prenatal diagnosis of an unborn child with an affected sibling, or for an individual who may have inherited or is a carrier of a known immunodeficiency gene defect. For some conditions, knowing the specific gene defect may help when one is assessing the prognosis and therapeutic options. Bone marrow transplantation for X-linked SCID (*IL2RG* gene defect) has been reported to be more successful than for other forms of SCID.[8] Knowledge of the specific gene defect also is useful for genetic counseling, most importantly to answer a common concern of the parents regarding the probability of having another child with a similar condition. Genetic studies for immunodeficiencies usually are used to confirm the diagnosis of DiGeorge syndrome, in which a deletion in chromosome 22 is identified by fluorescence in situ hybridization in approximately 95 percent of patients affected.[98]

MANAGEMENT

Management of an immunodeficient patient requires specialized care that may dictate recommendations according to the specific diagnosis. Hematopoietic cell transplantation is indicated for the most severe immunodeficiencies and necessitates careful individualized assessment of risks and benefits before proceeding with this treatment. One common therapeutic measure is replacement therapy with intravenous or subcutaneous immunoglobulins for patients with proven deficiency of IgG response,

TABLE 79-6 Key Concepts in the Management of Primary Immunodeficiencies

Immune function	T- and B-cell number and function should be assessed periodically
IgG replacement therapy	For patients with low IgG levels and poor antibody function
Immunizations	Live vaccines should not be administered to patients with immunodeficiency except for patients with complement deficiency and selective IgA deficiency
	Patients with complement deficiency may benefit from receiving pneumococcal and meningococcal vaccines because of their increased susceptibility to encapsulated organisms
	Household contacts of children with immunodeficiency should not receive oral poliovirus vaccines because of the risk of transmission to the immunodeficient child
	Other live vaccines (BCG, MMR, and varicella vaccine) may be administered to the household contact
	If the vaccine recipient develops a rash, contact with the immunodeficient child should be avoided[7]
Blood products	When needed, patients with immunodeficiencies should receive only irradiated, cytomegalovirus-negative, leukocyte-depleted blood products
Antibiotic prophylaxis	T-cell–deficient patients should take antibiotic prophylaxis for *Pneumocystis jiroveci*
	Antibiotic prophylaxis is recommended for dental and surgical procedures
	Patients with recurrent infections may benefit from antibiotic prophylaxis
Infectious diseases	Infections should be recognized promptly, and unusual pathogens should be considered
	Antibiotic therapy should be started early and discontinued cautiously
Diet and activity	Patients with immunodeficiency should have a regular diet and lifestyle but should be instructed to avoid eating raw food and playing in environments potentially highly contaminated with pathogens, including daycare centers
	Strict handwashing and reverse isolation may be indicated for patients with poor T-cell function

when presenting alone or in combination with cellular immunity defects. Other recommendations that apply to patients with immunodeficiency include the avoidance of contact with sick individuals and avoidance of live vaccines[6]; the use of irradiated, leukocyte-depleted, cytomegalovirus-negative blood products when needed; use of antibiotic prophylaxis; and prompt establishment of the diagnosis and provision of treatment of infections. Isolation in sterile environments is not recommended, except for patients with severe T-cell deficiency who are awaiting hematopoietic cell transplant, because of the severe impact on psychosocial development and the advances in the treatment and prevention of community-acquired infections (Table 79-6).

SELECTED PRIMARY ANTIBODY DEFICIENCIES

X-LINKED AGAMMAGLOBULINEMIA

Clinical Features

Boys with X-linked agammaglobulinemia (XLA), or Bruton disease, often are healthy during the first months of life because of the protective presence of transplacentally acquired maternal IgG. As maternal immunoglobulin disappears from the infant, chronic or recurrent infections develop.[25,82,112] Frequent episodes of otitis media, sinusitis, pneumonia, and diarrhea are most common, but infections are not limited to mucosal surfaces; bacteremia, meningitis, and osteomyelitis also may occur. The mean age at establishment of the diagnosis in a retrospective study of 96 patients with XLA was 2.5 years when there was a family history of the disease and 3.5 years when there was not.[112]

S. pneumoniae, Hib, S. aureus, and P. aeruginosa are the bacterial pathogens observed most frequently in the setting of XLA. Mycoplasma spp. infections also occur with increased frequency and have been implicated as a cause of a subacute, destructive arthritis.[107] Gastrointestinal infections may be caused by Salmonella, Shigella, Campylobacter, or rotavirus.[82,112] Chronic giardiasis with intestinal malabsorption has been reported.[75]

Increased incidence of vaccine-associated paralytic poliomyelitis also has been reported.[112] Children with XLA are susceptible to chronic enteroviral meningoencephalitis,[66] which is a severe complication, even with treatment using intrathecal and intravenous immunoglobulin therapy. Most reported cases have a fatal outcome.

Pathogenesis

The defective gene (BTK) maps to the midportion of the long arm of the X chromosome. The gene encodes a cytoplasmic protein-tyrosine kinase, the normal function of which is necessary for expansion of B-cell populations during their maturation.[105] Deleterious mutations of the gene have been found in all affected individuals studied. XLA results from developmental arrest of B-cell maturation because lack of the Bruton tyrosine kinase (BTK)–mediated signal. Consequently, blood, lymph nodes, and bone marrow contain markedly diminished numbers of B cells and plasma cells, resulting in hypogammaglobulinemia. Other components of the immune system are not affected.

Diagnosis

Because of the presence of transplacentally acquired maternal IgG, the determination of serum immunoglobulin for establishing the diagnosis of XLA in the child's first 6 months of life is unreliable. Infants with XLA also have low concentrations of other immunoglobulin isotypes (e.g., IgA, IgM), but defining values that clearly differentiate between infants with the disease and normal infants has been difficult. Establishing a definitive diagnosis during early infancy generally relies on immunophenotyping by flow cytometry to show the absence of B cells in peripheral blood. After an infant with XLA reaches 6 months of age, serum IgG concentrations usually are less than 100 mg/dL, and concentrations of other immunoglobulin isotypes are low or undetectable. Isohemagglutinins are absent, and specific antibodies are not produced in response to immunization or natural infection. Recurrent infections in male family members may suggest an X-linked condition. Definitive diagnosis is obtained by finding inactivating mutations in the BTK gene sequence.

Treatment and Prognosis

Lifetime immunoglobulin replacement therapy is indicated for all patients with XLA.[61,78] It decreases the frequency of serious infections, reduces the need for hospitalization, and may help to prevent the development of chronic lung disease with progressive decrease of lung function. The dose and frequency of administration of immunoglobulins are adjusted to produce serum IgG trough concentrations of at least 500 mg/dL. For most patients, intravenous immunoglobulins are required at doses of 400 to 600 mg/kg, given every 3 or 4 weeks.

Acute infections in patients with XLA should be treated promptly. Minor middle ear, sinus, and skin infections usually respond to oral antibiotics. Pneumonia and other serious focal or systemic infections should be treated initially with intravenous antibiotics. Empiric antibiotic therapy is directed against common bacterial pathogens, including S. pneumoniae, H. influenzae, and S. aureus. If possible, etiologic diagnosis should be obtained, particularly in cases of severe or chronic infection. Because serum IgG concentrations often decrease during acute infection, the serum IgG concentration should be measured, and additional doses of immunoglobulins may be indicated. Chronic pulmonary disease with bronchiectasis is an important cause of death of patients with XLA. Long-term antibiotic therapy, similar to that used in patients with cystic fibrosis, may be helpful in individual cases. Long-term survivors of XLA are at increased risk for developing lymphoid malignancies.[82]

IMMUNOGLOBULIN DEFICIENCY WITH INCREASED IgM

Clinical Features

Approximately 70 percent of cases of immunoglobulin deficiency with increased IgM (i.e., hyper-IgM syndrome) are associated with X-linked inheritance, due to CD40L gene defects, but autosomal recessive and dominant inheritance patterns also have been reported.[57] Patients with this disorder develop recurrent pyogenic infections during infancy as transplacentally acquired IgG wanes. Respiratory tract infections and chronic diarrhea with failure to thrive are common occurrences; septicemia, meningitis, and other serious systemic infections also occur.[60] Opportunistic infections, such as Pneumocystis jiroveci pneumonia, also are common occurrences.[113]

Half of patients with hyper-IgM syndrome have neutropenia. It can be intermittent, but it lacks the precise periodicity of cyclic neutropenia. Aphthous ulcers occur commonly. Perirectal ulcers and abscesses also have been reported. Hyperplasia of superficial and deep lymph nodes occur commonly, and intestinal nodular lymphoid hyperplasia may lead to malabsorption and protein-losing enteropathy. Autoimmune conditions, including arthritis and nephritis, have been described. The incidence of lymphoreticular malignancies is increased in these patients.[60,113]

Pathogenesis

Males with hyper-IgM syndrome may have mutations of a gene on the X chromosome that encodes the T-cell ligand (CD154, CD40L) for the B-cell surface molecule CD40.[4,9] Several patients with normal expression of CD40L but defects in the B-cell CD40 signaling pathway also have been described.[26] Interaction of CD40 with CD40L is essential to B-cell proliferation, isotype switching, and terminal differentiation of B cells to antibody-secreting plasma cells. Mutations in the activation-induced cytidine deaminase (AICD) and the uracil DNA glycosylase (UNG) genes have been found in patients with the autosomal recessive form of hyper-IgM syndrome.[68]

Diagnosis

Patients with hyper-IgM syndrome have a characteristic increase in serum IgM concentrations in association with low to absent concentrations of serum IgA and IgG. Serum IgM concentrations may exceed 1000 mg/dL; however, they can be within normal range. Circulating B cells expressing surface IgM are found in normal numbers, but only a few cells bear surface IgA or IgG. Antibody responses to immunization often are present but consist predominantly or exclusively of IgM because isotype switching does not occur. More than half of patients are diagnosed before they reach 1 year of age, and 90 percent of patients are diagnosed by the time they are 4 years old. Evaluation of boys with suspected immunoglobulin deficiency with increased IgM should include a determination of CD40L expression in activated T cells, which is done by flow cytometry.[9]

Treatment and Prognosis

Immunoglobulin replacement therapy and antibiotic prophylaxis are indicated.[78] Reports of patients treated successfully with HLA-identical bone marrow transplantation have been published.[102] Patients with hyper-IgM syndrome usually have a clinical course worse than that of patients with XLA. In addition, X-linked forms of hyper-IgM syndrome have increased morbidity and mortality compared with autosomal forms, possibly reflecting that the X-linked condition results from a T-cell defect, rather than a B-cell defect. Causes of mortality include infections other than respiratory, sclerosing cholangitis with liver disease often secondary to *Cryptosporidium parvum* infection, and malignancy.[113]

COMMON VARIABLE IMMUNODEFICIENCY

Clinical Features

Common variable immunodeficiency (CVID) includes a heterogeneous group of disorders with similar clinical manifestations, characterized by hypogammaglobulinemia with low or normal numbers of B cells, abnormal production of antibodies, recurrent infections, and a propensity for autoimmune conditions. Onset can occur at any time from infancy to old age,[27] but symptoms frequently begin during the second or third decades of life.[28]

The clinical manifestations of CVID are similar to those of XLA, with recurrent infections of the respiratory tract, bacteremia, meningitis, osteomyelitis, and septic arthritis. Patients frequently develop bronchiectasis and chronic lung disease. The most common infectious organisms are *S. pneumoniae, H. influenzae,* and *S. aureus*.[28] Many individuals with CVID have chronic diarrhea and intestinal malabsorption that have an infectious or autoimmune basis.[28] The inflammation induced by these conditions may result in protein-losing enteropathy and may exacerbate the underlying hypogammaglobulinemia. Organisms implicated in these gastrointestinal infections include *Giardia, Campylobacter, Salmonella,* and *Cryptosporidium*. Bacterial overgrowth syndrome commonly occurs. Patients with CVID present with increased frequency of ulcerative colitis, Crohn disease, atrophic gastritis with achlorhydria, viral or autoimmune chronic active hepatitis, and cholelithiasis.

Approximately 22 percent of patients with CVID develop autoimmune conditions, which include a chronic arthritis resembling juvenile rheumatoid arthritis; scleroderma, a lupus-like syndrome; hypothyroidism; and autoimmune neutropenia, anemia, and thrombocytopenia.[27,28] Malignancies, including lymphomas and gastric carcinoma, occur commonly among adults with CVID. A pseudolymphoma syndrome with lymphoid hyperplasia of the lung (i.e., lymphoid interstitial pneumonia) and intestine (i.e., nodular lymphoid hyperplasia), massive splenomegaly, and mediastinal adenopathy may be seen in patients with CVID.

Pathogenesis

The pathogenesis of CVID is poorly defined and may correspond to several different genetic defects that result in impaired antibody secretion. Bone marrow B-cell maturation is intact, and normal or low numbers of B cells are present in peripheral blood and lymph nodes, but production of antibody is impaired. Decreased or absent memory B cells is associated with severity of disease and development of autoimmune disorders and malig-

nancies.[2,20] Many patients with CVID seem to have an intrinsic B-cell defect that impairs the ability of these cells to differentiate into immunoglobulin-secreting plasma cells, but a variety of T-cell functional abnormalities, including decreased proliferation of lymphocytes to mitogens and antigens and reduced expression of cytokines, also have been described.[49,96] Most recently, inactivating mutations in the *TACI, ICOS,* and *CD19* genes have been reported individually in a small proportion of families with several members affected with CVID and IgA deficiency, providing a link between these two clinical syndromes and supporting the concept of a multiple etiology of CVID.[21]

Diagnosis

Quantitative immunoglobulin determination generally reveals a serum IgG concentration persistently less than 250 mg/dL, with comparable decreases in other immunoglobulin isotypes. Immunophenotyping of peripheral blood lymphocytes shows the presence of mature B cells expressing surface immunoglobulins, with a subset of patients lacking switched memory B cells. Antibody responses to immunizations are subnormal or absent.

Treatment and Prognosis

Treatment of patients with CVID is similar to treatment of patients with XLA. Immunoglobulin replacement therapy is indicated and has been shown to decrease the frequency of respiratory infections.[19] Antibiotic prophylaxis may be indicated as an adjunctive measure in patients who continue to develop infections despite having adequate serum IgG levels. Because of enteric protein loss, patients with CVID and enteropathy may require unusually large doses of immunoglobulin to maintain protective serum IgG concentrations. Chronic lung disease with bronchiectasis resulting from multiple pneumonias is the most frequent cause of morbidity and mortality.[28] Patients with absence of switched memory B cells are at risk of developing lymphoma, splenomegaly, and autoimmune complications.

IgA DEFICIENCY

Clinical Features

IgA deficiency is estimated to occur with a frequency of 1 in 500 individuals and is considered the most common immunodeficiency. Most individuals with IgA deficiency are clinically asymptomatic, however.[33,88] Some patients have frequent, noninvasive viral and bacterial infections of the respiratory tract, although most of these patients also have concomitant IgG2 subclass deficiency. Chronic diarrhea occurs with increased frequency, with *Giardia* being a pathogen commonly implicated. Infections in patients with IgA deficiency usually are less severe than infections observed in patients with XLA or CVID. Individuals with more severe or chronic infections often have another associated immunodeficiency, such as IgG subclass deficiency[80] or, rarely, ataxia telangiectasia.

Patients with IgA deficiency have a higher incidence of atopy than the general population. Autoimmune disorders, including systemic lupus erythematosus, rheumatoid arthritis, and pernicious anemia, and lymphoid and gastrointestinal malignancies are more prevalent in this population.

Pathogenesis

The pathogenesis of IgA deficiency has been compared with that of CVID. The fundamental defect in both disorders is a failure of B cells to differentiate into immunoglobulin-secreting plasma cells. Rare alleles of complement genes within major histocompatibility complex III on chromosome 6 have been associated strongly with the development of selective IgA deficiency and CVID, suggesting that these two disorders may be related.[109] Some individuals with selective IgA deficiency subsequently develop CVID. Inactivating mutations in *TACI* and *ICOS* genes have been found in families with members presenting with either of those conditions.[21]

Diagnosis

Selective IgA deficiency is diagnosed by a quantitative serum immunoglobulin determination showing subnormal concentration or absence of circulating IgA, in the presence of normal amounts of the other immunoglobulins. In interpreting test results, an important consideration is that serum IgA concentrations can be undetectable in normal infants younger than 6 to 9 months because of a possible maturational delay. This diagnosis is reliable only after the child reaches 4 years of age.

Treatment and Prognosis

Immunoglobulin replacement generally is not recommended in the management of patients with selective IgA deficiency. Although rarely reported, IgA-deficient patients are at risk for developing IgE-mediated anaphylactic reactions if the patient is sensitized to IgA and receives blood products containing IgA.[17]

Patients deficient in IgA respond adequately to vaccines unless they have concomitant IgG deficiency. Sinopulmonary infections in individuals with IgA deficiency often require unusually long courses of antibiotic therapy. Antibiotic prophylaxis for respiratory infections may be recommended if infections are recurrent. Parenteral antibiotic therapy sometimes is necessary for refractory cases of sinusitis or pneumonia.

IgG SUBCLASS DEFICIENCY

Clinical Features

The most common IgG subclass deficiency reported is IgG2, sometimes occurring in association with deficiency of IgG4 or IgA. The second most common is IgG3 deficiency, which may occur in association with IgG1 deficiency.[46,91] Many individuals with IgG subclass deficiencies are asymptomatic; others have recurrent or chronic bacterial infections, usually of the respiratory tract. Commonly implicated pathogens include *S. pneumoniae*, Hib, and other encapsulated bacteria. Children with selective IgG subclass deficiency usually do not have problems with intestinal malabsorption or autoimmunity.

Pathogenesis

The pathogenesis of IgG subclass deficiency is unknown. Genetic factors have been implicated by studies showing linkage to certain immunoglobulin allotypes.[46] T-cell immunity has been reported to be intact in patients with IgG subclass deficiency.

Diagnosis

A diagnosis of IgG subclass deficiency is supported by finding a marked decrease from age-adjusted normal values in the serum concentrations of one or more IgG subclasses, together with evidence of a functional impairment in antibody responses to immunizations. The total serum IgG concentration may be normal, decreased, or elevated as a result of a compensatory increase in production of unaffected IgG subclasses.

Children with low IgG2 subclass levels may respond poorly to polysaccharide vaccines.[106] Responses to protein antigens (e.g., tetanus toxoid) and protein-conjugated polysaccharide vaccines (e.g., Hib conjugate vaccines) also may be abnormal. In contrast, patients with IgG3 subclass deficiency may respond poorly to protein antigens, but responses to polysaccharides generally are normal. Assessment of the patient's antibody responses to vaccination with polysaccharide and protein antigens can help to establish the functional significance of an IgG subclass deficiency. Because of the age-dependent development of anti-polysaccharide antibody responses, such testing is unreliable in children younger than 2 years.

Treatment and Prognosis

Antibiotic prophylaxis of recurrent sinopulmonary infections and early and prompt treatment of infections form the cornerstone of management for symptomatic IgG subclass deficiency. Immunoglobulin replacement therapy is reserved for patients with abnormal antibody responses and a demonstrated propensity for frequent or chronic infections.[78] Because of the anecdotal evidence of the clinical benefit of this measure, the effectiveness and continued need for immunoglobulins should be reassessed periodically.

TRANSIENT HYPOGAMMAGLOBULINEMIA OF INFANCY

Clinical Features

Many infants come to medical attention because they have recurrent respiratory tract infections (e.g., otitis media, sinusitis) and serum immunoglobulin levels that are lower than laboratory normal ranges. Septicemia, meningitis, and other serious systemic infections are rare findings.[31,65]

Pathogenesis

Transient hypogammaglobulinemia of infancy is a developmental disorder with a delay in the physiologic maturation of immunoglobulin synthesis, resulting in prolongation of the relative hypogammaglobulinemia observed in most normal infants at 4 or 5 months of age, when most maternal immunoglobulins have cleared from the infant's circulation. Patients with transient hypogammaglobulinemia of infancy do not seem to have any inherent defects of B-cell maturation or function, or defects of specific antibody responses.

Diagnosis

Transient hypogammaglobulinemia of infancy is a diagnosis that can be made with certainty only in retrospect. Serum immunoglobulin concentrations may remain low in children until they are several years of age in some cases.[65] Circulating mature B-cell numbers are normal and generate normal antibody responses to diphtheria, tetanus, and pertussis vaccines.

Treatment and Prognosis

Infants with suspected transient hypogammaglobulinemia should be followed clinically, and serial serum immunoglobulin concentration measurements should be performed. Some of these children eventually are diagnosed with CVID, selective IgA deficiency, or another secondary immunodeficiency disorder. Because the condition is self-limited, and production of specific antibodies usually is normal, immunoglobulin replacement therapy is not indicated. Antibiotic prophylaxis for respiratory infections is indicated in cases with recurrent episodes of infection.

SELECTED PRIMARY CELLULAR AND COMBINED IMMUNODEFICIENCIES

DIGEORGE SYNDOME

Clinical Features

DiGeorge syndrome is a common genetic disorder that includes facial, cardiac, parathyroid, and thymic abnormalities.[98] Patients with DiGeorge syndrome may present early in infancy with findings unrelated to immunodeficiency. Congenital heart disease, particularly truncus arteriosus and interrupted aortic arch, usually is detected in the first few weeks of life. Neonatal hypoparathyroidism occurs in almost all infants with DiGeorge syndrome, and hypocalcemic seizures or tetany is a common presenting feature. Characteristic facial features include microstomia and micrognathia; hypertelorism; upturned nose; arched palate; posteriorly rotated and small, low-set ears with notched pinnae; and anti-mongoloid slant of the eyes (see Fig. 79–1). Hypothyroidism, esophageal atresia, tracheoesophageal fistula, and bifid uvula have been described.

Based on the degree of immunodeficiency, clinical manifestations may include predisposition to a wide variety of common and opportunistic infectious diseases. Common findings are recurrent or chronic pneumonias; chronic diarrhea; and candidiasis of the skin, mouth, or esophagus. Recurrent or severe herpesvirus infections (e.g., herpes simplex virus, cytomegalovirus); *P. jiroveci* pneumonia; and other opportunistic viral, fungal, protozoal, and mycobacterial infections occasionally are observed. Fatal graft-versus-host disease may occur if infants receive blood products containing viable lymphocytes during surgical correction of heart defects. Although DiGeorge syndrome is the most common of the cellular immunodeficiencies, with an incidence of 1 in 3000 live births, only a few patients with DiGeorge syndrome have clinically significant immunodeficiency (complete DiGeorge syndrome). Most patients develop adequate T-cell numbers and function by the time they reach 1 year of age and do not have an increased incidence of opportunistic infections (partial DiGeorge syndrome).[23,99] At Texas Children's Hospital, 20 percent of patients with DiGeorge syndrome and mild T-cell deficiency present with an increased incidence of respiratory infections.[23]

Pathogenesis

DiGeorge syndrome is classified as a developmental defect resulting from faulty embryologic development of the third and fourth branchial arches and their derivatives, including parathyroid glands, aortic arch structures, and thymus gland.[98] Partial deletions of chromosomes 22 and 10 are found in more than 90 percent of patients. Three groups of investigators simultaneously reported that they reproduced all the characteristic features of DiGeorge syndrome, working with mice models bearing the deletion of *Tbx-1*, a gene within the chromosome 22 critical region.[116] Whether the absence of this gene in humans is responsible for this syndrome is still not definitive.

Diagnosis

Hypocalcemia, congenital heart disease, and characteristic facies may lead to suspicion of DiGeorge syndrome in the newborn period. A deletion in chromosome 22q is detected by fluorescence in situ hybridization analysis. Lymphopenia varies, and severe T-cell deficiency is rare. Determination of T-cell number and a proliferative response to mitogens allows the clinician to make a better assessment of the degree of immunodeficiency. Quantitative serum immunoglobulin determinations often are normal, but antibody responses after immunization usually are

poor. Chest x-ray may show absence of the thymic shadow. A significant group of patients with DiGeorge syndrome are totally or partially thymectomized while heart surgery is performed for repair of characteristic conotruncal cardiac malformations.

Treatment and Prognosis

Initial management should focus on the treatment of hypocalcemia and the surgical correction of congenital heart disease. Immunoglobulin replacement therapy and antibiotic prophylaxis should be considered for patients with recurrent infections. Children with CD4+ lymphopenia or evidence of significant cellular immune dysfunction should receive *P. jiroveci* pneumonia prophylaxis. Infections should be recognized early and treated promptly. Only irradiated, cytomegalovirus-negative blood products and inactivated vaccines should be administered. Several small retrospective studies have suggested that children with partial DiGeorge syndrome and normal or only mildly decreased CD4+ T cell counts may receive vaccines without experiencing serious adverse events.[10,71,81] The safety of live vaccination has not been well established, however, and currently is not recommended. Therapeutic options being investigated for patients with DiGeorge syndrome and severe immunodeficiency include bone marrow transplantation and, experimentally, thymus transplantation.[64]

WISKOTT-ALDRICH SYNDROME

Clinical Features

Wiskott-Aldrich syndrome is an X-linked disorder classically characterized by recurrent infection, bleeding, and eczema. Only a few patients have this classic triad of features, however, and some patients have infectious manifestations alone.[76] Patients commonly present with recurrent otitis media or pneumonia caused by encapsulated bacteria (e.g., *S. pneumoniae*, *H. influenzae*). Septicemia, meningitis, and other serious systemic bacterial infections also may occur. Common opportunistic pathogens include *Candida*, cytomegalovirus, other herpesviruses, and *P. jiroveci*.

Individuals with Wiskott-Aldrich syndrome often have depressed platelet counts. A unique feature is the presence of small platelets (low mean platelet volume) in most cases. Consequently, bruises combined with gastrointestinal bleeding in the first months of life is are common presenting feature of Wiskott-Aldrich syndrome. Life-threatening gastrointestinal or intracranial hemorrhage also may occur. Eczematous lesions are generalized and prone to superinfection.

Patients with Wiskott-Aldrich syndrome have a high incidence of autoimmune disorders.[32] Hemolytic anemia, a juvenile rheumatoid arthritis–like condition, and large or small vessel vasculitis have been reported. Some patients develop autoimmune thrombocytopenia as disease progresses. Lymphoid malignancies, especially non-Hodgkin lymphomas involving the brain, have been reported.

Pathogenesis

The gene (*WASP*) that is mutated in patients with Wiskott-Aldrich syndrome[29] maps to the X chromosome. This gene encodes a protein that is expressed in lymphocytes and platelets and is involved in cytoskeletal organization and formation of pseudopodia. This defect results in failure to form an adequate immunologic synapse, resulting in poor cognate interaction between T cells and B cells.[18] T-cell morphologic and membrane abnormalities and signal transduction defects have been described.[69] X-linked thrombocytopenia without or with only mild immunodeficiency and eczema has been found to be caused by *WASP* mutations that allow partial protein expression.[108]

Diagnosis

Wiskott-Aldrich syndrome should be suspected in a boy with thrombocytopenia and small platelets. The presence of eczema supports the diagnosis. Serum immunoglobulin concentrations vary, with the most typical pattern showing normal IgG, increased IgA and IgE, and decreased IgM. Antibody responses to protein antigens (e.g., tetanus) usually are normal, but responses to polysaccharides (e.g., *S. pneumoniae*, Hib, isohemagglutinins) are absent.

Patients with Wiskott-Aldrich syndrome are anergic on delayed hypersensitivity skin testing. They have near-normal numbers of circulating T cells, and in vitro proliferative responses to mitogens could be normal. Responses to specific antigens are decreased, however. Monocytes exhibit abnormal chemotaxis and poor antibody-dependent cellular cytotoxicity. The determination of WAS protein expression and the sequencing of the *WASP* gene are available in specialized research laboratories.

Treatment and Prognosis

Bone marrow transplantation results in normalization of cellular immunity, specific antibody responses, and platelet count. It is the definitive treatment of choice; however, mortality is high if the donor is not a matched HLA sibling, or if multiple infections and organ damage have occurred. Splenectomy is indicated for severe thrombocytopenia and may improve the patient's quality of life. Daily antibiotic prophylaxis directed against *S. pneumoniae* and *H. influenzae* should be indicated for patients who have undergone splenectomy. Aspirin is contraindicated because it increases the risk of bleeding. Acute infections should be treated aggressively. Immunoglobulin replacement therapy is indicated for patients with recurrent bacterial infections.

The prognosis of Wiskott-Aldrich syndrome has improved in recent years, with some patients surviving to adulthood.[76] Infection, malignancy, and hemorrhage are the leading causes of death.

ATAXIA TELANGIECTASIA

Clinical Features

Ataxia telangiectasia is characterized by cerebellar ataxia, oculocutaneous telangiectases, variable immunodeficiency with frequent infections, and a high incidence of malignancy.[114] Neurologic signs and symptoms dominate the clinical picture. Ataxia usually becomes evident when the child is approximately 1 year old. Progressive choreoathetosis, myoclonic jerking movements, and oculomotor abnormalities develop subsequently, resulting in severe disability. Telangiectases appear on the bulbar conjunctivae, usually in patients 2 to 5 years old (see Fig. 79-2). They subsequently appear on the nasal bridge, ears, and other areas of sun exposure or trauma. Other cutaneous manifestations include café-au-lait spots, vitiligo, and prematurely gray hair.

Recurrent infections are a major feature of ataxia telangiectasia in most patients. Sinopulmonary infections predominate, but systemic infections are rare despite the immunologic abnormalities.[74] Organisms commonly implicated include *S. pneumoniae* and *H. influenzae*. Fifteen percent of patients with ataxia telangiectasia may develop neoplasias. Non-Hodgkin lymphomas and leiomyomas occur most frequently. Carcinomas (especially of the stomach) occur commonly among adults with ataxia telangiectasia.[114]

Pathogenesis

Ataxia telangiectasia is inherited in an autosomal recessive manner. The defective gene (*ATM*) responsible for the disorder has been identified and maps to chromosome 11.[86] One domain of the ATM protein seems to be important in numerous cellular responses, including cytokine signaling. Another region of the protein is involved in DNA repair. Disease manifestations result from a major defect in one or more DNA repair mechanisms. Breakage and rearrangements of chromosomes, including the T-cell receptor genes and immunoglobulin heavy-chain genes on chromosomes 7 and 14, may explain the observed immunodeficiency.

Diagnosis

A clinical diagnosis of ataxia telangiectasia is possible when the disease is fully manifested. Laboratory studies usually are needed for early diagnosis, however. Increased serum alpha-fetoprotein concentrations are observed in essentially all patients older than 6 months. Most patients have deficiencies in serum IgA and IgE. Specific antibody responses usually decline as the patient ages. Most patients have serum IgM in a monomeric 7S form, rather than the usual pentameric 19S molecule. Common manifestations of immunodeficiency include delayed hypersensitivity skin test anergy and decreased lymphocyte proliferative responses to mitogens and antigens. The sequencing of the *ATM* gene is available in specialized laboratories.

Treatment and Prognosis

No specific treatment is curative for ataxia telangiectasia because of the pathology involving multiple body systems. Infections should be treated promptly with oral or parenteral antibiotics. Continuous prophylactic antibiotic therapy may be beneficial for individual patients. Immunoglobulin replacement therapy is reserved for patients with recurrent infections and abnormal specific antibody responses.

The clinical course and prognosis of ataxia telangiectasia vary. Death from chronic pulmonary disease or malignancy occurs commonly.

SEVERE COMBINED IMMUNODEFICIENCY

Clinical Features

Infants with SCID generally present during the first few months of life with recurrent infections.[16,97] Newborns may present with a rash produced by a graft-versus-host reaction induced by maternal lymphocytes. Recurrent pneumonias, other respiratory tract infections, and persistent oral and cutaneous candidiasis are common, as are chronic diarrhea and failure to thrive. Septicemia and other serious systemic bacterial infections also occur. Causative organisms include routine pathogens (e.g., *S. pneumoniae*, Hib) and more unusual organisms. Life-threatening opportunistic infections, including *P. jiroveci* pneumonia, frequently occur early in infancy. Fatal Epstein-Barr virus–associated lymphocyte proliferative disease has been observed in bone marrow transplant recipients and untreated patients with SCID.[36]

Pathogenesis

SCID represents a heterogeneous group of genetic disorders having in common a profound immunodeficiency with failure of cellular and humoral immune function. Various types of SCID have been defined on the basis of enzymatic, genetic, and immunologic criteria (Table 79-7), including reticular dysgenesis, with

TABLE 79-7 Types of Severe Combined Immunodeficiency (SCID)

Type	Defect
Reticular dysgenesis	Stem cell
RAG1, RAG2 deficiency, Omenn syndrome	Rearrangement of B- and T-cell receptor genes
Artemis deficiency	Rearrangement of B- and T-cell receptor genes
DNA ligase IV	Rearrangement of B- and T-cell receptor genes
X-linked SCID (common gamma-chain deficiency)	Signaling for IL-2, IL-4, IL-7, IL-15, IL-21
JAK3 deficiency	Cytokine signaling
IL-7 receptor deficiency	Signaling for IL-7
CD3 δ or ε deficiency	CD3 signaling
CD45 deficiency	Signaling for CD45, cell activation
Adenosine deaminase deficiency	Metabolite (dATP) toxicity to lymphocytes
MHC class I deficiency	Defect in transporter proteins TAP-1, TAP-2
MHC class II deficiency	Defects in transcription factors RFXAP, RFX5, RFXANK, and transactivator CIITA

impaired lymphoid, myeloid, and erythroid differentiation; absence of T-cell and B-cell differentiation; selective defects of T-cell differentiation; and purine metabolism defects (e.g., adenosine deaminase deficiency [ADA]). Autosomal and X-linked recessive inheritance patterns have been recognized. Individuals with X-linked SCID have a defect in the gamma chain of the IL-2 receptor, and it is the genetic defect identified in approximately half of SCID patients.[16] This protein is a functional component of the receptors for IL-4, IL-7, IL-9, IL-15, and IL-21 receptors.[58,72,85] These functions help to explain why this defect has such a profound effect on lymphoid development and function.

Diagnosis

Infants with SCID typically lack palpable lymph nodes, visible tonsils, and radiographic evidence of a thymus gland. Lymphopenia often is identified.[97] Some patients have panhypogammaglobulinemia, whereas others have depressed concentrations of only one or two immunoglobulin isotypes. Antibody responses almost always are profoundly impaired or absent. Lymphocyte monoclonal phenotyping may reveal the presence of circulating mature B cells. Particularly in boys with X-linked SCID and JAK3-deficient SCID, B cells may account for all circulating lymphocytes. Circulating T cell counts are diminished (<10% of normal range) in most patients with SCID. Delayed hypersensitivity skin test anergy is found, and lymphocyte proliferative responses to mitogens and antigens are severely depressed. Testing for specific genetic defect should be pursued, and a genetic evaluation of immediate relatives for carrier status is recommended for genetic counseling purposes. Biochemical tests for ADA and purine nucleoside phosphorylase levels and enzymatic activities are available in specialized laboratories.

Treatment and Prognosis

Hematopoietic stem cell transplantation (HSCT) is the treatment of choice for most patients with SCID. Prognosis is poor for patients without therapy. HSCT performed with HLA-matched related donors has a survival rate of greater than 95 percent.[8] Most patients do not have such a donor available, however, and receive an HLA-haploidentical transplant. Survival rates with these donors vary from 50 to 75 percent at 5-year follow-up, according to the different transplant centers. This survival rate can increase to greater than 95 percent if the SCID is detected early and HSCT is performed before the infant reaches 3.5 months of age, likely because infections and organ damage are yet to occur at this early age. HLA-matched unrelated donors and HLA-matched cord blood have been used increasingly for different forms of SCID, accompanied with different chemotherapy regimens for myeloablation. Success rates are not uniform; they approximate 75 percent in the best transplant centers.

As an alternative because of the high mortality and morbidity associated with HSCT, French and British investigators have reported success in experimental gene therapy trials for X-linked SCID. Using autologous CD34+ stem cells carrying the correct version of the gene, the investigators were able to restore humoral and cellular immunity in 12 of 14 affected patients.[41,45] Four patients in the French trial developed leukemia that was caused partly by the gene therapy procedure. One of the patients died, and the other three responded to anti-leukemic chemotherapy and are alive and well.

Enzyme replacement[47] and gene therapy[13] have been used for treatment of SCID resulting from ADA deficiency. Polyethylene glycol–adenosine deaminase has shown efficacy to increase lymphocyte counts and provide adequate immunity in most affected patients. Some patients ultimately develop "resistance" to the drug in the form of eliciting neutralizing anti-ADA antibodies or simply showing a decrease of lymphocyte counts. Italian researchers have reported positive results of an experimental gene therapy trial for SCID caused by ADA deficiency with the restoration of cellular and humoral immunity in seven patients, in a treatment protocol that included withdrawal of exogenous ADA and reduced myeloablation.

MISCELLANEOUS CELLULAR IMMUNODEFICIENCIES

Many other disorders of cellular immunity have been described. Particularly noteworthy are disorders characterized for dysregulation of the immune system with autoimmune inflammation. X-linked lymphoproliferative syndrome represents a defect in control of Epstein-Barr virus infection. Mutations in the SLAM-associated protein (SAP), a factor involved in the signal transduction of T cells, have been identified to cause X-linked lymphoproliferative syndrome. The absence of this protein affects the interaction of T cells and B cells, leading to an inability to control B cell proliferation caused by Epstein-Barr virus infection.[42,87] Patients may present with severe and often fatal infectious mononucleosis or with B-cell lymphoma.

Chronic mucocutaneous candidiasis is a condition characterized by chronic, severe *Candida* spp. infection of mucous membranes, skin, and nails, often in association with autoimmune polyendocrinopathy, in which case it is termed *autoimmune polyendocrinopathy ectodermal dystrophy*.[1] T-cell numbers and function usually are normal, but most patients do not manifest delayed hypersensitivity skin test responses to *Candida*, and their lymphocytes fail to proliferate in response to *Candida* antigen in vitro. In cases with autoimmune polyendocrinopathy ectodermal dystrophy, deleterious mutations have been found in the Auto-Immune REgulator (*AIRE*) gene. This gene promotes the expression of many self-antigens in the thymus, facilitating the development of immune tolerance of the newly formed lymphocytes. IPEX (immunodeficiency, polyendocrinopathy, enteropathy, X-linked) is another autoimmune endocrinopathy with immunodeficiency. IPEX results from mutations in the *FoxP3* gene and is characterized by lack of T-regulatory cells and clinically by eczema, chronic diarrhea, diabetes mellitus, and other hormone deficiencies.[56]

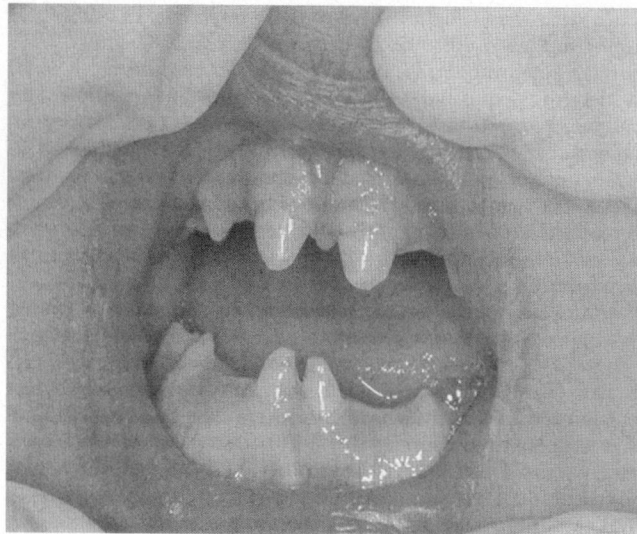

Figure 79–5 Conical teeth characteristic of incontinentia pigmentosa with immunodeficiency, resulting from defects in the *IKKb* gene (NEMO defect). (See companion Expert Consult web site for color version.)

Mutations in the interferon-γ receptor genes have been shown in patients with severe infections caused by atypical mycobacteria.[30,53,83] Patients with a mutation in the IL-12 receptor β2-chain gene or in the IL-12 gene also showed increased susceptibility to mycobacterial disease and disseminated nontuberculous mycobacterial infection.[5]

Deficiency in the nuclear factor-κB enhancing modulator (NEMO) is a newly recognized primary immunodeficiency caused by specific missense mutations in the *IKKG* (also known as *NEMO*) gene, located on chromosome Xq28. NEMO participates in signal transduction mediated by nuclear factor-κB. Most mutations in the NEMO gene are lethal for male fetuses, and female carriers of these mutations may present with incontinentia pigmenti. The surviving male patients with specific missense mutations present with anhidrotic ectodermal dysplasia, conical teeth (Fig. 79–5), low IgG, low IgA, normal or increased IgM levels, and poor T-cell proliferative responses to mitogen and antigen stimuli.[77,93,117]

PRIMARY COMPLEMENT DEFICIENCIES

CLINICAL FEATURES

Three types of complement function deficiencies can cause increased susceptibility to infections: deficiency of opsonic activity of complement proteins, deficiency of the complement lytic proteins, and deficiency of the mannose-binding lectin pathway.[110] Patients with deficiencies of early-acting complement components (e.g., C3, C1, C4, C2) are particularly susceptible to infection with encapsulated bacteria, including *S. pneumoniae* and *H. influenzae*; in addition, they have an increased risk of developing autoimmune disorders, such as systemic lupus erythematosus.[52] *Neisseria meningitidis* is the most important bacterial pathogen observed in patients with deficiencies of terminal complement components (C5 through C9). Recurrent episodes of septicemia and meningitis are especially common.[35,55,84] Although patients with deficiencies of late-acting complement components are at increased risk for developing meningococcal septicemia and meningitis, they seem to suffer lower rates of morbidity and mortality than immunologically normal individuals with systemic

meningococcal infection. The frequency of primary complement deficiencies in patients with invasive meningococcal disease is approximately 5 to 10 percent[7,67]; however, the likelihood of having complement deficiency increases dramatically (31%) among individuals who have had more than one episode of invasive disease. A deficiency of opsonization in children with recurrent pyogenic infections and failure to thrive led to the recognition of the mannose-binding lectin pathway deficiencies. The clinical characteristic of these patients is the increased frequency of pyogenic infections.[100]

PATHOGENESIS

Various gene defects are responsible for the many distinct primary complement deficiencies. The particular bacteria that cause infection may indicate the missing component in host defense. C3b, the major cleavage product of C3, is an important opsonic ligand that promotes ingestion and killing of bacteria. Consequently, patients with C3 deficiency have increased susceptibility to bacterial infections (e.g., *S. pneumoniae*, *H. influenzae*), for which opsonization is the primary mechanism of host defense.[84,110] Individuals with deficiencies of C1, C4, or C2 also have increased susceptibility to these encapsulated bacteria because these components are necessary for activation of C3 through the classic pathway. Activation of terminal complement components C5, C6, C7, C8, and C9 results in assembly of the membrane attack complex C5b-9, a multicomponent macromolecule capable of bactericidal activity. Only gram-negative bacteria are susceptible to this bactericidal effect. Infections in patients with deficiencies of terminal complement components are limited to gram-negative bacteria, such as *N. meningitidis*.

DIAGNOSIS

When the history of infections is suggestive, the screening test used for complement deficiencies is the CH_{50} assay, which depends on the activity of all numbered components of the classic complement pathway from C1 through C9. When CH_{50} test results suggest a complement component deficiency, specific immunochemical and functional testing can identify the deficient component.[111]

TREATMENT AND PROGNOSIS

No specific therapy exists for primary complement deficiencies. Meningococcal vaccine is recommended for children with terminal complement component deficiencies.[7] Antibiotic prophylaxis and vaccines for other encapsulated organisms may be beneficial.

PRIMARY PHAGOCYTE DEFICIENCIES

The primary phagocyte deficiencies are a heterogeneous group of disorders having in common a susceptibility for frequent infections, resulting from a decreased number of phagocytic cells (e.g., neutropenia) or because of impaired adhesion, chemotaxis, opsonization and phagocytosis, or intracellular killing (Table 79–8). Infections resulting from quantitative or qualitative phagocyte deficiencies tend to be prolonged and recurrent, with a response to antibiotic therapy that is slower than expected. Common pathogens include *S. aureus*, *P. aeruginosa*, enteric gram-negative bacteria, and certain fungi (e.g., *Candida* spp., *Aspergillus* spp.).

TABLE 79–8 Primary Phagocyte Deficiencies

Quantitative Defects
Infantile agranulocytosis
Familial granulocytopenia
Cyclic neutropenia

Qualitative Defects
Adhesion Defects
Leukocyte adhesion deficiency
  Type I, β-integrin deficiency
  Type II, fucose-transporter deficiency

Intracellular Killing Defects
Chronic granulomatous disease
  X-linked
  Autosomal recessive
Glucose-6-phosphate dehydrogenase deficiency
Myeloperoxidase deficiency
Chédiak-Higashi syndrome
Griscelli syndrome

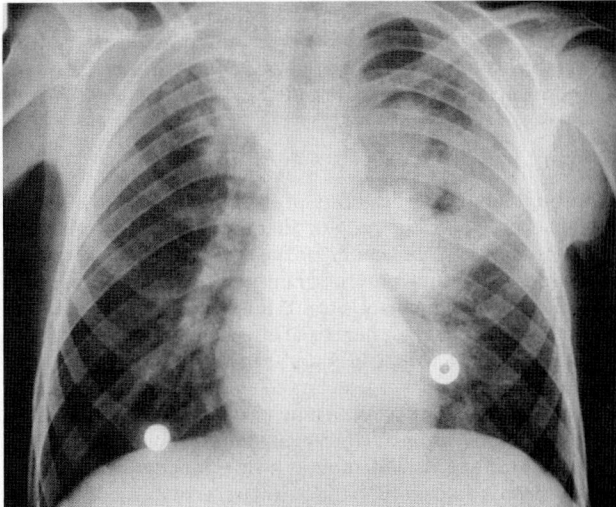

Figure 79–6 Chest radiograph of a 10-year-old boy with chronic granulomatous disease shows a left-sided pulmonary infiltrate and cavitary lung lesion. Biopsy revealed an *Aspergillus fumigatus* infection.

QUANTITATIVE PHAGOCYTE ABNORMALITIES

Primary quantitative phagocyte deficiencies can be observed as solitary defects or in association with other disorders (e.g., Shwachman syndrome). Infantile agranulocytosis (i.e., Kostmann syndrome) is an autosomal recessive disorder characterized by arrest of granulocyte maturation, markedly decreased numbers of circulating granulocytes, and severe infection. The more benign familial granulocytopenia syndrome manifests at various ages from infancy to adulthood, usually with indolent infections of the skin and soft tissues.

Cyclic neutropenia is an autosomal dominant defect of myelopoiesis, resulting from mutation in the leukocyte elastase (*ELA2*) gene, in which periodic disappearance of granulocytes from the circulation occurs.[11] Early granulocyte precursors are present in the bone marrow during periods of granulocytopenia, suggesting transient maturation arrest. Periods of granulocytopenia usually last 5 to 7 days and occur at 14- to 35-day intervals. The length of the cycle generally is constant for any given individual. Fever, malaise, aphthous stomatitis, and skin and soft tissue infections often are observed during periods of granulocytopenia.[94]

Some primary quantitative phagocyte deficiencies, particularly familial granulocytopenia and cyclic neutropenia, respond to therapy with recombinant granulocyte colony-stimulating factor.[39] Alternate-day corticosteroid therapy also has been used with some success in cyclic neutropenia.[115]

CHRONIC GRANULOMATOUS DISEASE

Clinical Features

Patients with CGD present with infections that begin during infancy and recur throughout the patient's life. Occasionally, patients have a mild course of disease and come to medical attention only during adolescence or adulthood.[70] History of suppurative lymphadenitis, soft tissue abscesses, pneumonia, lung abscess, hepatic abscess, and osteomyelitis suggest the presence of CGD. Perirectal abscesses may occur during early infancy. The physical findings of patients with CGD are nonspecific. Lymphadenopathy and hepatomegaly are common, and patients may have aphthous stomatitis. Infections in patients with CGD may progress with few symptoms, and the erythrocyte sedimentation rate and C-reactive protein may be useful to detect active infection.

Patients with CGD generally have infections caused by catalase-positive bacteria and fungi. *S. aureus* accounts for almost

one third of all infections of determined cause. *Nocardia, S. marcescens, Pseudomonas* spp., *Burkholderia cepacia,*[89] and certain enteric gram-negative bacilli also are common findings. *S. marcescens* osteomyelitis particularly is suggestive of the diagnosis of CGD. Fungi, especially *Aspergillus* spp., account for nearly one fifth of all defined infections in patients with CGD (Fig. 79-6).

Patients with CGD often have poor wound healing. Granulomatous obstructive lesions of the urinary[3] and gastrointestinal[62] tracts have been reported. Granulomatous bowel involvement resembles Crohn disease. Corticosteroid therapy may be effective in relieving these sometimes life-threatening lesions.[22] Boys with X-linked CGD may present with the McLeod blood phenotype, which results in difficulty crossmatching for blood transfusion and the potential for hemolytic transfusion reactions.[15]

Pathogenesis

X-linked and autosomal recessive forms of CGD have been described. The various gene defects result in abnormalities of membrane or cytosolic components of the nicotinamide adenine dinucleotide phosphate oxidase complex system.[89] Despite the genetic heterogeneity, all individuals with CGD have in common the failure of the cellular respiratory burst, which ordinarily accompanies phagocytosis and various soluble stimuli. Consequently, oxygen-derived microbicidal factors are not formed, and intracellular killing of phagocytized microorganisms is severely impaired. Catalase-negative microorganisms are killed normally because hydrogen peroxide can accumulate within the phagocytic vacuole.[24,95]

Diagnosis

The diagnosis of CGD historically has been made with the NBT dye test.[51] Neutrophils are stimulated in the presence of NBT, a soluble yellow dye that is reduced by cellular superoxide to formazan, an insoluble blue precipitate. Neutrophils from normal individuals show 100 percent reduction of NBT, asymptomatic carriers show 20 to 90 percent reduction, and patients with CGD show essentially no dye reduction. In patients with mild forms of the disease, the NBT test result may be normal. A more sensitive method to measure production of hydrogen peroxide is based on chemiluminescence of DHR on activation, detected by flow cytometry; this increasingly is used as a confirmatory test of the disease, replacing the NBT dye test.[50]

Treatment and Prognosis

Specific microbiologic diagnosis of infections should be established whenever possible. Empiric therapy is directed against the organisms known to be common causes of infection: *S. aureus*, *Pseudomonas* spp., and enteric gram-negative bacilli. Surgical drainage or débridement of sites of infection often is required. Anecdotal reports suggest beneficial effects of granulocyte transfusions in patients with CGD and serious bacterial or fungal infections. HSCT has been used successfully with HLA-matched related donors,[59,90] and gene therapy trials for X-linked CGD in humans resulted in gene-corrected, autologous granulocytes detectable for more than 30 months post-treatment, with resolution of chronic infections.[79] The oxidase activity of the gene-corrected cells had decreased progressively, however, by mechanisms of "gene silencing."[79]

Antibiotic prophylaxis with trimethoprim-sulfamethoxazole reduces the frequency of bacterial infections in patients with CGD.[63] Itraconazole and other antifungals given as prophylaxis may be effective for the prevention of *Aspergillus* infections, which usually are severe and difficult to eradicate.[40] The administration of interferon-γ, given by subcutaneous injection three times weekly, reduces the incidence of serious infections in CGD by two thirds without causing major deleterious side effects.[48] Patients should be educated about not performing activities that expose them to environments containing mold spores, such as mulching or raking leaves. The prognosis of CGD has improved remarkably during the past several decades, and now most patients survive to adulthood.

LEUKOCYTE ADHESION DEFICIENCY

Clinical Features

Patients with LAD have severe and recurrent bacterial infections of the skin and soft tissues, mucosal surfaces, and gastrointestinal tract, often beginning during early infancy.[104] Common pathogenic microorganisms include staphylococci and *Pseudomonas* spp. Infants with the severe phenotype may have delayed separation of the umbilical cord secondary to omphalitis. Cutaneous infections may become necrotic, resembling ecthyma gangrenosum or pyoderma gangrenosum. Poor wound healing also is observed. Individuals surviving infancy typically develop severe gingivitis and periodontitis with progressive alveolar bone loss (see Fig. 79-3).

Marked granulocytosis is a hallmark of LAD. Circulating granulocyte counts may range from 15,000/mm³ to 75,000/mm³, even in the absence of infection, and counts of 100,000/mm³ or greater are common during episodes of infection. Despite the presence of granulocytosis, formation of pus is poor because of impaired migration to tissues.

Pathogenesis

LAD type I is an autosomal recessive disorder that maps to chromosome 21q22.3. Neutrophils from individuals with LAD are defective in their expression of several surface glycoproteins known as the leukocyte integrin (CD11/CD18) complex. These molecules are crucial for adhesion-dependent functions, and their absence is responsible for defects in leukocyte adherence, chemotaxis, and phagocytosis. The severity of infectious complications of LAD is related directly to the degree of CD18 gene

expression. Patients with the severe clinical phenotype have undetectable expression of CD11/CD18 complexes on their phagocytes, whereas individuals with the moderate phenotype generally have 2 to 8 percent expression.

A second form of LAD has been described in two patients with craniofacial dysmorphism, neurologic deficits, recurrent respiratory infections, and marked granulocytosis.[34] Both individuals manifested the Bombay (hh) blood phenotype. In contrast to the neutrophils of patients with LAD type I, neutrophils from patients with LAD type II had normal surface expression of CD18. The molecular basis for the phagocyte dysfunction is a defect in the fucose transporter influencing the glycosylation of sialyl-Lewis X, a carbohydrate ligand for the endothelial adhesion molecules E-selectin and P-selectin. A third form of LAD has been described, characterized by a deficiency of all β integrins, resulting from a deficiency of Rap1 activation, a signal transduction necessary for integrin stabilization.[54]

Diagnosis

The diagnosis of LAD type I is made by flow cytometry using fluorescence-labeled monoclonal anti-CD11/CD18 antibody. In vitro studies reveal abnormalities of phagocyte adherence, chemotaxis, and phagocytosis. Individuals with LAD type II have similar phagocyte function abnormalities, with normal expression of CD18 and down-regulation of selectins. LAD type III is characterized by altered expression of all β integrins.

Treatment and Prognosis

Intercurrent bacterial infections in patients with LAD must be treated aggressively with prolonged courses of parenteral antibiotics. Antibiotic prophylaxis and universal hygiene measures are recommended. Although survival to adulthood is described, almost half of affected individuals die before reaching 2 years of age. Administration of fucose normalizes leukocyte function in LAD type II. Bone marrow transplantation offers the best hope for long-term survival.[103]

OTHER PRIMARY PHAGOCYTE DEFICIENCIES

A variety of other defects of phagocyte chemotaxis, phagocytosis, and intracellular killing have been described. Chédiak-Higashi syndrome is a rare autosomal recessive disorder characterized by partial oculocutaneous albinism, rotatory nystagmus, and peripheral neuropathy. Affected individuals develop recurrent serious or life-threatening infections caused by a wide variety of bacteria. In the accelerated phase of the illness, hepatosplenomegaly, lymphadenopathy, lymphocytic infiltration of multiple body organs, and unexplained febrile illnesses are common. Giant granules are found in numerous different cell types, including leukocytes, in the body. Neutrophils exhibit defective chemotaxis and abnormal bactericidal activity.

Hyperimmunoglobulinemia E (also known as hyper-IgE syndrome, Buckley syndrome, and Job syndrome) is characterized by markedly elevated serum IgE levels, eczema, recurrent staphylococcal abscesses, sinusitis, and otitis media. Coarse facial features are common. In addition to staphylococcal abscesses, recurrent pneumonia with bronchiectasis and pneumatoceles and mucocutaneous candidiasis are common. Other observed features include delay of shedding of primary dentition, recurrent bone fractures, scoliosis, and joint hyperextensibility. Hyper-IgE syndrome manifests with autosomal dominant inheritance and can be diagnosed with certainty only when the patient or family members present with the skeletal manifestations.[43] Missense mutations in STAT 3 gene have been found to cause this disease.[47a]

CONCLUSIONS

Primary immunodeficiencies are rare diseases, with an estimated minimal frequency of 1 in 10,000 live births for most conditions, although the actual incidence is unknown. Mutations in more than 120 genes have been identified to be responsible for primary immunodeficiencies, and several advances have clarified the immunopathogenesis of these conditions.

These diseases should be suspected and investigated in children who present with infections of unusual severity, frequency, or etiologic organisms and unexplained general symptoms, such as fever or failure to thrive. The initial immunologic screening consists of simple laboratory tests, and prompt referral to the clinical immunologist is warranted when a primary immunodeficiency is suspected. Management for these disorders has advanced during recent years to remarkably improved care, reflected in most immunodeficient patients surviving to adulthood. Curative treatment is available for severe immunodeficiencies in the form of allogeneic HSCT; however, it is not without considerable risk of mortality, and cure is not always optimal. Although still experimental, gene therapy has reached the stage of clinical trials for X-linked SCID, ADA-deficient SCID, and CGD, with successful and promising results.

REFERENCES

1. Ahonen, P., Myllarniemi, S., Sipila, I., et al.: Clinical variations of autoimmune polyendocrinopathy-candidiasis-ectoderm dystrophy (APECED) in a series of 68 patients. N. Engl. J. Med. *322*:1829-1836, 1990.
2. Alachkar, H., Taubenheim, N., Haeney, M. R., et al.: Memory switched B cell percentage but not serum immunoglobulin concentration is associated with clinical complications in children and adults with specific antibody deficiency and common variable immunodeficiency. Clin. Immunol. *120*:310-318, 2006.
3. Aliabadi, H., Gonzalez, R., and Quie, P. G.: Urinary tract disorders in patients with chronic granulomatous disease. N. Engl. J. Med. *321*:706-708, 1989.
4. Allen, R. C., Armitage, R. J., Conley, M. E., et al.: CD40 ligand gene defects responsible for X-linked hyper-IgM syndrome. Science *259*:990-993, 1993.
5. Altare, F., Durandy, A., Lammas, D., et al.: Impairment of mycobacterial immunity in human interleukin-12 receptor deficiency. Science *280*:1432-1435, 1998.
6. American Academy of Pediatrics: Active and passive immunization. *In* Pickering, L. K. (ed.): 2006 Red Book: Report of the Committee on Infectious Diseases. 27th ed. Elk Grove Village, IL, American Academy of Pediatrics, 2006, pp. 71-85.
7. American Academy of Pediatrics: Meningococcal infections. *In* Pickering, L. K. (ed.): 2006 Red Book: Report of the Committee on Infectious Diseases. 27th ed. Elk Grove Village, IL, American Academy of Pediatrics, 2006, pp. 452-460.
8. Antoine, C., Muller, S., Cant, A., et al.: Long-term survival and transplantation of hematopoietic stem cells for immunodeficiencies: Report of the European experience 1968-1999. Lancet *361*:553-560, 2003.
9. Aruffo, A., Farrington, M., Hollenbaugh, D., et al.: The CD40 ligand, gp39, is defective in activated T cells from patients with X-linked hyper-IgM syndrome. Cell *72*:291-300, 1993.
10. Azzari, C., Gambineri, E., Resti, M., et al.: Safety and immunogenicity of measles-mumps-rubella vaccine in children with congenital immunodeficiency (DiGeorge syndrome). Vaccine *23*:1668-1671, 2005.
11. Ballane-Chantellot, C., Clauin, S., Leblanc, T., et al.: Mutations in the ELA gene correlate with more severe expression of neutropenia: A study of 81 patients from the French neutropenia register. Blood *103*:4119-4125, 2004.
12. Bartlett, A. V., Moore, M., Gary, G. W., et al.: Diarrheal illness among infants and toddlers in day care centers, II: Comparison with day care homes and households. J. Pediatr. *107*:503-509, 1985.
13. Bordignon, C., Notarangelo, L. D., Nobili, N., et al.: Gene therapy in peripheral blood lymphocytes and bone marrow for adenosine deaminase immunodeficient patients. Science *270*:470-474, 1995.
14. Brimblecombe, F. S. W., Cruickshank, R., Masters, P. L., et al.: Family studies of respiratory infections. B. M. J. *1*:119, 1958.
15. Brzica, S. M., Jr., Pineda, A. A., Taswell, H. F., et al.: Chronic granulomatous disease and the McLeod phenotype: Successful treatment of infection with granulocyte transfusions resulting in subsequent hemolytic transfusion reaction. Mayo Clin. Proc. *52*:153-156, 1977.
16. Buckley, R. H.: Molecular defects in human severe combined immunodeficiency and approaches to immunoreconstitution. Annu. Rev. Immunol. *22*:625-655, 2004.
17. Burks, A. W., Sampson, H. A., and Buckley, R. H.: Anaphylactic reactions after gamma globulin administration in patients with hypogammaglobu-

18. linemia: Detection of IgE antibodies to IgA. N. Engl. J. Med. *314*:560-564, 1986.
18. Burns, S., Cory, G. O., Vainchenker, W., et al.: Mechanisms of WASp-mediated hematologic and immunologic disease. Blood *104*:3454-3462, 2004.
19. Busse, P. J., Razvi, S., and Cunningham-Rundles, C.: Efficacy of intravenous immunoglobulin in the prevention of pneumonia in patients with common variable immunodeficiency. J. Allergy Clin. Immunol. *109*:1001-1004, 2002.
20. Carsetti, R., Rosado, M. M., Donnano, S., et al.: The loss of IgM memory B cells correlates with clinical disease in common variable immunodeficiency. J. Allergy Clin. Immunol. *115*:412-417, 2005.
21. Castigli, E., and Geha, R. S.: Molecular basis of common variable immunodeficiency. J. Allergy Clin. Immunol. *117*:740-746, 2006.
22. Chin, T. W., Stiehm, E. R., Falloon, J., et al.: Corticosteroids in treatment of obstructive lesions of chronic granulomatous disease. J. Pediatr. *111*:349-352, 1987.
23. Chinen, J., Rosenblatt, H. M., Smith, E. O., et al.: Long-term assessment of T cell populations in DiGeorge syndrome. J. Allergy Clin. Immunol. *111*:573-579, 2003.
24. Cohen, M. S., Isturiz, R. E., Malech, H. L., et al.: Fungal infection in chronic granulomatous disease: The importance of the phagocyte in defense against fungi. Am. J. Med. *71*:59-66, 1981.
25. Conley, M. E., and Howard, V.: Clinical findings leading to the diagnosis of X-linked agammaglobulinemia. J. Pediatr. *141*:566-571, 2002.
26. Conley, M. E., Larche, M., Bonagura, V. R., et al.: Hyper IgM syndrome associated with defective CD40-mediated B cell activation. J. Clin. Invest. *94*:1404-1409, 1994.
27. Conley, M. E., Park, C. L., and Douglas, S. D.: Childhood common variable immunodeficiency with autoimmune disease. J. Pediatr. *108*:915-922, 1986.
28. Cunningham-Rundles, C., and Bodian, C.: Common variable immunodeficiency: Clinical and immunological features of 248 patients. Clin. Immunol. *92*:34-38, 1999.
29. Derry, J. M. J., Ochs, H. D., and Francke, U.: Isolation of a novel gene mutated in Wiskott-Aldrich syndrome. Cell *78*:635-644, 1994.
30. Dorman, S. E., Picard, C., Lammas, D., et al.: Clinical features of dominant and recessive interferon gamma receptor 1 deficiencies. Lancet *364*:2113-2121, 2004.
31. Dressler, F., Peter, H. H., Muller, W., et al.: Transient hypogammaglobulinemia of infancy. Acta Paediatr. Scand. *78*:767-774, 1989.
32. Dupuis-Girod, S., Medioni, J., Haddad, E., et al.: Autoimmunity in Wiskott-Aldrich syndrome: Risk factors, clinical features and outcome in a single center cohort of 55 patients. Pediatrics *111*:e622-e627, 2003.
33. Edwards, E., Razvi, S., and Cunningham-Rundles, C.: IgA deficiency: Clinical correlates and responses to pneumococcal vaccine. Clin. Immunol. *111*:93-97, 2004.
34. Etzioni, A., Sturla, L., Antonellis, A., et al.: Leukocyte adhesion deficiency (LAD) type II/carbohydrate deficient glycoprotein (CDG) II c founder effect in genotype/phenotype correlation. Am. J. Med. Genet. *110*:131-135, 2002.
35. Figueroa, J. E., and Densen, P.: Infectious diseases associated with complement deficiencies. Clin. Microbiol. Rev. *4*:359-395, 1991.
36. Filipovich, A. H., Mathur, A., Kamat, D., et al.: Lymphoproliferative disorders and other tumors complicating immunodeficiencies. Immunodeficiency *5*:91-112, 1994.
37. Fleisher, T. A., and Olivera, J. B.: Functional and molecular evaluation of lymphocytes. J. Allergy Clin. Immunol. *114*:227-234, 2004.
38. Fox, J. P., Hall, C. E., Cooney, M. K., et al.: The Seattle virus watch, II: Objectives, study population and its observation, data processing and summary of illnesses. Am. J. Epidemiol. *96*:270-285, 1972.
39. Frampton, J. E., Lee, C. R., and Faulds, D.: Filgrastim: A review of its pharmacological properties and therapeutic efficacy in neutropenia. Drugs *48*:731-760, 1994.
40. Gallin, J. I., Alling, D. W., Malech, H. L., et al.: Itraconazole to prevent fungal infections in chronic granulomatous disease. N. Engl. J. Med. *348*:2416-2422, 2003.
41. Gaspar, H. B., Parsley, K. L., Lowe, S., et al.: Gene therapy for X-linked severe combined immunodeficiency by use of a pseudotyped gammaretroviral vector. Lancet *364*:2181-2187, 2004.
41a. Geha, R. S., Notarangelo, L. D., Casanova, J. L., et al.: Primary immunodeficiency diseases: An update from the International Union of Immunological Societies Primary Immunodeficiency Diseases Classification Committee. J. Allergy Clin. Immunol. *120*:776-794, 2007.
42. Grierson, H., and Purtilo, D. T.: Epstein-Barr virus infections in males with the X-linked lymphoproliferative syndrome. Ann. Intern. Med. *106*:538-545, 1987.
43. Grimbacher, B., Holland, S. M., and Puck, J. M.: Hyper-IgE syndromes. Immunol. Rev. *203*:244-250, 2005.
44. Guerrant, R. L., Lohr, J. A., and Williams, E. K.: Acute infectious diarrhea, I: Epidemiology, etiology, and pathogenesis. Pediatr. Infect. Dis. *5*:353-359, 1986.
45. Hacein-Bey-Abina, S., LeDeist, F., Carlier, F., et al.: Sustained correction of X-linked severe combined immunodeficiency by ex vivo gene therapy. N. Engl. J. Med. *346*:1185-1193, 2002.
46. Hanson, L. A., Soderstrom, R., Nilssen, D. E., et al.: IgG subclass deficiency with or without IgA deficiency. Clin. Immunol. Immunopathol. *61*:S70-S77, 1991.
47. Hershfield, M. S.: Adenosine deaminase deficiency: Clinical expression, molecular basis and therapy. Semin. Hematol. *35*:291-297, 1998.

47a. Holland, S. M., De Leo, F. R., Elloumi, H. Z., et al.: STAT 3 mutations in the hyper IgE syndrome. N. Engl. J. Med. *357*:1608-1619, 2007.

48. International Chronic Granulomatous Disease Cooperative Study Group: A controlled trial of interferon gamma to prevent infection in chronic granulomatous disease. N. Engl. J. Med. *324*:509-516, 1991.

49. Isgro, A., Marzilai, M., Mezzaroma, I., et al.: Bone marrow clonogenic capability, and thymic output in patients with common variable immunodeficiency. J. Immunol. *174*:5074-5081, 2005.

50. Jirapongsanaruruk, O., Malech, H. L., Kuhns, D. B., et al.: Diagnostic paradigm for evaluation of male patients with chronic granulomatous disease, based on the dihydrorhodamine assay. J. Allergy Clin. Immunol. *111*:374-379, 2003.

51. Johnston, R. B.: Defects of neutrophils function. N. Engl. J. Med. *307*:434-436, 1982.

52. Jonsson, G., Truedson, L., Sturfelt, G., et al.: Hereditary C2 deficiency in Sweden, frequent occurrence of invasive infection, atherosclerosis and rheumatic disease. Medicine (Baltimore) *84*:23-34, 2005.

53. Jouanguy, E., Lanhamedi-Cherradi, S., Lammas, D., et al.: A human IFNGR1 small deletion hotspot associated with dominant susceptibility to mycobacterial infection. Nat. Genet. *21*:370-380, 1999.

54. Kinashi, T., Aker, M., Sokolovsky-Eisenberg, M., et al.: LAD III, a leukocyte adhesion deficiency syndrome associated with defective Rap 1 activation and impaired stabilization of integrin bonds. Blood *103*:1033-1036, 2004.

55. Kline, M. W.: Recurrent bacterial meningitis. Antibiot. Chemother. *45*:254-261, 1992.

56. LeBras, S., and Geha, R. S.: IPEX and the role of FoxP3 in the development and function of human Tregs. J. Clin. Invest. *116*:1473-1475, 2005.

57. Lee, W. I., Torgerson, T. R., Schumacher, M. J., et al.: Molecular analysis of a large cohort of patients with the hyper immunoglobulin M (IgM) syndrome. Blood *105*:1881-1890, 2005.

58. Leonard, W. J., Noguchi, I. M., Russell, S. M., et al.: The molecular basis of X-linked severe combined immunodeficiency: The role of interleukin-2 receptor gamma chain is a common gamma chain. Immunol. Rev. *138*:61-64, 1994.

59. Leung, T., Chik, K., Li, C., et al.: Bone marrow transplantation for chronic granulomatous disease: Long-term follow up and review of the literature. Bone Marrow Transplant. *24*:567-570, 1999.

60. Levy, J., Espanol-Boren, T., Thomas, C., et al.: The clinical spectrum of X-linked hyper-IgM syndrome. J. Pediatr. *131*:47-54, 1997.

61. Liese, J. G., Wintergerst, J., Tympner, K. D., et al.: High- vs low-dose immunoglobulin therapy in the long-term treatment of X-linked agammaglobulinemia. Am. J. Dis. Child. *146*:335-339, 1992.

62. Marciano, B. E., Rosenzweig, S. D., Kleiner, D. E., et al.: Gastrointestinal involvement in chronic granulomatous disease. Pediatrics *114*:462-468, 2004.

63. Margolis, D. M., Melnick, D. A., Alling, D. W., et al.: Trimethoprim-sulfamethoxazole prophylaxis in the management of chronic granulomatous disease. J. Infect. Dis. *162*:723-726, 1990.

64. Markert, M. L., Alexieff, M. J., Li, J., et al.: Postnatal thymus transplantation with immunosuppression as treatment for DiGeorge syndrome. Blood *104*:2574-2581, 2004.

65. McGeady, S. J.: Transient hypogammaglobulinemia of infancy: Need to reconsider name and definition. J. Pediatr. *110*:47-50, 1987.

66. McKinney, R. E., Jr., Katz, S. L., and Wilfert, C. M.: Chronic enteroviral meningoencephalitis in agammaglobulinemic patients. Rev. Infect. Dis. *9*:334-356, 1987.

67. Merino, J., Rodriguez-Valverde, V., Lamelas, J. A., et al.: Prevalence of deficits of complement components in patients with recurrent meningococcal infections. J. Infect. Dis. *148*:331, 1983.

68. Minegishi, Y., Lavoie, A., Cunningham-Rundles, C., et al.: Mutations in activation-induced cytidine deaminase in patients with hyper IgM syndrome. Clin. Immunol. *97*:203-210, 2000.

69. Molina, I. J., Kenney, D. M., Rosen, F. S., et al.: T cell lines characterize events in the pathogenesis of the Wiskott-Aldrich syndrome. J. Exp. Med. *176*:867-874, 1992.

70. Mouy, R., Fischer, A., Vilmer, E., et al.: Incidence, severity, and prevention of infections in chronic granulomatous disease. J. Pediatr. *114*:555-560, 1989.

71. Moylett, E. H., Wasan, A. N., Noroski, L. M., et al.: Live viral vaccines in patients with partial DiGeorge syndrome: Clinical experience and cellular immunity. Clin. Immunol. *112*:106-112, 2004.

72. Noguchi, M., Nakamura, Y., Russell, S. M., et al.: Interleukin-2 receptor gamma chain: A functional component of the interleukin-7 receptor. Science *262*:1877-1880, 1993.

73. Notarangelo, L. D., Casanova, J. L., Conley, M. E., et al. Primary immunodeficiency diseases: An update from the International Union of Immunological Societies Primary Immunodeficiencies Committee Meeting in Budapest, 2005. J. Allergy Clin. Immunol. *117*:883-896, 2006.

74. Nowak-Wegrzyn, A., Crawford, T. O., Winkelstein, J. A., et al.: Immunodeficiency and infections in ataxia-telangiectasia. J. Pediatr. *144*:505-511, 2004.

75. Ochs, H. D., Ament, M. E., and Davis, S. D.: Giardiasis with malabsorption in X-linked agammaglobulinemia. N. Engl. J. Med. *287*:341-342, 1972.

76. Ochs, H. D., and Thrasher, A. J.: The Wiskott-Aldrich syndrome. J. Allergy Clin. Immunol. *117*:725-738, 2006.

77. Orange, J. S., and Geha, R. S.: Finding NEMO: Genetic disorders of NF-kappaB activation. J. Clin. Invest. *112*:983-985, 2003.

78. Orange, J. S., Hossny, E. M., Weiler, C. R., et al.: Use of intravenous immunoglobulin in human disease: A review of the evidence by members of the Primary Immunodeficiency Committee of the American Academy of Allergy, Asthma and Immunology. J. Allergy Clin. Immunol. *117*:S525-S553, 2006.

79. Ott, M. G., Schmidt, M., Schwarzwaelder, K., et al: Correction of X-linked chronic granulomatous disease by gene therapy, augmented by insertional activation of MDS1-EVI1, PRDM16 or SETBP1. Nat. Med. *12*:401-409, 2006.

80. Oxelius, V. A., Laurell, A. B., Lindquist, B., et al.: IgG subclasses in selective IgA deficiency: Importance of IgG2-IgA deficiency. N. Engl. J. Med. *302*:1476-1477, 1981.

81. Perez, E. E., Bokszzanin, A., McDonald-McGinn, D., et al.: Safety of live viral vaccines in patients with chromosome 22q11.2 deletion syndrome (DiGeorge syndrome/velocardiofacial syndrome). Pediatrics *112*:e325, 2003.

82. Plebani, A., Soresina, A., Rondelli, R., et al.: Clinical, immunological and molecular analysis of a large cohort of patients with X-linked agammaglobulinemia: An Italian multicenter study. Clin. Immunol. *104*:221-230, 2002.

83. Rosenzweig, S. D., Dorman, S. E., Uzel, G., et al.: A novel mutation in IFN-gamma receptor 2 with dominant negative activity biological consequences of homozygous and heterozygous states. J. Immunol. *173*:4000-4008, 2004.

84. Ross, S. C., and Densen, P.: Complement deficiency states and infection: Epidemiology, pathogenesis and consequences of neisserial and other infections in an immune deficiency. Medicine (Baltimore) *63*:243-273, 1984.

85. Russell, S. M., Keegan, A. D., Harada, N., et al.: Interleukin-2 receptor gamma chain: A functional component of the interleukin-4 receptor. Science *262*:1880-1883, 1993.

86. Savitsky, K., Bar-Shira, A., Gilad, S., et al.: A single ataxia-telangiectasia gene with a product similar to PI-3 kinase. Science *268*:1749-1753, 1995.

87. Sayos, J., Wu, C., Morra, M., et al.: The X-linked lymphoproliferative disease gene product SAP regulates signal induced through the coreceptor SLAM. Nature *395*:462-469, 1998.

88. Schaffer, F. M., Monteiro, R. C., Volanakis, J. E., et al.: IgA deficiency. Immunodefic. Rev. *3*:15-44, 1991.

89. Segal, B. H., Leto, T. L., Gallin, J. I., et al.: Genetic, biochemical and clinical features of chronic granulomatous disease. Medicine (Baltimore) *79*:170-200, 2000.

90. Seger, R. A., Gungor, T., Belohradsky, B. H., et al.: Treatment of chronic granulomatous disease with myeloablative conditioning and an unmodified hematopoietic allograft: A survey of the European experience. Blood *100*:4344-4350, 2002.

91. Shackelford, P. G., Granoff, D. M., Polmar, S. H., et al.: Subnormal serum concentrations of IgG2 in children with frequent infections associated with varied patterns of immunologic dysfunction. J. Pediatr. *116*:529-538, 1990.

92. Siegel, S. R., Siegel, B., Sokoloff, B. Z., et al.: Urinary tract infection in infants and preschool children. Am. J. Dis. Child. *134*:369-372, 1980.

93. Smahi, A., Courtois, G., Vabres, P., et al.: Genomic rearrangement in NEMO impairs NF-kappaB activation and is a cause of incontinentia pigmenti. The International Incontinentia Pigmenti (IP) Consortium. Nature *405*:466-472, 2000.

94. Souid, A. K.: Congenital cyclic neutropenia. Clin. Pediatr. *34*:151-155, 1995.

95. Speert, D. P., Bond, M., Woodman, R. C., et al.: Infection with *Pseudomonas cepacia* in chronic granulomatous disease: Role of nonoxidative killing by neutrophils in host defense. J. Infect. Dis. *170*:1524-1531, 1994.

96. Spickett, G. P., Webster, A. D., and Farrant, J.: Cellular abnormalities in common variable immunodeficiency. Immunodefic. Rev. *2*:199-219, 1990.

97. Stephan, J. L., Vlekova, V., Le Deist, F., et al.: Severe combined immunodeficiency: A retrospective single-center study of clinical presentation and outcome in 117 cases. J. Pediatr. *123*:564-572, 1993.

98. Sullivan, K. E.: The clinical, immunological, and molecular spectrum of chromosome 22q11.2 deletion syndrome and DiGeorge syndrome. Curr. Opin. Allergy Clin. Immunol. *4*:505-512, 2004.

99. Sullivan, K. E., McDonald-McGinn, D., Driscoll, D. A., et al.: Longitudinal analysis of lymphocyte function and numbers in the first year of life in chromosome 22q11.2 deletion syndrome (DiGeorge syndrome/velocardiofacial syndrome). Clin. Diagn. Lab. Immunol. *6*:906-911, 1999.

100. Summerfield, J. A., Sumya, M., Levin, M., and Turner, M. W.: Association of mutations in mannose binding protein gene with childhood infection in consecutive hospital series. B. M. J. *314*:1229-1232, 1997.

101. Teele, D. W., Klein, J. O., Rosner, B., et al.: Epidemiology of otitis media during the first seven years of life in children in greater Boston: A prospective cohort study. J. Infect. Dis. *160*:83-94, 1989.

102. Thomas, C., deSaint Basile, G., Le Deist, F., et al.: Correction of X-linked hyper IgM syndrome by allogeneic bone marrow transplantation. N. Engl. J. Med. *333*:426-429, 1995.

103. Thomas, C., Le Deist, F., Cavazzana-Calvo, M., et al.: Results of allogeneic bone marrow transplantation in patients with leukocyte adhesion deficiency. Blood *86*:1629-1635, 1995.

104. Todd, R. F., III, and Freyer, D. R.: The CD11/18 leukocyte glycoprotein deficiency. Hematol. Oncol. Clin. North Am. *2*:13-31, 1988.

105. Tsukada, S., Saffran, D. C., Rawlings, D. J., et al.: Deficient expression of a B cell cytoplasmic tyrosine kinase in human X-linked agammaglobulinemia. Cell *72*:279-290, 1993.

106. Umetsu, D. T., Ambrosino, D. M., Quinti, I., et al.: Recurrent sinopulmonary infection and impaired antibody response to bacterial capsular polysaccharide antigen in children with selective IgG-subclass deficiency. N. Engl. J. Med. *313*:1247-1251, 1985.
107. Verbruggen, G., Debajer, S., Deforce, D., et al.: X-linked agammaglobulinemia and rheumatoid arthritis. Ann. Rheum. Dis. *64*:1075-1078, 2005.
108. Villa, A., Notarangelo, L., Mach, P., et al.: X-linked thrombocytopenia and Wiskott-Aldrich syndrome are allelic diseases with mutations in the WASP gene. Nat. Genet. *9*:414-417, 1995.
109. Volanakis, J. E., Zhu, Z. B., Schaffer, F. M., et al.: Major histocompatibility complex class III genes and susceptibility to immunoglobulin A deficiency and common variable immunodeficiency. J. Clin. Invest. *89*:1914-1922, 1992.
110. Walport, M. J.: Complement. N. Engl. J. Med. *344*:1058-1066, 2001.
111. Wen, L., Atkinson, J. P., and Giclas, P. C.: Clinical and laboratory evaluation of complement deficiency. J. Allergy Clin. Immunol. *113*:585-593, 2004.
112. Winkelstein, J. A., Marino, M. C., Lederman, H. M., et al.: X-linked agammaglobulinemia: Report on a United States registry of 201 patients. Medicine (Baltimore) *85*:193-202, 2006.
113. Winkelstein, J. A., Marino, M. C., Ochs, H., et al.: The X-linked hyper IgM syndrome: Clinical and immunological features of 79 patients. Medicine (Baltimore) *82*:373-384, 2003.
114. Woods, C. G., and Taylor, A. M.: Ataxia-telangiectasia in the British Isles: The clinical and laboratory features of 70 affected individuals. Q. J. M. *82*:169-179, 1992.
115. Wright, D. G., Fauci, A. S., Dale, D. C., et al.: Correction of human cyclic neutropenia and prednisolone. N. Engl. J. Med. *298*:295-300, 1978.
116. Yagi, H., Furutani, Y., Hamada, H., et al.: Role of TBX1 in human del22q11.2 syndrome. Lancet *362*:1366-1373, 2003.
117. Zonana, J., Elder, M. E., Schneider, L. C., et al.: A novel X-linked disorder of immune deficiency and hypohidrotic ectodermal dysplasia is allelic to incontinentia pigmenti and due to mutations in IKK-gamma (NEMO). Am. J. Hum. Genet. *67*:1555-1562, 2000.

CHAPTER 80

OPPORTUNISTIC INFECTIONS IN HEMATOPOIETIC STEM CELL TRANSPLANTATION

Christian C. Patrick

Hematopoietic stem cell transplantation (HSCT) involves the infusion of stem cells from a donor into a recipient who has received a special conditioning regimen for the procedure. In recent years, the term HSCT has replaced the traditional term bone marrow transplantation (BMT) because hematopoietic stem cells can be obtained from bone marrow, umbilical cord blood, and peripheral blood.[86,117] HSCT has become the standard treatment for many patients with hematologic malignances and solid tumors, as well as nonmalignant conditions such as primary immunodeficiencies, hemoglobinopathies, bone marrow failure syndromes, and a variety of genetic conditions, including inherited metabolic disorders.*

HSCT can be classified as syngeneic, autologous, or allogeneic, depending on the genetic match of the donor to the recipient of the stem cells. Syngeneic HSCT is transplantation of stem cells from an identical twin. In autologous HSCT, the patient's own stem cells harvested before ablative chemotherapy are transplanted. Autologous HSCT is used for patients who require marrow ablative chemotherapy to treat the underlying malignancy but have healthy bone marrow.[4] Allogeneic HSCT involves the transplantation of stem cells from a human leukocyte antigen (HLA)-matched sibling, an HLA-partially matched family member, or an HLA-matched unrelated donor.[4] In general, engraftment is faster for syngeneic and autologous transplantation when a total HLA match between the recipient and the donor exists. Allogeneic HSCT has a higher chance of success when completely HLA-matched sibling donors are used.

The three main sources of stem cells are bone marrow, peripheral blood, and cord blood. The different cell populations harvested from these sites can be correlated with complications. Peripheral blood progenitor cells from an allogeneic donor can increase the incidence of graft-versus-host disease (GHVD) secondary to an increase in T cells from the transplant.[30] Peripheral blood stem cells contain a high amount of CD34+ cells and an increased amount of T cells, which equates to quicker engraftment but an increased rate of GVHD.[30] Cord blood transplants allow less stringent matching of HLA haplotypes because mismatched cord blood stem cells are less likely to cause GVHD, but they have fewer CD34+ cells, which leads to slower engraftment.[159]

Infectious complications occurring after HSCT are somewhat predictable based on the underlying primary disease and the acquired immunodeficiencies that occur after transplantation.[96,134,142] Patients undergoing HSCT are at increased risk for infectious complications secondary to the acquired immunodeficiencies that occur after the procedure or secondary to medications (e.g., cyclosporine, steroids) used to treat complications of transplantation.[4] Infections are a major cause of morbidity and mortality and represent the most significant barrier to both immediate and long-term survival after HSCT.

Recovery of immune function after undergoing HSCT is a gradual process that takes place over the course of several months to years. Immune reconstitution after HSCT follows the normal pattern of immune ontogeny, with development from immature to mature immune functions. The general early immune mechanisms, such as phagocytic and cytotoxic functions, recover first, usually by post-transplant day 100, but the specialized functions of T and B lymphocytes may remain impaired for a year or even longer.[36,121]

These immune defects and the gradual recovery of host defenses cause infections to occur in three predictable time periods, as shown in Table 80–1. The first or pre-engraftment period begins with onset of the conditioning regimen and continues until engraftment, about 30 days after transplantation. This phase is characterized by profound neutropenia that lasts 3 to 4 weeks. Treatment with colony-stimulating factors can shorten the duration of this phase.[85,143] The middle or early engraftment period starts after resolution of the neutropenia with transplant engraftment and lasts until approximately 100 days after HSCT. The last or late engraftment period starts about 100 days after transplantation and is associated with selected deficits in both cellular and humoral immune responses and reticuloendothelial function.[134]

EPIDEMIOLOGY

Several risk factors place HSCT recipients at increased risk for acquiring infectious complications; however, there are significant differences in the relative risk for infection after HSCT, depending on the type of transplantation. The degree of immunosuppression is less with autologous HSCT because no risk for

*See references 4, 18, 27, 60, 74, 76, 89, 136, 152, 163.

TABLE 80-1   Temporal Association of Infections and Predominant Etiologic Agents after Hematopoietic Stem Cell Transplantation

Phase	Predominant Host Defect	Bacterial Infections	Fungal Infections	Viral Infections
Pre-engraftment (0-30 days)	Neutropenia	*Staphylococcus aureus* *Staphylococcus epidermidis* Viridans streptococci *Pseudomonas aeruginosa* Enterobacteriaceae *Escherichia coli* *Klebsiella pneumoniae* *Enterobacter* species	*Candida* species *Aspergillus* species	Herpes simplex virus
Early engraftment (31-100 days)	Cytotoxic and phagocytic functions	*S. aureus* *S. epidermidis* Viridans streptococci *P. aeruginosa* Enterobacteriaceae	*Candida* species *Aspergillus* species *Pneumocystis jiroveci*	Cytomegalovirus Adenovirus Respiratory viruses
Late engraftment (>100 days)	Cellular and humoral immunity	*Haemophilus influenzae* *Streptococcus pneumoniae*	*Candida* species	Varicella-zoster virus

TABLE 80-2   Diagnostic Evaluation of Patients Undergoing Hematopoietic Stem Cell Transplantation

Complete blood count with differential
Serology for Epstein-Barr virus, cytomegalovirus, human immunodeficiency virus, hepatitis B virus surface antigen, hepatitis C virus, rapid plasma reagin, and toxoplasmosis
Liver function tests
Renal function tests
Stool for ova and parasites
Skin testing with Mantoux purified protein derivative
Posteroanterior and lateral chest radiographs

GVHD exists. Preventive therapy against GVHD, which can include cyclosporine, methotrexate, steroids, and purging of T cells from the graft, increases the risk for development of infection. All these agents enhance the infection rate by depressing the cell-mediated immune response and, in the case of methotrexate, by disrupting mucosal barriers. The presence of GVHD increases the infection rate because it is associated with a delay in the return of normal immune function, prolonged immunodeficiency, and ulceration of the gastrointestinal tract.[4,49] The conditioning regimens for most allogeneic HSCT patients include concomitant total-body irradiation, which compromises the immune system and can cause severe mucositis. Diarrhea also is a very frequent complication in the first week after undergoing irradiation.

The serologic status of the donor and recipient is important as well because many infections in transplant recipients are caused by reactivation of previous infections. Serologic evaluation for cytomegalovirus (CMV), Epstein-Barr virus (EBV), hepatitis B virus, hepatitis C virus, human immunodeficiency virus, and toxoplasmosis should be performed on both donor and recipient before transplantation (Table 80-2).[96,147]

All HSCT recipients have a central venous catheter in place for administration of blood products, nutritional supplements, and medications, thus adding a potential site for development of infection.[115,123] The presence of other indwelling medical devices, such as a Foley catheter or a cerebrospinal fluid shunt, is associated with increased risk for the development of infection.

Knowledge of the epidemiology of the hospital and the transplantation unit allows the risk for acquiring environmental organisms to be assessed. Infection rates can be reduced by preventive strategies that inhibit aerosolization of organisms, such as the use of laminar air flow rooms or high-efficiency particulate air (HEPA)-filtered rooms.

CLINICAL MANIFESTATIONS AND APPROACH

The clinical approach to infections in a patient after HSCT is based on understanding the type of transplantation and the natural history of infections that can occur during each of the different at-risk periods based on immune reconstitution after transplantation. Such knowledge provides the framework for matching possible etiologic agents with the clinical syndromes noted during evaluation.[38,134]

INFECTIONS DURING THE PRE-ENGRAFTMENT PHASE

The pre-engraftment phase begins with the conditioning regimen, usually 7 to 10 days before the time of stem cell infusion, and continues to stem cell engraftment, usually 3 to 4 weeks after transplantation. Profound neutropenia is the major immune defect present during this stage of transplantation.[125,129,134] Evaluation of patients in this phase is similar to that of patients with neutropenia after chemotherapy.

Bacterial Infections

During the neutropenic period, bacterial infections are the most frequent infectious complication in HSCT recipients. These patients are at high risk for acquiring bacterial infection, similar to patients with cancer in whom chemotherapy-induced neutropenia develops.[25] Most infections result from invasion and colonization of the oral mucosa, gastrointestinal tract, or skin by the patient's endogenous flora.[109]

Catheter-related infections are common occurrences, and the spectrum of etiologic agents is similar to that in other chemotherapy-induced neutropenic patients. Among gram-positive organisms, *Staphylococcus aureus* and *Staphylococcus epidermidis* are isolated most frequently, with other gram-positive bacteria such as *Stomatococcus mucilaginosus* also being implicated.[70] Infection with *S. epidermidis* and other coagulase-negative staphylococci continues to occur as long as the central venous catheter remains in place.[32,42,115,123] Infection with viridans streptococci is associated with mucositis after chemotherapy and antibiotic prophylaxis with quinolones, and in some series these bacteria have replaced *Staphylococcus* spp. as the most common cause of bacteremia.[10,25,132,145,155]

Gram-negative bacterial infections develop after mucosal damage occurs as a result of translocation of bacteria from the intestinal lumen into the bloodstream. The organisms most frequently involved from this group are *Pseudomonas aeruginosa* and the Enterobacteriaceae, including *Escherichia coli*, *Klebsiella* spp., and *Enterobacter* spp., although other gram-negative organisms have been identified. *Enterobacter* spp. are especially worrisome because they display a high rate of an inducible β-lactamase, which limits the effect of front-line drugs such as the cephalosporins.

Fungal Infections

Fungal infections, predominantly with *Candida* spp., occur frequently in this phase.[83] *Aspergillus* spp. represent the second most common fungal infection during this time.[77] Less frequently, infections occur with the agents of mucormycosis (*Mucor*, *Rhizopus*, and *Absidia* spp.), *Trichosporon* spp., *Fusarium* spp., and other saprophytic fungi.[100,157] Fungal infections generally occur after a period of antibiotic therapy and correlate with the degree and duration of neutropenia.[59,106,107,158]

Candida spp. colonizing the gastrointestinal tract disseminate after mucosal injury, usually between 2 and 4 weeks after transplantation. Seeding of the portal circulation leads to hepatosplenic candidiasis manifested as fever and hepatosplenomegaly. Ultrasound or computed tomography reveals multiple round defects in the liver and spleen ("bull's eye" lesions). Candidal infections also can involve the lungs, kidneys, and central nervous system, where they can lead to meningitis or brain abscess.[83] Although *Candida albicans* is the most frequent *Candida* spp. causing candidemia, *Candida tropicalis* may be more aggressive.[59,158] Other *Candida* spp., including *Candida krusei*, have emerged as pathogens because of their resistance to the antifungal agent fluconazole, which is used as prophylaxis.[75,167]

Aspergillus spp., *Fusarium* spp., and the agents of mucormycosis use the respiratory tract as their portal of entry and generally are associated with sinopulmonary disease and dissemination to other sites, including the central nervous system.[1,15,37,52,106,107,113,176]

Viral Infections

Herpes simplex virus (HSV) infection usually is the result of reactivation in seropositive patients undergoing HSCT and is one of the most common viral infections in patients after HSCT.[97,164] Reactivation generally occurs in the form of oral and genital lesions. Oral lesions can be difficult to diagnose because lip involvement rarely occurs and the mucosal ulcers are similar to the mucositis caused by the conditioning regimen. HSV reactivation can be complicated by esophagitis, pneumonitis, and bacterial superinfection of skin lesions. Mortality is a rare event, and rapid diagnosis allows timely administration of therapy. The use of acyclovir prophylaxis in HSV-seropositive patients has decreased the incidence of this complication.[47]

Diarrhea after transplantation is related mostly to noninfectious causes, especially total-body irradiation, GVHD, and chemotherapy-related toxicity.[29,118] Viral gastroenteritis can occur throughout the transplant period. Etiologic agents to consider are rotavirus, coxsackievirus, and enteric adenovirus.[6,9,22,29,50,56,64,78] Generally, the enteric viruses are seasonal in their appearance. The course of these enteric infections can be very prolonged, especially with the adenoviruses. In approximately 5 percent of HSCT recipients, adenovirus infection develops and can become latent in lymphoid and renal tissue.[173] A recent study in adult transplant patients has shown that human metapneumovirus can occur during the pre-engraftment phase and cause upper and lower respiratory disease with high mortality rates.[44]

Hemorrhagic cystitis can occur throughout the transplantation period. This condition has several infectious and noninfectious causes (Table 80-3).[133] Chemotherapy-induced cystitis (e.g., high-dose cyclophosphamide) occurs soon after the conditioning regimen. Later in the transplantation period, GVHD can

TABLE 80–3 Differential Diagnosis of Hemorrhagic Cystitis after Hematopoietic Stem Cell Transplantation

Infectious Causes

Bacterial
Mainly gram-negative enteric rods associated with urinary tract infection

Fungal
Urinary tract infection
Fungus ball

Viral
Adenovirus
Polyomaviruses BK and JC
Herpesviruses: cytomegalovirus, herpes simplex virus

Noninfectious Causes
Chemotherapy-induced (e.g., cyclophosphamide)
Graft-versus-host disease
Mechanical trauma from a Foley catheter

be a contributing cause. The most common infectious causes of hemorrhagic cystitis are adenovirus and the polyomaviruses BK or JC.[2,6,24,48,73] Adenoviral infections can be systemic with associated pneumonitis, hepatitis, and renal insufficiency.[64] Allogeneic transplantation and the use of total-body irradiation are risk factors for acquisition of adenovirus infection.[64] BK viremia has been shown to correlate with hemorrhagic cystitis by polymerase chain reaction (PCR) analysis.[48] Of note, shedding of polyomaviruses in urine may occur in as many as 44 percent of HSCT patients without any clinical symptoms. HSV and CMV also have been associated with hemorrhagic cystitis.

INFECTIONS DURING THE EARLY ENGRAFTMENT PHASE

The risk for infection decreases after stem cell engraftment occurs. However, severe abnormalities in host defense still exist. The general early immune functions, such as phagocytic and cytotoxic cells, recover first, followed by the cellular and humoral arms of the immune system.[121,134] Another factor that influences immunologic recovery is the presence of acute GVHD.

Bacterial Infections

Bacterial infections continue to occur in this phase as a complication of indwelling central venous catheters or as a complication of acute GVHD and are accompanied by skin and gastrointestinal tract breakdown. The same organisms that cause illness during the neutropenic phase can produce illness in this phase.[10,42]

Fungal Infections

Fungal infections still occur during this phase, with *Candida* and *Aspergillus* spp. being the prominent pathogens. Systemic candidal infections usually occur earlier than aspergillosis.[37,59,158] Fungal pathogens other than *C. albicans*, *Aspergillus fumigatus*, and *Aspergillus flavus* are increasing in prevalence.[125]

Development of brain abscess after HSCT usually occurs during this phase and, in contrast to immunocompetent hosts, is caused mainly by fungal pathogens. The most common etiologic agents of brain abscess in transplant recipients are *Aspergillus* and *Candida* spp. Despite initiation of aggressive antifungal and surgical therapy, the outcome of this complication after HSCT is very poor.[1,63]

In the past, *Pneumocystis jiroveci* pneumonia occurred in 5 to 10 percent of allogeneic HSCT recipients during this phase. However, the routine use of trimethoprim-sulfamethoxazole prophylaxis has decreased its incidence significantly. Patients with *P. jiroveci* pneumonia usually have hypoxemia, dyspnea, cough, fever, and bilateral infiltrates.[154] The treatment of choice is trimethoprim-sulfamethoxazole.

Viral Infections

In the past, CMV infections predominated during this phase, but their incidence has decreased since the routine use of prophylactic ganciclovir was initiated. CMV infection generally occurs between 40 and 50 days after the transplantation. Most commonly, it results from reactivation in seropositive patients, but it also can occur in seronegative patients who receive their stem cells from a seropositive donor. The immunomodulatory effects of CMV infection, especially in a CMV-seronegative recipient of a CMV-seropositive donor, place the patient at high risk for developing bacterial and fungal infection.[112] The clinical manifestations of CMV infection vary from asymptomatic infection to the constellation of fever, hepatitis, and leukopenia to life-threatening diseases such as esophagitis, interstitial pneumonitis, and encephalitis.[46,175]

Pneumonia continues to be a common problem after HSCT, and the outcome still is poor.[40] Pulmonary infiltrates in an HSCT recipient must be distinguished from infectious processes or noninfectious pulmonary complications after HSCT (Table 80–4). Diffuse alveolar hemorrhage is manifested as gradually worsening dyspnea and repeated bloody aspirates from bronchoscopic examination.[69] Idiopathic interstitial pneumonitis is a process of widespread alveolar damage characterized clinically by varying degrees of respiratory failure and diffuse interstitial infiltrates in the absence of infection.[91] Idiopathic interstitial pneumonitis occurs in two peaks, one in the first few weeks and the other near the end of the early engraftment period. It is thought to be

related to the chemotherapy and total-body irradiation used in the conditioning regimen and has a high mortality rate.

Viral respiratory infections may occur throughout the transplantation period but are more severe during the early engraftment period. Etiologic agents include respiratory syncytial virus, human parainfluenza viruses 1 to 4, influenza viruses A and B, adenovirus, rhinoviruses, and nonpolio enteroviruses.[64,66,165,166] Distinctive features of respiratory viral infections in immunocompromised hosts include a high frequency of nosocomial acquisition, prolonged persistence of infection, a higher rate of progression to pneumonia, and high mortality rate in association with the infection.[95]

Respiratory viral infections occur throughout the year in HSCT recipients, although seasonal variations in the type of respiratory viral infection are similar to those seen in the general pediatric population, with respiratory syncytial virus and influenza viruses predominating during the winter and human parainfluenza viruses during the spring and summer.[95]

The differential diagnosis of jaundice and increase in liver enzymes after HSCT is very broad (Table 80–5) and presents a challenge in distinguishing infectious from noninfectious causes of hepatic disease. Two major noninfectious causes of liver disease after HSCT are GVHD of the liver and hepatic veno-occlusive disease.[49,104] The latter is a complication related to the conditioning regimen and is characterized by weight gain, hepatomegaly, and direct hyperbilirubinemia without elevation of liver enzymes.[104] The differential diagnosis of infectious causes includes viral hepatitis with any of the hepatitis viruses from A through C, as well as other hepatotropic viruses such as CMV, EBV, adenovirus, HSV, and varicella-zoster virus (VZV).[51,64,80,84,147]

EBV can reactivate after HSCT and cause EBV-associated lymphoproliferative disease. This disease is manifested as fever, hepatosplenomegaly, and lymphadenopathy and can progress to lymphoma. These EBV lymphomas are of donor origin and can occur for as long as 6 months after HSCT.[94]

Protozoan Infections

Toxoplasmosis is an infrequent, but almost always fatal, infection after HSCT. It usually occurs 2 to 6 months after transplantation and in most cases is the result of reactivation of a previous infection. The brain is the organ most frequently affected. Cerebral toxoplasmosis is manifested as neurologic focal signs, fever, seizures, headache, and altered mental status. Imaging of the central nervous system typically shows multiple lesions in both hemi-

---

TABLE 80–4 Differential Diagnosis of Pneumonitis after Hematopoietic Stem Cell Transplantation

Infectious Causes

Bacterial
Enterobacteriaceae
Legionella pneumophila
Staphylococcus aureus
Chlamydia trachomatis
Mycoplasma hominis

Fungal
Aspergillus spp.
Candida spp.
Pneumocystis jiroveci
Mucormycosis

Viral
Cytomegalovirus
Human parainfluenza viruses 1 to 4
Respiratory syncytial virus
Influenza viruses A and B
Adenovirus
Rhinovirus
Nonpolio enteroviruses
Human herpesvirus 6

Noninfectious Causes
Radiation
Chemotherapy (e.g., bleomycin)
Bronchiolitis obliterans organizing pneumonia
Underlying malignancy
Pulmonary edema
Diffuse alveolar hemorrhage
Idiopathic interstitial pneumonitis
Pulmonary vascular disease

See references 6, 9, 52, 54, 64, 89, 93, 158, 159, 160.

TABLE 80–5 Differential Diagnosis of Hepatitis after Hematopoietic Stem Cell Transplantation

Infectious Causes

Bacterial
Cholestatic liver injury secondary to septicemia

Viral
Hepatitis viruses A to D
Herpes simplex virus
Epstein-Barr virus
Cytomegalovirus
Adenovirus
Varicella-zoster virus
Echovirus
Human herpesvirus 6

Noninfectious Causes
Acute graft-versus-host disease
Veno-occlusive disease secondary to sepsis chemotherapy (e.g., cyclosporine)
Drug-induced (e.g., acetaminophen)
Parenteral hyperalimentation

spheres and basal ganglia with peripheral enhancement after infusion of contrast medium.[102,103,141]

Dermatologic Manifestations

Rash is a common symptom after HSCT and can occur in any phase after transplantation.[99] The differential diagnosis is broad and includes both infectious and noninfectious causes (Table 80–6). Noninfectious causes include acute GVHD, chemotherapy-induced toxicity, and drug eruptions, most commonly caused by the β-lactam antibiotics used for empiric treatment of febrile neutropenia. Because the etiology of these lesions generally is indistinguishable on a clinical basis, skin biopsy is helpful in determining the diagnosis.

Infectious skin disorders after HSCT may be secondary to bacterial, fungal, or viral causes (see Table 80–6). Embolic lesions can be a manifestation of systemic bacterial or fungal infection, especially with *C. tropicalis*, *Aspergillus* spp., and *Fusarium* spp.[15,137] Lesions are tender and usually papular but can be purpuric, nodular, or necrotic and scattered on the trunk and extremities.

Primary infection with human herpesvirus type 6 after HSCT generally is associated with self-limited clinical symptoms, including a diffuse maculopapular rash. Asymptomatic reactivation with human herpesvirus type 6 appears to be a common occurrence after allogeneic HSCT. Human herpesvirus type 6 might have a possible role in pneumonitis, meningoencephalitis, and bone marrow dysfunction after HSCT.[23,26,81] Human parvovirus B19 is another cause of erythroderma after HSCT, as well as a rare cause of anemia.[138]

INFECTIONS DURING THE LATE ENGRAFTMENT PHASE

The late engraftment period is characterized by decreased risk for the development of infection, especially in autologous transplant recipients because they have more rapid recovery of immune function. During this phase, the central venous catheter usually is removed and immunosuppressive therapy to prevent GVHD is discontinued. Most recipients are outpatients at this point, and educating recipients and their families to avoid environmental exposure to opportunistic pathogens is very important.

Serious infections still can occur, particularly in patients with chronic GVHD or inadequate stem cell engraftment. Chronic GVHD predisposes patients to infection by delaying recovery of the immune system and its effects on target organs; in addition,

---

TABLE 80–6 Differential Diagnosis of Rash after Hematopoietic Stem Cell Transplantation

Infectious Causes

Bacterial
Embolic lesions of systemic gram-negative bacteremia
Cellulitis of central venous catheter exit site or tunnel infections

Fungal
Focal dermatitis (*Candida* species and superficial dermatophytes)
Embolic lesions of systemic fungal disease (*Aspergillus* and *Fusarium* species)

Viral
Varicella-zoster virus
Herpes simplex virus
Human herpesvirus type 6
Human parvovirus B19

Noninfectious Causes
Graft-versus-host disease
Chemotherapy
Drug-induced (e.g., β-lactam antibiotics)
Radiation for conditioning therapy

---

the steroid therapy that patients receive likewise predisposes them to infection. Moreover, the cellular and humoral arms of the immune system are not recovered fully at this stage, thus placing the patient at risk for the development of infection. Most defects in immune function resolve by 1 year after transplantation.[114,131]

Bacterial Infections

Encapsulated bacteria, including *Haemophilus influenzae* type b, *Neisseria* spp., and *Streptococcus pneumoniae*, are the predominant causes of bacterial infection not related to catheters during this phase. These infections are secondary to deficient opsonization activity and decreased function of the reticuloendothelial system.[114]

Viral Infections

The predominant viral infection contracted during this period is caused by VZV, which occurs in 25 to 40 percent of pediatric HSCT recipients. Most infections represent reactivation, and risk factors include both acute and chronic GVHD, as well as allogeneic transplantation. VZV infection usually is characterized by localized vesicles in a dermatomal distribution. Disseminated infection occurs more frequently with VZV than with HSV, especially in patients with GVHD.[65,88,97]

DIAGNOSIS AND LABORATORY FINDINGS

The most important diagnostic evaluation is a complete physical examination because it can identify a site of infection that may be missed by laboratory tests. Sites requiring special attention include the skin, the oral mucosa to look for ulcers and thrush, the nares to look for necrotic lesions suggestive of invasive mold infection, the sinuses to look for tenderness, the chest, the abdomen, and the perianal area. All suspicious lesions should be cultured. Signs of infection may be subtle in patients who are neutropenic because inflammation is minimal.

The diagnostic approach should be guided by knowledge of which organisms are frequent pathogens during the specific phase after the transplantation (see Table 80–1). Except for microbiologic evaluations, laboratory tests are of limited value. Blood cultures for bacteria, fungi, and viruses should be obtained for any febrile episode. Use of the Wampole isolator blood culture system (Wampole Laboratories, Cranbury, NJ) may increase the yield of fungal pathogens and can help in establishing the diagnosis of central line infections by the use of quantitative cultures. Urine cultures are indicated in the presence of hemorrhagic cystitis or if the patient has a Foley catheter in place. Evaluation of cerebrospinal fluid should be reserved for patients with neurologic signs and symptoms.

Diagnosis of mold infections depends on tissue histology and culture of samples obtained by bronchoscopy, bronchoalveolar lavage, paranasal sinus washings, lung biopsy, or skin biopsy because these organisms are not recovered routinely from blood cultures. Recent improvements in antigen-based tests, including galactomannan and 1-3-β-D-glucan, allow establishing the diagnosis and noninvasive monitoring of antifungal therapy, although the false-positive rate appears to be higher in infected children than in adults.[144,149,174] Fungal surveillance cultures are not indicated for asymptomatic HSCT patients.[128] Additionally, Gram stain, acid-fast stains, and other special stains can be useful in identifying microorganisms early in the infectious process.

Nasopharyngeal swabs or washes for viral culture and direct fluorescent antibody testing are helpful for identifying respiratory viruses in patients with upper respiratory tract symptoms. Shell vial assay is a rapid viral diagnostic technique used for a variety of viruses, including CMV, adenovirus, and respiratory viruses. The base of vesicular skin lesions should be scraped and the cells examined by direct fluorescent antibody stain with specific monoclonal antibodies to confirm the diagnosis of either HSV or VZV infection.

Nucleic acid detection, such as with PCR, has shown usefulness in the rapid diagnosis of certain pathogens, including adenovirus, CMV, EBV, human herpesvirus type 6, and parvovirus B19.[12,23,26,87] Additionally, quantification of viruses has allowed the response to therapy to be evaluated. Blood assays to detect viral antigens such as pp65 also have been used for establishing the diagnosis of CMV infection.[11,13]

Serologic testing is useful for diagnosing toxoplasmosis, *Bartonella henselae*, and fungal infections such as histoplasmosis and blastomycosis. However, serologic assays have limited value because patients are immunosuppressed and immunoglobulin therapy is administered to most patients.

Other laboratory tests are of limited value. Complete blood counts are useful to determine engraftment status. Liver and renal function tests can provide evidence of disease from an infectious agent or can indicate noninfectious causes of hepatic or renal disease such as chemotherapy or GVHD.

Performance of radiology studies should be based on assessment of the patient. A chest roentgenogram should be part of the work-up of a febrile, neutropenic patient and any patient with respiratory symptoms. Computed tomography scans of the paranasal sinuses, chest, and abdomen are helpful in evaluating and monitoring patients with invasive fungal disease.[37] Ultrasound examination can be used to diagnose abdominal problems such as typhlitis. Neuroimaging studies should be reserved for patients with neurologic signs and symptoms.

MANAGEMENT AND THERAPY

The initial management of HSCT recipients with fever and neutropenia is similar to that of cancer patients with chemotherapy-induced fever and neutropenia.[79,124,129] A standardized antibiotic regimen should be developed to ensure adequate coverage of organisms identified by the hospital's environment and to allow the hospital's staff to compare outcomes of patients. Empiric antibiotic therapy directed against the predominant pathogens should be started after obtaining appropriate samples for culture.[79] One approach consists of an empiric antibiotic regimen of ceftazidime with or without vancomycin, a combination that provides adequate therapy for gram-positive cocci and gram-negative bacteria. If *P. aeruginosa* is suspected, an aminoglycoside should be added. Other approaches using cefepime or quinolones have shown equal efficacy.[16,17]

The choice of any specific antimicrobial therapy should take into account the transplantation center's spectrum of organisms, the patient's surveillance isolates, and the antibiotic susceptibility pattern within the community and hospital. If fever persists after 3 or more days, re-evaluation of the patient may lead to modification of the antibiotic regimen.[79]

THERAPY FOR FUNGAL INFECTIONS

Empiric amphotericin B is recommended for the treatment of occult fungal disease in patients who remain persistently febrile after 5 to 7 days of antibiotic therapy, without identification of a bacterial cause.[79] The introduction of expanded-spectrum triazoles and cell wall–active agents such as echinocandins has changed the antifungal armamentarium.

Amphotericin B has been the traditional drug of choice for *Candida* infection, but recent data support the use of liposomal amphotericin B and itraconazole, which have similar clinical efficacy with reduced toxicity.[119,146,160,172] Voriconazole has become the agent of choice for the treatment of invasive aspergillosis in immunocompromised hosts.[33,71] Posaconazole, a triazole, will probably be the best option for the treatment of Zygomycetes. Caspofungin, an echinocandin active against *Candida* and *Aspergillus*, is available only in an intravenous formulation and probably is relegated to a second-line agent.[161] However, interaction with other drugs may impair its use in HSCT recipients. Combination therapy may be potentially antagonistic, but the efficacy of any of these combinations has not been established.[105] Fluconazole has activity against most *Candida* spp. and exhibits good penetration of the central nervous system.[40]

Surgery plays a prominent role in the treatment of mold infections, especially in neutropenic patients. However, the outcome of invasive mold infections in HSCT patients remains dismal.

THERAPY FOR VIRAL INFECTIONS

Treatment of viral infections is started once the diagnosis is established, if therapy is available. Acyclovir is the recommended therapy for both HSV and VZV infections. Famciclovir and valacyclovir also can be used to treat HSV infections, but they are available only for oral administration. CMV pneumonitis is treated with a combination of intravenous gamma-globulin and ganciclovir. In the case of acyclovir-resistant HSV or ganciclovir-resistant CMV infection, foscarnet is the drug of choice.[111] Cidofovir also has been used for CMV infection.[93]

Respiratory syncytial virus infections have been treated with aerosolized ribavirin and more recently with respiratory syncytial virus immunoglobulin.[34,35,45] Aerosolized ribavirin also has been used for the treatment of human parainfluenza virus infection.[41,45]

Intravenous ribavirin has been used for the treatment of adenovirus hemorrhagic cystitis, with anecdotal success.[20,53] More recently, cidofovir treatment of adenoviral infections has been associated with clinical improvement, as well as viral clearance in cultures and PCR analysis.[14,87,110,173]

The recommended therapy for infection with influenza A virus includes oral amantadine or rimantadine. Their efficacy, particularly in the treatment of severe disease, has not been established in immunocompromised hosts. Both drugs also are useful as prophylaxis for influenza A virus infection.[68] Zanamivir and oseltamivir, both neuraminidase inhibitors, appear promising for the treatment of both influenza A and B virus infection, but data are lacking regarding their use in pediatric immunocompromised patients.[68]

Adoptive immunotherapy by transferring virus-specific cytotoxic T lymphocytes to patients who have undergone allogeneic HSCT has proved to be useful in treating CMV and EBV infection and in reconstituting immune dysfunction selectively against these viruses.[72,130,162]

PREVENTION OF INFECTIONS AFTER TRANSPLANTATION

Measures to prevent infectious complications are a high priority for all HSCT recipients. Regular hand hygiene remains the best strategy for prevention of infections in HSCT recipients. Every HSCT recipient should undergo a dental evaluation before conditioning to assess oral health and any needed dental procedures should be performed to decrease the risk for the development of oral complications and infections after transplantation.[31,132] Strong effort should be made to enforce published guidelines for preventing indwelling catheter–related infections.[113,123]

The Centers for Disease Control and Prevention recently published extensive guidelines for the prevention of opportunistic infections in HSCT recipients that go beyond the scope of this chapter.[21] A brief review of preventive strategies, including targeted antimicrobial prophylaxis, prevention of exposure, enhancement of immune reconstitution with colony-stimulating factors, and active and passive immunization, is presented here.

ANTIMICROBIAL PROPHYLAXIS

Antimicrobial prophylaxis must be weighed against the toxicity and the drug interactions of the prophylactic agent. Prophylaxis against *P. jiroveci* infection with trimethoprim-sulfamethoxazole is started after engraftment and is taken orally three times a week for 6 months after transplantation. For patients with intolerance to sulfa-containing medications, other options for prophylaxis include atovaquone, dapsone, or inhaled pentamidine.[90,98] Quinolone prophylaxis has been the major antibiotic class used to prevent bacterial infections, but breakthrough infections are problematic.[108]

Administration of fluconazole or itraconazole for 75 to 100 days after HSCT is associated with persistent protection against disseminated candidal infections and candidiasis-related death; in a randomized, placebo-controlled trial, these drugs resulted in an overall survival benefit in allogeneic HSCT recipients.[101,169] However, emergence of resistant pathogens such as *C. krusei* and some strains of *C. albicans* has complicated the routine use of fluconazole.[18] Low-dose amphotericin B is similar in efficacy to fluconazole in preventing fungal infections, but the latter is tolerated better.[171] The use of aerosolized amphotericin B to prevent *Aspergillus* infection needs further study.[74,140] In some centers voriconazole is used for prophylaxis.

Antiviral prophylaxis is indicated to prevent infections with herpesviruses during high-risk periods. Acyclovir has been used to prevent reactivation of HSV in seropositive transplant recipients during the neutropenic phase after transplantation. This strategy can reduce the incidence of reactivation of HSV in seropositive recipients from 80 to 5 percent during the first month after transplantation.

Strategies used to prevent CMV infection include prophylactic and preemptive therapy. Prophylactic therapy is administered to all recipients at risk for acquiring CMV infection and is used routinely for allogeneic transplant recipients when the donor is CMV-seropositive.[57,139] Ganciclovir is the agent of choice for prophylaxis of CMV infection.[57,58] Ganciclovir usually is given for 3 to 4 months after engraftment; however, its use has been associated with neutropenia.[57,135] Preemptive therapy is administered only to recipients who have evidence of CMV replication based on plasma PCR or pp65 antigenemia.[11,13] Primary CMV infection also can be prevented in CMV-seronegative HSCT recipients by transfusing blood products that are leukocyte filtered and seronegative for CMV.[148]

ISOLATION MEASURES

The use of laminar air flow protection for HSCT patients is controversial, and, although some studies have proved its effectiveness, it is very expensive.[39] HEPA filtration is associated with similar efficacy as laminar air flow in preventing airborne pathogens such as *Aspergillus* spp. Major indications for strict isolation of patients include colonization with resistant bacteria, viral respiratory infections, and disseminated VZV infection.[13,126]

COLONY-STIMULATING FACTORS

The use of granulocyte and granulocyte-macrophage colony-stimulating factors in stem cell transplant recipients is safe and effective in reducing the period of neutropenia after HSCT.[85,143,153] A meta-analysis of children receiving chemotherapy has shown a significant reduction in febrile neutropenic episodes, documented

infections, and length of hospitalizations.[151] However, there has been a report of an increase in myeloid leukemia or myelodysplastic syndrome in patients with acute lymphocytic leukemia receiving granulocyte colony-stimulating factor.[127] These growth factors also appear to be safe and effective in transplant recipients who do not show engraftment 3 to 4 weeks after transplantation.

ACTIVE IMMUNIZATION

Immunizations should be part of the routine follow-up care of HSCT recipients. Most allogeneic and a large proportion of autologous and syngeneic transplant recipients lose their immunity to vaccine-preventable diseases. The degree that immunity is lost depends on multiple factors, including the donor's immunity, the type of transplant, the interval since the transplant, the presence of GVHD, and the use of immunosuppressive medication.[3] Moreover, transplant recipients are at increased risk for acquiring infections with encapsulated bacteria, such as *H. influenzae* type b and *S. pneumoniae*, for which vaccines are available.[7,55] For all these reasons, reimmunization of HSCT recipients between the first and second year after transplantation is very important.[92,142] When immunizing transplant recipients, recent administration of immunoglobulin must be kept in mind because it may interfere with the response to vaccinations.

An optimal schedule for administering vaccinations to pediatric patients after HSCT has not been established. Some experts will reimmunize HSCT recipients without performing serologic titers for specific antigens, such as diphtheria and tetanus, whereas others obtain titers 1 year after transplantation and provide vaccinations accordingly.[170] A schedule for immunization of HSCT recipients based on the recommendations of the Centers for Disease Control and Prevention Advisory Committee on Immunization Practices and the Infectious Diseases Committee of the American Academy of Pediatrics is presented in Table 80–7.[3,21] Specific recommendations probably will change as further data become available.

Immunizations can be started 12 months after HSCT as long as the patient has no persistent complications such as chronic GVHD and is not receiving immunosuppressive therapy. If the patient is younger than 7 years old, diphtheria and tetanus toxoids (DT) or diphtheria and tetanus toxoids with acellular pertussis vaccine (DTaP) can be used for diphtheria and tetanus.[120,156] For patients older than 7 years of age, immunization with DT at 12, 14, and 24 months after transplantation elicits an immune response.

H. influenzae type b vaccine is included in the first round of immunizations 12 months after HSCT. Boosters of these vaccines are given 14 and 24 months after transplantation.[7,62,122,156]

TABLE 80–7 Immunizations in Patients after Hematopoietic Stem Cell Transplantation

Recommended Time after HSCT	Immunizations
12 mo	Td,* IPV, Hib, pneumococcal, meningococcal hepatitis B
14 mo	Td, IPV, Hib, pneumococcal, hepatitis B
24 mo	Measles-mumps-rubella,† varicella, Td, IPV, Hib pneumococcal and hepatitis B

*DTaP or DT if the patient is younger than 7 years; Tdap if >11 years of age and indicated.

†Do not use live virus vaccines for patients who have active chronic graft-versus-host disease or who are receiving immunosuppressive therapy.

Td and DT, diphtheria and tetanus toxoids; DTaP, diphtheria and tetanus toxoids and acellular pertussis vaccine; Hib, Haemophilus influenzae type b vaccine; IPV, inactivated polio vaccine.

Immunization with the 23-valent pneumococcal vaccine is recommended 12 and 24 months after transplantation.[3,5,21] The second dose is not a booster dose but provides a second opportunity for immunization in patients who failed to respond to the first dose.[3]

The measles-mumps-rubella vaccine (MMR) should be given 24 months after transplantation to both autologous and allogeneic HSCT patients. It should not be given to patients with chronic GVHD or to those receiving steroids or any other form of immunosuppressive therapy.[82] The live attenuated varicella vaccine should be avoided in patients less than 24 months after HSCT.[3] Of note, a report using an inactivated varicella vaccine has shown efficacy in autologous transplant recipients.[67]

Only the inactivated polio vaccine should be given to HSCT patients. This vaccine should be administered 12, 14, and 24 months after transplantation.

The inactivated influenza vaccine (subvirion or purified surface antigen vaccines) should be given 6 months after HSCT and yearly thereafter in early autumn. Children younger than 9 years old who are receiving influenza vaccine for the first time require two doses given 1 month apart. Children younger than 12 years old should receive only split-virus influenza vaccine.[3,21,43,68] Live attenuated influenza vaccine should not be given.

Vaccination for hepatitis A is not recommended routinely but may be considered 12 months or more after HSCT for patients with chronic liver disease or chronic GVHD, for those living in areas endemic for hepatitis A, and for those in areas experiencing outbreaks. Hepatitis A immunization is given in two doses 6 to 12 months apart.[3,21]

Use of hepatitis B vaccine is unclear, but administration 12, 14, and 24 months after HSCT is reasonable with serologic follow-up.

Health care workers and household contacts of HSCT recipients should have immunity to or be immunized against hepatitis A, influenza, polio, measles, mumps, rubella, and varicella.[3,21,142]

PASSIVE IMMUNIZATION

Intravenous immunoglobulin commonly has been administered in the first months after allogeneic HSCT to prevent infections and acute GVHD and is approved by the Food and Drug Administration.[8,19,116] The use of intravenous immunoglobulin in conjunction with ganciclovir after transplantation has been shown to decrease the incidence of CMV pneumonia, as well as bacterial infections and interstitial pneumonia.[150,168] The optimal dose is not known. However, two meta-analyses have drawn divergent conclusions regarding the efficacy of intravenous immunoglobulin.[8,28,61]

The indications for passive immunization with specific immunoglobulin preparations, such as hepatitis B, rabies, and tetanus vaccines, in transplant recipients are similar to those in otherwise healthy individuals.[3,21] Patients with tetanus-prone wounds sustained during the first year after transplantation should be given tetanus immunoglobulin, regardless of their tetanus immunization status.[3] Passive immunization with varicella-zoster immunoglobulin is recommended for susceptible patients with known exposure to varicella.[3]

REFERENCES

1. Abbasi, S., Shenep, J. L., Hughes, W. T., et al.: *Aspergillus* in children with cancer: A 34-year experience. Clin. Infect. Dis. 29:1210-1219, 1999.
2. Akiyama, H., Kurosu, T., Sakashita, C., et al.: Adenovirus is a key pathogen in hemorrhagic cystitis associated with bone marrow transplantation. Clin. Infect. Dis. 32:1325-1330, 2001.
3. American Academy of Pediatrics: Immunization in special clinical circumstances: Hematopoietic stem cell and other transplant recipients. *In* Pickering,

L. (ed.): Red Book: 2006 Report of the Committee on Infectious Diseases. 27th ed. Elk Grove Village, IL, American Academy of Pediatrics, 2006, pp. 78-80.
4. Armitage, J. O.: Bone marrow transplantation. N. Engl. J. Med. 330:827-838, 1994.
5. Avanzini, M., Carra, A., Maccario, R., et al.: Antibody response to pneumococcal vaccine in children receiving bone marrow transplantation. J. Clin. Immunol. 15:137-144, 1995.
6. Baldwin, A., Kingman, H., Darville, M., et al.: Outcome and clinical course of 100 patients with adenovirus infection following bone marrow transplantation. Bone Marrow Transplant. 26:1333-1338, 2000.
7. Barra, A., Cordonnier, C., Presiosi, M., et al.: Immunogenicity of *Haemophilus influenzae* type B conjugate vaccine in allogeneic bone marrow recipients. J. Infect. Dis. 166:1021-1028, 1992.
8. Bass, E. B., Powe, N. R., Goodman, S. N., et al.: Efficacy of immune globulin in preventing complications of bone marrow transplantation: A meta-analysis. Bone Marrow Transplant. 12:273-282, 1993.
9. Biggs, D. D., Toorkey, B. C., Carrigan, D. R., et al.: Disseminated echovirus infection complicating bone marrow transplantation. Am. J. Med. 88:421-425, 1990.
10. Bochud, P.-Y., Eggiman, P. H., Calandra, T., et al.: Bacteremia due to viridans streptococcus in neutropenic patients with cancer: Clinical spectrum and risk factors. Clin. Infect. Dis. 18:25-31, 1994.
11. Boeckh, M., Bowden, R. A., Gooley, T., et al.: Successful modification of a pp65 antigenemia-based early treatment for prevention of cytomegalovirus disease in allogeneic marrow transplant recipients. Blood 93:1781-1782, 1999.
12. Boeckh, M., Gallez-Hawkins, G. M., Myerson, D., et al.: Plasma polymerase chain reaction for cytomegalovirus DNA after allogeneic bone marrow transplantation: Comparison with polymerase chain reaction using peripheral blood leukocytes, pp65 antigenemia, and viral culture. Transplantation 64:108-113, 1997.
13. Boeckh, M., Gooley, T. A., Myerson, D., et al.: Cytomegalovirus pp65 antigenemia-guided early treatment with ganciclovir versus ganciclovir at engraftment after allogeneic bone marrow transplantation: A randomized double-blind study. Blood 10:4063-4071, 1996.
14. Bordigoni, P., Carret, A.-S., Venard, V., et al.: Treatment of adenovirus infections in patients undergoing allogeneic hematopoietic stem cell transplantation. Clin. Infect. Dis. 32:1290-1297, 2001.
15. Boutati, E. I., and Anaissie, E. J.: *Fusarium*, a significant emerging pathogen in patients with hematologic malignancy: Ten years' experience at a cancer center and implications for management. Blood 90:999-1008, 1997.
16. Bow, E. J., Rotstein, C., Noskin, G. A., et al. A randomized, open-label, multicenter comparative study of the efficacy and safety of piperacillin-tazobactam and cefepime for the empirical treatment of febrile neutropenic episodes in patients with hematologic malignancies. Clin. Infect. Dis. 43:447-459, 2006.
17. Bucaneve, G., Micozzi, A., Menichetti, F., et al.: Levofloxacin to prevent bacterial infections in patients with cancer and neutropenia. N. Engl. J. Med. 353:977-987, 2005.
18. Buckley, R. H., Schiff, S. E., Schiff, R. I., et al.: Hematopoietic stem-cell transplantation for the treatment of severe combined immunodeficiency. N. Engl. J. Med. 340:508-516, 1999.
19. Casper, J. T., Sedmak, G., and Harrie, R. E.: Intravenous immunoglobulin: Use in pediatric bone marrow transplantation. Semin. Hematol. 29(Suppl. 2): S100-S105, 1992.
20. Cassano, W. F.: Intravenous ribavirin therapy for adenovirus cystitis after allogeneic bone marrow transplantation. Bone Marrow Transplant. 7:247-248, 1991.
21. Centers for Disease Control and Prevention, Infectious Disease Society of America, American Society of Blood and Marrow Transplantation: Guidelines for preventing opportunistic infections among hematopoietic stem cell transplant recipients. M. M. W. R. Recomm. Rep. 49(RR-10)1-128, 2000.
22. Chakrabart, S., Mautner, V., Osman, H., et al.: Adenovirus infections following allogeneic stem cell transplantation: Incidence and outcome in relation to graft manipulation, immunosuppression, and immune recovery. Blood 100:1619-1627, 2002.
23. Chan, P. K. S., Peiris, J. S. M., Yuen, K. Y., et al.: Human herpesvirus-6 and human herpesvirus-7 infections in bone marrow transplant recipients. J. Med. Virol. 53:295-305, 1997.
24. Childs, R., Sanchez, C., Engler, H., et al.: High incidence of adeno- and polyomavirus-induced hemorrhagic cystitis in bone marrow allotransplantation for hematological malignancy following T cell depletion and cyclosporine. Bone Marrow Transplant. 22:889-893, 1998.
25. Collin, B. A., Leather, H. L., Wingard, J. R., and Ramphal, R.: Evolution, incidence and susceptibility of bacterial bloodstream isolates from 519 bone marrow transplant patients. Clin. Infect. Dis. 33:947-953, 2001.
26. Cone, R. W., Huang, M.-L. W., Corey, L., et al.: Human herpes virus 6 infections after bone marrow transplantation: Clinical and virologic manifestations. J. Infect. Dis. 179:311-318, 1999.
27. Copelan, E. A.: Hematopoietic stem-cell transplantation. N. Engl. J. Med. 354:1813-1826, 2006.
28. Cordonnier, C., Chevret, S., Legrand, M., et al.: Should immunoglobulin therapy be used in allogeneic stem-cell transplantation? A randomized, double-blind, dose effect, placebo-controlled, multicenter trial. Ann. Intern. Med. 139:8-18, 2003.

29. Cox, G. J., Matsui, S. M., Lo, R. S., et al.: Etiology and outcome of diarrhea after marrow transplantation: A prospective study. Gastroenterology 107:1398-1407, 1994.

30. Cutler, C., Giri, S., Jeyapalan, S., et al.: Acute and chronic graft-versus-host disease after allogeneic peripheral-blood stem-cell and bone marrow transplant: A meta-analysis. J. Clin. Oncol. 19:3685-3691, 2001.

31. da Fonseca, M. A.: Pediatric bone marrow transplantation: Oral complications and recommendations for care. Pediatr. Dent. 20:386-394, 1998.

32. Dell'Orto, M. G., Rovelli, A., Barzaghi, A., et al.: Febrile complications in the first 100 days after bone marrow transplantation in children: A single center's experience. Pediatr. Hematol. Oncol. 14:335-347, 1997.

33. Denning, D. W., Ribaud, P., Milpied, N., et al.: Efficacy and safety of voriconazole in the treatment of acute invasive aspergillosis. Clin. Infect. Dis. 34:563-571, 2002.

34. DeVincenzo, J. P., Hirsch, R. L., Fuentes, R. J., and Top, F. H., Jr.: Respiratory syncytial virus immune globulin treatment of lower respiratory tract infection in pediatric patients undergoing bone marrow transplantation: A compassionate use experience. Bone Marrow Transplant. 25:161-165, 2000.

35. DeVincenzo, J. P., Leombuno, D., Soiffer, R. J., and Siber, G. R.: Immunotherapy of respiratory syncytial virus pneumonia following bone marrow transplantation. Bone Marrow Transplant. 17:1051-1056, 1996.

36. de Vries, E., van Tol, M. J. D., Langlois van den Bergh, R., et al.: Reconstitution of lymphocyte subpopulations after pediatric bone marrow transplantation. Bone Marrow Transplant. 25:267-275, 2000.

37. Drakos, P. E., Nagler, A., Or, R., et al.: Invasive fungal sinusitis in patients undergoing bone marrow transplantation. Bone Marrow Transplant. 12:203-208, 1993.

38. Dykewicz, C. A.: Summary of the guidelines for preventing opportunistic infections among hematopoietic stem cell transplant recipients. Clin. Infect. Dis. 33:139-144, 2001.

39. Dykewicz, C. A.: Hospital infection control in hematopoietic stem cell transplant recipients. Emerg. Infect. Dis. 7:263-267, 2001.

40. Edwards, J. E., Jr., Bodey, G. P., Bowden, R. A., et al.: International conference for the development of a consensus on the management and prevention of severe candidal infections. Clin. Infect. Dis. 25:43-59, 1997.

41. Elizaga, J., Olavarria, E., Apperley, J. F., et al.: Parainfluenza virus 3 infection after stem cell transplant: Relevance to outcome of rapid diagnosis and ribavirin treatment. Clin. Infect. Dis. 32:413-418, 2001.

42. Engelhard, D., Elishoov, H., Strauss, N., et al.: Nosocomial coagulase-negative staphylococcal infections in bone marrow transplantation recipients with central vein catheter: A 5-year prospective study. Transplantation 61:430-434, 1996.

43. Engelhard, D., Nagler, A., Hardan, I., et al.: Antibody response to a two-dose regimen of influenza vaccine in allogeneic T cell–depleted and autologous BMT recipients. Bone Marrow Transplant. 11:1-5, 1993.

44. Englund, J. A., Boeckh, M., Kuypers, J., et al.: Brief communication: Fatal human metapneumovirus infection in stem-cell transplant recipients. Ann. Intern. Med. 144:344-349, 2006.

45. Englund, J. A., Piedra, P. A., and Whimbey, E.: Prevention and treatment of respiratory syncytial virus and parainfluenza viruses in immunocompromised patients. Am. J. Med. 102(3A):S61-S70, 1997.

46. Enright, H., Haake, R., Weisdorf, D., et al.: Cytomegalovirus pneumonia after bone marrow transplantation. Transplantation 55:1339-1346, 1993.

47. Epstein, J. B., Ransier, A., Sherlock, C. H., et al.: Acyclovir prophylaxis of oral herpes virus during bone marrow transplantation. Eur. J. Cancer B Oral. Oncol. 32:158-162, 1996.

48. Erard, V., Storer, B., Corey, L., et al.: BK virus in hematopoietic stem cell transplant recipients: Frequency, risk factors, and association with postengraftment hemorrhagic cystitis. Clin. Infect. Dis. 39:1861-1865, 2004.

49. Ferrara, J. L. M., and Deeg, H. J.: Graft versus host disease. N. Engl. J. Med. 324:667-674, 1991.

50. Flomenberg, P., Babbitt, J., Drobyski, W. R., et al.: Increasing incidence of adenovirus disease in bone marrow transplant recipients. J. Infect. Dis. 169:775-781, 1994.

51. Frickhofen, N., Wiesneth, M., Jainta, C., et al.: Hepatitis C virus infection is a risk factor for liver failure from veno-occlusive disease after bone marrow transplantation. Blood 83:1998-2004, 1994.

52. Gamis, A. S., Gudnason, T., Giebink, G. S., et al.: Disseminated infection with Fusarium in recipients of bone marrow transplants. Rev. Infect. Dis. 13:1077-1088, 1991.

53. Gavin, P. J., and Katz, B. Z.: Intravenous ribavirin treatment for severe adenovirus diseases in immunocompromised children. Pediatrics 110:e9-e17, 2002.

54. Ghosh, S., Champlin, R., Couch, R., et al.: Rhinovirus infections in myelosuppressed adult blood and marrow transplant recipients. Clin. Infect. Dis. 29:528-532, 1999.

55. Giebink, G. S., Warkentin, P. I., Ramsay, N. K. C., et al.: Titers of antibody to pneumococci in allogeneic bone marrow transplant recipients before and after vaccination with pneumococcal vaccine. J. Infect. Dis. 166:1021-1028, 1992.

56. González, Y., Martino, R., Badell, I., et al.: Pulmonary enterovirus infections in stem cell transplant recipients. Bone Marrow Transplant. 23:511-513, 1999.

57. Goodrich, J. M., Bowden, R. A., Fisher, L., et al.: Ganciclovir prophylaxis to prevent cytomegalovirus disease after allogeneic marrow transplant. Ann. Intern. Med. 118:173-178, 1993.

58. Goodrich, J. M., Mori, M., Gleaves, C. A., et al.: Early treatment with ganciclovir to prevent cytomegalovirus disease after allogeneic bone marrow transplantation. N. Engl. J. Med. 325:1601-1607, 1991.

59. Goodrich, J. M., Reed, E. C., Mori, M., et al.: Clinical features and analysis of risk factors for invasive candidal infection after marrow transplantation. J. Infect. Dis. 164:731-740, 1991.

60. Gratwohl, A., Hermans, J., Baldomero, H., et al.: Indications for haematopoietic precursor cell transplants in Europe. Br. J. Haematol. 92:35-43, 1996.

61. Guglielmo, B. J., Wong-Beringer, A., Linker, C. A.: Immune globulin therapy in allogeneic bone marrow transplant: A critical review. Bone Marrow Transplant. 13:499-510, 1994.

62. Guinan, E. C., Molrine, D. C., Antin, J. H., et al.: Polysaccharide conjugate vaccine response in bone marrow transplant recipients. Transplantation 57:677-684, 1994.

63. Hagensee, M. E., Bauwens, J. E., Kjos, B., et al.: Brain abscess following marrow transplantation: Experience at the Fred Hutchinson Cancer Research Center, 1984-1992. Clin. Infect. Dis. 19:402-408, 1994.

64. Hale, G. A., Heslop, H. E., Krance, R. A., et al.: Adenovirus infection after pediatric bone marrow transplantation. Bone Marrow Transplant. 23:277-282, 1999.

65. Han, C. S., Miller, W., Haake, R., et al.: Varicella zoster infection after bone marrow transplantation: Incidence, risk factors and complications. Bone Marrow Transplant. 13:277-283, 1994.

66. Harrington, R. D., Hooton, T. M., Hackman, R. C., et al.: An outbreak of respiratory syncytial virus in a bone marrow transplant center. J. Infect. Dis. 165:987-993, 1992.

67. Hata, A., Asanuma, H., Rinki, M., et al.: Use of inactivated varicella vaccine in recipients of hematopoietic-cell transplants. N. Engl. J. Med. 347:26-34, 2002.

68. Hayden, F. G.: Prevention and treatment of influenza in immunocompromised patients. Am. J. Med. 102(3A):S55-S60, 1997.

69. Heggen, J., West, C., Olson, E., et al.: Diffuse alveolar hemorrhage in pediatric cell transplant patients. Pediatrics 109:965-971, 2002.

70. Henwick, S., Koehler, M., and Patrick, C. C.: Complications of bacteremia due to Stomatococcus mucilaginosus in neutropenic children. Clin. Infect. Dis. 17:667-671, 1993.

71. Herbrecht, R., Denning, D. W., Patterson, T. F., et al.: Voriconazole versus amphotericin B for primary therapy on invasive aspergillosis. N. Engl. J. Med. 347:408-415, 2002.

72. Heslop, H. E., Ny, C. Y. C., Li, C., et al.: Long-term restoration of immunity against Epstein-Barr virus by infection by adoptive transfer of gene-modified virus-specific T lymphocytes. Nat. Med. 2:551-555, 1996.

73. Hierholzer, J. C.: Adenovirus in the immunocompromised host. Clin. Microbiol. Rev. 5:262-274, 1992.

74. Hong, R.: Bone marrow transplantation. Adv. Pediatr. 40:101-124, 1993.

75. Hoppe, J. E., Klingebiel, T., and Niethammer, D.: Selection of Candida glabrata in pediatric bone marrow transplant recipients receiving fluconazole. Pediatr. Hematol. Oncol. 11:207-210, 1994.

76. Horwitz, M. E.: Stem-cell transplantation for inherited immunodeficiency disorders. Pediatr. Clin. North Am. 47:1371-1387, 2000.

77. Hovi, L., Saarinen-Pihkala, U. M., Vettenranta, K., and Saxen, I. L.: Invasive fungal infections in pediatric bone marrow transplant recipients: Single center experience of 10 years. Bone Marrow Transplant. 9:999-1004, 2000.

78. Howard, D. S., Phillips, G. L., III, Reece, D. E., et al.: Adenovirus infections in hematopoietic stem cell transplant recipients. Clin. Infect. Dis. 29:1494-1501, 1999.

79. Hughes, W. T., Armstrong, D., Bodey, G. P., et al.: Guidelines for the use of antimicrobial agents in neutropenic patients with cancer. Clin. Infect. Dis. 34:730-751, 2002.

80. Johnson, J. R., Egaas, S., Gleaves, C. A., et al.: Hepatitis due to herpes simplex virus in marrow transplant recipients. Clin. Infect. Dis. 14:38-45, 1992.

81. Kadakia, M. P., Rybka, W. B., Stewart, J. A., et al.: Human herpes virus 6: Infection and disease following autologous and allogeneic bone marrow transplantation. Blood 87:5341-5354, 1996.

82. King, S. M., Saunders, E. F., Petric, M., and Gold, R.: Responses to measles, mumps and rubella vaccine in paediatric bone marrow transplant recipients. Bone Marrow Transplant. 17:633-636, 1996.

83. Klingspor, L., Stintzing, G., Fasth, A., and Tollemar, J.: Deep Candida infection in children receiving allogeneic bone marrow transplants: Incidence, risk factors and diagnosis. Bone Marrow Transplant. 17:1043-1049, 1996.

84. Kolho, E., Ruutu, P., and Ruutu, T.: Hepatitis C in BMT patients. Bone Marrow Transplant. 11:119-123, 1993.

85. Lau, A. S., Lehman, D., Geertsma, F. R., et al.: Biology and therapeutic uses of myeloid hematopoietic growth factors and interferons. Pediatr. Infect. Dis. J. 15:563-575, 1996.

86. Laughlin, M. J.: Umbilical cord blood for allogeneic transplantation in children and adults. Bone Marrow Transplant. 27:1-6, 2001.

87. Legrand, F., Berrebi, D., Houhou, N., et al.: Early diagnosis of adenovirus infection and treatment with cidofovir after bone marrow transplantation in children. Bone Marrow Transplant. 27:621-625, 2001.

88. Leung, T. F., Chik, K. W., Li, C. K., et al.: Incidence, risk factors and outcome of varicella-zoster virus infection in children after haematopoietic stem cell transplantation. Bone Marrow Transplant. 25:167-172, 2000.

89. Leung, W., Pitts, N., Burnette, K., et al.: Allogeneic bone marrow transplantation for infants with acute leukemia or myelodysplastic syndrome. Bone Marrow Transplant. 27:717-722, 2001.

90. Link, H., Vöhringer, H.-F., Wingen, F., et al.: Pentamidine aerosol prophylaxis of *Pneumocystis carinii* pneumonia after BMT. Bone Marrow Transplant. 11:403-406, 1993.

91. Ljungman, P.: Respiratory virus infections in bone marrow transplant recipients: The European perspective. Am. J. Med. 102(3A):S44-S47, 1997.

92. Ljungman, P., Cordonnier, C., de Bock, R., et al.: Immunizations after bone marrow transplantation: Results of the European group for blood and marrow transplantation. Bone Marrow Transplant. 15:455-460, 1995.

93. Ljungman, P., Deliliers, G. L., Platzbecker, U., et al.: Cidofovir for cytomegalovirus infection and disease in allogeneic stem cell transplant recipients. Blood 97:388-392, 2001.

94. Lucas, K. G., Pollok, K. E., and Emanuel, D. J.: Post-transplant EBV induced lymphoproliferative disorders. Leuk. Lymphoma 25:1-8, 1996.

95. Luján-Zilbermann, J., Benaim, E., Tong, X., et al.: Respiratory virus infections in pediatric hematopoietic stem cell transplantation. Clin. Infect. Dis. 33:962-968, 2001.

96. Luján-Zilbermann, J., and Patrick, C. C.: Infections in patients undergoing hematopoietic stem cell transplantation. *In* Patrick, C. C. (ed.): Clinical Management of Infections in Immunocompromised Infants and Children. Philadelphia, Lippincott Williams & Wilkins, 2001, pp. 195-211.

97. Maltezou, H. C., Kafetzis, D. A., Abisaid, D., et al.: Viral infections in children undergoing hematopoietic stem cell transplant. Pediatr. Infect. Dis. J. 19:307-312, 2000.

98. Maltezou, H. C., Petropoulos, D., Choroszy, M., et al.: Dapsone for *Pneumocystis carinii* prophylaxis in children undergoing bone marrow transplantation. Bone Marrow Transplant. 20:879-881, 1997.

99. Manzoni, A. P. S., Kruse, R. L., Troian, C., et al.: Skin changes in pediatric transplant patients. Pediatr. Transplant. 10:210-214, 2006.

100. Marr, K. A., Carter, R. A., Crippa, F., et al.: Epidemiology and outcome of mould infections in hematopoietic stem cell transplant recipients. Clin. Infect. Dis. 34:909-917, 2002.

101. Marr, K. A., Seidel, K., Slavin, M. A., et al.: Prolonged fluconazole prophylaxis is associated with persistent protection against candidiasis-related death in allogeneic marrow transplant recipients: Long-term follow-up of a randomized, placebo-controlled trial. Blood 96:2055-2061, 2000.

102. Martino, R., Maertens, J., Bretagne, S., et al.: Toxoplasmosis after hematopoietic stem cell transplantation. Clin. Infect. Dis. 31:1188-1194, 2000.

103. Maschke, M., Dietrich, U., Prumbaum, M., et al.: Opportunistic CNS infections after bone marrow transplantation. Bone Marrow Transplant. 23:1167-1176, 1999.

104. McDonald, G. B., Hinds, M. S., Fischer, L. D., et al.: Veno-occlusive disease of the liver and multiorgan failure after bone marrow transplantation: A cohort study of 335 patients. Ann. Intern. Med. 118:255-267, 1993.

105. Meletiadis, J., Petraitis, V., Petraitiene, R., et al.: Triazole-polyene antagonism in experimental invasive pulmonary aspergillosis: In vitro and in vivo correlation. J. Infect. Dis. 194:1008-1018, 2006.

106. Morrison, V. A., Haake, R. J., and Weisdorf, D. J.: The spectrum of non-*Candida* fungal infections following bone marrow transplantation. Medicine (Baltimore) 72:78-89, 1993.

107. Morrison, V. A., and McGlave, P. B.: Mucormycosis in the BMT population. Bone Marrow Transplant. 11:383-388, 1993.

108. Mullen, C. A.: Ciprofloxacin in treatment of fever and neutropenia in pediatric cancer patients. Pediatr. Infect. Dis. 22:1138-1142, 2003.

109. Mullen, C. A., Nair, J., Sandesh, S., and Chan, K. W.: Fever and neutropenia in pediatric hematopoietic stem cell transplant patients. Bone Marrow Transplant. 25:59-65, 2000.

110. Muller, W. J., Levin, M. J., Shin, Y. K., et al.: Clinical and in vitro evaluation of cidofovir for treatment of adenovirus infection in pediatric hematopoietic stem cell transplant recipients. Clin. Infect. Dis. 41:1812-1816, 2005.

111. Naik, H. R., Siddique, N., and Chandrasekar, P. H.: Foscarnet therapy for acyclovir-resistant herpes simplex virus 1 infection in allogeneic bone marrow transplant recipients. Clin. Infect. Dis. 21:1514-1515, 1995.

112. Nichols, W., Corey, L., Gooley, T., et al.: High risk of death due to bacterial and fungal infection among CMV seronegative recipients of stem cell transplantation from seropositive donors (D+/R–): Evidence for "indirect" effects of primary CMV infection. J. Infect. Dis. 185:273-282, 2002.

113. Nucci, M., Marr, K. A., Queiroz-Telles, F., et al.: *Fusarium* infection in hematopoietic stem cell transplant recipients. Clin. Infect. Dis. 38:1237-1242, 2004.

114. Ochs, L., Shu, X. O., Miller, J., et al.: Late infections after allogeneic bone marrow transplantation: Comparison of incidence in related and unrelated donor transplant recipients. Blood 86:3979-3986, 1995.

115. O'Grady, N. P., Alexander, M., Dellinger, E. P., et al.: Guidelines for the prevention of intravascular catheter–related infections. Pediatrics 110:e51-e75, 2002.

116. Orange, J. S., Hossny, E. M., Weiler, C. R., et al.: Use of intravenous immunoglobulin in human disease: A review of evidence by members of the Primary Immunodeficiency Committee of the American Academy of Allergy, Asthma and Immunology. J. Allergy Clin. Immunol. 117(Suppl. 4):S525-S553, 2006.

117. Ottinger, H. D., Beelen, D. W., Scheulen, B., et al.: Improved immune reconstitution after allotransplantation of peripheral blood stem cells instead of bone marrow. Blood 88:2775-2779, 1996.

118. Papadopoulou, A., Nathavitharana, K. A., Williams, M. D., et al.: Diarrhea and weight loss after bone marrow transplantation in children. Pediatr. Hematol. Oncol. 11:601-611, 1994.

119. Pappas, P. G., Rex, J. H., Sobel, J. D., et al.: Guidelines for treatment of candidiasis. Clin. Infect. Dis. 38:161-189, 2004.

120. Parkkali, T., Olander, R., Ruutu, T., et al.: A randomized comparison between early and late vaccination with tetanus toxoid vaccine after allogeneic BMT. Bone Marrow Transplant. 19:933-938, 1997.

121. Parkman, R., and Weinberg, K.: Immunological reconstitution following bone marrow transplantation. Immunol. Rev. 157:73-78, 1997.

122. Pauksen, K., Hammarström, V., Ljungman, P., et al.: Immunity to poliovirus and immunization with inactivated poliovirus vaccine after autologous bone marrow transplantation. Clin. Infect. Dis. 18:547-552, 1994.

123. Pearson, M. L.: Guidelines for prevention of intravascular device–related infections. Part I. Intravascular device–related infections: An overview. Am. J. Infect. Control 24:262-293, 1996.

124. Pfaller, M. A., Pappas, P. G., and Wingard, J. R.: Invasive fungal pathogens: Current epidemiological trends. Clin. Infect. Dis. 43:S3-S14, 2006.

125. Picazo, J. J.: Management of the febrile neutropenic patient: A consensus conference. Clin. Infect. Dis. 39:S1-S6, 2004.

126. Raad, I., Abbas, J., and Whimbey, E.: Infection control of nosocomial respiratory viral disease in the immunocompromised host. Am. J. Med. 102(3A):S48-S52, 1997.

127. Relling, M. V., Boyett, J. M., Blanco, J. G., et al.: Granulocyte colony-stimulating factor and the risk of secondary myeloid malignancy after etoposide treatment. Blood 101:3862-3867, 2003.

128. Riley, D. K., Pavia, A. T., Beatty, P. G., and Denton, D.: Surveillance cultures in bone marrow transplant recipients: Worthwhile or wasteful? Bone Marrow Transplant. 15:469-473, 1995.

129. Rolston, K. V. I.: The Infectious Diseases Society of America 2002 guidelines for the use of antimicrobial agents in patients with cancer and neutropenia: Salient features and comments. Clin. Infect. Dis. 39:S44-S48, 2004.

130. Rooney, C. M., Smith, C., Ng, C. Y., et al.: Use of gene modified virus specific T lymphocytes to control Epstein-Barr-virus–related lymphoproliferation. Lancet 345:9-13, 1995.

131. Roy, V., Ochs, L., and Weisdorf, D.: Late infections following allogeneic bone marrow transplantation: Suggested strategies for prophylaxis. Leuk. Lymphoma 26:1-15, 1997.

132. Ruescher, T. J., Sodeifi, A., Scrivani, S. J., et al.: The impact of mucositis on alpha-hemolytic streptococcal infection in patients undergoing autologous bone marrow transplantation for hematologic malignancies. Cancer 82:2275-2281, 1998.

133. Russell, S. J., Vowels, M. R., and Vale, T.: Hemorrhagic cystitis in pediatric bone marrow transplant patients: An association with infective agents, GVHD and prior cyclophosphamide. Bone Marrow Transplant. 13:533-539, 1994.

134. Sable, C. A., and Donowitz, G. R.: Infections in bone marrow transplant recipients. Clin. Infect. Dis. 19:273-284, 1994.

135. Salzberger, B., Bowden, R. A., Hackman, R. C., et al.: Neutropenia in allogeneic marrow transplant recipients receiving ganciclovir for prevention of cytomegalovirus disease: Risk factors and outcome. Blood 90:2502-2508, 1990.

136. Sanders, J. E.: Bone marrow transplantation for pediatric malignancies. Pediatr. Clin. North Am. 44:1005-1020, 1997.

137. Schimmelpfennig, C., Naumann, R., Zuberbier, T., et al.: Skin involvement as the first manifestation of systemic aspergillosis in patients after allogeneic hematopoietic cell transplantation. Bone Marrow Transplant. 27:753-755, 2001.

138. Schleuning, M., Jager, G., Holler, E., et al.: Human parvovirus B19–associated disease in bone marrow transplantation. Infection 27:114-117, 1999.

139. Schmidt, G. M., Horak, D. A., Niland, J. C., et al.: A randomized, controlled trial of prophylactic ganciclovir for cytomegalovirus pulmonary infection in recipients of allogeneic bone marrow transplants. N. Engl. J. Med. 324:1005-1011, 1991.

140. Schwartz, S., Behre, G., Heinemann, V., et al.: Aerosolized amphotericin B inhalations as prophylaxis of invasive *Aspergillus* infections during prolonged neutropenia: Results of a prospective randomized multicenter trial. Blood 93:3654-3661, 1999.

141. Slavin, M. A., Meyers, J. D., Remington, J. S., et al.: *Toxoplasma gondii* infection in bone marrow transplant recipients: A 20-year experience. Bone Marrow Transplant. 13:549-557, 1994.

142. Singhal, S., and Mehta, J.: Reimmunization after blood or marrow stem cell transplantation. Bone Marrow Transplant. 23:637-646, 1999.

143. Smith, T. J., Khatcheressian, J., Lyman, G. H., et al.: 2006 update of recommendations for the use of white blood cell growth factors: An evidence-based clinical practice guideline. J. Clin. Oncol. 24:3187-3205, 2006.

144. Steinbach, W. J.: Pediatric aspergillosis. Disease and treatment differences in children. Pediatr. Infect. Dis. J. 24:358-364, 2005.

145. Steiner, M., Villablanca, J., Kersey, J., et al.: Viridans streptococcal shock in bone marrow transplant patients. Am. J. Hematol. 42:354-358, 1993.

146. Stevens, D. A., Kan, V. L., Judson, M. A., et al.: Practice guidelines for diseases caused by *Aspergillus*. Clin. Infect. Dis. 30:696-709, 2000.

147. Strasser, S. I., and McDonald, G. B.: Hepatitis viruses and hematopoietic stem cell transplantation: A guide to patient and donor management. Blood 93:1127-1136, 1999.

148. Strauss, R. G.: Leukocyte-reduction to prevent transfusion-transmitted cytomegalovirus infections. Pediatr. Transplant. 3:S19-S22, 1999.

149. Sulahian, A., Touratier, S., and Ribaud, P.: False-positive test for *Aspergillus* antigenemia related to concomitant administration of piperacillin and tazobactam. N. Engl. J. Med. *349*:2366-2367, 2003.

150. Sullivan, K. M., Kopecky, K. J., Jocom, J., et al.: Immunomodulatory and antimicrobial efficacy of intravenous immunoglobulin in bone marrow transplantation. N. Engl. J. Med. *323*:705-712, 1990.

151. Sung, L., Nathan, P. C., Lange, B., et al.: Prophylactic granulocyte colony-stimulating factor and granulocyte-macrophage colony-stimulating factor decrease febrile neutropenia after chemotherapy in children with cancer: A meta-analysis of randomized controlled trials. J. Clin. Oncol. *22*:3350-3356, 2004.

152. Trigg, M. E.: Hematopoietic stem cells. Pediatrics *113*:1051-1057, 2004.

153. Trigg, M. E., Peters, C., and Zimmerman, M. B.: Administration of recombinant human granulocyte-macrophage colony-stimulating factor to children undergoing allogeneic marrow transplantation: A prospective, randomized, double-masked, placebo-controlled trial. Pediatr. Transplant. *4*:123-131, 2000.

154. Tuan, I. Z., Dennison, D., and Weisdorf, D. J.: *Pneumocystis carinii* pneumonitis following bone marrow transplantation. Bone Marrow Transplant. *10*:267-272, 1992.

155. Valteau, D., Hartmann, O., Brugieres, L., et al.: Streptococcal septicaemia following autologous bone marrow transplantation in children treated with high-dose chemotherapy. Bone Marrow Transplant. 7:415-419, 1991.

156. Vance, E., George, S., Guinan, E. C., et al.: Comparison of multiple immunization schedules for *Haemophilus influenzae* type b-conjugate and tetanus toxoid vaccines following bone marrow transplantation. Bone Marrow Transplant. *22*:735-741, 1998.

157. Vartivarian, S. E., Anaissie, E. J., and Bodey, G. P.: Emerging fungal pathogens in immunocompromised patients: Classification, diagnosis and management. Clin. Infect. Dis. *17*:S487-S491, 1993.

158. Verfaille, C., Weisdorf, D. J., Haake, R. J., et al.: *Candida* infections in bone marrow transplant recipients. Bone Marrow Transplant. *8*:177-184, 1991.

159. Wagner, J. E., Barker, J. N., DeFor, T. E., et al.: Transplantation of unrelated donor umbilical cord blood in 102 patients with malignant and nonmalignant diseases: Influence of CD34 cell dose and HLA disparity on treatment-related mortality and survival. Blood *100*:1611-1618, 2002.

160. Walsh, T. J., Finberg, R. W., Arndt, C., et al.: Liposomal amphotericin B for empirical therapy in patients with persistent fever and neutropenia. N. Engl. J. Med. *340*:764-771, 1999.

161. Walsh, T. J., Teppler, H., Donowitz, G. R., et al.: Caspofungin versus liposomal amphotericin B for empirical antifungal therapy in patients with persistent fever and neutropenia. N. Engl. J. Med. *351*:1391-1402, 2004.

162. Walter, E. A., Greenberg, P. D., Gilbert, M. J., et al.: Reconstitution of cellular immunity against cytomegalovirus in recipients of allogeneic bone marrow

by transfer of T-cell clones from the donor. N. Engl. J. Med. *333*:1038-1044, 1995.

163. Walters, M. C., Patience, M., Leisenring, W., et al.: Bone marrow transplantation for sickle cell disease. N. Engl. J. Med. *330*:827-838, 1996.

164. Wasserman, R., August, C. S., and Plotkin, S. A.: Viral infections in pediatric bone marrow transplant patients. Pediatr. Infect. Dis. J. 7:109-115, 1988.

165. Wendt, C. H., Weisdorf, D. J., Jordan, M. C., et al.: Parainfluenza virus respiratory infection after bone marrow transplantation. N. Engl. J. Med. *326*:921-926, 1992.

166. Whimbey, E., Champlin, R. E., Couch, R. B., et al.: Community respiratory virus infections among hospitalized adult bone marrow transplant recipients. Clin. Infect. Dis. *22*:778-782, 1996.

167. Wingard, J. R., Merz, W. G., Rinaldi, M. G., et al.: Increase in *Candida krusei* infection among patients with bone marrow transplantation and neutropenia treated prophylactically with fluconazole. N. Engl. J. Med. *325*:1274-1277, 1991.

168. Winston, D. J., Ho, W. G., Lin, C.-H., et al. Intravenous immunoglobulin for prevention of interstitial pneumonia after bone marrow transplantation. Ann. Intern. Med. *106*:12-18, 1987.

169. Winston, D. J., Maziarz, R. T., and Chandrasekar, P. H.: Intravenous and oral itraconazole versus intravenous and oral fluconazole for long-term antifungal prophylaxis in allogeneic hematopoietic stem-cell transplant recipients. A multicenter, randomized trial. Ann. Intern. Med. *138*:705-713, 2003.

170. Wolfe, S., and Bhatt, A.: Evolving recommendations for vaccinating the immunocompromised patient. J. Public Health Management Practice *11*:566-570, 2005.

171. Wolff, S. N., Fay, J., Stevens, D., et al.: Fluconazole vs low-dose amphotericin B for the prevention of fungal infections in patients undergoing bone marrow transplantation: A study of the North American Marrow Transplant Group. Bone Marrow Transplant. *25*:853-859, 2000.

172. Wong-Beringer, A., Jacobs, R. A., and Guglielmo, B. J.: Lipid formulations of amphotericin B: Clinical efficacy and toxicities. Clin. Infect. Dis. *27*:603-618, 1998.

173. Yusuf, U., Hale, G. A., Carr, J., et al.: Cidofovir for the treatment of adenoviral infection in pediatric hematopoietic stem cell transplant patients. Transplantation *81*:1398-1404, 2006.

174. Zaas, A. K., and Alexander, B. D.: Galactomannan and advances in fungal diagnostics. Curr. Opin. Organ Transplant. *10*:307-311, 2005.

175. Zaia, J. A.: Epidemiology and pathogenesis of cytomegalovirus disease. Semin. Hematol. *27*:S5-S10, 1990.

176. Zaoutis, T. E., Heydon, K., Chu, J. H., et al.: Epidemiology, outcomes, and costs of invasive aspergillosis in immunocompromised children in the United States, 2000. Pediatrics *117*:e711-716, 2006.

CHAPTER 81

INFECTIONS IN PEDIATRIC HEART TRANSPLANTATION

Sheldon L. Kaplan

Each year in the United States, more than 350 children undergo heart transplantation,[66] and infection is an important cause of morbidity and some mortality in these patients. The Registry of the International Society for Heart and Lung Transplantation found that for children who underwent heart transplantation between 1992 and 2004, non-cytomegalovirus (CMV) infection was the cause of mortality in 14 percent of patients in the first 30 days after receiving transplants, peaked at 16.4 percent for 30 days to 1 year after transplantation, and thereafter accounted for 4.3 to 8.6 percent of deaths until more than 5 years after transplantation.[17] The Pediatric Heart Transplant Study Group prospectively collected data from 22 pediatric centers in the United States from January 1993 to December 1994 on 332 children younger than 18 years (mean age, 5.5 years) who had undergone heart transplantation.[123] One or more infections (276 total) occurred in 41 percent of the patients (mean follow-up time, 11.8 months) for an average of 0.84 infections per patient; 22 percent had one infection, 8 percent had two infections, and 11 percent had three or more infections during the study period (Table 81–1). In a similar multicenter study in adults who had undergone heart transplantation between January 1990 and June 1991, infec-

TABLE 81–1 Types of Infections Encountered in 332 Children after Heart Transplantation in a Multi-Institutional Study*

Type	No.
Bacterial (total)	**164**
Coagulase-negative staphylococci	25
Enterobacter species	21
Pseudomonas aeruginosa	16
Viral	
Cytomegalovirus	51
Varicella-zoster virus	11
Respiratory syncytial virus	10
Herpes simplex	6
Other viruses	8
Fungal	**19**
Candida species	12
Pneumocystis carinii	7

*276 infections in 136 patients.
Data from Schowengerdt, K. O., Naftel, D., Seib, P. M., et al.: Infection after pediatric heart transplantation: Results of a multiinstitutional study. J. Heart Lung Transplant. 16:1207-1216, 1997.

tions developed in 31 percent of 814 patients, with 22 percent having one infection and 9 percent having two or more infections.[91] Bacterial infections were the most common type of infection occurring after transplantation in pediatric and adult patients.

Immunosuppressive therapy for children who have undergone heart transplantation usually consists of some combination of cyclosporine or tacrolimus, mycophenolate mofetil or azathioprine, and corticosteroids. Induction immunosuppression may include interleukin-2 receptor antibodies; OKT3 is now being used less frequently.[29,152] Cyclosporine and tacrolimus predominantly block the effect of interleukin-2 on T cells, an action resulting in a diminished T-cell response to mitogen stimulation.[53] The infections seen in heart transplant patients outside the postoperative period generally are a result of this block in T-cell function. Because the types of infections seen in these patients vary with the time elapsed since transplantation, this chapter is organized in such a manner.

PRETRANSPLANTATION EVALUATION

Several infectious agents may be transmitted to the patient via the transplanted organ or can become "reactivated" after transplantation. Determining the antibody status of the recipient and the donor against selected microorganisms (CMV, Epstein-Barr virus [EBV], *Toxoplasma gondii*) helps physicians anticipate or diagnose infections that develop after transplantation. A reasonable pretransplant evaluation for children is outlined in Table 81–2. The child's immunization status is documented, and vaccinations are completed when possible (i.e., hepatitis B vaccine or *Streptococcus pneumoniae*). The Committee on Infectious Diseases of the American Academy of Pediatrics recommends that for immunized children older than 12 months who are scheduled to undergo solid organ transplantation, serologic tests be performed for rubeola, mumps, rubella, and varicella to determine whether protective titers are present.[4] If possible, appropriate vaccines should be administered at least 1 month before the patient undergoes transplantation. Evidence of selected active infections is a contraindication for transplantation. Chemoprophylaxis should be considered strongly for children with a positive tuberculin skin test (purified protein derivative). Dental status also is assessed.

In addition to having the routine pretransplant evaluation as outlined in Table 81–2, each patient should be screened carefully for selected infections appropriate to the individual circumstances. If surgery is planned during the respiratory disease season and the patient has respiratory symptoms just before having surgery, screening for influenza virus or respiratory syncytial virus (RSV) by rapid techniques may facilitate prescribing

---

TABLE 81–2   Evaluation of Children before Heart Transplantation

Serology
   Cytomegalovirus
   Epstein-Barr virus
   Toxoplasma gondii
   Human immunodeficiency virus
   Hepatitis A, B, and C
   Rubeola, mumps, rubella, varicella*
Cultures
   Nasopharyngeal, stool, or tracheal aspirates†
Skin tests
   Purified protein derivative
Freezing of an extra aliquot of serum
Review of the child's immunization status

*For children who are >12 mo old and previously immunized.
†See text for an explanation.

---

antiviral therapy postoperatively. In areas where community-acquired methicillin-resistant *Staphylococcus aureus* (MRSA) is an important cause of infection, performing surface cultures to detect MRSA colonization may modify the choice of antibiotics used for surgical prophylaxis.[64] Applying mupirocin intranasally may influence the rate of postoperative MRSA infections.[98] Children from resource-poor countries may harbor *Salmonella* or intestinal parasites asymptomatically, and these organisms can cause serious infection after the child undergoes transplantation. Preoperative stool cultures for enteropathogens and examination of the stool for parasites may alert the clinician that these pathogens are present and could be the etiology of postoperative infections.

If the patient is being mechanically ventilated before undergoing transplantation, review of recent tracheal aspirate cultures may help in the selection of empiric antibiotics for initial treatment of suspected nosocomial sepsis or pneumonia. Pretransplant infections associated with procedures such as implantation of ventricular assist devices may require prolonged antibiotic therapy after transplantation is performed.[85,131] These infections typically are caused by common nosocomial pathogens and are not a contraindication to undergoing heart transplantation.

SURGICAL PROPHYLACTIC ANTIBIOTICS

Prophylactic antibiotics typically are administered to patients undergoing heart transplantation surgery. For each institution, selection of prophylactic antibiotics should be based partly on the organisms isolated from postoperative wound infections in that center and the antimicrobial susceptibility of these organisms. Cefazolin generally is a reasonable choice for prophylaxis, unless MRSA is a nosocomial pathogen of concern, in which case vancomycin is suggested.[20] In areas where MRSA is a common community pathogen, vancomycin or some other antibiotic active against MRSA might be considered instead of cefazolin, as determined by preoperative surveillance cultures. Routine use of extended-spectrum cephalosporins is discouraged because it may lead to colonization of the patient by antibiotic-resistant, gram-negative organisms that hyperproduce β-lactamase, such as *Enterobacter cloacae*. Recommendations for the duration of prophylactic antibiotic treatment in these patients are not definite, but some centers continue prophylactic antibiotics for 2 to 5 days or more postoperatively, or until all lines and chest tubes have been removed.

IMMEDIATE POSTOPERATIVE INFECTIONS

COMMON INFECTIONS

During the month after the patient undergoes heart transplantation, the types of infections encountered are the same as those complicating major thoracic surgery. Pneumonia and bacteremia are the most common postoperative infections. The frequency of bacteremia and the distribution of organisms are similar in children and adults after undergoing heart transplantation.[91,123] In a multi-institutional pediatric study, the risk of development of any infection was 25 percent 1 month after transplantation. Overall, 60 episodes of bacteremia occurred in the 136 patients who became infected, and the bloodstream was the most common site of bacterial infection.[123] Lung abscesses and mediastinitis are seen less frequently. Familiarity with the organisms and the antimicrobial susceptibility of isolates recovered from other children in the intensive care units (ICUs) in which these patients receive care helps direct the initial selection of empiric antibiotics.

Postoperative bacteremia is related predominantly to the indwelling lines required for monitoring and infusion of medication. *S. aureus*; coagulase-negative staphylococci; *Enterococcus* spp.; and gram-negative enteric organisms such as *Enterobacter* spp., *Pseudomonas aeruginosa*, *Klebsiella* spp., and *Escherichia coli* are the most common causes of nosocomial bacteremia in the pediatric ICU.[113] Other foci of infection, such as pneumonia or mediastinitis, also may result in bacteremia.[11,49] Vancomycin plus an aminoglycoside is a typical empiric antibiotic combination for suspected bacteremia in patients with central lines in place and without focal evidence of infection. Vancomycin therapy should be discontinued as soon as possible if an organism requiring the administration of vancomycin is not isolated.[110] A bacterial line infection may be eradicated successfully without removing the line, but the line should be removed if blood cultures remain positive or the patient's clinical condition deteriorates.[121] Fungemia, generally with *Candida albicans* or other *Candida* spp., also may be associated with line-related infections. Central lines complicated by fungemia should be removed immediately.[39] Centrally placed lines must be removed as soon as practical so that catheter-associated infections can be prevented.

As in other critically ill children, pneumonia is a particularly common occurrence in heart transplant patients because of the operative site and requirements for intubation and mechanical ventilation. During the first postoperative week, definite bacterial pneumonia developed in 3 of 22 children (14%) in an early study from Pittsburgh.[57] In the pediatric multi-institutional study, 56 bacterial lung infections were identified, 24 of which developed in patients maintained on a ventilator at the time of transplantation.[123] Nosocomial pneumonia caused by gram-negative bacilli such as *Pseudomonas* and *Enterobacter* or *S. aureus* is especially common in this setting.[113] Daily chest radiographs taken until the patient is released from the ICU may identify pneumonitis before it is clinically suspected. Gram stain and culture of a tracheal aspirate can help guide therapy for lobar pneumonia.

A broad-spectrum combination of antibiotics, such as an extended-spectrum penicillin with a β-lactamase inhibitor (i.e., piperacillin-tazobactam or ticarcillin-clavulanate) plus an aminoglycoside, usually is initiated until a pathogen or pathogens are identified. Empiric therapy should be based on the antibiotic susceptibility patterns of the common nosocomial pathogens in the specific ICU in which the patient is receiving care. Vancomycin also should be considered if MRSA is part of the resident flora in the ICU. Computed tomography (CT) of the chest may detect basilar and retrocardiac pneumonia, which may not be visualized readily by conventional chest radiographs. CT or ultrasound generally is helpful in assessing the size or characteristics of pleural effusions that may require drainage.

If interstitial pneumonitis is encountered, a more aggressive approach to determining an etiology is warranted. Bronchoscopy with bronchoalveolar lavage should be considered strongly. In children who have pulmonary infiltrates after undergoing heart transplantation, flexible bronchoscopy is more useful for establishing a fungal or viral etiology as opposed to a bacterial cause of pneumonia because most patients have received broad-spectrum antibiotics before undergoing the procedure.[140] Lavage fluid is pooled and processed for bacteria including mycobacteria, viruses, fungi, and protozoa by using culture techniques and special stains. *Legionella* may be an important consideration in some centers.[19,111] Noninfectious causes of pulmonary infiltrates in these children include pulmonary edema, atelectasis, hemorrhage, and adult respiratory distress syndrome.

Urinary tract infections (UTIs) also are common occurrences in the month after undergoing heart transplantation. Urinary catheterization and the immunosuppressive agents contribute to the risk for developing a UTI. Gram-negative enteric organisms (*E. coli*, *K. pneumoniae*, *P. aeruginosa*, and *Enterobacter* spp.), enterococci, and *Candida* spp. are isolated most commonly. Removal of the catheter as soon as possible minimizes the potential for development of a UTI, which has occurred in approxi-

mately 10 percent of adults. In the multicenter pediatric study, the urinary tract was the site of 16 bacterial infections.[123] In addition, UTIs developed in three children (14%) in Pittsburgh during the 2 to 3 weeks after undergoing transplantation.[57]

The broad-spectrum antibiotics used to treat the bacterial complications of transplantation promote *Candida* infection of the urinary tract. Along with removal of the urinary catheter, short-course intravenous amphotericin B for 10 days or less or fluconazole with careful dosing because of drug interactions with cyclosporine and tacrolimus is an option for treating candidal cystitis.[27,43,74,103] In some patients, a urine culture positive for *Candida* is a clue that a disseminated *Candida* infection is present and that further investigation is necessary to exclude the involvement of other organs, especially the kidneys.

Risk factors for early infection in the pediatric multi-institutional study were younger recipient age (particularly <6 months), mechanical ventilation at the time of transplantation, positive donor CMV serology with a CMV-negative recipient, and longer donor ischemic time.[123]

STERNAL WOUNDS AND MEDIASTINITIS

Sternal wound infections and mediastinitis occur in less than 5 percent of adult patients receiving modern immunosuppressive therapy for heart transplantation.[70,91,92] Most of these infections occur during the first postoperative month, usually within the first 2 weeks, and are superficial. Almost all are caused by bacteria. Staphylococci and other gram-positive bacteria generally are responsible for 50 percent of cases, and the remainder are caused by a variety of gram-negative bacilli.[94] Surgical wound infections developed in eight children in the pediatric multi-institution study, although the site of the infection was not noted.[123] Over a 15-year period, 15 (0.2%) children at Texas Children's Hospital, Houston, Texas, developed mediastinitis after undergoing cardiac surgery; 2 children had undergone heart transplantation.[144] At another children's hospital, between 1995 and 2003, 3 percent (5 of 165) of children undergoing heart and lung transplantation developed mediastinitis.[81]

Postoperative bleeding requiring re-exploration is a risk factor for development of mediastinitis. Fever, incisional pain, and an unstable sternum suggest mediastinitis; however, patients may have no specific evidence of infection, including fever. The white blood cell count may be elevated. A pericardial effusion frequently is detected with the development of mediastinitis, and pericardiocentesis may yield purulent material. CT of the chest may show a fluid collection or abscess within the mediastinum and can detect sternal osteomyelitis. Most cases of mediastinitis are caused by *S. aureus*, coagulase-negative staphylococci, or gram-negative bacteria. Median sternotomy wound infections after repair of a congenital heart lesion occur in less than 1 percent of children in large centers. Mediastinitis caused by gram-negative bacilli in association with pneumonia and bacteremia developed in 3 of the 22 children in the Pittsburgh series;[57] each occurred within 2 weeks postoperatively. Two of the three patients died. *Candida* spp. caused both cases of mediastinitis in the two children after heart transplantation. Long and colleagues[81] reported that the mediastinitis that developed in the five patients who had undergone heart and lung transplantation was caused by *E. coli*, *Torulopsis glabrata*, *Aspergillus fumigatus*, *Burkholderia cepacia*, vancomycin-resistant enterococcus.

A superficial median sternotomy wound infection not associated with an unstable sternum can be treated by local drainage of the infected subcutaneous tissue and administration of appropriate antibiotics.[34] Vacuum-assisted closure may be an important aid in addition to antibiotics.[1] A more aggressive approach is required for more serious infections associated with an unstable sternum, mediastinitis, or osteomyelitis of the sternum.[23,34,70]

Adequate drainage and débridement of the area are crucial, and any involved wires should be removed. Mediastinal drains usually are kept in place for several days. Some authorities recommend irrigating the drains with povidone-iodine, but the duration of irrigation is uncertain. A reoperation after the initial drainage procedure may be necessary. Pending culture results, antibiotic therapy is directed against *S. aureus* and gram-negative bacilli. A 4- to 6-week course of antibiotics usually is recommended. Antifungal therapy is initiated if a yeast or fungus is noted on Gram or special stains or isolated from cultures. Careful attention given to surgical technique to minimize postoperative bleeding and early withdrawal of chest and mediastinal tubes placed intraoperatively decrease the incidence of these potentially fatal infections.

OTHER INFECTIONS ENCOUNTERED DURING THE FIRST POSTOPERATIVE MONTH

Herpes Simplex

Herpes simplex infections of the oral mucosa and other superficial surfaces are common after heart transplantation. Oral herpes simplex was observed in 21 percent (11 of 53) of children undergoing transplantation at Stanford.[14] In the pediatric multi-institutional study, only six episodes of herpes simplex infection were noted. Visceral involvement is unusual, although it may develop.[78] Herpes simplex infections typically occur approximately 13 days (range 0 to 4 months) after transplantation and are reactivation processes, not newly acquired infections.[107] A decrease in lymphocyte transformation in response to viral antigen in vitro may explain the increased rate of infection that occurs in the first 12 weeks post-transplantation. In a large randomized study comparing azathioprine with mycophenolate mofetil in adult heart transplant recipients who also were receiving cyclosporine and steroids, herpes simplex infection occurred more commonly in the group treated with mycophenolate mofetil (23% versus 16%, $p < .05$).[36] Institution of antiviral therapy for herpes simplex infection is warranted in these immunocompromised patients. The most common antiviral agent for herpes simplex is acyclovir, which can be administered orally or intravenously. Valacyclovir dosing in children has not been established, and a suspension is unavailable.

Some authorities recommend providing prophylactic acyclovir for heart transplant recipients who are seropositive for herpes simplex.[52] Acyclovir is given intravenously during the perioperative period and then orally for 30 days. Other physicians suggest that because labial or oral herpes simplex is treated so easily, a prophylactic approach is not warranted. In view of concern related to toxicity, drug interactions, and the possibility of resistance developing, I favor the approach that targets treatment after a mucocutaneous lesion is noted.

Legionella pneumophila

Legionella pneumophila infection should be included in the differential diagnosis for fever, respiratory symptoms, and pulmonary infiltrates that develop after heart transplantation.[25] *Legionella* pneumonia can develop during the first postoperative month, but the frequency with which this infection occurs varies among transplant centers. Although legionnaires' disease is an uncommon occurrence in children, nosocomial infections have been documented in a children's hospital, and immunosuppression is a risk factor.[19,22] Appropriate cultures and direct fluorescent antibody stains for *Legionella* should be performed on sputum, other respiratory secretions (obtained by invasive techniques), pleural fluid, or lung tissue to detect this pathogen in a timely fashion. A *Legionella* urinary antigen test is available for serogroup 1 antigens and is quite sensitive.[141]

Macrolides should be considered for empiric therapy if *Legionella* is a serious consideration in children with nosocomial pneumonia. Erythromycin or azithromycin is provided for 2 weeks to complete therapy. Macrolides interact with many of the immunosuppressive agents administered to these patients, however. Quinolones also are quite active against *Legionella* and avoid many of these interactions; in adult transplant patients, they have become the agents of choice.[141] The use of quinolones should be considered for pediatric organ transplant recipients in whom infection with *L. pneumophila* is suspected.[26] In hospitals caring for patients with transplants, routine surveillance culture of the hospital water supply is recommended.

Respiratory Syncytial Virus

Ten episodes of RSV infection were noted in the pediatric multi-institutional study.[123] RSV can be acquired in the hospital soon after undergoing transplantation or can be acquired in the community before undergoing surgery or after discharge. Too few patients in whom RSV infection developed after they underwent heart transplantation have been described to comment on the clinical features. Two children in the early Pittsburgh study were noted to be infected with RSV, both infections occurring on postoperative day 10. Rapidly progressive patchy infiltrates on chest radiographs developed in one child after undergoing heart-lung transplantation, and the second child had only mild upper respiratory symptoms.[49] Tachypnea, cough, fever, wheezing, and the use of accessory muscles occurred commonly in the 18 pediatric liver transplant recipients from Pittsburgh with RSV infection.[106] Radiographic changes included interstitial and lobar infiltrates, atelectasis, and pleural effusion in 12 patients. Two patients required mechanical ventilation after the onset of symptoms related to RSV infection occurred; three others were intubated before acquiring RSV infection and subsequently had complicated courses.

Morbidity and mortality rates related to RSV infection are increased in otherwise immunocompetent children with congenital heart disease, especially when associated with pulmonary hypertension.[84] Because RSV can be acquired in the hospital, RSV infection should be considered in a young transplant patient with respiratory symptoms and fever, especially during the colder months.[59] RSV infection is documented by culture or by rapid detection of RSV infection by enzyme-linked immunosorbent assay or fluorescent antibody testing of respiratory secretions.

The decision to administer ribavirin to these patients is based primarily on the severity of the illness. In a small group of children with underlying bronchopulmonary dysplasia or congenital heart disease, aerosolized ribavirin seemed to be associated with more rapid improvement than that in patients given placebo.[60] Administration of aerosolized ribavirin to a heart transplant recipient with proved or suspected moderate to severe RSV infection is reasonable. As is the case with children requiring mechanical ventilation because of severe RSV lower respiratory tract infection, however, the efficacy of ribavirin in this situation is unknown.[137] The 2006 *Red Book* states, "A decision about ribavirin administration should be made on the basis of the particular clinical circumstances and the experience of the physician."[7,109]

The monoclonal antibody palivizumab was found to be safe, well tolerated, and effective in preventing serious RSV infections in young children with hemodynamically significant congenital heart disease in a large multicenter randomized, double-blind, placebo-controlled trial.[41] Although no specific recommendations have been made regarding the use of palivizumab in children who have undergone heart or other organ transplantation, it would be reasonable to administer it to children 24 months or younger after they undergo heart transplantation and especially postoperatively when the patient is stable.[102,108] The combination of ribavirin and RSV immunoglobulin has been administered to pediatric bone marrow transplant recipients with RSV lower respiratory tract infection.[31] The outcome in these patients was improved over that of historical controls, but no randomized trials have been conducted. RSV immunoglobulin was not efficacious in treating RSV lower respiratory tract infection in children with congenital heart disease who were younger than 2 years.[114] Although palivizumab reduced the concentration of RSV in the tracheal aspirates of children with respiratory failure caused by RSV, its efficacy in treatment is unknown.[86]

INFECTIONS BETWEEN THE FIRST AND SIXTH POSTOPERATIVE MONTHS

CYTOMEGALOVIRUS

CMV is the virus that most frequently infects immunosuppressed cardiac transplant patients. Asymptomatic or symptomatic infections are noted most commonly between the first and sixth months after undergoing transplantation and rarely after the seventh month. In adult series, 12 to 90 percent of patients had evidence of CMV infection postoperatively.[33,55,91] In the multi-institutional pediatric study, 51 episodes of CMV infection occurred in 332 patients and accounted for 60 percent of the viral infections, with a peak occurrence in the second month after transplantation.[123] CMV infection occurred more frequently in older children than in infants. In another study, infants younger than 120 days had CMV infection and disease less commonly than did infants older than 120 days after undergoing heart transplantation.[46] Maternal antibody to CMV may have been protective in the younger infants. In the Pittsburgh series, seven children (32%) had CMV infections, with onset occurring at a mean of 33 days post-transplant (range 23 to 43 days).

CMV infection in transplant recipients occurs in three or four possible settings. In a seronegative recipient, primary CMV infection is acquired through the transplanted heart, through blood transfusions from seropositive donors, or from the community. Seropositive recipients can have reactivation of latent CMV infection or be re-infected with a second strain of CMV from the heart or from blood products derived from seropositive donors.[24] The exact site within the donor heart where CMV may reside in a latent form is unknown, but it may be either cardiac cells or leukocytes that remain within the donor heart. When primary CMV infection is acquired from the donor organ, CMV disease tends to be more severe than if CMV infection is acquired from blood or blood products.[155]

Several risk factors for development of CMV infection after undergoing organ transplantation are recognized. Donor and recipient serologic status and the immunosuppressive regimen are the most significant risk factors for acquiring CMV infection after undergoing heart transplantation. Gorensek and colleagues[55] found that positive recipient CMV serology before transplantation and a larger than average dose of corticosteroids were significant risk factors for acquiring CMV infection. Among the group of patients with CMV infection, positive recipient serology was associated with asymptomatic infection, and excessive steroid dosing was a risk factor for acquiring symptomatic CMV infection. CMV tissue invasion occurred more commonly in patients receiving mycophenolate mofetil compared with azathioprine.

The clinical manifestations of CMV infection vary. Patients may seroconvert, or a latent infection may be reactivated, as determined by positive cultures, but these patients have no symptoms attributable to the CMV infection. Fever, leukopenia, and thrombocytopenia are common postoperative manifestations of systemic CMV infection. Patients may complain of arthralgias, myalgias, and nonspecific abdominal pain. Atypical lymphocytes are noted more commonly in adult than pediatric patients. CMV infection can cause hepatitis, pneumonitis, retinitis, myocarditis,

and gastrointestinal disease, including colitis.[33,40,42,54,55,69,130] The retinitis may be asymptomatic or associated with complaints such as floaters or scotomata. Ophthalmologic screening for CMV retinitis is recommended for all patients 3 to 4 months after cardiac transplantation.[42]

Of the tissues invaded by CMV, involvement of the lung leads to the greatest mortality rate—13 percent in one study.[73] CMV pneumonitis is characterized by fever, hypoxemia, and, usually, diffuse interstitial infiltrates, although lobar consolidation may occur.[129] Pulmonary infections with other viruses or with bacteria or *Pneumocystis carinii* and other pathologic processes (infarction) may coexist with CMV pneumonitis. Gastritis, gastric ulceration, duodenitis, esophagitis, pyloric perforation, and colonic hemorrhage can be documented by endoscopy. In the multi-institutional pediatric study, the lung or gastrointestinal tract was the site of CMV infection in 13 (lung) and 6 (gastrointestinal tract) episodes.[123] Death related to CMV in the pediatric study occurred in 6 percent. In the 2005 Heart Transplant Registry report, CMV accounted for 2.5 percent of deaths in the 30 to 365 days after transplant, 0.5 percent of deaths 1 to 3 years after transplant, and zero deaths after 3 years.[17]

The diagnosis of CMV infection can be based on changes in antibody titer to CMV in paired sera run in parallel with the use of established tests or on changes in CMV IgM results. Isolation of CMV or detection of CMV DNA from a variety of sources, such as urine, blood, bronchial washings, or tissues, also establishes that CMV infection is present. In a seronegative recipient, the possibility of active CMV infection can be anticipated by periodic monitoring of CMV serology and cultures. Whether the CMV infection is causing a symptomatic or invasive illness is more difficult to establish. Histopathologic evidence of CMV infection, such as typical viral inclusions or detection of antigen in tissue by special stains, is required to confirm organ involvement by CMV, although this criterion often is not considered a requirement for clinical trials of preventive measures for CMV disease. Cultures of the buffy coat are positive more frequently in patients with symptomatic than in patients with asymptomatic CMV infection; in patients with primary CMV infection and lung involvement, CMV cultures tend to be positive earlier in the postoperative period than in patients who do not have lung involvement.[55] CMV antigen-positive leukocytes detected by monoclonal antibodies to the early antigen of CMV were found 10 to 28 days before increases in CMV antibody occurred in five patients with active CMV infection.[148] Polymerase chain reaction (PCR) can detect DNA from CMV in blood and other tissues readily and with great sensitivity.[45] The antigen and PCR techniques have been used for early detection of CMV infection so that preemptive antiviral therapy can be initiated.[35]

In addition to the CMV infection syndromes, CMV infection itself seems to affect the transplant recipient adversely in other ways. Symptomatic or asymptomatic CMV infection is associated with a higher rate of graft rejection or graft loss, a greater risk of development of fungal infection, more frequent and earlier graft atherosclerosis, and a significantly lower survival rate than occur in patients who do not have CMV infection.[45,116] In the multi-institutional study, CMV-positive donor serology in conjunction with CMV-negative recipient serology was a risk factor for the acquisition of earlier infection with any organism.[123]

CMV infection of the wide variety of cells that it invades leads to the activation of protein synthesis and the production of multiple immunologically active molecules, including cytokines, especially tumor necrosis factor-α, which adds to the immune deficits induced by the immunosuppressive agents.[45,75] Allograft injury or rejection may be associated with CMV infection of the transplanted organ itself.[45]

Successful treatment or suppression of visceral CMV disease by ganciclovir, a nucleoside analogue active in vitro against CMV, requires a timely diagnosis. Ganciclovir has been shown to alter

CMV disease favorably in heart transplant patients, along with allowing a reduction in immunosuppressive therapy, when possible.[71] The standard approach for treating symptomatic CMV infection is administration of 2 to 3 weeks of intravenous ganciclovir, although the optimal duration of this therapy and the need for maintenance oral doses are unclear.[117] The dose is 5 mg/kg every 12 hours with careful monitoring of hematologic parameters and renal function if renal function initially is normal. Modification of the dose is necessary if renal function is impaired. Viremia should be cleared before discontinuing therapy.[45] The most common adverse reactions to ganciclovir are neutropenia, thrombocytopenia, impaired renal function, seizures, and other central nervous system (CNS) abnormalities.

The role of CMV hyperimmunoglobulin in treating CMV infection in these patients requires further study. After bone marrow transplantation, the addition of CMV immunoglobulin to ganciclovir may be superior to ganciclovir alone in treating CMV pneumonia.[38,112]

In one pediatric study, symptomatic CMV disease developed in five children after they had undergone heart transplantation; each had blood cultures and PCR positive for CMV.[48] Four were treated with ganciclovir for 14 days; one received ganciclovir for 30 days. All received CMV-IgG (150 mg/kg) weekly for 3 weeks. Symptomatic CMV disease was treated successfully in each case.

If possible, prevention of CMV infection in heart transplant recipients is optimal. Only seronegative blood should be used for transfusions when the recipient and the donor are seronegative. Careful control of immunosuppressive therapy, especially with corticosteroids, may help avoid the acquisition of some infections. In the situation of a seronegative recipient of a heart from a seropositive donor, prophylactic administration of CMV immunoglobulin may be useful in some patients. In one study involving the prevention of CMV disease, ganciclovir was compared with CMV immunoglobulin (misoprostol [Cytotec]) in 31 CMV-seropositive heart transplant recipients in whom OKT3 monoclonal antibody was used for early immunoprophylaxis.[2] CMV disease and visceral involvement occurred more frequently in the group given CMV immunoglobulin (40%) than in the group given ganciclovir (6%; $p = .03$). CMV-IgG would be expected to be more beneficial in recipients who are CMV-seronegative.

In one large randomized double-blind, placebo-controlled trial of CMV-seropositive transplant recipients, ganciclovir significantly reduced the incidence of CMV illness during the first 120 days after heart transplantation (9% versus 46% in controls, $p < .001$).[89] No differences were noted between the study groups for seronegative recipients. Combining ganciclovir and CMV-IgG for prophylaxis of high-risk seronegative recipients of hearts from seropositive donors has resulted in mixed findings. Avery[11] found that the combination was not particularly effective; symptomatic CMV syndrome developed in 50 percent of patients. Garjarski and associates[48] provided CMV-IgG (150 mg/kg intravenously at weeks 0, 2, 4, 6, and 8 and 100 mg/kg intravenously at weeks 12 and 16) plus ganciclovir (5 mg/kg every 12 hours intravenously for weeks 1 and 2 and 6 mg/kg/day intravenously at weeks 3 and 4) to 19 children who were recipients of heart transplants from CMV-seropositive donors. CMV disease occurred in 3 of the 10 children who were CMV-seronegative and in 1 of the 10 recipients who were seropositive. Adverse effects of these agents were not reported.

In the study from Stanford, high-risk recipients received CMV-IgG immediately after undergoing transplantation (150 mg/kg administered within 72 hours after transplantation, followed by 100 mg/kg at weeks 2, 4, 6, and 8 and 50 mg/kg at weeks 12 and 16).[146,147] In addition, ganciclovir was administered intravenously immediately after transplantation at a dose of 5 mg/kg every 12 hours for 14 days, followed by 6 mg/kg/day for

the next 2 weeks. These patients were compared with a historical control group at the same institution that received ganciclovir in the 2 to 3 years before CMV-IgG was used. The 27 recipients treated prophylactically with ganciclovir and CMV-IgG had a higher disease-free incidence of CMV, a lower incidence of rejection, and a higher survival rate than those of the historical cohort treated with ganciclovir alone. The combination looks promising for prevention of CMV disease in high-risk heart transplant recipients but requires a randomized trial before the combination can be recommended routinely.

CMV resistant to ganciclovir may emerge as a result of ganciclovir prophylaxis or treatment.[13] Foscarnet or cidofovir is an alternative agent in this situation.

In a meta-analysis of CMV prevention strategies for post-transplantation CMV disease, Small and associates[136] concluded that universal prophylaxis and preemptive approaches are equally effective in reducing the incidence of CMV disease.

EPSTEIN-BARR VIRUS

EBV may cause a spectrum of diseases, including a mononucleosis-like syndrome, polyclonal lymphoproliferation, or monoclonal lymphoproliferation, usually of B cells, in pediatric heart transplant recipients. The transplanted organ is thought to be the most frequent source of EBV. Post-transplantation lymphoproliferative disorders (PTLDs) refer to B-cell expansion that may be localized, nodal, extranodal, or widely disseminated. The largest series of children who have undergone heart transplantation is from Pittsburgh; in this series, PTLD developed in 7.7 percent (6 of 78) of pediatric heart transplant recipients.[18] A major risk factor for the subsequent development of PTLD was being seronegative for EBV before undergoing transplantation. PTLD developed in one third of seronegative recipients of thoracic organs who acquired primary EBV infection (10 of 30). PTLD developed in none of the children who were seropositive before transplantation. Almost all these cases occurred within 1 year of transplantation.

In another series, 19 children were EBV-seropositive and 31 were EBV-seronegative before undergoing heart transplantation. PTLD developed in 1 of 19 patients who were seropositive before undergoing transplantation and in 12 of 19 who became seropositive after transplantation.[157] It did not develop in any of the 12 recipients who remained EBV-seronegative. In contrast to the Pittsburgh experience, the mean time to confirmation of PTLD was 29 months (range 3 to 72 months).

Webber and associates[153] reviewed the experience with PTLD after heart transplantation among 1184 primary organ recipients in 19 centers from 1993 to 2002. Fifty-six patients (5%) developed PTLD a mean of 23.8 months post-transplantation.

Symptoms of PTLD may include fever, malaise, sore throat, and lymphadenopathy. Some children may have splenomegaly, CNS symptoms such as lethargy or seizures, or gastrointestinal complaints.[15,18] Concurrent opportunistic infections are common. Nodules in the lung may be noted on chest radiographs.

The diagnosis of PTLD requires biopsy of involved tissue showing lymphoid proliferation with an immunoblastic component. Molecular techniques typically detect EBV nucleic acids in tissue. EBV serology also is helpful. Quantitative measurement of EBV DNA and RNA in peripheral blood is used to detect primary infection or reactivation at a very early time point and to monitor viral loads serially over time to detect PTLD in the most timely manner.[115] When reported as EBV copies per 10^5 peripheral blood lymphocytes, patients with PTLD typically have viral loads between 500 and 5000, which are much greater than the loads detected in normal latency.

Management generally involves decreasing the immunosuppressive regimen or discontinuing it temporarily. Anti-CD20 antibody (rituximab) is a commercially available monoclonal antibody that specifically binds to the CD20 antigen of normal and malignant B cells and results in antibody-dependent and complement-dependent cytotoxicity. Rituximab has been administered to children with PTLD after they have undergone solid organ transplantation, with some success.[126] Antiviral therapy with acyclovir or ganciclovir also is administered. Some centers administer ganciclovir, acyclovir, or intravenous gamma-globulin for prevention of PTLD, although no prospective studies have confirmed that such an approach is efficacious.[56]

TOXOPLASMA GONDII

An increased incidence of toxoplasmosis is apparent in recipients of heart transplants compared with other organ transplants, although it remains an uncommon infection after heart transplantation.[138] In the pediatric multi-institutional study, toxoplasmosis was not mentioned. *T. gondii* has a predilection for muscle and can be transmitted to the recipient from the heart of a seropositive donor. Active *T. gondii* infections may occur in donor hearts.[118] Less commonly, reactivation of old infection occurs in the recipient. The greatest risk for acquisition of toxoplasmosis occurs in a seronegative recipient of a heart from a seropositive donor. Clinical symptoms usually develop after the first postoperative month and generally within 3 months of transplantation.[61,83,90] Fever alone may be the only clinical manifestation. Dissemination of the parasite to the CNS may lead to signs and symptoms of meningoencephalitis, such as lethargy, seizures, coma, and hemiparesis. Chorioretinitis may result in diminished visual acuity. A sepsislike picture, pneumonia, and cutaneous lesions are unusual manifestations.[10]

CT or magnetic resonance imaging of the brain may detect ring-enhancing mass lesions, which typically are multiple and in periventricular locations. Definitive diagnosis of CNS toxoplasmosis requires the demonstration of tachyzoites or cysts in tissue by biopsy or at necropsy. Serologic tests help monitor seronegative patients for seroconversion and allow a more aggressive approach to be taken to the early diagnosis of toxoplasmosis.[135] *T. gondii* has been seen on endomyocardial biopsy specimens routinely obtained to monitor for rejection.[82]

Therapy for toxoplasmosis with pyrimethamine and sulfadiazine may lead to recovery; these drugs also should be administered if the patient seroconverts.[47] Prophylactic administration of pyrimethamine to seronegative recipients of hearts from seropositive donors is recommended.[156] Prophylactic trimethoprim-sulfamethoxazole also seems to be protective in this high-risk situation.[12,94] Spiramycin is not a useful prophylactic agent.[135]

ASPERGILLUS FUMIGATUS

A. fumigatus is the non-*Candida* fungal infection most commonly reported outside the immediate postoperative period in most series and may be noted first at necropsy.[104] In an early Stanford series, *Aspergillus* infections (four pulmonary, four disseminated) occurred in 8 of 72 (11%) cyclosporine-treated patients 12 to 45 days postoperatively.[65] In a follow-up report, 54 *Aspergillus* infections developed in 620 consecutive heart transplant recipients between 1980 and 1996.[94] Most commonly, *Aspergillus* infections were in the lung (*n* = 31) or were disseminated (*n* = 17). The median time to onset was 52 days. Disseminated aspergillosis was the most common infectious episode responsible for the highest mortality rates in this series. One child in Pittsburgh had disseminated aspergillosis.[57] In the multi-institutional study, seven non-*Candida* fungal infections occurred: *Aspergillus*

spp., two; *Cryptococcus*, *Rhizopus*, and *Rhizomucor*, one each; and unspecified, two.[123] All patients with disseminated infection died.

CNS invasion occurs in many patients with pulmonary aspergillosis, and aspergillosis is the most common cause of brain abscess in organ transplant recipients.[61,93,133] Alterations in mental status occur most frequently, and seizures may occur in 40 percent of cases. On CT scans of the head, multifocal lesions are seen commonly and show a predilection for the junction of the gray and white matter. Mediastinitis and endocarditis are other manifestations of invasive aspergillosis.[79,127] Although isolation of *Aspergillus* from respiratory secretions in a patient with pneumonitis does not establish a diagnosis, aspergillosis is so difficult to establish firmly and is so frequently fatal that treatment should be considered seriously based on this culture alone.

Voriconazole is the agent of choice for invasive aspergillosis.[63] The prospective administration of the combination of voriconazole and caspofungin has been found to be superior to liposomal amphotericin B in historic control solid organ transplant patients with invasive aspergillosis.[134] Itraconazole should not be used for aspergillosis in heart transplant recipients now that superior agents are available.[96] Caspofungin alone also may be beneficial in some patients.[9] Performing surgical drainage and débridement is important for managing most infections.[24] Some type of drainage procedure is indicated if CNS aspergillosis is documented or suspected, although the response to therapy with amphotericin B generally is dismal. In some centers, inhalation of aerosolized amphotericin B (20 mg in sterile water three times per day) has been used prophylactically throughout the hospital stay to prevent the acquisition of invasive aspergillosis.[81] Liposomal amphotericin B may provide an alternative therapy for patients failing treatment with or intolerant of conventional amphotericin B for other mycoses.[37,150]

INFECTIONS AFTER THE SIXTH POSTOPERATIVE MONTH

NOCARDIA ASTEROIDES

A dry cough, fever, and the presence of a solitary pulmonary nodule or abscess on a chest radiograph are characteristic of infection with *N. asteroides*.[77,132] Although pulmonary nodules are characteristic of *Nocardia*, *Aspergillus* and CMV can be associated with nodules as well.[95] Some patients are asymptomatic despite having an abnormal chest radiograph. Infection with *Nocardia* was noted in only 3 percent of cyclosporine-treated patients in the early Stanford series.[65] The median time to the onset of infection was 225 days. A similar incidence of lung nodules or masses secondary to *Nocardia* was noted in a series from New York.[62] In the follow-up Stanford series, 23 episodes of *Nocardia* infection (3.7%) occurred, 19 in the lung.[94] The median onset of infection in the second series was 147 days. *Nocardia* infections are rare in pediatric heart transplant recipients.

Nocardia is isolated best from direct lung tissue specimens, but it may be cultured from bone, skin, or other sites of involvement as well. If a cutaneous skin lesion of *Nocardia* is recognized, other sites should be evaluated promptly for involvement.[51] The formation of single or multiple abscesses in the CNS may result from hematogenous dissemination.[61] Seizures may develop after invasion of brain parenchyma.

The drug of choice for treating *N. asteroides* infection is a sulfonamide. Prolonged administration (average 10 months) generally leads to clearing of the pulmonary lesions. Minocycline is an alternative therapy.[105] The incidence of *Nocardia* infection has declined with the introduction of routine prophylaxis with trimethoprim-sulfamethoxazole.

PNEUMOCYSTIS CARINII

P. carinii pneumonia has been reported in approximately 3 to 4 percent of heart transplantation recipients during the post-cyclosporine era.[44,58,65] In the multi-institutional study, *P. carinii* was noted in seven children (2.1%).[123] Fever, a nonproductive cough, and tachypnea are typical symptoms; hypoxemia is characteristic. The chest radiograph classically shows a diffuse interstitial infiltrate that can progress rapidly. The most expeditious method of documenting *P. carinii* pneumonia in children is methenamine silver or specific antibody staining of fluid or tissue obtained by bronchoalveolar lavage or lung biopsy. Co-infection with CMV or other pathogens occurs commonly.

Treatment of *Pneumocystis* pneumonia in a pediatric heart transplant recipient is identical to that for other immunocompromised children. Use of trimethoprim-sulfamethoxazole prophylaxis for at least 4 months after transplantation has decreased markedly the incidence of this infection in recipients of heart transplants.[100]

STREPTOCOCCUS PNEUMONIAE

S. pneumoniae is an important community-acquired pathogen in heart transplant recipients, who are at increased risk for acquiring this organism.[3] In the multi-institutional pediatric study, two episodes of pneumococcal infection were recorded.[123] During a 10-year period, 9 (11%) of 80 cardiac transplant patients in Little Rock, Arkansas, had 12 episodes of pneumococcal bacteremia.[142] Over an 11-year period, 4 of 105 children undergoing heart transplantation in Toronto had systemic pneumococcal infections.[145] In the follow-up series from Stanford, seven pulmonary infections with *S. pneumoniae* were reported.[94] In an eight-center pediatric surveillance study spanning 5 years, pneumococcal infection developed in 10 patients after a median time from transplantation of 17 months (range, 5-76 months).[125] Three of the 10 patients had two episodes, and one patient had three episodes of pneumococcal infection. The median age of the 10 patients at the time of the first pneumococcal infection was 26 months (range, 15-89 months). The pneumococcal serotypes of the isolates from these patients were the same as noted in healthy children and generally would be covered by the 23-valent pneumococcal vaccine or the 7-valent pneumococcal conjugate vaccine.

OTHER VIRUSES

Influenza and parainfluenza viruses can cause serious infections at any time after transplantation, but especially in the immediate postoperative period.[8,87] Additional risk factors for development of severe disease leading to death are young age and augmentation of immunosuppression. Fever, cough, rhinorrhea, and pharyngitis are typical symptoms of upper respiratory infections. More serious manifestations include adult respiratory distress syndrome; a requirement for intubation and mechanical ventilation; a sepsis-like picture; or CNS symptoms such as headache, photophobia, and lethargy. Viral infection may enhance the likelihood of allograft rejection occurring.

For influenza A infection, oseltamivir, amantadine, or rimantadine should be considered in younger children older than 12 months of age with a heart transplant because of their enhanced predisposition for severe or complicated influenza infection.[5] In older children, zanamivir or oseltamivir is indicated. Experience with these agents in patients with solid organ transplants is limited, however.[119] Early antiviral treatment of influenza in bone marrow transplant recipients was associated with decreased progression to pneumonia and shortened viral shedding in one study.[97]

Parvovirus B19 infection is recognized to cause severe anemia associated with low or no reticulocytes in recipients of heart transplants, similar to the red blood cell suppression in other immunosuppressed patients.[99] In one child, severe pneumonia developed in association with fever and a blanching maculopapular rash involving the face, trunk, and extremities.[68] The parvovirus B19 genome also has been detected in myocardial biopsy specimens of children experiencing cardiac allograft rejection. Of six children described in one report, one had a diffuse rash and two had persistent rejection despite receiving aggressive therapy.[124] In a series of children from Loma Linda who underwent myocardial biopsy for possible rejection, parvovirus genome was detected in 5 of 553 biopsy samples taken from 149 children.[128] Intravenous immunoglobulin is beneficial for the treatment of anemia related to parvovirus B19, but its efficacy in treating pneumonia or possible allograft rejection is unknown.

Varicella virus infection remains a common childhood illness that can cause life-threatening disease in immunocompromised children. In a group of 28 children younger than 10 years old at the time of undergoing heart transplantation who had been monitored for at least 1 year between 1986 and 1999, 14 cases of primary infection with varicella-zoster virus were identified.[32] The mean time post-transplant was 3 years (range, 9 months to 7.5 years). All children were seronegative at the time of transplantation. These children were treated successfully with either parenteral followed by oral acyclovir or oral valacyclovir (mean dose 77 mg/kg/day) for 7 days. Only one child had recurrent varicella, and none had zoster. Routine administration of varicella vaccine to young children helps to decrease most concerns about varicella developing after organ transplantation because of herd protection. Some patients do lose serologically measured immunity to varicella after undergoing transplantation, although the significance of this loss is unclear.[151]

Adenovirus has been associated with serious infections after solid organ transplantation. Among 28 children with solid organ transplants (9 heart) and adenoviral infections, the most common symptoms were fever, diarrhea, vomiting, and abdominal pain.[28] Infection occurred a median of 1.6 months after transplantation. Only two of these patients received antiviral therapy, and all survived the infection. Cidofovir may be beneficial in some patients with disseminated infection, especially of the lungs, or increasing viral loads determined by PCR.[66]

IMMUNOSUPPRESSIVE AGENTS AND ANTIBIOTICS

Cyclosporine and tacrolimus have improved the success of organ transplantation considerably. Generally, the incidence of infection seems to be less since the introduction of cyclosporine than with the earlier immunosuppressive regimens, although morbidity and morality rates remain high in heart transplant recipients.[62] Cyclosporine serum levels are monitored carefully to ensure that concentrations associated with optimal immunosuppression and minimal adverse effects are maintained. Some antibiotics interfere with the pharmacokinetics of cyclosporine or tacrolimus, which may lead to an increase or decrease in their levels.[21,76,101,120,122,139,143] Table 81–3 outlines these interactions. Because cyclosporine and tacrolimus are nephrotoxic, the antimicrobial agents (amphotericin B, aminoglycosides, acyclovir, ceftazidime) administered to heart transplant recipients may be additive; renal function must be monitored carefully.

TABLE 81-3 Effect of Various Antibiotics on Cyclosporine/
Tacrolimus Levels

Increase Cyclosporine/ Tacrolimus Level	Decrease Cyclosporine/Tacrolimus Level
Clarithromycin	Sulfadiazine
Azithromycin	Rifampin
Erythromycin	Trimethoprim-sulfamethoxazole
Ketoconazole	? Nafcillin
Fluconazole	? Isoniazid
Voriconazole	? Ciprofloxacin (counteracts
Itraconazole	immunosuppression)
Caspofungin	

IMMUNIZATIONS

No specific guidelines exist for the immunization of children after they have received a heart transplant, although studies examining the immunogenicity of selected vaccines in this population are being conducted. A prudent approach is to follow the recommendations that the Committee on Infectious Diseases of the American Academy of Pediatrics has developed for immunizing immunosuppressed children.[4] Ideally, the patient will have received the recommended routine vaccines before undergoing transplantation.

Children who have received transplants before reaching 2 to 3 years of age do not respond to the pneumococcal polysaccharide vaccine as well as do children who are older when they receive a transplanted heart, even though the vaccine is administered several years after they receive the transplant.[50] An impairment in immunoglobulin isotype switching from IgM to IgG and especially IgG2 seems to result from the immunosuppressive therapy that these children are receiving.[49] In one study, the antibody response of children aged 2 to 18 months old following solid organ transplantation was compared with age-matched children to the 7-valent pneumococcal conjugate vaccine (PCV7) followed by the 23-valent polysaccharide vaccine (PV23) 2 months later.[80] The antibody levels achieved were significantly higher in the controls, and a second dose of PCV7 given 2 months after the administration of the first PCV7 dose did not lead to higher antibody levels.

For previously unimmunized transplant recipients aged 2 to 18 years old, conjugate pneumococcal vaccine is recommended, followed by the 23-valent pneumococcal vaccine at least 2 to 12 months later. Ideally, children will have completed their PCV7 series before undergoing transplantation.[6] Ongoing immunosuppression seems to prevent maturation of the response to polysaccharide antigens in younger children, which it is hoped that the conjugate vaccine can overcome. The 23-valent pneumococcal vaccine is less immunogenic in adults after they have undergone heart transplantation than it is in healthy controls.

Antibodies to the influenza vaccine develop in most children, but previous exposure predicts a better response.[88] Annual administration of influenza vaccine seems to be safe and immunogenic in children after they have undergone solid organ transplantation. In one study, low-level histologic rejection occurred after the administration of influenza vaccine.[16] In a later study, the administration of inactivated influenza vaccine was not associated with an increased risk of rejection.[154] Depending on the time of year and the approximate date of transplantation, influenza vaccination is appropriate for the patient and all household contacts and health care workers to whom the patient might be exposed. The live-attenuated influenza vaccine is not recommended for individuals receiving immunosuppressive therapy or their close contacts.

After transplantation has been performed and after immunosuppressive therapy has been initiated, administration of live viral vaccines is contraindicated. The enhanced inactivated polio vaccine should be given to the child and to normal siblings. Measles, mumps, rubella, and varicella vaccines can be given to the siblings. Diphtheria, tetanus, and acellular pertussis inactivated vaccines should be given at the routine booster schedule, although antibody responses may not be equivalent to those observed in normal children. Varicella vaccine should be administered before transplantation is performed if varicella antibody is not detected at the pretransplant evaluation in a child aged 12 months or older. Whether the antibody response data generated in children with leukemia during maintenance chemotherapy can be applied to heart transplant recipients who must continue daily immunosuppressive therapy is unclear.

REFERENCES

1. Agarwal, J. P., Ogilvie, M., Wu, L. C., et al.: Vacuum-assisted closure for sternal wounds: A first-line therapeutic management approach. Plast. Reconstr. Surg. 116:1035-1040, 2005.
2. Aguado, J. M., Gomez-Sanchez, M. A., Lumbreras, C., et al.: Prospective randomized trial of efficacy of ganciclovir versus that of anti-cytomegalovirus (CMV) immunoglobulin to prevent CMV disease in CMV-seropositive heart transplant recipients treated with OKT3. Antimicrob. Agents Chemother. 39:1643-1645, 1995.
3. Amber, I. J., Gilbert, E. M., Schiffman, G., and Jacobson, J. A.: Increased risk of pneumococcal infections in cardiac transplant recipients. Transplantation 49:122-125, 1990.
4. American Academy of Pediatrics: Immunization in special clinical circumstances. In Pickering, L. K., Baker, C. J., Long, S. S., McMillan, J. A. (eds.): Red Book: Report of the Committee on Infectious Diseases. 27th ed. Elk Grove Village, IL, American Academy of Pediatrics, 2006, pp. 80-81.
5. American Academy of Pediatrics: Influenza. In Pickering, L. K., Baker, C. J., Long, S. S., McMillan, J. A. (eds.): Red Book: Report of the Committee on Infectious Diseases. 27th ed. Elk Grove Village, IL, American Academy of Pediatrics, 2006, pp. 401-411.
6. American Academy of Pediatrics. Pneumococcal infections. In Pickering, L. K., Baker, C. J., Long, S. S., McMillan, J. A. (eds.): Red Book: Report of the Committee on Infectious Diseases. 27th ed. Elk Grove Village, IL, American Academy of Pediatrics, 2006, pp. 525-537.
7. American Academy of Pediatrics: Respiratory syncytial virus. In Pickering, L. K., Baker, C. J., Long, S. S., McMillan, J. A. (eds.): Red Book: Report of the Committee on Infectious Diseases. 27th ed. Elk Grove Village, IL, American Academy of Pediatrics, 2006, pp. 560-566.
8. Apalsch, A. M., Green, M., Ledesma-Medina, J., et al.: Parainfluenza and influenza virus infections in pediatric organ transplant recipients. Clin. Infect. Dis. 20:394-399, 1995.
9. Arkin, S., Lozano-Chui, M., Paetnick, V., and Rex, J. H.: In vitro synergy of caspofungin and amphotericin B against Aspergillus and Fusarium spp. Antimicrob. Agents Chemother. 46:245-247, 2002.
10. Arnold, S. J., Kinney, M. C., McCormick, S., et al.: Disseminated toxoplasmosis: Unusual presentation in the immunocompromised host. Arch. Pathol. Lab. Med. 121:869-873, 1997.
11. Avery, R. K.: Prevention and treatment of cytomegalovirus infection and disease in heart transplant recipients. Curr. Opin. Cardiol. 13:122-129, 1998.
12. Baden, L. R., Katz, J. T., Franck, L., et al.: Successful toxoplasmosis prophylaxis after orthotopic cardiac transplantation with trimethoprim-sulfamethoxazole. Transplantation 75:339-343, 2003.
13. Baldanti, F., Simoncini, L., Sarasini, A., et al.: Ganciclovir resistance as a result of oral ganciclovir in a heart transplant recipient with multiple human cytomegalovirus strains in blood. Transplantation 66:324-329, 1998.
14. Baum, D., Bernstein, D., Starnes, V. A., et al.: Pediatric heart transplantation at Stanford: Results of a 15-year experience. Pediatrics 88:203-214, 1991.
15. Bernstein, D., Baum, D., Berry, G., et al.: Neoplastic disorders after pediatric heart transplantation. Circulation 88:230-237, 1993.
16. Blumberg, E. A., Fitzpatrick, J., Stutman, P. C., et al.: Safety of influenza vaccine in heart transplant recipients. J. Heart Lung Transplant. 17:1075-1080, 1998.
17. Boucek, M. M., Edwards, L. B., Keck, B. M., et al.: Registry of the International Society for Heart and Lung Transplantation: Eighth Official Pediatric Report—2005. J. Heart Lung Transplant. 24:968-982, 2005.
18. Boyle, G. J., Michaels, M. G., Webber, S. A., et al.: Transplantation lymphoproliferative disorders in pediatric thoracic organ recipients. J. Pediatr. 131:309-313, 1997.
19. Brady, M. T.: Nosocomial legionnaires' disease in a children's hospital. J. Pediatr. 115:46-50, 1989.

20. Bratzler, D. W., and Houck, P. M., for the Surgical Infection Prevention Guidelines Writers Workgroup: Antimicrobial Prophylaxis for Surgery: An Advisory Statement from the National Surgical Infection Prevention Project. Clin. Infect. Dis. *38*:1706-1715, 2004.

21. Campana, C., Regazzi, M. B., Buggia, I., and Molinaro, M.: Clinically significant drug interactions with cyclosporine: An update. Clin. Pharmacokinet. *30*:141-179, 1996.

22. Carlson, N. C., Kuskie, M. R., Dobyns, E. L., et al.: Legionellosis in children: An expanding spectrum. Pediatr. Infect. Dis. J. *9*:133-137, 1990.

23. Carrier, M., Hudon, G., Paquet, E., et al.: Mediastinal and pericardial complications after heart transplantation: Not-so-unusual postoperative problems? Cardiovasc. Surg. *2*:395-397, 1994.

24. Chou, S.: Cytomegalovirus infection and reinfection transmitted by heart transplantation. J. Infect. Dis. *155*:1054-1056, 1987.

25. Chow, J. W., and Yu, V. L.: *Legionella*: A major opportunistic pathogen in transplant recipients. Semin. Respir. Infect. *13*:132-139, 1998.

26. Committee on Infectious Diseases: The use of systemic fluoroquinolones. Pediatrics *118*:1287-1292, 2006.

27. Como, J. A., and Dismukes, W. E.: Oral azole drugs as systemic antifungal therapy. N. Engl. J. Med. *330*:263-272, 1994.

28. de Mezerville, M. H., Tellier, R., Richardson, S., et al.: Adenoviral infections in pediatric transplant recipients: A hospital-based study. Pediatr. Infect. Dis. J. *25*:815-819, 2006.

29. Deng, M. C.: Cardiac transplantation. Heart *87*:177-184, 2002.

30. Denning, D. W., and Stevens, D. A.: Antifungal and surgical treatment of invasive aspergillosis: Review of 2,121 published cases. Rev. Infect. Dis. *12*:1147-1201, 1990.

31. DeVincenzo, J. P., Hirsch, R. L., Fuentes, R. J., and Top, F. H., Jr.: Respiratory syncytial virus immune globulin treatment of lower respiratory tract infection in pediatric patients undergoing bone marrow transplantation—a compassionate use experience. Bone Marrow Transplant. *25*:161-165, 2000.

32. Dodd, D. A., Burger, J., Edwards, K. M., and Dummer, J. S.: Varicella in a pediatric heart transplant population on nonsteroidal maintenance immunosuppression. Pediatrics *108*:e80, 2001.

33. Dummer, J. S., White, L. T., Ho, M., et al.: Morbidity of cytomegalovirus infection in recipients of heart or heart-lung transplants who received cyclosporine. J. Infect. Dis. *152*:1182-1191, 1985.

34. Edwards, M. S., and Baker, C. J.: Median sternotomy wound infections in children. Pediatr. Infect. Dis. *2*:105-109, 1983.

35. Egan, J. J., Lomax, J., Barber, L., et al.: Preemptive treatment for the prevention of cytomegalovirus disease in lung and heart transplant recipients. Transplantation *65*:747-752, 1998.

36. Eisen, H. J., Kobashigawa, J., Keogh, A., et al.: Three-year results of a randomized, double-blind, controlled trial of mycophenolate mofetil versus azathioprine in cardiac transplant recipients. J. Heart Lung Transplant. *24*:517-525, 2005.

37. Ellis, M., Spence, D., de Pauw, B., et al.: An EORTC international multicenter randomized trial (EORTC Number 19923) comparing two dosages of liposomal amphotericin B for treatment of invasive aspergillosis. Clin. Infect. Dis. *27*:1406-1412, 1998.

38. Emanuel, D., Cunningham, I., Jules-Elysee, K., et al.: Cytomegalovirus pneumonia after bone marrow transplantation successfully treated with the combination of ganciclovir and high-dose intravenous immune globulin. Ann. Intern. Med. *109*:777-782, 1988.

39. Epps, S. C., Troutman, J. L., and Gutman, L. T.: Outcome of treatment of candidemia in children whose central catheters were removed or retained. Pediatr. Infect. Dis. J. *8*:99-104, 1989.

40. Etheridge, S. P., Bolman, R. H., and Braunlin, E. A.: Cytomegalovirus colitis in a pediatric heart transplant patient. Clin. Transplant. *8*:409-412, 1994.

41. Feltes, T. F., Cabalka, A. K., Meissner, H. C., et al.: Palivizumab prophylaxis reduces hospitalization due to respiratory syncytial virus in young children with hemodynamically significant congenital heart disease. J. Pediatr. *143*:532-540, 2003.

42. Fishburne, B. C., Mitrani, A. A., and Davis, J. L.: Cytomegalovirus retinitis after cardiac transplantation. Am. J. Ophthalmol. *125*:104-106, 1998.

43. Fisher, J. F., Chew, W. H., Shadomy, S., et al.: Urinary tract infections due to *Candida albicans*. Rev. Infect. Dis. *4*:1107-1118, 1982.

44. Fishman, J. A.: *Pneumocystis carinii* and parasitic infections in transplantation. Infect. Dis. Clin. N. Am. *9*:1005-1074, 1995.

45. Fishman, J. A., and Rubin, R. H.: Infection in organ-transplant recipients. N. Engl. J. Med. *338*:1741-1751, 1998.

46. Fukushima, N., Gundry, S. R., Razzouk, A. J., and Bailey, L. L.: Cytomegalovirus infection in pediatric heart transplantation. Transplant. Proc. *25*:1423-1425, 1993.

47. Gallino, A., Maggiorini, M., Kiowoski, W., et al.: Toxoplasmosis in heart transplant recipients. Eur. J. Clin. Microbiol. Infect. Dis. *15*:389-393, 1996.

48. Garjarski, R. J., Rosenblatt, H. M., Denfield, S. W., et al.: Outcomes among pediatric heart transplant recipients after dual-therapy cytomegalovirus prophylaxis. Tex. Heart Inst. J. *24*:97-104, 1997.

49. Gennery, A. R., Cant, A. J., Baldwin, C. I., and Calvert, J. E.: Characterization of the impaired antipneumococcal polysaccharide antibody production in immunosuppressed pediatric patients following cardiac transplantation. J. Clin. Immunol. *21*:43-50, 2001.

50. Gennery, A. R., Cant, A. J., Spickett, G. P., et al.: Effect of immunosuppression after cardiac transplantation in early childhood on antibody response to polysaccharide antigen. Lancet *351*:1778-1781, 1998.

51. Gentry, L. O., Zeluff, B., and Kielhofner, M. A.: Dermatologic manifestations of infectious diseases in cardiac transplant patients. Infect. Dis. Clin. N. Am. *8*:637-654, 1994.

52. Gold, D., and Corey, L.: Acyclovir prophylaxis for herpes simplex virus infection. Antimicrob. Agents Chemother. *31*:361-367, 1987.

53. Goldman, M. H., Barnhart, G., Mohanakumar, T., et al.: Cyclosporine in cardiac transplantation. Surg. Clin. North Am. *65*:637-659, 1985.

54. Gonwa, T. A., Capehart, J. E., Pilcher, J. W., and Alivizatos, P. A.: Cytomegalovirus myocarditis as a cause of cardiac dysfunction in a heart transplant recipient. Transplantation *47*:197, 1989.

55. Gorensek, M. J., Stewart, R. W., Keys, T. F., et al.: A multivariate analysis of the risk of cytomegalovirus infection in heart transplant recipients. J. Infect. Dis. *157*:515-522, 1988.

56. Green, M., Reyes, J., Webber, S., and Rowe, D.: The role of antiviral and immunoglobulin therapy in the prevention of Epstein-Barr virus infection and post-transplant lymphoproliferative disease following solid organ transplantation. Transpl. Infect. Dis. *3*:97-103, 2001.

57. Green, M., Wald, E. R., Fricker, F. J., et al.: Infections in pediatric orthotopic heart transplant recipients. Pediatr. Infect. Dis. J. *8*:87-93, 1989.

58. Gryzan, S., Paradis, I. L., Zeevi, A., et al.: Unexpectedly high incidence of *Pneumocystis carinii* infection after lung heart transplantation: Implications for lung defense and allograft survival. Am. Rev. Respir. Dis. *137*:1268-1274, 1988.

59. Hall, C. B., Douglas, R. G., Jr., Geiman, J. M., and Messner, M. K.: Nosocomial respiratory syncytial virus infections. N. Engl. J. Med. *293*:1343-1346, 1975.

60. Hall, C. B., McBride, J. T., Gala, C. L., et al.: Ribavirin treatment of respiratory syncytial viral infection in infants with underlying cardiopulmonary disease. J. A. M. A. *254*:3047-3051, 1985.

61. Hall, W. A., Martinez, A. J., Dummer, J. S., et al.: Central nervous system infections in heart and heart-lung transplantation recipients. Arch. Neurol. *46*:173-177, 1989.

62. Haramati, L. B., Schulman, L. L., and Austin, J. H.: Lung nodules and masses after cardiac transplantation. Radiology *188*:491-497, 1993.

63. Herbrecht, R., Denning, D. W., Patterson, T. F., et al.: Voriconazole versus amphotericin B for primary therapy of invasive aspergillosis. N. Engl. J. Med. *347*:408-415, 2002.

64. Herold, B. C., Immergluck, L. C., Maranan, M. C., et al.: Community-acquired methicillin-resistant *Staphylococcus aureus* in children with no identifying predisposing risk. J. A. M. A. *279*:593-598, 1998.

65. Hofflin, J. M., Potasman, I., Baldwin, J. C., et al.: Infectious complications in heart transplant recipients receiving cyclosporine and corticosteroids. Ann. Intern. Med. *106*:209-216, 1987.

66. Hoffman, J. A.: Adenoviral disease in pediatric solid organ transplant recipients. Pediatr. Transplant. *10*:17-25, 2006.

67. International Society for Heart and Lung Transplantation Registry. 18th Annual Report. Available at www.ishlt.org.

68. Janner, D., Bork, J., Baum, M., and Chinnock, R.: Severe pneumonia after heart transplantation as a result of human parvovirus B19. J. Heart Lung Transplant. *13*:336-338, 1994.

69. Kaplan, C. S., Peterson, E. A., Icenogle, T. B., et al.: Gastrointestinal cytomegalovirus infection in heart and heart-lung transplant recipients. Arch. Intern. Med. *149*:2095-2100, 1989.

70. Karwande, S. V., Renlund, D. G., Olsen, S. L., et al.: Mediastinitis in heart transplantation. Ann. Thorac. Surg. *54*:1039-1045, 1992.

71. Keay, S., Petersen, E., Icenogle, T., et al.: Ganciclovir treatment of serious cytomegalovirus infection in heart and heart-lung transplant recipients. Rev. Infect. Dis. *10*(Suppl. 3):563-572, 1988.

72. Kim, J. H., and Perfect, J. R.: Infection and cyclosporine. Rev. Infect. Dis. *11*:677-690, 1989.

73. Kirklin, J. K., Naftel, D. C., Levine, T. B., et al.: Cytomegalovirus after heart transplantation: Risk factors for infection and death: A multiinstitutional study. J. Heart Lung Transplant. *13*:394-404, 1994.

74. Kohn, D. B., Uehling, D. T., Peters, M. E., et al.: Short-course amphotericin B therapy for isolated candiduria in children. J. Pediatr. *10*:310-313, 1987.

75. Koskinen, P. K., Kallio, E. A., Tikkanen, J. M., et al.: Cytomegalovirus infection and cardiac allograft vasculopathy. Transpl. Infect. Dis. *1*:115-126, 1999.

76. Kramer, M. R., Marshall, S. E., Denning, D. W., et al.: Cyclosporine and itraconazole interaction in heart and lung transplant recipients. Ann. Intern. Med. *113*:327-329, 1990.

77. Krick, J. A., Stinson, E. B., and Remington, J. S.: *Nocardia* infection in heart transplant patients. Ann. Intern. Med. *82*:18-26, 1975.

78. Kusne, S., Schwartz, M., Breinig, M. K., et al.: Herpes simplex virus hepatitis after solid organ transplantation in adults. J. Infect. Dis. *163*:1001-1007, 1991.

79. Levin, T., Suh, B., Beltramo, D., and Samuel, R.: *Aspergillus* mediastinitis following orthotopic heart transplantation: Case report and review of the literature. Transpl. Infect. Dis. *6*:129-131, 2004.

80. Lin, P. L., Michaels, M. G., Green, M., et al.: Safety and immunogenicity of the American Academy of Pediatrics—recommended sequential pneumococ-

cal conjugate and polysaccharide vaccine schedule in pediatric solid organ transplant recipients. Pediatrics *116*:160-167, 2005.

81. Long, C. B., Sha, S. S., Lautenbach, E., et al.: Postoperative mediastinitis in children: Epidemiology, microbiology and risk factors for gram-negative pathogens. Pediatr. Infect. Dis. J. *24*:315-319, 2005.

82. Luft, B. J., Billingham, M., and Remington, J. S.: Endomyocardial biopsy in the diagnosis of toxoplasmic myocarditis. Transplant. Proc. *83*:1871-1873, 1986.

83. Luft, B. J., Naot, Y., Araujo, F. G., et al.: Primary and reactivated *Toxoplasma* infection in patients with cardiac transplants, clinical spectrum and problems in diagnosis in a defined population. Ann. Intern. Med. *99*:27-31, 1983.

84. MacDonald, N. E., Hall, C. B., Suffin, S. C., et al.: Respiratory syncytial viral infection in infants with congenital heart disease. N. Engl. J. Med. *307*:397-400, 1982.

85. Malani, P. N., Dyke, D. B. S., Pagini, F. D., and Chenoweth, C. E.: Nosocomial infections in left ventricular device recipients. Clin. Infect. Dis. *34*:1295-1300, 2002.

86. Malley, R., DeVincenzo, J., Ramilo, O., et al.: Reduction of respiratory syncytial virus (RSV) in tracheal aspirates in intubated infants by use of humanized monoclonal antibody to RSV F protein. J. Infect. Dis. *178*:1555-1561, 1998.

87. Mauch, T. J., Bratton, S., Myers, T., et al.: Influenza B virus infection in pediatric solid organ transplant recipients. Pediatrics *94*:225-229, 1994.

88. Mauch, T. J., Crouch, N. A., Freese, D. K., et al.: Antibody response of pediatric solid organ transplant recipients to immunization against influenza virus. J. Pediatr. *127*:957-960, 1995.

89. Merigan, T. C., Renlund, D. G., Keay, S., et al.: A controlled trial of ganciclovir to prevent cytomegalovirus disease after heart transplantation. N. Engl. J. Med. *326*:1182-1186, 1992.

90. Michaels, M. G., Wald, E. R., Fricker, F. J., et al.: Toxoplasmosis in pediatric recipients of heart transplants. Clin. Infect. Dis. *14*:847-851, 1992.

91. Miller, L. W., Naftel, D. C., Bourge, R. C., et al.: Infection after heart transplantation: A multi-institutional study. J. Heart Lung Transplant. *13*:981-993, 1994.

92. Miller, R., Ruder, J., Karwande, S. V., and Burton, N. A.: Treatment of mediastinitis after heart transplantation. J. Heart Transplant. *5*:477-479, 1986.

93. Montero, C. G., and Martinez, A. J.: Neuropathy of heart transplantation: 23 cases. Neurology *36*:1149-1154, 1986.

94. Montoya, J. G., Giraldo, L. F., Efron, B., et al.: Infectious complications among 620 consecutive heart transplant patients at Stanford University Medical Center. Clin. Infect. Dis. *33*:629-640, 2001.

95. Muñoz, P., Palomo, J., Guembe, P., et al.: Lung nodular lesions in heart transplant recipients. J. Heart Lung Transplant. *19*:660-667, 2000.

96. Nanas, J. N., Saroglou, G., Anastasian-Nana, M. I., et al.: Itraconazole for the treatment of pulmonary aspergillosis in heart transplant recipients. Clin. Transplant. *12*:30-34, 1998.

97. Nichols, W. G., Guthrie, K. A., Corey, L., and Boeckh, M.: Influenza infections after hematopoietic stem cell transplantation: risk factors, mortality, and the effect of antiviral therapy. Clin. Infect. Dis. *39*:1300-1306, 2004.

98. Nicholson, M. R., and Huesman, L. A.: Controlling the usage of intranasal mupirocin does impact the rate of *Staphylococcus aureus* deep sternal wound infections in cardiac surgery patients. Am. J. Infect. Control *34*:44-48, 2006.

99. Nour, B., Green, M., Michaels, M., et al.: Parvovirus B19 infection in pediatric transplant patients. Transplantation *56*:835-838, 1993.

100. Olsen, S. L., Renlund, D. G., O'Connell, J. B., et al.: Prevention of *Pneumocystis carinii* pneumonia in cardiac transplant recipients by trimethoprim-sulfamethoxazole. Transplantation *56*:359-362, 1993.

101. Osowski, C. L., Dix, S. P., Lin, S. L., et al.: Evaluation of the drug interaction between intravenous high-dose fluconazole and cyclosporine or tacrolimus in bone marrow transplant patients. Transplantation *61*:1268-1272, 1996.

102. Palivizumab, a humanized respiratory syncytial virus monoclonal antibody, reduces hospitalization from respiratory syncytial virus infection in high-risk infants. The IMpact-RSV Study Group. Pediatrics *102*:531-537, 1998.

103. Pappas, P. G., Rex, J. H., Sobel, J. D., et al.: Guidelines for treatment of candidiasis. Clin. Infect. Dis. *38*:161-189, 2004.

104. Paya, C. V.: Fungal infections in solid-organ transplantation. Clin. Infect. Dis. *16*:677-688, 1993.

105. Peterson, E. A., Nash, M. L., Mammana, R. B., and Copeland, J. G.: Minocycline treatment of pulmonary nocardiosis. J. A. M. A. *250*:930-932, 1983.

106. Pohl, C., Green, M., Wald, E. R., and Ledesma-Medina, J.: Respiratory syncytial virus infections in pediatric liver transplant recipients. Clin. Infect. Dis. *165*:166-169, 1992.

107. Pollard, R. B., Arvin, A. M., Gambert, P., et al.: Specific cell-mediated immunity and infections with herpes viruses in cardiac transplant recipients. Am. J. Med. *73*:679-687, 1982.

108. Prevention of respiratory syncytial virus infections: Indications for the use of palivizumab and update on the use of RSV-IGIV. American Academy of Pediatrics and Committee on Infectious Diseases and Committee on Fetus and Newborn. Pediatrics *102*:1211-1216, 1998.

109. Reassessment of the indications for ribavirin therapy in respiratory syncytial virus infections. American Academy of Pediatrics Committee on Infectious Diseases. Pediatrics *97*:137-140, 1996.

110. Recommendation for preventing the spread of vancomycin resistance. Hospital Infection Control Practices Advisory Committee (PICPAC). Infect. Control Hosp. Epidemiol. *16*:105-113, 1995.

111. Redd, S. C., Schuster, D. M., Quan, J., et al.: Legionellosis in cardiac transplant recipients: Results of a nationwide study. J. Infect. Dis. *158*:651-653, 1988.

112. Reed, E. C., Bowden, R. A., Dandliker, P. S., et al.: Treatment of cytomegalovirus pneumonia with ganciclovir and intravenous cytomegalovirus immunoglobulin in patients with bone marrow transplants. Ann. Intern. Med. *109*:783-788, 1988.

113. Richards, M. J., Edwards, J. R., Culver D. H., et al.: Nosocomial infections in pediatric intensive care units in the United States. Pediatrics *103*:e39, 1999.

114. Rodriguez, W. J., Gruber, W. C., Welliver, R. C., et al.: Respiratory syncytial virus (RSV) immune globulin intravenous therapy for RSV lower respiratory tract infection in infants and young children at high risk for severe RSV infections. Pediatrics *99*:454-461, 1997.

115. Rowe, D. T., Webber, S., Schauer, E. M., et al.: Epstein-Barr virus load monitoring: Its role in the prevention and management of post-transplant lymphoproliferative disease. Transpl. Infect. Dis. *3*:79-87, 2001.

116. Rubin, R. H.: The indirect effects of cytomegalovirus infection on the outcome of organ transplantation. J. A. M. A. *261*:3607-3609, 1989.

117. Rubin, R. H.: Prevention and treatment of cytomegalovirus disease in heart transplant patients. J. Heart Lung Transplant. *19*:731-735, 2000.

118. Ryning, F. W., McLeod, R., Maddox, J. C., et al.: Probable transmission of *Toxoplasma gondii* by organ transplantation. Ann. Intern. Med. *90*:47-49, 1979.

119. Sable, C. A., and Hayden, F. G.: Orthomyxoviral and paramyxoviral infections in transplant recipients. Infect. Dis. Clin. N. Am. *9*:987-1003, 1994.

120. Sadaba, B., Lopez de Ocariz, A., Jr., Quiroga, J., and Cienfuegos, J. A.: Concurrent clarithromycin and cyclosporine A treatment. J. Antimicrob. Chemother. *42*:393-395, 1998.

121. Salzman, M. B., and Rubin, L. G.: Intravenous catheter-related infections. Adv. Pediatr. Infect. Dis. *10*:337-368, 1995.

122. Sands, M., and Brown, R. B.: Interactions of cyclosporine with antimicrobial agents. Rev. Infect. Dis. *11*:691-697, 1989.

123. Schowengerdt, K. O., Naftel, D., Seib, P. M., et al.: Infection after pediatric heart transplantation: Results of a multiinstitutional study. The Pediatric Heart Transplant Study Group. J. Heart Lung Transplant. *16*:1207-1216, 1997.

124. Schowengerdt, K. O., Ni, J., Denfield, S. W., et al.: Association of parvovirus B19 genome in children with myocarditis and cardiac allograft rejection: Diagnosis using the polymerase chain reaction. Circulation *96*:3549-3554, 1997.

125. Schutze, G. E., Mason, E. O., Jr., Wald, E. R., et al.: Pneumococcal infections in children after transplantation. Clin. Infect. Dis. *33*:16-21, 2001.

126. Serinet, M. O., Jacquemin, E., Habes, D., et al.: Anti-CD20 monoclonal antibody (rituximab) treatment for Epstein-Barr virus-associated, B-cell lymphoproliferative disease in pediatric liver transplant recipients. J. Pediatr. Gastroenterol. Nutr. *34*:389-393, 2002.

127. Sherman-Weber, S., Axelrod, P., Suh, B., et al.: Infective endocarditis following orthotopic heart transplantation: 10 cases and a review of the literature. Transpl. Infect. Dis. *6*:165-170, 2004.

128. Shiral, G. S., Ni, J., Chinnock, R. E., et al.: Association of viral genome with graft loss in children after cardiac transplantation. N. Engl. J. Med. *344*:1498-1503, 2001.

129. Shulman, L. L.: Cytomegalovirus pneumonitis and lobar consolidation. Chest *91*:558-601, 1978.

130. Shuster, L. D., Cox, G., Bhatia, P., and Miner, P. B., Jr.: Gastric mucosal nodules due to cytomegalovirus infection. Dig. Dis. Sci. *34*:103-107, 1989.

131. Simon, D., Fischer, S., Grossman, A., et al.: Left ventricular assist device-related infection: treatment and outcome. Clin. Infect. Dis. *40*:1108-1115, 2005.

132. Simpson, G. L., Stinson, E. B., Egger, M. J., and Remington, J. S.: Nocardial infections in the immunocompromised host: A detailed study in a defined population. Rev. Infect. Dis. *3*:492-508, 1981.

133. Singh, N., and Husain, S.: Infections of the central nervous system in transplant recipients. Transpl. Infect. Dis. *2*:101-111, 2000.

134. Singh, N., Limaye, A. P., Forrest, G., et al.: Combination of voriconazole and caspofungin as primary therapy for invasive aspergillosis in solid organ transplant recipients: A prospective, multicenter, observational study. Transplantation *81*:320-326, 2006.

135. Sluiters, J. F., Balk, A. H. M. M., Essed, C. E., et al.: Indirect enzyme-linked immunoassay for immunoglobulin G and four immunoassays for immunoglobulin M to *Toxoplasma gondii* in a series of heart transplantation recipients. J. Clin. Microbiol. *27*:529-535, 1989.

136. Small, L. N., Lau, J., and Snydman, D. R.: Preventing post-organ transplantation cytomegalovirus disease with ganciclovir: A meta-analysis comparing prophylactic and preemptive therapies. Clin. Infect. Dis. *43*:869-880, 2006.

137. Smith, D. W., Frankel, L. R., Mathers, L. H., et al.: A controlled trial of aerosolized ribavirin in infants receiving mechanical ventilation for severe respiratory syncytial virus infection. N. Engl. J. Med. *325*:24-29, 1991.

138. Spiers, G. E., Hakim, M., Calne, R. Y., and Wreghitt, T. G.: Relative risk of donor-transmitted *Toxoplasma gondii* infection in heart, liver and kidney transplant recipients. Clin. Transplant. *2*:257-260, 1988.

139. Stamatakis, M. K., and Richards, J. G.: Interaction between quinupristin/dalfopristin and cyclosporine. Ann. Pharmacother. *31*:576-578, 1997.

140. Stokes, D. C., Shenep, J. L., Parham, D., et al.: Role of flexible bronchoscopy in the diagnosis of pulmonary infiltrates in pediatric patients with cancer. J. Pediatr. 115:561-567, 1989.
141. Stout, J. E., and Yu, V. L.: Legionellosis. N. Engl. J. Med. 337:682-687, 1997.
142. Stovall, S. H., Ainley, K. A., Mason, E. O., Jr., et al.: Invasive pneumococcal infections in pediatric cardiac transplant patients. Pediatr. Infect. Dis. J. 20:946-950, 2001.
143. Theisen, K.: Sulfadiazine therapy for toxoplasmosis in heart transplant recipients decreases cyclosporine concentration. Clin. Invest. 70:752-754, 1992.
144. Tortoriello, T. A., Friedman, J. D., McKenzie, E. D., et al.: Mediastinitis after pediatric cardiac surgery: A 15-year experience at a single institution. Ann. Thorac. Surg. 76:1655-1660, 2003.
145. Tran, L., Hébert, D., Dipchand, A., et al.: Invasive pneumococcal disease in pediatric organ transplant recipients: A high risk population. Pediatr. Transplant. 9:183-186, 2005.
146. Valantine, H. A.: Prevention and treatment of cytomegalovirus disease in thoracic organ transplant: Evidence for a beneficial effect of hyperimmune globulin. Transplant. Proc. 27(Suppl. 1):49-57, 1995.
147. Valantine, H. A., Luikart, H., Doyle, R., et al.: Impact of cytomegalovirus hyperimmune globulin on outcome after cardiothoracic transplantation: A comparative study of combined prophylaxis with CMV hyperimmune globulin plus ganciclovir versus ganciclovir alone. Transplantation 72:1647-1652, 2001.
148. Van der Bij, W., Van Dijk, R. B., Van Son, W. J., et al.: Antigen test for early diagnosis of active cytomegalovirus infection in heart transplant recipients. J. Heart Transplant. 7:106-109, 1988.
149. Wagener, M. W., and Yu, V. L.: Bacteremia in transplant recipients: A prospective study of demographics, etiologic agents, risk factors and outcomes. Am. J. Infect. Control 20:239-247, 1992.
150. Walsh, T. J., Hiemenz, J. W., Seibel, N. L., et al.: Amphotericin B lipid complex for invasive fungal infections: Analysis of safety and efficacy in 556 cases. Clin. Infect. Dis. 26:1383-1396, 1998.
151. Warmington, L., Lee, B. E., and Robinson, J. L.: Loss of antibodies to measles and varicella following solid organ transplantation in children. Pediatr. Transplant. 9:311-314, 2005.
152. Webber, S. A., McCurry, K., and Zeevi, A.: Heart and lung transplantation in children. Lancet 368:53-69, 2006.
153. Webber, S. A., Naftel, D. C., Fricker, F. J., et al.: Lymphoproliferative disorders after paediatric heart transplantation: A multi-institutional study. Lancet 367:233-239, 2006.
154. White-Williams, C., Brown, R., Kirklin, J., et al.: Improving clinical practice: Should we give influenza vaccinations to heart transplant patients? J. Heart Lung Transplant. 25:320-325, 2006.
155. Wreghitt, T.: Cytomegalovirus infections in heart and heart-lung transplant recipients. J. Antimicrob. Chemother. 23(Suppl. E):49-60, 1989.
156. Wreghitt, T. G., Gray, J. J., Pavel, P., et al.: Efficacy of pyrimethamine for the prevention of donor-acquired Toxoplasmosis gondii infection in heart and heart-lung transplant patients. Transplant. Int. 5:197-200, 1992.
157. Zangwill, S. D., Hsu, D. T., Kichuk, M. R., et al.: Incidence and outcome of primary Epstein Barr virus infection and lymphoproliferative disease in pediatric heart transplant recipients. J. Heart Lung Transplant. 17:1161-1166, 1998.

CHAPTER 82

INFECTIONS IN PEDIATRIC LUNG TRANSPLANTATION

Jill A. Hoffman

The first pediatric lung transplant was reported to the International Society for Heart and Lung Transplantation (ISHLT) in 1986, and by the end of 2005, a total of 963 transplants had been reported to the registry.[446] In addition, living lobar transplantation (LLT) is being performed at some centers as a way to address the shortage of available organs,[395,408,461] but it still accounts for less than 10 percent of all pediatric lung transplants.[446] At Children's Hospital Los Angeles (CHLA), the first pediatric LLT was performed in 1993 on a 13-year-old boy with cystic fibrosis (CF). He received lobes from each of his parents and survived for 5 years, unfortunately succumbing to renal failure while waiting for a kidney transplant.[461] Fifty-three LLT procedures (34% of total lung transplants) have been performed on pediatric patients at CHLA.[40]

The primary indication for lung transplantation in the pediatric population is CF. Most pediatric transplants, 56 percent regardless of age and almost 70 percent of transplants in 12- to 17-year-old patients, were performed for this diagnosis. By age, most pediatric transplant recipients are adolescents (>60%).[446] The most common diagnoses were complex congenital heart disease in infants younger than 1 year of age undergoing lung transplantation and primary pulmonary hypertension in children aged 1 to 5 years. Since 2000, approximately 66 pediatric lung transplants have been performed annually at 27 centers.[446]

Infectious morbidity and mortality rates remain high for lung transplant recipients (LTRs) and are probably greater than for most other solid organ transplant recipients (SOTRs).[8] This high incidence results from constant communication of the lungs and fresh bronchial anastomosis (BA) with the environment and from the high preoperative microbial burden of patients who constitute the majority of recipients of pediatric lung transplants.

Denervation of the transplanted lung, interruption of the bronchial and lymphatic circulation, abnormal cough reflexes, and impaired mucociliary clearance also probably play roles.[8] In addition, these patients receive relatively high-dose, long-term immunosuppression; at 5 years, most patients still are maintained on tacrolimus (60% of patients) and corticosteroids (98% of patients).[446] In the first year after lung transplantation at CHLA, the overall incidence of infection was 0.24 episode per patient per month, or 2.88 infections per patient per year.[237] Fifty-five percent of all infections occurred in the first month after transplantation, with infections becoming much less frequent thereafter (Tables 82–1 and 82–2).[237] A summary of the causes of infection in this cohort during the first year after transplantation is presented in Tables 82–3 and 82–4.[237]

The additional indirect impact of infections on the outcome of LTRs also is recognized. Cytomegalovirus (CMV) and probably other viruses, as well as bacterial infections, have been implicated in immunologically mediated processes leading to bronchiolitis obliterans syndrome (BOS) or chronic graft dysfunction, acute rejection, graft loss, and death.[8]

The overall survival of pediatric LTRs as reported to the ISHLT is 74, 59, 49.5, and 30 percent at 1, 3, 5, and 10 years, respectively, similar to that of adult recipients.[446] There is no difference in survival according to donor lung source, living versus deceased.[33,408,446] Infection is the single most common cause of death from 1 month to 1 year after transplantation (44%), and it remains a significant cause of death in all periods through 5 years after transplantation.[446] BOS causes approximately 40 percent of deaths after the first year. Graft failure accounts for a third of deaths in the first month and 8 to 20 percent thereafter.[446] In the series of 75 pediatric transplants at CHLA (12 heart-lung, 18 cadaveric, 45 LLTs), the mortality rate

TABLE 82–1   Timetable of Infections for Pediatric Lung Transplant Recipients

Time of Initial Evaluation	Infection/Pathogen	Comments
0–1 Month	Wound, respiratory tract, line/bloodstream, and urinary tract infections	Related to the surgical procedure: *Candida*, *Staphylococcus* species, *Pseudomonas* species
	HSV stomatitis	Reactivation
	CMV infection	
	HHV-6?	
	Bronchial anastomosis (*Aspergillus*)	
	Other: rabies, West Nile virus, lymphocytic choriomeningitis virus, endemic mycoses	Unusual pathogens preexisting in the recipient or in the donor graft
1–6 Months	CMV disease	Onset of opportunistic infections from immunosuppression
	EBV	
	Aspergillus	
	Mycobacterium tuberculosis	
	Pneumocystis jiroveci	
	Endemic mycoses	
	HHV-6	
	Respiratory tract, line/bloodstream, and urinary tract infections	Continued bacterial (*Pseudomonas*) and candidal infections common through 3–4 months
	Respiratory viruses	Community-acquired infections
>6 Months	Respiratory viruses	Community-acquired infections
	Persistent *Pseudomonas*, *Burkholderia cepacia*, and *Aspergillus* infections	Persistence of organisms from cystic fibrosis in the proximal airways and sinuses
	Opportunistic infections:	Patients receiving continuous high-level immunosuppression or therapy for steroid-resistant rejection, CMV infection
	Pneumocystis jiroveci	
	Cryptococcosis	
	Nontuberculous mycobacteria	
	EBV/PTLD	
	Herpes zoster	

CMV, cytomegalovirus; EBV, Epstein-Barr virus; HHV, human herpesvirus; HSV, herpes simplex virus; PTLD, post-transplant lymphoproliferative disease.
Adapted from Rubin, R. H., Ikonen, T., Gummert, J. F., and Morris, R. E.: The therapeutic prescription for the organ transplant recipient: The linkage of immunosuppression and antimicrobial strategies. Transpl. Infect. Dis. 1:39, 1999.

TABLE 82–2   Timing of Infections in 75 Pediatric Lung Transplant Recipients at Childrens Hospital Los Angeles

Months after Transplantation	% of Episodes
0–1	55
1–3	18
3–6	13
6–9	8
9–12	7

TABLE 82–3   Etiology of Infections in 75 Pediatric Lung Transplant Recipients in the First Postoperative Month at Childrens Hospital Los Angeles

Etiology	Number of Episodes
Pseudomonas, respiratory tract	22
Candida, respiratory tract	13
Herpes stomatitis	12
Cytomegalovirus infection	10
Aspergillus infection of the respiratory tract, bronchial anastomosis	4

TABLE 82–4   Etiology of Infections in 75 Pediatric Lung Transplant Recipients in the First Year at Childrens Hospital Los Angeles

Etiology	% of Total Infections
Bacterial infections	55
Pseudomonas spp.	18 (35% of bacterial infections)
Viral	27
Cytomegalovirus	12 (42% of viral infections)
Fungal	16
Candida	10
Aspergillus	4

was 18.6 percent at 1 year, 50 percent of which was attributed to infection.[237]

IMMUNOSUPPRESSION AND TIMING OF INFECTION

An understanding of the mechanisms and effects of immunosuppressive therapy is fundamental to predicting the timing and types of infections that occur after transplantation, and several excellent reviews are available.[349,352] This predictability of certain infections has facilitated establishing more timely diagnosis and determining strategies for preventive antimicrobial therapy.[127] Historically, the mainstay of therapy has included corticosteroids and combinations of the following medications: azathioprine, the calcineurin inhibitors (CNIs) cyclosporine and tacrolimus, sirolimus, mycophenolate mofetil (MMF), and polyclonal and monoclonal antibodies. In recent years, substitution of MMF and tacrolimus for azathioprine and cyclosporine, respectively, has become standard, and "steroid-sparing therapy" also is gaining favor. These regimens may provide a superior cost-benefit ratio in terms of prevention of rejection and risk of infection. A general time line of the occurrence of specific infectious agents in pediatric LTRs is presented in Table 82–1.

OVERVIEW OF INFECTIONS AND ANTIBIOTIC USE IN SOLID ORGAN TRANSPLANTATION

The "therapeutic prescription," as described by Rubin and colleagues,[352] for successful organ transplantation requires a careful balance between immunosuppression and the use of antimicrobials therapeutically, prophylactically, or preemptively to manage the risk of rejection versus infection. A transplant recipient's risk for developing infection is determined by multiple factors, including (1) the technical skill of the surgeon; (2) the quality of perioperative care; (3) the net state of immunosuppression; (4) the patient's infectious exposure, including that from the community, hospital, and donor grafts; (5) the underlying condition of the patient (e.g., colonization in CF); and (6) the virulence of the organisms. Preventive/prophylactic strategies can alter these patterns, most notably for CMV and fungal infections, and delay their appearance past the expected time periods.[350] In sum, these considerations indicate that although a standard set of antimicrobials can be prescribed, they must be tailored closely to the risks, exposure, and immunosuppression of each individual.[353]

General principles of infection and therapy have been proposed by Rubin and Marty [353] and include the recognition that a transplant recipient is likely to have a greater microbial load and more advanced infection at the time of diagnosis, thereby requiring longer therapy with greater potential for drug toxicity. Early establishment of the diagnosis and provision of therapy are paramount to a successful outcome. Furthermore, a broader range of organisms must be considered. Although a common practice in medicine is to assume a single diagnosis for a given manifestation, a recognized caveat is that transplant recipients may have "simultaneous and sequential" infections.[353] In fact, many infectious processes are influenced directly by proceeding or concurrent events. The prototype of this interaction is the immunomodulating effect of CMV infection such that alterations in the cytokine/chemokine milieu, T-lymphocyte subsets and function, neutrophil activity, and activation of endothelial cells emerge. The result of these derangements is further immunosuppression, enhanced production of virus, and subsequent increased susceptibility to additional infections. Other putative immunomodulating viruses include human herpesvirus-6 (HHV-6), Epstein-Barr virus (EBV), and the hepatitis viruses.[353,373]

Length of therapy depends on consideration of the degree of current immunosuppression and location of the infection. In general, experts suggest treating until all signs and symptoms of infection are gone, followed by a "buffer period" of weeks to months, depending on the infection.[353] Finally, drug interactions and toxicities, which may be synergistic, must be taken into consideration when prescribing medications in these complex patients.[265,352]

SITES OF INFECTION

THORACIC CAVITY: RESPIRATORY TRACT INFECTIONS, INCLUDING PNEUMONIA AND ANASTOMOTIC SITE INFECTIONS

The vast majority (80%) of infections in LTRs occur in the thorax—lung, mediastinum, pleural space[132]—with 35 to 66 percent of all infections being manifested as pneumonia.[8] In the CHLA cohort of patients during the first 12 months after transplantation, 62 percent of all infections were pneumonia.[237] The onset of pneumonia in LTRs appears in a bimodal pattern, with most cases occurring in the first postoperative month. A second, albeit smaller group has late (<6 to 12 months) recurrent episodes of gram-negative pneumonia associated with a poor outcome. The immunologic consequences of these infections in some

patients may include bronchiolitis obliterans with organizing pneumonia (BOOP), which is characterized by inflammation and fibrotic granulation tissue of the small airways extending into the alveoli. The mortality rate of patients with BOOP is high (50%), and those who survive appear to be at an increased risk for developing BOS (41%).[8,69,132]

Unique to lung transplantation are BA infections, most of which are fungal and caused by *Aspergillus* and sometimes *Candida* species.[162,176,217,298,318] The BA is susceptible to such infections for a variety of reasons. Anatomically, the post-transplant bronchus is relatively devascularized, with the blood supply flowing retrograde from the pulmonary arterial circulation; neovascularization from collaterals takes as long as 1 month to occur. In the interim, the bronchus may experience ischemia and subsequent necrosis and sloughing of bronchial epithelium. Evolving surgical techniques have diminished this risk of ischemia in recent years. This environment is optimal for developing infection caused by saprophytic flora, such as *Aspergillus*, present in ambient air to which the airways are in direct contact. In addition, local reaction to suture material, postoperative corticosteroid use, and immunosuppressive therapy have a negative impact on healing and increase the patient's susceptibility to infection. As a result of this early tenuous anatomy, infections at this site are most likely to occur within the first 2 to 3 months after surgery.[76,162,176,298,300] BA infections rarely can lead to early catastrophic complications, such as dehiscence and hemorrhage. They are linked to substantial late bronchial complications, including dehiscence, bronchial stenosis, malacia, and retransplantation.[294,298]

Some studies have demonstrated that pretransplant isolation of *Aspergillus* spp. has not been found to be a risk factor for the development of *Aspergillus* infection after transplantation.[199,300,323] Others suggest that patients with CF and perioperative *Aspergillus* colonization may be at heightened risk for the development of early BA infection. Although the numbers are small, the authors speculate that the presence of *Aspergillus* at the site of the fresh, devascularized anastomosis renders it more vulnerable.[300] Postoperative isolation of *Aspergillus* from airways appears to identify patients at risk for the later development of BA abnormalities.[76,176,294,298] The overall incidence of airway infections, complications, or both ranges from 5 to 25 percent.[76,162,176,216,298] The mortality rate associated with BA infection and its complications is reported to be 2 to 7 percent.[176,298] Finally, one small study evaluating the effect of early sirolimus-based immunosuppression on the rate of rejection described poor wound healing and anastomotic complications in an unexpectedly high number of patients treated with sirolimus, which resulted in changes in immunosuppression strategies at that institution.[158]

BLOODSTREAM INFECTIONS

The second most common site of infection is the bloodstream. Two recent studies have looked specifically at the epidemiology of bloodstream infections (BSIs) in pediatric and adult LTRs.[91,315] Both studies found that BSI occurred in approximately 25 percent of transplant recipients, with staphylococci, *Pseudomonas aeruginosa*, and *Candida* spp. being the most common organisms identified. Late infections in both groups consisted of a wide range of gram-negative organisms. Both studies demonstrated that post-transplant BSI, especially early (<30 days) BSI in children and candidal BSI in both populations, was associated significantly with mortality. In the pediatric population, most BSI was related to central venous catheters and was not secondary to other sites of infection (5% with pneumonia, sternal wound, ruptured subglottic cysts). These infections were most likely to occur in the first 7 days after transplantation. In adult transplant recipients, BSI largely was associated with pulmonary infections. Specifically, *P. aeruginosa* bacteremia was more likely to develop in adult patients with CF (20% of the transplant cohort) than in patients with other indications. *Burkholderia cepacia* and *Staphylococcus aureus* BSI was seen in similar frequency in non-CF patients. In addition, BSI in patients with CF was associated with a decreased risk for death when compared with other LTRs with similar infections, possibly because antimicrobials active against resistant gram-negative organisms were being administered at the time that the infection developed. In children, *Pseudomonas* BSI was not associated with the diagnosis of CF (45% of the transplant cohort), nor with any outcome measures in this study.

Empiric therapy in patients with suspected BSI should include agents active against staphylococcal and pseudomonal spp., with a low threshold for adding antifungal therapy. Furthermore, the need for indwelling central catheters should be assessed routinely, and catheters should be removed as soon as clinically feasible.

SELECTED PATHOGENS

BACTERIA

Pseudomonas aeruginosa and *Burkholderia cepacia* Complex

P. aeruginosa and *B. cepacia* play prominent roles in postoperative infections in patients with CF, the majority of pediatric LTRs. Despite the removal of colonized lung tissue with the procedure, the proximal airways and sinuses remain colonized and a source of infection postoperatively in the immunosuppressed transplant recipients. In patients with multidrug-resistant (MDR) organisms, this concern is heightened. MDR, gram-negative organisms have been defined as those resistant to all agents in two or more classes of effective drugs[357] (e.g., resistance to all aminoglycosides, β-lactams, fluoroquinolones). *B. cepacia* complex organisms are resistant to aminoglycosides intrinsically, having high rates of resistance to β-lactams, inducible resistance to fluoroquinolones, and resistance to colistin and polymyxin.[53]

As lung transplantation was emerging as a treatment option, patients with MDR organisms generally were excluded.[299] Such exclusion was based on data suggesting that pretransplant infection with MDR *P. aeruginosa* and *B. cepacia* complex diminished the chance of survival and, therefore, was considered a (relative) contraindication to transplantation.[213,262,388]

More recent data have documented that the presence of preoperative MDR and even pan-resistant *P. aeruginosa*, but not *Burkholderia cenocepacia*, may not have an impact on survival; these patients may be more likely to acquire postoperative infections, but they generally respond to treatment without increases in mortality rates.[22,107,128,199,299] The most recent ISHLT guidelines for selection of LTRs list "colonization with highly resistant or highly virulent bacteria, fungi, or mycobacteria" as a relative contraindication.[309] Additionally, it acknowledges that although "certain resistant pathogens may increase risk of poor outcome . . . it is not possible currently to identify absolute contraindications based on either the type of organisms or the pattern of antibiotic resistance." Despite the status of the immunocompromised host, the relatively low virulence of some of these organisms, the new healthy lung epithelium and improved airway function of the transplanted lungs, the aggressive use of antimicrobials during and after the procedure, and discordance between in vitro susceptibilities and in vivo efficacy may account for the diminished influence that MDR organisms have on the outcomes of transplant recipients.[29]

Recent analysis has shown that *B. cepacia* complex represents a group of nine related species that possess variable pathogenic potential in abnormal hosts.[240,241] Misidentification of *B. cepacia* complex organisms at the genus (*Alcaligenes*, *Stenotrophomonas*,

and *Pseudomonas* most commonly) and species levels is a common occurrence.[240,271] This information is critical to evaluating patients considering transplantation and, in postoperative care, to assessing their risk for developing invasive disease.[240] There are species-specific differences in antimicrobial resistance and virulence. Several putative virulence/transmissibility factors that have been identified for *B. cenocepacia* (formerly genomavar III, ET-12 strain)[240] include quorum sensing,[389] cable pili (*cbl*A) for enhanced binding to respiratory epithelium,[359] increased neutrophil recruitment with suboptimal activation of polymorphonuclear neutrophils and macrophages,[358] and production of exopolysaccharides that inhibit neutrophil chemotaxis and scavenge reactive oxygen species.[56]

In the United States, *B. cepacia* complex is present in 3.2 percent of the CF population, with *B. cenocepacia* accounting for 50 percent of cases. In Canada, 15 percent harbor *B. cepacia* complex,[70] and as many as 80 percent of cases involve *B. cenocepacia*.[99] Some controversy continues regarding performing transplantation on patients who have *B. cenocepacia*. Data demonstrate increased morbidity and mortality rates associated with this organism in nontransplanted patients with CF[195,228,229,255] and in LTRs,[23,70,100,240] although successful transplantation has been accomplished in several centers.[70,101,237]

One of the largest and best characterized reports of *B. cepacia* complex in LTRs comes from the Toronto Lung Transplant Program, which documented that from 1988 to 1995, 15 of 28 (54%) patients with preoperative sputum positive for *B. cepacia* (genomavar III, ET-12) died after undergoing transplantation of causes related to this infection, whereas 4 of 25 (16%) *B. cepacia*–negative patients died. The 1-year survival rate for colonized patients was 67 percent versus 92 percent for those without colonization. Of note, 60 percent of *B. cepacia*–related deaths took place in the first 3 months after transplantation, with the additional deaths occurring between 14 and 48 months post-transplantation as a result of infection associated with BOS. Of the 13 surviving patients, 4 had complications related to *B. cepacia*, including abscess and empyema, and were successfully treated medically and surgically. In all surviving patients (34 total), the rate of BOS in the *B. cepacia* group (46%) was comparable to that in the *B. cepacia*–negative group (48%).[70]

More recently, the Toronto center has had improved mortality statistics with the use of 2 to 3 weeks of aggressive antimicrobial therapy, including tobramycin (intravenous, inhaled), ceftazidime, chloramphenicol, and trimethoprim-sulfamethoxazole (TMP-SMX), and a reduction in immunosuppressive therapy. Only one of five transplant patients with MDR *B. cepacia* has died of *B. cepacia*/BOS since this regimen was implemented. One other patient survived a postoperative *B. cepacia* abscess, and three additional patients remained *B. cepacia*–negative and clinically stable.[70]

In vitro synergy or multiple combination bactericidal testing (MCBT) for MDR or pan-resistant gram-negative organisms has been suggested to facilitate the use of effective multidrug regimens.[1,2,53,224,357] In vitro testing can identify combinations of antimicrobials that inhibit bacterial growth. How these data translate to patient care, however, has yet to be fully demonstrated. Recent published data did not reveal better outcomes, specifically the time to the next exacerbation, when using combination therapy to treat CF patients infected with MDR bacteria.[2] In this report, study patients received two-drug combinations based on MCBT, but these patients did not necessarily have MDR/pan-resistant organisms, nor had they failed conventional therapy. Extrapolating these results to LTRs with MDR organisms is difficult. The CHLA has been using MCBT from the University of Ottawa since 2001; our experience suggests that this approach, with as many three or four drugs used in combination, is helpful for managing preoperative and postoperative patients with MDR/pan-resistant organisms, including *B. cepacia* complex.[237] Clearly, additional data are needed to assess this approach for LTRs with MDR organisms.

Optimal therapy for infections caused by these gram-negative organisms is not known. Therapy should be tailored to susceptibility studies. The duration of therapy requires individualization but generally is no less than 2 weeks, and treatment should be continued for a significant period after the signs and symptoms of infection have resolved. Combination therapy (two or three drugs) usually is recommended. For *P. aeruginosa*, an extended-spectrum, antipseudomonal β-lactam and an aminoglycoside, if renal status allows, with or without aerosolized tobramycin, can be used. Aerosolized tobramycin can deliver drug levels above the minimal inhibitory concentrations (MICs) of resistant organisms directly to the lungs and thereby reduce the bacterial burden with minimal systemic toxicity.[141] Aerosolized tobramycin should not be used as single therapy in transplant recipients at risk for dissemination. Colistin in either an aerosol or intravenous formulation may be helpful for pan-resistant organisms, but renal toxicity may preclude its systemic use. For *B. cepacia*, combinations that include ceftazidime, meropenem, TMP-SMX, tetracyclines, quinolones, and chloramphenicol may be used.[185] A protocol using aerosolized aztreonam has shown some benefit at CHLA.[124,145,462] Therapy is initiated in patients identified with *B. cepacia* complex, preoperatively if possible, and continued through the first year after transplantation. Preliminary data suggest that outcomes are similar to those of patients who are colonized with susceptible *Pseudomonas* organisms. Further investigation is needed in this promising area of therapy.

Other Gram-Negative Organisms

Infections with other gram-negative organisms, including extended-spectrum, β-lactamase–producing organisms (*Escherichia coli* and *Klebsiella pneumoniae*), have been described in other transplant populations, such as pediatric liver or intestinal transplantation, and notably in outbreak situations.[152,337] No data exist on rates in pediatric LTRs. Some increased risk related to antimicrobial exposure, infection control practices, stays in intensive care units, and hospitalization is likely.[289] Carbapenems (meropenem, imipenem) generally are considered the drugs of choice for extended-spectrum, β-lactamase–producing organisms, especially for empiric therapy.

Mycobacterium tuberculosis

M. tuberculosis (MTB) remains an important pathogen in SOTRs. As noted by many authors, it behaves as an opportunistic infection in these patients in that its frequency is greatly increased in comparison to the normal population (up to 74-fold in some U.S. studies), it has diverse manifestations with high rates of extrapulmonary disease, and mortality rates are high (20-40%).[290,351,383] Most cases of MTB arise from reactivation of latent infection, although acquired cases are seen, especially in pediatrics.[269,287,425] Multiple cases of donor-derived MTB infection, including pulmonary MTB in LTRs[340] and extrapulmonary MTB in renal and liver transplants, have been documented.[150] In addition, nosocomial transmission to transplant recipients has occurred.[193]

Important differences appear to exist in the epidemiology of MTB infection in different transplant populations and for adults versus pediatric patients. Most data are available for the former, who are more likely to have reactivation of latent disease and higher rates of liver toxicity with therapy. In the United States and Europe, MTB infections occur most frequently in LTRs (2-6.5%), followed by liver (0.9-2.3%) and heart (1-1.4%) recipients.[383] Studies of MTB infection in SOTRs, including small numbers of children, suggest that most cases occur within the first post-transplant year, with a median time of 9 months

for all SOTRs and 3.5 months for LTRs. Risk factors for early MTB infection include allograft rejection; receipt of OKT3 or anti–T-cell antibodies, which also predict dissemination; and previous exposure to MTB, with radiographic evidence of old infection or a history of a positive tuberculin skin test (TST). Co-infection with CMV, mycoses, *Pneumocystis jiroveci*, and *Nocardia* has been associated with the development of disease.[287,290] As would be expected, most manifestations include pulmonary disease (71%), with interstitial infiltrates, nodules, effusion, and cavities seen on imaging studies. Extrapulmonary disease (16%) includes a wide variety of gastrointestinal (GI) disease and skin, musculoskeletal, genitourinary, lymph node, and central nervous system (CNS) involvement. In one study, a third of patients had disseminated disease, 91 percent of whom were febrile as compared with 64 percent of those with localized disease.[383] Significant predictors of mortality, which was 17 percent for LTRs, were disseminated disease, previous rejection, and receipt of OKT3 or anti–T-cell antibodies.[383]

Several studies have investigated mycobacterial infections in LTRs.[46,202,257,287] Two of the studies were conducted in countries with a low endemicity of MTB, Australia and North America (rates of MTB, 5 to 15/100,000), and two in Spain (rates of MTB, 25 to 49/100,000). Rates of MTB in LTRs in the two former studies were less than 1 percent,[202,257] but they were 2.6 percent and 6.4 percent (500-fold higher than the national average) in the Spanish studies.[46,287] Indeed, nontuberculous mycobacterial (NTM) infections were more common than were MTB infections in the first two reports, whereas NTM infection was encountered only once in the Spanish study. No deaths from mycobacterial disease were reported in three studies,[46,202,257] but the mortality rate was 43 percent in the final report.[287]

Few data exist on MTB in pediatric SOTRs and none in LTRs in particular. Two small series of MTB in pediatric liver transplants have been published.[269,425] Initial symptoms included fever in most patients. Pulmonary findings were most common. Pediatric patients may be seen later than adults after transplantation (median of 8 months versus 4 months) as a result of differences in acquisition of disease.[425] TST results were negative or minimal in all patients. A 5-mm induration (two patients) should be considered positive in an immunocomprised patient with compatible symptoms.[18] Furthermore, screening of family members was very useful in both series of patients, thus suggesting that as for immunocompetent children, the index case of exposure is in the home. Invasive diagnostic procedures were needed to confirm the diagnosis in most patients. No deaths were directly attributable to MTB. An additional case report of MTB complex disease in a pediatric renal transplant recipient highlights another potential difference between pediatric and adult cases.[73] *Mycobacterium bovis* disease, which can be indistinguishable from MTB but often is manifested as abdominal disease, developed in this child. It usually is acquired from the ingestion of unpasteurized milk products from infected cows. It appears to be distinctly more common in children and, in the United States, is seen most often in children who have immigrated from or visited countries where *M. bovis* is endemic in cattle, such as Mexico.[88] The importance of recognizing this infection is its inherent resistance to pyrazinamide and the implications that this resistance has for therapy.

Diagnosis of MTB in the transplant setting can be challenging because symptoms may be nonspecific, such as fever of unknown origin, or unusual, such as abdominal manifestations; co-infections also may modify the signs and symptoms. Delayed-type hypersensitivity often is suppressed in transplant candidates and recipients, thus rendering TST unreliable. Moreover, just a minority of patients undergo skin testing before transplantation. Consequently, a high index of suspicion is required, and frequently, aggressive diagnostic techniques, such as bronchoscopy, laparoscopy, and tissue biopsy, are needed.[269,299,425]

Several new methods are available for culture-based diagnosis. Broth-based culture systems coupled with DNA probes allows rapid (2 or 3 weeks for positive and negative smears, respectively) establishment of a diagnosis.[314,363] In addition, culture-based diagnostics are the only widely available methods by which to assess susceptibility. Technologies for the rapid detection of MDR organisms are still experimental.[24,363,412] Two commercially available kits are available in the United States for diagnosis based on nucleic acid amplification (NAA) assays.[314] They are approved for smear-positive (MTD, GenProbe; Amplicor, Roche) and smear-negative samples (MTD), but there is still some debate on the optimal use of these tests. The American Thoracic Society and the Centers for Disease Control and Prevention have published recommendations,[19,65,363] although they have not been studied in transplant recipients or pediatric populations specifically. Newer modalities such as the microscopic-observation drug susceptibility (MODS) assay may allow rapid, inexpensive diagnosis and susceptibility testing in countries with limited resources.[190,286,314] Finally, new tests exist for the detection of latent MTB: the "QuantiFERON-TB Gold," a whole-blood enzyme-linked immunosorbent assay (ELISA), and "T-SPOT. TB," an ex-vivo enzyme-linked immunospot (ELISpot) assay.[267,339,363] Both assays rely on interferon production from peripheral blood mononuclear cells in response to MTB antigens. The advantage of these tests is they may allow MTB to be distinguished from NTM infection and bacille Calmette-Guérin (BCG) vaccine response. In adults, these tests have higher specificity than TST does, especially with regard to BCG, and may be most useful in low-endemic, high-income settings.[267,313,394] However, their use in young children and immunocompromised patients has not been fully evaluated.[313,394]

Specific guidelines exist for the treatment of MTB in children infected with human immunodeficiency virus (HIV).[15] None is available for pediatric SOTRs, and the optimal therapy has not been defined.[41] Clearly complicating factors include liver toxicity from single- and multiple-drug regimens and drug interactions, most notably between rifampin and CNIs. Isoniazid (INH) alone and in combination with other first-line drugs, such as rifampin and pyrazinamide, can lead to toxicity requiring discontinuation of all or some of these drugs and the need to institute new regimens.[290,383] Drug toxicity is most notable in adult liver transplant recipients. Liver biopsy may be necessary to distinguish drug toxicity from rejection or hepatic granuloma from MTB infection.[290,351,383] Pediatric patients generally tolerate first-line therapy, with occasional need for reduced dosage and rarely discontinuation.[73,269,425]

The use of rifampin in SOTRs remains controversial. Significant morbidity of MTB from graft dysfunction and loss can be due to the simultaneous use of rifampin with CNIs. Rifampin lowers serum levels of cyclosporine and tacrolimus considerably, as well as decreases steroid levels somewhat, via induction of cytochrome P-450. Some authors argue that rifampin can be used successfully with increased CNI dosing and careful monitoring of CNI serum levels.[257,425] Others suggest that a longer duration of therapy (up to 50%) with rifampin-free/INH-containing regimens has a comparable outcome without the risk of rejection and potential graft loss, and they do not recommend the use of rifampin.[46,290] Most authors agree that regimens should contain INH if at all possible.[46,287,290,383] If rifampin-free regimens are used, therapy should be prolonged to a minimum of 12 to 18 months.[46,383] Ethambutol and second-line therapies (aminoglycosides and quinolones) may be considered if a first-line drug cannot be used.[290,351] If both INH and rifampin are not used, therapy should be continued for 2 to 3 years.[350]

Recommendations for chemoprophylaxis of MTB infection are similarly without consensus. Some authors suggest that all SOTRs with a positive TST of 5-mm or greater induration be treated with INH. They reason that the morbidity and mortality from MTB and the potential risk for nosocomial transmission from unidentified patients are high enough to warrant the risk of hepatotoxicity.[383] Others use a staged approach in which INH therapy is initiated in LTRs and other non–liver transplant recipients as soon as possible but deferred in liver recipients until liver function is stable.[290] A third strategy is active surveillance, with initiation of INH only if additional risk factors are present, such as recent conversion, exposure to active MTB, recipient or donor with a history of MTB without adequate therapy, or the existence of significant abnormalities on chest radiographs.[351]

Nontuberculous Mycobacterial Infections

NTM infections are more common occurrences in LTRs in areas where MTB is not endemic, including the United States.[110] NTM organisms are divided into slowly growing species, *Mycobacterium avium* complex (MAC), *Mycobacterium kansasii*, *Mycobacterium marinum*, and *Mycobacterium ulcerans*, and rapid growers, *Mycobacterium fortuitum* group, *Mycobacterium abscessus*, and *Mycobacterium chelonae*.[16] Patients with chronic lung disease and CF in particular have a high incidence of NTM colonization. As many as 24 percent of patients with CF are colonized with NTM organisms, most commonly *M. abscessus* or MAC.[121,305,308,330] The contribution of these organisms to progression of lung disease in pretransplant patients still is being defined.[87,121,156,166,305-307] In one center, 20 percent of patients with end-stage CF referred for transplantation were colonized with NTM organisms, which were isolated from 14 percent of CF LTRs. The prevalence of post-transplant invasive disease was approximately 3 percent.[66] Most authors do not consider that the presence of NTM infection before transplantation should serve as an exclusion to transplantation, but these organisms clearly are responsible for serious and fatal post-transplant infections.[66,74,110,202,257,360,410]

Clinical manifestations of NTM infection in lung transplantation vary by organism and include pulmonary, cutaneous, and disseminated disease.[110] In a survey of transplant centers regarding *M. abscessus* infection in LTRs, the majority had pulmonary infections, followed by skin involvement; several patients had both. Disease occurred at a median of 18.5 months after transplantation (1-110 months). Pulmonary disease may be manifested as chronic cough, sputum production, and fatigue. Skin infections may involve surgical sites (sternal wounds) and the extremities.[66,257] Painful, erythematous cutaneous or subcutaneous nodules may develop into abscesses and ulcerate.[74]

Diagnosis requires a high level of suspicion. Cutaneous lesions should be subjected to biopsy for histology, special stains, and culture. The differential diagnosis includes fungal and nocardial infections. These organisms are ubiquitous, and differentiating respiratory colonization from infection may be difficult. The diagnosis of NTM infection should be entertained, with a low threshold for performing bronchoalveolar lavage (BAL) or biopsy for any unexplained or unresolving pleuropulmonary disease.[110,157] The American Thoracic Society has published diagnostic criteria that include signs and symptoms present after the treatment of other possible diseases, such as radiologic evidence of progressive pulmonary disease, including infiltrates, cavities, nodules or bronchiectasis, and bacteriologic evidence of NTM infection, generally on multiple respiratory specimens or on biopsy.[157]

Providing therapy for NTM infection may be difficult and depends on the species isolated. Most authors recommend combination therapy that includes a macrolide. For MAC, therapy with a macrolide, ethambutol, and rifampin, with or without an aminoglycoside, depending on the severity of disease, is recommended.[157] Therapy for *M. abscessus* is undefined because this organism is notoriously resistant to many antimicrobials. Even regimens based on in vitro susceptibilities may not produce a cure. Combinations that include a macrolide, amikacin, and cefoxitin or a carbapenem, based on susceptibility testing, are general recommendations. Acquired resistance mutations to clarithromycin and amikacin can occur.[157] The duration of therapy is prolonged and depends on the patient's clinical, radiologic, and microbiologic response, but the suggested minimum duration is 12 to 18 months. Reduction of immunosuppression, surgical excision or débridement, and treatment of co-infections may improve the outcome.[74] Relapses are not uncommon. Consideration of lifelong suppression is recommended by some experts for patients with a high burden of disease and persistently high levels of immunosuppression.[110] Most patients who can complete long-term therapy improve (32% cleared their infection, 36% improved); minimal response to therapy was seen in 23 percent of LTRs.[116] Fatal infections occur rarely.[74,360,410] Drug interactions between macrolides and rifampin and CNIs and sirolimus occur. Both can lower serum levels of immunosuppressive drugs and trigger rejection.

The optimal management of patients infected or colonized with NTM organisms before transplantation is debated. A report of 146 patients with CF who underwent lung transplantation found a highly significant association between pretransplant isolation of *M. abscessus* and post-transplant disease, thus suggesting that these patients remain colonized in respiratory tree sites above the anastomosis. The hilar lymph nodes in two patients were positive for *M. abscessus*, thus suggesting other potential reservoirs.[66] Given the concern for emergence of resistance and toxicity related to long-term therapy, prolonged antimycobacterial therapy cannot be recommended for all patients. Some centers opt for pretransplant or peritransplant prophylaxis, whereas others observe for evidence of disease.[110]

FUNGAL INFECTIONS

Aspergillus

Aspergillus infections remain a major challenge to the success of lung transplantation. Manifestations range from semi-invasive tracheobronchitis and BA infections (up to 60% of infections) to invasive pulmonary disease (30%) and, rarely, dissemination to extrapulmonary sites, including the CNS (10%).[139,376] The published incidence of invasive *Aspergillus* (IA) infections varies considerably and probably reflects differences in dates of publication, patient populations that included adults and children, underlying disease such as CF, net state of immunosuppression, use of prophylactic measures, local issues of exposure (e.g., construction), and rates of rejection and viral infection, among others. In addition, distinguishing between isolation of *Aspergillus* from airway cultures versus true invasive disease may be difficult. Despite these caveats, rates of IA infection in LTRs are the highest among SOTRs. Studies suggest that invasive disease occurs in 3 to 33 percent of LTRs, although rates of colonization/isolation of *Aspergillus* may be considerably higher. In most cases, colonization appears to be transient and does not lead to invasive disease.[57,139,148,173,273,283,285,300,376]

Infections usually develop 1 to 6 months after transplantation and are a major cause of death during this time period.[217,273,283,376] Early infections, those that develop less than 3 months after transplantation, are more likely to be tracheobronchitis or BA site infections, whereas invasive pulmonary or disseminated aspergillosis occurs more often in late-onset infections.[376,390] Patients who require retransplantation or have BA infection may present in the first month.[76,162,176,283]

Recent studies have identified different risk factors for the bimodal pattern of the development of IA.[139,375] Risk factors for early disease in LTRs include *Aspergillus* colonization in the 6 months before transplantation or early post-transplant colonization, a complicated postoperative period, and CMV disease.[57,139,173,189,285,300] Corroboration of the importance of CMV is

the observation that a significant decrease in IA was associated with the use of prophylactic ganciclovir in heart transplant recipients. This decrease no doubt reflects the immunomodulating effects of the virus on host immune status.[347,437] Patients in whom IA infection developed later than 3 months after transplantation were older (<50 years); "overimmunosuppressed" with the use of sirolimus, tacrolimus, or both for chronic or refractory graft rejection or dysfunction; or both older and overimmunosuppressed.[139,378] In both the early and late groups, IA was associated with renal failure and repeated bacterial infections.

Aspergillus fumigatus causes the majority of disease, although non-*fumigatus* species are becoming more common.[57,273] Such species include *Aspergillus flavus*, *Aspergillus niger*, *Aspergillus nodularis*, *Aspergillus ustus*, and *Aspergillus terreus*. This change may be important because of the recognized potential for differences in antifungal susceptibility of some non-*fumigatus* species. For example, *A. terreus* is innately resistant to amphotericin B, and *A. ustus* has diminished susceptibility to the azoles.[32]

Clinical findings in patients with pulmonary disease are largely nonspecific and may include cough, shortness of breath, and hypoxia, although chest pain and occasionally hemoptysis may raise clinical suspicion of IA.[84,272] Symptoms are seen more commonly in patients with diffuse disease than in those with focal or nodular disease.[95] Although fever is a common early manifestation of IA in neutropenic hematology patients,[95] it occurred in only 15 percent of LTRs with *Aspergillus* infection and usually more often in patients with disseminated (50%) or invasive pulmonary disease (20%) than in those with tracheobronchial or BA infections (0%).[376] Lack of fever also has been documented in other studies of non-neutropenic patients with IA.[84,272] Patients with disseminated disease may have involvement of the sinuses, orbits, musculoskeletal system (osteomyelitis), ophthalmologic structures, cutaneous sites, and CNS. Symptoms of CNS disease may include headache, sinus pain, cranial nerve abnormalities, seizures, changes in mental status, or other focal neurologic findings.[32,95,148]

The radiologic manifestation of IA in LTRs is highly variable.[95,104,369,414] Chest radiographs are highly insensitive and nonspecific for IA. Computed tomography (CT) of the chest has become an integral part of early diagnostic strategies and has been incorporated into recent definitions of invasive fungal infections in immunocompromised hosts.[25] On chest CT scans of neutropenic adults, large nodules and cavitary lesions are common findings.[25,95,155] In addition, much has been made of the early "halo sign," a macronodule surrounded by a perimeter of ground-glass opacity (edema and hemorrhage), and the later "air crescent sign," a crescent-shaped air interface between viable lung and infarcted tissue at the periphery of a nodule, seen with recovery and return of neutrophils. These findings are considered highly suggestive, though not pathognomonic, of IA.[25,59,155] Unfortunately, these findings are seen less commonly in LTRs and in children in general. Multiple ill-defined pulmonary nodules were the most common findings in adult LTRs, with approximately half demonstrating halo signs. Cavitation was rarely seen, and no air crescent signs were observed.[84,104] In a review of immunocompromised children with IA, radiographic findings were highly variable and included consolidations and small nodular masses and effusions, with little evidence of cavitation and no halo or crescent signs.[414]

The gold standard for diagnosis of IA is the demonstration of small hyaline, septate, dichotomously branched hyphae in tissue with evidence of associated tissue damage or positive cultures from a normally sterile body site in the face of signs and symptoms of invasive disease in an immunocompromised host.[25,32,95,179] Blood cultures rarely are positive and, therefore, are not helpful. Unfortunately, obtaining adequate tissue specimens in a timely manner frequently is not possible. An immunocompromised patient with neutropenia or taking steroids may not exhibit obvious signs or symptoms of invasive disease until late in the course of infection.[6] Additionally, these patients often are deemed too ill to undergo the invasive procedures necessary to obtain tissue for culture.[384] Therefore, the diagnosis is established late in the course of the disease or at autopsy. Indeed, frequently it is not established but is based on radiology and host factors.

Early diagnosis is thought to be critical to improving the outcome of patients with IA, especially now with the availability of more active therapeutic agents and the possibility of combination therapy. In addition to early and frequent CT scanning in high-risk patients, especially those who do not respond to broad-spectrum antibiotics, several recent advances have been achieved in molecular/non–culture-based approaches to establishing a diagnosis. The most widely used and well characterized of these modalities is the Platelia *Aspergillus* serum galactomannan antigen, detected by double-sandwich ELISA.[276,277,403,452,454] This test detects very small amounts of a polysaccharide cell wall component of *Aspergillus* and other fungal species that is released into blood with invasive growth in tissues. A positive test (<0.5 ng/mL) requires confirmation by a second sample for diagnosis. False-positive tests have been documented, notably in patients receiving piperacillin-tazobactam,[3,26,246,250,382,406,435,444] which may be related to cross reactions to *Penicillium* spp.–derived semisynthetic penicillins,[404] although this theory has not been proved conclusively. In general, false-positive tests result in transient and low-positive findings.[276,452] Pediatric patients appear to have higher rates of false positivity,[175,342,405] but the mechanism for this observation remains unclear. Previous antifungal therapy has been shown to decrease the sensitivity of the assay.[258,261,342]

In controlled trials, twice-a-week galactomannan screening of very-high-risk adults with hematologic malignancies and hematopoietic stem cell transplant (HSCT) recipients had high sensitivity and specificity and allowed the diagnosis of IA to be established, often many days before the development of fever and CT findings, with the potential for initiating early therapy.[252-254,258] The addition of galactomannan testing to early CT scans also was found to be helpful in establishing the diagnosis of IA.[55,251,342] The galactomannan assay has been incorporated into recent diagnostic criteria for the diagnosis of IA in immunocompromised patients with cancer and in HSCT recipients.[25] To date, no studies have documented a survival advantage in patients with early diagnosis by galactomannan testing.

In SOTRs and non-neutropenic patients, this test appears to be less sensitive.[129,183,223,327,426] For example, twice-a-week screening of 70 consecutive LTRs, with IA documented in 17.1 percent, revealed a sensitivity of 30 percent and a specificity of 95 percent.[183] False-negative results occurred most commonly in patients with tracheobronchitis, followed by pulmonary disease, versus patients with disseminated disease. Two of five patients with pulmonary *Aspergillus* and negative tests had received antifungals previously. False-positive results occurred in 36 tests on 14 patients, with a median value of 0.868; consecutive positive tests were seen in 5 patients. The majority of these results occurred in the first 2 weeks after transplantation. None of these patients was receiving piperacillin-tazobactam.

Finally, use of the galactomannan assay for specimens other than serum is being evaluated for cerebrospinal fluid (CSF) and BAL fluid.[35,208,247,292,361,436] Assays on these fluids appear to be more sensitive and to offer some advantage in certain patient populations, such as non-neutropenic SOTRs, although controlled clinical trials have not been published. False-positive galactomannan results have been linked to the use of Plasmalyte (Baxter) for lavage fluid instead of normal saline.[163] The product contains gluconate, which is produced by fermentation in *A. niger* and results from contamination of small amounts of galactomannan by this process.

Several other molecular-based methods for detection that are being investigated include the Fungitell beta-glucan assay, which measures a cell wall component found in many fungi, including *Aspergillus* and *Candida* spp., and, like the galactomannan assay, does not detect zygomycetes.[201,284,301,310,325] It is approved by the Food and Drug Administration (FDA) and is available in kit form. Cross-reacting glucan-containing material occurs commonly in the environment, and false-positive tests have been demonstrated in patients maintained on dialysis or exposed to gauze and with gram-positive bacteremia. In addition, false-positive results are associated with the use of some antimicrobials and with sample manipulation, thus suggesting that laboratory contamination is possible.[106,179,264,325,328,454]

The *Aspergillus* polymerase chain reaction (PCR) remains nonstandardized, but most assays rely on detection of fungal sequences of 18S or 28S rRNA or mitochondrial genes in whole blood, plasma, serum, or BAL fluid.* More recent protocols have used real-time PCR, which allows rapid, automated, quantitative, and reliable results, with less chance of contamination.† Clinical information is limited on both these methods. No studies have been published on the use of these tests in SOTRs, but some show promise in febrile neutropenic cancer patients and HSCT recipients. The optimal clinical specimen and PCR protocol have yet to be established.

Several studies have compared the use of these three methods.[48,52,201,292,325,361] No reproducible results suggest that one test is convincingly or consistently better than the others. Several authors suggest that combining two methodologies may improve diagnostic reliability.[48,85,109,281,292,325,361]

Despite historically poor outcomes of IA in immunocompromised patients, new mold-active therapies appear to be improving mortality figures.[40] The Infectious Diseases Society of America (IDSA) practice guidelines for *Aspergillus* infections, published in 2008, recommends therapy with voriconazole as primary therapy for most patients,[445a] as it has demonstrated superiority.[27,97,174] Additionally, voriconazole has shown promise for treatment of CNS disease, which historically has been uniformly fatal.[174,364,442] Lipid formulations of amphotericin B can be recommended as alternative therapy for patients unable to receive voriconazole. For patients refractory to or intolerant of primary therapy, lipid formulations of amphotericin B, itraconazole, and caspofungin are FDA approved for treatment of IA. Other antimicrobials that have activity against *Aspergillus* include posaconazole and other echinocandins, although these are not approved for this indication.

Most data on the use of voriconazole for IA involved adult HSCT recipients and patients with leukemia, although some studies contained small numbers of pediatric patients and SOTRs. The paucity of data in these groups is important for several reasons. The optimal dosing for pediatric patients remains unclear, and much higher doses than currently recommended probably may be tolerated and beneficial.[396,441] This dosing information is currently under investigation.[396] In addition, several important drug interactions occur with medications routinely used in SOTRs. The most important of these interactions involve tacrolimus and sirolimus, in which concomitant use with voriconazole can lead to decreased metabolism, via cytochrome P-450 3A4/5 (CYP3A4/5), and result in greatly increased serum levels of the immunosuppressant.[354] The use of tacrolimus can be controlled safely by reducing the dose by 50 percent generally and monitoring daily levels.[354,424] The effect of voriconazole on sirolimus levels is even more pronounced, and it is labeled as an absolute contraindication by the manufacturer.[354,356] Several case reports/small series describe the use of these two drugs together, with significant dose reduction of sirolimus (up to 90%) and close follow-up of serum sirolimus levels.[263,266,356] The second azole to be approved for use by the FDA recently is posaconazole, which

*See references 51, 118, 165, 168, 196, 226, 244, 386, 420, 460.
†See references 47, 67, 86, 197, 198, 201, 207, 292, 361, 392, 457, 458.

is available only in an oral formulation. Currently, based on several randomized multicenter studies, it is licensed for prophylaxis of invasive fungal disease in patients with fever and neutropenia and those with chronic graft-versus-host disease.[82,418] Posaconazole also has been used for the treatment of *Aspergillus* in patients refractory or intolerant of other therapy, most of these patients having received an amphotericin product or itraconazole.[215,365,443] The use of posaconazole as primary therapy for IA currently is being investigated. Azoles are generally well tolerated. Unique events associated with voriconazole include transient visual disturbances (photopsia) and cutaneous photosensitivity. Both drugs have been associated with hepatic toxicity, which can be fatal.[108,174]

The polyenes AmBD and its lipid formulation (LFAB) are active against *Aspergillus* spp., except for *A. terreus*, and exert their activity on the cell membrane. AmBD was the "gold standard for serious fungal infections for almost 40 years" but now has been supplanted by newer, more effective and less toxic agents, including the azoles, echinocandins, and LFAB. The recent consensus suggests that LFAB may be more effective than AmBD is in certain settings and is clearly less toxic. LFAB and posaconazole are the most broad-spectrum antifungals and are the only agents active against zygomycetes.[108] One of these drugs should be used singly or in combination if the diagnosis of a zygomycelial infection, which can be clinically indistinguishable from IA and equally fatal, is being considered.

Echinocandins have a unique mode of activity; they inhibit the biosynthesis of 1,3-β-glucan in the fungal cell wall, which is absent in mammalian cells, thus offering a high therapeutic index.[108] Moreover, fewer notable drug interactions have occurred. Initial reports suggested that concomitant use of caspofungin, the first licensed echinocandin, with cyclosporine caused increased hepatotoxicity, although subsequent studies did not substantiate this interaction.[108,260] Caspofungin has been demonstrated to be useful in and has been licensed for the treatment of IA in patients refractory to or intolerant of other therapies[249] and for empiric antifungal therapy in patients with fever and neutropenia.[445] Several studies have addressed the safety, efficacy, and dosing of caspofungin in pediatric patients.[130,159,278,302,440] All studies have found caspofungin to be safe and well tolerated in children, even neonates. As was seen with voriconazole, extrapolation of pediatric dosing from adult dosing led to underdosing of caspofungin, which has been revised on the basis of pediatric pharmacokinetic data.[440] No prospective data on the efficacy of caspofungin for IA in immunocompromised pediatric patients have been published, although two small retrospective studies (64 and 25 patients), consisting mostly of children with leukemia, showed promising results with caspofungin, either alone for less aggressive disease or in combination with voriconazole for first-line therapy.[159,278] A second echinocandin, micafungin, also has been licensed recently for prophylaxis of *Candida* infections in HSCT recipients and for treatment of esophageal candidiasis.[103,421] Randomized, controlled data on the use of micafungin for primary treatment of IA are lacking. Several reports of high-risk patients (HSCT recipients, hematologic malignancy) suggest that it is useful, either alone or in combination, in the setting of refractory IA.[68,96,209] Some studies included small numbers of children, who appeared to have similar success rates. In an assessment of its safety, tolerability, and pharmacokinetics in febrile, neutropenic children, dose-limiting toxicity did not occur with doses of 4 mg/kg/day or lower, and young children cleared the drug up to 1.5 times faster than older children and adults did.[367] Optimal dosing regimens are still under investigation. A final echinocandin, anidulafungin, has been approved for the treatment of candidal infection.[423] It also has potent in vitro activity against *Aspergillus*. A unique property of anidulafungin is that its pharmacokinetics is similar across a variety of patient populations, including children, which suggests that dose adjustments are not

necessary. The drug appears to have an excellent safety profile, with minimal drug-drug interactions. Its use in the treatment of IA has yet to be defined, but most likely it will be similar to other echinocandins.

Combination therapy remains controversial. Advantages of combination therapy include possible synergistic interaction of two drugs with different targets, lower doses leading to less toxicity, greater spectrum of activity, and decreased potential for the development of resistance.[234] Potential disadvantages include antagonistic antifungal activity, increased overall drug interactions, enhanced toxicity when adding new agents, and great increases in cost.[194,288,434]

Preclinical data from in vitro and animal studies investigating the use of combinations of antifungal agents against *Aspergillus* are generally promising.[194,288,397,399,434] Complexities and differences in methodologies used to determine in vitro efficacy, experimental design, and animal models confound interpretation of the data and render extrapolating to patients difficult.[288,397,399,453]

The comparator to combination therapy in most clinical data to date is primary therapy with LFAB, not voriconazole, which is now considered the drug of choice for IA. Combination treatment also has been studied for salvage therapy in patients who have already failed therapy; however, most studies are retrospective.[96,211,212,248,259,297,320,377,399] Preferred combinations include azoles (voriconazole or posaconazole) with echinocandins (caspofungin or micafungin).

A single prospective multicenter observational study has evaluated combination therapy in SOTRs.[377] Forty transplant recipients (13 lung transplants, or 33%) received voriconazole and caspofungin as primary therapy for IA (2003 to 2005); 47 patients (9 lung transplants, or 19%) received LFAB (1999 to 2002). A trend toward decreased mortality rates at 90 days in the combination group was noted, and subset analysis demonstrated that in transplant recipients with renal failure or *A. fumigatus* infection, combination therapy was associated with improved 90-day survival ($p = 0.04$ and $p = 0.03$, respectively). No patient required discontinuation because of side effects or intolerance. These authors note that currently, "combination therapy constitutes our standard for the therapy of invasive aspergillosis."[291] Data from prospective, randomized trials in which voriconazole is compared with combinations that include voriconazole still are needed to evaluate first-line therapy. Many authors recommend caution in using combination therapy before the results of controlled, prospective investigations are available, even though they acknowledge that widespread use of combination therapy already is evident.[30,194,288,397,399,434]

No definitive data are available on how long to treat IA, although the natural history of disease, assessment of risk factors, and the state and length of immunosuppression, along with investigations on response to therapy and animal studies, can inform us on regimens most likely to be effective. Clearly, one must balance the risk of incomplete therapy and recurrent disease with the dangers of increased toxicity and expense from prolonged therapy. One thoughtful approach, based on these many variables, suggests use of the "most effective therapy first for 10 to 12 weeks, or for at least 4 to 6 weeks beyond resolution of all clinical and radiographic abnormalities, whichever is longer."[372] Length of therapy should be individualized, and factors such as recovery from neutropenia or other immunocompromised state, extent of disease, presence of graft-versus-host disease, and co-infections (e.g., CMV) predict poorer outcome and slower response and probably will prolong duration of therapy for patients with these comorbid findings.

In terms of adjunctive therapy, surgery may be recommended for cutaneous and soft tissue infections,[171] for lesions on the great vessels or major airways to prevent massive hemoptysis[37,58,60,312] in patients with endophthalmitis[447] and osteomyelitis,[205] and for removal of remove of residual lesions before hematopoietic stem cell transplantation is performed. Immunomodulatory strategies that improve host immune response, in theory, are attractive adjuvant therapies. Alveolar macrophages, polymorphonuclear neutrophils, and pulmonary dendritic cells are critical first-line defenses against IA.[344] Therefore, modalities that improve the number or function of these cells may improve outcome. Decreasing the use of immunosuppression and steroids as much as possible should be the goal in transplant recipients with IA. Additional strategies, including enhancement of T_H1 immune responses, exogenous administration of colony-stimulating factors (granulocyte colony-stimulating factor [G-CSF], granulocyte-macrophage colony-stimulating factor [GM-CSF]) or cytokines (interferon-γ) to activate or recruit phagocytes (or both), G-CSF donor-primed white blood cell transfusions, and augmentation of innate pathogen recognition pathways (toll-like receptors, pentraxins), all still are investigational.[137,140,343,366,398,400] Finally, vaccine strategies and adoptive immunotherapy have shown promise in animal models of IA and await further refinement and clinical trials.[43-46,64,366]

When *Aspergillus* causes invasive disease, mortality rates are high (30% to 100%) and notably so for invasive and disseminated forms of the infection.[57,139,273,390] In a review of English language articles on *Aspergillus* infections in LTRs, the overall mortality rate was 53 percent (59/112), 24 percent (9/38) for tracheobronchial or BA infections, 82 percent (18/22) in patients with invasive pulmonary disease, and 67 percent (2/3) for disseminated invasive infection.[376] These published data are on adult patients (19-64 years old) and reflect the limited therapeutic options previously available (before the advent of extended-spectrum azoles and echinocandins). Somewhat surprisingly, several studies in which the mortality of IA in neutropenic patients was compared with that of non-neutropenic patients found a comparable or higher incidence of mortality in the latter group.[84,272] Authors speculate that a lower index of suspicion may delay establishing the diagnosis and that suboptimal monitoring or lack of the use of *Aspergillus* active fungal prophylaxis may lead to high mortality rates.

Despite the lack of controlled trials, two surveys document that most lung transplant centers in the United States and worldwide use prophylactic or preemptive systemic antifungals (itraconazole or amphotericin formulations), aerosolized amphotericin formulations, or both in patients with preoperative or postoperative isolation of airway *Aspergillus*.[113,188] Because *Aspergillus* infections are acquired through the lungs and most infections are pulmonary, attaining high pulmonary drug levels via aerosolization and limiting systemic toxicity are attractive options for prevention.[384] Several nonrandomized, non–placebo-controlled trials have suggested a reduction in IA infections with the use of aerosolized amphotericin formulations.[61,111,112,176,283,285,316,338] A single retrospective study incorporating the use of voriconazole prophylaxis in LTRs has been published.[184] This study compared targeted itraconazole prophylaxis, with or without inhaled amphotericin, in patients colonized by *Aspergillus* preoperatively or postoperatively with universal voriconazole for a minimum of 4 months. The rate of IA at 1 year was 1.5 percent in patients receiving voriconazole versus 23.5 percent in the other group. In addition, there was a significant delay in *Aspergillus* colonization in patients receiving voriconazole, thereby permitting healing of the BA, and a considerable decrement in immunosuppressive therapy in most patients by that time. Abnormalities in liver enzymes were common findings; twice as many patients had to discontinue antifungal therapy in the voriconazole group because of side effects. All liver enzymes returned to normal within 2 months of terminating therapy. Finally, interactions with CNIs need to be managed by decreasing doses and monitoring serum levels of tacrolimus. Based on two phase III studies, posaconazole appears to be the drug of choice for prophylaxis of invasive fungal infections in certain high-risk patient populations.[82,418] The generalizability of these findings to SOTRs has not been examined.

Further randomized, multicenter studies are needed to clarify which agents and prophylactic strategies are most effective.

Prevention of IA through environmental controls also is important.[319,324,336] Cases of IA in transplant recipients can be nosocomial or community acquired. Most germane to prevention is air control inasmuch as both epidemic IA and sporadic IA correlate with concentrations of *Aspergillus* in the air.[5] A protective hospital environment should consist of high-efficiency particulate air (HEPA) filtration, positive air pressure, high air exchange rate, properly sealed rooms, and removal of carpets, plants, and water-damaged ceiling and floor tiles.[83,116,164,324,413] In addition, the environment and air should be monitored frequently for changes in particulates and fungal spores. Patients should be wearing "fit-tested" masks (N95) when leaving protected environments, effort should be made to have construction barriers in place, and patient transport routes should be adjusted accordingly if construction is occurring in the hospital and clinics.[319] When patients are discharged home, they should be counseled to avoid certain high-risk exposure to agents such as dust and mold if possible.[324]

Candida

Candida infections in LTRs often occur early, within the first month, in the form of BSI; urinary tract infections, especially if indwelling catheters remain in place; respiratory tract infections (tracheitis); pneumonia; and, rarely, BA site infections. Although colonization of the respiratory tract is a common occurrence, primary invasive candidal pneumonia is not. Invasion usually occurs when comorbid conditions are present.[217] Rarely, disseminated disease of abdominal organs and the CNS occurs.[321] The source of infection usually is endogenous, although contributions from donor organs also are possible. Risk factors for candidal infections in transplant recipients include surgical complications, use of broad-spectrum antibiotics, CMV infection, and indwelling foreign bodies.[217,321]

The diagnosis of candidal infection can be challenging and requires differentiating colonization from infection because *Candida* spp. are ubiquitous, especially in the upper GI and respiratory tracts. Although the diagnosis of most candidal infections is made by culture, these techniques are insensitive and, except for blood culture, nonspecific. If recovery of *Candida* spp. from BAL fluid is associated with respiratory symptoms or deterioration of lung function (e.g., increased sputum production), treatment should be considered, although other causes such as rejection and co-infections should be taken into account. *Candida* in the blood should be treated, and indwelling catheters should be removed as soon as feasible. Organisms should be identified to the species level because of species-specific susceptibility profiles. Early germ tube determination can confirm the presence of *Candida albicans*, and a negative test can alert the physician to the presence of non-*albicans* species, which may have an impact on the choice of antifungal agent.[321] Newer molecular probes, such as PNA FISH, can identify *C. albicans* rapidly from positive blood cultures.[7]

The Fungitell beta-glucan assay measures a cell wall component of many fungi, including *Candida* spp., and, therefore, is not specific for *Candida*. It has been FDA-approved as an adjunct for the diagnosis of invasive *Candida*, although its role in the early diagnosis of these infections is under investigation.[321] Use of the serum galactomannan antigen assay and PCR techniques shows some promise, but these techniques are still experimental, and the ubiquity of *Candida* increases concern about contamination with PCR.[133,321] The usefulness of these tests in LTRs with candidal infections is currently unknown.

The choice of agent for the treatment of *Candida* infections has become more complicated; non-*albicans Candida* spp. are becoming more prevalent, as are azole-resistant *C. albicans* isolates.[321,336] *Candida krusei* is innately resistant to fluconazole and itraconazole, whereas *Candida glabrata* has variable susceptibility to these drugs. Voriconazole and posaconazole are likely to be effective. Treatment failures have been noted with the use of echinocandin therapy for *Candida parapsilosis* infections, and some *Candida lusitaniae* strains may be resistant to polyene antifungals.[108] Putative risk factors for infections with these organisms include widespread use of fluconazole, prolonged pretransplant hospitalization, and long-term use of broad-spectrum antibiotics. The choice of initial antifungal therapy should be based on azole exposure, susceptibility profiles, dominant species at the institution caring for the patient, comorbid conditions, sites of involvement, and the use of other medications that might have significant drug-drug interactions.[321] Fluconazole is appropriate for *C. albicans* infections in moderately ill patients. For severely ill or hemodynamically unstable patients or for those with suspected or proven *C. glabrata* or *C. krusei* infection, the use of LFAB or an echinocandin is preferred. Alternative agents include the newer azoles voriconazole and posaconazole. Duration of therapy, as with other infections, should be individualized, but treatment should be continued for at least several weeks after the last positive culture has been obtained and the signs and symptoms have resolved.[322] As noted earlier for *Aspergillus* infections, issues of dosing in pediatrics with the newer antifungals and drug-drug interactions should be considered. Several excellent resources are available for detailed treatment algorithms.[321,322,391] Updated IDSA guidelines for the treatment of candidal infections are expected in 2007. Antifungal susceptibility testing should be considered on non-*albicans Candida* spp. and for *C. albicans* infections that are refractory to conventional therapy. Interpretive breakpoints are available for most common antifungals, although those for the echinocandins still are being determined.[6,13,321]

Cryptococcus

Though relatively rare, cryptococcosis is the third most common fungal infection seen in solid organ transplantation, after *Aspergillus* and *Candida*.[430] Disease can be newly acquired, reactivated from latent disease, or derived from the donor organ.[147,187,464] Although meningitis generally is thought to be the most common manifestation of cryptococcal disease,[187,464] two recent studies suggest that in SOTRs, CNS disease and pulmonary disease are equally common occurrences.[374,430,433] Disseminated disease also is a common finding (61% of cases) and is most likely to be seen in liver transplant recipients and least likely in LTRs.[374] Infection occurs less frequently in pediatric patients than in adults[385] and more commonly in the northeastern United States than in other locations.[430] It is most common in heart and liver transplant recipients and least common in LTRs.[430,433,464] Additional unique properties of cryptococcal infections appear to be seen in the SOTR population, notably an intriguing relationship between the immunosuppressive regimen and clinical findings. A review of published reports of cryptococcal infections in transplant recipients and a prospective multicenter study suggest that patients receiving CNI-based immunosuppressive therapy were less likely to acquire CNS disease and had lower mortality rates.[187,374] A proposed mechanism for protection of this site is the temperature-dependent antifungal activity of CNIs, which suppresses fungal growth at 37° C but not at 24° C, coupled with the high level of CNS penetration by tacrolimus.[187] Additionally, these authors suggest that cutaneous infections may appear more like bacterial cellulitis than the typical molluscum contagiosum–like lesions seen in HIV-infected patients.[187,385] Finally, an immune reconstitution syndrome that correlates with the evolving host response to infection also has been described in SOTRs with cryptococcosis,[381] and it may be associated with allograft loss, as described in renal transplant recipients.[380]

The diagnosis can be made by culture, visualization of encapsulated yeast with India ink or other special stains, and cryptococcal capsular polysaccharide antigen in serum or CSF.[72] Serum cryptococcal antigen is most reliable for CNS and disseminated disease but not for pulmonary infection.[430,433]

The mainstay of therapy for severe, disseminated disease with CNS involvement remains combination induction therapy with an amphotericin-containing regimen plus flucytosine.[355,379] Therapy should continue for an extended period because relapses are well documented, especially in HIV-infected patients. The risk of relapse in SOTRs and the optimal length of therapy are not known. Suppressive therapy with fluconazole for 6 to 12 months has been suggested after induction therapy.[355] Duration of treatment less than 6 months has been associated with an increased rate of relapse.[379] Management of elevated intracranial pressure also should be considered.[72] For less severe disease localized to the lungs, fluconazole alone may be adequate.[355,379] Mortality rates vary by site of infection and type of transplant and possibly by immunosuppressive regimen. The overall mortality rate for cryptococcal disease in SOTRs is 14 to 30 percent. The highest rates are seen in liver and kidney transplant recipients with disseminated disease or fungemia, or both (20-70%). The lowest mortality rates (3-13%) are seen in localized pulmonary disease.[374,433,464]

Pneumocystis jiroveci (Formerly Pneumocystis carinii)

Pneumocystis pneumoniae (PCP) infections are caused by the renamed fungal pathogen *Pneumocystis jiroveci*.[402] PCP has been associated notably with defects in T-cell immunity, as in HIV infection, in patients with leukemia, and with the immunosuppression used in SOTRs. It also is described in patients with other immune defects, including those associated with steroid use and radiation therapy, neutropenia, and congenital immunodeficiency.[341] Serologic data suggest universal, albeit asymptomatic, infection occurs by the time the patient is 4 years of age. In most cases, symptomatic PCP in an immunocompromised host is thought to be reactivation of latent infection, although person-to-person transmission also may occur.[93]

Heart-lung recipients and LTRs are at increased risk for developing infection, with reported attack rates of 6.5 to 43 percent without prophylaxis, up to a 10-fold increase from heart transplants alone.[341] Higher rates of infection in LTRs have been associated with CMV co-infection, use of cyclosporine and steroids, and receipt of therapy for rejection. In addition, cases can occur many years after transplantation. Therefore, many experts suggest the benefit of long-term and perhaps lifelong prophylaxis, especially if additional risk factors are ongoing.[332,341] The drug of choice for prophylaxis remains TMP-SMX, and its use is associated with dramatic decreases in the incidence of PCP infection. Additional benefits of this drug include prevention of many community-acquired respiratory, GI, and urinary tract pathogens and protection against most *Toxoplasma gondii* and *Nocardia* infections. Multiple regimens exist, and 3-day/wk dosing appears to be as effective as is daily dosing in all populations studied. Toxicity remains an issue for some patients and includes bone marrow suppression, decreased renal function, hepatitis, and rash/Stevens-Johnson syndrome, which may be severe. Alternative regimens exist for patients intolerant of TMP-SMX, but they should be considered second line because of breakthrough PCP infection or diminished coverage of non-PCP pathogens mentioned earlier. Such alternatives include pentamidine, dapsone, atovaquone, and clindamycin/pyrimethamine. Details of these regimens have been reviewed recently.[341]

PCP infection is manifested as progressive dyspnea, cough, tachypnea, chest pain, and cyanosis over the course of days to weeks. In addition, fevers, sweats, and flulike symptoms may be prominent. Hypoxia and shortness of breath, in the context of normal or minimal findings on chest radiographs, are common findings. Steroids and CNIs may alter the signs and symptoms and render early diagnosis more difficult to establish. The diagnosis is confirmed by identification of *P. jiroveci* in respiratory samples or lung tissue. Immunofluorescent staining of organisms with monoclonal antibodies is the technique of choice; Gomori methenamine silver nitrate, which stains cyst forms only (5-10% of the total organisms), is the most reliable staining method.[332] BAL fluid and tissue obtained by open lung biopsy are preferred specimens because they have the highest diagnostic yield.[341] Newer molecular techniques, including PCR, are promising but are nonstandardized and not commercially available.[114,238]

The mainstay of therapy for severe PCP infection remains high-dose TMP-SMX for 14 to 21 days.[126] Therapy can be continued through mild adverse events, such as rash and minimal perturbations in transaminases and complete blood counts. Dose reduction, desensitization, or both may be helpful, and renal dosing should be implemented if renal dysfunction is present. Steroids may be added for severe disease.[332] For patients intolerant of TMP-SMX or those less seriously ill, alternative therapies can be used. Second-line drugs are dapsone with trimethoprim, atovaquone, and intravenous pentamidine. Third-line therapies include trimetrexate, clindamycin/primaquine, and pyrimethamine/sulfadiazine, as well as several others under study.[126] Relapse in patients without acquired immunodeficiency syndrome (AIDS) is an uncommon occurrence with TMP-SMX therapy if a reduction in immunosuppression can be accomplished and co-infections such as CMV do not occur.[126]

Endemic Mycoses

Cases of endemic mycoses—histoplasmosis, blastomycosis, and coccidioidomycosis—causing disease in SOTRs have been reported. Infection may be caused by latent reactivated disease or by donor-derived and newly acquired infections. Because of the nonspecific findings, latency of these organisms, increased worldwide travel, and organ procurement from different parts of the country, infections in transplant recipients may be difficult to recognize, especially if they occur in nonendemic areas.

Coccidioidomycosis, caused by *Coccidioides immitis* and *Coccidioides posadasii*, is the endemic mycosis most commonly seen after transplantation. It occurs in as many as 9 percent of SOTRs in endemic areas of the southwestern United States (especially California and Arizona), northern Mexico, and Central America.[40] Unlike histoplasmosis and blastomycosis, pretransplant infection poses an increased risk for development of post-transplant disease. In addition, if secondary prophylaxis is not given, the mortality rate is very high (70%).[40] Pulmonary infections may be accompanied by an acute onset of respiratory symptoms and fever and progress rapidly to respiratory failure. Nonspecific symptoms of anorexia, weight loss, and fatigue may herald extrapulmonary disease. Dissemination to bones, skin, and the CNS occurs commonly. The time of highest risk appears to be in the first 3 months after transplantation, with the majority of infections occurring by 1 year. Donor-derived coccidioidomycosis has been established in LTRs and liver and renal organ recipients.[280,415,463] None of the patients had evidence of pretransplant coccidioidomycosis, and none lived or traveled to endemic areas. Several of the donors had documented epidemiologic risk factors. These patients all had fulminant pulmonary or disseminated infection within the first 2 weeks after undergoing transplantation. Three of the four infections were fatal.

The diagnosis of coccidioidomycosis can be made definitively by culture, usually from respiratory samples or urine and rarely from blood or CSF.[20] Histopathologic evaluation may reveal large spherules with the presence of endospores. Serologic tests also are available and include tube-precipitin antigen (IgM), which can be detected early in disease, and complementation fixation (IgG), which arises later in the course of infection and is helpful in monitoring response to therapy.[20,40] Immunocompromised patients

may have negative serologic findings. Skin testing for delayed hypersensitivity no longer is available in the United States. The optimal therapy for SOTRs with coccidioidomycosis is unknown. Most experts suggest that patients with rapidly progressive, nonmeningeal disease should receive amphotericin B–based therapy until stabilized, followed by a prolonged course of azole therapy (fluconazole, itraconazole, possibly voriconazole or posaconazole). For meningitis, high-dose azoles are indicated, probably lifelong. Patients with evidence of previous infection should receive secondary prophylaxis with azole therapy for a minimum of 6 to 12 months after undergoing transplantation.[20,40,135]

Histoplasmosis capsulatum infection is a rare occurrence after transplantation, even in patients with presumed pretransplant infection. Cases have been observed in conjunction with outbreaks in areas hyperendemic for histoplasmosis, the Mississippi and Ohio River valleys and Central America.[419] Two cases of histoplasmosis in renal transplant recipients were linked by molecular typing to donor-derived disease.[236] Manifestations include pulmonary, mediastinal, inflammatory, and disseminated syndromes with or without CNS involvement.[455] The diagnosis can be made by culture, histopathology, serology, or antigen detection.[455] In immunosuppressed patients with disseminated disease, urine antigen detection and culture appear to be the most useful (sensitivity of 80%).[451] Long-term therapy (3 to 4 months) with LFAB generally is recommended for immunocompromised patients with disseminated or CNS involvement, followed by 6 to 12 months of itraconazole or posaconazole.[450,455] Monitoring antigen levels is beneficial to assess response to therapy and relapse.[451]

Blastomycosis dermatitidis, the causative agent of blastomycosis, appears to be even more uncommon in the post-transplant setting. Indeed, it is a rare event in series of fungal infections in immunocompromised patients, including patients with AIDS, even in endemic areas of the south central and north central United States. Several case reports of post-transplant disease have been described. Manifestations can involve pulmonary, cutaneous, and disseminated disease with or without CNS involvement.[200,368] Most immunocompromised patients should receive an amphotericin-containing regimen until stabilized, followed by a prolonged course (6-12 months) of an azole. Most data are available for itraconazole, although voriconazole and posaconazole also may be effective.[71,200]

Emerging non-*Aspergillus* Mycelial Fungi

The impact of non-*Aspergillus* mycelial fungi is currently unknown for LTRs. Published reports suggest that these mold infections are becoming increasingly common. These organisms include non-*Aspergillus* hyalohyphomycetes, or hyaline hyphae without pigment (*Scedosporium apiospermum*, *Fusarium* spp.); phaeohyphomycetes, or dematiaceous pigmented molds (*Cladophialophora bantaina*, *Scedosporium prolificans*, *Exophiala jeanselmei*, *Pyrenochaeta romeroi*, *Cladosporium* spp.); and zygomycetes, or nonseptated hyphae (*Rhizopus* spp., *Mucor* spp.). All have been described in SOTRs.[182] Many of these organisms have unique susceptibility profiles and thus are less amenable to conventional antifungal agents. The newer azoles, voriconazole and posaconazole, show some promise for therapy.[108] Indeed, these infections may be more likely to be disseminated and fatal than those caused by *Aspergillus* spp.[182]

VIRAL INFECTIONS

Cytomegalovirus

The epidemiology of CMV in SOTRs has changed in recent years. Advances in diagnosis and in preemptive and prophylactic strategies and therapy have decreased the impact of early CMV in transplant populations. However, it remains one of the most important pathogens in SOTRs, with wide-ranging effects on morbidity and mortality. The source of infection can be endogenous reactivation, or it can be carried by the donor graft or leukocyte-containing blood products and cause primary infection or re-infection. Rarely, primary infection may be acquired from the community.[346]

The publication of definitions has helped standardize studies on rates of CMV and the impact of therapy.[242] The effects of the virus have both profound direct and indirect consequences.[242,346,466] Direct effects of the virus range from CMV infection, which can be detected by viremia (culture positive), antigenemia (pp65 in leukocytes), and DNAemia or RNAemia (generally by PCR), to true end-organ disease. The diagnosis of end-organ disease, such as pneumonitis, GI disease, hepatitis, and CNS disease, requires signs or symptoms of disease at that site with detection of CMV by culture, histopathology, immunohistochemical staining, or in situ hybridization. Except for CNS disease, detection by PCR is not sufficient for establishing the diagnosis because it is probably too sensitive and may signify transient viremia. In addition, the identification of co-pathogens is important and may confound the diagnosis. CMV syndrome with fever, neutropenia, or thrombocytopenia (or any combination) and detection of CMV in blood also have been defined in SOTRs.[242]

The indirect, immunomodulatory effects of CMV appear to have broad-reaching consequences, as mentioned previously. Epidemiologically, CMV has been associated with dysfunction and rejection of the graft, accelerated atherosclerosis (heart transplant), secondary infections, and BOS.[242,467]

The incidence of CMV infection in LTRs is higher than that in other SOTRs. The reasons are multifactorial but include intense immunosuppression, high levels of CMV latency, viral load, and recurrence associated with the lung and its transplantation.[31,468] The incidences of infection and disease are reported to be 54 to 92 percent without prophylaxis[468] and 30 to 86 percent with various different strategies, thus pointing to the difficulty in identifying the optimal regimen.[467] The greatest risk factor for developing CMV infection is donor/recipient (D/R) mismatch, with D+/R− having the highest rate of infection, although infection does occur in D+/R+ and rarely in D−/R− matches.[89] Other risks include the use of antilymphocyte antibody and blood-product transfusion.[468] A study of pediatric LTRs reported that CMV viremia developed in 23 percent of 194 patients.[89] CMV prophylaxis was given to all D+ or R+ patients and consisted of 42 days of intravenous ganciclovir. The median time at onset was 80 days. A first episode of viremia was associated with retransplantation or death between days 90 and 365. Early viremia, before 42 days, was not associated with mortality. This study did not find an association between viremia and BOS, but patients with viremia were statistically more likely to experience two or more episodes of acute rejection.

A combination of tools can be used to reduce the incidence of CMV infection. The use of CMV-negative or leukocyte-free blood products for CMV-negative recipients is standard practice in most transplant centers and has been shown to reduce infection rates. Matching of D/R serologic status probably would reduce infection rates but also would limit the donor pool for R− recipients significantly and is not considered to be indicated. The final strategies use different regimens of antivirals to suppress replication and immunoglobulin products for enhanced passive immunity.[467] These regimens can be prophylactic, in which all patients at risk are treated for a certain period, or preemptive, in which highly sensitive screening techniques, antigenemia (pp65) or DNAemia, are used to identify patients needing therapy. To complicate matters, regimens can include multiple antivirals such as intravenous ganciclovir or acyclovir, and/or oral ganciclovir,

acyclovir, or valganciclovir for various periods. A recent international survey of pediatric lung transplant centers reported variable approaches to reducing the incidence of CMV infection.[90] All centers used prophylactic ganciclovir or valganciclovir, generally based on serostatus stratification; the duration of therapy ranged from 3.5 weeks to indefinitely, but most used 12 weeks. In addition, 50 percent of responding centers used CMV intravenous immunoglobulin (IVIG) with variable schedules. One center used a combination of prophylaxis followed by preemption using antigenemia. Although most centers used active surveillance of antigenemia for detection of CMV, PCR also was used, and one center used viral culture. The monitoring regimen also varied considerably.

A consensus of evidence-based recommendations by an expert advisory group has been published recently.[468] The recommendations are as follows: 1. All D+ or R+ LTRs should be considered for prophylaxis. 2a. Prophylaxis with valganciclovir for at least 100 days significantly reduces CMV infection. Some limited data suggest that longer duration (up to 180 days) may reduce infection rates further.[142,469] 2b. Combination prophylaxis with CMV IVIG should be considered, if available, because evidence suggests that its use may reduce infection rates further.[466,469] 3. Monitoring should be performed every 2 weeks for the first 6 months after transplantation to assess for breakthrough viremia and disease. Whole-blood quantitative PCR is the method of choice and should be validated at each center. If a preemptive approach is being used, monitoring should be performed more frequently. 4. Breakthrough disease should be treated with ganciclovir, 5 mg/kg every 12 hours for up to 21 days, until the viral load is below detection. Immunosuppression should be reduced if possible. 5. Infection that occurs after the initial prophylaxis has been stopped should be treated with ganciclovir or valganciclovir until the viral load is below detection. 6. Resistance should be considered in patients with breakthrough viremia, recurrent infections, or poor response to therapy. Genotypic analysis should be performed on isolates recovered from these patients. Foscarnet is the drug of choice, with or without ganciclovir, for possible resistant strains. Of note is that valganciclovir is not FDA-approved for prophylaxis in LTRs, although it is for other SOTRs. Available data suggest that it is safe and effective in LTRs as well.[181,469] Data in pediatric patients are lacking. These authors believe that the data are stronger for the safety and efficacy of prophylaxis than for preemptive strategies, although they acknowledge that some centers have used the latter approach effectively.

Epstein-Barr Virus/Post-transplant Lymphoproliferative Disorder

The disease manifestations of primary EBV infection in SOTRs range from uncomplicated mononucleosis to conditions indistinguishable from malignant lymphoma. Early lesions of EBV-driven lymphoproliferation, such as the plasmacytic hyperplasia, are seen in mononucleosis-like syndromes, within the context of normal tissue architecture. The term post-transplantation lymphoproliferative disease (PTLD) generally is reserved for proliferation of EBV-positive immunoblasts and atypical lymphocytes associated with effacement or destruction of normal tissue architecture. These disorders can be classified further into polymorphic or monomorphic PTLD and finally malignant lymphomas that may contain clonal chromosomal abnormalities. These tumors are characterized by rapid and progressive growth despite a reduction in immunosuppression. Fatal non-PTLD viral syndromes can occur in SOTRs as well.[154] The reader is referred to several excellent, in-depth reviews on these topics.[154,335,409]

The manifestation of EBV/PTLD is varied and depends on the site of involvement, which may be intrathoracic, extrathoracic (abdominal, head and neck, CNS), or disseminated and intranodal or extranodal.[235] Often, PTLD is seen in the allograft, as with lung, liver, and intestinal transplantation.[154] Signs and symptoms of PTLD can be nonspecific, such as fever of unknown origin, malaise, weight loss, and sore throat.[42] Abdominal pain, GI bleeding, intestinal obstruction and perforation, allograft dysfunction such as changes in respiratory status in LTRs, diffuse lymphadenopathy on physical examination or CT, or hepatosplenomegaly should raise the index of suspicion for PTLD. Focal neurologic findings also can be seen with CNS disease. An additional challenge is to differentiate allograft rejection from PTLD; both entities in LTRs may be characterized by allograft dysfunction with diffuse consolidation on imaging, without obvious lymphadenopathy or a mass. Because the therapies for these two conditions are diametrically opposed, increasing or decreasing immunosuppression, this distinction obviously is critical.[154,335]

Risk factors for the development of PTLD have been identified.[42,79] Pretransplant EBV seronegativity (as a surrogate marker for the risk of development of post-transplant primary EBV infection) is probably the most important predisposing factor for the development of PTLD. Because primary EBV infection occurs almost universally in children, older individuals are already immune and young children undergoing transplantation are, therefore, at greatest risk. In addition, concomitant CMV infection or CMV mismatch before transplantation increases the risk for developing PTLD. Patients at highest risk by type of transplant include recipients of lung and intestinal organs. This risk is probably multifactorial and includes more intense immunosuppressive regimens and transplantation of large amounts of lymphoid tissue with the graft, thereby increasing recipients' potential exposure to donor-derived EBV. The published incidence of PTLD in pediatric LTRs ranges from 7.7 to 26.3 percent.[42,79,329] Certain immunosuppressive regimens, such as the use of OKT3 and polyclonal antilymphocyte antibodies and possibly tacrolimus in pediatric patients, are linked to the development of PTLD. Many experts acknowledge that the overall intensity of immunosuppression, not a specific agent, is most important in defining the risk for development of PTLD.

PTLD most often occurs within 12 months after transplantation.[42] Late PTLD has been documented and appears to have specific properties, including an increased incidence in older recipients, long duration of immunosuppression, EBV-negative disease, and poorer prognosis.[79,120,227]

The diagnosis of PTLD requires a high index of suspicion. The gold standard is histopathologic examination of tissue from either excisional or fine-needle biopsy. Specimens should be processed by pathologists familiar with the morphologic classifications, and ancillary tests that may be helpful include staining for EBV-encoded RNA 2 by in situ hybridization (EBERS) and the presence of CD20, which has implications for therapy.[335] Imaging also can be used for presumptive diagnosis, to guide biopsy, and for follow-up.[329,370] In LTRs, CT of the chest may reveal discrete nodules, airspace consolidation, or mediastinal lymphadenopathy. Extrathoracic involvement is less common but may include abdominal lymphadenopathy, liver/spleen lesions, and a thickened bowel wall. On head and neck imaging, the cervical lymph nodes, pharynx, orbit, sinus, and rarely the brain are found to be involved occasionally.

Patients at the highest risk for mortality are those in whom primary EBV infection develops early after transplantation is performed; therefore, every effort should be made to identify these patients. Pretransplant serologic assessment of donors and recipients for both EBV and CMV can alert physicians to most of these high-risk patients, as donor/recipient mismatch of either virus appears to play an important role.[42,79] Once identified, these patients should be monitored carefully by PCR for evidence of primary infection, and careful examination and use

of CT scanning for early diagnosis of disease should be included. Several strategies have been used for the prevention of EBV/PTLD in high-risk patients.[154,335] The use of EBV-negative donors, though probably effective, would reduce the donor pool substantially and generally is not advocated. The use of prophylactic antiviral therapy has not been proved to prevent the development of PTLD. Although these agents are active against the lytic viral infection that proceeds PTLD, they are not active in the latent viral phase that characterizes PTLD. Acyclovir and ganciclovir often are used for prevention of CMV, and historical comparisons of the incidence of PTLD in certain high-risk patients receiving them suggest some benefit[92]; however, PTLD has developed in some patients while receiving these antiviral agents. The use of IVIG is similarly a potential, but unproven strategy and is currently undergoing evaluation.[154]

Preemptive strategies aimed at identifying primary infection by blood PCR monitoring have received significant attention.[29,36,151,154,335,345,401,417] In these protocols, high-risk patients undergo EBV quantitative viral load monitoring at frequent intervals, usually weekly, to identify increases associated with infection, a prerequisite for the development of EBV/PTLD. Many issues remain regarding the use of EBV viral load.[151,153,335] For example, these assays are not standardized and therefore are difficult to compare among institutions. Many questions are raised: Which compartment is most revealing and should be sampled—peripheral blood lymphocytes, whole blood, or serum? Is there a threshold level at which therapy should be instituted? How does serostatus affect the sensitivity and specificity of viral loads? Additionally, not all patients with EBV/PTLD have elevated viral loads, and viral loads may be elevated without evidence of disease; therefore, these assays lack specificity. Although these assays are now widely used at transplant centers, further controlled studies are necessary to optimize their use in immunocompromised patients.

When patients with high viral loads are identified, several therapeutic options are available; however, few controlled trials of these interventions have been performed, and the optimal timing and use of each are unknown at this time.[151,336] All experts agree on immediate reduction or cessation, if possible, of immunosuppressive regimens. Most patients with nonmalignant lesions will respond to this maneuver alone. The use of antiviral agents has become routine, though without proven benefit. Patients with a persistently high viral load should be evaluated aggressively for the presence of PTLD on examination and imaging, and suspicious lesions should undergo biopsy for the diagnosis of EBV/PTLD. When the diagnosis of PTLD is made, ideally, immunosuppression should be discontinued, the optimal duration of which is uncertain. Re-initiation of immunosuppressive agents usually is prompted by rejection or clear evidence of clinical and virologic response. Surgical resection and local radiation therapy may be beneficial for localized disease and in the event of GI involvement.

Monoclonal B-cell antibody therapy is now an attractive option for CD20$^+$ lesions not responsive to a reduction in immunosuppression.[335] The currently available product is an anti-CD20 antibody (rituximab). Initial retrospective data reported complete remission rates of 62.5 percent,[282] and these data have been corroborated in several prospective trials.[39,119,303] This therapy generally is well tolerated, although long-term hypogammaglobulinemia is a common occurrence in recipients. In addition, severe CMV and hepatitis B and C infections, as well as parvovirus B19–induced aplasia and enteroviral meningoencephalitis, have been associated with its use.[334] Detailed recommendations for the initial approach to pediatric transplant recipients with EBV/PTLD have been published.[151] For refractory disease, cytotoxic chemotherapy may be indicated. Other investigational therapies include anticytokine therapy (anti–interleukin-6), adoptive immunotherapy (EBV-specific cytotoxic T lymphocytes, lymphokine-activated killer cells), and boosting of the host immune response (interferon-α). Vaccine technology is in progress.[151,334]

Other Herpesviruses: Herpes Simplex Viruses 1 and 2, Varicella-Zoster Virus, Human Herpesviruses 6, 7, and 8

Infections with herpes simplex virus (HSV) 1 and 2 are common occurrences in SOTRs, and in older children and adults, HSV usually is a reactivation disease manifested as orolabial or genital disease.[311] Primary disease occurs in young children who contract the infection from viral shedding of close contacts. In LTRs, serious or disseminated disease such as esophagitis, hepatitis, and pneumonitis can occur.[387] Infections tend to occur early, within the first month after transplantation, unless prophylaxis is used. As with other herpesviruses, concomitant infection with CMV is not an uncommon event. The diagnosis can be made clinically when typical lesions are present. Culture and PCR technology can be helpful for unusual manifestations. Prophylactic strategies with ganciclovir or acyclovir for CMV can prevent HSV. Intravenous acyclovir and oral valacyclovir and famciclovir are effective therapies for localized mucocutaneous disease. More severe disease should be treated with intravenous formulations only. Resistance of HSV in SOTRs is rare, but when it occurs, it should be treated with foscarnet.[311]

Primary varicella-zoster virus (VZV) infection can occur in pediatric LTRs, as can reactivation of previous disease leading to herpes zoster. No data on VZV infections in SOTRs have been published since the widespread use of varicella vaccine (Varivax), but, presumably, rates of infection after transplantation are low. Patients should be screened for evidence of immunity, and seronegative transplant candidates should receive varicella vaccine, optimally at least 6 weeks before transplantation.[311] If the vaccine does not prevent disease, it may mitigate development of severe disease. In addition, susceptible family members also should receive vaccine. Exposure in postoperative patients should be treated with a high-titer varicella immunoglobulin preparation if available or IVIG within 96 hours of exposure. Additionally, some experts recommend the use of prophylactic acyclovir if exposure such as household or intimate contact is likely to lead to development of disease or is revealed past the window for immunoglobulin prophylaxis to be effective. Varicella vaccine, which is an attenuated live viral product, generally is not recommended in post-transplant recipients at this time. Limited data suggest that it is safe and may ameliorate disease in some immunocompromised patient populations, such as those with leukemia, HIV infection, or renal transplants.[54] Detailed recommendations for prophylaxis are given in the American Academy of Pediatrics *Red Book*.[17]

Patients taking steroids, especially during the incubation period, are at increased risk for the development of severe disease. Hemorrhagic and disseminated disease, including encephalitis, hepatitis, and pneumonitis, can occur in immunocompromised patients.

Herpes zoster is a common event in adult transplant recipients; rates in children have not been published for SOTRs. A recent study of SOTRs aged 16 to 74 years found a 15 percent incidence of herpes zoster in LTRs, with a mean time to onset of 14 months and a median of 9 months (9 days-5.8 years).[149] The diagnosis is made clinically and with the use of viral culture or PCR techniques if necessary. Infections should be treated with intravenous acyclovir and pain control. Steroids should be diminished if possible.

HHV-6 is an emerging opportunistic viral pathogen. Seropositivity reaches nearly 100 percent in early childhood, and HHV-6 is responsible for febrile illnesses with or without GI or upper respiratory symptoms, febrile seizures, roseola (exanthema subitum, sixth disease), and asymptomatic infection in normal infants and young children.[9] Therefore, disease in all but the very youngest transplant recipients probably represents reactivation. Several studies have documented HHV-6 by PCR or culture (or both) in a majority (66-90%) of apparently asymptomatic adult LTRs.[192,231] Reactivation of HHV-6 can occur in the setting of CMV antiviral prophylaxis. These infections occur early after transplantation (median of 6 and 18 days), and most are without obvious clinical manifestations that could be ascribed to HHV-6 alone. In immunocompromised patients, HHV-6 appears to exert direct and indirect effects on the host. It probably is responsible for rare cases of encephalitis, hepatitis, pneumonitis, febrile illnesses, and bone marrow suppression.[231] The presence of HHV-6 alone or as a cofactor to CMV may augment the immunomodulatory effects and increase the risk associated with fungal and other infections, as well as allograft rejection, BOS, and mortality.[192,275,296]

Many questions regarding HHV-6 in this population remain unanswered. PCR of peripheral blood lymphocytes is the most sensitive method for detection of virus, but it cannot differentiate between latent and active virus. Routine monitoring of asymptomatic patients is not recommended. Data are insufficient to recommend prophylactic or preemptive therapies, although the virus is susceptible to achievable levels of ganciclovir, foscarnet, and cidofovir. Finally, which patients should be treated remains unclear. Treatment with ganciclovir, foscarnet, or cidofovir may be considered in patients with compatible syndromes if other causes are eliminated. Whether asymptomatic patients with documented HHV-6 infection would benefit from therapy with regard to the indirect effects of the virus remains unknown.[5]

The role of HHV-7 and HHV-8 in SOTRs is undefined. HHV-7 is similar to HHV-6 in normal hosts, although it appears to be less prevalent and occurs later in life. Symptomatic disease is less well characterized, but it may be responsible for similar syndromes seen with HHV-6 in normal children and transplant recipients.[311] Evidence of HHV-8 infection in normal children is rare. It is associated with Kaposi sarcoma in immunocompromised patients, as well as body cavity lymphomas, PTLD, and Castleman disease.[10] It also may be associated with fever and bone marrow suppressive syndromes of donor origin in transplant recipients.[245]

Community-Acquired Respiratory Viruses: Respiratory Syncytial Virus, Parainfluenza Virus, Human Metapneumovirus, Influenza, and Adenovirus

The paramyxoviruses respiratory syncytial virus (RSV), parainfluenza virus (PIV), and human metapneumovirus (hMPV) are common causes of upper and lower respiratory tract disease in normal children; symptoms range from congestion and rhinorrhea to laryngeal tracheobronchitis (croup), bronchiolitis, and pneumonia.[12-14] Disease can be severe and persistent in immunocompromised patients, although the exact impact of these viruses on LTRs is not well studied. Co-infection and sequential infection with other respiratory viruses, including CMV, probably occurs.[143] Importantly, transmission occurs from person to person, from exposure to nasopharyngeal secretions, from infected individuals, and from fomites. Consideration should be given to screen recipients for incubating respiratory viruses before they undergo transplantation, especially if high levels of circulating virus are present in the community or illness is present in family members, or both. Strict adherence to hospital infection control practices is most important in reducing nosocomially acquired disease from visitors and health care workers. Patients and their families should be counseled on avoidance of exposure and on good handwashing practices when discharged from the hospital.[81]

RSV can cause severe lower respiratory tract disease in LTRs. Although most infections resolve, with or without therapy, fatal cases have been reported, as have long-term declines in pulmonary function.[38,143,268,448] The diagnosis can be made by rapid antigen-detection kits, standard viral culture, or more rapid shell vial culture methods, and some centers offer PCR detection; the preferred specimen is nasal washings, although in adults with lower tract disease, BAL fluid is recommended.[14,81] Risk factors for poor outcome in immunocompromised patients include neutropenia, lymphopenia, age younger than 1 year, underlying lung disease, and augmented immunosuppression.[81] High mortality rates in HSCT recipients have led to prevention and treatment strategies that can serve as models for care in SOTRs,[102,144,456] though they are not without controversy because no controlled data exist.[38,146] Supportive care remains the mainstay of therapy. For children with upper tract disease and risk factors or lower tract disease, aerosolized ribavirin should be considered. In addition, because outcomes, even in treated HSCT recipients, are poor with ribavirin alone, some experts suggest combination therapy with RSV IVIG or monoclonal antibody (palivizumab) for immunocompromised patients with significant infections.[38,81,407] Effective prophylaxis with palivizumab and RSV IVIG has been achieved in young infants with lung disease.[160,274] Care must be taken when extrapolating to other patient populations, given the unexpected results of some studies in infants with complex congenital heart disease who are administered RSV IVIG[371] but not pavilizumab.[123] Some experts would consider the use of immunoprophylaxis in young infants undergoing organ transplantation during the RSV season.[81]

hMPV was described in healthy young children in 2001. It appears to have signs and symptoms similar to those of RSV, and almost universal infection probably occurs by 5 years of age.[422,459] The impact of hMPV on immunocompromised patients is as yet uncharacterized, in part because it has been identified relatively recently and diagnostic tests are not widely available. The virus can be cultured, but reverse transcriptase PCR appears to be the test of choice. Antigen assays are not yet available.[12] When found in adult LTRs with upper and lower respiratory tract symptoms, it usually is a single pathogen or co-pathogen.[143,225] In addition, it has been associated with episodes of allograft rejection and mortality.[225] Therapy is supportive, with treatment of co-pathogens if identified.

PIV (types 1 to 4) is isolated frequently as a cause of upper respiratory infections and croup in normal children.[13] PIV can cause severe lower tract infection in immunocompromised patients, including respiratory failure in LTRs, most notably caused by serotype 3.[21,431,449] Though rarely fatal in adults, persistent declines in pulmonary function and acute allograft rejection are important consequences of PIV infection.[268,431,449] A retrospective study on PIV in pediatric SOTRs (liver, small bowel, lung, heart, kidney) found significant age-related morbidity and mortality.[21] Although 44 percent of all patients with PIV had upper respiratory infections, only 11 percent of children younger than 1 year old had limited disease. A 16 percent mortality rate was associated with PIV, and predictors of mortality included age younger than 6 months, infection occurring less than 3 months after transplantation, and augmented immunosuppression. Infection in these children occurred in the context of community outbreaks. The diagnosis can be made most rapidly by antigen detection; culture isolation can take weeks. Respiratory secretions obtained from nasal washings or BAL fluid can be used.[38] No proven therapy for PIV in LTRs is available. Intravenous and aerosolized ribavirin has been used in immunocompromised hosts, but without randomized controlled data or clear evidence of efficacy.[38,268]

Despite available immunoprophylaxis and chemoprophylaxis, influenza viruses A and B remain an important cause of morbidity in the normal population and lead to a considerable rate of mortality in the very young and the elderly.[11] Transplant recipients are at risk for acquiring community-acquired infection during the yearly epidemics, as well as nosocomial infection from visitors, hospital workers, and other transplant recipients as a result of outbreaks occurring in the inpatient setting.[256,348,429] Influenza infection is relatively rare in SOTRs—4.2 percent of adult LTRs over the course of a 10-year-period and 2.6 percent of pediatric SOTRs over a similar period[21,38]—but LTRs appear to be at a uniquely high risk of acquiring infection. In the adult study, the incidence was 41.8 cases per 1000 person-years for adult LTRs versus 2.8 and 4.3 per 1000 in liver and kidney transplant recipients, respectively.[432] The authors speculate that optimal protection from influenza infection afforded by serum and secretory antibodies in the respiratory tract are altered in LTRs, thereby leading to higher attack rates.

In addition to the usual symptoms of acute onset of malaise, fever, myalgias, and respiratory symptoms, GI symptoms also may be prominent.[136] Most pediatric SOTRs with influenza had minimal disease consisting of upper respiratory symptoms, although 3 of 13 patients (23%) died.[21] In these children, steroid bolus and OKT3 therapy given within a week of diagnosis of infection were associated with mortality. Transplant recipients may be at increased risk for acquiring secondary bacterial infections and nonpulmonary complications such as hepatitis, myocarditis, and aseptic meningitis.[38,432]

Influenza is unique among the respiratory viruses in that both vaccine and chemoprophylatic strategies are available, as are several effective therapies. Unfortunately, immunosuppressed patients may not respond well to influenza vaccine, and, if disease is not recognized promptly, the effectiveness of therapy for established disease may not be optimal. Studies on the immunogenicity of influenza vaccine in pediatric SOTRs are more encouraging than in adult reports, which have documented poor response, especially when associated with MMF or sirolimus, and occasional association with acute rejection.[54,167] In pediatric renal transplant recipients, response was similar to that of normal controls, without evidence of rejection,[117,134] although in pediatric heart transplant recipients protective antibody responses were not achieved until three doses of vaccine were administered.[4] The current recommendation is that influenza vaccine be administered yearly to all SOTRs and those awaiting transplantation, as well as to household contacts and caretakers.[11,54,81] Chemoprophylaxis can be administered to patients who have not been vaccinated or who have not had sufficient time to respond to vaccination, especially if influenza is circulating in the community. Agents that are approved for prophylaxis of influenza A in children older than 1 year include amantadine and rimantadine, although resistance commonly is reported to these antivirals, and oseltamivir, which is additionally active against influenza B.[11,429]

The diagnosis of influenza can be made by rapid antigen testing, which is highly sensitive in ill children, though less so in adults with a lower burden of disease. PCR techniques, including multiplex assays for detection of multiple respiratory viruses in one sample, are currently under development but are not yet widely available.[80,131,222,411]

Most experts would recommend therapy with antiviral agents in an LTR with suspected (community epidemic with compatible symptoms) or proven influenza, although their utility in such patient populations has yet to be defined.[38] The choice of agent depends on the type of virus (A or B) and information about resistance. The neuraminidase inhibitors oseltamivir and zanamivir are currently favored because of their broad spectrum of activity and less reported resistance.[81,429] Some would consider the addition of aerosolized ribavirin for severe lower tract disease.[81] The implications of pandemic influenza, including higher disease burdens and mortality and longer duration of viral shedding with considerable potential for spread of disease, for those who already have undergone transplantation and those awaiting transplants probably would be significant. These authors speculate that transplantation under these circumstance probably would be curtailed.[220]

Despite recent interest, published data on adenovirus (AdV) infections in pediatric SOTRs are limited, and most describe infection in liver transplant recipients. The majority of information on AdV in pediatric immunocompromised hosts comes from those undergoing hematopoietic stem cell transplantation. AdV infections in SOTRs appear to be more common occurrences in young pediatric than adult transplant recipients[94,279,304] because young transplant recipients may remain naïve to many of the 51 recognized serotypes. AdV infections have multiple putative sources, including the donor organ, reactivation from latency in host tissues, and infection acquired from the community or nosocomially.[62,210,270,279,331]

Cases of acute, disseminated, and fatal disease have been described in cardiothoracic transplant recipients. In LTRs, infections occur in the early post-transplant period and often cause disease in the graft in the form of necrotizing pneumonia.[49,304] AdV has been associated with graft dysfunction, BOS, retransplantation, and death.[50]

Several methods that are used for the identification of AdV include culture, direct identification of antigens, and serology, as well as histologic examination of tissues for the presence of AdV inclusions and immunohistochemical staining.[75,81] Viral isolation by culture can be expedited by centrifugation in shell vial assays and immunofluorescent staining with adenoviral monoclonal antibodies, although viral serotyping cannot be done with this method. Direct identification of AdV antigens, usually performed on respiratory specimens, can be achieved by radioimmunoassay, immunofluorescence, or ELISA techniques, which are rapid and specific but less sensitive than culture.

Detection of virus with culture techniques and direct antigen detection are insensitive in identifying patients at risk for the development of disseminated disease. In addition, cultures may take a week or longer, and neither method may detect low levels of circulating virus. PCR is emerging as a powerful tool for detection of AdV in body fluids and tissues and for serotyping.[115,161,170,232,239,362] The virus's ability to establish latency can render interpreting the presence of virus or viral DNA in clinical specimens a challenge.[138,233] A single determination of the presence of AdV by PCR in immunocompromised patients may be nonspecific and perhaps misleading. As with other important viruses that establish latency, quantitative viral load patterns appear to be more informative with regard to the pathogenic role of AdV in these patient populations. Studies in pediatric HSCT recipients support the use of blood PCR surveillance as a method to identify patients at risk for disseminated disease.[78,115,161,170,232,239,362,439] These methods have not been validated in LTRs.

The optimal therapy for AdV has not been determined. Supportive care and reduction of immunosuppression are the mainstays of therapy currently recommended.[81] Recent data suggest that administration of cidofovir may be helpful in severely ill patients with disseminated disease and rising viral loads.[63,178,230,243,438,465] Use of this agent may be associated with significant renal toxicity,[169,230,333] and use of modified dosing regimens has been investigated with some success.[63,178,293,438] Strategies involving adoptive immunotherapy also may be feasible and efficacious in the future. Data on these therapeutic modalities have been reviewed recently.[177]

Although a detailed discussion is beyond the scope of this chapter, the link between respiratory viruses and BOS or chronic allograft dysfunction should be addressed briefly. BOS is a progressive condition, without good treatment options, and the greatest impediment to long-term survival for LTRs. It affects 50 percent of patients alive 5 years after transplantation and is the leading cause of death in adult and pediatric LTRs 1 year after transplantation.[416,446] Although the exact mechanisms are still being determined, the final common pathway is epithelial injury and intraluminal proliferation of fibroblasts leading to air flow obstruction.[186,203,427] Stimulation of T cells and release of cytokines and chemokines by viruses are leading candidates for the initiation of these pathways. Many studies have linked viral infections, such as CMV, AdV, RSV, PIV, and others, often working in concert, to the development of BOS.[122,136,219,317,428,431] The role of these agents has yet to be proved, although it is biologically plausible.[186] Reduction of BOS remains an incentive for the continued development of preventive strategies against these viral infections.

ZOONOSES: RABIES, WEST NILE VIRUS, LYMPHOCYTIC CHORIOMENINGITIS VIRUS, AND *BORDETELLA*

Isolation of unusual pathogens often is a sign of an unexpected environmental exposure.[28,352] This statement is epitomized by the recent reports of SOTRs with uncommon zoonotic infections.[214] In the case of donor-derived rabies, lymphocytic choriomeningitis virus, and West Nile Virus infections, multiple cases were traced to a donor or donors with retrospectively assessed exposures or risk factors (or both).[125,172,191,393] West Nile virus in SOTRs also has been community acquired,[206,221] and cases of *Bordetella bronchiseptica* in transplant recipients have been traced to sick pet dogs.[34,77,295] These cases are humbling in many respects. Many of these infections have no established therapy and, as expected, are associated with increased morbidity and mortality in SOTRs.[98,125,206,221,295] Therefore, prevention is of utmost importance. These cases advise us to counsel our post-transplant recipients on avoidance of potentially infectious exposures, such as sick pets and arthropod vectors of diseases.[214,218,295] Undeniably, they remind us of the almost limitless pathogens that may befall SOTRs, including those not yet described. These cases have newly informed the policies for reporting suspected donortransmitted conditions and opened a new dialogue on how screening procedures of organ and blood donors are conducted.[105,125,180,204]

REFERENCES

1. Aaron, S. D., Ferris, W., Henry, D.A., et al.: Multiple combination bactericidal antibiotic testing for patients with cystic fibrosis infected with *Burkholderia cepacia*. Am. J. Respir. Crit. Care Med. *161*:1206, 2000.
2. Aaron, S. D., Vandemheen, K. L., Ferris, W., et al.: Combination antibiotic susceptibility testing to treat exacerbations of cystic fibrosis associated with multiresistant bacteria: A randomised, double-blind, controlled clinical trial. Lancet *366*:463, 2005.
3. Adam, O., Auperin, A., Wilquin, F., et al.: Treatment with piperacillin-tazobactam and false-positive *Aspergillus* galactomannan antigen test results for patients with hematological malignancies. Clin. Infect. Dis. *38*:917, 2004.
4. Admon, D., Engelhard, D., Strauss, N., et al.: Antibody response to influenza immunization in patients after heart transplantation. Vaccine *15*:1518, 1997.
5. Alberti, C., Bouakline, A., Ribaud, P., et al.: Relationship between environmental fungal contamination and the incidence of invasive aspergillosis in haematology patients. J. Hosp. Infect. *48*:198, 2001.
6. Alexander, B., and Pfaller, M. A.: Contemporary tools for the diagnosis and management of invasive mycoses. Clin. Infect. Dis. *43*:S15, 2006.
7. Alexander, B. D.: Diagnosis of fungal infection: New technologies for the mycology laboratory. Transpl. Infect. Dis. *4*(Suppl. 3):32, 2002.
8. Alexander, B. D., and Tapson, V. F.: Infectious complications of lung transplantation. Transpl. Infect. Dis. *3*:128, 2001.
9. American Academy of Pediatrics: Human herpesvirus 6 and 7. *In* Pickering, L. K., Baker, C. J., Long, S. S., and McMillan, J. A. (eds.): Red Book: 2006 Report of the Committee on Infectious Diseases. 27th ed. Elk Grove Village, IL, American Academy of Pediatrics, 2006, p. 375.
10. American Academy of Pediatrics: Human herpesvirus 8. *In* Pickering, L. K., Baker, C. J., Long, S. S., and McMillan, J. A. (eds.): Red Book: 2006 Report of the Committee on Infectious Diseases. 27th ed. Elk Grove Village, IL, American Academy of Pediatrics, 2006, p. 377.
11. American Academy of Pediatrics: Influenza. *In* Pickering, L. K., Baker, C. J., Long, S. S., and McMillan, J. A. (eds.): Red Book: 2006 Report of the Committee on Infectious Diseases. 27th ed. Elk Grove Village, IL, American Academy of Pediatrics, 2006, p. 401.
12. American Academy of Pediatrics: Human metapneumovirus. *In* Pickering, L. K., Baker, C. J., Long, S. S., and McMillan, J. A. (eds.): Red Book: 2006 Report of the Committee on Infectious Diseases. 27th ed. Elk Grove Village, IL, American Academy of Pediatrics, 2006, p. 460.

13. American Academy of Pediatrics: Parainfluenza viral infections. *In* Pickering, L. K., Baker, C. J., Long, S. S., and McMillan, J. A. (eds.): Red Book: 2006 Report of the Committee on Infectious Diseases. 27th ed. Elk Grove Village, IL, American Academy of Pediatrics 2006, p. 479.

14. American Academy of Pediatrics: Respiratory syncytial virus. *In* Pickering, L. K., Baker, C. J., Long, S. S., and McMillan, J. A. (eds.): Red Book: 2006 Report of the Committee on Infectious Diseases. 27th ed. Elk Grove Village, IL, American Academy of Pediatrics, 2006, p. 560.

15. American Academy of Pediatrics: Tuberculosis. *In* Pickering, L. K., Baker, C. J., Long, S. S., and McMillan, J. A. (eds.): Red Book: 2006 Report of the Committee on Infectious Diseases. 27th ed. Elk Grove Village, IL, American Academy of Pediatrics, 2006, p. 678.

16. American Academy of Pediatrics: Diseases caused by notuberculous mycobacteria. *In* Pickering, L. K., Baker, C. J., Long, S. S., and McMillan, J. A. (eds.): Red Book: 2006 Report of the Committee on Infectious Diseases. 27th ed. Elk Grove Village, IL, American Academy of Pediatrics, 2006, p. 698.

17. American Academy of Pediatrics: Varicella-zoster infections. *In* Pickering, L. K., Baker, C. J., Long, S. S., and McMillan, J. A. (eds.): Red Book: 2006 Report of the Committee on Infectious Diseases. 27th ed. Elk Grove Village, IL, American Academy of Pediatrics, 2006, p. 711.

18. American Academy of Pediatrics Committee on Infectious Diseases: Screening for tuberculosis in infants and children. Pediatrics 93:131, 1994.

19. American Thoracic Society: Rapid diagnostic tests for tuberculosis: What is the appropriate use? American Thoracic Society Workshop. Am. J. Respir. Crit. Care Med. 155:1804, 1997.

20. Anstead, G. M., and Graybill, J. R.: Coccidioidomycosis. Infect. Dis. Clin. North Am. 20:621, 2006.

21. Apalsch, A. M., Green, M., Ledesma-Medina, J., et al.: Parainfluenza and influenza virus infections in pediatric organ transplant recipients. Clin. Infect. Dis. 20:394, 1995.

22. Aris, R. M., Gilligan, P. H., Neuringer, I. P., et al.: The effects of panresistant bacteria in cystic fibrosis patients on lung transplant outcome. Am. J. Respir. Crit. Care Med. 155:1699, 1997.

23. Aris, R. M., Routh, J. C., LiPuma, J. J., et al.: Lung transplantation for cystic fibrosis patients with *Burkholderia cepacia* complex. Survival linked to genomovar type. Am. J. Respir. Crit. Care Med. 164:2102, 2001.

24. Arnold, C., Westland, L., Mowat, G., et al.: Single-nucleotide polymorphism–based differentiation and drug resistance detection in *Mycobacterium tuberculosis* from isolates or directly from sputum. Clin. Microbiol. Infect. 11:122, 2005.

25. Ascioglu, S., Rex, J. H., de Pauw, J., et al.: Defining opportunistic invasive fungal infections in immunocompromised patients with cancer and hematopoietic stem cell transplants: An international consensus. Clin. Infect. Dis. 34:7, 2002.

26. Aubry, A., Porcher, R., Bottero, J., et al.: Occurrence and kinetics of false-positive *Aspergillus* galactomannan test results following treatment with beta-lactam antibiotics in patients with hematological disorders. J. Clin. Microbiol. 44:389, 2006.

27. Baden, L. R., Katz, J. T., Fishman, J. A., et al.: Salvage therapy with voriconazole for invasive fungal infections in patients failing or intolerant to standard antifungal therapy. Transplantation 76:1632, 2003.

28. Baden, L. R., and Rubin, R. H.: The sentinel chicken revisited: The impact of West Nile virus infection on transplant patients. Transplantation 77:356, 2004.

29. Bakker, N. A., van Imhoff, G. W., Verschuuren, E. A., et al.: Presentation and early detection of post-transplant lymphoproliferative disorder after solid organ transplantation. Transpl. Int. 20:207, 2007.

30. Bal, A. M.: Combination antifungal therapy in solid organ transplant recipients. Transplantation 82:291, 2006.

31. Balthesen, M., Messerle, M., and Reddehase, M. J.: Lungs are a major organ site of cytomegalovirus latency and recurrence. J. Virol. 67:5360, 1993.

32. Barnes, P. D., and Marr, K. A.: Aspergillosis: Spectrum of disease, diagnosis, and treatment. Infect. Dis. Clin. North Am. 20:545, 2006.

33. Barr, M. L., Schenkel, F. A., Bowdish, M. E., et al.: Living donor lobar lung transplantation: Current status and future directions. Transplant. Proc. 37:3983, 2005.

34. Bauwens, J. E., Spach, D. H., Schacker, T. W., et al.: *Bordetella bronchiseptica* pneumonia and bacteremia following bone marrow transplantation. J. Clin. Microbiol. 30:2474, 1992.

35. Becker, M. J., Lutgeburg, E. J., Cornelissen, J. J., et al.: Galactomannan detection in computerized tomography–based broncho-alveolar lavage fluid and serum in haematological patients at risk for invasive pulmonary aspergillosis. Br. J. Haematol. 121:448, 2003.

36. Benden, C., Aurora, P., Burch, M., et al.: Monitoring of Epstein-Barr viral load in pediatric heart and lung transplant recipients by real-time polymerase chain reaction. J. Heart Lung Transplant. 24:2103, 2005.

37. Bernard, A., Caillot, D., Couaillier, J. F., et al.: Surgical management of invasive pulmonary aspergillosis in neutropenic patients. Ann. Thorac. Surg. 64:1441, 1997.

38. Billings, J. L., Hertz, M. I., and Wendt, C. H.: Community respiratory virus infections following lung transplantation. Transpl. Infect. Dis. 3:138, 2001.

39. Blaes, A. H., Peterson, B. A., Bartlett, N., et al.: Rituximab therapy is effective for posttransplant lymphoproliferative disorders after solid organ transplantation: Results of a phase II trial. Cancer 104:1661, 2005.

40. Blair, J. E., and Logan, J. L.: Coccidioidomycosis in solid organ transplantation. Clin. Infect. Dis. 33:1536, 2001.

41. Blumberg, H. M., Burman, W. J., Chaisson, R. E., et al.: American Thoracic Society/Centers for Disease Control and Prevention/Infectious Diseases Society of America: Treatment of tuberculosis. Am. J. Respir. Crit. Care Med. 167:603, 2003.

42. Boyle, G. J., Michaels, M. G., Webber, S. A., et al.: Posttransplantation lymphoproliferative disorders in pediatric thoracic organ recipients. J. Pediatr. 131:309, 1997.

43. Bozza, S., Gaziano, R., Lipford, G. B., et al.: Vaccination of mice against invasive aspergillosis with recombinant *Aspergillus* proteins and CpG oligodeoxynucleotides as adjuvants. Microbes Infect. 4:1281, 2002.

44. Bozza, S., Montagnoli, C., Gaziano, R., et al.: Dendritic cell–based vaccination against opportunistic fungi. Vaccine 22:857, 2004.

45. Bozza, S., Perruccio, K., Montagnoli, C., et al.: A dendritic cell vaccine against invasive aspergillosis in allogeneic hematopoietic transplantation. Blood 102:3807, 2003.

46. Bravo, C., Roldan, J., Roman, A., et al.: Tuberculosis in lung transplant recipients. Transplantation 79:59, 2005.

47. Bretagne, S., and Costa, J. M.: Towards a molecular diagnosis of invasive aspergillosis and disseminated candidosis. F. E. M. S. Immunol. Med. Microbiol. 45:361, 2005.

48. Bretagne, S., Costa, J. M., Bart-Delabesse, E., et al.: Comparison of serum galactomannan antigen detection and competitive polymerase chain reaction for diagnosing invasive aspergillosis. Clin. Infect. Dis. 26:1407, 1998.

49. Bridges, N. D., Mallory, G. B., Huddleston, C. B., et al.: Lung transplantation in infancy and early childhood. J. Heart Lung Transplant. 15:895, 1996.

50. Bridges, N. D., Spray, T. L., Collins, M. H., et al.: Adenovirus infection in the lung results in graft failure after lung transplantation. J. Thorac. Cardiovasc. Surg. 116:617, 1998.

51. Buchheidt, D., Baust, C., Skladny, H., et al.: Detection of *Aspergillus* species in blood and bronchoalveolar lavage samples from immunocompromised patients by means of 2-step polymerase chain reaction: Clinical results. Clin. Infect. Dis. 33:428, 2001.

52. Buchheidt, D., Hummel, M., Schleiermacher, D., et al.: Prospective clinical evaluation of a LightCycler-mediated polymerase chain reaction assay, a nested-PCR assay and a galactomannan enzyme-linked immunosorbent assay for detection of invasive aspergillosis in neutropenic cancer patients and haematological stem cell transplant recipients. Br. J. Haematol. 125:196, 2004.

53. Burns, J. L., and Saiman, L.: *Burkholderia cepacia* infections in cystic fibrosis. Pediatr. Infect. Dis. J. 18:155, 1999.

54. Burroughs, M., and Moscona, A.: Immunization of pediatric solid organ transplant candidates and recipients. Clin. Infect. Dis. 30:857, 2000.

55. Busca, A., Locatelli, F., Barbui, A., et al.: Usefulness of sequential *Aspergillus* galactomannan antigen detection combined with early radiologic evaluation for diagnosis of invasive pulmonary aspergillosis in patients undergoing allogeneic stem cell transplantation. Transplant. Proc. 38:1610, 2006.

56. Bylund, J., Burgess, L. A., Cescutti, P., et al.: Exopolysaccharides from *Burkholderia cenocepacia* inhibit neutrophil chemotaxis and scavenge reactive oxygen species. J. Biol. Chem. 281:2526, 2006.

57. Cahill, B. C., Hibbs, J. R., Savik, K., et al.: *Aspergillus* airway colonization and invasive disease after lung transplant. Chest 112:1160, 1997.

58. Caillot, D., Casasnovas, O., Bernard, A., et al.: Improved management of invasive pulmonary aspergillosis in neutropenic patients using early thoracic computed tomographic scan and surgery. J. Clin. Oncol. 15:139, 1997.

59. Caillot, D., Couaillier, J. F., Bernard, A., et al.: Increasing volume and changing characteristics of invasive pulmonary aspergillosis on sequential thoracic computed tomography scans in patients with neutropenia. J. Clin. Oncol. 19:253, 2001.

60. Caillot, D., Mannone, L., Cuisenier, B., et al.: Role of early diagnosis and aggressive surgery in the management of invasive pulmonary aspergillosis in neutropenic patients. Clin. Microbiol. Infect. 7(Suppl. 2):54, 2001.

61. Calvo, V., Borro, J. M., Morales, P., et al.: Antifungal prophylaxis during the early postoperative period of lung transplantation. Valencia Lung Transplant Group. Chest 115:1301, 1999.

62. Cames, B., Rahier, J., Burtomboy, G., et al.: Acute adenovirus hepatitis in liver transplant recipients. J. Pediatr. 120:33, 1992.

63. Carter, B. A., Karpen, S. J., Quiros-Tejeira, R. E., et al.: Intravenous cidofovir therapy for disseminated adenovirus in a pediatric liver transplant recipient. Transplantation 74:1050, 2002.

64. Cenci, E., Mencacci, A., Bacci, A., et al.: T cell vaccination in mice with invasive pulmonary aspergillosis. J. Immunol. 165:381, 2000.

65. Centers for Disease Control and Prevention: Update: Nucleic acid amplification tests for tuberculosis. M. M. W. R. Morb. Mortal. Wkly. Rep. 49(26):593, 2000.

66. Chalermskulrat, W., Sood, N., Neuringer, I. P., et al.: Non-tuberculous mycobacteria in end stage cystic fibrosis: Implications for lung transplantation. Thorax 61:507, 2006.

67. Challier, S., Boyer, S., Abachin, E., et al.: Development of a serum-based Taqman real-time PCR assay for diagnosis of invasive aspergillosis. J. Clin. Microbiol. 42:844, 2004.

68. Chandrasekar, P. H., and Sobel, J. D.: Micafungin: A new echinocandin. Clin. Infect. Dis. 42:1171, 2006.

69. Chaparro, C., Chamberlain, D., Maurer, J., et al.: Bronchiolitis obliterans organizing pneumonia (BOOP) in lung transplant recipients. Chest 110:1150, 1996.

70. Chaparro, C., Maurer, J., Gutierrez, C., et al.: Infection with *Burkholderia cepacia* in cystic fibrosis: Outcome following lung transplantation. Am. J. Respir. Crit. Care Med. *163*:43, 2001.

71. Chapman, S. W., Bradsher, R. W., Jr., Campbell, G. D., Jr., et al.: Practice guidelines for the management of patients with blastomycosis. Infectious Diseases Society of America. Clin. Infect. Dis. *30*:679, 2000.

72. Chayakulkeeree, M., and Perfect, J. R.: Cryptococcosis. Infect. Dis. Clin. North Am. *20*:507, 2006.

73. Chen, S. F., and Gutierrez, K.: *Mycobacterium bovis* disease in a pediatric renal transplant patient. Pediatr. Infect. Dis. J. *25*:564, 2006.

74. Chernenko, S. M., Humar, A., Hutcheon, M., et al.: *Mycobacterium abscessus* infections in lung transplant recipients: The international experience. J. Heart Lung Transplant. *25*:1447, 2006.

75. Cherry, J. D.: Adenoviruses. *In* Feigin, R. D., Cherry, J. D., Demmler, G. J, and Kaplan, S. L. (eds.): Textbook of Pediatric Infectious Diseases. 5th ed., Vol. 2. Philadelphia, W. B. Saunders, 2004, p. 1843.

76. Choong, C. K., Sweet, S. C., Zoole, J. B., et al.: Bronchial airway anastomotic complications after pediatric lung transplantation: Incidence, cause, management, and outcome. J. Thorac. Cardiovasc. Surg. *131*:198, 2006.

77. Choy, K. W., Wulffraat, N. M., Wolfs, T. F., et al.: *Bordetella bronchiseptica* respiratory infection in a child after bone marrow transplantation. Pediatr. Infect. Dis. J. *18*:481, 1999.

78. Claas, E. C., Schilham, M. W., de Brouwer, C. S., et al.: Internally controlled real-time PCR monitoring of adenovirus DNA load in serum or plasma of transplant recipients. J. Clin. Microbiol. *43*:1738, 2005.

79. Cockfield, S. M.: Identifying the patient at risk for post-transplant lymphoproliferative disorder. Transpl. Infect. Dis. *3*:70, 2001.

80. Coiras, M. T., Aguilar, J. C., Garcia, M. L., et al.: Simultaneous detection of fourteen respiratory viruses in clinical specimens by two multiplex reverse transcription nested-PCR assays. J. Med. Virol. *72*:484, 2004.

81. Community-acquired respiratory viruses. Am. J. Transplant. *4*(Suppl. 10):105, 2004.

82. Cornely, O. A., Maertens, J., Winston, D. J., et al.: Posaconazole vs. fluconazole or itraconazole prophylaxis in patients with neutropenia. N. Engl. J. Med. *356*:348, 2007.

83. Cornet, M., Levy, V., Fleury, L., et al.: Efficacy of prevention by high-efficiency particulate air filtration or laminar airflow against *Aspergillus* airborne contamination during hospital renovation. Infect. Control. Hosp. Epidemiol. *20*:508, 1999.

84. Cornillet, A., Camus, C., Nimubona, S., et al.: Comparison of epidemiological, clinical, and biological features of invasive aspergillosis in neutropenic and nonneutropenic patients: A 6-year survey. Clin. Infect. Dis. *43*:577, 2006.

85. Costa, C., Costa, J. M., Desterke, C., et al.: Real-time PCR coupled with automated DNA extraction and detection of galactomannan antigen in serum by enzyme-linked immunosorbent assay for diagnosis of invasive aspergillosis. J. Clin. Microbiol. *40*:2224, 2002.

86. Costa, C., Vidaud, D., Olivi, M., et al.: Development of two real-time quantitative TaqMan PCR assays to detect circulating *Aspergillus fumigatus* DNA in serum. J. Microbiol. Methods *44*:263, 2001.

87. Cullen, A. R., Cannon, C. L., Mark, E. J., et al.: *Mycobacterium abscessus* infection in cystic fibrosis. Colonization or infection? Am. J. Respir. Crit. Care Med. *161*:641, 2000.

88. Dankner, W. M., and Davis, C. E.: *Mycobacterium bovis* as a significant cause of tuberculosis in children residing along the United States–Mexico border in the Baja California region. Pediatrics *105*:E79, 2000.

89. Danziger-Isakov, L. A., DelaMorena, M., Hayashi, R. J., et al.: Cytomegalovirus viremia associated with death or retransplantation in pediatric lung-transplant recipients. Transplantation *75*:1538, 2003.

90. Danziger-Isakov, L. A., Faro, A., Sweet, S., et al.: Variability in standard care for cytomegalovirus prevention and detection in pediatric lung transplantation: Survey of eight pediatric lung transplant programs. Pediatr. Transplant. *7*:469, 2003.

91. Danziger-Isakov, L. A., Sweet, S., Delamorena, M., et al.: Epidemiology of bloodstream infections in the first year after pediatric lung transplantation. Pediatr. Infect. Dis. J. *24*:324, 2005.

92. Darenkov, I. A., Marcarelli, M. A., Basadonna, G. P., et al.: Reduced incidence of Epstein-Barr virus–associated posttransplant lymphoproliferative disorder using preemptive antiviral therapy. Transplantation *64*:848, 1997.

93. de Boer, M., Bruijnesteijn van Coppenraet, L., Gaasbeek, A., et al.: An outbreak of *Pneumocystis jiroveci* pneumonia with 1 predominant genotype among renal transplant recipients: Interhuman transmission or a common environmental source? Clin. Infect. Dis. *44*:1143, 2007.

94. de Mezerville, M. H., Tellier, R., Richardson, S., et al.: Adenoviral infections in pediatric transplant recipients: A hospital-based study. Pediatr. Infect. Dis. J. *25*:815, 2006.

95. Denning, D. W.: Invasive aspergillosis. Clin. Infect. Dis. *26*:781, 1998.

96. Denning, D. W., Marr, K. A., Lau, W. M., et al.: Micafungin (FK463), alone or in combination with other systemic antifungal agents, for the treatment of acute invasive aspergillosis. J. Infect. *53*:337, 2006.

97. De Pauw, B. E., and Donnelly, J. P.: Prophylaxis and aspergillosis—has the principle been proven? N. Engl. J. Med. *356*:409, 2007.

98. DeSalvo, D., Roy-Chaudhury, P., Peddi, R., et al.: West Nile virus encephalitis in organ transplant recipients: Another high-risk group for meningoencephalitis and death. Transplantation *77*:466, 2004.

99. De Soyza, A., and Corris, P. A.: Lung transplantation and the *Burkholderia cepacia* complex. J. Heart Lung Transplant. *22*:954, 2003.

100. De Soyza, A., McDowell, A., Archer, L., et al.: *Burkholderia cepacia* complex genomovars and pulmonary transplantation outcomes in patients with cystic fibrosis. Lancet *358*:1780, 2001.

101. De Soyza, A., Morris, K., McDowell, A., et al.: Prevalence and clonality of *Burkholderia cepacia* complex genomovars in UK patients with cystic fibrosis referred for lung transplantation. Thorax *59*:526, 2004.

102. DeVincenzo, J. P., Hirsch, R. L., Fuentes, R. J., et al.: Respiratory syncytial virus immune globulin treatment of lower respiratory tract infection in pediatric patients undergoing bone marrow transplantation—a compassionate use experience. Bone Marrow Transplant. *25*:161, 2000.

103. de Wet, N., Llanos-Cuentas, A., Suleiman, J., et al.: A randomized, double-blind, parallel-group, dose-response study of micafungin compared with fluconazole for the treatment of esophageal candidiasis in HIV-positive patients. Clin. Infect. Dis. *39*:842, 2004.

104. Diederich, S., Scadeng, M., Dennis, C., et al.: *Aspergillus* infection of the respiratory tract after lung transplantation: Chest radiographic and CT findings. Eur. Radiol. *8*:306, 1998.

105. Dietzschold, B., and Koprowski, H.: Rabies transmission from organ transplants in the USA. Lancet *364*:648, 2004.

106. Digby, J., Kalbfleisch, J., Glenn, A., et al.: Serum glucan levels are not specific for presence of fungal infections in intensive care unit patients. Clin. Diagn. Lab. Immunol. *10*:882, 2003.

107. Dobbin, C., Maley, M., Harkness, J., et al.: The impact of pan-resistant bacterial pathogens on survival after lung transplantation in cystic fibrosis: Results from a single large referral centre. J. Hosp. Infect. *56*:277, 2004.

108. Dodds Ashley, E., Lewis, R., Lewis, J. S., et al.: Pharmacology of systemic antifungal agents. Clin. Infect. Dis. *43*:S28, 2006.

109. Donnelly, J. P.: Polymerase chain reaction for diagnosing invasive aspergillosis: Getting closer but still a ways to go. Clin. Infect. Dis. *42*:487, 2006.

110. Doucette, K., and Fishman, J. A.: Nontuberculous mycobacterial infection in hematopoietic stem cell and solid organ transplant recipients. Clin. Infect. Dis. *38*:1428, 2004.

111. Drew, R.: Potential role of aerosolized amphotericin B formulations in the prevention and adjunctive treatment of invasive fungal infections. Int. J. Antimicrob. Agents *27*(Suppl. 1):36, 2006.

112. Drew, R. H., Dodds Ashley, E., Benjamin, D. K., Jr., et al.: Comparative safety of amphotericin B lipid complex and amphotericin B deoxycholate as aerosolized antifungal prophylaxis in lung-transplant recipients. Transplantation *77*:232, 2004.

113. Dummer, J. S., Lazariashvili, N., Barnes, J., et al.: A survey of anti-fungal management in lung transplantation. J. Heart Lung Transplant. *23*:1376, 2004.

114. Durand-Joly, I., Chabe, M., Soula, F., et al.: Molecular diagnosis of *Pneumocystis pneumonia*. F. E. M. S. Immunol. Med. Microbiol. *45*:405, 2005.

115. Echavarria, M., Forman, M., van Tol, M. J., et al.: Prediction of severe disseminated adenovirus infection by serum PCR. Lancet *358*:384, 2001.

116. Eckmanns, T., Ruden, H., and Gastmeier, P.: The influence of high-efficiency particulate air filtration on mortality and fungal infection among highly immunosuppressed patients: A systematic review. J. Infect. Dis. *193*:1408, 2006.

117. Edvardsson, V. O., Flynn, J. T., Deforest, A., et al.: Effective immunization against influenza in pediatric renal transplant recipients. Clin. Transplant. *10*:556, 1996.

118. Einsele, H., Hebart, H., Roller, G., et al.: Detection and identification of fungal pathogens in blood by using molecular probes. J. Clin. Microbiol. *35*:1353, 1997.

119. Elstrom, R. L., Andreadis, C., Aqui, N. A., et al.: Treatment of PTLD with rituximab or chemotherapy. Am. J. Transplant. *6*:569, 2006.

120. Epstein-Barr virus and lymphoproliferative disorders after transplantation. Am. J. Transplant. *4*(Suppl. 10):59, 2004.

121. Esther, C. R., Jr., Henry, M. M., Molina, P. L., et al.: Nontuberculous mycobacterial infection in young children with cystic fibrosis. Pediatr. Pulmonol. *40*:39, 2005.

122. Faul, J. L., Akindipe, O. A., Berry, G. J., et al.: Influenza pneumonia in a paediatric lung transplant recipient. Transpl. Int. *13*:79, 2000.

123. Feltes, T. F., Cabalka, A. K., Meissner, H. C., et al.: Palivizumab prophylaxis reduces hospitalization due to respiratory syncytial virus in young children with hemodynamically significant congenital heart disease. J. Pediatr. *143*:532, 2003.

124. Fernandez, D. J., Torronters, S. R., Pineda, M. M., Ramos, M. C., and Sanchez, G.: Inhaled aztreonam therapy in patients with cystic fibrosis colonized with *Pseudomonas aeruginosa*. Spanish Ann. Pediatr. *40*, 1994

125. Fischer, S. A., Graham, M. B., Kuehnert, M. J., et al.: Transmission of lymphocytic choriomeningitis virus by organ transplantation. N. Engl. J. Med. *354*:2235, 2006.

126. Fishman, J. A.: Treatment of infection due to *Pneumocystis carinii*. Antimicrob. Agents Chemother. *42*:1309, 1998.

127. Fishman, J. A., and Rubin, R. H.: Infection in organ-transplant recipients. N. Engl. J. Med. *338*:1741, 1998.

128. Flume, P. A., Egan, T. M., Paradowski, L. J., et al.: Infectious complications of lung transplantation. Impact of cystic fibrosis. Am. J. Respir. Crit. Care Med. *149*:1601, 1994.

129. Fortun, J., Martin-Davila, P., Alvarez, M. E., et al.: *Aspergillus* antigenemia sandwich-enzyme immunoassay test as a serodiagnostic method for invasive aspergillosis in liver transplant recipients. Transplantation 71:145, 2001.

130. Franklin, J. A., McCormick, J., and Flynn, P. M.: Retrospective study of the safety of caspofungin in immunocompromised pediatric patients. Pediatr. Infect. Dis. J. 22:747, 2003.

131. Freymuth, F., Vabret, A., Cuvillon-Nimal, D., et al.: Comparison of multiplex PCR assays and conventional techniques for the diagnostic of respiratory virus infections in children admitted to hospital with an acute respiratory illness. J. Med. Virol. 78:1498, 2006.

132. Frost, A. E.: Role of infections, pathogenesis, and management in lung transplantation. Transplant. Proc. 31:175, 1999.

133. Fungal infections. Am. J. Transplant. 4(Suppl. 10):110, 2004.

134. Furth, S. L., Neu, A. M., McColley, S. A., et al.: Immune response to influenza vaccination in children with renal disease. Pediatr. Nephrol. 9:566, 1995.

135. Galgiani, J. N., Ampel, N. M., Blair, J. E., et al.: Coccidioidomycosis. Clin. Infect. Dis. 41:1217, 2005.

136. Garantziotis, S., Howell, D. N., McAdams, H. P., et al.: Influenza pneumonia in lung transplant recipients: Clinical features and association with bronchiolitis obliterans syndrome. Chest 119:1277, 2001.

137. Garlanda, C., Hirsch, E., Bozza, S., et al.: Non-redundant role of the long pentraxin PTX3 in anti-fungal innate immune response. Nature 420:182, 2002.

138. Garnett, C. T., Erdman, D., Xu, W., et al.: Prevalence and quantitation of species C adenovirus DNA in human mucosal lymphocytes. J. Virol. 76:10608, 2002.

139. Gavalda, J., Len, O., San Juan, R., et al.: Risk factors for invasive aspergillosis in solid-organ transplant recipients: A case-control study. Clin. Infect. Dis. 41:52, 2005.

140. Gaziano, R., Bozza, S., Bellocchio, S., et al.: Anti–*Aspergillus fumigatus* efficacy of pentraxin 3 alone and in combination with antifungals. Antimicrob. Agents Chemother. 48:4414, 2004.

141. Geller, D. E., Pitlick, W. H., Nardella, P. A., et al.: Pharmacokinetics and bioavailability of aerosolized tobramycin in cystic fibrosis. Chest 122:219, 2002.

142. Gerbase, M. W., Dubois, D., Rothmeier, C., et al.: Costs and outcomes of prolonged cytomegalovirus prophylaxis to cover the enhanced immunosuppression phase following lung transplantation. Chest 116:1265, 1999.

143. Gerna, G., Vitulo, P., Rovida, F., et al.: Impact of human metapneumovirus and human cytomegalovirus versus other respiratory viruses on the lower respiratory tract infections of lung transplant recipients. J. Med. Virol. 78:408, 2006.

144. Ghosh, S., Champlin, R. E., Englund, J., et al.: Respiratory syncytial virus upper respiratory tract illnesses in adult blood and marrow transplant recipients: Combination therapy with aerosolized ribavirin and intravenous immunoglobulin. Bone Marrow Transplant. 25:751, 2000.

145. Gibson, R. L., Retsch-Bogart, G. Z., Oermann, C., et al.: Microbiology, safety, and pharmacokinetics of aztreonam lysinate for inhalation in patients with cystic fibrosis. Pediatr. Pulmonol. 41:656, 2006.

146. Glanville, A. R., Scott, A. I., Morton, J. M., et al.: Intravenous ribavirin is a safe and cost-effective treatment for respiratory syncytial virus infection after lung transplantation. J. Heart Lung Transplant. 24:2114, 2005.

147. Goldman, D. L., Khine, H., Abadi, J., et al.: Serologic evidence for *Cryptococcus neoformans* infection in early childhood. Pediatrics 107:E66, 2001.

148. Gordon, S. M., and Avery, R. K.: Aspergillosis in lung transplantation: Incidence, risk factors, and prophylactic strategies. Transpl. Infect. Dis. 3:161, 2001.

149. Gourishankar, S., McDermid, J. C., Jhangri, G. S., et al.: Herpes zoster infection following solid organ transplantation: Incidence, risk factors and outcomes in the current immunosuppressive era. Am. J. Transplant. 4:108, 2004.

150. Graham, J. C., Kearns, A. M., Magee, J. G., et al.: Tuberculosis transmitted through transplantation. J. Infect. 43:251, 2001.

151. Green, M: Management of Epstein-Barr virus–induced post-transplant lymphoproliferative disease in recipients of solid organ transplantation. Am. J. Transplant. 1:103, 2001.

152. Green, M., and Barbadora, K.: Recovery of ceftazidime-resistant *Klebsiella pneumoniae* from pediatric liver and intestinal transplant recipients. Pediatr. Transplant. 2:224, 1998.

153. Green, M., and Webber, S. A.: EBV viral load monitoring: Unanswered questions. Am. J. Transplant. 2:894, 2002.

154. Green, M., and Webber, S.: Posttransplantation lymphoproliferative disorders. Pediatr. Clin. North Am. 50:1471, 2003.

155. Greene, R. E., Schlamm, H. T., Oestmann, J. W., et al.: Imaging findings in acute invasive pulmonary aspergillosis: Clinical significance of the halo sign. Clin. Infect. Dis. 44:373, 2007.

156. Griffith, D. E.: Emergence of nontuberculous mycobacteria as pathogens in cystic fibrosis. Am. J. Respir. Crit. Care Med. 167:810, 2003.

157. Griffith, D. E., Aksamit, T., Brown-Elliott, B. A., et al.: An official ATS/IDSA statement: Diagnosis, treatment, and prevention of nontuberculous mycobacterial diseases. Am. J. Respir. Crit. Care Med. 175:367, 2007.

158. Groetzner, J., Kur, F., Spelsberg, F., et al.: Airway anastomosis complications in de novo lung transplantation with sirolimus-based immunosuppression. J. Heart Lung Transplant. 23:632, 2004.

159. Groll, A. H., Attarbaschi, A., Schuster, F. R., et al.: Treatment with caspofungin in immunocompromised paediatric patients: A multicentre survey. J. Antimicrob. Chemother. 57:527, 2006.

160. Groothuis, J. R.: Role of antibody and use of respiratory syncytial virus (RSV) immune globulin to prevent severe RSV disease in high-risk children. J. Pediatr. 124:S28, 1994.

161. Gu, Z., Belzer, S. W., Gibson, C. S., et al.: Multiplexed, real-time PCR for quantitative detection of human adenovirus. J. Clin. Microbiol. 41:4636, 2003.

162. Hadjiliadis, D., Howell, D. N., Davis, R. D., et al.: Anastomotic infections in lung transplant recipients. Ann. Transplant. 5:13, 2000.

163. Hage, C. A., Reynolds, J. M., Durkin, M., et al.: Plasmalyte as a cause of false positive *Aspergillus* galactomannan in bronchoalveolar lavage fluid. J. Clin. Microbiol. 45:676-677, 2007.

164. Hahn, T., Cummings, K. M., Michalek, A. M., et al.: Efficacy of high-efficiency particulate air filtration in preventing aspergillosis in immunocompromised patients with hematologic malignancies. Infect. Control Hosp. Epidemiol. 23:525, 2002.

165. Halliday, C., Hoile, R., Sorrell, T., et al.: Role of prospective screening of blood for invasive aspergillosis by polymerase chain reaction in febrile neutropenic recipients of haematopoietic stem cell transplants and patients with acute leukaemia. Br. J. Haematol. 132:478, 2006.

166. Hayes, D., Jr.: *Mycobacterium abscessus* and other nontuberculous mycobacteria: Evolving respiratory pathogens in cystic fibrosis: A case report and review. South. Med. J. 98:657, 2005.

167. Hayney, M. S., Welter, D. L., Francois, M., et al.: Influenza vaccine antibody responses in lung transplant recipients. Prog. Transplant. 14:346, 2004.

168. Hebart, H., Loffler, J., Reitze, H., et al.: Prospective screening by a panfungal polymerase chain reaction assay in patients at risk for fungal infections: Implications for the management of febrile neutropenia. Br. J. Haematol. 111:635, 2000.

169. Hedderwick, S. A., Greenson, J. K., McGaughy, V. R., et al.: Adenovirus cholecystitis in a patient with AIDS. Clin. Infect. Dis. 26:997, 1998.

170. Heim, A., Ebnet, C., Harste, G., et al.: Rapid and quantitative detection of human adenovirus DNA by real-time PCR. J. Med. Virol. 70:228, 2003.

171. Heinz, T., Perfect, J., Schell, W., et al.: Soft-tissue fungal infections: Surgical management of 12 immunocompromised patients. Plast. Reconstr. Surg. 97:1391, 1996.

172. Hellenbrand, W., Meyer, C., Rasch, G., et al.: Cases of rabies in Germany following organ transplantation. Euro. Surveill. 10:E050224.6, 2005.

173. Helmi, M., Love, R. B., Welter, D., et al.: *Aspergillus* infection in lung transplant recipients with cystic fibrosis: Risk factors and outcomes comparison to other types of transplant recipients. Chest 123:800, 2003.

174. Herbrecht, R., Denning, D. W., Patterson, T. F., et al.: Voriconazole versus amphotericin B for primary therapy of invasive aspergillosis. N. Engl. J. Med. 347:408, 2002.

175. Herbrecht, R., Letscher-Bru, V., Oprea, C., et al.: *Aspergillus* galactomannan detection in the diagnosis of invasive aspergillosis in cancer patients. J. Clin. Oncol. 20:1898, 2002.

176. Herrera, J. M., McNeil, K. D., Higgins, R. S., et al.: Airway complications after lung transplantation: Treatment and long-term outcome. Ann. Thorac. Surg. 71:989, 2001.

177. Hoffman, J. A.: Adenoviral disease in pediatric solid organ transplant recipients. Pediatr. Transplant. 10:17, 2006.

178. Hoffman, J. A., Shah, A. J., Ross, L. A., et al.: Adenoviral infections and a prospective trial of cidofovir in pediatric hematopoietic stem cell transplantation. Biol. Blood Marrow Transplant. 7:388, 2001.

179. Hope, W. W., Walsh, T. J., and Denning, D. W.: Laboratory diagnosis of invasive aspergillosis. Lancet Infect. Dis. 5:609, 2005.

180. Humar, A: Screening for West Nile virus: More uncertainty. Am. J. Transplant. 4:1217, 2004.

181. Humar, A., Doucette, K., Kumar, D., et al.: Assessment of adenovirus infection in adult lung transplant recipients using molecular surveillance. J. Heart Lung Transplant. 25:1441, 2006.

182. Husain, S., Alexander, B. D., Munoz, P., et al.: Opportunistic mycelial fungal infections in organ transplant recipients: Emerging importance of non-*Aspergillus* mycelial fungi. Clin. Infect. Dis. 37:221, 2003.

183. Husain, S., Kwak, E. J., Obman, A., et al.: Prospective assessment of Platelia *Aspergillus* galactomannan antigen for the diagnosis of invasive aspergillosis in lung transplant recipients. Am. J. Transplant. 4:796, 2004.

184. Husain, S., Paterson, D. L., Studer, S., et al.: Voriconazole prophylaxis in lung transplant recipients. Am. J. Transplant. 6:3008, 2006.

185. Husain, S., and Singh, N.: *Burkholderia cepacia* infection and lung transplantation. Semin. Respir. Infect. 17:284, 2002.

186. Husain, S., and Singh, N.: Bronchiolitis obliterans and lung transplantation: Evidence for an infectious etiology. Semin. Respir. Infect. 17:310, 2002.

187. Husain, S., Wagener, M. M., and Singh, N.: *Cryptococcus neoformans* infection in organ transplant recipients: Variables influencing clinical characteristics and outcome. Emerg. Infect. Dis. 7:375, 2001.

188. Husain, S., Zaldonis, D., Kusne, S., et al.: Variation in antifungal prophylaxis strategies in lung transplantation. Transpl. Infect. Dis. 8:213, 2006.

189. Husni, R. N., Gordon, S. M., Longworth, D. L., et al.: Cytomegalovirus infection is a risk factor for invasive aspergillosis in lung transplant recipients. Clin. Infect. Dis. 26:753, 1998.

190. Iseman, M. D., and Heifets, L. B.: Rapid detection of tuberculosis and drug-resistant tuberculosis. N. Engl. J. Med. *355*:1606, 2006.

191. Iwamoto, M., Jernigan, D. B., Guasch, A., et al.: Transmission of West Nile virus from an organ donor to four transplant recipients. N. Engl. J. Med. *348*:2196, 2003.

192. Jacobs, F., Knoop, C., Brancart, F., et al.: Human herpesvirus-6 infection after lung and heart-lung transplantation: A prospective longitudinal study. Transplantation *75*:1996, 2003.

193. Jereb, J. A., Burwen, D. R., Dooley, S. W., et al.: Nosocomial outbreak of tuberculosis in a renal transplant unit: Application of a new technique for restriction fragment length polymorphism analysis of *Mycobacterium tuberculosis* isolates. J. Infect. Dis. *168*:1219, 1993.

194. Johnson, M. D., MacDougall, C., Ostrosky-Zeichner, L., et al.: Combination antifungal therapy. Antimicrob. Agents Chemother. *48*:693, 2004.

195. Jones, A. M., Dodd, M. E., Govan, J. R., et al.: *Burkholderia cenocepacia* and *Burkholderia multivorans*: Influence on survival in cystic fibrosis. Thorax *59*:948, 2004.

196. Jones, M. E., Fox, A. J., Barnes, A. J., et al.: PCR-ELISA for the early diagnosis of invasive pulmonary *Aspergillus* infection in neutropenic patients. J. Clin. Pathol. *51*:652, 1998.

197. Jordanides, N. E., Allan, E. K., McLintock, L. A., et al.: A prospective study of real-time panfungal PCR for the early diagnosis of invasive fungal infection in haemato-oncology patients. Bone Marrow Transplant. *35*:389, 2005.

198. Kami, M., Fukui, T., Ogawa, S., et al.: Use of real-time PCR on blood samples for diagnosis of invasive aspergillosis. Clin. Infect. Dis. *33*:1504, 2001.

199. Kanj, S. S., Tapson, V., Davis, R. D., et al.: Infections in patients with cystic fibrosis following lung transplantation. Chest *112*:924, 1997.

200. Kauffman, C. A.: Endemic mycoses: Blastomycosis, histoplasmosis, and sporotrichosis. Infect. Dis. Clin. North Am. *20*:645, 2006.

201. Kawazu, M., Kanda, Y., Nannya, Y., et al.: Prospective comparison of the diagnostic potential of real-time PCR, double-sandwich enzyme-linked immunosorbent assay for galactomannan, and a (1→3)-beta-D-glucan test in weekly screening for invasive aspergillosis in patients with hematological disorders. J. Clin. Microbiol. *42*:2733, 2004.

202. Kesten, S., and Chaparro, C.: Mycobacterial infections in lung transplant recipients. Chest *115*:741, 1999.

203. Khalifah, A. P., Hachem, R. R., Chakinala, M. M., et al.: Respiratory viral infections are a distinct risk for bronchiolitis obliterans syndrome and death. Am. J. Respir. Crit. Care Med. *170*:181, 2004.

204. Kiberd, B. A., and Forward, K.: Screening for West Nile virus in organ transplantation: A medical decision analysis. Am. J. Transplant. *4*:1296, 2004.

205. Kirby, A., Hassan, I., and Burnie, J.: Recommendations for managing *Aspergillus* osteomyelitis and joint infections based on a review of the literature. J. Infect. *52*:405, 2006.

206. Kleinschmidt-DeMasters, B. K., Marder, B. A., Levi, M. E., et al.: Naturally acquired West Nile virus encephalomyelitis in transplant recipients: Clinical, laboratory, diagnostic, and neuropathological features. Arch. Neurol. *61*:1210, 2004.

207. Klingspor, L., and Jalal, S.: Molecular detection and identification of *Candida* and *Aspergillus* spp. from clinical samples using real-time PCR. Clin. Microbiol. Infect. *12*:745, 2006.

208. Klont, R. R., Mennink-Kersten, M. A., and Verweij, P. E.: Utility of *Aspergillus* antigen detection in specimens other than serum specimens. Clin. Infect. Dis. *39*:1467, 2004.

209. Kohno, S., Masaoka, T., Yamaguchi, H., et al.: A multicenter, open-label clinical study of micafungin (FK463) in the treatment of deep-seated mycosis in Japan. Scand. J. Infect. Dis. *36*:372, 2004.

210. Koneru, B., Jaffe, R., Esquivel, C. O., et al.: Adenoviral infections in pediatric liver transplant recipients. J. A. M. A. *258*:489, 1987.

211. Kontoyiannis, D. P., Boktour, M., Hanna, H., et al.: Itraconazole added to a lipid formulation of amphotericin B does not improve outcome of primary treatment of invasive aspergillosis. Cancer *103*:2334, 2005.

212. Kontoyiannis, D. P., Hachem, R., Lewis, R. E., et al.: Efficacy and toxicity of caspofungin in combination with liposomal amphotericin B as primary or salvage treatment of invasive aspergillosis in patients with hematologic malignancies. Cancer *98*:292, 2003.

213. Kotloff, R. M., and Zuckerman, J. B.: Lung transplantation for cystic fibrosis: Special considerations. Chest *109*:787, 1996.

214. Kotton, C. N.: Zoonoses in solid-organ and hematopoietic stem cell transplant recipients. Clin. Infect. Dis. *44*:857, 2007.

215. Krishna, G., Sansone-Parsons, A., Martinho, M., et al.: Posaconazole plasma concentrations in juvenile patients with invasive fungal infection. Antimicrob. Agents Chemother. *51*:812, 2007.

216. Kshettry, V. R., Kroshus, T. J., Hertz, M. I., et al.: Early and late airway complications after lung transplantation: Incidence and management. Ann. Thorac. Surg. *63*:1576, 1997.

217. Kubak, B. M.: Fungal infection in lung transplantation. Transpl. Infect. Dis. *4*(Suppl. 3):24, 2002.

218. Kumar, D., Drebot, M. A., Wong, S. J., et al.: A seroprevalence study of West Nile virus infection in solid organ transplant recipients. Am. J. Transplant. *4*:1883, 2004.

219. Kumar, D., Erdman, D., Keshavjee, S., et al.: Clinical impact of community-acquired respiratory viruses on bronchiolitis obliterans after lung transplant. Am. J. Transplant. *5*:2031, 2005.

220. Kumar, D., and Humar, A.: Pandemic influenza and its implications for transplantation. Am. J. Transplant. *6*:1512, 2006.

221. Kumar, D., Prasad, G. V., Zaltzman, J., et al.: Community-acquired West Nile virus infection in solid-organ transplant recipients. Transplantation *77*:399, 2004.

222. Kuypers, J., Wright, N., Ferrenberg, J., et al.: Comparison of real-time PCR assays with fluorescent-antibody assays for diagnosis of respiratory virus infections in children. J. Clin. Microbiol. *44*:2382, 2006.

223. Kwak, E. J., Husain, S., Obman, A., et al.: Efficacy of galactomannan antigen in the Platelia *Aspergillus* enzyme immunoassay for diagnosis of invasive aspergillosis in liver transplant recipients. J. Clin. Microbiol. *42*:435, 2004.

224. Lang, B. J., Aaron, S. D., Ferris, W., et al.: Multiple combination bactericidal antibiotic testing for patients with cystic fibrosis infected with multiresistant strains of *Pseudomonas aeruginosa*. Am. J. Respir. Crit. Care Med. *162*:2241, 2000.

225. Larcher, C., Geltner, C., Fischer, H., et al.: Human metapneumovirus infection in lung transplant recipients: Clinical presentation and epidemiology. J. Heart Lung Transplant. *24*:1891, 2005.

226. Lass-Florl, C., Aigner, J., Gunsilius, E., et al.: Screening for *Aspergillus* spp. using polymerase chain reaction of whole blood samples from patients with haematological malignancies. Br. J. Haematol. *113*:180, 2001.

227. Leblond, V., Davi, F., Charlotte, F., et al.: Posttransplant lymphoproliferative disorders not associated with Epstein-Barr virus: A distinct entity? J. Clin. Oncol. *16*:2052, 1998.

228. Ledson, M. J., Gallagher, M. J., Corkill, J. E., et al.: Cross infection between cystic fibrosis patients colonised with *Burkholderia cepacia*. Thorax *53*:432, 1998.

229. Ledson, M. J., Gallagher, M. J., Jackson, M., et al.: Outcome of *Burkholderia cepacia* colonisation in an adult cystic fibrosis centre. Thorax *57*:142, 2002.

230. Legrand, F., Berrebi, D., Houhou, N., et al.: Early diagnosis of adenovirus infection and treatment with cidofovir after bone marrow transplantation in children. Bone Marrow Transplant. *27*:621, 2001.

231. Lehto, J. T., Halme, M., Tukiainen, P., et al.: Human herpesvirus-6 and -7 after lung and heart-lung transplantation. J. Heart Lung Transplant. *26*:41, 2007.

232. Leruez-Ville, M., Minard, V., Lacaille, F., et al.: Real-time blood plasma polymerase chain reaction for management of disseminated adenovirus infection. Clin. Infect. Dis. *38*:45, 2004.

233. Leung, T. F., Chik, K. W., Li, C. K., et al.: Incidence, risk factors and outcome of varicella-zoster virus infection in children after haematopoietic stem cell transplantation. Bone Marrow Transplant. *25*:167, 2000.

234. Lewis, R. E., and Kontoyiannis, D. P.: Rationale for combination antifungal therapy. Pharmacotherapy *21*:149S, 2001.

235. Lim, G. Y., Newman, B., Kurland, G., et al.: Posttransplantation lymphoproliferative disorder: Manifestations in pediatric thoracic organ recipients. Radiology *222*:699, 2002.

236. Limaye, A. P., Connolly, P. A., Sagar, M., et al.: Transmission of *Histoplasma capsulatum* by organ transplantation. N. Engl. J. Med. *343*:1163, 2000.

237. Linsangan, L. C., Hoffman, J. A., Woo, M. S., MacLaughlin, E. F., et al.: Infectious complications in pediatric lung and heart lung transplantation, including living donors. *In* Los Angeles, Childrens Hospital Los Angeles, Keck School of Medicine, University of Southern California, 2006. Unpublished data.

238. Linssen, C. F., Jacobs, J. A., Beckers, P., et al.: Inter-laboratory comparison of three different real-time PCR assays for the detection of *Pneumocystis jiroveci* in bronchoalveolar lavage fluid samples. J. Med. Microbiol. *55*:1229, 2006.

239. Lion, T., Baumgartinger, R., Watzinger, F., et al.: Molecular monitoring of adenovirus in peripheral blood after allogeneic bone marrow transplantation permits early diagnosis of disseminated disease. Blood *102*:1114, 2003.

240. LiPuma, J. J.: *Burkholderia cepacia* complex: A contraindication to lung transplantation in cystic fibrosis? Transpl. Infect. Dis. *3*:149, 2001.

241. Lipuma, J. J.: Update on the *Burkholderia cepacia* complex. Curr. Opin. Pulm. Med. *11*:528, 2005.

242. Ljungman, P., Griffiths, P., and Paya, C.: Definitions of cytomegalovirus infection and disease in transplant recipients. Clin. Infect. Dis. *34*:1094, 2002.

243. Ljungman, P., Ribaud, P., Eyrich, M., et al.: Cidofovir for adenovirus infections after allogeneic hematopoietic stem cell transplantation: A survey by the Infectious Diseases Working Party of the European Group for Blood and Marrow Transplantation. Bone Marrow Transplant. *31*:481, 2003.

244. Loeffler, J., Hebart, H., Brauchle, U., et al.: Comparison between plasma and whole blood specimens for detection of *Aspergillus* DNA by PCR. J. Clin. Microbiol. *38*:3830, 2000.

245. Luppi, M., Barozzi, P., Schulz, T. F., et al.: Bone marrow failure associated with human herpesvirus 8 infection after transplantation. N. Engl. J. Med. *343*:1378, 2000.

246. Machetti, M., Furfaro, E., and Viscoli, C.: Galactomannan in piperacillin-tazobactam: How much and to what extent? Antimicrob. Agents Chemother. *49*:3984, 2005.

247. Machetti, M., Zotti, M., Veroni, L., et al.: Antigen detection in the diagnosis and management of a patient with probable cerebral aspergillosis treated with voriconazole. Transpl. Infect. Dis. *2*:140, 2000.

248. Maertens, J., Glasmacher, A., Herbrecht, R., et al.: Multicenter, noncomparative study of caspofungin in combination with other antifungals as salvage therapy in adults with invasive aspergillosis. Cancer *107*:2888, 2006.

249. Maertens, J., Raad, I., Petrikkos, G., et al.: Efficacy and safety of caspofungin for treatment of invasive aspergillosis in patients refractory to or intolerant of conventional antifungal therapy. Clin. Infect. Dis. *39*:1563, 2004.

250. Maertens, J., Theunissen, K., Verhoef, G., et al.: False-positive *Aspergillus* galactomannan antigen test results. Clin. Infect. Dis. *39*:289, 2004.

251. Maertens, J., Theunissen, K., Verhoef, G., et al.: Galactomannan and computed tomography–based preemptive antifungal therapy in neutropenic patients at high risk for invasive fungal infection: A prospective feasibility study. Clin. Infect. Dis. *41*:1242, 2005.

252. Maertens, J., Van Eldere, J., Verhaegen, J., et al.: Use of circulating galactomannan screening for early diagnosis of invasive aspergillosis in allogeneic stem cell transplant recipients. J. Infect. Dis. *186*:1297, 2002.

253. Maertens, J., Verhaegen, J., Demuynck, H., et al.: Autopsy-controlled prospective evaluation of serial screening for circulating galactomannan by a sandwich enzyme-linked immunosorbent assay for hematological patients at risk for invasive aspergillosis. J. Clin. Microbiol. *37*:3223, 1999.

254. Maertens, J., Verhaegen, J., Lagrou, K., et al.: Screening for circulating galactomannan as a noninvasive diagnostic tool for invasive aspergillosis in prolonged neutropenic patients and stem cell transplantation recipients: A prospective validation. Blood *97*:1604, 2001.

255. Mahenthiralingam, E., Vandamme, P., Campbell, M. E., et al.: Infection with *Burkholderia cepacia* complex genomovars in patients with cystic fibrosis: Virulent transmissible strains of genomovar III can replace *Burkholderia multivorans*. Clin. Infect. Dis. *33*:1469, 2001.

256. Malavaud, S., Malavaud, B., Sandres, K., et al.: Nosocomial outbreak of influenza virus A (H3N2) infection in a solid organ transplant department. Transplantation *72*:535, 2001.

257. Malouf, M. A., and Glanville, A. R.: The spectrum of mycobacterial infection after lung transplantation. Am. J. Respir. Crit. Care Med. *160*:1611, 1999.

258. Marr, K. A., Balajee, S. A., McLaughlin, L., et al.: Detection of galactomannan antigenemia by enzyme immunoassay for the diagnosis of invasive aspergillosis: Variables that affect performance. J. Infect. Dis. *190*:641, 2004.

259. Marr, K. A., Boeckh, M., Carter, R. A., et al.: Combination antifungal therapy for invasive aspergillosis. Clin. Infect. Dis. *39*:797, 2004.

260. Marr, K. A., Hachem, R., Papanicolaou, G., et al.: Retrospective study of the hepatic safety profile of patients concomitantly treated with caspofungin and cyclosporin A. Transpl. Infect. Dis. *6*:110, 2004.

261. Marr, K. A., Laverdiere, M., Gugel, A., et al.: Antifungal therapy decreases sensitivity of the *Aspergillus* galactomannan enzyme immunoassay. Clin. Infect. Dis. *40*:1762, 2005.

262. Marshall, S. E., Kramer, M. R., Lewiston, N. J., et al.: Selection and evaluation of recipients for heart-lung and lung transplantation. Chest *98*:1488, 1990.

263. Marty, F. M., Lowry, C. M., Cutler, C. S., et al.: Voriconazole and sirolimus coadministration after allogeneic hematopoietic stem cell transplantation. Biol. Blood Marrow Transplant. *12*:552, 2006.

264. Marty, F. M., Lowry, C. M., Lempitski, S. J., et al.: Reactivity of (1→3)-beta-D-glucan assay with commonly used intravenous antimicrobials. Antimicrob. Agents Chemother. *50*:3450, 2006.

265. Marty, F. M., and Rubin, R. H.: The prevention of infection post-transplant: The role of prophylaxis, preemptive and empiric therapy. Transpl. Int. *19*:2, 2006.

266. Mathis, A. S., Shah, N. K., and Friedman, G. S.: Combined use of sirolimus and voriconazole in renal transplantation: A report of two cases. Transplant. Proc. *36*:2708, 2004.

267. Mazurek, G. H., Jereb, J., Lobue, P., et al.: Guidelines for using the QuantiFERON-TB Gold test for detecting *Mycobacterium tuberculosis* infection, United States. M. M. W. R. Recomm. Rep. *54*(RR-15):49, 2005.

268. McCurdy, L. H., Milstone, A., and Dummer, S.: Clinical features and outcomes of paramyxoviral infection in lung transplant recipients treated with ribavirin. J. Heart Lung Transplant. *22*:745, 2003.

269. McDiarmid, S. V., Blumberg, D. A., Remotti, H., et al.: Mycobacterial infections after pediatric liver transplantation: A report of three cases and review of the literature. J. Pediatr. Gastroenterol. Nutr. *20*:425, 1995.

270. McLaughlin, G. E., Delis, S., Kashimawo, L., et al.: Adenovirus infection in pediatric liver and intestinal transplant recipients: Utility of DNA detection by PCR. Am. J. Transplant. *3*:224, 2003.

271. McMenamin, J. D., Zaccone, T. M., Coenye, T., et al.: Misidentification of *Burkholderia cepacia* in US cystic fibrosis treatment centers: An analysis of 1,051 recent sputum isolates. Chest *117*:1661, 2000.

272. Meersseman, W., Vandecasteele, S. J., Wilmer, A., et al.: Invasive aspergillosis in critically ill patients without malignancy. Am. J. Respir. Crit. Care Med. *170*:621, 2004.

273. Mehrad, B., Paciocco, G., Martinez, F. J., et al.: Spectrum of *Aspergillus* infection in lung transplant recipients: Case series and review of the literature. Chest *119*:169, 2001.

274. Meissner, H. C., Welliver, R. C., Chartrand, S. A., et al.: Immunoprophylaxis with palivizumab, a humanized respiratory syncytial virus monoclonal antibody, for prevention of respiratory syncytial virus infection in high risk infants: A consensus opinion. Pediatr. Infect. Dis. J. *18*:223, 1999.

275. Mendez, J. C., Dockrell, D. H., Espy, M. J., et al.: Human beta-herpesvirus interactions in solid organ transplant recipients. J. Infect. Dis. *183*:179, 2001.

276. Mennink-Kersten, M. A., Donnelly, J. P., and Verweij, P. E.: Detection of circulating galactomannan for the diagnosis and management of invasive aspergillosis. Lancet Infect. Dis. *4*:349, 2004.

277. Mennink-Kersten, M. A., and Verweij, P. E.: Non–culture-based diagnostics for opportunistic fungi. Infect. Dis. Clin. North Am. *20*:711, 2006.

278. Merlin, E., Galambrun, C., Ribaud, P., et al.: Efficacy and safety of caspofungin therapy in children with invasive fungal infections. Pediatr. Infect. Dis. J. *25*:1186, 2006.

279. Michaels, M. G., Green, M., Wald, E. R., et al.: Adenovirus infection in pediatric liver transplant recipients. J. Infect. Dis. *165*:170, 1992.

280. Miller, M. B., Hendren, R., and Gilligan, P. H.: Posttransplantation disseminated coccidioidomycosis acquired from donor lungs. J. Clin. Microbiol. *42*:2347, 2004.

281. Millon, L., Piarroux, R., Deconinck, E., et al.: Use of real-time PCR to process the first galactomannan-positive serum sample in diagnosing invasive aspergillosis. J. Clin. Microbiol. *43*:5097, 2005.

282. Milpied, N., Vasseur, B., Parquet, N., et al.: Humanized anti-CD20 monoclonal antibody (rituximab) in post transplant B-lymphoproliferative disorder: A retrospective analysis on 32 patients. Ann. Oncol. *11*(Suppl. 1):113, 2000.

283. Minari, A., Husni, R., Avery, R. K., et al.: The incidence of invasive aspergillosis among solid organ transplant recipients and implications for prophylaxis in lung transplants. Transpl. Infect. Dis. *4*:195, 2002.

284. Miyazaki, T., Kohno, S., Mitsutake, K., et al.: Plasma (1→3)-beta-D-glucan and fungal antigenemia in patients with candidemia, aspergillosis, and cryptococcosis. J. Clin. Microbiol. *33*:3115, 1995.

285. Monforte, V., Roman, A., Gavalda, J., et al.: Nebulized amphotericin B prophylaxis for *Aspergillus* infection in lung transplantation: Study of risk factors. J. Heart Lung Transplant. *20*:1274, 2001.

286. Moore, D. A., Evans, C. A., Gilman, R. H., et al.: Microscopic-observation drug-susceptibility assay for the diagnosis of TB. N. Engl. J. Med. *355*:1539, 2006.

287. Morales, P., Briones, A., Torres, J. J., et al.: Pulmonary tuberculosis in lung and heart-lung transplantation: Fifteen years of experience in a single center in Spain. Transplant. Proc. *37*:4050, 2005.

288. Mukherjee, P. K., Sheehan, D. J., Hitchcock, C. A., et al.: Combination treatment of invasive fungal infections. Clin. Microbiol. Rev. *18*:163, 2005.

289. Multiply antibiotic-resistant gram-negative bacteria. Am. J. Transplant. *4*(Suppl. 10):21, 2004.

290. Munoz, P., Rodriguez, C., and Bouza, E.: *Mycobacterium tuberculosis* infection in recipients of solid organ transplants. Clin. Infect. Dis. *40*:581, 2005.

291. Munoz, P., Singh, N., and Bouza, E.: Treatment of solid organ transplant patients with invasive fungal infections: Should a combination of antifungal drugs be used? Curr. Opin. Infect. Dis. *19*:365, 2006.

292. Musher, B., Fredricks, D., Leisenring, W., et al.: *Aspergillus* galactomannan enzyme immunoassay and quantitative PCR for diagnosis of invasive aspergillosis with bronchoalveolar lavage fluid. J. Clin. Microbiol. *42*:5517, 2004.

293. Nagafuji, K., Aoki, K., Henzan, H., et al.: Cidofovir for treating adenoviral hemorrhagic cystitis in hematopoietic stem cell transplant recipients. Bone Marrow Transplant. *34*:909, 2004.

294. Nathan, S. D., Shorr, A. F., Schmidt, M. E., et al.: *Aspergillus* and endobronchial abnormalities in lung transplant recipients. Chest *118*:403, 2000.

295. Ner, Z., Ross, L. A., Horn, M. V., et al.: *Bordetella bronchiseptica* infection in pediatric lung transplant recipients. Pediatr. Transplant. *7*:413, 2003.

296. Neurohr, C., Huppmann, P., Leuchte, H., et al.: Human herpesvirus 6 in bronchoalveolar lavage fluid after lung transplantation: A risk factor for bronchiolitis obliterans syndrome? Am. J. Transplant. *5*:2982, 2005.

297. Nivoix, Y., Zamfir, A., Lutun, P., et al.: Combination of caspofungin and an azole or an amphotericin B formulation in invasive fungal infections. J. Infect. *52*:67, 2006.

298. Nunley, D. R., Gal, A. A., Vega, J. D., et al.: Saprophytic fungal infections and complications involving the bronchial anastomosis following human lung transplantation. Chest *122*:1185, 2002.

299. Nunley, D. R., Grgurich, W., Iacono, A. T., et al.: Allograft colonization and infections with pseudomonas in cystic fibrosis lung transplant recipients. Chest *113*:1235, 1998.

300. Nunley, D. R., Ohori, P., Grgurich, W. F., et al.: Pulmonary aspergillosis in cystic fibrosis lung transplant recipients. Chest *114*:1321, 1998.

301. Odabasi, Z., Mattiuzzi, G., Estey, E., et al.: Beta-D-glucan as a diagnostic adjunct for invasive fungal infections: Validation, cutoff development, and performance in patients with acute myelogenous leukemia and myelodysplastic syndrome. Clin. Infect. Dis. *39*:199, 2004.

302. Odio, C. M., Araya, R., Pinto, L. E., et al.: Caspofungin therapy of neonates with invasive candidiasis. Pediatr. Infect. Dis. J. *23*:1093, 2004.

303. Oertel, S. H., Verschuuren, E., Reinke, P., et al.: Effect of anti-CD 20 antibody rituximab in patients with post-transplant lymphoproliferative disorder (PTLD). Am. J. Transplant. *5*:2901, 2005.

304. Ohori, N. P., Michaels, M. G., Jaffe, R., et al.: Adenovirus pneumonia in lung transplant recipients. Hum. Pathol. *26*:1073, 1995.

305. Oliver, A., Maiz, L., Canton, R., et al.: Nontuberculous mycobacteria in patients with cystic fibrosis. Clin. Infect. Dis. *32*:1298, 2001.

306. Olivier, K. N.: The natural history of nontuberculous mycobacteria in patients with cystic fibrosis. Paediatr. Respir. Rev. *5*(Suppl. A):S213, 2004.

307. Olivier, K. N., Weber, D. J., Lee, J. H., et al.: Nontuberculous mycobacteria. II: Nested-cohort study of impact on cystic fibrosis lung disease. Am. J. Respir. Crit. Care Med. *167*:835, 2003.

308. Olivier, K. N., Weber, D. J., Wallace, R. J., Jr., et al.: Nontuberculous mycobacteria. I: Multicenter prevalence study in cystic fibrosis. Am. J. Respir. Crit. Care Med. *167*:828, 2003.

309. Orens, J. B., Estenne, M., Arcasoy, S., et al.: International guidelines for the selection of lung transplant candidates: 2006 update—a consensus report from the Pulmonary Scientific Council of the International Society for Heart and Lung Transplantation. J. Heart Lung Transplant. 25:745, 2006.

310. Ostrosky-Zeichner, L., Alexander, B. D., Kett, D. H., et al.: Multicenter clinical evaluation of the (1→3) beta-D-glucan assay as an aid to diagnosis of fungal infections in humans. Clin. Infect. Dis. 41:654, 2005.

311. Other herpesviruses: HHV-6, HHV-7, HHV-8, Hsv-1 and -2, and VZV. Am. J. Transplant. 4(Suppl. 10):66, 2004.

312. Pagano, L., Ricci, P., Nosari, A., et al.: Fatal haemoptysis in pulmonary filamentous mycosis: An underevaluated cause of death in patients with acute leukaemia in haematological complete remission. A retrospective study and review of the literature. Gimema Infection Program (Gruppo Italiano Malattie Ematologiche dell'Adulto). Br. J. Haematol. 89:500, 1995.

313. Pai, M., Kalantri, S., and Dheda, K.: New tools and emerging technologies for the diagnosis of tuberculosis: Part I. Latent tuberculosis. Expert Rev. Mol. Diagn. 6:413, 2006.

314. Pai, M., Kalantri, S., and Dheda, K.: New tools and emerging technologies for the diagnosis of tuberculosis: Part II. Active tuberculosis and drug resistance. Expert Rev. Mol. Diagn. 6:423, 2006.

315. Palmer, S. M., Alexander, B. D., Sanders, L. L., et al.: Significance of blood stream infection after lung transplantation: Analysis in 176 consecutive patients. Transplantation 69:2360, 2000.

316. Palmer, S. M., Drew, R. H., Whitehouse, J. D., et al.: Safety of aerosolized amphotericin B lipid complex in lung transplant recipients. Transplantation 72:545, 2001.

317. Palmer, S. M., Jr., Henshaw, N. G., Howell, D. N., et al.: Community respiratory viral infection in adult lung transplant recipients. Chest 113:944, 1998.

318. Palmer, S. M., Perfect, J. R., Howell, D. N., et al.: Candidal anastomotic infection in lung transplant recipients: Successful treatment with a combination of systemic and inhaled antifungal agents. J. Heart Lung Transplant. 17:1029, 1998.

319. Panackal, A. A., Dahlman, A., Keil, K. T., et al.: Outbreak of invasive aspergillosis among renal transplant recipients. Transplantation 75:1050, 2003.

320. Pancham, S., Hemmaway, C., New, H., et al.: Caspofungin for invasive fungal infections: Combination treatment with liposomal amphotericin B in children undergoing hemopoietic stem cell transplantation. Pediatr. Transplant. 9:254, 2005.

321. Pappas, P. G.: Invasive candidiasis. Infect. Dis. Clin. North Am. 20:485, 2006.

322. Pappas, P. G., Rex, J. H., Sobel, J. D., et al.: Guidelines for treatment of candidiasis. Clin. Infect. Dis. 38:161, 2004.

323. Paradowski, L. J.: Saprophytic fungal infections and lung transplantation—revisited. J. Heart Lung Transplant. 16:524, 1997.

324. Patterson, J. E., Peters, J., Calhoon, J. H., et al.: Investigation and control of aspergillosis and other filamentous fungal infections in solid organ transplant recipients. Transpl. Infect. Dis. 2:22, 2000.

325. Pazos, C., Ponton, J., Del Palacio, A.: Contribution of (1→3)-beta-D-glucan chromogenic assay to diagnosis and therapeutic monitoring of invasive aspergillosis in neutropenic adult patients: A comparison with serial screening for circulating galactomannan. J. Clin. Microbiol. 43:299, 2005.

326. Pfaller, M. A., and Diekema, D. J.: Epidemiology of invasive candidiasis: A persistent public health problem. Clin. Microbiol. Rev. 20:133, 2007.

327. Pfeiffer, C. D., Fine, J. P., and Safdar, N.: Diagnosis of invasive aspergillosis using a galactomannan assay: A meta-analysis. Clin. Infect. Dis. 42:1417, 2006.

328. Pickering, J. W., Sant, H. W., Bowles, C. A., et al.: Evaluation of a (1→3)-beta-D-glucan assay for diagnosis of invasive fungal infections. J. Clin. Microbiol. 43:5957, 2005.

329. Pickhardt, P. J., Siegel, M. J., Hayashi, R. J., et al.: Posttransplantation lymphoproliferative disorder in children: Clinical, histopathologic, and imaging features. Radiology 217:16, 2000.

330. Pierre-Audigier, C., Ferroni, A., Sermet-Gaudelus, I., et al.: Age-related prevalence and distribution of nontuberculous mycobacterial species among patients with cystic fibrosis. J. Clin. Microbiol. 43:3467, 2005.

331. Pinchoff, R. J., Kaufman, S. S., Magid, M. S., et al.: Adenovirus infection in pediatric small bowel transplantation recipients. Transplantation 76:183, 2003.

332. *Pneumocystis jiroveci* (formerly *Pneumocystis carinii*). Am. J. Transplant. 4(Suppl. 10):135, 2004.

333. Polis, M. A., Spooner, K. M., Baird, B. F., et al.: Anticytomegaloviral activity and safety of cidofovir in patients with human immunodeficiency virus infection and cytomegalovirus viruria. Antimicrob. Agents Chemother. 39:882, 1995.

334. Preiksaitis, J. K.: New developments in the diagnosis and management of posttransplantation lymphoproliferative disorders in solid organ transplant recipients. Clin. Infect. Dis. 39:1016, 2004.

335. Preiksaitis, J. K., and Keay, S.: Diagnosis and management of posttransplant lymphoproliferative disorder in solid-organ transplant recipients. Clin. Infect. Dis. 33(Suppl. 1):S38, 2001.

336. Raviv, Y., Kramer, M. R., Amital, A., et al.: Outbreak of aspergillosis infections among lung transplant recipients. Transpl. Int. 20:135, 2007.

337. Rebuck, J. A., Olsen, K. M., Fey, P. D., et al.: Characterization of an outbreak due to extended-spectrum beta-lactamase–producing *Klebsiella pneumoniae* in a pediatric intensive care unit transplant population. Clin. Infect. Dis. 31:1368, 2000.

338. Reichenspurner, H., Gamberg, P., Nitschke, M., et al.: Significant reduction in the number of fungal infections after lung, heart-lung, and heart transplantation using aerosolized amphotericin B prophylaxis. Transplant. Proc. 29:627, 1997.

339. Richeldi, L.: Rapid identification of *Mycobacterium tuberculosis* infection. Clin. Microbiol. Infect. 12(Suppl. 9):34, 2006.

340. Ridgeway, A. L., Warner, G. S., Phillips, P., et al.: Transmission of *Mycobacterium tuberculosis* to recipients of single lung transplants from the same donor. Am. J. Respir. Crit. Care Med. 153:1166, 1996.

341. Rodriguez, M., and Fishman, J. A.: Prevention of infection due to *Pneumocystis* spp. in human immunodeficiency virus–negative immunocompromised patients. Clin. Microbiol. Rev. 17:770, 2004.

342. Rohrlich, P., Sarfati, J., Mariani, P., et al.: Prospective sandwich enzyme-linked immunosorbent assay for serum galactomannan: Early predictive value and clinical use in invasive aspergillosis. Pediatr. Infect. Dis. J. 15:232, 1996.

343. Roilides, E., Lyman, C. A., Panagopoulou, P., et al.: Immunomodulation of invasive fungal infections. Infect. Dis. Clin. North Am. 17:193, 2003.

344. Romani, L.: Immunity to fungal infections. Nat. Rev. Immunol. 4:1, 2004.

345. Rowe, D. T., Webber, S., Schauer, E. M., et al.: Epstein-Barr virus load monitoring: Its role in the prevention and management of post-transplant lymphoproliferative disease. Transpl. Infect. Dis. 3:79, 2001.

346. Rubin, R. H.: Cytomegalovirus in solid organ transplantation. Transpl. Infect. Dis. 3(Suppl. 2):1-5, 2001.

347. Rubin, R. H.: Overview: Pathogenesis of fungal infections in the organ transplant recipient. Transpl. Infect. Dis. 4(Suppl. 3):12, 2002.

348. Rubin, R. H.: Influenza and the transplant recipient. Transpl. Infect. Dis. 4:175, 2002.

349. Rubin, R. H.: Infections in the organ transplant patient. In Rubin, R. H., and Young, L. S. (eds.): Clinical Approach to Infection in the Compromised Host. 4th ed. New York. Kluwer Academic/Plenum Publishers, 2002, p. 573.

350. Rubin, R. H.: Temporal aspects of transplant infectious disease. Transpl. Infect. Dis. 5:63, 2003.

351. Rubin, R. H.: Management of tuberculosis in the transplant recipient. Am. J. Transplant. 5:2599, 2005.

352. Rubin, R. H., Ikonen, T., Gummert, J. F., et al.: The therapeutic prescription for the organ transplant recipient: The linkage of immunosuppression and antimicrobial strategies. Transpl. Infect. Dis. 1:29, 1999.

353. Rubin, R. H., and Marty, F. M.: Principles of antimicrobial therapy in the transplant patient. Transpl. Infect. Dis. 6:97, 2004.

354. Saad, A. H., DePestel, D. D., and Carver, P. L.: Factors influencing the magnitude and clinical significance of drug interactions between azole antifungals and select immunosuppressants. Pharmacotherapy 26:1730, 2006.

355. Saag, M. S., Graybill, R. J., Larsen, R. A., et al.: Practice guidelines for the management of cryptococcal disease. Infectious Diseases Society of America. Clin. Infect. Dis. 30:710, 2000.

356. Sadaba, B., Campanero, M. A., Quetglas, E. G., et al.: Clinical relevance of sirolimus drug interactions in transplant patients. Transplant. Proc. 36:3226, 2004.

357. Saiman, L., Mehar, F., Niu, W. W., et al.: Antibiotic susceptibility of multiply resistant *Pseudomonas aeruginosa* isolated from patients with cystic fibrosis, including candidates for transplantation. Clin. Infect. Dis. 23:532, 1996.

358. Sajjan, U., Thanassoulis, G., Cherapanov, V., et al.: Enhanced susceptibility to pulmonary infection with *Burkholderia cepacia* in Cftr(–/–) mice. Infect. Immun. 69:5138, 2001.

359. Sajjan, U., Wu, Y., Kent, G., et al.: Preferential adherence of cable-piliated *Burkholderia cepacia* to respiratory epithelia of CF knockout mice and human cystic fibrosis lung explants. J. Med. Microbiol. 49:875, 2000.

360. Sanguinetti, M., Ardito, F., Fiscarelli, E., et al.: Fatal pulmonary infection due to multidrug-resistant *Mycobacterium abscessus* in a patient with cystic fibrosis. J. Clin. Microbiol. 39:816, 2001.

361. Sanguinetti, M., Posteraro, B., Pagano, L., et al.: Comparison of real-time PCR, conventional PCR, and galactomannan antigen detection by enzyme-linked immunosorbent assay using bronchoalveolar lavage fluid samples from hematology patients for diagnosis of invasive pulmonary aspergillosis. J. Clin. Microbiol. 41:3922, 2003.

362. Schilham, M. W., Claas, E. C., van Zaane, W., et al.: High levels of adenovirus DNA in serum correlate with fatal outcome of adenovirus infection in children after allogeneic stem-cell transplantation. Clin. Infect. Dis. 35:526, 2002.

363. Schluger, N. W.: Changing approaches to the diagnosis of tuberculosis. Am. J. Respir. Crit. Care Med. 164:2020, 2001.

364. Schwartz, S., Ruhnke, M., Ribaud, P., et al.: Improved outcome in central nervous system aspergillosis, using voriconazole treatment. Blood 106:2641, 2005.

365. Segal, B. H., Barnhart, L. A., Anderson, V. L., et al.: Posaconazole as salvage therapy in patients with chronic granulomatous disease and invasive filamentous fungal infection. Clin. Infect. Dis. 40:1684, 2005.

366. Segal, B. H., Kwon-Chung, J., Walsh, T. J., et al.: Immunotherapy for fungal infections. Clin. Infect. Dis. 42:507, 2006.

367. Seibel, N. L., Schwartz, C., Arrieta, A., et al.: Safety, tolerability, and pharmacokinetics of micafungin (FK463) in febrile neutropenic pediatric patients. Antimicrob. Agents Chemother. 49:3317, 2005.

368. Serody, J. S., Mill, M. R., Detterbeck, F. C., et al.: Blastomycosis in transplant recipients: Report of a case and review. Clin. Infect. Dis. 16:54, 1993.

369. Shreeniwas, R., Schulman, L. L., Berkmen, Y. M., et al.: Opportunistic bronchopulmonary infections after lung transplantation: Clinical and radiographic findings. Radiology 200:349, 1996.

370. Siegel, M. J., Lee, E. Y., Sweet, S. C., et al.: CT of posttransplantation lymphoproliferative disorder in pediatric recipients of lung allograft. A. J. R. Am. J. Roentgenol. 181:1125, 2003.

371. Simoes, E. A., Sondheimer, H. M., Top, F. H., Jr., et al.: Respiratory syncytial virus immune globulin for prophylaxis against respiratory syncytial virus disease in infants and children with congenital heart disease. The Cardiac Study Group. J. Pediatr. 133:492, 1998.

372. Singh, N.: Treatment of opportunistic mycoses: How long is long enough? Lancet Infect. Dis. 3:703, 2003.

373. Singh, N.: Interactions between viruses in transplant recipients. Clin. Infect. Dis. 40:430, 2005.

374. Singh, N., Alexander, B. D., Lortholary, O., et al.: Cryptococcus neoformans in organ transplant recipients: Impact of calcineurin-inhibitor agents on mortality. J. Infect. Dis. 195:756, 2007.

375. Singh, N., Avery, R. K., Munoz, P., et al.: Trends in risk profiles for and mortality associated with invasive aspergillosis among liver transplant recipients. Clin. Infect. Dis. 36:46, 2003.

376. Singh, N., and Husain, S.: Aspergillus infections after lung transplantation: Clinical differences in type of transplant and implications for management. J. Heart Lung Transplant. 22:258, 2003.

377. Singh, N., Limaye, A. P., Forrest, G., et al.: Combination of voriconazole and caspofungin as primary therapy for invasive aspergillosis in solid organ transplant recipients: A prospective, multicenter, observational study. Transplantation 81:320, 2006.

378. Singh, N., Limaye, A. P., Forrest, G., et al.: Late-onset invasive aspergillosis in organ transplant recipients in the current era. Med. Mycol. 44:445, 2006.

379. Singh, N., Lortholary, O., Alexander, B. D., et al.: Antifungal management practices and evolution of infection in organ transplant recipients with Cryptococcus neoformans infection. Transplantation 80:1033, 2005.

380. Singh, N., Lortholary, O., Alexander, B. D., et al.: Allograft loss in renal transplant recipients with Cryptococcus neoformans associated immune reconstitution syndrome. Transplantation 80:1131, 2005.

381. Singh, N., Lortholary, O., Alexander, B. D., et al.: An immune reconstitution syndrome–like illness associated with Cryptococcus neoformans infection in organ transplant recipients. Clin. Infect. Dis. 40:1756, 2005.

382. Singh, N., Obman, A., Husain, S., et al.: Reactivity of Platelia Aspergillus galactomannan antigen with piperacillin-tazobactam: Clinical implications based on achievable concentrations in serum. Antimicrob. Agents Chemother. 48:1989, 2004.

383. Singh, N., and Paterson, D. L.: Mycobacterium tuberculosis infection in solid-organ transplant recipients: Impact and implications for management. Clin. Infect. Dis. 27:1266, 1998.

384. Singh, N., and Paterson, D. L.: Aspergillus infections in transplant recipients. Clin. Microbiol. Rev. 18:44, 2005.

385. Singh, N., Rihs, J. D., Gayowski, T., et al.: Cutaneous cryptococcosis mimicking bacterial cellulitis in a liver transplant recipient: Case report and review in solid organ transplant recipients. Clin. Transplant. 8:365, 1994.

386. Skladny, H., Buchheidt, D., Baust, C., et al.: Specific detection of Aspergillus species in blood and bronchoalveolar lavage samples of immunocompromised patients by two-step PCR. J. Clin. Microbiol. 37:3865, 1999.

387. Smyth, R. L., Higenbottam, T. W., Scott, J. P., et al.: Herpes simplex virus infection in heart-lung transplant recipients. Transplantation 49:735, 1990.

388. Snell, G. I., de Hoyos, A., Krajden, M., et al.: Pseudomonas cepacia in lung transplant recipients with cystic fibrosis. Chest 103:466, 1993.

389. Sokol, P. A., Sajjan, U., Visser, M. B., et al.: The CepIR quorum-sensing system contributes to the virulence of Burkholderia cenocepacia respiratory infections. Microbiology 149:3649, 2003.

390. Sole, A., Morant, P., Salavert, M., et al.: Aspergillus infections in lung transplant recipients: Risk factors and outcome. Clin. Microbiol. Infect. 11:359, 2005.

391. Spellberg, B. J., Filler, S. G., and Edwards, J. E., Jr.: Current treatment strategies for disseminated candidiasis. Clin. Infect. Dis. 42:244, 2006.

392. Spiess, B., Buchheidt, D., Baust, C., et al.: Development of a LightCycler PCR assay for detection and quantification of Aspergillus fumigatus DNA in clinical samples from neutropenic patients. J. Clin. Microbiol. 41:1811, 2003.

393. Srinivasan, A., Burton, E. C., Kuehnert, M. J., et al.: Transmission of rabies virus from an organ donor to four transplant recipients. N. Engl. J. Med. 352:1103, 2005.

394. Starke, J. R.: Interferon-gamma release assays for diagnosis of tuberculosis infection in children. Pediatr. Infect. Dis. J. 25:941, 2006.

395. Starnes, V. A., Bowdish, M. E., Woo, M. S., et al.: A decade of living lobar lung transplantation: Recipient outcomes. J. Thorac. Cardiovasc. Surg. 127:114, 2004.

396. Steinbach, W. J.: Pediatric aspergillosis: Disease and treatment differences in children. Pediatr. Infect. Dis. J. 24:358, 2005.

397. Steinbach, W. J.: Combination antifungal therapy for invasive aspergillosis—is it indicated? Med. Mycol. 44(Suppl.):373, 2006.

398. Steinbach, W. J., and Stevens, D. A.: Review of newer antifungal and immunomodulatory strategies for invasive aspergillosis. Clin. Infect. Dis. 37(Suppl. 3):S157, 2003.

399. Steinbach, W. J., Stevens, D. A., and Denning, D. W.: Combination and sequential antifungal therapy for invasive aspergillosis: Review of published in vitro and in vivo interactions and 6281 clinical cases from 1966 to 2001. Clin. Infect. Dis. 37(Suppl. 3):S188, 2003.

400. Stevens, D. A., Kan, V. L., Judson, M. A., et al.: Practice guidelines for diseases caused by Aspergillus. Infectious Diseases Society of America. Clin. Infect. Dis. 30:696, 2000.

401. Stevens, S. J., Verschuuren, E. A., Pronk, I., et al.: Frequent monitoring of Epstein-Barr virus DNA load in unfractionated whole blood is essential for early detection of posttransplant lymphoproliferative disease in high-risk patients. Blood 97:1165, 2001.

402. Stringer, J. R., Beard, C. B., Miller, R. F., et al.: A new name (Pneumocystis jiroveci) for Pneumocystis from humans. Emerg. Infect. Dis. 8:891, 2002.

403. Stynen, D., Goris, A., Sarfati, J., et al.: A new sensitive sandwich enzyme-linked immunosorbent assay to detect galactofuran in patients with invasive aspergillosis. J. Clin. Microbiol. 33:497, 1995.

404. Stynen, D., Sarfati, J., Goris, A., et al.: Rat monoclonal antibodies against Aspergillus galactomannan. Infect. Immun. 60:2237, 1992.

405. Sulahian, A., Boutboul, F., Ribaud, P., et al.: Value of antigen detection using an enzyme immunoassay in the diagnosis and prediction of invasive aspergillosis in two adult and pediatric hematology units during a 4-year prospective study. Cancer 91:311, 2001.

406. Sulahian, A., Touratier, S., and Ribaud, P.: False positive test for Aspergillus antigenemia related to concomitant administration of piperacillin and tazobactam. N. Engl. J. Med. 349:2366, 2003.

407. Swedish Consensus Group: Management of infections caused by respiratory syncytial virus. Scand. J. Infect. Dis. 33:323, 2001.

408. Sweet, S. C.: Pediatric living donor lobar lung transplantation. Pediatr. Transplant. 10:861, 2006.

409. Taylor, A. L., Marcus, R., and Bradley, J. A.: Post-transplant lymphoproliferative disorders (PTLD) after solid organ transplantation. Crit. Rev. Oncol. Hematol. 56:155, 2005.

410. Taylor, J. L., and Palmer, S. M.: Mycobacterium abscessus chest wall and pulmonary infection in a cystic fibrosis lung transplant recipient. J. Heart Lung Transplant. 25:985, 2006.

411. Templeton, K. E., Scheltinga, S. A., Beersma, M. F., et al.: Rapid and sensitive method using multiplex real-time PCR for diagnosis of infections by influenza A and influenza B viruses, respiratory syncytial virus, and parainfluenza viruses 1, 2, 3, and 4. J. Clin. Microbiol. 42:1564, 2004.

412. Tenover, F. C.: Rapid detection and identification of bacterial pathogens using novel molecular technologies: Infection control and beyond. Clin. Infect. Dis. 44:418, 2007.

413. Thio, C. L., Smith, D., Merz, W. G., et al.: Refinements of environmental assessment during an outbreak investigation of invasive aspergillosis in a leukemia and bone marrow transplant unit. Infect. Control Hosp. Epidemiol. 21:18, 2000.

414. Thomas, K. E., Owens, C. M., Veys, P. A., et al.: The radiological spectrum of invasive aspergillosis in children: A 10-year review. Pediatr. Radiol. 33:453, 2003.

415. Tripathy, U., Yung, G. L., Kriett, J. M., et al.: Donor transfer of pulmonary coccidioidomycosis in lung transplantation. Ann. Thorac. Surg. 73:306, 2002.

416. Trulock, E. P., Edwards, L. B., Taylor, D. O., et al.: Registry of the International Society for Heart and Lung Transplantation: Twenty-third official adult lung and heart-lung transplantation report—2006. J. Heart Lung Transplant. 25:880, 2006.

417. Tsai, D. E., Nearey, M., Hardy, C. L., et al.: Use of EBV PCR for the diagnosis and monitoring of post-transplant lymphoproliferative disorder in adult solid organ transplant patients. Am. J. Transplant. 2:946, 2002.

418. Ullmann, A. J., Lipton, J. H., Vesole, D. H., et al.: Posaconazole or fluconazole for prophylaxis in severe graft-versus-host disease. N. Engl. J. Med. 356:335, 2007.

419. Vail, G. M., Young, R. S., Wheat, L. J., et al.: Incidence of histoplasmosis following allogeneic bone marrow transplant or solid organ transplant in a hyperendemic area. Transpl. Infect. Dis. 4:148, 2002.

420. Van Burik, J. A., Myerson, D., Schreckhise, R. W., et al.: Panfungal PCR assay for detection of fungal infection in human blood specimens. J. Clin. Microbiol. 36:1169, 1998.

421. van Burik, J. A., Ratanatharathorn, V., Stepan, D. E., et al.: Micafungin versus fluconazole for prophylaxis against invasive fungal infections during neutropenia in patients undergoing hematopoietic stem cell transplantation. Clin. Infect. Dis. 39:1407, 2004.

422. van den Hoogen, B. G., de Jong, J. C., Groen, J., et al.: A newly discovered human pneumovirus isolated from young children with respiratory tract disease. Nat. Med. 7:719, 2001.

423. Vazquez, J. A., and Sobel, J. D.: Anidulafungin: A novel echinocandin. Clin. Infect. Dis. 43:215, 2006.

424. Venkataramanan, R., Zang, S., Gayowski, T., et al.: Voriconazole inhibition of the metabolism of tacrolimus in a liver transplant recipient and in human liver microsomes. Antimicrob. Agents Chemother. 46:3091, 2002.

425. Verma, A., Dhawan, A., Wade, J. J., et al.: Mycobacterium tuberculosis infection in pediatric liver transplant recipients. Pediatr. Infect. Dis. J. 19:625, 2000.

426. Verweij, P. E., Weemaes, C. M., Curfs, J. H., et al.: Failure to detect circulating Aspergillus markers in a patient with chronic granulomatous disease and invasive aspergillosis. J. Clin. Microbiol. 38:3900, 2000.

427. Vilchez, R. A., Dauber, J., and Kusne, S.: Infectious etiology of bronchiolitis obliterans: The respiratory viruses connection—myth or reality? Am. J. Transplant. 3:245, 2003.

428. Vilchez, R. A., Dauber, J., McCurry, K., et al.: Parainfluenza virus infection in adult lung transplant recipients: An emergent clinical syndrome with implications on allograft function. Am. J. Transplant. 3:116, 2003.

429. Vilchez, R. A., Fung, J., and Kusne, S.: The pathogenesis and management of influenza virus infection in organ transplant recipients. Transpl. Infect. Dis. 4:177, 2002.

430. Vilchez, R. A., Fung, J., and Kusne, S.: Cryptococcosis in organ transplant recipients: An overview. Am. J. Transplant. 2:575, 2002.

431. Vilchez, R. A., McCurry, K., Dauber, J., et al.: The epidemiology of parainfluenza virus infection in lung transplant recipients. Clin. Infect. Dis. 33:2004, 2001.

432. Vilchez, R. A., McCurry, K., Dauber, J., et al.: Influenza virus infection in adult solid organ transplant recipients. Am. J. Transplant. 2:287, 2002.

433. Vilchez, R., Shapiro, R., McCurry, K., et al.: Longitudinal study of cryptococcosis in adult solid-organ transplant recipients. Transpl. Int. 16:336, 2003.

434. Viscoli, C.: Combination therapy for invasive aspergillosis. Clin. Infect. Dis. 39:803, 2004.

435. Viscoli, C., Machetti, M., Cappellano, P., et al.: False-positive galactomannan Platelia *Aspergillus* test results for patients receiving piperacillin-tazobactam. Clin. Infect. Dis. 38:913, 2004.

436. Viscoli, C., Machetti, M., Gazzola, P., et al.: *Aspergillus* galactomannan antigen in the cerebrospinal fluid of bone marrow transplant recipients with probable cerebral aspergillosis. J. Clin. Microbiol. 40:1496, 2002.

437. Wagner, J. A., Ross, H., Hunt, S., et al.: Prophylactic ganciclovir treatment reduces fungal as well as cytomegalovirus infections after heart transplantation. Transplantation 60:1473, 1995.

438. Wallot, M. A., Dohna-Schwake, C., Auth, M., et al.: Disseminated adenovirus infection with respiratory failure in pediatric liver transplant recipients: Impact of intravenous cidofovir and inhaled nitric oxide. Pediatr. Transplant. 10:121, 2006.

439. Walls, T., Hawrami, K., Shingadia, D., et al.: Polymerase chain reaction in the management of disseminated adenovirus infection after stem cell transplantation. Pediatr. Infect. Dis. J. 23:1167, 2004.

440. Walsh, T. J., Adamson, P. C., Seibel, N. L., et al.: Pharmacokinetics, safety, and tolerability of caspofungin in children and adolescents. Antimicrob. Agents Chemother. 49:4536, 2005.

441. Walsh, T. J., Karlsson, M. O., Driscoll, T., et al.: Pharmacokinetics and safety of intravenous voriconazole in children after single- or multiple-dose administration. Antimicrob. Agents Chemother. 48:2166, 2004.

442. Walsh, T. J., Lutsar, I., Driscoll, T., et al.: Voriconazole in the treatment of aspergillosis, scedosporiosis and other invasive fungal infections in children. Pediatr. Infect. Dis. J. 21:240, 2002.

443. Walsh, T. J., Raad, I., Patterson, T. F., et al.: Treatment of invasive aspergillosis with posaconazole in patients who are refractory to or intolerant of conventional therapy: An externally controlled trial. Clin. Infect. Dis. 44:2, 2007.

444. Walsh, T. J., Shoham, S., Petraitiene, R., et al.: Detection of galactomannan antigenemia in patients receiving piperacillin-tazobactam and correlations between in vitro, in vivo, and clinical properties of the drug-antigen interaction. J. Clin. Microbiol. 42:4744, 2004.

445. Walsh, T. J., Teppler, H., Donowitz, G. R., et al.: Caspofungin versus liposomal amphotericin B for empirical antifungal therapy in patients with persistent fever and neutropenia. N. Engl. J. Med. 351:1391, 2004.

445a. Walsh, T. J., Anaissie, E. J., Denning, D. W., et al.: Treatment of *Aspergillus*: Clinical practice guidelines of the Infectious Disease Society of America. Clin. Infect. Dis. 46:327-360, 2008.

446. Waltz, D. A., Boucek, M. M., Edwards, L. B., et al.: Registry of the International Society for Heart and Lung Transplantation: Ninth official pediatric lung and heart-lung transplantation report—2006. J. Heart Lung Transplant. 25:904, 2006.

447. Weishaar, P. D., Flynn, H. W., Jr., Murray, T. G., et al.: Endogenous *Aspergillus* endophthalmitis. Clinical features and treatment outcomes. Ophthalmology 105:57, 1998.

448. Wendt, C. H.: Community respiratory viruses: Organ transplant recipients. Am. J. Med. 102:31, 1997.

449. Wendt, C. H., Fox, J. M., and Hertz, M. I.: Paramyxovirus infection in lung transplant recipients. J. Heart Lung Transplant. 14:479, 1995.

450. Wheat, J., Sarosi, G., McKinsey, D., et al.: Practice guidelines for the management of patients with histoplasmosis. Infectious Diseases Society of America. Clin. Infect. Dis. 30:688, 2000.

451. Wheat, L.: Current diagnosis of histoplasmosis. Trends Microbiol. 11:488, 2003.

452. Wheat, L. J.: Rapid diagnosis of invasive aspergillosis by antigen detection. Transpl. Infect. Dis. 5:158, 2003.

453. Wheat, L. J.: Combination therapy for aspergillosis: Is it needed, and which combination? J. Infect. Dis. 187:1831, 2003.

454. Wheat, L. J.: Antigen detection, serology, and molecular diagnosis of invasive mycoses in the immunocompromised host. Transpl. Infect. Dis. 8:128, 2006.

455. Wheat, L. J.: Histoplasmosis: A review for clinicians from non-endemic areas. Mycoses 49:274, 2006.

456. Whimbey, E., Champlin, R. E., Englund, J. A., et al.: Combination therapy with aerosolized ribavirin and intravenous immunoglobulin for respiratory syncytial virus disease in adult bone marrow transplant recipients. Bone Marrow Transplant. 16:393, 1995.

457. White, P. L., Barton, R., Guiver, M., et al.: A consensus on fungal polymerase chain reaction diagnosis? A United Kingdom–Ireland evaluation of polymerase chain reaction methods for detection of systemic fungal infections. J. Mol. Diagn. 8:376, 2006.

458. White, P. L., Linton, C. J., Perry, M. D., et al.: The evolution and evaluation of a whole blood polymerase chain reaction assay for the detection of invasive aspergillosis in hematology patients in a routine clinical setting. Clin. Infect. Dis. 42:479, 2006.

459. Williams, J. V., Harris, P. A., Tollefson, S. J., et al.: Human metapneumovirus and lower respiratory tract disease in otherwise healthy infants and children. N. Engl. J. Med. 350:443, 2004.

460. Williamson, E. C., Leeming, J. P., Palmer, H. M., et al.: Diagnosis of invasive aspergillosis in bone marrow transplant recipients by polymerase chain reaction. Br. J. Haematol. 108:132, 2000.

461. Woo, M. S., MacLaughlin, E. F., Horn, M. V., et al.: Living donor lobar lung transplantation: The pediatric experience. Pediatr. Transplant. 2:185, 1998.

462. Woo, M. S., Perez, E., Horn, M. V., et al.: Post-operative use of aerosolized aztreonam in cystic fibrosis patients colonized with *Burkholderia cepacia* prior to lung transplantation. J. Heart Lung Transplant. 23:S78, 2004.

463. Wright, P. W., Pappagianis, D., Wilson, M., et al.: Donor-related coccidioidomycosis in organ transplant recipients. Clin. Infect. Dis. 37:1265, 2003.

464. Wu, G., Vilchez, R. A., Eidelman, B., et al.: Cryptococcal meningitis: An analysis among 5,521 consecutive organ transplant recipients. Transpl. Infect. Dis. 4:183, 2002.

465. Yusuf, U., Hale, G. A., Carr, J., et al.: Cidofovir for the treatment of adenoviral infection in pediatric hematopoietic stem cell transplant patients. Transplantation 81:1398, 2006.

466. Zamora, M. R.: Use of cytomegalovirus immune globulin and ganciclovir for the prevention of cytomegalovirus disease in lung transplantation. Transpl. Infect. Dis. 3(Suppl. 2): 49-52, 2001.

467. Zamora, M. R.: Cytomegalovirus and lung transplantation. Am. J. Transplant. 4:1219, 2004.

468. Zamora, M. R., Davis, R. D., and Leonard, C.: Management of cytomegalovirus infection in lung transplant recipients: Evidence-based recommendations. Transplantation 80:157, 2005.

469. Zamora, M. R., Nicolls, M. R., Hodges, T. N., et al.: Following universal prophylaxis with intravenous ganciclovir and cytomegalovirus immune globulin, valganciclovir is safe and effective for prevention of CMV infection following lung transplantation. Am. J. Transplant. 4:1635, 2004.

CHAPTER

83

OPPORTUNISTIC INFECTIONS IN LIVER AND INTESTINAL TRANSPLANTATION

Michael D. Green ⊙ Marian G. Michaels

For more than 20 years, liver transplantation has been established as an effective treatment of end-stage liver disease in children. Improved surgical techniques and the availability of new and more potent immunosuppressive regimens have led to enhanced short- and long-term survival rates that now approach or exceed 80 percent. In response to these excellent results, more children

are being referred for liver transplantation, and increasing numbers of pediatric centers routinely perform this procedure. More recently, intestinal transplantation, performed as an isolated procedure or in combination with the liver or other organs, also is gaining expanded acceptance as treatment of refractory intestinal failure in children, particularly those who experience progressive liver failure as a result of hyperalimentation-induced liver disease. Although this newer procedure has been performed routinely at only a limited number of centers, an increasing number of transplant programs are beginning to offer intestinal transplantation.

Infectious complications have been a significant cause of morbidity and mortality in children undergoing liver transplantation since this procedure gained initial acceptance in the 1980s. However, improvements in immune suppression management along with the increasing availability of new antimicrobial agents and diagnostic tools have resulted in improved treatment regimens that have reduced the impact of infectious complications on these children. The introduction of intestinal transplantation brought with it many of the same infectious complications seen after liver transplantations, as well as a number of infectious issues that appear to be unique to this procedure. The experience garnered from the treatment of patients undergoing liver and other organ transplant procedures has been translated effectively to the management of infections occurring after intestinal transplantation. Although development of increasingly effective treatment strategies is of great benefit to the children undergoing these procedures, emphasis also focuses on the development of strategies aimed at prevention of infectious complications in children undergoing abdominal transplantation. This chapter provides a general overview of the problem of infections that develop after liver transplantation and intestinal transplantation in children.

PREDISPOSING FACTORS

Liver transplantation and intestinal transplantation are associated with a set of technical and medical conditions that predispose one to a unique set of infectious complications. The abdomen is a common site of infection in patients undergoing both these procedures,[29,77] almost certainly as a result of local ischemic injury and bleeding as well as potential soilage with contaminated material.[59] Additional factors predisposing recipients to infection can be divided into those that exist before transplantation and those secondary to intraoperative and post-transplant activities.

PRETRANSPLANT FACTORS

The underlying illnesses leading to transplantation may be associated with intrinsic risk factors for the development of infection. Some disorders may have required palliative surgery that increases the technical difficulty of the transplant procedure and may be associated with an enhanced risk for the development of post-transplant infection.[25] For example, in children undergoing liver transplantation for biliary atresia, a Kasai procedure (choledo-chojejunostomy) may have been performed previously and predisposed them to recurrent episodes of bacterial cholangitis before transplantation, thereby increasing the likelihood of colonization with multiple antibiotic–resistant bacteria, which can cause infection after transplantation. Similarly, children undergoing liver transplantation for cystic fibrosis may have an increased risk for the development of invasive aspergillosis if they were colonized with this pathogen before receiving the transplant. Complications of end-stage liver disease (as part of a primary liver disease or as a consequence of hyperalimentation in patients with intestinal insufficiency) also may predispose the patient to the development of infection after undergoing transplantation. A history of one or more episodes of spontaneous bacterial peritonitis before transplantation in patients with ascites has been associated with an increased rate of bacterial infection developing after liver transplantation[120] and could be expected in patients with liver disease associated with intestinal insufficiency. Finally, children undergoing intestinal transplantation experi-

ence frequent episodes of gastrointestinal-associated bloodstream infections. Recurrent exposure to antimicrobials to treat these episodes of bacteremia increases the likelihood that colonization and disease with multiply resistant bacterial and fungal pathogens will occur after transplantation. Risks for the occurrence of bacterial translocation after intestinal transplantation, with resultant bloodstream infection, include the presence of a colon graft,[21] hospitalization before transplantation, and treatment with mycophenolate mofetil.[77]

Age, another important pretransplant factor, is a major determinant of susceptibility to certain agents, severity of expression of infection, and immune maturation. Young children undergoing abdominal transplantation may experience moderate to severe infection with certain viral (e.g., respiratory syncytial virus [RSV]) or bacterial (coagulase-negative staphylococci) pathogens, as opposed to the milder illness experienced by adult recipients infected with these pathogens. In contrast, infections caused by certain pathogens, such as *Cryptococcus neoformans*, are seldom manifested before young adulthood.[124] Age also is an important factor governing clinical expression of infection with cytomegalovirus (CMV) and Epstein-Barr virus (EBV). When transplants are performed in young patients, a high likelihood exists that they will be seronegative for CMV and EBV and, therefore, susceptible to primary infection, which is more severe than that caused by reactivation.[11,60,96]

Donor-related issues represent another set of pretransplant factors. Transplant recipients are at risk for acquiring infections that may be active or latent within the donor at the time of organ harvesting. The best described examples of donor-associated infections are CMV and EBV.[10,12,19,96] Infections caused by CMV and EBV have been more severe after intestinal transplantation than after transplantation of other organs. This difference may be due to the fact that the intestine is an organ rich in lymphoid tissue, which may result in transmission of a larger viral load from the donor than with other graft types. Similarly, adenovirus has been isolated more commonly from pediatric recipients of intestinal transplants than from other organs, which also may be related to donor transmission in the accompanying lymphoid tissue.[83,92] Although the frequencies of some donor-associated pathogens (e.g., human immunodeficiency virus [HIV],[30] hepatitis B, hepatitis C) have decreased substantially with better diagnostic screening tests,[5] recent evidence now demonstrates donor-associated transmission of West Nile virus and rabies.[67,112] Because organs from a single donor often go to disparate sites, it is important for the recipient center to report back to United Network for Organ Sharing (UNOS) any unusual infections that possibly could have come from the donor.

INTRAOPERATIVE FACTORS

Operative factors unique to liver transplantation may predispose the recipient to infectious complications. For example, liver transplant recipients undergoing Roux-en-Y choledochoduodenostomy experience more infectious episodes than do those who undergo choledochocholedochostomy with T-tube drainage.[70,102] However, usually only the former option is performed in children undergoing liver transplantation because of the small size of their bile ducts. For combined liver-intestinal transplantation, evolution to en bloc replacement of the liver and intestine avoids the need for performing an additional biliary anastomosis and minimizes the risk of development of infection related to biliary complications. Prolonged operative time (>12 hours) during the initial transplant procedure has been associated with an increased risk for developing infection after transplantation[36,70] and probably is a surrogate marker for the technical difficulty of the surgery. Intraoperative events, such as contamination of the operative field, also predispose the recipient to postoperative infections.

Finally, inability to close the abdomen after the transplant has been performed, as a result of size discrepancy or intraoperative complications, appears to increase the risk for development of postoperative infections.

POST-TRANSPLANT FACTORS

Technical problems, immunosuppression, the presence of indwelling cannulas, and nosocomial exposure are major postoperative risk factors for the development of infectious complications. Thrombosis of the hepatic artery is the most serious technical problem after liver transplantation and predisposes the recipient to the development of areas of necrotic liver, hepatic abscesses, and bacteremia.[99,102] Bile duct strictures, developing as a sequela of a thrombosed hepatic artery and ischemia or as a result of technical difficulties, may predispose the recipient to the development of cholangitis.[102] Retransplantation represents a high risk for the development of intra-abdominal infection after intestinal transplantation.[77]

Immunosuppression is the critical postoperative factor predisposing to the development of infection in all transplant recipients. Immunosuppressive regimens have evolved in an attempt to achieve more specific control of rejection with the least impairment of immunity. Thus, this evolution is aimed not only at improved control of rejection but also at a decreased rate of morbidity and mortality from infections. The use of cyclosporine-based regimens has resulted in a decreased incidence of infections in renal and cardiac transplant recipients.[29,61,89] The introduction of tacrolimus has allowed many patients to be managed without steroids.[49,118] Although reported rates of infection have been similar in liver transplant recipients treated with either tacrolimus or cyclosporine, an apparent decrease in morbidity and mortality rates, especially from viral pathogens, has been noted with tacrolimus.[2,49] In contrast to these results, some centers have reported an increased rate of EBV-associated post-transplant lymphoproliferative disease (PTLD) in patients receiving tacrolimus.[24] However, data from the University of Pittsburgh suggest that the short- and long-term incidence of EBV-associated PTLD appears to be similar in pediatric liver transplant recipients treated with either cyclosporine or tacrolimus.[15]

Children undergoing intestinal transplantation require a higher baseline level of immunosuppression than do patients undergoing most other solid organ transplant procedures.[96] With this increased level of immunosuppression has come an increased risk for the development of infection. In an effort to overcome this risk, numerous alternative immunosuppressive strategies have been explored. Looking at one such alternative strategy, Loinaz and colleagues[77] found an increased risk for the development of bacterial infection after intestinal transplantation with both mycophenolate mofetil and daclizumab.

Treatment of rejection with additional or higher doses of immunosuppressants increases the risk for development of invasive and potentially fatal infection. Of particular concern is the use of antilymphocyte preparations, especially OKT3, which often is indispensable in the management of rejection refractory to steroids.[10,36,70] Newer antilymphocyte antibodies (e.g., thymoglobulin) also are likely to be associated with an increased risk for the development of infection.

The prolonged use of indwelling cannulas at any site is an important cause of infection throughout the postoperative course. The presence of central venous catheters is a cause of bacteremia after transplantation. This is a particularly important consideration for children undergoing intestinal transplantation, for which maintenance of long-term central venous access has been required for prolonged periods after transplantation. Urinary

tract infections and bacterial pneumonia are associated with the use of urethral catheters and prolonged nasotracheal or endotracheal intubation, respectively.[36,70]

Nosocomial exposure constitutes the final group of postoperative risk factors. Transplant recipients, especially children, may be exposed to many common viral pathogens (e.g., rotavirus, RSV, or influenza) while hospitalized. In addition, all transplant recipients are at risk for exposure to transfusion-associated pathogens (e.g., hepatitis B, hepatitis C, HIV). Finally, the presence in the hospital of heavy areas of contamination with pathogenic fungi, such as *Aspergillus*, may increase the risk for acquisition of invasive fungal disease in these patients. The rate of fungal colonization increases during times of hospital reconstruction. Implementation of infection control policies aimed at the local epidemiology of circulating infections is paramount.

TIMING OF INFECTIONS

The time of onset of infection with various pathogens after transplantation tends to be predictable. Most clinically important infections occur within the first 180 days after transplantation.[46,70] The timing of infections can be divided into three intervals: early (0-30 days after transplantation), intermediate (30-180 days after transplantation), and late (>180 days after transplantation). In addition, some infections may occur throughout the postoperative course. These divisions, though arbitrary, generally are useful in approaching a patient with fever after undergoing transplantation and can be used as a guide to the differential diagnosis. An overview of the infectious complications occurring during each of these time periods is provided in Tables 83–1 to 83–3 and is summarized in the following sections.

EARLY INFECTIONS (0 TO 30 DAYS)

Early infections tend to be associated with preexisting conditions and surgical manipulation (Table 83–1). In general, they are caused by either bacteria or yeast. Bacterial infections are particularly common developments after intestinal transplantation and have been reported in up to 90 percent of recipients.[62,77,116] As many as half of these early infectious complications may develop in the first 2 weeks after the patient has undergone abdominal transplantation.[9] Cholangitis or spontaneous bacterial peritonitis occurring at or near the time of liver transplantation may lead to the development of intra-abdominal infection after the procedure. Herpes simplex infection also can reactivate and cause early symptomatic disease,[70] although reactivation is an uncommon occurrence in children. Technical difficulties (e.g., thrombosis of the hepatic artery or portal vein, biliary strictures) predispose recipients to early development of bacterial infections. Likewise, the development of bile leaks and bowel perforations is associated with polymicrobial intra-abdominal infections, primarily consisting of enteric bacteria and *Candida* species, in the first month after transplantation.[38] Bacteremia may be seen in intestinal transplant recipients in association with the presence of central venous catheters, intestinal rejection, or PTLD involving the intestine.[41,107] Finally, re-exploration of the abdomen has been linked to increased rates of fungal infection.[70]

INTERMEDIATE PERIOD (31 TO 180 DAYS)

The intermediate period (Table 83–2) is the typical time of onset of infections associated with donor transmission (either organ or blood products), reactivated viruses, and opportunistic infections. CMV infection peaks in incidence during this time.[10,70] However,

TABLE 83–1 Differential Diagnosis of Infectious Complications during the Early Period (0 to 30 Days) after Pediatric Liver and Intestinal Transplantation

Clinical Syndrome	Associated Pathogens
Wound infection	*Staphylococcus aureus*
Superficial	Enterococci
Deep	Enterobacteriaceae
	Candida species
Intra-abdominal infection	Enterobacteriaceae
Peritonitis	Enterococci
Intra-abdominal abscess	*Candida* species
Intrahepatic abscess (isolated liver and liver-intestine transplants) with or without bacteremia	
Bloodstream infection associated with	
Central venous catheters	Coagulase-negative staphylococci
	Enterococci
	S. aureus
	Candida species
Hepatic artery thrombosis (isolated liver transplant only)	Enterobacteriaceae
	Enterococci
	Candida species
Intestinal rejection (intestine only)	Enterobacteriaceae
	Enterococci
	Candida species
Bacterial cholangitis (isolated liver transplant only)	Enterobacteriaceae
	Enterococci
	Candida species
Urinary tract infection	Enterobacteriaceae
	Enterococci
	Candida species
Ventilator-associated pneumonia	Enterobacteriaceae
	Enterococci
	S. aureus
	Candida species
Nosocomial acquisition of common community pathogens	Respiratory syncytial virus
	Parainfluenza virus
	Influenza virus
	Rotavirus
Noninfectious causes	Rejection
	Drug fever

TABLE 83–2 Differential Diagnosis of Infectious Complications during the Intermediate Period (31 to 180 Days) after Pediatric Liver and Intestinal Transplantation

Clinical Syndrome	Associated Pathogens
Viral syndrome	CMV
Fever, leukopenia, thrombocytopenia ±Atypical lymphocytosis	EBV
Hepatitis	CMV
	EBV
	Adenovirus
	Hepatitis B
	Hepatitis C
Enteritis	CMV
	EBV
	Rotavirus
	Adenovirus
	Clostridium difficile
PTLD	EBV
Bacterial cholangitis*	Enterobacteriaceae
	Enterococci
	Candida species
Pneumonia	*Streptococcus pneumoniae*
	CMV
	Adenovirus
	RSV
	Parainfluenza
	Influenza
	Pneumocystis jiroveci
	Aspergillus fumigatus
Bacteremia†	Enterobacteriaceae
	Enterococcus
	Candida species
Adenopathy	EBV/PTLD
Pulmonary nodules	EBV/PTLD
	A. fumigatus

*Typically only seen in isolated liver transplant recipients and usually associated with the presence of technical complications (e.g., biliary stricture).
†Seen in intestinal transplant recipients in association with the presence of central venous catheters, intestinal rejection, or PTLD involving the intestine.
CMV, cytomegalovirus; EBV, Epstein-Barr virus; PTLD, post-transplant lymphoproliferative disease.

TABLE 83–3 Differential Diagnosis of Infectious Complications during the Late Period (>180 Days) after Pediatric Liver and Intestinal Transplantation

Clinical Syndrome	Associated Pathogens
Bacterial cholangitis*	Enterobacteriaceae
	Enterococci
	Candida species
PTLD	EBV
Bacteremia†	Enterobacteriaceae
	Enterococcus
	Candida species
Varicella/zoster	Varicella-zoster virus

*Usually associated with the presence of technical complications (e.g., biliary stricture).
†Seen in intestinal transplant recipients in association with the presence of central venous catheters, intestinal rejection, or PTLD involving the intestine.
EBV, Epstein-Barr virus; PTLD, post-transplant lymphoproliferative disease.

if CMV prophylaxis is instituted, disease from this virus may occur after 180 days. The intermediate period also is when many patients begin to have EBV-associated PTLD[60] and *Pneumocystis jiroveci* (formerly *P. carinii*) pneumonia (PCP).[70]

LATE INFECTIONS (>180 DAYS)

Late infections developing after abdominal transplantation (Table 83–3) are less well characterized than those of other periods because patients usually have been discharged from the transplant center to their respective homes, which often are quite far away. This renders accumulating accurate data on these late infections difficult. Nonetheless, problems such as recurrent episodes of bacterial cholangitis in liver transplant recipients (typically associated with underlying problems of the biliary tree), bacteremia associated with intestinal graft rejection, and PTLD (in both groups of patients)[78] occur in this period. In addition, children who are at high risk for the development of CMV disease and have been maintained on prophylaxis may have the onset of CMV disease delayed to the late period.[17]

INFECTIONS OCCURRING THROUGHOUT THE POSTOPERATIVE COURSE

Iatrogenic factors are important causes of bacterial and fungal infection at all times but predominantly in the early transplant period. Central venous lines are maintained for a variable time; the risk of infection developing persists for the entire period that the catheter remains in place. This problem is particularly important for recipients of intestinal transplants, in whom central line access is maintained until the graft is fully functional. Similarly, the presence of urethral catheters and endotracheal tubes also increases the risk for the development of infections whenever they are in use.

Nosocomial acquisition of community viruses, such as RSV, rotavirus, and influenza A or B, can occur at any time after transplantation. These viruses spread easily in hospital environments from personnel or other hospitalized patients to transplant recipients. It is, therefore, important to modify diagnostic considerations according to local epidemiologic considerations.

BACTERIAL AND FUNGAL INFECTIONS

Bacterial and fungal pathogens are important causes of morbidity and occasionally mortality in children undergoing liver or intestinal transplantation (or both). With the exception of infections related to the use of indwelling catheters, sites of bacterial infection tend to occur at or near the transplanted organ. Accordingly, the intra-abdominal space is an important site of infection after any of the abdominal transplant procedures. Adding to the complexity of management of bacterial infections in children undergoing abdominal transplantation is the fact that recovery of multiply antibiotic-resistant bacteria is occurring increasingly frequently. Outbreaks of colonization and disease caused by vancomycin-resistant *Enterococcus faecium* and extended-spectrum β-lactamase (ESBL)-producing *Klebsiella pneumoniae* have been reported in pediatric liver and intestinal transplant recipients.[40,42] These multiply resistant bacteria have been transmitted from patient to patient, thus prompting the imposition of strict infection control procedures. Reports of multiply resistant strains of *Enterobacter cloacae* associated with de-repression of a chromosomally located, broad-spectrum, β-lactamase enzyme have identified this very resistant organism as an important pathogen after liver transplantation.[20] More recently, isolates of *E. cloacae* identified to also be carrying ESBL enzymes have been recovered from our intestinal transplant candidates and recipients and, as a result, have limited our antimicrobial alternatives even further. The increasing prevalence of these multiply antibiotic-resistant organisms limits the therapeutic options available for the treatment of bacterial infections that occur after abdominal transplantation; in some cases, effective antimicrobials may be unavailable to treat these complications. Knowledge of the results of previous cultures and local antimicrobial resistance patterns is critical in choosing initial empiric antibiotic therapy in these patients to maximize their outcomes.

LIVER TRANSPLANTATION

Bacterial and fungal infections are common early problems after liver transplantation.[22,23,57,62,122,130] Rates of bacterial infection of 40 to 70 percent have been reported from multiple series.[49,70,102] Bacteremia often occurs in association with intra-abdominal infection or with the use of central venous catheters, but it can develop without an obvious source. Enteric gram-negative organisms account for more than half of these episodes. Bacterial infections involving the abdomen or surgical wound are common developments in most series. Infectious complications of the transplanted liver also occur. The most important complication is hepatic abscess associated with hepatic artery or portal vein thrombosis, often accompanied by persistent bacteremia. However, the introduction of frequent surveillance Doppler studies early after transplantation to monitor for the development of thrombosis, coupled with the use of operative thrombectomy

and thrombolysis, has essentially eliminated the development of hepatic abscesses in this population.

Ascending cholangitis is a common occurrence after liver transplantation and usually is associated with biliary abnormalities. This diagnosis typically is made on clinical grounds in a patient with fever and biochemical evidence of biliary inflammation. Enteric gram-negative bacteria and enterococcal species predominate. However, because this clinical picture can be identical to that of acute graft rejection, liver biopsy should be performed to differentiate these processes. A cholangiogram is performed to assess the status of the biliary tract in patients with proven cholangitis.

As many as 40 percent of children undergoing liver transplantation may contract a fungal infection during the first year after the procedure.[122] *Candida* spp. are the most common fungal pathogens, and infection usually is associated with an intra-abdominal focus or indwelling catheter. Infections caused by *Candida* spp. usually are recognized in the first month after transplantation, with *Candida* peritonitis most likely occurring in the first 2 weeks after liver transplantation in association with a bile leak or bowel perforation. Other risk factors associated with the development of *Candida* infection include a prolonged duration of intubation after transplantation, hepatic artery thrombosis, volume of blood transfused, and exposure to steroids within the 3 months before the transplant procedure. Recovery of *Candida* from a Jackson-Pratt drain in the early postoperative period may be the first indication of either of these two technical complications and may occur before the onset of clinical symptoms of intra-abdominal infection.[40] Accordingly, recovery of *Candida*, alone or in combination with enteric bacteria, should prompt initiation of antimicrobial therapy and aggressive evaluation for the presence of these complications. Early initiation of treatment is particularly important, given an attributable mortality rate of up to 33 percent for candidal infections in pediatric liver transplant recipients.[40] The availability of fluconazole and the newer echinocandin antifungal agents (e.g., caspofungin and micafungin) has increased the number of therapeutic options for the treatment of *Candida* infection. However, acquired or inherent resistance to the azoles is an increasing concern, as are drug-drug interactions between azoles and echinocandins with both cyclosporine and tacrolimus.

Episodes of invasive aspergillosis are uncommon occurrences but can be fatal.[50] Children undergoing liver transplantation for cystic fibrosis are at particular risk for infection with *Aspergillus*.[121] We have observed early disseminated disease in children with cystic fibrosis undergoing liver transplantation, which has prompted the use of perioperative antifungal prophylaxis in liver recipients with cystic fibrosis and a history of recovery of *Aspergillus* before transplantation. Because data defining the precise duration of prophylaxis necessary to protect against this complication are not available, prophylactic treatment has ranged from 1 month of intravenous amphotericin to prolonged use of an oral azole agent (e.g., itraconazole or voriconazole). The availability of newer antifungal agents, including the advanced-generation azoles (voriconazole and posaconazole), as well as the echinocandins, has increased the number and complexity of therapeutic options for the treatment of aspergillosis in children undergoing liver transplantation. A summary of a suggested approach to the diagnosis and management of fungal infections that occur after liver transplantation in children is provided in Table 83–4.

INTESTINAL TRANSPLANTATION

A relatively small number of children have undergone intestinal transplantation. Many have received combined liver and intestine or multivisceral transplants. Bacterial infection occurs frequently in these patients.[41,106] One recent series reported that as many as

TABLE 83-4   Overview of Diagnosis and Management of Fungal Infections after Liver and Intestinal Transplantation in Children

	Candida—Noninvasive (Mucositis, Dermatitis and Cystitis)	Candida—Invasive	Aspergillus	Cryptococcus	Others (Histoplasma, Mucor, Fusarium, Blastomycetes, Alternaria, etc.)
Frequency*	Common	Common	Uncommon	Rare	Rare
Diagnostic Tests	Clinical examination Culture Gram stain	Culture Gram stain Histology	Culture Gram stain Histology Radiographic staging[¶]	Culture Antigen test India ink stain Histology CSF examination	Culture Histology Antigen testing (when appropriate)
Treatment					
Primary	Nystatin	Amphotericin B[†]	Amphotericin B[†]	Amphotericin B[†]	Amphotericin B[†]
Secondary	Clotrimazole Topical amphotericin B[‡]	Fluconazole[‡,¶] Echinocandin therapy** 5-Flucytosine[††]	Echinocandin therapy** Itraconazole[§,‡‡,§§] Voriconazole[§,¶¶] 5-Flucytosine[††]	Fluconazole[§,¶] 5-Flucytosine[††]	Azole therapy (for susceptible organisms)[§]
Adjunctive	Fluconazole[§,‖]	Removal of central lines	Surgical resection		Surgical débridement
Duration of therapy	Dependent on the rate of clearance	Dependent on the rate of clearance: minimum of 14 days	Dependent on the rate of clearance: minimum of 4 weeks, usually 8-12 weeks	Minimum of 6-8 weeks Many would continue with fluconazole indefinitely	Dependent on the rate of clearance
Follow-up	Clinical examination Repeat urine analysis/cultures	Dependent on the clinical scenario	Dependent on the clinical scenario	Clinical examination Antigen testing Repeat culture of the appropriate source (sputum, CSF, urine) Radiographs if relevant	Clinical examination Antigen testing Repeat culture of the appropriate source (sputum, CSF, urine) Radiographs if relevant

*Common, greater than 5 percent; uncommon, 1 to 5 percent; rare, less than 1 percent.
[†]Amphotericin B is dosed at 0.75 to 1.0 mg/kg/day; lipid formulations are used if renal failure is present.
[‡]Topical amphotericin B for bladder wash for noninvasive candiduria. Ultrasound of the kidneys is recommended to determine that no invasive disease is present.
[§]Azole use must be accompanied by close follow-up of levels of cyclosporine or tacrolimus. In general, tacrolimus dosing should be cut in half when using a standard dose of fluconazole.
[¶]Radiographic staging includes computed tomography of head, chest, and abdomen.
[‖]Fluconazole is the alternative first-line drug for invasive disease if the species is known to be sensitive to fluconazole and the patient is clinically stable. Fluconazole is dosed at 6 to 12 mg/kg/day based on the severity of infection.
**The use of either of the approved echinocandins (caspofungin or micafungin) may be an appropriate alternative for the treatment of invasive candidiasis, candidemia, and aspergillosis. Dose adjustments may be necessary in the face of impaired liver function. Monitoring of tacrolimus levels is indicated because these agents may decrease tacrolimus levels.
[††]5-Flucytosine should not be used alone but is synergistic when used in conjunction with amphotericin B. Flucytosine is dosed at 100 to 150 mg/kg/day divided every 6 hours.
[‡‡]Itraconazole can be used long-term for patients who have been treated for invasive Aspergillus, but in general it is not recommended as first-line therapy.
[§§]Itraconazole absorption can be erratic. Accordingly, monitoring of itraconazole levels is recommended. Itraconazole is dosed at 3 to 5 mg/kg/day as a single dose. Dosing adjustment based on monitoring of levels is recommended. Adjustment of cyclosporine or tacrolimus dosing should be individualized.
[¶¶]Voriconazole levels should be checked in patients treated with oral therapy.
CSF, cerebrospinal fluid.

92 percent of children undergoing intestinal transplantation experienced an average of 2.9 episodes of bacterial infection per patient.[77] In more than 80 percent of these patients, the first bacterial infection occurred during the first 2 months after receiving the transplant. Bacteremia, which can be explained in part by disruption of the mucosal barrier associated with harvest injury or intestinal allograft rejection, is a common finding.[41,106] Coagulase-negative staphylococci and enterococci and gram-negative enteric bacilli account for most episodes. As noted earlier, antibiotic resistance is seen commonly in recovered pathogens. In our experience, episodes of gut-associated bacteremia frequently are responsible for secondary infection of central venous catheters, and persistent positive cultures are produced even after resolution of clinical symptoms. Accordingly, treatment strategies aimed at preserving the catheter (e.g., antibiotic lock therapy) may need to be implemented in conjunction with systemic antibiotics to achieve a sustained clinical cure.

Intra-abdominal and wound infections also are seen commonly in this population; they occur in more than a third of patients and typically are detected during the first month after transplantation. Gram-negative enteric pathogens, which frequently demonstrate multiple-antibiotic resistance, as well as enterococci (often exhibiting vancomycin resistance), are the most common organisms associated with these complications.

Recurrent laparotomy has been identified as a risk factor for intra-abdominal infection. One unique aspect of intestinal transplantation is the potential inability to achieve abdominal wall closure. Although failure to close the abdominal wall is an obvious risk for the development of intra-abdominal infection, the use of abdominal mesh as part of an effort to resolve difficult abdominal wall closure also has been associated with the development of superficial and deep wound infection.[28] Successful treatment of mesh-related infections may require removal of the mesh to obtain a sustained clinical cure.

Another important site of infection is the intestine itself. *Clostridium difficile* enteritis can be accompanied by a pattern of fever, abdominal pain, and diarrhea that easily can be mistaken for graft rejection or viral infection caused by CMV, EBV, and adenovirus. Accordingly, the diagnosis of *C. difficile* enteritis must be considered in any child in whom fever and changes in stool output are noted. In one small series, *C. difficile* enteritis was diagnosed in nearly 10 percent of children undergoing intestinal transplantation.[129] The frequent exposure to antibiotics and prolonged hospital stays that children undergoing intestinal transplantation experience are major risk factors for the development of this complication. Standard treatment with oral metronidazole is the recommended first-line therapy. However, prolonged therapy or oral vancomycin might be necessary for patients who experience relapse or recurrent episodes after primary treatment.

Candidemia also may occur in any of the settings in which bloodstream infections are observed after intestinal transplantation. Although the majority of episodes of candidemia take place in the first 3 to 6 months after transplantation, episodes may occur later. Intra-abdominal infection with *Candida* also is observed, typically as part of a polymicrobial infection related to technical problems occurring during the initial transplant surgery or subsequent laparotomies.

Invasive mycoses caused by fungal pathogens other than *Candida* seldom are observed. Rare infections with *Aspergillus*, *Alternaria*, and *Scedosporium* spp. have occurred in children undergoing intestinal transplantation at our institution. In general, these children have been receiving high levels of immune suppression, and the outcome of these infections has been poor. Guidelines for the diagnosis and management of fungal infection in children undergoing intestinal transplantation are provided in Table 83-4.

VIRAL INFECTIONS

Viral pathogens, especially herpesviruses, are a major source of morbidity and mortality after solid organ transplantation. Patterns of disease associated with individual viral pathogens generally are similar among all transplant recipients. However, frequency, mode of manifestation, and relative severity can differ according to the type of organ transplanted and the serologic status of the recipient.

CYTOMEGALOVIRUS

CMV continues to be the most common and one of the most important viral pathogens seen after organ transplantation in children. CMV infection can be asymptomatic or symptomatic and may be due to primary infection (from either the donor graft or blood products), reactivation of latent infection, or superinfection with a different CMV strain in a previously seropositive child. Before the use of prophylaxis, the incidence of symptomatic CMV infection was reported to be as high as 22 percent in adult[53] and 40 percent in pediatric[10] liver transplant recipients. Use of ganciclovir prophylaxis has resulted in a decreased rate and severity of CMV disease.[44] Intestinal transplantation was introduced after ganciclovir became available and, therefore, has been able to take advantage of using ganciclovir both as prophylaxis and as treatment. Nonetheless, CMV disease can be very severe after intestinal transplantation and has a high rate of recurrence.[12,71] Primary CMV infection, typically acquired from the donor organ (or passenger donor leukocytes that accompany the organ), is associated with the greatest degree of morbidity and mortality.[39,44] Accordingly, CMV-seronegative recipients of organs from CMV-seropositive donors are considered at high risk for the development of CMV disease. Reactivation of or superinfection with CMV tends to result in milder illness after liver transplantation but still can be severe after intestinal transplantation.[11,13] CMV disease appears to be more likely to develop in CMV-seropositive recipients of CMV-seropositive donor organs than in seropositive recipients of seronegative donor organs.[39] Patients treated with unusually high doses of immunosuppressants, especially antilymphocyte antibody preparations, experience an increased rate of CMV disease regardless of previous immunity.[10,70]

Symptomatic CMV disease typically occurs between 1 and 3 months after transplantation. An important note is that the use of prophylactic regimens may delay the onset of CMV disease.

A characteristic constellation of fever (which may be high-grade, prolonged, and hectic) and hematologic abnormalities (including leukopenia, atypical lymphocytosis, and thrombocytopenia) frequently is seen. This "CMV syndrome" occurs in 25 to 50 percent of patients with symptomatic CMV infection. Invasive CMV disease is characterized by visceral organ involvement; common sites include the gastrointestinal tract, liver, and lungs. CMV hepatitis appears to be the most common site in liver transplant recipients, whereas CMV enteritis is a frequent finding in intestinal transplant recipients. CMV chorioretinitis is a rare development in organ transplant recipients.

The diagnosis of CMV disease may be confirmed by positive buffy coat culture, pp65 antigenemia assay,[117] or the presence of CMV DNA in the blood of a patient with a compatible clinical syndrome.[71] However, clinicians must be aware that the results of viral culture of urine and even bronchoalveolar lavage specimens are difficult to interpret in previously infected patients because CMV frequently is shed asymptomatically in these secretions. Similarly, the presence of pp65 antigen and CMV DNA in blood can be misleading because these assays often are positive in asymptomatic patients. The specificity of this approach may be improved by quantitative determination of pp65 antigen or CMV DNA. Because of the lack of specificity of these assays, histologic examination of involved organs to confirm the presence of CMV is critical when the diagnosis of invasive CMV is being entertained.

Antiviral agents with activity against CMV (e.g., ganciclovir, foscarnet, and cidofovir) have improved the survival of transplant recipients with CMV disease. Fatal, disseminated CMV disease occurred in 19 percent of infected children[10] and 5 percent of infected adults undergoing liver transplantation in the preganciclovir era.[105] For clinical CMV disease, ganciclovir therapy is given in conjunction with reduction of immunosuppression unless evidence of rejection is present. Clinical response usually occurs 5 to 7 days after initiation of therapy. Baseline immunosuppression levels typically are restored at the time of initial clinical response or upon recognition of rejection. Recent evidence supports serial monitoring of CMV load in peripheral blood as a guide to the duration of treatment of CMV disease.[26,104] The role of CMV hyperimmune globulin in combination with ganciclovir for the treatment of CMV disease is controversial, although some evidence of improved outcome has been reported in the treatment of CMV pneumonia in adult liver transplant recipients.[37] Finally, because of the relatively high rates of nephrotoxicity associated with their use, foscarnet and cidofovir should be restricted to patients with apparent or proven resistance to ganciclovir.

In approximately 25 percent of patients treated with ganciclovir for an initial episode of symptomatic CMV disease, one or more episodes of recurrent CMV disease will develop.[104,114] Recurrences are observed approximately 1 month after the initial infectious episode occurs and may be associated with invasive disease. More commonly, however, these recurrent episodes tend to be milder than is the initial episode. Factors associated with an increased risk for the development of recurrent CMV disease include being a CMV-seronegative recipient of a CMV-seropositive organ, having disseminated CMV disease, and having a history of multiple treatment courses for rejection.[104] In addition, one center has demonstrated a correlation between the height of the CMV viral load in peripheral blood leukocytes before treatment and also at the end of treatment and the likelihood of recurrent CMV disease developing.[104] These results are the basis for the recommendation to use the results of CMV viral load measurement to guide the duration of therapy for CMV disease.[26] A summary of our suggested approach to the diagnosis and management of CMV infection is provided in Table 83-5.

TABLE 83–5 Overview of Diagnosis and Management of Viral Infections after Liver and Intestinal Transplantation in Children

	Cytomegalovirus	Epstein-Barr Virus	Respiratory Syncytial Virus	Influenza	Parainfluenza	Adenovirus
Frequency*	Common	Common	Uncommon	Uncommon	Uncommon	Liver: uncommon Intestine: common
Diagnostic tests	Culture pp65 antigen Histology	EBV PCR Histology Serology	NP aspirate for antigen detection and culture	NP aspirate for antigen detection and culture	NP aspirate for culture	Viral culture Histology
Treatment						
Primary	Ganciclovir (5 mg/kg bid)	Decrease IS	Supportive care	Supportive care	Supportive care	Decrease IS
Secondary	Foscarnet[†] Cidofovir		Aerosolized ribavirin	Amantadine Rimantadine Zanamivir Oseltamivir		IV ribavirin
Adjunctive	Decrease IS CMV IVIG	Ganciclovir IVIG	RSV IVIG Decrease IS	Decrease IS	Decrease IS	IVIG
Duration of therapy	Site-dependent	Individualized	Individualized	Individualized	Individualized	Individualized
Follow-up	Monitor pp65 antigen or CMV PCR (treat until negative)	Monitor EBV PCR Repeat imaging studies if positive at outset	None	None	None	None

*Common, frequency greater than 5 percent; uncommon, frequency of 1 to 5 percent; rare, frequency of less than 1 percent.
[†]Foscarnet is used for CMV infection when ganciclovir resistance is suspected or proven. Experience from patients infected with human immunodeficiency virus suggests that a synergistic benefit will be obtained from the combined use of both of these agents when ganciclovir resistance is present.
CMV, cytomegalovirus; EBV, Epstein-Barr virus; IS, immune suppression; IVIG, intravenous immunoglobulin; NP, nasopharyngeal; PCR, polymerase chain reaction; RSV, respiratory syncytial virus.

EPSTEIN-BARR VIRUS

EBV infection, including EBV-associated PTLD, is an important cause of morbidity and mortality after liver transplantation and intestinal transplantation,[60,81,113,119,128] particularly in children undergoing intestinal transplantation, who experience the highest rates of EBV-related disease among transplant recipients.[91]

Symptomatic EBV infection in general and PTLD in particular most commonly occur in transplant recipients experiencing primary EBV infection, especially those who receive organs from seropositive donors. Accordingly, children undergoing transplantation are disproportionately affected by EBV when compared with their adult counterparts.[51] In as many as 80 percent of children who are EBV-seronegative before undergoing liver transplantation, primary EBV infection will develop after this procedure.[108,111] Although primary infection occurs in the vast majority of seronegative patients, clinical disease develops in less than a third of these children.[108,111] In one study, PTLD developed in 4 percent of children undergoing solid organ transplantation and 10 percent of children with primary EBV infection between 1 month and 5 years after transplantation[60]; 75 percent of cases occurred during the first postoperative year in patients receiving cyclosporine-based immune suppression. The cumulative incidence can be as high as 12 to 20 percent by 7 to 12 years after liver transplantation.[78,87]

Pediatric recipients of intestinal transplants appear to behave differently from children undergoing other types of organ transplantation in that the rate of EBV disease, including PTLD, appears to be similar in both patients who are EBV-seronegative and those who are EBV-seropositive before undergoing intestinal transplantation. Rates of EBV disease and PTLD after intestinal transplantation as high as 30 to 40 percent were reported during the initial experiences with intestinal transplantation. More recently, these rates have declined to approximately 10 percent as a result of improved immune suppression regimens and EBV-monitoring protocols. However, these rates still remain higher than those seen in other organ recipients.

A wide spectrum of EBV disease is recognized and includes nonspecific viral illness, mononucleosis, and PTLD, including lymphoma. Histologic evaluation is important in differentiating among these categories; manifestations can evolve in individual patients, and asymptomatic seroconversion also occurs. Variation in severity and extent of disease is related to the degree of immunosuppression and adequacy of the host immune response. Although EBV disease and PTLD may affect many different clinical sites, the tendency of EBV disease is to involve the transplanted organ. Thus, EBV hepatitis and PTLD of the liver are observed more commonly in liver transplant recipients.[18] Similarly, the intestine is the most frequently observed site of involvement of EBV disease in intestinal transplant recipients. Of interest, involvement of sites beyond the gastrointestinal tract is an uncommon occurrence in intestinal transplant recipients.

The onset of viral syndrome, mononucleosis, and PTLD takes place primarily within the first year, whereas lymphoma tends to occur later. Immunosuppressive regimens based on the use of tacrolimus appear to have induced a shift in the timing of PTLD; only rare cases develop more than 18 months after transplantation.[16,128] This pattern of timing of EBV disease and PTLD appears to apply to all pediatric organ recipients, including children undergoing liver or intestinal transplantation. However, the impact of newer immunosuppressive agents and regimens on EBV disease remains to be determined.

The diagnosis of EBV-associated PTLD is made on the basis of clinical, laboratory, and histopathologic examination and should be suspected in patients with protracted fever, exudative tonsillitis, lymphadenopathy, organomegaly, leukopenia, or atypical lymphocytosis.[46,91] Gastrointestinal involvement should be suspected in patients with persistent fever and diarrhea. Accordingly, EBV must be considered in the differential diagnosis of rejection in intestinal transplant recipients. Serologic diagnosis often is confounded by the presence of passive antibody acquired at the time of transplantation or during subsequent transfusions. Detection of increased EBV viral load in peripheral blood by polymerase chain reaction (PCR) has gained wide acceptance as a means of predicting the risk for or presence of EBV or PTLD.[48,69,91,97,100] Though extremely sensitive, these assays are limited by their lack of specificity; they often are elevated in asymptomatic patients.[3] Accordingly, every effort should be made to confirm the diagnosis of EBV or PTLD histologically. Occult sites of PTLD are assessed by performance of computed tomography of the chest and abdomen. Palpable nodes or lesions (or both) identified by radiographic surveillance should undergo biopsy. Endoscopic evaluation should be considered in patients with diarrheal illnesses and elevated viral loads. Histologic evaluation for typical features may be augmented through use of the Epstein-Barr–encoded RNA (EBER) probe.[95] Use of the EBER probe may be particularly helpful in differentiating between the presence of rejection and EBV infection in intestinal transplant recipients.

Management of patients with PTLD is controversial.[14,16,46,91] Reduction of immunosuppression is recommended widely. Antiviral agents typically are used,[54,55,98] although their role has not been studied formally. Reduction of immunosuppression, alone or in combination with antiviral agents, results in an approximate 67 percent cure rate of EBV disease and PTLD. The potential impact of monoclonal antibodies,[33] interferon,[103] and chemotherapy[35] awaits formal clinical trials. Resection of tumor also may be of value for patients with lymphoma. Recent experience has focused on several novel approaches to the management of EBV disease and PTLD. These newer strategies generally have been used for patients who fail to respond to reduction of immune suppression (with or without the use of antiviral agents). Rituximab, an anti-CD20 antibody, has been used increasingly for the treatment of EBV disease. Experience to date suggests that as many as two thirds of patients who fail initial withdrawal of immunosuppression will respond to a 4-week course of this agent.[47] However, relapse of EBV disease has been observed in 20 to 25 percent of treated patients 6 to 8 months after completion of therapy, at the time that rituximab no longer is present in the body. An alternative, chemotherapy-based approach for patients who fail to respond to initial reduction or withdrawal of immunosuppression also has been proposed.[52] This strategy, which uses modified doses of cyclophosphamide and prednisone, likewise has achieved success in approximately two thirds of treated patients. Unfortunately, as with rituximab, relapse of PTLD has been seen in 22 percent of treated patients, and outright treatment failures have occurred in patients with fulminant disease. Definitive studies comparing these two second-line therapies are needed to determine the best option for children who fail to respond to initial therapeutic modification of immunosuppression. A summary of our suggested approach and management of EBV/PTLD is provided in Table 83–5.

OTHER HERPESVIRUSES

Other herpesviruses also can be hazardous after transplantation. Herpes simplex can reactivate early after surgery or after augmentation of immunosuppression. Prophylaxis with acyclovir has been beneficial in these situations. A summary of the suggested approach to the diagnosis and management of infection with herpes simplex virus is provided in Table 83–5. Varicella in nonimmune transplant recipients can lead to disseminated fatal disease[82] and should be treated early and aggressively with intravenous acyclovir.

More recently, interest has focused on determining what role, if any, the recently recognized human herpesvirus-6 (HHV-6) and HHV-7 may play in causing disease in organ transplant recipients in general and abdominal transplant recipients in particular. Several groups of investigators have identified a potential interaction between the development of HHV-6 and HHV-7 and CMV infection in organ transplant recipients.[65,84] Reactivation of

HHV-6 infection after liver transplantation has been associated with the development of an increased CMV viral load in peripheral blood, as well as a greater likelihood of symptomatic CMV disease developing.[65] In addition, some investigators have suggested that some or all of the symptoms typically associated with CMV syndrome (e.g., fever, leukopenia) in patients with proven CMV infection may be attributable in part to HHV-6 or HHV-7. Studies in children have suggested that infection with HHV-6 alone is a relatively common cause of unexplained fever in pediatric liver transplant recipients.[126,127] Interest also has begun to focus on what role, if any, HHV-8 may have in causing infection and disease in organ transplant recipients, particularly recipients from countries with moderate to high rates of HHV-8 prevalence, such as Africa, the Middle East, and the Carribean.[86] The full spectrum of disease caused by these newer viruses and their potential therapies remain to be determined.

ADENOVIRUS

Adenovirus has been reported to be the third most important virus affecting pediatric liver transplant recipients; it was found in 10 percent of our series of 484 children undergoing liver transplantation under cyclosporine-based immunosuppression.[85] Symptomatic disease (ranging from self-limited fever, gastroenteritis, or cystitis to devastating illness with necrotizing hepatitis or pneumonia) occurred in more than 60 percent of infected patients. Infection developed within the first 3 months after transplantation. The frequency of invasive adenovirus infection after pediatric liver transplantation appears to have decreased markedly with the use of tacrolimus-based immunosuppression.[50] In a more recent report, McLaughlin and colleagues[85] found that only 4.2 percent of pediatric liver recipients receiving tacrolimus-based therapy had adenovirus disease. This rate is in contrast to a significantly higher incidence of adenovirus infection of 20.8 percent in pediatric intestinal transplant recipients at the same institution. The increased prevalence of adenovirus in intestinal transplant recipients is illustrated further by the report of Pinchoff and colleagues,[92] who found adenovirus in all 14 of their pediatric intestinal transplant recipients. However, this exceptionally high rate might be attributable to the fact that viral cultures were performed as part of routine screening of graft biopsy specimens and not all of the patients were symptomatic. In both these studies, high volume of stool output, alone or in the presence of fever, was the most common symptom found in the patients.

Presumptively diagnosing infection caused by adenovirus in pediatric abdominal transplant recipients is very difficult inasmuch as fever, hepatitis, and pneumonia may be due to a variety of other pathogens and high volume of stool output after intestinal transplantation is nonspecific and can occur with rejection as well. The presence of high-grade fever and symptoms suggestive of adenovirus infection should prompt obtaining serial cultures for viruses (including adenovirus) or PCR investigation and evaluation of graft biopsy tissue. Unexplained elevations in hepatocellular enzymes suggestive of hepatitis should warrant consideration of liver biopsy. Similarly, an increase in stool output, with or without fever, should prompt endoscopic evaluation of the intestinal allograft. Histologic examination for the presence of adenoviral inclusions, as well as immunohistochemical staining of biopsy specimens from either site, should be undertaken to help confirm this diagnosis.

Unfortunately, no definitive treatment is available for adenoviral infection at this time. The most important component of therapy is supportive care along with a decrease in immunosuppression. The role of antiviral agents is unproven. A small number of case reports describe the use of ribavirin[8,68,76,83,88] and ganciclovir[125] in the treatment of single patients with adenoviral infection after undergoing solid organ or bone marrow transplantation. In vitro evidence supports the theoretical role of ribavirin but not that of ganciclovir in the treatment of these infections. In addition to these published reports, an adult lung transplant recipient with disseminated adenovirus type 7 improved after treatment with cidofovir and pooled, high-titer immunoglobulin against RSV (Respigam) along with decreased immunosuppression.[43] Several other case reports have described the successful use of cidofovir for the treatment of adenoviral disease in a bone marrow transplant recipient, as well as a patient with acquired immunodeficiency syndrome.[56,96] A single case report also raised the possibility of a role for intravenous immunoglobulin (IVIG) as treatment of adenovirus infection.[27] Unfortunately, no conclusive evidence of the efficacy of these antiviral agents or IVIG can be drawn from these reports. A summary of a suggested approach to the diagnosis and management of adenovirus infection is provided in Table 83-5.

COMMON COMMUNITY-ACQUIRED VIRUSES

Although the course of illness has been poorly documented, most children who undergo liver and intestinal transplantation experience the usual respiratory viruses and gastrointestinal illness without significant problems. However, infection by influenza, parainfluenza, or RSV leads to more severe disease in young children, especially if the infection occurs soon after transplantation and during periods of maximal immunosuppression.[6,31,66,93] Likewise, transplant recipients may have prolonged viral shedding even after resolution of symptoms. A summary of suggested strategies for the diagnosis and management of these community-acquired viruses can be found in Table 83-5.

OTHER VIRUSES

Other viruses, including both donor-associated viral infections (e.g., hepatitis B and C) and community-acquired viral pathogens (e.g., enterovirus, rotavirus) are relatively uncommon causes of infection or disease after abdominal transplantation. Suggested approaches to the diagnosis and management of each of these viral pathogens are provided in Table 83-5.

OPPORTUNISTIC INFECTIONS

P. jiroveci is a well-documented cause of pneumonia in immunocompromised patients, including liver and intestinal transplant recipients. Prophylactic trimethoprim-sulfamethoxazole (TMP-SMX) is safe, inexpensive, and effective.[64] Use of this strategy has eliminated PCP in these patients at our center. Alternative prophylactic regimens for sulfa-allergic patients include aerosolized pentamidine (for patients >5 years of age)[74] or dapsone.[63]

Tuberculosis (TB) is a particular concern in immunosuppressed hosts, including recipients of liver and intestinal transplants. The incidence of TB after liver transplantation in Europe and the United States has been reported to range from 0.9 to 2.3 percent, with most cases reported in adults.[106,121] In contrast, TB may develop in as many as 15 percent of organ transplant recipients in areas of high-level endemicity.[106] However, development of TB after pediatric liver transplantation is an extremely uncommon event, with only 11 cases reported thus far.[79,106,121] To date, no cases have been reported in recipients of intestinal transplants. The development of TB in solid organ transplant recipients is associated with mortality rates ranging from 25 to 40 percent, with additional morbidity and mortality associated with the development of rejection in patients receiving antituberculous therapy.[106,121] The diagnosis of TB in transplant recipients is

complicated by the fact that extrapulmonary disease occurs frequently and purified protein derivative (PPD) testing is likely to be unreliable after transplantation. Management of TB in liver transplant recipients is difficult because of both the side effects of antituberculous agents and their potential interactions with immunosuppressive agents.[106,121] Limited published experience in pediatric liver transplant recipients suggests that most infections caused by *Mycobacterium tuberculosis* in all probability are due to a primary infection, often associated with family contacts who have positive skin tests.[79,121] In contrast, experience with adult transplant recipients suggests that the development of TB is more likely to be due to reactivation of latent TB.[58,106,121] Despite the limited published information describing TB in these patients, transplant recipients known to have a positive PPD test or who come from an area endemic for TB appear to be at increased risk for symptomatic reactivation after transplantation.[58,121] Similar data are not available for recipients of intestinal transplants. Additional factors predisposing to the development of TB after transplantation include severe hepatic failure at the time of transplantation, aggressive anti-rejection therapy, and HIV infection.[58,115] Experience with adult renal transplant recipients suggests that even though the risk appears to be greatest in patients who received inadequate or no previous TB therapy,[75,78] it also can occur in patients who received appropriate anti-TB therapy in the pretransplant period.[75,78,94] Although TB has been encountered only rarely in pediatric liver transplant recipients[121] and not in intestinal recipients, screening for TB by history and PPD testing, along with review of a chest radiograph for lesions consistent with healed TB, is highly recommended. Patients with a positive TB history or a positive PPD test, or both, should receive isoniazid for 6 to 12 months after undergoing transplantation, although some experts recommend continuing isoniazid indefinitely while patients remain on immunosuppression. Attempts at establishing a more definitive diagnosis are indicated for patients from endemic areas with a negative PPD test but a suspicious chest radiograph. Careful evaluation for evidence of side effects, particularly hepatotoxicity, is recommended, and isoniazid is discontinued if unacceptable toxicity is identified.

Additional potential opportunistic infections include cryptococcosis, coccidioidomycosis, and histoplasmosis, although these pathogens have not been reported frequently in pediatric liver or intestinal transplant recipients. Previous infection with these pathogens is common in geographic areas where they are endemic. Because patients often travel to transplant centers distant from their homes, it is imperative that transplant physicians be aware of the local environmental risks for each patient. Experience with coccidioidomycosis in transplant recipients suggests that a minimum of 4 months of antifungal therapy, such as fluconazole, should be given to transplant recipients with this history.[53] Similarities between coccidioidomycosis and other fungal pathogens suggests that similar strategies may be necessary for patients with a positive history of previous fungal infection with pathogens known to recur after resolution of the primary infection.

MANAGEMENT

PRETRANSPLANT EVALUATION

Pretransplant evaluation is helpful in the management of infectious complications in liver and intestinal transplant recipients. A complete history and physical examination should be performed with particular attention given to previous infections, immunizations, and drug allergies. Attention should be paid to a history of infection with multiply antibiotic-resistant bacteria, which may provide guidance for any future empiric treatment that may be required after transplantation. An intermediate-strength tuberculin skin test should be performed on all patients.

We recommend serologic evaluation of all candidates for CMV; EBV; varicella; herpes simplex virus; hepatitis A, B, and C; and HIV. Serologic tests on the donor should include HIV, hepatitis B and C viruses, CMV, and EBV. Donors positive for HIV or hepatitis B virus should be excluded. The use of organs from donors positive for hepatitis C probably would be contraindicated except in the circumstance in which the recipient also is positive for hepatitis C. Knowledge of donor and recipient status for these viruses allows one to anticipate infection, identify patients who might benefit from prophylactic regimens, and narrow the differential diagnosis in a patient with fever.

PROPHYLACTIC REGIMENS

Prophylactic regimens vary among transplant centers. These strategies have been divided into perioperative and long-term prophylaxis and often evolve to reflect the infectious complications seen at individual institutions.

Perioperative prophylaxis is used to prevent intraoperative sepsis and wound infection. It is based on individual patient characteristics and the expected normal flora. We consider piperacillin-tazobactam an appropriate agent for perioperative prophylaxis. If sepsis is suspected in the donor, antibiotics are chosen to cover organisms identified from the donor, and treatment usually is extended to a therapeutic course of 10 to 14 days. In the absence of proven or suspected infection in the donor, perioperative prophylaxis generally is limited to the first 48 hours after transplantation.

Considerations regarding long-term prophylaxis against infections occurring beyond the perioperative period include the risk and severity of infection, as well as the toxicity, cost, and efficacy of a given prophylactic strategy. Nystatin is recommended for all pediatric transplant recipients in an effort to prevent oropharyngeal candidiasis. TMP-SMX is used to prevent PCP. Although some centers recommend using TMP-SMX for only the first 6 months after liver transplantation, anecdotal experience of PCP occurring long after patients receive their transplants and the relative safety of this agent have led us to recommend its use indefinitely after liver and intestinal transplantation in children.

The frequency and severity of CMV infections in transplant recipients prompt consideration of prophylactic strategies, and optimization of the target population and timing of interventions require further study.[7,26,32,90,101,123] Potential roles exist for intravenous and oral ganciclovir[34,42,72] and oral valganciclovir.[109,110] Currently, we recommend the use of intravenous ganciclovir alone (for varying durations) for liver and low-risk intestinal transplant recipients (recipient CMV-positive before transplantation or donor and recipient seronegative) and ganciclovir plus IVIG with a high titer of antibody against CMV for high-risk (donor CMV-positive/recipient CMV-negative) intestinal transplant recipients if it is available. At the present time, oral valganciclovir is an alternative to prophylaxis with intravenous ganciclovir for adolescents. Pharmacokinetic studies of dosing of oral valganciclovir suspension in children after transplantation are ongoing. On completion of these studies, the use of valganciclovir suspension probably will be of merit as an alternative to intravenous treatment in younger children.

Serial monitoring of the blood CMV viral load with either the pp65 antigen assay or quantitative CMV PCR as an indicator for the use of preemptive antiviral therapy has been proposed as an alternative to these chemoprophylactic and immunoprophylactic strategies.[45] In this approach, only patients demonstrating increased risk because of increased viral load are treated with intravenous or oral ganciclovir. Although this strategy has gained acceptance at some centers, experience in pediatric transplant recipients in general and abdominal transplant recipients in particular remains limited. The use of viral load monitoring after completion of chemoprophylaxis is gaining increasing acceptance.

The growing recognition of the importance of EBV infection in pediatric organ transplant recipients has led to an interest in the prevention of EBV infection and PTLD. Numerous strategies (e.g., immunoprophylaxis, monitoring, and preemptive therapy) are being explored,[47,80] the efficacy of these approaches has not been established. The use of viral load monitoring to inform preemptive reductions in immunosuppression appears to be the most promising of these strategies.[73,80] Because reduction of immune suppression is not always possible for intestinal transplant recipients with a rising EBV load, preemptive intravenous ganciclovir and IVIG have been used in addition to reduction of immune suppression (when possible) for this cohort of patients. Although prospective comparative data are not available, the use of this strategy appears to have resulted in a decreased risk for disease and better outcome than in historical controls who were not managed with this strategy.[41]

SUMMARY

Infections remain an important problem after liver and intestinal transplantation. Knowledge of the type, timing, and predisposing risk factors for these infectious complications allows for timely and appropriate diagnosis and management.

REFERENCES

1. Abedi, M. R., Linde, A., Christensson, B., et al.: Preventive effect of IgG from EBV-seropositive donors on the development of posttransplant lymphoproliferative disease in SCID mice. Int. J. Cancer 71:624-629, 1997.
2. Alessiani, M., Kusne, S., Martin, F. M., et al.: Infections with FK 506 immunosuppression: Preliminary results with primary therapy. Transplant. Proc. 22:44-46, 1990.
3. Allen, U., Hebert, D., Petric, M., et al.: Utility of semiquantitative polymerase chain reaction for Epstein-Barr virus to measure virus load in pediatric organ transplant recipients with and without posttransplant lymphoproliferative disease. Clin. Infect. Dis. 33:145-150, 2001.
4. Andrews, W., Fyock, B., Gray, S., et al.: Pediatric liver transplantation: The Dallas experience. Transplant. Proc. 19:3267-3276, 1987.
5. Angelis, M., Cooper, J. T., and Freeman, R. B.: Impact of donor infections on orthotopic liver transplantation. Liver Transpl. 9:451-462, 2003.
6. Apalsch, A. M., and Green, M.: Influenza and parainfluenza virus infections in pediatric organ transplant recipients. Clin. Infect. Dis. 20:394-399, 1995.
7. Balfour, H. H., Chace, B. A., Stapleton, J. T., et al.: A randomized, placebo controlled trial of oral acyclovir for the prevention of cytomegalovirus disease in recipients of renal allografts. N. Engl. J. Med. 320:1381-1387, 1989.
8. Boger-Arav, R., Echavarria, M., Forman, M., et al.: Clearance of adenoviral hepatitis with ribavirin therapy in a pediatric liver transplant recipient. Pediatr. Infect. Dis. J. 19:1097-1100, 2000.
9. Bouchut, J. C., Stamm, D., Boillot, O., et al.: Postoperative infectious complications in paediatric liver transplantation: A study of 48 transplants. Paediatr. Anaesth. 11:93-98, 2001.
10. Bowman, J. S., Green, M., Scantlebury, V. P., et al.: OKT3 and viral disease in pediatric liver transplant recipients. Clin. Transpl. 5:294-300, 1991.
11. Breinig, M. K., Zitelli, B., Starzl, T. E., and Ho, M.: Epstein-Barr virus, cytomegalovirus, and other viral infections in children after liver transplantation. J. Infect. Dis. 156:273-279, 1987.
12. Bueno, J., Green, M., Kocoshis, S., et al.: Cytomegalovirus infection after intestinal transplantation in children. Clin. Infect. Dis. 25:1078-1083, 1997.
13. Burroughs, M., Sobanjo, A., Florman, S.. et al.: Cytomegalovirus matching does not predict symptomatic disease in intestinal transplantation. Transplant. Proc. 34:946-947, 2002.
14. Cacciarelli, T. V., Green, M., Jaffe, R., et al.: Management of posttransplant lymphoproliferative disease in pediatric liver transplant recipients receiving primary tacrolimus (FK506) therapy. Transplantation 66:1047-1052, 1998.
15. Cacciarelli, T. V., Jaffe, R., Green, M., et al.: A decreased incidence of posttransplant lymphoproliferative disorder (PTLD) in pediatric liver transplant recipients under primary tacrolimus (FK506) therapy. Abstract 289. Program and Abstracts of the 16th Annual Scientific Committee of the American Society for Transplant Physicians, Chicago, 1997, p. 157.
16. Cacciarelli, T. V., Reyes, J., Jaffe, R., et al.: Primary tacrolimus (FK 506) therapy and the long-term risk of posttransplant lymphoproliferative disease in pediatric liver transplant recipients. Pediatr. Transplant. 5:359-364, 2001.

17. Campbell, A. L., and Herold, B. C.: Strategies for the prevention of cytomegalovirus infection and disease in pediatric liver transplantation recipients. Pediatr. Transplant. 8:619-627, 2004.

18. Cao, S., Cox, K., Esquivel, C. O., et al.: Posttransplant lymphoproliferative disorders and gastrointestinal manifestations of Epstein-Barr virus infection in children following liver transplantation. Transplantation 66:851-856, 1998.

19. Cen, H., Breinig, M. C., Atchinson, R. W., et al.: Epstein-Barr virus transmission via the donor-organ in solid-organ transplantation: Polymerase chain reaction and restriction fragment length polymorphism analogue of IR2, IR3, IR4. J. Virol. 65:976-980, 1991.

20. Chow, J. W., Fine, M. J., Shlaes, D. M., et al.: *Enterobacter* bacteremia: Clinical features and emergence of antibiotic resistance during therapy. Ann. Intern. Med. 115:585-590, 1991.

21. Cicalese, L., Sileri, P., Green, M., et al.: Bacterial translocation in clinical intestinal transplantation. Transplantation 71:1414-1417, 2001.

22. Cienfugos, J. A., Dominguez, R. M., Tamelchoff, P. J., et al.: Surgical complications in the postoperative period of liver transplantation in children. Transplant. Proc. 16:1230-1235, 1984.

23. Colonna, J. O., Winston, D. J., Brill, J. E., et al.: Infectious complications in liver transplantation. Arch. Surg. 123:360-364, 1988.

24. Cox, K. L., Lawrence-Miyasaki, L. S., Garcia-Kennedy, R., et al. An increased incidence of Epstein-Barr virus infection and lymphoproliferative disorder in young children on FK506 after pediatric liver transplantation. Transplantation 59:524-529, 1995.

25. Cuervas-Mons, V., Rimola, A., Van Thiel, D. H., et al.: Does previous abdominal surgery alter the outcome of pediatric patients subjected to orthotopic liver transplantation. Gastroenterology 90:853-857, 1986.

26. Cytomegalovirus. In: Guidelines for the Prevention and Management of Infectious Complications of Solid Organ Transplantation. Eds: Green, M., Avery, R. K., and Preiksaittis, J. Am. J. Transplant. 4(Suppl. 10):51-58, 2004.

27. Dagan, R., Schwartz, R. H., Insel, R. A., and Menegua, M. A.: Severe diffuse adenovirus 7a pneumonia in a child with combined immunodeficiency: Possible therapeutic effect of human immune serum containing specific neutralizing antibodies. Pediatr. Infect. Dis. J. 3:246-251, 1984.

28. Di Benedetto, F., Lauro, A., Masetti, M., et al.: Use of prosthetic mesh in difficult abdominal wall closure after small bowel transplantation in adults. Transplant. Proc. 37:2272-2274, 2005.

29. Dummer, J. S., Hardy, A., Poorsattar, A., and Ho, M.: Early infections in kidney, heart and liver transplant recipients on cyclosporine. Transplantation 36:259-267, 1983.

30. Dummer, J. S., Siegfried, E., Breinig, M. K., et al.: Infection with human immunodeficiency virus in the Pittsburgh transplant population. Transplantation 47:134-139, 1989.

31. Englund, J. E., and Whimbey, E. E.: Community-acquired respiratory viruses after hematopoietic stem cell or solid organ transplantation. In Bowden, R. A., Ljungman, P., and Paya, C. V. (eds.): Transplant Infections. 2nd ed. Baltimore, Lippincott Williams & Wilkins, 2003, pp. 367-398.

32. Fehir, K. M., Decker, T., Samo, T., et al: Immune globulin (GAMMAGARD) prophylaxis of CMV infections in patients undergoing organ transplantation and allogeneic bone marrow transplantation. Transplant. Proc. 21:3107-3109, 1989.

33. Fischer, A., Blanche, S., Le Bidois J., et al.: Anti–B-cell monoclonal antibody in the treatment of severe B-cell lymphoproliferative syndrome following bone marrow and solid-organ transplantation. N. Engl. J. Med. 324:1451-1456, 1991.

34. Gane, E., Saliba, F., Valdecasas, G. J., et al.: Randomized trial of efficacy and safety of oral ganciclovir in prevention of cytomegalovirus disease in livertransplant recipients. Lancet 350:1729-1733, 1997.

35. Garrett, T. J., Chadburn, A., Barr, M. L., et al.: Posttransplantation lymphoproliferative disorders treated with cyclophosphamide-doxorubicin-vincristine-prednisone chemotherapy. Cancer 72:2782-2785, 1993.

36. George, D. L., Arnow, P. M., Fox, A. S., et al.: Bacterial infection as a complication of liver transplantation: Epidemiology and risk factors. Rev. Infect. Dis. 13:387-396, 1991.

37. George, M. J., Snydman, D. R., Werner, B. G., et al.: Use of ganciclovir plus cytomegalovirus immune globulin to treat CMV pneumonia in orthotopic liver transplant recipients. Transplant. Proc. 25(Suppl. 4):22-24, 1993.

38. Gladdy, R. A., Richardson, S. E., Davies, H. D., and Superina, R. A.: *Candida* infection in pediatric liver transplant recipients. Liver Transpl. Surg. 5:16-24, 1999.

39. Green, M.: Vancomycin resistant enterococci: Impact and management in pediatrics. Adv. Pediatr. Infect. Dis. 13:257-277, 1998.

40. Green, M., and Barbadora, K.: Recovery of ceftazidime-resistant *Klebsiella pneumoniae* from pediatric liver transplant recipients. Pediatr. Transplant. 2:224-230, 1998.

41. Green, M., Bueno, J., Sigurdsson, L., et al.: Unique aspects of the infectious complications of intestinal transplantation. Curr. Opin. Organ Transplant. 4:361-367, 1999.

42. Green, M., Kaufmann, M., Wilson, J., and Reyes, J.: Comparison of intravenous ganciclovir followed by oral acyclovir with intravenous ganciclovir alone for prevention of cytomegalovirus and Epstein-Barr virus disease after liver transplantation in children. Clin. Infect. Dis. 25:1344-1349, 1997.

43. Green, M., and Michaels, M.: Infectious complications after solid-organ transplantation. Adv. Pediatr. Infect. Dis. 7:181-204, 1992.

44. Green, M., and Michaels, M.: Adenovirus, parvovirus B19 and papillomavirus. In Bowden, R. A., Ljungman, P., and Paya, C. (eds.): Transplant Infections. Philadelphia, Lippincott-Raven, 1998, pp. 287-294.

45. Green, M., and Michaels, M.: Preemptive therapy of cytomegalovirus disease in pediatric transplant recipients. Pediatr. Infect. Dis. J. 19:875-877, 2000.

46. Green, M., Michaels, M. G., Webber, S. A., et al.: The management of Epstein-Barr virus associated post-transplant lymphoproliferative disorders in pediatric solid-organ transplant recipients. Pediatr. Transplant. 3:271-281, 1999.

47. Green, M., Reyes, J., and Rowe, D.: New strategies in the prevention and management of Epstein-Barr virus infection and posttransplant lymphoproliferative disease following solid organ transplantation. Curr. Opin. Organ Transplant. 3:143-147, 1998.

48. Green, M., Reyes, J., Webber, S., et al.: The role of viral load in the diagnosis, management, and possible prevention of Epstein-Barr virus–associated posttransplant lymphoproliferative disease following solid organ transplantation. Curr. Opin. Organ Transplant. 4:292-296, 1999.

49. Green, M., Tzakis, A., Reyes, J., et al.: Infectious complications of pediatric liver transplantation under FK 506. Transplant. Proc. 23:3038-3039, 1991.

50. Green, M., Wald, E. R., Tzakis, A., et al.: Aspergillosis of the central nervous system in a pediatric liver transplant recipient and review of the literature. Rev. Infect. Dis. 13:653-657, 1991.

51. Green, M., Weinfeld, A., Mazariegos, G., and Reyes, J.: Short-course intravenous ganciclovir prophylaxis against cytomegalovirus disease following liver transplantation in children. Pediatr. Transplant. 2(Suppl. 1):75, 1998.

52. Gross, T. G., Bucuvalas, J. C., Park, J. R., et al.: Low-dose chemotherapy for Epstein-Barr Virus–positive post-transplantation lymphoproliferative disease in children after solid organ transplantation. J. Clin. Oncol. 23:6481-6488, 2005.

53. Hall, K. A., Copeland, J. G., Zukoski, C. F., et al.: Markers of coccidiomycosis prior to cardiac or renal transplantation and risk of recurrent infection. Transplantation 55:1422-1425, 1993.

54. Hanto, D., Frizzera, G., Gajl-Peczalska, K., and Simmons, R.: Epstein-Barr virus, immunodeficiency, and B cell lymphoproliferation. Transplantation 39:461-470, 1985.

55. Hanto, D. W., Frizzera, G., Gajl-Peczalska, K. J., et al.: Epstein-Barr virus–induced B-cell lymphoma after renal transplantation: Acyclovir therapy and transition from polyclonal to monoclonal B-cell proliferation. N. Engl. J. Med. 306:913-918, 1982.

56. Hedderwick, S. A., Greenson, J. K., McGaughy, V. R., et al.: Adenovirus cholecystitis in a patient with AIDS. Clin. Infect. Dis. 28:997-999, 1998.

57. Hiatt, J. R., Ament, M. E., Berquist, M. E., et al.: Pediatric liver transplantation at UCLA. Transplant. Proc. 19:3282-3288, 1987.

58. Higgins, R., Kusne, S., Reyes, J., et al.: *Mycobacterium tuberculosis* after liver transplantation: Management and guidelines for prevention. Clin. Transplant. 6:81-90, 1992.

59. Ho, M., and Dummer, J. S.: Risk factors and approaches to infection in transplant recipients. In Mandell, G. L., Douglas, R. G., Jr., and Bennett, J. E. (eds.): Principles and Practice of Infectious Diseases. 3rd ed. New York, Churchill Livingstone, 1990.

60. Ho, M., Jaffe, R., Miller, G., et al.: The frequency of Epstein-Barr virus infection and associated lymphoproliferative syndrome after transplantation and its manifestations in children. Transplantation 45:719-727, 1988.

61. Hofflin, J. M., Potasman, I., Baldwin, J. C., et al: Infectious complication in heart transplant recipients receiving cyclosporine and corticosteroids. Ann. Intern. Med. 106:209-216, 1987.

62. Hollenbeak, C. S., Alfrey, E. J., Sheridan, K., et al.: Surgical site infections following pediatric liver transplantation: Risks and costs. Transplant. Infect. Dis. 5:72-78, 2003.

63. Hughes, W. T., Kennedy, W., Dugdale, M., et al.: Prevention of *Pneumocystis carinii* pneumonitis in AIDS patients with weekly dapsone. Lancet 2:1066, 1990.

64. Hughes, W. T., Rivera, G. K., Schell, M. J., et al.: Successful intermittent chemoprophylaxis for *Pneumocystis carinii* pneumonitis. N. Engl. J. Med. 316:1627-1632, 1987.

65. Humar, A., Malkan, G., Moussa, G., et al.: Human herpesvirus-6 is associated with cytomegalovirus reactivation in liver transplant recipients. J. Infect. Dis. 181:1450-1453, 2000.

66. Ison, M. G., and Hayden, F. G.: Viral infections in immunocompromised patients: What's new with respiratory viruses? Curr. Opin. Infect. Dis. 15:355-367, 2002.

67. Iwamoto, M., Jernigan, D. B., Guashch, A., et al.: West Nile Virus in Transplant Recipients Investigation Team. Transmission of West Nile virus from an organ donor to four transplant recipients. N. Engl. J. Med. 348:2196-2203, 2003.

68. Kapelushnik, J., Or, R., Delukina, A., et al.: Intravenous ribavirin therapy for adenovirus gastroenteritis after bone marrow transplantation. J. Pediatr. Gastroenterol. Nutr. 21:110-112, 1995.

69. Kenagy, D. N., Schlessinger, Y., Weck, K., et al.: Epstein-Barr virus DNA in peripheral blood leukocytes of patients with post-transplant lymphoproliferative disease. Transplantation 60:547-554, 1995.

70. Kusne, S., Dummer, J. S., Singh, N., et al.: Infection after liver transplantation. An analysis of 101 consecutive cases. Medicine (Baltimore) 67:132-143, 1988.

71. Kusne, S., Manez, R., Frye, B. L., et al.: Use of DNA amplification for diagnosis of cytomegalovirus enteritis after intestinal transplantation. Gastroenterology *112*:1121-1128, 1997.

72. Kusne, S., Shapiro, R., and Fung, J.: Prevention and treatment of cytomegalovirus infection in organ transplant recipients. Transplant. Infect. Dis. *1*:187-203, 1999.

73. Lee, T. C., Savoldo, B., Rooney, C. M., et al.: Quantitative EBV viral loads and immunosuppression alterations can decrease PTLd incidence in pediatric liver transplant recipients. Am. J. Transplant. *5*:2222-2228, 2005.

74. Leoung, G. S., Feigal, D. W., Montgomery, B., et al.: Aerosolized pentamidine for prophylaxis against *Pneumocystis carinii* pneumonia. N. Engl. J. Med. *323*:769-775, 1990.

75. Lichenstein, I. H., and MacGregor, R. R.: Mycobacterial infections in renal transplant recipients: Report of five cases and review of the literature. Rev. Infect. Dis. *5*:216-226, 1983.

76. Liles, W. C., Cushing, H., Holt, S., et al.: Severe adenovirus nephritis following bone marrow transplantation: Successful treatment with intravenous ribavirin. Bone Marrow Transplant. *14*:663-664, 1993.

77. Loinaz, C., Kato, T., Nishida, S., et al.: Bacterial infections after intestine and multivisceral transplantation. The experience of the University of Miami (1994-2001). Hepatogastroenterology *58*:234-242, 2006.

78. Malatack, J. J., Gartner, J. C., Urbach, A. H., and Zitelli, B. J.: Orthotopic liver transplantation, Epstein-Barr virus, cyclosporine and lymphoproliferative syndrome—a growing concern. J. Pediatr. *118*:667-675, 1991.

79. Malhorta, K. K., Dash, S. C., Dhawan, I. K., et al.: Tuberculosis and renal transplantation—observations from an endemic area. Postgrad. Med. J. *62*:359-362, 1986.

80. McDiarmid, S. V., Blumberg, D. A., Remotti, H., et al.: Mycobacterial infections after pediatric liver transplantation: A report of three cases and review of the literature. J. Pediatr. Gastroenterol. Nutr. *20*:425-431, 1995.

81. McDiarmid, S. V., Jordan, S., Lee, G. S., et al.: Prevention and pre-emptive therapy of post-transplant lymphoproliferative disease in pediatric liver recipients. Transplantation *66*:1604-1611, 1998.

82. McGregor, R. S., Zitelli, B. J., Urbach, A. H., et al.: Varicella in pediatric orthotopic liver transplant recipients. Pediatrics *83*:256-261, 1989.

83. McLaughlin, G. E., Delis, S., Kashimawo, L., et al.: Adenovirus infection in pediatric liver and intestinal transplant recipients: Utility of DNA detection by PCR. Am. J. Transplant. *3*:224-228, 2003.

84. Mendez, J. C., Dockrell, D. H., Espy, M. J., et al.: Human beta-herpesvirus interactions in solid-organ transplant recipients. J. Infect. Dis. *183*:179-184, 2001.

85. Michaels, M., Green, M., Wald, E. R., and Starzl, T. E.: Adenovirus infection in pediatric orthotopic liver transplant recipients. J. Infect. Dis. *165*:170-174, 1992.

86. Michaels, M. G., and Jenkins, F.: Human herpesvirus 8: Is it time for routine surveillance in pediatric solid organ transplant recipients to prevent the development of Kaposi's sarcoma? Pediatr. Transplant. 7:1-3, 2003.

87. Migliazza, L., Lopez, S. M., Murcia, J., et al.: Long-term survival expectancy after liver transplantation in children. J. Pediatr. Surg. *35*:5-7, 2000.

88. Murphy, G. F., Wood, D. P., McRoberts, J. W., and Henslee-Downey, P. J.: Adenovirus-associated hemorrhagic cystitis treated with intravenous ribavirin. J. Urol. *149*:565-566, 1993.

89. Najarian, J. S., Fryd, D. S., Strand, M., et al.: A single institution, randomized, prospective trial of cyclosporine versus azathioprine–antilymphocyte globulin for immunosuppression in renal allograft recipients. Ann. Surg. *201*:142-157, 1985.

90. Paya, C. V.: Prevention of cytomegalovirus disease in recipients of solid-organ transplants. Clin. Infect. Dis. *32*:596-603, 2001.

91. Paya, C., Fung, J. J., Nalesnik, M. A., et al.: Epstein-Barr virus–induced posttransplant lymphoproliferative disorders. Transplantation *68*:1517-1525, 1999.

92. Pinchoff, R. J., Kaurfman, S. S., Magid, M. S., et al.: Adenovirus infection in pediatric small bowel transplantation recipients. Transplantation.*76*:183-189, 2003.

93. Pohl, C., Green, M., and Wald, E. R.: RSV infection after pediatric liver transplantation. J. Infect. Dis. *165*:166-169, 1992.

94. Quinibi, W., Al-Sibai, M. B., Taher, S., et al.: Mycobacterial infection after renal transplantation: Report of 14 cases and review of the literature. Q. J. Med. *282*:1039-1060, 1990.

95. Randhawa, P. S., Jaffe, R., Demetris, A. J., et al.: Expression of Epstein-Barr virus–encoded small RNA (by the EBER-1 gene) in liver specimens from transplant recipients with post-transplantation lymphoproliferative disease. N. Engl. J. Med. *327*:1710-1714, 1992.

96. Reyes, J., Mazariegos, G. V., Bond, G. M., et al.: Pediatric intestinal transplantation: Historical notes, principles and controversies. Pediatr. Transplant. 6:193-207, 2002.

97. Ribaud, P., Scieux, C., Freymuth, F., et al.: Successful treatment of adenovirus disease with intravenous cidofovir in an unrelated stem-cell transplant recipient. Clin. Infect. Dis. *28*:690-691, 1999.

98. Riddler, S. A., Breinig, M. C., and McKnight, J. L. C.: Increased levels of circulating Epstein-Barr virus–infected lymphocytes and decreased EBV nuclear antigen antibody responses are associated with the development of posttransplant lymphoproliferative disease in solid-organ transplant recipients. Blood *84*:972-984, 1994.

99. Rollins, N. K., Andrews, W. S., Currino, G., et al.: Infected bile lakes following pediatric liver transplantation: Non-surgical management. Radiology *166*:169-171, 1988.

100. Rowe, D. T., Qu, L., Reyes, J., et al.: Use of quantitative competitive PCR to measure Epstein-Barr virus genome load in peripheral blood of pediatric transplant recipients with lymphoproliferative disorders. J. Clin. Microbiol. *35*:1612-1615, 1997.

101. Saliba, F., Arulnaden, J. L., Gugenheim, J., et al.: CMV hyperimmune globulin prophylaxis after liver transplantation: A prospective randomized controlled study. Transplant. Proc. *21*:2260-2262, 1989.

102. Schroter, G. P. J., Hoelscher, M., Putnam, C. W., et al.: Infections complicating orthotopic liver transplantation. Arch. Surg. *111*:1337-1347, 1976.

103. Shapiro, R. S., Chauvenet, A., McGuire, W., et al.: Treatment of B-cell lymphoproliferative disorders with interferon alpha and intravenous gamma globulin. N. Engl. J. Med. *318*:1334, 1988.

104. Sia, I. G., Wilson, J. A., Groettum, C. M., et al.: Cytomegalovirus (CMV) DNA load predicts relapsing CMV infection after solid organ transplantation. J. Infect. Dis. *181*:717-720, 2000.

105. Singh, N., Dummer, S., Kusne, S., et al.: Infections with cytomegalovirus and other herpesviruses in 121 liver transplant recipients: Transmission by donated organ and the effect of OKT3 antibodies. J. Infect. Dis. *155*:202-206, 1988.

106. Singh, N., Paterson, D. L.: *Mycobacterium tuberculosis* infection in solid-organ transplant recipients: Impact and implications for management. Clin. Infect. Dis. *27*:1266-1277, 1998.

107. Sigurdsson, L., Reyes, J., Kocoshis, S. A., Mazariegos, G., et al.: Bacteremia after intestinal transplantation in children correlates temporally with rejection or gastrointestinal lymphoproliferative disease. Transplantation *70*:302-305, 2000.

108. Smets, F., Bodeus, M., Goubau, P., et al.: Characteristics of Epstein-Barr virus primary infection in pediatric liver transplant recipients. J. Hepatol. *32*:100-104, 2000.

109. Snydman, D. R., Werner, B. G., Dougherty, N. N., et al.: Cytomegalovirus immune globulin prophylaxis in liver transplantation. A randomized, double-blind, placebo-controlled trial. Ann. Intern. Med. *119*:984-991, 1993.

110. Snydman, D. R., Werner, B. G., Heinze-Lacey, B., et al.: Use of cytomegalovirus immune globulin to prevent cytomegalovirus disease in renal-transplant recipients. N. Engl. J. Med. *317*:1049-1054, 1987.

111. Sokal, E. M., Antunes, H., Beguin, C., et al.: Early signs and risk factors for the increased incidence of Epstein-Barr virus–related posttransplant lymphoproliferative diseases in pediatric liver transplant recipients treated with tacrolimus. Transplantation *64*:1438-1442, 1997.

112. Srinivasan, A., Burton, E. C., Kuehnert, M. J., et al.: Transmission of rabies virus from an organ donor to four transplant recipients. N. Engl. J. Med. *352*:1103-1111, 2005.

113. Starzl, T. E., Porter, K. A., Iwatsuki, S., et al.: Reversibility of lymphomas and lymphoproliferative lesions developing under cyclosporin-steroid therapy. Lancet *1*:583-587, 1984.

114. Stratta, R. J., Shaefer, M. S., Markin, R. S., et al.: Clinical patterns of cytomegalovirus disease after liver transplantation. Arch. Surg. *124*:1443-1450, 1989.

115. Strernecik, M., Ferrell, S., Asher, N., et al.: Mycobacterial infection after liver transplantation: A report of three cases and review of the literature. Clin. Transplant. *6*:55-61, 1992.

116. Sudan, D. L., Chinnakotla, S., Horslen, S., et al.: Basiliximab decreases the incidence of acute rejection in intestinal transplantation. Transplant. Proc. *34*:940-941, 2002.

117. The, T. H., van der Ploeg, M., van der Berg, A., et al.: Direct detection of cytomegalovirus in peripheral blood leukocytes—a review of the antigenemia assay and polymerase chain reaction. Transplantation *54*:193-198, 1992.

118. Todo, S., Fung, J. J., Starzl, T. E., et al.: Liver, kidney, and thoracic organ transplantation under FK 506. Ann. Surg. *212*:295-307, 1990.

119. Touraine, J. L., Bosi, E., El Yafi, M. S., et al.: The infectious lymphoproliferative syndrome in transplant recipients under immunosuppressive treatment. Transplant. Proc. *17*:96-98, 1985.

120. Ukah, F. O., Merhave, H., and Kramer, D.: Early outcome of liver transplantation in patients with a history of spontaneous bacterial peritonitis. Transplant. Proc. *25*:1113-1115, 1993.

121. Verma, A., Dhawan, A., Wade, J. J., et al.: *Mycobacterium tuberculosis* infections in pediatric liver transplant recipients. Pediatr. Infect. Dis. J. *19*:625-630, 2000.

122. Verma, A., Wade, J. J., Cheeseman, P., et al.: Risk factors for fungal infection in paediatric liver transplant recipients. Pediatr. Transplant. *9*:220-225, 2005.

123. Winston, D. J., Wirin, D., Shaked, A., and Busuttil, R. W.: Randomized comparison of ganciclovir and high-dose acyclovir for long-term cytomegalovirus prophylaxis in liver transplant recipients. Lancet *246*:69-74, 1995.

124. Wittner, M.: Cryptococcosis. *In* Feigin, R. D., and Cherry, J. D. (eds.): Textbook of Pediatric Infectious Diseases. 2nd ed. Philadelphia, W. B. Saunders, 1987.

125. Wreghitt, T. G., Gray, J. J., Ward, K. N., et al.: Disseminated adenovirus infection after liver transplantation and its possible treatment with ganciclovir. J. Infect. *19*:88-89, 1989.

126. Yoshikawa, T., Ihira, M., Furukawa, H., et al.: Four cases of human herpesvirus 6 variant B infection after pediatric liver transplantation. Transplantation *65*:1266-1269, 1998.

127. Yoshikawa, T., Ihira, M., Suzuki, K., et al.: Human herpesvirus 6 infection after living related liver transplantation. J. Med. Virol. *62*:52-59, 2000.
128. Younes, B. S., McDiarmid, S. V., Hargas, J. H., et al.: The effect of immunosuppression on posttransplant lymphoproliferative disease in pediatric liver transplant patients. Transplantation *70*:94-99, 2000.
129. Ziring, D., Tran, R., Edelstein, S. et al.: Infectious enteritis after intestinal transplantation: Incidence, timing, and outcome. Transplantation *79*:702-709, 2005.
130. Zitelli, B. J., Gartner, J. C., Malatach, J. J., et al.: Pediatric liver transplantation: Patient evaluation and selection, infectious complications, and life-style after transplantation. Transplant. Proc. *19*:3309-3316, 1987.

CHAPTER 84

OPPORTUNISTIC INFECTIONS IN KIDNEY TRANSPLANTATION

Gail J. Demmler-Harrison

Renal transplantation is the therapy of choice for end-stage renal disease (ESRD) in children and adolescents.[139] It is successful in 90 percent of recipients and allows most children the best opportunities for normal growth and development and an almost normal lifestyle.[74,142,221] Despite the overall success of renal transplantation, infection remains the major cause of morbidity, graft loss, and mortality in renal transplant recipients.[50,214] Newer and more effective immunosuppressive regimens have reduced the rates and hospitalizations for graft rejection after renal transplantation, but rates and hospitalizations for bacterial and viral infections seem to be unchanged or increasing.[53,143,185] Prednisone-free maintenance immunosuppressive combinations with tacrolimus, mycophenolate mofetil, and sirolimus help maintain graft function, but they also may increase the risk for development of post-transplantation lymphoproliferative disorders (PTLD) and invasive fungal diseases.[104]

These infections can be managed successfully if detected early and treated appropriately.[104] This chapter presents a general approach to renal transplant recipients from the perspective of the infectious disease specialist. Specific, detailed information regarding the diagnosis and management of each particular pathogen can be found in the respective chapters in the section of this textbook dedicated to infections with specific microorganisms.

PRE-TRANSPLANT EVALUATION

The role of the pediatric infectious disease specialist in the care of a renal transplant recipient ideally begins during the pre-transplantation period.[168,169] Before the patient undergoes transplantation, a thorough history and physical examination should be performed, with a focus on evaluation for evidence of an active infection that may require immediate therapy or, rarely, preclude transplantation (Table 84-1). The history should be comprehensive but focus on the details of any history of previous infections that may re-emerge during the post-transplant period, including urinary tract infections (UTIs); mucocutaneous diseases such as herpes simplex virus (HSV); systemic illnesses such as tuberculosis; chronic infections such as hepatitis B virus (HBV), hepatitis C virus (HCV), or human immunodeficiency virus (HIV); and diarrheal diseases. Infection with HIV previously was regarded as a reason to exclude a potential recipient from undergoing rental transplantation. More recent successes with highly active antiretroviral therapy have improved long-term survival in HIV-infected pediatric patients, however, and have led clinicians, research scientists, and family members themselves to investigate the role of renal transplantation as a treatment for ESRD.[60,167]

Renal transplant candidates undergo peritoneal dialysis or hemodialysis, so a history of previous dialysis catheter–associated

TABLE 84-1 Guidelines for Pre-transplant Evaluation in Pediatric Kidney Transplant Candidates

History
Past infectious diseases
Routine childhood illnesses
Travel to, birth or residence in areas endemic for fungal or parasitic diseases
Tuberculosis exposure
Animal exposure
Diet preferences and water resources
Vaccinations
Reactions or allergies to antimicrobials
Current or past immunosuppression

Physical
Search for active or latent focus of infection
Nutritional status

Laboratory and Other Testing
PPD
Chest radiograph
Urinalysis and urine culture
Viral serology for HSV, CMV, EBV, VZV, human *Erythrovirus* (human parvovirus B19), HAV, HBV, HCV, HIV, BK virus, WNV, and others depending on the history
Baseline HSV, CMV and EBV DNA PCR or CMV antigenemia, parvovirus B19, HCV, BK virus if seropositive or post-transplant monitoring is anticipated
Fungal and parasitic testing if travel or exposure history positive; sputum or stool tests as indicated

Anticipatory Guidance
Update vaccines
Counsel regarding measures to reduce infection risk
Consider antimicrobial prophylaxis if at risk

CMV, cytomegalovirus; EBV, Epstein-Barr virus; HAV, hepatitis A virus; HBV, hepatitis B virus; HCV, hepatitis C virus; HIV, human immunodeficiency virus; HSV, herpes simplex virus; PCR, polymerase chain reaction; PPD, purified protein derivative; VZV, varicella-zoster virus; WNV, West Nile virus.

infections should be documented, and any current infection should be treated and eliminated before transplantation is performed. Another focus of the history should include an exposure history for the patient's country of origin or foreign travel, especially to areas endemic for organisms such as *Strongyloides stercoralis*, *Coccidioides immitis*, *Blastomyces dermatitidis*, or *Histoplasma capsulatum* and for diseases such as malaria and tuberculosis.[87,185] Other important exposures include blood product transfusions; exposure to animals or plants; well water as a source of drinking water; and dietary habits, especially consumption of raw or undercooked eggs or meat or unpasteurized dairy products.[168,169]

In children, a careful history of routine childhood illnesses, including varicella, measles, mumps, and rubella, should be documented.[107]

The immunization history of the patient should be documented carefully and, if needed or indicated, updated before the patient undergoes transplantation. Ideally, children with chronic renal disease should be fully immunized before progression to ESRD, for optimal immune response and protection during outbreaks of vaccine-preventable diseases.[41] Vaccinations against tetanus, pertussis, and diphtheria; polysaccharide vaccines, such as those against pneumococcus and *Haemophilus influenzae* type B; inactivated vaccines against polio and hepatitis A; and recombinant vaccines, such as those for hepatitis B, may be given or updated at any time before transplantation is performed.[28,208,220] Meningococcal vaccine is indicated routinely now for specific age groups and for special outbreak situations. The live varicella vaccine is recommended for renal transplant candidates who have not had varicella; it should be given at least 2 to 4 weeks before transplantation is performed.[238] Measles, mumps, rubella vaccine should be administered even earlier, preferably months before the patient undergoes transplantation. In addition, annual influenza vaccine and a tetanus booster every 10 years are recommended for patients who are renal transplant candidates or recipients.

If the child is unable to be fully immunized before undergoing transplantation, the routine immunization schedule for the inactivated vaccines may be reinstituted after immunosuppression is decreased, approximately 6 to 12 months after an uncomplicated transplant procedure.[28,208,220] Live virus vaccines should be avoided in the post-transplant period in most instances. Reports of safe and effective vaccination with varicella vaccine in selected post-transplant patients have been published, however.[26,34,71,161,162] Close contacts and family members of renal transplant candidates and recipients also should be fully immunized and should receive the annual influenza vaccine.[10] Other important points in the pre-transplant evaluation history include allergies or reactions to medications, especially antibiotics, and the use of immunosuppressive agents.

Pre-transplant laboratory and diagnostic imaging evaluations for most renal transplant candidates should include a tuberculin skin test, chest radiograph, urinalysis, and urine culture for bacteria. Baseline renal and liver function tests also should be performed.

Serologic screening of the transplant recipient's status regarding organisms that may reactivate in the recipient or infect the recipient via the donor organ should be performed; such screening should include tests for HSV; cytomegalovirus (CMV); varicella-zoster virus (VZV); Epstein-Barr virus (EBV); human *Erythrovirus* (human parvovirus B19); syphilis; toxoplasmosis; hepatitis A, B, and C viruses; and HIV. Transplant recipients who are seropositive for HSV or CMV usually receive antiviral prophylaxis during the peritransplant period, whereas recipients seropositive for EBV may undergo post-transplant monitoring. It may be helpful to save an aliquot of the recipient's (and donor's) serum in case unusual circumstances occur, such as infection with West Nile virus (WNV). In CMV-seropositive transplant candidates, baseline CMV antigenemia or quantitative DNA polymerase chain reaction (PCR) may be useful, and in EBV-seropositive candidates, detection of EBV DNA by quantitative PCR may be helpful to document pre-transplant viral load, especially if post-transplant virologic monitoring is to be performed. Other laboratory tests or imaging studies may be useful, depending on the patient's exposure history and physical examination.

The pre-transplant evaluation also is an opportunity for the infectious disease specialist to counsel the patient and family about measures that may reduce the transplant recipient's risk for development of infectious disease complications post-transplant. Patients who have an exposure, or even a suspected exposure, to

varicella (chickenpox) or zoster (shingles) should contact their physicians immediately to see whether passive immunoprophylaxis with varicella-zoster immunoglobulin or post-exposure antiviral therapy with acyclovir or valacyclovir is indicated. Plans for foreign travel to remote areas also should be discussed with the physician. The transplant recipient should consume only thoroughly cooked meat and seafood and thoroughly washed fresh fruits and vegetables. In addition, drinking water should be pure. Transplant recipients should avoid, if possible, changing cat litter boxes, aquariums, and birdcages and should avoid close contact with people who have viral respiratory illnesses. Finally, medical attention should be sought if fever occurs, especially if it is significant or persistent.

POST-TRANSPLANT INFECTIOUS COMPLICATIONS

Infections occurring in the post-transplant period can be grouped into three main time frames: the first month post-transplant (early), 2 to 6 months post-transplant (middle), and 6 months post-transplant and onward (late).[187,204] Although almost any organism or pathogen can infect a transplant recipient at any time, these time periods provide the clinician with a guide to the organisms and disease processes most commonly encountered (Table 84–2).

INFECTIONS OCCURRING DURING THE EARLY POST-TRANSPLANT PERIOD

Infections occurring during the first month after renal transplantation has been performed usually are bacterial.[193] Common sites of early infections include the wound, urinary tract, lungs, and indwelling intravascular catheters.[174]

Wound Infections

As with any surgical procedure, wound infections may develop in a renal transplant recipient. They occur in approximately 2 percent of renal transplant recipients and range in severity from a superficial wound infection, easily treated with wound care and antimicrobial therapy, to deep perinephric abscesses that may be difficult to treat and result in transplant nephrectomy.[188,193] Wound infections are more likely to occur in patients with technical problems associated with the transplant surgery, including urinary leaks, vesicoureteral reflux, wound hematomas, or lymphoceles.[148,239] Malnutrition during the pre-transplant period may impair wound healing and predispose the patient to development of wound infection.

Open Penrose drains may increase the likelihood of introducing microorganisms into the wound, whereas closed suction drainage, such as with a Jackson-Pratt drain, may reduce this risk. In addition, prompt removal of all drains, usually within 5 days in most uncomplicated cases, and administration of prophylaxis with perioperative antibiotics may decrease the incidence of wound infections; such measures are performed routinely in most renal transplant centers. The regimen usually is aimed at uropathogens and staphylococci. One dose generally is given pre-transplant, and the regimen is continued for only 24 hours post-transplant.

The diagnosis of a wound infection should be suspected if erythema, warmth, or discharge is present at the wound site or if an unexplained fever develops. Fluid may drain from the wound persistently, or a fluid collection or abscess may be seen on imaging of the deeper operative sites. The patient will be receiving immunosuppressive agents, however, and the findings may be unusual, or the symptoms may be blunted. Any fluid or pus

TABLE 84–2   Timetable for the Occurrence of Common Infections and Usual Pathogens after Kidney Transplantation

Early Period
Wound infections
UTI
Bacteremia and sepsis syndrome
Pneumonia
HSV
HBV
Human *Erythrovirus* (human parvovirus B19)
WNV
Seasonal viruses
Drug reactions

Middle Period
Herpesviruses
   CMV
   EBV
   VZV
   HHV types 6, 7, and 8
Polyomaviruses
   JC virus
   BK virus
Papillomaviruses
Adenoviruses
Human *Erythrovirus* (human parvovirus B19)
Listeria monocytogenes
Mycobacterium tuberculosis
Atypical mycobacteria
Nocardia
Fungal diseases
Pneumocystis carinii
Parasitic diseases

Late Period
Community-acquired respiratory viruses and bacterial pathogens
UTI
Streptococcus pneumoniae
CMV
EBV
VZV
HBV
HCV
HIV/AIDS

AIDS, acquired immunodeficiency syndrome; CMV, cytomegalovirus; EBV, Epstein-Barr virus; HBV, hepatitis B virus; HCV, hepatitis C virus; HHV, human herpesvirus; HIV, human immunodeficiency virus; HSV, herpes simplex virus; UTI, urinary tract infection; VZV, varicella-zoster virus; WNV, West Nile virus.

obtained should be stained and cultured for bacterial, mycobacterial, and fungal organisms. Organisms most likely to be identified as causes of wound infection include staphylococci (*Staphylococcus aureus*, especially methicillin-resistant *S. aureus*, but also coagulase-negative staphylococci), streptococci, and gram-negative enteric organisms. Unusual, multidrug-resistant, or health care–associated bacterial pathogens and yeast, such as *Candida albicans*, also may cause wound infections post-transplant. In addition, case reports of wound and perinephric fluid collections infected with *Mycoplasma hominis* have been published.[206]

Appropriate antimicrobial therapy, initially broad-spectrum and then ultimately tailored to the isolated organism and its susceptibility pattern, should be administered. The duration of appropriate antimicrobial therapy usually is 10 to 14 days, or until the wound infection has resolved and the patient has been afebrile for 3 to 5 days. Deep abscesses or unusual organisms may require longer therapy.

Urinary Tract Infections

UTIs are common developments after renal transplantation and may affect 35 to 79 percent of renal transplant recipients.[116,239]

Post-transplant UTIs are associated with acute and chronic graft dysfunction and may threaten renal graft survival.[2,11,30,48,106,151,213] They may occur during the early, middle, or late post-transplant period. A UTI that occurs during the early or early/middle post-transplant period often is a severe illness complicated by pyelonephritis, urosepsis, metastatic foci of infection, allograft dysfunction, rejection, and relapse.[152,189] UTIs occurring in the early post-transplant period are associated more often with graft loss than are UTIs that occur later.[48]

The risk for developing an invasive UTI after undergoing renal transplantation seems to be increased in patients with prolonged bladder catheterization (most catheters can be removed during the first few days post-transplant), dysfunctional bladder, ureterovesical disorders with reflux, malnutrition, underlying disorders, renal stones, obstructive uropathy, or a contaminated cadaveric kidney.[2,168] Surgical complications, such as hematoma, reflux, or obstruction at the urinary anastomosis, or inability of the bladder to empty completely are associated with UTIs. In addition, young infants, especially infants who have vesicoureteral reflux, seem to have a high incidence of complicated UTIs post-transplant.[152] Procedures that address the etiology and correct underlying physiologic and anatomic abnormalities of the bladder and ureters should be performed before transplantation to avoid or lessen development of complications associated with these problems.[2,11,30,213] Newer surgical techniques allow children with reconstructed bladders to undergo successful renal transplantation with minimal risk for post-transplant development of UTIs.[148,189]

The organisms most commonly isolated from patients with early-onset UTIs include not only the typical gram-negative enteric bacteria, but also enterococci, staphylococci, and *Pseudomonas aeruginosa*. Unusual organisms, such as *Streptococcus mitis*, *Serratia marcescens*, and *Corynebacterium urealyticum*, also can be found. Antimicrobial therapy should be tailored to the susceptibility pattern of the organism isolated from the urine. Because 30 percent of patients experiencing a UTI during the early post-transplant period may have recurrent UTIs, a prolonged 6-week course of antibiotics usually is recommended to reduce the risk of developing a relapsing kidney infection.[148,189] Antimicrobial prophylaxis may reduce the risk of developing a UTI. Trimethoprim-sulfamethoxazole administered for the first 4 months after renal transplantation is effective in preventing most UTIs and can provide cross-cover prophylaxis against *Pneumocystis carinii* pneumonia and other diseases.[69]

Pneumonia

Pneumonia can occur during the first month after renal transplantation and often is associated with prolonged endotracheal intubation. Gram-positive and gram-negative bacterial pathogens acquired from normal oropharyngeal flora and unusual or health care–associated multidrug-resistant organisms predominate during the early post-transplant period.[169] *Legionella pneumophila* and unusual *Legionella* spp., such as *Legionella micdadei*, *Legionella bozemanae*, and *Legionella dumoffii*, also have caused outbreaks of serious, life-threatening pneumonia in transplant recipients in some centers.[29,39,115,169] *P. carinii* can cause pneumonia in a transplant recipient during the early post-transplant period, but more often it is associated with disease after the first month post-transplant.[89] Rare or unusual pathogens, such as *Rhodococcus equi*, may cause pneumonia in these patients.[128]

Patients with pneumonia usually present with fever, chills, chest pain, malaise, change in tracheal secretions, cough, dyspnea, tachypnea, change in ventilatory status, rales or rhonchi on auscultation of the lungs, and pulmonary infiltrates on chest radiograph. Pneumonia may be complicated by pleural effusion, empyema, or pulmonary abscess, and death may occur if pneumonia is severe and not diagnosed and treated promptly.

Treatment with antibiotics effective against the bacterial pathogens isolated from culture of tracheal aspirates, bronchoalveolar lavage fluid, or lung tissue is appropriate.

Bacteremia, Fungemia, and Sepsis

Bacteremia, fungemia, and sepsis occurring during the early post-transplant period often are associated with indwelling catheters.[167] The urinary tract, surgical wound, or transplanted or native kidney also may be a source.[138] Usual bacterial organisms such as coagulase-negative staphylococci or *S. aureus*, unusual bacterial organisms, and yeasts such as *C. albicans* and other *Candida* spp. may be involved. *Listeria monocytogenes* also may cause primary bacteremia or sepsis at any time after a kidney transplantation has been performed, but the greatest risk occurs during the early period. Complications include meningitis, and 10 percent of these patients may die.[150,199] Renal transplant recipients also are at increased risk for development of bacteremia with *Salmonella* nontyphoidal species.[47,100,167]

Complications such as UTI, graft infection, peritonitis, abscesses, and meningitis can occur, and recurrences are common. Therapy for bacteremia, sepsis, or its complications is tailored to the susceptibility pattern of the organism isolated from the patient's blood. The duration of therapy for uncomplicated bacteremia usually is 10 to 14 days, but a longer course of treatment may be indicated if abscesses occur or an unusual organism is isolated. Removal of the indwelling catheter may be necessary to clear persistent bacteremia, and abscesses and other foci of infection should be drained.

Other Bacterial Diseases

Pediatric renal transplant recipients also seem to be at increased risk for development of antibiotic-associated colitis caused by *Clostridium difficile*.[232] Infection of a lymphocele with *Pasteurella multocida* has been reported, as has systemic infection with *Bartonella henselae*.[3,37,52,132,167] A high index of suspicion always must be maintained when evaluating a transplant recipient for infection because the immunosuppression required to maintain the transplanted kidney predisposes the recipient to development of infection with unusual organisms.

Viral Infections

HERPES SIMPLEX VIRUS

HSV is the most common virus encountered during the early post-transplant period, although antiviral prophylaxis significantly reduces the risk of this infection.[56,57] It occurs less frequently in pediatric (8%) than in adult renal transplant recipients (30%).[167,168] Most HSV infections encountered post-transplant are due to reactivation of the recipient's strain; however, primary or recurrent infection acquired from the renal allograft may occur, and primary infection from person-to-person transmission has been documented.[56,167,168,189]

Post-transplant HSV infection may be asymptomatic or associated with disease, most frequently oral ulcers in pediatric patients.[83] Genital and perianal ulcers may occur in adolescents and adults. Rarely, HSV may cause disseminated cutaneous lesions or zosteriform eruptions. HSV esophagitis may be manifested as dysphagia, refusal to eat, irritability, and substernal chest pain, and it may complicate oral HSV disease, especially if the oral mucosa has been traumatized by orogastric or nasogastric tubes. Acute, severe hepatitis with hepatic necrosis, often accompanied by hypotension and disseminated intravascular coagulation, also can occur. Tracheobronchitis and pneumonitis may occur as a result of HSV, primarily in patients with pneumonia caused by another pathogen and whose mucosa has been trauma-

tized by endotracheal intubation. It is often severe and life-threatening, even with appropriate supportive care and antiviral therapy.[167] Encephalitis also has been reported in renal transplant recipients.[79]

The diagnosis is made by isolation of HSV in cell culture or detection of viral antigen by immunofluorescence or viral DNA by PCR in the end-organ involved. Detection or isolation of HSV in body secretions may represent asymptomatic shedding or disease and should be correlated clinically. Treatment with acyclovir is recommended for patients with disease, and HSV-seropositive transplant recipients should receive acyclovir or valacyclovir prophylaxis during the peritransplant period to prevent development of HSV infection. Most patients receiving ganciclovir, valganciclovir, foscarnet, or cidofovir for CMV prophylaxis also are protected against HSV.

OTHER VIRUSES

Seasonal viruses, especially winter respiratory viruses such as respiratory syncytial virus, influenza viruses, parainfluenza viruses, and adenoviruses; winter diarrhea viruses, such as rotavirus; and late summer/early fall viruses, such as the enteroviruses, can infect the transplant recipient during the early post-transplant period and cause disease. Such infections may be acquired from the family or the community, or they may occur from health care-associated exposures. The illness associated with these viruses typically is not as severe as the illness seen with the herpes family of viruses or adenoviruses.

Renal transplant recipients who are chronically infected with HBV or HCV may experience liver dysfunction during the early transplant period, but the late post-transplant period, beyond the first year, carries the greatest risk for progression of liver disease to cirrhosis. If a renal transplant recipient acquires HBV soon after undergoing transplantation, acute hepatitis can develop, often with death from liver failure.[46,167]

Non-infectious Causes of Fever

The most common non-infectious cause of fever in the first post-transplant month is allograft rejection.[188] Fever often is the first sign of rejection, especially in children, and rejection should be considered if an infectious source of the fever is not identified. Another common non-infectious cause of fever early after transplantation is antilymphocyte antibody therapy (OKT3). The first two or three doses of OKT3 produce a release of cytokines, which cause fever and chills. In most patients, these symptoms resolve after the third dose. Other non-infectious causes of fever during this period include drug reactions and pulmonary emboli.

INFECTIONS OCCURRING DURING THE MIDDLE POST-TRANSPLANT PERIOD

The cumulative effects of immunosuppression begin to be revealed during the period 2 to 6 months after transplantation. If a significant amount of antirejection therapy is required for multiple episodes of rejection, the effects may be more pronounced. Such immunosuppression allows classic opportunistic pathogens, such as CMV, *P. carinii*, *Toxoplasma gondii*, *L. monocytogenes*, *Aspergillus*, and *Nocardia*, to evade immune surveillance and cause disease.[89,167,231,233] Reactivation of organisms previously infecting the transplant recipient or the donor allograft, including *Mycobacterium tuberculosis*, HBV, HCV, HIV, *H. capsulatum*, and *C. immitis*, also may cause disease. In addition, an occult bacterial focus of infection that was not adequately identified and treated pre-transplant may become apparent at this time and cause significant disease.[188]

Herpesviruses

The herpes family of viruses (HSV types 1 and 2, CMV, EBV, VZV, and human herpesvirus [HHV] types 6, 7, and 8) share the biologic properties of latency, reactivation, cell association, and oncogenicity, which renders them the most important group of pathogens that affect renal transplant recipients.[167,194] HSV is more important during the early post-transplant period, whereas the other herpes family members are important causes of morbidity and mortality during the middle and late post-transplant periods.[90]

CYTOMEGALOVIRUS

CMV may cause primary infection in a CMV-seronegative transplant recipient through a renal allograft or blood product transfusion from a seropositive donor.[16,45,186] Person-to-person transmission within the family or close community also is possible. Recurrent CMV infection develops in seropositive transplant recipients if the recipient's CMV strain becomes reactivated. The renal allograft from a seropositive donor also can be a source of re-infection to the recipient and produce active CMV infection or disease.[36,84] CMV infection in renal transplant recipients may cause silent or asymptomatic infection; end-organ diseases such as hepatitis, esophagitis, colitis, encephalitis, vasculitis, and retinitis; and systematic disease with persistent fever and leukopenia. A case report also linked CMV infection with post-transplant occurrence of atypical hemolytic-uremic syndrome that resolved with plasma exchange and ganciclovir antiviral therapy.[160] It has been linked in some studies to allograft dysfunction and nephropathy.

CMV also causes depressed cell-mediated immunity and impaired alveolar macrophage function, rendering the host more vulnerable to other opportunistic infections, such as fungal disease and *P. carinii* pneumonia, and it serves as a cofactor for other viruses, such as EBV and HHV-6 and HHV-7.[111,163,175,216,217] In addition, CMV is associated with acute and chronic rejection and allograft nephropathy and decreased long-term patient survival.[1,58,121,167,186]

Disease caused by CMV can be documented by isolation of CMV from blood or tissue; detection of CMV antigen pp65 in circulating leukocytes; or detection of CMV DNA by PCR or similar assays in blood, bronchoalveolar fluid, or tissue.[21,22,171,176,186] Isolation of CMV in urine or saliva documents active infection but has little significance in predicting disease; serologic tests may document seroconversion in primary infections but generally should be reserved for pre-transplant screening only. Most transplant patients at risk for acquiring CMV disease (i.e., CMV-seropositive recipients [D$^+$/R$^+$] or CMV-seronegative recipients [D$^+$/R$^-$] who received a renal allograft from a seropositive donor) should be monitored by viral surveillance, usually by testing blood weekly for CMV antigen pp65 or for CMV DNA by PCR.[20,94]

Detection of significant levels of the virus by quantitative or semiquantitative assay, or an increase from baseline levels, usually predicts CMV disease.[217] Reduction of immunosuppression, along with preemptive antiviral therapy, generally is indicated and results in a decrease or resolution of CMV levels detected in blood.[7,22,40,43,77,81,129] Despite receiving adequate antiviral therapy, some patients have persistently positive CMV DNA by PCR, however, which should be interpreted within the clinical context.[21] In some patients who otherwise appear well, the DNA may be fragmented and nonreplicating, whereas in other patients with persistent symptoms, a strain of CMV resistant to one or more antiviral agents may be the cause.

The antiviral agents currently available for the treatment of CMV disease and preemptive therapy for positive CMV markers include ganciclovir, valganciclovir, foscarnet, and cidofovir.[230] For renal transplant patients with moderate to severe CMV-

associated disease, 2 to 3 weeks of therapy with intravenous ganciclovir usually is adequate to treat disease; however, patients with CMV retinitis or repeat episodes of rejection may require maintenance therapy, usually with oral ganciclovir or valganciclovir.[101,134,153] Asymptomatic or mild CMV infections may respond to oral ganciclovir or valganciclovir administered for 1 to 3 months.[135,149] Preemptive therapy should be continued throughout the period of immunosuppression in patients who are severely immunosuppressed and at risk for development of CMV disease and recurrence (D$^+$/R$^-$).[81,94,135,149] Foscarnet and cidofovir have significant renal toxicity and should be used with extreme caution in renal transplant recipients. Prophylaxis for CMV disease is indicated in high-risk transplant recipients (D$^+$/R$^-$); options include intravenous CMV immune globulin, oral and intravenous acyclovir and ganciclovir, and oral valacyclovir and valganciclovir.[25,66,77,124,153,198,205,226]

EPSTEIN-BARR VIRUS

EBV infection in children who have received a renal transplant may be asymptomatic or may be associated with a variety of different syndromes, including a nonspecific viral syndrome, mononucleosis, smooth muscle tumors (leiomyoma), post-transplant PTLD, and lymphoma.[23,24,54,88,96] Infection and disease may occur after primary and recurrent EBV infection, but primary infection is more likely to occur and produce PTLD in younger children than in adults who have received solid organ transplants.[35,96] EBV disease may affect 10 percent of pediatric renal transplant recipients and may develop 1 month to 5 or more years post-transplant, with the risk accumulating every year of post-transplant survival.[50,200]

Knowledge about post-transplant EBV infection and disease is evolving; as graft survival has improved, with more intense immunosuppressive regimens that preserve graft function, and other opportunistic infections such as HSV, CMV, and *P. carinii* being successfully managed, EBV has emerged as a formidable obstacle to successful solid organ transplantation in children.[23,49,51,54,86,109,200] The estimated overall risk for development of serious life-threatening EBV-associated illness is at least 4 percent and increases to 10 percent in children who experience a primary infection with EBV after undergoing renal transplantation.[49,96] Other risk factors for PTLD in children who have received solid organ transplants include receipt of antilymphocyte therapy such as OKT3 for rejection; receipt of tacrolimus, sirolimus, or mycophenolate mofetil, rather than cyclosporine, for immunosuppression; and CMV or EBV donor/recipient (D$^+$/R$^-$) mismatch.[51,103,104]

Nonspecific viral syndromes and mononucleosis occur during the earlier post-transplant period, whereas lymphoma and leiomyoma are more likely to be a manifestation during the late post-transplant period.[25,54,70,86] Uncomplicated post-transplant mononucleosis is characterized by the self-limited illness of fever, pharyngitis, cervical adenopathy, and splenomegaly. The signs and symptoms of PTLD vary but often include persistent fever, weight loss, and generalized adenopathy.[96] The disease frequently is multisystemic and progressive, and involvement of the neck, chest, lungs, gastrointestinal tract, liver, spleen, eyes, and brain, as well as lesions, may be detected by computed tomography of the head, neck, chest, and abdomen.[4,5,168,195] The renal allograft also may be involved and show dysfunction. Lymphoma may be manifested as solid tumors in the renal allograft, lung, liver, spleen, brain, and soft tissues.[70,88] Smooth muscle tumors (leiomyoma) frequently are multicentric and multifocal; they often occur in lung, liver, and spleen but also may occur in unusual locations, including the brain and renal allograft.[23,86,95]

Laboratory diagnosis of post-transplant, EBV-associated disease is based on detection by PCR of EBV DNA in circulating lymphocytes.[5,43,62] Quantitative or semiquantitative PCR assays may show increasing or persistently high copies of EBV DNA in the circulating lymphocytes of patients who are at risk for developing PTLD.[5,85,184] If end-organ disease is observed, the diagnosis can be confirmed histopathologically by detection by PCR of EBV DNA in tissue or by in situ hybridization with an EBV-encoded RNA probe.[4,217]

The diseases associated with EBV also may be classified in the laboratory as polyclonal or monoclonal. Polyclonal illnesses seem to be more benign than are monoclonal diseases, which often are associated with chromosomal abnormalities and malignant transformation.[168] The virus cannot be cultivated by routine means; when studied by special culture techniques, EBV has been found frequently in the oropharyngeal secretions of seropositive transplant recipients and is not predictive of EBV-associated disease.[168,184] Similarly, serologic approaches to establishing the diagnosis of EBV infection post-transplant also are nonspecific and difficult to interpret in most patients, unless the recipient clearly has seroconverted during the post-transplant period.

Aggressive or intense treatment of uncomplicated EBV-associated viral syndrome or mononucleosis usually is unnecessary because these illnesses seem to be self-limited in most patients. Immunosuppression may be reduced, and acyclovir may be administered; the patient should be monitored carefully. If symptoms in the patient or EBV DNA levels in the blood persist or increase, PTLD should be suspected, and the diagnosis should be confirmed.[211,218]

Treatment of established PTLD is challenging.[82] Mortality rates are high, and the best results seem to occur if the disease is diagnosed by quantitative PCR viral-load monitoring and serial imaging studies and treated aggressively.[217] Preemptive therapy instituted when viral surveillance monitoring detects an increase in EBV DNA in circulating lymphocytes before end-organ disease is evident also may be helpful in some patients.[43,134] Reduction in immunosuppression remains the most widely recommended strategy, but a variety of regimens have been studied as well.

Antiviral agents such as acyclovir and ganciclovir seem to reduce EBV replication early in the course of the disease process and may halt the progression of disease in some patients.[51,169,230] Antiviral agents are ineffective, however, against latent EBV or cells that have been transformed by the virus. Interferon-α, immunoglobulin, and anti–CD20 monoclonal antibody preparations such as rituximab have been used successfully in patients with established PTLD. Experimental protocols evaluating adoptive immunotherapy in transplant recipients are under way. In addition, some experts suggest that administration of intense anti-CMV therapy with ganciclovir and CMV hyperimmune globulin may improve chances of survival in certain patients with PTLD because CMV may serve as a cofactor in progression of disease caused by other members of the herpes family.[1,16,24,163,203,216] Treatment of patients with lymphoma or leiomyoma includes a reduction in immunosuppression, chemotherapy, radiation therapy, and surgical resection of tumors.

VARICELLA-ZOSTER VIRUS

VZV can cause primary (varicella, chickenpox) or reactivation (zoster, shingles) disease in a renal transplant recipient.[168,204] Infection with VZV can occur at any time but does so most often during the middle post-transplant period. Patients present with fever and painful or pruritic vesicular skin lesions.[153] Hepatitis, encephalitis, acute or chronic recurrent cerebral vasculitis and vasculopathy, and pneumonia also may occur, even in the absence of skin lesions, especially in an immunocompromised host.[97] Varicella occurs more frequently in children, and zoster occurs more frequently in adolescent and adult transplant recipients.[35]

In contrast to other herpes family viruses, VZV almost always is transmitted person-to-person or by aerosol in health care, family, and community settings; it rarely, if ever, has been linked to the transplanted allograft.[141,168] Before the advent of routine immunization and antiviral therapy, infection with VZV was a major cause of morbidity and mortality in children receiving solid organ transplants.[35,64,189] Untreated primary varicella may continue for several weeks and result in visceral dissemination, pneumonitis, hepatic necrosis, encephalitis, vasculitis with stroke, disseminated intravascular coagulation, hemorrhagic skin lesions, and death.[64,169,194] Zoster in solid organ transplant recipients may remain localized to a dermatome, but it often disseminates beyond the dermatomal distribution and produces widespread skin lesions and even visceral dissemination.

The diagnosis of VZV disease often is clinical, but it should be confirmed by isolation of VZV from fresh, vesicular skin lesions or detection of viral antigen by direct immunofluorescence assay on cells obtained by scraping the base of the skin lesion.[169] Tzanck smear may show multinucleated giant cells, suggesting a viral infection, but it cannot differentiate VZV from HSV. Other pathogens, especially HSV, may mimic VZV disease, so establishing an accurate viral diagnosis is important. VZV also may be detected by PCR-based DNA detection methods, which also may distinguish wild-type strains from OKA vaccine strain of VZV; VZV PCR tests may be performed by reference and research laboratories. Establishing a serologic diagnosis of active VZV infection is difficult. Routine serologic screening performed in the pre-transplant period identifies patients who are seronegative and at risk for developing primary infection with VZV.

Treatment of established VZV disease should be instituted as early as possible during the course of the illness because survival is improved if treatment begins before the fifth day of illness.[64] Acyclovir is recommended for most renal transplant recipients experiencing either primary infection with varicella or zoster with dissemination; it is administered intravenously in high doses (500 mg/m^2 per dose every 8 hours if renal function is normal or adjusted for renal function as needed) for 5 to 10 days, or until new lesions have ceased to occur for 24 to 48 hours, old lesions have crusted, the fever has resolved, and disease has abated.[26,161,168,230] Uncomplicated zoster or very mild primary varicella may be treated with oral acyclovir, famciclovir, or valacyclovir, provided that the patient is monitored carefully for clinical response. Ganciclovir, foscarnet, or cidofovir also provide cross-cover protection for most VZV strains, if these antiviral agents are being administered for difficult CMV infections.

Prevention of post-transplant VZV disease can be accomplished by several effective strategies, which should be discussed during the pre-transplant evaluation. Transplant recipients who were seronegative for VZV during the pre-transplant evaluation should receive varicella vaccine before undergoing transplantation, if possible.[71,112,238] Pre-transplant varicella vaccination is safe, beneficial, and cost-effective when administered to pediatric renal transplant candidates and in selected renal transplant recipients post-transplant.[26,34,71,72,161]

Seronegative, unimmunized transplant recipients who are exposed to varicella or zoster during the post-transplant period should receive passive immunoprophylaxis with varicella-zoster immunoglobulin. Preemptive therapy with oral acyclovir also is recommended by some experts in this situation because varicella-zoster immunoglobulin does not prevent, but only attenuates, the postexposure disease process. Finally, acyclovir, valacyclovir, ganciclovir, and valganciclovir administered prophylactically to transplant recipients who are seropositive for HSV or CMV also may provide protection against VZV disease.[124,168]

HUMAN HERPESVIRUSES 6, 7, AND 8

HHV-6, HHV-7, and HHV-8 also infect renal transplant recipients by primary infection and by reactivation.[32,33,37,61,92,187,188,203] Infection with these viruses becomes evident during the middle post-transplant period, but their roles in specific disease processes are unclear.[169,197,212] HHV-6 and HHV-7 may act as cofactors in the progression of a disease, especially diseases caused by CMV and EBV.[61,111,153,163,216] HHV-8 is associated with Kaposi sarcoma post-transplant in severely immunosuppressed adult renal transplant recipients, but it has not been appreciated as a major opportunistic pathogen in pediatric renal transplant recipients to date.[32,35,63,168,181,193] HHV-8 may be transmitted through the renal allograft or by blood product transfusion, or it can become reactivated in the recipient post-transplant.[181]

Polyomaviruses and Papillomaviruses

POLYOMAVIRUSES

Human polyomaviruses (JC, BK, and SV40) frequently infect children and are present in urine and stool.[224,225] They can be detected in the urine of 33 to 58 percent of renal transplant recipients and detected serologically in 56 percent, and they are found histopathologically and by PCR in blood, body fluids, and tissue in 8 to 13 percent.* Knowledge about the roles that these viruses play in the outcome of renal transplant patients is evolving.

The JC and BK polyomaviruses seem to have a significant impact on adult and pediatric renal transplant recipients.[18,73,133,154-156,182,190] BK virus has been implicated in various syndromes, including ureteral stenosis, hemorrhagic or chronic cystitis, interstitial nephritis with graft failure, allograft nephropathy (BK-associated nephropathy [BKAN]), and rejection, in renal transplant recipients.[18,38,95,98,155,166,176,188,190] Disease associated with these viruses most often occurs during the middle and late post-transplant periods. BK virus may be asymptomatic or cause increasing serum creatinine levels, cystitis, tubular necrosis, graft dysfunction, or allograft rejection.[179] Risk factors for BKAN seem to include BK serostatus at the time of transplant, greater immunosuppression with use of mycophenolate mofetil, and concurrent CMV infection.[59,75,76,91,127]

BK virus often is detected in urine by the presence of "decoy cells," which are cells containing intranuclear viral inclusions, or more recently by quantitative PCR assays that detect and quantify BK viral DNA. BK viruria precedes BK viremia, which precedes BK nephropathy.[93] Patients with BK-associated nephropathy may have BK viral DNA detected in the urine, blood, or plasma, and renal biopsy specimens may show characteristic viral inclusions. Most recently, quantitative PCR viral surveillance in blood or plasma has been shown in renal transplant recipients to be useful in predicting the development of BK nephropathy and in guiding preemptive antiviral and immunosuppressive strategies.

Pediatric kidney transplant recipients who have increasing BK viremia levels should be managed preemptively with carefully monitored reduction of immunosuppression to prevent development of more serious complications of BKAN and graft rejection. This strategy usually results in reduction and then clearance of BK viremia and development of BK-specific cellular immunity coincident with BK virus clearance.[127] Treatment of established BKAN includes a reduction in immunosuppression. Cidofovir has activity against BK virus and has been used anecdotally to treat severe disease caused by BKAN.[93,230]

JC virus causes a rare syndrome called *progressive multifocal leukoencephalopathy*. It may be diagnosed by viral DNA detection using PCR-based assays available in reference and research laboratories or histopathologically by brain biopsy or autopsy examination. Successful treatment options for progressive multifocal leukoencephalopathy caused by JC virus are very limited, and most, if not all, patients die of progressive encephalopathy.

PAPILLOMAVIRUSES

Human papillomaviruses are common viruses that infect healthy children, adolescents, and adults. Adult renal transplant recipients are at increased risk for development of human papillomavirus–associated disease, such as cervical cancer and anogenital papillomas, whereas pediatric patients may develop numerous disfiguring warts post-transplant, especially if they require severe immunosuppression.[158,168,188] Malignant transformation of cutaneous warts caused by high-risk types has been documented.[188] Treatment options are limited but include physical removal of papillomas with laser and cryotherapy and careful reduction of immunosuppression. Information on the use of human papillomavirus vaccines in patients with ESRD or renal transplant recipients has not been published at this time.

Adenoviruses

Adenoviruses may infect pediatric renal transplant recipients at any time, but they are most likely to cause significant disease during the middle post-transplant period. They continue to emerge as a significant pathogen in pediatrics, including transplant recipients. They do not seem to play as important a role in renal transplant outcome, however, as do other viruses, such as the herpes family of viruses, and they currently are not as prominent in renal transplant recipients as they are in other transplant recipients, such as recipients of liver, lung, bone marrow, or stem cell transplants.[80,137,159,168,169] Nonetheless, infections with adenoviruses in pediatric renal transplant recipients, when they occur, can be serious and include hemorrhagic cystitis, diarrhea, allograft nephropathy, pneumonia, hepatitis, and disseminated disease with multisystemic involvement.[19,110,188,214,233,235]

The diagnosis is made by isolation of the virus in respiratory secretions, stool, urine, blood, or tissue. Rapid diagnosis may be accomplished within 30 to 60 minutes, using a rapid immunochromatographic assay that detects adenovirus antigens in eye secretions, respiratory samples, urine, and stool. Viral DNA also may be detected by PCR or quantitative PCR available in reference or research laboratories, and characteristic changes may be seen by histopathology in tissue. Adenovirus serotyping by neutralization assays and genotyping by PCR sequence-based assays are available in reference laboratories.[80] Treatment of serious adenoviral disease primarily is supportive. Immunosuppression also may be reduced, when possible. Antiviral agents, such as ribavirin, ganciclovir, and cidofovir, have activity against adenoviruses. Clinical reports of use of these agents in children with serious adenovirus disease post-transplant are published, but clinical trials documenting efficacy have not been performed.[31]

Human *Erythrovirus* (Human Parvovirus B19)

Human *Erythrovirus* (human parvovirus B19) has been reported to cause acute and chronic infection, manifesting as chronic anemia, red blood cell aplasia, and pancytopenia in renal transplant recipients.* It also has been implicated in collapsing glomerulopathy and thrombotic microangiopathy in renal transplant recipients.[228] Unusual manifestations, such as hepatic necrosis or central nervous system infection with vasculitis, also have been reported.[15,17,118,119] Transmission most likely is person-to-person; however, some reports indicate that the virus may be transmitted

---

*See references 6, 55, 59, 67, 68, 73, 75, 76, 91, 93, 95, 98, 127, 147, 154-156, 164, 166, 176, 177, 190, 219.

---

*See references 9, 14, 15, 17, 118, 126, 131, 144, 165, 209, 228, 234.

by blood product transfusion or in the renal allograft.[14,15,117] More recent reports suggest that the role that this virus plays in the outcome of renal transplant recipients may be more important than previously recognized, but systemic studies in pediatric patients have not been done.[14]

The diagnosis of acute infection with human parvovirus B19 is supported by parvovirus B19–specific IgG seroconversion; detection of parvovirus B19–specific IgM antibodies in serum; or detection of viral DNA in plasma, blood, body fluids, bone marrow, or tissue. The virus is not cultivatable in clinical virology laboratories that use routine cell cultures, but laboratories using special erythroid precursor cell lines may be able to cultivate parvovirus B19 for research purposes. No specific antiviral therapy is available, but anecdotal experience and case reports support a beneficial role for intravenous immunoglobulin and carefully monitored reduction in immunosuppression as management strategies to resolve parvovirus B19 viremia and associated end-organ disease.[149]

WEST NILE VIRUS

WNV is a single-stranded RNA flavivirus that has emerged as an important pathogen worldwide. It usually is transmitted by mosquitoes and causes a febrile illness, viral meningoencephalomyelitis, and acute flaccid paralysis in the normal host. Renal transplant recipients may become infected with WNV that is transmitted by the organ donor, by blood product transfusions, or naturally from mosquitoes.[44,102,112,180,227] Infection with WNV may manifest in the early post-transplant period if it is transmitted by the graft or blood products and, because of immunosuppression, produce severe febrile illnesses, seizures with status epilepticus, encephalitis, paralysis, and movement disorders. Death also may occur.[44] A high index of suspicion is required, and if WNV is suspected, serum and CSF should be sent for WNV-specific IgG and IgM antibody testing. The virus also may be isolated in special cell cultures and detected by reverse transcriptase PCR-based assays. Immunohistochemical staining may show WNV proteins in tissues from biopsy or autopsy examination. Outcome in renal transplant recipients with WNV disease improves with early establishment of the diagnosis and carefully managed reduction of immunosuppression.[180]

Mycoplasma

Mycoplasma spp. commonly infect school-aged children. Children and adolescents who undergo renal transplantation also may experience respiratory tract infections with *Mycoplasma pneumoniae* and *M. hominis*. The infection also may disseminate to extrapulmonary sites, causing hepatitis, septic arthritis, or perinephric fluid collections in pediatric renal transplant recipients.[108,136,206] *Mycoplasma* spp. may be detected using special biphasic culture media or PCR-based assays. Serologic diagnosis is difficult to accomplish, owing to cross-reactivity of antigens producing the possibility of false-positive reactions in some patients. Antimicrobial therapy with macrolide antibiotics, along with carefully managed reduction of immunosuppression, may be beneficial in selected patients.[108,136]

Bacterial and Mycobacterial Diseases

Bacteria that commonly produce disease in renal transplant recipients during the middle post-transplant period include *L. monocytogenes*, which often causes sepsis or meningitis.[168,199] Routine bacterial illnesses that were not identified and properly treated during the pre-transplant period also may emerge at this time and cause abscesses, sepsis syndrome, and death.

Mycobacterial disease caused by *M. tuberculosis* may occur at any time post-transplantation, but it occurs most frequently during the middle post-transplant period.[122,125,168,178] *M. tuberculosis* causes disease in approximately 1 percent of renal transplant recipients in the developed continents, such as North America and Europe, and in 15 percent of renal transplant recipients in developing countries with a high prevalence of tuberculosis, such as India or Pakistan.[105,168,178,185,191,192] Tuberculosis may develop in renal transplant recipients as a result of primary and reactivation infection in almost any site, and transmission from the renal allograft and reactivation in the native kidney have occurred.[114,145,146,185] *M. tuberculosis* may cause various diseases, including pulmonary infiltrates, cavitary lesions, adenopathy, cutaneous lesions, bone and joint disease, liver or spleen granulomata, and meningitis. Fever frequently occurs, and miliary or disseminated disease may occur, especially in young children.

Because the purified protein derivative (PPD) test is negative in most renal transplant recipients with active tuberculosis, the diagnosis is determined best by detection of acid-fast bacilli in smears from tissue or sputum and by isolation of *M. tuberculosis* in cultures of gastric aspirates, sputum, tracheal secretions, spinal fluid, or tissue.[125,168] The presence of granulomata in tissue also strongly suggests the diagnosis of tuberculosis.

Treatment of tuberculosis in a renal transplant recipient usually includes isoniazid, rifampin, and pyrazinamide for 1 year, although shorter courses may be acceptable in some patients.[122,168] Other antituberculous drugs may be added to or substituted for this standard regimen, depending on the disease process, the susceptibility pattern of the organism, and potential drug interactions. Because many antituberculosis drugs are excreted by the kidney, doses may need to be adjusted in a renal transplant recipient. Because rifampin may interact with cyclosporine, levels of cyclosporine should be monitored closely to avoid rejection of the allograft.[157] If a history of tuberculosis exposure is elicited during the pre-transplant evaluation, the transplant candidate should be evaluated for tuberculosis, including having a PPD and chest radiograph.[145,146,178] All close contacts also should be investigated for evidence of having tuberculosis. Treatment is recommended if disease is discovered, and prophylaxis with isoniazid is indicated for most patients who have a recently positive PPD on pre-transplant evaluation.[122,168,169,192,237] A transplant recipient who receives an allograft from a donor with a history of tuberculosis or a positive PPD also may be a candidate for prophylaxis with isoniazid post-transplant.[122,168,169]

Atypical mycobacteria are ubiquitous nontuberculous mycobacteria that can infect and produce disease in renal transplant recipients. They can cause disease during the middle post-transplant period and so are included here. Their effects usually do not become evident, however, until many years after the patient has undergone transplantation, during the late post-transplant period.[42,146,170] Atypical mycobacteria that have been documented to cause disease in solid organ transplant recipients include *Mycobacterium kansasii*, *Mycobacterium avium-intracellulare*, *Mycobacterium fortuitum*, *Mycobacterium xenopi*, *Mycobacterium haemophilum*, *Mycobacterium marinum*, *Mycobacterium chelonae*, *Mycobacterium abscessus*, *Mycobacterium gastri*, *Mycobacterium scrofulaceum*, and *Mycobacterium thermoresistibile*.[105,168,169]

A high index of suspicion is necessary to detect these elusive pathogens. They should be considered as the cause of disease in patients with persistent cutaneous ulcers, abscesses, adenopathy, pulmonary nodules, chronic wound infections, or bone and joint disease after negative routine bacterial cultures have been obtained, and the patient has failed to respond to standard antimicrobial therapy.[188] Disseminated, multisystem disease also can occur. Environmental sources of atypical mycobacteria include contaminated dialysis equipment, soil, and contaminated water in aquariums and pools. The diagnosis is established by isolation of nontuberculous mycobacteria in fluid or tissue. Granulomata are not observed consistently in tissue, and acid-fast stains may be negative.[188] Atypical nontuberculous mycobacteria are difficult to treat, and treatment must be individualized to each patient. Strategies include reduction of immunosuppression and surgical débridement of localized disease. Antimicrobial therapy based on in vitro susceptibility testing of the isolate also should be administered, often for a prolonged period.

Nocardia

Nocardia asteroides is the most common *Nocardia* spp. causing illness in renal transplant recipients; however, other, more unusual *Nocardia* spp., including *Nocardia transvalensis, Nocardia brasiliensis, Nocardia nova, Nocardia otitidiscaviarum,* and *Nocardia farcinica,* also have been shown to cause disease in solid organ transplant recipients.[168,169,233] The most common manifestations of nocardial disease in transplant recipients are fever, cough, and pulmonary infiltrates.[233] Pleural effusion, pulmonary nodules, and cavitary lesions also may occur. Cutaneous infection, adenitis, arthritis, meningitis with brain abscesses, and infection of the renal allograft also may occur. *Nocardia* spp. can be seen on Gram and modified acid-fast stains of sputum, bronchoalveolar lavage fluid, abscess fluid, and tissue. They can be isolated on routine media but may take longer than conventional bacteria to grow. Prolonged treatment with sulfonamides, alone or in combination with trimethoprim, is recommended. Amikacin and other antimicrobials may be added in selected patients with severe disease, provided that renal function is monitored closely.[188] Trimethoprim-sulfamethoxazole prophylaxis for UTI and *P. carinii* also may be effective in preventing disease caused by *Nocardia*.

Fungal Diseases

Fungal infections occur infrequently in renal transplant recipients relative to other solid organ transplant recipients.[168,169,188] This lower rate of infection probably is related to technical procedures performed at the time of transplantation and the lower level of immunosuppression required to maintain most renal allografts.[188] When they do occur, however, fungal infections often are serious and life-threatening.[87,90,99] Fungal disease in a renal transplant recipient usually is manifested in one of two ways: (1) pulmonary or disseminated disease caused by one of the environmental mycoses, such as *H. capsulatum* or *C. immitis,* or (2) opportunistic infection with fungi that rarely cause disease in a normal host, such as *Candida* spp., *P. carinii, Aspergillus* spp., *Cryptococcus neoformans, Nocardia* spp., and others.[87,201]

Travel to endemic areas increases a transplant recipient's risk for development of histoplasmosis and coccidioidomycosis and may be identified during the pre-transplant evaluation. Factors that increase a transplant recipient's risk for acquisition of opportunistic fungal disease include underlying conditions such as diabetes mellitus, repeated episodes of rejection, long-term administration of steroids, prolonged use of antibiotics, and CMV infection. Similar to tuberculosis, invasive fungal disease can be a result of primary infection or reactivation infection with secondary dissemination.[188]

P. carinii, currently classified as a fungus, may cause pneumonia in 10 percent of solid organ transplant recipients, most often during the first 6 months post-transplant.[8,168,169] It seems to occur more commonly in children than in adults and usually causes fever, dyspnea, tachypnea, hypoxemia, and a nonproductive cough.[57,168] Interstitial pulmonary infiltrates are typical findings, but almost any radiographic picture can be observed, and pneumothorax is common in severe disease. The diagnosis can be suspected clinically but is documented best by organisms being shown in lung biopsy specimens; bronchoalveolar lavage may provide the diagnosis in some patients.

Treatment with high-dose oral or intravenous trimethoprim-sulfamethoxazole for 14 to 21 days is used most often. Intravenous pentamidine may be administered to selected patients, but

renal function should be monitored carefully.[188] Corticosteroids may be helpful in treating severe disease if given early in the course. Low-dose oral trimethoprim-sulfamethoxazole provides effective prophylaxis against *P. carinii* pneumonia and UTIs and usually is administered to renal transplant recipients for at least 6 months post-transplant.[69] Transplant recipients experiencing repeated episodes of rejection, allograft dysfunction, or CMV disease may require a longer period of prophylaxis.[168,169] Aerosolized pentamidine is an alternative prophylaxis strategy for some patients.[188]

Candida spp., especially *C. albicans,* are the opportunistic fungi most frequently isolated in renal transplant recipients.[168,169] Other *Candida* spp. isolated include *Candida krusei, Candida glabrata,* and *Candida tropicalis.* Most fungal infections caused by *Candida* spp. occur during the first 2 months post-transplant, usually at the site of indwelling intravascular and urinary catheters.[188] Esophagitis, abscesses, and arthritis also can develop, and endocarditis with metastatic foci can occur if the fungemia persists. Other opportunistic fungi such as *Aspergillus* most often cause sinusitis and pulmonary disease, and, because of its angioinvasive nature, *Aspergillus* often disseminates and causes lesions in the liver, spleen, and brain.[168,169,201,202]

A thorough search for metastatic foci always should be undertaken when a primary focus of invasive fungal disease is documented. *C. neoformans* usually causes cutaneous lesions or abscesses and pneumonia with pleural effusion, but meningitis, arthritis, and pyelonephritis also can occur.[168,169,196] Exposure to soil or bird droppings provides an epidemiologic clue to the diagnosis. In addition, the Zygomycetes, including *Rhizopus, Mucor, Rhizomucor,* and *Absidia* spp., can cause disease in solid organ transplant recipients.[201,202] They most often cause cutaneous, rhinocerebral, or pulmonary disease or brain abscesses in renal transplant patients. Cutaneous and soft tissue infections, wound infections, and gastrointestinal disease with perforation also have been described. The Zygomycetes, similar to *Aspergillus,* are angioinvasive and disseminate via the bloodstream to cause disease, which often is severe. A variety of unusual fungi, such as *Paecilomyces, Fusarium,* and *Bipolaris,* have been shown to cause cutaneous infection, usually at the site of indwelling catheters, and *Hansenula anomala* reportedly has caused UTI in a renal transplant recipient.[78]

The endemic dimorphic fungi include *H. capsulatum, C. immitis, B. dermatitidis,* and *Paracoccidioides brasiliensis.* Infection with these organisms can occur anytime after the patient has undergone transplantation but usually occurs during the intermediate post-transplant period.[215] These organisms usually are noted in renal transplant recipients who reside in endemic areas. Histoplasmosis is endemic in the central part of the United States and many foreign countries, and nosocomial outbreaks have occurred during hospital construction projects. Fever, chills, and cough are the usual initial signs. Skin lesions, hepatosplenomegaly, and meningitis also can occur. Pancytopenia often is present as well, and the organism frequently is found in the bone marrow of patients with disseminated disease. Coccidioidomycosis is endemic in the southwestern portion of the United States and northern Mexico. It usually is manifested as fever, cough, and pulmonary infiltrates, but extrapulmonary dissemination frequently occurs. Blastomycosis is endemic in the southern United States, along the Mississippi and Ohio River valleys, and in the Great Lakes area. It is a rare development after renal transplantation, but most often causes lung and skin lesions. Paracoccidioidomycosis rarely has been reported in renal transplant recipients.[210]

The diagnosis of invasive fungal disease is established best by isolating the fungus from sputum or tracheal aspirate, bone marrow, tissue, or fluid. *C. neoformans* also may be isolated from urine. Fungal serology and tests for cryptococcal antigen may support the diagnosis.[210]

Fungal identification and susceptibility testing now can be performed in reference laboratories and should be used to guide therapy whenever possible. Amphotericin B usually is used to treat most invasive fungal disease in transplant recipients, and the deoxycholate, lipid complex, or liposomal forms can be used, provided that renal function is monitored closely.[123] Flucytosine may have additive or synergistic effects against many yeasts and fungi. The azole antifungal agents are not nephrotoxic and are used in renal transplant recipients whenever possible. Many *Candida* spp. are susceptible to fluconazole, although resistance is emerging in all *Candida* spp. and is present in a high percentage of *C. krusei* and *C. glabrata*. Itraconazole and voriconazole may be effective against other fungi, such as *Aspergillus*. Voriconazole has emerged as a treatment of choice for most *Aspergillus* infections. Itraconazole should be used with caution, however, because it has variable oral absorption and may interact with cyclosporine.[215] Caspofungin also has activity against most *Candida* spp. and a variety of opportunistic fungi, including *Aspergillus*. Currently, experience using the newest triazole, posaconazole, and the newest echinocandin, micafungin, in pediatric renal transplant recipients is limited.

Surgical resection or drainage of abscesses, avascular cavities, or effusions may be required to treat some forms of invasive fungal disease of the lungs, liver, or spleen. Carefully monitored reduction in immunosuppression also may help the host recover from invasive fungal disease.

Parasitic Infections

The parasites most commonly encountered in renal transplant recipients during the intermediate post-transplant period are *T. gondii*, *S. stercoralis*, and *Trypanosoma cruzi*.[65,168] These infections occur most often in adults. Children also may be infected with routine parasites such as *Enterobius vermicularis*, *Ascaris*, *Giardia*, and others pre-transplant. Other parasitic infections that may be found in renal transplant recipients include leishmaniasis, schistosomiasis, and malaria. Renal transplant recipients seem to be at much lower risk for acquisition of parasitic diseases than are other solid organ transplant recipients.

T. gondii usually occurs as a result of reactivation of latent disease in the donor allograft or recipient.[130] It is encountered most frequently in heart transplant recipients, but any solid organ recipient, including renal, may be affected. Clinical manifestations of infection with *T. gondii* include focal meningoencephalitis, brain abscesses, pneumonia, myocarditis, pericarditis, hepatitis, and retinochoroiditis.[140,207,215,222] The diagnosis may be made by demonstration of the organism in tissue by histopathology, detection of DNA by PCR in body fluids or tissue, or serologically by detection of high titers of IgG and specific IgM antibody to *T. gondii*. Treatment with pyrimethamine, sulfadiazine, and folinic acid usually is recommended; however, some patients also may respond to clindamycin. Routine prophylaxis with trimethoprim-sulfamethoxazole for UTI and *P. carinii* infection may help prevent disease with *T. gondii*.

S. stercoralis is an important pathogen in adult transplant recipients, but it is rarely, if ever, a significant problem in pediatric patients. Because *S. stercoralis* can be maintained in the human intestinal tract for decades, it can disseminate and cause serious disease in transplant recipients who were infected pre-transplant. A complete blood count for eosinophilia should be obtained, and stool and other specimens should be examined for rhabditiform larvae if the pre-transplant evaluation reveals travel to endemic areas. Thiabendazole should be given before transplantation is performed if *S. stercoralis* infection has been documented or is suspected. *T. cruzi*, the cause of Chagas disease, rarely has been transmitted by renal transplantation.[65,120]

INFECTIONS OCCURRING DURING THE LATE POST-TRANSPLANT PERIOD

Infections occurring 6 months or more after the patient has undergone renal transplantation usually are less severe than infections experienced in the earlier periods, especially if the level of immunosuppressive therapy is low and the allograft is functioning well.[187] Constant vigilance for health care–associated and community-acquired viral and bacterial diseases and unusual infections should continue, however.

Chronic rejection or repeated episodes of acute rejection complicated by allograft dysfunction predispose the patient to development of more serious opportunistic infections, similar to infections encountered during the first 6 months post-transplant. UTIs that develop during this period, in contrast to UTIs in the early post-transplant period, usually are benign and may be treated with conventional antimicrobial therapy in most instances, if they do not seem to threaten the function of the allograft or the patient's survival. Patients also may experience community-acquired infections with respiratory viruses, such as influenza virus and respiratory syncytial virus, and with bacteria, especially *Streptococcus pneumoniae* (pneumococcus) or *S. aureus*. These common community-acquired bacterial pathogens may be resistant to usual β-lactam antibiotics.[208,220] In addition, patients vaccinated with 7-valent or 23-valent pneumococcal vaccines still may acquire invasive pneumococcal disease with emerging, non-vaccine serotypes, such as 19A and 3A. These serotypes often are also multidrug-resistant. Opportunistic viral infections encountered during this period are zoster or, rarely, CMV retinitis.[149] The risk for developing PTLD also persists during this late post-transplant period.

Renal transplant recipients may be chronically infected with HBV or HCV pre-transplant. Increased risk of mortality from fulminant hepatitis with hepatic failure may occur during the early pre-transplant period, and chronic liver disease, cirrhosis, and liver failure may be seen 10 years or more after renal transplantation has been performed in hepatitis B surface antigen (HBsAg)–positive recipients.[236] All transplant recipients who are not immune to HBV should receive HBV vaccine before transplantation.[229] Most experts agree that renal allografts from HBsAg-positive donors should not be used, but the decision to perform renal transplantation in recipients who are HBsAg-positive is controversial and must be made on an individualized basis.

Renal transplant recipients who are infected with HCV pre-transplant usually do well during the early post-transplant period, but long-term survival is poorer than in recipients who are not infected with HCV. Not only can chronic liver disease develop, but also membranoproliferative glomerulonephritis has been reported in renal transplant recipients infected with HCV.[27] Despite these risks, however, most experts do not consider infection with HCV a contraindication for renal transplantation in patients with ESRD.[173] Hepatitis G virus also has been detected in the serum of renal transplant recipients, and at least one association with membranous glomerulonephritis has been reported.[12,13] The role of HGV in clinical disease in renal transplant recipients is not established, however.

HIV may be transmitted by kidney transplantation despite routine screening of donors of blood and organs.[117,183] A transplant recipient also may become infected with HIV after undergoing transplantation.[168] Shortly after a patient has undergone transplantation, HIV infection may cause fever and a mononucleosis-like syndrome. Complications of acquired immunodeficiency syndrome may develop during the late transplant period. HIV-infected patients with ESRD traditionally have been excluded from receiving renal transplantation. More recent advances in HIV therapy have caused some experts to reconsider this policy on an individual basis, however.[168]

REFERENCES

1. Acott, P., Lee, S., Bitter-Suermann, H., et al.: Infection concomitant with pediatric renal allograft rejection. Transplantation 62:689, 1996.
2. Adams, J., Mehls, O., and Wiesel, M.: Pediatric renal transplantation and the dysfunctional bladder. Transpl. Int. 17:596, 2004.
3. Ahsan, N., Holman, M., Riley, T., et al.: Peliosis hepatis due to *Bartonella henselae* in transplantation: A hemato-hepato-renal syndrome. Transplantation 65:1000, 1998.
4. Al-Atlar, L., Berrocal, A., Warman, R., et al.: Diagnosis by PCR of ocular post transplant lymphoproliferative disease after pediatric renal transplantation. Am. J. Ophthalmol. 137:569, 2004.
5. Allen, U., Herbert, D., Pedric, M., et al.: Utility of semiquantitative polymerase chain reaction for Epstein-Barr virus to measure virus load in pediatric organ transplant recipients with and without post-transplant lymphoproliferative disease. Clin. Infect. Dis. 33:145, 2001.
6. Andrews, S., Shas, K., Daniel, R., et al.: A serologic investigation of BK virus and JC virus infections in recipients of renal allografts. J. Infect. Dis. 158:176, 1988.
7. Anglicheau, D., Lautrette, A., Scieux, C., et al.: Efficacy and safety of lowering immunosuppression to treat CMV infection in renal transplant recipients with valacyclovir prophylaxis: a pilot study. Nephrol. Dial. Transplant. 18:1654, 2003.
8. Arend, S., Westendrop, R., Kroon, F., et al.: Rejection treatment and cytomegalovirus infection as risk factors for *Pneumocystis carinii* pneumonia in renal transplant recipients. Clin. Infect. Dis. 22:920, 1996.
9. Ashan, N., Holman, M., Gocke, C., et al.: Pure red cell aplasia due to parvovirus B19 infection in solid organ transplantation. Clin. Transplant. 11:265-270, 1997.
10. Avery, R.: Infections and immunizations in organ transplant recipients: A preventive approach. Cleve. Clin. J. Med. 61:386, 1994.
11. Barrero, R., Fij, J., Fernandez-Hurtado, M., et al.: Vesicoureteral reflux after kidney transplantation in children. Pediatr. Transpl. 11:498, 2007.
12. Berthoux, P., Dejean, C., Cecillon, S., et al.: High prevalence of hepatitis G (HGV) infection in renal transplantation. Nephrol. Dial. Transplant. 13:2909, 1998.
13. Berthoux, P., Laurent, B., Cecillon, S., et al.: Membrane proliferative glomerulonephritis and subendothelial deposits (type 1) associated with hepatitis G virus infection. Am. J. Nephrol. 19:513, 1999.
14. Bertoni, E., Rosati, A., Zanazzi, M., et al.: Aplastic anemia due to B19 parvovirus infection in cadaveric renal transplant recipients: An underestimated infectious disease in the immune compromised host. J. Nephrol. 10:152, 1997.
15. Bertoni, E., Rosati, A., Zanazzi, M., et al.: Unusual incidence of aplastic anemia due to B-19 parvovirus infection. Transplant. Proc. 29:818, 1997.
16. Betts, R., Freeman, R., Douglas, R., et al.: Clinical manifestations of renal allograft derived primary cytomegalovirus infection. Am. J. Dis. Child. 131:759, 1977.
17. Bilge, I., Sadkoglu, B., Emre, S., et al.: Central nervous system vasculitis secondary to parvovirus B19 infection in a pediatric renal transplant patient. Pediatr. Nephrol. 20:529, 2005.
18. Binet, I., Nickeleit, V., Hirsch, H., et al.: Polyomavirus disease under new immunosuppressive drugs: A cause of renal graft dysfunction and graft loss. Transplantation 67:918, 1999.
19. Blohme, L., Nyberg, S., Jeansson, S., et al.: Adenovirus infection in a renal transplant patient. Transplant. Proc. 24:295, 1992.
20. Boland, G., deGast, G., Hene, R., et al.: Early detection of active cytomegalovirus (CMV) infection after heart and kidney transplantation by testing for immediate early antigenemia and influence of cellular immunity on the occurrence of CMV infection. J. Clin. Microbiol. 28:2069, 1990.
21. Boom, R., Sol, C., Schuurman, T., et al.: Human cytomegalovirus DNA in plasma and serum specimens of renal transplant recipients is highly fragmented. J. Clin. Microbiol 40:4105, 2002.
22. Boom, R., Sol, C., Weel, J., et al.: A highly sensitive assay for the detection and quantitation of human cytomegalovirus DNA in serum and plasma by PCR and electrochemiluminescence. J. Clin. Microbiol. 37:1489, 2000.
23. Boudjemaa, S., Boman, F., Guigonis, V., et al.: Brain involvement in multicentric Epstein-Barr virus-associated smooth muscle tumors in a child after kidney transplantation. Virchows Arch 444:387, 2004.
24. Brenig, M., Zitelli, B., Starzl, T., et al.: Epstein-Barr virus, cytomegalovirus, and other viral infections in children after liver transplantation. J. Infect. Dis. 156:273, 1987.
25. Brennam, D., Garlock, K., Singer, G., et al.: Prophylactic oral ganciclovir compared with deferred therapy for control of cytomegalovirus in renal transplant recipients. Transplantation 64:1843, 1997.
26. Breyer, M., Tete, M., Guest, G., et al.: Varicella-zoster in children after kidney transplantation: Long-term results of vaccination. Pediatrics 99:35, 1997.
27. Brunkhorst, R., Kliem, V., and Koch, K.: Recurrence of membranoproliferative glomerulonephritis after renal transplantation in a patient with chronic hepatitis C. Nephron 72:465, 1996.
28. Burroughs, M., and Moscona, A.: Immunization of pediatric solid organ transplant candidates and recipients. Clin. Infect. Dis. 30:857, 2000.
29. Campins, M., Ferrer, A., Callis, L., et al.: Nosocomial Legionnaire's disease in a children's hospital. Pediatr. Infect. Dis. J. 19: 228, 2000.
30. Capizzi, A., Zanon, G., Zachello, G., et al.: Kidney transplantation in children with reconstructed bladders. Transplantation 15:1113, 2004.
31. Carter, B., Karpen, S., Quiros-Tejeiro, R., et al.: Intravenous cidofovir treatment for disseminated adenovirus in a pediatric liver transplant recipient. Transplant 74:1050, 2002.
32. Caterino-de-Araujo, A., Magri, M., Santos-Fortuna, E., et al.: Human herpesvirus-8 infection in hemodialysis patients from Sao Paulo, Brazil: Preliminary results. Transplant. Proc. 39:3044, 2007.
33. Cattani, P., Capuano, M., Graffeo, R., et al.: Kaposi's sarcoma associated with previous human herpesvirus 8 infection in kidney transplant recipients. J. Clin. Microbiol. 39:506, 2001.
34. Chaves-Ido, S., Lopes, M., deSouza, V., et al.: Seroprevalence of antibody against varicella zoster virus and response to the varicella vaccine in pediatric renal transplant patients. Pediatr. Transplant. 9:192, 2005.
35. Chavez, B., Gillingham, K., and Mata, A.: Complications by age in primary pediatric renal transplant recipients. Pediatr. Nephrol. 11:399, 1997.
36. Chou, S.: Acquisition of donor strains of cytomegalovirus by renal transplant recipients. N. Engl. J. Med. 314:1418, 1986.
37. Cline, M., Cummings, O., Goldman, M., et al.: Bacillary angiomatosis in a renal transplant recipient. Transplantation 67:296, 1999.
38. Coleman, D., MacKenzie, E., Gardner, S., et al.: Human polyomavirus (BK) infection and ureteric stenosis in renal allograft recipients. J. Clin. Pathol. 31:338, 1978.
39. Colombo, J., Sammut, P., Langnas, A., et al.: The spectrum of *Pneumocystis carinii* infection after liver transplant in children. Transplantation 54:621, 1992.
40. Conti, D., Freed, B., Singh, T., et al.: Preemptive ganciclovir therapy in cytomegalovirus-positive renal transplant recipients. Arch. Surg. 130:1217, 1995.
41. Cortesa, M., Jordan, H. T., Cums, A. T., et al.: Mumps vaccine performance among university students during a mumps outbreak. Clin. Infect. Dis. 46:1172, 2008.
42. Costa, J., Meyers, A., Botha, J., et al.: Mycobacterial infections in recipients of kidney allografts: A seventeen-year experience. Acta Med. Port. 1:51, 1988.
43. Crompton, C., Cheung, C., Conjon, I., et al.: Epstein-Barr virus surveillance after renal transplantation. Transplantation 57:1182, 1994.
44. Cushing, M., Brat, D., Mosunijac, M., et al.: Fatal West Nile virus encephalitis in a renal transplant recipient. Am J. Clin. Pathol. 121:26, 2004.
45. Danziger-Isakov, L., and Storch, G.: Prevention and treatment of cytomegalovirus infections in solid organ transplant recipients. Pediatr. Infect. Dis. J. 21:431, 2002.
46. Davis, C., Gretch, D., and Carithers, R.: Hepatitis B and transplantation. Infect. Dis. Clin. North Am. 9:925, 1995.
47. Dhar, J., Al-Khader, A., Al-Sulaiman, M., et al.: Non-typhoidal *Salmonella* in renal transplant recipients: A report of twenty cases and review of the literature. Q. J. M. 78:235, 1991.
48. Dharnidharka, V., Agodoa, L., and Abbott, K.: Effects of urinary tract infection on outcomes after renal transplantation in children. Clin. J. Am. Soc. Nephrol. 2:100, 2007.
49. Dharnidharka, V., and Araya, C.: Post-transplant lymphoproliferative disease. Pediatr. Nephrol. 2007.
50. Dharnidharka, V., and Harmon, W.: Management of pediatric postrenal transplantation infections. Semin. Nephrol. 21:521, 2001.
51. Dharnidharka, V., Ho, P., Stablein, D., et al.: Mycophenolate, tacrolimus, and post-transplant lymphoproliferative disorder: A report of the North American Pediatric Renal Transplant Cooperative Study. Pediatr. Transplant. 6:396, 2002.
52. Dharnidharka, V., Richard, G., Neiberger, R., et al.: Cat scratch disease and acute rejection after pediatric renal transplantation. Pediatr. Transplant. 6:327, 2002.
53. Dharnidharka, V., Stablein, D., and Harmon, W.: Post-transplant infections now exceed acute rejection as cause for hospitalization: A report of the NAPRTCS. Am. J. Transplant. 4:384, 2004.
54. Dionne, J., Carter, J., Matsell, D., et al.: Renal leiomyoma associated with EBV in a pediatric transplant patient. Am. J. Kidney Dis. 46:351, 2005.
55. Drachenberg, C., Beskow, C., Cangno, C., et al.: Human polyomavirus in renal allograft biopsies: Morphological findings and correlation with urine cytology. Hum. Pathol. 30:970, 1999.
56. Dummer, J., Armstrong, J., Somers, J., et al.: Transmission of infection with herpes simplex virus by renal transplantation. J. Infect. Dis. 155:202, 1987.
57. Dummer, J., Hardy, A., Poorsattar, A., et al.: Early infections in kidney, heart and liver transplant recipients on cyclosporine. Transplantation 36:259, 1983.
58. Durlik, M., Siennicka, J., Litwinska, B., et al.: Clinical manifestations and diagnosis of cytomegalovirus infection in renal allograft recipients. Transplant. Proc. 33:1237, 2001.
59. Elldemir, O., Chang, I., Schecter, M., et al.: BK-virus associated hemorrhagic cystitis in a pediatric lung transplant recipient. Pediatr. Transplant. 11:807, 2007.
60. El Sayegh, S., Keller, M., Huprikar, S., et al.: Solid organ transplantation in HIV-infected recipients. Pediatr. Transplant. 8:214, 2004.
61. Emery, V.: Human herpesviruses 6 and 7 in solid organ transplant recipients. Clin. Infect. Dis. 32:1357, 2001.
62. Falco, D., Nepomuceno, R., Karm, S., et al.: Identification of Epstein-Barr virus-specific CD8+ T lymphocytes in the circulation of pediatric transplant recipients. Transplantation 74:501, 2002.

63. Fargie, D., Lebbe, C., Marjanovic, Z., et al.: Human herpesvirus-8 and other risk factors for Kaposi's sarcoma in kidney transplant recipients. Transplantation 67:1236, 1999.

64. Feldhoff, C., Balfour, H., Simmons, R., et al.: Varicella in children with renal transplants. J. Pediatr. 98:25, 1981.

65. Ferraz, A., and Figueiredo, J.: Transmission of Chagas disease through transplanted kidney: Occurrence of the acute form of the disease in two recipients from the same donor. Rev. Inst. Med. Trop. Sao Paulo 35:461, 1993.

66. Flechner, A., Avery, R., Fisher, R., et al.: A randomized prospective controlled trial of oral acyclovir versus oral ganciclovir for cytomegalovirus prophylaxis in high-risk kidney transplant recipients. Transplantation 66:1682, 1998.

67. Fogazzi, G., Cantu, M., and Saglembeni, L.: Decoy cells in the urine due to polyomavirus BK infection easily seen by phase-contrast microscopy. Nephrol. Dial. Transplant. 16:1496, 2001.

68. Fogeda, M., Munoz, M., Luque, A., et al.: Cross-sectional study of BK-virus infection in pediatric kidney transplant recipients. Pediatr. Transplant. 11:394, 2007.

69. Fox, B., Sollinger, H., Belzer, F., et al.: A prospective, randomized, double-blind study of trimethoprim-sulfamethoxazole for prophylaxis of infection in renal transplantation: Clinical efficacy, absorption, trimethoprim-sulfamethoxazole effects on the microflora, and the cost-benefit of prophylaxis. Am. J. Med. 89:255, 1990.

70. Frias, C., Lauzurica, R., Vaquero, M., et al.: Determination of Epstein-Barr virus in post transplant T-cell lymphoma in a kidney transplant recipient: Case report and review. Clin. Infect. Dis. 30:576, 2006.

71. Furth, S., and Fivush, B.: Varicella vaccination in pediatric kidney transplant candidates. Pediatr. Transplant. 6:97, 2002.

72. Furth, S., Hogg, R., Tarver, J., et al.: Varicella vaccination in children with chronic renal failure: A report of the SW Pediatric Nephrology Study Group. Pediatr. Nephrol. 18:33, 2003.

73. Gardner, S., MacKenzie, E., Smith, C., et al.: Prospective study of the human polyoma viruses BK and JC and cytomegalovirus in renal transplant recipients. J. Clin. Pathol. 37:578, 1984.

74. Giessling, M., Muller, D., Winkelman, B., et al.: Kidney transplantation in children and adolescents. Transplant. Proc. 39:2197, 2007.

75. Ginevri, F., Azzi, A., Hirsch, H., et al.: Prospective monitoring of polyomavirus BK replication and impact on pre-emptive intervention in pediatric kidney transplant recipients. Am. J. Transplant. 7:2727, 2007.

76. Ginevri, F., DeSantis, R., Comoli, P., et al.: Polyomavirus BK infection in pediatric kidney-allograft recipients: A single center analysis of incidence, risk factors and novel therapeutic approaches. Transplantation 75:1266, 2003.

77. Ginevri, F., Losurdo, G., Fontana, I., et al.: Acyclovir plus CMV immuno-globulin prophylaxis and early therapy with ganciclovir are effective and safe in CMV high-risk renal transplant pediatric recipients. Transpl. Int. 11(Suppl. 1):130, 1998.

78. Girardi, M., Glusac, E., and Imaedo, S.: Subcutaneous *Fusarium* foot abscess in a renal transplant patient. Cutis 63:67, 1999.

79. Gomez, E., Melon, S., Aguado, S.: Herpes simplex virus encephalitis in a renal transplant patient: Diagnosis by polymerase chain reaction detection of HSV DNA. Am. J. Kidney Dis. 30:423, 1997.

80. Gray, G., McCarthy, T., Lebeck, M., et al.: Genotype prevalence and risk factors for severe clinical adenovirus infections, United States 2004-2006. Clin. Infect. Dis. 45:1120, 2007.

81. Green, M., and Michaels, M.: Pre-emptive therapy of CMV disease in pediatric transplant recipients. Pediatr. Infect. Dis. J. 19:875, 2000.

82. Green, M., Michaels, M., Webber, S., et al.: The management of Epstein-Barr virus associated post-transplant lymphoproliferative disorders in pediatric solid-organ transplant recipients. Pediatr. Transplant. 3:271, 1999.

83. Greenberg, M., Friedman, H., Cohen, S., et al.: A comparative study of herpes simplex infections in renal transplant and leukemia patients. J. Infect. Dis. 156:280, 1987.

84. Grundy, J., Super, M., Sweney, P., et al.: Symptomatic cytomegalovirus infection in seropositive kidney recipients: Reinfection with donor virus rather than reactivation of recipient virus. Lancet 2:132, 1988.

85. Gupta, M., Filler, G., Kovesi, T., et al.: Quantitative tissue polymerase chain reaction for Epstein-Barr virus in pediatric solid organ recipients. Am. J. Kidney Dis. 41:212, 2003.

86. Haddu, T., Andre, J., Bourguard, R., et al.: Long-term followup of Epstein-Barr virus viremia in pediatric recipients of renal transplants. Pediatr. Nephrol. 20:76, 2005.

87. Hall, K., Copeland, J., Zuloski, C., et al.: Markers of coccidioidomycosis prior to cardiac or renal transplant and risk of recurrent disease. Transplantation 55:1422, 1993.

88. Hanto, D., Frizzera, G., Gajl-Peczaiska, K., et al.: Epstein-Barr virus induced B-cell lymphoma after renal transplantation. N. Engl. J. Med. 306:913, 1982.

89. Hardy, A., Wajszczuk, C., Suffredini, F., et al.: *Pneumocystis carinii* pneumonia in renal transplant recipients treated with cyclosporine and steroids. J. Infect. Dis. 149:143, 1984.

90. Harman, W.: Opportunistic infection in children following renal transplantation. J. Pediatr. Nephrol. 5:118, 1991.

91. Haysom, L., Rosenberg, A., Kainer, G., et al.: BK virus infection in an Australian pediatric renal transplant population. Pediatr. Transplant. 8:480, 2004.

92. Herbein, G., Strasswimmer, J., Alteiri, M., et al.: Longitudinal study of human herpesvirus 6 infection in organ transplant recipients. Clin. Infect. Dis. 22:171, 1996.

93. Herman, J., van Ranst, M., Snoeck, R., et al.: Polyomavirus infection in pediatric renal transplant recipients: Evaluation using a quantitative real-time PCR technique. Pediatr. Transplant. 8:485, 2004.

94. Hibberd, P., Tolkoff-Rubin, N., Conti, D., et al.: Pre-emptive ganciclovir therapy to prevent cytomegalovirus disease in cytomegalovirus antibody-positive renal transplant recipients: A randomized controlled trial. Ann. Intern. Med. 123:18, 1995.

95. Hirsch, H.: Polyomavirus BK nephropathy: A (re-) emerging complication in renal transplantation. Am. J. Transplant. 2:25, 2002.

96. Ho, M., Jaffe, R., Miller, G., et al.: The frequency of Epstein-Barr virus infection and associated lymphoproliferative syndrome after transplantation and its manifestations in children. Transplantation 45:719, 1988.

97. Hovens, M., Vaessen, N., Sijpkens, Y., et al.: Unusual presentation of central nervous system manifestations of varicella-zoster virus vasculopathy in renal transplant recipients. Transpl. Infect. Dis. 9:237, 2007.

98. Howard, D., Smith, S., Butterly, M., et al.: Diagnosis and management of BK polyomavirus interstitial nephritis in renal transplant recipients. Transplantation 68:1279, 1999.

99. Howard, R., Simmons, R., and Najarian, J.: Fungal infections in renal transplant recipients. Ann. Surg. 188:598, 1978.

100. Huang, J., Huang, C., Lai, M., et al.: *Salmonella* infection in renal transplant recipients. Transplant. Proc. 26:2147, 1994.

101. Humar, A., Gillingham, K., Payne, W., et al.: Association between cytomegalovirus disease and chronic rejection in kidney transplant recipients. Transplantation 68:1879, 1999.

102. Iwamoto, M., Jernigan, D., Guasch, A., et al.: Transmission of West Nile virus from an organ to four transplant recipients. N. Engl. J. Med. 348:2196, 2003.

103. Jamil, B., Nicholls, K., Becker, G., et al.: Influence of anti-rejection therapy on the timing of cytomegalovirus disease and other infections in renal transplant recipients. Clin. Transplant. 114:14, 2000.

104. Jensen, S., Jackson, E., Riley, L., et al.: Tacrolimus-based immunosuppression with steroid withdrawal in pediatric kidney transplantation—4 year experience at a moderate volume center. Pediatr. Transplant. 7:11, 2003.

105. Jie, T., Matas, A., Gilliingham, K., et al.: Mycobacterial infection after kidney transplant. Transplant. Proc. 37:937, 2005.

106. John, U., and Kemper, M.: Urinary tract infections in children after renal transplantation. Pediatr. Nephrol. 23:16, 2008.

107. Kalman, S., Bakkaloglu, S., Ozkaya, O., et al.: Measles: A rare communicable disease in a child with renal transplantation. Pediatr. Transplant. 6:432, 2002.

108. Kalman, S., Kurekci, A., Gak, F., et al.: *Mycoplasma pneumoniae* infection in a child after renal transplant. Pediatr. Transplant. 18:493, 2004.

109. Karakayali, H., Emiroglu, R., Arslan, G., et al.: Major infectious complications after kidney transplantation. Transplant. Proc. 33:1816, 2001.

110. Keswani, M., and Moudgli, A.: Adenovirus-associated hemorrhagic cystitis in a pediatric renal transplant recipient. Pediatr. Transplant. 11:568, 2007.

111. Kidd, I., Clark, D., Sabin, C., et al.: Prospective study of human beta-herpesviruses following renal transplantation: Association with HHV-7 and CMV co-infection with CMV disease and increased rejection. Transplantation 69:2400, 2000.

112. Kitai, I., King, S., Gafni, A., et al.: An economic evaluation of varicella vaccine for pediatric liver and kidney transplant recipients. Clin. Infect. Dis. 17:441, 1993.

113. Kleinschmidt-Demasters, B., Marder, B., Levi, M., et al.: Naturally acquired West Nile virus encephalomyelitis in transplant recipients: Clinical, laboratory, diagnostic and neuropathologic features. Arch. Neurol. 61:1210, 2004.

114. Klemperer, J., Wang, J., Hartman, B., and Stubenbord, W.: *Mycobacterium tuberculosis* infection of a native polycystic kidney following renal transplantation. Transplantation 66:118, 1998.

115. Knirsch, C., Jakob, K., Schoonmaker, D., et al.: An outbreak of *Legionella micdadei* pneumonia in transplant patients: Evaluation, molecular epidemiology and control. Am. J. Med. 108:290, 2000.

116. Krieger, J., Brem, A., and Kaplan, M.: Urinary tract infection in pediatric renal transplantation. Urology 15:362, 1980.

117. Kumar, P., Pearson, J., Martin, D., et al.: Transmission of human immunodeficiency virus by transplantation of a renal allograft with development of the acquired immunodeficiency syndrome. Ann. Intern. Med. 106:244, 1987.

118. Laurenz, M., Winkelman, B., Roigas, J., et al.: Severe parvovirus B 19 encephalopathy after renal transplantation. Pediatr. Transplant. 10:978, 2006.

119. Lee, P., Hung, C., Lei, H., et al.: Parvovirus B 19-related acute hepatitis in an immunosuppressed kidney transplant. Nephrol. Dial. Transplant. 15:1486, 2000.

120. Leiguarda, R., Roncoroni, A., Taratuto, L., et al.: Acute central nervous system infection by *Trypanosoma cruzi* (Chagas disease) in immunosuppressed patients. Neurology 40:830, 1990.

121. Lewis, R., Johnson, P., Golden, D., et al.: The adverse impact of cytomegalovirus infection on clinical outcome in cyclosporine-prednisone treated renal allograft recipients. Transplantation 45:353, 1988.

122. Lichenstein, I., and MacGregor, R.: Mycobacterial infections in renal transplant recipients: Report of five cases and review of the literature. Rev. Infect. Dis. 5:216, 1983.

123. Linden, P., Williams, P., and Chann, K.: Efficacy and safety of amphotericin B lipid complex (ABLC) in solid-organ transplant recipients with invasive fungal infections. Clin. Transplant. 14:329, 2000.

124. Lowance, D., Neumayer, H.-H., Legendre, C., et al.: Valacyclovir for the prevention of cytomegalovirus disease after renal transplantation. N. Engl. J. Med. 340:1462, 1999.

125. Malhorta, K., Dash, S., Dhawan, I., et al.: Tuberculosis and renal transplantation: Observations from an endemic area. Postgrad. Med. J. 62:359, 1986.

126. Marchand, S., Tchernia, G., Hiesse, C., et al.: Human parvovirus B19 infection in organ transplant recipients. Clin. Transplant. 13:17, 1999.

127. Marinelli, K., Bagnarelli, P., Gaffi, G., et al.: PCR real time assays for the early detection of BK virus-DNA in immune compromised patients. New Microbiol. 30:275, 2007.

128. Marsh, H., Bowler, I., and Watson, C.: Successful treatment of *Rhodococcus equi* pulmonary infection in a renal transplant recipient. Ann. R. Coll. Surg. Engl. 82:107, 2000.

129. Mas, V., Alvarellos, T., Albano, S., et al.: Utility of cytomegalovirus viral load in renal transplant patients in Argentina. Transplantation 67:1050, 2000.

130. Mason, J., Ordelheide, K., Grames, G., et al.: Toxoplasmosis in two renal transplant recipients from a single donor. Transplantation 44:588, 1987.

131. Mathias, R.: Chronic anemia as a complication of parvovirus B19 infection in a pediatric kidney transplant recipient. Pediatr. Nephrol. 11:355, 1997.

132. Mayo, R., and Lipschultz, D.: An interesting case of failed renal transplant complicated by a lymphocoele infected with *Pasteurella multocida* and a review of the literature. Am. J. Nephrol. 16:361, 1996.

133. McCormick, W., Schochet, S., Sailes, H., et al.: Progressive multifocal leukoencephalopathy in renal transplant recipients. Arch. Intern. Med. 136:829, 1976.

134. McDiarmid, S., Jordan, S., Geoffrey, S., et al.: Prevention and preemptive therapy of post-transplant lymphoproliferative disease following solid organ transplantation. Transplantation 68:1604-1611, 1998.

135. Melgosa-Hinojosa, M., Garcia-Mesegher, C., Pena-Garcia, F., et al.: Preemptive treatment with oral ganciclovir for pediatric renal transplantation. Clin. Nephrol. 61:246, 2004.

136. Mian, A., Farney, A., and Mendley, S.: *Mycoplasma hominis* septic arthritis in a pediatric renal transplant recipient: Case report and review of the literature. Am. J. Transplant. 5:103, 2005.

137. Michaels, M., Green, M., and Wald, E.: Adenovirus infection in pediatric orthotopic liver transplant recipients. J. Infect. Dis. 165:170, 1992.

138. Miemois-Foley, J., Paunio, M., and Lyytikainen, O.: Bacteremia among kidney transplant recipients: A case-control study of risk factors and short-term outcome. Scand. J. Infect. Dis. 32:69, 2000.

139. Mir, S., Erdogan, H., Serdaroglu, E., et al.: Pediatric renal transplantation: Single center experience. Pediatr. Transplant. 9:56, 2005.

140. Mocelin, A., Brandina, P., Gordan, J., et al.: Immunosuppression and circulating *Trypanosoma cruzi* in a kidney transplant recipient. Transplantation 23:163, 1977.

141. Molyneaux, P., Parker, S., Khan, I., et al.: Use of genomic analysis of varicella zoster virus to investigate suspected varicella-zoster transmission within a renal unit. J. Clin. Virol. 36:76, 2006.

142. Morris, P.: Transplantation—a medical miracle of the 20th century. N. Engl. J. Med. 23:2678, 2004.

143. Moudgil, A., and Puliyanda, D.: Induction therapy in pediatric renal transplant recipients: An overview. Paediatr. Drugs 9:323, 2007.

144. Moudgil, A., Snidban, H., Nast, C., et al.: Parvovirus B19 infection-related complications in renal transplant recipients: Treatment with intravenous immune globulin. Transplantation 64:1847, 1997.

145. Mourad, G., Soulillou, J., Chong, G., et al.: Transmission of *Mycobacterium tuberculosis* with renal allografts. Nephron 41:82, 1985.

146. Mrowka, C., Heintz, B., Reul, J., et al.: Cerebral tuberculoma 11 years after renal transplantation. Am. J. Nephrol. 18:557, 1998.

147. Muller, A., Beck, B., Theilemann, K., et al.: Detection of polyomaviruses BK and JC in children with kidney disease and renal transplant recipients. Pediatr. Infect. Dis. J. 24:778, 2005.

148. Munoz, P.: Management of urinary tract infections and lymphocele in renal transplant recipients. Clin. Infect. Dis. 33(Suppl. 1):53, 2001.

149. Murray, B., and Subramaniam, J.: Late cytomegalovirus infection after oral ganciclovir prophylaxis in renal transplant recipients. Transpl. Infect. Dis. 6:3, 2004.

150. Mylonakis, E., Hohmann, E., and Calderwood, S.: Central nervous system infection with *Listeria monocytogenes*: 33 years experience at a general hospital and review of 776 episodes from the literature. Medicine (Baltimore) 77:313, 1998.

151. Nahas, T., and Antonopoulos, I.: Comparison of renal transplant outcomes in children with or without bladder dysfunction: A customized approach equals the difference. J. Urol. 179:712, 2008.

152. Neuhaus, T., Schwobel, M., Schlumpf, R., et al.: Pyelonephritis and vesiculoureteral reflux after renal transplant in young children. J. Virol. 157:1400, 1997.

153. Nichols, J., Becker, G., and Walker, R.: Influence of anti-rejection therapy on the timing of cytomegalovirus disease and other infections in renal transplant recipients. Clin. Transplant. 14:14, 2000.

154. Nickeleit, V., Hirsch, H., Binet, I., et al.: Polyomavirus infection of renal allograft recipients from latent infection to manifestations of disease. J. Am. Soc. Nephrol. 10:1080, 1999.

155. Nickeleit, V., Hirsch, H., Zeiler, M., et al.: BK-virus nephropathy in renal transplant-tubular necrosis, MHC-class II expression, and rejection in a puzzling game. Nephrol. Dial. Transplant. 15:324, 2000.

156. Nickeleit, V., Klimkait, T., Binet, I., et al.: Testing for polyomavirus type BK DNA in plasma to identify renal-allograft recipients with viral nephropathy. N. Engl. J. Med. 342:1309, 2000.

157. Offermann, G., Keller, F., and Molzahn, M.: Low cyclosporin A blood levels and acute graft rejection in a renal transplant recipient during rifampin treatment. Am. J. Nephrol. 5:385, 1985.

158. Ogunbiyi, O., Scholefield, J., Raftery, A., et al.: Prevalence of anal human papillomavirus infection and intraepithelial neoplasia in renal allograft recipients. Br. J. Surg. 81:365, 1994.

159. Ohori, N., Michaels, M., Jaffe, R., et al.: Adenovirus pneumonia in lung transplant recipients. Hum. Pathol. 26:1073, 1995.

160. Olie, K., Goodshop, T., Verlaak, R., et al.: Posttransplantation CMV-induced recurrence of atypical hemolytiuc uremic syndrome associated with a factor H mutation: Successful treatment with intensive plasma exchanges and ganciclovir. Am. J. Kidney Dis. 45:e12, 2005.

161. Olson, A., Shope, T., and Flynn, J.: Pre-transplant varicella vaccination is cost-effective in pediatric renal transplantation. Pediatr. Transplant. 5:44, 2001.

162. Ortega-Sanchez, I. R.: Economics of an adolescent meningococcal conjugate vaccination catch-up campaign in the United States. Clin. Infect. Dis. 46:1-13, 2008.

163. Osman, H., Peiris, J., Taylor, C., et al.: Cytomegalovirus disease in renal allograft recipients: Is human herpesvirus 7 a co-factor for disease progression? J. Med. Virol. 48:295-301, 1996.

164. Pahari, A., and Rees, L.: BK virus-associated renal problems. Pediatr. Nephrol. 18:643, 2003.

165. Pamidi, S., Friedman, K., Kampalath, B., et al.: Human parvovirus B19 infection presenting as persistent anemia in renal transplant recipients. Transplantation 69:2666, 2000.

166. Pappo, O., Demetris, A., Raikow, R., et al.: Human polyoma virus infection of renal allografts: Histopathologic diagnosis, clinical significance, and literature review. Mod. Pathol. 9:105, 1996.

167. Patel, K., Heman, M., Williams, P., et al.: Long-term effectiveness of highly active antiretroviral therapy on the survival of children and adolescents with HIV infection: A 10-year perspective. Clin. Infect. Dis. 46:1751, 2008.

168. Patel, R.: Infections in recipients of kidney transplants. Infect. Dis. Clin. North Am. 15:1, 2001.

169. Patel, R., and Paya, C.: Infections in solid-organ transplant recipients. Clin. Microbiol. Rev. 10:86, 1997.

170. Patel, R., Roberts, G., Keating, M., et al.: Infections due to nontuberculous mycobacteria in kidney, heart and liver transplant recipients. Clin. Infect. Dis. 19:263, 1994.

171. Patel, R., Smith, T., Espy, M., et al.: Detection of cytomegalovirus DNA in sera of liver transplant recipients. J. Clin. Microbiol. 32:1431, 1994.

172. Pellegrin, I., Garrigue, I., and Ekouevi, E.: New molecular assays to predict occurrence of CMV disease in renal transplant recipients. J. Infect. Dis. 182:36, 2000.

173. Pereira, B., Natov, S., Bouthot, B., et al.: Effects of hepatitis C infection and renal transplantation on survival in end-stage renal disease. The New England Organ Bank Hepatitis C Study Group. Kidney Int. 53:1374, 1998.

174. Peterson, P., Balfour, H., Fryd, D., et al.: Fever in renal transplant recipients: Causes, prognostic significance and changing patterns at the University of Minnesota Hospital. Am. J. Med. 71:345, 1981.

175. Pirsch, J.: Cytomegalovirus infection and posttransplant lymphoproliferative disease in renal transplant recipients: Results of the U.S. multicenter FK506 Kidney Transplant Study Group. Transplantation 68:1203, 1999.

176. Priftakis, P., Bogdanovic, G., Tyden, G., et al.: Polyomaviruria in renal transplant patients is not correlated to the cold ischemia period or to rejection episodes. J. Clin. Microbiol. 38:406, 2000.

177. Puliyanda, D., Toyoda, M., Traum, A., et al.: Outcome of management strategies for BK virus replication in pediatric renal transplant recipients. Pediatr. Transplant. 12:180, 2008.

178. Quinibi, W., Al-Sibai, M., Taher, S., et al.: Mycobacterial infection after renal transplant: Report of 14 cases and review of the literature. Q. J. M. 77:1039, 1991.

179. Randhawa, P., Finkelstein, S., Scantlebury, V., et al.: Human polyomavirus-associated interstitial nephritis in the allograft kidney. Transplantation 67:103, 1999.

180. Ravindra, K., Freifeld, A., Kalil, A., et al.: West Nile-associated encephalitis in recipients of renal and pancreas transplants: Case series and literature review. Clin. Infect. Dis. 38:1257, 2004.

181. Regamey, N., Tamm, M., Wernli, M., et al.: Transmission of human herpesvirus 8 infection from renal-transplant donors to recipients. N. Engl. J. Med. 339:1358, 1998.

182. Reznik, M., Halleux, J., Urbain, E., et al.: Two cases of progressive multifocal leukoencephalopathy after renal transplantation. Acta Neuropathol. Suppl. 7:189, 1981.

183. Ribot, S., and Eslami, H.: HIV infection in kidney transplant recipients. N. Engl. J. Med. 39:597, 1992.

184. Riddler, S., Brenig, M., and McKnight, J.: Increased levels of circulating Epstein-Barr virus (EBV)-infected lymphocytes and decreased EBV nuclear antigen antibody responses are associated with the development of post transplant lymphoproliferative disease in solid-organ transplant recipients. Blood 3:972, 1994.

185. Rizvi, S., Naqvi, S., Hussain, Z., et al.: Living-related pediatric renal transplantation: A single-center experience from a developing country. Pediatr. Transplant. 6:101, 2002.

186. Robinson, L., Hilinski, J., Graham, F., et al.: Predictors of cytomegalovirus disease among pediatric transplant recipients within one year of renal transplantation. Pediatr. Transplant. 6:111, 2002.

187. Rubin, R.: Infectious disease complications of renal transplantation. Kidney Int. 44:221, 1993.

188. Rubin, R.: Infection in the organ transplant recipient. *In* Rubin, R. H., and Young, L. S. (eds.): Clinical Approach to Infection in the Compromised Host. 3rd ed. New York, Plenum Medical, 1994, pp. 629-705.

189. Rubin, R., Wolfson, J., Cosimi, A., and Tolkoff-Rubin, N.: Infection in the renal transplant recipient. Am. J. Med. 70:405, 1981.

190. Saitoh, K., Sugae, N., Koike, N., et al.: Diagnosis of childhood BK virus cystitis by electron microscopy and PCR. J. Clin. Pathol. 46:773, 1993.

191. Sakhuja, V., Jha, V., Varma, P., et al.: The high incidence of tuberculosis among renal transplant recipients in India. Transplantation 61:211, 1996.

192. Sayiner, A., Ece, T., Duman, S., et al.: Tuberculosis in renal transplant recipients. Transplantation 68:1268, 1999.

193. Schmaldienst, S., and Horl, W.: Bacterial infection after renal transplantation. Nephron 75:140, 1997.

194. Scroggs, M., Wolfe, J., Bollinger, R., et al.: Causes of death in renal transplant recipients. Arch. Pathol. Lab. Med. 111:983, 1987.

195. Sebire, N., Malone, M., Risdon, R., et al.: Epstein-Barr virus-associated lymphoproliferative disease presenting as gastrointestinal lesions in childhood. Pediatr. Dev. Pathol. 8:88, 2005.

196. Shaariah, W., Morad, Z., and Suleiman, A.: Cryptococcosis in renal transplant recipients. Transplant. Proc. 24:1898, 1992.

197. Sheldon, J., Henry, S., Mourad, M., et al.: Human herpes virus 8 infection in kidney transplant patients in Belgium. Nephrol. Dial. Transplant. 15:1443, 2000.

198. Shen, G., Alfrey, E., Knoppel, C., et al.: Eradication of cytomegalovirus reactivation disease using high-dose acyclovir and targeted intravenous ganciclovir in kidney and kidney/pancreas transplantation. Transplantation 64:931, 1997.

199. Shorter, G., and Weil, R.: *Listeria monocytogenes* infection after renal transplantation. Arch. Intern. Med. 137:1395, 1977.

200. Shroft, R., and Ross, L.: The post-transplantation lymphoproliferative disorders: A literature review. Pediatr. Nephrol. 19:369, 2004.

201. Singh, N.: Invasive mycoses in organ transplant recipients: Controversies in prophylaxis and management. J. Antimicrob. Agents Chemother. 45:749, 2000.

202. Singh, N., Gayowski, T., Singh, T., et al.: Invasive gastrointestinal zygomycosis in a liver transplant recipient: Case report and review of zygomycosis in solid-organ transplant recipients. Clin. Infect. Dis. 20:617, 1995.

203. Smith, S., Butterly, D., Alexander, B., et al.: Viral infections after renal transplantation. Am. J. Kidney Dis. 37:659, 2001.

204. Snydman, D. R.: Epidemiology of infections after solid-organ transplantation. Clin. Infect. Dis. 33(Suppl. 1):5, 2001.

205. Snydman, D., Werner, B., Heinze-Lacey, B., et al.: Use of cytomegalovirus immune globulin to prevent cytomegalovirus disease in renal-transplant recipients. N. Engl. J. Med. 317:1049, 1987.

206. Souweine, B., Mathevon, T., Bret, L., et al.: Successful treatment of infection due to *Mycoplasma hominis* with streptogramins in a renal transplant patient: Case report and review. Clin. Infect. Dis. 26:1233, 1998.

207. Speirs, G., Hakim, M., and Wreghitt, T.: Relative risk of donor-transmitted *Toxoplasma gondii* infection in heart, liver, and kidney transplant recipients. Clin. Transplant. 2:257, 1988.

208. Stovall, S., Ainley, K., Mason, E., et al.: Invasive pneumococcal infection in pediatric cardiology transplant patients. Pediatr. Infect. Dis. J. 20:946, 2001.

209. Sturm, I., Watschinger, B., Geissler, K., et al.: Chronic parvovirus B 19 infection-associated pure red cell anemia in a kidney transplant recipient. Nephrol. Dial. Transplant. 11:1367, 1996.

210. Sugar, A., Restrepo, A., and Stevens, D.: Paracoccidioidomycosis in the immune suppressed host: Report of a case and review of the literature. Am. Rev. Respir. Dis. 129:340, 1984.

211. Suzuki, T., Karzum, I., Okubo, Y., et al.: Epstein-Barr virus DNA load and seroconversion in pediatric renal transplantation with tacrolimus immunosuppression. Pediatr. Transplant. 11:749, 2002.

212. Szende, B., Toth, A., Perner, F., et al.: Clinicopathologic aspects of 8 Kaposi's sarcomas among 1009 renal transplant patients. Gen. Diagn. Pathol. 143:209, 1997.

213. Taghizadeh, A., Desai, D., Lederman, S., et al.: Renal transplantation or bladder augmentation first? A comparison of complications and outcomes in children. B. J. U. Int. 100:1365, 2007.

214. Their, M., Holmberg, C., Lautenschlager, I., et al.: Infections in pediatric kidney and liver patients after perioperative hospitalization. Transplantation 69:1617, 2000.

215. Tolkoff-Rubin, N., and Rubin, R.: Opportunistic fungal and bacterial infections in the renal transplant recipient. J. Am. Soc. Nephrol. 2(Suppl. 12):264, 1992.

216. Tong, C., Bakran, A., Williams, H., et al.: Association of human herpesvirus 7 with cytomegalovirus disease in renal transplant recipients. Transplantation 70:213, 2000.

217. Tong, C., Cuevas, L., Williams, H., et al.: Use of laboratory assays to predict cytomegalovirus disease in renal transplant recipients. J. Clin. Microbiol. 36:2681, 1998.

218. Toyoda, M., Moudgil, A., Warady, B., et al.: Clinical significance of peripheral blood Epstein-Barr viral load monitoring using PCR in renal transplant recipients. Pediatr. Transplant. 12:778, 2008.

219. Toyoda, M., Puliyanda, D., Amat, N., et al.: Co-infection of polyomavirus BK and cytomegalovirus (CMV) in renal transplant recipients. Transplantation 80:198, 2005.

220. Tran, L., Hebert, D., Dipchand, A., et al.: Invasive pneumococcal disease in pediatric solid organ transplant recipients: A high risk population. Pediatr. Transplant. 9:183, 2005.

221. Travis, L., and Kalia, A.: Renal transplantation in children: Experience of 23 years at the Children's Renal Center of the University of Texas Medical Branch at Galveston. J. Tex. Med. 87:50, 1991.

222. Tsanaclis, A., and deMorais, C.: Cerebral toxoplasmosis after renal transplantation: Case report. Pathol. Res. Proc. 181:339, 1986.

223. Umekawa, T., and Kurita, T.: Acute glomerulonephritis by adenovirus type 11 with and without type 37 after kidney transplantation. Urol. Int. 56:114, 1996.

224. Vanchiere, J., Nicome, R., Greer, J., et al.: Frequent detection of polyomaviruses in stool samples from hospitalized children. J. Infect. Dis. 192:658, 2005.

225. Vanchiere, J., White, Z., and Butel, J.: Detection of BK virus and Simian virus 40 in the urine of healthy children. J. Med. Virol. 75:447, 2005.

226. Varga, M., Remport, A., Hidvegi, M., et al.: Comparing CMV prophylaxis in renal transplantation: Single center experience. Transpl. Infect. Dis. 7:63, 2005.

227. Wadie, H., Alangaden, G., Sillix, D., et al.: West Nile virus encephalitis: An emerging disease in renal transplant recipients. Clin. Transplant. 18:753, 2004.

228. Waldman, M., and Kopp, J.: Parvovirus B-19-associated complications in renal transplant recipients. Nat. Clin. Pract. Nephrol. 3:540, 2007.

229. Watkins, S., Alexander, S., Brewer, E., et al.: Response to recombinant hepatitis B vaccine in children and adolescents with chronic renal failure. Am. J. Kidney Dis. 40:365, 2002.

230. Waugh, S., Pillay, D., Carrington, D., et al.: Antiviral prophylaxis and treatment (excluding HIV therapy). J. Clin. Microbiol. 25:241, 2002.

231. Weiland, D., Ferguson, R., Peterson, P., et al.: Aspergillosis in 25 renal transplant patients. Ann. Surg. 198:622, 1983.

232. West, M., Pirenne, J., Chavers, B., et al.: *Clostridium difficile* colitis after kidney and kidney-pancreas transplantation. Clin. Transplant. 13:318, 1999.

233. Wilson, J., Turner, H., Kirchner, K., et al.: Nocardial infections in renal transplant recipients. Medicine (Baltimore) 68:38, 1989.

234. Wong, T., Chan, P., Leung, C., et al.: Parvovirus B19 infection causing red cell aplasia in renal transplantation on tacrolimus. Am. J. Kidney Dis. 34:1132, 1999.

235. Yagisawa, T., Takahashi, K., Yamaguchi, Y., et al.: Adenovirus induced nephropathy in kidney transplant recipients. Transplant. Proc. 21:2097, 1989.

236. Yagisawa, T., Toma, H., Tanabe, K., et al.: Long-term outcome of renal transplantation in hepatitis B surface antigen-positive patients in cyclosporine era. Am. J. Nephrol. 17:440, 1997.

237. Yildiz, A., Sever, M., Turkman, A., et al.: Tuberculosis after renal transplant: Experience of one Turkish center. Nephrol. Dial. Transplant. 13:1872, 1998.

238. Zamora, I., Simon, J., DaSilva, M., et al.: Attenuated varicella vaccine in children with renal transplants. Pediatr. Nephrol. 8:190, 1994.

239. Zaontz, M., Hatch, D., and Firlit, C.: Urological complications in pediatric renal transplantation: Management and prevention. J. Urol. 140:1123, 1988.

CHAPTER 85

INFECTIONS RELATED TO PROSTHETIC OR ARTIFICIAL DEVICES

Ram Yogev ✪ Tina Q. Tan

The development of biomaterials used in the manufacturing of temporary or permanent implantable prosthetic devices has been one of the greatest advances in modern medicine.[64,85,86] These devices have become an integral and important part of the current practice of medicine and have improved considerably the lives

and health of countless patients. In the United States, the number and types of permanent prosthetic devices implanted to replace diseased or damaged body parts has increased substantially during the last several decades. An estimated 3 million or more people in the United States currently have some type of long-term bio-

TABLE 85–1   Temporary or Permanent Implantable Devices Currently in Use

Temporary Devices
Intravascular catheters
Urinary catheters
Endotracheal and tracheostomy tubes

Permanent Devices
Central nervous system shunts
Deep-brain stimulators
Peritoneal dialysis catheters
Orthopedic prostheses (artificial hip, knee, and other joints; screws, pins, plates, and rods)
Intracardiac and intravascular prostheses (heart valves, vascular grafts)
Ventricular assist devices
Pacemakers and defibrillators
Ocular prostheses (artificial globes, intraocular lenses, ocular explants)
Implantable pump devices (baclofen, insulin)
Cochlear implant devices
Tissue expander devices

medical implant.[80,322,377] Table 85–1 is a listing of the implantable prosthetic devices in use today.

One of the major medical complications associated with the use of implantable prosthetic devices is infection, which may result in serious tissue destruction and dysfunction of the prosthetic device or in local and systemic consequences that may be life-threatening. In most cases, these infections are very difficult to cure with antimicrobial agents alone, and removal of the device usually is required for resolution of the infection.

INTERACTION OF THE HOST WITH A PROSTHETIC DEVICE

The prosthetic devices currently in use are composed of a variety of biomaterials, including cobalt-chromium-molybdenum alloy, titanium alloy, and complex polymers such as polytetrafluoroethylene, silicone, and polyethylene, which in general are chosen for their inert, nonreactive, and nontoxic qualities. The interplay of both implant and host factors determines the risk of acquiring and the severity of infection. The human body has numerous well-developed defense mechanisms to protect it against possible invasion by various microorganisms. Such mechanisms include cellular and humoral immune systems, anatomic barriers, and an elaborate network of cells that phagocytize and destroy invading organisms. The presence of a foreign body may compromise one or more of these defenses and elicit a complex acute or chronic inflammatory response (or both) from the host. Many of these devices breach cutaneous and mucosal barriers, thereby creating a direct route by which bacteria and fungi may invade. In addition, implanted devices may alter the local immunity of the host directly or indirectly.[18,85,322,377,389]

Shortly after being implanted, hydrophobic polymeric materials such as polyethylene, Dacron, polydimethylsiloxane, and polyether urethanes become coated with a layer of host proteins such as plasma and interstitial fluid proteins (fibronectin, albumin, laminin, collagen, immunoglobulin G, fibrinogen) that bind to and are absorbed readily into the surface of the implant.[21,291,377] This protein layer (especially fibrinogen) has a major influence on the body's response to and the biocompatibility of the implant. The presence of fibrinogen attracts a large number of phagocytic cells (neutrophils, monocytes/macrophages) to the implant; these cells interact with the implant surface and initiate an acute inflammatory response.[85,377] Some of these host proteins also serve as

a receptor for various colonizing microorganisms. Collagen, laminin, and fibrinogen have been reported to play a role in adherence of bacteria,[393] whereas fibronectin has been found to be the major receptor for gram-positive cocci, especially *Staphylococcus aureus*.[314,382]

Chronic inflammatory responses, also known as *foreign body reactions*, are seen around many types of biomaterial implants and arise from interactions among the protein-coated surfaces of the implant and host tissues and adhering phagocytic cells such as macrophages and foreign body giant cells. These interactions may result in degradation and damage to the implant from the continuous generation of toxic catabolites and release of inflammatory mediators such as hydrolases, activated complement components, tumor necrosis factor (TNF), interleukins, prostaglandins, coagulation factors, and plasminogen activator by the phagocytic cells.[375,377,389]

INTERACTION OF MICROORGANISMS WITH A PROSTHETIC DEVICE

Once a prosthetic device is implanted, the surface of the device provides a potential area for adherence and multiplication of bacteria. Adherence is a complex process that involves electrostatic attachment of the bacteria to the surface of the implant, bacterial mechanisms that function specifically in attachment, and host-derived substances that coat the prosthetic device and serve as receptors for various bacteria. Bacteria arrive at the surface of the implant by many different routes: they may be inoculated at the time of implantation, the patient may have episodes of transient bacteremia, the device may be exposed by local trauma or infection, or the device may be implanted within an area in which the organism is part of the normal flora.[80,85]

Adherence of bacteria to the surface of an implant is influenced by numerous different factors, including the material used to make the device, the source of the device material (adherence is greater with synthetic material than with biomaterial), the surface of the device (irregular more than regular, textured more than smooth, hydrophobic more than hydrophilic), and the shape of the device.[80] Cell surface molecules or structures known as adhesins also play a role in adherence by attaching or binding an organism to specific receptors on implant surfaces; different bacteria use different adhesins to attach to and colonize medical implants. For example, *Staphylococcus epidermidis* uses proteinaceous autolysin and capsular polysaccharide intercellular adhesin for initial adherence to the implant surface and for adherence of bacteria to each other. These bacteria also produce a biofilm that increases cell-to-cell association and allows accumulation of bacteria.[330] *Streptococcus pyogenes* uses lipoteichoic acid as its adhesin, whereas *S. aureus* uses both lipoteichoic acid and host-tissue ligands (e.g., fibronectin, fibrinogen, collagen) for adherence. Binding of *S. aureus* to host-tissue ligands is mediated by genetically defined microbial surface proteins known as *microbial surface components recognizing adhesive matrix molecules* (MSCRAMM).[81] *Escherichia coli* and other bacteria use fimbriae as an adhesin to mediate binding to receptors on the surfaces of target cells.

Bacteria also can protect themselves from host defenses by synthesizing and excreting numerous complex polysaccharides, known as glycocalyces, that function either as part of the bacterial capsule or as the slime layer. This slime layer is known to play a major role in keeping an organism attached to an implant surface by coalescing with the polysaccharides of other bacteria and with host products to produce a thick, adherent, and somewhat impenetrable biofilm.[390] The biofilm functions by trapping nutrients and protecting the organism from phagocytosis, antimicrobial agents, and competing microflora. It also plays a role in inhibiting the response to chemotactic stimuli, increases both *N*-formyl-methionyl-leucyl-phenylalanine (FMLP)-induced superoxide generation and release of specific granules, and impairs natural killer cell function while also altering the composition of T-lymphocyte cell subpopulations.[136,184,390] Therefore, the biofilm aids bacteria in evading host cellular and humoral defense mechanisms and thereby allows the organism to colonize and infect an implanted device effectively.

Substantial progress has been made in our understanding of the pathogenesis, prevention, and treatment of foreign body infections; this increased knowledge has resulted in a dramatic decrease in the morbidity associated with these infections, as well as subsequent improvement in the patient's quality of life. In the following sections we discuss specific device-related infections and the suggested treatment and management of these infections.

TISSUE EXPANDERS

The use of soft tissue expansion in reconstructive surgery was reported in the literature first in 1957, and since that time it has been used widely for the correction of multiple problems in plastic and reconstructive surgery in the adult and pediatric populations.[12,19] These expanders consist of an alloplastic prosthesis with a filling port that is implanted into a subcutaneous pocket. The expander is filled with saline through the filling port at various intervals to create adequate expansion of the skin. In children, tissue expansion is used most commonly to provide coverage for skin defects caused by burns, trauma, hemangiomas, and other congenital deformities.[237]

The most common complication of tissue expansion is infection of the subcutaneous expander pocket, usually with skin organisms introduced during insertion of the expander. Cellulitis of the overlying skin and hematogenous or lymphatic seeding of the expander pocket are seen as well but occur much less frequently.[12,123,171,235,237,272] In several pediatric case series, the infection rate ranged from 3.4 to 11 percent.[123,237] *S. aureus*, *S. epidermidis*, and group A streptococci are the microorganisms recovered most commonly from these infections.[123,171,236,237] Less commonly, nontypable *Haemophilus influenzae*,[237] *Pseudomonas aeruginosa*, *E. coli*, and *Actinomyces* spp.[252] have been isolated from infections of expander pockets.[236]

In cases of infection of subcutaneous pockets, treatment consists of removal of the tissue expander, débridement and drainage of the subcutaneous pocket, and administration of intravenous antibiotic therapy tailored to the organism isolated. For cellulitis of the overlying skin of an expander pocket, treatment with intravenous antibiotics but without removal of the tissue expander has been shown to be successful.[12]

The most common empiric antimicrobial therapeutic regimen consists of a first-generation cephalosporin or an extended-spectrum, penicillinase-resistant penicillin. For all of the infections of prosthetic devices discussed in the chapter, empiric antistaphylococcal coverage should include agents effective against community strains of methicillin-resistant *S. aureus* (MRSA) if warranted by their frequency in the area.

Therapy is tailored once the organism has been identified and its antibiotic susceptibility has been determined.

COCHLEAR IMPLANTS

During the last several decades, cochlear implantation has emerged as one of the best methods of providing auditory rehabilitation for the profoundly deaf (congenital or acquired). The goal of this surgery in young children is to provide hearing that is adequate to facilitate the development of receptive and expressive language. The surgical technique involves the creation of a C-shaped flap in the postauricular and parietal-occipital scalp skin areas, elevation of the flap, implantation of a multichannel

prosthesis, and insertion of an electrode array into the cochlea through openings drilled into the temporal bone.[68,71,230]

The most common infectious complications associated with these implants are cellulitis of the overlying skin flap, meningitis, otitis media, and delayed cochlear implant infections leading to extrusion of the implant.* Rates of infection range from 0.3 to 0.5 percent for meningitis, 2 to 3 percent for cellulitis of the skin flap and delayed cochlear implant infections, to 36 percent for otitis media. The reported cases of meningitis have occurred either in association with leakage of cerebrospinal fluid (CSF) in persons with a malformed cochlea who undergo cochlear implantation or as a consequence of intracranial spread of a developing middle ear infection along the electrode pathway. In June 2002, the U.S. Food and Drug Administration received numerous reports of bacterial meningitis in children with cochlear implants who were younger than 6 years old when they received the implants. The most common causative organism identified was *Streptococcus pneumoniae*, followed by nontypable and type b *H. influenzae*. The incidence of pneumococcal meningitis in this group of patients was calculated to be 138.2 cases per 100,000 person-years—more than 30 times the incidence in the same-aged cohort in the general population. This increased incidence of meningitis was found to be associated strongly with the use of a cochlear implant with a positioner (a wedge-shaped insert that facilitates transmission of the electrical signal by pushing the electrode against the medial wall of the cochlea) in conjunction with the presence of radiographic evidence of a malformation of the inner ear and leakage of CSF. Cochlear implants with a positioner were voluntarily recalled in the United States in July 2002, although removal of existing implants containing a positioner was not recommended; use of appropriate vaccination against *S. pneumoniae* and type b *H. influenzae* was strongly recommended.[17,131,321] Children with cochlear implants may have a higher risk for the development of middle ear infections because of several factors, including the naturally high incidence of acute otitis media (AOM) in this population, the presence of a foreign body in the area of the infection, and the potential for spread of the infection into the cochlea along the electrode pathway. In a study of 50 children who received cochlear implants between 1991 and 1995, researchers found that children prone to the development of otitis media before undergoing implantation were at higher risk for developing postimplantation AOM but responded well to routine oral antimicrobial therapy. The overall prevalence and the severity of AOM were not found to be increased in children with cochlear implants.[227]

In cases of cellulitis of the skin flap, intravenous antimicrobial therapy commonly consists of a first-generation cephalosporin or an extended-spectrum, penicillinase-resistant penicillin to provide coverage for *S. aureus* and group A streptococci. Empiric antimicrobial therapy for meningitis usually consists of vancomycin and a third-generation cephalosporin that is tailored to the organism isolated. For delayed development of cochlear implant infections, therapy consists of removal of the implant and administration of intravenous antibiotics.

OCULAR PROSTHESES

This group of prosthetic devices includes artificial globes used primarily for cosmetic purposes, orbital implants, ocular explants, intraocular lenses (IOLs), and contact lenses.

ORBITAL IMPLANTS

Orbital implants are made of hydroxyapatite or porous polyethylene and frequently are used in orbital reconstruction after

---

*See references 32, 69-71, 82, 158, 159, 168, 175, 176, 227, 277, 289.

enucleation or evisceration surgery. Infection of these implants is a rare event, with only a handful of cases reported in the literature.* Patients most commonly complain of anophthalmic socket pain, discomfort, and irritation while wearing an artificial globe. Papillary conjunctivitis of the socket with exudate and sometimes dehiscence of the overlying conjunctiva also may be seen.[125,261] Infection may develop months to years after placement of the implant, and severity ranges from cellulitis to the development of an abscess around the implant itself.

Radiographic studies that can aid in the detection of these types of infection include technetium 99m–labeled leukocyte scintigraphy, which is most useful in detecting early low-grade graft infection,[186] and computed tomography (CT) and magnetic resonance imaging (MRI), which are useful later in the course of the infection to detect the presence of abscesses and structural tissue changes. Gram-positive cocci, primarily *S. aureus* and coagulase-negative staphylococci (CoNS), are the organisms associated most commonly with these infections; however, *H. influenzae, S. pneumoniae,* alpha-hemolytic streptococci, *Capnocytophaga, Pseudomonas,* and *Aspergillus fumigatus* have been cultured as well.[321,365,419,427] To cure the infection effectively, treatment involves both removal of the implant and institution of topical and parenteral antibiotic therapy directed against the organism isolated. Empiric therapy directed against gram-positive organisms may be started initially until the results of culture and sensitivity testing are available. The most common empiric regimens include a first-generation cephalosporin, a second-generation cephalosporin, or an extended-spectrum, penicillinase-resistant penicillin.

INTRAOCULAR LENSES

Insertion of polymethyl methacrylate (PMMA) IOLs at the time of removal of a cataract is the standard surgical therapy for this disorder. Even though the rate of postoperative infection of IOLs is low (ranging from 0.10% to 0.30%), the infection usually is serious and results in endophthalmitis and permanent loss of vision.[187,206] The predisposing factor for infection is bacterial adhesion to IOLs during their insertion. After adhesion is accomplished, the bacteria replicate, congregate, and form multiple layers of microcolonies that represent a biofilm in which the bacteria are embedded in a layer of slime. The major pathogens associated with this infection are *S. aureus* and *S. epidermidis,* which account for 90 percent of all isolates, although gram-negative bacilli, fungi, *Chlamydia trachomatis,* and rapidly growing mycobacteria are isolated on occasion.[6,93,206,239,348,428] IOL-associated endophthalmitis is a serious infection that is difficult to diagnose and treat.[412] In a few cases, use of topical and systemic antibiotics alone has been successful in eradicating the infection, but in most cases surgical débridement and systemic antibiotics are required for cure. Empiric therapy for these infections consists of an extended-spectrum, penicillinase-resistant penicillin, a second-generation cephalosporin, or, in some instances, clindamycin or vancomycin. In cases of fungal endophthalmitis, treatment with the later-generation azoles alone and in combination with an echinocandin has been shown to have clinical success[93]; in rapidly growing mycobacterial endophthalmitis combinations of topical and intravenous antibiotics to which the organism is susceptible have been used for treatment.[239]

CONTACT LENSES

Primarily three different types of contact lenses are available. Hard lenses are made of PMMA, a substance that is impermeable

*See references 3, 67, 126, 158, 165, 186, 187, 192, 206, 261, 426.

to water and gas. This type of lens is designed to be worn only during waking hours because it limits oxygen flow to the cornea to that present in tears. Gas-permeable hard lenses are composed of silicone, cellulose acetate butyrate, or PMMA-silicone co-polymers; they allow gas but not fluid to pass through the lens. Hydrophilic or soft lenses are made of a cross-linked hydrogel polymer or copolymer and consist of between 38 and 85 percent water by weight; these lenses are permeable to both gas and water and allow the user to wear them continuously. However, for all these types of lenses, infection may result in damage to the corneal epithelium.

The two main infections that occur in association with contact lenses are conjunctivitis and keratitis.[55] The causative bacteria seen most commonly with these infections are *S. aureus,* streptococci, *Pseudomonas* spp. (found in improperly stored cleansing solutions), and fungi. Improper cleaning of soft or hydrophilic lenses may cause them to become a source of infection when bacteria penetrate the lens matrix. Treatment usually consists of removal of the lens and application of topical antibiotics. To prevent the development of infections associated with contact lenses, users should adhere strictly to the manufacturer's suggested guidelines for wearing and cleaning the lenses.

A rare and often devastating infection associated with the use of contact lenses is infection with the fresh-water protozoan *Acanthamoeba.*[67,157,261,367] This organism contaminates the lens when sterility of the cleansing solutions is not maintained; it usually is associated with users who prepare their own solutions. *Acanthamoeba* is very difficult to eradicate because it is not susceptible to standard antiparasitic agents, and it produces a chronic keratitis that can be complicated by corneal perforation and loss of the eye. Corneal transplantation may be necessary in many cases to restore vision.[157,367]

LEFT VENTRICULAR ASSIST DEVICES

The development plus use of mechanical circulatory assist devices has grown very rapidly in the last decade, especially with the shortage of available donor hearts. Such devices have improved considerably the hemodynamic status and quality of life of patients with heart failure who are awaiting cardiac transplantation. Figure 85–1 shows a left ventricular assist device (LVAD), a pneumatically driven pump located outside the heart that draws blood from an inflow cannula in the left ventricular apex and ejects the blood through an outlet into the ascending aorta. Within the pump are several sections of Dacron graft material and two trileaflet porcine valves in the inflow and outflow positions to ensure that blood flow is unidirectional. The pump is encased in titanium and implanted via an extended median sternotomy into the left rectus sheath. A percutaneous driveline connects to an exterior power pack for venting or for pneumatic actuation and exits the body, after passing through a subcutaneous tunnel, in the left lower quadrant. The interior surface of the pump is textured to prevent the formation of thrombi and encourage the deposition of a biologic pseudo-intimal lining. Once the device is implanted, in most cases it cannot be removed without performing concurrent cardiac transplantation.[154,193,243,245,288]

The approach taken by many centers for infection of an LVAD includes both preventive and interventional steps that are instituted before, during, and after implantation. Preventive strategies are focused on prevention of infections related primarily to the driveline and device pocket through the use of clean implantation techniques and limited traffic in the operating room in which the procedure is being performed. Antibiotic prophylaxis usually is given for 48 hours near the time of implantation of the LVAD and may include intravenous trimethoprim-sulfamethoxazole, rifampin, and fluconazole, along with the application of mupirocin ointment to the nares. Additional

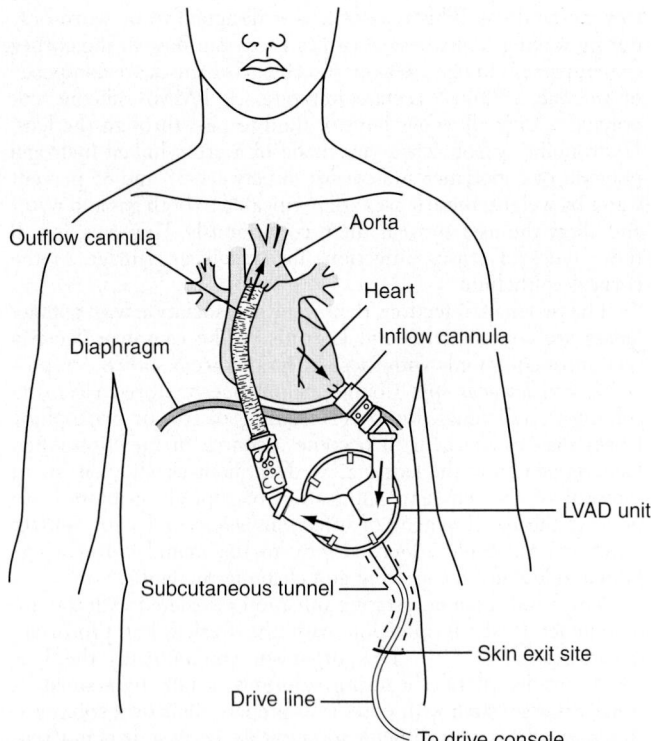

Figure 85–1 Left ventricular assist device (LVAD). *(Adapted from Fisher, S. A., Trenholme, G. M., Costanzo, M. R., and Piccione, W.: Infectious complications in left ventricular assist device recipients. Clin. Infect. Dis. 24:18-23, 1997.)*

preventive measures include soaking the surfaces of the LVAD in vancomycin and gentamicin for 30 minutes before placing it, irrigating the device pocket with povidone-iodine (Betadine), and meticulously placing the subcutaneous tunnel in the appropriate position. Postoperative care with sterile and semi-sterile dressing changes around the driveline is emphasized.[105,163,355]

Despite the preventive measures taken, infection, thromboembolism, and hemorrhage at the time of implantation remain the most common complications associated with the use of mechanical circulatory support devices. Of these complications, infection has the most significant impact on morbidity and mortality.[116] Predisposing factors for development of device-related infections in these patients include contact of blood with the prosthetic surfaces, device-related pockets and cavities, transcutaneous drivelines, and power cables; extent of surgery necessary for implantation; hemorrhage; reoperation; frequent occurrence of multiple organ dysfunction or failure; duration of mechanical circulatory support; poor health; and comorbid conditions. The incidence of infection in patients on LVAD support for longer than 60 days is reported to be two times higher than that in patients with an LVAD in place for less than 30 days; initial episodes of infection after 90 days are rare.[271,306,354] In addition, some evidence indicates that implantation of an LVAD itself may lead to defects in cellular immunity secondary to an aberrant state of T-cell activation that predisposes LVAD recipients to the development of candidal and other systemic infections.[11,128,174,306] The incidence of infection after implantation of an LVAD is reported to range between 13 and 80 percent, with most studies documenting an infection rate of 30 to 50 percent.* Most series report that the device pocket and drivelines are the device-related sites that account for most of the infections. Placement of the LVAD

*See references 14, 105, 114, 163, 244, 246, 298, 346, 373, 414.

in the abdominal cavity instead of the preperitoneal area has been shown to decrease the chance for development of infection.[271]

Driveline infections are thought to result from a lack of integration of tissue around the driveline that allows the driveline to move and irritate surrounding tissues, which can result in an infection in the exit site and, in some cases, bacteremia. Such infections generally are defined by pain, erythema, warmth, drainage, or purulent discharge at the driveline exit site in the presence of a positive culture. Bacteremia developing after implantation of a pump and infections of the pump itself are additional reported complications.[14,244] In a study of 205 patients who underwent placement of LVADs at the Cleveland Clinic, positive blood cultures were noted in 52 percent, infections of the driveline site occurred in 22 percent, and infections of the pump pocket developed in 9.2 percent.[193] Sun and colleagues[373] reported their experience with 95 patients who underwent insertion of an LVAD. Twenty-six (27%) of these patients experienced device-related infections involving the driveline, device pocket, or blood-contacting surfaces; 15 of the 26 (57.7%) had infections of the driveline site. Persistent bacteremia and progression of infection of the device pocket and driveline site can lead to the serious infection of LVAD endocarditis, which mimics prosthetic valve endocarditis, is very difficult to treat, and is associated with a high mortality rate. LVAD endocarditis is defined as positive cultures of the LVAD surface in conjunction with clinical signs and symptoms of infection during LVAD support. Manifestations of this condition are varied and range from persistent fever and bacteremia or fungemia to cerebral thromboembolism, LVAD inlet obstruction with hemorrhage, or LVAD outflow graft rupture.[14] In a report by Weyland and associates[414] of 27 patients who underwent insertion of LVADs, infections of the driveline developed in 8 (30%) of the 27 recipients, and LVAD endocarditis, defined as positive cultures from the pump chamber, was found in 12 (44%) of the patients; 8 of the 12 (67%) died of endocarditis.

Despite a high potential for the development of serious morbidity after placement of an LVAD, studies have shown that the presence of an infection after insertion of an LVAD does not seem to have very much influence on eventual cardiac transplantation and post-transplant outcome. During a 5-year period, Argenziano and coworkers[14] compared the effect that infection after insertion of an LVAD had on mortality, the development of LVAD endocarditis, and eventual heart transplantation. The study found that infection subsequently developed in 29 of 60 (48%) patients who underwent insertion of an LVAD. The most frequent sites of infection were the blood (27%), LVAD driveline (13%), LVAD surface (13%), and central venous catheter (10%); these sites thus represented 63 percent of all infections.[11,14] The overall mortality rate, the rate of successful cardiac transplantation, and the rate of infection after transplantation were not influenced by the presence of infection during LVAD support.[14] In another study, Sinha and colleagues[355] reviewed their experience with 86 patients who received LVADs; device-related infections developed in 6 patients, 5 (83%) of whom had infections of the pocket. This study also found that that the presence of infection during LVAD support did not influence successful cardiac transplantation or patient survival after transplantation.

MICROBIOLOGY OF LEFT VENTRICULAR ASSIST DEVICE INFECTIONS

Numerous organisms have been isolated from LVAD infections. In most series, *S. aureus*, *S. epidermidis*, and *Enterococcus* spp. are the organisms most commonly isolated from these infections, usually within the first 4 weeks after implantation. Other organisms such as *Enterobacter*, *P. aeruginosa*, *Serratia marcescens*, other gram-negative organisms, and polymicrobial organisms were seen more commonly later in the clinical course.[14,87,105,130,163,242,244,355,414] Fungal infections (e.g., *Candida albicans*) were reported as well and were responsible for only approximately 16 percent of the infections.[87,163,242] However, colonization with fungi occurs in 35 to 39 percent of patients with LVADs.[128] Investigators suggested that treatment with broad-spectrum antibiotics (common in these patients) rendered them more susceptible to the development of fungal infection. When a fungal LVAD infection is suspected, signs of thrush, esophagitis, retinal changes, peripheral embolization, and unexplained decrease in LVAD output should be investigated. The presence of yeast on Gram stain of the fluid surrounding the device and ultrasound showing increasing amounts of fluid around the device can be used to help in confirming the diagnosis.[128] Management of these infections, especially LVAD endocarditis, presents a major challenge, given that the device usually cannot be removed unless simultaneous heart transplantation is performed; moreover, if transplantation is accomplished, multiple issues regarding the immunosuppressed condition of the patient are raised. In most cases, management involves a prolonged course (usually 4 to 6 weeks) of aggressive antimicrobial or antifungal therapy (or both) appropriate for the organism or organisms isolated, with meticulous attention given to skin care around the driveline exit site; débridement, drainage, surgical revision, and irrigation with povidone-iodine of infected wound sites; or in certain instances, replacement of the LVAD unit or cardiac transplantation before completing antibiotic therapy if a donor heart becomes available and all blood cultures are negative.[105,163,244]

EXTRACORPOREAL MEMBRANE OXYGENATION CIRCUITS

Extracorporeal membrane oxygenation (ECMO) is the method used most commonly for treating severe cardiac and pulmonary failure in neonates and children. Almost 1 percent of all children treated by open heart surgery will undergo ECMO. In addition to these postcardiotomy patients, a growing number of children receive ECMO for acute decompensation of myocarditis or cardiomyopathy. ECMO also is used to support children after sudden cardiac arrest when conventional closed or open heart massage is unsuccessful. In children, perfusion through the neck venoarterial vessels is the preferred method, but the trans-sternal approach is used when direct decompression of the distended left ventricle is required. Although the overall survival rate of children managed by ECMO has improved in recent years, it still is only 50 to 70 percent,[23,408] in contrast to 88 percent in neonates treated for respiratory failure.[9,313] Multiple cardiac and noncardiac factors are associated with increased morbidity and mortality rates. Patients with a single ventricle or residual cardiac defect after surgery have a less favorable ECMO outcome.[34,79,202] Renal dysfunction, multiple organ system failure, initiation of ECMO in the operating room, blood product transfusion, mediastinal bleeding, ECMO circuit problems, and duration of ECMO for longer than 10 days also were predictors of increased risk of mortality.[202,260] The presence of infection (mostly nosocomial) while being supported by ECMO was associated with increased mortality rates.[207,260,315,431] Of interest, none of the patients who had a positive blood culture in the first 24 hours of ECMO survived.[262]

The same organisms that cause LVAD-associated infections also are associated with ECMO infections.[47,260] The distribution of these pathogens is similar to their distribution in other patients with infections treated in the intensive care unit, except for an increase in the incidence of *Enterobacter* and *Acinetobacter* infections.[47]

The signs and symptoms of infection often are subtle and nonspecific. Fever develops in only half of these patients. The value of tachycardia and elevated cardiac output also is limited because these patients frequently are tachycardic with increased cardiac output caused by a systemic inflammatory response (e.g., complement; cytokines such as TNF, interleukin-1 [IL-1], and IL-6), which is characteristic of cardiopulmonary bypass procedures.[257] For the same reason, leukocytosis (unless developing acutely) and an elevated erythrocyte sedimentation rate (ESR) should be interpreted with caution. Consequently, a high index of suspicion with random surveillance of blood and urine cultures and chest radiographs (to rule out pneumonia) is needed to identify these infections.

Most patients undergoing ECMO are treated with multiple broad-spectrum antibiotics. This practice probably is one of the reasons for the increased incidence of multidrug-resistant, gram-positive (e.g., *Enterococcus*) and gram-negative bacteria, as well as fungal (e.g., *Candida*), infections. In addition, many of these patients will be colonized with these same bacteria. Therefore, if a deep bronchial suction or urine culture (performed routinely) becomes positive but without supporting evidence of infection (e.g., increased white blood cell [WBC] count, fever), serious effort to distinguish between colonization and infection should be made before initiating an unnecessary change in antimicrobial therapy. If a decision to treat is made, appropriate coverage for both gram-positive and gram-negative organisms should be chosen. If blood, urine, and bronchial cultures remain negative and the patient's condition is not improving or the culture becomes positive for a fungus, antifungal therapy should be added.

PERMANENT CARDIAC PACEMAKER AND IMPLANTABLE CARDIOVERTER-DEFIBRILLATOR INFECTIONS

PERMANENT CARDIAC PACEMAKER INFECTIONS

Cardiac pacemakers were developed in the late 1950s, and since that time the field of cardiac pacing has made great strides with regard to the development and design of multiple types of pacemakers and the implantation of millions of devices into both adults and children worldwide. In the United States alone, the number of patients who have permanent pacemakers is estimated to be greater than 1 million.[95,403] The two types of permanent pacemaker generators in use include those with transvenous electrodes and those with epicardial electrodes. Both types are implanted in either the chest or the abdominal wall; pacemakers with epicardial electrodes are the ones used most commonly in the pediatric population.[403]

Infection is the most common medical complication of implantation of permanent pacemakers, with reported rates ranging from 0.13 percent to as high as 20 percent and a mortality rate of 27 to 66 percent.[36,49,62,95,113] An estimated 25 percent of cardiac pacemaker–associated infections develop within 1 to 2 months of placement of the device, but delays of up to 12 months may occur before diagnosis is established. However, since the 1980s, the incidence of infection associated with permanent pacemakers has decreased significantly because of improved surgical techniques and better design of the devices themselves; most series since that time report infection rates no higher than 5.7 percent.[13,36,95,156]

Studies have shown that infections of permanent cardiac pacemakers seem to occur more commonly in patients with both local and systemic underlying medical problems, especially diabetes mellitus or an underlying malignancy, or in those who are undergoing treatment with corticosteroids, anticoagulants, or other types of immunosuppressive therapy.[60,313] Other well-characterized independent risk factors include surgery related to any part of the pacemaker (especially replacement of a battery or upgrade of the pacemaker),[60,149,150,156,210] the presence of a hematoma after implantation,[50,60,153,201] temporary transvenous pacing,[156,268] and operative time.[268] Multiple (two or more) pacemaker insertions and physician inexperience with insertion also represent significant risks for development of infection.[149]

Infections of permanent cardiac pacemakers are subdivided into different groups depending on the specific site of involvement and whether they are early infections (<1 to 2 months after implantation) or late infections (>2 months after implantation). The different groups include (1) local inflammation, infection, and the formation of an abscess in the generator pocket or subcutaneous portion of the lead, or in both sites; (2) secondary infection involving either the generator or the electrodes (including pacemaker endocarditis)[13,50,95,201]; (3) fever plus associated bacteremia, with or without concomitant infective endocarditis, in a patient without any apparent focus of infection[13,95]; and (4) mediastinitis, pericarditis, bronchopleural cutaneous fistulas, and mixed infections.[95]

The generator pocket and the subcutaneous portions of the leads (transvenous and epicardial) are the most common sites of infection. In a case series of permanent pacemaker–associated infections, Choo and associates[60] reported that abscesses in the generator pocket were present in 72 percent of the patients and were the only manifestation of infection in almost 40 percent. Infections of the pocket often are difficult to diagnose and may develop at any time after implantation; however, most tend to develop early and frequently are the result of contamination by skin flora at the time of the procedure.[258] Late infection usually occurs as a consequence of erosion of the device through the subcutaneous tissue and skin. The infection may remain localized to the pocket or may spread to the adjacent electrodes and lead to the development of bacteremia.[26,36] Infection of transvenous pacemaker leads may occur in as many as 17 percent of patients who receive permanent pacemakers. These infections often are not apparent initially but have been associated with significant morbidity and mortality. Bluhm[36] and others[140] reported a 25.3 percent mortality rate in 1734 patients with permanent pacemakers who had retained infected transvenous leads. Infection generally develops along the subcutaneous portion of the leads and, if unrecognized, may progress centrally and result in sustained bacteremia, endocarditis, or both.[36,140] Infections of the leads tend to occur later than infections of the pocket, with the median time of occurrence being 7 to 8 months after implantation of the pacemaker.[36,37] Endocarditis as a complication of unrecognized infected transvenous leads usually develops an average of 37 months after placement of the pacemaker.[263] Infections of permanent epicardial leads generally occur as a complication of infections of the generator pocket, skin erosion, or direct contamination at the time of placement. However, in contrast to infections of the transvenous leads, infections of the epicardial leads usually result in only local symptoms; rarely, they may lead to more severe disseminated disease such as pericarditis, mediastinitis, bronchopleural cutaneous fistulas, bacteremia, or sepsis.[26]

Clinical Findings

Diagnosing a pacemaker-associated infection can be difficult because of its nonspecific symptomatology, and months may elapse after the onset of symptoms before the diagnosis is established. Symptoms may be confined to a local area or may be more widespread with the development of bacteremia or other systemic effects. Fever (84-100%) and chills (75-84%) are considered the most common systemic symptoms and are indicators of local infection, especially if they occur after the second postoperative day in association with other signs; however, they may be the only clinical manifestation in more than a third of

patients.[50,201,259,263,269,416] Early infections are more likely to be accompanied by both local and systemic clinical findings and are manifested more commonly as infections of the generator pocket, bacteremia, or septicemia[50,217,229,432]; late infections, on the other hand, typically cause vague symptoms that evolve over the course of time and usually are lead-related infections and endocarditis.[60,194,210,397]

Infections of the generator pocket typically cause local swelling (21%), erythema (34%), pain (32%), drainage (through an incompletely healed incision or fistulous tract) over or adjacent to the generator pocket (25%), and warmth (11.5%).[62] Sterile breakdown of the pacemaker pocket develops in an estimated 5 percent of patients with permanent pacemakers, and skin or soft tissue erosion over the electrodes occurs in an additional 2 to 4 percent. Because these complications are associated with a high risk for the subsequent development of infections, the presence of any erosion is considered a potential indicator of device-related infection, especially if the erosion occurs more than 24 months after placement of the pacemaker, at which time the infection rate may be as high as 80 percent.[33,138,143] Pacemaker-related endocarditis is a relatively rare complication that occurs in 0.05 to 0.5 percent of cases after implantation of a pacemaker. Such endocarditis is associated with a mortality rate as high as 34 percent in some series.[50,115,170,201] It tends to be a late complication; only 27 to 36 percent of patients are seen within 6 to 12 weeks after the last procedure at the pacemaker implant site, with symptoms developing in most patients a mean of 25 months after the last procedure at the implant site. The diagnosis of pacemaker-related endocarditis is difficult to establish, and usually a delay in making the diagnosis, with a mean interval of 5 to 8 months after the onset of symptoms, occurs.[50,201] Pulmonary symptoms are found in 20 to 45 percent of patients with pacemaker-related infections and may consist of bronchitis, lung abscess, pneumonia, or pulmonary embolism; these symptoms are seen more commonly in late-onset infection and in patients with intravenous lead–related infection.[50,201]

A variety of laboratory and imaging studies may be performed to aid in establishing the diagnosis of a pacemaker-related infection. An elevated ESR is found in 82 to 97 percent of patients, and peripheral leukocytosis is seen in 50 to 66 percent. The presence of a collection of fluid around the device as seen on ultrasound is suggestive of device-related infection. Gallium scanning may be performed in an attempt to determine the nature of the fluid (inflammatory versus infectious). Transthoracic echocardiography has emerged as a major tool in diagnosis; studies have shown that this test was able to demonstrate vegetations and other lesions on the electrodes, ventricular endocardium, and tricuspid valve in 90 to 96 percent of patients with pacemaker-related infections.[50,201,397]

Microbiology

Staphylococci (S. aureus and CoNS) are the most common causes of pacemaker-related infections, and they account for more than 85 percent of such infections; however, a wide variety of organisms have been isolated.[13,36,50,51,60,201,217,397] A higher proportion of S. aureus is isolated from early infections, whereas CoNS are isolated more commonly from late infections.[36,78,217] An increasing number of these organisms are methicillin-resistant. Other gram-positive organisms such as viridans streptococci, other streptococci, enterococci, Listeria, and Corynebacteria have been isolated as well, but each causes less than 1 percent of cases. Gram-negative organisms such as E. coli, Proteus, Enterobacter cloacae, P. aeruginosa, Klebsiella, and S. marcescens are isolated from 5 to 20 percent of device-related infections. In addition, Candida, Aspergillus, and other fungi have been isolated rarely; however, infections with these organisms generally are associated with poor clinical outcomes.[13,50,69,72,201,205,262,397,416,417]

Management and Treatment of Infection

Appropriate therapy for pacemaker-related infections is tailored to the specific clinical situation and depends on several different factors: (1) whether the infection is limited to the generator pocket or subcutaneous electrodes without bacteremia, (2) whether bacteremic pacemaker-related endocarditis is present with or without involvement of the subcutaneous electrodes, and (3) what organism is involved.

If the infection is limited to the generator pocket or subcutaneous electrodes, optimal treatment consists of both medical and surgical intervention in which all the parts of the infected device are removed. Studies have shown that failure to remove completely all portions of the infected device results not only in failure to cure the infection but also in higher mortality rates.[51,60,324,400] The patient is given parenteral antimicrobial therapy, and an exchange of the pacing system with total removal of the infected device and simultaneous insertion of a new pacemaker at a different site is performed surgically. The infected subcutaneous pocket is drained, débrided, and packed open, and local wound care is instituted. Initial antibiotic therapy should provide coverage for both staphylococci and gram-negative bacteria; therapy is tailored once the organism is identified and its antibiotic susceptibility is known. Typical regimens include vancomycin plus an aminoglycoside for a duration of 2 to 4 weeks, or oxacillin or nafcillin plus an aminoglycoside may be used. In certain instances, a new pacemaker cannot be placed at the time of removal of the infected device; in such situations, a period of temporary transvenous pacing is instituted until a new pacemaker can be implanted.[217]

The consensus approach to the management of pacemaker-related endocarditis and bacteremia involves removal of both the generator unit and the electrodes in conjunction with prolonged administration of parenteral antibiotic therapy designed to treat endocarditis (usual duration, 4-6 weeks). Mortality rates may be as high as 50 percent for patients in whom total removal of the pacemaker unit is not performed.[13,50,51,201] If the electrodes have been in place for longer than 18 months or large vegetations (>10 mm) are associated with them, extraction of the electrodes by traction may be difficult and risky to perform, so surgical extraction by cardiotomy may be necessary. In patients who require a pacemaker, temporary transvenous pacing may be implemented until a new permanent pacemaker can be placed. Antimicrobial therapy targeted at the causative organism should be administered for a minimum of 2 weeks, and sterility of blood cultures should be ensured before a new pacemaker generator and electrode are placed. Typical empiric therapy consists of vancomycin plus gentamicin and rifampin; therapy may be tailored once the organism has been identified and its antibiotic susceptibility is known.

INFECTION OF IMPLANTABLE CARDIOVERTER-DEFIBRILLATORS

The first implantable cardioverter-defibrillator (ICD) was placed in 1980, and during the last several decades it has become a successful therapeutic modality for the treatment of patients (both adults and children) with life-threatening ventricular arrhythmias. Older devices required surgical placement of a pulse generator, extrapericardial or epicardial defibrillation patches, and a transvenous rate-sensing electrode. The systems placed today use a rate-sensing lead that is implanted transvenously, a superior vena cava coil electrode, and additional subcutaneous or epicardial electrodes all connected to a pulse generator that is placed subcutaneously or submuscularly and usually is located in a pocket created in the abdominal region.[195,362,420]

Infection is the most serious complication of placement of an ICD.[50,211] Infection rates associated with placement of ICDs

ranged from 1 to 7 percent.[13,363,383] However, infection rates have decreased substantially with the advent of transvenous non–thoracotomy-placed systems, with rates ranging from 0.8 to 1.5 percent.[127,286,357] Several risk factors that have been identified as increasing the likelihood for development of infection include steroid use, diabetes, malignancy, and renal failure.[35] Most ICD-related infections are clinically apparent within 3 to 6 months after placement, with infections of the generator pocket, subcutaneous patch wound site, or epicardial patches or bacteremia and endocarditis being the most common manifestations. An increased WBC count and ESR, anemia, and microscopic hematuria are the most common laboratory findings. Echocardiography may be helpful in half of the cases. Infection of the generator pocket or subcutaneous patch wound site usually causes local findings of pain, erythema, and collection and drainage of fluid from the site. Occasionally, these patients also may be bacteremic or hypotensive. In contrast, infection of the epicardial patches generally results in more systemic symptoms, bacteremia, or pericarditis.[286] The diagnosis of ICD-related infection typically is made on clinical grounds and confirmed by culture of the fluid or drainage around the device.

Microbiology

S. aureus and CoNS are the major pathogens seen with ICD-related infections, and they account for 60 to 80 percent of cases.[211,286,336,363] However, a broad spectrum of other gram-positive, gram-negative, and fungal organisms, including *P. aeruginosa*, corynebacteria, streptococci, *E. coli*, *Klebsiella*, *Bacteroides fragilis*, *Propionibacterium acnes*, atypical mycobacteria, and *Candida* spp., have been isolated from ICD-related infections. Polymicrobial infections may occur in the generator pocket.[211,336,357]

Management

To eliminate ICD-related infections effectively, optimal management involves a combination of medical and surgical interventions, especially if the patient is bacteremic or has systemic findings or if the causative organism is *S. aureus*. Several studies have suggested that conservative management (i.e., antibiotic therapy without removal of the hardware) may be sufficient. However, such an approach should be tried in cases in which only the generator pocket is infected (management may consist of the administration of parenteral antibiotics, wound care, and removal of only the generator portion of the device, with implantation of another generator at a different site) or in patients whose condition prevents removal of the entire device. In these situations, treatment of the ICD-related infection should include a prolonged course of parenteral antibiotics, followed by continuous suppressive oral antibiotic therapy.[286,386] The optimal management of ICD-related infections is parenteral antibiotics and removal of the entire ICD system.[13,62,211,336] The duration of antibiotic therapy varies from 2 to several weeks.

PROSTHETIC JOINT AND ORTHOPEDIC IMPLANT INFECTIONS

The implantation of prosthetic joints along with the use of other implantable orthopedic devices (e.g., pins, screws, plates, rods, external fixators, Ilizarov apparatus) has improved the quality of life greatly and restored function to patients suffering from debilitating bone and joint disease, tumor, or injury. Based on conservative estimates, millions of people worldwide have some form of prosthetic joint or other implantable orthopedic device. Of the possible complications associated with implantation, infection is the second most common cause of prosthetic joint failure.[10] It occurs in 1 to 13 percent of cases[213] and results in postoperative prosthesis failure, chronic pain, immobility, and, in some cases, loss of the affected limb or, in the worst-case scenario, loss of life.[2,31,90,119,366] The health care cost in the United States for treating a single infection of a prosthetic joint is estimated to be more than $50,000, with an extrapolated expenditure of greater than $100 million per year nationwide.[28,152,344,366]

Prosthetic joints and implantable orthopedic devices may become infected by two major mechanisms: (1) the prosthetic device may be contaminated by microorganisms at the time of implantation, either as a result of airborne contamination in the operating room or by direct inoculation at the time of surgery, or (2) the prosthetic device may become infected as a result of hematogenous seeding from bacteremia or by direct contiguous spread from an infection adjacent to the prosthesis. Twenty to 40 percent of infections of prosthetic joints arise by hematogenous seeding, with the remainder occurring as a result of airborne or direct inoculation.[1,41,220,221,233] Infections may remain asymptomatic for years before symptoms become apparent, and usually a long delay occurs between onset of the infection and the appearance of symptoms and confirmation of the diagnosis. The overall rate of infection of prosthetic joints has been shown to be highest in the first 6 months postoperatively, with a steady decline occuring after this time. The incidence rate for infection of total-hip and total-knee arthroplasties during the first 2 years postoperatively is reported to be 5.9 infections per 1000 joint-years; in contrast, during postoperative years 2 to 10, it is 2.3 infections per 1000 joint-years.[366] The risk of acquiring infection and the incidence of infection depend on the anatomic location of the implanted orthopedic device or prosthetic joint, with the hips having the highest risk followed in descending order by the knees, elbows, shoulders, wrists, and ankles.[65,143,317,371] For implantable orthopedic devices, rates of infection range from 2 to 30 percent.[234,396,422]

RISK FACTORS

Numerous factors have been identified as increasing a patient's risk for developing infection of a prosthetic joint or orthopedic implant. These factors include rheumatoid arthritis, diabetes mellitus, obesity, poor nutritional status, the use of steroids, immunocompromised status, psoriasis, hemophilia, sickle-cell hemoglobinopathy, solid-organ transplant, dialysis-dependent renal failure, joint dislocation, and extremes of age.* In addition, previous surgery at the site of the prosthesis or implant also increases the risk of acquiring an infection. For example, several studies showed that the risk of deep infection developing in patients undergoing revision of a hip or knee arthroplasty was twofold to eightfold higher than that in patients with primary arthroplasty.[312,316,425] The relative risk for the development of prosthesis-related infections in patients with poor healing and wound complications increases from 13- to 20-fold after total-knee replacement and from 22- to 52-fold after total-hip replacement.[425]

The implanted metal prosthetic device and the PMMA cement that binds the prosthetic device to adjacent bone also predispose the joint space and bone to infectious processes, given that both are foreign bodies. In vitro studies have shown that the unpolymerized form of PMMA cement predisposes to infection by inhibiting phagocytic, lymphocytic, and complement function; the risk of acquiring infection seems to be enhanced further once the cement has polymerized in the body.[300,301] Cementless prostheses have been designed in an attempt to overcome the problem of infection associated with the PMMA cement. For certain orthopedic implants, the integrity of the skin is compromised chronically, thus providing ready access to organisms from the external environment.

*See references 31, 41, 109, 124, 139, 148, 182, 226, 292, 312, 370.

MICROBIOLOGY

More than 65 percent of infections associated with prosthetic joints and implanted orthopedic devices are caused by *S. aureus*, CoNS, beta-hemolytic streptococci, viridans streptococci, and enterococci. Antibiotic resistance in these organisms is increasing, and multiple different strains of staphylococci may be present in a single prosthetic joint infection.[173,180,234,337,396,421] Less commonly, aerobic gram-negative bacilli, including *E. coli*, *Proteus mirabilis*, *Klebsiella* spp., *Salmonella* spp., *S. marcescens*, other Enterobacteriaceae, and *P. aeruginosa*, may cause infection. In addition, 4 to 10 percent of infections are caused by anaerobic organisms such as peptostreptococci and *Bacteroides* spp.; polymicrobial infections occur in approximately 12 percent of cases.[173] Infections with fungi, particularly *Candida*, *Aspergillus*, and *Penicillium* spp., or with mycobacteria (i.e., *Mycobacterium tuberculosis*, *Mycobacterium avium* complex [MAC], and other rapidly growing mycobacteria) also have been described.[20,30,41,236,385] Rarely, a wide spectrum of other organisms, including *Corynebacterium*, *Propionibacterium*, *Bacillus* spp., and *Mycoplasma hominis*, have been reported to cause infection.[41] Zoonotic bacteria such as *Brucella* spp., *Yersinia* spp., and *Pasteurella* spp. rarely can cause infection and should be considered in the correct epidemiologic setting.[236]

Certain clinic situations may predispose a patient to particular organisms as the cause of infection. Pyogenic skin infections commonly result in staphylococcal and streptococcal infections of prosthetic joints, whereas infections of the teeth and gums are frequent causes of viridans streptococcal and anaerobic infections in prostheses. Genitourinary and gastrointestinal tract procedures or infections frequently are associated with enterococcal and gram-negative bacillary infections of prostheses.[41]

CLINICAL MANIFESTATIONS

The clinical findings and the severity of symptoms seen with infections of prosthetic joints are highly variable and determined primarily by three factors: (1) the route of infection—the hematogenous route versus direct inoculation; (2) the virulence of the infecting pathogen—*S. aureus* and, to a lesser extent, beta-hemolytic streptococci and gram-negative bacilli seem to be particularly virulent pathogens capable of producing a fulminant clinical picture, whereas infection with organisms such as CoNS is associated with a more chronic, indolent course; and (3) the nature of the tissue in which the microorganism proliferates—hematomas, seromas, ischemic wounds, and the tissues of diabetic patients and those receiving steroids all enhance the ability of the bacteria to proliferate and spread, thereby promoting the development of a more deep-seated fulminant infection.

The most common initial symptom is joint pain, which occurs in 95 percent of cases. Such pain can range from an acute fulminant illness with erythema, severe joint pain, swelling (38%), high fever (43%), and systemic symptoms to, more frequently, a chronic, slowly increasing pain in the joint that may be associated with the formation of a cutaneous draining sinus (32%) but no systemic symptoms.[173] The presence of constant joint pain is more indicative of infection than is the presence of pain occurring only with movement or weight bearing, which is indicative of mechanical loosening and inflammation.[139]

For implantable orthopedic devices, the most common initial symptom of infection is erythema, swelling, pain, or drainage from the area around and adjacent to the implant. Local symptoms also may be associated with fever, especially if the device is extensive or deep-seated.

DIAGNOSTIC STUDIES

Laboratory screening tests commonly used to diagnose infection of a prosthetic joint or implanted orthopedic device are the peripheral WBC count, C-reactive protein (CRP), and the ESR. Elevation of one or more of these factors may help support the diagnosis of an infection.[22,360]

The principal radiologic studies used for detection of an infected prosthetic joint include plain radiographs, arthrograms or sinograms, and radioisotope scans (indium and technetium diphosphate). Abnormalities that may be suggestive of infection and can be seen on plain radiographs include radiolucency at the bone-cement interface, motion and changes in position of the prosthetic components, evidence of osteomyelitis, cement fractures, and periosteal reaction. Intra-articular injection of dye (arthrogram or sinogram—in the presence of a sinus tract) may demonstrate abnormal communication between the joint space and the bone-cement interface. These radiographic abnormalities are present in approximately 50 percent of infected prostheses.[77,139,231] Nuclear scans with indium or technetium diphosphate may be used to detect periprosthetic inflammation. Both these scanning techniques are very sensitive but lack specificity. Technetium diphosphate (^{99m}Tc) shows increased uptake in areas of bone with an enhanced blood supply or increased metabolic activity. Increased uptake normally is seen around uninfected prostheses within the first 6 months after implantation; positive findings after this time are abnormal and reflect inflammation (which could be due to a variety of causes) but not specifically infection.[94,160,191,287] Indium 111–labeled leukocyte scanning has been shown to have a specificity of only 50 to 80 percent for knee and hip prosthetic infections.[278] In contrast, ^{99m}Tc-labled ciprofloxacin (which probably binds to live bacteria at the infection site) was shown to be 94 percent sensitive and 83 percent specific for the diagnosis of chronic infection.[359] Use of this technique allowed 11 of 12 infections of prosthetic joints to be identified, whereas ^{99m}Tc-WBC scintigraphy was positive in only seven patients.[359] CT and MRI are not used routinely in the evaluation of a patient with a suspected infection of a prosthetic implant because of the large amount of imaging artifact created by prosthetic devices.[40,256]

Aspiration of joint fluid for culture and culture of tissue obtained intraoperatively are the optimal ways of establishing a specific diagnosis of infection of a prosthetic joint. Although joint fluid findings indicative of an infectious process are a high leukocyte count (consisting mainly of polymorphonuclear leukocytes [PMNs]), a high protein content, and a low glucose concentration, these changes are not specific for bacterial infection and are present in only some patients. Nonetheless, infection should be suspected if there are five or more neutrophils per high-power field in a periprosthetic specimen.[360] The fluid obtained should be cultured for a variety of organisms; Gram stain is positive in a third of the cases, and a causative pathogen can be identified in only two thirds of patients.[297,361] Intraoperative cultures should include, if possible, any purulent discharge, devitalized bone, and tissue from the bone-cement interface. Vortexing or bath sonication (or both) of the explanted prosthesis may increase the yield.[294] Histopathologic examination of this tissue usually reveals an infiltration of PMNs consistent with an acute inflammatory reaction but not specific for infection.[141] More rapid, specific, and sensitive tests (e.g., in situ hybridization, immunofluorescence, polymerase chain reaction) are needed to differentiate between noninfectious inflammation and bacterial infection.

TREATMENT

Successful treatment of an infected prosthetic joint involves extensive surgical débridement of all devitalized bone and tissue, removal of the prosthesis and all associated cement, and prolonged parenteral antibiotic therapy.[22] For optimal results, the débridement should be performed within 1 to 2 weeks.[213] Microbiologic cure has been found to correlate well with the extent of débridement and the completeness of removal of all residual methylmethacrylate cement.[52] Historically, attempts at simple surgical débridement without removal of the prosthetic device in conjunction with parenteral antibiotic therapy have been successful in only 20 percent of cases, with relapse rates being as high as 88 percent by 2 to 4 years after therapy.[107,338,418] However, recent studies have shown that in patients with a short duration of prosthetic joint infection caused by penicillin-susceptible streptococci, débridement and antibiotic therapy alone appear to be sufficient, with a low risk of relapse.[251]

Two protocols have been used for the treatment of these infections. A two-stage surgical procedure with prolonged parenteral antibiotic therapy has been shown to be one of the most successful treatment regimens with the best functional results. The first stage involves complete removal of the prosthesis and cement followed by a 6-week regimen of antibiotic therapy empirically chosen to cover the most likely organism and then tailored once the organism has been identified and its antibiotic susceptibility known. The second stage involves reimplantation of a new prosthetic device at the end of the antibiotic course. Success rates with this procedure range from 53 to 100 percent.[104,119,124,222,270] An alternative method of therapy involves a one-stage exchange operation in which the infected prosthetic device and cement are removed, all devitalized tissue and bone are débrided, and a new prosthesis is reimplanted immediately, followed by 6 weeks of parenteral antibiotic therapy. Antibiotic-impregnated (either tobramycin or gentamicin) methylmethacrylate cement is used in these situations, and success rates range from 33 to 80 percent.[46,53,97,148,253,319,388] This procedure is appropriate only for patients with infections caused by less virulent microorganisms because of the high failure rates seen when a more virulent organism such as S. aureus or a gram-negative bacillus is the cause of the infection.[106]

The Ilizarov method allows simultaneous treatment of infection, bone and joint deformities, bone loss, and shortening of the limb. This device includes proximal and distal circular external rings with wires passing through the bone and soft tissue from one side of the limb to the other. The wires are placed in several planes and orientations to stabilize the bone. The rings are connected with threaded rods and nuts to allow for lengthening or shortening of the limb. Although this method is used more often for the treatment of bone nonunion or bone loss with or without infection,[265,290,296,350] David and colleagues[83] used this technique successfully to treat 12 patients who failed total-knee arthroplasty because of infection. Wound infection and chronic osteomyelitis caused by infection of the wire tract occur infrequently and should be treated by débridement of the infected soft tissue and curettage of the infected bone.

Currently, a two-stage prosthetic removal-reimplantation procedure coupled with the incorporation of antibiotic-impregnated cement during reinsertion of the implant, in combination with a 6-week antibiotic regimen, is the mainstay of therapy for infections of prosthetic joints.[120,270] Selection of antibiotics should take into account the recent increase in methicillin resistance among staphylococci for the following reasons: MRSA infections of the prosthetic joint result in a higher incidence of treatment failure than do infections with methicillin-susceptible S. aureus, and the former result in longer durations of hospitalization and a low survival rate free of treatment failure.[332] Thus, vancomycin (with and without rifampin) should be the initial drug of choice for gram-positive bacteria until the susceptibility of the infecting organism is known. Recent reports of treatment failures (even with vancomycin susceptibility within the treatment range [i.e., 2 to 4 µg/mL])[169,379] suggest that other antibiotics (e.g., trimethoprim-sulfamethoxazole, linezolid) should be considered. Several reports have shown that linezolid is a reasonable alternative that results in control of the infection.[394]

For infected implanted orthopedic devices, the success of therapy is based on total removal of the device together with parenteral antibiotic therapy. In cases in which the foreign body cannot be removed, extended parenteral antibiotic therapy should be instituted and continued until the device can be removed. The duration of therapy varies with the severity of the infection and ranges from several weeks to several years.

CENTRAL NERVOUS SYSTEM SHUNTS

Infection is a major cause of morbidity in children who undergo CSF shunting procedures. Such procedures are performed to divert CSF in symptomatic hydrocephalic patients and are used commonly in patients with anatomic abnormalities (e.g., meningomyelocele and Chiari malformations), in premature newborns with intraventricular hemorrhage or intracranial infections (e.g., congenital cytomegalovirus, congenital toxoplasmosis, bacterial meningitis), and in patients with central nervous system (CNS) tumors or head trauma. Usually, the proximal end of the shunt is placed in the frontal or fourth ventricle and the distal end is inserted into the peritoneal cavity (i.e., ventriculoperitoneal [VP] shunt). Other compartments such as the right atrium (i.e., ventriculoatrial [VA] shunt), the pleural cavity, or the gallbladder can be used to place the distal end. CSF shunts are prone to complications, with a 10-year failure rate greater than 50 percent.[88,305] The most common complication is mechanical (such as obstruction or overdrainage from siphoning), followed by shunt-related infection. The incidence of shunt-related infection varies considerably, from 0.3 to 12 percent.[45,61,74,99,147,197,208,395] These infections increase morbidity rates and, in some cases, significantly affect patients' outcomes.[25] Recent understanding of some of the factors that contribute to the development of these infections has helped reduce their incidence.[61,102,198,409]

EPIDEMIOLOGY

Almost two thirds of shunt-related infections occur within 1 month after placement of the shunt, and 90 percent of infections are manifested within 6 months.[146,204,248] The incidence of shunt-related infections is significantly higher in infants in the first 6 months of life than in older children.[98,310,398] The infection rate is even higher in newborns with intraventricular hemorrhage who undergo shunting in the first week of life[7] and in premature infants.[208,249] Reasons for the increased incidence of shunt-related infection in very young patients are multifactorial. Several mechanisms that have been suggested include delayed wound healing, higher skin density of bacteria that are more resistant to antibiotics and more adherent to the shunt than in older children, longer duration of hospitalization, surgical technique, and increased exposure to antibiotics just before the shunt is placed.

No significant difference in infection rate is seen in patients with VP or VA shunts,[284,352] but a lower infection rate was noted in those with lumboperitoneal or cholecystic shunts. An increased risk of development of infection was reported for shunts placed immediately after removal of a previously infected shunt, probably because of incomplete eradication of bacteria.[99,199,346] Several other factors, including the underlying cause of the hydrocephalus,[98] the surgeon's experience,[66,196] previous shunt infection,[249] the duration of surgery, the number of people in the operating room, operative technique (e.g., prophylactic antibiotics, skin preparation, shaveless operation),[166] operative time, open surgery to insert the abdominal catheter versus direct puncture of the

abdominal wall with a trocar, and postoperative CSF leakage,[208] have been reported to be associated with an increased incidence of shunt-related infection. Although a trend toward more shunt-related infections has been reported with these factors, it has not been demonstrated consistently. A few studies suggest that tapping the shunt may result in an infection, with an incidence ranging from negligible to greater than 30 percent in premature infants with shunts tapped multiple times.[45]

ETIOLOGY

Staphylococcal species are the most common cause of shunt-related infection, with CoNS (e.g., *S. epidermidis*, *Staphylococcus capitis*, *Staphylococcus hominis*, *Staphylococcus lugdunensis*)[96] being isolated in 25 to 70 percent of cases (Table 85–2).[96,204,264,352] *S. aureus*, the second most common gram-positive bacterium, is responsible for 10 to 40 percent of cases. Streptococci (e.g., viridans, group B or C, *S. pyogenes*, *S. pneumoniae*, enterococci) are identified less commonly (3% to 7%). Other gram-positive bacteria such as *Propionibacterium*[381] and *Corynebacterium* (diphtheroids)[15,137] are isolated as well. The seemingly increased incidence of shunt-related infections caused by these two groups of bacteria probably is the result of poor culture technique (e.g., failure to use anaerobic culture media, less than 5 to 7 days' incubation period) or misinterpretation of culture results (e.g., culture contamination) leading to under-reporting (or both).

Gram-negative bacteria (e.g., *E. coli*, *Klebsiella* spp., *Proteus* spp.) together are the cause of 5 to 25 percent of shunt-related infections.[364] *Pseudomonas* spp. and *Acinetobacter* spp. are reported as well, but less frequently. Shunt-related infections caused by gram-negative bacteria occur more commonly in patients with myelomeningocele and those in whom the distal part of the VP shunt is inserted into the peritoneal cavity via a percutaneous trocar (i.e., with an inadvertently perforated intestinal tract). Many other etiologic agents, including fungi (e.g., *Candida*,[76,122,133] *Histoplasma*,[342] *Cryptococcus*,[172] *Torulopsis*[405]), *Pasteurella multocida*,[214] *Neisseria* spp.,[167,372] *S. marcescens*,[44] nontuberculous myco-

TABLE 85–2 Pathogens Causing Cerebrospinal Fluid Shunt Infection

Pathogens	Incidence (%)
Gram-Positive Bacteria	
Staphylococcus, coagulase-negative (e.g., *Staphylococcus epidermidis*, *Staphylococcus capitis*, *Staphylococcus hominis*, *Staphylococcus warneri*, *Staphylococcus lugdunensis*, *Staphylococcus haemolyticus*)	25-70
Staphylococcus aureus	10-40
Streptococci (e.g., *Streptococcus pyogenes*, group B or C streptococci, Enterococcus, *Streptococcus pneumoniae*)	3-7
Propionibacterium species	Rare
Corynebacterium species	1-2
Gram-Negative Bacteria	
Escherichia coli	5-25
Klebsiella species	5-10
Proteus species	2-6
Pseudomonas species	2-4
Acinetobacter species	1-3
Other gram-negative bacteria (e.g., *Neisseria* species, *Haemophilus influenzae*, *Pasteurella*)	<1
Fungi	<1
Candida species	
Histoplasma	
Cryptococcus	
Torulopsis	

bacteria,[56] and others, have been reported less commonly as causing shunt-related infections. With the increase in the number of patients who are immunocompromised for various reasons (e.g., neutropenia, chronic intravenous catheters, prolonged administration of broad-spectrum antibiotics, hyperalimentation), the incidence of these rare infections will increase. Bacteria that traditionally cause meningitis, such as *H. influenzae*,[323,369] *S. pneumoniae*,[283] and *Neisseria meningitidis*,[215] were reported as causing shunt-related infections. Whether these cases were isolated shunt-related infections or extension of meningitis into the ventricular system (i.e., ventriculitis) is not clear. Therefore, if such bacteria are isolated from a suspected shunt and the patient has a communicating hydrocephalus, lumbar puncture should be performed to rule out meningitis.

PATHOGENESIS

Several observations suggest that most CNS shunt–related infections are caused by inoculation of the organism during surgery or contamination of the device by ward personnel during manipulation.[91,310,406] These observations include the facts that common skin flora (e.g., CoNS, *S. aureus*) are the pathogens most frequently encountered, most of the infections occur within the first few weeks after surgery, and irrigation of the system is a risk factor for the development of infection. Another common mechanism (occurring with gram-negative bacterial infections) is retrograde progression of bacteria from the gastrointestinal tract (i.e., bowel perforation)[164,328] or from the urinary tract (in the case of a ventriculo-ureteral shunt).[118] Other mechanisms by which shunts become infected include (1) hematogenous infection in which a distant site of infection produces bacteremia leading to a shunt infection (this type of infection occurs quite rarely and in most cases represents meningitis with secondary infection of the shunt, such as *S. pneumoniae* or *N. meningitidis* CNS infection in patients with a shunt) and (2) wound or skin infection (e.g., cellulitis, decubitus ulcer), with direct extension from the infection site to the shunt.

The predominant role of CoNS and *S. aureus* in CNS shunt–related infection is the result of their being the major constituents of normal cutaneous flora, especially in young children,[218,347] and their having the ability to adhere directly to the shunt (e.g., *S. epidermidis*) or to host proteins covering the shunt (e.g., *S. aureus*). In addition, CoNS (and some *S. aureus* strains) produce large amounts of extracellular slime (i.e., biofilm) that completely covers the organism.[42] More than 60 percent of staphylococci isolated from infected shunts produce biofilm.[84,101,142] The biofilm of *S. epidermidis* is a mixture of teichoic acid and protein.[170] Production of biofilm also was reported in corynebacterial infection, which may explain the increasing importance of this bacterium in CNS shunt–related infections.[74] The biofilm facilitates attachment of these organisms to the surface of the shunt and protects the bacteria from the host's immune defenses (i.e., reduces phagocytosis). Once the organisms are attached to the shunt material, they are extremely difficult to remove except by completely replacing the shunt. In addition, penetration of antibiotic into the biofilm is variable, and the biofilm antagonizes the antimicrobial activity of some antibiotics (e.g., vancomycin).[89,103] The importance of production of biofilm for the establishment of shunt-related infection caused by CoNS was shown by Younger and colleagues,[429] who found that 88 percent of the CoNS strains isolated from true shunt-related infections produced slime. Moreover, infections caused by nonadherent organisms were significantly more likely to be cured by antibiotics alone (without removal of the colonized shunt) than were infections caused by adherent organisms. Similarly, Diaz-Mitoma[84] and coworkers found that both obstruction of VP shunts and failure to cure the infection with antibiotics alone occurred more frequently when

infectious episodes were caused by biofilm-producing CoNS. Therefore, complete removal of the shunt should be considered in patients with CoNS or *S. aureus* infection because biofilm-producing organisms may not be treated effectively when the shunt is in situ.

S. aureus infection is established primarily by the production of adhesin proteins. The most important proteins are fibronectin-binding (finb A and finb B) and fibrinogen-binding (Clf A and Clf B) proteins.[110] The ability to bind to fibronectin is very common in isolated strains of *S. aureus*, and its efficiency depends on the amount of finb A and finb B expressed on the cell surface of the individual isolate. The two fibrinogen-binding proteins attach to different parts of the host ligand, which suggests that they are acting synergistically or allow the bacteria to adhere to the ligand even during unfavorable conditions (e.g., antibodies against one of them).

The immature humoral immune system of young infants is not likely to explain the increased incidence of shunt-related infections in patients younger than 6 months old because these infants mount antistaphylococcal antibody responses that are comparable to those of older children.[310] Although levels of immunoglobulins and complement proteins are lower in this young group, levels of these proteins normally are very low in the CSF of older individuals (CSF levels of IgG and IgA are between 0.25% and 0.5% of those in serum). In addition, the types of bacteria causing CNS shunt–related infections are not associated commonly with humoral immunodeficiency states, thus suggesting that humoral protection is less important in CNS shunt–related infections. Little is known about the possible role of reduced tissue immunity in these infections.

The foreign body nature of the shunt apparatus plays an important role in the local host defense defect.[39] Electron-microscopic findings demonstrate irregularities in catheters that allow microorganisms to be buried in the catheter. In addition, the function of neutrophils is suboptimal because phagocytic and bactericidal activities are reduced as a result of the loss of lysosomal contents. Therefore, even when pathogens are phagocytized, they may not be killed and are protected from antibiotics that do not penetrate the cell membrane.

Other mechanisms that may contribute to shunt-related infections include (1) abnormal CSF flow (not being absorbed by the venous sinuses, thought to be important for prevention of infection in the CNS) and (2) interruption of the blood-brain barrier by the shunt catheter, with the creation of a direct tract between the subcutaneous tissues and the ventricles resulting in significant compromise in host defenses.[406]

CLINICAL MANIFESTATIONS

The initial signs and symptoms of most patients with shunt-related infections are nonspecific and include mild to moderate fever, malaise, irritability, nausea, vomiting, vague abdominal pain, and headache. With such nonspecific findings, the physician must be careful to differentiate between the possibility of a shunt-related infection and an intercurrent viral or bacterial infection of the upper respiratory, urinary, or gastrointestinal tract. Examination of the CSF (from a shunt tap) may be of help (see "Diagnosis"). Only a minority of patients have the classic signs and symptoms of CNS inflammation, such as a stiff neck, bulging fontanelle, change in mental status, cranial nerve palsy, or papilledema. In some patients the shunt tract may be infected, with evidence of cellulitis or dehiscence (or both) of the surgical wounds. Tenderness, edema, or erythema along the tract itself may be the only sign.

The type of shunt affects the nature of the infection. For example, VP shunt–related infections may cause symptoms and signs confined to the abdominal cavity, such as abdominal pain, tenderness (with or without guarding), intestinal obstruction,[325] or spontaneous bacterial peritonitis.[121] Rarely, a distal shunt-related infection will be manifested as frank ascites as a result of CSF malabsorption.[209] A relatively common complication of VP shunts is an inflammatory peritoneal exudate that may lead to CSF loculation and the subsequent formation of a peritoneal pseudocyst.[8,326] These pseudocysts often are palpable and can be visualized by ultrasonography or CT. Bacteria are isolated in a third of cases, suggesting that infection may play a role in the pathogenesis of pseudocysts. In most cases, however, a high index of suspicion is required because the initial symptoms frequently are abdominal only, with no signs of shunt malfunction.

A unique complication of patients with VA shunts is the development of immune complex disease such as "shunt nephritis" (a form of acute glomerulonephritis), arthritis, or rash. In most of these cases, the infecting organism has been *S. epidermidis*, but other bacteria such as *Corynebacterium* can cause this complication.[38] In the case of shunt nephritis, the patient has fever, edema, malaise, hepatosplenomegaly, hypocomplementemia, anemia, azotemia, hematuria, and proteinuria.[78] Pathologic findings consist of mesangial hypercellularity and granular deposits of immunoglobulins and complement along the glomerular membrane. Rarely, arthritis may be the initial symptom because it may develop by the same immunologic mechanisms that cause nephritis.[216]

DIAGNOSIS

Although shunt-related infections are not common occurrences, the nonspecific signs and symptoms and the insidious onset in many cases render establishing a diagnosis very difficult. Therefore, any patient with a CNS shunt and fever without an obvious source should be suspected of having a shunt-related infection, especially if the symptoms continue for longer than a week. A higher index of suspicion for shunt-related infection is needed in young patients, in whom fever develops within 3 to 6 months after placement of the shunt. The only definitive diagnostic test is direct observation and culture of CSF. Tapping the shunt or sampling fluid in direct contact with the shunt should be performed if no signs or symptoms of increased intracranial pressure (ICP) are noted. CT of the head is recommended before the tap is done if such symptoms exist. The shunt tap should be performed with utmost attention given to sterile technique. The tap should be done by a neurosurgeon or physician who is familiar with the technique and the underlying hardware.

When percutaneous needle aspiration is performed, the area around the shunt reservoir should be scrubbed with antiseptic soap and the surrounding hair shaved (2 inches in each direction). The scalp area should be prepared by repeated application (at least three times) of povidone-iodine solution followed by alcohol. A 21- or 23-gauge butterfly needle is placed into the reservoir (or valve if no reservoir is present). Measurement of opening pressure can help in diagnosing a distal malfunction (i.e., increased pressure) or proximal shunt obstruction (i.e., less than expected pressure). CSF sample aliquots then should be allowed to drip into sterile vials. Gentle aspiration of CSF sometimes is performed if no fluid returns spontaneously. If only a few drops of CSF can be obtained, the more important tests, Gram stain and culture, should be performed first. Culturing the shunt wound, blood, or CSF obtained by lumbar puncture (which usually is not communicating with the ventricular fluid) often is unrevealing, misleading, or both. Although bacteremia frequently is present in patients with VA shunts and may help in diagnosing the etiologic agent, blood cultures generally are negative in patients with all other shunts (e.g., VP or pleural shunts). In

addition, CoNS are the most common contaminants of blood cultures, and, therefore, interpreting a positive blood culture in these patients would be difficult.

CSF should be tested for glucose concentration, differential cell count, Gram stain, and culture. Protein concentration is requested often, but it is of very limited help in evaluating the presence or absence of an infection because high protein levels are found in many patients with shunt malfunction and no infection. In contrast, normal protein levels have been reported in many patients with shunt-related infections. A low glucose level suggests an infection, but one should confirm that the CSF sample was not diluted before the test was performed. Some physicians use saline to get a better flow of CSF (because of an occluded tube), which may affect the biochemical results. Of importance is to note that in many cases of shunt-related infection, the glucose level is within the normal range. Usually, pleocytosis with a predominance of PMNs is indicative of a shunt-related infection. Although in some cases the finding of a positive CSF culture is interpreted as a shunt-related infection despite a normal WBC count (<10 WBCs/mm³), the absence of clinical symptoms (e.g., fever) in many of these patients suggests that the positive culture probably represents colonization or contamination. Other cells such as mononuclear cells[204,364] or eosinophils[247,384,399] may predominate during an infection. If eosinophilia is the predominant cellular response, an allergy to the shunt (e.g., silicone[183]) or the materials used for sterilization (e.g., ethylene oxide[307]) or intraventricular administration of antibiotics (e.g., gentamicin,[255] vancomycin[135]) should be considered.

Interpretation of the WBC count should be done cautiously if the red blood cell count is high because the increased number of WBCs can be the result of blood spilling into CSF without any infection or be part of the inflammatory response to the presence of blood (i.e., chemical ventriculitis). A positive Gram stain with an increased CSF WBC count or reduced glucose level (or both) is helpful in making the diagnosis of a shunt-related infection. A negative Gram stain does not exclude an infection, and one should wait for the results of culture. Ventricular fluid always should be cultured anaerobically as well as aerobically. Although most bacteria causing shunt-related infections grow within 48 to 78 hours, cultures should be held for 7 days (if still negative) for fastidious organisms such as *Propionibacterium*. The possibility of contamination or colonization of the shunt without infection should be considered when the culture is positive but other CSF parameters are normal. If such a scenario occurs and bacteria are growing only from one sample (e.g., a shunt tap) and not from follow-up cultures (i.e., from extraventricular drainage), a shorter course of therapy (see later) may be sufficient.

Blood cultures, a peripheral complete blood count (CBC), and ultrasound of the abdomen (for VP shunts) are of limited value. For example, although 90 percent of patients with VA shunt-related infection will have a positive blood culture, less than 10 percent of patients with other shunt-related infections will have a positive culture. In addition, in more than a third of patients with shunt-related infections, no elevation in the peripheral WBC count was found. Some investigators suggest that blood but not CSF CRP levels may be helpful in establishing the diagnosis of shunt-related infection when other concurrent infections (e.g., sinusitis, pneumonia) were excluded.[212,340] One suggestion is that if the CRP level is less than 7 mg/L, the shunt should not be removed because no infection is present. More data are needed to verify this observation. In patients with a VA shunt–related infection, measurement of serum anti-staphylococcal antibodies or the C3 and C4 components of the complement cascade may aid in establishing the diagnosis.[25,334] The triad of fever, abnormal CSF WBC count, and greater than 5 percent eosinophilia is highly predictive of a shunt-related infection.

TREATMENT

A variety of medical and surgical approaches to treatment of an infected shunt have been suggested.[415] Regimens include (1) the use of antibiotics alone (systemically, with or without intraventricular administration) without replacement of the shunt; (2) removal of the infected shunt followed by immediate insertion of a new shunt and the administration of systemic or intraventricular antibiotics, or both; (3) removal of the infected shunt and insertion of an extraventricular device (EVD) to monitor the patient's response to the accompanying antibiotic therapy, with a new shunt inserted only when the ventricular system is sterilized; (4) removal of the infected shunt followed by a stereotactic third ventriculostomy and administration of antibiotics; and (5) externalization of only the distal (e.g., peritoneal) catheter along with the administration of systemic or intraventricular antibiotics, or both.

The use of antibiotics alone without surgery was justified by the need to maintain CSF drainage and avoid costly operations and lengthy duration of hospital stay. The low success rate of this approach (33%) and the higher mortality rate associated with it suggest that it should not be used (Table 85-3). Of interest, the failure rate was much higher with infections caused by slime-producing organisms than with infections caused by non–slime-producing bacteria.[84] Only in shunted patients with purulent meningitis caused by *S. pneumoniae*, *N. meningitidis*, or *H. influenzae* did the administration of systemic antibiotics alone without removal of the shunt seem to be an acceptable option.[215,288,323,369]

Combining immediate replacement of the infected shunt with a new shunt and antibiotic therapy has a higher rate of success (70%, see Table 85-3) than does the use of antibiotics alone. Nonetheless, it is less effective than removal of the infected shunt accompanied by insertion of an EVD and administration of antibiotic therapy (88% success rate, see Table 85-3). A decision analysis of 17 studies reached the same conclusion and suggested that "this treatment option has the highest cure rate and the lowest failure and mortality rates."[339] In addition, lack of the ability to monitor when the ventricular fluid is sterilized results in a longer period of systemic antibiotic therapy (e.g., 4 to 8 weeks), which may lead to an increase in iatrogenic infections and cost. Some surgeons suggest removing the shunt and delaying replacement (i.e., a few days after removal to allow sterilization of the shunt's tract), but this approach is associated with increased morbidity.[108,407]

For infection that involves only the distal part of the shunt (e.g., pseudocyst, appendicitis,[295] erythema or swelling along the shunt tract, surgical wound infection), externalization of only the distal end of the shunt along with the administration of antibiotic therapy is recommended by some neurosurgeons. Potential advantages of this technique include (1) diversion of CSF from an infected area to avoid ascending infection, (2) maintenance of CSF flow to prevent increased ICP, (3) the ability to perform frequent CSF sampling, and (4) the capability of monitoring therapy. The disadvantage is that early infection or colonization of the proximal portion of the shunt may be obscured by the antibiotic treatment and become active after discontinuation of therapy and reinsertion of the distal part.

Internal shunting by a third ventriculostomy (with avoidance of a prosthetic device) was shown to be effective in managing patients with refractory shunt-related infections who have a noncommunicating hydrocephalus, patent subarachnoid space, and adequate CSF absorption.[108,185,264,275,352] Shunt independence for extended periods was documented in many patients without myelomeningocele. The success rate is lower in those with myelomeningocele or hemorrhage or after meningitis. Disadvantages of this technique include increased morbidity (e.g., hypothalamic injury, subarachnoid hemorrhage), technical difficulty in younger children, and, if the stereotactic technique is used, cost and availability of the necessary equipment.

The most effective treatment of shunt-related infections is to remove the entire infected shunt and insert an EVD to control ICP and monitor the infection (i.e., provide CSF access). After

---

TABLE 85-3   Shunt Infection Cure Rates in Relation to the Therapeutic Approach

Author	Antibiotics Alone*	Antibiotics and Immediate Replacement with a New Shunt	Antibiotics, Removal of the Shunt, and Insertion of an EVD
Schoenbaum[338a]	5/30†		25/26
Nelson[275]	10/13		46/46
Salmon[333]		5/10	
Sells[345]	1/8	1/6	9/9
James[179]	3/10		9/10
Venes[392]		6/9	3/3
James[178]	4/11	11/13	16/17
Wald[404]	15/20		
Mates[238]	7/8		
Shurtleff[351]	2/27	6/20	19/19
Morrice[266]	4/14	19/23	14/18
Nicholas[276]			
Frame[112]	8/11	21/27	
Forward[108]	8/15	2/2	13/13
Luthardt[228]	1/17		
O'Brien[281]	11/11	15/19	9/9
Walters[406]	13/92	11/21	44/71
Swayne[376]			19/20
Ronan[327]	3/4	4/7	21/22
Stamos[364]			23/23
Morissette[264]	3/6		3/3
Younger[429]	4/11	42/46	
Total (success rate)	**102/308 (33%)**	**143/203 (70%)**	**273/309 (88%)**

*With and without intraventricular antibiotics.
†Number cured/number treated.
EVD, extraventricular device.

antibiotic therapy has been successful, a new shunt is placed. With this approach, treatment success is very high (see Table 85-3), with more rapid clearance of the infection and a shorter duration of therapy. The choice of intravenous antibiotic depends on local patterns of antimicrobial susceptibility and the ability of the antibiotic to penetrate the blood-brain barrier. With the increasing rate of methicillin-resistant staphylococci, vancomycin should be used as initial therapy while awaiting bacteriologic identification and the results of antibiotic sensitivity testing. Effort should be made to discontinue vancomycin as soon as the infecting bacteria are found to be sensitive to the semisynthetic penicillins so that the chance of the bacteria becoming resistant to vancomycin is reduced. In addition, even if in vitro data suggest that the bacteria are highly sensitive to the first-generation cephalosporins (e.g., cephalothin, cefazolin, cephapirin), they should not be used because they penetrate the blood-brain barrier poorly. Linezolid has been used successfully in a few cases of shunt infection.[54] This drug has a good CSF penetration, with concentrations above the minimal inhibitory concentration (MIC) of most gram-positive bacteria, including MRSA. It is also effective against bacteria living in biofilms. The limited data available suggest that linezolid should be considered cautiously when vancomycin fails or cannot be given.

To achieve more consistent and efficient eradication of bacteria, the CSF drug level should be at least 10 times higher than the MIC of the pathogen. Therefore, the dosage of antibiotic or antibiotics and the dosing interval should be maximized (i.e., "meningeal schedule"). If the selected antibiotic does not clear the infection within 2 to 3 days and no improvement occurs in CSF biochemical and WBC parameters (i.e., seemingly no control of the infection), measurement of the bactericidal titer of ventricular fluid should be considered. To determine bactericidal titer, 1 mL of CSF (if CSF production is >5 mL/hr) at the expected peak antibiotic level (i.e., 2 to 3 hours after the antibiotic is given parenterally) is diluted serially with culture media to produce dilutions of 1:2, 1:4, 1:8, and 1:16. To these dilutions, an equal amount of medium with 10^5 colonies per milliliter of the offending bacteria is added (the final CSF dilution is 1:4, 1:8, 1:16, and 1:32). After 24 hours of incubation, the tubes are observed for turbidity, which reflects the growth of bacteria. If no turbidity is seen in the 1:8 and 1:16 or higher dilution tubes, the CSF level of the antibiotic probably is sufficient, and continued growth of bacteria from CSF may be caused by colonization of the EVD or contamination. On the other hand, if turbidity is noted in the tube with less than a 1:8 dilution (i.e., a 1:4 dilution), the CSF level of antibiotic may not be sufficient to combat the infection, and the addition of another antibiotic or change to a different antibiotic is warranted.

In vitro synergy studies can help determine the best drug combination. Rifampin should be considered as one of the drugs in the combination for gram-positive bacteria for three reasons. First, most staphylococci are still sensitive to this antibiotic and their MIC usually is 10-fold lower (i.e., 0.05 µg/mL) than that of other anti-staphylococcal drugs (e.g., vancomycin, 0.5 µg/mL). Unfortunately, the use of rifampin alone may be followed rapidly by rifampin-resistant variants because they already are present in small numbers in any staphylococcal population. Second, rifampin penetrates CSF well and easily achieves a greater than 10-fold level over the MIC of most staphylococci. Third, rifampin has demonstrated good bactericidal activity even when staphylococci were embedded in slime. In contrast, staphylococcal slime inhibits the antimicrobial activity of vancomycin.[103]

Selection of the initial antibiotic before culture results are known can be based on the patient's clinical and CSF findings. An algorithm for initial antibiotic therapy before CSF culture results are available is presented in Figure 85-2. This algorithm should not be used for neonates or immunocompromised patients with suspected shunt-related infections because they often have

less severe clinical symptoms and CSF response. The decision-making process starts with assessment of the patient's clinical condition. Usually, patients with infection in the CNS are only mildly symptomatic, whereas patients with *S. aureus* or gram-negative bacterial infection often are more seriously ill.

The next step is evaluation of the Gram stain. If the Gram stain is positive for gram-positive bacteria (e.g., *Staphylococcus, Streptococcus*), the drug of choice is vancomycin. If the Gram stain shows gram-negative bacteria, the drug of choice is cefotaxime or ceftriaxone. Treatment with an aminoglycoside is acceptable, but the outcome seems to be less favorable because of poorer penetration into CSF.[364] If the Gram stain is negative, other CSF parameters (e.g., WBC count and glucose) should be examined. If either is abnormal and the patient is not severely sick, vancomycin alone should be started because the chance of having a gram-negative infection is low.[364]

In contrast, if the patient is more seriously ill, coverage for gram-negative bacteria should be added (e.g., cefotaxime or ceftriaxone). In nontoxic patients with normal CSF parameters and no distal symptoms (e.g., peritonitis, wound or tract infection), antibiotic therapy can be withheld until the results of culture are known. On the other hand, if distal signs or symptoms exist, therapy is tailored according to the site. In patients with skin involvement, vancomycin is the drug of choice, whereas in febrile patients with abdominal symptoms, the combination of cefotaxime (or ceftriaxone) and clindamycin (to cover both gram-positive and anaerobic bacteria) is preferred.

Direct instillation of antibiotics into the ventricular system to increase their levels is recommended by some experts. Unfortunately, the suggested doses for intraventricular treatment have been determined empirically on only a small number of patients, and their pharmacokinetics and pharmacodynamics have not been studied well. This therapy is not without hazard, especially when the recommended doses often are much higher than those found to cause neurotoxicity.[200,356,411,413] Pleocytosis and eosinophilia also have occurred in patients receiving intraventricular vancomycin[224] or gentamicin.[255] In addition, preservative-containing preparations should be checked for appropriateness for intraventricular instillation. Limited pharmacokinetic data suggest that clearance of the instilled intraventricular antibiotic is sufficiently slow to allow once-daily administration. If possible, the EVD should be closed for 30 to 60 minutes after the drug is administered. If the EVD cannot be closed and the amount of CSF drainage exceeds 7 to 10 mL/hr, the frequency of intraventricular antibiotic instillation should be increased to twice daily.

Antibiotics commonly recommended for intravenous and intraventricular use according to the etiologic agent are shown in Table 85-4. A recent small study in adults showed that administration of 10 mg of vancomycin intraventricularly once daily was safe and achieved levels above 5 µg/mL (the recommended CSF trough level needed to achieve cure) for up to 21 hours.[303] Because of the potential toxicity of the empirically recommended intraventricular antibiotic doses and the unpredictability of CSF levels, irrigation of the ventricular system with a known concentration of an antibiotic solution is preferred when systemic antibiotics fail to eradicate the bacteria. To achieve irrigation, two EVDs must be inserted to produce a continuous flow of solution. The concentration of antibiotic in the solution should be equal to the highest safe plasma level when the drug is given intravenously. For example, for treating gram-negative bacteria sensitive to amikacin, amikacin at a dose of 30 to 40 mg/L of saline solution (producing a concentration of 30 to 40 µg/mL) is recommended. Gentamicin at a dose of 10 to 12 mg/L (using a special intrathecal preparation) is an acceptable alternative when the gentamicin MIC for the bacteria is less than 1 µg/mL. The antibiotic solution is administered through one EVD at a rate of 10 mL/hr, and the second EVD is left open to drain the fluid and to remove debris and pus from the ventricles.

PATIENT CONDITION

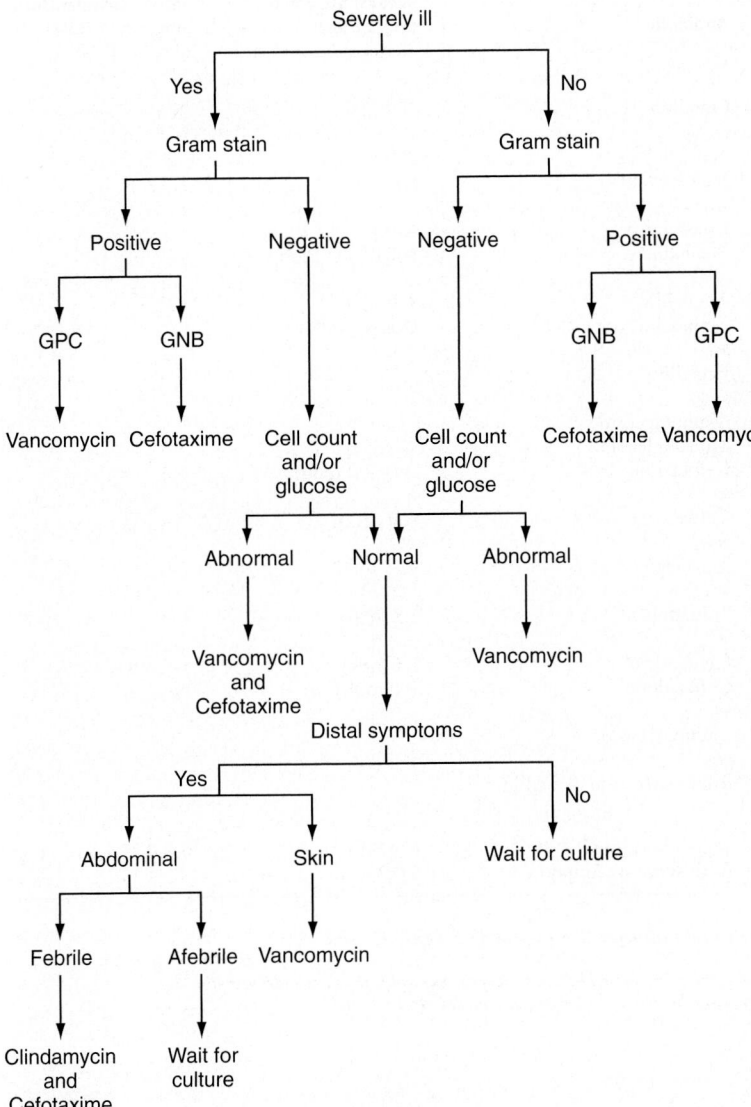

Figure 85–2 Algorithm for selection of antibiotic therapy before culture results are known. GNB, gram-negative bacillus; GPC, gram-positive coccus.

When antibiotic therapy is completed, abnormal CSF findings such as low glucose or mildly elevated protein or cell counts should not delay reshunting. The duration of treatment is empiric and depends on the etiologic agent, the CSF parameters at initial evaluation, and the time to sterilization. In our institution, we found the following schedule to be successful. If CSF parameters are *normal* but culture yields CoNS only from the operating room (i.e., the initial sample), therapy should be given for only 3 to 4 days. If subsequent cultures also are positive, therapy should continue until negative cultures have been obtained for 7 days. If CSF parameters are *abnormal* in the operating room and culture is positive *only* from that specimen, therapy should continue for 7 days. If subsequent samples show abnormal CSF findings and positive cultures, therapy should be extended until negative cultures have been obtained for 10 days.

A longer duration of antibiotic therapy is recommended with other bacteria (e.g., *S. aureus*, gram-negative bacteria). If culture is positive *only* on samples from the *operating room* and CSF findings are normal, treatment should be given until negative cultures have been obtained for 7 days. In all other situations, therapy should continue until negative cultures have been achieved for

10 days. Reshunting should take place immediately at the end of treatment. No benefit is found in observing the patient for a time without antibiotics for relapse of the infection.[409]

COMPLICATIONS

Shunt-related infections are associated with increased morbidity and mortality rates. Patients with shunt-related infection have an increase in shunt-related operations, which contributes to the increased morbidity and cost. In addition, these patients have been shown to have an increase in mortality rates in comparison to patients without shunt-related infection.[356] Even when the original infection is treated successfully, secondary infection (or contamination) of the EVD occurs in 5 to 10 percent of cases. To minimize the risk of development of a secondary infection, a sterile closed-drainage system should be maintained carefully. Only trained personnel should be allowed to drain CSF samples from the system, and injections into the system should be avoided. Continuous external drainage of CSF also causes loss of electrolytes and fluid. Therefore, routine assessment of serum

TABLE 85–4   Recommended Intravenous and Intraventricular Antibiotic Therapy for Shunt Infection according to the Etiologic Agent

Etiologic Agent	Antibiotic	Intravenous Dose (mg/kg/day)	Intraventricular Dose (mg/day, 1 Dose)
Bacteria			
Staphylococcus aureus or coagulase-negative staphylococci			
Methicillin-sensitive	Oxacillin*,†	200 (q8h)	NA
	or		
	Nafcillin*,†	200 (q8h)	50-75
Methicillin-resistant	Vancomycin†	60 (q8h)	5-10
	or		
	Linezolid	15 (q12)	
Streptococcal species	Penicillin*	400,000 U (q6h)	—
or	*or*		
Diphtheroids	Ampicillin*	400 (q6h)	10-25
Enterococcus faecalis	Ampicillin*	Doses as above	
	or		
	Penicillin*		NA
	plus		
	Aminoglycoside‡		
Anaerobic bacteria	Metronidazole	30 (q8h)	NA
Escherichia coli, Klebsiella, Proteus, Enterobacter	Cefotaxime	200-300 (q6h)	NA
	or		
	Ceftriaxone	100 (q12h)	NA
	or		
	Amikacin§	22.5 (q8h)	2-8
	or		
	Tobramycin§	7.5 (q8h)	1-4
	or		
	Gentamicin§	7.5 (q8h)	1-4
Pseudomonas species	Ceftazidime	200 (q8h)	NA
	or		
	Aminoglycoside		
	plus		
	Broad-spectrum penicillin		
Fungi			
Candida species	Amphotericin B¶	1 (q24h)	0.1-0.25
	AmBisome or Amphotec	5 (q24h)	

In patients allergic to penicillin, use vancomycin.
†*If cerebrospinal fluid levels are not sufficient and the bacteria are sensitive to rifampin, add rifampin, 20 mg/kg/day divided every 12 hours.*
‡*See doses (for the specific aminoglycoside) for treatment of E. coli below.*
§*The addition of a broad-spectrum penicillin (e.g., piperacillin or ticarcillin, 300 to 400 mg/kg/day divided every 6 hours) may add to the bactericidal activity.*
¶*If ventricular fluid remains positive after 5 to 7 days of therapy with amphotericin, add flucytosine (150 mg/kg/day divided every 6 hours).*
NA, not available.

electrolytes once or twice weekly is recommended, and the total daily amount of drained CSF should be replaced. Recurrent shunt-related infection after completion of treatment is common, with two thirds of such infections being caused by the same organism.[197] Unusual complications of ventricular shunt infections include brain abscess and subdural empyema.[100,402]

PROGNOSIS

Long-term morbidity occurring after a shunt-related infection includes seizures, psychomotor retardation, and cognitive deficiency. The intelligence quotient (IQ) scores of children with myelomeningocele who had a shunt-related infection were found to be significantly lower (mean IQ, 72) than the scores of children with shunts but no infection (mean IQ, 95).[250] A trend was observed in which younger children with shunt-related infections had a lower IQ than older children with shunt-related infections did, especially if the infection was caused by gram-negative bacteria. In addition, shunt-related infection adversely affected school performance.[398] With appropriate combined medical and surgical therapy, the mortality rate from shunt-related infection

is low, but any episode of shunt-related infection appears to increase the probability of another episode developing.

PREVENTION

Preventive measures to reduce the incidence of shunt-related infection include attention to preoperative and intraoperative technique and the prophylactic use of antibiotics. Bactericidal shampoos (e.g., chlorhexidine) should be used to reduce the bacterial density of the scalp before surgery is performed. Shaving the scalp seems to be a risk factor, so shaveless surgery should be considered.[166] During the operation, only essential personnel should be present, and the skin should be cleaned with a fat solvent, followed by solutions that reduce the number of bacteria (elemental tincture of iodine, 20 ppm, is preferred over 10% povidone-iodine, which contains <1 ppm free iodine)[58] or their ability to adhere to the shunt (bacitracin A).[134] Careful attention should be paid to surgical technique, with contact between the shunt and the skin being avoided. A detailed preoperative protocol developed by Choux and associates[61] has reduced the infection rate from greater than 7 percent to less than 1 percent. This protocol emphasizes a shorter operating time, less operating room staff and traffic, and fewer manipulations of the shunt. Even though several investigators were able to reduce the infection rate by using measures similar to those suggested by Choux and coworkers,[59,198] other studies have failed to show that all the factors emphasized by Choux and associates have a positive effect on the infection rate.[305,310] Although a few recent studies suggested that use of an antibiotic-impregnated shunt significantly reduces the incidence of shunt infections in comparison to the use of a standard shunt,[132,343] no significant reduction in the overall shunt-related infection rate was observed in other studies.[151,189] Large prospective, randomized studies are needed to evaluate the real contribution of an antibiotic-impregnated shunt to the reduction in infection rate.

Multiple studies have examined the effect of prophylactic antibiotics for the shunt insertion procedure on reducing the infection rate. Major variations in study design and the number of patients in each study preclude arriving at definitive conclusions. Previous meta-analyses of well-designed studies suggest that the use of prophylactic antibiotics is associated with a significant reduction in the incidence of infections *if* the baseline rate of shunt-related infections is greater than 5 percent.[145] If the infection rate is lower than 5 percent, prophylactic antibiotics are *not* recommended. A recent meta-analysis of 2134 patients (in 17 trials) found a statistically significant benefit for either systemic antibiotic prophylaxis (15 studies) or antibiotic-impregnated catheters (2 studies) in reducing the incidence of shunt-related infections.[318] The choice of antibiotics should be based on the local antibiotic sensitivity pattern of the pathogens commonly causing shunt-related infections in that area. Preferably, prophylaxis should be started 8 to 12 hours before surgery to allow higher levels of drug to accumulate in skin tissue than would do so if treatment were given just before the operation. The duration of prophylaxis should not exceed 24 to 36 hours. Further studies are needed to identify factors important in the development of shunt-related infections so that better techniques can be developed to further reduce or even eliminate this devastating complication of CNS shunting.

INTRACRANIAL PRESSURE MONITORS

Monitoring of ICP has become an important part of the evaluation, treatment, and management of children with a variety of intracranial pathologic processes,[225] including congenital anomalies (e.g., cranial or craniofacial dysostosis), metabolic diseases (e.g., Reye syndrome), trauma, intraventricular or subarachnoid hemorrhage, intracranial infections (e.g., encephalitis), and other ischemic or hypoxic insults. Several studies have demonstrated the therapeutic and prognostic benefit of monitoring ICP in children with high ICP[111,181,219,380]; nonetheless, this procedure is not without complications such as hematoma, bleeding, leakage of CSF, and infection. Infections for which monitoring of ICP is used include ventriculitis, meningitis, brain abscess, subdural empyema, skin infection, and cranial bone infections.[201,224,241,273,423]

Several methods are available for monitoring ICP. Intraventricular placement of a catheter with the distal end connected to a pressure transducer is the method used most frequently because of its accuracy and ease of calibration. This procedure also allows drainage of CSF for biochemical or dynamic testing. Disadvantages of ventriculostomy are penetration of the meninges and brain, technical difficulties if the ventricles are small, and greater risk for the development of infection. Other methods used to monitor ICP include a subdural bolt or catheter (only the meninges are penetrated, but the brain remains intact), an epidural transducer (the dura remains intact), and a continuous intraparenchymal monitor (i.e., a fiberoptic cable is inserted through the

dura into the brain parenchyma, not intraventricularly). Although both the epidural transducer and the intraparenchymal monitor have fewer complications (e.g., infection) than the intraventricular devices do, they are prone to inaccuracy, which limits their use. Selection of the appropriate ICP-monitoring method depends on the patient's condition and the risk associated with the procedure.[232]

EPIDEMIOLOGY

Assessing the true infection rate of ICP monitoring devices is very difficult, mainly because the methods used to define infection (i.e., inclusion and exclusion criteria) and antibiotic use vary widely among reported studies. The incidence of infection ranged from less than 1 percent to 40 percent, with an average incidence of 8.8 percent.[63,73,223,233,346,368,401] A much higher rate of infection was reported in patients who had devices that penetrated the meninges[18,162,273] than in those who had parenchymal monitors.[311]

Multiple factors were suggested as increasing the risk for development of ICP device–related infection (Table 85–5). Patients with intracerebral hemorrhage usually do not have a higher risk for acquiring infection than do those without such hemorrhage. In contrast, if the bleeding is intraventricular, the incidence of infection increases dramatically.[241] The rate of infection also is higher in patients with open head trauma than in those with closed head trauma or intracranial malignancy.[168] Neurosurgical operations contributed significantly to the risk of acquiring infection,[241,374] and the same was noted if ICP was greater than 20 mm Hg.[241]

Interruption of the monitoring system's integrity (e.g., in-line stopcocks, number of times that the system was open, blockage of drainage, and irrigation) was identified by several investigators as increasing patients' risk of acquiring infection.[18,241,254,280] The effect of the duration of monitoring on the risk for infection is controversial, especially in patients with ventriculostomy catheters. Although several studies found a correlation between the length of time that the monitoring device was in place and the infection rate,[18,162,190,273] some investigators found no relationship with the duration of monitoring.[282,358,374,422] The different conclusions probably were the result of differences in the populations studied, the types of devices used to measure ICP, the definitions of infection, and analyses of the data. One critical review of the

TABLE 85–5   Risk Factors for Infection of Devices for Monitoring Intracranial Pressure

Factors Associated with Increased Risk for Infection
Intraventricular hemorrhage
ICP >20 mm Hg
Open head trauma
Neurosurgical procedure/operation
Perforation of the dura
Duration of catheterization
Problems with the system
Disconnections
Leaks
Irrigations
Blockage

Factors Not Associated with Increased Risk for Infection
Head trauma
Intracerebral hemorrhage
Intracranial malignancy
Underlying disease
Drainage of cerebrospinal fluid
Previous ICP monitoring device in the intensive care unit
ICP device dressing changes
ICP device component changes

literature found a correlation between the duration of ICP monitoring and the rate of infections.[223]

The need to replace the device at a certain time has been challenged. Analysis of the outcome in 584 patients (receiving 712 ventriculostomy catheters) who had 61 infections showed a steady increase in the daily incidence of infection, with a peak occurring at day 10. The average time until the onset of infection was 6.8 days.[162] In addition, replacing the ventriculostomy catheter before day 5 did not affect the daily rate of infection. The authors concluded that the lowest rate of infection occurred in the first 4 days of monitoring but that replacement of the catheter by day 5 did not reduce the infection rate, which continued to rise until day 10. The authors recommended that "ICP monitoring [devices] should be removed as quickly as possible," but if "prolonged monitoring is required, there appears to be no benefit from or need for catheter exchange."[162]

Several potential risk factors for ICP monitor–related infections that do not increase the infection rate are shown in Table 85–5.

ETIOLOGY

In general, the microorganisms that cause infections related to ICP monitoring devices are the same as those causing CNS shunt–related infections (see Table 85–2). The major difference is that gram-negative bacteria are isolated more often in ICP monitor-related infection than in CNS shunt–related infections. The more common bacteria include *Enterobacter* spp., *Klebsiella* spp., *S. marcescens*, and *Acinetobacter* spp. These bacteria are found in water and cause widespread colonization of hospitalized patients. Colonization of the respiratory tract is an especially common occurrence in patients in the intensive care unit and in those with serious underlying disease. Thus, these organisms are occurring increasingly frequently in ICP monitor–related infections. Few infections are caused by *Corynebacterium*, *Propionibacterium*, and fungi.[144]

CLINICAL MANIFESTATIONS

ICP monitor–related infections often occur in patients with an altered sensorium; therefore, the signs and symptoms of meningeal irritation usually are not present. The clinical diagnosis is complicated further by the fact that these patients frequently are critically ill and their signs and symptoms are caused by the underlying condition and are not a result of the ICP monitor–related infection. In addition, they may be receiving multiple antibiotics for other sources of infection (e.g., pneumonia, bacteremia, urinary tract infection), both nosocomial and non-nosocomial. Although fever is the most frequent indication of infection, the presence of infections or inflammatory processes at other body sites causes the predictive value of fever to be low. Therefore, providing close follow-up, having a high index of suspicion, and obtaining frequent cultures of CSF when available (e.g., ventriculostomy device) are recommended.

DIAGNOSIS

The predictive value of the peripheral WBC count and differential count is very low, and the only definitive diagnostic tests are the CSF WBC count and culture.[304] CSF biochemistry (i.e., protein and glucose) has a very low predictive value. Although a low glucose level may be of help in establishing the diagnosis, a normal level does not exclude the possibility of an infection. Calculation of the ratio of leukocytes to erythrocytes in CSF versus their ratio in peripheral blood was suggested as a potential

diagnostic tool for early infection.[302] Most patients with ICP monitor–related infection will have an increased CSF WBC count with a predominance of PMNs. In some cases, with low growth of bacteria, no elevation in CSF WBC counts (<10/mm³) was reported. Most of these cases were caused by CoNS. In such cases, if no other indicators of infection (e.g., clinical symptoms, low glucose) are present, the possibility that the positive cultures represent colonization or contamination should be considered before treatment is initiated.

TREATMENT AND PROPHYLAXIS

The same principles used for the management of CNS shunt–related infections can be applied to infections associated with ICP monitoring devices. The use of antibiotics alone without removal of the device may be adequate for the treatment of infections associated with devices placed in the subdural or epidural space, unless an abscess or empyema has formed. In the case of ventriculostomy, the infected device should be removed and appropriate antibiotic therapy instituted. Because gram-negative bacteria are almost as common as are gram-positive bacteria in causing ICP device-related infections, initial antibiotic therapy should include both vancomycin and cefotaxime or ceftazidime if the Gram stain is negative. When the etiologic agent is identified, the specific antibiotic or antibiotics can be chosen from those listed in Table 85–4. The duration of therapy depends on the etiologic agent and the CSF parameters. In patients with positive CSF culture but minimal CSF pleocytosis, if the CSF culture becomes negative immediately after removal of the catheter, therapy should be given for only 3 or 4 days because the cultures before removal of the catheter reflect colonization and not infection. If subsequent cultures are positive, therapy should continue for 10 days of negative cultures.

Removal of the ICP monitor (if longer than 5 days) and reinsertion at an alternate site was recommended as a prophylactic approach to reduce the infection rate. This recommendation is controversial, and several studies showed that routine changes of the ICP monitor did not reduce the risk for development of infection.[223,424]

Many physicians use prophylactic antibiotics for the duration of ICP monitoring in the hope of preventing infection. Unfortunately, the few studies that have evaluated the utility of antimicrobial agents in preventing such infections did not find any efficacy.[24,320] The optimal duration of antibiotic prophylaxis is controversial. Jacobs and Westerband[177] showed that patients who received prophylaxis had statistically significantly higher rates of septic morbidity and pneumonia. Yet a decreased rate of ICP monitor infection was reported in patients who received prophylaxis for the duration of the ICP monitoring.[309] Most studies found that the use of prophylaxis has no effect on infection rates. In addition, broad-spectrum antibiotic prophylaxis was associated with shifting to resistant gram-negative pathogens.[240]

INTRATHECAL PUMP INFUSION DEVICES

The intrathecal pump infusion system currently is used to infuse morphine to treat refractory pain,[285] to deliver baclofen (a γ-aminobutyric acid agonist), or to treat spasticity of spinal or cerebral origin.[4,16,297] In addition, patients with generalized dystonia also benefited from intrathecal baclofen.[5] More than 50,000 patients are being treated with implanted intrathecal pumps for pain or spasticity. Several pump systems are used. The simpler systems consist of an externalized catheter system similar to the Hickman catheter[89] or a subcutaneous reservoir system similar to an intravascular implanted port.[43] The more sophisticated systems include a programmable pump that usually is implanted in an abdominal subcutaneous pocket and connected via a subcutaneous catheter to the subarachnoid space.[27,43] An optional sideport in some of these implanted pumps allows aspiration of CSF from the subarachnoid space.

Complications of the intrathecal pump system are relatively rare events[129,391] and include mechanical problems with the catheter, such as breaking, kinking, dislodging, or leaking.[378] Skin necrosis also has been reported.[117,378] Complications (especially wound complications such as CSF fistula, dehiscence, granuloma formation, and infection) occur more frequently in children than in adults, probably because of their decreased muscle and subcutaneous tissue.[391] The pump itself is very durable and only very rarely causes a mechanical problem. Overdose that may result in coma, respiratory depression, apnea, cardiac conduction abnormalities, hypotension or hypertension, and abnormalities of the pupils was reported as well.[299] Intrathecal baclofen can induce both recurrent and new-onset seizures.[16,203] In addition, acute withdrawal syndrome was reported when treatment was stopped.[353] Infectious complications included suppuration at the exit site,[48,92,161,308] along the subcutaneous catheter (tunnel infection),[27,48,92,161] or around the pump.[27,48,57] Furthermore, more severe infections such as epidural abscess and meningitis also were reported.[29,48,75,92,274,335,430]

EPIDEMIOLOGY

The infection rate of intrathecal pump infusion devices ranges from 0 to 27 percent (median, 4%). Of note, in general the infection rate was lower in studies that included a larger number of patients. A more accurate description of the incidence would be the infection rate per 1000 catheter-days, which ranged from 0 to 2.5. The infection rate was higher in patients with an externalized catheter (0.65 per 1000 catheter-days) than in those who had an implanted system (0.48 per 1000 catheter-days). Most of the infections occurred at the exit site, along the catheter, or in the subcutaneous pocket of the pump, but the infection in as many as 16 percent of cases involved the epidural space, the meninges, or both. The incidence of infections can be reduced by using the subfascial pump implementation technique and perioperative antibiotic prophylaxis.[267]

Infections occur more often within 2 to 4 weeks after insertion of the catheter, which suggests that the initial surgery to place the intrathecal pump system may be a risk factor. Byers and coworkers[48] found that the only risk factor associated with infection during this surgery was a prolonged duration of the procedure (i.e., >100 minutes). Multiple other factors, such as the patient's age, underlying diseases, immune deficiency, other concurrent infections (e.g., pneumonia), previous intrathecal catheter, number of pump refills, intraspinal anesthetics, surgeon's or anesthesiologist's experience with the procedure, and operative complications (e.g., operative loss of blood), were not associated significantly with an increased risk for the acquisition of infection.[48] Very thin or malnourished patients may be prone to wound dehiscence, which may increase their vulnerability to infection. In addition, patients with narrowed intervertebral spaces tended to have operations of longer duration, which puts them at risk for the development of infection.

ETIOLOGY

The most common bacteria causing intrathecal device–related infection are from the skin flora. CoNS and *S. aureus* lead the list, but *Streptococcus mitis*,[48,279] *Streptococcus* group G,[48] *Corynebacterium striatum*,[48] and *Enterococcus faecalis*[115] infections are observed as well. In addition, several studies have reported gram-negative bacteria as the cause of the pump-related infection. Such bacteria

include *P. aeruginosa*,[48,115] *Pseudomonas paucimobilis*,[297] *E. coli*,[92] and *Klebsiella pneumoniae*.[297] One case each of *C. albicans*,[92] *Mycobacterium* spp.,[92] and *Acinetobacter baumanii*[387] also has been reported. A rare case of baclofen vial contamination with the fungus *Wangiella* that caused infection was reported as well.[249,297]

CLINICAL MANIFESTATIONS

Clinical findings depend on the site of the infection. Patients with more severe infections (i.e., epidural abscess, meningitis) may have symptoms of these infections (e.g., fever, irritability, headache, nerve root pain, meningeal signs). In some patients, pain experienced during the injection may be the clue, but in many patients, a high level of awareness for possible infection is important because they will have nonspecific signs and symptoms.

Exit-site and superficial catheter-related infections usually cause local inflammation (e.g., swelling, redness), tenderness, and drainage. The more serious deep-tract (tunnel) infections are more difficult to assess. Visible inflammation along the tract or a soft fluctuant fluid collection around it may be the only clue. Fever is not always present.

DIAGNOSIS

Performing a complete physical and neurologic examination may be helpful in some cases. A routine CBC is relatively unhelpful because leukocytosis is not always present. MRI may be useful for diagnosing an epidural abscess and evaluating its extent. The only definitive diagnostic tests are Gram stain and culture of exudate/drainage from the exit site (if available) or an aspirate of the fluid collection along the catheter tract if tunnel infection is suspected or CSF for suspected meningitis. Irrigation of the epidural space with 1 or 2 mL of saline after removal of the pump filter (which should be sent for culture) may help in diagnosing an epidural abscess or empyema.

TREATMENT AND PROPHYLAXIS

If infection has occurred only at the exit site and the superficial catheter tract, local drainage with aggressive cleansing (i.e., topical antibiotics and antiseptics) but without removal of the catheter was suggested.[92] Unfortunately, more severe infections developed (e.g., deep-tunnel and epidural abscess) in some of these patients. In addition, failure of "catheter-sparing" treatment also was reported.[161,308] Therefore, removal of the catheter should be considered even for mild infections if they do not respond promptly to therapy. In patients with pocket, epidural, and meningeal infections, the intrathecal pump system should be removed as soon as possible and systemic antibiotic therapy initiated (for selection of drugs and doses, see Table 85–4). With the increasing rate of multidrug-resistant staphylococci and the low CSF levels of vancomycin (only 20% to 30% of serum levels), linezolid should be considered as an alternative. Linezolid has very good CSF penetration (60-70% of the serum level) and was effective in treating severe CNS infections,[331] including intrathecal infusion pump infection.[188] Although a few studies have reported clinical improvement (and sometimes cure) of tunnel infection or meningitis with the administration of intravenous antibiotics and retention of the catheter, in many cases, the infection recurred when the treatment was stopped.[48,92] A few reports suggest successful treatment of severe pump infections (including meningitis) without removal of the pump system.[29,43,115,308,335,391,430] In some of these cases, the pathogen was considered to be of low virulence (e.g., CoNS) or colonization. In most of these cases, however, instillation of antibiotics into the reservoir with cautious flushing of the catheter was combined with systemic antibiotics. In one protocol, "intrapump therapy is started by filling the pump to the total reservoir volume with a 5-mg vancomycin/185-µg baclofen/ml solution and programming the pump to deliver an initial volume of 1 mL per day and oral baclofen therapy is initiated to prevent withdrawal. Intravenous vancomycin therapy is used concomitantly and serum trough levels are drawn to optimize the dose and to avoid toxicity."[391] The main reason for the intrathecal administration of antibiotics is to increase the level of drug in CSF. Before antibiotics are added to the baclofen infusion, their compatibility with baclofen should be verified or tested (vancomycin is compatible and can be used safely according to Zed and associates[430]).

No guidelines exist on how to treat severe infections of intrathecal pump systems, but in most cases, removal of the pump system while systemic antibiotics are given and then reimplantation appear to be the treatment of choice. In rare cases in which removal of the pump will be detrimental to the patient, a trial of intrathecal administration of antibiotics may be justified, with close observation to ensure that the patient is not getting worse.

Although many physicians use perioperative (or longer) antibiotics for prophylaxis, their efficacy in preventing infection has not been proved. Therefore, prophylactic antibiotics should not be used or, if given, should not be administered for longer than 24 to 36 hours after the operation.

REFERENCES

1. Ahlberg, A., Carlsson, A. S., and Lindberg, L.: Hematogenous infection in total joint replacement. Clin. Orthop. Relat. Res. 137:69-75, 1978.
2. Ahnfelt, L., Herberts, P., Malchau, H., and Andersson, G. B.: Prognosis of total hip replacement. A Swedish multicenter study of 4,664 revisions. Acta Orthop. Scand. Suppl. 238:1-26, 1990.
3. Ainbinder, D. J., Haik, B. G., and Tellado, M.: Hydroxyapatite orbital implants abscess: Histological correlation of an infected implant following evisceration. Ophthal. Plast. Reconstr. Surg. 10:267-270, 1994.
4. Albright, A. L.: Baclofen in the treatment of cerebral palsy. J. Child Neurol. 11:77-83, 1996.
5. Albright, A. L., and Ferson, S.: Intrathecal baclofen therapy in children. Neurosurg. Focus 21:E3, 2006.
6. Altiparmak, U. E., Ozer, P. A., Ozkuyumcu, C., et al.: Postoperative endophthalmitis caused by Bacillus cereus and Chlamydia trachomatis. J. Cataract Refract. Surg. 33:1284-1287, 2007.
7. Ammirati, M., and Raimondi, A. J.: Cerebrospinal fluid shunt infections in children. Childs Nerv. Syst. 3:106-109, 1987.
8. Anderson, C. M., Sorrells, D. L., and Kerby, J. D.: Intra-abdominal pseudocysts as a complication of ventriculoperitoneal shunts: A case report and review of the literature. Am. J. Surg. 60:338-340, 2003.
9. Anderson, H. L., III, Attorri, R. J., Custer, J. R., et al.: Extracorporeal membrane oxygenation for pediatric cardiopulmonary failure. J. Thorac. Cardiovasc. Surg. 99:1011-1021, 1990.
10. Anguita-Alonso, P., Hanssen, A. D., and Patel, R.: Prosthetic joint infection. Expert Rev. Antiinfect. Ther. 3:797-804, 2005.
11. Ankersmit, H. J., Tugulea, S., Spanier, T., et al.: Activation-induced T-cell death and immune dysfunction after implantation of left-ventricular assist device. Lancet 354:550-555, 1999.
12. Antonyshyn, O., Gruss, J. S., Mackinnon, S. E., and Zuker, R.: Complications of soft tissue expansion. Br. J. Plast. Surg. 41:239-250, 1988.
13. Arber, N., Pras, E., Copperman, Y., et al.: Pacemaker endocarditis. Report of 44 cases and review of the literature. Medicine (Baltimore) 73:299-305, 1994.
14. Argenziano, M., Catanese, K. A., Moazami, N., et al.: The influence of infection on survival and successful transplantation in patients with left ventricular assist devices. J. Heart Lung Transplant. 16:822-831, 1997.
15. Arisoy, E. S., and Demmler, G. J.: Corynebacterium xerosis ventriculoperitoneal shunt infection in an infant: Report of a case and review of the literature. Pediatr. Infect. Dis. J. 12:536-538, 1993.
16. Armstrong, R. W., Steinbok, P., Cochrane, D. D., et al.: Intrathecally administered baclofen for treatment of children with spasticity of cerebral origin. J. Neurosurg. 87:409-414, 1997.
17. Arnold, W., Bredberg, G., Gstottner, W., et al.: Meningitis following cochlear implantation: Pathomechanisms, clinical symptoms, conservative and surgical treatments. O. R. L. J. Otorhinolaryngol. Relat. Spec. 64:382-389, 2002.
18. Aucoin, P. J., Kotilainen, H. R., Gantz, N. M., et al.: Intracranial pressure monitors. Epidemiologic study of risk factors and infections. Am. J. Med. 80:369-376, 1986.
19. Austad, E. D.: Evolution of the concept of tissue expansion. Facial Plast. Surg. 5:277-279, 1988.
20. Austin, K. S., Testa, N. N., Luntz, R. K., et al.: Aspergillus infection of total knee arthroplasty presenting as a popliteal cyst. Case report and review of the literature. J. Arthroplasty 7:311-314, 1992.
21. Baier, R. E., and Dutton, R. C.: Initial events in interactions of blood with a foreign surface. J. Biomed. Mater. Res. 3:191-206, 1969.
22. Barberan, J.: Management of infections of osteoarticular prosthesis. Clin. Microbiol. Infect. 12(Suppl 3):93-101, 2006.
23. Bartlett, R. H., Roloff, D. W., Custer, J. R., et al.: Extracorporeal life support—the University of Michigan experience. J. A. M. A. 283:904-908, 2000.
24. Bayston, R., Compton, C., and Richards, K.: Production of extracellular slime by coryneforms colonizing hydrocephalus shunts. J. Clin. Microbiol. 32:1705-1709, 1994.
25. Bayston, R., and Rodgers, J.: Role of serological tests in the diagnosis of immune complex disease in infection of ventriculoatrial shunts for hydrocephalus. Eur. J. Clin. Microbiol. Infect. Dis. 13:417-420, 1994.
26. Beeler, B. A.: Infections of permanent transvenous and epicardial pacemakers in adults. Heart Lung 11:152-156, 1982.
27. Benedetti, C., McDonald, J. S., Lingam, R., and Seitz, M.: Efficacy of a Port-a-Cath epidural system for cancer pain management. Abstract. Anesthesiology 77(3A):841, 1992.
28. Bengtson, S.: Prosthetic osteomyelitis with special reference to the knee: Risks, treatment and costs. Ann. Med. 25:523-529, 1993.
29. Bennett, M. I., Tai, Y. M. A., and Symonds, J. M.: Staphylococcal meningitis following Synchromed intrathecal pump implant: A case report. Pain 56:243-244, 1994.
30. Berbari, E., Hanssen, A., Duffy, M., et al.: Prosthetic joint infection due to Mycobacterium tuberculosis: A case series and review of the literature. Am. J. Orthop. 27:219-227, 1998.
31. Berbari, E. F., Hanssen, A. D., Duffy, M. C., et al.: Risk factors for prosthetic joint infection: Case-control study. Clin. Infect. Dis. 27:1247-1254, 1998.
32. Berkowitz, R. G., Franz, B. K. H., Shepherd, R. K., et al.: Pneumococcal middle ear infections and cochlear implantation. Ann. Otol. Rhinol. Laryngol. Suppl. 128:55-56, 1987.
33. Bernstein, A. D., and Parsonnet, V.: Survey of cardiac pacing and defibrillation in the United States in 1993. Am. J. Cardiol. 78:187-196, 1996.
34. Black, M. D., Coles, J. G., Williams, W. G., et al.: Determinants of success in pediatric cardiac patients undergoing extracorporeal membrane oxygenation. Ann. Thorac. Surg. 60:133-138, 1995.
35. Bloom, H., Heeke, B., Leon, A., et al.: Renal insufficiency and the risk of infection from pacemaker or defibrillator surgery. Pacing Clin. Electrophysiol. 29:142-145, 2006.
36. Bluhm, G.: Pacemaker infections. A clinical study with special reference to prophylactic use of some isoxazolyl penicillins. Acta Med. Scand. (Suppl.) 699:1-62, 1985.
37. Bluhm, G. L.: Pacemaker infections: A 2-year follow-up of antibiotic prophylaxis. Scand. J. Thorac. Cardiovasc. Surg. 19:231-235, 1985.
38. Bolton, W. K., Sande, M. A., Normansell, D. E., et al.: Ventriculojugular shunt nephritis with Corynebacterium bovis. Am. J. Med. 59:417-423, 1975.
39. Borges, L. F.: Host defenses. Neurosurg. Clin. North Am. 3:275-278, 1992.
40. Boutin, R., Brossman, J., Sartoris, D., et al.: Update on imaging of orthopedic infections. Orthop. Clin. North Am. 29:41-46, 1998.
41. Brause, B. D.: Prosthetic joint infections. Curr. Opin. Rheumatol. 1:194-198, 1989.
42. Braxton, E. E., Jr., Ehrlich, G. D., Hall-Stoodley, L., et al.: Role of biofilms in neurosurgical device-related infections. Neurosurg. Rev. 28:249-255, 2005.
43. Brazenor, G. A.: Long term intrathecal administration of morphine: A comparison of bolus injection via reservoir with continuous infusion by implanted pump. Neurosurgery 21:484-491, 1987.
44. Bremer, A. A., and Darouiche, R. O.: Ventriculoperitoneal shunt infection due to Serratia marcescens. J Infect. 50:138-141, 2005.
45. Bruinsma, N., Stobberingh, E. E., Herpers, M. J., et al.: Subcutaneous ventricular catheter reservoir and ventriculoperitoneal drain–related infection in preterm infants and young children. Clin. Microbiol. Infect. 6:202-206, 2000.
46. Buchholz, H. W., Elson, R. A., and Heinert, K.: Antibiotic-loaded acrylic cement: Current concepts. Clin. Orthop. Relat. Res. 190:96-108, 1984.
47. Burket, J. S., Bartlett, R. H., Vander Hyde, K., and Chenoweth, C. E.: Nosocomial infections in adult patients undergoing extracorporeal membrane oxygenation. Clin. Infect. Dis. 28:828-833, 1999.
48. Byers, K., Axelrod, P., Michael, S., and Rosen, S.: Infections complicating tunneled intraspinal catheter systems used to treat chronic pain. Clin. Infect. Dis. 21:403-408, 1995.
49. Cabell, C. H., Heidenreich, P. A., Chu, V. H., et al.: Increasing rates of cardiac device infections among Medicare beneficiaries: 1990-1999. Am. Heart J. 147:582-586, 2004.
50. Cacoub, P., Leprince, P., Nataf, P., et al.: Pacemaker infective endocarditis. Am. J. Cardiol. 82:480-484, 1998.
51. Camus, C., Leport, C., Raffi, F., et al.: Sustained bacteremia in 26 patients with a permanent endocardial pacemaker: Assessment of wire removal. Clin. Infect. Dis. 17:46-55, 1993.
52. Canner, G. C., Steinberg, M. E., Heppenstall, R. B., and Balderston, R.: The infected hip after total hip arthroplasty. J. Bone Joint Surg. Am. 66:1393-1399, 1984.

53. Carlsson, A. S., Josefsson, G., and Lindberg, L.: Revision with gentamicin-impregnated cement for deep infection in total hip arthroplasties. J. Bone Joint Surg. Am. 60:1059-1064, 1978.

54. Castro, P., Soriano, A., Escrich, C., et al.: Linezolid treatment of ventriculo-peritoneal shunt infection without implant removal. Eur. J. Clin. Microbiol. Infect. Dis. 24:603-606, 2005.

55. Chahipa, E., Swarhrick, H. A., Holden, B. A., and Sjostrand, J.: Severe corneal infections associated with contact lens wear. Ophthalmology 94:17-22, 1987.

56. Chan, K. H., Mann, K. S., and Seto, W. H.: Infection of a shunt by Mycobacterium fortuitum: Case report. Neurosurgery 29:472-474, 1991.

57. Cherry, D. A., Gourlay, G. K., Counsins, M. J., and Gannon, B. J.: A technique for the insertion of an implantable portal system for the long-term epidural administration of opioids in the treatment of cancer pain. Anaesth. Intensive Care 13:145-152, 1985.

58. Choi, S. H., McComb J. G., Levy, M. L., et al.: Use of elemental iodine for shunt infection prophylaxis. Neurosurgery 52:908-913, 2003.

59. Choksey, M. S., and Malik, I. A.: Zero tolerance to shunt infections: Can it be achieved? J. Neurol. Neurosurg. Psychiatry 75:87-91, 2004.

60. Choo, M. H., Holmes, D. R., Gersh, B. J., et al.: Permanent pacemaker infections: Characterization and management. Am. J. Cardiol. 48:559-564, 1981.

61. Choux, M., Genitori, L., Lang, D., and Lena, G.: Shunt implantation: Reducing the incidence of shunt infection. J. Neurosurg. 77:875-880, 1992.

62. Chua J. D., Wilkoff, B. L., Lee, I., et al.: Diagnosis and management of infections involving implantable electrophysiologic cardiac devices. Ann. Intern. Med. 133:604-608, 2000.

63. Clark, W. K., Mulbauer, M. S., Lowrey, R., et al.: Complications of intracranial pressure monitoring in trauma patients. Neurosurgery 25:20-24, 1988.

64. Cobb, D. K., High, K. P., Sawyer, R. G., et al.: A controlled trial of scheduled replacement of central venous and pulmonary-artery catheters. N. Engl. J. Med. 327:1062-1067, 1992.

65. Cobb, T. K., and Beckenbaugh, R. D.: Biaxial total wrist arthroplasty. J. Hand Surg. [Am.] 21:1011-1021, 1996.

66. Cochrane, D. D., Kestle, J. R. W.: The influence of surgical operative experience on the duration of first ventriculoperitoneal shunt infection. Pediatr. Neurosurg. 38:295-301, 2003.

67. Cohen, E. J., Buchanan, H. W., Laughrea, P. A., et al.: Diagnosis and management of Acanthamoeba keratitis. Am. J. Ophthalmol. 100:389-395, 1985.

68. Cohen, N. L.: Cochlear implant soft surgery: Fact or fantasy? Otolaryngol. Head Neck Surg. 117:214-216, 1997.

69. Cohen, N. L., and Hoffman, R. A.: Complications of cochlear implant surgery in adults and children. Ann. Otol. Rhinol. Laryngol. 100:708-711, 1991.

70. Cohen, N. L., and Hoffman, R. A.: Surgical complications of multichannel cochlear implants in North America. In Fraysse, B., and Deguine, O. (eds.): Cochlear Implants: New Perspectives. New York, Karger, 1993, pp. 70-74.

71. Cohen, N. L., Hoffman, R. A., and Stroschein, M.: Medical or surgical complications related to the nucleus multichannel cochlear implant. Ann. Otol. Rhinol. Laryngol. 97:8-13, 1988.

72. Cohen, T. J., Pons, V. G., Schwartz, J., and Griffin, J. C.: Candida albicans pacemaker site infection. Pacing Clin. Electrophysiol. 14:146-148, 1991.

73. Constantini, S., Cotev, S., Rappaport, Z. H., et al.: Intracranial pressure monitoring after elective intracranial surgery. J. Neurosurg. 69:540-544, 1988.

74. Cotton, M. F., Hartzenberg, B., Donald, P. R., and Burger, P. J.: Ventriculoperitoneal shunt infections in children: A 6-year study. S. Afr. Med. J. 79:139-142, 1991.

75. Crawford, M. E., Andersen, H., Augustenborg, G. A., et al.: Pain treatment on outpatient basis utilizing extradural opiates: A Danish multicentre study comprising 105 patients. Pain 16:41-47, 1983.

76. Cruciani, M., Di Perri, G., Molesini, M., et al.: Use of fluconazole in the treatment of Candida albicans hydrocephalus shunt infection. Eur. J. Clin. Microbiol. Infect. Dis. 11:957-961, 1992.

77. Cuckler, J. M., Star, A. M., Alavi, A., and Noto, R. B.: Diagnosis and management of the infected total joint arthroplasty. Orthop. Clin. North Am. 22:512-530, 1991.

78. Da Costa, A., Lelievre, H., Kirkorian, G. M., et al.: Role of preaxillary flora in pacemaker infections: A prospective study. Circulation 97:1791-1795, 1998.

79. Dalton, H. J., Siewers, R. D., Fuhrman, B. P., et al.: Extracorporeal membrane oxygenation for cardiac rescue in children with severe myocardial dysfunction. Crit. Care Med. 21:1020-1028, 1993.

80. Darouiche, R. O.: Device-associated infections: A macroproblem that starts with microadherence. Clin. Infect. Dis. 33:1567-1572, 2001.

81. Darouiche, R. O., Landon, G. C., Patti, G. M., et al.: Role of Staphylococcus aureus surface adhesions in orthopaedic device infections. J. Med. Microbiol. 46:75-79, 1997.

82. Daspit, C. P.: Meningitis as a result of cochlear implant: Case report. Otolaryngol. Head Neck Surg. 105:115-116, 1991.

83. David, R., Shtarker, H., Horesh, Z., et al.: Arthrodesis with the Ilizarov device after failed knee arthroplasty. Orthopedics 24:33-36, 2001.

84. Diaz-Mitoma, F., Hardin, G. K. M., Wilson, D. J., et al.: Clinical significance of a test for slime production in ventriculoperitoneal shunt infections caused by coagulase-negative staphylococci. J. Infect. Dis. 156:555-560, 1987.

85. Dickinson, G. M., and Bisno, A. L.: Infections associated with indwelling devices: Concepts of pathogenesis; infections associated with intravascular devices. Antimicrob. Agents Chemother. 33:597-601, 1989.

86. Dickinson, G. M., and Bisno, A. L.: Infections associated with indwelling devices: Infections related to extravascular devices. Antimicrob. Agents Chemother. 33:602-607, 1989.

87. Didisheim, P., Olsen, D. B., Farrar, D. J., et al.: Infections and thromboembolism with implantable cardiovascular devices. Trans. Am. Soc. Artif. Intern. Organs 35:54-70, 1994.

88. Di Rocco, C., Marchese, E., and Velardi, F.: A survey of the first complication of newly implanted CSF shunt devices for the treatment of nontumoral hydrocephalus. Childs Nerv. Syst. 10:321-325, 1994.

89. Downing, J. E., Busch, E. H., and Stedman, P. M.: Epidural morphine delivered by a percutaneous epidural catheter for outpatient treatment of cancer pain. Anesth. Analg. 67:1159-1161, 1988.

90. Duggan, J. M., Georgiadis, G. M., and Kleshinski, J. F.: Management of prosthetic joint infections. Infect. Med. 18:534-541, 2001.

91. Duhaime, A. C., Bonner, K., McGowan, K. L., et al.: Distribution of bacteria in the operating room environment and its relation to ventricular shunt infections: A prospective study. Childs Nerv. Syst. 7:211-214, 1991.

92. Du Pen, S. L., Peterson, D. G., Williams, A., and Bogosian, A. J.: Infection during chronic epidural catheterization: Diagnosis and treatment. Anesthesiology 73:905-909, 1990.

93. Durand, M. L., Kim, I. K., D'Amico, D. J., et al.: Successful treatment of Fusarium endophthalmitis with voriconazole and Aspergillus endophthalmitis with voriconazole plus caspofungin. Am. J. Ophthalmol. 140:552-554, 2005.

94. Duus, B. R., Boeckstyns, M., and Stadeager, C.: The natural course of radio-nuclide bone scanning in the evaluation of total knee replacement—a 2 year prospective study. Clin. Radiol. 41:341-343, 1990.

95. Eggimann, P., and Waldvogel, F.: Pacemaker and defibrillator infections. In Waldvogel, F. A., and Bisno, A. L. (eds.): Infections Associated with Indwelling Medical Devices. 3rd ed. Washington, D. C., A. S. M. Press, 2000, pp. 247-264.

96. Elliott, S. P., Yogev, R., and Shulman, S. T.: Staphylococcus lugdunensis: An emerging cause of ventriculoperitoneal shunt infections. Pediatr. Neurosurg. 35:128-130, 2001.

97. Elson, R.: One-stage exchange in the treatment of the infected total hip arthroplasty. Semin. Arthroplasty 5:137-141, 1994.

98. Enger, P. O., Svendsen, F., and Wester, K.: CSF shunt infections in children: Experiences from a population-based study. Acta Neurochir. 145:243-248, 2003.

99. Ersahin, Y., McLone, D. G., Storrs, B. B., et al.: Review of 3,017 procedures for the management of hydrocephalus in children. Concepts Pediatr. Neurosurg. 9:21-33, 1989.

100. Ersahin, Y., and Yurtseven, T.: Rare complications of shunt infection. Pediatr. Neurosurg. 40:90-92, 2004.

101. Etienne, J., Charpin, B., Grando, J., et al.: Characterization of clinically significant isolates of Staphylococcus epidermidis from patients with cerebrospinal fluid shunt infections. Epidemiol. Infect. 106:467-475, 1991.

102. Faillace, W. J.: A no-touch technique protocol to diminish cerebrospinal fluid shunt infection. Surg. Neurol. 43:344-350, 1995.

103. Farber, B. F., Kaplan, M. H., and Clogston, A. G.: Staphylococcus epidermidis extracted slime inhibits the antimicrobial action of glycopeptide antibiotics. J. Infect. Dis. 161:37-40, 1988.

104. Fehring, T. K., Calton, T. F., and Griffin, W. L.: Cementless fixation in 2-stage reimplantation for periprosthetic sepsis. J. Arthroplasty 14:175-181, 1999.

105. Fischer, S. A., Trenholme, G. M., Costanzo, M. R., and Piccione, W.: Infectious complications in left ventricular assist device recipients. Clin. Infect. Dis. 24:18-23, 1997.

106. Fitzgerald, R. H., and Jones, D. R.: Hip implant infection. Am. J. Med. 78(Suppl. 6B):225-228, 1986.

107. Fitzgerald, R. H., Nolan, D. R., Ilstrup, D. M., et al.: Deep wound sepsis following total hip arthroplasty. J. Bone Joint Surg. Am. 59:847-855, 1977.

108. Forward, K. R., Fewer, H. D., and Stiver, H. G.: Cerebrospinal fluid shunt infections: A review of 35 infections in 32 patients. J. Neurosurg. 59:389-394, 1983.

109. Foster, M. R., Heppenstall, R. B., Friedenberg, Z. B., and Hozack, W. J.: A prospective assessment of nutritional status and complications in patients with fractures of the hip. J. Orthop. Trauma 4:49-57, 1990.

110. Foster, T. J., and Hook, M.: Surface protein adhesins of Staphylococcus aureus. Trends Microbiol. 6:484-488, 1998.

111. Fouyas, I. P., Case, A. T. H., Thompson, D., et al.: Use of intracranial pressure monitoring in the management of childhood hydrocephalus and shunt-related problems. Neurosurgery 38:726-732, 1996.

112. Frame, P. T., and McLaurin, R. L.: Treatment of CSF shunt infections with intrashunt plus oral antibiotic therapy. J. Neurosurg. 60:354-360, 1984.

113. Frame, R., Brodman, R. F., Furman, S., et al.: Surgical removal of infected transvenous pacemaker leads. Pacing Clin. Electrophysiol. 16:2343-2348, 1993.

114. Frazier, O. H., Rose, E. A., Macmanus, Q., et al.: Multicenter clinical evaluation of the HeartMate 1000 IP left ventricular assist device. Ann. Thorac. Surg. 53:1080-1090, 1992.

115. Galloway, A., and Falope, F. Z.: Pseudomonas aeruginosa infection in an intrathecal baclofen pump: Successful treatment with adjunct intra-reservoir gentamicin. Spinal Cord 38:126-128, 2000.

116. Gandelman G., Frishman W. H., Wiese, C., et al.: Intravascular device infections. Cardiol. Rev. 15:13-23, 2007.

117. Gardner, B.: Intrathecal baclofen—a multicentre clinical comparison of the Medtronics Programmable, Cordis Sector, and constant infusion Infusaid drug delivery systems. Paraplegia 33:551-554, 1995.

118. Gardner, P., Leipzig, T., and Phillips, P.: Infections of central nervous system shunts. Symposium on infections of the central nervous system. Med. Clin. North Am. 69:297-314, 1985.

119. Garvin, K. L., and Hanssen, A. D.: Infection after total hip arthroplasty. Past, present, and future. J. Bone Joint Surg. Am. 77:1576-1588, 1995.

120. Garvin, K. L., Salvati, E. A., and Brause, B. D.: Role of gentamicin-impregnated cement in total joint arthroplasty. J. Bone Joint Surg. Am. 65:1081-1086, 1988.

121. Gaskill, S. J., and Marlin, A. E.: Spontaneous bacterial peritonitis in patients with ventriculoperitoneal shunts. Pediatr. Neurosurg. 26:115-119, 1997.

122. Geers, T. A., and Gordon, S. M.: Clinical significance of Candida species isolated from cerebrospinal fluid following neurosurgery. Clin. Infect. Dis. 28:1139-1147, 1999.

123. Gibstein, L. A., Abramson, D. L., Bartlett, R. A., et al.: Tissue expansion in children: A retrospective study of complications. Ann. Plast. Surg. 38:358-364, 1997.

124. Gillespie, W. J.: Infection in total joint replacement. Infect. Dis. Clin. North Am. 4:465-484, 1990.

125. Glasgow, B. J., Weinberg, D. A., Shorr, N., and Goldberg, R. A.: Draining cutaneous fistula associated with infections of hydroxyapatite orbital implant. Ophthal. Plast. Reconstr. Surg. 12:131-135, 1996.

126. Glatt, H. J., Googe, P. B., Powers, T., and Apple, D. J.: Anophthalmic socket pain. Am. J. Ophthalmol. 116:357-362, 1993.

127. Gold, M. R., Peters, R. W., and Johnson, J. W. Complications associated with pectoral implantation of cardioverter defibrillators. Pacing Clin. Electrophysiol. 20:208-211, 1997.

128. Goldberg, S. P., Baddley, J. W., Aaron, M. F., et al.: Fungal infections in ventricular assist devices. A. S. A. I. O. J. 46:S37-S40, 2000.

129. Gooch, J. L., Oberg, W. A., Grams, B., et al.: Complications of intrathecal baclofen pumps in children. Pediatr. Neurosurg. 39:1-6, 2003.

130. Gordon, S. M., Schmitt, S. K., Jacobs, M., et al.: Nosocomial bloodstream infections in patients with implantable left ventricular assist devices. Ann. Thorac. Surg. 72:725-730, 2001.

131. Govaerts, P. J., De Beukelaer, C., Daemers, K., et al.: Outcome of cochlear implantation at different ages from 0 to 6 years. Otol. Neurotol. 23:885-890, 2002.

132. Govender, S. T., Med, M., Nathoo, N., and Van Dellen, J. R.: Evaluation of an antibiotic-impregnated shunt system for the treatment of hydrocephalus. J. Neurosurg. 99:831-839, 2003.

133. Gower, D. J., Crone, K., Alexander, E., and Kelly, D. L.: Candida albicans shunt infection: Report of two cases. Neurosurgery 19:111-113, 1986.

134. Gower, D. J., Gower, V. C., Richardson, S. H., and Kelly, D. L.: Reduced bacterial adherence to silicone plastic neurosurgical prosthesis. Pediatr. Neurosci. 12:127-133, 1985.

135. Grabb, P. A., and Albright, A. I.: Intraventricular vancomycin–induced cerebrospinal fluid eosinophilia: Report of two patients. Neurosurgery 30:630-635, 1992.

136. Gray, E. D., Peters, G., Verstegen, M., and Regelmann, W. E.: Effect of extracellular slime substance from Staphylococcus epidermidis on the human cellular immune response. Lancet 1:365-367, 1984.

137. Greene, K. A., Clark, R. J., and Zabramski, J. M.: Ventricular CSF shunt infections associated with Corynebacterium jeikeium: Report of three cases and review. Clin. Infect. Dis. 16:139-141, 1993.

138. Griffith, M. J., Mounsey, J. P., Bexton, R. S., and Holden, M. P.: Mechanical, but not infective, pacemaker erosion may be successfully managed by reimplantation of pacemakers. Br. Heart J. 71:202-205, 1994.

139. Gristina, A. G., and Kolkin, J.: Total joint replacement and sepsis. J. Bone Joint Surg. Am. 65:128-134, 1993.

140. Grogler, F. M., Frank, G., Greven, G., et al.: Complications of permanent transvenous cardiac pacing. J. Thorac. Cardiovasc. Surg. 69:895-904, 1975.

141. Gruninger, R. P.: Diagnostic microbiology in bone and joint infections. In Gustilo, R. B. (ed.): Orthopaedic Infection: Diagnosis and Treatment. Philadelphia, W. B. Saunders, 1989, pp. 42-51.

142. Guevara, J. A., Zuccaro, G., Trevisan, B. S., and Denoya, C. D.: Bacterial adhesion to cerebrospinal fluid shunts. J. Neurosurg. 67:438-445, 1987.

143. Gutow, A. P., and Wolfe, S. W.: Infection following total elbow arthroplasty. Hand Clin. 10:521-529, 1994.

144. Hader, W. J., and Steinbok, P.: The value of routine cultures of the cerebrospinal fluid in patients with external ventricular drains. Neurosurgery. 46:1149-1155, 2000.

145. Haines, S. J., and Walters, B. C.: Antibiotic prophylaxis for cerebrospinal fluid shunts: A metaanalysis. Neurosurgery 34:87-92, 1994.

146. Hanekom, W., and Yogev, R.: Diagnosis and management of CSF shunt infections. Adv. Pediatr. Infect. Dis. 11:29-54, 1995.

147. Hanlo, P. W., Cinalli, G., Vandertop, W. P., et al.: Treatment of hydrocephalus determined by the European Orbis Sigma Valve II survey: A multicenter prospective 5 year shunt survival study in children and adults in whom a flow-regulating shunt was used. J. Neurosurg. 99:52-57, 2003.

148. Hanssen, A. D., and Rand, J. A.: Evaluation and treatment of infection at the site of a total hip or knee arthroplasty. J. Bone Joint Surg. Am. 80:910-922, 1998.

149. Harcombe, A. A., Newell, S. A., Ludman, P. F., et al.: Late complications following permanent pacemaker implantation or elective unit replacement. Heart 80:240-244, 1998.

150. Harjula, A., Jarvinen, A., Virtanen, K. S., and Mattila, S.: Pacemaker infections—treatment with total or partial pacemaker system removal. Thorac. Cardiovasc. Surg. 33:218-220, 1985.

151. Hayhurst, C., Cooke, R., Williams, D., et al.: The impact of antibiotic-impregnated catheters on shunt infection in children and neonates. Childs Nerv. Syst. on line, Oct. 26, 2007.

152. Hebert, C. K., Williams, R. E., Levy, R. S., and Barrack, R. L.: Cost of treating an infected total knee replacement. Clin. Orthop. Relat. Res. 331:140-145, 1996.

153. Heimberger, T. S., and Duma, R. J.: Infections of prosthetic heart valves and cardiac pacemakers. Infect. Dis. Clin. North Am. 3:221-245, 1989.

154. Helman, D. N., Morales, D. L., Edwards, N. M., et al.: Left ventricular assist device bridge-to-transplant network improves survival after failed cardiotomy. Ann. Thorac. Surg. 68:1187-1194, 1999.

155. Hickman, K. M., Mayer, B. L., and Muwaswes, M.: Intracranial pressure monitoring: Review of risk factors associated with infection. Heart Lung 19:84-90, 1990.

156. Hildick-Smith, D. J., Lowe, M. D., Newell, S. A., et al.: Ventricular pacemaker upgrade: Experience, complications and recommendations. Heart 79:383-387, 1998.

157. Hirst, L. W., Green, W. R., Merz, W., et al.: Management of Acanthamoeba keratitis: A case report and a review of the literature. Ophthalmology 91:1105-1111, 1984.

158. Hoffman, R. A.: Cochlear implant in the child under two years of age: Skull growth, otitis media, and selection. Otolaryngol. Head Neck Surg. 117:217-219, 1997.

159. Hoffman, R. A., and Cohen, N. L.: Complications of cochlear implant surgery. Ann. Otol. Rhinol. Laryngol. 104(Suppl. 166):420-422, 1995.

160. Hofmann, A. A., Wyatt, R. W., Daniels, A., et al.: Bone scans after total knee arthroplasty in asymptomatic patients. Cemented versus cementless. Clin. Orthop. Relat. Res. 251:183-188, 1990.

161. Hogan, Q., Haddox, J. D., Abram, S., et al.: Epidural opiates and local anesthetics for the management of cancer pain. Pain 46:271-279, 1991.

162. Holloway, K. L., Barnes, T., Choi, S., et al.: Ventriculostomy infections: The effect of monitoring duration and catheter exchange in 584 patients. J. Neurosurg. 85:419-424, 1996.

163. Holman, W. L., Murrah, C. P., Ferguson, E. R., et al.: Infections during extended circulatory support: University of Alabama at Birmingham experience. Ann. Thorac. Surg. 61:366-371, 1996.

164. Holt, R. J.: Bacteriological studies on colonised ventriculoatrial shunts. Dev. Med. Child Neurol. 12(Suppl. 22):83-87, 1970.

165. Hong, S. W., Paik, J. S., Kim, S. Y., et al.: A case of orbital abscess following porous orbital implant infection. Korean J. Ophthalmol. 20:234-237, 2006.

166. Horgan, M. A., and Piatt, J. H., Jr.: Shaving of the scalp may increase the rate of infection in CSF shunt surgery. Pediatr. Neurosurg. 26:180-184, 1997.

167. Hornyik, G., and Piatt, J. H., Jr.: Cerebrospinal fluid shunt infection by Neisseria sicca. Pediatr. Neurosurg. 21:189-191, 1994.

168. House, W. F., Luxford, W. M., and Courtney, B.: Otitis media in children following cochlear implant. Ear Hear. 6(Suppl.):24-26, 1985.

169. Howden, B. P., Johnson, P. D., Charles, P. G., and Grayson, M. L.: Failure of vancomycin for treatment of methicillin-resistant Staphylococcus aureus infections. Clin. Infect. Dis. 39:1544-1545, 2004.

170. Hussain, M., Wilcox, M. H., and White, P. J.: The slime of coagulase-negative staphylococci: Biochemistry and relation to adherence. F. E. M. S. Microbiol. Rev. 10:191-207, 1993.

171. Iconomou, T. G., Michelow, B. J., and Zuker, R. M.: Tissue expansion in the pediatric patient. Ann. Plast. Surg. 31:134-140, 1993.

172. Ingram, C. W., Haywood, H. B., III, Morris, V. M., et al.: Cryptococcal ventricular-peritoneal shunt infection: Clinical and epidemiological evaluation of two closely associated cases. Infect. Control Hosp. Epidemiol. 14:719-722, 1993.

173. Inman, R. D., Gallegos, K. V., Brause, P. B., et al.: Clinical and microbial features of prosthetic joint infection. Am. J. Med. 77:47-53, 1984.

174. Itescu, S., Ankersmit, J. H., Kocher, A. A., et al.: Immunobiology of left ventricular assist devices. Prog. Cardiovasc. Dis. 43:67-80, 2000.

175. Ito, J., Fujino, K., Okumura, T., et al.: Surgical difficulties and postoperative problems associated with cochlear implants. Ann. Otol. Rhinol. Laryngol. 104(Suppl. 166):425-426, 1995.

176. Jackler, R. K., O'Donoghue, G. M., and Schindler, R. A.: Cochlear implantation: Strategies to protect the implanted cochlea from middle ear infection. Ann. Otol. Rhinol. Laryngol. 95:66-70, 1986.

177. Jacobs, D. G., and Westerband, A.: Antibiotic prophylaxis for intracranial pressure monitors. Natl. Med. Assoc. 90:417-423, 1998.

178. James, H. E., Walsh, J. W., Wilson, H. D., and Connor, J. D.: Management of CSF shunt infection: A clinical experience. Monogr. Neurol. Sci. 8:75-77, 1982.

179. James, H. E., Walsh, J. W., Wilson, H. D., et al.: A prospective randomized study of therapy in cerebrospinal fluid shunt infection. Neurosurgery 7:459-463, 1980.

180. James, P. J., Butcher, I. A., Gardner, E. R., and Hamblen, D. L.: Methicillin-resistant Staphylococcus epidermidis in infection in hip arthroplasties. J. Bone Joint Surg. Br. 76:725-727, 1994.

181. Jenkins, J. G., Glasgow, J. F. T., Black, G. W., et al.: Reye's syndrome: Assessment of ICP monitoring. B. M. J. *294*:337-338, 1987.

182. Jensen, J. E., Jensen, T. G., Smith, T. K., et al.: Nutrition in orthopaedics. J. Bone Joint Surg. Am. *64*:1263-1272, 1982.

183. Jiminez, D. F., Keating, R., and Goodrich, J. T.: Silicone allergy in ventriculoperitoneal shunts. Childs Nerv. Syst. *10*:59-63, 1994.

184. Johnson, G. M., Lee, D. A., Regelmann, W. E., et al.: Interference with granulocyte function by *Staphylococcus epidermidis* slime. Infect. Immun. *54*:13-20, 1986.

185. Jones, R. F. C., Stening, W. A., Kwok, B. C. T., and Sands, T. M.: Third ventriculostomy for shunt infections in children. Neurosurgery *32*:855-859, 1993.

186. Jordan, D. R., Brownstein, S., and Shivinder, S. J.: Abscessed hydroxyapatite orbital implants: A report of two cases. Ophthalmology *103*:1784-1787, 1996.

187. Kaitreider, S. A., and Newman, S. A.: Prevention and management of complications associated with the hydroxyapatite implant. Ophthal. Plast. Reconstr. Surg. *12*:18-31, 1996.

188. Kallweit, U., Harzheim, M., Markleni, G., et al.: Successful treatment of methicillin-resistant *Staphylococcus aureus* meningitis using linezolid without removal of intrathecal infusion pump. J. Neurosurg. *107*:651-653, 2007.

189. Kan, P., and Kestle, J.: Lack of efficacy of antibiotic-impregnated shunt systems in preventing shunt infections in children. Childs Nerv. Syst. *23*:773-777, 2007.

190. Kanter, R. K., Weiner, L. B., Patti, A. M., et al.: Infectious complications and duration of intracranial pressure monitoring. Crit. Care Med. *13*:837-839, 1985.

191. Kantor, S. G., Schneider, R., Insall, J. N., and Becker, M. W.: Radionuclide imaging of asymptomatic versus symptomatic total knee arthroplasties. Clin. Orthop. Relat. Res. *260*:118-123, 1990.

192. Karsloglu, S., Serin, D., Simsek, I., et al.: Implant infection in porous orbital implants. Ophthal. Plast. Reconstr. Surg. *22*:461-466, 2006.

193. Kasirajan, V., McCarthy, P. M., Hoercher, K. J., et al.: Clinical experience with long-term use of implantable left ventricular assist devices: Indications, implantation, and outcomes. Semin. Thorac. Cardiovasc. Surg. *12*:229-237, 2000.

194. Kearney, R. A., Eisen, H. J., and Wolf, J. E.: Nonvalvular infections of the cardiovascular system. Ann. Intern. Med. *121*:219-230, 1994.

195. Kennergren, C.: Impact of implant techniques on complications with current implantable cardioverter-defibrillator systems. Am. J. Cardiol. *78*(Suppl. 5A):15-20, 1996.

196. Kestle, J. R. W., Cochrane, D. D., and Drake, J. M.: Shunt insertion in the summer: Is it safe? Pediatr. Neurosurg. *105*:165-168, 2006.

197. Kestle, J. R. W., Garton, H. J. L., Whitehead, W. E., et al.: Management of shunt infections: A multicenter pilot study. J. Neurosurg. *105*(3 Suppl.):177-181, 2006.

198. Kestle, J. R. W., Hoffman, H. J., Soloniuk, D., et al.: A concerted effort to prevent shunt infection. Childs Nerv. Syst. *9*:163-165, 1993.

199. Ketoff, J., Klein, R. L., and Maukkassa, K. F.: Ventricular cholecystic shunts in children. J. Pediatr. Surg. *32*:181-183, 1997.

200. Klibanov, O. M., Filicko, J. E., DeSimone, J. A., Jr., and Tice, D. S.: Sensorineural hearing loss associated with intrathecal vancomycin. Ann. Pharmacother. *37*:61-65, 2003.

201. Klug, D., Lacroix, D., Savoye, C., et al.: Systemic infection related to endocarditis on pacemaker leads: Clinical presentation and management. Circulation *95*:2098-2107, 1997.

202. Kocis, K. C.: Pediatric cardiac extracorporeal membrane oxygenation: Supporting life or prolonging death? Crit. Care Med. *28*:594-595, 2000.

203. Kofler, M., Kronenberg, M. F., Rifici, C., et al.: Epileptic seizures associated with intrathecal baclofen application. Neurology *44*:25-27, 1994.

204. Kontny, U., Höfling, B., and Gutjahr, P.: CSF shunt infections in children. Infection *21*:89-95, 1993.

205. Kramer, L., Rojas-Corona, R. R., Sheff, D., and Eisenberg, E. S.: Disseminated aspergillosis and pacemaker endocarditis. Pacing Clin. Electrophysiol. *8*:225-229, 1985.

206. Kristinsson, J. K., Sigurdsson, H., Sigfusson, A., et al.: Detection of orbital implant infection with technetium 99m–labeled leukocytes. Ophthal. Plast. Reconstr. Surg. *13*:256-258, 1997.

207. Kulik, T. J., Moler, F. W., Palmisano, J. M., et al.: Outcome-associated factors in pediatric patients treated with extracorporeal membrane oxygenator after cardiac surgery. Circulation *94*(Suppl. II):63-68, 1996.

208. Kulkarni, A. V., Drake, J. M., and Lamberti-Pasculli, M.: Cerebrospinal fluid shunt infection: A prospective study of risk factors. J. Neurosurg. *94*:195-201, 2001.

209. Kumar, R., Sahay, S., Gaur, B., and Singh, V.: Ascites in ventriculoperitoneal shunt. Indian J. Pediatr. *70*:859-864, 2003.

210. Kusumoto, F. M., and Goldschlager, N.: Cardiac pacing. N. Engl. J. Med. *334*:89-97, 1996.

211. Lai, K. K., and Fontecchio, S. A.: Infections associated with implantable cardioverter-defibrillators placed transvenously and via thoracotomies: Epidemiology, infection control, and management. Clin. Infect. Dis. *27*:265-269, 1998.

212. Lan, C. C., Wong, T. T., Chen, S. J., et al.: Early diagnosis of ventriculoperitoneal shunt infections and malfunctions in children with hydrocephalus. J. Microbiol. Immunol. Infect. *36*:47-50, 2003.

213. Lee, S. H., Oh, J. H., Lee, K. S., et al.: Infection after prosthetic reconstruction in limb salvage surgery. Int. Orthop. *26*:179-184, 2002.

214. Lee, T., Kerr, R. S., and Adams, C. B.: *Pasteurella multocida*: A rare case of shunt infection. Br. J. Neurosurg. *4*:237-239, 1990.

215. Leggiadro, R. J., Atluru, V. L., and Katz, S. P.: Meningococcal meningitis associated with cerebrospinal fluid shunts. Pediatr. Infect. Dis. J. *3*:489-490, 1984.

216. Legoupil, N., Ronco, P., and Berenbaum, F.: Arthritis-related shunt nephritis in an adult. Rheumatology *42*:698-699, 2003.

217. Lewis, A. B., Hayes, D. L., Holmes, D. R., Jr., et al.: Update on infections involving permanent pacemakers. Characterization and management. J. Thorac. Cardiovasc. Surg. *89*:758-763, 1985.

218. Leyden, J. J., McGinley, K. J., Mills, O. H., and Kligman, A. M.: Age-related changes in the resident bacterial flora of the human face. J. Invest. Dermatol. *65*:379-381, 1975.

219. Lidofsky, S. P., Bass, N. M., Prage, M. C., et al.: Intracranial pressure monitoring and liver transplantation for fulminant hepatic failure. Hepatology *16*:1-4, 1992.

220. Lidwell, O. M., Lowbury, E. J. L., Whyte, W., et al.: Effect of ultraclean air in operating rooms on deep sepsis in the joint after total hip or knee replacement: A randomized study. B. M. J. *250*:99-102, 1982.

221. Lidwell, O. M., Lowbury, E. J. L., Whyte, W., et al.: Airborne contamination of wounds in joint replacement operations: The relationship to sepsis rates. J. Hosp. Infect. *4*:111-131, 1983.

222. Lieberman, J. R., Callaway, G. H., Salvati, E. A., et al.: Treatment of the infected total hip arthroplasty with a two-stage reimplantation protocol. Clin. Orthop. Relat. Res. *301*:205-212, 1994.

223. Lozier, A. P., Sciacca, R. R., Romagnoli, M. F., and Connolly, E. S.: Ventriculostomy-related infections: A critical review of the literature. Neurosurgery *51*:170-182, 2002.

224. Luer, M. S., and Hatton, J.: Vancomycin administration into the cerebrospinal fluid: A review. Ann. Pharmacother. *27*:912-921, 1993.

225. Luerssen, T. G.: Intracranial pressure: Current status in monitoring and management. Semin. Pediatr. Neurol. *4*:146-153, 1997.

226. Luessenhop, C. P., Higgins, L. D., Brause, B. D., and Ranawat, C. S.: Multiple prosthetic infections after total joint arthroplasty. Risk factor analysis. J. Arthroplasty *11*:862-868, 1996.

227. Luntz, M., Hodges, A. V., Balkany, T., et al.: Otitis media in children with cochlear implants. Laryngoscope *106*:1403-1405, 1995.

228. Luthardt, T.: Bacterial infections in ventriculo-auricular shunt systems. Dev. Med. Child Neurol. *12*(Suppl. 22):105-109, 1970.

229. Lutwick, L. I., Vaghjimal, A., and Connolly, M. W.: Postcardiac surgery infections. Crit. Care Clin. *14*:221-250, 1998.

230. Luxford, W. M., and House, W. F.: House 3M cochlear implant: Surgical considerations. *In* Clark, G. M., and Busby, P. A. (eds.): International Cochlear Implant Symposium and Workshop-Melbourne, 1985. Ann. Otol. Rhinol. Laryngol. *96*(Suppl. 128):12-14, 1987.

231. Lyons, C. W., Berquist, T. H., Lyons, J. C., et al.: Evaluation of radiographic findings in painful hip arthroplasties. Clin. Orthop. Relat. Res. *195*:239-251, 1985.

232. Lyons, M. K., and Meyer, F. B.: Cerebrospinal fluid physiology and the management of increased intracranial pressure. Mayo Clin. Proc. *65*:684-707, 1990.

233. Maderazo, E. G., Judson, S., and Pasternak, H.: Late infections of total joint prostheses. A review and recommendations for prevention. Clin. Orthop. Relat. Res. *229*:131-142, 1988.

234. Mahan, J., Selgison, D., Henry, S. L., et al.: Factors in pin tract infections. Orthopedics *14*:305-308, 1991.

235. Manders, E. K., Schenden, M. J., Furrey, J. A., et al.: Soft-tissue expansion: Concepts and complications. Plast. Reconstr. Surg. *74*:493-507, 1984.

236. Marculescu, C. E., Berbari, E. F., Cockerill, F. R., III, and Osmon, D. R.: Fungi, mycobacteria, zoonotic and other organisms in prosthetic joint infection. Clin. Orthop. Relat. Res. *451*:64-72, 2006.

237. Mason, A. C., Davison, S. P., and Manders, E. K.: Tissue expander infections in children: Look beyond the expander pocket. Ann. Plast. Surg. *43*:539-541, 1999.

238. Mates, S., Glaser, J., and Shapiro, K.: Treatment of cerebrospinal fluid shunt infections with medical therapy alone. Neurosurgery *11*:781-783, 1982.

239. Matieli, L. C., De Freitas, D., Samparo, J., et al.: *Mycobacterium abscessus* endophthalmitis: Treatment dilemma and review of the literature. Retina *26*:826-829, 2006.

240. May, A. K., Fleming, S. B., Carpenter, R. O., et al.: Influence of broad-spectrum antibiotic prophylaxis on intracranial pressure monitor infections and subsequent infectious complications in head-injured patients. Surg. Infect. *7*:409-417, 2006.

241. Mayhall, C. G., Archer, N. H., Lamb, V. A., et al.: Ventriculostomy-related infections: A prospective epidemiologic study. N. Engl. J. Med. *310*:553-559, 1984.

242. McBride, L. R., Ruzevich, S. A., Pennington, D. G., et al.: Infectious complications associated with ventricular assist device support. Trans. Am. Soc. Artif. Intern. Organs *33*:201-202, 1994.

243. McCarthy, P. M., Portner, P. M., Oyer, P. E., et al.: Clinical experience with the Novacor ventricular assist system: Bridge-to-transplant and the transition to chronic application. J. Thorac. Cardiovasc. Surg. *102*:578-587, 1991.

244. McCarthy, P. M., Schmitt, S. K., Vargo, R. L., et al.: Implantable LVAD infections: Implications for permanent use of the device. Ann. Thorac. Surg. 61:359-365, 1996.

245. McCarthy, P. M., Smedira, N. O., Vargo, R. L., et al.: One hundred patients with the HeartMate left ventricular assist device: Evolving concepts and technology. J. Thorac. Cardiovasc. Surg. 115:904-912, 1998.

246. McCarthy, P. M., Wang, N., and Vargo, R.: Preperitoneal insertion of the HeartMate 1000 IP implantable left ventricular assist device. Ann. Thorac. Surg. 57:634-638, 1994.

247. McClinton, D., Carraccio, C., and Englander, R.: Predictors of ventriculo-peritoneal shunt pathology. Pediatr. Infect. Dis. J. 20:593-597, 2001.

248. McGirt, M. J., Leveque, J. C., Wellons, J. C., 3rd., et al.: Cerebrospinal fluid shunt survival and etiology of failures: A seven year institutional experience. Pediatr. Neurosurg. 36:248-255, 2002.

249. McGirt, M. J., Zaas, A., Fuchs, H. E., et al.: Risk factors for pediatric ventriculoperitoneal shunt infection and predictors of infectious pathogens. Clin. Infect. Dis. 36:858-862, 2003.

250. McLone, D. G., Czyzewski, D., Raimondi, A. J., and Sommers, R. C.: Central nervous system infections as a limiting factor in the intelligence of children with myelomeningocoele. Pediatrics 70:338-342, 1982.

251. Meehan, A. M., Osmon, D. R., Duffy, C. T., et al.: Outcome of penicillin-susceptible streptococcal prosthetic joint infection treated with debridement and retention of the prosthesis. Clin. Infect. Dis. 36:845-849, 2003.

252. Menderes, A., Ayden, O. E., Vayvada, H., et al.: Aerobic *Actinomyces* spp. infection with a silicone tissue expander: A case report. J. Plast. Reconstr. Aesthet. Surg. 59:560-561, 2006.

253. Miley, G. B., Scheller, A. D. J., and Turner, R. H.: Medical and surgical treatment of the septic hip with one-stage revision arthroplasty. Clin. Orthop. Relat. Res. 170:76-82, 1982.

254. Miller, J. D., Becker, D. P., Ward, J. D., et al.: Significance of intracranial hypertension in severe head injury. J. Neurosurg. 47:503-516, 1977.

255. Mine, S., Sato, A., Yamaura, A., et al.: Eosinophilia of the cerebrospinal fluid in a case of shunt infection: Case report. Neurosurgery 19:835-836, 1986.

256. Modic, M., Pflanze, W., Feiglin, D., and Belhobek, G.: Magnetic resonance imaging of musculoskeletal infections. Radiol. Clin. North Am. 24:247-258, 1986.

257. Mojcik, C. F., and Levy, J. H.: Aprotinin and the systemic inflammatory response after cardiopulmonary bypass. Ann. Thorac. Surg. 71:745-754, 2001.

258. Mokaddem, A., Bachraoui, K., Sdiri, W., et al.: Pacemaker infections. Tunis. Med. 80:509-514, 2002.

259. Molina, J. E.: Undertreatment and overtreatment of patients with infected antiarrhythmic implantable devices. Ann. Thorac. Surg. 63:504-509, 1997.

260. Montgomery, V. L., Strotman, J. M., and Ross, M. P.: Impact of multiple organ system dysfunction and nosocomial infections on survival of children treated with extracorporeal membrane oxygenation after heart surgery. Crit. Care Med. 28:526-531, 2000.

261. Moore, M. B., McCully, J. P., Luckenback, M., et al.: *Acanthamoeba* keratitis associated with soft contact lenses. Am. J. Ophthalmol. 100:396-403, 1985.

262. Moorman, J. R., Steinbergen, C., Durack, D. T., et al.: *Aspergillus* infection of a permanent ventricular pacing lead. Pacing Clin. Electrophysiol. 7:361-366, 1984.

263. Morgan, G., Ginks, W., Siddons, H., and Leatham, A.: Septicemia in patients with an endocardial pacemaker. Am. J. Cardiol. 44:221-224, 1979.

264. Morissette, I., Gourdeau, M., and Francoeur, J.: CSF shunt infections: A fifteen-year experience with emphasis on management and outcome. Can. J. Neurol. Sci. 20:118-122, 1993.

265. Mornadi, M., Zembo, M. M., and Ciotti, M.: Infected tibial pseudarthrosis: A 2-year follow-up on patients treated by the Ilizarov technique. Orthopedics 12:497-502, 1989.

266. Morrice, J. J., and Young, D. G.: Bacterial colonisation of Holter valves: A ten-year survey. Dev. Med. Child Neurol. 16(Suppl. 32):85-90, 1974.

267. Motta, F., Buonaguro, V., and Stignani, C.: The use of intrathecal baclofen pump implants in children and adolescents: Safety and complications in 200 consecutive cases. J. Neurosurg. 107(1 Suppl.):32-35, 2007.

268. Mounsey, J. P., Griffith, M. J., Tynan, M., et al.: Antibiotic prophylaxis in permanent pacemaker implantation: A prospective randomised trial. Br. Heart J. 72:339-343, 1994.

269. Muers, M. F., Arnold, A. G., and Sleight, P.: Prophylactic antibiotics for cardiac pacemaker implantation: A prospective trial. Br. Heart J. 46:539-544, 1981.

270. Murray, W. R.: Use of antibiotic-containing bone cement. Clin. Orthop. Relat. Res. 190:89-95, 1984.

271. Myers, T. J., Khan, T., and Frazier, O. H.: Infectious complications associated with ventricular assist systems. A. S. A. I. O. J. 46:S28-S36, 2000.

272. Nahabedran, M. Y., Tsangans, R., Momen, B., et al.: Infectious complications following breast reconstruction with expanders and implants. Plast. Reconstr. Surg. 112:467-476, 2003.

273. Narayan, R. K., Kishore, P. R. S., Becker, D. P., et al.: Intracranial pressure: To monitor or not to monitor? A review of our experience with severe head injury. J. Neurosurg. 56:650-659, 1982.

274. Naveira, F. A., Speight, K. L., and Rauck, R. L., et al.: Meningitis after injection of intrathecal baclofen. Anesth. Analg. 82:1297-1299, 1996.

275. Nelson, J. D.: Cerebrospinal fluid shunt infections. Pediatr. Infect. Dis. 3(Suppl.):30-32, 1984.

276. Nicholas, J. L., Kamal, I. M., and Eckstein, H. B.: Immediate shunt replacement in the treatment of bacterial colonisation of Holter valves. Dev. Med. Child Neurol. 12(Suppl. 22):110-113, 1970.

277. NIH consensus conference. Cochlear implants in adults and children. J. A. M. A. 274:1955-1961, 1995.

278. Nijhof, M. W., Oyen, W. J., van Kampen, A., et al.: Hip and knee arthroplasty infection. In 111-IgG scintigraphy in 102 cases. Acta Orthop. Scand. 68:332-336, 1997.

279. Nitescu, P., Hultman, E., Appelgren, L., et al.,: Bacteriology, drug stability and exchange of percutaneous delivery systems and antibacterial filters in long-term intrathecal infusion of opioid drugs and bupivacaine in "refractory" pain. Clin. J. Pain 8:324-337, 1992.

280. North, B., and Reilly, P.: Comparison among three methods of intracranial pressure recording. Neurosurgery 18:730-732, 1986.

281. O'Brien, M., Parent, A., and Davis, B.: Management of ventricular shunt infections. Childs Brain 5:304-309, 1979.

282. Ohrstrom, J. K., Skou, J. K., Ejlertsen, T., and Kosteljanetz, M.: Infected ventriculostomy: Bacteriology and treatment. Acta Neurochir. (Wien) 100:67-69, 1989.

283. O'Keeffe, P. T., and Bayston, R.: Pneumococcal meningitis in a child with a ventriculoperitoneal shunt. J. Infect. 22:77-79, 1991.

284. Olsen, L., and Frykberg, T.: Complications in the treatment of hydrocephalus in children. Acta Paediatr. Scand. 72:385-390, 1983.

285. Onofrio, B. M., and Yaksh, T. L.: Long-term pain relief produced by intrathecal morphine infusion in 53 patients. J. Neurosurg. 72:200-204, 1992.

286. O'Nunain, S., Perez, I., Roelke, M., et al.: The treatment of patients with infected implantable cardioverter-defibrillator systems. J. Thorac. Cardiovasc. Surg. 113:121-129, 1997.

287. Owen, R. J., Harper, W. M., Finlay, D. B., and Belton, I. P.: Isotope bone scans in patients with painful knee replacements: Do they alter management? Br. J. Radiol. 68:1204-1207, 1995.

288. Oz, M. C., Argenziano, M., Catanese, K. A., et al.: Bridge experience with long-term implantable left ventricular assist devices: Are they an alternative to transplantation? Circulation 95:1844-1852, 1997.

289. Page, E. L., and Eby, T. L.: Meningitis after cochlear implantation in Mondini malformation. Otolaryngol. Head Neck Surg. 116:104-106, 1997.

290. Paley, D., Chaludray, M., Pirone, M., et al.: Treatment of malunions and mal-nonunions of the femur and tibia by detailed preoperative planning and the Ilizarov techniques. Orthop. Clin. North Am. 21:667-679, 1990.

291. Pankowsky, D. A., Ziats, N. P., Topham, N. S., et al.: Morphologic characteristics of absorbed human plasma proteins on vascular grafts and biomaterials. J. Vasc. Surg. 11:599-606, 1990.

292. Papagelopoulos, P. J., Hay, J. E., Galanis, E., and Morrey, B. F.: Infection around joint replacements in patients who have a renal or liver transplantation. J. Bone Joint Surg. Am. 80:607-608, 1998.

293. Papo, I., and Caruselli, G.: Long-term intracranial pressure monitoring in comatose patients suffering from head injuries: A critical survey. Acta Neurochir. (Wien) 39:187-200, 1977.

294. Patel, R., Osmon, D. R., and Hanssen, A. D.: The diagnosis of prosthetic joint infection: Current techniques and emerging technologies. Clin. Orthop. Relat. Res. 437:55-58, 2005.

295. Patrick, D., Marcotte, P., and Garber, G. E.: Acute abdomen in the patient with a ventriculoperitoneal shunt. Can. J. Surg. 33:37-40, 1990.

296. Pearson, R. L., and Perry, C. R.: The Ilizarov technique in the treatment of infected tibial nonunions. Orthop. Rev. 18:609-626, 1989.

297. Penn, R. A.: Intrathecal baclofen for spasticity of spinal origin. Seven years of experience. J. Neurosurg. 77:236-240, 1992.

298. Pennington, D. G., McBride, L. R., Peigh, P. S., et al.: Eight years' experience with bridging to cardiac transplantation. J. Thorac. Cardiovasc. Surg. 107:472-481, 1994.

299. Perry, H. E., Wright, R. O., Shannon, M. W., et al.: Baclofen overdose: Drug experimentation in a group of adolescents. Pediatrics 101:1045-1048, 1998.

300. Petty, W.: The effect of methylmethacrylate on bacterial inhibiting properties of normal human serum. Clin. Orthop. Relat. Res. 132:266-277, 1978.

301. Petty, W.: The effect of methylmethacrylate on bacterial phagocytosis and killing by human polymorphonuclear leukocytes. J. Bone Joint Surg. Am. 60:752-757, 1978.

302. Pfausler, B., Beer, R., Engelhardt, K., et al.: Cell index—a new parameter for the early diagnosis of ventriculostomy (external ventricular drainage)-related ventriculitis in patients with intraventricular hemorrhage? Acta Neurochir. (Wien). 146:477-481, 2004.

303. Pfausler, B., Spiss, H., Beer, R., et al.: Treatment of staphylococcal ventriculitis associated with external cerebrospinal fluid drains: A prospective randomized trial of intravenous compared with intraventricular vancomycin therapy. J. Neurosurg. 98:1040-1044, 2003.

304. Pfisterer, W., Muhlbauer, M., Czech, T., and Reinprecht, A.: Early diagnosis of external ventricular drainage infection: Results of a prospective study. J. Neurol. Neurosurg. Psychother. 74:929-932, 2003.

305. Piatt, J. H.: Cerebrospinal fluid shunt failure: Late is different from early. Pediatr. Neurosurg. 23:133-136, 1995.

306. Piccione, W.: Left ventricular assist device implantation: Short and long-term surgical complications. J. Heart Lung Transplant. 19:S89-S94, 2000.

307. Pittman, T., Williams, D., Rathore, M., et al.: The role of ethylene oxide allergy in sterile shunt malfunctions. Br. J. Neurosurg. 8:41-43, 1994.

308. Plummer, J. L., Cherry, D. A., Cousins, M. J., et al.: Long-term spinal administration of morphine in cancer and non-cancer pain: A retrospective study. Pain *44*:215-220, 1991.

309. Poon, W. S., Ng, S., and Wai, S.: CSF antibiotic prophylaxis for neurosurgical patients with ventriculostomy: A randomized study. Acta Neurochir. Suppl. (Wien) *71*:146-148, 1998.

310. Pople, I. K., Bayston, R., and Hayward, R. D.: Infection of cerebrospinal fluid shunts in infants: A study of etiological factors. J. Neurosurg. *77*:29-36, 1992.

311. Pople, I. K., Mulbauer, M. S., Sanford, R. A., et al.: Results and complications of intracranial pressure monitoring in 303 children. Pediatr. Neurosurg. *23*:64-69, 1995.

312. Poss, R., Thornhill, T. S., Ewald, F. C., et al.: Factors influencing the incidence and outcome of infection following total joint arthroplasty. Clin. Orthop. Relat. Res. *182*:117-126, 1984.

313. Preventing pacemaker infections. Lancet *1*:537-538, 1986.

314. Proctor, R. A.: The staphylococcal fibronectin receptor: Evidence for its importance in invasive infections. Rev. Infect. Dis. *9*(Suppl.):335-340, 1987.

315. Raithel, S. C., Pennington, D. G., Boegner, E., et al.: Extracorporeal membrane oxygenation in children after cardiac surgery. Circulation *86*(Suppl. II):305-310, 1992.

316. Rand, J. A., and Fitzgerald, R. H., Jr.: Diagnosis and management of the infected total knee arthroplasty. Orthop. Clin. North Am. *20*:201-210, 1989.

317. Rand, J. A., Morrey, B. F., and Bryan, R. S.: Management of the infected total joint arthroplasty. Orthop. Clin. North Am. *15*:491-504, 1984.

318. Ratilal, B., Costa, J., and Sampaio, C.: Antibiotic prophylaxis for surgical introduction of intracranial ventricular shunts. Cochrane Database Syst. Rev. *3*:CD005365, 2006.

319. Raut, V. V., Orth, M. S., Orth, M. C., et al.: One stage revision arthroplasty of the hip for deep gram negative infection. Int. Orthop. *20*:12-14, 1996.

320. Rebuck, J. A., Murray, K. R., Rhoney, D. H., et al.: Infection related to intracranial pressure monitors in adults: Analysis of risk factors and antibiotic prophylaxis. J. Neurol. Neurosurg. Psychiatry *69*:381-384, 2000.

321. Reefhuis, J., Honein, M. A., Whitney, C. G., et al.: Risk of bacterial meningitis in children with cochlear implants. N. Engl. J. Med. *349*:435-445, 2003.

322. Reid, G.: Bacterial colonization of prosthetic devices and measures to prevent infection. New Horizons *6*(Suppl. 2):58-63, 1998.

323. Rennels, M. B., and Wald, E. R.: Treatment of *Haemophilus influenzae* type b meningitis in children with cerebrospinal fluid shunts. J. Pediatr. *97*:424-426, 1980.

324. Rettig, G., Doenecke, P., Sen, L., et al.: Complications with retained transvenous pacemaker electrodes. Am. Heart J. *98*:587-594, 1979.

325. Reynolds, M., Sherman, J. O., and McLone, D. G.: Ventriculoperitoneal shunt infection masquerading as an acute surgical abdomen. J. Pediatr. Surg. *18*:951-954, 1983.

326. Roitberg, B. Z., Tomita, T., and McLone, D. G.: Abdominal cerebrospinal fluid pseudocyst: A complication of ventriculoperitoneal shunt in children. Pediatr. Neurosurg. *29*:267-273, 1998.

327. Ronan, A., Hogg, G. G., and Klug, G. L.: Cerebrospinal fluid shunt infections in children. Pediatr. Infect. Dis. J. *14*:782-786, 1995.

328. Rubin, R. C., Ghatak, N. R., and Kisudhipan, P.: Asymptomatic perforated viscus and gram-negative ventriculitis as a complication of valve-regulated ventriculoperitoneal shunts. J. Neurosurg. *37*:616-618, 1972.

329. Rubinstein, J. T., Gantz, F. J., and Parkinson, W. S.: Management of cochlear implant infections. Am. J. Otol. *20*:46-49, 1999.

330. Rupp, M. E., Ulphani, J. S., Fey, P. D., et al.: Characterization of the importance of polysaccharide intercellular/hemagglutinin of *Staphylococcus epidermidis* in the pathogenesis of biomaterial-based infection in a mouse foreign body infection model. Infect. Immun. *67*:2627-2632, 1999.

331. Rupprecht, T. A., and Pfister, H. W.: Clinical experience with linezolid for the treatment of central nervous system infections. Eur. J. Neurol. *12*:536-542, 2005.

332. Salgado, C. D., Dash, S., Cantey, J. R., and Marculescu, C. E.: Higher risk of failure of methicillin-resistant *Staphylococcus aureus* prosthetic joint infections. Clin. Orthop. Relat. Res. *461*:48-53, 2007.

333. Salmon, J. H.: Adult hydrocephalus: Evaluation of shunt therapy in 80 patients. J. Neurosurg. *37*:423-428, 1972.

334. Samtleben, W., Bauriedel, G., Bosch, T., et al.: Renal complications of infected ventriculoatrial shunts. Artif. Organs *17*:695-701, 1993.

335. Samuel, M., Finnerty, G. T., and Rudge, P.: Intrathecal baclofen pump infection treated by adjuvant intrareservoir antibiotic instillation. J. Neurol. Neurosurg. Psychiatry *57*:1146-1147, 1994.

336. Samuels, L. E., Samuels, F. L., Kaufman, M. S., et al.: Management of infected implantable cardiac defibrillators. Ann. Thorac. Surg. *64*:1702-1706, 1997.

337. Sanderson, P. J.: Infection in orthopaedic implants. J. Hosp. Infect. *18*(Suppl. A):367-375, 1991.

338. Schoifet, S. D., and Morrey, B. F.: Treatment of infection after total knee arthroplasty by débridement with retention of the components. J. Bone Joint Surg. Am. *72*:1383-1390, 1990.

338a. Schoenbaum, S. C., Gardner, P., and Shillito, J.: Infections of cerebrospinal fluid shunts: Epidemiology, clinical manifestations, and therapy. J. Infect. Dis. *131*:543-552, 1975.

339. Schreffler, R. T., Schreffler, A. J., and Wittler, R. R.: Treatment of cerebrospinal fluid shunt infections: A decision analysis. Pediatr. Infect. Dis. J. *21*:632-636, 2002.

340. Schuhmann, M. U., Ostrowski, K. R., Draper, E. J. et al.: The value of C-reactive protein in the management of shunt infections. J. Neurosurg. *103*(3 Suppl.):223-230, 2005.

341. Schultz, M., Moore, K., and Foote, A. W.: Bacterial ventriculitis and duration of ventriculostomy catheter insertion. J. Neurosci. Nurs. *25*:158-164, 1993.

342. Schwartz, J. G., Tio, F. O., and Fetchick, R. J.: Filamentous *Histoplasma capsulatum* involving a ventriculoatrial shunt. Neurosurgery *18*:487-490, 1986.

343. Sciubba, D. M., Lin, L. M., Woodworth, G. F., et al.: Factors contributing to the medical costs of cerebrospinal fluid shunt infection treatment in pediatric patients with standard shunt components compared with those in patients with antibiotic impregnated components. Neurosurg. Focus *22*:E9, 2007.

344. Sculco, T. P.: The economic impact of infected total joint arthroplasty. Instr. Course Lect. *42*:349-356, 1993.

345. Sells, C. J., Shurtleff, D. B., and Loeser, J. D.: Gram-negative cerebrospinal fluid shunt–associated infections. Pediatrics *59*:614-618, 1977.

346. Selman, W. R., Spetzler, R. F., Wilson, C. B., and Grollmus, J. W.: Percutaneous lumboperitoneal shunt: Review of 130 cases. Neurosurgery *6*:255-257, 1980.

347. Selwyn, S., and Ellis, H.: Skin bacteria and skin disinfection reconsidered. B. M. J. *1*:136-140, 1972.

348. Sharma, N. S., Ooi, J. L., Downie, J. A., et al.: Corneal perforation and intraocular lens prolapse in *Serratia marcescens* endophthalmitis. Clin. Exp. Ophthalmol. *35*:381-382, 2007.

349. Sharma, N. S, Ooi, J. L, Maloof, T. C, et al.: Culture-proven *Aspergillus fumigatus* infection in a primary hydroxyapatite orbital implant. Clin. Exp. Ophthalmol. *35*:294-295, 2007.

350. Shtarker, H., David, R., Stolero, J., et al.: Treatment of open tibial fractures with primary suture and Ilizarov fixation. Clin. Orthop. Relat. Res. *335*:268-274, 1997.

351. Shurtleff, D. B., Foltz, E. L., Weeks, R. D., and Loeser, J.: Therapy of *Staphylococcus epidermidis*: Infections associated with cerebrospinal fluid shunts. Pediatrics *53*:55-62, 1974.

352. Shurtleff, D. B., Stuntz, J. T., and Hayden, P. W.: Experience with 1201 cerebrospinal fluid shunt procedures. Pediatr. Neurosci. *12*:49-57, 1986.

353. Siegfried, R. N., Jacobson, L., and Chabal, C.: Development of an acute withdrawal syndrome following the cessation of intrathecal baclofen in a patient with spasticity. Anesthesiology *77*:1048-1050, 1992.

354. Simon, D., Fischer, S., Grossman, A., et al.: Left ventricular assist device–related infection: Treatment and outcome. Clin. Infect. Dis. *40*:1108-1115, 2005.

355. Sinha, P., Chen, J. M., Flannery, M., et al.: Infections during left ventricular assist device support do not affect posttransplant outcomes. Circulation *102*(Suppl. III):194-199, 2000.

356. Smith, E., Butler, W., and Barker, F. G., 2nd.: In-hospital mortality rates after ventriculoperitoneal shunt procedures in the United States, 1998 to 2000: Relation to hospital and surgeon volume of care. J. Neurosurg. *100*(2 Suppl.):90-97, 2004.

357. Smith, P. N., Vidaillet, H. J., Hayes, J. J., et al.: Infections with nonthoracotomy implantable cardioverter defibrillators: Can these be prevented? Pacing Clin. Electrophysiol. *21*:42-55, 1998.

358. Smith, R. W., and Alksne, J. F.: Infections complicating the use of external ventriculostomy. J. Neurosurg. *44*:567-570, 1976.

359. Sonmezoglu, K., Sonmezoglu, M., Halac, M., et al.: Usefulness of ^{99m}Tc-ciprofloxacin (Infecton) scan in diagnosis of chronic orthopedic infections: Comparative study with ^{99m}Tc-HMPAO leukocyte scintigraphy. J. Nucl. Med. *42*:567-574, 2001.

360. Spangehl, M., Masri, B., O'Connell, J., and Duncan, C.: Prospective analysis of preoperative and intraoperative investigations for the diagnosis of infection at the sites of 202 revision total hip arthroplasties. J. Bone Joint Surg. Am. *81*:672-683, 1999.

361. Spangehl, M. J., Younger, A. S. E., Masri, B. A., et al.: Diagnosis of infection following total hip arthroplasty. J. Bone Joint Surg. Am. *79*:1578-1588, 1997.

362. Spencer, M., and Bird, Q.: Device-related nonintravascular infections. Crit. Care Nurs. Clin. North Am. *7*:685-693, 1995.

363. Spinler, S. A., Nawarskas, J., Foote, E. F., et al.: Clinical presentation and analysis of risk factors for infectious complications of implantable cardioverter-defibrillator implantations at a university medical center. Clin. Infect. Dis. *26*:1111-1116, 1998.

364. Stamos, J. K., Kaufman, B. A., and Yogev, R.: Ventriculoperitoneal shunt infections with gram-negative bacteria. Neurosurgery *33*:858-862, 1993.

365. Stark, W. J., Worthen, D. M., Holladay, J. T., et al.: The FDA report on intraocular lenses. Ophthalmology *90*:311-317, 1983.

366. Steckelberg, J. M., and Osmon, D. R.: Prosthetic joint infections. *In* Waldvogel, F. A., and Bisno, A. L. (eds.): Infections Associated with Indwelling Medical Devices. 3rd ed. Washington, D. C., A. S. M. Press, 2000, pp. 173-209.

367. Stehr-Green, J., Bailey, T. M., Brandt, F. H., et al.: *Acanthamoeba* keratitis in soft contact lens wearers. J. A. M. A. *258*:57-60, 1987.

368. Stenager, E., Gerner-Smidt, P., and Kock-Jensen, C.: Ventriculostomy-related infections—an epidemiological study. Acta Neurochir. *83*:20-23, 1986.

369. Stern, S., Bayston, R., and Hayward, R. J.: *Haemophilus influenzae* meningitis in the presence of cerebrospinal fluid shunts. Childs Nerv. Syst. *4*:164-166, 1988.

370. Stern, S. H., Insall, J. N., Windsor, R. E., et al.: Total knee arthroplasty in patients with psoriasis. Clin. Orthop. Relat. Res. *248*:108-111, 1989.

371. Stewart, M. P. M., and Kelly, I. G.: Total shoulder replacement in rheumatoid disease: 7-13 year followup of 37 joints. J. Bone Joint Surg. Br. 79:68-72, 1997.

372. Stotka, J. L., Rupp, M. E., Meier, F. A., et al.: Meningitis due to *Neisseria mucosa*: Case report and review. Rev. Infect. Dis. 13:837-841, 1991.

373. Sun, B. C., Catanese, K. A., Spanier, T. B., et al.: 100 Long-term implantable left ventricular assist devices: The Columbia Presbyterian interim experience. Ann. Thorac. Surg. 68:688-694, 1999.

374. Sundbärg, G., Kjällquistt, A., Lungberg, N., and Pontén, U.: Complications due to prolonged ventricular fluid pressure recordings in clinical practice. *In* Borck, M., and Dietz, H. (eds.): Intracranial Pressure: Experimental and Clinical Aspects. Berlin, Springer-Verlag, 1972, pp. 348-352.

375. Sutherland, K., Mahoney, J. R., II, Coury, A. J., and Eaton, J. W.: Degradation of biomaterials by phagocyte-derived oxidants. J. Clin. Invest. 92:2360-2367, 1993.

376. Swayne, R., Rampling, A., and Newsom, S. W. B.: Intraventricular vancomycin for treatment of shunt-associated ventriculitis. J. Antimicrob. Chemother. 19:249-253, 1987.

377. Tang, L., and Eaton, J. W.: Inflammatory responses to biomaterials. Am. J. Clin. Pathol. 103:466-471, 1995.

378. Teddy, P., Jamous, A., Gardner, B., et al.: Complications of intrathecal baclofen delivery. Br. J. Neurosurg. 6:115-118, 1992.

379. Tenover, F. C., and McDonald, L. C.: Vancomycin-resistant staphylococci and enterococci: Epidemiology and control. Curr. Opin. Infect. Dis. 18:300-305, 2005.

380. Thompson, D. N., Malcolm, G. P., Jones, B. M., et al.: Intracranial pressure in single-suture craniosynostosis. Pediatr. Neurosurg. 22:235-239, 1995.

381. Thompson, T. P., and Albright, A. L.: *Propionibacterium acnes* infections of cerebrospinal fluid shunts. Childs Nerv. Syst. 14:378-380, 1998.

382. Toy, P. T. C. Y., Lai, L. W., Drake, T. A., and Sande, M. A.: Effect of fibronectin on adherence of *Staphylococcus aureus* to fibrin thrombi in vitro. Infect. Immun. 48:83-86, 1985.

383. Trappe, H. J., Pfitzner, P., and Klein, H.: Infections after cardioverter-defibrillator implantation: Observations in 335 patients over 10 years. Br. Heart J. 73:20-24, 1995.

384. Tung, H., Raffel, C., and McComb, J. G.: Ventricular cerebrospinal fluid eosinophilia in children with ventriculoperitoneal shunts. J. Neurosurg. 75:541-544, 1991.

385. Tunkel, A. R., Thomas, C. Y., and Wispelwey, B.: *Candida* prosthetic arthritis: Report of a case treated with fluconazole and review of the literature. Am. J. Med. 94:100-103, 1993.

386. Turkisher, V., Priel, I., and Dan, M.: Successful management of an infected implantable cardioverter defibrillator with oral antibiotics and without removal of the device. Pacing Clin. Electrophysiol. 20:2268-2270, 1997.

387. Ubogu, E. E., Lindenberg, J. R., and Werz, M. A.: Transverse myelitis associated with *Acinetobacter baumanii* intrathecal pump catheter–related infection. Reg. Anesth. Pain Med. 28:470-474, 2003.

388. Ure, K. J., Amstutz, H. C., Nasser, S., and Schmalzried, T. P.: Direct-exchange arthroplasty for the treatment of infection after total hip replacement. An average ten-year follow-up. J. Bone Joint Surg. Am. 80:961-968, 1998.

389. Vaudaux, P., Francois, P., Lew, D. P., and Waldvogel, F. A.: Host factors predisposing to and influencing therapy of foreign body infections. *In* Waldvogel, F. A., and Bisno, A. L. (eds.): Infections Associated with Indwelling Medical Devices. 3rd ed. Washington, D. C., A. S. M. Press, 2000, pp. 1-26.

390. Vaudaux, P. E., Zulian, G., Huggler, E., and Waldvogel, F. A.: Attachment of *Staphylococcus aureus* to polymethylmethacrylate increases its resistance to phagocytosis in foreign body infection. Infect. Immun. 50:472-477, 1985.

391. Vender, J. R., Hester, S., Waller, J. L., et al.: Identification and management of intrathecal baclofen pump complications: A comparison of pediatric and adult patients. J. Neurosurg. 104:9-15, 2006.

392. Venes, J. L.: Control of shunt infection: Report of 150 consecutive cases. J. Neurosurg. 45:311-314, 1976.

393. Vercellotti, G. M., McCarthy, J. D., Lindholm, P., et al.: Extracellular matrix proteins (fibronectin, laminin and type IV collagen) bind and aggregate bacteria. Am. J. Pathol. 120:13-21, 1985.

394. Vercillo, M., Patzakis, M. J., Holtom, P., and Zalavras, C. G.: Linezolid in the treatment of implant-related chronic osteomyelitis. Clin. Orthop. Relat. Res. 461:40-43, 2007.

395. Vernet, O., Campiche, R., and de Tribolet, N.: Long-term results after ventriculoatrial shunting in children. Childs Nerv. Syst. 9:253-255, 1993.

396. Vertullo, C. J., Duke, P. F., and Askin, G. N.: Pin-site complications of the halo thoracic brace with routine pin re-tightening. Spine 22:2514-2516, 1997.

397. Victor, F., DePlace, C., Camus, C., et al.: Pacemaker lead infection: Echocardiographic features, management, and outcome. Heart 81:82-87, 1999.

398. Vinchon, M., and Dhellemmes P.: Cerebrospinal fluid shunt infection: Risk factors and long-term follow-up. Childs Nerv. Syst. 22:692-697, 2006.

399. Vinchon, M., Vallee, L., Prin, L., et al.: Cerebrospinal fluid eosinophilia in shunt infections. Neuropediatrics 23:235-240, 1992.

400. Vogt, P. R., Sagdic, K., Lachat, M., et al.: Surgical management of infected permanent transvenous pacemaker systems: Ten year experience. J. Card. Surg. 11:180-186, 1996.

401. Voldby, B., and Enevoldsen, E. M.: Intracranial pressure changes following aneurysm rupture. Part 1: Clinical and angiopathic correlations. J. Neurosurg. 56:186-196, 1982.

402. Vougioukas, V. I., Feuerhake, F., Hubbe, U., et al.: Latent abscess formation adjacent to a non-functioning intraventricular catheter. Childs Nerv. Syst. 19:119-121, 2003.

403. Wade, J. S., and Cobbs, C. G.: Infections in cardiac pacemakers. Curr. Clin. Top. Infect. Dis. 9:44-61, 1988.

404. Wald, S. L., and McLaurin, R. L.: Cerebrospinal fluid antibiotic levels during treatment of shunt infections. J. Neurosurg. 52:41-46, 1980.

405. Walter, E. B., Jr., Gingras, J. L., and McKinney, R. E., Jr.: Systemic *Torulopsis glabrata* infection in a neonate. South. Med. J. 83:837-838, 1990.

406. Walters, B. C.: Cerebrospinal fluid shunt infection. Neurosurg. Clin. North Am. 3:387-401, 1992.

407. Walters, B. C., Hoffman, H. J., Hendrick, E. B., and Humphreys, R. P.: Cerebrospinal fluid shunt infection: Influences on initial management and subsequent outcome. J. Neurosurg. 60:1014-1021, 1984.

408. Walters, H. L., III, Hakimi, M., Rice, M. D., et al.: Pediatric cardiac surgical ECMO: Multivariate analysis of risk factors for hospital death. Ann. Thorac. Surg. 60:329-337, 1995.

409. Wang, K. C., Lee, H. J., Sung, J. N., and Cho, B. K.: Cerebrospinal fluid shunt infection in children: Efficiency of management protocol, rate of persistent shunt colonization, and significance of "off-antibiotics" trial. Childs Nerv. Syst. 15:38-44, 1999.

410. Wang, R. C., Parisier, S. C., Weiss, M. H., et al.: Cochlear implant flap complications. Ann. Otol. Rhinol. Laryngol. 99:791-795, 1990.

411. Watanabe, I., Hodges, G. R., Dworzack, D. L., et al.: Neurotoxicity of intrathecal gentamicin: A case report and experimental study. Ann. Neurol. 4:564-572, 1978.

412. Weber, D. J., Hofman, K. L., Thoft, R. A., and Baker, A. S.: Endophthalmitis following intraocular lens implantation. Rev. Infect. Dis. 8:12-80, 1986.

413. Weiss, M. H., Kurze, T., and Nulsen, F. E.: Antibiotic neurotoxicity: Laboratory and clinical study. J. Neurosurg. 41:486-489, 1974.

414. Weyland, M., Hermann, M., Kondruweit, M., et al.: Clinical impact of infections of left ventricular assist device recipients: The importance of site and organism. Transplant. Proc. 29:3327-3329, 1997.

415. Whitehead, W. E., and Kestle, J. R. W.: The treatment of cerebrospinal fluid shunt infections. Pediatr. Neurosurg. 35:205-210, 2001.

416. Wilhelm, M. J., Schmid, C., Hammel, D., et al.: Cardiac pacemaker infection: Surgical management with and without extracorporeal circulation. Ann. Thorac. Surg. 64:1707-1712, 1997.

417. Wilson, H. A., Jr., Downes, T. R., Julian, J. S., et al.: *Candida* endocarditis, a treatable form of pacemaker infection. Chest 103:283-284, 1993.

418. Wilson, M. G., Kelley, K., and Thornhill, T. S.: Infection as a complication of total knee-replacement arthroplasty. Risk factors and treatment in sixty-seven cases. J. Bone Joint Surg. 72:878-883, 1990.

419. Wilson, M. W., Wobig, J. L., and Dailey, R. A.: Infection of a porous polyethylene orbital implant with *Capnocytophaga*. Ophthal. Plast. Reconstr. Surg. 14:398-402, 1998.

420. Wilson, W. R., Greer, G. E., and Grubb, B. P.: Implantable cardioverter-defibrillators in children: A single-institutional experience. Ann. Thorac. Surg. 65:775-781, 1998.

421. Wimmer, C., Gluch, H., Franzreb, M., and Ogon, M.: Predisposing factors for infection in spine surgery: A survey of 850 spinal procedures. J. Spinal Disord. 11:124-128, 1998.

422. Winfield, J. A., Rosenthal, P., Kanter, R. K., et al.: Duration of intracranial pressure monitoring does not predict daily risk of infectious complications. Neurosurgery 33:424-431, 1993.

423. Winn, H. R., Dacey, R. G., and Jane, J. A.: Intracranial subarachnoid pressure recording: Experience with 650 patients. Surg. Neurol. 8:41-47, 1977.

424. Wong, G. K. C., Poon, W. S., Wai, S., et al.: Failure of regular external ventricular drain exchange to reduce cerebrospinal fluid infection: Result of a randomized controlled trial. J. Neurol. Neurosurg. Psychother. 73:759-761, 2002.

425. Wymenga, A. B., van Horn, J. R., Theeuwes, A., et al.: Perioperative factors associated with septic arthritis after arthroplasty. Prospective multicenter study of 362 knee and 2,651 hip operations. Acta Orthop. Scand. 63:665-671, 1992.

426. Yar, J. R., Seo, J. H., Kim, Y. H., et al.: Six cases of bacterial infection in porous orbital implants. Jpn. J. Ophthalmol. 47:512-518, 2003.

427. Yeh, L. K., Kao, S. C., Tsai, C. C., et al.: [Delayed-onset of *Pseudomonas* infection in a hydroxyapatite orbital implant: A case report.] Chung Hua I Hsueh Tsa Chih [Chinese Medical Journal] 62:832-837, 1999.

428. Yildiran, S. T., Mutlu, F. M., Sarachi, M. A., et al.: Fungal endophthalmitis caused by *Aspergillus ustus* in a patient following cataract surgery. Med. Mycol. 44:665-669, 2006.

429. Younger, J. J., Christensen, G. D., Bartley, D. L., et al.: Coagulase-negative staphylococci isolated from cerebrospinal fluid shunts: Importance of slime production, species identification, and shunt removal to clinical outcome. J. Infect. Dis. 156:548-554, 1987.

430. Zed, P. J., Stiver, G., Devonshire, V., et al.: Continuous intrathecal pump infusion of baclofen with antibiotic drugs for treatment of pump-associated meningitis. J. Neurosurg. 92:347-349, 2000.

431. Ziomek, S., Harrell, J. E., Fasules, J. W., et al.: Extracorporeal membrane oxygenation for cardiac failure after congenital heart operation. Ann. Thorac. Surg. 54:861-868, 1992.

432. Zipes, D. P., and Roberts, D.: Results of the international study of the implantable pacemaker cardioverter-defibrillator. A comparison of epicardial and endocardial lead systems. Circulation 92:59-65, 1995.

INFECTIONS RELATED TO CRANIOFACIAL SURGICAL PROCEDURES

Marc A. Mazade

Advances in plastic and reconstructive surgery have created the opportunity for surgeons to offer patients with complications of facial neoplasia, craniosynostosis, fibrous dysplasia, Crouzon syndrome, Apert syndrome, Treacher Collins syndrome, craniofacial clefts, and other anomalies relief from associated mechanical complications and restoration of a more normal cosmetic appearance. Operative procedures to address these problems involve cranial vault remodeling or reconstruction (or both) or advancement of the midface and maxillary block and, occasionally, correction of malocclusion by repositioning of the mandible. The overall incidence of infection associated with these procedures was 14.7 percent in one study,[10] but it varies greatly and may range from 3 to 45 percent, depending on the number of procedures attempted during a single anesthetic regimen, the duration of surgery, and the structures involved. A review published in 2005 demonstrated a rate of 3.2 infections per 100 craniofacial surgical procedures and found that surgical duration longer than 426 minutes, closure of skin under tension, use of bovine pericardium, and the presence of more than four surgeons in the operating suite were common risks for development of infection.[24] Many patients suffering infection were categorized as having complicated diagnoses.

PROCEDURES AND OSTEOTOMIES

Some familiarity with a few of the more common procedures in craniofacial surgery, beyond basic craniotomy and cranial vault remodeling, is necessary to understand the pathogenesis of associated infectious complications. Although every patient has a unique set of problems, several corrective procedures are used frequently and then are modified as specifically needed for each circumstance.

In young children with midfacial retrusion, frontofacial monoblock advancement may be performed.[17] This procedure involves detachment and advancement of the entire facial bony mask, excluding the mandible. Exposure for this procedure commonly requires a large frontal craniotomy, the bone from which may be shaped to complete the repair or used as needed to form a suitable foundation to which the advanced block can be secured. Retraction of the frontal lobes is necessary to provide access to the roof of the orbits, and much of the procedure is performed intracranially. The boundaries of the advancement block are formed by osteotomies performed horizontally along the lower portion of the frontal bone and posteriorly along the roof of the orbits, vertically along the lateral and medial inferior walls and horizontally along the inferior walls of the orbits, and vertically through the zygomatic arches, with subsequent dissection and pterygomaxillary disjunction. Finally, a frontoethmoidal osteotomy divides the posterior portion of the nasal septum to free the monoblock so that it can be advanced and secured in place, perhaps by wiring it anteriorly to a slightly fore-tilted strip of frontal bone and stabilizing it laterally with wired-in strips of calvarial bone grafts to bridge gaps in the zygomatic arches. Bone blocks in the pterygomaxillary area help to hold the maxillary portion forward. The temporary dead space created in the anterior cranial fossa after this procedure eventually is obliterated in a growing, developing child, although its persistence is problematic in some patients.[23] This intracranial procedure is associated with an inherent risk of developing meningitis, which is associated less frequently with the extracranial procedures described later, although meningitis still may occur.[21]

A subcranial Le Fort III osteotomy sometimes is used for the treatment of midface retrusion in children.[11,17] Exposure is provided through a coronal incision, but craniotomy is not necessary. Neither the orbital roof nor any portion of the frontal bone is advanced with this procedure. Osteotomies are required to free part of the medial, lateral, and inferior walls of the orbit and the nasal bridge, and the remainder of the block is freed by pterygopalatine disjunction and osteotomies of the zygomatic arch and posterior nasal septum. The entire inferior orbital and nasomaxillary unit is brought forward, and interposition grafts, hydroxyapatite, microplates, and wires secure the block in the advanced position. An intraoral stab incision may be required for pterygopalatine disjunction. As in the frontofacial advancement, split calvarial bone grafts bridge the space in the zygomatic arches.

If further advancement of the maxilla is desired, a subsequent Le Fort I osteotomy, which is an isolated maxillary advancement procedure that changes the position of the upper teeth, is performed.[11,14,17] This entirely intraoral procedure involves making various buccal sulcus and upper vestibular incisions. The palate and maxillary arch are freed for advancement by transverse osteotomies at the level of the nasal floor, through the nasal septum, and then posteriorly.

Another procedure that may be performed in some cases of Treacher Collins syndrome is the integrale (simultaneous midfacial and mandibular osteotomies).[17] In this complicated procedure requiring a tracheostomy, the midface osteotomies exclude the temporal, lateral walls of the orbits from the advanced block. In addition, C-shaped or inverted V-shaped osteotomies through the mandibular rami with placement of the interposition bone grafts and wiring provide advancement of the mandible. Split calvarial bone grafts subsequently reestablish the zygomatic arches. Incidentally, the bone grafts are harvested either by performing a true craniotomy or by removing the outer cortical bone table from the donor site.

More thorough descriptions of these and other operations, such as facial bipartition, are provided in the referenced texts,[11,17] to which the reader is referred for a better grasp of the inherent risks of bacterial contamination from intraoral, sinus, and skin sources that are specific to each craniofacial procedure. Nonetheless, suffice it that the infections encountered usually are caused by bacteria that are resident or pathogenic in the clean-contaminated sites through which incisions and osteotomies are performed and that each additional site that is surgically violated increases the risk of developing an infection.

Many reconstructive materials are used for various procedural applications. Some materials include bone autograft and solvent-treated allograft, titanium plates, and alloplasts such as polymethylmethacrylate (PMMA) and hydroxyapatite cements, some of which readily accept bone ingrowth. In an effort to limit postoperative infection, antibiotics such as tobramycin sometimes are mixed into hydroxyapatite cements, which are released into the surrounding field within the first 24 hours of placement.[15] Efficacy data regarding prevention of infection using this practice are not widely available.

EPIDEMIOLOGY

Infections that may be encountered include cellulitis and dehiscence of the wound, infection of subgaleal fluid, osteomyelitis, focal soft tissue abscesses, epidural abscesses,[23,24] and septicemia. In many instances, infection permeates the entire operative field and encompasses any number of these specific entities.[10] Donor bone graft sites may be involved in some instances. Bacteria may infect the wound or soft tissue area, may spread by contiguous extension through cortical bone during long periods of contact, or may extend through osteotomies that have disrupted the integrity of the periosteum and cortical bone barriers. Additionally, surgical alteration of the local blood supply to the cranial bones through disruption of medullary channels and removal of the adherent periosteum, as well as the presence of hardware required to secure the bony structures in their new locations, can render infection difficult to treat. Repeated or prolonged hospitalizations for previous surgical procedures, often for co-morbid conditions such as syndactyly, gastroesophageal reflux, or dysphagia, result in colonization of the skin and sinopulmonary tracts and subsequent postoperative infection with multidrug-resistant bacteria. Attempts to reduce the incidence of infection have made the use of parenteral prophylactic perioperative antibiotic regimens for 2 to 5 days commonplace.

The development of meningitis always is a concern when craniofacial procedures are performed. The presence of a cerebrospinal fluid leak is a predisposing factor, and meningitis may be manifested years after the procedure in the case of a leak.[21] However, the dura provides a significant barrier to infection when painstaking neurosurgical technique is applied during repair. In fact, no cases of meningitis were identified from a combined report of complications after 567 procedures spanning 6.5 years at Medical City Dallas Hospital and at the Division of Plastic Surgery at the University of Pennsylvania in Philadelphia, primarily for cranial vault remodeling.[9] Similarly, meningitis was not identified from an earlier report of 170 transcranial operations spanning 10 years at the South Australian Cranio-Facial Unit in which 53 accidental dural tears occurred and 32 planned dural openings were performed.[8] Nonetheless, meningitis has been documented to occur in association with a frontal abscess with osteomyelitis, subgaleal fluid infection, and contamination of cerebrospinal fluid drains.[10]

The Australian group just mentioned documented an average operative time of 10.5 hours for patients in whom a postoperative infection developed, 2.5 hours longer than operations on patients in whom an infection did not develop.[8] However, these observations were confounded by variables such as type of procedure and whether the procedure was a primary or subsequent operation. Longer and more complicated monoblock advancement procedures have been associated with infection rates as high as 45 percent,[10] whereas anterior cranial vault remodeling may be associated with infection rates as low as 2.5 percent.[9] In staged or subsequent procedures, the dura encountered during primary craniofacial procedures is manipulated more easily and has better vascularization than does the scarred dura encountered in more complicated and laborious secondary procedures, which are associated with higher rates of infection.[9] Additionally, craniofacial postoperative infections develop in infants far less frequently than in adults.[8,9] Whether this age difference is a reflection of the types of surgeries performed in infants or other microbial or host factors is not clear. Of the common procedures, infection remains a relatively rare complication of the less complicated Le Fort I maxillary osteotomy. In a large review of outcomes of 1000 such procedures, only 1.1 percent developed abscess or related infection.[12]

As experience in craniofacial surgery has grown, the reduction in the frequency of infection has been attributed to shortened operative time, attempts to avoid entrance into the contaminated

sinus cavities (an easier task in young children, in whom the sinuses often are still poorly developed), and mucosal repair at the end of surgery.[22] The mean time to diagnosis of infection is approximately 10 days.[10]

MICROBIOLOGY

Organisms causing infection include flora of the skin such as *Candida albicans*, *Staphylococcus aureus*, *Staphylococcus epidermidis*, beta-hemolytic streptococci, and *Propionibacterium acnes*. Resident flora of the oropharynx such as *Bacteroides* spp., *Corynebacterium* spp., various alpha-hemolytic streptococci, *Streptococcus pneumoniae*, *Morganella morganii*, *Eikenella corrodens*, *Haemophilus influenzae*, and *Haemophilus parainfluenzae* can be causative, as can nosocomial gram-negative bacilli such as *Pseudomonas aeruginosa*, *Escherichia coli*, *Klebsiella* spp., and *Acinetobacter calcoaceticus*.[6,9,24] Procedures that disrupt the oropharynx and sinus cavities are more apt to be complicated by polymicrobial infections. Procedures that do not violate these spaces are more inclined to be complicated solely by infection with skin flora. The frequency of infection with *Candida* spp. may rival the frequency of infection with more common bacteria.[9,23,24]

PREOPERATIVE PREPARATION, INTRAOPERATIVE IRRIGATION, AND PERIOPERATIVE ANTIBIOTIC THERAPY

Because wounds created during craniofacial surgery fall between the clean-contaminated category and the contaminated category,[6,7] giving attention to the treatment of dental caries, periodontal disease, and acute sinusitis is prudent before embarking on procedures involving intraoral incisions and trans-sinus osteotomies.[21] Protocols for the administration of perioperative antibiotics and for preoperative preparation of the oral cavity have been developed. Many of these protocols involve irrigation of the oral cavity with povidone-iodine (Betadine) solutions. Nonetheless, the sinus cavities do not lend themselves to preoperative antiseptic washing. Some surgeons make use of intraoperative antibiotic-containing irrigants to help reduce the incidence of infection. These irrigants may be flushed over the intact cranium after subperiosteal exposure and again before skin closure. Other surgeons prefer to use a solution of one part povidone-iodine to four parts saline for intraoperative irrigation.[21] No strong evidence supports any one approach over others for reducing infection.[10]

The choice and duration of perioperative antibiotics vary among surgical centers and their surgical teams. Antibiotic regimens may consist of the following: penicillin; ampicillin-sulbactam; a first-, second-, or third-generation cephalosporin; clindamycin; or any two of these drugs in combination.[6,7,9,10,12] Erythromycin is used in penicillin-allergic patients in some centers.[1]

Continuation of antibiotics may be necessary for 0 to 5 days postoperatively. The optimal duration of treatment is not clear. Higher infection rates occurred in some centers that tried restricting antibiotics to intraoperative use only.[1] Reports from one orthognathic surgical center showed a 10-fold reduction in infection rates with a 5-day antibiotic regimen in comparison with a single-day regimen.[2] Furthermore, isolation of a few infecting organisms that were susceptible in vitro to an antibiotic given 6 hours preoperatively until 48 hours postoperatively suggested that longer durations of treatment with postoperative antibiotics are needed for patients with more heavily contaminated wounds.[6] Some advocates of a shorter duration of treatment with perioperative antibiotics suggested that longer administration of perioperative antibiotics contributes to infection with gram-negative organisms or may result in infection with more resistant gram-negative bacilli such as *P. aeruginosa* or other pathogens such as *C. albicans*.[7-10]

Nonetheless, although the use of antibiotics indeed selects for these organisms, many single-organism infections occurring after initiation of antibiotics would have been polymicrobial were it not for intraoperative and immediate postoperative treatment. From an infectious disease perspective, continuation of antibiotics beyond the intraoperative period is similar to treatment of an open fracture and not very much like antibiotic prophylaxis in the traditional sense. Perhaps better stated is that the use of intraoperative antibiotics and immediate postoperative treatment may kill bacteria that have contaminated operative sites, including surgically fractured bone.

POSTOPERATIVE FEVER

Pyrexia is thought to be a normal physiologic response to craniofacial surgery. In a study of 136 transcranial surgical procedures performed for nonsyndromic craniosynostosis, postoperative temperatures of 38° C or higher were encountered in 76 percent of subjects, and hyperpyrexia exceeding 39° C was encountered in 11 percent. Temperature elevations usually are encountered in the first 48 hours but occasionally occur up to 5 days postoperatively.[18] Close clinical evaluation is warranted in all cases of pyrexia.

EVALUATION

Signs of postoperative craniofacial surgical infection include the following: fever (although not in all cases)[18]; the rapid development of unilateral local soft tissue warmth, tenderness, and erythema; and rapid recurrence of swelling.[5] Reasons for the delay in establishing the diagnosis and for providing definitive treatment of some infections are multifactorial. Postoperative swelling may persist for some time, often improving and worsening in dependent areas according to the patient's sleeping or resting position. Periorbital tissues are particularly prone to fluctuations in swelling. Violaceous discoloration and bruising of the overlying skin may complicate assessment further. In addition, the overall facial appearance of the child may be so altered by the surgical intervention that parents may not recognize subtle signs of infection immediately. In some instances, large distances may separate the child from the craniofacial surgery referral center after discharge from the hospital, and the surgeon must rely on verbal descriptions of the child's postoperative appearance from concerned caregivers. Therefore, patients who live far from the referral center should be educated that prompt local medical evaluation along with a phone call to the craniofacial surgeon at the referral center can assist in early diagnosis, determination of bacteriology by needle aspiration, and initiation of preliminary treatment during travel back to the referral center. Prescription of oral antibiotics in the hope of preserving the tenuous bone grafts without aspiration may render the interpretation of subsequent surgical culture results difficult.

Evaluation of extraocular movement may be limited by the age of the child, by postoperative swelling, and, frequently, by the limited capacity of the patient to comply interactively with the examination. Few operations, however, limit the ability to assess the presence of meningismus. Some patients may exhibit lassitude, lethargy, or increased irritability, subtle signs in children who have limited capacities to communicate.

The wound, often a coronal incision, should be examined closely. Purulent or seropurulent wound drainage or persistent serous wound drainage usually is indicative of underlying soft tissue and possibly bone infection, although infection may not be limited to the structures located directly beneath an area of wound dehiscence.[5] Drainage at one location along a wound may be the result of inflammatory fluids that originate elsewhere and are following a hydrodynamic gravity flow pattern or an established route to a low-pressure efflux portal at a nonhealing area of the wound, especially when the infection has become well established. Similarly, fluid collections in suborbital areas of the face such as the malar or submalar areas may suggest a local abscess when, in fact, the primary site of infection is cranial and the collection is only a dependent pool.

Laboratory abnormalities may be subtle. Leukocytosis may be present. The erythrocyte sedimentation rate has been shown to peak approximately 5 days after major orthopedic surgery and to decline slowly and irregularly for a period of 3 to 9 weeks, but it provides little diagnostic value initially.[3,13,19] C-reactive protein (CRP) levels peak within 2 to 3 days but usually normalize within 21 postoperative days.[3,13,16,19] Because an abrupt increase in CRP may be indicative of infection, some orthopedic centers monitor CRP levels to assist in early detection of infection after elective procedures such as total-joint replacement and spinal surgery.[13,19] Similarly, monitoring serial CRP levels is helpful when trying to discriminate between infection and shifting postoperative dependent swelling and in assessing the response to therapy in a craniofacial surgical patient.

Needle aspiration of underlying fluid collections is the best primary means of diagnosing infection, especially if significant residual postoperative swelling has rendered clinical assessment of a particular area difficult. In most instances, needle aspiration cultures are superior to surface cultures of wound drainage, which often yield coagulase-negative staphylococci of uncertain significance. However, cultures of wound drainage sometimes grow obvious pathogens and may be helpful.

Diagnostic imaging such as computed tomography with contrast or magnetic resonance imaging may identify occult fluid collections, but diagnosing bone infection, especially in the flat bones of the cranium, is difficult with these modalities. Not infrequently, focal enhancement of the meninges in regions where the cranium has been manipulated is noted on postoperative imaging. Corresponding postoperative cerebral gliosis also can be difficult to differentiate from cerebritis developing near an area of infection above the dura. Serial weekly or biweekly imaging can provide a means of performing ongoing evaluation of these abnormalities inasmuch as neurologic manifestations of cerebritis in the frontal lobes may not be elucidated easily. Surgical exploration of suspected areas of infection remains the most helpful source of diagnostic information regarding infection.

TREATMENT

Management of infections complicating craniofacial procedures is primarily surgical. Open débridement, inspection and scraping of contiguous bone, and copious pressurized saline irrigation are essential. The value of adding antibiotics to the irrigant is questionable. Some physicians argue that irrigation with povidone-iodine may devitalize tissues that participate in the healing process and should not be used, whereas other physicians avoid using povidone-iodine irrigation because of concern about systemic iodine absorption.[9] Removal of all hardware provides the best chance for eradicating the infection, but occasionally, as in the case of procedures that involve maxillary distraction devices, removing all the hardware initially is impractical. Furthermore, distraction pins may dislodge as the integrity of the bone is compromised by infection.[20]

Placement of several drains ensures an opportunity for drainage of what otherwise would remain sequestered focal soft tissue fluid collections. Continuous subgaleal flow-through irrigation with saline at a rate of 15 to 30 mL/hr (with or without antibiotic additives) is an adjunctive measure instituted by some surgeons; other surgeons question the advisability of this approach.[9] Removal of devitalized bone and of any bone grafts in the infected surgical bed is an unpopular but necessary part of treatment. Failure to do so may result in multifocal osteomyelitis, possible meningitis or cerebritis, and persistence of chronic infection with potentially multidrug-resistant organisms.

Reluctance by the surgical team to excise infected bone aggressively and widely and to remove devitalized bone is understandable because the initial surgical procedure itself involves extensive planning, operative time, and anesthetic risk. In addition, interposition grafts may provide architectural platforms for the advanced structures, and successful treatment of these infections was reported in some surgical centers in which the initial bony débridement was limited to areas of visibly apparent osteitis.[9]

With regard to post-craniotomy wound infections, traditional dogma suggested operative débridement and complete removal of devitalized bone flaps followed by delayed cranioplasty.[4] However, some patient groups may fare better with attempted preservation of bone flap with minor surgical débridement and systemic antibiotic therapy. Within a small group of five patients who had undergone craniotomy without a history of previous craniotomy, radiation therapy, or skull-base surgery, operative débridement accompanied by culture and susceptibility data-driven systemic antibiotic therapy successfully treated infection with a mean of 35 ± 20 months of follow-up. Several other patients required second-look operations with more débridement, but they did not require removal of the bone flap and were cured. In the same study, the two other subjects had undergone more extensive craniofacial surgery and had recurrent infection requiring removal of the bone flap at 2 months after presentation in one patient and at 29 months in the other one, respectively; this finding bears out the concern that contamination of the bone flap can result in persistent, long-standing infection.[4]

As an advisor, the infectious disease consultant should point out evidence of persistent infection, suggest the possibility of deeper or more serious infection when concern arises, alert the surgical team when a point of failure of medical therapy has been reached, and emphasize that antimicrobial therapy is only an adjuvant to bony débridement and copious intraoperative irrigation, which may improve the outcome and limit the spread of infection. Recurrent wound dehiscence and continued wound drainage should prompt thorough exploration of the soft tissues and bone for evidence of osteomyelitis or retained hardware, including wires. Advanced infection in devitalized bone cannot be treated effectively in situ, and often entire bone plates must be removed, with cranioplasty performed months later.

For infections that complicate procedures not involving the oropharynx or sinus cavities, an antistaphylococcal antibiotic such as vancomycin, cefazolin, or nafcillin may be an appropriate empiric antibiotic choice pending the results of intraoperative drainage and débridement cultures. A third-generation cephalosporin with or without an aminoglycoside may be considered if the risk of developing an infection with a nosocomial pathogen is high because of prolonged hospitalization or persistent tracheal colonization with gram-negative bacilli such as *Pseudomonas*[8] or if infection of the central nervous system threatens. Infections complicating procedures involving the oropharynx or sinuses often are caused by organisms resistant to the perioperative prophylactic antibiotic chosen.[6] Thus, it may be reasonable to consider antibiotic therapy with clindamycin or metronidazole when a cephalosporin has been used or treatment with a second- or third-generation cephalosporin or ampicillin-sulbactam when

clindamycin has been used prophylactically. The duration of antibiotic therapy must be individualized to each case. A period of 6 weeks of antibiotic therapy has been suggested for patients with suspected osteomyelitis.[21]

REFERENCES

1. Acebal-Bianco, F., Vuylsteke, P. L., Mommaerts, M. Y., and De Clercq, C. A.: Perioperative complications in corrective facial orthopedic surgery: A 5-year retrospective study. J. Oral Maxillofac. Surg. *58*:754-760, 2000.
2. Bentley, K. C., Head, T. W., and Aiello, G. A.: Antibiotic prophylaxis in orthognathic surgery: A 1-day versus 5-day regimen. J. Oral Maxillofac. Surg. *57*:226-230, 1999.
3. Bilgen, O., Atici, T., Durak, K., et al.: C-reactive protein values and erythrocyte sedimentation rates after total hip and total knee arthroplasty. J. Int. Med. Res. *29*:7-12, 2001.
4. Bruce, J. N., and Bruce, S. S.: Preservation of bone flaps in patients with post-craniotomy infections. J. Neurosurg. *98*:1203-1207, 2003.
5. Carson, B. S., and Dufresne, C. R.: Surgical complications. *In* Dufresne, C. R., Carson, B. S., and Zinreich, S. J. (eds.): Complex Craniofacial Problems: A Guide to Analysis and Treatment. New York, Churchill Livingstone, 1992, pp. 467-487.
6. Clayman, G. L., Raad, I. I., Hankins, P. D., and Weber, R. S.: Bacteriologic profile of surgical infection after antibiotic prophylaxis. Head Neck *15*:526-531, 1993.
7. Conover, M. A., Kaban, L. B., and Mulliken, J. B.: Antibiotic prophylaxis for major maxillocraniofacial surgery. J. Oral Maxillofac. Surg. *43*:865-870, 1985.
8. David, D. J., and Cooter, R. D.: Craniofacial infection in 10 years of transcranial surgery. Plast. Reconstr. Surg. *80*:213-225, 1987.
9. Fearon, J. A., Yu, J., Bartlett, S. P., et al.: Infections in craniofacial surgery: A combined report of 567 procedures from two centers. Plast. Reconstr. Surg. *100*:862-868, 1997.
10. Israele, V., and Seigel, J. D.: Infectious complications of craniofacial surgery in children. Rev. Infect. Dis. *11*:9-15, 1989.
11. Kawamoto, H. K., Jr., and Cohen, S. R.: Aesthetic Le Fort I, II, and III. *In* Ousterhout, D. K. (ed.): Aesthetic Contouring of the Craniofacial Skeleton. Boston, Little, Brown, 1991, pp. 487-499.
12. Kramer, F. J., Baethge, C., Swennen, G., et al.: Intra- and perioperative complications of Le Fort I osteotomy: A prospective evaluation of 1000 patients. J. Craniofac. Surg. *15*:971-977, 2004.
13. Larsson, S., Thelander, U., and Friberg, S.: C-reactive protein (CRP) levels after elective orthopedic surgery. Clin. Orthop. Relat. Res. *275*:237-242, 1992.
14. Mason, R. M., and Georgiade, N. G.: Facial osteotomies. *In* Georgiade, N. G., Georgiade, G. S., Riefkohl, R., and Barwick, W. (eds.): Essentials of Plastic, Maxillofacial, and Reconstructive Surgery. Baltimore, Williams & Wilkins, 1987, pp. 332-340.
15. Pietrzak, W. S., and Eppley, B. L.: Antibiotic elution from hydroxyapatite cement cranioplasty materials. J. Craniofac. Surg. *16*:228-233, 2005.
16. Rosahl, S. K., Gharabaghi, A., Zink, P. M., and Samii, M.: Monitoring of blood parameters following anterior cervical fusion. J. Neurosurg. *92*(Suppl.):169-174, 2000.
17. Stratoudakis, A. C.: An outline of craniofacial anomalies and principles of their correction. *In* Georgiade, N. G., Georgiade, G. S., Riefkohl, R., and Barwick, W. (eds.): Essentials of Plastic, Maxillofacial, and Reconstructive Surgery. Baltimore, Williams & Wilkins, 1987, pp. 299-331.
18. Takagi, S., Anderson, P. J., and David, D. J.: Pyrexia after transcranial surgery. J. Craniofac. Surg. *17*:202-204, 2006.
19. Thelander, U., and Larsson, S.: Quantitation of C-reactive protein levels and erythrocyte sedimentation rate after spinal surgery. Spine *17*:400-404, 1992.
20. Van der Meulen, J., Wolvius, E., Van der Wal, K., et al.: Prevention of halo pin complications in post-cranioplasty patients. J. Craniomaxillofac. Surg. *33*:145-149, 2005.
21. Whitaker, L. A.: Problems and complications in craniofacial surgery. *In* Goldwyn, R. M. (ed.): The Unfavorable Result in Plastic Surgery: Avoidance and Treatment. 2nd ed. Boston, Little, Brown, 1984, pp. 229-250.
22. Whitaker, L. A., Munro, I. R., Salyer, K. E., et al.: Combined report of problems and complications in 793 craniofacial operations. Plast. Reconstr. Surg. *64*:198-203, 1979.
23. Wolfe, S. A.: The monoblock frontofacial advancement: Outcome after retrofrontal epidural abscess. *In* Craniofacial Surgery. Proceedings of the Sixth International Congress of the International Society of Cranio-Facial Surgery. Bologna, Italy, Munduzzi, 1995, pp. 211-213.
24. Yeung, L. C., Cunningham, M. L., Allpress, A. L., et al.: Surgical site infections after pediatric intracranial surgery for craniofacial malformation: Frequency and risk factors. Neurosurgery *56*:733-738, 2005.

INFECTIONS IN BURN PATIENTS

Janak A. Patel ⊕ Natalie Williams-Bouyer

According to the American Burn Association, approximately 500,000 persons are treated for burns every year in the United States; of these, approximately 40,000 are hospitalized and approximately 4000 die from the burn injury.[4] Improvement in the rate of burn-associated mortality is a direct result of advancement in burn care, comprising developments in fluid resuscitation, wound care, early excision and grafting, nutritional support, infection control, and antimicrobial therapy. The mortality rates and lengths of stay of burned children have been reduced greatly in the past several decades. In the 1960s, the likelihood of survival was only 50 percent for pediatric patients with burns covering 35 to 44 percent of the total body surface area (TBSA), and few children with burns covering more than 45 percent of TBSA survived. The average length of stay was 103 days. In 2008, the LA$_{50}$ (lethal burn size for 50% of patients) for children exceeded 95 percent of TBSA, and the average length of hospital stay for most serious burn injuries can be expected to be only 0.5 days per percent TBSA that is burned. Since 1998, the mortality rate at the Shriners Burns Hospital for Children (Galveston, Texas) has ranged from 1 to 3 percent.

BURN WOUND

1. **Burn wound depth:** Burn wounds are categorized by their depth (Fig. 87–1).[42]

a. *First-degree burns* consist of epidermal damage only. These wounds are painful and erythematous resulting from local vasodilation. They heal spontaneously, usually without forming scars, within 7 days.

b. *Second-degree burns* are injuries with partial thickness and are further categorized as *superficial* or *deep*. The epidermis and superficial portions of the dermis are injured in superficial second-degree burns. These wounds are painful and often result in formation of blisters. Healing occurs via epithelial migration from the wound edges, hair follicles, and sebaceous glands. Relatively little scarring occurs, and reepithelization occurs within 2 weeks. Deep second-degree burns are much more serious. The majority of the dermis is destroyed, leaving the bases of the epidermal appendages spared. The nerve endings also are destroyed, rendering the wound insensate. Blisters usually are not present owing to the thicker formation of eschar. These wounds are treated as full-thickness injuries. Reepithelialization is tenuous and slow. The protracted inflammatory phase often results in excessive deposition of collagen and extensive scarring.

c. *Third-degree burns* are full-thickness injuries to the skin. Healing occurs by contraction and reepithelialization from the edges of the wound. As with deep second-degree burns, these wounds are insensate and without blistering. Infants and young children have a much thinner dermal layer to their skin, resulting in increased propensity for deeper burn injury. Treatment for third-degree burns is with excision and skin grafting.

d. *Fourth-degree burns* extend into the deep tissue, which includes muscle, bone, and viscera. Treatment is débridement and possible amputation. Closure of these wounds may vary from primary closure post amputation to skin grafting and possibly flap reconstruction.

2. **Cytologic findings:** The effects of extreme heat on the skin lead to cellular and subcellular impairment. The determin-

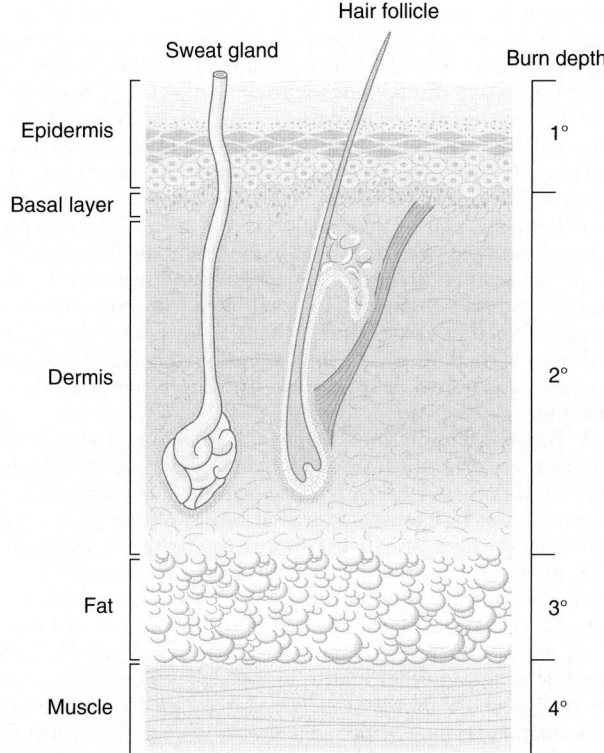

Figure 87–1 The burn wound depth. (See companion Expert Consult web site for color version.) *(With permission from Greenhalgh, D.: Wound healing. In Herndon, D. N. [ed.]: Total Burn Care. Philadelphia, WB Saunders, 2007, p. 579 [Fig. 46.1]).*

ing factors of how severe a burn will be are the temperature, the length of exposure, and the actual burning agent. Moritz and Henrique[83] showed that the skin is able to withstand temperatures up to 40° C (104° F) for relatively long periods of time before an injury becomes apparent.[83] Increase in temperature leads to cell membrane dysfunction as ion channels are disrupted, resulting in sodium and water intake. As temperatures exceed 45° C, protein denaturation supersedes the cell's reparative capabilities and oxygen radicals are liberated. Plasma membrane necrosis has been observed in cells exposed to 45° C for 1 hour. Other cytologic findings in thermal injury include the redistribution of solid and fluid components of the cell nuclei. Imbibition of fluid results in nuclear swelling, rupture of membranes, and pyknosis. As denaturation proceeds, vital cellular metabolic processes are injured. If enzyme activity is decreased to less than 50 percent of its normal level, cell death occurs. In lesser degrees of enzyme impairment, cell recovery may be possible.

3. **Local tissue changes:** Local burn injury is classically described by Jackson[54] in three concentric zones. As temperature increases, protein denaturation results in coagulation. The protein architecture is destroyed and new aberrant macromolecules are formed. The central area of a burn wound is that which is in direct contact with the source of heat. Cell necrosis is com-

plete and is called the *zone of coagulation*. Cellular recovery is impossible, and the severity of injury decreases from the surface to the deeper levels. This zone is called the *burn eschar*. At the peripheral margins of the zone of coagulation, a less injured zone is present. The cells in this *zone of stasis* show direct injury from the heat, but the damage is not lethal. However, blood flow becomes progressively impaired to this area. Ischemia to the already compromised cells may lead to necrosis and conversion to dead eschar. Circulatory impairment occurs via adherence of neutrophils to the vessel wall, deposition of fibrin, formation of platelet microthrombus, vasoconstriction, and endothelial swelling. Heat-compromised erythrocytes lose their ability to deform, and their passage through microvessels is impeded. The circulatory embarrassment may be delayed for up to 24 hours, and the ischemia may progress for up to 48 hours after the burn has occurred. If stasis conditions are minimal, the injury may be halted and cell recovery may occur within 1 week. However, this tissue is fragile, and further insults such as infection, hypovolemia, pressure, and over-resuscitation can lead to further necrosis. Finally, the *zone of hyperemia* lies peripheral to the zone of stasis. This zone sustains minimal injury and often recovers within 7 to 10 days. Notable vasodilation is caused by potent vasoactive mediators secondary to the inflammatory response. Complete recovery is expected in this zone barring further trauma or infection.

4. **Burn inflammation:** Many of the above processes are either part of or result from the inflammatory process. Cellular infiltration, initiated by local inflammatory mediators such as prostanoids and leukotrienes, as well as proinflammatory cytokines from the burn wound, begins with the arrival of neutrophils at 4 to 5 days postburn, followed by macrophages.[106] The neutrophils further mediate damage by releasing oxygen free radicals.[36] Reestablishment of blood flow in the zone of stasis is yet another setting wherein oxygen free radicals are produced, leading to further injury. This phenomenon of ischemia-reperfusion injury occurs as oxygen is restored to the tissues.[59] Inflammation becomes prominent at 7 to 10 days. Consequently, blood flow is maximal at this stage, creating a troublesome and hazardous setting for surgical excision of the eschar. Along with local inflammatory responses, several systemic responses occur with burns of more than 15 percent of the TBSA.

5. **Inhalation injury:** Burn victims, especially those trapped in enclosed areas, injure the respiratory tract upon inhalation of toxic gases from surrounding burning materials. An actual thermal airway injury is quite rare. The upper airway is rather effective in cooling and warming inspired air. Also, air has a very low heat capacity. In order to have direct injury to the airway, the flames must come into direct contact with them. Injury to the oropharynx after inhalation of toxic gases resembles thermal injury elsewhere in the body.[1] Protein denaturation, release of inflammatory mediators, and increased cellular and microvascular permeability all occur, leading to airway edema and consequent obstruction of the airway.

The chemical injury from inhalation of toxic gases can damage the tracheobronchial tree. First, separation of ciliated epithelial cells from the basement membrane occurs.[11] Next, the circulation of blood to the lung, as well as to the bronchial tree, is increased due to vasodilation. Shortly thereafter, edema is evident. The inflammatory phase is followed by an exudative phase.[52] Furthermore, the protein component of this fluid is composed of lung lymph and induces bronchoconstriction. As postburn time increases, fibrin casts are formed from the exudates, resulting in obstruction of the airway. As the epithelium sloughs and formation of fibrin casts increases, susceptibility to infection also increases. Pneumonia leading to sepsis and death are well-known sequelae at this stage. Finally, formation of pseudomembranes proceeds and then squamous metaplasia follows.[92] Healing may

take weeks to initiate, and permanent damage to the airway (e.g., stenosis and formation of tracheal granulomas) may occur.

INFLAMMATORY AND IMMUNE RESPONSES IN BURNS

Intact human skin is vital for preservation of the host's protection against infection. A combination of impaired local and systemic host defenses and loss of the skin barrier are major factors responsible for the increased susceptibility to infections in patients with burns. The major elements initially contributing to the inflammatory response that occurs after burns are incurred include the plasma proteins, mast cells, tissue macrophages, and systemically recruited neutrophils and monocytes.

Alterations in the host defenses include induction of local and systemic cytokine synthesis, decreased immunoglobulin levels, changes in the concentration and activity of both the classical and alternative complement pathways, reduced levels of circulating plasma fibronectin, depressed serum opsonic activity, and impairment of the macrophages, lymphocytes, neutrophils, and the reticuloendothelial system. However, many mechanisms of immune alterations remain unknown; for example, an association of the volume of blood transfusions with increased mortality rates and infectious episodes in patients with major burns was observed in two reports.[56,92] The immunologic status of the burned patient has a measurable impact on survival, death, and major morbidity.

1. **The cytokine response:** After burn injury occurs, numerous cytokines are induced rapidly. Many cytokines correlate with the severity of the burn injury and the prognosis. Recent studies at our center have shown a specific pattern of systemic cytokine responses in children with thermal injury. Compared with unburned healthy children, children with burns covering more than 40 percent of TBSA had significant increases in serum levels of 15 cytokines and immunoregulatory molecules during the first week after incurring the thermal injury: interleukin (IL)-1β, IL-2, IL-4, IL-5, IL-6, IL-7, IL-8, IL-10, IL-12 p70, IL-13, IL-17, interferon gamma, monocyte chemoattractant protein-1 (MCP-1), macrophage inflammatory protein (MIP)-1β, and granulocyte colony-stimulating factor (G-CSF).[31] Granulocyte-macrophage colony-stimulating factor (GM-CSF) was significantly increased during the second week after burn occurred. Within 5 weeks, the serum concentrations of most cytokines decreased, approaching normal levels. In another study of children, serum IL-8, tumor necrosis factor (TNF), IL-6, IL-12p70, MCP-1, and GM-CSF were significantly increased in those with large burns.[56] In general, the notion was that the smaller the burn size, the lower the cytokine concentration.

In children with inhalation injury, the serum cytokine studies at enrollment showed significant reduction in level of IL-7 and elevation of IL-12p70, as compared with children without inhalation injury.[30] However, 5 to 7 days later, the levels were comparable. Host genetic factors also may affect the cytokine response in patients with burns. For example, single nucleotide polymorphisms for TNF-α (308G), Toll-like receptor 4 (+896G), IL-6 (174C), and CD14 (159C) were significantly associated with an increased risk for severe sepsis following burns.[7]

2. **Neutrophils:** Thermal injury induces neutropenia and myeloid maturation arrest despite elevated G-CSF levels.[108] The degree of neutropenia correlates with the reduction in bone marrow G-CSF receptor expression. The neutrophils of patients with burns also are functionally altered[84]: The expression of the Fc receptor is decreased, and intracellular killing capacity is depressed (this is a differential suppression, more for some organisms than others) and is accompanied by a brief increase in neutrophil respiratory burst response. Failure of initial alkalization

of the phagolysosome and alteration of subsequent kinetics of acidification also occur.[14] This depression of oxygen-independent bactericidal mechanism may impair the capacity of the neutrophil for intracellular killing after a thermal injury occurs. Expression of CD16 (Fc receptor [FcR], Fc immunoglobulin G [IgG] receptor) and CD11 (adhesion molecule) on neutrophils is impaired after a major injury occurs; this reduction appears to be related directly to the appearance of bacteremia or pneumonia.[5] These changes in expression of adhesion molecules, which is closely related to chemotaxis, may play a part in the failure of delivery of neutrophils in adequate numbers to the local site of a burn. Furthermore, a defect is present in actin polymerization in the neutrophils of patients with burns; as a basic mechanism of chemotaxis, it also may contribute to a failure of motility.

Generation of leukotrienes from the neutrophils of severely burned patients also is impaired and appears to be based on the availability, or lack of availability, of the metabolizable substrate-free arachidonic acid.[62] Because leukotriene B also is a potent neutrophil chemotactic agent, this impairment may further contribute to the failure of neutrophil function.

3. Complements: The fluid of the burn blister shows much lower opsonic activity for bacteria such as *Pseudomonas aeruginosa* than the patient's own serum.[90] A mild impairment of production of C3 and release by macrophages of burn patients in vitro also occurs. Systemically, both the classical and the alternative pathways are depleted, but the alternative pathway is more profoundly perturbed. After the development of bacteremia, additional complement activation and depletion occur.[115]

4. Macrophages: Suppression of the ability of the reticuloendothelial system to take up particulate material was among the original observations of burn immunology made in the 1960s. More recent reports, however, have described the demonstration of a differentially increased uptake of colloid in alveolar macrophages compared with other organs, perhaps indicating alveolar macrophage activation. Macrophages and monocytes appear to be activated in a fashion similar to that of lymphocytes after thermal injury occurs. Activation of macrophages, as measured by the serum neopterin level, is increased after thermal injury occurs.[6] This activation is confirmed by increased expression of the monocyte cell surface antigens C3b and iC3b.[82] At the same time, expression of human leukocyte antigen (HLA)-DR, HLA-DQ, and HLA-DP by monocytes is reduced, and these class II antigens are obligatory for many cell-mediated immunologic processes, thereby implying that a possible loss of function of monocytes occurs after thermal injury.[39] Production of C3 by macrophages is suppressed in patients with burns, but the synthetic ability for key cytokines such as IL-6 is increased.[126]

Peripheral blood monocytes are superstimulated to produce large amounts of IL-1, leading to exhaustion of the function on monocytes.[73] Reduced production of IL-1 by monocytes was found in patients with complicated organ injury, multiorgan failure, and systemic infection. Blood monocytes of patients with burns produce significantly more IL-10 at 7 to 10 days after burn injury, which correlates significantly with subsequent septic events.[61]

5. T lymphocytes and cell-mediated immunity: Early studies of T cells in patients with burns showed a variety of changes: impairment in mitogenic and antigenic responsiveness of lymphocytes, suppression of graft-versus-host reactivity related to the size of the burn, suppression of delayed cutaneous sensitivity tests, and diminution in both numbers of peripheral lymphocytes and concentration of thoracic duct lymphocytes. Whether the failure of T cell functions is due to an intracellular defect related to thermal injury, the result of "overuse," or indirectly the result of down-regulation by the cytokine cascade or other products of the inflammatory reaction remains controversial.

Analysis of peripheral blood T cells supports the theory that, rather than an absolute reduction in CD4 and an increase in CD8

cells, a redistribution of lymphocyte traffic may occur.[91] Suppression in the numbers of the total population of lymphocytes is the only consistent overall change. Further, not only does lymphocyte traffic between stores of central lymphocytes and the peripheral blood occur after a thermal injury, but the responsiveness of these populations of lymphocytes also vary according to the site; for example, splenic lymphocytes of experimentally burned animals remain most profoundly depressed in response to antigenic stimulation, compared with the peripheral blood and other organs.[25] In addition, in peripheral blood, the appearance of "activation" antigens on CD4 and CD8 cells (HLA-DR, IL-2 receptor [IL-2R], and transferrin receptor) is depressed significantly as early as 1 day after burn injury occurs.[75]

Addition of recombinant IL-2 does not appear to reverse the suppression of the appearance of surface markers such as IL-2R in burned patients, although it does not improve the response of natural killer (NK) cells to stimulation.[34] In experimental preparations, at least some of the observed T-cell suppression can be alleviated by early removal of the burn wound, thereby creating one further argument for promptly closing the burn wound.[45]

6. B lymphocytes and humoral immunity: The function of B cells after the occurrence of a thermal injury is less well documented than is that of macrophages or T cells. The expression of this major histocompatibility complex is impaired and, therefore, some diminution of B-cell function can be expected as a result of diminished recognition of antigenic presentation.[87] Under the influence of stress-induced corticosteroids, the number of circulating B cells is relatively increased compared with T cells in peripheral blood.[58] Spontaneous cytokine (IL-4 and IL-2)-induced expression of the activation antigen CD23 is reduced significantly during the second to fifth week after burn injury occurs.[103]

If the products of B-cell activation, namely the immunoglobulins, are measured in vivo, the results are somewhat difficult to interpret because of the increased catabolism of protein and the leakage through the burn wound. Briefly, marked diminution of serum IgG concentration, total and all subclasses, is present; these levels return to normal between 10 and 14 days after the burn injury has occurred. Extremely low levels of IgG on admission (300-400 mg/dL) are predictors of a poor prognosis. Levels of IgM and IgA appear to be relatively unaffected. Overall, the defective production of immunoglobulin after a thermal injury occurs appears to be a factor of macrophage/lymphocyte interaction rather than a failure of intrinsic activity by B cells.[29]

BURN WOUND MICROBIOLOGY

A working knowledge of the common flora of burn wounds is essential to appropriately tailor therapy. Pathogens peculiar to thermal injuries are basically no different from the normal flora of the environment. Table 87–1 shows the types of microorganisms found in various body tissues and secretions as either normal flora or as pathogens. However, the organisms that predominate as causative agents of infections of burn wounds in any burn-treatment facility change over the course of time. Gram-positive organisms prevail in the early postburn period and then are replaced by gram-negative bacteria and fungi.[27]

1. Gram-positive bacteria: The gram-positive predominance is consistent with the normal inhabitants of the skin prior to the thermal injury. *Staphylococcus* spp., *Micrococcus* spp., *Streptococcus* spp., *Pediococcus* spp., and *Enterococcus* spp. are gram-positive cocci commonly encountered in burn wounds. Erol and associates[27] recently demonstrated that coagulase-negative staphylococci and *Staphylococcus aureus* were the most prevalent isolates in admission cultures, followed by diphtheroids. These organisms can be life-threatening as invasive infections or simply be locally

TABLE 87-1   Tissue Association of Microorganisms Most Commonly Found in Burn Wound Infection*

Organism	Soft Tissue Skin	Upper Respiratory	Lower Respiratory	Endocardial	Gastrointestinal	Urogenital	Bone and Joint
Staphylococcus aureus	NF, P	P, NF	P	P	P	NF, P	P
Staphylococcus epidermidis	NF, P	NF, P	P	P	P	NF, P	P
Other *Staphylococci* spp.	NF	NF, P	P	P	NF, P	NF, P	P
Streptococcus pyogenes	P, NF	P, NF	P	P	P	P	P
Other *Streptococci* spp.	NF	NF	P	P	NF	NF, P	P
Enterococcus spp.	P	P	P	P	NF, P	NF, P	P
Escherichia coli	NF, P	NF, P	P	P	NF, P	NF, P	P
Klebsiella pneumoniae	NF, P	NF, P	P	P	NF, P	NF, P	P
Enterobacter cloacae	NF, P	NF, P	P	P	NF, P	NF, P	P
Enterobacter aerogenes	NF, P	NF, P	P	P	NF, P	NF, P	P
Proteus spp.	NF, P	P	P	P	NF, P	NF, P	P
Serratia marcescens	NF, P	(–)	P	P	P	P	P
Other enterics	NF, P	NF, P	P	P	NF, P	P	P
Pseudomonas aeruginosa	P	NF, P	P	P	NF, P	P	P
Acinetobacter spp.	NF	NF	P	(–)	NF	NF	P
Candida albicans	NF	NF	P	P	NF	P, NF	P

NF, normal flora; P, pathogens; (–), normally not found, but these organisms should not be ignored when encountered.
Modified from Heggers, J.: Microbiology for surgeons. In Kerstein, M. D. (ed.): Management of Surgical Infections. Mt Kisco, NY, Futura Publishing, 1980, pp. 27-55.

TABLE 87-2   Bacteria Isolated from 304 Acute Care Pediatric Burn Patients Admitted to Shriners Burns Hospitals for Children—Galveston, Texas (January 2006 to December 2006)

Gram-Positive Organisms	No. (%) of Isolates
Methicillin-resistant *Staphylococcus epidermidis*	196 (23.7)
Methicillin-resistant *Staphylococcus aureus*	152 (18.4)
Enterococcus faecium	119 (14.4)
Methicillin-sensitive *S. epidermidis*	84 (10.2)
Methicillin-sensitive *S. aureus*	82 (9.9)
Enterococcus faecalis	80 (9.7)
Other gram-positives*	113 (13.7)
Total no. of gram-positive isolates	**826**
Gram-Negative Organisms	
Carbohydrate Fermenters (Enterics)	
Escherichia coli	103 (17.4)
Enterobacter cloacae	67 (11.3)
Klebsiella pneumoniae	66 (11.1)
Other fermentors†	132 (22.3)
Noncarbohydrate Fermenters	
Pseudomonas aeruginosa	122 (20.6)
Acinetobacter spp.	48 (8.2)
Stenotrophomonas maltophia	16 (2.7)
Other nonfermentors‡	38 (6.4)
Total no. of gram-negative isolates	**592**
Total no. of bacterial isolates	**1418**
Gram-positive organisms (%)	**(58.3)**
Gram-negative organisms (%)	**(41.7)**

Includes other Staphylococcus, Enterococcus spp.; Micrococcus, Pediococcus and Streptococcus spp.
†*Includes other Enterobacter, Klebsiella, Serratia, Proteus, and Citrobacter spp.*
‡*Includes other Aeromonas and Achromobacter spp.*

colonized. Table 87–2 shows the distribution of gram-positive bacteria at Shriners Burns Hospital for Children in Galveston, Texas, which receives pediatric burn patients from all over the world. For the year 2006, the gram-positive cocci accounted for 58.3 percent of bacterial isolates. Within this group, the staphylococci are more prevalent (62.2%) than are the enterococci, which account for 24.1 percent. Among staphylococci, a predominance of methicillin-resistant (42.1%) versus methicillin-sensitive (20.1%) isolates was noted. The rate of staphylococcal methicillin resistance has increased in this patient population

since 2000. This increase is reflective of a worldwide emergence of such antimicrobial resistance in both hospitalized-acquired and community-acquired infections.

Because of such resistance patterns, Cook[21] stresses the importance of microbial surveillance and epidemiologic studies. This approach is thought to reduce the prevalence of methicillin-resistant *S. aureus* (MRSA), yet it may be inadequate for eradicating or preventing outbreaks. Minimizing transmission and infection is emphasized. However, Reardon and colleagues[95] suggest that this process is time-consuming and requires extensive resources for little gain. Colonization with methicillin-sensitive *S. aureus* and MRSA in 86 patients was studied and found to have no significant changes on length of stay, number of operations, or mortality between these two organisms. However, the presence of either type of *S. aureus* significantly increased the number of surgical procedures performed and the lengths of stay. Many burn units report frequent colonization of burn patients with toxic shock toxin (TSS-1)–producing strains of staphylococci; however, their presence does not correlate well with increased morbidity or mortality rates.[20]

In the past, group A β-hemolytic *Streptococcus* frequently was the cause of epidemics in burn units, but it seldom is encountered today because of the frequent emperic use of antibiotics for manipulations of burn wounds. Other β-hemolytic streptococci belonging to groups B, C, E, F, and G can be encountered as well.[71] Significant infection-control vigilance still is necessary, as occasional clusters of outbreaks of group A streptococcal infection continue to be reported.[43,98] Fortunately, group A *Streptococcus* remains uniformly sensitive to penicillins; hence, prophylaxis and treatment are easily accomplished.

Although enterococcal infections (*Enterococcus faecalis* and *Enterococcus faecium*) account for only 24.1 percent of burn-wound infections caused by gram-positive bacteria (see Table 87–2), a significant cause for concern is the emergence of vancomycin-resistant *Enterococcus* (VRE) in burn units.[67,69] Although additional morbidity associated with VRE itself is not clear, when it occurs as a polymicrobial bacteremia, a mortality rate as high as 20 percent has been noted.[69]

Other gram-positive bacilli include the aerobic *Corynbacterium* spp. and *Listeria* spp., as well as the spore-forming *Bacillus* spp. (aerobe) and *Clostridium* spp. (anaerobe). *Bacillus* and *Clostridium* spp. are associated with burn wounds that have come in contact with contaminated soil. In avascular muscle injuries (e.g., electrical injuries or crush injuries combined with burns), the risk for developing tetanus *(Clostridium tetani)* is high[68] and has led to the practice of using tetanus immunoprophylaxis and booster vaccines.[105]

2. Gram-negative bacteria: The presence of the gram-negative bacteria in burn wounds is due in part to translocation of the bacteria from the gastrointestinal tract of the patients.[8] In a study of children with burns at our center, patients with large wounds (>50% TBSA) were found to have significantly higher colonization with their fecal gram-negative bacteria than were those with smaller wounds.[32] At our center, although the gram-negative bacteria account for only 41.7 percent of the total bacterial isolates of the wound, they represent a formidable adversary (see Table 87–2). The majority of this group are extended β-lactam–resistant (EBLR) bacteria. Although the carbohydrate fermenting enterics seem to account for 62.1 percent of the gram-negative isolates as a whole, *P. aeruginosa*, a nonfermentor, is the most common gram-negative pathogen in burned patients. Other important gram-negative bacteria include the Enterobacteriaceae such as *Escherichia coli, Enterobacter cloacae, Klebsiella pneumonia*, and *Serratia marcescens*. The Enterobacteriaceae also are encountered as a cause of nosocomial pneumonia in patients with inhalation injury who are on ventilators, and they are a cause of urinary tract infection in patients with indwelling urinary catheters. *Acinetobacter*, an increasingly more common cause of gram-negative infections, has been found more frequently in burned patients with glucose intolerance or preexisting diabetes mellitus.[33] *Acinetobacter* infections also are found more often in patients with more severe burns and comorbidities.[3]

Even without invasive infections, gram-negative bacteria have been implicated in systemic inflammatory diseases, including shock and disseminated intravascular coagulation, secondary to the circulation of bacterial endotoxin from the gut and the burn wound.[64,74] Often gut decontamination is instituted to reduce the incidence of endotoxin-mediated disease.

3. Fungi: Until the advent of topical antimicrobials and systemic antibiotics, fungal infections were not common developments in patients with burns. The burn wound is the site most commonly infected, although fungemia and dissemination to the respiratory tract in patients on ventilators and to the urinary tract in patients with indwelling catheters are encountered frequently. *Candida* spp. are the most common fungal colonizers of the wound (Table 87–3); however, less than 20 percent of patients develop widespread candidiasis. Overall, the rate of candidemia in the burn population is 3 to 5 percent, and burn-wound invasion has a comparable rate. A study of burned children at our center showed that those developing candidemia did so during the first week postburn and 7 days after excision of burn eschar.[24] One hypothesis is that massive burns with immunosuppression are further suppressed by repeated surgical intervention, anesthesia, and perioperative use of broad-spectrum antibiotics, further predisposing these patients to early development of *Candida* septicemia. With early recognition of invasion of burn wounds by

TABLE 87–3 Medically Important Fungi Isolated from 304 Acute Care Pediatric Burn Patients Admitted to Shriners Burns Hospitals for Children—Galveston, Texas (January 2006 to December 2006)

Organism	No. (%) of Isolates
Candida species	86 (83.5)
Fusarium species	6 (5.8)
Trichosporon beigelii	5 (4.9)
Rhizomucor species	2 (1.9)
Aspergillus species	2 (1.9)
Geotrichum species	1 (1.0)
Curvularia species	1 (1.0)
Total no. of fungal isolates	**103**

routine biopsies, wound swabs, and early amphotericin therapy, the mortality rate has been reduced to less than 10 percent, as compared with 60 to 90 percent reported in earlier series.[104]

Unlike *Candida*, true fungal infections caused by *Aspergillus, Penicillium, Rhizopus, Mucor, Rhizomucor, Fusarium*, and *Curvularia* occur early in the hospital course, specifically in those exposed to the spores on the ground or in water at the time the injury occurred. Once colonized, broad nonbranching hyphae extend into subcutaneous tissue and stimulate an inflammatory response. Vascular invasion occurs frequently and often is accompanied by thrombosis and avascular necrosis, which is clinically observed as rapidly advancing dark discolorations of the wound margin. Systemic dissemination occurs with invasion of the vasculature.

4. Viruses: Linnemann and MacMillan[72] performed a retrospective survey of serum for viral antibodies in pediatric burn patients, 22 percent had fourfold increases in antibodies to cytomegalovirus (CMV), 8 percent had increases to herpes simplex virus (HSV) and to Epstein-Barr virus, and 5 percent had increases in antibodies to varicella-zoster virus (VZV). None of the patients had evidence of adenovirus or hepatitis B virus infection. On the basis of these observations, a prospective study of viral infections, using both serologic and viral culture techniques, was performed. This study showed that CMV infection developed in 33 percent of the children; herpes simplex infection in 25 percent, and adenovirus infection in 17 percent. CMV infections developed in all of the most severely burned children, and both primary and reactivation infections were observed. Most primary CMV infections that develop during treatment for burns are likely to occur from transfusion of blood products. CMV infection typically occurs approximately 1 month after the burn occurs and clinically presents as fever of unknown origin with lymphocytosis; however, it rarely alters the patient's clinical course.[23] Kealey and colleagues[60] have shown that 56 percent of burned patients who initially were seropositive for CMV had a fourfold or greater rise in CMV antibodies as evidence of CMV reactivation. These patients tended to be younger, to have a larger burn area, and to have a longer hospital stay. No patient who experienced CMV infection, whether primary or reactivated, had serious complications attributable to CMV. On the basis of these observations, despite the availability of anti-CMV agents such as ganciclovir and valganciclovir, treatment for CMV infection remains controversial.[96]

Since the screening of blood began, hepatitis C virus (HCV) has been an important risk. Coursaget and colleagues[22] screened 45 burn patients for anti-HCV antibodies, at the time of burn injury and more than 6 months postburn. HCV infection was detected in 18 percent of these patients, as a consequence of the numerous transfusions of blood or blood derivatives used during the postburn treatment. Five patients displayed evidence of anti-C100, anti-C33c, and anti-core antibodies together; two patients had only anti-C100 and anti-C33c antibodies, and the last one showed only anti-core antibodies. Chronic hepatitis was observed in 83 percent of HCV infections. Kinetics of appearance of anti-HCV antibodies varied among patients. Anti-core generally is the first to be detected at high levels; however, in at least one case, it was detected only 2.5 months after C100 and C33c antibodies were detected. The incidence of HCV using polymerase chain reaction (PCR) technique to detect the viral genome has not been evaluated in burn patients. Nonetheless, the current blood banking procedures have decreased the transmission of HCV by blood products.

Another transfusion-related agent is human immunodeficiency virus (HIV), which has become extremely rare as a result of the screening of donors that began in 1987 in the United States. However, significant risk existed prior to that period. A retrospective review of burned children at our center who had received blood/blood products between 1978 and 1985 identified

52 patients at risk for developing HIV infection.[100] More than 50 percent of the identified population had received three or more units of blood/blood products during their acute hospital stay. A total of 214 patients (36.8%) were tested for HIV seroconversions: five tested HIV-positive by enzyme-linked immunosorbent assay (ELISA) and four were confirmed by Western blot, yielding a 1.9 percent incidence. The four confirmed patients received two to nine total body blood volume turnovers during their postburn period in the hospital. HIV may affect the outcome of burn wound injury. A study of Malawian children showed that with burns affecting 11 to 30 percent of the body surface area, HIV-positive children had a mortality rate approximately twice that of the of HIV-negative children.[55]

HSV is of significant concern in burn units because it is a dermatopathologic virus. A review of the literature suggests that patients younger than 10 years of age were at greater risk of acquiring an HSV infection when the size of the burn wound was greater than 15 percent of TBSA.[46] However, the role of HSV in the healing of wounds is unclear. Bourdarias and colleagues[15] showed that in 11 patients with burns, local areas of active epidermal regeneration were affected most often. Acyclovir therapy was not used, and the duration of hospitalization was normal when compared with other children. Nonetheless, HSV in lungs may worsen morbidity. Byers and associates[17] showed that the relative risk for developing HSV infection was higher for cases with adult respiratory distress syndrome but not with pneumonia. Disseminated HSV infection also can be fatal.[17]

Another dermatopathologic virus is VZV. Mini-epidemics of VZV have occurred within pediatric burn units.[122] With the routine VZV vaccination of young children (1 to 2 years of age) in the United States, the outbreaks of varicella in burn units are now uncommon. The characteristic fluid-filled lesions appear in partial-thickness burns that are healed or healing, as well as in uninjured epithelium and mucous membranes. The vesicles are much more destructive in the injured than uninjured skin and may present as hemorrhagic, oozing pockmarks that are prone to development of secondary infection and subsequent scarring. Neovascularized skin grafts may be lost; therefore, further grafting procedures should be delayed until the lesions are quiescent.

The morbidity due to respiratory virus infections, particularly in those with inhalation injury, has not been studied well. More than 100 pediatric burn patients at our center were tested for respiratory syncytial virus (RSV) during the winter seasons of 1995 and 1996 (unpublished observations). Only six patients were found to be positive for RSV, with one death (1% mortality rate).

5. **Parasites:** Parasitic infestation also is seen especially in children from the developing world. Because many patients in our center originate from Mexico, where such infestation is endemic, parasitemia has been found to complicate burn injuries. Parasites that are asymptomatic in sites such as the intestinal tract and the respiratory tract can become symptomatic as a result of the stress of a burn injury. At the Shriners Burns Hospital for Children in Galveston, Texas, we have described three cases of ascaris pneumonitis that exacerbated the smoke-induced lung injury.[47] In 2006 the parasites isolated most frequently were *Giardia lamblia* and *Blastocystis homini.*

CLINICAL MANIFESTATIONS OF INFECTION

LOCAL SIGNS

An open burn wound is a favorable target for bacterial colonization. The progression from simple eschar colonization to the invasive process is favored by a series of factors related to the patient, such as extension and depth of the burn, age, presence of previous disease, and local conditions of the wound; to the microorganism such as density, motility, toxins and antimicrobial resistance; to iatrogenic causes such as prosthetic devices; and to the nosocomial spread of bacteria. It is essential to recognize the early signs of infection of a local burn wound by examining the wound at least once a day.

The local signs of burn wound infection include black or dark brown focal areas of discoloration, conversion of partial-thickness injury to full-thickness necrosis, hemorrhagic discoloration of subcutaneous tissue, enhanced sloughing of burned tissue or eschar, and purplish discoloration or edema of skin around the margins of the wound. Presence of *Pseudomonas* infection can lead to ecthyma gangrenosa and green pigmentation of subcutaneous fat. In fungal infection, centrifugal advance of subcutaneous edema with central ischemic necrosis and hemorrhagic saponification of subcutaneous fat in fungal infection can be seen. In viral infection, vesicular lesions in healing or healed partial-thickness burns and crusted serrated margins of partial-thickness burns may be observed.

SYSTEMIC SIGNS

Progression from local to systemic invasion can occur rapidly, which correlates with the size of the burn wound, the extent of environmental contamination, and the surgical procedures. Early recognition of systemic invasion is critical to avoid the high rates of mortality. Many of the signs of sepsis resemble complications of the burn itself; for example, fevers, tachycardia, shock, and elevated or depressed neutrophil count can occur in burned patients with or without infection. However, certain patterns of clinical signs and symptoms may help recognize the systemic bacterial invasion (Table 87–4).[35] A rise in levels of C-reactive protein serum has been found useful in predicting systemic infection, although increases in the first 2 days after the burn or the day after surgery may occur without infection.[86] When sepsis did occur, it always was preceded by increased levels of C-reactive protein approximately 2 days before the patient was deemed septic clinically. Elevated levels of certain cytokines may be useful markers, but they largely remain research tools.

TABLE 87–4 Signs and Symptoms of Progression from Local Invasion to Systemic Illness*

Gram-Negative Sepsis	Gram-Positive Sepsis
Burn wound biopsy >10⁵ organisms/g tissue and/or histologic tissue invasion	Same
Rapid onset, well to ill in 8-12 hr	Gradual
Temp. 37-39°C, can be normal, followed by hypothermia (34°-35°C), plus decrease in WBC	Temp. >40°C
WBC may be elevated	WBC 20-50 × 10³, hematocrit decrease
Ileus	Same
Decreased blood pressure and urinary output	Same
Wounds develop focal gangrene, satellite lesions away from burn wound	Macerated wounds, Ropy and tenacious exudate
Mental obtundation	Anorexic and irrational

Five or more signs or symptoms are definitive diagnostic parameters.
Modified from reference 35.
WBC, white blood cell count.

INFECTION COMPLICATIONS

Other than the primary infection of the burned skin, several types of infectious complications in the burned patients have been recognized. Bacteremia is a frequent complication. Surgical burn wound manipulations are responsible for development of bacteremias in approximately 50 percent of cases, but routine instrumentation and intravascular catheter devices also can cause bacteremia.[13,44] The risk of developing bacteremia also correlates with the TBSA affected by burns; Sasaki and colleagues[101] showed that those patients with a positive blood culture had an average total body surface area injury of 47 percent, whereas those with a 26 percent injury had negative blood cultures. TSS caused by TSS toxin–producing strains of *S. aureus* has been identified in acutely burned children. Childs and colleagues[20] found that 13 percent of children developed a toxic shock–like illness; however, its effect on overall burn mortality was not clear.

Subacute bacterial endocarditis is a risk associated with persistent bacteremia caused by any cause, including repeated instrumentation, surgical intervention, and placement of central venous catheters.[12,18] *S. aureus* and gram-negative bacilli are the most frequent cause. In most cases, the antemortem diagnosis rarely is suspected in burned children.[2,12] In addition to causing local valvular damage, infected vegetations may dislodge septic emboli. Suppurative thrombophlebitis occurs at the site of the insertion of the catheter. It may occur in as many as 5 percent of patients with burns covering 20 percent of the TBSA.[109]

Suppurative chondritis occurs in patients with full-thickness burn of the ear. Because of the auricle's relatively low level of blood supply, chondritis frequently follows the progression of tissue ischemia, usually 3 to 5 weeks after burn injury occurs.[80] *P. aeruginosa* and *S. aureus* are the most common pathogens. However, with use of mafenide acetate as a topical agent, the incidence of suppurative chondritis has decreased significantly.

Suppurative sinusitis is seen in patients with long-term nasotracheal intubation. In one study, 8 percent of patients with burns who had nasotracheal intubation for more than 7 days developed sinusitis.[16] Pneumonia may occur with or without inhalation injury, although those with inhalation injury have a substantially higher risk.[107] Bronchopneumonia is the most common type of pulmonary infection, usually occurring in the second week of burn injury. Predisposing factors are size of the burn wound (hematogenous spread), aspiration, presence of tracheostomy or nasotracheal tube (nosocomial spread from burn wound), existence of inhalation injury, and disturbances of fluid and electrolyte balances. Currently, most infection-related deaths in burned patients are caused by pneumonia rather than wound infection.[107]

Urinary tract infection occurs in association with prolonged and often unnecessary catharization.[102] Osteomyelitis can occur when bones are exposed by the burn or by open fracture accompanying the burn; from extension of infection from a septic joint, introduction of organisms along traction pins, and internal fracture fixation devices; or by bacteremia. However, clinically significant osteomyelitis in burned patients is rare.[28] Septic arthritis occurs when a joint is exposed by a burn or by removal of burn eschar.[28] The joints most frequently exposed are the knee, the elbow, the proximal interphalangeal joints of the hand, and the metacarpophalangeal joints on the dorsal surfaces of the hand. The incidence of septic arthritis is obscured by its frequent association with signs and symptoms of severe burns that rarely are separable. Rarely in burns, a joint may become infected from adjacent metaphysical osteomyelitis. In children, most joints can be salvaged. Adult joints are less resilient.

Central nervous system infections in burned patients include meningitis, microabscesses, and septic infarcts. In one review, *Candida* spp., *S. aureus*, and *P. aeruginosa* caused almost 80 percent of infections, occurring most frequently in patients with extensive burns with wound infection or endocarditis.[123]

MICROBIOLOGIC INVESTIGATIONS

The three major approaches to determine burn wound infection are (1) quantitative burn wound cultures (BWCs), (2) histologic assessment of bacterial invasion, and (3) bronchioalveolar lavage (BAL).

1. **Quantitative BWC by biopsy:** Teplitz[112] demonstrated that quantitative bacterial counts of BWCs correlated with histologic specimens showing invasion or colonization. Burn wound infection (often referred to as "burn wound sepsis" in surgical literature) is suspected when proliferating microorganisms exceed 10^5/g tissue and when there is invasion of subjacent unburned tissue has occurred (Fig. 87–2). The presence of microorganisms within the necrotic eschar cannot be considered evidence of burn wound infection. Furthermore, although a bacterial count of 10^5/g tissue is likely to indicate bacterial invasion, this is not invariably true. Only the histologic sections can indicate the level of infection. Therefore, BWCs always should be accompanied by histologic sections from the same area.[93,94]

At the time that surgery is performed, the potentially infected tissues should be excised with a punch biopsy (Fig. 87–3) and divided into equal aliquots.[50] One aliquot should be placed into saline and delivered to the microbiology section for quantitative assessment. These biopsies are weighed aseptically, homogenized in a sterile tube in 3 mL of sterile saline. Known dilutions of the homogenate then are plated using precalibrated loops (10 μL) onto blood agar, colistin-neomycin agar, MacConkey agar, and Sabourands agar for identification in the initial dilutions of 0.1 mL with a 1-mL sterile pipette. After 24 hours, the number of colonies are counted and the quantitative wound culture (QWC) is calculated according to the following formula.

$$\text{Colony forming unit (CFU)} \times \text{g of tissue} = \frac{number\ of\ colonies \times volume \times dilution}{\text{weight of biopsy in grams}}$$

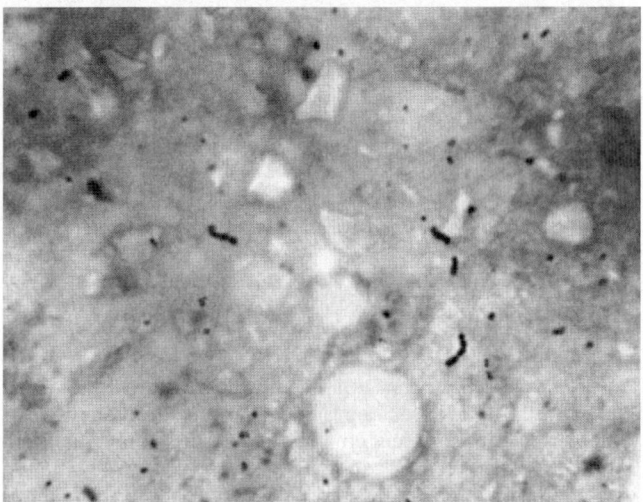

Figure 87–2 Photomicrograph of a homogenized biopsy stained with Gram stain. Gram-positive cocci are seen (cultures grew group A *Streptococcus* at >10^5 colony-forming units/gram tissue). *(With permission from Hunsicker, L., Heggers, J. P., Patel, J. A.: Infections in burn patients. In Patrick, C. C. [ed.]: Clinical Management of Infections in Immunocompromised Infants and Children. 2nd ed. Philadelphia, Lippincott Williams & Wilkins, 2001, p. 338 [Fig. 16.2]).*

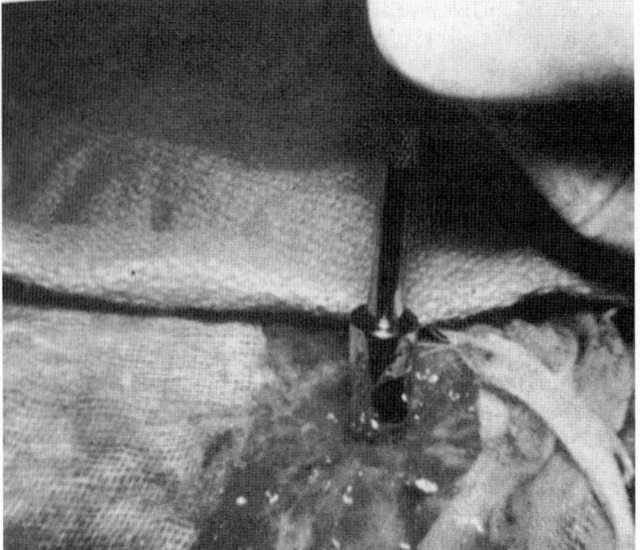

Figure 87–3 Photograph showing the use of a 6-mm punch for collecting a skin biopsy for tissue histology and quantitative culture. *(With permission from Hunsicker, L.; Heggers, J. P.; Patel, J. A.: Infections in burn patients. In Patrick, C. C.: Clinical Management of Infections in Immunocompromised Infants and Children. 2nd ed. Philadelphia, Lippincott Williams & Wilkins, 2001, p. 339 [Fig. 16.3]).*

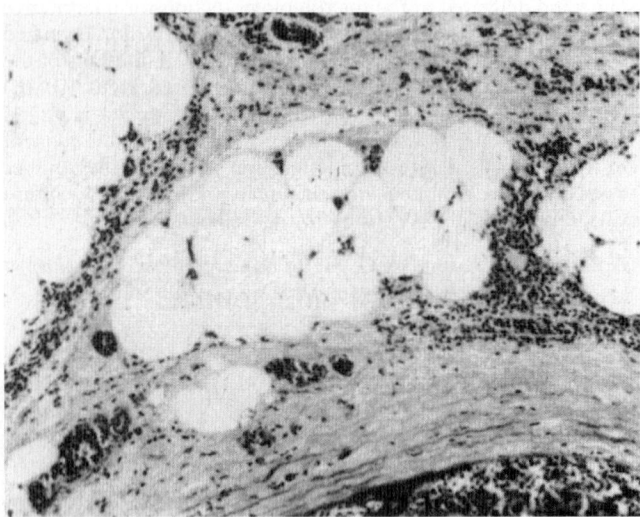

Figure 87–4 Photomicrograph of a cross-section of tissue stained with hematoxylin and eosin showing invasion of *Pseudomonas aeruginosa*. *(With permission from Hunsicker, L., Heggers, J. P., Patel, J. A.: Infections in burn patients. In Patrick, C. C. [ed.]: Clinical Management of Infections in Immunocompromised Infants and Children. 2nd ed., Lippincott Williams & Wilkins, 2001, p. 338 [Fig. 16.4]).*

Despite the dependence on quantitative tissue cultures, reliability of this procedure has been questioned because of the high degree of variability in quantitative counts. In a study published in 1981, Woolfrey and colleagues[124] found that when biopsy samples were divided and cultured separately, only 38 percent of paired quantitative results agreed within the same $\log_{10}$ unit, whereas 44 percent differed by +2 $\log_{10}$ units or more.

2. **Histologic procedures:** Standard histologic procedures, as well as cyrostat examination, are necessary.[94] The tissues should be examined for morphologic changes and for the presence of pathogens. Many bacterial and fungal pathogens can be identified by staining with Gram stain and Gomori–methamine silver stains (Fig. 87–4). More specialized stains may be necessary

TABLE 87–5 Staging of Microbial Status of the Burn Wound by Biopsy Histology*

Stage I: colonization
A. Superficial: microorganisms present only on burn wound surface
B. Penetrating: variable depth of microbial penetration of eschar
C. Proliferating: variable level of microbial proliferation at nonviable-viable tissue interphase (subeschar space)

Stage II: invasion
A. Microinvasion: microorganisms present in viable tissue immediately subjacent to subeschar space
B. Deep invasion: penetration of microorganisms to variable depth and expanse within viable subcutaneous tissue
C. Microvascular involvement: microorganisms within small blood vessels and lymphatics (thrombosis of vessels common)

Modified from reference 94.

to identify other fastidious bacteria and fungi. Tzanck stain can be used to identify inclusion bodies suggestive of invasion of HSV or VZV. Viral-specific antibodies also can be used to detect these viruses by immunohistochemistry. The microbial status of the burn wound (i.e., colonization or invasion), as assessed by histologic examination of a biopsy specimen, can be graded on the basis of the density and depth of penetration of microorganisms (Table 87–5).[94]

3. **BAL:** BAL fluid needs to be collected by personnel experienced in the evaluation of patients with inhalation injury who are at risk for developing airway edema and obstruction. Ventilator-associated pneumonia can be diagnosed if 10^4 or more organisms/mL are cultured. In a study reported by Wahl and colleagues,[118] BAL eliminated the unnecessary antibiotic treatment of 21 percent of patients. In winter months, BAL fluids also can be processed for prevalent respiratory viruses such as RSV and influenza by rapid antigenic detection by immunoassays that are within the capability of most laboratories, or by culture that requires specialized virology laboratory.

PREVENTION AND TREATMENT OF INFECTION

Care of the wound is the mainstay of burn therapy. The goal is to minimize infection and facilitate healing of the burn wound. Wound care addresses both partial- and full-thickness burn injuries until all wounds are closed.

1. **Wound dressing:** The superficial epidermal layer provides a barrier to microorganisms while the deeper lipid epidermal layer provides protection against loss of water vapor. In full-thickness burns, the eschar may extend beyond the skin into the subcutaneous fat and muscle. Closure of the wound cannot occur until the eschar is removed. Bacterial proteases lead to eschar pseudo-separation and are slowed with antiseptic therapies. Then, the eschar is allowed to fragment and slough, with resultant decreased size. This process is called *wound contraction*. This can also be excised and skin grafted. Full-thickness skin grafts have the least contraction rates. Deep dermal wounds allowed to heal spontaneously lead to hypertrophic scarring. Compression garments are used for prevention and treatment.

When approaching burn wound care, a plan must first be decided. Outer burn dressings provide comfort, metabolic enhancement, and protection. First, superficial burns are exquisitely sensitive to air currents, as are deeper burns after some healing. Also, dressings provide splinting and drainage containment. Next, occlusive dressings help eliminate shivering, cold stress, and evaporative heat loss. In open, granulating wounds, loss of water vapor is maximal. Finally, the protective component deals with the control of topical organisms. Supplies consist of large 9 × 9-inch burn gauze, Kerlex wraps, Ace wraps, and topical antimicrobials. Gentle cleansing of the wound and daily débridement also are important. Buttock burn wounds should be examined carefully and frequently for the presence of deep stool staining, an ominous predictor of burn wound sepsis and death.[97] Such wounds should be emergently excised.

2. Topical antimicrobials: Topical antimicrobial agents are used extensively in burned patients. Most patients with stage I and stage II A and B wounds (Table 87–5) can be treated with topical or subeschar antimicrobials alone.

Silver sulfadiazine (Silvadene, SSD, Thermazine, Flamazine, Burnazine): Silver sulfadiazine is a 1 percent water-soluble cream combining sulfadiazine with silver (Ag^+). The Ag^+ ion binds with the DNA of an organism and consequently releases the sulfonamide that interferes with the intermediary metabolic pathway of the microbe. It is most effective against *P. aeruginsosa*, the gram-negative enteric bacteria, and *C. albicans*. *S. aureus*, and some strains of *Klebsiella* spp. have been less effectively controlled.[35] Antimicrobial effectiveness has been observed to last for up to 24 hours. More frequent changes are required if a creamy exudate forms on the wound. The benefits of this topical agent are its ease of use and its ability to reduce pain. It has some tissue-penetrating ability, but it is limited to the epidermis.

Silver sulfadiazine can be used separately or in combination with other antibacterials or enzymatic escharotomy compounds. It can be combined with nystatin, which enhances the antifungal activity of this agent. By itself, silver sulfadiazine has been shown to retard wound healing; however, in conjunction with nystatin or *Aloe vera*, the wound-retardant effect is reversed.

Cerium nitrate–silver sulfadiazine (Flammacerium): The lanthanide salt cerium nitrate has been added to silver sulfadiazine since the 1970s and has been shown to have increased bacterio-stastic effect in large burn wounds. The antimicrobial spectrum is similar to that of silver nitrate. Methemoglobinemia has been seen only rarely, and no associated electrolyte disturbances occur. Only minimal cerium absorption has been noted in patients with large burns treated for weeks. No complications were noted. Its use is somewhat limited because it is not commercially available in the United States. It is, however, available in several western European countries. Koller and Orsag[63] studied the effects of cerium sulfadiazine in 20 burn patients and found it to be safe and effective in the treatment of deep, extensive burn wounds. Caution is advised for use of sulfadiazine products as cases of *P. aeruginosa* resistance to sulfadiazine have been reported.[49]

Silver nitrate: Silver nitrate is available as a 0.5 percent solution that does not injure the regenerating epithelium in the wound and provides bacteriostatic effect against *S. aureus*, *E. coli*, and *P. aeruginosa*.[35] Silver nitrate is most effective when the wound is cleansed carefully of all emollients and other debris. Multilayered coarse mesh dressings should be placed over the wound and saturated with the silver nitrate solution. Like silver sulfadiazine, silver nitrate has limited penetration because the Ag^+ ion is bound rapidly to the body's natural anions such as Cl^-. Because it is hypotonic in nature, it can cause osmolar dilution, resulting in hyponatremia and hypochloremia. Serum electrolytes should be monitored very carefully.

Notable detriments to the use of silver nitrate include its high expense and light sensitivity. Furthermore, it also requires special handling because if it is allowed to dry or if it is covered with an impervious dressing, hyperpyrexia could occur. *Klebsiella, Providencia*, and other *Enterobacteriaceae* spp. are not as susceptible to it as are other bacteria. *E. cloacae* and other nitrate-positive bacteria can cause methemoglobinemia by converting nitrite to nitrate.

Mafenide acetate (Sulfamylon): Mafenide acetate is available both in a 10 percent water-soluble cream or a 5 percent solution and has more substantial bacteriologic data to support its efficacy than do any of the other topical antimicrobials.[66,78] It has been shown to be effective against a broad range of microorganisms, especially against all strains of *P. aeruginosa* and *Clostridium* spp.[101] After a wound has been cleansed of debris, mafenide acetate is applied to the wound like "butter." The treated burn surface is left exposed for maximal antimicrobial potency. The cream is applied a minimum of twice a day and can be reapplied as needed. The 5 percent solution is applied every 8 hours.

Additionally, mafenide acetate has the ability to permeate burn eschar and thereby reduce the risk of bacterial colonization of a deep burn wound, and it is especially effective after the dead tissue is removed from the granulating bed. Unfortunately, several detrimental aspects are associated with the use of mafenide acetate. Protracted use with the low environmental pH favors the growth of *C. albicans*. Mafenide acetate is converted to *p*-sulfamyl vanzoic acid by monamine oxidase, which is a carbonic anhydrase inhibitor; it subsequently causes metabolic acidosis in the patient. Another detrimental problem is that it is painful when applied to superficial, partial-thickness burns with intact free nerve endings. Also, its requirement to remain uncovered for antimicrobial activity may be considered a disadvantage when a dressing is required.

Membrane dressings: Acticoat and Aquacel are silver-coated dressings that have a broad antibacterial activity. Compared with silver nitrate or silver sulfadiazine use, Acticoat and Aquacel have been found easier to apply, were associated with less pain on removal, and have faster rates of reepithelialization.[19,114] Mepitel is another gridlike, silicone-coated, nylon dressing used in partial-thickness burn wounds. Gotschall and colleagues[40] found this product to decrease the pain experienced during dressing change, the time needed for the wound to heal, and the overall duration of the hospital stay as compared with silver sulfadiazine. This study did not find any difference in the incidence of infections between Mepitel and silver sulfadiazine treatments.

Topical antibiotics: Several topical antibiotics have been tried in the management of burn infections. These agents are highly discouraged in the setting of a burn unit because of rapid emergence of resistance:

a. Gentamicin sulfate: It is available as a 0.1 percent water-soluble cream and is chemically similar to the other aminoglycosides, such as kanamycin and neomycin. It has a broad spectrum of antimicrobial activity. It is used for its activity against *P. aeruginosa;* however, its topical use is highly limited because of the high level of gentamicin resistance in burn units.

b. Bacitracin/polymyxin: This antibiotic combination has little or no effect on localized infections of burn wounds.

c. Nitrofurantoin: It is used topically as adjunctive therapy in patients with second- and third-degree burns. With good eschar penetration, it can be used in the treatment of invasive burn wound infections with sensitive agents. The drug presents some advantages for the ambulatory patient. Tissue granulation begins sooner and crusts separate more rapidly.

d. Mupirocin (Bactroban): Studies at our center have shown mupirocin to be superior to silver sulfadiazine in treating methicillin-susceptible *S. aureus* (MSSA) or MRSA infection.[110] Although mupirocin is weaker against gram-negative bacteria, it is also comparable to silver sulfadiazine and mafenide acetate against *P. aeruginosa*, *E. coli*, and *K. pneumonia*.

Nystatin (Mycostatin, Nilstat): Studies at our center have noted that combining nystatin and silver sulfadiazine or nitrofurantoin results in effective prevention of local and systemic *Candida* infections, as well as burn wound sepsis.[48] However, in combination therapy of silver sulfadiazine and nystatin, mafenide acetate actually loses its antimicrobial activity. Therefore, use of nystatin with mafenide acetate is discouraged. Our investigators also have studied concentrated nystatin powder on the effect of angioinvasive fungi (*Fusarium, Aspergillus*) refractory to systemic amphotericin B and serial excisions, including amputations.[10] A concentrated form of nystatin (6,000,000 units/g) was used as dry aerosol every 6 hours and wet to dry dressings laid overtop. Within 14 days, all four of the children studied recovered, with the eradication of their invasive fungal infections. Also, all areas previously autografted underneath the nystatin powder healed nicely.

Sodium Hypochlorite (0.025% Heggers Solution): Currently, the most effective topical antibacterial agent for cleansing a wound is sodium hypochlorite (NaOCl). It transcends the topical antimicrobial effects and tissue toxicity of such products as povidone-iodine, acetic acid, and hydrogen peroxide. The efficacy of NaOCl has been determined to be at a concentration of 0.025 percent, which is bactericidal, nontoxic to fibroblasts, and does not inhibit wound healing, provided buffers are used.[51] It is a broad-spectrum antiseptic and is bactericidal for *P. aeruginosa*, *S. aureus* (MRSA and MSSA), enterococci, and other gram-negative and gram-positive organisms.[101]

Povidone-iodine (Betadine): The active antimicrobial component in this compound is the iodine. It has a broad spectrum of antibacterial and antifungal activities. However, there are disadvantages that limit its use in a burn center. It is painful when applied and is inactivated by wound exudates. Renal dysfunction and acidosis have been noted in association with systemic absorption when applied to open wounds.[65]

Chlorhexidine: Chlorhexidine when combined with 0.5 percent silver nitrate has efficacy similar to that of silver sulfadiazine.[70] Some variants of this product have broader antimicrobial activities, but pain experienced by patients on application has limited its use. Unlike the sulfonamides, plasma-mediated resistance has not occurred.

Subeschar antibiotics: Moncrief[81] has described the technique of subeschar antibiotic infusion. It is used upon microbial invasion into unburned tissue, when topical therapies have not been effective, or in cases in which treatment has been delayed. The most common drugs used are tobramycin, gentamicin, and kanamycin. However, development of antimicrobial resistance is likely substantial, so subeschar infusion of antibiotics should be used infrequently. The antibiotic solution is administered via multiple needle infusions by subcutaneous lysis. The results of this technique are more rapid separation of eschar. The fluid infusion limit is 2000 mL (adult dose) and should be accounted for in patient's fluid requirements. The infusion fluid should consist of 0.25 to 0.45 N saline to avoid salt overload. Lactated Ringer solution should be avoided because some of the drugs are incompatible with calcium. Erythromycin has been studied but is too painful to use. Colistin, novobiocin, and cephaloridine have been used but found to be ineffective.

3. **Systemic anti-infective agents:** Drug pharmacokinetics are significantly altered in the burned patient and show significant inter- and intrapatient variation.[121] In 1976, altered aminoglycoside pharmacokinetics and the need for increased dosage in burned patients were reported, but despite this early study, a review of the currently available literature shows that for many drugs there is a paucity of information to support current dosage recommendations, specifically in children of various age groups. In addition, many reports are based on small numbers of patients, and even in larger studies, no standardization of the study population exists with regard to the important variables known to affect drug handling. For the subpopulation of burned patients who eliminate drugs extremely rapidly, a concern exists over the adequacy of antibiotic dosing. Researchers have suggested that antibiotic serum concentrations be measured for all drugs in every patient to ascertain whether a significant problem exists with dosing.

Whereas stage I and stage II A and B wounds (see Table 87–6) can be treated with topical or subeschar antimicrobials alone, stage II C wounds require the immediate institution of systemic anti-infective agents. Systemic agents also are indicated for the treatment of various systemic infectious complications as discussed earlier. Detailed information on selection of the appropriate systemic antimicrobials for specific bacterial, fungal, and viral pathogens is available in other chapters of this book. Nonetheless, the following general principles can help guide the use of antimicrobial therapy:

a. Each antimicrobial agent must be selected for its specificity for the microbe present.

b. Such decisions should be made on appropriately collected culture and susceptibility data.

c. Colonizing flora should be distinguished from those responsible for inflammation and invasion.

d. The time, dosage, route of administration, and duration of treatment should be in accordance with what is required to make the organism nonpathogenic.

e. The need for broad-spectrum antibiotics should be balanced with the risk of promoting fungal infections.

Treatment of multidrug-resistant, gram-negative bacteria: This issue deserves specific mention because it most severely affects the burn units. In many centers, pan-resistant *P. aeruginosa* strains and *Acinetobacter* spp. are identified frequently. In these cases, colistin and polymyxin B often remain the only susceptible antimicrobial agents. In a recent study, Goverman and colleagues[41] summarized their experience in 14 children treated with intravenous colistin: favorable response was obtained in 79 percent and the overall mortality rate was 14 percent. Both colistin and polymyxin B are associated with significant elevation in serum creatinine or renal failure in 15 to 25 percent of recipients. Neurotoxicity in children is an infrequent occurrence. Intravenous and/or aerosol polymyxin B, doxycycline, and ampicillin/sulbactam (the active component is thought to be sulbactam) have been tried in multidrug-resistant *Acinetobacter* infections as well.[88] Other studies have demonstrated in vitro susceptibility of multidrug-resistant *Acinetobacter* to various synergistic combinations of antimicrobials, including carbapenems, colistin, rifampin, tigecycline, and ampicillin-sulbactam.[38,53,125] The clinical utility of these combinations against pan-resistant *Acinetobacter* remains to be determined.

4. **Antibiotic prophylaxis:** Prophylactic use of antibiotics remains a highly controversial topic in the literature. Penicillin prophylaxis is used commonly in many burn centers during outbreaks of group A streptococcal infections.[43,98] Prophylactic antibiotics also are used before surgical manipulation or instrumentation because the risk of developing bacteremia is as high as 50 percent. The choice of perioperative antibiotics is dependent on the knowledge of existing microorganisms, which are present not only on injured skin but also in the wound that is ready for surgery. Nonetheless, carefully controlled studies are necessary to identify the value of prophylactic antibiotics. In a placebo-controlled study of cefazolin use in burned children, researchers found that in children with less than 35 percent burn, cefazolin was not necessary, and in those with 35 percent burn or more, it was not effective.[99] In a retrospective review study, antibiotic prophylaxis was not associated with any reduction in the rate of wound infection; instead, the duration of hospitalization was found to be longer.[26]

5. **Wound excision and grafting:** Studies at our center have shown that early excision of wounds leads to significantly decreased rates of bacterial colonization and wound infection.[9] A meta-analysis of six trials found that early excision of burns is beneficial in reducing mortality (in patients without inhalational injury) and length of hospital stay. The only drawback is the greater volume of blood loss.[89]

6. **Gut support and decontamination:** The gut microflora have been implicated in the development of multiorgan failure when the gut barrier fails. Hence, one theory is that early enteral feeding of the gut, which promotes function of the gut barrier, is important for preventing multiorgan failure. A decontaminated gut with nonabsorbable, broad-spectrum antibiotics might dimin-

ish the impact of failure of the gastrointestinal barrier. Although the suggestion has been made that the rate of pneumonia may be decreased by such maneuvers, no apparent impact on mortality rates have been noted.[75] Overall, convincing human data on the beneficial effect of enteral feeding and decontamination of the gut on sepsis and multiorgan failure are lacking.

7. **Immunomodulators:** In view of the intricate relationship between altered immune defenses in burned patients and increased susceptibility to infections, various types of immunotherapies have been tried in burned patients. In an Italian study, treatment with intravenous pooled immunoglobulins (IVIG) was found to have a beneficial effect on septic phenomena and recovery.[79] However, in two U.S. studies, no change in rates of infection or mortality was shown. Overall, the beneficial role of IVIG as prophylaxis or treatment remains unproven.[85,119] In a German study, prophylaxis with intravenous *Pseudomonas* immunoglobulin did not appear to be beneficial to burned patients in general; however, it was shown to be effective in burned patients with inhalation injury.[111] In a South African study, prophylaxis with high-titer anti-lipopolysaccharide immunoglobulin G (IgG) reduced the incidence of burn wound infection but did not affect mortality.[57] Benefits of plasmapheresis or fresh frozen plasma infusion have not been proven.

INFECTION CONTROL

Hospital-acquired infections in burn patients are common occurrences. In burned children, wound infections, ventilator-related pulmonary infections, central-line bacteremias, and catheter-associated urinary tract infections are the most common nosocomial infections.[102,120] The rates of infections may be lower than those seen in adults, but urinary tract infections occur more frequently in children.[102] In a German study of children with burns, the overall infection rate was 59.7 nosocomial infections per 1000 inpatient days, and the device-associated infections per 1000 device days were 55.2 for pneumonia, 8.9 for primary bloodstream infections, and 41.7 for urinary tract infections.[37] The incident density of burn wound infections was 18.5 per 1000 inpatient days, which was associated with the percentage of TBSA of the burn wound. On the other hand, the rate of device-associated infections was not associated with the percentage of TBSA.

Surveillance of infection in a burned patient is performed to implement prompt treatment on the basis of surveillance cultures and antimicrobial sensitivities at the earliest sign of invasion. Such surveillance requires cultures of sputum, urine, and wounds about three times weekly; however, the need for such cultures and the frequency of monitoring remain controversial. Additional infection control measures involve surveillance of spread of pathogens among burned patients of a unit. In dealing with the burn wound, strict infectious disease precautions must be maintained to prevent contamination and worsening infection in these already immunocompromised patients.

In the past, poor handwashing and shared hydrotherapy tubs were the source of many infections, some of which were life-threatening. Strict enforcement of handwashing and use of gowns, gloves, and masks have led to decreased rates of patient contamination. Also, disposable hydrotherapy tub liners are used without the risk of patient-to-patient transmission of infections.[113] Besides this, isolation of burned patients in a single room compared with an open ward scenario has dramatically affected infection rates. McManus and colleagues[77] studied this measure in 2519 patients and found significantly lower incidence and mortality rates associated with gram-negative bacteremia in the isolated patients. Also, the open ward bacterial isolates showed significantly more antimicrobial resistance compared with those of the patients in isolation.

Additional infection control measures include the use of germicidal solutions to clean daily all of the hardware, such as intravenous poles and pumps, monitoring equipment, bedside tables, and beds in patients' rooms. Upon discharge of the patient, the whole room, including floors, walls, ceilings, and mattresses, needs to be cleaned with germicidal solutions. Air filters should be monitored repeatedly for fungal and bacterial growth.

Lai and colleagues[67] studied the effects of strict isolation of patients with VRE, the use of vancomycin, and the cost-to-benefit analysis of barrier precautions. Their findings showed that pharyngeal swabs were poor for surveillance but that rectal swabs were more useful. Also, vancomycin-use guidelines were adhered by 85 percent of the staff. The overall cost for these implementations, including the barrier supplies and cleaning protocols, was $11,000. Nonetheless, VRE was not eradicated. On the other hand, van Rijn and colleagues[116] have shown that isolation in a quarantine unit was highly effective in preventing outbreaks of multidrug-resistant bacteria.

REFERENCES

1. Abdi, S., Herndon, D. N., McGuire, J., et al.: Time course of alterations in lung lymph and bronchial blood flows after inhalation injury. J. Burn Care Rehabil. *11*:510-515, 1990.
2. Albertson, S., Greenhalgh, D. G., Breeden, M. P., et al.: Cardiac abnormalities in children with burns: An autopsy analysis. J. Burn Care Rehabil. *15*:401-404, 1994.
3. Albrecht, M. C., Griffith, M. E., Murray, C. K., et al.: Impact of *Acinetobacter* infection on the mortality of burn patients. J. Am. Coll. Surg. *203*:546-550, 2006.
4. American Burn Association. Factsheet. *http://www.ameriburn.org/resources_factsheet.php* (9/20/2007).
5. Babcock, G. F., Alexander, J. W., and Warden, G. D.: Flow cytometric analysis of neutrophil subsets in thermally injured patients developing infection. Clin. Exp. Immunol. *54*:117-125, 1990.
6. Balogh, D., Lammer, H., Kornberger, E., et al.: Neopterin plasma levels in burn patients. Burns *18*:185-188, 1992.
7. Barber, R. C., Chang, L. Y., Arnoldo, B. D., et al.: Innate immunity SNPs are associated with risk for severe sepsis after burn injury. Clin Med Res *4*:250-255, 2006.
8. Baron, P., Traber, L. D., Traber, D. L., et al.: Gut failure and translocation following burn and sepsis. J. Surg. Res. *57*:197-204, 1994.
9. Barret, J. P., and Herndon, D. N.: Effects of burn wound excision on bacterial colonization and invasion. Plast. Reconstr. Surg. *111*:744-750, 2003.
10. Barrett, J. P., Ramzy, P. I., Heggers, J. P., et al.: Topical nystatin powder in severe burns: A new treatment for angioinvasive fungal infections refractory to other topical and systemic agents. Burns *25*:505-508, 1999.
11. Barro, R. E., Wang, C. Z., Cox, R. A., et al.: Cellular sequence of tracheal repair in sheep post smoke inhalation injury. Lung *170*:331-338, 1992.
12. Baskin, T. W., Rosenthal, A., and Pruitt, B. A.: Acute bacterial endocarditis: A silent source of sepsis in the burn patient. Ann. Surg. *184*:618, 1976.
13. Beard, C. H., Ribeiro, C. D., and Jones, D. M.: The bacteremia associated with burns surgery. Br. J. Surg. *62*:638-641, 1975.
14. Bjerknes, R., and Vindenes, H.: Neutrophil dysfunction after thermal injury-alteration of phagolysosomal acidification in patients with large burns. J. Trauma *15*:71-81, 1989.
15. Bourdarias, B., Perro, G., Cutillas, M., et al.: Herpes simplex virus infection in burned patients: Epidemiology of 11 cases. Burns *22*:287-290, 1996.
16. Bowers, B. L., Purdue, G. F., and Hunt, J. L.: Paranasal sinusitis in burn patients following nasotracheal intubation. Arch. Surg. *126*:1411-1412, 1991.
17. Byers, R. J., Hasleton, P. S., Quigley, A., et al.: Pulmonary herpes simplex in burns patients. Eur. Respir. J. *9*:2313-2317, 1996.
18. Cartotto, R. C., Macdonald, D. B., and Wasan, S. M.: Acute bacterial endocarditis following burns: Case report and review. Burns *24*:363-373, 1998.
19. Caruso, D. M., Foster, K. N., Blome-Eberwein, S. A., et al.: Randomized clinical study of Hydrofiber dressing with silver or silver sulfadiazine in the management of partial-thickness burns. J. Burn Care Rehabil. *27*:298-309, 2006.
20. Childs, C., Edwards-Jones, V., Heathcote, D. M., et al.: Patterns of *Staphylococcus aureus* colonization, toxin production, immunity and illness in burned children. Burns *20*:514-521, 1994.
21. Cook, N.: Methicillin-resistant *Staphylococcus aureus* versus the burn patient. Burns *24*:91-98, 1998.
22. Coursaget, P., Lesage, G., Simpson, B., et al.: Incidence of hepatitis C virus infection in burn patients: Detection of anti-C100, anti-C33c and anti-Core antibodies. Biomed Pharmacother *45*: 445-449, 1991.
23. Deepe, G. S., Jr., MacMillan, B. C., and Linnemann, C. C., Jr.: Unexplained fever in burned patients due to cytomegalovirus infection. JAMA *248*:2299-2301, 1982.

24. Desai, M. H., Herndon, D. N., and Abston, S.: *Candida* infection in massively burned patients. J. Trauma 27:1186-1188, 1987.
25. Dietich, E. A., Xu, D., and Qi, L.: Different lymphocyte compartments respond differently to mitogenic stimulation after thermal injury. Ann. Surg. 211:72-77, 1990.
26. Ergün, O., Celik, A., Ergün, G., et al.: Prophylactic antibiotic use in pediatric burn units. *Eur J Pediatr Surg* 14:422-426, 2004.
27. Erol, S., Altoparlak, U., Akcay, M. N., et al.: Changes in microbial flora and wound colonization in burned patients. Burns 30:357-361, 2004.
28. Evans, E. B.: Musculoskeletal changes secondary to thermal burns. *In* Herndon, D. N. (ed.): Total Burn Care, London, W. B. Saunders, 2007, pp. 652-666.
29. Faist, E., Ertel, W., Baker, C. C., et al.: Terminal B-cell maturation and immunoglobulin (Ig) synthesis in vitro in patients with major injury. J. Trauma 29:2-9, 1989.
30. Finnerty, C. C., Herndon, D. N., and Jeschke, M. G.: Inhalation injury in severely burned children does not augment the systemic inflammatory response. Crit. Care 11:R22, 2007.
31. Finnerty, C. C., Herndon, D. N., Przkora, R., et al.: Cytokine expression profile over time in severely burned pediatric patients. Shock 26:13-19, 2006.
32. Fleming, R. Y., Zeigler, S. T., Walton, M. A., et al.: Influence of burn size on the incidence of contamination of burn wounds by fecal organisms. J. Burn Rehabil. 12:510-515, 1991.
33. Furniss, D., Gore, S., Azadian, B., et al.: *Acinetobacter* is associated with acquired glucose intolerance in burn patients. J. Burn Care Rehabil. 26:405-408, 2005.
34. Gadd, M. A., Hansbrough, J. F., Hoyt, D. B., et al.: Defective T-cell surface antigen expression after mitogen stimulation: An index of lymphocyte dysfunction after controlled murine injury. Ann. Surg. 29:112-118, 1989.
35. Gallagher, J. J., Williams-Bouyer, N., Villarreal, C., et al.: Treatment of infections in burns. In Total Burn Care: Herndon, D. N. (ed.): Philadelphia, W. B. Saunders, 2007, p. 143.
36. Gasser, H., Paul, E., Redl, H., et al.: Loss of plasma antioxidants after burn injury. Circ. Shock 34:13, 1991. Abstract.
37. Gastmeier, P., Weigt, O., Sohr, D., and Rüden, H.: Comparison of hospital-acquired infection rates in paediatric burn patients. J. Hosp. Infect. 52:161-165, 2002.
38. Giamarellos-Bourboulis, E. J., Xirouchaki, E., and Giamarellou, H.: Interactions of colistin and rifampin on multidrug-resistant *Acinetobacter baumannii*. Diagn. Microbiol. Infect. Dis. 40:117-120, 2001.
39. Gibbons, R. A., Martinez, O. M., Lim, R. C., et al.: Reduction in HLA-DR, HLA-DQ, and HLA-DP expression by Leu-M3+ cells. Clin. Exp. Immunol. 75:371-375, 1989.
40. Gotschall, C. S., Morrison, M. I., and Eichelberger, M. R.: Prospective, randomized study of the efficacy of Mepitel on children with partial-thickness scalds. J. Burn Care Rehabil. 19:279-283, 1998.
41. Governan, J., Weber, J. M., Keaney, T. J., et al.: Intravenous colistin for the treatment of multi-drug resistant, gram-negative infection in the pediatric burn population. J. Burn Care Res. 28:421-426, 2007.
42. Greenhalgh, D.: Wound healing. In Herndon, D. N. (ed.): Total Burn Care. Philadelphia, W. B. Saunders, 2007, pp. 578-559.
43. Gruteke, P., van Belkum, A., Schouls, L. M., et al.: Outbreak of group A streptococci in a burn center: Use of pheno- and genotypic procedures for strain tracking. J. Clin. Microbiol. 34:114-118, 1996.
44. Hamory, B. H.: Nosocomial sepsis related to intravascular access. Crit. Care Nurs. J. 11:58-65, 1989.
45. Hansbrough, J. F., Zapata-Sirvent, R., and Hoyt, D.: Postburn immune suppression: An inflammatory response to the burn wound? J. Trauma 30:671-675, 1990.
46. Hayden, F. G., Himmel, H. N., and Heggers, J. P.: Herpes virus infections in burn patients. Chest 106(Suppl):15S-21S, 1994.
47. Heggers, J. P., Muller, M. J., Elwood, E., and Herndon, D. N.: Ascariasis pneumonitis: A potentially fatal complication in smoke inhalation injury. Burns 21:149-151, 1995.
48. Heggers, J. P., Robson, M. C., Herndon, D. N., and Desai, M. H.: The efficacy of nystatin combined with topical microbial agents in the treatment of burn wound sepsis. J. Burn Care Rehabil. 10:508-511, 1989.
49. Heggers, J. P., and Robson, M. C.: The emergence of silver sulfadiazine resistant *Pseudomonas aeruginosa*. Burns 5:184-187, 1978.
50. Heggers, J. P., and Robson, M. C. (eds.): Quantitative Bacteriology: Its Role in the Armamentarium of the Surgeon. 1st ed. Boca Raton, FL, CRC Press, 1991, pp. 1-139.
51. Heggers, J. P., Sazy, J. A., Stenberg, B. D., et al.: Bactericidal and wound healing properties of sodium hypochlorite. The 1991 Lindberg Award. J. Burn Care Rehab. 12:420-424, 1991.
52. Herndon, D. N., Traber, L. D., Linares, H., et al.: Etiology of the pulmonary pathophysiology associated with inhalation injury. Resuscitation 14:43-59, 1986.
53. Higgins, P. G., Wisplinghoff, H., Stefanik, D., et al.: In vitro activities of the beta-lactamase inhibitors clavulanic acid, sulbactam, and tazobactam alone or in combination with beta-lactams against epidemiologically characterized multidrug-resistant *Acinetobacter baumannii* strains. Antimicrob. Agents Chemother. 48:1586-1592, 2004.
54. Jackson, D. M.: The diagnosis of the depth of burning. Br. J. Surg. 40:588-596, 1953.
55. James, J., Hofland, H. W., Borgstein, E. S., et al.: The prevalence of HIV infection among burn patients in a burn unit in Malawi and its influence on outcome. Burns 29:55-60, 2003.
56. Jeschke, M. G., Mlcak, R. P., Finnerty, C. C., et al.: Burn size determines the inflammatory and hypermetabolic response. Crit. Care 11:R90, 2007.
57. Jones, E. B.: Prophylactic anti-lipopolysaccharide freeze-dried plasma in major burns: A double blind controlled trial. Burns 21:267-272, 1995.
58. Kagan, R. J., Bratescu, A., Jonason, O., et al.: The relationship between the percentage of circulating B cells, corticosteroid levels, and other immunologic parameters in thermally injured patients. J. Trauma 29:208-213, 1989.
59. Kaufman, T., Neuman, R. A., and Weinberg, A.: Is postburn dermal ischemia enhanced by oxygen free radicals? Burns 15:291-294, 1989.
60. Kealey, G. P., Bale, J. F., Strauss, R. G., et al.: Cytomegalovirus infection in burn patients. J. Burn Care Rehabil. 8:543-545, 1987.
61. Kelly, J. L., Lyons, A., Soberg, C. C., et al.: Anti-interleukin-10 antibody restores burn-induced defects in T-cell function. Surgery 122:146-152, 1997.
62. Killer, M., Konig, W., Brom, J., et al.: Studies on the mechanisms of granulocyte dysfunctions in severely burned patients—evidence for altered leukotriene generation. J. Trauma 29:435:45, 1989.
63. Koller, J., and Orsag, M.: Our experience with the use of cerium sulphadiazine in the treatment of extensive burns. Acta. Chir. Plast. 40:73-75, 1998.
64. Konigova, R., Konickova, Z., and Bouska, I.: Clinical forms of endotoxin in burns. Scand. J. Plast. Reconstr. Surg. 13:61-62, 1979.
65. Krizek, T. J., Davis, J. H., DesPrez, J. D., et al.: Topical therapy of burns—experimental evaluation. Plast. Reconstr. Surg. 39:248, 1967.
66. Kucan, J. O., and Smoot, E. C.: Five percent mafenide acetate solution in the treatment of thermal injuries. J. Burn Care Rehabil. 14:158-153, 1993.
67. Lai, K. K., Kelley, A. L., Melvin, Z. S., et al.: Failure to eradicate vancomycin-resistant enterococci in a university hospital and the cost of barrier precautions. Infect. Control Hosp. Epidemiol. 19:647-652, 1998.
68. Larkin, J. M., and Moylan, J. A.: Tetanus following a minor burn. J. Trauma 15:546-548, 1975.
69. Law, E. J., Blecher, K., and Still, J. M.: Enterococcal infection as cause of morbidity and mortality in patients with burns. J. Burn Care Rehabil. 15:236-239, 1994.
70. Lawrence, J. C., Cason, J. S., and Kidson, A.: Evaluation of phenoxetol-chlorhexidine cream as prophylactic agent in burns. Lancet 24:524-525, 1982.
71. Lesseva, M., Girgitzova, B. P., and Bojadjiev, C.: Beta-hemolytic streptococcal infections in burned patients. Burns 20:422-425, 1994.
72. Linnemann, C. C., Jr., and MacMillan, B. G.: Viral infections in pediatric burn patients. Am. J. Dis. Child. 135:750-753, 1981.
73. Liu, X. S., Yang, Z. C., Luo, Z. H., et al.: Clinical significance of the change in blood monocyte interleukin-1 production in vitro in severely burned patients. Burns 20:302-306, 1994.
74. Ljunghusen, O., Lundahl, J., Nettelblad, H., et al.: Endotoxemia and complement activation after severe burn injuries—effect on leukocytes, soluble selectins, and inflammatory cytokines. Inflammation 20:229-241, 1996.
75. Mackie, D. P., van Hertum, W. A., Schumburg, T., et al.: Prevention of infection in burns: Preliminary experience with selective decontamination of the digestive tract in patients with extensive injuries. J. Trauma 32:570-575, 1992.
76. Maldonado, M. D., Venturoli, A., Franco, A., et al.: Specific changes in peripheral blood lymphocyte phenotype from burn patients: Probable origin of the thermal injury-related lymphocytopenia. Burns 17:188-192, 1991.
77. McManus, A. T., Mason, A. D., Jr., McManus, W. F., and Pruitt, B. A., Jr.: A decade of reduced gram-negative infections and mortality associated with improved isolation of burned patients. Arch. Surg. 129:1306-1309, 1994.
78. Mendelson, J. A.: The management of burns under conditions of limited resources using topical aqueous Sulfamylon (mafenide) hydrochloride spray. J. Burn Care Rehabil. 18:238-244, 1997.
79. Mian, E. U., Gianfaldoni, R., and Mian, M.: The use of intravenous immunoglobulins in patients with severe burns. Clin. Ther. 141:75-81, 1992.
80. Mills, D. C., II, Roberts, L. W., Mason, A. D., Jr., et al.: Suppurative chondritis: Its incidence, prevention, and treatment in burn patients. Plast. Reconstr. Surg. 82:267-276, 1988.
81. Moncrief, J. A.: Topical antibacterial treatment of the burn wound. In Artz, C. P., Moncrief, J. A., and Pruitt, B. A., Jr. (eds.): Burns: A Team Approach. Philadelphia, W. B. Saunders, 1979, pp. 250-269.
82. Moore, F. D., Jr., and Davis, C. F.: Monocyte activation after burns and endotoxemia. J. Surg. Res. 46:350-354, 1989.
83. Moritz, A. R., and Henrique, F. C., Jr.: Studies of thermal injury: The relative importance of time and surface temperature in the causation of cutaneous burns. Am. J. Pathol. 23:695-720, 1947.
84. Munster, A. M.: Alterations of the host defense mechanism in burns. Surg. Clin. North Am. 50:1217-1225, 1970.
85. Munster, A. M., Moran, K. T., Thupari, J., et al.: Prophylactic intravenous immunoglobulin replacement in high-risk burn patients. J. Burn Care Rehabil. 8:376-380, 1987.
86. Neely, A. N., Smith, W. L., and Warden, G. D.: Efficacy of a rise in C-reactive protein serum levels as an early indicator of sepsis in burned children. J. Burn Care Rehabil. 19:102-105, 1998.

87. Noelle, R. J., and Snow, E. C.: T helper cell-dependent B cell activation. FASEB J. *5*:2770-2776, 1991.
88. Obritsch, M. D., Fish, D. N., MacLaren, R., et al.: Nosocomial infections due to multidrug-resistant *Pseudomonas aeruginosa*: Epidemiology and treatment options. Pharmacotherapy *25*:1353-1364, 2005.
89. Ong, Y. S., Samuel, M., and Song, C.: Meta-analysis of early excision of burns. Burns *32*:145-150, 2006.
90. Ono, Y., Kunii, O., Suzuki, H., et al.: Opsonic activity of sera and blister fluid from severely burned patients evaluated by a chemiluminescence method. Microbiol. Immunol. *38*:373-377, 1994.
91. Organ, B. C., Antonacci, A. C., Chio, J., et al.: Changes in lymphocyte number and phenotype in seven lymphoid compartments after thermal injury. Ann. Surg. *210*:78-89, 1988.
92. Palmieri, T. L., Caruso, D. M., Foster, K. N., et al.: Effect of blood transfusion on outcome after major burn injury: A multicenter study. Crit. Care Med. *34*:1062-1067, 2006.
93. Parks, D. H., Linares, H. A., and Thompson, P. D.: Surgical management of burn wound sepsis. Surg. Gynecol. Obstet. *153*:374-376, 1982.
94. Pruitt, B. A., and Foley, F. D.: The use of biopsies in burn patient care. Surgery *73*:887-897, 1973.
95. Reardon, C. M., Brown, T. P., Stephenson, A. J., et al.: Methicillin-resistant *Staphylococcus aureus* in burns patients—Why all the fuss? Burns *24*:393-397, 1998.
96. Rennekampff, H. O., and Hamprecht, K.: Cytomegalovirus infection in burns: A review. J. Med. Microbiol. *55*:483-487, 2006.
97. Renz, B. M., and Sherman, R.: Exposure of buttock burn wounds to stool in scald-abused infants and children: Stool-staining of eschar and burn wound sepsis. Am. Surg. *59*:379-383, 1993.
98. Ridgway, E. J., and Allen, K. D.: Clustering of group A streptococcal infections on a burn unit: Important lessons in outbreak management. J. Hosp. Infect. *25*:173-182, 1993.
99. Rodgers, G. L., Fisher, M. C., Lo, A., et al.: Study of antibiotic prophylaxis during burn wound débridement in children. J. Burn Care Rehabil. *18*:342-346, 1997.
100. Rutan, R. L., Bjarnason, D. L., Desai, M. H., et al.: Incidence of HIV seroconversion in paediatric burn patients. Burns *18*:216-219, 1992.
101. Sasaki, T. M., Welch, O. W., Herndon, D. N., et al.: Burn wound manipulation induced bacteremia. J. Trauma *19*:46-48, 1979.
102. Schlager, T., Sadler, J., Weber, D., et al.: Hospital-acquired infections in pediatric burn patients. South Med. J. *87*:481-448, 1994.
103. Schluter, B., Konig, W., Koller, M., et al.: Differential regulation of T- an B-lymphocyte activation in severely burned patients. J. Trauma *31*:239-246, 1991.
104. Sheridan, R. L., Weber, J. M., Budkevich, L. G., et al.: Candidemia in pediatric patients with burns. J. Burn Care Rehabil. *16*:440-443, 1995.
105. Sherman, R. T.: The prevention and treatment of tetanus in the burn patient. Surg. Clin. North Am. *50*:1277-1281, 1970.
106. Shilling, J. A.: Burn healing. Physiol. Rev. *48*:374-423, 1968.
107. Shiranin, K. Z., Pruitt, B. A., Jr., and Mason, A. D., Jr.: The influence of inhalation injury and pneumonia on burn mortality. Ann. Surg. *205*:82-87, 1987.
108. Shoup, M., Weisenberger, J. M., Wang, J. L., et al.: Mechanisms of neutropenia involving myeloid maturation arrest in burn sepsis. Ann. Surg. *228*:112-122, 1998.
109. Stein, J. M., and Pruitt, B. A., Jr.: Suppurative thrombophlebitis: A lethal iatrogenic disease. N. Engl. J. Med. *282*:1452-1455, 1970.
110. Strock, L. L., Lee, M., Rutan, R. L., et al.: Topical bactroban (Mupirocin): Efficacy in treating MRSA wounds infected with methicillin-resistant staphylococci. J. Burn Care Rehabil. *11*:454-459, 1990.
111. Stuttmann, R., Hebebrand, D., Hartert, M., et al.: [Prevention with pseudomonas immune globulin in burn injury patients with inhalation trauma: Does it have an effect on lung function and outcome]? Klin. Wochenschr. *69*(Suppl 26):168-177, 1991.
112. Teplitz, C.: The pathology of burns and the fundamentals of burn wound sepsis. *In* Artz, C. P., Moncrief, J. A., and Pruitt, B. A., Jr. (eds.): Burns—A Team Approach. Philadelphia, W. B. Saunders, 1979, pp. 45.
113. Tredget, E. E., Shankowsky, H. A., Joffe, A. M., et al.: Epidemiology of infections with *Pseudomonas aeruginosa* in burn patients: The role of hydrotherapy. Clin. Infect. Dis. *15*:941-949, 1992.
114. Tredget, E. E., Shankowsky, H. A., Groeneveld, A., et al.: A matched-pair, randomized study evaluating the efficacy and safety of Acticoat silver-coated dressing for the treatment of burn wounds. J. Burn Care Rehabil. *19*:531-537, 1998.
115. Utoh, J., Utsunomiya, T., Imamura, T., et al.: Complement activation and neutrophil dysfunction in burned patients with sepsis—a study of two cases. Jpn. J. Surg. *19*:462-467, 1989.
116. van Rijn, R. R., Kuijper, E. C., and Kreis, R. W.: Seven-year experience with a "quarantine and isolation unit" for patients with burns. A retrospective analysis. Burns *23*:345-348, 1997.
117. Vindenes, H. A., and Bjerknes, R.: Impaired actin polymerization and depolymerization in neutrophils from patients with thermal injury. Burns *23*:131-136, 1997.
118. Wahl, W. L., Ahrns, K. S., Brandt, M. M., et al: Bronchoalveolar lavage in diagnosis of ventilator-associated pneumonia in patients with burns. J. Burn Care Rehabil. *26*:57-61, 2005.
119. Waymack, J. P., Jenkins, M. E., Alexander, J. W., et al.: A prospective trial of prophylactic intravenous immune globulin for the prevention of infections in severely burned patients. Burns *15*:71-76, 1989.
120. Weber, J. M., Sheridan, R. L., Pasternack, M. S., et al.: Nosocomial infections in pediatric patients with burns. Am. J. Infect. Control *25*:195-201, 1997.
121. Weinbren, M. J.: Review: Pharmacokinetics of antibiotics in burn patients. J. Antimicrob. Chemother. *44*:319-327, 1999.
122. Weintrub, W. H., Lilly, A. B., and Randolph, J. G.: A chickenpox epidemic in a pediatric burn unit. Surgery *76*:490-494, 1974.
123. Winkelman, M. D., and Galloway, P. G.: Central nervous system complications of thermal burns. A postmortem study of 139 patients. Medicine (Baltimore) *71*:271-283, 1992.
124. Woolfrey, B. F., Fox, J. M., and Quall, C. O.: An evaluation of burn wound quantitative microscopy. I. Quantitative eschar cultures. Am. J. Pathol. *75*:532-537, 1981.
125. Yoon, J., Urban, C., Terzian, C., et al.: In vitro double and triple synergistic activities of Polymyxin B, imipenem, and rifampin against multidrug-resistant *Acinetobacter baumannii*. Antimicrob. Agents Chemother. *48*:753-757, 2004.
126. Zhou, D., Munster, A. M., and Winchurch, R. A.: Inhibitory effects of interleukin 6 on immunity: Possible implications in burns. Arch. Surg. *127*:65-68, 1992.

UNCLASSIFIED INFECTIOUS DISEASES

CHAPTER

88

KAWASAKI DISEASE

Stanford T. Shulman

Kawasaki disease is a multisystem acute febrile vasculitic syndrome of unknown (presumably infectious) origin that affects predominantly infants and young children. The diagnosis is based on characteristic clinical features (Table 88–1). Serious complications include coronary arteritis, coronary artery aneurysms and stenoses, coronary thrombosis leading to myocardial infarction, and, very rarely, rupture of a coronary aneurysm. Kawasaki disease has become the leading cause of acquired heart disease in children in most developed countries including the United States and Japan.[364,365] It has been reported in children of all racial groups and from all continents. Although the origin of Kawasaki disease remains unknown and a specific diagnostic test is lacking, establishing a timely diagnosis is very important because administration of intravenous immunoglobulin (IVIG) and aspirin before the 10th day of illness generally has a dramatic effect on the clinical manifestations and markedly reduces the likelihood of development of coronary abnormalities (see the later sections on treatment).[99,238,247,250-252,322,367]

Synonyms for Kawasaki disease include *Kawasaki syndrome* and *mucocutaneous lymph node syndrome* (MCLS, MLNS, or MCLNS). It also has been referred to as *lymphomucocutaneous syndrome* and similar terms. An earlier term used in autopsy reports was *infantile periarteritis nodosa* (IPAN), which is pathologically indistinguishable from fatal Kawasaki disease. The International Classification of Diseases (ICD-9) designates the condition as both Kawasaki disease and mucocutaneous lymph node syndrome (acute) (febrile) (infantile) under rubric 446.1. Before 1983, the National Library of Medicine listed Kawasaki disease publications under various subject headings, particularly "Lymphatic Diseases." Since 1984, publications have been listed under "Mucocutaneous Lymph Node Syndrome," a term very rarely used today.

HISTORY

The illness now bearing his name was first recognized as a clinical entity in 1961 by Dr. Tomisaku Kawasaki, who subsequently became Chairman of the Department of Pediatrics at Tokyo's Japan Red Cross Medical Center. Between 1961 and 1967, Kawasaki identified 50 infants and young children who manifested a distinctive constellation of signs that included prolonged high fever, unilateral cervical lymphadenopathy, bilateral conjunctival injection, a polymorphous erythematous rash, changes of the mucosa of the upper respiratory tract, and edema and erythema of the extremities, with subsequent desquamation of the finger and toes. Although the syndrome was impressive, its signs were nonspecific. Laboratory tests ruled out other disorders. A series of the first seven cases was presented by Kawasaki at the 61st Chiba General Meeting of the Japan Pediatric Society in 1962.[158] Convinced that he was observing a distinct clinical syndrome,

Kawasaki published a report of his experience with 50 cases of "febrile oculo-oro-cutaneo-acrodesquamatous syndrome with or without acute nonsuppurative cervical lymphadenitis" in 1967.[159,160,162] Other Japanese physicians quickly recognized the syndrome after Kawasaki's report, although considerable discussion ensued about whether it was a distinct entity or an illness such as Stevens-Johnson syndrome.[161]

Cardiac involvement in this illness was suspected first in 1968, when Yamamoto and Kimura reported an infant with Kawasaki disease who had transient tachycardia with a gallop rhythm, cardiomegaly, and minor abnormalities on the electrocardiogram (ECG).[394] In 1970, Kawasaki succeeded in obtaining funding to establish the Research Committee of Mucocutaneous Lymph Node Syndrome, sponsored by the Japanese Ministry of Health and Welfare, which was organized with Dr. Fumio Kosaki as chair.[162] In the first national survey of this committee, four autopsied and six non-autopsied cases of children who had died of coronary artery complications after having apparent Kawasaki disease were identified.[175] These children were predominantly younger than 2 years of age and had died suddenly within 30 days of onset of disease, with evidence of coronary aneurysms and acute thrombosis. The first biennial national epidemiologic survey was conducted by this committee in 1970 under the leadership of Dr. I. Shigematsu and was published in 1972.[317] By this time, it had become well established that some patients who recovered apparently uneventfully from this acute illness were at risk for sudden cardiac death, with findings of acute myocardial infarction secondary to thrombosis within coronary arteries damaged by a severe vasculitic process.[175]

In 1971, physicians at the University of Hawaii who were unaware of the Japanese experience began to recognize patients with an unusual Reiter syndrome–like illness. When information about Kawasaki disease was published in the English-language literature,[162] the illness in Hawaii was recognized clearly as Kawasaki disease. Information exchanged between Japanese and U.S. investigators led to the 1974 publication of English-language articles by both groups[162,221,222] and triggered worldwide recognition of cases. In the early 1970s, death from myocardial infarction was reported to occur in approximately 2 percent of cases of Kawasaki disease; more recent data reflect much lower mortality rates of less than 0.1 percent.[120,241,400] With the availability of echocardiography in the late 1970s, researchers determined that 20 to 25 percent of patients will develop evidence of coronary artery abnormalities.[147]

In the decades before Kawasaki recognized the clinical features of the illness, many individual reports of fatal coronary arteritis in children (usually labeled IPAN) were published in the non-Japanese pediatric and pathology literature.[54,77,234,271,283,290] Clinical details of these cases generally are highly suggestive of Kawasaki disease, and the pathologic features of IPAN are indistinguishable from those of Kawasaki disease, as demonstrated

TABLE 88-1 Diagnostic Criteria for Kawasaki Disease

Fever for at least 5 days*
   PLUS
Presence of four of the following features:
   Bilateral conjunctival injection
   Polymorphous exanthem
   Changes in the lips and oral cavity (erythema, cracking of lips;
     oropharyngeal erythema; strawberry tongue)
   Peripheral extremity changes (erythema and swelling of hands and
     feet; later periungual desquamation, Beau lines)
   Cervical lymphadenopathy (≥1.5 cm in diameter)
   Exclusion of other diseases with similar features

Note: The finding of fever plus three criteria in the presence of coronary abnormalities qualifies.
In the presence of classic features, experienced clinicians may be able to establish the diagnosis before the fifth day of illness.

conclusively by Landing and Larson in 1977.[184] Almost 100 years before Kawasaki's description was published, Samuel Gee of St. Bartholomew's Hospital in London in 1871 reported the case of a 7-year-old boy who at death ("following scarlatinal dropsy") had three coronary aneurysms, each filled with a fresh clot; histologic examination of that patient's cardiac tissue is compatible with inactive Kawasaki disease with extensive coronary myointimal proliferation and fibrosis.[103,327] Shibuya and colleagues identified cases of illnesses compatible with Kawasaki disease that occurred in Japan up to 2 decades before Kawasaki's description was published.[316] Likely, patients with Kawasaki disease in previous decades were misdiagnosed as having measles, scarlet fever, rubella, or other once common conditions, and reductions in the numbers of cases of those illnesses helped to facilitate recognition of Kawasaki disease.[161]

Kawasaki's clinical description of the syndrome has remained the foundation of diagnosis and the basis of the clinical and epidemiologic case definitions in use today (see Table 88-1). The American Heart Association Committee on Rheumatic Fever, Bacterial Endocarditis, and Kawasaki disease published guidelines for the management of patients with incomplete (or atypical) Kawasaki disease (see later).[252]

EPIDEMIOLOGY

SOURCES OF EPIDEMIOLOGIC DATA

As with most notifiable diseases, passive reporting of Kawasaki disease cases is incomplete. Passive surveillance data may help to monitor secular trends and to identify epidemics, but these data are of little value in estimating the incidence of disease. Outbreak investigations are more sensitive in determining local disease incidence, and they enable investigators to study potential risk factors.

In the absence of a confirmatory diagnostic test, the epidemiologic case definitions of Kawasaki disease are strict and exclude from surveillance data other exanthematous conditions that could dilute "true" cases and thus could obscure secular trends. However, the original epidemiologic case definitions were not intended for clinical application, a very important point since effective treatment became available. Thus, less strict application of clinical case criteria is appropriate for management of patients. Clinicians must be aware that children often present with clinical illnesses that do not completely fulfill the diagnostic criteria for Kawasaki disease but who are nonetheless at risk for having coronary artery sequelae and therefore warrant therapy. These patients generally are considered to have *incomplete* or *atypical* Kawasaki disease.[28,91,252,299] Incomplete presentations of Kawasaki disease are particularly common occurrences in young infants in whom clinical signs often are subtle or fleeting but who are at

the highest risk for development of coronary artery abnormalities.[40,293] In the United States, the Centers for Disease Control and Prevention (CDC) case definition usually is used for epidemiologic purposes, and the American Heart Association published an algorithm to aid in the diagnosis of incomplete (atypical) Kawasaki disease.[252] The current Japanese diagnostic guidelines were revised for the fifth time and also reflect the importance of incomplete cases.[16]

INCIDENCE RATES

The incidence of Kawasaki disease varies throughout the world and reflects primarily the racial composition of various countries. Rates in Japan have climbed steadily, with an annual rate of 151 per 100,000 children younger than 5 years of age in 2002 (17th National Survey)[400] and as high as 175 per 100,000 children younger than 5 years.[34] In countries with predominantly white populations, the rate is approximately 15 per 100,000 children younger than 5 years of age.[128]

GENDER

In virtually all population-based studies in many countries, the ratio of male to female patients with Kawasaki disease approximates 1.5:1.[400,402] In addition, serious and fatal complications also are significantly more common findings among male patients with Kawasaki disease compared with female patients.[241,401] Examination of fatal Japanese cases indicated almost three times as many Kawasaki-related fatalities among male patients compared with female patients, with a higher ratio in infancy.[241] The basis for the preponderance of Kawasaki disease in male patients and for the even greater predominance of serious coronary artery disease in male patients with Kawasaki disease remains unclear. Of interest is that a male predominance is observed in many infectious diseases.

RACE OR ETHNIC BACKGROUND

The first cases of Kawasaki disease were recognized in Japanese children and in Hawaiian children of predominantly Japanese ethnicity, and subsequent data consistently supported higher rates in those of Asian background. Annual incidence rates in Japan have climbed steadily to more than 150 cases per 100,000 children younger than 5 years of age,[400] from 102.6 in 1995 and 108 in 1996, reaching 184.6 in 2005-2006,[243a] and are among the highest in the world, exceeded only by rates for Japanese-American children in Hawaii (≈197/100,000 <5 years).[129] In epidemic years in Japan, the annual age-specific incidence rates have reached or exceeded 200 per 100,000 children younger than 5 years of age.[396] Incidence rates in white children in many communities are much lower, most often approximating 10 to 15 per 100,000 children younger than 5 years.[60,128,329] Surveys in countries with almost exclusively white populations often yield rates of 5 to 10 cases per 100,000 children younger than 5 years of age.[29,32,45,121,276,333] In Washington state, ethnic group–specific incidence rates per 100,000 children younger than 5 years of age were estimated to be 33.3 for Asian Americans, 23.4 for blacks, and 12.7 for whites.[60] In Hawaii, with its complex racial-ethnic make-up, data showed the overall annual incidence to be 45 per 100,000 children younger than 5 years of age.[129] The yearly incidence for Japanese children in Hawaii approaches 200 cases per 100,000 children, and for whites it is 35 per 100,000, with intermediate rates for those of native Hawaiian and Chinese, Filipino, and other Asian ancestry.[129] In New Zealand, differences in incidence between white and Polynesian children were not apparent,[104] but in Singapore, a higher rate of Kawasaki disease in Chinese children compared with Malay children was suggested.[253] Extrapolation of data from surveys of U.S. hospitals with large children's services led to estimates of approximately 2500 cases per year in the United States from 1984 to 1993,[364,365] with other estimates as high as 5000 cases annually.[34] A study of Kawasaki disease in the United States identified approximately 4200 hospitalizations in the year 2000, with highest rates among Asian and Pacific Islanders, lowest in whites, and intermediate in blacks and Hispanics.[128] Recent data from Japan indicated that a steady increase to more than 10,000 patients with Kawasaki disease diagnosed yearly has occurred,[243a] with occasional local clusters rather than the nationwide outbreaks as seen in 1979, 1982, and 1985 to 1986.[400]

The higher rates of Kawasaki disease in those of Japanese and some other Asian backgrounds suggest a genetic rather than an environmental basis, as supported by increased rates among third- and fourth-generation immigrants from Japan to Hawaii.[129] The increased incidence of Kawasaki disease among siblings and parents of patients (see later) also supports a genetic predisposition.[383,399] The genetic basis is complex in that no single human leukocyte antigen (HLA) is common to most patients with Kawasaki disease. Early reports that Kawasaki disease was associated with HLA-Bw 22 (or subtype Bw 54)[157,177,217] were not confirmed by subsequent studies in Japan, Hong Kong, or Boston, where HLA-Bw 51 and HLA-B 44 were found to be more common.[46,178] HLA-Bw 51 also was increased in a series of Israeli patients.[164] A small Maryland study suggested that the A2 B44 Cw5 haplotype was a risk factor for epidemic Kawasaki disease.[146] Studies of HLA major histocompatibility complex (MHC) class II genes have detected no clear association.[19,81] Immunoglobulin allotypic markers were studied as possible genetic markers for Kawasaki disease.[330] The kappa chain allotype Km1, which is very common in Asian populations, and the combination of Km1 with Gm heterozygosity were present in significantly greater proportions of white patients with Kawasaki disease than in the control white population. In addition, the haplotype G1m(a), G3m(t) was found significantly more often in Japanese and Japanese-American patients with Kawasaki compared with race-matched control populations. This study supports a complex genetic basis for susceptibility to Kawasaki disease.[330] Susceptibility has been linked to other allelic variations in small studies, but larger and more definitive studies are in progress.[35] Transmission disequilibrium studies involving children with Kawasaki disease and their parents may provide better insights into the genetic basis of susceptibility, with functional polymorphisms in the inositol triphosphate kinase-3 gene[268a] and in a network of gene single nucleotide polymorphisms.[32a]

AGE

Kawasaki disease occurs almost exclusively in children. In the United States and Japan, adult cases are quite rare, although some reports of adults diagnosed by accepted diagnostic criteria have been published.* Many of these adult patients have been infected with human immunodeficiency virus (HIV).[141] Many of the early reported adult cases, however, appear to have been associated with toxic shock syndrome or drug hypersensitivity reactions. Perhaps the best-documented adult case was that of a 31-year-old Japanese man (confirmed by Dr. Kawasaki) who later developed bilateral coronary artery aneurysms.[343] Because the signs and symptoms are nonspecific, adults suspected to have Kawasaki disease should be evaluated carefully for infectious, toxic, and other possible causes of illness.

The distribution of Kawasaki disease by age in childhood is characteristic. The disease occurs most frequently in young children: 50 percent are younger than 2 years of age, 80 percent are

younger than 5 years of age, and cases seldom occur in those older than 12 years of age.[128,336,400] Infants in the first 3 to 6 months of life have a low incidence of Kawasaki disease, but the incidence rises rapidly from that point. In the United States, the peak age is approximately 15-18 months, whereas more recent data from Japan identified 26 percent as younger than 1 year old, 89 percent as younger than 5 years, and the peak age incidence as 9 to 11 months of age.[400] In Hawaii, 29 percent of cases are in children younger than 1 year old, and 85 percent of patients are younger than 5 years.[129] The lower peak age in Japan and perhaps in Hawaii may reflect better recognition of Kawasaki disease in infants, in whom Kawasaki disease may be more difficult to diagnose, or it may indicate a biologic difference. The age-incidence curve may be helpful in elucidating risk factors for developing Kawasaki disease. Such a pattern is compatible with highly transmissible infectious agents, particularly respiratory agents, and suggests possible transplacental immunity. The features of 28 patients with Kawasaki disease who were aged 8 years and older at the time of diagnosis at our Chicago institution were reported.[336] Delays in establishing the diagnosis and in providing treatment were common occurrences and were at least partially related to the prominence of arthritic and gastrointestinal symptoms in this population. We recently cared for a 19-year-old woman with classic Kawasaki disease.

Japanese mortality data suggest that fatality rates are approximately three times higher in children younger than 1 year old at the time of onset of disease, compared with older children, and that fatalities occur predominantly in the first several months after onset of Kawasaki disease.[399] The overall mortality rate in Japan has dropped from the initial report of approximately 2 percent to more recent Japanese estimates of approximately 0.08 percent.[399] Male patients account for a disproportionate number of deaths in infants and older children.[120,243,399] Long-term mortality rates in a large Japanese Kawasaki disease cohort study were increased over background rates, particularly during and shortly after the acute stage of illness.[241,243]

RECURRENT KAWASAKI DISEASE

A recurrence of Kawasaki disease is defined generally as a new episode of illness meeting clinical criteria for Kawasaki disease that begins at least 3 months after the initial episode and after inflammatory markers such as the erythrocyte sedimentation rate or serum C-reactive protein level have normalized. The frequency of recurrences after first cases of Kawasaki disease in Japan was estimated to be approximately 1.9 percent during a 3-year follow-up period, with approximately 0.07 percent of patients experiencing a third episode.[240] This corresponds to a rate of 5.21 per 1000 person-years for one or more recurrences.[240] With longer follow-up, recurrence rates in Japan may approach 3 percent.[401] Data from the United States suggest a recurrence rate of approximately 2 percent.[23] Recurrences occur most frequently within the first 2 years after the initial episode, especially in male patients and in children who have their initial episode before reaching their second birthday.[240] The frequency of recurrences in Chicago appears to be approximately 1 percent, although recurrences were documented in about 2 percent of Hawaiian cases from 1996 to 2000,[129] a finding possibly reflecting a racial difference. The true recurrence rate will be determined only when a specific diagnostic test becomes available for Kawasaki disease and thus minimizes recognition bias.

FAMILY CASES

Simultaneous or sequential cases of Kawasaki disease in siblings, twins, or other family contacts also have been reported,

---

*See references 12, 42, 44, 76, 109, 141, 191, 226, 278, 282, 313.

particularly during outbreaks in Japan.[86,132,215,402] Japanese epidemiologists have documented secondary sibling cases in approximately 1 percent of cases, a rate that is approximately 10 times greater than that in the general child population.[86] However, such figures are difficult to interpret because they may be influenced by recognition and reporting biases. Sibling cases are reported to occur more frequently in twins than in non-twins. Only three sibling pairs were recognized in approximately 1300 Chicago patients, and none were reported in 400 children in Los Angeles.[213] A report from two U.S. medical centers noted 18 families with multiple affected Kawasaki disease patients, including 9 families with 2 affected siblings and 9 with Kawasaki disease in 2 generations or in multiple affected members.[64]

EPIDEMICS AND OUTBREAKS

Japanese investigators noted large nationwide outbreaks of Kawasaki disease in 1979, 1982, and 1985 to 1986, with wavelike spread occurring from one prefecture (state) to the next, suggesting an infectious origin.[242,395,397] The 1982 Japanese epidemic started simultaneously in four areas and spread outward from each region, similar to the way that epidemic influenza spreads in Europe and America.[242,395] In the 1985 to 1986 Japanese epidemic, investigators identified epidemic "waves" that spread outward from an initial focus in the Tokyo metropolitan area and extended simultaneously northward and southward to involve most of the country within approximately 4 months.[242,395,397] A similar but less distinctive pattern of interprefectural progression in waves was noted in the 1982 Japanese epidemic. Within the northern Tohoku District, for example, Kawasaki disease spread from prefecture to prefecture over a period of approximately 7 months.[395] Korean epidemics were detected 7 and 15 months after the Japanese epidemics of 1979 and 1985 to 1986, respectively.[190,395] More localized outbreaks also have been observed. In the United States and elsewhere, community-wide outbreaks have been documented beginning in 1977.[24] Investigation of outbreaks provides opportunities to study potential risk and etiologic factors. Clustering of cases within families, schools, or neighborhoods is quite unusual, even during large-scale epidemics. Japanese investigators have associated epidemics with a significantly increased likelihood of second cases occurring in families, fatalities, and recurrent cases, but the implications of these findings are uncertain. It is striking that since 1986 no further nationwide Japanese outbreaks have been identified, a finding suggesting that the epidemiology of Kawasaki disease may have changed.[399,404]

GEOGRAPHY

Kawasaki disease has been diagnosed throughout the United States and Japan and in virtually all developed and many developing countries on all continents, including temperate and tropical zones.[32,45,78,210,279,305,307,374] No striking rural-urban differences have been noted. Elevation, longitude, and latitude have not been implicated. Travel histories of patients are unremarkable, although an anecdotal report of a 7-month-old infant in Australia documented Kawasaki disease onset 17 days after leaving Japan during that country's 1982 epidemic.[333]

SEASONALITY

In Japan, Kawasaki disease occurs year round but is most prevalent in the winter and spring, with peaks usually occurring in December or January, with a lower peak in June, and the lowest number of cases in October.[36,398,401] In the United States and

other temperate areas, the number of cases peaks in the winter and early spring and is least in late summer; nonetheless, cases occur throughout the year.[25,128,213,284] Winter predominance has been observed in at least some Southern Hemisphere countries. That sporadic cases are recognized year round is somewhat different from the pattern usually observed with highly transmissible respiratory viral diseases, incidences of which peak sharply in the winter and spring (e.g., measles, rubella, influenza).

COMMUNICABILITY

Although little direct evidence exists that Kawasaki disease is transmissible from person to person, considerable circumstantial evidence supports an infectious origin. Secondary or co-primary cases in families occur but are not common. Several outbreak investigations found a higher rate of antecedent respiratory tract illness in patients with Kawasaki disease compared with matched controls.[24,375] This finding is of particular interest in view of the finding that immunoglobulin A (IgA) plasma cells infiltrate the proximal respiratory tract in fatal cases of Kawasaki disease, and it supports a respiratory mode of spread of an inciting agent (see later).[300] A history of previous exposure of children with Kawasaki disease to food or objects from Japan or elsewhere in Asia is a common factor, but the ubiquity of such exposures renders interpreting the data difficult. Japanese family data suggest that sibling cases cluster either on the same day as the index case or 7 days later.[86] Because these results are based on questionnaire data, however, the possibility of ascertainment bias is great; thus, determining the degree to which Japanese familial cases represent co-primary or secondary cases is difficult.

OTHER RISK FACTORS

In addition to demographic risk factors for Kawasaki disease, specific exposures that could be related to an etiologic agent have been linked to the disorder by some epidemiologic investigations. As noted earlier, a history of more frequent recent antecedent respiratory illnesses in cases compared with controls was documented in the early 1980s.[24] Because many viral agents are prevalent in the winter and spring, when Kawasaki disease is most prevalent, "background" isolation of various viruses from patients and from matched controls is expected.

Other past Kawasaki disease associations include exposure to recent carpet cleaning or shampooing, exposure to house dust mites, and residence near bodies of water. The association of Kawasaki disease with exposure to recently cleaned or shampooed carpets was observed in some reports,[27,79,110,131,264,275,284,286] but not in others.[59,209,230,284,291,292,366] In three carpet shampoo-associated clusters investigated by the CDC, the exposures clustered significantly in the 2- to 4-week interval before onset of disease, with few exposures in the 2-week interval immediately preceding the onset. The significance of a possible association with shampoo is unclear, because it is absent entirely in many well-studied outbreaks, and carpets are relatively uncommon in Japan.[59,230] Conceivably, rug shampooing could lead to aerosolization of a microbial or sensitizing agent present in the carpet, such as mites or microbial agents. A possible link between Kawasaki disease and house dust mites (chiefly *Dermatophagoides farinae* and *D. pteronyssinus*), initially proposed as an allergic hypothesis,[100] gained support when the presence of mites and mite antigens in carpets was realized. A Japanese group reported *Rickettsia*-like bodies in the digestive systems of mites in house dust of patients with Kawasaki disease.[115] Other investigators suggested that Kawasaki disease could result from an infectious agent in dust mites.[85] However, counts of dust mites were not significantly different in the houses of case and control patients,[110,135] and no evidence of increased anti-mite IgE, IgG, or antibodies to *D. pteronyssinus* was found in patients with Kawasaki disease.[110,142]

In a small number of outbreaks, CDC investigators found that patients with Kawasaki disease lived closer to "bodies of water" compared with control patients.[286,287] However, other studies, including one in Washington State, did not find living in proximity to water to be a risk factor.[60]

ETIOLOGY

The origin of Kawasaki disease remains unknown. However, clinical and epidemiologic features strongly suggest that the disease has an infectious cause. A self-limited, generally nonrecurring illness manifested by fever, rash, enanthem, conjunctival injection, and cervical adenitis fits well with an infectious cause. The epidemiologic features noted earlier, including the age distribution (Fig. 88–1), the winterspring seasonality, the occurrence of community outbreaks with wavelike geographic spread, and apparent epidemic cycles, resemble those of a transmissible disease of childhood. The laboratory features, including leukocytosis with a "left shift," elevated acute-phase reactants, and pyuria, also suggest infection. Vasculitis with inflammatory cell infiltration (including IgA plasma cells)[300] may be infectious or may represent an immune reaction to infection. A very attractive

hypothesis is that Kawasaki disease is caused by a ubiquitous infectious agent that produces clinically apparent disease only in selected, genetically predisposed individuals, particularly Asians. Its rarity in the first few months of life and in older children and adults suggests an agent to which virtually all adults are immune and from which very young infants are protected by passive maternal antibody. Consistent with this hypothesis is the paucity of evidence of person-to-person spread of Kawasaki disease, because most infections would be asymptomatic, and only a very few of those infected would develop clinical features of Kawasaki disease. This would be analogous to acute poliomyelitis, the relatively uncommon complication of poliovirus infection that occurs in only approximately 1 in 200 of those infected. However, efforts to identify an infectious agent of Kawasaki disease using conventional bacterial and viral culture and serologic methods, as well as inoculation of primates, mice, and guinea pigs, have failed to yield an infectious cause.[326]

Two major theories to explain the etiology of Kawasaki disease have gained prominence in the past decade: the specific respiratory pathogen theory[295] and the superantigen theory.[201] A very long list of microorganisms, including bacteria, leptospires, spirochetes, fungi, chlamydia, rickettsiae, and viruses, have been suggested at one time or another to cause Kawasaki disease, without confirmation.[303] Chlamydial studies eliminated this possibility.[116,314,337] The hypothesis that Kawasaki disease may be

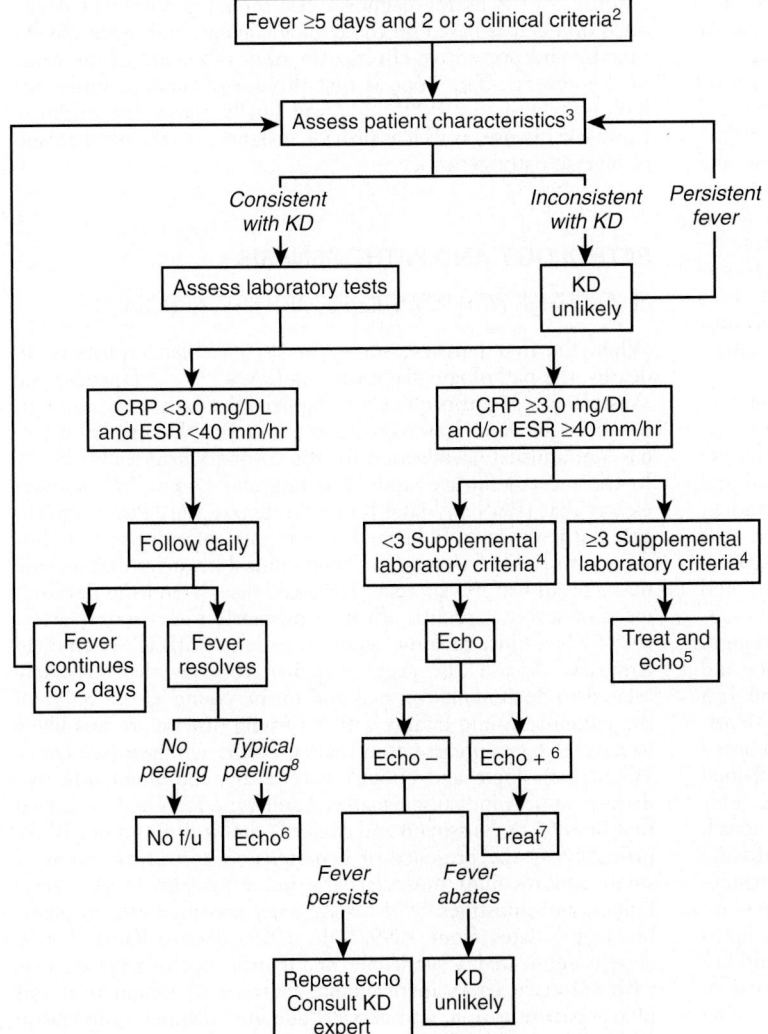

Figure 88–1 Evaluation of suspected incomplete Kawasaki disease (KD). *1,* In the absence of a gold standard for diagnosis, this algorithm cannot be evidence based but rather represents the informed opinion of the expert committee. Consultation with an expert should be sought anytime assistance is needed. *2,* Infants up to 6 months old on day 7 or later of fever without any other explanation should undergo laboratory testing and, if evidence of systemic inflammation is found, an echocardiogram, even if the infants have no clinical criteria. *3,* Patient characteristics suggesting Kawasaki disease are listed in Table 88–1. Characteristics suggesting disease other than Kawasaki disease include exudative conjunctivitis, exudative pharyngitis, discrete intraoral lesions, bullous or vesicular rash, or generalized adenopathy. Consider alternative diagnoses (see Table 88–2). *4,* Supplemental laboratory criteria include albumin less than or equal to 3.0 g/dL, anemia for age, elevation of alanine aminotransferase, platelets after 7 day 450,000/mm³ or greater, white blood cell count 15,000/mm³ or higher, and urine with 10 or more white blood cells/high-power field. *5,* The patient can be treated before an echocardiogram is performed. *6,* Echocardiogram is considered positive for purposes of this algorithm if any of three conditions are met: Z score of left anterior descending (LAD) or right coronary artery (RCA) 2.5 or greater, coronary arteries meet Japanese Ministry of Health criteria for aneurysms, or ≥3 other suggestive features exist, including perivascular brightness, lack of tapering, decreased left ventricular function, mitral regurgitation, pericardial effusion, or Z scores in LAD or RCA of 2 to 2.5. *7.* If the echocardiogram is positive, treatment should be given to children within 10 days of fever onset and to those beyond day 10 with clinical and laboratory signs (C-reactive protein [CRP], erythrocyte sedimentation rate [ESR]) of ongoing inflammation. *8,* Typical peeling begins under nail bed of fingers and then toes. See the text for further details. f/u, follow-up. *(Newburger, J. W., Takahashi, M., Gerber, M. A., et al.: Diagnosis, treatment, and long-term management of Kawasaki disease. (American Heart Association Scientific Statement). Circulation 110:2747-2771, 2004.)*

caused by *Rickettsia*-like agents also seems very unlikely.[143] *Yersinia*, particularly *Yersinia pseudotuberculosis*, causes a systemic illness resembling Kawasaki disease in selected areas of Japan,[50,188,310] but convincing evidence of an etiologic link between *Yersinia* and Kawasaki disease is lacking, despite the use of newer molecular tools.[357]

That Kawasaki disease may be caused by a novel retrovirus was suggested when two groups reported reverse transcriptase activity in cultured peripheral blood mononuclear cells from patients with acute Kawasaki disease.[37,325] Other studies failed to confirm this finding.[223,268] Serologic studies for the retroviruses HIV-1, human T-cell lymphotropic virus types I and II, simian immunodeficiency virus, and feline T-cell lymphotrophic virus have been negative,[254,268,285,301] although features resembling Kawasaki disease have been described in adults with HIV infection.[141]

The hypothesis that Kawasaki disease may be the result of a bacterial superantigenic toxin was suggested because of possible selective expansion of $V\beta_2$ and $V\beta_8$ T-cell receptor families among circulating mononuclear cells.[1] Superantigens such as bacterial toxins bind to MHC class II molecules on monocytes and B cells and to the T-cell receptor, with resultant activation of large numbers of immunoreactive cells with release of inflammatory cytokines. Superantigens potentially cause expansion of autoreactive T cells.[123,176] Features of immune cell activation characterize the acute phase of Kawasaki disease. Toxic shock syndrome and Kawasaki disease share the features of fever, rash, conjunctival infection, and convalescent desquamation to some degree, but differences are present, such as the rarity of hypotension in Kawasaki disease and the absence of maculopapular or erythema multiforme–like rashes in toxic shock syndrome.[117,277] Although one group of investigators reported selective expansion of the $V\beta_2$ and $V\beta_8$ T-cell receptor families in acute Kawasaki disease,[1,2,56] this finding was not confirmed by others.[3,256,280,376] Although 11 of 16 studied patients with Kawasaki disease and only 1 of 15 controls were colonized with toxic shock syndrome toxin I (TSST-I)–producing staphylococci,[201] *Staphylococcus aureus* colonization rates, including by TSST-I–producing staphylococci, were not significantly different among patients with Kawasaki disease and controls in other studies.[202,211,370] That most studies failed to show *any* disturbance of Vβ T-cell receptor expression in Kawasaki disease substantially challenges the superantigen hypothesis.[61]

More recent work indicated that the immune response in Kawasaki disease is oligoclonal (antigen driven, i.e., a response to a conventional antigen) rather than polyclonal (as typically found in superantigen-driven responses), with both B-cell and T-cell oligoclonality demonstrated.[51,302] In a series of studies, Rowley and colleagues[298,300] demonstrated that IgA plasma cells infiltrate peribronchial, coronary arterial, and other tissues in patients who have died of Kawasaki disease in the acute stage and that the IgA plasma cells are oligoclonal,[302] findings strongly suggesting an immune response driven by a conventional agent. Using the techniques of modern molecular biology, Rowley and colleagues[295] synthesized oligoclonal antibodies from the IgA genes from a fatal acute-stage case of Kawasaki disease and identified an antigen in acute Kawasaki disease (but not control) bronchial epithelial cells and in a subset of macrophages in inflamed acute Kawasaki disease tissues, including coronary arteries. This antigen was localized to distinctive perinuclear, primarily apical, intracytoplasmic "spheroidal bodies" in acute Kawasaki disease ciliated bronchial epithelium. Light microscopic and transmission electron microscopic studies showed that the bodies are homogeneous electron-dense perinuclear inclusion bodies up to 1.4 μg in diameter that contain both protein and RNA and are consistent with aggregates of viral proteins and RNA, possibly related to the etiologic agent of Kawasaki disease.[296] The specific agent is still under very active investigation.

Reports of an association between a novel human coronavirus (dubbed HCoV-NH but later shown to be HCoV-NL63) appeared in 2005,[75] thus raising the possibility that this virus could be the agent observed by Rowley and colleagues noted earlier. However, several additional studies from four countries were unable to confirm any relationship between Kawasaki disease and this agent,[22,47,67,72,318] and Rowley's synthetic antibodies do not bind to HCoV-NL63.

Researchers have suggested that Kawasaki disease may be an immunologic response triggered by any of several different microbial agents. Consistent with this hypothesis is documented infection by different microorganisms in different individual cases, failure to detect a single microbiologic or environmental agent after 4 decades of study, and analogies to other multifactorial syndromes (e.g., aseptic meningitis). However, this hypothesis is difficult to reconcile with the distinctive clinical and laboratory pictures of Kawasaki disease, with its epidemiologic features such as epidemics and wavelike geographic spread, and with the studies of Rowley and colleagues.[295,296]

Efforts to associate Kawasaki disease with exposure to drugs[130] or to such environmental pollutants as toxins, pesticides, chemicals, and heavy metals have failed. However, clinical similarities between Kawasaki disease and acrodynia (mercury poisoning) are notable.[15,269]

Clearly, conventional culture and serologic methodologies have failed to yield the causative agent of Kawasaki disease. In addition, establishing the diagnosis can be difficult, particularly in young infants and in those with incomplete or atypical presentations.[28,40,299] A useful diagnostic test probably cannot be developed unless it is based on the etiologic agent, and more specific therapy and preventive efforts also await discovery of the cause of this disease. The hope is that the use of modern molecular biology techniques[295,296,298,302,324] will finally clarify the origin of Kawasaki disease, as well as provide insights into the mechanisms of disease pathogenesis.

PATHOLOGY AND PATHOGENESIS

RELATIONSHIP WITH INFANTILE PERIARTERITIS NODOSA

When the first Japanese survey in 1970 yielded reports of 10 deaths, the pathologic diagnosis was IPAN.[139,163,175] Japanese and Western investigators quickly recognized the pathologic similarities between fatal Kawasaki disease and IPAN, long known to have an unusual predilection for the coronary arteries.[4,20,21,359-362] In the most definitive study, Landing and Larson[184,189] showed clearly that IPAN and fatal Kawasaki disease were indistinguishable pathologically. Published case reports of autopsies of children with IPAN frequently contain clinical histories that include many or all features of acute Kawasaki disease and the development of severe vasculitis affecting primarily the coronary arteries.[290] The failure of some reported patients with IPAN to meet Kawasaki disease case criteria applied retrospectively is likely related to documentation bias and to the young age of many of the patients. Young infants with Kawasaki disease are less likely to have a classic presentation than are older children (see later). When pathologic and clinical criteria are combined, the two diseases appear indistinguishable. Adult-type PAN was described first in 1866 by Kussmaul and Maier,[183] and it differs from IPAN primarily by the presence of hypertension and involvement of small and medium muscular arteries, especially in the lung, kidney, and intestines.[88,184,361,362] An early recorded case of possible IPAN dates from 1899.[180] In 1959, Munro-Faure[234] very clearly delineated a syndrome of infantile necrotizing arteritis with coronary artery involvement, fever, rash, conjunctival and pharyngeal infection, and cervical adenitis, distinct from classic PAN. Roberts and Fetterman[290] and others expanded on these observations to define a distinct clinical-pathologic syndrome of IPAN shortly before Kawasaki recognized the clinical syndrome.[159,160]

Coronary artery aneurysms were described as early as the early 19th century, with a male-to-female ratio of roughly 3:1, including a male preponderance in childhood cases. Childhood death from multiple coronary artery aneurysms was known to occur at least as early as 1871, as reported by Samuel Gee.[103] The cardiac specimen from this case, formalin fixed for more than 120 years in the pathology museum at St. Bartholomew's Hospital, London, recently was sectioned and examined histologically. We found that the coronary arteries showed the characteristic histologic findings of inactive Kawasaki disease and IPAN.[327] Whether these early cases with childhood coronary artery aneurysms truly represented early examples of Kawasaki disease is not certain; details of the clinical histories usually were scant.[103,283] What is clear, however, is that most of these cases greatly resemble (and very likely do, in fact, represent) Kawasaki disease.[54,77,234,283] From the features of many such early case reports, a reasonably accurate picture of Kawasaki disease as recognized today emerges. It is highly likely that in the decades before the introduction of the measles vaccine in the 1960s, cases of Kawasaki disease were misdiagnosed as measles, scarlet fever, drug hypersensitivity, or other common conditions.

PATHOLOGIC FEATURES OF KAWASAKI DISEASE

Cardiac death in Kawasaki disease generally occurs in the subacute or convalescent stages of illness.[241,243] Autopsy findings usually reveal evidence of active or inactive vasculitis, which is most severe in the medium-sized arteries, with a marked predilection for the coronary arteries.[8,9,87,184,353,361,362] Small arterioles, larger arteries, capillaries, and veins also are affected to a lesser extent.[9,88] In more than 80 percent of fatal cases in the acute stage, the immediate cause of death is acute thrombosis of inflamed coronary arteries, with resultant myocardial infarction. In a few early deaths, pancarditis with inflammation of the atrioventricular conduction system apparently caused a fatal arrhythmia or intractable congestive heart failure, whereas small numbers of other deaths may have been associated with acute coronary rupture, usually within a few weeks of the onset of illness. Deaths that occur months to years after the acute episode of Kawasaki disease often are secondary to coronary stenosis, with or without thrombosis with myocardial ischemia, or, very rarely, to rupture of a coronary aneurysm. In some patients with coronary artery abnormalities (usually patients with quite severe coronary disease), aneurysms of other major medium-sized arteries, including the brachial, renal, and iliac arteries, also may be present. Although phlebitis may be found, vascular inflammation more typically and more severely affects medium-sized musculoelastic arteries in their extraparenchymal portions. In the acute stage of Kawasaki disease, systemic inflammatory changes also are evident in many other organs, including myocardium, pericardium, cardiac valves, cerebrospinal fluid, lung, lymph nodes, pancreas, spleen, joints, and liver.[10,88]

In the early stages of the vasculitis of Kawasaki disease, edema of endothelial cells with nuclear degeneration and mild adventitial inflammation are seen.[8,87,359] Mononuclear cells predominate even in the acute stage of Kawasaki disease, and neutrophils also are prominent in the first 10 days after onset.[354] In more severely involved vessels such as the coronary arteries, panvasculitis is present, with inflammation of the endothelium, the media with edema and necrosis of smooth muscle cells, and the adventitia. Fragmentation and destruction of elastin and collagen fibers and the internal and external elastic laminae are seen in severely affected vessels.[8] These changes eventually obscure the various layers of the wall. Structural integrity may be lost, resulting in an aneurysm. In larger arteries with vasa vasorum, inflammation is seen in and around these vessels.[8]

Within 1 to 2 months after the onset of Kawasaki disease, inflammatory cells disappear, and fibrous connective tissue, collagen and elastic fibers begin to form within the vessel wall. The intima proliferates and thickens. In time, the vessel wall may become stenotic, and occlusion by stenosis or by superimposed thrombus can result. Calcification may occur, and intraluminal thrombus may become organized, remodeled, and recanalized.[8,245,309,349,350] Several groups investigated the mechanisms of vascular remodeling in Kawasaki disease. Suzuki and colleagues[351] showed by immunohistochemistry that active remodeling continues for at least several years after the onset of Kawasaki disease, with luxuriant intimal proliferation and neoangiogenesis. Extensive expression of vascular growth factors, including vascular endothelial growth factor (VEGF) within smooth muscle cells, was evident particularly in newly formed microvessels in the intima.[351] Gavin and colleagues[102] showed the prominence of matrix metalloproteinases in this process, particularly within the intima and media. Suzuki and associates[352] found evidence of inflammatory changes in the intact coronary artery of a child who died 13 months after having Kawasaki disease and who had no evidence of coronary artery involvement during the acute stage.

Fujiwara and associates[89,90] identified significant atrioventricular conduction system lesions in 5 of 10 autopsy specimens, with a strong correlation found between findings on the ECG, especially PQ prolongation, and acute inflammation of the atrioventricular conduction system. Severe acute changes were most pronounced at 21 to 31 days after onset. In a unique study of 201 right ventricular endomyocardial biopsies in uncomplicated acute Kawasaki disease, Yutani and associates[406,407] noted some degree of myocarditis and cellular infiltration, ranging from very mild (subclinical) to quite severe myocardial inflammation, in all 201 patients studied.

A histologic/immunochemical study examined the intercostal arteries to compare the nature and developmental processes of lesions with those of the coronary arteries.[214] Although similar lesions were seen, the lesions appeared somewhat later in the intercostal arteries.

The precise nature of the inflammatory infiltrate in the vessel wall or myocardium has been studied. Terai and colleagues[368] demonstrated helper (CD4) T cells and monocytes/macrophages in the arterial wall of one patient with fatal acute Kawasaki disease, as well as expression of class II MHC antigen (an activation marker) in coronary vascular endothelium, findings supporting the importance of immune responses in this form of vasculitis. Terai[371] also reported evidence of eosinophils in epicardial microvessel lesions in acute Kawasaki disease leading to death.

Rowley and colleagues[298] demonstrated the presence of many plasma cells of the IgA isotype in the vascular walls of patients who died in the acute stage. These investigators also showed that the IgA plasma cells are oligoclonal (i.e., they appear to be responding in an antigen-driven process)[302] and that they can be observed also in peribronchial, pancreatic, and renal tissues.[300] A predominance of CD8 cytotoxic/suppressor T cells over CD4 helper T cells in seven of eight acute-stage deaths also was observed in our laboratory by immunohistochemistry.[31] Takahashi[354] reported CD68+ monocytes and macrophages to be most prominent in acute Kawasaki disease, but CD3+ cells (T cells), CD20+ cells (B cells), and neutrophils also were present in autopsy specimens of children who died in the first month of the illness.

Other less commonly reported pathologic findings include renal infarcts and glomerular histologic changes, possible evidence of immune complex deposition,[304] including mesangial deposition of IgM and C3, and multifocal periglomerular infiltration of lymphocytes and IgA plasma cells.[300] Changes have been noted in other arteries, the thymus, and lymph nodes. Tanaka[359] described thymic atrophy and nondiagnostic lymph node changes at autopsy (although most patients likely had been treated with steroids). Naoe and colleagues[246] reported lymph node biopsies to show thrombotic arteriolitis, severe lymphadenitis with necrosis, and postcapillary venules with endothelial cell and reticular cell hyperplasia. Other reports described early lymph node biopsies showing multiple foci of necrosis and fibrin thrombi within the microvasculature, as well as T-zone hyperplasia, B-zone macrophage infiltration, and immunoblast proliferation.[108] Rowley and colleagues[300] identified IgA plasma cells not only in vascular and renal tissues but also in pancreatic and peribronchial locations. Miura and associates[228] found prominent macrophage infiltration of pancreatic acini and islets in 3 of 10 fatal cases.

CLINICAL MANIFESTATIONS

CLINICAL PHASES OF ILLNESS

The clinical course of Kawasaki disease can be divided into acute, subacute, and late or convalescent phases. The *acute* febrile phase begins with fever, rash, conjunctival injection, "strawberry" tongue, red swollen lips, edema and erythema of the hands and feet, lymphadenitis, and sometimes aseptic meningitis and mild hepatic dysfunction. Young children often are quite irritable. Evidence of myocarditis, rarely including congestive heart failure or arrhythmias, may develop during this time. Pericardial effusion, mitral regurgitation, or depressed myocardial function may be detected by echocardiogram. Without aspirin and IVIG treatment, the acute phase generally lasts for 8 to 30 days (mean, 11 days). After defervescence, the physical findings rapidly disappear, but during this *subacute* phase, the child may remain irritable and anorectic, with decreased activity. Some conjunctival injection may persist. Arthritis or arthralgia, mainly of larger joints, may develop in the subacute phase. Desquamation of fingers and toes, typically beginning in the periungual region, and thrombocytosis are very common manifestations during this period. The subacute phase persists until the child has returned to his or her normal state of health at approximately 3 to 6 weeks after the onset of fever, with normalization of inflammatory markers. The time of greatest risk of sudden death occurring from acute coronary artery thrombosis in patients with coronary lesions is during the subacute phase and the early convalescent phase. The *convalescent* phase begins when all clinical signs and symptoms have disappeared and inflammatory markers are normal, usually at about 6 to 8 weeks after onset.

When manifested completely, Kawasaki disease is a distinctive clinical entity with a fairly predictable course.[57,252] However, children who do not fulfill the criteria for diagnosis of Kawasaki disease, in fact, may have the illness and are at risk of developing complications, particularly coronary artery disease (see "Incomplete or Atypical Kawasaki Disease" later).[252,299] The principal clinical diagnostic criteria are presented in Table 88–1. Kawasaki disease should be considered in the differential diagnosis of infants and children with fever for at least 5 days associated with two or more of the five classic features: generalized polymorphous erythematous rash, conjunctival injection, characteristic changes of the lips and mouth, bilateral redness and swelling of the hands and feet, or unilateral nonfluctuant cervical lymph node enlargement greater than 1.5 cm.[252] All features are not necessarily present at the same time. A diagnosis of typical Kawasaki disease, according to accepted clinical criteria (see Table 88–1), is made in patients with fever and at least four of the five clinical criteria and with exclusion of other illnesses that mimic Kawasaki disease. Each of the five clinical features is present in 80 to 90 percent of patients with typical cases, except cervical lymphadenopathy, which is present in approximately 50 percent

of patients. The most commonly encountered diseases to be excluded are as follows: (1) febrile exanthems, presumably viral, including measles; (2) acute streptococcal and staphylococcal infections; and (3) drug hypersensitivity reactions. Japanese diagnostic guidelines for Kawasaki disease are similar to the U.S. guidelines with rare exception; they consider fever and the other five major features to be six equal criteria and require at least five of those six criteria for diagnosis. Thus, a child could have no fever but all five other criteria and be considered a typical case by the Japanese criteria. The Japanese criteria also accept a course of fever lasting less than 5 days if it is shortened by early IVIG treatment.[16]

Certain scoring systems using clinical and laboratory features have been developed, primarily in Japan.[13,119,172,244] The goal of these systems generally has been to identify those patients with Kawasaki disease at highest risk for development of coronary abnormalities and who, therefore, would benefit most from receiving IVIG therapy, as well as those at low risk for coronary changes who could be spared IVIG treatment. This practice is decreasing in Japan because no such scoring system appears sufficiently sensitive and specific to enable selective therapy (i.e., to allow non-treatment of patients predicted to be at low risk for development of coronary abnormalities). Patients who are at greatest risk are as follows: those younger than 1 year old; male patients; those with prolonged or recurrent fever; and those with anemia, hypoalbuminemia, hyponatremia, and thrombocytopenia. Nonetheless, we recommend that all patients diagnosed with Kawasaki disease within the first 10 days after onset of disease and those diagnosed later who are still manifesting significant inflammation be treated with IVIG and aspirin.[252] Newer scoring systems have been developed to help predict those patients who are likely to be unresponsive to IVIG therapy, but confirmation is necessary.[172]

In Kawasaki disease, fever typically is high-spiking and remittent, with peak temperatures generally exceeding 39° C (102° F) and in many cases exceeding 40° C (104° F). Unless treated with aspirin or IVIG, fever persists for a mean of 11 days,[125] but it may continue for 3 to 4 weeks, rarely longer. In patients treated with 80 to 100 mg/kg/day of aspirin and a single 2 g/kg dose of IVIG, fever generally resolves within 1 to 2 days.[249]

Bilateral painless vascular infection of the bulbar conjunctivae, clearly more severe than infection of the palpebral conjunctivae and sparing the limbic region around the cornea, generally is seen in the first week of illness, usually beginning shortly after onset of fever. It generally is not associated with exudate, conjunctival edema, or corneal ulceration, thus distinguishing the eye findings of Kawasaki disease from purulent conjunctivitis and from Stevens-Johnson syndrome. Mild acute iridocyclitis or anterior uveitis, which may be noted by slit-lamp examination, resolves rapidly and only rarely is associated with photophobia or eye pain.[33,105,187,265,332] Less common ocular findings include superficial punctate keratitis, vitreous opacities, vitreous and chorioretinal inflammation, lateral rectus palsy, periorbital vasculitis, and papilledema and other optic disk changes.[11,80,137,391]

Changes of the mouth and lips consist of the following: (1) erythema, dryness, fissuring, peeling, cracking, and bleeding of the lips; (2) a strawberry tongue indistinguishable from that associated with streptococcal scarlet fever, with erythema and prominent papillae; and (3) diffuse erythema of the oropharyngeal mucosae. Oral ulcerations, pharyngeal exudates, and Koplik spots are rarely, if ever, found in Kawasaki disease and when present help to exclude the diagnosis.

Changes in the extremities are among the most distinctive features of Kawasaki disease. The hands and feet become indurated and swollen with stretched, shiny skin, sometimes with painful induration. The palms and soles become erythematous, often with an abrupt change to normal skin at the wrist and ankle. Infants and young children frequently refuse to hold objects or to bear weight. In the subacute phase, a distinctive pattern of periungual desquamation of fingers and toes may occur from 2 weeks to 2 months after onset of Kawasaki disease in 50 to 70 percent of affected patients. Beau lines, which are transverse grooves across the nails, may appear at the nail base 1 to 2 months after a case of acute Kawasaki disease and may grow out over several months.

The erythematous rash associated with Kawasaki disease may take many forms. Most common is a nonspecific, diffuse, macular-papular, primarily truncal erythematous rash. Occasionally, diffuse scarlatiniform erythroderma, urticaria, or an erythema multiforme–like rash with target lesions develops. Vesicles and bullae are not seen, although very fine pustules occur rarely. Perineal erythema and then desquamation are quite common manifestations in diapered as well as toilet-trained children in the acute stage of illness. Rashes in Kawasaki disease tend to be most prominent on the trunk, with perineal accentuation, but they frequently also involve the face and extremities.

Cervical lymphadenopathy is the least common of the principal diagnostic criteria, but it sometimes is the dominant clinical feature along with fever.[335] It usually is unilateral and confined to the anterior cervical triangle. To fulfill diagnostic criteria, the enlarged node or mass of nodes exceeds 1.5 cm, is not fluctuant, usually is not associated with erythema of the overlying skin, and is not tender or only moderately tender. Lymphadenopathy generally is benign and transient. Clinicians should be aware that children with suspected acute cervical adenitis that is unresponsive to antibiotic therapy may have Kawasaki disease. Because other features of Kawasaki disease often are present but overlooked, Kawasaki disease should be considered in febrile children with suspected acute bacterial cervical adenitis that is unresponsive to antibiotics and without an alternate diagnosis.[335] The ultrasound appearance of lymph nodes in Kawasaki disease has been described as similar to that of acute Epstein-Barr virus (EBV) infection and distinct from bacterial adenitis.[363] The absence of changes on imaging (e.g., ultrasound or computed tomography [CT]) suggesting suppuration of such lesions should strengthen the suspicion of possible Kawasaki disease in this setting. Impressive cervical adenopathy in patients with Kawasaki disease generally resolves remarkably promptly after administration of appropriate therapy.

The associated features of Kawasaki disease reflect its multisystemic nature (Table 88–2). Sterile pyuria as a manifestation of urethritis, occasionally with meatitis, is found in approximately half of patients. Arthritis appearing during the first week of illness can be polyarticular or oligoarticular, including the small interphalangeal joints as well as large weight-bearing joints, with a prevalence of approximately 7.5 percent.[111] Arthrocentesis manifesting during this early phase yields purulent-appearing fluid, with a mean white blood cell count of 125,000 to 300,000/mm³, normal glucose levels, and negative Gram stain and bacterial cultures. Arthritis developing after the 10th day of illness has a predilection for large weight-bearing joints, especially the knees and ankles, with a somewhat lower synovial fluid white blood cell count.[125] Gastrointestinal complaints occur in approximately one third of patients with acute cases; these complaints may be severe, leading to laparotomy, and they include nausea, abdominal pain, and some diarrhea. These findings may be related to hydropic gallbladder, pancreatitis, or appendicular vasculitis.[14,408] Obstructive jaundice and acute hydrops of the gallbladder are not uncommon findings, whereas mild to moderate elevations of serum transaminases occur in almost half of patients. Central nervous system involvement including aseptic meningitis occurs in almost half of patients.[62] Transient unilateral lower motor neuron facial nerve palsy occurs rarely,[281] as does sensorineural hearing loss.[345] Characteristic extreme irritability is very common, especially in young infants. Reactivation of inflammation at the site of a previous bacillus Calmette-Guérin (BCG) vaccination coincident with

TABLE 88–2 Associated Noncardiac Features of Kawasaki Disease

Musculoskeletal System
Arthritis or arthralgia

Central Nervous System
Aseptic meningitis
Facial nerve palsy
Marked irritability
Sensorineural hearing loss

Gastrointestinal System
Hydrops of gallbladder
Abdominal pain, diarrhea
Hepatic dysfunction, obstructive jaundice
Pancreatitis

Genitourinary System
Urethritis, meatitis

Respiratory System
Pulmonary infiltrates, nodules
Preceding respiratory illness

Other
Erythema and induration of bacille Calmette-Guérin vaccine site
Anterior uveitis (mild)
Peripheral gangrene (young infants)
Desquamating groin rash
Flare of atopic dermatitis or psoriasis

acute Kawasaki disease is a common finding in Japan, where BCG is used widely,[331] and we observed a child in whom a BCG site and purified protein derivative (PPD) test site reactivated with acute Kawasaki disease.[371a] Some patients experience a flare of atopic dermatitis or psoriasis during or after experiencing acute Kawasaki disease.[30,71] Various pulmonary manifestations of Kawasaki disease, including isolated pulmonary nodules,[84] pleural effusions, acute respiratory distress syndrome,[273] and pulmonary infiltrates,[384] all of which are interesting in view of the increased numbers of IgA plasma cells found in respiratory tract tissue, have been observed.[298,300]

By far, the most important associated feature of Kawasaki disease is cardiac involvement. Cardiac manifestations can be prominent in acute Kawasaki disease, and they certainly are the major cause of long-term morbidity and mortality. In addition to the coronary artery abnormalities that develop in 20 to 25 percent of untreated children, pericardial effusion and myocarditis with congestive heart failure, tachycardia, gallop rhythm, nonspecific changes on the ECG, or arrhythmia may occur.[147,150,152,252] An imperfect correlation exists between clinically apparent cardiac involvement and echocardiographic evidence of coronary abnormalities, although in the pre-IVIG era, echocardiographic evidence of mitral regurgitation or pericardial effusion in the acute stage was shown to be predictive of subsequent coronary abnormalities.[106] Acute Kawasaki disease may involve pericardium, myocardium, endocardium, coronary arteries, and cardiac valves. Clinical and auscultatory features may include a hyperdynamic precordium, tachycardia out of proportion for the child's age and temperature, a gallop rhythm, and a flow murmur. Some infants may manifest very low cardiac output, and ECG changes (ST-segment and T-wave changes, prolonged PR interval, and arrhythmias) may be present.

INCOMPLETE OR ATYPICAL KAWASAKI DISEASE

A substantial subset of children presents with illnesses that do not completely fulfill diagnostic criteria for Kawasaki disease but that include at least 5 days of fever and some features of the disease. Incomplete or atypical Kawasaki disease (incomplete is the preferred usage) is associated with a substantial risk for development of coronary artery aneurysms,[28,91,205,252,299] but it can be very difficult to diagnose. Incomplete Kawasaki disease occurs most frequently in young infants, who unfortunately are at greatest risk of developing coronary disease with Kawasaki disease,[40,293,299] and fatalities have occurred. The laboratory profile of incomplete cases is similar to that of classic cases, and laboratory results can increase or decrease the likelihood of the presence of Kawasaki disease in a particular patient. Echocardiographic findings in the acute stage, including perivascular brightness, coronary ectasia, decreased myocardial contractility, pericardial effusion, and mild mitral regurgitation, can support the diagnosis of Kawasaki disease. Individual manifestations of Kawasaki disease in young infants tend to be more subtle than those in older children and can be fleeting.[252,293] Kawasaki disease should be considered in the differential diagnosis of prolonged fever in infants because patients are described in whom such fevers are virtually the sole manifestation of Kawasaki disease.

A committee of the American Heart Association developed an algorithm to assist in the evaluation of patients with suspected incomplete Kawasaki disease (see Fig. 88–1), with emphasis placed on clinical assessment and measurement of acute-phase reactants (C-reactive protein [CRP], erythrocyte sedimentation rate [ESR]) in patients with 5 or more days of fever and two or three features of Kawasaki disease, or in infants 6 months old or younger with 7 days or more of fever without other explanation.[252] In addition to elevated ESR (≥40 mm/hour) and CRP (≥3.0 mg/dL), a set of six supplementary laboratory criteria that can be useful in this regard is as follows: albumin, 3.0 g/dL or less; anemia for age; increased alanine transaminase (ALT); platelets after day 7 of more than 450,000/mm^3; white blood cell counts of 15,000/mm^3 or more; and 10 or more white blood cells/high-power field in the urine.

Retrospective diagnosis of Kawasaki disease often is based on finding coronary abnormalities by echocardiogram, although the real goal is to identify patients with incomplete Kawasaki disease before detection of coronary changes. The existence of these patients again emphasizes the need to identify the etiologic agent of Kawasaki disease so that a diagnostic test can be developed. When possible, patients with illnesses suggesting incomplete Kawasaki disease should be referred to physicians with considerable experience in making the diagnosis.

LABORATORY FINDINGS

A specific diagnostic test for Kawasaki disease is not available and awaits discovery of the etiologic agent of the illness (Table 88–3). The laboratory features of Kawasaki disease, albeit quite nonspecific, are nonetheless characteristic of the illness. Leukocytosis,

TABLE 88-3 Laboratory Features of Kawasaki Disease

Leukocytosis with neutrophilia
Elevated erythrocyte sedimentation rate
Elevated C-reactive protein (and other acute-phase reactants)
Anemia
Thrombocytosis after week 1
Sterile pyuria
Hypoalbuminemia
Hyponatremia
Elevated serum transaminases, gamma-glutamyltransferas
Plasma lipid abnormalities
Cerebrospinal fluid pleocytosis
Synovial fluid pleocytosis

especially with neutrophilia, is typical in the acute stage, with a predominance of immature and mature granulocytes. White blood cell counts in excess of 30,000/mm^3 occur in approximately 5 percent of patients and in excess of 15,000/mm^3 in approximately 50 percent. Leukopenia is quite rare. Toxic granulations and Döhle bodies occasionally are seen on peripheral blood smear.[26] Anemia may develop, usually with normocytic red blood cell indices, particularly in patients with more prolonged duration of active inflammation. Severe hemolytic anemia requiring transfusions occurs but is unusual and usually can be related to IVIG therapy.[53,323] Curiously, Kawasaki's first patient in 1961 (and only rare subsequent patients) manifested Coombs-positive hemolytic anemia.[159,327]

Elevation of acute-phase reactants such as ESR, CRP, and alpha$_1$-antitrypsin is nearly universal in Kawasaki disease, with the ESR usually returning to normal by 6 to 10 weeks after illness onset. CRP values rise and fall much more quickly than do ESR values. Additionally, IVIG therapy per se leads to elevation of the ESR (but not CRP) for several weeks, and, thus, it is of limited value in assessing the degree of inflammatory activity in IVIG-treated patients; CRP or other acute-phase reactants clearly are superior for this purpose.

A very characteristic feature of the later phases of illness is thrombocytosis, with platelet counts ranging from 500,000 to more than 1,000,000/mm^3. Thrombocytosis rarely is present in the first week of illness, usually appears in the second week, and peaks in the third week, with a gradual return to normal by 4 to 8 weeks after onset in uncomplicated cases. The mean peak platelet count is approximately 700,000/mm^3. In one study, infants younger than 1 year old with fever without a source who had platelet counts greater than 800,000/mm^3 were 17 times more likely to be diagnosed with Kawasaki disease ultimately than were infants with platelet counts lower than 800,000/mm^3.[255] No differences exist in chromium-65–labeled autologous platelet survival between cases and controls, and little correlation exists between thrombocytosis and increased platelet aggregation. The latter situation has been detected in patients with Kawasaki disease from a few days until a year after onset.[155,392] The rare patients with thrombocytopenia in the acute stage of Kawasaki disease, most often young patients, appear to be at increased risk for development of coronary artery disease and myocardial infarction.[257,259] The mechanism of thrombocytopenia appears to be consumptive coagulopathy.[259]

Plasma lipids are markedly perturbed in acute Kawasaki disease, with depression of plasma cholesterol, high-density lipoprotein (HDL) cholesterol, and apolipoprotein A-I (apo A-I).[43,248,308] Similar changes are observed in other conditions associated with an acute-phase response.[43] Marked appearance of serum amyloid A (SAA) protein in plasma, associated with HDL3-like lipoprotein particles, is seen acutely.[43] Cabana and colleagues[43] also showed that total cholesterol, HDL cholesterol, apoA-I, and triglyceride levels normalize over the course of several weeks, and that SAA disappears from plasma. The core composition of HDL normalizes more slowly than do plasma HDL cholesterol and apoA-I levels, a finding suggesting that Kawasaki disease has a profound effect on the lipoprotein profile acutely and a more subtle sustained effect on HDL composition.

Mild to moderate elevations in serum transaminase levels are present in as many as 40 percent of patients, and mild hyperbilirubinemia occurs in approximately 10 percent.[38] Plasma gamma-glutamyl transpeptidase levels are elevated in most patients.[372] Hypoalbuminemia and hyponatremia[386] are associated with more prolonged and more severe disease. Hypoalbuminemia appears to indicate more severe and more prolonged acute disease.[119] Urinalysis reveals intermittent mild to moderate sterile pyuria in approximately one third of patients, although suprapubic urine generally does not show pyuria, a finding suggesting urethritis.[63,221] In those children who undergo lumbar puncture,

evidence of aseptic meningitis, with a predominance of mononuclear cells, normal glucose, and normal to mildly elevated
protein levels, is a common finding.[62]

Laboratory tests, even though nonspecific, can provide diagnostic support in patients with clinical features that are suggestive, but not diagnostic, of Kawasaki disease[252] and may aid in
prediction of nonresponder patients.[172] A moderately to markedly
elevated CRP (>3.0 mg/dL) or ESR (>40 mm/hour), almost universal in Kawasaki disease, is an uncommon finding in viral exanthems and hypersensitivity reactions. Platelet counts higher than
450,000 mm³ usually are present in patients with Kawasaki disease
after the seventh day of illness. In cases of incomplete Kawasaki
disease associated with coronary abnormalities, thrombocytosis
and elevated ESR are very common events in the acute stage.
Clinical experience suggests that Kawasaki disease is very unlikely
if platelet counts and a full panel of acute-phase inflammatory
reactants (e.g., ESR, CRP) are essentially normal after the seventh
day of illness.

IMMUNOLOGIC FINDINGS

Studies of children with acute Kawasaki disease reveal widespread
immune perturbations[328] and have focused on immune activation,
endothelial activation, and vascular infiltration with a variety
of immune cells. Evidence of marked immune activation is
present and is reflected by increased levels of a wide variety of
pro-inflammatory cytokines, including tumor necrosis factor-α
(TNF-α), interferon-γ, interleukin-1 (IL-1), IL-2, IL-4, IL-6,
IL-8, IL-10, and soluble IL-2 receptor.* Increased chemokine
and selectin activity also have been reported in acute Kawasaki
disease.[358,389] The most intense immune activation and cytokine
production occur during the acute and early subacute phases, the
period of most intense vascular inflammation and of aneurysm
formation. The immune perturbations subside as the illness
resolves either spontaneously[197] or more promptly in response to
anti-inflammatory therapy, and the benefit of therapy appears to
result from immune modulating effects, although precise details
are lacking.[194,321]

In acute Kawasaki disease, serum IgG levels are lower than
normal for age,[251] whereas in the subacute stage, polyclonal elevation of all immunoglobulin classes generally is found.[204] Serum
IgE and IgM levels particularly are frequently elevated.[179,181] The
increase in serum immunoglobulins is associated with a very high
proportion of circulating activated B cells,[168] which is reversed by
aspirin/IVIG treatment.[196] Shingadia and colleagues[320] found
decreased numbers of circulating B lymphocytes and plasma cells
with surface or cytoplasmic IgA in the acute and subacute stages
of Kawasaki disease, thus complementing the finding of IgA
plasma cell infiltration in tissues.[298,300]

Circulating immune complexes can be detected in the
subacute and convalescent (but not the acute) stages; these complexes appear to be unrelated to the development of coronary
abnormalities by virtue of their time course of detection[124,204,206,212,266,270,306,387] and to be unaffected by IVGG
infusions.[212] Some investigators have detected IgA in these
immune complexes.[266] Most circulating IgG immune complexes
in Kawasaki disease contain IgG1 and IgG3 antibodies,[206] with
Fc portions that bind to monocytes and platelets. Immune complexes in Kawasaki disease may promote aggregation of platelets,
with release of vasoactive factors.[206]

Several autoantibodies have been found in Kawasaki disease
sera, but antinuclear antibody and rheumatoid factor are very
uncommon findings. Antibodies to type III collagen have been
detected,[171] but without clear relation to coronary complications.

*See references 17, 70, 94, 127, 165, 167, 185, 186, 197, 207, 208, 216,
218, 219, 301.

Some acute-phase sera contain IgM anti-myosin antibodies
directed against epitopes that differ from those reactive with
acute rheumatic fever sera, a finding suggesting a possible relationship with myocarditis in Kawasaki disease.[55] Both IgM and
IgG anti-neutrophil cytoplasmic antibodies (ANCAs)[288,312,334]
and anti-myeloperoxidase antibodies[288] have been reported in
Kawasaki disease. Several reports have noted IgM or IgG antiendothelial cell antibodies in Kawasaki disease, which may injure
endothelial cells directly or participate in complement-mediated
injury or in antibody-mediated cytotoxic reactions.[145,195,198-200]
Among the endothelial cell antigens of interest are adhesion
molecules such as intercellular adhesion molecule-1 (ICAM-1),
vascular cell adhesion molecule-1 (VCAM-1), E-selectin, P-
selectin, and endothelin, all of which may be up-regulated in
Kawasaki disease.[35,93,166,232,261] The precise role of immunologic
reactions to endothelial cells in the pathogenesis of Kawasaki
disease is unclear; Miura and colleagues[229] found focal but not
widespread expression of VCAM-1 or E-selectin on endothelial
cells of acute Kawasaki disease coronary arteries, especially in
areas of neovascularization. However, the temporal correlation
of immune activation and endothelial cell activation with secretion of monocyte chemoattractant protein-1 (MCP-1)[35,200,368] and
the development of coronary abnormalities and their suppression
by IVIG are consistent with an immune stimulant that triggers
an immune response leading to vascular damage in part through
cytokine-induced exposure of endothelial epitopes, inflammatory
cell infiltration, myointimal proliferation, matrix metalloproteinase release, and other mechanisms resulting in vascular wall
damage.[102,315] A less than optimal animal model of Kawasaki
disease induced by injected cell wall fragments of *Lactobacillus
casei* has been reported.[193]

Investigation of the distribution of circulating T cells in acute
and subacute Kawasaki disease has yielded conflicting results that
range from no significant change in distribution of CD3, CD4,
CD8, and CD19 cells at any stage of illness[51] to significant
decreases in circulating CD8[203,369] or CD4[369] numbers acutely. An
immunohistochemistry study of eight autopsied acute-stage
Kawasaki hearts found activated T cells, a predominance of CD8
cells and macrophages, but no B cells,[31] whereas Terai and colleagues'[368] study of one autopsied child showed predominance of
activated CD4 cells and macrophages as well as activated coronary endothelial cells. The presence of activated T cells in
peripheral blood in acute Kawasaki disease is controversial.

As discussed earlier under etiology, expansion of Vβ2 and Vβ8
T-cell receptor families in acute Kawasaki disease has been
reported,[1,2,56] but this finding has not been reproduced by other
investigators.[3,211,224,256,280,370,376] Such expansion would suggest the
possible role of a superantigen or could reflect clonal expansion
of certain Vβ families in response to a conventional antigen.
However, clonal expansion of CD8 T cells in acute Kawasaki
disease supports the hypothesis that a conventional antigen rather
than a superantigen is involved in the pathogenesis,[51,326] and compelling evidence of an oligoclonal IgA response in the vascular
wall also strongly supports this hypothesis.[302]

Evidence for activation of neutrophils in Kawasaki disease is
of interest because these cells, along with monocytes and macrophages, are postulated to mediate endothelial cell damage by
production of oxygen radicals.[258,354,382] Kawasaki disease also is
associated with widespread activation of monocytes and macrophages,[95-97] T lymphocytes,[98,311] and B lymphocytes.[168] Jejunal
mucosal changes similar to delayed-type hypersensitivity in the
epithelium and lamina propria, including decreases in CD8⁺ cells
and increases in CD4⁺ and HLA-DR⁺ cells, have been detected.[239]
Delayed hypersensitivity skin test responsiveness to *Candida*,
streptokinase/streptodornase, phytohemagglutinin, and PPD
(tuberculin) is suppressed during the acute stage of Kawasaki
disease but normalizes within 1 to 2 months.[403] Acute Kawasaki
disease is associated with inflammatory reactivation of previous

BCG vaccination sites, apparently reflecting both cellular and humoral responses.[405] We cared for a patient with acute Kawasaki disease and reactivation of a BCG site and the site of a recent tuberculin skin test.[371a] Plasma fibronectin levels are reported to be decreased early in illness but to rebound to high levels by the fourth week of illness.[319]

Circulating complement components C3 and C4 commonly are elevated, probably as acute reactants in the first several weeks of illness, and then normalize.[289] Nonetheless, complement appears to be activated through the classical pathway,[173] with high plasma C4D levels.[237]

Production of the chemoattractant leukotriene B$_4$ by polymorphonuclear cells is increased from 13 to 29 days after onset of Kawasaki disease,[114] and it may attract more inflammatory cells to the site. Leukotriene E$_4$ and prostaglandin E$_2$ also are elevated in Kawasaki disease,[92,192,220] as are increased platelet synthesis of thromboxane A$_2$ and plasma levels of thromboxane B$_2$.[126]

The strongest evidence of the importance of immunologic factors in the pathogenesis of vasculitis in Kawasaki disease is provided by the remarkably beneficial effect of IVIG on the acute febrile illness and the prevention of the development of coronary aneurysms.[238,247,251,262,321] It correlates with the effect of IVIG to reduce B-cell activation, more rapidly normalize T-cell activity, down-regulate cytokine secretion, and induce disappearance of endothelial cell activation antigens.[194,200] Potential mechanisms of the beneficial action of IVIG in Kawasaki disease include modulation of cytokine production, suppression of endothelial cell activation, inhibition of immunoglobulin production by a negative feedback mechanism, specific neutralization of an unknown etiologic agent or toxin, nonspecific blockade of a receptor for immune complexes, and augmentation of T-cell suppressor activity.[321]

TREATMENT IN THE ACUTE STAGE

INITIAL THERAPY

Patients diagnosed with Kawasaki disease should be admitted to hospital, undergo a baseline echocardiogram, and receive IVIG 2 g/kg over the course of 10 to 12 hours, with high-dose aspirin at 80 to 100 mg/kg/day in four divided doses (Table 88-4).[57,252] When administered by the 10th illness day, this regimen is highly effective in reducing the risk of development of coronary abnor-

---

TABLE 88-4   Treatment for Kawasaki Disease

Acute and Subacute Stages
IVIG, 2 g/kg infusion over 10-12 hr
  PLUS
Aspirin, 80-100 mg/kg/day in four divided doses (until 14th illness day and patient afebrile at least 3-4 days), then 3-5 mg/kg once daily for 6-8 wk
IVIG may be repeated if fever persists or recurs together with at least one classic sign of Kawasaki disease (see text for other alternative "rescue therapies")

Convalescent Stage
No coronary abnormalities: no therapy
Transient coronary abnormalities: aspirin, 3-5 mg/kg once daily at least until resolution of abnormalities
Persistent small to medium coronary aneurysms: aspirin, 3-5 mg/kg once daily
Giant or multiple small coronary aneurysms: aspirin, 3-5 mg/kg once daily, with or without clopidogrel, with warfarin or low-molecular-weight heparin for most patients
Coronary obstruction: thrombolytic therapy, surgical or interventional procedures

IVIG, intravenous immunoglobulin.

---

malities.[249] Because few data exist regarding therapy of patients treated later than the 10th illness day, the goal is to treat by day 10 whenever possible. Patients who are diagnosed after the 10th illness day and who are still febrile may benefit from therapy, but the ability to prevent coronary changes is less certain. IVIG and aspirin have been shown to prevent the development of giant coronary aneurysms[52,297] and to have direct benefits on cardiac function.[249] The mechanism of action of IVIG in Kawasaki disease is unknown. The single high-dose schedule is superior to the earlier regimen of 400 mg/kg/day IVIG for 4 days with high-dose aspirin with respect to rapidity of defervescence and normalization of acute-phase reactants.[247,251,252,262] The large single-dose infusion generally is well tolerated, even in patients with decreased myocardial function.[249] Patients should remain hospitalized until they have been afebrile for at least 24 hours, to ensure that they are available for re-treatment if necessary.

Whether treatment with IVIG and aspirin earlier than the fifth illness day leads to poorer outcomes remains unclear. Tse and colleagues[378] compared 89 children treated on or before the fifth day of illness with controls treated on illness day 6 to 9. These investigators found significantly fewer patients with coronary ectasia at 1 year after Kawasaki disease and shorter total fever duration in the former group, without differences in frequency of recrudescence, need for additional therapy, need of steroids, length of hospitalization, or development of coronary aneurysms within 3 months. Zhang and associates[409] also concluded that patients treated before the sixth illness day had a significantly lower risk of developing cardiac sequelae compared with patients treated later than the sixth day. In contrast, Muta and colleagues[235] evaluated 4731 patients treated on days 1 to 4 and 4020 treated on days 5 to 9 and found that patients treated earlier were somewhat more likely to require additional therapy (odds ratio, 1.12, 1.10 to 1.16); no significant differences in cardiac sequelae were found between groups. Another study also found that treatment before illness day 5 was associated with increased need for re-treatment but no difference in coronary outcome.[82]

Single infusions of IVIG at doses less than 2 g/kg have not been demonstrated to be as effective as 2 g/kg.[18,74] A comprehensive meta-analysis of all Japanese and North American IVIG treatment trials showed that the coronary artery outcome is correlated directly with the *total* dose per kilogram of IVIG administered, with 2 g/kg superior to 1.6 g/kg, which is superior to 1.2 and 1.0 g/kg; the initial dose of aspirin used did not appear to influence coronary outcome.[367] Another study confirmed this finding.[69]

Patients diagnosed after the 10th illness day who are still febrile or who manifest other signs of active disease may benefit from IVIG and aspirin therapy because this treatment may result in prompt clinical improvement, with subsidence of fever and other signs of inflammation. No evidence supports that this approach results in lower rates of development of coronary abnormalities, however. Patients beyond the 10th to 12th illness day who have become afebrile and have resolved features of Kawasaki disease without therapy are unlikely to benefit from IVIG. Such children should be treated instead with aspirin, 3 to 5 mg/kg once daily, and should be evaluated carefully by serial echocardiograms. In patients who have already developed coronary aneurysms and whose acute manifestations of illness have resolved, no evidence suggests a beneficial effect of IVIG.

Various brands of IVIG differ in manufacturing processes and, therefore, in composition (e.g., proportion of IgG monomers, presence of proteins other than IgG). Although adverse reaction rates differ among products, clinical efficacy does not seem to differ.[294] An exception is a report that showed IVIG prepared with β-propiolactone, which can affect the biologic activity of the Fc portion of IgG, to be less effective in Kawasaki disease.[377] Measles and varicella immunizations (but not others) should be deferred for 9 to 11 months after administration of high-dose IVIG because of impaired immune responses to these live virus vaccines.

The aspirin dosage for acute Kawasaki disease that is most thoroughly studied in the United States is 80 to 100 mg/kg/day in four doses. This therapy should be maintained until approximately the 14th day of illness (longer if necessary to ensure that the patient has been afebrile for ≥3 to 4 days) and then reduced to a daily dose of 3 to 5 mg/kg and continued until 2 to 3 months after onset of illness in those who have not developed coronary abnormalities.[252] Patients who develop coronary abnormalities should continue to take low-dose aspirin. High-dose aspirin is used for its anti-inflammatory activity, whereas the much lower doses inhibit platelet aggregation. Japanese clinicians generally use an intermediate anti-inflammatory dose of 30 to 50 mg/kg/day[182] because of perceived higher rates of untoward effects in Japan. Difficulty in achieving what are usually considered therapeutic anti-inflammatory serum salicylate levels during the acute phase of illness (20 to 25 mg/dL) may complicate aspirin treatment,[138] and selected refractory patients may require salicylate doses in excess of 100 mg/kg/day to achieve anti-inflammatory benefit. This situation probably reflects impaired absorption and bioavailability and enhanced salicylate clearance in acute Kawasaki disease.[174] An important note is that, with clinical improvement, patients with Kawasaki disease who are receiving very high doses can suddenly increase their salicylate absorption and may become salicylate toxic. Serum salicylate levels should be monitored if symptoms of vomiting, hyperpnea, tinnitus, lethargy, or striking liver function abnormalities develop in children receiving aspirin.

One study that randomized patients to receive salicylates at 80 to 100 mg/kg/day or 3 to 5 mg/kg/day for initial therapy (each regimen with 2 g/kg of IVIG) concluded that no difference in coronary outcome occurred, but a more prompt anti-inflammatory benefit was noted in the high-dose aspirin group.[225] In the absence of IVIG, aspirin therapy does not decrease the frequency of coronary abnormalities.[69] Reye syndrome has been reported rarely in children taking high-dose aspirin for Kawasaki disease, but whether low-dose aspirin poses this risk is unclear.[356]

The potential value of adding corticosteroid therapy to IVIG or aspirin for primary therapy was addressed in several trials.[250] For example, Jibiki and colleagues[140] compared 3 days of intravenous dexamethasone (0.3 mg/kg/day) plus heparin and IVIG, with subsequent low-dose aspirin, to IVIG plus higher-dose aspirin. These investigators found more prompt decreases in fever and inflammatory markers such as CRP in the dexamethasone-treated group, but no difference in rates of coronary abnormalities. Okada and associates[267] showed that the addition of intravenous prednisolone followed by a long taper of oral prednisolone to IVIG and aspirin was associated with shorter duration of fever and more prompt fall in CRP and circulating IL-2, IL-6, IL-8, and IL-10 levels. Inoue and colleagues[134] compared 88 patients treated with IVIG and aspirin with 90 patients who received in addition intravenous prednisolone (2 mg/kg/day in 3 divided doses) until afebrile and then orally until the CRP normalized, with a subsequent taper over 15 days, for a median of 23 days of steroids. The results indicated fewer coronary abnormalities, shorter durations of fever, more rapid decline in CRP level, and fewer initial treatment failures in the steroid recipients. Caution must be exercised in the interpretation of the findings of these Japanese trials because the IVIG regimens and aspirin doses differ from those used in the United States, and echocardiograms were not interpreted by investigators blinded to the treatment group.

The most definitive trial in this regard showed little if any direct benefit of the addition of a single dose of intravenous methylprednisolone (30 mg/kg) to the current IVIG and aspirin

regimen, with the possible exception of patients who failed to respond to standard therapy and who required retreatment.[250] This observation will require additional study.

RESCUE THERAPY FOR TREATMENT FAILURES

Most patients with acute Kawasaki disease respond promptly to treatment with IVIG and aspirin, with defervescence and subsidence of inflammatory manifestations occurring within 48 hours.[57,247,322] A subgroup of approximately 5 to 15 percent, however, fails to show significant clinical response; these patients remain febrile 24 to 48 hours after receiving IVIG, or they manifest only transient improvement, with recurrent fever and clinical evidence of inflammatory signs. These patients need additional anti-inflammatory therapy, and specific guidelines or controlled treatment trials do not exist. Of course, when treating apparently treatment-refractory patients, it is also prudent to reconfirm the diagnosis.

In these patients, administration of a second dose of 2 g/kg of IVIG generally is effective in suppressing disease activity.[83,252,344] In a retrospective study of 179 patients with Kawasaki disease, 89 percent responded to the first dose of IVIG, and 67 percent of the nonresponders responded to a second IVIG dose; thus, only 3 to 4 percent of these patients failed to respond after a second dose of IVIG.[118] Carefully increasing the dose of aspirin to 120 mg/kg/day or higher, with monitoring of serum levels, may be helpful. Some physicians recommend a course (usually 3 days) of intravenous pulse methylprednisolone at 30 mg/kg/day instead of a second dose of IVIG.[390] We generally reserve pulse steroid therapy for the quite rare patient with highly refractory acute disease, who has failed to respond to at least two doses of IVIG, because early Japanese data suggested that steroids may predispose to development of coronary disease.[155] In addition, a more recent study noted coronary dilatation shortly after pulse steroids were administered in three of nine treatment-refractory patients.[122] No direct comparison between repeat IVIG dosing and corticosteroids has been performed. In a few particularly treatment-refractory patients, we employed a slow oral steroid taper over the course of several months once inflammatory activity appeared to have been controlled.

Infliximab (Remicade), a monoclonal anti–TNF-α antibody, has been reported in an open-label experience to be effective in most patients with acute Kawasaki disease who are refractory to standard therapy[39]; this agent is being studied in a randomized trial of patients with refractory Kawasaki disease. Even less published experience exists regarding other therapies for IVIG-refractory Kawasaki disease. Cyclophosphamide with or without methotrexate has been used in a very small number of patients.[385]

PREDICTION OF TREATMENT FAILURES

Several attempts have been made to develop scoring systems to predict, at the time of initial presentation, those patients who are at increased risk for failure to respond to standard therapy[73,172] or to develop coronary lesions after therapy.[231] In a retrospective analysis of 193 patients, Mori and colleagues[231] found that elevations in white blood cell counts, neutrophil counts, and CRP levels after IVIG treatment predicted increased risk for subsequent development of coronary lesions. Egami and colleagues[73] compared 279 patients who responded to initial standard treatment with 41 patients who were treatment resistant. These investigators developed a scoring system giving 1 point each for age less than 6 months, treatment before 4 days of illness, platelet count less than or equal to 300,000/mm^3, and CRP 8 mg/dL or higher, and 2 points for ALT 80 IU/L or higher; a score of 3 points or higher identified the IVIG-resistant group with 78 percent sensitivity and 76 percent specificity.[73] A similar predictive scoring system for IVIG unresponsiveness was developed by Kobayashi and colleagues,[172] who gave two points each for day of illness at initial treatment 1 to 4 days, serum sodium less than 133 mmol/L, aspartate aminotransferase (AST) 100 IU/L or higher, and neutrophils 80 percent or greater, and two points each for CRP 10 mg/dL or higher, platelet count up to 300,000/mm³, and age ≤12 months; this provided 86 percent sensitivity and 67 to 68 percent specificity for patients with 4 or more points.

SEQUELAE OF KAWASAKI DISEASE

The major (and virtually the only) sequelae of Kawasaki disease are cardiovascular, particularly involving the coronary arteries. Therefore, appropriate cardiac imaging is critical for the evaluation of patients suspected to have acute Kawasaki disease and for their subsequent follow-up. Echocardiography is considered the ideal imaging modality because it is noninvasive and has high sensitivity and specificity for detection of abnormalities of the proximal left main, left anterior descending, circumflex, and right coronary arteries.[252] This procedure should be performed under the supervision of an echocardiographer experienced with children, and internal arterial diameters should be measured and compared with normal standards for body surface area.[252] The American Heart Association classifies coronary aneurysms as small (<5 mm), medium (5 to 8 mm), or giant (>8 mm), and de Zorzi and colleagues[65] showed that adjusting coronary dimensions for body surface area may identify more accurately those patients with enlarged coronaries. Giant coronary aneurysms, defined as having 8 mm or larger internal diameter, are associated with worse prognosis, and these patients require particularly close follow-up.[52] The sensitivity and specificity of echocardiography to identify coronary thrombi and coronary stenosis are unclear, and visualization of coronary vessels is more difficult as body size increases. Therefore, angiography, magnetic resonance angiography (MRA), and ultrafast CT may be useful for selected patients with Kawasaki disease.[252]

MANAGEMENT BEYOND THE ACUTE STAGE

Patients with Kawasaki disease should be re-evaluated within 2 weeks after hospital discharge and again approximately 6 to 8 weeks after onset of illness because echocardiography at these time points is most likely to detect coronary artery aneurysms should they develop. If a baseline study and these two follow-up echocardiograms fail to detect evidence of coronary abnormality, performing further echocardiograms probably is unnecessary,[381] although a 6- to 12-month follow-up echocardiogram is performed at many centers.[58,252] Low-dose aspirin therapy (3 to 5 mg/kg/day) can be discontinued after the 6- to 8-week follow-up echocardiogram unless evidence of coronary abnormalities is present. To reduce the theoretical (and extremely low) risk of Reye syndrome in patients receiving low-dose aspirin, clopidogrel can be substituted for aspirin for a brief time in patients who develop varicella or influenza. Clopidogrel also can be used in the rare patient who is allergic to, or intolerant of, aspirin.

CARDIAC COMPLICATIONS

MYOCARDIAL INFARCTION

Myocardial infarction is the most common cause of death in Kawasaki disease (Table 88–5). In a cooperative Japanese study

TABLE 88–5 Cardiac Abnormalities in Kawasaki Disease

Acute Stage
Pericardial effusion
Decreased myocardial function
Mitral regurgitation
Brightness of coronary artery wall
Enlargement (ectasia) of coronary arteries
Arrhythmia (rare)

Subacute Stage
Coronary aneurysms, irregularity, ectasia
Mitral or aortic regurgitation, or both (rare)
Coronary aneurysm rupture (very rare)
Myocardial infarction (rare)

Convalescent Stage
Persistent coronary aneurysms
Regressed coronary aneurysms (residual fibrosis)
Coronary artery stenosis
Coronary aneurysm rupture (very rare)
Myocardial infarction (rare)

of 195 cases, the first myocardial infarction usually occurred in the first year after onset of disease and was fatal in 22 percent and asymptomatic in 37 percent of these patients. Major symptoms were shock, vomiting, and abdominal pain, with chest pain complaints only from children older than 4 years of age. Of those patients who survived a first infarct, 16 percent had a second myocardial infarct.[149,151] Patients with giant (>8 mm) coronary aneurysms are at greatest risk for having infarcts. Most fatal infarctions were the result of obstruction of the left main coronary artery or both the right coronary and left anterior descending coronary arteries; survivors were most likely to have isolated right coronary involvement. Approximately half the survivors of acute myocardial infarction had one or more complications, including ventricular dysfunction, mitral regurgitation, and arrhythmias. Parents of all children with Kawasaki disease with coronary abnormalities should be instructed to seek emergency medical care if chest pain, dyspnea, lethargy, or syncope develops. Prompt fibrinolytic therapy should be attempted at a tertiary care center if acute coronary thrombosis is diagnosed.[148] The degree of reversibility of coronary thrombosis in children with Kawasaki disease may be somewhat less than that in adults with atherosclerotic disease. Late cardiac sequelae of Kawasaki disease may not manifest until adulthood.[154]

OTHER CARDIOVASCULAR COMPLICATIONS

Other cardiac complications include myocardial fibrosis, valvulitis, and coronary rupture. Some researchers have suggested that valvular disease occurs in as many as 1 percent of patients with Kawasaki disease; most of these cases result in mitral regurgitation.[5,170] Patients with well-documented aortic regurgitation also have been observed. At least one patient with Kawasaki disease developed severe aortic and mitral regurgitation that necessitated two valve replacements.[107] In an autopsy study, coronary rupture was a quite rare finding but was noted more commonly among older children who died of Kawasaki disease, whereas myocardial infarction was seen more commonly in younger fatal cases.[300]

Peripheral artery aneurysms develop in fewer than 1 percent of patients with Kawasaki disease, virtually always in those who have significant coronary abnormalities.[156,348] These abnormalities generally involve medium-sized muscular arteries, such as subclavian, brachial, axillary, iliac, or femoral arteries, and occasionally the hepatic or renal arteries or the abdominal aorta. In patients with Kawasaki disease who are undergoing their first coronary arteriography, abdominal aortography and subclavian arteriography are, therefore, recommended.[252]

PERIPHERAL GANGRENE

A rare but very serious complication in the acute febrile stage of Kawasaki disease is severe peripheral ischemia and dry gangrene of distal extremities.[373] Virtually all these patients have been young infants up to approximately 7 months of age with giant coronary aneurysms, and some have developed peripheral (especially axillary or iliac) arterial aneurysms as well. This complication is virtually unknown in Japan[161] and has been reported primarily in non-Asian children in North America.[68,373] Possible pathogenic mechanisms of peripheral gangrene include the following: severe arteritis of digital or other small peripheral arteries; arteriospasm of peripheral arteries, perhaps in association with severe vasculitis; thrombosis of inflamed or spastic arteries as a result of stasis and damaged endothelium; thrombosis of a more proximal aneurysm (especially axillary) with embolism distally; rarely, cardiogenic shock; and, most likely, a combination of these factors.[373,388] This process has led to amputations in a small number of infants. Therapy has been empiric, primarily because the precise mechanisms of disease are unclear, and has included aggressive use of anti-inflammatory agents, prostaglandin infusion, and anti-platelet, anti-coagulant, and vasodilation therapies.[68,373]

NONVASCULAR COMPLICATIONS

As many as 10 percent of patients with Kawasaki disease develop painful arthritis or arthralgia in the acute stage of disease, often in the ankles or elsewhere in the lower extremities, and they may require treatment with a nonsteroidal anti-inflammatory agent. Earlier-onset arthritis (≤10 days of illness) tends to be polyarticular, whereas later-onset arthritis involves primarily larger weight-bearing joints. We have used naproxen, usually 10 to 15 mg/kg/day divided into two or three doses, for several weeks with considerable success.

Abdominal pain and diarrhea in the early acute stage usually respond to intravenous hydration and supportive care. Acalculous distention (hydrops) of the gallbladder manifests clinically as right upper quadrant tenderness or a mass with or without obstructive jaundice and can be confirmed by ultrasonography.[338] Performing a cholecystectomy is not necessary. Hepatic involvement appears to be entirely self-limited and has not been associated with chronic liver disease.

Rare patients with Kawasaki disease develop hemophagocytic syndrome (HPS), also known as *macrophage activation syndrome* (MAS), as a complication. This syndrome manifests as persistent fever associated with cytopenias, hepatosplenomegaly, hepatic dysfunction, often hyperferritinemia, elevated serum lactate dehydrogenase, hypofibrinogenemia, and hypertriglyceridemia.[233,265,274] Therapy with high-dose prednisone or other immune modifiers are indicated for this rare but serious complication.

Rare events that occur in association with Kawasaki disease include sensorineural hearing loss,[345] transient unilateral facial nerve palsy,[101,281] and pneumonitis or pulmonary nodules.[84] We have cared for two older children who had sufficient abdominal findings to warrant performing appendectomies before establishing the diagnosis of Kawasaki disease. Consultation with a center that treats large numbers of patients with Kawasaki disease should be sought by the physician faced with rare or serious complications.

LONG-TERM FOLLOW-UP AND PROGNOSIS

Kawasaki disease normally is an acute and self-limited illness. However, cardiac abnormalities that develop when the disease is active may be progressive, and the prognosis clearly is related to the coronary artery status. Approximately 20 to 25 percent of patients not treated with IVIG develop coronary abnormalities that are detectable by two-dimensional echocardiography or angiography. The risk of development of coronary aneurysms is reduced to approximately 2 to 3 percent overall when IVIG is given in the first 10 days of illness.[247,251] However, the rates for coronary abnormalities for young infants are somewhat higher, even with timely IVIG therapy. Patients who develop moderate to severe coronary abnormalities are at risk of myocardial ischemia, myocardial infarction, and sudden death for at least 5 years after onset of illness.[151]

Children without apparent cardiac sequelae during the first month after onset of Kawasaki disease appear to return to their previous states of health, without cardiac signs or symptoms. However, some reports suggest the possibility of generalized endothelial dysfunction in patients with Kawasaki disease who never had coronary abnormalities. These dysfunctions include altered lipid metabolism,[43] increased brachial-radial artery mean pulse wave velocity,[49] lower myocardial flow reserve,[236] and abnormal endothelium-dependent brachial artery reactivity,[66,227,393] but the data conflict somewhat, and additional studies are needed.

Regression of small and medium aneurysms is a common occurrence. Overall, approximately half of all children with coronary aneurysms at 4 to 8 weeks after onset demonstrate regression by 1 to 2 years, with apparently normal vessels on angiography or echocardiography.[149] The likelihood that an aneurysm will regress is higher with smaller aneurysms, age younger than 1 year at the onset of Kawasaki disease, fusiform rather than saccular morphology, and involvement of a more distal coronary segment.[7,355] Regression of the internal diameter of the vessel to normal may occur by myointimal proliferation or by thrombus organization and recanalization.[87,309] If regression occurs, it generally does so within 2 years of the onset of disease.[152] Intravascular ultrasound studies show that thickened intima and media sometimes with calcifications are present in areas of regressed coronary aneurysms.[113,341] Regressed aneurysmal segments are histologically abnormal (intimal fibrosis) and have abnormal functional responses, with decreased vascular reactivity in response to exercise or pharmacologic agents such as isosorbide dinitrate or acetylcholine.[66,309,340] Only a small number of regressed aneurysms progress to stenosis.[153,340,347,350]

Functional abnormalities of coronary vessel endothelium relaxation have been reported years after the onset of Kawasaki disease[66,227] and warrant further investigation. Newer imaging methods have demonstrated vascular wall changes sometimes even in patients with no history of abnormalities in the acute phase. The meaning of these findings in patients thought to have escaped coronary abnormalities with acute Kawasaki disease and their long-term significance are uncertain.

Patients with giant coronary aneurysms are at the greatest risk for the development of significant stenosis with resultant myocardial ischemia.[133,156] The risk of significant stenosis, usually developing at the inlet or outlet of a moderate to large coronary aneurysm, shows a steady rise over 15 to 20 years of observation.[144,156,339,347] These markedly abnormal vessels are subject to calcification and thrombosis, which may lead to myocardial ischemia or infarction.

In 10- to 20-year follow-up studies of patients with Kawasaki disease, researchers found that the arteries most likely to develop stenosis are the right main and left anterior descending coronary arteries.[144,156,339,347,349] A limited number of studies of young adults with ischemic heart disease and history of diagnosed Kawasaki disease or a compatible clinical illness has been performed.[154] A survey of Japanese adult cardiologists identified 130 adult patients with coronary aneurysms detected by angiography to evaluate myocardial infarction or ischemia.[154] Twenty-one of these patients (mean age, 34 years; range, 20 to 63 years) had a history compatible with Kawasaki disease in childhood. These patients had severe coronary disease with myocardial infarction, angina pectoris, mitral regurgitation, arrhythmias, congestive heart failure, and need for coronary bypass grafting. This study indicates that the coronary artery sequelae of Kawasaki disease likely are important causes of ischemic heart disease in young adults. Fatty deposits and advanced changes resembling atherosclerotic disease sometimes have been found at autopsy of children with a history of Kawasaki disease who died of other causes.[353] This finding raises the important but unanswered question of whether patients with Kawasaki disease are at increased risk for developing premature atherosclerosis or of having a more severe form of this disease.

LONG-TERM MANAGEMENT

The risk of coronary artery thrombosis or stenosis that may result in myocardial ischemia and infarction remains the most important long-term clinical problem in the subset of patients with Kawasaki disease who develop significant coronary abnormalities (see Table 88–5). Patients with medium (6 to 8 mm) and giant (>8 mm) aneurysms are at substantial risk for development of stenosis years after having the acute illness, compared with patients with small aneurysms or no aneurysmal changes,[7,144,149,152,156,348,380] and patients with giant aneurysms are at the highest risk for thrombosis.[252] Echocardiography and electrocardiography are not sufficiently sensitive to detect stenotic lesions. Various stress tests for detection of reversible myocardial ischemia, including nuclear perfusion scans with exercise, exercise echocardiography, and stress echocardiography with agents such as dobutamine, dipyridamole, or adenosine, have been used in children to detect stenosis.[252,260,272] Newer techniques, including stress magnetic resonance imaging (stress MRI), are being developed. Coronary arteriography remains the most definitive method to determine the degree of stenosis and the adequacy of collateral circulation. Intravascular ultrasound is an effective method to evaluate vascular wall morphology in selected patients during angiography.[342,346] All patients with evidence of myocardial ischemia or infarction should be studied by angiography to determine the need for intervention.[252] Most experts agree that patients with moderate to severe coronary artery aneurysms, a single large aneurysm, or multiple aneurysms should have their coronary anatomy defined by angiography at least once after the acute stage of illness (after the inflammatory process has subsided) to define fully the extent of involvement and to identify potential sites of thrombotic or stenotic complications.[252] Because aneurysms can occur in non-coronary arteries, especially the subclavian, brachial, axillary, iliac, and femoral arteries, and occasionally in the abdominal aorta and renal arteries,[348] in patients with coronary abnormalities, abdominal aortography and subclavian arteriography are recommended for patients with Kawasaki disease who are undergoing coronary angiography the first time.[252]

PATIENTS WITH NO EVIDENCE OF CORONARY ARTERY ABNORMALITIES AT ANY TIME (RISK LEVEL I)

Patients who have never manifested coronary artery abnormalities have no need for aspirin or other anti-platelet medication beyond 2 to 3 months after onset of illness or for restriction of physical activities in the convalescent stage. Only routine pediatric follow-up beyond 1 year, with routine cardiovascular risk assessment, is indicated.

PATIENTS WITH TRANSIENT CORONARY ECTASIA OR DILATATION (RISK LEVEL II)

Patients with transient coronary artery abnormalities that resolve by 6 to 8 weeks should be treated with aspirin, 3 to 5 mg/kg/day, until resolution of abnormalities. No restrictions are indicated after 6 to 8 weeks, angiography is not indicated, and risk assessment and counseling are recommended at 3- to 5-year intervals.

PATIENTS WITH ISOLATED (SOLITARY) SMALL TO MEDIUM (3- TO 6-MM) CORONARY ANEURYSM IN ONE OR MORE CORONARY ARTERIES (RISK LEVEL III)

Patients with solitary small to medium coronary artery aneurysms should be maintained on daily low-dose aspirin (3 to 5 mg/kg) at least until regression is documented with annual echocardiographic follow-up. For patients younger than 11 years old, no restriction on physical activity is indicated, but for those 11 years old and older, physical activity should be guided by a biennial stress test or myocardial perfusion test. Angiography should be performed if stenosis or ischemia is suggested.

PATIENTS WITH ONE OR MORE LARGE (>6-MM) OR GIANT (>8-MM) CORONARY ANEURYSM, OR MULTIPLE (SEGMENTED) SMALLER OR COMPLEX ANEURYSMS WITHOUT OBSTRUCTION (RISK LEVEL IV)

Long-term anti-platelet therapy with aspirin (3 to 5 mg/kg once daily) or clopidogrel (1 mg/kg/day up to adult dose of 75 mg) is indicated for these children and should be continued indefinitely. Anti-coagulant therapy with warfarin, with the international normalized ratio (INR) maintained at approximately 2.0 to 2.5, should be added for patients with giant aneurysms because these patients are at substantial risk for having coronary thrombosis. Daily subcutaneous low-molecular-weight heparin is an alternative to warfarin. All such patients should be under the care of a pediatric cardiologist with experience in managing patients with Kawasaki disease. Cardiac evaluation with echocardiogram and ECG should be performed every 6 months, with stress testing performed approximately annually. Angiography should be performed 6 to 12 months after the patient has recovered from the acute stage of disease to define the coronary anatomy, and it should be repeated whenever symptoms or stress tests suggest the presence of myocardial ischemia. Physical activity should be regulated on the basis of annual stress test results and level of anti-coagulation, and strenuous athletics should be discouraged.

PATIENTS WITH CORONARY ARTERY OBSTRUCTION (RISK LEVEL V)

Patients with obstructive lesions or signs of ischemia should be evaluated urgently for possible intervention. Balloon angioplasty, rotablator angioplasty, coronary artery bypass grafting, stent placement, and even cardiac transplantation all have been employed for patients with Kawasaki disease and particularly serious coronary artery disease.[6,48,112,136,379] Researchers have shown that arterial bypass grafts are superior to venous grafts in these patients.[169] Balloon angioplasty procedures have been associated with high rates of recurrent stenosis in patients with Kawasaki disease and coronary stenosis.[6]

REFERENCES

1. Abe, J., Kotzin, B. L., Jujo, K., et al.: Selective expansion of T cells expressing T-cell receptor variable regions V beta 2 and V beta 8 in Kawasaki disease. Proc. Natl. Acad. Sci. U. S. A. *89*:4066-4070, 1992.

2. Abe, J., Kotzin, B. L., Meissner, C., et al.: Characterization of T cell repertoire changes in acute Kawasaki disease. J. Exp. Med. *177*:791-796, 1993.

3. Abe, J., Takeda, T., Ito, Y., et al.: TCR-V specificity of *Staphylococcus aureus* isolated from acute patients with Kawasaki syndrome. *In* Kato, H. (ed.): Kawasaki Disease. Amsterdam, Elsevier Science, 1995, pp. 127-132.

4. Ahlström, H., Lundström, N. R., Mortensson, W., et al.: Infantile periarteritis nodosa or mucocutaneous lymph node syndrome: A report of four cases and diagnostic considerations. Acta Paediatr. Scand. *66*:193-198, 1977.

5. Akagi, T., Kato, H., Inoue, O., et al.: Valvular heart disease in Kawasaki syndrome: Incidence and natural history. Am. Heart J. *120*:366-372, 1990.

6. Akagi, T., Ogawa, S., Ino, T., et al.: Catheter interventional therapy in Kawasaki disease. J. Pediatr. *137*:181-186, 2000.

7. Akagi, T., Rose, V, Benson, L. N., et al.: Outcome of coronary artery aneurysms after Kawasaki disease. J. Pediatr. *121*:689-694, 1992.

8. Amano, S., Hazama, F., and Hamashima, Y.: Pathology of Kawasaki disease. I. Pathology and morphogenesis of the vascular changes. Jpn. Circ. J. *43*: 633-643, 1979.

9. Amano, S., Hazama, F., and Hamashima, Y.: Pathology of Kawasaki disease. II. Distribution and incidence of the vascular lesions. Jpn. Circ. J. *43*:741-748, 1979.

10. Amano, S., Hazama, F., Kubagawa, H., et al.: General pathology of Kawasaki disease. Acta Pathol. Jpn. *30*:681-694, 1980.

11. Anand, S., and Yang, Y. C.: Optic disc changes in Kawasaki disease. J. Pediatr. Ophthalmol. Strabismus *41*:177-179, 2004.

12. Anderson, L. J., Morens, D. M., and Hurwitz, E. S.: Kawasaki disease in a young adult. Arch. Intern. Med. *140*:280-281, 1980.

13. Asai, T.: Evaluation method for the degree of seriousness in Kawasaki disease. Acta Paediatr. Jpn. *25*:170-175, 1983.

14. Asano, T., Sasaki, N., Yashiro, K., et al.: Acute pancreatitis with Kawasaki disease. Eur. J. Pediatr. *164*:180-181, 2005.

15. Aschner, M., and Aschner, J. L.: Mucocutaneous lymph node syndrome: Is there a relationship to mercury exposure? Am. J. Dis. Child. *143*:1133-1134, 1989.

16. Ayusawa, M., Sonobe, T., Uemura, S., et al.: Revision of diagnostic guidelines for Kawasaki disease (5th revised edition). Pediatr. Int. *47*:232-234, 2005.

17. Barron, K. S., Montalvo, J. F., Joseph, A. K., et al.: Soluble interleukin-2 receptors in children with Kawasaki syndrome. Arthritis Rheum. *33*: 1371-1377, 1990.

18. Barron, K. S., Murphy, D. J., Silverman, E. D., et al.: Treatment of Kawasaki syndrome: A comparison of two dosage regimens of intravenously administered globulins. J. Pediatr. *117*:638-644, 1990.

19. Barron, K. S., Silverman, E. D., Gonzales, J. C., et al.: Major histocompatibility complex class II alleles in Kawasaki syndrome: Lack of consistent correlation with disease or cardiac involvement. J. Rheumatol. *19*:1790-1793, 1992.

20. Becker, A .E.: Kawasaki disease. Lancet *1*:864, 1976.

21. Becker, A. E., Beekman, R. P., and van der Hal, A. L.: De infantiele polyarteritis nodosa en de ziekte van Kawasaki ("muco-cutaneous lymph node syndrome"): Twee verschillende ziekten of uitingen van een zelfde ziekteproces? Ned. Tijdschr. Geneeskd. *120*:2147-2151, 1976.

22. Belay, E. D., Erdman, D. D., Anderson, L. J., et al.: Kawasaki disease and human coronavirus. J. Infect. Dis. *192*:352-353, 2005.

23. Belay, E. D., Maddox, R. A., Holman, R. C., et al.: Kawasaki syndrome and risk factors for coronary artery abnormalities: United States, 1994-2003. Pediatr. Infect. Dis. J. *25*:245-249, 2006.

24. Bell, D. M., Brink, E. W., Nitzkin, J., et al.: Kawasaki syndrome: Description of two outbreaks in the United States. N. Engl. J. Med. *304*:1568-1575, 1981.

25. Bell, D. M., Morens, D. M., Holman, R. C., et al.: Kawasaki syndrome in the United States. Am. J. Dis. Child. *137*:211-224, 1983.

26. Birdi, N., Klassen, T., Quinlan, A., et al.: Role of the toxic neutrophil count in the early diagnosis of Kawasaki disease. J. Rheumatol. *26*:904-908, 1999.

27. Blum-Hoffmann, E., Hoffman, G. F., Wessel, A., et al.: Kawasaki syndrome: Association mit der exposition von teppichshampoo und erfolgreiche therapie mit immunoglobulinen in der zweiten krankheitswoche. Monatsschr. Kinderheilkd. *140*:273-276, 1992.

28. Boven, K., De Fraeff-Meeder, E. R., Spliet, W., et al.: Atypical Kawasaki disease: An often missed diagnosis. Eur. J. Pediatr. *151*:577-580, 1992.

29. Bronstein, D. E., Dille, A. N., Austin, J. P., et al.: Relationship of climate, ethnicity, and socioeconomic status to Kawasaki disease in San Diego County, 1994-1998. Pediatr. Infect. Dis. J. *19*:1087-1091, 2000.

30. Brosius, C. L., Newburger, J. W., Burns, J. C., et al.: Increased prevalence of atopic dermatitis in Kawasaki disease. Pediatr. Infect. Dis. J. *7*:863-866, 1988.

31. Brown, T. J., Crawford, S. E., Shulman, S. T., et al.: CD8 positive cells and macrophages infiltrate coronary artery aneurysms in acute Kawasaki disease. Pediatr. Res. *49*:13A, 2001.

32. Bülow, S. L., Hansen, U. S., Hansen, D., et al.: Kawasaki's syngdom: Forekomst i Danmark i perioden 1981-1990. Ugeskr. Laeger *156*:4813-4816, 1994.

32a. Burgner, D., Davila, S., Breunis, W. B., et al.: A genome-wide association study identifies novel and functionally related susceptibility loci for Kawasaki disease.

33. Burke, M. J., and Rennebohm, R. M.: Eye involvement in Kawasaki disease. J. Pediatr. Ophthalmol. Strabismus *18*:7-11, 1981.

34. Burns, J. C.: The riddle of Kawasaki disease. N. Engl. J. Med. *356*:659-661, 2007.

35. Burns, J. C., and Glodé, M. P.: Kawasaki syndrome. Lancet *364*:533-544, 2004.

36. Burns, J. C., Cayan, D. R., Tong, G., et al.: Seasonality and temporal clustering of Kawasaki syndrome. Epidemiology *16*:220-225, 2005.

37. Burns, J. C., Geha, R. S., Schneeberger, E. E., et al.: Polymerase activity in lymphocyte culture supernatants from patients with Kawasaki disease. Nature *323*:814-816, 1987.

38. Burns, J. C., Mason, W. H., Glodé, M. P., et al.: Clinical and epidemiologic characteristics of patients referred for evaluation of possible Kawasaki disease. J. Pediatr. *118*:680-686, 1991.

39. Burns, J. C., Mason, W. H., Hauger, S. B., et al.: Infliximab treatment for refractory Kawasaki syndrome. J. Pediatr. *146*:662-667, 2005.

40. Burns, J. C., Wiggins, J. W., Toews, W. H., et al.: Clinical spectrum of Kawasaki syndrome in infants younger than 6 months of age. J. Pediatr. *109*:759-763, 1986.

41. Burns, J. C., Shimizu, C., Gonzalez, E., et al.: Genetic variations in the receptor-ligand pair CCR5 and CCL31 are important determinants of susceptibility to Kawasaki disease. J. Infect. Dis. *192*:344-349, 2005.

42. Butler, D. F., Hough, D. R., Friedman, S. J., et al.: Adult Kawasaki syndrome. Arch. Dermatol. *123*:1356-1361, 1987.

43. Cabana, V. G., Gidding, S. S., Getz, G. S., et al.: Serum amyloid A and high density lipoprotein participate in the acute phase response of Kawasaki disease. Pediatr. Res. *42*:651-655, 1997.

44. Caron, G. A.: Kawasaki disease in an adult. JAMA *243*:430, 1980.

45. Casey, F., Craig, B., Shanks, D., et al.: Kawasaki disease: The Northern Ireland experience. Ir. J. Med. Sci. *162*:397-400, 1993.

46. Chang, C. C., Hawkins, B. R., Kao, H. K., et al.: Human leukocyte antigens in Southern Chinese with Kawasaki disease. Eur. J. Pediatr. *151*:866, 1992.

47. Chang, L.-Y., Chiang, B.-L., Kao, C.-L., et al.: Lack of association between infection with a novel coronavirus and Kawasaki disease in Taiwan. J. Infect. Dis. *193*:283-286, 2006.

48. Checci, P. A., Pahl, E., Shaddy, R., et al.: Cardiac transplantation for Kawasaki disease. Pediatrics *100*:695-699, 1997.

49. Cheung, Y. F., Yung, T. C., Tam, S. C., et al.: Novel and traditional cardiovascular risk factors in children after Kawasaki disease. J. Am. Coll. Cardiol. *43*:120-124, 2004.

50. Chiba, S., Kaneko, K., Hashimoto, N., et al.: *Yersinia pseudotuberculosis* and Kawasaki disease. Pediatr. Infect. Dis. J. *2*:494, 1983.

51. Choi, I., Chwae, Y., Shim, W., et al.: Clonal expansion of CD8 positive T cells in Kawasaki disease. J. Immunol. *159*:481-486, 1997.

52. Chung, K. J., and U. S. Multicenter Kawasaki Study Group: Incidence and prognosis of giant coronary artery aneurysms in Kawasaki disease. Circulation *80*(Suppl. II):II-282, 1989.

53. Comenzo, R. L., Malachowski, S. E., Meissner, H. C., et al.: Immune hemolysis, DIC, and serum sickness after large doses of IVIG for Kawasaki disease. J. Pediatr. *120*:926-928, 1992.

54. Crocker, D. W., Sobin, S., and Thomas, W. C.: Aneurysms of the coronary arteries: Report of three cases in infants and review of the literature. Am. J. Pathol. *33*:819-843, 1957.

55. Cunningham, M. W., Meissner, H. C., Heuser, J. S., et al.: Anti-human cardiac myosin autoantibodies in Kawasaki disease. J. Immunol. *163*:1060-1065, 1999.

56. Curtis, N., Zheng, R., Lamb, J. R., et al.: Evidence for a superantigen-mediated process in Kawasaki disease. Arch. Dis. Child. *72*:308-311, 1995.

57. Dajani, A. S., Taubert, K. A., Gerber, M. A., et al.: Diagnosis and therapy of Kawasaki disease in children. Circulation *87*:1776-1780, 1993.

58. Dajani, A. S., Taubert, K. A., Takahashi, M., et al.: Guidelines for long-term management of patients with Kawasaki disease. Circulation *89*:916-922, 1994.

59. Daniels, S. R., and Specker, B.: Association of rug shampooing and Kawasaki disease. J. Pediatr. *118*:485-488, 1991.

60. Davis, R. L., Waller, P. L., Mueller, B. A., et al.: Kawasaki syndrome in Washington State: Race-specific incidence rates and residential proximity to water. Arch. Pediatr. Adolesc. Med. *149*:66-69, 1995.

61. DeInocencio, J., and Hirsch, R.: The role of T cells in Kawasaki disease. Crit. Rev. Immunol. *15*:349-357, 1995.

62. Dengler, L. D., Capparelli, E. V., Bastian, J. F., et al.: Cerebrospinal fluid profile in acute Kawasaki disease. Pediatr. Infect. Dis. J. *17*:478-481, 1998.

63. Dennis, M. K., Ayoub, E. M., Graham, T., et al.: Mucocutaneous lymph node syndrome in Florida. J. Fla. Med. Assoc. *64*:21-26, 1977.

64. Dergun, M., Kao, A., Hauger, S., et al.: Familial occurrence of Kawasaki syndrome in North America. Arch. Pediatr. Adolesc. Med. *159*:876-881, 2005.

65. de Zorzi, A., Colan, S. D., Gauvreau, K., et al.: Coronary artery dimensions may be misclassified as normal in Kawasaki disease. J. Pediatr. *133*:354-358, 1998.

66. Dhillon, R., Clarkson, P., Donald, S. E., et al.: Endothelial dysfunction late after Kawasaki disease. Circulation *94*:2103-2106, 1996.

67. Dominguez, S., Anderson, M. S., Glodé, M. P., et al.: Blinded case-control study of the relationship between human coronavirus NL63 and Kawasaki disease. J. Infect. Dis. *194*:1697-1701, 2006.

68. Durall, A. L., Phillips, J. R., Weisse, M. E., et al.: Infantile Kawasaki disease and peripheral gangrene. J. Pediatr. *149*:131-133, 2006.
69. Durongpisitkul, K., Gururaj, V. J., Park, J. M., et al.: The prevention of coronary artery aneurysm in Kawasaki disease. Pediatrics *96*:1057-1061, 1995.
70. Eberhard, B. A., Anderson, U., Laxer, R. M., et al.: Evaluation of the cytokine response in Kawasaki disease. Pediatr. Infect. Dis. J. *14*:199-203, 1995.
71. Eberhard, B. A., Sundel, R. P., Newburger, J. W., et al.: Psoriatic eruption in Kawasaki disease. J. Pediatr. *137*:578-580, 2000.
72. Ebihara, T., Endo, R., Ma, X., et al.: Lack of association between New Haven coronavirus and Kawasaki disease. J. Infect. Dis. *192*:351, 2005.
73. Egami, K., Muta, H., Ishii, M., et al.: Prediction of resistance to IVIG treatment in patients with Kawasaki disease. J. Pediatr. *149*:237-240, 2006.
74. Engle, M. A., Fatica, N. S., Bussel, J. B., et al.: Clinical trial of single dose intravenous gamma globulin in Kawasaki disease: Preliminary report. Am. J. Dis. Child. *143*:1300-1304, 1989.
75. Esper, F., Shapiro, E. D., Weibel, C., et al.: Association between a novel human coronavirus and Kawasaki disease. J. Infect. Dis. *191*:499-502, 2005.
76. Everett, E. D.: Mucocutaneous lymph node syndrome (Kawasaki's disease) in adults. JAMA *242*:542-543, 1979.
77. Fager, D. B., Bigler, J. A., and Simonds, J. P.: Polyarteritis nodosa in infancy and childhood. J. Pediatr. *39*:65-79, 1951.
78. Falcini, F., Cimaz, R., Calabri, G. B., et al.: Kawasaki disease in northern Italy. Clin. Exp. Rheumatol. *20*:421-426, 2002.
79. Fatica, N. S., Ichida, F., Engle, M. A., et al.: Rug shampoo and Kawasaki disease. Pediatrics *84*:231-234, 1989.
80. Felz, M., Patni, A., Brooks, S., et al.: Periorbital vasculitis complicating Kawasaki syndrome in an infant. Pediatrics *101*:e9, 1998.
81. Fildes, N., Burns, J. C., Newburger, J. W., et al.: The HLA class II region and susceptibility to Kawasaki disease. Tissue Antigens *39*:99-101, 1992.
82. Fong, N. C., Hui, Y. W., Li, C. K., et al.: Evaluation of the efficacy of treatment of Kawasaki disease before day 5 of illness. Pediatr. Cardiol. *25*: 31-34, 2004.
83. Freeman, A. F., and Shulman, S. T.: Refractory Kawasaki disease. Pediatr. Infect. Dis. J. *23*:463, 2004.
84. Freeman, A. F., Crawford, S. E., Finn, L. S., et al.: Inflammatory pulmonary nodules in Kawasaki disease. Pediatr. Pulmonol. *36*:102-106, 2003.
85. Fujimoto, T., Kato, H., Ichiose, E., et al.: Immune complex and mite antigen in Kawasaki disease. Lancet *2*:980-981, 1982.
86. Fujita, Y., Nakamura, Y., Sakata, K., et al.: Kawasaki disease in families. Pediatrics *84*:666-669, 1989.
87. Fujiwara, H., and Hamashima, Y.: Pathology of the heart in Kawasaki disease. Pediatrics *61*:100-107, 1978.
88. Fujiwara, H., Fujiwara, T., Kao, T. C., et al.: Pathology of Kawasaki disease in the healed stage: Relationships between typical and atypical cases of Kawasaki disease. Acta Pathol. Jpn. *36*:857-867, 1986.
89. Fujiwara, H., Kawai, C., and Hamashima, Y.: Clinico-pathologic study of the conduction systems in 10 patients with Kawasaki's disease (mucocutaneous lymph node syndrome). Am. Heart J. *96*:744-750, 1978.
90. Fujiwara, T., Fujiwara, H., and Nakano, H.: Pathological features of coronary arteries in children with Kawasaki disease in which coronary arterial aneurysm was absent at autopsy: Quantitative analysis. Circulation *78*: 345-350, 1988.
91. Fukushige, J., Takahashi, N., and Ueda, Y.: Incidence and clinical features of incomplete Kawasaki disease. Acta Paediatr. *83*:1057-1060, 1994.
92. Fulton, D. R.: Effects of current therapy of Kawasaki disease on eicosanoid metabolism. Am. J. Cardiol. *61*:1323-1327, 1988.
93. Furukawa, S., Imai, K., Matsubara, T., et al.: Increased levels of ICAM-1 in Kawasaki disease. Arthritis Rheum. *35*:672-677, 1992.
94. Furukawa, S., Matsubara, T., Jujoh, K., et al.: Peripheral blood monocyte/macrophages and serum tumor necrosis factor in Kawasaki disease. Clin. Immunol. Immunopathol. *48*:247-251, 1988.
95. Furukawa, S., Matsubara, T., Jujoh, K., et al.: Reduction of peripheral blood macrophages/monocytes in Kawasaki disease by intravenous gamma globulin. Eur. J. Pediatr. *150*:43-47, 1990.
96. Furukawa, S., Matsubara, T., Motohashi T., et al.: Expression of Fc,R2/CD23 on peripheral blood macrophages/monocytes in Kawasaki disease. Clin. Immunol. Immunopathol. *56*:280-286, 1990.
97. Furukawa, S., Matsubara, T., and Yabuta, K.: Mononuclear cell subsets and coronary artery lesions in Kawasaki disease. Arch. Dis. Child. *67*:706-708, 1992.
98. Furumoto, H., Sakano, T., Tanabe, A., et al.: Serum soluble CD8 antigen level is not elevated in mucocutaneous lymph node syndrome (Kawasaki disease) in spite of an increase in serum soluble interleukin 2 receptors. Eur. J. Pediatr. *149*:448-449, 1990.
99. Furusho, K., Kamiya, T., Nakano, H., et al.: High-dose intravenous gamma globulin for Kawasaki disease. Lancet *2*:1055-1058, 1984.
100. Furusho, K., Ohba T., Soeda T., et al.: Possible role for mite antigen in Kawasaki disease. Lancet *2*:194-195, 1981.
101. Gallagher, P. G.: Facial nerve paralysis and Kawasaki disease. Rev. Infect. Dis. *12*:403-405, 1990.
102. Gavin, P. J., Crawford, S. E., Shulman, S. T., et al.: Systemic arterial expression of matrix metalloproteinases-2 and -9 in acute Kawasaki disease. Arterioscl. Thromb. Vasc. Biol. *23*:576-581, 2003.
103. Gee, S. J.: Aneurysms of the coronary arteries in a boy. St. Barth. Hosp. Rep. Lond. *7*:148, 1871.
104. Gentles, T. L., Clarkson, P. M., Trenholme, A. A., et al.: Kawasaki disease in Auckland, 1979-1988. N. Z. Med. J. *103*:389-391, 1990.
105. Germain, B. F., Moroney, J. D., Guggino, G. S., et al.: Anterior uveitis in Kawasaki disease. J. Pediatr. *97*:780-781, 1980.
106. Gidding, S. S., Duffy, C. E., Pajcic, S., et al.: Usefulness of echocardiographic evidence of pericardial effusion and mitral regurgitation in predicting coronary artery aneurysms. Am. J. Cardiol. *60*:76-79, 1987.
107. Gidding, S. S., Shulman, S. T., Ilbawi, M., et al.: Mucocutaneous lymph node syndrome (Kawasaki disease): Delayed aortic and mitral insufficiency secondary to active valvulitis. J. Am. Coll. Cardiol. *7*:894-897, 1986.
108. Giesker, D. W., Krause, P. J., Pastuszak, W. T., et al.: Lymph node biopsy for early diagnosis in Kawasaki disease. Am. J. Surg. Pathol. *6*:493-501, 1982.
109. Glanzer, J. M., Galbraith, W. B., and Jacobs, J. P.: Kawasaki disease in a 28-year-old man. JAMA *244*:1604-1606, 1980.
110. Glode, M. P., Brogden, R., Joffe, L. S., et al.: Kawasaki syndrome and house dust mite exposure. Pediatr. Infect. Dis. J. *5*:644-648, 1986.
111. Gong, G. W. K., McCrindle, B. W., Ching, J. C., et al.: Arthritis presenting during the acute phase of Kawasaki disease. J. Pediatr. *148*:800-805, 2006.
112. Gotteiner, N., Mavroudis, C., Backer, C. L., et al.: Coronary artery bypass grafting for Kawasaki disease. Pediatr. Cardiol. *23*:62-67, 2002.
113. Hamada, R., Uehara, R., and Fuyama, Y.: CT detection of coronary calcification in Kawasaki disease. *In* Kato, H. (ed.): Kawasaki Disease. Amsterdam, Elsevier Science, 1995, pp. 598-602.
114. Hamasaki, Y., and Miyazaki, S.: Leukotriene B$_4$ and Kawasaki disease. Acta Paediatr. Jpn. *33*:771-777, 1991.
115. Hamashima, Y., Tasaka, K., Hoshino, T., et al.: Mite-associated particles in Kawasaki disease. Lancet *2*:266, 1982.
116. Hammerschlag, M., Boman, J., and Rowley, A. H.: Failure to demonstrate *Chlamydia pneumoniae* in cardiovascular tissue from children with Kawasaki disease. Pediatr. Infect. Dis. J. *20*:76-77, 2001.
117. Hansen, R. C.: Staphylococcal scaled skin syndrome, toxic shock syndrome, and Kawasaki disease. Pediatr. Clin. North Am. *30*:533-544, 1983.
118. Han, R. K., Silverman, E. D., Newman, A., et al.: Management and outcome of persistent or recurrent fever after initial intravenous gamma globulin therapy in acute Kawasaki disease. Arch. Pediatr. Adolesc. Med. *154*:694-699, 2000.
119. Harada, K., Yamaguchi, H., Kato, H., et al.: Indication for IVGG in Kawasaki disease. *In* Takahashi, M., and Taubert, K. A. (eds.): Proceedings of Fourth International Symposium on Kawasaki Disease. Dallas, American Heart Association, 1993, pp. 459-462.
120. Hayasaka, S., Nakamura, Y., Yashiro, M., et al.: Analyses of fatal cases of Kawasaki disease in Japan. J. Epidemiol. *13*:246-250, 2003.
121. Harnden, A., Alves, B., and Sheikh, A.: Rising incidence of Kawasaki disease in England: Analysis of hospital admission data. BMJ *324*:1424-1425, 2002.
122. Hashino, K., Ishii., M., Iemura, M., et al.: Retreatment for immune globulin resistant Kawasaki disease. Pediatr. Int. *43*:211-217, 2001.
123. Herman, A., Kappler, J. W., Marrack, P., et al.: Superantigens: Mechanism of T cell stimulation and role in immunologic responses. Annu. Rev. Immunol. *9*:745-772, 1991.
124. Herold, B. C., Davis, A. T., Arroyave, C. M., et al.: Cryoprecipitates in Kawasaki syndrome: Association with coronary artery aneurysms. Pediatr. Infect. Dis. J. *7*:255-257, 1988.
125. Hicks, R. V., and Melish, M. E.: Kawasaki syndrome: Rheumatic complaints and analysis of salicylate therapy. Arthritis Rheum. *22*:621-622, 1979.
126. Hidaka, T., Nakano, M., Ueta, T., et al.: Increased synthesis of thromboxane A$_2$ by platelets from patients with Kawasaki disease. J. Pediatr. *102*:94-96, 1983.
127. Hirao, J., Hibi, S., Andoh, T., et al.: High levels of circulating IL-4 and IL-10 in Kawasaki disease. Int. Arch. Allergy Immunol. *112*:152-156, 1997.
128. Holman, R. C., Curns, A. T., Belay, E. D., et al.: Kawasaki syndrome: Hospitalizations in the U.S, 1997 and 2000. Pediatrics *112*:495-501, 2003.
129. Holman, R. C., Curns, A. T., Belay, E. D., et al.: Kawasaki syndrome in Hawaii. Pediatr. Infect. Dis. J. *24*:429-433, 2005.
130. Hurvitz, H., Branski, D., Gross-Kieselstein, E., et al.: Acetaminophen hypersensitivity resembling Kawasaki disease. Isr. J. Med. Sci. *20*:145-147, 1984.
131. Ichida, F., Fatica, N. S., O'Loughlin, J. E., et al.: Epidemiologic aspects of Kawasaki disease in a Manhattan hospital. Pediatrics *84*:235-241, 1989.
132. Imada, Y., Kawasaki, T., and Nakamura, Y.: Cousin cases of Kawasaki disease suggesting person-to-person transmission. Pediatrics *85*:1127, 1990.
133. Inoue, O., Akagi, T., and Kato, H.: Fate of giant coronary artery aneurysms in Kawasaki disease. Circulation *80*(Suppl. II):II-262, 1989.
134. Inoue, Y., Okada, Y., Shinohara, M., et al.: A multicenter prospective randomized trial of corticosteroids in primary therapy for Kawasaki disease. J. Pediatr. *149*:336-341, 2006.
135. Ishii, A., Yatani, T., Kato, H., et al.: Mite fauna, house dust, and Kawasaki disease. Lancet *2*:102-103, 1983.
136. Ishii, M., Ueno, T., Akagi, T., et al.: Guidelines for catheter intervention in coronary artery lesion in Kawasaki disease. Pediatr. Int. *43*:558-562, 2001.
137. Jacob, J. L., Polomeno, R. C., Chad, Z., et al.: Ocular manifestations of Kawasaki disease (mucocutaneous lymph node syndrome). Can. J. Ophthalmol. *17*:199-202, 1982.
138. Jacobs, J. C.: Salicylate treatment of epidemic Kawasaki disease in New York City. Ther. Drug Monit. *1*:123-130, 1979.
139. Japanese Kawasaki Disease Research Committee: Shonika Rinsho (Jpn. J. Pediatr.) *24*:2545-2559, 1971.

140. Jibiki, T., Terai, M., Kurosaki, T., et al.: Efficacy of IVIG therapy combined with dexamethasone for the initial treatment of acute Kawasaki disease. Eur. J. Pediatr. 163:229-233, 2004.
141. Johnson, R. M.: Kawasaki-like syndromes associated with HIV infection. Clin. Infect. Dis. 32:1628-1634, 2001.
142. Jordan, S. C., Platts-Mills, T. A., Mason, W., et al.: Lack of evidence for mite-antigen–mediated pathogenesis in Kawasaki disease. Lancet 1:931, 1983.
143. Kafetzis, D. A., Maltezou, H. C., Constantopoulou, I., et al.: Lack of association between Kawasaki syndrome and infection with Rickettsia conorii, Rickettsia typhi, Coxiella burnetii or Ehrlichia phagocytophila group. Pediatr. Infect. Dis. J. 20:703-706, 2001.
144. Kamiya, T., Suzuki, A., Ono, Y., et al.: Angiographic follow-up study of coronary artery lesion in the cases with a history of Kawasaki disease: With a focus on the follow-up more than 10 years after the onset of the disease. In Kato, H. (ed.): Kawasaki Disease. Amsterdam, Elsevier Science, 1995, pp. 569-573.
145. Kaneko, K., Savage, C. O., Pottinger, B. E., et al.: Antiendothelial cell antibodies can be cytotoxic to endothelial cells without cytokine pre-stimulation and correlate with ELISA antibody measurement in Kawasaki disease. Clin. Exp. Immunol. 98:264-269, 1994.
146. Kaslow, R. A., Bailowitz, A., Lin, F. Y. C., et al.: Association of epidemic Kawasaki syndrome with the HLA-A2, B44, Cw5 antigen combination. Arthritis Rheum. 28:938-940, 1985.
147. Kato, H.: Natural history of Kawasaki disease. In Shiokawa, Y. (ed.): Vascular Lesions of Collagen Diseases and Related Conditions. Baltimore, University Park Press, 1977, pp. 281-286.
148. Kato, H.: Intracoronary thrombolytic therapy in Kawasaki disease: Treatment and prevention of acute myocardial infarction. Prog. Clin. Biol. Res. 250:445-454, 1987.
149. Kato, H.: Long-term consequences of Kawasaki disease: Pediatrics to adults. In Kato, H. (ed.): Kawasaki Disease. Amsterdam, Elsevier Science, 1995, pp. 557-566.
150. Kato, H., and Ichinose, E.: Cardiovascular involvement in Kawasaki disease. Acta Paediatr. Jpn. 26:132-145, 1984.
151. Kato, H., Ichinose, E., and Kawasaki, T.: Myocardial infarction in Kawasaki disease. J. Pediatr. 108:923-928, 1986.
152. Kato, H., Ichinose, E., Yoshioka, F., et al.: Fate of coronary aneurysms in Kawasaki disease: Serial coronary angiography and long-term follow-up study. Am. J. Cardiol. 49:1758-1766, 1982.
153. Kato, H., Inoue, O., Akagi, T.: Kawasaki disease: Cardiac problems and management. Pediatr. Rev. 9:209-217, 1988.
154. Kato, H., Inoue, O., Kawasaki, T., et al.: Adult coronary artery disease probably due to childhood Kawasaki disease. Lancet 340:1127-1129, 1992.
155. Kato, H., Koike, S., and Yokoyama, T.: Kawasaki disease: Effect of treatment of coronary artery involvement. Pediatrics 63:175-179, 1979.
156. Kato, H., Sugimura, T., Akagi, T., et al.: Long-term consequences of Kawasaki disease. Circulation 94:1279-1285, 1996.
157. Kato, S., Kimura, M., Tsuji, K., et al.: HLA antigens in Kawasaki disease. Pediatrics 61:252-255, 1978.
158. Kawasaki, T.: Non-scarlet fever syndrome with desquamation. Chiba Igakukai Zasshi 38:279, 1962.
159. Kawasaki, T.: Acute febrile mucocutaneous syndrome with lymphoid involvement with specific desquamation of the fingers and toes in children. Jpn. J. Allergy 16:178-222, 1967 [English translation, Pediatr. Infect. Dis. J. 21:993-995, 2002].
160. Kawasaki, T.: Kawasaki disease. Asian Med. J. 32:497-506, 1989.
161. Kawasaki, T.: Personal communication, March, 2001.
162. Kawasaki, T., Kosaki, F., Okawa, S., et al.: A new infantile acute febrile mucocutaneous lymph node syndrome (MLNS) prevailing in Japan. Pediatrics 54:271-276, 1974.
163. Kawasaki, T., Kubo, N., Sakata, G., et al.: Two autopsy cases of infantile periarteritis nodosa and their clinical findings: In relation to Kawasaki disease. Chiryo J. Ther. 52:633-644, 1970.
164. Keren, G., Danon, Y. L., Orgad, S., et al.: HLA Bw 51 is increased in mucocutaneous lymph node syndrome in Israeli patients. Tissue Antigens 20:144-146, 1982.
165. Kim, D. S.: Serum interleukin-6 in Kawasaki disease. Yonsei Med. J. 33:183-188, 1992.
166. Kim, D. S., and Lee, K. Y.: Serum soluble E-selectin levels in Kawasaki disease. Scand J. Rheumatol. 23:283-286, 1995.
167. Kim, D. S., Lee, H. K., Noh, G. W., et al.: Increased serum IL-10 in Kawasaki disease. Yonsei Med. J. 37:125-130, 1996.
168. Kisimoto, T.: B-cell stimulatory factors (BSFs): Molecular structure, biological function, and regulation of expression. J. Clin. Immunol. 7:343-355, 1987.
169. Kitamura, S., Kamedo, Y., Sekit, S., et al.: Long-term outcome of myocardial revascularization in Kawasaki disease. J. Thorac. Cardiovasc. Surg. 197:663-674, 1994.
170. Kitamura, S., Kawashima, Y., Kawachi, K., et al.: Severe mitral regurgitation due to coronary arteritis of mucocutaneous lymph node syndrome. J. Thorac. Cardiovasc. Surg. 80:629-636, 1980.
171. Kobayashi, S., Wada, N., and Kubo, M.: Antibodies to native type III collagen in the serum of patients with Kawasaki disease. Eur. J. Pediatr. 151:183-187, 1992.
172. Kobayashi, T., Inoue, Y., Takeuchi, K., et al.: Prediction of IVIG unresponsiveness in patients with Kawasaki disease. Circulation 113:2606-2612, 2006.
173. Kohsaka, T., Abe, J., Asahina T., et al.: Classical pathway complement activation in Kawasaki syndrome. J. Allergy Clin. Immunol. 93:520-525, 1994.
174. Koren, G., Schaffer, F., Silverman, E. D., et al.: Determinants of low serum salicylates in patients with Kawasaki disease. J. Pediatr. 112:663-667, 1988.
175. Kosaki F, Kawasaki, T., Okawa S., et al.: Clinicopathological conference on 10 fatal cases with acute febrile mucocutaneous lymph node syndrome. Shonika Rinsho (Jpn. J. Pediatr.) 24:2545-2559, 1971.
176. Kotb, M.: Superantigens: A possible link between infection and autoimmunity. In Kato, H. (ed.): Kawasaki Disease. Amsterdam, Elsevier Science, 1995, pp. 111-119.
177. Krensky, A. M., Berenberg, W., Shanley, K., et al.: HLA antigens in mucocutaneous lymph node syndrome in New England. Pediatrics 67:741-744, 1981.
178. Krensky, A. M., Grady, S., Shanley, K. M., et al.: Epidemic and endemic HLA-B and DR associations in mucocutaneous lymph node syndrome. Hum. Immunol. 6:75-77, 1983.
179. Krous, H. F., Clausen, C. R., and Ray, C. G.: Elevated immunoglobulin E in infantile polyarteritis nodosa. Pediatrics 84:841-845, 1974.
180. Krzyszkowski, J.: Periarteritis nodosa. Przegl. Post. Nauk. Lek. (Warsaw) 38:30, 45, 58, 1899.
181. Kusakawa, S., and Heiner, D. C.: Elevated levels of immunoglobulin E in the acute febrile mucocutaneous lymph node syndrome. Pediatr. Res. 10:108-111, 1976.
182. Kusakawa, S., and Tatara, K.: Efficacies and risks of aspirin in the treatment of Kawasaki disease. Prog. Clin. Biol. Res. 20:401-413, 1987.
183. Kussmaul, A., and Maier, R.: Dtsch. Arch. Klin. Med. 1:484, 1866.
184. Landing, B. H., and Larson, E. J.: Are infantile periarteritis nodosa with coronary artery involvement and fatal mucocutaneous lymph node syndrome the same?: Comparison of 20 patients from North America with patients from Hawaii and Japan. Pediatrics 59:651-662, 1977.
185. Lang, B. A., Silverman, E. D., Laxer, R. M., et al.: Spontaneous tumor necrosis factor production in Kawasaki disease. J. Pediatr. 115:939-943, 1989.
186. Lang, B. A., Silverman, E. D., Laxer, R. M., et al.: Serum-soluble interleukin-2 receptor levels in Kawasaki disease. J. Pediatr. 116:592-596, 1990.
187. Lapointe, N., Chad, Z., Lacroix, J., et al.: Kawasaki disease: Association with uveitis in seven patients. Pediatrics 69:376-379, 1982.
188. Larsen, J. H.: Kawasaki disease: A yersiniosis? J. Infect. Dis. 160:900, 1989.
189. Larson, E. J.: Comparison of pathology of infantile periarteritis nodosa (IPN) with coronary artery disease in North America with Kawasaki disease (MCLS) in Hawaii and Japan. In Japan Medical Research Foundation (ed.): Vascular Lesions of Collagen Diseases and Related Conditions. Tokyo, University of Tokyo Press, 1977, pp. 322-334.
190. Lee, D. B.: Epidemiological survey of Kawasaki syndrome in Korea (1976-1984). J. Cath. Med. Coll. 38:13-19, 1985.
191. Lee, T., and Vaughan, D.: Mucocutaneous lymph node syndrome in a young adult. Arch. Intern. Med. 139:104-105, 1979.
192. Lee, T., Furukawa, S., Fukuda Y., et al.: Plasma prostaglandin E₂ level in Kawasaki disease. Prostaglandins Leukot. Essent. Fatty Acids 31:53-57, 1988.
193. Lehman, T. J. A., Warren, R., Gietl, D., et al.: Variable expression of Lactobacillus casei cell-wall–induced coronary arteritis: An animal model of Kawasaki's disease in selected inbred mouse strains. Clin. Immunol. Immunopathol. 48:108-118, 1988.
194. Leung, D. Y. M.: Immunomodulation by intravenous immune globulin in Kawasaki disease. J. Allergy Clin. Immunol. 84:588-594, 1989.
195. Leung, D. Y. M.: The potential role of cytokine-mediated vascular endothelial cell activation in the pathogenesis of Kawasaki disease. Acta Paediatr. Jpn. 33:739-744, 1991.
196. Leung, D. Y. M., Burns, J. C., Newburger, J. W., et al.: Reversal of lymphocyte activation in vivo in the Kawasaki syndrome by intravenous gammaglobulin. J. Clin. Invest. 79:468-472, 1987.
197. Leung, D. Y. M., Chu, E. T., Wood, N., et al.: Immunoregulatory T cell abnormalities in mucocutaneous lymph node syndrome. J. Immunol. 130:2002-2004, 1983.
198. Leung, D. Y. M., Collins, T., LaPierre, L. A., et al.: Immunoglobulin M antibodies present in the acute phase of Kawasaki syndrome lyse cultured vascular endothelial cells stimulated by gamma interferon. J. Clin. Invest. 77:1428-1435, 1986.
199. Leung, D. Y. M., Geha, R., and Newberger, J.: Two monokines, interleukin-1 and tumor necrosis factor, render cultured vascular endothelial cells susceptible to lysis by antibodies circulating during Kawasaki syndrome. J. Exp. Med. 164:1958-1972, 1986.
200. Leung, D. Y. M., Kurt-Jones, E., Newberger, J. W., et al.: Endothelial cell activation and high interleukin-1 secretion in the pathogenesis of acute Kawasaki disease. Lancet 2:1298-1302, 1989.
201. Leung, D. Y. M., Meissner, H. C., Fulton, D. R., et al.: Toxic shock syndrome toxin-secreting Staphylococcus aureus in Kawasaki syndrome. Lancet 342:1385-1388, 1993.
202. Leung, D. Y. M., Meissner, H. C., Shulman, S. T., et al.: Prevalence of superantigen-secreting bacteria in patients with Kawasaki disease. J. Pediatr. 140:742-746, 2002.
203. Leung, D. Y. M., Seigel, R. L., Grady, S., et al.: Immunoregulatory abnormalities in mucocutaneous lymph node syndrome. Clin. Immunol. Immunopathol. 23:100-112, 1982.
204. Levinsky, R., and Marshall, W. C.: Circulating immune complexes in mucocutaneous lymph node syndrome. Arch. Dis. Child. 54:240-245, 1979.

205. Levy, M., and Koren, G.: Atypical Kawasaki disease: Analysis of clinical presentation and diagnostic clues. Pediatr. Infect. Dis. J. *9*:122-126, 1990.

206. Li, C. R., Yang, X. Q., Shen, J., et al.: Immunoglobulin G subclasses in serum and circulating immune complexes in patients with Kawasaki syndrome. Pediatr. Infect. Dis. J. *9*:544-547, 1990.

207. Lin, C. Y., Lin, C. C., Hwang, B., et al.: Serial changes of serum interleukin-6, interleukin-8, and tumor necrosis factor alpha among patients with Kawasaki disease. J. Pediatr. *121*:924-926, 1992.

208. Lin, C. Y., Lin, C. C., Hwang, B., et al.: Cytokines predict coronary aneurysm formation in Kawasaki disease patients. Eur. J. Pediatr. *152*:309-312, 1993.

209. Lin, F. Y. C., Bailowitz, A., Koslowe, P., et al.: Kawasaki syndrome: A case-control study during an outbreak in Maryland. Am. J. Dis. Child. *139*:277-279, 1985.

210. Lynch, M., Holman, R. C., Mulligan, A., et al.: Kawasaki syndrome hospitalizations in Ireland, 1996-2000. Pediatr. Infect. Dis. J. *22*:959-962, 2003.

211. Marchette, N. J., Cao, Y., Kihara, S., et al.: Staphylococcal toxic shock syndrome toxin-1, one possible cause of Kawasaki syndrome. *In* Kato, H. (ed.): Kawasaki Disease. Amsterdam, Elsevier Science, 1995, pp. 149-155.

212. Mason, W., Jordan, S., Sakai, R., et al.: Lack of effect of gamma-globulin infusion on circulating immune complexes in patients with Kawasaki syndrome. Pediatr. Infect. Dis. J. *7*:94-99, 1988.

213. Mason, W., Schneider, T., and Takahashi, M.: The epidemiology and etiology of Kawasaki disease. Cardiol. Young *1*:196-205, 1991.

214. Masuda, H., Shozawa, T., Naoe, S., et al.: The intercostal artery in Kawasaki disease: A pathologic study of 17 autopsy cases. Arch. Pathol. Lab. Med. *110*:1136-1142, 1986.

215. Matsubara, T., Furukawa, S., Ino, T., et al.: A sibship with recurrent Kawasaki disease and coronary artery lesion. Acta Paediatr. *83*:1002-1004, 1994.

216. Matsubara, T., Furukawa, S., and Yabuta, K.: Serum levels of tumor necrosis factor, interleukin-2 receptor, and interferon-gamma in Kawasaki disease involved coronary artery lesions. Clin. Immunol. Immunopathol. *56*:29-36, 1990.

217. Matsuda, I., Hattori, S., Nagata, N., et al.: HLA antigens in mucocutaneous lymph node syndrome. Am. J. Dis. Child. *131*:1417-1418, 1977.

218. Maury, C. P., Salo, E., and Pelkonen, P.: Circulating interleukin-1 beta in patients with Kawasaki disease. N. Engl. J. Med. *312*:1670-1671, 1988.

219. Maury, C. P., Salo, E., and Pelkonen, P.: Elevated circulating tumor necrosis factor-alpha in patients with Kawasaki disease. J. Lab. Clin. Med. *113*:651-654, 1989.

220. Mayatepek, E., and Lehmann, W. D.: Increased generation of cysteinyl leukotrienes in Kawasaki disease. Arch. Dis. Child. *72*:526-527, 1995.

221. Melish, M. E., Hicks, R. M., and Larson, E. J.: Mucocutaneous lymph node syndrome (MCLS) in the U.S. Pediatr. Res. *8*:427, 1974.

222. Melish, M. E., Hicks, R. M., and Larson, E. J.: Mucocutaneous lymph node syndrome in the United States. Am. J. Dis. Child. *130*:599-607, 1976.

223. Melish, M. E., Marchette, N. J., Kaplan, J. C., et al.: Absence of significant RNA-dependent DNA polymerase activity in lymphocytes from patients with Kawasaki syndrome. Nature *337*:288-290, 1989.

224. Melish, M. E., Parsonett, J., and Marchette, N. J.: Kawasaki syndrome is not caused by toxic shock syndrome toxin-1 (TSST-1) positive staphylococci. Pediatr. Res. *35*:187A, 1994.

225. Melish, M. E., Takahashi, M., Shulman, S. T., et al.: Comparison of low dose aspirin versus high dose aspirin as an adjunct to IVGG for Kawasaki syndrome. Pediatr. Res. *31*:170A, 1992.

226. Milgrom, H., Palmer, E. L., Slovin, S. F., et al.: Kawasaki disease in a healthy young adult. Ann. Intern. Med. *92*:467-470, 1980.

227. Mitani, Y., Okada, Y., Inoue, M., et al.: Impaired endothelium dependent relaxation of angiographically normal coronary arteries in patients after Kawasaki disease in the long-term follow-up period. *In* Kato, H. (ed.): Kawasaki Disease. Amsterdam, Elsevier Science, 1995, pp. 587-591.

228. Miura, M., Garcia, F., Crawford, S. E., et al.: Macrophage infiltration of pancreatic acini and islets in acute Kawasaki disease. Pediatr. Infect. Dis. J. *22*:1106-1108, 2003.

229. Miura, M., Garcia, F. L., Crawford, S. E., et al.: Cell adhesion molecule expression in coronary artery aneurysms in acute Kawasaki disease. Pediatr. Infect. Dis. J. *23*:931-936, 2004.

230. Morens, D. M.: Kawasaki disease and rug shampooing. J. Pediatr. *120*:333-334, 1992.

231. Mori, M., Imagawa, T., Yasui, K., et al.: Predictors of coronary artery lesions after IVGG treatment in Kawasaki disease. J. Pediatr. *137*:177-180, 2000.

232. Morise, T., Takeuchi, Y., Takeda, R., et al.: Increased plasma endothelin levels in Kawasaki disease: A possible marker for Kawasaki disease. Angiology *44*:719-723, 1993.

233. Muise, A., Tallett, S. E., Silverman, E. D.: Are children with Kawasaki disease and prolonged fever at risk for macrophage activation syndrome? Pediatrics *12*:e495-e497, 2003.

234. Munro-Faure, H.: Necrotizing arteritis of the coronary vessels in infancy: Case report and review of the literature. Pediatrics *23*:914-926, 1959.

235. Muta, H., Ishii, M., Egami, K., et al.: Early IVGG treatment for Kawasaki disease: The nationwide surveys in Japan. J. Pediatr. *144*:496-499, 2004.

236. Muzik, O., Paridon, S. M., Singh, T. P., et al.: Quantification of myocardial blood flow and flow reserve in children with a history of Kawasaki disease and normal coronary arteries. J. Am. Coll. Cardiol. *28*:757-762, 1996.

237. Myones, B., Tomita, S., and Shulman, S. T.: Intravenous IgG administration is associated with a decrease in classical pathway activation products in Kawasaki disease. Arthritis Rheum. *34*(Suppl.):S44, 1991.

238. Nagashima, M., Matsushima, M., Matsuoka, H., et al.: High-dose gamma globulin therapy for Kawasaki disease. J. Pediatr. *110*:710-712, 1987.

239. Nagata, S., Yamashiro, Y., Maeda, M., et al.: Immunohistochemical studies on small intestinal mucosa in Kawasaki disease. Pediatr. Res. *33*:557-563, 1993.

240. Nakamura, Y., Hirose, K., Yanagawa, H., et al.: Incidence rate of recurrent Kawasaki disease in Japan. Acta Paediatr. *83*:1061-1064, 1994.

241. Nakamura, Y., Yanagawa, H., Harada, K., et al.: Mortality among persons with a history of Kawasaki disease in Japan: The fifth look. Arch. Pediatr. Adolesc. Med. *156*:162-165, 2002.

242. Nakamura, Y., Yanagawa, H., and Kawasaki, T.: Temporal and geographical clustering of Kawasaki disease in Japan. Prog. Clin. Biol. Res. *250*:19-32, 1987.

243. Nakamura, Y., Yanagawa, H., and Kawasaki, T.: Mortality among children with Kawasaki disease in Japan. N. Engl. J. Med. *326*:1246-1249, 1992.

243a. Nakamura, Y.: Forty-one years after the 1st report of Kawasaki Disease in Japan. Abstlos, Proceedings of Ninth International Kawasaki Disease Symposium. Taipei, April 2008.

244. Nakano, H., Ueda, K., Saito, A., et al.: Scoring method for identifying patients with Kawasaki disease at high risk of coronary artery aneurysms. Am. J. Cardiol. *58*:739-742, 1986.

245. Naoe, S., Shibuya, K., Takahashi, M., et al.: Pathological observations concerning the cardiovascular lesions in Kawasaki disease. Cardiol. Young *1*:212-220, 1991.

246. Naoe, S., Takahashi, K., and Masuda, H.: Kawasaki disease with particular emphasis on arterial lesions. Acta Pathol. Jpn. *41*:785-797, 1991.

247. Newburger, J. W., and U. S. Multicenter Kawasaki Study Group: A single infusion of intravenous gamma globulin compared to four daily doses in the treatment of acute Kawasaki syndrome. N. Engl. J. Med. *324*:1633-1639, 1991.

248. Newburger, J. W., Burns, J. C., Beiser, A. S., et al.: Altered lipid profile after Kawasaki disease. Circulation *85*:625-631, 1991.

249. Newburger, J. W., Sanders, S. P., Burns, J. C., et al.: Left ventricular contractility and function in Kawasaki disease. Circulation *79*:1237-1246, 1989.

250. Newburger, J. W., Sleeper, L. A., McCrindle, B. W., et al.: Randomized trial of pulse steroid therapy for primary treatment of Kawasaki disease. N. Engl. J. Med. *356*:663-675, 2007.

251. Newburger, J. W., Takahashi, M., Burns, J. C., et al.: The treatment of Kawasaki syndrome with intravenous gamma globulin. N. Engl. J. Med. *315*:341-347, 1986.

252. Newburger, J. W., Takahashi, M., Gerber, M. A., et al.: Diagnosis, treatment, and long-term management of Kawasaki disease. (American Heart Association Scientific Statement). Circulation *110*:2747-2771, 2004.

253. Ng, M. P., Wong, K. Y., Tan, C. L., et al.: Kawasaki disease: The Singapore experience. Ann. Acad. Med. *18*:15-18, 1989.

254. Nigro, G., and Midulla, M.: Retrovirus and Kawasaki disease. Lancet *2*:1045, 1986.

255. Nigrovic, L. E., Nigrovic, P. A., Harper, M. B., et al.: Extreme thrombocytosis predicts Kawasaki disease in infants. Clin. Pediatr. *45*:446-452, 2006.

256. Nishiyori, A., Sakaguchi, M., Kato, H., et al.: Toxic shock syndrome toxin 1 and V2 expression on T cells in Kawasaki disease. *In* Kato, H. (ed.): Kawasaki Disease. Amsterdam, Elsevier Science, 1995, pp. 139-143.

257. Niwa, K., Aotsuka, M., Karasawa, K., et al.: Thrombocytopenia: A risk factor for acute myocardial infarction during acute Kawasaki disease. Coron. Artery Dis. *6*:857-864, 1995.

258. Niwa, K., and Sohmiya, K.: Enhanced neutrophilic functions in mucocutaneous lymph node syndrome, with special reference to the possible role of increased oxygen intermediate generation in the pathogenesis of coronary thromboarteritis. J. Pediatr. *104*:56-60, 1984.

259. Nofech-Mozes, Y., and Garty, B.-Z.: Thrombocytopenia in Kawasaki disease. Pediatr. Hematol. Oncol . *20*:597-601, 2003.

260. Noto, N., Ayusawa, M., Karasawa, K., et al.: Dobutamine stress echocardiography for detection of coronary artery stenosis in children with Kawasaki disease. J. Am. Coll. Cardiol. *27*:1251-1256, 1996.

261. Ogawa, S., Zhang, J., Yuge, K., et al.: Increased plasma endothelin-1 concentration in Kawasaki disease. J. Cardiovasc. Pharmacol. *22*(Suppl. 8):S364-S366, 1993.

262. Ogino, H., Ogawa, M., Harima, Y., et al.: Clinical evaluation of gamma-globulin preparations for the treatment of Kawasaki disease. Prog. Clin. Biol. Res. *250*:555-556, 1987.

263. Ohga, K., Ooshima, A., Fukushige, J., et al.: Histiocytic haemophagocytosis in a patient with Kawasaki disease. Eur. J. Pediatr. *154*:539-541, 1995.

264. Ohga, K., Yamanaha, R., Kinumaki, H., et al.: Kawasaki disease and rug shampoo. Lancet *1*:930, 1983.

265. Ohno, S., Miyajima, T., Higuchi, M., et al.: Ocular manifestations of Kawasaki disease (mucocutaneous lymph node syndrome). Am. J. Ophthalmol. *93*:713-717, 1982.

266. Ohshio, G., Furukawa, F., Khine, M., et al.: High levels of IgA-containing circulating immune complex and secretory IgA in Kawasaki disease. Microbiol. Immunol. *31*:891-898, 1987.

267. Okada, Y., Shinohara, M., Kobayashi, T., et al.: Effect of corticosteroids in addition to IVIG on serum cytokine levels in acute Kawasaki disease. J. Pediatr. *143*:363-367, 2003.

268. Okamoto, T., Kuwabara, H., Shimotohno, K., et al.: Lack of evidence of retroviral involvement in Kawasaki disease. Pediatrics *81*:599, 1988.

268a. Onouchi, Y., Gunji, T., Burns, J. C., et al.: ITPKC Functional polymorphism associated with Kawasaki disease susceptibility and formation of coronary artery aneurysms. Nat. Genet. *40*:35-42, 2008.

269. Orlowski, J. P., and Mercer, R. D.: Urine mercury levels in Kawasaki disease. Pediatrics *66*:633-636, 1980.

270. Pachman, L. M., Herold, B. C., and Davis, A. T.: Immune complexes in Kawasaki syndrome: A review. Prog. Clin. Biol. Res. *250*:193-207, 1987.

271. Packard, M., and Wechsler, H. F.: Aneurysm of the coronary arteries. Arch. Intern. Med. *43*:1-14, 1929.

272. Pahl, E., Sehgal, R., Chrystof, D., et al.: Feasibility of exercise stress echocardiography for follow-up of children with coronary involvement secondary to Kawasaki disease. Circulation *91*:122-128, 1995.

273. Palmer, A. L., Walker, T., and Smith, J. C.: Acute respiratory distress syndrome in a child with Kawasaki disease. South. Med. J. *98*:1031-1033, 2005.

274. Palazzi, D. L., McClain, K. L., and Kaplan, S. L.: Hemophagocytic syndrome after Kawasaki disease. Pediatr. Infect. Dis. J. *22*:663-666, 2003.

275. Patriarca, P. A., Rogers, M. F., Morens, D. M., et al.: Kawasaki syndrome: Association with the application of rug shampoo. Lancet *2*:578-580, 1982.

276. Pelkonen, P., and Salo, E: Epidemiology of Kawasaki disease. Clin. Exp. Rheumatol. *12*(Suppl 10):S83-S85, 1994.

277. Person, J. R.: Kawasaki disease and staphylococcal exotoxins. Arch. Dermatol. *116*:986, 1980.

278. Phillips, W. G., and Marsden, J. R.: Adult Kawasaki syndrome. Br. J. Dermatol. *129*:330-333, 1993.

279. Pierre, R., Sue-Ho, R., and Watson, D.: Kawasaki syndrome in Jamaica. Pediatr. Infect. Dis. J. *9*:539-543, 2000.

280. Pietra, B. A., De Inocencio, J., Giannini, E. H., et al.: TCR V family repertoire and T cell activation markers in Kawasaki disease. J. Immunol. *153*:1881-1888, 1994.

281. Poon, L. K., Lun, K. S., Ng, Y. M.: Facial nerve palsy and Kawasaki disease (a review). Hong Kong Med. J. *6*:224-226, 2000.

282. Porneuf, M., Sotto, A., Barbuat, C., et al.: Kawasaki syndrome in an adult AIDS patient. Int. J. Dermatol. *35*:292-294, 1996.

283. Rae, M. V.: Coronary aneurysms with thrombosis in rheumatic carditis: Unusual occurrence accompanied by hyperleukocytosis in a child. Arch. Pathol. *24*:369-376, 1937.

284. Rauch, A. M.: Kawasaki syndrome: Critical review of U.S. epidemiology. Prog. Clin. Biol. Res. *250*:33-44, 1987.

285. Rauch, A. M., Fultz, P. N., and Kalyanaraman, V. S.: Retrovirus serology and Kawasaki syndrome. Lancet *1*:1431, 1987.

286. Rauch, A. M., Glode, M. P., Wiggins, J. W., et al.: Outbreak of Kawasaki syndrome in Denver, Colorado: Association with rug and carpet cleaning. Pediatrics *87*:663-669, 1991.

287. Rauch, A. M., Kaplan, S. L., Nihill, M. R., et al.: Kawasaki syndrome clusters in Harris County, Texas, and eastern North Carolina. Am. J. Dis. Child. *142*:441-444, 1988.

288. Rider, L. G., Wener, M. H., French, J., et al.: Autoantibody production in Kawasaki syndrome. Clin. Exp. Rheumatol. *11*:445-449, 1993.

289. Rieger, C. H., Kawasaki, T., Yanare, Y., et al.: Complement and protease inhibitors in Kawasaki disease. Eur. J. Pediatr. *140*:92-97, 1983.

290. Roberts, F. B., and Fetterman, G. H.: Polyarteritis nodosa in infancy. J. Pediatr. *63*:519-529, 1963.

291. Rogers, M. F.: Kawasaki syndrome. Am. J. Dis. Child. *140*:191, 1986.

292. Rogers, M. F., Kochel, R. L., Hurwitz, E. S., et al.: Kawasaki syndrome: Is exposure to rug shampoo important? Am. J. Dis. Child. *139*:777-779, 1985.

293. Rosenfeld, E. A., Corydon, K. E., and Shulman, S. T.: Kawasaki disease in infants less than one year of age. J. Pediatr. *126*:524-529, 1995.

294. Rosenfeld, E. A., Shulman, S. T., Corydon, K. E., et al.: Comparative safety and efficacy of two IVIG products in Kawasaki disease. J. Pediatr. *126*:1000-1003, 1995.

295. Rowley, A. H., Baker, S. C., Shulman, S. T., et al.: Detection of antigen in bronchial epithelium and macrophages in acute Kawasaki disease by use of synthetic antibody. J. Infect. Dis. *190*:856-865, 2004.

296. Rowley, A. H., Baker, S. C., Shulman, S. T., et al.: Cytoplasmic inclusion bodies are detected by synthetic antibody in ciliated bronchial epithelium during acute Kawasaki disease. J. Infect. Dis. *192*:1757-1766, 2005.

297. Rowley, A. H., Duffy, E., and Shulman, S. T.: Prevention of giant aneurysms in Kawasaki disease by intravenous gamma globulin therapy. J. Pediatr. *113*:290-294, 1988.

298. Rowley, A. H., Eckerley, C. A., Jack, H. M., et al.: IgA plasma cells in vascular tissue of patients with Kawasaki syndrome. J. Immunol. *159*:5946-5955, 1997.

299. Rowley, A. H., Gonzalez-Crussi, F., Gidding, S. S., et al.: Incomplete Kawasaki disease with coronary artery involvement. J. Pediatr. *110*:409-413, 1987.

300. Rowley, A. H., Shulman, S. T., Mask, C. A., et al.: IgA plasma cell infiltration in proximal respiratory tract, pancreas, kidney and coronary artery in acute Kawasaki disease. J. Infect. Dis. *182*:1183-1191, 2000.

301. Rowley, A. H., Shulman, S. T., Preble, O. T., et al.: Serum interferon concentrations and retroviral serology in Kawasaki syndrome. Pediatr. Infect. Dis. J. *7*:663-665, 1988.

302. Rowley, A. H., Shulman, S. T., Spike, B. T., et al.: Oligoclonal IgA response in the vascular wall in acute Kawasaki disease. J. Immunol. *166*:1334-1343, 2001.

303. Rowley, A. H., Wolinsky, S. M., Relman, D. A., et al.: Search for highly conserved viral and bacterial nucleic acid sequences corresponding to an etiologic agent of Kawasaki disease. Pediatr. Res. *36*:567-571, 1994.

304. Salcedo, J. R., Greenberg, L., and Kapur, S.: Renal histology of mucocutaneous lymph node syndrome. Clin. Nephrol. *29*:47-51, 1988.

305. Salo, E.: Kawasaki disease in Finland in 1982-1983. Scand. J. Infect. Dis. *25*:497-502, 1993.

306. Salo, E., Kekomaki, R., Pelkonen, P., et al.: Kawasaki disease: Monitoring of circulating immune complexes. Eur. J. Pediatr. *147*:377-380, 1988.

307. Salo, E., Pelkonen, P., and Pettay, O.: Outbreak of Kawasaki syndrome in Finland. Acta Paediatr. Scand. *75*:75-80, 1986.

308. Salo, E., Pesonen, E., and Viikari, J.: Serum cholesterol levels during and after Kawasaki disease. J. Pediatr. *119*:557-561, 1991.

309. Sasaguri, Y., and Kato, H.: Regression of aneurysms in Kawasaki disease: A pathologic study. Pediatrics *100*:225-231, 1982.

310. Sato, K., Ouichi, K., and Taki, M.: *Yersinia pseudotuberculosis* infection in children, resembling Izumi fever and Kawasaki syndrome. Pediatr. Infect. Dis. J. *2*:123-126, 1983.

311. Sato, N., Sagawa, K., Sasaguri, Y., et al.: Immunopathology and cytokine detection in the skin lesions of patients with Kawasaki disease. J. Pediatr. *122*:198-203, 1993.

312. Savage, C. O. S., Tizard, J., Jayne, D., et al.: Antineutrophil cytoplasm antibodies in Kawasaki disease. Arch. Dis. Child. *64*:360-363, 1989.

313. Saxe, N., Horak, K., and Goldblatt, J.: Mucocutaneous lymph node syndrome in a young adult. S. Afr. Med. J. *68*:1011-1013, 1980.

314. Schrag, S. J., Besser, R. E., Olson, C., et al.: Lack of association between Kawasaki syndrome and *Chlamydia pneumoniae* infection. Pediatr. Infect. Dis. J. *19*:17-22, 2000.

315. Senzaki, H.: The pathophysiology of coronary artery aneurysms in Kawasaki disease: Role of matrix metalloproteinases. Arch. Dis. Child. *91*:847-851, 2006.

316. Shibuya, N., Shibuya, K., Kato, H., et al.: Kawasaki disease before Kawasaki at Tokyo University Hospital. Pediatrics *110*:e17, 2002.

317. Shigematsu, I.: Epidemiology of mucocutaneous lymph node syndrome [Japanese]. Acta Paediatr. Jpn. *76*:696, 1972.

318. Shimizu, C., Shike, H., Baker, S. C., et al.: Human coronavirus NL63 is not detected in the respiratory tracts of children with acute Kawasaki disease. J. Infect. Dis. *192*:1767-1771, 2005.

319. Shimizu, S., Kuratsuji, T., and Ojima, T.: Plasma fibronectin concentrations in mucocutaneous lymph node syndrome. Arch. Dis. Child. *61*:72-74, 1986.

320. Shingadia, D., O'Gorman, M., Rowley, A. H., and Shulman, S. T.: Surface and cytoplasmic immunoglobulin expression in circulating B-lymphocytes in acute Kawasaki disease. Pediatr. Res. *50*:538-543, 2001.

321. Shulman, S. T.: IVGG therapy in Kawasaki disease: Mechanism(s) of action. Clin. Immunol. Immunopathol. *53*:5141-5146, 1989.

322. Shulman, S. T.: Management of Kawasaki syndrome: A consensus statement prepared by North American participants of the Third International Kawasaki Disease Symposium: Tokyo, Japan, December, 1988. Pediatr. Infect. Dis. J. *8*:663-667, 1989.

323. Shulman, S. T.: Hemolysis in Kawasaki disease (letter). Transfusion *31*:572, 1991.

324. Shulman, S. T.: A commentary on disease mechanism. *In* Takahashi, M., and Taubert, K. (eds.): Proceedings of the Fourth International Symposium on Kawasaki Disease. Dallas, American Heart Association, 1993.

325. Shulman, S. T., and Rowley, A. H.: Does Kawasaki disease have a retroviral etiology? Lancet *2*:545-546, 1986.

326. Shulman, S. T., and Rowley, A. H.: Advances in Kawasaki disease. Eur. J. Pediatr. *163*:285, 2004.

327. Shulman, S. T., and Rowley, A. H.: Kawasaki disease before the 1967 description by T. Kawasaki. Pediatr. Res. *47*:277A, 2000. Abstract.

328. Shulman, S. T., DeInocencio, J., and Hirsch, R.: Kawasaki disease. Pediatr. Clin. North Am. *42*:1205-1222, 1995.

329. Shulman, S. T., McAuley, J. B., Pachman, L. M., et al.: Risk of coronary abnormalities due to Kawasaki disease in an urban area with a small Asian population. Am. J. Dis.Child. *141*:420-425, 1987.

330. Shulman, S. T., Melish, M., Inoue, O., et al.: Immunoglobulin allotypic markers in Kawasaki disease. J. Pediatr. *122*:84-86, 1993.

331. Sinha, R., and Balakumar, T.: BCG reactivation: A useful diagnostic tool even for incomplete Kawasaki disease. Arch. Dis. Child. *90*:891, 2005.

332. Smith, L. B., Newburger, J. W., and Burns, J. C.: Kawasaki syndrome and the eye. Pediatr. Infect. Dis. J. *8*:116-118, 1989.

333. Smith, P. K., and Goldwater, P. N.: Kawasaki disease in Adelaide: A review. J. Paediatr. Child. Health *29*:126-131, 1993.

334. Soppi, E., Salo, E., and Pelkonen, P.: Antibodies against neutrophil cytoplasmic components in Kawasaki disease. APMIS *100*:269-272, 1992.

335. Stamos, J. K., Corydon, K., Donaldson J., et al.: Lymphadenitis as the dominant manifestation of Kawasaki disease. Pediatrics *93*:525-528, 1994.

336. Stockheim, J. A., Innocentini, N., and Shulman, S. T.: Kawasaki disease in older children and adolescents. J. Pediatr. *137*:250-252, 1994.

337. Strigl, S., Kutlin, A., Roblin, P. M., et al.: Is there an association between Kawasaki disease and *Chlamydia pneumoniae*? J. Infect. Dis. *181*:2103-2105, 2000.

338. Suddleson, E. A., Reid, B., Woolley, M. M., et al.: Hydrops of the gall bladder associated with Kawasaki syndrome. J. Pediatr. Surg. 22:956-959, 1987.

339. Sugimura, T., Kato, H., Inoue, O., et al.: Long-term consequences of Kawasaki disease: Serial coronary angiography and 10-20 years follow-up study. *In* Kato, H. (ed.): Kawasaki Disease. Amsterdam, Elsevier Science, 1995, pp. 574-579.

340. Sugimura, T., Kato, H., Inoue, O., et al.: Vasodilatory response of the coronary arteries after Kawasaki disease: Evaluation by intracoronary injection of isosorbide dinitrate. Pediatrics 121:684-688, 1992.

341. Sugimura, T., Kato, H., Inoue, O., et al.: Intravascular ultrasound of coronary arteries in children: Assessment of the wall morphology and the lumen after Kawasaki disease. Circulation 89:258-265, 1994.

342. Sugimura, T., Kato, H., Yokoi, H., et al.: Intravascular ultrasound study in Kawasaki disease: Assessment of coronary and systemic arterial pathology and application for coronary intervention. *In* Kato, H. (ed.): Kawasaki Disease. Amsterdam, Elsevier Science, 1995, p. 460.

343. Sugiura, K., Sakurai, K., Takamoto, T., et al.: Kawasaki disease in an adult [Japanese]. Intern. Med. 47:857-860, 1981.

344. Sundel, R., Burns, J. C., Baker, A., et al.: Gamma globulin re-treatment in Kawasaki disease. J. Pediatr. 123:657-659, 1998.

345. Sundel, R., Newburger, J. W., McGill, T., et al.: Sensorineural hearing loss associated with Kawasaki disease. J. Pediatr. 117:371-377, 1990.

346. Suzuki, A., Arakaki, Y., Sugiyama, H., et al.: Observation of coronary arterial lesion due to Kawasaki disease by intravascular ultrasound. *In* Kato, H. (ed.): Kawasaki Disease. Amsterdam, Elsevier Science, 1995, pp. 451-459.

347. Suzuki, A., Kamiya, T., Arakaki, Y., et al.: Fate of coronary aneurysms in Kawasaki disease. Am. J. Cardiol. 74:822-824, 1994.

348. Suzuki, A., Kamiya, T., Kuwahara, N., et al.: Coronary arterial lesions of Kawasaki disease: Cardiac catheterization findings of 1100 cases. Pediatr. Cardiol. 7:3-9, 1986.

349. Suzuki, A., Kamiya, T., Ono, Y., et al.: Follow-up study of coronary arterial lesions due to Kawasaki disease. Heart Vessels 3:159-165, 1987.

350. Suzuki, A., Kamiya, T., Ono, Y., et al.: Functional behavior and morphology of coronary artery wall in Kawasaki disease. J. Am. Coll. Cardiol. 27:291-296, 1996.

351. Suzuki, A., Miyagawa-Tomita, S., Komatsu, K., et al.: Active remodeling of the coronary arterial lesions in the late phase of Kawasaki disease. Circulation 101:2935-2941, 2000.

352. Suzuki, A., Miyagawa-Tomita, S., Komatsu, K., et al.: Immunohistochemical study of apparently intact coronary artery in a child after Kawasaki disease. Pediatr. Int. 46:590-596, 2004.

353. Takahashi, K., Naoe, S., Wakayama, M., et al.: Pathologic study of coronary aneurysms in adults who had Kawasaki disease in childhood. *In* Kato, H. (ed.): Kawasaki Disease. Amsterdam, Elsevier Science, 1995, pp. 592-597.

354. Takahashi, K., Oharaseki, T., Naoe, S., et al.: Neutrophilic involvement in the damage to coronary arteries in acute stage of Kawasaki disease. Pediatr. Int. 47:305-310, 2005.

355. Takahashi, M., Mason, W., and Lewis, A. B.: Regression of coronary aneurysms in patients with Kawasaki syndrome. Circulation 75:387-394, 1987.

356. Takahashi, M., Mason, W., Thomas, D., et al.: Reye syndrome following Kawasaki syndrome confirmed by liver histopathology. *In* Kato, H. (ed.): Kawasaki Disease: Proceedings of 5th International Kawasaki Disease Symposium, Fukuoka, Japan, 1995. New York, Elsevier, 1995, pp. 436-444.

357. Takeda, T., Abe, J., Yoshino K., et al.: Establishment of a novel superantigen produced by *Yersinia pseudotuberculosis* and its association with systemic Kawasaki disease–like symptoms. *In* Kato, H. (ed.): Kawasaki Disease. Amsterdam, Elsevier Science, 1995, pp. 193-199.

358. Takeshita, S., Dobashi, H., Nakatani, K., et al.: Circulating soluble selectins in Kawasaki disease. Clin. Exp. Immunol. 108:446-450, 1997.

359. Tanaka, N.: Kawasaki disease (acute febrile mucocutaneous lymph node syndrome) in Japan: Relationship with infantile periarteritis nodosa. Pathol. Microbiol. 43:204-218, 1975.

360. Tanaka, N., Naoe, S., and Kawasaki, T.: Pathological study of autopsy cases of MCLS: Relationship with infantile periarteritis nodosa. J. Jpn. Red Cross Cen. Hosp. 2:85-94, 1971.

361. Tanaka, N., Sekimoto, K., Fukushima, T., et al.: Pathological study of fatal MCLS cases of Kawasaki disease: Relationship with infantile polyarteritis nodosa. *In* Shiokawa, Y. (ed.): Vascular Lesions of Collagen Diseases and Related Conditions. Baltimore, University Park Press, 1977, p. 44.

362. Tanaka, N., Sekimoto, K., and Naoe, S.: Kawasaki disease: Relationship with infantile periarteritis nodosa. Arch. Pathol. Lab. Med. 100:81-86, 1976.

363. Tashiro, N., Matsubara, T., Uchida, M., et al.: Ultrasonographic evaluation of cervical nodes in Kawasaki disease. Pediatrics 109:e77, 2002.

364. Taubert, K. A., Rowley, A. H., and Shulman, S. T.: Seven-year national survey of Kawasaki disease and acute rheumatic fever. Pediatr. Infect. Dis. J. 13: 704-708, 1994.

365. Taubert, K. A., Rowley, A. H., and Shulman, S. T.: A 10-year (1984-1993) United States hospital survey of Kawasaki disease. *In* Kato, H. (ed.): Kawasaki Disease. Amsterdam, Elsevier Science, 1995, pp. 34-38.

366. Teixeira, O. H. P., and Quinn, A.: Kawasaki syndrome. Am. J. Dis. Child. 140:190-191, 1986.

367. Terai, M., and Shulman, S. T.: Prevalence of coronary artery abnormalities in Kawasaki disease is highly dependent on gammaglobulin dose but independent of salicylate dose. J. Pediatr. 131:888-893, 1997.

368. Terai, M., Kohno, Y., Namba, M., et al.: Class II major histocompatibility antigen expression on coronary arterial endothelium in a patient with Kawasaki disease. Hum. Pathol. 21:231-234, 1990.

369. Terai, M., Kohno, Y., Niwa, K., et al.: Imbalance among T-cell subsets in patients with coronary arterial aneurysms in Kawasaki disease. Am. J. Cardiol. 60:555-559, 1987.

370. Terai, M., Miwa, K., Williams, T., et al.: The absence of evidence of staphylococcal toxin involvement in the pathogenesis of Kawasaki disease. J. Infect. Dis. 172:558-561, 1995.

371. Terai, M., Yasukawa, K., Honda, T., et al.: Peripheral blood eosinophilia and eosinophil accumulation in coronary microvessels in acute Kawasaki disease. Pediatr. Infect. Dis. J. 21:777-780, 2002.

371a. Terp, S., Bar-Meir, M., Tan, T.: Inflammatory reaction at the site of a BCG vaccination scar in an adopted child. Clin. Infect. Dis. 45:487, 518-519, 2007.

372. Ting, E. C., Capparelli, E. V., Billman, G. F., et al.: Elevated gamma-GT concentrations in acute Kawasaki disease. Pediatr. Infect. Dis. J. 17:431-432, 1998.

373. Tomita, S., Chung, K., Mas, M., et al.: Peripheral gangrene associated with Kawasaki disease. Clin. Infect. Dis. 14:121-126, 1992.

374. Tourneux, P., Dufillot, D., Belloy, M., et al.: Epidemiologie de la maladie de Kawasaki en Guadeloupe. Presse Med. 34:25-28, 2005.

375. Treadwell, T. A., Maddox, R. A., Holman, R. C., et al.: Investigation of Kawasaki syndrome risk factors in Colorado. Pediatr. Infect. Dis. J. 21: 976-978, 2002.

376. Tristani-Fironzi, M., Kamango-Sollo, E. D., Sun, S., et al.: TCR V gene family repertoire and humoral immunity in Kawasaki syndrome. *In* Kato, H. (ed.): Kawasaki Disease. Amsterdam, Elsevier Science, 1995, pp. 200-205.

377. Tsai, M.-H., Huang, Y.-C., Yen, M.-H., et al.: Clinical responses of patients with Kawasaki disease to different brands of intravenous immunoglobulin. J. Pediatr. 148:38-43, 2006.

378. Tse, S. M. L., Silverman, E. D., McCrindle, B. W., et al.: Early treatment with IVIG in Kawasaki disease. J. Pediatr. 140:450-455, 2002.

379. Tsuda, E., and Kitamura, S.: National survey of coronary artery bypass grafting for coronary stenosis caused by Kawasaki disease in Japan. Circulation 110 (Suppl. II):II61-66, 2004.

380. Tsuda, E., Kamiya, T., Ono, Y., et al.: Incidence of stenotic lesions predicted by acute phase changes in coronary arterial diameter during Kawasaki disease. Pediatr. Cardiol. 26:73-79, 2005.

381. Tuohy, A. M. M., Tani, L. Y., Cetta, F., et al.: How many echocardiograms are necessary for follow-up evaluation of patients with Kawasaki disease? Am. J. Cardiol. 88:328-330, 2001.

382. Uchida, N., Asayama, K., Dobashi, K., et al.: Antioxidant enzymes and lipoperoxide in blood in patients with Kawasaki disease: Comparison with the changes in acute infections. Acta Paediatr. Jpn. 32:242-248, 1990.

383. Uehara, R., Yashiro, M., Nakamura, H., et al.: Kawasaki disease in parents and children. Acta Paediatr. 92:694-697, 2003.

384. Uziel, Y., Hashkes, P. J., Kassem, E., et al.: "Unresolving pneumonia" as the main manifestation of atypical Kawasaki disease. Arch. Dis. Child. 88:940-942, 2003.

385. Wallace, C. A., French, J. W., Kahn, S. J., et al.: Initial IVIG treatment failure in Kawasaki disease. Pediatrics 43:211-217, 2000.

386. Watanabe, T., Abe, Y., Sato, S., et al.: Hyponatremia in Kawasaki disease. Pediatr. Nephrol. 21:778-781, 2006.

387. Weindling, A. M., Levinsky, R. J., and Marshall, W. C.: Circulating immune complexes in mucocutaneous lymph node syndrome (Kawasaki disease). Arch. Dis. Child. 54:241-242, 1979.

388. Westphalen, M. A., McGrath, M. A., Kelly, W., et al.: Kawasaki disease with severe peripheral ischemia: Treatment with prostaglandin E$_1$ infusion. J. Pediatr. 112:431-433, 1988.

389. Wong, M., Silverman, E. D., and Fish, E. N.: Evidence for RANTES, MCP-1, and MIP-β in Kawasaki disease. J. Rheumatol. 24:1179-1185, 1997.

390. Wright, D. A., Newberger, J. W., Baker, A., et al.: Treatment of immune globulin-resistant Kawasaki disease with pulsed doses of corticosteroids. J. Pediatr. 128:146-149, 1996.

391. Wurzburger, B. J., and Avner, J. R.: Lateral rectus palsy in Kawasaki disease. Pediatr. Infect. Dis. J. 18:1029-1030, 1999.

392. Yamada, K., Fukumoto, T., Shinkai, A., et al.: The platelet function in acute febrile mucocutaneous lymph node syndrome and a trial of prevention for thrombosis by antiplatelet agent. Acta Hematol. Jpn. 41:791-802, 1978.

393. Yamakawa, R., Ishii, M., Sugimura, T., et al.: Coronary endothelial dysfunction after Kawasaki disease. J. Am. Coll. Cardiol. 31:1074-1080, 1998.

394. Yamamoto, T., and Kimura, J.: Acute mucocutaneous lymph node syndrome: A case associated with carditis [Japanese]. Jpn. J. Pediatr. 21:336-339, 1968.

395. Yanagawa, H.: Epidemiology of Kawasaki disease in Japan. Prog. Clin. Biol. Res. 250:5-17, 1987.

396. Yanagawa, H., Kawasaki, T., and Shigematsu, I.: Nationwide survey on Kawasaki disease in Japan. Pediatrics 80:58-62, 1987.

397. Yanagawa, H., Nakamura, Y., Yashiro, M., et al.: Nationwide epidemic of Kawasaki disease in Japan during winter of 1985-86. Lancet 2:1138-1139, 1986.

398. Yanagawa, H., Nakamura, Y., Yashiro, M., et al.: A nationwide incidence survey of Kawasaki disease in 1985-1986 in Japan. J. Infect. Dis. 158:1296-1301, 1988.

399. Yanagawa, H., Nakamura, Y., Yashiro, M., et al.: Results of the nationwide epidemiologic survey of Kawasaki disease in 1995 and 1996 in Japan. Pediatrics 102:e65, 1998.

400. Yanagawa, H., Nakamura, Y., Yashiro, M., et al.: Incidence of Kawasaki disease in Japan: The nationwide surveys of 1999-2002. Pediatr. Int. *48*:356-361, 2006.
401. Yanagawa, H., Yashiro, M., Nakamura, Y., et al.: Epidemiologic pictures of Kawasaki disease in Japan: From the nationwide incidence survey in 1991 and 1992. Pediatrics *95*:475-479, 1995.
402. Yanagawa, H., Yashiro, M., Nakamura, Y., et al.: Results of 12 nationwide epidemiological incidence surveys of Kawasaki disease in Japan. Arch. Pediatr. Adolesc. Med. *149*:779-783, 1995.
403. Yanase, Y., Takayama, J., Aso, S., et al.: Studies on serum immunoglobulins and delayed skin tests in patients with MCLS. Acta Paediatr. Jpn. *24*:408-409, 1982.
404. Yashiro, M., Nakamura, Y., Hirose, K., et al.: Surveillance of Kawasaki disease in Japan, 1984-1994. *In* Kato, H. (ed.): Kawasaki Disease. Amsterdam, Elsevier Science, 1995, pp. 15-21.
405. Yokota, S.: Heat shock protein as a predisposing and immunopotentiating factor in Kawasaki disease. Acta Paediatr. Jpn. *33*:756-764, 1991.
406. Yutani, C., Go, S., Kamiya, F., et al.: Cardiac biopsy of Kawasaki disease. Arch. Pathol. Lab. Med. *105*:470-473, 1981.
407. Yutani, C., Okano, K., Kamiya, T., et al.: Histopathological study on right endomyocardial biopsy of Kawasaki disease. Br. Heart J. *43*:589-592, 1980.
408. Zalian, F., Falcini, F., Zancan, L., et al.: Acute surgical abdomen as presenting manifestation of Kawasaki disease. J. Pediatr. *142*:731-735, 2003.
409. Zhang, T., Yanagawa, H., Oki, I., et al.: Factors related to the cardiac sequelae of Kawasaki disease one month after initial onset. Acta Paediatr. *91*:517-520, 2002.

CHRONIC FATIGUE SYNDROME

89

Leonard R. Krilov

"All cases are unique and very similar to others." T.S. Eliot, *The Cocktail Party*, 1949.

Chronic fatigue syndrome (CFS) is an illness complex characterized by a prolonged (>6 months) period of constant or intermittent debilitating fatigue in association with multiple, often nonspecific, symptoms that may include new-onset headaches, decreased ability to concentrate, recurrent complaints of sore throat and tender cervical or axillary lymphadenitis, reports of low-grade fever, diffuse muscle or joint pain, postexertional increase in fatigue, and unrefreshing sleep. To date, no specific cause for this syndrome has been identified, and, despite similar arrays of signs and symptoms, patients with CFS likely represent a heterogeneous population. Still, evaluation of groups of patients with this symptom complex has provided information about pathophysiologic changes occurring in patients with CFS, and potentially beneficial, although not curative, approaches to therapy for affected individuals have been developed.

In an attempt to provide a degree of uniformity as a basis for research into the evaluation of such patients, the U.S. Centers for Disease Control and Prevention (CDC) developed a definition of CFS in 1988.[38] These criteria were revised in 1994, with physical signs removed from the definition because they appeared to be unreliably documented in studies, and the required number of symptoms for the diagnosis of CFS decreased from 8 of a list of 11 to 4 of 8 components (Table 89–1).[33] These changes, being less restrictive, may serve to increase the sensitivity of the diagnosis, but they also decrease the specificity. However, these criteria are purely speculative in the absence of any gold standard or definitive diagnostic test for CFS. These 1994 criteria also suggest subdivisions of patients with CFS for research purposes and provide guidelines for non-research clinicians as well. Other international groups have generated similar definitions of CFS for evaluating this condition.[12,54,80]

The primary manifestations of CFS are severe fatigue of more than 6 months' duration that limits activity to less than 50 percent of premorbid function and the association of multiple other symptoms, as outlined in the case definitions of CFS.[33,38,54,80] These symptoms include new or more intense headaches, decreased ability to focus or concentrate, recurrent sore throats, a sensation of tender cervical or axillary lymph nodes, low-grade temperature elevations, myalgias and arthralgias, postexertional fatigue lasting longer than 24 hours, and sleep disturbances (hypersomnia or insomnia). The severity and persistence of these findings vary among individual patients with CSF. In addition, although not included in the case definitions, many patients report dizziness, especially with changes in position, feeling hot when others are cold or vice versa, chronic costochondritis, and a Raynaud-like phenomenon.

HISTORICAL OVERVIEW

In all likelihood, CFS is not a new illness. Numerous conditions with features comparable to those of CFS have appeared in the medical literature during the past several centuries.[91] Many of these descriptions attempted to associate an illness characterized by prolonged debilitating fatigue and numerous other symptoms with an infectious agent. They have included chronic brucellosis,[84] chronic enteroviral syndrome,[17,21,36] chronic candidiasis,[74] myalgic encephalomyelitis,[2] chronic mononucleosis (Epstein-Barr virus [EBV] infection),[3,40,96,97] human herpesvirus type 6 infection,[7,102] human herpesvirus type 7 infection,[26] chronic Lyme disease,[85] parvovirus B19 infection,[45] and a new retroviral infection.[23] Noninfectious conditions described with similarities to CFS include total allergy syndrome, hypoglycemia, neurasthenia, Iceland disease, Royal Free disease, and fibromyalgia rheumatica.[48] In addition to clinical similarity to CFS, all these conditions, at least at the time they were described, lacked a diagnostic test to confirm a definitive causative agent and, in their acute form, manifested with fatigue in association with multiple other complaints.

A review of the experience in the mid-1980s associated groups of patients with CFS-like illness with patients with chronic EBV infection.[3,40,96] These reports described elevated and aberrant

TABLE 89–1 Centers for Disease Control and Prevention 1994 Workshop Case Definition of Chronic Fatigue Syndrome

1. Fatigue (persistent or relapsing) that has new or definite onset, is of >6 months' duration, and leads to a substantial (>50%) reduction in level of activity
   PLUS
2. At least four of the following:
   Impaired memory or concentration
   Sore throat
   Tender lymph nodes: cervical or axillary
   Myalgias
   Arthralgias (multiple joints, without swelling or erythema)
   New onset (or in severity) of headaches
   Unrefreshing sleep (hypersomnia or insomnia)
   Postexertional fatigue lasting >24 hours
   AND
3. The absence of another diagnosis for the individual's signs and symptoms

Modified from Fukuda, K., Straus, S. E., Hickie, I., et al.: The chronic fatigue syndrome: A comprehensive approach to its definition and study. Ann. Intern. Med. 121:953-959, 1994.

patterns of EBV antibody responses in individuals with prolonged fatigue and multiple symptoms consistent with CFS. Acute infectious mononucleosis also often manifests with fatigue, fever, malaise, sore throat, lymphadenitis, and multiple systemic complaints, although typically in a more pronounced manner. Subsequent studies, however, revealed that the elevation or pattern of EBV antibody responses in such patients were not consistently different from findings in others who resolved symptoms of acute EBV infection.[60] Additionally, shedding of EBV in secretions was not increased in these individuals, and no association was found between viral shedding and severity of symptoms.[98] Furthermore, no response to the antiviral drug acyclovir occurred in a group of such patients in a placebo-controlled, double-blind, crossover study, in terms of improvement of clinical symptoms.[93] After these observations were made, the name *chronic fatigue syndrome* was chosen to define this illness,[38] at least until a specific cause or marker for this illness is identified.

Cameron and colleagues recently reported on a cohort of patients with prolonged fatigue after having infectious mononucleosis. These investigators demonstrated no difference in EBV load in eight patients with 6 months or more of disabling symptoms after the diagnosis of infectious mononucleosis was established, and again they demonstrated a lack of correlation between persistent symptoms and viremia or altered host responses to EBV.[10]

EPIDEMIOLOGY

The definitions of CFS allow for attempts to characterize the prevalence and demographic features of this condition. Still, given the vagaries of the symptom complex, possible variations in application of the diagnosis by different health care providers, and the potential differences within groups of people to seek medical attention for this condition, data reported on these issues may not be a complete representation of the epidemiology of this condition. CFS has been reported in all age groups, including children as young as 5 years of age, and in all ethnic, racial, and socioeconomic groups, but most CFS cases have been reported to occur in middle- to upper-class white women with a median age of 35 to 40 years.[47] Based on a study of physician-diagnosed patients from four cities using the 1988 case definition of CFS,[1] the CDC estimates a minimum prevalence rate of CFS of 2 to 10 cases per 100,000, or higher, in adults aged 18 years and older in the United States.[8,57,71] A population-based descriptive epidemiologic study conducted by the CDC in Kansas estimated the prevalence of CFS to be 235 per 100,000 persons and a 1-year incidence to be 180 per 100,000 persons.[75] Studies from outside the United States have reported similar or higher prevalence rates of CFS in adults.[27,54]

Although the CDC definition does not include age criteria for the diagnosis of CFS, the prevalence of CFS in the pediatric age range has not been studied well. Some researchers have suggested that the diagnosis of CFS should not be used in children, to avoid potential delay in making an alternative medical or psychological diagnosis.[70] However, many referral centers have reported groups of pediatric patients, primarily adolescents, with features and a clinical course similar to those reported in adults.[5,13,28,50,58,83] Furthermore, in these studies, missed or alternative diagnoses were not found, despite years of follow-up. Rimes and colleagues reported prevalence rates of CFS in an adolescent population similar to those reported in adults.[76]

In these pediatric studies, a predominance of female patients with a median age of 14 years at the time of diagnosis was noted. Additionally, these patients were from predominately middle- to upper-class families, and, as discussed later, their signs and symptoms at presentation (Table 89–2) and their course of illness were

TABLE 89-2 Symptoms Reported by 58 Children and Adolescents Evaluated for Chronic Fatigue Syndrome (1989 to 1994)

Symptom	No. of Patients	Percentage (%)
Fatigue	58	100
Headache	43	74
Sore throat	34	59
Abdominal pain	28	48
Fever	21	36
Impaired cognition	19	33
Myalgia	18	31
Diarrhea	17	29
Adenopathy	17	29
Anorexia	16	28
Nausea/vomiting	15	26
Congestion	13	22
Dizziness	10	17
Arthralgia	10	17
Otitis	6	10
Cough	6	10
Rash	5	9
Sweats	5	9
Chills	4	7
Depression	4	7

From Krilov, L. R., Fisher, M., Friedman, S. B., et al.: Course and outcome of chronic fatigue in children and adolescents. Pediatrics 102:360-366, 1998.

similar to those reported in adults with CFS. CDC studies suggest that the prevalence of CFS in adolescents approaches that reported in adults, but cases in children younger than 12 years of age occur much less commonly.[33] One suggestion is that a shorter duration of symptoms (3 to 4 months versus 6 months) may be appropriate for establishing the diagnosis of CFS in pediatric patients.[33,41] Multiple family members with CFS may be seen as well, but to date, evidence that CFS is contagious does not exist.

ETIOLOGY AND PATHOGENESIS

INFECTION

As noted previously, an infectious origin of CFS has not been demonstrated to date, and a single microorganism as the cause of CFS is unlikely. However, an acute infection appears possibly to play a role in precipitating CFS because most (as many as two thirds) patients with CFS relate a sudden onset of their symptoms to an acute infection, most often infectious mononucleosis. Lyme disease[56,85] and an influenza-like illness[39] also have been reported in association with the onset of CFS.

IMMUNOLOGIC DYSFUNCTION

A role for immunologic dysfunction in CFS has been suggested, based on numerous studies demonstrating abnormalities in lymphocyte function or cytokine production.[9,46,53,61,92,95,99] However, these findings have not been reproducible in different groups of patients with CSF. Some evidence suggests that nonspecific elevation of antibody titers and an increase in allergic symptoms occur in patients with CSF.[94] However, these findings are mild, and similar immunologic changes may be seen in other conditions, including depression. Individuals with CFS may report an increased frequency and duration of infections compared with their pre-CFS state, but they tend to be mostly routine viral illnesses. Neither unusual or opportunistic infection nor increased risk for developing malignant disease has been observed in these individuals. Intravenous immunoglobulin infusions have not demonstrated long-term clinical benefit when they are administered to patients with CFS and may cause significant adverse reactions.[55,69,90]

Some studies have focused on potential genetic markers of CFS using DNA microarray technology.[86] An analysis of cytokine gene polymorphisms in 80 Italian patients with a diagnosis of CFS assessed using the 1994 CDC definition reported significant difference in tumor necrosis factor and interferon-γ phenotypes compared with controls. The authors hypothesized a potential altered immunologic or inflammatory response based on these differences as potentially contributing to the pathogenesis of CFS.[11] An analysis of prolonged post-infectious fatigue in patients who had had mononucleosis identified certain genes involved in immune responses, and hormonal and neurologic pathways that were altered in a subset of patients with mononucleosis were associated with the development of prolonged fatigue.[10] The CDC has developed a molecular epidemiology program to standardize assays that can be applied to understanding the potential of alterations in gene expression in CFS (available at http://www.cdc.ncidod/diseases/cfs/publications/molecular_epi.htm; accessed 7/12/2007).

NEUROLOGIC FEATURES

Many patients with CFS report cognitive impairment manifest as a decreased ability to concentrate and focus, difficulty in processing information, and trouble with word recall. Complaints of headache (new onset or altered pattern) and other neurologic symptoms, such as paresthesias and dysequilibrium, also are reported commonly by patients with CFS.

Despite these complaints, physical examination does not reveal abnormal neurologic signs. Formal neuropyschometric testing also may not reveal objective abnormalities to the extent reported by the patient. Whether this discrepancy reflects a problem with testing methods or altered perception on the part of the individual is uncertain at this time.[7,66]

Magnetic resonance imaging (MRI) studies have been reported to show an increase in cerebral white matter abnormalities in patients with CFS.[7,65,78] Similarly, in many studies, single photon emission computed tomography (SPECT) scanning has demonstrated changes in perfusion in certain areas of the brain in patients with CFS.[19,30,79] In other studies, however, abnormalities specific to CFS have not been observed consistently, and methodologic concerns have been raised regarding the interpretation of abnormal findings cited previously.[18,37] An abnormality at the base of the fourth ventricle detected on focal computed tomography (CT) scan of the base of the brain and responding to neurosurgical intervention was reported in a group of patients with CFS,[35] but this defect is not seen on routine CT or magnetic resonance imaging (MRI) views, and this observation requires confirmation by other researchers before determining its significance for these patients. At present, imaging of the central nervous system is not indicated routinely in the evaluation of a patient with CFS.

ENDOCRINOLOGIC FACTORS

Subtle defects in the hypothalamic-pituitary-adrenal axis have been described in cohorts of patients with CFS. These abnormalities include decreased free urinary cortisol levels and exaggerated adrenal responsiveness to corticotropin infusion.[25] These changes are quantitatively minor, and mean values are still within normal for age and sex, thus rendering these values unreliable as a diagnostic test for CFS. Similar changes have been described in patients with fibromyalgia and post-traumatic stress disorder.

CARDIOVASCULAR FACTORS

In 1995, investigators at Johns Hopkins Hospital in Baltimore described a cohort of seven adolescents with chronic fatigue and autonomic dysfunction as assessed by tilt-table testing.[77] Furthermore, these patients reported improvement or resolution of symptoms, including fatigue, with treatment of their orthostatic intolerance. Further studies from this group demonstrated some component of orthostatic hypotension in 92 percent of patients with CFS.[6] Studies in groups of adults, in contrast, showed tilt-table test abnormalities in only 25 to 40 percent of patients.[31,82] Whether this finding reflects true age-related differences in this phenomenon in patients with CFS is uncertain, given potential methodologic differences in the performance of the tests.

The pattern of orthostatic intolerance among adolescents with CFS was characterized further by Stewart and colleagues and is consistent with the postural orthostatic tachycardia syndrome (POTS).[87-89] Symptoms of POTS may develop after an acute infectious illness or with severe deconditioning and include fatigue, light-headedness, impaired cognition, inappropriate sweating, headache, palpitations, nausea, vomiting, and tremulousness. These authors suggest that CFS may be an extreme expression of POTS in at least some cases.

The importance of these cardiovascular findings in CFS remains unsettled. Subjective components may contribute to defining a tilt-table test as abnormal because subjects are not blinded during these studies. Some healthy individuals also may experience hypotension during these tests. Further studies defining the effect of treatment of POTS on the course of CFS should help to answer this question. In this context, evaluation and therapy of orthostatic changes, especially if dizziness is a significant component of the patient's complaints, may be indicated.[109]

SLEEP PHYSIOLOGY

Sleep disturbances have been described in selected groups of patients with CFS, and some of these patients may be amenable to therapy.[52,73] However, no single pattern of sleep abnormality has been reported for these patients, and in our experience, the pattern of hypersomnia or insomnia tends to improve as the patient recovers.

PSYCHOLOGICAL COMPONENTS

Psychological factors have been considered in the origin and perpetuation of CFS. Adults with CFS have demonstrated a higher frequency of depression and other psychiatric disorders before the onset of their CFS compared with age-matched controls.[1,51] Certainly, many of the symptoms reported in CFS also are reported commonly in depression. They may include sleep disturbances, loss of energy, difficulty in concentrating, changes in appetite, and musculoskeletal complaints. Studies in children and adolescents with CFS also have shown significant psychological features, especially depression and somatization, compared with both healthy controls and those with other chronic illnesses (e.g., juvenile rheumatoid arthritis, cancer, cystic fibrosis).[13,14,41,67,104] Still, certain features of CFS argue against its being solely a variant of depression. Individuals with CFS do not have the mood-related symptoms reported in patients with clinical depression. These mood-related symptoms include negative affect, anhedonia, low self-esteem, and suicidal ideation. Furthermore, patients with CFS and their families have a firm belief that an infectious, immunologic, or other medical cause for their symptoms exists, and the patients desire a return to normal activities.

In considering the possible link between depression or psychological stress and CFS, several possible relationships may exist. Preexisting depression or stress may create a psychological vulnerability that allows for the development of CFS in combination with any of numerous other factors discussed previously. Studies have demonstrated a role for psychological factors predicting the response to mononucleosis and influenza.[39,43] Similar factors may be involved in the development of CFS. Alternatively, depression may be a physiologic consequence of the central nervous system changes that occur in those who develop CFS, just as decreased concentration and memory occur as part of the syndrome.[41,104] Furthermore, reactive depression may occur in these patients in response to the inability to participate in their usual activities and to absence from school and separation from friends. Finally, CFS may be, at least in some cases, a manifestation of separation anxiety or school phobia in which secondary gain, as a conversion reaction, is playing a major role. Certainly, at least a subset of adolescents and children with CFS in our experience does not appear eager to return to school or activities, and secondary gain may play a role in the perpetuation of their illness.[48]

In summary, each of these potential links between depression or stress and CFS likely plays a role, with the relative contribution of each feature varying for different people. This suggestion is consistent with the overall hypothesis that many different factors appear to contribute to the development and perpetuation of CFS. The relative contribution of these different features may vary from individual to individual and even for the same patient over the course of the illness. The assessment and management of the patient with CFS should attempt to consider these issues and their relative importance for that individual.

DIAGNOSIS, DIFFERENTIAL DIAGNOSIS, AND EVALUATION

The diagnosis of CFS is one of exclusion and requires a comprehensive history. In the pediatric population, this information is obtained best from the patient and parents. Additionally, we request that families bring prior medical records, test results, and pertinent school records, to facilitate a complete evaluation. This process may be lengthy because the details are complicated, long standing, and often a source of debate between the patient and parents. The history should focus on the onset of illness, the duration and severity of symptoms, prior evaluations (often multiple) as well as medical history before the illness, family history, academic performance, and social history. The physical examination of the individual with suspected CFS almost always is essentially normal despite the multitude of symptoms. Findings of mild pharyngeal erythema and cervical adenopathy commonly are reported. However, finding fever, weight loss, significant adenopathy, or organomegaly should alert the clinician to the possibility of an alternative diagnosis.

DeMeirleir and colleagues reported increased detection of a 37-kd, 2-5A-synthetase binding protein in peripheral blood mononuclear cells from patients with CFS compared with healthy controls.[24] These binding proteins are related to the ribonuclease L antiviral pathway of these cells. This finding requires further confirmation before it can be considered a potential diagnostic test for CFS. At present, no specific tests for diagnosing CFS exist, and laboratory testing is aimed primarily at eliminating other possible diagnoses. Most patients have undergone multiple laboratory tests before a diagnosis of CFS has been considered, but these tests may be repeated or completed as part of the initial CFS evaluation. Additionally, interpreting previously performed tests may be part of the initial patient assessment. Screening studies may include complete blood count with differential and platelets, erythrocyte sedimentation rate, hepatic and renal func-

tion studies, urinalysis, and thyroid function tests. Additional tests that may be indicated based on history and physical examination may include toxicology screening, human immunodeficiency virus serology, antinuclear antibody, rheumatoid factor, tuberculin skin test, and cortisol level. Serologic evaluations for EBV, Lyme disease, and group A streptococcal infection may be requested based on history and physical infection. In most instances, these tests are not indicated; however, they often are obtained before CFS is suspected, and they need to be appropriately reviewed or repeated as part of the initial evaluation for CFS. Screening radiographic studies may include a chest radiograph or imaging of the paranasal sinuses based on the patient's symptoms.

Elimination of every possible disorder that may cause a patient to experience prolonged fatigue is impossible, but when guided by history, physical examination, and laboratory screening tests as outlined previously, the clinician can make a reliable diagnosis of CFS. Follow-up for periods of 4 to 13 years for pediatric patients diagnosed with CFS have not identified cases of missed or alternative diagnoses for their complaints.[4,50] In general, the longer the duration and the greater the number of symptoms, the less the need for extensive laboratory evaluations to suggest the diagnosis of CFS. Conversely, alternative diagnoses should be considered if a single symptom dominates the clinical presentation or if physical examination or laboratory tests reveal significant abnormalities.

Psychosocial assessment is indicated for all children and adolescents presenting for CFS evaluation. The extent of such evaluation may be limited to assessment by primary care personnel or may include collaboration with a social worker, psychologist, or psychiatrist, based on the individual's needs and the comfort level of the examiner. Cardiopulmonary and neurologic evaluations may be used in some cases, both to consider possible alternative diagnoses and to assist in assessing factors that may be contributing to the symptoms of CFS.

MANAGEMENT

"One of the essential qualities of the clinician is interest in humanity, for the secret of care of the patient is in caring for the patient."

Dr. Francis Peabody, 1926 (wall plaque, lobby of the Massachusetts General Hospital, Boston)

Management of patients with CFS is aimed at providing a combination of supportive treatment and emotional support.[32] Such an approach is outlined in Table 89-3.

This process can be initiated during the initial evaluation, with a discussion of the diagnostic criteria for CFS and a review of previously obtained laboratory tests. The relationship between physical and psychological symptoms can be explained, and the patient and family can be reassured that symptoms are real, even if the symptoms have psychiatric components. Additionally, the patient and family can be advised that most children and adolescents with CFS do well over time[4,28,49,50] and have a better long-term outlook than that described for adults with CFS.[42,108] Furthermore, emphasizing the frequent ups and downs in symptoms that generally characterize the course of CFS is important in assisting the patient and family to develop coping skills. This assistance may include guidance on how to modify lifestyle most appropriately and how to set realistic schedules and goals. Studies from the United Kingdom suggest that formal cognitive-behavioral therapy[22,72,81,107] or graded exercise programs, or both, may be beneficial for patients with CFS.[15,34,105]

Many other therapies have been advocated by different groups for patients with CFS. These treatments may include supplements, such as essential fatty acids,[103] magnesium,[20] liver extract

TABLE 89–3   Approach to Management of Chronic Fatigue Syndrome in Children and Adolescents

Evaluation and explanation of the diagnosis, including overview of multifactorial components

Reassurance that symptoms are real

Anticipatory guidance regarding secondary problems, up-and-down course of syndrome, secondary gain

Coping skills: lifestyle modification, decreased stress, and realistic expectations and schedule

Cognitive behavioral approaches: gradual increases in activity, an exercise program, attention to sleep patterns, attention to nutrition

Psychological support for individual and family

Educational issues: return to classes, home tutors, neuropsychiatric testing as indicated

Relationship issues: friends and family

Follow-up plan: monitoring of physical symptoms and psychological issues, ongoing guidance and reassurance (follow-up visits every 4 to 6 weeks)

Minimize: shopping for a doctor; unnecessary testing; family strain; unconventional, unproven, or experimental therapies

Modified from Krilov, L. R., and Fisher, M.: Chronic fatigue syndrome in children and adolescents. Contemp. Pediatr. 19:61-68, 2002.

injections,[44] and vitamin and nutritional supplements,[59] as well as pharmacologic treatments, such as steroids,[16,62,68] reduced nicotinamide adenine dinucleotide,[100] antidepressants,[64,101] and growth hormone.[63] Homeopathic therapies, osteopathy, and massage therapy[29] also have been reported to be beneficial in the management of CFS. Most of these approaches have not been studied adequately to allow definitive comment on their potential benefit for a given patient. Still, the clinician should be aware of them, to help guide patients who are likely to hear about them from other patients or outside sources, including the Internet.[35,106,107]

PROGNOSIS AND FUTURE DIRECTIONS

CFS likely affects heterogeneous groups of patients, and a single cause or definitive treatment modality most likely will not be uncovered. Nonetheless, studying groups of such patients yields helpful information on the pathophysiology of this condition, and useful steps to address and alleviate symptoms for patients have been reported. In recognition of the significance of this entity, the CDC launched an awareness campaign, including the development of an Internet site for health care professionals and the public (http://www.cdc.gov.cfs; accessed 7/12/2007). In addition, long-term follow-up data demonstrating improvement over the course of time, especially in children and adolescents, without emergence of significant other conditions, are encouraging for patients, families, and clinicians caring for such individuals.

REFERENCES

1. Abbey, S. E., and Garfinkel, P. E.: Chronic fatigue syndrome and the psychiatrist. Can. J. Psychiatry 35:625-633, 1990.
2. Acheson, E. D.: The clinical syndrome variously called benign myalgic encephalomyelitis, Iceland disease and epidemic neuromyasthenia. Am. J. Med. 26:569-955, 1959.
3. Barnes, D. M.: Mystery disease at Lake Tahoe challenges virologists and clinicians. Science 234:541-542, 1986.
4. Bell, D. S., Jordan, K., and Robinson, M.: Thirteen-year follow-up of children and adolescents with chronic fatigue syndrome. Pediatrics 107:994-998, 2001.
5. Bell, K. M., Cookfair, D., Bell, D. S., et al.: Risk factors associated with chronic fatigue syndrome in a cluster of pediatric cases. Rev. Infect. Dis. 13(Suppl.): S320-S338, 1991.
6. Bou-Holaigah, I., Rowe, P. C., Kan, J., and Calkins, H.: The relationship between neurally mediated hypotension and the chronic fatigue syndrome. JAMA 274:961-967, 1995.
7. Buchwald, D., Cheney, P. R., Peterson, D. L., et al.: A chronic illness characterized by fatigue, neurologic and immunologic disorders, and active human herpesvirus type 6 infection. Ann. Intern. Med. 116:103-113, 1992.
8. Buchwald, D., Umali, P., Umali, J., et al.: Chronic fatigue and the chronic fatigue syndrome: Prevalence in a Pacific Northwest health care system. Ann. Intern. Med. 123:81-88, 1995.
9. Caligiuri, M., Murray, C., Buchwald, D., et al.: Phenotypic and functional deficiency of natural killer cells of patients with chronic fatigue syndrome. J. Immunol. 139:3306-3313, 1987.
10. Cameron, B., Galbraith, S., Zhang, Y., et al.: Gene expression correlates of post-infective fatigue syndrome after infectious mononucleosis. J. Infect. Dis. 196:56-66, 2007.
11. Carlo-Stella, N., Badulli, C., DeSilvestri, A., et al.: A first study of cytokine genomic polymorphisms in CFS: Positive association of TNF-857 and IFNγ 874 rare alleles. Clin. Exp. Rheumatol. 24:179-182, 2006.
12. Carruthers, B. M., Jain, A. K., DeMeirleir, K. L., et al.: Myalgic encephalomyelitis/chronic fatigue syndrome: Clinical working definition, diagnostic and treatment protocols. J. Chronic Fatigue Syndr. 11:7-36, 2003.
13. Carter, B. D., Edwards, J. F., Kronenberger, W. G., et al.: Case control study of chronic fatigue in pediatric patients. Pediatrics 95:179-186, 1995.
14. Carter, B. D., Kronenberger, W. G., Edwards, J. F., et al.: Differential diagnosis of chronic fatigue in children: Behavioral and emotional dimensions. Dev. Behav. Pediatr. 17:16-21, 1996.
15. Chambers, D., Bagnall, A. M., Hempel, S., and Forbes, C.: Interventions for the treatment, management and rehabilitation of patients with chronic fatigue syndrome/myalgic encephalitis: An updated systematic review. J. R. Soc. Med. 99:506-520, 2006.
16. Cleare, A. J., Heap, E., Malhi, G. S., Wessely S., et al.: Low-dose hydrocortisone in chronic fatigue syndrome: A randomized crossover trial. Lancet 353:455-458, 1999.
17. Clements, G. B., McGarry, F., Nairn, C., and Galbraith D. N.: Detection of enterovirus-specific RNA in serum: The relationship to chronic fatigue syndrome. J. Med. Virol. 45:156-161, 1995.
18. Cope, H., and David, A. S.: Neuroimaging in chronic fatigue. J. Neurol. Neurosurg. Psychiatry 60:471-473, 1996.
19. Costa, D. C., Tannock, C., and Brostoff, J.: Brainstem perfusion is impaired in chronic fatigue syndrome. Q. J. Med. 88:767-773, 1995.
20. Cox, I. M., Campell, M. J., and Dowson D.: Red blood cell magnesium and chronic fatigue syndrome. Lancet 337:757-760, 1991.
21. Cunningham, L., Bowles, N. E., Lane, R. J. M., et al.: Persistence of enteroviral RNA in chronic fatigue syndrome is associated with abnormal production of equal amounts of positive and negative strands of enteroviral RNA. J. Gen. Virol. 71:1399-1402, 1990.
22. Deale, A., Chalder, T., Marks, I., and Wessely, S.: Cognitive behavior therapy for chronic fatigue syndrome: A randomized controlled trial. Am. J. Psychiatry 154:408-414, 1997.
23. DeFritas, E., Hilliard, B., Cheney, P. R., et al.: Retroviral sequences related to human T-lymphotropic virus type II in patients with chronic fatigue immune dysfunction syndrome. Proc. Natl. Acad. Sci. U. S. A. 88:2922-2926, 1991.
24. DeMeirleir, K., Bisbal, C., Campine, I., et al.: A 37 kDa 2-5A binding protein as a potential biochemical marker for chronic fatigue syndrome. Am. J. Med. 108:99-105, 2000.
25. Demitrack, M. A., Dale, J. K., Straus, S. E., et al.: Evidence for impaired activation of the hypothalamic-pituitary-adrenal axis in patients with chronic fatigue syndrome. J. Clin. Endocrinol. Metab. 73:1224-1234, 1991.
26. DiLuca, D., Zorzenon, M., Mirandola, P., et al.: Human herpesvirus 6 and human herpesvirus 7 in chronic fatigue syndrome. J. Clin. Microbiol. 33:1660-1661, 1995.
27. Dowsett, E. G., and Colby, J.: Long-term sickness absence due to ME/CFS in UK schools: An epidemiological study with medical and educational implications. J. Chronic Fatigue Syndr. 3:29-42, 1997.
28. Feder, H. M., Dworkin, P. H., and Orkin, C.: Outcome of 48 pediatric patients with chronic fatigue: A clinical experience. Arch. Fam. Med. 3:1049-1055, 1994.
29. Field, T. M., Sunshine, W., Hernandez-Reif, M., et al.: Massage therapy effects on depression and somatic symptoms in chronic fatigue syndrome. J. Chronic Fatigue Syndr. 3:43-51, 1997.
30. Fischler, B., D'Haenen, H., Cluydts, R., et al.: Comparison of 99m Tc HMPAO SPECT scan between chronic fatigue syndrome, major depression and healthy controls: An exploratory study of clinical correlates of regional cerebral blood flow. Neuropsychobiology 34:175-183, 1996.
31. Freeman, R., and Komaroff, A. L.: Does the chronic fatigue syndrome involve the autonomic system? Am. J. Med. 102:357-362, 1997.
32. Fukuda, K., and Gantz, N. M.: Management strategies for chronic fatigue syndrome. Fed. Pract. 12:12-27, 1995.
33. Fukuda, K., Straus, S. E., Hickie, I., et al.: The chronic fatigue syndrome: A comprehensive approach to its definition and study. Ann. Intern. Med. 121:953-959, 1994.
34. Fulcher, K. Y., and White, P. D.: Randomised, double-blind, placebo-controlled trial of graded exercise in patients with chronic fatigue syndrome. BMJ 314:1647-1652, 1997.
35. Gantz, N. M., and Coldsmith, E. E.: Chronic fatigue syndrome and fibromyalgia resources on the World Wide Web: A descriptive journey. Clin. Infect. Dis. 32:938-948, 2001.

36. Gow, J. W., Behan, W. M. H., Simpson, K., et al.: Studies on enterovirus in patients with chronic fatigue syndrome. Clin. Infect. Dis. *18*(Suppl. 1): S126-S129, 1994.

37. Greco, A., Tannock, C., Brostoff, J., and Costa, D. C.: Brain MR in chronic fatigue syndrome. A. J. N. R. Am. J. Neuroradiol. *18*:1265-1269, 1997.

38. Holmes, G. P., Kaplan, J. E., Gantz, N. M., et al.: Chronic fatigue syndrome: A working case definition. Ann. Intern. Med. *108*:387-389, 1988.

39. Imboden, J. B., Canter, A., and Cluff, L. E.: Convalescence from influenza. Arch. Intern. Med. *108*:115-121, 1961.

40. Jones, J. F., Ray, C. G., Minnich, L. L., et al.: Evidence for Epstein-Barr virus infection in patients with persistent, unexplained illnesses: Elevated anti-early antigen antibodies. Ann. Intern. Med. *102*:1-7, 1985.

41. Joyce, E., Blumentahl, S., and Wessely, S.: Memory, attention, and executive function in chronic fatigue syndrome. J. Neurol. Neurosurg. Psychiatry *60*:495-503, 1996.

42. Joyce, J., Hotopf, M., and Wessely, S.: The prognosis of chronic fatigue and chronic fatigue syndrome: A systematic review. Q. J. Med. *90*:223-233, 1997.

43. Kasl, S. V., Evans, A. S., and Niederman, J. C.: Psychosocial risk factors in the development of infectious mononucleosis. Psychosom. Med. *41*:445-466, 1979.

44. Kaslow, J. E., Rucker, L., and Onishi, R.: Liver extract–folic acid–cyanocobalamin vs. placebo for chronic fatigue syndrome. Arch. Intern Med. *149*: 2501-2503, 1989.

45. Kerr, J.R., Bracewell, J., Laing, I., et al.: Chronic fatigue syndrome and arthralgia following parvovirus B19 infection. J. Rheumatol. *29*:595-602, 2002.

46. Klimas, N. G., Salvato, F. R., Morgan, R., and Fletcher, M. A.: Immunologic abnormalities in chronic fatigue syndrome. J. Clin. Microbiol. *28*:1403-1410, 1990.

47. Komaroff, A. L., Fagioli, L. R., Geiger, A. M, et al.: An examination of the working case definition of chronic fatigue syndrome. Am. J. Med. *100*:56-64, 1996.

48. Krilov, L. R.: Chronic fatigue syndrome. Pediatr. Ann. *24*:290-294, 1995.

49. Krilov, L. R., and Fisher, M.: Chronic fatigue syndrome in children and adolescents. Contemp. Pediatr. *19*:61-68, 2002.

50. Krilov, L. R., Fisher, M., Friedman, S. B., et al.: Course and outcome of chronic fatigue in children and adolescents. Pediatrics *102*:360-366, 1998.

51. Kruesi, D., Dale, J., and Straus, S. E.: Psychiatric diagnoses in patients who have chronic fatigue syndrome. J. Clin. Psychiatry *50*:53-56, 1989.

52. Krupp, L. B., Jandorf, L., Coyle, P. K., and Mendelson, W. B.: Sleep disturbance in chronic fatigue syndrome. J. Psychosom. Res. *37*:325-331, 1993.

53. Landay, A. L., Jessop, C., Lennette, E. T., and Levy, J. A.: Chronic fatigue syndrome: Clinical condition associated with immune activation. Lancet *338*:707-721, 1991.

54. Lloyd, A., Hickie, I., Boughton, C. R., et al.: Prevalence of chronic fatigue syndrome in an Australian population. Med. J. Aust. *153*:522-528, 1990.

55. Lloyd, A., Hickie, I., Wakefield, D., et al.: A double-blind, placebo-controlled trial of intravenous immunoglobulin therapy in patients with chronic fatigue syndrome. Am. J. Med. *89*:561-568, 1990.

56. MacDonald, K. L., Osterholm, M. T., LeDell, K. H., et al.: A case-controlled study to assess possible triggers and cofactors in chronic fatigue syndrome. Am. J. Med. *100*:548-554, 1996.

57. Marshall, G. S.: Report of a workshop on the epidemiology, natural history, and pathogenesis of chronic fatigue syndrome in adolescents. J. Pediatr. *134*:395-405, 1999.

58. Marshall, G. S., Gesser, R. M., Yamanishi, K., and Starr, S. E.: Chronic fatigue in children: Clinical features, Epstein-Barr virus and human herpesvirus 6 serology and long term follow-up. Pediatr. Infect. Dis. J. *10*:287-290, 1991.

59. Martin, R. W. Y., Ogston, S. A., and Evans, J. R.: Effects of vitamin and mineral supplementations on symptoms associated with chronic fatigue syndrome with coxsackie B antibodies. J. Nutr. Med. *4*:11-23, 1994.

60. Mawle, A. C., Nisenbaum, R., and Dobbins, J. G., et al.: Seroepidemiology of chronic fatigue syndrome: A case-control study. Clin. Infect. Dis. *21*: 1386-1389, 1995.

61. Mawle, A. C., Nisenbaum, R., Dobbins, J. G., et al.: Immune responses associated with chronic fatigue syndrome: A case-control study. J. Infect. Dis. *175*:136-141, 1997.

62. McKenzie, R., O'Fallon, A., Dale, J., et al.: Low-dose hydrocortisone for treatment of chronic fatigue syndrome: A randomized controlled trial. JAMA *280*:1061-1066, 1998.

63. Moorkens, G., Wynants, H., and Abs, R.: Effect of growth hormone treatment in patients with chronic fatigue syndrome. Growth Horm. IGF Res. *8*: 131-133, 1998.

64. Natelson, B. H., Cheu, J., Pareja, J., et al.: Randomized, double-blind, controlled placebo-phase in trial of low dose phenelzine in the chronic fatigue syndrome. Psychopharmacology *124*:226-230, 1996.

65. Natelson, B. H., Cohen, J. M., Brassloff, I., et al.: A controlled study of brain magnetic resonance imaging in patients with the chronic fatigue syndrome. J. Neurol. Sci. *120*:213-217, 1993.

66. National Institutes of Allergy Infectious Diseases: CFS. Available at http://www3.niaid.gov/topics/womensHealth.pdf.

67. Pelcovitz, D., Septimus, A., Friedman, S. B., et al.: Psychosocial correlates of chronic fatigue syndrome in adolescent girls. Dev. Behav. Pediatr. *16*:333-338, 1995.

68. Peterson, P. K., Pheley, A., Schreoppel, J., et al.: A preliminary placebo-controlled crossover trial of fludrocortisone for chronic fatigue syndrome. Arch. Intern. Med. *158*:908-914, 1998.

69. Peterson, P. K., Shepard, J., Macres, M., et al.: A controlled trial of intravenous immunoglobulin G in chronic fatigue syndrome. Am. J. Med. *89*: 554-560, 1990.

70. Plioplys, A. V.: Chronic fatigue syndrome should not be diagnosed in children. Pediatrics. *100*:270-271, 1997.

71. Price, P. K., North, C. S., Wessely, S., and Fraser, V. J.: Estimating the prevalence of chronic fatigue syndrome and associated symptoms in the community. Public Health Rep. *107*:514-522, 1992.

72. Prins, J., Bleijenberg, G., Bazelmans, E., et al.: Cognitive behaviour therapy for chronic fatigue syndrome: A multicentre randomized controlled trial. Lancet *357*:841-847, 2001.

73. Regestein, Q. R., and Monk, T. H.: Delayed sleep phase syndrome: A review of its clinical aspects. Am. J. Psychiatry *152*:602-608, 1995.

74. Renfro, L., Feder, H. M., Lane, T. J., et al.: Yeast connection among 100 patients with chronic fatigue. Am. J. Med. *86*:165-168, 1989.

75. Reyes, M., Nisenbsum, R., and Hoaglin, D.C.: Prevalence and incidence of chronic fatigue syndrome in Wichita, Kansas. Arch. Intern. Med. *163*: 1530-1536, 2003.

76. Rimes, K.A., Goodman, R., Hotopf, M., et al.: Incidence, prognosis, and risk factors for fatigue and chronic fatigue syndrome in adolescents: A prospective community study. Pediatrics *119*:e603-e609, 2007.

77. Rowe, P. C., Bou-Holaigah, I., Kan, J. S., and Calkins, H.: Is neurally mediated hypotension an unrecognized cause of chronic fatigue? Lancet *345*: 623-624, 1995.

78. Schwartz, R. B., Garada, B. M., Komaroff, A. L., et al.: Detection of intracranial abnormalities in patients with chronic fatigue syndrome: Comparison of MR imaging and SPECT. A. J. R. Am. J. Roentgenol. *162*:935-941, 1994.

79. Schwartz, R. B., Komaroff, A. L., Garada, B. M., et al.: SPECT imaging of the brain: Comparison of findings in patients with chronic fatigue syndrome, AIDS dementia complex, and major unipolar depression. A. J. R. Am. J. Roentgenol. *162*:943-951, 1994.

80. Sharpe, M.: A report—chronic fatigue syndrome: Guidelines for research. J. R. Soc. Med. *84*:118-121, 1991.

81. Sharpe, M., Hawton, K., Simkin, S., et al.: Cognitive behaviour therapy for the chronic fatigue syndrome: A randomized controlled trial. BMJ *312*:22-26, 1996.

82. Sisto, S. A., Tapp, W., Dristal, S., et al.: Vagal tone is reduced during paced breathing in patients with the chronic fatigue syndrome. Clin. Auton. Res. *5*:139-143, 1995.

83. Smith, M. S., Mitchell, J., Corey, L., et al.: Chronic fatigue in adolescents. Pediatrics *88*:195-202, 1991.

84. Spink, W. W.: What is chronic brucellosis? Ann. Intern. Med. *35*:358-374, 1951.

85. Steere, A. C., Taylor, E., McHugh, G. L., and Logigian, E. L.: The overdiagnosis of Lyme disease. JAMA *269*:1812-1816, 1993.

86. Steinau, M., Unger, E., Vernon, S., et al.: Differential display PCR of peripheral blood for biomarker discovery in chronic fatigue syndrome. J. Mol. Med. *82*:750-755, 2004.

87. Stewart, J. Autonomic nervous system dysfunction in adolescents with postural orthostatic tachycardia syndrome and chronic fatigue syndrome is characterized by attenuated vagal baroreflex and potentiated sympathetic vasomotion. Pediatr. Res. *48*:218-226, 2000.

88. Stewart, J. M., Gewitz, M. H., Weldon, A., and Munoz, J.: Patterns of orthostatic intolerance: The orthostatic tachycardia syndrome and adolescent chronic fatigue. J. Pediatr. *135*:218-225, 1999.

89. Stewart, J. M., Gewitz, M. H., Weldon, A., et al.: Orthostatic intolerance in adolescent chronic fatigue syndrome. Pediatrics *103*:116-121, 1999.

90. Straus, S. E.: Intravenous immunoglobulin treatment for the chronic fatigue syndrome. Am. J. Med. *89*:551-553, 1990.

91. Straus, S. E.: History of chronic fatigue syndrome. Rev. Infect. Dis. *13*(Suppl. 1):S2-S7, 1991.

92. Straus, S. E., Dale, J. K., Peter, J. B., and Dinarello, C. A.: Circulating lymphokine levels in the chronic fatigue syndrome. J. Infect. Dis. *160*:1085-1086, 1989.

93. Straus, S. E., Dale, D. K., Tobi, M., et al.: Acyclovir treatment of the chronic fatigue syndrome. N. Engl. J. Med. *319*:1692-1698, 1988.

94. Straus, S. E., Dale, J. K., Wright, R., and Metcalfe, D. D.: Allergy and the chronic fatigue syndrome. J. Allergy Clin. Immunol. *81*:791-795, 1988.

95. Straus, S. E., Fritz, S., Dale, J. K., et al.: Lymphocyte phenotype and function in the chronic fatigue syndrome. J. Clin. Immunol. *13*:30-40, 1993.

96. Straus, S. E., Tosato, G., Armstrong, G., et al.: Persisting illness in adults with evidence of Epstein-Barr infection. Ann. Intern Med. *102*:7-16, 1985.

97. Sumaya, C. V.: Serologic and virologic epidemiology of Epstein-Barr virus: Relevance to chronic fatigue syndrome. Rev. Infect. Dis. *13*(Suppl. 1): S19-S25, 1991.

98. Swanink, C. M., Van der Meer, J. W., Vercoulen, J. H., et al.: Epstein-Barr virus (EBV) and the chronic fatigue syndrome: Normal virus load in blood and normal immunologic reactivity in the EBV regression assay. Clin. Infect. Dis. *20*:1390-1392, 1995.

99. Swanink, C. M., Vercoulen, J. H., Galama, J. M., et al.: Lymphocyte subsets, apoptosis, and cytokines in patients with chronic fatigue syndrome. J. Infect. Dis. *173*:460-463, 1996.

100. Vollmer-Conna, U., Lloyd, A., Hickie, I., and Wakefield D.: Chronic fatigue syndrome: An immunological perspective. Aust. N. Z. J. Psychiatry 32:523-527, 1998.
101. Vercoulen, J., Swanink, C. M., Zitman, F. G., et al.: Randomised, double-blind, placebo-controlled study of fluoxetine in chronic fatigue syndrome. Lancet 347:858-861, 1996.
102. Wakefield, D., Lloyd, A., Dwyer, J., et al.: Human herpesvirus 6 and myalgic encephalomyelitis. Lancet 1:1059, 1988.
103. Warren, G., McKendrick, M., and Peet, M.: The role of essential fatty acids in chronic fatigue syndrome: A case-controlled study of red-cell membrane essential fatty acids (EFA) and a placebo-controlled treatment study with high-dose of EFA. Acta Neurol. Scand. 99:112-116, 1999.
104. Weardon, A. J., and Appleby, L.: Research on cognitive complaints and cognitive functioning in patients with chronic fatigue syndrome (CFS): What conclusions can we draw? J. Psychosom. Res. 41:197-211, 1996.
105. Wearden, A. J., Morriss, R. K., Mullis, R., et al.: Randomised, double-blind, placebo-controlled treatment trial of fluoxetine and graded exercise for chronic fatigue syndrome. Br. J. Psychiatry 172:485-492, 1998.
106. Wessely, S.: Chronic fatigue syndrome: Trials and tribulations. JAMA 286:1378-1379, 2001.
107. Whiting, P., Bagnall, A. M., Sowden, A. J., et al.: Interventions for the treatment and management of chronic fatigue syndrome: A systematic review. JAMA 286:1360-1368, 2001.
108. Wilson, A., Hickie, L., Lloyd, A., et al.: Longitudinal study of outcome of chronic fatigue syndrome. BMJ 308:756-759, 1994.
109. Wyller, V.B., Thaulow, E., Amlie, J.P.: Treatment of chronic fatigue and orthostatic intolerance with propranolol. J. Pediatr. 150:654-655, 2007.

INFECTIONS WITH SPECIFIC MICROORGANISMS

BACTERIAL INFECTIONS

CHAPTER 90

NOMENCLATURE FOR AEROBIC AND ANAEROBIC BACTERIA

David A. Bruckner

Table 90–1 represents an update of the current nomenclature, taxonomy, and classification of various microbial agents. Taxonomic methods have evolved from the use of biochemical testing to molecular characterization using 16S or 23S rRNA. Molecular methods have helped to define groupings of organisms and have led to considerable changes in bacterial nomenclature. The classification process is not complete until molecular and phenotypic descriptions of the studied taxa are provided. The primary purpose of nomenclature is to permit us to know as exactly as possible what another clinician, microbiologist, epidemiologist, or investigator is referring to when describing an organism responsible for infecting individuals or for causing an outbreak. The *International Code of Nomenclature of Bacteria*[20] includes rules on how to name bacteria and use the name. The most comprehensive taxonomic information available for bacteriologic classification can be found in *Bergey's Manual of Determinative Bacteriology*, ninth edition,[9] and in *Bergey's Manual of Systematic Bacteriology*,[7,8] volumes 1 through 4. Leading journals that contain up-to-date information on nomenclature and new species include *Anaerobe*, *International Journal of Systematic and Evolutionary Microbiology*, *Annales de Microbiologie* (Institut Pasteur), *Current Microbiology*, *Journal of Clinical Microbiology*, and *Systematic and Applied Microbiology*. An overview of validly published names can be obtained at http://www.bacterio.cict.fr or http://www.dsmz.de/microorganisms/bacterial_nomenclature.php.

Taxonomic ranks for naming bacterial organisms include kingdom, division, class, order, family, genus, species, and subspecies. All these ranks have official standing in nomenclature. Ranks below subspecies have no official standing but are used to indicate groups of strains or isolates that can be distinguished by some special characteristics (Table 90–2). Each taxonomic name should be represented by a nomenclature type. The species is represented by a type strain that is deposited in a recognized culture collection.

Nomenclature priorities for bacteriologic names date back to May, 1753. Because of difficulties in searching literature and limited available information on described species, approved lists of bacterial names were published in the *International Journal of Systematic Bacteriology* in 1980. Names not included on those lists have lost all standing in nomenclature status.

Historically, bacterial classification has been based on phenotypic characteristics. Multivariate analysis has played a large role in classification since the 1950s. This analysis used biochemical, cultural, and morphologic characteristics and susceptibilities to antibiotics and inorganic compounds to define the degrees of similarities among organisms. More recently, molecular techniques (e.g., DNA hybridization, rRNA-DNA hybridization, gene sequence analysis) have played a major role in determining phylogenetic relationships.

The DNA molecular weight for most bacteria is 1×10^9 to 8×10^9 daltons, enough to specify 1500 to 6000 genes. Using nucleic acid analysis, researchers have developed numerous parameters to determine taxonomic relationships. These parameters include genome size, mole percent guanine plus cytosine content, DNA relatedness under optimal and supraoptimal conditions for DNA reassociation, and rRNA oligonucleotide sequences. By correlating phenotypic results with DNA homology and rRNA sequence analysis, researchers have been able to select phenotypic tests that can be used more accurately to identify organisms belonging to specific groups.

The bacterial classification shown in Table 90–1 is based on the organism's morphologic and stain characteristics. Organisms included are those that often are associated with pathologic processes or that are medically significant. The current names are those either officially recognized or proposed for recognition and currently used in the literature.[1-21] The type species for *Salmonella* is *Salmonella enterica* rather than *Salmonella choleraesuis*, although in the United States, Public Health uses the genus *Salmonella* and the serovar for reporting purposes.[4]

Text continued on p. 1196

TABLE 90–1   Current Bacterial Nomenclature, Taxonomy, and Classification

I. Aerobic Gram-Positive Cocci
Characteristics: aerotolerant anaerobes that can occur singly or in pairs, tetrads, chains, or clusters; they can be catalase-positive or catalase-negative. Organisms positive for coagulase or clumping factor include *Staphylococcus aureus*, *Staphylococcus intermedius*, *Staphylococcus lugdunensis*, and *Staphylococcus schleiferi* subspecies *coagulans*.

Current Name	Synonym	Current Name	Synonym
Catalase-Positive Organisms		*Aerococcus viridans*	
Alloiococcus otitidis	*Alloiococcus otitis*	*Dolosicoccus paucivorans*	
Kocuria kristinae	*Micrococcus kristinae*	*Dolosigranulum pigrum*	
Kocuria rosea	*Micrococcus roseus*	*Enterococcus avium*	*Streptococcus avium*
Kocuria varians	*Micrococcus varians*		Group D *Enterococcus*
Kytococcus schroeteri		*Enterococcus caccae*	
Kytococcus sedentarius	*Micrococcus sedentarius*	*Enterococcus casseliflavus*	*Enterococcus flavescens*
Micrococcus luteus			*Streptococcus casseliflavus*
Micrococcus lylae		*Enterococcus cecorum*	*Streptococcus cecorum*
Nesterenkonia halobia	*Micrococcus halobius*	*Enterococcus dispar*	
Staphylococcus arlettae		*Enterococcus durans*	*Streptococcus durans*
Staphylococcus aureus subspecies *anaerobius*			Group D *Enterococcus*
Staphylococcus aureus subspecies *aureus*		*Enterococcus faecalis*	*Streptococcus faecalis*
Staphylococcus auricularis			Group D *Enterococcus*
Staphylococcus capitis subspecies *capitis*		*Enterococcus faecium*	*Streptococcus faecium*
Staphylococcus capitis subspecies *ureolyticus*			Group D *Enterococcus*
Staphylococcus caprae		*Enterococcus gallinarum*	*Streptococcus gallinarum*
Staphylococcus carnosus subspecies *carnosus*		*Enterococcus gilvus*	
Staphylococcus carnosus subspecies *utilis*		*Enterococcus hirae*	
Staphylococcus casei	*Staphylococcus succinus* subspecies *casei*	*Enterococcus italicus*	*Enterococcus saccharominimus*
Staphylococcus chromogenes	*Staphylococcus hyicus* subspecies *chromogenes*	*Enterococcus malodoratus*	
		Enterococcus mundtii	
Staphylococcus cohnii subspecies *cohnii*		*Enterococcus pallens*	
Staphylococcus cohnii subspecies *urealyticus*		*Enterococcus pseudoavium*	
Staphylococcus condimenti		*Enterococcus raffinosus*	
Staphylococcus delphini		*Facklamia hominis*	
Staphylococcus epidermidis	*Staphylococcus albus*	*Facklamia ignava*	
Staphylococcus equorum		*Facklamia languida*	
Staphylococcus felis		*Facklamia sourekii*	
Staphylococcus fleurettii		*Gemella bergeriae*	
Staphylococcus gallinarum		*Gemella haemolysans*	*Neisseria haemolysans*
Staphylococcus haemolyticus		*Gemella morbillorum*	*Streptococcus morbillorum*
Staphylococcus hominis subspecies *hominis*			*Peptostreptococcus morbillorum*
Staphylococcus hominis subspecies *novobiosepticus*		*Gemella sanguinis*	
Staphylococcus hyicus		*Globicatella sanguinis*	Salt-tolerant viridans streptococci
Staphylococcus intermedius			
Staphylococcus kloosii		*Granulicatella adiacens*	*Abiotrophia adiacens*
Staphylococcus lentus	*Staphylococcus sciuri* subspecies *lentus*		*Streptococcus adiacens* Nutritionally variant streptococci
Staphylococcus lugdunensis			
Staphylococcus lutrae		*Granulicatella elegans*	*Abiotrophia elegans*
Staphylococcus muscae			Nutritionally variant streptococci
Staphylococcus nepalensis			
Staphylococcus pasteuri		*Granulicatella para-adiacens*	
Staphylococcus piscifermentans		*Helcococcus kunzii*	
Staphylococcus pseudintermedius		*Helcococcus pyogenica*	
Staphylococcus saccharolyticus	*Peptococcus saccharolyticus*	*Helcococcus sueciensis*	
Staphylococcus saprophyticus subspecies *saprophyticus*	*Micrococcus* subgroup 3	*Ignavigranum ruoffiae*	
		Lactococcus garviae	*Streptococcus garvieae* Lancefield group N
Staphylococcus schleiferi subspecies *coagulans*			
Staphylococcus schleiferi subspecies *schleiferi*		*Lactococcus lactis*	
Staphylococcus sciuri subspecies *rodentium*		*Leuconostoc citreum*	
Staphylococcus sciuri subspecies *sciuri*		*Leuconostoc cremoris*	
Staphylococcus simulans		*Leuconostoc dextranicum*	
Staphylococcus succinus subspecies *succinus*		*Leuconostoc lactis*	
Staphylococcus vitulinus		*Leuconostoc mesenteroides*	
Staphylococcus warneri		*Leuconostoc pseudomesenteroides*	
Staphylococcus xylosus		*Oenococcus oeni*	*Leuconostoc oenos*
		Pediococcus acidilactici	
Catalase-Negative Organisms		*Pediococcus damnosus*	
Abiotrophia defectiva	*Streptococcus defectivus*	*Pediococcus dextrinicus*	
	Nutritionally variant streptococci	*Pediococcus equinus*	*Streptococcus equinus*
		Pediococcus parvulus	
Aerococcus christensenii		*Pediococcus pentosaceus*	
Aerococcus sanguicola	*Aerococcus sanguinicola*	*Streptococcus acidominimus*	
Aerococcus urinae			

TABLE 90–1 Current Bacterial Nomenclature, Taxonomy, and Classification—cont'd

Current Name	Synonym	Current Name	Synonym
Streptococcus bovis group	Group D streptococci	Peptoniphilus harei	Peptostreptococcus harei
Streptococcus alactolyticus		Peptoniphilus ivorii	Peptostreptococcus ivorii
Streptococcus bovis		Peptoniphilus lacrimalis	Peptostreptococcus lacrimalis
Streptococcus equines			
Streptococcus gallolyticus subspecies gallolyticus		Peptostreptococcus anaerobius	
		Peptostreptococcus indolicus	Peptococcus indolicus
Streptococcus gallolyticus subspecies macedonicus		Peptostreptococcus magnus	Peptococcus magnus
			Peptococcus variabilis
Streptococcus gallolyticus subspecies pasteurianus		Peptostreptococcus massiliae	
		Peptostreptococcus stomatis	
Streptococcus infantarius		Peptostreptococcus trisimilis	
Streptococcus milleri group	Viridans streptococci	Ruminococcus hansenii	Streptococcus hansenii
Streptococcus anginosus		Ruminococcus productus	Peptostreptococcus productus
Streptococcus constellatus			
Streptococcus intermedius			
Streptococcus mitis group	Viridans streptococci		
Streptococcus australis		**III. Aerobic Gram-Negative Cocci**	
Streptococcus infantis		**Characteristics: occur singly or in pairs or clumps; catalase and oxidase positive**	
Streptococcus mitis	Streptococcus mitior		
	Streptococcus sanguis II	Lautropia mirabilis	Sarcina mirabilis
Streptococcus oralis		Neisseria canis	
Streptococcus peroris		Neisseria bacilliformis	
Streptococcus pneumoniae	Diplococcus pneumoniae	Neisseria cinerea	Micrococcus cinereus
Streptococcus pseudopneumoniae			Neisseria pharyngis
Streptococcus mutans group	Viridans streptococci	Neisseria elongata subspecies elongata	Neisseria elongata
Streptococcus cricetus		Neisseria elongata subspecies glycolytica	Neisseria elongata
Streptococcus mutans		Neisseria elongata subspecies nitroreducens	Neisseria elongata
Streptococcus ratti			CDC group M-6
Streptococcus sobrinus		Neisseria flavescens	
Streptococcus pyogenes group		Neisseria gonorrhoeae	
Streptococcus agalactiae	Group B streptococci	Neisseria kochii	
Streptococcus canis		Neisseria lactamica	Neisseria lactamicus
Streptococcus dysgalactiae subspecies equisimilis	Group C streptococci	Neisseria meningitidis	
	Streptococcus equi	Neisseria mucosa	
	Streptococcus equi subspecies zooepidermidis	Neisseria parelongata	
		Neisseria polysaccharea	
	Streptococcus equisimilis	Neisseria sicca	
	Group G streptococci	Neisseria subflava biovar flava	Neisseria subflava
Streptococcus iniae	Streptococcus shiloi	Neisseria subflava biovar perflava	Neisseria subflava
Streptococcus porcinus		Neisseria subflava biovar subflava	Neisseria subflava
Streptococcus pyogenes	Group A streptococci	Neisseria weaveri	Moraxella sp. M-5
Streptococcus salivarius group	Viridans streptococci		CDC group M-5
Streptococcus salivarius			
Streptococcus thermophilus			
Streptococcus vestibularis		**IV. Anaerobic Gram-Negative Cocci**	
Streptococcus sanguinis group	Viridans streptococci	**Characteristics: occur in pairs or clumps**	
Streptococcus cristatus	Streptococcus crista		
Streptococcus gordonii		Acidaminococcus fermentans	
Streptococcus massiliensis		Anaeroglobus geminatus	
Streptococcus parasanguis		Megasphaera elsdenii	Peptostreptococcus elsdenii
Streptococcus sanguis		Megasphaera micronuciformis	
Streptococcus suis		Subdoligranulum variabile	
Tetragenococcus halophilus	Enterococcus solitarius	Veillonella atypica	
Vagococcus fluvialis		Veillonella dispar	
Weissella paramesenteroides	Leuconostoc paramesenteroides	Veillonella montpellierensis	
		Veillonella parvula	

II. Anaerobic Gram-Positive Cocci
Characteristics: occur singly or in pairs, chains, or clumps

Current Name	Synonym
Anaerococcus octavius	Peptostreptococcus octavius
	Peptostreptococcus prevotii
	Peptostreptococcus tetradius
Anaerococcus hydrogenalis	Peptostreptococcus hydrogenalis
	Peptostreptococcus lactolyticus
Gemella morbillorum	Streptococcus morbillorum
Micromonas micros	Peptostreptococcus micros
Peptococcus niger	Micrococcus niger
Peptoniphilus asaccharolyticus	Peptostreptococcus asaccharolyticus

V. Aerobic Gram-Positive Bacilli
Characteristics: rodlike; catalase-negative or -positive; some are acid-fast stain-positive, and some have branching. Only *Bacillus*, *Brevibacillus*, and *Brevibacterium* spp. produce spores.

Current Name	Synonym
Actinomadura latina	
Actinomadura madurae	
Actinomadura pelletieri	
Amycolata autotrophica	
Amycolatopsis orientalis	Nocardia orientalis
	Streptomyces orientalis
Arcanobacterium bernardiae	Actinomyces bernardiae
	CDC coryneform group 2
Arcanobacterium haemolyticum	Corynebacterium haemolyticum
Arcanobacterium pyogenes	Actinomyces pyogenes
	Corynebacterium pyogenes
Arthrobacter albus	

TABLE 90–1   Current Bacterial Nomenclature, Taxonomy, and Classification—cont'd

Current Name	Synonym	Current Name	Synonym
Arthrobacter creatinolyticus		*Corynebacterium minutissimum*	
Arthrobacter cumminsii		*Corynebacterium mucifaciens*	
Arthrobacter luteolus		*Corynebacterium nigricans*	CDC fermentive coryneform group 4
Arthrobacter nicotianae			
Arthrobacter oxydans		*Corynebacterium pilosum*	
Arthrobacter scleromae		*Corynebacterium propinquum*	CDC coryneform group ANF-3
Arthrobacter woluwensis			
Aureobacterium spp.	*Corynebacterium aquaticum*	*Corynebacterium pseudodiphtheriticum*	*Corynebacterium hofmanii*
		Corynebacterium pseudotuberculosis	
Aureobacterium resistens		*Corynebacterium resistens*	
Bacillus anthracis		*Corynebacterium riegelii*	
Bacillus cereus		*Corynebacterium sanguinis*	
Bacillus circulans		*Corynebacterium simulans*	
Bacillus coagulans		*Corynebacterium singulare*	
Bacillus licheniformis		*Corynebacterium striatum*	
Bacillus massiliensis		*Corynebacterium sundsvallense*	*Corynebacterium thomssenii*
Bacillus megaterium			*Rothia dentocarrosa*
Bacillus mycoides			
Bacillus pumilus		*Corynebacterium tuscaniae*	
Bacillus sphaericus		*Corynebacterium ulcerans*	
Bacillus subtilis		*Corynebacterium urealyticum*	*Corynebacterium* group D2
Bacillus thuringiensis			CDC coryneform group D2
Brevibacillus agri	*Bacillus agri*		
Brevibacillus brevis	*Bacillus brevis*		
Brevibacillus laterosporus	*Bacillus laterosporus*	*Corynebacterium xerosis*	
	Brevibacterium casei	*Curtobacterium* spp.	
	CDC coryneform groups B-1 and B-3	*Dermabacter hominis*	CDC fermentative coryneform groups 3 and 5
Brevibacterium epidermidis			
Brevibacterium mcbrellneri		*Dermatophilus congolensis*	*Actinomyces congolensis*
Brevibacterium otitidis		*Erysipelothrix rhusiopathiae*	*Erysipelothrix insidiosa*
Brevibacterium sanguinis		*Exiguobacterium acetylicum*	*Brevibacterium acetylicum*
Callatomonas turbata	*Oerskovia turbata*	*Exiguobacterium aurantiacum*	*Brevibacterium aurantiacum*
Cellulomonas hominis	CDC coryneform group A-3	*Gardnerella vaginalis*	*Haemophilus vaginalis*
Cellulosimicrobium cellulans	*Cellumonas cellulans*		*Corynebacterium vaginalis*
	Oerskovia xanthineolytica	*Gordonia aichiensis*	*Rhodococcus aichiensis*
	CDC coryneform groups A-1 and A-2		*Tsukamura aichiessii*
Corynebacterium accolens		*Gordonia bronchialis*	*Rhodococcus bronchialis*
Corynebacterium afermentans subspecies *afermentans*	CDC coryneform group ANF-1	*Gordonia polyisoprenivorans*	
		Gordonia rubropertincta	*Rhodococcus rubropertincta*
Corynebacterium afermentans subspecies *lipophilum*	CDC coryneform group ANF-1	*Gordonia sputi*	*Rhodococcus sputi*
			Rhodococcus chubuensis
Corynebacterium amycolatum	*Corynebacterium xerosis*	*Gordonia terrae*	*Rhodococcus terrae*
	Corynebacterium minutissimum	*Kurthia* spp.	
	Corynebacterium striatum	*Listeria bulgaria*	
	CDC coryneform groups F-2 and I-2	*Listeria grayi* subspecies *grayi*	*Listeria grayi*
		Listeria ivanovii subspecies *ivanovii*	*Listeria monocytogenes* serovar 5
Corynebacterium aquaticum			
Corynebacterium argentoratense		*Listeria ivanovii* subspecies *londoniensis*	
Corynebacterium aurimucosum	CDC fermentive coryneform group 4	*Listeria monocytogenes*	
		Microbacterium spp.	CDC coryneform groups A-4 and A-5
Corynebacterium auris	CDC coryneform group ANF-1	*Microbacterium arborescens*	CDC coryneform group A-4
Corynebacterium confusum		*Microbacterium imperiale*	CDC coryneform group A-4
Corynebacterium coyleae			
Corynebacterium diphtheriae		*Microbacterium lacticum*	
Corynebacterium durum		*Microbacterium oxydans*	
Corynebacterium falsenii		*Microbacterium phyllosphaerae*	
Corynebacteriun freneyi		*Mycobacterium abscessus*	*Mycobacterium chelonae* subspecies *abscessus*
Corynebacterium glucuronolyticum			
Corynebacterium imitans		*Mycobacterium africanum* subtype I	
Corynebacterium jeikeium	*Corynebacterium* group JK	*Mycobacterium africanum* subtype II	
	CDC coryneform group JK	*Mycobacterium alvei*	
		Mycobacterium arupense	
		Mycobacterium asiaticum	
		Mycobacterium aurum	
Corynebacterium kroppenstedtii		*Mycobacterium avium* subspecies *avium*	
Corynebacterium lipophiloflavum		*Mycobacterium avium* subspecies *paratuberculosis*	
Corynebacterium macginleyi	CDC coryneform group G-1	*Mycobacterium barassie*	
Corynebacterium matruchotii	*Bacterionema matruchotii*	*Mycobacterium bohemicum*	

TABLE 90–1   Current Bacterial Nomenclature, Taxonomy, and Classification—cont'd

Current Name	Synonym	Current Name	Synonym
Mycobacterium bovis		Mycobacterium triviale	
Mycobacterium branderi		Mycobacterium tuberculosis	
Mycobacterium brumae		Mycobacterium ulcerans	Mycobacterium buruli
Mycobacterium celatum		Mycobacterium vaccae	
Mycobacterium chelonae	Mycobacterium chelonae subspecies chelonae	Mycobacterium wolinskyi	
	Mycobacterium chelonei	Mycobacterium xenopi	
Mycobacterium chubuense		Nocardia abscessus	
Mycobacterium colombiense		Nocardia aoensis	
Mycobacterium conceptionense		Nocardia africana	
Mycobacterium confluentis		Nocardia anaemiae	
Mycobacterium conspicuum		Nocardia araoensis	
Mycobacterium cookii		Nocardia arthritidis	
Mycobacterium flavescens		Nocardia asiatica	
Mycobacterium fortuitum	Mycobacterium fortuitum subspecies fortuitum	Nocardia asteroides type IV	
	Mycobacterium fortuitum (third complex) sorbitol-positive biovariant	Nocardia asteroides type VI	
		Nocardia beijingensis	
		Nocardia brasiliensis	
		Nocardia brevicatena	Mycropolyspora brevicatena
		Nocardia camea	
		Nocardia carnea	
	Mycobacterium fortuitum (third complex) sorbitol-negative biovariant	Nocardia corynebacteroides	
		Nocardia cyriacigeorgica	Nocardia cyriacigeorgici
		Nocardia exalbida	
Mycobacterium gadium		Nocardia farcinica	
Mycobacterium gastri		Nocardia higoensis	
Mycobacterium genavense		Nocardia ignorata	
Mycobacterium goodii		Nocardia inohanensis	
Mycobacterium gordonae	Mycobacterium aquae	Nocardia kruczakiae	
Mycobacterium haemophilum		Nocardia mexicana	
Mycobacterium hassiacum		Nocardia niigatensis	
Mycobacterium heckeshornense		Nocardia nova	
Mycobacterium heidelbergense		Nocardia otitidiscaviarum	Nocardia caviae
Mycobacterium immunogenum		Nocardia paucivorans	
Mycobacterium intracellulare		Nocardia pneumoniae	
Mycobacterium interjectum		Nocardia pseudobrasiliensis	
Mycobacterium jacuzzii		Nocardia puris	
Mycobacterium kansasii		Nocardia sienata	Nocardia senatus
Mycobacterium kubicae		Nocardia testaceus	Nocardia testaceus
Mycobacterium lacticola		Nocardia thailandica	
Mycobacterium lentiflavum		Nocardia transvalensis	
Mycobacterium leprae		Nocardia vermiculata	
Mycobacterium mageritense		Nocardia veterana	
Mycobacterium maichiense		Nocardia vinacea	
Mycobacterium malmoense		Nocardia yamanashiensis	
Mycobacterium marinum	Mycobacterium balnei	Nocardiopsis dassonvillei	Actionmadura dassonvillei Nocardia dassonvillei
Mycobacterium massiliense		Nocardiopsis synnemataformans	Oerskovia turbata CDC coryneform groups A-3 and A-4
Mycobacterium microgenicum			
Mycobacterium microti			
Mycobacterium monacense		Paenibacillus alvei	Bacillus alvei
Mycobacterium mucogenicum	Mycobacterium chelonae–like organism (MCLO)	Paenibacillus amylolyticus	
		Paenibacillus macerans	Bacillus mascerans
		Paenibacillus massiliensis	
Mycobacterium moriokaense		Paenibacillus polymyxa	Bacillus polymyxa
Mycobacterium neoaurum		Paenibacillus sanguinis	
Mycobacterium nonchromogenicum		Paenibacillus stellifer	
Mycobacterium novocastrense		Parastreptomyces abscessus	
Mycobacterium parascrofulaceum		Rhodococcus equi	Corynebacterium equi
Mycobacterium peregrinum	Mycobacterium fortuitum biovar peregrinum	Rothia dentocariosa	Nocardia dentocariosus
		Rothia mucilaginosa	Stomatococcus mucilaginosus
Mycobacterium phlei			
Mycobacterium ratisbonense		Streptomyces anulatus	Streptomyces griseus
Mycobacterium scrofulaceum		Streptomyces lydicus	
Mycobacterium senegalense	Mycobacterium peregrinum type II	Streptomyces paraguayensis	
		Streptomyces sampsonii	
Mycobacterium sherrisii		Streptomyces somaliensis	
Mycobacterium shimoidei		Tropheryma whipplei	Tropheryma whippelii
Mycobacterium simiae	Mycobacterium habana	Tsukamurella inchonensis	
Mycobacterium smegmatis		Tsukamurella paurometabola	Gordona aurantiaca
Mycobacterium szulgai		Tsukamurella pulmonis	
Mycobacterium terrae		Tsukamurella tyrosinosolvens	
Mycobacterium thermoresistibile		Turicella otitidis	Rhodococcus aurantiacus
Mycobacterium triplex		Williamsia deligens	

TABLE 90-1   Current Bacterial Nomenclature, Taxonomy, and Classification—cont'd

Current Name	Synonym	Current Name	Synonym
VI. Anaerobic Gram-Positive Bacilli (Non–Spore-Forming)		*Eubacterium yurii* subspecies *margaretiae*	
Characteristics: may be long-branching bacilli or pleomorphic coccobacilli		*Eubacterium yurii* subspecies *schtitka*	
		Eubacterium yurii subspecies *yurii*	
		Holdemania filiformis	*Eubacterium* S14
Actinobaculum massiliae		*Lactobacillus acidophilus*	
Actinobaculum schaalii		*Lactobacillus brevis*	
Actinobaculum timonae		*Lactobacillus casei*	
Actinobaculum suis	*Actinomyces suis*	*Lactobacillus catenaforme*	
Actinobaculum urinale		*Lactobacillus colehominis*	
Actinomyces cardiffensis		*Lactobacillus crispatus*	
Actinomyces europaeus		*Lactobacillus fermentum*	
Actinomyces funkei		*Lactobacillus gasseri*	
Actinomyces georgiae	*Actinomyces* DO8	*Lactobacillus iners*	
Actinomyces gerencseriae	*Actinomyces israelii* serotype II	*Lactobacillus jensenii*	
		Lactobacillus leichmannii	
Actinomyces graevenitzii		*Lactobacillus oris*	
Actinomyces hongkongensis		*Lactobacillus paracasei* subspecies *paracasei*	
Actinomyces israelii		*Lactobacillus paraplantarum*	
Actinomyces meyeri		*Lactobacillus plantarum*	
Actinomyces nasicola		*Lactobacillus rhamnosus*	*Lactobacillus* GG
Actinomyces naeslundii		*Lactobacillus salivarius*	
Actinomyces neuii subspecies *anitratus*		*Lactobacillus vaginalis*	
Actinomyces neuii subspecies *neuii*	CDC coryneform group 1	*Mobiluncus curtisii* subspecies *curtisii*	
		Mobiluncus curtisii subspecies *holmesii*	
Actinomyces odontolyticus		*Mobiluncus mulieris*	*Falcivibrio grandis*
Actinomyces oricola		*Olsenella profuse*	
Actinomyces radicidentis		*Olsenella uli*	*Lactobacillus uli*
Actinomyces radingae	CDC coryneform group E; APL1	*Parascardovia denticolens*	*Bifidobacterium denticolens*
		Propionibacterium acnes	
Actinomyces turicensis	CDC coryneform group E; APL10	*Propionibacterium avidum*	
		Propionibacterium granulosum	
Actinomyces viscosus		*Propionibacterium lymphophilum*	
Anaerofustis haemolyticum		*Propionibacterium propionicus*	*Propionibacterium propionicum*
Anaerofustis stercorihominis			
Atopobium fossor	*Eubacterium fossor*		*Arachnia propionica*
Atopobium minutum	*Lactobacillus minutus*		*Actinomyces propionicus*
Atopobium parvulum	*Streptococcus parvulus*	*Pseudoramibacter alactolyticus*	*Eubacterium alactolyticum*
	Peptostreptococcus parvulus	*Scardovia inopinata*	*Bifidobacterium inopinatum*
Atopobium rimae	*Lactobacillus rimae*		*Bifidobacterium dentium*
Atopobium vaginae			*Eubacterium exigaum*
Bifidobacterium adolescentis		*Slackia exigua*	*Peptostreptococcus heliotrinreducens*
Bifidobacterium angulatum		*Slackia heliotrinireducens*	
Bifidobacterium bifidum			
Bifidobacterium breve		*Solobacterium moorei*	
Bifidobacterium catenulatum		*Varibaculum cambriensis*	
Bifidobacterium dentium	*Bifidobacterium appendicitis*		
		VII. Anaerobic Gram-Positive Bacilli (Spore-Forming)	
Bifidobacterium eriksonii		**Characteristics: broad, short bacilli with blunt ends. Most organisms readily produce spores, except *Clostridium perfringens*.**	
Bifidobacterium longum subspecies *infantis*	*Bifidobacterium infantis*		
Bifidobacterium longum subspecies *longum*	*Bifidobacterium longum*	*Clostridium absonum*	
Bifidobacterium pseudocatenulatum		*Clostridium aldenense*	
Collinsella aerofaciens	*Eubacterium aerofaciens*	*Clostridium amygdalinum*	
Cryptobacterium curtum		*Clostridium argentinense*	*Clostridium botulinum* group G
Dorea formicigenerans	*Eubacterium formicigenerans*		*Clostridium subterminale*
			Clostridium hastiforme
Dorea longicatena			*Clostridium barati*
Eggerthella hongkongensis		*Clostridium baratii*	*Clostridium paraperfringens*
Eggerthella lenta	*Eubacterium lentum*		
Eggerthella sinensis			*Clostridium perenne*
Eubacterium brachy			
Eubacterium combesii		*Clostridium bartlettii*	
Eubacterium contortum		*Clostridium bifermentans*	
Eubacterium infirmum		*Clostridium beijerinckii*	
Eubacterium limosum		*Clostridium bolteae*	
Eubacterium minutum	*Eubacterium tardum*	*Clostridium botulinum*	*Clostridium putrificum*
Eubacterium moniliforme		*Clostridium butyricum*	*Clostridium pseudotetanicum*
Eubacterium nitritogenes			
Eubacterium nodatum		*Clostridium cadaveris*	
Eubacterium saburreum		*Clostridium carnis*	
Eubacterium saphenum		*Clostridium celatum*	
Eubacterium sulci	*Fusobacterium sulci*	*Clostridium celerecrescens*	
Eubacterium tenue		*Clostridium citroniae*	
Eubacterium timidum		*Clostridium clostridioforme*	*Clostridium clostridiiforme*

TABLE 90–1   Current Bacterial Nomenclature, Taxonomy, and Classification—cont'd

Current Name	Synonym	Current Name	Synonym
Clostridium coccoides		*Citrobacter sedlakii*	*Citrobacter genomospecies 8*
Clostridium cochlearium	*Clostridium lentoputrescens*		*Citrobacter freundii*
Clostridium cocleatum		*Citrobacter werkmanii*	*Citrobacter genomospecies 7*
Clostridium difficile	*Clostridium difficilis*		*Citrobacter freundii*
Clostridium fallax	*Clostridium pseudofallax*	*Citrobacter youngae*	*Citrobacter genomospecies 5*
Clostridium ghonii	*Clostridium ghoni*		*Citrobacter freundii*
Clostridium glycolicum			
Clostridium haemolyticum	*Clostridium novyi* type		
Clostridium hastiforme		*Edwardsiella hoshinae*	
Clostridium hathewayi		*Edwardsiella tarda*	
Clostridium hiranonis		*Enterobacter aerogenes*	*Aerobacter aerogenes*
Clostridium histolyticum		*Enterobacter agglomerans* group	
Clostridium indolis		*Enterobacter amnigenus*	
Clostridium innocuum		*Enterobacter asburiae*	CDC enteric group 17
Clostridium irregulare	*Clostridium irregularis*	*Enterobacter cancerogenus*	*Enterobacter taylorae*
Clostridium leptum			*Erwinia cancerogena*
Clostridium limosum	CDC group P-1		CDC enteric group 19
Clostridium malenominatum			
Clostridium neonatale		*Enterobacter cowanii*	
Clostridium novyi		*Enterobacter cloacae*	
Clostridium oroticum	*Zymobacterium oroticum*	*Enterobacter gergoviae*	
Clostridium paraputrificum		*Enterobacter hormaechei* subspecies *hormaechei*	CDC enteric group 75
Clostridium perfringens	*Clostridium welchii*	*Enterobacter hormaechei* subspecies *oharae*	
	Welchia perfringens	*Enterobacter hormaechei* subspecies *steigerwaltii*	
Clostridium piliforme	*Bacillus piliformis*		
Clostridium putrefaciens		*Enterobacter intermedius*	*Enterobacter intermedium*
Clostridium ramosum	*Eubacterium filamentosum*	*Enterobacter kobei*	
	Ramibacterium ramosum	*Enterobacter sakazakii*	
	Actinomyces ramosus	*Erwinia persicinus*	
	Eubacterium ramosum	*Escherichia blattae*	
Clostridium scindens		*Escherichia coli*	
Clostridium septicum		*Escherichia fergusonii*	CDC enteric group 10
Clostridium sordellii		*Escherichia hermannii*	CDC enteric group 11
Clostridium sphenoides		*Escherichia vulneris*	CDC enteric group 1
Clostridium sporogenes	Nontoxigenic *Clostridium botulinum*	*Ewingella americana*	CDC enteric group 40
		Hafnia alvei	*Enterobacter hafniae*
Clostridium subterminale		*Klebsiella granulomatis*	*Calymmatobacterium granulomatis*
Clostridium symbiosum	*Fusobacterium symbiosum*		
	Fusobacterium biacutus	*Klebsiella ornithinolytica*	*Klebsiella oxytoca* ornithine positive
	Bacteroides symbiosus		
Clostridium tertium		*Klebsiella oxytoca*	
Clostridium tetani		*Klebsiella planticola*	*Klebsiella travisanii*
Filifactor alocis	*Fusobacterium alocis*	*Klebsiella pneumoniae* subspecies *ozaenae*	*Klebsiella ozaenae*
Filifactor villosus	*Clostridium villosum*	*Klebsiella pneumoniae* subspecies *pneumoniae*	*Klebsiella pneumoniae*
		Klebsiella pneumoniae subspecies *rhinoscleromatis*	
		Klebsiella terrigena	
		Kluyvera ascorbata	CDC enteric group 8
		Kluyvera cryocrescens	
		Kluyvera georgiana	CDC enteric group 36/37
			Kluyvera spp. group 3
Budvicia aquatica		*Leclercia adecarboxylata*	*Escherichia adecarboxylata*
Buttiauxella noackiae	CDC enteric group 59		CDC enteric group 41
Cedecea davisae	CDC enteric group 15	*Leminorella grimontii*	CDC enteric group 57
Cedecea lapagei		*Leminorella richardii*	
Cedecea neteri	*Cedecea* subspecies 4	*Moellerella wisconsensis*	CDC enteric group 46
Cedecea subspecies 3		*Morganella morganii* subspecies *morganii*	*Proteus morganii*
Cedecea subspecies 5		*Morganella morganii* subspecies *sibonii*	*Proteus morganii*
Citrobacter amalonaticus	*Levinea amalonatica*	*Pantoea agglomerans*	*Enterobacter agglomerans*
Citrobacter braakii	*Citrobacter freundii*	*Pantoea ananatis*	
Citrobacter farmeri	*Citrobacter amalonaticus* biogroup 1	*Pantoea dispersa*	
		Photorhabdus luminescens	*Xenorhabdus luminescens*
Citrobacter freundii	*Colobactrum freundii*	*Pragia fontium*	
Citrobacter gillenii	*Citrobacter genomospecies 10*	*Proteus hauseri*	*Proteus vulgaris* biogroup 3
	Citrobacter freundii		
Citrobacter koseri	*Citrobacter diversus*	*Proteus mirabilis*	
	Levinea malonatica	*Proteus penneri*	*Proteus vulgaris* biogroup 1
Citrobacter murliniae	*Citrobacter genomospecies 11*		
	Citrobacter freundii	*Proteus vulgaris*	*Proteus vulgaris* biogroup 2
Citrobacter rodentium	*Citrobacter genomospecies 9*	*Providencia alcalifaciens*	*Proteus inconstans*
	Citrobacter freundii	*Providencia heimbachae*	

VIII. Aerobic Gram-Negative Bacilli: Enterobacteriaceae

Characteristics: ferment sugars; are oxidase-negative; most reduce nitrate to nitrite. Diagnostic laboratories may report *Salmonella* serovars by name (e.g., *Salmonella typhi* or *Salmonella* serovar *typhi*).

TABLE 90–1   Current Bacterial Nomenclature, Taxonomy, and Classification—cont'd

Current Name	Synonym	Current Name	Synonym
Providencia rettgeri	*Proteus rettgeri*	*Aeromonas veronii* biotype *veronii*	
Providencia rustigianii	*Providencia alcalifaciens* biogroup 3	*Chromobacterium violaceum*	*Bacillus violaceus*
		Pasteurella aerogenes	
Providencia stuartii	*Proteus inconstans*	*Pasteurella bettyae*	CDC group HB-5
Rahnella aquatilis		*Pasteurella canis*	*Pasteurella multocida* biotype 6
Salmonella bongori	*Salmonella* subgroup 5		
Salmonella enterica		*Pasteurella dagmatis*	*Pasteurella* new sp. 1
Salmonella enterica subspecies *arizonae*	*Salmonella choleraesuis* subspecies *arizonae*		*Pasteurella* "gas"
	Salmonella subgroup 3a	*Pasteurella gallinarum*	
Salmonella enterica subspecies *diarizonae*	*Salmonella choleraesuis* subspecies *diarizonae*	*Pasteurella haemolytica*	
		Pasteurella multocida subspecies *gallicida*	*Pasteurella septica*
	Salmonella subgroup 3b	*Pasteurella multocida* subspecies *multocida*	
Salmonella enterica subspecies *enterica*	*Salmonella choleraesuis* subspecies *choleraesuis*	*Pasteurella multocida* subspecies *septica*	
		Pasteurella pneumotropica	
	Salmonella subgroup 1	*Pasteurella stomatis*	
Salmonella enterica subspecies *houtenae*	*Salmonella choleraesuis* subspecies *houtenae*	*Pasteurella*-like	CDC group EF-4
		Photobacterium damsela	
	Salmonella subgroup 4	*Plesiomonas shigelloides*	*Aeromonas shigelloides*
Salmonella enterica subspecies *indica*	*Salmonella choleraesuis* subspecies *indica*	*Vibrio alginolyticus*	*Vibrio parahaemolyticus* biotype 2
	Salmonella subgroup 6	*Vibrio carchariae*	
Salmonella enterica subspecies *salamae*	*Salmonella choleraesuis* subspecies *salamae*	*Vibrio cholerae*	*Vibrio comma*
		Vibrio cincinnatiensis	
	Salmonella subgroup 2	*Vibrio damsela*	CDC group EF-5
Serratia ficaria		*Vibrio fluvialis*	CDC group EF-6
Serratia fonticola		*Vibrio furnissii*	*Vibrio fluvialis* biogroup 2
Serratia grimesii	*Serratia liquefaciens*		
Serratia liquefaciens	*Enterobacter liquefaciens*	*Vibrio hollisae*	CDC group EF-13
Serratia marcescens			CDC enteric group 42
Serratia odorifera		*Vibrio metschnikovii*	CDC enteric group 16
Serratia plymuthica			*Vibrio cholerae* biovar *proteus*
Serratia proteamaculans subspecies *proteamaculans*	*Serratia liquefaciens*	*Vibrio mimicus*	*Vibrio cholerae* sucrose negative
Serratia proteamaculans subspecies *quinovora*	*Serratia liquefaciens*	*Vibrio parahaemolyticus*	
Serratia rubidaea		*Vibrio vulnificus*	CDC group EF-3
Shigella boydii	*Shigella* biogroup C		*Beneckea vulnifica*
Shigella dysenteriae	*Shigella* biogroup A		
Shigella flexneri	*Shigella* biogroup B		

X. Aerobic Gram-Negative Bacilli: Nonenterobacteriaceae; Nonfermentative
Characteristics: may or may not oxidize sugars; are catalase positive; are oxidase variable

Current Name	Synonym
Shigella sonnei	*Shigella* biogroup D
Tatumella ptyseos	CDC group EF-9
Trabulsiella guamensis	CDC enteric group 90
Yersinia aldovae	
Yersinia bercovieri	*Yersinia enterocolitica* biogroup 3b
Yersinia enterocolitica	*Pasteurella enterocolitica*
Yersinia frederiksenii	
Yersinia intermedia	
Yersinia kristensenii	
Yersinia mollaretii	*Yersinia enterocolitica* biogroup 3a
Yersinia pestis	*Pasteurella pestis*
Yersinia pseudotuberculosis	*Pasteurella pseudotuberculosis*
Yersinia rohdei	
Yokenella regensburgei	*Koserella trabulsii* CDC enteric group 45

Current Name	Synonym
Achromobacter piechaudii	*Alcaligenes piechaudii*
Achromobacter xylosoxidans subspecies *denitrificans*	*Alcaligenes denitrificans* *Alcaligenes xylosoxidans* subspecies *denitrificans* CDC group Vc
Achromobacter xylosoxidans subspecies *xylosoxidans*	*Alcaligenes xylosoxidans* *Alcaligenes xylosoxidans* subspecies *xylosoxidans* *Alcaligenes denitrificans* subspecies *xylosoxidans* *Achromobacter xylosoxidans* CDC groups IIIa and IIIb

IX. Aerobic Gram-Negative Bacilli: Nonenterobacteriaceae; Fermentative
Characteristics: ferment sugars; are oxidase-positive

Current Name	Synonym
Aeromonas allosaccharophila	
Aeromonas bestiarum	
Aeromonas caviae	
Aeromonas enteropelogenes	
Aeromonas hydrophila	*Pseudomonas hydrophila*
Aeromonas jandaei	
Aeromonas media	
Aeromonas popoffii	
Aeromonas salmonicida	
Aeromonas schubertii	
Aeromonas trota	
Aeromonas veronii biotype *sobria*	

Current Name	Synonym
Acidovorax delafieldii	*Pseudomonas delafieldii*
Acidovorax facilis	*Pseudomonas facilis*
Acidovorax temperans	*Pseudomonas temperans*
Acinetobacter baumannii	*Acinetobacter anitratus*
Acinetobacter baylyi	
Acinetobacter bouvetii	
Acinetobacter calcoaceticus	*Acinetobacter anitratus* *Acinetobacter calcoaceticus* subspecies *calcoaceticus*
Acinetobacter gerneri	
Acinetobacter grimontii	
Acinetobacter haemolyticus	*Acinetobacter anitratus*
Acinetobacter johnsonii	
Acinetobacter junii	*Acinetobacter anitratus*
Acinetobacter lwoffii	*Acinetobacter calcoaceticus* subspecies *lwoffi*

TABLE 90-1 Current Bacterial Nomenclature, Taxonomy, and Classification—cont'd

Current Name	Synonym	Current Name	Synonym
Acinetobacter parvus		*Methylobacterium mesophilicum*	
Acinetobacter radioresistens		*Methylobacterium organophilum*	
Acinetobacter schindleri		*Methylobacterium podarium*	
Acinetobacter tandoii		*Methylobacterium radiotolerans*	
Acinetobacter tjernbergiae		*Methylobacterium rhodesianum*	
Acinetobacter towneri		*Methylobacterium rhodinum*	
Acinetobacter ursingii		*Methylobacterium zatmanii*	
Agrobacterium radiobacter	*Agrobacterium tumefaciens* CDC group Vd-3	*Moraxella atlantae*	CDC group M-3
		Moraxella canis	
Alcaligenes faecalis subspecies *faecalis*	*Alcaligenes odorans* *Pseudomonas odorans* CDC group VI	*Moraxella catarrhalis*	*Branhamella catarrhalis* *Neisseria catarrhalis* *Moraxella liquefaciens*
Asaia bogorensis		*Moraxella lacunata*	
Azospirillum brasilense	*Roseomonas fauriae* CDC "pink coccoid" group	*Moraxella lincolnii*	
		Moraxella nonliquefaciens	
		Moraxella osloensis	
Balneatrix alpica		*Myroides odoratimimus*	
Bergeyella zoohelcum	*Weeksella zoohelcum* CDC group IIj	*Myroides odoratum*	*Chryseobacterium odoratum* *Flavobacterium odoratum* CDC group M-4f
Brevundimonas diminuta	*Pseudomonas diminuta* CDC group Ia	*Ochrobactrum anthropi*	*Achromobacter* spp. biotypes 1 and 2 CDC groups Vd-1, Vd-2
Brevundimonas vesicularis	*Pseudomonas vesicularis* *Corynebacterium vesiculare*		
Burkholderia ambifaria		*Ochrobactrum intermedium*	
Burkholderia anthina		*Oligella ureolytica*	CDC group IVe
Burkholderia cenocepacia		*Oligella urethralis*	*Moraxella urethralis* CDC group M-4
Burkholderia cepacia	*Pseudomonas cepacia* *Pseudomonas multivorans* *Pseudomonas kingae* CDC group EO-1	*Pandoraea apista*	
		Paracoccus yeeii	*Paracoccus yeeii* CDC group EO-2
Burkholderia dolosa			
Burkholderia gladioli	*Pseudomonas gladioli* *Pseudomonas marginata* *Pseudomonas mallei* *Actinobacillus mallei*	*Photorhabdus asymbiotica*	*Xenorhabdus luminescens*
		Pseudomonas aeruginosa	*Pseudomonas pyocyanea* *Bacterium aeruginosum*
Burkholderia mallei		*Pseudomonas alcaligenes*	
Burkholderia multivorans	*Burkholderia cepacia* genomovar II	*Pseudomonas chlororaphis*	*Pseudomonas aureofaciens*
		Pseudomonas fluorescens	
Burkholderia oklahomensis		*Pseudomonas luteola*	*Chryseomonas luteola* CDC group Ve-1
Burkholderia pseudomallei	*Pseudomonas pseudomallei*		
Burkholderia pyrrocinia		*Pseudomonas mendocina*	CDC group Vb-2
Burkholderia stabilis	*Burkholderia cepacia* genomovar IV	*Pseudomonas oryzihabitans*	*Flavimonas oryzihabitans* CDC group Ve-2
Burkholderia thailandensis		*Pseudomonas otitidis*	
Burkholderia vietnamiensis	*Burkholderia cepacia* genomovar V	*Pseudomonas pertucinogena*	*Bordetella pertussis* rough phase IV
Chryseobacterium gleum	*Flavobacterium gleum* CDC group IIb	*Pseudomonas pseudoalcaligenes*	*Pseudomonas alcaligenes* biotype B
Chryseobacterium indologenes	*Flavobacterium indologenes* CDC group IIb	*Pseudomonas putida*	
		Pseudomonas stutzeri	CDC group Vb-1
Chryseobacterium massiliae		*Pseudomonas stutzeri*–like	CDC group Vb-3
Chryseobacterium timonae		*Psychrobacter immobilis*	*Micrococcus cryophilus*
Comamonas terrigena	CDC group EF-19	*Psychrobacter phenylpyruvicus*	*Moraxella phenylpyruvicus* CDC group M-2
Comamonas testosteroni	*Pseudomonas testosteroni*		
Delftia acidovorans	*Comamonas acidovorans* *Pseudomonas acidovorans*	*Ralstonia* spp.	CDC group IVc-2
Elizabethkingia meningoseptica	*Chryseobacterium meningosepticum* *Flavobacterium meningosepticum* CDC group IIa	*Ralstonia pickettii*	*Burkholderia pickettii* *Pseudomonas pickettii* CDC groups Va-1, Va-2, Va-3 *Pseudomonas thomasii*
		Roseomonas cervicalis	CDC "pink coccoid" group
Elizabethkingia miricola	*Chryseobacterium miricola*		
Empedobacter brevis	*Flavobacterium breve*	*Roseomonas* genomospecies 4	CDC "pink coccoid" group
Flavobacterium group IIe	CDC group IIe		
Flavobacterium group IIh	CDC group IIh	*Roseomonas* genomospecies 5	CDC "pink coccoid" group
Flavobacterium group IIi	CDC group IIi		
Granulibacter bethesdensis		*Roseomonas* genomospecies 6	CDC "pink coccoid" group
Inquilinus limosus			
Laribacter hongkongensis		*Roseomonas gilardii* subspecies *gilardii*	
Massilia timonae		*Roseomonas gilardii* subspecies *rosea*	
Methylobacterium spp.		*Roseomonas mucosa*	
Methylobacterium aminovarans		*Shewanella algae*	
Methylobacterium extorquens		*Shewanella putrefaciens*	*Alteromonas putrefaciens* *Pseudomonas putrefaciens* CDC groups Ib-1, Ib-2
Methylobacterium fujisawaense			

TABLE 90–1   Current Bacterial Nomenclature, Taxonomy, and Classification—cont'd

Current Name	Synonym	Current Name	Synonym
Sphingobacterium mizutae	*Flavobacterium mizutaii*	*Desulfovibrio vulgaris*	
Sphingobacterium multivorum	*Flavobacterium multivorum*	*Dialister invisus*	
		Dialister pneumosintes	*Bacteroides pneumosintes*
	CDC group IIk-2	*Dichelobacter nodosus*	*Bacteroides nodosus*
Sphingobacterium spiritivorum	*Flavobacterium spiritivorum*	*Fusobacterium gonidiaformans*	
		Fusobacterium mortiferum	
	Sphingobacterium versatilis	*Fusobacterium naviforme*	
		Fusobacterium necrogenes	
	CDC group IIk-3	*Fusobacterium necrophorum* subspecies *funduliforme*	
Sphingobacterium thalpophilum	*Flavobacterium thalpophilum*	*Fusobacterium necrophorum* subspecies *necrophorum*	
Sphingobacterium yabuuchiae		*Fusobacterium nucleatum* subspecies *fusiforme*	
Sphingomonas parapaucimobilis		*Fusobacterium nucleatum* subspecies *nucleatum*	
Sphingomonas paucimobilis	*Pseudomonas paucimobilis*		
	CDC group IIk-1	*Fusobacterium nucleatum* subspecies *polymorphum*	
Sphingomonas sanguis		*Fusobacterium nucleatum* subspecies *vincentii*	
Sphingomonas yanoikuyae			
Stenotrophomonas africana		*Fusobacterium periodonticum*	
Stenotrophomonas maltophilia	*Xanthomonas maltophilia*	*Fusobacterium russii*	
	Pseudomonas maltophilia	*Fusobacterium sulci*	
Wautersiella falsenii		*Fusobacterium ulcerans*	
Weeksella virosa	*Flavobacterium genitale*	*Fusobacterium varium*	*Fusobacterium pseudonecrophorum*
	CDC group IIf		

XI. Anaerobic Gram-Negative Bacilli
Characteristics: may appear as rods with rounded ends, curved rods, coccobacilli, or slender, spindle-shaped rods with tapered ends. *Dialister* and *Johnsonella* belong to the *Clostridium* subphylum.

Current Name	Synonym	Current Name	Synonym
		Johnsonella ignava	
		Leptotrichia amnionii	
		Leptotrichia buccalis	
		Leptotrichia goodfellowii	
		Leptotrichia hofstadii	
		Leptotrichia shahii	
Alistipes finegoldii		*Leptotrichia trevisanii*	
Alistipes onderdonkii		*Leptotrichia wadei*	
Alistipes shahii		*Mitsuokella multacida*	*Mitsuokella multiacida*
Anaerobiospirillum succiniciproducens			*Bacteroides multiacidus*
Anaerobiospirillum thomasii			
Anaerorhabdus furcosus	*Bacteroides furcosus*	*Olsenella profuse*	
Anaerostipes caccae		*Olsenella uli*	
Atopobium parvulus		*Parabacteroides distasonis*	*Bacteroides distasonis*
Bacteroides caccae		*Parabacteroides goldsteinii*	*Bacteroides goldsteinii*
Bacteroides capillosus		*Parabacteroides merdae*	*Bacteroides merdae*
Bacteroides coagulans			*Bacteroides fragilis* T4-1
Bacteroides dorei		*Porphyromonas asaccharolytica*	*Bacteroides asaccharolyticus*
Bacteroides eggerthii			*Bacteroides melaninogenicus* subspecies *asaccharolyticus*
Bacteroides finegoldii			
Bacteroides forsythus			
Bacteroides fragilis		*Porphyromonas cangingivalis*	
Bacteroides fragilis group	True *Bacteroides*	*Porphyromonas canoris*	
Bacteroides intestinalis	*Bacteroides putredinis*	*Porphyromonas cansulci*	
	Alistipes putredinis	*Porphyromonas catoniae*	*Oribaculum catoniae*
	Bacteroides furcosus	*Porphyromonas circumdentaria*	
Bacteroides massiliae		*Porphyromonas crevioricanis*	
Bacteroides nordii		*Porphyromonas endodontalis*	*Bacteroides endodontalis*
Bacteroides ovatus		*Porphyromonas gingivalis*	*Bacteroides gingivalis*
Bacteroides putredinis		*Porphyromonas gingivicanis*	
Bacteroides pyogenes	*Bacteroides tectus*	*Porphyromonas ulae*	
Bacteroides salyersae		*Porphyromonas levii*	*Bacteroides levii*
Bacteroides splanchnicus			*Bacteroides melaninogenicus* subspecies *levii*
Bacteroides stercoris	*Bacteroides fragilis* subspecies a		
Bacteroides tectus	*Bacteroides tectum*	*Porphyromonas macacae*	*Bacteroides macacae*
Bacteroides thetaiotaomicron			*Porphyromonas salivosa*
Bacteroides uniformis	*Bacteroides corrodens*	*Porphyromonas salivosa*	
Bacteroides ureolyticus		*Porphyromonas somerae*	
Bacteroides vulgatus		*Prevotella bergensis*	
Bilophila wadsworthia		*Prevotella bivia*	*Bacteroides bivius*
Butyrivibrio fibrisolvens		*Prevotella buccae*	*Bacteroides buccae*
Catonella morbi			*Bacteroides ruminicola* subspecies *brevis*
Centipeda periodontii			*Bacteroides capillus*
Cetobacterium somerae			*Bacteroides pentosaceus*
Desulfobulbus spp.			
Desulfomonas pigra		*Prevotella buccalis*	*Bacteroides buccalis*
Desulfovibrio fairfieldensis		*Prevotella corporis*	*Bacteroides corporis*
Desulfovibrio desulfuricans			

TABLE 90–1   Current Bacterial Nomenclature, Taxonomy, and Classification—cont'd

Current Name	Synonym	Current Name	Synonym
Prevotella dentalis	*Mitsuokella dentalis*	*Bartonella koehleras*	
	Hallella seregens	*Bartonella quintana*	*Rochalimaea quintana*
Prevotella denticola	*Bacteroides denticola*	*Bartonella vinsonii*	*Rochalimaea vinsonii*
Prevotella disiens	*Bacteroides disiens*	subspecies *arupensis*	
Prevotella enoeca		*Bartonella vinsonii*	
Prevotella heparinolytica	*Bacteroides heparinolyticus*	subspecies *berkhoffii*	
Prevotella intermedia	*Bacteroides intermedius*	*Bartonella washoensis*	
	Bacteroides melaninogenicus subspecies *intermedius*	*Bordetella bronchiseptica*	CDC group IVa
		Bordetella hinzii	
		Bordetella holmesii	CDC group NO-2
Prevotella loescheii	*Bacteroides loescheii*	*Bordetella parapertussis*	
Prevotella massiliensis		*Bordetella pertussis*	
Prevotella melaninogenica	*Bacteroides melaninogenicus*	*Bordetella trematum*	
	Bacteroides melaninogenicus subspecies *melaninogenicus*	*Brucella abortus*	
		Brucella canis	
		Brucella melitensis	
		Brucella suis	
		Campylobacter coli	
Prevotella nigrescens	*Prevotella intermedia*	*Campylobacter concisus*	CDC group EF-22
Prevotella oralis	*Bacteroides oralis*	*Campylobacter curvus*	*Wolinella curva*
Prevotella oris	*Bacteroides oris*	*Campylobacter fetus* subspecies *fetus*	*Vibrio fetus*
	Bacteroides ruminicola subspecies *brevis*	*Campylobacter fetus* subspecies *venerealis*	
Prevotella oulorum	*Bacteroides oulorum*	*Campylobacter gracilis*	*Bacteroides gracilis*
	Prevotella oulora	*Campylobacter hominis*	
Prevotella pallens		*Campylobacter hyointestinalis* subspecies *hyointestinalis*	
Prevotella salivae			
Prevotella shahii		*Campylobacter jejuni* subspecies *doylei*	
Prevotella tannerae			
Prevotella veroralis	*Bacteroides veroralis*	*Campylobacter jejuni* subspecies *jejuni*	
Prevotella zoogleoformans	*Bacteroides zoogleoformans*		
Selenomonas artemidis		*Campylobacter lari*	*Campylobacter laridis*
Selenomonas dianae		*Campylobacter mucosalis*	
Selenomonas flueggei		*Campylobacter rectus*	*Wolinella recta*
Selenomonas infelix		*Campylobacter showae*	
Selenomonas noxia		*Campylobacter sputorum* subspecies *paraureolyticus*	
Selenomonas sputigena			
Sneathia sanguinegens	*Leptotrichia sanguinegens*	*Campylobacter sputorum* subspecies *sputorum*	
Sutterella wadsworthensis			
Synergistes cluster I		*Campylobacter upsaliensis*	
Synergistes cluster II		*Campylobacter ureolyticus*	*Bacteroides ureolyticus*
Tannerella forsythus	*Bacteroides forsythus*	*Capnocytophaga canimorsus*	CDC group DF-2
	Tannerella forsythensis	*Capnocytophaga cynodegmi*	CDC group DF-2
Tissierella praeacuta	*Bacteroides praeacutus*	*Capnocytophaga gingivalis*	CDC group DF-1
		Capnocytophaga granulosa	
		Capnocytophaga haemolytica	
		Capnocytophaga ochracea	CDC group DF-1
		Capnocytophaga sputigena	CDC group DF-1
		Cardiobacterium hominis	CDC group IId
		Cardiobacterium valvarum	
		Chlamydophila avium	
		Chlamydophila pneumoniae	*Chlamydia pneumoniae* TWAR
		Chlamydophila psittaci	*Chlamydia psittaci*
		Chlamydophila trachomatis	*Chlamydia trachomatis*
		Chromobacterium violaceum	
		Coxiella burnetii	
		Dysgonomonas capnocytophagoides	CDC group DF-3
		Dysgonomonas gadei	
		Ehrlichia spp.	Human granulocytic ehrlichiosis
		Ehrlichia canis	
		Ehrlichia chaffeensis	Human monocytic ehrlichiosis
		Ehrlichia ewingii	
		Ehrlichia sennetsu	
		Eikenella corrodens	CDC group HB-1
		Francisella philomiragia	*Yersinia philomiragia*
		Francisella tularensis biovar *mediaasiatica*	

XII. Aerobic Gram-Negative Fastidious Coccobacilli
Characteristics: small, curved or straight gram-negative bacilli or coccobacilli. They may require carbon dioxide and enriched media or special conditions for adequate growth.

Current Name	Synonym	
Actinobacillus arthritidis	*Actinobacillus lignieresii*	
Actinobacillus equuii		
Actinobacillus hominis		
Actinobacillus ureae	*Pasteurella ureae*	
Afipia broomeae		
Afipia clevelandensis		
Afipia felis		
Aggregatibacter actinomycetemcomitans	*Actinobacillus actinomycetemcomitans*	CDC groups HB-3, HB-4
Aggregatibacter aphrophilus	*Haemophilus aphrophilus*	CDC group HB-2
Aggregatibacter paraphrophilus	*Haemophilus paraphrophilus*	
Aggregatibacter segnis	*Haemophilus segnis*	
Arcobacter butzleri	*Campylobacter butzleri*	
Arcobacter cryaerophilus	*Campylobacter cryaerophila*	
Bartonella alsatica		
Bartonella bacilliformis		
Bartonella clarridgieae		
Bartonella elizabethae	*Rochalimaea elizabethae*	
Bartonella grahamii		
Bartonella henselae	*Rochalimaea henselae*	

TABLE 90–1 Current Bacterial Nomenclature, Taxonomy, and Classification—cont'd

Current Name	Synonym	Current Name	Synonym
Francisella tularensis biovar *novicida*	*Francisella novicida* *Pasteurella tularensis* *Bacterium tularense*	*Rickettsia helvetica* subspecies *mongolotimonae*	
Francisella tularensis biovar *palearctica*	*Francisella tularensis* type B *Bacterium tularense*	*Rickettsia helvetica* subspecies *sibirica* *Rickettsia honei*	
Francisella tularensis biovar *tularensis*	*Francisella tularensis* type A *Pasteurella tularensis* *Bacterium tularense*	*Rickettsia japonica* *Rickettsia marmionii* *Rickettsia massiliae* *Rickettsia parkeri*	
Haemophilus ducreyi		*Rickettsia prowazekii*	
Haemophilus haemolyticus		*Rickettsia rickettsii*	
Haemophilus influenzae	*Haemophilus aegyptius*	*Rickettsia sibirica*	
Haemophilus parahaemolyticus		*Rickettsia slovaca*	
Haemophilus parainfluenzae		*Rickettsia texiana*	
Helicobacter bilis		*Rickettsia typhi*	
Helicobacter cinaedi	*Campylobacter cinaedi*	*Streptobacillus moniliformis*	*Haverhillia multiformis*
Helicobacter bizzozeronii		*Suttonella indologenes*	*Kingella indologenes*
Helicobacter canadensis			
Helicobacter canis		**XIII. Mycoplasma (Pleuropneumonia-like Organisms [PPLO])**	
Helicobacter fennelliae	*Campylobacter fennelliae*	**Characteristics: small, highly pleomorphic organisms that are difficult to observe with routine stains; require complex medium for growth**	
Helicobacter heilmannii	*Gastrospirillum hominis*		
Helicobacter pullorum			
Helicobacter pylori	*Campylobacter pylori*	*Acholeplasma laidlawii*	
Helicobacter rappini	*Flexispira rappini*	*Mycoplasma amphoriforme*	
Helicobacter westmeadii		*Mycoplasma buccale*	
Helicobacter winghamensis		*Mycoplasma faucium*	
Kingella denitrificans	CDC group TM-1	*Mycoplasma fermentans*	*Mycoplasma incognitus*
Kingella kingae	*Moraxella kingae* *Moraxella kingii*	*Mycoplasma gallisepticum* *Mycoplasma genitalium*	
Kingella oralis		*Mycoplasma hominis*	
Kingella potus		*Mycoplasma lipophilum*	
Legionella anisa		*Mycoplasma orale*	
Legionella birminghamensis		*Mycoplasma penetrans*	
Legionella bozemanii	*Fluoribacter bozemanae*	*Mycoplasma pirum*	
Legionella cincinnatiensis		*Mycoplasma pneumoniae*	
Legionella dumoffii	*Fluoribacter dumoffii*	*Mycoplasma primatum*	
Legionella feeleii		*Mycoplasma salivarium*	
Legionella gormanii		*Mycoplasma spermatophilum*	
Legionella hackeliae		*Mycoplasma synoviae*	
Legionella israelensis		*Ureaplasma parvum*	
Legionella jordanis		*Ureaplasma urealyticum*	T-mycoplasma
Legionella lansingensis			
Legionella longbeachae		**XIV. Treponemataceae (Spiral Organisms)**	
Legionella maceachernii		**Characteristics: filamentous, spiral organisms that may or may not stain with usual laboratory stains; require complex media or animal host for growth**	
Legionella micdadei	*Tatlockia micdadei*		
Legionella oakridgensis			
Legionella pneumophila		*Borrelia afzelii*	
Legionella sainthelensi		*Borrelia andersonii*	
Legionella tucsonensis		*Borrelia anserina*	
Legionella wadsworthii		*Borrelia bissettii*	
Orientia tsutsugamushi	*Rickettsia tsutsugamushi*	*Borrelia burgdorferi*	
Rickettsia aeschlimannii		*Borrelia caucasica*	
Rickettsia africae		*Borrelia crocidurae*	
Rickettsia akari		*Borrelia duttoni*	
Rickettsia amblyommii		*Borrelia garinii*	
Rickettsia australis		*Borrelia hermsii*	
Rickettsia canadensis		*Borrelia hispanica*	
Rickettsia conorii subspecies *caspia*		*Borrelia japonica*	
Rickettsia conorii subspecies *conorii*		*Borrelia latyschewii* *Borrelia lonestari*	
Rickettsia conorii subspecies *indica*		*Borrelia lusitaniae* *Borrelia mazzottii*	
Rickettsia conorii subspecies *israelensis*		*Borrelia miyamti* *Borrelia parkeri*	
Rickettsia felis		*Borrelia persica*	
Rickettsia helvetica subspecies *heilongjiangensis*		*Borrelia recurrentis* *Borrelia spielmanii* *Borrelia tanukii* *Borrelia turdae* *Borrelia turicatae*	*Borrelia spielmani*

TABLE 90-1 Current Bacterial Nomenclature, Taxonomy, and Classification—cont'd

Current Name	Synonym	Current Name	Synonym
Borrelia valaisiana		*Leptospira interrogans* serogroup *pyrogenes*	
Borrelia venezuelensis		*Leptospira kirschneri*	
Brachyspira aalborgi		*Leptospira noguchii*	
Brachyspira intermedia	*Serpulina intermedia*	*Leptospira santarosai*	
Brachyspira murdochii	*Serpulina murdochii*	*Leptospira weilii*	
Brachyspira pilosicoli	*Serpulina pilosicoli*	*Spirillum minus*	*Spirillum minor*
Leptospira alexandria		*Treponema amylovorum*	
Leptospira borgpetersenii		*Treponema carateum*	
Leptospira broomii		*Treponema denticola*	
Leptospira fainei		*Treponema maltophilum*	
Leptospira inadai		*Treponema medium*	
Leptospira interrogans		*Treponema minutum*	
Leptospira interrogans serogroup *australis*		*Treponema pallidum* subspecies *endemicum*	*Treponema pallidum*
Leptospira interrogans serogroup *autumnalis*		*Treponema pallidum* subspecies *pallidum*	*Treponema pallidum*
Leptospira interrogans serogroup *ballum*		*Treponema pallidum* subspecies *pertenue*	*Treponema pertenue*
Leptospira interrogans serogroup *bataviae*		*Treponema parvum*	
Leptospira interrogans serogroup *bulgarica*		*Treponema pectinovorum*	
Leptospira interrogans serogroup *canicola*		*Treponema phagedenis*	
Leptospira interrogans serogroup *copenhageni*		*Treponema putidum*	
Leptospira interrogans serogroup *grippotyphosa*		*Treponema refringens*	
Leptospira interrogans serogroup *hardjo*		*Treponema skoliodontum*	
Leptospira interrogans serogroup *icterohaemorrhagiae*		*Treponema socranskii*	
Leptospira interrogans serogroup *pomona*		*Treponema vincentii*	

CDC, Centers for Disease Control and Prevention.

TABLE 90-2 Bacterial Ranks Below Subspecies

Preferred Name	Synonym	When Applied
Biovar features	Biotype	Special biochemical or physiologic features
Serovar	Serotype	Distinct antigenic features
Pathovar	Pathotype	Host-specific pathogenic features
Phagovar	Phagotype	Lysis by distinct bacteriophages
Morphovar	Morphotype	Special morphologic features

REFERENCES

1. Brenner, D. J., O'Connor, S. P., Winkler, H. H., et al.: Proposals to unify the genera *Bartonella* and *Rochalimaea*, with descriptions of *Bartonella quintana* comb. nov., *Bartonella vinsonii* comb. nov., *Bartonella henselae* comb. nov., and *Bartonella elizabethae* comb. nov., and to remove the family Bartonellaceae from the order Rickettsiales. Int. J. Syst. Bacteriol. *43*:777-786, 1993.
2. Brenner, F. W., Villar, R. G., Tauxe, R., et al.: *Salmonella* nomenclature. J. Clin. Microbiol. *38*:2465-2467, 2000.
3. Coykendall, A. L.: Classification and identification of the viridans streptococci. Clin. Microbiol. Rev. *2*:315-328, 1989.
4. Editor: Recent changes in *Salmonella* nomenclature: The need for clarification. Vet. J. *170*:275-277, 2005.
5. Facklam, R.: Newly described, difficult-to-identify, catalase-negative, gram-positive cocci. Clin. Microbiol. Newslett. *23*:1-7, 2001.
6. Farmer, J. J., III, Davis, B. R., Hickman-Brenner, F. W., et al.: Biochemical identification of new species and biogroups of Enterobacteriaceae isolated from clinical specimens. J. Clin. Microbiol. *21*:46-76, 1985.
7. Garrity, G. M. (ed.): Bergey's Manual of Systematic Bacteriology. New York, Springer, 2001 (Vol. 1), 2005 (Vol. 2).
8. Holt, J. G. (ed.): Bergey's Manual of Systematic Bacteriology. Vols. 3 and 4. Baltimore, Williams & Wilkins, 1989.
9. Holt, J. G., Krieg, N. R., Sneath, P. H. A., et al.: Bergey's Manual of Determinative Bacteriology. 9th ed. Baltimore, Williams & Wilkins, 1994.
10. Janda, W. M.: The corynebacteria revisited: New species, identification kits and antimicrobial susceptibility testing. Clin. Microbiol. Newslett. *21*:175-182, 1999.
11. Kawamura, Y., Hou, X., Sultana, F., et al.: Determination of 16S rRNA sequences of *Streptococcus mitis* and *Streptococcus gordonii* and phylogenetic relationships among members of the genus *Streptococcus*. Int. J. Syst. Bacteriol. *45*:406-408, 1995.
12. Kawamura, Y., Hou, X., Sultana, F., et al.: Transfer of *Streptococcus adjacens* and *Streptococcus defectivus* to *Abiotrophia* gen. nov. as *Abiotrophia adjacens* comb. nov. and *Abiotrophia defectiva* comb. nov., respectively. Int. J. Syst. Bacteriol. *45*:798-803, 1995.
13. McNeil, M. M., and Brown, J. M.: The medically important aerobic actinomycetes: Epidemiology and microbiology. Clin. Microbiol. Rev. *7*:357-417, 1994.
14. Palleroni, N. J., and Bradbury, J. F.: *Stenotrophomonas*, a new bacterial genus for *Xanthomonas maltophilia* (Hugh 1980) Swings et al. 1983. Int. J. Syst. Bacteriol. *43*:606-609, 1993.
15. Ruimy, R., Boiron, P., Boivin, V., et al.: A phylogeny of the genus *Nocardia* deduced from the analysis of small-subunit ribosomal DNA sequences, including transfer of *Nocardia amarae* to the genus *Gordona* as *Gordona amarae* comb. F. E. M. S. Microbiol. Lett. *123*:261-268, 1994.
16. Ruoff, K. L.: Recent taxonomic changes in the genus *Enterococcus*. Eur. J. Clin. Microbiol. Infect. Dis. *9*:75-79, 1990.
17. Shah, H. N., and Collins, M. D.: Proposal for reclassification of *Bacteroides asaccharolyticus*, *Bacteroides gingivalis*, and *Bacteroides endotalis* in a new genus, *Porphyromonas*. Int. J. Syst. Bacteriol. *38*:128-131, 1988.
18. Shah, H. N., and Collins, M. D.: *Prevotella*, a new genus, to include *Bacteroides melaninogenicus* and related species formerly classified in the genus, *Bacteroides*. Int. J. Syst. Bacteriol. *40*:205-208, 1990.
19. Shinnick, T. M., and Good, R. C.: Mycobacterial taxonomy. Eur. J. Clin. Microbiol. *13*:884-901, 1994.
20. Sneath, P. H. A.: International Code of Nomenclature of Bacteria: Bacteriological Code, 1990 Revision. Washington, D.C., American Society of Microbiology, 1992.
21. Stackebrandt, E., and Goebel, B. M.: Taxonomic note: A place for DNA-DNA reassociation and 16S rRNA sequence analysis in the present species definition in bacteriology. Int. J. Syst. Bacteriol. *44*:846-849, 1994.

Gram-Positive Cocci

CHAPTER

91

STAPHYLOCOCCUS AUREUS INFECTIONS (COAGULASE-POSITIVE STAPHYLOCOCCI)

Sheldon L. Kaplan ✪ Kristina G. Hulten ✪ Edward O. Mason

Staphylococcus aureus is a gram-positive coccus that occurs in pairs, chains, and grapelike clusters (Fig. 91–1). *S. aureus* is ubiquitous in nature and can be pathogenic for humans and animals. Staphylococci are nonmotile, aerobic, or facultative anaerobic and are readily cultivated on routine laboratory media.

These organisms are part of the normal human flora. *S. aureus* is responsible for an impressive variety of diseases ranging from minor skin and soft tissue infections to major life-threatening and fatal infections such as bacteremia, endocarditis, pericarditis, pneumonia, empyema, osteomyelitis, myositis, and septic arthritis.

On blood agar, *S. aureus* forms round, convex, shiny opaque colonies 1 to 4 mm in diameter, often with a zone of clear beta-hemolysis (Fig. 91–2) surrounding the colony. Production of pigment is variable, with strains exhibiting a yellow or golden pigment on primary isolation; yellow pigment actually is an *S. aureus* virulence factor.[132] *S. aureus* secretes free coagulase, the basis for the most definitive and most accepted method for identifying pathogenic staphylococci associated with human and animal infection. Free coagulase reacts with coagulase activator in plasma and converts fibrinogen to fibrin, with the formation of a fibrin clot. Coagulase also can be evaluated by testing for bound coagulase or clumping factor in a rapid slide test (Fig. 91–3). Clumping factor bound to the organism acts directly on fibrinogen and converts it to fibrin; it is detected by visible clumping or agglutination when a suspension is incubated with plasma. The bound coagulase test is used frequently in clinical laboratories and is faster than the tube coagulase test. However, the slide test for clumping factor may be falsely negative in 10 to 15 percent of cases. Thus, a negative slide coagulase test with an isolate that is highly suggestive of *S. aureus* should be confirmed with a tube coagulase test for free coagulase.[120,174] A limited number of biochemical reactions can differentiate *S. aureus* from other staphylococci (Table 91–1).

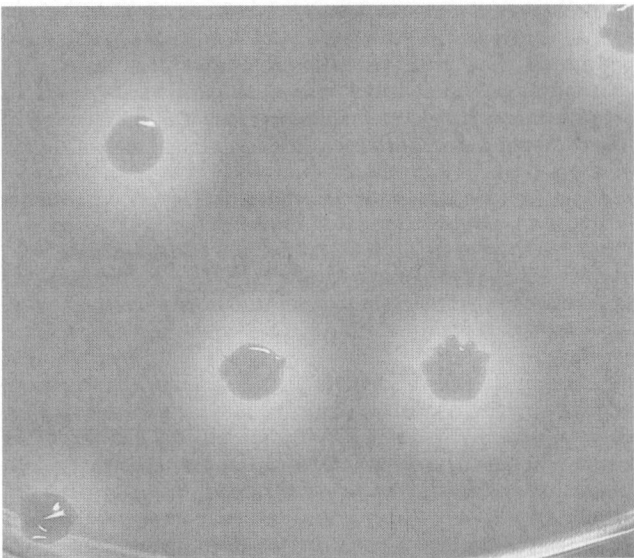

Figure 91–2 Typical hemolysis produced by *Staphylococcus aureus* on sheep blood agar. (See companion Expert Consult web site for color version.)

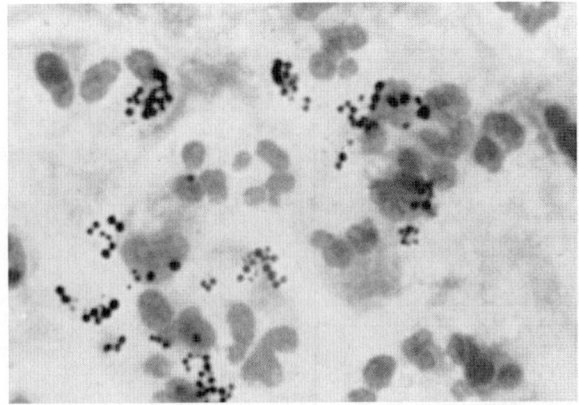

Figure 91–1 Staphylococci in pus. The organisms tend to form clusters, are round, and stain purple with Gram stain (positive), similar to bunches of grapes.

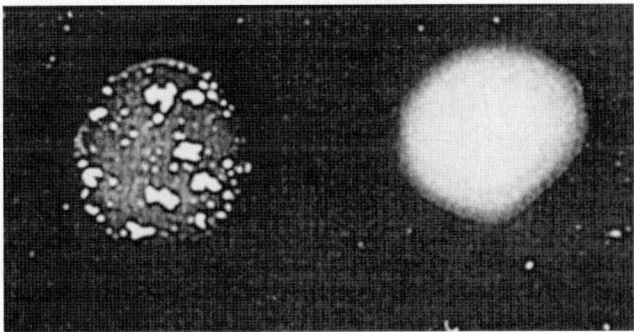

Figure 91–3 Bound (slide) coagulase test. A suspension of organisms is mixed with plasma. Immediate clumping (reaction on the *left*) indicates both the presence of bound coagulase and the fact that the organism is coagulase-positive.

STRUCTURE

CAPSULE

Capsule production often is considered a virulence factor and frequently is used by bacteria to hinder phagocytosis by the host.[159] Karakawa and colleagues described a scheme of eight *S. aureus* capsular types in 1982.[110] Subsequently, Sompolinsky and coworkers described three more serotypes, bringing the total number to 11.[199] Most *S. aureus* organisms are encapsulated to a varying degree (Fig. 91–4). Two serotypes (1 and 2) produce mucoid colonies on agar media but are rare among clinical isolates.[199] Serotypes 5 and 8 account for approximately 75 percent of strains recovered from infections in humans. In practice, strains that do not belong to serotypes 1, 2, 5, or 8 are referred to as *nontypeable*.[93] The role of capsule polysaccharide (CP) in virulence comes primarily from studies of CP5 and CP8 and is not completely clear. These studies show that inhibition of phagocytosis by capsule can result in persistence on surfaces but modulates adherence to endothelial surfaces.[159] A protein conjugate vaccine composed of CP5 and CP8 conjugated to nontoxic recombinant *Pseudomonas aeruginosa* exotoxin A (StaphVAX) initially appeared promising in prevention of *S. aureus* bacteremia in patients undergoing hemodialysis.[192] However, in a larger study, this vaccine was not found to be efficacious.[190]

PROTEIN A

Staphylococcal protein A, a major component of the cell wall of coagulase-positive staphylococci, has been found to bind to the Fc portion of immunoglobulin G (IgG). This binding is nonimmune. It differs from specific antigen-antibody reactions in that the reaction is nonspecific, although both precipitation and agglutination are observed. Protein A binds the IgG of many mammalian species. This property has rendered protein A a major reagent in many immune assays. Protein A also has been found to bind to platelets through the platelet gC1qr, a 33-kd cell protein[158] as well as to von Willebrand factor,[87] both of which may be important in the pathogenesis of endovascular infections caused by *S. aureus*. Protein A plays a central role in the pathogenesis of staphylococcal pneumonia in that TNFR1, a receptor for tumor necrosis factor-α (TNF-α), also is a receptor for protein A, and thus protein A is a principal staphylococcal proinflammatory factor in the lung.[74]

EXTRACELLULAR PRODUCTS

S. aureus elaborates a wide variety of extracellular toxins, many of which have potent biologic effects in the isolated state on intact animals, tissues, cells, and membranes. These toxins generally are thought to be responsible for the virulence of *S. aureus*, and the role of several of these products in staphylococcal infections has been proved definitively in humans. The important staphylococcal extracellular products include the following: alpha-, beta-, and delta-hemolysins; coagulases; leukocidin; hyaluronidase; staphylokinase; bacteriocins; the epidermolytic toxins; toxic shock syndrome toxin type I (TSST-I); and the enterotoxins.

Almost half of the known toxins and virulence genes in *S. aureus* are found in pathogenicity islands. These genetic clusters, commonly 15 to 20 kb in size, also contain genetic elements such as integrases and transposases. A high genetic instability is associated with many of these islands, and mosaic structures are common findings. Seven pathogenicity islands (νSa) have been associated with *S. aureus*.[68] Table 91–2 illustrates some of the features described for these islands, although allelic variations in gene content occur. All sequenced strains of *S. aureus* contain variations of the νSaα, νSaβ, and νSaγ.[47,68,94] In addition to the pathogenicity islands, virulence genes are also located on prophages (e.g., *lukS-PV* and *lukF-PV* on SLT).

TABLE 91–1 Identification of Staphylococci

Characteristics	*S. aureus*	*S. epidermidis*	*S. saprophyticus*
Coagulase	+	–	–
Acid aerobically from			
Sucrose	+	+	+
Trehalose	+	–	+
Mannitol	+	–	+
Phosphatase	+	+	–
Novobiocin	Sensitive	Sensitive	Resistant

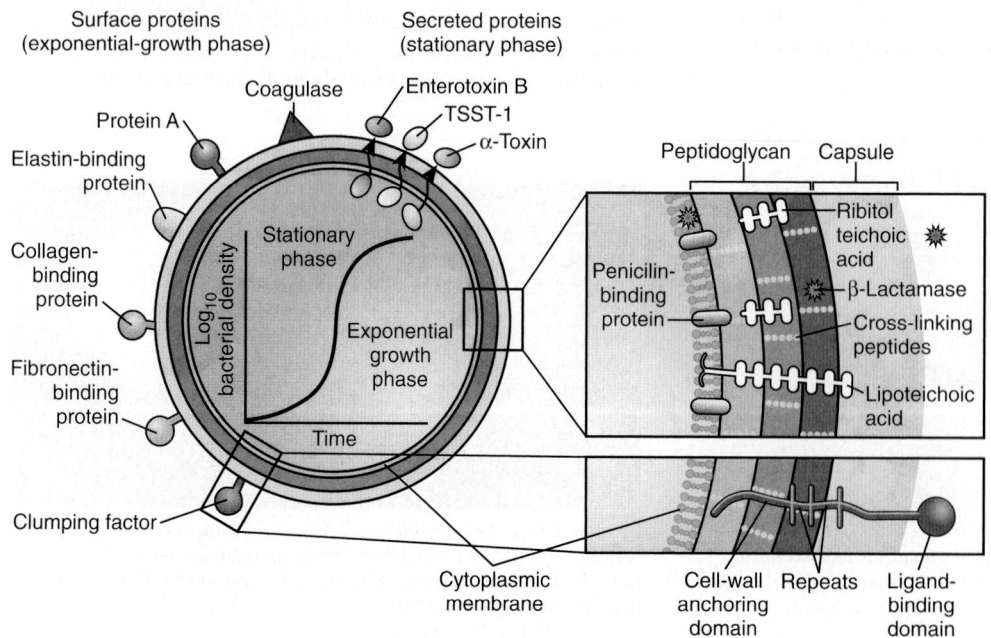

Figure 91–4 Structure of *Staphylococcus aureus*. TSST-1, toxic shock syndrome toxin type I. *(From Lowy, F. D.: Medical progress: Staphylococcus aureus infections. N. Engl. J. Med. 339:520-532, 1998.)*

TABLE 91–2 Pathogenicity Islands of *Staphylococcus aureus**

Island	Alleles	Genes	Reference
vSa1	SaPI1, SaPI3	*seb, tst, sek, seq, ear*	131
vSa2	SaPIbov	*tst, sec*	60
vSa3	SaPI3	Type I: *fhuD*; type II: *sel2, sec4, ear*	232
vSa4	SaPI2	Type I: *sel, sec3, tst*; Type II: 4 unknown ORFs	130
vSaα		Type I: *set 6-15, lpl 1-9*; Type II: *set 16-26, lpl 10-14* Type III: *set 1-5, lpl 2,7,8,11,13*	68, 235
vSaβ		Type I: *spl A-F, lukDE, ear*, epidermin gene cluster; Type II: *spl A-F, lukDE, ear, seg, sen, sei, sem, seo*, epidermin gene cluster	68
vSaγ		*set 1,3,4, eta*, phenol-soluble modulin,	68

Enterotoxins: seb, sec, seg, sei, sel, sem, sen, seo; exotoxins: set 1-26, toxic shock syndrome toxin I (tst), β-lactamase (ear), tandem lipoprotein (lpl), ferric hydroxamate uptake (fhuD), leukocidin (lukDE), serine protease (IA-F), exfoliative toxin A.
ORF, open reading frame.

HEMOLYSINS

Alpha-hemolysin is produced by most *S. aureus* isolates and is a classic pore-forming bacterial toxin. The purified toxin has impressive hemolytic, dermonecrotic, and lethal properties. Advances in protein purification have allowed pure toxin to be produced; this development, in turn, has led to a better understanding of its properties.

The protein interacts with and damages a variety of cell membranes, releases hemoglobin from erythrocytes of various mammalian and avian species, and is cytotoxic to numerous cell lines in tissue culture. It lyses rabbit and human platelets and disrupts lysosomes. It causes contraction in skeletal and vascular smooth muscle, an action that perhaps explains its property of causing localized dermal necrosis. In a rat model, alpha-toxin damages the air-blood barrier in vivo during *S. aureus* pneumonia.[143] Alpha-toxin forms pores in the membranes of endothelial cells; this process leads to vasoconstriction and increases vascular permeability, as well as having effects that cause apoptosis of numerous different cells.[49]

Injection of alpha-toxin is lethal to mammals and reptiles; death occurs within 2 to 5 minutes. Human death has been attributed to preformed alpha-toxin on at least one occasion. Anti–alpha-toxin can be demonstrated in physiologically normal persons; however, the level of anti–alpha-hemolysin is high in approximately 70 percent of patients with staphylococcal osteomyelitis.[208] In humans and experimental animals, the presence of anti–alpha-hemolysin neither modifies nor prevents staphylococcal infection.

The other hemolytic toxins, beta- and delta-hemolysin, also possess hemolytic and cytotoxic activities. In addition, beta-toxin produces lethal and dermonecrotic effects. Eighty to 100 percent of adults possess antibody to beta-hemolysin.

Despite evidence that these toxins are produced during infection, their roles in production of the typical staphylococcal tissue lesion remain unclear.[21,49] Although these toxins may be important in the establishment of infection by interacting with each other and with other biologically active staphylococcal products, this theory has not been proved; infection is not prevented by antitoxin antibody, and virulent staphylococci that lack one or more of these toxins are encountered.[197]

A recent in vitro study using proteomics (two-dimensional gel electrophoresis coupled with automated direct infusion-tandem mass spectrometry [ADI-MS/MS] analysis) showed that alpha-toxin was present in culture supernatants seven- to ninefold greater in the USA300 compared with the USA400 strain when grown at mid-exponential and stationary phases of growth.[31] Further studies of the way in which exotoxins influence strain-induced disease and host response are warranted.

LEUKOCIDIN

Although certain hemolysins are toxic to various leukocytes, the Panton-Valentine leukocidin (PVL) is the only known extracellular toxin that attacks the leukocyte exclusively.[166] It consists of two protein components, LukS-PV and LukF-PV, encoded by the genes *lukS-PV* and *lukF-PV* carried on a bacteriophage, that synergistically cause pores in polymorphonuclear leukocytes and macrophages.[26] Leukocidin injected into rabbits causes a striking fall in levels of circulating and bone marrow leukocytes, followed by marked granulocytosis; these changes occur without death of the rabbits. Leukocidin interacts with the membrane phospholipid and causes depolarization, increased permeability, and cell death. Local secretion of leukocidin may appear to confer an advantage to the staphylococcus by killing leukocytes and thereby preventing phagocytosis and intracellular killing. Levels of anti-leukocidin rise rapidly in the course of infection,[71,99] and some evidence indicates that infants and mothers with high levels of anti-leukocidin antibody are less likely to contract staphylococcal disease in high-risk epidemiologic situations.[17]

In early studies, only a few *S. aureus* isolates recovered from humans were *pvl*-positive.[171] Interest in PVL greatly increased following reports that *S. aureus* isolates carrying *pvl* genes were associated with severe furunculosis[41] and, particularly, necrotizing pneumonia in children and adolescents that frequently was fatal.[70,128] Furthermore, the independent emergence worldwide of community-acquired methicillin-resistant *S. aureus* (CA-MRSA) clones that generally carry the *pvl* genes led to further studies of the role of PVL in the pathogenesis of *S. aureus* infections.[215] The USA300 CA-MRSA clone especially has been linked to *pvl*.[150,151] In children with invasive *S. aureus* osteomyelitis, the presence of *pvl* genes was associated with greater local and systemic inflammation, longer duration of fever, greater frequency of positive blood cultures, and more frequent complications such as the development of chronic osteomyelitis or venous thrombosis.[24,140] Pulmonary manifestations also occurred more frequently among children with invasive *S. aureus* infections caused by *pvl*-positive isolates.[75] In adults with staphylococcal pneumonia, *pvl*-positive isolates were associated with increased rates of mortality.[134] Thus, the presence of *pvl* genes may be a marker for isolates capable of causing more severe disease.[56]

The contribution of PVL to the severity of *S. aureus* infections has been examined in mice using isogenic *pvl*-positive or *pvl*-negative isolates. One study found no difference in lethality for sepsis or abscess volume in a skin abscess model,[219] as well as no difference in the destruction of human neutrophils by the isogenic strains. The investigators concluded that PVL was not a major virulence determinant of CA-MRSA. The other study found that *pvl*-positive isolates caused much greater lung inflammation and necrosis in a mouse acute pneumonia model.[118] PVL was detected in the infected lung tissues. These investigators also discovered that staphylococcal protein A is more highly expressed in *pvl*-positive strains and postulated that PVL coupled with increased staphylococcal protein A could result in greater tissue inflammation than that found with *pvl*-negative strains. The discrepancy in these studies may be explained by the use of different *S. aureus* isolates as well as different models of infection.

Although the exact role of PVL in *S. aureus* infections has not been fully established, treatment measures directed against PVL have been proposed and include the preferred use of protein-inhibiting antibiotics rather than or in addition to bactericidal antibiotics to decrease production of PVL,[51,202] as well as adjunctive administration of intravenous immunoglobulin preparations containing antibody to PVL.[67]

ENZYMES

Staphylococci elaborate a variety of enzymes, including hyaluronidase, nuclease, proteases, lipase, catalase, lysozyme, and lactate dehydrogenase, that may play a role in the spread of infection in local tissues or the establishment of a nidus of infection. Other biologically active extracellular products, as yet unidentified, undoubtedly are produced by the staphylococcus. The potency and number of these weapons in the armamentarium of the coagulase-positive staphylococcus, in contrast to the small number of extracellular products associated with the much less virulent coagulase-negative staphylococcus, suggest that the synergistic action of these toxins and enzymes may explain the superior ability of coagulase-positive staphylococci to establish infection and cause tissue necrosis. Several extracellular toxins have been proved to have specific roles in staphylococcal infection or disease: the epidermolytic toxins, TSST-I, and the enterotoxins.

EPIDERMOLYTIC TOXINS

Two biochemically and immunologically distinct exotoxins, epidermolytic toxins A and B (epidermolysins, exfoliatins), can separate adjacent cell layers within the epidermis and can cause the various skin manifestations of the staphylococcal scalded skin syndrome (SSSS). The toxin acts extracellularly; it does not induce cell death directly or lysis of the cell membrane or elicit an inflammatory response. This toxin does not damage any organ or cell, except those of the upper epidermis.[53,127,147] These low-molecular-weight (≈24,000 d) protein exotoxins now are known to hydrolyze desmoglein-1, an important structural skin protein.[9] Exfoliatin toxin D has been described but has not been associated with bullous impetigo or SSSS.[231]

TOXIC SHOCK SYNDROME TOXIN TYPE I

TSST-I was discovered independently in 1981 by two research groups. It was documented to be an excellent marker for staphylococci associated with vaginal toxic shock syndrome (TSS), in which it correctly identified more than 90 percent of strains in blinded testing. In experimental animal models, purified TSST-I can induce the major physiologic changes of TSS: fever, mucous membrane suffusion, renal impairment, hepatic damage, hypocalcemia, lymphocytopenia, and hypotension. TSST-I can be detected in blood, pus, urine, and tissues during human and experimental model TSS. USA300, the major CA-MRSA clone in the United States, does not carry the gene encoding TSST-1.[151] TSS is discussed in Chapter 71.

ENTEROTOXINS

Multiple different staphylococcal exotoxins (enterotoxins A to Q) have been identified, and most of them cause emesis in primates.[49] The toxins are heat-stable and resist boiling. Therefore, once sufficient toxin has formed within food, even heating or boiling will not inactivate the toxin. Foods involved in outbreaks of food poisoning frequently have been inoculated by a lesion on the hand of a food handler in situations in which the food is then held at temperatures that allow bacterial growth (between 25° C and 60° C) to occur for some time before the food is served.

Foods implicated in particular are ham, salads with starch and mayonnaise, salami, poultry, cream sauces, pastries, and dairy products. The mode of action of enterotoxins is not understood completely, but vomiting appears to be induced through receptors in the abdominal viscera that lead to an emetic response.[29] Intravenous injection of purified enterotoxins in laboratory animals causes hypotension, cardiovascular collapse, and death. The significance of these properties of enterotoxins in naturally occurring human infections is unknown, although they may be linked to clinical syndromes, including TSS. Enterotoxin A often is elaborated with TSST-I in menstrual-associated TSS, but it also is elaborated without TSST-I in patients with septicemia in whom TSS does not develop. Staphylococcal enterotoxin B, most often isolated in phage group V organisms, is associated with local infections and pneumonia.[139] USA300 strains typically do not contain the genes encoding most enterotoxins, but they frequently have the genes for enterotoxins Q and K.[46] In contrast, USA400 isolates may carry many of the enterotoxin genes, including enterotoxin H, which is unique among the other S. aureus genomes.[14,156]

STAPHYLOCOCCUS AUREUS MSCRAMMs

Bacterial adherence to host tissues is mediated by numerous bacterial surface components or adhesins that recognize and bind to host extracellular matrix and cell surface molecules.[98] The subfamily of adhesins that bind to the extracellular matrix is known as Microbial Surface Components Recognizing Adhesive Matrix Molecules (MSCRAMMs). For S. aureus, important MSCRAMMs are protein A, fibronectin-binding proteins (A and B), clumping factors A and B (fibrinogen-binding proteins), and collagen-binding protein (cna).[63] Many other less well characterized adhesins also have been identified from the S. aureus genome.[181] The MSCRAMMs are linked to bacterial wall peptidoglycan following sortase cleavage of the LPXTG (LeuProX-ThrGly) motif that is a conserved C-terminal cell wall sorting signal among the adhesins.[36] Fibronectin-binding proteins play a role in S. aureus invasion into endothelial cells.[24,98] Collagen adhesin protein may contribute to the pathogenesis of S. aureus musculoskeletal infections,[52,164] although both animal studies and clinical studies are conflicting in this area.[100,184] USA300 CA-MRSA isolates do not carry the gene for cna, yet osteomyelitis is the most common CA-MRSA invasive infection in children.[140]

Clumping factor A has been the target for protective immunity in the prevention of S. aureus infections, and this approach has been successful in experimental models.[217] The safety and pharmacokinetics of an intravenous immunoglobulin preparation enriched for antibody to clumping factor A were established in low-birth-weight infants; however, a large randomized trial did not document efficacy in prevention of staphylococcal infections in this population.[53] A monoclonal antibody (tefibazumab [Aurexis]) directed against clumping factor A has undergone preliminary evaluation as adjunctive therapy of S. aureus bacteremia in adults.[224]

REGULATION

Bacterial pathogenesis is reliant on cell population, density-dependent gene expression. This quorum sensing acts to adjust the production of accessory genes (e.g., virulence genes), depending on the needs of the cell. Studies have shown that in low-density populations, when the bacterial cells are multiplying, accessory genes are either turned off or are expressed at a low level to the advantage of other genes, such as genes involved in cell wall formation. In high-density bacterial populations, expression of the accessory genes is increased. The accessory gene regulator, agr, is genus specific, and the effector molecule is a regulatory RNA molecule, named RNAIII. Many staphylococcal toxins and virulence factors are under the regulation of agr.[1,13,28] The staphylococcal accessory regulator, sar, is another global regulator in *S. aureus*. The effector peptide, SarA, is a DNA-binding protein. In animal models of infection, both RNAIII and Sar A have been shown to affect virulence. In addition to agr and sar, several other factors have been described that affect accessory gene regulation.[22] Thus, the complex network of regulatory operons that act on each other or directly on specific genes is not completely understood.

STAPHYLOCOCCAL L-FORMS AND SMALL-COLONY VARIANTS

L-forms are staphylococcal variants with impaired or absent cell walls. L-forms can be induced in vitro by growing staphylococci in hypertonic media, in the presence of the muralytic enzyme lysostaphin, or with the addition of antibiotics that inhibit the formation of cell walls, such as the penicillin-methicillin group, cycloserine, and vancomycin. These L-forms, or protoplasts, require hypertonic environments for survival, do not accept Gram stain, and are resistant to cell wall–inhibiting antibiotics. Under favorable conditions, L-forms revert to complete bacteria with cell walls.

Clinical interest in L-forms has arisen because of concern that antibiotics may induce these forms in vivo. L-forms then could persist in the host in a latent or less virulent phase and revert to a fully virulent state at some time when antibiotics no longer are present. Identification of L-forms in specimens from human infection or in infected animals treated with antibiotics has been reported exceedingly rarely, despite considerable effort.[220] The presence of latent L-forms remains an attractive hypothesis to explain the well-known tendency of staphylococcal infections to persist and recur. Despite extensive laboratory and clinical investigation, no evidence has demonstrated that L-forms are important causes of bacterial persistence in clinical infections.

Small-colony variants of *S. aureus* are isolates with atypical colony morphology, decreased hemolysis and pigmentation, decreased growth rate, and unusual biochemical characteristics that result in difficulty isolating and identifying these organisms.[216] Small-colony variants also have been implicated in persistent and recurrent *S. aureus* infections including osteomyelitis,[172] brain abscesses, and pulmonary infections in patients with cystic fibrosis.[104,188] Small-colony variants can persist intracellularly and often are more resistant to antibiotics than is the parent strain, and antibiotics that penetrate cells (e.g., rifampin) may be advantageous in their treatment.[173]

TYPING METHODS

Staphylococcal strains were characterized historically by bacteriophage typing (World Health Organization method).[18] In the 1990s, pulsed-field gel electrophoresis (PFGE) became the gold standard for strain typing used by both reference and research laboratories.[210] The method has proven to be reliable and reproducible, and the use of digital imaging and band analysis has enhanced the quality of inter-gel comparisons. The Centers for Disease Control and Prevention (CDC) used the PFGE method to define and interrelate staphylococcal clones circulating in the United States and designated these 11 clones USA100 to USA1100 (available through the Network on Antimicrobial Resistance of *Staphylococcus aureus* [NARSA] at http://www.narsa. net).[142]

Multilocus sequence typing (MLST) is a nucleotide sequence-based method, adapted from multilocus enzyme electrophoresis (MLEE). In MLST typing, the alleles at each locus of seven housekeeping genes (*arc*C, *aro*E, *glp*F, *gmk*, *pta*, *tpi*, and *yqi*L) are determined through polymerase chain reaction (PCR) amplification, nucleotide sequencing, and submission of sequence data through computer Web site to the MLST database (http://www.mlst.net).[54] In this database, strains can be compared with strains submitted by other investigators, and within-laboratory comparisons with control strains thus have become obsolete.

spa typing was developed based on the polymorphic X or the short sequence repeat (SSR) region of the protein A gene.[194] *spa* typing has some advantages over PFGE in terms of speed, interpretation, and exportability; the main limitation is the single locus-based design.[84] Less commonly used methods include repetitive element PCR (rep-PCR), restriction fragment length polymorphism (RFLP), and toxin typing.

STAPHYLOCOCCUS AUREUS CLONES IN THE HOSPITAL AND IN THE COMMUNITY

Of the methods mentioned earlier, MLST has been especially useful in dividing *S. aureus* strains into lineages (or clonal clusters). Frequently, these clones are described in the literature by their sequence type followed by the staphylococcal cassette chromosome *mec* (SCC*mec*) type (e.g., ST8-IV). Most human *S. aureus* strains belong to 1 of 10 independent lineages. Five major clonal clusters (CCs) that have been described to contain a majority of the human MRSA strains are CC5, CC8, CC22, CC30, and CC45. Of these, MRSA clones within the CC5 and CC8 clusters have been recognized as the main causes of hospital outbreaks worldwide.[38] Examples of widespread hospital MRSA clones are EMRSA15-ST22, EMRSA16 (ST36-II), the Archaic (ST250-I or 247-I), the Pediatric (ST5-IV), and the Brazilian (ST239-III) clones.[73]

Although a few hospital MRSA clones have circulated around the world, genetically distinct community clones have been reported from different geographic areas. Commonly, these strains contain the smaller SCC*mec* elements, type IV or V.[179] Why these different clones emerged in parallel at this point in time is unknown.

In the United States, the two most commonly described community MRSA clones are USA300-ST8 and USA400-ST1. USA400, originally described as MRSA strain MW2 and responsible for four pediatric deaths in Minnesota and North Dakota, has been observed more commonly in the Midwestern States.[10] USA300 is the strain most frequently reported causing community-acquired disease in both pediatric and adult settings in the United States. Like many other epidemic strains, it has been associated with a spectrum of disease presentations ranging from simple skin and soft tissue infections[105,108] to severe sepsis syndrome,[76] sometimes with a fatal outcome. USA300 is a highly virulent strain that has been distributed across the continent and has become the most prevalent cause of community-acquired infections in less than a decade.[151] It also has become the most common source of hospital-acquired *S. aureus* infection in many hospitals, where it has acquired one or more antibiotic resistance markers.[45,77,189] The special features and adaptability of this strain are discussed further in the genome section of this chapter.

MLST typing has enabled the ancestry of many of these clones to be traced phylogenetically. For example, phage type 80/81 (ST30-MSSA) was epidemic in the 1960s and is the likely ancestor to the widely circulated Southwest Pacific clone, ST30-MRSA-IV, which has been successful both as a colonizer and as a cause of diseases ranging from skin and soft tissue infections to invasive manifestations.[180] Similarly, the USA300 (ST8-MRSA-IV) clone is postulated to have descended from an archaic ST8-MSSA.[55]

S. aureus isolates are susceptible to lysis when they are exposed to bacteriophages. The particular pattern of bacteriophage lysis can be used to identify strains of staphylococci, but bacteriophage typing has been used primarily as an epidemiologic tool for identifying related strains in epidemics. An international system for identifying strains by bacteriophage typing has been established, but it is not widely used currently. Staphylococci of phage group 80/81 were widespread during the pandemic of staphylococcal disease in the late 1950s. At present, many different phage types are involved in staphylococcal disease.[180]

GENOMES

To date, nine genomes of *S. aureus* have been sequenced (Table 91–3). MW2,[14] FPR3757,[47] and TCH1516[90a] are the three CA-MRSA isolates with sequenced genomes, designated PFGE USA400 and USA300, respectively. *S. aureus* COL[68] is an early hospital-associated MRSA strain, and N315 and Mu50 are hospital-associated MRSA strains from Japan.[117] The Mu50 strain also has intermediate resistance to the glycopeptides(GISA/VISA). Strains 476[94] and NCTC8325[69] are methicillin-susceptible strains from the community and hospital environment, and EMRSA-16 is an MRSA strain that is a major hospital pathogen in Europe.[101] Genome sizes range from 2.8 to 2.9 Mb, and the structures of the chromosomes are well conserved. The core genome (the part of the genome that is the same in all strains) represents 75 percent of the genome.[129] Only approximately 40 to 50 percent of the predicted proteins have a known function.

EPIDEMIOLOGY

S. aureus isolates are responsible for both sporadic infections and epidemics of varying extent ranging from the intrafamily outbreaks of commonly encountered staphylococcal disease to large and often prolonged hospital-associated outbreaks, such as those emanating from a newborn nursery or a surgical service. Epidemic spread of staphylococci of phage type 80/81 was so widespread in hospitals worldwide in the period encompassing the mid-1950s through the early 1960s that it constituted a pandemic. Researchers have suggested that a few "epidemiologically virulent" strains, such as 80/81, are particularly capable of spreading widely and causing disease. Because we are largely ignorant of the factors responsible for pandemic spread, we cannot prevent or predict recurrence. Robinson and colleagues concluded that descendants of 80/81 have acquired methicillin resistance to emerge as a CA-MRSA clone, closely related to the southwest Pacific ST30 clone.[180]

Staphylococci may be transmitted by multiple routes, including contact with infected persons, contact with asymptomatic carriers, airborne spread, and contact with contaminated objects. Of these mechanisms, contact with a person who has a staphylo-coccal lesion appears to be particularly important in the spread of staphylococci. Persons with open draining lesions disseminate organisms into their environment and to others by direct contact. In a hospital, staphylococci may be spread from an infected patient to another on the hands of caretakers, such as physicians or nurses. Hospital personnel with mild or inapparent lesions, such as styes, furuncles, or paronychia, may themselves spread organisms. In family and small community outbreaks, multiple secondary cases frequently can be traced to an individual with a draining lesion. Secondary cases tend to appear for months after the initiating case within these small epidemiologic units.[200]

Staphylococci also may be spread by asymptomatic carriers who have staphylococci in one or more body sites, including the nose, skin, hair, nails, axillae, and perineum. At any one time, as many as 30 percent of individuals are colonized in their anterior nose with *S. aureus*.[114] The rate of nasal carriage of MRSA appears to have increased in the past decade. Nasal carriage of MRSA was 0.8 percent in 2001[157] and 9 percent in 2004[40] for children seen in an emergency center in Nashville, Tennessee. For children admitted to the hospital in Corpus Christi, Texas, in 2005, the rate of MRSA colonization was 22 percent.[6] Why nasal colonization of children by CA-MRSA has increased during the past decade is unclear but likely is related to unique properties of the major CA-MRSA clone, USA300.[47] Detailed studies have been performed to delineate factors regulating the carrier state and its establishment and perpetuation, as well as factors responsible for dispersion of organisms from carriers. Asymptomatic carriers may be a source of disease for themselves and for others. For example, a wound infection appears to be more likely to develop in a hospitalized patient who becomes a carrier than in a noncar-rier.[225] Much attention has been devoted to detecting and attempting to treat nasal carriers of staphylococci; however, studies of nursery outbreaks have indicated that nasal carriage is not as important as is hand transmission in the dispersal of staphylococci.[226] Transmission by hand contact can be minimized by effective handwashing.[72] The problem of hair carriage of staphylococci in operating room personnel has been minimized by using improved head coverings.

Staphylococci are widespread in the environment and can be cultured from clothing, carpets, toiletries (e.g., hairbrushes, razors), and virtually all environmental surfaces. Airborne dissemination of organisms is possible, particularly in operating rooms with poor ventilation and heavy traffic; improved methods of ventilating operating rooms may have reduced the rates of sepsis or colonization. Environmental staphylococci may serve as an important reservoir, but direct human-to-human transfer probably is a much more important means of transmission in epidemic situations than is airborne spread or contact with contaminated objects. This means of transmission is particularly true for spread of CA-MRSA among athletes.[112] Various methods that

TABLE 91–3 Complete Genomes of *Staphylococcus aureus*

Strain	Class	Meth	Van	ST	PFGE	SCC*mec*	PVL	*spa*	agr
COL	HA	R	S	250		I	Pos	YHGRMBQBLO	1
252/MRSA16	HA	R	S	36	200	II	Neg	WCKAKAOMQQQ	3
476	CA	S	S	30		N/A	Pos	UKJFKBPE	3
Mu50	HA	R	I	5	100	II	Pos	MDMGMK	3
MW2	CA	R	S	1	400	IV	Pos	UJJJJFE	3
N315	HA	R	S	5		II	Pos	MDMGMK	3
NCTC8325	HA	S	S	8		n/a	Pos	YHGGFMBQBLO	1
FPR3757	CA	R	S	8	300	IV	Pos	YHGFMBQBLO	1
TCH1516	CA	R	S	8	300	IV	Pos	YHGFMBQBLO	1

agr, accessory gene regulator; CA, community-acquired; HA, hospital acquired; I (under vancomycin), intermediated; meth, methicillin; N/A, not applicable; neg, negative; pos, positive; PVL, Panton Valentine leukocidin; PFGE, pulsed field gel electrophoresis USA pattern; R, resistant; S, susceptible; SCCmec, staphylococcal cassette chromosome; spa, spa type; ST, ST-sequence type; van, vancomycin.

are used to identify epidemiologic markers in nosocomial outbreaks of staphylococcal infection include molecular typing techniques, plasmid DNA analysis, restriction endonuclease fingerprinting of chromosome DNA, and rapid-field inversion gel electrophoresis. Molecular methods of typing offer adjunctive information useful in characterizing strains involved in outbreaks.[48,54]

The neonatal nursery has been an area of particular concern in the transmission of staphylococci. Until the 1980s, *S. aureus* was the major concern. During the pandemic of strain 80/81 disease, outbreaks of serious neonatal disease were commonplace, high colonization rates were found in infants on discharge from the nursery, and the subsequent incidence of disease in some outbreaks was as high as 50 to 70 percent. Skin disease and infant and maternal mastitis usually appear within 1 to 4 weeks after discharge. Staphylococcal pneumonia, far more common during that period than at present, may not be seen for months after delivery, even though the infecting strain was acquired in a hospital. During the experience with strain 80/81 disease, a particularly high staphylococcal attack rate was seen in the families of colonized infants. The same epidemiology has been noted for the USA300 CA-MRSA clone, which has been associated with staphylococcal infections in otherwise healthy newborns up through 30 days of life.[61] The mother in approximately 20 percent of cases had a presumed or concomitant *S. aureus* infection around the time of her infant's infection in one study.[61]

Various control measures were used successfully to terminate individual outbreaks during the 1980s. Measures to protect the infant from colonization and subsequent development of disease by establishing a barrier at the site of initial colonization included hexachlorophene bathing, application of antibiotic ointment to the umbilicus and circumcision site, and application of an antiseptic dye to the umbilicus. Another approach, deliberate colonization of the umbilicus with an interfering "avirulent" strain, was successful in controlling several epidemics but itself caused skin disease and, in one case, fatal septicemia.[193] Hexachlorophene bathing became a widespread practice during the period in which nosocomial staphylococcal infections were declining.[72,169] After approximately a decade of using hexachlorophene, researchers recognized that cutaneous absorption of hexachlorophene could result in potentially toxic hexachlorophene blood levels in infants, particularly premature ones, subjected to repeated daily baths over time. Brain stem abnormalities associated with the use of hexachlorophene were demonstrated in premature infants. For these reasons, controls were placed on the sale of hexachlorophene, and its routine use was discouraged in 1973. In one neonatal nursery outbreak of MRSA, the use of 0.3 percent triclosan (Bacti-Stat) was associated with cessation of an outbreak.[233]

Coincident with the widespread discontinuation of hexachlorophene bathing, but not necessarily causally related to it, was the reported increased incidence of nursery outbreaks of *S. aureus* disease. Many of these outbreaks were caused by epidermolytic toxin-producing strains of staphylococci belonging to phage group II. In these outbreaks, limited areas of bullous impetigo developed in most children within 1 to 4 weeks after discharge, and a few children showed the more dramatic manifestations of generalized exfoliative disease. Contemporary epidemics appear to have a much lower incidence of septicemia, pneumonia, and osteomyelitis and less potential for spread to other family members.

Patterns of crowding of infants and understaffing contribute to outbreaks. Active clinical and bacteriologic surveillance and cohorting of infants may be effective in reducing the number of outbreaks.[16,83]

The frequency of bacteremia related to intravenous catheters and prosthetic devices has increased considerably.[137,138] Methicillin-resistant staphylococci have become more prevalent in the community and are responsible for widespread nosocomial outbreaks of disease in hospitals.[25,29,39,43,57,113,186,204,223]

HOST DEFENSES

S. aureus is ubiquitous in the environment, and approximately 30 percent of the population can be classified as carriers. A major defense against staphylococcal infection is intact skin. Minor wounds frequently become colonized and infected and serve as portals to deeper, more significant staphylococcal infection. In some cases, the integumentary infection may be of major importance; in others, minor skin punctures may serve to introduce infection to distant internal sites. Burns, varicella virus and cutaneous herpesvirus infections, insect bites, minor lacerations or abrasions, primary skin diseases (e.g., atopic eczema), epidermolysis bullosa, and surgical wounds are important portals of entry for staphylococci. A deficiency in peptides (defensins and cathelicidins) important for innate immunity of skin against *S. aureus* has been shown in biopsied skin of patients with atopic dermatitis and likely contributes to the increased susceptibility of the skin to *S. aureus* infections in these patients.[115,163] In hospitalized patients, intravenous needles and catheters may be sources of staphylococcal infection.[137,138]

Foreign bodies reduce local resistance to staphylococcal engraftment and are important in the pathogenesis and perpetuation of infection. Noteworthy foreign bodies are cerebrospinal fluid shunts, prosthetic cardiac valves, nonabsorbable sutures, vascular prostheses (including arteriovenous shunts for hemodialysis), and orthopedic prostheses, nails, and wires. In neonates, the umbilicus and circumcision sites, which may be colonized within the first few hours of life and from which both local and distant infections may be established, are important portals of entry.

Viral respiratory diseases such as measles and influenza[82,170] predispose the individual to development of pulmonary infection, again predominantly by damaging the integrity of the barrier at the portal of entry. Disruption of the respiratory epithelium and impairment of ciliary motion and other local defenses may allow secondary staphylococcal invasion to occur.

Once the integumentary barrier has been breached, the polymorphonuclear leukocyte appears to be the most important line of defense. Successful phagocytosis involves chemotaxis, opsonization, and intracellular killing. The incidence of difficulty with staphylococcal infection is highest in patients with defects in this area of host defense. Granulocytopenia of any origin predisposes one to the development of infection, particularly with the host's endogenous bacteria, including staphylococci.[15]

Patients with disorders of neutrophil chemotaxis are particularly subject to the development of recurrent and severe staphylococcal infections. Patients with lazy leukocyte syndrome have recurrent respiratory infections, gingivitis, and stomatitis. Their leukocytes exhibit normal phagocytosis and intracellular killing but are deficient in both motility toward a chemotactic stimulant and random motility. Leukocyte adhesion deficiency is a rare autosomal recessive disorder of leukocytes in which patients suffer recurrent skin infections. Patients with Chédiak-Higashi syndrome have recurrent infection in association with neutrophils that are morphologically abnormal, with giant lysosomes present in decreased number.[230] Hyper-IgE syndrome or Job syndrome is associated with severe, recurrent staphylococcal infections of the subcutaneous and deep skin tissues. Even for patients without defects in neutrophil chemotaxis, approximately 60 percent of *S. aureus* isolates secrete the chemotaxis inhibitory protein of staphylococci (CHIPS), and almost all have the extracellular adherence proteins that interfere with neutrophil chemotaxis and extravasation.[62]

Once the staphylococcus and the leukocyte are close to one another, opsonization of the bacterium must proceed for phagocytosis to occur. Two systems for opsonization of staphylococci have been described. Serum from normal adults has good opsonic activity when unheated but generally is inactive after heating at 56° C for 1 hour. The heat lability of normal opsonin and the observation of normal or only slightly decreased opsonic activity in unheated sera from patients with agammaglobulinemia[227] indicate that the major opsonin is complement. A few sera, generally from patients convalescing from serious staphylococcal disease, contain heat-stable opsonins, presumably antibody directed at the staphylococcal cell wall components.[121] Therefore, either complement or antibody can provide opsonins for staphylococci; specific antibody is helpful but not required. The clinical correlate to these observations may be found in patients with defective defenses; patients with agammaglobulinemia and defective antibody generally have more severe problems with organisms other than staphylococci, whereas patients with deficiencies in complement components have been reported to have repeated and severe staphylococcal infections.[3,7,8,64,149,167]

Once the bacterium has been ingested, intracellular killing proceeds normally. Coagulase-positive staphylococci can survive within polymorphonuclear leukocytes for a considerably longer period than can coagulase-negative organisms.[148] Prolonged intracellular survival may be an important virulence factor separating coagulase-negative from coagulase-positive strains and may provide a mechanism whereby surviving organisms may be carried to distant body sites to establish metastatic foci of infection. Some S. aureus exotoxins outlined earlier, such as PVL, contribute to the ability of S. aureus to evade human neutrophils. In addition, many S. aureus genes are regulated upward or downward after being exposed to human neutrophils, and differences exist in gene expression among various strains in response to human innate host response that may account for differences in the ability of the isolate to cause infection.[218]

Patients with chronic granulomatous disease of childhood have an inborn error in intraleukocytic killing of catalase-positive bacteria and fungi. These patients have an early onset of recurrent purulent infections of the skin, subcutaneous tissue, lungs, and reticuloendothelial organs, particularly the liver, that often are caused by S. aureus.[176] The response of these patients to therapy is slow and poor, a finding further demonstrating the absolute necessity of an intact polymorphonuclear bactericidal system in host defense against staphylococci. In contrast to the primacy of polymorphonuclear defense against staphylococci, evidence for an important role of specific humoral and cellular immunity in host defense against staphylococci is either lacking or contradictory.

Specific antibody is not required for opsonization of unencapsulated strains of staphylococci. The opsonic activity of serum from patients recovering from staphylococcal endocarditis or other serious disease is greater than that in physiologically normal persons.[121,228] Despite the presence of humoral antibodies to cell wall teichoic acids and to various toxins and enzymes, which are found regularly in those convalescing from serious staphylococcal infection, the patient remains susceptible to recurrence of infection with the same strain of staphylococci.

Staphylococcal infections generally occur and progress in the presence of some degree of humoral immunity. Specific antibody to one or more staphylococcal components or products does not protect against infection. Clinical evidence from patients with deficient cell-mediated immunity (combined immunodeficiency, thymic aplasia, Nezelof syndrome) suggests that staphylococcal infections are not among the most important pathogens in these patients.

Present evidence, therefore, suggests that intact local skin and mucous membrane barriers are the most important defenses against the establishment of staphylococcal infection. Once infection is established, an intact polymorphonuclear response is essential for containment of the infection and clearance of the organisms.

PATHOGENESIS

Staphylococci cause disease by two mechanisms: direct invasion of tissues with liberation of toxins, which may have effects at sites distant from the focus of infection, and colonization. The hallmark of a staphylococcal lesion is the abscess. Local tissue destruction at the site of inoculation is followed rapidly by hyperemia and a vigorous inflammatory response marked by the accumulation of large numbers of polymorphonuclear leukocytes. Tissue necrosis in the center of the lesion occurs next. At the site of intensive hyperemia surrounding the lesion, a fibrin wall is formed. Liquefaction necrosis occurs centrally; the mature lesion consists of a fibrin wall surrounded by inflamed tissues enclosing a central core of pus consisting of organisms and leukocytes. Live bacteria may persist within these lesions for a considerable period of time. As pus accumulates, it may drain toward the skin surface or into adjacent tissues, where it forms sinus tracts and secondary abscesses. In the presence of an intact host inflammatory response, this type of reaction may be seen in diverse areas, including the skin and subcutaneous tissues, lymph nodes, joints, renal tissues, liver, parotid glands, muscles, lungs, and long bones.

In addition to local extension, S. aureus may disseminate hematogenously from this focus of infection, even from abscesses that are trivial in size. Hematogenous dissemination may result in infection of bones, joints, and heart valves. Given the ubiquitous nature of staphylococci, skin and wounds, which are the usual ports of entry, appear to be remarkably resistant to infection. This natural resistance is affected dramatically by the presence of foreign bodies within the wound, such as sutures and bits of soil or gravel. Natural resistance also is affected by the tissue compromise that develops after ecchymosis or hemorrhage occurs and by vascular insufficiency. Poor personal hygiene also predisposes to development of staphylococcal skin infection. Moist, macerated skin is invaded more easily and thus contributes to the increased frequency of staphylococcal skin infection in intertriginous areas and in tropical climates.

Toxigenic staphylococcal disease includes SSSS, TSS, and staphylococcal food poisoning. The major manifestations of these diseases are caused by the effects of specific toxins. Clinical manifestations of infections caused by S. aureus in children are discussed in several chapters, and the reader is referred to the specific infection of interest.

DIAGNOSIS

The diagnosis of significant staphylococcal infections should be pursued with vigor. Collections of pus, whether superficial or deep, should be aspirated or drained surgically for diagnostic and therapeutic purposes. Gram stain and culture should be performed. An aggressive approach to establishing the diagnosis of osteomyelitis by bone aspiration and bone biopsy provides an etiologic security that is helpful during the prolonged treatment phase that necessarily follows. When infection is associated with a foreign body, such as an intravenous catheter or suture, removal and culture of the foreign body help in determining the cause, and removal almost always is required for successful resolution of infection.

At least two blood cultures should be obtained before starting therapy for all serious infections. One need not wait for fever spikes or delay therapy to obtain specimens. Blood cultures frequently are negative in serious staphylococcal infection, a finding that demonstrates the need for performing other cultures. Blood cultures are positive in most cases of staphylococcal endocarditis, approximately half the cases of osteomyelitis and septic arthritis, and fewer than half the cases of pneumonia and deep-tissue abscesses. Measurement of nonspecific indicators of inflammation (e.g., erythrocyte sedimentation rate and C-reactive protein), although of limited value in establishing the diagnosis, can be helpful in monitoring the clinical course of infection and response to intervention. Accurate, sensitive serologic methods for determining a diagnosis of serious staphylococcal infection are not available.

Enterotoxins can be identified by a variety of methods. Immunoassay is used routinely but may lack the sensitivity required to detect levels seen in staphylococcal food poisoning. DNA oligonucleotide probes are highly sensitive, but their clinical utility is limited by the identification of nonexpressed genes.[160] Numerous molecular tests are available to identify MRSA rapidly once it is isolated in the microbiology laboratory and to detect MRSA colonization in patients at the time of hospital admission.[214]

TREATMENT

Successful treatment of staphylococcal infection depends on adequate drainage of collections of pus and the rational use of antibiotic therapy. (Strategies for clinical management of MRSA in the community are outlined in a document developed by the CDC and available at http://www.cdc.gov/ncidod/dhqp/pdf/ar/CAMRSA_ExpMtgStrategies.pdf.) Staphylococcal infections have a particular tendency to persist and recur; for these reasons, prolonged courses of antibiotic therapy usually is required for all but minor infections. Surgical drainage is extremely important and, in some patients with minor superficial abscesses, may be all that is required. In one study, an abscess less than 5 cm in diameter was associated with successful outcome of incision and drainage, regardless of whether the antibiotic administered was active against the isolated pathogen, which was CA-MRSA.[124] For most

infections, a course of antibiotic therapy administered after surgical drainage better ensures that the infection has been contained. In an adult study, antibiotics active against CA-MRSA were associated with significantly greater cures than achieved with agents not active against CA-MRSA in patients who had undergone incision and drainage of skin and soft tissue infections.[183] Failure to provide surgical drainage is an important reason for persistence or recurrence of organisms. Antibiotics cannot be expected to penetrate the avascular center of abscess cavities. When abscess cavities are undrained or when antibiotic therapy is discontinued before an area is sterilized, live bacteria may persist and disseminate to cause later recurrence at that site or at distant sites.

For moderate to severe staphylococcal infection, the patient should be hospitalized initially for intravenous therapy. This strategy ensures peak antibiotic levels, which may allow greater penetration into relatively avascular areas. Intramuscular injections rarely are indicated in children. Once the patient is afebrile, has negative blood culture, and shows definite evidence of clinical improvement, therapy can be completed with home administration of antibiotics or with oral agents, as deemed appropriate by the treating physicians.

ANTIBIOTICS FOR *STAPHYLOCOCCUS AUREUS* INFECTIONS

Since the mid-1960s, most *S. aureus* isolates from most sections of North America and Europe have been penicillinase producers and, therefore, are penicillin-resistant. When *S. aureus* isolates are likely to be the cause of infection, the most appropriate agents to administer for empiric treatment are based on the relative frequency of CA-MRSA isolates in the particular community. In areas where CA-MRSA isolates are not a concern, treatment with a penicillinase-resistant penicillin or cephalosporin should be initiated before isolating the bacteria and performing susceptibility testing (Tables 91–4 and 91–5). Methicillin-resistant organisms

TABLE 91–4   Therapy for Staphylococcal Infections in Infants and Children (Excluding Neonates)

Agent	Oral (Mild-Moderate Infection)		Parenteral (Moderate-Severe Infection)	
	Children <40 kg	Children >40 kg and Adults	Children <40 kg	Children >40 kg and Adults
Penicillins				
Oxacillin			150-200 mg/kg/24 hr in 4-6 doses q4-6h IV	4-8 g/24 hr in 4-6 doses q4-6h IV
Nafcillin			150-200 mg/kg/24 hr in 4-6 doses q4-6h IV	4-8 g/24 hr in 4-6 doses q4-6h IV
Cloxacillin	50-100 mg/kg/24 hr in 4 doses	2-4 g/24 hr in 4 doses		
Dicloxacillin	25-75 mg/kg/24 hr in 4 doses	1-2 g/24 hr in 4 doses		
Cephalosporins				
Cefazolin (Ancef, Kefzol)			75-100 mg/kg/24 hr in 3 doses q8h	4-6 g/24 hr in 3 doses
Cephalexin (Keflex)	25-100 mg/kg/24 hr in 4 doses	1-4 g/24 hr in 4 doses		
Cefadroxil (Duricef, Ultracef)	30 mg/kg/24 hr in 2 doses	1-2 g/24 hr in 2 doses		
Other Agents				
Erythromycin	35-50 mg/kg/24 hr in 4 doses	1-2 g/24 hr in 4 doses		
Clindamycin	20-40 mg/kg/24 hr in 3 doses	600-1200 mg/24 hr in 3-4 doses	30-40 mg/kg/24 hr q6-8h IV	600-3000 mg/24 hr q6-8h IV
Vancomycin			40-60 mg/kg/24 hr q6h drip over 1 hr or by continuous drip IV	1-2 g/24 hr q6h over 1 hr or by drip continuous IV
Linezolid (Zyvox)	10 mg/kg/dose q8h*	10 mg/kg/dose q12h†	10 mg/kg/dose q8h*	10 mg/kg/dose q12h†
Doxycycline	2-4 mg/kg/24 hr 1or 2 doses for children >7 yr of age	100-200 mg/24 hr		
Trimethoprim-sulfamethoxazole	8-12 mg/kg/24 hr of TMP in 2 doses	160 mg of TMP q12h		

*The dose for children younger than 12 years.
†The dose for children ≥12 years of age, not to exceed 600 mg/dose.
IV, intravenously; TMP, trimethoprim.

TABLE 91–5 Anti-staphylococcal Therapy in Neonates with Moderate to Severe Infection

Agent	Premature Infants (<2000 g)		Term Infants	
	<1 wk	1-4 wk	<1 wk	1-4 wk
Oxacillin or nafcillin IV	25-50 mg/kg/dose q12h	25-50 mg/kg/dose q8h	25-50 mg/kg/dose q12h	100-200 mg/kg/24 hr nafcillin IV in 4 doses
Linezolid IV	10 mg/kg q 8-12h*	10 mg/kg/dose q8h	10 mg/kg/dose q8h	10 mg/kg/dose q8h
Vancomycin IV	15 mg/kg/dose q12-24h†	15 mg/kg/dose q8-24h†	30 mg/kg/24 hr in 2 doses q12h†	45 mg/kg/24 hr in 3 doses q8h†

*For infants <34 weeks' gestation and <1 week of age, administer every 12 hours.
†Administer over a 1-hour period. Monitor serum concentrations during therapy.
IV, intravenously.

cannot be treated adequately with any β-lactam antibiotic, including cephalosporins. In some locations, methicillin resistance is widespread in community isolates; thus, alternative agents (discussed later) are indicated for empiric treatment. When a penicillin-resistant organism that is susceptible to oxacillin is isolated, the semisynthetic penicillinase-resistant penicillins are the drugs of choice. Oxacillin and nafcillin are available for parenteral use. Dicloxacillin and cephalexin are the preferred oral agents.

If clinical response appears to be slow, nothing is to be gained by switching to another antibiotic within this category. Instead, microbiologic data are reviewed, and the dose of antibiotic is rechecked to be certain it is correct. The patient is reassessed to be certain that all sites requiring drainage have been addressed, and compliance with therapy is addressed, especially if the antibiotics have been administered orally.

ALTERNATIVE DRUGS

The cephalosporin antibiotics are active against penicillinase-producing staphylococci and cause less irritation of veins with intravenous infusion than do penicillinase-resistant penicillins. A potential disadvantage lies in their broader spectrum of activity, which may promote superinfection with cephalosporin-resistant, gram-negative organisms in a debilitated patient with serious staphylococcal disease. Cephalosporins have been advocated widely for use in patients allergic to penicillin, but because of considerable cross-reactivity, they should be used extremely cautiously, if at all, in patients with a clear history of serious penicillin allergy or anaphylaxis. Among this group of antibiotics, cefazolin is the agent of choice for parenteral use.[168] It is well tolerated and can be administered every 8 hours intravenously. Serum concentrations of cefazolin are higher, and effective tissue levels appear to be easier to attain. Cefazolin also is associated with less bone marrow suppression than is nafcillin or oxacillin. The efficacy of the second- and third-generation cephalosporins against S. aureus is reduced. Therefore, these drugs, especially cefotaxime, ceftriaxone, and cefuroxime, should be given in addition to specific anti-staphylococcal agents if S. aureus is suspected strongly. Clindamycin and trimethoprim-sulfamethoxazole are alternative agents for patients who are seriously allergic to or intolerant of β-lactam antibiotics.[12,58,109]

The β-lactam resistance of MRSA is caused by the production of a novel penicillin-binding protein (PBP) designated PBP-2′ or 2a, which, unlike the intrinsic set of PBPs (PBP-1 to PBP-4) of S. aureus, has remarkably reduced binding affinities to β-lactam antibiotics. Despite the presence of otherwise inhibitory concentrations of β-lactam antibiotics, MRSA can continue to synthesize cell walls solely through the uninhibited activity of PBP-2′ or 2a.[111,141] PBP2′ or PBP2a is encoded by the mecA gene, which is carried by a unique mobile genetic element integrated into the S. aureus chromosome designated SCCmec.[92]

Some cases of MRSA actually may be caused by infection with S. aureus that lacks the mecA gene responsible for true methicillin resistance. The mechanism of resistance in these cases may be hyperproduction of β-lactamase.[102] Frequently in these cases, methicillin resistance is borderline, with minimal inhibitory concentrations (MICs) of 8 μg/mL or less. Hence, high doses of β-lactam antibiotics may be inhibitory. The clinical significance of these isolates is unknown.

STAPHYLOCOCCAL CASSETTE CHROMOSOME mec

SCCmec is a region spanning between 20 and 70 kilobases approximately 30 kb downstream from the chromosomal origin of replication. SCCmec contains the mecA gene encoding a PBP (PBP2a or PBP2′) with poor affinity to β-lactam antibiotics, thus allowing essential functions of cell wall formation to proceed in the presence of β-lactam antibiotics. The mecA gene is regulated by mecR1-mecI, in which activated mecR1 (signal transducer) inactivates mecI (repressor) through site-specific proteolytic cleavage, thereby initiating production of PBP2a or PBP2′. In vitro studies have suggested that the β-lactamase regulators blaR1-blaI may also be effective regulators of mecA.[146]

The SCCmec classification systems are based on several genetic elements including the class of mec and the ccr genes, which are recombination genes involved in the mobility of the genetic cassette. Other elements that may be present are IS431, IS1272, Tn554, pUB110, and pT181. SCCmec types II and III also contain other antibiotic resistance genes such as tet (tetracycline resistance). All strains contain a J(unk)-region of variable size and composition. Several schemes for SCCmec typing have been published.[116,161,162] Historically, nosocomial MRSA isolates contained the SCCmec types I to III, and when community isolates were first described, three new types (IV, V, and VI) were introduced. The smaller size (<30 kb) of SCCmec types IV to VI is thought to explain an increased mobility between strains. Because the community strains have been brought into the health care setting, SCCmec typing cannot be used reliably to predict whether an infection is related to health care or to the community.[77,88,189]

MRSA was described first within 1 year of the introduction of penicillinase-resistant penicillins.[97] Initial reports of infection appeared in England in the early 1960s and subsequently were followed by reports from other European countries.[119,203] In the United States, only sporadic cases were observed initially,[113,119] and not until 1968 was the first nosocomial outbreak described.[19] Since then, the prevalence of MRSA in the hospital setting has increased steadily. In a 1989 survey of U.S. hospitals, 97 percent reported the presence of MRSA.[25] The SCOPE (Surveillance and Control of Pathogens of Epidemiologic Importance) prospective surveillance project conducted between 1995 and 2001 identified more than 3400 episodes of nosocomial bacteremias in children. S. aureus accounted for 9 percent of isolates.[229] The proportion of S. aureus isolates that were MRSA increased from 10 percent in 1995 to 29 percent in 2001. Risk factors associated with development of infection or colonization with MRSA include recent or prolonged hospitalization, exposure to antibiotics, and stay in an intensive care unit.[133] Nosocomially acquired MRSA appears to be fully virulent, with in vitro characteristics similar to those of methicillin-susceptible staphylococci. It has equivalent virulence in studies of experimental infection in mice, and clinical studies confirm comparable mortality rates.[90,213] These strains characteristically are multiresistant and usually show little or no susceptibility to cephalosporins, aminoglycosides, erythromycin, clindamycin, and tetracyclines.[4,222] Strains that appear to be susceptible to cephalosporins by standard disk sensitivity tests are proved resistant in quantitative dilution tests. The clinical efficacy of cephalosporins against methicillin-resistant strains has been poor.[222]

Epidemic outbreaks of nosocomially acquired MRSA have been reported. In these outbreaks, nasopharyngeal colonization with MRSA often occurs before infection develops. A high rate of nasal and hand carriage has been observed in health care workers associated with units that have MRSA outbreaks.[153] The usual approach to outbreaks has been to emphasize handwashing between examining and caring for patients. Strict isolation in a private room generally is advocated.[154] Single-room isolation usually is impractical in neonatal and pediatric intensive care units, where isolation facilities are in short supply and a single MRSA-colonized patient may occupy a room for months. Strict adherence to universal precautions (body substance isolation) with all moist body fluids and strict handwashing between seeing patients appear to be rational alternatives to "strict isolation."[135] Intranasal application of mupirocin ointment has been found to be capable of eliminating nasal and hand carriage of both colonized patients and hospital staff.[178] Interventions to control outbreaks of MRSA in intensive care or other units are multifaceted, and the reader is referred to major guidelines for recommendations.[154,196]

Occasional cases of MRSA infection apparently acquired in the community were observed sporadically in the 1970s. However, these infections were from patients who were chronically ill, and many patients had a history of nursing home residence, recent admission to acute or chronic health care facilities, previous receipt of antibiotics, or intravenous drug abuse.[125,145,185,206] Hence, in these cases, infections usually were traceable to the hospital setting. By contrast, since the 1980s, cases of true CA-MRSA infection in patients without identified risk factors have appeared in the literature. The first reports in children arose from small MRSA outbreak investigations.[85] Subsequently, Rathore and Kline described three patients with deep-seated infections caused by MRSA acquired in the community.[177] In the 1990s, reports of CA-MRSA in patients without known risk factors continued to appear sporadically in the literature. However, most of the infections described occurred in adults.[79,122,152] Four pediatric deaths in Minnesota and North Dakota in the period 1997 to 1999 demonstrated the potential for severe disease resulting from CA-MRSA infections.[10] The landmark study describing the changing epidemiology of CA-MRSA in children was published in 1998.[89] Herold and colleagues performed a retrospective review of medical records and compared the frequency of *S. aureus* isolation in hospitalized children during two time periods: between 1988 and 1990 and between 1993 and 1995. The prevalence of CA-MRSA in children without identified risk factors was 25.9 times higher in 1993 to 1995 than in 1988 to 1990.[89] After the publication of this article, several reports of CA-MRSA in children without risk factors from different parts of the United States and many regions of the world appeared.[30,37,103,108,175,187,234] This explosive increase in reporting that occurred in just a few years suggests that clones of CA-MRSA have unique properties that allow rapid spread once these pathogens are introduced into the community.[106]

All reports of the clinical characteristics of CA-MRSA infection in children without risk factors document a predominance of superficial infections, including subcutaneous abscesses and cellulitis.[30,89,108,175] However, many children with abscesses require admission to the hospital for incision and drainage with the patient under anesthesia.[108] Invasive disease with CA-MRSA, including severe, life-threatening infection, has been increasing and accounted for about 5 percent of cases in children seeking care in an emergency center of a large children's hospital in Houston.[5,10,75,76,108]

Unlike hospital-acquired MRSA, CA-MRSA isolates usually are susceptible to most non–β-lactam antibiotics, including clindamycin, gentamicin, trimethoprim-sulfamethoxazole, and doxycycline or minocycline, in addition to vancomycin, daptomycin, and linezolid.[105] Erythromycin susceptibility is somewhat more variable; the proportion of susceptible isolates varied from 29 to 80 percent in various studies.[80,89,95,155] Macrolide (erythromycin, azithromycin, clarithromycin)-resistant strains remain susceptible to clindamycin if the macrolide resistance is caused by an efflux pump (MEF). However, resistance to clindamycin, lincosamide, and streptogramin B can be constitutive (macrolide-lincosamide-streptogramin B] MLS_B]) or inducible ($iMLS_B$). Both mechanisms can be detected with molecular methods and also reliably in the routine laboratory by the "D test" (Fig. 91–5).[59] In vitro as well as some in vivo evidence indicates that, in the presence of erythromycin resistance, *S. aureus* could become resistant to clindamycin during therapy with this antibiotic.[50,144,165,221] This phenomenon, $iMLS_B$ resistance, which consists of modification of the target rRNA of *S. aureus*, is mediated by the presence of the resistance-conferring *erm* (erythromycin resistance methylase) gene, which encodes a 23S rRNA methylase.[96,123] Although 14-membered ring macrolides such as erythromycin are the most potent inducers, lincosamides such as clindamycin also can act as weaker inducers.[123] This ability may have clinical relevance in the setting of infections in which the bacteria are not eliminated quickly and may be exposed to sub-inhibitory concentrations of clindamycin for any amount of time. Examples include therapy for undrained deep-seated abscesses or treatment of osteoarticular infections. In patients infected with a strain having the $iMLS_B$ resistance genotype and expressing

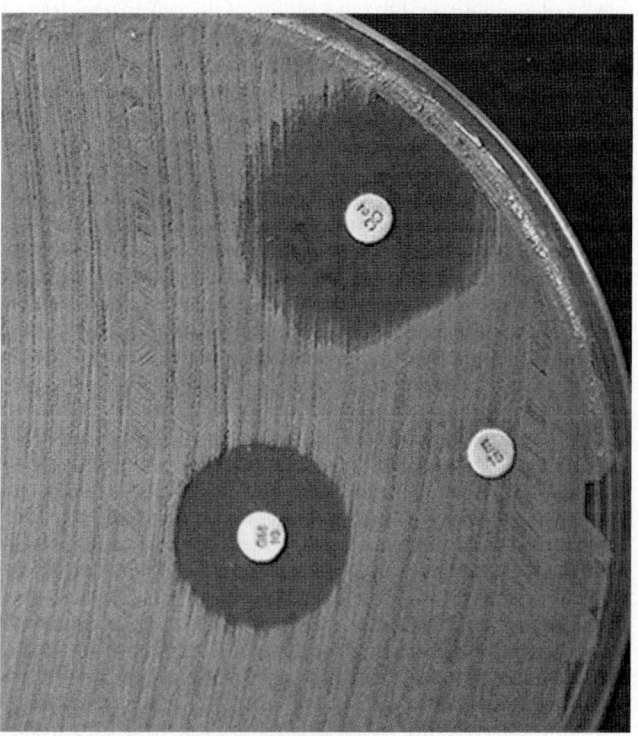

Figure 91–5 D test.

the erythromycin-resistant, clindamycin-susceptible phenotype, cases of clindamycin therapeutic failure have been reported.[66,126,195] Therefore, for MRSA isolates that are erythromycin-resistant and clindamycin-susceptible, detection of the presence of inducible MLS_B resistance should be performed by the disk approximation method, in which clindamycin- and erythromycin-impregnated disks are set 15 to 20 mm apart over Mueller-Hinton agar containing a standard inoculum of bacteria. After a 24-hour incubation period, if the zone of inhibition around the clindamycin disk is flattened or blunted (D shaped, as in Fig. 91–5) on the side facing the erythromycin disk, the isolate is classified as having an $iMLS_B$ resistance phenotype.[123]

Vancomycin, alone or together with an aminoglycoside or rifampin, is the drug of choice for serious MRSA infections. Linezolid, the first of a new family of antimicrobial agents known as oxazolidinones, has demonstrated significant activity against MRSA, vancomycin-resistant enterococci, and penicillin-resistant *S. pneumoniae*. It is available in both oral and intravenous formulations. Quinupristin-dalfopristin is an intravenous streptogramin antibiotic combination that has been found to be effective in the treatment of MRSA and vancomycin-resistant *Enterococcus faecium* infections in patients intolerant of therapy or in whom previous therapy failed. The frequent development of phlebitis with parenteral administration through a peripheral vein mandates the use of central venous access whenever possible. Both linezolid and quinupristin-dalfopristin are expensive, so their use should be restricted to situations for which other alternatives are not feasible. Daptomycin is another newer agent with the most rapidly bactericidal activity in vitro against MRSA.[27]

For severe infections caused by MRSA, the antibiotic of choice is vancomycin. In areas where CA-MRSA has been isolated from children without identified risk factors, severe, life-threatening infections suspected to be caused by *S. aureus* should be treated empirically with both nafcillin and vancomycin because nafcillin is a more active antibiotic than is vancomycin for the treatment of methicillin-susceptible isolates.[78] The addition of gentamicin should be considered for synergistic purposes. Antibiotic therapy can be adjusted subsequently after antibiotic susceptibility testing results are available. Clindamycin and linezolid are options for therapy depending on the susceptibility of the isolate, the desired route of administration, and the absence of endovascular involvement. Daptomycin is approved for serious *S. aureus* infections including bacteremia in adults, but pharmacokinetics and safety studies in children are lacking.[11,65] Tigecycline is another newer agent most useful for polymicrobial infections including MRSA in adults, but it has not been studied in children.[201] Nafcillin, oxacillin, and cefazolin are the recommended agents for treatment of severe MSSA infections.

For mild to moderate skin and soft tissue infections caused by CA-MRSA, empirical treatment may include other antibiotics such as clindamycin or trimethoprim-sulfamethoxazole. Doxycycline or minocycline are options for children older than 8 years of age.[182] If more than 90 percent of community *S. aureus* isolates are susceptible to clindamycin, this agent can be used for empiric treatment of moderately invasive infections, such as in children with osteomyelitis or pneumonia and empyema who do not require intensive care. This approach is not recommended when the clindamycin rate exceeds 10 percent of the CA-MRSA and CA-MSSA isolates combined.[44] Vancomycin or linezolid would be considerations in such circumstances.[107] Once an organism is isolated, therapy is modified based on susceptibility patterns. Nafcillin, oxacillin, and cefazolin are the preferred parenteral agents, and dicloxacillin and cephalexin are the preferred oral agents for moderate MSSA infections.

The origin of CA-MRSA is not known. The absence of health care exposure in patients harboring the bacterium, the unique antibiotic susceptibility characteristics of these isolates, and distinctive pulsed-field electrophoresis patterns that are different from the patterns of hospital-acquired MRSA isolates for a given institution suggest that the origin may be the community and that these isolates were not merely transferred from the hospital setting.[2,81] The unique combination of the gene complex and the much smaller SCC*mec* size than identified in the SCC*mec* of hospital-acquired MRSA also suggest a different origin.[136] Whether the origin is the hospital or the community, the changing epidemiology of MRSA is remarkably similar to the emergence of penicillin-resistant *S. aureus* that occurred in the 1940s and 1950s.[34] Finally, the increasing rate of isolation of MRSA will mandate the use of alternative antibiotics, which, in turn, may promote the development of additional resistance to other antibiotic classes, the most concerning of which is resistance to glycopeptide antibiotics such as vancomycin. Although vancomycin is the antibiotic of choice for severe MRSA infection, its use must remain monitored and controlled because clinical isolates with decreased susceptibility to this antibiotic, vancomycin- or glycopeptide-intermediate *S. aureus* (VISA or GISA), have been reported.[198]

In June of 2002, the first documented infection by vancomycin-resistant *S. aureus* (VRSA) in the United States was reported.[32] The isolate, obtained from a catheter exit site of a 40-year-old diabetic patient undergoing chronic dialysis, had high MICs for vancomycin (1024 µg/mL) and oxacillin (>16 µg/mL) but was susceptible to chloramphenicol, linezolid, minocycline, quinupristin-dalfopristin, and trimethoprim-sulfamethoxazole.[32,35] Since then, six additional isolates have been reported from Michigan, Pennsylvania, and New York.[33,209,212] All the VRSA strains are resistant to the glycopeptides by virtue of the *van*A gene found in the enterococci. VISA strains (MIC of 4 or 8 µg/mL) do not harbor the *van*A gene and are intermediately resistant to vancomycin because of a thickened cell wall containing vancomycin-binding dipeptides.[42,86,91] Vancomycin (and other glycopeptides) intermediate resistance detection in the laboratory is not detected by disk diffusion techniques and may not be consistently detected by automated systems.[211] In response to Clinical and Laboratory Standards Institute guidelines, microbiology laboratories have lowered the breakpoints for vancomycin susceptibility to 2 µg/mL or less, intermediate to 2 to 8 µg/mL, and resistant to 16 µg/mL or more. In actuality, very few *S. aureus* have MICs greater than 4 µg/mL.[209]

PREVENTION

Staphylococcal infections are so common that virtually everyone has had at least some minor encounters. Skin infections occur more commonly in tropical climates or during warm, humid weather in temperate areas and are likely to arise in moist areas of the body such as the axillae and skin creases. High standards of personal hygiene, careful cleaning, and adequate protection of abrasions and minor lacerations reduce the likelihood of skin infection developing.[207] Early attention given to minor infections in these small wounds with careful cleaning and antibiotic ointment may help to prevent more serious or invasive infections. We have been impressed repeatedly with the minor nature of the cutaneous source of infection in serious staphylococcal osteomyelitis, pneumonia, and endocarditis.

Person-to-person spread from an overt lesion is a major route for dissemination of infection within families, in hospitals, and in schools. A person with an infected, purulent wound should receive prompt treatment and be excused from school and from such occupations as hospital worker or food handler while the infection is open or draining. At home, special precautions should be taken in care and dressing of the wound. Disposable gauze pads should be used to wash and dry it, and towels and washcloths should not be shared with other members of the family. For children with recurrent infections or for families with multiple family members with infections, we have found that having the patients take a bath twice a week in water to which bleach (1 teaspoon/gallon of bath water) has been added decreases the frequency of recurrences.

To date, no vaccine has been successfully developed for the prevention of *S. aureus* infections.[191] As noted earlier, a vaccine targeting types 5 and 8 polysaccharide capsule initially appeared promising but was not efficacious in a larger study.[192] One trial using immune globulin enriched for antibody to clumping factor A failed to prevent staphylococcal infections in low-birth-weight infants,[23] and a monoclonal antibody directed against clumping factor A was investigated preliminarily in adults with *S. aureus* bacteremia.[224] A polyclonal IgG preparation containing high levels of antibody to *S. aureus* capsular polysaccharides 5 and 8 has been developed by collecting plasma from healthy donors immunized with StaphVAX.[20] The pharmacokinetics and safety of this product in very low-birth-weight infants were established in a phase II trial, but further development of this antibody preparation is questionable. The safety and pharmacokinetics of human chimeric monoclonal antibody directed against the lipoteichoic acid, an integral component of the cell wall of gram-positive organisms, including *S. aureus*, were evaluated in a phase II study in very low-birth-weight infants.[23] Whether this antibody (pagibaximab) will be efficacious in preventing invasive *S. aureus* infections in these infants is to be determined.

Perhaps taking advantage of the *S. aureus* genome with a reverse vaccinology approach will lead to a safe and efficacious vaccine.[205] Until such time, however, simple measures such as washing hands frequently, giving attention to skin breaks, and avoiding contact of obviously infected skin lesions are the most effective measures to prevent *S. aureus* infections.

REFERENCES

1. Abdelnour, A., Arvidson, S., Bremell, T., et al.: The accessory gene regulator (agr) controls *Staphylococcus aureus* virulence in a murine arthritis model. Infect. Immun. *61*:3879-3885, 1993.
2. Abi-Hanna, P., Frank, A. L., Quinn, J. P., et al.: Clonal features of community-acquired methicillin-resistant *Staphylococcus aureus* in children. Clin. Infect. Dis. *30*:630-631, 2000.
3. Abramson, N., Alper, C. A., Lachmann, P. J., et al.: Deficiency of C3 inactivator in man. J. Immunol. *107*:19-27, 1971.
4. Acar, J. F., Courvalin, P., and Chabbert, Y. A.: Methicillin-resistant staphylococcemia: Bacteriological failure of treatment with cephalosporins. Antimicrob. Agents Chemother. *10*:280-285, 1970.
5. Adem, P. V., Montgomery, C. P., Husain, A. N., et al.: *Staphylococcus aureus* sepsis and the Waterhouse-Friderichsen syndrome in children. N. Engl. J. Med. *353*:1245-1251, 2005.
6. Alfaro, C., Mascher-Denen, M., Fergie, J., and Purcell, K.: Prevalence of methicillin-resistant *Staphylococcus aureus* nasal carriage in patients admitted to Driscoll Children's Hospital. Pediatr. Infect. Dis. J. *25*:459-461, 2006.
7. Alper, C. A., Abramson, N., Johnston, R. B., Jr., et al.: Increased susceptibility to infection associated with abnormalities of complement-mediated functions and of the third component of complement (C3). N. Engl. J. Med. *282*:350-354, 1970.
8. Alper, C. A., Colten, H. R., Rosen, F. S., et al.: Homozygous deficiency of C3 in a patient with repeated infections. Lancet *2*:1179-1181, 1972.
9. Amagai, M., Matsuyoshi, N., Wang, Z. H., et al.: Toxin in bullous impetigo and staphylococcal scalded-skin syndrome targets desmoglein 1. Nat. Med. *6*:1275-1277, 2000.
10. Anonymous: From the Centers for Disease Control and Prevention: Four pediatric deaths from community-acquired methicillin-resistant *Staphylococcus aureus*—Minnesota and North Dakota, 1997-1999. JAMA *282*:1123-1125, 1999.
11. Arbeit, R. D., Maki, D., Tally, F. P., et al.: The safety and efficacy of daptomycin for the treatment of complicated skin and skin-structure infections. Clin. Infect. Dis. *38*:1673-1681, 2004.
12. Ardati, K. O., Thirumoorthi, M. C., and Dajani, A. S.: Intravenous trimethoprim-sulfamethoxazole in the treatment of serious infections in children. J. Pediatr. *95*:801-806, 1979.
13. Arvidson, S., and Tegmark, K.: Regulation of virulence determinants in *Staphylococcus aureus*. Int. J. Med. Microbiol. *291*:159-170, 2001.
14. Baba, T., Takeuchi, F., Kuroda, M., et al.: Genome and virulence determinants of high virulence community-acquired MRSA. Lancet *359*:1819-1827, 2002.
15. Baehner, R. L.: Neutrophil dysfunction associated with states of chronic and recurrent infection. Pediatr. Clin. North Am. *27*:377-401, 1980.
16. Baker, C. J.: Nosocomial septicemia and meningitis in neonates. Am. J. Med. *70*:698-701, 1981.
17. Banffer, J. R.: Anti-leucocidin and mastitis puerperalis. BMJ *2*:1224-1226, 1962.
18. Bannerman, T. L., Hancock, G. A., Tenover, F. C., and Miller, J. M.: Pulsed-field gel electrophoresis as a replacement for bacteriophage typing of *Staphylococcus aureus*. J. Clin. Microbiol. *33*:551-555, 1995.
19. Barrett, F. F., McGehee, R. F., Jr., and Finland, M.: Methicillin-resistant *Staphylococcus aureus* at Boston City Hospital: Bacteriologic and epidemiologic observations. N. Engl. J. Med. *279*:441-448, 1968.
20. Benjamin, D. K., Schelonka, R., White, R., et al.: A blinded, randomized, multicenter study of an intravenous *Staphylococcus aureus* immune globulin. J. Perinatol. *26*:290-295, 2006.
21. Bhakdi, S., and Tranum-Jensen, J.: Alpha-toxin of *Staphylococcus aureus*. Microbiol. Rev. *55*:733-751, 1991.
22. Blevins, J. S., Elasri, M. O., Allmendinger, S. D., et al.: Role of sarA in the pathogenesis of *Staphylococcus aureus* musculoskeletal infection. Infect. Immun. *71*:516-523, 2003.
23. Bloom, B., Schelonka, R., Kueser, T., et al.: Multicenter study to assess safety and efficacy of INH-A21, a donor-selected human staphylococcal immunoglobulin, for prevention of nosocomial infections in very low birth weight infants. Pediatr. Infect. Dis. J. *24*:858-866, 2005.
24. Bocchini, C. E., Hulten, K. G., Mason, E. O., Jr., et al.: Panton-Valentine leukocidin genes are associated with enhanced inflammatory response and local disease in acute hematogenous *Staphylococcus aureus* osteomyelitis in children. Pediatrics *117*:433-440, 2006.
25. Boyce, J. M.: Methicillin-resistant *Staphylococcus aureus*: Detection, epidemiology, and control measures. Infect. Dis. Clin. North Am. *3*:901-913, 1989.
26. Boyle-Vavra, S., and Daum, R. S.: Community-acquired methicillin-resistant *Staphylococcus aureus*: The role of Panton-Valentine leukocidin. Lab. Invest. *87*:3-9, 2007.
27. Bradley, J. S.: Newer antistaphylococcal agents. Curr. Opin. Pediatr. *17*:71-77, 2005.
28. Bronner, S., Monteil, H., and Prevost, G.: Regulation of virulence determinants in *Staphylococcus aureus*: Complexity and applications. F. E. M. S. Microbiol. Rev. *28*:183-200, 2004.
29. Brumfitt, W., and Hamilton-Miller, J.: Methicillin-resistant *Staphylococcus aureus*. N. Engl. J. Med. *320*:1188-1196, 1989.
30. Buckingham, S. C., McDougal, L. K., Cathey, L. D., et al.: Emergence of community-associated methicillin-resistant *Staphylococcus aureus* at a Memphis, Tennessee Children's Hospital. Pediatr. Infect. Dis. J. *23*:619-624, 2004.
31. Burlak, C., Hammer, C. H., Robinson, M. A., et al.: Global analysis of community-associated methicillin-resistant *Staphylococcus aureus* exoproteins reveals molecules produced in vitro and during infection. Cell. Microbiol. *9*:1172-1190, 2007.
32. Centers for Disease Control and Prevention: *Staphylococcus aureus* resistant to vancomycin—United States, 2002. M. M. W. R. Morb. Mortal. Wkly. Rep. *51*:565-567, 2002.
33. Centers for Disease Control and Prevention: Vancomycin-resistant *Staphylococcus aureus*—New York, 2004. M. M. W. R. Morb. Mortal. Wkly. Rep. *53*:322-323, 2004.
34. Chambers, H. F.: The changing epidemiology of *Staphylococcus aureus*? Emerg. Infect. Dis. *7*:178-182, 2001.
35. Chang, S., Sievert, D. M., Hageman, J. C., et al.: Infection with vancomycin-resistant *Staphylococcus aureus* containing the vanA resistance gene. N. Engl. J. Med. *348*:1342-1347, 2003.
36. Chavakis, T., Wiechmann, K., Preissner, K. T., and Herrmann, M.: *Staphylococcus aureus* interactions with the endothelium: The role of bacterial "secretable expanded repertoire adhesive molecules" (SERAM) in disturbing host defense systems. Thromb. Haemost. *94*:278-285, 2005.
37. Chavez-Bueno, S., Bozdogan, B., Katz, K., et al.: Inducible clindamycin resistance and molecular epidemiologic trends of pediatric community-acquired methicillin-resistant *Staphylococcus aureus* in Dallas, Texas. Antimicrob. Agents Chemother. *49*:2283-2288, 2005.
38. Cockfield, J. D., Pathak, S., Edgeworth, J. D., and Lindsay, J. A.: Rapid determination of hospital-acquired methicillin-resistant *Staphylococcus aureus* lineages. J. Med. Microbiol. *56*:614-619, 2007.
39. Coovadia, Y. M., Bhana, R. H., Johnson, A. P., et al.: A laboratory-confirmed outbreak of rifampicin-methicillin resistant *Staphylococcus aureus* (RMRSA) in a newborn nursery. J. Hosp. Infect. *14*:303-312, 1989.
40. Creech, C. B., Kernodle, D. S., Alsentzer, A., et al.: Increasing rates of nasal carriage of methicillin-resistant *Staphylococcus aureus* in healthy children. Pediatr. Infect. Dis. J. *24*:617-621, 2005.
41. Cribier, B., Prevost, G., Couppie, P., et al.: *Staphylococcus aureus* leukocidin: A new virulence factor in cutaneous infections? An epidemiological and experimental study. Dermatology *185*:175-180, 1992.
42. Cui, L., Murakami, H., Kuwahara-Arai, K., et al.: Contribution of a thickened cell wall and its glutamine nonamidated component to the vancomycin resistance expressed by *Staphylococcus aureus* Mu50. Antimicrob. Agents Chemother. *44*:2276-2285, 2000.
43. Dacre, J., Emmerson, A. M., and Jenner, E. A.: Gentamicin-methicillin-resistant *Staphylococcus aureus*: Epidemiology and containment of an outbreak. J. Hosp. Infect. *7*:130-136, 1986.

44. David, M. Z., Crawford, S. E., Boyle-Vavra, S., et al.: Contrasting pediatric and adult methicillin-resistant *Staphylococcus aureus* isolates. Emerg. Infect. Dis. *12*:631-637, 2006.

45. Davis, S. L., Rybak, M. J., Amjad, M., et al.: Characteristics of patients with healthcare-associated infection due to SCC*mec* type IV methicillin-resistant *Staphylococcus aureus*. Infect. Control Hosp. Epidemiol. *27*:1025-1031, 2006.

46. Diep, B. A., Carleton, H. A., Chang, R. F., et al.: Roles of 34 virulence genes in the evolution of hospital- and community-associated strains of methicillin-resistant *Staphylococcus aureus*. J. Infect. Dis. *193*:1495-1503, 2006.

47. Diep, B. A., Gill, S. R., Chang, R. F., et al.: Complete genome sequence of USA300, an epidemic clone of community-acquired methicillin-resistant *Staphylococcus aureus*. Lancet *367*:731-739, 2006.

48. Diep, B. A., Perdreau-Remington, F., and Sensabaugh, G. F.: Clonal characterization of *Staphylococcus aureus* by multilocus restriction fragment typing, a rapid screening approach for molecular epidemiology. J. Clin. Microbiol. *41*:4559-4564, 2003.

49. Dinges, M. M., Orwin, P. M., and Schlievert, P. M.: Exotoxins of *Staphylococcus aureus*. Clin. Microbiol. Rev. *13*:16-34, 2000.

50. Drinkovic, D., Fuller, E. R., Shore, K. P., et al.: Clindamycin treatment of *Staphylococcus aureus* expressing inducible clindamycin resistance. J. Antimicrob. Chemother. *48*:315-316, 2001.

51. Dumitrescu, O., Boisset, S., Badiou, C., et al.: Effect of antibiotics on *Staphylococcus aureus* producing Panton-Valentine leukocidin. Antimicrob. Agents Chemother. *51*:1515-1519, 2007.

52. Elasri, M. O., Thomas, J. R., Skinner, R. A., et al.: *Staphylococcus aureus* collagen adhesin contributes to the pathogenesis of osteomyelitis. Bone *30*:275-280, 2002.

53. Elias, P. M., Fritsch, P., Dahl, M. V., and Wolff, K.: Staphylococcal toxic epidermal necrolysis: Pathogenesis and studies on the subcellular site of action of exfoliatin. J. Invest. Dermatol. *65*:501-512, 1975.

54. Enright, M. C., Day, N. P., Davies, C. E., et al.: Multilocus sequence typing for characterization of methicillin-resistant and methicillin-susceptible clones of *Staphylococcus aureus*. J. Clin. Microbiol. *38*:1008-1015, 2000.

55. Enright, M. C., Robinson, D. A., Randle, G., et al.: The evolutionary history of methicillin-resistant *Staphylococcus aureus* (MRSA). Proc. Natl. Acad. Sci. U. S. A. *99*:7687-7692, 2002.

56. Etienne, J.: Panton-Valentine leukocidin: A marker of severity for *Staphylococcus aureus* infection? Clin. Infect. Dis. *41*:591-593, 2005.

57. Eykyn, S. J.: Staphylococcal sepsis: The changing pattern of disease and therapy. Lancet *1*:100-104, 1988.

58. Feigin, R. D., Pickering, L. K., Anderson, D., et al.: Clindamycin treatment of osteomyelitis and septic arthritis in children. Pediatrics *55*:213-223, 1975.

59. Fiebelkorn, K. R., Crawford, S. A., McElmeel, M. L., and Jorgensen, J. H.: Practical disk diffusion method for detection of inducible clindamycin resistance in *Staphylococcus aureus* and coagulase-negative staphylococci. J. Clin. Microbiol. *41*:4740-4744, 2003.

60. Fitzgerald, J. R., Monday, S. R., Foster, T. J., et al.: Characterization of a putative pathogenicity island from bovine *Staphylococcus aureus* encoding multiple superantigens. J. Bacteriol. *183*:63-70, 2001.

61. Fortunov, R. M., Hulten, K. G., Hammerman, W. A., et al.: Community-acquired *Staphylococcus aureus* infections in term and near-term previously healthy neonates. Pediatrics *118*:874-881, 2006.

62. Foster, T. J.: Immune evasion by staphylococci. Nat. Rev. Microbiol. *3*:948-958, 2005.

63. Foster, T. J., and Hook, M.: Surface protein adhesins of *Staphylococcus aureus*. Trends Microbiol. *6*:484-488, 1998.

64. Fournier, B., and Philpott, D. J.: Recognition of *Staphylococcus aureus* by the innate immune system. Clin. Microbiol. Rev. *18*:521-540, 2005.

65. Fowler, V.G., Jr., Boucher, H. W., Corey, G. R., et al.: Daptomycin versus standard therapy for bacteremia and endocarditis caused by *Staphylococcus aureus*. N. Engl. J. Med. *355*:653-665, 2006.

66. Frank, A. L., Marcinak, J. F., Mangat, P. D., et al.: Clindamycin treatment of methicillin-resistant *Staphylococcus aureus* infections in children. Pediatr. Infect. Dis. J. *21*:530-534, 2002.

67. Gauduchon, V., Cozon, G., Vandenesch, F., et al.: Neutralization of *Staphylococcus aureus* Panton Valentine leukocidin by intravenous immunoglobulin in vitro. J. Infect. Dis. *189*:346-353, 2004.

68. Gill, S. R., Fouts, D. E., Archer, G. L., et al.: Insights on evolution of virulence and resistance from the complete genome analysis of an early methicillin-resistant *Staphylococcus aureus* strain and a biofilm-producing methicillin-resistant *Staphylococcus epidermidis* strain. J. Bacteriol. *187*:2426-2438, 2005.

69. Gillaspy, A. F., Worrell, V., Orvis, J., et al.: *The Staphylococcus aureus NCTC 8325 Genome*. Washington, D.C.: ASM Press, 2006.

70. Gillet, Y., Issartel, B., Vanhems, P., et al.: Association between *Staphylococcus aureus* strains carrying gene for Panton-Valentine leukocidin and highly lethal necrotising pneumonia in young immunocompetent patients. Lancet *359*:753-759, 2002.

71. Gladstone, G. P., Mudd, S., Hochstein, H. D., and Lenhart, N. A.: The assay of anti-staphylococcal leucocidal components (F and S) in human serum. Br. J. Exp. Pathol. *43*:295-312, 1962.

72. Gluck, L., and Wood, H. F.: Effect of an antiseptic skin-care regimen in reducing in reducing staphylococcal colonization in newborn infants. N. Engl. J. Med. *265*:1177-1181, 1961.

73. Gomes, A. R., Vinga, S., Zavolan, M., and de Lencastre, H.: Analysis of the genetic variability of virulence-related loci in epidemic clones of methicillin-

resistant *Staphylococcus aureus*. Antimicrob. Agents Chemother. *49*:366-379, 2005.

74. Gomez, M. I., Lee, A., Reddy, B., et al.: *Staphylococcus aureus* protein A induces airway epithelial inflammatory responses by activating TNFR1. Nat. Med. *10*:842-848, 2004.

75. Gonzalez, B. E., Hulten, K. G., Dishop, M. K., et al.: Pulmonary manifestations in children with invasive community-acquired *Staphylococcus aureus* infection. Clin. Infect. Dis. *41*:583-590, 2005.

76. Gonzalez, B. E., Martinez-Aguilar, G., Hulten, K. G., et al.: Severe staphylococcal sepsis in adolescents in the era of community-acquired methicillin-resistant *Staphylococcus aureus*. Pediatrics *115*:642-648, 2005.

77. Gonzalez, B. E., Rueda, A. M., Shelburne, S. A., III, et al.: Community-associated strains of methicillin-resistant *Staphylococcus aureus* as the cause of health-care-associated infection. Infect. Control Hosp. Epidemiol. *27*:1051-1056, 2006.

78. Gonzalez, C., Rubio, M., Romero-Vivas, J., et al.: Bacteremic pneumonia due to *Staphylococcus aureus*: A comparison of disease caused by methicillin-resistant and methicillin-susceptible organisms. Clin. Infect. Dis. *29*:1171-1177, 1999.

79. Gosbell, I. B., Barbagiannakos, T., Neville, S. A., et al.: Non-multiresistant methicillin-resistant *Staphylococcus aureus* bacteraemia in Sydney, Australia: Emergence of EMRSA-15, Oceania, Queensland and Western Australian MRSA strains. Pathology *38*:239-244, 2006.

80. Gottlieb, R. D., Shah, M. K., Perlman, D. C., and Kimmelman, C. P.: Community-acquired methicillin-resistant *Staphylococcus aureus* infections in otolaryngology. Otolaryngol. Head Neck Surg. *107*:434-437, 1992.

81. Groom, A. V., Wolsey, D. H., Naimi, T. S., et al.: Community-acquired methicillin-resistant *Staphylococcus aureus* in a rural American Indian community. JAMA *286*:1201-1205, 2001.

82. Hageman, J. C., Uyeki, T. M., Francis, J. S., et al.: Severe community-acquired pneumonia due to *Staphylococcus aureus*, 2003-04 influenza season. Emerg. Infect. Dis. *12*:894-899, 2006.

83. Haley, R. W., and Bregman, D. A.: The role of understaffing and overcrowding in recurrent outbreaks of staphylococcal infection in a neonatal special-care unit. J. Infect. Dis. *145*:875-885, 1982.

84. Hallin, M., Deplano, A., Denis, O., et al.: Validation of pulsed-field gel electrophoresis and spa typing for long-term, nationwide epidemiological surveillance studies of *Staphylococcus aureus* infections. J. Clin. Microbiol. *45*:127-133, 2007.

85. Hamoudi, A. C., Palmer, R. N., and King T. L.: Nafcillin resistant *Staphylococcus aureus*: A possible community origin. Infect. Control *4*:153-157, 1983.

86. Hanaki, H., Kuwahara-Arai, K., Boyle-Vavra, S., et al.: Activated cell-wall synthesis is associated with vancomycin resistance in methicillin-resistant *Staphylococcus aureus* clinical strains Mu3 and Mu50. J. Antimicrob. Chemother. *42*:199-209, 1998.

87. Hartleib, J., Kohler, N., Dickinson, R. B., et al.: Protein A is the von Willebrand factor binding protein on *Staphylococcus aureus*. Blood *96*:2149-2156, 2000.

88. Healy, C. M., Hulten, K. G., Palazzi, D. L., et al.: Emergence of new strains of methicillin-resistant *Staphylococcus aureus* in a neonatal intensive care unit. Clin. Infect. Dis. *39*:1460-1466, 2004.

89. Herold, B. C., Immergluck, L. C., Maranan, M. C., et al.: Community-acquired methicillin-resistant *Staphylococcus aureus* in children with no identified predisposing risk. JAMA *279*:593-598, 1998.

90. Hershow, R. C., Khayr, W. F., and Smith, N. L.: A comparison of clinical virulence of nosocomially acquired methicillin-resistant and methicillin-sensitive *Staphylococcus aureus* infections in a university hospital. Infect. Control Hosp. Epidemiol. *13*:587-593, 1992.

90a. Highlander, S. K., Hulten, K. G., Qin, X., et al.: Subtle genetic changes enhance virulence of methicillin resistant and sensitive *Staphylococcus aureus*. BMC Microbiol. *7*:99-113, 2007.

91. Hiramatsu, K., Hanaki, H., Ino, T., et al.: Methicillin-resistant *Staphylococcus aureus* clinical strain with reduced vancomycin susceptibility. J. Antimicrob. Chemother. *40*:135-136, 1997.

92. Hiramatsu, K., Katayama, Y., Yuzawa, H., and Ito, T.: Molecular genetics of methicillin-resistant *Staphylococcus aureus*. Int. J. Med. Microbiol. *292*:67-74, 2002.

93. Hochkeppel, H. K., Braun, D. G., Vischer, W., et al.: Serotyping and electron microscopy studies of *Staphylococcus aureus* clinical isolates with monoclonal antibodies to capsular polysaccharide types 5 and 8. J. Clin. Microbiol. *25*:526-530, 1987.

94. Holden, M. T., Feil, E. J., Lindsay, J. A., et al.: Complete genomes of two clinical *Staphylococcus aureus* strains: Evidence for the rapid evolution of virulence and drug resistance. Proc. Natl. Acad. Sci. U. S. A. *101*:9786-9791, 2004.

95. Hussain, F. M., Boyle-Vavra, S., Bethel, C. D., and Daum, R. S.: Current trends in community-acquired methicillin-resistant *Staphylococcus aureus* at a tertiary care pediatric facility. Pediatr. Infect. Dis. J. *19*:1163-1166, 2000.

96. Jenssen, W. D., Thakker-Varia, S., Dubin, D. T., and Weinstein, M. P.: Prevalence of macrolides-lincosamides-streptogramin B resistance and erm gene classes among clinical strains of staphylococci and streptococci. Antimicrob. Agents Chemother. *31*:883-888, 1987.

97. Jevons, M. P.: "Celbenin" resistant staphylococci. Br. Med. J. *1*:124-125, 1961.

98. Joh, D., Wann, E. R., Kreikemeyer, B., et al.: Role of fibronectin-binding MSCRAMMs in bacterial adherence and entry into mammalian cells. Matrix Biol. *18*:211-223, 1999.

99. Johanovsky, J.: [Importance of antileukocidin and antitoxin in immunity against staphylococcal infections.] Z. Immunitatsforsch. Allerg. Klin. Immunol. *116*:318-328, 1958.

100. Johansson, A, Flock, JI, and Svensson, O.: Collagen and fibronectin binding in experimental staphylococcal osteomyelitis. Clin. Orthop. Relat. Res. *382*:241-246, 2001.

101. Johnson, A. P., Aucken, H. M., Cavendish, S., et al.: Dominance of EMRSA-15 and -16 among MRSA causing nosocomial bacteraemia in the UK: Analysis of isolates from the European Antimicrobial Resistance Surveillance System (EARSS). J. Antimicrob. Chemother. *48*:143-144, 2001.

102. Jorgensen, J. H.: Mechanisms of methicillin resistance in *Staphylococcus aureus* and methods for laboratory detection. Infect. Control Hosp. Epidemiol. *12*:14-19, 1991.

103. Jungk, J., Como-Sabetti, K., Stinchfield, P., et al.: Epidemiology of methicillin-resistant *Staphylococcus aureus* at a pediatric healthcare system, 1991-2003. Pediatr. Infect. Dis. J. *26*:339-344, 2007.

104. Kahl, B., Herrmann, M., Everding, A. S., et al.: Persistent infection with small colony variant strains of *Staphylococcus aureus* in patients with cystic fibrosis. J. Infect. Dis. *177*:1023-1029, 1998.

105. Kaplan, S. L.: Implications of methicillin-resistant *Staphylococcus aureus* as a community-acquired pathogen in pediatric patients. Infect. Dis. Clin. North Am. *19*:747-757, 2005.

106. Kaplan, S. L.: Community-acquired methicillin-resistant *Staphylococcus aureus* infections in children. Semin. Pediatr. Infect. Dis. *17*:113-119, 2006.

107. Kaplan, S. L., Afghani, B., Lopez, P., et al.: Linezolid for the treatment of methicillin-resistant *Staphylococcus aureus* infections in children. Pediatr. Infect. Dis. J. *22*:S178-S185, 2003.

108. Kaplan, S. L., Hulten, K. G., Gonzalez, B. E., et al.: Three-year surveillance of community-acquired *Staphylococcus aureus* infections in children. Clin. Infect. Dis. *40*:1785-1791, 2005.

109. Kaplan, S. L., Mason, E. O., Jr., and Feigin, R. D.: Clindamycin versus nafcillin or methicillin in the treatment of *Staphylococcus aureus* osteomyelitis in children. South. Med. J. *75*:138-142, 1982.

110. Karakawa, W.W., and Vann, W. F.: Capsular polysaccharides of *Staphylococcus aureus*. Semin. Infect. Dis. *4*:285-293, 1982.

111. Katayama, Y., Ito, T., and Hiramatsu, K.: A new class of genetic element, staphylococcus cassette chromosome *mec*, encodes methicillin resistance in *Staphylococcus aureus*. Antimicrob. Agents Chemother. *44*:1549-1555, 2000.

112. Kazakova, S. V., Hageman, J. C., Matava, M., et al.: A clone of methicillin-resistant *Staphylococcus aureus* among professional football players. N. Engl. J. Med. *352*:468-475, 2005.

113. Klimek, J., Marsik, F. J., Bartlett, R.C., et al.: Clinical, epidemiologic and bacteriologic observations of an outbreak of methicillin-resistant *Staphylococcus aureus* at a large community hospital. Am. J. Med. *61*:340-345, 1976.

114. Kluytmans, J., van Belkum, A., and Verbrugh, H.: Nasal carriage of *Staphylococcus aureus*: Epidemiology, underlying mechanisms, and associated risks. Clin. Microbiol. Rev. *10*:505-520, 1997.

115. Komatsuzawa, H., Ouhara, K., Yamada, S., et al.: Innate defences against methicillin-resistant *Staphylococcus aureus* (MRSA) infection. J. Pathol. *208*:249-260, 2006.

116. Kondo, Y., Ito, T., Ma, X. X., et al.: Combination of multiplex PCRs for staphylococcal cassette chromosome *mec* type assignment: Rapid identification system for *mec*, *ccr*, and major differences in junkyard regions. Antimicrob. Agents Chemother. *51*:264-274, 2007.

117. Kuroda, M., Ohta, T., Uchiyama, I., et al.: Whole genome sequencing of methicillin-resistant *Staphylococcus aureus*. Lancet *357*:1225-1240, 2001.

118. Labandeira-Rey, M., Couzon, F., Boisset, S., et al.: *Staphylococcus aureus* Panton-Valentine leukocidin causes necrotizing pneumonia. Science *315*:1130-1133, 2007.

119. Lacey, R. W.: Genetic basis, epidemiology, and future significance of antibiotic resistance in *Staphylococcus aureus*: A review. J. Clin. Pathol. *26*:899-913, 1973.

120. Lairscey, R., and Buck, G. E.: Performance of four slide agglutination methods for identification of *Staphylococcus aureus* when testing methicillin-resistant staphylococci. J. Clin. Microbiol. *25*:181-182, 1987.

121. Laxdal, T., Messner, R. P., Williams, R. C., Jr., and Quie, P. G.: Opsonic, agglutinating, and complement-fixing antibodies in patients with subacute bacterial endocarditis. J. Lab. Clin. Med. *71*:638-653, 1968.

122. Layton, M. C., Hierholzer, W. J., Jr., and Patterson, J. E.: The evolving epidemiology of methicillin-resistant *Staphylococcus aureus* at a university hospital. Infect. Control Hosp. Epidemiol. *16*:12-17, 1995.

123. Leclercq, R., and Courvalin, P.: Bacterial resistance to macrolide, lincosamide, and streptogramin antibiotics by target modification. Antimicrob. Agents Chemother. *35*:1267-1272, 1991.

124. Lee, M. C., Rios, A. M., Aten, M. F., et al.: Management and outcome of children with skin and soft tissue abscesses caused by community-acquired methicillin-resistant *Staphylococcus aureus*. Pediatr. Infect. Dis. J. *23*:123-127, 2004.

125. Levine, D. P., Cushing, R. D., Jui, J., and Brown, W. J.: Community-acquired methicillin-resistant *Staphylococcus aureus* endocarditis in the Detroit Medical Center. Ann. Intern. Med. *97*:330-338, 1982.

126. Lewis, J. S., and Jorgensen, J. H.: Inducible clindamycin resistance in staphylococci: Should clinicians and microbiologists be concerned? Clin. Infect. Dis. *40*:280-285, 2005.

127. Lillibridge, C. B., Melish, M. E., and Glasgow, L. A.: Site of action of exfoliative toxin in the staphylococcal scaled-skin syndrome. Pediatrics *50*:728-738, 1972.

128. Lina, G., Piemont, Y., Godail-Gamot, F., et al.: Involvement of Panton-Valentine leukocidin-producing *Staphylococcus aureus* in primary skin infections and pneumonia. Clin. Infect. Dis. *29*:1128-1132, 1999.

129. Lindsay, J. A., and Holden, M. T.: *Staphylococcus aureus*: Superbug, super genome? Trends Microbiol. *12*:378-385, 2004.

130. Lindsay, J. A., Moore, C. E., Day, N. P., et al.: Microarrays reveal that each of the ten dominant lineages of *Staphylococcus aureus* has a unique combination of surface-associated and regulatory genes. J. Bacteriol. *188*:669-676, 2006.

131. Lindsay, J. A., Ruzin, A., Ross, H. F., et al.: The gene for toxic shock toxin is carried by a family of mobile pathogenicity islands in *Staphylococcus aureus*. Mol. Microbiol. *29*:527-543, 1998.

132. Liu, G. Y., Essex, A., Buchanan, J. T., et al.: *Staphylococcus aureus* golden pigment impairs neutrophil killing and promotes virulence through its antioxidant activity. J. Exp. Med. *202*:209-215, 2005.

133. Locksley, R. M., Cohen, M. L., Quinn, T. C., et al.: Multiply antibiotic-resistant *Staphylococcus aureus*: Introduction, transmission, and evolution of nosocomial infection. Ann. Intern. Med. *97*:317-324, 1982.

134. Lopez-Aguilar, C., Perez-Roth, E., Mendez-Alvarez, S., et al.: Association between the presence of the Panton-Valentine leukocidin-encoding gene and a lower rate of survival among hospitalized pulmonary patients with staphylococcal disease. J. Clin. Microbiol. *45*:274-276, 2007.

135. Lynch, P., Cummings, M. J., Roberts, P. L., et al.: Implementing and evaluating a system of generic infection precautions: Body substance isolation. Am. J. Infect. Control *18*:1-12, 1990.

136. Ma, X. X., Ito, T., Tiensasitorn, C., et al.: Novel type of staphylococcal cassette chromosome *mec* identified in community-acquired methicillin-resistant *Staphylococcus aureus* strains. Antimicrob. Agents Chemother. *46*:1147-1152, 2002.

137. Maki, D. G.: Nosocomial bacteremia: An epidemiologic overview. Am. J. Med. *70*:719-732, 1981.

138. Maki, D. G., Goldman, D. A., and Rhame, F. S.: Infection control in intravenous therapy. Ann. Intern. Med. *79*:867-887, 1973.

139. Marples, R. R., and Wieneke, A. A.: Enterotoxins and toxic-shock syndrome toxin-1 in non-enteric staphylococcal disease. Epidemiol. Infect. *110*:477-488, 1993.

140. Martinez-Aguilar, G., Avalos-Mishaan, A., Hulten, K., et al.: Community-acquired, methicillin-resistant and methicillin-susceptible *Staphylococcus aureus* musculoskeletal infections in children. Pediatr. Infect. Dis. J. *23*:701-706, 2004.

141. Matthews, P., and Tomasz, A.: Insertional inactivation of the *mec* gene in a transposon mutant of a methicillin-resistant clinical isolate of *Staphylococcus aureus*. Antimicrob. Agents Chemother. *34*:1777-1779, 1990.

142. McDougal, L. K., Steward, C. D., Killgore, G. E., et al.: Pulsed-field gel electrophoresis typing of oxacillin-resistant *Staphylococcus aureus* isolates from the United States: establishing a national database. J. Clin. Microbiol. *41*:5113-5120, 2003.

143. McElroy, M. C., Harty, H. R., Hosford, G. E., et al.: Alpha-toxin damages the air-blood barrier of the lung in a rat model of *Staphylococcus aureus*-induced pneumonia. Infect. Immun. *67*:5541-5544, 1999.

144. McGehee, R. F., Barrett, F. F., and Finland, M.: Resistance of *Staphylococcus aureus* to lincomycin, clinimycin, and erythromycin. Antimicrob Agents Chemother. *8*:392-397, 1968.

145. McGowan, J. E.: The impact of changing pathogens of serious infections in hospitalized patients. Clin. Infect. Dis. *31*(Suppl. 4):S124-S130, 2000.

146. McKinney, T. K., Sharma, V. K., Craig, W. A., and Archer, G. L.: Transcription of the gene mediating methicillin resistance in *Staphylococcus aureus* (*mecA*) is corepressed but not coinduced by cognate mecA and beta-lactamase regulators. J. Bacteriol. *183*:6862-6868, 2001.

147. Melish, M. E., Glasgow, L. A., and Turner, M. D.: The staphylococcal scalded-skin syndrome: Isolation and partial characterization of the exfoliative toxin. J. Infect. Dis. *125*:129-140, 1972.

148. Melly, M. A., Thomison, J. B., and Rogers, D. E.: Fate of staphylococci within human leukocytes. J. Exp. Med. *112*:1121-1130, 1960.

149. Miller, M. E., and Nilsson, U. R.: A familial deficiency of the phagocytosis-enhancing activity of serum related to a dysfunction of the fifth component of complement (C5). N. Engl. J. Med. *282*:354-358, 1970.

150. Mishaan, A. M., Mason, E. O., Jr., Martinez-Aguilar, G., et al.: Emergence of a predominant clone of community-acquired *Staphylococcus aureus* among children in Houston, Texas. Pediatr. Infect. Dis. J. *24*:201-206, 2005.

151. Moran, G. J., Krishnadasan, A., Gorwitz, R. J., et al.: Methicillin-resistant *S. aureus* infections among patients in the emergency department. N. Engl. J. Med. *355*:666-674, 2006.

152. Moreno, F., Crisp, C., Jorgensen, J. H., and Patterson, J. E.: Methicillin-resistant *Staphylococcus aureus* as a community organism. Clin. Infect. Dis. *21*:1308-1312, 1995.

153. Muder, R. R., Brennen, C., Wagener, M. M., et al.: Methicillin-resistant staphylococcal colonization and infection in a long-term care facility. Ann. Intern. Med. *114*:107-112, 1991.

154. Muto, C. A., Jernigan, J., Ostrowsky, B. E., et al.: SHEA guideline for preventing nosocomial transmission of multidrug-resistant strains of *Staphylococcus aureus* and enterococcus. Infect. Control Hosp. Epidemiol. *24*:362-386, 2003.

155. Naimi, T. S., LeDell, K. H., Boxrud, D. J., et al.: Epidemiology and clonality of community-acquired methicillin-resistant *Staphylococcus aureus* in Minnesota, 1996-1998. Clin. Infect. Dis. *33*:990-996, 2001.

156. Naimi, T. S., LeDell, K. H., Como-Sabetti, K., et al.: Comparison of community- and health care-associated methicillin-resistant *Staphylococcus aureus* infection. JAMA *290*:2976-2984, 2003.

157. Nakamura, M. M., Rohling, K. L., Shashaty, M., et al.: Prevalence of methicillin-resistant *Staphylococcus aureus* nasal carriage in the community pediatric population. Pediatr. Infect. Dis. J. *21*:917-922, 2002.

158. Nguyen, T., Ghebrehiwet, B., and Peerschke, E. I.: *Staphylococcus aureus* protein A recognizes platelet gC1qR/p33: A novel mechanism for staphylococcal interactions with platelets. Infect. Immun. *68*:2061-2068, 2000.

159. O'Riordan, K., and Lee, J. C.: *Staphylococcus aureus* capsular polysaccharides. Clin. Microbiol. Rev. *17*:218-234, 2004.

160. Okoji, C. N., Inglis, B., and Stewart, P. R.: Potential problems in the use of oligonucleotide probes for staphylococcal enterotoxin genes. J. Appl. Bacteriol. *74*:637-644, 1993.

161. Okuma, K., Iwakawa, K., Turnidge, J. D., et al.: Dissemination of new methicillin-resistant *Staphylococcus aureus* clones in the community. J. Clin. Microbiol. *40*:4289-4294, 2002.

162. Oliveira, D. C., and de Lencastre, H.: Multiplex PCR strategy for rapid identification of structural types and variants of the *mec* element in methicillin-resistant *Staphylococcus aureus*. Antimicrob. Agents Chemother. *46*:2155-2161, 2002.

163. Ong, P. Y., Ohtake, T., Brandt, C., et al.: Endogenous antimicrobial peptides and skin infections in atopic dermatitis. N. Engl. J. Med. *347*:1151-1160, 2002.

164. Palmqvist, N., Foster, T., Fitzgerald, J. R., et al.: Fibronectin-binding proteins and fibrinogen-binding clumping factors play distinct roles in staphylococcal arthritis and systemic inflammation. J. Infect. Dis. *191*:791-798, 2005.

165. Panagea, S., Perry, J. D., and Gould, F. K.: Should clindamycin be used as treatment of patients with infections caused by erythromycin-resistant staphylococci? J. Antimicrob. Chemother. *44*:581-582, 1999.

166. Panton, P. N., and Valentine, F. C. O.: Staphylococcal toxins. Lancet *1*:506-510, 1932.

167. Peterson, P. K., Quie, P. G., Kim, Y., et al.: Recognition of *Staphylococcus aureus* by human phagocytes: Signals and disguises of the bacterial surface. Scand. J. Infect. Dis. Suppl. *41*:67-78, 1983.

168. Pickering, L. K., O'Connor, D. M., Anderson, D., et al.: Comparative evaluation of cefazolin and cephalothin in children. J. Pediatr. *85*:842-847, 1974.

169. Plueckhahn, V. D.: Hexachlorophene and the control of staphylococcal sepsis in a maternity unit in Geelong, Australia. Pediatrics *51*:368-382, 1973.

170. Podewils, L. J., Liedtke, L. A., McDonald, L. C., et al.: A national survey of severe influenza-associated complications among children and adults, 2003-2004. Clin. Infect. Dis. *40*:1693-1696, 2005.

171. Prevost, G., Couppie, P., Prevost, P., et al.: Epidemiological data on *Staphylococcus aureus* strains producing synergohymenotropic toxins. J. Med. Microbiol. *42*:237-245, 1995.

172. Proctor, R. A., van Langevelde, P., Kristjansson, M., et al.: Persistent and relapsing infections associated with small-colony variants of *Staphylococcus aureus*. Clin. Infect. Dis. *20*:95-102, 1995.

173. Proctor, R. A., von Eiff, C., Kahl, B. C., et al.: Small colony variants: A pathogenic form of bacteria that facilitates persistent and recurrent infections. Nat. Rev. Microbiol. *4*:295-305, 2006.

174. Punsalang, A., Jr., Migneault, P. C., and Nolte, F. S.: Reliability of latex agglutination tests for identification of *Staphylococcus aureus* resistant to oxacillin. J. Clin. Microbiol. *24*:1104-1106, 1986.

175. Purcell, K., and Fergie, J.: Epidemic of community-acquired methicillin-resistant *Staphylococcus aureus* infections: A 14-year study at Driscoll Children's Hospital. Arch. Pediatr. Adolesc. Med. *159*:980-985, 2005.

176. Quie, P. G.: Chronic granulomatous disease of childhood. Adv. Pediatr. *16*:287-300, 1969.

177. Rathore, M. H., and Kline, M. W.: Community-acquired methicillin-resistant *Staphylococcus aureus* infections in children. Pediatr. Infect. Dis. J. *8*:645-647, 1989.

178. Reagan, D. R., Doebbeling, B. N., Pfaller, M. A., et al.: Elimination of coincident *Staphylococcus aureus* nasal and hand carriage with intranasal application of mupirocin calcium ointment. Ann. Intern. Med. *114*:101-106, 1991.

179. Robinson, D. A., and Enright, M. C.: Evolutionary models of the emergence of methicillin-resistant *Staphylococcus aureus*. Antimicrob. Agents Chemother. *47*:3926-3934, 2003.

180. Robinson, D. A., Kearns, A. M., Holmes, A., et al.: Re-emergence of early pandemic *Staphylococcus aureus* as a community-acquired methicillin-resistant clone. Lancet *365*:1256-1258, 2005.

181. Roche, F. M., Massey, R., Peacock, S. J., et al.: Characterization of novel LPXTG-containing proteins of *Staphylococcus aureus* identified from genome sequences. Microbiology *149*:643-654, 2003.

182. Ruhe, J. J., Monson, T., Bradsher, R. W., and Menon, A.: Use of long-acting tetracyclines for methicillin-resistant *Staphylococcus aureus* infections: Case series and review of the literature. Clin. Infect. Dis. *40*:1429-1434, 2005.

183. Ruhe, J. J., Smith, N., Bradsher, R. W., and Menon, A.: Community-onset methicillin-resistant *Staphylococcus aureus* skin and soft-tissue infections: Impact of antimicrobial therapy on outcome. Clin. Infect. Dis. *44*:777-784, 2007.

184. Ryding, U., Flock, J. I., Flock, M., et al.: Expression of collagen-binding protein and types 5 and 8 capsular polysaccharide in clinical isolates of *Staphylococcus aureus*. J. Infect. Dis. *176*:1096-1099, 1997.

185. Saravolatz, L. D., Markowitz, N., Arking, L., et al.: Methicillin-resistant *Staphylococcus aureus*: Epidemiologic observations during a community-acquired outbreak. Ann. Intern. Med. *96*:11-16, 1982.

186. Saravolatz, L. D., Pohlod, D. J., and Arking, L. M.: Community-acquired methicillin-resistant *Staphylococcus aureus* infections: A new source for nosocomial outbreaks. Ann. Intern. Med. *97*:325-329, 1982.

187. Sattler, C. A., Mason, E. O., Jr., and Kaplan, S. L.: Prospective comparison of risk factors and demographic and clinical characteristics of community-acquired, methicillin-resistant versus methicillin-susceptible *Staphylococcus aureus* infection in children. Pediatr. Infect. Dis. J. *21*:910-917, 2002.

188. Sendi, P., Rohrbach, M., Graber, P., et al.: *Staphylococcus aureus* small colony variants in prosthetic joint infection. Clin. Infect. Dis. *43*:961-967, 2006.

189. Seybold, U., Kourbatova, E. V., Johnson, J. G., et al.: Emergence of community-associated methicillin-resistant *Staphylococcus aureus* USA300 genotype as a major cause of health care-associated blood stream infections. Clin. Infect. Dis. *42*:647-656, 2006.

190. Shinefield, H. R.: Use of a conjugate polysaccharide vaccine in the prevention of invasive staphylococcal disease: Is an additional vaccine needed or possible? Vaccine *24*(Suppl. 2):S2-S9, 2006.

191. Shinefield, H. R., and Black, S.: Prospects for active and passive immunization against *Staphylococcus aureus*. Pediatr. Infect. Dis. J. *25*:167-168, 2006.

192. Shinefield, H., Black, S., Fattom, A., et al.: Use of a *Staphylococcus aureus* conjugate vaccine in patients receiving hemodialysis. N. Engl. J. Med. *346*:491-496, 2002.

193. Shinefield, H. R., Ribble, J. C., Eichenwald, H. F., et al.: Bacterial interference: Its effect on nursery-acquired infection with *Staphylococcus aureus*. V. An analysis and interpretation. Am. J. Dis. Child *105*:683-688, 1963.

194. Shopsin, B., Gomez, M., Montgomery, S. O., et al.: Evaluation of protein A gene polymorphic region DNA sequencing for typing of *Staphylococcus aureus* strains. J. Clin. Microbiol. *37*:3556-3563, 1999.

195. Siberry, G. K., Tekle, T., Carroll, K., and Dick, J.: Failure of clindamycin treatment of methicillin-resistant *Staphylococcus aureus* expressing inducible clindamycin resistance in vitro. Clin. Infect. Dis. *37*:1257-1260, 2003.

196. Siegel, J. D., Rhinehart, E., Jackson, M., et al.: Management of Multidrug-Resistant Organisms in Healthcare Settings. Am. J. Infect. Control *35*:S165-S193, 2007.

197. Smeltzer, M. S., Hart, M. E., and Iandolo, J. J.: Phenotypic characterization of xpr, a global regulator of extracellular virulence factors in *Staphylococcus aureus*. Infect. Immun. *61*:919-925, 1993.

198. Smith, T. L., Pearson, M. L., Wilcox, K. R., et al.: Emergence of vancomycin resistance in *Staphylococcus aureus*: Glycopeptide-Intermediate *Staphylococcus aureus* Working Group. N. Engl. J. Med. *340*:493-501, 1999.

199. Sompolinsky, D., Samra, Z., Karakawa, W. W., et al.: Encapsulation and capsular types in isolates of *Staphylococcus aureus* from different sources and relationship to phage types. J. Clin. Microbiol. *22*:828-834, 1985.

200. Steele, R. W., Ashcraft, E. W., Payton, T. S., and Eisenach, K. D.: Recurrent staphylococcal infection in a pediatric residential care facility. Am. J. Infect. Control *11*:217-220, 1983.

201. Stein, G. E., and Craig, W. A.: Tigecycline: A critical analysis. Clin. Infect. Dis. *43*:518-524, 2006.

202. Stevens, D. L., Ma, Y., Salmi, D. B., et al.: Impact of antibiotics on expression of virulence-associated exotoxin genes in methicillin-sensitive and methicillin-resistant *Staphylococcus aureus*. J. Infect. Dis. *195*:202-211, 2007.

203. Stewart, G. T., and Holt, R. J.: Evolution of natural resistance to the newer penicillins. Br. Med. J. *1*:308-311, 1963.

204. Storch, G. A., and Rajagopalan, L.: Methicillin-resistant *Staphylococcus aureus* bacteremia in children. Pediatr. Infect. Dis. *5*:59-67, 1986.

205. Stranger-Jones, Y. K., Bae, T., and Schneewind, O.: Vaccine assembly from surface proteins of *Staphylococcus aureus*. Proc. Natl. Acad. Sci. U. S. A. *103*:16942-16947, 2006.

206. Strausbaugh, L. J., Jacobson, C., Sewell, D. L., et al.: Methicillin-resistant *Staphylococcus aureus* in extended-care facilities: Experiences in a Veterans' Affairs nursing home and a review of the literature. Infect. Control Hosp. Epidemiol. *12*:36-45, 1991.

207. Taplin, D., Lansdell, L., Allen, A. M., et al.: Prevalence of streptococcal pyoderma in relation to climate and hygiene. Lancet *1*:501-503, 1973.

208. Taylor, A. G., Cook, J., Fincham, W. J., and Millard, F. J.: Serological tests in the differentiation of staphylococcal and tuberculous bone disease. J. Clin. Pathol. *28*:284-288, 1975.

209. Tenover, F. C., and Moellering, R. C., Jr.: The rationale for revising the Clinical and Laboratory Standards Institute vancomycin minimal inhibitory concentration interpretive criteria for *Staphylococcus aureus*. Clin. Infect. Dis. *44*:1208-1215, 2007.

210. Tenover, F. C., Arbeit, R. D., Goering, R. V., et al.: Interpreting chromosomal DNA restriction patterns produced by pulsed-field gel electrophoresis: Criteria for bacterial strain typing. J. Clin. Microbiol. *33*:2233-2239, 1995.

211. Tenover, F. C., Lancaster, M. V., Hill, B. C., et al.: Characterization of staphylococci with reduced susceptibilities to vancomycin and other glycopeptides. J. Clin. Microbiol. *36*:1020-1027, 1998.

212. Tenover, F. C., Weigel, L. M., Appelbaum, P. C., et al.: Vancomycin-resistant *Staphylococcus aureus* isolate from a patient in Pennsylvania. Antimicrob. Agents Chemother. *48*:275-280, 2004.

213. Thompson, R. L., Cabezudo, I., and Wenzel, R. P.: Epidemiology of nosocomial infections caused by methicillin-resistant *Staphylococcus aureus*. Ann.
Intern. Med. 97:309-317, 1982.
214. van Hal, S. J., Stark, D., Lockwood, B., et al.: MRSA detection: Comparison
of two molecular methods (IDI-MRSA® PCR assay and GenoType®
MRSA Direct PCR assay) with three selective MRSA agars (MRSA ID®,
MRSASelect® and CHROMagar MRSA) for infection control swabs. J. Clin.
Microbiol. 45:2486-2490, 2007.
215. Vandenesch, F., Naimi, T., Enright, M. C., et al.: Community-acquired
methicillin-resistant *Staphylococcus aureus* carrying Panton-Valentine leukocidin genes: Worldwide emergence. Emerg. Infect. Dis. 9:978-984, 2003.
216. Vaudaux, P., Kelley, W. L., and Lew, D. P.: *Staphylococcus aureus* small colony
variants: Difficult to diagnose and difficult to treat. Clin. Infect. Dis. 43:968-
970, 2006.
217. Vernachio, J. H., Bayer, A. S., Ames, B., et al.: Human immunoglobulin
G recognizing fibrinogen-binding surface proteins is protective against
both *Staphylococcus aureus* and *Staphylococcus epidermidis* infections in vivo.
Antimicrob. Agents Chemother. 50:511-518, 2006.
218. Voyich, J. M., Braughton, K. R., Sturdevant, D. E., et al.: Insights into mechanisms used by *Staphylococcus aureus* to avoid destruction by human neutrophils.
J. Immunol. 175:3907-3919, 2005.
219. Voyich, J. M., Otto, M., Mathema, B., et al.: Is Panton-Valentine
leukocidin the major virulence determinant in community-associated
methicillin-resistant *Staphylococcus aureus* disease? J. Infect. Dis. 194:1761-
1770, 2006.
220. Watanakunakorn, C.: Changing epidemiology and newer aspects of infective
endocarditis. Adv. Intern. Med. 22:21-47, 1977.
221. Watanakunakorn, C.: Clindamycin therapy of *Staphylococcus aureus* endocarditis: Clinical relapse and development of resistance to clindamycin, lincomycin
and erythromycin. Am. J. Med. 60:419-425, 1976.
222. Watanakunakorn, C.: Treatment of infections due to methicillin-resistant
Staphylococcus aureus. Ann. Intern. Med. 97:376-378, 1982.
223. Webster, J., and Faoagali, J. L.: Endemic methicillin-resistant *Staphylococcus
aureus* in a special care baby unit: A 2 year review. J. Paediatr. Child Health
26:160-163, 1990.
224. Weems, J. J., Jr., Steinberg, J. P., Filler, S., et al.: Phase II, randomized,
double-blind, multicenter study comparing the safety and pharmacokinetics
of tefibazumab to placebo for treatment of *Staphylococcus aureus* bacteremia.
Antimicrob. Agents Chemother. 50:2751-2755, 2006.
225. Wertheim, H. F., Melles, D. C., Vos, M. C., et al.: The role of nasal carriage
in *Staphylococcus aureus* infections. Lancet Infect. Dis. 5:751-762, 2005.
226. Williams, C. P., and Oliver, T. K., Jr.: Nursery routines and staphylococcal
colonization of the newborn. Pediatrics 44:640-646, 1969.
227. Williams, R. C., Jr., and Quie, P. G.: Opsonic activity of agammaglobulinemic
human sera. J. Immunol. 106:51-55, 1971.
228. Williams, R. C., Jr., Dossett, J. H., and Quie, P. G.: Comparative studies of
immunoglobulin opsonins in osteomyelitis and other established infections.
Immunology 17:249-265, 1969.
229. Wisplinghoff, H., Seifert, H., Tallent, S. M., et al.: Nosocomial bloodstream
infections in pediatric patients in United States hospitals: Epidemiology, clinical features and susceptibility. Pediatr. Infect. Dis. J. 22:686-691, 2003.
230. Wolff, S. M.: The Chediak-Higashi syndrome: Studies of host defenses. Ann.
Intern. Med. 76:293-306, 1972.
231. Yamasaki, O., Tristan, A., Yamaguchi, T., et al.: Distribution of the exfoliative toxin D gene in clinical *Staphylococcus aureus* isolates in France. Clin.
Microbiol. Infect. 12:585-588, 2006.
232. Yarwood, J. M., McCormick, J. K., Paustian, M. L., et al.: Characterization
and expression analysis of *Staphylococcus aureus* pathogenicity island 3:
Implications for the evolution of staphylococcal pathogenicity islands. J. Biol.
Chem. 277:13138-13147, 2002.
233. Zafar, A. B., Butler, R. C., Reese, D. J., et al.: Use of 0.3% triclosan (Bacti-
Stat) to eradicate an outbreak of methicillin-resistant *Staphylococcus aureus* in a
neonatal nursery. Am. J. Infect. Control 23:200-208, 1995.
234. Zaoutis, T. E., Toltzis, P., Chu, J., et al.: Clinical and molecular epidemiology
of community-acquired methicillin-resistant *Staphylococcus aureus* infections
among children with risk factors for health care-associated infection: 2001-
2003. Pediatr. Infect. Dis. J. 25:343-348, 2006.
235. Zheng, W. F., Tan, R. X., Yang, L., and Liu, Z. L.: Two flavones from
Artemisia giraldii and their antimicrobial activity. Planta Med. 62:160-162,
1996.

CHAPTER 92

COAGULASE-NEGATIVE STAPHYLOCOCCAL INFECTIONS

David Y. Hyun ☉ **Carina A. Rodriguez** ☉ **Christian C. Patrick** ☉ **Sheldon L. Kaplan**

Coagulase-negative staphylococci are among the most common
causative agents of nosocomial infections and are among the
bacteria most frequently isolated in the microbiology laboratory.
Their normal habitat includes skin and mucous membranes of
humans and animals. This ecologic niche hampers studies on this
group of bacteria because they also are frequent contaminants in
the clinical microbiology laboratory. Coagulase-negative staphylococci infections occur mainly in immunocompromised patients,
particularly those with indwelling medical devices.[160,178,203,249]
New epidemiologic and molecular techniques can be useful to
identify characteristics of strains in nosocomial outbreaks. Understanding the pathogenesis of infections caused by these organisms
has advanced, and several possible virulence factors have been
identified. The clinical spectrum of the disease is characterized
by a more indolent presentation when compared with other
gram-positive cocci. Removal of catheters or prosthetic devices
may be necessary for patients with persistent infections. Furthermore, effective therapy can be difficult to achieve because of the
high proportion of isolates resistant to antibiotics. This chapter
reviews the microbiology, epidemiology, pathogenesis, clinical
manifestations and diagnoses, and treatment of infections caused
by these ubiquitous organisms.

techniques for species definition existed. Rosenbach in 1884 used
the term *S. albus* for coagulase-negative staphylococci to denote
the white color imparted by the colony on an agar plate, in contrast to the pathogenic *Staphylococcus aureus*, which had a yellow
colony color.

In the 1960s, coagulase-negative staphylococci clearly were
identified in association with infections in certain patient populations. Coagulase-negative staphylococci were implicated as the
etiologic agent of infections in patients with atrioventricular
shunts and peritoneal catheters and in neonatal sepsis.[30,32,137,217]

During the 1960s, *Staphylococcus saprophyticus* was recognized
as a singular species and found to be a pathogen in urinary tract
infections. Additionally, *Staphylococcus epidermidis* supplanted *S.
albus* as a generic term for all coagulase-negative staphylococci
other than *S. saprophyticus*. The association of disease with coagulase-negative staphylococci highlighted the need for further
specification. Work in the 1970s focused on coagulase-negative
staphylococci biotyping (differentiation based on biochemical
reactions), and this work continues. Currently, more than 32
species of coagulase-negative staphylococci are recognized. Now
that individual species can be identified, *S. epidermidis* is used as
a specific species term.

HISTORICAL BACKGROUND

Staphylococcus albus was the descriptive term used to define all
coagulase-negative staphylococci before 1960 because so few

MICROBIOLOGY

Staphylococci are nonmotile, non–spore-forming, gram-positive
bacteria. The genus *Staphylococcus* is related most closely to the

newly described genus *Macrococcus*, and it has a relatively close relationship with the genera *Bacillus, Salinicoccus, Gamella, Listeria, Planococcus,* and *Brochothrix*.[129] Members of the genus *Staphylococcus* have a low DNA G + C content (30 to 39 mol %), whereas members of the genus *Micrococcus* have a G + C content within the range of 66 to 75 mol percent.[127] Staphylococci can be divided by the ability to produce or not produce coagulase, an extracellular enzyme that promotes the congealing of rabbit plasma. The thermonuclease reaction is particularly useful for rapidly differentiating *S. aureus* (positive) from other staphylococcal species (negative) and is more accurate than are tests based on coagulase production.[101] *S. aureus* also can be differentiated from most coagulase-negative staphylococci by the fermentation of mannitol. Currently, 32 species of staphylococci are recognized, 29 of which are coagulase-negative staphylococci, and are identified by the following criteria: (1) colony morphology, (2) oxygen requirements, (3) novobiocin resistance, (4) aerobic acid production from carbohydrates, and (5) selected liability to enzymatic activities.[127,129] Susceptibility to novobiocin is a convenient assay to differentiate *S. saprophyticus* from most coagulase-negative staphylococci from human specimens, including *S. epidermidis*. *S. saprophyticus*, the uncommon pathogen *Staphylococcus cohnii*, and the rare pathogen *Staphylococcus xylosus* are novobiocin resistant.[186] Commercial kits used to identify species of coagulase-negative staphylococci have various degrees of confidence: an identification is made 60 to 95 percent of the time, depending on the species. Most systems are developed to identify especially *S. epidermidis* and *S. saprophyticus* because these are the species clearly associated with clinical diseases.[189] Additionally, DNA-pairing studies have identified intraspecies differences with strains considered to be *S. epidermidis* by biotyping.[265]

Coagulase-negative staphylococci are prototypic gram-positive bacteria. The outermost structure is a cell wall composed primarily of peptidoglycan with teichoic acid molecules and an assortment of interspersed proteins. The teichoic acid has a glycerol backbone, compared with the ribitol of *S. aureus*.[167] Approximately 20 to 30 proteins are located within the cell wall; 15 to 20 of these are surface exposed and thus are able to interact with the host.[180]

S. epidermidis and other coagulase-negative staphylococci produce a capsule that appears to be a virulence factor in animal models.[106,168,261] However, its presence has been demonstrated in only 9 percent of fresh clinical isolates.[105] A glycocalyx or slime-layer substance, produced by most strains of *S. epidermidis*, is considered a virulence factor that inhibits phagocytosis.[39,41,52,53]

EPIDEMIOLOGY

Epidemiologic studies involving strain delineation of coagulase-negative staphylococci have proved difficult to perform because of the organism's commensal nature on the human body. *S. epidermidis* is the prominent species, accounting for 60 to 90 percent of all staphylococci recovered from humans. The ecologic niches of coagulase-negative staphylococci have allowed a classification, as shown in Table 92–1.

Coagulase-negative staphylococci, except for *S. saprophyticus*, cause primarily nosocomial infections. Antibiotic resistance of coagulase-negative staphylococci is a common occurrence because of selective antibiotic use in the hospital setting. In 1997, the National Nosocomial Infections Surveillance Report noted an 87 percent increase in the rate of oxacillin resistance among coagulase-negative staphylococci isolates from patients in intensive care units when compared with the same period 5 years earlier.[36] Coagulase-negative staphylococci gain access to the bloodstream primarily by breakdown of skin or mucocutaneous barriers, by following a prosthetic catheter tract, or through the hub of a central venous catheter. Two studies addressed the acquisition of

TABLE 92–1 Staphylococci That Are Part of the Normal Flora, Including Common Sites of Habitation and Pathogenic Potential

Species	Common Anatomic Site of Habitation	Pathogenic Potential
S. aureus	Nares	Common
S. epidermidis	Nares; axillae; skin of head, arms, and legs	Common
S. saprophyticus	Occasionally skin	Common
S. haemolyticus	Skin of head, arms, and legs	Uncommon
S. hominis	Axillae; skin of head, arms, and legs	Uncommon
S. lugdunensis	Widely distributed on body	Uncommon
S. simulans	Occasionally skin	Uncommon
S. cohnii	Occasionally skin	Uncommon
S. warneri	Occasionally skin	Uncommon
S. saccharolyticus	Rarely skin	Uncommon
S. caprae	Occasionally skin	Rare
S. capitis	Skin of head, face, ears, and arms	Rare
S. auricularis	Ears	Rare
S. schleiferi	? Skin	Rare
S. xylosus	Occasionally skin	Rare

Modified from Pfaller, M. A., and Herwaldt, L. A.: Laboratory, clinical, and epidemiological aspects of coagulase-negative staphylococci. Clin. Microbiol. Rev. 1:281-299, 1988.

TABLE 92–2 Current Methods of Epidemiologic Analysis of Coagulase-Negative Staphylococci

Conventional	Molecular
Biotyping[94,175]	Multilocus enzyme electrophoresis[166,239,249,267]
Colony morphology[127]	Plasmid analysis[8,127,172,173,213,214,236,253]
Antibiograms[91,92,127,136,149,155]	Chromosomal analysis[20,75,107]
Serology[1,182,263]	Polymerase chain reaction amplification[127]
Polypeptide analysis[31,33,44,57,239]	
Slime-layer production[40,47]	
Phage typing[39,50,175,176,230,234]	
Pyrolysis mass spectrometry[68]	

S. epidermidis as a colonizing organism in low-birth-weight neonates.[46,90] Both reports described rapid colonization, in which 75 percent of neonates were colonized by 2 weeks of age, but differed in their findings of increased production of slime-layer or antibiotic-resistant organisms with increased colonization time.[46,90] Although most infants acquire coagulase-negative staphylococci from environmental sources, including hospital personnel, a few are colonized by vertical transmission.[89,181]

Epidemiologic techniques are of paramount importance in coagulase-negative staphylococci infections to identify a strain causing either a common-source outbreak or repeated infections within an individual.[166,189,249] Techniques currently available are divided into conventional or molecular and are listed in Table 92–2. Conventional methods are fraught with poor standardization, sensitivity, and specificity. However, a combination of these techniques has been used for strain delineation. Genotyping by pulse-field gel electrophoresis (PFGE) has been shown to be highly discriminatory when investigating patterns of transmission and sources of outbreaks.[26,134,156,238,249] Random amplification of polymorphic DNA (RAPD) by polymerase chain reaction (PCR) also has been successful in identifying clonal outbreaks and transmissions. Although it is less discriminatory than is PFGE, RAPD

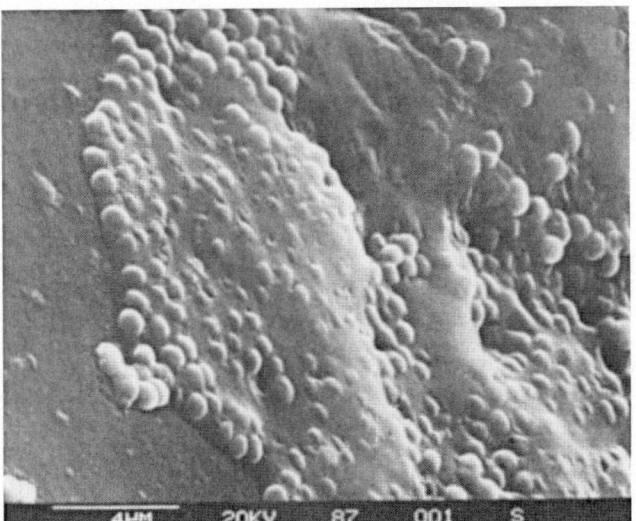

Figure 92–1 Scanning electron microscopy of slime-producing coagulase-negative staphylococci. *(From Peters, G., Locci, R., and Pulverer, G.: Adherence and growth of coagulase-negative staphylococci on surfaces of intravenous catheters. J. Infect. Dis. 146:479-482, 1982.)*

TABLE 92–3 Biofilm Formation

Mechanisms

Initial Attachment
Physicochemical forces (charge, van der Waals, hydrophobic interactions)
Staphylococcal surface proteins (SSP-1 and SSP-2)
Surface-associated autolysin (AtlE)
Capsular polysaccharide/adhesin (PS/A)
Host factor–binding proteins: fibrinogen-binding protein (Fbe); AtlE*
Adhesin/autolysin (Aas)†

Accumulation Process
Polysaccharide intercellular adhesin (PIA)
Capsular polysaccharide/adhesin (PS/A)
Accumulation-associated protein (AAP)

AtlE exhibits vitronectin-binding activity.
†*Aas binds fibronectin and hemaglutinates sheep erythrocytes.*
Data from Heilman, C., and Peters, G.: Biology and pathogenesis of Staphylococcus epidermidis. In Fischetti, V. A., Novick, R. P., Ferretti, J. J., et al. (eds.): Gram-Positive Pathogens. Washington, D.C., ASM Press, 2000, pp. 442-449.

is less costly and time-consuming.[23,195] Multilocus sequence typing (MLST) can be used to delineate clonal relationships between strains and has been used to identify predominant clones from a group of clinical isolates.[144,266]

Antimicrobial susceptibility testing is the method most readily available for typing using a phenotypic characteristic. Methicillin resistance is mediated by the *mecA* gene, which is carried on a chromosomal element called *staphylococcus chromosomal cassette mec* (SCC*mec*).[266] This mobile element is thought to be capable of horizontal transfer between species and to confer methicillin resistance in community-acquired *S. aureus*. Typing of SCC*mec* can be achieved by PCR.

PATHOGENESIS

Several risk factors for development of coagulase-negative staphylococci infection are caused by changes in host defense. Initial risk factors include a breakdown of the mucocutaneous barrier, immunosuppression,[64,119] and prior antibiotic therapy.[120,218] In addition, the presence of a prosthetic device, such as an indwelling central venous catheter, cerebrospinal fluid (CSF) shunt, or peritoneal dialysis catheter, increases the susceptibility to infection.[12,19,59,138] Opsonophagocytosis is the most important immune defense against coagulase-negative staphylococci.[64,120,227] An increased rate of infection has been noted in patients with a dysfunctional opsonophagocytosis system, including neonates[64,227] and patients receiving continuous ambulatory peritoneal dialysis.[77,120]

Biolfilm formation (Fig. 92–1 and Table 92–3) is considered to be a major virulence factor for *S. epidermidis* and other coagulase-negative staphylococci, especially in nosocomial and prosthetic device infections.[5,56,144,241,247] It consists of multiple layers of cells embedded in an amorphous extracellular material often referred to as *slime*. It provides a mechanism for staphylococci to evade antibiotics and host defense.[34,60,79,111,131,220,221,248,252]

Biofilm formation is initiated by attachment of the organism to a surface such as polystyrene.[144,145] This adhesion is mediated by cell wall teichoic acids[102] and proteins, including autolysins AltE (surface-associated autolysin) and Aae,[98,102,204,240] that interact and bind with extracellular matrix proteins such as fibronectin, fibrinogen, and vitronectin. Nonspecific electrostatic and hydrophobic interaction also promote attachment.[95,100,243] Initial

attachment is followed by accumulation of biofilm, which is primarily mediated by polysaccharide intercellular adhesin (PIA).[97,205] PIA also acts as a hemaglutinin[144,202] and protects the bacteria from phagocytosis and killing by human polymorphonuclear leucocytes.[222,252] The *ica*ADBC operon, which is found in both *S. epidermidis* and *S. aureus*, encodes enzymes necessary for PIA production.[97]

In numerous epidemiologic studies, the presence of the *ica* operon has been associated more frequently with *S. epidermidis* strains isolated from hospitalized patients with prosthetic device infections than with community strains isolated from healthy individuals. Eighty-one to 89 percent of isolates from hospitalized patients have been reported to carry the *ica* operon. In contrast, only 6 to 38 percent of community-acquired isolates were found to carry the *ica* operon.[67,130,244] The utility of *ica* operon detection in differentiating between invasive strains and commensal strains of *S. epidermidis* obtained from patients in neonatal intensive care units, bone marrow transplant units, and oncology units has been investigated. Although both groups of strains demonstrated high carriage rates of the *ica* operon, no significant difference was found.[27,51,183,198] However, higher proportions of invasive strains demonstrated biofilm production in quantitative assays compared with commensal strains.[27,198] Most of the commensal strains were biofilm-negative despite possessing the *ica* operon, a finding suggesting that regulation of gene expression plays a large role in virulence.

Numerous extracellular enzymes are produced by coagulase-negative staphylococci; an extracellular metalloprotease with elastase activity; a cysteine protease that degrades human secretory immunoglobulin A, immunoglobulin M, serum albumin, fibrinogen, and fibronectin; and an extracellular serine protease involved in epidermin processing.[96,251,254] Two lipases have been postulated to facilitate skin colonization.[96,251] Unlike *S. aureus*, which is capable of producing various cytolytic and superantigenic toxins, *S. epidermidis* produces very few toxins.[251] Delta toxin, an enteropathogenic toxin, encoded by the *hld* component of the regulatory system *agr*, has been linked to necrotizing enterocolitis in infants.[215] *S. epidermidis* also produces antibacterial peptides called *lantibiotics* that may play a role in bacterial interference on skin and mucous membranes and in the creation of an ecologic niche for *S. epidermidis*.[132]

S. saprophyticus can cause urinary tract infections in the absence of indwelling catheters.[132] Several virulence factors have been described to explain its pathogenic potential to adhere and persistently grow in the urinary tract. A surface-exposed protein with hemagglutinin and adhesive properties[74] and a surface fibrillar protein,[73] designated *ssp*, are associated with attachment to urinary tract epithelium. Urease production also has been associated with invasiveness of this organism by causing damage to bladder tissues.[71,72] The whole genome of *S. saprophyticus* has been sequenced and compared with *S. aureus* and *S. epidermidis*.[132] Analysis revealed a single, unique cell wall anchored protein with properties of hemagglutination and adherence to human bladder cells. A high population of ionic transport systems capable of providing osmotolerence in the highly variant ionic environment of urine also was demonstrated.

CLINICAL MANIFESTATIONS

Coagulase-negative staphylococci have been implicated in a variety of clinical infections in immunocompetent and immunocompromised patients (Table 92–4).[126,178,206] A basic difficulty in interpreting clinical studies of coagulase-negative staphylococci exists because of the different criteria used to define a clinically significant culture.[54] In neonates, immunocompromised patients, and patients with prosthetic implants, repeated isolation of the same phenotypic strain of coagulase-negative staphylococci from blood cultures facilitates interpretation. For catheter-related bacteremia, quantitative cultures from the catheter exhibit a five- to tenfold increase in the number of colony-forming units as compared with cultures from a peripheral vessel. The Committee on Infectious Diseases of the American Academy of Pediatrics suggested the following considerations to distinguish pathogenic from contaminant coagulase-negative staphylococci: (1) two or more positive blood cultures from different sites, (2) a positive culture from blood and another usually sterile site with identical or nearly identical antimicrobial susceptibility patterns, (3) growth in continuously monitored blood culture system within 15 hours of incubation, (4) clinical findings of infection in the patient, (5) an intravascular catheter that has been in place for 3 days or more, and (6) similar or identical genotypes among all isolates.[4]

Clinical presentation markedly differs from that of *S. aureus* infection. In general, infections caused by coagulase-negative

TABLE 92–4 Clinically Important Coagulase-Negative Staphylococcal Infections

Bacteremia
Neonates
Patients with leukemia and lymphoma
Bone marrow transplant recipients

Infections in Patients with Indwelling Medical Devices
Central venous catheters
Cerebrospinal fluid shunts
Peritoneal dialysis catheter
Prosthetic values

Other Infections
Prosthetic joints
Vascular grafts and prostheses
Hemodialysis shunt
Pacemaker
Scalp electrode

Native Valve Endocarditis
Urinary Tract Infections
Miscellaneous Infections
Endophthalmitis after ocular surgery
Postoperative wound infections
Osteomyelitis (sternal wound or hematogenous)
Toxic shock syndrome

Modified from Patrick, C. C.: Coagulase-negative staphylococci: Pathogens with increasing clinical significance. J. Pediatr. 116:497-507, 1990.

staphylococci are more indolent and can manifest with a subacute or even chronic course.

BACTEREMIA

Coagulase-negative staphylococci, particularly *S. epidermidis*, have become the major nosocomial pathogens in most studies.[54,197] The analysis of 6290 nosocomial infections, including 110,709 patients from 61 pediatric intensive care units in the United States during 1992 to 1997, showed that bloodstream infections were the most common types of nosocomial infection; coagulase-negative staphylococcus was the causative agent in 38 percent (717 of 1887) of the cases.[197] In a large surveillance study between 1995 and 2001 among 49 hospitals in the United States, coagulase-negative staphylococci were the most common cause of nosocomial bacteremias in pediatric patients and accounted for 43 percent of the isolates.[258] These infections occur primarily with the use of indwelling vascular catheters. In febrile, immunocompromised pediatric patients with cancer, coagulase-negative staphylococci can account for 35 percent of all positive blood culture isolates.[2,11,133]

NEONATAL BACTEREMIAS

Coagulase-negative staphylococci are the single most frequent cause of late-onset septicemia among premature infants, especially in low-birth-weight infants.[16,65,80,87,88,165,179] Table 92–5 lists the salient features from six large studies.[65,88,114,115,158,179] These infections are found predominantly in premature infants with a gestational age of less than 35 weeks who have an immature immune system, particularly in quantitative and qualitative neutrophil function.[35,227,257] The presence of indwelling peripheral or umbilical catheters has been implicated in approximately half of neonatal coagulase-negative staphylococci bacteremias.[16,88,164,175]

Signs and symptoms of coagulase-negative staphylococci bacteremia *usually* are subtle and most commonly include bradycardia, apnea, and temperature instability (see Table 92-5). Skin abscesses were noted in more than 40 percent of neonates with coagulase-negative staphylococci bacteremia in one study.[179] Frequency of fulminant late-onset sepsis caused by coagulase-negative staphylococcosis bacteremia is very low (1%).[118]

Laboratory studies usually are not helpful in identifying patients with coagulase-negative staphylococci bacteremia.[161] Leukocytosis is an inconsistent finding. Reports have conflicted about production of slime, a possible virulence factor, as a marker for infection.[88,179] One study successfully correlated quantitative blood cultures with specific clinical information to distinguish a true pathogen.[233] Peripheral blood cultures yielding more than 50 colony-forming units per milliliter occurred exclusively in infants with proven septicemia. In contrast, low colony counts were observed in both septicemia and culture contamination. Those patients with low colony counts and septicemia were more likely to have a central venous line or an abnormal hematologic value (leukocytosis, decreased platelets, or increased immature to total neutrophil ratio).[233]

Persistence of coagulase-negative staphylococci bacteremia (mean duration, 12 to 13 days), despite administration of adequate antibiotic therapy, was described in neonates.[122,179] This persistence was observed in patients with and without central venous catheters and in patients with normal findings on cardiac echocardiography. Neonates with persistent bacteremia had a significantly higher incidence of severe thrombocytopenia requiring platelet transfusions than did those with nonpersistent bacteremia.[122]

Rarely, coagulase-negative staphylococci meningitis has been reported in low-birth-weight neonates with normal CSF

TABLE 92–5   Salient Aspects of Six Studies of Coagulase-Negative Staphylococci Bacteremia in Neonates

Characteristics	Munson et al., 1982[158] (n = 27)	Fleer et al., 1983[65] (n = 30)	Hall et al., 1987[88] (n = 29)	Patrick et al., 1989[179] (n = 32)	Kacica et al., 1994[114] (n = 47)	Kallman et al., 1997[115] (n = 27)
Patient						
Mean birth weight (g)	1130	1564	1607	1172	1259	NR
Gestational age	28.9	32.1	31	28.6	29	<30
Central lines (%)	85	NR	34	19	NR	NR
TPN (%)	78	77 (20/26)	NR	91	81	NR
Clinical						
Apnea or bradycardia (%)	>50	100	62	78	NR	NR
Temperature instability (%)	<50	70	7	22	NR	NR
Tachycardia (%)	>50	100	NR	6	NR	NR
Mortality (%)	0	0 (0/13)	0	0	NR	7.4
Laboratory						
Slime production, patient isolates (%)	NR	NR	79	54 (6/13)	65	NR
Antibiotic susceptibility	100% S to cephalothin	100% S to cephalothin	83% S to methicillin; 100% S to vancomycin	100% S to vancomycin	48% S to oxacillin; 100% S to vancomycin	86% S to methicillin*; 55% S to methicillin†

*Period: 1981-1986.
†Period: 1987-1994.
NR, not reported; S, susceptible; TPN, total parenteral nutrition.

TABLE 92–6   Clinical Characteristics of Coagulase-Negative Staphylococcal Bacteremia in Patients with Childhood Cancer*

Characteristics	Friedman et al., 1984[69] (n = 150)	Langley and Gold, 1988[133] (n = 100)	Aledo et al., 1998[2] (n = 140)	Auletta et al., 1999[11] (n = 102)
Coagulase-negative staphylococci among total bacteremias (%)	12.7	35	31.4	35
Patients with central venous catheters (%)	32	53	95	95
Mortality (%)	10.5	38	<5	19
Patient isolates susceptible to				
Methicillin (%)	17	38	NR	NR
Vancomycin (%)	100	100	NR	NR

*Percentages are based on the number of episodes of coagulase-negative staphylococcal sepsis.
NR, not reported.

profiles.[85] Thus, CSF examination should be considered in neonates with coagulase-negative staphylococci bacteremia. Abnormal CSF findings or a positive CSF culture may influence the duration of therapy. Coagulase-negative staphylococci also have been implicated as etiologic agents of necrotizing enterocolitis,[84,215] although one report showed no association.[201]

LEUKEMIA AND LYMPHOMA

Immunocompromised patients with leukemia, lymphoma, or both are at risk for the development of coagulase-negative staphylococci bacteremia (Table 92–6).[2,11,69,133,190,191,219] The most common portals of entry are the gastrointestinal tract, where chemotherapy causes defects, and the skin in association with catheter devices. In several reports, coagulase-negative staphylococci were the isolates most commonly causing bacteremia in pediatric patients with cancer and accounted for 35 percent of all initial isolates.[2,11,133] One third of these patients did not have central venous catheters at the time of their bacteremia.[69]

RAPD analysis and PFGE of DNA macrorestriction fragments of blood culture coagulase-negative staphylococci isolates obtained from 40 neutropenic hemato-oncologic patients related to 61 episodes of Hickman catheter–related infections allowed the characterization of clonal coagulase-negative staphylococci types that successfully and persistently colonized patients; this finding confirmed that the skin flora was the likely source of catheter-related infections (CRIs) in 75 percent of the patients.[166]

Morbidity from coagulase-negative staphylococci bacteremia is appreciable because of the organism's acquisition of multiple antibiotic resistance, which requires the use of vancomycin or combination antibiotic therapy, with potentially toxic effects.[69,119,133,142,143,192,212] Mortality rates have varied from 0 to 11 percent.[69,133]

HEMATOPOIETIC STEM CELL TRANSPLANTATION

Coagulase-negative staphylococci have become the primary pathogen causing bacteremia in hematopoietic stem cell transplant recipients.[31,154] These episodes occur most often during periods of agranulocytosis before marrow engraftment,[31] and they can be fatal.[18] Most of these episodes are a result of the universal use of central venous catheters and the use of broad-spectrum antibiotics. Bacteremia that occurs during the neutropenic phase after hematopoietic stem cell transplantation appears to be associated with early death from invasive fungal infection.[232]

INDWELLING MEDICAL DEVICES

Central Venous Catheters

Infections associated with central venous catheters are caused primarily by coagulase-negative staphylococci, which also can cause infections in peripheral catheters composed of steel or polyethylene.[242] Central venous catheters often are used in children for long-term hyperalimentation or administration of medication.[104] Two types of devices are in common use: (1) Broviac and Hickman catheters, which have an external port, and (2) totally implanted vascular access devices.[29,99,200] Broviac and Hickman catheters have an exit site where the catheter enters the skin, whereas the totally implanted vascular devices have a subcutaneous tract; all three types have a Dacron cuff that promotes fibrosis, thereby limiting the trafficking of potential pathogens, and an insert site into the major vessel. Thus, infection can occur at the exit site, along the catheter tunnel, or at the catheter vessel insertion site. Totally implanted catheters (e.g., port-A-Cath) have the lowest rates of bacteremia (0 to 0.04 per 100 catheter days), followed by long-term Hickman or Broviac catheters (0.14 per 100 catheter days).[101] Infection at the vessel insertion site can lead to bacteremia or septic thrombophlebitis, with further complications caused by metastatic spread.[193]

Infectious complications involving central venous catheters have a variable reported frequency of 2.7 to 47 percent.[19,76,93,141,157,229,250] Coagulase-negative staphylococci are the pathogen in approximately half these cases. This variability depends on the definition of a CRI, the type of catheter used, and the presence of hyperalimentation fluid and lipid in the infusion.[146,221,223] The use of a guide wire for catheter placement or of a multilumen catheter leads to higher infection rates.[225]

S. epidermidis is the species associated most often with central venous CRIs; it is identified in approximately 70 percent of coagulase-negative staphylococci central venous CRIs.[19,93] This prevalence is not unexpected because the organism is the predominant species colonizing the skin.[128] Other implicated coagulase-negative staphylococci species include *Staphylococcus haemolyticus*, *Staphylococcus warneri*, and *Staphylococcus hominis*.[93]

Differentiating between a true infection caused by *S. epidermidis* and a contaminated specimen is difficult. Establishing the diagnosis depends on the patient's clinical status and the isolation of identical isolate strains in repeated cultures. Proper therapy, possibly including removal of a catheter, requires accurate diagnosis.[194] Additionally, distinguishing central venous catheter–related bacteremia from bacteremia not associated with a central venous catheter is important. The use of quantitative blood cultures using the DuPont isolator system has shown that catheter-related bacteremias have a 5- to 10-fold difference in bacterial concentration in blood cultures drawn through the catheter compared with peripheral cultures.[66,196] Maki and associates[147] determined that catheter-related bacteremia can be confirmed after removal of the catheter by rolling the distal 5 to 7 cm of the catheter on a culture plate and finding more than 15 colony-forming units.

Therapy for coagulase-negative staphylococci infections involving central venous catheters should include removal of the catheter if the catheter no longer is necessary. Exit-site infections usually can be managed without removing the catheter.[194] Approximately one third of tunnel tract infections can be managed without removing the catheter, but the remaining patients have continued bacteremia or relapse of their bacteremia that requires removal of their catheters. Catheters should be removed immediately if the patient's clinical status deteriorates. Duration of therapy depends on whether the catheter has been removed and on the patient's underlying immune status.

Central Nervous System Shunts

Central nervous system (CNS) shunts divert or shunt CSF to relieve hydrocephalus.[121] Other prosthetic devices within the CNS have been used to monitor ventricular pressure or to administer chemotherapy.[53] Initial shunts diverted CSF into the right atrium; this technique is used infrequently because of its high complication rate.[169] Ventriculoperitoneal shunts that divert CSF into the peritoneal cavity have been used since the 1960s because of their lower rate of mechanical complications.[121,159,169] However, the incidences of infection involving both the ventriculoperitoneal and the ventriculoatrial shunts are comparable.[121,169,224] Infection rates are higher in neonates. Coagulase-negative staphylococci account for 60 to 75 percent of all bacterial causes of shunt infections.[121,162,224]

The pathogenesis of CSF shunt infections occurs primarily at the insertion site by contamination of the catheter from the patient's skin flora[224] or during subsequent revisions, with a short-term infection rate of 13 percent and a 10-year infection rate of 27 percent.[199] Seventy percent of ventriculoperitoneal shunt infections occur within 2 months of placement of the shunt.[162] The pathogenesis of this infection appears to be similar to that of CRI, described in the pathogenesis section.

The diagnosis of CNS shunt infections caused by coagulase-negative staphylococci may be difficult to make, owing to the differentiation between a true infection and a contaminating organism. The Gram stain of ventricular fluid often is negative, but culture is sensitive. Subtle changes are noted in CSF and ventricular fluid cell counts or cytochemical findings.[262] Patients with ventriculoatrial shunts often have signs and symptoms compatible with septicemia and the additional complications of glomerulonephritis secondary to immune complexes. In patients with ventriculoperitoneal shunts, because of the distal placement of the catheter into the peritoneum, an intra-abdominal cyst may develop at the distal end of the catheter. Dysfunctions of the shunt secondary to development of infections often lead to signs and symptoms consistent with increased intracranial pressure. Standard therapy for ventriculoperitoneal shunt infections has been removal of the shunt system and administration of systemic antibiotics.[224,262,264]

Peritoneal Dialysis Catheters

Infection remains the most common complication of peritoneal dialysis, and *S. epidermidis* is the bacterial pathogen most commonly isolated,[83,187] representing as many as 50 percent of infecting organisms.[187] The pathogenesis of infections involving the peritoneal dialysis catheter is similar to that of CRIs, with infections involving the exit site, infections along the subcutaneous catheter tunnel, and peritonitis.[187] The prevalence of peritonitis in patients undergoing continuous ambulatory peritoneal dialysis is approximately 60 percent. Signs of peritonitis include fever, abdominal pain, and cloudy peritoneal dialysis; fever is variable. Removal of the catheter usually is not necessary for successful therapy but may be required in refractory cases or when the catheter malfunctions. Antibiotics are administered in the dialysis fluid, and systemic antibiotics also can be used.[62]

Prosthetic Devices

Coagulase-negative staphylococci are the second most common cause of prosthetic valve endocarditis; these pathogens account for 17 percent of contemporary cases.[255] The in-hospital mortality rate from prosthetic valve endocarditis is reported to be 26 percent. Commonly, coagulase-negative staphylococcus prosthetic valve endocarditis occurs within 60 days of implanting the device and is defined as early prosthetic valve endocarditis. It can occur in the first year after surgery, probably caused by inoculation of the organism at the time of surgery, as noticed by the multiresistant phenotype analysis from the isolates in these patients.[26] The condition finally leads to an abscess of the mechanical valve ring. No sign or symptom is consistently diagnostic of prosthetic valve endocarditis, but fever is the most common finding. Classic endocarditis findings such as peripheral emboli and multiple positive blood cultures may be lacking in coagulase-negative staphylococci endocarditis. Anemia is the abnormality identified most commonly by laboratory tests. Obtaining blood cultures is imperative in diagnosing prosthetic valve endocarditis. Therapy should include institution of vancomycin and rifampin or an aminoglycoside, with surgical intervention as indicated.[13]

Other Indwelling Medical Devices

Coagulase-negative staphylococci are involved in an expanded spectrum of infections involving indwelling medical devices.[52,81] They include infections of prosthetic joints,[63,116] vascular grafts,[14,55] hemodialysis shunts,[174,216,217] and pacemaker pockets.[38,108,148,185] Additionally, osteomyelitis secondary to S. epidermidis has been reported to occur after hemodialysis and in neonates after the use of a monitoring scalp electrode.[170]

NATIVE-VALVE ENDOCARDITIS

Native-valve endocarditis, along with S. saprophyticus urinary tract infection, is the only non-nosocomial infection caused by coagulase-negative staphylococci.[110] Approximately 7 percent of cases of native-valve endocarditis are caused by coagulase-negative staphylococcus, and S. epidermidis is the most frequently isolated species.[42] These infections usually are subacute and arise from transient bacteremia. Pathogenesis is thought to involve seeding of a previously damaged valve or endocarditis that previously had not been identified.[6,17]

Staphylococcus lugdunensis can cause acute, severe, and destructive endocarditis similar to S. aureus endocarditis,[246] with most favorable outcomes occurring in patients who undergo valve replacement.[48] Most patients with S. lugdunensis endocarditis have been older than 50 years of age. Native aortic or mitral valves are involved most frequently.[245] The perineum appears to have a high colonization rate of S. lugdunensis.[112]

SURGICAL SITE INFECTIONS

Coagulase-negative staphylococci are the second most common cause of postoperative surgical site infections, according to National Nosocomial Infections Surveillance Report survey data.[37] Most infections probably are caused by the patient's own endogenous skin flora, but outbreaks originating from operating room personnel have been reported.[26] Outbreaks of S. epidermidis surgical site infections, such as mediastinitis and endocarditis, among patients who have undergone cardiac valve replacements also have been reported.[25,195]

URINARY TRACT INFECTIONS

S. saprophyticus is the most common coagulase-negative staphylococcus that causes infections in both the upper and the lower urinary tracts.[135] These infections occur predominantly in young, healthy, sexually active women,[113,135,150] during late summer and fall, with a pattern similar to that of sexually transmitted diseases.[71] Recent sexual intercourse, outdoor swimming, and

occupational meat processing have been identified as risk factors.[71] S. epidermidis and other coagulase-negative staphylococci rarely cause urinary tract infections, but they have been noted to produce disease in older adults with urinary tract complications.[86,139,163] McDonald and Lohr[152] and Hall and Snitzer[87] described healthy children with pyelonephritis caused by S. epidermidis.

MISCELLANEOUS

Endophthalmitis secondary to S. epidermidis has been reported in patients undergoing ocular surgery or trauma.[15,28,188] Postoperative mediastinitis that develops after median sternotomy for open heart surgery can be caused by S. epidermidis.[24,58,82] Primary osteomyelitis secondary to coagulase-negative staphylococci is a rare occurrence in healthy children.[171] Staphylococcus caprae[226] and S. lugdunensis[211] have been linked to bone and joint infections. Coagulase-negative staphylococci have been implicated as a possible cause of toxic shock syndrome.[45]

TREATMENT

The treatment of coagulase-negative staphylococcal infections[2] depends on the patient's immunologic status, the presence of an indwelling medical device, and the results of antimicrobial susceptibility testing. Infections are more difficult to treat when they are associated with a thrombosed vessel or an intra-atrial thrombus. When an intravascular catheter becomes infected, the presence of vegetation or a thrombus in the heart or great vessels always should be considered.

Many coagulase-negative staphylococci, particularly S. epidermidis and S. haemolyticus, are resistant to many antimicrobiotics.[7,9,39,49,61,78,218,231,256] Methicillin resistance, especially, is prevalent in nosocomial infections and occurs in most cases.[208,228] Methicillin-resistant coagulase-negative staphylococcus has a high degree of resistance to other antibiotics, such as clindamycin, erythromycin, and gentamicin.[7]

The mechanism of methicillin resistance in coagulase-negative staphylococci is similar to that of S. aureus because of the production of an additional non-native penicillin-binding protein (PBP), PBP2a, encoded by the mecA gene.[96,103] PBP2a does not allow the correct binding of β-lactams to the bacterial cell wall. Phenotypic methicillin resistance can be difficult to detect because of the heterogeneous expression of the mecA gene by many strains of staphylococci.[103] S. aureus breakpoints have been seen to fail to detect many coagulase-negative staphylococci that contained the mecA gene involved in staphylococcal resistance. As a consequence, the Clinical and Laboratory Standards Institute in 2007 recommended specific breakpoints for coagulase-negative staphylococci (Table 92-7).[43] In some species other than S. epidermidis, the differentiation between mecA-negative and mecA-positive strains may not be possible by susceptibility methods,[238] and isolates may falsely be designated as oxacillin resistant. Detecting the mecA gene is an accurate method to predict resistance to oxacillin.[103] Testing of coagulase-negative staphylococci using oxacillin screen plate no longer is recommended because of its failure to detect many resistant strains.[238]

Coagulase-negative staphylococci (S. haemolyticus and S. epidermidis) were the first organisms in which acquired glycopeptide resistance was recognized in 1986.[218] In addition, S. epidermidis, S. haemolyticus, and S. hominis are more likely to be multiresistant to antimicrobial agents than are other coagulase-negative staphylococcal species. A prolonged course of vancomycin is a well-recognized risk factor for the emergence of strains with decreased susceptibility to glycopeptides.[21,260] Although they are uncommon

TABLE 92–7 Breakpoints for Antibiotic Susceptibility for Coagulase-Negative Staphylococci

MICs	Oxacillin-Susceptible	Oxacillin-Resistant	
CoNS	≤0.25 μg/mL	≥0.5 μg/mL	
S. aureus	≤2 μg/mL	≥4 μg/mL	

Zone Size	Oxacillin-Susceptible	Oxacillin-Intermediate	Oxacillin-Resistant
CoNS	≥18 mm	No intermediate zone	≤17 mm
S. aureus	≥13 mm	11-12 mm	≤10 mm

CoNS, coagulase-negative staphylococci; MICs, minimal inhibitory concentrations.
Data from Clinical and Laboratory Standards Institute: Performance testing for antimicrobial susceptibility testing, 17th informational supplement M100-S17, 2007.

occurrences, infections caused by these strains have been described and may become more common. To prevent or delay development of resistance, the Centers for Disease Control and Prevention published recommendations for the prudent use of vancomycin.[36] Decreased susceptibility occurs more frequently to teicoplanin than to vancomycin. The minimal inhibitory concentrations of teicoplanin usually fall over a wide range, whereas vancomycin minimal inhibitory concentrations tend to remain more stable over a narrower range within the limits of susceptibility.[21] The peptidoglycan of these strains is highly cross-linked, containing additional serine in place of glycine, an alteration that may interfere with glycopeptide binding.[96]

The mechanism for vancomycin-intermediate resistance of S. aureus and coagulase-negative staphylococci is unknown. Vancomycin-intermediate S. aureus and vancomycin-intermediate, coagulase-negative staphylococcal strains have thickened cell walls, as shown by electron microscopy. Vancomycin resistance may be related to an increased ability of these organisms to bind vancomycin at sites other than those to which they normally bind.[96]

For the few isolates that are established to be penicillin susceptible and β-lactamase negative, penicillin is a suitable drug. For organisms that are resistant to penicillin but susceptible to semisynthetic penicillins, nafcillin and oxacillin are the most active antibiotics.[189,209] A degree of cross-resistance exists between the semisynthetic penicillin-resistant penicillins and cephalosporins.[208] Thus, routine susceptibility testing can indicate that a strain is susceptible to a cephalosporin when, in fact, it is resistant.[83,136] Methicillin resistance means resistance to all β-lactam antibiotics.[109]

Vancomycin is the drug of choice for methicillin-resistant organisms and is recommended for treating severe infections.[3,124] Coagulase-negative staphylococci can exhibit heteroresistance, defined as a culture population comprising two subpopulations, one susceptible to methicillin and the other resistant.[208,260] Enhanced detection of this admixture of organisms can be obtained by change in the culture conditions.[153] If these strains are incubated overnight on plates of increasing concentrations of methicillin or vancomycin, a small fraction of the total population will be able to grow at much higher antibiotic concentrations. If these highly resistant subclones are recultured, they may maintain this high level of resistance, a finding suggesting a mutant strain. However, in some cases, the highly resistant subclone will revert to methicillin or vancomycin susceptibility when it is replated, even though it was grown from a single colony. No satisfactory model can explain the mechanism governing heterogeneous resistance. Strains of coagulase-negative staphylococci and S. aureus with heterogeneous resistance are stable in the absence of antibiotic selective pressure. These strains may con-

stitute 10 to 15 percent of any coagulase-negative staphylococci or S. aureus collection of isolates. In addition, to avoid overlooking these organisms, the clinical microbiology laboratory should attempt to optimize expression of resistance by culturing on salt-containing media at 30° C to 35° C.[207] The clinical significance of this heteroresistance in coagulase-negative staphylococci is unknown, but a study of S. aureus showed it did not affect outcome.[125]

The quinolones and teicoplanin have shown activity against coagulase-negative staphylococci and could be useful in therapy of highly selected multiresistant organisms.[140,221] Teicoplanin is significantly less active than is vancomycin against coagulase-negative staphylococci, in particular S. haemolyticus, and, to a lesser extent, S. epidermidis. Resistance to these agents also has been observed.[9,218,231,256]

Gentamicin and rifampin are active against coagulase-negative staphylococci, but rapid emergence of resistance has limited their use as single drugs.[39,151,209] These two antibiotics have been shown to be synergistic with vancomycin against methicillin-resistant, coagulase-negative staphylococci.[142] Additionally, rifampin has been used in neonates with persistent bacteremia to eradicate the organisms.[235] The association of vancomycin and rifampin is the mainstay of therapy for deep-seated, foreign body infections.

Excellent in vitro activity of quinupristin-dalfopristin, a streptogramin combination,[10] and linezolid, an oxazolidinone compound that inhibits bacterial growth through inhibition of protein synthesis,[206] has been shown against staphylococcal species tested, regardless of the resistance pattern, particularly resistance to methicillin. Linezolid is an option for vancomycin-intermediate susceptible isolates or for completing therapy with oral administration.[117] Daptomycin is a lipopeptide antibiotic with excellent in vitro activity against coagulase-negative staphylococci.[210]

PREVENTION

Preventing the development of coagulase-negative staphylococci infection is difficult because of these organisms' ubiquitous nature as predominant skin commensals. A 3-year analysis by molecular typing of coagulase-negative staphylococci nosocomial infections in a neonatal intensive care unit showed that many of the infections were caused by clonal dissemination and, thus, potentially were preventable by handwashing, thus reducing the transmission rate from staff to patient or from patient to patient.[249] Additionally, proper surgical techniques help to minimize these infections associated with installation of indwelling medical devices.

The effort toward developing catheters that are both inert and resistant to bacterial colonization adherence has increased; however, these attempts have been only marginally successful.[123,177,184] Catheters with antibiotics or disinfectants impregnated in their surfaces appear promising.[237] Prophylactic antibiotics are administered routinely for surgical procedures involving placement of a prosthetic device or material. However, the most appropriate agent to prevent infections caused by coagulase-negative staphylococci varies among institutions.[3] Vancomycin often is recommended for CSF shunt or prosthetic valve placement. Polyclonal antibody (intravenous gamma-globulin) and polyclonal antibody enriched for antibody to clumping factor A have not been found to be efficacious for preventing coagulase-negative staphylococcal infections in neonates.[22]

In reference to infection control policies, standard precautions should be used for methicillin-resistant, coagulase-negative staphylococci. For vancomycin-intermediate, coagulase-negative staphylococci, contact transmission precautions for multidrug-resistant organisms should be used.[4]

CONCLUSION

Coagulase-negative staphylococci, particularly *S. epidermidis*, are a major source of nosocomial infection in a variety of clinical situations. Most infections occur in patients who are immunosuppressed or have an indwelling medical device. Epidemiologic studies are difficult to perform because of the organisms' commensal existence, but newer molecular tools will help investigators to gain insight with regard to the epidemiology of these infections. The pathogenesis of coagulase-negative staphylococci infection is being defined in the context of a CRI. Therapy can be complex because of the usual presence of an indwelling medical device and the multiple antimicrobial resistance of the organisms.

REFERENCES

1. Aasen, J., and Oeding, P.: Antigenic studies on *Staphylococcus epidermidis*. Acta Pathol. Microbiol. Scand. 79:827-834, 1972.
2. Aledo, A., Hellr, G., Ren, L., et al.: Septicemia and septic shock in pediatric patients: 140 Consecutive cases on a pediatric hematology-oncology service. J. Pediatr. Hematol. Oncol. 20:215-221, 1998.
3. American Academy of Pediatrics: Antimicrobial prophylaxis. *In* Pickering, L. K., Baker, C. J., Long, S. S., McMillan, J. A. (eds.): Red Book: 2006 Report of the Committee on Infectious Diseases. 27th ed. Elk Grove Village, IL: American Academy of Pediatrics, 2006, pp. 829-836.
4. American Academy of Pediatrics: Staphylococcal infections. *In* Pickering, L. K. (ed.): 2006 Red Book: Report of the Committee on Infectious Diseases. 25th ed. Elk Grove Village, IL, American Academy of Pediatrics, 2006, pp. 602-603.
5. Ammendiola, M. G., Di Rosa, R., and Montanaro, L.: Slime production and expression of the slime-associated antigen by staphylococcal clinical isolates. J. Clin. Microbiol. 37:3235-3238, 1999.
6. Archer, G. L.: *Staphylococcus epidermidis* and other coagulase-negative staphylococci. *In* Mandell, G. L., Bennett. J. E., and Dolin, R. (eds.): Principles and Practice of Infectious Diseases. 5th ed. New York, Churchill Livingstone, 2000, pp. 2092-2100.
7. Archer, G. L., and Climo, M. W.: Antimicrobial susceptibility of coagulase-negative staphylococci. Antimicrob. Agents Chemother. 38:2231-2237, 1994.
8. Archer, G. L., Karchmer, A. W., Vishniavsky, N., et al.: Plasmid-pattern analysis for the differentiation of infecting from noninfecting *Staphylococcus epidermidis*. J. Infect. Dis. 149:913-920, 1984.
9. Arioli, V., and Pallanza, R.: Teicoplanin-resistant coagulase-negative staphylococci. Lancet 1:39, 1987.
10. Auckenthaler, R., Courvalin, P., Feer, C., et al.: In vitro activity of quinupristin/dalfopristin in comparison with five antibiotics against worldwide clinical isolates of staphylococci. Clin. Microbiol. Infect. 6:608-612, 2000.
11. Auletta, J., Riordan, M. A., and Nieder, M. L.: Infections in children with cancer: A continued need for the comprehensive physical examination. J. Pediatr. Hematol. Oncol. 21:501-508, 1999.
12. Baddour, L. M., Smalley, D. L., Kraus, A. P., Jr., et al.: Comparison of microbiologic characteristics of pathogenic and saprophytic coagulase-negative staphylococci from patients on continuous ambulatory peritoneal dialysis. Diagn. Microbiol. Infect. Dis. 5:197-205, 1986.
13. Baddour, L. M., Wilson, W. R., Bayer, A. S., et al.: Infective endocarditis: Diagnosis, antimicrobial therapy, and management of complications: a statement for healthcare professionals from the Committee on Rheumatic fever, Endocarditis, and Kawasaki Disease, Council on Cardiovascular Disease in the Young, and the Councils on Clinical Cardiology, Stroke, and Cardiovascular Surgery and Anesthesia, American Heart Association. Circulation 111:394-434, 2005.
14. Bandyk, D. F., Berni, G. A., Thiele, B. L., et al.: Aortofemoral graft infection due to *Staphylococcus epidermidis*. Arch. Surg. 119:102-108, 1984.
15. Baum, J. L.: Current concepts in ophthalmology: Ocular infections. N. Engl. J. Med. 299:28-31, 1978.
16. Baumgart, S., Hall, S. E., Campos, J. M., et al.: Sepsis with coagulase-negative staphylococci in critically ill newborns. Am. J. Dis. Child. 137:461-463, 1983.
17. Belik, J., Finn, G., Rivera, G., et al.: Successful management of bacterial endocarditis of the mitral valve due to *Staphylococcus epidermidis* in an immunocompromised host. Acta Paediatr. Scand. 69:731-734, 1980.
18. Bender, J. W., and Hughes, W. T.: Fatal *Staphylococcus epidermidis* sepsis following bone marrow transplantation. Johns Hopkins Med. J. 146:13-15, 1980.
19. Benezra, D., Kiehn, T. E., Gold, J. W., et al.: Prospective study of infections in indwelling central venous catheters using quantitative blood cultures. Am. J. Med. 85:495-498, 1988.
20. Bialkowska-Hobrzanska, H., Jaskor, D., and Hammerberg, O.: Evaluation of restriction endonuclease fingerprinting of chromosomal DNA and plasmid profile analysis for characterization of multiresistant coagulase-negative staphylococci in bacteremic neonates. J. Clin. Microbiol. 28:269-275, 1990.
21. Biavasco, F., Vignaroli, C., and Varaldo, P. E.: Glycopeptide resistance in coagulase-negative staphylococci. Eur. J. Clin. Microbiol. Infect. Dis. 19:403-417, 2000.
22. Bloom, B., Schelonka, R., Kueser, T., et al. Multicenter study to assess safety and efficacy of INH-A21, a donor-selected human staphylococcal immunoglobulin, for prevention of nosocomial infections in very low birth weight infants. Pediatr. Infect. Dis. J. 24:858-866, 2005.
23. Bogado, I., Limansky, A., Sutich, E., et al.: Molecular characterization of methicillin-resistant coagulase-negative staphylococci from a neonatal intensive care unit. Infect. Control Hosp. Epidemiol. 23:447-451, 2002.
24. Bor, D. H., Rose, R. M., and Modlin, J. F.: Mediastinitis after cardiovascular surgery. Rev. Infect. Dis. 5:885-896, 1983.
25. Bou, R., Peris, M., Perpinan, J., et al: A protracted outbreak of *Staphylococcus epidermidis* infections among patients undergoing valve replacement. Infect. Control Hosp. Epidemiol. 25:498-503, 2004.
26. Boyce, J. M., Potter-Bynoe, G., and Opal, S. M.: A common source outbreak of *Staphylococcus epidermidis* infections among patients undergoing cardiac surgery. J. Infect. Dis. 161:493-499, 1990.
27. Bradford, R., Abdul Manan, R., Daley, A. J., et al.: Coagulase-negative staphylococci in very-low-birth-weight infants: Inability of genetic markers to distinguish invasive strains from blood culture contaminants. Eur. J. Clin. Microbiol. Infect. Dis. 25:283-90, 2006.
28. Brinton, G. S., Topping, T. M., and Hyndiuk, R. A.: Posttraumatic endophthalmitis. Arch. Ophthalmol. 102:547-550, 1984.
29. Broviac, J. W., Cole, J. J., and Scribner, B. H.: A silicone rubber atrial catheter for prolonged parenteral alimentation. Surg. Gynecol. Obstet. 136:602-606, 1973.
30. Bruce, A. M., Lorber, J., Shedden, W. I. H., et al.: Persistent bacteremia following ventriculo-caval shunt operations for hydrocephalus in infants. Dev. Med. Child. Neurol. 5:461-470, 1963.
31. Buckner, C. D., Clift, R. A., Sanders, J. E., et al.: Protective environment for bone marrow transplant recipients: A prospective study. Ann. Intern. Med. 89:893-901, 1978.
32. Buetow, K. C., Klein, S. W., and Lane, R. B.: Septicemia in premature infants. Am. J. Dis. Child. 110:29-41, 1965.
33. Burnie, J. P., Lee, W., Matthews, R. C., et al.: Immunoblot fingerprinting of coagulase-negative staphylococci. J. Clin. Pathol. 41:103-110, 1988.
34. Bykowska, K., Ludwicka, A., and Wegrzynowicz, Z.: Anticoagulant properties of extracellular slime substance produced by *Staphylococcus epidermidis*. Thromb. Haemost. 54:853-856, 1985.
35. Cairo, M. S.: Neonatal neutrophil host defense: Prospects for immunologic enhancement during neonatal sepsis. Am. J. Dis. Child. 143:40-46, 1989.
36. Centers for Disease Control and Prevention, NNIS System: National Nosocomial Infections Surveillance (NNIS) report, data summary from October 1986-April 1997. Am. J. Infect. Control. 25:477-487, 1997.
37. Centers for Disease Control and Prevention, Hospital Infection Control Practices Advisory Committee (HICPAC): Recommendations for preventing the spread of vancomycin resistance. M. M. W. R. Morb. Mortal. Wkly. Rep. 44:1-13, 1995.
38. Choo, M. H., Holmes, D. R., Jr., Gersh, B. J., et al.: Permanent pacemaker infections: Characterization and management. Am. J. Cardiol. 48:559-564, 1981.
39. Christensen, G. D., Parisi, J. T., Bisno, A. L., et al.: Characterization of clinically significant strains of coagulase-negative staphylococci. J. Clin. Microbiol. 18:258-269, 1983.
40. Christensen, G. D., Simpson, W. A., Bisno, A. L., et al.: Adherence of slime-producing strains of *Staphylococcus epidermidis* to smooth surfaces. Infect. Immun. 37:318-326, 1982.
41. Christensen, G. D., Simpson, W. A., Bisno, A. L., et al.: Experimental foreign body infections in mice challenged with slime-producing *Staphylococcus epidermidis*. Infect. Immun. 40:407-410, 1983.
42. Chu, V., Cabell, C., Abrutyn, E., et al.: Native valve endocarditis due to coagulase-negative staphylococci: Report of 99 episodes from the International Collaboration on Endocarditis Merged Database. Clin Infect Dis. 39:1527-1530, 2004.
43. Clinical and Laboratory Standards Institute: Performance testing for antimicrobial susceptibility testing, 17th informational supplement. M100-S17, 2007.
44. Clink, J., and Pennington, T. H.: Staphylococcal whole-cell polypeptide analysis: Evaluation as a taxonomic and typing tool. J. Med. Microbiol. 23:41-44, 1987.
45. Crass, B. A., and Bergdoll, M. S.: Involvement of coagulase-negative staphylococci in toxic shock syndrome. J. Clin. Microbiol. 23:43-45, 1986.
46. D'Angio, C. T., McGowan, K. L., and Baumgart, S.: Surface colonization with coagulase-negative staphylococci in premature neonates. J. Pediatr. 114:1029-1034, 1989.
47. Davenport, D. S., Massanari, R. M., Pfaller, M. A., et al.: Usefulness of a test for slime production as a marker for clinically significant infections with coagulase-negative staphylococci. J. Infect. Dis. 153:332-339, 1986.
48. De Hondt, G., Ieven, M., and Vandermersch, C.: Destructive endocarditis caused by *Staphylococcus lugdunensis*: Case report and review of the literature. Acta Clin. Belg. 52:27-30, 1997.
49. Del Bene, V. E., John, J. F., Jr., Twitty, J. A., et al.: Antistaphylococcal activity of teicoplanin, vancomycin, and other antimicrobial agents: The significance of methicillin resistance. J. Infect. Dis. 154:349-352, 1986.

50. de Saxe, M. J., Crees-Morris, J. A., Marples, R. R., et al.: Evaluation of current phage-typing systems for coagulase-negative staphylococci. *In* Jeljaszewicz, J. (ed.): Staphylococci and Staphylococcal Infections. Stuttgart, Gustave Fischer Verlag, 1981, pp. 197-204.

51. de Silva, G. D., Kantzanou, M., Justice, A., et al.: The ica operon and biofilm production in coagulase-negative staphylococci associated with carriage and disease in a neonatal intensive care unit. J. Clin. Microbiol. *40*:382-388, 2002.

52. Dickinson, G. M., and Bisno, A. L.: Infections associated with indwelling devices: Concepts of pathogenesis. Infections associated with intravascular devices. Antimicrob. Agents Chemother. *33*:597-601, 1989.

53. Dickinson, G. M., and Bisno, A. L.: Infections associated with indwelling devices: Infections related to extravascular devices. Antimicrob. Agents Chemother. *33*:602-607, 1989.

54. Donowitz, L. C., Haley, C. E., Gregory, W. W., et al.: Neonatal intensive care unit bacteremia: Emergence of gram-positive bacteria as major pathogens. Am. J. Infect. Control *15*:141-147, 1987.

55. Dougherty, S. H., and Simmons, R. L.: Infections in bionic man: The pathobiology of infections in prosthetic devices. Parts I and II. Curr. Probl. Surg. *19*:217-319, 1982.

56. Drewry, D. T., Galbraith, L., Wilkinson, B. J., et al.: Staphylococcal slime: A cautionary tale. J. Clin. Microbiol. *28*:1292-1296, 1990.

57. Dryden, M. S., Talsania, H. G., Martin, S., et al.: Evaluation of methods for typing coagulase-negative staphylococci. J. Med. Microbiol. *37*:109-117, 1992.

58. Edwards, M. S., and Baker, C. J.: Median sternotomy wound infections in children. Pediatr. Infect. Dis. J. *2*:105-109, 1987.

59. Etienne, J., Brun, Y., and El Solh, N., et al.: Characterization of clinically significant isolates of *Staphylococcus epidermidis* from patients with endocarditis. J. Clin. Microbiol. *26*:613-617, 1988.

60. Farber, B. F., Kaplan, M. H., and Clogston, A. G.: *Staphylococcus epidermidis* extracted slime inhibits the antimicrobial action of glycopeptide antibiotics. J. Infect. Dis. *161*:27-40, 1990.

61. Fass, R. J., Helsel, V. L., Barnishan, J., et al.: In vitro susceptibilities of four species of coagulase-negative staphylococci. Antimicrob. Agents Chemother. *30*:545-552, 1986.

62. Fine, R. N., Salusky, I. B., Hall, T., et al.: Peritonitis in children undergoing continuous ambulatory peritoneal dialysis. Pediatrics *71*:806-809, 1983.

63. Fitzgerald, R. H., Jr., Nolan, D. R., Ilstrup, D. M., et al.: Deep wound sepsis following total hip arthroplasty. J. Bone Joint Surg. *59*:847-855, 1977.

64. Fleer, A., Gerards, L. J., Aerts, P., et al.: Opsonic defense to *Staphylococcus epidermidis* in the premature neonate. J. Infect. Dis. *152*:930-937, 1985.

65. Fleer, A., Senders, R. C., Visser, M. R., et al.: Septicemia due to coagulase-negative staphylococci in a neonatal intensive care unit: Clinical and bacteriological features and contaminated parenteral fluids as a source of sepsis. Pediatr. Infect. Dis. J. *2*:426-431, 1983.

66. Flynn, P. M., Shenep, J. L., Stokes, D. C., et al.: In situ management of confirmed central venous catheter-related bacteremia. Pediatr. Infect. Dis. J. *6*:729-734, 1987.

67. Frebourg, N. B., Lefebvre, S., Baert, S., and Lemeland, J. F.: PCR-based assay for discrimination between invasive and contaminating *Staphylococcus epidermidis* strains. J. Clin. Microbiol. *38*:877-880, 2000.

68. Freeman, R., Goodfellow, M., Ward, A. C., et al.: Epidemiological typing of coagulase-negative staphylococci by pyrolysis mass spectrometry. J. Med. Microbiol. *34*:245-248, 1991.

69. Friedman, L. E., Brown, A. E., Miller, D. R., et al.: *Staphylococcus epidermidis* septicemia in children with leukemia and lymphoma. Am. J. Dis. Child. *138*:715-719, 1984.

70. Galdbart, J. O., Allignet, J., Tung, H. S., et al.: Screening for *Staphylococcus epidermidis* markers discriminating between skin-flora strains and those responsible for infections of joint prostheses. J Infect Dis. *182*:351-355, 2000.

71. Gatermann, S., Crossley, K. B.: Urinary tract infections. *In* Crossley, K. B., and Archer, G. L. (eds.): The Staphylococci in Human Disease. New York, Churchill Livingstone, 1997, pp. 493-508.

72. Gatermann, S., John, J., and Marre, R.: *Staphylococcus saprophyticus* urease: Characterization and contribution to uropathogenicity in unobstructed urinary tract infections of rats. Infect. Immun. *57*:110-116, 1989.

73. Gatermann, S., Kreft, B., Marre, R., et al.: Identification and characterization of a surface-protein (Ssp) of *Staphylococcus saprophyticus*. Infect. Immun. *60*:1055-1060, 1992.

74. Gatermann, S., Meyer, H. G., and Wanner, G.: *Staphylococcus saprophyticus* hemagglutinin is a 160-kilodalton surface protein. Infect. Immun. *65*:4127-4132, 1992.

75. Goering, R. V., and Winters, M. A.: Rapid method for epidemiologic evaluation of gram-positive cocci by field inversion gel electrophoresis. J. Clin. Microbiol. *30*:577-580, 1992.

76. Goldman, D. A., and Pier, G. B.: Pathogenesis of infections relapsed to intravascular catheterization. Clin. Microbiol. Rev. *6*:176-192, 1993.

77. Gordon, D. L., Rice, J. L., and Avery, V. M.: Surface phagocytosis and host defense in the peritoneal cavity during continuous ambulatory peritoneal dialysis. Eur. J. Clin. Microbiol. Infect. Dis. *9*:191-197, 1990.

78. Graninger, W., Wenish, C., and Hasenhandl, M.: Treatment of staphylococcal infections. Curr. Opin. Infect. Dis. *8* (Suppl. 1):520-528, 1995.

79. Gray, E. D., Peters, G., Verstegen, M., et al.: Effect of extracellular slime substance from *Staphylococcus epidermidis* on the human cellular immune response. Lancet *1*:365-367, 1984.

80. Gray, J. E., Richardson, D. K., McCormick, M. C., et al.: Coagulase-negative staphylococcal bacteremia among very low birth weight infants: Relation to admission illness severity, resource use, and outcome. Pediatrics *95*:225-230, 1995.

81. Gristina, A. G.: Biomaterial-centered infection: Microbial adhesion versus tissue integration. Science *237*:1588-1595, 1987.

82. Grossi, E. A., Culliford, A. T., and Krieger, K. H., et al.: A survey of 77 major infectious complications of median sternotomy: A review of 7,949 consecutive operative procedures. Ann. Thorac. Surg. *40*:214-223, 1985.

83. Gruer, L. D., Bartlett, R., and Ayliffe, G. A. J.: Species identification and antibiotic sensitivity of coagulase-negative staphylococci from CAPD peritonitis. J. Antimicrob. Chemother. *13*:577-583, 1984.

84. Gruskay, J. A., Abbasi, S., Anday, E., et al.: *Staphylococcus epidermidis*–associated enterocolitis. J. Pediatr. *109*:520-524, 1986.

85. Gruskay, J., Harris, M. C., Costarino, A. T., et al.: Neonatal *Staphylococcus epidermidis* meningitis with unremarkable CSF examination results. Am. J. Dis. Child. *143*:580-582, 1989.

86. Gunn, B. A., and Davis, C. E., Jr.: *Staphylococcus haemolyticus* urinary tract infection in a male patient. J. Clin. Microbiol. *26*:1055-1057, 1988.

87. Hall, D. E., and Snitzer, J. A., III: *Staphylococcus epidermidis* as a cause of urinary tract infections in children. J. Pediatr. *124*:437-438, 1994.

88. Hall, R. T., Hall, S. L., Barnes, W. G., et al.: Characteristics of coagulase-negative staphylococci from infants with bacteremia. Pediatr. Infect. Dis. J. *6*:377-383, 1987.

89. Hall, S. L., Hall, R. T., Barnes, W. G., et al.: Relationship of maternal to neonatal colonization with coagulase-negative staphylococci. Am. J. Perinatol. *7*:384-388, 1990.

90. Hall, S. L., Riddell, S. W., Barnes, W. G., et al.: Evaluation of coagulase-negative staphylococcal isolates from serial nasopharyngeal cultures of premature infants. Diagn. Microbiol. Infect. Dis. *13*:17-23, 1990.

91. Hamilton-Miller, J. M. T., and Iliffe, A.: Antimicrobial resistance in coagulase negative staphylococci. J. Med. Microbiol. *19*:217-226, 1985.

92. Hamory, B. H., Parisi, J. T., and Hutton, J. P.: *Staphylococcus epidermidis*: A significant nosocomial pathogen. Am. J. Infect. Control *15*:59-74, 1987.

93. Haslett, T. M., Isenberg, H. D., Hilton, E., et al.: Microbiology of indwelling central intravascular catheters. J. Clin. Microbiol. *26*:696-701, 1988.

94. Hebert, G. A., Cooksey, R. C., Clark, N. C., et al.: Biotyping coagulase-negative staphylococci. J. Clin. Microbiol. *26*:1950-1956, 1988.

95. Heidrich, C., Hantke, K., Bierbaum, G., et al.: Identification and analysis of a gene encoding a Fur-like protein of *Staphylococcus epidermidis*. F. E. M. S. Microbiol. Lett. *140*:253-259, 1996.

96. Heilmann, C., and Peters, G.: Biology and pathogenesis of *Staphylococcus epidermidis*. *In* Fischetti, V. A., Novick, R. P., Ferretti, J. J., et al. (eds.): Gram-Positive Pathogens. Washington, D.C., ASM Press, 2000, pp. 442-449.

97. Heilmann, C., Schweitzer, O., Gerke, C., et al: Molecular basis of intercellular adhesion in the biofilm-forming *Staphylococcus epidermidis*. Mol. Microbiol. *20*:1083-91, 1996.

98. Heilmann, C., Thumm, G., Chhatwal, G. S., et al.: Identification and characterization of a novel autolysin (Aae) with adhesive properties from *Staphylococcus epidermidis*. Microbiology *149*:2769-78, 2003.

99. Hickman, R. O., Buckner, C. D., Clift, R. A., et al.: A modified right atrial catheter for access to the venous system in marrow transplant recipients. Surg. Gynecol. Obstet. *148*:871-875, 1979.

100. Hogt, A. H., Dankert, J., Hulstaert, C. E., et al.: Cell surface characteristics of coagulase-negative staphylococci and their adherence to fluorinated poly (ethyleneprophylene). Infect. Immun. *51*:294-301, 1986.

101. Huebner, J., and Goldman, D. A.: Coagulase negative staphylococci: Role as pathogens. Annu. Rev. Med. *50*:223-236, 2000.

102. Hussain, M., Heilmann, C., Peters, G., and Herrmann, M.: Teichoic acid enhances adhesion of *Staphylococcus epidermidis* to immobilized fibronectin. Microb. Pathog. *31*:261-70, 2001.

103. Hussain, Z., Stoakes, L., Garrow, S., et al.: Rapid detection of *mecA*- positive and *mecA*-negative coagulase-negative staphylococci by an anti-penicillin binding protein 2a slide latex agglutination test. J. Clin. Microbiol. *38*:2051-2054, 2000.

104. Iannacci, L., and Piomelli, S.: Supportive care for children with cancer: Guidelines of the Children's Cancer Study Group: Use of venous access lines. Am. J. Pediatr. Hematol. Oncol. *6*:277-281, 1984.

105. Ichiman, Y.: Applications of fluorescent antibody for detecting capsular substance in *Staphylococcus epidermidis*. J. Appl. Bacteriol. *56*:311-316, 1984.

106. Ichiman, Y., and Yoshida, K.: The relationship of capsular-type of *Staphylococcus epidermidis* to virulence and induction of resistance in the mouse. J. Appl. Bacteriol. *51*:229-241, 1981.

107. Izard, N. C., Hachler, H., Grehn, M., et al.: Ribotyping of coagulase-negative staphylococci with special emphasis on intraspecific typing of *Staphylococcus epidermidis*. J. Clin. Microbiol. *30*:817-823, 1992.

108. Jara, F. M., Toledo-Pereyra, L., Lewis, J. W., Jr., et al.: The infected pacemaker pocket. J. Thorac. Cardiovasc. Surg. *78*:298-300, 1979.

109. John, J. F., and McNeill, W. F.: Activity of cephalosporins against methicillin-susceptible and methicillin-resistant, coagulase-negative staphylococci: Minimal effect of beta-lactamases. Antimicrob. Agents Chemother. *17*:179-183, 1980.

110. Johnson, C. M., and Rhodes, K. H.: Pediatric endocarditis. Mayo Clin. Proc. 57:86-94, 1982.

111. Johnson, G. M., Lee, D. A., Regelmann, W. E., et al.: Interference with granulocyte function by *Staphylococcus epidermidis* slime. Infect. Immun. 54:13-20, 1986.

112. Jones, R.M., Jackson, M.A., Ong, C., and Lofland, G.K.: Endocarditis caused by *Staphylococcus lugdunensis*. Pediatr. Infect. Dis. J. 21:265-8,2002.

113. Jordan, P. A., Iravani, A., Richard, G. A., et al.: Urinary tract infection caused by *Staphylococcus saprophyticus*. J. Infect. Dis. 142:510-515, 1980.

114. Kacica, M. A., Horgan, M. J., Preston, K. E., et al.: Relatedness of coagulase-negative staphylococci causing bacteremia in low-birthweight infants. Infect. Control Hosp. Epidemiol. 15:658-662, 1994.

115. Kallman, J., Kihlstrom, E., and Schollin, J.: Increase of staphylococci in neonatal septicaemia: A fourteen-year study. Acta Paediatr. 86:533-538, 1997.

116. Kamme, C., and Lindberg, L.: Aerobic and anaerobic bacteria in deep infections after total hip arthroplasty: Differential diagnosis between infectious and non-infectious loosening. Clin. Orthop. 154:201-207, 1981.

117. Kaplan, S. L., Deville J. G., Yogev, R., et al. Linezolid versus vancomycin for treatment of resistant Gram-positive infections in children. Pediatr. Infect. Dis. J. 22:677-685, 2003.

118. Karlowicz, M., Buescher, S., and Surka, A.: Fulminant late-onset sepsis in a neonatal intensive care unit, 1988-1997, and the impact of avoiding empirical vancomycin therapy. Pediatrics 106:1387-1390, 2000.

119. Karp, J. E., Dick, J. D., Angelopulos, C., et al.: Empiric use of vancomycin during prolonged treatment-induced granulocytopenia: Randomized, double-blind, placebo-controlled clinical trial in patients with acute leukemia. Am. J. Med. 81:237-242, 1986.

120. Keane, W. F., Comty, C. M., Verbrugh, H. A., et al.: Opsonic deficiency of peritoneal dialysis effluent in continuous ambulatory peritoneal dialysis. Kidney Int. 25:539-543, 1984.

121. Keucher, T. R., and Mealey, J., Jr.: Long-term results after ventriculoatrial and ventriculoperitoneal shunting for infantile hydrocephalus. J. Neurosurg. 50:79-186, 1979.

122. Khashu, M., Osiovich, H., Henry, D. et al.: Persistent bacteremia and severe thrombocytopenia caused by coagulase-negative staphylococcus in a neonatal intensive care unit. Pediatrics 117:340-348, 2000.

123. Kingston, D., Seal, D., and Hill, I. D.: Self-disinfecting plastics for intravenous catheters and prosthetic inserts. J. Hyg. 96:185-198, 1986.

124. Kirby, W. M.: Vancomycin therapy in severe staphylococcal infections. Rev. Infect. Dis. 3(Suppl.):236-239, 1981.

125. Kline, M. W., Mason, E. O., Jr., and Kaplan, S. L.: Outcome of heteroresistant *Staphylococcus aureus* infections in children. J. Infect. Dis. 156:205-208, 1987.

126. Kloos, W. E., and Bannerman, T. L.: Update of clinical significance of coagulase-negative staphylococci. Clin. Microbiol. Rev. 7:117-140, 1994.

127. Kloos, W. E., and Bannerman, T. L.: *Staphylococcus* and *Micrococcus*. In Murray, P. R., Baron, E. J., Pfaller, A., et al. (eds.): Manual of Clinical Microbiology, 7th ed. Washington, D. C., American Society for Microbiology, 1999, pp. 264-282.

128. Kloos, W. E., and Musselwhite, M. S.: Distribution and persistence of *Staphylococcus* and *Micrococcus* species and other aerobic bacteria on human skin. Appl. Microbiol. 30:381-385, 1975.

129. Kloos, W. E., Ballard, D. N., George, C. G., et al.: Delimiting the genus *Staphylococcus* through description of *Micrococcus caseolyticus* gen. nov., comb. nov. and the new species *Macrococcus equipercicus* sp. nov., *Macrococcus bovicus* sp. nov., and *Macrococcus carouselicus* sp. nov. Int. J. Syst. Bacteriol. 48:859-877, 1998.

130. Kozitskaya, S., Olson, M. E., Fey, P. D., et al.: Clonal analysis of *Staphylococcus epidermidis* isolates carrying or lacking biofilm-mediating genes by multilocus sequence typing. J. Clin. Microbiol. 43:4751-7, 2005.

131. Kristinsson, K. G., Hastings, J. G., and Spencer, R. C.: The role of extracellular slime in opsonophagocytosis of *Staphylococcus epidermidis*. J. Med. Microbiol. 27:207-213, 1988.

132. Kuroda, M., Yamashita, A., Hirakawa, H., et al.: Whole genome sequence of *Staphylococcus saprophyticus* reveals the pathogenesis of uncomplicated urinary tract infection. Proc. Natl. Acad. Sci. U. S. A. 102:13272-13277, 2005.

133. Langley, J., and Gold, R.: Sepsis in febrile neutropenic children with cancer. Pediatr. Infect. Dis. J. 7:34-37, 1988.

134. Lark, R. L., VanderHyde, K., Deeb, G. M., et al.: An outbreak of coagulase-negative staphylococcal surgical-site infections following aortic valve replacement. Infect. Control Hosp. Epidemiol. 22:618-623, 2001.

135. Latham, R. H., Running, K., and Stamm, W. E.: Urinary tract infections in young adult women caused by *Staphylococcus saprophyticus*. JAMA 250:3063-3066, 1983.

136. Laverdiere, M., Peterson, P. K., and Verhoef, J.: In vitro activity of cephalosporins against methicillin-resistant coagulase-negative staphylococci. J. Infect. Dis. 137:245-250, 1978.

137. Levison, M. E., and Bush, L. M.: Peritonitis and other intra-abdominal infections. In Mandell, G. L., Bennett, J. E., and Dolin. R. (eds.): Principles and Practice of Infectious Diseases. New York, Churchill Livingstone, 2000, pp. 821-856.

138. Lew, D. P.: Physiopathology of foreign body infections. Eur. J. Cancer Clin. Oncol. 25:1379-1382, 1989.

139. Lewis, J. F., Brake, S. R., Anderson, D. J., et al.: Urinary tract infection due to coagulase-negative *Staphylococcus*. Am. J. Clin. Pathol. 77:736-739, 1982.

140. Low, D. E., McGeer, A., and Poon, R.: Activities of daptomycin and teicoplanin against *Staphylococcus haemolyticus* and *Staphylococcus epidermidis*, including evaluation of susceptibility testing recommendation. Antimicrob. Agents Chemother. 33:585-588, 1989.

141. Lowder, J. N., Lazarus, H. M., and Herzig, R. H.: Bacteremias and fungemias in oncologic patients with central venous catheters: Changing spectrum of infection. Arch. Intern. Med. 142:1456-1459, 1982.

142. Lowy, F. D., Chang, D. S., and Lash, P. R.: Synergy of combinations of vancomycin, gentamicin, and rifampin against methicillin-resistant, coagulase-negative staphylococci. Antimicrob. Agents Chemother. 23:932-934, 1983.

143. Lowy, F. D., Walsh, J. A., and Mayers, M. M.: Antibiotic activity in-vitro against methicillin-resistant *Staphylococcus epidermidis* and therapy of an experimental infection. Antimicrob. Agents Chemother. 16:314-321, 1979.

144. Mack, D., Davies, A. P., Harris, L. G., et al.: Microbial interactions in *Staphylococcus epidermidis* biofilms. Anal. Bioanal. Chem. 387:399-408, 2007.

145. Mack, D., Siemssen, N., and Laufs, R.: Parallel induction by glucose of adherence and a polysaccharide antigen specific for plastic-adherent *Staphylococcus epidermidis*: Evidence for functional relation to intracellular adhesion. Infect. Immun. 60:2048-2057, 1992.

146. Maki, D., Goldman, D., and Rhame, F. S.: Infection control in intravenous therapy. Ann. Intern. Med. 79:867-887, 1973.

147. Maki, D., Weise, C. E., and Safarin, H. W.: A semi-quantitative culture method for identifying intravenous-catheter-related infection. N. Engl. J. Med. 296:1305-1309, 1977.

148. Mansour, K. A., Kauten, J. R., and Hatcher, C. R., Jr.: Management of the infected pacemaker: Explanation, sterilization, and reimplantation. Ann. Thorac. Surg. 40:617-619, 1985.

149. Marples, R. R.: Laboratory assessment in the epidemiology of infections caused by coagulase-negative staphylococci. J. Med. Microbiol. 22:285-287, 1986.

150. Marrie, T. J., Kwan, C., and Noble, A.: *Staphylococcus saprophyticus* as a cause of urinary tract infections. J. Clin. Microbiol. 16:427-431, 1982.

151. Marsik, F. J., and Brake, S.: Species identification and susceptibility to 17 antibiotics of coagulase-negative staphylococci isolated from clinical specimens. J. Clin. Microbiol. 15:640-645, 1982.

152. McDonald, J. A., and Lohr, J. A.: *Staphylococcus epidermidis* pyelonephritis in a previously healthy child. Pediatr. Infect. Dis. J. 13:1155-1156, 1994.

153. McDougal, L. K., and Thornsberry, C.: New recommendations for disk diffusion antimicrobial susceptibility tests for methicillin-resistant (hetero-resistant) staphylococci. J. Clin. Microbiol. 19:482-488, 1984.

154. Meyers, J. D.: Infection in bone marrow transplant recipients. Am. J. Med. 81(Suppl. 1A):27-38, 1986.

155. Mickelsen, P. A., Plorde, J. J., Gordon, K. P., et al.: Instability of antibiotic resistance in a strain of *Staphylococcus epidermidis* isolated from an outbreak of prosthetic valve endocarditis. J. Infect. Dis. 152:50-58, 1985.

156. Milisavljevic, V., Wu, F., Cimmotti, J., et al.: Genetic relatedness of *Staphylococcus epidermidis* from infected infants and staff in the neonatal intensive care unit. Am. J. Infect. Control. 33:341-347, 2005.

157. Mirro, J., Jr., Rao, B. N., Stokes, D. C., et al.: A prospective study of Hickman/Broviac catheters and implantable ports in pediatric oncology patients. J. Clin. Oncol. 7:214-222, 1989.

158. Munson, D. P., Thompson, T. R., Johnson, D. E., et al.: Coagulase-negative staphylococci septicemia: Experience in a newborn intensive care unit. J. Pediatr. 101:602-605, 1982.

159. Murtagh, F., and Lehman, R.: Peritoneal shunts in the management of hydrocephalus. J. A. M. A. 202:1010-1014, 1967.

160. Nafziger, D. A., and Wenzel, R. P.: Coagulase-negative staphylococci: Epidemiology, evaluation, and therapy. Infect. Dis. Clin. North Am. 3:915-928, 1989.

161. Nataro, J. P., Corcoran, L., Zirin, S., et al.: Prospective analysis of coagulase-negative staphylococcal infections in hospitalized infants. J. Pediatr. 125:798-804, 1994.

162. Nelson, J. D.: Cerebrospinal fluid shunt infections. Pediatr. Infect. Dis. J. 3(Suppl.):S30-S32, 1984.

163. Nicolle, L. E., Hoban, S. A., and Harding, G. K. M.: Characterization of coagulase-negative staphylococci from urinary tract infections. J. Clin. Microbiol. 17:267-271, 1983.

164. Noel, G. J., and Edelson, P. J.: *Staphylococcus epidermidis* bacteremia in neonates: Further observations and the occurrence of focal infection. Pediatrics 74:832-837, 1984.

165. Noel, G. J., O'Loughlin, J. E., and Edelson, P. J.: Neonatal *Staphylococcus epidermidis* right-sided endocarditis: Description of five catheterized infants. Pediatrics 82:234-239, 1988.

166. Nouwen, J. L., van Belkum, A., de Marie, S., et al.: Clonal expansion of *Staphylococcus epidermidis* strains causing Hickman catheter–related infections in a hemato-oncologic department. J. Clin. Microbiol. 36:2696-2702, 1998.

167. Oeding, P.: Genus *Staphylococci*. In Gergan, T., and Norris, J. R. (eds.): Methods in Microbiology. Vol. 12. New York, Academic Press, 1978, pp. 130-133.

168. Ohshima, Y., Schumacher-Perdreau, F., and Peters, G.: Antiphagocytic effect of the capsule of *Staphylococcus simulans*. Infect. Immun. 58:1350-1354, 1990.

169. Olsen, L., and Frykberg, T.: Complications in the treatment of hydrocephalus in children: A comparison of ventriculoatrial and ventriculoperitoneal shunts in a 20-year material. Acta Paediatr. Scand. 72:385-390, 1983.

170. Overturf, G. D., and Balfour, G.: Osteomyelitis and sepsis: Severe complications of fetal monitoring. Pediatrics 55:244-247, 1975.
171. Paley, D., Moseley, C. F., Armstrong, P., et al.: Primary osteomyelitis caused by coagulase-negative staphylococci. J. Pediatr. Orthop. 6:622-626, 1986.
172. Parisi, J. T.: Coagulase-negative staphylococci and the epidemiological typing of Staphylococcus epidermidis. Microbiol. Rev. 49:126-139, 1985.
173. Parisi, J. T., and Hecht, D. W.: Plasmid profiles in epidemiologic studies of infections by Staphylococcus epidermidis. J. Infect. Dis. 141:637-643, 1980.
174. Parker, M. A., and Tuazon, C. U.: Cervical osteomyelitis: Infection due to Staphylococcus epidermidis in hemodialysis patients. JAMA 240:50-51, 1978.
175. Parisi, J. T., Lampson, B. C., Hoover, D. L., et al.: Comparison of epidemiologic markers for Staphylococcus epidermidis. J. Clin. Microbiol. 24:56-60, 1986.
176. Parisi, J. T., Talbot, H. W., Jr., and Skahan, J. M.: Development of a phage typing set for Staphylococcus epidermidis in the United States. Zentralbl. Bakteriol. [A] 241:60-67, 1978.
177. Pascual, A., Fleer, A., Westerdaal, N. A. C., et al.: Modulation of adherence of coagulase-negative staphylococci to Teflon catheters in vitro. Eur. J. Clin. Microbiol. 5:518-522, 1986.
178. Patrick, C. C.: Coagulase-negative staphylococci: Pathogens with increasing clinical significance. J. Pediatr. 116:497-507, 1990.
179. Patrick, C. C., Kaplan, S. L., Baker, C. J., et al.: Persistent bacteremia due to coagulase-negative staphylococci in low birth weight neonates. Pediatrics 84:977-985, 1989.
180. Patrick, C. C., Plaunt, M. R., Sweet, S. M., et al.: Defining Staphylococcus epidermidis cell wall proteins. J. Clin. Microbiol. 28:2757-2760, 1990.
181. Patrick, C. H., John, J. F., Levkoff, A. H., et al.: Relatedness of strains of methicillin-resistant coagulase-negative Staphylococcus colonizing hospital personnel and producing bacteremias in a neonatal intensive care unit. Pediatr. Infect. Dis. J. 11:935-940, 1992.
182. Pereira, A. T.: Coagulase-negative strains of Staphylococcus possessing antigen 51 as agents of urinary tract infection. J. Clin. Pathol. 15:252-253, 1962.
183. Persson, L., Strid, H., Tidefelt, U., and Soderquist, B.: Phenotypic and genotypic characterization of coagulase-negative staphylococci isolated in blood cultures from patients with haematological malignancies. Eur. J. Clin. Microbiol. Infect. Dis. 25:299-309, 2006.
184. Peters, G., and Pulverer, G.: Pathogenesis and management of Staphylococcus epidermidis "plastic" foreign body infections. J. Antimicrob. Chemother. 14(Suppl. D):67-71, 1984.
185. Peters, G., Saborowski, F., Locci, R., et al.: Investigations on staphylococcal infection of transvenous endocardial pacemaker electrodes. Am. Heart J. 108:359-365, 1984.
186. Peters, G., von Eiff, C., and Herrmann, M.: The changing pattern of coagulase-negative staphylococci as infectious pathogens. Curr. Opin. Infect. Dis. 8(Suppl. 1):512-519, 1995.
187. Peterson, P. K., Matzke, G., and Keane, W. F.: Current concepts in the management of peritonitis in patients undergoing continuous ambulatory peritoneal dialysis. Rev. Infect. Dis. 9:604-612, 1987.
188. Peyman, G. A., Carroll, C. P., and Raichand, M.: Prevention and management of traumatic endophthalmitis. Ophthalmology 87:320-324, 1980.
189. Pfaller, M. A., and Herwaldt, L. A.: Laboratory, clinical, and epidemiological aspects of coagulase-negative staphylococci. Clin. Microbiol. Rev. 1:281-299, 1988.
190. Pizzo, P. A., Hathorn, J. W., Hiemenz, J., et al.: A randomized trial comparing ceftazidime alone with combination antibiotic therapy in cancer patients with fever and neutropenia. N. Engl. J. Med. 315:552-558, 1986.
191. Pizzo, P. A., Ladisch, S., Simon, R. M., et al.: Increasing incidence of gram-positive sepsis in cancer patients. Med. Pediatr. Oncol. 5:241-244, 1978.
192. Ponce De Leon, S., and Wenzel, R. P.: Hospital-acquired bloodstream infections with Staphylococcus epidermidis: Review of 100 cases. Am. J. Med. 77:639-644, 1984.
193. Power, J., Wing, E. J., Talamo, T. S., et al.: Fatal bacterial endocarditis as a complication of permanent indwelling catheters: Report of two cases. Am. J. Med. 81:166-168, 1986.
194. Press, O. W., Ramsey, P. G., Larson, E. B., et al.: Hickman catheter infections in patients with malignancies. Medicine (Baltimore) 63:189-200, 1984.
195. Raimundo, O., Heussler, H., Bruhn, J. B., et al.: Molecular epidemiology of coagulase-negative staphylococcal bacteraemia in a newborn intensive care unit. J. Hosp. Infect. 51:33-42, 2002.
196. Raucher, H. S., Hyatt, A. C., and Barzilai, A.: Quantitative blood cultures in the evaluation of septicemia in children with Broviac catheters. J. Pediatr. 104:29-33, 1984.
197. Richards, M. J., Edwards, J. R., Culver, D. H., et al.: Nosocomial infections in pediatric intensive care units in the United States. Pediatrics 103:e39, 1999.
198. Rohde, H., Kalitzky, M., Kroger N., et al.: Detection of virulence-associated genes not useful for discriminating between invasive and commensal Staphylococcus epidermidis strains from a bone marrow transplant unit. J. Clin. Microbiol. 42:5614-5619, 2004.
199. Roos, K. L., and Scheld, W. M.: Central nervous system infections. In Crossley, K. B., and Archer, G. L. (eds.): The Staphylococci in Human Disease. New York, Churchill Livingstone, 1997, pp. 413-440.
200. Ross, M. N., Haase, G. M., and Poole, M. A.: Comparison of totally implanted reservoirs with external catheters as venous access devices in pediatric oncologic patients. Surg. Gynecol. Obstet. 167:141, 1988.

201. Rotbart, H. A., Johnson, Z. T., and Reller, L. B.: Analysis of enteric coagulase-negative staphylococci from neonates with necrotizing enterocolitis. Pediatr. Infect. Dis. J. 8:140-142, 1989.
202. Rupp, M. E., and Archer, G.: Hemagglutination and adherence to plastic by Staphylococcus epidermidis. Infect. Immun. 60:1055-1060, 1992.
203. Rupp, M. E., and Archer, G. L.: Coagulase-negative staphylococci: Pathogens associated with medical progress. Clin. Infect. Dis. 19:231-245, 1994.
204. Rupp, M. E., Fey, P. D., Heilmann, C., and Gotz, F.: Characterization of the importance of Staphylococcus epidermidis autolysin and polysaccharide intercellular adhesin in the pathogenesis of intravascular catheter-associated infection in a rat model. J. Infect. Dis. 183:1038-1042, 2001.
205. Rupp, M. E., Ulphani, J. S., Fey, P. D., and Mack, D.: Characterization of Staphylococcus epidermidis polysaccharide intercellular adhesin/hemagglutinin in the pathogenesis of intravascular catheter-associated infection in a rat model. Infect. Immun. 67:2656-2659, 1999.
206. Ryback, M. J., Cappelletty, D. M., Moldovan, T., et al.: Comparative in vitro activities and postantibiotic effects of the oxazolidinone compounds eperezolid (PNU-100592) and linezolid (PNU-100766) versus vancomycin against Staphylococcus aureus, coagulase-negative staphylococci, Enterococcus faecalis, and Enterococcus faecium. Antimicrob. Agents Chemother. 42:712-724, 1998.
207. Sabath, L. D.: Chemical and physical factors influencing methicillin-resistance of Staphylococcus aureus and Staphylococcus epidermidis. J. Antimicrob. Chemother. 3:S47-S51, 1977.
208. Sabath, L. D.: Reappraisal of the antistaphylococcal activities of first-generation (narrow-spectrum) and second-generation (expanded-spectrum) cephalosporins. Antimicrob. Agents Chemother. 33:407-411, 1989.
209. Sabath, L. D., Garner, C., Wilcox, C., et al.: Susceptibility of Staphylococcus aureus and Staphylococcus epidermidis to 65 antibiotics. Antimicrob. Agents Chemother. 9:962-969, 1976.
210. Sader, H. S., Streit, J. M., Fritsche, T. R., and Jones, R. N.: Antimicrobial susceptibility of Gram-positive bacteria isolated from European medical centers: Results of the Daptomycin Surveillance Programme (2002-2004). Clin. Microbiol. Infect. 12:844-852, 2006.
211. Sampathkumar, P., Osmon, D. R., and Cockerill, F. R.: Prosthetic joint infection due to Staphylococcus lugdunensis. Mayo Clin. Proc. 75:511-512, 2000.
212. Sattler, F. R., Foderaro, J. B., and Aber, R. C.: Staphylococcus epidermidis bacteremia associated with vascular catheters: An important cause of febrile morbidity in hospitalized patients. Infect. Control 5:279-283, 1984.
213. Schaberg, D. R., and Zervos, M. J.: Intergeneric and interspecies gene exchange in gram-positive cocci. Antimicrob. Agents Chemother. 30:817-822, 1986.
214. Schaberg, D. R., and Zervos, M.: Plasmid analysis in the study of the epidemiology of nosocomial gram-positive cocci. Rev. Infect. Dis. 8:705-712, 1986.
215. Scheifele, D. W., Bjornson, G. L., Dyer, R. A., et al.: Delta-like toxin produced by coagulase-negative staphylococci is associated with neonatal necrotizing enterocolitis. Infect. Immun. 55:2268-2273, 1987.
216. Scheretz, R. J., Falk, R. J., Huffman, K. A., et al.: Infections associated with subclavian Udall catheters. Arch. Intern. Med. 143:52-56, 1983.
217. Schimke, R. T., Black, P. H., Mark, V. H., et al.: Indolent Staphylococcus albus or aureus bacteremia after ventriculoatriostomy: Role of foreign body in its initiation and perpetuation. N. Engl. J. Med. 264:264-270, 1961.
218. Schwalbe, R. S., Stapleton, J. T., and Gilligan, P. H.: Emergence of vancomycin resistance in coagulase-negative staphylococci. N. Engl. J. Med. 316:927-931, 1987.
219. Shenep, J. L., Hughes, W. T., Robertson, P. K., et al.: Vancomycin, ticarcillin and amikacin compared with ticarcillin-clavulanate and amikacin in the empirical treatment of febrile, neutropenic children with cancer. N. Engl. J. Med. 319:1053-1058, 1988.
220. Sheth, N. K., Franson, T. R., Rose, H. D., et al.: Colonization of bacteria on polyvinyl chloride and Teflon intravascular catheters in hospitalized patients. J. Clin. Microbiol. 18:1061-1063, 1983.
221. Sheth, N. K., Franson, T. R., and Sohnle, P. G.: Influence of bacterial adherence to intravascular catheters on in vitro antibiotic susceptibility. Lancet 2:1266-1268, 1985.
222. Shiro, H., Muller, E., Gutierrez, N., et al.: Transposon mutants or Staphylococcus epidermidis deficient in elaboration of capsular polysaccharide/adhesion and slime are avirulent in a rabbit model or endocarditis. J. Infect. Dis. 169:1042-1049, 1994.
223. Shiro, H., Muller, E., Takeda, S., et al.: Potentiation of Staphylococcus epidermidis catheter-related bacteremia by lipid infusions. J. Infect. Dis. 171:220-224, 1995.
224. Shoenbaum, S. C., Gardner, P., and Shillito, J.: Infections of cerebrospinal fluid shunts: Epidemiology, clinical manifestations, and therapy. J. Infect. Dis. 131:543-552, 1975.
225. Shulman, R. J., Smith, E. O., Rahman, S., et al.: Single- vs double-lumen central venous catheters in pediatric oncology patients. Am. J. Dis. Child. 142:893-895, 1988.
226. Shuttleworth, R., Behme, R. J., McNabb, A., et al.: Human isolates of bone and joint infections. J. Clin. Microbiol. 35:2537-2541, 1997.
227. Schutze, G. E., Hall, M. A., Baker, C. J., et al.: Role of neutrophil receptors in opsonophagocytosis of coagulase-negative staphylococci. Infect. Immun. 59:2573-2578, 1991.
228. Siebert, W. T., Moreland, N., and Williams, T. W., Jr.: Methicillin-resistant Staphylococcus epidermidis. South. Med. J. 71:1353-1355, 1978.

229. Sitges-Serra, A., Puig, P., and Jaurrieta, E.: Catheter sepsis due to *Staphylococcus epidermidis* during parenteral nutrition. Surg. Gynecol. Obstet. *151*:481-483, 1980.
230. Skahan, J. M., and Parisi, J. T.: Development of a bacteriophage-typing set for *Staphylococcus epidermidis*. J. Clin. Microbiol. *6*:16-18, 1977.
231. Smith, J. A., Henry, D. A., Bourgault, A., et al.: Comparison of agar disk diffusion, microdilution broth, and agar dilution for testing antimicrobial susceptibility of coagulase-negative staphylococci. J. Clin. Microbiol. *25*:1741-1746, 1987.
232. Sparrelid, E., Hagglund, H., Remberger, M., et al.: Bacteraemia during aplastic phase after allogeneic bone marrow transplantation is associated with early death from invasive fungal infection. Bone Marrow Transplant. *22*:795-800, 1998.
233. St. Geme, J. W., III, Bell, L. M., Baumgart, S., et al.: Distinguishing sepsis from blood culture contamination in young infants with blood cultures growing coagulase-negative staphylococci. Pediatrics *86*:157-162, 1990.
234. Talbot, H. W., Jr., and Parisi, J. T.: Phage typing of *Staphylococcus epidermidis*. J. Clin. Microbiol. *3*:519-523, 1976.
235. Tan, T. Q., Mason, E. O., Jr., Ou, C. N., et al.: Use of intravenous rifampin in neonates with persistent staphylococcal bacteremia. Antimicrob. Agents Chemother. *37*:2401-2406, 1993.
236. Tan, T. Q., Musser, J. M., Shulman, R. J., et al.: Molecular epidemiology of coagulase-negative staphylococcus blood isolated from neonates with persistent bacteremia and children with central venous catheter infections. J. Infect. Dis. *169*:1393-1397, 1994.
237. Tebbs, S. E., and Elliott, T. S. J.: Modification of central venous catheter polymers to prevent in vitro microbial colonization. Eur. J. Clin. Microbiol. Infect. Dis. *13*:111-117, 1994.
238. Tenover, F. C., Jones, R. N., Swenson, B., et al.: Methods for improved detection of oxacillin resistance in coagulase-negative staphylococci: Results of a multicenter study. J. Clin. Microbiol. *37*:4051-4058, 1999.
239. Thomson-Carter, F. M., and Pennington, T. H.: Characterization of coagulase-negative staphylococci by sodium dodecyl sulfate-polyacrylamide gel electrophoresis and immunoblot analysis. J. Clin. Microbiol. *27*:2199-2203, 1989.
240. Timmermann, C. P., Fleer, A., Besnier, J. M., et al.: Characterization of a proteinaceous adhesion of *Staphylococcus epidermidis* which mediates attachment to polystyrene. Infect. Immun. *59*:4187-4192, 1991.
241. Tojo, M., Yamashita, N., Goldmann, D. A., et al.: Isolation and characterization of a capsular polysaccharide adhesion from *Staphylococcus epidermidis*. J. Infect. Dis. *157*:713-722, 1988.
242. Tully, J. L., Friedland, G. H., Baldini, L. M., et al.: Complications of intravenous therapy with steel needles and small-bore Teflon catheters: A comparative study. Am. J. Med. *70*:702-706, 1981.
243. Van Bronswijk, H., Verbrugh, H. A., Heezius, C. J. M., et al.: Heterogeneity in opsonic requirements of *Staphylococcus epidermidis*: Relative importance of surface hydrophobicity, capsules and slime. Immunology *67*:81-86, 1989.
244. Vandecasteele, S. J., Peetermans, W. E., Merckx, R., et al.: Reliability of the *ica, aap* and *atlE* genes in the discrimination between invasive, colonizing and contaminant *Staphylococcus epidermidis* isolates in the diagnosis of catheter-related infections. Clin. Microbiol. Infect. *9*:114-119, 2003.
245. Vandenesch, F., Etienne, J., Reverdy, M. E., and Eykyn, S. J.: Endocarditis due to *Staphylococcus lugdunensis*: report of 11 cases and review. Clin. Infect. Dis. *5*:871-876, 1993.
246. Vandenesch, F., Eykyn, S. J., and Etienne, J.: Infections caused by newly-described species of coagulase-negative staphylococci. Rev. Med. Microbiol. *6*:94-100, 1995.
247. Veenstra, G. J., Cremers, F. F. M., van Dijk, H., et al.: Ultrastructural organization and regulation of a biomaterial adhesion of *Staphylococcus epidermidis*. J. Bacteriol. *178*:537-541, 1996.
248. Venditti, M., Santini, C., Serra, P., et al.: Comparative in vitro activities of new fluorinated quinolones and other antibiotics against coagulase-negative *Staphylococcus* blood isolates from neutropenic patients, and relationship between susceptibility and slime production. Antimicrob. Agents Chemother. *33*:209-211, 1989.
249. Villari, P., Sarnataro, C., and Iacuzio, L.: Molecular epidemiology of *Staphylococcus epidermidis* in a neonatal intensive care unit over a three-year period. J. Clin. Microbiol. *38*:1740-1746, 2000.
250. Viscoli, C., Garaventa, A., Boni, L., et al.: Role of Broviac catheters in infections in children with cancer. Pediatr. Infect. Dis. J. *7*:556-560, 1988.
251. von Eiff, C., Peters, G., and Heilmann, C.: Pathogenesis of infections due to coagulase-negative staphylococci. Lancet Infect. Dis. *2*:677-685, 2002. Y. Vuong, C., Otto, M.: *Staphylococcus epidermidis* infections. Microbes Infect. *4*:481-489, 2002.
252. Vuong, C., Voyich, J. M., Fischer, E. R., et al.: Polysaccharide intercellular adhesin (PIA) protects *Staphylococcus epidermidis* against major components of the human innate immune system. Cell. Microbiol. *6*:269-275, 2004.
253. Wachsmuth, K.: Molecular epidemiology of bacterial infections: Examples of methodology and investigations of outbreaks. Rev. Infect. Dis. *8*:682-692, 1986.
254. Wadstrom, T., and Rozgonyi, F.: Virulence determinants of coagulase-negative staphylococci. *In* Mardh, P. A., and Schleifer, K. H. (eds.): Coagulase-Negative Staphylococci. Stockholm, Almquist and Wiksel International, 1986, pp. 123-130.
255. Wang, A., Athan, E., Pappas, P.A., et al. Contemporary clinical profile and outcome of prosthetic valve endocarditis. JAMA *297*:1354-1361, 2007.
256. Wilson, A. P. R., O'Hare, M. D., Felmingham, D., et al.: Teicoplanin-resistant coagulase-negative *Staphylococcus*. Lancet *2*:973, 1986.
257. Wilson, C. B.: Immunologic basis for increased susceptibility of the neonate to infection. J. Pediatr. *108*:1-12, 1986.
258. Wisplinghoff, H., Bischoff, T., Tallent, S. M., et al.: Nosocomial bloodstream infections in US hospitals: analysis of 24, 179 cases from a prospective nationwide surveillance study. Clin. Infect. Dis. *39*:309-317, 2004.
259. Wisplinghoff, H., Seifert, H., Tallent, S. M., et al.: Nosocomial bloodstream infections in pediatric patients in United States hospitals: epidemiology, clinical features and susceptibilities. Pediatr. Infect. Dis. J. *22*:686-691, 2003.
260. Wong, S. S., Ho, P. L., Woo, P. C., et al.: Bacteremia caused by staphylococci with inducible vancomycin heteroresistance. Clin. Infect. Dis. *29*:760-767, 1999.
261. Yamada, T., Ichiman, Y., and Yoshida, K.: Possible common biological and immunological properties for detecting encapsulated strains of *Staphylococcus epidermidis*. J. Clin. Microbiol. *26*:2167-2172, 1988.
262. Yogev, R.: Cerebrospinal fluid shunt infections: A personal view. Pediatr. Infect. Dis. J. *4*:113-118, 1985.
263. Yoshida, K., Umeda, A., Ichiman, T., et al.: Cross protection between a strain of *Staphylococcus epidermidis* and eight other species of coagulase-negative staphylococci. Can. J. Microbiol. *34*:913-915, 1988.
264. Younger, J. J., Christensen, G. D., Bartley, D. L., et al.: Coagulase-negative staphylococci isolated from cerebrospinal fluid shunts: Importance of slime production, species identification and shunt removal to clinical outcome. J. Infect. Dis. *156*:548-554, 1987.
265. Zakrzewska-Czerwinska, J., Mordarski, M., Goodfellow, M., et al.: Deoxyribonucleic acid relatedness amongst *Staphylococcus epidermidis* and *Staphylococcus saprophyticus* strains. Zentralbl. Bakteriol. Mikrobiol. Hyg. *269*:179-187, 1988.
266. Ziebuhr, W., Hennig, S., Eckart, M., et al.: Nosocomial infections by *Staphylococcus epidermidis*: How a commensal bacterium turns into a pathogen. Int. J. Antimicrob. Agents *28*(Suppl. 1):S14-S20, 2006.
267. Zimmerman, R. J., and Kloos, W. E.: Comparative zone electrophoresis of esterases of *Staphylococcus* species isolated from mammalian skin. Can. J. Microbiol. *22*:771-779, 1976.

CHAPTER 93

GROUP A, GROUP C, AND GROUP G BETA-HEMOLYTIC STREPTOCOCCAL INFECTIONS

Edward L. Kaplan ✿ Michael A. Gerber

GROUP A STREPTOCOCCAL INFECTIONS

Group A beta-hemolytic streptococci (*Streptococcus pyogenes*) are common pathogenic bacteria isolated from children. They are associated with a wide variety of infections and disease states (Fig. 93-1). Although uniformly sensitive to penicillin and still exquisitely sensitive to many other antibiotics, group A streptococcal infections present formidable clinical and public health problems for pediatricians and primary care physicians. Although most group A streptococcal infections are of short duration and relatively benign, they may be fulminant and life-threatening. The importance of group A streptococcal infections was reinforced in

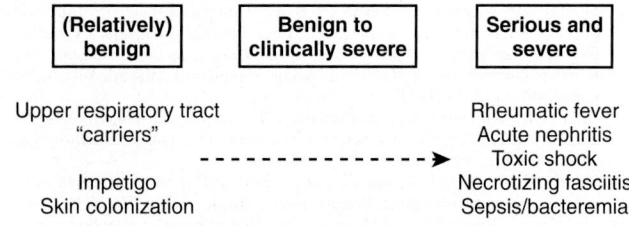

Figure 93–1 Spectrum of group A streptococcal infections.

the late 1990s by a resurgence of acute rheumatic fever in the United States[114] and the appearance of a group A streptococcal toxic shock syndrome (TSS) with very high morbidity and mortality rates.[153,154] Additionally, this bacterium is different from other pyogenic bacteria because of the potential for development of delayed, nonsuppurative sequelae (e.g., acute glomerulonephritis, acute rheumatic fever, reactive arthritis) to follow uncomplicated infections.

ORGANISM

S. pyogenes (group A streptococcus) is a gram-positive coccus, forming either short or long chains. Group A streptococci produce clear (beta) hemolysis on blood agar, a bacteriologic feature important in their recognition and in their differentiation from nonhemolytic (gamma) streptococci and from viridans (alpha) streptococci, which cause partial or green hemolysis on sheep blood agar. Although hemolysis is produced on culture plates containing blood from a variety of mammalian species, sheep or horse blood gives the clearest differentiation. Some strains of group A streptococci hemolyze red blood cells slowly or result in almost greenish hemolysis on the surface of blood agar plates incubated aerobically. These strains can be recognized by their ability to produce clear hemolysis under anaerobic conditions, which is achieved readily by routinely making a short cut or stab into the blood agar at the time of inoculation.[85] Incubation with carbon dioxide or in a candle jar also can be helpful in enhancing beta-hemolysis. Rare strains of group A streptococci are not hemolytic.[77,84]

Approximately 124 different types of group A streptococci have been recognized either on the basis of a series of serologically distinct surface proteins, the M proteins, or by sequencing of the *emm* gene, which encodes for M protein.[56,57,85,108] The M serotypes of streptococci associated with impetigo and pyoderma often are different from the serotypes associated with clinical pharyngitis, although a few M types have the capacity to produce both kinds of infection.[6] The M protein renders the group A streptococcus resistant to phagocytosis and is a major virulence factor for these organisms. Additional evidence indicates that more M-types exist that have not been identified yet; new *emm* sequences are continuing to be described (see http://www.cdc.gov/ncidod/biotech/strep/strepindex.htm).

The group A streptococcal cell is a complex structure. In rapidly dividing strains (e.g., young cultures, epidemic strains), the cell is covered with a hyaluronic acid capsule, which gives the colonies a mucoid or water drop appearance. Protruding from the cell surface and into the hyaluronic capsular layer are microscopic hairlike fimbriae, which are responsible for adherence of group A streptococci to epithelial cells. A basic chemical component of these fimbriae is lipoteichoic acid.[12] The M protein also is associated with these fimbriae.[60] Other surface proteins of interest are the T and R proteins, the serum opacity factor (SOF)

proteins, and proteins that bind nonspecifically to the Fc fragment of gamma-globulins. The function and the exact location of these other proteins on the surface of the organism have not been identified precisely. Strains of a particular M type generally are associated with a particular T agglutination pattern.[82] In strains producing serum opacity, the serologically specific SOR protein usually correlates closely with the M type of the strain. At present, more than 50 opacity factor–positive types of group A streptococci have been recognized; others undoubtedly have not been identified yet. All of these characteristics are useful in epidemiologic studies of streptococcal infections, either in an individual patient or in a community.

In addition to these surface proteins, the carbohydrate moiety responsible for group specificity (e.g., group A carbohydrate) is found in the cell wall in a position sufficiently superficial to permit reaction with antibody specifically directed toward it. The group A carbohydrate is a polymer of rhamnose units with side chains of *N*-acetylglucosamine, which is responsible for its group (e.g., A) specificity.[118] The structure providing rigidity for the cell wall is another large polymer, a peptidoglycan, consisting of glycan strands cross-linked by peptide bridges. Its role in the pathogenesis of infection remains incompletely defined.

Within the cell wall of the group A streptococcus lies the cell membrane, composed mainly of lipoprotein or lipid-protein complexes. This membrane is the outer surface of the osmotically fragile protoplasts or L forms of streptococci. These wall-less forms of group A streptococci are resistant to penicillin.[62]

Intracellular constituents of the group A streptococci include, in addition to DNA and RNA, many enzymes and hemolysins.[26] Plasmids have been identified that control resistance to certain antibiotics (e.g., erythromycin).[113] Bacteriophages play an important role in the genetics of group A streptococci, including the transfer of the determinants of antibiotic resistance and the control of pyrogenic exotoxin production.[169,174]

Group A streptococci produce and release into the surrounding medium numerous biologically active extracellular products. Some of these are toxic for human and other mammalian (eukaryotic) cells. Streptolysin O (the oxygen-labile hemolysin) and streptolysin S (the oxygen-stable hemolysin) injure cell membranes, not only lysing red blood cells, but also damaging other eukaryotic cells (including myocardial cells) and membranous subcellular organelles.[15] Streptolysin O is antigenic; streptolysin S is not. The latter hemolysin is bound loosely to the streptococcal cell and is released in a complexed, stable form with a variety of carrier molecules. The pyrogenic exotoxins resemble endotoxin in exhibiting a primary or intrinsic toxicity and a secondary toxicity resulting from the acquisition of host hypersensitivity.[103] The outbreak of streptococcal TSS, which became pronounced in the late 1990s, was reported to be associated with the reappearance of strains making pyrogenic exotoxin A, but many unanswered questions remain about the precise pathogenesis.[153] Group A streptococci also produce bacteriocins,[155] low-molecular-weight proteins that can kill a variety of other gram-positive bacterial species and may play a role in promoting infection or even persistence of colonization.

Many of the other extracellular products of group A streptococci are specific enzymes that do not seem to be directly toxic for mammalian or bacterial cells, but digest or initiate the breakdown of important biologic substrates. Included are the deoxyribonucleases (nucleases A, B, C, and D), the streptokinases (which activate the fibrinolytic or plasmin-plasminogen system), a hyaluronidase, an amylase, a proteinase, an esterase, a nicotinamide adenine dinucleotidase (NADase), and C5a peptidase. Several of these enzymes are antigenic (e.g., DNAse B, streptokinase, hyaluronidase, NADase, C5a peptidase). Among group A streptococcal surface virulence factors, C5A peptidase plays a major role by inactivating the complement chemotaxin C5A, reducing the early phagocytic response in allowing group A streptococci to become locally established. This extracellular product has been shown to be antigenic in animals and in humans.[34]

TRANSMISSION

Humans are the only known reservoir for group A streptococci. The mechanism of spread of streptococci from one person to another and from one body site to another varies according to the clinical manifestations of the infection. Epidemiologic studies of patients with streptococcal sore throat indicate that airborne routes of spread (by small droplet nuclei, dust) and environmental contamination (e.g., contaminated clothing or bedding) play little, if any, role in transmission of this kind of group A streptococcal infection.[132] Close personal contact is required for transmission of streptococcal pharyngitis to occur, apparently by direct projection of large droplets or by physical transfer of respiratory secretions containing the infectious bacteria. Spread within homes, school rooms, or crowded facilities such as military barracks is a common occurrence.[49] Residential nursing facilities also have proven to be highly susceptible to spread among staff members and patients.

Contaminated food or milk also may result in group A streptococcal infection of the throat, producing a common-source outbreak.[74] Salads containing hard-boiled eggs (e.g., egg salad) seem to be a special problem. Anal carriers have been identified as the source of contagion in several hospital outbreaks of streptococcal wound infections. Some studies have suggested that rectal or anal carriers may be more common than suspected.[104]

The period of greatest contagiousness of streptococcal pharyngitis and scarlet fever is during the acute stage of the illness. Most antibiotic therapies (especially penicillin) rapidly suppress the growth of group A streptococci and, if continued, most often eradicate them from the upper respiratory tract. A patient can be considered much less contagious after 24 hours of antimicrobial therapy. Most physicians concur that children can return to school by that time, especially if they are afebrile, with reduced risk of spread of the organism to close contacts.[150]

Although humans with active but subclinical infection also may contribute to the spread of group A streptococci, the role of throat "carriers" in the spread of this organism apparently is less important. Most secondary spread occurs during the first 2 weeks after acquisition occurs.[163] Rarely do streptococcal upper respiratory tract carriers spread the organism.[87] In contrast to carriage in the throat, which may persist for weeks or months, the prolonged presence of group A streptococci in the anterior nares is unusual.

In contrast to the upper respiratory tract, where group A streptococcus can establish infection readily on an intact epithelial surface, the production of streptococcal impetigo or pyoderma seems to be facilitated by prior disruption of the skin by trauma, insects, or some preexisting skin disorder. Group A streptococci may be found on the normal skin for several days to 2 weeks before infection develops,[59] requiring some other means of access. It does not seem likely that the source of infection for streptococcal skin infections is the upper respiratory tract. Group A streptococci causing impetigo may be found in the nose or throat, but they usually do not reach this site until several weeks after cutaneous infection has been established. One possible source is a skin lesion in another child, with spread occurring by direct contact. Some data suggest that spread may occur even by small flies that feed on such lesions.[11] The exact role of environmental contamination in the spread of streptococcal impetigo and pyoderma, and in secondary infection of wounds, burns, and eczema and other dermatoses, is unknown. The mechanism of transmission of erysipelas also is poorly understood, but may involve spread via the respiratory tract.

Measures to prevent spread of group A streptococcal infections vary in their effectiveness. Spread of throat or skin infection within a family often occurs before the index case is identified and isolated or treated. In epidemic situations, especially situations involving cases of rheumatic fever or acute nephritis, a culture survey with treatment of all individuals with positive cultures (mass prophylaxis) may be indicated. Reduction of crowding, especially in sleeping quarters, seems to be an effective long-term method of minimizing the incidence of transmission of streptococcal sore throat among some groups.

In families in which persistence or recurrence of streptococcal infection is a problem, simultaneous throat culture and culture of skin lesions of all members and treatment of all who have positive results have been successful in eradicating the organism. Some investigators have advocated a role for family pets (dogs) in transmission of streptococcal infections. Available data do not support such transmission as a common occurrence, however.[17,39,172] Control of environmental contamination would be expected to have little or no influence on the spread of group A streptococcal respiratory infections, although it possibly has an effect in controlling skin or wound infections. It also is suggested that family toothbrushes may have a role in the intrafamilial transmission of group A streptococci. More recent guidelines have suggested, however, that obtaining cultures of all family members in instances in which invasive group A streptococcal infections occur is not always necessary. Because of reported instances in which secondary cases have occurred, this guideline remains controversial.[132,136]

EPIDEMIOLOGY

Group A streptococci have a narrow range of hosts. They are one of the pathogenic bacteria identified almost exclusively in humans and only extremely rarely are found in other species.[108] In considering the epidemiology of group A streptococcal infections, one must recognize that significant differences exist between throat and skin infections.[133,164]

Streptococcal impetigo occurs with greatest frequency in preschool-aged children, whereas streptococcal pharyngitis predominantly is a disease of school-aged children. Outbreaks of streptococcal respiratory tract infections also have been observed in daycare centers.[149] On average, streptococcal respiratory infections occur at the rate of one every 3 to 5 years during childhood. One comprehensive long-term study suggested that the average child has three documented group A streptococcal infections (range of one to eight per child) before reaching age 13.[49] Among preschool and early school–aged children of certain populations, streptococcal impetigo is a recurrent problem.

The seasonal occurrence and geographic distribution are different for throat and skin infections. Tonsillitis and pharyngitis caused by streptococci are common occurrences in temperate and cold climates; streptococcal pyoderma and impetigo seem to occur with greater frequency in hot or tropical climates.[28] Streptococcal sore throat occurs more frequently in late autumn, winter, and early spring months. In tropical climates, pharyngeal colonization seems to occur more frequently during the rainy season. Streptococcal impetigo usually is a disease of the summer months in temperate climates, but it may occur with equal frequency year-round in tropical countries. In some tropical climates, groups C and G beta-hemolytic streptococci are isolated more frequently from the upper respiratory tract than is group A.[69] This finding has led some researchers to speculate about a possible etiologic role for groups C and G streptococci in the pathogenesis of rheumatic fever.[69]

PATHOGENESIS

No complete explanation is available for the predilection of certain body sites for infection by group A streptococci, or for the ability of strains of certain M types to produce pharyngitis or tonsillitis and of others to produce impetigo or pyoderma. In the establishment of throat infection, a primary requisite is a method of attachment to the epithelial cells of the pharynx. Group A streptococci attach by means of their fimbriae. To initiate an infection, group A streptococci also must compete with the resident pharyngeal flora, notably the alpha-hemolytic or viridans streptococci, which may interfere with the colonization of group A streptococci in the throat,[40] perhaps as a result of the production of a bacteriocin-like substance.[45] The relative importance of bacterial interference in preventing colonization of the human upper respiratory tract with group A streptococci is unclear, however. The influence of producers of a bacteriocin-like substance may be minimal in certain situations.[76]

In the production of impetigo, group A streptococci also must vie with other local bacterial flora. Removal of the normal flora increases the time of survival of group A streptococci applied to the skin.[3] Skin lipids, some of which are lethal for group A streptococci in vitro, also may provide a natural barrier against the establishment of streptococcal infection.

Invasion of the tissues by group A streptococci may be facilitated by a combination of bacteriologic properties. Damage to leukocytes and to fixed tissue cells may result from any of the several toxins produced, and the spread of infection may be aided by specific enzymes that attack hyaluronic acid and fibrin. M protein is antiphagocytic and contains a moiety that is cytotoxic in the presence of non–type-specific antibody.[14] The protective role of mucosal immunity remains incompletely defined. The hyaluronic acid capsule of group A streptococcus may serve as a camouflage because it resembles mammalian hyaluronic acid. In addition, several streptococcal substances (streptococcal pyrogenic exotoxins and peptidoglycan) have been shown to have endotoxin-like properties. A role for pyrogenic exotoxins has been postulated for streptococcal TSS and for necrotizing fasciitis.[152,153]

The factors responsible for the early host defense against group A streptococci (before the development of antibody) are incompletely understood. Type-specific antibody against M protein, which greatly promotes phagocytosis, usually is not detectable until 6 to 8 weeks after the infection has occurred[47]; its primary role may not be in the limitation or termination of active infection, but rather in the prevention of re-infection by the same serologic type. Reports indicate that type-specific immunity may be to specific strains within a given serotype, rather than to all strains within a given serotype.[46,161] The significance of this potentially important observation in the epidemiology of streptococcal infections and in the pathogenesis of nonsuppurative sequelae has not been defined fully. Surface phagocytosis, first by monocytes and later by polymorphonuclear leukocytes, may be the primary mechanism of defense in the early stages of infection.[141] In streptococcal skin infections, an increase in the leukotactic activity of polymorphonuclear leukocytes has been reported.[65]

Approximately 30 minutes after ingestion by a polymorphonuclear leukocyte has occurred, the streptococcus may be killed. Occasionally, the reverse occurs because of a phenomenon known as *leukotoxicity*, which apparently is related to the production of streptolysin S.[124] Degradation of the streptococcus within phagocytes or in tissues is a much slower process, suggesting that the human host may be unable to break down the streptococcal cell wall in an efficient manner.[65] This feature seems to be in contrast to the reported engulfment of group A streptococci by respiratory epithelial cells; in the latter instance, evidence suggests intracellular survival of the streptococci occurs, perhaps accounting

for the persistence of these organisms in individuals thought to be carriers.[109]

Spread of streptococci to the regional lymph nodes can occur, especially in infections of the pharynx and tonsils.[45] Bacteremia occurs in the absence of underlying systemic disease, such as leukemia or other malignancies,[52,68] but it is an uncommon occurrence in older children and adults. The reason for the apparent increase in prevalence of severe systemic group A streptococcal infections beginning in the 1980s and 1990s and continuing into the 21st century remains incompletely explained. Although certain M types seem to be isolated more frequently from such severe infections (e.g., M-1, M-3), these strains apparently are no different from similar M types causing uncomplicated infections. Many M/*emm* types have been recovered from patients with severe systemic infections.

The rash and other toxic manifestations of scarlet fever have been attributed to the development of hypersensitivity to the pyrogenic toxins.[119] Toxic manifestations that have been noted in group A streptococcal TSS also may result from a direct influence of the pyrogenic exotoxins on lymphokines, such as tumor necrosis factor.[152,153] Hypersensitivity to other streptococcal products also may contribute to the manifestations of streptococcal disease.

Theories abound about the pathogenetic mechanism leading to the development of the nonsuppurative complications of streptococcal infections, acute rheumatic fever, and acute glomerulonephritis. Most of these hypotheses invoke immunologic processes in one way or another.[75,119,159] A major impediment toward clarifying the pathogenetic mechanism responsible for the development of nonsuppurative sequelae has been the lack of an appropriate animal model for study.

CLINICAL MANIFESTATIONS

Streptococcal pharyngitis or tonsillitis usually is a short-lived clinical illness with a brief incubation period (12 hours to 4 days). It varies greatly in its severity, from a subclinical or almost subclinical form, occurring in 30 to 50 percent of infections, to a very toxic form with high fever, nausea, and vomiting. Extreme toxicity may occur more frequently in epidemic situations, especially food-borne outbreaks, suggesting the importance of the rapid passage of the infecting organism from person to person in determining the severity of infection. The onset is acute and may be marked by fever, sore throat, headache, or abdominal pain (more common in children). The tonsils and pharynx may appear inflamed or infected but may look pale in the presence of marked edema. Exudate is a common manifestation (50%-90%). It usually appears by the second day and typically is discrete and whitish yellow and may become confluent by the following day. Swollen, tender anterior cervical lymph nodes (adenitis) also can be observed in 30 to 60 percent of patients.

The clinical manifestations usually subside spontaneously in 3 to 5 days, unless suppurative complications (otitis media, sinusitis, peritonsillar abscess) develop. Patients who develop nonsuppurative sequelae have a latent period of 1 to 3 weeks during which they seem completely well. After streptococcal infection of the upper respiratory tract develops, the average latent period for acute glomerulonephritis is 10 days; for acute rheumatic fever, the average latent period is 18 days.[164]

An infantile form of streptococcal infection, referred to as *streptococcal childhood fever*, may take a more prolonged course, with chronic low-grade fever, generalized lymphadenopathy, and a persistent serous nasal discharge; little or no evidence of localized inflammation is present in the pharyngeal area. The term *streptococcosis*, which sometimes has been used to refer specifically to this infantile form, should be employed more correctly to indicate the broad spectrum of clinical pictures that change with age in a manner analogous to tuberculosis.[131]

Scarlet fever is a rare disease in infants. This observation may be because of the possibility of placental transfer of maternal antibody to the pyrogenic toxins. A more complete explanation may relate to a necessity for hypersensitization to these exotoxins to develop before this manifestation of streptococcal disease can be expressed.[99] In the mid-20th century, the severe toxic form of scarlet fever was a rare occurrence in most industrialized countries; milder forms of the illness were prevalent. In the late 1980s, numerous reports of an illness characterized by scarlet fever–like rash but with severe systemic manifestations, including fasciitis, myositis, adult respiratory distress syndrome, and very high mortality rate (up to 30%), became more prevalent in the United States.[22,91]

The characteristic rash is red and finely punctate, appearing initially on the trunk and spreading peripherally within several hours to several days to cover almost the entire body in full-blown cases. A typical feature of the rash is that it fades on pressure and almost always leads to desquamation. Linear red lines may develop in the skin folds of the joints (Pastia lines) or in other areas of the extremities. The strawberry tongue of scarlet fever has a swollen, red, and mottled appearance and eventually peels. A scarlatiniform rash also may occur with streptococcal impetigo and streptococcal wound infections. An enanthema of stippled, bright red or hemorrhagic spots may appear on the soft palate or the anterior pillars of the tonsillar fossae. Exudate and tender cervical nodes may be present as in streptococcal pharyngitis without a rash, but the pharyngeal signs sometimes are minimal.

Streptococcal impetigo may develop a few days to several weeks after deposition of the infecting strain on the normal skin; the average latent period is 10 days.[59] In contrast to pharyngitis, this form of group A streptococcal infection frequently is painless, and the patient usually is afebrile. The initial lesion is a superficial vesicle with little surrounding erythema. This lesion rapidly develops into a pustule and then into a thick, honey-colored crust; this stage may last for a few days to several weeks. Secondary infection with staphylococci is a common development in the pustular and crust stages.[44,48] Removal of the crusts by trauma or as part of local therapy reveals a moist or purulent undersurface in the earlier stages. The infection does not involve the dermis. On healing, depigmentation may be seen, but permanent scarring rarely occurs. The lesions develop most frequently on the lower extremities but may occur on other exposed portions of the body, such as the upper extremities and the face.

Acute poststreptococcal glomerulonephritis may develop after impetigo or other forms of cutaneous streptococcal infection produced by a nephritogenic strain have occurred; rheumatic fever has not been proven to be associated with group A streptococcal skin infections.[166] This concept has been challenged by investigators working in populations in which group A streptococcal upper respiratory tract infections are rare compared with streptococcal pyoderma; these populations have very high incidence rates for acute rheumatic fever.[28] At present, however, a role for group A streptococcal skin infection in the pathogenesis of rheumatic fever remains unproven. The latent period for acute nephritis is longer after a skin infection (average, 3 weeks) than after a throat infection (average, 10 days).[92] The serologic types associated with nephritis after skin infection usually differ from the types causing nephritis after throat infection.[164] M-12 has been the classic nephritogenic serotype associated with pharyngitis, whereas serotypes such as M-49, M-55, and M-57 have been associated more frequently with nephritis occurring after skin infection.[164]

Impetigo and more nondescript forms of streptococcal pyoderma may be superimposed on scabies, eczema, other dermatoses, burns, and wounds, which afford a means of access through the cutaneous barrier. Ecthyma is a more deep-seated and chronic form of streptococcal pyoderma found predominantly in tropical climates.[1]

Erysipelas is an unusual type of streptococcal infection involving the skin and sometimes the adjacent mucous membranes. It is an elevated erythematous lesion, sometimes exhibiting blebs filled with yellowish fluid, which may crust over after rupture. The lesion is characterized by a well-demarcated advancing border, more reddened and edematous than is the central area, which may fade and become more normal in appearance as the lesion progresses. Erysipelas most often involves the face (especially in children), the extremities, or the body. The lesion may surround a surgical or traumatic wound, an area of dermatosis, or the umbilical stump in a newborn infant. Erysipelas tends not to spread from one body region to another. In erysipelas, the onset is acute and often is accompanied by the manifestations of systemic toxicity characteristic of other febrile forms of streptococcal infection. The lesion may last for a few days to several weeks. Relapses are common occurrences, with recurrences frequently at the same body site.

In addition to the infections described earlier, group A streptococci may produce a variety of other clinical pictures. Other infections associated with upper respiratory tract infections by these organisms include otitis media, retropharyngeal abscess, sinusitis, mastoiditis, pneumonia, and empyema. Beta-hemolytic streptococci are recoverable from approximately 50 percent of patients with peritonsillar abscess and may act in concert with anaerobic bacteria in the production of this clinical picture.[61] Acute puerperal sepsis, now a rare development, classically has been associated with group A streptococci. Outbreaks of omphalitis, bacteremia, and meningitis in nurseries continue to be reported occasionally.[156] Fatal gangrene,[66] disseminated intravascular coagulopathy,[80] and purpura fulminans[38] may be associated with infection by group A streptococci. These bacteria also are a common cause of perianal cellulitis and vaginitis in children.[4,104] Subpectoral abscesses and empyemas may develop as complications of streptococcal infections of the thumb and index finger as a result of the lymphatic drainage of that part of the hand.[4] Septic complications of varicella, including varicella gangrenosa,[25,148] osteomyelitis (especially in infants),[70] hand-foot syndrome,[71] blistering distal dactylitis,[72] necrotizing fasciitis, and TSS, are associated with beta-hemolytic streptococci. Some investigators have suggested that streptococcal infections may be responsible for episodes of acute guttate psoriasis.[8]

STREPTOCOCCAL UPPER RESPIRATORY TRACT CARRIER STATE

A puzzling aspect of the relationship of group A streptococci and the human host is the streptococcal "carrier" state. Not only does it represent a diagnostic and a therapeutic enigma for clinicians and public health authorities, but also the theoretical implications relating to pathogenesis of nonsuppurative sequelae are intriguing.[87] Data in the literature suggest that group A upper respiratory tract carriers are less dangerous to others because carriers only rarely spread the organism to close contacts. In addition, the risk of developing nonsuppurative sequelae, such as rheumatic fever, seems to be significantly reduced in carriers.[88] The epidemiologic and immunologic reasons for establishment and continuation of the carrier state are not understood.

Much of this confusion has resulted from the definition of the carrier state. In contrast to true infection, in which the patient has the presence of an organism and evidence of a host immune response, group A streptococcal upper respiratory tract carriers may harbor the organism in the upper respiratory tract for prolonged periods without evidence of an immunologic response, as measured by an increase in antibody to streptococcal antigens.[87]

The explanation for this prolonged persistence of group A streptococci in the upper respiratory tract is unknown. Whether it is attributable to bacterial or host factors is unexplained. Hypotheses have been proposed to explain persistence of the organism in the upper respiratory tract. Bacterial data suggest that internalization of the group A streptococci into epithelial cells may explain their ability to continue to survive. Researchers have seen in vitro that stationary phase organisms are internalized easily by epithelial cells, and others have associated internalization with the presence of fibronectin-binding proteins in specific strains of group A streptococci.[109,122] Because of the inability of penicillin to penetrate the epithelial cell and to eradicate the organism from the carrier, this is an attractive explanation for clinical findings.[94]

For clinicians, the carrier has proven to be particularly problematic.[82,168] The ability to identify prospectively carriers and to separate them from individuals with bona fide upper respiratory tract infections, and the reported difficulty of eradicating the organism from the upper respiratory tract of carriers remains a perplexing and frustrating problem, especially considering that 5 to 20 percent of children may carry group A streptococci in their upper respiratory tract during the late autumn, winter, and early spring.

IMMUNOLOGIC RESPONSE

The numerous somatic constituents and extracellular products of group A streptococci, most of which are antigenic, accounts for the complex nature of the host immune response after group A streptococcal infection develops. Humoral and cellular immune responses have been studied, the former more thoroughly than the latter.[167]

Skin and in vitro tests suggest that most adults are hypersensitive to a variety of streptococcal antigenic preparations, whereas infants more often are nonreactive. Lymphocyte transformation responses to most streptococcal substances probably are specific in nature, resulting from prior sensitization. Some studies indicate, however, that a nonspecific (mitogenic) response may occur with certain extracellular and cellular fractions. Inhibition of migration of leukocytes has been shown with fractions of streptococcal culture supernates and with cell membrane and cell wall fractions.[135,144] Some evidence from research in humans suggests that the cellular immune response to a streptococcal extracellular antigen is controlled genetically.[67,144]

In humans, humoral immune responses have been shown to numerous somatic components of the group A streptococcal cell. Of particular interest are antibodies to the group A carbohydrate that serologically are cross-reactive with the glycoprotein of human and bovine heart valves and antibodies to protein components of the group A cell wall or cell membrane that have been reported to be cross-reactive with the sarcolemma of heart muscle.[9]

Antibody to the M protein (type-specific antibody) is of special importance because it is the basis of immunity and protection against re-infection with the same serologic type.[13,107,163] Type-specific antibody may be transferred across the placenta from mother to fetus.[176] The development of type-specific antibody can be inhibited partially by prompt administration of penicillin for the streptococcal infection.[42]

Humoral antibodies to specific streptococcal extracellular products can be shown readily by neutralization assays.[21] These assays have been especially useful as a more precise method of defining streptococcal infection in clinical and epidemiologic studies and of documenting the occurrence of a preceding streptococcal infection in patients with a suspected nonsuppurative complication.

The anti-streptolysin O assay is the streptococcal antibody test used most frequently.[145] Because streptolysin O also is produced by group C and G streptococci, the test is not specific for

TABLE 93–1 Upper Limits of Normal for Anti-streptolysin O and Anti-deoxyribonuclease B for Children 2 to 12 Years Old

Age (yr)	Mean Titer ASO	ULN ASO	Mean Titer Anti-DNaseB	ULN Anti-DNase B
2	52	160	46	240
3	52	120	30	60
4	52	120	49	240
5	56	160	58	320
6	72	240	76	480
7	87	240	126	640
8	110	240	166	640
9	117	240	186	640
10	126	320	166	640
11	129	320	204	800
12	141	320	219	480

Anti-DNAse B, anti-deoxyribonuclease B; ASO, anti-streptolysin O; ULN, upper limits of normal.
From Kaplan, E. L., Rothermel, C. D., and Johnson, D. R.: Antistreptolysin O and anti-deoxyribonuclease B titers: Normal values for children ages 2-12 in the United States. Pediatrics 101:86-88, 1998.

group A infection. The antistreptolysin O response can be feeble in patients with streptococcal impetigo or pyoderma[93]; its usefulness for this latter condition is limited. In contrast, the anti-deoxyribonuclease B (anti-DNAse B) and the anti-hyaluronidase responses are reliable after skin and throat infections have occurred.[93]

Another antibody test, the Streptozyme agglutination test, is based on antibody agglutination of erythrocytes coated with a mixture of streptococcal extracellular antigens. It has the theoretical appeal of simplicity, speed, and reaction with numerous streptococcal antigens.[78] Peak titers for an immune response as measured by the Streptozyme test have been shown within the first 7 to 10 days after onset of infection,[125] whereas neutralizing antibody titers to streptolysin O (3-6 weeks) or anti-DNAse B (6-8 weeks) do not peak until later. Because of documented problems of standardization of this reagent (variable results may be obtained with different lots) and because of problems with group specificity, this test should be interpreted with caution.[97,167] Some studies have indicated problems in interpretation of this test, and the World Health Organization has recommended that it not be used.[5]

Antibody titers reported by clinical immunology laboratories may vary. Upper limits of normal are higher for children than for adults, and these values, even for the same age group, are higher in some populations than in others. Interpretation of antibody titers for clinical purposes must take these factors into consideration.[145] Often, values given by laboratories for upper limits of normal are determined using adult sera; these values often are much too low to be used in a pediatric population. Table 93–1 gives results of normal levels of antibody titers in children 2 to 12 years old.[99]

DIAGNOSIS AND DIFFERENTIAL DIAGNOSIS

In patients presenting with acute pharyngitis or tonsillitis, the clinician must rely on a combination of the clinical appearance, identification of the organism, and epidemiologic findings to confirm the probability of group A streptococcal infection. The clinical difficulty is compounded because most of the clinical manifestations of streptococcal pharyngitis can be associated with a variety of other etiologic agents.[19] Group A streptococci often are found in the throats of normal children and in children whose clinical findings are due to one of these other agents (see also Chapter 10).[165] Exudative sore throat may be caused by many viruses, *Corynebacterium diphtheriae*, gonococci, and groups C and G in addition to group A streptococci.[19] The clinical syndrome associated with *Arcanobacterium haemolyticus* can be quite similar and clinically confusing.

Viral pharyngitis may closely mimic streptococcal pharyngitis, which can be ruled out only by the absence of a positive culture for group A streptococci. In children, the white blood cell count may be elevated in viral infections, but a low count renders it unlikely that the infection is streptococcal. The C-reactive protein test is only marginally useful in the acute phase of the illness.[101]

Because most streptococcal infections are short-term illnesses and antibody responses can be slow in appearing, streptococcal antibody titers are useful only retrospectively in diagnosing acute group A streptococcal infection. Little or no reason exists to use streptococcal antibody titers in the management of acute pharyngitis. In addition to their primary role in supporting the diagnosis of nonsuppurative complications (acute nephritis and acute rheumatic fever), however, occasionally they may be useful clinically in diagnosing infections in which obtaining cultures from the primary site is difficult (e.g., streptococcal pneumonia or osteomyelitis) or the infections have been treated or partially treated with antibiotics. The presence of an elevated streptococcal antibody titer does not, by itself, confirm a diagnosis of rheumatic fever, however. A more reliable approach is to use an increase in titer to confirm group A streptococcal infection.

Numerous clinical schemes have been proposed for differentiating streptococcal from nonstreptococcal pharyngitis, but none of them is entirely satisfactory in making this distinction or in differentiating streptococcal carriers with an intervening nonstreptococcal pharyngitis from individuals with active streptococcal disease.[86,165] Clinical manifestations that are most suggestive of a group A streptococcal cause include the scarlatiniform rash (which, however, occasionally is associated with staphylococcal, rather than streptococcal, infection), excoriated nares (especially in infants), tender (not merely enlarged) anterior cervical lymph nodes, and a history of close contact with a well-documented case of group A streptococcal infection. The presence of cough, hoarseness, or conjunctivitis renders the diagnosis of streptococcal pharyngitis unlikely. Exudative pharyngitis in infants usually is nonstreptococcal in etiology.[2] In addition, numerous clinical scoring systems have been found to be helpful to the clinician in some circumstances, but even they are not entirely reliable.[168]

Cultures may yield invalid results unless they are obtained and processed carefully. For cultures of the throat, the affected areas (tonsils and posterior pharynx) should be rubbed firmly with the rayon or cotton culture swab. Impetiginous lesions should be cleansed with alcohol, and the vesicle should be punctured or the crust lifted by a sterile needle so that purulent material or the moist base can be touched by the swab.[85] Group A streptococci sometimes can be recovered even from dry crusted lesions if the swab is moistened with culture broth before touching the exposed base of the lesion. Because streptococcal impetigo lesions commonly contain secondarily invading staphylococci, which may overgrow and obscure the colonies of streptococci, cultures should be examined carefully with a hand lens; alternatively, gentian violet or other inhibitors of normal flora may be incorporated on the blood agar plates as an inhibitor of staphylococci.

Presumptive differentiation of group A from other hemolytic streptococci can be achieved by the sensitivity of group A streptococci (but relatively few of other hemolytic streptococci) to bacitracin, but only when tested by a disk designed specifically for this purpose.[85] Definite identification of group A streptococci can be accomplished by several serologic or immunologic techniques, including (1) extraction of the organism by boiling in hydrochloric acid or by several other extraction methods with examination of the resulting extract in a precipitin test, (2) fluorescent antibody test on isolated colonies or broth cultures, and (3) agglutination of the organisms by group-specific antisera bound to protein A–containing staphylococci.

Numerous rapid techniques for direct identification of group A streptococci from the upper respiratory tract are available commercially. Direct and rapid identification of group A streptococcal antigens from throat swabs (e.g., latex agglutination, enzyme-linked immunosorbent assay) has become quite popular. The specificity of these tests usually is very good, but published reports indicate that the sensitivity varies widely.[90,146] Guidelines promote a back-up throat culture if a rapid antigen detection test is negative.[20] These techniques employ extraction of the group-specific carbohydrate from the cell wall of the organism. Available data suggest that the specificity for these tests generally is greater than 90 percent, but the sensitivity ranges from less than 60 percent to greater than 90 percent.[90]

The advantages of these tests include the ability to identify group A streptococci rapidly and to treat the patient at the time the patient is in the physician's office or emergency department. This advantage has appeal, especially in view of the data suggesting that in children, the more quickly the patient is treated, the more rapid is the clinical response.[134] Studies also have shown that rapid antigen detection tests can be useful in the detection of group A streptococci in streptococcal pyoderma-like lesions.[95]

Data suggest that the sensitivity of rapid antigen detection tests is improved, leading to the suggestion that a positive rapid antigen detection test is sufficient proof of group A infection, but that a negative rapid antigen detection test should be confirmed with a conventional throat culture on sheep blood agar. The throat culture remains a "gold standard" for identifying group A streptococci in the upper respiratory tract. Although they rarely are encountered, false-positive rapid antigen detection tests also have been documented, owing to a cross-reaction with antigens present in some *Streptococcus milleri*.[88] Just as with any other laboratory test, a "learning curve effect" exists with streptococcal rapid antigen detection tests.[98]

On clinical findings alone, it generally is safer to make a diagnosis of streptococcal impetigo than it is to make a diagnosis of streptococcal pharyngitis. Impetigo in which staphylococci are the primary invader generally is bullous rather than vesicular in type, and on rupture of the vesicle a crust appears that is paper-thin and white, rather than thick and honey-colored. Some confusion may result from reports of cultures performed on patients with primary streptococcal impetigo. Staphylococci, often present as secondary invaders, may overgrow the streptococci, which consequently may be missed, unless the colonies are well isolated and the bacteriologist has an unusually sharp eye, or unless a culture medium inhibitory for staphylococci is used.

The vesicles of varicella infection may resemble those of streptococcal impetigo superficially, but they are less transient, are surrounded by a red areola, are more centripetal in distribution (tending to involve the trunk and the proximal portions of the extremities), frequently itch, occur in crops, and often are accompanied by constitutional symptoms. The crusts are not as thick as are those of streptococcal impetigo. The lesions of chickenpox can be infected with streptococci secondarily, and varicella has been identified as an important risk factor in the development of severe and invasive group A streptococcal infections.

PROGNOSIS

Patients with streptococcal sore throat or streptococcal impetigo recover spontaneously. A very few may develop suppurative complications, and an occasional patient may have a nonsuppurative sequela, particularly in industrialized countries. There is more chance of developing complications in socially and economically disadvantaged populations.

In the general population, the risk of developing rheumatic fever after an untreated bona fide group A streptococcal infection of the upper respiratory tract has been shown to be approximately 3 percent under epidemic conditions but is apparently considerably less (about 0.3%) in endemic situations,[147] owing partly to differences in definition of infection.[100] Patients who have had one attack of rheumatic fever are at high risk of a rheumatic fever recurrence when re-infected with group A streptococci. There seems to be no risk of developing rheumatic fever after having a streptococcal infection only of the skin, but this concept has been challenged if not yet substantiated.[28]

The risk of acute glomerulonephritis depends on whether the infection is caused by a nephritogenic strain. With a nephritogenic strain, the attack rate is about 10 to 15 percent, and acute glomerulonephritis can occur after either throat or skin infection.[164]

In contrast to the usual short, often benign course of throat and superficial skin infections, streptococcal cellulitis spreads rapidly locally and to the regional lymph nodes and bloodstream. In immunosuppressed patients and patients with streptococcal infection superimposed on leukemia, lymphoma, or other malignancies, bacteremia may develop, and patients may have serious life-threatening problems. Patients with puerperal sepsis, neonatal infection, streptococcal toxic shock–like syndrome, or gangrene owing to group A streptococci also have a high mortality rate despite timely administration of and high doses of penicillin therapy.[153]

The prognosis for complete recovery in patients with group A streptococcal TSS and in patients with necrotizing fasciitis varies. Morbidity and mortality rates have been reported to be greater in adults, especially the elderly, than in pediatric patients. Several series reported a mortality rate of at least 30 percent in patients with TSS.[154] The mortality rate with necrotizing fasciitis can be even greater.[152,153]

TREATMENT

Although group A streptococci generally are susceptible to many antibiotics,[37,53,117] penicillin remains the drug of choice for treatment except in patients allergic to it.[20] No clinical isolates of group A streptococci have been identified yet that are resistant to penicillin.[112] Although tolerance to penicillin has been described in group A streptococci, its clinical significance has not been determined.[102]

Eradicating group A streptococci from the upper respiratory tract (especially from carriers) with penicillin or other antibiotics sometimes is difficult.[89,95] This observation has not been explained adequately, but possible explanations include the presence of β-lactamase–producing organisms in the upper respiratory tract, the presence of group A streptococci tolerant to penicillin, and the production by certain of the normal upper respiratory tract flora of inhibitory substances that reduce persistence of the organism. In addition, some evidence suggests that persistence frequently is associated with the upper respiratory tract carrier state.[105] The presence of intracellular group A streptococci also has been noted in this regard.

Erythromycin remains the drug of choice in patients allergic to penicillin. Resistance to erythromycin is a rare occurrence in many countries (<5%). More recent data from Europe, where macrolides are widely used, show resistance rates in some countries of greater than 30 percent. In some countries, noticeable increases in resistance to macrolide by group A streptococci has been associated with increased use of macrolides. Although the prevalence of macrolide-resistant group A streptococci generally has been low in North America and of little clinical significance,[73,173] isolated examples have shown the ability of the organism to become resistant to macrolides.[115] The incidence was high in Japan in the 1960s,[50] and this observation also has been noted in Finland.[143] The use of broad-spectrum antibiotics for group A streptococcal infections has no advantage and potential disadvantages.[6-20] Group A streptococci most frequently are resistant to tetracyclines and the sulfonamides. β-lactamase–resistant antibiotics have been advocated in some studies[23]; a role for production of β-lactamase by normal flora in penicillin treatment failures has not been clarified yet.

Some reports have pointed out that cephalosporins may be more efficacious than is penicillin, especially in carriers. This form of oral therapy has been recommended by some clinicians.[30,31]

In the treatment of bona fide streptococcal sore throat, the group A streptococcus must be eradicated to prevent the development of acute rheumatic fever.[32] Many guidelines recommend administration of 10 days of oral penicillin V, or erythromycin for a penicillin-allergic individual, as being optimal for eradication.[20] Administration of a single intramuscular injection of benzathine penicillin G (1,200,000 U in adults and in children weighing >60 lb; 600,000 U in children weighing <60 lb) is one method of accomplishing this objective. If a combination of benzathine penicillin and procaine penicillin is used, the total dosage should be based on the amount of benzathine penicillin used.

If oral medication (penicillin or erythromycin) is used, the parent must be impressed with the importance of continuing the medication for a full 10 days. Oral penicillin V (250 mg two to three times a day) has been the treatment of choice for children. Many pediatricians prefer amoxicillin because of its taste. For adolescents, 250 mg given either three or four times a day or 500 mg twice a day has been suggested.[20] More recent studies have reported that amoxicillin given once daily (750 to 1000 mg) is as effective as is amoxicillin given twice daily (two doses of 375 mg or 500 mg) in eradicating group A streptococci in children.

In patients with a suspected allergy to penicillin, erythromycin (in adults, 250 mg four times a day; in children, 40 mg/kg/day in four doses, not to exceed the adult dose) has been used.[43] Two other macrolide/azalide preparations, azithromycin and clarithromycin, have been used as substitutes for erythromycin. The exact dose of erythromycin varies with the preparation used (e.g., stearate, estolate). Other antibiotics that have been used successfully in the therapy of group A beta-hemolytic streptococcal pharyngitis or tonsillitis include clindamycin, amoxicillin, a mixture of amoxicillin with clavulanic acid, and other cephalosporins. For patients who have *not* had an immediate type reaction to penicillin, many clinicians feel safe using a first-generation cephalosporin.

The problem of patient adherence to a 10-day course of oral antibiotics is well recognized. Because of this problem, several antibiotics have been approved for short-course therapy (<10 days) for treatment of group A streptococcal pharyngitis. These antibiotics include some cephalosporins and one of the newer macrolides/azalides. Some studies show equivalence of short-course therapy to 10 full days of conventional penicillin V oral therapy. Because of conflicting data, some guidelines still promote caution in using short-course therapy for the treatment of group A streptococcal upper respiratory tract infection.[20]

In patients with strong clinical or epidemiologic evidence of streptococcal infection, the physician may decide to begin therapy before the result of the throat culture is available. If oral antibiotic therapy is used for initiating treatment, the therapy may be continued or discontinued, depending on the culture report. Alternatively, an intramuscular injection of benzathine penicillin G may be administered at that time if the laboratory culture report is positive for group A streptococci. For patients who may not return for a culture report, or who may be difficult to contact, making an immediate clinical judgment whether to prescribe penicillin therapy may be important. In these situations, the use of the rapid direct techniques for detection of group A streptococci is advantageous. Because such patients also may be less reliable with respect to completing a course of oral therapy, the use of intramuscular benzathine penicillin G may be preferable. Even if the decision to treat or not to treat must be made on clinical grounds, throat cultures can be useful in indicating to the physician the current prevalence and clinical features of streptococcal and nonstreptococcal respiratory illnesses. Intramuscular benzathine penicillin G also is advantageous in epidemic situations.

At one time, obtaining repeat throat cultures after completion of oral therapy was thought to be appropriate to ensure that the group A streptococci had been eradicated. Studies have shown that many penicillin treatment failures seem to occur in carriers of group A streptococci in the upper respiratory tract.[87] In areas where rheumatic fever has not reappeared, re-culturing asymptomatic individuals routinely after they have received antibiotic therapy usually is unnecessary unless unusual epidemiologic circumstances (a rheumatic individual in the household or epidemic streptococcal disease in the community) exist. Other regimens that have been used for treating patients with persistently positive cultures include clindamycin, a mixture of amoxicillin and clavulanic acid, and rifampin along with either an injection of benzathine penicillin G or 10 days of oral penicillin.[20]

For patients who show a repeated clinical pattern of treatment failure, determining the serologic group and type of the strains recovered may be helpful to ascertain whether the isolates are the same or are different M protein types. Such testing is not done routinely in hospital laboratories, however, and in those circumstances contact with a state health department or streptococcal research laboratory would be required. It is important in "problem" families, in which intrafamilial spread is problematic, to culture the throats of all members of the family simultaneously and to treat all family members with positive results. The main problem of the persisting carrier is that this carrier status may complicate the interpretation of throat cultures obtained at the time of future nonstreptococcal respiratory tract infections.

Some researchers have suggested that the rapid treatment of group A streptococcal upper respiratory tract infection tends to promote recurrent streptococcal infections in the future because of the suppression of the type-specific antibody response. Some studies have shown no difference, however, in the frequency of recurrences of streptococcal infections whether therapy is started on diagnosis or delayed 48 hours.[63]

In contrast to group A streptococcal pharyngitis or tonsillitis, no authoritative guidelines have been developed for the treatment of streptococcal impetigo.[170] The effectiveness of hygienic measures and local skin care (removal of crusts and use of antibacterial soaps) probably depends on the thoroughness and perseverance with which they are carried out. These measures and the use of local antimicrobial ointments can be sufficient for the management of patients with only a few lesions. Systemic antibiotics have been associated with rapid clearing of the lesions, however. Oral or parenteral penicillin or oral erythromycin (in the amounts prescribed for the treatment of streptococcal pharyngitis) should be administered to patients with more severe or persistent infections. In the absence of microbiologic data, many clinicians use antibiotics that are effective against streptococci and staphylococci. First-generation cephalosporins and semisynthetic penicillins also are effective. Antibiotic therapy probably does help prevent the spread of streptococcal impetigo in family members. In an era when methicillin-resistant *Staphylococcus aureus* are common findings, special care must be exercised when selecting antibiotic therapy.

Whether penicillin or other antibiotic treatment reduces the risk of development of acute nephritis is unclear.[171] One study suggests that penicillin therapy may reduce the risk of this complication occurring in patients with streptococcal sore throat caused by a nephritogenic strain.[151] No definitive proof that penicillin treatment reduces the frequency of acute nephritis after treatment of skin infections exists, however. Clinical experience indicates that patients with cutaneous infections caused by a nephritogenic strain of group A streptococci may develop this complication despite receiving adequate penicillin therapy.[92]

Otitis media or cervical adenitis caused by group A streptococci usually responds to regimens prescribed for treatment of streptococcal sore throat. Patients with peritonsillar abscess require surgical drainage in addition to vigorous parenteral antibiotic therapy. Patients with more serious infections (e.g., mastoiditis, pneumonia, empyema) also should be given intensive systemic therapy. Patients with meningitis, arthritis, or osteomyelitis require high-dose intravenous penicillin administered for a long time (see Chapters 37 and 61). Patients with streptococcal TSS and patients with necrotizing fasciitis may be treated with parenteral penicillin, but more recent evidence suggests that clindamycin combined with penicillin has advantages.[152] In patients allergic to penicillin, clindamycin is an excellent alternative. Because of cross-reactions with penicillin, the cephalosporins always should be used cautiously in penicillin-allergic patients, especially in patients who have had immediate-type reactions.

PREVENTION

Antimicrobial agents have been helpful in controlling group A streptococcal infections and their sequelae, but they do not provide an encompassing solution for this group of diseases, either in industrialized countries or in the developing world—hence the "resurgence" of rheumatic fever and the appearance of streptococcal TSS in the United States during the 1980s and 1990s. Penicillin's greatest impact has been on the prevention of recurrences of rheumatic fever (see Chapter 35).[18] Prevention of first attacks of rheumatic fever is a problem of greater dimensions because it involves detection, diagnosis, and appropriate treatment in the general population. One cost-effective program can be developed from well-conceived secondary prevention programs in defined rheumatic patients and perhaps from primary prevention programs in school-aged children, especially programs in socially and economically disadvantaged populations.[127]

The prevention of spread by isolation, limiting the density of the population, and antibiotic treatment of known cases is discussed in the section on transmission (see earlier). Mass penicillin prophylaxis has been used in epidemics with a well-defined streptococcal etiology,[24] but in actual practice, the epidemic often is subsiding by the time a large-scale prophylactic effort can be mounted. Intramuscular benzathine penicillin G is very effective for this purpose.[24] The dose is the same as recommended for treating streptococcal pharyngitis. In populations in which streptococcal infections occur at epidemic or near-epidemic levels over a long period of time (e.g., certain military populations), it may be necessary to repeat the injections of benzathine penicillin at monthly intervals and to administer them to all new arrivals.

Although guidelines for management of contacts of patients with severe streptococcal infections are available, and routine surveillance cultures among family members and close contacts are not recommended universally,[132] this approach remains controversial because of documented secondary cases in families.[136] In the family studies carried out several decades ago, researchers found that approximately 25 percent of family contacts harbored the organisms in families where an index case was identified.[49] Because of documented instances in which secondary cases have occurred, some clinicians choose to culture close contacts and to use long-acting benzathine penicillin, long-acting benzathine penicillin plus rifampin, or clindamycin to treat individuals who are positive for group A streptococci. The effectiveness of such regimens has not been studied; contacts need to be monitored closely even after being treated.

The question of the possible advantages of tonsillectomy for the prevention of streptococcal infections and their sequelae also has not been settled by well-controlled studies. Available information indicates that tonsillectomy may reduce the frequency of clinically apparent streptococcal infections,[128] perhaps rendering it less likely that these patients receive appropriate treatment.[33] One study indicates, however, that recurrences are more frequent in individuals who have had rheumatic fever and who have large tonsils.[58]

The inability of antibiotics to influence significantly the epidemiology of group A streptococcal infections and their sequelae consistently and favorably is reflected by the concentration of sequelae occurring more recently in middle-class populations with ready access to medical care.[160] Control measures would be much more effective if a group A streptococcal vaccine were available. Several different approaches to streptococcal vaccines that are being investigated include a multivalent, type-specific vaccine based on M-protein type, a vaccine based on conserved regions of the M-protein that are present in all M-protein types, and a third group of candidate vaccines that are based on immunity to extracellular or somatic antigens of the organism not associated with M protein. Early studies in animals have shown immunogenicity in several of these candidate vaccines, and some vaccines based on type-specific immunity have undergone early clinical trials in humans. Although one cannot make a prediction with certainty, the availability of a cost-effective group A streptococcal vaccine to the general public still does not seem imminent. Large-scale clinical trials in different geographic areas and among different populations are required ultimately to determine safety and efficacy.

GROUP C AND GROUP G STREPTOCOCCAL INFECTIONS

ORGANISMS

The characterization of beta-hemolytic streptococci on the basis of group-specific carbohydrate antigens is complicated by the presence of similar antigens among streptococci that, on the basis of biochemical and genetic testing, have been shown to be different species. Organisms that possess either the group C or group G Lancefield antigens can be divided into groups based on colony size. The strains that produce small or minute colonies (<0.5 mm in diameter) have been placed in the *Streptococcus anginosus* group (classified as *Streptococcus milleri* by British taxonomists). Although these small-colony-forming strains of group C and group G streptococci may produce human infections, with abscesses being the most common form, they also are found as commensals and have considerably less pathogenic potential than do the large-colony-forming group C and group G streptococci. Despite the existence of these groupable, beta-hemolytic strains, members of the *S. anginosus* species group are considered to be viridans group streptococci, most of which display alpha-hemolytic or nonhemolytic reactions.

In contrast, the strains that produce large-sized colonies (≥5 mm in diameter) have been referred to as true or large-colony-forming group C or group G streptococci, depending on the nature of their carbohydrate antigen. The heterogeneity of large-colony streptococci with the Lancefield group C or group G polysaccharides has produced considerable confusion, however. The taxonomic classification of these streptococci still is unsettled, and more changes are likely to occur before a universally accepted scheme is established; however, at least three species

have been found in human infections: *Streptococcus dysgalactiae* subsp. *equisimilis*, *Streptococcus equi* subsp. *zooepidemicus*, and *Streptococcus canis*.[54,137,140]

Most group C streptococci are beta-hemolytic on blood agar plates, but all types of hemolysis have been observed. Group C streptococci are aerobic, facultatively anaerobic, coprophilic, and catalase-negative organisms. Rhamnose-*N*-acetylgalactosamine is the group C antigenic determinant in the cell wall. Traditionally, four species possessing this determinant have been differentiated on the basis of their ability to ferment various carbohydrates: *S. equisimilis*, *S. zooepidemicus*, *S. equi*, and *S. dysgalactiae*. More recent genetic studies have led, however, to the reclassification of group C streptococci into two species— *S. dysgalactiae* and *S. equi*—each with two subspecies. Although most group C streptococci are resistant to bacitracin, at least a third (in one study, 62%) of group C streptococci are bacitracin-sensitive.[7]

S. dysgalactiae subsp. *equisimilis* is the species of group C streptococci and group G streptococci that most often colonizes and causes infections in humans.[54] The actual frequency is unknown, however, because clinical laboratories do not perform phenotypic tests on group C or group G streptococcal isolates other than the hemolytic reaction and the Lancefield group determinations. *S. dysgalactiae* subsp. *equisimilis* has been isolated from the nose, throat, and genital tract of asymptomatic children and adults and from the umbilicus of asymptomatic newborns. This species produces streptokinase and streptolysin O, and infection may elicit an antibody response to these extracellular antigens similar to that seen with a group A streptococcal infection.

S. dysgalactiae subsp. *equisimilis* are pyogenic streptococci that are similar to *S. pyogenes* with respect to some virulence traits. They express homologues of the M virulence protein of *S. pyogenes* that are antiphagocytic (encoded by the *emm* gene), and some strains contain superantigen genes first characterized in *S. pyogenes*.[111,129] The *emm* genes of *S. dysgalactiae* subsp. *equisimilis* isolates with either the group C or the group G Lancefield antigen can be used for sequence-based typing. Pulsed-field gel electrophoresis also can be used to identify specific stains. This organism can cause infections in a variety of domestic animals (e.g., horses, cattle, pigs, chickens). *S. dysgalactiae* subsp. *dysgalactiae* has not been found to cause human infections but does cause a serious mastitis in cows and a suppurative polyarthritis in lambs.

S. equi subsp. *zooepidemicus* possess the group C Lancefield antigen and can cause significant, often epidemic, infections in domestic animals (e.g., horses, cattle, pigs, sheep), but it is an uncommon pathogen in humans. Most human infections have been associated with consumption of homemade cheese or unpasteurized cow's milk. *S. equi* subsp. *equi* possess the group C Lancefield antigen and have not been found to cause human infections but do cause a serious and highly contagious respiratory disease in horses, known as *strangles*.

Most group G streptococci are beta-hemolytic on blood agar plates. L-rhamnose is the group G antigenic determinant in the cell wall. Most of the group G streptococci isolated from human infections are thought to be *S. dysgalactiae* subsp. *equisimilis*. *S. canis* with the group G Lancefield antigen also cause infections in humans.

Several schemes for typing group G streptococci have been described based on biochemical properties or bacteriocin typing. Although no association between particular types and infections in humans has been identified, these schemes have been useful in distinguishing human from animal strains and in epidemiologic investigations. T-typing and M-typing schemes similar to those used for group A streptococci also have been devised for group G streptococci. Newer methods, such as *emm*-typing, pulsed-field gel electrophoresis, and multilocus enzyme electrophoresis, also are being used to type specific strains of group G streptococci.[16,129] Although most group G streptococci are resistant to bacitracin, various reports have determined that 8 to 67 percent of group G streptococci are bacitracin-sensitive.[140]

In addition to M protein, human isolates of group G streptococci share other virulence factors with group A streptococci, such as a streptokinase, a hyaluronidase, and a C5a peptidase. Group G streptococci also produce a streptolysin that is similar antigenically to the streptolysin O produced by group A streptococci. Patients with group G streptococcal infections may show a significant increase in levels of antistreptolysin O titers.

EPIDEMIOLOGY

Group C streptococci are an uncommon cause of human infections but more commonly are pathogenic in animals. Humans infected with this organism often have had some animal contact. Group C and group G streptococci often can be part of the normal human flora of the nasopharynx, skin, or genital tract. Group C streptococci also can be cultured from the umbilicus of asymptomatic newborns and from routine puerperal vaginal cultures. Group G streptococci also can be cultured from the gastrointestinal tract. The low virulence of group C and group G streptococci is indicated by the fact that most humans infected with either of these organisms have some underlying medical disorder (e.g., diabetes mellitus, malignancy, alcohol abuse, immunosuppression).[29,106]

CLINICAL MANIFESTATIONS

The clinical features of group C and group G streptococcal pharyngitis are similar to those of group A streptococcal pharyngitis and include fever, mild to moderate sore throat, pharyngeal exudate, and cervical adenitis.[110] In temperate climates, 1 to 18 percent of asymptomatic individuals have been reported to harbor group C streptococci in the upper respiratory tract. The proportion of carriers among individuals living in the tropics is even greater.[69,126] Such carrier rates render establishing the etiologic role of group C streptococci in acute pharyngitis difficult. Several earlier studies compared the isolation rates of group C streptococci from patients with acute pharyngitis with rates in asymptomatic controls; the results were contradictory.[7,35] Several more recent investigations have established a strong epidemiologic association between group C streptococci and endemic acute pharyngitis. In two investigations, group C streptococci were isolated significantly more often from college students with acute pharyngitis than from asymptomatic controls.[157,158] In the other investigation, group C streptococci were isolated significantly more often from adults who came to an emergency department with acute pharyngitis (6%) than from asymptomatic controls (1.4%).[121]

In addition to endemic pharyngitis, group C streptococci can cause epidemic food-borne pharyngitis after contaminated products, such as unpasteurized cow's milk, have been ingested. Epidemics have been reported from Great Britain, Romania, the United States, and Israel.[7,35] In one report of a milk-borne epidemic of pharyngitis caused by *S. equi* subsp. *zooepidemicus*, approximately one third of the patients developed signs of acute glomerulonephritis.[51] This outbreak was related to the consumption of unpasteurized milk from cattle with mastitis. No cases of acute rheumatic fever occurred. More recently, a large outbreak of acute glomerulonephritis in Brazil was attributed to the consumption of unpasteurized cheese containing *S. equi* subsp. *zooepidemicus*.[10] Family outbreaks of group C streptococcal pharyngitis and an outbreak in a residential school for boys also have been described.

Group C streptococci also have been reported as the cause of numerous other uncommon infections, including skin and soft tissue infections, septic arthritis, osteomyelitis, pneumonitis, infective endocarditis, bacteremia and septicemia, meningitis, epiglottitis, pericarditis, urinary tract infections, and sinusitis. These organisms also have been associated with epidemic and nonepidemic cases of puerperal sepsis and endometritis.[81] Several reports have suggested that an association exists between group C streptococci and reactive arthritis and a toxic shock–like syndrome.[54,79]

Some studies have reported that 1 to 23 percent of asymptomatic individuals may carry group G streptococci in their upper respiratory tract. As with group C streptococci, the carrier rates of group G streptococci seem to be even higher in the tropics.[69,126] Such carrier rates also render establishing the etiologic role of group G streptococci in acute pharyngitis difficult. Several studies have been performed comparing the isolation rates of group G streptococci from patients with acute pharyngitis with rates from asymptomatic controls. The results of these studies showed little difference in the isolation rates, suggesting that group G streptococci may not play an important role in endemic acute pharyngitis. Few of these studies were adequately controlled, prospective investigations, however, and in many of them, the incidence of group G streptococci in the symptomatic group was so low as to preclude any possibility of showing a statistically significant difference.

Support for an etiologic role of group G streptococci in acute pharyngitis comes primarily from anecdotes, small case clusters, and a few large outbreaks, most of which were food-borne. To date, several food-borne outbreaks of group G streptococcal pharyngitis, all of which occurred in semiclosed populations, including one outbreak at a college cafeteria, have been reported.[116] In the first reported respiratory outbreak of group G streptococcal pharyngitis in the United States, McCue[120] described 68 cases of acute pharyngitis on a college campus seen during a 9-day period in 1981. The possibility of food-borne spread could not be eliminated completely but seemed unlikely, and airborne droplet transmission seemed to be the most likely mechanism of spread.

Despite the evidence supporting the etiologic role of group G streptococci in epidemic pharyngitis, the role of group G streptococci in acute, endemic pharyngitis remains unclear. Previous outbreaks of group G streptococcal pharyngitis had been reported in college-age or older patients, and all had occurred in semiclosed communities. A community-wide, respiratory outbreak of group G streptococcal pharyngitis in a pediatric population was described, however.[64] During a 6-month period, group G streptococci were isolated from 56 of 222 (25%) consecutive children with acute pharyngitis seen at a private pediatric office. Results of DNA fingerprinting of the group G streptococcal isolates suggested that 75 percent of them were the same strain. The patients with group G streptococcal pharyngitis were comparable to patients with group A streptococcal pharyngitis with respect to clinical findings, antistreptolysin O titer response, and clinical response to antibiotic therapy. Patients with group G streptococci were significantly older, however. The findings suggested that antibiotic therapy may have an impact on the clinical course of group G streptococcal pharyngitis. These findings lend support to the belief that group G streptococci may be a more important cause of acute, endemic pharyngitis than was recognized previously.

The actual role of group C and group G streptococci in acute pharyngitis may be underestimated for several reasons. Anaerobic incubation increases the yield of these organisms, but most clinicians do not use anaerobic incubation for throat cultures routinely.[142] Because clinicians generally disregard beta-hemolytic streptococci that are bacitracin-resistant (and most strains of group C and group G streptococci are bacitracin-resistant), many group C and group G streptococci would be missed.

Acute rheumatic fever has not been described as a complication of either group C or group G streptococcal pharyngitis, and although there have been reports attempting to link acute glomerulonephritis with group G streptococcal pharyngitis, the evidence is anecdotal, and a causal relationship has not been established.[130,137] Although acute glomerulonephritis has been reported as a complication of group C streptococcal pharyngitis, it is extremely unusual.[10,51,123] The primary reason to identify either group C or group G streptococci as the etiologic agent of acute pharyngitis is to initiate antibiotic therapy that may reduce the clinical impact of the illness. No convincing evidence as yet has emerged from controlled studies of a clinical response to antibiotic therapy in patients with acute pharyngitis and either group C or group G streptococci isolated from the upper respiratory tract.

Group G streptococci also have been reported to be an uncommon cause of puerperal sepsis, and they occasionally may cause a neonatal infection that is clinically very similar to early-onset group B streptococcal infections. Other infections occasionally caused by group G streptococci include bacteremia, endocarditis, septic arthritis, osteomyelitis, pneumonia, erysipelas and other skin and soft tissue infections, and meningitis.[55,81] Group G streptococci also have been associated with a toxic shock–like syndrome.[54,162]

TREATMENT

Penicillin is the antibiotic of choice for treating infections caused by either group C or group G streptococci.[139] Some strains of group C and group G streptococci have been shown to be tolerant to penicillin in laboratory studies, but the clinical significance of this finding is unknown.[123,138] Synergism in producing in vitro killing of group C and group G streptococci has been shown with gentamicin and various β-lactam antibiotics, but no controlled trials have been performed to establish the clinical significance of this finding. Group C and group G streptococci also are susceptible to most β-lactam antibiotics and to macrolides, vancomycin, clindamycin, and chloramphenicol. Pharyngitis usually is treated in a manner similar to that for group A streptococcal upper respiratory infections. More severe infection requires parenteral therapy.

REFERENCES

1. Allan, A. M., Taplin, D., and Twigg, L.: Cutaneous streptococcal infections in Vietnam. Arch. Dermatol. 104:271-280, 1971.
2. Alpert, J. J., Pickering, M. R., and Warren, R. J.: Failure to isolate streptococci from children under the age of 3 years with exudative tonsillitis. Pediatrics 38:663-666, 1966.
3. Aly, R., Maibach, H. I., Shinefield, H. R., et al.: Survival of pathogenic microorganisms on human skin. J. Invest. Dermatol. 58:205-210, 1972.
4. Amren, D. P.: Unusual forms of streptococcal disease. In Wannamaker, L. W., and Matsen, J. M. (eds.): Streptococci and Streptococcal Diseases: Recognition, Understanding, and Management. New York, Academic Press, 1972, pp. 545-556.
5. Anonymous: Evaluation of the Streptozyme test for streptococcal antibodies. Bull. W. H. O. 64:504, 1986.
6. Anthony, B. F., Kaplan, E. L., Wannamaker, L. W., et al.: The dynamics of streptococcal infections in a defined population of children: Serotypes associated with skin and respiratory infections. Am. J. Epidemiol. 104:652-666, 1976.
7. Arditi, M., Shulman, S. T., Davis, A. T., et al.: Group C beta-hemolytic streptococcal infections in children: Nine pediatric cases and review. Rev. Infect. Dis. 11:34-45, 1989.
8. Asboe-Hansen, G.: Psoriasis in childhood. In Farber, E. M., and Cox, A. J. (eds.): Psoriasis. Proceedings of the International Symposium, Stanford University. Stanford, Stanford University Press, 1971, pp. 53-59.
9. Ayoub, E. M.: Cross-reacting antibodies in the pathogenesis of rheumatic myocardial and valvular disease. In Wannamaker, L. W., and Matsen, J. M.

(eds.): Streptococci and Streptococcal Diseases: Recognition, Understanding, and Management. New York, Academic Press, 1972, pp. 451-464.
10. Balter, S., Benin, A., Pinto, W. L., et al.: Epidemic nephritis in Nova Serrana, Brazil. Lancet 355:1776-1780, 2000.
11. Bassett, D. C. J.: Hippelates flies and acute nephritis. Lancet 1:503, 1967.
12. Beachey, E. H., and Ofek, I.: Epithelial cell binding of group A streptococci by lipoteichoic acid on fimbriae denuded of M protein. J. Exp. Med. 143:759-771, 1976.
13. Beachey, E. H., Seyer, J. M., Dale, J. B., et al.: Type-specific protective immunity evoked by synthetic peptide of Streptococcus pyogenes M protein. Nature 292:457-459, 1981.
14. Beachey, E. H., and Stollerman, G. H.: Mediation of cytotoxic effects of streptococcal M protein by non-type-specific antibody in human sera. J. Clin. Invest. 52:2563-2570, 1973.
15. Bernheimer, A. W.: Hemolysins of streptococci: Characterization and effects on biological membranes. In Wannamaker, L. W., and Matsen, J. M. (eds.): Streptococci and Streptococcal Diseases: Recognition, Understanding, and Management. New York, Academic Press, 1972, pp. 19-31.
16. Bert, F., Branger, C., and Lambert-Zechovsky, N.: Pulsed-field gel electrophoresis is more discriminating than multilocus enzyme electrophoresis and random amplified polymorphic DNA analysis for typing pyogenic streptococci. Curr. Microbiol. 34:226-229, 1997.
17. Biberstein, E. L., Brown, C., and Smith, T.: Serogroups and biotypes among beta-hemolytic streptococci of canine origin. J. Clin. Microbiol. 11:558-561, 1980.
18. Bisno, A. L.: Therapeutic strategies for the prevention of rheumatic fever. Ann. Intern. Med. 86:494-496, 1977.
19. Bisno, A. L.: Acute pharyngitis: Etiology and diagnosis. Pediatrics 97:949-954, 1996.
20. Bisno, A. L., Gerber, M. A., Gwaltney, J. M., Jr., et al.: Group A streptococcal pharyngitis: Diagnosis and management. A Practice Guideline. Infectious Diseases Society of America. Clin. Infect. Dis. 35:113-125, 2002.
21. Bisno, A. L., and Stollerman, G. H.: Streptococcal antibodies in the diagnosis of rheumatic fever. In Cohen, A. S. (ed.): Laboratory Diagnostic Procedures in the Rheumatic Diseases. Boston, Little, Brown, 1975, pp. 207-263.
22. Breiman, R. F., David, J. P., Facklam, R. R., et al.: Defining the group A streptococcal TSS: Rationale and consensus definition. J. A. M. A. 269:390-391, 1993.
23. Brook, I.: The role of beta-lactamase-producing bacteria in the persistence of streptococcal tonsillar infection. Rev. Infect. Dis. 6:601-607, 1984.
24. Brundage, J. F., Gunzenhauser, J. D., Longfield, J. N., et al.: Epidemiology and control of acute respiratory diseases with emphasis on group A beta-hemolytic streptococcus: A decade of U.S. Army experience. Pediatrics 97:964-970, 1996.
25. Bullowa, J. G. M., and Wishik, S. M.: Complications of varicella: Their occurrence among 2,534 patients. Am. J. Dis. Child. 49:923-926, 1935.
26. Calandra, G. B., Whitt, R. S., and Cole, R. M.: Relationship of cellular potential hemolysin in group A streptococci to extracellular streptolysin S. Infect. Immun. 13:813-817, 1976.
27. Campo, R. E., Schultz, D. R., and Bisno, A. L.: M proteins of group G streptococci: Mechanisms of resistance to phagocytosis. J. Infect. Dis. 171:601-606, 1995.
28. Carapetis, J. R., Currie, B. J., and Kaplan, E. L.: The epidemiology and prevention of group A streptococcal infections: Acute respiratory tract infections, skin infections and their sequelae at the close of the twentieth century. Clin. Infect. Dis. 28:205-210, 1999.
29. Carmeli, Y., Schapiro, J. M., Neeman, D., et al.: Streptococcal group C bacteremia: Survey in Israel and analytic review. Arch. Intern. Med. 155:1170-1176, 1996.
30. Casey, J. R., and Pichichero, M. E.: Meta-analysis of cephalosporins versus penicillin for treatment of group A streptococcal tonsillopharyngitis in adults. Clin. Infect. Dis. 38:1526-1534, 2004.
31. Casey, J. R., and Pichichero, M. E.: Meta-analysis of cephalosporin versus penicillin treatment of group A streptococci. Pediatrics 113:866-882, 2004.
32. Catanzaro, F. J., Rammelkamp, C. H., Jr., and Chamovitz, R.: Prevention of rheumatic fever by treatment of streptococcal infections, II: Factors responsible for failures. N. Engl. J. Med. 259:51-57, 1958.
33. Chamovitz, R., Rammelkamp, C. H., Jr., Wannamaker, L. W., et al.: The effect of tonsillectomy on the incidence of streptococcal respiratory disease and its complications. Pediatrics 26:355-367, 1960.
34. Chen, C. C., and Clearly, P. P.: Complete nucleotide sequence of the streptococcal C5a peptidase gene of Streptococcus pyogenes. J. Biol. Chem. 265:3161-3167, 1990.
35. Cimolai, N., Elford, R. W., Bryan, L., et al.: Do the beta-hemolytic non-group A streptococci cause pharyngitis? Rev. Infect. Dis. 10:587-601, 1988.
36. Collins, C. M., Kimura, A., and Bisno, A. L.: Group G streptococcal M protein exhibits structural features analogous to those of class I M protein of group A streptococci. Infect. Immun. 60:3689-3696, 1992.
37. Coonan, K. M., and Kaplan, E. L.: In vitro susceptibility of recent North American group A streptococcal isolates to eleven oral antibiotics. Pediatr. Infect. Dis. J. 13:630-635, 1994.
38. Crawford, S. E., and Riddler, J. G.: Purpura fulminans. Am. J. Dis. Child. 97:197-201, 1959.
39. Crowder, H. R., Dorn, C. R., and Smith, R. E.: Group A Streptococcus in pets and group A streptococcal disease in man. Int. J. Zoonoses 5:45-54, 1978.

40. Crowe, C. C., Sanders, W. E., Jr., and Longley, S.: Bacterial interference, II: Role of the normal throat flora in prevention of colonization by group A *Streptococcus*. J. Infect. Dis. *128*:527-532, 1973.
41. Cunningham, M. W., and Beachey, E. H.: Peptic digestion of streptococcal M protein, I: Effect of digestion at suboptimal pH upon the biological and immunochemical properties of purified M protein extracts. Infect. Immun. *9*:244-248, 1974.
42. Daikos, G., and Weinstein, L.: Streptococci bacteriostatic antibody in patients treated with penicillin. Proc. Soc. Exp. Biol. Med. *78*:160-163, 1951.
43. Dajani, A. S., Bisno, A. L., Chung, K. J., et al.: Prevention of rheumatic fever: A statement for health professionals by the Committee on Rheumatic Fever, Endocarditis and Kawasaki Disease of the Council on Cardiovascular Disease in the Young, the American Heart Association. Pediatr. Infect. Dis. J. *8*:263-266, 1989.
44. Dajani, A. S., Ferrieri, P., and Wannamaker, L. W.: Endemic superficial pyoderma in children. Arch. Dermatol. *108*:517-522, 1973.
45. Dajani, A. S., Garcia, R. E., and Wolinsky, E.: Etiology of cervical lymphadenitis in children. N. Engl. J. Med. *268*:1329-1333, 1963.
46. De Malmanche, S. A., and Martin, D. R.: Protective immunity to the group A streptococcus may be only strain specific. Med. Microbiol. Immunol. *183*:299-306, 1994.
47. Denny, F. W., Jr., Perry, W. D., and Wannamaker, L. W.: Type-specific streptococcal antibody. J. Clin. Invest. *36*:1092-1100, 1957.
48. Dillon, H. C., Jr.: Impetigo contagiosa: Suppurative and non-suppurative complications, I: Clinical, bacteriologic, and epidemiologic characteristics of impetigo. Am. J. Dis. Child. *115*:530-541, 1968.
49. Dingle, J. H., Badger, G. F., and Jordan, W. S., Jr. (eds.): Illness in the Home. Cleveland, The Press of Western Reserve University, 1964.
50. Dixon, J. M., and Lipinski, A. E.: Infections with beta-hemolytic streptococcus resistant to lincomycin and erythromycin and observations on zonal-pattern resistance to lincomycin. J. Infect. Dis. *130*:351-356, 1974.
51. Duca, E., Teodorovici, G., Radu, C., et al.: A new nephritogenic streptococcus. J. Hyg. *67*:691-698, 1969.
52. Dudding, B., Humphrey, G. B., and Nesbit, M. E.: Beta-hemolytic streptococcal septicemias in childhood leukemia. Pediatrics *43*:359-364, 1969.
53. Eickhoff, T. C., and Finland, M.: In vitro susceptibility of group A beta hemolytic streptococci to 18 antibiotics. Am. J. Med. Sci., *249*:261-268, 1965.
54. Ekelund, K., Skinhaj, P., Madsen, J., and Konradsen, H. B.: Invasive group A, B, C and G streptococcal infections in Denmark 1999-2002: Epidemiological and clinical aspects. Clin. Microbiol. Infect. *11*:569-576, 2005.
55. Eriksson, B., Jorup-Ronstrom, C., Karkkonen, K., et al.: Erysipelas: Clinical and bacteriologic spectrum and serological aspects. Clin. Infect. Dis. *23*:1091-1098, 1996.
56. Facklam, R.: What happened to the streptococci: Overview of taxonomic and nomenclature changes. Clin. Microbiol. Rev. *15*:613-630, 2002.
57. Facklam, R. F., Martin, D. R., Lovgren, M., et al.: Extension of the Lancefield classification for group A streptococci by addition of 22 new M protein gene sequence types from clinical isolates: *emm* 103 to *emm* 124. Clin. Infect. Dis. *34*:28-38, 2002.
58. Feinstein, A. R., and Levitt, M.: The role of tonsils in predisposing to streptococcal infections and recurrences of rheumatic fever. N. Engl. J. Med. *282*:285-291, 1970.
59. Ferrieri, P., Dajani, A. S., Wannamaker, L. W., et al.: Natural history of impetigo, I: Site sequence of acquisition and familial patterns of spread of cutaneous streptococci. J. Clin. Invest. *51*:2851-2862, 1972.
60. Fischetti, V. A.: Streptococcal M protein: molecular design and biological behavior. Clin. Microbiol. Rev. *2*:285, 1989.
61. Flodstrom, A., and Hallander, H. O.: Microbiological aspects on peritonsillar abscesses. Scand. J. Infect. Dis. *8*:157-160, 1976.
62. Freimer, E. H.: Studies of L forms and protoplasts of group A streptococci, II: Chemical and immunological properties of the cell membrane. J. Exp. Med. *117*:377-399, 1963.
63. Gerber, M. A., Deleo, K., Randolph, M. F., et al.: Lack of impact of early antibiotic therapy for streptococcal pharyngitis on recurrence rates. J. Pediatr. *117*:853-858, 1990.
64. Gerber, M. A., Randolph, M. F., Martin, N. J., et al.: Community-wide outbreak of group G streptococcal pharyngitis. Pediatrics *87*:598-603, 1991.
65. Ginsburg, I., and Sela, M. N.: The role of leukocytes and their hydrolases in the persistence, degradation, and transport of bacterial constituents in tissues: Relation to chronic inflammatory processes in staphylococcal, streptococcal, and mycobacterial infections and in chronic periodontal disease. C. R. C. Crit. Rev. Microbiol. *4*:249-322, 1976.
66. Graybill, J. R., Pierson, D. N., and Charache, P.: Tissue antibiotic penetration in streptococcal gangrene. Johns Hopkins Med. J. *133*:45-50, 1973.
67. Greenberg, L. J., Gray, E. D., and Yunis, E. J.: Association of HL-A 5 and immune responsiveness in vitro to streptococcal antigens. J. Exp. Med. *141*:935-943, 1975.
68. Hable, K. A., Horstmeier, C., Wold, A., et al.: Hemolytic streptococcemia: Bacteriologic and clinical: Group A study of 44 cases. Mayo Clin. Proc. *48*:336-339, 1973.
69. Haidan, A., Talay, S. R., Rohde, M., et al.: Pharyngeal carriage of group C and group G streptococci and acute rheumatic fever in an Aboriginal population. Lancet *356*:1167-1169, 2000.
70. Hall, J. E., and Silverstein, E. A.: Acute hematogenous osteomyelitis. Pediatrics *31*:1033-1038, 1963.
71. Haltalin, K. C., and Nelson, J. D.: Hand-foot syndrome due to streptococcal infection. Am. J. Dis. Child. *109*:156-159, 1965.
72. Hays, G. C., and Mullard, J. E.: Blistering distal dactylitis: A clinically recognizable streptococcal infection. Pediatrics *56*:129-131, 1975.
73. Henderson, R. J., Bares, G. J., Rambin, E. D., et al.: Typing and plasmid analysis of clinical isolates of group A beta hemolytic streptococcus with increased resistance to erythromycin. Clin. Res. *38*:55A, 1990.
74. Hill, H. R., Zimmerman, R. A., Reid, G. V., et al.: Food-borne epidemic of streptococcal pharyngitis at the United States Air Force Academy. N. Engl. J. Med. *280*:917-921, 1969.
75. Hosein, B., McCarty, M., and Fischetti, V. A.: Amino acid sequence and physicochemical similarities between streptococcal M protein and mammalian tropomyosin. Proc. Natl. Acad. Sci. U. S. A. *76*:3765-3768, 1976.
76. Huskins, W. C., and Kaplan, E. L.: Inhibitory substances produced by *Streptococcus salivarius* and colonization of the upper respiratory tract with group A streptococci. Epidemiol. Infect. *102*:401-412, 1989.
77. James, L., and McFarland, R. B.: An epidemic of pharyngitis due to a non-hemolytic group A *Streptococcus* at Lowry Air Force Base. N. Engl. J. Med. *284*:750-752, 1971.
78. Janeff, J., Janeff, D., Taranta, A., et al.: A screening test for streptococcal antibodies. Lab. Med. *2*:38-40, 1971.
79. Jansen, T. L., Janssen, M., and de Jong, A. J.: Reactive arthritis associated with group C and group G beta-hemolytic streptococci. J. Rheumatol. *25*:1126-1130, 1998.
80. Jewett, J. F.: Coagulopathy syndrome due to streptococci. N. Engl. J. Med. *289*:43-44, 1973.
81. Johnson, C. C., and Tunkel, A. R.: Viridans streptococci and groups C and G streptococci. *In* Mandell, G. L., Bennett, J. E., and Dolin, R. (eds.): Principles and Practice of Infectious Diseases. 5th ed. New York, Churchill Livingstone, 2000, pp. 2167-2183.
82. Johnson, D. R., and Kaplan, E. L.: A review of the correlation of T-agglutination patterns and M-protein typing and opacity factor production in the identification of group A streptococci. J. Med. Microbiol. *38*:311-315, 1993.
83. Johnson, D. R., and Kaplan, E. L.: False positive rapid antigen detection tests: Reduced specificity in the absence of group A streptococci in the upper respiratory tract. J. Infect. Dis. *183*:1135-1137, 2001.
84. Johnson, D. R., Kaplan, E. L., and Ferrieri, P.: Pharyngitis-associated M-12 group A *Streptococcus* satellite strain: Association with *Neisseria subflava*. Pediatr. Infect. Dis. J. *8*:800-802, 1989.
85. Johnson, D. R., and Kaplan, E. L. (World Health Organization Collaborating Center for Reference and Research on Streptococci; Minneapolis, MN); and Sramek, J., Motlova, J., Bicova, R., et al. (World Health Organization Collaborating Center for Reference and Research on Streptococci; Prague, Czech Republic): Laboratory Diagnosis of Group A Streptococcal Infections: A Laboratory Manual. Geneva, Switzerland, World Health Organization, 1996.
86. Kaplan, E. L.: Unresolved problems in diagnosis and epidemiology of streptococcal infection. *In* Wannamaker, L. W., and Matsen, J. M. (eds.): Streptococci and Streptococcal Diseases: Recognition, Understanding, and Management. New York, Academic Press, 1972, pp. 557-570.
87. Kaplan, E. L.: The group A streptococcal upper respiratory tract carrier state: An enigma. J. Pediatr. *97*:337-345, 1980.
88. Kaplan, E. L.: Group A streptococcal carriers and contacts: (When) is retreatment necessary? *In* Shulman, S. (ed.): Management of Pharyngitis in an Era of Declining Rheumatic Fever. Columbus, OH, Ross Conference of Pediatric Research, 1984, p. 92.
89. Kaplan, E. L.: Benzathine penicillin G for treatment of group A streptococcal pharyngitis: A reappraisal in 1985. Pediatr. Infect. Dis. *4*:592-596, 1985.
90. Kaplan, E. L.: The rapid identification of group A beta-hemolytic streptococci in the upper respiratory tract: Current status. Pediatr. Clin. North Am. *35*:535-542, 1988.
91. Kaplan, E. L.: Global assessment of rheumatic fever and rheumatic heart disease at the close of the century: Influences and dynamics of populations and pathogens: A failure to realize prevention? T. Duckett Jones Memorial Lecture. Circulation *88*:1964-1972, 1993.
92. Kaplan, E. L., Anthony, B. F., Chapman, S. S., et al.: Epidemic acute glomerulonephritis associated with type 49 streptococcal pyoderma, I: Clinical and laboratory findings. Am. J. Med. *48*:9-27, 1970.
93. Kaplan, E. L., Anthony, B. F., Chapman, S. S., et al.: The influence of the site of infection on the immune response to group A streptococci. J. Clin. Invest. *49*:1405-1414, 1970.
94. Kaplan, E. L., Chhatwal, G. S., and Rohde, M.: Reduced ability of penicillin to eradicate ingested group A streptococci from epithelial cells: Clinical and pathogenetic implications. Clin. Infect. Dis. *43*:1398-1406, 2006.
95. Kaplan, E. L., and Johnson, D. R.: Unexplained reduced efficacy of oral penicillin V and intramuscular benzathine penicillin G in the eradication of group A streptococci from children with acute pharyngitis. Pediatrics *108*:1180-1186, 2001.
96. Kaplan, E. L., Johnson, D. R., Nanthapisud, P., et al.: A comparison of group A streptococcal serotypes isolated from the upper respiratory tract in the USA and Thailand: Implications. Bull. W. H. O. *70*:433-437, 1992.
97. Kaplan, E. L., and Kunde, C.: Quantitative evaluation of variation in composition of the streptozyme agglutination reagent for detection of antibodies to group A streptococcal extracellular antigens. J. Clin. Microbiol. *14*:678-680, 1981.

98. Kaplan, E. L., Reid, H. F., Johnson, D. R., et al.: Rapid antigen detection in the diagnosis of group A streptococcal pyoderma: Influence of a "learning curve effect" on sensitivity and specificity. Pediatr. Infect. Dis. J. 8:591-593, 1989.

99. Kaplan, E. L., Rothermel, C. D., and Johnson, D. R.: Antistreptolysin O and anti-deoxyribonuclease B titers: Normal values for children ages 2-12 in the United States. Pediatrics 101:86-88, 1998.

100. Kaplan, E. L., Top, F. H., Jr., Dudding, B. A., et al.: Diagnosis of streptococcal pharyngitis: Differentiation of active infection from the carrier state in the symptomatic child. J. Infect. Dis. 123:490-501, 1971.

101. Kaplan, E. L., and Wannamaker, L. W.: C-reactive protein in streptococcal pharyngitis. Pediatrics 60:28-32, 1977.

102. Kim, K. S.: Clinical perspectives on penicillin tolerance. J. Pediatr. 112:509-514, 1988.

103. Kim, Y. B., and Watson, D. W.: Streptococcal exotoxins: Biological and pathological properties. In Wannamaker, L. W., and Matsen, J. M. (eds.): Streptococci and Streptococcal Diseases: Recognition, Understanding, and Management. New York, Academic Press, 1972, pp. 33-50.

104. Kokx, N. P., Comstock, J. A., and Facklam, R. R.: Streptococcal perianal disease in children. Pediatrics 80:659-663, 1987.

105. Krause, R. M., and Rammelkamp, C. H., Jr.: Studies of the carrier state following infection with group A streptococci. J. Clin. Invest. 41:575, 1962.

106. Kristensen, B., and Schonheyder, H. C.: A 13-year survey of bacteraemia due to beta-haemolytic streptococci in a Danish county. J. Med. Microbiol. 43:63-67, 1995.

107. Lancefield, R. C.: Current knowledge of type-specific M antigens of group A streptococci. J. Immunol. 89:307-313, 1962.

108. Lancefield, R. C.: Group A streptococcal infections in animals: Natural and experimental. In Wannamaker, L. W., and Matsen, J. M. (eds.): Streptococci and Streptococcal Diseases: Recognition, Understanding, and Management. New York, Academic Press, 1972, pp. 313-326.

109. LaPenta, D., Rubens, C., Chi, E., and Cleary, P. P.: Group A streptococci efficiently invade human respiratory epithelial cells. Proc. Natl. Acad. Sci. U. S. A. 91:12115-12119, 1994.

110. Lindboek, M., Hoiby, E. A., Lermark, G., et al.: Clinical signs in sore throat platients with large colony variant beta-haemolytic streptococci groups C or G versus group A. Br. J. Gen. Pract. 55:615-619, 2005.

111. Lopardo, H. A., Vidal, P., Sparo, M., et al.: Six month multicenter study of invasive infections due to Streptococcus pyogenes and Streptococcus dysgalactiae subsp. equisimilis in Argentina. J. Clin. Microbiol. 43:802-807, 2005.

112. Macris, M., Hartman, N., Murray, B., et al.: Studies of the continuing susceptibility to penicillin of group A streptococcal strains isolated over a period spanning eight decades. Pediatr. Infect. Dis. J. 17:377-381, 1998.

113. Malke, H., Jacob, H. E., and Storl, K.: Characterization of the antibiotic resistance plasmid ERL1 from Streptococcus pyogenes. Mol. Gen. Genet. 144:333-338, 1976.

114. Markowitz, M., and Kaplan, E. L.: Reappearance of rheumatic fever. In Barness, L. A. (ed.): Advances in Pediatrics. Chicago, Year Book Medical Publishers, 1989, pp. 39-66.

115. Martin, J. M., Green, M., Barbadora, K. A., and Wald, E. R.: Erythromycin-resistant group A streptococci in schoolchildren in Pittsburgh. N. Engl. J. Med. 346:1200-1206, 2002.

116. Martin, N. J., Kaplan, E. L., Gerber, M. A., et al.: Comparison of epidemic and endemic group G streptococci by restriction enzyme analysis. J. Clin. Microbiol. 28:1881-1886, 1990.

117. Matsen, J. M., and Coghlan, C. R.: Antibiotic testing and susceptibility patterns of streptococci. In Wannamaker, L. W., and Matsen, J. M. (eds.): Streptococci and Streptococcal Diseases: Recognition, Understanding, and Management. New York, Academic Press, 1972, pp. 189-204.

118. McCarty, M.: The streptococcal cell wall. Harvey Lectures 65:73-96, 1971.

119. McCarty, M.: Theories of pathogenesis of streptococcal complications. In Wannamaker, L. W., and Matsen, J. M. (eds.): Streptococci and Streptococcal Diseases: Recognition, Understanding, and Management. New York, Academic Press, 1972, pp. 517-526.

120. McCue, J. D.: Group G streptococcal pharyngitis: Analysis of an outbreak at a college. J. A. M. A. 248:1333-1336, 1982.

121. Meier, F. A., Centor, R. M., Graham, L., Jr., et al.: Clinical and microbiological evidence for endemic pharyngitis among adults due to group C streptococci. Arch. Intern. Med. 150:825-829, 1990.

122. Neeman, R., Keller, N., Barzilai, A., et al.: Prevalence of internalization-associated gene, prtF1, among persisting group A streptococcus strains isolated from asymptomatic carriers. Lancet 352:1974-1977, 1998.

123. Nicholson, M. L., Ferdinand, L., Sampson, J. S., et al.: Analysis of immunoreactivity to a Streptococcus equi subsp. zooepidemicus M-like protein to confirm an outbreak of poststreptococcal glomerulonephritis, and sequences of M-like proteins from isolates obtained from different host species. J. Clin. Microbiol. 38:4126-4130, 2000.

124. Ofek, I., Bergner-Rabinowitz, S., and Ginsburg, I.: Oxygen-stable hemolysins of group A streptococci, VII: The relation of the leukotoxic factor to streptolysin S. J. Infect. Dis. 122:517-522, 1970.

125. Ofek, I., Kaplan, O., Bergner-Rabinowitz, S., et al.: Antibody tests in streptococcal pharyngitis: Streptozyme versus conventional methods. Clin. Pediatr. 12:341-344, 1973.

126. Ogunbi, O., Lasi, Q., and Lawal, S. F.: An epidemiological study of beta-hemolytic streptococcal infections in a Nigerian (Lagos) urban population.

In Haverkorn, M. J. (ed.): Streptococcal Disease and the Community. Amsterdam, Excerpta Medica, 1974, pp. 282-284.

127. Pantell, R. H.: Cost-effectiveness of pharyngitis management and prevention of rheumatic fever. Ann. Intern. Med. 86:497-499, 1977.

128. Paradise, J. L.: Etiology and management of pharyngotonsillitis in children: A current review. Ann. Otol. Rhinol. Laryngol. 155:51-57, 1992.

129. Pinho, M. D., Melo-Cristino, J., Rameriz, M.; and the Portuguese Group for the Study of Streptococcal Infections: Clonal relationships between invasive and noninvasive Lancefield group C and group G streptococci and emm-specific differences in invasiveness. J. Clin. Microbiol. 44:841-846, 2006.

130. Poon-King, T., Mohammed, I., Cox, R., et al.: Recurrent epidemic nephritis in South Trinidad. N. Engl. J. Med. 277:728-733, 1967.

131. Powers, G. F., and Boisvert, P. L.: Tuberculosis and streptococcosis. Yale J. Biol. Med. 15:517-530, 1943.

132. Prevention of Invasive Group A Streptococcal Infections Workshop Participants: Prevention of invasive group A streptococcal disease among household contacts of case patients and among postpartum and postsurgical patients. Clin. Infect. Dis. 2002.

133. Rammelkamp, C. H., Jr.: Epidemiology of streptococcal infections. Harvey Lectures 51:113-142, 1957.

134. Randolph, M. F., Gerber, M. A., DeMeo, K. K., et al.: Effect of antibiotic therapy on the clinical course of streptococcal pharyngitis. J. Pediatr. 106:870-875, 1985.

135. Read, S. E., Fischetti, V. A., Utermohlen, V., et al.: Cellular reactivity studies to streptococcal antigens: Migration inhibition studies in patients with streptococcal infections and rheumatic fever. J. Clin. Invest. 54:439-450, 1974.

136. Recco, R., Cortes, H., Zaman, M. M., et al.: Intra-familial transmission of life-threatening group A streptococcal infection. Epidemiol. Infect. 2002.

137. Reid, H. F., Bassett, D. C., Poon-King, T., et al.: Group G streptococci in healthy school-children and in patients with glomerulonephritis in Trinidad. J. Hyg. 94:61-68, 1985.

138. Rolston, K. V., Chandrasekar, P. H., and LeFrock, J. L.: Antimicrobial tolerance in group C and group G streptococci. J. Antimicrob. Chemother. 13:389-392, 1984.

139. Rolston, K. V., LeFrock, J. L., and Schell, R. F.: Activity of nine antimicrobial agents against Lancefield group C and group G streptococci. Antimicrob. Agents Chemother. 22:930-932, 1982.

140. Ruoff, K. L., Whiley, R. A., and Beighton, D.: Streptococcus. In Murray, P. R., Baron, E. J., Pfaller, M. A., et al. (eds.): Manual of Clinical Microbiology. 8th ed. Washington, D.C., ASM Press, 2003, pp. 405-421.

141. Sawyer, W. D., Smith, M. R., and Wood, W. B., Jr.: The mechanisms by which macrophages phagocyte encapsulated bacteria in the absence of antibody. J. Exp. Med. 100:417-424, 1954.

142. Schwartz, R. H., Gerber, M. A., and McCoy, P.: Effect of atmosphere of incubation on the isolation of group A streptococci from throat cultures. J. Lab. Clin. Med. 106:88-92, 1985.

143. Seppala, H., Nissinen, A., Jarvinen, H., et al.: Resistance to erythromycin in group A streptococci. N. Engl. J. Med. 326:292-297, 1992.

144. Seravalli, E., and Taranta, A.: Lymphocyte transformation and macrophage migration inhibition by electrofocused and gel-filtered fractions of group A streptococcal filtrate. Cell. Immunol. 14:366-375, 1974.

145. Shet, A., and Kaplan, E. L.: The clinical use and interpretation of group A streptococcal antibody tests: A practical approach for the pediatrician or primary care physician. Pediatr. Infect. Dis. J. 21:420-426, 2002.

146. Shulman, S. T.: Streptococcal pharyngitis: Diagnostic considerations. Pediatr. Infect. Dis. J. 13:567-571, 1994.

147. Siegel, A. C., Johnson, E. E., and Stollerman, G. H.: Controlled studies of streptococcal pharyngitis in a pediatric population, I: Factors related to the attack rate of rheumatic fever. N. Engl. J. Med. 265:559-566, 1961.

148. Smith, E. W., Garson, A., Jr., Boyleston, J. A., et al.: Varicella gangrenosa due to group A beta-hemolytic Streptococcus. Pediatrics 57:306-310, 1976.

149. Smith, T. D., Wilkinson, V., and Kaplan, E. L.: Group A Streptococcus-associated upper respiratory tract infections in a day-care center. Pediatrics 83:380-384, 1989.

150. Snellman, L. W., Stang, H. J., Stang, J. M., et al.: Duration of positive throat cultures for group A streptococci after initiation of antibiotic therapy. Pediatrics 91:1166-1170, 1993.

151. Stetson, C. A., Rammelkamp, C. H., Jr., Krause, R. M., et al.: Epidemic acute nephritis: Studies on etiology, natural history and prevention. Medicine 34:431-450, 1955.

152. Stevens, D. L.: Streptococcal toxic-shock syndrome: Spectrum of disease, pathogenesis, and new concepts in treatment. Emerg. Infect. Dis. 1:69-78, 1995.

153. Stevens, D. L.: Life-threatening streptococcal infections: Scarlet fever, necrotizing fasciitis, myositis, bacteremia, and streptococcal TSS. In Stevens, D. L., and Kaplan, E. L. (eds.): Streptococcal Infections: Clinical Aspects, Microbiology, and Molecular Pathogenesis. New York, Oxford University Press, 2000, pp. 163-179.

154. Stevens, D. L., Tanner, M. H., Winship, J., et al.: Severe group A streptococcal infections associated with a toxic shock-like syndrome and scarlet fever toxin A. N. Engl. J. Med. 321:1-7, 1989.

155. Tagg, J. R., Dajani, A. S., Wannamaker, L. W., et al.: Group A streptococcal bacteriocin: Production, purification, and mode of action. J. Exp. Med. 138:1168-1183, 1973.

156. Tancer, M. L., McManus, J. E., and Bellotti, G.: Group A, type 33, beta-hemolytic streptococcal outbreak on a maternity and newborn service. Am. J. Obstet. Gynecol. *103*:1028-1033, 1969.

157. Turner, J. C., Hayden, G. F., Kiselica, D., et al.: Association of group C beta-hemolytic streptococci with endemic pharyngitis among college students. J. A. M. A. *264*:2644-2647, 1990.

158. Turner, J. C., Hayden, G. F., Lobo, M. C., et al.: Epidemiologic evidence for Lancefield group C beta-hemolytic streptococci as a cause of exudative pharyngitis in college students. J. Clin. Microbiol. *35*:1-4, 1997.

159. Veasy, L. G., and Hill, H. R.. Immunologic and clinical correlations in rheumatic fever and rheumatic heart disease. Pediatr. Infect. Dis. J. *16*:400-407, 1997.

160. Veasy, L. G., Tani, L. Y., and Hill, H. R.: Persistence of acute rheumatic fever in the intermountain area of the United States. J. Pediatr. *124*:9-16, 1994.

161. Villasenor-Sierra, A., McShan, W. M., Salmi, D., et al.: Variable susceptibility to opsonophagocytosis group A streptococcus M-1 strains by human immune sera. J. Infect. Dis. *180*:1921-1928, 1999.

162. Wagner, J. G., Schlievert, P. M., Assimacopoulos, A. P., et al.: Acute group G streptococcal myositis associated with streptococcal TSS: Case report and review. Clin. Infect. Dis. *23*:1159-1161, 1996.

163. Wannamaker, L. W.: The epidemiology of streptococcal infections. *In* McCarty, M. (ed.): Streptococcal Infections. New York, Columbia University Press, 1954, pp. 157-175.

164. Wannamaker, L. W.: Differences between streptococcal infections of the throat and of the skin, I. N. Engl. J. Med. *282*:23-31, 1970.

165. Wannamaker, L. W.: Perplexity and precision in the diagnosis of streptococcal pharyngitis. Am. J. Dis. Child. *124*:352-358, 1972.

166. Wannamaker, L. W.: The chain that links the heart to the throat. Circulation *48*:9-18, 1973.

167. Wannamaker, L. W.: Immunology of streptococci. *In* Good, R. A., Nahmias, A. J., and O'Reilly, R. J. (eds.): Comprehensive Immunology: Immunology of Human Infection. New York, Plenum, 1981, pp. 47-72.

168. Wannamaker, L. W.: Diagnosis of pharyngitis: Clinical and epidemiologic features. *In* Shulman, S. (ed.): Management of Pharyngitis in an Era of Declining Rheumatic Fever. Columbus, OH, Ross Conference on Pediatric Research, 1984, p. 25.

169. Wannamaker, L. W., Almquist, S., and Skjold, S.: Intergroup phage reactions and transduction between group C and group A streptococci. J. Exp. Med. *137*:1338-1353, 1973.

170. Wannamaker, L. W., and Ferrieri, P.: Streptococcal infections: Updated. Disease-A-Month, pp. 1-40, 1975.

171. Weinstein, L., and Le Frock, J.: Does antimicrobial therapy of streptococcal pharyngitis or pyoderma alter the risk of glomerulonephritis? J. Infect. Dis. *124*:229-231, 1971.

172. Wesley, T. B., Johnson, D. R., Diesch, S. L., et al.: Do beta hemolytic streptococci in the upper respiratory tract (URT) of household dogs constitute a significant zoonotic threat? Abstracts of the Interscience Conference on Antibiotics and Chemotherapy, 1995.

173. Wittler, R. R., Yamada, S. M., Bass, J. W., et al.: Penicillin tolerance and erythromycin resistance of group A beta-hemolytic streptococci in Hawaii and the Philippines. Am. J. Dis. Child. *144*:587-589, 1990.

174. Zabriskie, J. B.: The role of temperate bacteriophage in the production of erythrogenic toxin by group A streptococci. J. Exp. Med. *119*:761-779, 1964.

175. Zaoutis, T., Schneider, B., Steele, M. L., and Klein, J. D.: Antibiotic susceptibility of group C and group G streptococci isolated from patients with invasive infections: Evidence of vancomycin tolerance among group G serotypes. J. Clin. Microbiol. *37*:3380-3383, 1999.

176. Zimmerman, R. A., and Hill, H. R.: Placental transfer of group A type-specific streptococcal antibody. Pediatrics *43*:809-814, 1969.

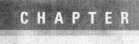

CHAPTER 94

GROUP B STREPTOCOCCAL INFECTIONS

Pia S. Pannaraj ⦿ Carol J. Baker

HISTORY

The organism we know as group B *Streptococcus*, or *Streptococcus agalactiae*, was isolated first by Nocard in 1887[233] and for decades was recognized as a cause of bovine mastitis[220] but not human infection. Serologic techniques for differentiating beta-hemolytic streptococci were developed by Lancefield,[173] who also described isolation of group B streptococci from parturient women in 1935.[174] In that same year, Congdon[82] included one fatal puerperal case of group B streptococcal sepsis and pneumonia in a report of streptococcal infections associated with childbirth. The significance of this organism as a human pathogen was reported first by Fry[115] in 1938, who described three cases of fatal puerperal sepsis. Group B streptococcal infections continued to be reported sporadically until the 1960s, when maternal and neonatal infections increasingly were ascribed to this pathogen.[68,101,147] In the 1970s, group B *Streptococcus* emerged as the predominant organism causing bacteremia and meningitis in neonates.[12,26,113,150,241] The incidence of neonatal infection remained stable, with reported attack rates ranging from 0.2 to 5.4 per 1000 live births, until the late 1990s, when maternal intrapartum chemoprophylaxis gained wide acceptance and incidence rates fell.[33,75,280] Invasive infection also occurs beyond the neonatal period in pregnant women, nonpregnant adults with underlying medical conditions, and elderly persons.[95,103,235,311]

MICROBIOLOGY

ISOLATION AND IDENTIFICATION

Group B streptococci are facultative gram-positive diplococci that grow on a variety of bacteriologic media. Colonies are 3 to 4 mm in diameter, grayish white, flat, and somewhat mucoid. Colonies are surrounded by a narrow zone of beta-hemolysis that for some strains is detectable only when the colony is lifted from the agar. Nonhemolytic strains account for 1 to 2 percent of isolates and may cause human disease.[12,269] Definitive identification of group B streptococci relies on detection of the group B-specific antigen, a carbohydrate cell wall antigen common to all strains. The standard method, as described by Lancefield,[173] requires acid treatment of the bacteria to solubilize the carbohydrate group B antigen, followed by capillary precipitation with hyperimmune rabbit serum. Several newer methods using hyperimmune antisera have been developed, but latex agglutination is used widely because of the commercial availability of test kits, the ease of performing the assay, and the specificity of the results when organisms in pure culture are tested.[292] Other laboratory methods for presumptive identification include testing for resistance to bacitracin or trimethoprim-sulfamethoxazole, hydrolysis of sodium hippurate broth, failure to hydrolyze bile esculin, production of orange pigment when cultured under certain conditions, and CAMP (Christie, Atkinson, Munch, Peterson) testing. CAMP is an acronym of the names of the authors who first described the production of CAMP factor by group B streptococci in the presence of the beta-toxin of *Staphylococcus aureus* that results in synergistic hemolysis on sheep blood agar.[81]

SEROLOGIC CLASSIFICATION AND ANTIGENIC STRUCTURE

Group B streptococci possess two carbohydrate cell wall antigens, the group B-specific antigen and type-specific capsular polysaccharide. Group B streptococci are classified into serotypes based on type-specific capsular polysaccharides. Nine such polysaccharides are characterized: Ia, Ib, and II to VIII. The type-specific polysaccharides of group B streptococci are repeating units of five to seven monosaccharides (glucose, galactose, glucosamine, and *N*-acetylneuraminic acid). All the characterized polysaccharides include an *N*-acetylneuraminic acid (sialic acid) residue, which is important in the pathogenesis of type III human infection and perhaps other types.[31,287,325] Despite structural relatedness, antibody directed against the capsular polysaccharide of one type does not provide cross-protection against other capsular polysaccharide types.[175,317,328] A few strains isolated from patients with systemic infection contain type-specific capsular polysaccharide genes by genotypic methods but produce very low levels of capsule or have modified capsular structures that do not react with hyperimmune sera to the characterized capsular polysaccharides.[260] These strains are called *nontypeable*.

Further differentiation of type Ia strains was based on the presence or absence of a protein antigen known as C, which led to the nomenclature of Ia and Ia/c serotypes. The C protein also is present in many other serotypes except type III strains and consists of two components, alpha (trypsin resistant), found in 70 percent of non–type III capsular polysaccharide isolates, and beta (trypsin sensitive), found in approximately 20 percent of isolates.[109,157,202]

Pili, an essential virulence factor in many gram-negative pathogens such as adhesins, was discovered in group B streptococci, and its role in pathogenesis is being studied.[179] Analyses of the group B *Streptococcus* genome sequenced in 2002 will provide further insights into its antigenic structure, genes contributing to its virulence, and targets for treatment.[123,305]

EXTRACELLULAR PRODUCTS

Several bacterial products are elaborated by group B streptococci. Type-specific capsular polysaccharide is released from cells, and the amount elaborated has been correlated with virulence.[169,338] These soluble polysaccharides inhibit opsonophagocytic killing in vitro, thereby providing a mechanism for the documented increase in virulence.[181] Most strains possess C5a-ase, an enzyme of the serine esterase class that inactivates complement component C5a.[144] Because C5a is a potent chemoattractant for neutrophils, this enzyme helps the bacteria to evade the host immune system by hindering the accumulation of neutrophils at the site of infection. The beta-hemolysin elaborated by group B streptococci was characterized in 1980, but only more recently has its role in virulence been explored through the creation of nonhemolytic and hyperhemolytic mutants.[205,322] Expression of beta-hemolysin correlated with tissue damage in an in vivo arthritis model,[256] activation of neutrophil signaling pathways in brain endothelium leading to development of meningitis,[92] and increased virulence in pulmonary infection in rats and rabbits.[140,232] Other bacterial products of group B streptococci, including CAMP factor,[163] lipoteichoic acid,[228,229] pigment,[303] hippuricase, neuraminidase, hyaluronidase,[111,213] and nucleases,[110] have been described, but the contributions of these substances to pathogenesis are not clear.

ANTIMICROBIAL SUSCEPTIBILITY

To date, human isolates of group B streptococci have remained uniformly susceptible to penicillin G. However, approximately 10-fold greater concentrations are required for inhibition and killing of group B streptococci than for group A streptococci. Group B streptococci also are susceptible to other β-lactam agents, cephalosporins, vancomycin, and carbapenems. The prevalence of resistance to the macrolides (erythromycin, clindamycin, clarithromycin) is increasing; from 1970 to 1990, it was reported in 3.4 to 7.4 percent of isolates, but more recent studies

reported resistance to erythromycin in 17 to 29 percent of isolates and resistance to clindamycin in 7 to 26 percent.[55,86,107,186] Resistance is related to the presence of *ermTR*, *ermB*, or *mefA* genes.[86] Macrolide resistance is highest in type V strains.[186] Ninety-five percent of strains are resistant to tetracycline, and resistance to bacitracin, nalidixic acid, trimethoprim-sulfamethoxazole, and metronidazole is uniform.[249] Low-level gentamicin resistance is typical, but when gentamicin is combined with either penicillin G or ampicillin, synergistic killing of group B streptococci occurs in vitro and in vivo.[275,276,300]

As many as 5 to 17 percent of group B streptococcal isolates have been reported to be tolerant to penicillin.[48,167] Expression of tolerance requires laboratory conditions that promote a greater than 16-fold discrepancy between minimal inhibitory concentrations and minimal bactericidal concentrations. Tolerant strains are characterized in vitro by delayed penicillin killing, similar rates of killing by penicillin whether growth is exponential or stationary, an additive rather than a synergistic response to the combination of penicillin and gentamicin, and deficient autolysis. The clinical significance, if any, of these laboratory-induced properties remains unknown.[22,166,290]

EPIDEMIOLOGY

MATERNAL COLONIZATION

Asymptomatic colonization occurs at vaginal, rectal, urethral, and pharyngeal sites in one third of healthy young women.[52,217] Much effort has been exerted trying to define groups of women at enhanced risk for colonization with group B streptococci. Factors found to be associated with vaginal acquisition include African-American ethnicity, multiple sex partners, frequent sexual intercourse, male-to-female oral sex, tampon use, and infrequent hand washing.[52,203,217] Women younger than 20 years of age have higher prevalence of colonization.[14,29] Several studies have found significantly higher colonization rates among African Americans,[71,143,217] whereas others found higher rates in Hispanics.[263] Asians have the lowest colonization rates.[71,217]

Maternal vaginal or rectal colonization rates during pregnancy vary from 18 to 35 percent in reported studies.[19,23,59,88,93,212,249,263] These rates relate to the body sites sampled, microbiologic techniques employed, and the period of gestation in which the cultures are performed. Specimens from the distal portion of the vagina yield group B streptococci more frequently than do specimens from the proximal vagina or cervix.[197] Concomitant sampling of the rectal site results in a 10 percent increase in detection over culturing the vaginal site alone.[19,88] Several investigators have suggested the gastrointestinal tract as the principal reservoir for this organism, and, not uncommonly, the rectal site is the only one that yields group B streptococci.[19,88,148,249] The urinary tract is an important site of infection (asymptomatic bacteriuria) because it is a surrogate for a high or "heavy" (>10^5 colony-forming units per milliliter) genital inoculum and a marker of increased risk for development of early-onset sepsis in neonates.[225,334] Bacteriuria mandates therapy during pregnancy.[278]

The manner in which swab specimens from the vagina and rectum are processed also is important in accurately assessing colonization.[74] Anogenital culture swabs collected by patients themselves are as accurate as those performed by physicians.[307] Swabs can be placed in transport media at environmental temperatures for as long as 96 hours.[278] Specimens then should be placed in a selective antibiotic-containing broth medium, rather than on solid media, because solid media fail to detect as many as 50 percent of group B streptococcal carriers.[27,30] The addition of antibiotics to the broth limits the growth of competing flora, especially gram-negative enteric organisms, and enhances detection.[23,27,30,209] Todd-Hewitt broth with gentamicin and nalidixic acid (selective broth medium)[27] or with colistin (Lim broth)[185] and nalidixic acid is recommended for detection of group B streptococcal colonization.[278] After overnight incubation, the broth is subcultured onto a 5 percent sheep blood agar plate and is processed conventionally.

Ninety-two percent of culture-positive women are identified if lower vaginal and rectal cultures are obtained at a single visit with correct laboratory detection methods.[94] The proximity to delivery affects the accuracy of predicting colonization at delivery. Cultures obtained at 35 and 37 weeks' gestation predict colonization at delivery with 87 percent sensitivity and 96 percent specificity.[59,248,337]

INFANT COLONIZATION

Colonization and infection in the neonate are associated significantly with the presence of group B streptococci in the maternal genital tract at delivery. Vertical transmission from colonized mothers to their infants occurs in 41 to 72 percent of cases (mean, ~50%).[7,15,23,57,93,143,212,340] Only 1 to 12 percent (mean, ~5%) of colonized infants are born to noncolonized mothers.[15,23,93,212,340] Acquisition is presumed to occur either by the ascending route through ruptured membranes or from contact with the organism in the genital tract during parturition. Heavy maternal inocula in the genital tract ($>10^5$ colony-forming units per milliliter) greatly increases the rates of vertical transmission to neonates and rates of heavy infant colonization.[9,15,59,148,159] Other factors associated with increased colonization rates in infants include prolonged rupture of membranes (>12 to 18 hours)[15,143] and vaginal delivery.[143] Maternal intrapartum antibiotic therapy substantially diminishes the vertical transmission of group B streptococci.[7,57,60,143,341] The body sites in neonates most likely to yield group B *Streptococcus* are the rectum and throat, findings reflecting replication of organisms at the respiratory or gastrointestinal tract sites after the ingestion of infected amniotic fluid or genital secretions.[143]

Horizontal transmission from nosocomial and community sources has been described.[1,93,118,234] Infant-to-infant or colonized staff member–to-infant spread may occur through hands of hospital personnel, but epidemics are unusual.[93,234] The rate of community acquisition, presumably by an oral-fecal route, appears to be low.[118,285] Breast milk also has been proposed as a mode of transmission for late-onset infection; most reported cases involved a mother with postpartum mastitis.[50,171,265]

INCIDENCE OF DISEASE

Before the widespread use of maternal intrapartum chemoprophylaxis to prevent early-onset disease, reported attack rates for group B streptococcal disease in infants ranged from 1.8 to 4.0 per 1000 live births.[235,323,343] Early-onset disease (onset within the first week of life) accounted for approximately 80 percent of cases.[280] Late-onset disease (onset between 7 days and 3 months of life) rates ranged from 0.3 to 1.8 per 1000 live births.[89,241] With the 2002 guidelines for universal screening of pregnant women at 35 to 37 weeks' gestation and administering of intrapartum chemoprophylaxis to carriers, the incidence of early-onset disease decreased to 0.3 cases per 1000 live births in 2004, a finding representing a decline of 81 percent from 1990.[75,280] However, the incidence of late-onset disease has remained unchanged.[75] Approximately 30 percent of cases of early-onset disease and up to 55 percent of those of late-onset and late, late-onset disease now occur in preterm infants.[188,280,283] Late, late-onset group B streptococcal disease occurs in infants older than 3 months of age and accounts for 7 to 13 percent of childhood group B streptococcal infections.[151,280,336] Affected infants typically were born

before 34 weeks' gestation or have an underlying immunodeficiency or concomitant infection with human immunodeficiency virus (HIV).[87,151,336] Case-fatality rates for all infants with group B streptococcal disease have dropped from 46 percent in the 1970s to 6.5 percent in 2004.[75,156]

Group B streptococcal disease also is a common finding in pregnant women, with clinical manifestations that include urinary tract infection (usually asymptomatic bacteriuria but also cystitis or pyelonephritis), intra-amniotic infection, postpartum endometritis (often with bacteremia), and puerperal sepsis.[240,283,342] Occasionally, meningitis, septic thrombophlebitis, and other serious complications occur.[342] Attack rates of 2 per 1000 deliveries have been reported, and 28 percent of maternal cases are associated with pregnancy loss or birth of an infant with early-onset group B streptococcal disease.[240,342] Nonpregnant women and men account for 68 percent of invasive group B streptococcal disease in adults.[103] These patients typically are more than 65 years old or have underlying medical conditions, including diabetes mellitus, malignant disease (especially breast cancer), HIV infection, liver disease, stroke and other neurologic disorders, decubitus ulcers, and neurogenic bladder.[103,154,235,311]

RISK FACTORS FOR INFANT DISEASE

Vertical transmission is a prerequisite for the development of invasive, early-onset infection.[23,211,241] Evidence suggests that approximately 50 percent of late-onset infections also occur after vertical transmission.[89] The degree of colonization or inoculum also increases the likelihood of infant disease; heavily colonized mothers are more likely to have infants with invasive infection, and heavily colonized infants are more likely to have either early- or late-onset disease.[59,89,159,184] Other maternal factors associated with the development of early-onset disease include delivery before 37 weeks' gestation, premature rupture of membranes (rupture of membranes before onset of labor) or rupture of membranes more than 18 hours before delivery at any gestation, and intrapartum fever.[12,58,59,89,113,241] Women colonized with group B *Streptococcus* also have a higher incidence of premature rupture of membranes and preterm labor, a finding suggesting a causal relationship between group B streptococci and events leading to preterm birth.[6,210,214,262] Other maternal factors associated with an increased attack rate of early-onset infection are African-American ethnicity, age younger than 20 years, history of previous fetal loss, history of urinary tract infection with group B streptococci, and primiparity.[282,283] Late-onset disease also is associated with young maternal age and African-American ethnicity.[283] Siblings of infected infants who are the product of a multiple pregnancy (e.g., twins, triplets) have enhanced risk for development of early- and late-onset group B streptococcal disease.[98,242]

CAPSULAR POLYSACCHARIDE TYPES CAUSING DISEASE

Reports from the 1970s indicated that the group B streptococcal capsular polysaccharide types colonizing pregnant women and neonates were divided fairly evenly among types I, II, and III.[24,327,329] The current distribution of capsule polysaccharide types in invasive disease from multiple North American studies[84,134,187,324,342] is shown in Figure 94–1. Serotypes Ia and III are the most common cause of early-onset infection, whereas serotype III is the most common cause of late-onset infection. In Europe, type III predominates in both early- and late-onset disease.[112,308,324] Serotype III is implicated in 80 to 93 percent of meningitis cases, either as a focus of early-onset disease or as a manifestation of late-onset infection (80 to 93%).[24,26,329] Capsular polysaccharide type V emerged in the 1990s.[53,71,143,266] Type V causes both early- and late-onset infant disease and is the

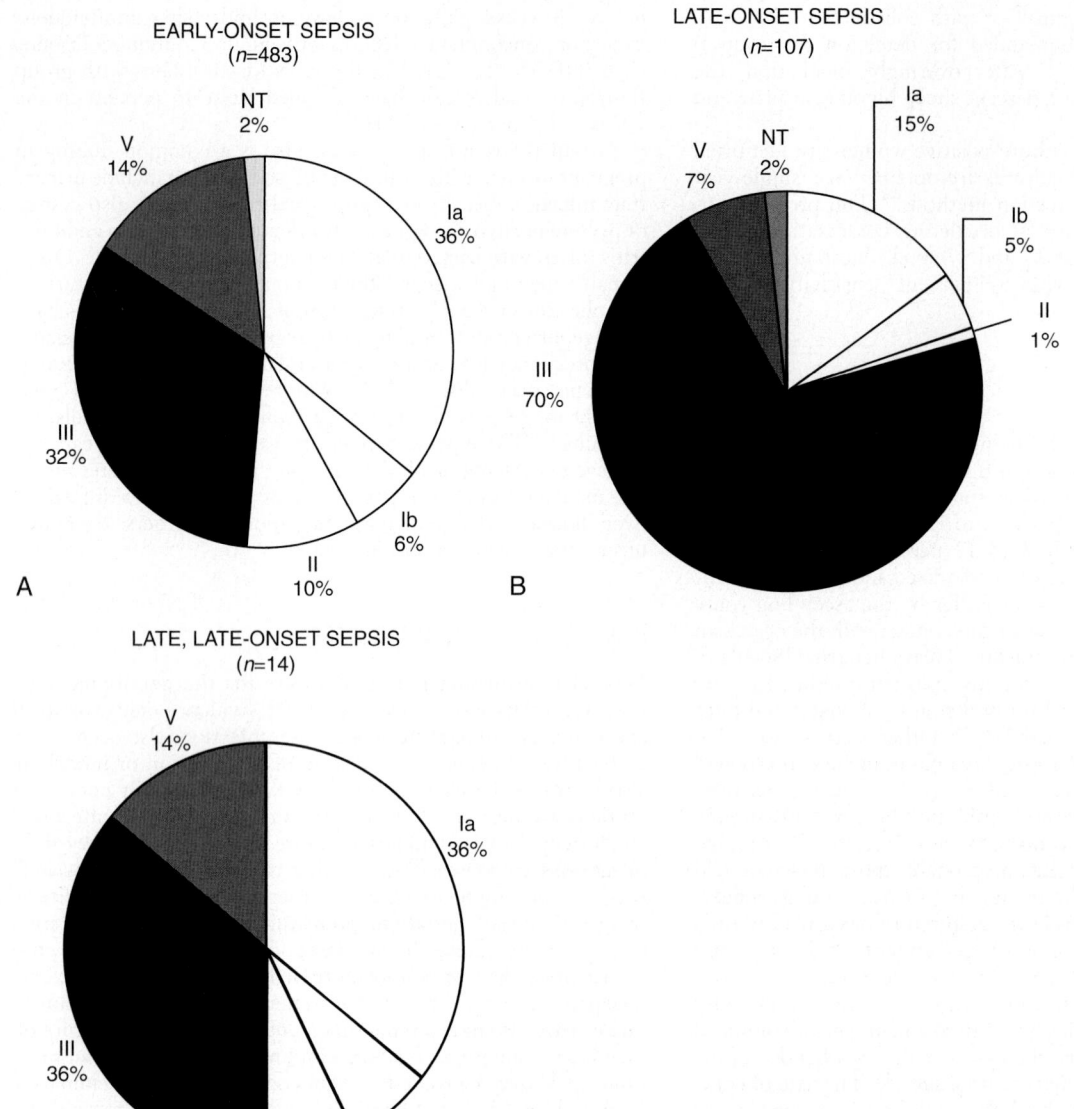

Figure 94–1 Serotype distribution of invasive group B streptococcal strains causing early-onset (**A**), late-onset (**B**), and late, late-onset (**C**) disease in infants.[53,84,134,187,342] NT, nontypeable.

type most commonly isolated from adults with invasive disease.[53,266] In Japan, types VI and VIII are the most common isolates from pregnant women.[172] The least common serotypes causing human disease are types Ib/c, IV, VI, VII, and VIII.

PATHOGENESIS

For pediatricians, group B streptococcal disease predominantly afflicts neonates, a predilection that results from a unique combination of maternal, bacterial, and host factors. Figure 94–2 shows a simplified flow chart of group B streptococcal transmission. First, an organism carried by an asymptomatically colonized mother is transmitted vertically to her neonate. Evidence suggests that this transmission may occur in utero shortly before birth or during parturition. This continuum in time of acquisition is reflected in the time of onset of symptoms; infected neonates often are ill at or within 12 hours of birth (≤90% of cases), whereas others may not have evidence of disease for a few days.[26,283] The organism successfully colonizes approximately 50

percent of all infants born to group B streptococcal carriers, yet disease develops in only 1 to 2 percent of these infants.[12,281,325] A breach in the delicate interplay of maternal, infant, and bacterial factors allows the organism to invade. Once invasion occurs, a combination of host defenses and therapeutic interventions may halt the progression of disease, or the infant's defenses may fail and the disease may progress and result in tissue damage or death.

MATERNAL FACTORS

The bacterial inoculum in the maternal genital tract determines the likelihood that the organism will be transmitted vertically. Infants born to heavily colonized women are more likely to be colonized themselves and are more likely to have early-onset disease.[9,15,59,89,148,159] Infants delivered before 37 weeks of gestation have an increased risk for development of early-onset disease.[211,262] Heavy maternal colonization may induce preterm delivery,[211,262] and disease is more likely to develop in the infant in this setting

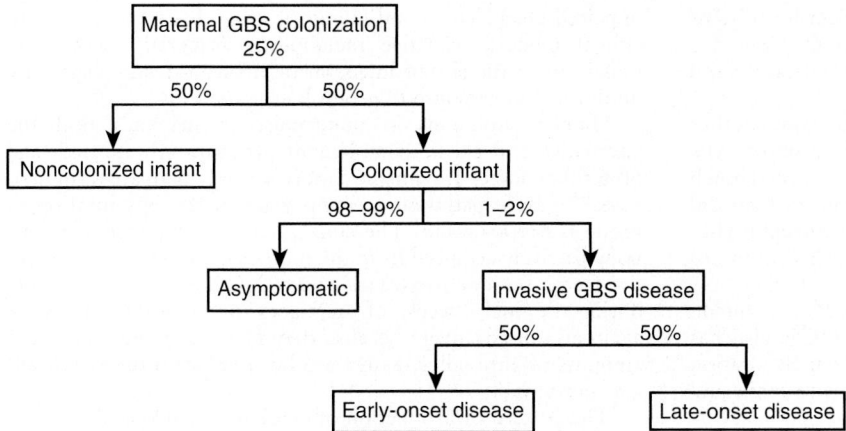

Figure 94–2 Flow chart of vertical transmission and disease manifestation of group B streptococcal disease in the era of intrapartum chemoprophylaxis.

of high bacterial inoculum and immunologic immaturity. Invasive disease also has been reported in term neonates delivered by elective cesarean section with intact membranes, but this is a rare event.[12,101,240]

In addition to bacterial inoculum, another critical maternal factor is the concentration of serum antibody to the serotype-specific polysaccharide capsule of the colonizing strain of group B *Streptococcus* at delivery. Antibody to the type-specific capsular polysaccharide is protective against the homologous serotype in the mouse model of lethal infection; antibody to the group B polysaccharide is not.[176] Baker and associates[28,32] determined that invasive disease with type III group B streptococci occurred primarily in infants born to women with low serum concentrations of antibodies directed against the type III capsular polysaccharide. Several other investigators also reported a correlation between low concentrations of antibody to types Ia, Ib, II, and III capsular polysaccharide in maternal delivery sera and the occurrence of early- and late-onset group B streptococcal infant disease.[125,127] A correlation between antibody concentration and maternal age may explain the epidemiologic association of young maternal age and increased likelihood of neonatal disease.[13] Animal models have demonstrated that antibody directed against the alpha or beta determinants of C protein is protective,[176,218] but definitive human studies are lacking. Invasive disease, but not colonization, elicits immunoglobulin M (IgM) and IgG antibodies to beta C protein in humans.[236] Antibody to other protein determinants in some serotypes has been postulated to be partially protective. Titers of antibody to R protein were found to be higher in maternal serum from mothers colonized with R protein–bearing strains whose infants were healthy than from mothers whose infants were ill; such antibodies were protective in a mouse model against type II, but not type III strains.[189,190] Presence of maternal antibody to Rib also was associated with protection in neonates against Rib-expressing group B streptococcal strains.[178]

BACTERIAL FACTORS

To colonize the genital tract or cause disease effectively, the organisms must be able to adhere to host tissue. Group B streptococci adhere well to many types of epithelium, including vaginal epithelium and chorioamnionic membranes.[116,196,293,302] Type III strains adhere more avidly to vaginal cells than do other serotypes in vitro.[56] Furthermore, invasive strains adhere better to epithelial tissue than colonizing strains do.[138] This capacity to adhere to and possibly invade chorioamnionic cells may explain the association of group B streptococcal colonization with preterm labor and premature rupture of membranes.[145] If a breach occurs in the

membranes, the bacteria can multiply in amniotic fluid.[139] After transmission and colonization occur, the capacity of the bacteria to adhere to neonatal epithelial cells may allow them to invade and disseminate. The lung, after aspiration of infected maternal fluids, is a frequent initial site of infection in a newborn with early-onset disease. Group B streptococci can adhere to and invade respiratory epithelial cell lines.[272] In addition, they can invade endothelial cells, which may be a mechanism for some of the pathologic features of disseminated disease.[121]

Several different factors may confer adherence properties of group B streptococci including bacterial cell wall component lipoteichoic acid[229] or surface proteins.[67,302] One study showed that translocation across epithelial barriers was mediated by alpha C protein binding to host cell surface glycosaminoglycan.[42] Several proteins with potential roles in adherence and invasion were identified by detecting up-regulation during cell invasion using proteomics and include an undefined surface antigen, penicillin-binding protein 2b, glyceraldehydes-3-phosphate dehydrogenase, and an iron-binding protein.[158] Mouse antisera to these five proteins inhibited binding of group B streptococci to cervical epithelial cells. Translocation also may occur by a paracellular route.[296] Adherence to and invasion of the microvascular endothelial cells of the blood-brain barrier has been associated with proper anchoring of lipoteichoic acid,[91] beta-hemolysin/cytolysin,[92] fibrinogen binding protein FbsA,[304] and the newly discovered pilus proteins.[199]

A well-defined virulence structure of group B streptococci is the capsular polysaccharide. Mouse virulent strains are able to synthesize greater amounts of surface-bound type-specific polysaccharide than avirulent strains.[169,338] An unencapsulated mutant, created by inserting a transposon into the gene regulating capsule expression, has significantly less virulence in neonatal rats than does the parent type III strain.[273] As with other encapsulated organisms, the capsule is thought to confer virulence primarily by interfering with opsonophagocytosis.[181] In vitro, the capsule of type III group B streptococci has been shown to prevent the deposition of C3,[207] and the presence of the terminal sialic acid residue on the repeating unit of the polysaccharide is crucial to this interference.[99] Removal of sialic acid residues from the polysaccharide leads to diminished virulence, and a desialylated mutant loses virulence when compared with the parent strain.[326] Furthermore, the presence of this sialic acid moiety prevents activation of the alternative complement pathway, the predominant pathway used by the human host when minimal type-specific antibody is present.[99] In addition, when bacteria grow in the presence of human serum, the quantity of sialic acid increases, thereby potentiating its contribution to virulence.[244] Opsonization may be affected by cell surface components other than capsular sialic acid. C protein also lends relative resistance to opsonization to strains bearing the antigen.[157,244] Beta-hemolysin/cytolysin contributes to cytolysis and apoptosis of phagocyte while protecting group B streptococci by the linked carotenoid pigment against oxidative damage.[194]

Sialic acid residues on the capsule may interfere with another component of the immune system. In a serum-free system, the desialylated mutant of type III group B streptococci elicited much larger quantities of leukotriene B$_4$ from macrophages than did the parent strain.[270] Leukotriene B$_4$ is a potent neutrophil chemoattractant, so this effect may result in diminished influx of effector cells. Similarly, C5a-ase may disable C5a, another host product capable of eliciting neutrophil influx. By enhancing phagocytosis and killing of group B streptococci, C5a also has direct stimulatory effects on neutrophils.[301] Bacterial elaboration of C5a-ase may affect both the accumulation of neutrophils and the efficiency of neutrophil function.

Once invasive infection is established, ongoing replication and digestion of bacteria can instigate host inflammatory responses that may be deleterious. Neonates recovering from group B streptococcal disease have circulating immune complexes for a prolonged period of time, and immune complexes can contribute to end-organ damage.[312] Additionally, immune complexes containing group B streptococcal components elicit inflammatory mediators such as leukotriene B$_4$ and interleukin-6 (IL-6). The cytokine response to gram-positive pathogens is not delineated as clearly as is that to gram-negative bacteria, partly because of the greater heterogeneity in structure of the latter.[54] Both group B and type III capsular polysaccharides induce the release of IL-6 from monocytes[296]; group B antigen also causes the release of tumor necrosis factor-α (TNF-α).[314] As with other gram-positive pathogens, the cell walls of group B streptococci contain peptidoglycan and lipoteichoic acid. Peptidoglycans from other gram-positive organisms elicit a variety of proinflammatory cytokines such as TNF-α, IL-1, IL-6, and granulocyte colony-stimulating factor.[90,142,264] Lipoteichoic acid also induces the release of IL-1β, IL-6, and TNF-α.[49,164] Group B streptococcal cell wall components likewise exert similar effects. Elaboration of these cytokines has been implicated in the clinical and hemodynamic effects of sepsis.[54] Specifically, blockade of IL-1 activity by administration of an IL-1 receptor antagonist in a piglet model of group B streptococcal sepsis ameliorated systemic hypotension and prolonged survival.[315]

INFANT HOST FACTORS

Neonates have several domains of immune dysfunction that affect their ability to mount a sufficient defense against group B streptococci. Neutrophils are the primary effector cell in host defense against extracellular bacterial pathogens, and neutrophils from neonates have many functional abnormalities.[182] The generation of chemotactic activity in neonatal serum in response to group B streptococci is diminished, as is the release of chemotactic factors by neonatal monocytes.[10,11,271] Thus, the diminished ability of neutrophils to migrate is amplified by a diminished level of chemotactic stimulation. Phagocytosis and bacterial killing also are impaired when opsonic activity is poor, as is the usual pattern in neonates with sepsis.[182] The neutrophil storage pools of neonates rapidly become depleted during invasive infection, thereby leading to profound neutropenia,[80] an ominous prognostic indicator.[245] These defects in neonatal neutrophils are even more pronounced in infants born prematurely.[182]

Cells of the monocyte/macrophage lineage also may play a role in host defense against group B streptococci, especially in the lungs, where the alveolar macrophage is the first effector cell to encounter pathogens. Defects in the functions of these cells have been described in neonates. Cord blood monocytes have impaired phagocytosis and killing of group B streptococci.[206] In animal models, oxidative metabolism, bacterial uptake, and migration to the site of infection by neonatal macrophages are diminished in response to group B streptococci.[208,284,286]

Humoral immunity is compromised in neonates. Both the alternative and classic complement pathways are affected, and preterm neonates are impaired more severely than are term neonates.[85,97] Both pathways are important in the opsonization of group B streptococci.[33] The concentration of type-specific antibody passively acquired from the mother is an important protective factor. Because passive transfer of IgG increases dramatically during the final 8 weeks of pregnancy, premature neonates are again at a disadvantage because they may not receive sufficient amounts of antibodies if they are born before protective levels are transferred.[79]

The pattern of production of cytokines by neonatal immune cells frequently is altered when compared with that of adults. For example, in response to group B streptococci, the level of TNF-α and IL-6[313] released by neonatal monocytes is increased relative to adults,[314,330] and IL-6[313] but levels of IL-8 and leukotriene B$_4$ are decreased.[271,277] IL-12 and interferon-γ are associated with improved outcome in an animal model of group B streptococcal infection, but lower quantities of these mediators are released by neonatal mononuclear cells.[162,201] Cytokine networks are important both in the manifestations of sepsis and in the stimulation of an appropriate immune response, so alterations in expression of cytokines may affect the neonate's response to this pathogen both clinically and immunologically.

CLINICAL MANIFESTATIONS

EARLY-ONSET DISEASE

Group B *Streptococcus* remains the leading cause of neonatal sepsis, and it accounts for 40 to 50 percent of early-onset sepsis cases.[40,51,152] The bimodal distribution of group B streptococcal infections corresponding to age of neonates and young infants was described first in 1973 and now is divided into two types, termed *early-* and *late-onset disease*.[26,113] The syndromes of early- and late-onset disease differ in epidemiologic characteristics, pathogenesis, clinical findings, and prognosis. Their major clinical features are detailed in Table 94–1. Early-onset disease is defined as onset of infection in the first 6 days of life, but most neonates (61-95%) become ill within the first 24 hours of life (median, 1 hour).[58,64,283] Premature infants often are ill at birth or within 6 hours of birth and account for 17 to 32 percent of neonates with early-onset group B streptococcal disease.[20,75,257,280,283] In very-low-birth-weight infants, group B *Streptococcus* has dropped to the second most common cause of early-onset sepsis, after *Escherichia coli*, since the implementation of intrapartum antibiotic chemoprophylaxis.[298]

Early-onset disease often occurs in the setting of maternal complications, including labor before 37 weeks' gestation, prolonged rupture of membranes for more than 12 hours, intrapartum fever greater than 100.4° F, chorioamnionitis, and early postpartum febrile morbidity.[25,45,58,59,89,323] In one study, infants born to a mother with one or more of these risk factors were 12.5 times more likely to develop early-onset group B streptococcal disease compared with those born to a mother with no risk factors.[58] Term infants can develop group B streptococcal disease without definable maternal risk factors except vaginal/rectal colonization.[33] In another study, 76 percent of mothers of infants with early-onset disease had deliveries complicated by at least one of the foregoing identifiable risk factor or was known to be a group B *Streptococcus* carrier.[257]

The three most frequent clinical manifestations are bacteremia without a focus, pneumonia, and meningitis.[12,323,336] The

TABLE 94–1   Features of Group B Streptococcal Disease in Infants

Feature (References)	Early-Onset Disease	Late-Onset Disease	Late, Late-Onset Disease
Age at onset (58, 64, 283)	≤6 days; mean, 8 hr; median, 1 hr	7-89 days; mean, 36 days; median, 27 days	≥90 days
Infants affected (75, 132, 283, 323)	Premature neonates, births after maternal obstetric complications	Term infants predominate	Premature neonates <32 wk gestation, immunodeficiency
Clinical findings (33)	Acute respiratory distress, apnea, and hypotension common	Fever, irritability, nonspecific signs, occasionally fulminant	Fever, irritability, nonspecific signs
Manifestations (12, 21, 96, 113, 323, 336)	Bacteremia (40-55%), pneumonia (30-45%), meningitis (6-15%)	Bacteremia without a focus (55%), meningitis (35%), osteoarthritis (~5%), cellulitis/ adenitis (~2%)	Bacteremia without a focus, focal infections as in late-onset disease
Case-fatality rate (75, 280, 283, 323, 336)	5-15%	2-6%	<5%

presentation for each may range from shock and respiratory failure at delivery to a healthy infant who has infection detected during evaluation because of maternal risk factors known to increase the risk for development of invasive infection.[257,323] Respiratory distress, including apnea, grunting respirations, tachypnea, and cyanosis, is the most common initial manifestation in all forms of early-onset group B streptococcal disease.[20,26,113,316,336] Other signs include lethargy, poor feeding, abdominal distention, pallor, jaundice, tachycardia, and hypotension. Fever usually is present in term neonates, but preterm infants often are normothermic or hypothermic.[323] Administration of intrapartum antibiotic prophylaxis to the mother does not alter the findings in infants, in whom early-onset disease develops despite administration of prophylaxis; most still become clinically ill in the first 24 hours of life.[40,64]

Bacteremia without a focus is present in 27 to 87 percent of neonates with early-onset disease.[283,323,336] Signs of septicemia, such as respiratory distress and poor perfusion, often are present, especially in neonates born at less than 37 weeks' gestation.[323] Bacteremia in healthy-appearing term infants also may develop, and in one series it occurred in 22 percent of cases.[150,323,336] These infants probably remained healthy because of early evaluation and institution of empiric antimicrobial therapy.[323] More often, bacteremic infants are mildly ill and have fever and nonspecific signs that should prompt bacteriologic evaluation. Bacteremia also frequently accompanies pneumonia and meningitis.

Radiographic findings of pulmonary involvement include infiltrates suggestive of congenital pneumonia, small pleural effusions, a pattern similar to that of hyaline membrane disease or respiratory distress syndrome, and increased vascular markings as seen in transient tachypnea of the newborn; radiographs also may appear normal despite abnormal pulmonary signs.[183,192,316] In preterm neonates, the findings frequently are identical to those of respiratory distress syndrome, and at autopsy, hyaline membranes containing bacteria and minimal inflammatory infiltrates have been described.[2,316]

Meningitis is documented in 6 to 15 percent of neonates with early-onset disease (Fig. 94–3).[283,323,332] As a rule, no signs specifically indicate its presence; this situation underscores the need to evaluate all neonates with presumed early-onset disease for the possibility of meningeal involvement.[323,332] Early in the course, the cerebrospinal fluid (CSF) white blood cell count may be normal despite isolation of group B streptococci.[14] Again, respiratory distress is the most frequent clinical finding.[26,323] Seizures rarely are the initial feature but do occur in as many as 50 percent of affected neonates early in the course of therapy; often these seizures are focal and subtle.[26] Postmortem evaluation of infants who die of early-onset group B streptococcal meningitis reveals

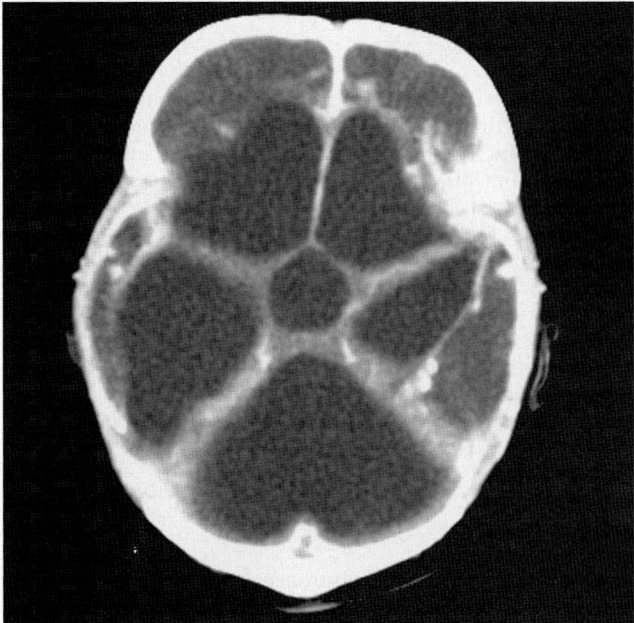

Figure 94–3 Head computed tomography scan at 6 weeks of age from a term infant with early-onset group B streptococcal (GBS) meningitis shows significant loss of normal brain matter.

hemorrhage, prominent basilar involvement, and abundant bacteria with relatively sparse inflammation.[113]

LATE-ONSET DISEASE

Late-onset disease is defined as infection in infants 7 to 90 days of age, and it primarily affects term infants with an unremarkable maternal history and early neonatal course.[26,89] However, more recent case series suggested that late-onset infection develops in a larger proportion of infants born quite prematurely (<34 weeks' gestation).[188] Bacteremia without a focus and meningitis are the two most common manifestations of late-onset disease.[113,117,336] Osteoarticular infections and cellulitis are additional clinical foci.[21,96,336] Whereas early-onset disease most frequently occurs acutely with apnea and hypotension, late-onset disease often is manifested by fever, irritability, and other nonspecific signs.[33] More fulminant, rapidly progressive cases do occur, however.[26]

Meningitis is a frequent complication, occurring in 35 to 40 percent of late-onset disease cases.[26,323,336] Late-onset meningitis most typically manifests with fever and lethargy, although respiratory distress, coma, and shock also may occur.[26] Classic signs of meningitis, such as a bulging fontanelle and nuchal rigidity, occur more commonly in neonates with late-onset than early-onset meningitis. Subdural effusions develop in as many as 20 percent of cases, but subdural empyema is a rare occurrence.[12,26,242] Infants who die of late-onset meningitis have purulent leptomeningitis at postmortem examination.[113]

Sequelae occur in 20 to 30 percent of survivors of early- and late-onset meningitis. These sequelae include mental retardation, spastic quadriplegia, cortical blindness, deafness, uncontrolled seizures, hydrocephalus, and speech and language delay.[100,318] Signs at admission that are correlated with a high likelihood of a poor outcome include hypotension, coma or semicoma, status epilepticus, neutropenia, CSF protein levels greater than 300 mg/dL, and high concentrations of bacterial capsular polysaccharide antigen in CSF.[39,100,245]

LATE, LATE-ONSET DISEASE

Contemporary studies show increasing incidence of group B streptococcal infection in infants older than 3 months of age, defined as late, late-onset disease.[151,280,336] These infections tend to occur in infants who were born extremely prematurely and whose corrected age is less than 3 months.[151,280,336] Late, late-onset disease also occurs in children co-infected with HIV and those with immunodeficiencies,[87,151,336] a finding supporting the recommendation that immunodeficiency be considered in any child infected beyond the usual period of risk.[87] The clinical manifestations in these older infants are similar to those in patients with typical late-onset infection; bacteremia without a focus and meningitis are the most common clinical features.[87,151] Endocarditis and central venous catheter infection also have been noted.[151]

SEPTIC ARTHRITIS AND OSTEOMYELITIS

Osteoarthritis occurs in approximately 5 percent of infants with late-onset infection.[336] Among neonates and young infants with osteomyelitis, group B streptococci have been identified as the causal agent in 7 to 38 percent of cases.[96,333] The osteoarticular disease usually is more indolent than is the osteomyelitis caused by other etiologic agents in young infants. Diagnosis usually is established after a mean of 9 days of findings at a mean age of 31 days.[33,96] Decreased motion of the involved extremity and pain with manipulation are common signs. Warmth and redness are uncommon findings but have been described.[96] Systemic signs and symptoms, including fever, are unusual manifestations.[96,214]

Group B *Streptococcus* has a predilection for the proximal humerus.[96] The femur is the second most commonly affected bone. Involvement of more than one bone is an unusual finding.[96] However, involvement of the adjacent joint is described.[214] Blood cultures infrequently are positive, unlike neonatal osteomyelitis caused by other etiologic agents. A lytic lesion often is seen on radiographs at first evaluation (Fig. 94–4). This observation suggests that lytic lesions may be a late phenomenon that develops after seeding of the metaphysis during an episode of asymptomatic, early-onset bacteremia several weeks before presentation.[33]

The mean age at diagnosis in infants who have septic arthritis without osteomyelitis is 20 days. The clinical picture typically is acute, with a mean of 2 days of abnormal findings before diag-

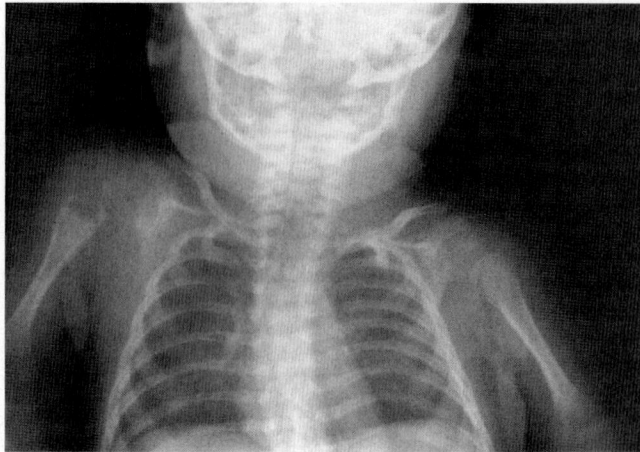

Figure 94–4 Radiograph of the right arm of a 26-day-old infant with a 2-day history of diminished movement of that extremity. A well-defined, lytic lesion is present in the proximal end of the humerus. Necrotic material from this area was débrided surgically and grew group B streptococci on culture. *(Courtesy of Morven S. Edwards, M.D.)*

nosis is established. The lower extremities are involved most often, with the hip joint predominating. Infants typically present with local joint signs in the absence of systemic symptoms.[215]

CELLULITIS/ADENITIS

In one case series, 2 percent of late-onset group B streptococcal infections were associated with cellulitis/adenitis syndrome.[336] Diagnosis is made at a mean age of 5 weeks, with a preponderance of cases in male patients.[21] Typical presentation includes fever, irritability, poor feeding, and swelling of the affected soft tissue area. Enlarged adjacent lymph nodes become palpable within a few days. The most frequent sites of cellulitis are the face and neck,[21,136,243] with enlarged lymph nodes in the submandibular area. Ipsilateral otitis media was noted in four of five infants with facial or submandibular cellulitis in one case series.[139] Less commonly affected areas reported include the genital or inguinal region (Fig. 94–5), the hand, and the prepatellar bursa.[21,33,61] Aspiration of the affected area of cellulitis often yields group B streptococci, and concomitant bacteremia almost always is present.

OTHER MANIFESTATIONS

Nearly every organ has been reported to be a site of group B streptococcal infection in young infants. Table 94–2 lists these reported unusual manifestations of early- and late-onset disease.

RECURRENT INFECTIONS

Second (and sometimes third) episodes of group B streptococcal infection occur in approximately 1 to 2 percent of cases after early- and late-onset infection.[128] In a case series from Houston, the mean age at recurrence was 44 days, and the mean duration between the first course of therapy and recurrence was 19 days.[128] Molecular epidemiologic techniques have indicated that most, but not all, of these recurrent infections are caused by the strain implicated in the first episode; this finding suggests that persistent mucosal colonization after treatment of the first episode is followed by invasion of the bloodstream.[227] Contaminated breast

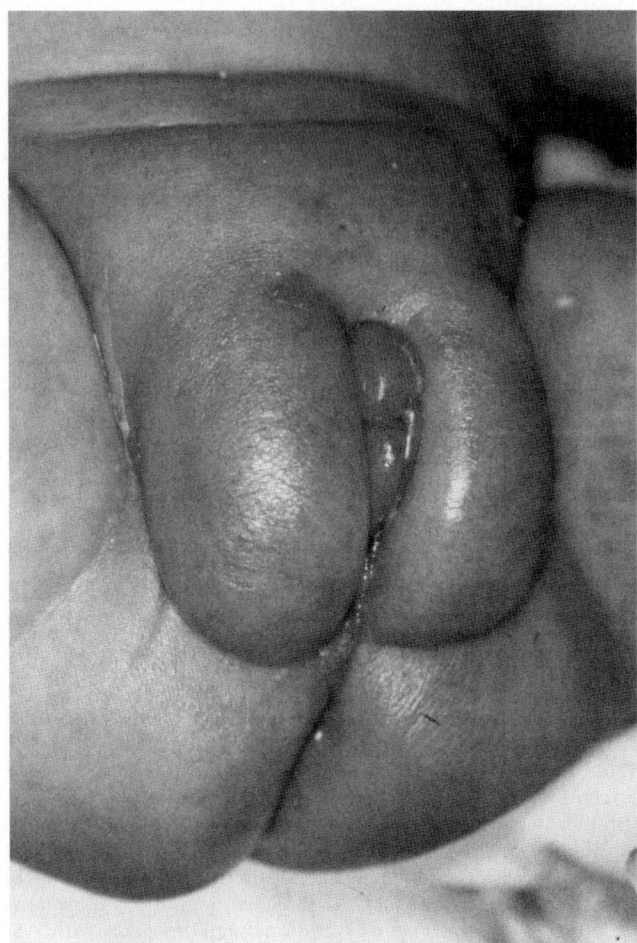

Figure 94–5 This 3-month-old female infant who was born after 28 weeks' gestation had fever, lethargy, swelling of the external genitalia, and erythema that extended to the lower part of the abdomen and the thigh. Blood culture grew type Ib/c group B streptococci. *(Courtesy of Morven S. Edwards, M.D.)*

TABLE 94–2 Unusual Clinical Manifestations of Group B Streptococcal Disease in Infants and Children

Site and Manifestation	References
Brain	
Abscess	290
Cerebritis	168
Chronic meningitis	295
Diabetes insipidus	198
Eosinophilic meningitis	221
Subdural empyema	106
Ventriculitis	222
Eye	
Conjunctivitis	16, 113, 254
Endophthalmitis	129, 180
Ear and Sinus	
Ethmoiditis	150
Otitis media/mastoiditis	21, 274, 288
Cardiovascular/Hematologic	
Asymptomatic bacteremia	117, 150, 261
Endocarditis	8, 43, 149, 234, 321
Myocarditis	44
Mycotic aneurysm	3
Pericarditis	133
Respiratory Tract	
Epiglottitis	339
Supraglottitis	191
Tracheitis	240
Pleural empyema	150, 294
Skin and Soft Tissue	
Breast abscess	230, 265
Bursitis	63
Cellulitis/adenitis	21, 136, 150, 177, 243, 331
Dactylitis	114
Fasciitis	124, 259
Impetigo neonatorum	46, 170, 193
Purpura fulminans	153, 195
Omphalitis	47, 155, 336
Rhabdomyolysis	310
Scalp abscess	104, 132
Abdomen	
Adrenal abscess	18, 72, 319
Delayed-onset diaphragmatic hernia	17, 41, 251, 299
Gallbladder distention	246
Peritonitis	70, 76
Urinary Tract	
Renal abscess	319, 335
Urinary tract infection	297, 336

Adapted from Baker, C. J., Nizet V, and Edwards, M. S.: Group B streptococcal infections. In Remington, J. S., and Klein, J. O. (eds.): Infectious Diseases of the Fetus and Newborn Infant. 6th ed. Philadelphia, W. B. Saunders, 2005, pp. 403-464.

milk also has been implicated as a source of recurrent infection.[171] No specific risk factors are evident in these infants, but most of them are born prematurely.[128]

DIAGNOSIS AND DIFFERENTIAL DIAGNOSIS

LABORATORY STUDIES

The diagnosis of group B streptococcal infection is confirmed by isolation of this pathogen from a normally sterile body site including blood, CSF, pleural fluid, bone aspirate, joint fluid, or soft tissue. Cultures of the skin, umbilicus, or mucous membranes do not have clinical significance. Tracheal aspirate cultures that grow group B streptococci indicate neonatal colonization but do not prove pulmonary invasion (pneumonia). Rather, isolation of the organism from blood (or in rare circumstances, lung tissue or the pleural space) is required.

Meningitis in early-onset disease is clinically indistinguishable from bacteremia without a focus, and 10 to 38 percent of neonates with meningitis have negative blood culture results,[332] so lumbar puncture is necessary to determine the presence or absence of meningeal involvement. Lumbar punctures also are indicated in patients with a focal site of group B streptococcal infection resulting from its propensity for involving the CNS. For example, group B streptococci grew from CSF cultures in 24 percent of infants with cellulitis/adenitis who underwent lumbar puncture.[5] One study found that if selected criteria were used instead of routine lumbar punctures, the diagnosis of bacterial meningitis would have been missed or delayed in 17 percent of infants.[332]

Several methods for detecting group B polysaccharide antigen in body fluid specimens have been developed. These techniques include countercurrent immunoelectrophoresis, latex particle agglutination, and enzyme immunoassay.[39,131,226,247,267]

The advantages of these methods are their simplicity, rapidity, and ability to detect antigen, even after cultures are rendered sterile by antimicrobial therapy. The disadvantage is the frequency of false-positive results, especially when they are used to "screen" asymptomatic infants for sepsis.[247] Studies also have shown false-negative results from specimens from infants with subsequent death from group B streptococcal disease.[231]

CSF has had detectable group B antigen in 72 to 89 percent of neonates with meningitis; serum is much less likely to be positive. The only specimens recommended for antigen testing are blood and CSF; urine specimens should not be tested because they are unreliable. Antigen testing should not be used as a substitute for bacterial culture. Their proper use should be limited to the setting of symptomatic infants in whom rapid diagnosis may alter therapy or allow proper tailoring of antibiotic choice, for example, a sick neonate with CSF pleocytosis and previous antibiotic administration. These tests are never useful in infants who appear healthy.

A limited study of real-time polymerase chain reaction (PCR) to detect DNA in blood of eight neonates with culture-proven group B streptococcal sepsis showed positive corresponding results.[160] However, larger, prospective studies are required to evaluate sensitivity and specificity.

The white blood cell count of a neonate with proven group B streptococcal sepsis may reflect leukopenia, neutropenia, or leukocytosis.[204,245,316] Manroe and associates[204] found the ratio of absolute immature neutrophils to absolute total neutrophils (I:T index) to be the most reliable index for distinguishing respiratory distress caused by group B streptococcal infection from that with a noninfectious origin. Most infected neonates had an elevation greater than 0.20 (91% versus 4% of uninfected infants). Other markers of inflammation such as C-reactive protein may also rise with acute infection and decrease in response to therapy.[250,255]

DIFFERENTIAL DIAGNOSIS

The signs and symptoms of early-onset group B streptococcal disease are clinically indistinguishable from neonatal sepsis caused by other bacterial pathogens such as *E. coli* and *Listeria monocytogenes*. The timing may be somewhat different, with group B streptococcal disease appearing earlier and leading to death earlier in fatal cases.[267] The prominence of respiratory signs in early-onset disease has led to confusion with noninfectious causes of respiratory distress such as transient tachypnea of the newborn, persistent fetal circulation, and respiratory distress syndrome.[2,20,245,316] Clinical features that suggest group B

streptococcal infection include a history of prolonged rupture of membranes, apnea, shock in the first 24 hours of life, a 1-minute Apgar score of 5 or less, and rapid progression of pulmonary disease.[2,20,316]

The differential diagnosis of late-onset disease depends on the focus of infection. Meningitis in infants of this age also is caused by *Streptococcus pneumoniae*, *Neisseria meningitidis*, *Listeria monocytogenes*, *Haemophilus influenzae* (type b and nontypeable), and viruses. If the results of Gram stain analysis of CSF are inconclusive, other potential pathogens should be considered when therapy is selected. The findings of osteomyelitis may be subtle; refusal to move the arm may be ascribed to neuromuscular disease or Erb palsy.[96] Careful physical examination usually reveals tenderness over the involved area, and radiographs generally show a lytic defect in the metaphyses.[96] If the organism is isolated from a bone aspirate, the diagnosis is definitive. Finally, as seen in Table 94-2, many unusual manifestations of group B streptococcal infection have been described, so this organism should be included in the differential diagnosis of any focal infection occurring in the age group at risk.

TREATMENT

EMPIRIC TREATMENT

The antimicrobial regimens recommended for the treatment of group B streptococcal infection in infants are summarized in Table 94–3. Penicillin G remains the drug of choice because susceptibility is uniform. In the usual circumstance, however, antimicrobial therapy for group B streptococcal infection is started before culture results are known. Initial empiric therapy for early-onset disease would include ampicillin and gentamicin for the treatment of neonatal pathogens in addition to group B streptococci. Irrespective of gestational age, neonates with suspected meningitis and those whose clinical condition will not permit lumbar puncture should receive high doses of ampicillin (300 mg/kg/day) plus gentamicin.[12] This combination is more effective than is either ampicillin or penicillin G alone in killing most group B streptococcal strains in vitro[275] and in vivo.[300] For suspected late-onset disease, the usual initial therapy includes intravenous ampicillin in combination with cefotaxime or ceftriaxone.[252] If an infant is receiving empiric vancomycin therapy and group B streptococcal meningitis has not been excluded, penicillin G or ampicillin should be added to the regimen because vancomycin is inhibitory in vitro rather than bactericidal, and CSF concentrations may not exceed the minimal inhibitory concentration if a high inoculum of group B streptococci is present.[33]

TABLE 94–3 Treatment of Group B Streptococcal Infections in Infants

Focus of Infection	Antibiotic	Daily Dose	Duration
Suspected meningitis (initial empiric therapy)	Ampicillin *plus* gentamicin	300-400 mg/kg 7.5 mg/kg	Until cerebrospinal fluid is sterile
Suspected sepsis* (initial empiric therapy)	Ampicillin *plus* gentamicin	150-200 mg/kg	Until bloodstream is sterile
Meningitis	Penicillin G	450,000-500,000 units/kg	14 days minimum[†]
Bacteremia	Penicillin G	200,000 units/kg	10 days
Arthritis	Penicillin G	200,000-300,000 units/kg	2-3 wk
Osteomyelitis	Penicillin G	200,000-300,000 units/kg	3-4 wk
Endocarditis	Penicillin G	400,000 units/kg	4 wk[‡]

Assumes that lumbar puncture has been performed and the cerebrospinal fluid has no abnormalities.
[†]*Should be extended to 21 days or longer if ventriculitis, cerebritis, subdural empyema, or other suppurative complications occur.*
[‡]*In combination with low-dose gentamicin for the first 14 days.*

SPECIFIC TREATMENT

Once group B streptococci have been identified in cultures of blood, CSF, or other normally sterile body sites and blood and CSF cultures are shown to be sterile, penicillin G alone should be used to complete therapy. Recommendations concerning the optimal dose and duration have varied, but they should be dictated by the focus and severity of the infection (see Table 94–3). Several issues should be considered when selecting the appropriate dose: (1) the usual minimal bactericidal concentration of penicillin for group B streptococci ranges from 0.04 to 0.8 µg/mL,[165] (2) only 10 percent of penicillin serum levels reach the CSF, (3) the inoculum of group B streptococci in the CSF of infants with meningitis may reach 10^7 to 10^8 colony-forming units per milliliter,[105] and (4) high doses of penicillin G and ampicillin are safe in neonates.[33] To ensure rapid bacterial killing, especially in infants with meningitis, relatively high doses of penicillin are recommended for both early- and late-onset infections.

The infant with meningitis should undergo a second lumbar puncture 24 to 48 hours into therapy to document CSF sterility.[33] Infants with continued positive CSF cultures may have very high inoculum, ventriculitis with obstruction, severe infection with cerebritis and vasculitis, subdural empyema, or septic thrombophlebitis, or they may be receiving an insufficient dose of antibiotics; in this circumstance, appropriate studies should be initiated to determine which of these conditions is present. When CSF sterility and penicillin G susceptibility are verified, penicillin G alone is given for a minimum of 14 days.[252] Longer treatment is indicated if the course is severe, the infant has ventriculitis, or CSF sterilization is delayed. Another lumbar puncture to evaluate CSF cell count and protein should be considered at the anticipated completion of therapy. Findings of polymorphonuclear cells greater than 30 percent or protein higher than 200 mg/dL may warrant further diagnostic evaluation and longer duration of therapy.[33] In addition, a contrast-enhanced computed tomography scan of the head should be performed near completion of therapy in complicated cases, including infants who have prolonged fever (>5 days), cerebritis, abscess, subdural empyema, or venous thrombosis. Such complications often correlate with neurologic abnormalities that lead to a poor prognosis for complete central nervous system recovery.[100,318]

Infants with bacteremia without a focus should receive intravenous therapy for a total of 10 days.[252] A shorter duration has not been documented to be efficacious, and relapses, although rare, have been reported in these circumstances.[65,320] Patients with septic arthritis, osteomyelitis, or endocarditis should be treated for the durations summarized in Table 94–3. Oral therapy has no place in the management of infants with group B streptococcal disease.[33,252] Alternative agents such as the cephalosporins and vancomycin are active against group B streptococci in vitro.[107,186] The efficacy of these agents is unknown, however, and these drugs are not recommended in most circumstances.

SUPPORTIVE TREATMENT

The importance of prompt, vigorous, and careful supportive therapy in the successful treatment of infant group B streptococcal infections cannot be overemphasized. Neonates with early-onset disease accompanied by pneumonia should be suspected of having early respiratory failure, and ventilatory support should be initiated before the onset of apnea, septic shock, or frank respiratory failure occurs. Persistent metabolic acidosis and delayed capillary refill should prompt treatment for shock. All patients with signs of impending respiratory or circulatory failure or meningitis should be treated in an intensive care unit. When present, hypoxemia, severe anemia, and acidosis should be corrected, and seizures should be controlled with anticonvulsants. In addition, fluid and electrolyte status should be monitored meticulously. Surfactant should be used as per nursery protocol; improved gas exchange is seen in infected premature neonates who receive surfactant, although the response is slower than in patients with respiratory distress syndrome.[141] Finally, if an infant has persistent pulmonary hypertension or if conventional ventilatory therapy has failed, extracorporeal membrane oxygenation may be considered, if available.

ADJUNCTIVE TREATMENT

Adjunctive treatment of life-threatening group B streptococcal disease is aimed at correcting poor host defenses and is being investigated. Such treatment includes intravenous human immunoglobulin, monoclonal antibodies to group B streptococcal polysaccharide antigen, leukocyte transfusion, and growth factors such as granulocyte colony-stimulating factor and granulocyte-monocyte colony-stimulating factor for neutropenia.[69,78,122] The efficacy of these agents has not been established, and, although they may be used occasionally, they should be considered experimental.

RECURRENT INFECTIONS

In the few infants who experience a recurrence, suppurative foci, HIV infection, or humoral immune deficiency should be excluded or treated. Immunoglobulin levels should be determined to exclude humoral immune deficiency. Although it may be too early to document humoral immune deficiency unequivocally, total IgG usually is significantly lower than would be expected for age in weeks.[128] Tube dilution susceptibility of isolates from the first and recurrent episodes should be determined to ensure in vitro susceptibility to penicillin. If the reason for the recurrence remains unknown, persistent mucous membrane colonization with group B streptococci probably is the source.[227] β-Lactam antibiotics, even when administered by the parenteral route, do not eradicate group B streptococcal colonization reliably.[239] Some studies have shown the benefit of rifampin (20 mg/kg/day) to eradicate mucosal group B streptococcal colonization when given orally during the last 4 days of parenteral therapy.[128,219] However, a more recent study showed failure of rifampin to eradicate group B streptococcal colonization in infants.[108]

PROGNOSIS

The outcome of group B streptococcal disease is related closely to the severity and site of infection at initial evaluation. Improved outcomes after early-onset infection have resulted from greater awareness among pediatricians and improved obstetric management. Improvements in obstetrics include the use of intrapartum antibiotic prophylaxis in women at risk for delivering an infant with early-onset group B streptococcal infection. However, the mortality rate remains substantial at 2 to 8 percent, especially in neonates born at less than 37 weeks' gestation, in whom the mortality rate often exceeds 20 percent.[75,281]

Little information is available on the long-term prognosis of survivors of group B streptococcal sepsis without meningitis. In infants with septic shock, the development of periventricular leukomalacia has been reported and associated with neurodevelopmental sequelae.[102] However, the frequency of this association is not known.

For infants with early- or late-onset meningitis, 20 to 30 percent will have permanent neurologic sequelae, and 20 percent of these impaired survivors have global mental retardation, cortical blindness, hearing loss, spasticity, or paresis.[100,135,318] Whether these rates reported over 20 years ago can be applied to infants currently being treated is unknown. Improvements in both specific and supportive therapy may have diminished the frequency of lasting impairments.

To date, the prognosis for infants with osteoarticular or soft tissue infections with group B streptococci has been excellent.[21,96] However, omission of early surgical intervention for infections that involve either the hip or shoulder joints may result in epiphyseal injury.

PREVENTION

The continuing magnitude and severity of group B streptococcal disease and its attendant mortality and morbidity have led to investigations aimed at its prevention. Several general approaches have been proposed: maternal chemoprophylaxis to decrease transmission, infant chemoprophylaxis to decrease colonization, and immunoprophylaxis to increase protection against disease.

CHEMOPROPHYLAXIS

Maternal Chemoprophylaxis

Epidemiologic studies during the 1980s showed that women with group B streptococcal colonization during pregnancy had greater than 25 times likelihood of delivering infants with early-onset disease compared with women with negative prenatal cultures.[278] The idea to give antibiotic therapy to the mother to prevent vertical transmission to her fetus was suggested first by Franciosi and colleagues.[113] The first strategy to be evaluated was antenatal treatment of group B streptococcal maternal carriers with oral or intramuscular penicillin. This method temporarily suppresses colonization density but does not eradicate it or interrupt vertical transmission of group B streptococci to neonates.[119,130,258]

The next strategy, maternal intrapartum chemoprophylaxis, has been demonstrated to be efficacious in the prevention of vertical transmission of group B streptococci from colonized mothers to their neonates, the development of early-onset disease, and maternal febrile morbidity. Infants are less frequently colonized with group B *Streptococcus* if they are born to mothers treated with ampicillin during labor than to mothers not given antibiotics.[59,60,341] Several controlled trials involving thousands of

deliveries indicated that intrapartum penicillin G or ampicillin given intravenously to group B streptococcal carriers during labor prevents early-onset disease in neonates.[57,211,309] Early-onset infection occurred in 0 to 1.1 percent of infants whose mothers received intrapartum ampicillin compared with 5 to 9 percent of infants of mothers in the groups not receiving treatment. A large trial involving more than 50,000 live births in Australia showed similar results.[120]

In 1996, guidelines supported by the Centers for Disease Control and Prevention (CDC), the American College of Obstetricians and Gynecologists, and the American Academy of Pediatrics recommended a risk-based approach or culture-based approach.[278] The risk-based approach was based on the presence of one of more of the following: premature labor at less than 37 weeks' gestation, prolonged rupture of membranes (>18 hours), group B streptococcal bacteriuria, intrapartum fever (≥100.4° F [38° C]), or delivery of a previous infant with group B streptococcal infection. The culture-based approach required intrapartum chemoprophylaxis for all women with positive vaginal and rectal cultures routinely obtained at 35 to 37 weeks' gestation regardless of risk factors. Use of these methods to define women who were candidates for intrapartum chemoprophylaxis led to a 70 percent decline in the incidence of early-onset group B streptococcal disease.[75,280]

In 2002, a population-based study compared the two approaches and found the culture-based approach to be 50 percent more effective than the risk-based approach in preventing early-onset group B streptococcal disease.[279] Sixty-two percent of infants with early-onset disease were born to mothers who did not have any clinical risk factors. Therefore, revised guidelines published by the CDC in 2002 recommended universal vaginal and rectal screening cultures of all pregnant women between 35 and 37 weeks of gestation, with intrapartum chemoprophylaxis for all women identified as group B streptococcal carriers.[278] The risk-based approach was to be reserved for any women in labor whose colonization status is unknown. Colonization during a previous pregnancy is not an indication for intrapartum chemoprophylaxis. Women with group B *Streptococcus* isolated from urine in any concentration during pregnancy should receive intrapartum chemoprophylaxis, because these women usually are heavily colonized. Women who previously gave birth to an infant with invasive group B streptococcal disease always should receive chemoprophylaxis. An algorithm of these current guidelines is shown in Figure 94–6.

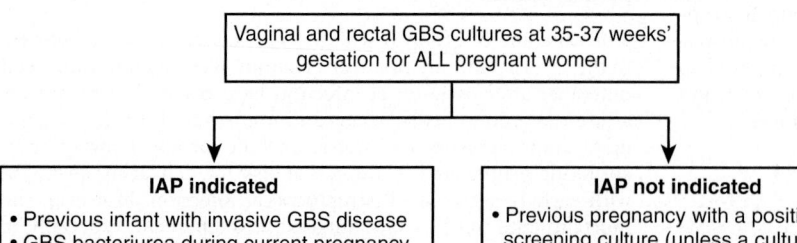

Figure 94–6 Recommendations for intrapartum antimicrobial prophylaxis (IAP) to prevent early-onset group B streptococcal (GBS) disease using a universal culture screening strategy. (*Adapted from Centers for Disease Control and Prevention: Prevention of perinatal group B streptococcal disease: Revised guidelines from CDC. M. M. W. R. Morb. Mortal. Wkly. Rep. 51:1-22, 2002.*)

Vaginal and rectal GBS cultures at 35-37 weeks' gestation for ALL pregnant women

IAP indicated
- Previous infant with invasive GBS disease
- GBS bacteriurea during current pregnancy
- Positive GBS screening culture during current pregnancy (unless planned cesarean section in absence of labor or membrane rupture)
- Unknown GBS status AND any of the following:
  - Delivery at <37 weeks' gestation
  - Membrane rupture >18 hours
  - Intrapartum fever ≥ 100.4° F (38° C)*

IAP not indicated
- Previous pregnancy with a positive GBS screening culture (unless a culture was positive during current pregnancy)
- Planned cesarean section in absence of labor or membrane rupture
- Negative vaginal and rectal GBS screening culture in late gestation, regardless of intrapartum risk factors

*If chorioamnionitis is suspected, broad-spectrum antimicrobial therapy that includes an agent active against GBS should replace GBS IAP.

Optimal culture techniques are discussed earlier in the chapter. Many rapid tests are being studied because they offer the advantage of detecting colonization status in women who present for preterm labor or who have not had prenatal care. These tests include latex agglutination, optical immunoassay, DNA hybridization, enzyme immunoassay, Islam starch medium tests, and PCR.[146] With the exception of PCR, all tests showed poor sensitivity or specificity compared with the standard culture method and are not sufficiently accurate to aid in decision making concerning intrapartum antibiotic prophylaxis. None of these tests can replace routine culture at this time. A prospective multicenter study evaluated a real-time PCR assay that gave results in 40 minutes.[83] Compared with intrapartum culture, the PCR assay had a sensitivity of 94 percent and a specificity of 96 percent.

Maternal chemoprophylaxis begins at hospital admission for delivery or at rupture of membranes and consists of intravenous penicillin G (initial dose, 5 million units; subsequent doses, 2.5 million units every 4 hours recommended for intrapartum chemoprophylaxis).[278] Although penicillin is preferred because of its narrow spectrum of activity, ampicillin (initial dose, 2 g; subsequent doses, 1 g every 4 hours) can be given as an alternative. For women who are allergic to penicillin, intrapartum chemoprophylaxis must take into account increasing resistance rates to clindamycin and erythromycin.[55,86] Women at low risk of developing anaphylaxis should be given cefazolin (initial dose, 2 g; subsequent doses, 1 g every 8 hours). Women at high risk of developing anaphylaxis should have susceptibility testing performed on their isolates obtained during screening at 35 to 37 weeks of gestation. If the isolate is susceptible, clindamycin (900 mg every 8 hours) or erythromycin (500 mg every 6 hours) can be used. If susceptibility testing is not available, the results are not known,

or the isolate is resistant to clindamycin and erythromycin, vancomycin (1 g every 12 hours) can be given as the alternative. The efficacy of the latter two regimens is not known.

Since the widespread adoption of chemoprophylaxis, the incidence of early-onset disease has plummeted.[75,280] Racial disparities in early-onset disease have declined significantly.[73,280] Opportunities to prevent early-onset disease still are missed, however, because of laboratory practices,[74] hospital or procedural errors in communication of the screening results, or failure to administer intrapartum chemoprophylaxis to a mother known to be colonized.[257] The incidence of late-onset disease remains unaffected by intrapartum chemoprophylaxis.[75]

Management of an infant born to a mother given intrapartum penicillin G prophylaxis depends on the clinical findings at birth, the gestational age, and the timing of doses administered to the mother (Fig. 94-7). Amniotic fluid levels of penicillin that will kill group B streptococci are not achieved until at least 3 hours after administration of the first dose.[62] If the infant appears healthy, has a gestational age of 35 weeks or more, and has a mother given at least one dose of intrapartum chemoprophylaxis at least 4 hours before delivery, neither diagnostic evaluation nor empiric antimicrobial therapy will be required. However, to ensure their ongoing stability, such infants should be observed in the hospital for at least 48 hours. Keeping the infant hospitalized through day of life 2 has been challenging because the associated expense affects the cost-to-benefit ratio of intrapartum prophylaxis.[223] However, an analysis of all live births in the state of Florida for the years 1992 through 1994 demonstrated a 115 percent increase in the rate of readmission for group B streptococcal infection in infants discharged on day of life 1; this finding supports the recommendation to observe infants for 48 hours.[126]

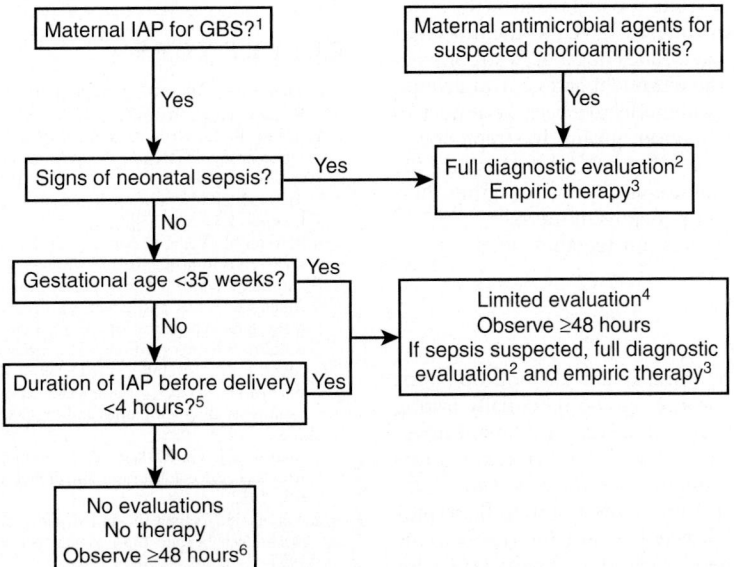

Figure 94-7 Empiric management of a newborn exposed to intrapartum antimicrobial prophylaxis (IAP) for group B streptococcal (GBS) infection. *1,* When no maternal intrapartum prophylaxis for GBS was administered despite the presence of an indication, data are insufficient on which to recommend a single management strategy. *2,* Includes complete blood cell count (CBC) and differential, blood culture, and chest radiograph if respiratory abnormalities are present. When signs of sepsis are present, a lumbar puncture, if feasible, should be performed. *3,* Duration of therapy varied depending on results of blood culture, cerebrospinal fluid findings, if obtained, and clinical course of the infant. If laboratory results and clinical course do not indicate bacterial infection, duration may be as short as 48 hours. *4,* CBC and differential and blood culture. *5,* Applies only to penicillin, ampicillin, or cefazolin and assumes recommended dosing regimens. *6,* A healthy-appearing infant who was at least 38 weeks' gestation at delivery and whose mother received at least 4 hours of IAP before delivery may be discharged home after 24 hours if other discharge criteria have been met and a person able to comply fully with instructions for home observation will be present. If any one of these conditions is not met, the infant should be observed in the hospital for at least 48 hours and until criteria for discharge are achieved. (*Adapted from Centers for Disease Control and Prevention: Prevention of perinatal group B streptococcal disease: Revised guidelines from CDC. M. M. W. R. Morb. Mortal. Wkly. Rep. 51:1-22, 2002.*)

Neonates with signs of sepsis are evaluated and treated empirically for sepsis. Healthy-appearing neonates who either are born at less than 35 weeks' gestation or are born to women given no intrapartum chemoprophylaxis or a single dose of intrapartum chemoprophylaxis less than 4 hours before delivery should undergo limited laboratory evaluation (complete blood count and blood culture) and observation in the hospital for 48 hours without therapy. However, if the subsequent clinical course or the laboratory results suggest infection, full diagnostic evaluation and therapy is initiated.

Concern that widespread use of intrapartum ampicillin use will result in a greater incidence of ampicillin-resistant neonatal infection has been supported by some case series.[161,216] Development of penicillin- or ampicillin-resistant group B streptococci has not been seen.[77] In most studies, incidence rates of *E. coli* and other gram-negative pathogens have remained stable.[4,161,216,268] The rate of ampicillin-resistant *E. coli* infections is increasing in preterm infants. However, rates of ampicillin resistance in term neonates before and after widespread intrapartum chemoprophylaxis are the same.

Infant Chemoprophylaxis

The two controlled trials evaluating neonatal prophylaxis reached contradictory conclusions.[256,289] In the first trial, more than 16,000 newborns received either intramuscular penicillin G or topical tetracycline (prophylaxis for gonococcal ophthalmia neonatorum) within an hour of birth during alternating weeks.[289] In penicillin-treated newborns, the incidence of proven early-onset group B streptococcal disease was less common, but death rates were similar, and an increase in the number of penicillin-resistant infections in the penicillin group was noted. In the second controlled study, blood cultures were obtained before initiation of penicillin therapy, and rates of group B streptococcal bacteremia were similar in the treatment and control groups.[256] In this study of nearly 1200 neonates weighing 2000 g or less at birth, intramuscular penicillin (or no treatment) was given in the first hour of life and was continued for 3 days. Rates of group B streptococcal bacteremia were similar in the treatment and control groups. Penicillin prophylaxis probably was ineffective because almost 90 percent of neonates with early-onset group B streptococcal disease were bacteremic immediately after birth. The results of the second study are supported by numerous observations, thus indicating that early-onset disease often begins in utero.[60,241,253,281,282] Infant chemoprophylaxis currently is not recommended.[278]

IMMUNOPROPHYLAXIS

Although efforts to implement intrapartum chemoprophylaxis further are ongoing, the most promising and potentially lasting method for prevention of both early- and late-onset infant infections is immunoprophylaxis. This approach remains investigational, and several reviews have summarized the rationale.[25,137,237] It is based on the observation that immunity to group B streptococci correlates with antibody directed against the type-specific capsular polysaccharides of these organisms. These IgG class antibodies and complement promote opsonization, phagocytosis, and bacterial killing of group B streptococci and protect animals against lethal challenge.[238,325] Thus, provision of protective levels of type-specific immunity to the infant could be achieved through active immunization of the mother. Baker and associates[36] immunized women at a mean gestation of 31 weeks with purified type III polysaccharide vaccine. Although the immune response was not optimal (63%), placental transport of maternal antibodies was 90 percent in neonates born to women who did respond to vaccination, and most of these infants had protective levels of antibodies in their sera at 3 months of age. A more recent study

immunizing women with a type III polysaccharide-tetanus toxoid conjugate reported a 95 percent immune response, with persistence of opsonophagocytic antibodies at 2 months of age in 100 percent of infants born to maternal responders.[38] Other studies immunizing nonpregnant adults with purified capsular polysaccharide-tetanus toxoid conjugate vaccines showed the safety and immunogenicity of these vaccines.[34,35,37]

Availability of the complete genome sequences for group B *Streptococcus* has led to the discovery of many potential surface proteins and secreted proteins that can be expressed in recombinant form and used for production of antibodies.[200,306] A set of proteins shared by the disease-causing serotypes theoretically can be used in combination to create a vaccine capable of providing protection against multiple serotypes. Group B streptococcal pili with at least one of the pilus islands present in all sequenced group B streptococcal genomes may be included in a future vaccine.[66]

Because most pregnant women (estimated at 85-90%) have nonprotective levels of these antibodies in their sera at delivery, active immunization of childbearing-age women before or during pregnancy would optimize strategy to induce high maternal antibody levels. Human studies have demonstrated efficient antibody transfer to the neonate.[36,38] Transfer of high levels of maternal antibody would provide protection of the neonates from early- and late-onset group B streptococcal disease. In addition, immunization also would offer protection for the mother against preterm deliveries and fetal loss caused by group B streptococcal infection. Finally, vaccination of elderly or nonpregnant adults with defined medical conditions could reduce the disease burden significantly. Because immunoprophylaxis should be the most cost-effective and beneficial prevention strategy for group B streptococcal disease,[224,291] it should be promoted by physicians, public health officials, parents, pharmaceutical manufacturers, and legislators.

REFERENCES

1. Aber, R. C., Allen, N., Howell, J. T., et al.: Nosocomial transmission of group B streptococci. Pediatrics 58:346-353, 1976.
2. Ablow, R. C., Driscoll, S. G., Effmann, E. L., et al.: A comparison of early-onset group B streptococcal neonatal infection and the respiratory-distress syndrome of the newborn. N. Engl. J. Med. 294:65-70, 1976.
3. Agarwala, B. N.: Group B streptococcal endocarditis in a neonate. Pediatr. Cardiol. 9:51-53, 1988.
4. Alarcon, A., Pena, P., Salas, S., et al.: Neonatal early onset *Escherichia coli* sepsis: Trends in incidence and antimicrobial resistance in the era of intrapartum antimicrobial prophylaxis. Pediatr. Infect. Dis. J. 23:295-299, 2004.
5. Albanyan, E. A., and Baker, C. J.: Is lumbar puncture necessary to exclude meningitis in neonates and young infants: Lessons from group B streptococcus cellulitis-adenitis syndrome. Pediatrics 102:985-986, 1998.
6. Alger, L. S., Lovchik, J. C., Hebel, J. R., et al.: The association of *Chlamydia trachomatis*, *Neisseria gonorrhoeae*, and group B streptococci with preterm rupture of the membranes and pregnancy outcome. Am. J. Obstet. Gynecol. 159:397-404, 1988.
7. Allardice, J. G., Baskett, T. F., Seshia, M. M. K., et al.: Perinatal group B streptococcal colonization and infection. Am. J. Obstet. Gynecol. 142:617-620, 1982.
8. Alsoub, H., Najma, F., and Robida, A.: Group B streptococcal endocarditis in children beyond the neonatal period. Pediatr. Infect. Dis. J. 16:418-420, 1997.
9. Ancona, R. J., Ferrieri, P., and Williams, P. P.: Maternal factors that enhance the acquisition of group B streptococci by newborn infants. J. Med. Microbiol. 13:273-280, 1980.
10. Anderson, D. C., Hughes, B. J., Edwards, M. S., et al.: Impaired chemotaxigenesis by type III group B streptococci in neonatal sera: Relationship to diminished concentration of specific anticapsular antibody and abnormalities of serum complement. Pediatr. Res. 17:496-502, 1983.
11. Anderson, D. C., Hughes, B. J., and Smith, C. W.: Abnormal mobility of neonatal polymorphonuclear leukocytes. J. Clin. Invest. 59:810-818, 1981.
12. Anthony, B. F., and Okada, D. M.: The emergence of group B streptococci in infections of the newborn infant. Annu. Rev. Med. 28:355-369, 1977.
13. Anthony, B. F., Concepcion, I. E., Concepcion, N. F., et al.: Relation between maternal age and serum concentration of IgG antibody to type III group B streptococci. J. Infect. Dis. 170:717-720, 1994.

14. Anthony, B. F., Okada, D. M., and Hobel, C. J.: Epidemiology of group B *Streptococcus*: Longitudinal observations during pregnancy. J. Infect. Dis. *137*:524-530, 1978.

15. Anthony, B. F., Okada, D. M., and Hobel, C. J.: Epidemiology of the group B *Streptococcus*: Maternal and nosocomial sources for infant acquisitions. J. Pediatr. *95*:431-436, 1979.

16. Armstrong, J. H., Zacarias, F., and Rein, M. F.: Ophthalmia neonatorum: A chart review. Pediatrics *57*:884-892, 1976.

17. Ashcraft, K. W., Holder, T. M., Amoury, R. A., et al.: Diagnosis and treatment of right Bochdalek hernia associated with group B streptococcal pneumonia and sepsis in the neonate. J. Pediatr. Surg. *18*:480-485, 1983.

18. Atkinson, G. O., Kodroff, M. B., Gay, B. B., et al.: Adrenal abscess in the neonate. Radiology *155*:101-104, 1985.

19. Badri MS, Zawaneh S, Cruz AC., et al.: Rectal colonization with group B *Streptococcus*: Relation to vaginal colonization of pregnant women. J. Infect. Dis. *135*:308-312, 1977.

20. Baker, C. J.: Early onset group B streptococcal disease. J. Pediatr. *93*:124-125, 1978.

21. Baker, C. J.: Group B streptococcal cellulitis/adenitis in infants. Am. J. Dis. Child. *136*:631-633, 1982.

22. Baker, C. J.: Antibiotic susceptibility testing in the management of an infant with group B streptococcal meningitis. Pediatr. Infect. Dis. J. *6*:1073-1074, 1987.

23. Baker, C. J., and Barrett, F. F.: Transmission of group B streptococci among parturient women and their neonates. J. Pediatr. *83*:919-925, 1973.

24. Baker, C. J., and Barrett, F. F.: Group B streptococcal infections in infants: The importance of the various serotypes. JAMA *230*:1158-1160, 1974.

25. Baker, C. J., and Kasper, D. L.: Group B streptococcal vaccines. Rev. Infect. Dis. *7*:458-467, 1985.

26. Baker, C. J., Barrett, F. F., Gordon, R. C., et al.: Suppurative meningitis due to streptococci of Lancefield group B: A study of 33 infants. J. Pediatr. *82*:724-729, 1973.

27. Baker, C. J., Clark, D. J., and Barrett, F. F.: Selective broth medium for isolation of group B streptococci. Appl. Microbiol. *26*:884-885, 1973.

28. Baker, C. J., Edwards, M. S., and Kasper, D. L.: Role of antibody to native type III polysaccharide of group B *Streptococcus* to infant infection. Pediatrics *68*:544-549, 1981.

29. Baker, C. J., Goroff, D. K., Alpert, S., et al.: Vaginal colonization with group B *Streptococcus*: A study in college women. J. Infect. Dis. *135*:392-397, 1977.

30. Baker, C. J., Goroff, D. K., Alpert, S. L., et al.: Comparison of bacteriological methods for the isolation of group B *Streptococcus* from vaginal cultures. J. Clin. Microbiol. *4*:46-48, 1976.

31. Baker, C. J., Kasper, D. L., and Davis, C. E.: Immunochemical characterization of the native type III polysaccharide of group B streptococcus. J. Exp. Med. *143*:258-270, 1976.

32. Baker, C. J., Kasper, D. L., Tager, I. B., et al.: Quantitative determination of antibody to capsular polysaccharide in infection with type III strains of group B *Streptococcus*. J. Clin. Med. *59*:810-811, 1977.

33. Baker, C. J., Nizet, V., and Edwards, M. S.: Group B streptococcal infections. *In* Remington, J. S., and Klein, J. O. (eds.): Infectious Diseases of the Fetus and Newborn Infant. 6th ed. Philadelphia, W. B. Saunders, 2005, pp. 403-464.

34. Baker, C. J., Paoletti, L. C., Rench, M. A., et al.: Immune response of healthy women to 2 different group B streptococcal type V capsular polysaccharide-protein conjugate vaccines. J. Infect. Dis. *189*:1103-1112, 2004.

35. Baker, C. J., Paoletti, L. C., Wessels, M. R., et al.: Safety and immunogenicity of capsular polysaccharide-tetanus toxoid conjugate vaccines for group B streptococcal types Ia and Ib. J. Infect. Dis. *179*:142-150, 1999.

36. Baker, C. J., Rench, M. A., Edwards, M. S., et al.: Immunization of pregnant women with a polysaccharide vaccine of group B *Streptococcus*. N. Engl. J. Med. *319*:1180-1185, 1988.

37. Baker, C. J., Rench, M. A., Fernandez, M., et al.: Safety and immunogenicity of a bivalent group B streptococcal conjugate vaccine for serotypes II and III. J. Infect. Dis. *188*:66-73, 2003.

38. Baker, C. J., Rench, M. A., and McInnes, P.: Immunization of pregnant women with group B streptococcal type III capsular polysaccharide-tetanus toxoid conjugate vaccine. Vaccine *21*:3468-3472, 2003.

39. Baker, C. J., Webb, B. J., Jackson, C. V., et al.: Countercurrent immunoelectrophoresis in the evaluation of infants with group B streptococcal disease. Pediatrics *65*:1110-1114, 1980.

40. Baltimore, R. S., Huie, S. M., Meek, J. I., et al.: Early-onset neonatal sepsis in the era of group B streptococcal prevention. Pediatrics *108*:1094-1098, 2001.

41. Banagale, R. C., and Watter, J. H.: Delayed right-sided diaphragmatic hernia following group B streptococcal infection: A discussion of its pathogenesis, with a review of the literature. Hum. Pathol. *14*:67-69, 1983.

42. Baron, M. J., Bolduc, G. R., Goldberg, M. B., et al.: Alpha C protein of group B *Streptococcus* binds host cell surface glycosaminoglycan and enters cells by an actin-dependent mechanism. J. Biol. Chem. *279*:24714-24723, 2004.

43. Barton, C. W., Crowley, D. C., Uzardk, K., et al.: A neonatal survivor of group B beta-hemolytic streptococcal endocarditis. Am. J. Perinatol. *1*:214-215, 1984.

44. Bateman, A. C., Richards, M., and Pallett, A. P.: Fatal myocarditis associated with a Lancefield group B streptococcus. J. Infect. *36*:354-355, 1998.

45. Becroft, D. M. O., Farmer, K., Mason, G. H., et al.: Perinatal infections by group B β-haemolytic streptococci. Br. J. Obstet. Gynaecol. *83*:960-966, 1976.

46. Belgaumkar, T. K.: Impetigo neonatorum congenita due to group B beta-hemolytic *Streptococcus* infection. J. Pediatr. *86*:982-983, 1975.

47. Bergqvist, G., Hurvall, B., Thal, E., et al.: Neonatal infections caused by group B streptococci. Scand. J. Infect. Dis. *3*:209-212, 1971.

48. Betriu, C., Gomez, M., Sanchez, A., et al.: Antibiotic resistance and penicillin tolerance in clinical isolates of group B streptococci. Antimicrob. Agents Chemother. *38*:2183-2186, 1994.

49. Bhakdi, S., Klonisch, T., Nuber, P., et al.: Stimulation of monokine production by lipoteichoic acids. Infect. Immun. *59*:4616-4620, 1991.

50. Bingen, E., Denamur, E., Lamvert-Zechovsky, N., et al.: Analysis of DNA restriction fragment length polymorphism extends the evidence for breast milk transmission in *Streptococcus agalactiae* late-onset infection. J. Infect. Dis. *165*:569-573, 1992.

51. Bizzarro, M. J., Raskind, C., Baltimore, R. S., et al.: Seventy-five years of neonatal sepsis at Yale:1928-2003. Pediatrics *116*:595-602, 2005.

52. Bliss, S. J., Manning, S. D., Tallman, P., et al.: Group B streptococcus colonization in male and nonpregnant female university students: A cross-sectional prevalence study. Clin. Infect. Dis. *34*:184-190, 2002.

53. Blumberg, H. M., Stephens, D. S., Modansky, M., et al.: Invasive group B streptococcal disease: The emergence of serotype V. J. Infect. Dis. *173*:365-373, 1996.

54. Bone, R. C.: Gram-positive organisms and sepsis. Arch. Intern. Med. *154*:26-34, 1994.

55. Borchardt, S. M., DeBusscher, J. H., Tallman, P. A., et al.: Frequency of antimicrobial resistance among invasive and colonizing group B streptococcal isolates. BMC Infect. Dis. *6*:57-64, 2006.

56. Botta, G. A.: Hormonal and type-dependent adhesion of group B streptococci to human vaginal cells. Infect. Immun. *25*:1084-1086, 1979.

57. Boyer, K. M., and Gotoff, S. P.: Prevention of early-onset neonatal group B streptococcal disease with selective intrapartum chemoprophylaxis. N. Engl. J. Med. *314*:1665-1669, 1986.

58. Boyer, K. M., Gadzala, C. A., Burd, L. I., et al.: Selective intrapartum chemoprophylaxis of neonatal group B streptococcal early-onset disease. I. epidemiologic rationale. J. Infect. Dis. *148*:795-801, 1983.

59. Boyer, K. M., Gadzala, C. A., Kelly, P. D., et al.: Selective intrapartum chemoprophylaxis of neonatal group B streptococcal early-onset disease. II. Predictive value of prenatal cultures. J. Infect. Dis. *148*:802-809, 1983.

60. Boyer, K. M., Gadzala, C. A., Kelly, P. D., et al.: Selective intrapartum chemoprophylaxis of neonatal group B streptococcal early-onset disease. III. Interruption of mother-to-infant transmission. J. Infect. Dis. *148*:810-816, 1983.

61. Brady, M. T.: Cellulitis of the penis and scrotum due to group B *Streptococcus*. J. Urol. *137*:736-737, 1987.

62. Bray, R. E., Boe, R. W., and Johnson, W. L.: Transfer of ampicillin into fetus and amniotic fluid from maternal plasma in late pregnancy. Am. J. Obstet. Gynecol. *96*:965-967, 1966.

63. Brian, M. J., O'Ryan, M., and Waagner, D.: Prepatellar bursitis in an infant caused by group B *Streptococcus*. Pediatr. Infect. Dis. J. *11*:502-503, 1992.

64. Bromberger, P., Lawrence, J. M., Braun, D., et al.: The influence of intrapartum antibiotics on the clinical spectrum of early-onset group B streptococcal infection in term infants. Pediatrics *106*:244-250, 2000.

65. Broughton, D. D., Mitchell, W. G., Grossman, M., et al.: Recurrence of group B streptococcal infection. J. Pediatr. *89*:183-185, 1976.

66. Buccato, S., Maione, D., Rinaudo, C. D., et al.: Use of *Lactococcus lactis* expressing pili from group B streptococcus as a broad-coverage vaccine against streptococcal disease. J. Infect. Dis. *194*:331-340, 2006.

67. Bulgakova, T. N., Grabovskaya, K. B., Roc, M., et al.: The adhesin structures involved in the adherence of group B streptococci to human vaginal cells. Folia Microbiol. (Praha) *31*:394-401, 1986.

68. Butter, M. N. W., and DeMoor, C. E.: *Streptococcus agalactiae* as a cause of meningitis in the newborn, and of bacteremia in adults. Antonie Van Leeuwenhoek *33*:439-450, 1967.

69. Cairo, M. S., Plunkett, J. M., Nguyen, A., et al.: Effect of stem cell factor with and without granulocyte colony-stimulating factor on neonatal hematopoiesis: In vivo induction of newborn myelopoiesis and reduction of mortality during experimental group B streptococcal sepsis. Blood *80*:96-101, 1992.

70. Callanan, D. O., and Harris, G. G.: Group B streptococcal infection in children with liver disease. Clin. Pediatr. (Phila.) *21*:99-100, 1982.

71. Campbell, J. R., Hillier, S. L., Krohn, M. A., et al.: Group B streptococcal colonization and serotype-specific immunity in pregnant women at delivery. Obstet. Gynecol. *96*:498-503, 2000.

72. Carty, A., and Stanley, P.: Bilateral adrenal abscesses in a neonate. Pediatr. Radiol. *1*:63-64, 1973.

73. Centers for Disease Control and Prevention: Diminishing racial disparities in early-onset neonatal group b streptococcal disease: United States, 2000-2003. M. M. W. R. Morb. Mortal. Wkly. Rep. *53*:502-505, 2004.

74. Centers for Disease Control and Prevention: Laboratory practices for prenatal group B streptococcal screening: Seven states, 2003. M. M. W. R. Morb. Mortal. Wkly. Rep. *53*:506-509, 2004.

75. Centers for Disease Control and Prevention: Early-onset and late-onset neonatal group B streptococcal disease: United States, 1996-2004. M. M. W. R. Morb. Mortal. Wkly. Rep. *54*:1205-1208, 2005.

76. Chadwick, E. G., Shulman, S. T., and Yogev, R.: Peritonitis as a late manifestation of group B streptococcal disease in newborns. Pediatr. Infect. Dis. J. *2*:142-143, 1983.

77. Chen, K. T., Puopolo, K. M., Eichenwald, E. C., et al.: No increase in rates of early-onset neonatal sepsis by antibiotic-resistant group B streptococcus in the era of intrapartum antibiotic prophylaxis. Am. J. Obstet. Gynecol. 192:1167-1171, 2005.

78. Christensen, K. K., and Christensen, P.: Intravenous gamma-globulin in the treatment of neonatal sepsis with special reference to group B streptococci and pharmacokinetics. Pediatr. Infect. Dis. J. 5 (Suppl.):S189-S192, 1986.

79. Christensen, K. K., Christensen, P., Duc, G., et al.: Correlation between serum antibody-levels against group B streptococci and gestational age in newborns. Eur. J. Pediatr. 142:86-88, 1984.

80. Christensen, R. D., and Rothstein, G.: Exhaustion of mature marrow neutrophils in neonates with sepsis. J. Pediatr. 96:316-318, 1980.

81. Christie, R., Atkins, N. E., and Munch-Petersen, E.: A note on a lytic phenomenon shown by group B streptococci. Aust. J. Exp. Biol. Med. Sci. 22:197-200, 1944.

82. Congdon, P. M.: Streptococcal infection in childbirth and septic abortion. Lancet 2:1287-1288, 1935.

83. Davies, H. D., Miller, M. A., Faro, S., et al.: Multicenter study of a rapid molecular-based assay for the diagnosis of group B *Streptococcus* colonization in pregnant women. Clin. Infect. Dis. 39:1129-1135, 2004.

84. Davies, H. D., Raj, S., Adair, C., et al.: Population-based active surveillance for neonatal group B streptococcal infections in Alberta, Canada: Implications for vaccine formulation. Pediatr. Infect. Dis. J. 20:879-884, 2001.

85. Davis, C. A., Vallota, E. H., and Forristal, J.: Serum complement levels in infancy: Age-related changes. Pediatr. Res. 13:1043-1046, 1979.

86. Desjardins, M., Delgaty, K. L., Ramotar K., et al.: Prevalence and mechanisms of erythromycin resistance in group A and group B streptococcus: Implications for reporting susceptibility results. J. Clin. Microbiol. 42:5620-5623, 2004.

87. DiJohn, D., Krasinski, K., and Lawrence, R.: Very late onset of group B streptococcal disease in infants infected with the human immunodeficiency virus. Pediatr. Infect. Dis. J. 9:925-928, 1990.

88. Dillon, H. C., Gray, E., Pass, M. A., et al.: Anorectal and vaginal carriage of group B streptococci during pregnancy. J. Infect. Dis. 145:794-799, 1982.

89. Dillon, H. C., Khare, S., and Gray, B. M.: Group B streptococcal carriage and disease: A 6-year prospective study. J. Pediatr. 110:31-36, 1987.

90. Dokter, W. H. A., Dijkstra, A. J., Koopmans, S. B., et al.: G(AnH) MTetra, a naturally occurring 1,6-anhydro muramyl dipeptide, induces granulocyte colony-stimulating factor expression in human monocytes: A molecular analysis. Infect. Immun. 62:2953-2957, 1994.

91. Doran, K. S., Engelson, E. J., Khosravi, A., et al.: Blood-brain barrier invasion by group B *Streptococcus* depends upon proper cell-surface anchoring of lipoteichoic acid. J. Clin. Invest. 115:2499-2507, 2005.

92. Doran, K. S., Liu, G. Y., and Nizet, V.: Group B streptococcal beta-hemolysin/cytolysin activates neutrophil signaling pathways in brain endothelium and contributes to development of meningitis. J. Clin. Invest. 112:736-744, 2003.

93. Easmon, C. S. F., Hastings, M. J. G., Clare, A. J., et al.: Nosocomial transmission of group B *Streptococci*. BMJ 283:459-561, 1981.

94. Easmon, C. S. F., Hastings, M. J. G., Neill, J., et al.: Is group B streptococcal screening during pregnancy justified? Br. J. Obstet. Gynaecol. 92:197-201, 1985.

95. Edwards, M. S., and Baker, C. J.: Group B streptococcal infections in elderly adults. J. Infect. Dis. 41:839-847, 2005.

96. Edwards, M. S., Baker, C. J., and Wagner, M. L., et al.: An etiologic shift in infantile osteomyelitis: The emergence of the group B *Streptococcus*. J. Pediatr. 93:578-583, 1978.

97. Edwards, M. S., Buffone, G. J., Fuselier, P. A., et al.: Deficient classical complement pathway activity in newborn sera. Pediatr. Res. 17:685-688, 1983.

98. Edwards, M. S., Jackson, C. V., and Baker, C. J.: Increased risk of group B streptococcal disease in twins. JAMA 245:2044-2046, 1981.

99. Edwards, M. S., Kasper, D. L., Jennings, H. J., et al.: Capsular sialic acid prevents activation of the alternative complement pathway by type III, group B streptococci. J. Immunol. 128:1278-1283, 1982.

100. Edwards, M. S., Rench, M. A., Haffar, A. A. M., et al.: Long-term sequelae of group B streptococcal meningitis in infants. J. Pediatr. 106:717-722, 1985.

101. Eickhoff, T. C., Klein, J. O., Daly, A. L., et al.: Neonatal sepsis and other infections due to group B beta-hemolytic streptococci. N. Engl. J. Med. 271:1221-1228, 1964.

102. Faix, R. G., and Donn, S. M.: Association of septic shock caused by early-onset group B streptococcal sepsis and periventricular leukomalacia in the preterm infant. Pediatrics 76:415-419, 1985.

103. Farley, M. M., Harvey, C., Stull, T., et al.: A population-based assessment of invasive disease due to group B *Streptococcus* in nonpregnant adults. N. Engl. J. Med. 328:1807-1811, 1993.

104. Feder, H. M., MacLean, W. C., and Moxon, R.: Scalp abscess secondary to fetal scalp electrode. J. Pediatr. 89:808-809, 1976.

105. Feldman, W. E.: Concentrations of bacteria in cerebrospinal fluid of patients with bacterial meningitis. J. Pediatr. 88:549-552, 1976.

106. Ferguson, L., and Gotoff, S. P.: Subdural empyema in an infant due to group B beta-hemolytic *Streptococcus*. Am. J. Dis. Child. 131:97, 1977.

107. Fernandez, M., Hickman, M. E., and Baker, C. J.: Antimicrobial susceptibilities of group B streptococci isolated between 1992 and 1996 from patients with bacteremia or meningitis. Antimicrob. Agents Chemother. 42:1517-1519, 1998.

108. Fernandez, M., Rench, M. A., Albanyan, E. A., et al.: Failure of rifampin to eradicate group B streptococcal colonization in infants. Pediatr. Infect. Dis. J. 20:371-376, 2001.

109. Ferrieri, P., and Flores, A. E.: Surface protein expression in group B streptococcal invasive isolates. Adv. Exp. Med. Biol. 418:635-637, 1997.

110. Ferrieri, P., Gray, E. D., and Wannamaker, L. W.: Biochemical and immunological characterization of the extracellular nucleases of group B streptococci. J. Exp. Med. 151:56-68, 1980.

111. Ferrieri, P., Wannamaker, L.,W., and Nelson, J.: Localization and characterization of the hippuricase activity of group B streptococci. Infect. Immun. 7:747-752, 1973.

112. Fluegge, K., Supper, S., Siedler, A., et al.: Serotype distribution of invasive group B streptococcal isolates in infants: Results from a nationwide active laboratory surveillance study over 2 years in Germany. Clin. Infect. Dis. 40:760-763, 2003.

113. Franciosi, R. A., Knostman, J. D., and Zimmerman, R. A.: Group B streptococcal neonatal and infant infections. J. Pediatr. 82:707-718, 1973.

114. Frieden, I. J.: Blistering dactylitis caused by group B streptococci. Pediatr. Dermatol. 6:300-302, 1989.

115. Fry, R. M.: Fatal infections by haemolytic *Streptococcus* group B. Lancet 1:199-201, 1938.

116. Galask, R. P., Varner, M. W., Petzold, C. R., et al.: Bacterial attachment to the chorioamnionic membranes. Am. J. Obstet. Gynecol. 148:915-928, 1984.

117. Garcia Pena, B. M., Harper, M. B., and Gleisher, G. R.: Occult bacteremia with group B streptococci in an outpatient setting. Pediatrics 102:67-72, 1998.

118. Gardner, S. E., Mason, E. O., and Yow, M. D.: Community acquisition of group B *Streptococcus* by infants of colonized mothers. Pediatrics 66:873-875, 1980.

119. Gardner, S. E., Yow, M. D., Leeds, L. J., et al.: Failure of penicillin to eradicate group B streptococcal colonization in the pregnant woman. Am. J. Obstet. Gynecol. 135:1062-1065, 1979.

120. Garland, S. M., and Fliegner, J. R.: Group B *Streptococcus* and neonatal infections: The case for intrapartum chemoprophylaxis. Aust. N. Z. J. Obstet. Gynaecol. 31:119-122, 1991.

121. Gibson, R. L., Lee, M. K., Soderland, C., et al.: Group B streptococci invade endothelial cells: Type III capsular polysaccharide attenuates invasion. Infect. Immun. 61:478-485, 1993.

122. Givner, L. B.: Human immunoglobulins for intravenous use: Comparison of available preparations for group B streptococcal antibody levels, opsonic activity, and efficacy in animal models. Pediatrics 86:995-962, 1990.

123. Glaser, P., Rusniok, C., Buchrieser, C., et al.: Genome sequence of *Streptococcus agalactiae*, a pathogen causing invasive neonatal disease. Mol. Microbiol. 45:1499-1513, 2002.

124. Goldberg, G. N., Hansen, R. C., and Lynch, P. J.: Necrotizing fasciitis in infancy: Report of three cases and review of the literature. Pediatr. Dermatol. 2:55-63, 1984.

125. Gotoff, S. P., Papierniak, C. K., Klegerman, M. E., et al.: Quantitation of IgG antibody to the type-specific polysaccharide of group B *Streptococcus* type Ib in pregnant women and infected infants. J. Pediatr. 105:628-630, 1984.

126. Graven, M. A., Cuddeback, J. K., and Wyble, L.: Readmission for group B streptococci or *Escherichia coli* infection among full-term, singleton, vaginally delivered neonates after early discharge from Florida hospitals for births from 1992 through 1994. J. Perinatol. 19:19-25, 1999.

127. Gray, B. M., Pritchard, D. G., and Dillon, H. C.: Seroepidemiological studies of group B *Streptococcus* type II. J. Infect. Dis. 151:1073-1080, 1985.

128. Green, P. A., Singh, K. V., Murray, B. E., et al.: Recurrent group B streptococcal infections in infants: Clinical and microbiologic aspects. J. Pediatr. 125:931-938, 1994.

129. Greene, G. R., Carroll, W. L., Morozumi, P. A., et al.: Endophthalmitis associated with group B streptococcal meningitis in an infant. Am. J. Dis. Child. 133:752, 1979.

130. Hall, R. T., Barnes, W., Krishnan, L., et al.: Antibiotic treatment of parturient women colonized with group B streptococci. Am. J. Obstet. Gynecol. 124:630-634, 1976.

131. Hamoudi, A. C., Marcon, M. J., Cannon, H. J., et al.: Comparison of three major antigen detection methods for the diagnosis of group B streptococcal sepsis in neonates. Pediatr. Infect. Dis. J. 2:432-435, 1983.

132. Handrick, W., Spencker, F. B., and Kunzel, R.: [Scalp infection caused by B-streptococci in a newborn infant following internal cardiotocography.] Zentrabl. Gynakol. 106:1544-1546, 1984.

133. Harper, I. A.: The importance of group B streptococci as human pathogens in the British Isles. J. Clin. Pathol. 24:438-441, 1971.

134. Harrison, L. H., Elliott, J. A., Dwyer, D. M., et al.: Serotype distribution of invasive group B streptococcal isolates in Maryland: Implications for vaccine formulation. J. Infect. Dis. 177:998-1002, 1998.

135. Haslam, R. H. A., Allen, J. R., Dorsen, M. M., et al.: The sequelae of group B β-hemolytic streptococcal meningitis in early infancy. Am. J. Dis. Child. 131:845-849, 1977.

136. Hauger, S. B.: Facial cellulitis: An early indicator of group B streptococcal bacteremia. Pediatrics 67:376-377, 1981.

137. Healy, C. M., and Baker, C. J.: Prospects for prevention of childhood infections by maternal immunization. Curr. Opin. Infect. Dis. 19:271-276, 2006.

138. Helmig, R., Halaburt, J. T., Uldbjerg, N., et al.: Increased cell adherence of group B streptococci from preterm infants with neonatal sepsis. Obstet. Gynecol. 76:825-828, 1990.
139. Hemming, V. G., Nagarajan, K., Hess, L. W., et al.: Rapid in vitro replication of group B *Streptococcus* in term human amniotic fluid. Gynecol. Obstet. Invest. 19:124-129, 1985.
140. Hensler, M. E., Liu, G. Y., Sobczak, S., et al.: Virulence role of group B *Streptococcus* beta-hemolysin/cytolysin in a neonatal rabbit model of early-onset pulmonary infection. J. Infect. Dis. 191:1287-1291, 2005.
141. Herting, E., Gefeller, O., Land, M., et al.: Surfactant treatment of neonates with respiratory failure and group B streptococcal infection. Pediatrics 106:957-964, 2000.
142. Heumann, D., Barras, C., Severin A., et al.: Gram-positive cell walls stimulate synthesis of tumor necrosis factor alpha and interleukin-6 by human monocytes. Infect. Immun. 62:2715-2721, 1994.
143. Hickman, M. E., Rench, M. A., Ferrieri, P., and Baker, C. J.: Changing epidemiology of group B streptococcal colonization. Pediatrics 104:203-209, 1999.
144. Hill, H. R., Bohnsack, J. F., Morris, E. Z., et al.: Group B streptococci inhibit the chemotactic activity of the fifth component of complement. J. Immunol. 141:3551-3556, 1988.
145. Hillier, S. L., Krohn, M. A., Thwin, S. S., et al.: The association of high-density vaginal colonization by group B *Streptococcus* and preterm birth. Presented at the 35th Annual Meeting of the Interscience Conference on Antimicrobial Agents and Chemotherapy, San Francisco, 1995, p. 322. Abstract K189.
146. Honest, H., Sharma, S., and Khan, K. S.: Rapid tests for group B streptococcus colonization in laboring women: A systematic review. Pediatrics 117:1055-1066, 2006.
147. Hood, M., Janney, A., and Dameron, G.: Beta hemolytic *Streptococcus* group B associated with problems of the perinatal period. Am. J. Obstet. Gynecol. 82:809-818, 1961.
148. Hoogkamp-Korstanje, J. A. A., Gerards, L. J., and Cats, B. P.: Maternal carriage and neonatal acquisition of group B streptococci. J. Infect. Dis. 145:800-803, 1982.
149. Horigome, H., Ikada, Y., Hirano, T., et al.: Group B streptococcal endocarditis in infancy with a giant vegetation on the pulmonary valve. Eur. J. Pediatr. 153:140-141, 1994.
150. Howard, J. B., and McCracken, G. H.: The spectrum of group B streptococcal infections in infancy. Am. J. Dis. Child. 128:815-818, 1974.
151. Hussain, S. M., Luedtke, G. S., Baker, C. J., et al.: Invasive group B streptococcal disease in children beyond early infancy. Pediatr. Infect. Dis. J. 14:278-281, 1995.
152. Hyde, T. B., Hilger, T. M., Reigold, A., et al.: Trends in incidence and antimicrobial resistance of early-onset sepsis: Population-based surveillance in San Francisco and Atlanta. Pediatrics 110:690-695, 2002.
153. Isaacman, S. H., Heroman, W. M., and Lightsey, A. L.: Purpura fulminans following late-onset group B beta-hemolytic streptococcal sepsis. Am. J. Dis. Child. 138:915-916, 1984.
154. Jackson, L. A., Hilsdon, R., Farley, M. M., et al.: Risk factors for group B streptococcal disease in adults. Ann. Intern. Med. 123:415-420, 1995.
155. Jacobs, M. R., Koornhof, H J., and Stein, H.: Group B streptococcal infections in neonates and infants. S. Afr. Med. J. 54:154-158, 1978.
156. Jeffery, H., Mitchison, R., Wigglesworth, J. S., et al.: Early neonatal bacteraemia. Arch. Dis. Child. 52:683-686, 1977.
157. Johnson, D. R., and Ferrieri, P.: Group B streptococcal Ibc protein antigen: Distribution of two determinants in wild-type strains of common serotypes. J. Clin. Microbiol. 19:506-510, 1984.
158. Johri, A. K., Margarit, I., Broenstrup, M., et al.: Transcriptional and proteomic profiles of group B *Streptococcus* type V reveal potential adherence proteins associated with high-level invasion. Infect. Immun. 75:1473-1483, 2007.
159. Jones, D. E., Kanarek, K. S., and Lim, D. V.: Group B streptococcal colonization patterns in mothers and their infants. J. Clin. Microbiol. 20:438-440, 1984.
160. Jordan, J. A., and Durso, M. B.: Real-time polymerase chain reaction for detecting bacterial DNA directly from blood of neonates being evaluated for sepsis. J. Mol. Diagn. 7:55-581, 2005.
161. Joseph, T. A., Pyati, S. P., and Jacobs, N.: Neonatal early-onset *Escherichia coli* disease. The effect of intrapartum ampicillin. Arch. Pediatr. Adolesc. Med. 152:35-40, 1998.
162. Joyner, J L., Augustine, N. H., Taylor, K. A., et al.: Effects of group B streptococci on cord and adult mononuclear cell interleukin-12 and interferon-gamma mRNA accumulation and protein secretion. J. Infect. Dis. 182:974-977, 2000.
163. Jürgens, D., Sterzik, B., and Fehrenbach, F. J.: Unspecific binding of group B streptococcal cocytolysin (CAMP factor) to immunoglobulins and its possible role in pathogenicity. J. Exp. Med. 165:720-732, 1987.
164. Keller, R., Fischer, W., Keist, R., et al.: Macrophage response to bacteria: Induction of marked secretory and cellular activities by lipoteichoic acids. Infect. Immun. 60:3664-3672, 1992.
165. Kim, K. S.: Antimicrobial susceptibility of group B streptococcus. Antimicrob. Agents Chemother. 35:83-89, 1985.
166. Kim, K. S.: Clinical perspectives on penicillin tolerance. J. Pediatr. 112:214-216, 1988.
167. Kim, K. S., and Anthony, B. F.: Penicillin tolerance in group B streptococci isolated from infection neonates. J. Infect. Dis. 144:411-419, 1981.
168. Kim, K. S., Kaye, K. L., Itabashi, H. H., et al.: Cerebritis due to group B *Streptococcus*. Scand. J. Infect. Dis. 14:305-308, 1982.
169. Klegerman, M. E., Boyer, K. M., Papierniak, C. K., et al.: Type-specific capsular antigen is associated with virulence in late-onset group B streptococcal type III disease. Infect. Immun. 44:124-129, 1984.
170. Kline, A., and O'Donnell, E.: Group B *Streptococcus* as a cause of neonatal bullous skin lesions. Pediatr. Infect. Dis. J. 12:165-166, 1993.
171. Kotiw, M., Zhang, G. W., Daggard, G., et al.: Late-onset and recurrent neonatal group B streptococcal disease associated with breast-milk transmission. Pediatr. Dev. Pathol. 6:251-256, 2003.
172. Lachenauer, C. S., Kasper, D. L., Shimada, J., et al.: Serotypes VI and VIII predominate among group B streptococci isolated from pregnant Japanese women. J. Infect. Dis. 179:1030-1033, 1999.
173. Lancefield, R. C.: A serological differentiation of human and other groups of hemolytic streptococci. J. Exp. Med. 57:571-595, 1933.
174. Lancefield, R. C., and Hare, R.: The serological differentiation of pathogenic and non-pathogenic strains of hemolytic streptococci from parturient women. J. Exp. Med. 61:335-349, 1935.
175. Lancefield, R. C., and Hare, R.: Two serologic types of group B hemolytic streptococci with related, but not identical, type-specific substances. J. Exp. Med. 67:25-40, 1938.
176. Lancefield, R. C., McCarty, M., and Everly, W. N.: Multiple mouse-protective antibodies directed against group B streptococci. J. Exp. Med. 142:165-179, 1975.
177. Lang, M. E., Vaudry, W., and Robingson, J. L.: Case report and literature review of late-onset group B streptococcal disease manifesting as necrotizing fasciitis in preterm infants: Is this a new syndrome? Clin. Infect. Dis. 37:e132-e135, 2003.
178. Larsson, C., Lindroth, M., Nordin, P., et al.: Association between low concentrations of antibodies to protein alpha and Rib and invasive neonatal group B streptococcal infection. Arch. Dis. Child. Fetal Neonatal Ed. 91:F403-F408, 2006.
179. Lauer, P., Rinaudo, C. D., Soriani, M., et al.: Genome analysis reveals pili in group B *Streptococcus*. Science 309:105, 2005.
180. Lee, S. Y., and Chee, S. P.: Group B *Streptococcus* endogenous endophthalmitis: Case reports and review of the literature. Ophthalmology 109:1879-86, 2002.
181. Levy, N. J., Nicholson-Weller, A., Baker, C. J., et al.: Potentiation of virulence by group B streptococcal polysaccharides. J. Infect. Dis. 149:851-860, 1984.
182. Lewis, D. B., and Wilson, C. B.: Developmental immunology and role of host defenses in neonatal susceptibility to infection. *In* Remington, J. S., and Klein, J. O. (eds.): Infectious Diseases of the Fetus and Newborn Infant. 6th ed. Philadelphia, W. B. Saunders, 2005, pp. 87-210.
183. Lilien, L. D., Harris, V. J., and Pildes, R. S.: Significance of radiographic findings in early-onset group B streptococcal infection. Pediatrics 60:360-365, 1977.
184. Lim, D. V., Kanarek, K. S., and Peterson, M. E.: Magnitude of colonization and sepsis by group B streptococci in newborn infants. Curr. Microbiol. 7:99-101, 1982.
185. Lim, D. V., Morales, W. J., and Walsh, A. F.: Lim group B Strep broth and coagglutination for rapid identification of group B streptococci in preterm pregnant women. J. Clin. Microbiol. 25:452-453, 1987.
186. Lin, F. Y., Azimi, P. H., Weisman, L. E., et al.: Antibiotic susceptibility profiles for group B streptococci isolated from neonates, 1995-1998. Clin. Infect. Dis. 31:76-79, 2000.
187. Lin, F. Y., Clemens, J. D., Azimi, P. H., et al.: Capsular polysaccharide types of group B streptococcal isolates from neonates with early-onset sepsis. J. Infect. Dis. 177:790-792, 1998.
188. Lin, F. Y., Weisman, L. E., Troendle, J., et al.: Prematurity is the major risk factor for late-onset group B *Streptococcus* disease. J. Infect. Dis. 188:267-271, 2003.
189. Lindén, V.: Mouse-protective effect of rabbit anti-R-protein antibodies against group B streptococci type II carrying R-protein. Acta Pathol. Microbiol. Immunol. Scand. [B] 91:145-151, 1983.
190. Lindén, V., Christensen, K. K., and Christensen, P.: Correlation between low levels of maternal IgG antibodies to R protein and neonatal septicemia with group B streptococci carrying R protein. Int. Arch. Allergy Appl. Immunol. 71:168-172, 1983.
191. Lipson, A., Kronick, J. B., Tewfik, L., et al.: Group B streptococcal supraglottitis in a 3-month-old infant. Am. J. Dis. Child. 140:411-412, 1986.
192. Long, W. A., Lawson, E. E., Harned, H. S., et al.: Pleural effusion in the first days of life: A prospective study. Am. J. Perinatol. 1:190-194, 1984.
193. Lopez, J. B., Gross, P., and Boggs, T R.: Skin lesions in association with β-hemolytic *Streptococcus* group B. Pediatrics 58:859-860, 1976.
194. Lui, G. Y., Doran, K. S., Lawrence, T., et al.: Sword and shield: Linked group B streptococcal beta-hemolysin/cytolysin and carotenoid pigment function to subvert host phagocyte defense. Proc. Natl. Acad. Sci. U. S. A. 101:14491-14496, 2004.
195. Lynn, N. J., Pauly, T. H., and Desai, N. S.: Purpura fulminans in three cases of early-onset neonatal group B streptococcal meningitis. J. Perinatol. 11:144-146, 1991.
196. Mårdh, P. A., and Weström, L.: Adherence of bacteria to vaginal epithelial cells. Infect. Immun. 13:661-666, 1976.

197. MacDonald, S. W., Manuel, F. R., and Embil, J. A.: Localization of group B beta-hemolytic streptococci in the female urogenital tract. Am. J. Obstet. Gynecol. *133*:57-59, 1979.

198. MacGilvray, S. S., and Billow, M.: Diabetes insipidus as a complication of neonatal group B streptococcal meningitis. Pediatr. Infect. Dis. J. *9*:742-743, 1990.

199. Maisey, H. C., Hensler, M., Nizet, V., et al.: Group B streptococcal pilus proteins contribute to adherence to and invasion of brain microvascular endothelial cells. J. Bacteriol. *189*:1464-1467, 2007.

200. Malone, D., Margarit, I., Rinaudo, C. D., et al.: Identification of a universal group B streptococcus vaccine by multiple genome screen. Science *309*:148-150, 2005.

201. Mancuso, G., Cusumano, V., Genovese, F., et al.: Role of interleukin 12 in experimental neonatal sepsis caused by group B streptococci. Infect. Immun. *65*:3731-3735, 1997.

202. Manning, S. D., Ki, M., Marrs, C. F., et al.: The frequency of genes encoding three putative group B streptococcal virulence factors among invasive and colonizing isolates. BMC Infect. Dis. *6*:116, 2006.

203. Manning, S. D., Tallman, P., Baker, C. J., et al.: Determinants of co-colonization with group B streptococcus among heterosexual college couples. Epidemiology *13*:533-539, 2002.

204. Manroe, B. L., Rosenfeld, C. R., Weinberg, A. G., et al.: The differential leukocyte count in the assessment and outcome of early-onset neonatal group B streptococcal disease. J. Pediatr. *91*:632-637, 1977.

205. Marchlewicz, B. A., and Duncan, J. L.: Properties of a hemolysin produced by group B streptococci. Infect. Immun. *30*:805-813, 1980.

206. Marodi, L., Leijh, P. C. J., and Van Furth, R.: Characteristics and functional capacities of human cord blood granulocytes and monocytes. Pediatr. Res. *18*:1127-1131, 1984.

207. Marques, M. B., Kasper, D. L., Pangburn, M K., et al.: Prevention of C3 deposition by capsular polysaccharide is a virulence mechanism of type III group B streptococci. Infect. Immun. *60*:3986-3993, 1992.

208. Martin, T. R., Rubens, C. E., and Wilson, C. B.: Lung antibacterial defense mechanisms in infant and adult rats: Implications for the pathogenesis of group B streptococcal infections in the neonatal lung. J. Infect. Dis. *157*:91-100, 1988.

209. Mason, E. O., Wong, P., and Barrett, F. F.: Evaluation of four methods for detection of group B streptococcal colonization. J. Clin. Microbiol. *4*:429-431, 1976.

210. Matorras, R., Garcia-Perea, A., Omenaca, F., et al.: Group B *Streptococcus* and premature rupture of membranes and preterm delivery. Gynecol. Obstet. Invest. *27*:14-18, 1989.

211. Matorras, R., Garcia-Perea, A., Omenaca, F., et al.: Intrapartum chemoprophylaxis of early-onset group B streptococcal disease. Eur. J. Obstet. Gynecol. Reprod. Biol. *40*:57-62, 1991.

212. Matorras, R., Garcia-Perea, A., Usandizaga, J. A., et al.: Natural transmission of group B *Streptococcus* during delivery. Int. J. Gynaecol. Obstet. *30*:99-103, 1989.

213. McClean, D.: The capsulation of streptococci and its relation to diffusion factor (hyaluronidase). J. Pathol. Bacteriol. *53*:13-27, 1941.

214. McDonald, H., Vigneswaran, R., and O'Loughlin, J. A.: Group B streptococcal colonization and preterm labour. Aust. N. Z. J. Obstet. Gynaecol. *29*:291-293, 1989.

215. Memon, I. A., Jacobs, N. M., Yeh, T. F., et al.: Group B streptococcal osteomyelitis and septic arthritis. Am. J. Dis. Child. *133*:921-923, 1979.

216. Mercer, B. M., Carr, T. L., Beazley, D. D., et al.: Antibiotic use in pregnancy and drug-resistant infant sepsis. Am. J. Obstet. Gynecol. *181*:816-821, 1999.

217. Meyn, L. A., Moore, D. M., Hillier, S. L., et al.: Association of sexual activity with colonization and vaginal acquisition of group B *Streptococcus* in nonpregnant women. Am. J. Epidemiol. *155*:949-957, 2002.

218. Michel, J. L., Madoff, L. C., Kling, D E., et al.: Cloned alpha and beta C-protein antigens of group B streptococci elicit protective immunity. Infect. Immun. *59*:2023-2028, 1991.

219. Millard, D. D., Bussey, M. E., Shulman, S. T., et al.: Multiple group B streptococcal infections in a premature infant: Eradication of nasal colonization with rifampin. Am. J. Dis. Child. *139*:964-965, 1985.

220. Minett, F. C., Stableforth, A. W., and Edwards, S. J.: Studies on bovine mastitis. 1. The bacteriology of mastitis. J. Comp. Pathol. *42*:213-231, 1929.

221. Miron, D., Snelling, L. K., Josephson, S. L., et al.: Eosinophilic meningitis in a newborn with group B streptococcal infection. Pediatr. Infect. Dis. J. *12*:966-967, 1993.

222. Miyairi, I., Causey, K. T., DeVincenzo, J. P., et al.: Group B streptococcal ventriculitis: A report of three cases and literature review. Pediatr. Neurol. *34*:395-399, 2006.

223. Mohle-Boetani, J. C., Lieu, T. A., Ray, G. T., et al, for the Neonatal GBS Prevention Working Group: Preventing neonatal group B streptococcal disease: Cost-effectiveness in a health maintenance organization and the impact of delayed hospital discharge for newborns who received intrapartum antibiotics. Pediatrics *103*:703-710, 1999.

224. Mohle-Boetani, J. C., Schuchat, A., Plikaytis, B. D., et al.: Comparison of prevention strategies for neonatal group B streptococcal infection: A population-based economic analysis. JAMA *270*:1442-1448, 1993.

225. Moller, M., Thomsen, A. C., Borch, K., et al.: Rupture of fetal membranes and premature delivery associated with group B streptococci in urine of pregnant women. Lancet *2*:69-70, 1984.

226. Morrow, D. L., Kline, J. B., Douglas, S. D., et al.: Rapid detection of group B streptococcal antigen by monoclonal antibody sandwich enzyme assay. J. Clin. Microbiol. *19*:457-459, 1984.

227. Moylett, E. H., Fernandez, M., Rench, M. A., et al.: A 5-year review of recurrent group B streptococcal disease: Lessons from twin infants. Clin. Infect. Dis. *30*:282-287, 2000.

228. Nealon, T. J., and Mattingly, S. J.: Association of elevated levels of cellular lipoteichoic acids of group B streptococci with human neonatal disease. Infect. Immun. *39*:1243-1251, 1983.

229. Nealon, T. J., and Mattingly, S. J.: Role of cellular lipoteichoic acids in mediating adherence of serotype III strains of group B streptococci to human embryonic, fetal, and adult epithelial cells. Infect. Immun. *43*:523-530, 1984.

230. Nelson, J. D.: Bilateral breast abscess due to group B *Streptococcus*. Am. J. Dis. Child. *130*:567, 1976.

231. Nightingale, S. L., and the Food and Drug Administration: Safety alert regarding risk of misdiagnosis of group B streptococcal infection. JAMA *277*:1343, 1997.

232. Nizet, V., Gibson, R. L., and Rubens, C. E.: The role of group B streptococci beta-hemolysin expression in newborn lung injury. Adv. Exp. Med. Biol. *418*:627-630, 1997.

233. Nocard, M.: Sur une mammite contagieuse des vaches laitières. Ann. Inst. Pasteur *1*:109-127, 1887.

234. Noya, FJD, Rench, M. A., Metzger, TG., et al.: Unusual occurrence of an epidemic of type Ib/c group B streptococcal sepsis in a neonatal intensive care unit. J. Infect. Dis. *155*:1135-1144, 1987.

235. Opal, S. M., Cross, A., Palmo, M., et al.: Group B streptococcal sepsis in adults and infants: Contrasts and comparisons. Arch. Intern. Med. *148*:641-645, 1988.

236. Pannaraj, P. S., Kelly, J. K., Madoff, L. C., et al.: Group B *Streptococcus* bacteremia elicits beta C protein-specific IgM and IgG in humans. J. Infect. Dis. *195*:353-356, 2007.

237. Paoletti, L. C., and Madoff, L. C.: Vaccines to prevent neonatal GBS infection. Semin. Neonatol. *7*:315-323, 2002.

238. Paoletti, L. C., Wessels, M. R., Rodewald, A. K., et al.: Neonatal mouse protection against infection with multiple group B streptococcal serotypes by maternal immunization with a tetravalent GBS polysaccharide-tetanus toxoid conjugate vaccine. Infect. Immun. *62*:3236-3243, 1994.

239. Paredes, A. B., Wong, P., and Yow, M. D.: Failure of penicillin to eradicate the carrier state of group B *Streptococcus* in infants. J. Pediatr. *89*:191-193, 1976.

240. Pass, M. A., Gray, B. M., and Dillon, H. C.: Puerperal and perinatal infections with group B streptococci. Am. J. Obstet. Gynecol. *143*:147-152, 1982.

241. Pass, M. A., Gray, B. M., Khare, S., et al.: Prospective studies of group B streptococcal infections in infants. J. Pediatr. *95*:437-443, 1979.

242. Pass, M. A., Khare, S., and Dillon, H. C.: Twin pregnancies: Incidence of group B streptococcal colonization and disease. J. Pediatr. *97*:635-637, 1980.

243. Patamasucon, P., Siegel, J. D., and McCracken, G. H.: Streptococcal submandibular cellulitis in young infants. Pediatrics *67*:378-380, 1981.

244. Payne, N. R., and Ferrieri, P.: The relation of the Ib/c protein antigen to the opsonization differences between strains of type II group B streptococci. J. Infect. Dis. *151*:672-681, 1985.

245. Payne, N. R., Burke, B. A., Day, D. L., et al.: Correlation of clinical and pathologic findings in early onset neonatal group B streptococcal infection with disease severity and prediction of outcome. Pediatr. Infect. Dis. J. *7*:836-847, 1988.

246. Peevy, K. J., and Wiseman, H. J.: Gallbladder distention in septic neonates. Arch. Dis. Child. *57*:75-76, 1982.

247. Perkins, M. D., Mirrett, S., and Reller, L. B.: Rapid bacterial antigen detection is not clinically useful. J. Clin. Microbiol. *33*:1486-1491, 1995.

248. Persson, K., Bjerre, B., Elfström, L., et al.: Longitudinal study of group B streptococcal carriage during late pregnancy. Scand. J. Infect. Dis. *19*:325-329, 1987.

249. Persson, K., and Forsgren, A.: Antimicrobial susceptibility of group B streptococci. Eur. J. Clin. Microbiol. *5*:165-167, 1986.

250. Philip, A. G.: Response of C-reactive protein in neonatal group B streptococcal infection. Pediatr. Infect. Dis. *4*:145-148, 1985.

251. Philipps, A. F., Bierney, J. P., and Crowe, C. P.: Neonatal radiology: Acquired diaphragmatic hernia with group B streptococcal pneumonia. J. Perinatol. *15*:160-162, 1995.

252. Pickering, L. K., Baker, C. J., Long, S. S., and McMillan, J. A. (eds.): Red Book: 2006 Report of the Committee on Infectious Diseases, 27th ed. Elk Grove Village, IL: American Academy of Pediatrics, 2006, pp. 620-627.

253. Platt, M. W., Correa, N., and Mold, C.: Growth of group B streptococci in human serum leads to increased cell surface sialic acid and decreased activation of the alternative complement pathway. Can. J. Microbiol. *40*:99-105, 1994.

254. Poschl, J. M., Hellstern, G., Bauer, R. P., et al.: Ophthalmia neonatorum caused by group B *Streptococcus*. Scand. J. Infect. Dis. *34*:921-922, 2002.

255. Pourcyrous, M., Bada, H. S., Korones, S. B., et al.: Significance of serial C-reactive protein responses in neonatal infection and other disorders. Pediatrics *92*:431-435, 1993.

256. Puliti, M., Nizet, V., von Hunolstein C., et al.: Severity of group B streptococcal arthritis is correlated with beta-hemolysin expression. J. Infect. Dis. *182*:824-832, 2000.

257. Puopolo, K. M., Madoff, L. C., and Eichenwald, E. C.: Early-onset group B streptococcal disease in the era of maternal screening. Pediatrics 115:1240-1246, 2005.

258. Pyati, S. P., Pildes, R. S., Jacobs, N. M., et al.: Penicillin in infants weighing two kilograms or less with early-onset group B streptococcal disease. N. Engl. J. Med. 308:1383-1389, 1983.

259. Ramamurthy, R. S., Srinivasan, G., and Jacobs, N. M.: Necrotizing fasciitis and necrotizing cellulitis due to group B Streptococcus. Am. J. Dis. Child. 131:1169-1170, 1977.

260. Ramaswamy, S. V., Ferrieri, P., Flores, A. E., et al.: Molecular characterization of nontypeable group B Streptococcus. J. Clin. Microbiol. 44:2398-2403, 2006.

261. Ramsey, P. G., and Zwerdling, R.: Asymptomatic neonatal bacteremia. N. Engl. J. Med. 295:225, 1977.

262. Regan, J. A., Chao, S., and James, L. S.: Premature rupture of membranes, preterm delivery, and group B streptococcal colonization of mothers. Am. J. Obstet. Gynecol. 141:184-186, 1981.

263. Regan, J. A., Klebanoff, M. A., and Nugent, R. P.: The epidemiology of group B streptococcal colonization in pregnancy. Obstet. Gynecol. 77:604-610, 1991.

264. Reisenfeld-Orn, I., Wolpe, S., Garcia-Bustos, J. F., et al.: Production of interleukin-1 but no tumor necrosis factor by human monocytes stimulated with pneumococcal cell surface components. Infect. Immun. 57:1890-1893, 1989.

265. Rench, M. A., and Baker, C. J.: Group B streptococcal breast abscess in a mother and mastitis in her infant. Obstet. Gynecol. 73:875-877, 1989.

266. Rench, M. A., and Baker, C. J.: Neonatal sepsis caused by a new group B streptococcal serotype. J. Pediatr. 122:638-640, 1993.

267. Rench, M. A., Metzger, T. G., and Baker, C. J.: Detection of group B streptococcal antigen in body fluids by a latex-coupled monoclonal antibody assay. J. Clin. Microbiol. 20:852-854, 1984.

268. Rentz, A. C., Samore, M. H., Stoddard, G. J., et al.: Risk factors associated with ampicillin-resistant infection in newborns in the era of group B streptococcal prophylaxis. Arch. Pediatr. Adolesc. Med. 158:556-560, 2004.

269. Roe, M. H., Todd, J. K., and Favara, B. E.: Non-hemolytic group B streptococcal infections. J. Pediatr. 89:75-77, 1976.

270. Rowen, J. L., Smith, C. W., and Edwards, M. S.: Capsule delays elaboration of leukotriene B$_4$ (LTB$_4$) by monocytes stimulated with type III group B streptococci. Abstract. Pediatr. Res. 37:187, 1995.

271. Rowen, J. L., Smith, C. W., and Edwards, M. S.: Group B streptococci elicit leukotriene B$_4$ and interleukin-8 from human monocytes: Neonates exhibit a diminished response. J. Infect. Dis. 172:420-426, 1995.

272. Rubens, C. E., Smith, S., Hulse, M., et al.: Respiratory epithelial cell invasion by group B streptococci. Infect. Immun. 60:5157-5163, 1992.

273. Rubens, C. E., Wessels, M. R., Heggen, L. M., et al.: Transposon mutagenesis of type III group B Streptococcus: Correlation of capsule expression with virulence. Proc. Natl. Acad. Sci. U. S. A. 84:7208-7212, 1987.

274. Sapir-Ellis, S., Johnson, A., and Austin, T. L.: Group B streptococcal meningitis associated with otitis media. Am. J. Dis. Child. 130:1003-1004, 1976.

275. Schauf, V., Deveikis, A., Riff, L., et al.: Antibiotic-killing kinetics of group B streptococci. J. Pediatr. 89:194-198, 1976.

276. Scheld, W. M., Alliegro, G. M., Field, M. R., et al.: Synergy between penicillins and low concentrations of gentamicin in experimental meningitis due to group B streptococci. J. Infect. Dis. 146:100, 1982.

277. Schibler, K. R., Trautman, M. S., Liechty, K. W., et al.: Diminished transcription of interleukin-8 by monocytes from preterm neonates. J. Leukoc. Biol. 53:399-403, 1993.

278. Schrag, S. J., Gorwitz, R., Fultz-Butts, K., et al.: Prevention of perinatal group B streptococcal disease: Revised guidelines from CDC. M. M. W. R. Recomm. Rep. 51:1-22, 2002.

279. Schrag, S. J., Zell, E. R., Lynfield, R., et al.: A population-based comparison of strategies to prevent early-onset group B streptococcal disease in neonates. N. Engl. J. Med. 347:233-239, 2002.

280. Schrag, S. J., Zywicki, S., Farley, M. M., et al.: Group B streptococcal disease in the era of intrapartum antibiotic prophylaxis. N. Engl. J. Med. 342:15-20, 2000.

281. Schuchat, A.: Group B streptococcal disease in newborns: A global perspective on prevention. Biomed. Pharmacother. 49:19-25, 1995.

282. Schuchat, A., Deaver-Robinson, K., Plikaytis, B. D., et al.: Multistate case-control study of maternal risk factors for neonatal group B streptococcal disease. Pediatr. Infect. Dis. J. 13:623-629, 1994.

283. Schuchat, A., Oxtoby, M., Cochi S., et al.: Population-based risk factors for neonatal group B streptococcal disease: Results of a cohort study in metropolitan Atlanta. J. Infect. Dis. 162:672-677, 1990.

284. Schuit, K. E., and DeBasio, R.: Kinetics of phagocyte response to group B streptococcal infections in newborn rats. Infect. Immun. 28:319-324, 1980.

285. Shannon, D., Neighbors, K., Tallman, P. A., et al.: Prevalence of group B Streptococcus colonization and potential for transmission by casual contact in healthy young men and women. Clin. Infect. Dis. 39:380-388, 2004.

286. Sherman, M. P., and Lehrer, R. I.: Oxidative metabolism of neonatal and adult rabbit lung macrophages stimulated with opsonized group B streptococci. Infect. Immun. 47:26-30, 1985.

287. Shigeoka, A. O., Rote, N. S., Santos, J. I., et al.: Assessment of the virulence factors of group B streptococci: Correlation with sialic acid content. J. Infect. Dis. 147:857-863, 1983.

288. Shurin, P. A., Howie, V. M., Pelton, S. I., et al.: Bacterial etiology of otitis media during the first six weeks of life. J. Pediatr. 92:893-896, 1978.

289. Siegel, J. D., McCracken, G. H., Threlkeld, N., et al.: Single-dose penicillin prophylaxis of neonatal group B streptococcal disease. Lancet 1:1426-1430, 1982.

290. Siegel, J. D., Shannon, K. M., and De Passe, B. M.: Recurrent infection associated with penicillin-tolerant group B streptococci: A report of two cases. J. Pediatr. 99:920-924, 1981.

291. Sinha, A., Lieu, T. A., Paoletti, L. C., et al.: The projected health benefits of maternal group B streptococcal vaccination in the era of chemoprophylaxis. Vaccine 23:3187-95, 2005.

292. Slifkin, M., and Pouchet-Melvin, G. R.: Evaluation of three commercially available test products for serogrouping beta-hemolytic streptococci. J. Clin. Microbiol. 11:249-255, 1980.

293. Sobel, J. D., Myers, P., Levison, M. E., et al.: Comparison of bacterial and fungal adherence to vaginal exfoliated epithelial cells and human vaginal epithelial tissue culture cells. Infect. Immun. 35:697-701, 1982.

294. Sokal, M. M., Nagaraj, A., Fisher, B. J., et al.: Neonatal empyema caused by group B beta-hemolytic Streptococcus. Chest 81:390-391, 1982.

295. Sokol, D. M., Demmler, G. J., and Baker, C. J.: Unusual presentation of group B streptococcal ventriculitis. Pediatr. Infect. Dis. J. 9:525-527, 1990.

296. Soriani, M., Santi, I., Taddel, A., et al.: Group B Streptococcus crosses human epithelial cells by a paracellular route. J. Infect. Dis. 193:241-50, 2006.

297. St. Laurent-Gagnon, T., and Weber, M. L.: Urinary tract Streptococcus group B infection in a 6-week-old infant. JAMA 140:1269, 1978.

298. Stoll, B. J., Hansen, N., Fanaroff, A. A., et al.: Changes in pathogens causing early-onset sepsis in very-low birth weight infants. N. Engl. J. Med. 347:240-247, 2002.

299. Suresh, B. R., Rios, A., Brion, L. P., et al.: Delayed onset right-sided diaphragmatic hernia secondary to group B streptococcal infection. Pediatr. Infect. Dis. J. 10:166-168, 1991.

300. Swingle, H. M., Bucciarelli, R. L., and Ayoub, E. M.: Synergy between penicillins and low concentrations of gentamicin in the killing of group B streptococci. J. Infect. Dis. 152:58-66, 1985.

301. Takahashi, S., Nagano, Y., Nagano, N., et al.: Role of C5a-ase in group B streptococcal resistance to opsonophagocytic killing. Infect. Immun. 63:4764-4769, 1995.

302. Tamura, G. S., Kuypers, J. M., Smith, S., et al.: Adherence of group B streptococci to cultured epithelial cells: Roles of environmental factors and bacterial surface components. Infect. Immun. 62:2450-2458, 1994.

303. Tapsall, J. W.: Pigment production by Lancefield-group B streptococci (Streptococcus agalactiae). J. Med. Microbiol. 21:75-81, 1986.

304. Tenenbaum, T., Bloier, C., Adam, R., et al.: Adherence to and invasion of human brain microvascular endothelial cells are promoted by fibrinogen-binding protein FbsA of Streptococcus agalactiae. Infect. Immun. 73:4404-4409, 2005.

305. Tettelin, H., Masignani, V., Cieslewicz, M. J., et al.: Complete genome sequence and comparative genomic analysis of an emerging human pathogen, serotype V Streptococcus agalactiae. Proc. Natl. Acad. Sci. U. S. A. 99:12391-12396, 2002.

306. Tettelin, H., Masignani, V., Cieslewicz, M. J., et al.: Genome analysis of multiple pathogenic isolates of Streptococcus agalactiae: Implications for the microbial "pan-genome." Proc. Natl. Acad. Sci. U. S. A. 102:13950-13955, 2005.

307. Torok, P. G., and Dunn, J. R.: Self-collection of antepartum anogenital group B streptococcus cultures. J. Am. Board Fam. Pract. 13:107-110, 2000.

308. Tribels-Smeulders, M., Kimpen, J., Kollee, L., et al.: Serotypes, genotypes, and antibiotic susceptibility profiles of group B streptococci causing neonatal sepsis and meningitis before and after introduction of antibiotic prophylaxis. Pediatr. Infect. Dis. J. 25:945-948, 2006.

309. Tuppurainen, N., and Hallman, M.: Prevention of neonatal group B streptococcal disease: Intrapartum detection and chemoprophylaxis of heavily colonized parturients. Obstet. Gynecol. 73:583-587, 1989.

310. Turner, M. C., and Naumburg, E. G.: Acute renal failure in the neonate: Two fatal cases due to group B streptococci with rhabdomyolysis. Clin. Pediatr. (Phila.) 25:189-190, 1987.

311. Tyrrell, G. J., Senzilet, L. D., Spika, J. S., et al.: Invasive disease due to group B streptococcal infection in adults: Results from a Canadian, population-based, active laboratory surveillance study—1996. J. Infect. Dis. 182:168-173, 2000.

312. Vallejo, J. G., Baker, C. J., and Edwards, M. S.: Demonstration of circulating group B streptococcal immune complexes in neonates with meningitis. J. Clin. Microbiol. 32:2041-2045, 1994.

313. Vallejo, J. G., Baker, C. J., and Edwards, M. S.: Interleukin-6 production by human neonatal monocytes stimulated by type III group B streptococci. J. Infect. Dis. 174:332-337, 1996.

314. Vallejo, J. G., Baker, C. J., and Edwards, M. S.: The role of bacterial cell wall and capsule in the induction of tumor necrosis factor alpha by type III group B streptococci. Infect. Immun. 64:5042-5046, 1996.

315. Vallette, J. D., Goldberg, R. N., Suguihara, C., et al.: Effect of an interleukin-1 receptor antagonist on the hemodynamic manifestations of group B streptococcal sepsis. Pediatr. Res. 38:704-708, 1995.

316. Vollman, J. H., Smith, W. L., Ballard, E. T., et al.: Early onset group B streptococcal disease: Clinical, roentgenographic, and pathologic features. J. Pediatr. 89:199-203, 1976.

317. von Hunolstein, C., D'Ascenzi, S., Wagner, B., et al.: Immunochemistry of capsular type polysaccharide and virulence properties of type VI *Streptococcus agalactiae* (group B streptococci). Infect. Immun. *61*:1272-1280, 1993.

318. Wald, E. R., Bergman, I., Taylor, H. G., et al.: Long-term outcome of group B streptococcal meningitis. Pediatrics 77:217-221, 1986.

319. Walker, K. M., and Coyer, W. F.: Suprarenal abscess due to group B *Streptococcus.* J. Pediatr. *94*:970-971, 1979.

320. Walker, S. H., Santos, A. Q., and Quintero, B. A.: Recurrence of group B III streptococcal meningitis. J. Pediatr. *89*:187-188, 1976.

321. Weinberg, A. G., and Laird, W. P.: Group B streptococcal endocarditis detected by echocardiography. J. Pediatr. *92*:334-336, 1978.

322. Weiser, J. N., and Rubens, C. E.: Transposon mutagenesis of group B *Streptococcus* beta-hemolysin biosynthesis. Infect. Immun. *55*:2314-2316, 1987.

323. Weisman, L. E., Stoll, B. J., Cruess, D. F., et al.: Early-onset group B streptococcal sepsis: A current assessment. J. Pediatr. *121*:428-433, 1992.

324. Weisner, A. M., Johnson, A. P., Lamagni, T. L., et al.: Characterization of group B streptococci recovered from infants with invasive disease in England and Wales. Clin. Infect. Dis. *38*:1203-1208, 2004.

325. Wessels, M. R., Paoletti, L. C., Kasper, D. L., et al.: Immunogenicity in animals of a polysaccharide-protein conjugate vaccine against type III group B *Streptococcus.* J. Clin. Invest. *86*:1428-1433, 1990.

326. Wessels, M. R., Rubens, C. E., Benedí, V. J., et al.: Definition of a bacterial virulence factor: Sialylation of the group B streptococcal capsule. Proc. Natl. Acad. Sci. U. S. A. *86*:8983-8987, 1989.

327. Wilkinson, H. W.: Analysis of group B streptococcal types associated with disease in human infants and adults. J. Clin. Microbiol. 7:176-179, 1978.

328. Wilkinson, H. W.: Detection of group B streptococcal antibodies in human sera by radioimmunoassay: Concentrations of type-specific antibodies in sera of adults and infants infected with group B streptococci. J. Clin. Microbiol. 72:194-201, 1978.

329. Wilkinson, H. W., Facklam, R. R., and Wortham, E. C.: Distribution by serological type of group B streptococci isolated from a variety of clinical material over a five-year period (with special reference to neonatal sepsis and meningitis). Infect. Immun. *8*:228-235, 1973.

330. Williams, P. A., Bohnsack, J. F., Augustine, N. H., et al.: Production of tumor necrosis factor by human cells in vitro and in vivo, induced by group B streptococci. J. Pediatr. *123*:292-300, 1993.

331. Wirth, J., Raymond, J., and Lapillonne, A.: Unusual report of diaper rash in a premature infant with group B streptococcal infection. Pediatr. Infect. Dis. J. *25*:750-751, 2006.

332. Wiswell, T. E., Baumgart, S., Gannon, C. M., et al.: No lumbar puncture in the evaluation for early neonatal sepsis: Will meningitis be missed? Pediatrics *95*:803-806, 1995.

333. Wong, M., Isaacs, D., Howman-Giles, R., et al.: Clinical and diagnostic features of osteomyelitis occurring in the first three months of life. Pediatr. Infect. Dis.. J *14*:1047-1053, 1995.

334. Wood, E. G., and Dillon, H. C.: A prospective study of group B streptococcal bacteriuria in pregnancy. Am. J. Obstet. Gynecol. *140*:515-520, 1981.

335. Woods, C. R., and Edwards, M. S.: Renal abscess caused by group B *Streptococcus.* Clin. Infect. Dis. *18*:662-662, 1994.

336. Yagupsky, P., Menegus, M. A., and Powell, K. R.: The changing spectrum of group B streptococcal disease in infants: An eleven-year experience in a tertiary care hospital. Pediatr. Infect. Dis. J. *10*:801-808, 1991.

337. Yancey, M. K., Schuchat, A., Brown, L. K., et al.: The accuracy of late antenatal screening cultures in predicting genital group B streptococcal colonization at delivery. Obstet. Gynecol. *88*:811-815, 1996.

338. Yeung, M. K., and Mattingly S. J.: Biosynthetic capacity for type-specific antigen synthesis determines the virulence of serotype III strains of group B streptococci. Infect. Immun. *44*:217-221, 1984.

339. Young, N., Finn, A., and Powell, C.: Group B streptococcal epiglottitis. Pediatr. Infect. Dis. J. *15*:95-96, 1996.

340. Yow, M. D., Leeds, L. J., Thompson, P. K., et al.: The natural history of group B streptococcal colonization in the pregnant woman and her offspring. I. Colonization studies. Am. J. Obstet. Gynecol. *137*:34-38, 1980.

341. Yow, M. D., Mason, E. O., Leeds, L. J., et al.: Ampicillin prevents intrapartum transmission of group B *Streptococcus.* JAMA *241*:1245-1247, 1979.

342. Zaleznik, D. F., Rench, M. A., Hillier, S. L., et al.: Invasive disease due to group B *Streptococcus* in pregnant women and neonates from diverse population groups. Clin. Infect. Dis. *30*:276-281, 2000.

343. Zangwill, K. M., Schuchat, A., and Wenger, J. D.: Group B streptococcal disease in the United States, 1990: Report from a multistate active surveillance system. M. M. W. R. C. D. C. Surveill. Summ. *41*:25-32, 1992.

CHAPTER 95

ENTEROCOCCAL AND VIRIDANS STREPTOCOCCAL INFECTIONS

B. Keith English ☉ Jerry L. Shenep

ENTEROCOCCAL INFECTIONS

The enterococci are gram-positive ovoid bacteria that are related closely to the streptococci but now are known to be phylogenetically distinct and make up the genus *Enterococcus*. These organisms are found in the normal bowel flora of humans and many animals and commonly are isolated from environmental sources. Enterococci generally are considered to be of low virulence but have been known to cause human infection for more than 100 years (reviewed by Murray[164]). These ubiquitous bacteria have become recognized increasingly as important causes of both nosocomial and community-acquired infection in adults[62,152,153,164,166,168,180,185] and children,* yet the role of *Enterococcus* spp. as a pathogen (or co-pathogen) in certain clinical settings, particularly intra-abdominal and pelvic infections, often remains uncertain.

Enterococci are intrinsically resistant to many antimicrobial agents (including the cephalosporins, oxacillin, clindamycin, and the aminoglycosides). Since the emergence of high-level aminoglycoside resistance in *Enterococcus* spp. more than 35 years ago,[157] increasing percentages of these organisms have acquired clinically significant resistance to β-lactam antibiotics and to vancomycin and other glycopeptides, as well as to aminoglycosides. Vancomycin-resistant enterococcal (VRE) infections, especially those caused by vancomycin-resistant *Enterococcus faecium* (VREF), are of particular concern because VREF isolates frequently are resistant to other bactericidal antimicrobial agents.[166,168] The dramatic increase in nosocomial VRE infections[62,166,180] has resulted in failure of antimicrobial therapy[125] and has inspired comparisons with the pre-antibiotic period[5] and even speculation about a "post-antimicrobial era."[44] Fortunately, new classes of antimicrobials active against most VRE isolates have become available recently, but pediatric experience with these agents is limited, and enterococci resistant to these agents already have been detected (see later). Concern about the continued nosocomial spread of VRE isolates and the documented transfer of vancomycin resistance determinants to *Staphylococcus aureus*[27,28,242,252] has led to the development of stringent hospital infection control guidelines designed to interrupt the spread of vancomycin-resistant organisms.[193] Although the impact of VRE infections in children has been less dramatic, increasing numbers of pediatric centers are reporting infections caused by these organisms.*

---

*See references 18, 19, 20, 30, 61, 117, 132, 159, 180, 194, 199, 202, 215, 216, 220, 221.

*See references 18, 30-38, 58, 59, 78, 91, 132, 159, 193, 202.

MICROBIOLOGY

The genus *Enterococcus* consists of gram-positive cocci that are catalase-negative and occur singly, in pairs, and in short chains. Morphologically, enterococci are indistinguishable from streptococci and traditionally were classified as members of the genus *Streptococcus*. Sherman's early classification scheme[222] divided the streptococci into four groups: pyogenic, viridans, lactic, and enterococcal. By the Lancefield criteria, enterococci were classified as group D streptococci, along with the "nonenterococcal" *Streptococcus bovis* group. However, recent genetic evidence has indicated that the enterococci are sufficiently different from the streptococci to merit establishment of a separate genus.[68]

Figure 95–1 is a scheme for the differentiation of enterococci from other gram-positive cocci. Catalase-negative gram-positive cocci that have been isolated from human sources include the streptococci, the enterococci, *Lactococcus* spp., *Leuconostoc* spp., *Pediococcus* spp., and *Gemella* spp. Most enterococci produce no (gamma) or partial (alpha) hemolysis on blood agar; differentiation between enterococci and certain alpha-hemolytic or nonhemolytic streptococci and other nonstreptococcal gram-positive cocci may require a series of biochemical tests.[67,68] Clinical laboratories may identify an organism presumptively on a primary isolation plate as an enterococcus based on colony morphology, Gram stain, and the pyrrolidonyl arylamidase (PYR) test. Most enterococci produce PYR, as do *Streptococcus pyogenes* and nutritionally variant streptococci (*Abiotrophia*), but not other streptococci. The PYR test is particularly useful for differentiating enterococci from group D streptococci and *Leuconostoc* spp. (see Fig. 95–1). *S. pyogenes* and *Abiotrophia* spp. are distinguished easily from enterococci by colony morphology, hemolysis, and special growth requirements.

Enterococci are able to hydrolyze esculin in the presence of 40 percent bile salts; of the true streptococci, only group D streptococci (*S. bovis* group) and approximately 5 to 10 percent of viridans streptococci share this characteristic.[68] Enterococci are facultatively anaerobic and grow under harsh conditions that inhibit the growth of streptococci; growth in 6.5 percent sodium chloride at 45° C is a useful confirmatory test. Enterococci produce leucine aminopeptidase, as do streptococci, lactococci, pediococci, and some *Gemella* strains. The presence of group D streptococcal antigen is of limited value because the *S. bovis* group, most pediococci, and half of the clinical *Leuconostoc* spp. isolates share this antigen.[68]

Occasional clinical isolates of *Leuconostoc* spp., *Pediococcus* spp., and *Lactococcus* spp. may be difficult to distinguish from the enterococci. Some strains of *Leuconostoc* spp. and *Pediococcus* spp. may grow in 6.5 percent NaCl at 45° C, but they are PYR-negative. Lactococci are PYR-positive, and some isolates will grow in 6.5 percent NaCl; however, most lactococci fail to grow (or grow very slowly) at 45° C. Consequently, definitive confirmation of an organism as an enterococcus may require complete identification to the species level. Molecular techniques allow rapid, reliable identification and speciation of enterococci,[50,57,60] but currently they are available only in the research setting.

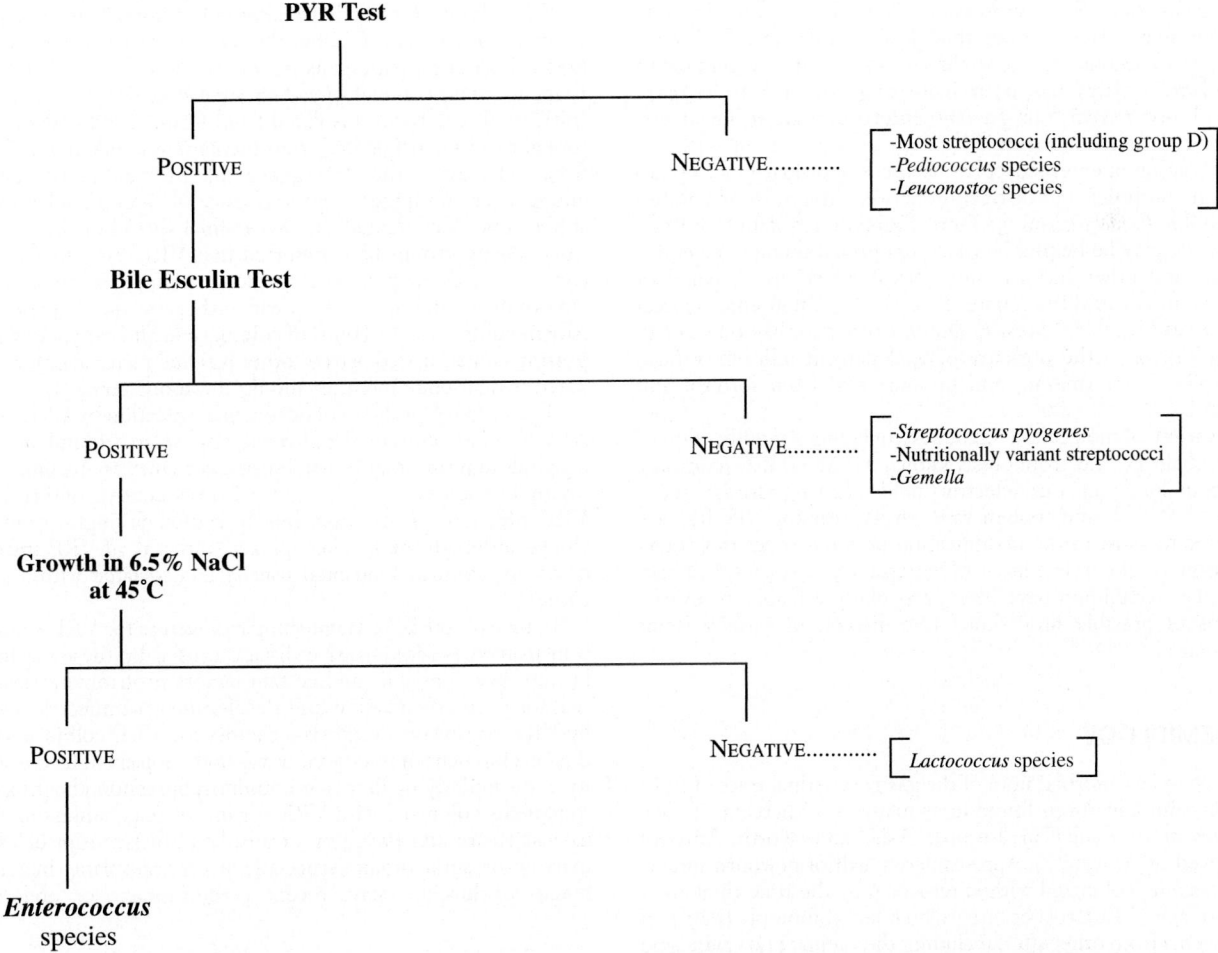

Figure 95–1 Differentiation of enterococci from other catalase-negative, gram-positive cocci. PYR, pyrrolidonyl arylamidase.

TABLE 95–1 *Enterococcus* Species

Typical Enterococci (PYR⁺)
E. faecalis
E. faecium
E. avium
E. casseliflavus
E. durans
E. raffinosus
E. gallinarum
E. malodoratus
E. hirae
E. mundtii
E. pseudoavium
E. dispar
E. flavescens
E. sulfureus

Atypical Enterococci (PYR⁻)
E. cecorum
E. columbae
E. saccharolyticus

PYR, pyrrolidonyl arylamidase.

The genus *Enterococcus* now includes at least 14 "typical" species and 3 additional "atypical" species (the latter are PYR-negative and grow very slowly in the presence of 6.5% NaCl) (Table 95–1). However, most human clinical isolates are either *Enterococcus faecalis* (50-90%) or *E. faecium* (5-37%), although clusters of human infection caused by *Enterococcus raffinosus*,[33] *Enterococcus casseliflavus*,[172] *Enterococcus avium*,[184] and *Enterococcus durans*[216] and occasional human infections attributable to *Enterococcus gallinarum*, *Enterococcus mundtii*, and *Enterococcus flavescens* have been reported.[66] Even though *E. faecalis* and *E. faecium* continue to account for most clinical isolates, the percentage of *E. faecium* isolates has been increasing, and relatively more "other" (non-*faecalis*, non-*faecium*) enterococci are being identified by clinical laboratories.[110,112,138]

Speciation of enterococci has been useful primarily for epidemiologic purposes, but distinction between the more antibiotic-susceptible *E. faecalis* and the more antibiotic-resistant (see later) *E. faecium* may be helpful in selecting optimal therapy for endocarditis and other serious enterococcal infections. A panel of biologic tests can differentiate these two common enterococcal species readily.[68,118,164] Most *E. faecalis* isolates (unlike those of *E. faecium*) grow in the presence of 0.04 percent tellurite, reduce tetrazolium to formazan, and produce acid from sorbitol and glycerol.

A variety of molecular techniques, including a modification of pulsed-field gel electrophoresis known as the CHEF (contour-clamped homogeneous electric field electrophoresis) technique[39,40,56,160,255] and polymerase chain reaction (PCR), are available to assist in the identification of enterococci and determination of the relatedness of enterococcal isolates.[60] These molecular techniques have been particularly valuable in investigations of possible nosocomial transmission of multiresistant enterococci.[39,40,57,60,68,160,182,205,255]

EPIDEMIOLOGY

Enterococci are normal flora of the gastrointestinal tract of most humans and have been found in as many as 97 percent of fecal samples from adults in Europe, Asia, and North America (reviewed by Murray[164]). Approximately half of newborn infants have become colonized with enterococci by the time they are 1 week of age.[175] Enterococci are isolated less commonly (<20% of specimens) from other sites, including the vagina, oral cavity, and skin. These organisms also are common inhabitants of the bowel

flora of many animals and frequently are present in soil, water, and food. Enterococci are hardy organisms and may persist for long periods on environmental surfaces, thereby contributing to potential nosocomial spread of these bacteria.

Human infection caused by enterococci was reported before the beginning of the 20th century, but the initial reports included patients with infections that seldom are associated with enterococci today: enteritis, meningitis, and appendicitis (reviewed by Murray[164]). The ubiquitous presence of enterococci in fecal samples led to the mistaken impression that these organisms cause enteritis and food poisoning. Enterococci are isolated commonly as part of mixed flora in intra-abdominal and pelvic infections, but the contribution of these organisms to the pathogenesis of such infections remains uncertain.[81,173] However, enterococci were identified as pathogens causing urinary tract infection and endocarditis as early as 1906,[4] with later confirmation by many studies. Subsequently, enterococci have been documented to cause invasive infection in neonates,[56,77,121] patients with malignancies,[85,86,159,221] recipients of bone marrow and solid organ transplants,[9,116,119,183,210] burn victims,[127] patients with indwelling catheters,[9,51,153,164,185,199] and other immunosuppressed or debilitated patients.[30,153,164,185,199]

In general, enterococcal infections occur less frequently in children (outside the neonatal period) than in adults, and enterococci are less common causes of pediatric (versus adult) urinary tract infection[259] and endocarditis.[231] Much of the published experience with enterococcal infection in children focuses on the neonatal period,[47,56,140,194] and some evidence suggests that late-onset (but not early-onset) neonatal enterococcal infection may be increasing in frequency.[39,56] Relatively few series of pediatric enterococcal infection have been published.[14,17,22,39,51,85,202]

Enterococci recently have emerged as important nosocomial agents, and they rank as either the second or third most common hospital-acquired pathogens in this country.[62,103,152,180,200,211,261,262] Evidence of nosocomial spread of enterococci is relatively recent. Initially, all enterococci isolated from hospitalized patients were thought to have originated from the patient's endogenous bowel flora. However, the emergence of multiantibiotic-resistant enterococci prompted the performance of careful epidemiologic studies that documented the nosocomial spread of these organisms.* Many groups have reported that VRE and other enterococcal isolates may persist for long periods of time in the environment and may be spread either by direct patient-to-patient contact via the hands of colonized health care personnel[194] or from contaminated beds or other hospital material or contaminated patient equipment, including thermometers.[18,117,132,153]

The growing problem of nosocomial infection by VRE organisms is multifactorial; the diversity of isolates found in many hospitals indicates that resistant organisms may be introduced via multiple sources.[39,61,78,161,167,199,221] Consequently, outbreaks of VRE infection in institutions may be caused by single or multiple clones, although the first recognized outbreak of VRE infection or colonization in a hospital usually is associated with a single clone.[30,78]

In many reports, distinguishing risk factors for VRE colonization from those for invasive disease caused by these organisms has not been possible, and certain factors probably increase the risk for both colonization and development of infection caused by VRE organisms. Major risk factors for VRE colonization or the development of infection, or for both, appear to be the severity of the underlying illness or immunosuppression; the proximity to patients colonized with VRE organisms (e.g., admission to an intensive care unit [ICU] or a transplant unit); receipt of a bone marrow or solid organ (especially liver) transplant; increasing length of hospital stay; recent cardiothoracic or abdominal

---

*See references 10, 11, 40, 87, 93, 194, 199, 200, 202, 229, 251, 262.

surgery; the presence of indwelling central venous or urinary catheters; and previous treatment with vancomycin, broad-spectrum antibiotics (particularly those lacking appreciable anti-enterococcal activity, such as the third-generation cephalosporins), or agents with broad anti-anaerobic activity.* Patients infected with human immunodeficiency virus (HIV) also appear to be at higher risk for the development of VRE bacteremia.[9] Factors contributing to nosocomial spread of these organisms probably differ from those responsible for the gradual overall increase in resistant strains.[199]

Since the first report of a vancomycin-resistant isolate in 1988,[128] infection and colonization with VRE bacteria in the United States have been observed primarily in the ICUs of large teaching hospitals.[166,168,180] For example, data reported to the National Nosocomial Infection Surveillance (NNIS) system of the Centers for Disease Control and Prevention (CDC) from January 1989 through March 1993 revealed no vancomycin resistance in hospitals with fewer than 200 beds, a resistance rate of 1.8 percent in hospitals with 200 to 500 beds, and a rate of 3.6 percent in hospitals with more than 500 beds.[180] A 1995 report from the multicenter *Enterococcus* Study Group analyzed 1936 isolates collected from 97 laboratories in 47 states during the last quarter of 1992 and generally confirmed the findings of the NNIS survey.[110] However, VRE infections are not limited to ICUs. A 1999 report from the Surveillance and Control of Pathogens of Epidemiologic Importance (SCOPE) group's ongoing surveillance of nosocomial bloodstream infections in 49 U.S. hospitals revealed no overall differences in rates of vancomycin resistance in enterococci isolated from patients located in critical care versus hospital ward settings.[62] Fortunately, VRE infections have occurred much less frequently in children than in adults, and overall rates of vancomycin resistance in enterococci isolated from children's hospitals remain very low. However, increasing numbers of pediatric centers have reported VRE infections.*

In the United States, VRE isolates generally have not been detected in environmental sources or in patients who have not had exposure to hospitals,[166] with rare exceptions.[30] However, the ecology of VRE organisms in Europe differs: they have been detected in the feces of nonhospitalized patients and healthy volunteers in several European studies, with rates of VRE colonization as high as 28 percent in adults living in some parts of Belgium (reviewed by Murray[166,168]). The more widespread occurrence of VRE strains in Europe probably was related to the use of oral glycopeptides such as avoparcin in animal feed and the oral administration of bacterial preparations (possibly contaminated with resistant enterococci) to humans and animals for therapeutic purposes.[166-168]

Initial reports of VRE organisms in the United States were clustered in the northeast region, particularly New York, Maryland, and Pennsylvania,[180] and geographic differences in rates of VRE colonization and infection persist. However, subsequent reports indicate that VRE strains are found in most parts of the United States[109,138] and that rates of vancomycin resistance among enterococci isolated from patients in this country generally are higher than those found in isolates from Canada, western Europe, or Latin America.[108,111,138] The reasons for these geographic differences remain uncertain, but the high rates of resistance in the United States may be related to the marked increase in the use of vancomycin in this country during the past 3 decades.[120]

PATHOGENESIS AND VIRULENCE

Enterococci are organisms of low virulence, and their ubiquitous presence in the human gastrointestinal tract probably has con-

tributed to both the spurious association of these organisms with some illnesses (e.g., enteritis) and the failure to recognize other situations in which enterococci are true pathogens (e.g., immunosuppressed and debilitated patients, neonates). When compared with organisms such as *S. pyogenes* and *S. aureus*, enterococci are much less virulent in animal models of infection,[104,152] but they are capable of causing disease at a higher inoculum.

Enterococci rarely cause primary cellulitis or abscesses, although these organisms are isolated frequently as components of polymicrobial wound infections and intra-abdominal and pelvic infections. The contribution of enterococci to the pathogenesis of these polymicrobial infections remains uncertain.[81,173] In animal models, synergy between enterococci and a variety of other organisms (particularly anaerobes) can be demonstrated, but enterococci injected alone have little propensity to cause either peritonitis or subcutaneous infection.[104,105,164,181] Many clinical trials have concluded that provision of anti-enterococcal therapy generally is not necessary to effect a cure of human intra-abdominal and pelvic infections, even though *Enterococcus* frequently (14-33% of cases) is isolated from primary peritoneal cultures.[81]

Enterococci are an important cause of urinary tract infections in adults (particularly in elderly men, patients with structural abnormalities of the urinary tract, and those with indwelling urinary catheters), but they are associated less frequently with urinary tract infections in children.[7,259] Enterococci also are important but less frequent (than in adults) causes of bacterial endocarditis in children.[151,231]

Adherence of bacteria to tissue is a necessary first step in the pathogenesis of both urinary tract infection and endocarditis, and evidence suggests that pathogenic enterococci produce factors that mediate adherence to urinary epithelial cells and endocardial tissue (reviewed by Jett and colleagues[104] and Johnson[105]). Enterococcal adhesins include an enterococcal surface protein known as aggregation substance[36,123] and surface carbohydrates. Lipoteichoic acid, an important adhesin for *S. pyogenes*, does not appear to mediate adherence of enterococci,[228] but it may trigger the host inflammatory response to these organisms.[238] Recent studies have implicated an enterococcal surface protein, Esp, in biofilm formation by *E. faecalis*.[24,240] In addition, many virulent *E. faecalis* isolates express a cytolysin in the presence of target cells.[43,48]

Nosocomial enterococcal bacteremia in adults frequently is associated with urinary tract and wound infections, but catheter-related bacteremia is of increasing importance. Enterococcal bacteremia without a source occurs relatively more commonly in children,[17,199] although Bonadio[14] reported that many children with enterococcal bacteremia had an identifiable focus of infection. Enterococcal bacteremia occurs more frequently in patients with severe underlying disease and may be life-threatening. However, the precise contribution of enterococcal bacteremia to morbidity and mortality in severely ill patients remains controversial. Adult ICU patients with enterococcal bacteremia have a very high mortality rate,[83] and some early studies suggested that isolation of *Enterococcus* from blood merely serves to identify a very high-risk group of patients.[164] In several studies, clearance of VRE organisms from blood was not associated with a reduced mortality rate in this high-risk population. In other studies, spontaneous resolution of VRE bacteremia has been reported, thus suggesting that transient VRE bacteremia or pseudobacteremia (or both) may occur.[246] However, a series of recent studies has clearly associated vancomycin resistance with an increased risk for mortality in certain patients and has demonstrated that effective anti-enterococcal therapy reduces the mortality rate in patients with VRE bacteremia.[53,54,61,97,168,185] Taken together, these findings indicate that at least a subset of high-risk patients with VRE bacteremia are at risk for the development of significant morbidity and mortality directly related to the infection.

---

*See references 14, 17, 47, 56, 77, 121, 140, 147, 194, 226.

CLINICAL MANIFESTATIONS

Enterococcal infections generally occur less frequently in children than in adults, but *Enterococcus* is a relatively frequent cause of neonatal infections.[56] The types of infections caused by enterococci in children are similar to those in adults,[14,17,51,199] although enterococcal bacteremia may be associated with fewer sequelae in children.[51] In children, as well as in adults, enterococci have become increasingly important nosocomial pathogens.[17,39,147,152,180,200,262] They are important causes of endocarditis, urinary tract infection, and bacteremia (particularly catheter-related bacteremia) in pediatric patients, and these organisms commonly are isolated as components of polymicrobial wound, intra-abdominal, and pelvic infections in children.[14,17,153,164] Meningitis[234] and septic arthritis[192] are rare manifestations of enterococcal infection. Respiratory infections caused by enterococci are extremely uncommon occurrences, although many neonates with enterococcal infection have pulmonary symptoms.[55]

URINARY TRACT INFECTION

Urinary tract infections are the most common enterococcal infections in adults,[153] and enterococci are important urinary pathogens in children.[52] Most enterococcal urinary tract infections occur in elderly men after they have undergone urinary catheterization, instrumentation, or both.[70,162] Enterococci are infrequent (<5% of isolates) causes of cystitis and pyelonephritis in otherwise healthy children, infants, and neonates[7,259] and are infrequent causes of urinary tract infection in young women.[164] However, some centers are reporting an increasing incidence of both community-acquired and nosocomial urinary tract infection caused by enterococci.[70]

Most enterococcal urinary tract infections in children[7,52,134] and adults[70,152] are nosocomial. Risk factors for the development of urinary tract infection by *Enterococcus* include indwelling urinary catheters, instrumentation of the urinary tract, structural abnormalities of the urinary tract, and previous broad-spectrum antimicrobial therapy.[162,164] The increasing problem of nosocomial enterococcal urinary tract infection[70] is compounded by the growing problem of multiantibiotic-resistant enterococci.[180]

The genitourinary tract reportedly is the most common entry site leading to enterococcal bacteremia in adults,[83,124] but it is implicated much less frequently in the cause of enterococcal bacteremia in children.[14,17,51] Christie and colleagues reported that urosepsis was the cause of 12 percent of episodes of nosocomial enterococcal bacteremia in one children's hospital,[39] but Das and Gray[51] failed to detect any cases of urosepsis in 75 consecutive cases of enterococcal bacteremia in another pediatric hospital during a 3-year period. Other complications of enterococcal urinary tract infection in adults include prostatitis and perinephric abscess.[153]

ENDOCARDITIS

Enterococcal endocarditis was reported first in 1906,[4] and these organisms are important causes of native- and prosthetic-valve endocarditis in children and adults.[2,150,197] Either normal or previously damaged valves may be involved. Enterococci cause approximately 5 to 20 percent of cases of native-valve endocarditis in adults (excluding cases in intravenous drug users),[150] approximately 6 to 7 percent of prosthetic-valve endocarditis,[150,243] and approximately 5 to 10 percent of endocarditis in intravenous drug users.[164] Enterococcal endocarditis in intravenous drug users generally involves the aortic or mitral valves, unlike staphylococcal endocarditis in this setting, which usually involves the tricuspid

valve.[164] As with other enterococcal infections, *E. faecalis* causes most cases of endocarditis.

Enterococcal endocarditis primarily is a disease of older men, and the genitourinary tract is the most commonly identified source of the initial bacteremia. Enterococci are relatively less frequent causes of endocarditis in children—less than 5 percent of cases in most series.[106,107,230,231,239,263] Typically, enterococcal endocarditis occurs after a subacute course that is clinically indistinguishable from that caused by streptococci.[150] Although the enterococcus is a common neonatal pathogen,[56] reports of neonatal enterococcal endocarditis are extremely rare.[239] The prognosis of enterococcal prosthetic-valve endocarditis is somewhat better than that of native-valve endocarditis caused by these organisms.[2,197] Aortic-valve involvement is associated with increased rates of morbidity and mortality.[150] Endocarditis rarely complicates nosocomial enterococcal bacteremia.[142,164,185] Consequently, VRE-associated endocarditis is a rare development, although a number of cases have been reported recently.[233]

BACTEREMIA

Enterococcal bacteremia often represents a conundrum. Bacteremia in severely ill hospitalized patients, particularly that caused by VRE organisms, is associated with considerable morbidity and mortality. However, only a portion of that morbidity and mortality can be attributed directly to enterococcal bacteremia *per se*. Nosocomial enterococcal bacteremia frequently occurs as a component of polymicrobial bacteremia, with 21 to 45 percent of bloodstream isolates of *Enterococcus* being accompanied by one or more other pathogens.[51,142,185,224] As many as half of cases of catheter-related enterococcal bacteremia are polymicrobial.[147,185] Many,[90,142] but not all,[96,147] series of patients with enterococcal bacteremia have reported increased mortality rates in patients with polymicrobial bacteremia (including *Enterococcus*) versus isolated enterococcal bacteremia. Mortality in adults with nosocomial enterococcal bacteremia has ranged from 23 to 46 percent,[142,143,185] but patients at risk for the acquisition of nosocomial enterococcal bacteremia are severely ill and have a poor prognosis independent of the bacteremic event. However, hospital-acquired enterococcal infections can be life-threatening,[61,164,185,189] and specific therapy does appear to reduce the overall mortality rate.[61,97,185] Furthermore, a recent meta-analysis concluded that vancomycin resistance is independently correlated with increased mortality in patients with enterococcal bloodstream infections.[53,54] Nonetheless, many episodes of enterococcal bacteremia in high-risk patients apparently resolve in the absence of specific therapy.[97,246] The mortality rate associated with enterococcal bacteremia in children has been lower than that reported in adults in most studies but has ranged from 7.5 percent[51] to 12 percent[17] to 20 percent[14] to 26 percent,[39] depending on the population studied.

In adults, many cases of enterococcal bacteremia are associated with a primary focus, most commonly a urinary tract infection.[55,85] In contrast, few children with enterococcal bacteremia have urosepsis, and most episodes of enterococcal bacteremia in children have not been associated with any identifiable focus.[17,199] However, Christie and coworkers identified a primary focus in 21 of 57 children (37%) with nosocomial enterococcal bacteremia, including 7 patients with urosepsis and 6 with peritonitis.[39] Many children with enterococcal bacteremia do have underlying disease involving the gastrointestinal or respiratory tract.[14,17] Central venous catheter–related enterococcal bacteremia is a growing problem in both children[14,17,39,51,56,185] and adults.[82,185] In earlier series, infections of vascular catheters were reported to account for only 2 to 14 percent of cases of enterococcal bacteremia (reviewed by Graninger and Ragette[83]), but more recent reports have implicated intravascular devices in as many as 22 to 28 percent of these episodes in adults and children.[51,185]

Most episodes of enterococcal bacteremia do not lead to endocarditis,[142,164,185] and endocarditis is particularly uncommon in the setting of nosocomial enterococcal bacteremia. Maki and Agger[142] identified only one case of endocarditis in 118 episodes of hospital-acquired enterococcal bacteremia, whereas endocarditis was diagnosed in 12 of 35 patients with community-acquired enterococcal bacteremia.

INTRA-ABDOMINAL INFECTIONS

Most of the published information about the role of *Enterococcus* in intra-abdominal and pelvic infections comes from series of adult patients. Enterococci commonly are isolated as components of polymicrobial infections involving the abdomen or pelvis,[81] and animal models suggest that these organisms can play a synergistic role in the pathogenesis of such infections.[104] However, evidence that the addition of specific anti-enterococcal therapy improves the outcome of human intra-abdominal and pelvic infections, even when enterococci are isolated from peritoneal cultures, is not compelling.[81]

Children with enterococcal bacteremia frequently have underlying conditions related to the gastrointestinal tract.[14,17,39] Bonadio reported five cases of enterococcal bacteremia in previously healthy infants with gastroenteritis, six cases associated with bowel obstruction, and one case associated with acute appendicitis without perforation.[14] Boulanger and coworkers[17] identified underlying conditions affecting the gastrointestinal system in 8 of 32 pediatric patients, but they were unable to specifically implicate any of these conditions as the source of the bacteremia. Das and Gray detected underlying chronic gastrointestinal pathology (short-gut syndrome, congenital anomalies of the gastrointestinal tract, ulcerative colitis, chronic liver disease) in fully a third (25 of 75) of pediatric patients with enterococcal bacteremia.[51]

MENINGITIS

Enterococci are rare causes of bacterial meningitis in adults and children. Stevenson and colleagues[234] found only four cases of enterococcal meningitis among 493 episodes (0.8%) of bacterial meningitis in adults, and they identified an additional 90 cases in a literature search of the interval from 1966 to 1992. These authors reviewed 16 published cases of enterococcal meningitis in children: 11 of these 16 pediatric cases were complications of central nervous system (CNS) trauma or surgery, but 4 children (3 of the 4 were neonates) had primary meningitis.[234] Enterococci are uncommon but well-recognized causes of infection involving cerebrospinal fluid (CSF) shunts and related devices.[122,170,214] Meningitis rarely complicates nosocomial bacteremia in adults,[142,185] but it has been reported more frequently in children (particularly neonates) with bacteremia. For example, meningitis developed in 7 percent (4 of 57) of episodes of nosocomial enterococcal bacteremia in children in Cincinnati[39] and in 15 percent (4 of 26) of premature neonates with late-onset enterococcal sepsis in Houston.[56]

Stevenson and associates found that most adults with enterococcal meningitis were immunocompromised (most were receiving steroids) or had a history of CNS trauma or surgery (or both).[234] Enterococcal meningitis has been reported in an adult patient with HIV infection who had completed a course of steroids for presumed *Pneumocystis* pneumonia.[187] Although many children with enterococcal meningitis do have a history of CNS trauma or surgery or are premature infants, most do not have other identifiable predisposing conditions or a history of immunosuppressive therapy.

As with the majority of enterococcal infections, most isolates from CSF are *E. faecalis*, but meningitis and ventriculoperitoneal shunt infections caused by *E. faecium* also have been reported in children.[170,171]

NEONATAL INFECTIONS

Enterococci are important neonatal pathogens,* and the published experience with neonatal enterococcal infections constitutes much of the pediatric experience with these organisms. Although several large series of neonatal sepsis included few cases of enterococcal infection (reviewed by Klein and Marcy[121]), many centers have reported that *Enterococcus* is a relatively frequent cause of neonatal bacteremia. Siegel and McCracken[226] found that enterococci were second only to group B streptococci as causes of neonatal sepsis at Parkland Hospital in Dallas from 1974 to 1977, with an incidence rate of approximately 1.0 case per 1000 live births. Gladstone and colleagues[77] reported that *Enterococcus* caused 18 of 270 (6.7%) episodes of neonatal sepsis at Yale–New Haven Hospital during the period 1979 to 1988, which ranked fourth in incidence behind group B streptococci (64 cases, 23.7%), *Escherichia coli* (46 cases, 17.0%), and coagulase-negative staphylococci (36 cases, 13.3%). During the 1990s, reports from Houston,[57] Cincinnati,[39] and New York City[147] documented sharp increases in the rate of late-onset neonatal infection with enterococci in both hospitalized high-risk premature neonates and infants[57,147] and otherwise healthy term newborns with "community-acquired" infection.[57]

Enterococci cause both early-onset (<7 days of age) and late-onset (>7 days of age) neonatal sepsis. Early-onset disease is indistinguishable from that caused by other neonatal pathogens, but it tends to be less severe.[56] Rates of early-onset disease have remained relatively stable; however, several centers are reporting increasing rates of late-onset infection. Dobson and Baker identified 56 neonates with enterococcal sepsis during a 10-year period at Jefferson Davis Hospital in Houston; 18 of 56 (32%) had early-onset sepsis, 26 of 56 (46%) had late-onset sepsis, and 12 of 56 (21%) had sepsis associated with necrotizing enterocolitis (2 early onset, 10 late onset).[56] In this study 25 of the 26 (96%) infants with late-onset enterococcal sepsis were premature infants. Christie and colleagues[39] identified 83 cases of enterococcal bacteremia between 1986 and 1992 at Children's Hospital of Cincinnati; 58 of the 83 episodes occurred in neonates. Most cases (57 of 83, 68.7%) were nosocomial, but many (26 of 83, 31.3%) were community acquired. Young infants (<3 months of age) accounted for almost all (24 of 26, 92.3%) of the community-acquired episodes and for many (34 of 57, 59.6%) of the nosocomial infections. Bonadio[14] and Boulanger and colleagues[17] also have reported community-acquired enterococcal bacteremia in young infants.

McNeeley and associates[147] identified 138 episodes of enterococcal bacteremia in a New York City neonatal ICU during a 20-year period and reviewed 100 of the episodes in detail. These authors noted a sharp increase in the rate of enterococcal bacteremia during the second decade (1984 to 1994) of this study and found that most cases occurred in older infants; during this decade, the mean age at onset was 44.7 days (versus 16.1 days during the first decade of the study), and 65 percent (51 of 78) of the episodes occurred after the infants reached 30 days of age. Most of the infections occurred in neonates with indwelling central venous catheters (77%), and more than half of the patients had evidence of gastrointestinal disease (necrotizing enterocolitis in 33% and abdominal distention in an additional 21%). The

---

*See references 5, 29, 30, 32, 47, 61, 69, 78, 89, 91, 117, 129, 139, 153, 161, 164, 166, 168, 174, 196, 199, 202.

overall mortality rate in this study was 28 percent, although many of the deaths were not attributed to the enterococcal infection. Most (64%) of the episodes of enterococcal bacteremia in this series were polymicrobial.[147]

Nosocomial outbreaks of enterococcal infection, including VRE infection, have been reported in several neonatal units in the United States.[39,47,140,194] Indwelling central venous catheters, necrotizing enterocolitis, and intra-abdominal surgery are important predisposing factors for the development of nosocomial enterococcal bacteremia in neonates, whereas the genitourinary tract is implicated much less frequently as a source.[39,147]

Enterococcal bacteremia in neonates and young infants has been associated with diarrhea[14,56] and with respiratory disease,[14,56] although a causative role for *Enterococcus* in the pathogenesis of gastroenteritis or pneumonia remains undefined. Enterococci rarely cause urinary tract infections in neonates,[14,39,56,147] but nosocomial and community-acquired cases have been reported. Enterococci have been noted to cause a variety of other neonatal infections, including focal skin and soft tissue infections such as scalp abscess,[56] brain abscess,[201] omphalitis,[56] and conjunctivitis.[250]

Most enterococcal infections in neonates are caused by *E. faecalis*, but outbreaks of infection with *E. faecium* have been reported.[47] In the series from Cincinnati reported by Christie and associates and consisting largely of neonates, 82 percent of enterococcal isolates were *E. faecalis* and 14 percent were *E. faecium*.[39] McNeeley and colleagues reported the isolation of *E. faecalis* from 94 of 100 patients and *E. faecium* from 15 of 100 patients in their series (both organisms were isolated from 9 of the patients).[147] Six of the *E. faecium* isolates were resistant to vancomycin, and all six patients with VRE bacteremia died, although only one death appeared to be related directly to the VRE infection.

SEPTIC ARTHRITIS

Enterococci rarely have been reported to cause septic arthritis, but they can infect native or prosthetic joints. Raymond and colleagues[192] reported a case of enterococcal septic arthritis involving a prosthetic hip and reviewed an additional 18 cases from the literature. Eleven of these 19 episodes involved prosthetic joints (2 hips, 9 knees), and 8 involved native joints; only 1 of the 8 individuals with native-joint arthritis had an underlying abnormality of the joint. In 7 of the 19 episodes, enterococcus was isolated from synovial fluid along with a second organism (3 with coagulase-negative staphylococci, 1 with group B streptococci, 1 with *Pseudomonas*, 1 with *Streptococcus*, and 1 with *Kingella kingae*). Only one pediatric case was identified: a 21-month-old girl with septic arthritis of the wrist whose joint aspirate grew *Enterococcus* spp. and *K. kingae*.[225]

DIAGNOSIS

Enterococcal infections usually are diagnosed by isolation of *Enterococcus* from a culture of blood or another normally sterile site. As discussed earlier, enterococci are ubiquitous inhabitants of the human gastrointestinal tract, and isolation of these organisms from stool or surface cultures is not evidence of invasive infection. Although enterococci are uncommon blood culture contaminants, transient bacteremia or pseudobacteremia (or both) may be caused by these organisms.[97,246]

More problematic is the interpretation of a positive culture for enterococcus as a component of polymicrobial infections, particularly intra-abdominal and pelvic infections. In this setting, the role of the enterococcus in pathogenesis is uncertain, and therapeutic regimens that do not include anti-enterococcal agents

usually suffice to effect a clinical cure.[81] However, rare cases of breakthrough enterococcal bacteremia have been reported with these regimens, and one study found a decreased rate of abdominal surgical wound infections when anti-enterococcal coverage was provided in a prophylactic regimen.[253]

ANTIMICROBIAL SUSCEPTIBILITY AND RESISTANCE

The increasing importance of *Enterococcus* as a human pathogen, especially in the nosocomial setting,[62,112,147,152,164,180,200,261,262] is of particular concern because of the concomitant development of antimicrobial resistance by these organisms. Furthermore, antibiotic resistance probably has played a critical role in allowing the organism to persist and eventually cause disease in high-risk patients despite its relatively low virulence.

Some enterococci have acquired high-level resistance to all three classes of antimicrobial agents that have been used to treat life-threatening enterococcal infections—β-lactams, aminoglycosides, and glycopeptides. This acquired resistance has occurred in the context of intrinsic (usually lower-level) resistance of enterococci to many antibiotics, and physicians have been confronted with the possibility that invasive disease caused by these organisms might not respond to any available antibiotics. Some enterococci also have acquired resistance to recently developed agents (e.g., quinupristin-dalfopristin, linezolid, daptomycin) that are active against most antibiotic-resistant gram-positive cocci (see later).

INTRINSIC RESISTANCE

β-Lactam Antibiotics

Relative resistance to β-lactam antibiotics is an intrinsic characteristic of enterococci that occurs even in human populations without previous exposure to antibiotics[154]; such resistance is due to the lower affinity of enterococcal (versus streptococcal) penicillin-binding proteins, especially PBP-5.[153,256] In general, the minimal inhibitory concentration (MIC) of penicillin for most *E. faecalis* isolates (2 to 8 µg/mL) is at least 10 to 100 times higher than that of most streptococci, and *E. faecium* is even more resistant (MIC of 8 to 32 µg/mL or higher).[164] Ampicillin is the most active of the β-lactam antibiotics against enterococci, with average MIC values approximately twofold lower than those for penicillin.[153,164] Nafcillin generally is less active than is penicillin, and methicillin is much less active (MIC > 50 µg/mL for *E. faecalis*), as are carbenicillin and ticarcillin. Importantly, enterococci exposed to β-lactam antibiotics rapidly become tolerant of the killing effects of these agents.[153,164] Along with intrinsic resistance to these agents, tolerance limits the utility of β-lactam monotherapy for the treatment of endocarditis or other severe enterococcal infections.

Imipenem has some activity against *E. faecalis* but is much less active against *E. faecium*.[153,164] None of the cephalosporins currently available has clinically useful activity against the enterococci, and frequent use of broad-spectrum cephalosporins and imipenem has been identified as a risk factor for the acquisition of nosocomial enterococcal infection.

Aminoglycosides

Enterococci are intrinsically resistant to all aminoglycosides because of diminished uptake of these drugs. For most *E. faecalis* isolates, the MIC for gentamicin or tobramycin ranges from 8 to 64 µg/mL, and that for streptomycin ranges from 12 to 250 µg/mL.[149,186,244] Moellering and colleagues first demonstrated that the addition of a cell wall–active antibiotic results in dramatically increased aminoglycoside uptake by enterococci[156,266] and that combinations of β-lactam and aminoglycoside antibiotics can lead to synergistic killing of these organisms. All *E. faecium* strains exhibit higher MICs (than *E. faecalis* does) to certain aminoglycosides, including tobramycin, netilmicin, kanamycin, and sisomicin, and these aminoglycosides do not exhibit synergy with β-lactam antibiotics against *E. faecium*.[34,164]

Other Antibiotics

Under carefully standardized laboratory conditions, enterococci are inhibited by the combination of trimethoprim and sulfamethoxazole (TMP-SMX). However, *Enterococcus* isolates should be considered resistant to TMP-SMX because these organisms are capable of using exogenous folinic acid to evade the antimicrobial action of TMP-SMX.[265] TMP-SMX fails to eradicate enterococci in animal models of infection,[31,88] and breakthrough enterococcal bacteremia has occurred in patients being treated with TMP-SMX for enterococcal urinary tract infection.[80] Enterococci also are intrinsically resistant to clindamycin, a drug with excellent activity against many other gram-positive cocci. Most enterococci have a clindamycin MIC of 12.5 to 100 μg/mL.[164] As with low-level β-lactam resistance, clindamycin resistance is found in enterococcal isolates from human populations with no previous antibiotic exposure.[154]

ACQUIRED RESISTANCE

Enterococci have acquired resistance to antibiotics by the acquisition of both narrow– and broad–host range plasmids and via the exchange of conjugative transposons (reviewed by Murray[164]). Resistance mediated by broad–host range plasmids is of particular concern because glycopeptide resistance encoded by broad–host range plasmids has been transferred to staphylococci in vitro[176] and in vivo.[27,28,242,252]

High-Level Resistance to Aminoglycosides

Intrinsic resistance of enterococci to aminoglycosides is caused by poor drug uptake by these organisms and can be overcome effectively both in vitro and in vivo by the addition of cell wall–active antibiotics. In contrast, high-level resistance to aminoglycosides is mediated either by the acquisition of plasmids encoding aminoglycoside-modifying enzymes (affecting all aminoglycosides via several different enzymes) or by ribosomal mutations (streptomycin only). High-level aminoglycoside resistance is of great clinical importance because it eliminates synergism between the affected aminoglycoside or aminoglycosides and β-lactam or glycopeptide antibiotics.[34,164,186] All *E. faecium* strains produce a chromosomally encoded aminoglycoside acetyltransferase that eliminates synergistic killing between cell wall–active antibiotics and certain aminoglycosides (including tobramycin, kanamycin, netilmicin, and sisomicin),[34] but it does not result in high-level resistance to these compounds. Consequently, these particular aminoglycosides should not be used to treat infections caused by *E. faecium*.

Enterococci with high-level resistance (MIC usually ≥2000 μg/mL) to streptomycin, kanamycin, and several other aminoglycosides (excluding gentamicin) were identified more than 35 years ago[157] and were widely prevalent in the United States by the mid-1970s.[23] High-level resistance to streptomycin occurs via two mechanisms, ribosomal mutation or enzymatic modification by 6′-adenylyltransferase. Initial reports of high-level resistance to kanamycin were associated with the production of 3′-phosphotransferase.[34,164]

Horodniceanu and colleagues first reported high-level resistance to gentamicin in *E. faecalis* in 1979,[99] and this resistance was

shown later to be mediated by a fusion enzyme containing both 6′-acetyltransferase and 2″-phosphotransferase activity. Expression of this fusion enzyme conferred resistance to all clinically useful aminoglycosides except streptomycin.[129,130] Enterococci expressing this fusion protein usually have gentamicin MICs that are 2000 μg/mL or higher. Thus, enterococci expressing this fusion enzyme and the 6′-adenylyltransferase mediating streptomycin resistance (or chromosomally mediated streptomycin resistance) are highly resistant to all available aminoglycosides and generally fail to be killed synergistically by any combination of β-lactam antibiotics and aminoglycosides. Strains of *E. faecalis* resistant to both streptomycin and gentamicin (and thus to all aminoglycosides) were detected first in Houston, Bangkok, and Santiago in 1983.[149,164] Subsequently, strains of *E. faecalis*, *E. faecium*, and other enterococci resistant to gentamicin, streptomycin, or both (or all) aminoglycosides have become increasingly prevalent[82,108,110,111,138,186] (Table 95–2). Although high-level resistance to both streptomycin and gentamicin was described first in *E. faecalis*, it now is at least as common in *E. faecium*.[110]

Enterococci resistant to all aminoglycosides have been isolated at an increasing rate from clinical specimens. Jones and colleagues and the *Enterococcus* Study Group[109] found that fully 20 percent of 1936 enterococcal isolates from late 1992 (from 97 participating laboratories in 47 states) exhibited high-level resistance to both gentamicin and streptomycin. Low and associates and the SENTRY Antimicrobial Resistance Surveillance Program[138] reported similar rates of high-level resistance to both gentamicin and streptomycin from 1997 to 1999 (see Table 95–2). Almost a third (32.8%) of enterococci collected by the SENTRY group from 1997 to 2005 were highly resistant to gentamicin.[111] Many medical centers in the United States now report that most enterococcal isolates exhibit high-level resistance to all aminoglycosides.[168]

Several new aminoglycoside-resistant genes were identified in enterococci during the late 1990s (reviewed by Chow[34]). Some enterococci produce three or more enzymes. Strains expressing some of the recently described resistant genes may fail to exhibit synergy between gentamicin and β-lactams despite MICs below those usually associated with high-level resistance. For example, the aph (2″)-Ic gene[37] found in clinical isolates of both *E. faecalis* and *E. faecium* results in gentamicin MICs of approximately 256 to 384 μg/mL, lower than the standard screening cutoff for high-level resistance to gentamicin (500 μg/mL). Nonetheless, these organisms are resistant to ampicillin-gentamicin synergism and would not be detected by standard screening methods.

High-Level Resistance to β-Lactams and Production of β-Lactamase

The mechanisms of resistance to penicillin, ampicillin, and other β-lactam antibiotics differ among enterococcal species. The high-level β-lactam resistance (ampicillin MIC ≥ 16 μg/mL) of *E. faecium*[19,87,146] and some other non-*faecalis* enterococcal strains[19] has increased considerably during the past decade and is mediated by additional alterations in PBPs, particularly PBP-5.[71,87,198] Thus, high-level resistance to ampicillin and other β-lactams in *E. faecium* (and other non-*faecalis* strains) represents an exaggerated form of intrinsic β-lactam resistance. *E. faecalis* isolates also are intrinsically resistant to β-lactams (though less so than *E. faecium*), but little change has occurred in the level of this resistance in recent years. However, some strains of *E. faecalis*[110,165,169] and *E. faecium*[46] have acquired clinically significant resistance to ampicillin and penicillin via the plasmid-mediated, constitutive production of a β-lactamase enzyme identical to that of *S. aureus*.[267] β-Lactamase–producing strains of *E. faecalis* and *E. faecium* will not be detected by routine susceptibility testing because of a pronounced inoculum effect. Therefore, enzymatic methods

TABLE 95–2   Antimicrobial Resistance Patterns of Enterococci (United States)

Agents	Gordon et al.[82] (July 1988–April 1989)			Jones et al.[110] (Enterococcus Study Group) (October 1992–December 1992)		
	E. faecalis (N = 632) (%)	E. faecium (N = 58) (%)	Total (N = 705) (%)	E. faecalis (N = 1428) (%)	E. faecium (N = 306) (%)	Total (N = 1936) (%)
Ampicillin resistance (MIC ≥ 16 µg/mL)	0*	41†	4	0.6-0.7‡	58.7-59.3	12
Streptomycin high-level resistance (MIC > 2000 µg/mL)	14	33	16	31.5	55.7	36
Gentamicin high-level resistance (MIC > 500 µg/mL)	11	2	10	26.0	30.8	27
Vancomycin resistance (MIC > 4 µg/mL)	0.3	0	0.3	2.0	21.9	5.6

*However, 11 of 632 (1.7%) E. faecalis isolates were β-lactamase producers.
†No β-lactamase–producing strains were identified.
‡Only two β-lactamase–producing isolates were identified.

such as the nitrocefin test must be used to screen for β-lactamase–producing strains.[118,165] Fortunately, such strains remain very uncommon.[153]

Glycopeptide Resistance

Enterococci resistant to vancomycin were identified first in 1988[128,247] and rapidly have become a major nosocomial problem. Data collected by the NNIS of the CDC revealed a dramatic increase in the rate of vancomycin resistance in nosocomial isolates of *Enterococcus* during the interval 1989 to 1993.[180] The NNIS survey documented a 26-fold increase in vancomycin resistance among all nosocomial isolates (from 0.3% of enterococcal isolates in 1989 to 7.9% in 1993) and a 34-fold increase in vancomycin resistance among isolates obtained from adult patients in ICUs (from 0.4% of isolates in 1989 to 13.6% in 1993). Rates of vancomycin resistance in enterococci continued to increase during the next decade (see Table 95–2). The NNIS reported that fully 25 percent of enterococci associated with nosocomial infections in adult patients in ICUs in the United States were resistant to vancomycin in 1999 and 2000; by 2003 to 2004, approximately 30 percent of the enterococcal isolates from these patients were vancomycin-resistant (*http://www.cdc .gov/ncidod/dhqp/pdf/ar/ICU_RESTrend1995-2004.pdf*). Isolates of *E. faecium* are particularly likely to be vancomycin-resistant. Jones and colleagues in the SENTRY Antimicrobial Resistance Surveillance Program reported that 69.4 percent of 1512 U.S. bloodstream isolates of *E. faecium* collected between 1997 and 2005 were resistant to vancomycin.[111] Similarly, Wisplinghoff and colleagues in the SCOPE surveillance study found that 60 percent of U.S. bloodstream isolates of *E. faecium* collected between 1995 and 2002 were resistant to vancomycin, whereas only 3 percent of *E. faecalis* bloodstream isolates were vancomycin-resistant.[261]

Enterococci were the second most common organisms associated with pediatric bloodstream infections in both the 1992-1997 NNIS database[200] and in the pediatric component of the 1995-2001 SCOPE survey.[261] However, VRE organisms were detected much less frequently in these pediatric patients; only 11 percent of *E. faecium* and 1 percent of *E. faecalis* bloodstream isolates (of 357 total enterococcal isolates) obtained from pediatric patients in the SCOPE study were vancomycin-resistant.[262] This finding is important because vancomycin-resistant isolates, particularly those of *E. faecium*, also may exhibit high-level resistance to both β-lactam antibiotics and aminoglycosides, thus rendering treatment of these infections extremely challenging.*

Vancomycin resistance among enterococci is phenotypically and genotypically heterogeneous[6,78,167,168] and may or may not be

associated with resistance to other glycopeptides, including teicoplanin. Five major phenotypes of vancomycin resistance (VanA, VanB, VanC, VanD, and VanE) have been characterized. The VanA and VanB phenotypes are most common, and both are transferable. The VanA phenotype is characterized by high-level resistance to vancomycin and teicoplanin, whereas strains with the VanB phenotype exhibit variable levels of resistance to vancomycin but not teicoplanin.[6,78,167,168] The VanC phenotype is limited to *E. gallinarum* and *E. casseliflavus* and is associated with constitutive, low-level, chromosomally mediated (nontransferable) resistance to vancomycin but not teicoplanin and is not transferable.[78,167,168,199] VanD and VanE phenotypes occur uncommonly and are not transferable.

High-level resistance to both vancomycin and teicoplanin (the VanA phenotype) is found primarily in strains of *E. faecium*, whereas most vancomycin-resistant strains of *E. faecalis* express the VanB phenotype and remain susceptible to teicoplanin. Jones and associates and the *Enterococcus* Study Group found that 10 of 11 (91%) vancomycin-resistant strains of *E. faecalis* remained susceptible to teicoplanin (VanB phenotype) whereas 49 of 62 (79%) vancomycin-resistant strains of *E. faecium* were resistant to teicoplanin (VanA phenotype).[110]

The biochemical mechanisms responsible for the major vancomycin-resistant phenotypes are the subject of intense study (reviewed by Murray[168] and Gold[78]). Both VanA and VanB phenotypes are mediated by homologous enzymes that catalyze the formation of an altered, vancomycin-resistant depsipeptide that is incorporated into cell wall peptidoglycan.[6,168,199] The *vanA* and *vanB* gene clusters share functional similarities but are regulated quite differently.[78,168] VanA resistance is transferable by either transposition (e.g., via the transposon Tn1546) or conjugative plasmids. VanB resistance often is encoded by chromosomal DNA but may be transferred by at least two different transposons (Tn1547 and Tn5382).[78,168] Vancomycin induces the production of enzymes encoded by both the *vanA* and *vanB* gene clusters, whereas teicoplanin induces VanA but not VanB enzymes.[78]

The peculiar phenomenon of infection caused by vancomycin-dependent enterococci has been described. Fraimow and colleagues[72] reported a urinary tract infection attributable to a strain of *E. faecalis* that would grow only in the presence of vancomycin, and Green and coworkers[89] reported breakthrough bacteremia with a vancomycin-dependent strain of *E. faecium* occurring during therapy for bacteremia. These organisms are progeny of VanA or VanB enterococci that undergo mutations preventing them from growing in the absence of glycopeptides.

Other Antibiotics

Recently licensed antimicrobials active against most antibiotic-resistant, gram-positive cocci (including VRE organisms) include

---

*See references 18, 74, 91, 113, 132, 159-161, 196, 199, 202, 220, 221.

Edmond et al.[62] (April 1995–April 1998) (Bloodstream Isolates)			Low et al.[138] (SENTRY Antimicrobial Surveillance Program) (1997-1999)	Jones, et al.[111] (SENTRY Antimicrobial Resistance Surveillance (1997-2005)
E. faecalis (*N* = 598) (%)	*E. faecium* (*N* = 303) (%)	Total (*N* = 1354) (%)	Total enterococcal Isolates (*N* = 2303) (%)	*E. faecium* (*N* = 1512) (%)
2.7	81.1	NA	24	89
NA	NA	NA	40	NA
NA	NA	NA	31	32.8
3.2	50.5	17.7	17	69.4

quinupristin-dalfopristin, linezolid, and daptomycin. Enterococcal isolates resistant to each of these new agents already have been identified, although overall resistance rates remain very low in the United States.

Streptogramins are protein synthesis inhibitor antibiotics and are natural combinations of two chemically unrelated molecules (referred to as streptogramin A and B, respectively).[137] Quinupristin-dalfopristin is a streptogramin agent that is active against *E. faecium* (including most strains of VREF) but lacks activity against *E. faecalis* at clinically achievable concentrations.[45] An early study found that more than 95 percent of 875 initial patient isolates of VREF were susceptible to quinupristin-dalfopristin,[65] but both emergence of resistance to this agent[155,207] and superinfection with *E. faecalis* and other organisms[35,260] have been reported during therapy with this drug. Multiple molecular mechanisms, including the expression of modifying enzymes (acetyltransferases), active transport via an efflux pump, and activation of the target site, account for resistance to quinupristin, dalfopristin, or both.[96] In the United States, overall rates of enterococcal resistance to quinupristin-dalfopristin remain low, in the range of 1 to 2 percent in most areas.[96] However, resistance to quinupristin-dalfopristin was observed in 10 percent of *E. faecium* isolates obtained from European patients in one recent survey.[55]

The oxazolidinones are a novel class of synthetic protein synthesis inhibitors that act to inhibit the formation of ribosomal initiation complexes in bacteria.[41] Linezolid, the first oxazolidinone antimicrobial approved for human use, is active against both *E. faecalis* and *E. faecium*, including VRE isolates. Initial studies demonstrated virtually uniform activity of this agent against clinical isolates of enterococci,[16,64,179] with 100 percent of 180 strains (representing multiple resistance profiles) inhibited by linezolid concentrations of 1 to 4 μg/mL in one study.[64] Furthermore, initial in vitro studies suggested that the development of resistance would occur very rarely.[41,112,268] However, resistance to linezolid has been reported in several patients receiving prolonged courses of therapy with this drug[79,144,151,217] and in some patients who have not previously received the agent,[15] and it has been associated with clinical failures.[79] Resistance to linezolid is conferred by single nucleotide changes in varying numbers of copies of the bacterial genes encoding 23S ribosomal RNA.[151] Resistance increases in strains containing multiple copies of these mutations.[144,151] Although some centers have reported increasing rates of linezolid resistance in VRE isolates[151] and nosocomial spread of linezolid-resistant VRE strains,[95] overall rates of linezolid resistance in enterococci remain low. For example, only 0.9 percent of 1512 U.S. bloodstream isolates of *E. faecium* collected from 1997 to 2005 by the SENTRY group were resistant to linezolid.[111]

Daptomycin is a novel cyclic lipopeptide antimicrobial that exhibits rapid, concentration-dependent bactericidal activity against gram-positive pathogens, including methicillin-resistant *S. aureus* (MRSA) and VRE strains.[26,232] Daptomycin has a novel method of action in which binding to bacterial membranes and triggering of rapid depolarization of membrane potential lead to inhibition of protein and nucleic acid synthesis.[1,74] Daptomycin was found to have potent activity against a panel of VRE isolates from the United States and Europe—all 75 VRE isolates tested (55 *E. faecium*, 20 *E. faecalis*) were susceptible to this agent.[206] Daptomycin also was reported to be active against a collection of VRE strains resistant to linezolid or quinupristin-dalfopristin.[3] However, daptomycin resistance has developed during therapy with this agent,[135,163,204] although resistance rates remain very low. The mechanism or mechanisms responsible for daptomycin resistance are not known.

TESTING FOR ANTIMICROBIAL RESISTANCE IN ENTEROCOCCI

All enterococci isolated from cultures of blood, CSF, or other normally sterile sites (with the possible exception of urine) should be tested for resistance to β-lactam antibiotics (ampicillin or penicillin, or both, including a test for β-lactamase production), vancomycin, and high levels of aminoglycosides (streptomycin and gentamicin)[68,193,199] by using the methodology and interpretative guidelines published by the Clinical and Laboratory Standards Institute (CLSI).[42] For multiantibiotic-resistant isolates, testing for susceptibility to alternative agents, including linezolid and daptomycin, should be performed.

Testing of enterococci for ampicillin (or penicillin) resistance must involve determination of the MIC of these agents and a test for β-lactamase production.[42] Jones and colleagues and the *Enterococcus* Study Group compared three techniques that are used commonly to determine the ampicillin MIC of enterococcal isolates—disk diffusion, broth microdilution, and E-test strips—and found excellent agreement among the three methods.[109] Enterococcal isolates with an ampicillin or penicillin MIC of 16 μg/mL or greater are considered resistant to these agents.[42] β-Lactamase-producing enterococci cannot be detected by these methods but are identified routinely by performance of the chromogenic nitrocefin assay.[237]

High-level resistance to gentamicin and streptomycin usually may be detected by either agar dilution (high-level resistance to gentamicin, MIC > 500 μg/mL; high-level resistance to streptomycin, MIC > 2000 μg/mL) or broth microdilution (high-level resistance to gentamicin, MIC > 500 μg/mL; high-level resistance to streptomycin, MIC > 1000 μg/mL).[42,235,237] These isolates also may be identified by disk diffusion with the use of high-content aminoglycoside disks (120-μg gentamicin disk, 300-μg streptomycin disks, ≥10-mm zone = susceptible)[237] or high-range E-test strips.[109,209] However, the recent identification of novel genes encoding gentamicin resistance in both *E. faecalis* and *E. faecium* has raised concern about continued use of the 500-μg/mL cutoff for detection of high-level resistance to gentamicin (reviewed by Chow[34]). These enterococcal isolates are not killed synergistically by combinations of ampicillin/penicillin and gentamicin, even though gentamicin MICs are 256 to 384 μg/mL. If these isolates become more widely prevalent, modification of the standard screening procedures for high-level aminoglycoside resistance may be required.

Commercially available automated antimicrobial susceptibility testing methods may fail to detect vancomycin resistance in enterococci, particularly the VanB phenotype of moderate resistance,[241] although newer versions of these systems appear to be much more reliable.[76,248] Routine disk diffusion testing is more dependable but requires an extended incubation time and the use of transmitted light for examination of zone size to be highly accurate.[236,241] Agar dilution screening using brain-heart infusion agar supplemented with 6 μg/mL vancomycin reliably identifies VRE strains,[42,237,254] as does the standard broth microdilution method.[110,241] E-test glycopeptide strips are a useful alternative to the more cumbersome broth dilution methodology.

THERAPY FOR ENTEROCOCCAL INFECTIONS

Before the emergence of VRE infection as a major nosocomial problem in high-risk patients, the optimal management of serious enterococcal infections (especially endocarditis) was well established. Successful treatment of enterococcal endocarditis required the administration of combination therapy consisting of a cell wall–active agent (usually ampicillin) and an aminoglycoside (gentamicin or streptomycin). Combination therapy also was recommended for other potentially life-threatening enterococcal infections (e.g., sepsis, meningitis) based on the extensive experience with endocarditis. Other enterococcal infections, including urinary tract infections, responded well to monotherapy with a variety of antimicrobials.

In contrast, the optimal therapy for many infections caused by VRE strains remains uncertain. Older agents such as chloramphenicol are no longer used.[177,188,195] Several new agents (quinupristin-dalfopristin, linezolid, daptomycin) have been used for the treatment of VRE infections in adults. However, only one of these antibiotics (linezolid) has been approved for use in children, and enterococci resistant to these new agents already have been detected.[96,150,163] In addition, the prognosis for patients with VRE infections (including bacteremia) often is related more closely to the underlying disease than to the infection, thus complicating the management of these high-risk patients.

TREATMENT OF INFECTIONS CAUSED BY ANTIBIOTIC-SUSCEPTIBLE ENTEROCOCCI

Any discussion of the treatment of serious enterococcal infection must begin with a review of the large experience in the treatment of enterococcal endocarditis. The difficulty of treating enterococcal endocarditis has been apparent since early reports showed that penicillin alone failed to cure as many as two thirds of patients with enterococcal endocarditis but was highly effective in the treatment of streptococcal endocarditis (reviewed by Murray[164]). The early failures of penicillin therapy stimulated studies of the in vitro and in vivo effects of β-lactam antibiotics on enterococci; these studies led to the discovery that enterococci were "tolerant" of the killing effects of cell wall–active agents and provided evidence that bactericidal therapy was required to cure bacterial endocarditis reliably.

For more than half a century, standard therapy for enterococcal endocarditis has included an aminoglycoside plus a cell wall–active agent. Hunter[101] first reported clinical evidence of

synergism between penicillin and streptomycin in the treatment of enterococcal endocarditis in 1947, and this synergism subsequently was confirmed for combinations of penicillin or ampicillin and streptomycin or gentamicin both in vitro and in vivo (reviewed by Murray[164]). Moellering and Weinberg[156] first demonstrated that synergy between β-lactams and aminoglycosides was a consequence of increased aminoglycoside uptake by enterococci exposed to cell wall–active agents. Glycopeptides and aminoglycosides also exhibit in vitro and in vivo synergy against "susceptible" (not expressing high-level resistance) strains of enterococci.[98,151]

The preferred therapy for endocarditis caused by "susceptible" strains of enterococci in both adults[13,151,153,197,257] and children[49,231] consists of combination therapy with parenteral ampicillin (or penicillin G) plus parenteral gentamicin (or streptomycin) for a minimal duration of 4 to 6 weeks. Patients with severe penicillin allergy should be treated with vancomycin plus gentamicin or streptomycin. Selected adult patients with a short duration of symptoms and an uncomplicated course may be treated with 4-week regimens[257,258]; most other patients, including those with mitral-valve involvement, a longer duration of symptoms (especially those with symptoms for >3 months), or prosthetic-valve endocarditis, probably should receive 6-week courses of therapy.[151,257] Interestingly, several reports indicate that the prognosis of enterococcal prosthetic-valve endocarditis is better than that of native-valve disease, perhaps because of the generally shorter duration of symptoms before the diagnosis is made.[151,197] Many patients with prosthetic-valve endocarditis caused by enterococci can be cured without surgery. Rice and colleagues[197] reported a 69 percent cure rate with medical therapy in patients with enterococcal endocarditis involving prosthetic valves.

The general consensus, based on experience with enterococcal endocarditis, is that other life-threatening enterococcal infections, including meningitis and septicemia, should be treated with bactericidal regimens.[152,164,234] The duration of therapy for uncommon enterococcal infections such as meningitis must be individualized, although 2- to 3-week courses of antibiotics have been reported to cure enterococcal meningitis.[234] The optimal treatment of enterococcal bacteremia, particularly that occurring in the nosocomial setting, remains controversial.

The prognosis for these patients varies widely and often is related more closely to the underlying disease than to the enterococcal infection. In adults, single-drug regimens generally are successful in the treatment of enterococcal bacteremia, thus indicating that bactericidal therapy often is not required in all cases.[152,164]

Considerable clinical experience supports the routine use of single-drug therapy for uncomplicated enterococcal urinary tract infection and for soft tissue infection caused by enterococci. Urinary tract infections by susceptible strains of enterococci generally respond promptly to ampicillin, penicillin, nitrofurantoin, or vancomycin.[152,162,164]

TREATMENT OF INFECTIONS CAUSED BY ANTIBIOTIC-RESISTANT ENTEROCOCCI (INCLUDING VANCOMYCIN-RESISTANT ENTEROCOCCI)

Unfortunately, the emergence of enterococci with clinically significant resistance to aminoglycosides, β-lactams, and glycopeptides has complicated the management of endocarditis and other serious infections caused by these organisms to a considerable extent. This discussion focuses on the management of endocarditis caused by drug-resistant enterococci because the need to provide bactericidal therapy has been well established in this setting. The general principles probably apply to the management of other life-threatening enterococcal infections (see earlier).

Endocarditis caused by enterococci with high-level resistance to either streptomycin or gentamicin may be treated by substituting the other aminoglycoside in a combination regimen, but isolation of strains with high-level resistance to both aminoglycosides means that no available aminoglycoside will provide synergistic killing in concert with cell wall–active agents.[151,164] No reliably bactericidal regimen is available for the treatment of endocarditis caused by these strains, even if the isolates remain susceptible to other classes of antimicrobials. Based on animal studies, some experts recommend prolonged treatment (8 to 12 weeks or more) with high-dose intravenous ampicillin given by continuous infusion in this situation (if the isolate is susceptible).[63,153] Surgical excision of infected valves may be required in such patients.[197]

Endocarditis and other serious infections caused by enterococci resistant to β-lactam antibiotics also are increasing in frequency.[87] Endocarditis caused by enterococci (usually *E. faecium*) highly resistant to β-lactams may be treated with vancomycin plus an aminoglycoside (if the strain is susceptible to vancomycin). Endocarditis caused by β-lactamase–producing strains of *E. faecalis* (or rarely, *E. faecium*) would be expected to respond to ampicillin-sulbactam because this combination is highly effective in animal models.[63] Higher-dose or continuous-infusion ampicillin may be effective in the treatment of endocarditis caused by some strains of enterococci that are "resistant" to ampicillin by current guidelines (MIC ≥ 16 µg/mL) because sustained plasma concentrations in excess of 100 µg/mL may be achieved with these regimens.[168] However, even high-dose ampicillin therapy probably will fail to cure endocarditis caused by enterococci with ampicillin MICs greater than 64 µg/mL.[21,78]

Enterococci resistant to vancomycin may remain susceptible to teicoplanin (VanB phenotype). Teicoplanin with or without the addition of an aminoglycoside has been used successfully in the treatment of serious enterococcal infections caused by susceptible isolates,[213] including some cases of endocarditis[190,213] and meningitis.[136] However, teicoplanin is not available in the United States, treatment of endocarditis with this agent has been associated with both treatment failure and relapse,[190,213] and high-level teicoplanin resistance may develop even without exposure to the drug.[92] Endocarditis caused by VanB strains of enterococci should be treated with high-dose ampicillin plus gentamicin or streptomycin if resistance to these agents is not present.

Similarly, endocarditis caused by enterococci highly resistant to both vancomycin and teicoplanin (VanA phenotype) but susceptible to β-lactams should be treated with ampicillin plus an aminoglycoside (if high-level resistance to aminoglycosides is not present). Unfortunately, the VanA phenotype is associated primarily with strains of *E. faecium*, which increasingly are resistant to β-lactams.[71,87,109] Endocarditis caused by enterococci highly resistant to both glycopeptides and β-lactams is especially difficult to treat. Combinations of ampicillin and vancomycin are not bactericidal against these isolates but may[223] or may not[29] provide additive or synergistic inhibition in vitro. If high-level resistance to aminoglycosides is not present, triple-combination therapy with a β-lactam, a glycopeptide, and an aminoglycoside may achieve bactericidal activity; such combinations are reported to be highly effective in animal models of endocarditis caused by ampicillin- and vancomycin-resistant *E. faecium*.[25] For endocarditis caused by enterococci exhibiting high-level resistance to both gentamicin and streptomycin along with resistance to β-lactams and glycopeptides, no proven effective therapies are available.

Newer Options for Treatment of Vancomycin-Resistant Enterococcal Infections

Three new antimicrobials with activity against most VRE strains recently have been licensed: quinupristin-dalfopristin, linezolid, and daptomycin. Of these drugs, only linezolid has been approved for use in children.

The streptogramin antibiotic quinupristin-dalfopristin[137] was approved by the Food and Drug Administration (FDA) in September 1999 for the treatment of adults with infections caused by VREF. This agent is not approved for the treatment of *E. faecalis* infections, nor for pediatric use. Although time-kill curves indicate that quinupristin-dalfopristin is not reliably bactericidal against strains of *E. faecium*,[45] it may provide bactericidal activity against some multiresistant clinical isolates.[141,170,207] Quinupristin-dalfopristin has been reported to effect clinical cures of several serious infections caused by multiresistant *E. faecium*, including ventriculoperitoneal shunt infections in two patients,[170,245] an infected aortic graft in one patient,[210] and VREF peritonitis in a series of adults.[141] Several case series suggest that treatment with quinupristin-dalfopristin reduces the mortality rate associated with VREF bacteremia in adults[131,155,260] and children.[84,133,249] Clinical response to quinupristin-dalfopristin has been reported in approximately 74 to 80 percent of patients with VREF bacteremia.[84,155,249,260] The lack of a consistent bactericidal effect may limit the utility of this agent in the treatment of endocarditis and other life-threatening infections. Therapy with quinupristin-dalfopristin for 10 weeks was reported to cure one patient with VREF endocarditis, although bacteremia persisted until the eighth week of therapy.[75] A second patient with VREF endocarditis failed treatment with 2 weeks of quinupristin-dalfopristin monotherapy but was cured by treatment with a combination of quinupristin-dalfopristin, doxycycline, and rifampin.[145] Other patients with VREF endocarditis have failed to respond to quinupristin-dalfopristin.[8,155]

Quinupristin-dalfopristin therapy generally has been tolerated fairly well in both adults and children, although a high rate of venous phlebitis in recipients has led to a recommendation that the agent be administered through a central venous catheter. Myalgias and arthralgias are other commonly reported side effects of this agent. The potential utility of quinupristin-dalfopristin for the treatment of pediatric patients is limited by its venous toxicity, its lack of a consistent bactericidal effect against VREF, and its lack of clinically useful activity against *E. faecalis*.[45]

Linezolid, the first oxazolidinone antibiotic, was approved by the FDA in April 2000 for the treatment of selected infections caused by antibiotic-resistant, gram-positive bacteria in adults, including those caused by VRE strains (*E. faecium* or *E. faecalis*). In December 2002, the FDA approved this agent for the treatment of pediatric patients with pneumonia, skin and skin structure infections, and VREF infections. Linezolid is available in both parenteral and oral formulations (with comparable bioavailability). Linezolid is active against many antibiotic-resistant, gram-positive pathogens, including MRSA, penicillin-resistant *S. pneumoniae*, and vancomycin-resistant isolates of both *E. faecium* and *E. faecalis*.[16,41,64,179] This agent is bacteriostatic against most susceptible organisms, including the enterococci, but it does exhibit bactericidal activity against some strains of pneumococci. Initial studies demonstrated virtually uniform activity of linezolid against clinical isolates of enterococci.[16,64,179]

Linezolid has been reported to effect both bacteriologic and clinical cure in patients with life-threatening VRE infections, including endocarditis,[8,12,32,233] bacteremia,[32,148,178] and meningitis,[219,264] although clinical experience with this agent in the treatment of endocarditis or meningitis remains limited. Several patients, including those with endocarditis[8] and persistent VREF bacteremia, who responded to linezolid therapy previously had failed therapy with quinupristin-dalfopristin.[148] Linezolid therapy has been reported to cure several patients with VRE endocarditis,[8,12,32,233] including 10 of 22 patients in one study[12] and all of 3 patients who received at least 6 weeks of the drug in another report.[233] These results are encouraging, but enthusiasm for the use of linezolid to treat serious VRE infection must be tempered by its generally bacteriostatic activity and the potential for increasing resistance to this agent. Pediatric experience with linezolid is limited, but the drug was demonstrated to be well tolerated and as effective as vancomycin in the treatment of children with serious gram-positive infections in a large multicenter trial.[114]

Linezolid generally has been tolerated well in both adults and children,[41,73,208] with fewer side effects occurring than with quinupristin-dalfopristin. Adverse effects most frequently reported in patients receiving linezolid have included nausea, diarrhea, and headache in adults and diarrhea and vomiting in children.[73] Reversible myelosuppression has been reported in adults.[73] Longer courses of linezolid therapy have been associated with more serious adverse effects, including optic neuropathy that usually is reversible and peripheral neuropathy that may be irreversible.[102,203]

Daptomycin is a novel cyclic lipopeptide antimicrobial that exhibits rapid, concentration-dependent bactericidal activity against enterococci, including VRE strains.[26,232] It was approved by the FDA in September 2003 for the treatment of adult patients with complicated skin and soft tissue infections caused by gram-positive bacteria, including staphylococci, streptococci, and vancomycin-susceptible strains of *E. faecalis*. Daptomycin is available in an intravenous formulation. It is not approved for use in children, and pediatric experience with the drug is very limited. Daptomycin should not be used for the treatment of pneumonia because it is inactivated by pulmonary surfactant.[227]

The published experience with daptomycin therapy in patients with VRE bloodstream infections is limited. Half (11 of 22) of the patients with VRE bacteremia or endocarditis treated with daptomycin summarized in three recent reports were cured.[126,189,218] Additional studies are under way, and pediatric trials are needed.

Numerous other promising new antibiotics with in vitro activity against VRE isolates recently have been licensed for use in adults (e.g., the glycylcycline antibiotic tigecycline) or are being evaluated in clinical trials. Agents in clinical trials include the lipoglycopeptides oritavancin and telavancin, as well as new members of the oxazolidinone and streptogramin classes of antibiotics.

PREVENTION OF ENTEROCOCCAL INFECTIONS

The explosive increase in nosocomial infections caused by vancomycin-resistant and multiantibiotic-resistant enterococci[61,180] has rendered prevention of enterococcal infections, particularly those caused by VRE strains, a public health priority in the United States.[30,78,168,193,220] In 1995, the Hospital Infection Control Practices Advisory Committee (HICPAC) recommended a series of overlapping strategies designed to prevent the development of serious enterococcal infections.[193] These strategies are aimed at simultaneous interruption of the considerable increase in vancomycin resistance in enterococci and prevention of nosocomial infection with these organisms. Implementation of such strategies has been reported to reduce or eliminate the transmission of VRE organisms in health care facilities.[182] However, overall rates of nosocomial infection by VRE continued to increase in the United States from 1995 to 2004 (*http://www.cdc.gov/ncidod/dhqp/pdf/ar/ICU_RESTrend1995-2004.pdf*), perhaps because the HICPAC guidelines have been followed inconsistently (reviewed by Cetinkaya and colleagues[30]).

REVERSING THE TREND TOWARD VANCOMYCIN AND MULTIPLE-ANTIBIOTIC RESISTANCE IN ENTEROCOCCI

The use of vancomycin[193,212,220] and treatment with broad-spectrum antibiotics, including the third-generation cephalosporins and carbapenems,[61,86,161,166,173,196] are risk factors for

colonization and the development of infection with VRE strains. Consequently, the HICPAC and the CDC have recommended that all hospitals, even those at which VRE organisms have not been isolated, should (1) develop a comprehensive antimicrobial utilization plan, (2) oversee surgical prophylaxis, and (3) develop institution-specific guidelines for the proper use of vancomycin.[193]

Efforts to eliminate unnecessary use of vancomycin are of critical importance[193,220] but may be inadequate unless the use of other classes of antimicrobials is reduced as well (see later). In 1995, the HICPAC provided recommendations regarding the acceptable and appropriate use of vancomycin (Table 95–3), as well as recommendations regarding situations in which vancomycin use should be discouraged[193] (Table 95–4). These recom-

---

TABLE 95–3   Situations in Which Vancomycin Use Is Appropriate or Acceptable

Treatment

Treatment of serious infections caused by β-lactam–resistant, gram-positive microorganisms

Treatment of gram-positive infections in patients with serious allergies to β-lactams

Treatment of antibiotic-associated colitis only when it fails to respond to metronidazole or is severe and potentially life-threatening

Prophylaxis

Endocarditis prophylaxis after certain procedures in high-risk patients according to the American Heart Association guidelines

Prophylaxis for major surgical procedures involving implantation of prosthetic materials or devices (single-dose prophylaxis usually is adequate)

Modified from Recommendations for preventing the spread of vancomycin resistance: Recommendations of the Hospital Infection Control Practices Advisory Committee (HICPAC). M. M. W. R. Recomm. Rep. 44(RR-12):1-13, 1995.

TABLE 95–4   Situations in Which Vancomycin Use Should Be Discouraged

Treatment

Empiric therapy for febrile neutropenic patients (unless there is presumptive evidence of an infection caused by gram-positive organisms, such as a Hickman catheter exit-site infection, and the local prevalence of methicillin-resistant *Staphylococcus aureus* strains is substantial)

Treatment of an isolated, single blood culture positive for coagulase-negative *Staphylococcus*

Treatment (chosen for dosing convenience) of infections caused by β-lactam–susceptible, gram-positive microorganisms in patients with renal failure

Continued empiric use of presumed infection in patients whose cultures are negative for β-lactam–resistant gram-positive microorganisms

Primary treatment of antibiotic-associated diarrhea

Eradication of methicillin-resistant *S. aureus* colonization

Prophylaxis

Routine surgical prophylaxis except in patients with life-threatening allergy to β-lactams

Systemic or local prophylaxis for infection of indwelling intravascular catheters

Routine prophylaxis for very-low-birth-weight infants

Routine prophylaxis for dialysis patients

Use of vancomycin solution for topical application or irrigation

Selective decontamination of the gastrointestinal tract

Modified from Recommendations for preventing the spread of vancomycin resistance: Recommendations of the Hospital Infection Control Practices Advisory Committee (HICPAC). M. M. W. R. Recomm. Rep. 44(RR-12):1-13, 1995.

mendations remain useful, but the recent emergence of community-acquired MRSA infections[94,100,115] has resulted in increased empiric and definitive use of vancomycin for a HICPAC-approved indication: "treatment of serious infections caused by β-lactam–resistant, gram-positive microorganisms."[193]

In addition, efforts should be undertaken to reduce the unnecessary use of broad-spectrum antibiotics and certain agents with potent anti-anaerobic activity, particularly in settings with high rates of nosocomial infection (such as ICUs). These efforts are necessary because many studies indicate that nonglycopeptide antibiotics also exert selective pressure for VRE strains and that limitation of the use of vancomycin alone has only a modest effect on reducing VRE colonization and infection (reviewed by Rice[196]). Exposure to agents with broad-spectrum activity (but lacking anti-enterococcal activity), such as the extended-spectrum cephalosporins, appears to predispose to colonization with VRE organisms,[59,196] whereas exposure to antimicrobials with potent anti-anaerobic activity (even if they are also active against enterococci) may promote high-density, prolonged VRE colonization (by eliminating gut anaerobes that may interfere with colonization by VRE strains).[58,191,196]

PREVENTING AND CONTROLLING THE SPREAD OF NOSOCOMIAL INFECTION BY VANCOMYCIN-RESISTANT ENTEROCOCCI

The increasing prevalence of *Enterococcus* in nosocomial infections is related to the intrinsic and acquired antimicrobial resistance of these organisms, but the factors leading to increased antibiotic resistance in enterococci are not identical to those that predispose to enterococcal colonization or infection, or both. Enterococcal infections are concentrated increasingly in debilitated and immunocompromised patients, including those with malignancies, recipients of bone marrow and solid organ transplants, burn victims, premature neonates, and critically ill patients with indwelling intravascular catheters. Consequently, special attention should be paid to potential outbreaks of VRE infection in hospital wards caring for these high-risk patients.[30]

Efforts to prevent the spread of VRE colonization or infection (or both) probably will be more successful if the VRE isolates are confined to a few patients in a single area of the hospital. Widespread colonization with VRE strains may precede identification of infections by these organisms. Therefore, all hospitals should implement active VRE surveillance and formulate a multidisciplinary plan to prevent nosocomial spread of VRE strains if such organisms are identified. In hospitals that have not isolated VRE strains, periodic antimicrobial susceptibility testing should be performed on enterococcal isolates from all sources, particularly from high-risk patient populations such as those in intensive care or transplant units. If VRE organisms are identified, a comprehensive plan to prevent nosocomial spread of these bacteria should be instituted immediately. The HICPAC guidelines summarized the essential elements of such a plan.[193] Hospital infection control staff and clinical staff must be notified promptly when VRE strains are isolated from a clinical sample, and isolation precautions should be implemented immediately to prevent patient-to-patient transmission of VRE organisms. These precautions include gown and glove isolation, vigorous handwashing, dedicated use of noncritical patient items such as thermometers and stethoscopes, and prompt surveillance of any possibly exposed patients for VRE colonization. Additional measures may be necessary in hospitals with endemic or continued VRE transmission despite implementation of the aforementioned measures.[193] Ostrowsky and colleagues[182] reported that an active infection control program that included surveillance cultures and prompt isolation of infected patients successfully reduced the spread of VRE strains in health care facilities throughout the Sioux land region of Iowa, Nebraska, and South Dakota.

Once VRE organisms become endemic in a hospital unit, achieving complete eradication is very difficult. The duration of VRE colonization in individual patients may be weeks or months,[30,159] although spontaneous resolution of colonization occurs frequently.[30,158] Attempts to eradicate colonization in individual patients generally have been unsuccessful.[30,158] Consequently, the measures recommended by HICPAC and others are directed at preventing the initial establishment of VRE strains in hospitals. Implementation of these policies will require the involvement of hospital pharmacy and therapeutics committees, quality assurance programs, and medical staff. Ongoing monitoring of the efficacy of these programs will be required.

REFERENCES

1. Alborn, W. E., Jr., Allen, N. E., and Preston, D. A.: Daptomycin disrupts membrane potential in growing *Staphylococcus aureus*. Antimicrob. Agents Chemother. 35:2282-2287, 1991.
2. Alminrante, B., Tornos, M., Gurgui, M., et al.: Prognosis of enterococcal endocarditis. Rev. Infect. Dis. 13:1248-1249, 1991.
3. Anastasiou, D. M., Thorne, G. M., Luperchio, S. A., and Alder, J. D.: In vitro activity of daptomycin against clinical isolates with reduced susceptibilities to linezolid and quinupristin-dalfopristin. Int. J. Antimicrob. Agents 28:385-388, 2006.
4. Andrewes, F. W., and Horder, T. J.: A study of the streptococci pathogenic for man. Lancet 2:708-713, 1906.
5. Armstrong, D., Neu, H., Peterson, L. R., et al.: The prospects of treatment failure in the chemotherapy of infectious diseases in the 1990s. Microb. Drug Resist. 1:1-4, 1995.
6. Arthur, M., and Courvalin, P.: Genetics and mechanisms of glycopeptide resistance in enterococci. Antimicrob. Agents Chemother. 37:1563-1571, 1993.
7. Ashkenazi, S., Even-Tov, S., Samra, Z., et al.: Uropathogens of various childhood populations and their antibiotic susceptibility. Pediatr. Infect. Dis. J. 10:742-746, 1991.
8. Babcock, H. M., Ritchie, D. J., Christiansen, E., et al.: Successful treatment of vancomycin-resistant *Enterococcus* endocarditis with oral linezolid. Clin. Infect. Dis. 32:1373-1375, 2001.
9. Bhavnani, S. M., Drake, J. A., Forrest, A., et al.: A nationwide, multicenter, case-control study comparing risk factors, treatment, and outcome for vancomycin-resistant and -susceptible enterococcal bacteremia. Diagn. Microbiol. Infect. Dis. 36:145-158, 2000.
10. Bingen, E. H., Denamur, E., and Lambert-Zechovsky, N. Y.: Evidence for the genetic unrelatedness of nosocomial vancomycin-resistant *Enterococcus faecium* strains in a pediatric hospital. J. Clin. Microbiol. 29:1888, 1991.
11. Bingen, E., Lambert-Zechousky, N., Mariane-Kurkdjian, P., et al.: Bacteremia caused by a vancomycin-resistant enterococcus. Pediatr. Infect. Dis. J. 8:475-476, 1989.
12. Birmingham, M. C., Rayner, C. R., Meagher, A. K., et al.: Linezolid for the treatment of multidrug-resistant, Gram-positive infections: Experience from a compassionate use program. Clin. Infect. Dis. 36:159-168, 2003.
13. Bisno, A. L., Dismukes, W. E., Durack, D. T., et al.: Antimicrobial treatment of infective endocarditis due to viridans streptococci, enterococci, and staphylococci. J. A. M. A. 261:1471-1477, 1989.
14. Bonadio, W. A.: Group D streptococcal bacteremia in children: Clin. Pediatr. (Phila.) 32:20-24, 1993.
15. Bonora, M. G., Ligozzi, M., Luzzani, A., et al.: Emergence of linezolid resistance in *Enterococcus faecium* not dependent on linezolid treatment. Eur. J. Clin. Microbiol. Infect. Dis. 25:197-198, 2006.
16. Bostic, G. D., Perri, M. B., Thal, L. A., et al.: Comparative in vitro and bactericidal activity of oxazolidinone antibiotics against multidrug-resistant enterococci. Diagn. Microbiol. Infect. Dis. 30:109-112, 1998.
17. Boulanger, J. M., Ford-Jones, E. L., and Matlow, A. G.: Enterococcal bacteremia in a pediatric institution: A four year review. Rev. Infect. Dis. 13:847, 1991.
18. Boyce, J. M., Opal, S. M., and Chow, J. W.: Outbreak of multi-drug resistant *Enterococcus faecium* with transferable vanB class vancomycin resistance. J. Clin. Microbiol. 32:1148-1153, 1994.
19. Boyce, J. M., Opal, S. M., Potter-Bynoe, G., et al.: Emergence and nosocomial transmission of ampicillin-resistant enterococci. Antimicrob. Agents Chemother. 36:1032-1039, 1992.
20. Brown, A. E., de Lancastre, H., Henning, K., et al.: Epidemic nosocomial vancomycin-resistant *Enterococcus faecium* (VREF) on a pediatric oncology unit. Presented at the 33rd Annual Meeting of the Infectious Diseases Society of America, San Francisco, 1995.
21. Bush, L., Calman, J., Cherney, C. L., et al.: High-level penicillin resistance among isolates of enterococci: Implications for treatment of enterococcal infections. Ann. Intern. Med. 110:515-520, 1989.

22. Butler, K. M.: Enterococcal infection in children. Semin. Pediatr. Infect. Dis. *17*:128-139, 2006.
23. Calderwood, S. A., Wennersten, C., and Moellering, R. C., Jr.: Resistance to six aminoglycosidic aminocyclitol antibiotics among enterococci: Prevalence, evolution, and relationship to synergism with penicillin. Antimicrob. Agents Chemother. *12*:401-405, 1977.
24. Carniol, K., and Gilmore, M. S.: Signal transduction, quorum-sensing, and extracellular protease activity in *Enterococcus faecalis* biofilm formation. J. Bacteriol. *186*:8161-8163, 2004.
25. Caron, F., Pestel, M., Kitzis, M. D., et al.: Comparison of different β-lactam–glycopeptide-gentamicin combinations for and experimental endocarditis caused by highly β-lactam–resistant and highly glycopeptide-resistant isolate of *Enterococcus faecium*. J. Infect. Dis. *171*:106-112, 1995.
26. Carpenter, C. F., and Chambers, H. F.: Daptomycin: Another novel agent for treating infections due to drug-resistant gram-positive pathogens. Clin. Infect. Dis. *38*:994-1000, 2004.
27. Centers for Disease Control and Prevention (CDC): *Staphylococcus aureus* resistant to vancomycin—United States, 2002. M. M. W. R. Morbid. Mortal. Weekly Rep. *51*(26):565-567, 2002.
28. Centers for Disease Control and Prevention (CDC): Brief report: Vancomycin-resistant *Staphylococcus aureus*—New York, 2004. M. M. W. R. Morbid. Mortal. Weekly Rep. *53*(15):322-333, 2004.
29. Cercenado, E., Eliopoulos, G. M., Wennersten, C. B., et al.: Absence of synergistic activity between ampicillin and vancomycin against highly vancomycin-resistant enterococci. Antimicrob. Agents Chemother. *36*:2201-2203, 1992.
30. Cetinkaya, Y., Falk, P., and Mayhall, C. G.: Vancomycin-resistant enterococci. Clin. Microbiol. Rev. *13*:686-707, 2000.
31. Chenoweth, C. E., Robinson, K. A., and Schaberg, D. R.: Efficacy of ampicillin versus trimethoprim-sulfamethoxazole in a mouse model of lethal enterococcal peritonitis. Antimicrob. Agents Chemother. *34*:1800-1802, 1990.
32. Chien, J. W., Kucia, M. L., and Salata, R. A.: Use of linezolid, an oxazolidinone, in the treatment of multidrug-resistant gram-positive bacterial infections. Clin. Infect. Dis. *30*:146-151, 2000.
33. Chirurgi, V. A., Oster, S. E., Goldberg, A. A., et al.: Ampicillin-resistant *Enterococcus raffinosus* in an acute-care hospital: Case-control study and antimicrobial susceptibilities. J. Clin. Microbiol. *29*:2663-2665, 1991.
34. Chow, J. W.: Aminoglycoside resistance in enterococci. Clin. Infect. Dis. *31*:586-589, 2000.
35. Chow, J. W., Davidson, A., Sanford, E., 3rd, et al.: Superinfection with *Enterococcus faecalis* during quinupristin/dalfopristin therapy. Clin. Infect. Dis. *24*:91-92, 1997.
36. Chow, J. W., Thal, L. A., Perri, M. B., et al.: Plasmid-associated hemolysin and aggregation substance production contributes to virulence in experimental enterococcal endocarditis. Antimicrob. Agents Chemother. *37*:2474-2477, 1993.
37. Chow, J. W., Zervos, M. J., Lerner, S. A., et al.: A novel gentamicin resistance gene in *Enterococcus*. Antimicrob. Agents Chemother. *41*:511-514, 1997.
38. Christenson, J. C., Korgenski, E. K., Jenkins, E., et al.: Detection of vancomycin-resistant enterococci colonization in a children's hospital. Am. J. Infect. Control *26*:569-571, 1998.
39. Christie, C., Hammond, J., Reising, S., et al.: Clinical and molecular epidemiology of enterococcal bacteremia in a pediatric teaching hospital. J. Pediatr. *125*:392-399, 1994.
40. Clark, N. C., Cooksey, R. C., Hill, B. C., et al.: Characterization of glycopeptide-resistant enterococci from U.S. hospitals. Antimicrob. Agents Chemother. *37*:2311-2317, 1993.
41. Clemett, D., and Markham, A.: Linezolid. Drugs *59*:815-827, 2000.
42. Clinical and Laboratory Standards Institute: Performance Standards for Antimicrobial Susceptibility Testing: Sixteenth Informational Supplement. CLSI document M100-S16, No. 3, Vol. 26. Wayne, PA, CLSI, 2006, pp. 96, 124-127.
43. Coburn, P. S., Pillar, C. M., Jett, B. D., et al.: *Enterococcus faecalis* senses target cells and in response expresses cytolysin. Science *306*:2270-2272, 2004.
44. Cohen, M.: Epidemiology of drug resistance: Implications for a post-antibiotic era. Science *257*:1050-1055, 1992.
45. Collins, L. A., Malanoski, G. J., Eliopoulos, G. M., et al.: In vitro activity of RP59500, an injectable streptogramin antibiotic, against vancomycin-resistant gram-positive organisms. Antimicrob. Agents Chemother. *37*:598-601, 1993.
46. Coudron, P. E., Markowitz, S. M., and Wong, E. S.: Isolation of a beta-lactamase–producing, aminoglycoside-resistant strain of *Enterococcus faecium*. Antimicrob. Agents Chemother. *36*:1125-1126, 1992.
47. Coudron, P. E., Mayhall, C. G., and Facklam, R. R.: *Streptococcus faecium* outbreak in a neonatal intensive care unit. J. Clin. Microbiol. *20*:1044, 1984.
48. Cox, C. R., Coburn, P. S., and Gilmore, M. S.: Enterococcal cytolysin: A novel two component peptide system that serves as a bacterial defense against eukaryotic and prokaryotic cells. Curr. Protein Pept. Sci. *6*:77-84, 2005.
49. Dajani, A. S.: Infective endocarditis. *In* Kaplan, S. L. (ed.): Current Therapy in Pediatric Infectious Diseases. 3rd ed. St. Louis, Mosby–Year Book, 1993, pp. 129-133.
50. Daly, J. A., Clifton, N. L., and Seskin, K. C.: Use of rapid, nonradioactive DNA probes in culture confirmation tests to detect *Streptococcus agalactiae*, *Haemophilus influenzae*, and *Enterococcus* spp. from pediatric patients with significant infections. J. Clin. Microbiol. *29*:80, 1991.
51. Das, I., and Gray, J.: Enterococcal bacteremia in children: A review of seventy-five episodes in a pediatric hospital. Pediatr. Infect. Dis. J. *17*:1154-1158, 1998.
52. Davies, H., Jones, E., Sheng, R., et al.: Nosocomial urinary tract infections at a pediatric hospital. Pediatr. Infect. Dis. J. *11*:349-354, 1992.
53. DiazGranados, C. A., and Jernigan, J. A.: Impact of vancomycin resistance on mortality among patients with neutropenia and enterococcal bloodstream infection. J. Infect. Dis. *191*:588-595, 2005.
54. DiazGranados, C. A., Zimmer, S. M., Klein, M., and Jernigan, J. A.: Comparison of mortality associated with vancomycin-resistant and vancomycin-susceptible enterococcal bloodstream infections: A meta-analysis. Clin. Infect. Dis. *41*:327-333, 2005.
55. Deshpande L. M., Fritsche, T. R., Moet, G. J., et al.: Antimicrobial resistance and molecular epidemiology of vancomycin-resistant enterococci from North America and Europe: A report from the SENTRY antimicrobial surveillance program. Diagn. Microbiol. Infect. Dis. *58*:163-170, 2007.
56. Dobson, S. R. M., and Baker, C. J.: Enterococcal sepsis in neonates: Features by age of onset and occurrence of focal infection. Pediatrics *85*:165, 1990.
57. Donabedian, S., Chow, J. W., Shales, D. M., et al.: DNA hybridization and contour-clamped homogeneous electric field electrophoresis for identification of enterococci to the species level. J. Clin. Microbiol. *33*:141-145, 1995.
58. Donskey, C. J., Chowdhry, T. K., Hecker, M. T., et al.: Effect of antibiotic therapy on the density of vancomycin-resistant enterococci in the stool of colonized patients. N. Engl. J. Med. *343*:1925-1932, 2000.
59. Donskey, C. J., Hanrahan, J. A., Hutton, R. A., et al.: Effect of parenteral antibiotic administration on the establishment of colonization with vancomycin-resistant *Enterococcus faecium* in the mouse gastrointestinal tract. J. Infect. Dis. *181*:1830-1833, 2000.
60. Dutka-Malen, S., Evers, S., and Courvalin, P.: Detection of glycopeptide resistance genotypes and identification to the species level of clinically relevant enterococci by PCR. J. Clin. Microbiol. *33*:24-27, 1995.
61. Edmond, M. B., Ober, J. F., Weinbaum, D. L., et al.: Vancomycin-resistant *Enterococcus faecium* bacteremia: Risk factors for infection. Clin. Infect. Dis. *20*:1126-1133, 1995.
62. Edmond, M. B., Wallace, S. E., McClish, D. K., et al.: Nosocomial bloodstream infections in United States hospitals: A three-year analysis. Clin. Infect. Dis. *29*:239-244, 1999.
63. Eliopoulos, G. M., Thauvin-Eliopoulos, C., and Moellering, R. C., Jr.: Contribution of animal models in the search for effective therapy for endocarditis due to enterococci with high-level resistance to gentamicin. Clin. Infect. Dis. *15*:58-62, 1992.
64. Eliopoulos, G. M., Wennersten, C. B., Gold, H. S., et al.: In vitro activities in new oxazolidinone antimicrobial agents against enterococci. Antimicrob. Agents Chemother. *40*:1745-1747, 1996.
65. Eliopoulos, G. M., Wennersten, C. B., Gold, H. S., et al.: Characterization of vancomycin-resistant *Enterococcus faecium* isolates from the United States and their susceptibility in vitro to dalfopristin-quinupristin. Antimicrob. Agents Chemother. *42*:1088-1092, 1998.
66. Facklam, R. R., and Collins, M. D.: Identification of *Enterococcus* species isolated from human infections by a conventional test scheme. J. Clin. Microbiol. *27*:731-734, 1989.
67. Facklam, R., Pigott, N., Franklin, R., et al.: Evaluation of three disk tests for identification of enterococci, leuconostocs, and pediococci. J. Clin. Microbiol. *33*:885-887, 1995.
68. Facklam, R. R., and Sahm, D. R.: *Enterococcus. In* Murray, P. R., Baron, E. J., Pfaller, M. A., et al. (eds.): Manual of Clinical Microbiology. 6th ed. Washington, D.C., American Society for Microbiology, 1995, pp. 308-314.
69. Fasola, E. L., Moody, J. A., Shanholtzer, C. J., et al.: Bactericidal action of gentamicin against enterococci that are sensitive, or exhibit low- or high-level resistance to gentamicin. Diagn. Microbiol. Infect. Dis. *19*:57-60, 1994.
70. Felmingham, D., Wilson, A. P., Quintant, A. L., et al.: *Enterococcus* species in urinary tract infection. Clin. Infect. Dis. *15*:295-301, 1992.
71. Fontana, R., Amalfitano, G., Rossi, L., et al.: Mechanisms of resistance to growth inhibition and killing by β-lactam antibiotics in enterococci. Clin. Infect. Dis. *15*:486-489, 1992.
72. Fraimow, H. S., Jungkind, D. L., Lander, D. W., et al.: Urinary tract infection with an *Enterococcus faecalis* isolate that requires vancomycin for growth. Ann. Intern. Med. *121*:22-26, 1994.
73. French, G.: Safety and tolerability of linezolid. J. Antimicrob. Chemother. *51*(Suppl. S2):ii45-ii53.
74. Fuchs, P. C., Barry, A. L., and Brown, S. D.: In vitro bactericidal activity of daptomycin against staphylococci. J. Antimicrob. Chemother. *49*:467-470, 2002.
75. Furlong, W. B., and Rakowski, T. A.: Therapy with RP 59500 (quinupristin/dalfopristin) for prosthetic valve endocarditis due to enterococci with VanA/VanB resistance patterns. Clin. Infect. Dis. *25*:163-164, 1997.
76. Garcia-Garrote, F., Cercenado, E., and Bouza, E.: Evaluation of a new system, VITEK 2, for identification and antimicrobial susceptibility testing of enterococci. J. Clin. Microbiol. *38*:2108-2111, 2000.
77. Gladstone, I. J., Ehrenkranz, R. A., Edberg, S. C., et al.: A ten-year review of neonatal sepsis and comparison with the previous fifty-year experience. Pediatr. Infect. Dis. J. *9*:819-825, 1990.
78. Gold, H.: Vancomycin-resistant enterococci: Mechanisms and clinical observations. Clin. Infect. Dis. *33*:210-219, 2001.

79. Gonzales, R. D., Schreckenberger, P. C., Graham, M. B., et al.: Infections due to vancomycin-resistant *Enterococcus faecium* resistant to linezolid. Lancet *357*:1179, 2001.

80. Goodhard, G. L.: In vivo vs. in vitro susceptibility of *Enterococcus* to trimethoprim-sulfamethoxazole. J. A. M. A. *252*:2748-2749, 1984.

81. Gorbach, S. L.: Intraabdominal infections. Clin. Infect. Dis. *17*:961-967, 1993.

82. Gordon, S., Swenson, J. M., Hill, B. C., et al.: Antimicrobial susceptibility patterns of common and unusual species of enterococci causing infections in the United States: Enterococcal Study Group. J. Clin. Microbiol. *30*:2373-2378, 1992.

83. Graninger, W., and Ragette, R.: Nosocomial bacteremia due to *Enterococcus faecalis* without endocarditis. Clin. Infect. Dis. *15*:49-57, 1992.

84. Gray, J. W., Darbyshire, P. J., Beath, S. V., et al.: Experience with quinupristin/dalfopristin in treating infections with vancomycin-resistant *Enterococcus faecium* in children. Pediatr. Infect. Dis. J. *19*:234-238, 2000.

85. Gray, J. W., and George, R. H.: Experience of vancomycin-resistant enterococci in a children's hospital. J. Hosp. Infect. *45*:11-18, 2000.

86. Gray, J. W., Pedler, S., Kernahan, J., et al.: Enterococcal superinfection in paediatric oncology patients treated with imipenem. Lancet *13*:1487-1488, 1992.

87. Grayson, M. L., Eliopoulos, G. M., Wennersten, C. B., et al.: Increasing resistance to beta-lactam antibiotics among clinical isolates of *Enterococcus faecium*: A 22-year review at one institution. Antimicrob. Agents Chemother. *35*:2180-2184, 1991.

88. Grayson, M. L., Thauvin-Eliopoulos, C., Eliopoulos, G. M., et al.: Failure of trimethoprim-sulfamethoxazole therapy in experimental enterococcal endocarditis. Antimicrob. Agents Chemother. *34*:1792-1794, 1990.

89. Green, M., Shlaes, J. H., Barbadora, K., et al.: Bacteremia due to vancomycin-dependent *Enterococcus faecium*. Clin. Infect. Dis. *20*:712-714, 1995.

90. Gullberg, R. M., Homann, S. R., and Phair, J. P.: Enterococcal bacteremia: Analysis of 75 episodes. Rev. Infect. Dis. *11*:74-85, 1989.

91. Handwerger, S., Raucher, B., Altarac, D., et al.: Nosocomial outbreak due to *Enterococcus faecium* highly resistant to vancomycin, penicillin and gentamicin. Clin. Infect. Dis. *16*:750-755, 1993.

92. Hayden, M. K., Trenholme, G. M., Schultz, J. E., et al.: In vivo development of teicoplanin resistance in a VanB *Enterococcus faecium* isolate. J. Infect. Dis. *167*:1224-1227, 1993.

93. Henning, K. J., Delencastre, H., Eagan, J., et al.: Vancomycin-resistant *Enterococcus faecium* on a pediatric oncology ward: Duration of stool shedding and incidence of clinical infection. Pediatr. Infect. Dis. J. *15*:848-854, 1996.

94. Herold, B. C., Immergluck, L. C., Maranan, M. C., et al.: Community-acquired methicillin-resistant *Staphylococcus aureus* in children with no predisposing factors. J. A. M. A. *279*:593-598, 1998.

95. Herrero, I. A., Issa, N. C., and Patel, R.: Nosocomial spread of linezolid-resistant vancomycin-resistant *Enterococcus faecium*. N. Engl. J. Med. *346*:867-869, 2002.

96. Hershberger, E., Donabedian, S., Konstantinou, K., and Zervos, M. J.: Quinupristin-dalfopristin resistance in gram-positive bacteria: Mechanism of resistance and epidemiology. Clin. Infect. Dis. *38*:92-98, 2004.

97. Hoge, C. W., Adams, J., Buchanan, B., et al.: Enterococcal bacteremia: To treat or not to treat, a reappraisal. Rev. Infect. Dis. *13*:600-605, 1991.

98. Hook, E. W. I., Roberts, R. B., and Sande, M. A.: Antimicrobial therapy of experimental endocarditis. Antimicrob. Agents Chemother. *8*:564-570, 1975.

99. Horodniceanu, T., Bougueleret, T., El-Solh, N., et al.: High-level, plasmid-borne resistance to gentamicin in *Streptococcus faecalis* subsp. *zymogenes*. Antimicrob. Agents Chemother. *16*:686-689, 1979.

100. Hunt, C., Dionne, M., Delorme, M., et al.: Four pediatric deaths from community-acquired methicillin-resistant *Staphylococcus aureus*: Minnesota and North Dakota, 1997-1999. M. M. W. R. Morb. Mortal. Wkly. Rep. *48*:707-710, 1999.

101. Hunter, T. H.: Use of streptomycin in treatment of bacterial endocarditis. Am. J. Med. *2*:436-442, 1947.

102. Javaheri, M., Khurana, R. N., O'Hearn, T. M., et al.: Linezolid-induced optic neuropathy: A mitochondrial disorder? Br. J. Ophthalmol. *91*:111-115, 2007.

103. Jarvis, W. R., and Martone, W. J.: Predominant pathogens in hospital infections. J. Antimicrob. Chemother. *29*(Suppl. A):19-24, 1992.

104. Jett, B. D., Huycke, M. M., and Gilmore, M. S.: Virulence of enterococci. Clin. Microbiol. Rev. *7*:462-478, 1994.

105. Johnson, A. P.: The pathogenicity of enterococci. J. Antimicrob. Chemother. *33*:1083-1089, 1994.

106. Johnson, D. H., Rosenthal, A., and Nadas, A. S.: Bacterial endocarditis in children under 2 years of age. Am. J. Dis. Child. *129*:183-186, 1975.

107. Johnson, D. H., Rosenthal, A., and Nadas, A. S.: A forty-year review of bacterial endocarditis in infants and children. Circulation *51*:581-588, 1975.

108. Jones, M. E., Draghi, D. C., Thornsberry, C., et al.: Emerging resistance among bacterial pathogens in the intensive care unit—a European and North American Surveillance study (2000-2002). Ann. Clin. Microbiol. Antimicrob. *3*:1-11, 2004.

109. Jones, R. N., Erwin, M. E., and Anderson, S. C.: Emerging multiply resistant enterococci among clinical isolates. II. Validation of the e-test to recognize glycopeptide-resistant strains. Diagn. Microbiol. Infect. Dis. *21*:95-100, 1995.

110. Jones, R. N., Sader, H. S., Erwin, M. E., and Anderson, S. C.: Emerging multiply resistant enterococci among clinical isolates. I. Prevalence data from

111. Jones, R. N., Turnidge, J., Sader, H. S., et al.: Evolutionary trends in antimicrobial resistance in *E. faecium* bacteremia: Report from the SENTRY Antimicrobial Surveillance Program (1997-2005). Abstract C2-208. Presented at the 46th Interscience Conference on Antimicrobial Agents and Chemotherapy, San Francisco, September 27-30, 2006.

112. Kaatz, G. W., and Seo, S. M.: In vitro activities of oxazolidinone compounds U100592 and U100766 against *Staphylococcus aureus* and *Staphylococcus epidermidis*. Antimicrob. Agents Chemother. *40*:799-801, 1996.

113. Kaplan, A. H., Gilligan, P. H., and Facklam, R. R.: Recovery of resistant enterococci during vancomycin prophylaxis. J. Clin. Microbiol. *26*:1216-1218, 1988.

114. Kaplan, S. L., Deville, J. G., Yogev, R., et al. for the Linezolid Pediatric Study Group: Linezolid versus vancomycin for treatment of resistant gram-positive infections in children. Pediatr. Infect. Dis. J. *22*:677-685, 2003.

115. Kaplan, S. L., Hulten, K. G., Gonzalez, B. E., et al.: Three-year surveillance of community-acquired *Staphylococcus aureus* infections in children. Clin. Infect. Dis. *40*:1785-1791, 2005.

116. Kapur, D., Dorsky, D., Feingold, J. M., et al.: Incidence and outcome of vancomycin-resistant enterococcal bacteremia following autologous peripheral blood stem cell transplantation. Bone Marrow Transplant. *25*:147-152, 2000.

117. Karanfil, L. V., Murphy, M., and Josephson, A.: A cluster of vancomycin-resistant *Enterococcus faecium* in an intensive care unit. Infect. Control Hosp. Epidemiol. *13*:195-200, 1993.

118. Kaufhold, A., and Ferrieri, P.: The microbiologic aspects, including diagnosis, of beta-hemolytic streptococcal and enterococcal infections. Infect. Dis. Clin. North Am. *7*:235-256, 1993.

119. Kirkpatrick, B. D., Harrington, S. M., Smith, D., et al.: An outbreak of vancomycin-dependent *Enterococcus faecium* in a bone marrow transplant unit. Clin. Infect. Dis. *29*:1268-1273, 1999.

120. Kirst, H. A., Thompson, D. G., and Nicas, T. I.: Historical yearly usage of vancomycin. Antimicrob. Agents Chemother. *42*:1303-1304, 1998.

121. Klein, J. O., and Marcy, S. M.: Bacterial sepsis and meningitis. In Remington, J. S., and Klein, J. O. (eds.): Infectious Diseases of the Fetus and Newborn Infant. 4th ed. Philadelphia, W. B. Saunders, 1995, pp. 835-890.

122. Koorevaar, C. T., Scherpenzeel, P. G., Neijens, H. J., et al.: Childhood meningitis caused by enterococci and viridans streptococci. Infection *20*:118-121, 1992.

123. Kreft, B., Marre, R., Schramm, U., et al.: Aggregation substance of *Enterococcus faecalis* mediates adhesion to cultured renal tubular cells. Infect. Immun. *60*:25-30, 1992.

124. Krieger, J. N., Kaiser, D. L., and Wenzel, R. P.: Urinary tract etiology of bloodstream infections in hospitalized patients. J. Infect. Dis. *146*:719-723, 1983.

125. Kunin, C.: Resistance to antimicrobial drugs: A worldwide calamity. Ann. Intern. Med. *118*:557-561, 1993.

126. Kvirikadze, N., Suseno, N., Vescio, T., et al.: Daptomycin for the treatment of vancomycin-resistant *Enterococcus faecium* bacteremia. Scand. J. Infect. Dis. *38*:290-292, 2006.

127. Law, E. J., Blecher, K., and Still, J. M.: Enterococcal infections as a cause of mortality and morbidity in patients with burns. J. Burn. Care Rehabil. *15*:236-239, 1994.

128. LeClercq, R., Derlot, E., Duval, J., et al.: Plasmid-mediated resistance to vancomycin and teicoplanin in *Enterococcus faecium*. N. Engl. J. Med. *319*:157-161, 1988.

129. LeClercq, R., Dutka-Malen, S., Brisson-Noel, A., et al.: Resistance of enterococci to aminoglycosides and glycopeptides. Clin. Infect. Dis. *15*:495-501, 1992.

130. LeClercq, R., Dutka-Malen, S., Brisson-Noel, A., et al.: Resistance of enterococci to aminoglycosides and glycopeptides. Letter. Clin. Infect. Dis. *16*:331, 1993.

131. Linden, P. K., Pasculle, A. W., McDevitt, D., et al.: Effect of quinupristin/dalfopristin on the outcome of vancomycin-resistant *Enterococcus faecium* bacteraemia: Comparison with a control cohort. J. Antimicrob. Chemother. *39*:145-151, 1997.

132. Livornese, L. L., Jr., Dias, S., Samel, C., et al.: Hospital-acquired infection with vancomycin-resistant *Enterococcus faecium* transmitted by electronic thermometers. Ann. Intern. Med. *117*:112-116, 1992.

133. Loeffler, A. M., Drew, R. H., Perfect, J. R., et al.: Safety and efficacy of quinupristin/dalfopristin for treatment of invasive gram-positive infections in pediatric patients. Pediatr. Infect. Dis. J. *21*:950-956, 2002.

134. Lohr, J. A., Donowitz, L. G., and Sadler, J. E., III: Hospital-acquired urinary tract infection. Pediatrics *83*:193-199, 1989.

135. Long, J. K., Choueiri, T. K., Hall, G. S., et al.: Daptomycin-resistant *Enterococcus faecium* in a patient with acute myeloid leukemia. Mayo Clin. Proc. *80*:1215-1216, 2005.

136. Losonsky, G., Wolf, A., Schwalbe, R., et al.: Successful treatment of meningitis due to multiply resistant *Enterococcus faecium* with a combination of intrathecal teicoplanin and intravenous antimicrobial agents. Clin. Infect. Dis. *19*:163-165, 1994.

137. Low, D. E.: Quinupristin/dalfopristin: Spectrum of activity, pharmacokinetics, and initial clinical experience. Microb. Drug Resist. *1*:223-234, 1995.

138. Low, D. E., Keller, N., Barth, A., et al.: Clinical prevalence, antimicrobial susceptibility, and geographic resistance patterns of enterococci: Results from

the SENTRY Antimicrobial Surveillance Program, 1997-1999. Clin. Infect. Dis. *32*(Suppl.):133-145, 2001.

139. Low, D. E., Willey, B. M., and McGeer, A. J.: Multidrug-resistant enterococci: A threat to the surgical patient. Am. J. Surg. *169*(Suppl.):8-12, 1995.

140. Luginbuhl, L. M., Rotbart, H. A., Facklam, R. R., et al.: Neonatal enterococcal sepsis: Case-control study and description of an outbreak. Pediatr. Infect. Dis. J. *6*:1022-1030, 1987.

141. Lynn, W. A., Clutterbuck, E., Want, S., et al.: Treatment of CAPD-peritonitis due to glycopeptide-resistant *Enterococcus faecium* with quinupristin/dalfopristin. Lancet *344*:1025-1026, 1994.

142. Maki, D. G., and Agger, W. A.: Enterococcal bacteremia: Clinical features, the risk of endocarditis, and management. Medicine (Baltimore) *67*:248-269, 1988.

143. Malone, D. A., Wagner, R. A., Myers, J. P., et al.: Enterococcal bacteremia in two large community teaching hospitals. Am. J. Med. *81*:601-606, 1986.

144. Marshall, S. H., Donskey, C. J., Hutton-Thomas, R., et al.: Gene dosage and linezolid resistance in *Enterococcus faecium* and *Enterococcus faecalis*. Antimicrob. Agents Chemother. *46*:3334-3336, 2002.

145. Matsumura, S., and Simor, A. E.: Treatment of endocarditis due to vancomycin-resistant *Enterococcus faecium* with quinupristin/dalfopristin, doxycycline, and rifampin: A synergistic drug combination. Clin. Infect. Dis. *27*:1554-1556, 1998.

146. McCarthy, A., Victor, G., Ramotar, K., et al.: Risk factors for acquiring ampicillin-resistant enterococci and clinical outcomes at a Canadian tertiary-care hospital. J. Clin. Microbiol. *32*:2671-2676, 1994.

147. McNeeley, D. F., Saint-Louis, F., and Noel, G. J.: Neonatal enterococcal bacteremia: An increasingly frequent event with potentially untreatable pathogens. Pediatr. Infect. Dis. J. *15*:800-805, 1996.

148. McNeil, S. A., Clark, N. M., Chandrasekar, P. H., et al.: Successful treatment of vancomycin-resistant *Enterococcus faecium* bacteremia with linezolid after failure of treatment with Synercid (quinupristin/dalfopristin). Clin. Infect. Dis. *30*:403-404, 2000.

149. Mederski-Samoraj, B. D., and Murray, B. E.: High-level resistance to gentamicin in clinical isolates of enterococci. J. Infect. Dis. *147*:751-757, 1983.

150. Megran, D. W.: Enterococcal endocarditis. Clin. Infect. Dis. *15*:63-71, 1992.

151. Meka, V. G., and Gold, H. S.: Antimicrobial resistance to linezolid. Clin. Infect. Dis. *39*:1010-1015, 2004.

152. Moellering, R. C., Jr.: Emergence of *Enterococcus* as a significant pathogen. Clin. Infect. Dis. *14*:1173-1176, 1992.

153. Moellering, R. C., Jr.: *Enterococcus* species, *Streptococcus bovis*, and *Leuconostoc* species. *In* Mandell, G. L., Bennett, J. E., and Dolin, R. (eds.): Principles and Practice of Infectious Diseases. 6th ed., Philadelphia, Elsevier Churchill Livingstone, 2005.

154. Moellering, R. C., Jr., and Krogstad, D. J.: Antibiotic resistance in enterococci. *In* Schlessinger, D. (ed.): Microbiology—1979. Washington, D.C., American Society for Microbiology, 1979, pp. 293-298.

155. Moellering, R. C., Jr., Linden, P. K., Reinhardt, J., et al.: The efficacy and safety of quinupristin/dalfopristin for the treatment of infections caused by vancomycin-resistant *Enterococcus faecium*: Synercid Emergency-Use Study Group. J. Antimicrob. Chemother. *44*:251-261, 1999.

156. Moellering, R. C., Jr., and Weinberg, A. N.: Studies on antibiotic synergism against enterococci. II. Effect of various antibiotics on the uptake of C14-labeled streptomycin by enterococci. J. Clin. Invest. *50*:2580-2584, 1971.

157. Moellering, R. C., Jr., Wennersten, C., and Medrek, T.: Prevalence of high-level resistance to aminoglycosides in clinical isolates of enterococci. Antimicrob. Agents Chemother. *1*:335-340, 1970.

158. Mondy, K. E., Shannon, W., and Mundy, L. M.: Evaluation of zinc bacitracin capsules versus placebo for enteric eradication of vancomycin-resistant *Enterococcus faecium*. Clin. Infect. Dis. *33*:473-476, 2001.

159. Montecalvo, M. A., Horowitz, H., and Gedris, C.: Outbreak of vancomycin-, ampicillin-, and aminoglycoside-resistant *Enterococcus faecium* bacteremia in an adult oncology unit. Antimicrob. Agents Chemother. *38*:1363-1367, 1994.

160. Moreno, F., Grota, P., Crisp, C., et al.: Clinical and molecular epidemiology of vancomycin-resistant *Enterococcus faecium* during its emergence in a city in southern Texas. Clin. Infect. Dis. *21*:1234-1237, 1995.

161. Morris, J. G., Jr., Shay, D. K., Hebden, J. N., et al.: Enterococci resistant to multiple antimicrobial agents, including vancomycin. Ann. Intern. Med. *123*:250-259, 1995.

162. Morrison, A. J., Jr., and Wenzel, R. P.: Nosocomial urinary tract infections due to enterococcus: Ten years' experience at a university hospital. Arch. Intern. Med. *146*:1549-1551, 1986.

163. Munoz-Price, L. S., Lolans, K., and Quinn, J. P.: Emergence of resistance to daptomycin during treatment of vancomycin-resistant *Enterococcus faecalis* infection. Clin. Infect. Dis. *41*:565-566, 2005.

164. Murray, B. E.: The life and times of the enterococcus. Clin. Microbiol. Rev. *3*:46-65, 1990.

165. Murray, B. E.: Beta-lactamase–producing enterococci. Antimicrob. Agents Chemother. *36*:2355-2359, 1992.

166. Murray, B. E.: Editorial response: What can we do about vancomycin-resistant enterococci. Clin. Infect. Dis. *20*:1134-1136, 1995.

167. Murray, B. E.: Diversity among multidrug-resistant enterococci. Emerg. Infect. Dis. *4*:37-47, 1998.

168. Murray, B. E.: Vancomycin-resistant enterococcal infections. N. Engl. J. Med. *342*:710-721, 2000.

169. Murray, B. E., and Mederski-Samoraj, B.: Transferable beta-lactamase: A new mechanism for in vitro penicillin resistance in *Streptococcus faecalis*. J. Clin. Invest. *72*:1168, 1983.

170. Nachman, S. A., Verma, R., and Egnor, M.: Vancomycin-resistant *Enterococcus faecium* shunt infection in an infant: An antibiotic cure. Microb. Drug Resist. *1*:95-96, 1995.

171. Nagai, K., Yuge, K., Ono, E., et al.: *Enterococcus faecium* meningitis in a child. Pediatr. Infect. Dis. J. *13*:1016-1017, 1994.

172. Nauschuetz, W. F., Trevino, S. B., Harrison, L. S., et al.: *Enterococcus casseliflavus* as an agent of nosocomial bloodstream infections. Med. Microbiol. Lett. *2*:102-108, 1993.

173. Nichols, R. L., and Muzik, A. C.: Enterococcal infections in surgical patients: The mystery continues. Clin. Infect. Dis. *15*:72-76, 1992.

174. Nicoletti, G., and Stefain, S.: Enterococci: Susceptibility patterns and therapeutic options. Eur. J. Clin. Microbiol. Infect. Dis. *14*(Suppl.):33-37, 1995.

175. Noble, C. J.: Carriage of group D streptococci in the human bowel. J. Clin. Pathol. *31*:1182-1186, 1978.

176. Noble, W. C., Virani, Z., and Cree, R.: Cotransfer of vancomycin and other resistance genes from *Enterococcus faecalis* NCTC12201 to *Staphylococcus aureus*. F. E. M. S. Microbiol. Lett. *93*:195-198, 1992.

177. Norris, A. H., Reilly, J. P., Edelstein, P. H., et al.: Chloramphenicol for the treatment of vancomycin-resistant enterococcal infections. Clin. Infect. Dis. *20*:1137-1144, 1995.

178. Noskin, G. A., Siddiqui, F., Stosor, V., et al.: Successful treatment of persistent vancomycin-resistant *Enterococcus faecium* bacteremia with linezolid and gentamicin. Clin. Infect. Dis. *28*:689-690, 1999.

179. Noskin, G. A., Siddiqui, F., Stosor, V., et al.: In vitro activities of linezolid against important gram-positive bacterial pathogens including vancomycin-resistant enterococci. Antimicrob. Agents Chemother. *43*:2059-2062, 1999.

180. Nosocomial enterococci resistant to vancomycin-United States, 1989-1993. M. M. W. R. Morb. Mortal. Wkly. Rep. *42*(30):597-599, 1993.

181. Onderdonk, A. B., Bartlett, J. G., Louie, T. J., et al.: Microbial synergy in experimental intra-abdominal abscess. Infect. Immun. *12*:22-26, 1976.

182. Ostrowsky, B. E., Trick, W. E., Sohn, A. H., et al.: Control of vancomycin-resistant enterococcus in health care facilities in a region. N. Engl. J. Med. *344*:1427-1433, 2001.

183. Patel, R., Allen, S. L., Manahan, J. M., et al.: Natural history of vancomycin-resistant enterococcal colonization in liver and kidney transplant recipients. Liver Transpl. Surg. *7*:27-31, 2001.

184. Patel, R., Keating, M. R., Cockerill, F. R., et al.: Bacteremia due to *Enterococcus avium*. Clin. Infect. Dis. *17*:1006-1011, 1993.

185. Patterson, J. E., Sweeney, A. H., Simms, M., et al.: An analysis of 110 serious enterococcal infections, epidemiology, antibiotic susceptibility, and outcome. Medicine (Baltimore) *74*:191-200, 1995.

186. Patterson, J. E., and Zervos, M. J.: High-level gentamicin resistance in enterococcus: Microbiology, genetic basis, and epidemiology. Rev. Infect. Dis. *12*:644, 1990.

187. Patton, W. N., Bienz, N., Franklin, I. M., et al.: Enterococcal meningitis in an HIV positive hemophilic patient. J. Clin. Pathol. *44*:608-609, 1991.

188. Perez Mato, S., Robinson, S., and Begue, R. E.: Vancomycin-resistant *Enterococcus faecium* meningitis successfully treated with chloramphenicol. Pediatr. Infect. Dis. J. *18*:483-484, 1999.

189. Poutsiaka, D. D., Skiffington, S., Miller, K. B., et al.: Daptomycin in the treatment of vancomycin-resistant *Enterococcus faecium* bacteremia in neutropenic patients. J. Infect. *54*:567-571, 2007.

190. Presterl, E., Graninger, W., and Georgopoulos, A.: The efficacy of teicoplanin in the treatment of endocarditis caused by gram-positive bacteria. J. Antimicrob. Chemother. *31*:755-766, 1993.

191. Pultz, N. J., Stiefel, U., Subramanyan, S., et al.: Mechanisms by which anaerobic microbiota inhibit the establishment in mice of intestinal colonization by vancomycin-resistant *Enterococcus*. J. Infect. Dis. *191*:949-956, 2005.

192. Raymond, N. J., Henry, J., and Workowski, K. A.: Enterococcal arthritis: Case report and review. Clin. Infect. Dis. *21*:516-522, 1995.

193. Recommendations for preventing the spread of vancomycin resistance: Recommendations of the Hospital Infection Control Practices Advisory Committee (HICPAC). M. M. W. R. Recomm. Rep. *44*(RR-12):1-13, 1995.

194. Rhinehart, E., Smith, N. E., Wennersten, C., et al.: Rapid dissemination of beta-lactamase–producing, aminoglycoside-resistant *Enterococcus faecalis* among patients and staff on an infant-toddler surgical ward. N. Engl. J. Med. *323*:1814-1818, 1990.

195. Ricaurte, J. C., Boucher, H. W., Turett, G. S., et al.: Chloramphenicol treatment for vancomycin-resistant *Enterococcus faecium* bacteremia. Clin. Microbiol. Infect. 7:17-21, 2001.

196. Rice, L. B.: Emergence of vancomycin-resistant enterococci. Emerg. Infect. Dis. 7:183-187, 2001.

197. Rice, L. B., Calderwood, S. B., Eliopoulos, G. M., et al.: Enterococcal endocarditis: A comparison of prosthetic and native valve disease. Rev. Infect. Dis. *13*:1-7, 1991.

198. Rice, L. B., Carias, L. L., Hutton-Thomas, R., et al.: Penicillin-binding protein 5 and expression of ampicillin resistance in *Enterococcus faecium*. Antimicrob. Agents Chemother. *45*:1480-1486, 2001.

199. Rice, L. B., and Shlaes, D. M.: Vancomycin resistance in the enterococcus. Pediatr. Clin. North Am. *42*:601-618, 1995.

200. Richards, M. J., Edwards, J. R., Culver, D. H., et al. for the National Nosocomial Infections Surveillance System: Nosocomial infections in pediatric intensive care units in the United States. Pediatrics 103:e39, 1999.
201. Ries, M., Deeg, K. H., Heininger, U., et al.: Brain abscesses in neonates—report of three cases. Eur. J. Pediatr. 152:745-746, 1993.
202. Rubin, L. G., Tucci, V., Cercenado, E., et al.: Vancomycin-resistant Enterococcus faecium in hospitalized children. Infect. Control Hosp. Epidemiol. 13:700-705, 1992.
203. Rucker, J. C., Hamilton, S. R., Bardenstein, D., et al.: Linezolid-induced toxic optic neuropathy. Neurology 66:595-598, 2006.
204. Sabol, K., Patterson, J. E., Lewis, J. S., II, et al.: Emergence of daptomycin resistance in Enterococcus faecium during daptomycin therapy. Antimicrob. Agents Chemother. 49:1664-1665, 2005.
205. Sader, H. S., Pfaller, M. A., Tenover, F. C., et al.: Evaluation and characterization of multiresistant Enterococcus faecium from 12 U.S. medical centers. J. Clin. Microbiol. 31:2840-2842, 1994.
206. Sader, H. S., Streit, J. M., Fritsche, T. R., and Jones, R. N.: Antimicrobial activity of daptomycin against multidrug-resistant gram-positive strains collected worldwide. Diagn. Microbiol. Infect. Dis. 50:201-204, 2004.
207. Sahgal, V. S., Urban, C., Mariano, N., et al.: Quinupristin/dalfopristin (RP 59500) therapy for vancomycin-resistant Enterococcus faecium aortic graft infection: Case report. Microb. Drug Resist. 1:245-247, 1995.
208. Saiman, L., Goldfarb, J., Kaplan, S. A., et al.: Safety and tolerability of linezolid in children. Pediatr. Infect. Dis. J. 22:S193-S200, 2003.
209. Sanchez, M. L., Barrett, M. S., and Jones, R. N.: The E-test applied to susceptibility tests of gonococci, multiply resistant enterococci, and Enterobacteriaceae producing potent beta-lactamases. Diagn. Microbiol. Infect. Dis. 15:459-462, 1992.
210. Sastry, V., Brennan, P. J., Levy, M. M., et al.: Vancomycin-resistant enterococci: An emerging pathogen in immunosuppressed transplant recipients. Transplant. Proc. 27:954-955, 1995.
211. Schaberg, D. R., Culver, D. H., and Gaynes, R. P.: Major trends in the microbial etiology of nosocomial infection. Am. J. Med. 91(Suppl. 3B):72-75, 1991.
212. Schaberg, D. R., Dillon, W. I., Terpenning, M. S., et al.: Increasing resistance of enterococci to ciprofloxacin. Antimicrob. Agents Chemother. 36:2533-2535, 1992.
213. Schmit, J.: Efficacy of teicoplanin for enterococcal infections: 63 cases and review. Clin. Infect. Dis. 15:302-306, 1992.
214. Schoenbaum, S. C., Gardner, P., and Shillito, J.: Infections of cerebrospinal fluid shunts: Epidemiology, clinical manifestations, and therapy. J. Infect. Dis. 131:543-552, 1975.
215. Schuster, F., Graubner, U. B., Schmid, I., et al.: Vancomycin-resistant-enterococci—colonization of 24 patients on a pediatric oncology unit. Klin. Padiatr. 210:261-263, 1998.
216. Schwartz, M., Slavoski, L., Dash, G., et al.: Nosocomial outbreak of multiresistant Enterococcus durans (VRED): Description of the epidemiology and antimicrobial sensitivity testing. Abstract 68. Presented at the 33rd Annual Meeting of the Infectious Diseases Society of America, San Francisco, 1995.
217. Seedat, J., Zick, G., Klare, I., et al.: Rapid emergence of resistance to linezolid during linezolid therapy of an Enterococcus faecium infection. Antimicrob. Agents Chemother. 50:4217-4219, 2006.
218. Segreti, J. A., Crank, C. W., and Finney, M. S.: Daptomycin for the treatment of gram-positive bacteremia and infective endocarditis: A retrospective case series of 31 patients. Pharmacotherapy 26:347-352, 2006.
219. Shaikh, Z. H., Peloquin, C. A., and Ericsson, C. D.: Successful treatment of vancomycin-resistant Enterococcus faecium meningitis with linezolid: Case report and literature review. Scand. J. Infect. Dis. 33:375-379, 2001.
220. Shay, D. K., Goldman, D. A., and Jarvis, W. R.: Reducing the spread of antimicrobial-resistant microorganisms: Control of vancomycin-resistant enterococci. Pediatr. Clin. North Am. 42:703-716, 1995.
221. Shay, D. K., Maloney, S. A., Montecalvo, M., et al.: Epidemiology and mortality risk of vancomycin-resistant enterococcal bloodstream infections. J. Infect. Dis. 172:993-1000, 1995.
222. Sherman, J. M.: The streptococci. Bacteriol. Rev. 1:3-97, 1937.
223. Shlaes, D. M., Etter, L., and Gutmann, L.: Synergistic killing of vancomycin-resistant enterococci of classes A, B, and C by combinations of vancomycin, penicillin and gentamicin. Antimicrob. Agents Chemother. 35:776-779, 1991.
224. Shlaes, D. M., Levy, J., and Wolinsky, E.: Enterococcal bacteremia without endocarditis. Arch. Intern. Med. 141:578-581, 1981.
225. Shuler, T. E., Riddle, C. D., Jr., and Potts, D. W.: Polymicrobic septic arthritis caused by Kingella kingae and Enterococcus. Orthopedics 13:254-256, 1990.
226. Siegel, J. S., and McCracken, G. H., Jr.: Group D streptococcal infections. J. Pediatr. 93:542-543, 1978.
227. Silverman, J. A., Mortin, L. I., Vanpraagh, A. D., et al.: Inhibition of daptomycin by pulmonary surfactant: In vitro modeling and clinical impact. J. Infect. Dis. 191:2149-2152, 2005.
228. Simpson, W. A., Courtney, H. S., and Ofek, I.: Interactions of fibronectin with streptococci: The role of fibronectin as a receptor for Streptococcus pyogenes. Rev. Infect. Dis. 9(Suppl.):351-359, 1987.
229. Singh-Naz, N., Sleemi, A., Pikis, A., et al.: Vancomycin-resistant Enterococcus faecium colonization in children. J. Clin. Microbiol. 37:413-416, 1999.
230. Stanton, B. F., Baltimore, R. S., and Clemens, J. D.: Changing spectrum of infective endocarditis in children. Am. J. Dis. Child 138:720-725, 1984.
231. Starke, J. R.: Infective endocarditis. In Feigin, R. D., Cherry, J. D., Demmler, G. J., and Kaplan, S. L. (eds.): Textbook of Pediatric Infectious Diseases. 5th ed. Philadelphia, W. B. Saunders, 2004, pp. 355-380.
232. Steenbergen, J. N., Alder, J., Thorne, G. M., and Tally, F. P.: Daptomycin: A lipopeptide antibiotic for the treatment of serious gram-positive infections. J. Antimicrob. Chemother. 55:283-288, 2005.
233. Stevens, M. P., and Edmond, M. B.: Endocarditis due to vancomycin-resistant enterococci: Case report and review of the literature. Clin. Infect. Dis. 41:1134-1142, 2005.
234. Stevenson, K. B., Murray, E. W., and Sarubbi, F. A.: Enterococcal meningitis: Report of four cases and review. Clin. Infect. Dis. 18:233-239, 1994.
235. Swenson, J. M., Clark, N. C., Ferraro, M. J., et al.: Development of a standardized screening method for detection of vancomycin-resistant enterococci. J. Clin. Microbiol. 32:1700-1704, 1994.
236. Swenson, J. M., Ferraro, M. J., Sahm, D. F., et al.: New vancomycin disk diffusion breakpoints for enterococci. The National Committee for Clinical Laboratory Standards Working Group on enterococci. J. Clin. Microbiol. 30:2525-2528, 1992.
237. Swenson, J. M., Hindler, J. A., and Peterson, L. R.: Special tests for detecting antibacterial resistance. In Murray, P. R., Baron, E. J., Pfaller, M. A., et al. (eds.): Manual of Clinical Microbiology. 6th ed. Washington, D.C., American Society for Microbiology, 1995, pp. 1356-1367.
238. Takada, H., Kawabata, Y., Arakaki, R., et al.: Molecular and structural requirements of a lipoteichoic acid from Enterococcus hirae ATCC 9790 for cytokine-inducing, antitumor, and antigenic activities. Infect. Immun. 63:57-65, 1995.
239. Teixeira, O. H., and Francis, C. K.: Enterococcal endocarditis in early infancy. Can. Med. Assoc. J. 127:612-613, 1982.
240. Tendolkar, P. M., Baghdayan, A. S., Gilmore, M. S., and Shankar, N.: Enterococcal surface protein, Esp, enhances biofilm formation by Enterococcus faecalis. Infect. Immun. 72:6032-6039, 2004.
241. Tenover, F. C., Swenson, J. M., O'Hara, C. M., et al.: Ability of commercial and reference antimicrobial susceptibility testing methods to detect vancomycin resistance in enterococci. J. Clin. Microbiol. 33:1524-1527, 1995.
242. Tenover, F. C., Weigel, L. M., Appelbaum, P. C., et al.: Vancomycin-resistant Staphylococcus aureus isolate from a patient in Pennsylvania. Antimicrob. Agents Chemother. 48:275-280, 2004.
243. Threlkeld, M. G., and Cobbs, C. G.: Infectious disorders of prosthetic valves and intravascular devices. In Mandell, G. L., Bennett, J. E., and Dolin, R. (eds.): Principles and Practices of Infectious Diseases. 4th ed. New York, Churchill Livingstone, 1995, pp. 783-793.
244. Tofte, R. W., Solliday, J., and Crossley, K. B.: Susceptibilities of enterococci to twelve antibiotics. Antimicrob. Agents Chemother. 25:532-533, 1984.
245. Tush, G. M., Huneycutt, S., Phillips, A., et al.: Intraventricular quinupristin/dalfopristin for the treatment of vancomycin-resistant Enterococcus faecium shunt infection. Clin. Infect. Dis. 26:1460-1461, 1998.
246. Urdaneta, M., Hollis, F., and Sperber, S. J.: Vancomycin resistant enterococci in the blood: Do we need to treat? Abstract 65. Presented at the 33rd Annual Meeting of the Infectious Diseases Society of America, San Francisco, 1995.
247. Uttley, A. H., Collins, C. H., Naidoo, J., et al.: Vancomycin-resistant enterococci. Letter. Lancet 1:57-58, 1988.
248. van Den Braak, N., Goessens, W., van Belkum, A., et al.: Accuracy of the VITEK 2 system to detect glycopeptide resistance in enterococci. J. Clin. Microbiol. 39:351-353, 2001.
249. Verma, A., Dhawan, A., Philpott-Howard, J., et al.: Glycopeptide-resistant Enterococcus faecium infections in paediatric liver transplant recipients: Safety and clinical efficacy of quinupristin/dalfopristin. J. Antimicrob. Chemother. 47:105-108, 2001.
250. Verma, M., Chatwal, J., and Varughese, P.: Neonatal conjunctivitis: A profile. Indian Pediatr. 31:1357-1361, 1994.
251. von Baum, H., Schehl, J., Geiss, H. K., et al.: Prevalence of vancomycin-resistant enterococci among children with end-stage renal failure: Mid-European Pediatric Peritoneal Dialysis Study Group. Clin. Infect. Dis. 29:912-916, 1999.
252. Weigel, L. M., Donlan, R. M., Shin, D. H., et al.: High-level vancomycin-resistant Staphylococcus aureus (VRSA) associated with a polymicrobial biofilm. Antimicrob. Agents Chemother. 51:231-238, 2007.
253. Weigelt, J. A., Easley, S. M., Thal, E. R., et al.: Abdominal surgical wound infection is lowered with improved perioperative Enterococcus and Bacteroides therapy. J. Trauma 34:579-584, 1993.
254. Willey, B. M., Kreiswirth, B. N., Simor, A. E., et al.: Detection of vancomycin resistance in enterococcus species. J. Clin. Microbiol. 30:1621-1624, 1992.
255. Willey, B. M., McGeer, A. J., Ostrowski, M. A., et al.: The use of the molecular typing techniques in the epidemiologic investigation of resistant enterococci. Infect. Control Hosp. Epidemiol. 15:548-556, 1994.
256. Williamson, R., LeBouguenec, C., Gutmann, L., et al.: One or two low affinity penicillin-binding proteins may be responsible for the range of susceptibility of Enterococcus faecium to benzylpenicillin. J. Gen. Microbiol. 131:1933-1940, 1985.
257. Wilson, W. R., Karchmer, A. W., Dajani, A. S., et al.: Antibiotic treatment of adults with infective endocarditis due to streptococci, enterococci, staphylococci, and HACEK microorganisms: American Heart Association. J. A. M. A. 274:1706-1713, 1995.
258. Wilson, W. R., Wilkowske, C. J., Wright, A. J., et al.: Treatment of streptomycin-susceptible and streptomycin-resistant enterococcal endocarditis. Ann. Intern. Med. 100:816-823, 1984.

259. Winberg, J., Anderson, H. J., and Bergstrom, T.: Epidemiology of symptomatic urinary tract infection in childhood. Acta Paediatr. Scand. Suppl. 252:1, 1974.

260. Winston, D. J., Emmanouilides, C., Kroeber, A., et al.: Quinupristin/dalfopristin therapy for infections due to vancomycin-resistant *Enterococcus faecium*. Clin. Infect. Dis. 30:790-797, 2000.

261. Wisplinghoff, H., Bischoff, T., Tallent, S. M., et al.: Nosocomial bloodstream infections in U.S. hospitals: Analysis of 24,179 cases from a prospective nationwide surveillance study. Clin. Infect. Dis. 39:309-317, 2004.

262. Wisplinghoff, H., Seifert, H., Tallent, S. M., et al.: Nosocomial bloodstream infections in pediatric patients in United States hospitals: Epidemiology, clinical features and susceptibilities. Pediatr. Infect. Dis. J. 22:686-691, 2003.

263. Zakrzewski, T., and Keith, J. D.: Bacterial endocarditis in infants and children. J. Pediatr. 67:1179-1193, 1965.

264. Zeana, C., Kubin, C. J., Della-Latta, P., et al.: Vancomycin-resistant *Enterococcus faecium* meningitis successfully managed with linezolid: Case report and review of the literature. Clin. Infect. Dis. 33:477-482, 2001.

265. Zervos, M. J., and Schaberg, D. S.: Reversal of the in vitro susceptibility of enterococci to trimethoprim-sulfamethoxazole by folinic acid. Antimicrob. Agents Chemother. 28:446-448, 1985.

266. Zimmerman, R. A., Moellering, R. C., Jr., and Weinberg, A. N.: Mechanism of resistance to antibiotic synergism in enterococci. J. Bacteriol. 105:873-879, 1971.

267. Zscheck, K. K., and Murray, B. E.: Genes involved in the regulation of beta-lactamase production in enterococci and staphylococci. Antimicrob. Agents Chemother. 37:1966-1970, 1993.

268. Zurenko, G. E., Yagi, B. H., Schaadt, R. D., et al.: In vitro activities of U-100592 and U-100766, novel oxazolidinone antibacterial agents. Antimicrob. Agents Chemother. 40:839-845, 1996.

VIRIDANS STREPTOCOCCAL INFECTIONS

A group of *Streptococcus* spp. known as viridans, alpha-hemolytic, or oral streptococci are ubiquitously present on the oral mucosa of virtually all humans. These organisms are important pathogens in children and adults alike and cause infections ranging from caries and bacterial endocarditis in immunocompetent hosts to fatal sepsis in neutropenic persons.

Each of the terms applied to this group is wanting. Not all members of the *alpha-hemolytic* streptococci are alpha-hemolytic, some being gamma-hemolytic (nonhemolytic) or even beta-hemolytic. *Streptococcus pneumoniae*, which is alpha-hemolytic, is considered to be a separate group. The term *viridans streptococci*

likewise is inadequate because it is derived from the Latin *viridis*, or green, and refers to the sheen caused by partial hemolysis around alpha-hemolytic colonies on sheep blood agar. The term *oral streptococci* circumvents the dilemma of outliers in the hemolytic classification schema, but it also is confusing because viridans streptococci are found in sites other than the oral cavity and nonviridans streptococcal species frequently are present in the oral cavity. In accordance with the American Society for Microbiology's most recent efforts in this field,[219] the term *viridans streptococci* will be used here in referring to this diverse group of bacteria in recognition that the member organisms typically, but not invariably are alpha-hemolytic. Also of emphasis is that viridans does not refer to a species of streptococci but rather to a group of species, erroneous references to "*Streptococcus viridans*" notwithstanding.[238]

Streptococci have been reclassified on the basis of molecular and genetic studies[55,219]; this reclassification adds to the clinical confusion, at least temporarily. For example, under the new classification system, certain small-colony, beta-hemolytic streptococci, including some that are in Lancefield group A, now are considered to be viridans streptococci. The hope is that classification based on molecular relatedness eventually will lead to a clearer understanding of the infectious diseases associated with these organisms. One should recognize, however, that the current knowledge of viridans streptococcal infections is based predominantly on study of the alpha-hemolytic members of the viridans group.

MICROBIOLOGY

Streptococci are gram-positive, catalase-negative bacteria that are spherical or ovoid and less than 2 μm in diameter. They are facultatively anaerobic and nonmotile and do not produce spores or gas. Some strains require an atmosphere enriched with carbon dioxide (5%). The enterococci (distinguished by their ability to grow in 6.5% sodium chloride) and lactococci (formerly Lancefield group N streptococci) once were considered to be streptococci but now are classified as separate genera.

Figure 95-2 is a schema for classifying the clinically important streptococcal species. Hemolysis of blood agar remains a key tool

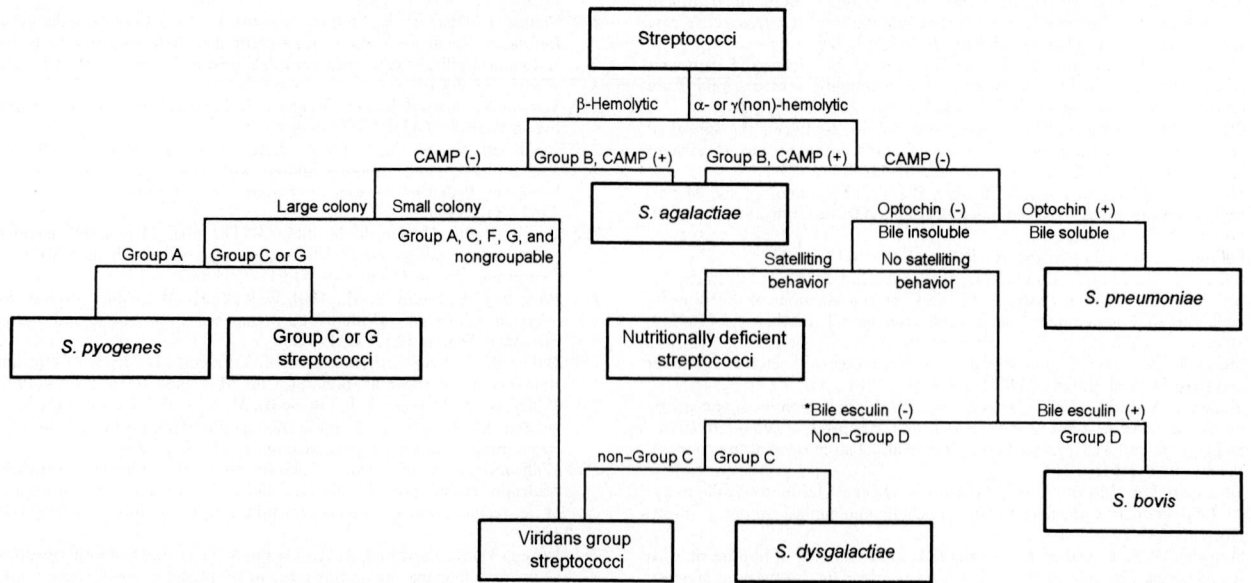

*Occasional viridans streptococcal strains are positive or weakly positive.

Figure 95-2 Schema for the identification of clinically important streptococcal species. Viridans group species are, in general, those remaining after identification of other streptococcal species. CAMP, Christie, Atkins, and Munch-Peterson test.

for classifying streptococci. Strains that are beta-hemolytic are characterized further according to colony size and Lancefield group (a serologic classification system based on cell wall carbohydrate). Group B *Streptococcus agalactiae* strains typically can be identified by beta-hemolysis and a positive result of the CAMP (Christie, Atkins, and Munch-Peterson) test[219]; however, some strains of *S. agalactiae* that are alpha- or gamma-hemolytic also are recognized by a positive CAMP test result.

Large-colony, beta-hemolytic, group A streptococci make up the species *Streptococcus pyogenes*. Other large-colony, beta-hemolytic streptococci occasionally are pathogenic, and most of them are group C or G streptococci. Small-colony, beta-hemolytic streptococci, including groups A, C, G, and F and nongroupable strains, partially constitute the *Streptococcus milleri* group of organisms within the viridans streptococci group. Among the alpha- or gamma-hemolytic streptococci, *S. agalactiae* (group B streptococci) and *S. pneumoniae* generally are identified by positive results on the CAMP test and optochin test, respectively. Bile solubility confirms an optochin-susceptible isolate as *S. pneumoniae*.

Nutritionally deficient streptococci are recognized by a requirement for the presence of a second bacterial species (*Staphylococcus aureus* typically is used in testing) to maintain growth on agar. These streptococci generally will grow in blood culture media in the absence of the reduced form of nicotinamide adenine dinucleotide (NADH) produced by a second bacterial species and may demonstrate some growth on agar in the absence of other bacteria. Nutritionally deficient streptococci once were classified as viridans streptococci, but more recent studies have classified these organisms in a new genus: *Abiotrophia adjacens* and *Abiotrophia defectiva*.[132] Excluding *Enterococcus* spp., streptococci that are alpha- or gamma-hemolytic, possess Lancefield group D antigen, and are bile esculin–positive may be identified tentatively as *Streptococcus bovis*. Though once included among viridans streptococci, this species now is classified separately from the viridans group.

Strains of one species of group C streptococci, *Streptococcus dysgalactiae*, are alpha- or gamma-hemolytic. These strains also must be distinguished from the viridans group of streptococci. A former streptococcal species included in the viridans group, *Streptococcus morbillorum*, was reclassified as *Gemella morbillorum*.[136] The remaining streptococcal organisms tentatively may be identified as viridans group streptococci. Thus, in practice, viridans streptococci continue to be characterized by the absence of features that distinguish the other major streptococcal pathogens. No characteristics can be used to confirm the identity of viridans streptococci definitively in the standard microbiology laboratory.

Classification of species within the viridans streptococci group also has been challenging. Over the years, several schemata that have been developed include those of Carlsson,[41] Coleman and Williams,[51] Facklam,[85] Ruoff and Kunz,[220,221] and Coykendall.[55] All these classification schemata lack reliable markers for member species and therefore result in inconsistent classification of clinical isolates. Consequently, efforts to characterize the clinical features of infections according to individual species of viridans streptococci have had marginal results. Molecular and polymerase chain reaction (PCR)-based taxonomies have been used to classify viridans streptococci,[4,55,183,218,290] but these techniques generally are not available in the clinical laboratory. Given the current flux in the taxonomy of these organisms, a simplified, practical approach to classifying viridans streptococci as outlined in Table 95–5 has been advocated.[219] The biochemical tests available in many clinical microbiology laboratories can be used to assign clinical isolates to one of five groups that encompass the 14 clinically important viridans streptococcal species listed in Table 95–5. Rapid molecular and PCR-based tests are available for tentative identification of individual viridans streptococcal species[89,98,189,221]; however, at this time, identification of precise species has little clinical significance except as an epidemiologic tool.

EPIDEMIOLOGY

Viridans streptococci are the predominant microorganisms in the oral flora of humans. These organisms also are found commonly in other areas of the upper respiratory tract, throughout the gastrointestinal tract, and in the female genital tract. Occasionally, viridans streptococci are found as members of the skin flora.

Viridans streptococci begin colonizing neonates shortly after birth. By 1 month of age, virtually all infants are colonized with at least one species of viridans streptococci.[186] The mix of colonizing viridans streptococcal species varies with ontogeny. For example, *Streptococcus mutans*, a species that plays an important role in the development of caries, rarely is found in predentate children but commonly is present after the eruption of teeth.[42,73,256] The ecology of other viridans streptococcal species also appears to be affected by the eruption of teeth.[43,73,239,256] In addition to these temporal factors in the colonization of infants and children, viridans streptococci have species-specific predilections for

TABLE 95–5   Simplified Classification Schema for Viridans Streptococci

Group	Species	Hemolysis	Sorbitol	Arginine	Voges-Proskauer	Mannitol	Esculin
S. milleri	S. anginosus	α, β, γ	–	+	+	±	±
	S. constellatus					–	
	S. intermedius					±	
S. mutans	S. mutans	β, γ, α	+	–	+	+	+
	S. sobrinus						
	S. rattus						
	S. cricetus						
S. salivarius	S. salivarius	γ, α	–	–	+	–	+
	S. vestibularis						
S. sanguis	S. sanguis	a	–	+	–	–	+
	S. gordonii						+
	S. parasanguis						±
	S. crista						+
S. mitis	S. mitis*	a	–	–	–	–	–

Previously included S. mitis, S. sanguis II, and S. oralis.
Data from Coykendall, A. L.: Classification and identification of the viridans streptococci. Clin. Microbiol. Rev. 2:315-328, 1989; and Ruoff, K. L.: Streptococcus. In Murray, P. R., Baron, E. J., Pfaller, M. A., et al. (eds.): Manual of Clinical Microbiology. 6th ed. Washington, D.C., American Society for Microbiology, 1995, pp. 299-307.

certain anatomic areas of the oral cavity and pharynx. For example, *Streptococcus sanguis* is the predominant isolate of the buccal mucosa but rarely is found on the dorsum of the tongue, where *Streptococcus mitis* is the predominant species.[93] Diet also may affect the viridans streptococcal ecology. For example, consumption of sugar-containing beverages and the low pH that can result from carbohydrate intake favor colonization with caries-producing *S. mutans*.[106,254]

Little is known about the transmission of viridans streptococci, but studies of the transmission of *S. mutans* within families indicate that intrafamily transmission commonly occurs.[3,110,222] Toothbrushes may be an important vehicle of transmission of viridans streptococci in children.[153] The hands of hospital personnel, especially those with skin disorders such as eczema, also may be a vehicle of transmission of viridans streptococci.[48] In addition, dental records have been suggested as a vehicle in the transmission of viridans streptococci.[56]

Viridans streptococci have an important role in the ecology of the oral flora in that they protect against potentially more invasive pathogens by resistance to colonization with these organisms.[17,97] This mechanism has been demonstrated by a double-blind study in which patients who had received antibiotic therapy for group A streptococcal pharyngitis were treated with either a preparation that contained four species of viridans streptococci or a placebo. In the treated group, none of 17 patients experienced recurrence of group A streptococcal pharyngitis. In contrast, pharyngitis recurred in 7 (37%) of 19 patients in the placebo group.[211] A second double-blind, placebo-controlled multicenter trial by the same group confirmed the finding of the first study.[212] Viridans streptococci also may have a role in resistance to colonization by pathogens such as methicillin-resistant *S. aureus* (MRSA) in the oral cavity of infants[269]; nontypeable *Haemophilus influenzae*, *S. pneumoniae*, and *Moraxella catarrhalis* at the eustachian tube orifice[255]; and *Neisseria gonorrhoeae* in the female genital tract.[162] In addition to competition for mucosal adherence sites, viridans streptococci produce hydrogen peroxide and bacteriocins that are bactericidal to certain competing bacteria and may contribute to resistance to colonization.[57,59,270,275] Conversion of hydrogen peroxide to ozone in the oral cavity may play a role in the resistance to colonization by other bacterial species and *Candida*.[268]

PATHOGENESIS

Viridans streptococci are organisms of low virulence that usually cause nonpyogenic infection when they do cause infection. They are involved most often in localized infections of the sinuses and oral cavity, including the teeth, in which the tissues are invaded directly by colonizing organisms. Caries is a disease of teeth that develops over a period of years, often in association with *S. mutans* infection. Viridans streptococci also have a role in a variety of gingival diseases, possibly including gingival hyperplasia accompanying the chronic administration of phenytoin. In an experimental animal model, phenytoin-induced gingival hyperplasia was enhanced in rats infected with *Streptococcus sobrinus* when compared with uninfected control animals.[175] Occasionally, viridans streptococci, usually organisms of the *S. milleri* group, cause pyogenic infections, including abscesses in the brain, lung, and abdomen. An intriguing, but preliminary study suggested that viridans streptococcal–related dental disease is associated with the subsequent development of coronary artery heart disease.[146] Viridans streptococci are among the microorganisms isolated from atherosclerotic plaque, although the role of these microbes in the pathogenesis of atherosclerosis has not been determined.[47] Typically, viridans streptococci cause life-threatening infection only in settings in which the oral mucosa is disrupted and the host's mechanisms of clearance are compro-

mised, such as in patients with neutropenia or cardiac-valve disease.

The preponderance of viridans streptococci in the oral flora rather than its virulence accounts for the domination of viridans streptococci in infections originating from the mouth. In a study of 36 children who underwent extraction of normal or abscessed teeth, 11 (30%) had postextraction positive blood cultures.[245] In all 11, viridans streptococci were isolated exclusively. Bacteremia occurred more commonly after removal of diseased teeth (37%), but it also occurred after removal of normal teeth (23%).

A separate study of 58 children who underwent dental extraction included 26 who received penicillin, amoxicillin, or erythromycin prophylaxis because of a risk of endocarditis developing.[54] Bacteremia was detected in only 9 (35%) of the 26 children who received prophylaxis and in 20 (63%) of 32 children who did not (*p* < 0.05). In this study, viridans streptococci accounted for 37 percent of the blood isolates, strict anaerobes accounted for 26.5 percent, and a variety of organisms accounted for the remainder. The number of colony-forming units per milliliter of blood ranged from 2 to 12. Even within a single colony-forming unit, more than one bacterial species sometimes was found after subculture.

Although these two studies were dissimilar in the diversity of organisms isolated, both indicated that viridans streptococci are the organisms most likely to invade the blood after trauma to the oral cavity. Also reflecting the predominance of these organisms in oral and salivary flora, bacteremia with viridans streptococci occurs commonly during orthodontic banding[84] and dilation of esophageal strictures.[296]

The ability of viridans streptococci to bind to oral mucosa, tooth surfaces, and dental plaque via interaction of specific microbial and host "receptors" accounts for the preferential colonization of the oral cavity by these organisms.[273] This interaction also helps explain localization of the various viridans streptococcal species to distinct anatomic sites, as well as the involvement of ontologic factors in colonization. The precise nature of bacterial adherence to the oral mucosa is not defined but appears to involve streptococcal lipoteichoic acid.[118] Through release of modulin protein I/II, viridans streptococci induce the expression of adhesion molecules such as E-selectin and intercellular (ICAM-1) and vascular cell (VCAM-1) adhesion molecules on endothelial cells, promote transendothelial migration of neutrophils in vitro, and induce release of cytokines in epithelial (interleukin-6 [IL-6]) and endothelial cells (IL-6 and IL-8).[277,278] The host's immunologic status also may be an important determinant of adherence and subsequent invasion. For example, immunocompetent persons produce secretory IgA to *S. mutans*,[11] and such antibody is capable of preventing caries.[169] Viridans streptococci within the biofilm present in dental plaque are at least 500 times more resistant to antibiotic treatment than predicted on the basis of their susceptibility in culture medium; therefore, this finding suggests that antibiotic treatment cannot eradicate viridans streptococci from dental plaque, even temporarily.[140]

At the University of Texas M. D. Anderson Cancer Center in Houston, the incidence of viridans streptococcal bacteremia increased extraordinarily between 1972 and 1989, from 1 to 47 cases per 10,000 admissions.[75] Analysis of risk factors associated with viridans streptococcal bacteremia indicated that prophylactic administration of trimethoprim-sulfamethoxazole (TMP-SMX) or a fluoroquinolone, profound neutropenia, and the administration of antacids or histamine type 2 receptor antagonists each significantly predisposed patients to the development of bacteremia.[75] Presumably, administration of the implicated antibiotics and antacids favored the overgrowth of viridans streptococci and their proliferation throughout the gastrointestinal tract, which in turn would favor the development of viridans streptococcal bacteremia in an immunocompromised host, especially if the mucosal barrier was disrupted by cytotoxic chemotherapy and the host was neutropenic. Of note, administration of cytarabine (cytosine arabinoside or ara-C) was not associated with viridans streptococcal sepsis in this study despite being identified as a major risk factor in many other studies.[28,29,39,67,123,157,167,205]

The ability to adhere to damaged cardiac valves and vegetations is a principal factor in the predominance of viridans streptococcal endocarditis. Strains of viridans streptococci carried by healthy children adhered less well to buccal and endocardial cells than did disease-producing strains isolated from children with endocarditis.[229,230] Lipoteichoic acid is thought to help mediate adhesion of viridans streptococci to endocardium, and penicillin prophylaxis may be effective in part because of its reduction of lipoteichoic acid on the bacterial cell surface.[148]

The ability of antibiotics to alter the surface properties of bacteria, even when the bacteria are resistant to the bactericidal action of the drug, may be an important determinant in the effectiveness of prophylactic antibiotics.[148,236] In the host, fibronectin is an important determinant of binding of viridans streptococci to damaged endothelium. Viridans streptococci do not bind to soluble fibronectin, but a reactive domain becomes available for binding when the fibronectin molecule is immobilized, as is the case in endocarditis.[147] Mutant viridans streptococci that cannot bind to fibronectin were significantly less virulent in an animal model of endocarditis.[147]

The ability of viridans streptococci to induce platelet aggregation also may be involved in the pathogenesis of endocarditis.[90,154] In viridans streptococci–challenged, anticoagulated rabbits, only microscopic vegetations developed despite fulminant sepsis. In contrast, viridans streptococci–challenged, non-anticoagulated animals tended to have large vegetations and a subacute course.[121] These findings are concordant with those of a separate study in which viridans streptococci–challenged thrombocytopenic rabbits had a greater density of bacteria within vegetations than did nonthrombocytopenic control animals; these results suggest that platelets limit progression of the disease.[250] Surprisingly, neutropenia appears to have little effect on susceptibility to endocarditis in animal models but affects containment of the infection.[165,166]

In neutropenic patients with cancer and in patients who have received bone marrow transplants, viridans streptococci cause septic shock and adult respiratory distress syndrome (ARDS). Viridans streptococci also induce nephritis.[5,259] In these circumstances, little is known about the mechanisms involved. Viridans streptococci produce no endotoxin, and specific exotoxins have not been identified. Nonetheless, products of these organisms can activate complement[173] and induce the production of tumor necrosis factor-α (TNF-α) and TNF-β; IL-1, IL-2, IL-6, and IL-8; interferon-γ; and nitric oxide.[18,80,112,161,182,240,242,253] Strains isolated from patients with sepsis were found to be more active in inducing TNF-β and IL-8 production than were colonizing strains isolated from healthy subjects.[243] In a study of two neutropenic patients with fatal viridans streptococcal sepsis, high blood levels of IL-6 were detected, especially late in the course, whereas IL-1 and TNF-α blood levels were not remarkable.[78] Viridans streptococcal lipoteichoic acid induces cytokine and nitric oxide production in vitro,[80,173] but the clinical significance of these observations is not known. In contrast to group A streptococci isolated from patients with septic shock, viridans streptococci isolated from the blood of pediatric cancer patients with septic shock do not express superantigens in vitro.[180] Thus, intravenous immunoglobulin, which has been suggested as an adjuvant therapy for group A streptococcal shock, may not be effective in patients with viridans streptococcal sepsis.

CLINICAL MANIFESTATIONS

The viridans streptococcal species are a diverse group of bacteria, and consequently, a variety of clinical manifestations are associated with the infections that they cause. Typically, the viridans streptococci cause nonpyogenic infections such as bacteremia and endocarditis, whereas the *S. milleri* group, also referred to as the *Streptococcus intermedius* group, tends to cause invasive pyogenic infections, including bone infections, brain abscesses, appendicitis, and pulmonary and abdominal abscesses.[176]

SEPSIS IN IMMUNOCOMPROMISED HOSTS

For obscure reasons, during the past 2 or 3 decades the relative incidence of gram-positive bacterial infections, especially viridans streptococcal infection, has increased in immunocompromised hosts. In 1978, viridans streptococci first were perceived as an important cause of sepsis in neutropenic patients with cancer when 29 episodes in adults and children at the National Cancer Institute[192] and 6 episodes in children at the M. D. Anderson Cancer Center[117] were reported. Before these reports, the significance of blood isolates of viridans streptococci in this setting generally was not appreciated. The fact that no deaths occurred in the original National Cancer Institute series or in a subsequent series from that center[216] suggested that viridans streptococci produce a benign bacteremia similar to that seen with coagulase-negative staphylococci. In contrast, three of the six children at M. D. Anderson died. Several other centers in Europe and North America have reported fulminant, sometimes fatal viridans streptococcal sepsis in patients with cancer and in those who have received transplants.* Overall, the death rate associated with viridans streptococcal sepsis has ranged from 0 to 50 percent, with most centers reporting mortality rates of approximately 10 percent. In some centers, viridans streptococci are the most common cause of fatal sepsis.[21,28,105] The incidence of viridans streptococcal sepsis appears to be higher in children than in adults.[160,248]

The oral cavity is the most common portal of entry in immunocompromised hosts. Catheter-related viridans streptococcal bacteremia is an unusual occurrence. However, because administration of antacid is a risk factor,[75] the lower gastrointestinal tract probably is a portal of entry in some patients. Several factors predispose patients to the development of viridans streptococcal sepsis. Profound neutropenia clearly is a predisposing factor,[28,75] although viridans streptococcal bacteremia occasionally develops in patients with cancer and absolute neutrophil counts greater than 1000 cells/mm³. Mucositis, especially oral mucositis, is a definitive risk factor.[28,29,75,105,157,167] Cytarabine appears to be a risk factor even beyond its predisposition to produce clinically evident mucositis,[28,29,39,67,79,123,157,167,205] although at least one study has not found this association.[99] The use of prophylactic TMP-SMX or quinolones also is an important risk factor.[28,29,49,75,105,188] The observation that the administration of acyclovir may decrease the incidence of viridans streptococcal bacteremia in transplant patients suggests that herpes simplex virus infection may be a risk factor as well.[206] Allogeneic bone marrow transplantation likewise has been associated with an increased risk for the development of viridans streptococcal sepsis, with a greater than fourfold increase in the mortality rate.[157] An association between the development of viridans streptococcal sepsis and menstruation has been noted.[75]

The hallmark clinical feature of viridans streptococcal sepsis in an immunocompromised host is fever that typically is high, occurs in the presence of neutropenia and mucositis, and frequently lasts for several days after viable organisms are cleared from the blood. Most patients recover uneventfully. However, fulminant septic shock may occur. Shock may appear early,

---

*See references 10, 13, 21, 28, 29, 39, 50, 52, 75, 105, 107, 114, 141, 157, 160, 188, 203, 205, 235, 241, 248, 281.

although it often is delayed for 2 or 3 days after the onset of sepsis, and it occurs despite prompt sterilization of blood by effective antibiotics.[248] ARDS frequently occurs in severe cases, usually 2 or 3 days after the initial bacteremia.[10,75,120,257] Focal complications, including pneumonia and meningitis, are uncommon occurrences. Rash and palmar desquamation may be present but are not common manifestations.[75] For unexplained reasons, the incidence of aspergillosis is increased after the development of viridans streptococcal sepsis in children with cancer.[181]

Several studies have implicated *S. mitis* as a more pathogenic species of viridans streptococci with a predilection to cause shock and ARDS in patients with cancer,[10,29,50,71,111,163,248,257] but other studies have not found a clear relationship between clinical features and species.[75] *S. mitis* isolated from cancer patients with sepsis also has been found to be more resistant to antibiotics than other species of viridans streptococci isolated from the same patient population are.[111]

NEONATAL SEPSIS, MENINGITIS, AND OTHER INFECTIONS

Viridans streptococci are normal inhabitants of the female genital tract and are a common cause of chorioamnionitis and subsequent abortion,[9] as well as a frequent cause of neonatal sepsis and meningitis.[1,25,34,94,145,174,284] Viridans streptococci ordinarily do not colonize newborns' skin and should not be dismissed as contaminants when isolated from normally sterile sites.[1] In some newborn centers, the incidence of viridans streptococcal bacteremia and meningitis has approached or exceeded that attributable to group B streptococci, although viridans streptococcal infections tend to be less severe.[34,174] *Streptococcus oralis* (*S. mitis*) caused more than half of the cases in one study.[284] The portal of entry of the organism generally is unknown in this setting, but a fetal scalp electrode was implicated in one case.[95] Unusual manifestations in newborns include pharyngitis and epiglottitis,[31] endocarditis,[164] and conjunctivitis.[138]

ENDOCARDITIS

Viridans streptococci are a common cause of endocarditis at all ages because of the organism's ability to adhere to diseased endocardium and its frequent implication in bacteremia during dental procedures and routine mouth care. A recent study at a teaching hospital in Finland found that starting in 1995, *S. aureus* became more prevalent than viridans streptococci as a cause of endocarditis[113]; however, a study from Minnesota found no significant change in the etiology of endocarditis from 1970 to 2000, with viridans streptococci being the most common cause throughout.[263] Viridans streptococci tend to cause subacute endocarditis; blood cultures may be positive only intermittently. *S. sanguis* and *S. mitis* are the species identified most commonly.[68,201,207,251,286] Complications of viridans streptococcal endocarditis include septic pulmonary emboli, congestive heart failure, pericarditis, myocardial abscess, meningitis, osteomyelitis, and glomerulonephritis.[139,201] The shock and ARDS that develop in immunocompromised patients do not occur in immunocompetent patients with endocarditis.

PNEUMONIA

Pulmonary infiltrates frequently complicate viridans streptococcal sepsis in neutropenic hosts. In most cases, these infiltrates represent ARDS, not primary pneumonia. However, several cases of primary viridans streptococcal pneumonia that developed in previously healthy persons have been reported.[96,104,155,177,198,226] In some cases the diagnosis was supported by multiple isolates of

viridans streptococci obtained from blood in the absence of endocarditis. The incidence of viridans streptococcal pneumonia may be underestimated significantly because tracheal isolates of viridans streptococci usually are discounted as contaminants and tracheal isolates probably do represent contamination of the specimen with oral flora in many cases.[213] Given the increasing incidence of viridans streptococcal infection and the escalating prevalence of antibiotic resistance among these organisms, clinicians should consider viridans streptococci as a potential cause of pneumonia when they are isolated in the absence of other pathogens.

OSTEOMYELITIS AND SEPTIC ARTHRITIS

Viridans streptococci are unusual causes of osteomyelitis and septic arthritis. Extension of an oral infection into the mandible or maxilla is the most common circumstance in which viridans streptococci cause osteomyelitis,[185] but vertebral osteomyelitis caused by these organisms has been described on several occasions.[2,38,62,217,271,282] Infection of the long bones[204] and septic arthritis[14] occur infrequently.

CARIES

Although caries was recognized as an infectious disease in 1890 by workers trained in Robert Koch's laboratory, its infectious nature still is not accepted universally.[8,12,72] Evidence that *S. mutans* is the major cause of caries in children and adults alike is substantial,[8,12,32,233,258,267,274] but other viridans streptococci and *Actinomyces* spp. also have cariogenic potential.[233,274] *S. mutans*, which colonizes the oral cavity only after the eruption of teeth, has a predilection for the dental surfaces, metabolizes sucrose, and produces a strong acid that weakens the mineral matrix of teeth and allows the organisms to penetrate the structure of the teeth.[44,233] Fluoridation of the water supply has been credited with strengthening tooth enamel, thereby fostering resistance to the harsh acids produced by *S. mutans*.[233] Fluoride has potent antibacterial action against *S. mutans*, particularly at low pH.[44,276] Thus, fluoridation of water supplies may represent, albeit in a unique form, the most widespread and successful use of antibacterial prophylaxis. Topical treatments also provide protection against the cariogenic actions of *S. mutans* and in some circumstances depend on the antibacterial action of fluoride.[116,262,272,294] Short courses of oral antibiotics can reduce colonization with *S. mutans* substantially and may be an important adjunct to the treatment of caries.[247] Specially designed culture systems are available to detect the presence and measure the concentration of *S. mutans* in plaque and thus permit the effects of therapy to be monitored.[32,283] Because the development of cavities typically requires a few years of infection, opportunity to interrupt the pathogenesis of this disease is ample.[8]

ABSCESSES AND OTHER INFECTIONS

The suppurative infections produced by viridans streptococci typically are caused by the *S. milleri* group: *Streptococcus anginosus*, *Streptococcus constellatus*, and *S. intermedius*. Like *S. aureus*, members of this group resist killing by polymorphonuclear leukocytes and stimulate less chemotaxis than other viridans streptococci do.[280] Because *S. milleri* bacteria inhabit the upper respiratory tract and the gastrointestinal tract and are relatively invasive, these organisms cause sinusitis, otitis media, meningitis, and abdominal abscesses and often are present in brain abscesses.[24,53,77,170,172,176,224] *S. milleri* group organisms may infect the brain via a hematogenous route that originates in the oral cavity or intestinal tract or by direct invasion through the upper respiratory tract. Sepsis in non-neutropenic patients occurs uncommonly, usually in association with an intra-abdominal source.[151,224]

Among other unusual infections caused by viridans streptococci was a large outbreak of pharyngitis caused by S. mitis accompanied by a toxic shock–like syndrome in half of the cases.[150] Meningitis resulting from both hematogenous and direct spread has been observed in healthy adults.[149] Iatrogenic meningitis caused by contamination with oral viridans streptococci may complicate lumbar puncture or other central nervous system procedures.[82,228,291] Lung abscesses caused by viridans streptococci may result from the aspiration of saliva.[128,198] Empyema and mediastinitis are other reported thoracic infections associated with viridans streptococci.[19,128] Myositis complicated by rhabdomyolysis in children with leukemia has been reported.[225] Viridans streptococci also are found occasionally in liver abscesses,[16,91,100] peritonitis,[23] and appendicitis.[193]

DIAGNOSIS

Infections caused by viridans streptococci cannot be distinguished clinically from infections caused by other gram-positive and gram-negative bacteria. Collection of adequate culture specimens is essential for establishing the diagnosis. Viridans streptococcal infections typically are diagnosed by culture of blood or other normally sterile tissue. The organisms may be present in low concentration. A volume of 30 mL of blood has been suggested as the optimal volume for culture in an adult-sized patient.[232] The addition of agents that neutralize the antibacterial effects of fresh blood, such as sodium polyanethole sulfonate, significantly improves the yield of blood cultures.[231] Chemotherapeutic agents may interfere with the detection of viridans streptococci in blood.[187]

Viridans streptococci normally are not part of the skin flora and ordinarily should not be considered contaminants. Viridans streptococci have been reported to cross-react with S. pneumoniae Omniserum, and this cross-reaction has the potential to lead to false-positive results of the Omniserum test.[120]

ANTIBIOTIC SUSCEPTIBILITY

In the past, viridans streptococci have been considered penicillin-sensitive. Today, penicillin-resistant and penicillin-tolerant viridans streptococci are found worldwide as causes of sepsis, endocarditis, meningitis, and other infections, including conjunctivitis of the newborn.* Penicillin resistance occurs commonly, particularly in patients receiving long-term penicillin therapy,[7,26,184,246,249] although even short courses of antibiotics may predispose patients to colonization with resistant viridans streptococci.[83,101,171] Infection with penicillin-resistant viridans streptococci is associated with a higher mortality rate than infection with penicillin-susceptible strains is.[64,244] Antibiotic resistance may develop in all species of viridans streptococci, although S. mutans rarely exhibits resistance.[127]

Resistance to a variety of antibiotic classes has developed during the past 2 decades,[196] although resistance still is an uncommon finding in patients who live in the community and have not been treated recently with antibiotics.[292] Resistance to cephalosporins is widespread, with the general pattern of susceptibility being the following: cefotaxime and ceftriaxone usually are more active than cefepime and cefuroxime, both of which are more active than ceftazidime and cephalexin.[65,156,190,287] Previous cepha-

losporin therapy is a risk factor for cephalosporin resistance, an observation with particular relevance for patients with cancer.[36,133] Resistance to fluoroquinolones, especially ciprofloxacin and ofloxacin, is a common finding.[46,60,63,134,227,290] Levofloxacin has better activity against viridans streptococci than the older fluoroquinolones do, and the newer agents garenoxacin, gatifloxacin, and moxifloxacin have enhanced activity against most gram-positive pathogens, including viridans streptococci.[208-210] However, resistance develops rapidly when patients receive quinolones prophylactically—levofloxacin, gatifloxacin, and moxifloxacin included.[197,260] At the Mayo Clinic in Rochester, Minnesota, viridans streptococcal sepsis developed in 6 (16%) of 37 transplant patients receiving levofloxacin prophylaxis (3 experienced shock); blood isolates were resistant to levofloxacin, as well as the newer quinolones gatifloxacin and moxifloxacin.[202] Resistance was associated with mutations in the quinolone resistance-determining region of GyrA or ParC. Resistance of viridans streptococci to aminoglycosides,[131] tetracycline,[60,65,290] TMP-SMX,[60,63,65,290] clindamycin,[63,266,290] erythromycin,[33,60,63,65,290] other macrolide antibiotics,[6] and vancomycin[237] also has been reported.

Resistance of viridans streptococci to penicillin appears to involve chromosomally mediated alterations in the organisms' PBPs.[200,295] Initially, researchers suspected that genes conferring penicillin resistance might have been acquired from S. pneumoniae.[70] Subsequent studies, however, indicated that penicillin resistance may have evolved first in S. mitis and that S. pneumoniae acquired genes mediating penicillin resistance from this and other closely related viridans streptococcal species.[45,69,195] Quinolone resistance determinants also are transmitted efficiently between viridans streptococci and S. pneumoniae,[126] and the mef(E) gene that confers resistance to macrolides is transmitted readily from viridans streptococci to S. pyogenes.[129]

The clinical impact of the development of penicillin resistance among viridans streptococci has been far-reaching. The emergence of penicillin-resistant viridans streptococci incidentally may be encouraging the development of vancomycin-resistant enterococci because of the increased use of vancomycin to prevent and treat viridans streptococcal infection in patients with cancer.

Overall, vancomycin is the antibiotic with the most reliable activity against viridans streptococci. Teicoplanin also has been used successfully to treat patients with endocarditis caused by viridans streptococci.[288] Daptomycin, dalbavancin, quinupristin-dalfopristin, and linezolid are active in vitro against most clinical isolates of viridans streptococci.[137,223,285]

TREATMENT

Empiric antibiotic therapy for viridans streptococci should be based on the local pattern of antibiotic susceptibility among recent clinical isolates. Antimicrobial susceptibility testing of viridans streptococcal isolates is necessary. Limited data indicate that antibiotic susceptibility testing performed with the E-test correlates well with agar dilution susceptibility testing.[214] Although vancomycin-resistant clinical isolates currently are very rare findings, inclusion of vancomycin in susceptibility testing is advisable. For infections other than endocarditis and meningitis, single-antibiotic therapy usually is preferred. An exception is infection in neutropenic patients with cancer because restricting antibiotic therapy to drugs active against gram-positive bacteria exclusively may predispose these patients to the development of gram-negative bacterial infections.[191] Some investigators have advocated reserving vancomycin for neutropenic patients with shock or ARDS,[265] whereas others have advocated inclusion of vancomycin in the initial empiric therapy for patients with fever and neutropenia.[76,235] Viridans streptococcal sepsis may occur in neutropenic

---

*See references 30, 35, 74, 87, 103, 119, 138, 144, 194, 200.

patients despite ongoing antibiotic therapy with β-lactam agents to which the infecting organisms are susceptible in vitro[233]; the fact that this phenomenon has not been observed with vancomycin therapy supports the use of this antibiotic for the treatment of viridans streptococcal sepsis in neutropenic patients.

Combination therapy often is advocated for the treatment of viridans streptococcal endocarditis[27,92,159,279] and may be considered for the treatment of meningitis, especially when the infecting organism is tolerant of penicillin.[81] Combinations of either penicillins and aminoglycosides or vancomycin and aminoglycosides are used most commonly. Penicillin and vancomycin are thought to increase uptake of aminoglycosides, thereby leading to synergistic bactericidal activity.[293] However, a recent meta-analysis of five clinical trials failed to identify any overall improvement in the outcome of patients who had endocarditis and were treated with β-lactam and aminoglycoside combination therapy versus β-lactam monotherapy.[86] Vancomycin monotherapy has been used to treat patients with penicillin-resistant viridans streptococcal endocarditis successfully,[122] and endocarditis also has been treated successfully with linezolid[179] or ceftriaxone[234] monotherapy.

Frequent dosing of antibiotics generally has been recommended; however, viridans streptococci exposed to penicillin or cephalosporin plus aminoglycoside combinations appear to be susceptible to a post-antibiotic effect.[40,135,142] Consequently, longer dosing intervals may be satisfactory, but data are insufficient currently to support a recommendation. Viridans streptococcal endocarditis usually is treated for 4 to 6 weeks; the duration of therapy for infections at other sites has not been studied but generally can be guided by site-specific practice and individual clinical response.

In the treatment of endocarditis, penetration of antibiotics into the fibrin vegetation may be impeded markedly. Viridans streptococci produce an exopolysaccharide composed predominantly of dextran, which may limit penetration. Experimental studies indicate that the degree of exopolysaccharide production by viridans streptococcal strains affects the success rate of antimicrobial therapy.[199] In accord with this observation, administration of dextranase to animals with experimental viridans streptococcal endocarditis enhances antibiotic efficacy.[168] In the future, such adjuvant therapies designed to reduce the size or density of valvular vegetations may offer promise for patients not helped by conventional antibiotic therapy for endocarditis.

Another setting in which adjuvant therapy may be considered is viridans streptococcal sepsis in neutropenic patients who have received cytarabine chemotherapy. One uncontrolled trial suggested that the early addition of high doses of corticosteroids to the antimicrobial therapeutic regimen may reduce the incidence of associated ARDS and death.[66] However, data are insufficient to recommend this approach routinely.

PREVENTION

Attempts to prevent viridans streptococcal infection have focused on three distinct settings: prevention of caries, prevention of endocarditis, and prevention of sepsis in neutropenic patients with cancer. Efforts have been successful in the former two settings. However, the emergence of penicillin-resistant viridans streptococci and concern about the possible emergence of vancomycin resistance highlight the need for new approaches to prevent infection with these ubiquitous organisms. In developing such methods, investigators should not forget that the resistance to colonization provided by viridans streptococci can protect the host from more virulent pathogens (see "Epidemiology").

The incidence of caries in the United States has been reduced sharply by fluoridation of water supplies, inclusion of fluoride in toothpaste, and modification of diet (e.g., use of sugar substi-

tutes). Fluoride acts as an antibacterial agent that also strengthens resistance of the teeth to invasion by bacteria. The use of dental varnishes, gels, and rinses that contain fluoride or other antibacterial agents such as chlorhexidine or vancomycin may be beneficial in selected cases.[88,130,158,178]

The American Heart Association has led a successful effort to prevent the development of endocarditis by systemic antibiotic prophylaxis of patients with known endocardial defects who are undergoing dental procedures.[58] These efforts are aimed especially at preventing viridans streptococcal endocarditis, and penicillin is the antibiotic used most commonly. The mechanism or mechanisms by which antibiotic prophylaxis prevents endocarditis are not understood completely. In animals, endocarditis can be prevented by the administration of bacteriostatic antibiotics and by maintenance of serum levels of bactericidal antibiotics that are well below the minimal inhibitory concentration for the colonizing viridans streptococci.[102] Vancomycin has been observed to prevent the development of vancomycin-tolerant *S. sanguis* endocarditis in experimentally challenged animals without reducing the incidence or level of bacteremia; thus, antibiotics may prevent endocarditis by reducing bacterial adherence to endocardium.[20] This hypothesis is supported by a study in which bacteremia, in some cases with antibiotic-resistant organisms, developed in 21 percent of children receiving antibiotic prophylaxis, but endocarditis rarely occurred.[115] However, studies in animals have indicated that the probability of preventing endocarditis is correlated with the antibiotic susceptibility of the challenging streptococcal strains.[115]

Prophylaxis should be targeted carefully[264] and administered immediately before dental procedures are initiated. Increased numbers of antibiotic-resistant viridans streptococci can be detected within 6 hours of administration of antibiotic treatment, and they persist for 9 days or longer.[143] Experimental studies of the prevention of endocarditis by the administration of antibiotics *after* challenge with bacterial inocula have yielded inconsistent results,[22,125,152] and the clinical utility of this approach is not known. Topical treatment with vancomycin or chlorhexidine has been advocated as an adjuvant to prevent the development of endocarditis, but the efficacy of this approach has not been proved.[252,289]

In recent years, viridans streptococcal infections have become a major problem in neutropenic patients with cancer and in recipients of bone marrow transplants. Because penicillin-resistant viridans streptococci are widespread, some cancer centers include vancomycin in the initial empiric antibiotic regimen for neutropenic patients with unexplained fever.[235] In addition, despite concern about the possibility of inducing vancomycin-resistant bacterial strains, physicians managing bone marrow transplant units are administering intravenous vancomycin prophylactically to high-risk patients in an effort to prevent the development of viridans streptococcal sepsis; the results of an observational cohort study support this practice.[124]

Two noncontrolled trials of oral vancomycin paste[15] or vancomycin mouthwash[37] in children who were receiving cytotoxic chemotherapy suggested efficacy in the prevention of viridans streptococcal infection. However, increased colonization and infection with vancomycin-resistant enterococci are a predictable consequence of increased vancomycin use, which has prompted the Centers for Disease Control and Prevention (CDC) to recommend that empiric vancomycin therapy be avoided when feasible and has led investigators to explore alternatives to the empiric or prophylactic use of vancomycin.

In a comparative trial, penicillin prophylaxis was superior to TMP-SMX prophylaxis in preventing viridans streptococcal infections in patients with cancer despite extensive colonization with penicillin-resistant streptococci.[109] In other studies, oral administration of penicillin or roxithromycin, a macrolide antibiotic, also appeared to reduce the incidence of viridans streptococcal infection in patients with cancer in comparison to historical controls.[61,215,244] In contrast, in a study of prophylactic administration of ampicillin to patients receiving autologous bone marrow transplants, no reduction in the incidence of viridans streptococcal sepsis occurred, whereas the incidence of penicillin resistance increased.[26] Increased penicillin resistance associated with penicillin prophylaxis has been noted in other prophylactic trials as well.[244] The CDC does not recommend the routine use of penicillin prophylaxis in patients receiving bone marrow transplants.[108]

Levofloxacin prophylaxis currently is used commonly to prevent bacterial infections in adults with cancer, but viridans streptococci rapidly develop quinolone resistance, a point of concern.[261] Innovative prophylactic methods and carefully designed clinical trials are needed to identify effective prophylactic measures, especially for patient cohorts at high risk such as children receiving chemotherapy for acute myeloid leukemia.

REFERENCES

1. Adams, J. T., and Faix, R. G.: *Streptococcus mitis* infection in newborns. J. Perinatol. *14*:473-478, 1994.
2. Adeotoye, O., and Kupfer, R.: *Streptococcus viridans* vertebral osteomyelitis. J. R. Soc. Med. *92*:306-307, 1999.
3. Alaluusua, S.: Transmission of mutans streptococci. Proc. Finn. Dent. Soc. *87*:443-447, 1991.
4. Alam, S., Brailsford, S. R., Whiley, R. A., et al.: PCR-based methods for genotyping viridans group streptococci. J. Clin. Microbiol. *37*:2772-2776, 1999.
5. Albini, B., Nisengard, R. J., Glurich, I., et al.: *Streptococcus mutans*–induced nephritis in rabbits. Am. J. Pathol. *118*:408-418, 1985.
6. Alcaide, F., Carratala, J., Linares, J., et al.: In vitro activities of eight macrolide antibiotics and RP-59500 (quinupristin-dalfopristin) against viridans group streptococci isolated from blood of neutropenic cancer patients. Antimicrob. Agents Chemother. *40*:2117-2120, 1996.
7. Alvarez, M., Alvarez, M. E., Maiz, L., et al.: Antimicrobial susceptibility profiles of oropharyngeal viridans group streptococci isolates from cystic fibrosis and non-cystic fibrosis patients. Microb. Drug Resist. *4*:123-128, 1998.
8. Anderson, M. H., Molvar, M. P., and Powell, L. V.: Treating dental caries as an infectious disease. Oper. Dent. *16*:21-28, 1991.
9. Ariel, I., and Singer, D. B.: *Streptococcus viridans* infections in midgestation. Pediatr. Pathol. *11*:75-83, 1991.
10. Arning, M., Gehrt, A., Aul, C., et al.: Septicemia due to *Streptococcus mitis* in neutropenic patients with acute leukemia. Blut *61*:364-368, 1990.
11. Arnold, R. R., Mestecky, J., and McGhee, J. R.: Naturally occurring secretory immunoglobulin A antibodies to *Streptococcus mutans* in human colostrum and saliva. Infect. Immun. *14*:355-362, 1976.
12. Asikainen, S., and Alaluusua, S.: Bacteriology of dental infections. Eur. Heart. J. *14*(Suppl. K):43-50, 1993.
13. Awada, A., van der Auwera, P., Meunier, F., et al.: Streptococcal and enterococcal bacteremia in patients with cancer. Clin. Infect. Dis. *15*:33-48, 1992.
14. Barbadillo, C., Trujillo, A., Cuende, E., et al.: Septic arthritis due to *Streptococcus viridans*. Clin. Exp. Rheumatol. *8*:520-521, 1990.
15. Barker, G. J., Call, S. K., and Gamis, A. S.: Oral care with vancomycin paste for reduction in incidence of alpha-hemolytic streptococcal sepsis. J. Pediatr. Hematol. Oncol. *17*:151-155, 1995.
16. Bateman, N. T., Eykyn, S. J., and Phillips, I.: Pyogenic liver abscess caused by *Streptococcus milleri*. Lancet *1*:657-659, 1975.
17. Beck, A.: Interference by an alpha-hemolytic *Streptococcus* of beta-hemolytic pathogenic streptococci. Inflammation *3*:463-465, 1979.
18. Benabdelmoumene, S., Dumont, S., Petit, C., et al.: Activation of human monocytes by *Streptococcus mutans* serotype f polysaccharide: Immunoglobulin G Fc receptor expression and tumor necrosis factor and interleukin-1 production. Infect. Immun. *59*:3261-3266, 1991.
19. Berlot, G., Tomasini, A., Cioffi, V., et al.: Fatal *Streptococcus viridans* descending mediastinitis: Case report and review of the literature. Eur. J. Emerg. Med. *4*:111-114, 1997.
20. Bernard, J. P., Francioli, P., Glauser, M.: Vancomycin prophylaxis of experimental *Streptococcus sanguis*: Inhibition of bacterial adherence rather than bacterial killing. J. Clin. Invest. *68*:1113-1116, 1981.
21. Berner, R., Sauter, S., Duffner, U., et al.: Bacteremic episodes in pediatric oncologic patients, especially caused by the *Streptococcus viridans* group. Klin. Padiatr. *210*:256-260, 1998.
22. Berney, P., and Francioli, P.: Successful prophylaxis of experimental streptococcal endocarditis with single-dose amoxicillin administered after bacterial challenge. J. Infect. Dis. *161*:281-285, 1990.
23. Bert, F., Noussair, L., Lambert-Zechovsky, N., et al.: Viridans group streptococci: An underestimated cause of spontaneous bacterial peritonitis in cirrhotic patients with ascites. Eur. J. Gastroenterol. Hepatol. *17*:929-933, 2005.
24. Bertrand, B., Rombaux, P., Eloy, P., et al.: Sinusitis of dental origin. Acta Otorhinolaryngol. Belg. *51*:315-322, 1997.
25. Bignardi, G. E., and Isaacs, D.: Neonatal meningitis due to *Streptococcus mitis*. Rev. Infect. Dis. *11*:86-88, 1989.
26. Bilgrami, S., Feingold, J. M., Dorsky, D., et al.: *Streptococcus viridans* bacteremia following autologous peripheral blood stem cell transplantation. Bone Marrow Transplant. *21*:591-595, 1998.
27. Bisno, A. L., Dismukes, W. E., Durack, D. T., et al.: Antimicrobial treatment of infective endocarditis due to viridans streptococci, enterococci, and staphylococci. J. A. M. A. *261*:1471-1477, 1989.
28. Bochud, P. Y., Calandra, T., and Francioli, P.: Bacteremia due to viridans streptococci in neutropenic patients: A review. Am. J. Med. *97*:256-264, 1994.
29. Bochud, P. Y., Eggiman, P., Calandra, T., et al.: Bacteremia due to viridans *Streptococcus* in neutropenic patients with cancer: Clinical spectrum and risk factors. Clin. Infect. Dis. *18*:25-31, 1994.
30. Boenning, D. A., Nelson, L. P., and Campos, J. M.: Relatively penicillin-resistant *Streptococcus sanguis* endocarditis in an adolescent. Pediatr. Infect. Dis. J. *7*:205-207, 1988.
31. Bos, A. P., Fetter, W. P., Baerts, W., et al.: Streptococcal pharyngitis and epiglottitis in a newborn infant. Eur. J. Pediatr. *151*:874-875, 1992.
32. Bratthall, D.: Mutans streptococci: Dental, oral and global aspects. J. Indian Soc. Pedod. Prev. Dent. *9*:4-12, 1991.
33. Bromberg, K., Orson, J. M., Triedman, R., et al.: Erythromycin-resistant *Streptococcus viridans* in oral flora with prolonged erythromycin therapy. Ann. Intern. Med. *93*:931-932, 1980.
34. Broughton, R. A., Krafka, R., and Baker, C. J.: Non–group D alpha-hemolytic streptococci: New neonatal pathogens. J. Pediatr. *99*:450-454, 1981.
35. Bruckner, L., and Gigliotti, F.: Viridans group streptococcal infections among children with cancer and the importance of emerging antibiotic resistance. Semin. Pediatr. Infect. Dis. *17*:153-160, 2006.
36. Bruckner, L. B., Korones, D. N., Karnauchow, T., et al.: High incidence of penicillin resistance among alpha-hemolytic streptococcus isolated from the blood of children with cancer. J. Pediatr. *140*:20-26, 2002.
37. Brunet, A. S., Ploton, C., Galambrun, C., et al.: Low incidence of sepsis due to viridans streptococci in a ten-year retrospective study of pediatric acute myeloid leukemia. Blood Cancer *47*:765-772, 2006.
38. Buchman, A. L.: *Streptococcus viridans* osteomyelitis with endocarditis presenting as acute onset lower back pain. J. Emerg. Med. *8*:291-294, 1990.
39. Burden, A. D., Oppenheim, B. A., Crowther, D., et al.: Viridans streptococcal bacteraemia in patients with haematological and solid malignancies. Eur. J. Cancer *27*:409-411, 1991.
40. Buxbaum, A., and Georgopoulos, A.: Postantibiotic effect of ceftriaxone and gentamicin alone and in combination on *Klebsiella pneumoniae, Pseudomonas aeruginosa* and *Streptococcus viridans*. Infection *24*:459-464, 1996.
41. Carlsson, J.: A numerical taxonomic study of human oral streptococci. Odontol. Rev. *19*:137-160, 1968.
42. Caufield, P. W., Cutter, G. R., and Dasanayake, A. P.: Initial acquisition of mutans streptococci by infants: Evidence for a discrete window of infectivity. J. Dent. Res. *72*:37-45, 1993.
43. Caufield, P. W., Dasanayake, A. P., Li, Y., et al.: Natural history of *Streptococcus sanguinis* in the oral cavity of infants: Evidence for a discrete window of infectivity. Infect. Immun. *68*:4018-4023, 2000.
44. Caufield, P. W., and Wannemuehler, Y. M.: In vitro susceptibility of *Streptococcus mutans* 6715 to iodine and sodium fluoride, singly and in combination, at various pH values. Antimicrob. Agents Chemother. *22*:115-119, 1982.
45. Chalkley, L., Schuster, C., Potgieter, E., et al.: Relatedness between *Streptococcus pneumoniae* and viridans streptococci: Transfer of penicillin resistance determinants and immunological similarities of penicillin-binding proteins. F. E. M. S. Microbiol. Lett. *69*:35-42, 1991.
46. Chambers, H. F., Xiang, Q., Liu, Q., et al.: Efficacy of levofloxacin for experimental aortic-valve endocarditis in rabbits infected with viridans group streptococcus or *Staphylococcus aureus*. Antimicrob. Agents Chemother. *43*:2742-2746, 1999.
47. Chiu, B.: Multiple infections in carotid atherosclerotic plaques. Am. Heart J. *138*(Suppl.):534-536, 1999.
48. Church, D. L., and Bryant, H. E.: Investigation of a *Streptococcus viridans* pseudobacteremia epidemic at a university teaching hospital. Infect. Control Hosp. Epidemiol. *10*:416-421, 1989.
49. Classen, D. C., Burke, J. P., Ford, C. D., et al.: *Streptococcus mitis* sepsis in bone marrow transplant patients receiving oral antimicrobial prophylaxis. Am. J. Med. *89*:441-446, 1990.
50. Cohen, P., Donnelly, J. P., Worsley, A. M., et al.: Septicaemia caused by viridans streptococci in neutropenic patients with leukaemia. Lancet *2*:1452-1454, 1983.
51. Coleman, G., and Williams, R. E. A.: Taxonomy of some human viridans streptococci. *In* Wannamaker, L. W., and Matsen, J. M. (eds.): Streptococci and Streptococcal Diseases: Recognition, Understanding, and Management. New York, Academic Press, 1972, pp. 282-299.
52. Collin, B. A., Leather, H. L., Wingard, J. R., et al.: Evolution, incidence, and susceptibility of bacterial bloodstream isolates from 519 bone marrow transplant patients. Clin. Infect. Dis. *33*:947-953, 2001.

53. Corson, M. A., Postlethwaite, K. P., and Seymour, R. A.: Are dental infections a cause of brain abscess? Case report and review of the literature. Oral Dis. 7:61-65, 2001.

54. Coulter, W. A., Coffey, A., Saunders, I. D., et al.: Bacteremia in children following dental extraction. J. Dent. Res. 69:1691-1695, 1990.

55. Coykendall, A. L.: Classification and identification of the viridans streptococci. Clin. Microbiol. Rev. 2:315-328, 1989.

56. Crompton, N., Griffiths, B. M., Wilson, M., et al.: The transfer of bacteria to, and survival on, dental records. Microbios 99:181-187, 1999.

57. Dajani, A. S., Law, D. J., Bollinger, R. O., et al.: Ultrastructural and biochemical alterations effected by viridin B, a bacterocin of alpha-hemolytic streptococci. Infect. Immun. 14:776-782, 1976.

58. Dajani, A. S., Taubert, K. A., Wilson, W., et al.: Prevention of bacterial endocarditis: Recommendations by the American Heart Association. Clin. Infect. Dis. 25:1448-1458, 1997.

59. Dajani, A. S., Tom, M. C., and Law, D. J.: Viridins, bacteriocins of alpha-hemolytic streptococci: Isolation, characterization, and partial purification. Antimicrob. Agents Chemother. 9:81-88, 1976.

60. de Azavedo, J. C., Trpeski, L., Pong-Porter, S., et al.: In vitro activities of fluoroquinolones against antibiotic-resistant blood culture isolates of viridans group streptococci from across Canada. Antimicrob. Agents Chemother. 43:2299-2301, 1999.

61. Dekker, A. W., Rozenberg-Arska, M., and Verdonck, L. F.: Prevention of bacteremias caused by alpha-hemolytic streptococci by roxithromycin in patients treated with intensive cytotoxic treatment. Hamatol. Bluttransfusion 33:551-554, 1990.

62. Demers, C., Tremblay, M., and Lacourciere, Y.: Acute vertebral osteomyelitis complicating Streptococcus sanguis endocarditis. Ann. Rheum. Dis. 47:333-336, 1988.

63. Diekema, D. J., Beach, M. L., and Pfaller, M. A.: Antimicrobial resistance in viridans group streptococci among patients with and without the diagnosis of cancer in the USA, Canada and Latin America. Clin. Microbiol. Infect. 7:152-157, 2001.

64. Docze, A., Mraz, M., Grey, E., et al.: Penicillin resistance in viridans streptococcal bacteremia is related with high mortality. Scand. J. Infect. Dis. 35:916-917, 2003.

65. Doern, G. V., Ferraro, M. J., Brueggemann, A. B., et al.: Emergence of high rates of antimicrobial resistance among viridans group streptococci in the United States. Antimicrob. Agents Chemother. 40:891-894, 1996.

66. Dompeling, E. C., Donnelly, J. P., Raemaekers, J. M., et al.: Pre-emptive administration of corticosteroids prevents the development of ARDS associated with Streptococcus mitis bacteremia following chemotherapy with high-dose cytarabine. Ann. Hematol. 69:69-71, 1994.

67. Donnelly, J. P., Dompeling, E. C., Meis, J. F., et al.: Bacteremia due to oral viridans streptococci in neutropenic patients with cancer: Cytostatics are a more important risk factor than antibacterial prophylaxis. Clin. Infect. Dis. 20:469-470, 1995.

68. Douglas, C. W., Heath, J., Hampton, K. K., et al.: Identity of viridans streptococci isolated from cases of infective endocarditis. J. Med. Microbiol. 39:179-182, 1993.

69. Dowson, C. G., Coffey, T. J., Kell, C., et al.: Evolution of penicillin resistance in Streptococcus pneumoniae: The role of Streptococcus mitis in the formation of a low-affinity PBP2B in S. pneumoniae. Mol. Microbiol. 9:635-643, 1993.

70. Dowson, C. G., Hutchison, A., Woodford, N., et al.: Penicillin-resistant viridans streptococci have obtained altered penicillin-binding protein genes from penicillin-resistant strains of Streptococcus pneumoniae. Proc. Natl. Acad. Sci. U. S. A. 87:5858-5862, 1990.

71. Dwyer, R., and Ringertz, S.: Viridans streptococci in blood cultures. Can we see any patterns of species related to patient category? Review of 229 cases of positive cultures with viridans streptococci. A. P. M. I. S. 105:972-974, 1997.

72. Edelstein, B. L.: The medical management of dental caries. J. Am. Dent. Assoc. 125(Suppl.):31-39, 1994.

73. Edwardsson, S., and Mejare, B.: Streptococcus milleri (Guthof) and Streptococcus mutans in the mouths of infants before and after tooth eruption. Arch. Oral Biol. 23:811-814, 1978.

74. Elliott, R. H., and Dunbar, J. M.: Antibiotic sensitivity of oral alpha-haemolytic Streptococcus from children with congenital or acquired cardiac disease: A prolonged survey. Br. Dent. J. 142:283-285, 1977.

75. Elting, L. S., Bodey, G. P., and Keefe, B. H.: Septicemia and shock syndrome due to viridans streptococci: A case-control study of predisposing factors. Clin. Infect. Dis. 14:1201-1207, 1992.

76. Elting, L. S., Rubenstein, E. B., Rolston, K. V. I., et al.: Outcomes of bacteremia in patients with cancer and neutropenia: Observations from two decades of epidemiological and clinical trials. Clin. Infect. Dis. 25:247-259, 1997.

77. Eng, R. H., Mangia, A. J., Smith, S. M., et al.: Meningitis following bacteremia with Streptococcus sanguis. N. Y. State J. Med. 89:625-626, 1989.

78. Engel, A., Kern, P., and Kern, W. V.: Levels of cytokines and cytokine inhibitors in the neutropenic patient with alpha-hemolytic streptococcus shock syndrome. Clin. Infect. Dis. 23:785-789, 1996.

79. Engelhard, D., Elishoov, H., Or, R., et al.: Cytosine arabinoside as a major risk factor for Streptococcus viridans septicemia following bone marrow transplantation: A 5-year prospective study. Bone Marrow Transplant. 16:565-570, 1995.

80. English, B. K., Patrick, C. C., Orlicek, S. L., et al.: Lipoteichoic acid from viridans streptococci induces the production of tumor necrosis factor and nitric oxide by murine macrophages. J. Infect. Dis. 174:1348-1351, 1996.

81. Entenza, J. M., Caldelari, I., Glauser, M. P., et al.: Importance of genotypic and phenotypic tolerance in the treatment of experimental endocarditis due to Streptococcus gordonii. J. Infect. Dis. 175:70-76, 1997.

82. Enting, R. H., de Gans, J., Blankevoort, J. P., et al.: Meningitis due to viridans streptococci in adults. J. Neurol. 244:435-438, 1997.

83. Erickson, P. R., and Herzberg, M. C.: Emergence of antibiotic resistant Streptococcus sanguis in dental plaque of children after frequent antibiotic therapy. Pediatr. Dent. 21:181-185, 1999.

84. Erverdi, N., Kadir, T., Ozkan, H., et al.: Investigation of bacteremia after orthodontic banding. Am. J. Orthod. Dentofacial Orthop. 116:687-690, 1999.

85. Facklam, R. R.: Physiological differentiation of viridans streptococci. J. Clin. Microbiol. 5:184-201, 1977.

86. Falagas, M. E., Matthalou, D. K., and Bliziotis, I. A.: The role of aminoglycosides in combination with a beta-lactam for the treatment of bacterial endocarditis: A meta-analysis of comparative trials. J. Antimicrob. Chemother. 57:639-647, 2006.

87. Farber, B. F., Eliopoulos, G. M., Ward, J. I., et al.: Multiply resistant viridans streptococci: Susceptibility to beta-lactam antibiotics and comparison of penicillin-binding protein patterns. Antimicrob. Agents Chemother. 24:702-705, 1983.

88. Fine, J. B., Harper, D. S., Gordon, J. M., et al.: Short-term microbiological and clinical effects of subgingival irrigation with an antimicrobial mouthrinse. J. Periodontol. 65:30-36, 1994.

89. Flynn, C. E., and Ruoff, K. L.: Identification of "Streptococcus milleri" group isolates to the species level with a commercially available rapid test system. J. Clin. Microbiol. 33:2704-2706, 1995.

90. Ford, I., Douglas, C. W., Preston, F. E., et al.: Mechanisms of platelet aggregation by Streptococcus sanguis, a causative organism in infective endocarditis. Br. J. Haematol. 84:95-100, 1993.

91. Ford, J. M., and DuBois, R. E.: Multiloculated hepatic abscess caused by alpha-hemolytic Streptococcus. South. Med. J. 77:514-516, 1984.

92. Francioli, P. B., and Glauser, M. P.: Synergistic activity of ceftriaxone combined with netilmicin administered once daily for treatment of experimental streptococcal endocarditis. Antimicrob. Agents Chemother. 37:207-212, 1993.

93. Frandsen, E. V., Pedrazzoli, V., and Kilian, M.: Ecology of viridans streptococci in the oral cavity and pharynx. Oral Microbiol. Immunol. 6:129-133, 1991.

94. Fraser, J. J., Jr., Marks, M. I., and Welch, D. F.: Neonatal sepsis and meningitis due to alpha-hemolytic Streptococcus. South. Med. J. 76:401-402, 1983.

95. Freedman, R. M., and Baltimore, R.: Fatal Streptococcus viridans septicemia and meningitis: Relationship to fetal scalp electrode monitoring. J. Perinatol. 10:272-274, 1990.

96. Freitas, M., Casteio, A., Petty, G., et al.: Viridans streptococci causing community acquired pneumonia. Arch. Dis. Child. 91:779-780, 2006.

97. Fujimori, I., Kikushima, K., Hisamatsu, K., et al.: Interaction between oral alpha-streptococci and group A streptococci in patients with tonsillitis. Ann. Otol. Rhinol. Laryngol. 106:571-574, 1997.

98. Garnier, F., Gerbaud, G., Courvalin, P., et al.: Identification of clinically relevant viridans group streptococci to the species level by PCR. J. Clin. Microbiol. 35:2337-2341, 1997.

99. Gassas, A., Grant, R., Richardson, S., et al.: Predictors of viridans streptococcal shock syndrome in bacteremic children with cancer and stem cell transplant recipients. J. Clin. Oncol. 22:1222-1227, 2004.

100. George, S., Wadhera, A., Mersich, K., et al.: Liver abscess due to Streptococcus sanguis. Clin. Infect. Dis. 22:191-192, 1996.

101. Ghaffar, F., Friedland, I. R., Katz, K., et al.: Increased carriage of resistant non-pneumococcal alpha-hemolytic streptococci after antibiotic therapy. J. Pediatr. 135:618-623, 1999.

102. Glauser, M. P., and Francioli, P.: Successful prophylaxis against experimental streptococcal endocarditis with bacteriostatic antibiotics. J. Infect. Dis. 146:806-810, 1982.

103. Goldfarb, J., Wormser, G. P., and Glaser, J. H.: Meningitis caused by multiply antibiotic-resistant viridans streptococci. J. Pediatr. 105:891-895, 1984.

104. Goolam Mahomed, A., Feldman, C., Smith, C., et al.: Does primary Streptococcus viridans pneumonia exist? S. Afr. Med. J. 82:432-434, 1992.

105. Graber, C. J., de Almeida, K. N., Atkinson, J. C., et al.: Dental health and viridans streptococcal bacteremia in allogeneic hematopoietic stem cell transplant recipients. Bone Marrow Transplant. 27:537-542, 2001.

106. Grindefjord, M., Dahllof, G., Wikner, S., et al.: Prevalence of mutans streptococci in one-year-old children. Oral Microbiol. Immunol. 6:280-283, 1991.

107. Groot-Loonen, J. J., van der Noordaa, J., de Kraker, J., et al.: Alpha-hemolytic streptococcal septicemia with severe complications during neutropenia in childhood cancer. Pediatr. Hematol. Oncol. 4:323-328, 1987.

108. Guidelines for preventing opportunistic infections among hematopoietic stem cell transplant recipients. M. M. W. R. Recomm. Rep. 49(RR-10):1-125, 2000.

109. Guiot, H. F., van der Meer, J. W., van den Broek, P. J., et al.: Prevention of viridans-group streptococcal septicemia in oncohematologic patients: A controlled comparative study on the effect of penicillin G cotrimoxazole. Ann. Hematol. 64:260-265, 1992.

110. Hamada, S., Masuda, N., and Kotani, S.: Isolation and serotyping of *Streptococcus mutans* from teeth and feces of children. J. Clin. Microbiol. *11*:314-318, 1980.

111. Han, X. Y., Kamana, M., and Rolston, K. V.: Viridans streptococci isolated by culture from blood of cancer patients: Clinical and microbiologic analysis of 50 cases. J. Clin. Microbiol. *44*:160-165, 2006.

112. Hanage, W. P., and Cohen, J.: Stimulation of cytokine release and adhesion molecule expression by products of viridans streptococci. J. Infect. Dis. *185*:357-367, 2002.

113. Heiro, M., Helenius, H., Makila, S., et al.: Infective endocarditis in a Finnish teaching hospital: A study on 326 episodes treated during 1980-2004. Heart *92*:1457-1462, 2006.

114. Henslee, J., Bostrom, B., Weisdorf, D., et al.: Streptococcal sepsis in bone marrow transplant patients. Lancet *1*:393, 1984.

115. Hess, J., Dankert, J., and Durack, D.: Significance of penicillin tolerance in vivo: Prevention of experimental *Streptococcus sanguis* endocarditis. J. Antimicrob. Chemother. *11*:555-564, 1983.

116. Hirschfeld, Z., Friedman, M., Golomb, G., et al.: New sustained release dosage form of chlorhexidine for dental use: Use for plaque control in partial denture wearers. J. Oral Rehabil. *11*:477-482, 1984.

117. Hoecker, J. L., Pickering, L. K., Groschel, D., et al.: *Streptococcus salivarius* sepsis in children with malignancies. J. Pediatr. *92*:337-338, 1978.

118. Hogg, S. D., and Manning, J. E.: Inhibition of adhesion of viridans streptococci to fibronectin-coated hydroxyapatite beads by lipoteichoic acid. J. Appl. Bacteriol. *65*:483-489, 1988.

119. Holbrook, W. P., Olafsdottir, D., Magnusson, H. B., et al.: Penicillin tolerance among oral streptococci. J. Med. Microbiol. *27*:17-22, 1988.

120. Holmberg, H., Danielsson, D., Hardie, J., et al.: Cross-reactions between alpha-streptococci and Omniserum, a polyvalent pneumococcal serum, demonstrated by direct immunofluorescence, immunoelectroosmophoresis, and latex agglutination. J. Clin. Microbiol. *21*:745-748, 1985.

121. Hook, E. W., III, and Sande, M. A.: Role of the vegetation in experimental *Streptococcus viridans* endocarditis. Infect. Immun. *10*:1433-1438, 1974.

122. Hsu, R. B., and Lin, F. Y.: Effect of penicillin resistance on presentation and outcome of nonenterococcal streptococcal infective endocarditis. Cardiology *105*:234-239, 2006.

123. Inoue, S., Boyer, D., and Gordon, R.: Interstitial pneumonia and alpha-hemolytic *Streptococcus* sepsis in a child with malignancy who recently received cytosine arabinoside. Pediatr. Infect. Dis. J. *9*:598-600, 1990.

124. Jaffe, D., Jakubowski, A., Sepkowitz, K., et al.: Prevention of peritransplantation viridans streptococcal bacteremia with early vancomycin administration: A single-center observational cohort study. Clin. Infect. Dis. *39*:1625-1632, 2004.

125. James, J., MacFarlane, T. W., McGowan, D. A., et al.: Failure of postbacteraemia delayed antibiotic prophylaxis of experimental rabbit endocarditis. J. Antimicrob. Chemother. *20*:883-885, 1987.

126. Janoir, C., Podglajen, I., Kitzis, M. D., et al.: In vitro exchange of fluoroquinolone resistance determinants between *Streptococcus pneumoniae* and viridans streptococci and genomic organization of the parE-parC region in *S. mitis*. J. Infect. Dis. *180*:555-558, 1999.

127. Jarvinen, H., Tenovuo, J., and Huovinen, P.: In vitro susceptibility of *Streptococcus mutans* to chlorhexidine and six other antimicrobial agents. Antimicrob. Agents Chemother. *37*:1158-1159, 1993.

128. Jerng, J. S., Hsueh, P. R., Teng, L. J., et al.: Empyema thoracis and lung abscess caused by viridans streptococci. Am. J. Respir. Crit. Care Med. *156*:1508-1514, 1997.

129. Jonsson, M., and Swedberg, G.: Macrolide resistance can be transferred by conjugation from viridans streptococci to *Streptococcus pyogenes*. Int. J. Antimicrob. Agents *28*:101-103, 2006.

130. Jordan, H. V., and De Paola, P. F.: Effect of a topically applied 3 percent vancomycin gel on *Streptococcus mutans* on different tooth surfaces. J. Dent. Res. *53*:115-120, 1974.

131. Kaufhold, A., and Potgieter, E.: Chromosomally mediated high-level gentamicin resistance in *Streptococcus mitis*. Antimicrob. Agents Chemother. *37*:2740-2742, 1993.

132. Kawamura, Y., Hou, X. G., Sultana, F., et al.: Transfer of *Streptococcus adjacens* and *Streptococcus defectivus* to *Abiotrophia* gen. nov. as *Abiotrophia adiacens* comb. nov. and *Abiotrophia defectiva* comb. nov., respectively. Int. J. Syst. Bacteriol. *45*:798-803, 1995.

133. Kennedy, H. F., Gemmell, C. G., Bagg, J., et al.: Antimicrobial susceptibility of blood culture isolates of viridans streptococci: Relationship to a change in empirical antibiotic therapy in febrile neutropenia. J. Antimicrob. Chemother. *47*:693-696, 2001.

134. Kerr, K. G., Armitage, H. T., and McWhinney, P. H.: Activity of quinolones against viridans group streptococci isolated from blood cultures of patients with haematological malignancy. Support Care Cancer *7*:28-30, 1999.

135. Kikuchi, K., Enari, T., Minami, S., et al.: Postantibiotic effects and postantibiotic sub-MIC effects of benzylpenicillin on viridans streptococci isolated from patients with infective endocarditis. J. Antimicrob. Chemother. *34*:687-696, 1994.

136. Kilpper-Balz, R., and Schleifer, K.-H.: Transfer of *Streptococcus morbillorum* to the genus *Gemella* as *Gemella haemolysans*. Int. J. Syst. Bacteriol. *38*:442-443, 1988.

137. Klastersky, J.: Role of quinupristin/dalfopristin in the treatment of gram-positive nosocomial infections in haematological or oncological patients. Cancer Treat. Rev. *29*:431-440, 2003.

138. Kontiainen, S., and Sivonen, A.: Multiply resistant *Streptococcus mitis* isolated from conjunctival exudate of newborns. Eur. J. Clin. Microbiol. *6*:53-55, 1987.

139. Kurland, S., Enghoff, E., Landelius, J., et al.: A 10-year retrospective study of infective endocarditis at a university hospital with special regard to the timing of surgical evaluation in *S. viridans* endocarditis. Scand. J. Infect. Dis. *31*:87-91, 1999.

140. Larsen, T., and Fiehn, N. E.: Resistance of *Streptococcus sanguis* biofilms to antimicrobial agents. A. P. M. I. S. *104*:280-284, 1996.

141. Leblanc, L., Leverger, G., Arlet, G., et al.: Frequency and severity of systemic infections caused by *Streptococcus mitis* and *sanguis* II in neutropenic children. Pathol. Biol. (Paris) *37*:459-464, 1989.

142. Lee, S. Y.: Postantibiotic effects and postantibiotic sub-MIC effects of amoxicillin on *Streptococcus gordonii* and *Streptococcus sanguis*. J. Chemother. *12*:379-384, 2000.

143. Leviner, E., Tzukert, A. A., Benoliel, R., et al.: Development of resistant oral viridans streptococci after administration of prophylactic antibiotics: Time management in the dental treatment of patients susceptible to infective endocarditis. Oral Surg. Oral Med. Oral Pathol. *64*:417-420, 1987.

144. Levy, C. S., Kogulan, P., Gill, V. J., et al.: Endocarditis caused by penicillin-resistant viridans streptococci: 2 cases and controversies in therapy. Clin. Infect. Dis. *33*:577-579, 2001.

145. Lilien, L. D., Wilks, A. K., and Yeh, T. F.: *Streptococcus sanguis* biotype II meningitis in a premature infant. Clin. Pediatr. (Phila.) *21*:465, 1982.

146. Loesche, W. J., Schork, A., Terpenning, M. S., et al.: Assessing the relationship between dental disease and coronary heart disease in elderly U.S. veterans. J. Am. Dent. Assoc. *129*:301-311, 1998.

147. Lowrance, J. H., Baddour, L. M., and Simpson, W. A.: The role of fibronectin binding in the rat model of experimental endocarditis caused by *Streptococcus sanguis*. J. Clin. Invest. *86*:7-13, 1990.

148. Lowy, F. D., Chang, D. S., Neuhaus, E. G., et al.: Effect of penicillin on the adherence of *Streptococcus sanguis* in vitro and in the rabbit model of endocarditis. J. Clin. Invest. *71*:668-675, 1983.

149. Lu, C. H., Chang, W. N., and Chang, H. W.: Adults with meningitis caused by viridans streptococci. Infection *29*:305-309, 2001.

150. Lu, H. Z., Weng, X. H., Zhu, B., et al.: Major outbreak of toxic shock–like syndrome caused by *Streptococcus mitis*. J. Clin. Microbiol. *41*:3051-3055, 2003.

151. Macaluso, A., Simmang, C., and Anthony, T.: *Streptococcus sanguis* bacteremia and colorectal cancer. South. Med. J. *91*:206-207, 1998.

152. Malinverni, R., Bille, J., and Glauser, M. P.: Single-dose rifampin prophylaxis for experimental endocarditis induced by high bacterial inocula of viridans streptococci. J. Infect. Dis. *156*:151-157, 1987.

153. Malmberg, E., Birkhed, D., Norvenius, G., et al.: Microorganisms on toothbrushes at day-care centers. Acta Odontol. Scand. *52*:93-98, 1994.

154. Manning, J. E., Hume, E. B., Hunter, N., et al.: An appraisal of the virulence factors associated with streptococcal endocarditis. J. Med. Microbiol. *40*:110-114, 1994.

155. Marrie, T. J.: Bacteremic community-acquired pneumonia due to viridans group streptococci. Clin. Invest. Med. *16*:38-44, 1993.

156. Marron, A., Carratala, J., Alcaide, F., et al.: High rates of resistance to cephalosporins among viridans-group streptococci causing bacteraemia in neutropenic cancer patients. J. Antimicrob. Chemother. *47*:87-91, 2001.

157. Marron, A., Carratala, J., Gonzalez-Barca, E. et al.: Serious complications of bacteremia caused by viridans streptococci in neutropenic patients with cancer. Clin. Infect. Dis. *31*:1126-1130, 2000.

158. Marsh, P. D.: Antimicrobial strategies in the prevention of dental caries. Caries Res. *27*(Suppl. 1):72-76, 1993.

159. Martinez, F., Martin-Luengo, F., Garcia, A., et al.: Treatment with imipenem of experimental endocarditis caused by penicillin-resistant *Streptococcus sanguis*. J. Antimicrob. Chemother. *33*:1201-1207, 1989.

160. Martino, R., Subira, M., Manteiga, R., et al.: Viridans streptococcal bacteremia and viridans streptococcal shock syndrome in neutropenic patients: Comparison between children and adults receiving chemotherapy or undergoing bone marrow transplantation. Clin. Infect. Dis. *20*:476-477, 1995.

161. Matsushita, K., Fujimaki, W., Kato, H., et al.: Immunopathological activities of extracellular products of *Streptococcus mitis*, particularly a superantigenic fraction. Infect. Immun. *63*:785-793, 1995.

162. McBride, M. E., Duncan, W. C., and Knox, J. M.: Bacterial interference of *Neisseria gonorrhoeae* by alpha-haemolytic streptococci. Br. J. Vener. Dis. *56*:235-238, 1980.

163. McWhinney, P. H., Gillespie, S. H., Kibbler, C. C., et al.: *Streptococcus mitis* and ARDS in eutropenic patients. Lancet *337*:429, 1991.

164. Mecrow, I. K., and Ladusans, E. J.: Infective endocarditis in newborn infants with structurally normal hearts. Acta Paediatr. *83*:35-39, 1994.

165. Meddens, M. J., Thompson, J., Eulderink, F., et al.: Role of granulocytes in experimental *Streptococcus sanguis* endocarditis. Infect. Immun. *36*:325-332, 1982.

166. Meddens, M. J., Thompson, J., Mattie, H., et al.: Role of granulocytes in the prevention and therapy of experimental *Streptococcus sanguis* endocarditis in rabbits. Antimicrob. Agents Chemother. *25*:263-267, 1984.

167. Menichetti, F., Del Favero, A., Guerciolini, R., et al.: Viridans streptococci septicemia in cancer patients: A clinical study. Eur. J. Epidemiol. 3:316-318, 1987.

168. Mghir, A. S., Cremieux, A. C., Jambou, R., et al.: Dextranase enhances antibiotic efficacy in experimental viridans streptococcal endocarditis. Antimicrob. Agents Chemother. 38:953-958, 1994.

169. Michalek, S. M., McGhee, J. R., Mestecky, J., et al.: Ingestion of *Streptococcus mutans* induces secretory immunoglobulin A and caries immunity. Science 192:1238-1240, 1976.

170. Michel, R. S., DeFlora, E., Jefferies, J., et al.: Recurrent meningitis in a child with inner ear dysplasia. Pediatr. Infect. Dis. J. 11:336-338, 1992.

171. Mogi, A., Nishi, J. I., Yoshinaga, M., et al.: Increased prevalence of penicillin-resistant viridans group streptococci in Japanese children with upper respiratory infection treated by beta-lactam agents and in those with oncohematologic diseases. Pediatr. Infect. Dis. J. 16:1140-1144, 1997.

172. Molina, J. M., Leport, C., Bure, A., et al.: Clinical and bacterial features of infections caused by *Streptococcus milleri*. Scand. J. Infect. Dis. 23:659-666, 1991.

173. Monefeldt, K., Helgeland, K., and Tollefsen, T.: In vitro activation of the classical pathway of complement by a streptococcal lipoteichoic acid. Oral Microbiol. Immunol. 9:70-76, 1994.

174. Moomjian, A. S., Sokal, M. M., and Vijayan, S.: Pathogenicity of alpha-hemolytic streptococci in the neonate. Am. J. Perinatol. 1:319-321, 1984.

175. Morisaki, I., Mihara, J., Kato, K., et al.: Phenytoin-induced gingival overgrowth in rats infected with *Streptococcus sobrinus* 6715. Arch. Oral Biol. 35:753-758, 1990.

176. Murray, H. W., Gross, K. C., Masur, H., et al.: Serious infections caused by *Streptococcus milleri*. Am. J. Med. 64:759-764, 1978.

177. Nascimento-Carvalho, C. M., Brandileone, M. C., Guerra, M. L., et al.: Do viridans streptococci cause pneumonia in children? Pediatr. Infect. Dis. J. 20:726-728, 2001.

178. Newbrun, E.: Preventing dental caries: Breaking the chain of transmission. J. Am. Dent. Assoc. 123:55-59, 1992.

179. Ng, K. H., Lee, S., Yip, S. F., et al.: A case of *Streptococcus mitis* endocarditis successfully treated by linezolid. Hong Kong Med. J. 11:411-413, 2005.

180. Ohuoba, E. F., Kansal, R. G., Hayden, R. T., et al.: Failure of viridans group streptococci causing bacteremia in pediatric oncology patients to express superantigens. J. Pediatr. Hematol. Oncol. 28:627-629, 2006.

181. Okamoto, Y., Ribeiro, R. C., Srivastava, D. K., et al.: Viridans streptococcal sepsis: Clinical features and complications in childhood acute myeloid leukemia. J. Pediatr. Hematol. Oncol. 25:696-703, 2003.

182. Orlicek, S. L., Branum, K. C., English, B. K., et al.: Viridans streptococcal isolates from patients with septic shock induce tumor necrosis factor-alpha production by murine macrophages. J. Lab. Clin. Med. 130:515-519, 1997.

183. Pan, Y. P., Li, Y., and Caufield, P. W.: Phenotypic and genotypic diversity of *Streptococcus sanguis* in infants. Oral Microbiol. Immunol. 16:235-242, 2001.

184. Parrillo, J. E., Borst, G. C., Mazur, M. H., et al.: Endocarditis due to resistant viridans streptococci during oral penicillin chemoprophylaxis. N. Engl. J. Med. 300:296-300, 1979.

185. Parrish, L. C., Kretzschmar, D. P., and Swan, R. H.: Osteomyelitis associated with chronic periodontitis: A report of three cases. J. Periodontol. 60:716-722, 1989.

186. Pearce, C., Bowden, G. H., Evans, M., et al.: Identification of pioneer viridans streptococci in the oral cavity of human neonates. J. Med. Microbiol. 42:67-72, 1995.

187. Peiris, V., and Oppenheim, B. A.: Antimicrobial activity of cytotoxic drugs may influence isolation of bacteria and fungi from blood cultures. J. Clin. Pathol. 46:1124-1125, 1993.

188. Persson, L., Vikerfors, T., Sjoberg, L., et al.: Increased incidence of bacteraemia due to viridans streptococci in an unselected population of patients with acute myeloid leukaemia. Scand. J. Infect. Dis. 32:615-621, 2000.

189. Peterson, E. M., Shigei, J. T., Woolard, A., et al.: Identification of viridans streptococci by three commercial systems. Am. J. Clin. Pathol. 90:87-91, 1988.

190. Pfaller, M. A., and Jones, R. N.: In vitro evaluation of contemporary beta-lactam drugs tested against viridans group and beta-haemolytic streptococci. Diagn. Microbiol. Infect. Dis. 27:151-154, 1997.

191. Pizzo, P. A., Ladisch, S., and Ribichaud, K.: Treatment of gram-positive septicemia in cancer patients. Cancer 45:206-207, 1980.

192. Pizzo, P. A., Ladisch, S., and Witebsky, F. G.: Alpha-hemolytic streptococci: Clinical significance in the cancer patient. Med. Pediatr. Oncol. 4:367-370, 1978.

193. Poole, P. M., and Wilson, G.: *Streptococcus milleri* in the appendix. J. Clin. Pathol. 30:937-942, 1977.

194. Potgieter, E., Carmichael, M., Koornhof, H. J., et al.: In vitro antimicrobial susceptibility of *viridans* streptococci isolated from blood cultures. Eur. J. Clin. Microbiol. Infect. Dis. 11:543-546, 1992.

195. Potgieter, E., and Chalkley, L. J.: Reciprocal transfer of penicillin resistance genes between *Streptococcus pneumoniae*, *Streptococcus mitior* and *Streptococcus sanguis*. J. Antimicrob. Chemother. 28:463-465, 1991.

196. Prabhu, R. M., Piper, K. E., Baddour, L. M., et al.: Antimicrobial susceptibility patterns among viridans group streptococcal isolates from infective endocarditis patients from 1971 to 1986 and 1994 to 2002. Antimicrob. Agents Chemother. 48:4463-4465, 2004.

197. Prabhu, R. M., Piper, K. E., Litzow, M. R., et al.: Emergence of quinolone resistance among viridans group streptococci isolated from the oropharynx of neutropenic peripheral blood stem cell transplant patients receiving quinolone antimicrobial prophylaxis. Eur. J. Clin. Microbiol. Infect. Dis. 24:832-838, 2005.

198. Pratter, M. R., and Irwin, R. S.: Viridans streptococcal pulmonary parenchymal infections. J. A. M. A. 243:2515-2517, 1980.

199. Pulliam, L., Dall, L., Inokuchi, S., et al.: Effects of exopolysaccharide production by viridans streptococci on penicillin therapy of experimental endocarditis. J. Infect. Dis. 151:153-156, 1985.

200. Quinn, J. P., DiVincenzo, C. A., Lucks, D. A., et al.: Serious infections due to penicillin-resistant strains of viridans streptococci with altered penicillin-binding proteins. J. Infect. Dis. 157:764-769, 1988.

201. Rapeport, K. B., Giron, J. A., and Rosner, F.: *Streptococcus mitis* endocarditis: Report of 17 cases. Arch. Intern. Med. 146:2361-2363, 1986.

202. Razonable, R. R., Litzow, M. R., Khaliq, Y., et al.: Bacteremia due to viridans group streptococci with diminished susceptibility to levofloxacin among neutropenic patients receiving levofloxacin prophylaxis. Clin. Infect. Dis. 34:1469-1474, 2002.

203. Reed, E., Arneson, M., Vaughan, W., et al.: *Streptococcus viridans* (SV): A significant cause of neutropenic fever (NF) that caused death in some patients not empirically treated for gram-positive (GP) bacteria. Proc. Annu. Meet. Am. Soc. Clin. Oncol. 9:A1239, 1990.

204. Ribner, B. S., and Freimer, E. H.: Osteomyelitis caused by viridans streptococci. Arch. Intern. Med. 142:1739, 1982.

205. Richard, P., Amador Del Valle, G., Moreau, P., et al.: Viridans streptococcal bacteraemia in patients with neutropenia. Lancet 345:1607-1609, 1995.

206. Ringden, O., Heimdahl, A., Lonnqvist, B., et al.: Decreased incidence of viridans streptococcal septicaemia in allogeneic bone marrow transplant recipients after the introduction of acyclovir. Lancet 1:744, 1984.

207. Roberts, R. B., Krieger, A. G., Schiller, N. L., et al.: Viridans streptococcal endocarditis: The role of various species, including pyridoxal-dependent streptococci. Rev. Infect. Dis. 1:955-966, 1979.

208. Rolston, K. V. I., Frisbee-Hume, S., LeBlanc, B., et al.: In vitro antimicrobial activity of moxifloxacin compared to other quinolones against recent clinical bacterial isolates from hospitalized and community-based cancer patients. Diagn. Microbiol. Infect. Dis. 47:441-449, 2003.

209. Rolston, K. V. I., Vaziri, I., Frisbee-Hume, S., et al.: In vitro antimicrobial activity of gatifloxacin compared with other quinolones against clinical isolates from cancer patients. Chemotherapy 50:214-220, 2004.

210. Rolston, K. V. I., Yadegarynia, D., Kontoyiannis, D. P., et al.: The spectrum of gram-positive bloodstream infections in patients with hematologic malignancies, and the in vitro activity of various quinolones against gram-positive bacteria isolated from cancer patients. Int. J. Infect. Dis. 10:223-230, 2006.

211. Roos, K., Holm, S. E., Grahn, E., et al.: Alpha-streptococci as supplementary treatment of recurrent streptococcal tonsillitis: A randomized placebo-controlled study. Scand. J. Infect. Dis. 25:31-35, 1993.

212. Roos, K., Holm, S., Grahn-Hakansson, E., et al.: Recolonization with selected alpha-streptococci for prophylaxis of recurrent streptococcal pharyngotonsillitis—a randomized placebo-controlled multicentre study. Scand. J. Infect. Dis. 28:459-462, 1996.

213. Rose, H. D.: Viridans streptococcal pneumonia. J. A. M. A. 245:32, 1981.

214. Rosser, S. J., Alfa, M. J., Hoban, S., et al.: E test versus agar dilution for antimicrobial susceptibility testing of viridans group streptococci. J. Clin. Microbiol. 37:26-30, 1999.

215. Rozenberg-Arska, M., Dekker, A., Verdonck, L., et al.: Prevention of bacteremia caused by alpha-hemolytic streptococci by roxithromycin (RU-28 965) in granulocytopenic patients receiving ciprofloxacin. Infection 17:240-244, 1989.

216. Rubin, M., Hathorn, J. W., Marshall, D., et al.: Gram-positive infections and the use of vancomycin in 550 episodes of fever and neutropenia. Ann. Intern. Med. 108:30-35, 1988.

217. Rubin, M. M., Sanfilippo, R. J., and Sadoff, R. S.: Vertebral osteomyelitis secondary to an oral infection. J. Oral Maxillofac. Surg. 49:897-900, 1991.

218. Rudney, J. D., and Larson, C. J.: Identification of oral mitis group streptococci by arbitrarily primed polymerase chain reaction. Oral Microbiol. Immunol. 14:33-42, 1999.

219. Ruoff, K. L.: *Streptococcus. In* Murray, P. R., Baron, E. J., Pfaller, M. A., et al. (eds.): Manual of Clinical Microbiology. 6th ed. Washington, D.C., American Society for Microbiology, 1995, pp. 299-307.

220. Ruoff, K. L., and Kunz, L. J.: Identification of viridans streptococci isolated from clinical specimens. J. Clin. Microbiol. 15:920-925, 1982.

221. Ruoff, K. L., and Kunz, L. J.: Use of the Rapid STREP system for identification of viridans streptococcal species. J. Clin. Microbiol. 18:1138-1140, 1983.

222. Saarela, M., von Troil-Linden, B., Torkko, H., et al.: Transmission of oral bacterial species between spouses. Oral Microbiol. Immunol. 8:349-354, 1993.

223. Sader, H. S., Streit, J. M., Fritsche, T. R., et al.: Antimicrobial susceptibility of gram-positive bacteria isolated from European medical centres: Results of the Daptomycin Surveillance Programme (2002-2004). Clin. Microbiol. Infect. 12:844-852, 2006.

224. Salavert, M., Gomez, L., Rodriguez-Carballeira, M., et al.: Seven-year review of bacteremia caused by *Streptococcus milleri* and other viridans streptococci. Eur. J. Clin. Microbiol. Infect. Dis. 15:365-371, 1996.

225. Sandlund, J. T., Howard, S. C., Hijiya, N., et al.: Myositis complicating viridans streptococcal sepsis in childhood leukemia. Pediatr. Blood Cancer 44:277-279, 2005.

226. Sarkar, T. K., Murarka, R. S., and Gilardi, G. L.: Primary *Streptococcus viridans* pneumonia. Chest 96:831-834, 1989.

227. Schmitz, F. J., Fisher, A., Boos, M., et al.: Quinolone-resistance mechanisms and in vitro susceptibility patterns among European isolates of *Streptococcus mitis*, *Streptococcus sanguis*, and *Streptococcus pneumoniae*. Eur. J. Clin. Microbiol. Infect. Dis. 20:219-222, 2001.

228. Schneeberger, P. M., Janssen, M., and Voss, A.: Alpha-hemolytic streptococci: A major pathogen of iatrogenic meningitis following lumbar puncture. Case reports and a review of the literature. Infection 24:29-33, 1996.

229. Schollin, J.: Adherence of alpha-hemolytic streptococci to human endocardial, endothelial and buccal cells. Acta Paediatr. Scand. 77:705-710, 1988.

230. Schollin, J., and Danielsson, D.: Bacterial adherence to endothelial cells from rat heart, with special regard to alpha-hemolytic streptococci. A. P. M. I. S. 96:428-432, 1988.

231. Shanson, D. C., Thomas, F. D., and Johnstone, D.: Improving detection of "viridans *Streptococcus*" bacteraemia by adding sodium polyanethol sulphonate to blood cultures. J. Clin. Pathol. 38:1346-1348, 1985.

232. Shanson, D. C., Thomas, F., and Wilson, D.: Effect of volume of blood cultured on detection of *Streptococcus viridans* bacteraemia. J. Clin. Pathol. 37:568-570, 1984.

233. Shaw, J. H.: Causes and control of dental caries. N. Engl. J. Med. 317:996-1004, 1987.

234. Shelburne, S. A., 3rd., Greenberg, S. B., Aslam, S., et al.: Success ceftriaxone therapy of endocarditis due to penicillin non-susceptible viridans streptococci. J. Infect. 54:e99-e101, 2007.

235. Shenep, J. L., Hughes, W. T., Roberson, P. K., et al.: Vancomycin, ticarcillin, and amikacin compared with ticarcillin-clavulanate and amikacin in the empirical treatment of febrile, neutropenic children with cancer. N. Engl. J. Med. 319:1053-1058, 1988.

236. Shibl, A. M.: Effect of antibiotics on adherence of microorganisms to epithelial cell surfaces. Rev. Infect. Dis. 7:51-65, 1985.

237. Shlaes, D. M., Marino, J., and Jacobs, M. R.: Infection caused by vancomycin-resistant *Streptococcus sanguis* II. Antimicrob. Agents Chemother. 25:527-528, 1984.

238. Shulman, S. T.: *Streptococcus viridans*—not! Am. J. Dis. Child. 47:611, 1993.

239. Smith, D. J., Anderson, J. M., King, W. F., et al.: Oral streptococcal colonization of infants. Oral Microbiol. Immunol. 8:1-4, 1993.

240. Soell, M., Holveck, F., Scholler, M., et al.: Binding of *Streptococcus mutans* SR protein to human monocytes: Production of tumor necrosis factor, interleukin 1, and interleukin 6. Infect. Immun. 62:1805-1812, 1994.

241. Sotiropoulos, S. V., Jackson, M. A., Woods, G. M., et al.: Alpha-streptococcal septicemia in leukemic children treated with continuous or large dosage intermittent cytosine arabinoside. Pediatr. Infect. Dis. J. 8:755-758, 1989.

242. Soto, A., Evans, T. J., and Cohen, J.: Proinflammatory cytokine production by human peripheral blood mononuclear cells stimulated with cell-free supernatants of viridans streptococci. Cytokine 8:300-304, 1996.

243. Soto, A., McWhinney, P. H., Kibbler, C. C., et al.: Cytokine release and mitogenic activity in the viridans streptococcal shock syndrome. Cytokine 10:370-376, 1998.

244. Spanik, S., Trupl, J., Kunova, A., et al.: Viridans streptococcal bacteraemia due to penicillin-resistant and penicillin-sensitive streptococci: Analysis of risk factors and outcome in 60 patients from a single cancer centre before and after penicillin is used for prophylaxis. Scand. J. Infect. Dis. 29:245-249, 1997.

245. Speck, W. T., Spear, S. S., Krongrad, E., et al.: Transient bacteremia in pediatric patients after dental extraction. Am. J. Dis. Child. 130:406-407, 1976.

246. Sprunt, K., Redman, W., and Leidy, G.: Penicillin-resistant alpha streptococci in pharynx of patients given oral penicillin. Pediatrics 42:957-968, 1968.

247. Staves, E., and Tinanoff, N.: Decline in salivary *S. mutans* levels in children who have received short-term antibiotic therapy. Pediatr. Dent. 13:176-178, 1991.

248. Steiner, M., Villablanca, J., Kersey, J., et al.: Viridans streptococcal shock in bone marrow transplantation patients. Am. J. Hematol. 42:354-358, 1993.

249. Stimmel, H. M., Orchen, J. J., Skaff, D. M., et al.: Penicillin-resistant alpha-hemolytic streptococci in children with heart disease who take penicillin daily. A. S. D. C. J. Dent. Child. 48:29-32, 1981.

250. Sullam, P. M., Frank, U., Yeaman, M. R., et al.: Effect of thrombocytopenia on the early course of streptococcal endocarditis. J. Infect. Dis. 168:910-914, 1993.

251. Sussman, J. I., Baron, E. J., Tenenbaum, M. J., et al.: Viridans streptococcal endocarditis: Clinical, microbiological, and echocardiographic correlations. J. Infect. Dis. 154:597-603, 1986.

252. Svinhufvud, L. B., Heimdahl, A., and Nord, C. E.: Effect of topical administration of vancomycin versus chlorhexidine on alpha-hemolytic streptococci in oral cavity. Oral Med. 66:304-309, 1988.

253. Takada, H., Kawabata, Y., Tamura, M., et al.: Cytokine induction by extracellular products of oral viridans group streptococci. Infect. Immun. 61:5252-5260, 1993.

254. Takahashi, N., Horiuchi, M., and Yamada, T.: Effects of acidification on growth and glycolysis of *Streptococcus sanguis* and *Streptococcus mutans*. Oral Microbiol. Immunol. 12:72-76, 1997.

255. Tano, K., Olofsson, C., Grahn-Hakansson, E., et al.: In vitro inhibition of *S. pneumoniae*, nontypable *H. influenzae* and *M. catarrhalis* by alpha-hemolytic streptococci from healthy children. Int. J. Pediatr. Otorhinolaryngol. 47:49-56, 1999.

256. Tappuni, A. R., and Challacombe, S. J.: Distribution and isolation frequency of eight streptococcal species in saliva from predentate and dentate children and adults. J. Dent. Res. 72:31-36, 1993.

257. Tasaka, T., Nagai, M., Sasaki, K., et al.: *Streptococcus mitis* septicemia in leukemia patients: Clinical features and outcome. Intern. Med. 32:221-224, 1993.

258. Thibodeau, E. A., and O'Sullivan, D. M.: Salivary mutans streptococci and incidence of caries in preschool children. Caries Res. 29:148-153, 1995.

259. Thorig. L., Daha, M. R., Eulderink, F., et al.: Experimental *Streptococcus sanguis* endocarditis: Immune complexes and renal involvement. Clin. Exp. Immunol. 40:469-477, 1980.

260. Timmers, G. J., Dijstelbloem, Y., Simoons-Smit, A. M., et al.: Pharmacokinetics and effects on bowel and throat microflora of oral levofloxacin as antibacterial prophylaxis in neutropenic patients with haematological malignancies. Bone Marrow Transplant. 33:847-853, 2004.

261. Timmers, G. J., Simoons-Smit, A. M., Leidekker, M. E., et al.: Levofloxacin vs. ciprofloxacin plus phenethicillin for the prevention of bacterial infections in patients with haematological malignancies. Clin. Microbiol. Infect. 13:497-503, 2007.

262. Tinanoff, N.: Review of the antimicrobial action of stannous fluoride. J. Clin. Dent. 2:22-27, 1990.

263. Tleyjeh, I. M., Steckelberg, J. M., Murad, H. S., et al.: Temporal trends in infective endocarditis: A population-based study in Olmsted County, Minnesota. J. A. M. A. 293:3022-3028, 2005.

264. Tong, D. C., and Rothwell, B. R.: Antibiotic prophylaxis in dentistry: A review and practice recommendations. J. Am. Dent. Assoc. 131:366-374, 2000.

265. Tunkel, A. R., and Sepkowitz, K. A.: Infections caused by viridans streptococci in patients with neutropenia. Clin. Infect. Dis. 34:1524-1529, 2002.

266. Tuohy, M., and Washington, J. A.: Antimicrobial susceptibility of viridans group streptococci. Diagn. Microbiol. Infect. Dis. 29:277-280, 1997.

267. Twetman, S., Mattiasson, A., Varela, J. R., et al.: Mutans streptococci in saliva and dental caries in children living in a high and a low fluoride area. Oral Microbiol. Immunol. 5:169-171, 1990.

268. Uehara, Y., Agematsu, K., Kikuchi, K., et al.: Secretory IgA, salivary peroxidase, and catalase-mediated microbicidal activity during hydrogen peroxide catabolism in viridans streptococci: Pathogen coaggregation. J. Infect. Dis. 194:98-107, 2006.

269. Uehara, Y., Kikuchi, K., Nakamura, T., et al.: Inhibition of methicillin-resistant *Staphylococcus aureus* colonization of oral cavities in newborns by viridans group streptococci. Clin. Infect. Dis. 32:1399-1407, 2001.

270. Uehara, Y., Kikuchi, K., Nakamura, T., et al.: H_2O_2 produced by viridans group streptococci may contribute to inhibition of methicillin-resistant *Staphylococcus aureus* colonization of oral cavities in newborns. Clin. Infect. Dis. 32:1408-1413, 2001.

271. Ullman, R. F., Strampfer, M. J., and Cunha, B. A.: *Streptococcus mutans* vertebral osteomyelitis. Heart Lung 17:319-321, 1988.

272. Ullsfoss, B. N., Ogaard, B., Arends, J., et al.: Effect of a combined chlorhexidine and NaF mouthrinse: An in vivo human caries model study. Scand. J. Dent. Res. 102:109-112, 1994.

273. van Houte, J.: Bacterial adherence in the mouth. Rev. Infect. Dis. 5(Suppl. 4):659-669, 1983.

274. van Houte, J.: Role of micro-organisms in caries etiology. J. Dent. Res. 73:672-681, 1994.

275. van Loveren, C., Buijs, J. F., and ten Cate, J. M.: Similarity of bacteriocin activity profiles of mutans streptococci within the family when the children acquire the strains after the age of 5. Caries Res. 34:481-485, 2000.

276. van Loveren, C., Van de Plassche-Simons, Y. M., De Soet, J. J., et al.: Acidogenesis in relation to fluoride resistance of *Streptococcus mutans*. Oral Microbiol. Immunol. 6:288-291, 1991.

277. Vernier, A., Diab, M., Soell, M., et al.: Cytokine production by human epithelial and endothelial cells following exposure to oral viridans streptococci involves lectin interactions between bacteria and cell surface receptors. Infect. Immun. 64:3016-3022, 1996.

278. Vernier-Georgenthum, A., al-Okla, S., Gourieux, B., et al.: Protein I/II of oral viridans streptococci increases expression of adhesion molecules on endothelial cells and promotes transendothelial migration of neutrophils in vitro. Cell. Immunol. 187:145-150, 1998.

279. Vicente, M. V., Olay, T., and Rodriguez, A.: Experimental endocarditis caused by *Streptococcus sanguis*: Single and combined antibiotic therapy. Antimicrob. Agents Chemother. 20:10-14, 1981.

280. Wanahita, A., Goldsmith, E. A., Musher, D. M., et al.: Interaction between human polymorphonuclear leukocytes and *Streptococcus milleri* group bacteria. J. Infect. Dis. 185:85-90, 2002.

281. Watanakunakorn, C., and Pantelakis, J.: Alpha-hemolytic streptococcal bacteremia: A review of 203 episodes during 1980-1991. Scand. J. Infect. Dis. 25:403-408, 1993.

282. Weber, M., Gubler, J., Fahrer, H., et al.: Spondylodiscitis caused by viridans streptococci: Three cases and a review of the literature. Clin. Rheumatol. 18:417-421, 1999.

283. Weinberger, S. J., and Wright, G. Z.: A comparison of *S. mutans* clinical assessment methods. Pediatr. Dent. 12:375-379, 1990.

284. West, P. W., Al-Sawan, R., Foster, H. A., et al.: Speciation of presumptive viridans streptococci from early onset neonatal sepsis. J. Med. Microbiol. 47:923-928, 1998.

285 Westling, K., Julander, I., Ljungman. P., et al.: Viridans group streptococci in blood culture isolates in a Swedish university hospital: Antibiotic susceptibility and identification of erythromycin resistance genes. Int. J. Antimicrob. Agents 28:292-296, 2006.

286. Westling, K., Ljungman, P., Thalme, A., et al.: Streptococcus viridans septicaemia: A comparison study in patients admitted to the departments of infectious diseases and haematology in a university hospital. Scand. J. Infect. Dis. 34:316-319, 2002.

287. Wilcox, M. H., Winstanley, T. G., Douglas, C. W., et al.: Susceptibility of alpha-haemolytic streptococci causing endocarditis to benzylpenicillin and ten cephalosporins. J. Antimicrob. Chemother. 32:63-69, 1993.

288. Wilson, A. P., and Gaya, H.: Treatment of endocarditis with teicoplanin: A retrospective analysis of 104 cases. J. Antimicrob. Chemother. 38:507-521, 1996.

289. Wilson, M., Patel, H., and Fletcher, J.: Susceptibility of biofilms of Streptococcus sanguis to chlorhexidine gluconate and cetylpyridinium chloride. Oral Microbiol. Immunol. 11:188-192, 1996.

290. Wisplinghoff, H., Reinert, R. R., Cornely, O., et al.: Molecular relationships and antimicrobial susceptibilities of viridans group streptococci isolated

from blood of neutropenic cancer patients. J. Clin. Microbiol. 37:1876-880, 1999.

291. Yaniv, L. G., and Potasman, I.: Iatrogenic meningitis: An increasing role for resistant viridans streptococci? Case report and review of the last 20 years. Scand. J. Infect. Dis. 32:693-696, 2000.

292. Yap, R. L., Mermel, L. A., and Maglio, J.: Antimicrobial resistance of community-acquired bloodstream isolates of viridans group streptococci. Infection 34:339-341, 2006.

293. Yee, Y., Farber, B., and Mates, S.: Mechanism of penicillin-streptomycin synergy for clinical isolates of viridans streptococci. J. Infect. Dis. 154:531-534, 1986.

294. Zickert, I., Emilson, C. G., Ekblom, K., et al.: Prolonged oral reduction of Streptococcus mutans in humans after chlorhexidine disinfection followed by fluoride treatment. Scand. J. Dent. Res. 95:315-319, 1987.

295. Zito, E. T., and Daneo-Moore, L.: Transformation of Streptococcus sanguis to intrinsic penicillin resistance. J. Gen. Microbiol. 134:1237-1249, 1988.

296. Zuccaro, G., Richter, J. E., Rice, T. W., et al.: Viridans streptococcal bacteremia after esophageal stricture dilation. Gastrointest. Endosc. 48:568-573, 1998.

CHAPTER 96

PNEUMOCOCCAL INFECTIONS

Ronald Dagan ✤ David Greenberg ✤ Michael R. Jacobs ✤ Brandon Lane Phillips

The pneumococcus (*Streptococcus pneumoniae*) continues to be a leading cause of morbidity and mortality in persons of all ages. Most children experience some form of pneumococcal infection (e.g., otitis media or pneumonia), and sepsis or meningitis develops in some cases. Despite more than a century of research, many of the aspects of pneumococcal disease remain obscure. The continued frequency and severity of pneumococcal disease, coupled with the knowledge that antimicrobial therapy invariably does not prevent illness or death, and the high and still increasing prevalence of strains of pneumococci resistant to antimicrobial agents serve to underscore the need for better understanding of pneumococcal infections. Currently, attention is concentrated on efforts to prevent these infections by the development and use of appropriate vaccines.

HISTORY

Pasteur and Sternberg, working independently in 1880 and 1881, discovered the pneumococcus. Pasteur called the organism *microbe septicémique de la salive*, and Sternberg called it *Micrococcus pasteri*. Each researcher recovered pneumococci from rabbits injected with human saliva. Friedlander demonstrated pneumococci in tissue from humans with pneumonia in 1882 and, in the following year, found them in most cases of acute pneumonia. Friedlander described both the characteristic capsule and colonial morphologic features of pneumococci and, in 1884, recovered pneumococci from the blood of patients with pneumonia for the first time. During the next few years, pneumococci were found in virtually all types of infection, including meningitis and otitis media. By 1890, researchers had established the pneumococcus as the most common cause of acute pneumonia, and, hence, the term *pneumococcus* emerged. In addition, the pneumococcus became recognized as a principal cause of meningitis and other serious infections.

During the next decade, researchers immunized animals with cell-free filtrates of pneumococci, demonstrated that serum from immune animals could protect against experimental pneumococcal infection, deduced the role of immunity in promoting phagocytosis, and noted agglutination of pneumococci by serum from immune animals. In 1897, Pane treated humans suffering from

pneumonia with serum from such animals. By 1900, researchers had laid the foundation for immunotherapy for pneumococcal pneumonia, the only effective treatment until the advent of chemotherapy.

During the next few years, investigators noted that agglutination of pneumococci appeared to depend on the strain isolated. In 1910, Neufeld and Haendel classified pneumococci into several discrete serotypes on the basis of the appearance of capsular swelling (the quellung reaction). Only strains exposed to homologous serum showed capsular swelling. Their work made possible all subsequent epidemiologic investigations of pneumococcal infection, immunotherapy with type-specific serum, and the development of vaccines.

After these discoveries were made, researchers concentrated on several aspects of pneumococcal disease, including identification of additional serotypes and their roles in disease, production and clinical use of antisera, and development of pneumococcal vaccines.

In 1926, the pneumococcus was called *Diplococcus pneumoniae* because it usually appears in pairs. In 1974, it was renamed *Streptococcus pneumoniae* because it forms long chains when grown in liquid medium. The original classification of pneumococci was limited to types I, II, III, and IV (others). Currently, 90 serotypes have been identified, and certain serotypes have proved to be more virulent than others, with virulence depending, to some extent, on the species of animal infected.

The use of antisera for the treatment of pneumococcal pneumonia proved strikingly effective when type-specific sera were administered. As early as 1913, Cole and associates showed that treatment with antisera lowered fatality rates from 25 to 30 percent to 10.5 percent. In addition to allergic reactions, difficulties associated with this treatment included the necessity of identifying the causative serotype, the need for the earliest possible administration of antisera, and the availability of antisera to only types I, II, and III. White compared the efficacy of early antisera therapy and found that 403 of 1614 (25.0%) who did not receive any therapy died, 32 of 377 (8.5%) who received therapy within 3 days of onset died, and 24 of 127 (18.9%) who received therapy 4 or more days after onset died. Unfortunately, therapy with antisera had no beneficial effect on other pneumococcal infections such as meningitis and endocarditis. Despite these drawbacks, the use of antisera soon became widespread. The advent of chemotherapy—first sulfa compounds, then penicillin—was followed by a precipitous decline in the use of antisera. Antimicrobial agents killed or inhibited pneumococci, regardless of serotype, and cured patients with previously incurable localized infections.[778]

Coincident with research resulting in the general use of antisera came research into the efficacy of pneumococcal vaccines. Proof of efficacy lagged, and indisputable evidence of protection induced by vaccination was not available until 1945. The ability of pneumococci to cause epidemic pneumococcal pneumonia in young men crowded into army camps or gold mines allowed large-scale trials to be performed. Highlights of the development of effective vaccines include the trial of Wright and associates[789] in South Africa beginning in 1911. Using a vaccine made with whole, killed pneumococci, this trial produced inconclusive results. Many trials followed, with some showing trends toward protection. In 1923, Heidelberger and Avery[317] published their classic article in which they stated that protective antibodies were reactive with surface capsular polysaccharides. In 1930, Francis and Tillett[238] showed capsular polysaccharides to be immunogenic for humans. Ekwurzel and colleagues[203] used a vaccine containing such polysaccharides during 1933 to 1937 and showed it to be effective. Smillie and associates used a preparation of serotype 1 polysaccharide to abort a hospital epidemic of pneumonia at State Hospital in Worcester, Massachusetts.[694]

Although many of these studies suggested that specific pneumococcal polysaccharide antigens could confer protection against severe pneumococcal infection, not until 1945, in a trial performed on U.S. Army and Air Force recruits, were they finally proved by MacLeod and associates[485] to do so. This trial showed vaccination to be strikingly effective in preventing pneumococcal pneumonia caused by serotypes contained in the vaccine but not in preventing disease caused by other serotypes, thus showing serotype-specific protection.

Regrettably, interest in vaccination waned rapidly with the general availability of penicillin, and manufacturers voluntarily withdrew their vaccines from the market. This unfortunate attitude persisted for the next 2 decades until the inability of chemotherapy to prevent many deaths from pneumococcal disease

was recognized.[42] The rapid development and spread of antibiotic resistance among many clinically important strains further emphasized that prevention could be more effective than treatment for pneumococcal disease. Fortunately, a few farsighted individuals continued to maintain surveillance of the serotypes causing human disease, and their work allowed the reintroduction of pneumococcal vaccines. The current status of vaccines is discussed later in this chapter.

Interested readers should consult both White's *The Biology of Pneumococcus* and Heffron's *Pneumonia, with Special Reference to Pneumococcus Lobar Pneumonia*, as well as a comprehensive review by Watson and colleagues, for a complete account of the long and fascinating history of this organism.[316,774,778]

THE ORGANISM, HOST DEFENSE MECHANISMS, AND PATHOGENESIS

STRUCTURE OF THE PNEUMOCOCCUS

Pneumococcal cells are surrounded by a trilamellar, lipopolysaccharide, cytoplasmic membrane that has two electron-dense bands, each 25 to 30 Å wide. A cell wall surrounding the plasma membrane has two bands—an inner 30- to 40-Å-wide band and an outer 60- to 80-Å-wide band. Numerous bridges connect the cell wall and the plasma membrane. The polysaccharide capsule covers the cell wall in encapsulated strains and is seen as a wider, less structured band.[735] A schematic representation of the major structural components and selected cell wall components is shown in Figure 96–1.

Cell Wall Structure

The predominant structural components of the pneumococcal cell wall are peptidoglycan, teichoic acid (TA), lipoteichoic acid (LTA), and several choline-bound proteins. Choline is a lipid that is an essential growth factor for *S. pneumoniae*.

PEPTIDOGLYCAN. Peptidoglycan, which accounts for approximately half of the cell wall mass, is a cell wall polymer

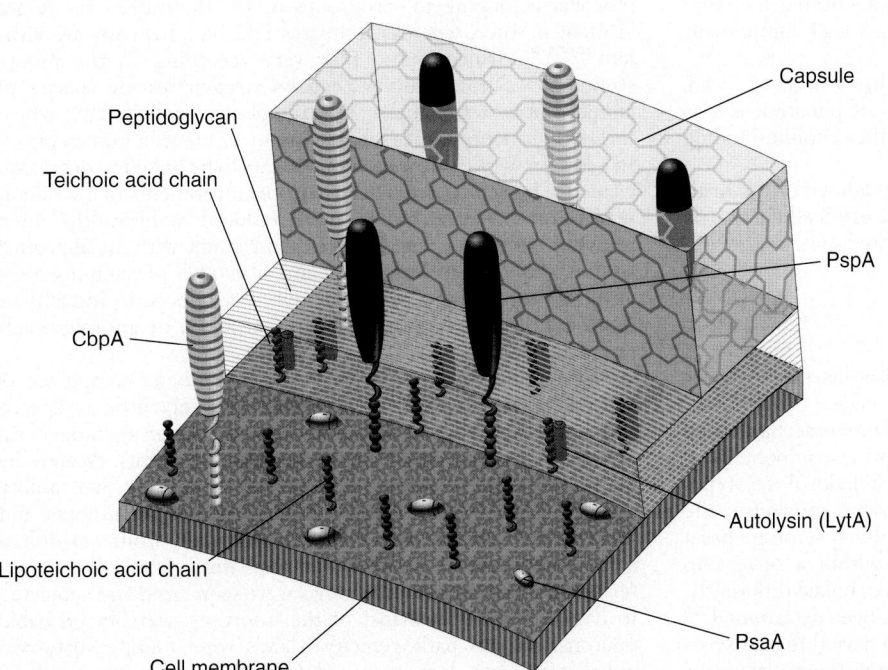

Peptidoglycan

Teichoic acid chain

CbpA

Lipoteichoic acid chain

Cell membrane

Capsule

PspA

Autolysin (LytA)

PsaA

Figure 96–1 Schematic three-dimensional representation of the major structural components of the cell membrane, cell wall, and capsule of *Streptococcus pneumoniae*. The locations of selected major virulence factors of the organism are shown as well. Chains of lipoteichoic acid are attached to cell membrane glycolipid, whereas surface proteins, such as PspA and CbpA, in turn are attached to the lipoteichoic acid chains via phosphocholine links. Chains of teichoic acid are attached to the peptidoglycan layer via phosphodiester bonds. Autolysin (LytA) is attached to teichoic acid chains via phosphocholine links. PsaA is found on the outer surface of the cell membrane. *(Adapted from references 229, 349, 740. Copyright Michael R. Jacobs, used with permission.)*

linked by stem peptides to form a complex, three-dimensional structure.[670] Stem peptides are formed when transpeptidases (also known as *penicillin-binding proteins* [PBPs]) link pentapeptide chains into linear stem peptides in penicillin-susceptible strains.[670] However, in non–penicillin-susceptible strains, branched and other variant stem peptides are produced.

LIPOTEICHOIC ACID. LTA also is known as *pneumococcal Forssman (F) antigen.* The LTA of pneumococci possesses identical repeat and chain structures linked to a cell membrane glycolipid that anchors LTA to the cell.[229,230] Phosphocholine is attached to saccharide residues. PspA and other proteins (see later) also are attached to choline residues on LTA.

TEICHOIC ACID. TA, also known as *pneumococcal C polysaccharide,* has a chain structure similar to that of LTA, except that the saccharide differs. TA chains are attached to the cell wall peptidoglycan. Some phosphocholine residues of both LTA and TA are expressed on the cell wall surface, where they are thought to serve three functions: (1) activation of the pneumococcal autolysin (LytA) enzyme, which is responsible for the autolysis of pneumococci; (2) binding of the choline-binding domain of LytA to choline on TA, which may regulate the activity of LytA; and (3) a function associated with transformability (choline-deficient cells lack transformability).[683]

SURFACE PROTEINS. Pneumococci have several surface proteins, with the four most important being *pneumococcal surface protein A* (PspA), *pneumococcal surface adhesin A* (PsaA), *choline-binding protein A* (CbpA), and *hyaluronate lyase* (Hyl).

PspA is a cell wall protein with a molecular size of 67 to 99 kd that is bound to TA and LTA by phosphocholine links.[373] This protein extends through the cell wall and capsule to the surface of the organism.[794] PspA exists in various antigenic forms, and epitopes within one PspA molecule can recombine into different types.[97] However, PspA variants usually are sufficiently cross-reactive that immunization with one PspA serotype elicits immunity to other PspA serotypes.

PsaA is a 37-kd surface protein thought to be anchored to the cell membrane and associated with magnesium and zinc transport.[187] It appears to be a lipoprotein and is common to virtually all *S. pneumoniae* isolates.[606] Considerable variation in the amino acid sequences of PsaA from different strains has been detected.[570] The relationship of this protein to other cell wall components has not been determined.[721]

CbpA is a protein similar to PspA and has a mass of 75 kd. It is an adhesin involved in the adherence of pneumococci to cytokine-activated human cells.[632] Several other choline-binding proteins also have been identified.

Hyl is a hyaluronidase that results in breakdown of the hyaluronan and chondroitin sulfate present in the extracellular matrix of human tissues.[373] It is bound to peptidoglycan in the cell wall.

Capsule

The capsule of pneumococci consists of polysaccharides that vary in the make-up of monosaccharides, the sequence of monosaccharides in polysaccharides, the linkage of monosaccharides to each other, and the presence of nonsaccharide components.[732] Currently, 90 serotypes consisting of 25 individual serotypes and 65 serogroups grouped into 21 serogroups are known (see the section "Microbiology" later) (Table 96–1). Each serotype has a specific capsular structure, and serotypes within a serogroup often have the same oligosaccharide sequences linked differently. The capsular structure of many serotypes has been determined.[250] Several epidemic clones have been shown to have different serotypes, and extensive genetic changes involving the replacement

of entire cassettes of genes related to capsule production are required for capsular switching to take place.[604]

Genetics and the Pneumococcal Genome

The pneumococcal genome has been mapped recently, and 90 to 95 percent of its DNA sequences are known. The genome has been estimated to be 2.0 to 2.1 megabases (Mb) in size, approximately half that of *Escherichia coli.*[51,192] The locations of more than 100 genes, including 20 tRNA synthetase and 20 ribosomal protein genes, have been mapped. Genes involved in cell wall synthesis also have been identified.

S. pneumoniae is a naturally transformable bacterium, which means that it is able to take up single-stranded DNA from its environment and incorporate this exogenous DNA into its genome. This process is known as *transformational recombination.*[521,703] Recombination is a powerful means of genome evolution and provides a great degree of genome flexibility to this organism. Transformation occurs only at high cell densities (10^5 to 10^8 colony-forming units per milliliter), and a peptide pheromone quorum-sensing signal called *activator* or *competence factor* is required.[602] This factor also is termed *competence-stimulating peptide.*

The genes associated with capsule synthesis have been characterized for several serotypes as well. The complete nucleotide sequence of 24 of these genes of several *S. pneumoniae* serotypes has been determined,[35,249] as has the genetic basis for the structural diversity of capsule polysaccharides within *S. pneumoniae* serogroups.[517,518] The abundance of transposable elements at the gene locus favors genetic variability of the capsule.[249]

VIRULENCE FACTORS

Animal models of pneumococcal infection have provided considerable insight into the pathogenesis of disease and the association of virulence factors with disease. However, the pneumococcus is primarily a human pathogen, and the host defenses of animal models can vary significantly from those in humans. For example, pneumococci adhere to human but not to rabbit polymeric immunoglobulin receptor (pIgR).[802] Additionally, virulence in mice varies considerably with the strain of pneumococcus: pneumococci belonging to serogroups 6, 14, 19, and 23 rarely are virulent in mice, whereas serotypes 1, 2, and 3 usually are virulent.[60,95,434] Virulence also may vary according to the mouse strain.[1,45,729] Some serotypes can be virulent to one species of animal but not to others. An example is serotype 19F, which rarely is virulent in mice[45] but is highly virulent in guinea pigs.[40] In addition, penicillin resistance appears to be linked to decreased virulence by virtue of the fact that isogenic mutants of a virulent, penicillin-susceptible strain were reduced significantly when transformed into a penicillin-resistant strain with an abnormal *pbp2x* gene.[614] Therefore, many animal models of pneumococcal virulence may not be representative of virulence in humans or representative of all pneumococcal serotypes or antimicrobial-resistant strains.

Although the polysaccharide capsule has been recognized as the major determinant of virulence, relatively little is known about the molecular basis of the pathogenesis of pneumococcal disease. A library of 1786 pneumococcal mutants created by insertion-duplication mutagenesis was analyzed for their ability to survive and replicate in murine models of pneumonia and bacteremia.[440] One hundred eighty-six mutant strains exhibited attenuated virulence; 56 of these strains were genetically characterized, and genomic DNA inserts were sequenced and subjected to database searches. Most of the insertions were in probable operons, but no pathogenicity islands were found. Forty-two novel virulence loci were identified. Five strains showed

TABLE 96–1 Capsular Serotypes of *Streptococcus pneumoniae*

Serogroup	Danish Serotype	U.S. Serotype	Serogroup	Danish Serotype	U.S. Serotype
	1	1	Group 22	22A	63
	2	2		22F	22
	3	3	Group 23	23A	46
	4	4		23B	64
	5	5		23F	23
Group 6	6A	6	Group 24	24A	65
	6B	26		24B	60
Group 7	7A	7		24F	24
	7B	48	Group 25	25A	NA
	7C	50		25F	25
	7F	51		27	27
	8	8	Group 28	28A	79
Group 9	9A	33		28F	28
	9L	49		29	29
	9N	9		31	31
	9V	68	Group 32	32A	67
Group 10	10A	34		32F	32
	10B	NA	Group 33	33A	40
	10C	NA		33B	42
	10F	10		33C	39
Group 11	11A	43		33D	NA
	11B	76		33F	70
	11C	53		34	41
	11D	NA	Group 35	35A	47, 62
	11F	11		35B	66
Group 12	12A	83		35C	61
	12B	NA		35F	35
	12F	12		36	36
	13	13		37	37
	14	14		38	71
Group 15	15A	30		39	69
	15B	54		40	45
	15C	77	Group 41	41A	74
	15F	15		41F	38
Group 16	16A	NA		42	80
	16F	16		43	75
Group 17	17A	78		44	81
	17F	17		45	72
Group 18	18A	44		46	73
	18B	55	Group 47	47A	84
	18C	56		47F	52
	18F	18		48	82
Group 19	19A	57			
	19B	58			
	19C	59			
	19F	19			
	20	20			
	21	21			

mutations in genes involved in gene regulation, cation transport, or stress tolerance; the virulence of these strains was shown to be highly attenuated in a murine respiratory tract infection model. Additional experiments also suggest that induction of competence for genetic transformation has a role in virulence.[440] This approach has revealed several previously unrecognized genes required for virulence.

A similar genomic approach was used to look for genes coding for surface-localized proteins that could be targets for protective humoral immunity. By exploiting the whole genome sequence of *S. pneumoniae*, researchers found 130 open-reading frames encoding proteins with secretion motifs or similarity to predicted virulence factors.[787] Mice were immunized with 108 of these proteins, and 6 conferred protection against disseminated pneumococcal infection. Each of the six protective antigens showed broad strain distribution and immunogenicity in human infections. Some of these proteins have been identified as LytB, LytC, and a cell

wall–anchored serine protease. Another genomic-based study used a genomic expression library of *S. pneumoniae* screened with convalescent-phase serum for immunoreactive proteins.[805] Six known and 17 unknown pneumococcal proteins were detected. Five of the known proteins, including PspA and SpsA (CbpA), were surface-located virulence factors, and 8 of the unknown proteins were putative membrane proteins. Use of these genomic approaches for the identification of novel microbial targets to elicit a protective immune response has been validated, and these new antigens may play roles in the development of improved vaccines against *S. pneumoniae*.

CAPSULE. The capsule is the major determinant of virulence in pneumococci. It prevents phagocytosis by polymorphonuclear leukocytes (PMNs) and macrophages, thereby allowing unrestricted extracellular multiplication of the organism. Because the pneumococcus has 90 antigenically distinct serotypes, production of anticapsular antibody in response to one serotype provides protection against only that serotype or serogroup, whereas non-encapsulated strains are considerably less virulent.[527] The importance of the capsule as a virulence factor is emphasized by the fact that protection from pneumococcal infection can be achieved by capsular-specific antibodies. Despite the large number of additional virulence factors (see the following paragraphs), the capsule remains the single most important determinant of virulence in avoiding host defenses after the epithelial barriers have been breached. Other virulence factors are important in breaching host defenses such as epithelial barriers.

NEURAMINIDASES. Neuraminidases are enzymes that cleave terminal sialic acid residues from glycolipids, glycoproteins, and oligosaccharides on eukaryotic cell surfaces; such cleavage may unmask cell surface receptors for pneumococcal adhesins.[570] The neuraminidase NanA has been implicated in the ability of *S. pneumoniae* to colonize and persist in the nasopharynx and middle ear.[736] A second neuraminidase, NanB, has much weaker activity than NanA does but exhibits optimal activity at pH 5, whereas NanA is most active at pH 7.[570]

PNEUMOLYSIN. Pneumolysin is a 53-kd cytoplasmic protein produced by all pneumococci. It is essential for the initial binding to membrane cholesterol and the interaction leading to subsequent membrane damage.[46] Functions of pneumolysin include the following:

1. Pore formation in host epithelial cell membranes. Pneumolysin binds to cholesterol in host epithelial cell membranes, where oligomers of pneumolysin molecules assemble to form 35- to 45-nm pores in the cell membrane, which results in lysis of the targeted cell. Pneumolysin is, therefore, cytotoxic to epithelial cells, and it also slows ciliary beating of bronchial epithelial cells and disrupts the tight junctions between epithelial cells. In addition, pneumolysin disrupts alveolar epithelial cells and the alveolar-capillary boundary, thereby facilitating entry of pneumococci into the bloodstream and through the blood-brain barrier.[269,806]
2. Effects on phagocytic and immune cell function. Pneumolysin attracts neutrophils in the early phases of disease and lymphocytes at a later stage.
3. Direct activation of the complement system. Expression of pneumolysin by pneumococci reduces serum complement levels and serum opsonic activity.[11]
4. Promotion of nitric oxide (NO) production by macrophages. NO is produced by an inducible NO synthase (iNOS) during inflammation as an essential element of antimicrobial defense, but it also can contribute to host-induced tissue damage.[93]

SURFACE-LOCATED CHOLINE-BINDING PROTEINS. The virulence of members of the choline-binding protein (Cbp) family and two recently described cell wall hydrolases, LytB and LytC, has been characterized.[281] Cbp-, LytB-, and LytC-deficient mutants show significantly reduced colonization of the nasopharynx. The following proteins of the Cbp family and their virulence mechanisms have been described:

1. *PspA* is a serologically variable protein that has undergone extensive recombination.[332] It is thought to exert its virulence function in systemic infection by interfering with deposition of the complement component C3b onto pneumococci or by blocking recruitment of the alternative pathway, thereby reducing the effectiveness of complement receptor–mediated pathways of clearance.[739] PspA recently has been shown to bind to lactoferrin, an iron-sequestering glycoprotein found in mucosal secretions, when the level of free extracellular iron is not sufficient for the

growth of pneumococci. This binding is thought to overcome the iron limitation at mucosal surfaces and might represent a potential virulence mechanism for colonization of mucosal surfaces.[303]

2. CbpA, or *SpsA*, is a surface protein adhesin that acts as a bridging element between pneumococci and host-cell glycoconjugates on cytokine-activated host cells.[304] This process is thought to be associated with change from nasopharyngeal colonization to invasion of epithelial and endothelial cells.[632] One mechanism by which this process occurs, wherein CbpA binds to the pIgR of human epithelial cells, has been described.[800] The pneumococcus co-opts the transcytosis machinery and gains entry into and across airway epithelial cells. This process is a novel example of a pathogen co-opting the transcytosis machinery to promote translocation across a mucosal barrier.[384]

3. *PsaA* is a surface protein that also is associated with virulence via adhesion to epithelial cells.[605]

4. *Pneumococcal histidine-containing protein A (PhpA)* is a 20-kd protein with putative proteolytic activity against the human complement component C3. PhpA is a potential candidate for use as a vaccine against systemic pneumococcal disease and otitis media.[802]

5. The *pneumococcal histidine triad (Pht)* proteins PhtA, PhtB, PhtD, and PhtE constitute a novel family of homologous surface proteins associated with virulence; they are also potential vaccine candidates.[7] Although antibodies targeting PhtA, PhtB, or PhtD are protective, the function of these proteins remains unknown. The number of histidine and tyrosine residues in these proteins suggests that they may be involved in metal or nucleoside binding.

PHASE VARIATION. Phase variation in the colonial opacity of *S. pneumoniae* has been implicated as a factor in bacterial adherence, colonization, and invasion.[776] On clear media, colonies can appear as opaque or translucent when viewed under magnification with oblique, transmitted light. All strains of *S. pneumoniae* are thought to be capable of phase variation. Opaque colonies are less likely to autolyze, contain less TA but more PspA in their cell walls, and colonize the nasopharynx poorly in animal models but are more virulent when inoculated into sterile sites. Conversely, translucent colonies are more likely to autolyze, contain more TA but less PspA in their cell walls, and colonize the nasopharynx well but are less virulent when inoculated into sterile sites. Translucent colonies become umbilicated as a result of autolysis, whereas opaque colonies remain dome-shaped.

PHOSPHORYLCHOLINE ESTERASE. This enzyme has activity that removes phosphorylcholine residues from cell wall TA and LTA.[759] Inactivation of the gene encoding for the enzyme in pneumococcal strains caused a change in colony morphology from translucent (colonizing) to opaque (virulent) and a striking increase in virulence in the intraperitoneal mouse model. Phosphorylcholine esterase therefore appears to be a regulatory element involved in the interaction of *S. pneumoniae* with its host.[759]

PNEUMOCOCCAL AUTOLYSIN. Pneumococcal autolysin (LytA) is a 36-kd cell wall protein attached to choline residues on TA and LTA. It is associated with unlinking of cell wall glycan from stem peptides during cell remodeling and division. Autolysin initially was considered to be a significant virulence factor, but more recent work has shown that it plays only a minor role and that immunization with autolysin does not provide protection.[570]

CELL WALL STEM PEPTIDES. The peptidoglycan of gram-positive bacteria triggers the release of cytokine from peripheral blood mononuclear cells.[489] However, 100 to 1000 times more gram-positive peptidoglycan than gram-negative lipopolysaccharide endotoxin is required to release the same amount of cytokine. Simple stem peptides were 10-fold less active than was undigested peptidoglycan in stimulating tumor necrosis factor (TNF). In contrast, complex branched peptides such as tripeptides were at least 100-fold more potent than was the native material. These complex branched peptides represented 2 percent or less of the total material, but their activity in stimulating TNF was almost equal to that of endotoxin.

IRON TRANSPORT. The availability of iron is a major requirement for the growth and survival of many organisms, including *S. pneumoniae*. Two *S. pneumoniae* genetic loci, *pit1* and *pit2*, which encode homologues of ABC iron transporters, are required for uptake of iron by this organism.[105] Virulence in mouse models of pulmonary and systemic infection is attenuated moderately with a *pit2*-disrupted strain and attenuated strongly with a *pit1/pit2*-disrupted strain.

IgA PROTEASE. IgA proteases belong to a family of proteins used by a diverse group of bacteria, including *S. pneumoniae*, for colonization and invasion. IgA1 protease allows bacteria to cleave human IgA1 in the hinge region. The exact role of these enzymes in bacterial pathogenesis is not understood completely, but they are important in bacterial colonization of mucosal membranes in the presence of secretory IgA antibodies by causing local IgA deficiency.[401] The IgA protease genes of *S. pneumoniae* and *Streptococcus mitis* show extensive polymorphism, which results in enzymes with considerable antigenic diversity.[591]

PHOSPHOGLUCOMUTASE. Phosphoglucomutase is an enzyme that is necessary in one of the early steps in capsular polysaccharide synthesis, and *S. pneumoniae* mutants lacking this enzyme do not produce a capsule and are avirulent in immunocompetent but not in immunosuppressed mice.[307] Other metabolic pathways also are thought to be affected by this enzyme.

FREE OXYGEN RADICALS. Release of free oxygen radicals has been implicated in the pathogenesis of otitis media by *S. pneumoniae*, and antibiotic killing of bacteria leads to the release of further free oxygen radicals, which results in tissue damage despite the administration of appropriate antibiotic therapy.[719] Reactive oxygen intermediates also mediate brain injury in bacterial meningitis.[38,477]

NADH OXIDASE. Reduced nicotinamide adenine dinucleotide (NADH) oxidase has been shown to be a virulence factor necessary for *S. pneumoniae* infection. The basis of NADH oxidase as a virulence factor is the conversion of O_2 to H_2O. If O_2 is not reduced fully, it can form superoxide anion (O_2^-) and hydrogen peroxide (H_2O_2), both of which can be toxic to cells.[796]

PYRUVATE OXIDASE. Pyruvate oxidase decarboxylates pyruvate to acetyl phosphate plus H_2O_2 and CO_2 and appears to be associated with regulation of the multiple adhesive properties of pneumococci.[702] A pneumococcal mutant lacking the gene encoding pyruvate kinase showed a greater than 70 percent loss of the ability to attach to all cell types.

PLASMINOGEN BINDING AND PENETRATION OF THE BASEMENT MEMBRANE. Binding of plasminogen plus penetration of the basement membrane is thought to be an essential step in the pathogenesis of bacterial meningitis.[199] Most strains adhere to reconstituted basement membrane, as well as to its purified laminin and collagen IV components, and to bound plasminogen. Penetration of the basement membrane was

achieved within 3 to 4 hours in the presence of plasminogen, whereas without plasminogen, no penetration occurred.

HYALURONIDASE. Virtually all pneumococcal strains produce the enzyme hyaluronidase, a 107-kd protein. Models used to simulate human meningitis generally involve the direct intracerebral route of infection. However, intranasal inoculation would provide a more realistic model, and it recently was achieved by intranasal administration of *S. pneumoniae* with hyaluronidase. This model induced meningitis in 50 percent of inoculated mice, whereas meningitis did not develop in any of the mice inoculated without hyaluronidase. Hyaluronidase was found to facilitate pneumococcal invasion of the bloodstream after colonization of the upper respiratory tract. This murine model mimics important features of human disease, which allows the model to be used to study issues related to the pathophysiology and treatment of pneumococcal meningitis.[804]

PEPTIDOGLYCAN *N*-ACETYLGLUCOSAMINE DEACETYLASE A. The glucosamine and muramic acid residues of the pneumococcal cell wall traditionally are regarded as being *N*-acetylated. However, more than 80 percent of the glucosamine and 10 percent of the muramic acid residues have been shown to be deacetylated, thereby explaining the resistance of peptidoglycan to the hydrolytic action of lysozyme, a muramidase that cleaves the glycan backbone.[758] A gene that encodes for peptidoglycan *N*-acetylglucosamine deacetylase A has been identified. This gene may, therefore, contribute to pneumococcal virulence by providing protection against host lysozyme, which is known to accumulate in high concentration at sites of infection.

PHAGES. Whereas transformation is recognized as occurring in pneumococci, another mechanism of DNA transfer in pneumococci is transduction of DNA carried by bacteriophages (lysogeny). A high proportion (76% of 791 isolates) of clinical isolates of pneumococci were found to carry multiple copies of LytA, thus indicating the widespread occurrence of lysogeny in pneumococci.[603] The LytA hybridization pattern of a strain has been found to be stable during extensive serial culturing; it is specific for the clonal type of the strain and can be used as a molecular epidemiologic marker.[671] In addition, phage DNA integrated into the pneumococcal genome acts as an integrase to facilitate the introduction of foreign genes into the pneumococcal chromosome.[270]

TOLERANCE. The ability of *S. pneumoniae* to escape lysis and killing by vancomycin and penicillin, a property termed *tolerance*, has been described recently.[324] Among 116 clinical isolates of pneumococci, 3 percent and 8 percent were tolerant to vancomycin and penicillin, respectively. Tolerance may contribute to treatment failure, particularly in meningitis, in which bactericidal activity is critical for eradication. A vancomycin- and cephalosporin-tolerant strain of *S. pneumoniae*, the Tupelo strain, has been isolated from the cerebrospinal fluid (CSF) of a patient in whom recrudescence of meningitis developed despite treatment with vancomycin and a third-generation cephalosporin.[503] The defect leading to tolerance in this strain involves the control pathway for triggering of autolysis.

HOST DEFENSE MECHANISMS

Although anticapsular antibody is the most prominent protective mechanism against pneumococcal infection, many host responses to infection occur and many other factors are associated with protection against disease.[527] Pneumococcal infection and disease have been modeled in several animal species. Most are models of sepsis arising from intravenous or intraperitoneal inoculation of bacteria, and only a few were designed to study disease arising from intranasal infection. Chinchillas provide the only animal model of middle ear pneumococcal infection in which the disease can be produced by very small inocula injected into the middle ear or intranasally. This model, developed at the University of Minnesota in 1975, has been used to study pneumococcal pathogenesis at a mucosal site, the immunogenicity and efficacy of pneumococcal capsular polysaccharide vaccine antigens, and the kinetics and efficacy of antimicrobial drugs.[265]

ANTICAPSULAR SERUM IgG ANTIBODY. IgG to the capsular polysaccharide of *S. pneumoniae* is thought to provide the greatest degree of protection against systemic pneumococcal disease, as well as limited protection against colonization. The reference method for measurement of antibody is the opsonophagocytosis assay, which involves serial dilutions of serum, viable pneumococci, complement, and viable PMNs incubated together for 1 hour.[626] An infant mouse assay system for assessment of protective concentrations of human serum pneumococcal anticapsular antibodies correlated well with opsonophagocytic titer but not with naturally occurring IgG antibody concentrations or IgG produced in response to nonconjugated polysaccharide vaccines, as determined by enzyme-linked immunosorbent assay (ELISA).[379,532] However, the ELISA method of serotype-specific antibody assay with absorption of cross-reacting antibody to cell wall polysaccharides does correlate well with protection after vaccination with conjugated vaccine, and it is the method used most commonly to predict serotype-specific immunity.[27,749,750] The development of a phagocytosis assay based on flow cytometry has not overcome the limitations of the ELISA method and is inferior to the opsonophagocytosis method.[371] Investigation of polymorphisms in the variable region of IgG that affect protective function has indicated that the capsular polysaccharide antibody repertoire in adults is derived from memory B-cell populations that have switched class and undergone extensive hypermutation.[483] Functionally disparate anticapsular polysaccharide antibodies can arise within individuals both by activation of independent clones and by intraclonal somatic mutation, which illustrates the complexity of assaying and interpreting serum capsular polysaccharide antibody levels.

ANTICAPSULAR IgA ANTIBODY. The role of IgA in the control of invasive mucosal pathogens such as *S. pneumoniae* is understood poorly. Human pneumococcal capsular polysaccharide–specific IgA initiates dose-dependent killing of *S. pneumoniae* in the presence of complement and phagocytes. The majority of specific IgA in serum is of the polymeric form, and the efficiency of killing initiated by this polymeric form exceeds that of monomeric IgA–initiated killing. In the absence of complement, specific IgA induces minimal bacterial adherence, uptake, and killing. Killing of *S. pneumoniae* by resting phagocytes with immune IgA requires complement, predominantly via the C2-independent alternative pathway, which in turn requires factor B but not calcium. Pneumococcal capsule–specific IgA may have distinct roles in effecting the clearance of pneumococci in the presence or absence of inflammation, and the polymeric form may control pneumococcal infections locally and after the pathogen's entry into the bloodstream by several mechanisms.[367]

PHAGOCYTOSIS AND LEUKOCYTE IgG RECEPTORS. IgG-mediated phagocytosis by PMNs is the main defense against *S. pneumoniae*. Two leukocyte IgG receptors, FcγRIIa and FcγRIIIb, are expressed constitutively on PMNs. Blocking experiments have shown that FcγRIIa is crucial for opsonophagocytosis of serum-opsonized *S. pneumoniae*. In adults, serum-induced phagocytic activity depends mainly on antipneumococcal IgG2 antibodies.[370,623] However, in infants and young children, the main response to pneumococcal conjugate vaccines occurs in the

IgG1 subclass.[26,205,755] Investigators have suggested that IgG1 subclass antibodies are at least as highly functional as is IgG2.[205] Recruitment and function of neutrophils also are important host defenses. In a pneumococcal infection model in immunocompetent and immunodeficient mice intranasally infected with *S. pneumoniae* type 2, immunocompetent BALB/c mice were resistant and immunodeficient CBA/Ca mice were susceptible to infection. BALB/c mice recruited significantly more neutrophils in the lungs, and inflammatory lesions were visible much earlier than in CBA/Ca mice.[271]

ANTIBODIES TO SURFACE PROTEINS AND PNEUMOLYSIN. PspA, PsaA, and pneumolysin are common to virtually all pneumococcal isolates. The development of antibodies to PspA, PsaA, and pneumolysin as a result of pneumococcal infection and carriage in young children was determined by measurement of serum antibodies to these proteins by ELISA in children at ages 6, 12, 18, and 24 months and in their mothers. All age groups were shown to produce antibodies to the three proteins, which increased with age and were associated strongly with pneumococcal exposure as a result of carriage or acute otitis media (AOM).[605] IgA to PspA, PsaA, and pneumolysin has been detected by ELISA in the saliva of children aged 6 to 24 months.[685] This finding was associated with pneumococcal carriage and otitis media.

Serum antipneumolysin IgG at the time of hospital admission has been found to be higher in patients with nonbacteremic pneumococcal pneumonia than in those with bacteremic pneumococcal pneumonia or uninfected control subjects.[531] Serum antipneumolysin IgG levels also rose significantly during convalescence in patients with bacteremic pneumonia, and the levels attained were equal to those observed in nonbacteremic patients. Children aged 6 to 24 months were shown to produce antibodies to pneumolysin, and antibody concentrations increased with age and were associated strongly with pneumococcal exposure, whether by carriage or infection such as AOM.[605] Infants also have been shown to mount a specific antibody response to pneumolysin during AOM.[606]

DEFENSE MECHANISMS OF THE SPLEEN. The spleen is the principal organ that clears pneumococci from the bloodstream.[527] Opsonized particles are removed from the circulation by the liver, but with decreasing opsonization, the spleen increasingly assumes the role of clearance. The slow passage of blood through the spleen and the prolonged contact time with reticuloendothelial cells in the cords of Billroth and the splenic sinuses allow time for the removal of nonopsonized particles. Overwhelming pneumococcal infection occurs in children and adults whose spleens have been removed or do not function normally. Pneumococcal disease progresses so rapidly in such individuals that pneumonia is not detectable clinically or by chest radiographs, although it is seen at autopsy. The increase in the incidence of pneumococcal bacteremia and meningitis in children with sickle-cell disease is due largely to splenic dysfunction.

VITAMIN A. The association of nasopharyngeal colonization with *S. pneumoniae* and vitamin A supplementation in infants in an area with endemic vitamin A deficiency in southern India showed that neonatal vitamin A supplementation delayed the age at which colonization occurs; therefore, it may play a role in lowering morbidity rates associated with pneumococcal disease.[139]

C-REACTIVE PROTEIN. C-reactive protein (CRP) is a normal constituent of human serum that is synthesized by hepatocytes and induced by proinflammatory cytokines. The function of this acute-phase reactant includes activation of complement and enhancement of opsonophagocytosis. CRP binds to phosphorylcholine, a constituent of eukaryotic membranes that also is found on the cell surface of the major bacterial pathogens of the human respiratory tract, including *S. pneumoniae* and *Haemophilus influenzae*. CRP is present in inflamed (0.17 to 42 mg/mL) and uninflamed (<0.05 to 0.88 mg/mL) secretions from the human respiratory tract in sufficient quantities to have an antimicrobial effect. In addition, the CRP gene was expressed in human respiratory epithelial cell cultures. The complement-dependent bactericidal activity of normal nasal airway surface fluid and sputum was abolished when the secretions were pretreated to remove CRP. Human respiratory epithelial cells are capable of expressing CRP, and this protein may contribute to bacterial clearance in the human respiratory tract.[282]

PLATELET-ACTIVATING FACTOR RECEPTORS OF AIRWAY EPITHELIAL CELLS. Adherence of pneumococci to cultured human tracheal epithelial cells increased after exposure to acid and decreased after exposure to a specific inhibitor of the receptor for platelet-activating factor.[348] Exposure to acid thus may stimulate the adherence of *S. pneumoniae* to airway epithelial cells via increases in platelet-activating factor receptors. The clinical significance of these findings is not clear.[348]

CYTOKINES. Polymorphonuclear granulocytes, which provide a major defense against *S. pneumoniae* infection, are attracted to and activated by various cytokines, including interleukin-1β (IL-1β), IL-6, TNF-α, IL-8, IL-10, IL-12, interferon-γ, and granulocyte-macrophage colony-stimulating factor.[36] The inflammatory response in bacterial meningitis also is mediated by TNF-α and IL-1, which are produced in the subarachnoid space by cells such as leukocytes, astrocytes, and microglia.[559] Inoculation of pneumococcal cell wall components directly into the CSF of rabbits also results in the induction of an inflammatory response with pleocytosis and increased levels of CSF TNF-α and IL-1.[283] Both TNF-α and IL-1α have been shown to increase mucosal adhesion of pneumococci to tracheal epithelium in a chinchilla trachea whole-organ perfusion model.[737]

Respiratory Viral Infections. The role of respiratory viral infection in predisposing the host to secondary bacterial infection, including pneumonia, empyema, and lung abscess, is well recognized.[462] The lungs of immunocompetent mice infected with influenza A virus on day 1 and *S. pneumoniae* on day 8 demonstrate greater *S. pneumoniae* colony counts, more extensive neutrophil infiltration, and higher lung levels of IL-1β and TNF-α after exposure to *S. pneumoniae* than do the lungs of control mice not pre-infected with influenza virus.[462]

L-ASCORBIC ACID (VITAMIN C). Degradation of the connective tissue component hyaluronic acid by the hyaluronate lyase produced by *S. pneumoniae* is inhibited competitively by L-ascorbic acid (vitamin C).[465] One L-ascorbic acid molecule was found to bind to the active site of the enzyme. The high concentration of L-ascorbic acid in human tissues probably provides a low level of natural resistance to pneumococcal invasion by this mechanism.

LEUKOTRIENES. Leukotrienes are produced by macrophages and are considered important for antibacterial defense in the lung. Leukotrienes comprise a group of highly potent lipid mediators synthesized by the enzyme 5-lipoxygenase. Multidrug-resistance protein 1 (mrp1) is a transmembrane protein responsible for the cellular extrusion of leukotrienes from macrophages. In a mouse pneumonia model, mrp1-deficient mice display diminished growth of pneumococci in the lungs and low mortality by a mechanism that involves increased release of leukotriene B₄.[661] Pneumococci also induce the production of leukotrienes in

the middle ear, which has been related to up-regulation of two genes that govern the lipoxygenase pathway.[469]

HUMAN ALVEOLAR MACROPHAGE BINDING AND PHAGOLYSOSOMES. Human alveolar macrophages are the major resident phagocytic cells of the lung. After contact with macrophages, bacteria enter phagosomes, which gradually acquire the characteristics of terminal phagolysosomes, with incorporation of lysosome-associated membrane protein. Opsonization with serum containing immunoglobulin resulted in significantly greater binding of pneumococci to macrophages than did opsonization with immunoglobulin-depleted serum.[279] Binding, intracellular localization, and killing of pneumococci by macrophages all are increased significantly by opsonization with serum containing immunoglobulin, complement, or both.

INTRACELLULAR KILLING. Once pneumococci undergo phagocytosis by "professional" phagocytes (leukocytes and macrophages), they are killed.[527] However, researchers have shown that pneumococci can enter and survive inside A549 cells, a human lung alveolar carcinoma (type II pneumocyte) cell line.[720] Not all clinical *S. pneumoniae* isolates were capable of penetrating these cells, and the presence of a polysaccharide capsule also reduced their capacity to penetrate A549 cells significantly. The intracellular activity of various antibiotics against pneumococci in A549 cells showed that in the presence of antibiotics for 18 hours, more than 98 percent of the A549 cells were viable and less than 3 percent of the pneumococci that initially were phagocytosed could be detected intracellularly after exposure to peak serum concentrations of penicillin G, azithromycin, moxifloxacin, trovafloxacin, rifampin, and telithromycin.[494] In the absence of antibiotics, pneumococci were phagocytosed efficiently but then paradoxically went on to kill all the A549 cells within 18 hours. The clinical significance of these findings is unknown.

COMPLEMENT. The second component of complement (C2) is an important factor associated with host defense against encapsulated organisms. Homozygous deficiency of C2 is the deficiency of complement most commonly inherited. Although C2 deficiency can be asymptomatic, patients usually have either autoimmune disease or recurrent pyogenic infection caused by encapsulated bacteria such as *S. pneumoniae*, *H. influenzae* type b (Hib), and *Neisseria meningitidis*. An association between C2 deficiency and IgG subclass deficiency also has been described previously.[37] *S. pneumoniae* challenge of mice deficient in the third component of complement (C3) results in a 2000-fold increase in organism load in the bloodstream in comparison to controls.[130] Binding of pneumococcal CbpA to epithelially produced C3 results in adhesion of pneumococci to type II pulmonary epithelial cells. CbpA-deficient pneumococcal mutants and lysates, therefore, fail to bind C3 and demonstrate a moderate decrease in adhesion to type II pulmonary epithelial cells, thus confirming the interaction of CbpA and C3 in adhesion.[696]

POLYMERIC IMMUNOGLOBULIN RECEPTOR. pIgR plays a crucial role in mucosal immunity against microbial infection by transporting polymeric immunoglobulins such as IgA across the mucosal epithelium. Polymeric IgA consists of two IgA molecules joined by a small polypeptide J chain. The J chain shows high affinity for the glycoprotein pIgRs of epithelial cells, which are responsible for externalization of polymeric IgA across cell membranes.[376] However, pIgR also can act as a "Trojan horse" and participate in the pathogenesis of invasive pneumococcal disease as pIgR binds to a major pneumococcal adhesin, CbpA.[800] Expression of pIgR in human nasopharyngeal cells greatly enhances pneumococcal adherence and invasion; this effect is abolished either by insertional knockout of CbpA in pneumococci or by antibodies against either pIgR or CbpA.

BASIC FIBROBLAST GROWTH FACTOR. Basic fibroblast growth factor is a neurotrophic factor in the central nervous system that is expressed at high levels in response to seizure or stroke. It also occurs in pneumococcal meningitis, as shown in experimental bacterial meningitis in mice and in children with bacterial meningitis.[341] Patients with meningitis in whom major sequelae or death occurred had much higher levels of CSF basic fibroblast growth factor than did those who survived. In patients with bacterial meningitis who survived, basic fibroblast growth factor decreased significantly in CSF after 24 to 50 hours of administration of antibiotic therapy. However, its biologic role in the pathophysiology of bacterial meningitis is not known.

GRANULOCYTE COLONY-STIMULATING FACTOR. In a limited study of 22 non-neutropenic adult patients with pneumococcal meningitis, granulocyte colony-stimulating factor (G-CSF), in addition to cefotaxime and dexamethasone, was administered subcutaneously for 6 days. All patients survived, and in only one patient did a complication develop (bilateral hearing deficit). Improvement of inflammation indices in CSF was rapid.[182] However, controlled clinical trials are needed. In a rabbit meningitis model, G-CSF increased the percentage of granulocytes in blood but not in CSF and increased CSF TNF-α and IL-1β concentrations.[658] However, G-CSF did not reduce the density of apoptotic neurons in the dentate gyrus of the hippocampus. A second study in a rabbit meningitis model used longer pretreatment with G-CSF and showed more positive results.[558] G-CSF pretreatment attenuated meningeal inflammation and enhanced systemic killing of bacteria. Pretreatment with recombinant human G-CSF in a murine model of pneumococcal pneumonia resulted in improved survival with low, but not high, bacterial inocula. Therefore, the benefits of using G-CSF are limited inasmuch as pneumococci already have recruited large numbers of neutrophils in the lungs by this time.[176]

INTRACELLULAR SIGNALING PATHWAYS. Pneumococcal cell walls activate multiple intracellular signaling pathways in microglial brain cells, with induction of an outwardly rectifying K+ channel; suppression of the constitutively expressed inwardly rectifying K+ current; and release of TNF-α, IL-6, IL-12, and other inflammatory mediators.[596] The presence of serum strongly facilitated these effects. The mechanisms involved in microglial activation by pneumococcal cell walls were different from those activated by gram-negative lipopolysaccharide.

LACTOFERRIN. Human lactoferrin is an iron-binding glycoprotein that is particularly prominent in exocrine secretions and leukocytes and also is found in serum, especially during inflammation. It is able to sequester iron from microbes and has immunomodulatory functions, including inhibition of both activation of complement and production of cytokines. Binding of human lactoferrin to the surface of *S. pneumoniae* depends entirely on PspA.[298] Prevention of the binding of lactoferrin to pneumococcal PspA could be an important host defense mechanism.

MANNOSE-BINDING LECTIN. Mannose-binding lectin (MBL) is a key mediator of innate host immunity that activates the complement pathway and directly opsonizes some infectious pathogens. Mutations in three codons in the MBL gene have been identified, and individuals homozygous for a mutant genotype have very little or no serum MBL. In a study conducted in the United Kingdom of 229 patients in whom *S. pneumoniae* was isolated from sterile sites, 28 (12%) were homozygous for MBL codon variants versus only 18 of 353 (5%) controls (odds ratio, 2.59; 95% confidence interval, 1.39 to 4.83).[638]

PATHOGENESIS OF DISEASE

To cause disease, pneumococci, like other extracellular bacterial pathogens, must adhere to mammalian cells, replicate in situ, be carried to and replicate in parts of the body that normally are free of them, escape phagocytosis, and damage tissue by causing inflammation or producing substances that directly damage cells and, in some cases, invade the bloodstream.[527] As discussed earlier, the vast array of virulence mechanisms available to pneumococci are countered by numerous host defense mechanisms, although some host responses facilitate infection.

Even though colonization with a pneumococcal strain can progress to disease, it usually does not occur, and the development of anticapsular type-specific antibodies occurs within 30 days,[287,288,529,530] at least in older children and adults. If organisms find their way into the eustachian tubes, sinuses, or bronchi, clearance mechanisms, chiefly ciliary action, lead to their rapid removal. After the development of humoral immunity, colonization with a strain may persist for 1 to 12 months, during which time disease may occur in contiguous sites, but the host is protected from invasive disease by circulating type-specific anticapsular IgG. Loss of colonization with a strain is followed, after a variable colonization-free interval, by colonization with a different serotype. Because 90 antigenically distinct serotypes exist, this cycle of colonization accompanied by the development of humoral immunity occurs many times.

Progression of colonization to disease usually requires the combination of two events: first, acquisition of a serotype to which the host is not immune and, second, a concurrent respiratory viral infection, chronic damage to respiratory epithelium (e.g., smoking or occupational exposure), allergy, or other conditions that result in the development of disease rather than just colonization.[527] Many of these concurrent conditions initiate cytokine activation of the respiratory epithelium, which facilitates increased adhesion of pneumococci to respiratory epithelial cells, as well as invasion of these cells.[462] Mechanisms by which cytokine activation results in these effects include expression of platelet-activating factor and pIgR as discussed earlier. This combination of factors leads to a higher density of colonizing organisms and enables pneumococci to cause infection, including pneumonia, acute exacerbations of chronic bronchitis, sinusitis, otitis media, and mastoiditis, in contiguous respiratory tract sites. Adherence of *S. pneumoniae* to host cells involves an array of surface adhesin molecules such as CbpA, PspA, PspC, Hyl, Ply, PsaA, and both neuraminidases. As discussed earlier, these proteins are involved in interactions with the host complement system (PspA), degradation of hyaluronan of the extracellular matrix (Hyl), lysis of cholesterol-containing membranes (pneumolysin), and binding of metals (divalent cations) such as Mn^{2+} or Zn^{2+} (PsaA), followed by their transport inside the cytoplasm of pneumococci.

Additionally, transepithelial and transendothelial transport of organisms into the bloodstream results in bacteremia, and subsequent transport across other epithelial cells leads to infection of noncontiguous sites such as the leptomeninges, peritoneum, and joint spaces. Such infection occurs in nonimmune hosts by virtue of the fact that pneumococci are able to escape ingestion and killing by host phagocytic cells in the absence of type-specific antibody because the capsule is the major determinant of virulence. *S. pneumoniae* produces few toxins and largely causes disease by its capacity to replicate in host tissues and generate an intense inflammatory response. Cell wall TA and peptidoglycan stimulate the production of cytokines (IL-1, IL-6, IL-8, and TNF) and activate complement by the alternative pathway. The polysaccharide capsule also activates the alternative complement pathway in vitro. Such activation is associated with the release of C5a, a potent attractant for PMNs. The classic complement pathway also is activated by antibody to cell wall polysaccharides in the absence of anticapsular antibody, and an intense inflammatory response fueled by vigorous activation of both the alternative and classical complement pathways accompanies pneumococcal infection of an immunologically naive host.[527] The disease process is largely a result of this inflammation, and its severity is in direct proportion to its intensity. Pneumolysin also is associated with the severity of disease, and injection of pneumolysin into rat lung causes all the histologic findings of pneumonia, whereas immunization of mice with pneumolysin before infection or challenge with pneumolysin knockout pneumococci is associated with a significant reduction in virulence.[49,221] Numerous other factors contribute to the ability of strains to cause disease and to the severity of disease, as discussed under virulence mechanisms.

A 2006 study evaluated 189 isolates from blood or CSF, 3200 isolates from middle ear fluid, and 348 isolates from the conjunctiva of children aged younger than 36 months with pneumococcal infection. A positive association with invasive pneumococcal disease was demonstrated for serotypes 1, 5, and 12F; with AOM for serotypes 1, 3, 5, 12F, 19A, and 19F; and with acute conjunctivitis for serotype 3 and nontypeable *S. pneumoniae*.[678]

Although pneumococci most commonly cause bacteremia, otitis media, pneumonia, and meningitis, they can produce disease in virtually any organ. Before the advent of immunotherapy and chemotherapy, such "unusual" infections were relatively common. Today, they are less so.

Survival of a patient with a pneumococcal disease depends on numerous variables, including the site of infection, the underlying disease, and the patient's age. Before the advent of chemotherapy, pneumococcal meningitis was universally fatal, whereas pneumococcal pneumonia killed approximately 25 percent of patients. Austrian and Gold[42] in 1964 dramatically illustrated the role of age and underlying disease when their survey of mortality associated with bacteremic pneumococcal pneumonia destroyed the complacency produced by the use of antimicrobial agents. The aged and infirm were likely to die despite receiving immediate and appropriate therapy with penicillin. Today, normal children rarely die of pneumococcal disease; thus, the prognosis must be related to the likelihood of permanent sequelae occurring. Pneumococci do not cause necrosis in pulmonary tissue, and survivors rapidly regain normal pulmonary function.[372] Many children recovering from pneumococcal meningitis are found to have neurologic sequelae. Some investigators suggest that the first attack of pneumococcal otitis media in some way predisposes the individual to subsequent attacks of otitis media.[338]

Before the availability of antimicrobial agents, recovery of a patient with pneumococcal pneumonia depended on the development of type-specific antibody. Although serum and white blood cells (WBCs) from nonimmune children kill pneumococci, probably by activation of the alternative complement pathway, they do so slowly. The importance of this pathway is illustrated best by the inability of children with sickle-cell disease to handle pneumococcal infection.[186,378,572] These children and others with asplenia may die rapidly despite the administration of prompt, vigorous therapy.[382,406,666]

MICROBIOLOGY

S. pneumoniae is a gram-positive coccus that replicates in pairs and chains in liquid medium. The shape of the individual organism is a lanceolate coccus, usually in pairs with the long axis forming a straight line. Elongated or pointed forms are common findings.

Pneumococci are cultured readily on blood and chocolate agar media, as well as in suitable liquid culture media for isolation from blood. Isolates are facultative anaerobes, and most strains require atmospheric enrichment with 5 to 10 percent CO_2 for primary isolation[41]; occasional strains are strict anaerobes. Strains can be adapted for growth without CO_2 supplementation by repeated subculture. Detection of nasopharyngeal carriage of pneumococci is a problem because of the presence of other flora; the use of antimicrobial-containing media, such as blood agar supplemented with gentamicin (5 µg/mL), has led to improvements in isolation of pneumococci, particularly resistant strains.[574,599] However, the sensitivity of current in vitro methods is poor in comparison to the sensitivity of mouse inoculation, although not all serotypes are virulent in mice.[330,423]

IDENTIFICATION OF PNEUMOCOCCI

Pneumococci usually are identified readily by standard features such as colonial morphology, alpha-hemolysis, negative catalase reaction, optochin susceptibility, bile solubility, and specific reactions with antisera to capsular polysaccharides.[353] *S. pneumoniae* produces an autolytic intracellular enzyme, LytA, that causes the organism to autolyze rapidly when grown on artificial media. Bile salts accelerate this natural autolytic process by combining with the pneumococcal cell and activating its autolysin. Strains with atypical features, such as rounded rather than flat or concentrically ringed colonies, optochin resistance, or lack of capsules, do occur and can result in misidentification of such strains as viridans streptococci. Atypical strains are more likely to be encountered from normal flora sites and with penicillin-resistant strains.

Strains with optochin zones greater than 14 mm can be identified presumptively as pneumococci, strains with 7- to 14-mm zones require confirmation by bile solubility, and strains with no zone usually are not *S. pneumoniae*. However, incubation in carbon dioxide has been recognized for a long time as decreasing the size of the zone around optochin disks, and incubation in room air generally results in an increase in zone size if the strain is a pneumococcus or a decrease if the strain is a member of the viridans group of streptococci.[600] Optochin-resistant variants of pneumococci can occur and usually are seen as a subpopulation within the zone of inhibition of an optochin disk, and optochin-resistant mutants can be selected by passage of strains in the presence of optochin.[525] Strains with equivocal optochin zones or atypical colonial morphology can be tested for bile solubility, either directly by placing a drop of bile salt solution (10% sodium deoxycholate) onto colonies and observing for lysis of the colonies or by suspension of organisms in a bile salt solution with a bile salt–free control. Care must be taken in the tube bile solubility test to avoid obtaining false-positive results, which can be caused by the organism suspension being too light or by organisms being suspended in broth rather than saline.[353]

Identification of the capsular polysaccharide serotype or serogroup also is useful in characterizing strains and confirming the identity of problem strains. Such identification is performed by the capsular swelling technique, in which equal volumes of an organism suspension, 0.3 percent methylene blue dye solution, and antiserum are mixed on a glass slide, covered with a coverslip, and read at 1000× magnification by phase-contrast microscopy. Alternatively, organism suspensions can be dried on slides and antiserum and methylene blue dye solution mixed on a coverslip, which then is placed on the slide. The polysaccharide capsule of the pneumococcal organism binds with type-specific antiserum, and organisms can be seen to clump or agglutinate; the resulting change in the refractive index of antibody-coated capsule causes the capsule to appear swollen. Currently, antisera to each serotype or serogroup are available commercially, and factoring antisera to subtype serogroups are available from Statens Serum Institut, Copenhagen, Denmark. The numbering system for the 90 pneumococcal serotypes is shown in Table 96–1.

Currently, 90 serotypes have been identified and are divided into 25 individual serotypes and 21 serogroups in the Danish classification, which now is used universally.[323] Most serotypes have one antigenic determinant, whereas serogroups have one or more antigenic determinants common to the group and one or more determinants unique to each serotype. Serotypes within a serogroup usually are identified by the serogroup number followed by a letter indicating the serotype to which a strain belongs in the Danish system, or they are identified by a unique number in the U.S. system. Except for serogroups 6 and 9, the letters in the Danish system are F for the first subtype, followed by A, B, and so on. Each serogroup contains 2 to 5 related types, and the 21 serogroups include 65 individual subtypes. Serotype numbers 26 and 30 are not in use. Omniserum containing antibodies to all 90 serotypes is available and can be used to confirm the identity of isolates as pneumococci. Because many serotypes or serogroups are included in this reagent, reactions may not always be optimal and usually are stronger in pool or monovalent reagents. Nine antiserum pools classified from A to I, each containing four to seven serotypes or serogroups, also are available and can be used to identify strains in a group of serotypes before individual serotype or serogroup reagents are tested. Other methods of capsular typing, such as latex agglutination, coagglutination, and capillary precipitation, can be used, but these methods are not available commercially.

The ability of a polymerase chain reaction (PCR) method to identify the capsular serotype of pneumococci has been developed on the basis of polymorphisms in two genes common to the different capsule loci.[441] In a limited study, the correct serotype or serogroup was identified in 92 of 93 strains, but this method did not differentiate serotype 6A from 6B strains. PCR holds promise as a noncultural method for determining serotype.

DETECTION OF CLONALITY

In addition to phenotypic features, such as serotype and antimicrobial resistance markers, the various DNA fingerprint methods for epidemiologic typing of *S. pneumoniae* that have been applied include ribotyping, BOX fingerprinting with the BOX repetitive sequence of *S. pneumoniae* used as a DNA probe, PCR fingerprinting with a primer homologous to the enterobacterial repetitive intergenic consensus sequence, pulsed-field gel electrophoresis of large DNA fragments digested by restriction enzymes, and restriction fragment end labeling to detect restriction fragment length polymorphisms of small DNA fragments.[325,504] The discriminatory power of the individual techniques differed significantly. BOX fingerprinting, pulsed-field gel electrophoresis, and restriction fragment end labeling provided the highest degree of discriminatory power. Ribotyping, BOX fingerprinting, and restriction fragment end labeling were very suitable techniques for computerized data analysis. Pulsed-field gel electrophoresis of large DNA fragments digested by restriction enzymes such as Sma1 is the method used most frequently. Descriptions and nomenclature for the 16 major pneumococcal clones that have contributed to the increase in antimicrobial resistance worldwide were published recently.[504]

DIAGNOSIS OF PNEUMOCOCCAL DISEASE

Definitive diagnosis of pneumococcal infection is based on recovery of pneumococci from the site of infection or documentation of pneumococcal bacteremia, whereas presumptive diagnosis is based on detection of pneumococcal cellular components, such as capsular polysaccharide, and on species-specific DNA and RNA sequences from the site of infection or from remote sites such as urine.[353] Definitive diagnosis is confounded in many instances by the need for invasive procedures to obtain specimens (e.g., from the middle ear space) and by nasopharyngeal carriage

of pneumococci when sputum is cultured. Pneumococci almost invariably are isolated from CSF in pneumococcal meningitis, even in patients receiving oral antibiotics.[635] However, establishing the diagnosis of pneumococcal pneumonia is more challenging because sputum rarely is available from children and direct lung puncture is performed very infrequently. Detection of pneumococcal bacteremia to confirm the diagnosis of pneumococcal pneumonia or other localized infection is valuable, but it does not occur frequently and the actual prevalence of bacteremic pneumococcal pneumonia in children is not known,[728] although a recent study suggests that the prevalence is approximately 17 percent (11/64).[509] Therefore, pediatricians must use other methods to diagnose pneumococcal pneumonia. Signs and symptoms significantly associated with bacteremic pneumococcal pneumonia in children include high temperature (>38.9° C [>102° F]), leukocytosis (>15,000/mm³), and lobar or segmental consolidation.[728] However, the frequency with which these findings are associated with nonbacteremic pneumococcal pneumonia is not known.

With the widespread deployment of pneumococcal vaccine, occult bacteremia caused by *S. pneumoniae* occurs less commonly. The likelihood that a positive blood culture will be a false-positive result is increased if the WBC count is less than 15,000/mm³, the time for the blood culture to become positive exceeds 24 hours, or the Gram stain result is suggestive of a contaminant.[655] Overall, the frequency with which positive blood cultures are obtained from children with occult bacteremia has declined in comparison to the pre-pneumococcal vaccine era and has declined precipitously since the era before the deployment of vaccine for Hib.

Direct examination of Gram-stained smears of clinically appropriate material remains the fastest diagnostic method and can be augmented if necessary by direct demonstration of capsular swelling of organisms in the presence of anticapsular antisera. The availability of antigen-detection systems that can be used in urine, serum, CSF, and other specimens, such as capsular antigen detection by counterimmunoelectrophoresis and latex agglutination with polyvalent pneumococcal reagent, generally has not improved patient management because of the low sensitivity and specificity of these methods and the fact that they usually are positive only when a Gram stain also is positive. The concentration of pneumococcal capsular antigen in saliva was evaluated by latex agglutination in a study consisting of children with community-acquired pneumonia and healthy controls. None of the children with pneumonia in this study had a positive blood culture, and pneumococcal capsular antigen was detected in the saliva of 27 percent of children with pneumonia versus 17 percent of controls. More cases (20%) than controls (2%) had a pneumococcal capsular antigen titer of 10 or greater ($p < 0.01$). Quantitative measurement of pneumococcal capsular antigen in saliva may be valuable in helping make an etiologic diagnosis in children with pneumonia, but its sensitivity is poor and it is confounded by false-positive results caused by pneumococcal carriage.[233]

A rapid (15-minute) immunochromatographic membrane test to detect pneumococcal polysaccharide capsular antigen in urine samples (Binax NOW) has been developed and was evaluated in the diagnosis of bacteremic and nonbacteremic pneumococcal pneumonia. Urine samples were studied in 51 patients with bacteremic and nonbacteremic pneumonia caused by *S. pneumoniae*; the pneumonia was diagnosed by blood culture, and pneumococcal polysaccharide capsular antigen was detected by counterimmunoelectrophoresis in urine samples. Pneumococcal antigen was detected in urine by the immunochromatographic membrane test in 41 of 51 patients with pneumococcal pneumonia (80.4%), including 23 of 28 bacteremic cases (82.1%) and 18 of 23 nonbacteremic cases (78.3%). Antigen also was detected in 7 of 16 patients with a diagnosis of presumptive pneumococcal pneumonia (43.7%) and in 1 of the 16 patients with pneumonia but in whom no pathogen was identified. The specificity of the immunochromatographic membrane test was 97.2 percent, but its sensitivity was only approximately 80 percent, thus limiting its value.[191] Furthermore, the usefulness of this test is questionable because the antigen was detected in the urine in 30 of 138 (22%) healthy children with nasopharyngeal carriage of *S. pneumoniae* versus only 3 of 71 (4%) noncarriers (*p* < 0.001).[302] Thus, the test was shown to be often positive in healthy pneumococcal carriers.

One recent study found that immunochromatographic testing for *S. pneumoniae* in CSF was both 100 percent sensitive and specific. The simplicity of the test and the longevity of the CSF antigen even after treatment suggest potential utility of this method in identifying *S. pneumoniae* meningitis in resource-poor countries with widespread prehospital antimicrobial use.[646] Another study showed immunochromatographic testing to be more sensitive than culture in detecting *S. pneumoniae* as the causative agent in thoracic empyema.[587]

Newer molecular-based methods for establishing the diagnosis of pneumococcal disease include the use of DNA probes to detect pneumolysin, autolysin, and PsaA protein, but considerable practical problems must be overcome before these methods will be applicable clinically.[173] Examples include a commercial method involving real-time PCR for simultaneous detection of *N. meningitidis*, *H. influenzae*, and *S. pneumoniae* in patients suspected of having meningitis and septicemia. This method is based on detection of the pneumolysin gene for *S. pneumoniae* and uses a single-tube, 5′-nuclease multiplex PCR assay on samples of CSF, plasma, serum, and whole blood. Amplified products are monitored with sequence-specific, fluorescent dye–labeled probes. The sensitivity of using clinical samples (CSF, serum, plasma, and whole blood) from culture-confirmed cases of *S. pneumoniae* infection was 91.8 percent. The multiplex assay also was used to test a large number of culture-negative samples, which resulted in the detection of numerous cases of meningococcal, *H. influenzae*, and pneumococcal disease that had not been detected by culture.[141] However, whether these results are true positives or false positives is not known, and in another study, although the sensitivity of PCR amplification of the pneumolysin gene in the serum and CSF of infants and children with culture-proven pneumococcal bacteremia and meningitis was 100 percent, the specificity was poor, with 17 percent of healthy controls having positive results.[173] The prevalence of false-positive reactions was highest (33%) in 2-year-old children, the age group with the highest rate of nasopharyngeal carriage of pneumococci. Therefore, although PCR of serum and CSF is a sensitive test for the detection of *S. pneumoniae* in these sites, its high rate of positivity in healthy controls as a result of nasopharyngeal carriage limits its utility in detecting systemic pneumococcal infection.[173]

Another rapid PCR method involving the use of a set of primers that amplify 273 base pairs of the autolysin gene has been developed to identify *S. pneumoniae*. In addition, three sets of primers were designed to amplify a 240–base pair fragment of the PBP-2B gene (*pbp2b*) of penicillin-susceptible *S. pneumoniae* and two common *pbp2b* mutations present in penicillin-resistant *S. pneumoniae* in order to simultaneously identify the penicillin susceptibility of strains. The autolysin gene was identified in all 1062 clinical isolates of *S. pneumoniae* evaluated. In addition, 98.9 percent of 621 penicillin-susceptible isolates were shown to have DNA fragments amplified by the penicillin-susceptible primers, whereas 72.1 percent of 441 penicillin-resistant isolates were detected by the penicillin-resistant *S. pneumoniae* primers.[741] Although further refinement of this method is required, this study has shown that it is possible to identify pneumococci and differentiate penicillin-susceptible from penicillin-resistant *S. pneumoniae* by applying PCR and a combination of primers to detect the susceptible *pbp2b* gene, resistant *pbp2b* gene mutations, and the autolysin gene. In another study, a 208–base pair region

of the pneumolysin gene was amplified by PCR in blood specimens from hospitalized children with pneumonia. Whole blood, buffy coat, or plasma samples from 67 children (44%) tested positive by PCR. The sensitivity was 100 percent in 11 culture-confirmed children, and the specificity was 95 percent in control subjects. Age, previous administration of oral antibiotic therapy, and pneumococcal nasopharyngeal colonization did not influence the PCR results, which were more specific than were serologic and urinary antigen testing.[509]

A gene probe for the gene encoding the PsaA protein also has been developed on the basis of PCR assay. PsaA was confirmed to be present in representative strains of all 90 serotypes of *S. pneumoniae*. The specificity of the assay was verified by the lack of signal from analysis of heterologous bacterial species (*n* = 30) and genera (*n* = 14), including viridans group streptococci. The potential of the assay for clinical application was shown by its ability to detect pneumococci in culture-positive nasopharyngeal specimens.[520]

SUSCEPTIBILITY TESTING

Susceptibility testing of pneumococci has been well standardized, and testing can be performed by determination of the minimal inhibitory concentration (MIC) and, for selected agents, by disk diffusion.[356] MICs can be performed by macrodilution or microdilution in cation-supplemented Mueller-Hinton broth enhanced with 5 percent whole defibrinated sheep or horse blood or 5 percent lysed and centrifuged horse blood.[537] If sulfonamides are tested, only the latter supplement should be used to avoid the presence of sulfonamide antagonists. MICs also can be determined by dilution in Mueller-Hinton agar supplemented as just described; agar dilution generally is regarded as the reference method for pneumococci and often is used for developmental work.[353]

Many systems based on frozen or dried microdilution trays are available commercially and used extensively for surveillance testing.[354] As with any system, commercial microdilution panels should be validated and used with appropriate quality controls.

A new method for determination of MICs, the E-test (A. B. Biodisk, Solna, Sweden), is much simpler to use than are the other methods for MIC determination. The E-test consists of a calibrated antibiotic-impregnated plastic strip that is applied to the surface of an inoculated agar plate. An antibiotic gradient is produced that results in an elliptical zone of inhibition after incubation. The MIC is read at the point where the ellipse of inhibition meets the strip. Evaluation of the E-test has shown that this method generally is reliable, although problems are encountered with some agents because acidification of the medium occurs during incubation of the plates in CO_2, which is required to ensure the growth of clinical isolates. Agents particularly affected are macrolides and some quinolones.

Disk diffusion also has been standardized well for testing pneumococci against selected agents. Distinction between susceptible and resistant strains is accomplished readily by using the current National Committee for Clinical Laboratory Standards (NCCLS) method involving macrolides, tetracycline, chloramphenicol, trimethoprim-sulfamethoxazole, and clindamycin.[353] For testing penicillin and other β-lactams, disk diffusion is used best as a screening method with 1-μg oxacillin disks that have a susceptible cutoff zone of 20 mm or larger. Strains with zones of 20 mm or larger are fully susceptible to penicillin and other β-lactams. However, strains with zones that are less than 20 mm need to have MICs of penicillin and other appropriate β-lactams determined.[537] Penicillin-susceptible strains with MICs of 0.06 μg/mL usually screen out with resistant strains.

Although interpretative categories for clarifying the significance of MIC values are available, many limitations to the currently available NCCLS pneumococcal breakpoints exist, particularly for agents that can be administered in multiple-dosing regimens and by multiple routes of administration and that are used for infections in different body sites. Breakpoints for parenteral β-lactam agents generally are based on the use of agents in meningitis, whereas those of oral β-lactam agents are based on nonmeningeal infections such as otitis media.[537] Nonmeningeal breakpoints for some parenteral β-lactam agents were introduced in 2002, which to some extent will avoid the use of non–β-lactam agents for serious nonmeningeal pneumococcal infections. These breakpoint changes classify strains previously interpreted as intermediate in sensitivity to penicillin G, cefotaxime, and ceftriaxone as susceptible if the agents are administered parenterally to treat pneumonia and other nonmeningeal infections. Pharmacokinetic and pharmacodynamic parameters recently have been shown to correlate with clinical outcome and offer a more rational approach to predicting antimicrobial efficacy and determining clinically relevant susceptibility breakpoints.[145,150,361]

ANTIBIOTIC RESISTANCE

Mechanisms of Antibiotic Resistance

RESISTANCE TO β-LACTAM DRUGS. Widespread resistance to β-lactam and other drug classes has evolved in the most common pathogens, including *S. pneumoniae*. Although pneumococci are naturally transformable organisms, β-lactamase production never has been described in this organism. Instead, a much more complex resistance mechanism has evolved in *S. pneumoniae* that is mediated by sophisticated restructuring of the targets of the β-lactams, the PBPs, and by other newly described mechanisms.[300] The PBP targets in penicillin-resistant strains of *S. pneumoniae* are modified, low-binding affinity versions of the native PBPs. PBP targets may be modified by mutation or by transformation and homologous recombination with DNA from the PBP genes of viridans streptococci. The level of resistance is determined by how many and to what extent targets are modified.[120] Restructuring of PBPs is mediated by stepwise alterations in PBPs. The high-molecular-weight PBPs—types 1A, 2X, and 2B—that usually are detected in *S. pneumoniae* are involved in transpeptidase activity and play an important role in resistance.[301] Alterations in PBP-2B are associated with low-level resistance to penicillin, and alterations in PBP-2X mediate low-level resistance to cephalosporins. The additional alterations in PBP-1A raise penicillin MICs to 1 μg/mL or greater and cefotaxime MICs to 0.5 μg/mL or greater. Genomic comparison between *S. pneumoniae* and commensal *S. mitis* and *Streptococcus oralis* strains has documented the mosaic nature of PBPs among these species, with pneumococci acquiring their altered PBP genes from *S. mitis* and *S. oralis*.[299] Many other mosaic gene clusters not associated with penicillin resistance also have been found.[255] The capacity to produce branched cell wall stem peptides encoded by altered *murM* and *murN* genes, as well as altered PBPs, is required for expression of penicillin resistance in *S. pneumoniae*.[224] The *fibA* and *fibB* genes, which are homologous to the *Staphylococcus aureus femA/B* genes required for expression of methicillin resistance in this organism, encode proteins involved in the formation of interpeptide bridges and also are required for expression of PBP-mediated penicillin resistance.[775] Other mechanisms of β-lactam resistance have been described in laboratory mutants and in a clone of Hungarian pneumococcal strains with notably high levels of β-lactam resistance (penicillin MIC, 16 μg/mL; cefotaxime MIC, 4 μg/mL).[300,695]

RESISTANCE TO NON–β-LACTAM DRUGS. The molecular and genetic mechanisms of resistance to macrolides, chloram-phenicol, tetracycline, fluoroquinolones, and trimethoprim-sulfamethoxazole in *S. pneumoniae* also have been determined. Resistance genes for several agents are carried on a transposon, Tn1545.[144] It confers resistance to three antimicrobial classes—kanamycin (*aphA-3*), macrolide-lincosamide-streptogramin B–type antibiotics (*ermB*), and tetracycline (*tetM*). This transposon has been conjugated and transposed to the chromosome of *Enterococcus faecalis*, oral streptococci, and *Listeria monocytogenes*. The properties of this transposon account for the sudden emergence, rapid dissemination, and stabilization of resistance to multiple antibiotics in *S. pneumoniae* in the absence of plasmids.

Resistance mechanisms include the production of chloramphenicol acetyltransferase, an enzyme capable of catalyzing the conversion of chloramphenicol to nonfunctional derivatives. Chloramphenicol acetyltransferase is encoded by a chloramphenicol acetyltransferase (*cat*) gene identical to the *cat* gene from the *S. aureus* plasmid pC194. Tetracycline resistance occurs through ribosomal protection encoded by the genes *tetM* and *tetO*. The tetM and tetO proteins are thought to cause tetracycline to be released from the ribosome. Resistance to fluoroquinolones primarily involves mutations in the DNA gyrase gene *gyrA* and in the topoisomerase IV genes *parC* and *parE*, as well as an efflux mechanism that affects some fluoroquinolones. Resistance to trimethoprim is mediated through a single amino acid substitution in the chromosomal dihydrofolate reductase gene of *S. pneumoniae*, which is thought to disrupt the bond with trimethoprim without affecting the action of dihydrofolate reductase. Sulfonamide resistance appears to result from repetitions of one or two amino acids in the chromosomal dihydropteroate synthase.[782]

Two major mechanisms have been described for resistance to erythromycin. Co-resistance to macrolides, clindamycin, and streptogramin B–type antibiotics is a result of modification of the ribosome through methylation of an adenine residue in domain V of the 23S rRNA. Methylation is encoded by a methylase gene, *ermB* (previously called *ermAM*). Resistance to 14- and 15-membered macrolides (erythromycin, azithromycin, and clarithromycin) but not to 16-membered macrolides (roxithromycin, josamycin, and spiramycin), ketolides, or clindamycin is a result of efflux of the antibiotic from the cell; such resistance is encoded by the gene *mefE* in *S. pneumoniae* and appears to be emerging rapidly as the predominant mechanism of resistance to erythromycin in many countries.[255] Other macrolide resistance mechanisms that have been described recently include mutations in position 2059 of the 23S rRNA and in genes encoding ribosomal protein L4.[717]

VANCOMYCIN TOLERANCE. Although vancomycin resistance has not been described in pneumococci, antibiotic tolerance, or the ability of bacteria to survive but not grow in the presence of antibiotics, has been described. It has been shown to be caused by loss of function of the VncS histidine kinase of a two-component gene expression sensor-regulator system in *S. pneumoniae* that produces tolerance to vancomycin and other classes of antibiotics.[543]

Evolution of Antibiotic Resistance among Pneumococci

Pneumococci initially were susceptible to many antimicrobial agents, but they became resistant with varying degrees of rapidity to many of these agents. The earliest example was the development of resistance to optochin (ethylhydrocupreine) when this agent was used experimentally in mice in the early part of the 20th century. With the introduction of sulfonamides in 1939, pneumococci similarly exhibited an ability to acquire resistance in experimental infections in mice, as well as in a human case of meningitis.[418] Sulfonamide resistance was identified sporadically thereafter, and a trimethoprim-sulfamethoxazole–resistant strain was recognized first in 1972. Trimethoprim-sulfamethoxazole resistance subsequently has become widespread in virtually all serotypes throughout the world, including developing countries, and resistance to this agent is greater than that to any other antimicrobial class worldwide.[328] Tetracycline resistance emerged in the 1960s and chloramphenicol resistance in 1970. However, little attention was paid to the development of resistance in this species until 1977, when isolates resistant to several antimicrobial classes, including penicillins, chloramphenicol, tetracyclines, macrolides, clindamycin, and trimethoprim-sulfamethoxazole, were detected in South Africa.[29,360] Subsequently, multiresistant clones of pneumococci have spread throughout many regions of the world. Noteworthy is that multiresistant clones are confined mostly to serotype 14 and serogroups 6, 9, 19, and 23.[179] Whereas resistance to penicillins occurs in a stepwise fashion and can be overcome by using β-lactams with appropriate pharmacokinetics, resistance to other drug classes usually is absolute, and distinct populations of strains are found to be susceptible and resistant to agents such as macrolides, clindamycin, tetracyclines, trimethoprim-sulfamethoxazole, and chloramphenicol. Unlike enterococci, resistance to vancomycin has not developed in pneumococci yet, although vancomycin-tolerant strains have been detected.[52,324]

Cross-resistance among *S. pneumoniae* to macrolides and other classes of antibiotics usually increases with increasing MICs to penicillin[357] (Fig. 96–2). Whereas only 6 percent of penicillin-susceptible pneumococci are resistant to macrolides and 14 percent to trimethoprim-sulfamethoxazole, approximately half of the penicillin-intermediate isolates were resistant to these agents. In the case of penicillin-resistant strains, three quarters were resistant to macrolides, 90 percent to trimethoprim-sulfamethoxazole, and 28 percent to clindamycin. However, this pattern is not the case in all countries, and at least one multiresistant clone resistant to chloramphenicol, tetracycline, erythromycin, clindamycin, and trimethoprim-sulfamethoxazole has remained susceptible to penicillin.[184,716]

Strains of *S. pneumoniae* were exquisitely susceptible to penicillin (MICs of 0.01 to 0.03 μg/mL) when this agent initially was used clinically in the 1940s and 1950s, and this MIC range is referred to as the baseline activity of penicillin against *S. pneumoniae*.[353] Evolution of resistance to this class of agents was noted first when a few strains of *S. pneumoniae* were isolated in the 1960s in Australia and New Guinea. These strains had decreased susceptibility to penicillin, with MICs of 0.1 to 0.25 μg/mL, approximately 10-fold higher than the MICs of baseline strains. Strains

with penicillin MICs of 2 to 4 μg/mL, approximately 100-fold higher than, the baseline strains, were isolated in South Africa in 1977, and, subsequently, strains with even higher MICs (16 μg/mL, approximately 1000-fold higher than baseline strains) were described in Hungary.[695] Pneumococci conventionally are classified as penicillin-susceptible if the MICs are 0.06 μg/mL or less, intermediate if the MICs are 0.12 to 1.0 μg/mL, and resistant if the MICs are 2.0 μg/mL or greater. This classification is useful mainly in characterizing strains as fully susceptible to β-lactams if susceptible or as having decreased susceptibility if intermediate or resistant. Strains with such decreased susceptibility are better referred to as β-lactam drug-challenged because the mechanism of resistance can be overcome if the pharmacokinetics of the β-lactam drug used in serum or at the site of infection exceeds the MIC for 40 to 50 percent of the dosing interval.[146] Similar variations in MIC ranges are seen with all β-lactams, although MIC ranges for many β-lactams are much higher than that for penicillin itself. Agents such as ampicillin, amoxicillin, cefotaxime, and ceftriaxone have MIC ranges similar to that of penicillin, whereas agents such as cefazolin, cefaclor, cefprozil, ceftazidime, and cefixime have much higher MIC ranges. For example, the baseline activity of cefaclor against *S. pneumoniae* is 0.5 to 1 μg/mL, which is a concentration approximately 20- to 30-fold higher than that required for penicillin to inhibit the most susceptible strains. Changes in susceptibility that occur over the course of time were illustrated in a study of recent versus archived otitis media strains. In this study, the MIC_{90} for cefaclor against archived isolates was 1 μg/mL, whereas the MIC_{90} against recent isolates was greater than 64 μg/mL.[355] A few agents, such as imipenem and meropenem, have slightly lower MIC ranges than those of penicillin. Currently, 50 to 60 percent of pneumococci in the United States are penicillin-susceptible, 15 to 20 percent are penicillin-intermediate, and 20 to 30 percent are penicillin-resistant. The proportions of strains in each group vary considerably throughout the world.

Resistance to macrolides in strains of *S. pneumoniae* was noted first in 1964 and was detected sporadically in the United States until it became widespread in the latter half of the 1990s.[328,344,418] The baseline activity of macrolides (0.03 μg/mL) and MIC distributions (1000-fold concentration range, 0.03 to >32 μg/mL) against *S. pneumoniae* are somewhat similar to those of penicillin. The MIC distribution of macrolides is trimodal, with strains being exquisitely susceptible (erythromycin MIC, ≤0.03 μg/mL) or highly resistant (erythromycin MIC, ≥32 μg/mL) or demonstrating intermediate resistance (MICs of 1 to 16 μg/mL).[216] These distributions closely correlate with macrolide ribosomal methylase and efflux resistance mechanisms. The prevalence of macrolide resistance and reports of clinical failure resulting from strains with efflux and ribosomal methylase resistance mechanisms continue to increase.* Some authors, however, have argued that isolates with efflux-mediated resistance could be susceptible to the high intracellular concentrations that these agents achieve in phagocytic cells and in epithelial lining fluid of the alveoli.[18,398] However, no clinical or animal data support these arguments for extracellular pathogens such as *S. pneumoniae*, whereas considerable clinical and animal data support the use of current breakpoints.[50,145,146,512] The rising incidence of macrolide-resistant pneumococci was directly proportional to the increasing use of macrolides in various communities and age groups.[251,344,586] In a recent report, 18 to 23 percent of pneumococci from the United States were macrolide-resistant[328,733] as compared with 10 percent from Canada, 11 percent from Latin America, 20 percent from Europe, and 39 percent from the Asia-Pacific region.[328]

Strains with multiple antibiotic resistance have greater selective advantages than do strains resistant to just one antibiotic because the opportunity for positive selection is increased as the

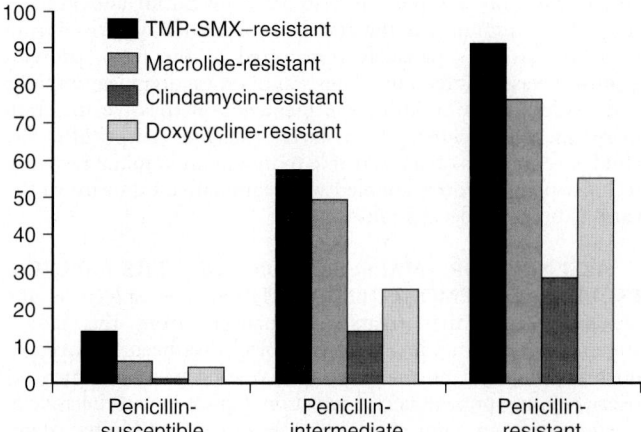

Figure 96–2 Pneumococci often are resistant to several drug classes, and cross-resistance to macrolides and other classes of antibiotics increases as minimal inhibitory concentrations of penicillin increase. TMP-SMX, trimethoprim-sulfamethoxazole.[357,687]

---

*See references 80, 232, 351, 399, 479, 480, 516, 586, 651, 773.

number of drug classes to which isolates are resistant increases.[419] Exposure to different classes of antibiotics allows more opportunity for selective advantage to a multiple antibiotic–resistant organism than to a monoresistant strain, which must wait to encounter the one antibiotic to which it is resistant and is likely to be killed by agents of other antibiotic classes. Thus, the increasing prevalence of antibiotic-resistant pneumococci is associated with the increasing prevalence of multidrug-resistant strains.[779] Therefore, one is not surprised that the use of one class of antibiotics (mainly macrolides and trimethoprim-sulfamethoxazole) can be associated with an increase in resistance to other classes of antibiotics (mainly β-lactam drugs).[5,30,169,277] Many authorities now think that antibiotic agents such as the newer macrolides (e.g., clarithromycin and azithromycin) and trimethoprim-sulfamethoxazole are stronger promoters of antibiotic resistance among *S. pneumoniae* strains than are the β-lactam drugs.[30,169,251,277,586] Researchers also have suggested that among the β-lactam drugs, cephalosporins are stronger promoters of resistance in *S. pneumoniae* than are the aminopenicillins.[251,650]

Although many strains are resistant to tetracyclines and macrolides, they are susceptible to the new tetracycline derivatives, the glycylcyclines, as well as to streptogramins, ketolides, glycopeptides, and rifampin. Many strains are resistant to trimethoprim-sulfamethoxazole worldwide, with more than 40 percent being resistant in the United States. Fluoroquinolones with antipneumococcal activity (e.g., gatifloxacin, levofloxacin, moxifloxacin) are active against most strains of *S. pneumoniae*; however, in several countries where fluoroquinolones have been prescribed widely, clinically relevant levels of resistance have been described.[122,328,613] No doubt, antibiotic resistance will continue to evolve and challenge us.

EPIDEMIOLOGY

Pneumococcal infection remains a serious problem at the beginning of the 21st century in both the developed and developing worlds. It still is a leading cause of death worldwide and a very important cause of morbidity in all countries.

In the United States, since the introduction of Hib vaccination, *S. pneumoniae* has become the leading cause of bacteremia and bacterial meningitis and has remained a major cause of otitis media. This organism causes more deaths than does any other vaccine-preventable organism.[252] The burden of pneumococcal disease in the United States has been estimated to be 125,000 to 500,000 cases of pneumonia, 50,000 cases of bacteremia, 3000 cases of meningitis, and 7 million cases of otitis media, with 40,000 deaths occurring annually.[56,315,594] In the developing world, pneumococcal infections are among the leading causes of death in children younger than 2 years old, with the estimated 1.2 million deaths per year accounting for 9 percent of all deaths.[409]

The only reservoir of *S. pneumoniae* is the human nasopharynx. From there, the organism can (1) enter the bloodstream and cause invasive infections such as sepsis and meningitis and infections in remote foci such as joints, bones, and soft tissues; (2) spread to adjacent mucosal tissue and cause mucosal infections such as otitis media, sinusitis, and pneumonia; and (3) be transmitted by direct contact and through aerosols to other individuals.[154] Acquisition and nasopharyngeal carriage of *S. pneumoniae* are associated with the occurrence of pneumococcal AOM,[210,442,478,799] bacteremia,[286,448,473,497] and pneumonia.[330]

The most common diseases caused by *S. pneumoniae* are related to the upper respiratory tract (mainly otitis media, conjunctivitis, and sinusitis). The least common are invasive infections such as bacteremia and meningitis, whereas pneumonia is of intermediate frequency. Figure 96–3 shows the difference in the order of magnitude of these diseases. The yearly incidence of invasive infections is reported to be less than 10 to greater than

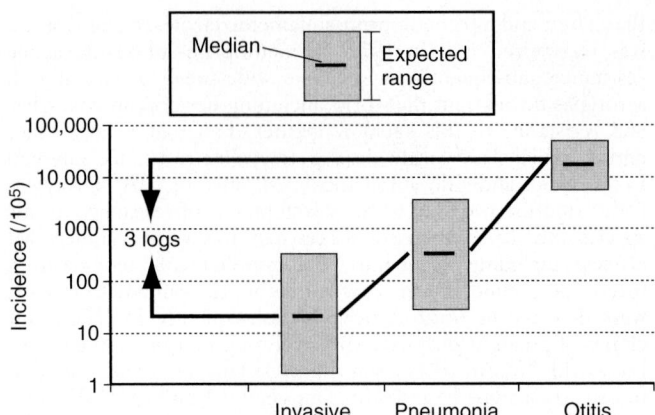

Figure 96–3 Relative incidence of pneumococcal invasive infections, pneumonia, and otitis media in children. The figure is based on estimates from global data that have been published or presented at meetings. The *horizontal line* in each box presents the estimated average value and the upper and lower limits of the presumed range.

1000 per 100,000 children younger than 5 years old in various populations. The incidence of pneumonia usually is reported as a few dozen to a few thousand per 100,000 children younger than 5 years of age. Pneumococci are responsible for 25 to 50 percent of cases of otitis media in children, which translates to more than 10,000 per 100,000 children younger than 5 years old. Thus, pneumococcal otitis media is roughly up to 1000-fold more common than is invasive pneumococcal infection, and pneumococcal pneumonia is 10- to 100-fold more common than is invasive infection.

RISK FACTORS FOR PNEUMOCOCCAL INFECTION

In general, decreased host defenses, especially in humoral immunity, or increased exposure to the organism can be considered the main risk factors for acquiring pneumococcal infection. Risk factors can be divided into various categories, although such division is arbitrary because numerous predisposing conditions can be present.

YOUNG AGE. Young age is perhaps the most important risk factor for acquiring pneumococcal infection because natural immunity is highly age-dependent. One of the best demonstrations of the relationship between age and immunity to pneumococcal infection was published in 1932 by Sutliff and Finland (Fig. 96–4). Immunity in the first few months of life, derived from maternal antibody passively transferred to the fetus, protects against invasive infection. These antibodies disappear rapidly, and, within a few months, the incidence of invasive infection increases. The incidence then starts to decline sharply after the child is 18 months of age and able to mount an immune response to most pneumococci, coupled with cumulative exposure to the various pneumococcal strains.

ABSENCE OR MALFUNCTION OF THE SPLEEN, INCLUDING HEMOGLOBINOPATHIES. The spleen is the principal organ that clears pneumococci from the bloodstream.[710,769] Patients in whom the spleen has been removed or does not function normally are at risk for the development of overwhelming pneumococcal infection. Children with invasive *S. pneumoniae* from eight children's hospitals in the United States were studied during the period 1993 to 1999. Of 2581 cases, 1 percent occurred either in children with congenital asplenia or in children who had undergone surgical splenectomy.[662] The mortality rate was high (6/22 [27%]), especially in those with meningitis.

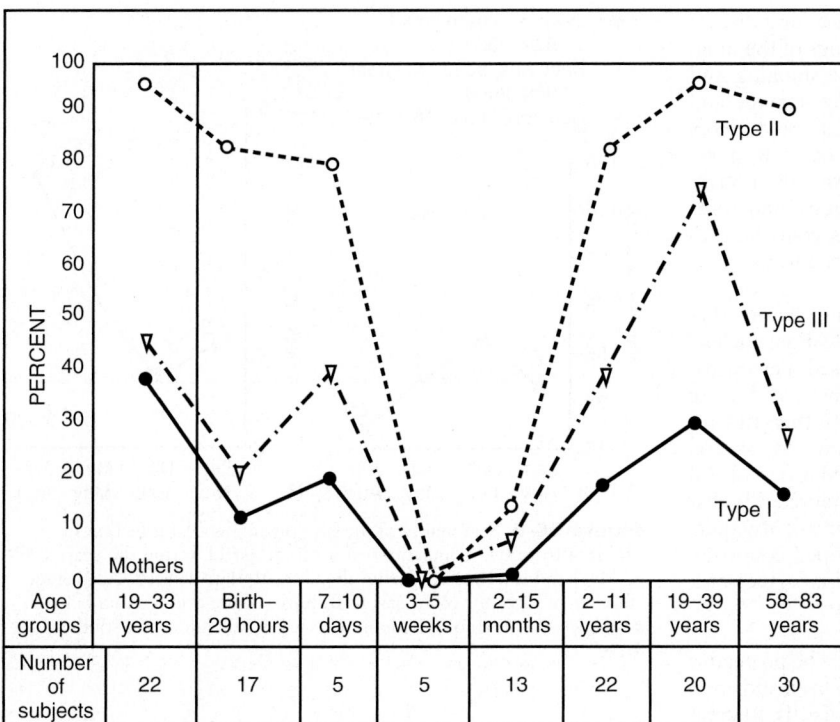

Figure 96–4 Percentage of subjects in different age groups whose blood is pneumococcidal.

Splenic malfunction is considered to be the most important reason for the increased incidence and severity of pneumococcal bacteremia in sickle-cell disease and other sickle hemoglobinopathies (e.g., hemoglobin SC disease or S-β-thalassemia).[569,571,662,797] Although the incidence of pneumococcal infection in children with hemoglobin SC disease is lower than in persons with sickle-cell disease, it is higher than in healthy children.[439,738] The incidence of overall bacterial sepsis in other hemoglobinopathies (e.g., S-β-thalassemia) is estimated to be intermediate between that for hemoglobin SC and hemoglobin SS disease.[560] The high risk for the development of pneumococcal infection in persons with sickle-cell disease is thought to be due to the combination of low levels of circulating antibodies, splenic dysfunction, and complement deficiency, which results in decreased clearance of encapsulated bacteria from the bloodstream.[571,784] Although the use of prophylactic penicillin has reduced the risk for acquiring pneumococcal disease, children younger than 5 years old with sickle-cell disease still have increased rates of invasive disease (range, 1230 to 1500/100,000 population).[226,569,788,797]

DEFECTIVE ANTIBODY FORMATION. As reviewed in the "Pathogenesis" and "Prevention" sections of this chapter, defective antibody production against pneumococcal polysaccharides is the rule for most serotypes in individuals younger than 18 months old and may be seen at even older ages for some serotypes. However, at all ages, conditions associated with reduced antibody formation constitute a high risk for acquiring pneumococcal infection in comparison to peers. Such conditions are congenital agammaglobulinemia, acquired common variable hypogammaglobulinemia,[147] selective IgG subclass deficiency,[746] and secondary defective antibody production in diseases such as malignancies and human immunodeficiency virus (HIV) infection. HIV infection predisposes individuals to the acquisition of secondary bacterial infection by several mechanisms, but defective antibody production is the most important factor in pneumococcal infection. The ability to produce antipneumococcal capsular antibody is inversely proportional to the peripheral blood CD4+ lymphocyte count, especially if it falls below 500/mm^3.[368,625] S. pneumoniae is the most common cause of invasive bacterial infection in HIV-infected children; it accounts for 35 to 50 percent of such episodes, with the relative risk of acquiring disease being 3- to 22-fold higher than that in children without HIV infection.[22,64,214,239,487,515] In one study, the incidence of invasive pneumococcal disease was 6.1 cases per 100 patient-years in HIV-infected children through the age of 7 years.[495]

DEFECTS IN COMPLEMENT. Congenital or acquired deficiencies in C1, C2, and C4 may be associated with increased susceptibility to pneumococcal infection, although cases documenting these associations are rare.[222]

NEUTROPENIA OR NEUTROPHIL DYSFUNCTION. The primary neutropenias, such as cyclic neutropenia, as well as secondary ones, such as drug-induced neutropenia and aplastic anemia, are associated with an increased incidence of severe pneumococcal infection. In some neutrophil dysfunction states, such as seen in alcoholism, liver cirrhosis, glucocorticoid treatment, and renal insufficiency, an increased incidence of pneumococcal infection is found. However, the incidence is not increased in other granulocyte dysfunction syndromes such as leukocyte adhesion deficiency syndromes[19] and chronic granulomatous disease.[248] In chronic granulomatous disease, although intracellular bacterial killing by polymorphonuclear WBCs is defective, the absence of catalase renders the pneumococcus susceptible to interaction between its endogenous H_2O_2 and myeloperoxidase and the halides present in PMNs.

DIABETES MELLITUS. Diabetes is associated with a high incidence of pneumococcal infection in adults.[113,213,601,772] However, because diabetes can predispose to pneumococcal infection by several mechanisms, some of which are found only in adults, whether diabetes mellitus in children also is a risk factor for the development of pneumococcal infection is not clear.

CONDITIONS ASSOCIATED WITH DECREASED PULMONARY CLEARANCE. Inflammatory conditions such as asthma, chronic bronchitis, and chronic obstructive lung disease predispose to the development of bacterial infections of the lung, including pneumococcal pneumonia. Both active smoking and passive smoking are associated with chronic lung damage and inflammation and have been shown to be important risk factors for development of serious pneumococcal infection.[545] Respiratory viral infections also contribute to decreased pulmonary clearance. However, as described in the "Pathogenesis" and "Prevention" sections of this chapter, viral infections contribute to pneumococcal infection by several additional mechanisms.

CROWDING. Crowding contributes to many factors that increase the risk for acquiring pneumococcal infection, including viral infections, poor hygiene, and increased person-to-person transmission of *S. pneumoniae*. Attendance at daycare centers was the most important risk factor for acquiring invasive pneumococcal infection in children and infants in several studies.[68,124,261,463,608,718] In a recent population-based, case-control study, adults aged 18 to 64 years who lived in households that included children attending daycare were at greater risk of acquiring invasive pneumococcal infection.[545] In developed countries, attendance at daycare centers is also the most important risk factor for acquiring AOM, including pneumococcal otitis.[535,637,744]

NON–BREAST-FEEDING. Breast-feeding may be protective against pneumococcal infection. Human milk has been shown to block the attachment of pneumococci to pharyngeal cells, whereas bovine milk demonstrated only a weak effect.[305] This antibacterial effect could be mediated through several components of the immune system, including secretory IgA, lactoferrin, and lysozyme. Some authors have suggested that breast-feeding protects against otitis media,[24,104,197,744] but others have failed to show this effect.[58] Studies in the United States demonstrated a protective effect of breast-feeding against invasive pneumococcal infection in children in the general population[463] and in Alaskan natives.[261] In Finland, in contrast, no such protective effect was seen.[718]

GENETIC VARIATION IN MANNOSE-BINDING LECTIN. Approximately 5 percent of the population in Europe and North America and an even larger population in many developing countries are homozygous for MBL codon variants. These subjects have a greater than 2.5-fold increased risk for the acquisition of pneumococcal infection than do those who do not have this variant or are only heterozygous for this variant.[638]

MALE GENDER. Males are affected more often than are females in most studies on pneumococcal disease, including studies on pneumococcal bacteremia, pneumonia, meningitis, and otitis media.* The reason for the male preponderance is not understood.

SEASONALITY. The occurrence of pneumococcal infection is related to season. Clustering of invasive infections, pneumonia, and otitis media occurs from September to October through April to May in the Northern Hemisphere (with the opposite picture in the Southern Hemisphere), with peaks usually occurring from December through February.† Variation in the seasonality of carriage of pneumococci also occurs and is lowest in the summer months.[290,476] This seasonality probably is related, at least in part, to two factors: (1) it parallels the seasonal variations in viral respiratory infections, which play an important role in predisposing to pneumococcal carriage and infection, and (2) the peak pneumococcal infection season coincides with attendance at

---

*See references 92, 103, 112, 153, 207, 240, 350, 360, 701, 726.
†See references 98, 153, 207, 243, 285, 286, 288, 387, 405, 411, 522, 706, 754.

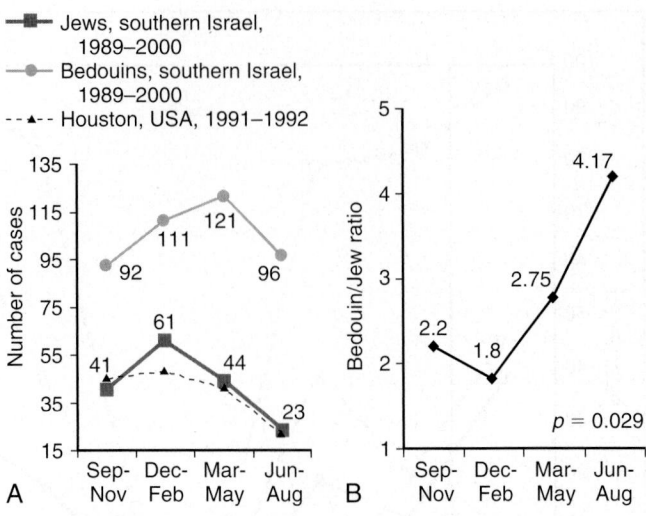

Figure 96–5 Seasonality of invasive pneumococcal infection in children from two populations in southern Israel during the years 1989 to 2000 and in Houston during the years 1991 to 1992.[405] **A,** Average number of cases for each season. **B,** Ratio of the average number of cases per season among Bedouin versus Jewish children in southern Israel.

school and daycare centers, which often excludes the summer months. However, many issues regarding seasonality remain unclear, as exemplified by data from an ongoing surveillance of invasive infections in southern Israel, where two different populations live side by side and have two distinct seasonal patterns (Fig. 96–5). In this example, the Jewish population in southern Israel, with a lifestyle equivalent to that of a middle/lower social class Western population, has a seasonality of invasive pneumococcal infection similar to that of developed populations, as represented in Figure 96–5 by children from Houston, Texas.[413] In contrast, the Bedouin population in southern Israel, a population in transition from semi-nomadism to a Western lifestyle and who live in crowded and poor hygienic conditions with a high birth rate and a disease pattern similar to that in the developing world,[464] does not demonstrate a clear pattern of seasonality. The relative abundance of cases in the spring and summer is speculated to be related to the peak of diarrheal illness in this population.[464] Further understanding of seasonality patterns may contribute to prevention of pneumococcal disease in the future.

NASOPHARYNGEAL CARRIAGE

Because acquisition and carriage of *S. pneumoniae* are associated with infection, that the higher incidence of pneumococcal infection in children than adults is associated with a higher incidence of nasopharyngeal carriage is not surprising. In various parts of the world, the carriage rate is approximately 5 to 10 percent in adults but can reach levels greater than 90 percent under various circumstances in infants and young children. Virtually all individuals carry pneumococci belonging to several serotypes during their lifetime. In a study conducted in the United States,[321] the prevalence of nasopharyngeal carriage in preschool children was 38 to 60 percent versus 29 to 35 percent and 9 to 25 percent in elementary school and junior high-school students, respectively. The prevalence in adults with no children at home was 6 percent. In studies in closed populations such as kibbutzim in Israel[87] or a poor and crowded black community in southern Israel,[160] the same differences between children and adults were noted.

Contact with young carriers increases the carriage rates in older children and adults. In the United States, although adults with no children had a carriage rate of 6 percent, the carriage rate increased to 29 percent when children were present at home. Similarly, primary school–aged children who have siblings younger than 2 years old carried *S. pneumoniae* more often than did those without young siblings.[481] In a study in Costa Rica, mother-child paired cultures showed an increased prevalence of carriage: from 6 percent at 1 month of age to 39 percent at 12 months of age. At the same time, carriage in mothers increased from 0 to 9.8 percent, thus confirming the influence of infants on adult carriage.[757] In Finland, the increased prevalence of carriage in mothers, fathers, and siblings when the index child grew older resulted in increased rates of pneumococci in the family.[459] In a Swedish study, the observed average duration of carriage was longer in children who had family carriers of the same serotype and, therefore, was suggestive of rapid recirculation in the family.[202]

Acquisition of *S. pneumoniae* may occur during the very first days of life. In infants aged 2 months, the prevalence of carriage ranges from less than 15 percent in some developed countries[23,82,171,286,459,476] to greater than 60 percent in developing countries.[138,241,284,498,514] Colonization peaks toward the second to third year of life.[171,290,320] The relationship of age to carriage is not understood, but it depends, at least in part, on the development of specific anticapsular antibodies.[288,289] In toddlers vaccinated with a pneumococcal conjugate vaccine, nasopharyngeal acquisition of new *S. pneumoniae* serotypes was related inversely to serum levels of specific antipolysaccharide IgG antibodies.[158] In another study, the presence of both circulating IgG and secretory IgA antibodies to the surface pneumococcal protein PsaA was associated with a lower prevalence of nasopharyngeal pneumococcal carriage.[397,605,685] A 2004 study showed that mucosal anticapsular IgA developed in response to colonization in preschool-aged children, regardless of vaccination status.[83,800] This phenomenon has been hypothesized to contribute to the falling carriage rates observed with increasing age.[801] The relative role of innate immunity with increasing age is not clear.

Crowding is an important factor that facilitates the spread of *S. pneumoniae*. Therefore, one is not surprised that in the developed world, the nasopharyngeal carriage rate and spread are highest in infants and toddlers attending daycare centers, with levels exceeding 90 percent in some studies,* followed by those living with one or more sibling at home.[23,171,481,595,753] In addition, the viral infections that are very prevalent in infants and toddlers attending daycare centers enhance colonization of the nasopharynx with *S. pneumoniae*.[290,476,763] The combination of young age, poor hygienic behavior, and increased incidence of respiratory viral infections renders daycare centers the ideal site for promotion and spread of *S. pneumoniae*. In addition, because of widespread antibiotic use, carriage of antibiotic-resistant *S. pneumoniae* is highest in daycare center attendees.[†] Daycare centers, thus, are a nucleus of high carriage of *S. pneumoniae*, particularly antibiotic-resistant strains. This nucleus is then responsible for the dissemination of such resistant organisms to other children, mainly to young siblings of daycare center attendees.[156,171]

The duration of carriage depends on age and serotype and may be related to additional factors such as antibiotic treatment, the immune status of the child, and other unknown factors. Carriage lasts longer in infants and young toddlers than in older children and adults.[159,202,288] In a study in Sweden,[202] infants were colonized for an average of 30 days, and after 3 months, 17 percent were carrying the same organism. In a study in the United States in adults, individual serotypes usually persisted for 2 to 4 weeks. The study showed that the first pneumococcal

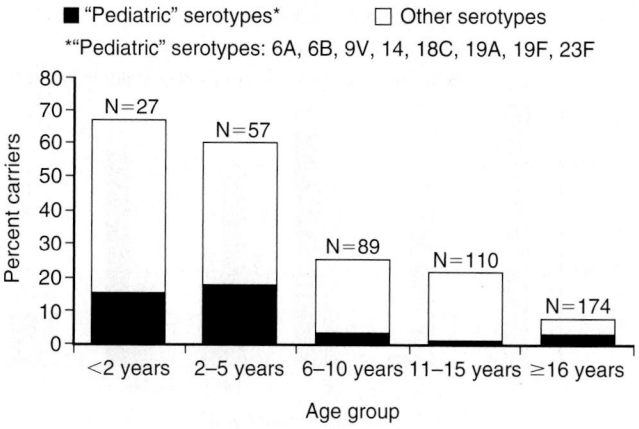

Figure 96–6 Nasopharyngeal carriage of *Streptococcus pneumoniae* in a closed black community living in crowded conditions in southern Israel. (*Adapted from Dagan, R., Gradstein, S., Belmaker, I., et al.: An outbreak of Streptococcus pneumoniae type 1 in a closed community in southern Israel. Clin. Infect. Dis. 30:319-321, 2000.*)

serotype that colonizes infants (typically before they reach 6 months of age) can be detected for as long as 12 months (mean, 4 months).[288]

The relationship between the ability of a specific serotype to colonize the nasopharynx of a child and its ability to cause respiratory or invasive infection is not clear. Some serotypes, such as 6A, 6B, 9V, 14, 18C, 19A, 19F, and 23F, are among the most frequent colonizers in infants and young children in most parts of the world and thus often are considered "pediatric" serotypes.[90,160] Some of these "pediatric" serotypes, such as serotypes 6B and 23F, also are less immunogenic than are others, especially in children younger than 2 years old, but some can show a reduced response even late in childhood. These serotypes are acquired frequently by infants and young children and often are carried for a prolonged period. After the child reaches the age of 2 years, carriage of these "pediatric" serotypes declines rapidly. Although pneumococcal carriage decreases overall with age, the proportion of the "nonpediatric" serotypes increases with age. This phenomenon is demonstrated in Figure 96–6.

In contrast to the "pediatric" serotypes, serotypes such as 1, 5, 7F, and 12 are carried infrequently and are eliminated from the nasopharynx rapidly. However, these serotypes are able to cause disease and even epidemics.[160,331,526,529,694] The different distribution of serotypes among colonized children, children with invasive infections, and adults with pneumonia is exemplified in Figure 96–7.

Although most colonization occurs without the development of disease, some prospective, longitudinal studies have suggested that most systemic infections develop soon after colonization by a new pneumococcal serotype.[210,286,288] Carriers are protected from invasive disease by the development of circulating antibodies. However, such antibodies do not always protect against invasion of contiguous sites, and other studies have shown that a substantial number of pneumococcal otitis media cases occur at any time during nasopharyngeal colonization by a specific serotype.[43,714]

The epidemiology of nasopharyngeal carriage of antibiotic-resistant pneumococci is important. The most significant promoter of carriage of antibiotic-resistant *S. pneumoniae* is antibiotic use.* Prolonged carriage of azithromycin-resistant *S. pneumoniae* was observed after a single dose of azithromycin was administered to Australian aboriginals for the treatment of trachoma.[443]

---

*See references 23, 84, 135, 159, 171, 274, 541, 595, 648, 791.
†See references 73, 159, 171, 185, 274, 400, 611, 648, 649, 715, 748, 791.

---

*See references 30, 33, 133, 159, 171, 195, 256, 419, 422, 595, 799.

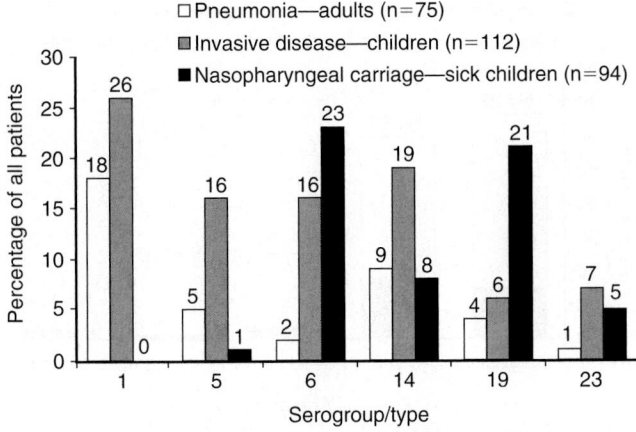

Figure 96–7 Distribution of selected serogroups/serotypes in *Streptococcus pneumoniae* isolates from adults with pneumonia, children with invasive infection, and nasopharyngeal specimens from sick children in Kenya. (*Adapted from Scott, J. A. G., Hall, A. J., Hannington, A., et al.: Serotype distribution and prevalence of resistance to benzylpenicillin in three representative populations of Streptococcus pneumoniae isolates from the coast of Kenya. Clin. Infect. Dis. 27:1442-1450, 1998.*)

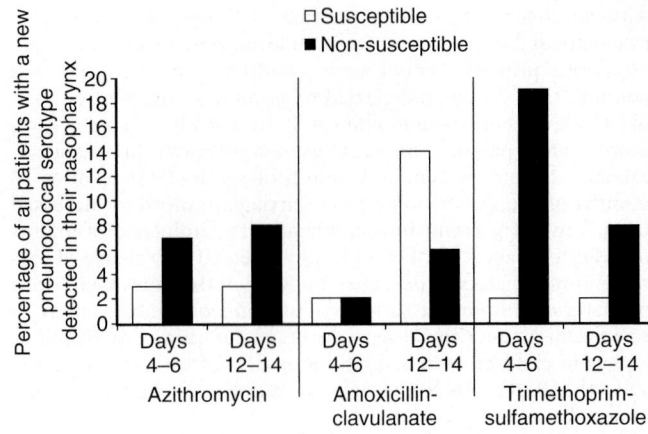

Figure 96–8 Nasopharyngeal acquisition of new pneumococcal serotypes during antibiotic treatment of acute otitis media based on susceptibility or resistance to the antimicrobial that was administered. Material for culture was obtained 3 to 5 days and 11 to 13 days after initiation of treatment. The regimens were azithromycin, 10 mg/kg as a single dose on day 1, followed by 5 mg/kg once daily for an additional 4 days; amoxicillin-clavulanate, 45/6.6 mg/kg/day in two divided doses for 10 days; and trimethoprim-sulfamethoxazole, 8/40 mg/kg/day in two divided doses for 10 days.[169]

Prophylaxis with amoxicillin increased the carriage of penicillin-resistant *S. pneumoniae*.[101] An association between trimethoprim-sulfamethoxazole prophylaxis and nasopharyngeal colonization with both trimethoprim-sulfamethoxazole– and penicillin-resistant *S. pneumoniae* has been demonstrated.[5,30,169]

A series of prospective studies revealed some of the early processes that occur in the nasopharynx during and in the immediate post-treatment period in cases of AOM caused by antibiotic-resistant *S. pneumoniae*.[133,137,148,167,169] These events can be summarized as follows: (1) most drugs studied had a substantial effect on the nasopharyngeal flora and eradicated or reduced the carriage of pneumococci that were susceptible to the drugs; (2) little, if any effect was seen when the organism had reduced susceptibility to the drugs administered; (3) some drugs, such as azithromycin and trimethoprim-sulfamethoxazole, appeared to promote colonization with resistant *S. pneumoniae*; and (4) β-lactam drugs with higher activity against *S. pneumoniae* in general and against non-penicillin-susceptible *S. pneumoniae* in particular, such as amoxicillin-clavulanate and cefuroxime axetil, decreased colonization better than did drugs with poor antipneumococcal activity, such as cefaclor, cefpodoxime, and cefixime.

Even more intriguing than the differential effect of various drugs on carriage of *S. pneumoniae* is the ability of these agents to alter nasopharyngeal colonization. Such alteration occurs by selection of pneumococcal strains that were masked by other organisms or selection of strains that were acquired after initiation of treatment, as was exemplified when children suffering from trachoma received one dose of azithromycin and were monitored for nasopharyngeal carriage of *S. pneumoniae*.[443] Before treatment, 68 percent were colonized with *S. pneumoniae*, but only 1 percent had azithromycin-resistant *S. pneumoniae*. Within 2 to 3 weeks after they received treatment, colonization decreased to 29 percent, but 16 percent were colonized with azithromycin-resistant *S. pneumoniae*. Two months later, 78 percent were colonized with *S. pneumoniae* and 27 percent with azithromycin-resistant *S. pneumoniae*. The prevalence of pneumococcal colonization and azithromycin susceptibility returned to pre-exposure values only after 6 months. In another study, cultures performed shortly after initiation of treatment and immediately after cessation of treatment showed that new serotypes, either susceptible or resistant to the treatment drug, appeared in 21, 24, and 31 percent of those treated with azithromycin, amoxicillin-clavulanate, and

trimethoprim-sulfamethoxazole, respectively[169] (Fig. 96–8). The proportion of new strains of pneumococci resistant to these drugs was 15, 8, and 27 percent, respectively.

A study looking at more than 31,000 *S. pneumoniae* isolates between 2000 and 2003 found that 29.4, 22.5, and 0.9 percent were resistant to erythromycin, penicillin, and levofloxacin, respectively. Thirty-one percent of the isolates exhibited multidrug resistance. Among macrolide-resistant isolates, *mefA* was the most prevalent resistant gene identified. Ninety percent of isolates that contained both the *mefA* and the *ermB* resistance genes were resistant to penicillin, tetracycline, or trimethoprim-sulfamethoxazole. However, 98.6 percent of those isolates were susceptible to levofloxacin.[374]

Prolonged and low-dose antibiotic regimens are suggested to be important contributors to promotion of carriage and spread of antibiotic-resistant *S. pneumoniae*.[136,294,329,482,659]

One of the serious problems with pneumococcal strains clearly is the emergence of resistance to more than one antibiotic class.[355] This phenomenon explains why the use of one antibiotic may result in carriage of *S. pneumoniae* resistant not only to the antibiotic to which the host was exposed but also to other, unrelated classes of antibiotics. In 1993, approximately a fifth of the pneumococcal strains in Iceland were not penicillin-susceptible and 80 percent of them were multidrug-resistant. When the risk for carriage of penicillin-resistant *S. pneumoniae* was investigated, a clear association was found not only with use of β-lactam drugs but also with the use of trimethoprim-sulfamethoxazole and erythromycin.[30] Other authors likewise have shown an association between the use of trimethoprim-sulfamethoxazole and carriage of penicillin-resistant *S. pneumoniae*.[82,507]

When a group of children who did not carry trimethoprim-sulfamethoxazole–resistant *S. pneumoniae* were studied longitudinally during therapy for AOM,[169] carriage of trimethoprim-sulfamethoxazole–resistant *S. pneumoniae* was found in 23 percent of patients by day 6 and in 33 percent by day 40. Additionally, non–penicillin-susceptible *S. pneumoniae* was carried at these times by 26 and 43 percent of children, respectively. This remarkable promotion of colonization with penicillin-resistant strains by trimethoprim-sulfamethoxazole treatment occurred because many strains were resistant to both penicillin and trimethoprim-sulfamethoxazole.

Mass chemoprophylaxis and therapeutic campaigns now are being conducted in different regions against a variety of diseases, which raises concern about the widespread development of resistance. Examples are mass azithromycin treatment campaigns to eradicate trachoma, mass sulfadoxine-pyrimethamine (Fansidar) treatment (shown to be associated with an increased rate of resistance to trimethoprim-sulfamethoxazole in pneumococci),[218] increasing use of trimethoprim-sulfamethoxazole for prophylaxis of patients infected with HIV, and mass treatment with fluoroquinolones and tetracyclines after exposure to *Bacillus anthracis*.

The dramatic change in nasopharyngeal flora after initiation of antibiotic therapy has two important consequences. First, the phenomenon described earlier predisposes patients to new acquisition of infection with more resistant organisms.[157] Antibiotic treatment not only can increase nasopharyngeal carriage of antibiotic-resistant *S. pneumoniae* but also can induce superinfection of the middle ear with a resistant strain within a few days.[167] Second, the increased prevalence of antibiotic-resistant *S. pneumoniae* in the nasopharynx may increase transmission in crowded conditions such as extended families and daycare centers.[171,262,274,320,595,627,791] A recent study found that reducing the number of antibiotic prescriptions written in a French community resulted in an 18 percent decrease in colonization ($p < 0.05$). Physicians participating in the study were instructed not to write prescriptions for presumed viral respiratory tract infections even with purulent rhinitis. In addition, the physicians were asked to document actual streptococcal pharyngitis with an antigen test.[295] Therefore, the widespread use of antibiotics is likely to be responsible for the increase in antibiotic-resistant *S. pneumoniae*, especially in crowded populations, thus creating a vicious cycle that is difficult, if not impossible, to overcome (Fig. 96–9). The presence of this vicious cycle poses a real challenge to society.

Since the use of pneumococcal vaccine has become widespread in the United States, the serotypes found most commonly in nasopharyngeal colonization have been replaced by nonvaccine serotypes. A study evaluating nasopharyngeal colonization in 16 Massachusetts communities during 2001 to 2004 showed a decrease in serotypes found in the PCV-7 vaccine from 36 percent to 14 percent along with an increase in non–PCV-7 serotypes from 34 percent to 55 percent.[342] Another study showed that 25 percent of children colonized with pneumococci carried antibiotic-resistant, nonvaccine serotypes, including serotypes 19A and 35B, rarely detected before introduction of the pneumococcal conjugate vaccine. Seven percent of the 19A isolates tested in the study were resistant to all oral agents tested (penicillin, amoxicillin, cefuroxime, ceftriaxone, azithromycin, and trimethoprim/sulfamethoxazole), and 12 percent of the 35B isolates were not susceptible to penicillin or cefuroxime.[359]

INVASIVE PNEUMOCOCCAL DISEASE

Although invasive pneumococcal infections occur far less commonly in early childhood than does pneumonia or otitis media, they are an important cause of morbidity and mortality during childhood worldwide. Pneumococci are more common than are Hib and *N. meningitidis* as causes of bacteremia in most countries and rank second after Hib or third after *N. meningitidis* in causing bacterial meningitis. Pneumococci are estimated to be responsible for 25 to 50 percent of cases of bacterial meningitis in children in the United States,[660] Europe,[140] and Africa.[575]

The incidence and severity of invasive pneumococcal disease vary in different populations. Figure 96–10 exemplifies the differences in incidence in various populations by age group. Several

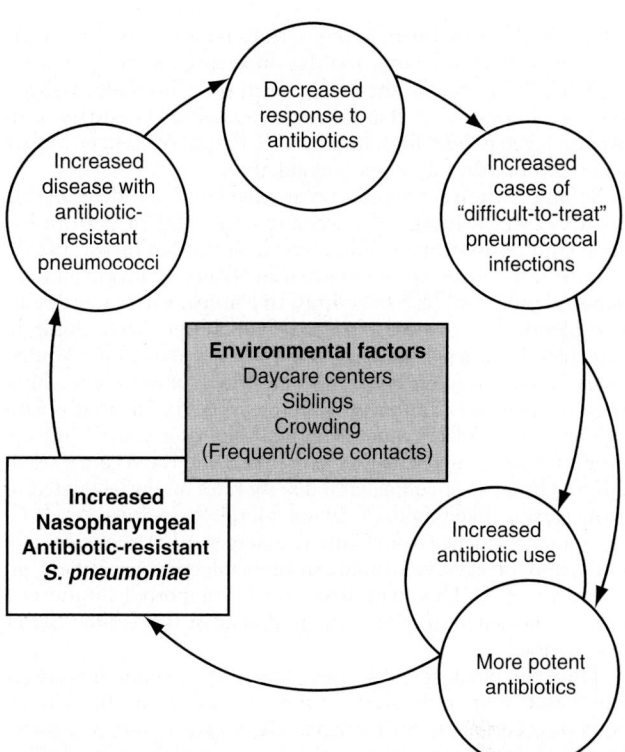

Figure 96–9 Chain of events that create a vicious cycle in which antibiotic treatment increases the carriage of antibiotic-resistant pneumococci, which cause more disease with resistant organisms. This situation results in reduced response to antibiotic treatment and an increase in the number of "difficult-to-treat" cases. As a result, the use of antibiotics is increased, especially more potent ones, thus again promoting a further increase in nasopharyngeal carriage of antibiotic-resistant pneumococci.

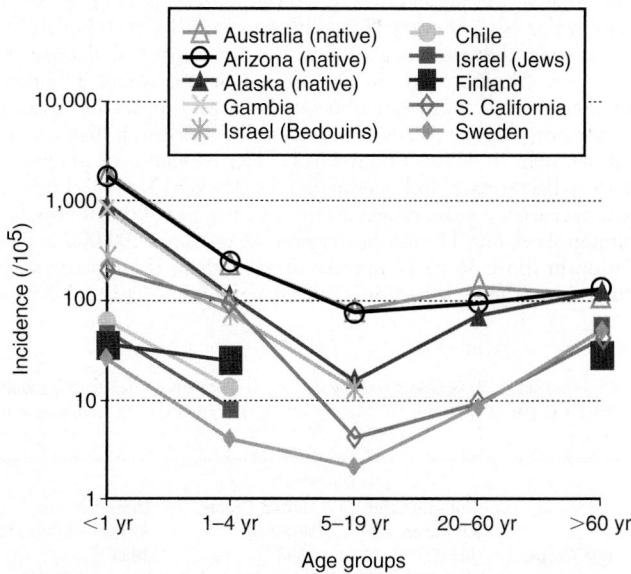

Figure 96–10 Age-specific incidence of invasive pneumococcal disease in various populations. Data were obtained from various presentations and publications.

important points can be drawn from this figure: (1) an age-dependent pattern exists that is similar in all populations: the highest rate is in infants, the rate decreases rapidly toward the age of 5 years, and then it increases again toward the age of 60 years, with a second peak occurring in persons older than 65; (2)

a marked difference exists among various populations in the incidence of invasive infection, and this difference can be up to 100-fold; and (3) in general, the incidence in the more industrialized countries is lower than that in less industrialized countries or in less privileged populations, but the U.S. figures seem to be higher than those of other developed populations.

Because invasive pneumococcal infections are detected by blood culture in most cases, variations in rates of performing blood cultures in young children could be responsible, at least in part, for differences in the reported incidence of invasive pneumococcal infection.[217,312] In contrast to Europe, where most pediatric blood isolates were obtained from hospitalized children, many blood cultures are performed on outpatients in the United States.[312] This difference arises because U.S. practice guidelines recommend blood cultures for children aged 3 to 36 months with high fever and WBC counts of 15,000/mm³ or greater.[53] Indeed, several European investigators have noted that the recent rises in reported invasive pneumococcal disease rates might be related to an increasing likelihood of taking blood for culture.[48,387,539,697] Preliminary evidence from Chile also suggests that a considerable proportion of relatively mild invasive infections routinely go unrecognized.[438] This hypothesis can be supported by the fact that the incidence of meningitis is similar in the United States and Europe.[312]

Thus, the incidence of invasive infection in children younger than 5 to 6 years in western Europe (e.g., Finland, the United Kingdom, Germany, Switzerland, Denmark, Spain) was lower than 25 cases per 100,000 population per year in various studies; in Chile, Australia, and New Zealand, it was 25 to 60 per 100,000; and during the same period in the United States, the range was approximately 65 to 75 cases per 100,000.[312] In contrast, the incidence of pneumococcal meningitis in these countries was similar: 3.6 per 100,000 in the United States versus a mean of 4.6 per 100,000 in Europe (range, 2.1 to 7.0).[312]

Differences in the incidence of invasive pneumococcal infection among populations are not due solely to different blood culture practices because true significant differences can be found within the same country. This difference can be exemplified by comparing the incidence of invasive pneumococcal disease in different ethnic groups in the United States, where a higher incidence of invasive pneumococcal disease occurs in African Americans, Alaskan Natives, and specific American Indian populations than in whites (Table 96–2). The incidence of pneumococcal bacteremia and meningitis in Alaskan Native children younger than 5 years ranges from 598 cases per 100,000 population in those 6 to 11 months of age to 56 cases per 100,000 population in those 36 to 47 months of age, which is approximately four times the incidence in similarly aged non–Alaskan Native/

non–American Indian children.[115] The highest incidence for any ethnic group in the United States is found in Navajo and Apache populations living on reservations in the southwestern United States. The incidence in children aged 1 to 2 years in these populations is 557 to 2396 per 100,000.[142,549] Among children younger than 5 years, the incidence of invasive pneumococcal disease in African American children in the United States is two to three times higher than that in white children of the same age.[61,94,309,622] In a case-control study of risk factors for the development of invasive disease in young children, the association of race with disease risk was not statistically significant in an analysis that controlled for socioeconomic status.[463] However, other studies have reported persistence of increased risk even when controlling for income.[94,123,223,309,322] The reasons for the increased incidence in some populations in comparison to others in the United States are unclear.

In other geographic regions, differences among populations also can be observed, again being higher in populations that live in underprivileged conditions, which raises the question of the importance of genetic versus environmental risk factors. In southern Israel, the incidence of pneumococcal invasive infection during the first year of life in Bedouin infants (a population with a lifestyle, birth rate, and general disease incidence similar to that of the developing world) was 270 cases per 100,000 versus 53 per 100,000 in Jewish infants (a population with standards of living comparable to the middle/low social class in the developed world) ($p < 0.001$).[240] This difference also was found in children aged 1 to 4 years: 75 and 21 cases per 100,000, respectively ($p < 0.001$). In New Zealand, when Maoris, Pacific Islanders, and others were compared, incidence rates of invasive pneumococcal disease in the first year of life per 100,000 population were 153, 276, and 52, respectively. The respective rates in children younger than 5 years were 67, 117, and 36 per 100,000, respectively.[760]

Studies on the incidence of invasive pneumococcal infection in developing regions are scanty. In one study in The Gambia, the annual incidence in children younger than 1 and 5 years was 554 and 240 per 100,000, respectively.[554] Another study in The Gambia documented the incidence of invasive pneumococcal infection to be 224, 139, and 82 cases per 100,000 children during the first, second, and third years of life, respectively.[747] *S. pneumoniae* plays a more important role in the acquisition of meningitis in developing countries than in developed countries. Reports from several African countries show that *S. pneumoniae* accounts for 20 to 50 percent of all cases.[575] Data from many other developing populations, especially from countries in Southeast Asia, are lacking but are needed because data from Africa cannot be extrapolated to other developing parts of the world.

TABLE 96–2 Incidence (Cases/100,000 Population) of Invasive Pneumococcal Disease in Selected U.S. Pediatric Populations—Selected Years

Age Group	United States, All Races, 1998[593]	United States, Whites, 1998[593]	United States, African Americans, 1998[593]	Alaska, Natives, 1986-1990[178]	Alaska, Natives, 1986-1997[115]	Navajo American Indians, 1989-1996[549]	Apache American Indians, 1983-1990[142]
0-5 mo	73.4	60.9	163.5	624*	276.8	629*	1820*
6-11 mo	227.8	178.2	542.2	↓	597.7	↓	↓
12-23 mo	184.2	137.2	440.7	↓	453.0	557	↓
24-35 mo	64.7	54.6	116.4	98*	125.2	73*	227*
36-47 mo	26.7	23.9	46.1	↓	56.2	↓	↓
48-59 mo	14.3	9.1	20.6	↓	73.2	↓	↓
5-9 yr	5.7	4.8	9.3	23	—	—	54
10-19 yr	2.9	2.5	4.8	5	—	—	35
All ages	23.2	19.7	49.7	—	—	63	207

Average of all age groups indicated by arrows.

The fatality rate of pneumococcal meningitis is higher than that of meningitis caused by other organisms.[575] Mortality rates for invasive pneumococcal infection in developed populations vary between less than 2 percent and 6.6 percent.[153,180,293,511,622,760] In contrast, in the developing world, mortality rates for invasive pneumococcal infection, including meningitis, vary from 19 percent in South Africa[343] to as high as 67 percent in Mali and Niger.[573,575]

Most invasive pneumococcal diseases in children are caused by a limited number of pneumococcal serotypes. However, despite the many studies reporting on serotypes or serogroups published or presented thus far, the data are not yet complete. Data on serotypes are important, especially with regard to the question of coverage of the various conjugate vaccines, as discussed in the section on prevention in this chapter. The extensive literature was summarized by Hausdorff and colleagues[310,311] in two review articles. The results of their exhaustive review, despite showing many gaps in our knowledge, did lead to certain conclusions (Fig. 96–11): (1) in children younger than 5 years, the great majority of invasive infections are covered by the 11 serotypes that will be included in future conjugate vaccines (or the cross-reacting serotypes in the same serogroup [serogroups 1, 3, 4, 5, 6, 7, 9, 14, 18, 19, 23]); (2) in some regions, 4 serogroups not present in the 7-valent vaccine (serogroups 1, 3, 5, and 7) are of great importance; (3) in older children and adults (mainly those older than 18 years), the 7-valent vaccine often covers only a minority of cases, whereas the 11-valent vaccine covers a greater percentage; and (4) the 23-valent nonconjugate vaccine provides considerably wider coverage than the conjugate vaccines do, although it may not be immunogenic in infants, young children, or immunocompromised hosts.

A recent study evaluating the invasiveness of different *S. pneumoniae* serotypes found that serotypes 4, 14, 7F, 9V, and 18C were associated with rates of greater than 20 invasive pneumococcal disease cases per 100,000 acquisitions, whereas serotypes 23F, 6A, 19F, 16F, 6B, and 15B/C were associated with fewer than 10 invasive pneumococcal disease cases per 100,000 acquisitions. The study also found an inverse relationship between the duration of carriage and the likelihood of causing invasive disease ($p < 0.0001$).[690]

Since the PCV-7 vaccine was introduced, the rate of invasive pneumococcal disease in young infants has decreased significantly.[588] In a study involving eight U.S. children's hospitals, the incidence of invasive pneumococcal disease has decreased more than 75 percent in children younger than 24 months. Replacement of vaccine serotypes by nonvaccine serotypes was noted, particularly serogroups 15 and 33.[278,393] Furthermore, penicillin resistance has increased among nonvaccine serogroups.[393] A study in northern California clinics showed an 84 percent reduction in *S. pneumoniae* bacteremia and a 67 percent reduction in overall bacteremia since routine vaccination was implemented. In this same study, a third of the pathogens identified in positive blood cultures were *E. coli*, a third were nonvaccine serotype *S. pneumoniae*, and the remaining third were mostly *S. aureus*, *Salmonella*, *N. meningitidis*, or *Streptococcus pyogenes*.[326] Despite the use of pneumococcal vaccine, children younger than 1 year and children with comorbid illnesses such as malignancy, HIV infection, immune deficiency, or nephrotic syndrome continue to remain at risk for acquiring invasive pneumococcal disease.[340]

Serotype 19A is, at present, the most important cause of invasive pneumococcal disease by replacement serotypes since the widespread use of pneumococcal vaccine, and it is becoming increasingly drug-resistant. Between July 1999 and June 2004, the overall rate of invasive pneumococcal disease decreased from 23.3 to 13.1 cases/100,000 population ($p < 0.00001$); during this same period, the rate of invasive pneumococcal disease caused by serotype 19A in children younger than 5 years old increased from 2.6 to 6.5 cases/100,000 population.[562]

In the first 3 years after routine vaccination with heptavalent pneumococcal conjugate vaccine was introduced, the incidence of overall invasive pneumococcal disease decreased 67 percent in Alaska Native children younger than 2 years old. However, between 2001 to 2003 and 2004 to 2006, an 82 percent increase occurred in the rate of invasive disease in Alaska Native children younger than 2 years old. Since 2004, the invasive pneumococcal disease rate caused by nonvaccine serotypes has increased 140 percent in comparison to the prevaccine period.[686]

Many reasons, such as differences in living conditions and socioeconomic status and genetic differences among populations, can be cited for the diversity of serotype/serogroup distribution in populations. However, Hausdorff and associates[312] suggest that the differences in serotype/serogroup distribution among various geographic regions may be related to differences in the testing and reporting practices of various countries. Some serotypes/serogroups may be associated with more severe disease than others are. In regions where blood cultures are performed for mildly ill children, such as the United States, the predominance of serogroups such as 6, 9, 14, 18, 19, and 23 can be accentuated, whereas serotypes such as 1, 3, 5, and 7F, which are found in more severe disease, appear to be less important. The importance of having local data on serotype coverage for evaluating disease burden that can be prevented by vaccination always should be considered.

PNEUMONIA

In adults, *S. pneumoniae* is by far the predominant cause of community-acquired bacterial pneumonia. However, this cause is more difficult to assess in children because obtaining bacteriologic specimens such as sputum from infants and young children is difficult. Blood cultures usually are positive in less than 5 percent of the children with any pneumonia and, thus, cannot provide an accurate representation of the pathogens in childhood pneumonia. Nasopharyngeal cultures, as well as antigen detection and PCR, also are difficult to correlate with bacterial pneumonia (see the section on diagnosis). Studies using lung aspirates are helpful but scant,[761] and most of the recent studies were performed in one developing country (The Gambia). However, data derived from these studies show an important role of *S. pneumoniae* as a causative agent of pneumonia in children.[8,234-236,673]

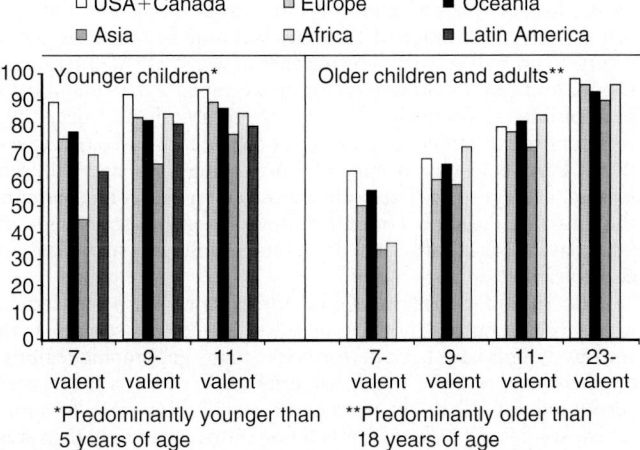

Figure 96–11 Coverage of 7-valent, 9-valent, and 11-valent conjugate pneumococcal vaccines and 23-valent nonconjugated pneumococcal polysaccharide vaccine in younger children (predominantly 5 years of age) and older children and adults (predominantly >18 years of age) in various regions of the world.[310,311]

In a recent study conducted in Finland, transthoracic needle aspiration disclosed an etiology in 18 of 26 patients from whom a representative sample specimen was obtained.[762] Of these patients, 10 of 26 (38%) had lung aspirate cultures positive for *S. pneumoniae*, and 1 additional child had a positive blood culture for *S. pneumoniae*. An additional six patients (23%) had a positive PCR test. Thus, in total, 17 of 26 (65%) had at least one test that was positive for *S. pneumoniae*.

Studies with the newly developed pneumococcal conjugate vaccines in children suggest that the role of *S. pneumoniae* in lower respiratory infections in general and pneumonia in particular may be more important than previously demonstrated. In a study in California,[71] administration of a 7-valent conjugate pneumococcal vaccine reduced the number of cases of clinical pneumonia in children younger than 3.5 years by 6.0 percent ($p = 0.13$) (intention-to-treat analysis). A reduction in the incidence of pneumonia of 8.9 percent ($p = 0.03$) was found in patients who had clinical features of pneumonia and had a chest radiograph performed, regardless of the findings. The incidence of pneumonia was reduced by 22.7 percent in patients with a positive finding on the chest radiograph (defined as parenchymal infiltrates, consolidation or effusion [or both], but not perihilar infiltrates only). In South Africa, administration of three doses of 9-valent conjugate pneumococcal vaccine reduced the incidence of radiologically proven pneumonia by 22.1 percent ($p = 0.049$) in children younger than 2 years old (Klugman, K., and Madhi, S.: Data presented at the Third International Symposium on Pneumococci and Pneumococcal Diseases, May 2002, Alaska). This ability of a pneumococcal vaccine to reduce the incidence of clinical and radiologically documented pneumonia suggests that (1) *S. pneumoniae* is the causative agent in most cases of pneumonia, with consolidation being seen in infants and toddlers in the population studied, and (2) *S. pneumoniae* is a causative agent in many cases usually considered to be viral. Supportive evidence for the latter suggestion can be derived from a study conducted in Israeli toddlers attending daycare centers.[174] In these toddlers, a 9-valent pneumococcal vaccine reduced the incidence of lower respiratory disease, including bronchiolitis, cough, and pneumonia, by 16 percent and reduced antibiotic treatment days for these entities by 47 percent. More studies are being undertaken to investigate the potential of pneumococcal conjugate vaccines to reduce the incidence of pneumonia and other lower respiratory tract infections in developing populations (Native Americans and those in The Gambia and the Philippines).

Although pneumonia usually is not a fatal disease in developed countries, it is an important cause of morbidity and hospitalization. Pneumococcal infections are thought to be rare causes of serious lower respiratory tract disease requiring hospitalization in children younger than 6 months.[181] However, *S. pneumoniae* is an important cause of hospitalization for community-acquired pneumonia in older children.[131,189,258,429,542,640]

In developing countries, acute respiratory infections in general and pneumonia in particular are the leading causes of morbidity and mortality.[505] The mortality rate from respiratory infections in developing countries is estimated to be 10- to 30-fold higher than that in developed countries.[6,461] In addition, of the 15 million children younger than 5 years old who die annually, an estimated 4 million die of pneumonia.[296,461] When obtained, rates of positive sputum culture for *S. pneumoniae* in developing countries can be as high as 88 percent in children.[63] Using a variety of methods, including antigen detection, cultures from blood, sputum, and pleural and lung aspirates, and antipneumococcal antibody testing, a series of investigations in The Gambia associated *S. pneumoniae* with severe acute lower respiratory tract infection in 20 percent of hospitalized infants and in 61 percent of children aged 1 to 9 years.[235,236] In another study in The Gambia[234] conducted on ambulatory children younger than 5 years old with lower respiratory tract infections, *S. pneumoniae* was associated

with 8.6 percent of all cases of clinical acute lower respiratory tract infection, 12.3 percent of episodes of radiologically proven acute lower respiratory tract infection, and 28.0 percent of episodes of lobar pneumonia. Despite the limitations of these diagnostic tests, these results demonstrate the importance of *S. pneumoniae* in severe respiratory infection.

No accurate information exists about the pneumococcal serotypes involved in pneumonia in infants and young children. The only accurate data are for bacteremic pneumococcal pneumonia. In these cases, the serotype distribution is not different from that for other invasive infections. However, the bacteremic cases represent only a minority of pneumococcal pneumonia cases, and one cannot extrapolate these data to nonbacteremic cases. The finding of an impressive reduction in pneumonia after the use of a conjugate pneumococcal vaccine, as reviewed earlier, suggests that most pneumonia cases in the population studied are pneumococcal and caused by serotypes included in the vaccine.

OTITIS MEDIA

Otitis media is the diagnosis that accounts for most office visits in pediatric clinics in the United States. It results in more than 15 million visits per year.[425,706] In the United States, 10 percent of children have one or more episodes of otitis media by the time that they are 3 months of age, approximately 60 percent by 1 year of age, and more than 80 percent by 3 years of age.[412,727] More recent statistics show even higher figures: a study involving 2253 infants in the Pittsburgh area showed that 48 percent had one or more episodes of otitis media between 2 and 6 months of age, 79 percent between 2 and 12 months of age, and 91 percent by 24 months of age.[566] Finnish studies in the 1980s showed an incidence of 0.47 to 1.05 episodes per year in infants aged 0 to 12 months.[394,598,688] Otitis media often is not perceived as a severe problem in developing countries, but community studies have shown perforation of the tympanic membrane in 0.4 to 6.1 percent and mastoiditis in 0.19 to 0.74 percent of all children.[62] Although serious complications rarely occur, the economic cost of otitis media is estimated at more than $3.5 billion each year in the United States.[254,706] During 1996, approximately 500,000 tympanostomy tubes were placed in children's ears in the United States.[536] AOM also is the leading reason for prescribing antibiotics to children.[593]

In a prospective study conducted in southern Israel that examined the burden of AOM on patients and their families,[291] the average number of days of severe crying, temperature higher than 38° C, loss of appetite, and insomnia was 2.9, 7.8, 7.0, and 6.6, respectively. An average of 18.6 days was required for a family to return to normal activity. The number of visits, use of emergency rooms, and care by otolaryngologists averaged 2.6, 0.3, and 0.35 per episode, respectively. The average antibiotic and over-the-counter drug treatment days per episode were 9.1 and 6.6, respectively. Parents lost an average of 1.6 working days, and children lost an average of 3.5 daycare days per episode. The parents thought that during a 1-month follow-up period, an average of 18.6 days were nonroutine days versus only 3.4 such days in controls.

The role of *S. pneumoniae* in otitis media has been studied extensively. During the last decades, numerous studies with various designs have been performed in many geographic regions. *S. pneumoniae* was the major bacterial cause of otitis media and accounted for 25 to 60 percent of cases.* However, in some recent studies, *H. influenzae* was found more commonly than was *S. pneumoniae* in AOM.[161,257,402] *H. influenzae* is a rare finding in

---

*See references 72, 77, 162, 183, 195, 206, 264, 358, 377, 402, 410, 484, 528, 629.

first episodes of AOM, but it becomes increasingly common from the third episode onward, whereas *S. pneumoniae* is a common finding in all episodes.[402]

Although the cost of each AOM episode may be relatively low when compared with other infections caused by *S. pneumoniae*, the highest overall cost in all pneumococcal infections is due to otitis media because of the large number of episodes.[466] The estimated cost for meningitis was 11,081 U.S. dollars per case in 1997, for bacteremia it was $2313, and for pneumonia with consolidation it was $1464. In contrast, for simple otitis media, the cost was $294 per episode, and for complex otitis media it was $1339 per episode. The cost of tympanostomy tube placement was $2390 per case. The estimated annual cost in the United States was $3 to $5 billion for simple pneumococcal otitis media and approximately $1.3 billion for complex pneumococcal otitis media. In contrast, the annual cost of pneumococcal meningitis was approximately $9 million, that of pneumococcal bacteremia was $35 million, and that of pneumococcal pneumonia was $113 million.

Antibiotic resistance in *S. pneumoniae* strains causing otitis media is rising sharply, and in some countries, resistance to at least one antibiotic class (in most cases penicillin and other β-lactams) is now the rule, not the exception. Figure 96–12 exemplifies the rapidity of the increase in antibiotic resistance among *S. pneumoniae* isolates from the middle ear fluid of children with AOM in France and Israel in the last decade. A well-established fact is that higher antibiotic resistance rates are found in pneumococci from patients with nonresponsive AOM and recurrent AOM, in whom recent antibiotic treatment is common, as well as in daycare center attendees.[55,73,135,157,164,458,583,799] In children younger than 18 months old, the prevalence of antibiotic-resistant *S. pneumoniae* in AOM is higher than that in older age groups.[55,73,159,358]

Studies of pneumococcal serotypes causing AOM in the last 60 years have demonstrated relatively similar patterns, with the most common serotypes being 6A, 6B, 9V, 14, 19A, 19F, and 23F.[43,73,114,157,225,257,556,577,680] (Fig. 96–13). As mentioned in the section on bacteriology, these serotypes also are the most frequent antibiotic-resistant serotypes. Furthermore, the great majority of highly penicillin-resistant and multiply-resistant *S. pneumoniae* belong to five serotypes (6B, 9V, 14, 19F, 23F) and, to a lesser extent, to related serotypes (6A and 19A).[157,380] This finding is somewhat reassuring with regard to vaccination because the serotypes most frequently associated with otitis media are included in the PCV-7 vaccine. The serotypes included in the PCV-7 vaccine are 4, 6B, 9V, 14, 18C, 19F, and 23F. A recent study found that 60 to 70 percent of all *S. pneumoniae* isolates that caused AOM in children in the 6- to 59-month age range were represented in the PCV-7 vaccine.[313] Most of the data with regard to AOM are obtained from studies involving middle ear puncture (tympanocentesis or myringotomy) or spontaneously draining ears; therefore, the spectrum of cases studied probably could be skewed toward the most severe cases or treatment failures.

Immunization with conjugate pneumococcal vaccine is associated with replacement of vaccine serotypes by other serotypes. Widespread immunization with conjugate vaccine may increase the importance of some nonvaccine serotypes while decreasing that of the serotypes included in the vaccine. A study in children showed a shift in pneumococcal colonization toward nonvaccine serotypes (11, 15 and 23B)[86] and an increase in *S. aureus*–related AOM after immunization.[85]

CLINICAL SYNDROMES

S. pneumoniae can spread from the nasopharynx, which is its natural niche, to adjacent mucosal surfaces and cause mucosal infections such as AOM, sinusitis, and pneumonia, or it can

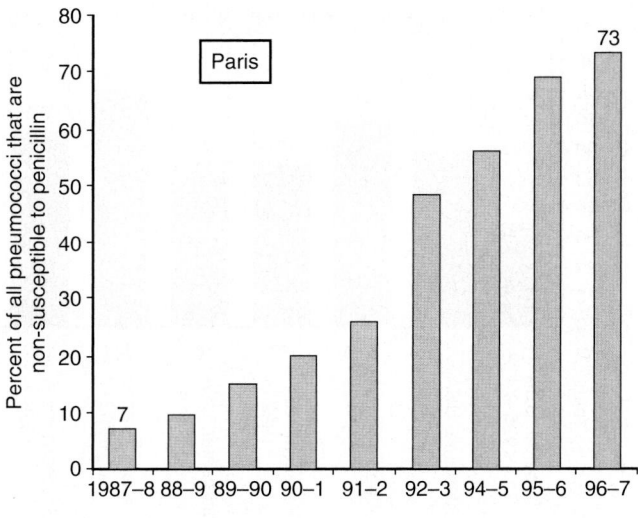

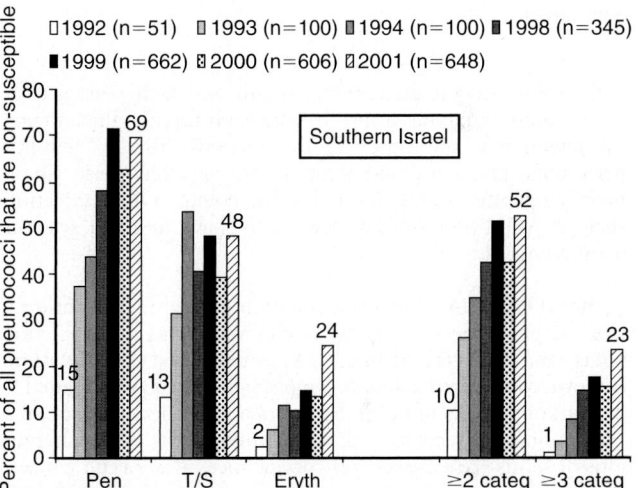

Figure 96–12 Rate of increase in non–antibiotic-susceptible pneumococci isolated from middle ear fluid during acute otitis media episodes in France and Israel during a 10-year period. **Top**, Non–penicillin-susceptible *Streptococcus pneumoniae* in Paris from 1987 through 1997. A 10-fold increase in resistance to penicillin occurred during this period.[259] **Bottom**, Non–penicillin-susceptible *S. pneumoniae* isolated from middle ear fluid during acute otitis media episodes in children in southern Israel from 1992 through 2001.[168] Categ, antibiotic drug category; Eryth, erythromycin; Pen, penicillin; T/S, trimethoprim-sulfamethoxazole. (Data from 1999 to 2001 are unpublished.)

invade the bloodstream. Infection may spread from the bloodstream to other sites and cause sepsis or meningitis or result in focal infection in heart valves, bones, joints, and soft tissues and within the peritoneal cavity. In rare cases, such as after penetrating trauma or fracture of the base of the skull, pneumococci can invade the brain directly from the upper respiratory tract. Organisms also can spread through the fallopian tubes to the peritoneal cavity after colonizing the perineum.

The clinical signs and symptoms of patients with pneumococcal infection are diverse. In general, invasive diseases such as bacteremia and meningitis are manifested as fever with temperatures that can exceed 40° C.[47] A peripheral blood leukocyte count of greater than 15,000/mm³ can be found in most patients with bacteremia, and in one study, the average WBC count was 20,000/mm³, with a range of 16,100 to 24,600/mm³.[47] In patients

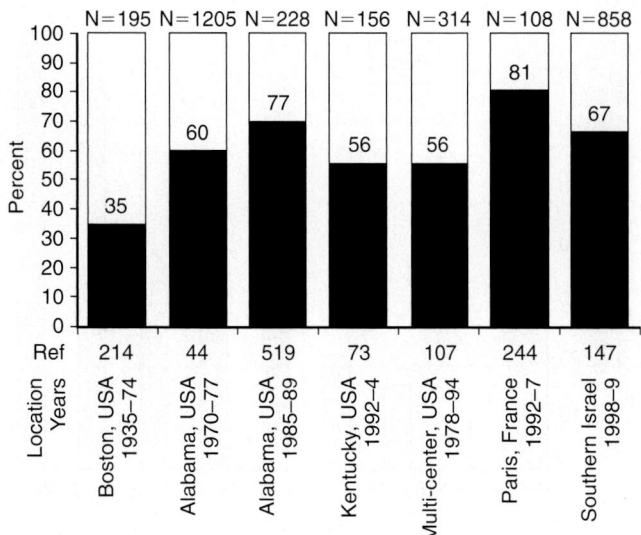

Figure 96–13 Relative proportion of serotypes 6A, 6B, 9V, 14, 19A, 19F, and 23F as a group in relation to all other serotypes causing acute otitis media.

with pneumococcal pneumonia, cough and tachypnea are the most common manifestations besides high fever.[722] Pneumococcal pneumonia and other focal infections such as cellulitis, peritonitis, and bone and joint infections often cause similar high temperatures and elevated WBC counts. Other infections such as AOM and sinusitis frequently have minimal systemic manifestations.

BACTEREMIA. The most common clinical manifestation of invasive pneumococcal disease in children younger than 3 years old is *occult bacteremia*, defined as a positive blood culture without a known focus of infection. *S. pneumoniae* caused an estimated 90 percent of all cases of occult bacteremia after the introduction of Hib conjugated vaccine.[446] Severe complications such as meningitis or sepsis are relatively rare occurrences after occult bacteremia—approximately 6 percent of all cases.[10] The risk for the development of occult bacteremia is related to age, with approximately 75 percent of all patients being between 3 and 24 months of age.[362] Signs and symptoms vary among patients with occult bacteremia. In most patients with pneumococcal bacteremia, fever appears within 24 hours after the diagnosis has been made. In one study, initial diagnoses at the time of occult bacteremia were AOM in 43 percent of patients, fever without a source in 30 percent, and viral infection in 22 percent.[47] Forty-one (8.7%) patients had complications: persistent bacteremia developed in 4 percent, meningitis in 1.7 percent, pneumonia in 1.7 percent, and cellulitis in 2.5 percent.

Febrile patients with focal infections such as otitis media or upper respiratory tract infection have a lower incidence of bacteremia than do febrile patients without an obvious source of infection (3.3% vs. 9.9%, respectively).[501] The height of the fever is associated with a greater risk for the development of bacteremia, with temperatures above 40° C being associated with a 25 percent risk.[57] A higher peripheral WBC count (>15,000/mm³) also is associated with the presence of occult bacteremia.[365,437] These findings can help in categorizing high- and low-risk patients for the presence of occult bacteremia.

Occult bacteremia resolves spontaneously without complication in most children. However, complications such as meningitis, pneumonia, osteomyelitis, arthritis, cellulitis, and fulminant sepsis develop in approximately 10 percent of patients.[446] The case-fatality rate usually is low and generally less than 1 percent in children without underlying immunologic problems.[392,622]

Persistent bacteremia and new focal infections were associated with higher temperature (mean of 38.8° C vs. 37.7° C), greater elevation in WBC count (18,900/mm³ vs. 14,900/mm³), age younger than 20 months, and no antibiotic treatment being prescribed during the initial visit.[47]

MENINGITIS. *S. pneumoniae* is either the most frequent or the second most frequent (after *N. meningitidis*) cause of bacterial meningitis in countries in which routine vaccination against Hib has been introduced. *S. pneumoniae* most commonly invades the meninges via the bloodstream.[198] However, in rare cases it can invade the meninges directly, especially after penetrating trauma or fracture of the base of the skull.[660] Patients with underling conditions such as CSF leak, HIV infection, sickle-cell anemia, or asplenia are predisposed to the development of pneumococcal meningitis.[31]

The initial signs and symptoms are variable, and a rapid onset (<24 hours of illness) occurs in less than 20 percent of children with pneumococcal meningitis.[89] Patients commonly have the typical signs of meningitis, including fever, nuchal rigidity, irritability or lethargy, and poor feeding. The anterior fontanelle often is bulging. The duration of meningeal signs before admission averages 28 hours but can be as short as 4 hours and as long as 52 hours. Seizures develop in approximately a quarter of patients. Decreased consciousness and septic shock occur in 11 and 16 percent, respectively.[31]

In one study, the mean total CSF WBC count was 1136/mm³, whereas it was 4612/mm³ with Hib disease and in *N. meningitidis* disease it reached 5476/mm³.[657] In another study, significantly higher median blood leukocyte counts, lower median CSF protein concentrations, and higher CSF glucose concentrations were found in children with meningitis caused by penicillin-resistant *S. pneumoniae* isolates than in patients with penicillin-susceptible *S. pneumoniae*.[227] However, in a different study, patients with penicillin-susceptible *S. pneumoniae* did not differ from those with non–penicillin-susceptible *S. pneumoniae* with regard to blood and CSF leukocyte counts and CSF glucose or protein concentrations.[110]

Children with CSF pleocytosis are admitted routinely to the hospital and treated with antibiotics, although few have bacterial meningitis. Patients are at very low risk for acquiring bacterial meningitis in the post–pneumococcal vaccine era if they lack all of the following criteria: (1) positive CSF Gram stain, (2) CSF absolute neutrophil count of at least 1000 cells/μL, (3) CSF protein of at least 80 mg/dL, (4) peripheral absolute neutrophil count of at least 10,000 cells/μL, and (5) a history of seizure before or at the time of evaluation.[540]

The course of pneumococcal meningitis can be associated with prolonged fever that can last for more than 10 days or with secondary fever higher than 38° C that occurs at least 1 day after the primary fever has resolved.[89] This course can be attributed to complications of the primary infection, such as subdural effusion or empyema, but these events are now relatively rare. More commonly, secondary fever is related to intercurrent conditions such as urinary tract infection, otitis media, phlebitis, pneumonia, drug fever, or a nosocomial viral infection.[177] In patients treated with corticosteroids in the first 2 to 4 days, a second spike of fever can be seen after discontinuation of the steroids.[582,597] The outcome of patients with prolonged or secondary fever is similar to that of other patients with pneumococcal meningitis.[208]

The outcome and long-term complications of pneumococcal meningitis include severe hearing loss (in as many as 46% of patients), seizures, learning or mental difficulties, or paralysis (in as many as 22%).[31] Patients with *S. pneumoniae* meningitis have a higher mortality rate and are at greater risk for the development of neurologic sequelae than are patients with *N. meningitidis* or Hib infection.[389,538] The mortality rate varies from 6.3 to 20 percent.[198,392,660] A peripheral WBC count of less than 5000/mm³ at initial evaluation was recognized as a poor prognostic factor with a high mortality rate.[428] A trend toward a higher mortality rate also was noted if the CSF WBC count was less than 1000/mm[3].[428] A similarly poor outcome can be predicted in patients with pneumococcal meningitis when low CSF glucose concentrations (<1.11 mmol/L)[237] or high CSF protein concentrations (>250 mg/dL) are present.[428]

A recent study evaluating outcomes of pneumococcal meningitis in pediatric patients in the intensive care unit over a 12-year period revealed a hospital mortality rate of 49 percent (24 of 49 patients) and neurologic deficits in 47 percent of survivors.[770]

Recent studies have shown that patients who have severe to profound hearing loss with cochlear implants are more than 30 times more likely than children in the general U.S. population to acquire pneumococcal meningitis. Children with implants with positioners were at a higher risk than were those with other implant models. The higher risk of bacterial meningitis developing continued for 24 months after implantation.[66,610]

Delayed sterilization of CSF cultures after antimicrobial treatment also has been associated with a poorer outcome.[444]

PNEUMONIA. Pneumococcal pneumonia in its classic form is manifested as an acute illness with rigors, fever with temperatures often exceeding 40° C, general malaise with a productive cough, dyspnea, and chest pain. However, the signs and symptoms may be subtle in young infants. Fever and cough occur in 90 and 70 percent of all patients, respectively. Lethargy, emesis, rhinorrhea, abdominal pain, and chest pain occur in 10 to 50 percent of patients.[722] Pneumococcal pneumonia can have an atypical and incomplete course, without respiratory symptoms, and in some cases even an absence of fever or the presence of extrathoracic manifestations. Severe abdominal pain with or without vomiting may be the only initial symptom, especially in left lower lobe pneumonia. Irritation of the meninges in cases of upper lobe pneumonia may elicit meningeal signs without meningitis.

When serologically diagnosed pneumococcal pneumonia was compared with pneumonia caused by respiratory syncytial virus (RSV), the serologically diagnosed pneumococcal pneumonia overlapped with RSV pneumonia. However, pneumococcal pneumonia was associated significantly less often with tachypnea (17% vs. 45%, respectively) and a high WBC count (mean of 20,800/mm[3] vs. 12,000/mm[3], respectively), as well as a higher CRP level (mean of 137 vs. 28 mg/L, respectively). Alveolar infiltrates were found in 76 versus 15 percent of chest radiographs, respectively.[381] Children with bacteremic pneumococcal pneumonia appeared ill more often than did those with serologically proven pneumococcal pneumonia without bacteremia (79% vs. 50%, respectively), and they had typical pneumococcal pneumonia with high fever, leukocytosis, and lobal infiltrates on chest radiographs more often (70% vs. 34%, respectively).

Pleural effusion can be found in as many as 40 percent of patients with pneumococcal pneumonia, but only approximately 10 percent have a significant amount of effusion and only approximately 2 percent exhibit empyema.[467] These patients can have a pleural friction rub, abdominal pain, chest pain, and dullness on percussion. In patients with pleural effusion, fever persists longer than in patients with pneumonia but without pleural effusion despite adequate treatment.[722]

In one study conducted in Salt Lake City during the years 1993 to 1999, 153 of 540 (28%) children hospitalized with community-acquired pneumonia had empyema.[117] Pathogenic bacteremia, 26 (41%) cases of which were caused by *S. pneumoniae*, was detected in 64 (42%) of the patients. In nine additional patients, gram-positive cocci were revealed by Gram stain but did not grow in culture. *S. pneumoniae* was the most common pathogen identified in patients with empyema. When compared with patients who had pneumonia only, patients with empyema

were more likely to be aged 3 years or older, to have had fever for 7 days or longer, to have varicella, and to have received antibiotics and ibuprofen before admission to the hospital.

Another study in Utah after widespread use of the PCV-7 vaccine found that pneumococcal parapneumonic empyema was more common. Serotype 1 was the most common cause, but serotypes 3 and 19A also were prevalent.[116]

CRP, the erythrocyte sedimentation rate, and the peripheral blood absolute neutrophil count are significantly higher in pneumococcal pneumonia than in viral pneumonia.[430] Blood culture is positive in no more than 10 percent of patients with pneumococcal pneumonia.[773] Children with bacteremic pneumococcal pneumonia usually have a high temperature and leukocytosis on admission, with peripheral WBC counts exceeding 15,000/mm[3], similar to those without bacteremia.[734] Body temperature, CRP, the erythromycin sedimentation rate, and leukocyte counts are of limited value in differentiating pneumococcal from nonpneumococcal pneumonia in individual patients.

No strict radiologic definition of pneumococcal pneumonia in children is accepted broadly. The classic chest radiographic finding in pneumococcal pneumonia is thought to be an alveolar infiltrate, usually confined to one lobe or a part of it.[557] Such infiltrates are thought to be present in approximately 85 percent of all cases. In studies performing lung aspiration in cases of radiologically proven lobar infiltrates, the proportion of patients in whom *S. pneumoniae* was detected was high.[212,761,768] In most instances in which patients with lobar consolidation were studied, the predominant bacterial pathogen was *S. pneumoniae*.[8] In addition, a 63 percent reduction in incidence of pneumonia with alveolar infiltrates was demonstrated in a study using this definition when children were vaccinated with a 7-valent pneumococcal conjugated vaccine versus placebo,[71] thus suggesting a major role of *S. pneumoniae* when alveolar infiltrates are present.

A recent study found that the incidence of human metapneumovirus (hMPV) lower respiratory tract infection was reduced by 45 percent (p < 0.002) and the incidence of clinical pneumonia was reduced by 55 percent (p < 0.003) in non–HIV-infected children who had received three doses of conjugate pneumococcal vaccine. In fully vaccinated HIV-infected children, the incidence of hMPV-associated lower respiratory tract infection was reduced by 53 percent and that of clinical pneumonia by 65 percent.[486]

In the pre-antibiotic era, the natural course of pneumococcal pneumonia consisted of 7 to 9 days of a stationary phase of symptoms followed by worsening of the systemic signs ("pre-crisis") and subsequently, in those who recovered, defervescence, sweating, polyuria, and a brief febrile attack ("post-crisis").[39,557] Today, long-term complications are rare developments, and the mortality rate is extremely low—less than 1 percent even in cases of bacteremic pneumonia.[392]

OTITIS MEDIA. *S. pneumoniae* causes 25 to 60 percent of cases of AOM.* The bacteriologic outcome of *S. pneumoniae* AOM is less favorable than is the outcome of AOM caused by other organisms when untreated or treated inappropriately.[414,528,555] A recent study found that as many as 79 percent of patients with pneumococcal AOM developed the disease in association with newly acquired carriage of pneumococcus.[713] Also recognized is that commonly used oral antibiotics are not as effective as they were in the past because of the increased antibiotic resistance among *S. pneumoniae* isolates.[149,150,152]

Some studies have suggested that pneumococcal AOM is more severe than that caused by other pathogens. In addition, a suggestion was made in 1970 that AOM caused by *S. pneumoniae*

---

*See references 72, 77, 162, 195, 206, 264, 358, 377, 402, 410, 484, 528, 629.

was accompanied more frequently by pain and fever than was AOM caused by other pathogens.[337] Moreover, on the first day of diagnosis, WBC counts in the middle ear fluid of patients with *S. pneumoniae* AOM were significantly higher than those in the case of AOM caused by other bacterial pathogens.[100] *S. pneumoniae* AOM was associated with significantly higher fever and more redness of the tympanic membrane than was AOM caused by *H. influenzae* or *Moraxella catarrhalis*.[624] The presence of *S. pneumoniae* in the nasopharynx during a case of otitis media was associated with a higher tympanic membrane severity score and higher rates of persistent symptoms on day 5, persistence of tympanic membrane abnormalities on day 28, and recurrence before day 28.[211,306] Spontaneous remission of the infection occurs less commonly in patients with pneumococcal AOM than in those with other pathogens.[335]

MASTOIDITIS. In the pre-antibiotic era, acute mastoiditis was the most common complication of otitis media and was observed in as many as 20 percent of cases without appropriate treatment. The infectious process may lead to reabsorption of the bony septa of mastoid air cells and subsequently to the formation of empyema and anatomic loss of the air-cell system.[231] *S. pneumoniae* is the most common cause of acute mastoiditis in children and accounts for 25 to 46 percent of all culture-proven cases.[272,333] A recent international study suggested that in countries in which otitis media cases are seldom treated with antibiotics, the rate of mastoiditis is greater than in those in which antibiotic treatment of otitis is the rule.[752]

SINUSITIS. The true incidence of pneumococcal sinusitis in children is unknown. It is estimated to be present in 10 percent of all upper respiratory tract infections, but the diagnosis usually is subjective.[765] *S. pneumoniae* is the pathogen most commonly isolated from patients with sinusitis, and it causes 35 to 42 percent of all bacterial cases.[767] The disease can occur at any age, and clinical signs and symptoms depend on the maturation of the different sinuses affected. The ethmoid and maxillary sinuses are the sites most commonly involved in children younger than 5 years old. Sinusitis is manifested initially as a viral infection, followed by a nasal discharge that frequently is purulent and accompanied by cough. The symptoms are aggravated at night because of postnasal drip from the sinus to the pharynx and larynx. Malodorous breath can be noted, as can vomiting.[347,385] In cases of sinusitis, isolation of *S. pneumoniae* from the nasal discharge strongly suggests its involvement at the site of infection.

CONJUNCTIVITIS. Bacterial conjunctivitis often is purulent and tends to be bilateral more frequently than is the case with viral conjunctivitis.[764] *S. pneumoniae* causes 12 to 32 percent of all cases of bacterial conjunctivitis.[75,268,777]

The syndrome of "conjunctivitis-otitis" was described first in 1982.[81] *H. influenzae* is the most common pathogen and can be isolated in as many as 73 percent of cases from the conjunctiva and the middle ear concomitantly. This rate is higher than the rate when conjunctivitis is present without AOM.[81]

In one study in the United States, the rate of non–penicillin-susceptible *S. pneumoniae* in isolates taken from children with bacterial conjunctivitis was 28 percent, with most isolates being fully resistant.[75]

A recent study in Minnesota evaluated 735 children with conjunctivitis in two cities. Forty-nine percent of positive cultures were *S. pneumoniae*. All isolates were nontypeable. Pulsed-field gel electrophoresis identified three clonal groups, with 84 percent of the isolates belonging to one clonal group. Multilocus sequence typing revealed that isolates had the same multilocus sequence type as that of isolates from a 2002 pneumococcal disease outbreak at a New England college. It has been suggested that certain pneumococcal strains have a predilection for causing

conjunctivitis.[108] Another study suggested that the absence of a capsule might provide *S. pneumoniae* with a selective virulence advantage in conjunctivitis.[590]

BONE AND JOINT INFECTIONS. Septic arthritis caused by *S. pneumoniae* is a relatively rare condition that accounts for 2.2 to 9.7 percent of all cases.[297,641] Its main initial clinical features are single or multiple swollen, warm, and painful joints. The joints most commonly involved are the knee and the ankle.[349] In one study, the mean duration of symptoms before hospitalization was 2 days, and patients were hospitalized for an average of 11 days. The mean peripheral WBC count was 20,600/mm³, the erythrocyte sedimentation rate usually was greater than 90 mm/hr, and the CRP concentration generally was higher than 100 mg/L. *S. pneumoniae* can be isolated from synovial fluid or blood in most patients.[641] The outcome is favorable in the majority of cases unless underlying diseases or sepsis occurs concomitantly.[349]

SOFT TISSUE INFECTIONS. *S. pneumoniae* is an uncommonly recognized etiologic agent of soft tissue infections, but it can cause serious infections of soft tissues, especially in patients with connective tissue diseases such as systemic lupus erythematosus. Other risk factors are HIV infection and corticosteroid treatment. The organism can be isolated from the infected tissue, as well as from blood.[188] *S. pneumoniae* can cause facial cellulitis as well. Periorbital infection can spread and cause infection of the orbit (orbital cellulitis or abscess) manifested as proptosis and ophthalmoplegia, but these sequelae are rare occurrences and usually a complication of purulent sinusitis, or they occur after bacteremia in infants and young children without another apparent source.[674] Most patients are younger than 3 years of age and previously were healthy. Fever and peripheral WBC counts higher than 15,000/mm³ can be observed in most patients, and blood cultures frequently are positive. Overall, response to therapy generally is good, and patients usually recover.[273]

PERITONITIS. The term *primary peritonitis* is associated with organisms that spread from the blood or via the lymphatic system to the peritoneal cavity and cause infection. Primary peritonitis is a rare condition that accounts for only 17 percent of all cases of peritonitis, and *S. pneumoniae* is the major pathogen in primary peritonitis and is responsible for 38 percent of all cases.[280] Primary pneumococcal peritonitis should be considered in the differential diagnosis of children with an acute abdominal syndrome.[242] This condition can be associated with underlying medical conditions such as nephrotic syndrome, immunocompromised status, or sickle-cell disease.[280] Colonization of the perineum and subsequent spread via the fallopian tube to the peritoneal cavity have been suggested to be important sources in young girls.[689] Indeed, 87 percent of all patients with pneumococcal primary peritonitis are females,[669] in contrast to other invasive infections, for which a male preponderance is observed.[3,15,92,103,112,207,240,350,701,726] Most of the patients are between 4 and 10 years of age.[669] Symptoms include diffuse abdominal pain, fever, vomiting, and diarrhea. Abdominal tenderness can be maximal in the right lower quadrant, which can lead to confusing it with acute appendicitis. In some cases, *S. pneumoniae* can be isolated as the only cause of peritonitis secondary to appendicitis.[319] Cultures should include blood, peritoneal fluid, and a vaginal swab. Some patients need laparotomy or laparoscopy to exclude other pathologies such as appendicitis or a tubo-ovarian abscess.[689] Morbidity and mortality rates can be high when the period without treatment exceeds 1 week, but in most cases the outcome is favorable when treated adequately.[669]

ENDOCARDITIS. Infection of native valves can lead to distal embolization and heart failure as a result of valve destruction. Cases of *S. pneumoniae* endocarditis, including those caused by non–penicillin-susceptible strains, were reported with involvement of the aortic and mitral valves.[683] The triad of pneumococcal meningitis, pneumonia, and endocarditis was described first by Osler, but this triad also is known as *Austrian syndrome*. Today, this entity is an uncommon occurrence because the incidence of *S. pneumoniae* endocarditis has decreased significantly from 10 to 15 percent of all endocarditis cases in the pre-antibiotic era to less than 3 percent today.[352,522,724]

Only 32 cases of pediatric pneumococcal endocarditis have been reported in the English medical literature since 1900. A fourth of them have been reported since 1990. Clinical features differed from adult cases, with mitral-valve involvement being more frequent and Osler's triad rarely present in children. A history of congenital heart disease was the only identifiable risk factor. Medical therapy alone resulted in a high mortality rate that was improved in a group of patients receiving combined medical and surgical interventions.[127]

PERICARDITIS. In the pre-antibiotic era, *S. pneumoniae* was the pathogen most commonly isolated from purulent pericarditis in children. These infections were common complications of pneumococcal pneumonia. After the introduction of antibiotics, pneumococcal cases decreased from 51 to 9 percent of all pericarditis cases and occurred mainly in adults.[275,643] Currently, infections of the pericardium are rare findings in children and often are related to underlying medical conditions such as immunodeficiency.[578]

INFECTION IN IMMUNOCOMPROMISED HOSTS. Patients with functional asplenia, including those with hemoglobinopathies, are at high risk for the acquisition of invasive pneumococcal infection. In a study of 19 asplenic patients with invasive pneumococcal infection, the clinical findings included fever (86%), shock (27%), petechiae or purpura (27%), disseminated vascular coagulopathy (18%), and respiratory distress (18%). Clinical illness included bacteremia alone (52%), meningitis (26%), bacteremia with otitis/sinusitis (13%), and bacteremia with pneumonia (9%). The mortality rate was 32 percent. No association was noted between antimicrobial resistance and mortality.[662]

HIV-infected children with pneumonia usually have the typical symptoms of fever, shortness of breath, and productive cough associated with pleuritic pain. The chest radiograph shows unilobar or multilobar infiltrates, and peripheral WBC counts often are elevated. A comparison between HIV-infected and non–HIV-infected children with community-acquired pneumonia showed no significant differences between groups with regard to the duration of hospitalization and mortality rates.[488] In contrast, when only patients from the aforementioned groups infected with isolates belonging to the "pediatric serotype group" (see the sections on epidemiology and prevention) were compared, marked differences, such as a higher rate of pneumonia with or without concurrent meningitis in the HIV-infected group and a higher rate of septic shock without focus in the non-HIV-infected group, were observed.[488] Recurrence of pneumococcal infection within 6 months from the initial episode is common in patients infected with HIV, particularly children.[260] Most HIV-infected patients recover without significant sequelae, and the clinical course of their systemic infection does not appear to be markedly different from that in healthy children.[369]

Patients with immunodeficiency disorders consisting of antibody and complement deficiencies are at high risk for acquisition of invasive and recurrent pneumococcal infection.[369] Children with nephrotic syndrome have a particularly increased risk for the development of pneumococcal peritonitis, mainly during relapse of their renal disease.[220] Other underlying diseases such as hematologic malignancies, diabetes mellitus, and cirrhosis, as well as conditions such as alcoholism, are associated with an increased risk for the development of pneumococcal bacteremia and other invasive diseases, mainly in adults.[369]

Children with sickle-cell disease are prone to the development of overwhelming *S. pneumoniae* bacteremia and sepsis; in children younger than 3 years of age, the incidence of bacteremia is 6.1 events per 100 patient-years, and the case-fatality rate is 24 percent for *S. pneumoniae* sepsis.[798]

Transplant recipients have been recognized for some time as being at high risk for the development of invasive pneumococcal disease. Of 42 children who had undergone bone marrow or solid organ transplantation and became infected with *S. pneumoniae*, 8 (19%) had two or more pneumococcal infections.[663] Solid organ recipients were more likely to have recurrent invasive disease than were recipients of bone marrow transplants. Death occurred in 2 of 42 recipients (5%). Cardiac transplant patients have an incidence of 39 cases of invasive pneumococcal infection per 1000 patients per year,[709] the highest risk of which occurs in African American heart transplant recipients who undergo transplantation because of idiopathic dilated cardiomyopathy.

TREATMENT

Penicillin G is the parenteral drug of choice for disease caused by penicillin-susceptible *S. pneumoniae* strains (defined as those with a penicillin MIC < 0.1 μg/mL). The usual doses of penicillin G result in serum concentrations that exceed this level in blood and most other body fluids for an adequate period. Penicillin G is the most common parenteral drug used for the treatment of pneumococcal infection, with doses ranging from 50,000 U/kg/day for minor infections to 300,000 U/kg/day for meningitis. For penicillin-susceptible strains, other parenteral β-lactams such as ampicillin, cefuroxime, cefotaxime, and ceftriaxone provide no advantage over penicillin G, even for serious infections. Macrolides and cephalosporins are an alternative treatment for penicillin-allergic patients if regional data do not show macrolide and cephalosporin resistance. Other agents such as clindamycin, tetracycline, and trimethoprim-sulfamethoxazole are active against *S. pneumoniae*, but resistance to these agents is increasing rapidly in most parts of the world.

In many regions, treatment of non–penicillin-susceptible *S. pneumoniae* has become a challenge, and reports of treatment failure have increased, especially in patients with invasive multidrug-resistant *S. pneumoniae* infection.[691] Rates of antibacterial resistance are highest in infants and decrease with increasing patient age.[106] Because isolates of *S. pneumoniae* that are resistant to penicillin frequently are resistant to other drug classes such as cephalosporins (mainly oral), macrolides, and trimethoprim-sulfamethoxazole,[779] the challenge of treatment is becoming complex.

The critical time for treatment of severe pneumococcal infection is during the first few hours after initial evaluation of the patient, before culture results are available and, thus, before knowledge of the presence or susceptibility of the pathogen is obtained. Therefore, the choice of antibiotics must rely on considerations based on the most recent epidemiologic data and the clinical status of the child, as well as the site of infection. Furthermore, because treatment is empiric, the choice of antibiotics must take into account other potential pathogens. Knowledge of the patient's antimicrobial use in the 3 months before infection developed is crucial for determining the appropriate therapy for a patient who has a possible pneumococcal infection.[751]

The proportion of *S. pneumoniae* isolates from U.S. pediatric patients covered by the PCV-7 vaccine decreased substantially in the 4 years after the vaccine was introduced. Resistance to commonly used antibiotics, including β-lactams and macrolides, as well as multidrug-resistant strains, also increased significantly among respiratory tract isolates of nonvaccine serotypes.[215]

Because treatment of pneumococcal infection is not necessarily similar in each of the clinical entities, specific details are provided for each clinical entity separately.

BACTEREMIA. Results of studies are conflicting with regard to the role of antibiotic treatment of occult pneumococcal bacteremia. In one study, the bacteremia resolved without any need for parenteral antibiotic treatment in 95.7 percent of patients.[12] No significant difference was found between amoxicillin and placebo recipients regarding complications such as meningitis in bacteremic patients, but faster reduction of fever and improvement in clinical appearance were observed in the group treated with amoxicillin.[366] A meta-analysis showed that rates of serious bacterial infection and meningitis did not differ between children treated with oral antibiotics and those treated with parenteral antibiotics.[634] In contrast, in another meta-analysis conducted by the same authors, treated patients had fewer serious bacterial infections than did untreated patients (3.3% versus 9.7%), and meningitis developed in only 0.8 percent of the treated group versus 2.7 percent of the untreated group.[636] In one study, the rate of persistent pneumococcal bacteremia was significantly higher in patients receiving no therapy for pneumococcal bacteremia than in those receiving either oral or parenteral treatment. A higher prevalence of persistent bacteremia in the orally treated group than in the parenterally treated group also was noted.[47] Thus, in patients suspected of having occult bacteremia, treatment with a β-lactam drug can be initiated, especially if the patient looks toxic or has a high fever. However, if the patient has been immunized with both Hib and pneumococcal conjugate vaccines, does not look toxic, and has no predisposing risk factors such as immunodeficiency, the risk of significant bacteremia resulting in complications is extremely low, and in this case, withholding treatment is reasonable.[792]

For proven *S. pneumoniae* bacteremia in a previously healthy child who is not critically ill, treatment, including oral amoxicillin, amoxicillin-clavulanate, second-generation oral cephalosporins, or parenteral third-generation cephalosporins such as ceftriaxone, can be initiated at the usually recommended dosages.[91] In most cases of penicillin-susceptible and penicillin-intermediate *S. pneumoniae* (penicillin MICs ≤1.0 µg/mL), most parenteral and some oral β-lactam antibiotic agents achieve serum concentrations that exceed the MIC of the organism for an adequate period.[421] The exceptions are drugs such as loracarbef, cefaclor, and cefixime, which have little activity against non–penicillin-susceptible *S. pneumoniae*.

In studies looking at the outcome of children with bacteremia caused by non–β-lactam–susceptible *S. pneumoniae* (not susceptible to penicillin, cefuroxime, or ceftriaxone), no difference in outcome was observed when compared with those with susceptible organisms.[126,392,684] However, in critically ill infants and children with invasive *S. pneumoniae* infection, initial antimicrobial therapy should include a third-generation cephalosporin (cefotaxime or ceftriaxone) alone or with vancomycin. Vancomycin should be discontinued as soon as antimicrobial susceptibility test results demonstrate effective alternative agents.[14,731] For children with severe hypersensitivity to β-lactam antibiotics (i.e., penicillins and cephalosporins), initial management of a potential pneumococcal infection could include clindamycin or vancomycin, in addition to antimicrobial drugs for other potential pathogens, as indicated.

MENINGITIS. Penicillin G, 250,000 to 400,000 U/kg/day, is an excellent treatment regimen for meningitis caused by penicillin-susceptible pneumococci, and ceftriaxone, 100 mg/kg/day, or cefotaxime, 300 mg/kg/day, is an excellent choice for meningitis caused by *S. pneumoniae* susceptible to these drugs.[14] However, treatment failures have been reported in penicillin- and ceftriaxone-nonsusceptible pneumococcal meningitis in patients,

as well as in animal models.[245,246] Therefore, because of the increased prevalence of penicillin-, cefotaxime-, and ceftriaxone-resistant *S. pneumoniae*, combination therapy consisting of vancomycin (60 mg/kg/day) and cefotaxime (300 mg/kg/day) or ceftriaxone (100 mg/kg/day) should be administered initially to all children 1 month of age or older with definite or probable bacterial meningitis. One recent study showed that delaying administration of the first dose of vancomycin until 2 or more hours after the first dose of parenteral cephalosporin has been administered was associated with a decrease the incidence of hearing loss related to the use of vancomycin.[111] This finding requires confirmation. However, vancomycin does not need to be used if compelling evidence indicates that the cause is an organism other than *S. pneumoniae* (e.g., gram-negative diplococci on a CSF smear or during an outbreak of meningococcal disease).[14] Vancomycin should not be given alone because bactericidal concentrations in CSF are difficult to sustain, clinical experience to support its use as monotherapy is minimal, and clinical failure and inadequate CSF drug concentrations have been reported.[9,756] Therapy should be modified after the organism has been isolated and based on the results of susceptibility testing. If the organism is susceptible to the β-lactam agent being used, vancomycin use should be discontinued. Antibiotic treatment in proven pneumococcal meningitis should not be shorter in duration than 10 days, and in complicated cases with a suspected focus, it may need to be provided for an even longer period.

When appropriately treated, the clinical manifestations and outcomes of meningitis caused by non–antibiotic-susceptible pneumococci are not significantly different from those caused by antibiotic-susceptible pneumococci.[31,110,227,723]

The combination of ceftriaxone and rifampin in an animal meningitis model had a bactericidal effect in meningitis caused by ceftriaxone-resistant *S. pneumoniae*.[567] The addition of rifampin to vancomycin after 24 to 48 hours of therapy should be considered in the following cases if the isolate is susceptible to rifampin: (1) when the patient's clinical condition has worsened despite therapy with vancomycin and cefotaxime or ceftriaxone, (2) when the subsequent Gram-stained smear or culture of CSF indicates failure to eradicate or substantially reduce the number of organisms, or (3) when the organism has an unusually high cefotaxime or ceftriaxone MIC (>4 µg/mL).[14] Although rifampin resistance is a rare event, rifampin should not be given as monotherapy because resistance may develop during therapy.[731]

Other β-lactam antimicrobial agents that can be used for the treatment of pneumococcal meningitis include meropenem (120 mg/kg/day) and cefepime (150 mg/kg/day).[390,644,645]

In patients with severe hypersensitivity to β-lactam antibiotics (i.e., penicillins and cephalosporins), the combination of vancomycin and rifampin should be considered.[246]

Chloramphenicol (75 to 100 mg/kg/day) is an acceptable alternative to β-lactam antibiotics in patients hypersensitive to these drugs. However, for unknown reasons, failure occurred in a patient with non–penicillin-susceptible pneumococcal meningitis treated with chloramphenicol.[244] Thus, treatment with chloramphenicol should be reserved for patients with β-lactam hypersensitivity who have pneumococcal meningitis caused by penicillin-susceptible strains.

Much debate has ensued on the role of dexamethasone as adjunctive therapy for pneumococcal meningitis. On the one hand, it might exert a positive effect in decreasing inflammatory reactions, but on the other hand, the same decrease in inflammation may reduce penetration of antibiotic agents into CSF. A meta-analysis of three randomized, double-blind, placebo-controlled studies combined with one retrospective study demonstrated a potential benefit of reducing hearing loss and neurologic sequelae after having pneumococcal meningitis.[656] Some studies had suggested a beneficial effect on pneumococcal meningitis when dexamethasone was given for 2 days with or before administration of parenteral antibiotics.[506] Thus, for infants and children aged 6 weeks and older, adjunctive therapy with dexamethasone should be considered after weighing the potential benefits and potential risks. When given in the recommended dosages to children with meningitis treated with dexamethasone, CSF concentrations of vancomycin, ceftriaxone, cefotaxime, and rifampin usually are adequate to treat meningitis caused by most strains of *S. pneumoniae*, but in some parts of the world, the CSF concentration of the drugs might be inadequate because of the high MIC values of ceftriaxone and cefotaxime. Dexamethasone may lead to decreased fever and a misleading impression of clinical improvement, even though CSF sterilization may not have been achieved. In some cases, after discontinuation of the steroids, secondary fever may develop, which also can be misleading and give the impression of a nonresponsive case and lead to use of additional lumbar punctures or other procedures.[208]

Repeat lumbar puncture should be considered after 24 to 48 hours of therapy if the following apply: (1) the organism is not susceptible to penicillin, (2) the results of cefotaxime and ceftriaxone susceptibility testing are not yet available, (3) the patient's condition has not improved or has worsened, or (4) the child has received dexamethasone, which might interfere with the ability to interpret a clinical response, such as the resolution of fever.[14,208]

PNEUMONIA. *S. pneumoniae* accounts for most cases of bacterial pneumonia in children. Thus, empiric treatment of pneumonia should cover this pathogen despite the fact that an organism-specific diagnosis seldom is established in children with pneumonia. Oral treatment with a β-lactam antibiotic such as amoxicillin, cefuroxime axetil, or amoxicillin-clavulanate is an appropriate option for the first-line treatment of ambulatory community-acquired pneumonia in children younger than 5 years old in most countries.[315]

In most cases of pneumonia caused by non–penicillin-susceptible *S. pneumoniae*, the outcome is favorable if the penicillin MIC is between 0.1 and 2.0 μg/mL and treatment consists of standard doses of parenteral penicillin G (100,000 to 300,000 U/mg/day), oral amoxicillin or amoxicillin-clavulanate (40 to 50 mg/kg/day), or cefuroxime (30 to 50 mg/kg/day).[315,722] No difference in outcome was found between patients with community-acquired pneumococcal pneumonia treated with oral amoxicillin-clavulanate and those treated with parenteral ceftriaxone.[633]

For immunocompetent hospitalized patients who are not critically ill on admission, parenteral treatment with β-lactam antibiotics such as cefuroxime, cefotaxime, or ampicillin (with or without β-lactamase inhibitors) is an appropriate option because both *S. pneumoniae* and most other potential organisms are covered.[315]

In adult and pediatric patients with pneumococcal pneumonia treated with standard regimens of parenteral penicillin G or a cephalosporin, the outcome was similar when patients infected with penicillin- or cephalosporin-resistant organisms were compared with those infected with susceptible organisms.[91,119,209,219,391,519,563,771,790]

In one retrospective cohort study, adult patients with bacteremic pneumonia caused by isolates that were not penicillin-susceptible had a significantly greater risk of dying in the hospital and of having more suppurative complications than did patients with susceptible isolates.[508] However, the mortality rate was not significantly different after adjustment for baseline differences in severity of illness. A population-based active surveillance study of pneumococcal disease in the United States found that 12 percent of 5837 cases were fatal.[219] In this study, a higher mortality rate was noted after the fourth hospital day in patients with invasive pneumococcal pneumonia caused by isolates with penicillin MICs of 4 μg/mL or greater. However, potential limitations of this study included absence of data on the severity of illness at initial evaluation, as well as lack of information on the antibiotics used.

Treatment failure and breakthrough meningitis were reported in a patient who was infected with highly resistant *S. pneumoniae* (penicillin MIC of 2 μg/mL, cefuroxime MIC of 2 μg/mL, and cefotaxime MIC > 8 μg/mL) and treated with cefotaxime and cefuroxime.[109] Because of such cases, some authorities recommend that in critically ill patients with highly resistant *S. pneumoniae*, vancomycin (or in older patients, fluoroquinolones active against *S. pneumoniae*) be added initially to third-generation cephalosporins.[315]

In a series of 32 children with pleural empyema caused by *S. pneumoniae*, those with non–penicillin-susceptible strains were significantly younger and more frequently had been treated previously with antibiotics than were children with penicillin-susceptible strains.[561] However, no significant differences were found between the two groups in the duration of fever and tachypnea, need for surgical treatment, presence of bacteremia, mean duration of therapy, or length of hospital stay.[561] In cases of pleural fluid or empyema in patients infected with highly resistant organisms, vancomycin or rifampin may be added if no clinical response is achieved within 48 to 72 hours.[91]

For β-lactam–allergic patients, macrolides are favored.[390] However, in some areas, macrolide resistance occurs commonly and may lead to treatment failure.[232,344,399,479,480,516,711,773] Breakthrough pneumococcal bacteremia has been reported during treatment with clarithromycin or azithromycin for community-acquired pneumonia.[399]

Drugs that are not appropriate for treating critically ill patients with pneumococcal pneumonia are the first-generation cephalosporins, ceftazidime, and ticarcillin because most penicillin-resistant *S. pneumoniae* also are resistant to these drugs.[190,565] Trimethoprim-sulfamethoxazole is not recommended because of the high prevalence of resistance to this drug.[315]

The duration of treatment is related to the clinical findings, clinical response to treatment, and underlying diseases of the patient and generally is 7 to 14 days. For hospitalized patients, 5 to 7 days of parenteral treatment followed by 7 days of oral therapy is recommended,[91,364] but many clinicians use a shorter course of 7 to 10 days total.

OTITIS MEDIA. Antibiotics are the standard of care for the treatment of AOM in the United States and in many other countries. Although antibiotic therapy is required in only 20 to 30 percent of all cases of AOM, most patients are treated with antibiotics because these cases cannot be identified quickly and easily.[415] As with other infections, the main goal of antibiotic therapy is to eradicate the causative pathogens from middle ear fluid.[166,386,453,631]

S. pneumoniae is responsible for 30 to 50 percent of all cases of acute bacterial otitis media, and it is the least likely pathogen to resolve without the administration of appropriate antibiotic treatment.[624] After 2 to 7 days, if not treated, approximately 50 percent of all *H. influenzae* organisms are eradicated spontaneously, but less than 20 percent of pneumococci are eradicated spontaneously in AOM.[334] Therefore, *S. pneumoniae* generally is considered the most important organism against which antibiotic treatment should be directed in AOM.

Studies in which tympanocentesis is performed before treatment and a second tympanocentesis procedure during treatment to document bacteriologic efficacy ("double-tympanocentesis" bacteriologic outcome studies) have demonstrated that pharmacodynamic models can predict bacteriologic outcome.[146,163] Studies have shown that the increasing resistance of *S. pneumoniae* to various drugs has increased the complexity of antibiotic treatment of otitis media. In addition to having activity against antibiotic-resistant pneumococci, a drug appropriate for empiric treatment of AOM should be active against the two other main pathogens of otitis media, namely, *H. influenzae* and *M. catarrhalis*. Table 96–3 summarizes the activity of drugs used commonly against otitis media pathogens, with the pharmacodynamic properties (the relationship between the drug concentration in plasma and the concentration at the site of infection) and the MIC of the drug to the infecting organism taken into account. The in vitro activity of oral agents has not always been predictive of their in vivo activity because of incorrect or unavailable interpretative breakpoints, but this deficiency has been rectified for *S. pneumoniae* in the United States since 2000.

Most of the drugs used for the treatment of AOM belong to the β-lactam and macrolide classes; these drugs act against pathogens by a "time-dependent killing" mechanism,[79,146] which means that an effective dosing regimen for AOM would require that the unbound plasma concentration exceed the MICs of the drug against the causative pathogens for at least 40 to 50 percent of the dosing interval. Although the drug exerts its effect in the middle ear cavity, penetration of the drug into this space is driven by the unbound plasma concentration, which is in equilibrium with the extracellular fluid compartment of tissues and sites such as the middle ear space.

For penicillin-susceptible *S. pneumoniae*, most β-lactam drugs (with the exception of penicillin V and the first-generation oral

cephalosporins) reach that goal and are appropriate drugs for otitis media caused by penicillin-susceptible *S. pneumoniae*.

In the case of non–penicillin-susceptible *S. pneumoniae*, on the other hand, the picture is different. The most active oral β-lactam drugs against penicillin-intermediate isolates are amoxicillin and amoxicillin-clavulanate (clavulanate has no effect on pneumococci, but it is used often to empirically add coverage against β-lactamase–producing organisms). However, most of the oral cephalosporins, with the exception of cefuroxime axetil, cefpodoxime proxetil, and cefprozil, cannot reach the goal of unbound plasma concentrations exceeding the MIC$_{90}$ values for most penicillin-intermediate organisms for 40 to 50 percent of the dosing interval and thus are not appropriate for the treatment of AOM in areas where penicillin-intermediate strains occur commonly.[146,195] For fully penicillin-resistant *S. pneumoniae* strains, of the β-lactam drugs commonly used against AOM, only high-dose amoxicillin (80 to 100 mg/kg/day), amoxicillin-clavulanate (80 to 100 mg/kg/day of the amoxicillin component), and intramuscular ceftriaxone (50 mg/kg/day) reach plasma or middle ear fluid concentrations that are above the MIC values for an appropriate duration. A recent study found that 90 mg/kg of amoxicillin (given as amoxicillin-clavulanate) significantly decreased nasopharyngeal colonization when compared with 45 mg/kg

TABLE 96–3 In Vivo Activity of Antibiotic Drugs in Common Use for the Treatment of AOM That Are Effective against the Major AOM Pathogens*

	Antimicrobial Activity					
	Streptococcus pneumoniae[†]			*Haemophilus influenzae*		*Moraxella catarrhalis*
Drug	Penicillin-Susceptible	Penicillin-Intermediate	Penicillin-Resistant	β-Lactamase–Negative	β-Lactamase–Positive	
Amoxicillin, 40-50 mg/kg/day	+++	+++	+	++	−	−
Amoxicillin, 80-90 mg/kg/day	+++	+++	+++	+++	−	−
Amoxicillin-clavulanate, 45/6.4 mg/kg/day	+++	++	+	++	++	+++
Amoxicillin-clavulanate, 90/6.4 mg/kg/day	+++	+++	++	+++	+++	+++
Cefaclor	+++	−	−	+	+	++
Cefdinir	+++	+	−	++	+++	+++
Cefixime	++	−	−	+++	+++	+++
Cefpodoxime proxetil	+++	++	+	+++	+++	+++
Cefprozil	+++	++	+	−	−	++
Ceftriaxone (50 mg/kg/day)—1 day	+++	++	+	+++	+++	+++
Ceftriaxone (50 mg/kg/day)—3 days	+++	+++	+++	+++	+++	+++
Cefuroxime axetil	+++	++	+	++	++	+++
Clindamycin	+++	++[‡]	++[‡]	−	−	−
Erythromycin-azithromycin-clarithromycin	+++	++[‡]	−[‡]	+/−	+/−	++
TMP-SMX	++	−[‡]	−[‡]	++	++	++

S. pneumoniae		
	Macrolide-Susceptible	Macrolide-Resistant
Clindamycin	+++	+
Erythromycin-azithromycin-clarithromycin	+++	−
	TMP-SMX–Susceptible	TMP-SMX–Resistant
TMP-SMX	+++	−

*In vitro activity, pharmacodynamic properties, and, if available, the results of bacteriologic outcome studies are taken into account.
[†]*Penicillin-susceptible (MICs ≤ 0.06 μg/mL), penicillin-intermediate (MICs of 0.1 to 1 μg/mL), penicillin-resistant (MICs ≥ 2 μg/mL).*
[‡]*When Streptococcus pneumoniae is not penicillin-susceptible, the prevalence of macrolide, clindamycin, and TMP-SMX resistance among the strains is higher than in penicillin-susceptible ones. This rate can be very high in penicillin-resistant S. pneumoniae. (See "Bacteriology.")*
+++, Appropriate; ++, may not be appropriate for some strains; +, frequent bacteriologic failures are likely; −, usually associated with bacteriologic failure.
AOM, acute otitis media; MICs, minimal inhibitory concentrations; TMP-SMX, trimethoprim-sulfamethoxazole.

$(p = 0.0261).$[102] To eradicate *S. pneumoniae* with penicillin MICs of 2.0 μg/mL or higher, an amoxicillin or amoxicillin-clavulanate dose of 80 to 100 mg/kg/day (divided into two or three doses) is necessary.[161,453,667]

Among the parenteral cephalosporins, ceftriaxone and cefotaxime have the lowest MICs, but high-level resistance of *S. pneumoniae* to these agents has been reported.[700] Intramuscular ceftriaxone (50 mg/kg/day) given once daily for 1 to 3 days is effective for pneumococcal otitis caused by penicillin-susceptible strains. For otitis caused by non–penicillin-susceptible *S. pneumoniae*, 3 days of treatment may be required.[456,457]

Resistance to macrolides is significant and affects bacteriologic and clinical outcomes in AOM.[28,52,165] All macrolides are efficacious against otitis caused by macrolide-susceptible *S. pneumoniae*. Efficacy was shown for erythromycin,[336] clarithromycin,[334] and azithromycin.[165] However, when the organism is resistant to macrolides, these drugs are not effective because the MIC is too high to be exceeded by drug concentrations at the site of infection, which has been demonstrated best for azithromycin[162,165] but can be generalized to other macrolides. In one child, pneumococcal bacteremia and meningitis were reported to have developed during azithromycin therapy for otitis media.[351]

Clindamycin is active against most non–penicillin-susceptible *S. pneumoniae* strains and may be used to treat pneumococcal AOM that does not respond to β-lactam antibiotics. However, prospective, controlled studies on the bacteriologic and clinical efficacy of clindamycin in the treatment of AOM have not been performed. Furthermore, as described in the section on microbiology, an increasing proportion of *S. pneumoniae* isolates resistant to macrolides also are resistant to clindamycin.

Trimethoprim-sulfamethoxazole no longer is an appropriate choice for empiric treatment of AOM because of the high prevalence of resistance to this drug among *S. pneumoniae* strains in many regions. In the case of AOM caused by *S. pneumoniae* resistant to trimethoprim-sulfamethoxazole, the effect of this drug is no better than that of placebo.[452]

Treatment of nonresponsive AOM (cases refractory to one or more courses of antibiotics) was studied in double-tympanocentesis studies, with bacteriologic outcome being the major endpoint.[415] Cefaclor, cefixime, loracarbef, ceftibuten, azithromycin, and trimethoprim-sulfamethoxazole clearly have been shown to be ineffective against nonsusceptible pneumococci and no longer can be recommended for the empiric treatment of nonresponsive AOM.[195] Second-line treatment preferably should be based on the results of middle ear fluid cultures and pathogen susceptibility tests.

For patients with clinically defined treatment failure after receiving 3 to 5 days of initial therapy, suitable second-line agents active against non–penicillin-susceptible pneumococci, as well as β-lactamase–producing *H. influenzae* and *M. catarrhalis*, should be administered. Three antibiotic drugs fulfill these criteria: amoxicillin-clavulanate, intramuscular ceftriaxone, and, to a lesser extent, cefuroxime axetil.[72,195,502] In these cases, amoxicillin-clavulanate should be given at 80 to 100 mg/kg/day of the amoxicillin component. Intramuscular ceftriaxone given for 3 days was found to be superior to a 1-day regimen in cases caused by penicillin-resistant *S. pneumoniae*.[457] A recent study found that gatifloxacin, 10 mg/kg once daily, was as effective and well tolerated in children with AOM treatment failure or recurrent otitis media.[675] Use of gatifloxacin was not associated with the development of arthropathy, and, in fact, an observational study of more than 6000 children treated with fluoroquinolones found the incidence of joint disorders comparable to that after treatment with erythromycin.[793]

Erythromycin-sulfisoxazole, clarithromycin, and azithromycin may be used as alternatives in penicillin-allergic patients.[454] One recent study found that azithromycin was as effective as was high-dose amoxicillin for the treatment of children with AOM

and that rates of adverse events were lower and compliance improved with the simplified single dosing regimen.[32] However, macrolide resistance among middle ear *S. pneumoniae* isolates has been increasing steadily.[496] Therefore, in such cases, tympanocentesis is recommended either before initiation of treatment or after 48 to 72 hours of treatment if no clinical response is observed.

The recommended duration of treatment usually is 10 days for most antibiotic drug regimens in children younger than 2 years.[416] Recent studies suggest that a shorter treatment course (5 to 7 days) may be adequate, at least for a subgroup of children older than 2 years of age with uncomplicated otitis.[435,580,584] However, data evaluating the bacteriologic outcome and clinical efficacy of shortened antibiotic treatment of AOM are not complete in children younger than 2 years old, children with severe or complicated AOM, and those with a history of recurrent or chronic otitis media, although such studies are being undertaken. Clinical studies suggest that 5 to 7 days of treatment may not be adequate for these groups of patients.[134,136,196,585] Children attending daycare centers are at particular risk of having a poor response and recurrence if treated for 5 rather than 10 days.[135] Therefore, until the results of more studies are available, shortened antibiotic treatment in AOM cannot be recommended for children younger than 2 years old, children with severe or complicated AOM, children with chronic or recurrent AOM, and children attending daycare centers.[136,151]

Prophylactic use of amoxicillin or trimethoprim-sulfamethoxazole at half the therapeutic dose may reduce the number of new episodes significantly in patients with recurrent AOM.* However, this approach may promote carriage of drug-resistant *S. pneumoniae* and lead to the development of new infections with resistant organisms.[164] Thus, antibiotic prophylaxis is not recommended except in children with frequently recurrent AOM episodes, defined as three or more documented episodes in 6 months or four or more in 12 months.[455]

Although most non–penicillin-susceptible *S. pneumoniae* are included in PCV-7, AOM caused by these strains will not disappear completely. Therefore, clinicians must continue to consider non–penicillin-susceptible pneumococci when prescribing antibiotics for AOM.[308]

SINUSITIS. Although studies on the bacteriology of acute sinusitis are sparse, they suggest that the pathogens causing sinusitis are similar to those causing AOM. Acute bacterial sinusitis usually is a complication of viral rhinosinusitis and occurs in 0.5 to 2 percent of cases. In a study comparing antimicrobial therapy with placebo for the treatment of children with a clinical and radiographic diagnosis of acute bacterial sinusitis, children receiving antimicrobial therapy recovered more quickly and more often than did those receiving placebo.[766] Thus, antimicrobial agents that are effective for the treatment of AOM also are likely to be effective and are recommended for acute sinusitis.[14,550,687,765]

In the selection of appropriate therapy for bacterial sinusitis, physicians should consider the following parameters: (1) the severity of disease: mild (healthy patients with 10 days of persistent anterior and posterior rhinorrhea and fatigue), moderate (patients with 10 days of nasal congestion in whom a low-grade fever developed during the past 3 days, as well as increasing unilateral tenderness over the frontal or maxillary sinuses that becomes aggravated while the patient bends forward), or severe (life-threatening infection); (2) antibiotic use during the 4 to 6 weeks before the onset of infection, which is an important risk factor for the selection of resistant organisms; (3) age younger than 5 years; (4) attendance at a daycare center; and (5) underlying condition predisposing to invasive infection, such as immunocompromised status.

---

*See references 65, 318, 413, 493, 499, 579, 592, 618, 630, 783.

Amoxicillin is recommended for the initial treatment of children who have uncomplicated acute bacterial sinusitis that is of mild severity, do not attend daycare centers, and have not been treated recently with an antimicrobial.[132] If the patient is allergic to amoxicillin, cefdinir, cefuroxime axetil, or cefpodoxime can be used (if the allergic reaction was not a type I hypersensitivity reaction). In children with serious allergic reactions, macrolides or clindamycin can be used in an effort to select an antimicrobial of an entirely different class.[132] In patients with disease moderate in severity or those attending daycare, therapy should be initiated with high-dose amoxicillin-clavulanate. Parenteral antibiotic treatment should be considered in patients with severe disease. For patients with mild or moderate disease who are not improving after receiving 72 hours of treatment, therapy should be changed to amoxicillin-clavulanate unless this agent was used initially, in which case treatment options are very limited.[132,363] In addition, re-evaluation of deteriorating or nonresponsive patients may include computed tomography, fiberoptic endoscopy, or sinus aspiration with culture.[687]

Acute sinusitis should be treated for 7 days after improvement is noted and for at least 10 to 14 days.[550] However, the duration of treatment has not been studied adequately and, therefore, is arbitrary.

CONJUNCTIVITIS. When compared with placebo, topical therapy with polymyxin-bacitracin ointment has been shown to reduce the duration of symptoms by half and to achieve a 2.5-fold increase in the rate of bacteriologic eradication after 8 to 10 days of therapy (31% vs. 79%, respectively).[267] Polymyxin B-trimethoprim, applied four times daily for 1 week, also can be an effective broad-spectrum therapy for nonsevere conjunctivitis, although the coverage against gram-positive organisms provided by trimethoprim is less than optimal for some species. Aminoglycoside drops (0.3% gentamicin or 0.3% tobramycin) are inherently less active against gram-positive organisms and have a low therapeutic-to-toxic ratio as topical agents. Neomycin-polymyxin B–gramicidin drops or neomycin–polymyxin B–bacitracin ointment provides broad-spectrum coverage, but neomycin poses a 10 percent risk for hypersensitivity reactions such as contact dermatitis.[764]

Most organisms causing conjunctivitis are susceptible to chloramphenicol.[75,621] However, significant public and professional concern regarding the use of chloramphenicol eyedrops has been raised because of the associated risk of development of bone marrow aplasia.[99,125]

Increased resistance to polymyxin B–sulfamethoxazole for the treatment of conjunctivitis caused by *S. pneumoniae* in children was reported recently. Topical tetracycline and fluoroquinolones are active against penicillin-resistant *S. pneumoniae* and are considered suitable for the treatment of patients with conjunctivitis that is not responsive to the other treatment.[75]

BONE AND JOINT INFECTIONS. In a review of 13 cases of septic arthritis or osteomyelitis caused by penicillin-susceptible *S. pneumoniae*,[4] the drug used most commonly was penicillin, followed by ampicillin. Nafcillin and cefotaxime also were used to treat these patients. In addition, three patients with non–penicillin-susceptible *S. pneumoniae* were treated with combinations of vancomycin and cefotaxime or ceftriaxone for septic arthritis and osteomyelitis.

Rifampin and clindamycin also were used to treat a patient with septic arthritis of the left hip and osteomyelitis of the proximal end of the femur caused by highly resistant *S. pneumoniae* (penicillin and cefotaxime MICs of 8 μg/mL); this patient also experienced prolonged fever (21 days). The patient had been treated initially with cefotaxime and nafcillin, as well as with drainage and irrigation of the infected site.[4]

The duration of treatment with parenteral antibiotics in patients with *S. pneumoniae* bone infection varied from 14 to 196 days and, in those with joint infection, from 12 to 67 days.[4,54] Parenteral treatment may be followed by oral antibiotic therapy once the patient has improved considerably.

ENDOCARDITIS. *S. pneumoniae* endocarditis is a rare event that accounts for less than 3 percent of all cases of endocarditis.[352,524,724] Cases caused by penicillin-resistant *S. pneumoniae* have been reported exclusively in adults.[683] Treatment is based on a combination of antibiotics and surgery because *S. pneumoniae* endocarditis is associated with rapid destruction of heart valves. Parenteral second- or third-generation cephalosporins are recommended as initial treatment, and the addition of vancomycin is advised in patients with penicillin- or cephalosporin-resistant organisms.[420] Newer fluoroquinolones may serve as an alternative treatment in older patients.[683]

TREATMENT OF PNEUMOCOCCAL INFECTION IN IMMUNOCOMPROMISED HOSTS. Children with underlying conditions such as HIV infection, nephrotic syndrome, sickle-cell disease, other congenital hemoglobinopathies, or congenital immunoglobulin deficiencies, as well as children receiving immunosuppressive drugs and those with congenital or acquired asplenia, are at increased risk for acquiring *S. pneumoniae* infection in general and infection with drug-resistant organisms in particular.[346,488,664,731] The results of two studies[665,740] suggested that in HIV-infected adults, the outcome is worse in patients with nonsusceptible *S. pneumoniae* than in those with susceptible *S. pneumoniae*. However, both studies had limitations that preclude arriving at firm conclusions. In regions where penicillin-resistant *S. pneumoniae* occurs commonly, consideration should be given to initiating therapy with vancomycin and cefotaxime or ceftriaxone in critically ill patients until susceptibility results are available; subsequent therapy should be based on these results and the patient's clinical course.

For infants with sickle-cell anemia, oral penicillin prophylaxis against invasive *S. pneumoniae* disease should be initiated as soon as the diagnosis is established, preferably by the time that the infant is 2 months of age. Although the efficacy of antimicrobial prophylaxis has been proved only in patients with sickle-cell anemia, other asplenic children at particularly high risk, such as those with malignant neoplasms or thalassemia, also should receive daily chemoprophylaxis. In general, antimicrobial prophylaxis (in addition to immunization) should be considered strongly for all asplenic children younger than 5 years old and for at least 1 year after they undergo splenectomy.[13]

The age at which chemoprophylaxis is discontinued often is empiric. Based on a multicenter study, prophylactic penicillin can be discontinued in children with sickle-cell anemia who are receiving regular medical attention and have not had a severe *S. pneumoniae* infection or surgical splenectomy when they reach approximately 5 years of age.[13] The appropriate duration of prophylaxis for children with asplenia caused by other conditions is unknown. Some experts continue administering prophylaxis throughout childhood and into adulthood for high-risk patients with asplenia.[13]

For antimicrobial prophylaxis, oral penicillin V (125 mg twice a day for children younger than 5 years old and 250 mg twice a day for children 5 years and older) usually is recommended. Some experts recommend amoxicillin (20 mg/kg/day). Breakthrough infections caused by drug-resistant *S. pneumoniae* may occur. Therefore, parents should be aware that all febrile illnesses are potentially serious in immunocompromised children and that immediate medical attention should be sought because the initial signs and symptoms of fulminant bacteremia can be subtle.[13]

In addition to receiving chemoprophylaxis, children aged 2 years and older who are at increased risk of acquiring invasive *S. pneumoniae* infection should be immunized with a pneumococcal conjugate vaccine followed by a 23-valent nonconjugate polysaccharide vaccine 2 months or longer after the last dose of the conjugate vaccine is taken.[593] Indications for immunization are the following: (1) sickle-cell disease; (2) functional or anatomic asplenia; (3) nephrotic syndrome or chronic renal failure; (4) conditions associated with immunosuppression, such as organ or bone marrow transplantation, drug therapy, or cytoreduction therapy (including long-term systemic corticosteroid therapy); (5) HIV infection; and (6) CSF leaks.[14] For details on immunization, see the section on prevention.

MISCELLANEOUS INFECTIONS. Other infections, such as primary peritonitis and orbital cellulitis, should be treated with antibiotic agents that are recommended for bacteremia. Parenteral penicillin, ampicillin and cefotaxime, or ceftriaxone is suitable treatment in most cases, and the addition of vancomycin for drug-resistant *S. pneumoniae* is recommended. Treatment should be adjusted according to susceptibility results.[731]

PREVENTION

Prevention of pneumococcal infection in all ages is, without doubt, a more effective approach to reducing the burden of pneumococcal disease than any successful treatment modality is. In general, prevention can be divided into nonimmunologic and immunologic strategies (immunoprophylaxis).

NONIMMUNOLOGIC STRATEGIES

This category includes interventions that aim at (1) reducing risk factors predisposing to the development of pneumococcal infection, (2) providing chemical substances (e.g., antibiotics) to abort or prevent pneumococcal colonization or disease, and (3) modifying anatomic abnormalities that predispose to the development of pneumococcal infection.[417]

A factor that is important not only for pneumococcal infection but also for many other serious bacterial infections is the need to improve general health and nutrition worldwide, particularly in developing countries. Many risk factors for the acquisition of pneumococcal infection that can be alleviated include poor living conditions, overcrowding, poor hygiene, malnutrition, and a high prevalence of viral infections, particularly respiratory viruses, measles, and HIV. In the developed world, carriage of pneumococci, especially antibiotic-resistant strains that result in sporadic infections as well as outbreaks, is related to daycare attendance and is proportional to the number of children per group.[124,135,168,171,463,608,718] Therefore, reducing the number of children per group in daycare centers and developing alternative forms of childcare may reduce the rate of pneumococcal morbidity.

The importance of passive smoking (namely, being in close contact with smokers in the same household) has been highlighted as a risk factor for the development of pneumococcal disease.[545] Thus, effort to prevent smoking in the home may have an important role in the prevention of pneumococcal infection. Breast-feeding may protect against some infections related to *S. pneumoniae*, such as otitis media.[23,104,197,628,744] Therefore, breast-feeding should be encouraged, especially in families in which otitis media occurs commonly, although the precise role of prolonged breast-feeding in protecting against pneumococcal infection has not been established.

Antimicrobial chemoprophylaxis is used predominantly for two indications: prevention of recurrent AOM and prevention of

pneumococcal sepsis in children with anatomic or functional asplenia. Data now exist to support the common practice of prescribing regular doses of penicillin for children with asplenia or sickle-cell disease.[253] Chemoprophylaxis is used commonly for the prevention of middle ear infections. Controlled clinical trials have compared antimicrobial chemoprophylaxis with placebo, surgery, or historical controls.[76] Various antibiotics were tested (either as ongoing daily prophylaxis or as intermittent treatment during viral infections). Most of the studies, but not all, showed a benefit of chemoprophylaxis over controls, especially for amoxicillin, ampicillin, sulfonamides, and trimethoprim-sulfamethoxazole.* However, those studies were performed before the era of increased antibiotic resistance in *S. pneumoniae*. The dosing schedule recommended for prophylaxis usually is half the daily therapeutic dose given once a day, but the optimal dosing regimen has not been defined.

The potential benefits of otitis media chemoprophylaxis have been weighed against the ability of chemoprophylaxis to alter the nasopharyngeal flora, foster colonization with resistant organisms, and thereby compromise the long-term efficacy of the prophylactic drug and contribute to the propagation of resistant organisms throughout the community. As a result, the practice of otitis media chemoprophylaxis has been reduced greatly. In one study,[101] prophylaxis with amoxicillin induced a dramatic increase in the carriage of penicillin-resistant *S. pneumoniae*, as well as increased carriage of other resistant pathogens. The fear of increasing resistance led the Committee on Infectious Diseases of the American Academy of Pediatrics to issue a warning against the widespread use of otitis media prophylaxis and to state in its recent report that "Antimicrobial prophylaxis should be reserved for control of recurrent acute otitis media, defined by 3 or more distinct and well-documented episodes during a period of 6 months or 4 or more episodes during a period of 12 months."[15]

Surgical otitis media prophylaxis by myringotomy and insertion of tympanostomy tubes or adenoidectomy (with or without tonsillectomy) has been recommended for otitis-prone children.[411] Some authorities now prefer this modality to the chemoprophylactic approach because it is not associated with altered flora. However, surgical risks also need to be considered.

A novel approach to prevention of pneumococcal disease is the potential use of oligosaccharides to prevent attachment of organisms, including *S. pneumoniae*, to the respiratory mucosa. Because colonization of the respiratory mucosa can result in local and systemic disease, as well as spread to other individuals, prevention of colonization is a reasonable approach to prevent disease. Human milk oligosaccharides can prevent attachment of *S. pneumoniae* and other organisms to the mucosa of the respiratory tract[19,803] and have been shown to interfere with the establishment and progression of experimental pneumococcal pneumonia in infant rats.[345] Natural oligosaccharides act as decoys in mucosa (also in saliva, tears, urine, sweat, and breast milk) and bind the carbohydrate-binding proteins of the microbial pathogens and thereby prevent mucosal attachment.[417] Despite this promise, a large-scale study examining the efficacy of such an oligosaccharide (3'-sialyllacto-*N*-neoteratose) given intranasally as prophylaxis for AOM and nasopharyngeal carriage of bacteria failed to show any beneficial effect on either outcome.[745]

Other experiments conducted in Finland showed that xylitol (a five-carbon sugar alcohol used extensively as a sweetener in toothpaste, chewing gum, and various foods) inhibited the growth of streptococci, including *S. pneumoniae*, in vitro[426,427] and prevented the development of otitis media in daycare center attendees when provided as chewing gum, lozenges, or syrup.[742,743]

---

*See references 65, 318, 413, 493, 499, 579, 592, 618, 630, 783.

Whether this approach eventually will develop into a practical strategy to prevent respiratory infections caused by *S. pneumoniae* and other organisms is not clear. Obviously, the concept of reducing nasopharyngeal colonization and thereby the number of episodes of bacterial respiratory infection through competitive inhibition remains "cutting-edge" medicine. Additional new agents, altered doses, or the existing agents or different methods of administration still should be studied.[576]

IMMUNOPROPHYLAXIS

As discussed in the section on pathogenesis in this chapter, *S. pneumoniae* infections typically are opportunistic infections complicating viral respiratory infection. Recent advances in the development of vaccines against respiratory viruses, especially influenza virus, RSV, and parainfluenza virus, could, therefore, reduce the incidence and severity of pneumococcal infection by reducing these preceding viral infections. Some of these vaccines are expected to be licensed and widely used in the next decade. Inactivated influenza vaccines are licensed already and used in children. The expected addition of live attenuated influenza vaccines may herald a new era in the prevention of influenza disease in children.

The reader is referred to the sections on the structure of the pneumococcus, virulence factors, and host defense mechanisms in this chapter for an understanding of the basis for the immune-based strategy of prevention of disease.

Unconjugated Capsular Polysaccharide Vaccines

Efforts to prevent pneumococcal infection by providing specific immunity started more than 100 years ago, as described in the section on history. That both passive immunization (administration of specific antibodies) and active immunization can protect against many pneumococcal infections is well established.

Passively administered serotype-specific antibodies can protect animals and humans against diseases caused by pneumococci. Administration of antisera was associated with improved clinical outcome, including reduced mortality rates.[118] Human immunoglobulins can prevent experimental pneumococcal bacteremia in mice[128,639] and otitis media in chinchillas.[679] The finding of low cord blood IgG antibodies, mainly of the IgG1 subset, is predictive of early-onset AOM in infancy.[59,474,647] In several clinical studies, bacterial polysaccharide immune globulin (BPIG) obtained by immunizing healthy adults with a 14-valent pneumococcal vaccine (in addition to group C meningococcal and Hib polysaccharide vaccines) decreased the prevalence of AOM[654,680] and invasive infection[682] in children. High-dose BPIG administered to infant rats resulted in high serum concentrations of serotype-specific IgG against serotype 3 (geometric mean concentrations of 8.2 and 1.4 µg/mL on days 1 and 7, respectively) and, consequently, protection against nasopharyngeal carriage of this serotype.[492]

Immunization with pneumococcal polysaccharide antigens, mainly in adults, has been studied for a long time. First, hexavalent polysaccharide vaccines were introduced in the late 1940s, followed by 14-valent vaccines in the late 1970s and 23-valent vaccines in the early 1980s. The last, produced by several manufacturers, contains 25 µg of purified, nonconjugated polysaccharide antigens per dose for serotypes 1, 2, 3, 4, 5, 6B, 7F, 8, 9N, 9V, 10A, 11A, 12F, 14, 15B, 17F, 18C, 19A, 19F, 20, 22F, 23F, and 33F. These 23 serotypes account for approximately 90 percent of the serotypes responsible for invasive pneumococcal infection in all age groups in both developed and developing countries.[17,310,311,619,698] The 23-valent polysaccharide vaccines are tolerated well by healthy children for primary[447,668] or repeated

immunization.[88] However, the presence of preexisting antibodies was associated with an increased incidence of adverse events at the site of infection in adults but less pronounced effects in children.[78,432,552]

Generally speaking, these bacterial polysaccharide-based vaccines are poorly immunogenic in infants and toddlers for important disease-causing serotypes, which is to be expected because bacterial capsular polysaccharides induce antibody production primarily by T-cell–independent mechanisms that still are not fully developed in this age group.[615] Polysaccharide-specific IgG concentrations are relatively high in very young infants because they are acquired transplacentally and consist mainly of IgG1. Nasopharyngeal colonization with various serotypes of *S. pneumoniae* results in the natural production of serotype-specific antibodies.[107,314,730,786] The immune response to pneumococcal polysaccharides is serotype-dependent, and some serotypes commonly associated with disease are especially poor immunogens until the child reaches the age of approximately 5 years.[194] Serotypes 6A, 6B, 12, 19A, 19F, and 23F are examples of this phenomenon.[170,194,431,447,460,599,699,730,786] As for other species, the IgG subclasses that are produced after exposure to polysaccharide antigens are mainly IgG2 and IgG4.[468] A second dose of polysaccharide vaccine does not provide a booster effect and even may result in a reduced immune response when compared with the response after the first dose, which may suggest an antigenic tolerance effect.[78,754]

Children with certain underlying conditions that predispose to the development of pneumococcal infection respond more poorly to pneumococcal polysaccharide vaccines than do otherwise normal children. Published studies of children with recurrent respiratory tract infections,[204,327,652,653] HIV infection,[34,263,581] sickle-cell disease,[67,754] splenectomy,[3,612] malignancies,[609] and chronic renal disease[247,630,642,703] all have demonstrated this phenomenon.

In addition to a relatively poor systemic immune response, the polysaccharide vaccines have been shown to induce only minimal mucosal immune responses. Serotype-specific antibodies to pneumococcal serotypes 6A, 14, 18C, and 23F were measured in the sera and middle ear effusions of 14 children who had received a 14-valent pneumococcal capsular polysaccharide vaccine and in controls.[431] Serotype-specific antibody concentrations in middle ear effusions correlated with serum concentrations and generally were higher in pneumococcal vaccine recipients than in control vaccine recipients. IgM class antibodies frequently were seen only in the serum samples, thus suggesting that antibodies diffuse into the middle ear space rather than being synthesized in situ in response to the vaccine. This finding refutes previous theories that local production of antibodies occurs in the middle ear after vaccination.[433,692,693]

Limited data exist regarding the efficacy of polysaccharide pneumococcal vaccines in preventing disease in infants and children. A large study conducted in Papua New Guinea on more than 7000 children showed a reduction in mortality rates from acute lower respiratory tract disease.[449,616,617] In this study the effect was dramatic: a 59 percent reduction in mortality rates in all children vaccinated (5 months to 5 years of age) and a 50 percent reduction in children vaccinated before they reached 2 years of age. However, the vaccine did not protect against nonfatal disease. In the United States, researchers have suggested that the polysaccharide vaccines would be 62 percent effective in preventing invasive pneumococcal disease caused by vaccine serotypes in children aged 2 to 5 years.[226] The effectiveness of polysaccharide pneumococcal vaccines in preventing otitis media is not clear. Several studies have shown some reduction in the incidence of otitis media in vaccinated children,[339,490] but other studies have failed to show this effect.[193,394,725] No effect of the use of polysaccharide pneumococcal vaccine on pneumococcal nasopharyngeal carriage could be demonstrated.[160,170]

The aforementioned data on T-cell–independent polysaccharide pneumococcal vaccines clearly show that the benefit in children was at best marginal.

Conjugated Capsular Polysaccharide Vaccines

In contrast to the T-cell–independent nature of the immune response that occurs after the administration of bacterial polysaccharides, when these polysaccharides are conjugated to protein, the antibody response changes to a T-cell–dependent one.[44,200,396,620,681,705] These conjugate vaccines induce helper T cells to stimulate polysaccharide-specific B cells that not only produce antibodies but also mature into memory cells (Fig. 96–14). Polysaccharide–protein conjugate products characteristically are immunogenic in infancy and result in the production of high concentrations of antibodies. These antibodies have improved functional capacity (determined by avidity and opsonization assays), are long lasting, and induce a brisk and rapid elevation in highly functional antigen-specific antibodies with re-exposure (booster effect).[205]

The development of pneumococcal conjugate vaccines initially used the technology developed for Hib conjugate vaccines. Increasing experience and challenges have led to modifications

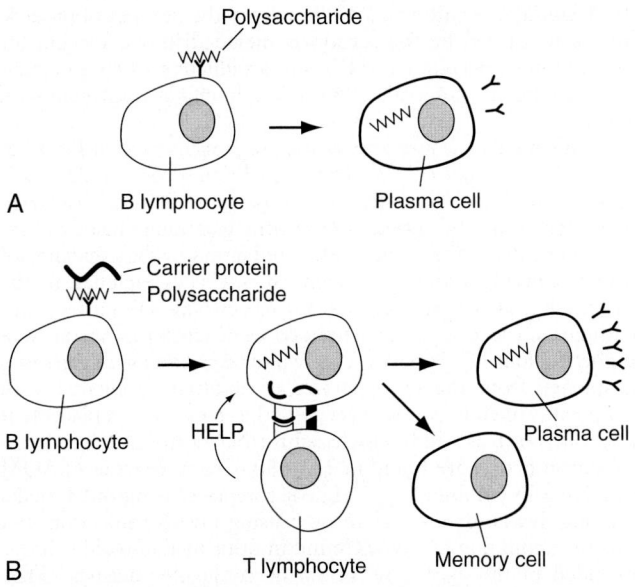

A
Polysaccharide
B lymphocyte
Plasma cell

B
Carrier protein
Polysaccharide
B lymphocyte
HELP
T lymphocyte
Plasma cell
Memory cell

Figure 96–14 T-cell–independent (**A**) and T-cell–dependent (**B**) antibody responses to polysaccharide or polysaccharide–protein conjugate antigens. (*From Eskola, J., and Anttila, M.: Pneumococcal conjugate vaccines. Pediatr. Infect. Dis. J. 18:543-551, 1999.*)

of that technology, the development of new technologies, and the addition of new protein carriers. Studies were initiated first on monovalent pneumococcal conjugate vaccines. Currently, this technology has brought about vaccines with 7 to 13 different conjugated pneumococcal polysaccharide antigens. Table 96–4 shows the pneumococcal conjugate vaccines that are licensed in at least one country, are being tested in phase III efficacy studies, or are in advanced phase II (safety and immunology) stages. The rationale for choosing among the 7-, 9-, 11-, or 13-valent conjugate vaccines is presented in the section on epidemiology in this chapter.

The main target populations for the development of conjugate pneumococcal vaccines were infants and young children. Conjugate pneumococcal vaccines have been studied in these target populations since the early 1990s. Pneumococcal conjugate vaccines have been found to be safe and well-tolerated. The reactions reported usually were local ones, such as pain, redness, and swelling at the injection site. The incidence of fever and irritability was somewhat higher than reported in studies with the Hib conjugate vaccines or hepatitis B vaccines, perhaps because these vaccines represent 7 to 11 separate monovalent vaccines administered together as opposed to the monovalent Hib conjugate vaccine or hepatitis B vaccine. The 7-valent pneumococcal vaccine conjugated to CRM$_{197}$ protein (PnCRM7) was found to be safe even when administered to low-birth-weight and preterm infants.[677]

The conjugate vaccines tested were able to elicit a T-cell–dependent immune response in normal infants and toddlers, namely, priming with immunologic memory and maturation of the functional antibody response, as measured by the predominance of IgG1 subclass antibodies, opsonophagocytic activity assays, and antibody avidity assays.[205,217] The immunogenicity of one vaccine (PnCRM7) also was studied in various high-risk groups. It was immunogenic in children with sickle-cell disease,[544,552,754] HIV infection,[407,408,419,534] solid organ transplants,[471] or allogeneic bone marrow transplants,[513] as well as in Alaska Natives and American Indians.[510] A 9-valent CRM (PnCRM9) pneumococcal vaccine also was immunogenic in children with sickle-cell disease.[276]

Determining the efficacy of pneumococcal vaccines is complex. Pneumococci cause a range of clinical diseases, and, therefore, several end-points of efficacy trials should be considered. The end-points thought to be of most importance in evaluating pneumococcal vaccines have been (1) prevention of invasive pneumococcal disease as defined by isolation of pneumococci from a normally sterile site (e.g., bacteremia or septicemia, meningitis, osteomyelitis/septic arthritis, and soft tissue infections); (2) prevention of mucosal infections such as otitis media, sinusitis, and nonbacteremic pneumonia; and (3) reduction of nasopharyngeal colonization, which in turn results in a reduction in spread of the organisms (the biologic basis for indirect effects, also known as *herd immunity*).

TABLE 96–4 Pneumococcal Conjugate Vaccines That Are Licensed in at Least One Country, Are Being Tested in Phase III Trials, or Are in Advanced Stages of Phase II Development

Vaccine	Valency	Pneumococcal Polysaccharides	Carrier Protein	Manufacturer
PnOMPC7	7-valent	4, 6B, 9V, 14, 18C, 19F, 23F	Meningococcal outer-membrane protein complex	Merck Research Laboratories
PnCRM7	7-valent	4, 6B, 9V, 14, 18C, 19F, 23F	CRM$_{197}$ protein	Wyeth Pharmaceuticals
PnCRM9	9-valent	1, 4, 5, 6B, 9V, 14, 18C, 19F, 23F	CRM$_{197}$ protein	Wyeth Pharmaceuticals
PncT/D	11-valent	1, 3, 4, 5, 6B, 7F, 9V, 14, 18C, 19F, 23F	A mixture of tetanus and diphtheria toxoids	Aventis Pasteur
Pn-PD	11-valent	1, 3, 4, 5, 6B, 7F, 9V, 14, 18C, 19F, 23F	*Haemophilus influenzae*—protein D	GlaxoSmithKline
PnCRM13	13-valent	1, 3, 4, 5, 6A, 6B, 7F, 9V, 14, 18C, 19A, 19F, 23F	CRM$_{197}$ protein	Wyeth Pharmaceuticals

By mid-2001, the 7-valent pneumococcal CRM vaccine had been licensed in the United States and in more than 30 other countries. The vaccine's trade name is Prevnar in the United States and Prevenar in other countries. In the United States, the Committee on Infectious Diseases of the American Academy of Pediatrics has made the following recommendations with regard to pneumococcal conjugate vaccines. PCV-7 is recommended for routine administration as a four-dose series for infants at ages 2, 4, 6, and 12 to 15 months; catch-up immunization is recommended for all children up to 23 months of age. The PCV-7 vaccine may given along with other age-appropriate childhood immunizations in a separate syringe and at a separate injection site. Infants of very low birth weight may be immunized when they reach a chronologic age of 6 to 8 weeks, regardless of their calculated gestational age. The PCV-7 vaccine also is recommended for all children younger than 60 months who are at high risk of acquiring invasive pneumococcal infection (patients with sickle-cell disease, asplenia, HIV/acquired immunodeficiency syndrome, diabetes, cancer, liver disorders, lung diseases, and cardiac diseases). For some high-risk children, supplemental protection should be given by administration of the PPV23 vaccine. The only contraindication to receiving the vaccine is a serious allergic reaction to a previous dose of this vaccine or one of its components. Children with minor illnesses such as colds may be vaccinated.[16]

In the United States, the practice of giving three primary doses and a booster dose is known as a "3 + 1 schedule." Some countries routinely immunize with fewer doses. Some countries give two primary doses and a booster, a "2 + 1 schedule," whereas others give three primary doses without a booster, a "3 + 0 schedule." Some serotypes, namely serotypes 6B and 23F,[395] produce less antibody when a two–primary dose series is used as opposed to a three–primary dose series.[475] One study found that three infant doses with a booster were more protective against vaccine-type disease than were two doses alone ($p = 0.0323$).[781] The booster dose may play a role in reducing nasopharyngeal carriage; therefore, absence of a booster dose may decrease indirect protection.[475]

Widespread use of the vaccine in the United States began in the first half of the year 2000. Such widespread use has provided additional data on the safety of PnCRM7. Common side effects of the vaccine include redness, tenderness, or swelling at the site of injection, fever, fussiness, drowsiness, rashes, and urticaria.[785] Furthermore, the incidence of invasive pneumococcal disease has decreased sharply in infants and toddlers and even in their household contacts.[70,676,780]

Three efficacy studies with the end-point of a reduction in the number of invasive infections were completed by mid-2002, two with PnCRM7 and one with the PnCRM9 vaccine. The first study was a prospective double-blind study of 37,868 healthy infants in northern California to whom either the PnCRM7 vaccine or a control vaccine was administered at 2, 4, 6, and 12 to 15 months of age.[69] The vaccine was 97.4 percent efficacious (95% confidence interval, 82.7-99.9%) against invasive disease caused by the serotype included in the vaccine in fully vaccinated infants and 93.9 percent efficacious (95% confidence interval, 79.6-98.5%) in partially vaccinated infants. No evidence of an increase in invasive disease caused by serotypes that were not included in the vaccine was detected, and thus the overall effect was a reduction in total invasive pneumococcal disease by 89.1 percent (95% confidence interval, 73.7-95.8%). This trial was the pivotal efficacy one that led to U.S. licensure of the vaccine by the Food and Drug Administration in February 2000 and subsequent licensure in many other countries. Additional analysis[677] has shown that the vaccine was as effective in the subset of low-birth-weight and premature infants as it was in the full study cohort.

A second large-scale efficacy study with the PnCRM7 vaccine was conducted among American Indian (Navajo and White Mountain Apache) children in the United States. This population has rates of invasive pneumococcal infection that are approximately five times those of the general U.S. population.[142,549] In a double-blind, community-randomized study, infants and young children aged 2 months to 2 years received the PnCRM7 vaccine or a control vaccine.[551] A total of 8292 infants from 43 communities were enrolled; of these, 8091 lived in 38 communities that were randomized to the pneumococcal or the control vaccine. During the study period, two cases of invasive pneumococcal infection caused by the serotypes included in the vaccine occurred in the vaccine group versus eight in the control group. After controlling for community randomization, the primary efficacy of the vaccine was 76.8 percent (95% confidence interval, 9.4-95.1%), and the intent-to-treat efficacy was 86.4 percent (95% confidence interval, 11-96.1%). These results are not statistically different from those of the trial in northern California.

A third efficacy study was conducted with the PnCRM9 vaccine among black infants in South Africa. In a double-blind, randomized, placebo-controlled study, PnCRM9 was administered to children at the ages of 6, 10, and 14 weeks according to the World Health Organization's Expanded Programme on Immunization. The infants were monitored until they reached 2 years of age, and the study was completed by the end of 2001. The intent-to-treat analysis showed a reduction of 82.5 percent (95% confidence interval, 39.0-96.7%) in the number of invasive infections caused by the serotypes included in the vaccine for children not infected with HIV and a reduction of 65.4 percent (95% confidence interval, 23.8-85.7%) in children infected with HIV.[424]

Otitis media is caused by various organisms in addition to *S. pneumoniae* (mainly *H. influenzae* [usually untypeable], *M. catarrhalis*, and, less frequently, *S. pyogenes* and enteric bacteria). Therefore, a positive evaluation of conjugate pneumococcal vaccines must demonstrate not only a reduction in the incidence of disease caused by the pneumococcal serotypes included in the vaccine but also a parallel increase in episodes caused by other pathogens, especially the pneumococci of serotypes not present in the vaccine. The latter were shown to be isolated with increased frequency from the nasopharynx of children vaccinated with conjugate pneumococcal vaccine (the so-called replacement phenomenon), as will be discussed further in the section.

Pneumococci are found in 25 to 50 percent of cases of AOM occurring in children.[77,378,484] The serotypes causing otitis media are not always identical to those causing invasive infection, but the most common serotypes found in otitis media worldwide are included in the 7-, 9-, or 11-valent conjugate vaccines. They include serotypes 3, 6B, 9V, 14, 19F, and 23F.[74,114,157,394] Serotypes 6A and 19A also are important causes of otitis media.[157,206] These two serotypes are not included in the vaccine, but cross-protection of serotype 6A by antibodies to serotype 6B has been demonstrated.[2,25,159,206,266,548,568] The pneumococcal serotypes included in the various vaccine formulations would account for 50 to 85 percent of all serotypes causing otitis media. Assuming 100 percent efficacy of pneumococcal conjugate vaccines against the serotypes included in the vaccines and no increase in otitis media caused by other pneumococcal serotypes or other pathogens, conjugate pneumococcal vaccines could reduce the incidence of all causes of otitis media by at most 10 to 25 percent. The results of analysis of four efficacy/effectiveness studies confirmed these expectations.

The northern California study, conducted primarily to determine efficacy of the PnCRM7 conjugate vaccine against invasive pneumococcal infection,[69] also looked at the reduction in the number of clinic visits for otitis media in 18,927 pneumococcal vaccine recipients and 18,941 control meningococcal vaccine recipients at the ages of 2, 4, 6, and 12 to 15 months. During the 30-month follow-up period, a total of 73,041 visits related to otitis media and 52,789 distinct episodes of otitis media had occurred in the study population. Of those, 5451 subjects had frequent episodes of otitis media (three episodes in 6 months or four episodes in 1 year). The pneumococcal vaccine reduced the number of clinically diagnosed otitis media episodes by 7 percent (95% confidence interval, 4.1-7.9%). The effectiveness of the PnCRM7 vaccine against frequent otitis media was 9.3 percent (95% confidence interval, 3.0-15.1%) when three episodes in 6 months or four in 12 months were counted, and it was 22.8 percent (95% confidence interval, 6.7-36.2%) when a frequency of five episodes in 6 months or six in 12 months was considered. Children who received the pneumococcal conjugate vaccine were 20.1 percent (95% confidence interval, 1.5-35.2%) less likely to require placement of a pressure-equalizing tube than controls were. This study was not designed to evaluate the effect of conjugate pneumococcal vaccine on otitis media as a primary outcome, and, therefore, no attempts were made to standardize or validate the clinical diagnoses of otitis media. Hence, the study was able to assess only the effect of PnCRM7 vaccine on otitis media as it is diagnosed and managed in the routine clinical setting. As a result, the authors were not able to examine the efficacy of the vaccine against otitis media caused by pneumococcal serotypes included in the vaccine, except for cultures performed on fluid obtained from spontaneously draining ears. In 23 children, culture of fluid from spontaneously draining ears was positive for pneumococci of the vaccine serotypes, with a 66 percent calculated efficacy against disease caused by serotypes included in the vaccine. However, its efficacy against clinically diagnosed otitis media indicated that the vaccine reduced morbidity attributed to otitis media and medical services used for the management of clinical otitis.

A second study, conducted in Finland, looked at the efficacy of PnCRM7 vaccine against AOM in general and more specifically against otitis media caused by serotypes in the conjugate pneumococcal vaccine under study.[206] A total of 1662 infants were enrolled and randomized in a double-blind manner to receive either the PnCRM7 vaccine or a hepatitis B vaccine at the ages of 2, 4, 6, and 12 months. The clinical diagnosis of AOM was based on predefined criteria, and bacteriologic diagnosis was based on culture of middle ear fluid obtained by myringotomy. The children were monitored through 24 months of age. A total of 2596 episodes of AOM occurred in children who had received three doses of vaccine by the time that they reached 6 months of age. The efficacy of the vaccine in reducing cases caused by the serotypes included in the vaccine was 57 percent (95% confidence interval, 46-67%). The PnCRM7 vaccine also provided cross-protection against serotypes 6A and 19A. The efficacy of the vaccine in reducing all culture-confirmed pneumococcal infections (including serotypes not included in the vaccine) was 34 percent (95% confidence interval, 24% to 45%). However, the vaccine was not effective against nonvaccine pneumococcal serotypes that are not cross-reactive with the ones included in the vaccine. The vaccine also was ineffective against otitis media caused by *H. influenzae* and *M. catarrhalis*, and a trend toward an increase in the incidence of otitis media among vaccinated children (replacement disease phenomenon) was noted. Thus, the overall high protection provided against the serotypes included in the vaccine was offset partially by an increase in the number of episodes of otitis media caused by other serotypes of pneumococci and other pathogens. The overall reduction in the number of episodes of AOM of any cause in the pneumococcal vaccine group was 6 percent (95% confidence interval, -4-16%). This difference did not reach statistical significance, but it was within the expected range when all theoretical considerations listed earlier were taken into account, and it also was strikingly similar

to the 7 percent reduction in the number of cases of otitis media observed in the California study.[69] In addition, similar to the California study, by the time that they reached the age of 4 to 5 years, the vaccinated subjects had undergone tympanostomy tube placement at a rate that was reduced by 39 percent (95% confidence interval, 4% to 61%) in comparison to controls.[564]

A third study was conducted by the same Finnish group in parallel with the study just described, but this time with a different 7-valent vaccine (serotypes 4, 6B, 9V, 14, 18C, 19F, and 23F conjugated to the meningococcal outer-membrane protein complex [OMPC]—PnOMPC7).[403,404] In this randomized, double-blind, controlled trial, 1666 children were randomized to receive either PnOMPC7 or hepatitis B vaccine at 2, 4, and 6 months of age. At 12 months of age, approximately 22 percent of the PnOMPC7 conjugate vaccine recipients received a nonconjugate 23-valent polysaccharide vaccine as a booster, and the others received a fourth dose of PnOMPC7. Follow-up continued through 24 months of age. The methodology was similar to that described earlier for the PnCRM7 conjugate vaccine, including cultures for the diagnosis of otitis media episodes. A total of 2709 otitis media episodes occurred in evaluable children who had completed their three-dose schedule, 360 of which were caused by pneumococci of the serotypes included in the vaccine. The efficacy of the vaccine in reducing the number of cases of otitis media caused by the serotypes included in the vaccine was 56 percent (95% confidence interval, 44-66%). In reducing the number of all pneumococcal otitis media episodes, the efficacy was 25 percent (95% confidence interval, 11-37%). However, no overall reduction in the number of episodes of otitis media was seen because of an increase in the number of episodes caused by nonvaccine serotype pneumococci and other nonpneumococcal organisms (replacement disease).

The results of the two studies in Finland and the study in northern California are strikingly consistent. They all have shown that (1) the efficacy of the two conjugate vaccines tested thus far in the prevention of otitis media caused by pneumococcal serotypes included in the vaccine was greater than 50 percent and that efficacy on the order of magnitude observed for invasive infections (i.e., 90%) cannot be achieved against otitis media, (2) replacement otitis media with pneumococci not included in the vaccine and other organisms such as *H. influenzae* and *M. catarrhalis* occurs and reduces the overall efficacy of the pneumococcal conjugate vaccines against otitis media, and (3) better protection is provided against episodes of more severe otitis media and recurrent otitis media than against simple otitis media. The more severe and recurrent otitis media episodes often are associated with pneumococcal serotypes 6B, 9V, 14, 19F, and 23F, which tend to persist both in the nasopharynx and in the middle ear. These serotypes also tend to be more resistant to antibiotics.[157,380]

A fourth study was conducted in toddlers attending daycare centers in southern Israel. In this double-blind study, the efficacy of a 9-valent CRM conjugate pneumococcal vaccine (PnCRM9) in reducing nasopharyngeal carriage of *S. pneumoniae* and respiratory infections was compared with that of a control vaccine. This study showed, in conjunction with an extensive reduction in carriage of the serotypes included in the vaccine, especially serotypes 6B, 9V, 14, 19F, and 23F,[155,159,174] a 17 percent (95% confidence interval, -0.2-33%) reduction in the number of cases of otitis media and a 20 percent (95% confidence interval, 14-36%) reduction in antibiotic use for otitis media.[174] These findings support the notion that conjugate pneumococcal vaccines can reduce the morbidity of otitis media, not only by reducing the number of episodes or reducing the severity of otitis media in general but also by selectively reducing otitis media in high-risk groups such as attendees at daycare centers.

TABLE 96–5   Studies* on the Effect of Conjugate Pneumococcal Vaccine on Carriage of *Streptococcus pneumoniae* and Antibiotic-Resistant *S. pneumoniae*

Author	Conjugate Vaccine (Valence)	Site	Age (mo) at Vaccination	Reduction in Serotypes Included in the Vaccine	Reduction in Resistant Pneumococci	Increase in Nonvaccine Serotypes
Dagan[170]	PnOMPC7	Israel	12-18	Yes	Yes	No
Dagan[172]	PnT, PnD (4-valent)	Israel	2, 4, 6	Yes	Yes	+/−
Obaro[546]	PnCRM5	The Gambia	2, 3, 4	Yes	ND	Yes
Kristinsson[436]	PnT, PnD (8-valent)	Iceland	3, 4, 6	Yes	ND	Yes
Mbelle[500]	PnCRM9	South Africa	1.5, 2.5, 3.5	Yes	Yes	Yes
Edwards[201]	PnCRM9	USA	2, 4, 6, 12	Yes	ND	Yes
Dagan[175]	PnT/D (11-valent)	Israel	2, 4, 6, 12	Yes	Yes	No
Dagan[155,159]	PnCRM9	Israel	12-35	Yes	Yes	Yes
O'Brien[548]	PnCRM7	USA (Native American)	2, 4, 6, 12-15	Yes	ND	Yes
Kilpi[404]	PnCRM7	Finland	2, 4, 6, 12	Yes	ND	ND

PnOMPC, 7-valent pneumococcal vaccine conjugated to the outer-membrane complex of Neisseria meningitidis B; PnT, pneumococcal vaccine conjugated to tetanus toxoid; PnD, pneumococcal vaccine conjugated to diphtheria toxoid; PnT/D, pneumococcal vaccine conjugated to a mixture of tetanus and diphtheria toxoid; PnCRM, pneumococcal vaccine conjugated to CRM$_{197}$ protein (PnCRM5, 5-valent; PnCRM7, 7-valent; PnCRM9, 9-valent).

Since the use of PCV-7 has become common practice, several studies have shown that the PCV-7 vaccine is not extremely efficacious in decreasing the total number of children who have AOM because of an increase in cases caused by nonvaccine serotypes or other organisms.[707,708] The vaccine should be promoted because of its primary indication of preventing invasive pneumococcal disease and not decreasing the incidence of AOM.[375] However, some papers have reported a decline in the number of visits to primary care physicians for AOM[292] by up to 19 percent.[475] Another study found that the incidence of tympanostomy tube placement decreased by 24 percent after introduction of the vaccine.[228]

Protection against pneumococcal pneumonia by the conjugate pneumococcal vaccines was shown in the PnCRM7 vaccine efficacy trial conducted in northern California.[69,71] However, pneumococcal pneumonia cases are associated only infrequently with bacteremia, and the PnCRM7 vaccine should provide protection against these invasive episodes to the same degree as they do against all other invasive episodes. Because most cases of pneumonia are nonbacteremic, the great majority remain without a clear bacteriologic diagnosis. In these cases, the role of *S. pneumoniae* can be demonstrated indirectly if the use of a vaccine significantly reduces the occurrence of pneumonia cases. Thus, the conjugate pneumococcal vaccines can be used as surrogates to estimate more accurately the proportion of pneumonia cases attributable to vaccine serotype pneumococci.

In the northern California study conducted on 37,868 infants given the PnCRM7 vaccine, all clinically diagnosed episodes of pneumonia identified through hospital, outpatient, and emergency records were collected.[71] In total, 3711 clinical episodes of pneumonia that occurred before the children reached the age of 3.5 years were identified; the efficacy of the PnCRM7 vaccine in reducing the incidence of disease (intent-to-treat analysis) was 6.0 percent (95% confidence interval, 1.5-11.0%). Of the 3711 clinical episodes, a chest radiograph was obtained in 2249 episodes, and among these children, vaccine efficacy was 8.9 percent (95% confidence interval, 0.9-16.3%). Of the 2249 children in whom a chest radiograph was obtained, 737 had a positive chest radiograph (defined as parenchymal infiltrates, consolidation or effusion [or both], but not perihilar infiltrates alone). In these 737 patients, efficacy was 22.7 percent (95% confidence interval, 8.7-34.5%). These findings have some limitations because they were not derived from a study in which the primary objective was to evaluate protection against pneumonia. However, the findings suggest two important points: (1) many cases of clinically and radiologically proven pneumonia in children are caused by *S. pneumoniae* by virtue of the fact that vaccination was associated

with a marked reduction in not only the "classic" lobar pneumonia usually associated with *S. pneumoniae* but also clinical pneumonia, with negative or minimal findings on the chest radiograph, and (2) the 22.7 percent efficacy observed for pneumonia with radiologically documented findings suggests that at least in the developed world where Hib vaccines are used widely, *S. pneumoniae* causes a high proportion of pneumonia with parenchymal infiltrates.

A recent study from South Africa showed that administration of three doses of PnCRM9 at the ages of 6, 10, and 14 weeks reduced the incidence of radiologically proven pneumonia by 22.1 percent (95% confidence interval, 0.1-39.5%) in children who were not infected with HIV.[424]

Additional supportive evidence that *S. pneumoniae* may play a more important role in respiratory infections than usually attributed to this pathogen can be derived from a study in southern Israel involving toddlers aged 12 to 35 months who attended daycare centers.[174] In this study, 263 children were randomized to receive either PnCRM9 vaccine or a control vaccine (meningococcus CRM conjugate) in a double-blind fashion. The children were monitored for 5556 child-months. A total of 906 episodes of non–otitis media upper respiratory tract infection were reported, for an efficacy estimate of 15 percent (95% confidence interval, 4-24%); 596 episodes of lower respiratory tract problems occurred, including bronchiolitis, cough, and pneumonia, and the efficacy of pneumococcal vaccine was 16 percent (95% confidence interval, 2-28%). For these two clinical illness categories, children received a total of 3678 days of antibiotics. A reduction of 10 percent in the number of days that antibiotics were given for upper respiratory tract infections was achieved, as was a reduction of 47 percent for lower respiratory tract problems in the pneumococcal vaccine group ($p < 0.001$ versus control children). The incidence of bronchiolitis and pneumonia, often regarded as viral in this age group, was decreased significantly by the administration of this conjugate pneumococcal vaccine, thus suggesting that *S. pneumoniae* plays a role as a pathogen or co-pathogen for these entities.

As stated earlier, control of nasopharyngeal carriage of pneumococci is the key to managing pneumococcal disease and person-to-person spread of *S. pneumoniae*. The nonconjugate pneumococcal vaccines do not have a significant effect on carriage of *S. pneumoniae* in children and adults.[170,485] In contrast, the conjugate vaccines do have a significant effect on carriage.* Table 96–5 shows the studies conducted and published thus far to

---

*See references 155, 159, 170, 172, 175, 201, 436, 500, 546, 548.

document the effect of pneumococcal vaccines on carriage of *S. pneumoniae*. Despite variations in the nature of the conjugate vaccines, populations, and the ages at which the vaccines were administered, a significant reduction in carriage of the serotypes included in the vaccine clearly was observed in all studies. However, in most of the studies, a "replacement" phenomenon occurred: an increase in the carriage of *S. pneumoniae* serotypes not included in the vaccine was observed in conjunction with a decrease in the carriage of serotypes included in the vaccine. Although this replacement phenomenon is remarkable, its clinical significance is not clear. In theory, such a phenomenon could be simply an artifact of "unmasking," in which nonvaccine serotypes are detected more readily in vaccinees than in controls because the vaccine serotypes are not present. However, the use of mathematic modeling and testing in controlled vaccine studies strongly suggests that a true "replacement phenomenon" does exist in which non–vaccine-type pneumococci truly are replacing vaccine-type pneumococci.[472] This suggestion is supported by the observation of an increase in the incidence of otitis media caused by organisms not included in the vaccine after vaccination with PnCRM7 and PnOMPC7 in Finland.[206,403]

The reduction in nasopharyngeal carriage of vaccine serotypes of pneumococci is important because it certainly will reduce the spread of these serotypes. Two studies in different settings clearly have shown the existence of this phenomenon. In one double-blind comparative study conducted in southern Israel, toddlers attending daycare centers were vaccinated with a PnCRM9 vaccine or a control vaccine.[156] In this study, attendees at daycare centers and their younger siblings who stayed home were monitored after the daycare attendees were vaccinated. A marked reduction in the incidence of vaccine-type pneumococcal carriage was seen in the young siblings of those who were vaccinated with the PnCRM9 vaccine when compared with siblings of the controls.[156]

In a second study, Navajo and White Mountain Apache children younger than 2 years old were randomized according to their community of residence to receive either PnCRM7 or meningococcus C conjugate vaccine. Nasopharyngeal swabs were cultured for *S. pneumoniae* from 598 nonimmunized infants residing in both vaccinated (by PnCRM7 vaccine) and control communities.[547] A 24 percent reduction in carriage of vaccine-associated serotypes was noted in vaccinated infants residing in the PnCRM7 communities versus those living in control vaccine communities. The reduction was found both in infants who lived with a PnCRM7-vaccinated sibling and in those who did not have direct contact with a PnCRM7-vaccinated child. This study demonstrated the indirect protective effect of pneumococcal vaccination on those in the household.

Because most antibiotic-resistant *S. pneumoniae* strains belong to only a few serotypes that are included in the conjugate pneumococcal vaccines or are related to these serotypes (see the section on epidemiology and microbiology), vaccines are expected to reduce disease, carriage, and spread of antibiotic-resistant *S. pneumoniae* and may have an impact on the use of antibiotics. Indeed, in all vaccine studies that investigated the effect of conjugate vaccines on nasopharyngeal carriage of antibiotic-resistant *S. pneumoniae*, a reduction in carriage of such strains was observed[155,170,172,175,500] (Table 96–5). Furthermore, the use of conjugate vaccines reduced the use of antibiotics in two prospective double-blind studies. In a study conducted in northern California, administration of the PnCRM7 vaccine reduced the use of antibiotics by 5.3 percent in patients given vaccines versus controls; the reduction was 5.0 percent for drugs generally used as first-line agents (such as amoxicillin and ampicillin) and 11.2 percent for those often used as second-line agents (cephalosporins, amoxicillin-clavulanate, and azithromycin) (Black, S., Shinefeld, H.: Presented at the 19th Annual Meeting of the European Society for Pediatric Infectious Diseases, April 26 to 28, 2001,

Istanbul, Turkey). In another study performed in toddlers attending daycare centers in southern Israel, the PnCRM9 conjugate vaccine reduced the use of antibiotics in vaccine recipients versus controls by 20 percent,[174] in parallel with the reduction in carriage of antibiotic-resistant *S. pneumoniae* and respiratory diseases. The reduction in both these factors may contribute to reducing antibiotic resistance in the community. However, the overall effect remains to be determined.

Although invasive infections are the most dramatic part of the pneumococcal disease spectrum, respiratory infections such as otitis media occur far more frequently.[466] In a study investigating current estimates of pneumococcal disease burden, clinical outcome, and vaccine efficacy, researchers estimated that for each annual U.S. birth cohort, routine use of a 7-valent vaccine could prevent 12,000 cases of pneumococcal bacteremia and meningitis, 53,000 cases of pneumococcal pneumonia, and more than 1 million clinical cases of otitis media per year.[466]

Pneumonia has a greater impact globally than do otitis media or even invasive infections because of the high mortality rate in children in the developing world.[63,296,461] However, it is more difficult to study because it does not occur as commonly as does otitis media, and bacteriologic documentation rarely is available for this entity in children.

Thus, the protection conferred by the conjugate pneumococcal vaccines with regard to reduction in the number of episodes of otitis media, pneumonia, and other mucosal infections, if proven by additional studies, could have an even greater impact on the burden of disease than on prevention of invasive infections.

Potential Future Vaccines and Future Strategies

Studies have been conducted to determine whether immunization of pregnant women with pneumococcal conjugate or nonconjugate vaccines can protect their offspring from acquiring pneumococcal diseases during their first few months of life, before they achieve immunity through active vaccination. This suggestion is based on studies that have shown that naturally acquired IgG antibodies are transferred transplacentally to the fetus readily,[21,129,143] and clinical studies of maternal immunization with pneumococcal polysaccharide vaccines have resulted in similar observations.[450,553,672] In experimental studies, a correlation has been demonstrated between higher concentrations of vaccine-specific antibodies at birth and greater response to specific serotypes after subsequent active immunization in the offspring of vaccine recipients.[445,470] In one study, administration of a conjugate pneumococcal vaccine to pregnant women[523] resulted not only in efficient transplacental passage of vaccine-induced pneumococcal antibodies (mainly of the IgG1 subtype) but also in prevention of pneumococcal carriage in the offspring of vaccinated mothers. A recent Cochrane review found no evidence that pneumococcal vaccination administered during pregnancy reduces the risk for neonatal infection. Although the data did suggest an effect in reducing pneumococcal colonization in infants by the time they reached 16 months of age, no evidence was found of this effect in infants at 2 months of age or by 7 months of age.[121] A recent study in New Guinea found that breast milk IgA was 1.1 to 1.8 times higher in women immunized with pneumococcal polysaccharide vaccine than in unimmunized women for 6 months post partum.[451] Thus, maternal immunization during pregnancy may prove to be a successful strategy to protect against pneumococcal infection in early infancy, but additional serotypes need to be included in these vaccines.

Adding more polysaccharide capsular antigens to the conjugate pneumococcal vaccines to increase serotype coverage is being investigated. In addition, much effort is being invested in combining the present conjugate pneumococcal vaccine with other childhood vaccines to be given in the same syringe in order to reduce the number of injections needed to immunize infants.

Despite the great potential benefit of the pneumococcal conjugate vaccines, they have two important limitations: (1) inclusion of a limited number of serotypes, which results not only in noncoverage of some other important serotypes causing disease but also in potential replacement disease by serotypes not related to the vaccine, and (2) their high price as a result of complex production and quality control processes.

Many of the proteins mentioned in the section on pathogenesis appear to be suitable antigens for candidate vaccines, and such vaccines that include proteins immunogenic in infants are being developed. The main drawback of protein vaccines is the antigenic variability of many pneumococcal proteins. However, some of the most important proteins considered essential for bacterial virulence have epitopes that are common to many pneumococcal strains. Among these proteins are pneumolysin, PspA, and PsaA.[96] Plasma concentrations of antibodies to these proteins increase with age and are associated strongly with pneumococcal exposure, whether by carriage or infection such as AOM.[605] One suggestion is that antibodies to PsaA may prevent pneumococcal otitis media,[607] but such prevention has not been confirmed. Preliminary studies show that PspA and PsaA given as single antigens or as a mixture of antigens are immunogenic and protective in mice and safe and immunogenic in humans.[533] Further studies in humans were expected to begin in 2002. Other candidate protein vaccines are being investigated in animals, but as of mid-2002, they had not yet been administered to humans. An additional novel approach to providing immunization against *S. pneumoniae* infection is to immunize subjects with killed whole-cell *S. pneumoniae* intranasally with an adjuvant. This approach was studied in animal models and showed promising results.[491]

During the next decade, other pneumococcal vaccine prototypes probably will be discovered and developed. Whether they will equal or surpass the beneficial effects of the pneumococcal conjugate vaccines remains to be seen.

REFERENCES

1. Aaberge, I. S., Eng, J., Lermark, G., et al.: Virulence of *Streptococcus pneumoniae* in mice: A standardized method for preparation and frozen storage of the experimental bacterial inoculum. Microb. Pathol. *18*:141-152, 1995.
2. Aaberge, I. S., Lovik, M., Hoogerhout, P., et al.: Pneumococcal type 6B conjugates differ in dependency on adjuvant and booster dose, and induce protection against type 6A as well as type 6. Poster 25. Presented at Pneumococcal Vaccines for the World 1998 Conference, Washington, D.C., 1998, p. 66.
3. Aaberge, I. S., Michaelsen, T. E., and Heier, H. E.: IgG subclass antibody responses to pneumococcal polysaccharide vaccine in splenectomized, otherwise normal, individuals. Scand. J. Immunol. *31*:711-716, 1990.
4. Abbasi, S., Orlicek, S. L., Almohsen, I., et al.: Septic arthritis and osteomyelitis caused by penicillin and cephalosporin-resistant *Streptococcus pneumoniae* in a children's hospital. Pediatr. Infect. Dis. J. *15*:78-83, 1996.
5. Abdel-Haq, N., Abuhammour, W., Asmar, B., et al.: Nasopharyngeal colonization with *Streptococcus pneumoniae* in children receiving trimethoprim-sulfamethoxazole prophylaxis. Pediatr. Infect. Dis. J. *18*:647-649, 1999.
6. Acute respiratory infections in under-fives: 5 million deaths a year. Lancet *2*:699-701, 1985.
7. Adamou, J. E., Heinrichs, J. H., Erwin, A. L., et al.: Identification and characterization of a novel family of pneumococcal proteins that are protective against sepsis. Infect. Immun. *69*:949-958, 2001.
8. Adegbola, R. A., Falade, A. G., Sam, B. E., et al.: The etiology of pneumonia in malnourished and well-nourished Gambian children. Pediatr. Infect. Dis. J. *13*:975-982, 1994.
9. Ahmed, A., Jafri, H., and Lutsar, I.: Pharmacodynamics of vancomycin for the treatment of experimental penicillin- and cephalosporin-resistant pneumococcal meningitis. Antimicrob. Agents Chemother. *43*:876-881, 1999.
10. Alario, A. J., Nelson, E. W., and Shapiro, E. D.: Blood cultures in the management of febrile outpatients late found to have bacteremia. J. Pediatr. *115*:195-199, 1989.
11. Alcantara, R. B., Preheim, L. C., and Gentry-Nielsen, M. J.: Pneumolysin-induced complement depletion during experimental pneumococcal bacteremia. Infect. Immun. *69*:3569-3575, 2001.
12. Alpern, E. R., Alessandrini, E. A., Bell, L. M., et al.: Occult bacteremia from a pediatric emergency department: Current prevalence, time to detection, and outcome. Pediatrics *106*:505-511, 2000.
13. American Academy of Pediatrics: *In* Pickering, L. K. (ed.): 2000 Red Book: Report of the Committee on Infectious Diseases. 25th ed. Elk Grove Village, IL, American Academy of Pediatrics, 2000, pp. 66-67.
14. American Academy of Pediatrics: *In* Pickering, L. K. (ed.): 2000 Red Book: Report of the Committee on Infectious Diseases. 25th ed. Elk Grove Village, IL, American Academy of Pediatrics, 2000, pp. 452-460.
15. American Academy of Pediatrics: *In* Pickering, L. K. (ed.): 2000 Red Book: Report of the Committee on Infectious Diseases. 25th ed. Elk Grove Village, IL, American Academy of Pediatrics, 2000, pp. 729-742.
16. American Academy of Pediatrics: *In* Pickering, L. K. (ed.): 2006 Red Book: Report of the Committee on Infectious Diseases. 27th ed. Elk Grove Village, IL, American Academy of Pediatrics, 2006, pp. 532-535.
17. American Academy of Pediatrics, Committee on Infectious Diseases: Policy statement: Recommendations for the prevention of pneumococcal infections, including the use of pneumococcal conjugate vaccine (Prevnar), pneumococcal polysaccharide vaccine, and antibiotic prophylaxis. Pediatrics *106*:362-366, 2000.
18. Amsden, G. W.: Pneumococcal macrolide resistance—myth or reality? J. Antimicrob. Chemother. *44*:1-6, 1999.
19. Anderson, B., Porras, O., Hanson, L. A., et al.: Inhibition of attachment of *Streptococcus pneumoniae* and *Haemophilus influenzae* by human milk and receptor oligosaccharides. J. Infect. Dis. *153*:232-237, 1986.
20. Anderson, D. C., Schmalstieg, F. C., Finegold, M. J., et al.: The severe and moderate phenotypes of heritable Mac-1, LFA-1 deficiency: Their quantitative definition and relation to leukocyte dysfunction and clinical features. J. Infect. Dis. *152*:668-689, 1985.
21. Anderson, P., Porcelli, S., and Pichichero, M.: Natural maternal and cord serum antibodies to pneumococcal serotypes 6A, 14, 19F and 23F polysaccharides. Pediatr. Infect. Dis. J. *11*:677-679, 1992.
22. Andiman, W. A., Mezger, J., and Shapiro, E.: Invasive bacterial infections in children born to women infected with human immunodeficiency virus type 1. J. Pediatr. *124*:846-852, 1994.
23. Aniansson, G., Alm, B., Andersson, B., et al.: Nasopharyngeal colonization during the first year of life. J. Infect. Dis. *165*(Suppl.):38-42, 1992.
24. Aniansson, G., Alm, B., Andersson, B., et al.: A prospective cohort study on breast-feeding and otitis media in Swedish infants. Pediatr. Infect. Dis. J. *13*:183-188, 1994.
25. Anttila, M., Eklund, C., Eskola, J., and Kayhty, H.: Functional cross-reactivity of antibodies to pneumococcal capsular polysaccharides of serotypes 6A and 6B. Poster 16. Presented at Pneumococcal Vaccines for the World 1998 Conference, Washington, D.C., 1998, p. 66.
26. Anttila, M., Soininen, A., Nieminem, T., et al.: Contribution of serotype specific IgG concentration, subclass ratio, and relative avidity to opsonophagocytic activity against *Streptococcus pneumoniae*. Abstract 58. Presented at Pneumococcal Vaccines for the World 1998 Conference, Washington, D.C., 1998.
27. Anttila, M., Voutilainen, M., Jäntti, V., et al.: Contribution of serotype-specific IgG concentration, IgG subclasses, and relative antibody avidity of opsonophagocytic activity against *Streptococcus pneumoniae*. Clin. Exp. Immunol. *118*:402-407, 1999.
28. Appelbaum, P. C.: Epidemiology and in vitro susceptibility of drug-resistant *Streptococcus pneumoniae*. Pediatr. Infect. Dis. J. *15*:932-934, 1996.
29. Appelbaum, P. C., Bhamjee, A., Scragg, J. N., et al.: *Streptococcus pneumoniae* resistant to penicillin and chloramphenicol. Lancet *2*:995-997, 1977.
30. Arason, V. A., Kristinsson, K. G., Sigurdsson, J. A., et al.: Do antimicrobials increase the carriage rate of penicillin resistant pneumococci in children? Cross sectional prevalence study. B. M. J. *313*:387-391, 1996.
31. Arditi, M., Mason, E. O., Bradley, J. S., et al.: Three-year multicenter surveillance of pneumococcal meningitis in children: Clinical characteristics, and outcome related to penicillin susceptibility and dexamethasone use. Pediatrics *102*:1087-1097, 1998.
32. Arguedas, A., Emparanza, P., Schwartz, R. H., et al.: A randomized, multicenter, double blind, double dummy trial of single dose azithromycin versus high dose amoxicillin for treatment of uncomplicated acute otitis media. Pediatr. Infect. Dis. J. *24*:153-161, 2005.
33. Arnold, K. E., Leggiadro, R. J., Breiman, R. F., et al.: Risk factors for carriage of drug-resistant *Streptococcus pneumoniae* among children in Memphis, Tennessee. J. Pediatr. *128*:757-764, 1996.
34. Arpadi, S. M., Back, S., O'Brien, J., and Janoff, E. N.: Antibodies to pneumococcal capsular polysaccharides in children with human immuno-deficiency virus infection given polyvalent pneumococcal vaccine. J. Pediatr. *125*:77-79, 1994.
35. Arrecubieta, C., Lopez, R., and Garcia, E.: Molecular characterization of cap3a, a gene from the operon required for the synthesis of the capsule of *Streptococcus pneumoniae* type 3: Sequencing of mutations responsible for the unencapsulated phenotype and localization of the capsular cluster on the pneumococcal chromosome. J. Bacteriol. *176*:6375-6383, 1994.
36. Arva, E., and Andersson, B.: Induction of phagocyte-stimulating and Th1-promoting cytokines by in vitro stimulation of human peripheral blood mononuclear cells with *Streptococcus pneumoniae*. Scand. J. Immunol. *49*:417-423, 1999.
37. Attwood, J. T., Williams, Y., and Feighery, C.: Impaired IgG responses in a child with homozygous C2 deficiency and recurrent pneumococcal septicaemia. Acta Paediatr. *90*:99-101, 2001.

38. Auer, M., Pfister, L. A., Leppert, D., et al.: Effects of clinically used antioxidants in experimental pneumococcal meningitis. J. Infect. Dis. *182*:347-350, 2000.

39. Austrian, R.: Pneumonia in the later years. J. Am. Geriatr. Soc. *29*:481-489, 1981.

40. Austrian, R.: The enduring pneumococcus: Unfinished business and opportunities for the future. *In* Tomasz A. (ed.): *Streptococcus pneumoniae:* Molecular Biology and Mechanisms of Disease. Larchmont, NY, Mary Ann Liebert, Inc., 2000, pp. 3-7.

41. Austrian, R., and Collins, P.: Importance of carbon dioxide in the isolation of pneumococci. J. Bacteriol. *92*:1281-1284, 1966.

42. Austrian, R., and Gold, J.: Pneumococcal bacteremia with a special reference to bacteremic pneumococcal pneumonia. Ann. Intern. Med. *60*:759-776, 1964.

43. Austrian, R., Howie, V. M., and Ploussard, J. H.: The bacteriology of pneumococcal otitis media. Johns Hopkins Med. J. *14*:104-111, 1977.

44. Avery, O. T.: Chemoimmunological studies on conjugated carbohydrate proteins: II. Immunological specificity of synthetic sugar-protein antigens. J. Exp. Med. *50*:533-550, 1929.

45. Azoulay-Dupuis, E., Rieux, V., and Muffat-Joly, M.: Relationship between capsular type, penicillin susceptibility, and virulence of human *Streptococcus pneumoniae* isolates in mice. Antimicrob. Agents Chemother. *44*:1575-1577, 2000.

46. Baba, H., Kawamura, I., Kohda, C., et al.: Essential role of domain 4 of pneumolysin from *Streptococcus pneumoniae* in cytolytic activity as determined by truncated proteins. Biochem. Biophys. Res. Commun. *281*:37-44, 2001.

47. Bachur, R., and Harper, M. B.: Reevaluation of outpatients with *Streptococcus pneumoniae* bacteremia. Pediatrics *105*:502-509, 2000.

48. Baer, M., Vuento, R., and Vesikari, T.: Increase in bacteraemic pneumococcal infections in children. Lancet *345*:661, 1995.

49. Balachandran, P., Hollingshead, S. K., Paton, J. C., and Briles, D. E.: The autolytic enzyme LytA of *Streptococcus pneumoniae* is not responsible for releasing pneumolysin. J. Bacteriol. *183*:3108-3116, 2001.

50. Ball, P.: Therapy for pneumococcal infection at the millennium: Doubts and certainties. Am. J. Med. *107*(Suppl.):77-85, 1999.

51. Baltz, R. H., Norris, F. H., Matsushima, P., et al.: DNA sequence sampling of the *Streptococcus pneumoniae* genome to identify novel targets for antibiotic development. Microb. Drug Resist. *4*:1-9, 1998.

52. Baquero, F., and Loza, E.: Antibiotic resistance of microorganisms involved in ear, nose and throat infections. Pediatr. Infect. Dis. J. *13*(Suppl.):9-14, 1994.

53. Baraff, L. J., Bass, J. W., Fleisher, G. R., et al.: Practice guideline for the management of infants and children 0-36 months of age with fever without source. Pediatrics *92*:1-12, 1993.

54. Bardley, J. S., Kaplan, S. L., Tan, T. Q., et al.: Pediatric pneumococcal bone and joint infections. Pediatrics *102*:1376-1382, 1998.

55. Barry, B., Gehanno, P., Blumen, M., and Boucot, I.: Clinical outcome of acute otitis media caused by pneumococci with decreased susceptibility to penicillin. Scand. J. Infect. Dis. *26*:446-452, 1994.

56. Bartlett, J. G., and Mundy, L. M.: Community-acquired pneumonia. N. Engl. J. Med. *333*:1618, 1995.

57. Bass, J. W., Steele, R. W., Wittler, R. R., et al.: Antimicrobial treatment of occult bacteremia: A multicenter cooperative study. Pediatr. Infect. Dis. J. *12*:466-473, 1993.

58. Bauchner, H., Leventhal, J. M., and Shapiro, E. D.: Studies of breastfeeding and infections: How good is the evidence? J. A. M. A. *256*:887-892, 1996.

59. Becken, E. T., Daly, K. A., Lindgreen, B. R., et al.: Low cord blood pneumococcal antibody concentrations predict more episodes of otitis media. Arch. Otolaryngol. Head Neck Surg. *127*:517-522, 2001.

60. Bedos, J. P., Rolin, O., Bouanchaud, D. H., et al.: Relationship between virulence and resistance to antibiotics in pneumococci. Contribution of experimental data obtained in an animal model. Pathol. Biol. (Paris) *39*:984-990, 1991.

61. Bennett, N. M., Buffington, J., and LaForce, F. M.: Pneumococcal bacteremia in Monroe County, New York. Am. J. Public Health *82*:1513-1516, 1992.

62. Berman, S.: Otitis media in developing countries. Pediatrics *96*:126-131, 1995.

63. Berman, S., and Mcintosh, K.: Selective primary health care: Strategies for control of disease in developing world. Acute respiratory infections. Rev. Infect. Dis. 7:674-691, 1985.

64. Bernstein, L. J., Krieger, B. Z., Novick, B., et al.: Bacterial infection in the acquired immunodeficiency syndrome of children. Pediatr. Infect. Dis. J. *4*:472-475, 1985.

65. Biedel, C. S.: Modification of recurrent otitis media by short-term sulfonamide therapy. Am. J. Dis. Child. *132*:681-683, 1978.

66. Biernath, K. R., Reefhuis, J., Whitney, C. G., et al.: Bacterial meningitis among children with cochlear implants beyond 24 months after implantation. Pediatrics *117*:284-289, 2006.

67. Bjornson, A. B., Falletta, J. M., Verter, J. I., et al.: Serotype-specific immunoglobulin G antibody responses to pneumococcal polysaccharide vaccine in children with sickle cell anemia: Effects of continued penicillin prophylaxis. J. Pediatr. *129*:828-835, 1996.

68. Black, S., Shinefield, H., Elvin, L., and Schwalbe, J.: Pneumococcal epidemiology in childhood in a large HMO population. Abstract 1031. Pediatr. Res. *35*:174, 1994.

69. Black, S., Shinefield, H., Fireman, B., et al.: Efficacy, safety and immunogenicity of heptavalent pneumococcal conjugate vaccine in children. Pediatr. Infect. Dis. J. *19*:187-195, 2000.

70. Black, S., Shinefield, H., Hansen, J., et al.: Post-licensure evaluation of the effectiveness of seven valent pneumococcal conjugate vaccine. Pediatr. Infect. Dis. J. *20*:1105-1107, 2001.

71. Black, S., Shinefield, H., and Ling, S.: Efficacy against pneumonia of heptavalent conjugate pneumococcal vaccine (Wyeth Lederle) in 37,868 infants and children: Expanded data analysis including duration of protection. Presented at the 20th Annual Meeting of the European Society for Paediatric Infectious Diseases (ESPID), Vilnius, Lithuania, 2002, p. 127.

72. Block, S. L.: Causative pathogens, antibiotic resistance and therapeutic considerations in acute otitis media. Pediatr. Infect. Dis. J. *16*:449-456, 1997.

73. Block, S. L., Harrison, C. J., Hedrick, J. A., et al.: Penicillin-resistant *Streptococcus pneumoniae* in acute otitis media: Risk factors, susceptibility patterns and antimicrobial management. Pediatr. Infect. Dis. J. *14*:751-759, 1995.

74. Block, S. L., Hedrick, J. A., and Harrison, C. J.: Pneumococcal serotypes from acute otitis media in rural Kentucky. Abstract 1185. Presented at the 39th Interscience Conference on Antimicrobial Agents and Chemotherapy (ICAAC), San Francisco, 1999, p. 677.

75. Block, S. L., Hedrick, J., Tyler, R., et al.: Increasing bacterial resistance in pediatric acute conjunctivitis (1997-1998). Antimicrob. Agents Chemother. *44*:1650-1654, 2000.

76. Bluestone, C. D., and Klein, J. O.: Otitis Media in Infants and Children. 2nd ed. Philadelphia, W. B. Saunders, 1995, pp. 188-191.

77. Bluestone, C. D., Stephenson, J. S., and Martin, L. M.: Ten-year review of otitis media pathogens. Pediatr. Infect. Dis. J. *11*(Suppl.):7-11, 1992.

78. Blum, M. D., Dagan, R., Mendelman, P. M., et al.: A comparison of multiple regimens of pneumococcal polysaccharide–meningococcal outer membrane protein complex conjugate vaccine and pneumococcal polysaccharide vaccine in toddlers. Vaccine *18*:2359-2367, 2000.

79. Blumer, J. L.: Implications of pharmacokinetics in making choices for the management of acute otitis media. Pediatr. Infect. Dis. J. *17*:565-570, 1998.

80. Bochud, P. Y., Calandra, T., Moreillon, P., et al.: Breakthrough *Streptococcus pneumoniae* meningitis during clarithromycin therapy for acute otitis media. Eur. J. Clin. Microbiol. Infect. Dis. *20*:136-137, 2001.

81. Bodor, F. F.: Conjunctivitis-otitis syndrome. Pediatrics *69*:695-698, 1982.

82. Bodwell Dunlap, M., and Stimson Harbery, H.: Host influence on upper respiratory flora. N. Engl. J. Med. *255*:640-646, 1956.

83. Bogaert, D., Veenhoven, R. H., Ramdin, R., et al: Pneumococcal conjugate vaccination does not induce a persisting mucosal IgA response in children with recurrent otitis media. Vaccine. *23*:2607-2613, 2005.

84. Bogaert, D., Engelen, M. N., Timmers-Reker, A. J. M., et al.: Pneumococcal carriage in children in the Netherlands: A molecular epidemiological study. J. Clin. Microbiol. *39*:3316-3320, 2001.

85. Bogaert, D., van Belkum, A., Sluijter, M., et al.: Colonisation by *S. pneumoniae* and *S. aureus* in healthy children. Lancet *363*:1871-1872, 2004.

86. Bogaert, D., Veenhoven, H., Sluijter, M., et al.: Molecular epidemiology of pneumococcal colonization in response to pneumococcal conjugate vaccination in children with recurrent otitis media. J. Clin. Microbiol. *43*:74-83, 2005.

87. Borer, A., Meirson, H., Peled, N., et al.: Antibiotic-resistant pneumococci carried by young children do not appear to disseminate to adult members of a closed community. Clin. Infect. Dis. *33*:436-444, 2001.

88. Borgono, J. M., Mclean, A. A., and Vella, P. P.: Vaccination and revaccination with polyvalent pneumococcal polysaccharide vaccines in adults and infants. Proc. Soc. Exp. Biol. Med. *157*:148-154, 1978.

89. Bosu, B. K., and Harper, M. B.: Fever interval before diagnosis, prior antibiotic treatment, and clinical outcome for young children with bacterial meningitis. Clin. Infect. Dis. *32*:556-572, 2001.

90. Box, Q. T., Cleveland, R. T., and Willard, C. Y.: Bacterial flora of the upper respiratory tract. 1. Comparative evaluation by anterior nasal, oropharyngeal, and nasopharyngeal swabs. Am. J. Dis. Child. *102*:293-301, 1961.

91. Bradley, J. S., Kaplan, S. L., Klugman, K. P., and Leggiadro, R. J.: Consensus: Management of infections in children caused by *Streptococcus pneumoniae* with decreased susceptibility to penicillin. Pediatr. Infect. Dis. J. *14*:1037-1041, 1995.

92. Bratton, L., Teele, D. W., and Klein, J. O.: Outcome of unsuspected pneumococcemia in children not initially admitted to the hospital. J. Pediatr. *90*:703-706, 1977.

93. Braun, J. S., Novak, R., Gao, G., et al.: Pneumolysin, a protein toxin of *Streptococcus pneumoniae*, induces nitric oxide production from macrophages. Infect. Immun. *67*:3750-3756, 1999.

94. Breiman, R. F., Spika, J. S., Navarro, V. J., et al.: Pneumococcal bacteremia in Charleston County, South Carolina: A decade later. Arch. Intern. Med. *150*:1401-1405, 1990.

95. Briles, D. E., Crain, M. J., Gray, B. M., et al.: Strong association between capsular type and virulence for mice among human isolates of *Streptococcus pneumoniae*. Infect. Immun. *60*:111-116, 1992.

96. Briles, D. E., Hollingshead, S. K., Nabors, G. S., et al.: The potential for using protein vaccines to protect against otitis media caused by *Streptococcus pneumoniae*. Vaccine *19*(Suppl.):87-95, 2000.

97. Briles, D. E., Tart, R. C., Swiatlo, E., et al.: Pneumococcal diversity: Considerations for new vaccine strategies with emphasis on pneumococcal surface protein A (pspA). Clin. Microbiol. Rev. *11*:645-657, 1998.

98. Brimblecombe, F. S. W., Cruickshank, R., Masters, P. L., et al.: Family studies of respiratory infections. B. M. J. *1*:119-128, 1958.

99. Brodsky, E., Biger, Y., Zeidan, Z., and Schneider, M.: Topical application of chloramphenicol eye ointment followed by fatal bone marrow aplasia. Isr. J. Med. Sci. *25*:54, 1989.

100. Broides, A., Leibovitz, E., Dagan, R., et al.: The cytology of middle ear fluid during acute otitis media. Pediatr. Infect. Dis. J. *21*:57-60, 2002.

101. Brook, I., and Gober, A. E.: Prophylaxis with amoxicillin or sulfisoxazole for otitis media: Effect on the recovery of penicillin-resistant bacteria from children. Clin. Infect. Dis. *22*:143-145, 1996.

102. Brook, I., and Gober, A. E.: Eradication of *S. pneumoniae* in the nasopharyngeal flora of children with acute otitis media after amoxicillin-clavulanate therapy. Antimicrob. Agents Chemother. *48*:1419-1421, 2004.

103. Broome, C. V., Facklam, R. R., Austrian, R., et al.: Epidemiology of pneumococcal serotypes in the United States, 1978-1979. J. Infect. Dis. *141*:119-123, 1980.

104. Brown, C. E., and Magnuson, B.: On the physics of the infant feeding bottle and middle ear sequela: Ear disease in infants can be associated with bottle feeding. Int. J. Pediatr. Otorhinolaryngol. *54*:13-20, 2000.

105. Brown, J. S., Gilliland, S. M., and Holden, D. W.: A *Streptococcus pneumoniae* pathogenicity island encoding an ABC transporter involved in iron uptake and virulence. Mol. Microbiol. *40*:572-585, 2001.

106. Brown, S. D., and Farrell, D. J. Antibacterial susceptibility among *S. pneumoniae* isolated from paediatric and adult patients as part of PROTEKT US study in 2001-2002. J. Antimicrob. Chemother. *54*(Suppl. S1):i23-i29, 2004.

107. Brussow, H., Baensch, M., and Sidoti, J.: Seroprevalence of immunoglobulin M (IgM) and IgG antibodies to polysaccharides of *Streptococcus pneumoniae* in different age groups of Ecuadorian and German children. J. Clin. Microbiol. *30*:2765-2771, 1992.

108. Buck, J. M., Lexau, C., Shapiro, M., et al.: A community outbreak of conjunctivitis caused by nontypeable *S. pneumoniae* in Minnesota. Pediatr. Infect. Dis. J. *25*:906-911, 2006.

109. Buckingham, S. C., Brown, S. P., and Joaquin, V. H.: Breakthrough bacteremia and meningitis during treatment with cephalosporins parenterally for pneumococcal pneumonia. J. Pediatr. *132*:174-176, 1998.

110. Buckingham, S. C., McCullers, J. A., Lujan-Zilbermann, J., et al.: Pneumococcal meningitis in children: Relationship of antibiotic resistance to clinical characteristics and outcomes. Pediatr. Infect. Dis. J. *20*:837-843, 2001.

111. Buckingham, S. C., McCullers, J. A., Luján-Zilbermann, J., et al.: Early vancomycin therapy and adverse outcomes in children with pneumococcal meningitis. Pediatrics *117*:1688-1694, 2006.

112. Burke, J. P., Klein, J. O., Gezon, H. M., and Finland, M.: Pneumococcal bacteremia. Review of 111 cases, 1957-1969, with special reference to cases with undetermined focus. Am. J. Dis. Child. *121*:353-359, 1971.

113. Burman, L. A., Norrby, R., and Trollfors, B.: Invasive pneumococcal infections: Incidence, predisposing factors, and prognosis. Rev. Infect. Dis. 7:133-142, 1985.

114. Butler, J. C., Breiman, R. F., Lipman, H. B., et al.: Serotype distribution of *Streptococcus pneumoniae* infections among pre-school children in the United States, 1978-1994: Implications for a conjugate vaccine. J. Infect. Dis. *171*:885-889, 1995.

115. Butler, J. C., Bulkow, K. R., Parks, D. J., and Parkinson, A. J.: Epidemiology of pneumococcal bacteremia and meningitis during the first 5 years of life in Alaska: Implications for conjugate pneumococcal vaccine use. Abstract 1058. Presented at the 39th Interscience Conference on Antimicrobial Agents and Chemotherapy (ICAAC), San Francisco, 1999, p. 672.

116. Byington, C. L., Korgenski, K., Daly, J., et al.: Impact of the pneumococcal conjugate vaccine on the pneumococcal parapneumonic empyema. Pediatr. Infect. Dis. J. *25*:250-254, 2006.

117. Byington, C. L., Spencer, L. Y., Johnson, T. A., et al.: An epidemiological investigation of a sustained high rate of pediatric parapneumonic empyema: Risk factors and microbiological associations. Clin. Infect. Dis. *34*:434-440, 2002.

118. Casadevall, A., and Scharff, M. D.: Serum therapy revisited: Animal models of infection and development of passive antibody therapy. Antimicrob. Agents Chemother. *38*:1695-1702, 1994.

119. Castillo, E. M., Rickman, L. S., Brodine, S. K., et al.: *Streptococcus pneumoniae*: Bacteremia in an era of penicillin resistance. Am. J. Infect. Control 28:239-243, 2000.

120. Chambers, H. F.: Penicillin-binding protein–mediated resistance in pneumococci and staphylococci. J. Infect. Dis. *179*(Suppl. 2):353-359, 1999.

121. Chaithongwongwatthana, S., Yamasmit, W., Limpongsanurak, S., et al.: Pneumococcal vaccination during pregnancy for preventing infant infection. Cochrane Database Syst. Rev. *1*:CD004903, 2006.

122. Chen, D. K., McGeer, A., de Azavedo, J. C., et al.: Decreased susceptibility of *Streptococcus pneumoniae* to fluoroquinolones in Canada. Canadian Bacterial Surveillance Network. N. Engl. J. Med. *341*:233-239, 1999.

123. Chen, F. M., Breiman, R. D., Farley, M., et al.: Geocoding and linking data from population-based surveillance and the US census to evaluate the impact of median household income on the epidemiology of invasive *Streptococcus pneumoniae* infections. Am. J. Epidemiol. *148*:1212-1218, 1998.

124. Cherian, T., Steinhoff, M. C., Harrison, L. H., et al.: A cluster of invasive pneumococcal disease in young children in child care. J. A. M. A. *271*:695-697, 1994.

125. Chloramphenicol-induced bone-marrow aplasia. N. Engl. J. Med. *277*:1035-1036, 1967.

126. Choi, E. H., and Lee, H. J.: Clinical outcome of invasive infections by penicillin-resistant *Streptococcus pneumoniae* in Korean children. Clin. Infect. Dis. *26*:1346-1354, 1998.

127. Choi, M., and Mailman, T. L.: Pneumococcal endocarditis in infants and children. Pediatr. Infect. Dis. J. *23*:166-171, 2004.

128. Chudwin, D. S.: Prophylaxis and treatment of pneumococcal bacteremia by immune globulin intravenous in a mouse model. Clin. Immunol. Immunopathol. *50*:62-71, 1989.

129. Chudwin, D. S., Wara, D. W., Schiffman, G., et al.: Maternal fetal transfer of pneumococcal capsular polysaccharide antibodies. Am. J. Dis. Child. *139*:378-380, 1985.

130. Circolo, A., Garnier, G., Fukuda, W., et al.: Genetic disruption of the murine complement C3 promoter region generates deficient mice with extrahepatic expression of C3 mRNA. Immunopharmacology *42*:135-149, 1999.

131. Claesson, B. A., Trollfors, B., Brolin, I., et al.: Etiology of community-acquired pneumonia in children based on antibody responses to bacterial and viral antigens. Pediatr. Infect. Dis. J. *8*:856-862, 1989.

132. Clinical practice guideline: Management of sinusitis. Pediatrics *108*:798-808, 2001.

133. Cohen, R., Bingen, E., Varon, E., et al.: Change in nasopharyngeal carriage of *Streptococcus pneumoniae* resulting from antibiotic therapy for acute otitis media in children. Pediatr. Infect. Dis. J. *16*:555-560, 1997.

134. Cohen, R., Levy, C., Boucherat, M., et al.: A multicenter, randomized, double-blind trial of 5 versus 10 days of antibiotic therapy for acute otitis media in young children. J. Pediatr. *133*:634-639, 1998.

135. Cohen, R., Levy, C., Boucherat, M., et al.: Characteristics and outcome of children with acute otitis media attending day care. Abstract 776. Presented at the 39th Interscience Conference on Antimicrobial Agents and Chemotherapy (ICAAC), San Francisco, 1999, p. 666.

136. Cohen, R., Levy, C., Boucherat, M., et al.: Five vs ten days of antibiotic therapy for acute otitis media in young children. Pediatr. Infect. Dis. J. *19*:458-463, 2000.

137. Cohen, R., Navel, M., Grunberg, J., et al.: One dose ceftriaxone vs. ten days of amoxicillin/clavulanate therapy for acute otitis media: Clinical efficacy and change in nasopharyngeal flora. Pediatr. Infect. Dis. J. *18*:403-409, 1999.

138. Coles, C. L., Kanungo, R., Rahmathullah, L., et al.: Pneumococcal nasopharyngeal colonization in young south Indian infants. Pediatr. Infect. Dis. J. *20*:289-295, 2001.

139. Coles, C. L., Rahmathullah, L., Kanungo, R., et al.: Vitamin A supplementation at birth delays pneumococcal colonization in south Indian infants. J. Nutr. *131*:255-261, 2001.

140. Connolly, M., and Noah, N.: Surveillance of Bacterial Meningitis in Europe, 1996. London, King's European Meningitis Surveillance Unit, King's College School of Medicine and Dentistry, 1997.

141. Corless, C. E., Guiver, M., Borrow, R., et al.: Simultaneous detection of *Neisseria meningitidis*, *Haemophilus influenzae*, and *Streptococcus pneumoniae* in suspected cases of meningitis and septicemia using real-time PCR. J. Clin. Microbiol. *39*:1553-1558, 2001.

142. Cortese, M. M., Wolff, M., Almeido-Hill, J., et al.: High incidence rates of invasive pneumococcal disease in the White Mountain Apache population. Arch. Intern. Med. *152*:2277-2282, 1992.

143. Costa Carvalho, B. T., Carneiro-Sampaio, M. M., Sole, D., et al.: Transplacental transmission of serotype specific pneumococcal antibodies in a Brazilian population. Clin. Diagn. Lab. Immunol. *6*:50-54, 1999.

144. Courvalin, P., and Carlier, C.: Transposable multiple antibiotic resistance in *Streptococcus pneumoniae*. Mol. Gen. Genet. *205*:291-297, 1986.

145. Craig, W. A.: Pharmacokinetics/pharmacodynamics parameters; rationale for antibacterial dosing of mice and men. Clin. Infect. Dis. *26*:1-10, 1998.

146. Craig, W. A., and Andes, D.: Pharmacokinetics and pharmacodynamics of antibiotics in otitis media. Pediatr. Infect. Dis. J. *15*:255-259, 1996.

147. Cunningham-Rundles, C.: Clinical and immunologic analyses of 103 patients with common variable immunodeficiency. J. Clin. Immunol. *9*:22-33, 1989.

148. Dabernat, H., Geslin, P., and Megraud, F.: Effects of cefixime or co-amoxiclav treatment on nasopharyngeal carriage of *Streptococcus pneumoniae* and *Haemophilus influenzae* in children with acute otitis media. J. Antimicrob. Chemother. *41*:253-258, 1998.

149. Dagan, R.: Can the choice of antibiotics for acute otitis media be logic? Eur. J. Clin. Microbiol. Infect. Dis. *17*:1-5, 1998.

150. Dagan, R.: Clinical significance of resistant organisms in otitis media. Pediatr. Infect. Dis. J. *19*:378-382, 2000.

151. Dagan, R.: Treatment of acute otitis media—challenges in the era of antibiotic resistance. Vaccine *19*(Suppl.):9-16, 2001.

152. Dagan, R., Abramson, O., Leibovitz, E., et al.: Impaired bacteriologic response to oral cephalosporins in acute otitis media caused by pneumococcus with intermediate resistance to penicillin. Pediatr. Infect. Dis. J. *15*:980-985, 1996.

153. Dagan, R., Engelhard, D., Piccard, E., and Engelhard, D. C.: Epidemiology of invasive childhood pneumococcal infections in Israel. J. A. M. A. *268*:3328-3332, 1992.

154. Dagan, R., and Fraser, D.: Conjugate pneumococcal vaccine and antibiotic-resistant *Streptococcus pneumoniae*: Herd immunity and reduction of otitis morbidity. Pediatr. Infect. Dis. J. *19*(Suppl.):79-88, 2000.

155. Dagan, R., Fraser, D., Janco, J., et al.: Reduction of resistant pneumococcal nasopharyngeal colonization in toddlers attending day care centers after vaccination with a 9-valent CRM$_{197}$ conjugate pneumococcal vaccine (PncCRM9). Abstract O-12. Presented at the 18th Annual Meeting of the European Society for Paediatric Infectious Diseases (ESPID), Noordwije, The Netherlands, 2000, p. 19.

156. Dagan, R., Givon-Lavi, N., Porat, N., et al.: Immunization of toddlers attending day care centers with a 9-valent conjugate pneumococcal vaccine reduces transmission of *Streptococcus pneumoniae* and antibiotic resistant *S. pneumoniae* to their young siblings. Abstract 687. Presented at the 40th Interscience Conference on Antimicrobial Agents and Chemotherapy (ICAAC), Toronto, 2000, p. 244.

157. Dagan, R., Givon-Lavi, N., Shkolnik, L., et al.: Acute otitis media caused by antibiotic-resistant *Streptococcus pneumoniae* in southern Israel: Implication for immunizing with conjugate vaccines. J. Infect. Dis. *181*:1322-1329, 2000.

158. Dagan, R., Givon-Lavi, N., Sikuler-Cohen, M., et al.: Type-specific antipolysaccharide IgG concentrations correlate with nasopharyngeal acquisition of vaccine serotype pneumococci in toddlers during a 2-year follow-up. Abstract 2040. Presented at the 41st Interscience Conference on Antimicrobial Agents and Chemotherapy (ICAAC), Chicago, 2001, p. 283.

159. Dagan, R., Givon-Lavi, N., Zamir, O., et al.: Reduction of nasopharyngeal carriage of *Streptococcus pneumoniae* after vaccination with a 9-valent pneumococcal conjugate vaccine in toddlers attending day care centers. J. Infect. Dis. *185*:927-936, 2002.

160. Dagan, R., Gradstein, S., Belmaker, I., et al.: An outbreak of *Streptococcus pneumoniae* type 1 in a closed community in southern Israel. Clin. Infect. Dis. *30*:319-321, 2000.

161. Dagan, R., Hoberman, A., Johnson, C., et al.: Bacteriologic and clinical efficacy of high-dose amoxicillin/clavulanate in children with acute otitis media. Pediatr. Infect. Dis. J. *20*:829-837, 2001.

162. Dagan, R., Johnson, C., McLinn, S., et al.: Bacteriologic and clinical efficacy of amoxicillin/clavulanate vs. azithromycin in acute otitis media. Pediatr. Infect. Dis. J. *19*:95-104, 2000.

163. Dagan, R., Klugman, K. P., Craig, W. A., and Baquero, F.: Evidence to support the rationale that bacterial eradication in respiratory tract infection provides guidance for antimicrobial therapy. J. Antimicrob. Chemother. *47*:129-140, 2001.

164. Dagan, R., Leibovitz, E., Cheletz, G., et al.: Antibiotic treatment in acute otitis media promotes superinfection with resistant *Streptococcus pneumoniae* carried before initiation of treatment. J. Infect. Dis. *183*:880-886, 2001.

165. Dagan, R., Leibovitz, E., Fliss, D. M., et al.: Bacteriologic efficacies of oral azithromycin and oral cefaclor in treatment of acute otitis media in infants and young children. Antimicrob. Agents Chemother. *44*:43-50, 2000.

166. Dagan, R., Leibovitz, E., Greenberg, D., et al.: Early eradication of pathogens from middle ear fluid during antibiotic treatment of acute otitis media is associated with improved clinical outcome. Pediatr. Infect. Dis. J. *17*:776-782, 1998.

167. Dagan, R., Leibovitz, E., Greenberg, D., et al.: Dynamics of pneumococcal nasopharyngeal colonization during the first days of antibiotic treatment in pediatric patients. Pediatr. Infect. Dis. J. *17*:880-885, 1998.

168. Dagan, R., Leibovitz, E., Leiberman, A., and Yagupsky, P.: Clinical significance of antibiotic resistance in acute otitis media and implication of antibiotic treatment on carriage and spread of resistant organisms. Pediatr. Infect. Dis. J. *19*(Suppl.):57-65, 2000.

169. Dagan, R., Leibovitz, E., Piglansky, L., and Yagupsky, P.: Effect of antibiotic treatment on pneumococcal nasopharyngeal carriage during and after acute otitis media: Comparison of 3 oral drugs. Abstract 1028. Presented at the 39th Interscience Conference on Antimicrobial Agents and Chemotherapy (ICAAC), San Francisco, 1999, p. 145.

170. Dagan, R., Melamed, R., Muallem, M., et al.: Reduction of nasopharyngeal carriage of pneumococci during the second year of life by a heptavalent conjugate pneumococcal vaccine. J. Infect. Dis. *174*:1271-1278, 1996.

171. Dagan, R., Melamed, R., Muallem, M., et al.: Nasopharyngeal colonization in southern Israel with antibiotic-resistant pneumococci during the first 2 years of life: Relation to serotypes likely to be included in pneumococcal conjugate vaccines. J. Infect. Dis. *174*:1352-1355, 1996.

172. Dagan, R., Muallem, M., Melamed, R., et al.: Reduction of pneumococcal nasopharyngeal carriage in early infancy after immunization with tetravalent pneumococcal vaccines conjugated to either tetanus toxoid or diphtheria toxoid. Pediatr. Infect. Dis. J. *16*:1060-1064, 1997.

173. Dagan, R., Shriker, O., Hazan, I., et al.: Prospective study to determine clinical relevance of detection of pneumococcal DNA in sera of children by PCR. J. Clin. Microbiol. *36*:669-673, 1998.

174. Dagan, R., Sikuler-Cohen, M., Zamir, O., et al.: Effect of a conjugate pneumococcal vaccine on the occurrence of respiratory infections and antibiotic use in day care center attendees. Pediatr. Infect. Dis. J. *20*:951-958, 2001.

175. Dagan, R., Zamir, O., Tirosh, N., et al.: Nasopharyngeal carriage of *Streptococcus pneumoniae* in toddlers vaccinated during infancy with an 11 valent pneumococcal vaccine conjugated to diphtheria and tetanus toxoids. Abstract 47. Presented at the 40th Interscience Conference on Antimicrobial Agents and Chemotherapy (ICAAC), Toronto, 2000, p. 236.

176. Dallaire, F., Ouellet, N., Simard, M., et al.: Efficacy of recombinant human granulocyte colony-stimulating factor in a murine model of pneumococcal pneumonia: Effects of lung inflammation and timing of treatment. J. Infect. Dis. *183*:70-77, 2001.

177. Daoud, A. S., Zaki, M., and al-Saleh, Q. A.: Prolonged and secondary fever in childhood bacterial meningitis. Eur. J. Pediatr. *149*:114-116, 1989.

178. Davidson, M., Parkinson, A. J., Bulkow, L. R., et al.: Epidemiology of invasive pneumococcal disease in Alaska, 1986-1990—ethnic differences and opportunities for prevention. J. Infect. Dis. *170*:368-376, 1994.

179. Davies, T., Goering, R. V., Lovgren, M., et al.: Molecular epidemiological survey of penicillin-resistant *Streptococcus pneumoniae* from Asia, Europe, and North America. Diagn. Microbiol. Infect. Dis. *34*:7-12, 1999.

180. Davis, C. W., and McIntyre, P. B.: Invasive pneumococcal infection in children, 1981-92: A hospital-based study. J. Paediatr. Child Health *31*:317-322, 1995.

181. Davis, H. D., Matlow, A., Petric, M., et al.: Prospective comparative study of viral, bacterial and atypical organisms identified in pneumonia and bronchiolitis in hospitalised Canadian infants. Pediatr. Infect. Dis. J. *15*:371-375, 1996.

182. de Lalla, F., Nicolin, R., and Lazzarini, L.: Safety and efficacy of recombinant granulocyte colony-stimulating factor as an adjunctive therapy for *Streptococcus pneumoniae* meningitis in non-neutropenic adult patients: A pilot study. J. Antimicrob. Chemother. *46*:843-846, 2000.

183. Del Beccaro, M. A., Mendelman, P. M., Inglis, A. F., et al.: Bacteriology of acute otitis media: A new perspective. J. Pediatr. *120*:81-84, 1992.

184. del Castillo, F., Ledesma, F., and García-Perea, A.: Penicillin-susceptible and erythromycin-resistant *Streptococcus pneumoniae* in children with acute mastoiditis. Eur. J. Clin. Microbiol. Infect. Dis. *20*:824-826, 2001.

185. De Lencastre, H. D., Kristinsson, K. G., Brito-Avo, A., et al.: Carriage of respiratory tract pathogens and molecular epidemiology of *Streptococcus pneumoniae* colonization in healthy children attending day care centers in Lisbon, Portugal. Microb. Drug Resist. *5*:19-29, 1999.

186. Dimitrov, N. V., Douwes, F. R., and Bartoletta, B.: Metabolic activity of polymorphonuclear leukocytes in sickle cell anemia. Acta Haematol. *47*:283-291, 1972.

187. Dintilhac, A., Alloing, G., Granadel, C., et al.: Competence and virulence of *Streptococcus pneumoniae*: Adc and PsaA mutants exhibit a requirement for Zn and Mn resulting from inactivation of putative ABC metal permeases. Mol. Microbiol. *25*:727-739, 1997.

188. DiNubile, M. J., Albornoz, M. A., and Stumacher, R. J.: Pneumococcal soft-tissue infections: Possible association with connective tissue diseases. J. Infect. Dis. *163*:897-900, 1991.

189. Djuretic, T., Ryan, M. J., Miller, E., et al.: Hospital admissions in children due to pneumococcal pneumonia in England. J. Infect. *37*:54-58, 1998.

190. Doern, G. V., Brueggemann, A., Holley, H. P., and Rauch, A. M.: Antimicrobial resistance of *Streptococcus pneumoniae* recovered from outpatients in the United States during the winter months of 1994 to 1995: Results of a 30-center national surveillance study. Antimicrob. Agents Chemother. *40*:1208-1213, 1996.

191. Dominguez, J., Gali, N., Blanco, S., et al.: Detection of *Streptococcus pneumoniae* antigen by a rapid immunochromatographic assay in urine samples. Chest *119*:243-249, 2001.

192. Dopazo, J., Mendoza, A., Herrero, J., et al.: Annotated draft genomic sequence from a *Streptococcus pneumoniae* type 19F clinical isolate. Microb. Drug Resist. *7*:99-125, 2001.

193. Douglas, R. M., and Miles, H. B.: Vaccination against *Streptococcus pneumoniae* in childhood: Lack of demonstrable benefit in young Australian children. J. Infect. Dis. *149*:861-869, 1984.

194. Douglas, R. M., Paton, J. C., and Duncan, S. J.: Antibody response to pneumococcal vaccination in children younger than five years of age. J. Infect. Dis. *148*:131-137, 1983.

195. Dowell, S. F., Butler, J. C., Giebink, G. S., et al.: Acute otitis media: Management and surveillance in an era of pneumococcal resistance—a report from the Drug-Resistant *Streptococcus pneumoniae* Therapeutic Working Group. Pediatr. Infect. Dis. J. *18*:1-9, 1999.

196. Dowell, S. F., Marcy, S. M., Philips, W. R., et al.: Otitis media: Principles of judicious use of antimicrobial agents. Pediatrics *101*(Suppl.):165-171, 1998.

197. Duncan, B., Ey, J., Holberg, C. J., et al.: Exclusive breast-feeding for at least 4 months protects against otitis media. Pediatrics *91*:867-872, 1993.

198. Eavery, R. D., Gao, Y., Schuknecht, H. F., and Gonzalez-Fineda, M.: Otologic features of bacterial meningitis of childhood. J. Pediatr. *136*:2025-2029, 1985.

199. Eberhard, T., Kronvall, G., and Ullberg, M.: Surface bound plasmin promotes migration of *Streptococcus pneumoniae* through reconstituted basement membranes. Microb. Pathog. *26*:175-181, 1999.

200. Eby, R.: Pneumococcal conjugate vaccines. Pharm. Biotechnol. *6*:695-718, 1995.

201. Edwards, K. M., Wandling, G., Palmer, P., and Decker, M. D.: Carriage of pneumococci among infants immunized with a 9-valent pneumococcal conjugate vaccine at 2, 4, and 6 months of age. Abstract 34. Presented at the 37th Annual Meeting of the Infectious Diseases Society of America (IDSA), Philadelphia, 1999, p. 28.

202. Ekdahl, K., Ahlinger, I., Hansson, H. B., et al.: Duration of nasopharyngeal carriage of penicillin-resistant *Streptococcus pneumoniae*: Experiences from the South Swedish pneumococcal intervention project. Clin. Infect. Dis. *25*:1113-1117, 1997.

203. Ekwurzel, G. M., Simmons, J. S., Dublin, L. I., et al.: Studies on immunizing substances in pneumococci. VIII. Report on field tests to determine prophylactic value of a pneumococcus antigen. Public Health Rep. *53*:1877-1893, 1938.

204. Epstein, M. M., and Gruskay, F.: Selective deficiency in pneumococcal antibody response in children with recurrent infections. Ann. Allergy Asthma Immunol. *75*:125-131, 1995.

205. Eskola, J., and Anttila, M.: Pneumococcal conjugate vaccines. Pediatr. Infect. Dis. J. *18*:543-551, 1999.

206. Eskola, J., Kilpi, T., Palmu, A., et al.: Efficacy of a pneumococcal conjugate vaccine against acute otitis media. N. Engl. J. Med. *344*:403-409, 2001.

207. Eskola, J., Takala, A. K., Kela, E., et al.: Epidemiology of invasive pneumococcal infections in children in Finland. J. A. M. A. *268*:3323-3327, 1992.

208. Esterle, T. M., and Edwards, K. M.: Concerns of secondary fever in *Streptococcus pneumoniae* meningitis in an era of increasing antibiotic resistance. Arch. Pediatr. Adolesc. Med. *150*:552-554, 1996.

209. Ewig, S., Ruiz, M., Torres, A., et al.: Pneumonia acquired in the community through drug-resistant *Streptococcus pneumoniae*. Am. J. Respir. Crit. Care Med. *159*:1835-1842, 1999.

210. Faden, H., Duffy, L., Wasielewski, R., et al.: Relationship between nasopharyngeal colonization and the development of otitis media in children. J. Infect. Dis. *175*:1440-1445, 1997.

211. Faden, H. S., Horomi, M., and Yamanaka, N.: The importance of *Streptococcus pneumoniae*: Colonization on the course of acute otitis media. Pediatric Academic Societies Annual Meeting. Abstract 1393. Pediatr. Res. *49*:244, 2001.

212. Falade, A. G., Mulholland, E. K., Adegbola, R. A., and Greenwood, B. M.: Bacterial isolates from blood and lung aspirate cultures in Gambian children with lobar pneumonia. Ann. Trop. Paediatr. *17*:315-319, 1997.

213. Fang, G. D., Fine, M., Orloff, J., et al.: New and emerging etiologies for community-acquired pneumonia with implications for therapy: A prospective multicenter study of 359 cases. Medicine (Baltimore) *69*:307-316, 1990.

214. Farley, J. J., King, J. C., Jr., Nair, P., et al.: Invasive pneumococcal disease among infected and uninfected children of mothers with human immunodeficiency virus infection. J. Pediatr. *124*:853-858, 1994.

215. Farrell, D. J., Klugman, K. P., and Pichichero, M.: Increased antimicrobial resistance among nonvaccine serotypes of *S. pneumoniae* in the pediatric population after the introduction of 7-valent pneumococcal vaccine in the United States. Pediatr. Infect. Dis. J. *26*:123-128, 2007.

216. Fasola, E. L., Bajaksouzian, S., Appelbaum, P. C., et al.: Variation in erythromycin and clindamycin susceptibilities of *Streptococcus pneumoniae* by four test methods. Antimicrob. Agents Chemother. *41*:129-134, 1997.

217. Fedson, D. S., Musher, D. M., and Eskola, J.: Pneumococcal vaccines. *In* Plotkin, S. A., and Orenstein, W. A. (eds.): Vaccines. 3rd ed. Philadelphia, W. B. Saunders, 1999, pp. 553-607.

218. Feikin, D. R., Dowell, S. F., Nwanyanwu, O. C., et al.: Increased carriage of trimethoprim/sulfamethoxazole-resistant *Streptococcus pneumoniae* in Malawian children after treatment for malaria with sulfadoxine/pyrimethamine. J. Infect. Dis. *181*:1501-1505, 2000.

219. Feikin, D. R., Schuchat, A., Kolczak, M., et al.: Mortality from invasive pneumococcal pneumonia in the era of antibiotic resistance, 1995-1997. Am. J. Public Health *90*:223-229, 2000.

220. Feldhoff, C., Kleine, L., and Bachmann, H.: Peritonitis and infection in children with idiopathic nephrotic syndrome. Klin. Padiatr. *200*:40-44, 1988.

221. Feldman, C., Munro, N. C., Jeffery, P. K., et al.: Pneumolysin induces the salient histologic features of pneumococcal infection in the rat lung in vivo. Am. J. Respir. Cell Mol. Biol. *5*:416-423, 1991.

222. Figueroa, J. E., and Densen, P.: Infectious diseases associated with complement deficiencies. Clin. Microbiol. Rev. *4*:359-395, 1991.

223. Filice, G. A., Van Etta, L. L., Darby, C. P., and Fraser, D. W.: Bacteremia in Charleston Country, South Carolina. Am. J. Epidemiol. *123*:128-136, 1986.

224. Filipe, S. R., and Tomasz, A.: Inhibition of the expression of penicillin resistance in *Streptococcus pneumoniae* by inactivation of cell wall muropeptide branching genes. Proc. Natl. Acad. Sci. U. S. A. *97*:4891-4896, 2000.

225. Finland, M., and Barnes, M.: Changes in occurrence of capsular serotypes of *Streptococcus pneumoniae* at Boston City Hospital during selected years between 1935 and 1974. J. Clin. Microbiol. *5*:154-166, 1977.

226. Fiore, A. E., Levine, O. S., Elliott, J. A., et al.: Effectiveness of pneumococcal polysaccharide vaccine for preschool-age children with chronic disease. Emerg. Infect. Dis. *5*:828-831, 1999.

227. Fiore, A. E., Moroney, J. F., Farley, M. M., et al.: Clinical outcomes of meningitis caused by *Streptococcus pneumoniae* in the era of antibiotic resistance. Clin. Infect. Dis. *30*:71-77, 2000.

228. Fireman, B., Black, S. B., Shinefield, H.R., et al: Impact of the pneumococcal conjugate vaccine on otitis media. Pediatr. Infect. Dis. J. 22:10-16, 2003.

229. Fischer, W.: Pneumococcal lipoteichoic and teichoic acid. *In* Tomasz, A. (ed.): *Streptococcus pneumoniae*: Molecular Biology and Mechanisms of Disease. Larchmont, NY, Mary Ann Liebert, Inc., 2000, pp. 155-177.

230. Fischer, W., Markwitz, S., and Labischinski, H.: Small-angle x-ray scattering analysis of pneumococcal lipoteichoic acid phase structure. Eur. J. Biochem. *244*:913-917, 1997.

231. Fliss, D. M., Leiberman, A., and Dagan, R.: Medical sequelae and complications of acute otitis media. Pediatr. Infect. Dis. J. *13*(Suppl.):34-40, 50-54, 1994.

232. Fogarty, C., Goldschmidt, R., and Bush, K.: Bacteremic pneumonia due to multidrug-resistant pneumococci in 3 patients treated unsuccessfully with azithromycin and successfully with levofloxacin. Clin. Infect. Dis. *31*:613-615, 2000.

233. Foo, R. L., Graham, S. M., Suthisarnsuntorn, U., et al.: Detection of pneumococcal capsular antigen in saliva of children with pneumonia. Ann. Trop. Paediatr. *20*:161-163, 2000.

234. Forgie, L. M., Campbell, H., Lloyd-Evans, N., et al.: Etiology of acute lower respiratory tract infections in children in a rural community in The Gambia. Pediatr. Infect. Dis. J. *11*:466-473, 1992.

235. Forgie, L. M., O'Neill, K. P., Lloyd-Evans, N., et al.: Etiology of acute lower respiratory tract infections in Gambian children: I. Acute lower respiratory tract infections in infants presenting at the hospital. Pediatr. Infect. Dis. J. *10*:33-41, 1991.

236. Forgie, L. M., O'Neill, K. P., Lloyd-Evans, N., et al.: Etiology of acute lower respiratory tract infections in Gambian children: II. Acute lower respiratory tract infections in children ages one to nine years presenting at the hospital. Pediatr. Infect. Dis. J. *10*:42-47, 1991.

237. Fortnum, H. M.: Hearing impairment after bacterial meningitis: A review. Arch. Dis. Child. *67*:1128, 1992.

238. Francis, T., Jr., and Tillett, W. S.: Cutaneous reactions in pneumonia. The development of antibodies following the intradermal injection of type-specific polysaccharide. J. Exp. Med. *52*:573-585, 1930.

239. Frankel, R. E., Virata, M., Hardalo, C., et al.: Invasive pneumococcal disease: Clinical features, serotypes, and antimicrobial resistance patterns in cases involving patients with and without human immunodeficiency virus infection. Clin. Infect. Dis. *23*:577-584, 1996.

240. Fraser, D., Givon-Lavi, N., Bilenko, N., and Dagan, R.: A decade (1989-1998) of pediatric invasive pneumococcal disease in two populations residing in one geographic location: Implications for vaccine choice. Clin. Infect. Dis. *33*:421-427, 2001.

241. Fredericksen, B., and Henrichsen, J.: Throat carriage of *Streptococcus pneumoniae* and *Streptococcus pyogenes* among infants and children in Zambia. J. Trop. Pediatr. *34*:114-117, 1988.

242. Freij, B. J., Votteler, T. P., and McCracken, G. H.: Primary peritonitis in previously healthy children. Am. J. Dis. Child. *138*:1058-1061, 1984.

243. Frenck, R. W., Jr., and Glezen, W. P.: Respiratory tract infections in children in day care. Semin. Pediatr. Infect. Dis. *1*:234-244, 1990.

244. Friedland, I. R., and Klugman, K. P.: Failure of chloramphenicol therapy in penicillin-resistant pneumococcal meningitis. Lancet *339*:405-408, 1992.

245. Friedland, I. R., and Klugman, K. P.: Cerebrospinal fluid bactericidal activity against cephalosporin-resistant *Streptococcus pneumoniae* in children with meningitis treated with high-dosage cefotaxime. Antimicrob. Agents Chemother. *41*:1888-1891, 1997.

246. Friedland, I. R., Paris, M., Ehrett, S., et al.: Evaluation of antimicrobial regimens for treatment of experimental penicillin- and cephalosporin-resistant pneumococcal meningitis. Antimicrob. Agents Chemother. *37*:1630-1636, 1993.

247. Fuchshuber, A., Kuhnemund, O., Keuth, B., et al.: Pneumococcal vaccine in children and young adults with chronic renal disease. Nephrol. Dial. Transplant. *11*:468-473, 1996.

248. Gallin, J. I., Buescher, E. S., and Seligmann, B. E.: Recent advances in chronic granulomatous disease. Ann. Intern. Med. *99*:657-674, 1983.

249. Garcia, E., Llull, D., and Lopez, R.: Functional organization of the gene cluster involved in the synthesis of the pneumococcal capsule. Int. Microbiol. *2*:169-176, 1999.

250. Garcia, E., and Lopez, R.: Molecular biology of the capsular genes of *Streptococcus pneumoniae*. F. E. M. S. Microbiol. Lett. *149*:1-10, 1997.

251. García-Rey, C., Aguilar, L., Baquero, F., et al.: Importance of local variations in antibiotic consumption and geographical differences of erythromycin and penicillin resistance in *Streptococcus pneumoniae*. J. Clin. Microbiol. *40*:159-164, 2002.

252. Gardner, P., and Schaffner, W.: Immunization of adults. N. Engl. J. Med. *328*:1252, 1993.

253. Gaston, M. H., Verter, J. I., Woods, G., et al.: Prophylaxis with oral penicillin in children with sickle cell anemia: A randomized trial. N. Engl. J. Med. *314*:1593-1599, 1986.

254. Gates, G. A.: Cost-effectiveness considerations in otitis media treatment. Otolaryngol. Head Neck Surg. *14*:525-530, 1996.

255. Gay, K., and Stephens, D. S.: Structure and dissemination of a chromosomal insertion element encoding macrolide efflux in *Streptococcus pneumoniae*. J. Infect. Dis. *184*:56-65, 2001.

256. Gehanno, P., Olivier, C., Boucot, I., et al.: Risk factors for nasopharyngeal carriage of penicillin-resistant *S. pneumoniae*. Abstract 160. Presented at the 15th Annual Meeting of the European Society for Paediatric Infectious Diseases (ESPID), Paris, 1997, p. 80.

257. Gehanno, P., Panaotopoulos, A., Barry, B., et al.: Microbiology of otitis media in the Paris, France, area from 1987 to 1997. Pediatr. Infect. Dis. J. *20*:570-573, 2001.

258. Gendrel, D., Raymond, J., and Moulin, F.: Etiology and response to antibiotic therapy of community-acquired pneumonia in French children. Eur. J. Clin. Microbiol. Infect. Dis. *16*:388-391, 1997.

259. Geslin, P., Buu-Hoi, A., Frémaux, A., and Acar, J. F.: Antimicrobial resistance in *Streptococcus pneumoniae*: An epidemiological survey in France, 1970-1990. Clin. Infect. Dis. *15*:95-98, 1992.

260. Gesner, M., Desiderio, D., Kim, M., and Kaul, A.: *Streptococcus pneumoniae* in human immunodeficiency virus type 1–infected children. Pediatr. Infect. Dis. J. *13*:697-703, 1994.
261. Gessner, B. D., Ussery, X. T., Parkinson, A. J., and Breiman, R. F.: Risk factors for invasive disease caused by *Streptococcus pneumoniae* among Alaska native children younger than two years of age. Pediatr. Infect. Dis. J. *14*:123-128, 1995.
262. Ghaffar, F., Friedland, I. R., and McCracken, G. H., Jr.: Dynamics of naso-pharyngeal colonization by *Streptococcus pneumoniae*. Pediatr. Infect. Dis. J. *18*:638-646, 1999.
263. Gibb, D., Spoulou, V., Giacomelli, A., et al.: Antibody responses to *Haemophilus influenzae* type b and *Streptococcus pneumoniae* vaccines in children with human immunodeficiency virus infection. Pediatr. Infect. Dis. J. *14*:129-135, 1995.
264. Giebink, G. S.: The microbiology of otitis media. Pediatr. Infect. Dis. J. *8*(Suppl.):18-20, 1989.
265. Giebink, G. S.: Otitis media: The chinchilla model. Microb. Drug Resist. *5*:57-72, 1999.
266. Giebink, G. S., Meier, J. D., Quartey, M. K., et al.: Immunogenicity and efficacy of *Streptococcus pneumoniae* polysaccharide–protein conjugate vaccines against homologous and heterologous vaccine serotypes in the chinchilla model. J. Infect. Dis. *173*:119-127, 1996.
267. Gigliotti, F., Hendly, J. O., Morgan, J., et al.: Efficacy of topical antibiotic therapy in acute conjunctivitis in children. J. Pediatr. *104*:623-626, 1984.
268. Gigliotti, F., Williams, W. T., Hayden, F. G., et al.: Etiology of acute conjunctivitis in children. J. Pediatr. *98*:531-536, 1981.
269. Gilbert, R. J., Heenan, R. K., Timmins, P. A., et al.: Studies on the structure and mechanism of a bacterial protein toxin by analytical ultracentrifugation and small-angle neutron scattering. J. Mol. Biol. *293*:1145-1160, 1999.
270. Gindreau, E., Lopez, R., and Garcia, P.: Mm1, a temperate bacteriophage of the type 23F Spanish/USA multiresistant epidemic clone of *Streptococcus pneumoniae*: Structural analysis of the site-specific integration system. J. Virol. *74*:7803-7813, 2000.
271. Gingles, N. A., Alexander, J. E., Kadioglu, A., et al.: Role of genetic resistance in invasive pneumococcal infection: Identification and study of susceptibility and resistance in inbred mouse strains. Infect. Immun. *69*:426-434, 2001.
272. Ginsburg, C. M., Rudoy, R., and Nelson, J. D.: Acute mastoiditis in infants and children. Clin. Pediatr. (Phila.) *19*:549-553, 1980.
273. Givner, L. B., Mason, E. O., Jr., Barson, W. J., et al.: Pneumococcal facial cellulitis in children. Pediatrics *106*:E61, 2000.
274. Givon-Lavi, N., Dagan, R., Fraser, D., et al.: Marked differences in pneumococcal carriage and resistance patterns between day care centers located within a small area. Clin. Infect. Dis. *29*:1274-1280, 1999.
275. Go, C., Asnis, D. S., and Saltzman, H.: Pneumococcal pericarditis since 1980. Clin. Infect. Dis. *27*:1338-1340, 1998.
276. Goldblatt, D., Akoto, A. Y., Ashton, L., et al.: Immunogenicity and the generation of immune memory following 9-valent pneumococcal conjugate vaccination in Ghanaian infants with sickle cell disease. Abstract 688. Presented at the 40th Interscience Conference on Antimicrobial Agents and Chemotherapy (ICAAC), Toronto, 2000, p. 245.
277. Goldstein, F. W.: Penicillin-resistant *Streptococcus pneumoniae*: Selection by both β-lactam and non–β-lactam antibiotics. J. Antimicrob. Chemother. *44*:141-144, 1999.
278. Gonzalez, B. E., Hulten, K. G., Lamberth, L., et al.: *Streptococcus pneumoniae* serogroups 15 and 33: An increasing cause of pneumococcal infections in children in the United States after the introduction of the pneumococcal 7-valent conjugate vaccine. Pediatr. Infect. Dis. J. *25*:301-305, 2006.
279. Gordon, S. B., Irving, G. R., Lawson, R. A., et al.: Intracellular trafficking and killing of *Streptococcus pneumoniae* by human alveolar macrophages are influenced by opsonins. Infect. Immun. *68*:2286-2293, 2000.
280. Gorensek, M. J., Lebel, M. H., and Nelson, J. D.: Peritonitis in children with nephrotic syndrome. Pediatrics *81*:849-856, 1988.
281. Gosink, K. K., Mann, E. R., Guglielmo, C., et al.: Role of novel choline binding proteins in virulence of *Streptococcus pneumoniae*. Infect. Immun. *68*:5690-5695, 2000.
282. Gould, J. M., and Weiser, J. N.: Expression of C-reactive protein in the human respiratory tract. Infect. Immun. *69*:1747-1754, 2001.
283. Granert, C., Raud, J., Waage, A., et al.: Effects of polysaccharide fucoidin on cerebrospinal fluid interleukin-1 and tumor necrosis factor alpha in pneumococcal meningitis in the rabbit. Infect. Immun. *67*:2071-2074, 1999.
284. Gratten, M., Gratten, H., Poli, A., et al.: Colonisation of *Haemophilus influenzae* and *Streptococcus pneumoniae* in the upper respiratory tract of neonates in Papua New Guinea: Primary acquisition, duration of carriage, and relationship to carriage in mothers. Biol. Neonate *50*:114-120, 1986.
285. Gray, B. M., Converse, G. M., III, and Dillon, H. C., Jr.: Serotypes of *Streptococcus pneumoniae* causing disease. J. Infect. Dis. *140*:979-983, 1979.
286. Gray, B. M., Converse, G. M., III, and Dillon, H. C., Jr.: Epidemiologic studies of *Streptococcus pneumoniae* in infants: Acquisition, carriage and infection during the first 24 months of life. J. Infect. Dis. *142*:923-933, 1980.
287. Gray, B. M., Converse, G. M., III, Huhta, N., et al.: Epidemiologic studies of *Streptococcus pneumoniae* in infants: Antibody response to nasopharyngeal carriage of types 3, 19, and 23. J. Infect. Dis. *144*:312-318, 1981.
288. Gray, B. M., and Dillon, H. C., Jr.: Epidemiological studies of *Streptococcus pneumoniae* in infants: Antibody to types 3, 6, 14, and 23 in the first two years of life. J. Infect. Dis. *158*:948-955, 1988.
289. Gray, B. M., and Dillon, H. C., Jr.: Natural history of pneumococcal infections. Pediatr. Infect. Dis. J. *8*(Suppl.):23-25, 1989.
290. Gray, B. M., Turner, M. E., Dillon, H. C., Jr.: Epidemiologic studies of *Streptococcus pneumoniae* in infants: The effects of season and age on pneumococcal acquisition and carriage in the first 24 months of life. Am. J. Epidemiol. *116*:692-703, 1982.
291. Greenberg, D., Bilenko, N., Fraser, D., et al.: Acute otitis media—burden of diseases on patient and family. Abstract 807. Presented at the 39th Annual Meeting of the Infectious Diseases Society of America (IDSA), San Francisco, 2001, p. 177.
292. Grijalva, C. G., Poehling, K. A., Nuorti, J. P., et al.: National impact of universal childhood immunization with pneumococcal conjugate vaccine on outpatient medical care visits in the United States. Pediatrics *118*:865-873, 2006.
293. Grimpel, E., and Floret, D.: [Pneumococcal bacteremia and sepsis in children: A multi-center study in France.] Mod. Mol. Infect. *24*:975-981, 1994.
294. Guillemot, D., Carbon, C., Balkau, B., et al.: Low dosage and long treatment duration of beta-lactam: Risk factors for carriage of penicillin-resistant *Streptococcus pneumoniae*. J. A. M. A. *279*:365-370, 1998.
295. Guillemot, D., Varon, E., Bernède, C., et al: Reduction of antibiotic use in the community reduces the rate of colonization with penicillin G–nonsusceptible *S. pneumoniae*. Clin. Infect. Dis. *41*:930-938, 2005.
296. Gwatkin, D. R.: How many die? A set of demographic estimates of the annual number of infant and child deaths in the world. Am. J. Public Health *70*:1286-1289, 1980.
297. Hadari, I., Dagan, R., Gedalia, A., et al.: Pneumococcal osteomyelitis. An unusual cluster of cases. Clin. Pediatr. (Phila.) *24*:143-145, 1985.
298. Hakansson, A., Roche, H., Mirza, S., et al.: Characterization of binding of human lactoferrin to pneumococcal surface protein A. Infect. Immun. *69*:3372-3381, 2001.
299. Hakenbeck, R., Balmelle, N., Weber, B., et al.: Mosaic genes and mosaic chromosomes: Intra- and interspecies genomic variation of *Streptococcus pneumoniae*. Infect. Immun. *69*:2477-2486, 2001.
300. Hakenbeck, R., Grebe, T., Zahner, D., et al.: Beta-lactam resistance in *Streptococcus pneumoniae*: Penicillin-binding proteins and non–penicillin-binding proteins. Mol. Microbiol. *33*:673-678, 1999.
301. Hakenbeck, R., Kaminski, K., Konig, A., et al.: Penicillin-binding proteins in beta-lactam–resistant *Streptococcus pneumoniae*. Microb. Drug Resist. *5*:91-99, 1999.
302. Hamer, D. H., Egas, J., Estrella, B., et al.: Assessment of the Binax NOW *Streptococcus pneumoniae* urinary antigen test in children with nasopharyngeal pneumococcal carriage. Clin. Infect. Dis. *34*:1025-1028, 2002.
303. Hammerschmidt, S., Bethe, G., Remane, P. H., et al.: Identification of pneumococcal surface protein A as a lactoferrin-binding protein of *Streptococcus pneumoniae*. Infect. Immun. *67*:1683-1687, 1999.
304. Hammerschmidt, S., Talay, S. R., Brandtzaeg, P., et al.: SpsA, a novel pneumococcal surface protein with specific binding to secretory immunoglobulin A and secretory component. Mol. Microbiol. *25*:1113-1124, 1997.
305. Hanson, L. A., Ahlstedt, S., Andersson, B., et al.: Protective factors in milk and the development of the immune system. Pediatrics *75*:172-176, 1985.
306. Harabuchi, Y., Kodama, H., and Faden, H.: Outcome of acute otitis media and its relation to clinical features and nasopharyngeal colonization at the time of diagnosis. Acta Otolaryngol. *121*:908-914, 2001.
307. Hardy, G. G., Magee, A. D., Ventura, C. L., et al.: Essential role for cellular phosphoglucomutase in virulence of type 3 *Streptococcus pneumoniae*. Infect. Immun. *69*:2309-2317, 2001.
308. Harrison, C. J.: Changes in treatment strategies for acute otitis media after full implementation of the pneumococcal seven valent conjugate vaccine. Pediatr. Infect. Dis. J. *22*:S120-S130, 2003.
309. Harrison, L. H., Dwyer, D. M., Billmann, L., et al.: Invasive pneumococcal infection in Baltimore, Md. Arch. Intern. Med. *160*:89-94, 2000.
310. Hausdorff, W. P., Bryant, J., Kloek, C., et al.: The contribution of specific pneumococcal serogroups to different disease manifestations: Implications for conjugate vaccine formulation and use, Part II. Clin. Infect. Dis. *30*:122-140, 2000.
311. Hausdorff, W. P., Bryant, J., Paradiso, P. R., and Siber, G. R.: Which pneumococcal serogroups cause the most invasive disease: Implications for conjugate vaccine formulation and use, Part I. Clin. Infect. Dis. *30*:100-121, 2000.
312. Hausdorff, W. P., Siber, G., and Paradiso, P. R.: Geographical differences in invasive pneumococcal disease rates and serotype frequency in young children. Lancet *357*:950-952, 2001.
313. Hausdorff, W. P., Yothers, G., Dagan, R., et al: Multinational study of pneumococcal serotypes causing acute otitis media in children. Pediatr. Infect. Dis. J. *21*:1008-1016, 2002.
314. Hazlewood, M., Nusrat, R., Kumararatne, D. S., et al.: The acquisition of anti-pneumococcal capsular polysaccharide *Haemophilus influenzae* type b and tetanus toxoid antibodies, with age, in the UK. Clin. Exp. Immunol. *93*:157-164, 1993.
315. Heffelfinger, J. D., Dowell, S. F., Jorgensen, J. H., et al.: Management of community-acquired pneumonia in the era of pneumococcal resistance: A report from the Drug-Resistant *Streptococcus pneumoniae* Therapeutic Working Group. Arch. Intern. Med. *160*:1399-1408, 2000.
316. Heffron, R.: Pneumonia with Special Reference to Pneumococcus Lobar Pneumonia. A Commonwealth Fund Book. Cambridge, MA, Harvard University Press, 1939.

317. Heidelberger, M., and Avery, O. T.: The soluble specific substance of pneumococcus. J. Exp. Med. 38:73, 1923.

318. Heikkinen, T., Ruuskanen, O., Ziegler, T., et al.: Short term use of amoxicillin-clavulanate during upper respiratory tract infection for prevention of acute otitis media. J. Pediatr. 126:313-316, 1995.

319. Heltberg, O., Korner, B., and Schouenborg, P.: Six cases of acute appendicitis with secondary peritonitis caused by Streptococcus pneumoniae. Eur. J. Clin. Microbiol. 3:141-143, 1984.

320. Henderson, F. W., Gilligan, P. H., Wait, K., and Goff, D. A.: Nasopharyngeal carriage of antibiotic-resistant pneumococci by children in group day care. J. Infect. Dis. 157:256-263, 1988.

321. Hendley, J. O., Sande, M. A., Stewart, P. M., and Gwaltney, J. M. J.: Spread of Streptococcus pneumoniae in families: I. Carriage rates and distribution of types. J. Infect. Dis. 132:55-61, 1975.

322. Henneberger, P. K., Galaid, E. I., and Marr, J. S.: Descriptive epidemiology of pneumococcal meningitis in New York City. Am. J. Epidemiol. 117:484-491, 1983.

323. Henrichsen, J.: Six newly recognized types of Streptococcus pneumoniae. J. Clin. Microbiol. 33:2759-2762, 1995.

324. Henriques Normark, B., Novak, R., Ortqvist, A., et al.: Clinical isolates of Streptococcus pneumoniae that exhibit tolerance of vancomycin. Clin. Infect. Dis. 32:552-558, 2001.

325. Hermans, P. W., Sluijter, M., Hoogenboezem, T., et al.: Comparative study of five different DNA fingerprint techniques for molecular typing of Streptococcus pneumoniae strains. J. Clin. Microbiol. 33:1606-1612, 1995.

326. Herz, A. M., Greenhow, T. L., Alcantara, J., et al.: Changing epidemiology of outpatient bacteremia in 3 to 36 month old children after the introduction of the heptavalent-conjugated pneumococcal vaccine. Pediatr. Infect. Dis. J. 25:293-300, 2006.

327. Hidalgo, H., Moore, C., Leiva, L. E., and Sorensen, R. U.: Preimmunization and postimmunization pneumococcal antibody titers in children with recurrent infections. Ann. Allergy Asthma Immunol. 76:341-346, 1996.

328. Hoban, D. J., Doern, G. V., Fluit, A. C., et al.: Worldwide prevalence of antimicrobial resistance in Streptococcus pneumoniae, Haemophilus influenzae, and Moraxella catarrhalis in the SENTRY antimicrobial surveillance program, 1997-1999. Clin. Infect. Dis. 32(Suppl. 2):81-93, 2001.

329. Hoberman, A., Paradise, J. L., and Cohen, R.: Duration of therapy for acute otitis media. Pediatr. Infect. Dis. J. 19:471-473, 2000.

330. Hodges, R. G., Macleod, C. M., and Berhnard, W. G.: Epidemic pneumococcal pneumonia: III. Pneumococcal carrier studies. Am. J. Hyg. 44:207-230, 1946.

331. Hoge, C. W., Reichler, M. R., Dominguez, E. A., et al.: An epidemic of pneumococcal disease in an overcrowded, inadequately ventilated jail. N. Engl. J. Med. 331:643-648, 1994.

332. Hollingshead, S. K., Becker, R., and Briles, D. E.: Diversity of PspA: Mosaic genes and evidence for past recombination in Streptococcus pneumoniae. Infect. Immun. 68:5889-5900, 2000.

333. Hoppe, J. E., Koster, S., Bootz, F., and Niethammer, D.: Acute mastoiditis—relevant once again. Infection 22:178-182, 1994.

334. Howie, V. M.: Eradication of bacterial pathogens from middle ear infections. Clin. Infect. Dis. 14(Suppl. 2):209-210, 1992.

335. Howie, V. M., and Ploussard, J. H.: The "in vivo sensitivity test"—bacteriology of middle ear exudate. Pediatrics 44:940-944, 1969.

336. Howie, V. M., and Ploussard, J. H.: Efficacy of fixed combination antibiotics versus separate components in otitis media. Clin. Pediatr. (Phila.) 11:205-214, 1972.

337. Howie, V. M., Ploussard, J. H., and Lester, R. L., Jr.: Otitis media: A clinical and bacteriological correlation. Pediatrics 45:29-35, 1970.

338. Howie, V. M., Ploussard, J. H., and Sloyer, J. L., Jr.: The "otitis prone" condition. Am. J. Dis. Child. 129:676-678, 1975.

339. Howie, V. M., Ploussard, J. H., Sloyer, J. L., and Hill, J. C.: Use of pneumococcal polysaccharide vaccine in preventing otitis media in infants: Different results between racial groups. Pediatrics 73:79-81, 1984.

340. Hsu, K., Pelton, S., Karumuri, S., et al.: Population-based surveillance for childhood invasive pneumococcal disease in the era of conjugate vaccine. Pediatr. Infect. Dis. J. 24:17-23, 2005.

341. Huang, C. C., Liu, C. C., Wang, S. T., et al.: Basic fibroblast growth factor in experimental and clinical bacterial meningitis. Pediatr. Res. 45:120-127, 1999.

342. Huang, S. S., Platt, R., Rifas-Shiman, S. L., et al.: Post-PCV7 changes in colonizing pneumococcal serotypes in 16 Massachusetts communities, 2001 and 2004. Pediatrics 116:e408-e413, 2005.

343. Hussey, G., Schaaf, H., Hanslo, D., et al.: Epidemiology of post-neonatal bacterial meningitis in Cape Town children. S. Afr. Med. J. 87:51-56, 1997.

344. Hyde, T. B., Gay, K., Stephens, D. S., et al.: Macrolide resistance among invasive Streptococcus pneumoniae isolates. J. A. M. A. 206:1857-1862, 2001.

345. Idanpaan-Heikkila, I., Simon, P. M., Zopf, D., et al.: Oligosaccharides interfere with the establishment and progression of experimental pneumococcal pneumonia. J. Infect. Dis. 176:704-712, 1997.

346. Ilyas, M., Roy, S., Abbasi, S., et al.: Serious infections due to penicillin-resistant Streptococcus pneumoniae in two children with nephrotic syndrome. Pediatr. Nephrol. 10:639-641, 1996.

347. Isaacson, G.: Sinusitis in childhood. Pediatr. Clin. North Am. 43:1297-1318, 1996.

348. Ishizuka, S., Yamaya, M., Suzuki, T., et al.: Acid exposure stimulates the adherence of Streptococcus pneumoniae to cultured human airway epithelial cells. Effects on platelet-activating factor receptor expression. Am. J. Respir. Cell Mol. Biol. 24:459-468, 2001.

349. Ispahani, P., Weston, V. C., Turner, D. P., and Donald, F. E.: Septic arthritis due to Streptococcus pneumoniae in Nottingham, United Kingdom, 1985-1998. Clin. Infect. Dis. 29:1450-1454, 1999.

350. Istre, G. R., Tarpay, M., Anderson, M., et al.: Invasive disease due to Streptococcus pneumoniae in an area with a high rate of relative penicillin resistance. J. Infect. Dis. 156:732-735, 1987.

351. Jackson, M. A., Burry, V. F., Olson, L. C., and Duthie, S. E.: Breakthrough sepsis in macrolide-resistant pneumococcal infection. Pediatr. Infect. Dis. J. 15:1049-1050, 1996.

352. Jackson, M. A., and Rutledge, J.: Pneumococcal endocarditis in children. Pediatr. Infect. Dis. 1:120-122, 1982.

353. Jacobs, M. R.: Treatment and diagnosis of infections caused by drug-resistant Streptococcus pneumoniae. Clin. Infect. Dis. 15:119-127, 1992.

354. Jacobs, M. R.: Emergence of antibiotic resistance in upper and lower respiratory tract infections. Am. J. Manag. Care 5(Suppl.):651-661, 1999.

355. Jacobs, M. R.: Increasing antibiotic resistance among acute otitis media pathogens and their susceptibility to oral agents based on pharmacodynamic parameters. Pediatr. Infect. Dis. J. 19(Suppl.):47-56, 2000.

356. Jacobs, M. R., and Appelbaum, P. C.: Streptococcus pneumoniae: Activity of newer agents against penicillin-resistant strains. Curr. Infect. Dis. Rep. 1:13-21, 1999.

357. Jacobs, M. R., Bajaksouzian, S., Zilles, A., et al.: Susceptibilities of Streptococcus pneumoniae and Haemophilus influenzae to 10 oral antimicrobial agents based on pharmacodynamic parameters: 1997 U.S. surveillance study. Antimicrob. Agents Chemother. 43:1901-1908, 1999.

358. Jacobs, M. R., Dagan, R., Appelbaum, P. C., and Burch, D.: Prevalence of antimicrobial-resistant pathogens in middle ear fluid: Multinational study of 917 children with acute otitis media. Antimicrob. Agents Chemother. 42:589-595, 1998.

359. Jacobs, M. R., Good, C. E., Sellner, T., et al.: Nasopharyngeal carriage of respiratory pathogens in children undergoing pressure equalization tube placement in the era of pneumococcal protein conjugate vaccine use: Laryngoscope 117:295-298, 2007.

360. Jacobs, M. R., Koornhof, H. J., Robins-Browne, R. M., et al.: Emergence of multiply resistant pneumococci. N. Engl. J. Med. 299:735-740, 1978.

361. Jacobs, M. R., and Weinberg, W.: Evidence-based guidelines for treatment of bacterial respiratory tract infections in the era of antibiotic resistance. Manag. Care Interface 14:68-80, 2001.

362. Jacobs, N. M., Lerdkachornsuk, S., and Metzger, W. I.: Pneumococcal bacteremia in infants and children: A ten-year experience at the Cook County Hospital with special reference to the pneumococcal serotypes isolated. Pediatrics 64:296-300, 1979.

363. Jacobs, R.: Judicious use of antibiotics for common pediatric respiratory infections. Pediatr. Infect. Dis. J. 19:938-943, 2000.

364. Jadavji, T., Law, B., Lebel, M. H., et al.: A practical guide for the diagnosis and treatment of pediatric pneumonia. C. M. A. J. 156(Suppl.):703-711, 1997.

365. Jaffe, D. M., and Fleisher, G. R.: Temperature and total white blood cell count as indicators of bacteremia. Pediatrics 87:670-674, 1991.

366. Jaffe, D. M., Tanz, R. R., Davis, A. T., et al.: Antibiotic administration to treat possible occult bacteremia in febrile children. N. Engl. J. Med. 317:1175-1180, 1987.

367. Janoff, E. N., Fasching, C., Orenstein, J. M., et al.: Killing of Streptococcus pneumoniae by capsular polysaccharide–specific polymeric IgA, complement, and phagocytes. J. Clin. Invest. 104:1139-1147, 1999.

368. Janoff, E. N., O'Brien, J., Thompson, P., et al.: Streptococcus pneumoniae colonization, bacteremia, and immune response among persons with human immunodeficiency virus infection. J. Infect. Dis. 167:49-56, 1993.

369. Janoff, E. N., and Rubins, J. B.: Invasive pneumococcal disease in the immunocompromised host. In Tomasz, A. (ed.): Streptococcus pneumoniae: Molecular Biology and Mechanisms of Disease. Larchmont, NY, Mary Ann Liebert, Inc., 2000, pp. 321-341.

370. Jansen, W. T., Breukels, M. A., Snippe, H., et al.: Fcγ receptor polymorphisms determine the magnitude of in vitro phagocytosis of Streptococcus pneumoniae mediated by pneumococcal conjugate sera. J. Infect. Dis. 180:888-891, 1999.

371. Jansen, W. T., Vakevainen-Anttila, M., Kayhty, H., et al.: Comparison of a classical phagocytosis assay and a flow cytometry assay for assessment of the phagocytic capacity of sera from adults vaccinated with a pneumococcal conjugate vaccine. Clin. Diagn. Lab. Immunol. 8:245-250, 2001.

372. Jay, S. J., Johanson, W. G., Jr., and Pierce, A. K.: The radiographic resolution of Streptococcus pneumoniae pneumonia. N. Engl. J. Med. 293:798-801, 1975.

373. Jedrzejas, M. J.: Pneumococcal virulence factors: Structure and function. Microbiol. Mol. Biol. Rev. 65:187-207, 2001.

374. Jenkins, S. G., Farrell, D. J., Patel, M., et al.: Trends in anti-bacterial resistance among S. pneumoniae isolated in the USA, 2000-2003: PROTEST US years 1-3. J. Infect. 51:355-363, 2005.

375. Jenson, H. B., and Baltimore, R. S.: Impact of pneumococcal and influenza vaccines on otitis media. Curr. Opin. Pediatr. 16:58-60, 2004.

376. Johansen, F. E., Braathen, R., and Brandtzaeg, P.: Role of J chain in secretory immunoglobulin formation. Scand. J. Immunol. 52:240-248, 2000.

377. Johnson, C. E., Carlin, S. A., Super, D. M., et al.: Cefixime compared with amoxicillin for treatment of acute otitis media. J. Pediatr. 119:117-122, 1991.

378. Johnson, R. B., Jr., Newman, S. L., and Struth, A. G.: An abnormality of the alternate pathway of complement activation in sickle-cell disease. N. Engl. J. Med. 288:803-808, 1973.

379. Johnson, S. E., Rubin, L., Romero-Steiner, S., et al.: Correlation of opsono-phagocytosis and passive protection assays using human anticapsular antibodies in an infant mouse model of bacteremia for *Streptococcus pneumoniae*. J. Infect. Dis. 180:133-140, 1999.

380. Joloba, M. L., Windau, A., Bajaksouzian, S., et al.: Pneumococcal conjugate vaccine serotypes of *Streptococcus pneumoniae* isolates and the antimicrobial susceptibility of such isolates in children with otitis media. Clin. Infect. Dis. 33:1489-1494, 2001.

381. Juvén, T., Mertsola, J., Toikka, P., et al.: Clinical profile of serologically diagnosed pneumococcal pneumonia. Pediatr. Infect. Dis. J. 20:1028-1033, 2001.

382. Kabins, S. A., and Lerner, C. C.: Fulminant pneumococcemia and sickle-cell anemia. J. A. M. A. 211:467-471, 1970.

383. Kadioglu, A., Gingles, N. A., Grattan, K., et al.: Host cellular immune response to pneumococcal lung infection in mice. Infect. Immun. 68:492-501, 2000.

384. Kaetzel, C. S.: Polymeric Ig receptor: Defender of the fort or Trojan horse? Curr. Biol. 11:R35-R38, 2001.

385. Kakish, K. S., Mahafza, T., Batieha, A., et al.: Clinical sinusitis in children attending primary care centers. Pediatr. Infect. Dis. J. 19:1071-1074, 2000.

386. Kaleida, P. H., Casselbrandt, M. L., Rockette, H. E., et al.: Amoxicillin or myringotomy or both for acute otitis media: Results of a randomized clinical trial. Pediatrics 87:466-474, 1991.

387. Kaltoft, M. S., Zeuthen, N., and Konradsen, H. B.: Epidemiology of invasive pneumococcal infections in children aged 0-6 years in Denmark: A 19-year nationwide surveillance study. Acta Paediatr. Suppl. 435:3-10, 2000.

388. Kaplan, B., Wandstrat, T. L., and Cunningham, J. R.: Overall cost in the treatment of otitis media. Pediatr. Infect. Dis. J. 16(Suppl.):9-11, 1997.

389. Kaplan, S. L.: Clinical presentations, diagnosis, and prognostic factors of bacterial meningitis. Infect. Dis. Clin. North Am. 13:579-594, 1999.

390. Kaplan, S. L., and Mason, E. O.: Management of infections due to antibiotic-resistant *Streptococcus pneumoniae*. Clin. Microbiol. Rev. 11:628-644, 1998.

391. Kaplan, S. L., Mason, E. O., Jr., Barson, W. J., et al.: Outcome of invasive infections outside the central nervous system caused by *Streptococcus pneumoniae* isolates nonsusceptible to ceftriaxone in children treated with beta-lactam antibiotics. Pediatr. Infect. Dis. J. 20:392-396, 2001.

392. Kaplan, S. L., Mason, E. O., Wald, E. R., et al.: Six year multicenter surveillance of invasive pneumococcal infections in children. Pediatr. Infect. Dis. J. 21:141-147, 2002.

393. Kaplan, S. L., Mason, E. O., Wald, E. R., et al.: Decrease of invasive pneumococcal infections in children among 8 children's hospitals in the United States after the introduction of the 7-valent pneumococcal conjugate vaccine. Pediatrics 113:443-449, 2004.

394. Karma, P., Pukander, J., and Sipila, M.: Prevention of otitis media in children by pneumococcal vaccination. Am. J. Otolaryngol. 6:173-184, 1985.

395. Käyhty, H., Åhman, H., Eriksson, K., et al.: Immunogenicity and tolerability of a heptavalent pneumococcal conjugate vaccine administered at 3, 5, and 12 months of age. Pediatr. Infect. Dis. J. 24:108-114, 2005.

396. Käyhty, H., and Eskola, J.: New vaccines for the prevention of pneumococcal infections. Emerg. Infect. Dis. 2:289-298, 1996.

397. Käyhty, H., Rapola, S., Simell, B., and Kilpi, T.: Development of serum and salivary antibodies to pneumococcal protein antigens PspA, PsaA and Ply in children. Abstract 018. Presented at the 2nd International Symposium on Pneumococci and Pneumococcal Diseases, Sun City, South Africa, 2000.

398. Kays, M. B., and Denys, G. A.: In vitro activity and pharmacodynamics of azithromycin and clarithromycin against *Streptococcus pneumoniae* based on serum and intrapulmonary pharmacokinetics. Clin. Ther. 23:413-424, 2001.

399. Kelley, M. A., Weber, D. J., Gilligan, P., et al.: Breakthrough pneumococcal bacteremia in patients being treated with azithromycin and clarithromycin. Clin. Infect. Dis. 31:1008-1011, 2000.

400. Kellner, J. D., and Ford-Jones, L.: *Streptococcus pneumoniae* carriage in children attending 59 Canadian child care centers. Toronto Child Care Centre Study Group. Arch. Pediatr. Adolesc. Med. 153:495-502, 1999.

401. Kilian, M., Reinholdt, J., Lomholt, H., et al.: Biological significance of IgA1 proteases in bacterial colonization and pathogenesis: Critical evaluation of experimental evidence. A. P. M. I. S. 104:321-338, 1996.

402. Kilpi, T., Herva, E., Kaijalainen, T., et al.: Bacteriology of acute otitis media in a cohort of Finnish children followed for the first two years. Pediatr. Infect. Dis. J. 20:654-662, 2001.

403. Kilpi, T. M., Palmu, A., Leinonen, M., et al.: Efficacy of a seven-valent pneumococcal conjugate vaccine against serotype-specific acute otitis media caused by *Streptococcus pneumoniae*. Abstract 689. Presented at the 40th Interscience Conference on Antimicrobial Agents and Chemotherapy (ICAAC), Toronto, 2000, p. 245.

404. Kilpi, T. M., Palmu, A., Leinonen, M., et al.: Effect of a 7-valent pneumococcal conjugate vaccine on acute otitis media due to vaccine serotypes after boosting with conjugate or polysaccharide vaccines. Abstract G-2036. Presented at the 41st Interscience Conference on Antimicrobial Agents and Chemotherapy (ICAAC), Chicago, 2001, p. 282.

405. Kim, P., Musher, D. M., Glezen, W. P., et al.: Association of invasive pneumococcal disease with season, atmospheric conditions, air pollution, and the isolation of respiratory viruses. Clin. Infect. Dis. 22:100-106, 1996.

406. King, H., and Schumacker, H. B., Jr.: Splenic studies. I. Susceptibility to infection after splenectomy performed in infancy. Ann. Surg. 136:239-242, 1952.

407. King, J. C., Vink, P. E., Farley, J. J., et al.: Comparison of the safety and immunogenicity of a pneumococcal conjugate with a licensed polysaccharide vaccine in human immunodeficiency virus and non–human immunodeficiency virus–infected children. Pediatr. Infect. Dis. J. 15:192-196, 1996.

408. King, J. C., Vink, P. E., Farley, J. J., et al.: Safety and immunogenicity of three doses of a five-valent pneumococcal conjugate vaccine in children younger than two years with and without human immunodeficiency virus infection. Pediatrics 99:575-580, 1997.

409. Klein, D. L.: Pneumococcal conjugate vaccines: Review and update. Microb. Drug Resist. 1:49-58, 1995.

410. Klein, J. O.: The microbiology of otitis media. In Wiet, R. J., and Coulthard, S. W. (eds.): Proceedings of the Second National Conference on Otitis Media. Columbus, OH, Ross Laboratories, 1979, pp. 43-46.

411. Klein, J. O.: The epidemiology of pneumococcal disease in infants and children. Rev. Infect. Dis. 3:246-253, 1981.

412. Klein, J. O.: Epidemiology of otitis media. Pediatr. Infect. Dis. J. 8(Suppl.):9, 1989.

413. Klein, J. O.: Preventing recurrent otitis: What role for antibiotics? Contemp. Pediatr. 11:44-60, 1994.

414. Klein, J. O.: Otitis media. Clin. Infect. Dis. 19:823-833, 1994.

415. Klein, J. O.: Clinical implications of antibiotic resistance for the management of acute otitis media. Pediatr. Infect. Dis. J. 17:1084-1089, 1998.

416. Klein, J. O.: Review of consensus reports on management of acute otitis media. Pediatr. Infect. Dis. J. 18:1152-1155, 1999.

417. Klein, J. O.: Nonimmune strategies for prevention of otitis media. Pediatr. Infect. Dis. J. 19(Suppl.):89-92, 2000.

418. Klugman, K. P.: Pneumococcal resistance to antibiotics. Clin. Microbiol. Rev. 3:171-196, 1990.

419. Klugman, K. P.: Antibiotic selection of multiply resistant pneumococci. Clin. Infect. Dis. 33:489-491, 2001.

420. Klugman, K. P., and Feldman, C.: Penicillin- and cephalosporin-resistant *Streptococcus pneumoniae*. Drugs 58:1-4, 1999.

421. Klugman, K. P., Friedland, I. R., and Bradley, J. S.: Bactericidal activity against cephalosporin-resistant *Streptococcus pneumoniae* in cerebrospinal fluid of children with acute bacterial meningitis. Antimicrob. Agents Chemother. 39:1988-1992, 1995.

422. Klugman, K. P., Koornhof, H. J., and Kuhnle, V.: Clinical and nasopharyngeal isolates of unusual multiply resistant pneumococci. Am. J. Dis. Child. 140:1186-1190, 1986.

423. Klugman, K. P., Koornhof, H. J., Wasas, A., et al.: Carriage of penicillin-resistant pneumococci. Arch. Dis. Child. 61:377-381, 1986.

424. Klugman, K. P., Madhi, S. A., Huebner, R. E., et al.: A trial of a 9-valent pneumococcal conjugate vaccine in children with and those without HIV infection. N. Engl. J. Med. 349:1341-1348, 2003.

425. Koch, H., and Dennison, N. J.: Office Visits to Pediatricians. Washington, DC, National Ambulatory Medical Care Service, National Center for Health Statistics, 1974.

426. Kontiokari, T., Svanberg, M., Mattila, P., et al.: Quantitative analysis of the effect of xylitol on pneumococcal nasal colonisation in rats. F. E. M. S. Microbiol. Lett. 178:313-317, 1999.

427. Kontiokari, T., Uhari, M., and Koskela, M.: Effect of xylitol on growth of nasopharyngeal bacteria in vitro. Antimicrob. Agents Chemother. 39:1820-1823, 1995.

428. Kornelisse, R. F., Westerbeek, C. M. L., Spoor, A. B., et al.: Pneumococcal meningitis in children: Prognostic indicators and outcome. Clin. Infect. Dis. 21:1390-1397, 1995.

429. Korppi, M., Heiskanen-Kosma, T., and Jalonen, E.: Aetiology of community-acquired pneumonia in children treated in hospital. Eur. J. Pediatr. 152:24-30, 1993.

430. Korppi, M., Heiskanen-Kosma, T., and Leinonen, M.: White blood cells, C-reactive protein and erythrocyte sedimentation rate in pneumococcal pneumonia in children. Eur. Respir. J. 10:1125-1129, 1997.

431. Koskela, M.: Antibody response of young children to parenteral vaccination with pneumococcal capsular polysaccharides: A comparison between antibody levels in serum and middle ear effusion. Pediatr. Infect. Dis. J. 5:431-434, 1986.

432. Koskela, M., Leinonen, M., and Haiva, V. M.: First and second dose antibody responses to pneumococcal polysaccharide vaccine in infants. Pediatr. Infect. Dis. J. 5:45-50, 1986.

433. Koskela, M., and Luotonen, J.: Recurrent pneumococcal otitis media: Presence of pneumococcal antigens and antibody in middle ear effusion compared with antibody levels in serum. In Lim, D. L., Bluestone, C. D., Klein, J. O., et al. (eds.): Recent Advances in Otitis Media with Effusion. New York, Marcel Decker, 1984, pp. 251-255.

434. Kostyukova, N. N., Volkova, M. O., Ivanova, V. V., et al.: A study of pathogenic factors of *Streptococcus pneumoniae* strains causing meningitis. F. E. M. S. Immunol. Med. Microbiol. 10:133-137, 1995.

435. Kozyrskyj, A. L., Hildes-Ripstein, G. E., Longstaffe, S. E., et al.: Treatment of acute otitis media with a shortened course of antibiotics: A meta-analysis. J. A. M. A. 279:1736-1742, 1998.

436. Kristinsson, K. G., Sigurdardottir, S. T., Gudnason, T., et al.: Effect of vaccination with octavalent protein conjugated pneumococcal vaccines on pneumococcal carriage in infants. Abstract G-5. Presented at the 37th Interscience

Conference on Antimicrobial Agents and Chemotherapy (ICAAC), Toronto, 1997, p. 193.

437. Kuppermann, N., Fleisher, G. R., and Jaffe, D. M.: Predictors of occult pneumococcal bacteremia in young febrile children. Ann. Emerg. Med. *31*:679-687, 1998.

438. Lagos, R., and Levine, M. M.: Prospective, population-based surveillance for ambulatory invasive pneumococcal disease in children in Santiago, Chile. Abstract 026. Presented at the Second International Symposium on Pneumococci and Pneumococcal Diseases, Sun City, South Africa, 2000.

439. Lane, P. A., Rogers, Z. R., Woods, G. M., et al.: Fatal pneumococcal septicemia in hemoglobin SC disease. J. Pediatr. *124*:859-862, 1994.

440. Lau, G. W., Haataja, S., Lonetto, M., et al.: A functional genomic analysis of type 3 *Streptococcus pneumoniae* virulence. Mol. Microbiol. *40*:555-571, 2001.

441. Lawrence, E. R., Arias, C. A., Duke, B., et al.: Evaluation of serotype prediction by cpsA-cpsB gene polymorphism in *Streptococcus pneumoniae*. J. Clin. Microbiol. *38*:1319-1323, 2000.

442. Leach, A. J., Boswell, J. B., Asche, V., et al.: Bacterial colonization of the nasopharynx predicts very early onset and persistence of otitis media in Australian Aboriginal infants. Pediatr. Infect. Dis. J. *13*:983-989, 1994.

443. Leach, A. J., Shelby-James, T. M., Mayo, M., et al.: A prospective study of the impact of community-based azithromycin treatment of trachoma on carriage and resistance of *Streptococcus pneumoniae*. Clin. Infect. Dis. *24*:356-362, 1997.

444. Lebel, M. H., and McCracken, G. H., Jr.: Delayed cerebrospinal fluid sterilization and adverse outcome of bacterial meningitis in infants and children. Pediatrics *83*:161-167, 1989.

445. Lee, C. J., Ching, E. D., and Vickers, J. H.: Maternal immunity and antibody response of neonatal mice to pneumococcal type 19F polysaccharide. J. Clin. Microbiol. *29*:1904-1909, 1991.

446. Lee, G. M., and Harper, M. B.: Risk of bacteremia for febrile young children in the post–*Haemophilus influenzae* type b era. Arch. Pediatr. Adolesc. Med. *152*:624-628, 1998.

447. Lee, H. J., Kang, J. H., Henrichsen, J., et al.: Immunogenicity and safety of a 23-valent pneumococcal polysaccharide vaccine in healthy children and in children at increased risk of pneumococcal infection. Vaccine *13*:1533-1538, 1995.

448. Lehmann, D., Gratten, M., and Montgomery, J.: Susceptibility of pneumococcal carriage isolates to penicillin provides a conservative estimate of susceptibility of invasive pneumococci. Pediatr. Infect. Dis. J. *16*:297-305, 1997.

449. Lehmann, D., Marshall, T. F., Riley, I. F., and Alpers, M. P.: Effect of pneumococcal vaccine on morbidity from acute lower respiratory tract infections in Papua New Guinean children. Ann. Trop. Paediatr. *11*:247-257, 1991.

450. Lehmann, D., Pomat, W. S., Combs, B., et al.: Maternal immunization with pneumococcal polysaccharide vaccine in the highlands of Papua New Guinea. Vaccine *20*:1837-1845, 2002.

451. Lehmann, D., Pomat, W. S., Riley, I. D., et al.: Studies of maternal immunisation with pneumococcal polysaccharide vaccine in Papua New Guinea. Vaccine *21*:3446-3450, 2003.

452. Leiberman, A., Leibovitz, E., and Piglansky, L.: Bacteriologic clinical efficacy of trimethoprim/sulfamethoxazole for the treatment of acute otitis media. Pediatr. Infect. Dis. J. *20*:260-264, 2001.

453. Leibovitz, E., and Dagan, R.: Antibiotic treatment for acute otitis media. Int. J. Antimicrob. Agents *15*:169-177, 2000.

454. Leibovitz, E., and Dagan, R.: Otitis media therapy and drug resistance—Part 1: Management principles. Infect. Med. *18*:212-216, 2001.

455. Leibovitz, E., and Dagan, R.: Otitis media therapy and drug resistance—Part 2: Current concepts and new directions. Infect. Med. *18*:263-270, 2001.

456. Leibovitz, E., Piglansky, L., and Raiz, S.: Bacteriologic efficacy of a three-day intramuscular ceftriaxone regimen in non-responsive acute otitis media. Pediatr. Infect. Dis. J. *17*:1126-1131, 1998.

457. Leibovitz, E., Piglansky, L., Raiz, S., et al.: Bacteriologic and clinical efficacy of one day versus three-day intramuscular ceftriaxone for treatment of non-responsive acute otitis media in children. Pediatr. Infect. Dis. J. *19*:1040-1045, 2000.

458. Leibovitz, E., Raiz, S., Piglansky, L., et al.: Resistance pattern of middle ear fluid isolates in acute otitis media recently treated with antibiotics. Pediatr. Infect. Dis. J. *17*:463-469, 1998.

459. Leino, T., Auranen, K., Jokinen, J., et al.: Pneumococcal carriage in children during their first two years: Important role of family exposure. Pediatr. Infect. Dis. J. *20*:1022-1027, 2001.

460. Leinonen, M., Sakkinen, A., and Kalliokoski, R.: Antibody response to 14-valent pneumococcal capsular polysaccharide vaccine in pre-school age children. Pediatr. Infect. Dis. J. *5*:39-44, 1986.

461. Leowski, J.: Mortality from acute respiratory infections in children under 5 years of age: Global estimates. World Health Stat. Q. *39*:138-144, 1986.

462. LeVine, A. M., Koeningsknecht, V., and Stark, J. M.: Decreased pulmonary clearance of *S. pneumoniae* following influenza A infection in mice. J. Virol. Methods *94*:173-186, 2001.

463. Levine, O. S., Farley, M., Harrison, L. H., et al.: Risk factors for invasive pneumococcal disease in children: A population-based case-control study in North America. Active Bacterial Core Surveillance Team. Pediatrics *103*(3):e28, 1999.

464. Levy, A., Fraser, D., Vardi, H., and Dagan, R.: Hospitalizations for infectious disease in Jewish and Bedouin children in southern Israel. Eur. J. Epidemiol. *14*:179-186, 1998.

465. Li, S., Taylor, K. B., Kelly, S. J., et al.: Vitamin C inhibits the enzymatic activity of *Streptococcus pneumoniae* hyaluronate lyase. J. Biol. Chem. *276*:15125-15130, 2001.

466. Lieu, T. A., Ray, G. T., Black, S. B., et al.: Projected cost-effectiveness of pneumococcal conjugate vaccination of healthy infants and young children. J. A. M. A. *283*:1460-1468, 2000.

467. Light, R. W., Girard, W. M., Jenkinson, S. G., and George, R. B.: Parapneumonic effusions. Am. J. Med. *60*:507-512, 1980.

468. Lim, P. L., and Lau, Y. L.: Occurrence of IGG subclass antibodies to ovalbumin, avidin, and pneumococcal polysaccharide in children. Int. Arch. Allergy Immunol. *104*:137-143, 1994.

469. Lin, J., Vambutas, A., Haruta, A., et al.: Pneumococcus activation of the 5-lipoxygenase pathway and production of glycoproteins in the middle ear of rats. J. Infect. Dis. *179*:1145-1151, 1999.

470. Lin, K. T., and Lee, C. J.: Immune response of neonates to pneumococcal polysaccharide protein conjugate. Immunology *46*:333-342, 1982.

471. Lin, P. L., Michaels, M. G., Green, M., et al.: Safety and immunogenicity of the American Academy of Pediatrics—recommended sequential pneumococcal conjugate and polysaccharide vaccine schedule in pediatric solid organ transplant recipients. Pediatrics *116*:160-167, 2005.

472. Lipsitch, M.: Interpreting results from trials of pneumococcal conjugate vaccines: A statistical test for detecting vaccine-induced increases in carriage of nonvaccine serotypes. Am. J. Epidemiol. *153*:85-92, 2001.

473. Lloyd-Evans, N., O'Dempsey, T. J. D., Baldeh, I., et al.: Nasopharyngeal carriage of pneumococci in Gambian children and in their families. Pediatr. Infect. Dis. J. *15*:866-871, 1996.

474. Lockhart, N. J., Daly, K. A., Lindgren, B. R., et al.: Low cord blood type 14 pneumococcal IgG1 but not IgG2 antibody predicts early infant otitis media. J. Infect. Dis. *181*:1979-1982, 2000.

475. Lockhart, S. P., Hackell, J. G., and Fritzell, B.: Pneumococcal conjugate vaccines: Emerging clinical information and its implications. Expert Rev. Vaccines *5*:553-564, 2006.

476. Loda, F. A., Collier, A. M., Glezen, W. P., et al.: Occurrence of *Diplococcus pneumoniae* in the upper respiratory tract of children. J. Pediatr. *87*:1087-1093, 1975.

477. Loeffler, J. M., Ringer, R., Hablutzel, M., et al.: The free radical scavenger alpha-phenyl-tert-butyl nitrone aggravates hippocampal apoptosis and learning deficits in experimental pneumococcal meningitis. J. Infect. Dis. *183*:247-252, 2001.

478. Long, S. S., Henretig, F. M., Teter, M. J., and McGowen, K. L.: Nasopharyngeal flora and acute otitis media. Infect. Immun. *41*:987-991, 1983.

479. Lonks, J., Garau, J., Gomez, L., et al.: Failure of macrolide antibiotic treatment in patients with bacteremia due to erythromycin-resistant *Streptococcus pneumoniae*. Clin. Infect. Dis. *35*:556-564, 2002.

480. Lonks, J. R., and Medeiros, A. A.: High rate of erythromycin and clarithromycin resistance among *Streptococcus pneumoniae* isolates from blood cultures from Providence, R.I. Antimicrob. Agents Chemother. *37*:1742-1745, 1993.

481. López, B., Cima, M. D., and Vázquez, F.: Epidemiological study of *Streptococcus pneumoniae* carriers in healthy primary-school children. Eur. J. Clin. Microbiol. Infect. Dis. *18*:771-776, 1999.

482. Low, D. E., and Scheld, W. M.: Strategies for stemming the tide of antimicrobial resistance. J. A. M. A. *279*:394-395, 1998.

483. Lucas, A. H., Moulton, K. D., Tang, V. R., et al.: Combinatorial library cloning of human antibodies to *Streptococcus pneumoniae* capsular polysaccharides: Variable region primary structures and evidence for somatic mutation of Fab fragments specific for capsular serotypes 6B, 14, and 23F. Infect. Immun. *69*:853-864, 2001.

484. Luotonen, J., Herva, E., Karma, P., et al.: The bacteriology of acute otitis media in children with special reference to *Streptococcus pneumoniae* as studied by bacteriological and antigen detection methods. Scand. J. Infect. Dis. *13*:177-183, 1981.

485. MacLeod, C. M., Hodges, R. G., Heidelberger, M., and Bernhard, W. G.: Prevention of pneumococcal pneumonia by immunization with specific capsular polysaccharides. J. Exp. Med. *82*:445-465, 1945.

486. Madhi, S. A., Ludewick, H., Kuwanda, L., et al.: Pneumococcal coinfection with human metapneumovirus. J. Infect. Dis. *193*:1236-1243, 2006.

487. Madhi, S. A., Petersen, K., Madhi, A., et al.: Increased disease burden and antibiotic resistance of bacteria causing severe community-acquired lower respiratory tract infections in human immunodeficiency virus type 1–infected children. Clin. Infect. Dis. *31*:170-176, 2000.

488. Madhi, S. A., Petersen, K., Madhi, A., et al.: Impact of human immunodeficiency virus type 1 on the disease spectrum of *S. pneumoniae* in South African children. Pediatr. Infect. Dis. J. *19*:1141-1147, 2000.

489. Majcherczyk, P. A., Langen, H., Heumann, D., et al.: Digestion of *Streptococcus pneumoniae* cell walls with its major peptidoglycan hydrolase releases branched stem peptides carrying proinflammatory activity. J. Biol. Chem. *274*:12537-12543, 1999.

490. Mäkela, P. H., Leinonen, M., Pukander, J., and Karma, P.: A study of the pneumococcal vaccine in prevention of clinically acute attacks of recurrent otitis media. Rev. Infect. Dis. *3*(Suppl.):124-132, 1981.

491. Malley, R., Lipsitch, M., Stack, A., et al.: Intranasal immunization with killed unencapsulated whole cells prevents colonization and invasive disease by capsulated pneumococci. Infect. Immun. *69*:4870-4873, 2001.

492. Malley, R., Stack, A. M., Ferretti, M. L., et al.: Anticapsular polysaccharide antibodies and nasopharyngeal colonization with *Streptococcus pneumoniae* in infant rats. J. Infect. Dis. *178*:878-882, 1998.

493. Mandel, E. M., Casselbrant, M. L., Rockette, H. E., et al.: Efficacy of antimicrobial prophylaxis for recurrent middle ear effusion. Pediatr. Infect. Dis. J. *15*:1074-1082, 1996.

494. Mandell, G. L., and Coleman, E. J.: Activities of antimicrobial agents against intracellular pneumococci. Antimicrob. Agents Chemother. *44*:2561-2563, 2000.

495. Mao, C., Harper, M., McIntosh, K., et al.: Invasive pneumococcal infections in human immunodeficiency virus–infected children. J. Infect. Dis. *173*:870-876, 1996.

496. Mason, E. O., Wald, E. R., Bradley, J. S., et al.: Macrolide resistance among middle ear isolates of *S. pneumoniae* observed at eight United States pediatric centers: Prevalence of M and MLS_B phenotypes. Pediatr. Infect. Dis. J. *22*:623-627, 2003.

497. Mastro, T. D., Ghafoor, A., Nomani, N. K., et al.: Antimicrobial resistance of pneumococci in children with acute lower respiratory tract infection in Pakistan. Lancet *337*:156-159, 1991.

498. Mastro, T. D., Nomani, N. K., Ishaq, Z., et al.: The use of nasopharyngeal isolates of *Streptococcus pneumoniae* and *Haemophilus influenzae* from children in Pakistan for surveillance for antimicrobial resistance. Pediatr. Infect. Dis. J. *12*:824-830, 1993.

499. Maynard, J. E., Fleshman, J. K., and Tschopp, C. F.: Otitis media in Alaskan Eskimo children: Prospective evaluation of chemoprophylaxis. J. A. M. A. *219*:597-599, 1972.

500. Mbelle, N., Huebner, R. E., Wasas, A. D., et al.: Immunogenicity and impact on nasopharyngeal carriage of a nonavalent pneumococcal conjugate vaccine. J. Infect. Dis. *180*:1171-1176, 1999.

501. McCarthy, P. L., Jekel, J. F., Stashwick, C. A., et al.: Further definition of history and observation variables in assessing febrile children. Pediatrics *67*:687-693, 1981.

502. McCracken, G. H., Jr.: Treatment of acute otitis media in an era of increasing microbial resistance. Pediatr. Infect. Dis. J. *17*:576-579, 1998.

503. McCullers, J. A., English, B. K., and Novak, R.: Isolation and characterization of vancomycin-tolerant *Streptococcus pneumoniae* from the cerebrospinal fluid of a patient who developed recrudescent meningitis. J. Infect. Dis. *181*:369-373, 2000.

504. McGee, L., McDougal, L., Zhou, J., et al.: Nomenclature of major antimicrobial-resistant clones of *Streptococcus pneumoniae* defined by the pneumococcal molecular epidemiology network. J. Clin. Microbiol. *39*:2565-2571, 2001.

505. McIntosh, K.: Community-acquired pneumonia. N. Engl. J. Med. *346*:429-437, 2002.

506. McIntyre, P. B., Berkey, C. S., King, S. M., et al.: Dexamethasone as adjunctive therapy in bacterial meningitis. A meta-analysis of randomized clinical trials since 1988. J. A. M. A. *278*:925-931, 1997.

507. Melander, E., Mölstad, S., Persson, K., et al.: Previous antibiotic consumption and other risk factors for carriage of penicillin-resistant *Streptococcus pneumoniae* in children. Eur. J. Clin. Microbiol. Infect. Dis. *17*:834-838, 1998.

508. Metlay, J. P., Hofman, J., Cetron, M. S., et al.: Impact of penicillin susceptibility on medical outcomes for adult patients with bacteremic pneumococcal pneumonia. Clin. Infect. Dis. *30*:520-528, 2000.

509. Michelow, I. C., Lozano, J., Olsen, K., et al.: Diagnosis of *Streptococcus pneumoniae* lower respiratory infection in hospitalized children by culture, polymerase chain reaction, serological testing, and urinary antigen detection. Clin. Infect. Dis. *34*:E1-E11, 2002.

510. Miernyk, K. M., Parkinson, A. J., Rudolph, K. M., et al.: Immunogenicity of a heptavalent pneumococcal conjugate vaccine in Apache and Navajo Indian, Alaska Native, and non-native American infants aged <2 years. Clin. Infect. Dis. *31*:34-41, 2000.

511. Miller, E., Waight, P., Efstratiou, A., et al.: Epidemiology of invasive and other pneumococcal disease in children in England and Wales 1996-1998. Acta Paediatr. Suppl. *435*:11-16, 2000.

512. Mitten, M. J., Meulbroek, J., Nukkala, M., et al.: Efficacies of ABT-773, a new ketolide, against experimental bacterial infections. Antimicrob. Agents Chemother. *45*:2585-2593, 2001.

513. Molrine, D., Antin, J., Guinan, E., et al.: Pneumococcal conjugate vaccine (PCV) elicits protective responses in allogeneic bone marrow transplant (BMT) recipients. Abstract G-2035. Presented at the 41st Interscience Conference on Antimicrobial Agents and Chemotherapy (ICAAC), Chicago, 2001, p. 282.

514. Montgomery, J. M., Lehmann, D., Smith, T., et al.: Bacterial colonization of the upper respiratory tract and its association with acute lower respiratory tract infections in Highland children of Papua New Guinea. Rev. Infect. Dis. *23*(Suppl.):1006-1016, 1990.

515. Moore, D., Nelson, M., and Henderson, D.: Pneumococcal vaccination and HIV infection. Int. J. S. T. D. A. I. D. S. *9*:1-7, 1998.

516. Moreno, S., Carcia-Leoni, M. E., Cercenado, E., et al.: Infections caused by erythromycin resistant *Streptococcus pneumoniae*: Incidence, risk factors, and response to therapy in a prospective study. Clin. Infect. Dis. *20*:1195-1200, 1995.

517. Morona, J. K., Miller, D. C., Coffey, T. J., et al.: Molecular and genetic characterization of the capsule biosynthesis locus of *Streptococcus pneumoniae* type 23F. Microbiology *145*:781-789, 1999.

518. Morona, J. K., Morona, R., and Paton, J. C.: Comparative genetics of capsular polysaccharide biosynthesis in *Streptococcus pneumoniae* types belonging to serogroup 19. J. Bacteriol. *181*:5355-5364, 1999.

519. Moroney, J. F., Fiore, A. E., and Harrison, L. H.: Clinical outcomes of bacteremic pneumococcal pneumonia in the era of antibiotic resistance. Clin. Infect. Dis. *33*:797-805, 2001.

520. Morrison, K. E., Lake, D., Crook, J., et al.: Confirmation of psaA in all 90 serotypes of *Streptococcus pneumoniae* by PCR and potential of this assay for identification and diagnosis. J. Clin. Microbiol. *38*:434-437, 2000.

521. Mortier-Barriere, I., Humbert, O., Martin, B., et al.: Control of recombination rate during transformation of *Streptococcus pneumoniae*: An overview. Microb. Drug Resist. *3*:233-242, 1997.

522. Mufson, M. A., Oley, G., and Hughey, D.: Pneumococcal disease in a medium-sized community in the United States. J. A. M. A. *248*:1486-1489, 1982.

523. Munoz, F. M., Englund, J. A., Cheesman, C. C., et al.: Maternal immunization with pneumococcal polysaccharide vaccine in the third trimester of gestation. Vaccine *20*:826-837, 2002.

524. Muñoz, P., Sainz, J., Rodríguez-Creixéms, M., et al.: Austrian syndrome caused by highly penicillin-resistant *Streptococcus pneumoniae*. Clin. Infect. Dis. *29*:1591-1592, 1999.

525. Munoz, R., Fenoll, A., Vicioso, D., et al.: Optochin-resistant variants of *Streptococcus pneumoniae*. Diagn. Microbiol. Infect. Dis. *13*:63-66, 1990.

526. Musher, D. M.: Pneumococcal outbreaks in nursing homes. N. Engl. J. Med. *38*:1915-1916, 1998.

527. Musher, D. M.: *Streptococcus pneumoniae*. *In* Mandell, G. L., Bennett, J. E., and Dolin, R. (eds.): Principles and Practice of Infectious Disease. 5th ed. Philadelphia, Churchill Livingstone, 2000, pp. 2128-2146.

528. Musher, D., and Dagan, R.: Is the pneumococcus the one and only in acute otitis media? Pediatr. Infect. Dis. J. *19*:399-400, 2000.

529. Musher, D. M., Groover, J. E., Reichler, M. R., et al.: Emergence of antibody to capsular polysaccharides of *Streptococcus pneumoniae* during outbreaks of pneumonia: Association with nasopharyngeal colonization. Clin. Infect. Dis. *24*:441-446, 1997.

530. Musher, D. M., Groover, J. E., Rowland, J. M., et al.: Antibody to capsular polysaccharides of *Streptococcus pneumoniae*: Prevalence, persistence, and response to revaccination. Clin. Infect. Dis. *17*:66-73, 1993.

531. Musher, D. M., Phan, H. M., and Baughn, R. E.: Protection against bacteremic pneumococcal infection by antibody to pneumolysin. J. Infect. Dis. *183*:827-830, 2001.

532. Musher, D. M., Phan, H. M., Watson, D. A., et al.: Antibody to capsular polysaccharide of *Streptococcus pneumoniae* at the time of hospital admission for pneumococcal pneumonia. J. Infect. Dis. *182*:158-167, 2000.

533. Nabors, G. S., Braun, P. A., Hermann, D. J., et al.: Immunization of healthy adults with a single recombinant pneumococcal surface protein A (PspA) variant stimulates broadly cross-reactive antibodies to heterologous PspA molecules. Vaccine *18*:1743-1754, 2000.

534. Nachman, S., Kim, S., King, J., et al.: Safety and immunogenicity of a heptavalent pneumococcal conjugate vaccine in infants with human immunodeficiency virus type 1 infection. Pediatrics *112*:66-73, 2003.

535. Nafstad, P, Hagen, J. A., Oie, L., et al.: Day care centers and respiratory health. Pediatrics *103*:753-758, 1999.

536. National Center for Health Statistics: Ambulatory Surgery in the United States, 1996. Hyattsville, MD, U.S. Department of Health and Human Services, Centers for Disease Control and Prevention, 1998 (advance data from Vital and Health Statistics, No. 300).

537. National Committee for Clinical Laboratory Standards: Performance standards for antimicrobial susceptibility testing. 11th Informational Suppl. Publication M100-S11. Wayne, PA, NCCLS, 2001.

538. Neuman, H. B., and Wald, E. R.: Bacterial meningitis in childhood at the children's hospital of Pittsburgh: 1988-1998. Clin. Pediatr. (Phila.) *40*:595-600, 2001.

539. Nielsen, S. V., and Henrichsen, J.: Incidence of invasive pneumococcal disease and distribution of capsular types of pneumococci in Denmark, 1989-1994. Epidemiol. Infect. *117*:411-416, 1996.

540. Nigrovic, L. E., Kuppermann, N., Macias, C. G., et al.: Clinical prediction rule for identifying children with cerebrospinal fluid pleocytosis at very low risk of bacterial meningitis. J. A. M. A. *297*:52-60, 2007.

541. Nilsson, P., and Laurell, M. H.: Carriage of penicillin-resistant *Streptococcus pneumoniae* by children in day-care centers during an intervention program in Malmö, Sweden. Pediatr. Infect. Dis. J. *20*:1144-1149, 2001.

542. Nohynek, H., Eskola, J., Laine, E., et al.: The causes of hospital-treated acute lower respiratory tract infection in children. Am. J. Dis. Child. *145*:618-622, 1991.

543. Novak, R., Henriques, B., Charpentier, E., et al.: Emergence of vancomycin tolerance in *Streptococcus pneumoniae*. Nature *399*:590-593, 1999.

544. Nowak-Wegrzyn, A. H., Winkelstein, J. A., Stover, B. M., et al.: Serum opsonic activity for *Streptococcus pneumoniae* types 6B and 14 in infants with sickle cell disease after immunization with pneumococcal protein conjugate vaccine. Pediatric Academic Societies Annual Meeting. Abstract 57. Pediatr. Res. *45*:11, 1999.

545. Nuorti, J. P., Butler, J. C., Farley, M. M., et al.: Cigarette smoking and invasive pneumococcal disease. N. Engl. J. Med. *342*:681-689, 2000.

546. Obaro, S. K., Adegbola, R. A., Banya, W. A., and Greenwood B. M.: Carriage of pneumococci after pneumococcal vaccination. Lancet *348*:272, 1996.

547. O'Brien, K. L., Bronsdon, M. A., Becenti, J., et al.: Ability of a seven valent pneumococcal conjugate vaccine to protect unvaccinated 2 month old infants against nasopharyngeal colonization. Abstract G-2032. Presented at the 41st Interscience Conference on Antimicrobial Agents and Chemotherapy (ICAAC), Chicago, 2001, p. 281.

548. O'Brien, K. L., Bronsdon, M., Carlone, G. M., et al.: Effect of a seven valent pneumococcal conjugate vaccine on nasopharyngeal (NP) carriage among native American infants. Pediatric Academic Societies Annual Meeting. Abstract 1463. Pediatr. Res. 49:256, 2001.

549. O'Brien, K. L., Croll, J., Parkinson, A. J., et al.: Active laboratory-based surveillance for invasive *Streptococcus pneumoniae* (pneumococcus) among Navajo people in the American southwest, 1989-1996. Abstract 1187. Presented at the 39th Interscience Conference on Antimicrobial Agents and Chemotherapy (ICAAC), San Francisco, 1999, p. 678.

550. O'Brien, K. L., Dowell, S. F., Schwartz, B., et al.: Acute sinusitis: Principle of judicious use of antimicrobial agents. Pediatrics 101:174-177, 1998.

551. O'Brien, K. L., Moulton, L., Reid, R. R., et al.: Invasive disease efficacy of a 7-valent pneumococcal conjugate vaccine among Navajo and White Mountain Apache children. Pediatric Academic Societies Annual Meeting. Abstract 1371. Pediatr. Res. 49:240, 2001.

552. O'Brien, K. L., Swift, A. J., Winkelstein, J. A., et al.: The safety and immunogenicity of heptavalent pneumococcal vaccine conjugated to CRM197 among infants with sickle cell disease. Pediatrics 106:965-972, 2000.

553. O'Demsey, T. D. J., McArdle, T., Ceesay, S. J., et al.: Immunization with a pneumococcal polysaccharide vaccine during pregnancy. Vaccine 14:963-970, 1996.

554. O'Dempsey, T. J., McArdle, T. F., Lloyd-Evans, N., et al.: Pneumococcal disease among children in a rural area of west Africa. Pediatr. Infect. Dis. J. 15:431-437, 1996.

555. Olson, L. C., and Jackson, M. A.: Only the pneumococcus. Pediatr. Infect. Dis. J. 18:849-850, 1999.

556. Orange, M., and Gray, B. M.: Pneumococcal serotypes causing disease in children in Alabama. Pediatr. Infect. Dis. J. 12:243-244, 1993.

557. Ort, S., Ryan, R. L., Barden, G., et al.: Pneumococcal pneumonia in hospitalized patients. J. A. M. A. 249:214-218, 1983.

558. Ostergaard, C., Benfield, T., Gesser, B., et al.: Pretreatment with granulocyte colony-stimulating factor attenuates the inflammatory response but not the bacterial load in cerebrospinal fluid during experimental pneumococcal meningitis in rabbits. Infect. Immun. 67:3430-3436, 1999.

559. Ostergaard, C., Yieng-Kow, R. V., Benfield, T., et al.: Inhibition of leukocyte entry into the brain by the selectin blocker fucoidin decreases interleukin-1 (IL-1) levels but increases IL-8 levels in cerebrospinal fluid during experimental pneumococcal meningitis in rabbits. Infect. Immun. 68:3153-3157, 2000.

560. Overturf, G. D.: Infections and immunizations of children with sickle cell disease. Adv. Pediatr. Infect. Dis. 14:191-218, 1999.

561. Paganini, H., Guiñazú, J. R., Hernández, C., et al.: Comparative analysis of outcome and clinical features in children with pleural empyema caused by penicillin-nonsusceptible and penicillin-susceptible *Streptococcus pneumoniae*. Int. J. Infect. Dis. 5:86-88, 2001.

562. Pai, R., Moore, M. R., Pilishvili, T., et al.: Postvaccine genetic structure of *S. pneumoniae* serotype 19A from children in the United States. J. Infect. Dis. 192:1988-1995, 2005.

563. Pallares, R., Linares, J., Vadillo, M., et al.: Resistance to penicillin and cephalosporin and mortality from severe pneumococcal pneumonia in Barcelona, Spain. N. Engl. J. Med. 333:474-480, 1995.

564. Palmu, A. A., Verho, J., Mäkelä, P. H., and Kilpi, T. M.: Long-term efficacy of the seven-valent PncCRM vaccine on otitis media. Presented at the 3rd International Symposium on Pneumococci and Pneumococcal Diseases, Anchorage, Alaska, 2002, p. 72.

565. Pankuch, G. A., Jacobs, M. R., and Appelbaum, P. C.: Susceptibilities of 200 penicillin-susceptible and -resistant pneumococci to piperacillin, piperacillin-tazobactam, ticarcillin, ticarcillin-clavulanate, ampicillin, ampicillin-sulbactam, ceftazidime, and ceftriaxone. Antimicrob. Agents Chemother. 38:2905-2907, 1994.

566. Paradise, J. L., Rockette, H. E., and Colborn, K.: Otitis media in 2253 Pittsburgh-area infants: Prevalence and risk factors during the first two years of life. Pediatrics 99:318-333, 1997.

567. Paris, M. M., Hickey, S. M., Uscher, M. I., et al.: Effect of dexamethasone on therapy of experimental penicillin- and cephalosporin-resistant pneumococcal meningitis. Antimicrob. Agents Chemother. 38:1320-1324, 1994.

568. Park, M. K., Sun, Y., Olander, J. V., et al.: The repertoire of human antibodies to the carbohydrate capsule of *Streptococcus pneumoniae* 6B. J. Infect. Dis. 174:75-82, 1996.

569. Pastor, P., Medley, F., and Murphy, T. V.: Invasive pneumococcal disease in Dallas County, Texas: Results from population-based surveillance in 1995. Clin. Infect. Dis. 26:590-595, 1998.

570. Paton, J. C., Berry, A. M., and Lock, R. A.: Molecular analysis of putative pneumococcal virulence proteins. Microb. Drug Resist. 3:1-10, 1997.

571. Pearson, H. A.: Prevention of pneumococcal disease in sickle cell anemia. J. Pediatr. 129:788-789, 1996.

572. Pearson, H. A., Cornelius, E. A., Schwartz, A. D., et al.: Transfusion-reversible functional asplenia in children with sickle-cell anemia. N. Engl. J. Med. 283:334-337, 1970.

573. Pécoul, B., Varaine, F., Keita, M., et al.: Long-acting chloramphenicol versus intravenous ampicillin for treatment of bacterial meningitis. Lancet 338:862-866, 1991.

574. Peled, N., and Yagupsky, P.: Improved detection of *Streptococcus pneumoniae* in middle ear fluid cultures by use of a gentamicin-containing medium. J. Clin. Microbiol. 37:3415-3416, 1999.

575. Peltola, H.: Burden of meningitis and other severe bacterial infections of children in Africa: Implications for prevention. Clin. Infect. Dis. 32:64-75, 2001.

576. Pelton, S.: Prevention of acute and recurrent otitis media. Lancet 356:1370-1371, 2000.

577. Pelton, S. I., and Klein, J. O.: The promise of immunoprophylaxis for prevention of acute otitis media. Pediatr. Infect. Dis. J. 18:926-935, 1999.

578. Perez Retortillo, J. A., Marco, F., Richard, C., et al.: Pneumococcal pericarditis with cardiac tamponade in a patient with chronic graft-versus-host disease. Bone Marrow Transplant. 21:299-300, 1998.

579. Perrin, J. M., Charney, E., MacWhinney, J. B., Jr., et al.: Sulfisoxazole as chemoprophylaxis for recurrent otitis media: A double-blind crossover study in pediatric practice. N. Engl. J. Med. 291:664-667, 1974.

580. Pessey, J. J., Gehanno, P., Thoroddsen, E., et al.: Short course therapy with cefuroxime axetil for acute otitis media: Results of a randomized multicenter comparison with amoxicillin/clavulanate. Pediatr. Infect. Dis. J. 18:854-859, 1999.

581. Peters, V. B., Diamant, E. P., Hodes, D. S., and Cimino, C. O.: Impaired immunity to pneumococcal polysaccharide antigens in children with human immunodeficiency virus infection immunized with pneumococcal vaccine. Pediatr. Infect. Dis. J. 13:933-934, 1994.

582. Pichard, E., Gillis, D., Aker, M., and Engelhard, D.: Rebound fever in bacterial meningitis: Role of dexamethasone dosage. Isr. J. Med. Sci. 30:408-411, 1994.

583. Pichichero, M. E.: Persistent acute otitis media: II. Antimicrobial treatment. Pediatr. Infect. Dis. J. 14:183-188, 1995.

584. Pichichero, M. E., and Cohen, R.: Shortened course of antibiotic therapy for acute otitis media, sinusitis and tonsillopharyngitis. Pediatr. Infect. Dis. J. 16:680-695, 1997.

585. Pichichero, M. E., Marscocci, S. M., Murphy, M. L., et al.: A prospective observational study of 5-, 7-, and 10-day antibiotic treatment for acute otitis media. Otolaryngol. Head Neck Surg. 124:381-387, 2001.

586. Pihlajamäki, M., Kotilainen, P., Kaurila, T., et al.: Macrolide-resistant *Streptococcus pneumoniae* and use of antimicrobial agents. Clin. Infect. Dis. 33:483-488, 2001.

587. Ploton, C., Freydiere, A. M., Benito, Y., et al.: *S. pneumoniae* thoracic empyema in children: Rapid diagnosis by using Binax NOW immunochromatographic membrane test in pleural fluids. Pathol. Biol. 54:498-501, 2006.

588. Poehling, K. A., Talbot, T. R., Griffin, M. R., et al.: Invasive pneumococcal disease among infants before and after introduction of pneumococcal conjugate vaccine. J. A. M. A. 295:1668-1674, 2006.

589. Pomat, W. S., Lehmann, D., Sanders, R. C., et al.: Immunoglobulin G antibody responses to polyvalent pneumococcal vaccine in children in the highlands of Papua New Guinea. Infect. Immun. 62:1848-1853, 1994.

590. Porat, N., Greenberg, D., Givon-Lavi, N., et al.: The important role of nontypeable *S. pneumoniae* international clones in acute conjunctivitis. J. Infect. Dis. 194:689-696, 2006.

591. Poulsen, K., Reinholdt, J., Jespersgaard, C., et al.: A comprehensive genetic study of streptococcal immunoglobulin A1 proteases: Evidence for recombination within and between species. Infect. Immun. 66:181-190, 1998.

592. Prellner, K., Fogle-Hansson, M., Jorgensen, F., et al.: Prevention of recurrent acute otitis media in otitis-prone children by intermittent prophylaxis with penicillin. Acta Otolaryngol. 114:182-187, 1994.

593. Preventing pneumococcal disease among infants and young children. Recommendations of the Advisory Committee on Immunization Practices (ACIP). M. M. W. R. Recomm. Rep. 49(RR-9):1-35, 2000.

594. Prevention of pneumococcal disease: Recommendations of the Advisory Committee on Immunization Practices (ACIP). M. M. R. W. Recomm. Rep. 46(RR-8):1-24, 1997.

595. Principi, N., Marchisio, P., Schito, G. C., and Mannelli, S.: Risk factors for carriage of respiratory pathogens in the nasopharynx of healthy children. Ascanius Project Collaborative Group. Pediatr. Infect. Dis. J. 18:517-523, 1999.

596. Prinz, M., Kann, O., Draheim, H. J., et al.: Microglial activation by components of gram-positive and -negative bacteria: Distinct and common routes to the induction of ion channels and cytokines. J. Neuropathol. Exp. Neurol. 58:1078-1089, 1999.

597. Prober, C. G.: The role of steroids in the management of children with bacterial meningitis. Pediatrics 95:29-31, 1995.

598. Pukander, J., Karma, P., and Sipila, M.: Occurrence and recurrence of acute otitis media among children. Acta Otolaryngol. (Stockh.) 94:479-486, 1982.

599. Radetsky, M., Istre, G., Johansen, T., et al.: Multiply resistant pneumococcus causing meningitis: Its epidemiology within a day-care centre. Lancet 2:771-773, 1981.

600. Ragsdale, A., and Sanford, J.: Interfering effect of incubation in carbon dioxide on the identification of pneumococci by optochin discs. Appl. Microbiol. 22:854-855, 1971.

601. Rahav, G., Toledano, Y., Engelhard, D., et al.: Invasive pneumococcal infections: A comparison between adults and children. Medicine (Baltimore) 76:295-303, 1997.

602. Ramirez, M., Morrison, D. A., and Tomasz, A.: Ubiquitous distribution of the competence related genes coma and comc among isolates of *Streptococcus pneumoniae*. Microb. Drug Resist. 3:39-52, 1997.

603. Ramirez, M., Severina, E., and Tomasz, A.: A high incidence of prophage carriage among natural isolates of *Streptococcus pneumoniae*. J. Bacteriol. 181:3618-3625, 1999.

604. Ramirez, M., and Tomasz, A.: Acquisition of new capsular genes among clinical isolates of antibiotic-resistant *Streptococcus pneumoniae*. Microb. Drug Resist. 5:241-246, 1999.

605. Rapola, S., Jäntti, V., Haikala, R., et al.: Natural development of antibodies to pneumococcal surface protein A, pneumococcal surface adhesin A, and pneumolysin in relation to pneumococcal carriage and acute otitis media. J. Infect. Dis. 182:1146-1152, 2000.

606. Rapola, S., Kilpi, T., Lahdenkari, M., et al.: Antibody response to the pneumococcal proteins pneumococcal surface adhesin A and pneumolysin in children with acute otitis media. Pediatr. Infect. Dis. J. 20:482-487, 2001.

607. Rapola, S., Kilpi, T., Lahdenkari, M., et al.: Do antibodies to pneumococcal surface adhesin A prevent pneumococcal involvement in acute otitis media? J. Infect. Dis. 184:577-581, 2001.

608. Rauch, A. M., O'Ryan, M., Van, R., and Pickering, L. K.: Invasive disease due to multiply resistant *Streptococcus pneumoniae* in a Houston, Tex, day-care center. Am. J. Dis. Child. 144:923-927, 1990.

609. Rautonen, J., Siimes, M. A., Lundstrom, U., et al.: Vaccination of children during treatment for leukemia. Acta Paediatr. 75:579-585, 1986.

610. Reefhuis, J., Honein, M. A., Whitney, C. G., et al.: Risk of bacterial meningitis in children with cochlear implants. N. Engl. J. Med. 349:435-445, 2003.

611. Reichler, M. R., Allphin, A. A., Breiman, R. F., et al.: The spread of multiply resistant *Streptococcus pneumoniae* at a day care center in Ohio. J. Infect. Dis. 166:1146-1153, 1992.

612. Reinert, R. R., Kaufhold, A., Kuhnemund, O., and Lutticken, R.: Serum antibody responses to vaccination with 23-valent pneumococcal vaccine in splenectomized patients. Int. J. Med. Microbiol. Virol. Parasitol. Infect. Dis. 281:481-490, 1994.

613. Resistance of *Streptococcus pneumoniae* to fluoroquinolones—United States, 1995-1999. M. M. W. R. Morb. Mortal. Wkly. Rep. 50(30):800-804, 2001.

614. Rieux, V., Carbon, C., and Azoulay-Dupuis, E.: Complex relationship between acquisition of β-lactam resistance and loss of virulence in *Streptococcus pneumoniae*. J. Infect. Dis. 184:66-72, 2001.

615. Rijkers, G. T., Sanders, E. A. M., Breukels, M. A., and Zegers, B. J. M.: Responsiveness of infants to capsular polysaccharides: Implications for vaccine development. Rev. Med. Microbiol. 7:3-12, 1996.

616. Riley, I. D., Lehmann, D., and Alpers, M. P.: Pneumococcal vaccine trials in Papua New Guinea: Relationships between epidemiology of pneumococcal infection and efficacy of vaccine. Rev. Infect. Dis. 13(Suppl.):S35-541, 1991.

617. Riley, I. D., Lehmann, D., Alpers, M. P., et al.: Pneumococcal vaccine prevents death from acute lower-respiratory-tract infections in Papua New Guinean children. Lancet 2:877-881, 1986.

618. Roark, R., and Berman, S.: Continuous twice daily or once daily amoxicillin prophylaxis compared with placebo for children with recurrent acute otitis media. Pediatr. Infect. Dis. J. 16:376-381, 1997.

619. Robbins, J. B., Austrian, R., Lee, C. J., et al.: Considerations for formulating the second-generation pneumococcal capsular polysaccharide vaccine with emphasis on the cross-reactive types within groups. J. Infect. Dis. 148:1136-1159, 1983.

620. Robbins, J. B., and Schneerson, R.: Polysaccharide-protein conjugates: A new generation of vaccines. J. Infect. Dis. 161:821-832, 1990.

621. Robert, P. Y., and Adenis, J. P.: Comparative review of topical ophthalmic antibacterial preparations. Drugs 61:175-185, 2001.

622. Robinson, K. A., Baughman, W., Rothrock, S. G., et al.: Epidemiology of invasive *Streptococcus pneumoniae* infections in the United States, 1995-1998. Opportunities for prevention in the conjugate vaccine era. J. A. M. A. 285:1729-1735, 2001.

623. Rodriguez, M. E., van der Pol, W. L., Sanders, L. A., et al.: Crucial role of FcγRIIa (CD32) in assessment of functional anti-*Streptococcus pneumoniae* antibody activity in human sera. J. Infect. Dis. 179:423-433, 1999.

624. Rodriguez, W. J., and Schwartz, R. H.: *Streptococcus pneumoniae* causes otitis media with higher fever and more redness of tympanic membrane than *Haemophilus influenzae* or *Moraxella catarrhalis*. Pediatr. Infect. Dis. J. 18:942-944, 1999.

625. Rodriguez-Barradas, M. C., Musher, D. M., Lahart, C., et al.: Antibody to capsular polysaccharides of *Streptococcus pneumoniae* after vaccination of human immuno-deficiency virus–infected subjects with 23-valent pneumococcal vaccine. J. Infect. Dis. 165:553-556, 1992.

626. Romero-Steiner, S., Libutti, D., Pais, L. B., et al.: Standardization of an opsonophagocytic assay for the measurement of functional antibody activity against *Streptococcus pneumoniae* using differentiated HL-60 cells. Clin. Diagn. Lab. Immunol. 4:415-422, 1997.

627. Rosén, C., Christensen, P., Hovelius, B., and Prellner, K.: A longitudinal study of the nasopharyngeal carriage of pneumococci as related to pneumococcal vaccination in children attending day-care centers. Acta Otolaryngol. (Stockh.) 98:524-532, 1984.

628. Rosen, I. A., Hakansson, A., and Aniansson, G.: Antibodies to pneumococcal polysaccharides in human milk: Lack of relationship to colonization and acute otitis media. Pediatr. Infect. Dis. J. 15:498-507, 1996.

629. Rosenblüt, A., Santolaya, M. E., González, P., et al.: Bacterial and viral etiology of acute otitis media in Chilean children. Pediatr. Infect. Dis. J. 20:501-507, 2001.

630. Rosenfeld, R. M.: What to expect from medical treatment of otitis media. Pediatr. Infect. Dis. J. 14:731-738, 1995.

631. Rosenfeld, R. M., Vertrees, J. E., Carr, J., et al.: Clinical efficacy of antimicrobial drugs for acute otitis media: Metaanalysis of 5400 children from thirty-three randomized trials. J. Pediatr. 124:355-367, 1994.

632. Rosenow, C., Ryan, P., Weiser, J. N., et al.: Contribution of novel choline-binding proteins to adherence, colonization and immunogenicity of *Streptococcus pneumoniae*. Mol. Microbiol. 25:819-829, 1997.

633. Roson, B., Carratala, J., Tubau, F., et al.: Usefulness of beta-lactam therapy for community-acquired pneumonia in the era of drug-resistant *Streptococcus pneumoniae*: A randomized study of amoxicillin-clavulanate and ceftriaxone. Microb. Drug Resist. 7:85-96, 2001.

634. Rothrock, S. G., Green, S. M., Harper, M. B., et al.: Parenteral vs oral antibiotics in the prevention of serious bacterial infections in children with *Streptococcus pneumoniae* occult bacteremia: A meta-analysis. Acad. Emerg. Med. 5:599-606, 1998.

635. Rothrock, S. G., Green, S. M., Wren, J., et al.: Pediatric bacterial meningitis: Is prior antibiotic therapy associated with an altered clinical presentation? Ann. Emerg. Med. 21:146-152, 1992.

636. Rothrock, S. G., Harper, M. B., Green, S. M., et al.: Do oral antibiotics prevent meningitis and serious bacterial infections in children with *Streptococcus pneumoniae* occult bacteremia? A meta-analysis. Pediatrics 99:438-444, 1997.

637. Rovers, M. M., Zielhuis, G. A., Ingels, K., et al.: Day-care and otitis media in young children: A critical overview. Eur. J. Pediatr. 158:1-6, 1999.

638. Roy, S., Knox, K., Segal, S., et al.: MBL genotype and risk of invasive pneumococcal disease: A case-control study. Lancet 359:1569-1573, 2002.

639. Rubin, L. G., Mardy, G. V., Pais, L., and Carlone, G.: Human anti-capsular concentration required for protection against experimental pneumococcal bacteremia. Abstract G47. Presented at the 35th Interscience Conference on Antimicrobial Agents and Chemotherapy (ICAAC), San Francisco, 1995, p. 166.

640. Ruuskanen, O., Nohynek, H., Ziegler, T., et al.: Pneumonia in childhood: Etiology and response to antimicrobial therapy. Eur. J. Clin. Microbiol. Infect. Dis. 11:217-223, 1992.

641. Ryan, M. J., Kavanagh, R., Wall, P. G., and Hazleman, B. L.: Bacterial joint infections in England and Wales: Analysis of bacterial isolates over a four year period. Br. J. Rheumatol. 36:370-373, 1997.

642. Rytel, M. W., Dailey, M. P., Schiffman, G., et al.: Pneumococcal vaccine immunization of patients with renal impairment. Proc. Soc. Exp. Biol. Med. 182:468-473, 1986.

643. Saenz, R. E., Sanders, C. V., Aldridge, K. E., and Patel, M. M.: Purulent pericarditis with associated cardiac tamponade caused by a *Streptococcus pneumoniae* strain highly resistant to penicillin, cefotaxime, and ceftriaxone. Clin. Infect. Dis. 26:762-763, 1998.

644. Saez-Llorens, X., Castano, E., Garcia, R., et al.: Prospective randomized comparison of cefepime and cefotaxime for treatment of bacterial meningitis in infants and children. Antimicrob. Agents Chemother. 39:937-940, 1995.

645. Saez-Llorens, X., and McCracken, G. H.: Antimicrobial and anti-inflammatory treatment of bacterial meningitis. Infect. Dis. Clin. North Am. 13:619-636, 1999.

646. Saha, S. K., Darmstadt, G. L., Yamanaka, N., et al.: Rapid diagnosis of pneumococcal meningitis: Implications for treatment and measuring disease burden. Pediatr. Infect. Dis. J. 24:1093-1098, 2005.

647. Salazar, J. C., Daly, K. A., Giebink, G. S., et al.: Low cord blood pneumococcal immunoglobulin G (IgG) antibodies predict early onset acute otitis media in infancy. Am. J. Epidemiol. 145:1048-1056, 1997.

648. Sá-Leão, R., Tomasz, A., Santos Sanches, I., et al.: Carriage of internationally spread clones of *Streptococcus pneumoniae* with unusual drug resistance patterns in children attending day care centers in Lisbon, Portugal. J. Infect. Dis. 182:1153-1160, 2000.

649. Sá-Leão, R., Tomasz, A., Santos Sanches, I., et al.: Genetic diversity and clonal patterns among antibiotic-susceptible and -resistant *Streptococcus pneumoniae* colonizing children: Day care centers as autonomous epidemiological units. J. Clin. Microbiol. 38:4137-4144, 2000.

650. Samore, M. H., Magill, M. K., Alder, S. C., et al.: High rates of multiple antibiotic resistance in *Streptococcus pneumoniae* from healthy children living in isolated rural communities: Association with cephalosporin use and intrafamilial transmission. Pediatrics 108:856-865, 2001.

651. Sanchez, C., Armengol, R., Lite, J., et al.: Penicillin-resistant pneumococci and community-acquired pneumonia. Lancet 339:988, 1992.

652. Sanders, L. A., Rijkers, G. T., Kuis, W., et al.: Defective antipneumococcal polysaccharide antibody response in children with recurrent respiratory tract infections. J. Allergy Clin. Immunol. 91:110-119, 1993.

653. Sanders, L. A., Rijkers, G. T., Tenbergen Meekes, A. M., et al.: Immunoglobulin isotype–specific antibody responses to pneumococcal polysaccharide vaccine in patients with recurrent bacterial respiratory tract infections. Pediatr. Res. 37:812-819, 1995.

654. Santosham, M., Reid, G., and Almeido-Hill, J.: Efficacy of bacterial polysaccharide immune globulin for prevention of bacteremia pneumococcal infections in Apache children. Abstract 1055. Pediatr. Res. 31:178, 1992.

655. Sard, B., Bailey, M. C., and Vinci, R.: An analysis of pediatric blood cultures in the postpneumococcal conjugate vaccine era in a community hospital emergency department. Pediatr. Emerg. Care 22:295-300, 2006.

656. Schaad, U. B., Kaplan, S. L., and McCracken, G. H.: Steroid therapy for bacterial meningitis. Clin. Infect. Dis. 20:685-690, 1995.

657. Schaad, U. B., Krucko, J., and Pfenninger, J.: An extended experience with cefuroxime therapy of childhood bacterial meningitis. Pediatr. Infect. Dis. 3:410-416, 1984.

658. Schmidt, H., Stuertz, K., Bruck, W., et al.: Intravenous granulocyte colony-stimulating factor increases the release of tumour necrosis factor and interleukin-1 beta into the cerebrospinal fluid, but does not inhibit the growth of Streptococcus pneumoniae in experimental meningitis. Scand. J. Immunol. 49:481-486, 1999.

659. Schrag, S. J., Peña, C., Fernández, J., et al.: Effect of short-course, high-dose amoxicillin therapy on resistant pneumococcal carriage. J. A. M. A. 286:49-56, 2001.

660. Schuchat, A., Robinson, K., Wenger, J. D., et al.: Bacterial meningitis in the United States in 1995. Active Surveillance Team. N. Engl. J. Med. 337:970-976, 1997.

661. Schultz, M. J., Wijnholds, J., Peppelenbosch, M. P., et al.: Mice lacking the multidrug resistance protein 1 are resistant to Streptococcus pneumoniae–induced pneumonia. J. Immunol. 166:4059-4064, 2001.

662. Schutze, G., Mason, E. O., Barson, W., et al.: Invasive pneumococcal infections in children with asplenia. Pediatr. Infect. Dis. J. 21:278-282, 2002.

663. Schutze, G. E., Mason, E. O., Wald, E. R., et al.: Pneumococcal infections in children after transplantation. Clin. Infect. Dis. 33:16-21, 2001.

664. Scott, J. A. G., Hall, A. J., Hannington, A., et al.: Serotype distribution and prevalence of resistance to benzylpenicillin in three representative populations of Streptococcus pneumoniae isolates from the coast of Kenya. Clin. Infect. Dis. 27:1442-1450, 1998.

665. Scott, J. A. G., Hall, A. J., Muyodi, C., et al.: Aetiology, outcome, and risk factors for mortality among adults with acute pneumonia in Kenya. Lancet 355:1225-1230, 2000.

666. Seeler, R. A., Metzger, W., and Mufson, M. A.: Diplococcus pneumoniae infections in children with sickle cell anemia. Am. J. Dis. Child. 123:8-10, 1972.

667. Seikel, K., Shelton, S., and McCracken, G. H.: Middle ear fluid concentrations of amoxicillin after large dosages in children with acute otitis media. Pediatr. Infect. Dis. J. 17:969-970, 1998.

668. Sell, S. H., Wright, P. F., and Vaughn, W. K.: Clinical studies of pneumococcal vaccines in infants: I. Reactogenicity and immunogenicity of two polyvalent polysaccharide vaccines. Rev. Infect. Dis. 3(Suppl.):97-107, 1981.

669. Sen, S., Lalitha, M. K., Fenn, A. S., and Mammen, K. E.: Primary peritonitis in children. Ann. Trop. Paediatr. 3:53-56, 1983.

670. Severin, A., Severina, E., and Tomasz, A.: Abnormal physiological properties and altered cell wall composition in Streptococcus pneumoniae grown in the presence of clavulanic acid. Antimicrob. Agents Chemother. 41:504-510, 1997.

671. Severina, E., Ramirez, M., and Tomasz, A.: Prophage carriage as a molecular epidemiological marker in Streptococcus pneumoniae. J. Clin. Microbiol. 37:3308-3315, 1999.

672. Shahid, N. S., Steinhoff, M. C., Hoque, S. S., et al.: Serum, breast milk, and infant antibody after maternal immunization with pneumococcal vaccine. Lancet 346:1252-1257, 1995.

673. Shann, F.: Etiology of severe pneumonia in children in developing countries. Pediatr. Infect. Dis. J. 5:247-252, 1986.

674. Shapiro, E. D., Wald, E. R., and Brozanski, B. A.: Periorbital cellulitis and paranasal sinusitis: A reappraisal. Pediatr. Infect. Dis. J. 1:91-94, 1982.

675. Sher, L., Arguedas, A., Husseman, M., et al.: Randomized, investigator-blinded, multicenter, comparative study of gatifloxacin versus amoxicillin/clavulanate in recurrent otitis media and acute otitis media treatment failure in children. Pediatr. Infect. Dis. J. 24:301-308, 2005.

676. Shinefield, H., Black, S., Elvin, L., et al.: Impact of the introduction of pneumococcal conjugate vaccine on the epidemiology of invasive disease in children less than five years of age within Northern California Kaiser Permanente (NCKP). Presented at the 20th Annual Meeting of the European Society for Paediatric Infectious Disease, Vilnius, Lithuania, 2002, p. 127.

677. Shinefield, H., Black, S., Ray, P., et al.: Efficacy, immunogenicity and safety of heptavalent pneumococcal conjugate vaccine in low birth weight and preterm infants. Pediatr. Infect. Dis. J. 21:182-186, 2002.

678. Shouval, D. S., Greenberg, D., Givon-Lavi, N., et al.: Site-specific disease potential of individual S. pneumoniae serotypes in pediatric invasive disease, acute otitis media and acute conjunctivitis. Pediatr. Infect. Dis. J. 25:602-607, 2006.

679. Shurin, P. A., Giebink, G. S., Wegman, D. G., et al.: Prevention of pneumococcal otitis media in chinchillas with human bacterial polysaccharide immune globulin. J. Clin. Microbiol. 26:755-759, 1988.

680. Shurin, P. A., Rehmus, J. M., Johnson, C. E., et al.: Bacterial polysaccharide immune globulin for prophylaxis of acute otitis media in high-risk children. J. Pediatr. 123:801-810, 1993.

681. Siber, G. R.: Pneumococcal disease: Prospects for a new generation of vaccines. Science 265:1385-1387, 1994.

682. Siber, G. R., Thompson, C., Raymond Reid, G., et al.: Evaluation of bacterial polysaccharide immune globulin for the treatment or prevention of Haemophilus influenzae type b and pneumococcal disease. J. Infect. Dis. 165(Suppl.):129-133, 1992.

683. Siegel, M., and Timpone, J.: Penicillin-resistant Streptococcus pneumoniae endocarditis: A case report and review. Clin. Infect. Dis. 32:972-974, 2001.

684. Silverstein, M., Bachur, R., and Harper, M. B.: Clinical implications of penicillin and ceftriaxone resistance among children with pneumococcal bacteremia. Pediatr. Infect. Dis. J. 18:35-41, 1999.

685. Simell, B., Korkeila, M., Pursiainen, H., et al.: Pneumococcal carriage and otitis media induce salivary antibodies to pneumococcal surface adhesin A, pneumolysin, and pneumococcal surface protein A in children. J. Infect. Dis. 183:887-896, 2001.

686. Singleton, R. J., Hennessy, T. W., Bulkow, L. R., et al.: Invasive pneumococcal disease caused by nonvaccine serotypes among Alaska Native children with high levels of 7-valent pneumococcal conjugate vaccine coverage. J. A. M. A. 297:1784-1792, 2007.

687. Sinus and Allergy Health Partnership: Antimicrobial treatment guidelines for acute bacterial rhinosinusitis. Otolaryngol. Head Neck Surg. 123:5-31, 2000.

688. Sipila, M., Pukander, J., and Karma, P.: Incidence of acute otitis media up to the age of 1½ years in urban infants. Acta Otolaryngol. (Stockh.) 104:138-145, 1987.

689. Sirotnak, A. P., Eppes, S. C., and Klein, J. D.: Tuboovarian abscess and peritonitis caused by Streptococcus pneumoniae serotype 1 in young girls. Clin. Infect. Dis. 22:993-996, 1996.

690. Sleeman, K., Griffiths, D., Shackley, F., et al.: Capsular serotype–specific attack rates and duration of carriage of S. pneumoniae in a population of children. J. Infect. Dis. 194:682-688, 2006.

691. Sloas, M. M., Barrett, F. F., Chesney, P. J., et al.: Cephalosporin treatment failure in penicillin- and cephalosporin-resistant Streptococcus pneumoniae meningitis. Pediatr. Infect. Dis. J. 11:662-666, 1992.

692. Sloyer, J. L., Jr., Howie, V. M., Ploussard, J. H., et al.: The immune response to acute otitis media in children. I. Serotypes isolated and serum and middle ear fluid antibody in pneumococcal otitis media. Infect. Immun. 9:1028-1032, 1974.

693. Sloyer, J. L., Jr., Ploussard, J. H., and Howie, V. M.: Efficacy of pneumococcal polysaccharide vaccine in preventing acute otitis media in infants in Huntsville, Alabama. Rev. Infect. Dis. 3(Suppl.):119-123, 1981.

694. Smillie, W. G., Warnock, G. H., and White, H. J.: A study of a type 1 pneumococcus epidemic at the state hospital at Worcester, Mass. Am. J. Public Health 28:293-302, 1938.

695. Smith, A. M., and Klugman, K. P.: Non–penicillin-binding protein mediated high-level penicillin and cephalosporin resistance in a Hungarian clone of Streptococcus pneumoniae. Microb. Drug Resist. 6:105-110, 2000.

696. Smith, B. L., and Hostetter, M. K.: C3 as substrate for adhesion of Streptococcus pneumoniae. J. Infect. Dis. 182:497-508, 2000.

697. Smith, M. D., Stuart, J. R., Andrews, N. J., et al.: Invasive pneumococcal infection in south and west England. Epidemiol. Infect. 120:117-123, 1998.

698. Sniadack, D. H., Schwartz, B., Lipman, H., et al.: Potential interventions for the prevention of childhood pneumonia: Geographic and temporal differences in serotype and serogroup distribution of sterile site pneumococcal isolates from children—implications for vaccine strategies. Pediatr. Infect. Dis. J. 14:503-510, 1995.

699. Soininen, A., Lahdenkari, M., Kilpi, T., et al.: Antibody response to pneumococcal capsular polysaccharides in children with acute otitis media. Pediatr. Infect. Dis. J. 21:186-192, 2002.

700. Spangler, S. K., Jacobs, M. R., Pankuch, G. A., and Appelbaum, P. C.: Susceptibility of 170 penicillin-susceptible and penicillin-resistant pneumococci to six oral cephalosporins, four quinolones, desacetylcefotaxime, Ro 23-9424 and RP 67829. J. Antimicrob. Chemother. 31:273-280, 1993.

701. Spanjaard, L., van der Ende, A., Rumke, H., et al.: Epidemiology of meningitis and bacteraemia due to Streptococcus pneumonia in the Netherlands. Acta Paediatr. Suppl. 435:22-26, 2000.

702. Spellerberg, B., Cundell, D. R., Sandros, J., et al.: Pyruvate oxidase, as a determinant of virulence in Streptococcus pneumoniae. Mol. Microbiol. 19:803-813, 1996.

703. Spika, J. S., Halsey, N. A., Le, C. T., et al.: Decline of vaccine-induced antipneumococcal antibody in children with nephrotic syndrome. Am. J. Kidney Dis. 7:466-470, 1986.

704. Steffen, S. E., and Bryant, F. R.: Purification and characterization of the RecA protein from Streptococcus pneumoniae. Arch. Biochem. Biophys. 382:303-309, 2000.

705. Stein, K. E.: Thymus-independent and thymus-dependent responses to polysaccharide antigens. J. Infect. Dis. 165(Suppl.):49-52, 1992.

706. Stool, S. E., and Field, M. J.: The impact of otitis media. Pediatr. Infect. Dis. J. 8(Suppl.):11-14, 1989.

707. Straetemans, M., Sanders, E. A. M., Veenhoven, R. H., et al.: Review of randomized controlled trials on pneumococcal vaccination for prevention of otitis media. Pediatr. Infect. Dis. J. 22:515-524, 2003.

708. Straetemans, M., Sanders, E. A. M., Veenhoven, R. H., et al.: Pneumococcal vaccines for preventing otitis media. Cochrane Database Syst. Rev. 1: CD001480, 2004.

709. Strovall, S. H., Ainley, K. A., Mason, E. O., et al.: Invasive pneumococcal infections in pediatric cardiac transplant patients. Pediatr. Infect. Dis. J. 20:946-950, 2001.

710. Styrt, B.: Infection associated with asplenia: Risks, mechanisms, and prevention. Am. J. Med. 88:33N-42N, 1990.

711. Sutcliffe, J., Tait-Kamradt, A., and Wondrack, L.: Streptococcus pneumoniae and Streptococcus pyogenes resistant to macrolides but sensitive to clindamycin: A

common resistance pattern mediated by an efflux system. Antimicrob. Agents Chemother. *40*:1817-1824, 1996.

712. Syriopoulou, V., Daikos, G. L., Soulis, K., et al.: Epidemiology of invasive childhood pneumococcal infections in Greece. Acta Paediatr. Suppl. *435*:30-34, 2000.

713. Syrjänen, R. K., Auranen, K. J., Leino, T. M., et al.: Pneumococcal acute otitis media in relation to pneumococcal nasopharyngeal carriage. Pediatr. Infect. Dis. J. *24*:801-806, 2005.

714. Syrjänen, R., Herva, E., Leino, T., et al.: Length of nasopharyngeal carriage of pneumococci before pneumococcal acute otitis media. FinOM Study Group, National Public Health Institute. Presented at the 19th Annual Meeting of the European Society for Paediatric Infectious Diseases (ESPID), Istanbul, Turkey, 2001, p. 6.

715. Syrogiannopoulos, G. A., Grivea, I. N., Beratis, N. G., et al.: Resistance patterns of *Streptococcus pneumoniae* from carriers attending day-care centers in southwestern Greece. Clin. Infect. Dis. *25*:188-194, 1997.

716. Syrogiannopoulos, G. A., Ronchetti, F., Dagan, R., et al.: Mediterranean clone of penicillin-susceptible, multidrug-resistant serotype 6B *Streptococcus pneumoniae* in Greece, Italy and Israel. Int. J. Antimicrob. Agents *16*:219-224, 2000.

717. Tait-Kamradt, A., Davies, T., Appelbaum, P. C., et al.: Two new mechanisms of macrolide resistance in clinical strains of *Streptococcus pneumoniae* from Eastern Europe and North America. Antimicrob. Agents Chemother. *44*:3395-3401, 2000.

718. Takala, A. K., Jero, J., Kela, E., et al.: Risk factors for primary invasive pneumococcal disease among children in Finland. J. A. M. A. *273*:859-864, 1995.

719. Takoudes, T. G., and Haddad, J., Jr.: Free radical production by antibiotic-killed bacteria in the guinea pig middle ear. Laryngoscope *111*:283-289, 2001.

720. Talbot, U. M., Paton, A. W., and Paton, J. C.: Uptake of *Streptococcus pneumoniae* by respiratory epithelial cells. Infect. Immun. *64*:3772-3777, 1996.

721. Talkington, D. F., Brown, B. G., Tharpe, J. A., et al.: Protection of mice against fatal pneumococcal challenge by immunization with pneumococcal surface adhesin a (PsaA). Microb. Pathog. *21*:17-22, 1996.

722. Tan, T. Q., Mason, E. O., Barson, W. J., et al.: Clinical characteristic and outcome of children with pneumonia attributable to penicillin-susceptible and penicillin-nonsusceptible *Streptococcus pneumoniae*. Pediatrics *102*:1369-1375, 1998.

723. Tan, T. Q., Schutze, G. E., Mason, E. O., and Kaplan, S. L.: Antibiotic therapy and acute outcome of meningitis due to *Streptococcus pneumoniae* considered intermediately susceptible to broad-spectrum cephalosporins. Antimicrob. Agents Chemother. *38*:918-923, 1994.

724. Taylor, S., and Sanders, C.: Unusual manifestations of invasive pneumococcal infections. Am. J. Med. *107*(Suppl.):12-27, 1999.

725. Teele, D. W., and Klein, J. O.: Use of pneumococcal vaccine for prevention of recurrent acute otitis media in infants in Boston. Rev. Infect. Dis. *3*(Suppl.):113-118, 1981.

726. Teele, D. W., Klein, J. O., and Rosner, B. A.: Epidemiology of otitis media in children. Ann. Otol. Rhinol. Laryngol. *89*(Suppl. 68):5-6, 1980.

727. Teele, D. W., Klein, J. O., and Rosner, B. A.: Epidemiology of otitis media during the first seven years of life in children in greater Boston: A prospective, cohort study. J. Infect. Dis. *160*:83-94, 1989.

728. Teele, D. W., Pelton, S. I., Grant, M. J., et al.: Bacteremia in febrile children under 2 years of age: Results of cultures of blood of 600 consecutive febrile children seen in a "walk-in" clinic. J. Pediatr. *87*:227-230, 1975.

729. Teitelbaum, R., Lifshitz, S., Ling, E., et al.: Vulnerability to *Streptococcus pneumoniae* infection: Difference between microbial strains and genetically determined host reponse in adult mice. Abstract 983. Presented at the 41st Interscience Conference on Antimicrobial Agents and Chemotherapy, Chicago, 2001, p. 52.

730. Temple, K., Greenwood, B., Inskip, H., et al.: Antibody response to pneumococcal capsular polysaccharide vaccine in African children. Pediatr. Infect. Dis. J. *10*:386-390, 1991.

731. Therapy for children with invasive pneumococcal infections. American Academy of Pediatrics Committee on Infectious Diseases. Pediatrics *99*:289-299, 1997.

732. Thijssen, M. J., Bijkerk, M. H., Kamerling, J. P., et al.: Synthesis of four spacer-containing "tetrasaccharides" that represent four possible repeating units of the capsular polysaccharide of *Streptococcus pneumoniae* type 6B. Carbohydr. Res. *306*:111-125, 1998.

733. Thornsberry, C., Sahm, D. F., Kelly, L. J., et al.: Regional trends in antimicrobial resistance among clinical isolates of *Streptococcus pneumoniae*, *Haemophilus influenzae*, and *Moraxella catarrhalis* in the United States: Results from the TRUST Surveillance Program, 1999-2000. Clin. Infect. Dis. *34*(Suppl.):4-16, 2002.

734. Toikka, P., Virkki, R., Mertsola, J., et al.: Bacteremic pneumococcal pneumonia in children. Clin. Infect. Dis. *29*:568-572, 1999.

735. Tomasz, A.: *Streptococcus pneumoniae*: Functional anatomy. *In* Tomasz, A. (ed.): *Streptococcus pneumoniae*: Molecular Biology and Mechanisms of Disease. Larchmont, NY, Mary Ann Liebert, Inc., 2000, pp. 9-21.

736. Tong, H. H., Blue, L. E., James, M. A., et al.: Evaluation of the virulence of a *Streptococcus pneumoniae* neuraminidase-deficient mutant in nasopharyngeal colonization and development of otitis media in the chinchilla model. Infect. Immun. *68*:921-924, 2000.

737. Tong, H. H., Fisher, L. M., Kosunick, G. M., et al.: Effect of tumor necrosis factor alpha and interleukin 1-alpha on the adherence of *Streptococcus pneumoniae* to chinchilla tracheal epithelium. Acta. Otolaryngol. *119*:78-82, 1999.

738. Toppley, J. M., Cupidore, L., Vaidya, S., et al.: Pneumococcal and other infections in children with sickle cell-hemoglobin C (SC) disease. J. Pediatr. *101*:176-179, 1982.

739. Tu, A. H., Fulgham, R. L., McCrory, M. A., et al.: Pneumococcal surface protein A inhibits complement activation by *Streptococcus pneumoniae*. Infect. Immun. *67*:4720-4724, 1999.

740. Turett, G. S., Blum, S., Fazal, B. A., et al.: Penicillin resistance and other predictors of mortality in pneumococcal bacteremia in a population with high human immunodeficiency virus seroprevalence. Clin. Infect. Dis. *29*:321-327, 1999.

741. Ubukata, K., Asahi, Y., Yamane, A., et al.: Combinational detection of autolysin and penicillin-binding protein 2B genes *of Streptococcus pneumoniae* by PCR. J. Clin. Microbiol. *34*:592-596, 1996.

742. Uhari, M., Kontiokari, T., and Kiemela, M.: A novel use of xylitol sugar in preventing acute otitis media. Pediatrics *102*:879-884, 1998.

743. Uhari, M., Kontiokari, T., Koskela, M., and Niemela, M.: Xylitol chewing gum in prevention of acute otitis media: Double-blind randomized trial. B. M. J. *313*:1180-1184, 1996.

744. Uhari, M., Mantysaari, K., and Niemela, M.: A meta-analytic review of the risk factors for acute otitis media. Clin. Infect. Dis. *22*:1079-1083, 1996.

745. Ukkonen, P., Varis, K., Jernsfors, M., et al.: Treatment of acute otitis media with an antiadhesive oligosaccharide: A randomized, double-blind, placebo-controlled trial. Lancet *356*:1398-1402, 2000.

746. Umetsu, D. T., Ambrosino, D. M., Quinti, I., et al.: Recurrent sinopulmonary infection and impaired antibody response to bacterial capsular polysaccharide antigen in children with selective IgG subclass deficiency. N. Engl. J. Med. *313*:1247-1251, 1985.

747. Usen, S., Adegbola, R., Mulholland, K., et al.: Epidemiology of invasive pneumococcal disease in the Western Region, The Gambia. Pediatr. Infect. Dis. J. *17*:23-28, 1998.

748. Ussery, X. T., Gessner, B. D., Lipman, H., et al.: Risk factors for nasopharyngeal carriage of resistant *Streptococcus pneumoniae* and detection of a multiply resistant clone among children living in the Yukon-Kuskokwin Delta Region of Alaska. Pediatr. Infect. Dis. J. *15*:986-992, 1996.

749. Väkeväinen, M., Eklund, C., Eskola, J., and Käyhty, H.: Cross-reactivity of antibodies to pneumococcal capsular polysaccharides of seroypes 6A and 6B evoked by different pneumococcal conjugate vaccines. J. Infect. Dis. *184*:789-793, 2001.

750. Väkeväinen, M., Jansen, W., Saeland, E., et al.: Are the opsonic activities of antibodies in infant sera measured by different pneumococcal phagocytic assays comparable? Clin. Diagn. Lab. Immunol. *8*:363-369, 2001.

751. Vanderkooi, O. G., Low, D. E., Green, K., et al.: Predicting antimicrobial resistance in invasive pneumococcal infections. Clin. Infect. Dis. *40*:1288-1297, 2005.

752. Van Zuijlen, D. A., Schilder, A. G. M., Van Balen, F. A. M., and Hoes, A. W.: National differences in incidence of acute mastoiditis: Relationship to prescribing patterns of antibiotics for acute otitis media? Pediatr. Infect. Dis. J. *20*:140-144, 2001.

753. Varon, E., Levy, C., De La Rocque, F., et al.: Impact of antimicrobial therapy on nasopharyngeal carriage of *Streptococcus pneumoniae*, *Haemophilus influenzae*, and *Branhamella catarrhalis* in children with respiratory tract infections. Clin. Infect. Dis. *31*:477-481, 2000.

754. Vernacchio, L., Neurfeld, E. J., MacDonald, K., et al.: Combined schedule of 7-valent pneumococcal conjugate vaccine followed by 23-valent pneumococcal vaccine in children and young adults with sickle cell disease. J. Pediatr. *133*:275-278, 1998.

755. Vidarsson, G., Sugurdardottir, S., Gudnason, T., et al.: Isotypes and opsonophagocytosis of pneumococcus type 6B antibodies elicited in infants and adults by an experimental pneumococcccus type 6B–tetanus toxoid vaccine. Infect. Immun. *66*:2866-2870, 1998.

756. Viladrich, P. F., Gudiol, F., Linares, J., et al.: Evaluation of vancomycin for therapy of adult pneumococcal meningitis. Antimicrob. Agents Chemother. *35*:2467-2472, 1991.

757. Vives, M., Garcia, M. E., Saenz, P., et al.: Nasopharyngeal colonization in Costa Rican children during the first year of life. Pediatr. Infect. Dis. J. *16*:852-858, 1997.

758. Vollmer, W., and Tomasz, A.: The pgdA gene encodes for a peptidoglycan N-acetylglucosamine deacetylase in *Streptococcus pneumoniae*. J. Biol. Chem. *275*:20496-20501, 2000.

759. Vollmer, W., and Tomasz, A.: Identification of the teichoic acid phosphorylcholine esterase in *Streptococcus pneumoniae*. Mol. Microbiol. *39*:1610-1622, 2001.

760. Voss, L., Lennon, D., Okesene-Gafa, K., et al.: Invasive pneumococcal disease in a pediatric population, Auckland, New Zealand. Pediatr. Infect. Dis. J. *13*:873-878, 1994.

761. Vuori-Holopainen, E., and Peltola, H.: Reappraisal of lung tap: Review of an old method for better etiologic diagnosis of childhood pneumonia. Clin. Infect. Dis. *32*:715-726, 2001.

762. Vuori-Holopainen, E., Salo, E., Saxén, H., et al.: Etiological diagnosis of childhood pneumonia by use of transthoracic needle aspiration and modern microbiological methods. Clin. Infect. Dis. *34*:583-590, 2002.

763. Wadowsky, R. M., Mietzner, S. M., Skoner, D. P., et al.: Effect of experimental influenza A virus infection on isolation of *Streptococcus pneumoniae* and other aerobic bacteria from the oropharynges of allergic and nonallergic adult subjets. Infect. Immun. *63*:1153-1157, 1995.

764. Wald, E. R.: Conjunctivitis in infants and children. Pediatr. Infect. Dis. J. *16*(Suppl.):17-20, 1997.

765. Wald, E. R.: Diagnosis and management of sinusitis in children. Semin. Pediatr. Infect. Dis. *9*:4-11, 1998.

766. Wald, E. R., Chiponis, D., and Ledesma-Medina, J.: Comparative effectiveness of amoxicillin and amoxicillin-clavulanate potassium in acute paranasal sinus infections in children: A double-blind, placebo-controlled trial. Pediatrics 77:795-800, 1986.

767. Wald, E. R., Milmoe, G. J., Bowen, A., et al.: Acute maxillary sinusitis in children. N. Engl. J. Med. *304*:749-754, 1981.

768. Wall, R. A., Corrah, P. T., Mabey, D. C. W., and Greenwood, B. M.: The etiology of lobar pneumonia in The Gambia. Bull. World Health Organ. *64*:553-558, 1986.

769. Wara, D. W.: Host defense against *Streptococcus pneumoniae*: The role of the spleen. Rev. Infect. Dis. *3*:299-309, 1981.

770. Wasier, A. P., Chevret, L., Essouri, S., et al.: Pneumococcal meningitis in a pediatric intensive care unit: Prognostic factors in a series of 49 children. Pediatr. Crit. Care *6*:568-572, 2005.

771. Watanabe, H., Sato, S., Kwakami, K., et al.: A comparative clinical study of pneumonia by penicillin-resistant and -sensitive *Streptococcus pneumoniae* in a community hospital. Respirology *5*:59-64, 2000.

772. Watanakunakorn, C., and Bailey, T. A.: Adult bacteremic pneumococcal pneumonia in a community teaching hospital, 1992-1996. A detailed analysis of 108 cases. Arch. Intern. Med. *157*:1965-1971, 1997.

773. Waterer, G. W., Jennings, S. G., and Wunderink, R. G.: The impact of blood cultures on antibiotic therapy in pneumococcal pneumonia. Chest *116*:1278-1281, 1999.

774. Watson, D. A., Musher, D. M., and Jacobson, J. W.: A brief history of the pneumococcus in biomedical research: A panoply of discovery. Clin. Infect. Dis. *17*:913-924, 1993.

775. Weber, B., Ehlert, K., Diehl, A., et al.: The fib locus in *Streptococcus pneumoniae* is required for peptidoglycan crosslinking and PBP-mediated beta-lactam resistance. F. E. M. S. Microbiol. Lett. *188*:81-85, 2000.

776. Weiser, J. N.: Phase variation in colony opacity by *Streptococcus pneumoniae*. Microb. Drug Resist. *4*:129-135, 1998.

777. Weiss, A., Brinser, J. H., and Nazar-Stewart, V.: Acute conjunctivitis in childhood. J. Pediatr. *122*:10-14, 1993.

778. White, B.: The Biology of Pneumococcus. Cambridge, MA, Commonwealth Fund, Harvard University Press, 1938.

779. Whitney, C. G., Farley, M. M., Hadler, J., et al.: Increasing prevalence of multidrug-resistant *Streptococcus pneumoniae* in the United States. N. Engl. J. Med. *343*:1917-1924, 2000.

780. Whitney, C. G., Farley, M. M., Hadler, J., et al.: Decline in invasive pneumococcal disease in the US in 2000: An effect on pneumococcal conjugate vaccine? Abstract G-2041. Presented at the 41st Interscience Conference on Antimicrobial Agents and Chemotherapy (ICAAC), Chicago, 2001, p. 284.

781. Whitney, C. G., Pilishvili, T., Farley, M. M., et al.: Effectiveness of seven-valent pneumococcal conjugate vaccine against invasive pneumococcal disease: A matched case control study. Lancet *368*:1495-1502, 2006.

782. Widdowson, C. A., and Klugman, K.: Molecular mechanisms of resistance to commonly used non–beta-lactam drugs in *Streptococcus pneumoniae*. Semin. Respir. Infect. *14*:255-268, 1999.

783. Williams, R. L., Chalmers, T. C., Stange, D. C., et al.: Use of antibiotics in preventing recurrent acute otitis media and in treating otitis media with effusion. A meta-analytic attempt to resolve the brouhaha. J. A. M. A. *370*:1344-1351, 1993.

784. Winkelstein, J. A., and Drachman, R. H.: Deficiency of pneumococcal serum opsonizing activity in sickle cell disease. N. Engl. J. Med. *279*:459-466, 1968.

785. Wise, R. P., Iskander, J., Pratt, R. D., et al.: Postlicensure safety surveillance for 7-valent pneumococcal conjugate vaccine. J. A. M. A. *292*:1702-1710, 2004.

786. Witt, C. S., Pomat, W., Lehmann, D., and Alpers, M. P.: Antibodies to pneumococcal polysaccharides in pneumonia and response to pneumococcal vaccination in young children in Papua New Guinea. Clin. Exp. Immunol. *83*:219-224, 1991.

787. Wizemann, T. M., Heinrichs, J. H., Adamou, J. E., et al.: Use of a whole genome approach to identify vaccine molecules affording protection against *Streptococcus pneumoniae* infection. Infect. Immun. *69*:1593-1598, 2001.

788. Wong, W. Y., Overturf, G. D., and Powars, D. R.: Infection caused by *Streptococcus pneumoniae* in children with sickle cell disease: Epidemiology, immunologic mechanisms, prophylaxis, and vaccination. Clin. Infect. Dis. *14*:1124-1136, 1992.

789. Wright, A. E., Morgan, W. P., Colebrook, L., et al.: Observations on prophylactic inoculation against pneumococcus infections, and on the results which have been achieved by it. Lancet *1*:87-95, 1914.

790. Wu, T.-T., Hsueh, P.-R., Lee, L.-N., et al.: Pneumonia caused by penicillin-nonsusceptible *Streptococcus pneumoniae*: Clinical characteristics, prognostic factors, and outcomes. J. Formos. Med. Assoc. *99*:18-23, 2000.

791. Yagupsky, P., Porat, N., Fraser, D., et al.: Acquisition, carriage and transmission of pneumococci with decreased antibiotic susceptibility in young children attending a day care facility in southern Israel. J. Infect. Dis. *177*:1003-1012, 1998.

792. Yamamoto, L. G.: Revising the decision analysis for febrile children at risk for occult bacteremia in a future era of widespread pneumococcal immunization. Clin. Pediatr. (Phila.) *40*:583-594, 2001.

793. Yee, C. L., Duffy, C., Gerbino, P. G., et al.: Tendon or joint disorders in children after treatment with floroquinolones or azithromycin. Pediatr. Infect. Dis. J. *21*:525-529, 2002.

794. Yother, J., Leopold, K., White, J., et al.: Generation and properties of a *Streptococcus pneumoniae* mutant which does not require choline or analogs for growth. J. Bacteriol. *180*:2093-2101, 1998.

795. Yother, J., and White, J. M.: Novel surface attachment mechanism of the *Streptococcus pneumoniae* protein PspA. J. Bacteriol. *176*:2976-2985, 1994.

796. Yu, J., Bryant, A. P., Marra, A., et al.: Characterization of the *Streptococcus pneumoniae* NADH oxidase that is required for infection. Microbiology *147*:431-438, 2001.

797. Zangwill, K. M., Vadheim, C. M., Vannier, A. M., et al.: Epidemiology of invasive pneumococcal disease in Southern California: Implications for the design and conduct of a pneumccoccal conjugate vaccine efficacy trial. J. Infect. Dis. *174*:752-759, 1996.

798. Zarkowsky, H. S., Gallagher, D., Gill, F. M., et al.: Bacteremia in sickle hemoglobinopathies. J. Pediatr. *109*:579-585, 1986.

799. Zenni, M. K., Cheatham, S. H., Thompson, J. M., et al.: *Streptococcus pneumoniae* colonization in the young child: Association with otitis media and resistance to penicillin. J. Pediatr. *127*:533-537, 1995.

800. Zhang, J. R., Mostov, K. E., Lamm, M. E., et al.: The polymeric immunoglobulin receptor translocates pneumococci across human nasopharyngeal epithelial cells. Cell *102*:827-837, 2000.

801. Zhang, Q., Arnaoutakis, K., Murdoch, C., et al.: Mucosal immune responses to capsular pneumococcal polysaccharides in immunized preschool children and controls with similar nasal pneumococcal colonization rates. Pediatr. Infect. Dis. J. *23*:307-313, 2004.

802. Zhang, Y., Masi, A. W., Barniak, V., et al.: Recombinant PhpA protein, a unique histidine motif–containing protein from *Streptococcus pneumoniae*, protects mice against intranasal pneumococcal challenge. Infect. Immun. *69*:3827-3836, 2001.

803. Zopf, D., and Roth, S.: Oligosaccharide anti-infective agents. Lancet *347*:1017-1021, 1996.

804. Zwijnenburg, P. J., van der Poll, T., Florquin, S., et al.: Experimental pneumococcal meningitis in mice: A model of intranasal infection. J. Infect. Dis. *183*:1143-1146, 2001.

805. Zysk, G., Bongaerts, R. J., ten Thoren, E., et al.: Detection of 23 immunogenic pneumococcal proteins using convalescent-phase serum. Infect. Immun. *68*:3740-3743, 2000.

806. Zysk, G., Schneider-Wald, B. K., Hwang, J. H., et al.: Pneumolysin is the main inducer of cytotoxicity to brain microvascular endothelial cells caused by *Streptococcus pneumoniae*. Infect. Immun. *69*:845-852, 2001.

CHAPTER

97

MISCELLANEOUS GRAM-POSITIVE COCCI

Randall G. Fisher

This chapter discusses relatively uncommon gram-positive cocci that are of importance because of their unusual antimicrobial sensitivities and because of their increasing recognition as pathogens in hospitalized patients. The reader is referred to a review of these organisms for more details.[16]

LEUCONOSTOC SPECIES

BACTERIOLOGY

Leuconostoc spp. are facultatively anaerobic, gram-positive cocci that usually appear in pairs or chains. They are catalase-negative,

Vogues-Proskauer–positive, and leucine aminopeptidase–positive. In addition, colonies often are alpha-hemolytic on blood agar and also may react with group D streptococcal antiserum. These properties are shared by viridans streptococci, with which *Leuconostoc* spp. often are confused.[18] They also may resemble enterococci, except that they are pyrrolidone carboxylyl peptidase–negative. Differences include the production of gas from glucose and high-level vancomycin resistance.

EPIDEMIOLOGY

Leuconostoc spp. are found commonly on plants, especially sugar cane and leafy vegetables. They also are present in dairy products and wine.[44] They are used in the food industry as starter cultures in food production.[30,55] Studies using culture methods have suggested that, although they occasionally are recovered from vaginal swabs in healthy individuals[48] and from mucosal surfaces in some hospitalized individuals,[26] *Leuconostoc* spp. are not part of the normal human flora.[3] However, a study of the acquisition of colonizing bacteria in the newborn gut involving phylogenetic analysis of 16S recombinant DNA sequences showed that *Leuconostoc citreum* generally was acquired by newborns on their first day of life. Case reports of pediatric infection began to appear in the 1980s.[12,27,29,41,60]

PATHOPHYSIOLOGY

Leuconostocs rarely are pathogenic. Underlying disease states or compromised immune system, gastrointestinal tract disease (especially short-gut syndrome), previous or current antibiotic therapy, venous or gastrointestinal tract access devices, recent invasive procedures, and infancy are thought to be risk factors.[14,15,26,44] Frequently, leuconostocs are isolated as part of a polymicrobial infection after a patient has been treated with vancomycin.[16] Of the first 21 cases reported in the English literature, 12 were in children, 10 of which occurred in patients younger than 1 year old. Documented portals of entry include central lines,[3,27] peritoneal dialysis and urinary catheters,[6] and gastrostomy tubes.[29] Contaminated enteral formula also has been implicated.[7,29,39] Occasional sporadic cases without a known risk factor have been described,[12,26] which underscores the pathogenic potential of *Leuconostoc* infection.

CLINICAL MANIFESTATIONS

Bacteremia, heralded by fever and usually leukocytosis in patients with the risk factors outlined earlier, is by far the most common clinical manifestation of *Leuconostoc* infection. Gastrointestinal disturbances, especially diarrhea, are common manifestations.[3] Infants are prone to emesis. *Leuconostoc* bacteremia, in association with cough and chest x-ray findings consistent with pneumonia, was reported in a child with acquired immunodeficiency syndrome (AIDS).[44] *L. citreum* has been isolated from the lung tissue of a 33-year-old patient with AIDS who also had *Pneumocystis carinii* pneumonia.[21] Small necrotic cavities scattered through both lungs were associated with gram-positive cocci in tissue. Patients with dental infections,[60] peritonitis,[22] osteomyelitis,[37] and meningitis[12,19] also have been described. Meningitis has been reported in an otherwise healthy 16-year-old patient and in a neonate with fatal infection despite high cerebrospinal fluid (CSF) bactericidal antibiotic titers.[12,19] A nosocomial cluster of five cases of urinary tract infection caused by *Leuconostoc pseudomesenteroides* (strictly a species of a new genus, *Weissella*)[11] has been reported,[6] as has a cluster of three cases of *Leuconostoc* septicemia in critically ill postsurgical patients.[51]

DIAGNOSIS

Cultures usually are positive within 24 to 48 hours. Leuconostocs are somewhat fastidious. Identification of vancomycin-resistant *Streptococcus* should raise suspicion of *Leuconostoc* infection and prompt additional biochemical studies,[44] including evaluation for the production of gas in MRS broth, failure to hydrolyze arginine, and delayed esculin hydrolysis.

TREATMENT

Treatment with relatively high doses of penicillin or ampicillin frequently is successful in eradicating infection. When possible, access devices should be removed. Leuconostocs are most sensitive to the primitive β-lactam antibiotics, especially penicillin and ampicillin, although penicillin tolerance is a common finding.[29,57] They also frequently are sensitive to erythromycin, cephalothin, and the aminoglycosides. *Leuconostoc* spp. are variably resistant to clindamycin and trimethoprim-sulfamethoxazole. Resistance increases with later generations of cephalosporins.[26,57] *Leuconostoc* spp. are intrinsically vancomycin-resistant because their pentapeptide cell wall precursors end in D-Ala-lactate rather than the usual D-Ala-alanine.[25] Vancomycin cannot bind the lactate. This mode of resistance is the same as that possessed by vancomycin-resistant enterococci. However, whereas resistance in enterococci is plasmid derived and transferable, in leuconostocs it is chromosomally mediated, constitutional, and not transferable.

PEDIOCOCCUS SPECIES

BACTERIOLOGY

Pediococci also are intrinsically vancomycin-resistant, facultatively anaerobic gram-positive cocci. They appear most characteristically in tetrads on Gram stain, although they may appear in pairs or clusters.[23] The genus name *Pediococcus* is derived from the Greek word *pedium*, which means "plane." The name, therefore, suggests that they are a genus of cocci that grow in a single plane. It is a misnomer, however, because pediococci are the only lactic acid bacteria that divide in two planes.[20] They are catalase- and oxidase-negative. They do not reduce nitrates, and no gas is produced in MRS broth.[53] They are pyrrolidone carboxylyl peptidase–negative.[16] Most isolates react with Lancefield group D streptococcal antibodies.[53] They are leucine aminopeptidase–positive, which distinguishes them from *Leuconostoc* spp.[17] They produce white, opaque, nonhemolytic colonies on sheep's blood agar. A new broth medium, a combination of 90 percent Iso-Sensitest broth and 10 percent deMan-Rogosa-Sharpe broth and called LAB susceptibility test medium, has been found to provide optimal support of growth and to yield the most accurate minimal inhibitory concentration values.[33]

Pediococci produce powerful bacteriocins, which are substances that kill other bacteria. The bacteriocins of pediococci are active against other gram-positive organisms in particular[10] but also are active against *Clostridium botulinum* spores,[40] some gram-negative organisms,[54] and *Listeria monocytogenes*. Reports have suggested that some species of *Pediococcus* have antifungal activity[35]; however, this activity in other studies has been found to be present only at low pH and has been attributed to acetic acid in the medium.[5]

EPIDEMIOLOGY

Like leuconostocs and other lactic acid bacteria, pediococci are found on plants, in dairy products, and in alcohol-containing beverages, where certain species are associated with spoilage.[58] They also are used in the formation of silage[53] and as starter cultures for some meat products. They are not thought to be part of the normal flora. They have been isolated from saliva and stool on rare occasion.[49] Though formerly thought to be nonpathogenic, they now are considered rare opportunistic pathogens with minimal virulence.

PATHOPHYSIOLOGY

Pediococci rarely are pathogenic. Many cases of blood isolates are found in patients without symptoms of infection or in polymicrobial cultures in which the significance of the isolate could not be assessed adequately.[36] One patient with a clinical picture of septic shock in whom the only organism recovered was *Pediococcus pentosaceus* has been reported.[13] Risk factors for bacteremia, with or without symptoms, appear to be the extremes of age, recent abdominal surgery or tube feeding, broad-spectrum antimicrobial therapy, and the presence of severe underlying disease states.[36] However, because the overall number of reported cases is small, the relative risks of these factors are uncertain.

CLINICAL MANIFESTATIONS AND DIAGNOSIS

Most patients either are asymptomatic or have fever as the only symptom. Six of the first 12 reported cases of *Pediococcus* bacteremia had concomitant pneumonia. Fifty-six percent of adult patients either were receiving tube feeding or had undergone abdominal surgery within 30 days of isolation of the organism.[36] The three reported pediatric cases occurred in infants, and all had underlying gastrointestinal tract anomalies. A 16-day-old infant with congenital jejunoileal atresia had undergone surgical repair just 8 days before being evaluated.[36] Her acute illness was characterized by emesis and a 200-g weight loss. She was afebrile when initially examined. The second patient was a 64-day-old infant with gastroschisis who had undergone two abdominal surgical procedures.[1] His fever reached 101.5° F, and his peripheral white blood cell count was 38,000 with a significant left shift. The third patient was a 3-month-old girl who had undergone surgical repair of gastroschisis on the first day of life.[2] Lethargy, direct hyperbilirubinemia, and a CSF pleocytosis were noted. Blood cultures grew *Pediococcus* spp., and the spinal fluid (obtained after initiation of antibiotics) was sterile. She responded to a 21-day course of ampicillin and gentamicin.

Pediococci are isolated frequently in localized infections, especially from abdominal sites, but they are virtually always part of a polymicrobial process. The relative importance of pediococci in these sites is difficult to assess. A case of *Pediococcus* bacteremic pneumonia was reported in a previously healthy pregnant woman.[50] Among 31 cases of *Pediococcus* infection submitted to the Centers for Disease Control and Prevention laboratory, 17 were from blood culture isolates (including 2 reported cases of endocarditis), and 4 strains were associated with urinary tract infections. Other sources included catheter tips, wounds, peritoneal fluid, CSF, lung, and bone.[16]

Diagnosis of infection with pediococci is established by identifying catalase-negative, vancomycin-resistant, gram-positive cocci in the characteristic tetrads. Many pediococci are misidentified initially as *Streptococcus equinus*, *Streptococcus constellatus*, or group D *Streptococcus*, not *Enterococcus*. Reported cases of pediococcal infection may, therefore, represent only a fraction of the total number of infections.

TREATMENT

Pediococci generally are susceptible to penicillin, ampicillin, imipenem, clindamycin, and first- and second-generation cephalosporins. Although both imipenem and penicillin are highly active against pediococci, they do not appear to be bactericidal. Pediococci are moderately resistant to the quinolones, tetracycline,[58] and trimethoprim-sulfamethoxazole.[47] Pediococci, like leuconostocs, are intrinsically resistant to vancomycin. Resistance is not plasmid-mediated, nor can it be transferred to other bacteria.[58] Sensitivity to ticarcillin and cefotaxime, when measured by agar dilution, is poor despite large zones of inhibition on disk susceptibility testing.[58] Occasionally, inducible resistance to erythromycin is found, although most isolates remain sensitive. Aminoglycoside sensitivity is variable.

AEROCOCCUS SPECIES

BACTERIOLOGY

The genus *Aerococcus* contains at least five species, but only two, *viridans* and *urinae*, have known clinical significance. In earlier papers, *A. urinae* was referred to as *Aerococcus*-like organism, or ALO.[9] Aerococci are catalase-negative, nonmotile, gram-positive cocci that appear preferentially in tetrads but sometimes in pairs or clusters. These relatively slow-growing organisms produce small, well-delineated, translucent, alpha-hemolytic colonies on blood agar.[8] They also are weakly bile esculin–positive and pyrrolidone carboxylyl peptidase–negative. They ferment mannose and mannitol.[45] Like enterococci, most aerococci will grow in 6.5 percent salt.[34]

EPIDEMIOLOGY

Aerococci are distributed throughout the world and are contaminants of air and dust.[28] They also have been found on meat, on raw vegetables, and in small numbers on human skin.[4] In hospitals, aerococci have been cultured from all areas, including operating suites and delivery rooms.[31] They also are found in salt water, where they cause a fatal disease in lobsters.[42]

Disease in humans is an uncommon event, and the organism usually is recovered from the bloodstream of patients with infective endocarditis. Most patients are elderly, but infection of infants and neonates also has been reported.[38,42] A rapidly fatal bacteremia has been described in patients with profound neutropenia.[32]

PATHOPHYSIOLOGY

In most circumstances, aerococci are saprophytic. The exact conditions that favor the development of infection have not been elucidated clearly. Some cases of *A. urinae* infection have occurred after genitourinary tract surgery. One case of septic arthritis developed after an elective abortion.[59] Immunocompromised patients are at higher risk, but infection in otherwise well persons has been described.[45] One report of meningitis in newborns found adherence of aerococci to inflammatory cells and suggested a role of as-yet-undefined adhesion factors.[38] Work in laboratory animals also has shown that a protease isolated from *A. viridans* cleaves the hemagglutinin of influenza virus and potentiates both viral replication and disease in mice.[52]

CLINICAL MANIFESTATIONS

Most cases of *A. viridans* bacteremia have been found in association with signs and symptoms of subacute infective endocarditis, although septic emboli and cardiac failure have not been described. In a recent series of four cases of *A. viridans* infective endocarditis, two of the patients required surgical intervention.[46] *A. urinae* causes urinary tract infection with dysuria and frequency, usually in the absence of fever.[8] *Aerococcus* infection in childhood is an uncommon occurrence. One case of bacteremia in a 1-month-old infant has been reported.[42] The patient had a 2-day history of loose stools, irritability, and drowsiness and on physical examination was noted to have mottled skin, circumoral cyanosis, and agitation. CSF and urine were normal, but blood cultures exhibited pure growth of *A. viridans*. No predisposing factors were identified.

Nathavitharana and associates[38] reported three cases of meningitis caused by *A. viridans*: a 7-month-old girl with jerking movements of the extremities, irritability, and a bulging fontanelle; a 5-month-old girl with fever, decreased appetite, and generalized convulsions; and a 24-month-old girl whose illness was manifested as fever, vomiting, and the neurologic signs of truncal ataxia, flaccidity, and hypoactive deep-tendon reflexes. All three patients had elevated CSF white blood cell counts with 55 to 93 percent segmented forms. Remarkably, all these patients had a history of prolonged illness (1 week to 2 months) before being evaluated, in contrast to patients with other causes of bacterial meningitis. No risk factors for infection were identified in any of these patients, who were thought to have normal immune function.

Swanson and colleagues[56] reported a case of penicillin-resistant *A. viridans* bacteremia in an 11-month-old girl receiving prophylactic penicillin for sickle-cell disease. The patient responded clinically to a 10-day course of therapy with cephalosporins.

Bone and joint infections and wound or other localized infections are exceedingly rare occurrences and not distinguishable from similar syndromes caused by more common organisms.

DIAGNOSIS

Careful observation of both appearance on Gram stain and growth in culture is key to establishing the diagnosis of aerococcal infection. On Gram stain, aerococci resemble staphylococci. On blood agar, they resemble viridans group streptococci. One series revealed that 1 percent of 719 cultures called streptococci actually were aerococci[43]; another study reclassified 3 percent of 168 cultures.[4] In one study of 24 alpha-hemolytic, nonenterococcal bacterial isolates from urine, standard identification methods were compared with 16S rRNA sequencing and special biochemical profiling. Thirteen of the isolates were aerococci; all were identified correctly by sequencing, but typical procedures failed to differentiate them from nonaerococcal isolates. Ciprofloxacin and trimethoprim susceptibility and the ability to grow at 45° C improved the discrimination of standard testing.[24] In their propensity toward tetrad formation, they mimic pediococci. However, all aerococci are vancomycin-sensitive. In their bile esculin hydrolysis and growth in 6.5 percent salt, they resemble enterococci; unlike enterococci, however, aerococci are pyrrolidone carboxylyl peptidase–negative and do not form chains.

TREATMENT

Aerococci generally are sensitive to penicillin, ampicillin, the cephalosporins, chloramphenicol, and the macrolides. They usually are intermediately susceptible or resistant to sulfonamides and aminoglycosides.[4,28] One report suggests that *A. viridans* and *A. urinae* have distinct antibiograms[34]; that is, *A. urinae* is more sensitive to penicillin and resistant to sulfonamides, whereas *A. viridans* is more resistant to penicillin and sensitive to the sulfonamides.[4] Individual case reports do not confirm these in vitro observations, and no large clinical trials of antimicrobial susceptibility have been conducted.

Acknowledgments

The author would like to thank Dr. William Gruber and Dr. Thomas Boyce for their invaluable assistance with earlier versions of this chapter.

REFERENCES

1. Atkins, J. T., Tillman, J., Tan, T. Q., et al.: *Pediococcus pentosaceus* catheter-associated infection an infant with gastroschisis. Pediatr. Infect. Dis. J. *13*:75-76, 1994.
2. Barton, L. L., Rider, E. D., and Coen, R. W.: Bacteremic infection with *Pediococcus*: Vancomycin-resistant opportunist. Pediatrics *107*:775-776, 2001.
3. Bernaldo de Quiros, J. C., Munoz, P., Cercenado, E., et al.: *Leuconostoc* species as a cause of bacteremia: Two case reports and a literature review. Eur. J. Clin. Microbiol. Infect. Dis. *10*:505-509, 1991.
4. Buu-Hoi, A., Branger, C., and Acar, J. F.: Vancomycin-resistant streptococci or *Leuconostoc* sp. Antimicrob. Agents Chemother. *28*:458-460, 1985.
5. Cabo, M. L., Braber, A. F., and Koenraad, P. M.: Apparent antifungal activity of several lactic acid bacteria against *Penicillium* discolor is due to acetic acid in the medium. J. Food Prot. *65*:1309-1316, 2002.
6. Cappelli, E. A., Barros, R. R., Camello, T. C., et al.: *Leuconostoc pseudomesenteroides* as a cause of nosocomial urinary tract infections. J. Clin. Microbiol. *37*:4124-4126, 1999.
7. Carapetis, J., Bishop, S., Davis, J., et al.: *Leuconostoc* sepsis in association with continuous enteral feeding: Two case reports and a review. Pediatr. Infect. Dis. J. *13*:816-823, 1994.
8. Christensen, J. J., Gutschik, E., Friis-Moller, A., et al.: Urosepticemia and fatal endocarditis caused by aerococcus-like organisms. Scand. J. Infect. Dis. *23*:717-721, 1991.
9. Christensen, J. J., Vibits, H., Ursing, J., et al.: *Aerococcus*-like organism, a newly recognized potential urinary tract pathogen. J. Clin. Microbiol. *29*:1049-1053, 1991.
10. Cintas, L. M., Rodriguez, J. M., Fernandez, M. F., et al.: Isolation and characterization of pediocin L50, a new bacteriocin from *Pediococcus acidilactici* with a broad inhibitory spectrum. Appl. Environ. Microbiol. *61*:2643-2648, 1995.
11. Collins, M. D., Samulis, J., Metaxopoulos, J., and Wallbanks, S.: Taxonomic studies on some *Leuconostoc*-like organisms from fermented sausages: Description of a new genus *Weissella* for the *Leuconostoc paramesenteroides* group of species. J. Appl. Bacteriol. *75*:595-603, 1993.
12. Coovadia, Y. M., Solwa, Z., and van den Ende, J.: Meningitis caused by vancomycin-resistant *Leuconostoc* sp. J. Clin. Microbiol. *25*:1784-1785, 1987.
13. Corcoran, G. D., Gibbons, N., and Mulvihill, T. E.: Septicaemia caused by *Pediococcus pentosaceus*: A new opportunistic pathogen. J. Infect. *23*:179-182, 1991.
14. Dhodapkar, K. M., and Henry, N. K.: *Leuconostoc* bacteremia in an infant with short-gut syndrome: Case report and literature review. Mayo Clin. Proc. *71*:1171-1174, 1996.
15. Espinoza, R., Kusne, S., Pasculle, A. W., et al.: *Leuconostoc* bacteremia after liver transplantation: Another cause of vancomycin resistant gram-positive infection. Clin. Transplant. *11*:322-324, 1997.
16. Facklam, R., and Elliott, J. A.: Identification, classification, and clinical relevance of catalase-negative, gram-positive cocci, excluding the streptococci and enterococci. Clin. Microbiol. Rev. *8*:479-495, 1995.
17. Facklam, R., Hollis, D., and Collins, M. D.: Identification of gram-positive coccal and coccobacillary vancomycin-resistant bacteria. J. Clin. Microbiol. *27*:724-730, 1989.
18. Facklam, R., Pigott, N., Franklin, R., et al.: Evaluation of three disk tests for identification of enterococci, leuconostocs, and pediococci. J. Clin. Microbiol. *33*:885-887, 1995.
19. Friedland, I. R., Snipelisky, M., and Khoosal, M.: Meningitis in a neonate caused by *Leuconostoc* sp. J. Clin. Microbiol. *28*:2125-2126, 1990.
20. Garvie, E. I.: Genus *Pediococcus*. In Sneath, P. H. A., Mair, N. S., Sharpe, M. E., and Holt, J. G. (eds.): Vol 2. Baltimore, The Williams & Wilkins Co., Bergey's Manual of Systematic Bacteriology. 1984, pp 1075-1079.
21. Giacometti, A., Ranaldi, R., Siquini, F. M., et al.: *Leuconostoc citreum* isolated from lung in AIDS patient. Lancet *342*:622, 1993.

22. Gillespie, R. S., Symons, J. M., and McDonald, R. A.: Peritonitis due to *Leuconostoc* species in a child receiving peritoneal dialysis. Pediatr. Nephrol. *17*:966-968, 2002.
23. Green, M., Barbadora, K., and Michaels, M.: Recovery of vancomycin-resistant gram-positive cocci from pediatric liver transplant recipients. J. Clin. Microbiol. *29*:2503-2506, 1991.
24. Grude, N., Jenkins, A., Tveten, Y., and Kristiansen, B. E.: Identification of *Aerococcus urinae* in urine samples. Clin. Microbiol. Infect. *9*:976-979, 2003.
25. Handwerger, S., Horowitz, H., Coburn, K., et al.: Infection due to *Leuconostoc* species: Six cases and review. Rev. Infect. Dis. *12*:602-610, 1990.
26. Handwerger, S., Pucci, M. J., Volk, K. J., et al.: Vancomycin-resistant *Leuconostoc mesenteroides* and *Lactobacillus casei* synthesize cytoplasmic peptidoglycan precursors that terminate in lactate. J. Bacteriol. *176*:260-264, 1994.
27. Hardy, S., Ruoff, K. L., Catlin, E. A., et al.: Catheter-associated infection with a vancomycin-resistant gram-positive coccus of the *Leuconostoc* sp. Pediatr. Infect. Dis. J. *7*:519-520, 1988.
28. Heilesen, A. M.: Septicaemia due to *Aerococcus urinae*. Scand. J. Infect. Dis. *26*:759-760, 1994.
29. Isenberg, H. D., Vellozzi, E. M., Shapiro, J., et al.: Clinical laboratory challenges in the recognition of *Leuconostoc* spp. J. Clin. Microbiol. *26*:479-483, 1988.
30. Jeppesen, V. F., and Huss, H. H.: Characteristics and antagonistic activity of lactic acid bacteria isolated from chilled fish products. Int. J. Food Microbiol. *18*:305-320, 1993.
31. Kerbaugh, M. A., and Evans, J. B.: *Aerococcus viridans* in the hospital environment. Appl. Microbiol. *16*:519-523, 1968.
32. Kern, W., and Vanek, E.: Aerococcus bacteremia associated with granulocytopenia. Eur. J. Clin. Microbiol. *6*:670-673, 1987.
33. Klare, I., Konstabel, C., Muller-Bertling, S., et al.: Evaluation of a new broth media for microdilution antibiotic susceptibility testing of lactobacilli, pediococci, lactococci, and bifidobacteria. Appl. Environ. Microbiol. *71*:8982-8986, 2005.
34. Kristensen, B., and Nielsen, G.: Endocarditis caused by *Aerococcus urinae*, a newly recognized pathogen. Eur. J. Clin. Microbiol. Infect. Dis. *14*:49-51, 1995.
35. Magnusson, J., Strom, K, Roos, S., et al.: Broad and complex antifungal activity among environmental isolates of lactic acid bacteria. F. E. M. S. Microbiol. Lett. *14*:126-135, 2003.
36. Mastro, T. D., Spika, J. S., Lozano, P., et al.: Vancomycin-resistant *Pediococcus acidilactici*: Nine cases of bacteremia. J. Infect. Dis. *161*:956-960, 1990.
37. Mulford, J. S., and Mills, J.: Osteomyelitis caused by *Leuconostoc* species. Aust N. Z. J. Surg. *69*:541-542, 1999.
38. Nathavitharana, K. A., Arseculeratne, S. N., Aponso, H. A., et al.: Acute meningitis in early childhood caused by *Aerococcus viridans*. Br. Med. J. (Clin. Res. Ed.) *286*:1248, 1983.
39. Noriega, F. R., Kotloff, K. L., Martin, M. A., et al.: Nosocomial bacteremia caused by *Enterobacter sakazakiki* and *Leuconostoc mesenteroides* resulting from extrinsic contamination of infant formula. Pediatr. Infect. Dis. J. *9*:447-449, 1990.
40. Okereke, A., and Montville, T. J.: Bacteriocin-mediated inhibition of *Clostridium botulinum* spores by lactic acid bacteria at refrigeration and abuse temperatures. Appl. Environ. Microbiol. *57*:3423-3428, 1991.
41. Park, H. K., Shim, S. S., Kim, S. Y., et al.: Molecular analysis of colonized bacteria in a human newborn infant gut. J. Microbiol. *43*:345-353, 2005.
42. Park, J. W., and Grossman, O.: *Aerococcus viridans* infection. Case report and review. Clin. Pediatr. (Phila.) *29*:525-526, 1990.
43. Parker, M. T., and Ball, L. C.: Streptococci and aerococci associated with systemic infection in man. J. Med. Microbiol. *9*:275-302, 1976.
44. Peters, V. B., Bottone, E. J., Barzilai, A., et al.: *Leuconostoc* species bacteremia in a child with acquired immunodeficiency syndrome. Clin. Pediatr. (Phila.) *31*:699-701, 1992.
45. Pien, F. D., Wilson, W. R., Kunz, K., et al.: *Aerococcus viridans* endocarditis. Mayo Clin. Proc. *59*:47-48, 1984.
46. Popescu, G. A., Benea, E., Mitache, E., et al.: An unusual bacterium, *Aerococcus viridans*, and four cases of infective endocarditis. J. Heart Valve Dis. *14*:317-319, 2005.
47. Riebel, W. J., and Washington, J. A.: Clinical and microbiologic characteristics of pediococci. J. Clin. Microbiol. *28*:1348-1355, 1990.
48. Rogosa, M., and Sharpe, M. E.: Species differentiation of human vaginal lactobacilli. J. Gen. Microbiol. *23*:197, 1960.
49. Ruoff, K. L., Kuritzkes, D. R., Wolfson, J. S., et al.: Vancomycin-resistant gram-positive bacteria isolated from human sources. J. Clin. Microbiol. *26*:2064-2068, 1988.
50. Sarma, P. S., and Mohanty, S.: *Pediococcus acidilactici* pneumonitis and bacteremia in a pregnant woman. J. Clin. Microbiol. *36*:2392-2393, 1998.
51. Scano, F., Rossi, L., Cattelan, A., et al.: *Leuconostoc* species: A case-cluster hospital infection. Scand. J. Infect. Dis. *31*:371-373, 1999.
52. Scheiblauer, H., Reinacher, M., Tashiro, M., et al.: Interactions between bacteria and influenza A virus in the development of influenza pneumonia. J. Infect. Dis. *166*:783-791, 1992.
53. Sire, J. M., Donnio, P. Y., Mesnard, R., et al.: Septicemia and hepatic abscess caused by *Pediococcus acidilactici*. Eur. J. Clin. Microbiol. Infect. Dis. *11*:623-625, 1992.
54. Skytta, E., Haikara, A., and Mattila-Sandholm, T.: Production and characterization of antibacterial compounds produced by *Pediococcus damnosus* and *Pediococcus pentosaceus*. J. Appl. Bacteriol. *74*:134-142, 1993.
55. Stiles, M. E.: Bacteriocins produced by *Leuconostoc* species. J. Dairy Sci. *77*:2718-2724, 1994.
56. Swanson, H., Cutts, E., and Lepow, M.: Penicillin-resistant *Aerococcus viridans* bacteremia in a child receiving prophylaxis for sickle-cell disease. Clin. Infect. Dis. *22*:387-388, 1996.
57. Swenson, J. M., Facklam, R. R., and Thornsberry, C.: Antimicrobial susceptibility of vancomycin-resistant *Leuconostoc*, *Pediococcus*, and *Lactobacillus* species. Antimicrob. Agents Chemother. *34*:543-549, 1990.
58. Tankovic, J., Leclercq, R., and Duval, J.: Antimicrobial susceptibility of *Pediococcus* spp. and genetic basis of macrolide resistance in *Pediococcus acidilactici* HM3020. Antimicrob. Agents Chemother. *37*:789-792, 1993.
59. Taylor, P. W., and Trueblood, M. C.: Septic arthritis due to *Aerococcus viridans*. J. Rheumatol. *12*:1004-1005, 1985.
60. Wenocur, H. S., Smith, M. A., Vellozzi, E. M., et al.: Odontogenic infection secondary to *Leuconostoc* species. J. Clin. Microbiol. *26*:1893-1894, 1988.

SUBSECTION 2

Gram-Negative Cocci

MORAXELLA CATARRHALIS

Barbara W. Stechenberg

Once thought to be an unimportant commensal organism in the human respiratory tract, *Moraxella catarrhalis* now is recognized as an important pathogen in respiratory tract diseases, particularly otitis, sinusitis, and lower tract disease. The initial paper by Ghon and Pfeiffer[25] published in 1902 described gram-negative cocci in sputum referred to as *Micrococcus catarrhalis*. Since then, the organism has undergone several changes in nomenclature, first to *Neisseria catarrhalis* because of its resemblance to other *Neisseria* organisms. In 1970, in recognition of the contributions of Sarah Branham, the name was changed to *Branhamella catarrhalis*.[11] More recently, that this organism should be a member of the genus *Moraxella* has become clear; thus, the name was changed to *M. catarrhalis*. With the transition in nomenclature, the last 2 decades have seen a parallel rebirth of this organism as a mucosal pathogen.

MICROBIOLOGY

M. catarrhalis is a gram-negative diplococcus that is morphologically indistinguishable from *Neisseria*. It has a tendency to resist decolorizing.[1] The organism is kidney-shaped, with the flat sides abutting each other. The size varies, but it may be larger than meningococcus or gonococcus. However, the resemblance on sputum Gram stain or conjunctival smear to gonococcus can be striking and clinically confusing.

The organism grows well on blood or chocolate agar and forms small, opaque, grayish colonies that are circular and non-hemolytic. They have poor adhesion to the agar surface, on which they act like hockey pucks when pushed over the surface of the agar plate.[17] The use of selective media such as modified Thayer-Martin or TV broth (Mueller-Hinton broth supplemented with trimethoprim and vancomycin) increases the likelihood of recovering *M. catarrhalis* from the complex flora of the mucosal surfaces.

Isolates of *M. catarrhalis* cannot use maltose, glucose, lactose, or sucrose as carbohydrate sources. *M. catarrhalis* is oxidase-positive and produces deoxyribonuclease. Valuable differentiating tests are hydrolysis of DNA and tributyrin. Several rapid tests such as butyrate hydrolysis, Tween 80 hydrolysis, and selective DNase agar have been described.[50,57] Fatty-acid analysis also has been used to identify atypical strains.

The surface of *M. catarrhalis* is composed of outer-membrane proteins, lipo-oligosaccharide, and pili. The organism does not appear to have a capsule, and the role of the pili is not defined well. Initial attempts to isolate outer-membrane proteins by detergent fractionation of cell envelopes were unsuccessful. By using a technique involving the collection of outer-membrane vesicles, which are released into the culture media, and then examination by sodium dodecyl sulfate–polyacrylamide gel electrophoresis (SDS-PAGE), Bartos and Murphy[6] identified eight proteins designated outer-membrane proteins A through H. The outer-membrane protein patterns of strains from diverse geographic and clinical sources were strikingly homogeneous.

Preliminary studies of the lipo-oligosaccharide of *M. catarrhalis* show that it is more antigenically conserved than are those of other gram-negative bacteria, thus rendering it a reasonable candidate for vaccine studies.[39,53] A recent study suggests that the lipo-oligosaccharide is not an adhesin, but its surface charge plays a critical role in the initial stage of attachment to human epithelial cells.[2]

Restriction endonuclease analysis has been used as an epidemiologic tool to distinguish strains of *M. catarrhalis*. Patterson and associates[42] used the technique to evaluate a nosocomial outbreak and to demonstrate the lack of association of other strains. Dickinson and coworkers[16] used a similar technique to study isolates from children with otitis media.

PATHOGENESIS

The ability of *M. catarrhalis* to produce disease, particularly in sequestered areas such as the ear and lung, indicates that this organism possesses virulence mechanisms that allow it not only to grow in these anatomic sites but also to produce pathologic effects. The presence of endotoxin in the *M. catarrhalis* outer membrane undoubtedly is important for its pathogenic potential, especially in situations in which inflammation plays a major role. Very little is known about the mechanisms involved in colonization and disease production. However, a subset of strains of *M. catarrhalis* associated with selected virulence traits suggests that some strains are more virulent than are others.[9,56]

A body of literature concerning the immune response to *M. catarrhalis* and the antigenic composition of this organism is accumulating rapidly.[12,13,34] Goldblatt and associates[26] demonstrated that children younger than 4 years old possess IgG1 and IgG2 that recognize an 82-kd outer-membrane protein exclusively but that older children mount an IgG3 response to a broad range of outer-membrane proteins. Faden and colleagues[23] developed a technique to measure opsonic antibody with the use of outer-membrane, antigen-coated beads. Convalescent sera opsonized homologous, antigen-coated sera significantly more often than acute sera did.

Unhanand and coworkers[52] used a murine model to study pulmonary clearance of *M. catarrhalis* from infected lungs. They investigated 10 strains and found marked variability in clearance rates and recruitment of phagocytic cells. With this model, Maciver and associates[36] actively immunized animals with the outer-membrane vesicles of *M. catarrhalis* and passively immunized animals with rabbit antiserum raised against these vesicles. Both experiments resulted in enhanced pulmonary clearance of both homologous and heterologous strains. The same model has been used to evaluate the role of a large, antigenically conserved protein of *M. catarrhalis* in pulmonary clearance, as well as the role of outer-membrane protein B in defense mechanisms of the lung.[30] The contribution of these proteins, as well as lipo-oligosaccharide, in host defense continues to unfold.

EPIDEMIOLOGY

M. catarrhalis is a normal inhabitant of the upper respiratory tract and is recovered exclusively from humans. The rate of colonization is highest in the early years and then declines steadily to less than 5 percent in adult life.[54] Prevalence studies report that as many as 50 percent of children are colonized with *M. catarrhalis*.[32,37] Faden and associates[22] monitored a large cohort of children from birth to 2 years of age. Sixty-six percent became colonized by the time that they reached 1 year of age, and 77.5 percent did so by 2 years of age. The frequency of nasopharyngeal colonization was higher during visits for otitis media than during well-child visits. Otitis-prone children were colonized by 6 months of age. Restriction endonuclease analysis showed marked heterogeneity, with children acquiring and eliminating many different strains over time.[22,42]

Numerous studies have documented the increased prevalence of *M. catarrhalis* as a pathogen in otitis media.[32,55] Shurin and colleagues[48] noted that isolation of *M. catarrhalis* from middle ear exudates increased from 6.4 percent between 1979 and 1980 to 26.5 percent between 1980 and 1982. A similar increase in *M. catarrhalis* as a pathogen in sinusitis has been reported.[58] In the pneumococcal conjugate vaccine (PCV7) era, a significantly higher proportion of PCV7-immunized children exhibit nasopharyngeal colonization with *M. catarrhalis*.[44]

Once colonization of the oropharynx occurs, colonization of the tracheobronchial tree may follow, but usually only if other risk factors are operative. In adults, such risk factors include previous cardiorespiratory disease, smoking, use of corticosteroids, use of immunosuppressive agents, malignancy, and intercurrent viral illnesses.[28,57] In children, many cases of pneumonia are associated with a preceding viral illness, prematurity, underlying lung disease, IgG deficiency, or other risk factors.

Nosocomial transmission has been well documented by DNA restriction endonuclease analysis.[14,42] In pediatric intensive care units, endotracheal intubation and frequent suctioning have been identified as risk factors for the development of pneumonia and bacterial tracheitis.[14,21]

Other interesting associations need to be investigated further. Seddon and associates[47] noted that colonization with *M. catarrhalis* occurred more commonly in asthmatic than in normal children. Whether the organism might be a trigger or pathogen in these children remains to be seen. Gottfarb and Brauner[27] found a high carriage rate of *M. catarrhalis* in children with severe persistent cough.

Infection with *M. catarrhalis* exhibits seasonality in both adults and children.[28,48,55] Infection is much more likely to occur in the winter and spring months.

CLINICAL MANIFESTATIONS AND DIAGNOSIS

Otitis media caused by *M. catarrhalis* is indistinguishable clinically from otitis caused by other pathogens such as *Streptococcus pneumoniae* and *Haemophilus influenzae*. *M. catarrhalis* may be isolated as a single agent or in combination with other organisms. In one study, children with *M. catarrhalis* were less likely to have a serum C-reactive protein level greater than 1.0 mg/dL than were children with either of the other two major pathogens.[55]

Because tympanocentesis usually is not performed in routine cases, the exact cause of an episode of acute otitis media generally is not known. One study found that *Moraxella* was an unusual organism as a single agent in children in whom acute otitis media had been treated recently.[29] Nonetheless, in a study of persistent otitis, Pichichero and Pichichero[43] demonstrated *Moraxella* in 7 percent of specimens. The spontaneous resolution rate of *M. catarrhalis* may be high,[4] and this fact should be considered when therapy is planned.

The clinical manifestations of acute sinusitis caused by *M. catarrhalis* are similar to those of other organisms; therefore, selection of antibiotics should be made with consideration of this organism as a potential pathogen.

Lower respiratory tract disease caused by *M. catarrhalis* may have a broad clinical spectrum; however, because sputum samples often are not available in children, many cases documented in the literature have been severe. Berg and Bartley[7] described five premature infants, all younger than 6 months old, in whom precipitous clinical deterioration developed after 2 to 4 days of a prodrome consisting of cough, tachypnea, and intercostal retractions. They all required assisted ventilation, which is common in young infants with severe pneumonia.[7,14,20] Some cases of *M. catarrhalis* pneumonia have been associated with bacteremia.

Underlying conditions such as leukemia, acquired immunodeficiency syndrome, and trauma have been reported to predispose a patient to the development of infection with *M. catarrhalis*.[37,59] An association with immunoglobulin deficiency has been demonstrated in some patients with disease caused by this organism.[12] In adults, *M. catarrhalis* pneumonia occurs more commonly in patients with human immunodeficiency virus infection, malignancy, or chronic lung problems.[26,57] The role of this organism in less severe manifestations probably is limited.[33]

Bacterial tracheitis caused by *M. catarrhalis* has been reported in both immunocompromised hosts and those with normal immune systems.[21]

M. catarrhalis also has been responsible for a wide variety of other infections. Urethritis caused by this organism can be mistaken for infection with *Neisseria gonorrhoeae*.[49] Several cases of conjunctivitis have been reported; when present in the newborn period, *M. catarrhalis* can mimic the ophthalmia neonatorum of *N. gonorrhoeae*.[51] The relationship of neonatal infections to maternal vaginal carriage of *Moraxella* has not been established.[41]

More severe infections with *M. catarrhalis* include meningitis and bacteremia, so this organism should be considered in appropriate circumstances, especially in immunocompromised children.

Children with *M. catarrhalis* bacteremia may have many different manifestations. Some patients have petechial or purpuric rashes, thus rendering the clinical picture indistinguishable from that of meningococcemia. Others have been neutropenic and have required mechanical ventilation.[8] Baron and Shapiro[5] reported two cases of unsuspected bacteremia in children with

nonspecific symptoms. Their manifestations were similar to those of children with occult pneumococcal bacteremia. An immunocompetent child with *M. catarrhalis* bacteremia and preseptal cellulitis has been reported.[46]

Meningitis can occur from hematogenous spread of *M. catarrhalis* from the nasopharynx or as a consequence of ventriculoperitoneal shunt placement or surgery. Rarely, suppurative arthritis has been seen in children and adults.[31,38] Endocarditis is a rare occurrence, as is peritonitis.

TREATMENT

In the past, *M. catarrhalis* was susceptible to all β-lactam antibiotics. In the late 1970s, however, β-lactamase–producing strains of *M. catarrhalis* were isolated in Europe. In the United States, a parallel increase in the frequency of isolation of β-lactamase–producing *M. catarrhalis* has been noted, so it is not unusual for a laboratory to report that more than 90 percent of strains are β-lactamase producers.

The β-lactamases BRO-1, BRO-2, and BRO-3 are of chromosomal origin. Laboratory detection of β-lactamase activity depends on the assay used; the chromogenic cephalosporin nitrocefin usually is recommended.[19] Polymerase chain reaction methods can be used. BRO-1 is the most common β-lactamase in North American strains.[15] The β-lactamase inhibitors clavulanic acid, sulbactam, and tazobactam are active against the enzymes produced by *Moraxella*. Most β-lactamase–positive isolates will respond to achievable concentrations of β-lactam/β-lactamase inhibitor antimicrobial combinations, cephalosporins, and cephamycins.[18,24] Because of the high prevalence of β-lactamase–producing strains, many laboratories choose not to do any such testing.

Among the oral cephalosporins active against β-lactamase–positive strains of *Moraxella*, the minimal inhibitory concentration increases twofold to fourfold in the presence of the β-lactamase BRO-1 but not the β-lactamase BRO-2; cefixime is more active than are the older cephalosporins.[40] Resistance to tetracycline (by the nontransferable tetB determinant) and erythromycin has been reported, but such resistance is a rare finding.[10,45]

In vitro, *M. catarrhalis* usually is susceptible to ampicillin-sulbactam, amoxicillin-clavulanate, erythromycin, azithromycin, clarithromycin, trimethoprim-sulfamethoxazole, tetracyclines, chloramphenicol, fluoroquinolones (e.g., ciprofloxacin), aminoglycosides, and second- or third-generation cephalosporins such as cefuroxime, cefprozil, cefpodoxime, cefixime, cefdinir, and loracarbef.[35] Levofloxacin also exhibits good activity against *M. catarrhalis*.[3] The *Moraxella* organism is resistant to clindamycin, vancomycin, and oxacillin.

PREVENTION

Prevention of nosocomial *M. catarrhalis* infection is dependent on sound practices of infection control, especially with regard to pulmonary toilet. Prevention of other infections with this organism has not been attempted, except for the use of prophylactic antibiotics for recurrent otitis media.

REFERENCES

1. Ainsworth, S. M., Nagy, S. B., Morgan, L. A., et al.: Interpretation of gram-stained sputa containing *Moraxella* (*Branhamella*) *catarrhalis*. Clin. Microbiol. 28:2559-2560, 1990.
2. Akgul, G., Erturk, A., Turkoz, M., et al.: Role of lipooligosaccharide in the attachment of *Moraxella catarrhalis* to human pharyngeal epithelial cells. Microbiol. Immunol. 49:931-935, 2005.

3. Arguedas, A., Dagan, R., Pichichero, M., et al.: An open-label, double tympanocentesis study of levofloxacin therapy in children with, or at high risk for, recurrent or persistent acute otitis media. Pediatr. Infect. Dis. J. 25:1102-1109, 2006.
4. Barnett, E. D., and Klein, J. O.: The problem of resistant bacteria for the management of acute otitis media. Pediatr. Clin. North Am. 42:509-518, 1995.
5. Baron, J., and Shapiro, E. D.: Unsuspected bacteremia caused by *Branhamella catarrhalis*. Pediatr. Infect. Dis. J. 4:100-101, 1985.
6. Bartos, L. C., and Murphy, T. F.: Comparison of the outer membrane proteins of 50 strains of *Branhamella catarrhalis*. J. Infect. Dis. 158:761-765, 1988.
7. Berg, R. A., and Bartley, D. L.: Pneumonia associated with *Branhamella catarrhalis* in infants. Pediatr. Infect. Dis. J. 6:569-573, 1987.
8. Bonadio, W. A.: *Branhamella catarrhalis* bacteremia in children. Pediatr. Infect. Dis. J. 7:738-739, 1988.
9. Bootsma, H. J., van der Heide, H. G., van de Pas, S., et al.: Analysis of *Moraxella catarrhalis* by DNA typing: Evidence of a distinct subpopulation associated with virulence traits. J. Infect. Dis. 181:1376-1387, 2000.
10. Brown, B. A., Wallace, R. J., Flanagan, C. W., et al.: Tetracycline and erythromycin resistance among clinical isolates of *Branhamella catarrhalis*. Antimicrob. Agents Chemother. 33:1631-1633, 1989.
11. Catlin, B. W.: Transfer of the organism named *Neisseria catarrhalis* to *Branhamella* gen. nov. Int. J. Syst. Bacteriol. 20:155-159, 1970.
12. Catlin, B. W.: *Branhamella catarrhalis*: An organism gaining respect as a pathogen. Clin. Microbiol. Rev. 3:293-320, 1990.
13. Chapman, A. J., Musher, D. M., Jonsson, S., et al.: Development of bactericidal antibody during *Branhamella catarrhalis* infection. J. Infect. Dis. 151:878-882, 1985.
14. Cook, P. P., Heent, D. W., and Syndman, D. R.: Nosocomial *Branhamella catarrhalis* in a pediatric intensive care unit: Risk factors for disease. J. Hosp. Infect. 13:299-307, 1989.
15. Deshpande, L. M., Sader, H. S., Fritsche, T. R., et al.: Contemporary prevalence of BRO beta-lactamases in *Moraxella catarrhalis*: Report from the SENTRY antimicrobial surveillance program (North America, 1997 to 2004). J. Clin. Microbiol. 44:3775-3777, 2006.
16. Dickinson, D. P., Loos, B. G., Dryja, D. M., et al.: Restriction fragment mapping of *Branhamella catarrhalis*: A new tool for studying the epidemiology of this middle ear pathogen. J. Infect. Dis. 158:208, 1988.
17. Doern, G. V.: *Branhamella catarrhalis*: Phenotypic characteristics. Am. J. Med. 88:335-355, 1990.
18. Doern, G. V., and Jones, R. N.: Antimicrobial susceptibility testing of *Haemophilus influenzae*, *Branhamella catarrhalis* and *Neisseria gonorrhoeae*. Antimicrob. Agents Chemother. 32:1747-1753, 1988.
19. Doern, G. V., and Tubert, A. T.: Detection of β-lactamase activity among clinical isolates of *Branhamella catarrhalis* with six different β-lactamase assays. J. Clin. Microbiol. 25:1380-1383, 1987.
20. Dyson, C., Poonyth, H. O., Watkinson, M., Rose, S. J.: Life threatening *Branhamella catarrhalis* pneumonia in young infants. J. Infect. 21:305-307, 1990.
21. Ernst, T. N., and Philp, M.: Bacterial tracheitis caused by *Branhamella catarrhalis*. Pediatr. Infect. Dis. J. 6:574, 1987.
22. Faden, H., Harabuchi, Y., Hong, J. J., et al.: Epidemiology of *Moraxella catarrhalis* in children during the first 2 years of life: Relationship to otitis media. J. Infect. Dis. 169:1312-1317, 1994.
23. Faden, H., Hong, J. J., and Pahade, N.: Immune response to *Moraxella catarrhalis* in children with otitis media: Opsonophagocytosis with antigen-coated latex beads. Ann. Otol. Rhinol. Laryngol. 103:522-524, 1994.
24. Fung, C.-P., Yeo, S.-F., and Livermore, D. M.: Susceptibility of *Moraxella catarrhalis* isolates to β-lactam antibiotics in relation to β-lactamase pattern. J. Antimicrob. Chemother. 33:215-222, 1994.
25. Ghon, A., and Pfeiffer, H.: Der Mikvococcus catarrhalis (R. Pfeiffer) als Krankheitserreger. Z. Klin. Med. 44:263-281, 1902.
26. Goldblatt, D., Turner, M. W., and Levinsky, R. J.: *Branhamella catarrhalis*: Antigenic determinants and the development of the IgG subclass response in childhood. J. Infect. Dis. 162:1128-1135, 1990.
27. Gottfarb, P., and Brauner, A.: Children with persistent cough: Outcome with treatment and role of *Moraxella catarrhalis*? Scand. J. Infect. Dis. 26:545-551, 1994.
28. Hager, H., Verghese, A., Alvarez, S., et al.: *Branhamella catarrhalis* respiratory infections. Rev. Infect. Dis. 9:1140-1149, 1987.
29. Harrison, C. J., Marks, J. I., and Welch, D. F.: Microbiology of recently treated acute otitis media compared with previously untreated acute otitis media. Pediatr. Infect. Dis. J. 4:641-646, 1985.
30. Helminen, M. E., Maciver, I., Paris, M., et al.: A mutation affecting expression of a major outer protein of *Moraxella catarrhalis* alters resistance and survival in vivo. J. Infect. Dis. 168:1194-1201, 1993.
31. Izraeli, S., Flasterstein, B., Shamir, R., et al.: *Branhamella catarrhalis* as a cause of suppurative arthritis. Pediatr. Infect. Dis. J. 8:256-257, 1989.
32. Klein, J. O.: Otitis media. Clin. Infect. Dis. 19:823-833, 1994.
33. Korppi, M., Katila, M. L., Jaaskelainen, J., et al.: Role of *Moraxella* (*Branhamella*) *catarrhalis* as a respiratory pathogen in children. Acta Paediatr. 81:993-996, 1992.
34. Leinonen, M., Luotonen, J., Herva, E., et al.: Preliminary serologic evidence for a pathogenic role of *Branhamella catarrhalis*. J. Infect. Dis. 144:570-574, 1981.
35. Lemmen, S. W., Anding, K., Engels, I., et al.: Bactericidal activity of clarithromycin and cefaclor against *Streptococcus pneumoniae* and *Moraxella catarrhalis* in healthy volunteers. J. Antimicrob. Chemother. 33:673-674, 1994.
36. Maciver, I., Unhanand, M., McCracken, G. H., et al.: Effect of immunization on pulmonary clearance of *Moraxella catarrhalis* in animal model. J. Infect. Dis. 168:469-472, 1993.
37. Marchant, C. D.: Spectrum of disease due to *Branhamella catarrhalis* in children with particular reference to acute otitis media. Am. J. Med. 88(Suppl. 5A):155-195, 1990.
38. Melendez, P. R., and Johnson, R. H.: Bacteremia and septic arthritis caused by *Moraxella catarrhalis*. Rev. Infect. Dis. 13:428-429, 1991.
39. Murphy, T. F.: The surface of *Branhamella catarrhalis*: A systematic approach to the surface antigens of an emerging pathogen. Pediatr. Infect. Dis. J. 8:575-577, 1989.
40. Nash, D. R., Flanagan, C., Steele, L. C., et al.: Comparison of the activity of cefixime and activities of other oral antibiotics against adult clinical isolates of *Moraxella* (*Branhamella*) *catarrhalis* containing BRO-1 and BRO-2 and *Haemophilus influenzae*. Antimicrob. Agents Chemother. 35:192-194, 1991.
41. Ohlsson, A., and Bailey, T.: Neonatal pneumonia caused by *Branhamella catarrhalis*. Scand. J. Infect. Dis. 17:225-228, 1985.
42. Patterson, J. E., Patterson, T. F., Farrel, P., et al.: Evaluation of restriction endonuclease analysis as an epidemiologic typing system for *Branhamella catarrhalis*. J. Clin. Microbiol. 27:994-946, 1989.
43. Pichichero, M. E., and Pichichero, C. L.: Persistent acute otitis media. I. Causative organisms. Pediatr. Infect. Dis. J. 14:178-183, 1995.
44. Revai, K., McCormick, D. P., Patel, J., et al.: Effect of pneumococcal conjugate vaccine in nasopharyngeal bacterial colonization during acute otitis media. Pediatrics 117:1823-1829, 2006.
45. Roberts, M. C., Pang, Y., Spencer, R. C., et al.: Tetracycline resistance in *Moraxella* (*Branhamella*) *catarrhalis*: Demonstration of two clonal outbreaks by using pulsed-field gel electrophoresis. Antimicrob. Agents Chemother. 35:2453-2455, 1991.
46. Rotta, A. T., and Asmar, B. I.: *Moraxella catarrhalis* bacteremia and preseptal cellulitis. South. Med. J. 87:541-542, 1994.
47. Seddon, P. C., Sunderland, D., O'Halloran, S. M., et al.: *Branhamella catarrhalis* colonization in preschool asthmatics. Pediatr. Pulmonol. 13:133-135, 1992.
48. Shurin, P. A., Marchant, C. D., Kim, C. H., et al.: Emergence of beta-lactamase–producing strains of *Branhamella catarrhalis* as important agents of otitis media. Pediatr. Infect. Dis. J. 2:34-38, 1983.
49. Smith, G.: *Branhamella catarrhalis* infection imitating gonorrhea in a man. N. Engl. J. Med. 326:1277, 1987.
50. Speeleveld, E., Fossepre, J. M., Gordts, B., and Van Landuyt, H. W.: Comparison of three rapid methods, tributyrin, 4-methylumbelliferyl butyrate, and indoxyl acetate, for rapid identification of *Moraxella catarrhalis*. J. Clin. Microbiol. 32:1362-1363, 1994.
51. Stull, T. L., and Stanford, E. J.: Pseudogonococcal ophthalmia neonatorum caused by *Branhamella catarrhalis*. Pediatr. Infect. Dis. J. 5:104-105, 1986.
52. Unhanand, M., Maciver, I., Ramilo, O., et al.: Pulmonary clearance of *Moraxella catarrhalis* in an animal model. J. Infect. Dis. 165:644-650, 1992.
53. Vaneechoutte, M., Verschraegen, G., Claeys, G., et al.: Serologic typing of *Branhamella catarrhalis* strains on the basis of lipopolysaccharide antigens. J. Clin. Microbiol. 28:182-187, 1990.
54. Vaneechoutte, M., Verschraegen, G., Claeys, G., et al.: Respiratory tract carrier rates of *Moraxella Branhamella catarrhalis* in adults and children and interpretation of the isolation of *Moraxella catarrhalis* from sputum. J. Clin. Microbiol. 28:2674-2680, 1990.
55. Van Hare, G. F., Shurin, P. A., Marchant, C. D., et al.: Acute otitis media caused by *Branhamella catarrhalis*: Biology and therapy. Rev. Infect. Dis. 9:16-27, 1987.
56. Verduin, C. M., Kools-Sijmons, M., van der Plas, J., et al.: Complement-resistant *Moraxella catarrhalis* forms a genetically distinct lineage with the species. F. E. M. S. Microbiol. Lett. 184:1-8, 2000.
57. Verghese, A., and Berk, S. L.: *Moraxella* (*Branhamella*) *catarrhalis*. Infect. Dis. Clin. North Am. 5:523-538, 1991.
58. Wald, E. R., Reilly, J. S., Casselbrant, M., et al.: Treatment of acute maxillary sinusitis in childhood: A comparative study of amoxicillin and cefaclor. J. Pediatr. 104:297-302, 1984.
59. Wong, V. K., and Ross, L. A.: *Branhamella catarrhalis* septicemia in an infant with AIDS. Scand. J. Infect. Dis. 20:559-560, 1988.

MENINGOCOCCAL INFECTIONS
99
Marsha S. Anderson ✧ Mary P. Glodé ✧ Arnold L. Smith

Epidemic meningococcal meningitis was described first by Gaspard Vieusseux in Geneva in the spring of 1805. In a monograph titled "The Disease Which Raged During the Spring of 1805," he wrote:

> It commences suddenly with prostration of strength, often extreme: the face is distorted, the pulse feeble. There appears a violent pain in the head, especially over the forehead; then there comes pain of the heart or vomiting of greenish material, stiffness of the spine, and in infants, convulsions. In cases which were fatal, loss of consciousness occurred. The course of the disease is very rapid, termination by death or by cure. In most of the patients who died in 24 hours or a little after, the body is covered with purple spots at the moment of death or very little time afterward.[200]

Today, Neisseria meningitidis continues to be a cause of endemic and epidemic disease. In the United States, approximately 1400 to 2800 cases occur each year, and 95 to 97 percent of these cases are sporadic.[10,170] In 2005 and 2006, 1904 and 1742 U.S. cases were reported to the Centers for Disease Control and Prevention (CDC), respectively.[35] However, epidemics in Brazil in the early 1970s and in Finland in 1975 serve as a reminder of the potential virulence of this organism. In São Paulo, Brazil, invasive meningococcal disease developed in almost 1 in every 300 inhabitants during the epidemic in a 1-year period.[49]

The reader is referred to several excellent reviews of meningococcal disease that have been published recently.[72,111,171]

MICROBIOLOGY

The Neisseria genus was named for Dr. Albert Neisser, who described the organism of gonorrhea in 1879. The genus Neisseria contains two species important in human disease, Neisseria gonorrhoeae and N. meningitidis. In addition, several species are part of the normal flora of humans and animals. Neisseria sicca, Neisseria lactamica, Neisseria subflava, Neisseria flavescens, Neisseria mucosa, Neisseria cinera, Neisseria polysacchreae, and Neisseria elongate are human commensals; they only occasionally cause human disease.[121]

N. meningitidis is a gram-negative coccus, usually less than 1 μm in diameter. It classically occurs in pairs, with adjacent sides flattened, similar to kidney beans. Occasionally, the organism divides into two planes at right angles to one another, which results in the formation of tetrads. The organisms are nonmotile and aerobic (but facultatively anaerobic), produce catalase and oxidase, and may be encapsulated. N. meningitidis oxidizes glucose and maltose to acid. This feature distinguishes it from N. gonorrhoeae, which oxidizes only glucose. However, certain rare strains of N. meningitidis have been reported that fail to produce acid from either glucose or maltose. Fresh isolates have complex nutritional requirements and grow best on chocolate or blood agar. Incubation in a humidified 10 percent carbon dioxide environment is not essential but enhances growth. Morphologically, the colonies are bluish gray in appearance and will produce beta-hemolysis after 48 to 72 hours of incubation on 5 percent horse blood agar.[24]

N. meningitidis can be transformed by DNA originating in other species of Neisseria. Thus, when a Neisseria spp. cohabiting the nasopharynx with N. meningitidis dies and releases its DNA, the co-resident meningococcus can take up the DNA and incorporate it into its genome. Although this sequence of events occurs very rarely, if the new DNA confers a selective advantage to the recipient meningococcus, the trait encoded by the incoming DNA may be retained in future progeny. This is the mechanism by which sulfonamide resistance and penicillin G resistance have arisen in N. meningitidis.[121] Many commensal Neisseria, which also inhabit the nasopharynx, are relatively resistant to penicillin G. DNA fragments from these commensal strains that encode penicillin resistance can be detected in penicillin-resistant N. meningitidis.[173] Transformation of new DNA into N. meningitidis also can introduce genes that modify the structure of the bacterium. Serotyping of groups A, B, and C meningococci has provided valuable macro-epidemiologic information.[71] Clearly, as a population develops immunity to one capsular polysaccharide, the organism is capable of acquiring DNA encoding for an alternative capsule. Switching from serogroup B to serogroup C has been observed in a population[188] and a contact of a case.[201] There also appears to be horizontal gene transfer from commensal Neisseria to N. meningitidis of genes whose products aid the bacterium in surviving in the host or are involved in housekeeping functions.[119] This phenomenon probably is responsible for the occasional report of commensal Neisseria causing meningitis.[6] In one case, the strain was a virulent meningococcus that acquired a gene for the synthesis of polysaccharide from sucrose; this additional property led it to be identified as N. subflava rather than N. meningitidis.

In addition to having the transformation route for varying the antigenic phenotype, meningococci also may exhibit phase variation, which allows variance of the number of surface antigens. Investigators have estimated that at least 65 genes in N. meningitidis, including porA, are subject to phase variation.[64,194] Capsule synthesis may be switched on and off by this mechanism.

Like other gram-negative bacteria, the outer and inner cell membranes of Neisseria are phospholipid bilayers. These membranes sandwich a layer of peptidoglycan. Lipo-oligosaccharide (LOS), which is similar to the lipopolysaccharide seen in gram-negative enteric bacteria, is associated with the outer leaflet of the outer cell membrane. Outer-membrane proteins, which function as porins, are an integral part of the outer membrane. Some of these outer-membrane proteins are opacity proteins and facilitate adherence and invasion.[138] Outside the outer membrane, meningococci possess a polysaccharide capsule that protects the organism from phagocytosis.

Meningococci also have pili, which seem to be important in some phases of adherence to host cells, colonization, and invasion. The genes that code for pili also can be turned on and off, so at times the organism may not express pili. This feature may help the meningococci detach and allow the organism to be transmitted to another site or another host.[87] Antigenic variation of pili by a cassette mechanism allows the bacterium to escape the host's immune system.[82] In addition, both outer-membrane proteins and lipo-oligopolysaccharide display antigenic differences by phase variation.

For epidemiologic purposes, meningococci are divided into serogroups, serotypes, and subtypes. Differences in capsular polysaccharides, outer-membrane proteins, and LOS constitute the basis for these classifications. The capsular polysaccharides are antigenic and the basis for serogroup designation. Thirteen serogroups currently are recognized: A, B, C, D, H, I, K, L, X, Y, Z, W-135, and 29E.[209] Serogroups A, B, C, Y, and W-135 are the most common causes of invasive disease worldwide.

Serotyping of organisms is based on antigenic differences in outer-membrane proteins called *porins*. Porins are protein channels in the outer membrane that permit nutrients and certain antibiotics to diffuse into the periplasmic space. A single locus encodes porin B, but two mutually exclusive alleles have antigenic differences. All meningococci have either antigenic class 2 or class 3 porin B. These differences permit serotyping. Differentiation of subtypes is based on antigenic differences in porin A. This highly variable antigen is called a class 1 outer-membrane protein. Multiple serotypes and subtypes have been identified. Antigenic specificity is achieved by the generation of monoclonal antibodies to the major protein (primarily class 2 or 3), LOS, and class 1 protein. The designation B:2a:P1.1:L3,7 indicates that the serogroup B strain is an "a" subtype of class 2 proteins, is a "one" of class 1 protein, and possesses two LOS antigens: 3 and 7.[77]

Type 2 protein antigen is isolated from more than 50 percent of cases in the United States and Canada and is an antigenic determinant in group B and C strains. These protein antigens not only are important as epidemiologic markers but also can induce protective bactericidal antibodies.[70]

EPIDEMIOLOGY

The incidence of meningococcal disease varies significantly by geographic location. Endemic disease, which occurs in developed countries such as the United States and Europe, ranges in incidence from 0.35 to 3.0 cases per 100,000 population per year.[30-32,170] The U.S. Active Bacterial Core Surveillance (ABC) system tracks invasive disease caused by encapsulated organisms in selected counties of 10 states geographically dispersed throughout the country. This reporting system covers a U.S. population of 39 million people. In 2005, the overall incidence of invasive meningococcal disease for the United States was estimated to be 0.35 per 100,000 population. Fifty-six percent of cases reported through the ABC system were meningitis with a fatality rate of 1.1 percent, and 31 percent of cases were bacteremia with a fatality rate of 15.1 percent. The rate of invasive disease was the same for African Americans and whites.[32]

In developing countries, the incidence is approximately 10 to 20 times higher than that in the United States (10-25 per 100,000 inhabitants per year).[80] The highest rate of meningococcal disease is found in a multicountry belt across sub-Saharan Africa, which has been termed the *meningitis belt*. Serogroup A meningococcal disease is prevalent there and occurs in epidemics during the dry season.[128] During epidemics, the incidence of meningococcal disease is as high as 1000 per 100,000 inhabitants (1%). Spread of clonal strains of group A meningococcus may be a factor in Africa's unusually high rate of epidemic disease. Clonal strains can migrate transcontinentally and cause epidemics, such as the clonal group A meningococcus designated electrophoretic type III-1 (ET III-1), which caused epidemics in China, Nepal, Saudi Arabia, Chad, and Kenya in the 1980s.[133,152]

International outbreaks of *N. meningitidis* infection occurred in 1987 and 2000 and were associated with Muslims making the annual pilgrimage to Mecca. The disease spread to persons of all nationalities represented, some of whom returned home before becoming ill.[133,156] In some cases, close contacts of travelers were infected. Several cases in U.S. citizens were attributed to the outbreaks. The 1987 outbreak was linked to serogroup A, whereas the 2000 outbreak was caused by serogroup W-135.[28,131,156] Saudi Arabia now requires meningococcal vaccine for travelers entering the country to participate in the annual pilgrimage to Mecca.[107]

Serogroups A, B, C, and Y account for more than 90 percent of meningococcal disease worldwide. Currently in the United States, serogroups B, C, and Y each accounts for approximately a third of the cases.[21,31] Serogroup A, which causes periodic epidemics in developing countries, is responsible for only occasional cases of meningococcal disease in the United States. Serogroup B usually causes sporadic disease but occasionally is associated with outbreaks.[29] Serogroup C, though also a cause of sporadic disease, has been associated with numerous outbreaks in the United States, Canada, and Europe.[96] In addition, school-related outbreaks of serogroup C meningococcal disease have been reported.[21,134,214] The incidence of serogroup C and serogroup Y disease has increased in the United States during the last few years as a result of antigenic shifts involving outer-membrane protein genes.[86] Disease caused by serogroup W-135 occurs infrequently and, like serogroup Y, has been associated with meningococcal pneumonia.[171,203] Recently, serogroup X has been identified as a predominant serogroup causing epidemic meningitis in Niger, with a case-fatality rate of 12.2 percent.[14]

In 2006, Brooks and colleagues reported on an analysis of 69 outbreaks of meningococcal disease that occurred in the United States from 1992 to 2002. Outbreak-associated cases represented less than 2 percent of the total cases of invasive disease. Additionally, outbreak-related cases were associated with a higher case-fatality rate than sporadic cases were (21% versus 11%; odds ratio, 3.3; 95% confidence interval, 2.0 to 5.5).[21]

Meningococcal disease in the United States peaks during the months November through March.[168,171] The highest attack rate is seen in February, and the lowest attack rate occurs in September. In Africa, epidemic disease occurs during the dry season and decreases once the rainy season starts.[152] Males and females are affected equally.

The risk of acquiring meningococcal disease is related inversely to age, with the highest rates of disease occurring in children younger than 1 year old.[31] As many as 49 percent of cases occur in children younger than 2 years old.[95] However, in epidemics, an age shift occurs, with older children, adolescents, and young adults more often being affected.[29] A progressive increase in the development of protective antibodies against meningococci occurs between the ages of 2 and 12 years. Neonates usually are protected by passive IgG transfer in utero if the mother has antimeningococcal antibody. In general, the development of bactericidal antibodies to meningococci increases in children at a rate of approximately 5 percent per year.[77]

The precise epidemiology of meningococcal disease was defined elegantly in a series of observations in New Jersey military recruits. An inverse correlation was noted between the age-related incidence of meningococcal disease in the United States and the prevalence of serum bactericidal activity against three pathogenic strains of *N. meningitidis*.[77,78] The investigators prospectively studied all incoming recruits to Fort Dix and demonstrated that those who lacked bactericidal activity to case strains had a 38 percent attack rate if they were exposed and acquired a pathogenic meningococcus strain.[77] Usually, nasopharyngeal carriage was an immunizing process. Carriage induced the formation of protective antibodies against homologous strains but also produced cross-reacting antibodies to heterologous strains of pathogenic meningococci. Antibody production typically was seen within 2 weeks of the acquisition of carriage.[77,78]

In addition to nasopharyngeal carriage, other processes may contribute to meningococcal antibody formation. Certain strains of cross-reacting bacteria, such as *Escherichia coli* and *Bacillus*, produce capsular polysaccharides that are immunologically identical to the capsules of meningococci serogroups A, B, and C. They represent a potential immunizing source against invasive meningococcal disease in the general population.[77,102,198]

Nasopharyngeal carriage of *N. meningitidis* is lowest in infants and children and highest in adolescents and young adults. One study determined that 2.4 percent of asymptomatic infants and children had a positive nasopharyngeal culture for *N. meningitidis* during a nonepidemic period.[123] A study of 1500 Norwegians found the carriage rate to be 32.7 percent in persons 20 to 24 years of age and 10 percent in individuals older than 25.[27] Other investigators have shown that approximately 20 percent of children harbor meningococcal species in their nasopharynx, but most of these isolates are atypical, nontypeable strains that ferment lactose in addition to glucose and maltose.[77,78]

Nasopharyngeal meningococcal carriage in household contacts of persons with documented meningococcal disease is approximately 10 percent.[123,144,164] Several studies have shown that the carriage rate increases if infants or children are in the home.[102,144] In one outbreak of serogroup C meningococcal disease, carriage rates were 37.8 percent in households with a case in an infant, 17.5 percent in households with a case in a child, and 6.9 percent in households with disease in an adult.[102]

Nasopharyngeal carriage is a common finding in those who have had household contact with an index case, and colonization can persist for weeks to months. Without chemoprophylaxis, as many as 35 percent of contacts become colonized by the eighth week. The median duration of carriage is 9 months.[123] However, in nearly 40 percent of individuals, it may exceed 16 months.[79] An association between smoking and an increased rate of meningococcal carriage has been demonstrated.[181,185] In addition, passive smoke has been implicated in increasing the risk for acquiring meningococcal disease in children younger than 5 years old by 7.5 times that of the general population.

The factors responsible for converting nasopharyngeal colonization to invasive disease have not been established firmly. Many people in whom invasive disease subsequently develops are colonized shortly before the illness begins. Probably, these individuals lack bactericidal antibody, and, for some reason, protective antibody does not develop after acquiring the pathogenic strain. Other risk factors associated with invasive disease include young age, crowding (new military recruits, college freshmen in dormitories),[23,127,159] lower socioeconomic class,[170] concurrent upper respiratory infections,[132,213] intimate kissing with multiple partners,[192] specific immune deficiencies (properdin or terminal complement),[65] functional or anatomic asplenia,[69] and active or passive smoking.[67,181]

Speculation regarding the role of other upper respiratory pathogens in meningococcal disease prompted several observations. The peak incidence of meningococcal infection has been noted to mirror the peaks of such agents as influenza and *Mycoplasma*. Several studies have shown an association between colonization or infection with respiratory viruses or *Mycoplasma* and an increased risk for development of meningococcal disease.[26,92,132,176] Simultaneous outbreaks of meningococcal and influenza or echovirus infections have been documented.[117,213] In addition, one study suggested that the incidence of meningococcal disease and the resultant morbidity and mortality increased in the 5 weeks after individuals had influenza-like syndromes.[132] Researchers have postulated that viral pathogens may affect the immune response temporarily and facilitate meningococcal disease. Also possible is that disruption of the normal respiratory epithelium occurs with viral infection and thereby increases the likelihood that colonizing meningococci might become invasive.[132] Preceding viral respiratory disease is not a prerequisite for the establishment of meningococcal carriage or disease; however, its occurrence may increase the risk for invasive meningococcal disease.

A variety of host genetic factors also may influence susceptibility to invasive meningococcal disease. Individuals with late complement component deficiencies (C5, C6, C7, C8, or C9) and properdin pathway deficiencies are at increased risk for acquiring meningococcal disease.[65] This defect usually is inherited, and other members of the family may have a history of meningococcal disease or repeated meningococcal infections. Acquired complement deficiencies associated with diseases such as systemic lupus erythematosus, nephrotic syndrome, and chronic liver disease

also are associated with an increased risk of acquiring meningococcal disease.[113] A Russian study found the incidence of complement deficiency in first episodes of meningococcal disease to be approximately 1 percent.[154] In Italy, the prevalence of complement deficiency in patients with meningococcal meningitis was 17 percent.[45] The decision of whom to screen for complement deficiency should be based partly on the prevalence of meningococcal disease in a given country. In countries where the incidence of meningococcal disease is high, complement deficiency is less likely to be found. In countries such as the United States, where the incidence is relatively low, complement screening may be justified.

The chance of finding a complement or alternative pathway (properdin) deficiency substantially increases in patients with recurrent meningococcal disease or with uncommon serogroups. The prevalence of complement or properdin deficiency in a patient infected with an unusual serogroup was found to range from 31 to 50 percent.[66,141] Therefore, screening all individuals with unusual serogroups is reasonable. CH_{50} testing generally is available and will screen for the combined activity of C1 to C9. If complement deficiency is found, the individual should receive the meningococcal vaccine. In addition, family members should be screened for complement deficiency, and all family members should be educated about the disease and immunized with quadrivalent polysaccharide or protein conjugate meningococcal vaccine. Most experts concur that the conjugate vaccine is preferred in the age groups for which the vaccine is licensed (2 to 55 years).

Some investigators have shown that although persons with complement deficiency are more at risk for acquiring meningococcal disease, the disease that they get often is mild. Meningococcal infection activates the complement system, and the LOS present in the bacterial outer membrane probably is responsible for the activation. In fatal cases, intense activation has continued until the time of death.[20] The case-fatality rate in complement-deficient individuals is approximately 3 percent.[172] Complement-deficient individuals are thought to be unable to maintain the high-level activation of the complement pathway and, therefore, have less severe disease.

Properdin deficiency, which impairs activation of the alternative complement pathway, is X-linked and has been associated with fulminant meningococcal disease.[51,66] The case-fatality rate in one kindred was 75 percent for persons with meningococcal disease.[12] Screening of individuals with exceptionally fulminant disease or those who have a family history of meningococcal infection should be considered. AP_{50} will screen for properdin deficiency in the alternative complement pathway. If a deficiency is documented, those individuals and their family members should receive the quadrivalent meningococcal vaccine to prevent disease caused by serogroups of meningococcus in the vaccine (conjugate vaccine is preferred in the age groups for which the vaccine is licensed, 2 to 55 years).

Mannose-binding lectin (MBL) is a pattern recognition receptor and a component of the innate immune system. Patients with meningococcal disease during childhood have a significantly increased incidence of structural mutations in the genes coding for MBL; such mutations lead to deficient MBL function when compared with healthy age-matched controls.[62] Similarly, mutations in genes coding for toll-like receptor 4 also may increase susceptibility to meningococcal disease. Human toll-like receptor 4 mutations are associated with susceptibility to invasive meningococcal disease in infancy.[61]

PATHOLOGY AND PATHOGENESIS

The mechanisms by which meningococci invade humans are understood only partially. We do know that encapsulated, typeable meningococci are virulent, whereas nonencapsulated strains are relatively nonpathogenic. Even among encapsulated strains, differences in virulence between case and carrier strains of *N. meningitidis* have been demonstrated in an animal model.[91] The presence of a polysaccharide capsule enhances invasiveness by resisting opsonization and subsequent phagocytosis.

The human nasopharynx is the only natural reservoir of *N. meningitidis*.[183] Once pathogenic meningococci have colonized the respiratory tract of susceptible persons, either they become invasive or antibody to the organism develops and confers immunity. Meningococci adhere to nonciliated, columnar epithelial cells in the nasopharynx via pili. Binding induces endocytosis of the organism into the epithelial cell, and the bacteria may penetrate the epithelial barrier via phagocytotic vacuoles.[182] If antibody is insufficient and invasion occurs, the individual may become bacteremic. Occasionally, unsuspected meningococcal bacteremia has been detected on blood culture and spontaneously cleared on a follow-up culture without antibiotics.[186] However, in most cases, such clearance does not occur, and the individual becomes progressively ill. Bacteria in blood may seed the meninges and cause meningitis.

Meningococci are gram-negative organisms, and LOS is a major component of the bacterial cell membrane. Meningococci release blebs from their surfaces that contain outer membrane laden with LOS. LOS is a potent endotoxin, and concentrations of LOS correlate with the severity of disease.[18-20] LOS induces the release of a host of inflammatory and anti-inflammatory mediators whose concentrations also are correlated with the severity of disease: tumor necrosis factor-α (TNF-α), interferon-γ, interleukin-1 (IL-1), IL-6, IL-8, IL-10, and IL-1 receptor antagonist.[75,114,195,196,205] TNF-α down-regulates thrombomodulin expression on endothelial cells, thereby leading to decreased activity of proteins S and C.[39,139] Like TNF-α, many of the mediators directly or indirectly contribute to the formation of a procoagulant state, which results in the formation of microthrombi characteristically found in the skin, digits, extremities, and organs.

Cytokines play an important role in development of the shock frequently seen in meningococcemia. Release of cytokines causes activation of neutrophils and up-regulation of adhesion molecules that may promote endothelial damage and capillary leakage.[59] Vasodilation also may occur secondary to increased production of nitric oxide by endothelial cells.[130] Subsequent compensatory vasoconstriction of splanchnic, skin, and renal vessels may not be sufficient to maintain adequate blood pressure. Endotoxin-related or cytokine-mediated cardiac dysfunction also may contribute to the development of heart failure and hypotension.[146] Profound capillary leakage in the pulmonary bed may lead to the development of acute respiratory distress syndrome.

The disseminated intravascular coagulation (DIC) commonly seen in meningococcemia also is thought to be a consequence of activation of the coagulation system by endotoxin.[167] Experimental work in animals has suggested a synergistic effect of meningococcal endotoxin and materials egested from leukocytes containing meningococci in the initiation of DIC.[53]

The pathologic purpuric lesions seen in fulminant meningococcal disease are similar to those that the generalized Shwartzman reaction induces in rabbits by endotoxin. Pathologically, these lesions show evidence of microthrombi in small dermal vessels, endothelial damage, and hemorrhage. Inflammatory vasculitis is mediated by up-regulation of endothelial adhesion molecules, activation of neutrophils, and effects of cytokines and bacterial endotoxin.[4,44,90] Circulating concentrations of endotoxin in patients with meningococcemia may be 50 to 100 times that of other gram-negative infections.[155] In addition, meningococcal endotoxin is more potent than is endotoxin from enteric bacilli.[46]

A pathologic study of 200 fatal meningococcal infections[85] illustrates the ability of the meningococcus to affect virtually any organ, either directly or indirectly. Approximately 40 percent of the patients had both meningococcemia and meningitis. Except for adults with meningitis, the average survival for all patients was 72 hours or less. The major organ systems involved at autopsy in these 200 cases were the heart, central nervous system (CNS), skin, mucous and serous membranes, and adrenals. Myocarditis developed in 78 percent of cases. Cutaneous hemorrhage occurred in 69 percent of the fatal infections and ranged from isolated petechiae to diffuse purpura. Acute meningitis was noted at autopsy in 68 percent, with brain abscesses found in two patients. In almost half the patients with acute meningococcemia, *N. meningitidis* was isolated from otherwise normal cerebrospinal fluid (CSF). Adrenal hemorrhage and necrosis were found in 48 percent of autopsy cases. Diffuse adrenal hemorrhage occurred in approximately 50 percent of adult cases and in more than 80 percent of pediatric cases. Focal areas of inflammation and petechial hemorrhage were seen in many other tissues, including the synovium, skeletal muscle, and the tracheobronchial tree. An association was noted between the pathologic findings and the infecting serogroup of *N. meningitidis*. Serogroup A infections most frequently were associated with encephalitis; serogroup B and C infections were associated with necrotizing myocarditis.

CLINICAL MANIFESTATIONS AND DIFFERENTIAL DIAGNOSIS

The spectrum of disease caused by *N. meningitidis* ranges from asymptomatic transient bacteremia, which clears spontaneously, to fulminant sepsis resulting in death only a few hours after the first symptoms occur.[186] In 2006, Kaplan and colleagues (U.S. Multicenter Meningococcal Surveillance Study Group) reviewed 159 episodes of invasive meningococcal disease seen at 10 children's hospitals in the United States between January 2001 and March 2005.[101] Meningitis was the most common manifestation of disease, seen in 70 percent of cases. Twenty-seven percent of children had bacteremia alone, and 4.4 percent had fulminant disease. Fifty-five percent of the children had petechiae, and 38 percent had purpura. Hypotension was present in 10 percent and thrombocytopenia in 6 percent on admission. The overall mortality rate was 8 percent, and it was significantly higher in children who were 11 years of age or older than in children younger than 11 years ($p < 0.001$). Hearing loss occurred in 12.5 percent of children with meningitis. Skin necrosis occurred in 9.4 percent of children, and 2.4 percent required skin grafts. One percent of children underwent amputations; one child lost all four limbs. Only one penicillin-intermediate isolate was identified in this study, and no penicillin-resistant isolates were found.

MENINGOCOCCEMIA/MENINGITIS

Serious or invasive disease usually is manifested in one of two ways: meningococcemia or meningitis (either with or without meningococcemia). It is important to consider other causes in the differential diagnosis of meningococcemia (Table 99–1).

The signs and symptoms of meningococcemia are variable. Early in the course, evidence of an upper respiratory infection, including coryza, pharyngitis, tonsillitis, and laryngitis, may be present. Patients generally are febrile, with complaints of headache, lethargy, and vomiting. Severe myalgia with muscle tenderness and joint pain also may be the initial complaint.[93] The typical patient with meningococcemia has a short history of upper respiratory symptoms, fever, and a hemorrhagic rash. Signs of severe circulatory collapse often develop. It is not unusual for purpura and shock to develop within hours of the onset of symptoms.

The skin manifestations of meningococcemia range from diffuse mottling to extensive purpuric lesions (Figs. 99–1 and

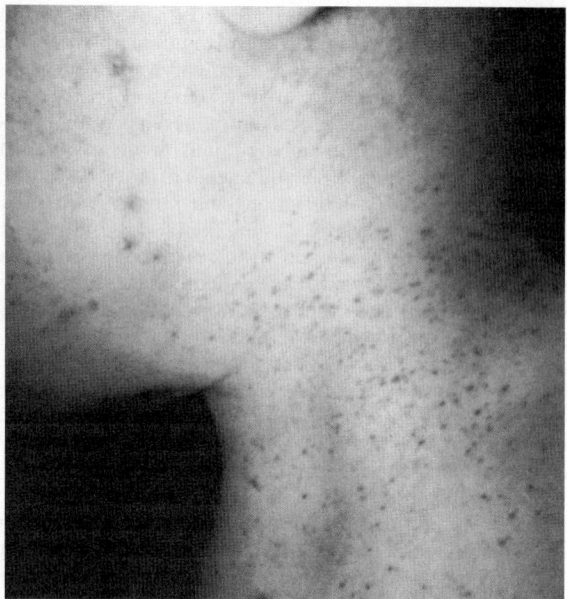

Figure 99–1 Petechial lesions are seen on the face and neck of a young child with meningococcemia.

TABLE 99-1   Differential Diagnosis of Meningococcemia

INFECTIOUS
Rocky Mountain spotted fever
Ehrlichia
Streptococcal pneumoniae sepsis
Haemophilus influenzae type b sepsis
Group A *Streptococcus* sepsis
Other bacterial sepsis with disseminated intravascular coagulation
  (i.e., enteric gram-negatives)
Subacute bacterial endocarditis
Gonococcemia
Rat-bite fever
Typhus
Secondary syphilis

NONINFECTIOUS
Henoch-Schönlein purpura
Idiopathic thrombocytopenic purpura
Collagen vascular disease
Neoplastic processes

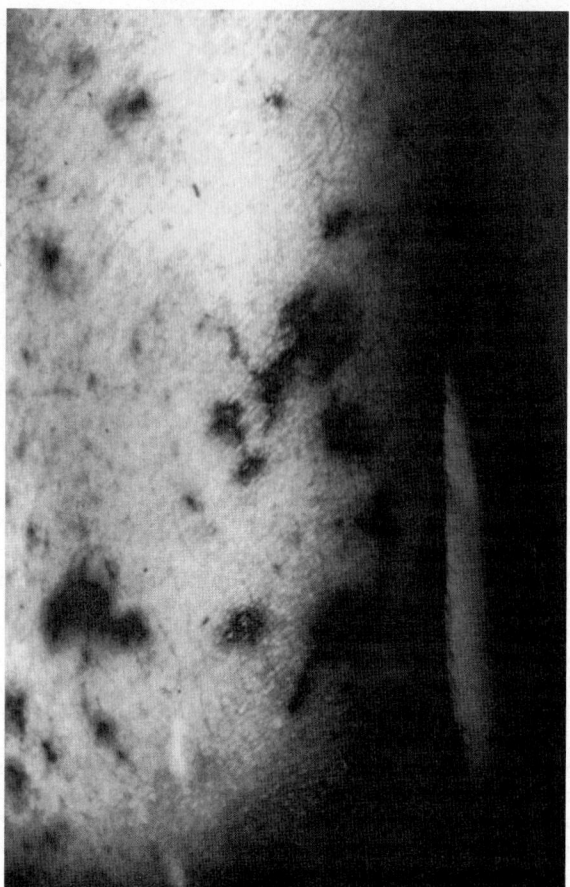

Figure 99–2 Extensive purpuric lesions occurring in a child with overwhelming meningococcemia and disseminated intravascular coagulation.

99–2). Unfortunately, some variation in the type of rash is seen. Petechiae or purpura is present in 50 to 60 percent of patients.[103,212] Maculopapular rash alone is reported in 10 to 13 percent of patients.[124,212] Twenty to 30 percent of children may have no rash at initial evaluation.[212] This variance renders differentiating meningococcemia from a viral exanthem particularly difficult. A pink macular rash resembling early varicella is another variant sometimes seen in children with meningococcemia; these lesions often are tender. They may occur in crops, as do petechiae, and are seen most frequently on the trunk and extremities.[55,89]

The finding of petechiae or purpura in a febrile child should increase the index of suspicion for meningococcemia or other serious disease (e.g., infectious, neoplastic, immunologic). Acral distribution of a rash, in particular, is worrisome for meningococcemia or another infectious vasculitic process. In two studies involving more than 200 patients with fever and petechiae (not purpura), 8 percent to 20.2 percent had invasive bacterial disease.[199,212] Seven to 10 percent of the total group had infections

caused by *N. meningitidis*. Therefore, obtaining blood cultures for most febrile patients with petechiae seems reasonable. Lumbar puncture should be performed if clinically indicated or if the blood culture ultimately is positive. Antibiotic therapy in these patients should include coverage for meningococcus.

Purpura is noted in 16 to 24 percent of patients.[157,168,212] When the purpura is extensive and accompanied by shock, it is referred to as *purpura fulminans*. Acquired deficiencies of protein S and protein C have been described in some patients with purpura fulminans.[157,158] One study showed a mortality rate of 50 percent in patients in whom purpura developed. Progressive purpura was accompanied by declining protein C levels, and the protein C level was related inversely to the clinical severity of the disease.[157]

Patients with meningitis often are febrile, with headache, vomiting, irritability, stiff neck, and sometimes seizures. They may have a history of lethargy, or they may be obtunded at initial evaluation. In neonates, physical findings of meningismus, such as the Kernig and Brudzinski signs, often are absent. The anterior fontanelle, if open, may be full and tense.

The most common neurologic complications of meningitis are hydrocephalus, cranial nerve palsy (especially hearing loss), subdural effusion or empyema, cerebral edema, cortical vein thrombosis, and cerebral infarction. Neurologic sequelae occur much more commonly in patients with meningitis, but complications such as cerebral infarction also can be seen in children with meningococcemia and shock.[145]

Cerebral edema and cranial nerve palsies may be seen initially or develop shortly thereafter. Sixth nerve or third nerve palsies are suggestive of increased intracranial pressure (ICP) and impending herniation, respectively. The development of either of these signs is indicative of an urgent intracranial process. Hearing loss occurs in 5 to 10 percent of patients with meningitis. Auditory testing should be performed after recovery on all patients with meningitis.

Subdural effusion or empyema should be considered in patients with fever persisting after 8 days of therapy, vomiting, or the development of signs of increased ICP after the initial few days of treatment. Drainage is recommended only if the effusion is infected (empyema) or is large enough to produce either focal neurologic signs or increased ICP.[145]

Vascular thrombosis, cerebral infarction, or both can be caused by arterial or venous thrombosis. Venous thrombosis is more common and generally is not seen before the second week. Hemorrhagic infarction of the brain then may occur. Cerebral infarction also may be seen in patients without arterial or venous thrombosis who present in shock with prolonged hypotension and cerebral ischemia. Cerebral infarction in these individuals is an early event.

Hydrocephalus occurs most frequently in young children and those with a delayed diagnosis or severe disease. It tends to occur 3 to 4 weeks after the onset of illness. Inflammation, with collagen deposition and proliferation of fibroblasts in the meninges, produces an obstruction to the flow of CSF. A progressive increase in head circumference should alert the clinician to the possibility of hydrocephalus.[145] Imaging (computed tomography, magnetic resonance imaging) studies are diagnostic.

Neonatal meningococcemia or meningitis (or the presence of both) is an uncommon finding but has been reported. In one report, a 2-week-old infant died after having a brief febrile illness with both CSF and blood cultures positive for meningococcus. Maternal endocervical colonization was documented. In addition, the mother's pharyngeal culture grew *N. meningitidis*.[99] If endocervical colonization by *N. meningitidis* is detected prenatally, treatment with antibiotics probably should be initiated in an attempt to eradicate colonization before delivery, or intrapartum antibiotics should be given. Ceftriaxone would seem to be a reasonable choice. Rifampin and ciprofloxacin are not advocated for use during pregnancy.

CHRONIC MENINGOCOCCEMIA

Chronic meningococcemia, first described in 1902, is defined as meningococcal septicemia without meningeal symptoms in which fever has persisted for at least a week before any antibiotic therapy is initiated.[57,143] Benoit[8] reviewed 148 cases of chronic meningococcemia in the United States in 1963; patients ranged in age from 3 months to 62 years. The major symptoms included fever and chills (present in 100% of patients), rash (93.2%), arthralgias (70.3%), and headache (61.5%). The patients generally did not appear toxic and were in good health before becoming infected. The mean duration of illness before diagnosis was 6 to 8 weeks (range, 1 to 40 weeks). Symptoms tended to be intermittent; the rash often appeared in association with fever and then disappeared over the next several days. Bacteremia also was intermittent in some patients. In the Benoit study, five blood cultures were obtained for the average patient before meningococci were isolated. However, after a blood culture yielded the organism, most subsequent cultures were positive. In children, some investigators report that the organism frequently is isolated in the first blood culture.[115] The arthralgias also tended to be intermittent in nature.

In Benoit's series,[8] localizing complications developed in almost 40 percent of the patients with chronic meningococcemia. The meninges were the most common site of localization, and meningitis developed in 15.5 percent of these patients. Other localized infections included carditis, nephritis, epididymitis, conjunctivitis, iritis, and retinitis. In only one instance was an organism recovered from the joint. The average duration of meningococcemia in patients with complications was 10.2 weeks, as opposed to 4 to 8 weeks in patients without any localization.

The diagnosis is established by identifying the organism in blood cultures. Antibiotic therapy results in prompt defervescence and dramatic recovery.

The pathophysiologic mechanisms permitting chronic meningococcemia remain unclear. No evidence exists that the organisms are less virulent than other meningococci are; thus, a defect in host immunity has been suggested. A hypersensitivity basis for this disease has been postulated, and researchers have theorized that the skin changes and arthritis may be secondary to antigen-antibody complexes.[143] In contrast to acute meningococcemia, bacteria almost never are found by biopsy or culture of skin lesions. The histology of the skin lesion is distinct from that seen in skin lesions of patients with acute meningococcemia.[8,85,143]

MENINGOCOCCAL PNEUMONIA

Meningococcal pneumonia occurs in conjunction with meningococcemia or meningitis in 8 to 15 percent of cases.[106] However, the meningococcus also can play a role as a primary respiratory pathogen.

Primary meningococcal pneumonia, once considered a rare disease, now is recognized as the most common form of meningococcal disease in certain military recruit populations and has been reported to be responsible for 4.5 percent of all cases of bacterial pneumonia in a general hospital population.[106,118]

Patients with preceding viral pneumonias are at risk for the development of meningococcal pneumonia; more than 100 cases of meningococcal pneumonia occurred during the influenza pandemic of 1918 and 1919. In addition to disease among military recruits, nosocomial acquisition of meningococcal pneumonia in hospitalized patients has been reported.[38]

The diagnosis of meningococcal pneumonia is difficult to establish because isolation of the organism from sputum does not distinguish a meningococcal carrier from an individual with meningococcal pneumonia. In addition, routine sputum cultures do not include media selective for the meningococcus. Blood cultures are positive in only 15 percent.[106]

Koppes and associates[106] reported on 68 cases of meningococcal pneumonia; diagnostic criteria included a compatible clinical syndrome and isolation of *N. meningitidis* from pleural fluid or blood. All 68 meningococcal pneumonia cases were group Y; during the same period, 10 cases of meningococcemia and 6 cases of meningitis caused by group Y occurred. The high ratio of pneumonia to meningitis in this study suggested that group Y organisms may be more likely than are other serogroups to cause pneumonia, and this finding has been substantiated by other investigators.[160,170] Pneumonia caused by group B or C meningococci has been reported, usually in association with meningococcemia or meningitis.[210]

Primary meningococcal pneumonia usually is associated with a gradual onset of symptoms and a history of an antecedent upper respiratory infection. Rales and fever are found in most patients, and 80 percent have pharyngitis. The radiograph often shows involvement of the lower lobes with patchy alveolar infiltrates. More than one lobe is involved in 40 percent of these patients. Twenty-five percent of them have pleural effusions. Petechiae, purpura, or shock was not present in any of the patients with pneumonia reported by Koppes and colleagues.[106]

The pathogenesis of this disease is thought to be pulmonary infection via inhalation of droplets. The epidemiologic importance of meningococcal pneumonia was emphasized in a report from the CDC that discussed nosocomial transmission of group Y *N. meningitidis* in oncology patients.[38] The index case had meningococcal pneumonia. Meningococcal bacteremia developed in one other patient in an adjacent room; in three additional patients, group Y *N. meningitidis* was isolated from nasopharyngeal cultures. Airborne dissemination seemed to be the mode of transmission. Respiratory isolation is indicated for a patient with suspected meningococcal pneumonia.

Penicillin therapy for penicillin-sensitive meningococcal pneumonia results in a prompt clinical response. Ninety-three percent of the patients reported by Koppes and colleagues[106] were afebrile after 3 days of therapy. Third-generation cephalosporins, such as ceftriaxone and cefotaxime, may be the current drugs of choice pending definitive identification.

OTHER MENINGOCOCCAL SYNDROMES

Conjunctivitis

Primary meningococcal conjunctivitis is indistinguishable clinically from acute bacterial conjunctivitis caused by other organisms. Usually, it is manifested in children as an acute onset of unilateral purulent conjunctivitis.[7] It has been reported in individuals aged 2 days to adulthood.[8] Gram stain of the purulent material typically shows gram-negative diplococci that sometimes may be confused with gonococcal conjunctivitis. Barquet and colleagues[7] showed that 44 percent of the isolates were serogroup B meningococci.

The complications of primary meningococcal conjunctivitis reported by Barquet and associates[7] included sepsis or meningitis in approximately 18 percent. The symptoms of systemic meningococcal disease occurred 3 to 96 hours after onset of the conjunctivitis (mean, 41 hours). In patients treated only with topical therapy when initially evaluated for conjunctivitis, systemic disease was 19 times more likely to develop than in patients treated with systemic therapy ($p = 0.001$). Ocular complications occurred in 15.5 percent of patients and included corneal ulcers (10.7%), keratitis, hemorrhage, and iritis.

Pharyngitis

The diagnosis of meningococcal pharyngitis is difficult to establish because, like group A beta-hemolytic streptococci, isolation of meningococcus from the pharynx does not establish that this organism is the etiologic agent. In fact, most individuals who harbor meningococci in their nasopharynx are asymptomatic carriers. However, Banks[5] noted overt nasopharyngitis in a third of patients with meningococcal sepsis or meningitis. Pizzi,[153] in describing a severe epidemic of meningococcal meningitis, noted that individuals with sore throats often had a pure culture of meningococci. Olcen and associates[144] performed cultures on family members of 21 consecutive patients with meningococcal disease and found that 61 percent of family members with a sore throat or other upper respiratory symptoms were meningococcal carriers, as opposed to 14 percent of asymptomatic family members.

On occasion, individuals in the community with symptomatic pharyngitis have cultures performed and the laboratory reports the growth of *N. meningitidis*. If the patient is febrile but otherwise appears well, we recommend obtaining blood for culture and administering intramuscular or intravenous ceftriaxone. If the blood culture is negative, the patient should be treated with an antibiotic that will eradicate the meningococcus (see "Chemoprophylaxis"). If the patient is afebrile and asymptomatic at the time that the culture results are obtained, we recommend eradication of the organism with one of the antibiotics suggested for chemoprophylaxis.

Arthritis

Meningococcal arthritis occurs primarily in adults. The overall incidence, as a complication of bacteremia, is approximately 2 to 14 percent.[81,212] There are two forms of meningococcal arthritis. The first is seen within the first few days of treatment and is characterized by severe arthralgias and few objective signs of joint inflammation. The pathogenesis of this arthritis has been suggested to be an inflammatory response to viable organisms that have seeded the synovium during the initial bacteremia. The second, more common form appears to be an immune complex phenomenon. It usually is noted 3 to 7 days after recognition of meningococcemia, often at a time when the patient appears to be improving from the meningitis or sepsis. The knee, wrist, elbow, and ankle joints are involved most commonly.[81]

In both forms, the arthritis usually is monarticular or oligoarticular with an effusion, minimal pain, erythema, and limitation of motion. Organisms seldom are cultured from the effusion; culture of joint fluid yields meningococci in less than 10 percent of cases. The exception is a child with suppurative arthritis on initial evaluation. In one study, 8 percent of patients with meningococcal infection had arthritis; 75 percent were culture-positive when culture was performed before receiving antibiotics.[210,212]

Synovial fluid leukocyte counts vary widely, but counts greater than $100,000/mm^3$ have been reported.[151] The appearance of arthritis often is accompanied by a rise in temperature; in 7 of 47 patients with arthritis, a characteristic skin lesion appeared at the same time.[82] These lesions began as skin hyperpigmentation but progressed to vesiculation and ulceration; biopsy showed vasculitis. Additional evidence of concurrent vasculitis is suggested by reports of episcleritis and mild proteinuria developing simultaneously with arthritis.[82]

On histologic examination, the synovium is infiltrated by mononuclear cells that contain IgM, C3, and meningococcal antigen,[82] which strongly suggests an immune complex–mediated disease. No specific therapy is indicated, and the arthritis resolves spontaneously. Controversy exists regarding the role of intermittent closed drainage of the joint space.[13] Permanent joint deformity is an uncommon feature of this disease that occurs in approximately 10 percent of cases.[175] Edwards and Baker[58] reported allergic complications of meningococcal disease in 10 percent of the 86 children monitored prospectively. More than 83 percent were serogroup B, although late-onset arthritis and vasculitis also have been reported with serogroup A and C disease.

Permanent joint damage is an unusual event that occurs in approximately 1.5 percent of patients with arthritis. Potential sequelae include ankylosis, decreased range of motion, and bone necrosis.[113]

Pericarditis and Myocarditis

Pericarditis occurs in 3 to 5 percent of cases as a complication of meningococcal disease, although one series reported a 19 percent incidence in 32 patients with meningococcal meningitis.[56,135] It generally occurs in patients with meningococcemia but has been reported as an isolated event without septicemia or meningitis.[88]

Pericarditis is presumed to be a late complication of meningococcal disease because clinical symptoms such as fever, dyspnea, or substernal chest pain (or even cardiac tamponade) usually do not appear until the fourth to seventh day of illness. However, several investigators have noted early evidence of pericarditis based on the electrocardiographic or roentgenographic data of patients examined at the time of hospital admission.

Because most symptomatic pericardial effusions develop late in the course of the illness, are serous in nature, and are sterile, the pathophysiologic mechanism is presumed to be an immune complex reaction. Uncontrolled studies report the successful use of steroids for the treatment of this complication.[101] However, one report documented pericarditis and the development of tamponade in a patient receiving steroids.[147]

The clinical course of meningococcal pericarditis usually is benign, but pericardial compression requiring pericardiocentesis can occur.[147] Early relapses also have been reported, but they were self-limited. Cases of constrictive pericarditis requiring pericardectomy have been reported.[147,177,204]

Myocarditis was noted at autopsy in 78 percent of patients with fatal meningococcal disease.[85] Myocarditis was seen most often in adults but was more severe when it occurred in children. Rosenblatt and colleagues[168] noted myocarditis at autopsy in 10 of 12 children with fatal meningococcal infection. Pathologic examination revealed collections of inflammatory cells in the myocardial interstitium and focal extravasation of erythrocytes with acute vasculitis. Abscesses and endocarditis were not seen. Inflammation occasionally may involve the atrioventricular node and has been reported as a cause of sudden death in a patient recovering from meningococcal meningitis.[166]

Miscellaneous Meningococcal Infections

Several unusual syndromes, including primary meningococcal pericarditis,[199] mesenteric adenitis,[109] peritonitis,[109] and genitourinary infections, have been reported.[63]

LABORATORY FINDINGS AND DIAGNOSIS

Wong and colleagues[212] reviewed 100 cases of meningococcal infection in children seen at their institution between 1985 and 1988. Leukopenia (white blood cell count <5000/mm^3) was present in 21 percent, and thrombocytopenia was noted in 14 percent. Fifty-five percent of patients had meningitis. Eleven percent of those with culture-positive meningitis had no CSF abnormalities detected on chemistry panels or examination.

Hyponatremia is seen in some patients with meningitis. Inappropriate secretion of antidiuretic hormone is the mechanism. In one study of 43 children with meningococcal meningitis, the syndrome of inappropriate secretion of antidiuretic hormone developed in 7 percent.[60]

Other laboratory abnormalities seen in patients with sepsis or shock include abnormal coagulation panels (DIC), acidosis, and abnormal liver function studies.

The gold standard for diagnosis is based on recovering the organism from blood, CSF, or petechiae. Blood culture alone is positive approximately 50 percent of the time in patients who have not received antibiotics.[212] Rapid diagnosis often can be made by Gram stain of CSF in patients with meningitis. Characteristic gram-negative diplococci are seen. Caution should be exercised in relying solely on the Gram stain to determine initial antibiotics. Broad-spectrum antibiotic therapy should be initiated pending identification of the organism by culture. Overdecolorized gram-positive cocci of *Streptococcus pneumoniae*, on occasion, have been confused with meningococci on Gram stain.

In patients who have skin lesions, a rapid presumptive diagnosis of meningococcemia frequently can be made by needle aspiration and Gram stain of a skin lesion. Needle aspiration yields gram-negative diplococci on the Gram-stained specimen in approximately 50 percent of patients with acute meningococcal infections.[197] Culture of the aspirate increases the yield further. Correlation of the Gram stain with clinical findings is important because disseminated gonococcal infection also may be accompanied by skin lesions that yield gram-negative diplococci on Gram stain.

Counterimmunoelectrophoresis and latex agglutination have been used to detect circulating antigen in the serum, CSF, and urine of patients with meningococcal disease.[207] Latex agglutinin tests using serum and urine are not recommended.[2] Cross-reactions with certain *E. coli* K1 (cause of neonatal meningitis) or *Bacillus* strains may occur. Latex agglutinin tests using CSF may be helpful in patients pretreated with antibiotics and with a compatible clinical syndrome.[2] These tests are of particular benefit in cases of partially treated meningococcal meningitis, in which culture and Gram stain may be negative.

Polymerase chain reaction (PCR), one of the newer tests for detection of *N. meningitidis*, may be very helpful in establishing the diagnosis in patients with partially treated meningococcemia or meningitis. Once antibiotics have been given, the chance that a blood culture will be positive decreases to less than 5 percent.[25] One study showed the sensitivity and specificity of PCR for *N. meningitidis* to be 91 percent with CSF specimens. Treatment with antibiotics before the test did not decrease the test's sensitivity or specificity.[140] Use of this test in confirming meningococcal infections in patients pretreated with antibiotics may be valuable in subsequent patient management, follow-up, and prompt institution of chemoprophylaxis in contacts. One report from the United Kingdom describes the use of a multiplex PCR assay for the simultaneous detection of *N. meningitidis*, *Haemophilus influenzae*, and *S. pneumoniae* from clinical samples of CSF and whole blood. Corless and colleagues[41] found that sensitivity for detection of the three organisms ranged from 88.4 percent to 91.8 percent with 100 percent specificity. Commercially available assays such as this would greatly facilitate establishing the etiologic diagnosis in children with sepsis or meningitis. Currently, meningococcal PCR is in use in the United Kingdom, but it is available in the United States only as a research test.

MORTALITY AND PROGNOSIS

The overall mortality associated with invasive meningococcal disease in the United States is 7 to 19 percent.[101,142,169,184] Numerous different scoring systems have been devised in an attempt to predict prognosis in patients with meningococcal disease. These scoring systems were reviewed in an article by Kirsch and colleagues.[105]

The Glasgow Meningococcal Septicaemia Prognostic Score (GMSPS) is a validated scoring system developed to assess clinically patients and facilitate admission of the most severely ill children to intensive care units.[178,189] This scoring system, which evaluates seven key items (hypotension, difference in skin core temperature, coma, acute deterioration, absence of meningismus, progressive purpura, and base deficit), has been used by many investigators to define criteria for entry into clinical trials.

In a review of 100 cases of meningococcal disease at the Los Angeles Children's Hospital, five features were identified that correlated with poor prognosis: shock or seizures on initial evaluation, hypothermia, total white blood cell count less than 5000/mm^3, platelet count less than 100,000/mm^3, and the development of purpura fulminans. The overall mortality in this series was 10 percent.[212]

Most prognostic scoring systems and clinical reviews agree that purpura fulminans and shock uniformly are poor prognostic signs. Individuals with only meningitis have a case-fatality rate lower than that of those with bacteremia or an isolate from another source (2% vs. 12%).[169] Presumably, this is a function of virulence of the organism, ability of the immune system to contain the infection, or both. Case-fatality rates also differ by serogroup and are higher in W-135 disease (21%) than in serogroups C (14%), Y (9%), or B (6%).[169]

Evidence suggests that a genetic component of host cytokine production may be associated with the severity of disease. Westendorp and coworkers[206] reported that families with low TNF production or high IL-10 production are at increased risk for having fatal outcomes of meningococcal disease. Recently, investigators have been studying variants of proinflammatory host genes (TNF-α, IL-1) to see whether polymorphisms in these genes might be linked to the severity of disease. Read and associates[163] found that homozygosis of certain alleles at the IL-1 locus increased the risk of death occurring in individuals with meningococcal disease and suggested that the IL-1 genotype may be associated with fatal outcomes.

TREATMENT

Therapy for meningococcal disease has evolved during the last century. In the early 1900s, treatment consisted of the administration of intravenous and intrathecal horse serum and CSF drainage. The mortality rate associated with this therapy was 26 percent.[89] The use of sulfonamides lowered the death rate to 5 or 10 percent.[83] With the emergence of sulfa-resistant strains, penicillin was added to the regimen and still may be used for susceptible meningococcal infections. In the late 1980s, reports began to appear of meningococci relatively resistant to penicillin. The mechanism of resistance is reduced binding affinity of penicillin-binding proteins. Relatively resistant strains have been reported in the United States, Canada, Europe, South Africa, Romania, and Croatia.[16,97,148,187,213] Isolates that are absolutely resistant to penicillin (minimal inhibitory concentration >1.0 µg/mL) have been documented from Spain and the United Kingdom.[148,187] Strains with resistance to fluoroquinolones also have been reported on rare occasion.[42,122] Non–ceftriaxone-susceptible strains have been reported from India.[122] Routine susceptibility testing of meningococcal strains is not currently recommended.

Genotypic and phenotypic studies of penicillin-resistant isolates from Spain revealed that the strains were genetically diverse and did not arise from a single clone.[215] In addition, Mendelman and colleagues[126] demonstrated that these strains have a penicillin-binding protein (PBP-3) with less penicillin-binding capacity than seen in sensitive strains. These strains appear to have arisen by the acquisition of segments of genes (by transformation) from the naturally resistant *Neisseria* commensals *N. flavescens* and *N. lactamica*.[180] The gene encoding PBP-2, *penA* in commensal *Neisseria*, encodes a protein that has less avidity for penicillin G. Transformation of *N. meningitidis* with *penA* from these strains leads to a slight decrease in penicillin G susceptibility; repeated transformation will yield a penicillin-resistant strain.

In 1988, penicillin-resistant meningococci also were reported from South Africa and the United Kingdom; these strains had acquired a gonococcal plasmid encoding for the production of β-lactamase.[187]

Prompt institution of antibiotic therapy for suspected meningococcal infection may be lifesaving. Children with fever and purpura should be considered to have meningococcemia until proved otherwise while recognizing that other pathogens may cause fever and purpura. A purpura fulminans–like manifestation also has been reported rarely to be caused by *Staphylococcus aureus*,[108] group A *Streptococcus*,[54] group B *Streptococcus*, and overt sepsis, with other organisms causing DIC. Antibiotics should be administered as soon as possible. A systematic review of the effectiveness of antibiotics given before admission concluded that "the data are consistent with benefit when a substantial proportion of cases are treated."[84] If possible, blood should be drawn for culture before antibiotics are administered, but collection of specimens should not delay such administration. A lumbar puncture can be performed in stable patients, but the procedure also should not delay the administration of antibiotics. CSF obtained after antibiotic therapy has been administered may be sterile, but pleocytosis will be apparent. In patients who are unstable or have significant coagulopathy, lumbar puncture should be deferred.

Shortly after receiving bactericidal antibiotics, some patients exhibit marked clinical deterioration, including hypotension and sometimes death. Rapid liberation of endotoxin (and resultant stimulation of cytokine release) from lysing organisms may be the cause of this phenomenon.[125]

The clinical features of *N. meningitidis* meningitis may be similar to those of meningitis caused by *S. pneumoniae* or *H. influenzae*. Empiric antibiotic therapy should, therefore, take into consideration the most likely pathogens. In children older than 1 month with meningitis, vancomycin plus cefotaxime (or vancomycin plus ceftriaxone) is an appropriate regimen until a definitive diagnosis has been established. Similarly, empiric therapy for children younger than 1 month includes ampicillin and cefotaxime, with consideration given to the addition of vancomycin.[171]

For penicillin-susceptible meningococcemia or meningitis, intravenous penicillin G, 250,000 to 300,000 U/kg/day (maximum, 12 million U/day) given in divided doses every 4 to 6 hours for 7 days, is effective.[2] Third-generation cephalosporins, ceftriaxone (100 mg/kg/day intravenously in two divided doses) or cefotaxime (200 mg/kg/day intravenously in three or four divided doses), also are effective. Cefotaxime or ceftriaxone is recommended for travelers from Spain, Italy, and parts of Africa because of reports of penicillin resistance in these areas.[2]

In confirmed cases of meningococcal disease, comparisons of penicillin G with ceftriaxone have shown ceftriaxone to be as efficacious. Necrotic skin lesions were seen more commonly in the penicillin group, but otherwise, complication and mortality rates were equivalent.[193] Meningococcal disease has been treated successfully with ceftriaxone intravenously in both once-a-day (80 to 100 mg/kg/day) and twice-a-day (100 mg/kg/day in two divided doses) dosing regimens.[193] Chloramphenicol is an alternative for penicillin-allergic patients. Currently, routine susceptibility testing of meningococcal isolates is not recommended. However, in selected cases in which the patient is not responding as expected, susceptibility testing may be warranted. With all cases of meningococcal disease, eradicating colonization of the index case is important (see "Chemoprophylaxis").

Administration of steroids to patients with septic shock and meningococcemia is controversial, but several studies have reported adrenal insufficiency (or partial adrenal insufficiency) in 10.3 to 16.9 percent of severely ill children with meningococcemia.[15,48,50,165] In those patients with Waterhouse-Friderichsen syndrome, treatment with steroids is indicated. However, treatment of meningococcal meningitis with steroids has been debated in the literature for years. Steroid proponents point to *H. influenzae* type b meningitis and *S. pneumoniae* studies, in which treatment with steroids decreases hearing loss and may reduce neurologic sequelae. They postulate that steroids, through anti-inflammatory effects, may decrease polymorphonuclear neutrophils, macrophages, and cytokines in the CNS and thus decrease CNS immune-mediated damage and hearing loss. Steroid opponents say that no conclusive studies show steroids to be of benefit in meningococcal meningitis and that risks include gastrointestinal ulceration, decreased penetration of antibiotics into the CNS (because of decreased meningeal inflammation), and steroid psychosis. If steroids are used, it seems prudent to administer them early (preferably close to the time that the first dose of antibiotics is administered). However, antibiotics should never be withheld while waiting for steroids to be given.

EXPERIMENTAL/ADJUNCTIVE THERAPIES

Many adjunctive and experimental therapies have been tried or are being evaluated presently. Anti-endotoxin therapies and infusion of protein C concentrate are the most recent additions (Table 99–2). Two anti-endotoxin therapies have been evaluated

TABLE 99–2   Recent Studies of Alternative Therapies for Severe Meningococcemia or Sepsis Syndrome

Year	Study	Authors	Randomized/Placebo Controlled	Eligible Patients	Patient Number (N)	Results
1997	Activated protein C	Smith, White, Vaughan, et al.[179]	No/No	3 months to 27 years old, severe meningococcemia with septic shock and purpura fulminans	12	0 deaths, 2 patients with amputations. Favorable results in comparison to the historical mortality rate of 50% in patients with shock, purpura fulminans, and Glasgow meningococcal septicemic prognostic score indicating an expected mortality of >80%
1999	HA-1A	Derkx, Wittes, and McCloskey[52]	Yes/Yes	3 months to 18 years old, petechiae or purpura, hypotension, toxicity, or end-organ dysfunction	269	No statistically significant reduction in 28-day mortality demonstrated. Mortality rate with HA-1A, 18%; with placebo, 28% ($p = 0.11$)
2000*	rBPI	Levin, Quint, Goldstein, et al.[116]	Yes/Yes	2 weeks to 18 years, petechiae or purpura, and severe disease	393	No statistically significant reduction in mortality (7.4% with rBPI, 9.9% with placebo). The treatment group had fewer amputations and a trend toward improved outcomes
2001†	Activated protein C	Bernard, Vincent, Laterre, et al.[9]	Yes/Yes	Severe sepsis (any organism, known or suspected) with organ dysfunction	1690	Significant reduction in mortality (30.8% with placebo versus 24.7% in the treatment group) and increased risk of bleeding in the treatment group
2005‡	Activated protein C	Nadel, Goldstein, Williams, et al.[137]	Yes/Yes	Pediatric patients with severe sepsis	477	Study stopped after review by Data Safety and Monitoring Committee. No difference in mortality or time to resolution of complete organ failure

Fifty-seven patients died before receiving drug or placebo (after randomization) and were not included in this analysis.
†*This study enrolled adults with severe clinical sepsis (meningococcemia not a criterion for entrance).*
‡*This study enrolled pediatric patients with severe clinical sepsis of all types.*
rBPI, recombinant bactericidal/permeability increasing protein.

in clinical trials: HA-1A and recombinant bactericidal/permeability increasing protein (rBPI). HA-1A, a human monoclonal antibody to endotoxin, was evaluated in a randomized, double-blind, placebo-controlled trial in 269 children with severe meningococcemia. Although the 28-day mortality rate in the treatment group was 18 percent as compared with 28 percent in the placebo group, this difference was not statistically significant ($p = 0.11$).[52] BPI is a naturally occurring protein in neutrophil azurophilic granules. BPI binds to and neutralizes the effects of endotoxin. Administration of rBPI was studied in 393 children with presumed meningococcal disease. There was no difference in mortality rates (7.4% with rBPI versus 9.9% with placebo). A trend in reduction of amputations in the treatment group that approached statistical significance ($p = 0.067$) was noted.[116]

Infusions of recombinant protein C concentrate have been studied in adults in a large randomized, placebo-controlled trial of 1690 patients with severe sepsis. A reduction in the mortality rate was demonstrated, but the treatment group had an increased risk of bleeding.[9] Smith and colleagues[179] compared 12 children with severe meningococcemia and purpura fulminans treated with protein C concentrate and historical controls. No deaths occurred in the treated patients versus a 50 percent rate in historical controls. A large study published in 2007 compared activated protein C with placebo in children with presumed meningococcal

infection. The study was terminated by the Data and Safety Monitoring Board because of a low likelihood of improved outcome in the treatment group.

Additional supportive measures such as prophylactic low-dose heparin are used by some clinicians.[208] Many investigators have studied the effect of heparin on survival and DIC in patients with meningococcemia, but no consistent beneficial effect on these parameters has been noted. Serious side effects directly attributed to heparin therapy have been reported rarely.[73] Difficulty adjusting the dose in small infants may lead to heparin intoxication. A retrospective chart review of 24 patients with purpura fulminans showed less necrosis of the digits and extremities in patients treated with heparin, but the results were not statistically significant.[110]

Many other experimental therapies have been attempted in patients with fulminant meningococcemia. Anecdotal reports or small case series describe the use of tissue plasminogen activator,[1,136] antithrombin III infusion,[37] topical nitroglycerin,[94,129] plasmapheresis,[36] and extracorporeal membrane oxygenation.[112] Continuous caudal block has been used to restore lower extremity perfusion.[190] Evidence is insufficient to state that any of these therapies has a significant impact on outcomes in meningococcal disease. Larger, multicenter studies are needed to evaluate efficacy.

CHEMOPROPHYLAXIS

The ability of *N. meningitidis* to spread from person to person and cause epidemic disease has been recognized since the 1800s. The secondary attack rate in households with an index case is approximately 1000 times the attack rate in the general population.[3,181] Household crowding and young age are factors that increase the secondary attack rate. The mode of transmission is direct contact with respiratory droplets or secretions. For these reasons, chemoprophylaxis is recommended for household contacts of an index case and for young daycare center contacts. Persons who have had significant contact with the oral secretions of an index case also should be considered for prophylaxis. Several epidemiologic studies suggest that casual acquaintances (such as school-aged classmates) are not at increased risk, although a number of authors have reported secondary cases in this population.[98,100] Prophylaxis is indicated for health care workers who have had intimate exposure to nasopharyngeal secretions (e.g., mouth-to-mouth resuscitation).[74] The period of communicability of the index patient is not well established. Most public health authorities recommend that persons in contact with the patient up to 7 days before the onset of illness be considered for prophylaxis. Prophylaxis should be instituted as soon as possible after identification of the index case. It is not necessary to wait for laboratory confirmation of a case if the clinical picture is most consistent with meningococcal infection. Nasopharyngeal cultures are not recommended because many nonpathogenic *Neisseria* spp. may colonize the nasopharynx.

The index patient should receive chemoprophylaxis before being discharged unless the patient has been treated with ceftriaxone (or cefotaxime). Bilukha and Rosenstein[9] reported that 4 of 14 (29%) patients with meningococcal infection treated with intravenous penicillin had positive cultures of the respiratory tract 1 week after completion of therapy.

Secondary cases originally were defined as cases occurring more than 24 but fewer than 31 days after onset in the index case. According to this definition, approximately 50 percent of secondary cases will develop in the first 7 days after occurrence in the index case. Prophylaxis must be initiated as soon as possible based on clinical findings in the index case (e.g., fulminant meningococcemia) or on laboratory culture data if the infection is manifested as bacterial meningitis, septic arthritis, or other disease.

The original drug used for chemoprophylaxis was sulfadiazine. However, a large percentage of strains now are resistant to sulfa. Table 99–3 lists four antibiotics that are highly effective in eradicating meningococcus from the nasopharynx. Rifampin generally is the drug of choice for chemoprophylaxis of children. It usually is tolerated well but has a number of side effects, including orange urine and sweat, orange staining of contact lenses, and stimulation of liver microsomal enzymes leading to a reduction in levels of other concurrent medications (e.g., oral contraceptives, anticoagulants, digoxin, phenytoin). The development of resistant strains has been reported rarely.[40] Ciprofloxacin, ceftriaxone, and rifampin have been evaluated in a randomized, comparative study.[43] All three drugs were highly effective in eradicating carriage. Ceftriaxone probably is the drug of choice for a pregnant contact and also may be indicated for children because a single intramuscular injection may result in greater compliance than do four doses of rifampin. Ciprofloxacin is contraindicated in individuals younger than 18 years old because of evidence of cartilage damage in juvenile beagles. Three cases of fluoroquinolone-resistant *N. meningitidis* disease were recently reported in North Dakota and Minnesota.[35a] Azithromycin was studied in a randomized, controlled trial that compared 500 mg of azithromycin given once orally with rifampin, 600 mg given twice daily orally for 2 days. Carriage was eradicated in 56 of 60 (93%) colonized adults treated with azithromycin versus 95 percent of the 59 colonized adults treated with rifampin.[76]

TABLE 99–3 Chemoprophylaxis Regimens for Eradication of *Neisseria meningitidis*

Drug	Age	Dose/Duration
Rifampin*	Children <1 month	5 mg/kg per dose PO bid for 2 days (4 doses)
	Children ≥1 month	10 mg/kg per dose PO bid for 2 days (4 doses)
	Adults	600 mg PO bid for 2 days (4 doses)
Ceftriaxone	Children <15 years	125 mg IM, single dose
	Children >15 years	250 mg IM, single dose
	Adults	250 mg IM, single dose
Ciprofloxacin†	Children	Not recommended
	Adults	500 mg PO, single dose
Azithromycin‡	Adults	500 mg PO, single dose (only studied in adults)

*Rifampin is not recommended for pregnant women (teratogenicity in laboratory animals). The reliability of oral contraceptives may be affected by rifampin therapy; therefore, alternative contraceptive measures should be used during and for the month after rifampin administration.
†Ciprofloxacin is not recommended for children, pregnant women, or lactating women. Three cases of fluoroquinolone-resistant N. meningitidis disease were reported in North Dakota and Minnesota. The CDC recommends the use of an alternative agent for chemoprophylaxis in affected counties.[35a]
‡Azithromycin is not currently listed in the Centers for Disease Control and Prevention's recommendations for prophylaxis.

As mentioned in the section on meningococcal vaccines, secondary disease also can be prevented by immunization of contacts. We recommend both immunization and chemoprophylaxis whenever possible (realizing that no protection against group B meningococci currently is provided by immunization).

The single most important element of chemoprophylaxis is education of contacts regarding the need for immediate medical attention if signs or symptoms of a febrile illness develop. No prophylactic strategy is 100 percent effective, and ill contacts should be evaluated medically with maintenance of a high suspicion for meningococcal disease.

MENINGOCOCCAL VACCINES

Primary prevention of meningococcal disease is essential for several reasons. The manifestation may be fulminant, with no opportunity for antibiotics to influence the course of the disease. Antibiotic-resistant strains now are recognized, and chemoprophylaxis of contacts is a cumbersome and often ineffective public health measure. Mass immunization offers the opportunity to prevent both endemic and epidemic disease worldwide.

Two vaccines, meningococcal polysaccharide vaccine and meningococcal conjugate vaccine, currently are licensed for prevention of meningococcal disease in the United States. Both vaccines are quadrivalent and contain antigens from serogroups A, C, Y, and W-135.

MENINGOCOCCAL POLYSACCHARIDE VACCINE

Meningococcal polysaccharide vaccine (MPSV4, Menomune) is a capsular polysaccharide vaccine licensed for use in individuals older than 2 years who are at increased risk for acquiring meningococcal disease. This vaccine was licensed in 1981 and has been the only meningococcal vaccine widely available in the United States until the licensing of meningococcal conjugate vaccine. MPSV4 has several limitations. First, children younger than 2 years old do not develop high levels of antibody to most pure polysaccharide antigens, so MPSV4 vaccination in young children is not reliably protective. Second, like other polysaccharide antigen–based vaccines, MPSV4 is unable to stimulate T-cell–dependent immunity to produce memory cells. Third, repeated boosting with MPSV4 has resulted in blunting of the antibody response, termed *hyporesponsiveness*.[17,120] Finally, meningococcal polysaccharide vaccines do not substantially decrease nasopharyngeal carriage. For these reasons, although MSPV4 remains licensed and available, most experts agree that meningococcal conjugate vaccines have significant advantages in indicated groups. MSPV4 is given subcutaneously as a single dose.

MENINGOCOCCAL CONJUGATE VACCINES

Meningococcal conjugate vaccines have been developed via technology similar to that used for the highly effective pneumococcal conjugate and *H. influenza*e type b conjugate vaccines. This technology couples polysaccharide antigens to a protein carrier. The United Kingdom has developed a monovalent serogroup C conjugate vaccine, and the U.S. vaccine is quadrivalent.

MENINGOCOCCAL CONJUGATE VACCINE IN THE UNITED KINGDOM. Meningococcal C conjugate vaccination in the United Kingdom has demonstrated efficacy,[161,191] ability to produce herd immunity (67% disease reduction in unvaccinated 1- to 17-year-olds),[162] and a 66 percent reduction in adolescent nasopharyngeal carriage. These studies and the dramatic reduction of disease in the United Kingdom after rollout of a comprehensive meningococcal vaccine program in children bolstered hopes that the MCV4 vaccine would have similar results.

MENINGOCOCCAL CONJUGATE VACCINE IN THE UNITED STATES. A meningococcal conjugate vaccine (MCV4, Menactra) was licensed by the U.S. Food and Drug Administration in 2005 for use in persons aged 11 to 55 years. This vaccine is a conjugate vaccine that couples polysaccharide capsular antigens (serogroups A, C, Y, W-135) to a diphtheria toxoid protein carrier. Protein conjugate vaccines stimulate both B- and T-cell–dependent immunity. The T-cell response leads to a good amnestic response.

The safety and immunogenicity of MCV4 were evaluated in adolescents and adults by several studies. In the United States, adolescent and adult immunogenicity studies comparing MCV4 and MPSV4 demonstrated no difference in the number of subjects (80%) achieving a fourfold rise in serum bactericidal antibody for all four serogroups.[104] Efficacy was inferred by demonstration of the development of serum bactericidal antibodies to each of the A, C, Y, and W-135 antigens at a level that was not inferior to the response generated by the polysaccharide vaccine (MPSV4).

The safety of MCV4 was evaluated before licensure in six clinical studies and included more than 7500 MCV4 vaccine participants and more than 3000 MPSV4 recipients. In general, the overall safety profile is similar to that of MPSV4. Local reactions occurred more commonly in the MCV4 group in both adolescents and adults; most reactions were graded as mild. The frequency of local reactions after MCV4 was similar to that reported after vaccination with tetanus and diphtheria toxoids (Td).[10,68] Some systemic symptoms (fever, headache, arthralgia, fatigue) were slightly more common in the MCV4 group than in the MPSV4 group, and most were mild in severity.

Close monitoring for potential adverse events has suggested a possible association between recent meningococcal conjugate vaccine receipt and Guillain-Barré syndrome (GBS). As of March 2007, 17 cases of GBS with onset occurring 2 to 33 days after administration of the vaccine have been reported through the Vaccine Adverse Event Reporting System since licensure of MCV4 in June 2005.[34] Researchers calculated the rate of GBS after MCV4 administration to be 0.20 per 100,000 person-months as compared with a background incidence rate of 0.11 per 100,000 person-months.[47] This study suggests that there *may* be a slightly higher risk of GBS developing in MCV4 recipients than in the general population. Because GBS is such a rare event, this association is difficult to study. The Advisory Committee for Immunization Practices (ACIP) and the American Academy of Pediatrics continue to recommend MCV4 because if the risk does exist, it is small. The observation that GBS has been reported rarely after meningococcal conjugate vaccine has been added to the Vaccine Information Statement for this vaccine.

Concomitant administration of Td and MCV4 produced similar frequencies of adverse events as did sequential administration (in which Td and MCV4 were separated by 28 days). Concomitant administration of Td and MCV4 did not result in decreased antibody titers of diphtheria, tetanus, or the meningococcal antibody responses. However, bactericidal antibody titers for serogroups C, Y, and W-135 were higher when MCV4 and Td were administered concomitantly versus sequentially (MCV4 given 28 days after Td). The clinical significance of this finding is unknown.[174] Diphtheria antibody titers were observed to be higher with concomitant administration of Td and MCV4 than with sequential administration. The clinical significance of this finding also is unknown.[174]

Meningococcal conjugate vaccine is administered intramuscularly (as opposed to MPSV4, which is administered subcutaneously). Since MCV4 has been licensed, there have been numerous reports of misadministration of it. The CDC studied 100 such cases and found that misadministration of MCV4 by the subcutaneous route still resulted in a protective immune response. Although this route of administration is not recommended for MCV4, persons who received the vaccine by this route do not need to be revaccinated.[33]

The duration of protection afforded by MCV4 is unknown. However, a study in adolescents compared persistence of serum bactericidal antibody for each of the four vaccine serogroups 3 years after vaccination with MPSV4 versus MCV4. MCV4 was associated with greater persistence of antibody titers to serogroups C and W-135 at 3 years than MSP4 was.[202]

Meningococcal conjugate vaccine studies are currently being conducted and analyzed in younger children. A U.S. study of the immunogenicity and safety of MCV4 in 2- to 10-year-old children showed higher seroconversion and antibody titers against all four vaccine serogroups in MCV4 recipients than in MPSV4 recipients ($p < 0.001$).[149] A follow-up study of these children at 23 to 36 months after receipt of MCV4 showed persistence of antibody activity, and a booster response was demonstrated by exposure to meningococcal polysaccharide antigens (small amount of MPSV4).[130]

RECOMMENDATIONS FOR USE OF MENINGOCOCCAL VACCINES

Table 99–4 summarizes recommendations of the ACIP for the use of vaccines to prevent meningococcal disease. Meningococcal vaccine is recommended for all U.S. children (who have not previously received it) at the 11- to 12-year-old pre-adolescent visit, with catch-up immunization of all older teens who have not received vaccine yet. The ACIP recommends that MCV4 be used as the preferred vaccine, but MPSV4 is an alternative.[10]

Entering college students who will be living in dormitories are at increased risk for acquiring meningococcal disease and should receive a dose of MCV4 if they have not been immunized previously (MCV4 preferred, MPSV4 is an alternative).[22] Other persons at increased risk for acquiring meningococcal disease and recommendations for vaccination are listed in Table 99–4.

TABLE 99–4   Current Recommendations for Meningococcal Vaccines in the U.S.

Age Group (Yr)	Recommendations for Healthy Persons	Recommendations for "At Risk Persons"*
0 to <2	No meningococcal vaccines are licensed in the U.S. for this age group. Phase III clinical trials of conjugate vaccines in progress.	No meningococcal vaccines are licensed in the U.S. for this age group.
2-10	Not routinely recommended	MCV4 intramuscularly[†] (preferred product) *or* MPSV4 subcutaneously[†]
11-18	Routine administration at 11-12 years recommended (catch up vaccination for older teens that have not previously been vaccinated): MCV4 intramuscularly (preferred product) or MPSV4 subcutaneously	MCV4 intramuscularly[†] (preferred product) *or* MPSV4 subcutaneously[†]
19-55	Not routinely recommended	MCV4 intramuscularly[†] (preferred product) *or* MPSV4 subcutaneously[†]

MCV4, meningococcal conjugate vaccine; MPSV4, meningococcal polysaccharide vaccine.
*"At risk persons" include: individuals with functional or anatomic asplenia, complement or properidin deficiency, travelers to areas where meningococcal disease is epidemic or hyperendemic, military recruits, college freshmen living in dormitories, persons infected with HIV, and military recruits.
†MCV4 is licensed for a single dose. Second doses of MCV4 are not currently recommended (studies pending). Persons who previously received MPSV4 and who continue to be "at risk" for meningococcal disease should receive a single dose of MCV4 three years after prior MPSV4 administration.

Persons 2 to 55 years of age who are at continued increased risk for acquiring meningococcal disease and previously have received MPSV4 should be vaccinated with a single dose of conjugate vaccine 3 years after receiving the last MPSV4 dose. Studies are currently under way regarding the issue of reimmunization with a second dose of conjugate vaccine in persons who remain at increased risk of acquiring meningococcal disease. Development of an immunogenic serogroup B meningococcal vaccine has been problematic because the polysaccharide capsule of group B meningococcus is not immunogenic in animals or humans. In 1983, Finnish investigators reported that horse antiserum to meningococcus group B reacted with glycoproteins isolated from human and rat brain.[11] Therefore, good immunogenic responses may not be achievable with group B polysaccharide antigen vaccines because the body may see these antigens as "self" antigens (similar to neural tissue). However, a serogroup B outer-membrane vesicle vaccine has been studied recently in 16- to 24-month-old children in New Zealand, and 75 percent demonstrated seroconversion after receiving three doses.[211]

Deeper understanding of the pathophysiologic mechanism of meningococcal disease and the bacterial structures critical for antigenicity and immunogenicity in humans is needed. A safe and effective vaccine that could induce protection against all encapsulated meningococci in all age groups is the ultimate goal.

REFERENCES

1. Aiuto, L., Barone, S., Cohen, P., et al.: Recombinant tissue plasminogen activator restores perfusion in meningococcal purpura fulminans. Crit. Care Med. 25:1079, 1997.
2. American Academy of Pediatrics: Red Book: Report on the Committee for Infectious Diseases. 27th ed. Elk Grove Village, IL, American Academy of Pediatrics, 2006.
3. Analysis of endemic meningococcal disease by serogroup and evaluation of chemoprophylaxis. J. Infect. Dis. 134:201, 1976.
4. Argenbright, L., and Barton, R.: Interactions of leukocyte integrins with intercellular adhesion molecule I in the production of inflammatory vascular injury in vivo. The Schwartzman reaction revisited. J. Clin. Invest. 89:259, 1992.
5. Banks, H.: Meningococcosis: A protean disease. Lancet 2:635, 1948.
6. Baraldes, M., Domingo, P., Barrio, J., et al.: Meningitis due to Neisseria subflava: Case report and review. Clin. Infect. Dis. 30:615, 2000.
7. Barquet, N., Gasser, I., Domingo, P., et al.: Primary meningococcal conjunctivitis: Report of 21 patients and review. Rev. Infect. Dis. 12:838, 1990.
8. Benoit, F.: Chronic meningococcemia. Medicine (Baltimore) 35:103, 1963.
9. Bernard, G., Vincent, J., Laterre, P., et al.: Efficacy and safety of recombinant human activated protein C for severe sepsis. N. Engl. J. Med. 344:699, 2001.
10. Bilukha, O. O., Rosenstein, N., National Center for Infectious Diseases, Centers for Disease Control and Prevention (CDC): Prevention and control of meningococcal disease. Recommendations of the Advisory Committee on Immunization Practices (ACIP). M. M. W. R. Recomm. Rep. 54(RR-7):1, 2005.
11. Bjune, G., Hoiby, E. A., Gronnesby, J. K., et al.: Effect of outer membrane vesicle vaccine against group B meningococcal disease in Norway. Lancet 338:1093, 1991.
12. Boger, W.: Fulminating meningococcemia. N. Engl. J. Med. 231:385, 1944.
13. Boger, W.: Purulent meningococcal arthritis. Am. J. Med. Sci. 208:708, 1944.
14. Boisier, P., Nicolas, P., Djibo, S., et al.: Meningococcal meningitis: Unprecedented incidence of serogroup X–related cases in 2006 in Niger. Clin. Infect. Dis. 44:657, 2007.
15. Bone, M., Diver, M., Selby, A., et al.: Assessment of adrenal function in the initial phase of meningococcal disease. Pediatrics 110:563, 2002.
16. Boras, A., Bozinovic, D., Tenover, F., et al.: First report of Neisseria meningitidis intermediately resistant to penicillin in Croatia. J. Clin. Microbiol. 39:823, 2001.
17. Borrow, R., Joseh, H., Andrews, N., et al.: Reduced antibody response to revaccination with meningococcal serogroup A polysaccharide vaccine in adults. Vaccine 19:1129, 2000.
18. Brandtzaeg, P., Halstensen, A., Kierulf, P., et al.: Molecular mechanisms in the compartmentalized inflammatory response presenting as meningococcal meningitis or septic shock. Microb. Pathog. 13:423-431, 1992.
19. Brandtzaeg, P., Kierulf, P., Gaustad, P., et al.: Plasma endotoxin as a predictor of multiple organ failure and death in systemic meningococcal disease. J. Infect. Dis. 159:195, 1989.
20. Brandtzaeg, P., Mollnes, T. E., and Kierulf, P.: Complement activation and endotoxin levels in systemic meningococcal disease. J. Infect. Dis. 160:58, 1989.
21. Brooks, R., Woods, C. W., Benjamin, D. K., Jr., et al.: Increased case-fatality rate associated with outbreaks of Neisseria meningitidis infection, compared with sporadic meningococcal disease, in the United States, 1994-2002. Clin. Infect. Dis. 43:49, 2006.
22. Bruce, M., Rosenstein, N., Capparella, J., et al.: Risk factors for meningococcal disease in college students. J. A. M. A. 286:688, 2001.
23. Brundage, J., and Zollinger, W.: Evolution of Meningococcal Disease Epidemiology in the U.S. Army. Vol. 1. Boca Raton, FL, CRC Press, 1987.
24. Buchanan, R., and Gibbons, N. (eds.): Bergey's Manual of Determinative Bacteriology. Baltimore, Williams & Wilkins, 1974, p. 427.
25. Cartwright, K., Reilly, S., White, D., et al.: Early treatment with parenteral penicillin in meningococcal disease. B. M. J. 305:143, 1992.

26. Cartwright, K. A., Jones, D. M., Smith, A. J., et al.: Influenza A and meningococcal disease. Lancet *338*:554, 1991.

27. Caugant, D. A., Hoiby, E. A., Magnus, P., et al.: Asymptomatic carriage of *Neisseria meningitidis* in a randomly sampled population. J. Clin. Microbiol. *32*:323, 1994.

28. Centers for Disease Control and Prevention: Meningococcal disease among travelers returning from Saudi Arabia. M. M. W. R. Morb. Mortal. Wkly. Rep. *36*(33):559, 1987.

29. Centers for Disease Control and Prevention: Serogroup B meningococcal disease—Oregon, 1994. M. M. W. R. Morb. Mortal. Wkly. Rep. *44*(7):121, 1995.

30. Centers for Disease Control and Prevention: Outbreaks of group B meningococcal disease—Florida, 1995 and 1997. M. M. W. R. Morb. Mortal. Wkly. Rep. *47*(39):833, 1998.

31. Centers for Disease Control and Prevention: Summary of Notifiable disease, U.S. 1999. M. M. W. R. Morb. Mortal. Wkly. Rep. *48*:1, 2001.

32. Centers for Disease Control and Prevention: Active Bacterial Core Surveillance Report, in Emerging Infections Program Network, *Neisseria meningitidis*, 2005, 2006.

33. Centers for Disease Control and Prevention: Inadvertent misadministration of meningococcal conjugate vaccine—United States, June-August 2005. M. M. W. R. Morb. Mortal Wkly. Rep. *55*(37):1016, 2006.

34. Centers for Disease Control and Prevention: Update: Guillain-Barré syndrome among recipients of Menactra meningococcal conjugate vaccine—United States, June 2005–September 2006. M. M. W. R. Morb. Mortal. Wkly. Rep. *55*(41):1120, 2006.

35. Centers for Disease Control and Prevention: Provisional cases of selected notifiable diseases, United States. M. M. W. R. Morb. Mortal. Wkly. Rep. *55*:1389, 2007.

35a. Centers for Disease Control and Prevention: Emergence of fluoroquinolone-resistant *Neisseria meningitidis*—Minnesota and North Dakota, 2007-2008. M. M. W. R. Morb. Mortal. Wkly. Rep. 57:173-175, 2008.

36. Churchwell, K., McManus, M., Kent, P., et al.: Intensive blood and plasma exchange for treatment of coagulopathy in meningococcemia. J. Clin. Apheresis *10*:171, 1995.

37. Cobroft, R., and Henderson, A.: Meningococcal purpura fulminans treated with antithrombin III concentrate: What is the optimal replacement therapy? Aust. N. Z. J. Med. *24*:575, 1994.

38. Cohen, M. S., Steere, A. C., Baltimore, R., et al.: Possible nosocomial transmission of group Y *Neisseria meningitidis* among oncology patients. Ann. Intern. Med. *91*:7, 1979.

39. Conway, E., and Rosenberg, R.: Tumor necrosis factor suppresses transcription of the thrombomodulin gene in endothelial cells. Mol. Cell. Biol. *8*:5588-5592, 1988.

40. Cooper, E., Ellison, R., Smith, G., et al.: Rifampin-resistant meningococcal disease in a contact patient given prophylactic rifampin. J. Pediatr. *108*:93, 1986.

41. Corless, C., Guiver, M., Borrow, R., et al.: Simultaneous detection of *Neisseria meningitidis*, *Haemophilus influenzae*, and *Streptococcus pneumoniae* in suspected cases of meningitis and septicemia using real-time PCR. J. Clin. Microbiol. *39*:1553, 2001.

42. Corso, A., Faccone, D., Miranda, M., et al.: Emergence of *Neisseria meningitidis* with decreased susceptibility to ciprofloxacin in Argentina. J. Antimicrob. Chemother. *55*:596, 2005.

43. Cuevas, L. E., Kazembe, P., Mughogho, G. K., et al.: Eradication of nasopharyngeal carriage of *Neisseria meningitidis* in children and adults in rural Africa: A comparison of ciprofloxacin and rifampicin. J. Infect. Dis. *171*:728, 1995.

44. Dahle, J.: Pathogenesis of hemorrhagic skin lesions in meningococcal disease. N. I. P. H. Ann. *6*:49, 1983.

45. D'Amelio, R., Agostoni, A., Biselli, R., et al.: Complement deficiency and antibody profile in survivors of meningococcal meningitis due to common serogroups in Italy. Scand. J. Immunol. *35*:589, 1992.

46. Davis, C. E., and Arnold, K.: Role of meningococcal endotoxin in meningococcal purpura. J. Exp. Med. *140*:159, 1974.

47. Davis, R.: Guillain-Barré syndrome among recipients of meningococcal conjugate vaccine (Menactra) June 2005–September 2006. Presented at a meeting of the Advisory Committee on Immunization Practices, Atlanta, 2006.

48. De Kleijn, E., Joosten, K., Van Rijn, B., et al.: Low serum cortisol in combination with high adrenocorticotrophic hormone concentrations are associated with poor outcome in children with severe meningococcal disease. Pediatr. Infect. Dis. J. *21*:330, 2002.

49. de Moraes, J. C., Perkins, B. A., Camargo, M. C., et al.: Protective efficacy of a serogroup B meningococcal vaccine in Sao Paulo, Brazil [published erratum appears in Lancet 1992 Dec 19-26;340(8834-8835):1554]. Lancet *340*:1074, 1992.

50. den Brinker, M., Joosten, K., Liem, O., et al.: Adrenal insufficiency in meningococcal sepsis: Bioavaialable cortisol levels and impact of interleukin-6 levels and intubation with etomidate on adrenal function and mortality. J. Clin. Endocrinol. Metab. *90*:5110, 2005.

51. Densen, P., Weiler, J. M., Griffiss, J. M., et al.: Familial properdin deficiency and fatal meningococcemia. Correction of the bactericidal defect by vaccination. N. Engl. J. Med. *316*:922, 1987.

52. Derkx, B., Wittes, J., and McCloskey, R.: Randomized, placebo-controlled trial of HA-1A, a human monoclonal antibody to endotoxin in children with meningococcal septic shock. Clin. Infect. Dis. *28*:770, 1999.

53. DeVoe, I. W., and Gilka, F.: Disseminated intravascular coagulation in rabbits: Synergistic activity of meningococcal endotoxin and materials egested from leucocytes containing meningococci. J. Med. Microbiol. *9*:451, 1976.

54. Dhodapkar, K., Corbacioglu, S., Chang, M. K., et al.: Purpura fulminans caused by group A beta-hemolytic *Streptococcus* sepsis. J. Pediatr. *137*:562, 2000.

55. Dickson, R., McKinnon, N., Magner, D., et al.: Meningococcal infection. Lancet *2*:631, 1941.

56. Dixon, L. M., and Sanford, H. S.: Meningococcal pericarditis in the antibiotic era. Mil. Med. *136*:433, 1971.

57. Dock, W.: Intermittent fever of seven months duration due to meningococcemia. J. A. M. A. *83*:399, 1924.

58. Edwards, M. S., and Baker, C. J.: Complications and sequelae of meningococcal infections in children. J. Pediatr. *99*:540, 1981.

59. Eley, B., and Levin, M.: Septic shock with special reference to meningococcal disease. Curr. Opin. Infect. Dis. 7:345, 1994.

60. Ellsworth, J., Marks, M. I., and Vose, A.: Meningococcal meningitis in children. C. M. A. J. *120*:155, 1979.

61. Faber, J., Meyer, C., Gemmer, C., et al.: Human toll-like receptor 4 mutations are associated with susceptibility to invasive meningococcal disease in infancy. Pediatr. Infect. Dis. J. *25*:80, 2006.

62. Faber, J., Schuessler, T. F., Finn, A., et al.: Age-dependent association of human mannose-binding lectin mutations with susceptibility to invasive meningococcal disease in childhood. Pediatr. Infect. Dis. J. *26*:243, 2007.

63. Faur, Y., Weisburd, M., and Wilson, M.: Isolation of *Neisseria meningitidis* from the genito-urinary tract and. J. Clin. Microbiol. *2*:178, 1975.

64. Feavers, I.: ABC of meningococcal diversity. Nature *404*:451, 2000.

65. Figueroa, J. E., and Densen, P.: Infectious diseases associated with complement deficiencies. Clin. Microbiol. Rev. *4*:359, 1991.

66. Fijen, C., Kuijper, E., Hannema, A. J., et al.: Complement deficiencies in patients over ten years old with meningococcal disease due to uncommon serogroups. Lancet *2*:585, 1989.

67. Fisher, M., Hedberg, K., Cardosi, P., et al.: Tobacco smoke as a risk factor for meningococcal disease. Pediatr. Infect. Dis. J. *10*:979, 1997.

68. Food and Drug Administration: Product Approval Information—Licensing Action, in U.S. Department of Health and human Services, Food and Drug Administration, Center for Biologics Evaluation and Research, 2005.

69. Francke, E., and Neu, H.: Postsplenectomy infection. Surg. Clin. North Am. *61*:135, 1981.

70. Frasch, C. E.: Role of protein serotype antigens in protection against disease due to *Neisseria meningitidis*. J. Infect. Dis. *136*(Suppl.):S84, 1977.

71. Frasch, C., Zollinger, W., and Poolman, J.: Serotype antigens of *Neisseria meningitidis* and a proposed scheme for design of serotypes. Rev. Infect. Dis. 7:504, 1985.

72. Gardner, P.: Prevention of meningococcal disease. N. Engl. J. Med. *355*:1466, 2006.

73. Gerard, P., Moriau, M., Bachy, A., et al.: Meningococcal purpura: Report of 19 patients treated with heparin. J. Pediatr. *82*:780, 1973.

74. Gilmore, A., Stuart, J., and Andrews, N.: Risk of secondary meningococcal disease in health-care workers. Lancet *356*:1654, 2000.

75. Girardin, E., Grau, G. E., Dayer, J. M., et al.: Tumor necrosis factor and interleukin-1 in the serum of children with severe infectious purpura. N. Engl. J. Med. *319*:397, 1988.

76. Girgis, N., Sultan, Y., Frenck, R. W., Jr., et al.: Azithromycin compared with rifampin for eradication of nasopharyngeal colonization by *Neisseria meningitidis*. Pediatr. Infect. Dis. J. *17*:816, 1998.

77. Goldschneider, I., Gotschlich, E. C., and Artenstein, M. S.: Human immunity to the meningococcus. I. The role of humoral antibodies. J. Exp. Med. *129*:1307, 1969.

78. Goldschneider, I., Gotschlich, E. C., and Artenstein, M. S.: Human immunity to the meningococcus. II. Development of natural immunity. J. Exp. Med. *129*:1327, 1969.

79. Greenfield, S., Sheehe, P. R., and Feldman, H. A.: Meningococcal carriage in a population of "normal" families. J. Infect. Dis. *123*:67, 1971.

80. Greenwood, B. M., Bradley, A. K., and Wall, R. A.: Meningococcal disease and season in sub-Saharan Africa. Lancet *2*:829, 1985.

81. Greenwood, B. M., Hassan-King, M., and Whittle, H. C.: Prevention of secondary cases of meningococcal disease in household contacts by vaccination. B. M. J. *1*:1317, 1978.

82. Greenwood, B., and Whittle, H.: The pathogenesis of meningococcal arthritis. *In* Dumonde. D., and Path, M. (eds.): Infection and Immunology in Rheumatic Diseases. Philadelphia, J. B. Lippincott, 1976, p. 119.

83. Haggerty, R., and Zaia, M.: Acute bacterial meningitis. Adv. Pediatr. *13*:129, 1964.

84. Hahné, S., Charlett, A., Purcell, B., et al.: Effectiveness of antibiotics given before admission in reducing mortality from meningococcal disease: Systematic review. B. M. J. *332*:1299, 2006.

85. Hardman, J.: Fatal meningococcal infections: The changing pathologic picture in the '60s. Mil. Med. *133*:951, 1968.

86. Harrison, L., Jolley, K., Shutt, K., et al.: Antigenic shift and increased incidence of meningococcal disease. J. Infect. Dis. *193*:1266, 2006.

87. Hart, C., and Rogers, T.: Meningococcal disease. J. Med. Microbiol. *39*:3, 1993.

88. Herman, R., and Rubin, H.: Meningococcal pericarditis without meningitis presenting as tamponade. N. Engl. J. Med. *290*:143, 1974.

89. Herrick, W.: Extrameningeal meningococcus infections. Arch. Intern. Med. *23*:409, 1919.

90. Hill, W., and Kinney, T.: The cutaneous lesions in acute meningococcemia. A clinical and pathologic study. J. A. M. A. *134*:513, 1947.

91. Holbein, B. E.: Differences in virulence for mice between disease and carrier strains of *Neisseria meningitidis*. Can. J. Microbiol. 27:738, 1981.

92. Hubert, B., Watier, L., Garnerin, P., et al.: Meningococcal disease and influenza-like syndrome: A new approach to an old question. J. Infect. Dis. *166*:542, 1992.

93. Inkelis, S., O'Leary, D., Wang, V., et al.: Extremity pain and refusal to walk in children with invasive meningococcal disease. Pediatrics *110*:e3, 2002.

94. Irazuzta, J., and McManus, M. L.: Use of topically applied nitroglycerin in the treatment of purpura fulminans. J. Pediatr. *117*:993, 1990.

95. Jackson, L., and Wenger, J.: Laboratory-based surveillance for meningococcal disease in selected areas: United States, 1989-1991. M. M. W. R. C. D. C. Surveill. Summ. *42*(2):21, 1993.

96. Jackson, L. A., Schuchat, A., Reeves, M. W., et al.: Serogroup C meningococcal outbreaks in the United States. An emerging threat. J. A. M. A. *273*:383, 1995.

97. Jackson, L. A., Tenover, F. C., Baker, C., et al.: Prevalence of *Neisseria meningitidis* relatively resistant to penicillin in the United States, 1991. Meningococcal Disease Study Group. J. Infect. Dis. *169*:438, 1994.

98. Jacobson, J. A., Camargos, P. A., Ferreira, J. T., et al.: The risk of meningitis among classroom contacts during an epidemic of meningococcal disease. Am. J. Epidemiol. *104*:552, 1976.

99. Jones, R. N., Slepack, J., and Eades, A.: Fatal neonatal meningococcal meningitis. Association with maternal cervical-vaginal colonization. J. A. M. A. *236*:2652, 1976.

100. Kaiser, A., Hennekens, C., Saslaw, M., et al.: Seroepidemiology and chemoprophylaxis of disease due to sulfonamide-resistant *Neisseria meningitidis* in a civilian population. J. Infect. Dis. *130*:217, 1974.

101. Kaplan, S., Schutze, G., Leake, J., et al.: Multicenter surveillance of invasive meningococcal infections in children. Pediatrics. *118*:4, 2006.

102. Kaspar, D., Winkelhake, J., and Zollinger, W.: Immunochemical similarity between polysaccharide antigens of *Escherichia coli* 07:K1(L):NM and group B *Neisseria meningitidis*. J. Immunol. *110*:262, 1973.

103. Kaufman, B., Levy, H., Zaleznak, B., et al.: Statistical analysis of 242 cases of meningococcus meningitis. Pediatrics 38:705, 1951.

104. Keyserling, H., Papa, T., Koranyi, K., et al.: Safety, immunogenicity, and immune memory of a novel meningococcal (groups A, C, Y, and W-135) polysaccharide diphtheria toxoid conjugate vaccine (MCV-4) in healthy adolescents. Arch. Pediatr. Adolesc. Med. *159*:907, 2005.

105. Kirsch, E., Barton, P., Kitchen, L., et al.: Pathophysiology, treatment and outcome of meningococcemia: A review and recent experience. Pediatr. Infect. Dis. J. *15*:967, 1996.

106. Koppe, J., Ellenbogen, E., and Gebhart, R.: Group Y meningococcal disease in United States Air Force recruits. Am. J. Med. *62*:661, 1977.

107. Kozarsky, P., Arguin, P., and Navin, A.: Health Information for International Travel 2005-2006. Atlanta, Department of Health and Human Services, 2006.

108. Kravitz, G., Dries, D., Peterson, M., Schlievert, P. M.: Purpura fulminans due to *Staphylococcus aureus*. Clin. Infect. Dis. 40:941, 2005.

109. Kunkel, M., Brown, L., Bauta, H., Iannini, P. B.: Meningococcal mesenteric adenitis and peritonitis in a child. Pediatr. Infect. Dis. J. *3*:327, 1984.

110. Kupperman, N., Inkelis, S., and Saladino, R.: The role of heparin in the prevention of extremity and digit necrosis in meningococcal purpura fulminans. Pediatr. Infect. Dis. J. *13*:867, 1994.

111. Leake, J., and Perkins, B.: Meningococcal disease: Challenges in prevention and management. Infect. Med. *17*:364, 2000.

112. Leclerc, F., Martinot, A., Cremer, R., Fourier, C.: ECMO for refractory cardiorespiratory failure due to meningococcal disease. Lancet *349*:1397, 1997.

113. Lehman, T. J., Bernstein, B., Hanson, V., et al.: Meningococcal infection complicating systemic lupus erythematosus. J. Pediatr. *99*:94, 1981.

114. Lehmann, A., Halstensen, A., Sornes, S., et al.: High levels of interleukin-10 during the initial phase of fulminant meningococcal septic shock. J. Infect. Dis. *171*:229, 1995.

115. Leibel, R., Fangman, J., and Ostrovsky, M.: Chronic meningococcemia in childhood. Am. J. Dis. Child. *127*:94, 1974.

116. Levin, M., Quint, P., Goldstein, B., et al.: Recombinant bactericidal/permeability-increasing protein (rBPI) as adjunctive treatment for children with severe meningococcal sepsis: A randomized trial. Lancet *356*:961, 2000.

117. Levitt, L., Bond, J., Hall, I., Jr., et al.: Meningococcal and ECHO-9 meningitis. Report of an outbreak. Neurology 20:45, 1970.

118. Lewis, J., Arnold, C., and Alexander, J.: Meningococcal pneumonia. Am. J. Clin. Pathol. *59*:388, 1973.

119. Linz, B., Schenker, M., Zhu, P., et al.: Frequent interspecific genetic exchange between commensal Neisseriae and *Neisseria meningitidis*. Mol. Microbiol. *36*:1049, 2000.

120. MacLennan, J., Obaro, S., Deeks, J., et al.: Immune response to revaccination with meningococcal A and C polysaccharides in Gambian children following repeated immunization during early childhood. Vaccine *17*:3086, 1999.

121. Maiden, M. C.: Population genetics of a transformable bacterium: The influence of horizontal genetic exchange on the biology of *Neisseria meningitidis*. F. E. M. S. Microbiol. Lett. *112*:243, 1993.

122. Manchanda, V., and Bhalla, P.: Emergence of non–ceftriaxone-susceptible *Neisseria meningitidis* in India. J. Clin. Microbiol. *44*:4290, 2006.

123. Marks, M. I., Frasch, C. E., and Shapera, R. M.: Meningococcal colonization and infection in children and their household contacts. Am. J. Epidemiol. *109*:563, 1979.

124. Marzouk, O., Thomson, A., Sills, J., et al.: Features and outcome in meningococcal disease presenting with maculopapular rash. Arch. Dis. Child. *66*:485, 1991.

125. Mellado, M., Rodriguez-Contreras, R., Mariscal, A., et al.: Effect of penicillin and chloramphenicol on the growth and endotoxin release by *N. meningitidis*. Epidemiol. Infect. *106*:283, 1991.

126. Mendelman, P., Campos, J., Chaffin, D., et al.: Relative penicillin G resistance in *Neisseria meningitidis* and reduced affinity of penicillin-binding protein 3. Antimicrob. Agents Chemother. *32*:706, 1988.

127. Meningococcal disease and college students. Recommendations of the Advisory Committee on Immunization Practices (ACIP). M. M. W. R. Recomm. Rep. *49*(RR-7):13, 2000.

128. Meningococcal Disease Update 2007. ProMed. Available at http://www.promedmail.org/pls/promed/f?p=2400:1202:10374748748848896256::NO::F2400_P1202_CHECK_DISPLAY,F2400_P1202_PUB_MAIL_ID:X,36797 (accessed April 6, 2007).

129. Meyer, M., Irazuzta, J., Tozibikian, H.: Topical nitroglycerin and pain in purpura fulminans. J. Pediatr. *134*:639, 1999.

130. Moncada, S., and Higgs, E.: Endogenous nitric oxide: Physiology, pathology and clinical relevance. Eur. J. Clin. Invest. *21*:361, 1991.

131. Moore, P. S., Harrison, L. H., Telzak, E. E., et al.: Group A meningococcal carriage in travelers returning from Saudi Arabia. J. A. M. A. *260*:2686, 1988.

132. Moore, P. S., Hierholzer, J., DeWitt, W., et al.: Respiratory viruses and mycoplasma as cofactors for epidemic group A meningococcal meningitis. J. A. M. A. *264*:1271, 1990.

133. Moore, P. S., Reeves, M. W., Schwartz, B., et al.: Intercontinental spread of an epidemic group A *Neisseria meningitidis* strain. Lancet *2*:260, 1989.

134. Morrow, H. W., Slaten, D. D., Reingold, A. L., et al.: Risk factors associated with a school-related outbreak of serogroup C meningococcal disease. Pediatr. Infect. Dis. J. *9*:394, 1990.

135. Morse, J., Oretsky, M., and Hudson, J.: Pericarditis as a complication of meningococcal meningitis. Ann. Intern. Med. 74:212, 1971.

136. Nadel, S., De Munter, C., Britto, J., et al.: Recombinant tissue plasminogen activator restores perfusion in meningococcal purpura fulminans. Crit. Care Med. *26*:971, 1998.

137. Nadel, S., Goldstein, B., Williams, M., et al.: Drotrecogin alfa (activated) in children with severe sepsis: A multicentre phase III randomized controlled trial. Lancet *369*:836, 2007.

138. Nassif, X., and So, M.: Interaction of pathogenic Neisseriae with nonphagocytic cells. Clin. Microbiol. Rev. *8*:376, 1995.

139. Nawroth, P., and Stern, D.: Modulation of endothelial cell hemostatic properties by tumor necrosis factor. J. Exp. Med. *320*:1165, 1986.

140. Ni, H., Knight, A., Cartwright, K., et al.: Polymerase chain reaction for diagnosis of meningococcal meningitis. Lancet *340*:1432, 1993.

141. Nielsen, H. E., Koch, C., Magnussen, P., et al.: Complement deficiencies in selected groups of patients with meningococcal disease. Scand. J. Infect. Dis. *21*:389, 1989.

142. Niklasson, P., Lundbergh, P., and Strandell, T.: Prognostic factors in meningococcal disease. Scand. J. Infect. Dis. *3*:17, 1971.

143. Ognibene, A., and Dito, W.: Chronic meningococcemia. Arch. Intern. Med. *114*:29, 1964.

144. Olcen, P., Kjellander, J., Danielsson, D., et al.: Epidemiology of *Neisseria meningitidis*; prevalence and symptoms from the upper respiratory tract in family members to patients with meningococcal disease. Scand. J. Infect. Dis. *13*:105, 1981.

145. Oppenheimer, E., and Rosman, N.: Bacterial meningitis in childhood: Neurologic complications and their management. Pediatr. Neurol. *287*:285, 1976.

146. Parillo, J.: Pathogenic mechanisms of septic shock. N. Engl. J. Med. *328*:307, 1993.

147. Penny, J., Grace, W., and Kennedy, R.: Meningococcal pericarditis. Am. J. Cardiol. *18*:281, 1966.

148. Perez-Trallero, E., Aldamiz-Echeverria, L., Perez-Yarza, E. G.: Meningococci with increased resistance to penicillin. Lancet *335*:1096, 1990.

149. Pichichero, M., Casey, J., Blatter, M., et al.: Comparative trial of the safety and immunogenicity of quadrivalent (A, C, Y, W-135) meningococcal polysaccharide–diphtheria conjugate vaccine versus quadrivalent polysaccharide vaccine in two- to ten-year-old children. Pediatr. Infect. Dis. J. *24*:57, 2005.

150. Pichichero, M., Papa, T., Blatter, M., et al.: Immune memory in children previously vaccinated with an experimental quadrivalent meningococcal polysaccharide diphtheria toxoid conjugate vaccine. Pediatr. Infect. Dis. J. *25*:995, 2006.

151. Pinals, R., and Ropes, M.: Meningococcal arthritis. Arthritis Rheum. 7:241, 1964.
152. Pinner, R. W., Onyango, F., Perkins, B. A., et al.: Epidemic meningococcal disease in Nairobi, Kenya, 1989. The Kenya/Centers for Disease Control (CDC) Meningitis Study Group. J. Infect. Dis. 166:359, 1992.
153. Pizzi, M.: A severe epidemic of meningococcus meningitis in Chile, 1941-2. Am. J. Public Health 34:231, 1944.
154. Platonov, A., Beloborodov, V., and Vershinina, I.: Meningococcal disease in patients with late complement deficiency: Studies in the U.S.S.R. Medicine (Baltimore) 72:374, 1993.
155. Poolman, J., van der Ley, P., and Tommassen, J.: Surface Structures and Secreted Products of Meningococci. Chichester, UK, Wiley, 1995.
156. Popovic, T., Sacchi, C. T., Reeves, M. W., et al.: Neisseria meningitidis serogroup W135 isolates associated with the ET-37 complex. Emerg. Infect. Dis. 6:428, 2000.
157. Powars, D., Larsen, R., Johnson, J., et al.: Epidemic meningococcemia and purpura fulminans with induced protein C deficiency. Clin. Infect. Dis. 17:254, 1993.
158. Powars, D., Rogers, Z., Patch, M., et al.: Purpura fulminans in meningococcemia: Association with acquired deficiencies of proteins C and S. N. Engl. J. Med. 317:571, 1987.
159. Prevention and control of meningococcal disease. Recommendations of the Advisory Committee on Immunization Practices (ACIP). M. M. W. R. Recomm. Rep. 49(RR-7):1, 2000.
160. Racoosin, J., Whitney, C., Conover, C., et al.: Serogroup Y meningococcal disease in Chicago, 1991-1997. J. A. M. A. 280:2094, 1998.
161. Ramsay, M., Andrews, N., Kaczmarski, E., et al.: Efficacy of meningococcal serogroup C conjugate vaccine in teenagers and toddlers in England. Lancet 357:195, 2001.
162. Ramsay, M., Andrews, N., Trotter, C., et al.: Herd immunity from meningococcal serogroup C vaccination in England: Database analysis. B. M. J. 326:365, 2003.
163. Read, R., Camp, N., Di Giovine, F., et al.: An interleukin-1 genotype is associated with fatal outcome of meningococcal disease. J. Infect. Dis. 182:1557, 2000.
164. Riedo, F. X., Plikaytis, B. D., and Broome, C. V.: Epidemiology and prevention of meningococcal disease. Pediatr. Infect. Dis. J. 14:643, 1995.
165. Riordan, F., Thomson, A., Ratcliffe, J., et al.: Admission cortisol and adrenocorticotrophic hormone levels in children with meningococcal disease: Evidence of adrenal insufficiency? Crit. Care Med. 27:2257, 1999.
166. Robboy, S.: Atrioventricular node inflammation: Mechanism of sudden death in protracted meningococcemia. N. Engl. J. Med. 286:1091, 1972.
167. Rodriguez-Erdmann, F.: Intravascular activation of the clotting system with phospholipids. Blood 26:541, 1965.
168. Rosenblatt, J., Ray, C., and Enquist, R. W.: Meningococcal infections in children: Observations on prognosis and therapy. Personal Communication, 1978.
169. Rosenstein, N. E., and Perkins, B. A.: Update on Haemophilus influenzae serotype b and meningococcal vaccines. Pediatr. Clin. North Am. 47:337, 2000.
170. Rosenstein, N. E., Perkins, B. A., Stephens, D. S., et al.: The changing epidemiology of meningococcal disease in the United States, 1992-1996. J. Infect. Dis. 180:1894, 1999.
171. Rosenstein, N. E., Perkins, B. A., Stephens, D. S., et al.: Meningococcal disease. N. Engl. J. Med. 344:1378, 2001.
172. Ross, S. C., and Densen, P.: Complement deficiency states and infection: Epidemiology, pathogenesis and consequences of neisserial and other infections in an immune deficiency. Medicine (Baltimore) 63:243, 1984.
173. Saez-Nieto, J., Lujan, R., Berron, S., et al.: Epidemiology and molecular basis of penicillin-resistant Neisseria meningitidis in Spain: A 5-year history (1985-1989). Clin. Infect. Dis. 1(Suppl.):S12, 1992.
174. Sanofi Pasteur: Meningococcal (Groups A, C, Y and W-135) Polysaccharide Diphtheria Toxoid Conjugate Vaccine. Sanofi Pasteur, Swiftwater, PA, 2006, p. 1.
175. Scheim, A.: Articular manifestations of meningococcic infections. Arch. Intern. Med. 62:963, 1938.
176. Scholten, R. J., Bijlmer, H. A., Tobi, H., et al.: Upper respiratory tract infection, heterologous immunisation and meningococcal disease. J. Med. Microbiol. 48:943, 1999.
177. Scott, L., Knox, D., Perry, L., et al.: Meningococcal pericarditis. Am. J. Cardiol. 29:104, 1972.
178. Sinclair, J., Skeoch, C., and Hallworth, D.: Prognosis of meningococcal septicaemia. Lancet 3:38, 1987.
179. Smith, O., White, B., Vaughn, D., et al.: Use of protein-C concentrate, heparin, and haemodiafiltration in meningococcus-induced purpura fulminans. Lancet 350:1590, 1997.
180. Spratt, B., Zhang, Q., Jones, D., et al.: Recruitment of a penicillin-binding protein gene from Neisseria flavescens during the emergence of penicillin-resistant Neisseria meningitidis. Proc. Natl. Acad. Sci. U. S. A. 86:315, 1989.
181. Stanwell-Smith, R. E., Stuart, J. M., Hughes, A. O., et al.: Smoking, the environment and meningococcal disease: A case control study. Epidemiol. Infect. 112:315, 1994.

182. Stephens, D., and Farley, M.: Pathogenic events during infection of the human nasopharynx with Neisseria meningitidis and Haemophilus influenzae. Rev. Infect. Dis. 12:22, 1991.
183. Stephens, D., Hoffman, L., and McGee, Z.: Interaction of Neisseria meningitidis with human nasopharyngeal mucosa: Attachment and entry into columnar epithelial cells. J. Infect. Dis. 148:369, 1983.
184. Stiehm, E., and Damrosch, D.: Factors in the prognosis of meningococcal infection. J. Pediatr. 68:457, 1966.
185. Stuart, J. M., Cartwright, K. A., Robinson, P. M., et al.: Effect of smoking on meningococcal carriage. Lancet 2:723, 1989.
186. Sullivan, T., and La Scolea, L.: Neisseria meningitidis bacteremia in children: Quantitation of bacteremia and spontaneous clinical recovery without antibiotic therapy. Pediatrics 80:63, 1987.
187. Sutcliffe, E. M., Jones, D. M., El-Sheikh, S., et al.: Penicillin-insensitive meningococci in the UK. Lancet 1:657, 1988.
188. Swartley, J., Marfin, A., Edupuganti, S., et al.: Capsule switching of Neisseria meningitidis. Proc. Natl. Acad. Sci. U. S. A. 94:271, 1997.
189. Thompson, A., Sills, J., and Hart, C.: Validation of the Glasgow meningococcal septicaemia prognostic score; a 10-year retrospective survey. Crit. Care Med. 19:26, 1991.
190. Tobias, J., Haun, S., Helfaer, M., et al.: Use of continuous caudal block to relieve lower extremity ischemia caused by vasculitis in a child with meningococcemia. J. Pediatr. 115:1019, 1989.
191. Trotter, C., Andrews, N., Kaczmarski, E., et al.: Effectiveness of meningococcal serogroup C conjugate vaccine 4 years after introduction. Lancet 364:365, 2004.
192. Tully, J., Viner, R., and Coen, P.: Risk and protective factors for meningococcal disease in adolescents: Matched cohort study. B. M. J. 332:445, 2006.
193. Tuncer, A., Gar, I., Ertem, U., et al.: Once daily ceftriaxone for meningococcemia and meningococcal meningitis. Pediatr. Infect. Dis. J. 7:711, 1988.
194. van de Ende, A., Hopman, C., and Dankert, J.: Multiple mechanism of phase variation of PorA in Neisseria meningitidis. Infect. Immun. 68:6685, 2000.
195. van der ven-Jongekrijg. J., van der ven-Jongekrijg. J., Demacker, P., et al.: Differential expression of proinflammatory cytokines and their inhibitors during the course of meningococcal infections. J. Infect. Dis. 169:157, 1994.
196. van Deuren, M., van der ven-Jongekrijg, J., Bartelink, A., et al.: Correlation between proinflammatory cytokines and anti-inflammatory mediators and the severity of disease in meningococcal infections. J. Infect. Dis. 172:632, 1995.
197. van Deuren, M., van Dijke, B., Koopman, R. J., et al.: Rapid diagnosis of acute meningococcal infections by needle aspiration or biopsy of skin lesions. B. M. J. 306:1229, 1993.
198. Vann, W., Liu, T., and Robbins, J.: Bacillus pumilus polysaccharide cross-reactive with meningococcal group A polysaccharide. Infect. Immun. 13:1654, 1976.
199. Van Nguyen, Z., Nguyen, E., Weiner, L.: Incidence of invasive bacterial disease in children with fever and petechiae. Pediatrics 74:77, 1984.
200. Vieusseux, G.: Memoire sur la maladie qui a regre a Geneve au printemps de 1805. J. Med. Chir. Pharm. 11:163, 1806.
201. Vogel, U., Claus, H., and Frosch, M.: Rapid serogroup switching in Neisseria meningitidis. J. Med. 342:219, 2000.
202. Vu, D. M., Welsch, J. A., Zuno-Mitchell, P., et al.: Antibody persistence 3 years after immunization of adolescents with quadrivalent meningococcal conjugate vaccine. J. Infect. Dis. 193:821, 2006.
203. Weightman, N. C., and Johnstone, D. J.: Three cases of pneumonia due to Neisseria meningitidis, including serogroup W135. Eur. J. Clin. Microbiol. Infect. Dis. 18:456, 1999.
204. Weis, E., and Silber, E.: Acute constrictive pericarditis. J. Pediatr. 58:548, 1961.
205. Westendorp, R., Langermans, J., de Bel, C., et al.: Release of tumor necrosis factor: An innate host characteristic that may contribute to the outcome of meningococcal disease. J. Infect. Dis. 171:1057, 1995.
206. Westendorp, R., Langermans, J., Huizinga, T., et al.: Genetic influence on cytokine production and fatal meningococcal disease. Lancet 349:170, 1997.
207. Whittle, H., Tugwell, P., Egler, L., et al.: Rapid bacteriologic diagnosis of pyogenic meningitis by latex agglutination. Lancet 2:619, 1974.
208. Wilson, F., and Morse, S.: Therapy of acute meningococcal infections: Early volume expansion and prophylactic low dose heparin. Am. J. Med. Sci. 264:445, 1972.
209. Winn, W., Jr., Allen, S., Janda, W., et al.: Koneman's Color Atlas and Textbook of Diagnostic Microbiology. Baltimore, Lippincott Williams & Wilkins, 2006.
210. Wolf, R., and Birbara, C.: Meningococcal infections at an army training center. Am. J. Med. 44:243, 1968.
211. Wong, S., Lennon, D., Jackson, C., et al.: New Zealand epidemic strain meningococcal B outer membrane vesicle vaccine in children aged 16-24 months. Pediatr. Infect. Dis. J. 26:345, 2007.
212. Wong, V., Hitchcock, W., and Mason, W.: Meningococcal infections in children: A review of 100 cases. Pediatr. Infect. Dis. J. 8:224, 1989.

213. Young, L., LaForce, F., Head, J., et al.: A simultaneous outbreak of meningococcal and influenza infections. N. Engl. J. Med. *287*:5, 1972.
214. Zangwill, K. M., Schuchat, A., Riedo, F. X., et al.: School-based clusters of meningococcal disease in the United States. Descriptive epidemiology and a case-control analysis. J. A. M. A. 277:389, 1997.

215. Zhang, Q., Jones, D., Saez-Nieto, J., et al.: Genetic diversity of penicillin-binding protein 2 genes of penicillin-resistant strains of *Neisseria meningitidis* revealed by fingerprinting of amplified DNA. Antimicrob. Agents Chemother. *34*:1523, 1990.

CHAPTER 100

GONOCOCCAL INFECTIONS

Charles R. Woods, Jr.

Gonorrhea, the foremost manifestation of human disease caused by *Neisseria gonorrhoeae* (the gonococcus), is one of the oldest known human diseases. Hippocrates called the disease "strangury" in the fifth and fourth centuries BCE. Galen coined the name *gonorrhea*, meaning "flow of semen," in the second century CE. The association of the disease with sexual activity was recognized, and sexual abstinence plus washing of the eyes of newborns was prescribed by Greco-Roman physicians for treatment of the disease. Gonorrhea also has been known as *clap* since the late 1300s. The origin of this term is unclear but may have derived from the Les Clapier district of Paris, where prostitutes were housed during the Middle Ages.[186,229]

After syphilis appeared in Europe in the late 15th century, the two diseases were thought to represent different manifestations of the same infection, and they often coexisted then as today. The description by Neisser of *N. gonorrhoeae* in stained smears of urethral and other exudates in 1879 and culture of the organism by Leistikow and Löffler in 1882 provided the foundation for modern understanding of the clinical spectrum of gonococcal diseases. The advent of safe and effective antimicrobial agents, first sulfonamides in 1936 and then penicillin in 1943, was the next major advance in combating gonorrhea.[186,229] Further understanding of the clinical aspects of the disease was facilitated by development of the Thayer-Martin medium in 1964.[322] Modern knowledge of the molecular pathogenesis of *N. gonorrhoeae* infection began in 1963 with the observation by Kellogg and colleagues that gonococcal strains with differences in colony morphology also varied in virulence.[188]

The potential reproductive sequelae of gonococcal infections (e.g., infertility), the ever-growing resistance to antimicrobial agents, and disproportionate case burdens in public clinics continue to cast *N. gonorrhoeae* infection as a major international public health problem.[57,213,276] The purpose of many current investigations remains the development of an effective vaccine.[81,308]

In infants, the gonococcus causes primarily ophthalmia neonatorum. Wound infections, including scalp abscess (often associated with fetal monitoring), funisitis, and vaginitis may occur. Infection can disseminate from any colonized or infected skin or mucous membrane site and may result in sepsis, meningitis, septic arthritis, or endocarditis. In prepubertal children, gonococcal infection usually involves the genital tract and almost always is transmitted sexually. Vaginitis is the most common manifestation. Extension to the upper genital tract in girls does occur but very seldom. Urethritis can develop in boys but rarely does so. Anorectal and tonsillopharyngeal infections also can occur in prepubertal children.

In adolescents, as in adults, the most common clinical manifestations are urethritis, endocervicitis, and salpingitis in females and urethritis in males. Epididymitis, bartholinitis, pelvic inflammatory disease (PID), and perihepatitis can occur as a result of extension from primary genital infections. Rectal and pharyngeal infections and disseminated disease, which may include reactive or septic arthritis, also are seen. Additional information on gonococcal infections is provided in Chapter 48.

EPIDEMIOLOGY OF GONOCOCCAL INFECTION

Gonococcal infections remain second only to *Chlamydia* infections in incidence among reportable diseases for 15- to 24-year-olds in the United States.[60,68] Gonococcal infections are relatively rare occurrences in Canada and much of western Europe but remain common in developing countries.[164] Rates of gonococcal infection in the United States and western and central Europe declined steadily in the 1980s and 1990s. Rates of gonorrhea increased in eastern Europe in the early 1990s.[326] These rates have declined but remain above those in other European regions.[342] Regions with higher rates of adult disease have higher numbers of pediatric cases,[109,131] a finding that reflects the adult origin of virtually all pediatric cases.

An estimated 1 million new cases of gonococcal infection occur annually in the United States, only approximately a third of which are reported. The 339,593 reported cases in the United States in 2005 (115.6 cases per 100,000 population) represented a slight increase in the national rate for the first time since 1999 (Fig. 100–1). This rate remains well above the Healthy People 2010 goal of 19 per 100,000. At least half the cases are thought to go undiagnosed or unreported. After World War II, reported cases of gonorrhea in the United States declined from 204 per 100,000 in 1950 to 129 per 100,000 in 1958. Rates rose in the 1960s and early 1970s, in association with changing sexual mores, before peaking at 472 per 100,000 in 1975. Gonococcal infections rarely are fatal (approximately four deaths per year in the United States), with death being caused by gonococcal sepsis.[58,60,65,213,276]

Adolescent females 15 to 19 years of age have the highest reported incidence of infection in the United States (625 cases per 100,000 in 2005). Among those aged 25 years and younger (including children), rates of gonorrhea are higher for females than for males. Rates for males are higher in those aged 25 years and older. Rates in African American adolescents of both genders greatly exceed those of white adolescents, and this trend continues into adulthood. The disparity between African Americans and non-Hispanic whites narrowed slightly from 26-fold in 2001 to 18-fold in 2005.[60,65]

Low socioeconomic status, early onset of sexual activity, unmarried marital status, and past gonococcal infections are risk factors for acquiring gonococcal infection, as are prostitution and illicit drug use.[16,39] Limited access to quality health care also may contribute to an increased prevalence of disease in impoverished populations.[65] The prevalence of gonococcal infection in adolescents attending private clinics probably is lower than that in those seeking care in publicly funded settings.[22] For women, the use of

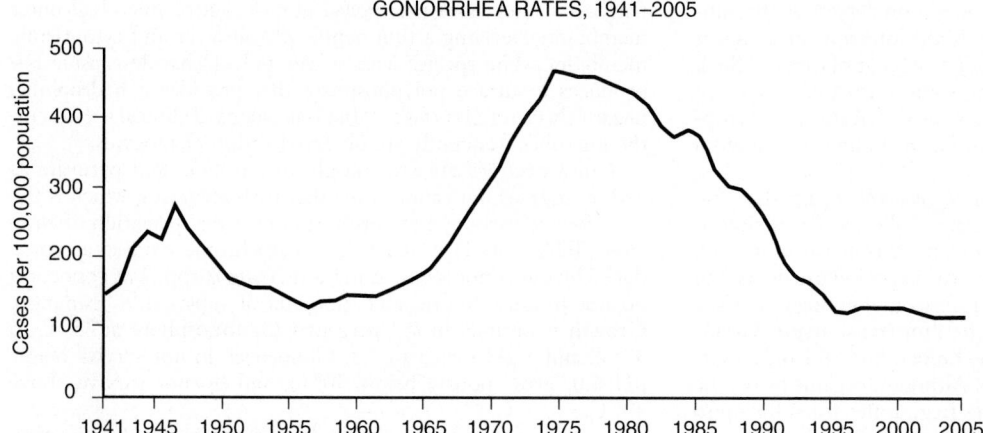

GONORRHEA RATES, 1941–2005

Figure 100–1 Rates of gonorrhea in the United States, 1941 to 2005. After a 74 percent decline from 1975 through 1997, overall gonorrhea rates have plateaued in recent years. Gonorrhea is substantially underdiagnosed and underreported. About twice as many new infections are estimated to occur each year as reported. (*From Centers for Disease Control and Prevention: Trends in reportable sexually transmitted diseases in the United States, 2005. December 2006. Available at* http://www.cdc.gov/std/stats/05pdf/trends-2005.pdf.)

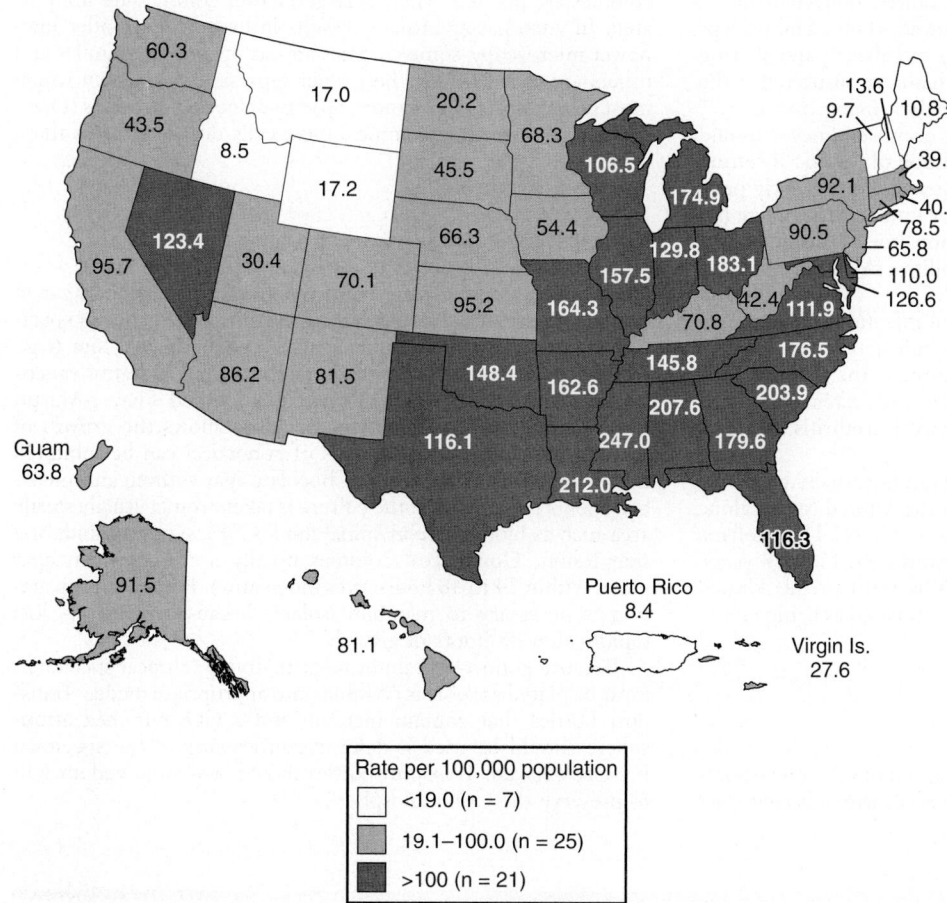

Figure 100–2 Rates of gonorrhea by state in the United States and outlying areas, 2005. (*From Centers for Disease Control and Prevention: Sexually Transmitted Disease Surveillance 2005 Supplement, Gonococcal Isolate Surveillance Project (GISP) Annual Report 2005. Atlanta, U.S. Department of Health and Human Services, Centers for Disease Control and Prevention, January 2007.*)

hormonal contraceptives may increase the risk of acquiring infection, whereas the use of spermicides or diaphragms appears to be at least partially protective.[210,211]

Rates of gonococcal infection among men who have sex with men (MSM) are lower than those in past years but remain higher than those among males who are exclusively heterosexual.[196] Among human immunodeficiency virus (HIV)-infected persons included in the Adult/Adolescent Spectrum of HIV Disease Project in the United States from 1991 to 1998, 9.5 cases occurred per 1000 person-years. A trend toward increasing rates of gonorrhea was noted during that period among MSM, whereas a decline occurred in those with heterosexual contact as their HIV

exposure risk.[112] In a prospective study from 2001 to 2003, the prevalence of pharyngeal gonorrhea among HIV-negative MSM was 5.5 percent; 92 percent of cases were asymptomatic.[227]

The southeastern United States continues to have rates of gonorrhea higher than those of other regions of the country, but rates per 100,000 population in the Southeast fell from 175 to 140 between 2001 and 2005 (Fig. 100–2). Rates in the western United States increased during this period from 72 to 82 per 100,000.[65] This increase occurred in all age, gender, and racial/ethnic groups, regardless of sexual orientation, and was explained only in part by increased testing and the use of more sensitive tests.[66]

Rates of gonorrhea are based primarily on detection of symptomatic infection. Asymptomatic chronic infection in adults is well documented and may account for 5 percent of cases.[164] Such persons can transmit the infection. Some untreated cases will resolve over the course of time. Data also indicate that asymptomatic infection occurs in children, including prepubertal children.[3,123,158,171]

Humans are the only reservoir of *N. gonorrhoeae*. Exudate and secretions from infected mucosal surfaces allow transmission to occur during the intimate contact of sexual acts, parturition, and, rarely, household exposure. The incubation period usually is 2 to 7 days. No evidence of airborne transmission of gonococci exists; contact with viable microbes is required for transmission. Gonococci survive on surfaces outside the human body for only short periods of time (probably minutes). Although organisms can be cultured from environmental sources (e.g., toilet seats) for up to 3 hours after artificial inoculation in large numbers, viable gonococci have not been recovered from random samplings in public restrooms.[133]

Gonococcal conjunctivitis can be acquired nonvenereally.[203] Vulvovaginitis potentially could be acquired when a child sleeps in the same bed with an infected family member,[133] and sharing of bath towels and other similar objects has been suspected as the cause of epidemics in prepubescent girls living together.[308] However, nonsexual transmission rarely occurs and never should be presumed without extensive investigation of the social setting of the infected child.[239] Although persistence of apparently perinatally acquired gonococcal infection for up to 1 year of age has been reported and fomite or maternal nonsexual transmission to young infants is plausible,[34] these possibilities should not be generalized beyond infancy.

The risk of a male acquiring urethral infection after a single episode of vaginal intercourse with an infected female is estimated to be 20 percent. With four exposures, the risk increases to 60 to 80 percent. The prevalence of infection in females named as sexual contacts of males with gonococcal urethritis has been reported to be 50 to 90 percent.[162,167]

The annual direct medical cost of treating sexually transmitted diseases (STDs), including HIV, in the United States alone has been estimated at $11 to $17 billion in 2003 U.S. dollars. Almost half of these costs accrue to persons aged 15 to 24 years. The reduction in gonorrhea and syphilis rates in the United States between 1990 and 2003 has been estimated as being equivalent to $5 billion during this period.[78]

MICROBIOLOGY

Neisseria spp. are aerobic, gram-negative, nonmotile, non–spore-forming cocci that occur in pairs (diplococci), with adjacent sides flattened. They have the typical gram-negative microbial outer membrane overlying a thin peptidoglycan layer and cytoplasmic membrane. The species lacks a true polysaccharide capsule but produces a surface polyphosphate that provides a hydrophilic, negatively charged surface.[246] In Gram stains of clinical specimens, the microbes frequently are observed within phagocytes.[303]

Gonococci are able to use glucose, lactate, and pyruvate as carbon sources but cannot use other carbohydrates, which is the basis for the carbohydrate utilization tests for speciation of *Neisseria* (Table 100–1). Catalase and cytochrome oxidase are produced by the gonococcus, as in most *Neisseria* spp., but gonococci do not produce appreciable amounts of superoxide dismutase. Growth is optimal in a 5 percent CO_2 atmosphere at 35° C to 37° C and a pH of 6.5 to 7.5. Gonococci do not survive below pH 6.0, grow poorly below 30° C, and do not survive above 40° C.

Neisseria spp. require enriched media, including free iron, to support their growth. Multiple colony types are evident when a single isolate is grown on clear agar. Small convex glistening colonies are piliated, whereas larger, flatter colonies are nonpiliated. In vitro passage usually results in loss of pili. Under low-power microscopy, some colonies appear opaque or granular and others are transparent. The former represent colonies in which most cells express one or more opacity-associated proteins (Opa), whereas in the latter colonies, most cells do not express these proteins.[37,42,188,310,318,319,331]

CULTURE FROM CLINICAL SPECIMENS

The organisms usually are cultured on chocolate blood agar in an atmosphere enriched by carbon dioxide. If the clinical specimen has been obtained from a highly contaminated site (e.g., rectum, cervix), a selective medium containing nystatin, vancomycin, trimethoprim, and colistin (e.g., modified Thayer-Martin medium) to suppress contaminating flora allows the growth of most *Neisseria* spp. A few strains of gonococci can be inhibited by vancomycin (see later).[37,225] Chocolate agar without antimicrobial agents is preferred if the culture is taken from a usually sterile area such as blood, cerebrospinal fluid (CSF), synovial fluid, or a skin lesion. Gonococcal colonies usually are evident on agar plates within 24 to 48 hours after inoculation. Frequent propagation is necessary to maintain isolates because viability is lost rapidly after 48 hours of growth.

Because gonococci cannot tolerate drying, clinical specimens must be plated as soon as possible onto appropriate media. Transport bottles that contain medium and a CO_2-enriched atmosphere should be used if definitive processing of the specimen must be delayed. Transport bottles should be maintained upright to preserve the CO_2 atmosphere.

TABLE 100–1 Biochemical Characteristics Differentiating Species of the Genus *Neisseria*

	N. gonorrhoeae	N. meningitidis	N. sicca	N. subflava	N. flavescens	N. mucosa	N. lactamica
Acid from							
Glucose	+	+	+	+	−	+	+
Maltose	−	+	+	+	−	+	−
Sucrose	−	−	+	±	−	+	−
Lactose	−	−	−	−	−	−	+
Polysaccharide produced from 5% sucrose	0	0	+	±	+	+	0
Reduction of							
Nitrate	−	−	−	−	−	+	−
Nitrite	−	±	+	+	+	+	+
Pigment	−	−	±	+	+	+	−
Extra CO_2 for growth	+	+	−	−	−	−	−

In addition to sugar fermentation patterns (see Table 100–1) and oxidase positivity, other biochemical reactions also can be used to differentiate between *Neisseria* spp. or confirm that an isolate is *N. gonorrhoeae*.[71] Enzyme substrate tests that identify the presence or absence of 1-hydroxyprolylaminopeptidase, gamma-glutamyl aminotransferase, and beta-galactosidase are available as an adjunctive means of confirmation.[97] Gonococci possess only the former. These reactions alone will not distinguish *N. gonorrhoeae* from several commensal *Neisseria* spp. Antigen-detection–based tests, including fluorescent antibody staining, also have been used to confirm the identity of an isolate as *N. gonorrhoeae*.[189] Tests based on detection of gonococcal nucleic acid sequences, which are being used increasingly for diagnostic purposes, also can be used to confirm the identify of gonococcal isolates from cultures (see "Diagnostic Testing" and "Medicolegal Issues" later).

GENETIC CHARACTERISTICS

Gonococci have a circular chromosome consisting of 2219 kilobases (kb), which is about half the size of the *Escherichia coli* genome.[107] The gonococcal genome has approximately 2250 predicted open-reading frames (ORFs).[35] The entire *N. gonorrhoeae* strain FA1090 has been sequenced. A macrorestriction map with the positions of many genetic markers has been available since 1991.[199,257] More than 1300 ORF sequences have been validated.[35]

Piliated gonococcal cells (the natural in vivo state) are competent for genetic transformation by exogenous DNA at all stages of growth.[25] Only homologous DNA is taken into the cell.[114] Gonococci are highly autolytic and release DNA in a biologically active form. Thus, different strains are able to exchange genetic material readily. Such exchange can lead to further genetic and phenotypic diversity, which helps maintain the species in its human hosts and facilitates transfer of chromosomal antibiotic resistance genes.[291]

A 36-kb conjugal plasmid is present in many gonococci. It efficiently mobilizes its own transfer and other non–self-mobilizable plasmids (e.g., the 4.5- and 7.5-kb penicillinase plasmids), but not chromosomal genes.[24,253,279] Extrachromosomal, non-plasmid DNA circles recently have been identified in wild-type gonococcal isolates. They may play a role in gene recombination, amplification of chromosomal genes, and transformation.[18]

Gonococci possess multiple restriction endonucleases and their corresponding DNA methylases.[317] No bacteriophages for *N. gonorrhoeae* are known, and no drug resistance transposon systems have been identified.[308] The species is relatively nonmutagenic and lacks photoreactivation and error-prone repair systems.[48]

STRAIN TYPING

The ability to differentiate one strain from another allows researchers to investigate the epidemiology of transmission of gonorrhea and assessment of virulence factors. Numerous methods have been applied to gonococci.

Auxotyping classifies strains according to their ability to grow or not grow in the absence of 11 specific compounds, including amino acids (e.g., arginine, proline), purines, pyrimidines (e.g., hypoxanthine, uracil), and other nutrients (e.g., thiamine). Approximately 20 auxotype phenotypes are recognized. Genetic studies have shown that multiple mutations in the same biochemical pathway can lead to the same phenotype, such that a single auxotype can represent many genotypes.[298] Auxotypes are stable in vitro, however, and organisms cultured from sexual partners are of a similar auxotype.[51,55] The auxotype of greatest

epidemiologic importance is designated arginine-, hypoxanthine-, and uracil-negative (AHU⁻). Such strains are unable to grow in the absence of these compounds. AHU⁻ strains typically are more resistant to killing by normal human serum, are more likely to cause asymptomatic infections in males, and are found more frequently in patients with disseminated infection.[117] AHU⁻ strains often are susceptible to vancomycin.[225]

Numerous serotyping schemes have been attempted,[72] but the best and most widely available serologic technique is based on antigenic heterogeneity of the porin protein (formerly called protein I) contained in the outer membrane of the gonococcus.[10,179,192,288,289] Two immunochemically distinct serogroups, PorA and PorB, exist and can be subdivided into serovars by using sets of monoclonal antibodies. Serovars remain stable in vitro and are designated IA-x or IB-x, where *x* is the numeral of the serovar. At least 26 IA and 31 IB serotypes have been identified.[62] Serotyping can be combined with auxotyping to further discriminate among gonococcal strains.[166,263] Limitations of auxotype-serovar classification include restricted supplies of reagents and batch-to-batch variation in monoclonal antibodies. In addition, common serovars can have such significant genetic diversity that this typing method may not provide sufficient discrimination for some epidemiologic evaluations.

Antimicrobial susceptibility patterns (antibiograms) have been used in the past as an adjunctive tool, but the usefulness of this method for long-term epidemiologic studies has been compromised by the ability of gonococci to transfer genetic elements for antibiotic resistance between strains.[308]

Genotyping methods have been applied to *N. gonorrhoeae* in the past 2 decades. Simple restriction endonuclease methods with rare cutting enzymes[122,262] have been supplanted by polymerase chain reaction (PCR)-based methods and pulsed-field gel electrophoresis (PFGE). Arbitrarily primed PCR (AP-PCR) has been used, but the reproducibility of this method can be problematic.[47,208] PFGE and Opa typing, which involves PCR primers that are able to generate DNA bands from each of the 11 *opa* genes, followed by restriction enzyme digestion, each appear to be able to produce higher discrimination among gonococcal isolates than does serotyping combined with AP-PCR.[208]

Sequencing of the *por* gene also appears to be highly discriminatory among strains,[87] and PCR amplification of the *por* gene with restriction enzyme digestion provides discrimination similar to that of combined auxotyping-serotyping.[111] Repetitive-element sequence-based PCR (rep-PCR), which uses longer primers than AP-PCR does and is a more reproducible method, correlates well with PFGE for analysis of gonococcal strains.[263] Rep-PCR is a rapid method that can be performed directly on colonies without having to purify microbial DNA, which is required with most other genotyping methods.[341]

PATHOGENESIS

A continuously expanding body of literature is devoted to the pathogenesis of *N. gonorrhoeae*. Gonococci are able to survive in the urethra in the face of hydrodynamic forces that tend to wash other microbes away and persist there despite close proximity and even attachment to the hoards of neutrophils that respond to their presence. These observations suggest that they have an ability to adhere to mucosal epithelia and evade the host's acute innate immune response. Individuals also can have repeated infections by the same gonococcal strain, thus suggesting that the organism can thwart established local immune responses, probably through frequent antigenic variation. The tissue damage that occurs in the fallopian tubes during salpingitis implies that one or more directly toxic moieties or factors can trigger a deleterious host response.[124,308] Much progress has been made in understanding the mechanisms that account for these properties.

Clinical studies have focused largely on the adaptation of organisms to specific anatomic areas (e.g., rectum, blood, endocervix) in older adolescents and adults. This information probably holds true for most infections in infants and children. Recent insight into the molecular pathogenesis of gonococcal infection has been derived from in vitro molecular studies involving cell lines and fallopian tube organ cultures and experimental infections in human males.[81,215,216,272] Currently, no adequate animal models of gonococcal infection exist.

After adhering to host epithelial cells, some gonococcal microbes are able to invade, replicate intracellularly inside phagosomes/vacuoles, and exit the basal (but not lateral) surface of the cell via exocytosis[216,221,237] (Fig. 100–3). Adjacent nonepithelial cells are sloughed, probably because of the toxicity of lipooligosaccharide (LOS) and peptidoglycans.[142] Mucosal cell damage and submucosal invasion are followed by an influx of neutrophils along with the formation of submucosal microabscesses and exudation of purulent material into the lumen of the infected organ.[339]

The vast majority of invading gonococci are ingested and killed by neutrophils. Gonococci are susceptible to the oxidative burst products of phagocytes, as well as to nonoxidative products such as cathepsin G.[52,296] A few gonococci are able to escape the innate and early adaptive immune responses such that infection and contagion can persist for weeks and sometimes months in the absence of treatment.

Adherence of gonococci to mucosal epithelial cells causes activation of nuclear factor κB and activator protein 1, which in turn leads to up-regulation and release of multiple cytokines and chemokines, including macrophage colony-stimulating factor, tumor necrosis factor-α (TNF-α), tumor growth factor-β, monocyte chemoattractant protein 1, interleukin-1β (IL-1β), IL-6, and IL-8.[238,266]

The initial steps in pathogenesis may result from the synergistic effects of pili, Opa proteins, and porin proteins.[19,144] Close interactions of *N. gonorrhoeae* with mucosal cells, erythrocytes, spermatozoa, and polymorphonuclear cells are well described. Species specificity is demonstrated by greater adherence of gonococci to human cells than to nonhuman cells. The best-characterized microbial factors are listed in Table 100–2 and discussed in the following sections.

TABLE 100–2 Pregnancy Complications and Outcomes of Mothers Who Were Infected with *Neisseria gonorrhoeae* at Delivery

Pregnancy Complications and Outcomes	Charles et al.[74] (N = 14)*	Sarrel and Pruett[290] (N = 37)	Israel et al.[175] (N = 39)	Amstey and Steadman[7] (N = 222)*	Edwards et al.[116] (N = 19)*	Handsfield and Holmes[154] (N = 12)*	Totals[†]
Normal or term infant	—	13 (35%)	30 (77%)	142 (64%)	7 (37%)	—	192/317 (61%)
Aborted	—	13 (35%)	1 (2%)	24 (11%)	—	—	38/298 (13%)
Perinatal death	—	3 (8%)	1 (2%)	15 (7%)	2 (11%)	—	21/317 (7%)
Premature	—	6 (16%)	5 (13%)	49 (22%)	8 (42%)	8 (67%)	76/329 (23%)
Perinatal distress	—	—	2 (5%)	—	2 (11%)	—	4/58 (7%)
Premature rupture of membranes	6 (43%)	8 (22%)	—	52 (23%)	12 (63%)	9 (75%)	87/304 (29%)

*Data were provided in which the outcomes of pregnancies of mothers not infected with N. gonorrhoeae were shown to be significantly more favorable.
†Percentages in all columns may sum to greater than 100 because pregnancies could have more than one of the listed outcomes.

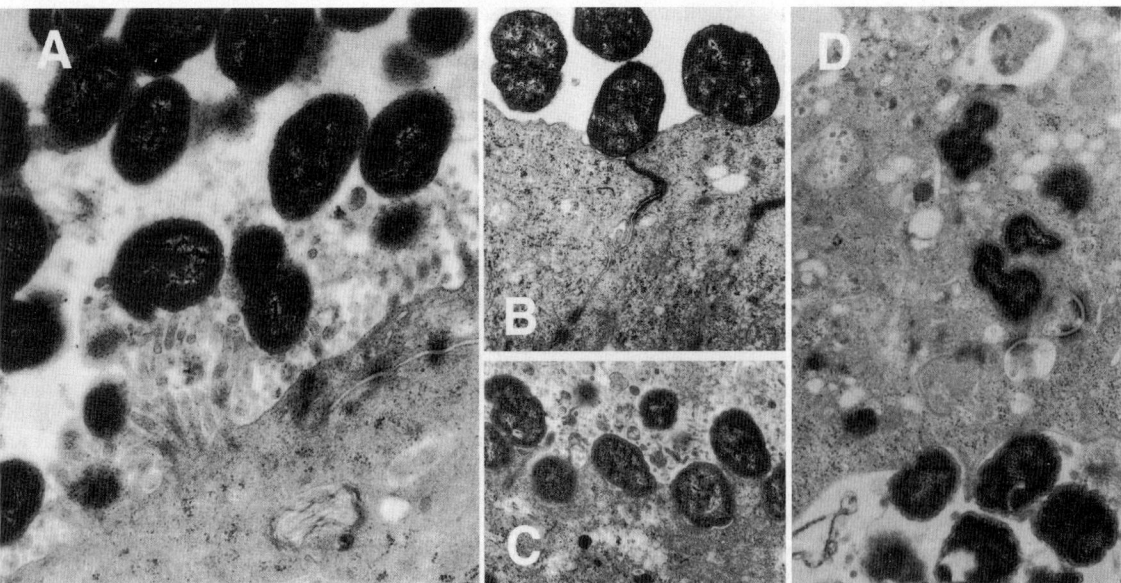

Figure 100–3 Electron micrographs of *Neisseria gonorrhoeae* (strain MS11) interactions with polarized T84 human epithelial cell monolayers. At early stages of infection, the microbes adhere to the apical plasma membrane as microcolonies. Adherent bacteria are surrounded by a matrix of microvilli (**A**). Bacteria subsequently disperse from the microcolony and adhere as a monolayer in which bacterial and host-cell membranes are tightly apposed (**B** and **C**). The region of contact between the bacteria and the host-cell membrane enlarges (**C**), with subsequent internalization of the microbes (**D**). Bacteria then traverse the host cell and exit via the basolateral membrane (**D**). (*Photographs by Magdalene So, from the* Annual Review of Cell and Developmental Biology, *Volume 16.* © *2000 by Annual Reviews.* www.AnnualReviews.org.)

VIRULENCE FACTORS

Characteristics of *N. gonorrhoeae* strains that appear to have a role in virulence include (1) pili, (2) opacity proteins, (3) porin protein, (4) the ability to survive in low iron environments, (5) IgA protease, (6) LOS, (7) cell wall peptidoglycan, and (8) reduction modifiable protein (Rmp). Many other gonococcal gene products and molecular systems have been identified, and a more detailed and complex understanding of virulence at the molecular level probably is forthcoming.

THE PRESENCE OF PILI. Gonococci are piliated predominantly in vivo and express type IV pili. Pili cover essentially the entire surface of the cell and are arranged in individual fibrils or fibrillar aggregates. Pili consist primarily of polymers of an 18-kd subunit now denoted as PilE. A single pilus is approximately 6 nm in diameter and up to several microns in length.[221] Each may contain thousands of PilE subunits.[44] The PilC protein is present in lower numbers in the pilus but appears to be the key pilus adhesin. PilC interacts with CD46 molecules, which are present on most human cells and serve as receptors for C3b, C4b, and measles and other viruses. PilC-CD46 attachment appears to be a key step in the initiation of microbial adherence to host cells.[45,185,190,283,285]

Binding of pili to a host-cell membrane induces at least two responses in the host cell: release of Ca^{2+} from intracellular stores[184] and cytoskeletal rearrangements with the formation of cortical plaques that represent an accumulation of actin, ezrin, and other phosphotyrosine-containing proteins.[219,220] The latter results in elongation of the microvilli that embrace the microbe. Formation of plaque appears to be induced by retraction of the attached pilus, and retraction is dependent on another pilus protein designated PilT.[222]

Gonococcal pili undergo both phase variation (switching from piliated to nonpiliated states) and high-frequency antigenic variation.[44] These variations occur during natural infection and in vitro passage.[293] Pili have a common N-terminal domain, semi-variable domains in the midportion, and two hypervariable regions in the carboxyl-terminal of the pilin protein subunit.[309] Relatively invariant regions occur between the variable domains. The pilin protein consists of 159 to 160 amino acids. A disulfide bridge is formed by cysteine residues at amino acids 121 and 151.

The genetic mechanism of pilus antigenic variation has been studied extensively. The chromosome contains either one or two complete pilin genes. The expressed gene contains an intact promoter region, a ribosome binding site, and a seven–amino acid signal sequence in addition to the pilin sequence. Scattered around the chromosome are six to eight loci that contain varying portions of the pilin sequence without the promoter region or the 5' end of the structural gene. Some loci may contain many incomplete pilin sequences arranged head to tail that differ slightly from one another. Movement of these sequences into the active expression site through nonreciprocal combination events results in antigenic variation of the pilus protein. If recombination leads to a faulty pilin subunit product that cannot be processed into a mature pilus, the progeny of that organism become nonpiliated (phase variation). Subsequent recombination events can allow reversion back to the piliated phase.[150,223,224,243,292,309,320]

In addition to promoting adhesion to epithelial cells, pili also provide a twitching motility, are involved in DNA transformation, and may play a role in resistance to ingestion by phagocytic cells.[221] The presence of pili, perhaps mediated through their promotion of adhesion, affects the activation of $CD4^+$ T-lymphocytes and the production of IL-10. This property may help gonococci diminish the T-cell response to their presence.[259]

OPACITY-ASSOCIATED PROTEINS. Opa proteins also influence adherence of the gonococcus to host cells. The isolation of particular Opa protein phenotypes from different anatomic sites or at different times during the menstrual cycle has suggested that these proteins contribute to the ability of the organism to succeed in a given niche. Opa proteins (formerly designated *protein II*) are a set of as many as 12 related proteins that are variably present in gonococcal outer membranes. Opa proteins are 24 to 28 kd in size and confer increased opacity to colonies of organisms by promoting adherence of the organisms to one another. A given strain has the capacity to make at least 10 different Opa proteins but appears to express no more than 5 at the same time. Some cells express no Opa proteins. Like pili, Opa proteins undergo both antigenic and phase variation. Both types of variations can occur within a single colony, so sector variations in opacity can be seen.[27,308,318,319]

Each *opa* gene is present as a complete gene with its own promoter and is transcribed at all times. Phase variation in expression occurs at the translational level. Each gene has a varying number of pentameric CTCTT repeat units adjacent to the ATG start codon. When the number of repeats is divisible by three, the transcribed mRNA is translationally in frame and the Opa protein is expressed. The number of pentameric repeats is subject to high-frequency variation. Antigenic variation results from recombinations between the two hypervariable regions in each of the *opa* genes.[86,313-315]

Two classes of host-cell receptors for Opa proteins have been identified. Heparan sulfate–proteoglycan (HSPG) receptors are present on epithelial cells and interact with one particular Opa protein variant (Opa_{50}). HSPG binding can stimulate the lipid hydrolysis enzymes phosphatidylcholine-specific phospholipase C and acid sphingomyelinase and thereby lead to clathrin-independent endocytosis. HSPG-Opa binding also can lead to interactions with serum factors such as vitronectin and fibronectin, which then mediate endocytosis via host-cell integrin receptors. The CD66 family is present on epithelial cells and neutrophils, recognizes many different Opa proteins, and mediates nonopsonic phagocytosis, a process distinct from antibody- and complement-mediated phagocytosis.[102,103,140,197,221,328]

PORIN PROTEIN. Formerly designated protein I, porin protein is the most common gonococcal outer-membrane protein. Porin is 34 to 36 kd, is exposed on the surface, exists as a trimer in the membrane, and is physically proximate to LOS and Rmp.[28,159] The trimer forms an anion-specific pore in the bacterial membrane that allows small water-soluble molecules to enter the cell.[343] The *por* locus has two alleles that encode chemically and immunologically distinct classes of porin protein—PorA and PorB—that are similar to porin proteins in other gram-negative bacteria. A given strain expresses only PorA or PorB, and many antigenic variants of both exist (thereby forming the basis for serotyping).[50,192]

The porin trimer appears to translocate into the host-cell membrane and is able to disrupt neutrophil degranulation, the oxidative burst, and phagosome maturation,[151,209,230] in addition to induction of apoptosis in epithelial cells and neutrophils in vitro.[234] Exposure to gonococcal porin protein induces the typical structural and biochemical changes seen in apoptotic cells.[233] Porin translocation permits rapid influx of Ca^{2+} into the host cell from the external environment.[234] Porin proteins also may play a role in endocytosis mediated by the binding of HSPG and Opa protein[19] and in down-regulation of complement by binding with C4b-binding protein.[265]

THE ABILITY TO USE IRON. Iron is an essential nutrient for *N. gonorrhoeae*, and in host tissues, iron is sequestered in hemin compounds as ferritin or is bound to lactoferrin or transferrin. The species does not produce any siderophores but relies on an iron-repressible system that scavenges iron from transferrin, lactoferrin, and hemoglobin. This system is composed of numerous proteins, some of which serve as receptors for the aforementioned iron-bearing ligands.[26,75,92,333] The ability to use iron from transferrin is a general property of pathogenic *Neisseria* spp. Transferrin- and lactoferrin-binding proteins are required for gonococci to cause experimental urethritis.[91]

IgA PROTEASE. All gonococci (and meningococci, but not nonpathogenic *Neisseria*) make a protease that cleaves both serum and secretory IgA1 (but not IgA2) at the hinge region with the release of Fab and Fc fragments. This protease may help the organism evade host IgA at the mucosal surface, especially early in secondary infections, when preexisting antibodies may be present. However, mutant strains without the IgA protease have limited ability to grow inside epithelial cells. The protease appears to cleave a host-cell intracellular protein (LAMP1) involved in phagosome compartmentalization.[205] IgA1 protease is not required for gonococci to cause experimental urethritis,[178] thus suggesting that its intraphagosome function may be more important in pathogenesis.

LIPO-OLIGOSACCHARIDE. Gonococci express LOS complexes of 3 to 7 kd on their cell surface. LOS consists of a lipid A moiety and a core polysaccharide composed of ketodeoxyoctanoic acid, heptose, glucose, galactose, glucosamine, galactosamine, or any combination of these constituents.[146] The lack of a long polymeric sugar attached to the core distinguishes LOS from the lipopolysaccharides of other gram-negative bacteria. The core sugar antigens of LOS are subject to intrastrain and interstrain variation, and a single strain may express as many as six variants of LOS.[105,145] Numerous genes are involved in LOS synthesis; these genes undergo high-frequency phase variation similar to *opa* genes.[139] LOS terminal sugars mimic the structure of certain human glycosphingolipids.[146]

Gonococci with predominately short LOS molecules appear to be more sensitive to killing by human serum but also more able to invade eukaryotic cells. Strains with longer LOS are more serum-resistant but noninvasive.[329] Longer LOS moieties are sialylated readily with host neuraminic acid by a bacterial sialyltransferase that appears to shield both LOS and porin molecules from antibody binding, thus providing protection from complement-mediated killing in serum.[33,334]

LOS from serum-sensitive strains is able to activate the classical complement pathway and may do so in the absence of antibody.[295] LOS induces the production of cytokines (TNF-α, IL-1β, IL-6, IL-8) by urethral epithelial cells[157] and can mediate host defensin-enhanced adherence to epithelial cells.[138]

CELL WALL PEPTIDOGLYCAN. Gonococci shed membrane fragments with peptidoglycan into their environment during exponential growth. Peptidoglycan monomers have numerous biologic properties, including activation of complement and modulation of mononuclear cell proliferation. These fragments also damage fallopian tube mucosa in organ culture, thus suggesting a pathogenic role for the compounds in invasive disease.[142,216]

REDUCTION MODIFIABLE PROTEIN. Rmp (formerly designated protein III) is an antigenically conserved, 30- to 31-kd protein that is present in all pathogenic *Neisseria*. Rmp is located proximate to LOS and porin in the outer membrane. Antibodies that bind to Rmp epitopes block the bactericidal effect of the complement-fixing IgM antibodies that recognize LOS. Women with preexisting anti-Rmp antibodies appear to be more susceptible to the development of infection than do those without such antibodies.[274,275,308]

RIBOSOMAL PROTEIN L12. Ribosomal protein L12 mimics the structure of human chorionic gonadotropin, the natural ligand for lutropin receptors. It is able to bind to lutropin receptors in the upper female genital tract, which may facilitate ascending infection in females.[115,312]

CHARACTERISTICS OF STRAINS CAUSING DISSEMINATED DISEASE

The increased virulence of some strains is suggested by observations such as a micro-epidemic of gonorrhea involving one asymptomatic infected male and eight female contacts.[154] Seven of the women were infected symptomatically, and four experienced disseminated infection. Clinical data repeatedly have shown that most infected women have asymptomatic infection and dissemination occurs relatively rarely.

Strains of *N. gonorrhoeae* obtained from adult patients with disseminated disease usually are less susceptible to the bactericidal activity of sera[38,83,272,273,297] (see discussion of LOS earlier). These strains have an atypical growth pattern on agar[226] that reflects the absence of Opa protein expression, which suggests that the genetic variation capacity described earlier allows adaptation to different niches and probably helps organisms elude the host response.[23] Unlike most gonococcal strains, many invasive strains (designated AHU⁻) require arginine, uracil, and hypoxanthine for growth.[191] A high degree of sensitivity to penicillin also has been characteristic of most strains from patients with disseminated disease.[338] *Many also are susceptible to vancomycin, which may prevent them from being detected in selective media but not in the usual media used for blood culture.*

HOST RESPONSE

The adult response to local and systemic infection with *N. gonorrhoeae* has been investigated extensively, but no such studies have been performed on infected children. Gonococcal infections usually are characterized by intense inflammation that involves neutrophilic and mononuclear granulocytes. The vast majority of gonococcal cells ingested by neutrophils are killed.[52] Gonococci are susceptible to the oxidative products produced by neutrophils but also can be killed efficiently by nonoxidative products such as cathepsin G.[296]

An intact complement system is essential for successful eradication of the organism. Persons with inherited or acquired complement deficiencies may be predisposed to contracting disseminated gonococcal infection, as is the case with meningococcal infection. Approximately 13 percent of patients with disseminated disease have complement deficiencies.[119,246]

Adherence of gonococci in vitro induces the activation of nuclear factor κB and activator protein 1, which leads to up-regulation of mRNA for and release of numerous cytokines and chemokines: macrophage colony-stimulating factor, TNF-α, tumor growth factor-β, monocyte chemoattractant protein 1, IL-1β, IL-6, and IL-8.[238] Intra-urethral challenge leads to increased levels of IL-8, IL-6, and TNF-α in urine before the onset of symptoms and in plasma at the onset of symptoms.[266]

Multiple episodes of gonorrhea may occur in a single individual in a short period of time and even may be caused by the same strain. The antigenic diversity and ease of altering the antigenicity of both pili and opacity proteins undoubtedly contribute to the insufficiency of the host response in preventing reinfection.

Circulating humoral antibody to the infecting strain is measured by an assay of bactericidal antibody and is present in most persons who have prolonged mucosal colonization with *N. gonor-*

rhoeae.[172,187] In addition, women in whom PID develops usually produce bactericidal antibody during the infection. IgA- and IgG-blocking antibodies against some gonococcal antigens appear to block killing of the bacteria mediated by otherwise bactericidal IgG and IgM antibodies (see Rmp information earlier).[272] Serum antibody responses are greater in patients with invasive disease (e.g., bacteremia, salpingitis).

Secretory IgA antibody is present in the urethral exudate of men with gonorrhea and in the genital secretions of women with gonorrhea.[247] The development of local IgA antibody occurs more rapidly and is more transient than is development of the serum bactericidal response. Microbial IgA1 protease is not required for infection but may play a role in reinfection.

A cellular immune response to gonococcal antigens in patients with uncomplicated gonorrhea has been demonstrated in vitro.[200] The significance of this response in controlling or preventing infection is unknown.

PERINATAL GONOCOCCAL INFECTIONS

Since the 1970s, health clinics have encouraged the routine screening of sexually active women for gonorrhea. Such screening is especially important during pregnancy, and rates of gonorrhea in pregnant women range from exceedingly low to approximately 10 percent. Adolescent girls have a higher prevalence of gonorrhea than do older women of child-bearing age, and this prevalence probably translates into higher rates of gonorrhea in pregnant adolescents. Rates of gonococcal infection in neonates reflect the frequency of infection in pregnant women. Recognition of gonorrhea early in pregnancy identifies a population at risk that should be monitored sequentially for reinfection throughout pregnancy.[180]

The spectrum of infection with *N. gonorrhoeae* appears to be similar in pregnant and nonpregnant women. Most women are asymptomatic. Pharyngeal infection seems to occur more commonly during pregnancy, perhaps reflecting altered sexual practices. One study reported that 39 percent of patients with *N. gonorrhoeae* at any site had concurrent involvement of the pharynx and that 30 percent had pharyngeal infection as the sole manifestation.[90] In adolescent girls, pregnancy and menstruation are associated with disseminated disease.[161]

Gonorrheal infection puts both the mother and infant at risk for the development of other forms of gonococcal disease. Pregnant women have an increased risk for the development of gonococcal septic arthritis, and most such cases occur during the third trimester or in the immediate postpartum period.[40,161] Although the incidence of gonococcal arthritis is low, many cases have occurred in pregnant adolescents.

Gonococcal PID and acute salpingitis also may complicate the pregnancy of an infected woman.[132] These complications usually occur during the first trimester and have been associated with a high rate of fetal loss. An increased incidence of postpartum fever in women with untreated gonorrhea likewise has been noted. A new mother with complications of peripartum gonorrhea may have difficulty providing care for her child.[175]

Maternal gonococcal infection has been associated with abnormalities in labor and delivery that may affect the infant adversely. Prolonged rupture of membranes, premature delivery, chorioamnionitis, funisitis, and a clinical diagnosis of sepsis occur frequently in infants with *N. gonorrhoeae* detected in the gastric aspirate during delivery.[7,116,153,280]

Hazards to the fetus posed by maternal gonorrhea include septic abortion, perinatal death, prematurity, perinatal distress, and premature rupture of membranes. Table 100–2 tabulates the proportions in six studies of infants born to infected mothers who experienced these problems. A controlled study in an area with a high prevalence of gonorrhea found that maternal infection with

N. gonorrhoeae was associated significantly with preterm birth and that 14 percent of preterm births in this population were attributable to gonococcal infection.[118]

GONOCOCCAL OPHTHALMIA NEONATORUM

Epidemiology

Researchers have recognized for centuries that ophthalmia neonatorum occurs in infants born to women with a vaginal discharge. Recommendations for flushing the eyes of a newborn commonly were given before the 20th century.[218] In the late 1800s, Neisser helped establish the relationship between the gonococcus and neonatal ophthalmia.

By 1881, Dr. Carl Sigmund Franz Credé had recognized that asymptomatic disease in the mother was a potential source of infection.[96] Gonorrhea was highly prevalent in Europe, and Credé described an increased incidence in patients from lower socioeconomic backgrounds. Mechanical cleansing of the birth canal failed to protect the infant from gonococcal ophthalmia neonatorum (GON), which was occurring in approximately 10 percent of newborns in major cities. The infection was the cause of a large proportion of admissions to schools for the blind.[17] Credé described the technique of instillation of 2 percent silver nitrate (AgNO₃) into the infant's conjunctival sac, which remains one method recommended for preventive procedures today.

By 1930, most states in the United States required that all newborns receive AgNO₃ prophylaxis (i.e., the Credé procedure). At present, prophylaxis of some form is required by most states. GON decreased as a cause of admission to schools for the blind in the United States, from an average of 24 percent from 1906 to 1911 to 0.5 percent from 1951 to 1955.

The worldwide decline in adult gonorrhea in the 1950s probably contributed to the decreased recognition of disease in newborns during that period. The incidence of GON rose in the 1960s and 1970s along with the increased incidence of gonorrhea in the general population and was very high in some developing nations.[197] In Los Angeles, California, the rate rose from 9 per 100,000 live births in 1957 to 1958 to 56 per 100,000 live births in 1962 to 1963. In a New York hospital between 1970 and 1973, a rate of 145 per 100,000 births was reported, and in a hospital in North Carolina during 1969 and 1970, a rate of 265 per 100,000 live births was proved by culture.[307] In the late 1970s and 1980s, GON again subsided in developed countries, but it has remained a major problem in underdeveloped nations.

Factors associated with higher rates of GON include lower socioeconomic class of the mother. An increased incidence of GON in infants of unwed mothers and mothers who have not had prenatal care also may exist.[304] Previous treatment of gonorrhea during pregnancy likewise is associated with an increased incidence of GON.[180]

The incidence of prematurity in infants with GON often is reported to be higher. Whether it is due to an adverse effect of gonorrhea on the pregnancy or because GON may be recognized more readily in premature infants has not been established. Premature rupture of membranes appears to increase the risk of GON occurring.

Prevention

Prophylaxis for GON has been accomplished mainly through the local instillation of either 1 percent AgNO₃ or one of several antimicrobial agents. In the United States, prophylaxis for GON is recommended for all infants immediately after birth and is required by law in most states. Prophylaxis regimens using a 1 percent solution of AgNO₃, 1 percent tetracycline ointment, or 0.5 percent erythromycin ophthalmic ointment have been considered equally effective for GON. Each is available in single-dose units, which are preferred over multidose tubes. One unit should be instilled into the eyes of every neonate as soon as possible after delivery. Installation may be delayed for as long as 1 hour to facilitate parent-infant bonding. Povidone-iodine 2.5 percent solution also may be effective, but this agent is not recommended for use in the United States at this time.[5] Bacitracin is not effective for prevention of GON.[141]

The efficacy of tetracycline and erythromycin in the prevention of tetracycline-resistant *N. gonorrhoeae* ophthalmia is unknown. Both probably are effective because of the high concentration of drug in these preparations. Studies of these agents for prevention of *Chlamydia trachomatis* ophthalmia have been conflicting. Povidone-iodine may be more effective in preventing *C. trachomatis* ophthalmia than is topical $AgNO_3$ or erythromycin is. None of these agents prevents chlamydial colonization of the nasopharynx. Some Western countries with low rates of gonococcal and chlamydial infection do not recommend routine ophthalmic prophylaxis.[5,149]

CURRENT PROPHYLAXIS RECOMMENDATIONS IN THE UNITED STATES. In the United States, the 2006 version of the Sexually Transmitted Diseases Treatment Guidelines of the Centers for Disease Control and Prevention (CDC) no longer includes the use of silver nitrate. This change reflects the lack of availability of this agent in the United States at that time and not concerns about safety or effectiveness. The recommended agents are erythromycin 0.5 percent ophthalmic ointment or tetracycline 1 percent ophthalmic ointment, either one administered as a single application to each eye as soon as possible after delivery. None of the topical agents prevents mother-to-infant transmission of *C. trachomatis*.[64]

SILVER NITRATE AND GONOCOCCAL OPHTHALMIA NEONATORUM. Numerous studies have compared the efficacy of $AgNO_3$ and no prophylaxis or prophylaxis with another agent in the prevention of GON, and these studies have been reviewed elsewhere.[76,248,281] Until the late 1900s, most studies of the efficacy of $AgNO_3$ were not randomized and did not document rates of perinatal gonococcal exposure in the infants studied. Such studies involved large numbers of infants and consistently have shown lower rates of GON in treated groups than in untreated controls. Observations of a decreased frequency of blindness from GON in the population during the last half century, even during periods of increased rates of gonorrhea in women of child-bearing age, further support the benefits of $AgNO_3$ prophylaxis.

In a randomized trial of Kenyan infants born to mothers with gonorrhea reported in 1988, rates of GON were 42 percent in the control group, 7 percent in the group treated with 1 percent $AgNO_3$ (83% reduction), and 3 percent in the group treated with 1 percent tetracycline (93% reduction). The two treatment arms were not statistically different.[199] In a randomized trial in the United States involving infants born to women without gonococcal infection, infants treated with 1 percent $AgNO_3$ had a 39 percent lower rate (statistically significant) of conjunctivitis of any type in the first 2 months of life than did infants receiving no prophylaxis. Infants treated with 0.5 percent erythromycin ointment in this trial had a 31 percent reduction in comparison to control infants, but this result was not statistically significant.[20]

The major advantages of the use of $AgNO_3$ for prophylaxis are the lack of allergic potential, the absence of development of bacterial resistance to the compound, and very low cost. Two outbreaks of erythromycin-resistant staphylococcal conjunctivitis in newborn nurseries have been associated with the use of erythromycin eye ointment as ocular prophylaxis, but the outbreaks remitted when $AgNO_3$ was substituted. Disadvantages include the occurrence of conjunctival irritation along with the develop-

ment of exudate in many babies and lack of effectiveness if infection already is established before drops are instilled into the eye. A solution of $AgNO_3$ that becomes concentrated may cause ophthalmic injury, but this problem largely has been alleviated by dispensing doses in ampules, which prevents evaporation.

Failure of $AgNO_3$ prophylaxis (as well as other agents for prevention of GON) does occur. Improper administration of $AgNO_3$ such that the solution does not reach the conjunctival sac, irrigation performed too quickly after instillation, and inadvertent omission of prophylaxis can lead to apparent failure. When gonococcal infection of the eye has begun before birth, $AgNO_3$ is not expected to prevent further progression. The increased risk of GON associated with premature rupture of membranes is due to exposure to and establishment of infection before actual delivery. In some cases of premature rupture of membranes, clinically apparent GON can be present at the time of birth.

Despite these problems, the use of 1 percent $AgNO_3$ remains a widely accepted, carefully evaluated, and safe form of GON prophylaxis. The occasional failure of $AgNO_3$ prophylaxis emphasizes that it is preferable to prevent GON through identification and treatment of pregnant women.

Clinical Features

The newborn eye is subject to colonization with numerous bacterial organisms that cause infections that usually are clinically mild, nonprogressive, and characterized by conjunctival discharge. The bacteria most commonly associated with conjunctival discharge are *Haemophilus influenzae*, *Streptococcus pneumoniae*, *Staphylococcus aureus*, *Neisseria cinerea*, *Klebsiella pneumoniae*, enterococci, and *C. trachomatis*.[110,195] Viral causes include herpes simplex virus and adenoviruses. In contrast, infection of the eye of a newborn with *N. gonorrhoeae* results in disease of a severity that, despite frequently being mild, can be rapidly destructive and lead to scarring and blindness. The chemical conjunctivitis that can result from $AgNO_3$ prophylaxis typically starts within 6 to 24 hours after administration and disappears within 24 to 48 hours.

Colonization during delivery is followed by an incubation period of 2 to 5 and usually less than 3 days, but cases occasionally may be recognized for 2 to 3 weeks after delivery.[130] A discharge typically develops that initially is watery but usually becomes thick and mucopurulent within a short time and may contain blood (Fig. 100–4). The disease generally is bilateral. Early findings include prominent edema of the conjunctivae and lids, followed by edema and later ulceration of the cornea or spread to wider areas in severe cases. Rapid arrest of the disease is essential because the degree of corneal involvement determines whether vision will be preserved. Some cases are self-limited and have benign outcomes, and occasional cases of asymptomatic GON have been discovered during routine screening.[261] Perforation of the globe and panophthalmitis can result from extensive local disease. The conjunctivae may serve as a portal of entry for gonococcal septicemia, arthritis, or other manifestations of invasive disease, but such events seldom occur.

A presumptive diagnosis may be made by demonstrating typical gram-negative diplococci by Gram stain of conjunctival exudate. Because other organisms also may cause exudative infection of the conjunctivae, laboratory confirmation of the diagnosis of GON depends on culture results of *N. gonorrhoeae*.

Invasive disease rarely occurs in association with GON. However, in the United States, the recommendation is that neonates with GON or any other manifestation of gonococcal infection have cultures performed on blood and CSF (as well as any local sites of infection) and be hospitalized pending culture results.[5]

GONOCOCCAL SCALP ABSCESS AND OTHER LOCAL INFECTIONS

Gonococcal infections of scalp wounds occur especially after fetal monitoring electrodes have been used on infants born to infected mothers.[99] The lesions may produce extensive local inflammatory disease and necrosis and can be a focus for disseminated infection. A scalp wound in a neonate should be cultured for gonococci, as well as other likely pathogens, which include *Staphylococcus* spp., group B streptococci, *H. influenzae*, and gram-negative enteric flora. Herpes simplex also may be present in areas of injury to the scalp of newborns. Overall, approximately 1 in 200 births that are monitored with fetal scalp electrodes has been complicated by infection at the monitoring site.[260]

Neonatal gonococcal vulvovaginitis, proctitis, rhinitis, funisitis, and urethritis have been described but are infrequent findings.[149] Gonococcal colonization of the oropharynx, gastric fluid, or both occurs relatively frequently in perinatally exposed infants, however. Pharyngeal colonization is present in as many as 35 percent of neonates who have GON.[127] A summary of selected studies on the incidence of neonatal gonococcal colonization and disease in exposed infants is presented in Table 100–3.

Infants with localized gonococcal infection at any site should have cultures obtained of blood and CSF, as well as the local site, and should be hospitalized pending the availability of culture results (see "Treatment" later).

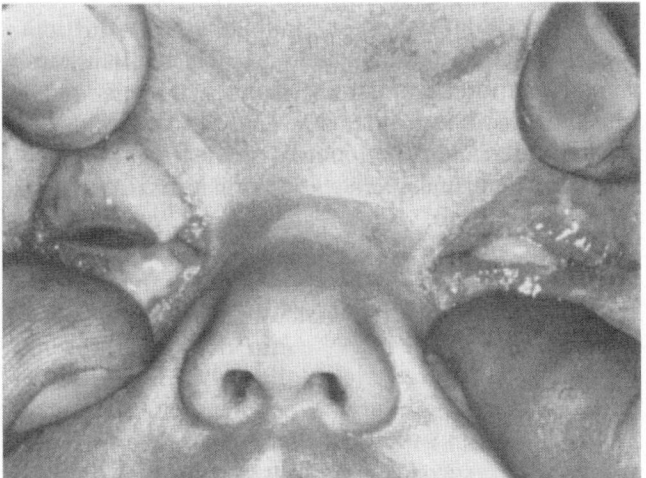

Figure 100–4 Gonococcal ophthalmia neonatorum. The usual clinical finding is bilateral conjunctivitis that becomes progressively purulent if untreated. (*From Gutman, L. T.: Gonococcal infections. Semin. Pediatr. Infect. Dis. 16:4, 2005.*)

SYSTEMIC DISEASE IN THE NEONATE

Disseminated disease occurs in 1 percent or less of infants who are perinatally exposed to gonococcal infection[13] (see Table 100–3). Septic arthritis is the most common form of disseminated gonococcal infection in neonates. Gonococcal arthritis of the newborn was described extensively between 1900 and 1930 by Cooperman[88,89] and Wehrbein,[332] and recent case reports suggest that the disease remains similar. Clinical findings usually become evident when the infant is 1 to 4 weeks old. Although a few infants with gonococcal arthritis will have evidence of GON or other sites of mucosal or skin infection at the time of onset of arthritis, most do not.

The signs and symptoms of gonococcal septic arthritis are similar to those of joint infection caused by other microbes in the neonatal period, including a predominance of polyarticular involvement. Infection most frequently involves the ankles, knees, wrists, and hands.[88] The hip may be infected with minimal signs other than pseudoparesis. Involvement of a joint may include suppurative arthritis, inflammatory disease of the periarticular structures, and tenosynovitis. Leukocytosis usually occurs, and most infants have a positive culture and compatible Gram stain results from the synovial fluid of the involved joint.[135]

In a hospital-associated outbreak of gonococcal polyarthritis that occurred in 1927, involvement of the joint was noted in 53 of 67 infected infants (79%). Other studies of outbreaks have indicated that perhaps 15 percent of children with gonorrhea acquire gonococcal arthritis. These rates probably are considerably higher than the estimated 1 to 3 percent incidence in adults and suggest an increased risk of dissemination in infants and children. For example, case reports have described gonococcal arthritis in both mother and newborn infant.[143] Prompt drainage of septic hips, along with initiation of antimicrobial therapy, is necessary because of the risk of development of aseptic necrosis of the femoral head. Long-term dysfunction from gonococcal infection of other joints seldom occurs.[89,149,163,193]

Although gonococcal sepsis can develop in neonates with or without associated septic arthritis, the bacteremic phase of spread to the joints from the initial sites of infection generally is clinically silent. Premature infants seem to be more at risk for the development of sepsis with bacteremia than term infants are. Meningitis has been documented but appears to be an exceedingly rare manifestation of neonatal gonococcal infection.[32,149,153] In the newborn period, the gastric aspirate may be cultured to determine colonization from a maternal source.

GONOCOCCAL DISEASE BEYOND THE NEONATAL PERIOD

LOWER GENITAL TRACT INFECTION IN PREPUBERTAL GIRLS

Gonococcal vaginitis or vulvovaginitis is the most common form of gonorrhea in prepubertal girls beyond the neonatal period. In

TABLE 100–3   Incidence of Neonatal Gonococcal Disease in Exposed Infants

Site of Neonatal Infection	Rate of Positive Cultures (%)	Population	Reference
Conjunctiva	0-10	Exposed infants who underwent AgNO₃ ocular prophylaxis	Edwards et al.,[116] Allen and Barrere,[4] Armstrong et al.,[11] Laga et al.[197]
	2-48	Exposed infants who had no ocular prophylaxis	Rothenberg,[281] Fransen et al.,[127] Laga et al.[197]
Orogastric fluid	26-40	Infants of infected mothers	Handsfield et al.,[153] Edwards et al.[116]
Oropharynx	35	Infants with gonococcal ophthalmia	Laga et al.[197]
Disseminated disease as a proportion of all neonatal gonorrhea	0-1 (rare)	Reported series of neonatal gonococcal disease	Folland et al.,[125] Tomeh and Wilfert,[323] Wald et al.,[330] Edwards et al.,[116] Fransen et al.[127]

contrast to that of postpubertal females, the anestrogenic vaginal mucosa of prepubertal girls creates an alkaline environment that is colonized and infected more readily with *N. gonorrhoeae*. Infection of the endocervix, urethra, paraurethral and Bartholin glands, and upper genital tract occurs only rarely.

Gonococcal vaginitis in prepubertal girls almost always is symptomatic, with vulvar erythema and a profuse vaginal discharge. The girl may complain of dysuria, urinary frequency, vulvar discomfort, or pain while walking.[235,297,300] Asymptomatic cases may occur but are uncommon.

Symptoms and signs should resolve promptly within a few days after treatment is initiated, but acute manifestations may persist for several weeks if the child is not treated. The natural course of disease is for the inflammation to subside and the discharge to become scant and seropurulent. Infection may resolve spontaneously but occasionally may persist until the girl reaches puberty.

Prepubertal vulvovaginitis can be caused by numerous irritative and infectious agents, including pinworms, foreign bodies, group A streptococci, *Neisseria meningitidis*, *Neisseria sicca*, and *Moraxella catarrhalis* (see also Chapter 48). Vulvovaginitis can mimic urinary tract infection, and pyuria can be seen on urinalysis with gonococcal and other causes of vulvovaginitis.[128,207]

Although ascending infection seldom occurs, it may result in salpingitis or peritonitis. One study found that 10 percent of girls with gonorrhea had signs compatible with peritonitis, including fever, diffuse abdominal pain, leukocytosis, and decreased bowel sounds.[46] Salpingitis and periappendicitis may cause findings similar to those of appendicitis. Therefore, perineal examination for vaginal irritation or discharge should be done before performing abdominal surgery in young girls.[12]

In children with gonorrheal infection of the genitourinary tract, concomitant anorectal and tonsillopharyngeal colonization is a common findng[240] because sexual abuse usually is the means of infection.

LOWER GENITAL TRACT INFECTION IN POSTMENARCHEAL FEMALES

Gonococcal infections in adolescent girls are similar to those in adults. The endocervix is the primary site of urogenital infection, although the external genitalia, urethra, vulvar mucosa, and vestibular glands also may be infected. Symptoms of acute infection usually begin 3 to 5 days after exposure with the development of a profuse, purulent vaginal discharge. The vulvar tissues are inflamed, with resultant pruritus and a burning sensation. Urethritis often is present initially and can lead to dysuria with urinary frequency and urgency. Urethral discharge can be seen but is much less prominent than in males. A purulent discharge from the vestibular and paraurethral glands also may be noted.

The endocervical mucosa is edematous, inflamed, and often friable. A profuse yellow-green discharge is present and detaches easily from the surface. The zone of endocervical ectopy that normally is present in as many as 50 percent of adolescents may appear bright red, does not bleed easily when touched with swabs, and should not be mistaken for cervicitis. Ectopy that appears swollen and friable suggests cervicitis. Nabothian inclusion cysts (transparent and grayish) also are normal findings.

Infection of the Bartholin (major vestibular) gland or paraurethral (Skene) gland ducts may develop during acute gonorrhea. Bartholin gland abscesses appear as large, circumscribed painful swellings of the dorsal aspect of the labium minus (see Fig. 48–12). They occur in 5 percent of females with endocervical gonorrhea.[269] Paraurethral duct abscesses (see Fig. 48–11) appear as small painful swellings in the urethrovaginal septum and may cause dysuria. Rupture into the urethra can create a urethral diverticulum. Bartholin gland or paraurethral duct abscesses

should be incised and drained, but small asymptomatic nodules do not require drainage.

If the gonococcal infection goes untreated, the acute symptoms generally subside in 8 to 10 weeks. Persisting acute symptoms are more likely to represent reinfection than chronic infection. Chronic urethritis, thickening of the vestibular glands and paraurethral ducts, and chronic cervicitis can occur. A secondary nonspecific vaginitis can develop as a result of irritation of the mucosa from persisting profuse endocervical discharge.

Mucopurulent cervicitis can be caused by *N. gonorrhoeae*, *C. trachomatis*, *Gardnerella vaginalis*, *Mycoplasma hominis*, *Ureaplasma urealyticum*, and group B streptococci. The overlap in clinical manifestations of infections caused by these microbes and the frequency of infection by two or more simultaneously preclude establishing the diagnosis by clinical findings alone.

Adolescents may be unaware of their infection, especially if they have a preexisting profuse discharge as a result of nonspecific vaginitis or trichomoniasis. Early recognition and treatment of lower genital tract gonococcal infection may prevent extension to and complications of upper genital tract infection. Therefore, sexually active adolescent females should be examined for gonococcal infection as part of their routine health care.[158,286]

A review of reported complications in 1232 cases of gonococcal vaginitis in the pre-antibiotic era revealed that 35 percent had urethritis, 19 percent had proctitis, and 6 percent had peritonitis.[21]

Urinalysis may provide clues to gonococcal infection in some cases. In a cross-sectional study of 296 sexually active females 14 to 22 years of age, gonorrhea or trichomoniasis was present in 65 percent who had sterile pyuria.[168]

UPPER GENITAL TRACT INFECTION IN POSTMENARCHEAL FEMALES

PID will develop in 10 to 17 percent of females with endocervical gonococcal infection. Conditions encompassed by the term PID include endometritis, parametritis, salpingitis, oophoritis, tubo-ovarian abscess, and pelvic peritonitis. PID can be caused by a variety of bacteria. Anaerobes, including *Bacteroides*, *Peptococcus*, and *Peptostreptococcus* spp., are the organisms usually recovered. *N. gonorrhoeae* is present in 25 to 50 percent of cases, similar to the proportion of cases from which *C. trachomatis* is recovered. Coliform organisms, *G. vaginalis*, *M. hominis*, *U. urealyticum*, and various streptococcal species also may be involved. PID develops when these organisms are able to ascend into the uterus, fallopian tubes, and beyond from the lower genital tract. Multiple species may be involved in a single episode. Gonococcal PID often occurs during or just after menses.[130,161] Identification of the specific microbial cause or causes of PID is complicated by the difficulty of obtaining fallopian tube specimens before initiating therapy.

Common findings in PID include an acute onset of lower abdominal pain with tenderness, fever, tenderness on lateral motion of the cervix, adnexal tenderness that generally is bilateral, and adnexal fullness. Vaginal discharge, urinary symptoms, and irregular vaginal bleeding also may be present. In moderate to severe cases, abdominal pain frequently is bilateral, exacerbated with movement, and continuous. Nausea, vomiting, marked abdominal tenderness, an abdomen that appears tense, and fever exceeding 39° C may be present. Such patients often appear to be ill and may have tachycardia consistent with the height of fever.[294] Leukocytosis and elevated erythrocyte sedimentation rates are common findings. Alternatively, PID may be clinically silent or cause only mild pain without discernible tenderness, vaginal discharge, or leukocytosis. Such mild cases can go unrecognized by patients and physicians.

Establishing the diagnosis of PID may be difficult, and the differential diagnosis includes numerous other lower abdominal conditions such as appendicitis, ectopic pregnancy, cholecystitis, mesenteric adenitis, pyelonephritis, and septic abortion. Sonography and pregnancy testing may be helpful in diagnostic decision making. No single symptom, sign, or laboratory finding is sensitive and specific for the diagnosis of PID. Combinations of findings can improve the sensitivity but do so at the expense of reduced specificity, and vice versa.

Initiation of empiric therapy for PID should be considered if the minimal criteria of lower abdominal tenderness, adnexal tenderness, and cervical motion tenderness all are present and no other cause for these findings is readily apparent. More elaborate evaluation may be needed in some cases because incorrect diagnosis and management might lead to unnecessary morbidity. Additional criteria that support the diagnosis of PID include an oral temperature higher than 38.3° C (101° F), an abnormal cervical or vaginal discharge, elevated erythrocyte sedimentation rate, increased C-reactive protein level, and laboratory documentation of cervical infection with *N. gonorrhoeae* or *C. trachomatis*. Some cases may require pursuit of definitive criteria for diagnosing PID, which include histopathologic evidence of endometritis on endometrial biopsy, transvaginal or abdominal ultrasonography or other imaging studies that show thickened fluid-filled fallopian tubes with or without free pelvic fluid or a tubo-ovarian abscess, and laparoscopic abnormalities consistent with PID.[59,176]

The outcome for fertility probably is improved with prompt and vigorous therapy. In the past, physicians have recommended that all adolescents suspected of having PID be hospitalized for therapy. More recently, inpatient observation and treatment have been recommended when a surgical emergency (e.g., ectopic pregnancy or appendicitis) cannot be excluded; when compliance with or tolerance of an outpatient treatment regimen and follow-up within 72 hours cannot be ensured; when the illness appears to be severe (e.g., pelvic or tubo-ovarian abscess, overt peritonitis); or when the patient is immunocompromised, is pregnant, or has failed to respond to outpatient therapy.[5] All courses of therapy should include treatment that is appropriate for *C. trachomatis* and other causes of PID, in addition to *N. gonorrhoeae*.

Complications of PID include tubo-ovarian abscess, perihepatitis (Fitz-Hugh-Curtis syndrome), future ectopic pregnancy, and infertility. Perihepatitis is characterized by right upper quadrant abdominal pain that may radiate to the shoulder. Nausea, fever, and other symptoms and signs of PID may be present as well. Leukocytosis occurs commonly, and liver enzymes are elevated in some cases. The differential diagnosis of perihepatitis includes pleuritis, cholelithiasis, subphrenic abscess, and perforated ulcers.[206]

An estimated 15 percent of women may become sterile after a single episode of PID and 50 percent after three infections. Because of scarring and fibrosis in the fallopian tube, patency is compromised and fertility is jeopardized.[53,120,121] PID in adolescents is particularly likely to result in infertility and ectopic pregnancy, and PID is the single most common cause of infertility in young women.[43,231] Between 1970 and 1980, the rate of ectopic pregnancies per 1000 live births increased from 4.8 to 14.5, and between 1975 and 1981, the rate of hospitalization of females 15 to 19 years of age for salpingitis was 4 per 100,000.[330] These increases correlated with rising rates of gonococcal infection in the affected populations. Data from several studies of gonococcal disease in adolescents are presented in Table 100–4.

Risk factors for the development of PID include young age at the time of acquisition of gonococcal disease or other STDs, a history of previous PID, multiple sexual partners, and the use of an intrauterine device (IUD) for contraception. The immature cervix may be at particular risk for progression to upper tract disease.[302] Disseminated gonococcal infection may accompany asymptomatic infection of an IUD,[84] and the rate of acute PID in those who use IUDs may be increased.

GENITAL TRACT INFECTION IN MALES

Gonococcal urethritis in prepubertal boys is a less frequent event than is vaginitis in girls because of gender differences in rates of sexual abuse. In children with gonorrheal infection of the genitourinary tract, concomitant anorectal and tonsillopharyngeal colonization is a frequent finding.[240]

Urethritis is the primary manifestation of gonococcal infection in males of all ages beyond the neonatal period. Even in young boys, the disease usually is symptomatic and resembles gonococcal urethritis in men.[95,132] Dysuria, purulent discharge, or both develop 2 to 7 days after exposure. Patients generally are afebrile. Purulence typically is greater than with nongonococcal urethritis, but symptoms often are mild enough that patients (or their parents) may delay seeking medical care for weeks. Associated inguinal adenopathy occurs rarely.

At least 5 percent of cases of gonococcal urethritis in males are asymptomatic, and asymptomatic infection can occur at all ages. Asymptomatic pyuria is a manifestation with which the pediatrician should be familiar.[100] It may be the only finding in some cases and should raise suspicion of gonococcal or chlamydial infection in boys who may have been sexually abused or in sexually active adolescent males.

Males with asymptomatic infection are a major reservoir for transmission to their sexual partners.[100,125] Untreated male urethral infection may persist for as long as 6 months.

Complications of gonococcal infection in males now occur much less frequently than in the pre-antibiotic era. Epididymitis is the most common complication. Unilateral swelling, pain, and erythema in the posterior aspect of the scrotum are the usual features. Fever may occur. If untreated, the infection may progress to involve the ipsilateral testis. Hydrocele may result from secretion of fluid into the potential space of the tunica vaginalis. Epididymitis can lead to testicular infarction, abscess, infertility, prostatitis, paraurethral abscesses, and penile lymphangitis, but these local complications are rare findings. Perihepatitis in males has been described but occurs extremely infrequently.[194]

TABLE 100–4 Prevalence of Gonorrhea and Other Sexually Transmitted Diseases in Clinics for Adolescents

Reference	Location	Total Clinic Population Studied	Gonorrhea (%)	Chlamydia Infection (%)	Other
Shafer et al., 1984[295]	California	366	15	4	*Trichomonas* infection
Golden et al., 1984[136]	New York	186	10	10	Syphilis, *Trichomonas* infection
Demetriou et al., 1984[106]	Oklahoma	839	14	—	
Mulcahy and Lacey, 1987[232]	Leeds	210	14	16	*Trichomonas* infection
Jamison et al., 1995[177]	Colorado	632	7	—	Human papillomavirus infection

DISSEMINATED DISEASE

Dissemination requires invasion of the bloodstream from local infection of the mucous membranes of the genital tract, rectum, pharynx, or conjunctiva. Bacteremia then can lead to infection of other sites. The risk of dissemination in children after mucosal infection appears to be higher than the 1 to 3 percent rate in adults. Dissemination in adults seems to be more common with asymptomatic infections, many of which are caused by AHU⁻ gonococcal strains (see "Pathogenesis" earlier).[189] Deficits in the complement system have been associated with disseminated disease in adults, but the frequency of such deficiencies in children is unknown.

As in neonates, gonococcal arthritis is the most common form of disseminated disease in older children, adolescents, and adults. The ankles, knees, wrists, and hands are involved most frequently. The clinical findings are not distinct from those of other microbial causes of septic arthritis. Polyarticular involvement occurs less frequently than in neonates.[93] Gram stain and synovial fluid cultures often are negative. Therefore, empiric coverage for *N. gonorrhoeae* must be considered when septic arthritis develops in a sexually active adolescent or a child who may have been sexually abused.

Typically, the patient has a single most severely affected joint, and associated myositis and tenosynovitis may be prominent findings. Gonococcal arthritis in older children and adolescents resembles that in adults and may be accompanied by cutaneous lesions (Fig. 100–5).[4] Osteomyelitis rarely occurs but has been reported in all age groups, usually in association with septic arthritis.[9]

Treatment of gonococcal arthritis depends on prompt recognition of the disease. Cultures of all mucous membranes (nasopharyngeal, rectal, vaginal or endocervical, conjunctival), blood culture, and aspiration of the involved joint should be performed. The local signs of gonococcal arthritis may not respond to antibiotic therapy for several days. Serial needle aspiration rather than open drainage usually is sufficient for relief of pain and recovery without sequelae (the hip may be an exception).

Gonococcemia is clinically silent generally but can cause a syndrome of migratory polyarthralgia, fever, and rash that precedes the onset of arthritis by several days to a week. The symptomatic course normally is only mild to moderate in severity.

Blood cultures often are negative by the time that care is sought. Gonococcemia-related symptoms may resolve after several days, even without treatment. Rare cases can resemble meningococcemia with purpura and fulminant sepsis with disseminated intravascular coagulopathy. These cases sometimes can be fatal.[253]

The skin lesions associated with gonococcemia usually are pustules on an erythematous base (Fig. 100–5), but petechiae, papules, and hemorrhagic bullae can develop. The development of skin lesions in conjunction with septic arthritis also has been called the arthritis-dermatitis syndrome. The lesions usually arise on the extremities and are fewer than 20 in number. Low-grade fever is most common, but high fever with shaking chills may occur. Tenosynovitis is present in a fourth of these patients. Leukocytosis, pyuria, and elevated liver enzyme test results may be seen. The resultant septic joints generally become clinically apparent during the second week after the onset of disseminated infection.

ANORECTAL GONORRHEA

Gonococcal anorectal infection (proctitis) frequently is asymptomatic but can be associated with pruritus, tenesmus, purulent discharge, or rectal bleeding. Rectal infection can occur as a result of rectal intercourse or inoculation from vaginal secretions. Approximately 40 percent of females with genital gonococcal infection have positive anorectal cultures. Rectal infection is an unusual finding in males who have not engaged in rectal intercourse.[311]

PHARYNGEAL GONORRHEA

Pharyngeal gonococcal infection in all age groups beyond the neonatal period is acquired by orogenital contact. Pharyngeal gonorrhea may be asymptomatic, without evidence of inflammation, or may cause an exudative tonsillopharyngitis that can mimic group A streptococcal or viral infection. Cervical adenopathy also may be present in some cases. In sexually abused children, the pharynx may be the only site of infection. It may be the sole culture-positive site in some cases of disseminated gonococcal infection, and pharyngeal infection possibly is a factor predis-

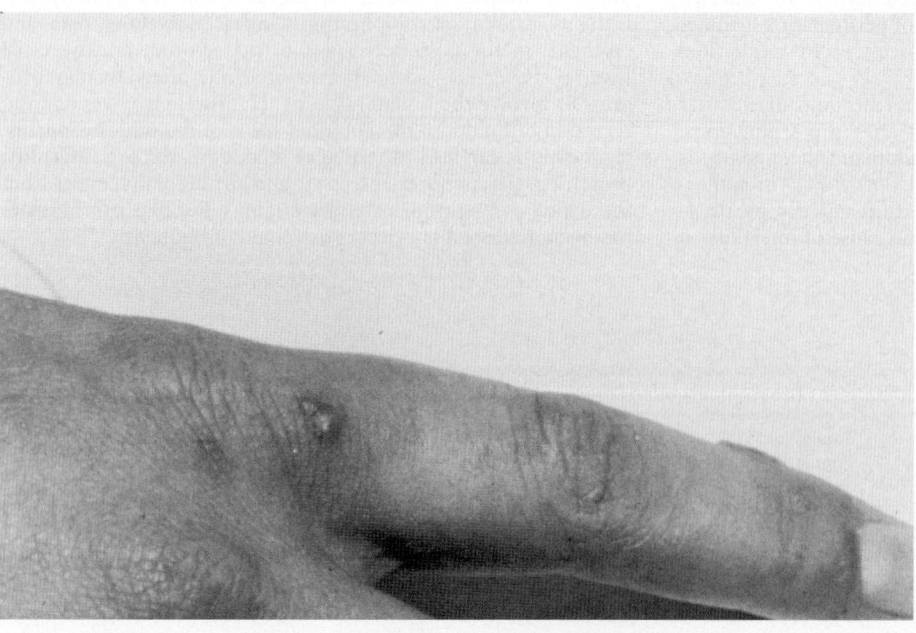

Figure 100–5 Skin lesion typical of the arthritis-dermatitis syndrome of disseminated gonococcal infection: necrotic pustule with an erythematous halo. (*Courtesy of Daniel P. Krowchuk, M.D.*)

posing to dissemination. Pharyngeal infection usually resolves spontaneously within 10 to 12 weeks but should be treated when recognized.

Throat cultures for *N. gonorrhoeae* should be considered in sexually active adolescents with pharyngitis, asymptomatic orogenital contacts of infected persons, patients with disseminated disease in whom other sites of initial infection are not readily apparent, and children who have been sexually abused.

Current treatment regimens for genital gonococcal infection are effective in eradicating gonococcal infection from the pharynx. Routine throat cultures for screening all sexually active adolescents are not cost-effective, but throat culture may be considered for those who give a history of frequently engaging in orogenital sexual activity.*

CONJUNCTIVITIS BEYOND INFANCY

Gonococcal ophthalmia occasionally is seen in children and adults. Direct inoculation of the eye can occur as a result of transmission of fomites from infected persons. Clinical findings typically include a profuse purulent discharge, chemosis, eyelid edema, keratitis, and fever. The initial ocular discharge may be watery before turning purulent. The acute phase may mimic orbital cellulitis. Untreated infection, as with neonates, can lead to corneal opacification, ulceration, and rupture of the globe with resultant visual loss. Some cases may be minimally symptomatic with a minimal inflammatory response and spontaneous resolution.[203,207,261]

OTHER FORMS OF GONOCOCCAL DISEASE

Gonococcal meningitis is a rare condition that may occur with or without associated signs of gonococcemia or septic arthritis. Pyomyositis of the biceps and soft tissue abscesses remote from the genital area have been reported. A gonococcal abscess arising in an area of blunt trauma to a hand has been described in an adolescent with associated endocervical infection.[137] Ventriculo-peritoneal shunt–associated infection, endocarditis, and myocarditis caused by *N. gonorrhoeae* have been reported in adults and can be expected to occur occasionally in children and adolescents.[161] These manifestations of gonococcal infection seldom are seen in children.

DIAGNOSTIC TESTING

Isolation of *N. gonorrhoeae* in culture remains the standard for diagnosing gonococcal infection, but non-culture, DNA-based tests have become widely used in recent years. Uses of these tests are listed in Table 100–5. Only culture should be used for rectal or pharyngeal specimens. Serologic tests based on complement fixation, latex agglutination, enzyme-linked immunosorbent assays, and other techniques have been developed, but the sensitivity of these methods is only about 70 percent, which limits their use primarily to studies of immune response and pathogenesis.[160,164,287]

A diagnosis of *N. gonorrhoeae* infection at any site should prompt evaluation for the presence of other common STDs, if not already done[286] (see also Chapter 48).

CULTURE

In adults, culture of clinical specimens is 80 to 95 percent sensitive when promptly inoculated and incubated. Cultures of adult

male urethral specimens, blood, and other normally sterile body sites tend to have sensitivities in the higher range.[164] Because false-positive cultures (with appropriate laboratory confirmation; see later) are not thought to occur, specificity and positive predictive values are 100 percent. Culture in adolescents and children probably has sensitivity similar to that of adults. Vaginal specimens are adequate for diagnosis in prepubertal girls, for whom obtaining endocervical specimens is unnecessary.

The use of selective media such as modified Thayer-Martin (which contains nystatin, vancomycin, and trimethoprim, and colistin) is required for culture of endocervical, rectal, and pharyngeal specimens to suppress contaminating flora. Selective or nonselective media (chocolate agar) can be used with equal sensitivity for male urethral cultures. Plating of specimens on both types of media may improve the sensitivity, but the incremental yield is small and probably not cost-effective for routine practice.[30,98,270]

Gonococcal colonies become evident on agar plates within 24 to 48 hours after inoculation. Isolates are considered presumptively positive if Gram stain shows gram-negative diplococci and colonies are oxidase-positive. Further testing that demonstrates the gonococcal phenotypic pattern of acid production from selected carbohydrates or a positive result by a nucleic acid method (or both; see later) is required for confirmation as *N. gonorrhoeae* (Table 100–5).[63]

Gonococci do not tolerate drying, so clinical specimens must be plated onto appropriate media as soon as possible. Transport bottles containing medium and a CO_2-enriched atmosphere should be used if definitive specimen processing will be delayed. Transport bottles should be maintained upright during inoculation to preserve the CO_2 atmosphere.

In sexually active females with endocervical gonococcal infection, the urethra, Bartholin gland ducts, and Skene gland ducts usually are infected also. Cultures of these sites may improve the overall yield/sensitivity, in part by avoiding the sampling errors that can occur with any single culture. However, the incremental yield is small enough to render obtaining such cultures unnecessary in routine clinical settings. Culture of the rectum and pharynx in females can be considered optional except when evaluating for sexual abuse.[30,182]

In sexually active males, sites to be cultured depend on the sexual practices and the anatomic sites exposed. Among MSM, rectal infection occurs almost as frequently as urethritis, and pharyngeal infection is not an uncommon finding.[36,164,217,227]

GRAM-STAINED SMEARS

In symptomatic males, a Gram stain of a urethral specimen that demonstrates polymorphonuclear leukocytes with intracellular gram-negative diplococci can be considered diagnostic of infection with *N. gonorrhoeae*. Gram stain in this population has greater than 99 percent specificity and greater than 95 percent sensitivity.[64] Negative Gram stain results are not sufficient to exclude the diagnosis of gonorrhea. Although nonpathogenic *Neisseria* spp. and *N. meningitidis* are morphologically indistinguishable from gonococci, the former rarely are cell-associated.

Gram stains of endocervical, pharyngeal, and rectal specimens are not recommended because of lower sensitivity in detection of infection at these sites. The specificity of a negative Gram stain appears to be at least 95 percent for specimens from the endocervix and rectum.[164,282]

Gram stains of eye exudates, joint fluid, and pustular fluid should be performed because the presence of gram-negative diplococci may help guide initial therapeutic interventions pending culture results.

---

*See references 1, 41, 73, 94, 104, 147, 165, 240, 250, 301, 335, 339.

TABLE 100–5 Laboratory Testing of Specimens for the Presence of *Neisseria gonorrhoeae*

Clinical Indication for Testing	Testing Method and Specimen Type
Suspected female genitourinary tract infection	1. Culture performed on an endocervical swab specimen (adolescents or adults) or vaginal swab specimen from prepubescent females* *If transport and storage conditions are not conducive to maintaining the viability of* N. gonorrhoeae, *a nucleic acid amplification test (NAAT) or nucleic acid hybridization test (NAHT) can be performed on an endocervical swab specimen*† (NAAT or NAHT generally is not acceptable for prepubescent children undergoing evaluation for sexual abuse) 2. NAAT performed on urine (generally not acceptable for prepubescent children undergoing evaluation for sexual abuse)
Suspected male urethral infection	1. Culture performed on an intraurethral swab specimen if collecting such a specimen is acceptable and transport and storage conditions are suitable for culture†,‡ 2. Gram stain of urethral discharge (positive if intracellular gram-negative diplococci are seen) 3. NAAT or NAHT performed on an intraurethral swab specimen if collecting such a specimen is acceptable 4. NAAT performed on urine
Suspected male or female rectal or pharyngeal infection	1. Culture performed on rectal or pharyngeal swab specimens* 2. No other tests recommended
Suspected gonococcal ophthalmia (neonatal or childhood) or disseminated infection	1. Culture performed on conjunctival exudate specimens, blood, synovial fluid, cerebrospinal fluid, or pustular skin lesions with the use of nonselective media (e.g. chocolate agar) 2. Gram stain on exudates or fluid samples (synovial, cerebrospinal fluid) can be useful as an initial point-of-care test that can help guide early treatment considerations pending culture results. Should be accompanied by culture

Scenario for Confirmatory Testing	Recommendations and Comments
Presumptively positive culture (identification in the laboratory of typical gram-negative, oxidase-positive diplococci consistent with *N. gonorrhoeae*)	1. Preferred methods for confirmation of *N. gonorrhoeae* are (a) acid production from carbohydrates§ or (b) positive NAHT results (use of molecular method to confirm culture results) 2. Requiring both methods to be positive ensures high specificity 3. If an isolate cannot be conclusively identified as *N. gonorrhoeae* at a local laboratory, it should be sent to a reference laboratory for confirmation (especially in cases of alleged sexual abuse, sexual assault, or rape)
Positive non-culture test (e.g., NAAT, NAHT)	1. Culture with confirmation as above is the preferred additional test after a positive non-culture test if specimen transport and storage conditions are suitable. Confirmatory testing is not routinely required unless medicolegal issues exist or there is need for antibiotic susceptibility testing 2. Competitive probe format after a positive NAHT (probe) test, but this approach theoretically is less likely to detect a false-positive result 3. A different NAAT as an additional test after NAAT or NAHT has received limited evaluation; certain NAATs sometimes cross-react with nongonococcal *Neisseria* species 4. Antibody tests that detect gonococcal antigens are not recommended for detection of *N. gonorrhoeae*

A selective medium (e.g., modified Thayer-Martin) should be used for culture of specimens from these sites.
†*Transport cultures with an enriched CO_2 atmosphere can be used in some situations.*
‡*Selective or nonselective media may be used.*
§*N. gonorrhoeae produces acid reactions with glucose but not maltose, lactose, sucrose, or fructose. The species also does not reduce nitrates or hydrolyze tributyrin.*
Compiled from Centers for Disease Control and Prevention: Screening tests to detect Chlamydia trachomatis and Neisseria gonorrhoeae infections—2002. M. M. W. R. Recomm. Rep. 51(RR-15):1-38, 2002.

NON-CULTURE DIAGNOSTICS

Non-culture diagnostic tests have become widely used in the United States for establishing a rapid diagnosis of gonococcal (and chlamydial) infection. Many offer the advantage of using urine samples rather than the more invasive swabs and also allow *C. trachomatis* to be evaluated with the same specimen. Numerous gonococcal antigen-detection tests have been developed, but they have been supplanted largely by nucleic acid detection methods.

Nonamplified DNA-DNA hybridization probe tests have been the non-culture tests used most commonly in the United States in recent years. These tests are based on a single-stranded DNA probe complementary to gonococcal rRNA. Sensitivities are about 95 percent (less than culture), with a specificity of 99 percent.[152,164,204,252] Nucleic acid amplification tests (NAATs) use standard PCR-based assay and actually are more sensitive than is culture (Table 100–5). False-positive reactions can occur as a result of the carry-over contamination that occurs during processing or because of occasional cross-reactions with commensal

Neisseria spp. that may be present in some clinical specimens. Specificities are generally greater than 98 percent. False-negative results can occur as a result of target sequence differences (or absence) in some gonococcal clones. NAATs can be used to evaluate first-void urine specimens, which permits screening for gonococcal infection in males and females when genital examination is impractical.[79,256,306,325,327,336]

NAATs and DNA probe tests can detect the presence of nonviable gonococcal microbes, thereby possibly reducing need for the stringent transport conditions often required for culture. Currently available NAATs are multiplex tests that also can detect *C. trachomatis*. NAATs generally are approved by the U. S. Food and Drug Administration for use with endocervical, vaginal, and urethral swab specimens and with urine specimens. They are not approved for rectal or pharyngeal specimens—culture remains the best testing method for detecting gonococcal infection at these sites.[64] Some NAATs can be used for conjunctival specimens.[5]

NAATs and DNA probe tests are adequate for rapid screening in clinical settings, and their results are adequate for making treatment decisions and public health case identifications. Culture remains the definitive test for medicolegal purposes (see the next section). In addition, because of ever-increasing resistance to the available antimicrobial agents, monitoring of gonococcal susceptibility by culture is necessary at the local level, at the very least in patients who do not respond to apparently adequate therapy.[63,336]

MEDICOLEGAL ISSUES RELATED TO DIAGNOSTIC TESTS

N. meningitidis and other members of the Neisseriaceae family are morphologically and often biochemically similar to *N. gonorrhoeae* and may be isolated from sites such as the vagina, blood, and nasopharynx.[108,113,337] Accurate identification of *Neisseria* organisms from any pediatric specimen is essential because misidentification of nongonococcal species as *N. gonorrhoeae* may lead to very serious social consequences for children and their families by precipitating concern regarding sexual abuse. Non-culture methods consistently identify more clinical specimens as positive than standard cultures do.[327] Determining whether such results indicate greater sensitivity, increased false positivity, or a combination of both has been difficult.

Because of this potential for obtaining false-positive results with non-culture NAAT or DNA probe tests, culture remains the medicolegal standard for children who require evaluation for suspected sexual victimization, including prepubertal girls with obvious vaginal discharge. Sequential testing using non-culture tests followed by culture if the former is positive has been proposed as a more sensitive approach than is culture alone.[251] Further study of this approach is required before it can be recommended for adoption.

The CDC also has defined three levels of diagnosis based on clinical and laboratory findings. They are more stringent than are the case definitions used for public health surveillance. A *suggestive diagnosis* is defined by presence of mucopurulent endocervical or urethral exudate and sexual exposure to a person with gonococcal infection. A *presumptive diagnosis* requires two of three criteria: (1) typical gram-negative *intracellular* diplococci on a Gram stain of urethral exudate from males or endocervical secretions; (2) growth of apparent *N. gonorrhoeae* from such specimens on culture medium, defined as typical colonial morphology, positive oxidase reaction, and typical gram-negative morphology; and (3) detection of *N. gonorrhoeae* by a non-culture laboratory test. A *definitive diagnosis* requires (1) isolation of *N. gonorrhoeae* from clinical specimens by culture, as in the second criterion for a presumptive diagnosis, and (2) confirmation of identity by biochemical, enzymatic, serologic, or nucleic acid testing (Table 100–5).[71]

PROPER COLLECTION OF CLINICAL SPECIMENS

Urethral exudate from males may be obtained by passing small swabs or bacteriologic loops 2 to 4 cm into the urethra.[155] Endocervical specimens from postpubertal females are obtained by speculum examination with swabs inserted 1 to 2 cm into the external os after the cervix has been cleansed of external exudate and vaginal secretions.[278] The swab should be rotated one full revolution and withdrawn. Self-obtained vaginal swabs also provide adequate specimens for non-culture methods.[305] This technique has been studied in adolescents. Vaginal specimens collected with tampons also can be used with non-culture methods.[321]

In prepubertal girls, cultures can be obtained from the vaginal introitus by gently swabbing the hymenal opening. Deeper insertion is not necessary. Swabs of exudates emanating from the urethral meatus or vaginal orifice also are sufficient for culture.

In persons with symptomatic anorectal infection, rectal specimens should be obtained by anoscopic means, which increases the sensitivity. In asymptomatic persons, rectal specimens can be procured by blindly inserting a swab 2 to 3 cm into the anal canal and applying lateral pressure to avoid entering any fecal mass. Swabs that are grossly contaminated with fecal matter should be discarded.[101,340]

When urine specimens can be used for non-culture methods, the first 15 to 30 mL of voided urine should be collected.[212,236] Collection of urine should be delayed at least 1 hour after the most recent void to maximize sensitivity. The posterior pharynx, tonsillar areas, and faucial pillars should be swabbed to obtain adequate specimens for the diagnosis of pharyngeal infection.[164]

ANTIMICROBIAL RESISTANCE AMONG GONOCOCCI

Gonococcal strains have been able to acquire resistance to antibiotics since the first agents were introduced. Sulfanilamide became available in 1936 and represented a major improvement over previous therapies that included local genital irrigation with solutions of silver nitrate or potassium permanganate.[255] Widespread resistance to sulfanilamide occurred by 1944. As successive agents have become available, multidrug-resistant strains are being seen with increasing frequency in many parts of the world. Ongoing analysis of gonococcal isolates for antibiotic susceptibility to the available antimicrobial agents remains essential for maintaining effective empiric therapeutic regimens.

In the 1940s, virtually all gonococcal isolates were highly susceptible to penicillin. Despite a gradual increase in the mean minimal inhibitory concentration (MIC) to penicillin from the mid-1950s through the mid-1970s, almost all strains had penicillin MICs of less than 0.5 μg/mL. This low-level resistance is mediated by alterations at a genetic locus called *penA* that result in modification of its product, penicillin-binding protein 2 (PBP-2). Two other loci designated *mtr*, which encodes an efflux pump that reduces concentrations of multiple antibiotics, and *penB*, which is an allele of *por*, the gene of the porin protein, also mediate low-level resistance to penicillins. *penB* encodes a porin with a mutation that decreases permeability to hydrophilic antibiotics.[134]

In 1976, strains of *N. gonorrhoeae* were discovered that had acquired plasmid-conferring resistance to penicillin through the production of penicillinase (a TEM-1 β-lactamase). These strains were found in many parts of the Far East and London, and in the former they constituted approximately 30 percent of the isolates in some cities. The strains caused the expected spectrum of clinical disease, and treatment with penicillin was not effective. Penicillinase-producing gonococci contain one of two closely related 5.3- or 7.2-kb plasmids (Pc^r) that carry a Tn2 transposon system. This plasmid appears to have been acquired from *Haemophilus ducreyi*.[8,49,77,258] In 1983, an outbreak of chromosomally mediated, penicillin-resistant (MICs of 2 to 4 μg/mL), non–penicillinase-producing gonococci was reported from North Carolina.[124] Such strains have been seen subsequently in other areas of the country.

Resistance to tetracycline antibiotics emerged in the 1980s and subsequently increased. Three chromosomal loci designated *mtr*, *penB*, and *tet* mediate low-level resistance. High-level resistance to tetracycline is conferred by *tetM*, which resides on a 38-kb plasmid (Tc^r) that is a derivative of the 36-kb conjugal plasmid. *tetM* produces a cytoplasmic protein that protects ribosomes from tetracycline. Tc^r gonococci can transfer this plasmid, as well as Pc^r, efficiently to other gonococcal strains.[228,308]

Spectinomycin resistance was described first in 1987 in U.S. military personnel in Korea. This agent had been introduced as the drug of choice there in 1981 because of high rates of penicillin resistance. Treatment failures actually began to occur in 1983. Resistance is chromosomally mediated and results in alteration of the ribosomal target site of the drug.[31,49] The widespread use of spectinomycin was associated with a decline in the rate of penicillin resistance.[31] Many gonococcal strains in some parts of the world also are resistant to streptomycin.[244]

Ciprofloxacin and other fluoroquinolone antibiotics became widely available for the treatment of gonococcal infection in the 1980s. Low-level resistance to fluoroquinolones is associated with mutations in the DNA gyrase gene *gyrA*, and high-level resistance has been linked to mutations in the topoisomerase gene *parC*.[174] Resistance to these agents has been noted since the early 1990s in areas of Southeast Asia.[126] In Hawaii in 1999, 9.5 percent of isolates were resistant to ciprofloxacin, but resistance elsewhere in the United States remained low at 0.2 percent.[61,62]

By the year 2000, fluoroquinolones no longer were recommended for initial treatment of gonococcal infection in Asia, the Pacific Islands, or Hawaii. In 2002 this recommendation was extended to the state of California and in 2004 to MSM throughout the United States. During the first 6 months of 2006, 13.3 percent of 3005 isolates collected through the CDC's Gonococcal Isolate Surveillance Project (GISP) were resistant to ciprofloxacin (and thus all other quinolone antibiotics). Among gonococcal isolates from MSM and heterosexual males from U.S. states other than California and Hawaii, ciprofloxacin-resistant rates were 30.7 and 5.1 percent, respectively. Therefore, as of April 2007, the CDC no longer recommends the use of fluoroquinolones for the treatment of gonococcal infections in the United States.[67]

In 1986, the CDC initiated the GISP to monitor the antimicrobial sensitivities of *N. gonorrhoeae* in STD clinics in 21 cities in the United States.[56] This system has been expanded to 27 sites.[62,68] In 1989, 13 percent of the *N. gonorrhoeae* isolates evaluated were resistant to penicillin, tetracycline, or both.[57] In 1999, such strains accounted for 28 percent of all isolates.[62] Rates of resistance to these two agents have fallen slightly in the United States since that time, with 9 percent being resistant to penicillin and 17 percent resistant to tetracycline in 2005.[68]

Strains resistant to azithromycin and erythromycin have been identified in the United States.[61] The distribution of azithromycin MICs has shifted upward in the last decade, although the proportion of strains that probably were resistant in 2005 was less than 3 percent.[68] Rifampin resistance is also high in some areas of the world.[244]

TREATMENT

Because of ever-changing gonococcal susceptibility patterns and variations in susceptibility in different international regions, practitioners must remain alert for modifications of treatment guidelines for their respective geographic locations. Indeed, based on the current patterns of antimicrobial resistance in prevalent *N. gonorrhoeae* strains in the United States, extended-spectrum, third-generation cephalosporins are the only remaining antibiotics routinely recommended as initial therapy in children and adults as of April 2007.

The recommendations for treatment of childhood gonorrhea in the United States discussed in this section and listed in Tables 100–6 and 100–7 are based on 2006 guidelines from the CDC[64,67,69] and the 2006 Report of the Committee on Infectious Diseases of the American Academy of Pediatrics.[5] The CDC guidelines are based on the stringent clinical efficacy criterion of an expected

TABLE 100–6 Treatment of Gonococcal Infections in the Neonatal Period

Disease Category	Treatment Regimen	Comments
Infants born to mothers with gonococcal infection	Ceftriaxone, 25 to 50 mg/kg IV or IM, not to exceed 125 mg (single dose) *or* Cefotaxime, 100 mg/kg IV or IM (single dose)	Ceftriaxone should be given cautiously to hyperbilirubinemic infants, especially premature ones
Gonococcal ophthalmia neonatorum (GON) or other focal sites of infection (i.e., rectum, pharynx, vagina, urethra)	Ceftriaxone, 25 to 50 mg/kg IV or IM, not to exceed 125 mg (single dose) *or* Cefotaxime, 100 mg/kg IV or IM (single dose)	Infants with GON should receive eye irrigation with saline solution immediately upon recognition and at frequent intervals subsequently until the discharge is eliminated. Topical agents alone are inadequate and unnecessary when recommended systemic antibiotics are given. Some experts prefer to continue parenteral therapy with one of these agents until blood (with or without cerebrospinal fluid) cultures have been negative for 48 to 72 hours
Disseminated gonococcal infection (septic arthritis, sepsis, meningitis) or scalp abscess	Ceftriaxone, 25 to 50 mg/kg IV or IM once daily for 7 days (10-14 days for meningitis) *or* Cefotaxime, dosed according to neonatal algorithms, IV or IM for 7 days (10-14 days for meningitis)	Cefotaxime is preferred for infants with hyperbilirubinemia who require more than a single dose of therapy. If meningitis is present, higher doses in the recommended ranges may be needed

Data largely compiled from Centers for Disease Control and Prevention: Sexually transmitted diseases treatment guidelines 2006. M. M. W. R. Recomm. Rep. 55(RR-11):1-94, 2006; and American Academy of Pediatrics: Gonococcal infections. In Pickering, L. K. (ed.): 2006 Red Book: Report of the Committee on Infectious Diseases. 27th ed. Elk Grove Village, IL, American Academy of Pediatrics, 2006, pp. 301-309.

TABLE 100–7   Treatment of Gonococcal Infections in Children beyond the Neonatal Period*,†

	Prepubertal Children Who Weigh <100 lb (45 kg)	Patients ≥8 Years Old and Who Weigh >100 lb (45 kg)
Uncomplicated Gonococcal Infections‡		
Vulvovaginitis	Ceftriaxone, 125 mg IM in a single dose	Ceftriaxone, 125 mg IM in a single dose¶
Endocervicitis	*Alternative regimen*	*or*
Urethritis	Spectinomycin,§ 40 mg/kg (maximum, 2 g)	Cefixime,¶ 400 mg orally in a single dose
Proctitis	IM in a single dose	*Alternative regimens*
Pharyngitis	(Cefixime has been used by some experts	Spectinomycin,§ 2 g IM in a single dose
	because it can be administered orally.	*or*
	There are no published data regarding	Single-dose cephalosporin regimens (see Note)
	safety or efficacy for this purpose)	
Conjunctivitis**	Ceftriaxone, 50 mg/kg (maximum, 1 g) IM in a single dose	Ceftriaxone, 1 g IM in a single dose
Disseminated Gonococcal Infection††,‡‡		
Arthritis, sepsis	Ceftriaxone, 50 mg/kg/day (maximum, 1 g/	Ceftriaxone, 1 g IV or IM every 24 hours for 24-48 hours
Arthritis-dermatitis syndrome	day) IV or IM once a day for 7 days§§	after clinical improvement, followed by cefixime,
		400 mg twice daily orally, or cefpodoxime, 400 mg
		twice daily orally to complete at least 7 days of total
		antimicrobial therapy§§
		Alternative regimens
		Cefotaxime, 1 g IV every 8 hours, or ceftizoxime, 1 g IV
		every 8 hours, with switch to oral therapy and duration
		as for ceftriaxone§§
		or
		Spectinomycin, 2 g IM every 12 hours
		or
		Fluoroquinolones if antimicrobial susceptibility can be
		documented by culture¶¶
Meningitis	Ceftriaxone, 50 mg/kg/day (maximum, 2 g/	Ceftriaxone, 1-2 g IV every 12 hr; for meningitis, the
Endocarditis	day) IV or IM given every 12 hr; for	duration is 10-14 days; for endocarditis, the duration is
	meningitis, the duration is 10-14 days;	at least 28 days
	for endocarditis, the duration is at least	
	28 days	
Epididymitis		Ceftriaxone, 250 mg IM in a single dose
Treatment of potential concurrent	Azithromycin, 20 mg/kg (maximum, 1 g) in	Doxycycline,¶¶ 100 mg orally twice a day for 7 days
C. trachomatis infection that has	a single dose	*or*
not been ruled out†	*or*	Azithromycin, 1 g orally in a single dose
	Erythromycin base or ethylsuccinate,	
	50 mg/kg/day (maximum, 2 g/day) in 4	
	divided doses for 14 days	

Note: Other single-dose cephalosporin therapies that are considered alternative treatment regimens for uncomplicated urogenital and anorectal gonococcal infections include ceftizoxime, 500 mg IM, or cefoxitin, 2 g IM, administered with probenecid, 1 g orally, or cefotaxime, 500 mg IM. Some evidence indicates that cefpodoxime, 400 mg, and cefuroxime axetil, 1 g, might be adequate oral alternatives. Ceftriaxone and cefixime are preferred.

*See text for discussion of treatment options for patients with allergies to the recommended regimens.

†In addition to the recommended treatment of gonococcal infection, therapy for Chlamydia trachomatis is recommended because of the common occurrence of co-infections with these microbes.

‡Hospitalization should be considered for children (1) who are unlikely to receive the prescribed treatment because of personal or parent/guardian failure to adhere to the regimen or (2) whose infection has not responded to outpatient therapy.

§Spectinomycin currently is not available in the United States. This agent is not recommended for the treatment of pharyngeal infections. If spectinomycin must be used for pharyngeal infection, follow-up cultures should be performed.

¶Alternative regimens for uncomplicated infections include spectinomycin (2 g IM in a single dose), ceftizoxime, cefotaxime, cefotetan, and cefoxitin. Spectinomycin is not recommended for pharyngitis.

¶Experience in adults suggests that cefixime can be considered for use in children with uncomplicated gonococcal infections, but few data are available to confirm its effectiveness for gonococcal infections in children.

**Eyes should be lavaged with saline initially and at regular intervals until secretions no longer continue to accumulate.

††Hospitalization is required. For older children and adolescents, parenteral therapy can be discontinued 24 to 48 hours after improvement occurs and the 7-day course completed with an appropriate oral antimicrobial agent. Cefotaxime also can be used for disseminated infections in children.

‡‡Persons with disseminated gonococcal infections also should receive one of the age-appropriate regimens for treatment of possible C. trachomatis co-infection listed in this table as part of treatment for persons with uncomplicated gonococcal infections.

§§Some experts advise a 10- to 14-day course of therapy for gonococcal sepsis or septic arthritis.

¶¶Fluoroquinolones are no longer recommended in the United States because of an increasing prevalence of antibiotic-resistant strains. Ciprofloxacin, ofloxacin, and levofloxacin are acceptable for use in adults and adolescents when gonococcal isolates have documented susceptibility. These agents generally are not used in children but may be considered depending on clinical circumstances and susceptibility of the infecting strain. Quinolones are contraindicated for women who are pregnant or nursing.

¶¶Doxycycline is not recommended for routine use in children younger than 8 years.

Data from Centers for Disease Control and Prevention: Sexually transmitted diseases treatment guidelines 2006. M. M. W. R. Recomm. Rep. 55(RR-11):1-94, 2006; Centers for Disease Control and Prevention: Updated recommended treatment regimens for gonococcal infections and associated conditions—United States, April 2007. Available at http://www.cdc.gov/std/treatment/2006/updated-regimens.htm (accessed May 2007); and American Academy of Pediatrics: Gonococcal Infections. In Pickering, L. K. (ed.): 2006 Red Book: Report of the Committee on Infectious Diseases. 27th ed. Elk Grove Village, IL, American Academy of Pediatrics, 2006, pp. 301-309.

95 percent efficacy with a lower bound of the 95 percent confidence interval of 95 percent or greater.[241] Children who are postpubertal or who weigh more than 45.4 kg (100 lb) may be treated with dosage regimens as defined for adults (including fluoroquinolones for infecting strains known to be susceptible to these agents).[64] The recommended regimens generally have not been studied in populations of prepubertal children with either uncomplicated or complicated gonococcal infection, but these regimens are likely to be highly effective in most cases, as they are for older adolescents and adults.

As of April 2007, recommendations for treating uncomplicated urogenital and anorectal gonorrhea in adolescents and adults in the United States are limited to a single 125-mg intramuscular dose of ceftriaxone or a single 400-mg oral dose of cefixime. Up-to-date information on treatment regimens for gonorrhea and other STDs can be obtained from the CDC website *http://www.cdc.gov/std/treatment.*[67,69]

In adults with an uncomplicated gonococcal infection at any site, 99 percent of cases are cured by ceftriaxone. As a general rule, children treated with ceftriaxone do not require follow-up cultures, but if other treatment regimens are used, follow-up cultures may be indicated. Cefixime has an antimicrobial spectrum similar to that of ceftriaxone. Experience in adults, including pregnant women,[267] suggests that oral cefixime may be considered for the treatment of uncomplicated gonococcal infections in children, provided that follow-up is ensured. The 400-mg oral dose in adults does not provide as high or as sustained a bactericidal concentration as that provided by a 125-mg parenteral dose of ceftriaxone, but clinical trials in adults with uncomplicated gonococcal infection have shown cure rates of 97 percent with cefixime.

Other parenteral cephalosporins that are safe and highly effective against uncomplicated gonococcal infection in adults—and probably in children as well—include cefotaxime, ceftizoxime, cefotetan, and cefoxitin. Some evidence indicates that cefpodoxime and cefuroxime axetil might be adequate oral alternatives in adults,[69] but no data have been reported regarding their use for gonococcal infections in children.

The fluoroquinolone antibiotics ciprofloxacin, ofloxacin, and levofloxacin have been used widely for treating gonococcal infection in adults. Cure rates for uncomplicated gonococcal infection with both agents exceed 98 percent in adults with susceptible isolates. These agents no longer are recommended for routine treatment of gonococcal infections in the United States and many other parts of the world because of substantial resistance rates.[67,69] They remain an option for adults and potentially for children in selected circumstances when the infecting gonococcal strain is known to be susceptible to them.

Resistance to spectinomycin remains rare in the United States, and this compound still is an effective alternative in most cases when other agents cannot be used.[5] However, spectinomycin remains unavailable in the United States at this time. Azithromycin may be useful in circumstances in which patients are unable to take standard regimens because of allergies, pregnancy, or concerns of age-related toxicity (e.g., dental staining with tetracyclines) or when no other alternatives are available.

PRESUMPTIVE TREATMENT OF CONCURRENT *CHLAMYDIA TRACHOMATIS* INFECTION

Persons with gonococcal infection, including children, are at high risk for acquiring concurrent chlamydial infection. Co-infections frequently occur and were present in 50 of 5877 students attending an urban U.S. high school in 1998 to 1999 who participated in a school-based screening program.[245] Among adolescents in 14 U.S. juvenile detention centers from 1997 through 2002, more

than 50 percent of the teens with gonorrhea were co-infected with *C. trachomatis*.[183] In adolescents, treatment of gonococcal cervicitis with drug regimens that are effective against gonococci but not *Chlamydia* has been associated with a high incidence of residual salpingitis in females and urethritis in males because of the ongoing presence of *C. trachomatis*.[254,268,271,294]

Therefore, treatment recommendations for gonococcal infections beyond the neonatal period include agents active against both organisms (Table 100–7). Neonates with gonococcal infections also should be evaluated for *C. trachomatis* co-infection. Penicillin, amoxicillin, ceftriaxone, or spectinomycin alone will fail to eradicate *C. trachomatis*. Trimethoprim-sulfamethoxazole, tetracycline, doxycycline, azithromycin, and erythromycin are effective in vitro and in many clinical forms of chlamydial disease.

TREATMENT OF INFANTS BORN TO MOTHERS WITH GONOCOCCAL INFECTION

Infants born to mothers with untreated gonorrhea are at high risk of acquiring infection (e.g., ophthalmia, disseminated gonococcal infection); consequently, even without overt signs of infection, such infants should be treated with a single injection of ceftriaxone (25 to 50 mg/kg intravenously or intramuscularly, not to exceed 125 mg). Ceftriaxone should be given cautiously to hyperbilirubinemic infants, especially premature ones (see Table 100–6). A single dose of cefotaxime (100 mg/kg intravenously or intramuscularly) is an acceptable alternative. Topical prophylaxis for neonatal ophthalmia is not adequate therapy for documented infections of the eye or other sites.

TREATMENT OF NEONATES WITH GONOCOCCAL INFECTION

Neonates with clinical evidence suggestive of gonococcal infection at any site (including the eye) should be evaluated for disseminated disease. The evaluation should include a thorough physical examination, especially of the joints. Exudate from the eyes or other sites of apparent local infection should be sent for Gram stain and culture on appropriate media. Blood and CSF generally should be cultured, and the infant should be admitted to the hospital for parenteral antibiotics and any needed supportive care. Most but not all experts recommend that CSF studies be performed even in afebrile, otherwise well-appearing infants whose only clinical manifestation is apparent GON.

The presence of typical gram-negative diplococci in Gram-stained specimens is sufficient justification to begin treatment of GON or gonococcal infection in other sites. The absence of gram-negative diplococci in Gram-stained specimens is not sufficient to abrogate presumptive treatment of GON in a neonate with conjunctival exudate.

Tests for concomitant *C. trachomatis* infection, HIV infection, and congenital syphilis should be performed in infants with gonococcal infection at any site. The mother and her partners should be evaluated for gonococcal infection (and other STDs) and treated according to the recommendations for gonococcal infection in adolescents and adults (see the next section).

Infants with GON can be treated with a single dose of ceftriaxone (25 to 50 mg/kg intravenously or intramuscularly, not to exceed 125 mg) (Table 100–6). This regimen also may be used for infants with other sites of nondisseminated gonococcal infection, including the rectum, pharynx, vagina, and urethra. A single dose of cefotaxime (100 mg/kg given intravenously or intramuscularly) is an alternative treatment of GON. Some experts prefer to continue parenteral therapy with one of these agents until blood cultures (with or without CSF cultures) have been negative for 48 to 72 hours. Infants with GON also should receive eye irrigation with saline solution immediately on recognition and at frequent intervals until the discharge is eliminated. Topical antimicrobial agents alone are inadequate and unnecessary when the recommended systemic antibiotics are given.[5,128,198]

Simultaneous infection with *C. trachomatis* should be considered a potential explanation for neonates who do not respond satisfactorily to the recommended treatment.

DISSEMINATED GONOCOCCAL INFECTION OR SCALP ABSCESS. The recommended therapy for gonococcal arthritis, scalp abscess, and sepsis is ceftriaxone (25 to 50 mg/kg intravenously or intramuscularly given once a day) for 7 days or cefotaxime for 7 days (50 mg/kg/day given intravenously or intramuscularly in two divided doses will be adequate for many infants; dose and interval adjustments may be needed depending on gestational and chronologic age and other clinical considerations). Cefotaxime is preferred for infants with hyperbilirubinemia. For gonococcal meningitis, treatment should be continued for 10 to 14 days, with consideration of the use of higher daily doses of these agents (see Table 100–6).

TREATMENT OF GONOCOCCAL INFECTIONS BEYOND THE NEONATAL PERIOD

Treatment recommendations based on weight for uncomplicated and complicated gonococcal infection are outlined in Table 100–7. Treatment recommendations for adolescents are the same as those for adults. For treatment recommendations for PID, see Tables 100–7 and 100–8. All treatment regimens include agents active against *C. trachomatis* in addition to *N. gonorrhoeae*. Treatment issues in a number of circumstances are discussed in more detail in the following text.

UNCOMPLICATED PHARYNGEAL GONORRHEA. Gonococcal infection of the pharynx is more difficult to eradicate than is infection of urogenital and anorectal sites. Chlamydial infection of the pharynx is an unusual occurrence, but genital co-infection may be present. A single dose of ceftriaxone (125 mg, intramuscularly) is the preferred treatment of uncomplicated pharyngeal gonococcal infection. A single dose of an oral fluoroquinolone may be used if the isolate is known to be susceptible to these agents. Spectinomycin is unreliable against *N. gonorrhoeae* in the pharynx; it eradicates the organism in only approximately 50 percent of cases. If spectinomycin is required because of allergies or contraindications to the other recommended treatments, pharyngeal culture should be performed 3 to 5 days after completion of therapy to verify eradication of the infection.

SEVERE ALLERGIES TO CEPHALOSPORINS. Selection of alternative antibiotic therapies for persons with a history of a

reaction to a cephalosporin must be guided by the severity of the reaction and the availability of suitable alternative regimens.[63] Azithromycin is probably the best available choice at this time for persons with documented severe allergies to penicillins or cephalosporins.[67,69] If circumstances permit delay in treatment until antibiotic susceptibility test results can be obtained, other agents such as fluoroquinolones or doxycycline may be used if the isolate is shown to be susceptible.

Azithromycin, 2 g orally, is effective against uncomplicated gonococcal infection in adolescents and adults, but it is expensive and frequently associated with gastrointestinal problems. Because of these issues and concern about rapid emergence of resistance, it is not recommended for routine use.[64] A single dose of 20 mg/kg (maximum, 1 g) is recommended for the treatment of chlamydial infection in children, but no dose recommendations for azithromycin are available for the treatment of gonococcal infection in children.[5]

Patients should be observed for at least 30 minutes after the ingestion of a dose of 2 g of azithromycin to monitor tolerance of the medication.[70] An oral dose of 1 g of azithromycin cures approximately 93 percent of uncomplicated gonococcal infections in adults. Though better tolerated, this dose is not sufficiently effective for routine use.

Spectinomycin (40 mg/kg given intramuscularly, with a maximal dose of 2 g) remains effective but no longer is available in the United States. Updated information regarding its potential availability can be obtained from the CDC website *http://www.cdc.gov/std/gonorrhea/org*.

INFECTION WITH HUMAN IMMUNODEFICIENCY VIRUS. Children and adolescents infected with HIV who acquire a gonococcal infection should receive the same treatment as persons without HIV infection.

CONCURRENT SYPHILIS INFECTION. A single dose of ceftriaxone is not adequate for treating syphilis. Longer courses of therapy are required (see Chapter 156). *Treponema pallidum* is not susceptible to fluoroquinolones or spectinomycin.

PREGNANCY. Pregnant women should not be treated with quinolone or tetracycline agents. Those unable to take one of the recommended cephalosporin regimens can be treated with spectinomycin. Azithromycin may be considered if the recommended cephalosporins or spectinomycin cannot be used.

FOLLOW-UP

The recommended regimens have such high cure rates that routine repeat testing for cure no longer is recommended.[59,64,80] Obtaining follow-up cultures may be prudent if alternative thera-

TABLE 100–8 Sexually Transmitted Diseases in Prepubertal Children Evaluated for Suspected Sexual Abuse

Reference	No. of Children Evaluated	Number (%) Who Had a Diagnosis of				
		Gonorrhea	Chlamydiosis	Syphilis	Trichomoniasis	Condylomata Acuminata
Wald et al., 1980[330]	189	28 (14.8%)	ND	ND	ND	ND
Rimsza and Niggemann, 1982[277]	285	21 (7.4%)	ND	0	ND	ND
White et al., 1983[335]	409	46 (10%)	ND	6 (5.5%)	4 (18%)	3 (5.6%)
Ingram et al., 1984[172]	50	10 (20%)	3 (6%)	ND	2 (4%)	ND
DeJong, 1986[104]	532	25 (4.7%)	ND	1 (0.2%)	ND	3 (0.6%)
Ingram et al., 1992[171]	1469	41 (2.8%)	17 (1.2%)	1 (0.1%)	3 (2%)	28 (2%)
Siegal et al., 1995[300]	855*	12 (1.4%)	11 (1.3%)	0	4 (0.5%)	ND
Muram et al., 1996[235]	865	12 (1.4%)	ND	ND	ND	ND

These children also were evaluated for HIV infection, and all were found to be uninfected.
ND, no data.

pies are used or adherence is uncertain. Children who receive treatment regimens other than ceftriaxone or who remain in at-risk environments for reinfection should have follow-up evaluations.[5]

Treatment failures can occur, and cultures should be repeated for antibiotic susceptibility testing when symptoms persist after treatment. This precaution may lead to recognition of an antibiotic-resistant strain that could have public health implications.

Apparent treatment failure usually is the result of reinfection. Reinfection may be associated with a higher risk for PID and other complications of gonococcal infection. Therefore, retesting in 3 months for reinfection (not test of cure) is advisable for sexually active adolescents and adults, regardless of whether patients think that their sex partners have been treated.[64]

GONOCOCCAL INFECTION AND SEXUAL ABUSE OF CHILDREN

When gonococcal infection or any other STD is identified in a prepubertal child or in adolescents who are not sexually active within their peer groups, sexual abuse must be considered to have occurred unless proved otherwise.[5] Nonsexual transmission never should be assumed without extensive investigation of the social setting of an infected child.[5,239] Isolation of *N. gonorrhoeae* in cultures from children should be reported to local public health authorities and also to child protective services to ensure that the child is not exposed to further abuse. Sexual abuse has been reported in approximately 10 percent of all self-reporting populations of girls during childhood in numerous studies, and rates in boys are around 3 percent.[14,284] Approximately 1 percent of children appear to experience serious forms of sexual abuse yearly.[6]

STDs occur in 3 to 20 percent of sexually abused children.[104,171,172,235,277,300,330,335] Gonococcal infections have been found in 5 to 7 percent of sexually abused children.[104] The absence of STDs does not rule out sexual abuse when other findings suggest that it has occurred. Table 100–8 summarizes the STD diagnoses from eight studies involving children who had been evaluated for suspected sexual abuse.

The prevalence and clinical manifestations of gonococcal infection in sexually abused children are determined by the prevalence of infection in the adults who constitute the population with whom the child resides, the age of the child, and the type and frequency of sexual contact.[251] Gonorrhea was the STD recognized most frequently in abused children when gonococcal infection was highly prevalent in the general population. As a result of improved control of gonorrhea in the 1980s, fewer pediatric cases have been recognized in the United States in recent years. Nonetheless, girls who are exposed to an infected male appear to have a high rate of acquired disease. In an outbreak in an orphanage, 53 of 95 abused girls were found to have contracted infection.[2]

Among prepubertal girls who have a vaginal discharge after being sexually abused, 9 to 11 percent have been found to have gonococcal infection. No cases of genital tract gonorrhea without discharge have been reported in prepubertal girls.[171,297,300] The oropharynx also is a common site of gonococcal infection associated with sexual abuse of children and may be the only site of infection in children forced to perform orogenital sexual acts with an infected abuser. Pharyngeal infection may be asymptomatic. Although few children who suffer sexual abuse subsequently contract an STD, the diagnosis of an STD is a very important indication that the child probably has been abused, and an STD may be the sole finding on physical examination.[169]

Children with suspected gonococcal infection (or suspected to have suffered sexual abuse) should undergo a thorough physical examination by someone familiar with the medicolegal and clinical aspects of sexually abused children. Genital, rectal, and pha-

ryngeal cultures should be obtained. Vaginal cultures are satisfactory in prepubertal girls. Endocervical cultures should be obtained only after puberty. Blood culture should be performed if disseminated disease is a consideration. Other sites (conjunctivae, joint fluid) should be cultured if clinically indicated. Cultures should be handled in a manner that will ensure legal acceptance if needed (see later).

Non-culture methods may be used in conjunction with—but not in lieu of—routine cultures to increase sensitivity in detecting gonococcal infection. These test results, when rapidly available, may permit more rapid initiation of therapy than possible with standard culture results.[251]

Selective criteria based on the observations that most sexually abused children do not have gonococcal infection or other STDs and that the vast majority of prepubertal girls with gonococcal infection will have clinical signs of vulvovaginitis have been developed to determine which children undergoing evaluation for sexual abuse should be tested for the presence of gonococcal infection and other STDs.[170,235,297,299,300] These criteria are (1) the known presence of any STD in the child, a sibling, another household member, a close associate of the child, or the apparent perpetrator or (2) a history or physical findings suggesting that oral, genital, or rectal contact has occurred.[170]

It is highly unlikely that a sexually abused child with gonococcal or chlamydial infection will be missed through the use of these criteria. Meanwhile, the number of potentially sexually abused children who must undergo culture is greatly decreased.[170,173] One caveat is that rectal and pharyngeal gonococcal infections in girls and boys and genital infections in boys often are asymptomatic, so these selective criteria may apply only to the issue of vaginal cultures in girls.[57]

All children with gonococcal infections (including neonates) should be evaluated for other STDs, including chlamydial disease, syphilis, hepatitis B, and HIV infection.[5,148,286]

The following are general issues for evaluation and management of children who may have been sexually abused:

1. Many institutions have a clinical service or clinician with training and skill in interviewing and examining children suspected of having experienced sexual abuse. Direct involvement by or consultation with persons with such expertise should be sought at the time of initial evaluation.[249]

2. If the child is symptomatic, all available and appropriate cultures and examinations should be completed before the child receives therapy. Because asymptomatic gonococcal infections occur commonly, strong consideration should be given to obtaining cultures from the rectum and oropharynx, even in the absence of symptoms, especially for children and adolescents who meet the selective criteria described earlier.[29,123,158]

3. A chain-of-custody policy that ensures proper handling, labeling, and delivery of diagnostic samples to the appropriate laboratory is essential for test results to be used in any court procedures when issues of the child's safety are being considered.

4. If sexual abuse is confirmed or suspected by the social history, physical findings, or laboratory results, the child should not be allowed to leave the evaluation site until the child's safety has been ensured. This determination usually is made by the local department of social services and may require involvement of law enforcement agencies. Temporary hospitalization of the child may be needed to permit sufficient time for any additional investigations to be performed. Reporting of suspected and confirmed cases to the social service of the county in which the child resides is required by child abuse reporting laws.

5. Most children who have been victims of sexual abuse will not have specific physical findings. Oral-genital contact is a common form of abuse, as are fondling and external genital contact. These forms of abuse may occur without physical signs of injury.

6. If the child is identified with an STD, other members of the family may be infected as well. Other female children are especially likely to be infected and should be examined.[123,131]

7. Internal pelvic examination of prepubertal children rarely is necessary unless there has been major trauma or there are concerns regarding foreign bodies. Internal examination of prepubertal girls should be performed by an experienced examiner with appropriate sedation or anesthesia.

8. Children often have compelling reasons to deny abuse and frequently do not disclose sexual abuse, even to skillful forensic interviewers.[202] Denial, therefore, is not compelling disproof of sexual abuse.

9. Sexual abuse of children can be a repeated event if the perpetrator has ongoing access to the child. If the child remains unprotected and the perpetrator has an STD, the child may be subject to recurrent episodes of that STD.[201]

10. Counseling with providers skilled in helping children who have been sexually abused should be part of long-term follow-up care. The likelihood of the child having serious emotional harm is greater when abuse has been more intrusive or violent, occurred repetitively over longer periods, or was committed by someone in a close relationship with the child;[85] Parents of victims also may need treatment and support.

11. Behavioral changes such as developmentally unusual sexual behavior or acting out can be a manifestation of child sexual abuse.[129] New onset of symptoms such as abdominal pain (which may lead to medical attention when it becomes persistent), enuresis, encopresis, sleep disturbances, and phobias can be manifestations of child sexual abuse. These issues also can arise from physical or emotional abuse or from non–abuse-related social stressors and do not indicate sexual abuse per se.[85]

PREVENTION AND CONTROL OF GONOCOCCAL INFECTIONS

All gonococcal infections must be reported to public health officials. Effort should be made to evaluate, counsel, and treat all sexual partners who were exposed to the index case within 60 days before the onset of symptoms or diagnosis in the index case. If a patient's last sexual intercourse occurred more than 60 days before the onset of symptoms, the most recent sexual partner of the patient should be evaluated and treated. Patients should be instructed to avoid engaging in sexual activity until therapy is completed and any symptoms have resolved.[69] Cases in prepubertal children must be investigated to identify the source of infection (and potential perpetrator of abuse).[5]

Condoms provide a high degree of protection against the acquisition and transmission of genital gonococcal infection.[181,324] Other barrier contraceptive measures and topical spermicidal and bactericidal agents likewise can reduce the likelihood of acquiring gonococcal (and chlamydial) infection.[15,54,214,316] Postexposure prophylactic antibiotics also reduce the risk of infection developing but are unlikely to be cost-effective.[156]

When patients, including infants with ophthalmia neonatorum,[5] with gonococcal infection are hospitalized, standard precautions are recommended.

PREVENTION OF NEONATAL INFECTION

Pregnant women should have an endocervical culture for *N. gonorrhoeae* as part of their initial prenatal care visit. A second culture late in the third trimester should be performed for those at high risk of exposure during pregnancy. Pregnant adolescents are at higher risk for contracting gonococcal infection than older women are. Treatment options are listed in Table 100–8. Fluo-

roquinolone and tetracycline antibiotics should not be used during pregnancy because of potential fetal toxicity.[5]

Infants born to mothers known to have active gonococcal infection are at risk of acquiring local and disseminated infection from colonization during birth. Such infants should be treated as listed in Table 100–7. Standard preventive measures for GON were described earlier.

VACCINE DEVELOPMENT

Research into the development of vaccines for gonococcal infection is ongoing. Although natural infection induces antibody responses directed primarily against pili, Opa, porin protein, and LOS, two factors render efforts to use these gonococcal components for vaccines a difficult challenge: (1) the rapid antigenic variation in gonococcal surface proteins and (2) the reality that natural genital infection does not induce a sufficient immune response to prevent later reinfection by the same strain. The development of a gonococcal vaccine shares the difficulties of similar efforts that are under way to produce nonpolysaccharide vaccines effective against serogroup B strains of *N. meningitidis*.[82,242]

Molecular analysis of gonococcal transferring binding proteins (Tbps) may have potential as vaccine antigens because of their exposure on the microbial surface. These proteins are expressed in all strains and have highly conserved gene sequences. Natural infection, however, generates little systemic or local antibody response to Tbps.[264] An oligosaccharide epitope (2C7 OS) of gonococcal LOS that is expressed on most strains and is widely conserved has been identified. A peptide that mimics the structure of 2C7 OS was able to induce antibodies in mice that possess dose-responsive complement-dependent bactericidal activity against 2C7+ strains.[242] This approach, as well as the potential use of combinations of recombinant antigens from multiple porin or Opa proteins, may have promise for future gonococcal vaccine development.

Acknowledgment

The author would like to acknowledge the contribution of Dr. Laura Gutman to this chapter through her authorship of this chapter in the first four editions of this textbook.

REFERENCES

1. Abbott, S. L.: Gonococcal tonsillitis-pharyngitis in a 5-year-old girl. Pediatrics *52*:287-289, 1973.
2. Ahmed, H. J., Ilardi, I., Antognoli, A., et al.: An epidemic of *Neisseria gonorrhoeae* in a Somali orphanage. Int. J. S. T. D. A. I. D. S. *3*:52-53, 1992.
3. Alexander, W. J., Griffith, H., Housch, J. G., et al.: Infections in sexual contacts and associates of children with gonorrhea. Sex. Transm. Dis. *11*:156-158, 1984.
4. Allen, J. H., and Barrere, L. E.: Prophylaxis of gonorrhea ophthalmia of the newborn. J. A. M. A. *141*:522-525, 1949.
5. American Academy of Pediatrics: Gonococcal infections. *In* Pickering, L. K. (ed.): 2006 Red Book: Report of the Committee on Infectious Diseases. 27th ed. Elk Grove Village, IL, American Academy of Pediatrics, 2006, pp. 301-309.
6. American Academy of Pediatrics Committee on Child Abuse and Neglect: Guidelines for the evaluation of sexual abuse of children. Pediatrics *87*:254-260, 1991.
7. Amstey, M. S., and Steadman, K. T.: Asymptomatic gonorrhea and pregnancy. J. Am. Vener. Dis. Assoc. *3*:14-16, 1976.
8. Anderson, B., Albritton, W. L., Biddle, J., and Johnson, S. R.: Common β-lactamase–specifying plasmid in *Haemophilus ducreyi* and *Neisseria gonorrhoeae*. Antimicrob. Agents Chemother. *25*:296-297, 1984.
9. Angevine, C. D., Hall, C. B., and Jacox, R. F.: A case of gonococcal osteomyelitis: A complication of gonococcal arthritis. Am. J. Dis. Child. *130*:1013-1014, 1976.

10. Apicella, M. A.: Serogrouping of *Neisseria gonorrhoeae*: Identification of four immunologically distinct acidic polysaccharides. J. Infect. Dis. *134*:377-383, 1976.
11. Armstrong, J. H., Zacarias, F., and Rein, M. F.: Ophthalmia neonatorum: A chart review. Pediatrics *57*:884-892, 1976.
12. Auman, G. L., and Waldenberg, L. M.: Gonococcal periappendicitis and salpingitis in a prepubertal girl. Pediatrics *58*:287-288, 1976.
13. Babl, F. E., Ram, S., Barnett, E. D., et al.: Neonatal gonococcal arthritis after negative prenatal screening and despite conjunctival prophylaxis. Pediatr. Infect. Dis. J. *19*:346-349, 2000.
14. Badgley, R. F., et al.: Sexual Offenses against Children. Ottawa, Canada, Minister of Supply and Services, 1984.
15. Barlow, D.: The condom and gonorrhea. Lancet *2*:811, 1977.
16. Barnes, R. C., and Holmes K. K.: Epidemiology of gonorrhea: Current perspectives. Epidemiol. Rev. *6*:1, 1984.
17. Barsam, P. C.: Specific prophylaxis of gonorrheal ophthalmia neonatorum: A review. N. Engl. J. Med. *274*:731-734, 1966.
18. Barten, R., and Meyer, T. F.: DNA circle formation in *Neisseria gonorrhoeae*: A possible intermediate in diverse genomic recombination processes. Mol. Gen. Genet. *264*:691-701, 2001.
19. Bauer, F. J., Rudel, T., Stein, M., and Meyer, T. F.: Mutagenesis of the *Neisseria gonorrhoeae* porin reduces invasion in epithelial cells and enhances phagocyte responsiveness. Mol. Microbiol. *31*:903-913, 1999.
20. Bell, T. A., Grayston, J. T., Krohn, M. A., et al.: Randomized trial of silver nitrate, erythromycin, and no eye prophylaxis for the prevention of conjunctivitis among newborns not at risk for gonococcal ophthalmitis. Pediatrics *92*:755-760, 1993.
21. Benson, R. A., and Weinstock, E.: Gonorrheal vaginitis in children: A review of the literature. Am. J. Dis. Child. *59*:1083-1096, 1940.
22. Best, D., Ford, C. A., and Miller, W. C.: Prevalence of *Chlamydia trachomatis* and *Neisseria gonorrhoeae* infection in pediatric private practice. Pediatrics *108*:e103, 2001.
23. Birji, M., and Everson, J. J.: Comparative virulence of opacity variance of *Neisseria gonorrhoeae* strain P9. Infect. Immun. *31*:965-970, 1981.
24. Biswas, G. D., Blackman, E. Y., and Sparling, P. F.: High-frequency conjugal transfer of a gonococcal penicillinase plasmid. J. Bacteriol. *143*:1318-1324, 1980.
25. Biswas, G. D., Sox, T., Blackman, E., and Sparling, P. F.: Factors affecting genetic transformation of *Neisseria gonorrhoeae*. J. Bacteriol. *129*:983-992, 1977.
26. Biswas, G. D., and Sparling, P. F.: Characterization of *lbpA*, the structural gene for a lactoferrin receptor in *Neisseria gonorrhoeae*. Infect. Immun. *63*:2958-2967, 1995.
27. Black, W. J., Schwalbe, R. S., Nachamkin, I., and Cannon, J. G.: Characterization of *Neisseria gonorrhoeae* protein II phase variation by use of monoclonal antibodies. Infect. Immun. *45*:453-457, 1984.
28. Blake, M. S., and Gotschlich, E. C.: Purification and partial characterization of the major outer membrane protein of *Neisseria gonorrhoeae*. Infect. Immun. *36*:277-283, 1982.
29. Bogaerts, J., Lepage, P., DeClercq, A., et al.: Etiology and outcome of acute pelvic inflammatory disease. J. Infect. Dis. *158*:510-517, 1988.
30. Bonin, P., Tanino, T. T., and Handsfield, H. H.: Isolation of *Neisseria gonorrhoeae* on selective and nonselective media in a sexually transmitted disease clinic. J. Clin. Microbiol. *92*:218-220, 1984.
31. Boslego, J. W., Tramont, E. C., Takafuji, E. T., et al.: Effect of spectinomycin use on the prevalence of spectinomycin-resistant and of penicillinase-producing *Neisseria gonorrhoeae*. N. Engl. J. Med. *317*:272-278, 1987.
32. Bradford, W. L., and Kelley, H. W.: Gonococcic meningitis in a newborn infant. Am. J. Dis. Child *46*:543-549, 1933.
33. Bramley, J., Demarco de Hormaeche, R., Constantinidou, C., et al.: A serum-sensitive, sialyltransferase-deficient mutant of *Neisseria gonorrhoeae* defective in conversion to serum resistance by CMP-NANA or blood cell extracts. Microb. Pathog. *18*:187-195, 1995.
34. Branch, G., and Paxton, R.: A study of gonococcal infections among infants and children. Public Health Rep. *80*:347-352, 1965.
35. Brettin, T., Altherr, M. R., Du, Y., et al.: Expression capable library for studies of *Neisseria gonorrhoeae*, version 1.0. B. M. C. Microbiol. *5*:50, 2005.
36. Bro-Jorgensen, A., and Jensen, T.: Gonococcal pharyngeal infections: Report of 110 cases. Br. J. Vener. Dis. *49*:491, 1973.
37. Bronson, J. E., Holmberg, I., Nygren, B., et al.: Vancomycin-sensitive strains of *Neisseria gonorrhoeae*: A problem for the diagnostic laboratory. Pont. J. Vener. Dis. *49*:452-453, 1973.
38. Brooks, F., Israel, K. S., and Petersen, B. H.: Bactericidal and opsonic activity against *Neisseria gonorrhoeae* in sera from patients with disseminated gonococcal infection. J. Infect. Dis. *134*:450-462, 1976.
39. Brooks, G. F., Darrow, W. W., and Day, J. A.: Repeated gonorrhea: An analysis of importance and risk factors. J. Infect. Dis. *137*:161-169, 1978.
40. Brown, D.: Gonococcal arthritis in pregnancy. South. Med. J. *66*:693-695, 1973.
41. Brown, R. T., Lossick, J. G., Mosure, D. J., et al.: Pharyngeal gonorrhea screening in adolescents: Is it necessary? Pediatrics *84*:623-625, 1989.
42. Brown, W. J., and Kraus, S. T.: Gonococcal colony types. J. A. M. A. *228*:862-863, 1974.
43. Brunham, R. C., Binns, B., Guijon, F., et al.: Etiology and outcome of acute pelvic inflammatory disease. J. Infect. Dis. *158*:510-517, 1988.

44. Buchanan, T. M.: Antigenic heterogeneity of gonococcal pili. J. Exp. Med. *151*:1470, 1975.
45. Buchanan, T. M.: Attachment role of gonococcal pili: Optimum conditions and quantitation of adherence of isolated pili to human cells in vitro. J. Clin. Invest. *61*:931, 1978.
46. Burry, V. F.: Gonococcal vulvovaginitis and possible peritonitis in prepubertal girls. Am. J. Dis. Child. *121*:536-537, 1971.
47. Camarena, J. J.: DNA amplification fingerprinting for subtyping *Neisseria gonorrhoeae* strains. Sex. Transm. Dis. *22*:128-136, 1995.
48. Campbell, L. A., and Yashin, R. E.: Mutagenesis of *Neisseria gonorrhoeae*: Absence or error-prone repair. J. Bacteriol. *106*:288-293, 1984.
49. Cannon, J. G., and Sparling, P. F.: The genetics of the gonococcus. Annu. Rev. Microbiol. *38*:111-133, 1984.
50. Carbonetti, N. H., Simnad, V. I., Seifert, H. S., et al.: Genetics of protein I of *Neisseria gonorrhoeae*: Construction of hybrid porins. Proc. Natl. Acad. Sci. U. S. A. *85*:6841-6845, 1988.
51. Carifo, K., and Catlin, B. W.: *Neisseria gonorrhoeae* autotyping: Differentiation of clinical isolates based on growth responses on chemically defined media. Appl. Microbiol. *26*:223-230, 1973.
52. Casey, S. G., Shafer, W. M., and Spitznagel, J. K.: *Neisseria gonorrhoeae* survive intraleukocytic oxygen-independent antimicrobial capacities of anaerobic and aerobic granulocytes in the presence of pyocin lethal for extracellular gonococci. Infect. Immun. *52*:384-389, 1986.
53. Cates, W.: Sexually transmitted organisms and infertility: The proof of the pudding. Sex. Transm. Dis. *11*:113-116, 1984.
54. Cates, W., Jr., Weisner, P. J., and Curran, J. W.: Sex and spermicides: Preventing unintended pregnancy and infection. J. A. M. A. *248*:1636-1637, 1982.
55. Catlin, B. W.: Nutritional profiles of *Neisseria gonorrhoeae*, *Neisseria meningitidis*, and *Neisseria lactamica* in chemically defined media and the use of growth requirements for gonococcal typing. J. Infect. Dis. *128*:178-194, 1973.
56. Centers for Disease Control and Prevention: Sentinel surveillance system for antimicrobial resistance in clinical isolates of *Neisseria gonorrhoeae*. M. M. W. R. Morb. Mortal. Wkly. Rep. *36*(35):585-586, 591-593, 1987.
57. Centers for Disease Control and Prevention: Plasmid-mediated antimicrobial resistance in *Neisseria gonorrhoeae*—United States, 1988 and 1989. M. M. W. R. Morb. Mortal. Wkly. Rep. *39*(17):284-293, 1990.
58. Centers for Disease Control and Prevention: Special focus: Surveillance for sexually transmitted diseases. M. M. W. R. C. D. C. Surveill. Summ. *42*(3):1-39, 1993.
59. Centers for Disease Control and Prevention: 1998 Guidelines for treatment of sexually transmitted diseases. M. M. W. R. Recomm. Rep. *47*(RR-1):1-116, 1998.
60. Centers for Disease Control and Prevention: Summary of notifiable diseases, United States, 1999. M. M. W. R. Morb. Mortal. Wkly. Rep. *48*(53):1-101, 1999.
61. Centers for Disease Control and Prevention: Fluoroquinolone-resistance in *Neisseria gonorrhoeae*, Hawaii, 1999, and decreased susceptibility to azithromycin in *N. gonorrhoeae*, Missouri, 1999. M. M. W. R. Morb. Mortal. Wkly. Rep. *49*(37):833-837, 2000.
62. Centers for Disease Control and Prevention: Sexually Transmitted Diseases Surveillance 1999 Supplement: Gonococcal Isolate Surveillance Project (GISP) Annual Report—1999. Atlanta, U.S. Department of Health and Human Services, Public Health Service, October 2000. Available at *http://www.cdc.gov/nchstp/dstd/Stats_Trends/99GISP/gisp99.pdf*.
63. Centers for Disease Control and Prevention: Screening tests to detect *Chlamydia trachomatis* and *Neisseria gonorrhoeae* infections—2002. M. M. W. R. Recomm. Rep. *51*(RR-15):1-38, 2002.
64. Centers for Disease Control and Prevention: Sexually transmitted diseases treatment guidelines 2006. M. M. W. R. Recomm. Rep. *55*(RR-11):1-94, 2006.
65. Centers for Disease Control and Prevention: Trends in Reportable Sexually Transmitted Diseases in the United States, 2005. December 2006. Available at *http://www.cdc.gov/std/stats/05pdf/trends-2005.pdf*.
66. Centers for Disease Control and Prevention: Increases in gonorrhea—eight western states, 2000-2005. M. M. W. R. Morb. Mortal. Wkly. Rep. *56*(10):222-225, 2007.
67. Centers for Disease Control and Prevention: Update to CDC's Sexually Transmitted Diseases Treatment Guidelines, 2006: Fluoroquinolones no longer recommended for treatment of gonococcal infections. M. M. W. R. Morb. Mortal. Wkly. Rep. *56*(14):332-336, 2007.
68. Centers for Disease Control and Prevention: Sexually Transmitted Disease Surveillance 2005 Supplement, Gonococcal Isolate Surveillance Project (GISP) Annual Report 2005. Atlanta, U.S. Department of Health and Human Services, Centers for Disease Control and Prevention, January 2007.
69. Centers for Disease Control and Prevention: Updated Recommended Treatment Regimens for Gonococcal Infections and Associated Conditions—United States, April 2007. Available at *http://www.cdc.gov/std/treatment/2006/updated-regimens.htm* (accessed May 2007).
70. Centers for Disease Control and Prevention: Alternatives to spectinomycin for the treatment of *Neisseria gonorrhoeae*. Available at *http://www. cdc.gov/std/spec-shortage.htm*.
71. Centers for Disease Control and Prevention: *N. gonorrhoeae*. Available at *http://www.cdc.gov.ncidod/dastlr/gcdir/NeIdent/Ngon.html*.

72. Centers for Disease Control and Prevention: *N. gonorrhoeae* serotyping. Available at *http://www.cdc.gov.ncidod/dastlr/gcdir/serotyp.htm*.

73. Chacko, M. R., Phillips, S., and Jacobson, M. S.: Screening for pharyngeal gonorrhea in the urban teenager. Pediatrics 70:620-623, 1982.

74. Charles, A. G., Cohen, S., Kass, M. B., et al.: Asymptomatic gonorrhea in prenatal patients. Am. J. Obstet. Gynecol. 108:595-599, 1970.

75. Chen, C. J., Sparling, P. F., Lewis, L. A., et al.: Identification and purification of a hemoglobin-binding outer membrane protein from *Neisseria gonorrhoeae.* Infect. Immun. 64:5008-5014, 1996.

76. Chen, J.-Y.: Prophylaxis of ophthalmia neonatorum: Comparison of silver nitrate, tetracycline, erythromycin, and no prophylaxis. Pediatr. Infect. Dis. 11:1026-1030, 1992.

77. Chen, S.-T., and Clowes, R. C.: Nucleotide sequence comparisons of plasmids pHD131, pJBl, pFA3, and pFA7 and p-lactamase expression in *Escherichia coli, Haemophilus influenzae,* and *Neisseria gonorrhoeae.* J. Bacteriol. 169:3124-3130, 1987.

78. Chesson, H. W., Gift, T. L., and Pulver, A. L. S.: The economic value of reductions in gonorrhea and syphilis incidence in the United States, 1990-2003. Prev. Med. 43:411-415, 2006.

79. Ching, S., Lee, H., Hook, E. W., 3rd, et al.: Ligase chain reaction for detection of *Neisseria gonorrhoeae* in urogenital swabs. J. Clin. Microbiol. 33:3111-3114, 1995.

80. Christian, C. W., Pinto-Martin, J. A., and McGowan, K. L.: The management of prepubertal children with gonorrhea. Clin. Pediatr. (Phila.) 34:415-418, 1995.

81. Cohen, M. S., and Cannon, J. G.: Human experimentation with *Neisseria gonorrhoeae*: Progress and goals. J. Infect. Dis. 179(Suppl. 2):375-379, 1999.

82. Cohen, M. S., Cannon, J. C., Jerse, A. E., et al.: Human experimentation with *Neisseria gonorrhoeae*: Rationale, methods, and implications for the biology of infection and vaccine development. J. Infect. Dis. 169:532-537, 1994.

83. Cohen, M. S., and Sparling, P. F.: Mucosal infection with *Neisseria gonorrhoeae.* J. Clin. Invest. 89:1699-1707, 1992.

84. Colin, M. J., and Weissmann, G.: Disseminated gonococcal infection and tenosynovitis from an asymptomatically infected intrauterine contraceptive device. N. Engl. J. Med. 294:598-599, 1976.

85. Committee on Child Abuse and Neglect, American Academy of Pediatrics: Guidelines for evaluation of sexual abuse of children: Subject review. Pediatrics 103:186-191, 1999.

86. Connell, T. D., Black, W. J., Kawula, T. H., et al.: Recombination among protein II genes of *Neisseria gonorrhoeae* generates new coding sequences and increases structural variability in the protein II family. Mol. Microbiol. 2:227-236, 1988.

87. Cooke, S. J., de la Paz, H., Poh., C. L., et al.: Variation within serovars of *Neisseria gonorrhoeae* detected by structural analysis of outer-membrane protein PIB and by pulsed-field gel electrophoresis. Microbiology 143:1415-1422, 1997.

88. Cooperman, M. B.: *Gonococcus* arthritis in infancy: A clinical study of forty-four cases. Am. J. Dis. Child. 33:932-948, 1927.

89. Cooperman, M. B.: End results of gonorrheal arthritis: A review of seventy cases. Am. J. Surg. 5:241-251, 1928.

90. Corman, L. C., Levison, M. E., Knight, R., et al.: The high frequency of pharyngeal gonococcal infection in a prenatal clinic population. J. A. M. A. 230:568-570, 1974.

91. Cornelissen, C. N., Kelley, M., Hobbs, M. M., et al.: The transferring receptor expressed by gonococcal strain FA 1090 is required for the experimental infection of human male volunteers. Mol. Microbiol. 27:611-616, 1998.

92. Cornelissen, C., and Sparling, P. F.: Iron piracy: Acquisition of transferrin-bound iron by bacterial pathogens. Mol. Microbiol. 14:843-850, 1994.

93. Coulter, K.: Migratory polyarthritis in a nine-year-old girl. Pediatr. Infect. Dis. J. 9:856-857, 1990.

94. Cramolini, G. M., and Litt, I. F.: The pharynx as the only positive culture site in an adolescent with disseminated gonorrhea. J. Pediatr. 100:644-646, 1982.

95. Crawford, G., Knapp, J. S., Hale, J., et al.: Asymptomatic gonorrhea in men caused by gonococci with unique nutritional requirements. Science 196:1352, 1977.

96. Credé, C. S. F.: Reports from the obstetrical clinic in Leipzig: Prevention of eye inflammation in the newborn. Am. J. Dis. Child. 121:3-4, 1971.

97. D'Amato, R. F., Eriquez, L. A., Tomfohrde, K. M., and Singerman, E.: Rapid identification of *Neisseria gonorrhoeae* and *Neisseria meningitidis* by using enzymatic profiles. J. Clin. Microbiol. 7:77-81, 1978.

98. Danielsson, D., and Johannisson, G.: Culture diagnosis of gonorrhea. A comparison of the yield with selective and non-selective gonococcal culture media inoculated in the clinic and after treatment of specimens. Acta Derm. Venereol. 53:75-80, 1973.

99. D'Auria, A., Tan, L., Kreitzer, M., et al.: Gonococcal scalp-wound infection. M. M. W. R. Morb. Mortal. Wkly. Rep. 24:115-116, 1975.

100. Dawar, S., and Hellerstein, S.: Gonorrhea as a cause of asymptomatic pyuria in adolescent boys. J. Pediatr. 81:357-358, 1972.

101. Deheragoda, P.: Diagnosis of rectal gonorrhea by blind anorectal swabs compared with direct vision swabs taken via a proctoscope. Br. J. Vener. Dis. 53:311, 1977.

102. Dehio, C., Gray-Owen, S. D., and Meyer, T. F.: The role of neisserial opa proteins in interactions with host cells. Trends Microbiol. 6:489-495, 1998.

103. Dehio, M., Gomez-Duarte, O. G., Dehio, C., and Meyer, T. F.: Vitronectin-dependent invasion of epithelial cells by *Neisseria gonorrhoeae* involves alpha (v) integrin receptors. F. E. B. S. Lett. 424:84-88, 1998.

104. DeJong, A. R.: Sexually transmitted diseases in sexually abused children. Sex. Transm. Dis. 13:123-126, 1986.

105. Demarco de Hormaeche, R., Jessop, H., and Senior, K.: Gonococcal variants selected by growth in vivo or in vitro have antigenically different LPS. Microb. Pathog. 4:289-297, 1988.

106. Demetriou, E., Sackett, R., Welch, D. F., et al.: Evaluation of an enzyme immunoassay for detection of *Neisseria gonorrhoea* in an adolescent population. J. A. M. A. 252:247-250, 1984.

107. Dempsey, J. F., Litaker, W., Madhure, T. L., et al.: Physical map of the chromosome of *Neisseria gonorrhoeae* FA1090 with locations of genetic markers. J. Bacteriol. 173:5476-5486, 1991.

108. Denison, M. R., Perlman, S., and Anderson, R. D.: Misidentification of *Neisseria* species in a neonate with conjunctivitis. Pediatrics 81:877-888, 1988.

109. Desenclos, J.-C. A., Garrity, D., and Wroten, J.: Pediatric gonococcal infection, Florida, 1984 to 1988. Am. J. Public Health 82:426-428, 1992.

110. Di Bartolomeo, S., Mirta, D. H., Janer, M., et al.: Incidence of *Chlamydia trachomatis* and other potential pathogens in neonatal conjunctivitis. Int. J. Infect. Dis. 5:139-143, 2001.

111. Dice, L. R.: Measure of the amounts of ecological association between species. Ecology 26:297-302, 1945.

112. Do, A. N., Hanson, D. L., Dworkin, M. S., et al.: Risk factors for and trends in gonorrhea incidence among persons infected with HIV in the United States. AIDS 15:1149-1155, 2001.

113. Dossett, J. H., Appelbaum, P. C., Knapp, J. S., et al.: Proctitis associated with *Neisseria cinerea* misidentified as *Neisseria gonorrhoeae* in a child. J. Clin. Microbiol. 21:575-577, 1985.

114. Dougherty, T. J., Asmus, A., and Tomasz, A.: Specificity of DNA uptake in genetic transformation of gonococci. Biochem. Biophys. Res. Commun. 86:97-104, 1979.

115. Edwards, J. L., and Apicella, M. A.: The molecular mechanisms used by *Neisseria gonorrhoeae* to initiate infection differ between men and women. Clin. Microbiol. Rev. 17:965-981, 2004.

116. Edwards, L. E., Barrada, M. I., Hamann, A. A., et al.: Gonorrhea in pregnancy. Am. J. Obstet. Gynecol. 132:637-641, 1978.

117. Eisenstein, B. I., Lee, T. J., and Sparling, P. F.: Penicillin sensitivity and serum resistance are independent attributes of strains of *Neisseria gonorrhoeae* causing disseminated gonococcal infection. Infect. Immun. 15:834-841, 1977.

118. Elliott, B., Brunham, R. C., Laga, M., et al.: Maternal gonococcal infection as a preventable risk factor for low birth weight. J. Infect. Dis. 161:531-536, 1990.

119. Ellison, R. T., III, Curd, J. G., Kholer, P. F., et al.: Underlying complement deficiency in patients with disseminated gonococcal infection. Sex. Transm. Dis. 14:201-204, 1987.

120. Eschenbach, D. A.: Acute pelvic inflammatory disease: Etiology, risk factors, and pathogenesis. Clin. Obstet. Gynecol. 19:147-169, 1976.

121. Eschenbach, D. A., Buchanan, T. M., Pollock, H. M., et al.: Polymicrobial etiology of acute pelvic inflammatory disease. N. Engl. J. Med. 293:166-171, 1975.

122. Falk, E. S., Danielsson, D., Bjornvatn, B., et al.: Genomic fingerprinting in the epidemiology of gonorrhea. Acta Derm. Venereol. 65:2235-2239, 1985.

123. Farrell, M. K., Billimire, M. E., Shamroy, J. A., et al.: Prepubertal gonorrhea: A multidisciplinary approach. Pediatrics 67:151-153, 1981.

124. Faruki, H., Kohmescher, R. N., McKinney, W. P., and Sparling, P. F.: A community-based outbreak of infection with penicillin-resistant *Neisseria gonorrhoeae* not producing penicillinase (chromosomally medicated resistance). N. Engl. J. Med. 313:607-611, 1985.

125. Folland, D. S., Burke, R. E., Hinman, A. R., et al.: Gonorrhea in preadolescent children: An inquiry into source of infection and mode of transmission. Pediatrics 60:153-156, 1977.

126. Forsyth, A., Moyes, A., and Young, H.: Increased ciprofloxacin resistance in gonococci isolated in Scotland. Lancet 356:1984-1985, 2000.

127. Fransen, I., Nsanze, H., Klaus, V., et al.: Ophthalmia neonatorum in Nairobi, Kenya: The roles of *Neisseria gonorrhoeae* and *Chlamydia trachomatis.* J. Infect. Dis. 153:862-869, 1986.

128. Frewen, T. C., and Bannatyne R. M.: Gonococcal vulvovaginitis in prepubertal girls. Clin. Pediatr. (Phila.) 18:491-493, 1979.

129. Friedrich, W. N., and Grambsch, P.: Child sexual behavior inventory: Normative and clinical comparisons. Psychol. Assess. 4:303-311, 1992.

130. Friendly, D. S.: Gonococcal conjunctivitis of the newborn. Clin. Prac. Child. Hosp. 25:1-9, 1969.

131. Geidinghagen, D. H., Hoff, G. L., and Biery, R. M.: Gonorrhea in children: Epidemiologic unit analysis. Pediatr. Infect. Dis. J. 11:973-974, 1992.

132. Genadry, R. R., Thompson, B. H., and Niebyl, J. R.: Gonococcal salpingitis in pregnancy. Am. J. Obstet. Gynecol. 126:512-513, 1976.

133. Gilbaugh, J. H., and Fuchs, P. C.: The gonococcus and the toilet seat. N. Engl. J. Med. 301:91-93, 1979.

134. Gill, M. J., Simjee, S., Al-Hattawi, K., et al.: Gonococcal resistance to β-lactams and tetracycline involves mutation in loop 3 of the porin encoded at the penB locus. Antimicrob. Agents Chemother. 42:2799-2803, 1998.

135. Glaser, S., Boxerbaum, B., and Kennell, J. H.: Gonococcal arthritis in the newborn: Report of a case and review of the literature. Am. J. Dis. Child. *112*:135-138, 1966.

136. Golden, N., Hammerschlag, M., Hewkoff, S., et al.: Prevalence of *Chlamydia trachomatis* cervical infections in female adolescents. Am. J. Dis. Child. *138*:562-564, 1984.

137. Gomperts, B. N., and White, L. K.: Gonococcal hand abscess. Pediatr. Infect. Dis. J. *19*:671-672, 2000.

138. Gorter, A. D., Oostrik, J., van der Lay, P., et al.: Involvement of lipooligo-saccharides of *Haemophilus influenzae* and *Neisseria meningitidis* in defensin-enhanced bacterial adherence to epithelial cells. Microb. Pathog. *34*:121-130, 2003.

139. Gotschlich, E. C.: Genetic locus for the biosynthesis of the variable portion of *Neisseria gonorrhoeae* lipooligosaccharide. J. Exp. Med. *180*:2181-2190, 1994.

140. Grassme, H., Gulbins, E., Brenner, B., et al.: Acidic sphingomyelinase mediates entry of *N. gonorrhoeae* into nonphagocytic cells. Cell *91*:605-615, 1997.

141. Greenberg, M., and Vandow, J. E.: Ophthalmia neonatorum: Evaluation of different methods of prophylaxis in New York City. Am. J. Public Health *51*:836-845, 1961.

142. Gregg, C. R., Melly, M. A., Hellerqvist, C. G., et al.: Toxic activity of puri-fied lipopolysaccharide as *N. gonorrhoeae* for human fallopian tube mucosa. J. Infect. Dis. *143*:432-439, 1983.

143. Gregory, J. E., Chisom, J. L., and Meadows, A. T.: Gonococcal arthritis in an infant. Br. J. Vener. Dis. *48*:306-307, 1972.

144. Griffiss, J. M., Lammel, C. J., Wang, J., et al.: *Neisseria gonorrhoeae* coordi-nately uses Pili and Opa to activate HEC-1-B cell microvilli, which causes engulfment of the gonococci. Infect. Immun. *67*:3469-3480, 1999.

145. Griffiss, J. M., O'Brien, J. P., Yamasaki, R., et al.: Physical heterogeneity of neisserial lipooligosaccharides reflects oligosaccharides that differ in apparent molecular weight, chemical composition, and antigenic expression. Infect. Immun. *55*:1792-1800, 1987.

146. Griffiss, J. M., Schneider, H., Mandrell, R. E., et al.: Lipooligosaccharides: The principal glycolipids of the neisserial outer membrane. Rev. Infect. Dis. *10*(Suppl. 2):287-295, 1988.

147. Groothuis, J. R., Bischoff, M. C., and Jauregui, L. E.: Pharyngeal gonorrhea in young children. Pediatr. Infect. Dis. J. *2*:99-101, 1983.

148. Gutman, L. T., Herman-Giddens, M. E., and McKinney, R. E., Jr.: Pediatric acquired immunodeficiency syndrome: Barriers to recognizing the role of child sexual abuse. Am. J. Dis. Child. *147*:775-780, 1993.

149. Gutman, L. T., and Holmes, K. K.: Gonococcal infections. *In* Remington, J. S., and Klein, J. O. (eds.): Infectious Diseases of the Fetus and Newborn Infant. 3rd ed. Philadelphia, W. B. Saunders, 1990.

150. Haas, R., Schwartz, H., and Meyer, T. F.: Release of soluble pilin antigen coupled with gene conversion in *Neisseria gonorrhoeae*. Proc. Natl. Acad. Sci. U. S. A. *84*:9079-9083, 1987.

151. Haines, K. A., Reibman, J., Tang, X. Y., et al.: Effects of protein I of *Neisseria gonorrhoeae* on neutrophil activation: Generation of diacylglycerol from phos-phatidylcholine via a specific phospholipase C is associated with exocytosis. J. Cell Biol. *114*:433-442, 1991.

152. Hale, Y. M., Melton, M. E., Lewis, J. S., and Willis, D. E.: Evaluation of the PACE 2 *Neisseria gonorrhoeae* assay by three public health laboratories. J. Clin. Microbiol. *31*:451-453, 1993.

153. Handsfield, H. H., Hodson, W. A., and Holmes, K. K.: Neonatal gonococcal infection. 1. Orogastric contamination with *Neisseria gonorrhoeae*. J. A. M. A. *225*:697-701, 1973.

154. Handsfield, H. H., and Holmes, K. K.: Microepidemic of virulent gonococcal infection. J. Am. Vener. Dis. Assoc. *1*:20-22, 1974.

155. Handsfield, H. H., Lipman, T. O., Harnisch, J. P., et al.: Asymptomatic gonorrhea in men: Diagnosis, natural course, prevalence and significance. N. Engl. J. Med. *290*:117-123, 1974.

156. Harrison, W. O., Hooper, R. R., Weisner, P. J., et al.: A trial of minocycline given after exposure to prevent gonorrhea. N. Engl. J. Med. *300*:1074-1078, 1979.

157. Harvey, H. A., Post, D. M. B., and Apicella, M. A.: Immortalization of human urethral epithelial cells: A model for the study of the pathogenesis of and the inflammatory cytokine response to *Neisseria gonorrhoeae* infection. Infect. Immun. *70*:5808-5815, 2002.

158. Hein, K., Marks, A., and Cohen, M. I.: Asymptomatic gonorrhea: Prevalence in a population of urban adolescents. J. Pediatr. *90*:634-635, 1977.

159. Hitchcock, P. J.: Analyses of gonococcal lipopolysaccharide in whole cell lysates by sodium dodecyl sulfate–polyacrylamide gel electrophoresis: Stable association of lipopolysaccharide with the major outer membrane protein (protein 1) of *Neisseria gonorrhoeae*. Infect. Immun. *46*:202, 1984.

160. Holmes, K. K., Buchanan T. M., Adam, J. L., and Aschenbach, D. A.: Is serol-ogy useful in gonorrhea? A critical analysis of factors influencing serodiagno-sis. *In* Brook, G. F., Gotschlich E. C., Sawyer, W. D., and Young, F. E. (eds.): Immunobiology of *Neisseria gonorrhoeae*. Washington, D.C., American Society for Microbiology, 1978, p. 370.

161. Holmes, K. K., Counts, G. W., and Beaty, H. N.: Disseminated gonococcal infection. Ann. Intern. Med. *74*:979-993, 1971.

162. Holmes, K. K., Johnson, D. W., and Trostle, H. J.: An estimate of the risk of men acquiring gonorrhea by sexual contact with infected females. Am. J. Epidemiol. *91*:170-174, 1970.

163. Holt, L. E.: Gonococcus infections in children with especial reference to their prevalence in institutions and means of prevention. N. Y. Med. J. *81*:521-527, 1905.

164. Hook, E. W., and Handsfield, H. H.: Gonococcal infections in the adult. *In* Holmes, K. K., Mårdh, P. A., Sparling, P. F., et al. (eds.): Sexually Transmitted Diseases. 3rd ed. New York, McGraw-Hill, 1999.

165. Hook, E. W., and Holmes, K. K.: Gonococcal infections. Ann. Intern. Med. *102*:229-243, 1985.

166. Hook, E. W., 3rd, Judson, F. N., Handsfield, H. H., et al.: Auxotype/serovar diversity and antimicrobial resistance of *Neisseria gonorrhoeae* in two mid-sized American cities. Sex. Transm. Dis. *14*:141-146, 1987.

167. Hooper, R. R., Reynolds, G. H., Jones, O. G., et al.: Cohort study of venereal disease: I. The risk of gonorrhea transmission from infected women to men. Am. J. Epidemiol. *108*:136-144, 1978.

168. Huppert, J. S., Biro, F., Lan, D., et al.: Urinary symptoms in adolescent females: STI or UTI? J. Adolesc. Health. *40*:418-424, 2007.

169. Ingram, D. L.: The gonococcus and the toilet seat revisited. Pediatr. Infect. Dis. *8*:191, 1989.

170. Ingram, D. L., Everett, V. D., Flick, L. A. R., et al.: Vaginal gonococcal cul-tures in sexual abuse evaluations: Evaluation of selective criteria for preteen-aged girls. Pediatrics *99*:e8, 1997.

171. Ingram, D. L., Everett, V. D., Lyna, P. R., et al.: Epidemiology of adult sexu-ally transmitted disease agents in children being evaluated for sexual abuse. Pediatr. Infect. Dis. J. *11*:945-950, 1992.

172. Ingram, D. L., Runyan, D. K., Collins, A. D., et al.: Vaginal *Chlamydia tracho-matis* infection in children with sexual contact. Pediatr. Infect. Dis. *3*:97-99, 1984.

173. Ingram, D. M., Miller, W. C., Schoenbach, V. J., et al.: Risk assessment for gonococcal and chlamydial infections in young children undergoing evalua-tion for sexual abuse. Pediatrics *107*:e73, 2001.

174. Ison, C. A., Woodford, P. J., Madders, H., and Claydon, E.: Drift in suscep-tibility of *Neisseria gonorrhoeae* to ciprofloxacin and emergence of therapeutic failure. Antimicrob. Agents Chemother. *42*:2919-2922, 1998.

175. Israel, K. S., Rissing, K. B., and Brooks, G. F.: Neonatal and childhood gono-coccal infections. Clin. Obstet. Gynecol. *18*:143-151, 1975.

176. Jacobson, L., and Westrom, L.: Objectivized diagnosis of acute pelvic inflam-matory disease. Am. J. Obstet. Gynecol. *105*:1088-1098, 1969.

177. Jamison, J. H., Kaplan, D. W., Hamman, R., et al.: Spectrum of genital human papillomavirus infection in a female adolescent population. Sex. Transm. Dis. *22*:236, 1995.

178. Johannsen, D. B., Johnston, D. M., Koymen, H. O., et al.: A *Neisseria gonor-rhoeae* immunoglobulin A1 protease mutant is infectious in the human chal-lenge model of urethral infection. Infect. Immun. *67*:3009-3013, 1999.

179. Johnston, K. H., Holmes, K. K., and Gotschlich, E. C.: The serological clas-sification of *Neisseria gonorrhoeae*. 1. Isolation of the outer membrane complex responsible for serotypic specificity. J. Exp. Med. *143*:741-758, 1976.

180. Jones, D. E. D., Brame, R. G., and Jones, C. P.: Gonorrhea in obstetric patients. J. Am. Vener. Dis. Assoc. *2*:30-32, 1976.

181. Judson, F. N., and Maltz, A. B.: A rational basis for the epidemiologic treat-ment of gonorrhea in a clinic for sexually transmitted diseases. Sex. Transm. Dis. *5*:89, 1978.

182. Judson, F. N., and Werness, B. A.: Combining cervical and anal-canal specimens for gonorrhea on a single culture plate. J. Clin. Microbiol. *12*:216, 1980.

183. Kahn, R. H., Mosure, D. J., Blank, S., et al.: *Chlamydia trachomatis* and *Neisseria gonorrhoeae* prevalence and coinfection in adolescents entering selected US juvenile detention centers, 1997-2002. Sex. Transm. Dis. *32*:255-259, 2005.

184. Kallstrom, H., Islam, M. S., Berggren, P. O., and Jonsson, A. B.: Cell signaling by the type IV pili of pathogenic *Neisseria*. J. Biol. Chem. *273*:21777-21782, 1998.

185. Kallstrom, H., Liszewski, M. K., Atkinson, J. P., and Jonsson A. B.: Membrane cofactor protein (MCP or CD46) is a cellular pilus receptor for pathogenic *Neisseria*. Mol. Microbiol. *25*:639-647, 1997.

186. Kampmeier, R. H.: Identification of the gonococcus by Albert Neisser. Sex. Transm. Dis. *5*:71, 1978.

187. Kasper, D. L., Rice, P. A., and McCormack, W. M.: Bactericidal antibody in genital infections due to *Neisseria gonorrhoeae*. J. Infect. Dis. *135*:243-251, 1977.

188. Kellogg, D. S., Peacock, W. L., Jr., Deacon, W. E., et al.: *Neisseria gonorrhoeae*: 1. Virulence genetically linked to clonal variation. J. Bacteriol. *85*:1274-1279, 1963.

189. Kellogg, J. A., and Orwig, L. K.: Comparison of Gonogen, Gono Gen II and Micro Trak Direct Fluorescent-Antibody Test with carbohydrate fermen-tation for confirmation of culture isolates of *Neisseria gonorrhoeae*. J. Clin. Microbiol. *33*:474-476, 1995.

190. Koomey, M.: Implications of molecular contacts and signaling initiated by *Neisseria gonorrhoeae*. Curr. Opin. Microbiol. *4*:53-57, 2001.

191. Knapp, J. S., and Holmes, K. K.: Disseminated gonococcal infections caused by *Neisseria gonorrhoeae* with unique nutritional requirements. J. Infect. Dis. *132*:204-208, 1975.

192. Knapp, J. S., Tam, M. R., Nowinski, R. C., et al.: Serological classification of *Neisseria gonorrhoeae* with use of monoclonal antibodies to gonococcal outer membrane protein I. J. Infect. Dis. *150*:44-48, 1984.

193. Kohen, D. P.: Neonatal gonococcal arthritis: Three cases and review of the literature. Pediatrics *53*:436-440, 1974.

194. Krieger, J. N.: Prostatitis, epididymitis, and orchitis. *In* Mandell, G. L., Douglas, R. G., and Bennett, J. E. (eds.): Principles and Practice of Infectious Disease. New York, Churchill Livingstone, 1985, pp. 745-748.
195. Krohn, M. A., Hillier, S. L., Bell, J. A., et al.: The bacterial etiology of conjunctivitis in early infancy. Am. J. Epidemiol. *138*:326-332, 1993.
196. Lafferty, W., Hughes, J. P., and Handsfield, H. H.: Sexually transmitted disease in men who have sex with men: Acquisition of gonorrhea and nongonococcal urethritis by fellatio and implications for STD/HIV prevention. Sex. Transm. Dis. *24*:272-278, 1997.
197. Laga, M., Meheus, A., and Piot, P.: Epidemiology and control of gonococcal ophthalmia neonatorum. Bull. World Health Organ. *67*:471-477, 1989.
198. Laga, M., Naamara, W., Brunham, R. C., et al.: Single-dose therapy of gonococcal ophthalmia neonatorum with ceftriaxone. N. Engl. J. Med. *315*:1382-1385, 1986.
199. Laga, M., Plummer, F. A., Piot, P., et al.: Prophylaxis of gonococcal and chlamydial ophthalmia neonatorum. N. Engl. J. Med. *318*:653-657, 1988.
200. Landolfo, P. J., Marrie, T. J., Nelson, N. A., and Ronald, A. R.: Cell-mediated immune response in gonococcal infection. Can. J. Microbiol. *27*:76-80, 1981.
201. Laras, L., Craighill, M., Woods, E. R., et al.: Epidemiologic observations of adolescents with *Neisseria gonorrhoeae* genital infections treated at a children's hospital. Adolesc. Pediatr. Gynecol. *7*:9-12, 1994.
202. Lawson, L., and Chaffin, M.: False negatives in sexual abuse disclosure interviews. J. Interpersonal Violence *7*:532-542, 1992.
203. Lewis, L. S., Glauser, T. A., and Joffe, M. D.: Gonococcal conjunctivitis in prepubertal children. Am. J. Dis. Child. *144*:546-548, 1990.
204. Limberger, R. J., Biega, R., Evancoe, A., et al.: Evaluation of culture and the Gen-Probe PACE 2 assay for detection of *Neisseria gonorrhoeae* and *Chlamydia trachomatis* in endocervical specimens transported to a state health laboratory. J. Clin. Microbiol. *30*:1162-1166, 1992.
205. Lin, L., Ayala, P., Larson, J., et al.: The *Neisseria* type 2 IgA1 protease cleaves LAMP1 and promotes survival of bacteria within epithelial cells. Mol. Microbiol. *24*:1083-1094, 1997.
206. Litt, I. F., and Cohen, M. I.: Perihepatitis associated with salpingitis in adolescents. J. A. M. A. *240*:1253, 1978.
207. Litt, I. F., Edberg, S. C., and Finberg, L.: Gonorrhea in children and adolescents: A current review. J. Pediatr. *85*:595-607, 1974.
208. Looveren, M. V., Ison, C. A., Ieven, M., et al.: Evaluation of the discriminatory power of typing methods for *Neisseria gonorrhoeae*. J. Clin. Microbiol. *37*:2183-2188, 1999.
209. Lorenzen, D. R., Gunther, D., Pandit, J., et al.: *Neisseria gonorrhoeae* porin modifies the oxidative burst of human professional phagocytes. Infect. Immun. *68*:6215-6222, 2000.
210. Louv, W. C., Austin H., Alexander, W., et al.: A clinical trial of nonoxynol-9 for preventing gonococcal and chlamydial infections. J. Infect. Dis. *158*:518-523, 1988.
211. Louv, W. C., Austin, H., Perlman, J., and Alexander, W. J.: Oral contraceptive use and the risk of chlamydial and gonococcal infection. Am. J. Obstet. Gynecol. *160*:396-402, 1989.
212. Luciano, A. A., and Grubin, L.: Gonorrhea screening: Comparison of three techniques. J. A. M. A. *243*:680-681, 1980.
213. Mascola, L., Albritton, W. L., Cates, W., et al.: Gonorrhea in American teenagers, 1960-1981. Pediatr. Infect. Dis. J. *2*:302-303, 1983.
214. McCormack, W. M., and Reynolds, G. H.: Effect of menstrual cycle and method of contraception on recovery of *Neisseria gonorrhoeae*. J. A. M. A. *247*:1292-1294, 1982.
215. McGee, Z. A., Johnson, A. P., and Taylor-Robinson, D.: Pathogenic mechanisms of *Neisseria gonorrhoeae*: Observations on damage to human fallopian tubes in organ culture by gonococci of colony type I or type 4. J. Infect. Dis. *143*:413-422, 1981.
216. McGee, Z. A., Stephens, D. S., Hoffman, L. H., et al.: Mechanisms of mucosal invasion by pathogenic *Neisseria*. Rev. Infect. Dis. *5*(Suppl. 4):708, 1983.
217. McMillan, A., and Young, H.: Gonorrhea in the homosexual man: Frequency of infection by culture site. Sex. Transm. Dis. *5*:146, 1978.
218. Mellin, G. W.: Ophthalmia neonatorum: Yesterday, today, tomorrow. Sight-Saver Rev. *31*:102-113, 1961.
219. Merz, A. J., Enns, C. A., and So, M.: Type IV pili of pathogenic *Neisseriae* elicit cortical plaque formation in epithelial cells. Mol. Microbiol. *32*:1316-1332, 1999.
220. Merz, A. J., and So, M.: Attachment of piliated, Opa⁻ and Opc⁻ gonococci and meningococci to epithelial cells elicits cortical actin rearrangements and clustering of tyrosine-phosphorylated proteins. Infect. Immun. *65*:4341-4349, 1997.
221. Merz, A. J., and So, M.: Interactions of pathogenic *Neisseriae* with epithelial cell membranes. Annu. Rev. Cell Dev. Biol. *16*:423-457, 2000.
222. Merz, A. J., So, M., and Sheetz, M. P.: Pilus retraction powers bacterial twitching motility. Nature *407*:98-102, 2000.
223. Meyer, T. F., Billyard, E., Haas, R., et al.: Pilus genes of *Neisseria gonorrhoeae*: Chromosomal organization and DNA sequence. Proc. Natl. Acad. Sci. U. S. A. *81*:6110-6114, 1984.
224. Meyer, T. F., Mlawer, N., and So, M.: Pilus expression in *Neisseria gonorrhoeae* involves chromosomal rearrangement. Cell *30*:45-52, 1982.
225. Mirrett, S., Reller, L. B., and Knapp, J. S.: *Neisseria gonorrhoeae* strains inhibited by vancomycin in selective media and correlation with auxotype. J. Clin. Microbiol. *14*:94-99, 1981.
226. Morello, J. A., Lerner, S. A., and Bohnhoff, M.: Characteristics of atypical *Neisseria gonorrhoeae* from disseminated and localized infections. Infect. Immun. *13*:1510-1516, 1976.
227. Morris, S. R., Klausner, J. D., Buchbinder, S. P., et al.: Prevalence and incidence of pharyngeal gonorrhea in a longitudinal sample of men who have sex with men: The EXPLORE study. Clin. Infect. Dis. *43*:1284-1289, 2006.
228. Morse, S. A., Johnson, S. R., Biddle, J. W., and Roberts, M. C.: High-level tetracycline resistance in *Neisseria gonorrhoeae* is result of acquisition of streptococcal term determinant. Antimicrob. Agents Chemother. *30*:664-670, 1986.
229. Morton, R. S. (ed.): Gonorrhoea. Vol. 9. *In* Major Problems in Dermatology. Philadelphia, W. B. Saunders, 1977.
230. Mosleh, I. M., Huber, L. A., Steinlein, P., et al.: *Neisseria gonorrhoeae* porin modulates phagosome maturation. J. Biol. Chem. *273*:35332-35338, 1998.
231. Mueller, B. A., Luz-Jimenez, M., Daling, J. R., et al.: Risk factors for tubal infertility. Sex. Transm. Dis. *19*:28-34, 1992.
232. Mulcahy, F. M., and Lacey, C. J. N.: Sexually transmitted infections in adolescent girls. Genitourin. Med. *63*:119-121, 1987.
233. Muller, A., Gunther, D., Brinkmann, V., et al.: Targeting of the pro-apoptotic VDAC-like porin (PorB) of *Neisseria gonorrhoeae* to mitochondria of infected cells. E. M. B. O. J. *19*:5332-5343, 2000.
234. Muller, A., Gunther, D., Dux, F., et al.: Neisserial porin (PorB) causes rapid calcium influx in target cells and induces apoptosis by the activation of cysteine proteases. E. M. B. O. J. *18*:339-352, 1999.
235. Muram, D., Speck, P. M, and Dockter, M.: Child sexual abuse examination: Is there a need for routine screening for *N. gonorrhoeae*? J. Pediatr. Adolesc. Gynecol. *9*:79-80, 1996.
236. Murray, E. S. Bentan, M. J., Coppola, S. R., et al.: New options for diagnosis and control of gonorrheal urethritis in males using uncentrifuged first voided urine (FVU) as a specimen for culture. Am. J. Public Health *69*:596-598, 1979.
237. Naumann, M., Rudel, T., and Meyer, T. F.: Host cell interactions and signaling with *Neisseria gonorrhoeae*. Curr. Opin. Microbiol. *2*:62-70, 1999.
238. Naumann, M., Wessler, S., Bartsch, C., et al.: *Neisseria gonorrhoeae* epithelial cell interaction leads to the activation of the transcription factors nuclear factor κB and activator protein 1 and the induction of inflammatory cytokines. J. Exp. Med. *186*:247-258, 1997.
239. Neinstein, L. S., Goldenring, J., and Carpenter, S.: Nonsexual transmission of sexually transmitted diseases: An infrequent occurrence. Pediatrics *74*:67-76, 1984.
240. Nelson, J. D., Mohs, E., Dajani, A. S., et al.: Gonorrhea in preschool- and school-age children: Report of the Prepubertal Gonorrhea Cooperative Study Group. J. A. M. A. *236*:1359-1364, 1976.
241. Newman, L. M., Moran, J. S., and Workowski, K. A.: Update on the management of gonorrhea in adults in the United States. Clin. Infect. Dis. *44*:S84-S101, 2007.
242. Ngampasutodol, J., Rice, P. A., Walsh, M. T., and Gulati, S.: Characterization of a peptide vaccine candidate mimicking an oligosaccharide epitope of *Neisseria gonorrhoeae* and resultant immune responses and function. Vaccine. *24*:157-170, 2006.
243. Nicolson, I. J., Perry, A. C., Virji, M., et al.: Localization of antibody-binding sites by sequence analysis of cloned pilin genes from *Neisseria gonorrhoeae*. J. Gen. Microbiol. *133*:825-833, 1987.
244. Noegel, A., and Gotschlich, E. C.: Isolation of a high molecular weight polyphosphate from *Neisseria gonorrhoeae*. J. Exp. Med. *157*:2049-2060, 1983.
245. Nsuami, M., Cammarata, C. L., Brooks, B. N., et al.: Chlamydia and gonorrhea co-occurrence in a high school population. Sex. Transm. Dis. *31*:424-427, 2004.
246. O'Brien, J. P., Goldenberg, D. L., and Rice, P. A.: Disseminated gonococcal infection: A prospective analysis of 49 patients and a review of pathophysiology and immune mechanisms. Medicine (Baltimore) *2*:395-406, 1983.
247. O'Reilly, R. J., Lee, L., and Welch, B. G.: Secretory IgA antibody responses to *Neisseria gonorrhoeae* in the genital secretions of infected females. J. Infect. Dis. *133*:113-125, 1976.
248. Oriel, J. D.: Ophthalmia neonatorum: Relative efficacy of current prophylactic practices and treatment. J. Antimicrob. Chemother. *14*:209-220, 1984.
249. Orr, D. P., and Preitto, S. V.: Emergency management of sexually abused children: The role of the pediatric resident. Am. J. Dis. Child. *133*:628-631, 1979.
250. Osborne, N. G., and Grubin, L.: Colonization of the pharynx with *Neisseria gonorrhoeae*. Sex. Transm. Dis. *6*:253-256, 1979.
251. Palusci, V. J., and Reeves, M. J.: Testing for genital gonorrhea infections in prepubertal girls with suspected sexual abuse. Pediatr. Infect. Dis. J. *22*:618-623, 2003.
252. Panke, E. S., Yang, L. I., Leist, P. A., et al.: Comparison of Gen-Probe DNA probe test and culture for the detection of *N. gonorrhoeae* in endocervical specimens. J. Clin. Microbiol. *29*:883-888, 1991.
253. Pasquariello, C. A., Plotkin, S. A., Rice, R. J., et al.: Fatal gonococcal septicemia. Pediatr. Infect. Dis. *4*:204-206, 1985.
254. Patamasucon, P., Rettig, P. J., and Nelson, J. D.: Cefuroxime therapy of gonorrhea and co-infection with *Chlamydia trachomatis* in children. Pediatrics *68*:534-538, 1981.
255. Pelouze, P. S.: Gonorrhea in the Male and Female. Philadelphia, W. B. Saunders, 1941.
256. Peralta, L., Durako, S. J., Ma, Y., et al.: Correlation between urine and cervical specimens for the detection of cervical *Chlamydia trachomatis* and *Neisseria gon-*

orrhoeae using ligase chain reaction in a cohort of HIV infected and uninfected adolescents. J. Adolesc. Health 29(Suppl.):87-92, 2001.

257. Perrin, A., Nassif, X., and Tinsley, C.: Identification of regions of the chromosome of *Neisseria meningitidis* and *Neisseria gonorrhoeae* which are specific to the pathogenic *Neisseria* species. Infect. Immun. 67:6119-6129, 1999.

258. Phillips, L.: P-lactamase–producing penicillin-resistant gonococcus. Lancet 2:656, 1976.

259. Plant, L. J., and Jonsson, A. B.: Type IV pili of *Neisseria gonorrhoeae* influence the activation of human CD4⁺ T cells. Infect. Immun. 74:442-448, 2006.

260. Plavidal, F. J., and Werch, A.: Fetal scalp abscess secondary to intrauterine monitoring. Am. J. Obstet. Gynecol. 125:65-68, 1976.

261. Podgore, J. K., and Holmes, K. K.: Ocular gonococcal infection with minimal or no inflammatory response. J. A. M. A. 246:242-243, 1981.

262. Poh, C. L., Khng, H. P., Lim, C. K., and Loh, G. K.: Molecular typing of *Neisseria gonorrhoeae* by restriction fragment length polymorphisms. Genitourin. Med. 68:106-110, 1992.

263. Poh, C. L., Ramachandran, V., and Tapsall, J.: Genetic diversity of *Neisseria gonorrhoeae* IB-2 and IB-6 isolates revealed by whole-cell repetitive element sequence-based PCR. J. Clin. Microbiol. 34:292-295, 1996.

264. Price, G. A., Hobbs, M. M., and Cornelissen, C. N.: Immunogenicity of gonococcal transferrin proteins during natural infections. Infect. Immun. 72:277-283, 2004.

265. Ram, S., Gulati, S., McQuillen, D. P., et al.: Interactions between *Neisseria gonorrhoeae* and C4b-binding protein: A molecular basis for gonococcal serum resistance. Abstract. Mol. Immunol. 36:297, 1999.

266. Ramsey, K. H., Schneider, H., Cross, A. S., et al.: Inflammatory cytokines produced in response to experimental human gonorrhea. J. Infect. Dis. 172:186-191, 1995.

267. Ramus, R. M., Sheffield, J. S., Mayfield, J. A., and Wendel, G. D.: A randomized trial that compared oral cefixime and intramuscular ceftriaxone for the treatment of gonorrhea in pregnancy. Am. J. Obstet. Gynecol. 185:629-632, 2001.

268. Rawstrom, S. A., Hammerschlag, M. R., Gullans, C., et al.: Ceftriaxone treatment of penicillinase-producing *Neisseria gonorrhoeae* infections in children. Pediatr. Infect. Dis. 8:445-448, 1989.

269. Rees E.: Gonococcal bartholinitis. Br. J. Vener. Dis. 43:150-156, 1967.

270. Reichart, C. A., Rupkey, L. M., Brady, W. E., and Hook, E. W., 3rd: Comparison of GC-Lect and modified Thayer-Martin media for isolation of *Neisseria gonorrhoeae*. J. Clin. Microbiol. 27:808-811, 1989.

271. Rettig, P. J., and Nelson, J. D.: Genital tract infection with *Chlamydia trachomatis* in prepubertal children. J. Pediatr. 99:206-210, 1981.

272. Rice, P. A., and Kasper, D. L.: Characterization of serum resistance of *Neisseria gonorrhoeae* that disseminate: Roles of blocking antibody in gonococcal outer membrane protein. J. Clin. Invest. 70:157-167, 1982.

273. Rice, P. A., McCormack, W. M., and Kasper, D. L.: Natural serum bactericidal activity against *N. gonorrhoeae* isolates from disseminated, locally invasive, and uncomplicated disease. J. Immunol. 124:2105-2109, 1980.

274. Rice, P. A., McQuillen, D. P., Gulati, S., et al.: Serum resistance of *Neisseria gonorrhoeae*. Does it thwart the inflammatory response and facilitate the transmission of infection? Ann. N. Y. Acad. Sci. 730:7-14, 1994.

275. Rice, P. A., Vayo, H. E., Tam, M. R., and Blake, M. S.: Immunoglobulin G antibodies directed against protein III block killing of serum-resistant *Neisseria gonorrhoeae* by immune serum. J. Exp. Med. 164:1735-1748, 1986.

276. Rice, R. J., Aral, S. O., Blount, J. H., et al.: Gonorrhea in the United States 1975-1989: Is the giant only sleeping? Sex. Transm. Dis. 14:83-87, 1987.

277. Rimsza, M. E., and Niggemann, E. H.: Medical evaluation of sexually abused children: A review of 311 cases. Pediatrics 69:8-14, 1982.

278. Ris, H. W., and Dodge, R. W.: Gonorrhea in adolescent girls in a closed population: Prevalence, diagnosis and treatment. Am. J. Dis. Child. 123:185, 1972.

279. Roberts, M., and Falkow, S.: Conjugal transfer of R plasmids in *Neisseria gonorrhoeae*. Nature 266:630-631, 1977.

280. Rothbard, M. J., Gregory, T., and Salerno, L. J.: Intrapartum gonococcal amnionitis. Am. J. Obstet. Gynecol. 121:565-566, 1975.

281. Rothenberg, R.: Ophthalmia neonatorum due to *Neisseria gonorrhoeae*: Prevention and treatment. Sex. Transm. Dis. 6(Suppl. 2):187-191, 1979.

282. Rothenberg, R. B., Simon, R., Chipperfield, E., and Catterall, R. D.: Efficacy of selected diagnostic tests for sexually transmitted diseases. J. A. M. A. 235:49-51, 1976.

283. Rudel, T., Scheurerpflug, I., and Meyer, T. F.: *Neisseria* PilC protein identified as type-4 pilus tip–located adhesin. Nature 373:357-359, 1995.

284. Russell, D. E. H.: The incidence and prevalence of intrafamilial and extrafamilial sexual abuse of female children. Child Abuse Negl. 7:133-142, 1983.

285. Rytkönen, A., Johansson, L., Asp, V., et al.: Soluble pilin of *Neisseria gonorrhoeae* interacts with human target cells and tissue. Infect. Immun. 69:6419-6426, 2001.

286. Sanders, J. M., Brookman, R. R., Brown, R. C., et al.: Committee on Adolescence: Role of the pediatrician in management of sexually transmitted diseases in children and adolescents. Pediatrics 79:454-456, 1987.

287. Sandstrom, E., and Danielsson, D.: A Survey of gonococcal serology. *In* Danielsson, D., Juhlin, L., and MPrdh, P.-A.: (eds.): Genital Infections and Their Complications. Stockholm, Almqvist & Wiksell, 1975, p. 253.

288. Sandström, E. G., and Danielsson, D.: Serology of *Neisseria gonorrhoeae*: Classification by coagglutination. Acta Pathol. Microbiol. Scand. 88:27-38, 1980.

289. Sandström, E. G., Knapp, J. S., and Buchanan, T. M.: Serology of *Neisseria gonorrhoeae*: W-antigen serogrouping by coagglutination and protein I serotyping by enzyme-linked immunosorbent assay both detect protein I antigens. Infect. Immun. 35:229-239, 1982.

290. Sarrel, P. M., and Pruett, K. A.: Symptomatic gonorrhea during pregnancy. Obstet. Gynecol. 32:670-673, 1968.

291. Sarubbi, F. A., Jr., and Sparling, P. F.: Transfer of antibiotic resistance in mixed cultures of *Neisseria gonorrhoeae*. J. Infect. Dis. 130:660-663, 1974.

292. Segal, E., Hagblom, P., Seifert, H. S., and So, M.: Antigenic variation of gonococcal pilus involves assembly of separated silent gene segments. Proc. Natl. Acad. Sci. U. S. A. 83:2177-2181, 1986.

293. Seifert, H. S., Wright, C. J., Jerse, A. E., et al.: Multiple gonococcal pilin antigenic variants are produced during experimental human infections. J. Clin. Invest. 93:2744-2749, 1994.

294. Shafer, M.-A. B., Irwin, C. E., and Sweet, R. L.: Acute salpingitis in the adolescent female. J. Pediatr. 100:339-350, 1982.

295. Shafer, W. M., Joiner, K., Guymon, L. F., et al.: Serum sensitivity of *Neisseria gonorrhoeae*: The role of lipopolysaccharide. J. Infect. Dis. 149:175-183, 1984.

296. Shafer, W., Onunka, V. C., and Martin, L. E.: Antigonococcal activity of human neutrophil cathepsin G. Infect. Immun. 54:184-188, 1986.

297. Shapiro, R. A., Schubert, C. J., and Siegel, R. M.: *Neisseria gonorrhea* infections in girls younger than 12 years of age evaluated for vaginitis. Pediatrics 104:e72, 1999.

298. Shinners, E. N., and Catlin, B. W.: Arginine and pyrimidine biosynthetic defects in *Neisseria gonorrhoeae* strains isolated from patients. J. Bacteriol. 151:295-302, 1982.

299. Sicoli, R. A., Losek, J. D., Hudlett, J. M., et al.: Indications for *Neisseria gonorrhoeae* cultures in children with suspected sexual abuse. Arch. Pediatr. Adolesc. Med. 149:86-89, 1995.

300. Siegel, R. M., Schubert, C. J., Myers, P. A., and Shapiro, R. A.: The prevalence of sexually transmitted diseases in children and adolescents evaluated for sexual abuse in Cincinnati: Rationale for limited STD testing in prepubertal girls. Pediatrics 96:1090-1094, 1995.

301. Silber, T. J., and Controni, G.: Clinical spectrum of pharyngeal gonorrhea in children and adolescents: A report of sixteen patients. J. Adolesc. Health Care 4:51-54, 1983.

302. Singer, A.: The uterine cervix from adolescence to the menopause. Br. J. Obstet. Gynaecol. 82:81-99, 1975.

303. Smith, A. L.: Principles of Microbiology. 10th ed. St. Louis, Mirror/Mosby, 1985.

304. Smith, J. A.: Ophthalmia neonatorum in Glasgow. Scott. Med. J. 14:272-279, 1969.

305. Smith, K., Harrington, K., Wingood, G., et al.: Self-obtained vaginal swabs for diagnosis of treatable sexually transmitted diseases in adolescent girls. Arch. Pediatr. Adolesc. Med. 155:676-679, 2001.

306. Smith, K. R., Ching, S., Lee, H., et al.: Evaluation of ligase chain reaction for use with urine for identification of *Neisseria gonorrhoeae* in females attending a sexually transmitted disease clinic. J. Clin. Microbiol. 33:455-457, 1995.

307. Snowe, R. J., and Wilfert, C. M.: Epidemic reappearance of gonococcal ophthalmia neonatorum. Pediatrics 57:110-114, 1973.

308. Sparling, P. F.: Biology of *Neisseria gonorrhoeae*. *In* Holmes, K. K., Mårdh, P. A., Sparling, P. F., et al. (eds.): Sexually Transmitted Diseases. 3rd ed. New York, McGraw-Hill, 1999.

309. Sparling, P. F., Cannon, J. G., and So, M.: Phase and antigenic variation of pili and outer membrane protein II of *Neisseria gonorrhoeae*. J. Infect. Dis. 153:196-201, 1986.

310. Sparling, P. F., and Yobs, A. R.: Colonial morphology of *Neisseria gonorrhoeae* isolated from males and females. J. Bacteriol. 93:513, 1967.

311. Speck, W. T., and Lawsky, A. R.: Symptomatic anorectal gonorrhea in an adolescent female. Am. J. Dis. Child. 122:438-439, 1971.

312. Spence, J. M., Tyler, R. E., Domaoal, R. A., et al.: L12 enhances gonococcal transcytosis of polarized Hec1B cells via the lutropin receptor. Microb. Pathog. 32:117-125, 2002.

313. Stern, A., Brown, M., Nickel, P., and Meyer, T. F.: Opacity genes in *Neisseria gonorrhoeae*: Control of phase and antigenic variation. Cell 47:61-71, 1986.

314. Stern, A., and Meyer, T. F.: Common mechanism controlling phase and antigenic variation in pathogenic *Neisseria*. Mol. Microbiol. 1:5-12, 1987.

315. Stern, A., Nickel, P., Meyer, T. F., and So, M.: Opacity determinants of *Neisseria gonorrhoeae*: Gene expression and chromosomal linkage to the gonococcal pilus gene. Cell 37:447-456, 1984.

316. Stone, K. M., Grimes, D. A., and Magder, L. S.: Personal protection against sexually transmitted diseases. Am. J. Obstet. Gynecol. 155:180-188, 1986.

317. Sullivan, K. M., MacDonald, H. J., and Saunders, J. R.: Characterization of DNA restriction and modification activities in *Neisseria* species. F. E. M. S. Microbiol. Lett. 44:389-393, 1987.

318. Swanson, J.: Studies on gonococcus infection: XIV. Cell wall protein differences among color/opacity colony variants of *Neisseria gonorrhoeae*. Infect. Immun. 21:292, 1978.

319. Swanson, J.: Colony opacity and protein II compositions of gonococci. Infect. Immun. 37:359, 1982.

320. Swanson, J., Robbins, K., Barrera, O., and Koomey, J. M.: Gene conversion variations generate structurally distinct pilin polypeptides in *Neisseria gonorrhoeae*. J. Exp. Med. 165:1016-1025, 1987.

321. Tabrizi, S. N., Paterson, B. A., Fairley, C. K., et al.: Comparison of tampon and urine as self-administered methods of specimen collection in the detec-

tion of *Chlamydia trachomatis*, *Neisseria gonorrhoeae* and *Trichomonas vaginalis* in women. Int. J. S. T. D. A. I. D. S. *9*:347-349, 1998.

322. Thayer, J. D., and Martin, J. E.: Selective medium for the cultivation of *N. gonorrhoeae* and *N. meningitidis*. Public Health Rep. *79*:49, 1964.
323. Tomeh, M. O., and Wilfert, C. M.: Venereal diseases of infants and children at Duke University Medical Center. N. C. Med. J. *34*:109-113, 1973.
324. Upchurch, D. M., Brady, W. E., Reichart, C. A., Hook, E. W., III: Behavioral contributions to acquisition and transmission of *Neisseria gonorrhoeae*. J. Infect. Dis. *161*:938-941, 1990.
325. Van Der Pol, B., Ferrero, D., Barrington, L. B., et al.: Multicenter evaluation of the BDProbe Tec ET system for detection of *Chlamydia trachomatis* and *Neisseria gonorrhoeae* in urine specimens, female endocervical swabs, and male urethral swabs. J. Clin. Microbiol. *39*:1008-1016, 2001.
326. Van Duynhoven, Y. T. H. P.: The epidemiology of *Neisseria gonorrhoeae* in Europe. Microbes Infect. *1*:455-464, 1999.
327. Van Dyck, E., Ieven, M., Pattyn, S., et al.: Detection of *Chlamydia trachomatis* and *Neisseria gonorrhoeae* by enzyme immunoassay, culture, and three nucleic acid amplification tests. J. Clin. Microbiol. *39*:1751-1756, 2001.
328. Van Putten, J. P., Duensing, T. D., and Cole, R. L.: Entry of opaA+ gonococci into Hep-2 cells requires concerted action of glycosaminoglycans, fibronectin and integrin receptors. Mol. Microbiol. *29*:369-379, 1998.
329. Van Putten, J. P. M., and Robertson, B. D.: Molecular mechanisms and implications for infection of lipopolysaccharide variation in *Neisseria*. Mol. Microbiol. *16*:847-853, 1995.
330. Wald, E. R., Woodward, C. L., Marston, G., et al.: Gonorrheal disease among children in a university hospital. Sex. Transm. Dis. *7*:41-43, 1980.
331. Walstad, D. L., Guymon, L. F., and Sparling, P. F.: Altered outer membrane protein in different colonial types of *Neisseria gonorrhoeae*. J. Bacteriol. *129*:1623-1627, 1977.
332. Wehrbein, H. L.: Gonococcus arthritis: A study of six hundred cases. Surg. Gynecol. Obstet. *49*:105-113, 1929.

333. West, S. E. H., and Sparling, P. F.: Response of *Neisseria gonorrhoeae* to iron limitation: Alterations in expression of membrane proteins without apparent siderophore production. Infect. Immun. *47*:388-394, 1985.
334. Wetzler, L. M., Barry, K., Blake, M. S., et al.: Gonococcal lipooligosaccharide sialylation prevents complement-dependent killing by immune sera. Infect. Immun. *60*:39-43, 1992.
335. White, S. T., Loda, F. A., Ingram, D. L., et al.: Sexually transmitted diseases in sexually abused children. Pediatrics *72*:16-21, 1983.
336. Whitley, D. M., Tapsall, J. W., and Sloots, T. P.: Nucleic acid amplification testing for *Neisseria gonorrhoeae*. J. Mol. Diagn. *8*:3-15, 2006.
337. Whittington, W. L., Rice, R. J., Biddle, J. W., et al.: Incorrect identification of *Neisseria gonorrhoeae* from infants and children. Pediatr. Infect. Dis. *7*:3-10, 1988.
338. Wiesner, P. J., Handsfield, H. H., and Holmes, K. K.: Low antibiotic resistance of gonococci causing systemic infection. N. Engl. J. Med. *288*:1221-1222, 1973.
339. Wiesner, P. J., Tronca, E., Bonin, P., et al.: Clinical spectrum of pharyngeal gonococcal infection. N. Engl. J. Med. *288*:181, 1973.
340. William, D. C., Felman, Y. M., and Riccardi, N. B.: The utility of anoscopy in the rapid diagnosis of symptomatic anorectal gonorrhea in men. Sex. Trans. Dis. *8*:16-17, 1981.
341. Woods, C. R., Versalovic, J., Koeuth, T., and Lupski, J. R.: Whole cell rep-PCR allows rapid assessment of clonal relationships of bacterial isolates. J. Clin. Microbiol. *31*:1927-1931, 1993.
342. World Health Organization: Trends in Sexually Transmitted Infections and HIV in the European Region, 1980-2005. Technical Briefing Document 01B/06, Copenhagen, September 12, 2006. Available at *http://www.euro.who.int/Document/RC56/etb01b.pdf* (accessed May 2007).
343. Young, J. D.-E., Blake, M., Mauro, A., and Cohn, Z. A.: Properties of the major outer membrane protein from *Neisseria gonorrhoeae* incorporated into model lipid membranes. Proc. Natl. Acad. Sci. U. S. A. *80*:3831-3835, 1983.

SUBSECTION 3
Gram-Positive Bacilli

DIPHTHERIA
Ralph D. Feigin ◦ Barbara W. Stechenberg ◦ Pratip K. Nag

Diphtheria is an acute infectious disease caused by *Corynebacterium diphtheriae* or, less commonly, *Corynebacterium ulcerans*. *Corynebacterium pseudotuberculosis*, which primarily causes infections in sheep and goats, is not discussed here because it only rarely causes a diphtheria-like disease in humans. Infection by toxigenic strains of *C. diphtheriae* causes disease that is mediated by the production of an extracellular protein. Nontoxigenic strains also can cause disease, but it is usually less severe.

Before the discovery of antitoxin at the turn of the 20th century, the "strangling angel of children," as diphtheria once was called, was a significant cause of mortality in children and adults.[104] Apparent reference to diphtheria can be traced to the 5th century B.C. in the works of Hippocrates, *Epidemics III*, case 7.[74] In 1821, it was recognized as a specific entity by Brettoneau, who suggested that the disease was caused by a germ and that it could be transmitted from person to person. Brettoneau coined the origin of the modern term *diphtheria* from the Greek root *diphthera*, which means "skin" or "hide."[46] In 1883, the causative agent was identified by Klebs in stained smears from diphtheritic membranes; in 1884, Löffler grew the organism on artificial media and showed that in guinea pigs it caused a fatal infection closely resembling human disease.

The toxin was purified in 1889 by Roux and Yersin, who found that toxin alone could cause the disease. Shortly thereafter, Behring and Kitasato discovered antitoxins when they immunized animals with toxins rather than bacteria. The use of antitoxin to treat children with diphtheria at the turn of the 20th century resulted in one of the largest decreases in mortality rates by a therapeutic intervention. In Germany alone, an estimated 45,000 lives were saved each year.[57]

ETIOLOGY

Corynebacteria (Klebs-Löffler bacilli) are irregularly staining, gram-positive, nonmotile, nonsporulating, pleomorphic bacilli.[49] The club-shaped appearance of the bacillus is not a true morphologic feature, but results from attempting to grow the bacillus on media that are nutritionally inadequate (Löffler media). The organism can be recovered most readily on media containing selective inhibitors that retard the growth of other microorganisms; a sheep blood agar–based medium containing fosfomycin (for selectivity) and Tindale medium (tellurite medium with cystine) are ideal.[39,40] *C. diphtheriae* and *C. ulcerans* grow on supplement-free blood agar, chocolate agar, and other standard media.[39]

Colonies of *C. diphtheriae* (with the exception of the lipophilic, gray *intermedius*) and *C. ulcerans* appear grayish white on Löffler medium. On tellurite medium, three diphtheria colony types can be distinguished: *mitis, gravis,* and *intermedius. Mitis* colonies are smooth, black, and convex; they do not ferment starch or glycogen and are hemolytic. *Gravis* colonies are gray, radially striate, and semirough; they ferment starch and glycogen and usually are not hemolytic. *Intermedius* colonies are small and smooth and have a black center; they do not ferment starch or glycogen and are not hemolytic. *C. ulcerans* colonies resemble *gravis* on Tindale medium but differ in that they are hemolytic. Similar to *gravis,* they ferment starch and glycogen. All diphtheria biotypes and *C. ulcerans* are characterized by cystinase activity and absence of pyrazinamidase activity. *C. ulcerans* may be distinguished from *C. diphtheriae* by its urease activity and ability to liquefy gelatin. Biotype *belfanti,* which does not occur in a toxigenic form, may be distinguished from the three potentially toxigenic diphtheria biotypes by its inability to reduce nitrate on Tindale medium and from *C. ulcerans* by its lack of production of urease.[39] Ribotyping and pulsed-field gel electrophoresis, both of which involve restriction digestion of genomic bacterial DNA followed by gel electrophoresis and Southern blotting, permit more specific typing within each diphtheria biotype and aid in the epidemiologic study of outbreaks.[36,91]

C. diphtheriae biotypes *intermedius, gravis,* and *mitis* and *C. ulcerans* all have been observed in a toxigenic form. *Intermedius* was the biotype isolated most commonly in the United States between 1971 and 1981. Of the strains isolated, *intermedius* was found to be toxigenic more often than was either *mitis* or *gravis.*[31] In the United Kingdom between 1993 and 1998, and similarly in other parts of Europe, the biovar *gravis* has represented most nontoxigenic isolates, followed by *mitis* and *belfanti.*[40] Of the four nontoxigenic isolates obtained during a surveillance study of a U.S. Northern Plains Native American Community in 1996, two were of biotype *mitis,* and two were *gravis.*[54] According to a United Kingdom diphtheria reference laboratory, between 1993 and 1998, the toxigenic isolates originating from Asia, Africa, and the Middle East were reported to be of the biotype *mitis* or *gravis,* with the exception of one *intermedius* isolate.[40] Golaz and associates[54] reported similar findings when they surveyed the different biotypes in South Dakota. A significant overall increase in the proportion of nontoxigenic isolates has been observed in Europe and Australia in recent years.[52] The reason for this increase is unclear, but one hypothesis is that increased immunity to toxigenic strains secondary to immunization has altered this epidemiology.

The complete genome sequence of *C. diphtheriae* biotype *gravis* has been elucidated.[28] The genome is approximately 2.48 Mb with a G+C content of 53 percent and has approximately 2320 predicted coding sequences. Metabolic analysis of the genome has revealed that *C. diphtheriae* has a complete set of enzymes for glycolysis, gluconeogenesis, pentose-phosphate pathways, anaerobic and aerobic respiration, amino acid biosynthesis, and purine nucleotide biosynthetic pathway. Most of the enzymes for the tricarboxylic acid cycle are present with the exception of an enzyme succinyl–coenzyme A (CoA) synthetase that catalyzes the conversion of succinate to succinyl-CoA. An alternative enzyme present in *C. diphtheriae* may fulfill this conversion, however. The pyrimidine pathway in *C. diphtheriae* lacks an enzyme that interferes with the production of cytidine; the pathway to the biosynthesis of thymidine is complete. The genome has revealed 13 regions that are unique to *C. diphtheriae* and may serve as pathogenicity islands.[28]

No functional or significant differences have been detected in the exotoxins elaborated by the three strains of *C. diphtheriae* or by *C. ulcerans.* Only strains that are lysogenic for beta-prophage or a closely related phage carrying the gene for toxin production produce diphtheria toxin. One or more *tox* gene sequences may exist in the bacterial genome, and the most highly toxigenic strains contain three or more copies.[77] Phage multiplication is not a prerequisite for the production of toxin. The capacity to synthesize toxin depends on genetic and nutritional factors. Toxin-producing cells apparently are cells in which spontaneous induction of the prophage to the phage occurs.[48] The most important factor controlling the yield of toxin is the concentration of inorganic iron in the culture medium.[34] Growth of *C. diphtheriae* in iron-deficient media prolongs the duration of induction lysis and is associated with a high yield of toxin. High concentrations of iron inhibit the production of toxin. Production of toxin also can be increased by the use of ultraviolet radiation. Conversion to a toxigenic strain occurs in nature, as has been shown by restriction enzyme studies of carriers of toxigenic and nontoxigenic strains in Manchester, England.

The ability of a strain of *C. diphtheriae* to elaborate diphtheria toxin can be shown by using several methods. In vivo studies involving necrosis of tissue in guinea pigs has been replaced by the widely used Elek[42] or modified Elek test.[45] Enzyme immunoassay[44] and polymerase chain reaction (PCR)[90] have been used to detect toxigenicity.

Diphtheria toxin is lethal to humans in an amount of approximately 130 µg/kg body weight. Cytoplasmic internalization of one molecule of toxin has been shown to cause cell death.[11] Toxigenic and nontoxigenic strains of *C. diphtheriae* can cause disease, but only strains that produce toxin cause disease with symptoms of myocarditis and neuritis.

EPIDEMIOLOGY

Asymptomatic human carriers serve as the reservoir for *C. diphtheriae.* Infection by *C. diphtheriae* is acquired by contact with either a carrier or an individual with active disease. The bacteria may be transmitted via droplets during coughing, sneezing, or talking. Rarely, transmission of *C. diphtheriae* occurs from skin lesions or fomites. Some reports suggest that skin carriers of *C. diphtheriae* are more infectious than are either nose or throat carriers and that skin carriers may serve as potential reservoirs for the initiation of epidemic spread.[12,63] In areas in which skin infections are endemic, levels of natural immunization may be high.[21] This phenomenon is illustrated particularly well in a survey of tetanus and diphtheria immunity in a rural Kenyan community, where age was not found to be predictive of immunity and no correlation was found between levels of antibody for tetanus and diphtheria.[72]

Person-to-person transmission of *C. ulcerans* is not known to occur, although *C. ulcerans* was isolated from the siblings of two patients reported in the United Kingdom between 1995 and 1997.[18] Cases of respiratory diphtheria caused by *C. diphtheriae* and by *C. ulcerans* have been documented in association with contaminated unpasteurized milk taken from cows with infected teats.[19,55,101] *C. diphtheriae* has been isolated from horses, dogs, and other domestic animals. *C. ulcerans* has been reported to infect ground squirrels in the United States, but transmission to humans has not been reported.[62,89]

According to World Health Organization reports, diphtheria is distributed worldwide and remains endemic in many developing areas of the world, including Asia, Africa, South America, and the Mediterranean regions.[20] Worldwide, diphtheria epidemics have occurred in a cyclical manner since the 16th century. The most recent epidemic began in 1990 in the Russian Federation, Ukraine, and the other newly independent states of the former Soviet Union.[23,103]

In the United States, the incidence and mortality rates from diphtheria in the 1920s were 140 to 150 cases per 100,000, with

13,000 to 15,000 deaths each year. The number of cases gradually declined to 15 per 100,000 population in 1945 with the extensive use of diphtheria toxoid vaccine. From 1970 through 1979, the average number of cases of diphtheria reported annually in the United States was 196.[8] From 1980 to 2004, only 57 cases of diphtheria were reported in the United States. Approximately 75 percent of the cases were in patients older than 15 years who were unimmunized or inadequately immunized.[8] From 1980 to 1995, only four fatal cases involving diphtheria and unimmunized children were reported.[14,83,92] In 1996, C. diphtheriae was isolated from a Native American population in South Dakota.[54] Only five cases of diphtheria have been reported since 2000. Maintenance of immunity in adults requires a booster vaccination every 10 years. The Centers for Disease Control and Prevention estimated in the mid-1990s that less than 50 percent of adults in the United States had received their 10-year boosters and that 40 to 50 percent of adults were susceptible to diphtheria.[81,92] In addition, the toxoid vaccine does not provide any protection against nontoxigenic strains.

The incidence peaks during the cooler autumn, winter, and spring months. Several epidemics, primarily in the southern United States, have occurred in late summer and fall and corresponded to a high prevalence of C. diphtheriae skin infections. Between the years 1971 and 1981, the incidence of diphtheria was highest in the western United States. A 100-fold greater incidence of diphtheria occurs in Native Americans than in the general population.[31] This difference may be attributable to socioeconomic factors more than to race.

Evidence that diphtheria is diagnosed more frequently in chronic alcoholics and the indigent than in the general population is significant. In a 1993-1994 outbreak in St. Petersburg, Russia, 69 percent of a total of 42 deaths occurred in individuals classified as chronic alcoholics.[94] Between 1972 and 1982, three outbreaks occurred in the indigent alcoholic population living in Seattle's Skid Road.[61] Cutaneous infections accounted for 86 percent of the 1100 total cases. The first outbreak was caused by a single toxigenic *intermedius* biotype clone, whereas the other two involved nontoxigenic *mitis* and *gravis* strains. The incidence was highest in winter and spring.

Native Americans also represent a disproportionate number of diphtheria cases, the reasons for which are unclear, but apparently infection is endemic in some closely knit communities. During 1974 and 1975, 27 percent of Native Americans in the Skid Road population were affected, compared with 5 percent of the white population. In 1996, a surveillance study was conducted in a Northern Plains American Indian community after C. diphtheriae was isolated from the skin of a resident of the community. The woman was a chronic alcoholic admitted to the hospital for detoxification and treatment of severe necrotizing leg ulcers, from which a toxigenic *mitis* biotype was isolated. In the following 4 months, 11 positive cultures were obtained from the community: 6 pharyngeal isolates from patients with pharyngitis, 1 ear isolate from a patient with suppurative otitis media, and 4 positive throat swabs from asymptomatic household contacts of the index cases. Of the 11 total isolates, 6 were biotype *mitis* and 5 were *gravis*; 9 isolates were toxigenic or weakly so. The two nontoxigenic isolates were biotype *gravis*. Ribotyping indicated that the isolates were related closely to each other genetically and to strains obtained from past cases from the same area; they were different from organisms obtained from other parts of the United States and from the former Soviet Union, where an ongoing epidemic was occurring at the time.[54,102]

A similar study was conducted in a Koorie (Aborigine) community in Victoria, Australia, in 1994, after three cases of nontoxigenic C. diphtheriae endocarditis were diagnosed in the community. After screening 359 asymptomatic (with the exception of 4 people who had chronic skin ulcers swabbed) contacts of the index cases, 12 produced positive cultures for nontoxigenic

C. diphtheriae. Five of them were of the same biovar *gravis* clone as the three index cases.[64]

A major epidemic began in 1990 in the new independent states of the former Soviet Union and spread throughout the area. Between 1990 and 1997, approximately 150,000 cases of diphtheria were reported, with approximately 4000 fatalities.[60,91] The epidemic was attributed to decreasing immunization rates and immunity in adults and children and to movement of large numbers of people during the collapse of the former Soviet Union.[23,103] Apparently multiple foci of infection existed across the continent. Most of the epidemic isolates from Ukraine and Russia were biotype *gravis*, but further molecular characterization of the *tox* genes from these areas revealed distinct epidemic strains in each location.[65] Superimposed over the steady increase in the number of cases from 1990 through 1994, a seasonal variation typical of the Northern Hemisphere also was observed, with a significant peak in the number of diagnoses occurring in October and November and a trough from April to July.[60]

A mass immunization program was initiated in Russia in 1993, with a resultant 10 percent decrease in the number of new cases reported between 1994 and 1995 (versus twofold to threefold increases in the number of cases each year for the preceding 3 years).[52] The World Health Organization also held training workshops and assembled laboratory kits to assist in establishing the proper diagnosis of diphtheria. As cases also began to appear in Europe with increasing frequency during this period, the European Working Group on Diphtheria (ELWGD) and reference laboratories were assembled to assist in an effort to increase routine screening for diphtheria. The ELWGD since has expanded and currently includes 20 participating countries, including representatives in Western and Eastern Europe, the United States, Australia, and Southeast Asia.[41]

PATHOGENESIS AND PATHOLOGY

Diphtheria is initiated by entry of C. diphtheriae into the nose or mouth, where the bacilli remain localized on the mucosal surfaces of the upper respiratory tract. Occasionally, the ocular or genital mucous membranes serve as the site of localization. The bacilli are unable to invade intact skin but may infect preexisting skin lesions. After a 2- to 4-day period of incubation, lysogenized strains may elaborate toxin.

Diphtheria toxin is secreted as a single polypeptide of 535 amino acids with a molecular weight of 58,342 D.[65] The toxin is composed of two subunits: a large B subunit that is involved in receptor binding and an A subunit that is the enzymatically active portion of the toxin. The toxin initially is absorbed onto the target cell membrane by binding a receptor on the cell surface and then undergoes receptor-mediated endocytosis. When it is in the endolysosomal complex, it undergoes a conformational change with subsequent release of the A subunit into the cytoplasm. The A subunit transfers an adenosine diphosphate (ADP)–ribosyl group from nicotinamide adenine dinucleotide (NAD) to elongation factor 2. This ADP-ribosylation inactivates elongation factor 2 and inhibits protein synthesis in the cell. Cholera and pertussis toxins also mediate target protein ribosylation by this mechanism. In addition to the inhibition of cellular protein synthesis, an independent mechanism of cytolysis has been described. In the presence of calcium and magnesium, diphtheria toxin has a nuclease-like activity that causes DNA fragmentation that results in cytolysis.[29,30,65,73]

Marked toxin-mediated tissue necrosis occurs in the vicinity of C. diphtheriae colonization and induces a robust local inflammatory response. The inflammatory response coupled with the necrotic tissue produces a patchy exudate that initially can be removed. As the infection progresses, the increased production of toxin causes a centrifugal widening of the area of infection, and eventually a fibrinous exudate develops. A tough adherent membrane results from coagulation of the exudate. The color of the pseudomembrane initially is white but over the course of time becomes dirty gray. Late in the course of the infection, green or black spots appear on the membrane, representing areas of necrosis. Histologic analysis of the pseudomembrane differs, based on the site of formation and maturation of the membrane. Analysis of the pharyngeal pseudomembrane shows fibrin; inflammatory cells, primarily composed of neutrophils, red blood cells, and colonies of organisms; and superficial epithelial cells.

With severe infections, significant vascular congestion, interstitial edema, fibrin exudate, and intense neutrophilic infiltration develop.[59] Profuse bleeding can occur when the membrane is torn off. The edematous tissue and the diphtheritic membrane may encroach on the airway. The membrane sloughs spontaneously during the recovery period, although sloughing can occur during the acute phase of the illness, leading to aspiration. Occasionally, secondary bacterial infection (classically caused by *Streptococcus pyogenes*) develops. Respiratory embarrassment or suffocation may occur, with involvement of the larynx or tracheobronchial tree. Bronchopneumonia may develop if the exudate enters the small airways and alveoli. Infection of these sites is an uncommon occurrence, however. Infections of the esophagus and stomach, with pseudomembranous lesions indistinguishable from lesions found in the respiratory tract, have been reported.[67]

Toxin produced at the site of infection is distributed throughout the body via the bloodstream and the lymphatics. This distribution occurs most readily when the pharynx and tonsils are covered by a diphtheritic membrane. Any organ or tissue can be damaged as a result of diphtheria toxin, but lesions of the heart, nervous system, and kidneys are particularly prominent. Clinical manifestations appear after a variable latent period of 10 to 14 days for myocarditis and 3 to 7 weeks for manifestations in the nervous system, such as peripheral neuritis. In a study of 102 patients who died of diphtheria caused by *C. diphtheriae*, the hearts appeared dilated, flabby, and pale, with a characteristic "streaky" appearance in the myocardium. The most prominent pathologic findings are necrosis and hyaline degeneration of the myocardium. The myocardium also appears edematous and is infiltrated with mononuclear cells with eosinophilic cytoplasm. In a significant proportion of cases, fatty accumulation in muscle fibers and the conducting system may be observed.[86] Burch and associates[22] showed mitochondrial damage with depletion of glycogen and accumulation of lipid droplets in the damaged myofibrils. Toxin may be observed within the myocardial cells with fluorescent antibody staining.[59] If the patient survives, muscle regeneration and interstitial fibrosis can be seen.

Peripheral neuropathy occurs secondary to *C. diphtheriae* infections. Histologic studies have shown that affected nerves have significant degeneration of myelin sheaths and axons. A toxic neuritis with fatty degeneration of paranodal myelin can be noted early in the disease course; segmental demyelination occurs later.[9] Axonal damage is secondary to the application of external pressure from the swollen Schwann cell cytoplasm and myelin.[76]

C. diphtheriae infections also can lead to necrosis and hyaline degeneration of the liver, which can lead to hypoglycemia. Adrenal hemorrhage and acute tubular necrosis of the kidney also have been known to occur secondary to *C. diphtheriae* infections.[59]

CLINICAL MANIFESTATIONS

The signs and symptoms of diphtheria depend on the site of infection, the immunization status of the host, and whether toxin has been distributed to the systemic circulation. The incubation period is 1 to 6 days (range, 1 to 10 days). Diphtheria can be classified clinically on the basis of the anatomic location of the initial infection and the diphtheritic membrane (nasal, pharyngeal/tonsillar, laryngeal or laryngotracheal, skin, and others) involved. More than one anatomic site may be involved simultaneously.

Nasal diphtheria initially resembles a common cold and is characterized by mild rhinorrhea and a paucity of systemic symptoms. Gradually, the nasal discharge becomes serosanguineous and then mucopurulent. A foul odor may be noticed, and careful inspection reveals a white membrane on the nasal septum. In severe cases, the infection may excoriate the nares and upper lip. Nasal diphtheria is a mild form of the disease because absorption of toxin usually is slow from this site. Frequently, delays in establishing an accurate diagnosis of nasal diphtheria occur because of the lack of systemic symptoms. The nasal form of the disease occurs most often in infants.

Pharyngeal and tonsillar diphtheria begin insidiously with anorexia, malaise, low-grade fever, and pharyngitis. Within 1 or 2 days, a membrane appears. The extent of membrane formation correlates with the immune status of the host; in some partially immune individuals, a membrane may not develop. The white or gray adherent membrane may cover the tonsils and pharyngeal walls and extend on to the uvula and soft palate or down on to the larynx and trachea. Attempts to remove the membrane are followed by bleeding. Cervical lymphadenitis varies. In some cases, it is associated with edema of the soft tissues of the neck and may be so severe that it gives the appearance of a "bull neck." In a 1970 epidemic, "erasure" edema of the neck was noted in patients with pharyngeal diphtheria.[80] Patients with erasure edema did not have a classic bull neck appearance, but the edema was characterized by obliteration of the sternocleidomastoid muscle border, the mandible, and the median border of the clavicle. The edema was brawny, pitting, warm to the touch, and tender to palpation. Erasure edema was noted in 29 percent of immunized patients and 30 percent of nonimmunized or inadequately immunized patients. It occurred most commonly in children older than 6 years and generally was associated with infection by the *gravis* or *intermedius* strain of *C. diphtheriae*.

The course of pharyngeal diphtheria depends on the degree of elaboration of the toxin and the extent of the membrane. In severe cases, respiratory and circulatory collapse may occur. The pulse rate is increased disproportionately to body temperature, which generally remains normal or slightly elevated. The palate may be paralyzed. This paralysis may be unilateral or bilateral and associated with difficulty swallowing and nasal regurgitation of swallowed fluids.[37] Stupor, coma, and death may occur within 7 to 10 days. In less severe cases, recovery may be slow and may be complicated by the development of myocarditis or neuritis. In mild cases, the membrane sloughs off in 7 to 10 days, and recovery is uneventful.

Laryngeal diphtheria generally reflects a downward extension of the membrane from the pharynx. Rarely, laryngeal diphtheria is primary and does not reflect an extension of disease from the pharynx. In these cases, toxicity and signs of toxemia generally are less prominent. Two cases of isolated diphtheritic tracheitis have been reported in the literature.[13,99] The clinical findings of laryngeal diphtheria are indistinguishable from other types of infectious croup. Noisy breathing, progressive stridor, hoarseness, and a dry barking cough may be noted. Suprasternal, subcostal, and supraclavicular retractions reflect severe laryngeal obstruction, which may be fatal unless alleviated. Occasionally, in a mild case, an acute and fatal obstruction may occur because of a partially detached piece of membrane that occludes the airway. In severe cases of laryngeal diphtheria, the membrane may extend downward and invade the entire tracheobronchial tree.

Cutaneous disease, in contrast to pharyngeal disease, is more common in warmer climates and often is caused by nontoxigenic strains. In some countries with tropical and subtropical climates, such as Uganda, Tanzania, Sri Lanka, and Samoa, *C. diphtheriae* has been isolated from 60 percent of skin lesions in children.[63] Cutaneous diphtheria is more contagious than is respiratory diphtheria. Cutaneous diphtheria may be an important source of person-to-person transmission of diphtheritic organisms and outbreaks in indigenous populations in which overcrowding and poor hygiene are important risk factors.[12,21,63] The skin lesions begin as vesicles or pustules that progress to typical ulcers with sharply defined borders, membranous bases, and surrounding erythema and edema. They may be covered with a dark pseudomembrane. The lesions occur most commonly on the legs, feet, and hands. For the first 1 to 2 weeks, the lesions are painful. Spontaneous healing generally takes 6 to 12 weeks, but lesions have been reported to persist for 1 year.[63]

Conjunctival, aural, and vulvovaginal diphtheria also may occur. Conjunctival lesions usually are limited to the palpebral conjunctiva, which appears red, edematous, and membranous. Rarely, conjunctival lesions have been associated with corneal erosion.[96] Diphtheria infections of the ear are characterized by the development of otitis externa with a persistent purulent and frequently foul-smelling discharge.

Clinical presentations other than typical diphtheria have been associated with isolation of the organism from patients with meningitis, endocarditis, osteomyelitis, and hepatitis. In most cases, these infections have occurred in patients with underlying problems, such as structural or valvular heart disease or intravenous drug use, or in individuals from poor socioeconomic backgrounds.[35,101]

Several cases of septic arthritis caused by nontoxigenic *C. diphtheriae* have been described.[1,58,101] Afghani and Stutman[1] reported the case of a 27-month-old child who had septic arthritis of the hip and skin lesions on the lower extremities. In this case, the skin lesions were presumed to be the portal of entry for nontoxigenic *C. diphtheriae*. Although the child had received four doses of diphtheria and tetanus toxoids and pertussis vaccines, immunization with toxoid does not provide protection against nontoxigenic strains of *C. diphtheriae*. In this case, the organism was sensitive to penicillin, cefuroxime, cephalothin, and clindamycin but was resistant to oxacillin, an antistaphylococcal antibiotic often used for the treatment of septic arthritis when the causative organism cannot be identified. A similar case was described in an immunocompetent, fully vaccinated 2-year-old child who had skin lesions from which *C. diphtheriae* was isolated. The skin lesions also were assumed to be the portal of entry for the organism because pan-sensitive *C. diphtheriae* were isolated from the skin and the articular aspirate.[58]

Within a 12-month period, in New South Wales, Australia, four cases of septic arthritis complicating endocarditis caused by the nontoxigenic *gravis* variety of *C. diphtheriae* were reported. In addition, the same strain caused three cases of endocarditis without the development of septic arthritis. Demographic distribution of these seven cases included a 12-year-old boy who died, five patients who were in their 20s, and a patient who was 49 years old. Three of the patients had underlying cardiac abnormalities, and one had a history of intravenous drug use.[101] This same clone of nontoxigenic *C. diphtheriae* was isolated from three patients in Koorie, an aborigine community in Victoria, Australia, who had with endocarditis and five asymptomatic contacts.[64] Two of the three patients with endocarditis were members of the same family, and one of them had a history of alcohol abuse. The third patient had a septic sternoclavicular joint, in addition to endocarditis, with isolation of the same organism. Nontoxigenic *C. diphtheriae* sepsis can lead to splenic and hepatic abscesses, as reported in a patient with chronic lymphocytic leukemia in British Columbia, Canada.[66]

Complications secondary to elaborated diphtheria toxin may affect any system, but myocarditis and involvement of the nervous system are most characteristic. Myocarditis may occur after mild and severe cases of diphtheria. Generally, it develops in patients in whom administration of antitoxin is delayed. Myocarditis most commonly appears in the second week of the disease, but it can appear as early as the first or as late as the sixth week of illness. Tachycardia, a muffled S_1, murmurs, and arrhythmias such as atrioventricular dissociation indicate myocardial involvement. Echocardiography may show left ventricular dysfunction.[3,56,75] Although some cases may result in cardiac failure, most myocardial complications are temporary.

Neurologic complications appear after a variable latent period. Approximately 75 percent of all patients with severe diphtheria develop neuropathies. The incidence of neurologic sequelae has been shown to correlate with the severity of respiratory symptoms; 20 percent of all patients with respiratory problems develop polyneuritis. Neurologic complications from diphtheria infections predominantly are bilateral, are motor rather than sensory, and usually resolve completely. Paralysis of the soft palate is the most common occurrence and generally appears in the third week. It is manifested by a nasal quality in the voice, nasal regurgitation, and difficulty swallowing. Ocular paralysis usually occurs around the fifth week of illness and is characterized by blurring of vision and difficulty with accommodation. Internal strabismus also may be noted. Paralysis of the diaphragm, peripheral neuropathy involving the limbs, and loss of deep tendon reflexes likewise are reported as complications of diphtheria. When they occur, along with an elevated cerebrospinal fluid protein, the syndrome is clinically indistinguishable from Guillain-Barré syndrome.

Rarely, 2 or 3 weeks after the onset of illness, involvement of the vasomotor centers results in hypotension and cardiac failure. Gastritis, hepatitis, nephritis, and hemolytic-uremic syndrome also have been reported as complications of diphtheria.[98]

Information on the effects, if any, of diphtheria on the fetus during pregnancy was unavailable until more recently. El Seed and associates[43] reported a case of pharyngeal diphtheria in a pregnant woman that occurred during the first trimester of pregnancy. Apart from vaginal bleeding, no complications of pregnancy were noted. Severe diphtheritic toxemia in the mother was characterized by quadriparesis, from which she fully recovered. A physically normal female infant was delivered at term. In this single case, severe diphtheritic toxemia during pregnancy was not associated with any teratogenic effect in the fetus and did not impair intrauterine fetal growth.

DIAGNOSIS

The diagnosis of diphtheria should be based on clinical findings because any delay in initiating therapy poses a serious risk to the patient. Isolation of the organism is used to confirm the clinical diagnosis. Material obtained from beneath the membrane, where organisms are concentrated most highly, or a portion of the membrane itself should be obtained for culture.[5,33]

C. diphtheriae is relatively resistant to drying. The use of a non-nutritive, moisture-reducing transport medium helps prevent the overgrowth of other microorganisms. The laboratory should be notified about the possibility of diphtheria so that appropriate culture media are inoculated. A Löffler slant, a tellurite plate, and a blood agar plate should be inoculated. Tellurite-containing media inhibit the growth of normal oral flora, allowing *C. diphtheriae* to grow into characteristic black colonies. Other corynebacteria, staphylococci, and yeast also can reduce tellurite and grow into black colonies.[14,33] Although examination of direct smears of colonies or diphtheritic lesions remains an important supplement to clinical examination, it often is inaccurate. Screening the colonies from the tellurite plate for catalase, urea, nitrate, pyrazinamidase, and cystinase is important. Most biotypes of

C. diphtheriae are catalase-positive, urease-negative, nitrate-positive (except biotype *belfanti*), pyrazinamidase-negative, and cystinase-positive.[39]

All diphtheria bacilli that are recovered should be tested for toxigenicity. In 1949, the Elek immunoprecipitation assay replaced in vivo testing for toxigenicity using guinea pigs or rabbits.[42] The Elek test is based on gel diffusion and immunoprecipitation of toxin, from organisms inoculated onto agar adjacent to an antitoxin-containing well. A strain that is positive for toxin is indicated by the formation of a precipitin band between the toxin and antitoxin.[40,42] The Elek test would take 48 hours to yield results on the toxigenic nature of a *C. diphtheriae* strain. A modified Elek test that consists of placement of an antitoxin-impregnated disk onto an agar plate surrounded by inoculates of clinical specimen and positive control has been described. Compared with the conventional Elek test, the modified test has the advantage of using "spot" inoculations of numerous colonies directly from the primary plate. In addition, the modified Elek test has fewer false-positive and false-negative results and yields results more rapidly (16 to 24 hours).[39]

A rapid enzyme immunoassay is another test available for the detection of diphtheria toxin. This method uses equine polyclonal antibody to capture the diphtheria toxin and an alkaline phosphatase-labeled monoclonal antibody to detect fragment A of the toxin. It is a rapid test that takes 3 hours and has a limit of detection of 100 pg/mL.[44]

Rapid testing for diphtheria toxin by PCR specific for the "A" or "B" portion of the toxin gene, *tox*, is sensitive and has produced positive results in specimens stored for 12 months before performance of the assay.[7,69,70,87,88,90] The absence of the *tox* gene by PCR excludes the diagnosis of diphtheria. PCR may give false-positive results, however, because it does not differentiate between partial or nonfunctional *tox* genes and functional *tox* gene products. An increasing number of cases of nontoxigenic diphtheria that are positive for *tox* gene by PCR have been reported from Ukraine and Russia.[53,78]

The immune status of patients can be determined by toxin neutralization in Vero cells.[85] This method is used frequently, although it is difficult to standardize and relies heavily on individual interpretation of results. Enzyme-linked immunosorbent assay is a more rapid and quite sensitive method, but it detects some nonspecific antibodies; when antitoxin levels are in the low range, the assay may generate falsely elevated results.[82] Finally, a delayed fluorescence immune assay method was developed by Aggerbeck and colleagues[2] in 1996 and has been reported to have good sensitivity, specificity, and reproducibility.[17] Levels of diphtheria antitoxin of 0.01 IU/mL or greater generally are accepted as protective. A skin-testing method, the Schick test, also has been used to assess immunity.

The Schick test was used previously to determine the immune status of the patient. It is not helpful in establishing an early diagnosis because it cannot be read for several days, and currently it is not widely used. In the Schick test, a measured amount of purified diphtheria toxin (0.1 mL) is injected subcutaneously. A hypersensitivity reaction indicates an inadequate presence of antitoxin. A toxoid control also is injected, in the opposite arm, to help distinguish between a reaction to toxin and a reaction to other antigens in the toxin preparation.

Other laboratory studies are of little diagnostic value. The white blood cell count may be normal or elevated. Rarely, anemia develops as a result of rapid hemolysis of red blood cells. Examination of cerebrospinal fluid may reveal a minimal elevation of protein and, rarely, a mild pleocytosis in patients with diphtheritic neuritis. Hypoglycemia, glucosuria, or both may occur and reflect hepatic toxicity. An elevation in blood urea nitrogen may develop in patients with acute tubular necrosis. An electrocardiogram should be obtained and may reveal ST-segment and T-wave changes or arrhythmias indicative of myocarditis.

DIFFERENTIAL DIAGNOSIS

Mild forms of nasal diphtheria in a partially immunized host may resemble the common cold. When the nasal discharge is more serosanguineous or purulent, nasal diphtheria must be distinguished from a foreign body in the nose, sinusitis, adenoiditis, or the snuffles of congenital syphilis. Careful examination of the nose with a nasal speculum, sinus radiographs, and appropriate serologic tests for syphilis are helpful in excluding these disorders.

Tonsillar or pharyngeal diphtheria must be differentiated from streptococcal pharyngitis. Generally, streptococcal pharyngitis is associated with more severe pain on swallowing, higher temperature, and a nonadherent membrane limited to the tonsils. In some patients, pharyngeal diphtheria and streptococcal pharyngitis coexist.

Tonsillar and pharyngeal diphtheria also must be differentiated from infectious mononucleosis (lymphadenopathy and splenomegaly are common findings, atypical lymphocytes are generally present, and heterophile antibody may be present), nonbacterial membranous tonsillitis (white blood cell count generally is low, throat cultures reveal normal flora, and the course is unaffected by antibiotics), primary herpetic tonsillitis (presence of gingivitis, stomatitis, and discrete lesions of the tongue and palate may be helpful), Vincent angina (may be indistinguishable), and thrush (constitutional symptoms are absent, and lesions are present on the buccal mucosa and tongue). Tonsillar and pharyngeal diphtheria also must be differentiated from blood dyscrasias such as agranulocytosis and leukemia (complete blood count and bone marrow study are helpful); post-tonsillectomy faucial membranes (membranes are stationary and do not spread); and oropharyngeal involvement by toxoplasmosis, *Arcanobacterium*, cytomegalovirus, tularemia, and salmonellosis (associated signs and symptoms and appropriate cultures and serologic tests may be diagnostic).[50]

Laryngeal diphtheria must be differentiated from spasmodic or nonspasmodic croup; acute epiglottitis; laryngotracheobronchitis; aspirated foreign bodies; peripharyngeal and retropharyngeal abscesses; and laryngeal papillomas, hemangiomas, or lymphangiomas. A careful history, followed by careful visualization in the hospital under controlled conditions, aids in making a correct diagnosis.

PREVENTION

Diphtheria is prevented on a community-wide basis most effectively by active immunization. Diphtheria toxoid is available in combination with tetanus toxoid as pediatric DT or adult Td and in combination with acellular pertussis as DTaP and Tdap. Combination regimens with DTaP and inactivated poliovirus and hepatitis B (Pediatrix) and inactivated poliovirus and *H. influenzae* type B (Pentacel) are also available. Pediatric formulations of diphtheria toxoid vaccines contain three to four times more diphtheria toxoid but the same tetanus toxoid compared with the adult formulations. Children younger than 7 years should be given the pediatric formulations of vaccine, whereas children older than 7 years should receive the adult Td. Two forms of Tdap are available: Boostrix, which is approved for children 10 to 18 years old, and Adacel, which is approved for individuals 11 to 64 years old.[24-27,38]

Primary immunization is carried out conveniently and effectively by giving diphtheria and tetanus toxoids and pertussis vaccine, DTaP, at 2, 4, and 6 months of age, with booster doses given at 15 to 18 months and again when the child is 4 to 6 years of age. Booster doses with adult-type diphtheria and tetanus toxoids adsorbed (Td) should be given at 10-year intervals to all immunized individuals. Current recommendations are to give

Tdap as the first booster dose in patients who are 11 to 12 years old. Td and Tdap contain 2 to 2.5 Lf (flocculation units) diphtheria toxoid per dose compared with 7 to 25 Lf in the pediatric diphtheria, tetanus toxoid, and pertussis vaccine preparations (DTaP, DT). Primary immunization of children older than 7 years may be performed with Td. Two doses are given intramuscularly at least 4 weeks apart, with a booster dose provided 1 year later. Children and adults who are severely immunocompromised or undergoing long-term hemodialysis should use the standard immunization schedule, although response may be suboptimal.[47,51,71]

Most local and systemic reactions to the diphtheria and tetanus toxoids and whole cell pertussis vaccine (DTP), including fever, were related to the pertussis component.[10,32] Administration of tetanus and diphtheria toxoids is not followed by the high incidence of reactions associated with the use of pediatric DTP vaccines. At least one study showed that 7.5 Lf toxoid can be given safely to adults without a higher risk of reactions occurring.[15] Primary immunization against diphtheria for infants with progressive neurologic disorders and completion of the primary immunization series in patients who had experienced an untoward reaction to an earlier DTP vaccine injection may be performed with diphtheria and tetanus toxoids rather than diphtheria and tetanus toxoids and pertussis vaccine.[4]

A report of 97 preterm infants who received diphtheria and tetanus toxoids and acellular pertussis vaccine (DTaP) (94 of these infants also received *Haemophilus influenzae* type b vaccine) showed that most infants tolerated the vaccination without side effects, although a subgroup of very-low-birth-weight infants (mean 873 g) had either recurrence or an increase in the number of apneic and bradycardic episodes in the 48 hours after receiving vaccination. The apneic and bradycardic episodes were present before immunization in every case.[97]

Booster doses of tetanus and diphtheria toxoids should be given at 10-year intervals to all immunized individuals. As mentioned earlier, levels of diphtheria antitoxin of 0.01 IU/mL or greater generally are accepted as protective.

Diphtheria immunization is not always followed by complete protection.[79] Immunization is directed against the phage-mediated toxin, not against infection. Fully immunized individuals may be carriers or may have disease caused by nontoxigenic strains. An investigation conducted during an epidemic in Texas showed no statistical difference in the risk of diphtheria infection developing in individuals with full, lapsed, inadequate, or no previous diphtheria immunization; however, a 30-fold increased risk of development of symptomatic diphtheria in individuals with no immunization and an 11.5-fold increase in individuals with inadequate immunization was noted.[84]

The most important health problem in the United States today is inadequate immunization of the population. Immunization rates in adults are poorer than those in infants and children because of failure to maintain adequate immunity through appropriate booster immunization. A 70 to 80 percent immunization level is thought to be required to prevent epidemic spread.[31]

Prevention of diphtheria also depends on management of the contacts of known cases of diphtheria and carriers of the organism and on isolation of patients to minimize the spread of disease. Individuals at risk of contracting the disease from the index case include those who have had close respiratory or physical contact or prolonged close proximity with the infected individual, including members of the index case's household.[18] Specifically, family members who share body towels and cups or eating utensils, share a bed or a bedroom with more than two people, or take a bath less than once a week have a significantly greater risk of contracting the disease from the infected patient. A history of eczema in the contact also has been associated with a significantly increased risk of contracting diphtheria from the index case.[93]

The patient is infectious until diphtheria bacilli no longer can be cultured from the site of infection. Two or three consecutive negative cultures at least 24 hours apart are required, and antibiotic therapy must be complete for 24 hours before the patient is released from isolation. If obtaining cultures is impossible, isolation may be ended after the completion of 14 days of appropriate antibiotic treatment.[6]

Cultures should be taken from the nose and throat of all close contacts, who should be kept under surveillance for 7 days (surveillance as an outpatient is acceptable).[5] Regardless of their immunization status, contacts should be treated with a single intramuscular dose of benzathine penicillin G (600,000 U for individuals weighing <30 kg and 1.2 million U for individuals weighing >30 kg) or a 7-day course of erythromycin, 40 to 50 mg/kg/day (maximum 2 g/day) divided into four doses.[5] The immune status of each contact should be determined; individuals for whom immune status is inadequate, including individuals who have had the primary series but more than 5 years has elapsed since they received their last booster dose, should receive an injection of diphtheria toxoid. In addition, patients with diphtheria should be immunized during convalescence because infection may not confer immunity.[6]

Asymptomatic carriers who previously were not immunized against diphtheria should have cultures taken, receive diphtheria toxoid and penicillin or erythromycin (as described earlier), and be seen daily by a physician. Asymptomatic contacts who are found to carry a toxigenic strain should be subjected to the same isolation and treatment measures as the index case.[6] If daily surveillance is impossible, benzathine penicillin is preferred over erythromycin for treatment because failure to adhere to an oral drug regimen is a concern. If a contact is experiencing symptoms when seen, treatment of diphtheria is indicated. It is important to initiate prophylactic therapy in contacts who have not been immunized, before the results of culture are received. Management of carriers is described in the next section. Contacts whose occupations involve close contact with unimmunized children or food handling (especially milk) should refrain from working until cultures are confirmed to be negative.[6]

TREATMENT

Treatment of diphtheria is predicated on neutralization of free toxin and eradication of *C. diphtheriae* or *C. ulcerans* by the use of antibiotics. Disease caused by *C. ulcerans* should be treated in the same manner as is disease caused by *C. diphtheriae*.[3,95] The decision to administer equine antitoxin should be based on the site and size of the membrane, the degree of toxicity, and the duration of illness.[16]

Antitoxin can neutralize circulating toxin or toxin that is absorbed onto cells, but is ineffective when cells have been penetrated. Early treatment is essential to limit tissue damage. An adequate dose of antitoxin must be administered intravenously as early as possible to neutralize all free toxins. A single dose is used to avoid the risk of developing sensitization from repeated doses of horse serum. Tests for sensitivity to horse serum must be performed before antitoxin is administered. For this purpose, 0.02 mL of a 1:1000 dilution of antitoxin in saline can be given intracutaneously. Positive (histamine) and negative (isotonic saline) controls should be applied similarly. A positive reaction consists of a wheal at least 3 mm larger than the negative control, with surrounding erythema at the site of injection, developing within 15 to 20 minutes, and necessitates desensitization. The histamine control must be positive if test results are to be considered valid. Alternatively, the test may be done with a drop of serum diluted 1:100 and applied to the site of a superficial scratch, prick, or puncture on the volar aspect of the forearm.

Controls should be applied and results interpreted as described for intracutaneous administration.[5]

If a patient has been shown to be sensitive to horse serum, the serum should be provided in a slowly increasing dosage given at 15-minute intervals. Several regimens have been used. One recommended regimen is as follows:[5]

- 0.1 mL of a 1:1000 dilution intravenously
- 0.3 mL of a 1:1000 dilution intravenously
- 0.6 mL of a 1:1000 dilution intravenously
- 0.1 mL of a 1:100 dilution intravenously
- 0.3 mL of a 1:100 dilution intravenously
- 0.6 mL of a 1:100 dilution intravenously
- 0.1 mL of a 1:10 dilution intravenously
- 0.3 mL of a 1:10 dilution intravenously
- 0.6 mL of a 1:10 dilution intravenously
- 0.1 mL undiluted intravenously
- 0.3 mL undiluted intravenously
- 0.6 mL undiluted intravenously
- 1 mL undiluted intravenously

The intravenous route for desensitization is considered safest because it offers good control, but protocols involving the intradermal, subcutaneous, and intramuscular routes also have been used frequently.[5]

If no reaction has occurred, the remaining material is given by slow intravenous infusion. Intravenous administration results in more rapid excretion of antitoxin into saliva, rendering it atoxic and preventing further absorption of toxin in the oropharynx, but it does not result in more rapid systemic elimination of antitoxin than intramuscular administration.[100] Reactions should be treated with aqueous epinephrine (1:1000) provided intravenously.

The antitoxin dosage is empiric. Pharyngeal or laryngeal disease of 48 hours' duration or less should be treated with 20,000 to 40,000 U, nasopharyngeal disease with 40,000 to 60,000 U, and severe pharyngeal or laryngeal diphtheria with 80,000 to 120,000 U of antitoxin. The last dose also should be given to patients with mixed clinical symptoms and to patients with brawny edema or disease of longer than 48 hours' duration. The value of antitoxin in the treatment of cutaneous disease is debated, but some experts recommend 20,000 to 40,000 U because toxic effects have been reported.[5]

Although antibiotics are not a substitute for treatment with antitoxin, they should be given when diphtheria is suspected clinically. Penicillin and erythromycin are still effective against most strains of *C. diphtheriae*. Penicillin and erythromycin also are effective in eradicating group A hemolytic streptococci, which may complicate 30 percent of cases of diphtheria. Treatment consists of a 14-day course of penicillin or erythromycin. Penicillin may be given as aqueous penicillin G, 100,000 to 150,000 U/kg/day in four divided doses intravenously, or as procaine penicillin, 25,000 to 50,000 U/kg/day (maximum of 1.2 million U) in two divided doses intramuscularly. Patients who are sensitive to penicillin should be given erythromycin in a daily dosage of 40 to 50 mg/kg (maximum of 2 g/day) in four divided doses for 14 days. When the patient is able to tolerate oral medications, erythromycin or penicillin V may be used in place of the intravenous antibiotics.[5]

Follow-up cultures should be obtained at least 2 weeks after antibiotic therapy is complete; if they are positive, erythromycin should be given for an additional 10 days.[5] Some resistance to erythromycin has been observed, but it is uncommon, and its epidemiologic significance is unknown.[5,6] Penicillin is recommended as first-line treatment in Vietnam, based on sensitivity data.[68] Amoxicillin, rifampin, and clindamycin provided in appropriate dosages also may be effective. Lincomycin and tetracycline have proved to be less effective, and cephalexin, oxacillin, and colistin have been shown to be ineffective against *C. diphtheriae*. The end-point of therapy is two to three consecutive negative cultures at least 24 hours apart. In addition to receiving antibiotic therapy, patients with diphtheria should be immunized during convalescence because infection may not confer immunity.[5]

The carrier state has been treated effectively with a single intramuscular dose of benzathine penicillin G (600,000 U for children weighing <30 kg or 1.2 million U for individuals weighing ≥30 kg) or oral erythromycin (40 to 50 mg/kg/day for children and 1 g/day for adults) for 7 to 10 days.[5] Carriers should have repeat pharyngeal cultures performed a minimum of 2 weeks after antibiotic therapy is complete; if the repeat cultures are positive, carriers should receive an additional course of antibiotics.

SUPPORTIVE TREATMENT

Bed rest is extremely important and should be required for 2 to 3 weeks. Serial electrocardiograms should be obtained two or three times each week for 4 to 6 weeks to detect myocarditis as early as possible. Absolute bed rest must be enforced if myocarditis is detected because sudden death has been precipitated by excessive activity. A patient with myocarditis may receive digitalization if congestive heart failure develops. Digitalization for arrhythmias caused by diphtheria may be contraindicated, however. In severe disease, prednisone, 1 to 1.5 mg/kg/day for 2 weeks, has been shown to lessen the incidence of myocarditis.

Hydration should be maintained, and a high-calorie liquid or soft diet should be provided. Secretions should be suctioned as needed to prevent aspiration. Palatal and pharyngeal paralysis increases the risk of aspiration occurring, so gavage via a nasogastric tube is indicated in these patients.

The quality of the voice and the gag reflex should be checked regularly for assessment of progression of the disease. Laryngeal diphtheria may require relief of obstruction with a tracheostomy. This procedure should be performed before the patient has become exhausted.

Adequate immunity does not develop in at least half of patients who recover from diphtheria, and they remain subject to reinfection. Immunization is indicated after the patient recovers.

PROGNOSIS

Many factors affect the prognosis in cases of diphtheria, the most important being the immunization status of the host. Morbidity and mortality rates are increased significantly in patients who are unimmunized or inadequately immunized. The rapidity with which medical care is sought and the diagnosis of diphtheria is suggested has a great impact on outcome. If specific treatment is provided on the first day of disease, the mortality rate may be reduced to less than 1 percent; delay in providing treatment until day 4 may be associated with a 20-fold increase in the mortality rate.

The virulence of the infecting organism and the location of infection are important prognostic factors. Infection with a nontoxigenic *C. diphtheriae* strain may cause disease but does not lead to myocarditis, neuritis, and other toxin-related phenomena. Toxigenic disease may vary from mild to severe. In cases of mild diphtheria, membrane sloughing and full recovery generally occur within 7 days. Disease caused by toxigenic *gravis* strains tends to be more severe and carries a poorer prognosis. Although diphtheria may affect the skin, nasopharynx, and other mucous membranes, involvement of the larynx heralds a more complicated course. Laryngeal diphtheria increases the risk of development of airway obstruction and promotes systemic absorption of the toxin. These patients require close monitoring of respiratory function and for involvement of other organ systems. Laryngeal diphtheria is more likely to be fatal in infants.

Few laboratory parameters indicate the severity of diphtheria. The development of amegakaryocytic thrombocytopenia and leukocytosis with counts of greater than 25,000 cells/mm^3 has been associated with a poor outcome.

The prognosis in a patient with diphtheria remains guarded until recovery is complete. At any time during the course of the illness, complications such as laryngeal obstruction, shock, and ventricular fibrillation may occur suddenly and unexpectedly. In patients with myocardial involvement, permanent damage to the heart, specifically fibrosis, may occur and lead to later complications. In addition, potentially severe neurologic manifestations, such as phrenic nerve paralysis, may appear late in the course of the disease.

Persistence of *C. diphtheriae* may be noted in the nasopharynx of 5 to 10 percent of convalescing patients. Recovery from diphtheria is followed by immunity that is demonstrable for at least 1 year after illness in 50 percent of patients. Second attacks are rare; nonetheless, immunization should be performed after the patient recovers.

Before the use of antitoxin and the availability of antibiotics, the mortality rate from diphtheria was 30 to 50 percent. Death was most common in children younger than 4 years old and was the result of suffocation. At present, the worldwide mortality rate is 5 to 10 percent, with no clear association with age.

REFERENCES

1. Afghani, B., and Stutman, H. R.: Bacterial arthritis caused by *Corynebacterium diphtheriae*. Pediatr. Infect. Dis. J. *12*:881-882, 1993.
2. Aggerbeck, H., Norgaard-Pedersen, B., and Heron, I.: Simultaneous quantitation of diphtheria and tetanus antibodies by double antigen, time-resolved fluorescence immunoassay. J. Immunol. Methods *190*:171-183, 1996.
3. Ahmad, N., Gainsborough, N., and Paul, J.: An unusual case of diphtheria and its complications. Hosp. Med. *61*:436-437, 2000.
4. American Academy of Pediatrics: Report of the Committee on Infectious Diseases. 22nd ed. Elk Grove Village, IL, American Academy of Pediatrics, 1991, pp. 195-199.
5. American Academy of Pediatrics: Diphtheria. *In* Pickering, L. K., Peter, G., Baker, L., et al. (eds.): 2000 Red Book: Report of the Committee on Infectious Diseases. 25th ed. Elk Grove Village, IL, American Academy of Pediatrics, 2000, pp. 230-234.
6. American Public Health Association: Diphtheria. *In* Chin, J. (ed.): Control of Communicable Diseases Manual. Washington, D.C., American Public Health Association, 2000, pp. 165-170.
7. Aravina-Roman, M., Bowman, R., and O'Neill, G.: Polymerase chain reaction for the detection of toxigenic *Corynebacterium diphtheriae*. Pathology *27*:71-73, 1995.
8. Atkinson, W., Hamborsky, J., McIntyre, L., and Wolfe, S. (eds.): Epidemiology and Prevention of Vaccine-Preventable Diseases. 9th ed. Washington, D.C., Public Health Foundation, 2006, pp. 57-68.
9. Baba, M., Gilliatt, R. W., Harding, A. E., and Reiners, K.: Demyelination following diphtheria toxin in the presence of axonal atrophy. J. Neurol. Sci. *64*:199-211, 1984.
10. Baraff, L. J., Manclark, C. R., Cherry, J. D., et al.: Analyses of adverse reactions to diphtheria and tetanus toxoids and pertussis vaccine by vaccine lot, endotoxin content, pertussis vaccine potency and percentage of mouse weight gain. Pediatr. Infect. Dis. J. *8*:502-507, 1989.
11. Battistini, A., Curatola, A. M., Gallinare, P., et al.: Inhibition of protein synthesis by diphtheria toxin induces a peculiar pattern of synthesized protein species. Exp. Cell Res. *176*:174-179, 1988.
12. Belsey, M. A., Sinclair, M., Roder, M. R., et al.: *Corynebacterium diphtheriae* skin infections in Alabama and Louisiana: A factor in the epidemiology of diphtheria. N. Engl. J. Med. *280*:135-141, 1969.
13. Berner, R., Leititis, J. U., Furste, H. O., and Brandis, M.: Bacterial tracheitis caused by *Corynebacterium diphtheriae*. Eur. J. Pediatr. *156*:207-208, 1997.
14. Bisgard, K. M., Hardy, I. R. B., Popovic, T., et al.: Respiratory diphtheria in the United States, 1980 through 1995. Am. J. Public Health *88*:787-791, 1998.
15. Bjorkholm, B., Granstrom, M., Wahl, M., et al.: Adverse reactions and immunogenicity in adults to regular and increased dosage of diphtheria vaccine. Eur. J. Clin. Microbiol. *6*:637-640, 1987.
16. Bjorkholm, B., Olling, S., Larsson, P., et al.: An outbreak of diphtheria among Swedish alcoholics. Infection *15*:354-358, 1987.
17. Bonin, E., Tiru, M., Hallander, H., and Bredberg-Raden, U.: Evaluation of single- and dual antigen delayed fluorescence immunoassay in comparison to an ELISA and the in vivo toxin neutralisation test for detection of diphtheria toxin antibodies. J. Immunol. Methods *230*:131-140, 1999.
18. Bonnet, J. M., and Begg, N. T.: Control of diphtheria: Guidance for consultants in communicable disease control. Commun. Dis. Public Health *2*:242-249, 1999.
19. Bostock, A. D., Gilbert, F. R., Lewis, D., and Smith, D. C.: *Corynebacterium ulcerans* infection associated with untreated milk. J. Infect. *9*:286-288, 1984.
20. Bowler, C. J., Mandal, B. K., Schlecht, B., et al.: Diphtheria: The continuing hazard. Arch. Dis. Child. *63*:194-195, 1988.
21. Bray, J. P., Burt, E. G., Potter, E. J., et al.: Epidemic diphtheria and skin infections in Trinidad. J. Infect. Dis. *126*:34-40, 1972.
22. Burch, G. E., Sun, S. C., Sohal, R. S., et al.: Diphtheritic myocarditis: A histochemical and electron microscopic study. Am. J. Cardiol. *21*:261-268, 1968.
23. Centers for Disease Control and Prevention: Diphtheria epidemic—new independent states of the former Soviet Union, 1990-1994. M. M. W. R. Morb. Mortal. Wkly. Rep. *44*:177-181, 1995.
24. Centers for Disease Control and Prevention: Use of diphtheria toxoid-tetanus toxoid-acelluar pertusis vaccine as a five-dose series. M. M. W. R. Morb. Mortal. Wkly. Rep. *49*(RR13):1-8, 2000.
25. Centers for Disease Control and Prevention: Notice to Readers: Food and Drug Administration approval of a fifth acellular pertussis vaccine for use among infants and young children—United States. M. M. W. R. Morb. Mortal. Wkly. Rep. *51*:574, 2002.
26. Centers for Disease Control and Prevention: Notice to Readers: FDA licensure of diphtheria and tetanus toxoids and acellular pertussis adsorbed, hepatitis B (recombinant), and poliovirus vaccine combined (PEDIARIX) for use in infants. M. M. W. R. Morb. Mortal. Wkly. Rep. *52*:203-204, 2003.
27. Centers for Disease Control and Prevention: Preventing tetanus, diphtheria, pertussis among adolescents: Use of tetanus, reduced diphtheria toxoid, and acellular pertussis vaccine. M. M. W. R. Morb. Mortal. Wkly. Rep. *55*(RR03):1-34, 2006.
28. Cerdeno-Tarraga, A. M., Efstratiou, A., Dover, L. G., et al.: The complete genome sequence and analysis of *Corynebacterium diphtheriae* NCTC13129. Nucl. Acid Res. *31*:6516-6523, 2003.
29. Chang, M. P., Baldwin, R. L., Bruce, C., and Wisnieski, B. J.: Second cytotoxic pathway of diphtheria toxin suggested by nuclease activity. Science *246*:1165, 1989.
30. Chang, M. P., Bramhall, J., Graves, S., et al.: Internucleosomal DNA cleavage precedes diphtheria toxin-induced cytolysis: Evidence that cell lysis is not a simple consequence of translation inhibition. J. Biol. Chem. *264*:15261-15267, 1989.
31. Chen, R. T., Broome, C. V., Weinstein, R. A., et al.: Diphtheria in the United States, 1971-1981. Am. J. Public Health *75*:1393-1397, 1985.
32. Cherry, J. D., Baraff, L. J., and Hewlett, E.: The past, present, and future of pertussis: The role of adults in epidemiology and future control. West. J. Med. *150*:319-328, 1989.
33. Clarridge, J. E., Popovic, T., and Inzana, T. J.: Diphtheria and other corynebacterial and coryneform infections. *In* Hausler, W. J., and Sussman, M. (eds.): Topley and Wilson's Microbiology and Microbial Infections. Vol. 3. New York, Oxford University Press, 1998, pp. 347-371.
34. Collier, R. J., and Kandel, J.: Structure and activity of diphtheria toxin, I: Thiol-dependent dissociation of a fraction of toxin into enzymatically active and inactive fragments. J. Biol. Chem. *246*:1496-1503, 1971.
35. Davidson, S., Rotem, Y., Bogkowski, B., and Rubinstein, E.: *Corynebacterium diphtheriae* endocarditis. Am. J. Med. Sci. *271*:351-353, 1976.
36. DeZoysa, A., Efstratiou, A., George, R. C., et al.: Molecular epidemiology of *Corynebacterium diphtheriae* from northwestern Russia and surrounding countries studied by using ribotyping and pulsed-field gel electrophoresis. J. Clin. Microbiol. *33*:1080-1083, 1995.
37. Dietze, W. E., and Sudderth, J. F.: Post-diphtheria polyneuritis: Three case reports. Laryngoscope *82*:765-770, 1972.
38. Diphtheria, tetanus and pertussis: Guidelines for vaccine prophylaxis and other preventive measures. M. M. W. R. Morb. Mortal. Wkly. Rep. *30*:392-407, 1981.
39. Efstratiou, A., Engler, K., Mazurova, I. K., et al.: Current approaches to the laboratory diagnosis of diphtheria. J. Infect. Dis. *181*(Suppl. 1):138-145, 2000.
40. Efstratiou, A., and George, R. C.: Laboratory guidelines for the diagnosis of infections caused by *Corynebacterium diphtheriae* and *C. ulcerans*. Commun. Dis. Public Health *2*:250-257, 1999.
41. Efstratiou, A., and Roure, C.: The European Laboratory Working Group on Diphtheria: A global microbiologic network. J. Infect. Dis. *181*(Suppl. 1):146-151, 2000.
42. Elek, S. D.: The plate virulence test for diphtheria. J. Clin. Pathol. *2*:250-258, 1949.
43. El Seed, A. M., Dafalla, A. A., and Abboud, O. I.: Fetal immune response following maternal diphtheria during pregnancy. Ann. Trop. Paediatr. *1*:217-219, 1981.
44. Engler, K. H., and Efstratiou, A.: A rapid ELISA for confirmation of diphtheria caused by toxigenic *Corynebacterium* spp. (abstract 1522). In Abstracts of the 8th European Congress of Clinical Microbiology and Infectious Diseases (Lausanne, Switzerland, May 1997). Clin. Microbiol. Infect. *3*(suppl 2):14, 1997.

45. Engler, K. H., Glushkevich, T. G., Mazurova, I. K., et al.: A modified Elek test for the detection of toxigenic corynebacteria. J. Clin. Microbiol. *35*:495-498, 1997.

46. English, P. C.: Diphtheria and theories of infectious disease: Centennial appreciation of the critical role of diphtheria in the history of medicine. Pediatrics 76:1-9, 1985.

47. Enke, B. U., Bokenkamp, A., Offner, G., et al.: Response to diphtheria and tetanus booster vaccination in pediatric renal transplant recipients. Transplantation *64*:237-241, 1997.

48. Freeman, V. J.: Studies on virulence of bacteriophage-infected strains of *Corynebacterium diphtheriae.* J. Bacteriol. *61*:675-688, 1951.

49. Funke, G., and Bernard, K.: Coryneform gram-positive rods. *In* Murray, P. R., Baron, E. J., Pfaller, M. A., et al. (eds.): Manual of Clinical Microbiology, 7th ed. Washington, D.C., ASM Press, 1999, pp. 319-340.

50. Gaston, D. A., and Zurowski, S. M.: *Arcanobacterium haemolyticum* pharyngitis and exanthem. Arch. Dermatol. *132*:61-64, 1996.

51. Ghio, L., Pedrazzi, C., Assael, B. M., et al.: Immunity to diphtheria and tetanus in a young population on a dialysis regimen or with a renal transplant. J. Pediatr. *130*:987-989, 1997.

52. Gilbert, L.: Infections with *Corynebacterium diphtheriae*—changing epidemiology and clinical manifestations. Commun. Dis. Intell. *21*:161-164, 1997.

53. Gluskevich, T. G., and Zherebko, G.: Study of the role of non-toxigenic *C. diphtheriae* strains on the aetiology of diphtheria in the Ukraine (abstract). *In:* Programme and Abstracts of the Fifth International Meeting of the European Laboratory Working Group on Diphtheria (Halkidiki, Greece, June 1998). London, Public Health Laboratory Service, 1998, p. 32.

54. Golaz, A., Lance-Parker, S., Welty, T., et al.: Epidemiology of diphtheria in South Dakota. S. D. J. Med. *53*:281-285, 2000.

55. Goldie, W., and Maddock, E. C. G.: A milk-borne outbreak of diphtheria. Lancet *1*:285-286, 1943.

56. Groundstroem, K. W. E., Molnar, G., and Lumio, J.: Echocardiographic follow-up of diphtheric myocarditis. Cardiology *87*:79-81, 1996.

57. Grundbacher, F. J.: Behring's discovery of diphtheria and tetanus antitoxins. Immunol. Today *13*:188-190, 1992.

58. Guran, P., Mollaret, H., Chatelain, R., et al.: [Septic arthritis due to a nontoxigenic diphtheria bacillus.] [French.] Arch. Fr. Pediat. *36*:926-929, 1979.

59. Hadfield, T., McEvoy, P., Polotsky, Y., et al.: The pathology of diphtheria. J. Infect. Dis. *181*(Suppl. 1):116-120, 2000.

60. Hardy, I. R. B., Dittmann, S., and Sutter, R. W.: Current situation and control strategies for resurgence of diphtheria in newly independent states of the former Soviet Union. Lancet *347*:1739-1744, 1996.

61. Harnisch, J. P., Tronca, E., Nolan, C. M., et al.: Diphtheria among alcoholic urban adults: A decade of experience in Seattle. Ann. Intern. Med. *111*:71-82, 1989.

62. Hart, R. J. C.: *Corynebacterium ulcerans* in humans and cattle in North Devon. J. Hyg. Camb. *92*:161-164, 1984.

63. Hofler, W.: Cutaneous diphtheria. Int. J. Dermatol. *30*:845-847, 1991.

64. Hogg, G. G., Strachan, J. E., Huayi, L., et al.: Non-toxigenic *Corynebacterium diphtheriae* biovar *gravis:* Evidence for an invasive clone in a south-eastern Australian community. M. J. Aust. *164*:72-75, 1996.

65. Holmes, R.: Biology and molecular epidemiology of diphtheria toxin and the *tox* gene. J. Infect. Dis. *181*(Suppl. 1):156-167, 2000.

66. Isaac-Renton, J. L., Boyko, W. J., Chan, R., and Crichton, E.: *Corynebacterium diphtheriae* septicemia. Am. J. Clin. Pathol. *75*:631-634, 1981.

67. Jennis, F., and Bale, P. M.: Fatal respiratory and gastric diphtheria in an adult. Med. J. Aust. *2*:760-762, 1966.

68. Kneen, R., Pham, N. G., Solomon, T., et al.: Penicillin vs. erythromycin in the treatment of diphtheria. Clin. Infect. Dis. *27*:845-850, 1998.

69. Kobaidze, K., Popovic, T., Nakao, H., and Quick, L.: Direct polymerase chain reaction for detection of toxigenic *Corynebacterium diphtheriae* strains from the Republic of Georgia after prolonged storage. J. Infect. Dis. *181*(Suppl. 1):152-155, 2000.

70. Komiya, T., Shibata, N., Ito, M., et al.: Retrospective diagnosis of diphtheria by detection of the *C. diphtheriae tox* gene in a formaldehyde-fixed throat swab using PCR and sequencing analysis. J. Clin. Microbiol. *38*:2400-2402, 2000.

71. Kreft, B., Klouche, M., Kreft, R., et al: Low efficiency of active immunization against diphtheria in chronic hemodialysis patients. Kidney Int. *52*:212-216, 1997.

72. Kurtzhals, J. A. L., Kjeldsen, K., Hey, A. S., et al.: Immunity to tetanus and diphtheria in rural Africa. Am. J. Trop. Med. Hyg. *56*:576-579, 1997.

73. Lessnick, S. L., Bruce, C., Baldwin, R. L., et al.: Does diphtheria toxin have nuclease activity? Science *250*:832-838, 1990.

74. Lloyd, G. E. R. (ed.): Hippocratic Writings. New York, Penguin Books, 1983, p. 118.

75. Loukoushkina, E. F., Bobko, P. V., Kolbasova, E. V., et al.: The clinical picture and diagnosis of diphtheritic carditis in children. Eur. J. Pediatr. *157*:528-533, 1998.

76. Lozhnikova , S. M., Pirogov, V. N., Piradov, M. A., et al.: Diphtheritic polyneuropath: Clinico-morphologic study. Arkh. Patol. *59*:11-17, 1997.

77. Lubran, M. M.: Bacterial toxins. Ann. Clin. Lab. Sci. *18*:58-71, 1988.

78. Mazurova, I. K., et al. Characterization of non-toxigenic *tox* bearing *Corynebacterium diphtheriae* in the waning Russian epidemic (abstract). *In:* Programme and Abstracts of the Fifth International Meeting of the European Laboratory Working Group on Diphtheria (Halkidiki, Greece, June 1998). London, Public Health Laboratory Service, 1998, p. 33.

79. McCloskey, R. V.: Diphtheria antitoxin titers in hospital workers after a single dose of adult-type diphtheria tetanus toxoid. Am. J. Med. Sci. *258*:209-213, 1969.

80. McCloskey, R. V., Eller, J. J., Green, M., et al.: The 1970 epidemic of diphtheria in San Antonio. Ann. Intern. Med. *75*:495-503, 1971.

81. Medical News and Perspectives: Diphtheria in Russia: A reminder of risk. J. A. M. A. *273*:1245, 1995.

82. Melville-Smith, M., and Balfour, A.: Estimation of *Corynebacterium diphtheriae* antitoxin in human sera: A comparison of an enzyme-linked immunosorbent assay with the toxin neutralisation test. J. Med. Microbiol. *25*:279-283, 1988.

83. Miller, L. W., Older, J. J., Drake, J., et al.: Diphtheria immunization: Effect upon carriers and the control of outbreaks. Am. J. Dis. Child. *123*:197-199, 1972.

84. Mirchamsy, H., Hamedi, H., Fatch, G., et al.: Oral immunization against diphtheria and tetanus infections by fluid diphtheria and tetanus toxoids. Vaccine *12*:1167-1172, 1994.

85. Miyamura, K., Nishio, S., Ito, A., et al.: Micro cell culture method for determination of diphtheria toxin and antitoxin titres using VERO cells, I: Studies on factors affecting the toxin and antitoxin titration. J. Biol. Stand. *2*:189-201, 1974.

86. Morales, A. R., Vichitbandha, P., Chandruang, P., et al.: Pathological features of cardiac conduction disturbances in diphtheric myocarditis. Arch. Pathol. *91*:1-7, 1971.

87. Nakao, H., and Popovic, T.: Development of a direct PCR assay for detection of the *diphtheria* toxin gene. J. Clin. Microbiol. *35*:1651-1655, 1997.

88. Natu, M., Borole, D., Shaikh, N., et al.: Comparative assessment of laboratory procedures: Diphtheria. Indian J. Pathol. Microbiol. *29*:31-35, 1986.

89. Olson, M. E., Goemans, I., Bolingbroke, D., and Lundberg, S.: Gangrenous dermatitis caused by *Corynebacterium ulcerans* in Richardson ground squirrels. J. Am. Vet. Med. Assoc. *193*:367-368, 1988.

90. Pallen, M. J., Hay, A. J., Puckey, L. H., et al.: Polymerase chain reaction for screening clinical isolates of corynebacteria for the production of diphtheria toxin. J. Clin. Pathol. *47*:353-356, 1994.

91. Popovic, T., Mazurova, I., Efstratiou, A., et al.: Molecular epidemiology of diphtheria. J. Infect. Dis. *181*(Suppl. 1):168-177, 2000.

92. Popovic, T., Wharton, M., Wenger, J. D., et al.: Are we ready for diphtheria? A report from the Diphtheria Diagnostic Workshop, Atlanta, 11 and 12 July 1994. J. Infect. Dis. *171*:765-767, 1995.

93. Quick, M. L., Sutter, R. W., Kobaidze, K., et al.: Risk factors for diphtheria: A prospective case-control study in the Republic of Georgia, 1995-1996. J. Infect. Dis. *181*(Suppl. 1):121-129, 2000.

94. Rakhmanova, A. G., Lumio, J., Groundstroem, K., et al.: Diphtheria outbreak in St. Petersburg: Clinical characteristics of 1860 adult patients. Scand. J. Infect. Dis. *28*:37-40, 1996.

95. Respiratory diphtheria caused by *Corynebacterium ulcerans*—Terre Haute, Indiana, 1996. M. M. W. R. Morb. Mortal. Wkly. Rep. *46*:330-332, 1997.

96. Rysselaere, M., and Vanneste, L.: Diphtheria of the eye. Bull. Soc. Belge Ophtalmol. *201*:89-92, 1982.

97. Sanchez, P. J., Laptook, A. R., Fisher, L., et al.: Apnea after immunization of preterm infants. J. Pediatr. *130*:746-752, 1997.

98. Sheth, K. J., and Sarff, L. D.: Hemolytic uremic syndrome associated with *Corynebacterium diphtheria* infection. Int. J. Pediatr. Nephrol. 7:17-20, 1986.

99. Suresh, G. K., Dhawan, A., and Kohli, V.: Tracheal diphtheria mimicking bacterial tracheitis. Pediatr. Infect. Dis. J. *11*:502, 1992.

100. Tasman, A., Minkenhof, J. E., Vink, H. H., et al.: Importance of intravenous injection of diphtheria antiserum. Lancet *1*:1299-1304, 1958.

101. Tiley, S. M., Kociuba, K. R., Heron, L. G., et al.: Infective endocarditis due to nontoxigenic *Corynebacterium diphtheriae*: Report of seven cases and review. Clin. Infect. Dis. *16*:271-275, 1993.

102. Toxigenic *Corynebacterium diphtheriae*—Northern Plains Indian Community, August-October 1996. M. M. W. R. Morb. Mortal. Wkly. Rep. *46*:506-510, 1997.

103. Vitek, C. R., and Wharton, M.: Diphtheria in the former Soviet Union: Reemergence of a pandemic disease. Emerg. Infect. Dis. *4*:539-550, 1998.

104. Wilson, G. S.: The necessity for a safe milk-supply. Lancet *2*:829-832, 1933.

ADDITIONAL READING

Barksdale, L.: *Corynebacterium diphtheriae* and its relatives. Bacteriol. Rev. *34*:378-422, 1970.

Pappenheimer, A. M., Jr.: Diphtheria toxin. *In* Ajl, S. J., Kadis, S., and Montie, T. C. (eds.): Microbial Toxins. Vol. 11B. New York, Academic Press, 1973.

Wood, W. B., Jr.: From Miasmas to Molecules. New York, Columbia University Press, 1961.

Zamiri, I.: *Corynebacterium. In* Collee, V. G., Fraser, A. G., Marmion, B. P., and Simmons, A. (eds.): Mackie and McCartney Practical Medical Microbiology. 14th ed. New York, Churchill Livingstone, 1996, pp. 299-307.

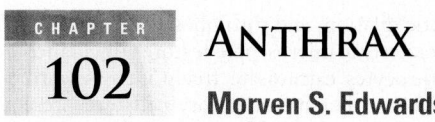

ANTHRAX
Morven S. Edwards

Anthrax is a toxigenic disease of herbivores for which humans are an incidental host. The term *anthrax*, derived from the Greek *anthrakos*, which means "coal," refers to the black eschar characteristic of cutaneous anthrax. The three clinical manifestations of anthrax are cutaneous, which accounts for 95 percent of infections in the United States; inhalational; and gastrointestinal. Each manifestation can occur in children,[22,30,42,48] and all can be complicated by meningitis.

HISTORICAL ASPECTS

Anthrax has been recognized since antiquity. The earliest reference to a disease thought to be anthrax is a description in *Exodus* of the plague that caused the death of all of the Egyptians' cattle.[7] Hippocrates described carbuncles that are thought to represent the cutaneous form of anthrax. An account of anthrax in animals is detailed in the third of the Roman poet Virgil's four *Georgics*.[39] In the early 17th century, an anthrax pandemic referred to as the "Black Bane" caused 60,000 human deaths in Europe.[7] By the 18th century, several excellent descriptions of the clinical disease in humans had been published.

Bacillus anthracis has a unique niche in the history of infectious diseases. The organism, seen microscopically by Delafond in 1838, was isolated and cultivated in 1877 by Koch, who showed its proliferation in vivo, establishing a model for the causation of infectious disease. In 1881, both Pasteur and Greenfield[45] showed that a live-attenuated anthrax bacillus vaccine protected against subsequent challenge in animals, demonstrating the efficacy of immunization for the prevention of an infectious disease. In the late 1800s, anthrax was proved to be the cause of woolsorter's disease, or inhalation anthrax, contracted by factory workers handling anthrax-contaminated animal hides.

During World War I, *B. anthracis* was manufactured as an agent for biologic warfare. Because anthrax is transmissible by the respiratory route, inhalational anthrax usually is fatal, and because *B. anthracis* spores are stable in the environment, anthrax continues to be a focus of biologic warfare research programs.[12] The accidental release of anthrax spores from a military research facility in Sverdlovsk in the former Soviet Union in 1979 resulted in at least 68 deaths from inhalational anthrax.[32] One estimate is that the aerosolized release of 100 kg of anthrax spores upwind of Washington, D.C., would result in 130,000 to 3 million deaths.[23]

The first confirmed outbreak associated with intentional anthrax release in the United States occurred in October and November 2001.[24] Anthrax spores were disseminated by mail, resulting in 5 deaths from inhalation and 22 total cases of cutaneous and inhalational anthrax. Envelopes containing anthrax spores were sent through the U.S. Postal Service to offices of newspaper and broadcast media and U.S. senators. The spores were "weaponized," or finely milled, and treated with chemicals to prevent clumping so that they dispersed when the envelopes were opened and leaked from sealed envelopes as they passed through mail sorting machines. A single anthrax strain was implicated. This outbreak has had a substantial impact on the health care system and has revealed the potential impact of a bioterrorism event on society.[5]

BACTERIOLOGY

B. anthracis is an aerobic, nonmotile, spore-forming rod in the family Bacillaceae. Optimal growth occurs at 36° C in nonselective media. Colonies are gray-white, rough, and flat and may have comma-shaped projections caused by the outgrowth of chains of bacilli from the edges of the colony, giving it a "Medusa head" appearance. Individual colonies are 4 to 5 mm in diameter with a ground-glass appearance and exhibit tenacity or a "beaten egg white" appearance when lifted with an inoculating loop.[16] A capsule, which is associated with virulence, can be delineated by electron microscopy. Encapsulation occurs with growth on enriched media. Gram stain of clinical material reveals large, square-ended, gram-positive rods singly or in short chains without a visible capsule. The equatorial or paracentral spores are invisible in smears fixed promptly after collection. After 24 to 48 hours of aerobic incubation, strands of rods are arranged in "boxcar" or "bamboo" fashion, and sporulation occurs. Small numbers of bacteria are pathogenic for mice, guinea pigs, and rabbits, and death usually occurs 2 to 5 days after inoculation. Currently, no method exists for serologically classifying strains of *B. anthracis*.

EPIDEMIOLOGY AND TRANSMISSION

Domestic herbivores—cattle, sheep, horses, goats, and swine—are the most important agricultural sources of anthrax, but all domestic and many wild animals can serve as hosts. Animals are infected by ingestion of spores from infected pastures. Spores germinate in vivo, and death, associated with massive septicemia, usually occurs in 1 or 2 days. Anthrax is endemic in areas where an animal-soil-animal cycle is established because the spores can survive indefinitely in a dry environment. Uncultivated soil with a pH greater than 6.0 and ambient temperature greater than 15.5° C provides an environment favorable for persistence of spores.[47]

An estimated 20,000 to 100,000 human cases of anthrax occur yearly worldwide.[40] Regions of high endemicity include South and Central America, southern Europe, eastern Europe, Asia, Africa, the Caribbean, and the Middle East. The number of human cases probably correlates with the enzootic status of the disease in livestock in these countries. Familial clustering can occur in association with exposure to diseased animals.[1,35] Children who live in endemic areas often contract cutaneous anthrax from direct animal contact.[34] More than half of 448 patients from the Gambia with cutaneous anthrax were younger than 15 years of age, and 11 percent were younger than 2 years.[20] In the United States, epizootics of anthrax occur in the lower Mississippi valley and in parts of California, Texas, Missouri, Nebraska, and South Dakota[49]; sporadic cases have been reported from almost every state. Cases of illness were identified in four states and in Washington, D.C., during the 2001 bioterrorism-related outbreak.

The incidence of human anthrax in the United States has decreased markedly since the early 1900s, when more than 100 cases were reported annually. Cutaneous infections are reported sporadically.[9] Cases often are associated with exposure to contaminated animal products in commercial preparations, but exposure to indigenous animal anthrax does occur in the United

States.[43] Two members of a farmer's family ate hamburgers made from an anthrax-infected steer in Minnesota in 2000. The family members received antibiotic prophylaxis and anthrax vaccine and remained well.[9]

Direct contact with contaminated animal meat or carcasses or with contaminated animal products, such as hides, hair, wool, bone meal, and animal feed, are sources of transmission of anthrax spores to humans. Children of industrial workers have acquired infection, presumably from contact with their parents' contaminated clothing.[7] Processed products, such as shaving brushes and saddle blankets, have been implicated as sources of infection. Cutaneous anthrax is transmitted by deposition of spores or bacilli into abrasions or cuts in the skin. Blood-sucking insects, including mosquitoes and stable flies, can be vectors.[31,46,47]

The specific mode of acquisition may be difficult to determine in children; in one child with cutaneous anthrax, the only potential exposure was proximity to a bone meal factory that he walked past on his way to school.[27] Tying the umbilicus with a dirty thread was the presumed portal of entry for a neonate with *B. anthracis* sepsis.[34] Rubbing with contaminated fingers or deposition by an insect vector can lead to cutaneous involvement of the eyelids.[51] Discharge from cutaneous lesions theoretically is infectious, but person-to-person transmission has not been confirmed. Skin-to-skin contact through his mother's exposure at her workplace was proposed as the route of transmission to an infant in the bioterrorism-related outbreak in the United States in 2001.[19] Maternal anthrax has been associated with preterm delivery.[25]

Inhalational anthrax results from inhalation of spores. The estimated infectious dose in humans is 8000 to 50,000 spores. Cases of inhalational anthrax in the United States have occurred in a weaver whose imported yarn was contaminated and in a drum maker whose imported hand-dried animal hide was contaminated with *B. anthracis*.[8,13] Eleven adults acquired inhalational anthrax during the 2001 bioterrorism outbreak of anthrax in the United States. Gastrointestinal anthrax is caused by ingestion of contaminated meat. A newborn was reported to have contracted anthrax meningitis from his mother, who was septicemic at the time of delivery.[20]

PATHOGENESIS AND PATHOLOGY

Anthrax toxicity results from the activity of three polypeptides—protective antigen, edema factor, and lethal factor—that combine to form two toxins, lethal toxin and edema toxin. Protective antigen is integral to the action of both toxins. Toxin entry into cells is initiated when protective antigen binds to membrane receptors of susceptible cells. Two related proteins, tumor endothelial marker 8 and capillary morphogenesis protein 2, function as receptors. Cleaved protective antigen oligomerizes, and a heptamer of protective antigen provides binding sites for edema factor or lethal factor. The complex is endocytosed as edema toxin or lethal toxin.

Edema factor is a calmodulin-dependent adenylate cyclase that increases intracellular cyclic adenosine monophosphate levels and is responsible for the massive edema that occurs in cutaneous anthrax.[28] Lethal factor is a zinc metalloproteinase that cleaves mitogen-activated protein kinase kinases so that they are unable to activate their downstream substrates, the mitogen-activated kinases.[18] Lethal factor stimulates production of tumor necrosis factor-α and interleukin-1β. The capsule of *B. anthracis* also contributes to virulence by inhibiting phagocytosis, and the toxins inhibit neutrophil priming by lipopolysaccharide, modulating the inflammatory response.[24,50]

Cutaneous infection is initiated when anthrax spores are ingested at the site of entry by macrophages, and germination occurs in skin tissues. Production of toxin results in local edema. Regional lymphangiitis and lymphadenopathy can occur.[15] Inter-

stitial edema, lymphatic dilation, and thrombosis and necrosis of blood vessels are characteristic microscopic features of cutaneous anthrax lesions. Erythrocytes extravasate freely into interstitial fluid. Few neutrophils or other inflammatory cells are present unless a lesion is infected secondarily. Hemorrhagic lymphadenitis involving regional lymph nodes occurs in all forms of anthrax.

In inhalation anthrax, spores entering the alveoli are phagocytosed by alveolar macrophages and dendritic cells and carried to hilar lymph nodes, where they germinate. Primary focal hemorrhagic necrotizing pneumonia can occur at the pulmonary portal of entry.[2] Massive hemorrhagic mediastinal lymphadenitis can block lymphatic drainage routes and can be causally related to the pulmonary edema and respiratory distress observed clinically.[48]

Gastrointestinal anthrax results from ingestion of spores or vegetative bacilli in contaminated meat. The primary sites of infection are the epithelium of the stomach or bowel wall.[6] Edema and small necrotic ulcers of the mucosa of the gastrointestinal tract, especially the ileum or cecum, are characteristic findings. Dissemination to the central nervous system can occur by hematogenous or lymphatic routes from any site of primary involvement. Hemorrhage involving the meninges and intense arteritis are uniform findings in patients who die of anthrax meningitis.

CLINICAL MANIFESTATIONS

CUTANEOUS ANTHRAX

The lesions of cutaneous anthrax occur mainly on exposed areas of the body. In one report, the distribution in young children was 52 percent of lesions on the head and neck, 28 percent on the trunk, and 20 percent on the extremities, whereas in older children, the distribution was 70 percent on the head and neck, 16 percent on the trunk, and 14 percent on the extremities.[22] Spores are introduced through abraded or injured skin. Children can have one or several lesions, and they are associated with regional adenitis.[29] After an incubation period of 2 to 5 days, a small, nontender, but frequently pruritic, papule develops at the site of inoculation. The lesion progresses to a serous or serosanguineous vesicle with surrounding nonpitting edema within 36 hours. Satellite vesicles, sometimes referred to as a "pearly wreath,"[51] may be seen occasionally.

The lesion undergoes central necrosis, with a black eschar left behind (Fig. 102–1).[38] The term *malignant edema* is used to describe severe lesions, particularly lesions involving the head and neck, which can be associated with systemic toxicity and occlusion of the airway. Small children can appear acutely ill with a temperature of 39° C to 40° C and leukocytosis with counts of 20,000 to 30,000 cells/mm[3].[19] Approximately 5 percent of patients are bacteremic. With appropriate therapy, the edema usually resolves within 2 to 3 days, but the central lesion continues its evolution unaffected. The eschar usually is 1 to 3 cm in diameter, with sharply defined margins seen 1 week to 10 days after onset. Separation of the eschar may take several weeks, and healing occurs with variable central scarring.[27]

INHALATIONAL ANTHRAX

Inhalational anthrax is a biphasic illness. Symptoms in the initial stage—malaise, low-grade fever, myalgia, and nonproductive cough—are nonspecific and resemble the symptoms of a respiratory viral illness or bronchitis. Adults who have inhalational anthrax are more likely to present with tachycardia, high hematocrit, low albumin, and sodium levels, and are less likely to present with myalgias, headache, and nasal symptoms than are by edema and enlargement of the cervical lymph nodes, dysphagia, and respiratory difficulty. Lesions on the tonsils or posterior oropharynx progress over 1 to 2 weeks from an area of edema to a pseudomembrane-covered ulcer. The oropharyngeal form of anthrax, although uncommon, has a more favorable prognosis than does intestinal anthrax.

Initial features of intestinal anthrax are fever, nausea, anorexia, vomiting, and diffuse abdominal pain that progresses rapidly to severe abdominal pain with rebound tenderness. Vomiting of blood-tinged or coffee ground-like material and melena are common symptoms and are secondary to ulceration of the intestinal mucosa.[6,24,33] The pain decreases, and massive ascites develops 24 to 48 hours after the onset of symptoms. Abdominal radiographs at this time show edematous loops of bowel and decreased air. If the abdomen is explored, findings include enlarged, erythematous mesenteric lymph nodes and straw-colored to purulent ascitic fluid in which organisms are readily visible.[3] Death usually occurs in association with significant blood loss, fluid and electrolyte imbalances, and subsequent shock. If the patient survives the acute illness, the edema and melena subside in 10 to 14 days.

MENINGITIS

Most reports of anthrax meningitis are associated with cutaneous disease, likely due to the higher frequency of cutaneous disease. Anthrax can disseminate to the meninges from any site of primary involvement. In the 2001 bioterrorism event, one adult with inhalation anthrax presented with meningitis, and several others had features suggestive of central nervous system involvement.[36] In a report of 70 patients with anthrax meningitis who ranged in age from newborn to 71 years, no primary focus could be found in 12 percent of patients.[21] Young and middle-aged men are affected most often as a consequence of occupational exposure.

Anthrax meningitis is characterized by a sudden onset and fulminant course. Initial symptoms include intense headache, nausea and vomiting, myalgia, chills, dizziness, and, occasionally, a petechial rash. Meningismus is usually, but not invariably, present because of the acuity of the course. Progressive neurologic deterioration with delirium, convulsions, and coma can occur in hours or over the course of 2 to 4 days. Overall survival has been only approximately 5 percent, but survival without apparent neurologic sequelae has been reported in at least three children, two of whom had cutaneous lesions at the time of diagnosis.[36,41,42,44]

Examination of cerebrospinal fluid reveals (1) gross or microscopic hemorrhage, (2) leukocytosis consisting predominantly of polymorphonuclear leukocytes, (3) elevated protein, and (4) depressed glucose levels. Gram-positive rods can be seen easily on smears of cerebrospinal fluid. Peripheral leukocytosis is a common finding, and the white blood cell count may be 60,000 to 80,000 cells/mm³. Blood cultures yield the organism in 70 percent, and cerebrospinal fluid cultures yield the organism in virtually 100 percent of patients.[20] Neuroimaging findings are notable for multiple hemorrhages in the ventricles, subarachnoid space, and deep gray matter.[36]

DIAGNOSIS AND DIFFERENTIAL DIAGNOSIS

B. anthracis can be visualized by direct smear and cultured from vesicular fluid or exudate from cutaneous lesions and from pleural fluid, blood, and cerebrospinal fluid in systemic infections. The commercially available QuickELISA Anthrax-PA Kit (Immunetics Inc., Boston, MA) can be used as a screening test.[4] Definitive diagnosis can be obtained through the Laboratory Response

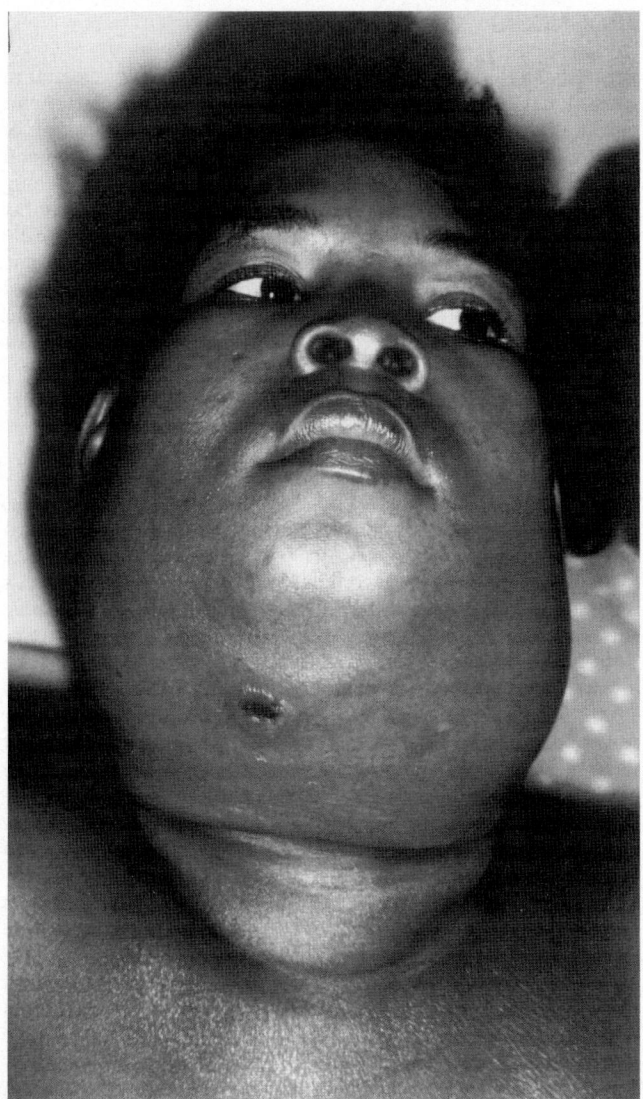

Figure 102–1 Cutaneous anthrax with associated massive submental edema. The lesion is located at the site of a small, initially trivial laceration that served as the portal of entry for the anthrax endospores. The patient received ampicillin and recovered completely. *(Courtesy of M. Thomas Casey, M.D.)*

adults who have influenza-like illnesses.[26] After several days of illness, dyspnea and stridor initiate onset of the second stage, which usually terminates fatally within 24 hours. Chest radiographs show a widened mediastinum with smooth borders and evidence of hemorrhagic mediastinitis and pleural effusions.[48] The pleural effusions often are large and usually contain bloody fluid. Pulmonary infiltrates usually are the result of superimposed bacterial infection. In the more recent cases from the United States, computed tomography scans of the chest showed the characteristic findings of hemorrhagic mediastinal and hilar lymph nodes and mediastinal edema and pleural effusions.[5]

GASTROINTESTINAL ANTHRAX

Gastrointestinal anthrax can manifest with oropharyngeal or intestinal manifestations. Each has an incubation period of 2 to 5 days after the ingestion of contaminated meat. The oropharyngeal form results in an oral or esophageal ulcer.[6,24,37] Presenting features include fever, severe sore throat, neck swelling caused

Network for Bioterrorism in each state. Time-resolved fluorescent assay, real-time polymerase chain reaction, serologic tests to detect antibodies against protective antigen, and tissue immunochemistry also are available through state health laboratories. The enzyme-linked immunosorbent assay used to detect IgG to *B. anthracis* protective antigen is highly sensitive, has good specificity, and yields a positive result 10 days after the onset of symptoms.[5]

The lesion of cutaneous anthrax must be differentiated from ecthyma gangrenosum and from ulcerative skin lesions with regional lymphadenopathy, including rat-bite fever, ulceroglandular tularemia, plague, glanders, scrub typhus, rickettsialpox, cowpox, and orf. Staphylococcal lymphangitis can be distinguished from anthrax by the discharge of purulent material and by the inflammatory response observed microscopically. Noninfectious causes of eschars include arachnoid bites and vasculitides.[24] The first stage of inhalational anthrax and the clinical features of the intestinal form are nonspecific, so a history of exposure is crucial for establishing the diagnosis. The mediastinal widening that occurs early in the course of inhalational anthrax can cause confusion with that seen in acute bacterial mediastinitis and in fibrous mediastinitis caused by *Histoplasma capsulatum*.[15] Gastrointestinal anthrax must be differentiated from other causes of acute abdominal illness and, if bleeding is present, from duodenal ulcer, typhoid, and intestinal tularemia. Anthrax meningitis must be differentiated from subarachnoid hemorrhage.[20]

TREATMENT

Most, but not all, strains of *B. anthracis* are susceptible to penicillin and tetracycline, but naturally resistant strains occur, and penicillin resistance can be induced. Resistance occurs sufficiently uncommonly in naturally occurring cutaneous disease that penicillin or tetracycline for 7 to 10 days is adequate treatment. Treatment for bioterrorism-associated cutaneous anthrax should be initiated with ciprofloxacin, 10 to 15 mg/kg every 12 hours (not to exceed 1 g/day) orally until susceptibility data are available. Doxycycline is an alternative antimicrobial for initial therapy. The dosage is 100 mg orally every 12 hours (children >8 years old) or 5 mg/kg/day in divided doses given every 12 hours (children ≤8 years old). Treatment should continue for 60 days in the context of bioterrorism-associated cutaneous anthrax.[4]

The initial regimen for treatment of inhalational anthrax, gastrointestinal anthrax, anthrax meningitis, or cutaneous anthrax if (1) systemic signs are present, (2) lesions are located on the head and neck, and (3) extensive edema is present should be ciprofloxacin intravenously (400 mg every 8-12 hours) or doxycycline intravenously (200 mg every 8-12 hours).[4,10,11] One or two additional antimicrobials should be administered intravenously with either ciprofloxacin or doxycycline as initial therapy until susceptibility testing is available. Other agents with in vitro activity include levofloxacin, gatifloxacin, penicillin, ampicillin, clindamycin, vancomycin, rifampin, imipenem, meropenem, clarithromycin, and chloramphenicol.[17] If the organism is determined to be susceptible to penicillin, penicillin may be administered at a dosage of 300,000 to 400,000 U/kg/day intravenously or 50,000 U/kg/day orally. Therapy should be continued for at least 60 days.

Supportive therapy includes attention to details of fluid and electrolyte balances, endotracheal intubation if indicated to maintain a patent airway, and local care for cutaneous lesions. Systemic steroids may reduce the severity of infections in patients with massive edema or meningitis.[42] A specific anthrax antitoxin is not available.

PROGNOSIS

Before penicillin was introduced, cutaneous anthrax was fatal in approximately 20 percent of patients. With effective treatment, the mortality rate is less than 1 percent. Cutaneous anthrax of the eyelid may be complicated by ectropion of the upper lid and corneal scarring with blindness.[51] Immunity probably is lifelong in most patients. Although second attacks of cutaneous anthrax have been recorded, they have not been confirmed serologically and usually are mild.[14,22] Fatality rates are high for systemic anthrax and range from 50 to 100 percent for gastrointestinal anthrax to virtually 100 percent for inhalation anthrax, but children who have survived these infections have no apparent sequelae.

PREVENTION

The only human anthrax vaccine licensed in the United States is BioThrax (BioPort Corporation, Lansing, MI), formerly known as *anthrax vaccine adsorbed*, which is prepared from a cell-free filtrate of *B. anthracis* that contains no dead or live bacteria.[12] It is an aluminum hydroxide–precipitated preparation of protective antigen from an attenuated, nonencapsulated anthrax strain. Routine vaccination is indicated for individuals engaged in work involving the production of quantities or concentrations of *B. anthracis* in culture and in activities involving a high potential for aerosol production. The primary immunization series consists of three subcutaneous injections at 0, 2, and 4 weeks and three booster vaccinations at 6, 12, and 18 months. To maintain immunity, an annual booster dose is recommended.[12]

The limited data available suggest that the best means of preventing inhalational anthrax after exposure to spores is administration of ciprofloxacin (10 to 15 mg/kg orally every 12 hours to a maximum of 500 mg orally every 12 hours) or doxycycline (100 mg orally every 12 hours for children >8 years old or 5 mg/kg/day in divided doses given every 12 hours for children ≤8 years old) in conjunction with a three-dose regimen of vaccine (given at 0, 2, and 4 weeks after exposure).[4] In the event of a biologic anthrax attack, children exposed to spores should receive ciprofloxacin as postexposure prophylaxis for 60 days. If penicillin sensitivity is established, prophylactic therapy can be changed to amoxicillin, 80 mg/kg divided into three doses taken every 8 hours (maximum dose 500 mg orally every 8 hours). Although no data in children are available, the vaccine probably would be safe and effective.[23]

Worldwide, anthrax is controlled through livestock immunization programs. Procedures to prevent the spread of anthrax in animals include disposal of contaminated carcasses by burning and annual vaccination of livestock in known enzootic areas. All suspected or proven cases of anthrax should be reported to public health officials. Hospitalized patients should be kept under isolation until the lesions are bacteriologically sterile. Contaminated dressings and clothing must be burned or sterilized, and the patient's room must be disinfected to destroy spores.

REFERENCES

1. Abdenour, D., Larouze, B., Dalichaouche, M., et al.: Familial occurrence of anthrax in eastern Algeria J. Infect. Dis. *155*:1083-1084, 1987.
2. Abramova, F. A., Grinberg, L. M., Yampolskaya, O. V., et al.: Pathology of inhalational anthrax in 42 cases from the Sverdlovsk outbreak of 1979. Proc. Natl. Acad. Sci. U. S. A. *90*:2291-2294, 1993.
3. Alizad, A., Ayoub, E. M., and Makki, N.: Intestinal anthrax in a two-year-old child. Pediatr. Infect. Dis. J. *14*:394-395, 1995.
4. American Academy of Pediatrics: Anthrax. *In* Pickering, L. K., Baker, C. J., Long, S. S., and McMillan, J. A. (eds.): Red Book: 2006 Report of the

Committee on Infectious Diseases. 27th ed. Elk Grove Village, IL, American Academy of Pediatrics, 2006, pp. 208-211.

5. Bartlett, J. G., Inglesby, T. V., Jr., and Borio, L.: Management of anthrax. Clin. Infect. Dis. *35*:851-858, 2002.

6. Beatty, M. E., Ashford, D. A., Griffin, P. M., et al.: Gastrointestinal anthrax: Review of the literature. Arch. Intern. Med. *163*:2527-2531, 2003.

7. Brachman, P. S.: Anthrax. Ann. N. Y. Acad. Sci. *174*:577-582, 1970.

8. Brachman, P. S.: Inhalation anthrax. Ann. N. Y. Acad. Sci. *353*:83-93, 1980.

9. Centers for Disease Control and Prevention: Human ingestion of *Bacillus anthracis*-contaminated meat—Minnesota, August 2000. M. M. W. R. Morb. Mortal. Wkly. Rep. *49*:813-832, 2000.

10. Centers for Disease Control and Prevention: Notice to readers: Update: Interim recommendations for antimicrobial prophylaxis for children and breastfeeding mothers and treatment of children with anthrax. M. M. W. R. Morb. Mortal. Wkly. Rep. *50*:1014-1016, 2001.

11. Centers for Disease Control and Prevention: Update: Investigation of bioterrorism-related anthrax and interim guidelines for exposure management and antimicrobial therapy, October 2001. M. M. W. R. Morb. Mortal. Wkly. Rep. *50*:909-919, 2001.

12. Centers for Disease Control and Prevention: Notice to readers: Use of anthrax vaccine in response to terrorism: Supplemental recommendations of the Advisory Committee on Immunization Practices. M. M. W. R. Morb. Mortal. Wkly. Rep. *51*:1024-1026, 2002.

13. Centers for Disease Control and Prevention: Inhalation anthrax associated with dried animal hides—Pennsylvania and New York City, 2006. M. M. W. R. Morb. Mortal. Wkly. Rep. *55*:280-282, 2006.

14. Christie, A. B.: The clinical aspects of anthrax. Postgrad. Med. J. *49*:565-570, 1973.

15. Dixon, T. C., Meselson, M., Guillemin, J., et al.: Anthrax. N. Engl. J. Med. *341*:815-826, 1999.

16. Doyle, R. J., Keller, K. F., and Ezzell, J. W.: Bacillus. *In* Lennette, E. H., Balows, A., Hauser, W. J., Jr., et al. (eds.): Manual of Clinical Microbiology. 4th ed. Washington, D.C., American Society for Microbiology, 1985, pp. 211-215.

17. Drago, L., De Vecchi, E., Lombardi, A., et al.: Bactericidal activity of levofloxacin, gatifloxacin, penicillin, meropenem and rokitamycin against *Bacillus anthracis* clinical isolates. J. Antimicrob. Chemother. *50*:1059-1063, 2002.

18. Duesbery, N. S., Webb, C. P., Leppla, S. H., et al.: Proteolytic inactivation of MAP-kinase-kinase by anthrax lethal factor. Science *280*:734-737, 1998.

19. Freedman, A., Afonja, O., Chang, M. W., et al.: Cutaneous anthrax associated with microangiopathic hemolytic anemia and coagulopathy in a 7-month-old child. J. A. M. A. *287*:869-874, 2002.

20. Gerhardt, P.: Cytology of *Bacillus anthracis*. Fed. Proc. *26*:1504-1517, 1967.

21. Haight, T. H.: Anthrax meningitis: Review of literature and report of two cases with autopsies. Am. J. Med. Sci. *224*:57-69, 1952.

22. Heyworth, B., Ropp, M. E., Voos, U. G., et al.: Anthrax in the Gambia: An epidemiological study. B. M. J. *4*:79-82, 1975.

23. Inglsby, T. V., Henderson, D. A., Bartlett, J. G., et al.: Anthrax as a biological weapon: Medical and public health management. J. A. M. A. *281*:1735-1745, 1999.

24. Inglesby, T. V., O'Toole, T., Henderson, D. A., et al.: Anthrax as a biological weapon, 2002: Updated recommendations for management. J. A. M. A. *287*:2236-2252, 2002.

25. Kadanali, A., Tasyaran, M. A., and Kadanali, S.: Anthrax during pregnancy: Case reports and review. Clin. Infect. Dis. *36*:1343-1346, 2003.

26. Kuehnert, M. J., Doyle, T. J., Hill, H. A., et al.: Clinical features that discriminate inhalational anthrax from other acute respiratory illnesses. Clin. Infect. Dis. *36*:328-336, 2003.

27. Lamb, R.: Anthrax. B. M. J. *1*:157-160, 1973.

28. Leppla, S. H.: *Bacillus anthracis* calmodulin dependent adenylate cyclase: Chemical and enzymatic properties and interactions with eucaryotic cells. Adv. Cyclic Nucleotide Protein Phosphorylation Res. *17*:189-198, 1984.

29. Maguiña, C., Flores del Pozo, J., Terashima, A., et al.: Cutaneous anthrax in Lima, Peru: Retrospective analysis of 71 cases, including four with a meningo-encephalitic complication. Rev. Inst. Med. Trop. S. Paulo *47*:25-30, 2005.

30. Manios, S., and Kavaliotis, I.: Anthrax in children: A long forgotten, potentially fatal infection. Scand. J. Infect. Dis. *11*:203-206, 1979.

31. McKendrick, D. R. A.: Anthrax and its transmission to humans. Cent. Afr. J. Med. *26*:126-129, 1980.

32. Meselson, M., Guillemin, J., Hugh-Jones, M., et al.: The Sverdlovsk anthrax outbreak of 1979. Science *266*:1202-1208, 1994.

33. Nalin, D. R., Sultana, B., Sahunja, R., et al.: Survival of a patient with intestinal anthrax. Am. J. Med. *62*:130-132, 1977.

34. Özkaya, E., Kirimi, E., Berktas, M., et al.: *Bacillus anthracis* sepsis in a newborn. Pediatr. Infect. Dis. J. *19*:487-488, 2000.

35. Seboxa, T., and Goldhagen, J.: Anthrax in Ethiopia. Trop. Geogr. Med. *41*:108-112, 1989.

36. Sejvar, J. J., Tenover, F. C., and Stephens, D. S.: Management of anthrax meningitis. Lancet Infect. Dis. *5*:287-295, 2005.

37. Sirisanthana, T., Navacharoen, N., Tharavichitkul, P., et al.: Outbreak of oral-pharyngeal anthrax: An unusual manifestation of human infection with *Bacillus anthracis*. Am. J. Med. Hyg. *33*:144-150, 1984.

38. Smego, R. A., Jr., Gebrian, B., and Desmangels, G.: Cutaneous manifestations of anthrax in rural Haiti. Clin. Infect. Dis. *26*:97-102, 1998.

39. Sternbach, G.: The history of anthrax. J. Emerg. Med. *24*:463-467, 2003.

40. Swartz, M. N.: Recognition and management of anthrax—an update. N. Engl. J. Med. *345*:1621-1626, 2001 (Erratum N. Engl. J. Med. *346*:634, 2002).

41. Tabatabaie, P., and Syadati, A.: *Bacillus anthracis* as a cause of bacterial meningitis. Pediatr. Infect. Dis. J. *12*:1035-1037, 1993.

42. Tahernia, A. C., and Hashemi, G.: Survival in anthrax meningitis. Pediatrics *50*:329-332, 1972.

43. Taylor, J. P., Dimmitt, D. C., Ezzell, J. W., et al.: Indigenous human cutaneous anthrax in Texas. South. Med. J. *86*:1-4, 1993.

44. Tengio, F. U.: Anthrax meningitis: Report of two cases. East Afr. Med. J. *50*:337-339, 1973.

45. Tigertt, W. D.: Anthrax. William Smith Greenfield, MD, FRCP, Professor Superintendent, The Brown Animal Sanatory Institution (1878-1881). Concerning the priority due to him for the production of the first vaccine against anthrax. J. Hyg. Camb. *85*:415-420, 1980.

46. Turell, M. J., Knudson, G. B.: Mechanical transmission of *Bacillus anthracis* by stable flies (*Stomoxys calcitrans*) and mosquitoes (*Aedes aegypti* and *Aedes taeniorhynchus*). Infect. Immun. *55*:1859-1861, 1987.

47. Van Ness, G. B.: Ecology of anthrax. Science *172*:1303-1307, 1971.

48. Vessal, K., Yeganehdoust, J., Dutz, W., et al.: Radiological changes in inhalation anthrax: A report of radiological and pathological correlation in two cases. Clin. Radiol. *26*:471-474, 1975.

49. Wolff, A. H., and Heimann, H.: Industrial anthrax in the United States. Am. J. Hyg. *53*:80-109, 1951.

50. Wright, G. G., and Mandell, G. L.: Anthrax toxin blocks priming of neutrophils by lipopolysaccharide and by muramyl dipeptide. J. Exp. Med. *164*:1700-1709, 1986.

51. Yorston, D., and Foster, A.: Cutaneous anthrax leading to corneal scarring from cicatricial ectropion. Br. J. Ophthalmol. *73*:809-811, 1989.

CHAPTER
103

BACILLUS CEREUS

Richard A. Oberhelman ❖ Thomas G. Cleary

Recognition of *Bacillus cereus* pathogenicity was delayed until clarification of the taxonomy of the genus *Bacillus* in the early 1950s. Multiple early reports of food poisoning and other infections including gastroenteritis, bacteremia-septicemia, cellulitis, ear and eye infections, endocarditis, and urinary tract infections that were attributed to *Bacillus subtilis* or to other *Bacillus* spp. probably were caused by *B. cereus*.[91] *B. cereus* can give rise to two distinct forms of food-borne diseases related to different toxins, the emetic and the diarrheal syndromes, and occasionally to localized and systemic disease.[36,53]

The diarrheal syndrome was recognized first by Hauge[43] in 1955 after four clinically similar outbreaks in Norway occurred. This common form of disease was related to a great variety of foods, such as meat and vegetable soup, poultry, pudding, sauce, pasta, cake, and milk. In 1974, Mortimer and McCann[69] described a vomiting syndrome associated with the consumption of fried rice in Chinese restaurants. Despite widespread recognition in Europe, *B. cereus* outbreaks have been reported infrequently in the United States. The first documented outbreak in the United States occurred in 1970.[66]

BACTERIOLOGY

Members of the genus *Bacillus* are aerobic or facultative anaerobic, gram-positive or gram-variable, spore-forming rods. They are distributed widely in the environment because of the high resistance of their endospores to extreme conditions, including heat, cold, desiccation, salinity, and radiation.[28,79] Based on the high variability in guanine and cytosine content (32 to 69%), the debate ensues regarding the classification of *Bacillus* spp.[96]

B. cereus belongs to the group of gram-positive rods that produce central or terminal ellipsoid or cylindric spores that do not distend the sporangia.[96] Studies of DNA-DNA hybridization and 16S and 23S rRNA sequencing and enzyme electrophoretic patterns have shown a close relationship among *B. cereus, Bacillus anthracis, Bacillus mycoides,* and *Bacillus thuringiensis*; these organisms are so closely related that they all may be considered variants of *B. cereus*. Differentiating, particularly between *B. cereus* and the insect pathogen *B. thuringiensis*, sometimes is difficult in the diagnostic laboratory. Polymerase chain reaction technology has been used for identifying species.[16]

B. cereus is a flagellated, motile, gram-positive rod, typically 1 to 1.2 μm in diameter by 3 to 5 μm in length. The organism sporulates freely on many media under well-aerated conditions, but vegetative cells also can grow anaerobically. It is able to metabolize glucose, fructose, and sucrose but not pentose and other sugar alcohols. It produces acid from glucose but not from arabinose, xylose, or mannitol. Starch hydrolysis and catalase production are similar to those of the other members of the genus. The presence of lipid globules or protoplasts is a characteristic that it shares with *Bacillus megaterium*.[54] Colonies on blood agar are large, flat, granular, and slightly green-tinged. *B. cereus* is differentiated from *B. anthracis* by motility, hemolysis, lack of lysis by gamma-phage, penicillin resistance, and absence of a capsule in *B. cereus*.[28] Identifying morphologic differentiation with nonmotile *B. cereus* strains and *B. anthracis* strains that are occasionally weakly hemolytic may be difficult.

Growth and multiplication of vegetative cells occur in a temperature range of 10° C to 50° C, with an optimum of 28° C to 35° C. Variations in toxin levels found in certain foods also can be related to pH levels, sugar content, the presence of other lactic acid bacteria, and aeration.[85,86] Some strains responsible for milk spoilage can grow at temperatures of 5° C,[54,79] but few strains are able to produce toxin at temperatures less than 7° C.[79] Ribosomal DNA characterization and genotyping based on the major cold shock protein homologue cspA have defined a novel species, *Bacillus weichenstephanensis*, which can grow at 4° C to 7° C, but not at 43° C.[56] These strains form a new fifth subgroup of *B. cereus* organisms described as psychrotolerant or psychrotropic, meaning they are able to grow at temperatures of 7° C and less.[55,75,87] Spore formation allows some *B. cereus* strains to survive pasteurization and heating.[55] More recently, a crystalline cell surface protein layer or "S-layer" has been described as a determinant of cell hydrophobicity. S-layer–producing cells are hydrophilic and able to bind to human matrix proteins, and presence of the S-layer in some *B. cereus* strains is associated with resistance to phagocytosis and increased radiation resistance against gamma irradiation.[53]

Serologic differentiation of *Bacillus* spp. is hampered by cross-reactive antigens and autoagglutination of spores caused by hydrophobic surface properties. Serologic typing based on the flagellar (H) antigen can be used during an outbreak to distinguish among strains and to determine the similarity of isolates obtained from humans with the strains isolated from suspect foods.[28] The serotype scheme is based on 42 H antisera raised against prototype strains. A common flagellar antigenic epitope has been suggested. Detection of the flagellar antigen by enzyme-linked immunosorbent assay is perhaps more sensitive than is detection by the agglutination method.[70] In addition to serology and biotyping (based on biochemical typing), plasmid analysis and phage typing have proved useful epidemiologically.[2,54,83,100] Techniques such as pyrolysis mass spectrometry and gas-liquid chromatography of whole-cell fatty acids are showing promise.[28]

Diagnosis of the rare extraintestinal infection is made by isolation from normally sterile sites (blood or tissue) after overnight incubation on nutrient or blood agar; clinical specimens from normally nonsterile sites (feces, vomitus) and food or environmental samples require selective techniques. Polymyxin B is used as a selective agent, and the lecithinase reaction of the organism on egg yolk and its inability to catabolize mannitol permit presumptive identification to be made with a variety of media: mannitol–egg yolk–polymyxin B, Kim and Goepfert medium, and polymyxin B–pyruvate–egg yolk–mannitol with bromothymol blue or bromocresol purple.[28]

EPIDEMIOLOGY

B. cereus in the spore and vegetative form is a ubiquitous organism found in soil, water, vegetation, and food products, especially cereals, dairy products, dried foods, spices, meat products, and vegetables.[54] The emetic syndrome typically is associated with cooked rice, usually fried, from Chinese restaurants.[52,69] Saving portions of boiled rice at room temperature overnight until required for frying previously was a common practice. Refrigerating boiled rice makes the grains stick together, which is less convenient for frying. The spores of *B. cereus* survive cooking and are capable of germination and outgrowth.[37,39] The optimal temperature for growth in boiled rice is 30° C to 37° C, although growth does occur during storage at 15° C to 43° C.[37] Most samples of uncooked rice contain multiple serotypes of *B. cereus*, and little difference occurs in the growth rate of the various serotypes in boiled rice at 22° C, but spores of serotype 1 strains are more resistant to heating at 95° C, which probably is the reason that this serotype usually is implicated in outbreaks.[72]

Starchy dried foods other than rice, such as cereals, frequently are contaminated.[15] Tortillas can be contaminated with the water used in preparation and from the hands of producers.[19] Specific foods incriminated in outbreaks in the United States include Chinese food (accounting for 50% of reported outbreaks between 1973 and 1987), followed by Mexican food, beef, fruits, and vegetables. Other foods implicated, particularly in the enterotoxin syndrome, include beef stew, turkey loaf, barbecued pork, macaroni and cheese, potatoes, spaghetti and other pastas, dairy and dried milk products, and seafoods.[27,35,46,50,53,59] In a study of 96 milk and milk product samples collected from retail shops in Nairobi, Kenya, 57 percent of samples were contaminated with *B. cereus* and 81 percent of the bacterial isolates (38 of 47) produced non-hemolytic enterotoxins, including 6 of 43 pasteurized milk products (43%).[71] Among the factors thought to contribute to the outbreaks, the most frequent were improper storage or holding temperature (94%), contaminated equipment (53%), inadequate cooking (32%), and poor personal hygiene (24%).[7]

Outbreaks of *B. cereus* have been recognized widely in Europe but rarely in the United States. In the Netherlands, *B. cereus* reportedly was the cause of 22.4 percent of food-borne disease outbreaks of known bacterial cause. Similarly, in Finland, it accounted for 11.9 percent of outbreaks. In most places, *B. cereus* is incriminated in 0.9 to 7 percent of outbreaks of food-related disease and 0.7 to 3 percent of cases.[54] In the United States between 1998 and 2002, *B. cereus* was identified as the cause of 37 of 6647 (0.6%) foodborne outbreaks reported to the Centers for Disease Control and Prevention, with a total of 571 cases and no deaths recorded.[62] The location of the outbreak is known for 24 of these outbreaks, and most of these (15 of 24 [62.5%]) occurred in commercial food outlets, such as restaurants, delicatessens, or workplace cafeterias. In outbreaks for which the implicated source was known, cereal products were the most common vehicle.[62] The susceptibility of children to this pathogen is evident from the report of an outbreak involving two daycare centers[52] and other reports that included neonates, children, and adolescents.[31,45,49,73,78,92,104] Only a small fraction of outbreaks are reported to the Centers for Disease Control and Prevention; small outbreaks of mild, brief illness are less likely to be reported. It is thought that 10^5 to 10^8 organisms per gram need to be ingested to cause the emetic syndrome and 10^5 to 10^7 cells or spores (total dose) ingested to cause the enterotoxin syndrome.[40]

For infections not related to food, groups at risk include neonates,[31,73] immunocompromised hosts,[4,20,30,39,45,49,83,89] intravenous drug abusers,[23,89] and patients with intravascular devices or artificial prostheses.[4,6,30,31,83,84] Studies in three different populations in South Africa and London, including school-aged children, found the organism in 18 to 43 percent of fecal samples.[95] The organism can be part of the normal intestinal flora. *B. cereus* does not persist in the intestine after ingestion.[34]

PATHOGENESIS

B. cereus produces an enormous range of extracellular metabolites, including peptides with antibiotic properties (biocerin, cerein, thiocillins), β-lactamases, hydrolases, nuclease, urease, and proteases.[91] Two different groups of toxins, known as diarrheal enterotoxins and emetic toxin, are responsible for the clinical syndromes of food poisoning.[64,97] Some strains may be able to produce both toxins based on the evidence that culture filtrates derived from strains isolated from emetic poisoning occasionally are able to produce a positive rabbit ileal loop assay.[79]

Biologic activities of diarrheal enterotoxins can be shown in multiple different assay systems. Three enterotoxins are produced. Purification plus isolation of multiple toxic fractions with some, but not all, of these activities has caused confusion.[28,90] Evaluation of the toxic activity of whole-cell suspension, cell-free culture filtrates, and the purified enterotoxin complex classically has included the rabbit ileal loop fluid accumulation assay, vascular permeability in rabbit skin, dermonecrosis and intestinonecrosis, mouse lethality, cytotoxicity, and hemolysis.[12,18,58,88,93,98] Hemolytic *B. cereus* enterotoxin has been characterized as a complex called *hemolysin BL* or *HBL*, composed of a binding component B (35 kd) and two lytic components, L1 and L2 (36 kd and 45 kd)[8]; all three are needed for fluid accumulation in the rabbit ileal loop.[10] Another *B. cereus* enterotoxin complex that is non-hemolytic and is composed of three distinct proteins has been described.[61] Several other single proteins with enterotoxic diarrhea–producing activity also have been described.[53]

The emetic toxin cereulide is a heat-stable (126° C for 90 minutes), ring-shaped peptide with a molecular weight of 1.2 kd[65]; it is stable between pH 2 and 11 and is protease-resistant. In contrast to the diarrheal toxins, it is preformed in foods, so the presence of living organisms at the time of ingestion is not necessary to cause symptoms.[36,91] Rice culture filtrates derived from emetic syndrome–associated strains cause cytoplasmic vacuolation and swollen mitochondria in HEp-2 cells, characteristics suggestive of uncoupling of oxidative phosphorylation.[76] Emetic activity occurs through the serotonin 5-HT$_3$ receptor and stimulation of the vagus afferent nerve.[1]

Among the multiple other substances with relevant activity, two groups are associated with local infection.[93,94] Cereolysin, or hemolysin I, is a thiol-activated cytolysin. Phospholipase C–like or lecithinase-like substances, including a sphingomyelinase and two hydrolases with preference for phosphatidylcholine and phosphatidylinositol, also exist. These enzymes induce the release of lysosomal enzymes from neutrophils that probably are involved in tissue damage, especially in wound and ocular infections.[28,106]

CLINICAL MANIFESTATIONS

FOOD POISONING

Diarrheal Syndrome

The enterotoxins preformed in food or produced in vivo in the intestine after the ingestion of bacilli cause profuse, watery, nonbloody diarrhea accompanied by abdominal pain and cramps, nausea, and, occasionally, vomiting or low-grade fever.[3,27,35,50,54,60,82] The typical incubation period is 8 to 16 hours, and the clinical characteristics resemble the food poisoning of *Clostridium perfringens*. The interval between ingestion and the onset of symptoms reflects the time required for production of toxin in the gut. The symptoms resolve within approximately 12 to 24 hours but occasionally can last 2 days to 2 weeks.[35] The diarrhea (3 to 10 bowel movements per day) rarely leads to dehydration in healthy individuals. In the elderly, bloody stools can occur.[35] The most prevalent flagellar H serotypes are 1, 2, 6, 8, 10, 12, and 19. Serotyping is available at research laboratories.[15,27,59,95]

Emetic Syndrome

The usual illness is characterized by a rapid onset (within 1 to 5 hours after the ingestion of contaminated food) of nausea, vomiting, and malaise, occasionally followed by diarrhea hours later.[69] Infrequently, the diarrhea is reported to last several days.[101] The short incubation reflects the ingestion of preformed emetic toxin.

EXTRAINTESTINAL INFECTIONS

Eye Infection

Keratitis, conjunctivitis, endophthalmitis, and panophthalmitis can be produced by *B. cereus*. Endophthalmitis that develops after the occurrence of penetrating wounds is caused by this organism in 27 to 46 percent of cases.[25,99] A history of soil contamination or the presence of a metal foreign body should raise clinical suspicion. Less frequently, corneal ulcers and surgical procedures are predisposing factors.[44,99] Exogenous endophthalmitis usually progresses rapidly, with deterioration of vision occurring in less than 48 hours. Severe pain is accompanied by chemosis, periorbital swelling, proptosis, and pus in the anterior chamber. The classic lesion is a corneal ring abscess, similar to that produced by *Pseudomonas* and *Proteus* spp. Endogenous cases may have subretinal exudation, retinal hemorrhage, and perivasculitis. Associated systemic symptoms are not unusual manifestations.[23] The outcome is poor, with almost half of patients left with visual acuity no better than simple light perception.[99] Many patients require enucleation. Endogenous ophthalmitis is associated with the use of illicit intravenous drugs or transfusion of contaminated blood products and subsequent bacteremic seeding of one eye.[23,83,89,99]

The pathogenesis of *B. cereus* on ocular tissue has been linked to the lecithinase activity of phospholipase C. A toxin fraction, hemolysin BL, which is formed by three separate components, produces similar destruction of retinal tissue in vitro and in animal experiments.[9] Its relationship with the diarrheal enterotoxin is unclear.[12]

Wound and Soft Tissue Infections

Wound infections of variable severity related to trauma, burns, or postsurgical complications occasionally are reported.[92-94,104] Because *Bacillus* is a common environmental contaminant, proof of the relevance of a *B. cereus* isolate is clearer if the organism is obtained from deep tissue in heavy pure growth. Severe infections in individuals involved in motor vehicle accidents can be complicated by necrotizing fasciitis and require extensive débridement.[104] Superficial, benignly infected wounds are common findings in the tropics.[29] Immunosuppressed patients may contract a severe gas gangrene–like infection with myonecrosis similar to disease caused by *Clostridium* spp.,[65] requiring amputation,[42] or a less severe primary cutaneous infection manifested by vesicles, pustules, or cellulitis.[45]

Skeletal Infections

Cases of chronic osteomyelitis occur rarely and result from accidental or surgical trauma. Radical débridement and antibiotic treatment are required.[83] Because *B. cereus* can be found as a co-pathogen with other more frequent pathogenic bacteria, resolution of symptoms is delayed until eradication of the organism.[78] Acute osteomyelitis may occur in drug abusers.[83,89]

Bacteremia and Septicemia

Bacteremia occurs with indwelling catheters and other foreign bodies, contaminated intravenous drugs (e.g., heroin), and blood products, particularly platelets.[17,30,107] Immunosuppression and impaired neutrophil killing, such as occur in individuals with neutropenia secondary to malignancy or chemotherapy and in neonates with immaturity of the immune system, are major contributors to morbidity in systemic *B. cereus* infection.[4,18,47,73,74] Disseminated intravascular coagulation, multiorgan failure, and a fulminant course may occur in neonates and compromised hosts. Intestinal perforation with abdominal infection in neonates also has been described.[38] Outbreaks of sepsis in newborn nurseries have been linked to contaminated ventilation balloon devices.[102] Endocarditis is an infrequent complication of bacteremia that usually occurs in intravenous drug abusers or individuals with a long-term intravascular device.[83,89] Vegetations can form over mechanical prosthetic valves or pacemaker wires, requiring their replacement.[83,84] Morbidity and mortality rates are high in patients with valvular heart disease. Fatal serosanguineous pericarditis in a patient undergoing hemodialysis has been reported.[32]

Pneumonia

Primary pulmonary disease rarely has been recorded. The manifestation can be subacute and consist of cough, fever, dyspnea, chest pain, and hemoptysis, with progression to necrotizing pneumonia, cavitation, and empyema. Pleural fluid may appear serosanguineous or sanguinopurulent.[13,47] Underlying predisposing conditions include leukemia, alcohol abuse, chronic hepatitis, and steroid use.[13,30,47,83] Multiorgan disease in premature neonates with necrotizing pneumonia usually is fatal.[51] Outbreaks of *B. cereus* pneumonia in neonates have been linked to contaminated ventilators.[41] Blood culture is positive in 75 percent of cases, followed by pleural fluid and sputum culture in 40 to 60 percent.[13] The pleural space may become contaminated with *B. cereus* by mishandling of the thoracic drainage system in patients with other causes of pleuritis.[48]

Infection of the Central Nervous System

Intracranial shunts and penetrating surgical or traumatic cranial wounds expose the central nervous system to environmental *B. cereus*.[31,81] Spinal anesthesia[30] was associated with *Bacillus* infection in the past. Contamination in the operating room through the linen is a potential source.[5,6] Premature neonates are susceptible to meningeal seeding by dissemination of intravascular infection related to catheters.[73] As in patients with other serious infections, patients who are immunosuppressed are at higher risk.[47] The

cerebrospinal fluid in *B. cereus* meningitis is purulent, with white blood cell counts of more than 1000/mm³, a predominance of polymorphonuclear leukocytes, and moderate increments in protein content. Gram stain is positive in 70 percent of cases. Multiple brain abscesses may result from hematogenous spread in patients with leukemia.[47,49] Sequelae include hydrocephalus and brain damage. Often, the infection is fatal unless caused by a contaminated spinal anesthetic, in which case the course is usually more benign.

Liver Failure

Fulminant hepatitis and rhabdomyolysis have been associated with the emetic toxin. The toxin inhibits hepatic mitochondrial fatty-acid oxidation. Liver changes include fatty infiltrates and midzonal necrosis.[63]

Pseudoinfections

Pseudoepidemics with *B. cereus* are a challenge for the clinical microbiologist.[67] Because these spore formers are so hardy, they are common laboratory contaminants. *Bacillus* spp. isolated from clinical specimens usually should be considered a contaminant, although their pathogenic potential is well known.[24,30,47,74,83,89,93,94] Pseudoinfections have been associated with contaminated blood culture media, syringes, blood culture analyzers, and fiberoptic bronchoscopes.[24] Colonization of umbilical cord stumps and eye surfaces by contaminated diapers may cause pseudo-outbreaks in nurseries.[105]

COMPLICATIONS

Death rarely ever results from the food-poisoning syndromes. Rapidly spreading wound infections may require amputation of extremities,[39] and ocular infections can lead to loss of vision with or without enucleation.[44,99,106] The risk of death in patients with septicemia, endocarditis, and meningitis is related to the underlying condition and severity of the disease.[4,45,68,73,84]

DIAGNOSIS

The laboratory finding of *B. cereus* in a foodstuff without quantitative cultures and without epidemiologic data is insufficient to establish its role in an outbreak.[101] In practice, appropriate specimens often either are unavailable or are submitted long after the incident, rendering their microbiologic significance questionable. During analysis of foods not involved in food-borne illness, the bacteria may be found in counts of 10^1 to 10^6 organisms per gram.[14,15,19,37,72,85] Diagnosis of the diarrheal form of *B. cereus* food poisoning is supported by the isolation of 10^5 or more organisms per gram from epidemiologically incriminated food.[68] The levels of *B. cereus* found in the implicated foods usually are in the range of 5×10^5 to 9.5×10^8 colony-forming units per gram. With the exception of milk, the products rarely appear to be spoiled, despite the bacteria's high density. Isolation of more than 10^5 organisms per gram in feces during an acute attack provides supportive evidence for the presumed diagnosis and confirms the association if the same serotype is isolated from incriminated food.

The organisms that produce emetic toxin are present in concentrations of 1×10^3 to 5×10^{10} colony-forming units per gram. Reheating may decrease or eliminate the organisms and leave the toxin intact, but render isolation of the organism difficult to accomplish.[28,101]

Commercial immunoassay kits (reversed passive latex agglutination test, enzyme-linked immunosorbent assay, and microslide

TABLE 103–1   Management and Complications Associated with *Bacillus cereus* Infections

Condition	Management	Complications
Food poisoning	Supportive measures; hydration	Usually none; liver failure rarely reported
Ocular	Systemic, topical, intravitreal antibiotics—vancomycin or clindamycin ± aminoglycosides; surgical—early vitrectomy	Severe decreased visual acuity, blindness, enucleation
Septicemia	Removal of IV device, foreign body; IV antibiotics (according to sensitivity)—vancomycin	Localization of infection—endophthalmitis, endocarditis, meningitis; death
Pneumonia/pleuritis	IV antibiotics; drainage of pleural space; resection of necrotic tissue	Death
Meningitis	IV antibiotics; removal of infected intracranial shunts or cerebrospinal fluid reservoirs	Hydrocephalus, brain damage, death
Wound/subcutaneous infection	IV antibiotics; surgical débridement	Amputation, death

IV, intravenous.

immunodiffusion assay) are available for the detection of *B. cereus* diarrheal toxin. The kits may detect a variety of proteins, however.[11,26] Experimental techniques based on the detection of genes for phospholipase C and sphingomyelinase by polymerase chain reaction have been developed for the identification of *B. cereus* in food products.[65]

The relevance of clinical isolates in extraintestinal syndromes can be assessed by the degree of growth (heavy versus scanty), the number of occasions that growth was obtained, the source of the material cultured, and predisposing or underlying conditions.[94] For suspected endophthalmitis, aqueous and vitreous samples should be obtained if possible before the initiation of antibiotics.[25]

TREATMENT

During a mild, self-limited attack of food poisoning, patients require only supportive therapy. Usually, oral fluid and electrolyte replacement is adequate (Table 103–1).[35]

No antibiotic therapy is required except in cases of non-gastrointestinal infection. The production of three different β-lactamases by most of the organisms renders penicillin derivatives, including third-generation cephalosporins, ineffective against *B. cereus*. Most strains are susceptible to chloramphenicol, vancomycin, clindamycin, aminoglycosides, erythromycin, tetracycline, imipenem, and ciprofloxacin.[4,21,93,94,103] Definitive antibiotic therapy should be based on the antibiogram susceptibility, but initial empiric therapy with clindamycin or vancomycin, with or without an aminoglycoside, is appropriate, pending susceptibility data.[4,13,24,49,78,104] Ciprofloxacin has been reported to be useful in the treatment of recurrent pneumonia and bacteremia[33] and may have advantages in the penetration of respiratory and eye secretions,[57] but other options for children younger than 18 years are preferred.

Immediate empiric coverage for *B. cereus* is indicated for endophthalmitis in groups at risk. Selection of the antibiotic and the appropriate means of administration are controversial.[25] Clindamycin and an aminoglycoside[106] or vancomycin[99] are the best options. Together with antibiotics administered parenterally, topical and periocular antibiotics are considered adjunctive therapy. In cases of penetrating trauma, early vitrectomy and intravitreal antibiotics (vancomycin in combination with amikacin) should be considered.[25,99]

Surgical débridement of necrotic tissue, drainage of closed-space infections, and prompt removal of foreign bodies and indwelling catheters are important aspects of successful therapy.[13,22,78] Some bacteremic patients may be cured by removal of the intravenous catheter only.[83]

PREVENTION AND CONTROL

Low-level contamination in food products is difficult to avoid, but proper food handling should diminish the proliferation of bacilli.[79] Practical precautions for handling cereals and rice include not preparing large quantities at a single time and maintaining the food at a hot temperature (>63° C) or cooling it quickly. The food must not be stored under warm conditions, especially in the range of 15° C to 50° C.[15,37]

REFERENCES

1. Agata, N., Ohta, M., Mori, M., and Isobe, M.: A novel dodecadepsipeptide, cereulide, is an emetic toxin of *Bacillus cereus*. F. E. M. S. Microbiol. Lett. *129*:17-20, 1995.
2. Ahmed, R., Sankar-Mistry, P., Jackson, S., et al.: *Bacillus cereus* phage typing as an epidemiological tool in outbreaks of food poisoning. J. Clin. Microbiol. *33*:636-640, 1995.
3. Baddour, L. M., Gala, S. M., Griffin, R., et al.: A hospital cafeteria-related food-borne outbreak due to *Bacillus cereus*: Unique features. Infect. Control *7*:462-465, 1986.
4. Banerjee, C., Bustamante, C. I., Wharton, R., et al.: *Bacillus* infections in patients with cancer. Arch. Intern. Med. *148*:1769-1774, 1988.
5. Barrie, D., Hoffman, P. N., Wilson, J. A., et al.: Contamination of hospital linen by *Bacillus cereus*. Epidemiol. Infect. *113*:297-306, 1994.
6. Barrie, D., Wilson, J. A., Hoffman, P. N., et al.: *Bacillus cereus* meningitis in two neurosurgical patients: An investigation into the source of the organism. J. Infect. *25*:291-297, 1992.
7. Bean, N. H., Griffin, P. M., Goulding, J. S., and Ivey, C. B.: Foodborne disease outbreaks, 5-year summary, 1983-1987. M. M. W. R. C. D. C. Surveill. Summ. *39*:15-55, 1990.
8. Beecher, D. J., and Macmillan, J. D.: Characterization of the components of hemolysin BL from *Bacillus cereus*. Infect. Immunol. *59*:1778-1784, 1991.
9. Beecher, D. J., Pulido, J. S., Barney, N. P., et al.: Extracellular virulence factors in *Bacillus cereus* endophthalmitis: Methods and implication of involvement of hemolysin BL. Infect. Immun. *63*:632-639, 1995.
10. Beecher, D. J., Schoeni, J. L., and Wong, A. C. L.: Enterotoxic activity of hemolysin BL from *Bacillus cereus*. Infect. Immunol. *63*:4423-4428, 1995.
11. Beecher, D. J., and Wong, A. C.: Identification and analysis of the antigens detected by two commercial *Bacillus cereus* diarrheal enterotoxin immunoassay kits. Appl. Environ. Microbiol. *60*:4614-4616, 1994.
12. Beecher, D. J., and Wong, A. C.: Improved purification and characterization of hemolysin BL, a hemolytic dermonecrotic vascular permeability factor from *Bacillus cereus*. Infect. Immun. *62*:980-986, 1994.
13. Bekemeyer, W. B., and Zimmerman, G. A.: Life threatening complications associated with *Bacillus cereus* pneumonia. Am. Rev. Respir. Dis. *131*:466-469, 1985.
14. Beuchat, L. R., Ma-Lin, C. F., and Carpenter, J. A.: Growth of *Bacillus cereus* in media containing plant seed materials and ingredients used in Chinese cookery. J. Appl. Bacteriol. *48*:397-407, 1980.
15. Blakey, L. J., and Priest, F. G.: The occurrence of *Bacillus cereus* in some dried foods including pulses and cereals. J. Appl. Bacteriol. *48*:397-407, 1980.
16. Brousseau, R., Saint-Onge, A., Prefontaine, G., et al.: Arbitrary primer polymerase chain reaction, a powerful method to identify *Bacillus thuringiensis* serovars and strains. Appl. Environ. Microbiol. *59*:114-119, 1993.

17. Bryce, E. A., Smith, J. A., Tweeddale, M., et al.: Dissemination of *Bacillus cereus* in an intensive care unit. Infect. Control Hosp. Epidemiol. *14*:459-462, 1993.

18. Burdon, A. L., Davis, J. S., and Wende, R. D.: Experimental infection of mice with *Bacillus cereus*: Studies of pathogenesis and pathologic changes. J. Infect. Dis. *117*:307-316, 1967.

19. Capparelli, E., and Mata, L.: Microflora of maize prepared as tortillas. Appl. Microbiol. *29*:802-806, 1975.

20. Christenson, J. C., Byington, C., Korgenski, E. K., et al.: *Bacillus cereus* infections among oncology patients at a children's hospital. Am. J. Infect. Control. *27*:543-546, 1999.

21. Conrod, J. D., Leadley, P. J., and Eickhoff, T. C.: Antibiotic susceptibility of *Bacillus* species. J. Infect. Dis. *123*:102-105, 1971.

22. Cotton, D. J., Gill, V. J., Marshal, D. J., et al.: Clinical features and therapeutic interventions in 17 cases of *Bacillus* bacteremia in an immunosuppressed patient population. J. Clin. Microbiol. *25*:672-674, 1987.

23. Cowan, C. L., Jr., Madden, W. M., Hatem, G. F., et al.: Endogenous *Bacillus cereus* panophthalmitis. Ann. Ophthalmol. *19*:65-68, 1987.

24. Cunha, B. A.: Pseudomeningitis: Another nosocomial headache. Infect. Control Hosp. Epidemiol. *9*:391-393, 1988.

25. David, D. B., Kirkby, G. R., and Noble, B. A.: *Bacillus cereus* endophthalmitis. Br. J. Ophthalmol. *78*:577-580, 1994.

26. Day, T. L., Tatani, S. R., Notermans, S., et al.: A comparison of ELISA and RPLA for detection of *Bacillus cereus* diarrhoeal enterotoxin. J. Appl. Bacteriol. *77*:9-13, 1994.

27. DeBuono, B. A., Brondum, J., Kramer, J. M., et al.: Plasmid, serotypic and enterotoxin analysis of *Bacillus cereus* in an outbreak setting. J. Clin. Microbiol. *26*:1571-1574, 1988.

28. Drobniewski, F. A.: *Bacillus cereus* and related species. Clin. Microbiol. Rev. *6*:324-338, 1993.

29. Dryden, M. S., and Kramer, J. M.: Toxigenic *Bacillus cereus* as a cause of wound infections in the tropics. J. Infect. *15*:207-212, 1987.

30. Farrar, W. E., Jr.: Serious infections due to "non-pathogenic" organisms of the genus *Bacillus*. Am. J. Med. *34*:134-141, 1963.

31. Feder, H. M., Garibaldi, R. A., Nurse, B. A., et al.: *Bacillus* species isolates from cerebrospinal fluid in patients without shunts. Pediatrics *82*:909-913, 1988.

32. Fricchione, L. F., Sepkowitz, D. V., Gradon, J. D., et al.: Pericarditis due to *Bacillus cereus* in an intravenous drug user. Rev. Infect. Dis. *13*:774, 1991.

33. Gascoigne, A. D., Richards, J., Gould, K., et al.: Successful treatment of *Bacillus cereus* infection with ciprofloxacin. Thorax *46*:220-221, 1991.

34. Ghosh, A. C.: Prevalence of *Bacillus cereus* in the faeces of healthy adults. J. Hyg. *80*:233-236, 1978.

35. Giannella, R. A., and Brasile, L.: A hospital food-borne outbreak of diarrhea caused by *Bacillus cereus*: Clinical, epidemiologic, and microbiologic studies. J. Infect. Dis. *139*:366-370, 1979.

36. Gilbert, R. J., and Kramer, J. M.: *Bacillus cereus* enterotoxins: Present status. Biochem. Soc. Trans. *12*:198-200, 1984.

37. Gilbert, R. J., Stringer, M. F., and Peace, T. C.: The survival and growth of *Bacillus cereus* in boiled and fried rice in relation to outbreaks of food poisoning. J. Hyg. *73*:433-444, 1974.

38. Girisch, M., Ries, M., and Zenker, M. et al.: Intestinal perforations in a premature infant caused by *Bacillus cereus*. Infection *31*:192-193, 2003.

39. Gonzalez, I, Lopez, M., Mazas, M., et al.: The effect of recovery conditions on the apparent heat resistance of *Bacillus cereus* spores. J. Appl. Bacteriol. *78*:548-554, 1995.

40. Granum, P. E., and Lund, T.: *Bacillus cereus* and its food poisoning toxins. F. E. M. S. Microbiol. Lett. *157*:223-228, 1997.

41. Gray, J., George, R. H., Durbin, G. M., et al.: An outbreak of *Bacillus cereus* respiratory tract infections on a neonatal unit due to contaminated ventilator circuits. J. Hosp. Infect. *41*:19-22, 1999.

42. Groschell, D., Burgess, M. A., and Bodey, G. P.: Gas gangrene-like infection with *Bacillus cereus* in a lymphoma patient. Cancer *37*:988-992, 1976.

43. Hauge, S.: Food poisoning caused by aerobic spore-forming bacilli. J. Appl. Bacteriol. *18*:591-595, 1955.

44. Hemadi, R., Zaltas, M., Paton, B., et al.: Bacillus-induced endophthalmitis: New series of 10 cases and review of the literature. Br. J. Ophthalmol. *74*:26-29, 1990.

45. Henrickson, K. J., Shenep, J. L., Flynn, P. M., et al.: Primary cutaneous *Bacillus cereus* infection in neutropenic children. Lancet *1*:601-603, 1989.

46. Holmes, J. R., Plunkett, T., Pate, P., et al.: Emetic food poisoning caused by *Bacillus cereus*. Arch. Intern. Med. *141*:766-767, 1981.

47. Ihde, D. C., and Armstrong, D.: Clinical spectrum of infection due to *Bacillus* species. Am. J. Med. *55*:839-846, 1973.

48. Jacobs, J. A., and Stobberingh, E. E.: Infection due to a contaminated thoracic drainage system. J. Hosp. Infect. *24*:23-28, 1993.

49. Jenson, H. B., Levy, S. R., Duncan, C., et al.: Treatment of multiple brain abscesses caused by *Bacillus cereus*. Pediatr. Infect. Dis. J. *8*:795-798, 1989.

50. Jephcott, A. E., Barton, B. W., Gilbert, R. J., et al.: An unusual outbreak of food poisoning associated with meals-on-wheels. Lancet *2*:129-130, 1977.

51. Jevon, G. P., Dunne, W. M., Hicks, M. J., et al.: *Bacillus cereus* pneumonia in premature neonates: A report of two cases. Pediatr. Infect. Dis. J. *12*:251-253, 1993.

52. Khodr, M., Hill, S., Perkins, L., et al.: *Bacillus cereus* food poisoning associated with fried rice at two child day care centers: Virginia, 1993. M. M. W. R. Morb. Mortal. Wkly. Rep. *43*:177-178, 1994.

53. Kotiranta, A., Lounatmaa, K., and Haapasalo, M.: Epidemiology and pathogenesis of *Bacillus cereus* infections. Microbes Infect. *2*:189-198, 2000.

54. Kramer, J. M., and Gilbert, R. J.: *Bacillus cereus* and other *Bacillus* species. *In* Doyle, M. P. (ed.): Foodborne Bacterial Pathogens. New York, Marcel Dekker, 1989, pp. 21-70.

55. Larsen, H. D., and Jorgensen, K.: Growth of *Bacillus cereus* in pasteurized milk products. Int. J. Food Microbiol. *46*:173-176, 1999.

56. Lechner, S., Mayr, R., Francis, K. P., et al.: *Bacillus weihenstephanensis* sp. nov. is a new psychrotolerant species of *Bacillus cereus* group. Int. J. Syst. Microbiol. *48*:1373-1382, 1998.

57. Lesk, M. R., Ammann, H., Marcil, G., et al.: The penetration of oral ciprofloxacin into the aqueous humor, vitreous and subretinal fluid of humans. Am. J. Ophthalmol. *115*:623-628, 1993.

58. Lettau, L. A., Benjamin, D., Cantrell, H. F., et al.: *Bacillus* species pseudomeningitis. Infect. Control Hosp. Epidemiol. *9*:394-398, 1988.

59. Luby, S., Jones, J., Dowda, H., et al.: A large outbreak of gastroenteritis caused by diarrheal toxin-producing *Bacillus cereus*. J. Infect. Dis. *167*:1452-1455, 1993.

60. Lund, B. M.: Foodborne disease due to *Bacillus* and *Clostridium* species. Lancet *336*:982-987, 1990.

61. Lund, T., and Granum, P. E.: Characterisation of a non-haemolytic enterotoxin complex from *Bacillus cereus* after a foodborne outbreak. F. E. M. S. Microbiol. Lett. *141*:151-156, 1996.

62. Lynch, M., Painter, J., and Woodruff, R.: Surveillance for foodbourne-disease outbreaks—United States, 1998-2002. M. M. W. R. Morb. Mortal. Wkly. Rep. *55*(SS-10):1-48, 2006.

63. Mahler, H., Pasi, A., Kramer, J. M., et al.: Fulminant liver failure in association with the emetic toxin of *Bacillus cereus*. N. Engl. J. Med. *336*:1142-1148, 1997.

64. Melling, J., Capel, B. J., Turnbul, P. C., et al.: Identification of a novel enterotoxigenic activity associated with *Bacillus cereus*. J. Clin. Pathol. *29*:938-940, 1976.

65. Meredith, F. T., Fowler, V. G., Gautier, M., et al.: *Bacillus cereus* necrotizing cellulitis mimicking clostridial myonecrosis: Case report and review of the literature. Scand. J. Infect. Dis. *29*:528-529, 1997.

66. Midura, T., Gerber, M., Wood, R., et al.: Outbreak of food poisoning caused by *Bacillus cereus*. Public Health Rep. *85*:45-48, 1970.

67. Morrell, R. M., Jr., and Wasilauskas, B. L.: Tracking laboratory contamination by using a *Bacillus cereus* pseudoepidemic as an example. J. Clin. Microbiol. *30*:1469-1473, 1992.

68. Morris, J. G., Jr.: *Bacillus cereus* food poisoning. Arch. Intern. Med. *141*:711, 1981.

69. Mortimer, P. R., and McCann, G.: Food poisoning episodes associated with *Bacillus cereus* in fried rice. Lancet *1*:1043-1045, 1974.

70. Murakami, T., Hiraoka, K., Mikami, T., et al.: Detection of *Bacillus cereus* flagellar antigen by enzyme-linked immunosorbent assay (ELISA). Microbiol. Immunol. *35*:223-234, 1991.

71. Ombui, J. N., and Nduhiu, J. G.: Prevalence of enterotoxigenic *Bacillus cereus* and its enterotoxins in milk and milk products in and around Nairobi. East Afr. Med. J. *82*:280-284, 2005.

72. Parry, J. M., and Gilbert, R. J.: Studies on the heat resistance of *Bacillus cereus* spores and growth of the organism in boiled rice. J. Hyg. *84*:77-82, 1980.

73. Patrick, C. C., Langston, C., and Baker, C. J.: *Bacillus* species infections in neonates. Rev. Infect. Dis. *111*:612-615, 1989.

74. Richard, V., Van der Auwera, P., Snoeck, R., et al.: Nosocomial bacteremia caused by *Bacillus* species. Eur. J. Clin. Microbiol. Infect. Dis. *7*:783-785, 1988.

75. Rowan, N. J., and Anderson, G. J.: Diarrheal enterotoxin production by psychrotropic *Bacillus cereus* present in reconstituted milk base infant formulae (MIF). Lett. Appl. Microbiol. *26*:161-165, 1998.

76. Sakurai, N., Koike, K. A., Irie, Y., et al.: The rice culture filtrate of *Bacillus cereus* isolated from emetic-type food poisoning causes mitochondrial swelling in a HEp-2 cell. Microbiol. Immunol. *38*:337-340, 1994.

77. Schraft, H., and Griffiths, M. W.: Specific oligonucleotide primers for detection of lecithinase-positive *Bacillus* spp. by PCR. Appl. Environ. Microbiol. *61*:98-102, 1995.

78. Schricker, M. E., Thompson, G. H., and Schreiber, J. R.: Osteomyelitis due to *Bacillus cereus* in an adolescent: Case report and review. Clin. Infect. Dis. *18*:863-867, 1994.

79. Schultz, F. J., and Smith, J. L.: *Bacillus*: Recent advances in *Bacillus cereus* food poisoning research. *In* Hui, Y. H., Gorham, J. R., and Murrel, K. D. (eds.): Foodborne Disease Handbook. New York, Marcel Dekker, 1994, pp. 29-62.

80. Shinagawa, K., Ueno, S., and Konuma, H., et al.: Purification and characterization of the vascular permeability factor produced by *Bacillus cereus*. J. Vet. Med. Sci. *53*:281-286, 1991.

81. Siegman-Igra, Y., Lavochkin, J., Schwartz, D., et al.: Meningitis and bacteremia due to *Bacillus cereus*: A case report and a review of *Bacillus* infections. Isr. J. Med. Sci. *19*:546-551, 1983.

82. Slaten, D. D., Oropeza, R. I., and Werner, S. B.: An outbreak of *Bacillus cereus* food poisoning: Are caterers supervised sufficiently? Public Health Rep. *107*:477-480, 1992.

83. Sliman, R., Rehm, S., and Shlaes, D. M.: Serious infections caused by *Bacillus* species. Medicine (Baltimore) *66*:218-223, 1987.

84. Steen, M. K., Bruno-Murtha, L. A., Chaux, G., et al.: *Bacillus cereus* endocarditis: Report of a case and review. Clin. Infect. Dis. *14*:945-946, 1992.

85. Sutherland, A. D.: Toxin production by *Bacillus cereus* in dairy products. J. Dairy Res. *60*:569-574, 1993.
86. Sutherland, A. D., and Limond, A. M.: Influence of pH and sugars on the growth and production of diarrhoeagenic toxin by *Bacillus cereus.* J. Dairy Res. *60*:575-580, 1993.
87. TeGiffel, M. C., Beumer, R. R., Granum, P. E., et al.: Isolation and characterization of *Bacillus cereus* from pasteurized milk in household refrigerators in the Netherlands. Int. J. Food Microbiol. *34*:307-318, 1997.
88. Thompson, N. E., Ketterhagen, M. J., Bergdoll, M. S., et al.: Isolation and some properties of an enterotoxin produced by *Bacillus cereus.* Infect. Immun. *43*:887-894, 1984.
89. Tuazon, C. U., Murray, H. W., Levy, C., et al.: Serious infections from *Bacillus* sp. J. A. M. A. *241*:1137-1140, 1979.
90. Turnbull, P. C.: Studies on the production of enterotoxins by *Bacillus cereus.* J. Clin. Pathol. *29*:941-948, 1976.
91. Turnbull, P. C.: *Bacillus cereus* toxins. Pharmacol. Ther. *13*:453-505, 1981.
92. Turnbull, P. C., French, T. A., and Dowsett, E. G.: Severe systemic and pyogenic infections with *Bacillus cereus.* B. M. J. *1*:1628-1629, 1977.
93. Turnbull, P. C., Jorgensen, K., Kramer, J. M., et al.: Severe clinical conditions associated with *Bacillus cereus* and the apparent involvement of exotoxins. J. Clin. Pathol. *32*:289-293, 1979.
94. Turnbull, P. C., and Kramer, J. M.: Non-gastrointestinal *Bacillus cereus* infections: An analysis of exotoxin production by strains isolated over a two year period. J. Clin. Pathol. *36*:1091-1096, 1983.
95. Turnbull, P. C., and Kramer, J. M.: Intestinal carriage of *Bacillus cereus*: Faecal isolation studies in three population groups. J. Hyg. *95*:629-638, 1985.
96. Turnbull, P. C., and Kramer, J. M.: *Bacillus. In* Murray, P. R., Baron, E. J., and Pfaller, M. A. (eds.): Manual of Clinical Microbiology. 6th ed. Washington, D.C., American Society for Microbiology, 1995, pp. 349-356.
97. Turnbull, P. C., Kramer, J. M., Jorgensen, K., et al.: Properties and production characteristics of vomiting, diarrheal and necrotizing toxins of *Bacillus cereus.* Am. J. Clin. Nutr. *32*:219-228, 1979.
98. Turnbull, P. C., Nottingham, J. F., and Ghosh, A. C.: A severe necrotic enterotoxin produced by certain food, food poisoning and other clinical isolates of *Bacillus cereus.* Br. J. Exp. Pathol. *58*:273-280, 1977.
99. Vahey, J. B., and Flynn, H. W., Jr.: Results in the management of *Bacillus* endophthalmitis. Ophthalmol. Surg. *22*:681-686, 1991.
100. Vaisanen, O. M., Mwaisumo, N. J., and Salkinoja-Salonen, M. S.: Differentiation of dairy strains of the *Bacillus cereus* group by phage typing, minimum growth temperature, and fatty acid analysis. J. Appl. Bacteriol. *70*:315-324, 1991.
101. Vandeloski, J., and Gensheimer, K. F.: *Bacillus cereus*: Maine. M. M. W. R. Morb. Mortal. Wkly. Rep. *35*:408-410, 1986.
102. Van Der Zwet, W. C., Parlevliet, G. A., Savelkoul, P. H., et al.: Outbreak of *Bacillus cereus* infections in a neonatal intensive care unit traced to balloons used in manual ventilation. J Clin. Microbiol. *38*:4131-4136, 2000.
103. Weber, D. J., Saviteer, S. M., Rutala, W. A., et al.: In vitro susceptibility of *Bacillus* spp to selected antimicrobial agents. Antimicrob. Agents Chemother. *32*:642-645, 1988.
104. Wong, M. T., and Dolan, M. J.: Significant infections due to *Bacillus* species following abrasions associated with motor vehicle-related trauma. Clin. Infect. Dis. *15*:855-857, 1992.
105. Young, E. J., Wallace, R. J., Ericsson, C. D., et al.: Panophthalmitis due to *Bacillus cereus.* Arch. Intern. Med. *140*:559-560, 1980.
106. Youngs, E. R., Roberts, C., Kramer, J. M., et al.: Dissemination of *Bacillus cereus* in a maternity unit. J. Infect. *10*:228-232, 1985.
107. Zaza, S., Tokars, J. I., Yomtovian, R., et al.: Bacterial contamination of platelets at a university hospital: Increased identification due to intensified surveillance. Infect. Control Hosp. Epidemiol. *15*:82-87, 1994.

ARCANOBACTERIUM HAEMOLYTICUM

CHAPTER 104

Natascha Ching

Arcanobacterium haemolyticum is a pleomorphic gram-positive coryneform rod that causes pharyngitis and exanthem in children and young adults.[18,37,41,46]

HISTORY

This diphtheroid was noted first by MacLean and colleagues[41] in association with exudative pharyngitis in American servicemen in the South Pacific during World War II. The organism originally was named *Corynebacterium haemolyticum* but was reclassified in 1986 as *A. haemolyticum* on the basis of phenetic, peptidoglycan, fatty acid, menaquinone, and DNA data.[16-18] The association between infection with *A. haemolyticum* and pharyngitis was observed repeatedly over the years, but a cause-and-effect relationship between the organism and illness has been established only more recently.[10,40,46]

ORGANISM

MICROBIOLOGY

A. haemolyticum is a gram-positive to gram-variable pleomorphic rod.[18,20,25,64,67] The laboratory characteristics are presented in Table 104-1. *A. haemolyticum* grows best at 37° C on a blood-enriched or serum-enriched medium with the addition of 5 percent carbon dioxide. Alternatively, it grows well anaerobically. On rabbit or human blood agar, colonies are pinpoint (0.5 mm) at 24 hours; they increase to 1 to 1.5 mm after 48 hours. At this time, a unique black opaque dot is noted in the center of the colony, and this dot remains on the agar when the colony is scraped away.

TABLE 104-1 Identification Characteristics of *Arcanobacterium haemolyticum*

Test or Characteristic	Finding
Catalase	Negative
Beta-hemolysis	Positive (narrow zone of slight hemolysis after 48 hr on sheep blood)
Nitrate reduction	Negative
Pigment production	White or gray
Urease	Negative
Gelatin hydrolysis	Negative
Motility	Negative
Esculin hydrolysis	Negative
Carbohydrate use	
Glucose	Positive
Maltose	Positive
Sucrose	Positive (requires rabbit serum for growth in peptone water)
Mannitol	Negative
Xylose	Negative

Data from Collins, M. D., and Cummins, C. S.: Genus Corynebacterium. In *Sneath, P. H. A., Main, N. S., Sharpe, M. E., et al. (eds.): Bergey's Manual of Systemic Bacteriology. Vol. 2. Baltimore, Williams & Wilkins, 1986, pp. 266-276.*

At 24 hours, a 1-mm zone of hemolysis develops around colonies grown on human or rabbit blood agar. The hemolytic zone increases to 3 to 5 mm by 48 hours. Growth and red blood cell hemolysis are minimal on horse and sheep blood agar. Because throat cultures usually are performed on sheep blood agar plates, the hemolytic activity of *A. haemolyticum* may be missed.

Colonies of *A. haemolyticum* can be of either the smooth or the rough biotypes on horse blood agar.[12] These biotypes also differ in their hemolysis and biochemical properties. Smooth colonies predominate in wound infections and frequently use sucrose and trehalose, are beta-hemolytic, and lack β-glucuronidase. Rough colonies are found almost exclusively in the respiratory tract and do not use sucrose and trehalose, are non-hemolytic, and are β-glucuronidase-positive.

A. haemolyticum resembles *Actinomyces pyogenes* (formerly *Corynebacterium pyogenes*), a common cause of bovine mastitis and a rare cause of skin ulcers in children.[33] These organisms can be differentiated by several means. *A. pyogenes* is able to hydrolyze gelatin and ferment xylose. In addition, *A. haemolyticum* has a positive reverse CAMP (Christie, Atkins, and Munch-Petersen) test in that it inhibits the beta-hemolysis of *Staphylococcus aureus*, whereas *A. pyogenes* shows slight enhancement of beta-hemolysis.[24] *A. haemolyticum*'s poor growth on tellurite medium and lack of catalase help distinguish it from *Corynebacterium diphtheriae*, which also causes pharyngitis.[29,35,37]

TOXIN PRODUCTION

A. haemolyticum liberates three toxins: phospholipase D (PLD), a hemolysin, and neuraminidase.[18] PLD is a dermonecrotic toxin that causes local hemorrhagic necrosis after intradermal inoculation in rabbits and guinea pigs; injection of PLD also is lethal in rabbits.[54] The PLD gene of *A. haemolyticum* has a high degree of homology to that of *Corynebacterium pseudotuberculosis*.[19,43] PLD has been shown to be involved in the virulence of *C. pseudotuberculosis*; PLD mutants are less pathogenic in experimental infections in goats.[42] The PLD of *C. pseudotuberculosis* is similar biochemically and shares some biologic activity with the PLD that is found in brown recluse spider venom and that plays a role in the venom's toxicity.[6,37] *A. haemolyticum* carries a gene similar to the gene encoding the erythrogenic toxin of *Streptococcus pyogenes*.[18]

ANTIMICROBIAL SUSCEPTIBILITY

Almost all *A. haemolyticum* strains are highly susceptible to erythromycin (minimal inhibitory concentration <0.06 μg/mL). Erythromycin is not bactericidal, however.[9,41,64] Carlson and colleagues[11] reported an *A. haemolyticum* isolate from a diabetic foot ulcer that was exceptionally resistant to macrolides, clindamycin, tetracycline, and ofloxacin. Waagner[64] noted that of 100 pharyngeal isolates, all were inhibited by concentrations of 0.25 μg/mL or less of penicillin G and by 1 μg/mL of penicillin V. Tolerance to penicillin has been observed, however.[41,51] In one study, the minimal bactericidal concentration-to-minimal inhibitory concentration ratio varied from 1:1 to 1:8.[41] In addition to being sensitive to penicillin and erythromycin, *A. haemolyticum* is sensitive to other β-lactams, clindamycin, chloramphenicol, azithromycin, vancomycin, ciprofloxacin, tetracyclines, and rifampin; most strains are resistant to sulfonamides and trimethoprim-sulfamethoxazole.[9,11,64]

Carlson[8] compared E Test (AB Biodisk, Sweden) and agar dilution methods for susceptibility testing of 12 antimicrobial agents in 70 *A. haemolyticum* isolates. E test and agar dilution method results for benzylpenicillin, clindamycin, erythromycin, imipenem, levofloxacin, rifampin, and vancomycin were in 100 percent agreement. Tetracycline, ciprofloxacin, and ofloxacin were in 97 to 99 percent agreement, but a lower percentage of agreement was found for cefotaxime and cefuroxime, 93 percent and 84 percent, respectively. Because there are no universal standards for the organism with regard to susceptible, intermediate, or resistant categories, results should be interpreted with caution for clinical care. Almuzara and colleagues[1] also evaluated the susceptibility of 19 strains of *A. haemolyticum* according to

National Committee for Clinical Laboratory Standards interpretative standards for aerobic organisms. Most isolates were susceptible to penicillin, cephalosporins, clindamycin, ciprofloxacin, vancomycin, and macrolides (erythromycin and azithromycin). Only 68 percent of isolates were found to be sensitive to tetracycline.

Although the Clinical and Laboratory Standards Institute has no standardized susceptibility testing method for *Arcanobacterium* spp., it has been suggested that the broth microdilution method used for testing *Corynebacterium* spp.[15] is appropriate for *Arcanobacterium* spp. (Janet Hindler, MCLS, UCLA Medical Center, Clinical Microbiology Laboratory, Los Angeles, CA, and Guido Funke, MD, Gartner & Colleagues Laboratories, Ravensburg, Germany, personal communication). This method involves testing in cation-adjusted Mueller-Hinton broth supplemented with lysed horse blood (2.5 to 5% v/v). Some investigators have used agar dilution or E test satisfactorily.[8]

A vancomycin-resistant *A. haemolyticum* isolated from stool during an outbreak of vancomycin-resistant enterococci has been described. It contained the *vanA* gene primarily found in *Enterococcus faecium*.[47] Two other case reports have described organisms resistant to ciprofloxacin[63] and tetracycline.[36]

EPIDEMIOLOGY

Although similar organisms are common causes of infection in animals, humans seem to be the primary host of *A. haemolyticum*.[56,64] The organism is isolated primarily from throat specimens in patients with pharyngitis,[41,46,64] although it also may be a commensal of human skin.[40] It likewise may be a commensal in the throat, but it often is overlooked because laboratories frequently do not differentiate diphtheroids, which are considered "normal flora." In addition, because *A. haemolyticum* often is found in polymicrobial respiratory infections with classic respiratory pathogens, including *S. pyogenes*, it sometimes is missed when these more classic pathogens are identified.[37]

Although no definitive data are available, person-to-person spread is assumed to be from the throat discharge of an infected individual to the throat of a susceptible host. Transmission could occur directly or indirectly by fomites. Secondary cases in families indicate that spread is from person to person rather than from an environmental source.[23,46]

In an 8-year study, the organism was found to be isolated from throat specimens in each year, with isolation rates varying from 0.2 to 0.7 percent.[46] The peak age for contracting illness caused by *A. haemolyticum* is during the second decade of life; in contrast, the peak age for developing pharyngitis caused by *S. pyogenes* is during the first decade of life.[23,41,46] In two studies, illnesses occurred more commonly in young women than in young men.[23,46] In a review of *A. haemolyticum* systemic and deep-seated infections, a preponderance of boys over girls was found among adolescents with no risk factors for development of invasive disease.[60] No seasonal prevalence has been reported.

Screening throat cultures for pharyngotonsillitis in northern Israel were performed in 518 patients aged 1 to 90 years old.[14] Only one culture was positive (0.2%) for *A. haemolyticum* compared with 26 percent recovery of group A streptococcus. The one case was in a 9-year-old patient, however, and only 58.7 percent of patients were aged 1 to 18 years old, the more common age of isolation for this organism.

PATHOGENESIS AND PATHOLOGY

Few data are available regarding pathogenesis and pathology. The dermonecrotic toxin probably plays a role in pharyngitis. Skin biopsy specimens were taken from the exanthem in two

TABLE 104–2 Signs and Symptoms in Children, Adolescents, and Young Adults with *Arcanobacterium haemolyticum* Infection

	Frequency (%)
Symptoms	
Sore throat	100
Rash	40-70
Pruritus	50
Fever	40-75
Hoarseness	60
Cough (nonproductive)	40-60
Vomiting	30
Signs	
Pharyngitis or tonsillitis	100
Exudative	50-70
Palatal petechiae	30
Glossitis	25
Cervical lymphadenitis	40-75
Rash	40-70
Scarlatiniform	50
Urticarial	5
Maculopapular	25

Data from references 23, 32, 41, 46, and 64.

patients, and both showed only a mild lymphohistiocytic perivascular infiltrate.[46] Cultures of both samples were negative, and no IgG, IgA, or IgM deposition was noted. These findings suggest that the rash may be toxin-mediated, similar to the rash in group A streptococcal infections.

A. haemolyticum has been found to persist intracellularly,[52] which might account for failure of penicillin treatment in some cases. In one study, 5 of 42 patients were found to have apparent dual infections with Epstein-Barr virus (EBV) and *A. haemolyticum*.[41] The authors of this study suggested that immunosuppression by the virus contributes to a more marked effect of the bacterial infection in the throat. With regard to the immune response to *A. haemolyticum*, paired acute and convalescent sera showed the development of a humoral response to four distinct cell wall–associated proteins on Western blot analysis in seven of eight patients with culture-confirmed infection.[49]

CLINICAL MANIFESTATIONS

PHARYNGITIS

Pharyngitis* is the most common finding in *A. haemolyticum* infection. Signs and symptoms associated with pharyngitis are listed in Table 104–2. The illness is indistinguishable from that caused by group A streptococci; frequently, it resembles EBV infectious mononucleosis. Several patients with typical infectious mononucleosis had laboratory evidence of infection with EBV and *A. haemolyticum*.[27,28,41] Peritonsillar abscess caused by *A. haemolyticum* has been reported on several occasions.[4,35,38,45] The most common exanthem is scarlatiniform, the onset of which occurs 1 to 4 days after the beginning of pharyngeal symptoms. The rash is most prominent on the extensor surfaces of the arms and legs (see Fig. 64–19). Circumoral pallor, which is seen with group A streptococcal scarlet fever, does not seem to occur with *A. haemolyticum* infection. The rash may progress to involve the chest and back; it usually spares the palms, soles, and face, and it rarely involves the abdomen and buttocks.

The rash frequently is pruritic and may be urticarial. Erythema multiforme has been described.[3] Gaston and Zurowski[26]

reported a 20-year-old man who had, in addition to pharyngitis, a rash involving mainly his hands and feet. His feet were swollen, and on the soles were erythematous macules, petechiae, and vesicles. His palms were tender, and 2- to 4-mm erythematous macular lesions that contained small central vesicles were present. Mehta[44] reported a 19-year-old woman who presented with pharyngitis and a pruritic rash on her arms and legs 4 days before evaluation. Physical examination revealed an erythematous, urticarial rash with large and small annular rings over the whole body with confluence on the upper thighs and smaller lesions in groups on distal dorsal parts of the hands and feet.

Carlson and colleagues[13] also reported a 19-year-old man who presented with a 2-day history of a pruritic exanthem on the upper back and chest, which spread centrifugally. The patient had pharyngitis that worsened to exudative tonsillitis, and a throat culture was positive for *A. haemolyticum*. He also had swollen fingers and worsening erythematous maculopapular exanthem over his trunk and proximal extremities. Pastia lines were observed on the third day. Two weeks after initiation of antimicrobial treatment and discharge, a mild late desquamation was noted on his palms and around his fingernails. The duration of the exanthem has not been described adequately in the literature. In one study, exanthem was noted to persist for longer than 2 days in 69 percent of patients.[46]

Occasionally, *A. haemolyticum* infection has been manifested as a grayish white pharyngeal pseudomembrane that has been confused with diphtheria.[3,29,31,35] *C. diphtheriae* and *A. haemolyticum* are diphtheroids that cannot be distinguished on Gram stain but can be differentiated by their biochemical properties.

SKIN INFECTIONS

In the initial report of infections with *A. haemolyticum* in 1946, MacLean and associates[41] noted pharyngitis in U.S. servicemen and skin infections in the native populations of the South Pacific Islands. Cutaneous infections have been observed mainly in tropical countries.[64] The most common manifestations are ulcerative lesions that resemble ecthyma. Cellulitis, wound infections, and paronychia all have been noted.[7,22,23,34,45,47,64,68] In wound infections, mixed infections with *A. haemolyticum* and other organisms are common.

Tan and colleagues[62] reported five cases of *A. haemolyticum* bacteremia associated with soft tissue infections in adults. These patients, two elderly bedridden patients with decubitus ulcers and three diabetic patients with foot ulcers with extensive involvement that required surgical débridement, had a history of soft tissue infections. Four patients also had *A. haemolyticum* isolated from the suspected soft tissue focus of infection. A 3-year retrospective review of clinical samples over the same period as the five reported cases revealed 25 isolates of *A. haemolyticum*. Isolates from wound infections or cellulitis or both were found in 96 percent of cases; 20 percent of those patients also had bacteremia. Cultures from nonsterile sites often were polymicrobial, but the authors reported that *A. haemolyticum* usually was the predominant isolate.

OTHER MANIFESTATIONS

Isolated instances of septicemia, brain abscess, meningitis, meningoencephalitis, orbital cellulitis, endocarditis, osteomyelitis, deep soft tissue infections, pleural empyema, cavitary pneumonia, pyothorax, Lemierre syndrome, and sinusitis have been attributed to *A. haemolyticum* infection.* Most of these serious infections

---

*See references 3, 10, 23, 26, 28, 29, 32, 40, 41, 46, 48, 50, 57-59, 64.

*See references 2, 5, 21, 24, 27, 28, 30, 36, 39, 53, 60, 62, 64-66, 69, 70.

occurred in adults and frequently were associated with underlying conditions, such as diabetes, a malignancy, or intravenous drug use. In a 1998 review of systemic and deep-seated infections caused by *A. haemolyticum*, Skov and associates[60] identified two groups of patients. The first group comprised middle-aged to elderly adults who were immunocompromised or had other known risk factors for development of serious infectious disease. The second group consisted of preteens to young adults with no known risk factors except for one individual receiving steroid treatment for EBV infection.

A pyothorax with multiloculated hydropneumothorax was reported in a 19-year-old man in India with no history of pharyngitis.[53] Pure growth of *A. haemolyticum* was obtained from the thoracentesis. Treatment consisted of a therapeutic thoracentesis and continued chest tube drainage for 1 month. Ceftriaxone and metronidazole were given for 1 month, and the patient had clinical and radiologic resolution.

A brain abscess was documented in an 18-year-old man in Venezuela with a history of multiple periodontal problems, including periodontitis, dental caries, and multiple teeth extractions.[63] The patient presented with headache, vomiting, and neurologic deficits in the left extremities. Computed tomography of the chest revealed a left-sided hypodense frontoparietal lesion with cystic, contrast ring enhancement; edema; and midline mass effect. When his neurologic status worsened, a craniotomy was performed, and aspiration of purulent material from the encapsulated mass revealed positive cultures with pure *A. haemolyticum* growth. Therapy consisted of ceftriaxone and metronidazole for 1 week, and he was switched after susceptibility testing to penicillin for 3 weeks. Limjoco-Antonio and colleagues[36] reported a 9-year-old girl who presented with a swollen right eye after incuring a blunt trauma. She had ethmoid and maxillary sinusitis and orbital cellulitis that required surgical drainage, débridement of a subperiosteal abscess, and a second procedure with external ethmoidectomy and endoscopic sinus surgery. Cultures from the ethmoid sinus grew *A. haemolyticum*. She was treated with ceftriaxone and clindamycin.

Younus and colleagues[70] reported Lemierre syndrome with co-infection of *A. haemolyticum* and *Fusobacterium necrophorum* bacteremia. A 21-year-old man presented with fever, sore throat, tenderness along the border of the left sternocleidomastoid muscle, crackles, a blanching maculopapular rash, sepsis, and worsening pulmonary symptoms. The initial blood culture had *F. necrophorum*, and repeat blood cultures from day of admission had *A. haemolyticum* before initiation of antimicrobial therapy. Computed tomography of the chest revealed multiple nodular densities in the lungs with evidence of central necrosis in one area. Therapy consisted of anticoagulation with heparin and initial antimicrobial therapy of gatifloxacin and metronidazole, which was switched to vancomycin and piperacillin-tazobactam for 2 weeks followed by an oral course of amoxicillin-clavulanic acid for 3 months; no surgical intervention was needed.

DIFFERENTIAL DIAGNOSIS

Pharyngitis caused by *A. haemolyticum* must be differentiated from all other causes of pharyngitis (see Chapter 10). Of particular importance is distinguishing *A. haemolyticum* pharyngitis from *S. pyogenes* pharyngitis. Such differentiation can be achieved with certainty only by specific culture. In *A. haemolyticum* infection, the rapid group A streptococcal antigen tests would be negative, as would the usual group A streptococcal culture. These negative tests in specimens from adolescents should suggest strongly the possibility of *A. haemolyticum* pharyngitis.

When exanthem occurs, the confusion with illness caused by *S. pyogenes* is more pronounced. In many cases, the rash in patients infected with *A. haemolyticum* is scarlatiniform. The lack of typical

circumoral pallor and a tendency for more discrete lesions in *A. haemolyticum* infection occasionally may help in establishing the clinical diagnosis. Other common causes of pharyngitis and exanthem in adolescents and young adults are *Mycoplasma pneumoniae* and EBV infections. As noted by Mackenzie and colleagues,[40] *A. haemolyticum* and EBV co-infections are common findings. Concurrent *M. pneumoniae* pneumonia and *A. haemolyticum* empyema and bacteremia have been reported in a previously healthy 20-year-old man.[61] Cutaneous infections, including subacute ulcerations, wound infections, cellulitis, and paronychia caused by *A. haemolyticum*, must be differentiated from cutaneous infections caused by other organisms, such as staphylococci and streptococci.

SPECIFIC DIAGNOSIS

A specific diagnosis is made by culturing *A. haemolyticum* from the pharynx, a skin lesion, or a sterile body site in invasive infections. Culturing is done best with rabbit or human blood agar and the addition of 5 percent carbon dioxide.[18,20,64,67] Horse or sheep blood agar, which generally is used for culture of *S. pyogenes*, is not satisfactory for the growth and identification of *A. haemolyticum*. Using biochemical identification systems such as the API (RAPID) Coryne strip (API bioMérieux, La-Balme-les-Grottes, France) or the Biolog system (Biolog, Hazelwood, CA) can help differentiate *A. haemolyticum* from other coryneform bacteria. The Biolog system can make the identification in 4 hours.[25]

TREATMENT

A. haemolyticum is highly sensitive to numerous antibiotics.[9,12,41,50,64] Although no specific treatment studies have been done, the experience in several large studies suggests that penicillin and erythromycin are effective.[9,32,41,46] Clinical failure with penicillin has been noted.[3,52,64] Erythromycin has been suggested for first-line therapy for certain indications, such as *A. haemolyticum* tonsillitis.[11] Carlson and coworkers[11] suggest using either a broad-spectrum β-lactam antibiotic or clindamycin or macrolides for serious systemic *A. haemolyticum* infection, although these authors acknowledge that macrolides do not provide anaerobic coverage. An alternative approach would be to use high-dose penicillin plus an aminoglycoside.[60,64]

PROGNOSIS

The prognosis in cases of *A. haemolyticum* pharyngitis is good, even in untreated patients. Invasive disease can be fatal, however, and peritonsillar abscess requires prompt surgical intervention and appropriate antimicrobial therapy.

REFERENCES

1. Almuzara, M. N., de Mier, C., Barberis, C. M., et al.: *Arcanobacterium hemolyticum*: Identification and susceptibility to nine antimicrobial agents. Clin. Microbiol. Infect. 8:828-829, 2002.
2. Altmann, G., and Bogokovsky, B.: Brain abscess due to *Corynebacterium haemolyticum*. Lancet 1:338-339, 1973.
3. Banck, G., and Nyman, M.: Tonsillitis and rash associated with *Corynebacterium haemolyticum*. J. Infect. Dis. 154:1037-1040, 1986.
4. Barnham, M., and Bradwell, R. A.: Acute peritonsillar abscess caused by *Arcanobacterium haemolyticum*. J. Laryngol. Otol. 106:1000-1001, 1992.
5. Ben-Yaacob, D., Waron, M., Boldur, I., et al.: Septicemia due to *Corynebacterium haemolyticum*. Isr. J. Med. Sci. 20:431-433, 1984.
6. Bernheimer, A. W., Campbell, B. J., and Forrester, L. J.: Comparative toxinology of *Loxosceles reclusa* and *Corynebacterium pseudotuberculosis*. Science 228:590-591, 1985.

7. Bowness, P., Bower, M., Montgomery, J., et al.: The bacteriology of skin sores in Goroka children. Papua New Guinea Med. J. *27*:83-87, 1984.

8. Carlson, P.: Comparison of the E test and agar dilution methods for susceptibility testing of *Arcanobacterium haemolyticum*. Eur. J. Clin. Microbiol. Infect. Dis. *19*:891-893, 2000.

9. Carlson, P., Kontiainen, S., and Renkonen, O. V.: Antimicrobial susceptibility of *Arcanobacterium haemolyticum*. Antimicrob. Agents Chemother. *38*:142-143, 1994.

10. Carlson, P., Kontianinen, S., Renkonen, O. V., et al.: *Arcanobacterium haemolyticum* and streptococcal pharyngitis in army conscripts. Scand. J. Infect. Dis. *27*:17-18, 1995.

11. Carlson, P., Korpela J., Walder M., et al.: Antimicrobial susceptibilities and biotypes of *Arcanobacterium haemolyticum* blood isolates. Eur. J. Clin. Microbiol. Infect. Dis. *18*:915-917, 1999.

12. Carlson, P., Lounatmaa, K., and Kontiainen, S.: Biotypes of *Arcanobacterium haemolyticum*. J. Clin. Microbiol. *32*:1654-1657, 1994.

13. Carlson, P., Seppanen, M., Tarvainen, K., et al.: Pharyngitis and exanthema caused by *Arcanobacterium haemolyticum*. Acta Derm. Venereol. *81*:143-144, 2001.

14. Chen, Y., Colodner, R., Chazan, B., and Raz, R.: Pharyngotonsillitis due to *Arcanobacterium haemolyticum* in northern Israel. Isr. Med. Assoc. J. *7*:241-242, 2005.

15. Clinical and Laboratory Standards Institute: Methods for Antimicrobial Dilution and Disk Susceptibility Testing of Infrequently Isolated or Fastidious Bacteria. Approved Guideline. CLSI document M45-A. Wayne, PA, Clinical and Laboratory Standards Institute, 2006.

16. Collins, M. D., and Cummins, C. S.: Genus *Corynebacterium*. *In* Sneath, P. H. A., Mair, N. S., Sharpe, M. E., et al. (eds.): Bergey's Manual of Systemic Bacteriology. Vol. 2. Baltimore, Williams & Wilkins, 1986, pp. 266-276.

17. Collins, M. D., Jones, D., and Schofield, G. M.: Reclassification of *Corynebacterium haemolyticum* (MacLean, Liebow and Rosenberg) in the genus *Arcanobacterium* gen. nov. as *Arcanobacterium haemolyticum* nom. rev., comb. nov. J. Gen. Microbiol. *128*:1279-1281, 1982.

18. Coyle, M. B., and Lipsky, B. A.: Coryneform bacteria in infectious diseases: Clinical and laboratory aspects. Clin. Microbiol. Rev. *3*:227-246, 1990.

19. Cuevas, W. A., and Songer, J. G.: *Arcanobacterium haemolyticum* phospholipase D is genetically and functionally similar to *Corynebacterium pseudotuberculosis* phospholipase D. Infect. Immun. *61*:4310-4316, 1993.

20. Cummings, L. A., Wu, W. K., Larson, A. M., et al.: Effects of media, atmosphere, and incubation time on colonial morphology of *Arcanobacterium haemolyticum*. J. Clin. Microbiol. *31*:3223-3226, 1993.

21. Dobinsky, S., Noesselt, T., Rucker, A, et al.: Three cases of *Arcanobacterium haemolyticum* associated with abscess formation and cellulitis. Eur. J. Clin. Microbiol. Infect. Dis. *18*:804-806, 1999.

22. Esteban, J., Zapardiel, J., and Soriano, F.: Two cases of soft-tissue infection caused by *Arcanobacterium haemolyticum*. Clin. Infect. Dis. *18*:835-836, 1994.

23. Fell, H. W. K., Nagington, J., Naylor, G. R. E., et al.: *Corynebacterium haemolyticum* infections in Cambridgeshire. J. Hyg. Camb. *79*:269-275, 1977.

24. Ford, J. G., Yeatts, R. P., and Givner, L. B.: Orbital cellulitis, subperiosteal abscess, sinusitis, and septicemia caused by *Arcanobacterium haemolyticum*. Am. J. Ophthalmol. *120*:261-262, 1995.

25. Funke, G., von Graevenitz, A., Clarridge, J. E., 3rd., et al.: Clinical microbiology of coryneform bacteria. Clin. Microbiol. Rev. *10*:125-159, 1997.

26. Gaston, D. A., and Zurowski, S. M.: *Arcanobacterium haemolyticum* pharyngitis and exanthem. Arch. Dermatol. *132*:61-64, 1996.

27. Givner, L. B., McGehee, D., Taber, L. H., et al.: Sinusitis, orbital cellulitis and polymicrobial bacteremia in a patient with primary Epstein-Barr virus infection. Pediatr. Infect. Dis. J. *3*:254-256, 1984.

28. Goudswaard, J., van de Merwe, D. W., van der Sluys, P., et al.: *Corynebacterium haemolyticum* septicemia in a girl with mononucleosis infectiosa. Scand. J. Infect. Dis. *20*:339-340, 1988.

29. Green, S. L., and LaPeter, K. S.: Pseudodiphtheritic membranous pharyngitis caused by *Corynebacterium haemolyticum*. J. A. M. A. *245*:2330-2331, 1981.

30. Jobanputra, R. S., and Swain, C. P.: Septicaemia due to *Corynebacterum haemolyticum*. J. Clin. Pathol. *28*:798-800, 1975.

31. Kain, K. C., Noble, M. A., Barteluk, R. L., et al.: *Arcanobacterium hemolyticum* infection: Confused with scarlet fever and diphtheria. J. Emerg. Med. *9*:33-35, 1991.

32. Karpathios, T., Drakonaki, S., Zervoudaki, A., et al.: *Arcanobacterium haemolyticum* in children with presumed streptococcal pharyngotonsillitis or scarlet fever. J. Pediatr. *121*:735-737, 1992.

33. Kotrajaras, R. P., Buddhavudhikral, S., Sukroongreung, S., et al.: Endemic leg ulcers caused by *Corynebacterium pyogenes* in Thailand. Int. J. Dermatol. *21*:407-409, 1982.

34. Kotrajaras, R., and Tagami, H.: *Corynebacterium pyogenes*: Its pathogenic mechanism in epidemic leg ulcers in Thailand. Int. J. Dermatol. *26*:45-50, 1987.

35. Kovatch, A. L., Schuit, K. E., and Michaels, R. H.: *Corynebacterium haemolyticum* peritonsillar abscess mimicking diphtheria. J. A. M. A. *249*:1757-1758, 1983.

36. Limjoco-Antonio, A. D., Janda, W. M., and Schreckenberger, P. C.: *Arcanobacterium haemolyticum* sinusitis and orbital cellulitis. Pediatr. Infect. Dis. J. *22*:465-467, 2003.

37. Linder, R.: *Rhodococcus equi* and *Arcanobacterium haemolyticum*: Two "coryneform" bacteria increasingly recognized as agents of human infection. Emerg. Infect. Dis. *3*:145-153, 1997.

38. Lipsky, B. A., Goldberger, A. C., Tompkins, L. S., et al.: Infections caused by nondiphtheria corynebacteria. Rev. Infect. Dis. *4*:1220-1235, 1982.

39. Locksley, R. M.: The lowly diphtheroid: Nondiphtheria corynebacterial infections in humans. West. J. Med. *137*:45-52, 1982.

40. Mackenzie, A., Fuite, L. A., Chan, F. T. H., et al.: Incidence and pathogenicity of *Arcanobacterium haemolyticum* during a 2-year study in Ottawa. Clin. Infect. Dis. *21*:177-181, 1995.

41. MacLean, P. D., Liebow, A. A., and Rosenberg, A. A.: A hemolytic corynebacterium resembling *Corynebacterium ovis* and *Corynebacterium pyogenes* in man. J. Infect. Dis. *79*:69-90, 1946.

42. McNamara P. J., Bradley G. A., and Songer J. G.: Targeted mutagenesis of the phospholipase D gene results in decreased virulence of *Corynebacterium pseudotuberculosis*. Mol. Microbiol. *12*:921-930, 1994.

43. McNamara, P. J., Cuevas, W. A., and Songer, J. G.: Toxic phospholipases D of *Corynebacterium pseudotuberculosis*, *C. ulcerans* and *Arcanobacterium haemolyticum*: Cloning and sequence homology. Gene *156*:113-118, 1995.

44. Mehta, C. L.: *Arcanobacterium haemolyticum*. J. Am. Acad. Dermatol. *48*:298-299, 2003.

45. Miller, R. A., and Brancato, F.: Peritonsillar abscess associated with *Corynebacterium haemolyticum*. West. J. Med. *140*:449-451, 1984.

46. Miller, R. A., Brancato, F., and Holmes, K. K.: *Corynebacterium haemolyticum* as a cause of pharyngitis and scarlatiniform rash in young adults. Ann. Intern. Med. *105*:867-872, 1986.

47. Montgomery, J.: The aerobic bacteriology of infected skin lesions in children of the Eastern Highlands Province. Papua New Guinea Med. J. *28*:93-103, 1985.

48. Moreno, M. M., Valle, V. A., and Aguillar, A. L.: Pharyngitis caused by *Arcanobacterium haemolyticum*. An. Esp. Pediatr. *30*:209-210, 1989.

49. Nyman, M., Alugupalli, K. R., Stromberg, S., et al.: Antibody response to *Arcanobacterium haemolyticum* infection in humans. J. Infect. Dis. *175*:1515-1518, 1997.

50. Nyman, M., and Banck, G.: The clinical picture in throat infections caused by *Corynebacterium haemolyticum*. Hygiea Swedish Med. Assoc. 109-110, 1984.

51. Nyman, M., Banck, G., and Thore, M.: Penicillin tolerance in *Arcanobacterium haemolyticum*. J. Infect. Dis. *161*:261-265, 1990.

52. Osterlund, A.: Are penicillin treatment failures in *Arcanobacterium haemolyticum* pharyngotonsillitis caused by intracellularly residing bacteria? Scand. J. Infect. Dis. *27*:131-134, 1995.

53. Parija, S. C., Kaliaperumal, V., Kumar, S. V., et al.: *Arcanobacterium haemolyticum* associated with pyothorax: Case report. B. M. C. Infect. Dis. *5*:68, 2005.

54. Patocka, F., Mara, M., Soucek, A., et al.: Observations on the biological properties of atypical haemolytic corynebacteria isolated from man as compared with *Corynebacterium haemolyticum*, *Corynebacterium pyogenes bovis* and *Corynebacterium ovis*. J. Hyg. Epidemiol. Microbiol. Imunol. *6*:1-12, 1962.

55. Power, E. G., Abdulla, Y. H., Talsania, H. G., et al.: *vanA* genes in vancomycin-resistant clinical isolates of *Oerskovia turbata* and *Arcanobacterium (Corynebacterium) haemolyticum*. J. Antimicrob. Chemother. *36*:595-606, 1995.

56. Roberts, R. J.: Isolation of *Corynebacterium haemolyticum* from a case of ovine pneumonia. Vet. Rec. *84*:490, 1969.

57. Robinson, B. E., and Murray, D. L.: *Corynebacterium haemolyticum* and pharyngitis. Ann. Intern. Med. *106*:778-779, 1987.

58. Ryan, W. J.: Throat infection and rash associated with an unusual corynebacterium. Lancet *2*:1345-1347, 1972.

59. Selander, B., and Ljungh, A.: *Corynebacterium haemolyticum* as a cause of nonstreptococcal pharyngitis. J. Infect. Dis. *154*:1041, 1986.

60. Skov, R. L., Sanden, A. K., Danchell, V. H., et al.: Systemic and deep-seated infections caused by *Arcanobacterium haemolyticum*. Eur. J. Clin. Microbiol. Infect. Dis. *17*:578-582, 1998.

61. Stacey, A., and Bradlow, A.: *Arcanobacterium haemolyticum* and *Mycoplasma pneumoniae* co-infection. J. Infect. *38*:41-42, 1999.

62. Tan, T. Y., Ng, S. Y., Thomas, H., and Chan, B. K.: *Arcanobacterium haemolyticum* bacteraemia and soft-tissue infections: Case report and review of the literature. J. Infect. *53*:e69-e74, 2006.

63. Vargas, J., Hernandez, M., Silvestri, C., et al.: Brain abscess due to *Arcanobacterium haemolyticum* after dental extraction. Clin. Infect. Dis. *42*:1810-1811, 2006.

64. Waagner, D. C.: *Arcanobacterium haemolyticum*: Biology of the organism and diseases in man. Pediatr. Infect. Dis. J. *10*:933-939, 1991.

65. Waller, K. S., and Wood, B. P.: Cavitary pneumonia due to *Arcanobacterium haemolyticum*. Am. J. Dis. Child. *145*:209-210, 1991.

66. Washington, J. A., Martin, W. J., and Spiekerman, R. E.: Brain abscess with *Corynebacterium haemolyticum*: Report of a case. Am. J. Clin. Pathol. *56*:212-215, 1971.

67. Wat, L. L., Fleming, C. A., Hodge, D. S., et al.: Selective medium for isolation of *Arcanobacterium haemolyticum* and *Streptococcus pyogenes*. Eur. J. Clin. Microbiol. Infect. Dis. *10*:443-446, 1991.

68. Wickremesinghe, R. S. B.: *Corynebacterium haemolyticum* infections in Sri Lanka. J. Hyg. Camb. *87*:271-277, 1981.

69. Worthington, M. G., Daly, B. D. T., and Smith, F. E.: *Corynebacterium haemolyticum* endocarditis on a native valve. South. Med. J. *78*:1261-1262, 1985.

70. Younus, F., Chua, A., Tortora, G., and Jimenez, V. E.: Lemierre's disease caused by co-infection of *Arcanobacterium haemolyticum* and *Fusobacterium necrophorum*: A case report. J. Infect. *45*:114-117, 2002.

105

ERYSIPELOTHRIX RHUSIOPATHIAE

Randall G. Fisher

Erysipelothrix rhusiopathiae (insidiosa) was identified definitively first by Rosenbach[29] in 1884 as a cause of the cutaneous disease erysipeloid. Although most commonly associated with localized skin infection in humans, this organism has been associated with sepsis,[13,27,37] chronic skin eruption,[9,16] and endocarditis.[3,13,21,22,28,37]

BACTERIOLOGY

E. rhusiopathiae is a slender, pleomorphic, gram-positive, unencapsulated rod that produces 0.1-mm bluish colonies on blood agar. On Gram staining, they may appear singly, in short chains, or, rarely, in long, branching filaments. Although they are gram-positive, they decolorize readily, sometimes producing a spotted appearance. Some strains produce alpha-hemolysis in 48 to 72 hours. Gelatin inoculated by stab inconsistently forms a "test-tube brush" or "pipe-cleaner pattern" appearance diagnostic for this organism.[13] *Erysipelothrix* is differentiated from morphologically similar *Listeria monocytogenes* and diphtheroids by the absence of motility and catalase production, and the presence of hydrogen sulfide production in triple-sugar iron medium.[13,37]

EPIDEMIOLOGY

First isolated from mice in 1880 by Koch, *Erysipelothrix* is a common commensal of wild and domestic mammals, birds, and fish.[13,37] The *Erysipelothrix* organism may lead a saphrophytic existence in soil. First identified by Loeffler in 1882 as the causative agent of swine erysipelas, it remains an important epidemic cause of disease in these animals, with losses greater than $25 million annually to this industry.[13] Sheep, rabbits, cattle, turkeys, and rats are subject to infection with this organism. *Erysipelothrix* has been recovered from wild moose and domestic emus.[5,20] *E. rhusiopathiae* survives salting and smoking procedures. Pieces of meat may contain the organism for 170 days after pickling, but exposure to moist heat for 15 minutes at 55° C[35] kills most strains.[13] Fish handlers, meat processors, poultry workers, veterinarians, abattoir workers, and food handlers are at risk for exposure to *Erysipelothrix*.[25] Isolates of the same serotype may show genetic diversity, so serotyping may not be completely reliable as an epidemiologic tool for tracking outbreaks.[6]

PATHOPHYSIOLOGY

Human infection is largely accidental and results from contamination of skin abrasions during handling of infected material. Males are infected more commonly than are females, perhaps because of an increased risk of exposure. The presence of an antiphagocytic capsule may be a virulence factor for *E. rhusiopathiae*.[32] In vitro study shows that encapsulated strains are poorly phagocytized by macrophages, unless immune serum is provided; ingested bacteria are able to replicate within the macrophage. The ability to survive and replicate within macrophages probably is due to failure of the encapsulated strains to induce the oxidative burst.[31] Disease usually is self-limited, most often involving the hands. Biopsy of skin lesions shows a marked inflammatory response. Difficulty of establishing bacteriologic confirmation has been attributed to the organism's location in the deep part of the pars reticularis of the corium.[7]

CLINICAL MANIFESTATIONS

Human disease typically manifests as a mild, localized cutaneous eruption; a more severe, generalized cutaneous form; or a septicemia often associated with endocarditis. Localized cutaneous infection, the erysipeloid of Rosenbach,[29] is the most common manifestation of *Erysipelothrix* disease.[25] After a 1- to 4-day incubation period, an acute localized lesion appears at the site of an abrasion contaminated with *E. rhusiopathiae*–colonized material. Slowly progressive, purplish red, painful induration is typical. Absence of suppuration and involution without desquamation help to distinguish this lesion from streptococcal or staphylococcal infection. Occasionally, the skin may show sharply circumscribed bluish red lesions, which are similar to the cutaneous manifestations in swine.[13,37] Fever and other constitutional symptoms are uncommon manifestations, occurring in less than 10 percent of cases, unless bacteremia supervenes.[9,25] Untreated infection usually is self-limited, with an average duration of 3 weeks.

Lymphangitis and adenitis occur in 10 percent of cases; in 20 percent of cases, progression of disease extends from lesions on the hand to the wrist and forearm.[17] In one case, a patient with type 2 diabetes was discovered at the time of surgery to have necrotizing fasciitis; *E. rhusiopathiae* was the predominant but not only organism isolated from surgical specimens.[33] A 7-week-old infant with localized *E. rhusiopathiae* infection of the knee without a known source of exposure has been reported,[19] and a 6-year-old girl with *Erysipelothrix* pyopneumothorax has been described.[26] Septic arthritis has been described in a healthy 18-year-old man in whom disease developed after he underwent arthroscopic knee surgery,[2] in association with infective endocarditis,[30] and in a patient with systemic lupus erythematosus and chronic monarthritis without associated systemic symptoms.[36]

Cutaneous eruptions rarely may occur in areas distant from the site of inoculation,[18] appearing as violaceous lesions with advancing pink borders. Bullous vesiculation has been described.[9] In 1921, Prausnitz[27] reported the first case of apparent septicemia in childhood, isolating the organism from the blood of a 10-year-old boy.

E. rhusiopathiae rarely is associated with the bite of a domestic dog or cat.[1] In one prospective study of infected domesticated animal–bite wounds, two patients who had cat-bite wounds infected with *E. rhusiopathiae* were identified.[34] Cultures were carefully processed and were performed in reference laboratories.

An uncommon but important complication of *Erysipelothrix* infection is endocarditis. Presumed or proven endocarditis accounts for 90 percent of serious *E. rhusiopathiae* infection.[12] Patients with congenital heart disease or heart valve damage secondary to acute rheumatic fever are at the greatest risk for development of endocarditis. However, previously normal heart valves can be infected.[13,21] Valvular and myocardial abscesses have been described.[24] In contrast to diphtheroid endocarditis, *E. rhusiopathiae* endocarditis usually does not involve prosthetic valves, and in contrast to *Bacillus* spp. endocarditis, it is not associated with intravenous drug abuse.[12] In a review of 1989 cases of endocarditis from 13 series,[3] *Erysipelothrix* was documented in two patients. *Erysipelothrix* endocarditis commonly involves the aortic or mitral valves or both. Overall mortality in reported cases is 38 percent, which is considerably higher than that associated with other pathogens of endocarditis.[11] Many patients with endocarditis are treated empirically with vancomycin, a drug to which all *Erysipelothrix* isolates are constitutively resistant.[15] No history or physical evidence of cutaneous lesions is found in 50 percent of cases of endocarditis, and history of exposure to contaminated material often is lacking. Although immunocompromised individuals[22] may be at increased risk, serious infection also occurs in otherwise normal hosts,[4,13,21] particularly in association with occupational exposure.

DIAGNOSIS

For localized disease, diagnosis depends largely on clinical appearance of the lesion in association with an appropriate history of exposure. Attempts to culture the organism from material collected by swab or aspirate of a local lesion almost always are unsuccessful, presumably because of the bacteria's location deep within the skin.[7,37] Biopsy specimens of affected skin cultured in broth generally yield the offending bacteria. Amplification and detection of *Erysipelothrix* DNA by polymerase chain reaction show promise in animal models of infection.[20] *Erysipelothrix* is isolated commonly from the blood of patients with septicemia or endocarditis and can be found in affected heart valves at autopsy or at the time of valve replacement.[9] A high index of suspicion is important for establishing the diagnosis of endocarditis. The organism has been misidentified as a viridans group streptococcus because of its pleomorphic coccoid appearance, alpha-hemolysis, and catalase-negative character. Abbreviated identification schema that do not include testing for hydrogen sulfide production sometimes lead to misidentification as *Lactobacillus* spp. or enterococci.[8]

TREATMENT

E. rhusiopathiae is exquisitely sensitive to penicillin. Most isolates also are sensitive to ceftriaxone.[10] Clindamycin or ciprofloxacin may be used for patients who are allergic to penicillin.[10] Localized disease usually can be treated with oral medication, but high parenteral doses occasionally are necessary, particularly for disseminated disease.[13] Treatment of endocarditis is similar to treatment of endocarditis caused by viridans streptococci. At least 12 million U of penicillin administered for 4 weeks has been curative in adult patients, but many cases have been treated for 6 weeks or longer. Concomitant administration of an aminoglycoside has been used in some cases. *Erysipelothrix* is resistant to vancomycin.[15] Prompt microbiologic differentiation of *E. rhusiopathiae* from other gram-positive organisms is important in guiding antimicrobial choice because vancomycin often is employed in empiric therapy for endocarditis. Hyperimmune serum, which at one time was advocated for therapy, is of little value. Risk of acquiring disease is minimized by protecting individuals exposed to potentially contaminated materials.

Acknowledgments

The author would like to thank Dr. William Gruber and Dr. Thomas Boyce for their invaluable assistance with earlier versions of this chapter.

REFERENCES

1. Abedini, S., and Lester, A.: [*Erysipelothrix rhusiopathiae* bacteremia after dog bite.] [Danish] Ugeskr Laeger. *159*:4400-4401, 1997.
2. Allianatos, P. G., Tilentzoglou, A. C., and Koutsoukou, A. D.: Septic arthritis caused by *Erysipelothrix rhusiopathiae* infection after arthroscopically assisted anterior cruciate ligament reconstruction. Arthroscopy *19*:E26, 2003.
3. Ben-Chetrit, E., Muiad, N., and Levo, Y.: Infective endocarditis caused by uncommon bacteria. Scand. J. Infect. Dis. *15*:179-183, 1983.
4. Callon, R. A. J., and Brady, P. G.: Toothpick perforation of the sigmoid colon: An unusual case associated with *Erysipelothrix rhusiopathiae* septicemia. Gastrointest. Endosc. *36*:141-143, 1990.
5. Campbell, G. D., Addison, E. M., Barker, I. K., et al.: *Erysipelothrix rhusiopathiae*, serotype 17, septicemia in moose (*Alces alces*) from Algonquin Park, Ontario. J. Wild. Dis. *30*:436-438, 1994.
6. Chooromoney, K. N., Hampson, D. J., Eamens, G. J., et al.: Analysis of *Erysipelothrix rhusiopathiae* and *Erysipelothrix tonsillarum* by multilocus enzyme electrophoresis. J. Clin. Microbiol. *32*:371-376, 1994.
7. Dhttman, G.: Schweinrotlauf und erysipeloid. Beitr. Klin. Chir. *123*:461-470, 1921.
8. Dunbar, S. A., and Clarridge, J. E., 3rd: Potential errors in recognition of *Erysipelothrix rhusiopathiae*. J. Clin. Microbiol. *38*:1302-1304, 2000.
9. Ehrlich, J. C.: *Erysipelothrix rhusiopathiae* infection in man. Arch. Intern. Med. *78*:565-577, 1944.
10. Fidalgo, S. G., Longbottom, C. J., and Riley, T. V.: Susceptibility of *Erysipelothrix rhusiopathiae* to antimicrobial agents and home disinfectants. Pathology *34*:462-465, 2002.
11. Fidalgo, S. G., and Riley, T. V.: Detection of *Erysipelothrix rhusiopathiae* in clinical and environmental samples. Methods Mol. Biol. *268*:199-205, 2004.
12. Gorby, G. L., and Peacock, J. E. J.: *Erysipelothrix rhusiopathiae* endocarditis: Microbiologic, epidemiologic, and clinical features of an occupational disease. Rev. Infect. Dis. *10*:317-325, 1988.
13. Grieco, M. H., and Sheldon, C.: *Erysipelothrix rhusiopathiae*. Ann. N. Y. Acad. Sci. *174*:523-532, 1970.
14. Griffiths, G. L., and Buller, N.: *Erysipelothrix rhusiopathiae* infection in semi-intensively farmed emus. Austr. Vet. J. *68*:121-122, 1991.
15. Johnson, A. P., Uttley, A. H., Woodford, N., et al.: Resistance to vancomycin and teicoplanin: An emerging clinical problem. Clin. Microbiol. Rev. *3*:280-291, 1990.
16. Klauder, J. V.: Erysipeloid as an occupational disease. J. A. M. A. *111*:1345-1348, 1938.
17. Klauder, J. V.: *Erysipelothrix rhusiopathiae* infection in swine and in human beings. Arch. Dermatol. Syph. *50*:151-159, 1944.
18. Kramer, M. R., Gombert, M. E., Corrado, M. L., et al.: *Erysipelothrix rhusiopathiae* endocarditis. South. Med. J. *75*:892, 1982.
19. Lacroix, J., Delage, G., and Mitchell, G.: Erysipeloid in an infant. J. Pediatr. *99*:745-746, 1981.
20. Makino, S., Okada, Y., Maruyama, T., et al.: Direct and rapid detection of *Erysipelothrix rhusiopathiae* DNA in animals by PCR. J. Clin. Microbiol. *32*:1526-1531, 1994.
21. Morris, C. A., Schwabacher, H., Lynch, P. G., et al.: Two fatal cases of septicaemia due to *Erysipelothrix insidiosa*. J. Clin. Pathol. *18*:614-617, 1965.
22. Muirhead, N., and Reid, T. M. S.: *Erysipelothrix rhusiopathiae* endocarditis. J. Infect. *2*:83-85, 1980.
23. Mutalib, A., Keirs, R., and Austin, F.: Erysipelas in quail and suspected erysipeloid in processing plant employees. Avian Dis. *39*:191-193, 1995.
24. Nandish, S., and Khandori, N.: Valvular and myocardial abscesses due to *Erysipelothrix rhusiopathiae*. Clin. Infect. Dis. *29*:1351-1352, 1999.
25. Nelson, E.: Five hundred cases of erysipeloid. Rocky Mountain Med. J. *52*:40-42, 1955.
26. Panhotra, B. R., Agarwal, K. C., Kumar, L., et al.: *Erysipelothrix rhusiopathiae* infection in a child: A case report with review of literature. Indian Pediatr. *16*:547-549, 1979.
27. Prausnitz, C.: Bakteriologische untersuchung über schweinrotlauf beim menschen. Zentralbl. Bakteriol. Mikrobiol. *85*:362, 1921.
28. Reboli, A. C., and Farrar, W. E.: *Erysipelothrix rhusiopathiae*: An occupational pathogen. Clin. Microbiol. Rev. *2*:354-359, 1989.
29. Rosenbach, F. J.: Experimentelle morphologische und klinische studie ber die (krankheitserregenden) mikroorganismen des erysipeloids, des erysipelroths und der muse muse. Z. Hyg. Infektionskrankheit. *63*:343-371, 1909.
30. Ruiz, M. E., Richards, J. S., Kerr, G. S., and Kan, V. L.: *Erysipelothrix rhusiopathiae* septic arthritis. Arthritis Rheum. *48*:1156-1157, 2003.
31. Shimoji, Y., Yokomizo, Y., and Mori, Y.: Intracellular survival and replication of *Erysipelothrix rhusiopathiae* within murine macrophages: Failure of induction of the oxidative burst of macrophages. Infect. Immun. *64*:1789-1793, 1996.
32. Shimoji, Y., Yokomizo, Y., Sekizaki, T., et al.: Presence of a capsule in *Erysipelothrix rhusiopathiae* and its relationship to virulence for mice. Infect. Immun. *62*:2806-2810, 1994.
33. Simionescu, R., Grover, S., Shekar, R., and West, B. C.: Necrotizing fasciitis caused by *Erysipelothrix rhusiopathiae*. South. Med. J. *96*:937-939, 2003.

34. Talan, D. A., Citron, D. M., Abrahamian, F. M., et al.: Bacteriologic analysis of infected dog and cat bites. Emergency Medicine Animal Bite Infection Study Group. N. Engl. J. Med. *340*:85-92, 1999.
35. Watarai, M., Sawada, T., Nakagomi, M., et al.: Comparison of etiological and immunological characteristics of two attenuated *Erysipelothrix rhusiopathiae* strains of serotypes 1a and 2. J. Vet. Med. Sci. *55*:595-600, 1993.

36. Wong, R. C., Kong, K. O., Lin, R. V., and Barkham, T.: Chronic monoarthritis of the knee in systemic lupus erythematosus. Lupus. *12*:324-326, 2003.
37. Woodbine, M.: *Erysipelothrix rhusiopathiae*: Bacteriology and chemotherapy. Bacteriol. Rev. *14*:161-178, 1947.

CHAPTER 106

LISTERIOSIS
Robert Bortolussi ⊙ Timothy Mailman

Listeria monocytogenes was described first by Murray and associates[105] in 1926 while they were investigating an epidemic of perinatal infection in laboratory rabbits. Human disease caused by *Listeria* was first published 3 years later, in 1929.[111] Neonatal infection was not described until 1936.[22] Since then, the organism has been isolated with increasing frequency from elderly individuals, pregnant women, immunocompromised individuals, and neonates. A large body of information has accumulated, and several comprehensive reviews have been published.[16,45,118,128] More recently, food-borne outbreaks of *Listeria* causing gastroenteritis have refocused attention on this organism.[6,112,124]

ORGANISM

Listeria is a regular, short, facultatively anaerobic, non–spore-forming, gram-positive rod that is motile and forms bluish gray colonies on nutrient agar. The genus is thought to be named in honor of Lister, the father of antiseptic technique. Of the six *Listeria* spp. (*L. monocytogenes, Listeria innocua, Listeria grayi, Listeria welshimeri, Listeria seeligeri,* and *Listeria ivanovii*), only *L. monocytogenes* and *L. ivanovii* have been reported to infect humans.[59,85] Various features of *L. monocytogenes* have been used to separate it from nonpathogenic *Listeria* spp. and other gram-positive rods.[130] The following four characteristics are used commonly for differentiation: (1) *Listeria* exhibits a characteristic tumbling motility at 25° C (77° F), with reduced motility at 37° C (98.6° F); (2) it grows with a narrow zone of beta-hemolysis (non-hemolytic strains exist but rarely appear in clinical material) and exhibits a rectangular area of increased hemolysis when streaked on blood agar in proximity to *Staphylococcus aureus* (Christie, Atkins, Munch-Peterson [CAMP] test); (3) it is catalase-positive; and (4) it ferments α-methyl-D-mannoside and L-rhamnose but not D-mylose.

Listeria organisms tolerate low temperatures, high salt concentrations, and high pH, which allows replication to occur in soil, water, sewage, manure, animal feed, and, more importantly, refrigerated foods. Cold enrichment procedures have been used to improve the isolation rate from clinical material, but generally they are not recommended.[12,45,128]

After the early work of Paterson,[113] Seeliger and Finger[131] performed an extensive serologic characterization of *L. monocytogenes*. At least 17 serotypes have been identified on the basis of somatic and flagellar antigens, but three (1/2a, 1/2b, 4b) account for most clinical isolates and are the serotypes most commonly found in food.[97,114]

TRANSMISSION

The factors involved in transmission are not well understood. Although contamination of food and human exposure to *Listeria* are common occurrences,[51] most infections are sporadic and have no epidemiologic explanation.[21,104,146] In investigations of outbreaks, a source that is linked to food often is discovered. An outbreak described by Schlech and colleagues[125] involving the consumption of *Listeria*-contaminated cabbage was the first investigation to prove that food-borne transmission can occur. Since then, numerous outbreaks have been linked to food, particularly contaminated dairy products.[45,66,86,124,145,146] Pate, pork, ready-cooked chicken, and hot dogs also have been implicated.[6,66,69,98,124,129] The incubation period for food-borne listeriosis is approximately 3 weeks. Molecular techniques involving polymerase chain reaction and multilocus enzyme electrophoresis are being used to track epidemic and sporadic strains found in food.[4,66,92,107,114,120]

EPIDEMIOLOGY

L. monocytogenes colonizes humans and a variety of mammals worldwide.[130] In the developed world, approximately 1 to 5 percent of the population carry the organism in their feces.[51,77] Nonetheless, listeriosis remains an uncommon infection. In the United States, estimates of its incidence range from 0.4 to 0.7 case per 100,000 population.[138] Listeriosis reported in the United States has a nonuniform age distribution, with most cases occurring in newborns and elderly individuals (Fig. 106–1). Although cases can occur in otherwise healthy subjects,[128,148] immunocompromised individuals with acquired immunodeficiency syndrome (AIDS), individuals with cancer (related to chemotherapy, particularly fludarabine), or organ transplant recipients are at significantly increased risk.[30,104,110,135] Other host factors associated with listeriosis include diabetes mellitus, renal failure requiring dialysis, hemochromatosis, and cirrhosis.

Perinatal attack rates during outbreaks are extremely high, reaching 1 to 2 percent of all deliveries.[125] Vertical transmission from mother to infant through the placenta is the mode of transmission for early-onset newborn infection; the epidemiologic factors contributing to late-onset infection are unknown. Nosocomial spread rarely has been reported in nursery outbreaks.[40,50,81,98,127]

PATHOGENESIS AND PATHOLOGY

The gross and microscopic findings in listeriosis are well documented. Although multiple granulomata are characteristic of disseminated disease, the basic pathologic change of suppurative inflammation is nonspecific.[75] Examination of the placenta of infants with early-onset infection reveals macroabscesses, funisitis, and villitis in most cases.[140]

L. monocytogenes is a facultative intracellular pathogen that has been used extensively to study cell-mediated immunity and the biochemical and pharmacologic abnormalities associated with

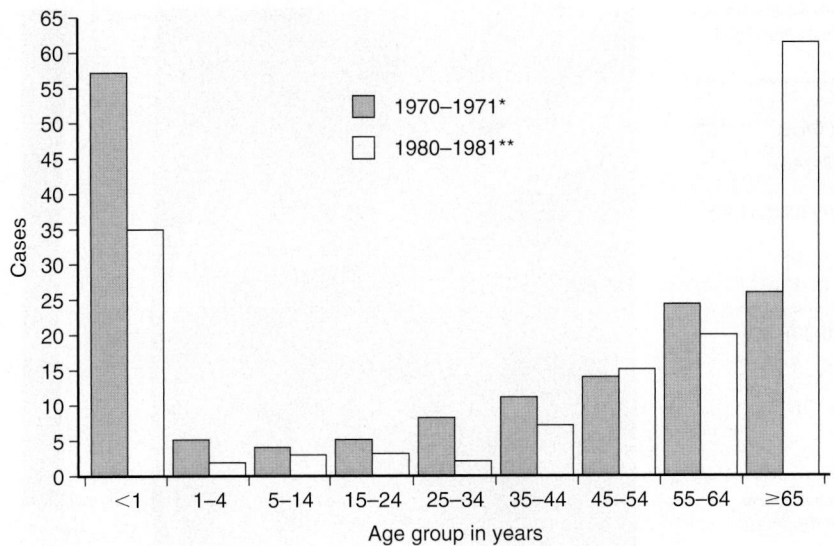

Figure 106–1 Human listeriosis cases by age group for the United States, 1970-1971 and 1980-1981. *(From Albritton, W. L., Cochi, S. L., and Feeley, J. C.: Overview of neonatal listeriosis. Clin. Invest. Med. 7:311-314, 1984.)*

* Age unknown for 63 cases
** Age unknown for 3 cases

infection.[7,13,64,78,93,96,137,151] Factors involved in mucosal colonization are crucial for invasion of the host to occur.[112] The cycle begins with adhesion to a eukaryotic cell and subsequent internalization. This process is mediated partly by an *L. monocytogenes* surface protein known as internalin[8,54,82] and its mammalian cell receptor, E-cadherin.[82] The internalin–E-cadherin interaction is necessary for the organism to cross the intestinal epithelium barrier. The intestinal mucosa is a depot for *Listeria*-specific effector CD8[+] T cells, which accumulate during and after infection.[63] Spread of the organism to the liver and bloodstream is the usual mode of infection. Resident hepatocytes, enterocytes, and fibroblasts are invaded by the organism. Intracellular bacteria are shielded from macrophage and polymorphonuclear phagocytic cells, permitting intracellular proliferation to occur.[27,43,56,70,79,117] Numerous virulence genes and their roles in the pathogenesis (internalization, vacuole escape, intracellular proliferation, and intercellular spread) are known to exist.[57,115] When inside the host cell, *Listeria* uses a hemolysin to escape into the cytoplasm.[116] The hemolysin secreted by *L. monocytogenes*, termed *listerolysin O*, has been purified, and its gene, *hly*, has been sequenced.[24,115] It is a pore-forming protein (antigenically similar to streptolysin O produced by group A streptococci) that causes lysis of host-cell vacuoles with the subsequent release of *Listeria* into the host cytoplasm. Monoclonal antibody to listerolysin O provides resistance to *Listeria* infection in a murine model of infection.[17,32,33] When in the cell, *Listeria* uses its ActA protein to promote actin polymerization for intracellular movement. The intracellular cycle is complete after escape from the host cell.[71,146]

The mechanism for passage through the placenta has provided new insights into pathogenic mechanisms in utero. In a transgenic mouse model that expresses human E-cadherin, the internalin–E-cadherin interaction was found to mediate crossing of the placental barrier by *L. monocytogenes*. The crucial role of internalin for placental passage was not present in a guinea pig model of perinatal infection model.[8] ActA-mediated, cell-to-cell spreading also plays a role in the vertical transmission of *Listeria* to the fetus in the murine model.[83]

For many years, immunity to *L. monocytogenes* and other facultative intracellular bacteria has been attributed almost exclusively to a repertoire of T cells and cytokines.[93,99] We now realize that phagocytic cells also play a role in resistance to *Listeria* infection.[31,88,152] Peak immunity to *Listeria* in adults is expressed after

5 to 6 days of infection, coinciding with the maximal T-cell responses.[15,76,99,33] Cytokines such as granulocyte colony-stimulating factor, tumor necrosis factor-α, and interleukin-6 (IL-6), IL-10, IL-12, IL-15, and IL-18 are induced and mediate clearance of *Listeria*.*

In newborn animals, susceptibility to *L. monocytogenes* is associated with delayed production of cytokines and activation of T cells and natural killer cells.[14,36,90] In particular, monocyte,[152] T-cell,[91] and natural killer cell activity[36,91] is immature in animal models. Delayed cytokine and cell activation processes seem to operate in humans.[65,152] Synthesis of tumor necrosis factor-α, interferon-γ, interferon-α, and IL-2, all of which modulate the immune response and macrophage activation, is deficient in newborns.[132,152] Pretreatment of newborn animals with interferon or inducers of interferon seems to enhance immune responsiveness and protects against *L. monocytogenes* infection.[16,20,24]

In older children and young adults, *Listeria* infection is rare; however, underlying diseases or medications that interfere with cell-mediated immunity may increase susceptibility.[30,133] Cyclosporine, which blocks production of cytokine, is associated with increased susceptibility.[62]

CLINICAL MANIFESTATIONS

Although a variety of clinical manifestations are described in *L. monocytogenes* infections, most pediatric infections occur in the first months of life. The initial clinical features are similar to those of the more prevalent group B streptococcal infection.[9] The serotype distribution of *L. monocytogenes* seems to depend on the age at onset. Serotypes 1a and 1b occur more commonly in the early-onset form of disease (<7 days of age), and serotype 4b occurs in the late-onset form (>7 days of age).[3]

The early-onset form of neonatal listeriosis usually is diagnosed within the first 24 hours of life, and affected infants have respiratory distress or pneumonia, septicemia, and, occasionally, meningitis (Table 106–1).[2,3,39,86,139,148] Mothers of these infants frequently have an influenza-like illness with fever, malaise, headache, gastrointestinal symptoms, or pharyngitis in the few days

---

*See references 28, 29, 73, 80, 87, 108, 109, 144, 149, 153.

TABLE 106–1 Features of Early-Onset and Late-Onset Neonatal Listeriosis*

	Early Onset[2,3,39,86,140]	Late Onset[3,41,74,128,148]
Age at onset (median in days)	<0.1 (<0.1-1.3)	28 (7-140)
Birth weight (median in g)	2250 (1800-2540)	3100 (3000-3150)
Percentage of isolates from		
Cerebrospinal fluid	5 (2-7)	63 (30-87)
Blood and cerebrospinal fluid	10 (6-26)	25 (13-40)
Blood alone	74 (45-88)	12 (0-30)
Other only[†]	5 (0-24)	0
Newborn and maternal	72 (54-93)	4 (0-8)
Percent mortality	38 (22-63)	3 (0-10)
Percentage with obstetric complications	63 (38-87)	3 (0-7)

*This table shows the median values and ranges of results from various publications.
†Sources other than blood and cerebrospinal fluid included cutaneous, gastric, throat, urine, and rectal sources.

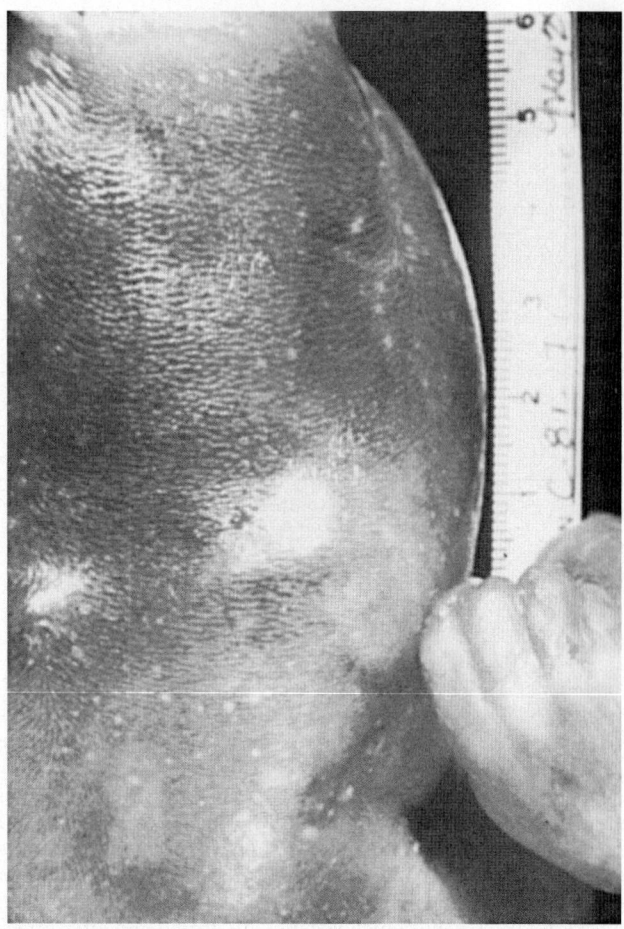

Figure 106–2 Typical pustular rash on the abdomen of a stillborn infant with listeriosis. Note the small pale granuloma measuring 1 to 3 mm and the dark erythema surrounding these lesions.

preceding delivery.[60,86] During labor, maternal fever and green-stained or brown-stained amniotic fluid may be seen.[2,84] More severely affected infants are infected in utero, born prematurely, and often critically ill at birth. Widespread microabscesses and macroabscesses may occur and are demonstrable externally as discrete roseolar or pustular lesions on the skin and pharynx. The rash has been termed *granulomatosis infantisepticum* (Fig. 106–2). Depression at birth, respiratory distress, apnea, lethargy, and fever are common manifestations; diarrhea, conjunctivitis, and myocarditis also have been described.[84] The respiratory symptoms may mimic symptoms of respiratory distress syndrome. Patchy bronchopneumonic infiltrates, probably caused by aspiration of infected amniotic fluid, may be seen on chest radiographs. In addition, intrauterine infection may result in spontaneous abortion or stillbirth.[60] Colonized asymptomatic adults and neonates have been reported, however.[126]

The late-onset form of neonatal listeriosis occurs less commonly than does the early-onset form and usually affects term infants, who appear healthy until the onset of meningitis or, less commonly, septicemia and colitis 1 to 8 weeks after birth.[3,41,60,74,81,127] Clinical manifestations of late-onset meningitis may be subtle and include fever, irritability, lethargy, and poor feeding.[74,127] Cerebrospinal fluid findings vary. Although pleocytosis usually is significant, not all infections have a polymorphonuclear cell predominance. The maternal history in these cases usually is negative. An outbreak of late-onset neonatal listeriosis associated with mineral oil, reported by Schuchat and associates,[127] provides insight into the pathophysiology of this disease. During the outbreak, infants were bathed at birth with mineral oil. A strain of *L. monocytogenes* identical to the one causing the outbreak was isolated from a mineral oil container in the delivery room. Despite intensive investigation, no other source of infection was identified. The incubation period before the development of symptoms was 5 days, and the median age at first positive culture was 7 days. The symptoms and signs in infants were those of the late-onset form of *Listeria* infection, including fever and meningitis, and, in 7 of 10 infants, a positive cerebrospinal fluid culture.

Immunocompromised patients can have a variety of clinical findings, most commonly meningitis or septicemia. Although patients receiving immunosuppressive therapy have a high incidence of infection, the clinical features are similar to those of non-immunosuppressed patients with *Listeria* infection.[133] Rhombencephalitis, brain abscess, arthritis, osteomyelitis, endocarditis, endophthalmitis, liver abscess, and peritonitis also have

been reported in adult patients.* Rarely, invasive listeriosis has been seen in children who are otherwise well.[94,97,128,148] *Listeria* also is recognized as a cause of febrile gastroenteritis.

DIAGNOSIS

Appropriate specimens for staining and culture vary with the clinical syndrome, but investigation of the usual sources, such as blood, cerebrospinal fluid, amniotic fluid, and genital tract secretions, is most productive. Because prompt recognition is essential, examination of Gram-stained material (ear, meconium, and placenta) from newborns is recommended in suspected, early-onset sepsis.[83] Pathologic specimens (e.g., biopsy material, placental or fetal tissue) may reveal the characteristic Gram-stain morphology and pathologic features, such as microabscesses and granulomata. Selective culture media, such as PALCAM (polymyxin B–acriflavine–lithium chloride–ceftazidime–esculin–mannitol agar) or modified Oxford agar, may be helpful for isolating from contaminated material, such as stool or vaginal secretions.[95,114] Laboratories undertaking primary isolation must be aware of the similarities between *L. monocytogenes* and frequently discarded "commensals."[97]

After 48 hours of incubation at 37° C on 5 percent sheep blood agar, colonies are gray with a narrow zone of beta-hemolysis. The appearance on Gram stain of short rods has been confused with lancet-shaped pneumococci. Traditionally,

*See references 1, 5, 19, 23, 35, 44, 52, 89, 94, 103, 106, 135.

identification is based on morphology; tumbling motility; beta-hemolysis; positive catalase, esculin, and CAMP tests; and carbohydrate use pattern. Commercial kits are available for the rapid identification of *Listeria* from culture. These kits include DNA probes, latex agglutination, and enzyme immunoassay methods.

Despite extensive attempts to develop serologic techniques for the diagnosis of listeriosis, none has proved satisfactory, and few centers attempt serodiagnosis.[10,61] At present, a confirmed diagnosis requires isolation of the organism.

Histologic diagnosis from pathologic material should be attempted if the organism is not cultured. Specific fluorescent antibody staining,[25] nucleic acid hybridization,[136] and polymerase chain reaction[4,67] generally are not available in the routine diagnostic laboratory, but they offer the potential for development in the future, especially in patients pretreated with antibiotics and for rapid food surveillance.

TREATMENT

Prompt administration of antibiotic therapy is needed to prevent death or severe sequelae caused by *Listeria* infection. Antibiotic resistance in *L. monocytogenes* is low.[53,150] The bactericidal activity of the antibiotics commonly used is influenced in vitro by such factors as size of inoculum, type of medium, and definition of end-points.[37,89] Similar to a few other bacteria, *L. monocytogenes* shows tolerance to some antibiotics in vitro; the minimal bactericidal concentration is more than fourfold the minimal inhibitory concentration.[37,102] The antibiotics commonly recommended for treatment—ampicillin, penicillin, erythromycin, and tetracycline—are bacteriostatic only at concentrations usually achieved in blood.[37,46,47,142,147] Relapse of *L. monocytogenes* infection after apparent therapeutic success has been documented in immunocompromised patients, suggesting that bactericidal regimens may be needed in such patients.[42,122]

Other antibiotics have been considered for possible therapy. Some studies have shown trimethoprim-sulfamethoxazole and rifampin to be effective in eradicating *Listeria* in vivo.[42,55,58,100,123] These drugs seem to be bactericidal and have been used successfully in a few cases of human listeriosis.[51,135] Rifampin and trimethoprim-sulfamethoxazole offer a theoretical advantage over other drugs because of their better intracellular penetration.[42] Many newer antibiotics, such as the quinolones, macrolides, and imipenem, have only moderate activity in vitro against *Listeria*. Most quinolone and macrolide antibiotics are bacteriostatic only, and in vivo studies with these agents are not promising.[101,121] In addition, *L. monocytogenes* is resistant to cephalosporin antibiotics.[37] Vancomycin has been used in a few penicillin-allergic and sulfa-allergic patients with some success, but experience with this drug is limited.[119]

Combinations of antibiotics for therapy and in vitro testing also have shown variable results. Ampicillin plus gentamicin has a synergistic effect on most *Listeria* strains.[34,100,141] Partial synergy seems to occur with combinations of ampicillin or vancomycin and rifampin, but combinations of penicillin G and rifampin have shown activity ranging from synergy to antagonism.[100] In an in vivo model of *L. monocytogenes* encephalitis, the combinations ampicillin/gentamicin and co-trimoxazole/rifampin were highly active against intracerebral bacteria.[11] Antagonism also seems to occur between some antibiotic combinations (erythromycin and penicillins, erythromycin and aminoglycosides, penicillin and chloramphenicol, and penicillin and tetracycline).[37,46,100] On the basis of results of in vitro susceptibility testing and in vivo models, ampicillin plus gentamicin has proved to be the most reliable synergistic combination and remains the recommended initial therapy for patients suspected to have listeriosis. Trimethoprim-sulfamethoxazole may be considered for use in non-perinatal listeriosis, particularly in the presence of penicillin allergy, but it

cannot be recommended for use in perinatal infections because of the concern of bilirubin toxicity developing with sulfonamides.[42] The duration of therapy depends on the clinical syndrome, the presence of underlying disease, and the response to treatment. In newborns, 2 weeks of antibiotic therapy usually seems to be adequate. Liposomal encapsulation also results in marked enhancement of the therapeutic activity of ampicillin.[8]

PROGNOSIS

Precise morbidity and mortality data for *L. monocytogenes* infection are unavailable. Maternal listeriosis may result in abortion or stillbirth. Fetal mortality rates probably are high with gestational listeriosis, although the relative risk of intrauterine death occurring is unknown. Convincing evidence that *L. monocytogenes* is associated with repeated abortions is lacking.[49]

Among reported cases of early-onset sepsis, the more recent mortality rate in North America is approximately 40 percent (see Table 106–1).[2,39] Most survivors seem to be normal.[38,39,139] Sequelae are related to the associated complications of prematurity, pneumonia, and sepsis; hydrocephalus and cerebral palsy also have been reported.[38,72] Early treatment of maternal disease would seem to affect fetal and neonatal outcome favorably.[39,72]

Late-onset *Listeria* meningitis has a mortality rate of less than 10 percent. The outcome after *Listeria* meningitis may be more favorable than the outcome associated with other types of bacterial meningitis.[74,148] Major sequelae are hydrocephalus and mental retardation. Beyond the newborn period, the outcome of listeriosis depends on the nature of any underlying disease and the availability of intensive medical care.

PREVENTION

The sporadic nature of the disease in North America emphasized the need for collaborative investigation and reporting of infections by physicians and veterinarians to public health authorities.[12,45] In the early 1990s, epidemiologists in the United States and Canada endorsed making listeriosis a notifiable disease.[114,138] Since then, the important role of food in the transmission of sporadic cases has been linked firmly.[128] Aggressive investigation of cases and close inspection and testing of food and food-handling facilities in the United States have been under way since the early 1990s.[92,138] By tracking strains of *L. monocytogenes* from patients' refrigerators to retail sources, specific foods have been identified. Strict adherence to regulations for pasteurization of raw milk is important to inactivate the organism and prevent listeriosis.[143] Contamination of food can occur during the preparation and processing of pasteurized milk products and ready-to-eat meat or poultry products. Recommendations for individuals at high risk, such as pregnant women and immunocompromised patients, include avoiding soft cheeses and delicatessen meats and avoiding reheating leftover foods or ready-to-eat foods (e.g., hot dogs).[114,138] Preventive strategies involving inspection of food and facilities and dissemination of recommendations and educational materials seem to have reduced the incidence of listeriosis in the developed nations.[4,48,138]

During an outbreak of *Listeria*, prompt investigation and treatment of pregnant women with a febrile "influenza-like" illness have been advocated.[12,72] The attack rate for late-onset disease in colonized infants is unknown, and no data show that treatment of colonized infants can either eradicate asymptomatic carriage or prevent infection. Careful attention given to the handling of infected infants in a neonatal unit in an attempt to prevent transmission is of the utmost importance for preventing nosocomial infection.[40,127]

REFERENCES

1. Ackermann, G., Schoen, H., Schaumann, R., et al.: Rapidly growing tumor-like brain lesion. Infection 29:278-279, 2001.
2. Ahlfors, C. E., Goetzman, B. W., Halsted, C. C., et al.: Neonatal listeriosis. Am. J. Dis. Child. 131:405-408, 1977.
3. Albritton, W. L., Wiggins, G. L., and Feeley, J. C.: Neonatal listeriosis: Distribution of serotypes in relation to age at onset of disease. J. Pediatr. 88:481-483, 1976.
4. Allmann, M., Hofelein, C., Koppel, E., et al.: Polymerase chain reaction (PCR) for detection of pathogenic microorganisms in bacteriological monitoring of dairy products. Res. Microbiol. 146:85-97, 1995.
5. Antal, E. A., Dietrichs, E., Loberg, E. M., et al.: Brain stem encephalitis in listeriosis. Scand. J. Infect. Dis. 37:190-194, 2005.
6. Aureli, P., Fiorucci, G. C., Caroli, D., et al.: An outbreak of febrile gastroenteritis associated with corn contaminated by Listeria monocytogenes. N. Engl. J. Med. 342:1236-1241, 2000.
7. Azri, S., and Renton, K. W.: Depression of murine hepatic mixed function oxidase during infection with Listeria monocytogenes. J. Pharmacol. Exp. Ther. 243:1089-1894, 1987.
8. Bakardjiev, A. I., Stacy, B. A., Fisher, S. J., and Portnoy, D. A.: Listeriosis in the pregnant guinea pig: A model of vertical transmission. Infect. Immun. 72:489-497, 2004.
9. Baker, C. J., and Barrett, F. F.: Group B streptococcal infections in infants: The importance of serotypes. J. A. M. A. 230:1158-1160, 1974.
10. Berche, P., Reich, K. A., Bonnichon, M., et al.: Detection of antilisterelysin O for serodiagnosis of human listeriosis. Lancet 335:624-627, 1990.
11. Blanot, S., Boumaila, C., and Berche, P.: Intracerebral activity of antibiotics against Listeria monocytogenes during experimental rhombencephalitis. J. Antimicrob. Chemother. 44:565-568, 1999.
12. Bortolussi, R.: An ongoing problem: Perinatal infection due to Listeria monocytogenes, an old pathogen reborn. J. Clin. Invest. Med. 7:213-215, 1984.
13. Bortolussi, R.: Neonatal listeriosis: Where do we go from here? Pediatr. Infect. Dis. 4:228-229, 1985.
14. Bortolussi, R., Campbell, N., and Krause, V.: Dynamics of Listeria monocytogenes type 4b infection in pregnant and infant rats. J. Clin. Invest. Med. 7:273-279, 1984.
15. Bortolussi, R., Issekutz, T., Burbridge, S., et al.: Neonatal host defence mechanisms against Listeria monocytogenes infection: The role of lipopolysaccharides and interferons. Pediatr. Res. 25:311-315, 1989.
16. Bortolussi, R., McGregor, D. D., Kongshavn, P. A. L., et al.: Host defence mechanism to perinatal and neonatal Listeria monocytogenes infection. Surv. Synth. Pathol. Res. 3:311-332, 1984.
17. Bouwer, H. G. A., Gibbins, B. L., Jones, S., et al.: Antilisterial immunity includes specificity to listeriolysin O (LLO) and non-LLO-derived determinants. Infect. Immun. 62:1039-1045, 1994.
18. Braun, L., Dramsi, S., Dehoux, P., et al.: InlB: An invasion protein in Listeria monocytogenes with a novel type of surface association. Mol. Microbiol. 25:285-294, 1997.
19. Brouwer, M. C., van de Beek, D., Heckenberg, S. G., et al.: Community-acquired Listeria monocytogenes meningitis in adults. Clin. Infect. Dis. 43:1233-1238, 2006.
20. Buchmeier, N. A., and Schreiber, R. D.: Immunology: Requirement endogenous interferon-production for resolution of Listeria monocytogenes infection. Proc. Natl. Acad. Sci. U. S. A. 82:7401-7408, 1985.
21. Buchner, L. H., and Schneirson, S. S.: Clinical and laboratory aspects Listeria monocytogenes infections. Am. J. Med. 45:904-921, 1968.
22. Burn, C. G.: Clinical and pathological features of an infection reused by new pathogen of the genus Listerella. Am. J. Pathol. 12:341-M, 1936.
23. Carvajal, A., and Frederiksen, W.: Fatal endocarditis due to Listeria monocytogenes. Rev. Infect. Dis. 10:616-623, 1988.
24. Chen, Y., Nakane, A., and Minagawa, T.: Recombinant murine gamma interferon induces enhanced resistance to Listeria monocytogenes infection in neonatal mice. Infect. Immun. 57:2345-2349, 1989.
25. Cherry, W. B., and Moody, M. D.: Fluorescent antibody techniques: Diagnostic microbiology. Bacteriol. Rev. 29:222-250, 1965.
26. Cossart, P.: The listeriolysin O gene: A chromosomal locus crucial for the virulence of Listeria monocytogenes. Infection 16(Suppl. 2):157-159, 1988.
27. Cowart, R. E., Lashmet, J., McIntosh, M. E., et al.: Adherence of virulent strain of Listeria monocytogenes to the surface of a hepatocaronoma cell line via lectin-substrate interaction. Arch. Microbiol. 153:282-286, 1990.
28. Deckert, M., Soltek, S., Geginat, G., et al.: Endogenous interleukin-10 required for prevention of a hyperinflammatory intracerebral immune response in Listeria monocytogenes meningoencephalitis. Infect. Immun. 69:4561-4571, 2001.
29. Desiderio, J. V., Kiener, P. A., Lin, P. F., et al.: Protection of mice against Listeria monocytogenes infection by recombinant human tumor necrose factor alpha. Infect. Immun. 57:1615-1617, 1989.
30. Doorduyn, Y., de Jager, C. M., van der Zwaluw, W. K., et al.: Invasive Listeria monocytogenes infections in the Netherlands, 1995-2003. Eur. J. Clin. Microbiol. Infect. Dis. 25:433-442, 2006.
31. Drevets, D. A: Dissemination of Listeria monocytogenes by infected phagocytes. Infect. Immun. 67:3512-3517, 1999.
32. Edelson, B. T., Cossart, P., and Unanue, E. R.: Cutting edge: Paradigm revisited: Antibody provides resistance to Listeria infection. J. Immunol. 163:4087-4090, 1999.
33. Edelson, B. T., and Unanue, E. R: Intracellular antibody neutralize Listeria growth. Immunity 14:503-512, 2001.
34. Edmiston, C. E., and Gordon, R. C.: Evaluation of gentamicin and penicillin as a synergistic combination in experimental murine listeriosis. Antimicrob. Agents Chemother. 16:862-863, 1979.
35. Ellis, L. C., Gitelis, S., and Huber, J. F.: Joint infections due to Listeria monocytogenes: Case report and review. Clin. Infect. Dis. 20:1548-1555, 1995.
36. Emoto, M., Miyamoto, M., Emoto, Y., et al.: A critical role of T-cell receptor gamma/delta cells in antibacterial protection in mice early in life. Hepatology 33:887-893, 2001.
37. Espaze, E. P., and Reynaud, A. E.: Antibiotic susceptibilities of Listeria in in vitro studies. Infection 16(Suppl. 2):160-164, 1988.
38. Evans, J. R., Allen, A. C., Bortolussi, R., et al.: Follow-up study survivors of fetal and early-onset neonatal listeriosis. J. Clin. Invest. Med. 7:329-334, 1984.
39. Evans, J. R., Allen, A. C., Stinson, D. A., et al.: Perinatal listeriosis: Report of an outbreak. Pediatr. Infect. Dis. 4:237-241, 1985.
40. Facinelli, B., Varaldo, P. E., Casolari, C., et al.: Cross-infection with Listeria monocytogenes confirmed by DNA fingerprinting. Lancet 2:1247-1248, 1988.
41. Filice, A. G., Cantrell, H. F., Smith, A. B., et al.: Listeria monocytogenes infection in neonates: Investigation of an epidemic. J. Infect. Dis. 138:17-23, 1978.
42. Forna, F., McConnell, M., Kitabire, F. N., et al.: Systematic review of the safety of trimethoprim-sulfamethoxazole for prophylaxis in HIV-infected pregnant women: Implications for resource limited settings. AIDS Rev. 8:24-36, 2006.
43. Gaillard, J.-L., Berche, P., Mounier, J., et al.: In vitro model of penetrate and intracellular growth of Listeria monocytogenes in the human enterocyte-like cell line caco-2. Infect. Immun. 55:2822-2829, 1987.
44. Gallagher, P. G., Amedia, C. A., and Watankunakom, C.: L. monocytogenes endocarditis in a patient on chronic hemodialysis, successfully treated with vancomycin amd gentamicin. Infection 14:125, 1986.
45. Gellin, B. G.: Listeriosis. J. A. M. A. 261:1313-1319, 1989.
46. Gordon, R. C., Barrett, F. F., and Clark, D. J.: Influence of several antibiotics, singly and in combination, on the growth of Listeria monocytogenes. J. Pediatr. 80:667-670, 1972.
47. Gordon, R. C., Barrett, F. F., and Yow, M. D.: Ampicillin treatment of listeriosis. J. Pediatr. 77:1067-1070, 1970.
48. Goulet, V., de-Valk, H., Pierre, O., et al.: Effect of prevention measures on incidence of human listeriosis, France, 1987-1997. Emerg. Infect. Dis. 7:983-989, 2001.
49. Gray, M. L., Seeliger, H. P. R., and Potel, J.: Perinatal infections due to Listeria monocytogenes: Do these affect subsequent pregnancies? Clin. Pediatr. (Phila.) 2:614-623, 1963.
50. Green, H. T., and Macaulay, M. B.: Hospital outbreak of Listeria monocytogenes septicemia: A problem of cross infection? Lancet 2:1039-1040, 1978.
51. Grif, K., Patscheider, G., Dierich, M. P., and Allerberger, F.: Incidence of fecal carriage of Listeria monocytogenes in three healthy volunteers: A one-year prospective stool survey. Eur. J. Clin. Microbiol. Infect. Dis. 22:16-20, 2003.
52. Harris, J. O., Marquez, J., Swerdloff, M. A., et al.: Listeria brain abscess in the acquired immunodeficiency syndrome. Arch. Neurol. 46:250, 1989.
53. Hansen, J. M., Gerner-Smidt, P., and Bruun, B.: Antibiotic susceptibility of Listeria monocytogenes in Denmark 1958-2001. A. P. M. I. S. 113:31-36, 2005.
54. Havell, E. A., Beretich, G. R., Jr., and Carter, P. B.: The mucosal phase of Listeria infection. Immunology 201:164-177, 1999.
55. Hawkins, A. E., Bortolussi, R., and Issekutz, A. C.: In vitro and in vivo activity of various antibiotics against Listeria monocytogenes type 4b. Clin. Invest. Med. 7:335-341, 1984.
56. Hess, C. B., Niesel, D. W., Cho, Y. J., et al.: Bacterial invasion of fibroblasts induces interferon production. J. Immunol. 138:3949-3953, 1987.
57. Hess, J., Gentschev, I., Szalay, G., et al.: Listeria monocytogenes p60 supports host cell invasion by an in vivo survival of attenuated Salmonella typhimurium. Infect. Immun. 63:2047-2053, 1995.
58. Hof, H., and Waldenmeier, G.: Therapy of experimental listeriosis: An evaluation of different antibiotics. Infection 16(Suppl. 2):171-174, 1988.
59. Holt, J. G., Krieg, N. R., Sneath, P. H. A., et al. (eds.): Bergey's Manual of Determinative Bacteriology. Baltimore, Williams & Wilkins, 1994, pp. 566-567.
60. Hood, M.: Listeriosis as an infection of pregnancy manifested in the newborn. Pediatrics 27:390-396, 1961.
61. Hudak, A. P., Lee, S. H., Issekutz, A. C., et al.: Comparison of three serological methods—enzyme-linked immunosorbent assay, complement fixation, and microagglutination—in diagnosis of human perinatal Listeria monocytogenes infection. Clin. Invest. Med. 7:349-354, 1984.
62. Hugin, A. W., Cerny, A., Wrann, M., et al.: Effect of cyclosporin A on immunity to Listeria monocytogenes. Infect. Immun. 52:12-17, 1986.
63. Huleatt, J. W., Pilip, I., Kerksiek, K., and Pamer, E. G.: Intestinal and splenic T cell responses to enteric Listeria monocytogenes infection: Distinct repertoires of responding CD8 T lymphocytes. J. Immunol. 166:4065-4073, 2001.
64. Inoue, S., Itagaki, S., and Amano, F.: Intracellular killing of Listeria monocytogenes in the J774.1 macrophage-like cell line and the lipopolysaccharide

(LPS)-resistant mutant LPS1916 cell line defective in the generation of reactive oxygen intermediates after LPS treatment. Infect. Immun. *63*:1876-1886, 1995.

65. Issekutz, T., Evans, J., and Bortolussi, R.: The immune response of human neonates to *Listeria monocytogenes* infection. Clin. Invest. Med. *7*:281-286, 1984.

66. Jacquet, C., Catimel, B., Brosch, R., et al.: Investigations related to the epidemic strain involved in the French listeriosis outbreak in 1992. Appl. Environ. Microbiol. *61*:2242-2246, 1995.

67. Jaton, K., Sahli, R., and Bille, J.: Development of polymerase chain reaction assays for detection of *Listeria monocytogenes* in clinical cerebrospinal fluid samples. J. Clin. Microbiol. *30*:1931-1936, 1992.

68. Jurado, R. L., Farley, M. M., Pereira, E., et al.: Increased risk of meningitis and bacteremia due to *Listeria monocytogenes* in patients with human immunodeficiency virus infection. Clin. Infect. Dis. *17*:224-227, 1993.

69. Kach, J., and Stark, K.: Significant increase in listeriosis in Germany—2001-2005. Eur. Surveill. *11*:85-88, 2006.

70. Karunasagar, I., Senghaas, B., Krohne, G., et al.: Ultrastructural study of *Listeria monocytogenes* entry into cultured human colonic epithelial cells. Infect. Immun. *62*:3554-3558, 1994.

71. Kathariou, S., Rocourt, J., Hof, H., et al.: Levels of *Listeria monocytogenes* hemolysin are not directly proportional to virulence in experimental infections of mice. Infect. Immun. *56*:534-536, 1988.

72. Katz, V. L., and Weinstein, L.: Antepartum treatment of *Listeria monocytogenes* septicemia. South. Med. J. *75*:1353-1354, 1982.

73. Kayashima, S., Tsuru, S., Hata, N., et al.: Therapeutic effect of granulocyte colony-stimulating factor (G-CSF) on the protection against *Listeria* infection in SCID mice. Immunology *80*:471-476, 1993.

74. Kessler, S. L., and Dejani, A. S.: *Listeria* meningitis in infants and children. Pediatr. Infect. Dis. J. *9*:61-62, 1990.

75. Klatt, E. C., Pavlova, Z., Teberg, A. J., et al.: Epidemic perinatal listeriosis at autopsy. Hum. Pathol. *17*:1278-1281, 1986.

76. Kohl, S., West, M. S., and Loo, L. S.: Defects in interleukin-2 stimulation of neonatal natural killer cytotoxicity to herpes simplex virus-infected cells. J. Pediatr. *112*:976-981, 1988.

77. Koneman, E. W., Allen, S., Janda, W. M., et al. (eds.): Color Atlas and Textbook of Diagnostic Microbiology. 5th ed. Philadelphia, Lippincott-Raven, 1997, pp. 664-667.

78. Kongshaven, P. A. A., and Skamene, E.: The role of natural resistance in protection of the murine host from listeriosis. Clin. Invest. Med. *7*:253-257, 1984.

79. Kuhn, M., and Goebel, W.: Identification of an extracellular protein of *Listeria monocytogenes* possibly involved m intracellular uptake by mammalian cells. Infect. Immun. *57*:55-61, 1989.

80. Langermans, J. A. M., Mayanski, D. M., Nibbering, P. H., et al.: Effect of IFN-γ and endogenous TNF on the histopathological changes in the liver of *Listeria monocytogenes*-infected mice. Immunology *81*:192-197, 1994.

81. Larsson, S., Cederberg, A., Ivarwon, S., et al.: *Listeria monocytogenes* causing hospital acquired enterocolitis and meningitis in newborn infants. B. M. J. *2*:473-474, 1978.

82. Lecuit, M.: Understanding how *Listeria monocytogenes* targets and crosses host barriers. Clin. Microbiol. Infect. *11*:430-643, 2005.

83. Le Monnier, A., Autret, N., Join-Lambert, O. F., et al.: ActA is required for crossing of the fetoplacental barrier by *Listeria monocytogenes*. Infect. Immun. *75*:950-957, 2007.

84. LeSouef, P. N., and Walters, B. N. J.: Neonatal listeriosis. Med. J. Aust. *2*:188-191, 1981.

85. Lessing, M. P., Curtis, G. D., and Bowler, L. C.: *Listeria ivanvii* infection. J. Infect. *29*:230-231, 1994.

86. Linnan, M. J., Mascola, L., Lou, X. D., et al.: Epidemic listeriosis associated with Mexican-style cheese. N. Engl. J. Med. *319*:823-828, 1988.

87. Liu, A., Simpson, R. J., and Cheers, C.: Role of interleukin-6 in T-cell activation during primary and secondary infection with *Listeria monocytogenes*. Infect. Immun. *63*:2790-2792, 1995.

88. Lopez, S., Marco, A.-J., Prats, N., and Czuprynaki, C. J.: Critical role of neutrophils in eliminating *Listeria monocytogenes* from the central nervous system during experimental murine listeriosis. Infect. Immun. *68*:4789-4791, 2000.

89. Louthrenoo, W., and Schumacher, H. R.: *Listeria monocytogenes* osteomyelitis complicating leukemia: Report and literature review of *Listeria* osteoarticular infections. J. Rheumatol. *17*:107-110, 1990.

90. Lu, C. Y.: The delayed ontogenesis of Ia-positive macrophages: Implications for host defense and self-tolerance in the neonate. Clin. Invest. Med. *7*:263-267, 1984.

91. Lu, C. Y., and Unanue, E. R.: Ontogeny of murine macrophages: Functions related to antigen presentation. Infect. Immun. *36*:169-175, 1982.

92. MacGowan, A. P., O'Donaghue, K., Nicholls, S., et al.: Typing of *Listeria* spp. by random amplified polymorphic DNA (RAPD) analysis. J. Med. Microbiol. *38*:322-327, 1993.

93. Mackaness, G. B.: The immunological basis of acquired cellular resistance. J. Exp. Med. *120*:105-119, 1964.

94. Massarotti, E. M., and Dinerman, H.: Septic arthritis due to *Listeria monocytogenes*: Report and review of the literature. J. Rheumatol. *17*:111-113, 1990.

95. McBride, M. E., and Girard, K. F.: Procedure for the selective isolation of *Listeria monocytogenes*. J. Lab. Clin. Med. *55*:153-157, 1960.

96. McCallum, R. E., and Sword, C. P.: Mechanisms of pathogenesis in *Listeria monocytogenes* infection, V: Early imbalance in host energy metabolism during experimental listeriosis. Infect. Immun. *5*:863-871, 1972.

97. McLaughlin, J.: Distribution of serovars of *Listeria monocytogenes* isolated from different categories of patients with listeriosis. Eur. J. Clin. Microbiol. Infect. Dis. *9*:210-213, 1990.

98. Mead, P. S., Dunne, E. F., Graves, L., et al.: Nationwide outbreak of listeriosis due to contaminated meat. Epidemiol. Infect. *134*:744-751, 2006.

99. Mercado, R., Vijh, S., Allen, S. E., et al.: Early programming of T cell populations responding to bacterial infection. J. Immunol. *165*:6833-6839, 2000.

100. Meyer, R. D., and Liu, S.: Determination of the effect of antimicrobics in combination against *Listeria monocytogenes*. Diagn. Microbiol. Infect. Dis. *6*:199-206, 1986.

101. Michelet, C., Leib, S. L., Bentue-Ferrer, D., and Tauber, M. G.: Comparative efficacies of antibiotics in a rat model of meningoencephalitis due to *Listeria monocytogenes*. Antimicrob. Agents Chemother. *43*:1651-1656, 1999.

102. Miguel-Yanes, J. M., Gonzalez-Ramallo, V. J., and Pastor, L.: Outcome of *Listeria monocytogenes* prosthetic valve endocarditis: As bad as it looks? Scand. J. Infect. Dis. *36*:709-711, 2004.

103. Mohan, I. C., Gordon, R. C., Beaman, T. C., et al.: Synergism of penicillin and gentamicin against *Listeria monocytogenes* in ex vivo hemodialysis culture. J. Infect. Dis. *135*:51-54, 1977.

104. Moore, R. M., and Zehmer, R. B.: Listeriosis in the United States, 1971. J. Infect. Dis. *127*:610-611, 1973.

105. Murray, M. G. D., Webb, R. A., and Swann, M. B. R.: A disease of rabbits characterized by large mononuclear leucocytosis, caused by a hitherto undescribed bacillus *Bacterium monocytogenes* (in. sp.). J. Pathol. Bacteriol. *29*:407-439, 1926.

106. Nadarajah, K., and Pritchard, C.: *Listeria monocytogenes* septic arthritis in a patient treated with etanercept for rheumatoid arthritis. J. Clin. Rheumatol. *11*:120-122, 2005.

107. Nadon, C. A., Woodward, D. L., Young, C., et al.: Correlations between molecular subtyping and serotyping of *Listeria monocytogenes*. J. Clin. Microbiol. *39*:2704-2707, 2001.

108. Nakane, A., Okamoto, M., Asano, M., et al.: An anti-CD3 monoclonal antibody protects mice against a lethal infection with *Listeria monocytogenes* through induction of endogenous cytokines. Infect. Immun. *61*:2786-2793, 1993.

109. Neighbors, M., Xu, X., and Barrat, F. J.: A critical role for interleukin 18 in primary and memory effector responses to *Listeria monocytogenes* that extends beyond its effects on interferon gamma production. J. Exp. Med. *194*:343-354, 2001.

110. Nieman, R. E., and Lorber, B.: Listeriosis in adults: A changing pattern: Report of eight cases and review of the literature, 1968-1978. Rev. Infect. Dis. *2*:207-227, 1980.

111. Nyfeldt, A.: Etiologie do la mononucleose infectieuse. Compt. Rend. Soc. Biol. *101*:590-591, 1929.

112. Ooi, S. T., and Lorber, B.: Gastroenteritis due to *Listeria monocytogenes*. Clin. Infect. Dis. *40*:1327-1332, 2005.

113. Paterson, J. S.: The antigenic structure of organisms of the genus *Listerella*. J. Pathol. Bacteriol. *51*:427-436, 1940.

114. Pinner, R. W., Schuchat, A., Swaminathan, B., et al.: Role of foods in sporadic listeriosis, II: Microbiologic and epidemiologic investigation. J. A. M. A. *267*:2046-2050, 1992.

115. Portnoy, D. A., Chakraborty, T., Goebel, W., et al.: Molecular determinants of *Listeria monocytogenes* pathogenesis. Infect. Immun. *60*:1263-1267, 1992.

116. Portnoy, D. A., Jacks, P. S., and Hinrichs, D. J.: Role of hemolysin for the intracellular growth of *Listeria monocytogenes*. J. Exp. Med. *167*:1459-1471, 1988.

117. Rakhmilevich, A. L.: Evidence for a significant role of CD⁴ T cells in adoptive immunity to *Listeria monocytogenes* in the liver. Immunology *82*:249-254, 1994.

118. Ramaswamy, V., Cresence, V. M., Rejitha, J. S., et al.: *Listeria*—review of epidemiology and pathogenesis. J. Microbiol. Immunol. Infect. *40*:4-13, 2007.

119. Renoult, T., Chabot, F., Aymard, B., et al.: Treatment of *Listeria* bacteremia with vancomycin. Rev. Infect. Dis. *13*:181-184, 1991.

120. Riedo, F. X., Pinner, R. W., de Lourdes Tosca, M., et al.: A point-source foodborne listeriosis outbreak: Documented incubation period and possible mild illness. J. Infect. Dis. *170*:693-696, 1994.

121. Rolston, K. V. I., and Bodey, G. P.: Activity of new antimicrobial agents against *Listeria monocytogenes*. Eur. J. Clin. Microbiol. *6*:686-688, 1987.

122. Saunders, B. D., Wiedmann, M., and Desjardins, M.: Recurrent *Listeria monocytogenes* infection: Relapse or reinfection with a unique strain confirmed by molecular subtyping. Clin. Infect. Dis. *33*:257-259, 2001.

123. Scheld, W. M.: Evaluation of rifampin and other antibiotics against *Listeria monocytogenes* in vitro and in vivo. Rev. Infect. Dis. *5*(Suppl. 3):593-599, 1983.

124. Schlech, W. F.: Foodborne listeriosis. Clin. Infect. Dis. *31*:770-775, 2000.

125. Schlech, W. F., Lavigne, P. M., Bortolussi, R. A., et al.: Epidemic listeriosis: Evidence for transmission by food. N. Engl. J. Med. *308*:203-206, 1983.

126. Schuchat, A.: Gastrointestinal carriage of *Listeria monocytogenes* in household contacts of patients with listeriosis. J. Infect. Dis. *167*:1261-1262, 1993.

127. Schuchat, A., Lizano, C., Broome, C. V., et al.: Outbreak of neonatal listeriosis associated with mineral oil. Pediatr. Infect. Dis. J. *10*:183-189, 1991.

128. Schuchat, A., Swaminathan, B., and Broome, C. V.: Epidemiology of human listeriosis. Clin. Microbiol. Rev. *4*:169-183, 1991.

129. Schwartz, B., Broome, C. V., Brown, G. R., et al.: Association of sporadic listeriosis with consumption of uncooked hot dogs and undercooked chicken. Lancet *2*:779-782, 1986.

130. Seeliger, H. P. R.: Listeriosis. New York, S. Karger, 1961.

131. Seeliger, H. P. R., and Finger, H.: Analytical serology of *Listeria*. In Kwapinski, J. B. G. (ed.): Analytical Serology of Microorganisms. New York, John Wiley & Sons, 1969, pp. 549-608.

132. Serushago, B., MacDonald, C., Lee, S. H. S., et al.: Interferon-α detection in cultures of newborn cells exposed to *Listeria monocytogenes*. J. Interferon Cytokine Res. *15*:633-635, 1995.

133. Skogberg, I. L., Syrjänen, J., Jahkola, M., et al.: Clinical presentation and outcome of listeriosis in patients with and without immunosuppressive therapy. Clin. Infect. Dis. *14*:815-821, 1992.

134. Spitzer, P. G., and Hammer, S. M.: Treatment of *Listeria monocytogenes* infection with trimethoprim-sulfamethoxazole: Case report and review of the literature. Rev. Infect. Dis. *8*:427, 1986.

135. Stamm, A. M., Dismukes, W. E., Simmons, B. P., et al.: Listeriosis in renal transplant recipients: Report of an outbreak and review of 102 cases. Rev. Infect. Dis. *4*:665-682, 1982.

136. Steinman, C. R.: Specific detection and semiquantitation of microorganisms in tissue by nucleic acid hybridization, I: Characterization of the method and application to model systems. J. Lab. Clin. Med. *86*:164-174, 1975.

137. Sword, C. P.: Mechanisms of pathogenesis in *Listeria monocytogenes* infection, I: The influence of iron. J. Bacteriol. *92*:536-542, 1966.

138. Tappero, J. W., Schuchat, A., Deaver, K. A., et al.: Reduction in the incidence of human listeriosis in the United States: Effectiveness of prevention efforts? J. A. M. A. *273*:1118-1122, 1995.

139. Teberg, A. J., Yonekura, M. L., Salminen, C., et al.: Clinical manifestations of epidemic neonatal listeriosis. Pediatr. Infect. Dis. J. *6*:817-820, 1987.

140. Topalovski, M., Yang, S. S., and Boonpassat, Y.: Listeriosis of the placenta: Clinicopathologic study of seven cases. Am. J. Obstet. Gynecol. *169*:616-620, 1993.

141. Traub, W. H.: Perinatal listeriosis. Chemotherapy *27*:423-431, 1981.

142. Tsai, Y. H., Hirth, R. S., and Leitner, F.: A murine model for listerial meningitis and meningoencephalomyelitis: Therapeutic evaluation or drugs in mice. Chemotherapy *26*:196-206, 1980.

143. Update—listeriosis and pasteurized milk. M. M. W. R. Morb. Mortal. Wkly. Rep. *37*:764-765, 1988.

144. van Furth, R., van Zwet, T. L., Buisman, A. M., et al.: Anti-tumor necrosis factor antibodies inhibit the influx of granulocytes and monocytes into an inflammatory exudate and enhance the growth of *Listeria monocytogenes* in various organs. Clin. Infect. Dis. *170*:234-237, 1994.

145. Vanllant, V., de Valk, H., Vaillant, V., et al.: Foodborne infections in France. Foodborne Pathog. Dis. *2*:221-232, 2005.

146. Varma, J. K., Samuel, M. C., Marcus, R., et al.: *Listeria monocytogenes* infection from foods prepared in a commercial establishment: A case-control study of potential sources of sporadic illness in the United States. Clin. Infect. Dis. *44*:529-530, 2007.

147. Vischer, W. A., and Rominger, C.: Rifampicin against experimental listeriosis in the mouse. Chemotherapy *24*:104-111, 1978.

148. Visintine, A. M., Oleske, J. M., and Nahmias, A. J.: *Listeria monocytogenes* infection in infants and children. Am. J. Dis. Child. *131*:393-397, 1977.

149. Wagner, R. D., Maroushek, H. M., Brown, J. F., et al.: Treatment with anti-interleukin-10 monoclonal antibody enhances early resistance to but impairs complete clearance of *Listeria monocytogenes* infection in mice. Infect. Immun. *62*:2345-2353, 1994.

150. Walsh, D., Duffy, G., Seridan, J. J., et al.: Antibiotic resistance among *Listeria monocytogenes*, in retail foods. J. Appl. Microbiol. *90*:517-522, 2001.

151. Wilder, M. S., and Sword, C. P.: Mechanisms of pathogenesis in *Listeria monocytogenes* infection, II: Characterization of listeriosis in the CD-1 mouse and survey of biochemical lesions. J. Bacteriol. *93*:531-542, 1967.

152. Yan, S. R., Qing, G., Byers, D. M., et al.: Role of MyD88 in diminished tumor necrosis factor alpha production by newborn mononuclear cells in response to lipopolysaccharide. Infect. Immun. *72*:1223-1229, 2004.

153. Zhan, Y., and Cheers, C.: Differential induction of macrophage-derived cytokines by live and dead intracellular bacteria in vitro. Infect. Immun. *63*:720-723, 1995.

CHAPTER

107   TUBERCULOSIS

Jeffrey R. Starke

Tuberculosis still ranks as one of the three most important infectious diseases in the world in terms of morbidity and mortality. Recognizable in skeletons from the Stone Age and in mummified corpses from the Egyptian Old Kingdom, tuberculosis became more widespread in western Europe after the plague years of the Middle Ages and the epidemic during the era of urbanization and industrialization in the 18th and 19th centuries.[153] At that time, scrofula affected more than half the young inhabitants of workhouses and orphanages.

As similar social trends developed outside Europe, tuberculosis followed. In the eastern cities of the United States (Boston, New York, and Philadelphia), the mortality rate from tuberculosis was about 400 per 100,000 population. With improving socioeconomic conditions, the mortality rate fell to 200 per 100,000 around 1900 and to 26 per 100,000 by 1950. Stress in all its forms—famine, war, rationing, long working hours, child labor, population displacement, crowded living and working conditions—favors the spread of tuberculosis in human beings, whereas years of peace and plenty favor its rapid decline.[152,463] The decrease in the Western world in the incidence of tuberculosis was accentuated by the discovery, development, and widespread use of antituberculosis drugs beginning in the late 1940s.

Another important factor leading to the decline of tuberculosis in Western countries was the recognition in the 1920s of the importance of bovine tuberculosis and its successful eradication as a public health problem in the United States by gradual slaughter of infected cattle and almost universal pasteurization of milk.

Tuberculosis was recognized as a clinical entity in the early 19th century by Schönlein, who first used the term *tuberculosis* in

1830, and by Laennec in Paris, among others. Credit for extensively detailed descriptions of the primary focus goes to Anton Ghon (1866-1936), professor of pathology in Prague. In 1882, Koch identified *Mycobacterium tuberculosis*. The special diagnostic tools essential to understanding the disease in children were provided by Escherich, who in 1898 set up the first diagnostic radiography for children; by von Pirquet, Mantoux, Mandel, and Moro, who developed tuberculin testing between 1907 and 1910; and by Meunier and DeLille, who in 1898 taught the usefulness of gastric lavage in children. Revealing, long-term studies on the natural history of tuberculosis in children and on chemotherapy and prevention came principally from Scandinavia (Wallgren, Ustvedt, Holm, Hyge) and the United States (Brailey, Hardy, Lincoln, Hsu, Ferrebee).

TERMINOLOGY: EXPOSURE, INFECTION, DISEASE[12]

The pathophysiologic process of tuberculosis is complicated, and the delay between acquisition of infection and manifestation of disease renders certain pathophysiologic events less distinct. This chapter considers three major stages of tuberculosis: exposure, infection, and disease.[561]

Exposure means that the child has had significant contact with an adult or adolescent with infectious pulmonary tuberculosis. The contact investigation—examination of individuals close to a person suspected of having tuberculosis by performing a tuberculin skin test, chest radiograph, and physical examination—is the most important activity in a community to prevent cases of tuberculosis in children.[10,50,234] The most frequent setting for exposure of a child is the household, but it can occur in a school, daycare center, or other closed setting.[136,227] In this stage, the tuberculin skin test result is negative, the chest radiograph is normal, and the child lacks signs or symptoms of disease. Some exposed children may have inhaled droplet nuclei infected with *M. tuberculosis* and have early infection, but the clinician cannot know it because delayed hypersensitivity to tuberculin—a positive skin test response—takes up to 3 months to develop. Children younger than 5 years old who are in the exposure stage should be treated to prevent the rapid development of disseminated or meningeal tuberculosis, which can occur before the skin test becomes reactive.[160,338,416,444,576]

Infection occurs when the individual inhales droplet nuclei containing *M. tuberculosis*, which becomes established intracellularly within the lung and associated lymphoid tissue. The hallmark of latent tuberculosis infection is a reactive tuberculin skin test. In this stage, the child has no signs or symptoms and the chest radiograph is either normal or reveals only granuloma or calcifications in the lung parenchyma or regional lymph nodes or in both tissues. In developed countries, virtually all children with tuberculosis infection should receive treatment, usually with isoniazid, to prevent the development of disease in the near or distant future.

Disease occurs when signs or symptoms or radiographic manifestations caused by *M. tuberculosis* become apparent. The word *tuberculosis* refers to disease. Not all infected individuals have the same risk of contracting disease. An immunocompetent adult with untreated tuberculosis infection has approximately a 5 to 10 percent lifetime risk for development of disease; half the risk exists in the first 2 to 3 years after infection occurs. Adults with tuberculosis infection who then become infected with human immunodeficiency virus (HIV) have a 5 to 10 percent annual risk for development of tuberculosis disease.[508] Historical studies have shown that disease, often serious, life-threatening forms, will develop within 1 to 2 years in as many as 40 percent of immunocompetent infants with untreated tuberculosis infection.

EPIDEMIOLOGY

INCIDENCE AND PREVALENCE

Between 20 and 45 percent of the world's population (approximately 2 billion people) are infected with *M. tuberculosis*, and more than 90 percent of new cases occur in the developing world, where resources are very limited. According to the World Health Organization (WHO), in 1997, only 32 percent of the world's population lived in areas where effective tuberculosis control programs were fully operational.[412] The WHO estimates that 8 million new cases and 2 million deaths from tuberculosis occur annually worldwide.[464,644] Approximately 11 percent (884,000) of new cases and about 5 percent of deaths are predicted to occur in children younger than 15 years.[295,405] Approximately 75 percent of childhood cases occur in the 22 highest burden countries. The inability to control tuberculosis despite the availability of effective, relatively inexpensive therapy is one of the greatest medical failures of our time.[210,560]

Between 1953, when reporting began, and 1985, the number of annually reported tuberculosis cases in the United States fell by 74 percent from 84,304 to 22,201.[92,93] In 1985, the overall case rate was approximately 10 per 100,000 population. At that time, the incidence curve flattened out, and for the first time since 1953, case numbers and rates increased to a peak of 26,673 cases in 1992. Between 1985 and 1992 in the United States, the total tuberculosis case numbers rose 20 percent.[92] During that same time, the number of pediatric tuberculosis cases rose 40 percent[264,612] (Fig. 107–1). Most experts cite four probable causes

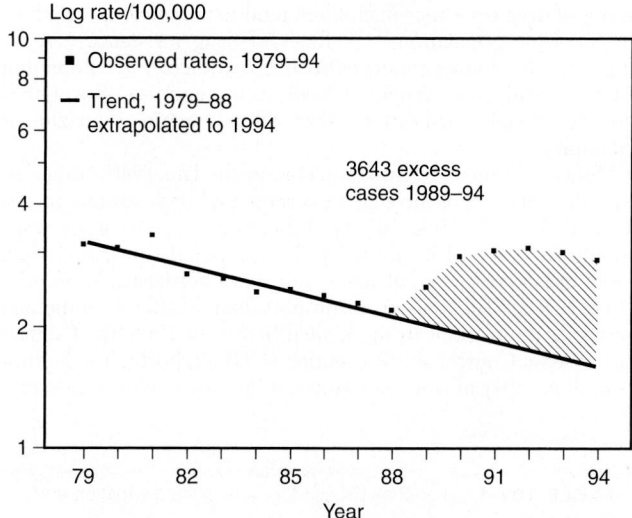

Figure 107–1 Observed and expected tuberculosis cases in children younger than 15 years old in the United States, 1979 to 1994.

for the increases: (1) the co-epidemic of HIV infection; (2) the increasing rates of tuberculosis in foreign-born individuals in the United States[71]; (3) the increased transmission among adults in congregate settings, including jails and prisons, nursing homes, homeless shelters, HIV treatment facilities, hospitals, and, rarely, schools;[35,38,52,376,442] and (4) a decline in the public health infrastructure in many areas of the country.[66,112,465,562] After several years of intense and expensive effort were expended, the number of tuberculosis cases in the United States declined again. In 2006, a total of 13,779 tuberculosis cases (4.6 cases per 100,000 population) were reported in the United States, a 21 percent decrease from 1999 and 48 percent decrease from 1992.[92] Rates have decreased consistently in the United States in all groups except immigrants from high-risk countries. However, the annual cost of tuberculosis in the United States still exceeds $1 billion.[65] An estimated 4 to 6 percent of the U.S. population, or approximately 11 million people, are infected with *M. tuberculosis*. This group represents a large reservoir from which cases of tuberculosis disease will emerge in the future if these individuals are not treated.[6] The resurgence of tuberculosis in the United States between 1985 and 1992 was associated with the emergence of multidrug-resistant tuberculosis (MDR-TB), strains that are resistant to at least isoniazid and rifampin and may be resistant to other antituberculosis medications as well.[654] MDR-TB is difficult and expensive to treat, and the mortality rates may be as high as 50 percent in complicated cases.[193,255] Since 1993, the incidence of resistance to isoniazid has remained stable, and the incidence of MDR-TB has decreased. In 2006, 8 percent of isolates were resistant to at least isoniazid, and 1 percent were resistant to at least isoniazid and rifampin (MDR-TB) in the United States.[92]

MDR-TB has become an important problem in many areas of the world.[159,654] Global surveys conducted between 1996 and 1998 in 58 geographic areas showed a median prevalence of MDR-TB of 1 percent, but the rates in some regions were alarming: 14 percent in Estonia, 10 percent in the Henan Province in China, and 9 percent in Latvia and parts of Russia.[171,654] There has been an emergence recently of extremely drug-resistant tuberculosis, isolates resistant to isoniazid, rifampin, fluoroquinolones, and at least one injectable drug.[514] In adults, drug resistance in *M. tuberculosis* often is secondary, the resistance emerging during therapy because treatment is inadequate or interrupted.[180] In children, drug resistance usually is primary in that the child is infected with a strain that already has become resistant.[413,494,496,591]

Rates of drug resistance in children tend to mirror those in adults in the same population.[567-569] Rates of drug resistance may be higher in developing countries because of difficulty in completing therapy, inadequate supply of medications, and use of over-the-counter cough medications that often contain isoniazid or rifampin.

Since treatment became available in the late 1940s, tuberculosis has been concentrated in certain high-risk groups in the United States[94] (Table 107–1). Tuberculosis occurs most commonly in areas with ethnically diverse populations, including large urban areas, coastal states, and states bordering Mexico[85,95] (Fig. 107–2). Tuberculosis disproportionately affects ethnic and minority populations in the United States. In 2006, the Centers for Disease Control and Prevention (CDC) reported the highest overall number of cases in Latinos, 4066 cases, but the case rate

TABLE 107–1 High-Risk Groups for Tuberculosis Infection and Disease

Groups at High Risk of Exposure or Infection
Close contacts of person with tuberculosis
Foreign-born persons from high-risk countries (Asia, Africa, Latin America, Russia, eastern Europe)
Residents and employees of high-risk congregate settings (correctional institutions, nursing homes, homeless shelters, hospitals serving high-risk populations, drug treatment centers)
Medically underserved, low-income populations
High-risk racial or ethnic minority populations
Injection drug users
Children exposed to adults in high-risk categories
Groups at Higher Risk for Disease Once Infected
Immunosuppressed patients, including HIV infected
Recent tuberculosis infection (within past 2 years)
Persons with certain medical conditions (diabetes mellitus, silicosis, cancer, end-stage renal disease, gastrectomy, body weight ≤90% of ideal)
Injection drug users
History of inadequately treated tuberculosis
Children ≤4 years, especially infants

was highest among Asians, with 25.6 cases per 100,000 population.[92,414]

During the 1990s, immigration from a high-prevalence country was the single largest risk factor for tuberculosis, with rates among foreign-born persons being four to six times higher than those for U.S.-born persons.[108] In 2006, the CDC reported that 50 percent of all cases occurred in foreign-born individuals.[92] Tuberculosis is endemic in most developing countries, and between 30 and 50 percent of recent immigrants to the United States have latent tuberculosis infection on entry into the country.[108,588] During the immigration process, adults are screened for tuberculosis disease with a chest radiograph, but skin testing to detect tuberculosis infection is not required. Children younger than 15 years receive neither a chest radiograph nor a tuberculin skin test.[506] Among children in the United States, being born in a country with a high rate of tuberculosis is the most important risk factor for having tuberculosis infection. Foreign-born adopted children also are at risk for having tuberculosis infection and disease.[179,309,482] People who enter the United States illegally may be unable or afraid to seek medical treatment, even when they are ill. Studies have shown that in most immigrants in whom tuberculosis develops, it does so within 5 years of immigration, thus indicating that many cases could be prevented if appropriate screening and treatment programs were conducted.

Other important risk factors for tuberculosis in adults include lower socioeconomic status, migrant work,[87] HIV infection, drug use, homelessness, travel to high-prevalence countries, history of incarceration, and occupations with exposure to high-risk populations (see Table 107–1). Children from high-risk population groups or children who have contact with adults in these groups may be at increased risk for development of tuberculosis infection.[359] Age has an important influence on tuberculosis case rates.[404] During 2006, 6 percent of cases in the United States occurred in children younger than 15 years, 11 percent in persons 15 to 24 years old, 34 percent in persons 25 to 44 years old, 29 percent in persons 45 to 64 years old, and 19 percent in persons older than 64 years.[92] The highest case rates among children are in those younger than 5 years. Children aged 5 to 14 years, the so-called favored age, have a consistently lower case rate than that of any other segment of the population.[353,404] In early childhood, the incidence is not significantly different in girls and boys, although adolescent girls generally experience higher rates of disease than adolescent boys do.[59]

The age at which tuberculosis disease initially develops currently varies among ethnic groups in the United States.[92] White persons develop tuberculosis more commonly as older adults, whereas African Americans and Hispanics have a higher incidence of disease as young adults or children (Fig. 107–3).[577] Many of the risk factors for development of tuberculosis, such as HIV

TB CASE RATES,* UNITED STATES, 2006

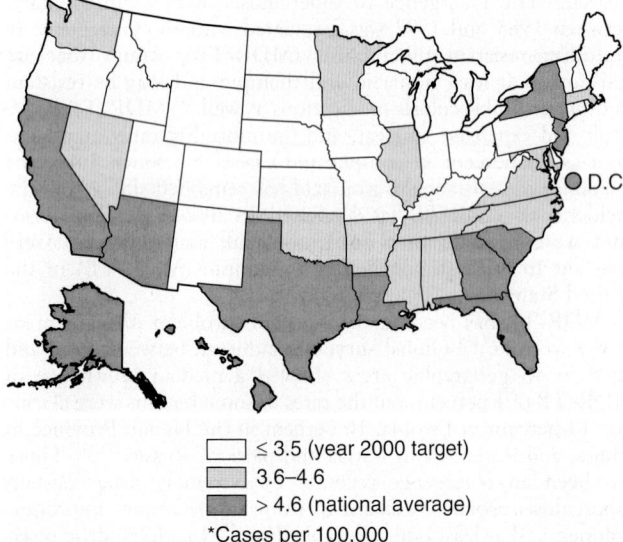

☐ ≤ 3.5 (year 2000 target)
▨ 3.6–4.6
■ > 4.6 (national average)
*Cases per 100,000

Figure 107–2 Tuberculosis case rates (cases per 100,000) by state, 2006. (*From Centers for Disease Control and Prevention: Reported Tuberculosis in the United States, 2006. Atlanta, GA, U.S. Department of Health and Human Services, CDC, October 2007.*)

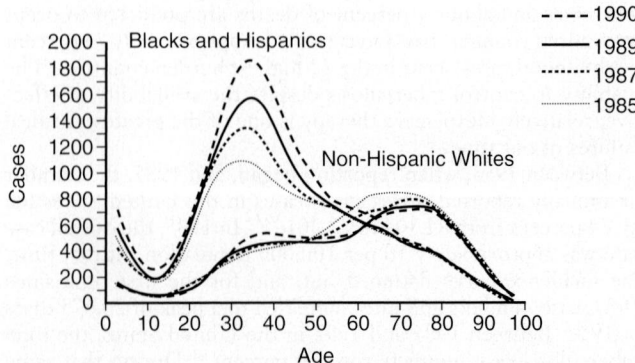

Figure 107–3 Tuberculosis cases in Hispanics and blacks versus non-Hispanic whites in the United States, 1985 to 1990.

infection, drug use, history of incarceration, and recent immigration, occur more commonly in young adults in their 20s, 30s, and 40s, a time when contact with children is more likely. Other factors, including recent immigration, socioeconomic status, high-risk behavior, and possibly genetic susceptibility, may influence the peak age distribution of tuberculosis among different groups.[349] Inherited susceptibility to tuberculosis may contribute to differences among various ethnic groups.[349] Laboratory animals and humans have been shown to differ in genetic susceptibility to tuberculosis.[343,511] In the United States, highly urbanized immigrants, such as Jews from European ghettos, fared much better than did their rural Irish and African counterparts, presumably because generations of exposure to tuberculosis in previous European epidemics had selected in favor of more resistant individuals.[454] As the disease spread to other continents, previously unexposed populations may have been more susceptible to tuberculosis and experienced higher rates of disease.

In some U.S. locales that have had recent increases in tuberculosis, the demographic groups with the greatest tuberculosis morbidity also have large numbers of HIV-infected persons.[104,226,401] The HIV epidemic has had a profound effect on the epidemiology of tuberculosis in children by two mechanisms[490]: (1) most important, in the United States, HIV-infected adults with tuberculosis may transmit *M. tuberculosis* to children in their environment, and tuberculosis disease will develop in some of them; and (2) important in many developing countries, children with HIV infection are at increased risk of progressing from asymptomatic tuberculosis infection to disease.[244,342] Several studies have demonstrated increased rates of childhood tuberculosis associated with increased rates of disease among HIV-infected adults in the community.[209,270] Tuberculosis probably is underdiagnosed in HIV-infected children, especially in the developing world, because of the similarity of its clinical manifestations with other opportunistic pulmonary diseases and the difficulty of confirming the diagnosis with the skin test or culture. All children with suspected tuberculosis disease should have HIV serotesting because the two infections are linked epidemiologically and many experts prolong treatment in HIV-infected children with tuberculosis.[204,640]

The site of manifestation of tuberculosis disease differs between adults and children. Although pulmonary disease is most common for all ages, extrapulmonary tuberculosis occurs more often in children.[404] Because HIV co-infection increases the risk for development of extrapulmonary disease, rates have increased in adults during the past 15 years. In general, 25 percent of pediatric cases are extrapulmonary, with 75 percent being pulmonary. In 1985, before widespread HIV infection occurred, 85 percent of adults had pulmonary disease and 15 percent had extrapulmonary disease. With the spread of HIV infection, these numbers have shifted, and in 2006, the CDC reported that 79 percent of all new cases, including those in adults and children, were pulmonary and 21 percent were extrapulmonary.[92] Comparison of the site of extrapulmonary disease in children and adults in 1985, before the acquired immunodeficiency syndrome (AIDS) epidemic, shows some important differences. First, approximately 70 percent of extrapulmonary tuberculosis in children involved the lymph nodes, as opposed to 25 percent in adults (Fig. 107–4). Second, tuberculous meningitis accounted for 13 percent of extrapulmonary disease in children versus 4 percent in adults. Genitourinary involvement occurred in 16 percent of adults, but it was a rare finding in children. Although the proportion of extrapulmonary cases in adults has increased as a result of the HIV-AIDS epidemic, extrapulmonary disease still occurs more commonly in children.

The global epidemiology of childhood tuberculosis is not well described.[405] In developing countries where the burden of disease is greatest, the only available diagnostic test often is an acid-fast smear of sputum, the result of which rarely is positive from

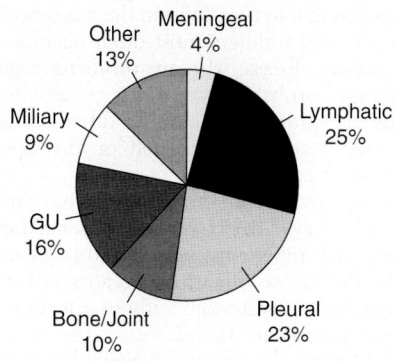

Extrapulmonary cases in adults

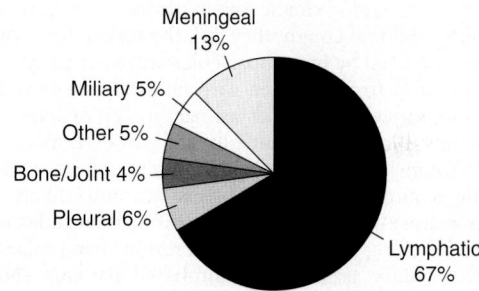

Extrapulmonary cases in children
<15 years of age

Figure 107–4 Extrapulmonary disease by site in adults and children in the United States. *(From the Centers for Disease Control and Prevention.)*

infants and children with pulmonary tuberculosis. In many developing countries, more than 50 percent of the population is younger than 18 years, so the true burden of childhood tuberculosis has been underestimated.

TRANSMISSION

Transmission of tuberculosis is from one human to another, usually through infected droplets of mucus that become airborne when an individual coughs, sneezes, or laughs.[103] The droplets dry and become droplet nuclei, which may remain suspended in air for hours. Only particles less than 10 μm in diameter are small enough to reach the alveoli.[476] Transmission sometimes occurs by direct contact with infected discharges (sputum, saliva, urine, or drainage from an open sinus or abscess); it occasionally occurs by means of heavily contaminated fomites, such as shoes, gastric lavage tubes, bronchoscopes, or syringes prepared by someone with positive sputum.[223] Rare cases of tuberculosis transmitted by a lung or kidney transplant have been reported.[381,400,473] Dogs may be a source of infection for children because dogs are susceptible to the human type of tubercle bacillus.[470]

The collective experience of many clinicians is that children usually are infected by an adult or adolescent in the immediate household, most often a parent, grandparent, older sibling, boarder, or household employee.[37] Casual extrafamilial contact is the source of infection much less often, but physicians, babysitters, schoolteachers, music teachers, school bus drivers, parishioners, nurses, gardeners, and candy store keepers have been implicated in individual cases and in hundreds of miniepidemics.[23,57,155,320,326,635] Attention has been drawn to the prevalence of active tuberculosis among residents of nursing homes for the elderly. Children visiting their grandparents have contracted tuberculosis in this setting. Within the household of an infectious adult, infants and toddlers most often become infected. Adults with pulmonary disease who are receiving regular, appropriate chemotherapy probably rarely infect children; much more dangerous are those with chronic tuberculous disease that is unrecognized, inadequately treated, or in relapse because of the development of resistance.

Wallgren[631] was the first to point out that children with tuberculosis rarely if ever infect other children. Many children with the disease have tuberculin-negative siblings and parents. Children with tuberculosis often have been cared for by their families or in hospitals and institutions without infecting their contacts.[399] When transmission of *M. tuberculosis* has been documented in children's hospitals, it almost invariably has come from an adult with undiagnosed pulmonary tuberculosis.[24,187,277,278,391,636] Adults accompanying a child with suspected tuberculosis disease should be screened as soon as possible for pulmonary tuberculosis.[61,82,107,279,280,559] In tuberculous children, tubercle bacilli in endobronchial secretions are relatively sparse, and cough is not characteristic of endothoracic tuberculosis or miliary disease. When young children cough, they lack the tussive force of adults. Specimens collected by bronchoalveolar lavage or early-morning gastric aspiration from children with clinically suspected tuberculosis seldom if ever have acid-fast bacilli seen on smears. Only approximately 40 percent eventually will grow *M. tuberculosis* by culture.[546] Young infants with congenital tuberculosis or advanced, postnatally acquired pulmonary disease are more likely to have smear- or culture-positive specimens (80%) than older children are.[493,613] Therefore, specimens and secretions from infants, children with cavitary lesions, and intubated patients should be handled as potentially infectious.[82,366] Most preadolescent children with tuberculosis, however, are not contagious and do not require isolation. Tuberculosis in adolescents may be more typical of adult-type reactivation disease, including the presence of cavitary lesions with smear- and culture-positive sputum. Children or adolescents who have symptomatic pulmonary tuberculosis with features of adult-type tuberculosis should be treated as potentially contagious until mycobacterial smears and cultures are negative.[74,120,175]

Children, nonetheless, play an extremely important role in the transmission of tuberculosis, not so much because they are likely to contaminate their immediate environment but rather because they may harbor a partially healed infection that lies dormant, only to be reactivated as infectious pulmonary tuberculosis many years later under the social, emotional, and physiologic stresses arising during adolescence, pregnancy, or old age. Thus, children infected with *M. tuberculosis* constitute a long-lasting reservoir of tuberculosis in the population.

The risk of infection developing in child contacts of adults receiving antituberculosis chemotherapy often is a matter of practical concern. Several studies reveal that most contacts are infected by the index case before the diagnosis is made and treatment is initiated. Although it is not possible to carry out a definitive clinical study, evidence indicates that patients receiving effective chemotherapy rarely transmit *M. tuberculosis*. Nonetheless, it seems prudent to avoid exposure of children to adults with positive sputum smears or positive cultures and to assume that adults positive by smear or culture remain infectious for at least several weeks after the start of therapy.

MYCOBACTERIOLOGY

The genus *Mycobacterium*, closely related by its cell wall antigens to the genera *Corynebacterium* and *Nocardia*, presently is classified in the order Actinomycetales and the family Mycobacteriaceae. Mycobacteria are nonmotile, non-spore-forming, pleomorphic, weakly gram-positive rods measuring 1 to 5 μm long, typically slender and slightly "bent." Some appear beaded, and some are clumped. In general, species pathogenic for humans are more acid fast, have more exacting nutritional requirements, grow more slowly, form less pigment, and are more sensitive to chemotherapeutic agents than are the saprophytic species.

The cell wall constituents of mycobacteria determine their most striking biologic properties. The cell walls contain 20 to 60 percent lipids by dry weight, largely bound to proteins and carbohydrates. These organisms are more resistant than are most others to light, alkali, acid, and the bactericidal action of antibodies. Their growth is slow, with a generation time of 14 to 24 hours, perhaps because of the slow metabolic exchange through the waxy "capsule." Their hydrophobic properties render them difficult to study.

Acid-fastness, that is, the capacity to form stable mycolate complexes with certain aryl methane dyes (specifically, carbolfuchsin, crystal violet, auramine, and rhodamine, which then are not removed readily even by rinsing with 95 percent ethanol plus hydrochloric acid), is the hallmark of mycobacteria. The cells appear red when stained with fuchsin (as with the Ziehl-Neelsen or Kinyoun stains), appear purple with crystal violet, or exhibit yellow-green fluorescence under ultraviolet light (when stained with auramine and rhodamine, as in Truant stain). Truant stain, in experienced hands, is considered the best stain for specimens expected to contain small numbers of organisms.

Identification of mycobacteria depends on their staining properties and on their biochemical and metabolic characteristics. Mycobacteria are obligate aerobes. On the whole, their growth requirements are simple. *M. tuberculosis* can grow in "classic" media, whose essential ingredients are egg yolk and glycerin (Löwenstein-Jensen, Petragnani, Dorset); often, a dye such as malachite green to inhibit contaminants; and, sometimes, potatoes, charcoal, and so on, which probably neutralize growth inhibitors. They also can grow in simple synthetic media, frequently with an admixture of asparagine, glutamate, or amino acid mixtures (Middlebrook 7H9, Tween-albumin). Once grown, they can be replated on media also containing antituberculosis drugs to determine drug susceptibility patterns. Isolation on solid media often takes 3 to 6 weeks, followed by another 2 to 4 weeks for drug susceptibility results. Improvements in laboratory methods have permitted more rapid culture, identification, and drug susceptibility testing of mycobacteria, such as by an automatic radiometric method known as the BACTEC (Becton-Dickinson, Towson, MD) method, in which a decontaminated, concentrated specimen is inoculated into a bottle of medium containing carbon 14–labeled palmitic acid as the substrate.[524] As mycobacteria metabolize the carbon 14–labeled palmitic acid, carbon dioxide 14 accumulates in the head space of the bottle, where radioactivity can be measured. Unfortunately, cross-contamination of bottles has been reported and has resulted in false-positive culture results.[154] The addition of appropriate dilutions of antituberculosis drugs permits an evaluation of drug susceptibility to be made. The time for identification and drug susceptibility testing can be reduced to 1 to 3 weeks, depending on the size of the inoculum.

Bacteriophage typing to determine the relatedness of isolates has advanced slowly. Progress is being made, however, in standardization of techniques, and phage typing already is of use in strain identification for epidemiologic purposes. However, a newer technique, restriction fragment length polymorphism analysis of mycobacterial DNA, has become a powerful tool for determining strain relatedness in both outbreaks and routine epidemiology of tuberculosis in a community.[8,529]

RESISTANCE AND IMMUNITY

Natural resistance to tuberculosis infection varies greatly among animal species; humans, guinea pigs, and rabbits are highly susceptible. However, Lurie[343] experimentally bred resistant rabbits and showed that although the virulent tubercle bacilli disseminated just as well in the resistant rabbits, multiplication within tissues was inhibited. Thus, the differences between resistant and susceptible rabbits appeared to lie in the ability of the resistant rabbits to produce an effective immune response, and this ability seemed to be controlled genetically.

Additional evidence that genetic factors influence susceptibility comes from data involving twins. Kallmann and Reisner[273] noted that when one homozygous twin suffered from tuberculosis, the other twin had a higher chance of being affected than was the case with heterozygous twins. Gender affects resistance, and females appear to be especially susceptible during adolescence. The negative nitrogen and calcium balance that can arise during adolescence may account in part for susceptibility at this age.[268]

Likewise, young age appears to predispose one to tuberculosis.[404,492,613] However, one cannot be sure that the apparent susceptibility is not due to a larger dose of bacteria because of more intimate contact between very young children and their infectors. Although diabetes mellitus affects the resistance of adults, whether it affects that of children is not clear. Many viral infections depress tuberculin reactivity, but only measles and perhaps influenza have been incriminated in lowering resistance to tuberculosis.[39,64,215,564,657] Unfortunately, natural resistance is ill-defined and poorly understood.

Cell-mediated immunity is regarded as most important in host defense against *M. tuberculosis*.[126,323,418] The T cell–mediated immune response involves a variety of cell subsets that are involved in numerous functions, including protection, delayed hypersensitivity, cytolysis, and establishment of memory immunity.[428] The functions also involve an array of cytokines, several of which direct cells of the monocyte-macrophage axis to contain and destroy the invading bacilli.[14,582] The exact role of individual cytokines is not yet clear, but an emerging concept is that much of the clinical response to the presence of *M. tuberculosis* is determined by the balance of the cellular-cytokine response, which to some degree is under genetic influence.[428] In general, T-helper 1 (T_H1) responses are more beneficial to the host than are T_H2 responses, but unfortunately, infants and young children have increased propensity to develop T_H2 responses to mycobacterial immunogens.[323] More details about the immune response to *M. tuberculosis* are emerging as new immunotherapies are developed. During the past decade, several monoclonal antibodies directed against tumor necrosis factor–α have been used to manage inflammatory bowel disease and rheumatologic disorders. Unfortunately, use of these agents, particularly infliximab, has been associated with a high incidence of serious tuberculosis in patients who had existing tuberculosis infection or who acquire it during treatment.[60,275,458] All immunocompromised patients, including those who will undergo any form of immunotherapy, should be evaluated carefully for tuberculosis infection or disease.

PATHOGENESIS

PORTAL OF ENTRY

The tubercle bacillus usually is inhaled. The observations of Riley[476] suggest that a single tubercle bacillus can initiate infection. Ghon, Kuedlich, and their associates (Table 107–2) reported that the primary focus found in 2114 autopsies on children was the lung in 95.93 percent of cases. Especially significant is that their study was done at a time when bovine tuberculosis, which

TABLE 107–2 Portal of Entry of Tubercle Bacilli

Respiratory (%)		Nonrespiratory (%)	
Lung	95.93*	Bowel	1.14
Tonsils	0.09	Skin	0.14
Nose	0.09	Eye	0.05
Middle ear	0.09	Parotid	0.05
Total†	**96.20**	**Total**	**1.38**

Of 2114 autopsies on children.
†*Undetermined, 2.4%.*
Data from Ghon, A., and Kuedlich, H.: Die Eintrittspforten der Infektion. In Engel, S., and Pirquet, C. (eds.): Handbuch der Kindertuberkulose. Stuttgart, Germany, Georg Thieme Verlag, 1930.

might have produced many primary gastrointestinal foci, was much more common than it is today. Ingestion probably accounts for a small percentage of primary pulmonary foci and for some gastrointestinal foci, particularly in infants who have consumed milk containing bovine tubercle bacilli. Contamination of a superficial skin or mucous membrane lesion, such as an abrasion of the sole of the foot or the elbow, insect bite, ritual circumcision, or infection of the vulva, may lead to infection. Infection by inoculation with a sputum-contaminated syringe has been reported in more recent years.[223] True congenital infection, although rare, may be a result of either lymphohematogenous spread in the mother during pregnancy or smoldering endometritis.[615]

INCUBATION PERIOD

The incubation period from the time that the tubercle bacillus enters the body until cutaneous sensitivity develops has been found to be 3 weeks to 3 months.[355] With both bacille Calmette-Guérin (BCG) and experimental infections, the incubation period is shorter when the inoculum is large, and clinical experience suggests that the same is true in humans. Debré, for example, noted long ago that tuberculosis acquired by an infant from its mother was likely to be much more severe than was an infection acquired from a visitor to the home. Animal experiments support this concept. The end of the incubation period coincides with the onset of tuberculin hypersensitivity and may be accompanied by a period lasting 1 to 3 weeks that Wallgren called fever of onset or fever of invasion. At this time, the tissue reaction intensifies throughout the primary complex and may permit the complex to be visible on x-ray films.

THE "TIMETABLE" OF TUBERCULOSIS

Wallgren's tremendous experience with tuberculous children in institutions permitted him to recognize and to describe the usual early course and timing of the initial infection and each of its best-known complications.[634] His timetable concept is an extremely useful one for clinicians because it permits a realistic prognosis, an understanding of what complications to look for and when, and a more productive approach to finding the infectious source case (Fig. 107–5).[355]

Symptomatic, massive lymphohematogenous spread (i.e., miliary or acute meningeal tuberculosis) is seen in only 0.5 to 3 percent of infected children. When it does occur, the usual onset is 2 to 6 months after initial infection. Endobronchial tuberculosis, possibly with segmental pulmonary lesions, develops slightly later on average. The metastatic lesions of bones and joints, which can be expected in 5 percent of untreated infected children, usually do not appear until approximately 1 year after infection

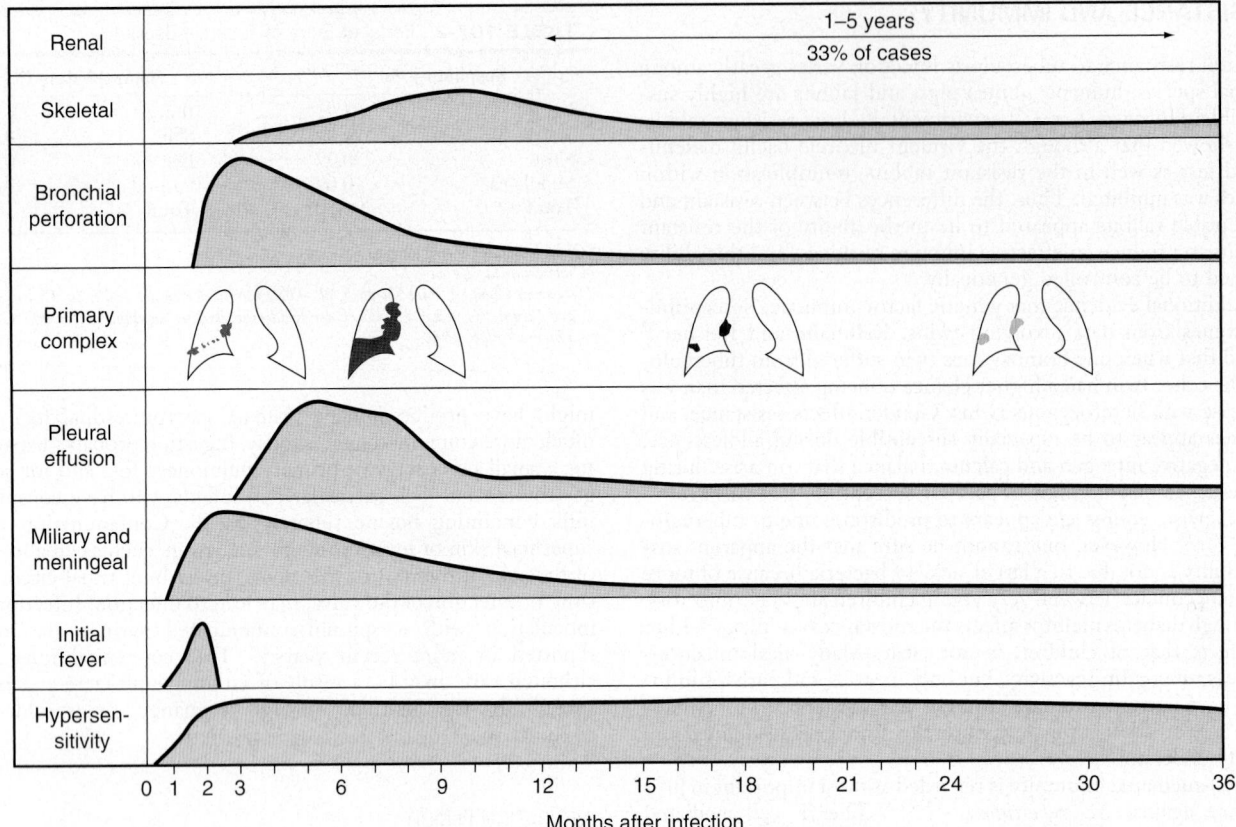

Figure 107-5 The timetable of tuberculosis.

TABLE 107-3   Median Age of Children* with Tuberculosis by Predominant Site of Involvement, United States, 1988

Site	No. of Cases (%)	Median Age (yr)
Pulmonary	1213 (77.5)	6
Lymphatic	209 (13.3)	5
Pleural	49 (3.1)	16
Meningeal	29 (1.9)	2
Bone or joint	19 (1.2)	8
Other	15 (1.0)	12
Miliary	14 (0.9)	1
Genitourinary	13 (0.8)	16
Peritoneal	4 (0.3)	13
Not stated	1 (0.1)	—
Total	1566 (100.0)	6

Younger than 20 years.

occurs, at the earliest. Renal lesions come later still, 5 to 25 years after initial infection. The relationship between the anatomic site of tuberculosis and the median age at onset in children is shown in Table 107-3. The interval between the acquisition of initial infection and the appearance of chronic pulmonary tuberculosis is extremely variable but can be months to decades, depending mainly on the age of the child at the time of infection. The interval is likely to be short in adolescents but much longer in infants.

In summary, the first 5 years after initial acquisition of tuberculosis infection in childhood, especially the first year, is when complications usually occur. Later in life, during times of stress, a previously silent or arrested lesion may reactivate and become dangerous to the patient as well as highly infectious to others.

CLINICAL FORMS OF TUBERCULOSIS IN CHILDREN

ENDOTHORACIC

Asymptomatic Tuberculosis Infection

Asymptomatic (or latent) infection can be defined as infection associated with tuberculin hypersensitivity and a positive tuberculin test result but with no striking clinical or radiographic manifestations. Computed tomography may reveal enlarged lymph nodes in the chest, even though the plain radiograph is normal.[19,132] On occasion, low-grade fever is found at the onset, usually by chance. If the child has been in recent contact with a person who has contagious tuberculosis and the tuberculin test result is positive, disease should be ruled out immediately with a chest radiograph and a thorough physical examination. Asymptomatic tuberculosis infection occurs more frequently in children of elementary school age than in adolescents or infants. Some 40 to 50 percent of infections in infants younger than 1 year and 80 to 95 percent in older children can be expected to cause no specific recognizable symptom or radiographic findings.[441] Gastric washings in these patients, even when performed with great care, yield a very low percentage of positive results.

A clinician making a diagnosis of tuberculosis infection in a child must assume, however, that the patient might be in the earliest stage of infection and at risk for the development of symptomatic disease in the near future.[355] A careful history and investigation of contacts should be undertaken immediately for determination, if possible, of the date of exposure. Chemotherapy must be started, and the patient closely monitored not only to detect any toxic effect of chemotherapy and to monitor adherence with treatment but also to be sure that disease does not develop.

The Endothoracic Primary Complex and Its Complications

The primary complex, described by Ghon,[188] includes three elements: the primary focus, lymphangitis, and regional lymphadenitis. This complex holds true for every primary infection, regardless of the portal of entry. Ghon noted that at least 70 percent of primary pulmonary foci are subpleural. Thus, pleurisy is almost a regular feature of the primary complex.

Evolution of the primary pulmonary focus begins with an acute inflammatory reaction around tubercle bacilli inhaled into an alveolus, with the localized alveolar consolidation varying from the size of a pea to the size of a walnut. Macrophages appear within hours in the inflammatory exudate and change into clusters of epithelioid cells to form tubercles. In turn, these tubercles may resolve and disappear, or central caseation consisting of incomplete cell autolysis may develop. The caseous lesion contains large numbers of multiplying tubercle bacilli that spread rapidly from the primary focus through the regional lymphatic vessels to the regional lymph nodes, with areas of inflammation being set up along the way that later may caseate and calcify.[452]

The primary pulmonary focus has been studied carefully by numerous investigators (Table 107–4). Plotting their locations on a normal chest radiograph creates a pattern resembling the scatter of birdshot on a paper target. Thus, all parts of the lung apparently are at equal risk of being seeded. The thought that the primary focus has a predilection for the lower fields of the lung probably arises from the fact that the lung is pyramid shaped, with more basilar than apical lung tissue.

Many investigators concur that 70 to 85 percent of primary infections are initiated by one focus.[188,585] In a study of 170 cases, Ghon[188] found two foci in 15 percent, three in 7 percent, four in 3 percent, and five in 2 percent. Multiple lung foci can result, although rarely, from the ingestion and inhalation of tubercle bacilli. This pattern of disease was shown clearly in the results of pathologic studies of the 71 infants who died in the Lübeck disaster of the 1930s, an incident in which 251 newborn infants mistakenly had been given live tubercle bacilli by mouth instead of BCG vaccine. Fifteen of the infants were found to have primary lung lesions at autopsy, and all 251 had primary intestinal lesions.

Although the lymphadenitis cannot be detected clinically and rarely is apparent even on radiographs, the hallmark of initial tuberculosis infection is the relatively large size and importance of the adenitis as opposed to the relatively insignificant size of the initial focus in the lung, skin, or elsewhere. The development of tuberculin hypersensitivity within 3 to 12 weeks after initial acquisition of infection enhances the cellular reaction throughout the primary complex, but with a particularly prominent effect on the primary focus and the regional lymph nodes. At this time, the

infection may spread along nearby lymphatic chains to involve more distant nodes. The lymphatic drainage of the lungs is outlined in Table 107–5; it occurs predominantly from left to right. One is not surprised, therefore, that the nodes in the right upper paratracheal area appear to be the ones most often affected. Many primary lesions are subpleural, and the lymphatic drainage of the apical pleura is to the cervical nodes. Moreover, the paratracheal chains have communications with both the deep cervical nodes and the abdominal nodes, as shown in Figure 107–6. Among 54 patients with the primary lesion in the right upper lobe, Blacklock found that 14 had involvement of the deep cervical nodes on the same side and three had involvement of the abdominal nodes.

Bronchial obstruction as a result of enlargement of the peribronchial lymph nodes was reported by Ghon[188] and others. Not until the 1920s did Wallgren[632] and others elucidate the role of these large nodes in producing the radiographic shadows variously called epituberculosis, collapse-consolidation, and segmental lesions that so often are seen in cases of childhood tuberculosis.[329,354,632] At the end of the incubation period, as tuberculin sensitivity develops, the hilar lymph nodes enlarge greatly, and in many cases, caseous foci appear within them. Acid-fast studies of smears and sections have confirmed that this caseum has few tubercle bacilli. As the nodes enlarge, they fre-

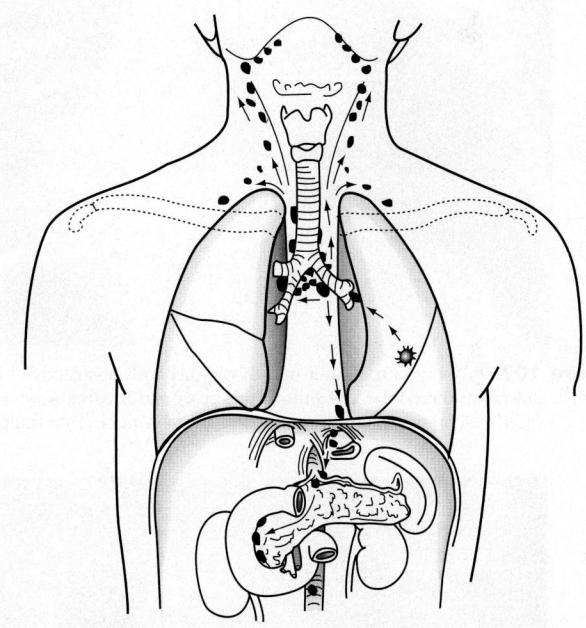

Figure 107–6 Schematic composite drawing illustrating wide lymphogenic spread of the tuberculosis infection from a primary pulmonary focus in the base of the left upper lobe. The infection extended cephalad to the submandibular nodes in the head and caudad as far as the pancreatic nodes in the abdomen. *(From Caffey, J.: Pediatric X-Ray Diagnosis. 7th ed. Chicago, Year Book, 1978.)*

TABLE 107–4 Location of the Primary Pulmonary Focus

Location	No. of Patients	%
Right upper lobe	138	27
Right middle lobe	40	7
Right lower lobe	107	20
Left upper lobe	122	24
Left lower lobe	104	20
Total	511	98

Data from Ghon, A., and Kuedlich, H.: Die Eintrittspforten der Infektion. In Engel, S., and Pirquet, C. (eds.): Handbuch der Kindertuberkulose. Stuttgart, Germany, Georg Thieme Verlag, 1930.

TABLE 107–5 Lymphatic Drainage of the Lung

Right upper lobe	→	Right paratracheal chain
Right middle lobe	→	Right and left paratracheal nodes
Right lower lobe	→	Subcarinal nodes
Left upper lobe	→	Left paratracheal nodes
Left lower lobe	→	Left paratracheal nodes
Lingula	→	Subcarinal nodes
Subcarinal nodes	→	Right paratracheal nodes

Based on data of Rouviere, quoted by Courtice, F. C., and Simmonds, W. J.: Physiological significance of lymph drainage of the serous cavities and lungs. Physiol. Rev. 34:419–442, 1954.

quently impinge on the neighboring regional bronchus and compress it and cause diffuse inflammation of its wall, even to the point of obstructing the lumen.[329,505,553] Daly and colleagues,[123] in their study of endobronchial tuberculosis in children at Bellevue, found this mechanism to be the cause of obstruction in half their patients. Other mechanisms of obstruction include damage to the bronchial cartilage leading to gradual (or, rarely, abrupt) perforation of the bronchus and the formation of plugs of semiliquid toothpaste-like caseum that partially or completely occludes the bronchus. In some cases, endobronchial granulomatous tissue forms around the stoma of the fistula and obstructs the lumen.

Three immediate results of bronchial obstruction are possible.

The first is sudden death by asphyxia, fortunately an extremely rare event.[311]

The second is obstructive hyperaeration (also called *obstructive emphysema*) of a lobar segment, a lobe, or even an entire lung.

This unusual result usually affects children younger than 2 years old, and it may be accompanied by wheezing. Physical examination generally is of little help; radiographs, best taken on expiration, show hyperaeration, which usually is not accompanied by mediastinal displacement, probably because of fixation by the tuberculous mediastinal nodes (Fig. 107–7). Aspiration of a foreign body always must be considered in the differential diagnosis. The obstruction ultimately resolves by itself; however, corticosteroids may be added to the chemotherapeutic regimen to hasten recovery.[406,407,602] Surgical removal of the obstructing nodes has been successful but rarely is performed.[129]

The third possible result of bronchial obstruction is the appearance of a segmental lesion, fan-shaped on a radiograph, representing mainly atelectasis and almost always involving the very segment occupied by the primary pulmonary focus[307,354,393] (Fig. 107–8). Actually, the radiographic opacity results from a combination of several elements: the primary pulmonary focus,

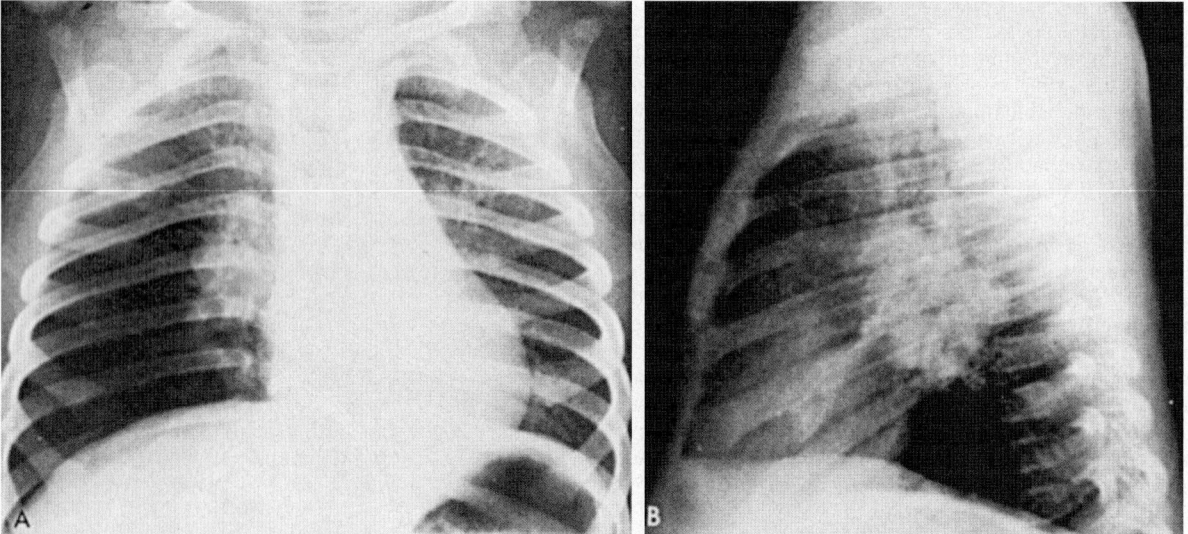

Figure 107–7 X-ray film of an 8-month-old girl with obstructive hyperaeration of the right lower lobe as a result of tuberculosis. **A,** Note the hyperlucent right lower lobe and shift of the heart and mediastinum away from the ball-valve obstruction to the left. **B,** Note the large hilar lymph nodes, which are compressing the right lower lobe bronchi. Tuberculosis should be considered in patients with hyperaeration of unknown etiology.

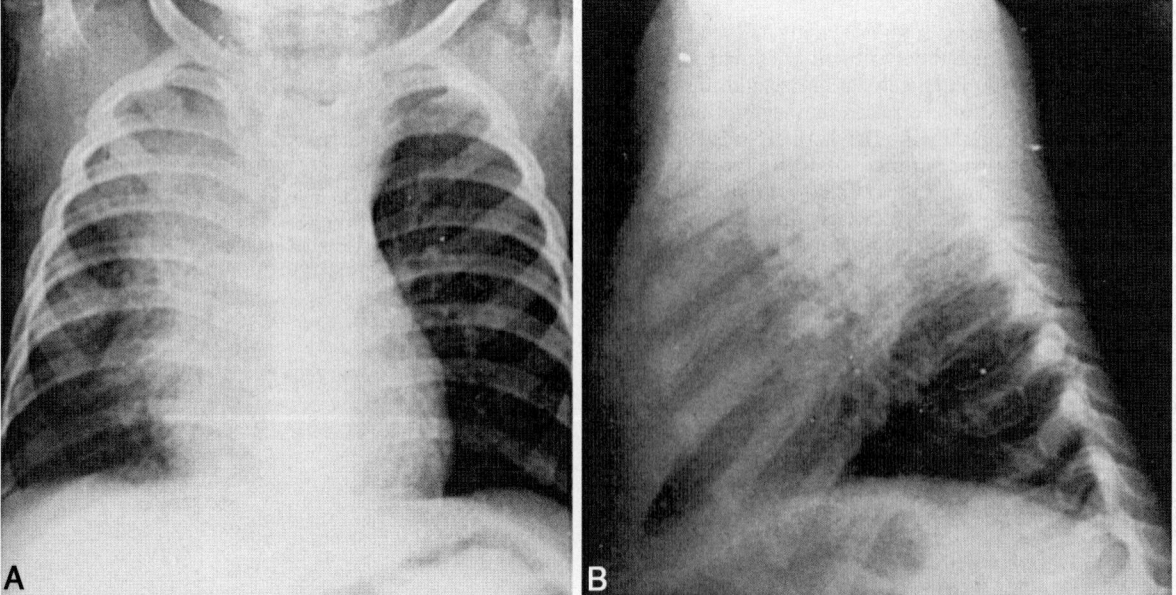

Figure 107–8 **A** and **B,** Radiographs of an 8-month-old boy with primary tuberculosis infection. The posteroanterior film shows collapse-consolidation of the right upper lobe, hilar and paratracheal adenopathy, and pleural reaction. Note the narrowed right bronchi.

the caseous material from an eroded bronchus, the inflammatory response elicited by the caseum, and atelectasis. In some instances, acute secondary infection plays a role. Children with secondary bacterial pneumonia often initially have high fever, cough, and rales; the signs and symptoms respond to conventional antibiotics, but the chest radiographic findings usually do not clear because of the underlying tuberculosis. The relative roles of these various elements often cannot be assessed; sometimes atelectasis is conspicuous, and, at other times, consolidation is the salient pathologic process, with the volume of the segment undiminished or even increased (hence the descriptive term *collapse-consolidation lesion*, preferred by some clinicians to the less accurate term *atelectasis*).

The percentage of infected children in whom segmental lesions develop has been estimated by several investigators. All agree that the younger the child, the more frequently collapse-consolidation lesions occur (Table 107–6). The segmental lesion is likely to form during the first 3 to 6 months after acquisition of infection (50 of 65 in Payne's series[441]). Multiple segmental lesions can occur simultaneously (18 of 160 children in Payne's experience). When multiple lesions develop, the segmental lesions usually form in one lung, but occasionally, the lobes or segments of both lungs are affected. Sometimes, segmental lesions and obstructive hyperaeration occur simultaneously. The physical signs and symptoms of segmental lesions—cough, rales, localized wheezing, egophony—are surprisingly meager but are seen more frequently in infants because of the smaller size of their airways.

Although segmental lesions and hyperaeration are the most common findings produced by enlarging thoracic lymph nodes, others occur. Enlarged peritracheal nodes may cause stridor and respiratory distress.[358] Subcarinal nodes may impinge on the esophagus and cause difficulty swallowing, followed occasionally by the formation of an esophageal diverticulum, or the nodes may rupture directly into the esophagus and produce a bronchoesophageal fistula. Enlarged lymph nodes may compress the subclavian vein and produce edema of the hand and arm, or they may erode major blood vessels, including the aorta. They also may rupture into the mediastinum and point in the left or more often the right supraclavicular fossa. Compression of the left recurrent laryngeal nerve has been reported. Compression of the left phrenic nerve leads to paralysis of the left leaf of the diaphragm in an estimated 0.1 to 0.3 percent of tuberculous children. Rupture into the pericardial sac is described later.

The late results of bronchial obstruction include the following possibilities: complete re-expansion of the lung and resolution of the radiographic findings; disappearance of the segmental lesion, with residual calcification of the primary focus or the regional lymph nodes; or scarring and progressive contraction of the lobe or segment, usually associated with bronchiectasis.[329,355] Permanent anatomic sequelae result from segmental lesions in approximately 60 percent of all cases, even though the abnormality usually is not apparent on plain radiographs. Cylindrical (rarely saccular) bronchiectasis, sometimes stenoses, and elongation or shortening can be demonstrated on bronchography. Fortunately, most of these abnormalities are asymptomatic in the upper lobes. However, secondary infection may occur in the middle and lower lobes and cause the middle lobe syndrome.[63] On occasion, the chronic vascularity that accompanies bronchiectasis leads to poor oxygen saturation during exercise and to restricted body growth. In addition, bronchogenic carcinoma may arise years later in the old scarred lesions remaining in the bronchus.

Calcification of the primary complex, when it appears, always results from caseation. In calcified caseum, as in bone, the predominant calcium salt is tribasic calcium phosphate. Calcification of caseous lesions occurs much more readily in children than in adults, probably because children's calcium and phosphorus plasma levels are higher. In the infants who were victims of the Lübeck disaster, autopsy showed calcification to be present as early as 58 days after the onset of massive infection. Payne,[441] in a study of calcification in 299 children from Newcastle-on-Tyne, reported calcification visible on the chest radiographs of one child within 6 months of infection, 38 within 12 months, 104 within 18 months, 165 within 24 months, 252 within 3 years, and 299 within 4 years.

Calcium usually is deposited as fine particles and creates a stippled effect (Fig. 107–9), but it may be deposited in large, even enormous masses. Calcification may persist without much change, or it may start resorbing within 5 years and eventually disappear completely. It occasionally progresses to ossification with the formation of true bone and functional bone marrow. Calcification, if it is visible at all on radiographs, most often involves the regional lymph nodes.[58] Sometimes, however, the primary pulmonary focus or the entire primary complex, including the lymphangitis, calcifies (Fig. 107–10).

Calcification took place in 75 to 80 percent of the 525 children with pulmonary tuberculosis monitored by Payne.[441] Currently, extensive calcification occurs uncommonly in the Western world, probably because tuberculous lesions treated early with isoniazid rarely caseate, and caseation is a prerequisite for calcification.

Pleural Effusion

Pleural effusion can be localized or generalized, unilateral or bilateral.[327] Localized pleural effusion so frequently accompanies the primary pulmonary focus that it is practically a component of the primary complex. All tuberculous serous effusions probably originate in the discharge of bacilli into the cavity from an adjacent lesion—in the case of the pleura, from a subpleural pulmonary focus or from subpleural caseous lymph nodes. The breakthrough may be small and the pleuritis localized and asymptomatic, or it may occur in the form of a generalized effusion, usually 3 to 6 months after infection occurs (Fig. 107–11). In 75 percent of Wallgren's[632] cases, later calcification of the pulmonary focus or regional lymph nodes proved the effusion to be on the same side as the original primary focus. Seemingly without logical explanation are the following clinical observations: tuberculous pleural effusion is a rare occurrence in children younger than 2 years and an uncommon one in children younger than 5 years (perhaps because sensitivity to tuberculin is lower in the very young), occurs more frequently in boys than in girls, almost never is associated with a segmental lesion, and rarely is associated with miliary tuberculosis.

The onset of pleurisy usually is abrupt and resembles bacterial pneumonia, with fever, chest pain, shortness of breath, and, on physical examination, dullness to percussion and diminished breath sounds. Fever may be high and, in untreated cases, last for several weeks. On occasion, differentiation of an effusion from an extensive pneumonic lesion is difficult; lateral decubitus radio-

TABLE 107–6 Percentage of Tuberculin Converters and Age at Which Segmental Lesions Develop

Age at Infection (yr)	Converters with Segmental Lesions		Total Converters (No.)
	Number	Pecent	
0–1	77	43	180
1–5	35	24	147
6–10	31	25	121
11–15	16	16	97
Total	159	29	545

After Payne, M., quoted by Miller, F. J. W., Seale, R. M. E., and Taylor, M. D.: Tuberculosis in Children. Boston, Little, Brown, 1963.

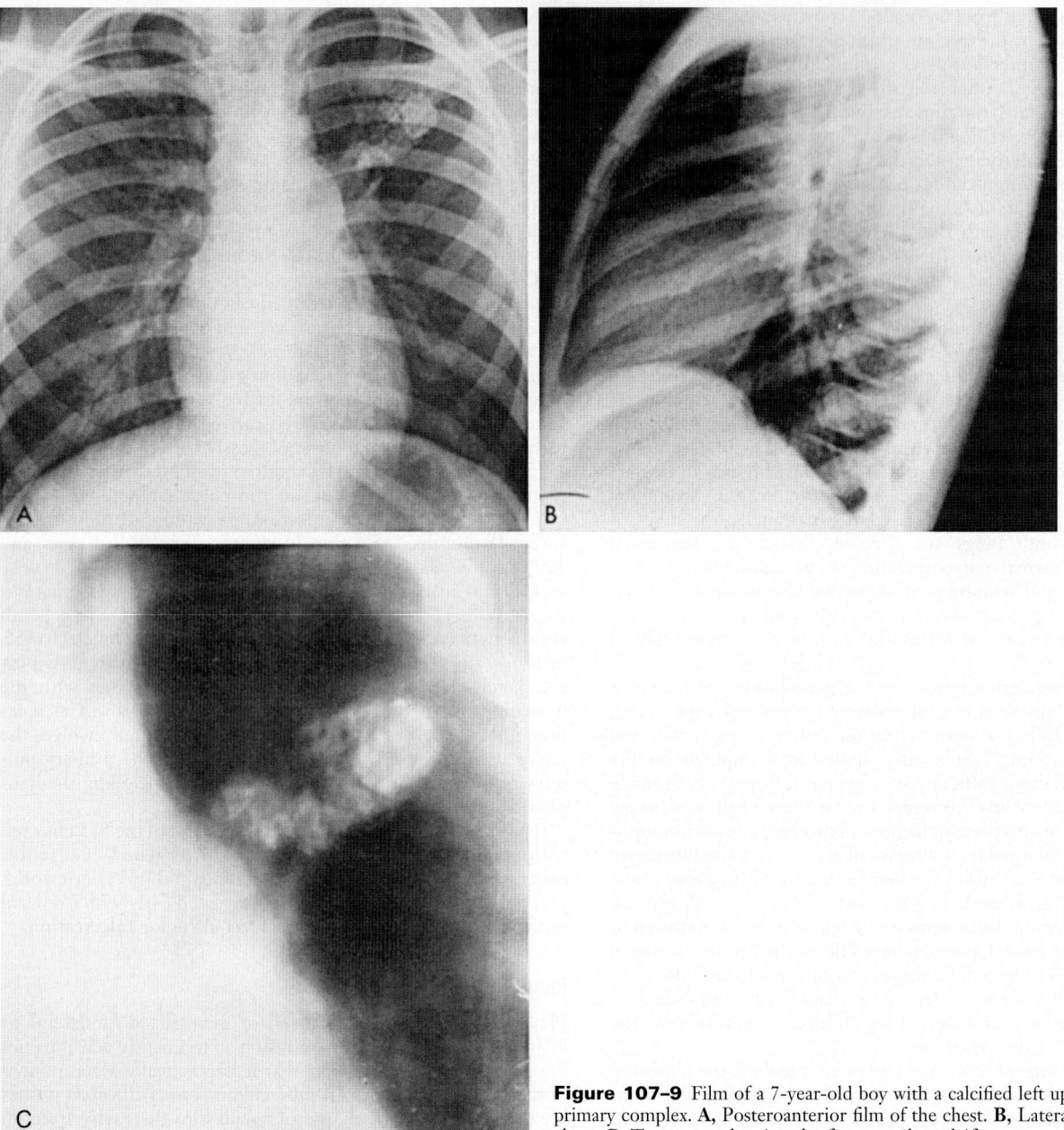

Figure 107–9 Film of a 7-year-old boy with a calcified left upper lobe, primary complex. **A,** Posteroanterior film of the chest. **B,** Lateral film of the chest. **C,** Tomogram showing the fine granular calcific pattern.

graphic views are helpful in confirming the presence of pleural fluid.

Thoracentesis is, of course, the essential diagnostic procedure. The puncture should be made in the area shown on the radiograph to have the greatest accumulation of fluid. No more than 30 mL of pleural fluid should be withdrawn; otherwise, the protein loss from this usually protein-rich fluid may be considerable. The fluid generally is greenish yellow, occasionally tinged with blood, with a specific gravity of 1.012 to 1.022, a high protein content, and often a low glucose level (<30 mg/dL), and it has several hundred white cells per cubic millimeter with a predominance of neutrophils or lymphocytes, depending on the age of the effusion. The cells in tuberculous pleural effusion are predominantly T lymphocytes, which are present in a higher proportion than in blood.[167,520] Tubercle bacilli generally are present in such small numbers that results from direct smears and cultures are likely to be disappointing; smears almost always are negative, and pleural fluid cultures are positive in less than 30 percent of cases. Pleural biopsy is a useful diagnostic procedure because both the finding of typical tubercles on histologic study and culture of the tissue are much more likely to establish the diagnosis than is culture of pleural fluid.[322]

The prognosis for children with tuberculous effusion always has been relatively good compared with that for other overt forms of tuberculosis, even in the days before chemotherapy.[331] Permanent impairment of pulmonary function is a surprisingly uncommon event after pleural effusion.[178] The development of scoliosis is a remote possibility and should be guarded against while the patient recovers.

Progressive Pulmonary Tuberculosis

In this serious complication of the primary complex, the primary pulmonary focus, instead of resolving or calcifying, enlarges steadily and develops a large caseous center. This center then

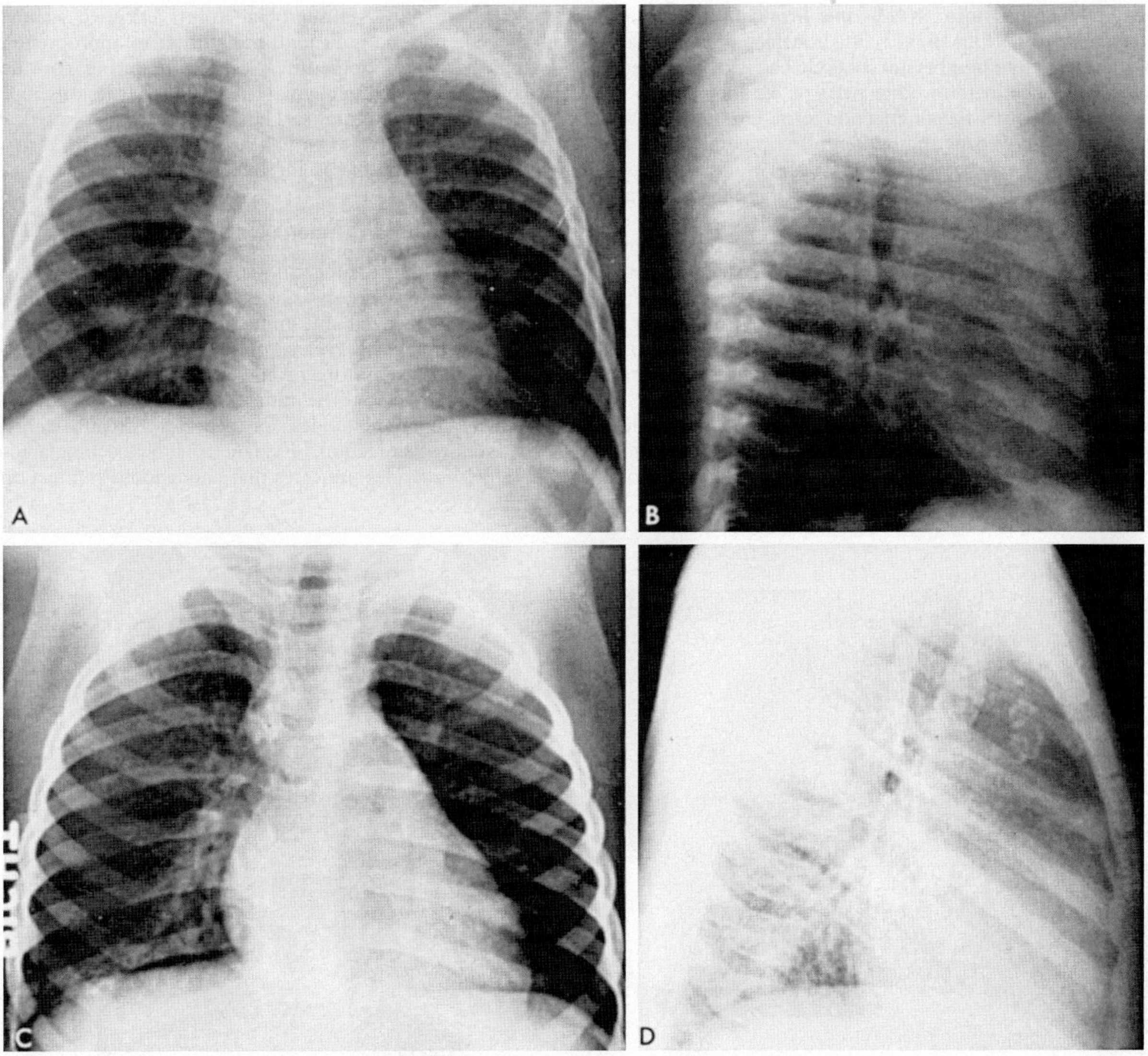

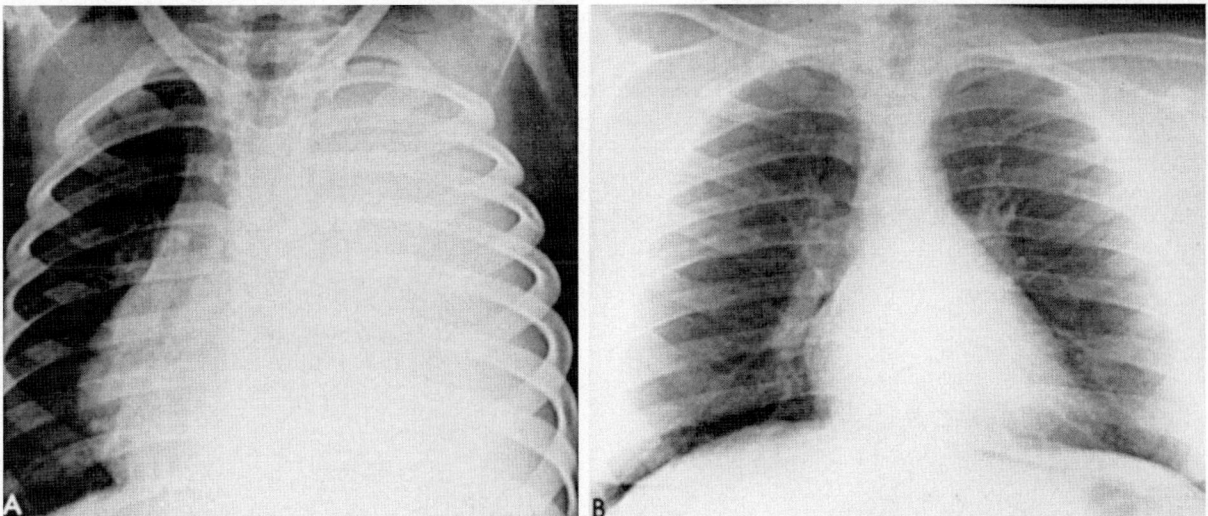

Figure 107–10 **A** and **B,** Radiographs of a 7-month-old girl with mild fullness of the right upper mediastinum and a hazy infiltrate in the right lower lobe. The result of a skin test for tuberculosis was positive. She was treated for tuberculosis and clinically improved. **C,** The same patient 3.5 years later has a calcified primary complex in the right upper and lower lobes over the diaphragm. **D,** The anterior location of the upper lobe complex is seen clearly on the lateral chest film.

Figure 107–11 Radiographs of a 5-year-old boy with massive left pleural effusion caused by tuberculosis. **A,** Posteroanterior film of the chest. **B,** The same patient 6 years later with a normal chest film and no physical complaint.

liquefies and empties into an adjacent bronchus to create a "primary cavity"[590,619] (Fig. 107–12); the liquefaction is associated with particularly large numbers of tubercle bacilli. The tubercle bacilli further disseminate to other parts of the lobe and to the entire lung, where other foci of infection form. On rare occasion, an enlarging primary focus ruptures into the pleural cavity and creates a pneumothorax, bronchopleural fistula, or caseous pyopneumothorax or into the pericardial sac or the mediastinum.

Whereas clinical symptoms often are minimal when the primary focus is uncomplicated, a progressive lesion often is accompanied by more severe fever, cough, malaise, and weight loss as well as classic signs of cavitation, such as egophony.[202,493] Before chemotherapy was available, the inability to contain the primary focus was associated with a grave outlook; 25 to 65 percent of patients thus affected died. Now, with appropriate treatment, the prognosis is good.

Distinguishing between progressive pulmonary tuberculosis and a simple tuberculous focus with a superimposed acute bacterial pneumonia caused by *Staphylococcus*, *Klebsiella*, or anaerobes may be difficult. Antimicrobial agents effective against these pathogens may be indicated, in addition to appropriate antituberculosis drugs. Sometimes, especially during convalescence from pulmonary parenchymal lesions, bullous lesions appear and persist for several months. They seem to be associated, in children as in adults, either with "tears" in damaged alveolar walls or with the emptying of caseum out of cavities.[367]

Chronic Pulmonary Tuberculosis

Chronic pulmonary tuberculosis, sometimes referred to as adult or reactivation tuberculosis, is the type of disease seen in pulmonary tissue sensitized and immunized by an earlier tuberculosis infection. For many years, ongoing debate centered around whether the lesions of chronic pulmonary tuberculosis, more localized than those of the initial tuberculous lesion and less likely to spread to lymph nodes and the bloodstream, were due to "endogenous reinfection." Evidence that has accumulated during subsequent decades indicates that endogenous reinfection is the

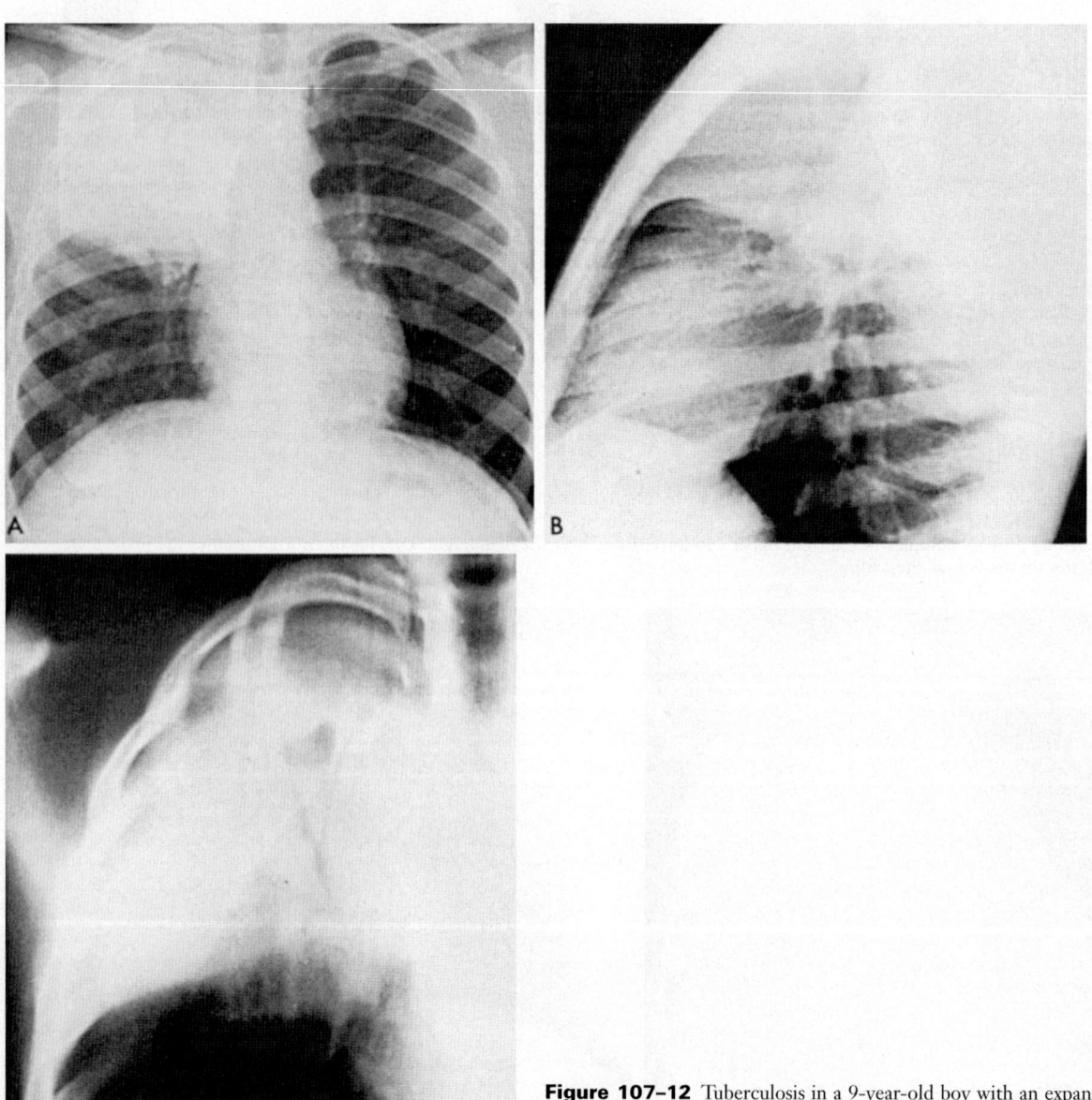

Figure 107–12 Tuberculosis in a 9-year-old boy with an expanding right upper lobe consolidation. **A,** Posteroanterior film of the chest. **B,** Lateral film of the chest. **C,** A tomogram shows an air bronchogram and a cystic cavitary lesion.

usual event.[565] However, reinfection with a different strain of *M. tuberculosis* has been documented and may be more common in areas where tuberculosis is prevalent.[530]

Careful long-term studies of children have revealed a continuum of involvement in many cases: first the primary focus, followed within a few years in some patients by infraclavicular small round foci in the lung apices that often were calcified (Assmann foci, Simon foci) and thought to result from hematogenous spread at the time of initial infection. Later, these foci disappear spontaneously or remain visible as tiny calcifications or as larger "round foci," which may, if untreated, progress to the typical lesions of chronic pulmonary tuberculosis.

Even before antituberculosis drugs were discovered, chronic pulmonary tuberculosis was a rare occurrence in children (6-7% in the series of Lincoln and colleagues[328] of closely monitored patients at Bellevue Hospital). It appears more frequently in children in the lower socioeconomic strata of society and more frequently in girls than in boys. Chronic pulmonary tuberculosis rarely develops in children who survive with a healed, untreated tuberculosis infection acquired before they have reached 2 years of age, but it is much more frequent in children who acquire their initial infection after reaching 7 years of age and particularly if they become infected close to the onset of puberty. In that case, the "adult" type of lesion often develops in the very lobe where the primary lesion occurred. In this situation, progressive pulmonary tuberculosis cannot be differentiated from chronic pulmonary tuberculosis. Now, with effective treatment, such differentiation is unimportant.[211]

Cough, fever of unknown origin, chest pain, hemoptysis, and supraclavicular adenitis are the most common clinical manifestations. Essential diagnostic procedures are the tuberculin skin test and appropriate chest radiographs, often including such special procedures as tomograms and lordotic views. An intense search for tubercle bacilli must be made in sputum, gastric washings, and, if necessary, secretions obtained by bronchoscopy.

Myocardial and Pericardial Tuberculosis

Tubercles often are found in the heart in miliary tuberculosis. Although it is exceedingly rare, myocardial caseation has been described, usually secondary to direct spread from mediastinal glands and accompanied by paroxysmal tachycardia or arrhythmias.[633]

Tuberculous pericarditis, although more common than symptomatic tuberculous myocarditis, occurred in only 0.4 percent of 2500 children monitored by Lincoln and Sewell[331] at Bellevue and in 4 percent of 200 children in Boyd's series.[56] It occurs more commonly in males than in females. In most cases, tuberculous pericarditis probably arises by direct invasion or by lymphatic drainage from caseous lymph nodes in the subcarinal area or from nodes close to the ductus arteriosus, with resulting exudation of hemorrhagic fluid and the development of granulation tissue on both the parietal and visceral surfaces of the pericardium.[477] Pericardial fluid may be serofibrinous or hemorrhagic; tubercle bacilli rarely are found on smears.[242] Sometimes, extensive fibrosis leads to obliteration of the pericardial sac, with the development, usually years later, of constrictive pericarditis.

The initial symptoms generally are nonspecific: low-grade fever, poor appetite, failure to gain weight, and, rarely, chest pain. On examination, a pericardial friction rub may be heard, or if a large effusion already is present, distant heart sounds, tachycardia, and a narrow pulse pressure may suggest the diagnosis. The diagnosis then is confirmed by radiography, echocardiography, electrocardiography, tuberculin skin test, and aspiration of fluid for culture. Before the advent of chemotherapy, approximately half the patients succumbed. Now, with appropriate drugs and possibly corticosteroids to diminish the size of the effusion[578] and also occasional partial pericardiectomy, the outlook is excellent.

Lymphohematogenous Spread

Tubercle bacilli from the lymphadenitis of the primary complex are disseminated during the incubation period in all cases of tuberculosis infection. The results of liver biopsy of young asymptomatic tuberculin converters (indicating recent infection) show that the liver always is involved.[106] Tubercle bacilli can reach deep, distant organs through the bloodstream or lymphatic channels. Autopsies on individuals who have died soon after development of initial infection show that bacilli often are deposited in the liver, spleen, skin, and apical pulmonary tissue.

The clinical picture produced by lymphohematogenous spread probably is determined by host susceptibility at the time of spread and by the quantity of tubercle bacilli released.[516,621] Three clinical forms can be recognized:

1. The lymphohematogenous spread may be occult, in which case it usually remains so, or it may be occult initially with metastatic, extrapulmonary lesions appearing months or years later (e.g., renal tuberculosis).[470]

2. So-called protracted hematogenous tuberculosis, rarely seen today, is characterized by high, spiking fever, marked leukocytosis, hepatomegaly and splenomegaly, and general glandular enlargement, sometimes with repeated evidence of metastatic seeding in the choroid, kidneys, and skin. Calcifications may appear subsequently, often in large numbers, in the pulmonary apices (Simon foci) and in the spleen, thus attesting to the earlier dissemination of tubercle bacilli through blood. The tuberculin skin test result usually is strongly positive. Bone marrow biopsy may confirm the clinical impression, but treatment often must be started on a presumptive basis. Although this type of tuberculosis in past years often ended tragically in tuberculous meningitis, today it is completely treatable if it is diagnosed in time.

3. The third form of lymphohematogenous spread, analogous to sepsis with pyogenic bacteria, is miliary tuberculosis.[244,516] It usually arises from discharge of a caseous focus, often a lymph node, into a blood vessel such as a pulmonary vein; it may be self-propagating, with repeated discharge arising at various sites. Most common during the first 2 to 6 months after infection in infancy, it can arise even in adults who have apparently well-healed, calcified lesions.[290,503]

Miliary disease provides a striking illustration of the difference in susceptibility of tissue to tubercle bacilli; tubercles tend to be larger and more numerous in the lung, spleen, liver, and bone marrow than in the heart, pancreas, and brain. The number of fixed intravascular phagocytes, as well as the relative tortuosity of the smaller blood vessels themselves, must play an important role in determining tissue susceptibility. In acute caseating miliary tuberculosis, the lesions are likely to be numerous and sometimes almost coalescent.

The clinical picture of miliary tuberculosis varies greatly, probably depending on the number of bacilli in the bloodstream. Sometimes, the patient is afebrile and appears to be well, and the condition is diagnosed by chance during contact investigation of another individual with infectious tuberculosis. The onset can be insidious, often occurring after the patient has had another precipitating infection. In rare cases, the onset is abrupt. Drowsiness, loss of weight and appetite, persistent fever, weakness, rapid breathing with a rustling sound on auscultation of the lungs, occasionally cyanosis, and almost always a palpable spleen are the clinical manifestations that lead the clinician to obtain a chest radiograph.

Usually within no more than 3 weeks after the onset of symptoms, tubercles, sometimes tiny and at times large, can be seen evenly distributed throughout both lung fields[427]; in the early stages, they often are detected best on a lateral view of the retrocardiac space (Fig. 107–13). The incidence of choroidal tuber-

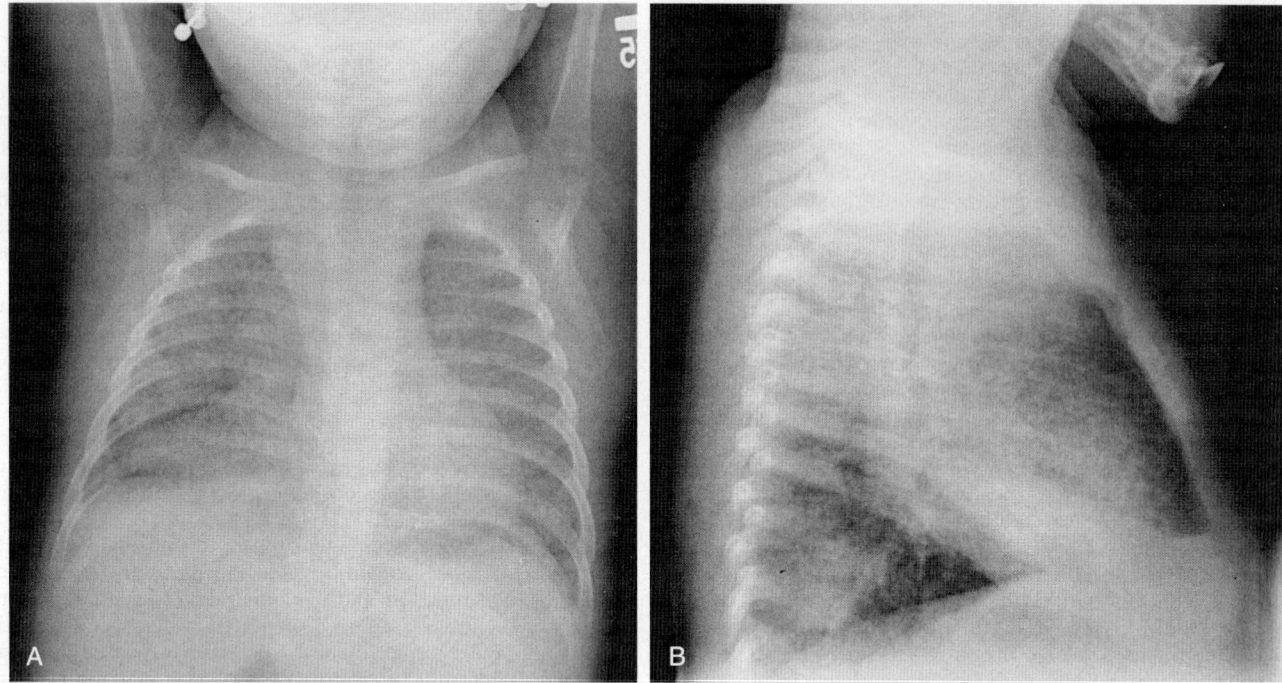

Figure 107–13 Miliary tuberculosis in an infant. The numerous tubercles can be seen on both the posteroanterior (**A**) and lateral (**B**) views.

cles varies greatly; it has been reported variously as 13 and 87 percent. Recurrent pneumothorax, subcutaneous emphysema, pneumomediastinum, and pleural effusion are less serious but well-recognized complications of miliary tuberculosis. Second attacks have been reported.[647] Cutaneous lesions, including painful nodules, papulonecrotic tuberculids, and purpuric lesions, may appear in crops.[286]

The diagnosis usually is established by means of the clinical picture and a chest radiograph. Sometimes it is confirmed by a liver or skin biopsy; by culture of *M. tuberculosis* from the gastric aspirate, urine, or bone marrow[106,214]; or by fiberoptic bronchoscopy and transbronchial biopsy.[67] Treatment usually is successful.

EXTRATHORACIC SPREAD

Central Nervous System Tuberculosis[558]

Tubercle bacilli are distributed by the bloodstream into all parts of the central nervous system (CNS) during lymphohematogenous spread.[330] Surprisingly, they do not multiply as well in nervous tissue as in other areas such as the lung. Thus, CNS tuberculosis, although an early manifestation of infection, usually does not appear simultaneously with miliary spread, but days later. The tubercle bacilli can affect the CNS in various ways[611,628] and produce tuberculous meningitis,[248,581] serous meningitis,[325,611] tuberculoma,[603,611] or tuberculous brain abscess, or it can affect mainly the spinal cord and cause spinal tuberculous leptomeningitis.[420]

Tuberculous meningitis arises from caseous foci, often very small ones, situated in the brain or meninges.[471] These lesions arise from hematogenous spread early in the infection.[143,260] In time, the caseous foci discharge tubercle bacilli directly into the subarachnoid space. The thick, gelatinous exudate lies in the meshes of the pia-arachnoid in the brain, where it infiltrates the walls of meningeal arteries and veins and produces inflammation, caseation, and obstruction; the exudate can extend along small

vessels into the cortex, where it causes occlusion and produces infarcts. This same exudate interferes with normal flow of cerebrospinal fluid in and out of the ventricular system and with absorption of the fluid by the pacchionian bodies. The predilection of the exudate for the base of the brain accounts for the frequent involvement of the third, sixth, and seventh nerves and the optic chiasm. The combination of vascular lesions producing infarcts,[321] interference with flow of cerebrospinal fluid resulting in hydrocephalus, and direct cranial nerve involvement, especially of the eye, causes the devastating damage that all too often results from tuberculous meningitis.[20]

Tuberculous meningitis has been estimated to develop in one of every 300 untreated infections.[258] Virtually never seen in infants younger than 4 months, it occurs most frequently in children younger than 6 years, usually appears within 2 to 6 months after initial infection, and accompanies miliary tuberculosis in approximately 50 percent of cases. Tuberculosis should be suspected as the cause of meningitis that is accompanied by cranial nerve involvement, hydrocephalus, or evidence of inflammation at the base of the brain.[616]

The onset of tuberculous meningitis usually is gradual and occurs during a period of approximately 3 weeks; in some cases, it seems to be precipitated by a viral infection, a fall, or a blow on the head. On occasion, the onset is abrupt and marked by a convulsion. A convenient approach is for the clinician to divide the course into three stages. The first stage is characterized by personality change, irritability, anorexia, listlessness, and some fever. After 1 or 2 weeks, the disease passes into the second stage, when signs of increased intracranial pressure and cerebral damage appear: drowsiness, stiff neck, cranial nerve palsies, inequality of the pupils, vomiting, tache cérébrale, absence of the abdominal reflexes, and convulsions that may be tonic or clonic, focal or generalized. The third stage is characterized by coma, irregular pulse and respirations, and rising fever. Papilledema occasionally is noted.

Aids in establishing the diagnosis are a history of contact with an adult who has tuberculosis (however, the family history of tuberculosis often is "negative" because the incubation period of meningitis is short and the contagious adult has not been discovered yet)[139]; a tuberculin skin test (positive result in only 50% of cases); positive tuberculin skin test results in siblings; a chest radiograph, which often reveals pulmonary disease; and changes in and the characteristic findings from spinal fluid. However, ventricular cerebrospinal fluid may be relatively normal because it is obtained proximal to the site of inflammation. The lumbar spinal fluid usually is clear and under substantially increased pressure. It will contain 50 to 500 white blood cells/mm³, with polymorphonuclear leukocytes predominant early and lymphocytes predominant later. The spinal fluid glucose level may be at the lower limits of normal if the patient is examined early in the second stage, and it falls by 5 mg or so each day; by the third stage, it usually is very low. The protein content may be normal at the time of the first spinal tap, but it rises steadily to very high concentrations, at which time a pellicle will develop on the fluid on standing. Tubercle bacilli may be found in the pellicle but are scarce at best. Only approximately 50 percent of cases of tuberculous meningitis in children can be confirmed by culture of spinal fluid. Gastric washings should be cultured, not only to confirm the diagnosis in retrospect but also to permit drug susceptibility testing of the organisms.[651]

Computed tomography or magnetic resonance imaging[17,20,203,423] is recommended for the evaluation of all patients with tuberculous meningitis. Both permit recognition and follow-up of tuberculomas,[610,646] infarction or vasculitis, and hydrocephalus that might require shunting.[20,119,265,572] Involvement of the basal ganglia often is a diagnostic clue for the presence of tuberculosis.[17] Profound abnormalities in the electrolyte pattern of intracellular and extracellular fluid and spinal fluid have been reported in patients with tuberculous meningitis. These abnormalities consist mainly of low sodium and chloride levels, with low or normal plasma potassium levels, accompanied by high sodium levels in red cells and skeletal muscle.[212] High levels of antidiuretic hormone (syndrome of "inappropriate" antidiuretic hormone secretion) may cause hypotonic expansion of the extracellular fluid. Because intense vomiting and dehydration usually accompany tuberculous meningitis, the electrolyte disturbances usually include severe hypochloremia. Salt wasting in the urine occurs in rare cases. Determination of the spinal fluid chloride concentration is useless because it merely reflects the plasma level.

A good prognosis depends on immediate initiation of treatment without awaiting epidemiologic and bacteriologic confirmation of the diagnosis.[243,484] Before chemotherapy was used, every case of true tuberculous meningitis was fatal within 3 to 4 weeks, whereas today, appropriate treatment during the first stage allows survival in nearly every case, although the patient's intelligence may never return to its previous level. When it is initiated during the second stage, treatment results in survival in 75 percent or more of patients. If patients are in coma when treatment is begun, they rarely recover unscathed. Very young age and the occurrence of convulsions generally are poor prognostic factors.[484,501] Hydrocephalus, usually of the communicating type, occurs frequently (38% in one series) and is largely responsible for poor outcomes. Relieving the hydrocephalus surgically appears to improve the sensorium, vision, and neurologic deficits. Studies support the early use of ventriculoperitoneal shunting in patients severely ill at the time of admission.[308,435] Infarcts caused by vasculitis also can leave catastrophic residua. The presence of drug-resistant tuberculous meningitis greatly worsens the prognosis,[431] as does co-infection with HIV.[618] The role of corticosteroids in the treatment of intracranial tuberculosis is discussed later in this chapter.

The long-term sequelae of tuberculous meningitis are numerous and include blindness, deafness, intracranial calcification, diabetes insipidus, obesity, paraplegia, and mental retardation.[501]

Serous tuberculous meningitis is an uncommon occurrence (13% of 500 cases in the experience of Udani and associates[611]). Apparently, it develops when a tuberculous focus close to the subarachnoid space causes a lymphocytic reaction in the subarachnoid space without the actual presence of tubercle bacilli.[655] In the days before the advent of chemotherapy, "serous" meningitis was differentiated readily from "true" tuberculous meningitis because the serous type was the only nonfatal form of tuberculous meningitis. Today, such differentiation no longer is possible because treatment is begun immediately, so true tuberculous meningitis does not develop.

Isolated tuberculoma is manifested clinically as a brain tumor.[26,128,140] As many as 30 percent of brain tumors are tuberculomas, depending on the incidence of tuberculosis in the particular population under study (in India, for instance). Tuberculomas occur most often in children younger than 10 years old and often are located at the base of the brain around the cerebellum.[630] In contrast, tuberculomas in adults more often are supratentorial. Headache, convulsions, fever, and other symptoms and signs usually associated with brain abscess or tumor also characterize tuberculoma. Only careful evaluation, including inquiry about exposure to tuberculosis, a tuberculin skin test, chest radiography, and computed tomography, will permit these cases to be recognized in time to begin appropriate chemotherapy before neurosurgical intervention is needed. The widespread use of neuroimaging has revealed that small, multiple tuberculomas are a frequent feature of tuberculous meningitis in infants and young children.[17,20] A phenomenon recognized fairly recently is a symptomatic intracranial tuberculoma appearing and enlarging during treatment of meningeal, miliary, and even pulmonary tuberculosis.[4,319,462,518,595] This phenomenon appears to be mediated immunologically; it usually responds to corticosteroids and does not necessitate a change in antituberculosis chemotherapy. In addition, some small children with severe pulmonary or disseminated tuberculosis have one or several tuberculomas but normal findings on spinal fluid evaluation.[139,261] Computed tomography or magnetic resonance imaging of the head should be performed whenever neurologic signs or symptoms accompany tuberculosis.

Tuberculous brain abscess is a rarely reported form of CNS tuberculosis that tends to occur at an older age than tuberculoma does.[303,641] On pathologic examination, the lesion lacks the giant-cell and granulomatous reaction associated with tuberculoma. Focal neurologic signs occur commonly. Computed tomography and magnetic resonance imaging, if used routinely in cases of tuberculous meningitis, may permit this type of abscess, which requires surgical intervention as well as chemotherapy, to be recognized more frequently. Intramedullary tuberculoma of the spinal cord is exceedingly rare.[266,345] It can be manifested as recurrent abdominal pain.[45,420]

Spinal tuberculous leptomeningitis occurs more often in older children and adults than in infants[340]; in the series of 500 cases studied by Udani and coworkers,[611] only 2 percent fell into this last age group. Protein levels in the spinal fluid are elevated substantially, and sometimes partial or total block may be noted on myelography. Exudate may completely surround the spinal cord.

Cutaneous Tuberculosis

The manifestations of cutaneous tuberculosis can be classified in children according to a modification of the earlier classifications designed for adults[301]: (1) lesions produced by inoculation from an exogenous source[448,517] in a previously uninfected child, in a previously infected child, or after inoculation with BCG vaccine; (2) lesions resulting from hematogenous dissemination[286]; (3) lesions arising from an endogenous source; and

(4) erythema nodosum. A newer classification has been proposed and perhaps is more useful for adults than for children.[44]

Skin lesions associated with the primary complex may be caused by direct inoculation of tubercle bacilli into a traumatized area, such as a lesion on the sole of a child's bare foot, a mosquito bite on the face, an abraded elbow, or the foreskin at the time of ritual circumcision. The initial skin focus usually is a small, painless nodule, sometimes with tiny satellite lesions that soon turn into indolent ulcers without surrounding inflammation. The most striking feature is regional lymphadenitis, which often is what convinces the patient to see a physician. Fever and systemic reactions generally are minimal; low-grade pyogenic infection and cat-scratch fever (*Bartonella* infection) always must be considered in the differential diagnosis. A strongly positive tuberculin skin test result usually is obtained. Needle aspiration and culture may differentiate disease caused by *M. tuberculosis* from that caused by environmental mycobacteria.

Scrofuloderma indicates tuberculosis of the skin overlying a caseous lymph node (most often in the cervical area) that has ruptured to the outside and left either a shallow ulcer or a deep sinus, sometimes surrounded by a cluster of nodules. In the past, scrofuloderma was a frequent manifestation of tuberculosis in children and usually left extensive scars. Today, it is a rare occurrence because the diagnosis generally is made before the node ruptures. Administration of chemotherapy often forestalls the need for surgical excision.

Manifestations that result from hematogenous dissemination are papulonecrotic tuberculids and tuberculosis verrucosa cutis. Papulonecrotic tuberculids[527] are miliary tubercles in the skin that usually appear as tiny papules with "apple-jelly" centers, most often on the trunk, thighs, and face. They frequently are similar to papular urticaria or early varicella lesions, or they may be confused with the skin lesions of Letterer-Siwe disease. Skin biopsy provides a reliable diagnosis. Lupus vulgaris is a rare form of chronic, indolent tuberculosis, usually on the face, that often seems to evolve from tuberculids, very rarely at the site of BCG inoculation.

Tuberculosis verrucosa cutis is a condition characterized by large (several centimeters in diameter) papulonecrotic tuberculids. The lesions usually appear on the arms, legs, or buttocks, suggesting that trauma may play some part in their causation. Fungal infection is the main consideration in the differential diagnosis.

Erythema nodosum formerly was a common manifestation of hypersensitivity to tuberculin. It occurs mostly in young teenage girls. Usually beginning with fever and systemic toxicity manifesting soon after initial infection develops, erythema nodosum is characterized by large, deep, painful, indurated nodules on the shins and sometimes on the thighs, elbows, and forearms. The nodules gradually change from light pink to a bruise-like color. Erythema nodosum is not specific for tuberculosis but also occurs with streptococcal and meningococcal infections, histoplasmosis, coccidioidomycosis, sarcoidosis, drug sensitivity reactions, and perhaps cat-scratch disease. Tuberculin hypersensitivity is pronounced in children with tuberculosis underlying erythema nodosum, and tuberculin skin testing should be performed with caution. These patients may or may not have associated tuberculous lesions, but some clinicians hold that these patients have a greater chance of suffering complications. Skin biopsy reveals only nonspecific changes regardless of cause and, therefore, is useless in establishing the diagnosis. Both fever and nodules clear within 2 or 3 weeks.

Skeletal Tuberculosis

Bone and joint tuberculosis can be expected in 1 to 5 percent of children whose initial infection with tubercle bacilli is untreated. Usually, the tubercle bacilli are disseminated to skeletal struc-

tures during lymphohematogenous spread of the initial infection.[31] The disease becomes symptomatic during the first 1 to 3 years after infection occurs. Each of the most frequently involved bones and joints has a characteristic "incubation period" (e.g., 1 month for dactylitis but about 30 months for tuberculosis of the hip). In very young children, blood flow through growing bone is intense; consequently, they suffer from skeletal tuberculosis more often than older children do. The lesion usually starts as an area of endarteritis in the metaphysis of the long bone, where the blood supply is particularly abundant; lesions can be single or multiple.[460,515] Bone infection can be initiated by two other mechanisms, particularly in the vertebrae: (1) direct extension through the lymphatics from a caseous paravertebral lymph node[68] and (2) direct local hematogenous or lymphatic extension from a neighboring bone. As bone is destroyed progressively by pressure necrosis and formation of a cold abscess, a nearby joint may become involved.[461,614,629]

The bones most often affected are the vertebrae.[426] In one study of 1074 patients with the disease, 440 had involvement of the vertebrae; 89, the knee; 81, the hip; and 51, the elbow.[608] The upper extremities and non–weight-bearing bones, such as the skull, clavicle, and mandible, rarely are involved.[213,216] Often a history of trauma is present and may play some part in activation of an underlying lesion or may serve simply to draw attention to the process.

Tuberculous spondylitis, or tuberculosis of the vertebrae, frequently affects the thoracic vertebrae, particularly the 12th one.[225] In one series of 64 cases of spinal tuberculosis in children, the lesions were in the thoracic area in 24 children, in the lumbar area in 19, and in both areas in 13. Cervical involvement is a rare finding.[238] Usually, two vertebrae are involved, but sometimes three, four, or even as many as 11 (usually contiguous, but at times with "skips") are affected. The body of the vertebra is affected far more often than the spinous processes or the arch.

The progression of tuberculous spondylitis, as seen on radiographs, is from slight narrowing of the disk space with only minimal disk involvement and slight collapse and "wedging" of the vertebral body; to marked narrowing of the disk space with collapse, wedging of the bodies, and resulting angulation of the spine (gibbus); to extensive destruction of the bodies with severe kyphosis (Pott disease).

Paravertebral abscess (Pott abscess), retropharyngeal abscess, psoas abscess, and neurologic lesions are serious complications to be expected in 10 to 30 percent of cases of spondylitis. Neurologic complications most often arise from cervical and lumbar vertebral lesions and consist of various degrees of neuroplegia, paraplegia, or even quadriplegia. The complications are caused by inflammation of the spinal cord secondary to a neighboring cold abscess, by caseum or granuloma in the extradural space, or by spinal vessel thrombosis.

The signs and symptoms of spondylitis include "night cries" and restless sleep, a low-grade daily fever, and a peculiar position (such as torticollis with cervical lesions) or gait. Findings on physical examination may include marked "guarding" because of dorsal muscle spasm, pain when the back is "pounded," a deformity (such as gibbus), or reflex changes (including clonus). On occasion, the presence of referred chest pain leads to discovery of a paravertebral abscess on the chest radiograph. With chemotherapy and, when necessary, surgery, the outlook for both eventual clinical healing and neural recovery is in the range of 80 to 90 percent, although patients may not gain their full expected height.

Tuberculosis of the knee can be divided into several clinical types[224]: effusion into the joint without bone erosion and with little restriction of motion; thickening and fibrosis of the synovial membrane without bone erosion but often with considerable restriction of motion; synovial disease and a bone focus but an intact joint space; and synovial disease with diminished range of motion.[629] Some degree of pain, stiffness, and limping, usually intermittent in milder cases, first calls attention to the problem.

Tuberculosis of the hip, in some series of patients more common than tuberculosis of the knee, should be considered in the differential diagnosis when a child refuses to walk or a limp develops. Today, when the disease still is limited at the time of discovery to the acetabulum or to the head of the femur and no intra-articular disease is present, good mobility of the joint usually can be preserved.

Tuberculous dactylitis (spina ventosa)[208] is the most common form of skeletal tuberculosis in infants. Endarteritis is followed by swelling (often painless), and cystic bone lesions are seen on radiographs. A cold abscess may form and drain spontaneously. The prognosis for recovery without deformity is surprisingly good and was so even before chemotherapy was available.

Tuberculous arthritis is a rare finding in children. Usually monarticular, it involves primarily the weight-bearing joints and only exceptionally the joints of the upper extremities. Bacterial cultures and histologic examination of the synovium establish the diagnosis.[629] Poncet disease is a rare form of rheumatic joint disease associated with tuberculosis; it is an exceedingly rare finding in children.[122] The diagnosis of skeletal tuberculosis should be considered immediately in any child who is known to have been infected with tubercle bacilli and in whom a bone or joint lesion develops and in any child with a persistent, not otherwise explained bone or joint lesion.[625] The differential diagnosis must include low-grade infections caused by *Staphylococcus, Haemophilus influenzae, Salmonella,* and *Brucella;* fungal infections; rheumatoid arthritis; malignant disease of bone; eosinophilic granuloma, particularly with skull or pelvic lesions; and osteochondrosis resulting from aseptic necrosis of bone, particularly Legg-Calvé-Perthes disease and tuberculosis of the hip.

Children with bone and joint tuberculosis usually react strongly to tuberculin. Although the number of tubercle bacilli in an active bone lesion is much lower than in a lung lesion, the organisms almost invariably can be recovered on culture, and a great effort to do so should be made by means of aspiration or open biopsy.[201]

Treatment of skeletal tuberculosis includes both chemotherapeutic and orthopedic interventions, the chemotherapeutic interventions by far the more important.[457] Orthopedic procedures can be used for several purposes: establishment of the diagnosis, evacuation of caseum and necrotic bone, immobilization of a joint, and reconstruction or strengthening of damaged bone. Since the advent of chemotherapy, any indicated surgical procedure can be performed without fear of subsequent development of sinus formation. However, the trend has been toward reliance on drug therapy with increasingly conservative surgical management. Controlled trials of treatment undertaken in different parts of the world (Southeast Asia) by the Medical Research Council Working Party on Tuberculosis of the Spine and others have demonstrated the remarkable effectiveness of ambulatory treatment with different regimens of chemotherapy in children and adults,[250,371-373] including short-course chemotherapy.[206]

Tuberculosis of the Superficial Lymph Nodes (Scrofula)

Striking enlargement of the superficial regional lymph nodes is an integral component of the primary tuberculous complex. The tonsillar and submandibular nodes are involved most often and probably represent extension from the paratracheal lymph nodes (and not from a primary lesion in the tonsil, as once was thought); occasionally, these nodes are involved when the primary lesion occurs in the mucous membranes of the mouth, a rare event. Enlarged supraclavicular nodes may accompany a primary pulmonary lesion in the upper lung fields. Enlarged axillary and epitrochlear nodes can result from a primary skin lesion of the elbow or hand, often a small, insignificant-looking area that has, however, been present for some time. Preauricular adenitis suggests a focus on the scalp or forehead or in the lacrimal sac, sometimes attributed to an insect bite. With inguinal adenitis, careful examination of the sole of the foot may reveal a small ulcer, often at the base of the toes.

When the superficial lymph nodes are involved early in the course of infection—the normal event—the enlargement usually is painless, and the node or nodes are rubbery and discrete.[360] Low-grade fever generally is present, sometimes unnoticed by the parents. On occasion, acute respiratory infections seem to precipitate or to aggravate superficial tuberculous lymphadenitis, and the patient has high fever, some local pain, and perilymphadenitis. Rarely, the patient is seen first with a fluctuant mass, and the overlying skin is shiny and erythematous.[124,550]

The diagnosis usually is not obvious, so it is wise in all cases of superficial cervical and supraclavicular lymphadenitis to perform a throat culture, radiography of the chest, and a Mantoux tuberculin test. If the node is fluctuant, it should be aspirated and cultured for mycobacteria as well as for pyogenic bacteria.[312] In preauricular, axillary, and inguinal adenitis, a possible primary skin lesion should be sought diligently. If a lesion is found, a biopsy should be performed, in addition to a tuberculin skin test, chest radiography, and a careful history.

Currently, in addition to pyogenic infection, cat-scratch disease, tularemia, malignant tumors, sarcoid, and infection caused by mycobacteria other than *M. tuberculosis* also must be considered as a possible cause.[30,306] If the adenitis is caused by infection with *M. tuberculosis,* the induration from a Mantoux tuberculin skin test usually is greater than 15 mm, whereas mycobacteria other than *M. tuberculosis* produce a less intense reaction. The key to distinguishing tuberculosis from infection by another mycobacterium generally is epidemiologic—has the child been exposed to tuberculosis?

Because infection with pyogenic bacteria often enhances mycobacterial adenitis, frequently a wise approach is to institute therapy with a conventional antibacterial agent while awaiting the results of the skin test, chest radiography, and cultures. If the adenitis persists and evidence of mycobacterial infection is elicited, antituberculosis drug therapy should be initiated and surgical excision seriously considered.[306,504] Surgical excision currently is the treatment of choice for adenitis caused by mycobacteria other than *M. tuberculosis.* In the case of lymphadenitis caused by *M. tuberculosis,* the response to antituberculosis drugs is likely to be good. On the other hand, the adenitis is more likely to extend down into the mediastinum and to be difficult to remove. Under these circumstances, surgical excision probably is unwise, whereas a few weeks of corticosteroid and antituberculosis therapy may be effective.[263,306]

Superficial tuberculous lymphadenitis sometimes occurs early in the course of lymphohematogenous spread, in which case it often is manifested as "general glandular enlargement" accompanied by swinging fever, malaise, and weight loss. The tuberculin test result almost always is positive in immunocompetent patients, and the tuberculin test should be included in the investigation of every patient with general glandular enlargement.

Finally, tuberculous adenitis, either localized or generalized, can occur in adolescents or young adults who were infected months or even years earlier, whose infection has been quiescent, and in whom the appearance of lymphadenitis heralds reactivation of the tuberculosis infection.[305]

Ocular Tuberculosis

Ocular tuberculosis is an uncommon finding in children.[136] When it does occur, the conjunctiva and the cornea are the areas most often involved.

The conjunctiva can serve as the initial portal of entry for tubercle bacilli, especially after trauma. Unilateral lacrimation and reddening may lead to the discovery of yellowish gray nodules, usually on the palpebral conjunctiva. Preauricular adenitis appears early; the submandibular and cervical nodes also may enlarge. A tuberculin skin test and biopsy with culture can be performed to confirm the diagnosis.

Phlyctenular conjunctivitis probably is one of the hypersensitivity phenomena of childhood tuberculosis. Tubercle bacilli have, on rare occasion, been isolated from the small, grayish, jelly-like nodules usually clustered on the limbus and surrounded by dilated conjunctival vessels. Pain and photophobia are intense, and the lesions may recur in crops for weeks and affect one or both eyes. In the differential diagnosis, foreign body, herpes simplex virus conjunctivitis, vernal conjunctivitis, and trachoma should be considered. Tuberculin sensitivity is likely to be pronounced, and 1 tuberculin unit of purified protein derivative (PPD) should be used in the initial tuberculin skin test. Fortunately, hydrocortisone drops are effective in controlling both a strong local reaction to the diagnostic tuberculin test and the discomfort from the underlying disease. The prognosis for complete recovery is excellent, provided the phlyctenules do not ulcerate and leave corneal scars. Systemic chemotherapy should be started immediately after the diagnostic procedures are completed.

Although tuberculosis of the ciliary body and iris has been reported rarely in children, tubercles of the choroid often have been found in patients with miliary tuberculosis (up to 70% of patients in some series) and occasionally in children with a seemingly uncomplicated infection.[394,424] Frequently multiple, the tubercles heal slowly with deposition of retinal pigment; residual scarring apparently can be prevented with steroid therapy. Tuberculous uveitis and tuberculosis manifested as an orbital mass are rare clinical entities.[519]

Tuberculosis of the Middle Ear

Tuberculosis of the middle ear is a relatively rare manifestation of the disease.[168,341,344,398,488] It occurs as a primary focus in the area of the eustachian tube (because of reflux up the tube) in neonates who have aspirated infected amniotic fluid or in older infants who have ingested tuberculous material. It can occur as a metastatic lesion in older children who have a primary focus elsewhere. If it is a primary focus, regional lymphadenitis involves the preauricular lymph node or the anterior cervical chain, and facial paralysis occurs frequently. The primary focus always is unilateral. Otorrhea is a common occurrence and painless but may become foul smelling because of bacterial contamination with enteric organisms. Older patients may complain of tinnitus and "funny noises." The eardrum often is damaged extensively. A large central perforation or several perforations are characteristic findings. A tuberculin skin test, biopsy, and careful cultures for tubercle bacilli are essential. Once greatly feared for the almost inevitable loss of hearing and the frequent occurrence of tuberculous meningitis, tuberculous otitis media now heals well with appropriate chemotherapy.[398]

Gastrointestinal and Abdominal Tuberculosis

Tuberculosis of the mouth occurred more commonly in the days of bovine tuberculosis than it does today; at that time, scrofula often represented a primary complex in the mouth or tonsils, with associated submandibular or cervical lymphadenitis.[380] A primary focus in the mouth generally consists of a painless ulcer or mass of granulation tissue around a tooth socket or in the gingivolabial sulcus, with enlarged submental or submandibular nodes. Primary tuberculosis of the tonsils begins as a painless swelling of one tonsil, sometimes with an ulcer or yellowish node and, of course,

enlargement of the regional lymph nodes. If tubercles found on histologic examination of a tonsil removed at tonsillectomy are unaccompanied by lymphadenitis, the lesion is considered a metastatic rather than a primary lesion. Tuberculosis of the esophagus occurs rarely if ever in children; sometimes, dysphagia is produced by a mass of mediastinal nodes, which may rupture into the lumen and later heal, possibly leaving an esophageal diverticulum.

Abdominal tuberculosis may occur after the ingestion of tubercle bacilli or as a part of generalized lymphohematogenous spread, but tuberculous enteritis always has been uncommon.[18,46,480,586,589] When tubercle bacilli penetrate the gut wall, they usually do so through the Peyer patches or the appendix, where they give rise to local ulcers followed by mesenteric lymphadenitis and sometimes peritonitis.[16] On occasion, especially in older children, tuberculous enteritis accompanies extensive pulmonary cavitation. Symptoms and signs include vague abdominal pain, intussusception, blood in the stool, and sinus formation after a seemingly routine appendectomy.

The spleen is seeded during the initial lymphohematogenous spread. Only rarely are the tubercles numerous and large enough to undergo caseation and to calcify.[296] The reticuloendothelial system of the liver is involved also. Symptoms rarely are manifested except in miliary tuberculosis, in which the liver may be enlarged markedly, or in congenital tuberculosis, in which both the liver and spleen usually are enlarged.[347]

Mesenteric lymphadenitis can arise as part of an intraabdominal primary complex or by extension from tuberculous thoracic or pelvic lymph nodes; often asymptomatic, it may be discovered later when calcified. It can cause ascites and dilatation of the superficial abdominal veins, but the symptom most frequently attributed to mesenteric lymphadenitis is colicky abdominal pain after exercise, probably because adhesions are stretched.

Tuberculous peritonitis can be a result of direct extension from a primary intestinal focus, adjacent mesenteric lymph nodes, or tuberculous salpingitis.[100,137,186] It may be "plastic" or accompanied by a serous effusion. On palpation, a mass of lymph nodes often can be felt, and the abdomen may have a characteristic "doughy" feeling. Paracentesis should be performed with care because the intestine may be immobilized by adhesions. Even with a large effusion, absorption usually occurs within a month. Malignant disease must, of course, be considered strongly in the differential diagnosis, and it may be necessary to obtain a biopsy specimen even if the tuberculin skin test result is positive. Laparoscopy frequently is useful, as is fine-needle aspiration[335] and ultrasonography.[276] The ascitic fluid–blood glucose ratio of the aspirated peritoneal fluid can be helpful in differentiating tuberculous peritonitis from ascites of other causes.[645]

Renal Tuberculosis

Renal tuberculosis is a late and uncommon complication of pulmonary disease; it rarely occurs less than 4 or 5 years after primary infection and is therefore likely to be diagnosed during adolescence.[162,531] However, tubercle bacilli can be recovered from the urine in many cases of miliary tuberculosis and some cases of pulmonary tuberculosis in young children. Hematogenous dissemination can give rise to tubercles in the glomeruli, with resultant caseating and sloughing but tiny lesions, which then discharge tubercle bacilli into the tubules. An encapsulated caseous mass occasionally develops in the zone between the renal pyramid and cortex; it may calcify in situ or discharge into the pelvis of the kidney and form a cavity analogous to a pulmonary cavity. Infection can be unilateral or bilateral and can spread downward to involve the bladder. Frequently, dysuria, hematuria, and "sterile" pyuria are the initial findings in the urine; they may occur grossly but often not until late in the course of a disease that causes strikingly few symptoms. Appropriate examination and culture of single early-morning urine specimens rarely fail to reveal tubercle bacilli. Intensive chemotherapy renders surgical intervention a rare necessity.[531] Urine from patients with renal tuberculosis is highly infectious, and such children should be isolated until their urine is sterile.

Dialysis- and Renal Transplant–Associated Tuberculosis

Infections are a common cause of morbidity and mortality in patients with end-stage renal disease. Depressed cellular immunity, as manifested by cutaneous anergy, delayed homograft rejection, and depressed lymphocyte count, has been demonstrated in uremic patients, whereas cell-mediated immunity appears to recover in stable patients treated by long-term hemodialysis. Thus, it is not surprising that tuberculosis occurs more frequently in patients maintained on dialysis than in the general population and that when it does become active, it does so before or early in the course of dialysis. Extrapulmonary involvement (mediastinal, meningeal, pleural, osseous, and renal) and miliary tuberculosis appear relatively frequently in this group. In these patients, fever of unknown origin should lead to suspicion of active tuberculosis.[15] Tuberculosis also can originate in the transplanted organ.[400,624]

Genital Tuberculosis

Tuberculosis of the genital tract is an uncommon finding in both sexes before puberty.[531] It usually arises as a metastatic lesion during lymphohematogenous spread and occasionally by direct extension from an adjacent lesion of bone, gut, or the urinary tract. Genital tuberculosis is a particular hazard for adolescent girls with tuberculosis infection. Frequently, other forms of tuberculosis associated with initial infection, such as a pleural effusion, also are present. The fallopian tubes are involved in 90 to 100 percent of cases, the endometrium in 50 percent, the ovaries in 20 to 30 percent, and the cervix in 2 to 4 percent.[498] With tubal involvement, peritoneal tuberculosis occurs frequently.

Lower abdominal pain and amenorrhea usually prompt the patient to seek medical care. A lower abdominal mass, free peritoneal fluid, and constitutional symptoms may or may not be present. Chemotherapy is effective, but infertility remains a potential sequela of the disease.

Tuberculosis of the external genitalia has been seen as a manifestation of child abuse.

Genital tuberculosis can occur in males as primary tuberculosis of the penis after ritual circumcision; many such instances were reported in the past.[228] Massive inguinal lymphadenopathy in a circumcised infant should arouse suspicion of a possible tuberculous etiology. Epididymitis or epididymo-orchitis can occur in early childhood.[196] These disorders are characterized by nodular, painless swelling of the scrotum and a dragging pain in the groin and have a gradual onset rather than the acute onset that results after trauma, torsion of the testis, mumps orchitis, or epididymitis associated with bacterial infection.

Inoculation Tuberculosis

More than 200 cases of syringe-transmitted tuberculosis have been described in the world literature.[223] It has become more common since the widespread use of injectable penicillin and routine childhood immunization and usually has been a result of contamination of the syringe or the solution by an individual with infectious sputum. If the recipient has not been infected previously, the lesion in the muscle or subcutaneous tissue will be the primary focus, and the regional lymph nodes will enlarge, caseate, and, under favorable circumstances, calcify. However, at least 10

infants thus infected have died as a result of generalized tuberculosis, and in others, bone tuberculosis has developed. If the recipient already is tuberculin positive, a tuberculous abscess will form without regional lymphadenitis. In this case, an injection abscess must be differentiated from a deep tuberculous abscess arising in the stage of hematogenous dissemination.

Perinatal Tuberculosis (Congenital and Postnatal)

Transmission of *M. tuberculosis* from mother to infant through the placenta or amniotic fluid has been reported in approximately 300 patients.[73] Infection of the placenta has been demonstrated, and tubercle bacilli have been grown from the tissues of stillborn infants and from living infants within a few days of birth. Perinatal tuberculosis can be acquired by the infant through one of several routes:

1. By transplacental spread through the umbilical vein from a mother with primary hematogenous tuberculosis occurring during pregnancy (i.e., true congenital tuberculosis). The liver is enlarged, enlarged lymph nodes may be present at the porta hepatis, and evidence of widespread miliary disease may be seen in the infant (i.e., the infant may have a primary liver complex or primary lung complexes).

2. By in utero aspiration of amniotic fluid infected from endometritis in the mother or from the placenta. This route of infection also constitutes true congenital tuberculosis. In both these situations, clinical onset of signs and symptoms is likely to be rapid (by 2 to 3 weeks of age) and to include failure to thrive, fever, respiratory distress, and hepatosplenomegaly.

3. By ingestion of infected amniotic fluid or secretions during delivery. This mechanism would seem to be less well documented than the first two routes, but it certainly is a possibility.

4. By inhalation of tubercle bacilli at or soon after birth from the mother, other relatives, or attendants with infectious pulmonary tuberculosis. This route is the most common mode of transmission to newborns.

5. By ingestion of infected breast milk or cow's milk.

One cannot always be sure of the type of infection in a particular neonate; only clear-cut evidence of a primary complex in the liver establishes a definite diagnosis of congenital tuberculosis. However, the presence of early forms of tuberculosis (such as pleural, miliary, or meningeal) in the mother during pregnancy or the puerperium also is strong evidence of true congenital tuberculosis in the infant.

Routes 4 and 5 are really "postnatally" acquired tuberculosis and need, for epidemiologic purposes, to be distinguished from routes 1, 2, and 3. Neonates with these types of tuberculosis usually lack striking clinical features until they are 1 or 2 months of age.

The diagnosis of perinatal tuberculosis is likely to be difficult to establish and often delayed.[318] Disease in the mother often is overlooked; the mother may have pleural effusion, fever of unknown origin, cough, endometritis, and other symptoms without the tuberculous etiology being recognized. The early symptoms and signs in the neonate likewise are overlooked frequently and may be similar to those caused by other congenital infections. Once the diagnosis is suspected, treatment should be started immediately, and diagnostic procedures should be carried out rapidly and aggressively.

The clinical manifestations vary, probably depending on the size of the infecting dose of bacilli and the site and size of the caseous lesions.[368,409] In many of the reported cases, tuberculosis disease was discovered only at autopsy.[241] Symptoms usually appeared during the second week of life and included loss of appetite and failure to gain weight, fever, nasal or ear discharge, cough, bronchopneumonia, jaundice, hepatomegaly, and splenomegaly occurring later.[73] Wasting has been noted frequently and, in one case, clearly was shown to be caused by hypoadrenocorticism.[392]

Because the result of the tuberculin skin test very rarely is positive in infants, demonstration of tubercle bacilli in gastric washings, middle ear fluid, lymph node biopsy specimens, skin biopsy specimens, bone marrow aspirate, endotracheal aspirate, or lung biopsy specimens is essential.[205] Examination of the placenta for organisms or characteristic histopathologic changes can be extremely helpful and should be done when tuberculosis is diagnosed in the mother around the time of delivery. Successful treatment of congenital tuberculosis has been reported by several investigators, although clinical response may be very slow, and extensive calcification of the lungs, liver, spleen, and muscles may result.[281,284,409,538,552]

Tuberculosis in Adolescents

Tuberculosis in adolescents has become relatively more important as the incidence of infection in childhood has lessened.[134,357,408,536] Logically, it should be considered in two ways: first, tuberculosis acquired as an initial infection during the adolescent years and, second, tuberculosis infection acquired in early life and reactivated during adolescence.[353,411] In actual practice, separating the two often is difficult or impossible, and most clinical reports and studies do not.

Tuberculosis in adolescents may occur exactly as it does in young children, or a classic primary complex may progress rapidly to chronic pulmonary tuberculosis while the hilar lymph node involvement characteristic of childhood tuberculosis remains present. The Medical Research Council in 1963 published a report of 504 cases of tuberculosis in adolescents, including 316 cases of pulmonary tuberculosis, 44 cases of pleural effusion, 44 with hilar lymph node enlargement, 6 cases of miliary and 5 of meningeal tuberculosis, 13 with bone and joint disease, and 8 with genitourinary tuberculosis. In a series of cases of primary tuberculosis in adults, Stead[565] included 11 adolescents, 5 with simple primary tuberculosis, 5 with pleurisy and effusion, and 1 with progressive pulmonary tuberculosis.

From the extensive clinical experience of Lincoln and Sewell[331] and others, several observations emerge. Tuberculosis infection in early infancy rarely leads to pulmonary tuberculosis in adolescence, perhaps because it has several years in which to heal, whereas tuberculosis infection acquired after 7 years of age and, in particular, acquired after 10 years of age is likely to progress. When M. tuberculosis is acquired during adolescence, chronic pulmonary tuberculosis may develop within 1 to 3 years. Moreover, the risk of acquiring pulmonary tuberculosis is two to six times greater for adolescent girls than for adolescent boys. In both sexes, the adolescent growth spurt is the time of greatest risk. The work of Johnston[268] suggests that the depressant effect of puberty on calcium and nitrogen retention, at least in girls, may be correlated with the failure of tuberculosis infection to heal.

Tuberculosis and Pregnancy

In the era before chemotherapy, whether pregnancy and tuberculosis affected each other adversely was an ongoing controversy. Since the advent of chemotherapy, however, the prognosis has improved greatly.[177] The main problems now are serious unrecognized tuberculosis in a pregnant woman, sometimes with a fatal outcome, and serious unrecognized disease in her infant. Another problem is whether pregnancy influences the risk of progression of tuberculosis infection to disease; the data are conflicting in this regard. Tuberculin skin testing probably is valid during pregnancy; chest radiographs (with shielding) should be obtained for all tuberculin-positive pregnant patients. Therapy, when indi-

cated, can safely include isoniazid (which crosses the placenta but apparently without ill effects), rifampin, and ethambutol. The safety of pyrazinamide in pregnancy has not been established, but a growing number of experts recommend it because anecdotal data have not shown it to be harmful to the mother or fetus. Streptomycin, because of fetal ototoxicity, is not recommended.[544] However, one study of seven pregnant women with multidrug-resistant tuberculosis showed no adverse effects on their newborns when mothers were treated with second-line drugs, including aminoglycosides.[150,521] Should a mother receiving antituberculosis therapy breast-feed?[545] It is probably safe for her to do so because the drugs, although found in milk, are present only in small amounts.

Tuberculosis and Human Immunodeficiency Virus Infection

In adults infected with both HIV and *M. tuberculosis*, the rate of progression from asymptomatic infection to disease is increased greatly.[491] The clinical manifestations of tuberculosis in HIV-infected adults are typical when the CD4+ cell count is higher than 500/mm^3. As the CD4+ cell count falls, manifestations become "atypical." Extrapulmonary foci occur in as many as 60 percent of profoundly immunocompromised patients.[27] Pulmonary cavities are rare findings; lower lobe infiltrates or nodules often accompanied by thoracic adenopathy are common occurrences, especially if the patient's tuberculosis infection is recent. Of course, many patients have a nonreactive tuberculin skin test. Sputum is less likely to be produced or to contain visible acid-fast organisms on stained smears; more invasive procedures, such as bronchoscopy, often are required to isolate *M. tuberculosis* and to rule out other causes of opportunistic lung disease.[361] Malabsorption of antituberculosis drugs in HIV-infected patients can lead to prolonged symptoms and disease.[446]

When tuberculosis develops in HIV-infected children, the clinical features tend to be fairly typical of childhood tuberculosis in immunocompetent children, although the disease often progresses more rapidly and the clinical manifestations are more severe.[53,97,105,164,289,395,434,598] Many children have sizeable pulmonary radiographic findings with minimal respiratory signs or symptoms. An increased tendency for extrapulmonary disease may be noted. Recurrent disease occurs more frequently in HIV-infected children.[497] Establishing the diagnosis can be very difficult; a diligent search for an infectious adult in the child's environment may yield the best clues to the correct diagnosis.[293] The prognosis generally is good if tuberculosis disease is not far advanced when the patient is diagnosed and appropriate antituberculosis drugs are available.[218]

The introduction of highly active antiretroviral therapy (HAART) into regions where tuberculosis is prevalent has had a profound effect on the epidemiology and clinical expression of both diseases. During the initial months of HAART, immune reconstitution can be complicated by adverse clinical phenomena in which either previously subclinical infections are "unmasked" or preexisting, partly treated opportunistic infections clinically deteriorate. These phenomena are referred to as the immune reconstitution inflammatory syndrome (IRIS).[555] Sometimes it is difficult to tell if a deterioration in the clinical course of a patient with an opportunistic infection who is started on HAART is due to IRIS, poor compliance with treatment for the opportunistic infection, or drug resistance.[314-316] Factors to be considered that suggest IRIS are temporal association (within 3 months of starting HAART), unusual clinical manifestations, unexpected clinical course, exclusion of alternative explanations, evidence of preceding immune restoration (rise in CD4 lymphocyte count), and fall in HIV viral load. In adults, the risk of developing IRIS in patients with tuberculosis who are started on HAART is greatest if they have extrapulmonary tuberculosis, high initial HIV viral loads and low CD4 lymphocyte counts, and rapid response to HAART.[54] Published reports of IRIS in children have been rare,[274,403,456,649] although anecdotal evidence from pediatric acquired immune deficiency clinics in Africa suggest it is becoming common as HAART is introduced to more children with HIV infection. IRIS in children has been associated with nontuberculous mycobacteria[456] and previous BCG vaccination.[299,455,523] The finding that IRIS occurs in children with tuberculosis and HIV infection who receive HAART is not surprising. For decades, so-called paradoxical reactions have been described in HIV-uninfected children with tuberculosis after antituberculosis therapy is started. The most common manifestations are fever, enlarging lymph nodes in the thorax or neck, and appearance or enlargement of tuberculomas in the brain, with or without accompanying meningitis.

The best management of IRIS is unknown. As with paradoxical reactions that cause tissue damage or obstruction, corticosteroids may be beneficial to "quiet" the local immune response, although no randomized clinical trials have been reported. The high frequency of IRIS associated with tuberculosis has led some experts to recommend delay of HAART until appropriate (for drug susceptibility pattern) antituberculosis chemotherapy has been given for at least 2 months.[324] No consensus on this approach has been reached, however, and data from children may indicate that they are more likely to die of complications of HIV than of tuberculosis when they are dually infected.[218]

DIAGNOSIS

HOW CHILDREN WITH TUBERCULOSIS ARE DISCOVERED

In the developing world, the only way that children with tuberculosis disease are discovered is passively, when they have a profound illness that is consistent with one manifestation of tuberculosis. Having an ill adult contact is an obvious clue to establishment of the correct diagnosis. The only available laboratory test usually is an acid-fast smear of sputum, which the child rarely produces. In many regions, chest radiography is not available. To aid in establishing the diagnosis, a variety of scoring systems based on available tests, clinical signs and symptoms, and known exposures have been devised.[379,638] However, no single clinical scoring system has been validated, and the sensitivity and specificity of these systems can be very low and lead to both overdiagnosis and underdiagnosis of tuberculosis.[288,379]

In industrial countries, children with tuberculosis usually are discovered in one of two ways.[148,291,492] Obviously, one way is to consider tuberculosis as the cause of a symptomatic illness.[485] Discovering an adult contact with infectious tuberculosis is an invaluable aid to establishing the diagnosis; the "yield" from a contact investigation usually is higher than that from cultures from the child.[36] Culture from the infectious adult case may yield the only drug susceptibility results for the child because cultures from children with tuberculosis frequently are negative. The second way is to discover a child with pulmonary tuberculosis during the contact investigation of an adult with tuberculosis.[362,388,547,576,579] Typically, the affected child has few or no symptoms, but investigation reveals a positive tuberculin skin test result and an abnormal chest radiograph. In some areas of the United States, as many as 50 percent of children with pulmonary tuberculosis are discovered in this manner, before significant symptoms have begun. The recent use of molecular epidemiology techniques has shown, however, occasional discordance between the isolate from the child and that from the presumed source, meaning that the real source of transmission to the child is undiscovered.[642,648] It is less common to find tuberculosis disease in a U.S.-born child as the result of a community-or school-based tuberculin skin testing program, although foreign-born children with tuberculosis may be found in this manner.[149,444]

TUBERCULIN SENSITIVITY AND THE SKIN TEST

Sensitization to tuberculin is induced by infection with living tubercle bacilli. Specific tuberculin sensitivity to either *M. tuberculosis* or other mycobacteria can be transferred in humans by injection of lymphocytes from sensitized donors and also by injection of certain purified mycobacterial protein antigens.

The time of appearance of sensitivity in animals after infection has occurred with tubercle bacilli depends on the number of tubercle bacilli in the infective dose and on the virulence (i.e., the rate of multiplication of the organisms), and such is also likely to be the case in humans.[28] For all practical purposes in humans, tuberculin reactivity seems to appear in 3 to 6 weeks, rarely a few days earlier, and occasionally as long as 3 months after initial infection.

The tuberculin sensitivity reaction has been studied best in the skin, although it can be elicited in any tissue of a sensitive subject (conjunctiva, lung, meninges, kidney, and so on) after tuberculoprotein has been injected. At first, an inflammatory reaction appears at the site of injection, with predominance of segmented neutrophils, followed by immigration of macrophages and T lymphocytes, until the entire area of induration consists of mononuclear cells.

The size of the induration depends on the amount of tuberculoprotein injected and the availability of sensitized T lymphocytes in sufficient number. Multiple tuberculin skin tests given simultaneously result in smaller individual reactions, probably because of a finite number of sensitized cells in the body. Corticosteroids,[55,346,499] adrenocorticotropic hormone, nitrogen mustard, irradiation, and viral infections such as measles, influenza, and mumps diminish tuberculin reactivity, perhaps simply by inducing lymphopenia.[561] The size of the induration seems to depend on at least two additional factors: the local behavior of the skin (the disappearance time for wheals of normal saline solution, the so-called Aldrich-McClure test, is accelerated during fever, pregnancy, cachexia, and extreme malnutrition) and the number of actively multiplying tubercle bacilli in the body, which can be demonstrated in animals and probably in humans as well. That still other factors must be involved is clear because 10 to 20 percent of immunocompetent patients with proven tuberculosis are tuberculin-negative during initial disease, with tuberculin sensitivity often regained during treatment.[450] Decreased T-lymphocyte blastogenesis has been demonstrated in some cases, and inhibition by B lymphocytes may play a role.

Temporary desensitization to tuberculin occurs most strikingly during measles and has been studied carefully. Full reactivity diminished during the incubation period and returned within approximately 1 month after appearance of the exanthem.[215] Influenza and administration of influenza and measles vaccines tend to depress sensitivity but rarely suppress it entirely.[64,657] Whether other viral diseases and vaccines regularly are less active in this regard and what the important factors may be are not known.[39] If a temporary desensitizing effect occurs in bacterial infections such as scarlet fever, it probably depends on factors such as hyperthermia and dehydration.

Sensitization to tuberculin as a result of infection with *M. tuberculosis* tends to persist undiminished for life.[161,207,235] The likelihood of disappearance of tuberculin sensitivity seems to be greater when the lesion is negligible. That low degrees of sensitivity to *M. tuberculosis* are induced by mycobacteria other than *M. tuberculosis* also is clear. Previous receipt of BCG vaccine can cause increased reactivity to tuberculin, but the association is weaker than many clinicians suspect.[9,78,339,396,510] Less than 50 percent of infants given BCG vaccination have a reactive tuberculin skin test at 9 to 12 months of age, and the great majority will have a nonreactive skin test by the time they are 5 years of age. Older children and adults who receive BCG vaccination have a reactive skin test and keep it longer, but by 10 to 15 years after vaccination, most individuals have lost tuberculin skin test reactivity.[114,378] Repeated administration of BCG vaccine can maintain tuberculin reactivity.[249] Repeated tuberculin skin tests in a person sensitized previously by BCG vaccination, infection with *M. tuberculosis*, or probably infection by an environmental mycobacterium may increase the reaction to subsequent tuberculin skin tests (called the booster phenomenon).[41,182,509,599]

The antigens currently used in tuberculin testing are crude extracts consisting of a mixture of many antigens, some species-specific, some shared among many species. Standardized, isolated, purified mycobacterial antigens are needed in clinical practice. The major antigen used in tuberculin testing is PPD, obtained from filtrates of heat-killed tubercle bacilli. Batch 49608, prepared by Dr. Florence Seibert in 1939, was designated by the WHO as the international standard tuberculin, the only one to be called PPD-S. All other PPD preparations are referred to simply as PPD or as PPD-T. However, each batch now must be stabilized with Tween 80 at 5 ppm to minimize adherence to glass and plastic and must be identified by manufacturer and lot number.

A tuberculin unit is the activity contained in a specified weight of PPD-S. The standard test dose, 5 tuberculin units, refers to the equivalence in biologic activity, determined in the guinea pig, of a commercial PPD preparation with that contained in 5 tuberculin units of PPD-S. Products labeled 1 tuberculin unit and 250 tuberculin units are calculated dilutions based on 5 tuberculin units. However, the potency of PPD doses varies from batch to batch.

The Mantoux test is the reference test. A graduated syringe and a 26- or 27-gauge needle are used to inject 0.1 mL of PPD into the most superficial layer of the epidermis of the forearm, which raises an immediate wheal (Fig. 107–14). Under optimal circumstances, the needle should not be withdrawn for a few seconds to minimize leakage. The reference test uses a dose of 5 tuberculin units. One tuberculin unit very rarely should be used, for example, if extreme hypersensitivity is suspected, as when a tuberculous eye lesion or erythema nodosum is present. The reading should be made at 48 to 72 hours, with the forearm slightly flexed. Any induration (not erythema) should be measured, preferably with calipers, and the diameter at right angles to the axis of administration recorded in millimeters. Use of the words "negative" and "positive" should be avoided because interpretation can change as more epidemiologic information becomes known. The previous widespread use of multiple-puncture tests led to the practice of allowing parents to interpret the results and to report them to the clinician. This practice assumes parental knowledge of and adherence to a broad range of motivational behavior and skills. No study has demonstrated that parents can read positive skin test results accurately, but that they may not correctly interpret or report positive results has been well documented.[101,102,199,233] Two studies have demonstrated that pediatric care providers tend to under-read Mantoux tuberculin skin tests.[77,285]

Several studies have shown great variability in readings of Mantoux tests.[33] Such variability can be minimized only by ongoing training of both testers and readers and by concentrating the responsibility of testing and reading to a small number of trained individuals.

The importance of the tuberculin test cannot be overemphasized as the main criterion for diagnosis of tuberculosis infection in an individual child. Only rarely is the tuberculin test response negative in an infected child, usually as a result of anergy from overwhelming infection, from viral infection, from HIV infection, from the use of immunosuppressive drugs, or because of factors not yet understood.[571] Anergy in tuberculosis can be selective for tuberculin; results of "control" skin tests may be positive but the Mantoux test result negative in a child with tuberculosis disease.[563]

The Mantoux test has a sensitivity and specificity of only approximately 95 percent.[239] When a test with these characteristics is applied to a population with a 90 percent prevalence of tuberculosis infection, the positive predictive value of the skin test is 99 percent, an excellent result. However, if the same test is applied to a population with only a 1 percent prevalence of infection, the positive predictive value drops to 15 percent; 85 percent of the "positive" results are false-positives created by biologic variability, nonspecific reactions, and infection with environmental mycobacteria. These false-positive results lead to unnecessary treatment, cost, and anxiety for the patient, family, and clinician. In short, the low sensitivity and specificity of the tuberculin skin test render the test undesirable for use in persons from low-prevalence groups. The trend in the United States is to reduce or to eliminate routine testing of low-risk children but to target children with specific risk factors for one-time or periodic tuberculosis skin testing.[10,90,389]

Several recently published studies have shown that a questionnaire can be used in the United States to identify children with significant risk factors for tuberculosis infection, who then can receive a tuberculin skin test.[183,337,430,483] Factors that consistently correlate with having a positive tuberculin skin test result include contact with a case of tuberculosis, other family members with a positive tuberculin skin test result, and foreign birth in or extensive travel to a high-prevalence country.[502]

The CDC and the American Academy of Pediatrics (AAP) have recommended varying the size of induration considered positive in various groups, according to their risk factors (Table 107–7), in an attempt to minimize the incidence of false-negative results in children most likely to have rapid progression of asymptomatic tuberculosis infection to disease and the false-positive results in persons with no known risk factors for tuberculosis. In general in the United States, previous receipt of BCG vaccine should not influence interpretation of the initial tuberculin skin test of a child.[267]

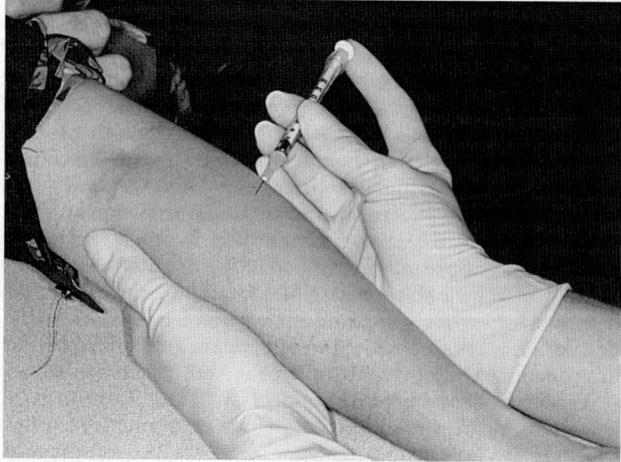

Figure 107–14 A useful technique for performing a Mantoux tuberculin skin test on a child. The needle is applied perpendicular to the long axis of the arm to attain better control.

INTERFERON RELEASE ASSAYS

Advances in molecular biology and genomics have led to use of alternatives to the tuberculin skin test.[432,472,554] Two new in vitro formats have been developed that measure interferon-γ release by sensitized lymphocytes after stimulation by *M. tuberculosis*

TABLE 107–7 Amount of Induration in Reaction to a Mantoux Tuberculin Skin Test Considered Positive (Indicating Probable Infection with *Mycobacterium tuberculosis*)

Reaction Size	Risk Factors
≥5 mm	Contact with infectious cases
	Abnormal chest radiograph
	HIV infection or other immunocompromise
≥10 mm	Birth or previous residence in a high-prevalence country
	Residence in long-term care or corrections facility
	Certain medical risk factors: diabetes mellitus, silicosis, renal disease
	Occupation in health care field, exposure to patients with tuberculosis
	Member of a local high-risk group
	Close contact with a high-risk adult (except health care workers)
	Age <4 years
≥15 mm	No risk factors

antigens. Both formats use two proteins—early secreted antigen target 6 and culture filtrate protein—that are found on *M. tuberculosis* and only a few fairly rare species of nontuberculous mycobacteria but not on the bacilli BCG or the *Mycobacterium avium* complex. The first test licensed in the United States was QuantiFERON-TB (Cellestis, Carnegie, Australia). The test measures whole-blood interferon production.

The second format licensed in the United States is the enzyme-linked immunospot (ELISPOT, T-SPOT.TB; Oxford Immunotec, Oxford, UK). This technique measures the number of mononuclear cells that produce interferon.

Both formats of interferon release assays have been studied primarily in adults.[432,472] In many clinical situations, these tests have a higher specificity than that of the tuberculin skin test, better correlation with surrogate measures of recent exposure to *M. tuberculosis* in low-incidence settings, and less cross-reactivity than does the tuberculin skin test because of previous BCG vaccination. Like the tuberculin skin test, interferon release assays cannot differentiate between tuberculosis infection and disease. Two clear advantages of the interferon release assays are the need for only one patient encounter (versus two with the tuberculin skin test) and the lack of possible boosting of the result, as the patient is not exposed to any biologic material.

Studies of interferon release assays in children are fewer for both ELISPOT[221,222,548] and QuantiFERON-TB.[22,117,173,606] Studies of child household contacts of adults with pulmonary tuberculosis have shown that children who previously received a BCG vaccination were more likely to have a positive tuberculin skin test result but a negative ELISPOT result.[173] A study from the Gambia showed an 83 percent agreement between tuberculin skin test and ELISPOT results in child household contacts, with a nonsignificant trend toward the ELISPOT being less sensitive than the tuberculin skin test.[25] In this study, previous BCG vaccination did not significantly affect the results of either test.

Although interferon release assays are becoming widely used[433] and are recommended by the CDC,[83] studies in adults have questioned their sensitivity even in patients with tuberculosis disease. At present, although the interferon release assays show great promise for improving the diagnosis of tuberculosis infection, too little is known about their characteristics in young children and immunocompromised hosts for their routine use to be recommended in these groups.

DIAGNOSTIC MYCOBACTERIOLOGY IN CHILDREN[487]

The demonstration of acid-fast bacilli in stained smears of sputum is presumptive evidence of pulmonary tuberculosis in most patients. However, in children, tubercle bacilli usually are relatively few in number. Gastric washings, which often are used in lieu of sputum, can be contaminated with acid-fast organisms from the mouth. However, fluorescence microscopy of gastric washings has been found to be useful, particularly in a setting where malnutrition and tuberculin-negative tuberculosis are rampant.[313] Tubercle bacilli in cerebrospinal fluid, pleural fluid, lymph node aspirate, and urine are sparse; thus, only rarely are direct-stained smears for tubercle bacilli of any use in pediatric practice.[573] Cultures for tubercle bacilli are of great importance, not only to confirm the diagnosis but increasingly to permit testing for drug susceptibility. If culture and drug susceptibility data are available from the associated adult case and the child has classic features of tuberculosis (positive skin test result, consistent abnormal chest radiograph), obtaining cultures from the child adds little to management.

Painstaking collection of specimens is essential for diagnosis of children because fewer organisms usually are present than in adults.[522] Gastric lavage should be performed in the very early morning, when the patient has had nothing to eat or drink for 8 hours and before the patient has a chance to wake up and start swallowing saliva, which could dilute the bronchial secretions that were brought up during the night and made their way into the stomach. The stomach contents should be aspirated first. Then, no more than 50 to 75 mL of sterile distilled water (not saline) should be injected through the stomach tube and the aspirate added to the first collection. The gastric acidity (poorly tolerated by tubercle bacilli) should be neutralized immediately. Concentration and culture should be performed as soon as possible after collection. However, even with optimal, in-hospital collection of three early-morning gastric aspirate samples, *M. tuberculosis* can be isolated from only 30 to 40 percent of children and 70 percent of infants with pulmonary tuberculosis.[69,563,613]

Bronchial secretions (sputum) produced by stimulation of a cough with an aerosol solution can be obtained commonly from older children.[76] The aerosol is heated in a nebulizer at 46° C to 52° C (114.8° F to 125.6° F) and administered to the patient for 15 to 30 minutes. This method gives good results and may be superior to gastric lavage both in yield of positive cultures and in acceptance by the patient.[76,517] Recent improvements in technique have led to improved induction of sputum in even young children, with culture yields as high as from inpatient gastric aspirates.[252,650] Nasopharyngeal aspiration also has been used.[429] The bronchial aspirate obtained at bronchoscopy often is thick, and the laboratory will process it with a mucolytic agent such as N-acetyl-L-cysteine. In most studies, the yield of *M. tuberculosis* from bronchoscopy specimens has been lower than from properly obtained gastric aspirates.[1,96]

Cerebrospinal fluid, pleural fluid, and synovial fluid (as much fluid as possible should be collected) usually are centrifuged, and the sediment is used for stained smear and culture. An overnight urine specimen should be obtained in the early morning and taken immediately to the laboratory for processing because the organisms tolerate the low pH of urine poorly. Lymph node aspirates and bits of biopsy tissue can be inoculated directly into a fluid medium such as Middlebrook 7H9.

Staining and examination of smears as well as inoculation of special media, incubation in a carbon dioxide environment, strain differentiation based on many cultural characteristics, and drug susceptibility testing require equipment, skills, and experience beyond those available in the usual clinic or hospital laboratory.[217] Thus, most laboratories depend on regional or reference laboratories for procedures beyond their scope.

Despite an enormous amount of research and thousands of publications on the subject, the only definite way to diagnose active tuberculosis is to demonstrate tubercle bacilli in tissues or secretions. No single species–specific antigen of *M. tuberculosis* ever has been identified. The search for quick, simple, inexpensive, specific, sensitive immunologic and chemical detection techniques is ongoing.

NUCLEIC ACID AMPLIFICATION

The main form of nucleic acid amplification studied in children with tuberculosis is polymerase chain reaction (PCR), which uses specific DNA sequences as markers for microorganisms.[163,352,390] Various PCR techniques, most using the mycobacterial insertion element IS6110 as the DNA marker for *M. tuberculosis* complex organisms,[11,81] have a sensitivity and specificity of more than 90 percent in comparison to sputum culture for detecting pulmonary tuberculosis in adults. However, test performance varies even among reference laboratories.[417,501] The test is relatively expensive, calls for fairly sophisticated equipment, and requires scrupulous technique to avoid cross-contamination of specimens. In the United States, it is approved for use only on acid-fast stain–positive specimens.

Evaluation of PCR in childhood tuberculosis has been limited. Compared with a clinical diagnosis of pulmonary tuberculosis in children, the sensitivity of PCR has varied from 25 to 83 percent, and specificity has varied from 80 to 100 percent.[133,390,440,451,533] PCR of gastric aspirates may be positive in a recently infected child even when the chest radiograph is normal, thus demonstrating the occasional arbitrariness of the distinction between tuberculosis infection and disease in children. PCR may have a useful but limited role in evaluating children for tuberculosis. A negative PCR analysis never eliminates tuberculosis as a diagnostic possibility, and a positive result does not confirm it. The major use of PCR will be in evaluating children with significant pulmonary disease when the diagnosis is not established readily by clinical or epidemiologic grounds. PCR may be particularly helpful in evaluating immunocompromised children with pulmonary disease, especially those with HIV infection, although published reports of its performance in such children are lacking. PCR also may aid in confirming the diagnosis of extrapulmonary tuberculosis, but only a few reports have been published.[194,351,383]

SEROLOGY AND ANTIGEN DETECTION

Despite hundreds of studies published during the past century, serology has found little place in the routine diagnosis of tuberculosis in adults or children.[125] Some studies have used enzyme-linked immunosorbent assay to detect antibodies to whole bacterial cells or to various purified or complex antigens of *M. tuberculosis* in children.[125,271,272] In general, both the sensitivity and specificity of the various tests have been unacceptably low.[42,245] Tests using the mycobacterial antigen A60 have shown both good and poor results in children.[131] No available serodiagnostic test for tuberculosis is adequate under various clinical conditions to be useful for children.

Detection of mycobacterial antigen has been evaluated in clinical samples from adults but rarely from children.[481] Most of these techniques require technically advanced equipment (such as high-pressure liquid chromatography apparatus) and expertise that are not available where tuberculosis in children is common.

TREATMENT

MANAGEMENT OF TUBERCULOUS CHILDREN

Treatment of cavitary tuberculosis in adults is one of the most scientifically accurate areas in all of medicine and one of the finest examples of international professional cooperation in all of history. Because tubercle bacilli in adult patients with tuberculosis can be seen and cultured, their numbers quantified, and the size of the cavities that they produce measured and because so many cases of tuberculosis exist in the world, researchers have been able to ask precise questions about treatment and to design prospective cooperative studies that yield accurate answers about the effect of individual drugs, multiple drug regimens, drug dosage, duration of chemotherapy, rest, and surgical procedures on the course of the disease. Although chemotherapy, without doubt, has been extremely effective in treating childhood tuberculosis, recommendations for treatment historically have been based to a great extent on analogy with adults, on "custom," and on "experience" because in children the tubercle bacilli are fewer in number and not readily accessible and the lesions are not as easy to evaluate as are cavities. However, during the past 3 decades, a large number of treatment trials for children have been reported, which has led to dramatic changes in the therapeutic approach to childhood tuberculosis.

As recently as the early 1980s, the recommended treatment duration for children with tuberculosis disease was 12 to 18 months. Although these regimens are effective when they are used properly, actual failure rates are high because of poor adherence during the long period of treatment. Newer regimens often are called short-course chemotherapy because treatment durations as short as 6 months are routinely successful. However, the key to the new approach is not the short duration but the intensive initial therapy with three or more antituberculosis drugs.

Antituberculosis Drugs (Tables 107–8 and 107–9)

Isoniazid (INH) is the mainstay of therapy for tuberculosis in children. Inexpensive, highly effective in preventing the multiplication of tubercle bacilli, of low molecular weight and therefore readily diffusible to all tissues in the body,[141] and relatively nontoxic to children, INH is one of the most nearly perfect drugs in the pediatrician's armamentarium. It can be administered orally, intramuscularly, or intravenously. When INH is taken orally, high plasma, sputum, and spinal fluid levels are reached within a few hours and persist for at least 6 to 8 hours.[310,425] Because of the slow multiplication of *M. tuberculosis*, the total daily dose can be given at one time. The usual level necessary to inhibit multiplication of tubercle bacilli is 0.02 to 0.05 μg/mL.

Human variation in the acetylation rate of INH to an inactive compound is known to be determined genetically.[365] Rapid acetylation occurs more frequently in black people and Asians than in whites. Although a simple method, specifically the use of a urine sample, now is available for classifying patients as slow or rapid inactivators of INH, the normal way of coping with the problem in children has been to give a sufficiently large dose of INH to ensure an adequate level even in rapid inactivators.[364,623]

The principal toxic effects of INH are peripheral neuritis and hepatitis. Peripheral neuritis resulting from competitive inhibition of pyridoxine utilization is a rare event in North American children because both milk and meat are the main dietary sources of pyridoxine.[48] In some well-nourished children, serum pyridoxine concentrations are depressed by INH, but clinical signs are not apparent.[445] In the case of most children, therefore, the use of supplementary pyridoxine is not necessary. However, in teenagers whose diets may be inadequate, in children from ethnic groups with low milk and meat intake, and in breast-fed babies,

TABLE 107-8 Commonly Used Drugs for the Treatment of Tuberculosis in Children

Drug	Dosage Forms	Daily Dose (mg/kg/day)	Twice-Weekly Dose (mg/kg/dose)	Maximal Daily Dose
Ethambutol	Tablets 100 mg 400 mg	20-25	50	2.5 g
Isoniazid*†	Scored tablets 100 mg 300 mg Syrup‡ 10 mg/mL	10-15†	20-30	Daily: 300 mg Twice weekly: 900 mg
Pyrazinamide	Scored tablets 500 mg	20-40	50	2 g
Rifampin*	Capsules 150 mg 300 mg Syrup Formulated in syrup from capsules	10-20	10-20	Daily: 600 mg Twice weekly: 900 mg
Streptomycin (IM administration)	Vials 1 g 4 g	20-40	20-40	

*Rifamate is a capsule containing 150 mg of isoniazid and 300 mg of rifampin. Two capsules provide the usual adult (>50 kg body weight) daily doses of each drug.
†When isoniazid is used in combination with rifampin, the incidence of hepatotoxicity increases if the isoniazid dose exceeds 10 mg/kg/day.
‡Most experts advise against the use of isoniazid syrup because of instability and a high rate of gastrointestinal adverse reaction (diarrhea, cramps).

TABLE 107-9 Drugs for Treatment of Drug-Resistant Tuberculosis in Children

Drugs	Dosage Forms	Daily Dosage (mg/kg/day)	Maximum Daily Dose
Capreomycin	Vials: 1 g	15-30 (IM)	1 g
Ciprofloxacin	Tablets 250 mg 500 mg 750 mg	Adults: 500-1500 mg in 2 divided doses	1.5 g
Clofazimine	Capsules 50 mg 100 mg	50-100 mg/day	200 mg
Cycloserine	Capsules 250 mg	10-20	1 g
Ethionamide	Tablets 250 mg	15-20 given in 2 or 3 divided doses	1 g
Kanamycin	Vials 75 mg/2 mL 500 mg/2 mL 1 g/3 mL	15-30 (IM)	1 g
Levofloxacin	Tablets 250 mg 500 mg 750 mg	Adults: 500-750 mg total/day	750 mg
p-Aminosalicylic acid	Packets: 4 g	200-300 given in 2 to 4 divided doses	12 g

pyridoxine supplementation (25 to 50 mg/day) is important. Peripheral neuritis, when it does occur, usually is manifested by "pins and needles" sensations in the hands and feet.

The risk for development of hepatotoxicity from INH, rare in children, increases in frequency with age.[34,80,298,333,402,422,459,551,566] Its cause is unclear.[300] Rapid acetylators are no more susceptible than are slow acetylators.[165,364] Simultaneous use of alcohol, phenytoin, piperazine, and especially rifampin (RIF) seems to increase the likelihood of hepatotoxicity.[80,304] Monitoring of aspartate aminotransferase and alanine aminotransferase activity sometimes reveals transient increases during treatment with INH, but the levels usually return spontaneously to normal without interruption of treatment. Liver enzyme abnormalities in adolescents receiving INH are common occurrences and usually disappear spontaneously, but severe hepatitis can occur.[184,334,436,539,617]

The possible occurrence of hepatitis raises the question of routine monitoring of liver enzyme levels once a month in all children receiving INH. The advantage of doing so has to be weighed not only against the expense but particularly against the difficulty of ensuring regular monthly visits if the patient and parents know that every clinic visit entails a venipuncture. Most experts prefer to substitute routine questions about appetite and well-being, determination of weight, and a check of the appearance of the sclera and the size of the liver.[70,444] Patients should be counseled to stop taking INH and to contact the clinician immediately if significant nausea, vomiting, abdominal pain, or jaundice occurs during the use of INH.

Allergic manifestations of INH hypersensitivity are extraordinarily rare. Convulsions have been reported after doses of 100 mg/kg or more, as in suicide attempts.[369,415,437,513]

The usual dosage in children is 10 to 20 mg/kg/day, to a maximum of 300 mg/day. INH is available in tablets of 100 and 300 mg. The original liquid preparation of INH in syrup was abandoned when investigators found that the drug was unstable in sucrose. A syrup of INH in sorbitol (10 mg/mL) is now on the market and appears to be satisfactory; however, it is unstable at 37° C (98.6° F) and should be kept cool. Significant gastrointestinal intolerance (nausea, diarrhea) develops in many children while they are taking the INH suspension. If tablets are used, they are crushed easily in a dessert spoon, to which then is added in the same spoon a vehicle such as applesauce, mashed banana, thawed undil frozen orange juice, or another palatable medium. The crushed tablets must never be added to the nursing bottle or offered in milk or water because they will be ingested only partially. If INH is given concurrently with RIF, the dose should not exceed 10 mg/kg/day.[422] If the intramuscular form is used, for example, in a child with meningitis who is vomiting, the daily dose is the same as the daily oral dose but usually is divided and given every 8 to 12 hours. INH can interact with several other drugs, particularly theophylline, and the dosage of each may need to be modified in a patient taking several drugs.[25] INH also can increase serum phenytoin levels by blocking its metabolism in the liver, thereby leading to toxicity.[382]

RIF is a semisynthetic drug derived from *Streptomyces mediterranei*. Active against a wide variety of both intracellular and extracellular organisms, it is more effective against mycobacteria than is any other drug except INH. Most clinical isolates are susceptible to 5 μg/mL or less. The drug is absorbed readily from the gastrointestinal tract in the fasting state; peak serum levels of 6 to 10 μg/mL are achieved within 2 hours, and the drug is distributed widely in body fluids and tissues, including spinal fluid. Excretion is mainly through the biliary tract; however, effective levels are achieved in the kidneys and urine. In many patients receiving RIF treatment, tears, saliva, urine, and stool turn orange as the result of a harmless metabolite, but patients always must be warned in advance. Drawbacks include the relatively high cost of treatment; the rare occurrence of explosive hypersensitivity reactions with hemolytic anemia, which, however, usually accompany intermittent (separated by weeks or months) rather than daily RIF therapy[190]; the occasional occurrence of leukopenia or thrombocytopenia while the patient is taking daily RIF[200]; the fact that RIF can render birth control pills inactive when both are used (an alternative method of birth control must be used); and finally—most serious of all for children—a "therapeutic orphan" clause in the United States for children younger than 5 years, which also means that no formulation is commercially available for young children. However, RIF easily can be made into a suspension for use in children.

RIF should be used alone only in treating tuberculosis infection with an INH-resistant organism. If one uses INH, 20 mg/kg, and RIF, 15 to 20 mg/kg, the incidence of hepatotoxicity is appreciable. Therefore, when the two are used together, one would be wise to approximate INH, 10 mg/kg, and RIF, 15 to 20 mg/kg. Rifamate is a capsule containing both INH (150 mg) and RIF (300 mg). Two capsules supply the usual adult (more than 50 kg) daily dose of each drug. Rifamate may be appropriate for older children and adolescents.[3] Rifater contains INH, RIF, and pyrazinamide (PZA) together in one pill in varying concentrations. Rifapentine is a new rifamycin with a very long half-life. Pharmacokinetic studies have been performed in adolescents, but no data on its effectiveness in adolescents or children have been published.[363]

PZA contributes to the killing of *M. tuberculosis*, particularly at a low pH, such as within macrophages.[486] The exact mechanism of action of PZA is a subject of controversy. PZA has no effect on extracellular tubercle bacilli in vitro but clearly contributes to the killing of intracellular bacilli. Primary resistance is very rare, except that *Mycobacterium bovis* is resistant. The drug diffuses readily into all areas, including spinal fluid.[166] The usual adult daily dose is 30 to 40 mg/kg. The adult dose is tolerated well by children, results in high cerebrospinal fluid concentrations, and clearly is effective in therapy trials for tuberculosis in children.[144,478,489,556] However, serum concentrations are lower in children than in adults taking a weight equivalent dose.[197] PZA appears to exert its maximal effect during the first 2 months of therapy. Hepatotoxicity can occur at high doses but rarely does at the usual dose. PZA routinely causes an increase in serum uric acid concentration by inhibiting its excretion through the kidneys. Toxic reactions in adults include flushing, cutaneous hypersensitivity, arthralgia, and overt gout; however, the considerable experience with this drug in children in Latin American countries, Hong Kong, and the United States has revealed few problems. It plays a major role in intensive, short-course treatment regimens.[191,556]

Ethambutol (EMB) has been used for many years as a companion drug for INH in adults. The usual oral dose is 20 mg/kg/day.[142] At this dose, the drug primarily is bacteriostatic, its major role being to prevent the emergence of resistance to other drugs. However, at doses of 25 mg/kg/day or 50 mg/kg given twice a week, EMB has some bactericidal action.[118,185] Unfortunately, at these higher doses, optic neuritis or red-green color blindness has occurred in some adults. Regular visual field and color chart testing should detect these reversible effects early. The incidence of ophthalmologic toxicity in children is extremely low, if it occurs at all.[142] It is used frequently and safely in children with life-threatening forms of tuberculosis or who are at risk for drug-resistant tuberculosis.

Ethionamide is an effective and well-tolerated drug in children at a dose of 15 to 20 mg/kg/day divided into two or three doses given after meals. Children rarely complain about its sulfurous taste, which is repulsive to adults. Related to INH, it likewise diffuses readily into spinal fluid.[145,146,240] Ethionamide is used in cases of drug-resistant tuberculosis and tuberculous meningitis. Unfortunately, no convenient pediatric dosage form is available.

Streptomycin (STM) is used in conjunction with INH and RIF in life-threatening forms of tuberculosis. It is bactericidal and tolerated well in children in the usual dose of 20 to 40 mg/kg/day intramuscularly up to 1 g. Usually, STM can be discontinued within 1 to 3 months if clinical improvement is definite, whereas the other two or three drugs are continued by mouth.

p-Aminosalicylic acid, either the sodium or the potassium salt, formerly was part of the standard treatment of tuberculosis. However, it is a purely bacteriostatic drug that has been superseded by more powerful drugs (RIF, PZA). It is used only for the treatment of drug-resistant tuberculosis.

Other antituberculosis drugs that may be needed for patients whose mycobacteria are resistant to INH or RIF are the aminoglycosides kanamycin, amikacin, and capreomycin, each of which has a spectrum of activity that differs from that of STM with respect to individual mycobacterial strains. Cycloserine and viomycin are other drugs sometimes used in patients with multidrug resistance. Clofazimine[259] and rifabutin (related to RIF) are newer drugs that have antimycobacterial activity but have been used mainly in children who have AIDS and are suffering from *M. avium-intracellulare* infection. Clofazimine also is used for infection with *Mycobacterium leprae*.

Several of the fluoroquinolones, especially levofloxacin and ciprofloxacin, have significant antituberculosis activity,[287,387] but they cannot be used routinely in children because of the possible destruction of growing cartilage seen in animal models. However, the dire consequences of drug-resistant tuberculosis lead many experts to use them successfully and with little apparent toxicity in children with MDR-TB disease.[246]

TABLE 107–10 In Vivo Location of *Mycobacterium tuberculosis*: A Model

	Population Size	Metabolism and Replication	pH	Most Effective Drugs
Cavity	10^7–10^9	Active and rapid	Neutral or alkaline	INH, RIF, STM
Closed caseous lesions	10^5–10^7	Slow and intermittent	Neutral	RIF, INH
Within macrophages	10^4–10^6	Very slow	Acid	PZA, RIF, INH

INH, isoniazid; PZA, pyrazinamide; RIF, rifampin; STM, streptomycin.

Microbiologic Basis for Treatment[384,537]

Laboratory observations of *M. tuberculosis* and the results of clinical therapy trials have led to a hypothesis concerning the actions of various drugs and drug combinations.[157,200,384,385] The tubercle bacillus can be killed only during replication, which occurs in organisms that are active metabolically. In one model, bacilli in a host exist in different populations (Table 107–10). They are active metabolically and replicate freely where oxygen tension is high and the pH is neutral or alkaline. Environmental conditions for growth are best within cavities, and such conditions can lead to a large bacterial population. Adults with reactivation-type pulmonary tuberculosis usually have all three populations of tubercle bacilli. Children with pulmonary tuberculosis and patients of all ages with only extrapulmonary tuberculosis are infected with a much smaller number of tubercle bacilli because the cavitary population is not present.

Naturally occurring drug-resistant mutant organisms occur within large populations of tubercle bacilli even before chemotherapy is started. All known genetic loci for drug resistance in *M. tuberculosis* are located on the chromosome; no plasmid-mediated resistance is known. The rate of resistance within populations of organisms is related to the rate of mutations at these loci.[375,584,587,592,652,653] Although a large population of bacilli as a whole may be considered drug susceptible, a subpopulation of drug-resistant organisms occurs at a fairly predictable rate. The mean frequency of these drug-resistant mutants is about 10^{-6} but varies among drugs: STM, 10^{-5}; INH, 10^{-6}; and RIF, 10^{-7}.[124] A cavity containing 10^9 tubercle bacilli has thousands of single drug–resistant mutant organisms, whereas a closed caseous lesion contains few if any resistant mutants.

The two microbiologic properties of population size and drug resistance mutation explain why single antituberculosis drugs cannot cure cavitary tuberculosis.[370] In the mid-1940s, STM alone was given to adults with cavitary pulmonary tuberculosis.[338] Within 3 months, 80 percent of patients had significant numbers of STM-resistant organisms. This phenomenon has been observed for every antituberculosis drug developed subsequently. However, the natural occurrence of resistance to one drug is independent of resistance to any other drug because the resistance loci are not linked. The chance of having even one organism "naturally" resistant to two drugs is on the order of 10^{-11} to 10^{-13}. Populations of this size in patients are extremely rare, and mutants naturally resistant to two drugs are nonexistent.

The population size of tubercle bacilli within a patient determines the appropriate therapy. For patients with large bacterial populations (adults with cavities or extensive infiltrates), many single drug–resistant mutants are present, and at least two antituberculosis drugs must be used.[127] Conversely, for patients with tuberculosis infection but no disease, the bacterial population is small (about 10^3 to 10^4 organisms), drug-resistant mutants are rare findings, and a single drug can be used. Children with pulmonary tuberculosis and patients of all ages with extrapulmonary tuberculosis have medium-sized populations in which drug-resistant mutants may or may not be present. In general, these patients should be treated with at least two drugs.

Some antituberculosis drugs, such as INH, RIF, and STM, are bactericidal against *M. tuberculosis*. Other drugs, including ethionamide, *p*-aminosalicylic acid, and low-dose EMB, are bacteriostatic. The earliest treatment regimens for tuberculosis combined the killing action of a bactericidal drug with a bacteriostatic drug that would suppress replication of drug-resistant mutant organisms. A small number of organisms survived despite administration of chemotherapy, and 18 to 24 months of treatment was necessary to permit host defenses to eliminate persisting organisms. Despite the prolonged treatment period, relapse rates were 5 to 15 percent, mostly a result of poor adherence to treatment.

The availability of RIF and the rediscovery of PZA in the early 1970s effected radical change in antituberculosis chemotherapy. These two drugs have the most potent sterilizing action, the ability to kill tubercle bacilli within lesions as quickly as possible. The addition of RIF to INH for the treatment of pulmonary tuberculosis leads to cure rates approaching 100 percent with only 9 months of treatment. The further addition of PZA shortens the necessary treatment duration to only 6 months.

TREATMENT OF THE STAGES OF TUBERCULOSIS

EXPOSURE

Children exposed to potentially infectious adults with pulmonary tuberculosis should begin treatment, usually with INH only, if the child is younger than 5 years or has other risk factors for the rapid development of tuberculosis disease, such as immunocompromise of some kind.[576,643] Failure to do so may result in the development of severe tuberculosis disease even before the tuberculin skin test becomes reactive; the "incubation period" of disease may be shorter than that for the skin test. The child is treated for a minimum of 3 months after contact with the infectious case is broken (by physical separation or by effective treatment of the case). After 3 months, the tuberculin skin test is repeated. If the second test result is positive, infection is documented and INH should be continued for a total duration of 9 months; if the second skin test result is negative, treatment can be discontinued. If the exposure was to a person with an INH-resistant but RIF-susceptible isolate, RIF is the recommended treatment.

Two special circumstances of exposure deserve attention. A difficult situation arises when exposed children are anergic because of HIV infection. These children are particularly vulnerable to rapid progression of tuberculosis, and it will not be possible to determine whether infection has occurred. In general, these children should be treated as though they have tuberculosis infection.

The second situation is potential exposure of a newborn to a mother (or other adult) with a positive tuberculin skin test result or, rarely, a nursery worker with contagious tuberculosis.[324,570] Management is based on further evaluation of the mother:

1. *The mother has a normal chest radiograph:* no separation of the infant and mother is required. Although the mother should receive treatment of tuberculosis infection and other household members should be evaluated for tuberculosis infection or disease, the infant needs no further work-up or treatment unless a case of disease is found.

2. *The mother has an abnormal chest radiograph:* the mother and child should be separated until the mother has been evaluated thoroughly. If the radiograph, history, physical examination, and analysis of sputum reveal no evidence of pulmonary tuberculosis in the mother, a reasonable assumption is that the infant is at low risk of acquiring infection. The radiographic abnormality is due to another cause or a quiescent focus of previous tuberculosis infection. However, if the mother remains untreated, contagious tuberculosis may develop later, and the infant will be exposed. Both the mother and infant should receive appropriate follow-up care, but the infant does not need treatment. If the radiograph and clinical history are suggestive of pulmonary tuberculosis, the child and mother should remain separated until both have begun appropriate chemotherapy. The infant should be evaluated for congenital tuberculosis. The placenta should be examined. If the mother has no risk factors for drug-resistant tuberculosis, the infant should receive INH and close follow-up care. The infant should have a tuberculin skin test at 3 or 4 months after the mother is judged to be contagious no longer; evaluation of the infant at this time follows the guidelines for other exposure of children. If no infection is documented at this time, repeating the tuberculin skin test in 6 to 12 months would be prudent. If the mother has tuberculosis caused by a multidrug-resistant isolate of *M. tuberculosis* or she has poor adherence to therapy, the child should remain separated from her until she is no longer contagious or the infant can be given BCG vaccine and be kept separated until the vaccine "takes" (marked by a reactive tuberculin skin test).

INFECTION

The recommendation for treatment of asymptomatic tuberculin-positive individuals is based on data from several well-controlled studies; it applies particularly to children and adolescents who are at high risk for the development of overt disease but at very low risk for development of the main toxic manifestation of INH therapy, which is hepatitis.[147,176,410,422,541] The large, carefully controlled U.S. Public Health Study of 1955, followed by others both in this country and abroad, demonstrated the favorable effect of 12 months of INH on the incidence of complications as a result of both lymphohematogenous and pulmonary spread.[237] The younger the tuberculin reactor, the greater the benefit.[116]

The American Thoracic Society and CDC,[13] recommend that INH treatment of tuberculosis infection be given to the following groups:

1. Household members and other close associates of potentially infectious tuberculosis cases. All contacts of any age with a Mantoux tuberculin skin test reading of 5 mm or greater and without a documented history of reaction in the past should be considered recently infected and receive therapy.

2. Newly infected people, regardless of age, who have had a tuberculin skin test conversion within the past 2 years.

3. People with HIV infection or at risk for development of HIV infection who have a reaction of 5 mm or greater to a Mantoux test.

4. People of any age with tuberculosis in the past who received inadequate treatment.

5. People of any age with a significant tuberculin reaction and an abnormal but stable chest radiograph.

6. People with significant tuberculin reactions who have special clinical situations, including silicosis, diabetes mellitus, prolonged corticosteroid therapy, immunosuppressive therapy, hematologic malignant disease, and end-stage renal disease.

7. All children and adolescents with a "positive" tuberculin skin test reaction or interferon release assay result.

The question arises regarding how long the protective effect can be expected to last. Comstock and associates,[113] in their final report on INH prophylaxis in Alaska, demonstrated the protective effect of 1 year of chemoprophylaxis to be 19 years at least. Hsu[236] described 2494 patients monitored for up to 30 years and showed that adequate drug prophylaxis prevented reactivation of tuberculosis infection during adolescence and into young adulthood. It seems reasonable to hope that the decreased risk of active tuberculosis after INH prophylaxis may in fact be lifelong in individuals infected with INH-susceptible tubercle bacilli. Failure of INH after exposure to INH-resistant *M. tuberculosis* has been documented. No controlled study of an alternative regimen has been reported. RIF alone is recommended and widely used, although failures have been reported.[336]

The dosage of INH to be used has had little study. Most investigators have used a regimen based on 4 to 8 mg/kg of body weight per day, usually taken all at once, for a period of 6 to 12 months. A dose of 5 mg/kg/day was found satisfactory in one study.[115] Most clinicians prescribe a dose of 10 to 15 mg/kg/day to a total of 300 mg/day for treatment of infection to be sure of achieving therapeutic levels even in patients who inactivate the drug rapidly by acetylation.

The duration of INH treatment initially was set arbitrarily at 12 months.[251] A large trial comparing regimens of daily INH taken for 12, 24, and 52 weeks with placebo for their ability to prevent tuberculosis disease was conducted in eastern Europe with adults who had old fibrotic lesions caused by tuberculosis. Therapy for 1 year was most effective, especially if the patients were adherent. However, therapy for 24 weeks afforded a fairly high level of protection. A subsequent analysis concluded that the 24-week duration of preventive therapy was more cost-effective for adults than was the 52-week duration.[540] Subsequently, many health departments have accepted 6 months of INH preventive therapy as their standard regimen for adults. However, the cost-effectiveness analysis does not apply to children. A recent review of all published studies concluded that the effectiveness of INH therapy increased up to 9 months' duration, but no additional benefit was achieved with a longer duration.[13] A duration of 9 months is recommended for children and adults by the AAP and CDC.[13] INH is taken daily under self-supervision or can be taken twice weekly under directly observed therapy. When the child is infected with an INH-resistant but RIF-susceptible strain of *M. tuberculosis*, RIF should be substituted for INH and given for 6 months' duration. If the infecting strain is resistant to both INH and RIF, usually two other drugs are used; an expert in tuberculosis should be consulted in this situation.

A shorter duration of effective treatment for tuberculosis infection is highly desirable to improve compliance and effectiveness.[359] In England, a 3- to 4-month course of INH plus RIF is used frequently. There have been published case-control series, and a recent meta-analysis of available data suggests that especially when compliance is considered, a 3- to 4-month course of INH plus RIF may be as effective as is a 9-month course of INH.[169] One small, randomized study also yielded favorable results with this regimen.[549] However, this regimen is not yet recommended by the CDC, AAP, or WHO.

DISEASE IN ADULTS

A shorter duration of antituberculosis chemotherapy is desirable for several reasons: it may be significantly less expensive than traditional therapy; the patient is exposed to potentially toxic drugs for shorter periods of time; more time and resources can be allotted to ensure adherence with treatment; and if a patient absconds from treatment, a greater likelihood will exist that bacteriologic cure already has been achieved as a result of the early and rapid sterilizing activity of the newer regimens.

A 9-month regimen of INH and RIF cures more than 98 percent of cases of drug-susceptible pulmonary tuberculosis in adults.[528] Both drugs are given daily for the first 2 weeks to 2 months and then can be given daily or twice weekly under directly observed therapy for the remaining 7 to 8 months with equivalent results and rates of adverse reactions. When it is given twice weekly, the RIF dose is the same as the daily dose, but the INH dose is increased to 900 mg in adults. Twice-weekly administration is supported by pharmacologic and animal model data determining the area-under-the-curve characteristics for these antituberculosis drugs. Unfortunately, durations of therapy with only INH and RIF for less than 9 months are unacceptable because failure and relapse rates exceed 10 percent.

When three or more antituberculosis drugs are used initially, treatment durations of 6 months are routinely successful.[109] Regimens using INH, RIF, PZA, and STM during the initial phase (2 months), followed by INH and RIF in the continuation phase (4 months), routinely yield cure rates greater than 98 percent and relapse rates below 4 percent.[21,525] If PZA is excluded from the initial phase, the rate of bacteriologic failure rises to 7 to 10 percent.[229] However, exclusion of STM does not affect cure or relapse rates appreciably.[229,542] Use of PZA beyond the first 2 months of therapy does not add any benefit.[230] Regimens of 4 months' total duration have unacceptably high relapse rates of 10 percent or greater.[262] On the basis of all reported studies, the American Thoracic Society and CDC currently recommend for the treatment of pulmonary tuberculosis in adults a 6-month regimen using INH, RIF, PZA, and EMB for 2 months, followed by 4 months of daily or twice-weekly doses of INH and RIF.[51,88]

CHEMOTHERAPY FOR CHILDREN

Clinical trials of antituberculosis drugs in children are difficult to perform, mostly because of the difficulty in obtaining positive cultures at diagnosis or relapse and the need for long-term follow-up.[556] Historically, recommendations for treating children with tuberculosis have been extrapolated from clinical trials of adults with pulmonary tuberculosis.[535] However, during the past 2 decades, a large number of clinical trials involving only children have been reported. In 1983, Abernathy and colleagues[2] reported successful treatment of 50 children with tuberculosis in Arkansas using INH and RIF daily for 1 month, then twice weekly for 8 months. The success rate virtually was 100 percent. Most pulmonary infiltrates cleared by the end of therapy, but hilar adenopathy usually was still present radiographically and then gradually cleared during a period of 2 to 3 years. Patients with only hilar adenopathy can be treated successfully with INH and RIF for 6 months.[256,467]

Several major studies of 6-month therapy in children with at least three drugs in the initial phase have been reported.[7,47,247,302,583,596,605] The regimen used most commonly was 6 months of INH and RIF supplemented during the first 2 months with PZA. The overall success rate has been greater than 98 percent and the incidence of clinically significant adverse reactions less than 2 percent. Regimens not using STM were as successful as those that included it. Use of twice-weekly medications (under directly observed therapy) during the continuation phase was as effective and safe as was daily administration. Three studies used twice-weekly therapy throughout the treatment regimen

with excellent success.[302,596,622] The 6-month, three-drug regimen is successful, tolerated well, and less expensive.[574,607] It also effects a cure faster, so the likelihood of successful treatment is greater if the child becomes nonadherent later in therapy.

EXTRAPULMONARY TUBERCULOSIS

Controlled treatment trials for various forms of extrapulmonary tuberculosis are rare. In most reports, extrapulmonary cases have been combined with pulmonary cases and often are not analyzed separately. Several of the 6-month, three-drug trials in children included extrapulmonary cases.[47,302] Most non–life-threatening forms of extrapulmonary tuberculosis respond well to a 9-month course of INH and RIF[156,158] or to a 6-month regimen including INH, RIF, and PZA.[254] One exception may be bone and joint tuberculosis, which may have a high failure rate when 6-month chemotherapy is used, especially if surgical intervention has not occurred.[156] Tuberculous meningitis usually is not included in trials of extrapulmonary tuberculosis therapy because of its serious nature and low incidence. Treatment with INH and RIF for 12 months generally is effective.[626] In the 1950s, Lorber[340] treated children with tuberculous meningitis for only 6 months with good results. A more recent study from Thailand showed that a 6-month regimen that included PZA for serious tuberculous meningitis led to fewer deaths and better outcomes than did longer regimens that did not contain PZA.[257] Most children are treated initially with four drugs (INH, RIF, PZA, and ethionamide or STM). Treatment with PZA and the fourth drug is stopped after 2 months, and INH and RIF are continued for a total of 6 to 9 months.[146]

DRUG-RESISTANT TUBERCULOSIS IN CHILDREN

The incidence of drug-resistant tuberculosis is increasing in the United States and the world because of poor adherence by the patient, the availability of some antituberculosis drugs in noncontrolled over-the-counter formulations, and poor management by physicians.[49,181,348,419] In the United States, approximately 10 percent of *M. tuberculosis* isolates are resistant to at least one drug.[86,92] Initial drug resistance rates of up to 80 percent have been noted in adults with pulmonary tuberculosis in some countries,[350] and rates of 20 to 30 percent are common findings. Resistance is most common to STM and INH and still is relatively rare to RIF.[130,231,386,656] Certain epidemiologic factors— disease in an Asian or Hispanic immigrant to the United States, homelessness in some communities, and history of previous antituberculosis therapy—correlate with drug resistance in adult patients.[5,29,439] Patterns of drug resistance in children tend to mirror those found in adult patients in the population.[84,475,495,512,543,567,569] Outbreaks of drug-resistant tuberculosis in children occurring at schools have been reported.[84,474] Individual cases also have been recognized. The key to determining drug resistance in childhood tuberculosis usually comes from the drug susceptibility results of the infectious adult contact case's isolate.

Therapy for drug-resistant tuberculosis is successful only when at least two bactericidal drugs are given to which the infecting strain of *M. tuberculosis* is susceptible.[72,193,438,494,593] If only one effective drug is given, secondary resistance will develop. When INH resistance is considered a possibility on the basis of epidemiologic risk factors or the identification of an INH-resistant source case isolate, an additional drug—usually EMB or STM— should be given initially to the child until the exact susceptibility pattern is determined and a more specific regimen can be designed.[584] Exact treatment regimens must be tailored to the specific pattern of drug resistance. The duration of therapy usually is extended to at least 9 to 12 months if either INH or RIF can be used and to at least 18 to 24 months if resistance to both drugs is present.[253] Children tend to tolerate second-line antituberculosis drugs well, and community-based treatment usually is successful.[151,397] On occasion, surgical resection of a diseased lung or lobe is required.[255,453] An expert in tuberculosis always should be involved in the management of children with drug-resistant tuberculosis infection or disease.

ADHERENCE AND DIRECTLY OBSERVED THERAPY

Nonadherence with drug treatment by patients is a major problem in control of tuberculosis because of the long-term nature of its treatment.[377,580,620,627] As treatment regimens become shorter in duration, adherence assumes an even greater importance.[43] Suspected cases of tuberculosis must be reported to the local health department so that it can perform the necessary contact investigations and assist both patients and health care providers in overcoming barriers to adherence. To comply, the patient and family must know what is expected of them through verbal and written instructions in the patient's first language. An assessment of potential nonadherence should be made at the beginning of therapy.[32] Missed appointments should be brought quickly to the attention of the responsible public health officials, who may be able to use incentives or enablers, behavior modification, or, rarely, confinement to ensure adherence. The success of twice-weekly therapy, especially after a period of daily administration of medications, allows directly observed therapy to be given by a health care professional in cases of proven or suspected nonadherence.[99,254] Most experts hold that twice-weekly medication should be administered only under the direct observation of a health care worker.[297,637] Direct observation means that a health care worker or other nonrelated third party (e.g., teacher, school nurse, social worker) is physically present while the patient ingests the medication. As many as 50 percent of patients taking long-term antituberculosis medications will have significant nonadherence, and its occurrence is not predictable by the physician. In most communities in the United States and in an increasing number of other nations, directly observed therapy is the standard of care for all patients with tuberculosis disease.[90,170] However, when directly observed therapy cannot be used, structured behavior interactions can increase compliance with treatment.[79,597]

SUMMARY OF TREATMENT RECOMMENDATIONS

1. A regimen of INH and RIF for 6 months, supplemented with PZA during the first 2 months, is standard therapy for children with drug-susceptible intrathoracic tuberculosis in the United States and Canada.

2. An alternative regimen is INH and RIF for 9 months. The disadvantages of this regimen include a longer duration, the potential for increased drug resistance during therapy, and less effectiveness if the patient absconds from treatment. This regimen should be used only if PZA cannot be tolerated.

3. After an initial 2 weeks to 2 months of daily drug administration, drugs can be given twice weekly under directly observed therapy with excellent effectiveness.[449] With patients for whom social or other restraints prevent reliable daily self-administration even during the initial phase of therapy, drugs can be given two or three times per week from the beginning under directly observed therapy.

4. In most cases, extrapulmonary tuberculosis can be treated with the same regimens as used for pulmonary tuberculosis,

although data for tuberculous meningitis and bone or joint disease are relatively lacking.

5. In cases of possible initial INH resistance, EMB or STM should be added to the initial phase of all regimens until drug susceptibilities are known.[87]

6. Optimal therapy for tuberculosis in children with HIV infection has not been established.[575] Most HIV-infected adults with tuberculosis respond well to antituberculosis drugs but may require longer durations of treatment.[269] Immunosuppressed children with tuberculosis, including those with HIV infection, should be treated with at least three drugs initially, and treatment should be continued for a minimum of 9 months. HIV testing is recommended for all infants and children with tuberculosis disease.

7. Tuberculosis disease occurring during pregnancy should be treated with a 9-month regimen of INH and RIF supplemented during the initial phase with EMB (STM should not be used). The use of PZA in pregnant patients is controversial although probably safe.

CORTICOSTEROIDS

Corticosteroids have a place in the treatment of patients with tuberculosis. They should never be used except under cover of effective antituberculosis drugs. Corticosteroids would be expected to be beneficial in situations in which the host inflammatory reaction is contributing to tissue damage or is impairing function.

Corticosteroids often are a useful addition to antituberculosis drugs if suppression of inflammatory reaction is desired, such as in the following situations[534]:

1. In patients with tuberculous meningitis in whom increased intracranial pressure is present.[600] The major actions are to reduce vasculitis, inflammation, and, ultimately, intracranial pressure. Not only is reduction of pressure desirable, but lowering of the pressure also probably favors the circulation of chemotherapeutic drugs through the brain and meninges.[174,189] One study demonstrated lower rates of mortality and long-term neurologic sequelae in patients with tuberculous meningitis treated with corticosteroids than in control patients not treated with steroids.[189]

2. In patients with acute pericardial effusion in whom tamponade is occurring. Relief of symptoms takes place within hours.[477,578]

3. In patients with pleural effusion, a shift of the mediastinum, and acute respiratory embarrassment.[317,537] The long-term course probably is the same with or without steroids, but symptomatic improvement usually is dramatic.

4. In patients with miliary tuberculosis if the inflammatory reaction is so severe that it produces alveolocapillary block with cyanosis.

5. In patients with enlarged mediastinal lymph nodes that are causing respiratory difficulty or a severe collapse-consolidation lesion, particularly in the middle or lower lobes, when bronchiectasis is likely to be a troublesome sequela.[407,408] Under either of these circumstances, a course of corticosteroids is warranted, with the realization that it will be more successful in a younger infection because inflammation characterizes the early stages of tuberculosis. If caseation already is advanced, steroids will be of little benefit.

The dosage of corticosteroids should be in the antiinflammatory range, that is, prednisone, 1 to 2 mg/kg/day for 4 to 6 weeks with gradual withdrawal. Some experts prefer dexamethasone, but no comparative trials have been published.

ACTIVITY

Activity need not be restricted in children with tuberculosis, except when a particular complication is inevitable (shortness of breath in pleural effusion, immobilization for a vertebral lesion). During the early months of treatment, patients probably should avoid engaging in competitive sports, excessive study, fatigue, and sunburn.

ISOLATION

Isolation should be maintained for children with cavitary lesions, productive cough with acid-fast, stain–positive sputum, draining sinuses, or renal tuberculosis until their secretions are negative on smear and preferably on culture. Young children are virtually noninfectious because they rarely cough and because their bronchial secretions contain few bacilli compared with those of adults with tuberculosis. Guidelines issued by the CDC state that most children with typical tuberculosis do not require isolation in the hospital.[82,399] Children with possible pulmonary tuberculosis should be treated as potentially infectious if they have a cavity or extensive upper lobe infiltrate, if they have a productive cough (especially if the sputum is acid-fast smear positive), or during high-risk procedures such as bronchoscopy.

FOLLOW-UP

Follow-up of children treated with antituberculosis drugs has become somewhat more streamlined in recent years. While receiving chemotherapy, the patient should be seen monthly, both to encourage regular intake of the prescribed drugs and to check, by a few simple questions (concerning appetite, well-being) and a few observations (weight gain; appearance of the skin and sclerae; palpation of the liver, spleen, and lymph nodes), that the disease is not spreading and that toxic effects of the drugs are not appearing.[639] Repeated chest radiographs should be obtained 1 to 2 months after the onset of chemotherapy to ascertain the maximal extent of disease before chemotherapy takes effect; thereafter, radiographs rarely are necessary.[292] Chemotherapy has been so successful that follow-up beyond its termination is not necessary, except for children with serious disease, such as tuberculous meningitis, or those with extensive residual chest radiographic findings at the end of chemotherapy.

CASE REPORTING

Every case of definite or suspected tuberculosis, by law,[89] must be reported immediately by telephone to the health authority[192] to ensure prompt contact investigation[234] and free antituberculosis drugs, which are available for diagnosed cases and for intimate contacts in almost every state of the United States and in many countries.

PREVENTION

Prevention of tuberculosis can be subdivided logically to consider the following circumstances:

1. Protection against exposure to the disease.
2. Use of antituberculosis drugs in tuberculin-negative individuals at high risk for development of infection.
3. Immunization of tuberculin-negative individuals.

Protection against exposure to disease is the ideal form of prevention.[356] It presupposes thorough pre-employment and ongoing case-finding programs among all who come in contact with children, including daycare center and school personnel, Sunday school personnel, music and art teachers, hospital nurses, babysitters, household servants, food handlers, beauticians, and barbers. Numerous epidemics, mini-epidemics, and mass exposures in newborn nurseries have been traced to such infected individuals.

IMMUNIZATION

Immunization against tuberculosis theoretically would be a tremendous boon to humanity, but in practice, it has been fraught with very great difficulty. Various strains of mycobacteria and diverse nonliving immunogenic fractions have been studied. The impossibility of standardizing vaccines in the early days, the lack of any clinically useful test reflecting the immune status of the individual, and the relatively slow course of the disease have handicapped epidemiologic studies considerably. Furthermore, the very lack of adequate scientific data has intensified national and individual emotional responses to the point that rational approaches to data gathering and interpretation are often impossible. Although the use of tuberculosis vaccines for control of tuberculosis has waned in recent years in industrialized countries because of the falling incidence of the disease, new interest in them has cropped up because of their beneficial effect in certain types of malignant disease. New insights into their mode of action may prove fruitful in the long run in understanding immunity to tuberculosis, as well as to neoplasia, and might lead to a greatly improved and clinically useful vaccine.

BCG was developed at the Institut Pasteur in Paris by Calmette and Guérin, who, starting in 1908, made 231 passages of a strain of *M. bovis* on a beef bile medium, thereby producing marked attenuation. Injected into laboratory animals, this strain was shown to increase resistance to challenge with virulent *M. tuberculosis*. In 1921, it first was administered orally to newborn infants and since then has been given to more than 4 billion people.

BCG vaccine attempts to replace the potentially dangerous primary infection with *M. tuberculosis* with an innocuous primary infection with the bacillus of Calmette and Guérin, thus activating host cell-mediated immunity with minimal chance of causing progressive disease so that an infection with *M. tuberculosis* will be of the "reinfection" type.[332]

Variations in strains and lack of standardization are basic problems in evaluating the results of immunization.[198,594] BCG was maintained for many years by serial passage at the Institut Pasteur and distributed to hundreds of laboratories all over the world. Not until 1966 did the WHO Expert Committee on Biological Standardization adopt formal requirements for the maintenance of frozen "seed lots" to minimize the inevitable mutations that have produced BCG vaccines with widely varying characteristics. Routine quality control measures carried out by the production laboratory include an identity test, a test for contamination, a safety test in guinea pigs, an estimate of the total bacillary mass, viability, and a test of heat stability. Periodic assessment of the allergenic capacity in humans is part of quality control testing. The WHO, through its International Reference Preparation for BCG vaccine and through quality control testing on request carried out in its several cooperating laboratories, has helped decrease the gross variations in BCG vaccine found until recent years.

Vaccination techniques and dosages are variable. Intradermal injection is the most precise technique. Multiple-puncture techniques are popular because they are easy, but reported results consistently are inferior to those obtained with intradermal injection. Oral vaccination, the original method of administration, largely has been abandoned because of poor results. The actual dose of BCG at present usually is approximately 10^6 culturable particles. Because in animals large doses produce better resistance to challenge than small ones do, the largest convenient dose is used. However, in neonates, who have a higher incidence of untoward reactions, the customary approach is to halve the dose generally used in older infants and children to prevent local complications.

The usual local reaction to intradermal BCG vaccine is the development of a papule at the site of vaccination, and this papule reaches its maximal diameter (10 to 20 mm) in the sixth week. A small crust that may form on the papule detaches at about this time, with only a small ulcer remaining that may discharge a surprising amount of pus. Most ulcers are healed by the 10th week. A small scar is visible in almost all BCG-vaccinated individuals. Enlargement of the regional lymph nodes occurs regularly and is painless, sometimes ending in calcification. Formation of an abscess with breakdown is a rare event, but it occurs more often in infants.

Untoward reactions to BCG rarely have been a problem.[609] Fatalities caused by progressive disease have been reported in no more than 60 vaccine recipients (of an estimated 3+ billion), usually (but not always) children with well-documented immunodeficiency.[75,135,172,195,443,447] No return of the attenuated strain to virulence has ever been noted. In countries where BCG is used routinely for immunization of neonates, osteomyelitis has been diagnosed in some 5 per 100,000 neonates. It usually becomes manifested when the child is between 5 and 33 months of age, when a tender swelling is noted near a joint; bone destruction is well localized and responds to conservative treatment. On the whole, BCG is one of the safest vaccines in use.

In many countries where BCG is given routinely, the incidence of HIV infection in adults and children is high.[62,479] Reports of local and systemic complications from BCG vaccine in HIV-infected people are increasing, but the true magnitude of the interaction is not known yet.[40,219,220,232,421,466] However, in more recent studies, the rate of adverse BCG reactions in HIV-infected children appears to be higher than thought previously.[219,220] In most cases, BCG complications occur shortly after vaccination, but in one man with AIDS, adenitis as a result of BCG occurred 30 years after inoculation.[469] Routine treatment of patients with previous BCG vaccination who subsequently become immunocompromised is not recommended, but the clinician should be aware of previous BCG vaccination if signs or symptoms of mycobacterial infection occur.

The effectiveness of revaccination has never been evaluated scientifically and is not recommended.

The efficacy of BCG vaccines in humans has been evaluated in several large, well-controlled studies (Table 107–11). Three of these trials showed excellent protection, two showed mediocre protection, and two showed little or no effect of BCG. Another study, not tabulated because its numbers are relatively small, is

the "experiment of nature" reported by Hyge[246a] in 1957. Hyge[246a] observed an epidemic of tuberculosis in a school for girls, where 105 girls initially were tuberculin negative, 130 were tuberculin positive, and 133 were BCG immunized. In this group, the total incidence of tuberculosis was 23 times as high in the tuberculin-negative as in the BCG-immunized girls. Explanations for these differences in outcomes among trials must be sought in the quality and characteristics of the BCG vaccine used in the particular trial, the possible immunizing effect (in Georgia and Alabama) of infections with other mycobacteria,[532] the possibly greater effectiveness of BCG vaccine in areas of high tuberculosis prevalence, and methodologic variations among the trials.

The most recent large study of BCG effectiveness is the Chingleput study, started in 1968 in Chingleput District near Madras, South India, an area where sensitization with environmental mycobacteria is prevalent. People of all ages were vaccinated with one of two BCG vaccines or a placebo; only the incidence of adult-type pulmonary tuberculosis in the three groups was compared (i.e., not the forms usually found in children). During the ensuing years, no difference in incidence was noted among the three groups.[20a] This disturbing result has been the subject of several WHO investigations because BCG is one of the vaccines recommended for all children in the Expanded Program of Immunization sponsored by the WHO itself.[468] Another study of neonatal vaccination with BCG in England reported very favorable results with BCG.[121]

A group at the Harvard School of Public Health reviewed all published studies of BCG efficacy in a meta-analysis.[111] Most published trials were not analyzed because of serious flaws in their experimental design or reporting. Among all trials and case-control studies included, the average protection against tuberculosis disease by various BCG preparations was 50 percent. The protective levels were higher for disease in children, particularly for meningitis and tuberculosis-associated death.[110,604] However, ascertainment bias and lack of standardized case definitions render the results of these analyses very difficult to interpret. The BCG vaccines prevent many cases of tuberculosis in children, but the effect is quite variable. That BCG vaccines are not an instrument of tuberculosis control also has become apparent because they do not prevent infection with *M. tuberculosis*, their protective effect is short-lived, and vaccination of infants does little to prevent future cases of contagious tuberculosis among adults in a community.

The role of BCG vaccine in the United States today is very limited. The Advisory Committee on Immunization Practices of the U.S. Public Health Service and the Advisory Council for the Elimination of Tuberculosis recommend BCG only for tuberculin-negative infants and children in the United States who (1) are at high risk for having intimate and prolonged exposure to persistently untreated or ineffectively treated adults with infectious pulmonary tuberculosis, cannot be removed from the source of infection, and cannot be prescribed long-term preventive

TABLE 107–11 Summary of Seven Large Controlled Trials of Bacillus Calmette-Guérin (BCG) Immunization Against Tuberculosis

Trial	Investigators	Intake Period	Vaccine Laboratory	Duration of Observation (yr)	% Protection from BCG
North America: Native Americans	Stein and Aronson, 1953	1935-1938	Phipps	9-11	80
Chicago: infants	Rosenthal et al., 1961	1937-1948	Tice	12-23	75
Britain: schoolchildren	Medical Research Council, 1971	1950-1952	Copenhagen	15	78
South India: rural population	Frimodt-Moller et al., 1964	1950-1955	Madras	2.5-7	60/31*
Puerto Rico: children	Palmer et al., 1958	1949-1951	New York State	5.5-7.5	31
Georgia, Alabama: population	Comstock and Palmer, 1966	1950	Tice	14	14
Georgia: schoolchildren	Comstock and Webster, 1969	1947	Tice	20	0

The initial estimate of efficacy was 60 percent. Subsequently, when follow-up was extended to 9 to 14 years, the efficacy figure declined to 31 percent.
Modified from Sutherland, quoted by Eickhoff, T. C.: The current status of BCG immunization against tuberculosis. Annu. Rev. Med. 28:411-423, 1977.

therapy or (2) continuously are exposed to people with tuberculosis resistant to INH and RIF.[91] A few experts, however, are more inclined toward the use of BCG in neonates who are at any risk of exposure to tuberculosis whatsoever.[282,283,526,601]

Contraindications to the use of BCG for prevention of tuberculosis include congenital immunodeficiency, known HIV infection (in the United States; the WHO recommends giving BCG to asymptomatic HIV-infected infants who reside in areas with high tuberculosis rates), leukemia, lymphoma, and generalized malignant disease as well as treatment with corticosteroids, alkylating agents, antimetabolites, and radiation.

SELECTED READINGS

American Thoracic Society/Centers for Disease Control and Prevention/Infectious Diseases Society of America: Controlling tuberculosis in the United States. Am. J. Respir. Crit. Care Med. 172:1169-1227, 2005.

Brailey, M. E.: Tuberculosis in White and Negro Children. II. The Epidemiologic Aspects of the Harriet Lane Study. Cambridge, MA, Harvard University Press, 1958.

Dubos, R., and Dubos, J.: The White Plague: Tuberculosis, Man and Society. Boston, Little, Brown, 1952. Reissued by Rutgers University Press, 1987.

Hardy, J. B.: Tuberculosis in White and Negro Children. I. The Roentgenologic Aspects of the Harriet Lane Study. Cambridge, MA, Harvard University Press, 1958.

Lincoln, E. M., and Sewell, E. M.: Tuberculosis in Children. New York, McGraw-Hill, 1963.

Raviglione, M. C. (ed.): Reichman and Hershfields' Tuberculosis: A Comprehensive International Approach, 3rd ed. New York, Informa Healthcare, 2006.

Reichman, L. B., and Hershfield, E. S. (eds.): Tuberculosis: A Comprehensive International Approach. New York, Marcel Dekker, 1999.

Seminars in Pediatric Infectious Disease, Vol. 10, No. 4, 1993. (Entire volume devoted to tuberculosis in children.)

REFERENCES

1. Abadco, D., and Steiner, P.: Gastric lavage is better than bronchoalveolar lavage for isolation of Mycobacterium tuberculosis in childhood pulmonary tuberculosis. Pediatr. Infect. Dis. J. 11:735-738, 1992.
2. Abernathy, R. S., Dutt, A. K., Stead, W. W., et al.: Short-course chemotherapy for tuberculosis in children. Pediatrics 72:801-806, 1983.
3. Acocella, G.: The use of fixed dose combinations in antituberculous chemotherapy: Rationale for their application in daily, intermittent and pediatric regimes. Bull. Int. Union Tuberc. Lung Dis. 65:77-83, 1990.
4. Afghani, B., and Lieberman, J. M.: Paradoxical enlargement or development of intracranial tuberculomas during therapy: Case report and review. Clin. Infect. Dis. 19:1092-1099, 1994.
5. Aitken, M. L., Sparks, R., Anderson, K., et al.: Predictors of drug resistant diseases: Mycobacterium tuberculosis. Am. Rev. Respir. Dis. 130:831-833, 1984.
6. Albisua, I., Artigao, F. B., Del Castillo, F., et al.: Twenty years of pulmonary tuberculosis in children: What has changed? Pediatr. Infect. Dis. J. 21:91-97, 2002.
7. Al-Dossary, F. S., Ong, L. T., Correa, A. G., and Starke, J. R.: Treatment of childhood tuberculosis with a six month directly observed regimen of only two weeks of daily therapy. Pediatr. Infect. Dis. J. 21:91-97, 2002.
8. Alland, D., Kolkut, G. E., Moss, A., et al.: Transmission of tuberculosis in New York City: An analysis by DNA fingerprinting and conventional epidemiologic methods. N. Engl. J. Med. 330:1710-1716, 1994.
9. Almeida, L. M. D., Barbieri, M. A., Da Paixao, A. C., et al.: Use of purified protein derivative to assess the risk of infection in children in close contact with adults with tuberculosis in a population with high Calmette-Guérin bacillus coverage. Pediatr. Infect. Dis. J. 20:1061-1065, 2001.
10. American Thoracic Society/Centers for Disease Control and Prevention/ Infectious Diseases Society of America: Controlling tuberculosis in the United States. Am. J. Respir. Crit. Care Med. 172:1169-1227, 2005.
11. American Thoracic Society: Rapid diagnostic tests for tuberculosis: What is the appropriate use? Am. J. Respir. Crit. Care Med. 15:1804-1814, 1997.
12. American Thoracic Society: Diagnostic standards and classification of tuberculosis in adults and children. Am. J. Respir. Crit. Care Med. 161:1376-1395, 2000.
13. American Thoracic Society and Centers for Disease Control and Prevention: Targeted tuberculin testing and treatment of latent tuberculosis infection. Am. J. Respir. Crit. Care Med. 161(Suppl.):221-247, 2000.
14. Anderson, P., Munk, M. E., Pollock, J. M., and Doherty, T. M.: Specific immune-based diagnosis of tuberculosis. Lancet 356:1099-1104, 2000.
15. Andrew, O. T., Schoenfeld, R. Y., Hopewell, P. C., et al.: Tuberculosis in patients with end-stage renal disease. Am. J. Med. 68:59-65, 1980.
16. Andronikou, S., Welman, C. J., and Kader, E.: The CT features of abdominal tuberculosis in children. Pediatr. Radiol. 32:75-81, 2002.
17. Andronikou, S., Smith, B., Hatherhill, M., et al.: Definitive neuroradiological diagnostic features of tuberculous meningitis in children. Pediatr. Radiol. 34:876-885, 2004.
18. Andronikou, S., and Wiesethaler, N.: Modern imaging of tuberculosis in children: Thoracic central nervous system and abdominal tuberculosis. Pediatr. Radiol. 34:861-875, 2004.
19. Andronikou, S., Joseph, E., Lucas, S., et al.: CT scanning for the detection of tuberculous mediastinal and hilar adenopathy in children. Pediatr. Radiol. 34:232-236, 2004.
20. Andronikou, S., Weiselthaler, N., Smith, B., et al.: Value of early followup CT in pediatric tuberculous meningitis. Pediatr. Radiol. 35:1092-1099, 2005.
20a. Anonymous: Fifteen year follow up of trial of BCG vaccines in south India for tuberculosis prevention. Tuberculosis Research Centre (ICMR), Chennai. Indian J. Med. Res. 110:56-69, 1999.
21. Aquinas, S. M.: Short-course therapy for tuberculosis. Drugs 24:118-132, 1982.
22. Arend, S. M., Thijsen, S., Leyton, E., et al.: Comparison of two interferon assays and tuberculin skin test for tracing tuberculosis contacts. Am. J. Respir. Crit Care. Med. 175:618-627, 2007.
23. Askew, G. L., Finelli, L., Hutton, M., et al.: Mycobacterium tuberculosis transmission from a pediatrician to patient. Pediatrics 100:19-23, 1997.
24. Aznar, J., Safi, H., Romero, J., et al.: Nosocomial transmission of tuberculosis infection in pediatrics wards. Pediatr. Infect. Dis. J. 14:44-48, 1995.
25. Baciewicz, A. M., and Self, T. H.: Isoniazid interactions. South. Med. J. 78:714-718, 1985.
26. Bagga, A., Kalra, V., and Ghai, O. P.: Intracranial tuberculoma evaluation and treatment. Clin. Pediatr. (Phila.) 27:487-490, 1988.
27. Barber, T. W., Craven, D. E., and McCabe, W. R.: Bacteremia due to Mycobacterium tuberculosis in patients with human immunodeficiency virus infection: A report of 9 cases and a review of the literature. Medicine (Baltimore) 69:375-383, 1990.
28. Barclay, W. R.: Does a positive tuberculin test indicate the presence of live tubercle bacilli? J. A. M. A. 232:755, 1975.
29. Barnes, P. F.: The influence of epidemiologic factors on drug resistance rates in tuberculosis. Am. Rev. Respir. Dis. 136:325-328, 1987.
30. Barton, L. L., and Feigin, R. D.: Childhood cervical lymphadenitis: A reappraisal. J. Pediatr. 84:846-852, 1974.
31. Bavadekan, A. V.: Osteoarticular tuberculosis in children. Prog. Pediatr. Surg. 15:131-151, 1982.
32. Bayer, R., and Wilkinson, D.: Directly observed therapy for tuberculosis: History of an idea. Lancet 345:1545-1548, 1995.
33. Bearman, J. E., Kleinman, H., Glyer, V. V., et al.: Study of variability in tuberculin skin reading. Am. Rev. Respir. Dis. 90:913-919, 1964.
34. Beaudry, P. H., Brickman, H. F., and Wise, M. B.: Liver enzyme disturbances during isoniazid chemoprophylaxis in children. Am. Rev. Respir. Dis. 110:581-584, 1974.
35. Beck-Sague, C., Dooley, S. W., Hutton, M. D., et al.: Hospital outbreak of multidrug-resistant Mycobacterium tuberculosis infections: Factors in transmission to staff and HIV-infected patients. J. A. M. A. 268:1280-1286, 1992.
36. Behr, M. A., Hopewell, P. C., Paz, E. A., et al.: Predictive value of contact investigation for identifying recent transmission of Mycobacterium tuberculosis. Am. J. Respir. Crit. Care Med. 158:465-469, 1998.
37. Behr, M. A., Warren, S. A., Salamon, H., et al.: Transmission of Mycobacterium tuberculosis from patients smear negative for acid-fast bacilli. Lancet 353:444-449, 1999.
38. Bellin, E. Y., Fletcher, D. D., and Safyer, S. M.: Association of tuberculosis infection with increased time in or admission to the New York City jail system. J. A. M. A. 269:2228-2231, 1993.
39. Belsey, M. A.: Tuberculosis and varicella infections in children. Am. J. Dis. Child. 113:444-448, 1967.
40. Besnard, M., Sauvion, S., Offredo, C., et al.: Bacillus Calmette-Guérin infection after vaccination of human immunodeficiency virus–infected children. Pediatr. Infect. Dis. J. 12:993-997, 1993.
41. Besser, R. E., Pakiz, B., Schulte, J., et al.: Risk factors for positive Mantoux tuberculin skin tests in children in San Diego, California: Evidence for boosting and possible food borne transmission. Pediatrics 108:305-310, 2001.
42. Beyazova, U., Rota, S., Ceuheroglu, C., et al.: Humoral immune response in infants after BCG vaccination. Tubercle Lung Dis. 76:248-253, 1995.
42. Beyers, N., Gie, R., Schaaf, H., et al.: Delay in the diagnosis, notification and initiation of treatment and compliance in children with tuberculosis. Tubercle Lung Dis. 75:260-265, 1994.
44. Beyt, B. E., Jr., Ortbals, D. W., Santa Cruz, D. J., et al.: Cutaneous mycobacteriosis: Analysis of 34 cases with a new classification of the disease. Medicine (Baltimore) 60:96-109, 1980.
45. Bhagwati, S. N.: Spinal intramedullary tuberculoma in children. Childs Brain 5:568, 1979.
46. Bhansali, S. K.: Abdominal tuberculosis: Experience with 300 cases. Am. J. Gastroenterol. 67:324-337, 1977.
47. Biddulph, J.: Short-course chemotherapy for childhood tuberculosis. Pediatr. Infect. Dis. J. 9:794-801, 1990.
48. Biehl, J. P., and Vilter, R. W.: Effects of isoniazid on pyridoxine metabolism. J. A. M. A. 156:1549-1552, 1954.

49. Bifani, P. J., Plikaytis, B. B., Kapur, V., et al.: Origin and interstate spread of a New York City multidrug-resistant *Mycobacterium tuberculosis* clone family. J. A. M. A. 275:452-457, 1996.
50. Bloch, A. B., and Snider, D. E., Jr.: How much tuberculosis in children must we accept? Am. J. Public Health 76:14-15, 1986.
51. Blumberg, H. M., Burman, W. J., Chaisson, R. E., et al.; American Thoracic Society/Centers for Disease Control and Prevention/Infectious Diseases Society of America: Treatment of tuberculosis. Am. J. Respir. Crit. Care Med. 167:603-662, 2003.
52. Blumberg, H. M., Watkins, D. L., Berschling, J. D., et al.: Preventing the nosocomial transmission of tuberculosis. Ann. Intern. Med. 122:658-663, 1995.
53. Blusse van Oud-Alblas, H. J., van Vliet, M. E., Kimpen, J. L., et al.: Human immunodeficiency virus infection in children hospitalized with tuberculosis. Ann. Trop. Paediatr. 22:115-123, 2002.
54. Bonnet, M. B., Pinoges, L. P., Varaine, F. V., et al.: Tuberculosis after HAART initiation in HIV-positive patients from five countries with a high tuberculosis burden. AIDS 20:1275-1279, 2006.
55. Bovornkitti, S., Kangsdal, P., Sathirapat, P., et al.: Reversion and reconversion rate of tuberculin skin test reactions in correlation with the use of prednisone. Dis. Chest 38:51-55, 1960.
56. Boyd, G. L.: Tuberculosis pericarditis in children. Am. J. Dis. Child. 86:293-300, 1953.
57. Braden, C. R.: Infectiousness of a university student with laryngeal and cavitary tuberculosis. Investigative team. Clin. Infect. Dis. 21:565-570, 1995.
58. Brailey, M. E.: Observations on the development of intrathoracic calcification in tuberculin-positive infants. Bull. Johns Hopkins Hosp. 61:258-271, 1937.
59. Brailey, M. E.: Tuberculosis in White and Negro Children. II. The Epidemiologic Aspects of the Harriet Lane Study. Cambridge, MA, Harvard University Press, 1958.
60. Brassand, P., Kezouh, A., and Suissa, S.: Antirheumatic drugs and the risk of tuberculosis. Clin. Infect. Dis. 43:717-722, 2006.
61. Bratcher, D. F., Stover, B. H., Lane, N. E., et al.: Compliance with national recommendations for tuberculosis screening and immunization of health care workers in a children's hospital. Infect. Control Hosp. Epidemiol. 21:338-340, 2000.
62. Braun, M. M., Byers, R. H., Heyward, W. L., et al.: Acquired immunodeficiency syndrome and extrapulmonary tuberculosis in the United States. Arch. Intern. Med. 150:1913-1916, 1990.
63. Brock, R. C.: Post-tuberculous bronchostenosis and bronchiectasis of the middle lobe. Thorax 5:5-39, 1950.
64. Brody, J. A., and McAlister, R.: Depression of tuberculin sensitivity following measles vaccination. Am. Rev. Respir. Dis. 90:607-611, 1964.
65. Brown, E. R., Miller, B., Taylor, W. R., et al.: Health-care expenditures for tuberculosis in the United States. Arch. Intern. Med. 155:1595-1600, 1995.
66. Brudney, K., and Dobkin, J.: Resurgent tuberculosis in New York City: Human immunodeficiency virus, homelessness and the decline of tuberculosis control programs. Am. Rev. Respir. Dis. 144:745-749, 1991.
67. Burk, J. R., Viroslav, J., and Bynum, L. J.: Miliary tuberculosis diagnosed by fiberoptic bronchoscopy and transbronchial biopsy. Tubercle 59:107-109, 1978.
68. Burke, H. E.: Pathogenesis of Pott's disease. Trans. Am. Clin. Climatol. Assoc. 59:122-137, 1948.
69. Burroughs, M., Beitel, A., Kawamura, A., et al.: Clinical presentation of tuberculosis in culture-positive children. Pediatr. Infect. Dis. J. 18:440-446, 1999.
70. Byrd, R. B., Horn, B. R., Solomon, D. A., et al.: Toxic effects of isoniazid in tuberculous chemoprophylaxis: Role of biochemical monitoring in 1,000 patients. J. A. M. A. 241:1239-1241, 1979.
71. Cain, K. P., Haley, C. A., Armstrong, L. R., et al.: Tuberculosis among foreign-born persons in the United States. Am. J. Respir. Crit. Care Med. 175:75-79, 2007.
72. Caminero, J. A.: Treatment of multidrug-resistant tuberculosis: Evidence and controversies. Int. J. Tuberc. Lung Dis. 10:829-837, 2006.
73. Cantwell, M., Shehab, Z., Costello, A., et al.: Brief report: Congenital tuberculosis. N. Engl. J. Med. 330:1051-1054, 1994.
74. Cardona, M., Bek, M. D., Mills, K., et al.: Transmission of tuberculosis from a seven-year-old child in a Sydney school. J. Paediatr. Child Health 35:375-378, 1999.
75. Carlgren, L. E., Hansson, C. G., Henricsson, L., et al.: Fatal BCG infection in an infant with congenital lymphocytopenic agammaglobulinemia. Acta Paediatr. Scand. 55:636-644, 1966.
76. Carr, D. T., Karlson, A. G., and Stilwell, G. G.: A comparison of cultures of induced sputum and gastric washings in the diagnosis of tuberculosis. Mayo Clin. Proc. 42:23-25, 1967.
77. Carter, E. R., and Lee, C. M.: Interpretation of the tuberculin skin test reaction by pediatric providers. Pediatr. Infect. Dis. J. 21:200-203, 2002.
78. Carvalho, A. C., Kritski, A. L., and De Reimer, K.: Tuberculin skin testing among BCG-vaccinated children who are household contacts. Int. J. Tuberc. Lung Dis. 5:297, 2001.
79. Cass, A. D., Talavera, G. A., Gresham, L. S., et al.: Structural behavioral intervention to increase children's abherence to treatment for latent tuberculosis infection. Int. J. Tuberc. Lung Dis. 9:415-420, 2005.
80. Casteels-Van Daele, M., Igodt-Ameye, L., Corbeel, L., et al.: Hepatotoxicity of rifampin and isoniazid in children. J. Pediatr. 86:739-741, 1975.
81. Cave, M., Eisenach, K., McDermott, P., et al.: IS6110: Conservation of sequence in the *Mycobacterium tuberculosis* complex and its utilization in DNA fingerprinting. Mol. Cell. Probes 5:73-80, 1991.
82. Centers for Disease Control and Prevention: Guidelines for preventing the transmission of *Mycobacterium tuberculosis* in health-care settings. M. M. W. R. Recomm. Rep. 54(RR-17):1-141, 2005.
83. Centers for Disease Control and Prevention: Guidelines for using the QuantiFERON-TB gold test for detecting *Mycobacterium tuberculosis* infection, United States. M. M. W. R. Morb. Mortal. Wkly. Rep. 54:49-55, 2005.
84. Centers for Disease Control and Prevention: Interstate outbreak of drug-resistant tuberculosis involving children—California, Montana, Nevada, Utah. M. M. W. R. Morb. Mortal. Wkly. Rep. 32:516-518, 1983.
85. Centers for Disease Control and Prevention: A strategic plan for the elimination of tuberculosis from the United States. M. M. W. R. Morb. Mortal. Wkly. Rep. 38:269-272, 1989.
86. Centers for Disease Control and Prevention: National action plan to combat multidrug-resistant tuberculosis. M. M. W. R. Recomm. Rep. 41(RR-11):5-48, 1992.
87. Centers for Disease Control and Prevention: Prevention and control of tuberculosis in migrant farm workers. Recommendations of the Advisory Council for the Elimination of Tuberculosis. M. M. W. R. Recomm. Rep. 41(RR-10):1-15, 1992.
88. Centers for Disease Control and Prevention: Initial therapy for tuberculosis in the era of multidrug resistance. M. M. W. R. Recomm. Rep. 42(RR-7):1-8, 1993.
89. Centers for Disease Control and Prevention: Tuberculosis control laws—United States, 1993. M. M. W. R. Recomm. Rep. 42(RR-15):1-28, 1993.
90. Centers for Disease Control and Prevention: Screening for tuberculosis and tuberculosis infection in high-risk populations. Recommendations of the Advisory Council for the Elimination of Tuberculosis. M. M. W. R. Recomm. Rep. 44(RR-11):19-34, 1995.
91. Centers for Disease Control and Prevention: The role of BCG vaccine in the prevention and control of tuberculosis in the United States: A joint statement by the Advisory Council for the Elimination of Tuberculosis and the Advisory Committee on Immunization Practices. M. M. W. R. Recomm. Rep. 45(RR-4):1-18, 1996.
92. Centers for Disease Control and Prevention: Reported tuberculosis in the United States, 2006. Atlanta, GA, U.S. Department of Health and Human Services, CDC, September 2007.
93. Centers for Disease Control and Prevention: Tuberculosis elimination revisited: Obstacles, opportunities, and a renewed commitment. Advisory Council for the Elimination of Tuberculosis (ACET). M. M. W. R. Recomm. Rep. 48(RR-9):1-13, 1999.
94. Centers for Disease Control and Prevention: Core Curriculum on Tuberculosis: What a Clinician Should Know. 4th ed. Atlanta, U. S. Department of Health and Human Services, 2000.
95. Centers for Disease Control and Prevention: Preventing and controlling tuberculosis along the U.S.-Mexican border. M. M. W. R. Recomm. Rep. 50(RR-1):1-27, 2001.
96. Chan, S., Abadco, D., and Steiner, P.: Role of flexible fiberoptic bronchoscopy in the diagnosis of childhood endobronchial tuberculosis. Pediatr. Infect. Dis. J. 13:506-509, 1994.
97. Chan, S., P., Birnbaum, J., and Rao, M.: Clinical manifestation and outcome of tuberculosis in children with acquired immunodeficiency syndrome. Pediatr. Infect. Dis. J. 15:443-447, 1996.
98. Chaulk, C. P., Moore-Rice, K., Rizzo, R., et al.: Eleven years of community-based directly observed therapy for tuberculosis. J. A. M. A. 274:945-951, 1995.
99. Chaulk, C. P., and Kazandijian, V. A.: Directly observed therapy for treatment completion of pulmonary tuberculosis. Consensus statement of the Public Health Tuberculosis Guidelines Panel. J. A. M. A. 279:943-948, 1998.
100. Chavalittamvong, B., and Talalak, P.: Tuberculous peritonitis in children. Prog. Pediatr. Surg. 15:161-167, 1982.
101. Cheng, T. L., Miller, E. B., Ottolini, M., et al.: Tuberculosis testing. Physician attitudes and practices. Arch. Pediatr. Adolesc. Med. 150:682-685, 1996.
102. Cheng, T. L., Ottolin, M., Getson, P., et al.: Poor validity of parent reading of skin test induration in a high risk population. Pediatr. Infect. Dis. J. 15:90-91, 1996.
103. Chin, D. P., Crane, C. M., Diul, M. Y., et al.: Spread of *Mycobacterium tuberculosis* in a community implementing recommended elements of tuberculosis control. J. A. M. A. 283:2968-2974, 2000.
104. Chintu, C., Bhat, G., Luo, C., et al.: Seroprevalence of human immunodeficiency virus type 1 infection in Zambian children with tuberculosis. Pediatr. Infect. Dis. J. 12:499-504, 1993.
105. Chintu, C., and Mwaba, P.: Tuberculosis in children with human immunodeficiency virus infection. Int. J. Tuberc. Lung Dis. 9:477-484, 2005.
106. Choremis, C., Vlachos, J., Vlachou, C. A., et al.: Needle biopsy of the liver in various forms of childhood tuberculosis. J. Pediatr. 62:203-207, 1963.
107. Christie, C. D. C., Contaniou, P., Marx, M. L., et al.: Low risk for tuberculosis in a regional pediatric hospital: Nine-year study of community rates and the mandatory employee tuberculin skin test program. Infect. Control Hosp. Epidemiol. 19:168-174, 1998.
108. Cohen, T., and Murray, M.: Incident tuberculosis among recent U.S. immigrants and exogenous reinfection. Emerg. Infect. Dis. 11:725-728, 2005.

109. Cohn, D. L., Catlin, B. J., Peterson, K. C., et al.: A 62-dose, 6-month therapy for pulmonary and extrapulmonary tuberculosis. Ann. Intern. Med. *112*:407-415, 1990.

110. Colditz, G., Berkey, C. S., Mosteller, F., et al.: The efficacy of bacillus Calmette-Guérin vaccination of newborns and infants in the prevention of tuberculosis: Meta-analysis of the published literature. Pediatrics *96*:29-35, 1995.

111. Colditz, G., Brewer, T., Berkey, C., et al.: Efficacy of BCG vaccine in the prevention of tuberculosis: Meta-analysis of the published literature. J. A. M. A. *271*:698-702, 1994.

112. Comstock, G. W.: Variability of tuberculosis trends in a time of resurgence. Clin. Infect. Dis. *19*:1015-1022, 1994.

113. Comstock, G. W., Baum, C., and Snider, D. E., Jr.: Isoniazid prophylaxis among Alaskan Eskimos: Final report of the Bethel isoniazid studies. Am. Rev. Respir. Dis. *119*:827-830, 1979.

114. Comstock, G. W., Edwards, L. B., and Nabangxang, H.: Tuberculin sensitivity eight to fifteen years after BCG vaccination. Am. Rev. Respir. Dis. *103*:572-575, 1971.

115. Comstock, G. W., Hammes, L. M., and Pio, A.: Isoniazid prophylaxis in Alaskan boarding schools: Comparison of two doses. Am. Rev. Respir. Dis. *100*:773-779, 1969.

116. Comstock, G. W., Livesay, V. T., and Woolpert, S. F.: Prognosis of a positive tuberculin reaction in childhood and adolescence. Am. J. Epidemiol. *99*:131-138, 1974.

117. Connell, T. G., Curtis, N, Ranganathan, S. C., and Buttery, J. P.: Performance of a whole blood interferon-gamma assay for detecting latent infection with *Mycobacterium tuberculosis* in children. Thorax *61*:616-620, 2006.

118. Crowle, A. J., Sbarbaro, J. A., Judson, F. N., et al.: The effect of ethambutol on tubercle bacilli within cultured human macrophages. Am. Rev. Respir. Dis. *132*:742-745, 1985.

119. Curless, R. G., and Mitchell, C. D.: Central nervous system tuberculosis in children. Pediatr. Neurol. *7*:270-274, 1991.

120. Curtis, A., Ridzon, R., Vogel, R., et al.: Extensive transmission of *Mycobacterium tuberculosis* from a child. N. Engl. J. Med. *341*:1491-1495, 1999.

121. Curtis, H. M., Bamford, F. N., and Leck, I.: Incidence of childhood tuberculosis after neonatal BCG vaccination. Lancet *1*:145-148, 1984.

122. Dall, L., Long, L., and Stanford, J.: Poncet's disease: Tuberculosis rheumatism. Rev. Infect. Dis. *11*:105-107, 1989.

123. Daly, J. F., Brown, D. S., Lincoln, E. M., et al.: Endobronchial tuberculosis in children. Dis. Chest *22*:380-398, 1952.

124. Dandapat, M. C., Mishra, B. M., Dash, S. P., et al.: Peripheral lymph node tuberculosis: Review of 80 cases. Br. J. Surg. *77*:911-912, 1990.

125. Daniel, T., and Debanne, S.: The serodiagnosis of tuberculosis and other mycobacterial diseases by enzyme-linked immunosorbent assay. Am. Rev. Respir. Dis. *135*:1137-1151, 1987.

126. Dannenberg, A. M., Jr.: Delayed-type hypersensitivity and cell-mediated immunity in the pathogenesis of tuberculosis. Immunol. Today *12*:228-234, 1991.

127. David, H. L.: Probability distribution of the drug-resistant mutants in unselected populations of *Mycobacterium tuberculosis*. Appl. Microbiol. *20*:810-814, 1970.

128. De Angelis, L. M.: Intracranial tuberculoma: Case report and review of the literature. Neurology *31*:1133-1136, 1981.

129. de Blic, J., Azevedo, I., Burren, C., et al.: The value of flexible bronchoscopy in childhood pulmonary tuberculosis. Chest *100*:188-192, 1991.

130. Debré, R., Noufflard, H., Brissaud, H. E., et al.: Infection of children by strains of tubercle bacilli initially resistant to streptomycin or to isoniazid. Am. Rev. Respir. Dis. *80*:326-331, 1959.

131. Delacourt, C., Gobin, J., Gaillard, J., et al.: Value of ELISA using antigen 60 for the diagnosis of tuberculosis in children. Chest *104*:393-398, 1993.

132. Delacourt, C., Mani, T. M., Bonnerot, V., et al.: Computed tomography with normal chest radiograph in tuberculous infection. Arch. Dis. Child. *69*:430-432, 1993.

133. Delacourt, C., Poveda, J. D., Churean, C., et al.: Use of polymerase chain reaction for improved diagnosis of tuberculosis in children. J. Pediatr. *126*:703-709, 1995.

134. de Pontual, L., Balu, L., Ovetchkine, P., et al.: Tuberculosis in adolescents. A French retrospective study of 52 cases. Pediatr. Infect. Dis. J. *25*:930-932, 2006.

135. Deeks, S. L., Clark, M., Scheifele, P., et al.: Serious adverse events associated with bacilli Calmette-Guérin vaccine in Canada. Pediatr. Infect. Dis. J. *24*:538-541, 2005.

136. Dewan, P. K., Banouvong, H., Abernathy, N., et al.: A tuberculosis outbreak in a private-home family child care center in San Francisco, 2002 to 2004. Pediatrics *117*:863-869, 2006.

137. Dineen, P., Homan, W. P., and Grafe, W. R.: Tuberculous peritonitis: 43 years' experience in diagnosis and treatment. Ann. Surg. *184*:717-722, 1976.

138. Dinning, W. J., and Mauston, S.: Cutaneous and ocular tuberculosis: A review. J. R. Soc. Med. *78*:576-581, 1985.

139. Doerr, C. A., Starke, J. R., and Ong, L. T.: Clinical and public health aspects of tuberculous meningitis in children. J. Pediatr. *127*:27-33, 1995.

140. Domingo, Z., and Peter, J. C.: Intracranial tuberculomas: An assessment of a therapeutic 4-drug trial in 35 children. Pediatr. Neurosci. *15*:161-167, 1989.

141. Donald, P. R., Gent, W. L., Seifart, H., et al.: Cerebrospinal fluid isoniazid concentrations in children with tuberculous meningitis: The influence of dosage and acetylation status. Pediatrics *89*:247-250, 1992.

142. Donald, P. R., Mahan, D., Maritz, J. S., and Qazi, S.: Ethambutol dosage for the treatment of children: Literature review and recommendations. Int. J. Tuberc. Lung Dis. *10*:1318-1330, 2006.

143. Donald, P. R., Schaaf, H. S., and Schoeman, J. F.: Tuberculous meningitis and miliary tuberculosis: The Rich Focus revisited. J. Infect. *50*:193-195, 2005.

144. Donald, P. R., and Seifart, H.: Cerebrospinal fluid pyrazinamide concentrations in children with tuberculous meningitis. Pediatr. Infect. Dis. J. *7*:469-471, 1988.

145. Donald, P. R., and Seifart, H. I.: Cerebrospinal fluid concentrations of ethionamide in children with tuberculous meningitis. J. Pediatr. *115*:483-486, 1989.

146. Donald, P. R., Schoeman, J. F., VanZyl, L. E., et al.: Intensive short-course chemotherapy in the management of tuberculous meningitis. Int. J. Tuberc. Lung Dis. *2*:704-711, 1998.

147. Dormer, B. A., Harrison, I., Swart, J. A., et al.: Prophylactic isoniazid protection of infants in a tuberculosis hospital. Lancet *2*:902-903, 1959.

148. Driver, C., Luallen, J., Good, W., et al.: Tuberculosis in children younger than five years old: New York City. Pediatr. Infect. Dis. J. *14*:117-121, 1995.

149. Driver, C. R., Valway, S. E., Cantwell, M. E., et al.: Tuberculin skin test screening of school children in the United States. Pediatrics *98*:97-102, 1996.

150. Drobac, P. C., del Castillo, H., Sweetland, A., et al.: Treatment of a multidrug-resistant tuberculous during pregnancy: Long-term follow-up of 6 children with intrauterine exposure to second-line agents. Clin. Infect. Dis. *40*:1689-1692, 2005.

151. Drobac, P. C., Mukherjee, J. S., Joseph, J. K., et al.: Community-based therapy for children with multidrug-resistant tuberculosis. Pediatrics *117*:2022-2028, 2006.

152. Drucker, E., Alcabes, P., Bosworth, W., et al.: Childhood tuberculosis in the Bronx, New York. Lancet *343*:1482-1485, 1994.

153. Dubos, R., and Dubos, J.: The White Plague: Tuberculosis, Man and Society. New Brunswick, NJ, Rutgers University Press, 1987.

154. Dunlap, N. E., Harris, R. H., Benjamin, W. H., Jr., et al.: Laboratory contamination of *Mycobacterium tuberculosis* cultures. Am. J. Respir. Crit. Care Med. *152*:1702-1704, 1995.

155. Dutt, A. K., Mehta, J. B., Whitaker, B. J., et al.: Outbreak of tuberculosis in a church. Chest *107*:447-452, 1995.

156. Dutt, A. K., Moers, D., and Stead, W. W.: Short-course chemotherapy for extrapulmonary tuberculosis. Ann. Intern. Med. *107*:7-12, 1986.

157. Dutt, A. K., and Stead, W. W.: Present chemotherapy for tuberculosis. J. Infect. Dis. *146*:698-704, 1982.

158. Dutt, A. K., and Stead, W. W.: Tuberculous pleural effusion: 6-month therapy with isoniazid and rifampin. Am. Rev. Respir. Dis. *145*:1429-1432, 1992.

159. Dye, C., Espinal, M. A., Watt, C. J., et al.: Worldwide incidence of multi-drug resistant tuberculosis. J. Infect. Dis. *185*:1197-1202, 2002.

160. Eamranond, P., and Jaramillo, E.: Tuberculosis in children: Reassessing the need for improved diagnosis in global control strategies. Int. J. Tuberc. Lung Dis. *5*:594-603, 2001.

161. Edwards, L. B., and Hardy, J. B.: Relation of the degree of sensitivity to tuberculin to the persistence of sensitivity and to prognosis in young children. Bull. Johns Hopkins Hosp. *78*:13-20, 1946.

162. Ehrlich, R. M., and Lattimer, J.: Urogenital tuberculosis in children. J. Urol. *105*:461-465, 1971.

163. Eisenach, K. D., Sifford, M. D., Cave, M. D., et al.: Detection of *Mycobacterium tuberculosis* in sputum samples using a polymerase chain reaction. Am. Rev. Respir. Dis. *144*:1160-1163, 1991.

164. Elenga, N., Kouakoussui, K. A., Bonard, D., et al.: Diagnosed tuberculosis during the follow-up of a cohort of human immunodeficiency virus–infected children in Abidjan, Café d'Ivoire. ANRS 1278 study. Pediatr. Infect. Dis. J. *24*:1077-1082, 2005.

165. Ellard, G. A.: Hepatic toxicity of isoniazid among rapid and slow acetylators of the drug. Am. Rev. Respir. Dis. *118*:628-629, 1978.

166. Ellard, G. A., Humphries, M. J., Gabriel, M., et al.: Penetration of pyrazinamide into the cerebrospinal fluid in tuberculous meningitis. B. M. J. *294*:284-285, 1987.

167. Ellner, J. J.: Pleural fluid and peripheral blood lymphocyte function in tuberculosis. Ann. Intern. Med. *89*:932-933, 1978.

168. Emmett, J. R., Fischer, N. D., and Biggers, W. P.: Tuberculous mastoiditis. Laryngoscope *87*:1157-1163, 1977.

169. Ena, J., and Valls, V.: Short-course therapy with rifampin plus isoniazid, compared with standard therapy with isoniazid, for latent tuberculosis infection: A meta-analysis. Clin. Infect. Dis. *40*:670-676, 2005.

170. Enarson, D. A.: The International Union Against Tuberculosis and Lung Disease model National Tuberculosis Programmes. Tubercle Lung Dis. *76*:95-99, 1995.

171. Espinal, M. A., Laszlo, A., Simonsen, L., et al.: Global trends in resistance to antituberculosis drugs. N. Engl. J. Med. *344*:1294-1303, 2001.

172. Esterly, J. R., Sturner, W. Q., Esterly, N. B., et al.: Disseminated BCG in twin boys with presumed chronic granulomatous disease of childhood. Pediatrics *48*:141-144, 1977.

173. Ewer, K., Decks, J., Alvarez, L., et al.: Comparison of T-cell based assay with tuberculin skin test for diagnosis of *Mycobacterium tuberculosis* infection in a school tuberculosis outbreak. Lancet *361*:1168-1173, 2003.

174. Excobar, J. A., Belsey, M. A., Dueñas, A., et al.: Mortality from tuberculous meningitis reduced by steroid therapy. Pediatrics 56:1050-1055, 1975.

175. Fennelly, K. P., and Nardell, E. A.: The relative efficacy of respirators and room ventilation in preventing occupational tuberculosis. Infect. Control Hosp. Epidemiol. 19:754-759, 1998.

176. Ferrebee, S. H.: Controlled chemoprophylaxis trials in tuberculosis: A general review. Adv. Tuberc. Res. 17:28-106, 1969.

177. Figueroa-Damian, R., and Arredondo-Garcia, J. L.: Neonatal outcome of children born to women with tuberculosis. Arch. Med. Res. 32:66-69, 2001.

178. Filler, J., and Porter, M.: Physiologic studies of the sequelae of tuberculous pleural effusion in children treated with antimicrobial drugs and prednisone. Am. Rev. Respir. Dis. 88:181-188, 1963.

179. Francis, J., Reed, A., Yohannes, F., et al.: Screening for tuberculosis among orphans in a developing country. Am. J. Prev. Med. 22:117-119, 2002.

180. Frieden, T. R., Fujiwara, P. I., Washko, R. M., et al.: Tuberculosis in New York City: Turning the tide. N. Engl. J. Med. 333:229-233, 1995.

181. Frieden, T. R., Sterling, T., Pablos-Mendez, A., et al.: The emergence of drug-resistant tuberculosis in New York City. N. Engl. J. Med. 328:521-526, 1993.

182. Friedland, I. R.: The booster effect with repeat tuberculin testing in children and its relationship to BCG vaccination. S. Afr. Med. 77:387-389, 1990.

183. Froehlich, H., Ackerson, L. M., and Morozumi, P. A.: Targeted testing of children for tuberculosis: Validation of a risk assessment questionnaire. Pediatrics 107:e54, 2001.

184. Gal, A. A., and Klatt, E. C.: Fatal isoniazid hepatitis in a child. Pediatr. Infect. Dis. J. 5:490-491, 1986.

185. Gangadharam, P. R. J., Pratt, P. F., Perumal, U. K., et al.: The effects of exposure time, drug concentration, and temperature on the activity of ethambutol versus Mycobacterium tuberculosis. Am. Rev. Respir. Dis. 141:1478-1482, 1990.

186. Gaur, S., Kesarwala, H., and Frenkel, L. D.: Tuberculous peritonitis in an adolescent female. Pediatr. Infect. Dis. J. 18:859-862, 1987.

187. George, R. H., Gully, P. R., Gill, O. N., et al.: An outbreak of tuberculosis in a children's hospital. J. Hosp. Infect. 8:129-142, 1986.

188. Ghon, A.: The Primary Lung Focus of Tuberculosis in Children. London, J. A. Churchill, 1916.

189. Girgis, N. I., Fariz, Z., Kilpatrick, M. E., et al.: Dexamethasone adjunctive treatment for tuberculous meningitis. Pediatr. Infect. Dis. J. 10:179-182, 1991.

190. Girling, D. J: Adverse reactions to rifampicin in antituberculosis regimens. J. Antimicrob. Chemother. 3:115, 1977.

191. Girling, D. J.: Role of pyrazinamide in primary chemotherapy for pulmonary tuberculosis. Tubercle 65:1-4, 1984.

192. Glassroth, J., Bailey, W. C., Hopewell, P. C., et al.: Why tuberculosis is not prevented. Am. Rev. Respir. Dis. 141:1236-1240, 1990.

193. Goble, M., Iseman, M. D., Madsen, L. A., et al.: Treatment of 171 patients with pulmonary tuberculosis resistant to isoniazid and rifampin. N. Engl. J. Med. 328:527-532, 1993.

194. Gomez, L. P., Morris, S. L., and Panduro, A.: Rapid and efficient detection of extra-pulmonary Mycobacterium tuberculosis by PCR analysis. Int. J. Tuberc. Lung Dis. 4:361-370, 2000.

195. Gonzalez, B., Moreno, S., Burdach, R., et al.: Clinical presentation of bacillus Calmette-Guérin infections in patients with immunodeficiency syndromes. Pediatr. Infect. Dis. J. 8:201-206, 1989.

196. Gorse, G. J., and Belshe, R. B.: Male genital tuberculosis: A review of the literature with instructive case reports. Rev. Infect. Dis. 7:511-524, 1985.

197. Graham, S. M., Bell, D. J., Nyirongo, S., et al.: Low levels of pyrazinamide and ethambutol in children with tuberculosis and impact of age, nutritional status, and human immunodeficiency virus infection. Antimicrob. Agents Chemother. 50:407-413, 2006.

198. Grange, J. M., Gibson, J., Osborn, T. W., et al.: What is BCG? Tubercle 64:129-139, 1983.

199. Graziani, A. L., and MacGregor, R. R.: Self-reading of tuberculin testing vs. physician reading. Infect. Dis. Clin. Pract. 4:72-74, 1995.

200. Grosset, J.: Bacteriologic basis for short-course chemotherapy for tuberculosis. Clin. Chest Med. 1:231-241, 1980.

201. Grosskopf, I., David, A., Charach, G., et al.: Bone and joint tuberculosis: A 10-year review. Isr. J. Med. Sci. 30:278-283, 1994.

202. Groussard, P., David, A., Charach, G., et al.: Expansile pneumonia in children caused by Mycobacterium tuberculosis: Clinical, radiological and bronchoscopic appearances. Pediatr. Pulmonol. 38:451-455, 2004.

203. Gupta, R., Gupta, S., Dingh, D., et al.: MR imaging and angiography in tuberculous meningitis. Neuroradiology 36:87-92, 1994.

204. Gutman, L., Moye, J., Zimmer, B., et al.: Tuberculosis in human immunodeficiency virus–exposed or -infected United States children. Pediatr. Infect. Dis. J. 13:963-968, 1994.

205. Hageman, J., Shulman, S., Schreiber, M., et al.: Congenital tuberculosis: Critical reappraisal of clinical findings and diagnostic procedures. Pediatrics 66:980-984, 1980.

206. Hannachi, J., Martin, M., Boulabal, F., et al.: Comparison of three daily short-course regimens in osteoarticular tuberculosis in Algiers. Bull. Int. Union Tuberc. 57:46-47, 1946.

207. Hardy, J. B.: Persistence of hypersensitivity to old tuberculin following primary tuberculosis in childhood: A long-term study. Am. J. Public Health 36:1417-1426, 1946.

208. Hardy, J. B., and Hartmann, J. R.: Tuberculous dactylitis in childhood. J. Pediatr. 30:146-156, 1947.

209. Harries, A. D.: Tuberculosis and human immunodeficiency virus infection in developing countries. Lancet 335:387-390, 1990.

210. Harries, A. D., Hargreaves, N. J., Graham, S., et al.: Childhood tuberculosis in Malawi: Nationwide case-finding and treatment outcomes. Int. J. Tuberc. Lung Dis. 6:424-431, 2002.

211. Harris, V. J., Dida, F., Lander, S. S., et al.: Cavitary tuberculosis in children. J. Pediatr. 90:660-661, 1977.

212. Harrison, H. E., Finberg, L., and Fleischman, E.: Disturbances of ionic equilibrium of intracellular and extracellular electrolytes in patients with tuberculous meningitis. J. Clin. Invest. 31:300-308, 1952.

213. Haygood, T., and Williamson, S.: Radiographic findings of extremity tuberculosis in childhood: Back to the future? Radiographics 14:561-570, 1994.

214. Heinle, E. W., Jr., Jensen, N. N., and Westerman, M. P.: Diagnostic usefulness of marrow biopsy in disseminated tuberculosis. Am. Rev. Respir. Dis. 91:701-705, 1965.

215. Helms, S., and Helms, P.: Tuberculin sensitivity during measles. Acta Tuberc. Scand. 35:166-171, 1956.

216. Heney, C., Baise, T., and Cohen, M. A.: Tuberculosis of the mandible: A case report. Pediatr. Infect. Dis. J. 7:74-76, 1988.

217. Hesseling, A. C., Schaaf, H. S., Gie, R. P., et al.: A critical review of diagnostic approaches used in the diagnosis of childhood tuberculosis. Int. J. Tuberc. Lung Dis. 6:1039-1045, 2002.

218. Hesseling, A. C., Westra, A. E., Werschkull, H., et al.: Outcome of HIV-infected children with culture-confirmed tuberculosis. Arch. Dis. Child. 90:1171-1174, 2005.

219. Hesseling, A. C., Rabie, H., Marais, B. J., et al.: Bacille Calmette-Guérin vaccine–induced disease in HIV-infected and HIV-uninfected children. Clin. Infect. Dis. 42:548-558, 2006.

220. Hesseling, A. C., Marais, B. J., Gie, R. P., et al.: The risk of disseminated bacille Calmette-Guérin (BCG) disease in HIV-infected children. Vaccine 25:14-18, 2007.

221. Hill, P. C., Brookes, R. H., Fox, A., et al.: Large-scale evaluation of enzyme-linked immunospot assay and skin test for diagnosis of Mycobacterium tuberculosis infection against a gradient of exposure in the Gambia. Clin. Infect. Dis. 38:966-973, 2004.

222. Hill, P. C., Brookes, R. H., Adetifa, M. O., et al.: Comparison of enzyme-linked immunospot assay and tuberculin skin test in healthy children exposed to Mycobacterium tuberculosis. Pediatrics 117:1542-1548, 2006.

223. Heycock, J. B., and Noble, T. C.: Four cases of syringe-transmitted tuberculosis. Tubercle 42:25-27, 1961.

224. Hoffman, E. B., Allin, J., Campbell, J. A., and Leisegang, F. M.: Tuberculosis of the knee. Clin. Orthop. 398:100-106, 2002.

225. Hoffman, E. B., Crosier, J. H., and Cremin, B. J.: Imaging in children with spinal tuberculosis. J. Bone Joint Surg. Br. 75:233-239, 1993.

226. Hoffman, N. D., Kelly, C., and Futterman, D.: Tuberculosis infection in human immunodeficiency virus–positive adolescents and young adults: A New York City cohort. Pediatrics 97:198-203, 1996.

227. Hoge, C., Fisher, L., Donnell, D., et al.: Risk factors for transmission of Mycobacterium tuberculosis in a primary school outbreak: Lack of racial difference in susceptibility to infection. Am. J. Epidemiol. 139:520-530, 1994.

228. Holt, L. E.: Tuberculosis acquired through ritual circumcision. J. A. M. A. 61:99-102, 1913.

229. Hong Kong Chest Service/British Medical Research Council Fifth Collaborative Study: Controlled clinical trial of five 6-month regimens of chemotherapy for pulmonary tuberculosis. Am. Rev. Respir. Dis. 136:1339-1342, 1987.

230. Hong Kong Chest Service/British Medical Research Council: Controlled trial of 2, 4 and 6 months of pyrazinamide in 6-month, three times weekly regimens for smear positive pulmonary tuberculosis, including an assessment of a combined preparation of isoniazid, rifampin and pyrazinamide: Results at 30 months. Am. Rev. Respir. Dis. 143:700-706, 1991.

231. Honore, N., and Cole, S.: Streptomycin resistance in mycobacteria. Antimicrob. Agents Chemother. 38:238-241, 1994.

232. Houde, C., and Dery, P.: Mycobacterium bovis sepsis in an infant with human immunodeficiency virus infection. Pediatr. Infect. Dis. J. 7:810, 1988.

233. Howard, T. P., and Soloman, D. A.: Reading the tuberculin skin test: Who, when and how? Arch. Intern. Med. 148:2457-2459, 1988.

234. Hsu, K. H. K.: Contact investigation: A practical approach to tuberculosis eradication. Am. J. Public Health 53:1761-1769, 1963.

235. Hsu, K. H. K.: Tuberculin reaction in children treated with isoniazid. Am. J. Dis. Child. 137:1090-1092, 1983.

236. Hsu, K. H. K.: Thirty years after isoniazid: Its impact on tuberculosis in children and adolescents. J. A. M. A. 251:1283-1285, 1984.

237. Hsu, K. H. K., and Starke, J. R.: Diagnosis and treatment of tuberculous infection. Semin. Pediatr. Infect. Dis. 4:283-290, 1993.

238. Hsu, L. C. S., and Leong, J. C. Y.: Tuberculosis of the lower cervical spine (C2 to C7). A report on 40 cases. J. Bone Joint Surg. Br. 66:1-5, 1984.

239. Huebner, R. E., Schein, M. F., and Bass, J. B.: The tuberculin skin test. Clin. Infect. Dis. 17:968-975, 1993.

240. Hughes, I. E., Smith, H., and Kane, P. O.: Ethionamide: Its passage into the cerebrospinal fluid in man. Lancet 1:616-617, 1962.

241. Hughesdon, M. R.: Congenital tuberculosis. Arch. Dis. Child. 21:121-138, 1946.

242. Hugo-Hamman, C. T., Scher, H., and DeMoor, M. M. A.: Tuberculous pericarditis in children: A review of 44 cases. Pediatr. Infect. Dis. J. *13*:13-18, 1994.

243. Humphries, M. J., Teoh, R., Lau, J., et al.: Factors of prognostic significance in Chinese children with tuberculous meningitis. Tubercle *71*:161-168, 1990.

244. Hussey, G., Chisholm, T., and Kibel, M.: Miliary tuberculosis in children: A review of 94 cases. Pediatr. Infect. Dis. J. *10*:832-836, 1991.

245. Hussey, G., Kibel, M., and Dempster, W.: The serodiagnosis of tuberculosis in children: An evaluation of an ELISA test using IgG antibodies to *M. tuberculosis*, strain H37RV. Ann. Trop. Paediatr. *11*:113-118, 1991.

246. Hussey, G., Kibel, M., and Parker, N.: Ciprofloxacin treatment of multiply drug-resistant extrapulmonary tuberculosis in a child. Pediatr. Infect. Dis. J. *11*:408-409, 1992.

246a. Hyge, T. V.: The efficacy of BCG-vaccination: Tuberculosis epidemic in a state school with an observation period of 12 years. Dan. Med. Bull. *4*:13-15, 1957.

247. Ibanez, S., and Ross, G.: Quimioterapia abreviada de 6 meses en tuberculosis pulmonar infantil. Rev. Chil. Pediatr. *51*:249-252, 1980.

248. Idriss, Z. H., Sinno, A., and Kronfol, N. M.: Tuberculous meningitis in childhood: Forty-three cases. Am. J. Dis. Child. *130*:364-367, 1976.

249. Ildirim, I., Hacimustafaoglu, M., and Ediz, B.: Correlation of tuberculin induration with the number of bacillus Calmette-Guérin vaccines. Pediatr. Infect. Dis. J. *14*:1060-1063, 1995.

250. Ingalhalikar, V. T., Deostale, D. A., and Abhyankar, V. K.: Nonimmobilization of surgically treated tuberculosis of spine in children. Prog. Pediatr. Surg. *15*:153-157, 1982.

251. International Union Against Tuberculosis Committee on Prophylaxis: Efficacy of various durations of isoniazid preventive therapy for tuberculosis: Five years of follow-up in the IUAT trial. Bull. World Health Organ. *60*:555-564, 1982.

252. Iriso, R., Mudido, P. M., Karamagi, C., et al.: The diagnosis of childhood tuberculosis in an HIV-endemic setting and the use of induced sputum. Int. J. Tuberc. Lung Dis. *9*:716-726, 2005.

253. Iseman, M. D.: Treatment of multidrug-resistant tuberculosis. N. Engl. J. Med. *329*:784-791, 1993.

254. Iseman, M. D., Cohn, D. L., and Sbarbaro, J. A.: Directly observed treatment of tuberculosis: We can't afford not to try it. N. Engl. J. Med. *328*:576-578, 1993.

255. Iseman, M. D., Madsen, L., Goble, M., et al.: Surgical intervention in the treatment of pulmonary disease caused by drug-resistant *Mycobacterium tuberculosis*. Am. Rev. Respir. Dis. *141*:623-625, 1990.

256. Jacobs, R. F., and Abernathy, R. S.: The treatment of tuberculosis in children. Pediatr. Infect. Dis. *4*:513-517, 1985.

257. Jacobs, R. F., Sunakorn, P., Chotpitayasunonah, T., et al.: Intensive short course chemotherapy for tuberculous meningitis. Pediatr. Infect. Dis. J. *11*:194-198, 1992.

258. Jaffe, I. P.: Tuberculous meningitis in childhood. Lancet *1*:738, 1982.

259. Jagannath, C., Reddy, M. V., Kailasam, S., et al.: Chemotherapeutic activity of clofazimine and its analogues against *Mycobacterium tuberculosis*. Am. J. Respir. Crit. Care Med. *151*:1083-1086, 1995.

260. Jain, S. K., Paul-Satyaseela, M., Lamichhane, G., et al.: *Mycobacterium tuberculosis* invasion and traversal across an in vitro human blood-brain barrier as a pathogenic mechanism for central nervous system tuberculosis. J. Infect. Dis. *193*:1287-1295, 2006.

261. Janner, D., Kirk, S., and McLeary, M.: Cerebral tuberculosis without neurologic signs and with normal cerebrospinal fluid. Pediatr. Infect. Dis. J. *19*:763-764, 2000.

262. Jasmer, R. M., Seaman, C. B., Gonzalez, L. C., et al.: Tuberculosis treatment outcomes. Am. J. Respir. Crit. Care Med. *170*:561-566, 2004.

263. Jawahar, M. S., Sivasubramanian, S., Vijayan, V. K., et al.: Short course chemotherapy for tuberculous lymphadenitis in children. B. M. J. *301*:359-362, 1990.

264. Jereb, J., Kelly, G., and Porterfield, D.: The epidemiology of tuberculosis in children. Semin. Pediatr. Infect. Dis. *4*:220-231, 1993.

265. Jinkins, J. R.: Computed tomography of intracranial tuberculosis. Neuroradiology *33*:126-135, 1991.

266. John, J. F., and Douglas, R. G.: Tuberculous arachnoiditis. J. Pediatr. *86*:235-237, 1975.

267. Johnson, H., Lee, B., Doherty, E., et al.: Tuberculin sensitivity and the BCG scar in tuberculosis contacts. Tubercle Lung Dis. *76*:122-125, 1995.

268. Johnston, J. A.: Nutritional Studies in Adolescent Girls and Their Relation to Tuberculosis. Springfield, IL, Charles C Thomas, 1953.

269. Jones, B. E., Otaya, M., Antoniskis, D., et al.: A prospective evaluation of antituberculosis therapy in patients with human immunodeficiency virus infection. Am. J. Respir. Crit. Care Med. *150*:1499-1502, 1994.

270. Jones, D., Malecki, J., Bigler, W., et al.: Pediatric tuberculosis and human immunodeficiency virus infection in Palm Beach County, Florida. Am. J. Dis. Child. *146*:1166-1170, 1992.

271. Kalish, S. B., Radiu, R. C., Phair, J. P., et al.: Use of an enzyme-linked immunosorbent assay technique in the differential diagnosis of active pulmonary tuberculosis in humans. J. Infect. Dis. *147*:523-530, 1983.

272. Kalish, S. B., Rodin, R. C., Levitz, D., et al.: Enzyme-linked immunosorbent assay method for IgG antibody to purified protein derivative in cerebrospinal fluid of patients with tuberculous meningitis. Ann. Intern. Med. *99*:630-633, 1983.

273. Kallmann, I. J., and Reisner, D.: Twin studies on the genetic factors in tuberculosis. Am. Rev. Tuberc. *47*:549, 1943.

274. Kampann, B., Tena-Coki, G. N., Nicol, M. P., et al.: Reconstruction of antimycobacterial immune responses in HIV-infected children receiving HAART. AIDS *20*:1011-1018, 2006.

275. Keane, J., Gershon, S., Wise, R., et al.: Tuberculosis associated with infliximab, a tumor necrosis factor-alpha neutralizing agent. N. Engl. J. Med. *345*:1098-1014, 2001.

276. Kedar, R. P., Shah, P. P., Shivde, R. S., et al.: Sonographic findings in gastrointestinal and peritoneal tuberculosis. Clin. Radiol. *49*:24-29, 1994.

277. Kellerman, S. E., Saiman, L., San Gabriel, P., et al.: Observational study of the use of infection control interventions for *Mycobacterium tuberculosis* in pediatric facilities. Pediatr. Infect. Dis. J. *20*:566-570, 2001.

278. Kellerman, S. E., Saiman, L., Soto-Irizarry, M., et al.: Costs associated with tuberculosis control programs at hospitals caring for children. Pediatr. Infect. Dis. J. *18*:604-608, 1999.

279. Kellerman, S. E., Simonds, D., Banerjee, S., et al.: APIC and CDC survey of *Mycobacterium tuberculosis* isolation and control practices in hospitals caring for children. Part I: Patient and family isolation policies and procedures. Am. J. Infect. Control *26*:478-482, 1998.

280. Kellerman, S. E., Simonds, D., Banergee, S., et al.: APIC and CDC survey of *Mycobacterium tuberculosis* isolation and control practices in hospitals caring for children. Part 2: Environmental and administrative controls. Am. J. Infect. Control *26*:483-487, 1998.

281. Kendig, E. L., Jr.: Tuberculosis in the very young: Report of three cases of infants less than one month of age. Am. Rev. Tuberc. *70*:161-165, 1954.

282. Kendig, E. L., Jr.: Prognosis of infants born of tuberculous mothers. Pediatrics *26*:97-100, 1960.

283. Kendig, E. L., Jr.: The place of BCG vaccine in the management of infants born of tuberculous mothers. N. Engl. J. Med. *281*:520-523, 1969.

284. Kendig, E. L., Jr., and Rodgers, W. L.: Tuberculosis in the neonatal period. Am. Rev. Tuberc. Pulm. Dis. *77*:418-422, 1958.

285. Kendig, E. L., Kirkpatrick, B. V., Carter, W. H., et al.: Underreading of the tuberculin skin test reaction. Chest *113*:1175-1177, 1998.

286. Kennedy, C., and Knowles, G. K.: Miliary tuberculosis presenting with skin lesions. B. M. J. *3*:356, 1975.

287. Kennedy, N., Fox, R., Kisyombe, G. M., et al.: Early bactericidal and sterilizing activities of ciprofloxacin in pulmonary tuberculosis. Am. Rev. Respir. Dis. *148*:1547-1551, 1993.

288. Khan, E. A., and Starke, J. R.: Diagnosis of tuberculosis in children: Increased need for better methods. Emerg. Infect. Dis. *1*:115-123, 1995.

289. Khouri, Y., Mastrucci, M., Hutto, C., et al.: *Mycobacterium tuberculosis* in children with human immunodeficiency virus type 1 infection. Pediatr. Infect. Dis. J. *11*:950-955, 1992.

290. Kim, J. H., Langston, A. A., and Gallis, H. A.: Miliary tuberculosis: Epidemiology, clinical manifestations, diagnosis and outcome. Rev. Infect. Dis. *12*:583-590, 1990.

291. Kimerling, M. E., Vaughn, E. S., and Dunlap, N. E.: Childhood tuberculosis in Alabama: Epidemiology of disease and indicators of program effectiveness, 1983 to 1993. Pediatr. Infect. Dis. J. *14*:678-684, 1995.

292. Kisembo, H. N., Kawooya, M. G., Zirembozi, G., and Okwera, A.: Serial chest radiographs in the management of children with a clinical suspicion of pulmonary tuberculosis. J. Trop. Pediatr. *47*:276-283, 2001.

293. Kiwanuka, J., Graham, S. M., Coulter, J. B., et al.: Diagnosis of pulmonary tuberculosis in children in an HIV-endemic area, Malawi. Ann. Trop. Paediatr. *21*:5-14, 2001.

294. Klausner, J. D., Ryder, R. W., Baende, E., et al.: *Mycobacterium tuberculosis* in household contacts of human immunodeficiency virus type 1–seropositive patients with active pulmonary tuberculosis in Kinshasa, Zaire. J. Infect. Dis. *168*:106-111, 1993.

295. Kochi, A.: The global tuberculosis situation and the new control strategy of the World Health Organization. Tubercle *72*:1-6, 1991.

296. Kohli, V., Kumar, L., and Kataria, S.: Multiple hepatosplenic tuberculous abscesses in an eight-year-old boy. Pediatr. Infect. Dis. J. *15*:178-179, 1996.

297. Kohn, M. R., Arden, M. R., Vasilakis, J., et al.: Directly observed preventive therapy: Turning the tide against tuberculosis. Arch. Pediatr. Adolesc. Med. *150*:727-729, 1996.

298. Kopanoff, D. E., Snider, D. E., and Caras, G. J.: Isoniazid-related hepatitis: A United States Public Health Service Cooperative Surveillance Study. Am. Rev. Respir. Dis. *117*:991-1001, 1978.

299. Kroidl, A., Huck, K., Weinspach, S., et al.: Immune reconstitution inflammatory syndrome (IRIS) due to bacille Calmette-Guérin (BCG) in an HIV-positive child. Scand. J. Infect. Dis. *38*:716-718, 2006.

300. Kumar, A., Misra, P. K., Mehotra, R., et al.: Hepatotoxicity of rifampin and isoniazid: Is it all drug-induced hepatitis? Am. Rev. Respir. Dis. *143*:1350-1352, 1991.

301. Kumar, B., Rai, R., Kaur, I., et al.: Childhood cutaneous tuberculosis: A study over 25 years from northern India. Int. J. Dermatol. *40*:26-32, 2001.

302. Kumar, L., Dhand, R., Singhi, P. D., et al.: A randomized trial of fully intermittent vs. daily followed by intermittent short-course chemotherapy for childhood tuberculosis. Pediatr. Infect. Dis. J. *9*:802-806, 1990.

303. Kumar, R., Pandery, C. K., Bose, N., and Sahay, S.: Tuberculosis brain abscess: Clinical presentation, pathophysiology and treatment (in children). Childs Nerv. Syst. *18*:118-123, 2002.

304. Kutt, H., Brennan, R., Dehejia, H., et al.: Diphenylhydantoin intoxication: A complication of isoniazid therapy. Am. Rev. Respir. Dis. *101*:377-384, 1970.

305. Lai, K. K., Stottmeier, K. D., Sherman, I. H., et al.: Mycobacterial cervical lymphadenopathy: Relation of etiologic agents to age. J. A. M. A. *251*:1286-1288, 1984.

306. Lake, A. M., and Oski, F. A.: Peripheral lymphadenopathy in childhood: Ten-year experience with excisional biopsy. Am. J. Dis. Child. *132*:357-359, 1978.

307. Lamont, A., Cremin, B., and Pettenet, B.: Radiologic patterns of pulmonary tuberculosis in the pediatric age group. Pediatr. Radiol. *16*:2-7, 1986.

308. Lamprecht, D., Schoeman, J., Donald, P., and Hartzenberg, H.: Ventriculoperitoneal shunting in childhood tuberculosis meningitis. Br. J. Neurosurg. *15*:119-125, 2001.

309. Lange, W. R., Warnock-Eckhart, E., and Bean, M. E.: Mycobacterium tuberculosis infection in foreign born adoptees. Pediatr. Infect. Dis. J. *8*:625-629, 1989.

310. Lanier, V. S., Russell, W. F., Jr., Heaton, A., et al.: Concentrations of active isoniazid in serum and cerebrospinal fluid of patients with tuberculosis treated with isoniazid. Pediatrics *21*:910-915, 1958.

311. Larmola, E.: Two cases of sudden death in infants recovering from primary tuberculosis. Acta Tuberc. Scand. *21*(Suppl.):67, 1949.

312. Lau, S. K., Kwan, S., Lee, J., et al.: Source of tubercle bacilli in cervical lymph nodes: A prospective study. J. Laryngol. Otol. *105*:558-561, 1991.

313. Laven, G. T.: Diagnosis of tuberculosis in children using fluorescence microscopic examination of gastric washings. Am. Rev. Respir. Dis. *115*:743-749, 1977.

314. Lawn, S. D., Bekker, L.-G., and Miller, R. F.: Immune reconstitution disease associated with mycobacterial infections in HIV-infected individuals receiving antiretrovirals. Lancet Infect. Dis. *5*:361-373, 2005.

315. Lawn, S. D., and Wood, R.: Incidence of tuberculosis during highly active antiretroviral therapy in high-income and low-income countries. Clin. Infect. Dis. *41*:1783-1786, 2005.

316. Lawn, S. D., Myer, L., Bekker, L. G., and Wood, R.: Tuberculosis-associated immune reconstitution disease: Incidence, risk factors and impact in an antiretroviral treatment service in South Africa. AIDS *21*:335-341, 2007.

317. Lee, C., Wang, W., Lan, R., et al.: Corticosteroids in the treatment of tuberculous pleurisy: A double-blind, placebo-controlled randomized study. Chest *94*:1256-1259, 1988.

318. Lee, L. H., Le Vea, C. M., and Graman, P. S.: Congenital tuberculosis in a neonatal intensive care unit: Case report, epidemiologic investigation and management of exposures. Clin. Infect. Dis. *27*:474-477, 1998.

319. Lees, A., Macleod, A., and Marshall, J.: Cerebral tuberculoma developing during treatment of tuberculous meningitis. Lancet *1*:1208-1211, 1980.

320. Leggiadro, R. J., Collery, B., and Dowdy, S.: Outbreak of tuberculosis in a family day care home. Pediatr. Infect. Dis. J. *8*:52-54, 1989.

321. Leiguarda, R., Berthier, M., Starkstein, S., et al.: Ischemic infarction in 25 children with tuberculous meningitis. Stroke *19*:200-204, 1988.

322. Levine, H., Metzger, W., Lacera, S., et al.: Diagnosis of tuberculous pleurisy by culture of pleural biopsy specimen. Arch. Intern. Med. *126*:269-271, 1970.

323. Lewinsohn, D. A., Gennaro, M. L., Scholuinck, L., and Lewinsohn, D. M.: Tuberculosis immunology in children: Diagnostic and therapeutic challenges and opportunities. Int. J. Tuberc. Lung Dis. *8*:658-674, 2004.

324. Light, I. J., Saidleman, M., and Sutherland, J. M.: Management of newborns after nursery exposure to tuberculosis. Am. Rev. Respir. Dis. *109*:415-419, 1974.

325. Lincoln, E. M.: Tuberculous meningitis in children: With special reference to serous meningitis. Am. Rev. Tuberc. *56*:75-94, 95-109, 1947.

326. Lincoln, E. M.: Epidemics of tuberculosis. Adv. Tuberc. Res. *14*:159-197, 1965.

327. Lincoln, E. M., Davies, P. A., and Bovornkitti, S.: Tuberculous pleurisy with effusion in children. Am. Rev. Tuberc. *77*:271-289, 1958.

328. Lincoln, E. M., Gilbert, L., and Morales, S. M.: Chronic pulmonary tuberculosis in individuals with known previous primary tuberculosis. Dis. Chest *38*:473-482, 1960.

329. Lincoln, E. M., Harris, L. C., Bovornkitti, S., et al.: Endobronchial tuberculosis in children. Am. Rev. Tuberc. Pulm. Dis. *77*:39-61, 1958.

330. Lincoln, E. M., Sabato, V. R., and Davies, P. A.: Tuberculous meningitis in children. J. Pediatr. *57*:807-823, 1960.

331. Lincoln, E. M., and Sewell, E. M.: Tuberculosis in Children. New York, McGraw-Hill, 1963.

332. Lindgren, I.: Pathology of tuberculous infection in BCG-vaccinated humans. Adv. Tuberc. Res. *14*:203-231, 1965.

333. Linna, O., and Uhari, M.: Hepatotoxicity of rifampicin and isoniazid in children treated for tuberculosis. Eur. J. Pediatr. *134*:227-229, 1980.

334. Litt, I. F., Cohen, M. I., and McNamara, H.: Isoniazid hepatitis in adolescents. J. Pediatr. *89*:133-135, 1976.

335. Liu, W. W., Chan, Y. L., Tseng, R., et al.: Childhood abdominal tuberculosis: The role of echo-guided fine-needle aspiration in its management. Surg. Endosc. *8*:326-328, 1994.

336. Livengood, J. R., Sigler, T. G., Foster, L. R., et al.: Isoniazid-resistant tuberculosis: A community outbreak and report of a rifampin prophylaxis failure. J. A. M. A. *253*:2847-2849, 1985.

337. Lobato, M., and Hopewell, P. C.: *Mycobacterium tuberculosis* infection after travel to or contact with visitors from countries with high prevalence of tuberculosis. Am. J. Respir. Crit. Care Med. *158*:1871-1875, 1998.

338. Lobato, M. N., Mohle-Boetani, J. C., and Royce, S. E.: Missed opportunities for preventing tuberculosis among children younger than five years of age. Pediatrics *106*:e75, 2000.

339. Lockman, S., Tappero, J. W., Kenyon, T. A., et al.: Tuberculin reactivity in a pediatric population with high BCG vaccination coverage. Int. J. Tuberc. Lung Dis. *3*:23-30, 1999.

340. Lorber, J.: Isoniazid and streptomycin in tuberculous meningitis. Lancet *1*:1140-1142, 1964.

341. Lucente, F. E., Tobias, G. W., Parisier, S. C., et al.: Tuberculous otitis media. Laryngoscope *88*:1107-1116, 1978.

342. Luo, C., Chintu, C., Bhat, G., et al.: Human immunodeficiency virus type-1 infection in Zambian children with tuberculosis: Changing seroprevalence and evaluation of a thiacetazone-free regimen. Tubercle Lung Dis. *75*:110-115, 1994.

343. Lurie, M. B.: Resistance to Tuberculosis: Experimental Studies in Native and Acquired Defense Mechanisms. Cambridge, MA, Harvard University Press, 1964.

344. MacAdam, A. M., and Rubio, T.: Tuberculous otomastoiditis in children. Am. J. Dis. Child. *131*:152-156, 1977.

345. MacDonnell, A. H., Baird, R. W., and Bronze, M. S.: Intramedullary tuberculomas of the spinal cord: Case report and review. Rev. Infect. Dis. *12*:432-439, 1990.

346. MacGregor, R. R., Sheagren, J. N., Lipsett, M. B., et al.: Alternate-day prednisone therapy: Evaluation of delayed hypersensitivity response, control of disease and steroid side effects. N. Engl. J. Med. *280*:1427-1431, 1969.

347. Maharaj, B., Leary, W. P., and Pudifin, D. J.: A prospective study of hepatic tuberculosis in 41 black patients. Q. J. Med. *242*:517-522, 1987.

348. Mahmoudi, A., and Iseman, M.: Pitfalls in the care of patients with tuberculosis: Common errors and their association with the acquisition of drug resistance. J. A. M. A. *270*:65-68, 1993.

349. Malik, S., Abel, L., Tooker, H., et al.: Alleles of *NRAMP-1* gene are risk factors for pediatric tuberculosis disease. Proc. Natl. Acad. Sci. U. S. A. *102*:12183-12188, 2005.

350. Manalo, F., Tan, F., Sbarbaro, J. A., et al.: Community-based short-course treatment of pulmonary tuberculosis in a developing nation: Initial report of an eight-month, largely intermittent, regimen in a population with a high prevalence of drug resistance. Am. Rev. Respir. Dis. *142*:1301-1305, 1990.

351. Mancao, M. Y., Nolte, F. S., Nahmias, A. J., et al.: Use of polymerase chain reaction for diagnosis of tuberculous meningitis. Pediatr. Infect. Dis. J. *13*:154-155, 1994.

352. Manjunath, N., Shankar, P., Rajan, L., et al.: Evaluation of a polymerase chain reaction for the diagnosis of tuberculosis. Tubercle *72*:21-27, 1991.

353. Marais, B. J., Gie, R. P., Schaaf, H. S., et al.: The clinical epidemiology of childhood pulmonary tuberculosis: A critical review of literature from the pre-chemotherapy era. Int. J. Tuberc. Lung Dis. *8*:278-285, 2004.

354. Marais, B. J., Gie, R. P., Schaaf, H. S., et al.: A proposed radiographic classification of childhood intra-thoracic tuberculosis. Pediatr. Radiol. *33*:886-894, 2004.

355. Marais, B. J., Gie, R. P., Schaaf, H. S., et al.: The natural history of childhood intra-thoracic tuberculosis: A critical review of the pre-chemotherapy literature. Int. J. Tuberc. Lung Dis. *8*:392-402, 2004.

356. Marais, B. J., Obihara, C. C., Warren, R. M., et al.: The burden of childhood tuberculosis: A public health perspective. Int. J. Tuberc. Lung Dis. *9*:1305-1313, 2005.

357. Marais, B. J., Gie, R. P., Hesseling, A. C., et al.: Adult-type pulmonary tuberculosis in children aged 10-14 years. Pediatr. Infect. Dis. J. *24*:743-744, 2005.

358. Marais, B. J., Gie, R. P., Hesseling, A. C., et al.: Radiographic signs and symptoms in children treated for tuberculosis. Possible implications for symptom-based screening in resource-limited settings. Pediatr. Infect. Dis. J. *25*:237-240, 2006.

359. Marais, B. J., Gie, R. P., Schaaf, H. S., et al.: Childhood pulmonary tuberculosis. Old wisdom and new challenges. Am. J. Respir. Crit. Care Med. *173*:1078-1090, 2006.

360. Marais, B. J., Wright, C. A., Schaaf, H. S., et al.: Tuberculous lymphadenitis as a cause of persistent cervical lymphadenopathy in children from a tuberculous endemic area. Pediatr. Infect. Dis. J. *25*:142-146, 2006.

361. Marais, B. J., Graham, S. M., Cotton, M. F., and Beyers, N.: Diagnostic and management challenges for childhood tuberculosis in the era of HIV. J. Infect. Dis. *196*(Suppl. 1):576-585, 2007.

362. Marks, S. M., Taylor, Z., Qualls, N. L., et al.: Outcomes of contact investigations of infectious tuberculosis patients. Am. J. Respir. Crit. Care Med. *162*:2033-2038, 2000.

363. Marshall, J. D., Abdel-Rahman, S., Johnson, K., et al.: Rifapentine pharmacokinetics in adolescents. Pediatr. Infect. Dis. J. *18*:882-888, 1999.

364. Martinez-Roig, A., Cami, J., Llorens-Terol, J., et al.: Acetylation phenotype and hepatotoxicity in the treatment of tuberculosis in children. Pediatrics *77*:912-915, 1986.

365. Mason, E., and Russell, D. W.: Isoniazid acetylation rates (phenotypes) of patients being treated for tuberculosis. Bull. World Health Organ. *45*:617-624, 1971.

366. Matlow, A. G., Harrison, A., Monteath, A., et al.: Nosocomial transmission of tuberculosis (TB) associated with a case of an infant with peritoneal TB. Infect. Control Hosp. Epidemiol. *21*:222-223, 2000.

367. Matsaniotis, N., Kattanis, C., Economou-Mavrou, C., et al.: Bullous emphysema in childhood tuberculosis. J. Pediatr. 71:703-708, 1967.

368. McCray, M. K., and Esterly, M. B.: Cutaneous eruptions in congenital tuberculosis. Arch. Dermatol. 117:460-464, 1981.

369. McKenzie, S. A., McNab, A. J., and Katz, G.: Neonatal pyridoxine responsive convulsions due to isoniazid therapy. Arch. Dis. Child. 51:567-568, 1976.

370. Medical Research Council Investigation: Streptomycin treatment of pulmonary tuberculosis. B. M. J. 2:769-782, 1948.

371. Medical Research Council Working Party on Tuberculosis of the Spine: Five-year assessment of controlled trials of inpatient and outpatient treatment and of plaster-of-paris jackets for tuberculosis of the spine in children on standard chemotherapy: Studies in Masan and Pusan, Korea. J. Bone Joint Surg. Br. 58:399-411, 1976.

372. Medical Research Council Working Party on Tuberculosis of the Spine: Five-year assessment of controlled trials of ambulatory treatment, débridement and anterior spinal fusion in the management of tuberculosis of the spine; studies in Bulawayo (Rhodesia) and in Hong Kong. J. Bone Joint Surg. Br. 60:163-177, 1978.

373. Medical Research Council Working Party on Tuberculosis of the Spine: Twelfth report: Controlled trial of short-course regimens of chemotherapy in the ambulatory treatment of spinal tuberculosis. J. Bone Joint Surg. Br. 75:240-248, 1993.

374. Mehta, J. B., and Bentley, S.: Prevention of tuberculosis in children: Missed opportunities. Am. J. Prev. Med. 8:283-286, 1992.

375. Meier, A., Kirschner, P., Bange, F., et al.: Genetic alterations in streptomycin-resistant *Mycobacterium tuberculosis*: Mapping of mutations conferring resistance. Antimicrob. Agents Chemother. 38:228-233, 1994.

376. Menzies, R., Fanning, A., Yuan, L., et al.: Tuberculosis among healthcare workers. N. Engl. J. Med. 332:92-98, 1995.

377. Menzies, R., Rocher, I., and Vissandjee, B.: Factors associated with compliance in treatment of tuberculosis. Tubercle Lung Dis. 74:32-37, 1993.

378. Menzies, R., and Vissandjee, B.: Effect of bacille Calmette-Guérin vaccination on tuberculin reactivity. Am. Rev. Respir. Dis. 141:621-625, 1992.

379. Migliori, G. B., Borghesi, A., Rossanigo, P., et al.: Proposal of an improved score method for the diagnosis of pulmonary tuberculosis in childhood in developing countries. Tubercle Lung Dis. 73:145-149, 1992.

380. Miller, F. J. W., Seale, R. M. E., and Taylor, M. D.: Tuberculosis in Children. Boston, Little, Brown, 1963, p. 214.

381. Miller, R. A., Lanza, L. A., Kline, J. N., et al.: *Mycobacterium tuberculosis* in lung transplant recipients. Am. J. Respir. Crit. Care Med. 152:374-376, 1995.

382. Miller, R. R., Porter, J., and Greenblatt, D. J.: Clinical importance of the interaction of phenytoin and isoniazid: A report from the Boston Collaborative Drug Surveillance Program. Chest 75:356-358, 1979.

383. Miorner, H., Sjobring, U., Nayak, P., et al.: Diagnosis of tuberculous meningitis: A comparative analysis of 3 immunoassays, an immune complex assay and the polymerase chain reaction. Tubercle Lung Dis. 76:381-386, 1995.

384. Mitchison, D. A.: Basic mechanisms of chemotherapy. Chest 76(Suppl.):771-781, 1979.

385. Mitchison, D. A.: The action of anti-tuberculous drugs in short-course chemotherapy. Tubercle 66:219-225, 1985.

386. Mitchison, D. A., and Nunn, A. J.: Influence of initial drug resistance on the response to short-course chemotherapy of pulmonary tuberculosis. Am. Rev. Respir. Dis. 133:423-428, 1986.

387. Mohanty, K. C., and Dhamgaye, T. M.: Controlled trial of ciprofloxacin in short-term chemotherapy for pulmonary tuberculosis. Chest 104:1194-1198, 1993.

388. Mohle-Boetani, J. C., and Flood, J.: Contact investigations and the continued commitment to control tuberculosis. J. A. M. A. 287:1040-1041, 2002.

389. Mohle-Boetani, J. C., Miller, B., Halpern, M., et al.: School-based screening for tuberculous infection: A cost benefit analysis. J. A. M. A. 274:613-619, 1995.

390. Montenegro, S., Gilman, R., Sheen, P., et al.: Improved detection of *Mycobacterium tuberculosis* in Peruvian children by use of a heminested IS6110 polymerase chain reaction assay. Clin. Infect. Dis. 3:16-23, 2003.

391. Moore, M., Schulte, J., Valway, S., et al.: Evaluation of transmission of *Mycobacterium tuberculosis* in a pediatric setting. J. Pediatr. 133:108-112, 1998.

392. Morens, D. M., Baublis, J. V., and Heidelberger, K. P.: Congenital tuberculosis and associated hypoadrenocorticism. South. Med. J. 72:160-161, 165, 1979.

393. Morrison, J. B.: Natural history of segmental lesions in primary pulmonary tuberculosis. Arch. Dis. Child. 48:90-98, 1973.

394. Morse, M. L., Karr, D. J., and Menddman, P. M.: Ocular tuberculosis in a five-month-old. Pediatr. Infect. Dis. J. 7:514-516, 1988.

395. Moss, W. J., Dedyo, T., Suarez, M., et al.: Tuberculosis in children infected with human immunodeficiency virus: A report of five cases. Pediatr. Infect. Dis. J. 11:114-120, 1992.

396. Mudido, P. M., Guwratudde, D., Nakakeeto, M. K., et al.: The effect of bacilli Calmette-Guérin vaccination at birth on tuberculin skin test reactivity in Ugandan children. Int. J. Tuberc. Lung Dis. 3:891-895, 1999.

397. Mukherjee, J. A., Joseph, K. S., Rich, M. L., et al.: Clinical and programmatic considerations in treatment of MDR-TB in children: A series of 16 patients in Lima, Peru. Int. J. Tuberc. Lung Dis. 7:637-644, 2003.

398. Mumtaz, M. A., Schwartz, R. H., Grundfast, K. M., et al.: Tuberculosis of the middle ear and mastoid. Pediatr. Infect. Dis. 2:234-236, 1983.

399. Munoz, F. M., Ong, L. T., Seavy, D., et al.: Tuberculosis among adult visitors of children with suspected tuberculosis and employees at a children's hospital. Infect. Control Hosp. Epidemiol. 23:568-572, 2002.

400. Munoz, P., Rodriguez, C., and Bouza, E.: *Mycobacterium tuberculosis* infection in recipients of solid organ transplants. Clin. Infect. Dis. 40:581-587, 2005.

401. Murray, J. F.: Cursed duet: HIV infection and tuberculosis. Respiration 57:210-220, 1990.

402. Nakajo, M. M., Rao, M., and Steiner, P.: Incidence of hepatotoxicity in children receiving isoniazid chemoprophylaxis. Pediatr. Infect. Dis. J. 8:649-650, 1989.

403. Narendran, G., Swaminathan, S., Sathish, S., and Rajosekaran, S.: Immune reconstitution syndrome in a child with TB and HIV. Indian J. Pediatr. 73:627-629, 2006.

404. Nelson, L. J., Schneider, E., Wells, C. D., and Moore, M.: Epidemiology of childhood tuberculosis in the United States, 1993-2001: The need for continued vigilance. Pediatrics 114:333-341, 2004.

405. Nelson, L. J., and Wells, C. D.: Global epidemiology of childhood tuberculosis. Int. J. Tuberc. Lung Dis. 8:636-647, 2004.

406. Nemir, R. L., Cardona, J., Lacoius, A., et al.: Prednisone therapy as an adjunct in the treatment of lymph node–bronchial tuberculosis in childhood: A double-blind study. Am. Rev. Respir. Dis. 88:189-198, 1963.

407. Nemir, R. L., Cardona, J., Vaziri, F., et al.: Prednisone as an adjunct in the chemotherapy of lymph node–bronchial tuberculosis in childhood: A double-blind study. II. Further term observation. Am. Rev. Respir. Dis. 95:402-410, 1967.

408. Nemir, R. L., and Krasinski, K.: Tuberculosis in children and adolescents in the 1980's. Pediatr. Infect. Dis. J. 7:375-379, 1988.

409. Nemir, R. L., and O'Hare, D.: Congenital tuberculosis. Am. J. Dis. Child. 139:284-287, 1985.

410. Nemir, R. L., and O'Hare, D.: Tuberculosis in children 10 years of age and younger: Three decades of experience during the chemotherapeutic era. Pediatrics 88:236-241, 1991.

411. Nemir, R. L., and Teichner, A.: Management of tuberculin reactors in children and adolescents previously vaccinated with BCG. Pediatr. Infect. Dis. 2:446-451, 1983.

412. Netto, E. M., Dye, C., and Raviglione, M. C.: Progress in global tuberculosis control 1995-1996, with emphasis on 22 high-incidence countries. Global Monitoring and Surveillance Project. Int. J. Tuberc. Lung Dis. 3:310-320, 1999.

413. Nivin, B., Nicholas, P., Gayer, M., et al.: A continuing outbreak of multidrug-resistant tuberculosis, with transmission in a hospital nursery. Clin. Infect. Dis. 26:303-307, 1998.

414. Nolan, C. M., and Elarth, A. M.: Tuberculosis in a cohort of Southeast Asian refugees. Am. Rev. Respir. Dis. 137:805-809, 1988.

415. Nolan, C. M., Elarth, A. M., and Barr, H. W.: Intentional isoniazid overdose in young Southeast Asian refugee women. Chest 93:803-806, 1988.

416. Nolan, R., Jr.: Childhood tuberculosis in North Carolina: A study of the opportunities for intervention in the transmission of tuberculosis in children. Am. J. Public Health 76:26-30, 1986.

417. Noordhoek, G., Kolk, A., Bjune, G., et al.: Sensitivity and specificity of PCR for detection of *Mycobacterium tuberculosis*: A blind comparison study among seven laboratories. J. Clin. Microbiol. 32:277-284, 1994.

418. North, R. J., and Jung, Y. L.: Immunity to tuberculosis. Annu. Rev. Immunol. 22:599-623, 2004.

419. Nunn, P., and Felten, M.: Surveillance of resistance to antituberculosis drugs in developing countries. Tubercle Lung Dis. 75:163-167, 1994.

420. Obaegbulam, S. C.: Spinal extraosseous extradural tuberculoma. Tubercle 58:97, 1977.

421. O'Brien, K., Ruff, A., Louis, M., et al.: Bacillus Calmette-Guérin complications in children born to HIV-1–infected women with a review of the literature. Pediatrics 95:414-418, 1995.

422. O'Brien, R. J., Long, M. W., Cross, F. S., et al.: Hepatotoxicity from isoniazid and rifampin among children treated for tuberculosis. Pediatrics 72:491-499, 1983.

423. Offenbacher, H., Fazekas, F., Schmidt. R., et al.: MRI in tuberculous meningoencephalitis: Report of four cases and review of the neuroimaging literature. J. Neurol. 238:340-344, 1991.

424. Olazabal, F.: Choroidal tubercles: A neglected sign. J. A. M. A. 200:104-107, 1967.

425. Olson, W. A., Pruitt, A. W., and Dayton, P. G.: Plasma concentration of isoniazid in children with tuberculous infections. Pediatrics 67:876-878, 1981.

426. Omari, B., Robertson, J. M., Nelson, R. J., et al.: Pott's disease: A resurgent challenge to the thoracic surgeon. Chest 95:145-150, 1989. (See also follow-up letters, Chest 96:955-956, 1989.)

427. Optican, R. J., Ost, A., and Ravin, C. E.: High-resolution computed tomography in the diagnosis of miliary tuberculosis. Chest 102:941-943, 1992.

428. Orme, I. M., Andersen, P., and Boom, W. H.: T cell response to *Mycobacterium tuberculosis*. J. Infect. Dis. 167:1481-1497, 1993.

429. Owens, S., Abdel-Rahman, I. E., Balyejusa, S., et al.: Nasopharyngeal aspiration for diagnosis of pulmonary tuberculosis. Arch. Dis. Child. 92:693-696, 2007. Epub ahead of print.

430. Ozuah, P. O., Ozuah, T. P., Stein, R. E. K., et al.: Evaluation of a risk assessment questionnaire used to target tuberculin skin testing in children. J. A. M. A. 285:451-453, 2001.

431. Padoyatchi, N., Bambar, S., Dawood, H., and Bobat, R.: Multidrug-resistant tuberculosis meningitis in children in Durban, South Africa. Pediatr. Infect. Dis. J. 25:147-150, 2006.

432. Pai, M., Kalantri, S., and Dheda, K.: New tools and emerging technologies for the diagnosis of tuberculosis: Part I. Latent tuberculosis. Expert Rev. Mol. Diagn. 6:413-422, 2006.

433. Pai, M., and Menzies, D.: Interferon-gamma release assays: What is their role in the diagnosis of active tuberculosis? Clin. Infect. Dis. 44:74-77, 2007.

434. Palme, I. B., Gudetta, B., Bruchfield, J., et al.: Impact of human immunodeficiency virus 1 infection on clinical presentation, treatment outcome and survival in a cohort of Ethiopian children with tuberculosis. Pediatr. Infect. Dis. J. 21:1053-1061, 2002.

435. Palur, R., Rajohekhar, V., Chandy, M. J., et al.: Shunt surgery for hydrocephalus in tuberculous meningitis: A long-term follow-up study. J. Neurosurg. 74:64-69, 1991.

436. Paluschi, V. J., O'Hare, D., and Lawrence, R. M.: Hepatotoxicity and transaminase measurement during isoniazid chemoprophylaxis in children. Pediatr. Infect. Dis. J. 14:144-148, 1995.

437. Parish, R. E., and Brownstein, D.: Emergency department management of children with acute isoniazid poisoning. Pediatr. Emerg. Care 2:88-90, 1986.

438. Park, M. M., Davis, A. L., Schluger, N. W., et al.: Outcome of MDR-TB patients, 1983-1993: Prolonged survival with appropriate therapy. Am. J. Respir. Crit. Care Med. 153:317-324, 1996.

439. Passannante, M., Gallagher, C., and Reichman, L.: Preventive therapy for contacts of multidrug-resistant tuberculosis: A Delphi study. Chest 106:431-434, 1994.

440. Pastrana, D. G., Torronteras, R., Caro, P., et al.: Comparison of Amplicor, in-house polymerase chain reactions and conventional culture for the diagnosis of tuberculosis in children. Clin. Infect. Dis. 32:17-22, 2001.

441. Payne, M., quoted by Miller, F. J. W., Seale, R. M. E., and Taylor, M. D.: Tuberculosis in Children. Boston, Little, Brown, 1963.

442. Pearson, M. L., Jereb, J. A., Frieden, T. R., et al.: Nosocomial transmission of multidrug-resistant *Mycobacterium tuberculosis*: A risk to patients and healthcare workers. Ann. Intern. Med. 117:191-196, 1992.

443. Pederson, F. K., Schiotz, P. O., Valerius, N. H., et al.: Fatal BCG infection in an immunocompetent girl. Acta Paediatr. Scand. 67:19-23, 1978.

444. Pediatric Tuberculosis Collaborative Group: Targeted tuberculin skin testing and treatment of latent tuberculosis infection in children and adolescents. Pediatrics 114:1175-1207, 2004.

445. Pellock, J. M., Howell, J., Kendig, E. L., Jr., et al.: Pyridoxine deficiency in children treated with isoniazid. Chest 87:658-661, 1985.

446. Peloquin, C. A., MacPhee, A. A., and Berning, S. E.: Malabsorption of antimycobacterial medications. N. Engl. J. Med. 329:1122-1123, 1993.

447. Peltola, H., Salmi, I., Vahvanen, V., et al.: BCG vaccination as a cause of osteomyelitis and subcutaneous abscess. Arch. Dis. Child. 59:157-161, 1984.

448. Pereira, C. A., Webber, B., and Orson, J. M.: Primary tuberculous complex of the skin. J. A. M. A. 235:942, 1976.

449. Perry, S., and Starke, J. R.: Adherence to prescribed treatment and public health aspects of tuberculosis in children. Semin. Pediatr. Infect. Dis. 4:291-298, 1993.

450. Pesanti, E.: The negative tuberculin skin test: Tuberculin, HIV and anergy panels. Am. J. Respir. Crit. Care Med. 149:1699-1709, 1994.

451. Pierre, C., Olivier, C., Lecossier, D., et al.: Diagnosis of primary tuberculosis in children by amplification and detection of mycobacterial DNA. Am. Rev. Respir. Dis. 147:420-424, 1993.

452. Pineda, P., Leung, A., Muller, N., et al.: Intrathoracic pediatric tuberculosis: A report of 202 cases. Tubercle Lung Dis. 74:261-266, 1993.

453. Pomerantz, M., Madsen, L., Goble, M., et al.: Surgical management of resistant mycobacterial tuberculosis and other mycobacterial pulmonary infections. Ann. Thorac. Surg. 52:1108-1112, 1991.

454. Pospelov, L. E., Matrakshin, A. G., Chernousova, L. N., et al.: Association of various genetic markers with tuberculosis and other lung disease in Tuvinian children. Tubercle Lung Dis. 77:77-80, 1996.

455. Puthanakit, T., Oberdorfen, P., Punjaisee, S., et al.: Immune reconstitution syndrome due to bacillus Calmette-Guérin after initiation of antiretroviral therapy in children with HIV infection. Clin. Infect. Dis. 41:1049-1052, 2005.

456. Puthanakit, T., Oberdorfen, P., Akarathum, N., et al.: Immune reconstitution syndrome after highly active antiretroviral therapy in human immunodeficiency virus–infected Thai children. Pediatr. Infect. Dis. J. 25:53-58, 2000.

457. Ramachondran, S., Clifton, I. J., Collyns, T. A., et al.: The treatment of spinal tuberculosis: A retrospective study. Int. J. Tuberc. Lung Dis. 9:541-544, 2005.

458. Rampton, D. S.: Preventing TB in patients with Crohn's disease needing infliximab or other anti-TNF therapy. Gut 54:1360-1362, 2005.

459. Rapp, R. S., Campbell, R. W., Howell, J. C., et al.: Isoniazid hepatotoxicity in children. Am. Rev. Respir. Dis. 118:794-796, 1978.

460. Rasool, M. N.: Osseous manifestations of tuberculosis in children. J. Pediatr. Orthop. 21:749-755, 2001.

461. Rasool, M., Govender, S., and Naidoo, K.: Cystic tuberculosis of bone in children. J. Bone Joint Surg. Br. 76:113-117, 1994.

462. Ravenscroft, A., Schoeman, J., and Donald, P. R.: Tuberculous granulomas in childhood tuberculous meningitis: Radiologic features and course. J. Trop. Pediatr. 47:5-12, 2001.

463. Raviglione, M. C., Rieder, H. L., Styblo, K., et al.: Tuberculosis trends in Eastern Europe and the former USSR. Tubercle Lung Dis. 75:400-416, 1994.

464. Raviglione, M. C., Snider, D., Jr., and Kochi, A.: Global epidemiology of tuberculosis: Morbidity and mortality of a worldwide epidemic. J. A. M. A. 273:220-226, 1995.

465. Reichler, M. R., Reves, R., Bur, S., et al.: Evaluation of investigations conducted to detect and prevent transmission of tuberculosis. J. A. M. A. 287:991-995, 2002.

466. Reichman, L. B.: Why hasn't BCG proved dangerous in HIV-infected patients? J. A. M. A. 261:3246, 1989.

467. Reis, F. J., Bedran, M. B., Mowra, J. A., et al.: Six-month isoniazid-rifampin treatment for pulmonary tuberculosis in children. Am. Rev. Respir. Dis. 142:996-999, 1990.

468. Report of a WHO Study Group: BCG vaccination policies. WHO Technical Report Series No. 652, 1980-1981.

469. Reynes, J., Perez, C., Lamaury, I., et al.: Bacille Calmette-Guérin adenitis 30 years after immunization in a patient with AIDS. J. Infect. Dis. 160:727, 1989.

470. Rich, A. R.: The Pathogenesis of Tuberculosis. 2nd ed. Springfield, IL, Charles C Thomas, 1951.

471. Rich, A. R., and McCordock, H. A.: The pathogenesis of tuberculous meningitis. Bull. Johns Hopkins Hosp. 52:5-35, 1933.

472. Richeldi, L.: An update on the diagnosis of tuberculosis infection. Am. J. Respir. Crit. Care Med. 174:736-742, 2006.

473. Ridgeway, A. L., Warner, G. S., Phillips, P., et al.: Transmission of *Mycobacterium tuberculosis* to recipients of single lung transplants from the same donor. Am. J. Respir. Crit. Care Med. 153:1166-1168, 1996.

474. Ridzon, R., Kent, J. H., Valway, S., et al.: Outbreak of drug-resistant tuberculosis with secondary-generation transmission in a high school in California. J. Pediatr. 131:863-868, 1997.

475. Riley, L. W., Arathoon, E., and Loverde, V. D.: The epidemiologic patterns of drug-resistant *Mycobacterium tuberculosis* infections: A community-based study. Am. Rev. Respir. Dis. 139:1282-1285, 1989.

476. Riley, R. L.: Airborne transmission. *In* Johnson, J. E. (ed.): Rational Therapy and Control of Tuberculosis. Gainesville, University of Florida Press, 1970.

477. Rooney, J. J., Crocco, J. A., and Lyons, H. A.: Tuberculous pericarditis. Ann. Intern. Med. 72:73-78, 1970.

478. Roy, V., Tekur, U., and Chopra, K.: Pharmacokinetics of pyrazinamide in children suffering from pulmonary tuberculosis. Int. J. Tuberc. Lung Dis. 3:133-137, 1999.

479. Ryder, R. W., Oxtoby, M. J., Mvula, M., et al.: Safety and immunogenicity of bacille Calmette-Guérin, diphtheria-tetanus-pertussis, and oral polio vaccines in newborn children in Zaire infected with human immunodeficiency virus type 1. J. Pediatr. 122:697-702, 1993.

480. Saczek, K. B., Schaaf, H. S., Vors, M., et al.: Diagnostic dilemmas in abdominal tuberculosis in children. Pediatr. Surg. Int. 17:111-115, 2001.

481. Sada, E., Aguilar, D., Torres, M., et al.: Detection of lipoarabinomannan as a diagnostic test for tuberculosis. J. Clin. Microbiol. 30:2415-2418, 1992.

482. Saiman, L., Aronson, J., Zhou, J., et al.: Prevalence of infectious diseases among internationally adopted children. Pediatrics 108:608-612, 2001.

483. Saiman, L., San Gabriel, P., Schultz, J., et al.: Risk factors for latent tuberculosis infection among children in New York City. Pediatrics 107:999-1003, 2001.

484. Saitah, A., Pong, A., Waecker, N. J., Jr., et al.: Prediction of neurologic sequelae in childhood tuberculous meningitis: A review of 20 cases and proposal of a novel scoring system. Pediatr. Infect. Dis. J. 24:207-212, 2005.

485. Salazar, G. E., Schmitz, T. L., Cama, R., et al.: Pulmonary tuberculosis in a developing country. Pediatrics 108:448-453, 2001.

486. Salfinger, M., Crowle, A., and Reller, L. B.: Pyrazinamide and pyrazinoic acid activity against tubercle bacilli in cultured human macrophages and in the BACTEC system. J. Infect. Dis. 162:201-207, 1990.

487. Salfinger, M., and Pfyfler, G. E.: The new diagnostic mycobacteriology laboratory. Eur. J. Clin. Microbiol. 13:961-979, 1994.

488. Saltzman, S. J., and Feigin, R. D.: Tuberculous otitis media and mastoiditis. J. Pediatr. 79:1004-1006, 1971.

489. Sanchez-Albisua, I., Vidal, M. L., Joya-Verde, G., et al.: Tolerance of pyrazinamide in short course chemotherapy for pulmonary tuberculosis in children. Pediatr. Infect. Dis. J. 16:760-763, 1997.

490. Sassan-Morokro, M., DeCock, K. M., Ackah, A., et al.: Tuberculosis and HIV infection in children in Abidjon, Cote d'Ivoire. Trans. R. Soc. Trop. Med. Hyg. 88:178-181, 1994.

491. Sathe, S. S., and Reichman, L. B.: Mycobacterial disease in patients infected with human immunodeficiency virus. Clin. Chest Med. 10:445-463, 1989.

492. Schaaf, H. S., Beyers, N., Gie, R. P., et al.: Respiratory tuberculosis in childhood: The diagnostic value of clinical features and special investigations. Pediatr. Infect. Dis. J. 14:189-194, 1995.

493. Schaaf, H. S., Gie, R. P., Beyers, N., et al.: Tuberculosis in infants less than 3 months of age. Arch. Dis. Child. 69:371-374, 1993.

494. Schaaf, H. S., Gie, R. P., Beyers, N., et al.: Primary drug-resistant tuberculosis in children. Int. J. Tuberc. Lung Dis. 4:1-7, 2000.

495. Schaaf, H. S., Gie, R. P., Beyers, N., et al.: Primary drug-resistant tuberculosis. Pediatr. Infect. Dis. J. 19:695-699, 2000.

496. Schaaf, H. S., Gie, R. P., Kennedy, M., et al.: Evaluation of young children in contact with adult multi-drug resistant pulmonary tuberculosis: A 30-month follow-up. Pediatrics 109:765-771, 2002.

497. Schaaf, H. S., Krook, S., Hollermans, D. W., et al.: Recurrent culture-confirmed tuberculosis in human immunodeficiency virus–infected children. Pediatr. Infect. Dis. J. 24:685-691, 2005.

498. Schaefer, G.: Tuberculosis in Obstetrics and Gynecology. Boston, Little, Brown, 1956.

499. Schick, B., and Dolgin, J.: The influence of prednisone on the Mantoux reaction in children. Pediatrics 31:856-859, 1963.

500. Schluger, N., Kinney, D., Harkin, T., et al.: Clinical utility of the polymerase chain reaction in the diagnosis of infections due to Mycobacterium tuberculosis. Chest 105:1116-1121, 1994.

501. Schoeman, J., Wait, J., Burger, M., et al.: Long-term followup of childhood tuberculous meningitis. Dev. Med. Child Neurol. 44:522-526, 2002.

502. Scholten, J. W., Fujiwara, P. I., and Frieden, T. R.: Prevalence and factors associated with tuberculosis infection among new school entrants, New York City, 1991-1993. Int. J. Tuberc. Lung Dis. 3:31-41, 1999.

503. Schuit, K. E.: Miliary tuberculosis in children. Am. J. Dis. Child. 133:583-585, 1979.

504. Schuit, K. E., and Powell, D. A.: Mycobacterial lymphadenitis in childhood. Am. J. Dis. Child. 132:675-677, 1978.

505. Schwartz, P.: Lymph node tuberculosis: A decisive factor in pulmonary pathology. Arch. Pediatr. 74:159-177, 201-218, 1957.

506. Schwartzman, K., and Menzies, D.: Tuberculosis screening of immigrants to low-prevalence countries. Am. J. Respir. Crit. Care Med. 161:780-789, 2000.

507. Sehgal, V. N., and Wagh, S. A.: Cutaneous tuberculosis. Int. J. Dermatol. 29:237-252, 1990.

508. Selwyn, P., Hartel, D., Lewis, V., et al.: A prospective study of the risk of tuberculosis among intravenous drug users with human immunodeficiency virus infection. N. Engl. J. Med. 320:545-550, 1989.

509. Sepulveda, R. L., Burr, C., Ferrer, X., et al.: Booster effect of tuberculosis testing in healthy 6-year-old school children vaccinated with bacille Calmette-Guérin at birth in Santiago, Chile. Pediatr. Infect. Dis. J. 7:578-582, 1988.

510. Sepulveda, R. L., Heiba, I. M., King, A., et al.: Evaluation of tuberculin reactivity in BCG-immunized siblings. Am. J. Respir. Crit. Care Med. 149:620-624, 1994.

511. Sepulveda, R. L., Heiba, I. M., Navarrete, C., et al.: Tuberculin reactivity after newborn BCG immunization in mono- and dizygotic twins. Tubercle Lung Dis. 75:138-143, 1994.

512. Shafer, R., Small, P., Larkin, C., et al.: Temporal trends and transmission patterns during the emergence of multidrug-resistant tuberculosis in New York City: A molecular epidemiologic assessment. J. Infect. Dis. 171:170-176, 1995.

513. Shah, B. R., Santucci, K., Sinert, R., et al.: Acute isoniazid neurotoxicity in an urban hospital. Pediatrics 95:700-704, 1995.

514. Shah, N. S., Wright, A., Bai, G. H., et al.: Worldwide emergency of extensively drug-resistant tuberculosis. Emerg. Infect. Dis. 13:380-387, 2007.

515. Shannon, F. B., Moore, M., Houkom, J. A., et al.: Multifocal cystic tuberculosis of bone. J. Bone Joint Surg. Am. 72:1089-1092, 1990.

516. Sharma, S. K., Mohan, A., Sharma, A., and Mitra, D. K.: Miliary tuberculosis: New insights into an old disease. Lancet Infect. Dis. 5:415-530, 2005.

517. Shata, A. M. A., Coulter, J. B. S., Parry, C. M., et al.: Sputum induction for the diagnosis of tuberculosis. Arch. Dis. Child. 74:535-537, 1996.

518. Shepard, W. E., Field, M. L., James, D. H., et al.: Transient appearance of intracranial tuberculomas during treatment of tuberculous meningitis. Pediatr. Infect. Dis. J. 5:599-601, 1986.

519. Sheridan, P. H., Edman, J. B., and Starr, S. E.: Tuberculosis presenting as an orbital mass. Pediatrics 67:874-875, 1981.

520. Shimokata, K., Kawachi, H., Kishumoto, H., et al.: Local cellular immunity in tuberculous pleurisy. Am. Rev. Respir. Dis. 126:822-824, 1982.

521. Shin, S., Guerra, D., Rich, M., et al.: Treatment of multidrug-resistant tuberculosis during pregnancy: A report of 7 cases. Clin. Infect. Dis. 15:996-1003, 2003.

522. Shingadia, D., and Novelli, V.: Diagnosis and treatment of tuberculosis in children. Lancet Infect. Dis. 3:624-632, 2003.

523. Siberry, G. K., and Tessema, S.: Immune reconstitution syndrome precipitated by bacille Calmette-Guérin after initiation of antiretroviral therapy. Pediatr. Infect. Dis. J. 25:648-649, 2006.

524. Siddiqi, S. H., Hwangbo, C. C., Silcox, V., et al.: Rapid radiometric methods to detect and differentiate Mycobacterium tuberculosis/M. bovis from other mycobacterial species. Am. J. Respir. Dis. 130:634-640, 1984.

525. Singapore Tuberculosis Service/British Medical Research Council: Five-year follow-up of a clinical trial of three 6-month regimens of chemotherapy given intermittently in the continuation phase in the treatment of pulmonary tuberculosis. Am. Rev. Respir. Dis. 137:1147-1150, 1988.

526. Sirinavin, S., Chotpitayasunondh, T., Suwanjutha, S., et al.: Efficacy of neonatal bacillus Calmette-Guérin vaccination against tuberculosis. Pediatr. Infect. Dis. J. 10:359-365, 1991.

527. Sloan, J. B.: Papulonecrotic tuberculid in a 9-year-old American girl: Case report and review of the literature. Pediatr. Dermatol. 7:191-195, 1990.

528. Slutkin, G., Schecter, G. F., and Hopewell, P. C.: The results of 9-month isoniazid-rifampin therapy for pulmonary tuberculosis under program conditions in San Francisco. Am. Rev. Respir. Dis. 138:1622-1624, 1988.

529. Small, P., Hopewell, P., Singh, S., et al.: The epidemiology of tuberculosis in San Francisco: A population-based study using conventional and molecular methods. N. Engl. J. Med. 330:1703-1709, 1994.

530. Small, P. M., Shafer, R. W., Hopewell, P. C., et al.: Exogenous reinfection with multidrug-resistant Mycobacterium tuberculosis in patients with advanced HIV infection. N. Engl. J. Med. 328:1137-1144, 1993.

531. Smith, A. M., and Lattimer, J. K.: Genitourinary tract involvement in children with tuberculosis. N. Y. State J. Med. 73:2325-2328, 1973.

532. Smith, D., Reeser, P., and Musa, S.: Does infection with environmental mycobacteria suppress the protective response to subsequent vaccination with BCG? Tubercle 66:17-23, 1985.

533. Smith, K. C., Starke, J. R., Eisenach, K., et al.: Detection of Mycobacterium tuberculosis in clinical specimens from children using a polymerase chain reaction. Pediatrics 97:155-160, 1996.

534. Smith, M. H. D.: The role of adrenal steroids in the treatment of tuberculosis. Pediatrics 22:774-776, 1958.

535. Smith, M. H. D.: What about short course and intermittent chemotherapy for tuberculosis in children? Pediatr. Infect. Dis. 1:298-303, 1982.

536. Smith, M. H. D.: Tuberculosis in children and adolescents. Clin. Chest Med. 10:381-395, 1989.

537. Smith, M. H. D., and Matsaniotis, N.: Treatment of tuberculous pleural effusions with particular reference to adrenal corticosteroids. Pediatrics 22:1074-1087, 1959.

538. Snider, D. E., Jr., and Block, A. B.: Congenital tuberculosis. Tubercle 65:81-82, 1984.

539. Snider, D. E., Jr., and Caras, G. J.: Isoniazid-associated hepatitis deaths: A review of available information. Am. Rev. Respir. Dis. 145:494-497, 1992.

540. Snider, D. E., Jr., Caras, G. J., and Kaplan, J. P.: Preventive therapy with isoniazid: Cost-effectiveness of different durations of therapy. J. A. M. A. 255:1579-1583, 1986.

541. Snider, D. E., Jr., and Farer, L. S.: Preventive therapy for tuberculous infection: An intervention in need of improvement. Am. Rev. Respir. Dis. 130:355-356, 1984.

542. Snider, D. E., Graczyk, J., Bek, E., et al.: Supervised six-month treatment of newly diagnosed pulmonary tuberculosis using isoniazid, rifampin, and pyrazinamide with and without streptomycin. Am. Rev. Respir. Dis. 130:1091-1094, 1984.

543. Snider, D. E., Jr., Kelly, G. D., Cauthen, G. M., et al.: Infection and disease among contacts of tuberculosis cases with drug-resistant and drug-susceptible bacilli. Am. Rev. Respir. Dis. 132:125-128, 1985.

544. Snider, D. E., Jr., Layde, P. M., Johnson, M. W., et al.: Treatment of tuberculosis during pregnancy. Am. Rev. Respir. Dis. 122:65-79, 1980.

545. Snider, D. E., Jr., and Powell, K. E.: Should women taking antituberculosis drugs breastfeed? Arch. Intern. Med. 144:589-590, 1984.

546. Somu, N., Swaminathan, S., Paramisivan, C. N., et al.: Value of bronchoalveolar lavage and gastric lavage in the diagnosis of pulmonary tuberculosis in children. Tuberc. Lung. Dis. 76:295-299, 1995.

547. Soren, K., Saiman, L., Irigoyen, M., et al.: Evaluation of household contacts of children with positive tuberculin skin tests. Pediatr. Infect. Dis. J. 18:949-955, 1999.

548. Soysal, A., Millington, K. A., Bakir, M., et al.: Effect of BCG vaccination on risk of Mycobacterium tuberculosis infection in children with household tuberculosis contact: A prospective community-based study. Lancet 366:1443-1451, 2005.

549. Spyridis, N. P., Spyridis, P. G., Gelesme, A., et al.: The effectiveness of a 9-month regimen of isoniazid alone versus 3- and 4- month regimens of isoniazid plus rifampin for treatment of latent tuberculosis infection in children: Results of an 11 year randomized study. Clin. Infect. Dis. 45:715-722, 2007.

550. Spyridis, P., Maltezou, H. C., Hantzakos, A., et al.: Mycobacterial cervical adenitis in children: Clinical and laboratory factors of importance for differential diagnosis. Scand. J. Infect. Dis. 33:362-366, 2001.

551. Spyridis, P., Sinaniotis, C., Papadea, I., et al.: Isoniazid liver injury during chemoprophylaxis in children. Arch. Dis. Child. 54:65-67, 1979.

552. Stallworth, J. R., Brasfield, D. M., and Tiller, R. E.: Congenital miliary tuberculosis proved by open lung biopsy specimen and successfully treated. Am. J. Dis. Child. 134:320-321, 1980.

553. Stansberry, S. D.: Tuberculosis in infants and children. J. Thorac. Imaging 5:17-27, 1990.

554. Starke, J. R.: Interferon-gamma release assays for diagnosis of tuberculosis infection in children. Pediatr. Infect. Dis. J. 25:941-942, 2006.

555. Starke, J. R.: New concepts in childhood tuberculosis. Curr. Opin. Pediatr. 19:306-313, 2007.

556. Starke, J. R.: Multidrug therapy for tuberculosis in children. Pediatr. Infect. Dis. J. 9:785-793, 1990.

557. Starke, J. R.: Current chemotherapy for tuberculosis in children. Infect. Dis. Clin. North Am. 6:215-238, 1992.

558. Starke, J. R.: Tuberculosis of the central nervous system in children. Semin. Pediatr. Neurol. 6:318-331, 1999.

559. Starke, J. R.: Transmission of Mycobacterium tuberculosis to and from children and adolescents. Semin. Pediatr. Infect. Dis. 12:115-123, 2001.

560. Starke, J. R.: Childhood tuberculosis: Ending the neglect. Int. J. Tuberc. Lung Dis. 6:373-374, 2002.

561. Starke, J. R., and Correa, A. G.: Management of mycobacterial infection and disease in children. Pediatr. Infect. Dis. J. 14:455-470, 1995.

562. Starke, J. R., Jacobs, R., and Jereb, J.: Resurgence of tuberculosis in children. J. Pediatr. *120*:839-855, 1992.

563. Starke, J. R., and Taylor-Watts, K. T.: Tuberculosis in the pediatric population of Houston, Texas. Pediatrics *84*:28-35, 1989.

564. Starr, S., and Berkovich, S.: Effects of measles, gammaglobulin-modified measles and vaccine measles on the tuberculin test. N. Engl. J. Med. *270*:386-391, 1964.

565. Stead, W. W.: Pathogenesis of a first episode of chronic pulmonary tuberculosis in man: Recrudescence of residuals of the primary infection or exogenous reinfection? Am. Rev. Respir. Dis. *95*:729-745, 1967.

566. Stein, M. T., and Liang, D.: Clinical hepatotoxicity of isoniazid in children. Pediatrics *64*:499-505, 1979.

567. Steiner, M., Steiner, P., and Schmidt, H.: Primary drug-resistant tuberculosis in children: A continuing study of the incidence of disease caused by primarily drug-resistant organisms in children observed between the years 1965 and 1968 at the Kings County Medical Center of Brooklyn. Am. Rev. Respir. Dis. *102*:75-82, 1970.

568. Steiner, P., and Rao, M.: Drug-resistant tuberculosis in children. Semin. Pediatr. Infect. Dis. *4*:275-282, 1993.

569. Steiner, P., Rao, M., and Mitchell, M.: Primary drug-resistant tuberculosis in children: Correlation of drug-susceptibility patterns of matched patient and source-case strains of *Mycobacterium tuberculosis*. Am. J. Dis. Child. *139*:780-782, 1985.

570. Steiner, P., Rao, M., Victoria, M. S., et al.: Miliary tuberculosis in two infants after nursery exposure: Epidemiologic, clinical, and laboratory findings. Am. Rev. Respir. Dis. *113*:267-271, 1976.

571. Steiner, P., Rao, M., Victoria, M. S., et al.: Persistently negative tuberculin reactions: Their presence among children culture positive for *Mycobacterium tuberculosis*. Am. J. Dis. Child. *134*:747-750, 1980.

572. Stevens, D. L., and Everett, E. D.: Sequential computerized axial tomography in tuberculous meningitis. J. A. M. A. *239*:642, 1978.

573. Stop TB Partnership Childhood TB Subgroup: Chapter 1: Introduction and diagnosis of tuberculosis in children. Int. J. Tuberc. Lung Dis. *10*:1091-1097, 2006.

574. Stop TB Partnership Childhood TB Subgroup: Chapter 2: Antituberculosis treatment in children. Int. J. Tuberc. Lung Dis. *10*:1205-1211, 2006.

575. Stop TB Partnership Childhood TB Subgroup: Chapter 3: Management of TB in the HIV-infected child. Int. J. Tuberc. Lung Dis. *10*:1331-1336, 2006.

576. Stop TB Partnership Childhood TB Subgroup: Chapter 4: Childhood contact screening and management. Int. J. Tuberc. Lung Dis. *11*:12-15, 2007.

577. Stout, J. E., Saharia, K. K., Nageswaron, S., et al.: Racial and ethnic disparities in pediatric tuberculosis in North Carolina. Arch. Pediatr. Adolesc. Med. *160*:631-637, 2006.

578. Strang, J. I. G., Kakaza, H. H. S., Gibson, D. G., et al.: Controlled trial of prednisolone as adjunct in treatment of tuberculous constrictive pericarditis in Transkei. Lancet *2*:1418-1422, 1987.

579. Sullama, P. M., Slutkin, G., and Hopewell, P. C.: The benefits of evaluating close associates of child tuberculin reactors from a high prevalence group. Am. J. Public Health *76*:1109-1111, 1986.

580. Sumartojo, E.: When tuberculosis treatment fails: A social behavior account of patient adherence. Am. Rev. Respir. Dis. *147*:1311-1320, 1993.

581. Sumaya, C. V., Simek, M., and Smith, M. H. D.: Tuberculous meningitis in children during the isoniazid era. J. Pediatr. *87*:43-49, 1975.

582. Swaminathan, S., Gong, J., Zhang, M., et al.: Cytokine production in children with tuberculous infection and disease. Clin. Infect. Dis. *28*:1290-1293, 1999.

583. Swaminathan, S., Raghavan, A., Duraipandian, M., et al.: Short-course chemotherapy for paediatric respiratory tuberculosis: 5-year report. Int. J. Tuberc. Lung Dis. *9*:693-696, 2005.

584. Swanson, D. S., and Starke, J. R.: Drug-resistant tuberculosis in pediatrics. Pediatr. Clin. North Am. *42*:553-581, 1995.

585. Sweany, H. C.: Studies on the pathogenesis of primary tuberculous infection. Am. Rev. Tuberc. *27*:559-588, 1933.

586. Tabrisky, J., Lindstrom, R. R., Peters, R., et al.: Tuberculous enteritis. Am. J. Gastroenterol. *63*:49-57, 1975.

587. Takiff, H., Salazar, L., Guerrero, C., et al.: Cloning and nucleotide sequence of *Mycobacterium tuberculosis* gyrA and gryB genes and detection of quinoline resistance mutations. Antimicrob. Agents Chemother. *38*:773-780, 1994.

588. Talbot, E. A., Moore, M., McCray, E., and Binkin, N. J.: Tuberculosis among foreign-born persons in the United States, 1993-1998. J. A. M. A. *284*:2894-2900, 2000.

589. Talwar, B. S., Talwar, R., Chowdhary, B., and Prasad, P.: Abdominal tuberculosis in children: An Indian experience. J. Trop. Pediatr. *46*:368-370, 2000.

590. Teeratkulpisarn, J., Lumbigagnon, P., Pairojkul, S., et al.: Cavitary tuberculosis in a young infant. Pediatr. Infect. Dis. J. *13*:545-546, 1994.

591. Teixeira, L., Perkins, M. D., Johnson, J. L., et al.: Infection and disease among household contacts of patients with multi-drug resistant tuberculosis. Int. J. Tuberc. Lung Dis. *5*:321-328, 2001.

592. Telenti, A., Imboden, P., Marchesi, F., et al.: Detection of rifampin-resistance mutations in *Mycobacterium tuberculosis*. Lancet *341*:647-650, 1993.

593. Telzak, E. E., Sepkowitz, K., Alpert, P., et al.: Multidrug-resistant tuberculosis in patients without HIV infection. N. Engl. J. Med. *333*:907-911, 1995.

594. tenDam, H. G.: Research on BCG vaccination. Adv. Tuberc. Res. *21*:79-106, 1984.

595. Teoh, R., Humphries, M. J., and Sister Gabriel O'Mahony: Symptomatic intracranial tuberculoma developing during treatment of tuberculosis: Report of 10 patients and review of the literature. Q. J. Med. *63*:449-460, 1987.

596. Te Water Naude, J. M., Donald, P. R., Hussey, G. D., et al.: Twice weekly vs. daily chemotherapy for childhood tuberculosis. Pediatr. Infect. Dis. J. *19*:405-410, 2000.

597. Thiam, S., LeFeure, A., Hane, F., et al.: Effectiveness of a strategy to improve adherence to tuberculosis treatment in a resource-poor setting. J. A. M. A. *297*:380-386, 2007.

598. Thomas, P., Bornschlegel, K., Singh, T. P., et al.: Tuberculosis in human immunodeficiency virus–infected and human immunodeficiency virus–exposed children in New York City. Pediatr. Infect. Dis. J. *19*:700-706, 2000.

599. Thompson, W. J., Glassroth, J. L., Snider, D. E., Jr., et al.: The booster phenomenon in serial tuberculin testing. Am. Rev. Respir. Dis. *119*:587-597, 1979.

600. Thwaites, G. E., Nguyen, D. B., Nguyen, H. D., et al.: Dexamethasone for the treatment of tuberculous meningitis in adolescents and adults. N. Engl. J. Med. *351*:1741-1751, 2004.

601. Tidjani, O., Amedome, A., and tenDam, H. G.: Protective effect of BCG vaccination of the newborn against childhood tuberculosis in an African community. Tubercle *67*:269-281, 1986.

602. Toppet, M., Malfroot, A., Derde, M. P., et al.: Corticosteroids in primary tuberculosis with bronchial obstruction. Arch. Dis. Child. *65*:1222-1226, 1990.

603. Traub, M., Colchester, A. C., Kingsley, D. P., et al.: Tuberculosis of the central nervous system. Q. J. Med. *53*:81-100, 1984.

604. Trunz, B. B., Fine, P., and Dye, C.: Effect of BCG vaccination on childhood tuberculous meningitis and miliary tuberculosis worldwide: A meta-analysis and assessment of cost-effectiveness. Lancet *367*:1173-1180, 2006.

605. Tsakalidis, D., Pratsidou, P., Hitoglou-Makedou, A., et al.: Intensive short course chemotherapy for treatment of Greek children with tuberculosis. Pediatr. Infect. Dis. J. *11*:1036-1042, 1992.

606. Tsiouris, S. J., Austin, J., Tora, P., et al.: Results of a tuberculosis-specific IFN-gamma assay in children at high risk for tuberculosis infection. Int. J. Tuberc. Lung Dis. *10*:939-941, 2006.

607. Tuberculosis in Children: Guidelines for diagnosis, prevention and treatment (Statement of the Scientific Committee of the International Union Against Tuberculosis and Lung Diseases). Bull. Int. Union Tuberc. Lung Dis. *66*:61-67, 1991.

608. Tuli, S. M.: Tuberculosis of the Spine. New Delhi, Amerind Publishing, 1975.

609. Turnbull, F. M., McIntyre, P. B., Achat, H. M., et al.: National study of adverse reactions after vaccination with bacille Calmette-Guérin. Clin. Infect. Dis. *34*:447-453, 2002.

610. Tyler, B., Bennett, H., and Kim, J.: Intracranial tuberculomas in a child: Computed tomographic scan diagnosis and nonsurgical management. Pediatrics *71*:952-954, 1983.

611. Udani, P. M., Parekh, U. C., and Dastur, D. K.: Neurological and related syndromes in CNS tuberculosis: Clinical features and pathogenesis. J. Neurol. Sci. *14*:341-357, 1971.

612. Ussery, X. T., Valway, S. E., McKenna, M., et al.: Epidemiology of tuberculosis among children in the United States. Pediatr. Infect. Dis. J. *15*:697-704, 1996.

613. Vallejo, J., Ong, L., and Starke, J.: Clinical features, diagnosis and treatment of tuberculosis in infants. Pediatrics *94*:1-7, 1994.

614. Vallejo, J., Ong, L. T., and Starke, J. R.: Tuberculous osteomyelitis of the long bones in children. Pediatr. Infect. Dis. J. *14*:542-546, 1995.

615. Vallejo, J. G., and Starke, J. R.: Tuberculosis and pregnancy. Clin. Chest Med. *13*:693-707, 1992.

616. Van den Bosch, A., Terken, M., Ypma, L., et al.: Tuberculous meningitis and miliary tuberculosis in young children. Trop. Med. Int. Health *9*:309-313, 2004.

617. Vanderhoof, J. A., and Ament, M. E.: Fatal hepatic necrosis due to isoniazid chemoprophylaxis in a 15-year-old girl. J. Pediatr. *88*:867-868, 1976.

618. vander Weert, E. M., Hertgers, N. M., Schaaf, H. S., et al.: Comparison of diagnostic criteria of tuberculous meningitis in human immunodeficiency virus–infected and uninfected children. Pediatr. Infect. Dis. J. *25*:65-69, 2006.

619. Van Hest, R., De Vries, G., Morbano, G., et al.: Cavitating tuberculosis in an infant. Pediatr. Infect. Dis. J. *23*:667-670, 2004.

620. Van Zyl, S., Marais, B. J., Hesseling, A. C., et al.: Adherence to antituberculosis chemoprophylaxis and treatment in children. Int. J. Tuberc. Lung Dis. *10*:13-18, 2006.

621. Van Zwanenberg, D.: Influence of the number of bacilli on the development of tuberculous disease in children. Am. Rev. Respir. Dis. *82*:31-44, 1960.

622. Varudkar, B. L.: Short-course chemotherapy for tuberculosis in children. Indian J. Pediatr. *52*:593-597, 1985.

623. Venkataraman, P., Menon, N. K., Nair, N. G. B., et al.: Classification of subjects as slow or rapid inactivators of isoniazid based on the ratio of urinary excretion of acetylisoniazid to isoniazid. Tubercle *53*:84-91, 1972.

624. Verma, A., Dhawan, A., Wade, J. J., et al.: *Mycobacterium tuberculosis* infection in pediatric liver transplant recipients. Pediatr. Infect. Dis. J. *19*:625-630, 2000.

625. Versfeld, G. A., and Soloman, A.: A diagnostic approach to tuberculosis of bones and joints. J. Bone Joint Surg. Br. *64*:446-449, 1982.

626. Visudhiphan, P., and Chiemchanya, S.: Tuberculous meningitis in children: Treatment with isoniazid and rifampin for twelve months. J. Pediatr. *114*:875-879, 1989.
627. Volmink, J., Matchaba, P., and Garner, P.: Directly observed therapy and treatment adherence. Lancet *355*:1345-1350, 2000.
628. Waeker, N. J., Jr., and Connor, J. D.: Central nervous system tuberculosis in children: A review of 30 cases. Pediatr. Infect. Dis. J. *9*:539-543, 1990.
629. Wallace, K., and Cohen, A. S.: Tuberculous arthritis: Report of two cases with review of biopsy and synovial fluid findings. Am. J. Med. *61*:277-282, 1976.
630. Wallace, R. C., Burton, E. M., Barrett, F. F., et al.: Intracranial tuberculosis in children: CT appearance and clinical outcome. Pediatr. Radiol. *21*:241-246, 1991.
631. Wallgren, A.: On contagiousness of childhood tuberculosis. Acta Paediatr. *22*:229-234, 1937.
632. Wallgren, A.: Pulmonary Tuberculosis in Adults and Children. New York, Thomas Nelson & Sons, 1939.
633. Wallgren, A.: Tuberculous heart disease. Acta Med. Scand. *196*(Suppl.):132-144, 1947.
634. Wallgren, A.: The time-table of tuberculosis. Tubercle *29*:245-251, 1948.
635. Washko, R., Robinson, E., Fehrs, L. J., et al.: Tuberculosis transmission in a high school choir. J. Sch. Health *68*:256-259, 1998.
636. Weinstein, J., Barrett, C., Baltimore, R., et al.: Nosocomial transmission of tuberculosis from a hospital visitor on a pediatrics ward. Pediatr. Infect. Dis. J. *14*:232-234, 1995.
637. Weis, S., Slocum, P., Blais, F., et al.: The effects of directly observed therapy on the rates of drug resistance and relapse in tuberculosis. N. Engl. J. Med. *330*:1179-1184, 1994.
638. Weismuller, M. M., Graham, S. M., Claessens, N. J. M., et al.: Diagnosis of childhood tuberculosis in Malawi: An audit of hospital practice. Int. J. Tuberc. Lung Dis. *6*:432-438, 2002.
639. Werhane, M. J., Snukst-Torbeck, G., and Schraufnagel, D. E.: The tuberculosis clinic. Chest *96*:815-818, 1989.
640. Whalen, C., Horsburgh, C., Hom, D., et al.: Accelerated course of human immunodeficiency virus infection after tuberculosis. Am. J. Respir. Crit. Care Med. *151*:129-135, 1995.
641. Whitener, D. R.: Tuberculous brain abscess. Arch. Neurol. *35*:148-155, 1978.
642. Wootten, S. H., Gonzalez, B. E., Pawlak, R., et al.: Epidemiology of pediatric tuberculosis using traditional and molecular techniques; Houston, Texas. Pediatrics *116*:1141-1147, 2005.
643. World Health Organization: Guidance for National Tuberculosis Programmes on the Management of Tuberculosis in Children. Geneva, World Health Organization, 2006.
644. World Health Organization: The World Health Report 1999. Making a Difference. Geneva, World Health Organization, 1999.
645. Wilkins, E. G. L.: Tuberculous peritonitis: Diagnostic value of the ascitic/blood glucose value. Tubercle *65*:47-52, 1984.
646. Witrak, B. J., and Ellis, G. T.: Intracranial tuberculosis: Manifestations on computerized tomography. South. Med. J. *78*:386-392, 1985.
647. Wright, F. W., and Hamilton, W. S.: Miliary tuberculosis twice. Br. J. Dis. Chest *68*:210-212, 1974.
648. Yeo, I. K. T., Tannenbaum, T., Scott, A. N., et al.: Contact investigation and genotyping to identify tuberculosis transmission to children. Pediatr. Infect. Dis. J. *25*:1037-1043, 2006.
649. Zampoli, M., Kilborn, T., and Eley, B.: Tuberculosis during early antiretroviral induced immune reconstitution in HIV-infected children. Int. J. Tuberc. Lung Dis. *11*:417-423, 2007.
650. Zar, H. J., Hanslo, D., Apollos, P., et al.: Induced sputum versus gastric lavage for microbiological confirmation of pulmonary tuberculosis in infants and young children: A prospective study. Lancet *365*:130-134, 2005.
651. Zarabi, M., Sane, S., and Girdany, B. R.: Chest roentgenogram in the early diagnosis of tuberculous meningitis in children. Am. J. Dis. Child. *121*:389-392, 1971.
652. Zhang, Y.: Genetic basis of isoniazid resistance of *Mycobacterium tuberculosis*. Rev. Microbiol. *144*:143-150, 1993.
653. Zhang, Y., Heym, B., Allen, B., et al.: Catalase-peroxidase gene and isoniazid resistance of *Mycobacterium tuberculosis*. Nature *358*:591-593, 1992.
654. Zignol, M., Hosseini, M. S., Wright, A., et al.: Global incidence of multidrug-resistant tuberculosis. J. Infect. Dis. *194*:479-485, 2006.
655. Zinneman, H. H., and Hall, W. H.: Transient tuberculous meningitis. Am. Rev. Respir. Dis. *114*:1185-1188, 1976.
656. Zitrin, C. M., and Lincoln, E. M.: Initial tuberculous infection due to drug-resistant organisms: With a review of the world literature on initial infection due to isoniazid-resistant tubercle bacilli. J. Pediatr. *58*:219-223, 1961.
657. Zweiman, B., Pappano, J. E., Jr., and Hildrath, E. A.: Effect of influenza vaccine administration on tuberculin skin sensitivity. Dis. Chest *52*:46-49, 1967.

OTHER MYCOBACTERIA

CHAPTER 108

J. Thomas Cross, Jr. ☙ Richard F. Jacobs

The definition of mycobacteria other than tubercle bacilli is quite confusing. Runyon,[135] in his address to the International Conference on Atypical Mycobacteria, probably defined them best: "Tubercle bacilli include *Mycobacterium tuberculosis*, *Mycobacterium bovis*, and *Mycobacterium africanum*. Together with *Mycobacterium microti* (not pathogenic for humans), these organisms constitute the tubercle bacillus complex." Any mycobacterium not listed in this group is considered to be in the "other" grouping. Mycobacteria other than those causing tuberculosis and leprosy were not recognized as causes of disease in humans until the 1950s.[165] The incidence of disease caused by these organisms remained stable until the acquired immunodeficiency syndrome (AIDS) epidemic began in the 1980s. The most common forms of the disease are chronic pulmonary disease resembling tuberculosis (occurring mainly in adults), cervical adenopathy in children, skin and soft tissue infection, and disseminated disease in immunocompromised individuals.[120] In the mid-1980s, the incidence of infections with atypical mycobacteria increased markedly, probably because of the increased number of immunocompromised patients (e.g., because of AIDS and organ transplantation) and the significant improvement in microbiologic methods for cultivating these organisms.[186,191]

EPIDEMIOLOGY

The atypical mycobacteria are ubiquitous in nature. They are found in soil, animals, milk,[42] and food. Of importance in some hospital-acquired infections or infections in immunocompromised hosts is the presence of the organisms in common tap water.[16,59,109,157] Exposure to environments (especially soil) colonized by these organisms seems to be important for acquisition of disease in children. Organisms commonly found in soil include *Mycobacterium scrofulaceum*, *Mycobacterium flavescens*, *Mycobacterium avium–intracellulare* (MAI), *Mycobacterium gastri*, *Mycobacterium terrae*, *Mycobacterium fortuitum*, and *Mycobacterium chelonae*. Water is an important source for all of the previously named organisms and for *Mycobacterium kansasii*, *Mycobacterium marinum*, *Mycobacterium gordonae*, and *Mycobacterium xenopi*.

In contrast, humans are the only known reservoirs for *M. tuberculosis*. In a survey from the Centers for Disease Control and Prevention (CDC), 35 percent of mycobacteria isolated in laboratories were nontuberculous.[53] MAI accounted for 66 percent of the nontuberculous isolates, followed by *M. fortuitum* (19%), *M. kansasii* (9%), and *M. scrofulaceum* (6%). These data were collected in 1980 before the present AIDS epidemic and before the rapid increase in the number and types of immunocompromised patients; therefore, current rates probably are much higher.

Geography also apparently has some bearing on the prevalence of these infections. The southeastern part of the United States has much higher rates in children than does the Northeast or the Northwest. *M. avium* complex (MAC) was seen most commonly along the coastal borders of the United States and in the states bordering Canada. The highest rates were seen in Hawaii (10.9 cases per 100,000 population), Connecticut (8.9 cases per 100,000 population), and Florida (8.4 cases per 100,000 population). High rates also were seen in Kansas and the desert

Southwest, however, showing the widespread nature of this organism in causing disease. In contrast, *M. kansasii* was seen most commonly in the Midwest of the United States and almost never was seen in the Southeast.[53] States with rates of *M. kansasii* greater than 0.75 case per 100,000 included Missouri, Illinois, Kentucky, Indiana, Kansas, Nebraska, Louisiana, Texas, Arizona, and Florida. North Carolina, a state with one of the highest rates of MAC (>4.8 cases per 100,000 population), had very few cases of *M. kansasii* (0 to 0.25 case per 100,000 population). *M. marinum* frequently was isolated from coastal areas, whereas *M. xenopi* was scattered across the United States, with 50 percent of cases being found in just three states (Connecticut, Wisconsin, and California).

For all the nontuberculous species, males and rural residents had a much higher incidence of infection.[141] Extrapolation of these rates to determine disease patterns is not without problems, however. The number of mycobacterial isolates could be skewed easily by the presence of multiple isolates from a single patient, or it may just represent colonization. Nonetheless, these rates can help predict which species of nontuberculous mycobacteria are most likely to be encountered in a particular geographic region while the physician awaits final identification and sensitivity testing on an isolated nontuberculous organism.

The site of isolation from the human source can be helpful in determining the type of mycobacteria that may be involved in the disease process. *M. avium* and *Mycobacterium intracellulare* are responsible for lymphadenitis, particularly in children. These two organisms also are responsible for pulmonary disease and disseminated disease to bones and occasionally to the meninges. *M. kansasii* is associated most commonly with infections of pulmonary origin and disseminated lesions in adults; rarely, it is associated with adenitis and skin granuloma in children. *M. scrofulaceum* also causes lymphadenitis in children, and *M. marinum* is responsible for skin granuloma and ulcers after exposure to certain salt-water beaches, swimming pools, and tropical fish tanks. The rapid growers (*M. fortuitum* and *M. chelonae*) rarely are responsible for pulmonary and disseminated disease in adults and children.

A familial immune defect predisposing to disseminated atypical mycobacterial infection in childhood has been reported.[96] The six children studied had disseminated infection with atypical mycobacteria and no obvious evidence of immunodeficiency. Clinical and immunologic features seem to indicate that these children acquire infections similar to Lsh/Ity/Bcg-susceptible mice. Ongoing studies to determine the defect may provide insight into the mechanisms by which certain children are susceptible to mycobacterial infections, whereas others exposed to the same environmental factors do not develop disseminated disease.

MICROBIOLOGY

Runyon and Timpe[133,134,165] in their monumental work on atypical mycobacteria suggested a useful classification system based on three characteristics of the organisms: production of pigment, rate of growth, and colonial characteristics. The four groups are as follows: group I—photochromogens, which produce bright yellow to red pigment in the presence of light; group II—scotochromogens, which produce yellow to orange pigment in the dark; group III—nonphotochromogens, which are nonpigment producers; and group IV—rapid growers, which generally grow in less than 1 week. Kubica[89] published an updated version of Runyon's classification in 1978, and it was useful for many years. Subsequently, a more "simplified" classification based on the growth rates of the organisms alone was proposed.[186]

The atypical mycobacteria still are differentiated by most clinical laboratories on the basis of various morphologic, physiologic, and biochemical characteristics (Tables 108–1 and 108–2). The difficulty with identifying many of these organisms is their slow growth rates with standard techniques. Beginning sensitivity testing as soon as an organism is cultivated and thought to be the responsible pathogen is useful because several months may be required for proper identification and susceptibility testing. Serologic tests can be helpful in identifying some of the

TABLE 108–1 Characteristics of Slow-Growing Pathogenic Mycobacteria

Organism	Growth Present (° C)			Growth Rate (Days)	Niacin	Nitrate Reduction	Pigment Dark	Pigment Light	Growth in 5% NaCl
	25	37	45						
Mycobacterium tuberculosis	−	+	−	12-28	+	+	−	−	−
Mycobacterium bovis	−	+	−	21-40	−	−	−	−	−
Photochromogens, Runyon group I									
Mycobacterium kansasii	+	+	−	10-21	−	+	−	+	−
Mycobacterium marinum	+	±	−	7-14	−	−	−	+	−
Scotochromogens, Runyon group II									
Mycobacterium scrofulaceum	+	+	−	10-28	−	−	+	+	−
Mycobacterium szulgai	+	+	−	12-28	−	+	+	+	−
Mycobacterium gordonae	+	+	−	10-28	−	−	+	+	−
Nonchromogens, Runyon group III									
Mycobacterium avium	+	+	+	10-21	−	−	−	−	−
Mycobacterium intracellulare	+	+	−	10-21	−	−	−	−	−
Mycobacterium ulcerans	−	−	+	28-60	−	−	−	−	?
Mycobacterium xenopi	−	+	−	14-28	−	−	−	−	−

TABLE 108–2 Characteristics of Rapid Mycobacterial Growers

Runyon Group IV	Optimal Temperature	Growth Rate	Niacin	Nitrate Reduction	Growth in 5% NaCl
Mycobacterium fortuitum	37° C	3-7 days	−	+	+
Mycobacterium abscessus	37° C	3-7 days	−	−	+
Mycobacterium chelonae	37° C	3-7 days	−	−	+

organisms.[35,90,133,168,176,186,187,191] In clinical medicine, they rarely are valuable, however, for establishing a diagnosis in an individual patient. A study using humoral immunoglobulins against mycobacterial antigens failed to diagnose tuberculosis or nontuberculous adenitis in children.[169]

Blood cultures for mycobacteria are best performed with the Isolator lysis-centrifugation system (Wampole Laboratories, Cranbury, NJ) or the radiometric BACTEC 13A blood culture bottle (Becton-Dickinson Diagnostic Instrument Systems, Cockeysville, MD).[1,81,82] Blood collected in ethylenediaminetetraacetic acid or coagulated blood is unacceptable. Body fluids such as cerebrospinal fluid, pleural fluid, and peritoneal fluid can be inoculated directly into BACTEC or Septi-Chek (Becton-Dickinson) broth, particularly if only small volumes are available. Gene probes became commercially available in the late 1980s. They involve DNA probes complementary to species-specific sequences of rRNA for the identification of *M. tuberculosis*, MAC, *Mycobacterium gordonae*, and *M. kansasii* (AccuProbe; Gen-Probe, San Diego, CA).[55]

Polymerase chain reaction (PCR) assay has been evaluated for the routine detection of *M. tuberculosis* in the clinical laboratory and compared with fluorochrome smear and culture. Two large studies compared PCR with the standard technique and found that the sensitivity of PCR assay was 84 percent in both studies.[28,50] In another study, a multiplex PCR assay for immediate identification of various *Mycobacterium* spp. was shown to be 97.9 percent sensitive and 96.9 percent specific.[87] The PCR testing offered by commercial laboratories at present is not approved by the U.S. Food and Drug Administration for in vitro diagnosis. The sensitivity and specificity of this test vary widely among laboratories.[118]

MANIFESTATIONS OF NONTUBERCULOUS MYCOBACTERIAL INFECTION IN CHILDREN

LYMPHADENITIS

Lymphadenitis is the most common manifestation of atypical mycobacterial infection in children. It also can occur rarely in adults.[37,94,101] All nodes in the cervical chain can be affected, but the nodes of the submandibular region seem to be the ones most commonly involved.[39] The parotid gland also can be affected.[32] The differential diagnosis frequently centers on deciding whether a malignant process versus a nonmalignant process is present. Nonmalignant processes to consider include mononucleosis, bacterial adenitis, cat-scratch disease, toxoplasmosis, and *M. tuberculosis* infection.

Most mycobacterial cases of lymphadenitis are caused by the nontuberculous organisms. The clinician also must consider the possibility of *M. tuberculosis*, however.[30] No clinical features help the clinician discern between nontuberculous mycobacterial infection and tuberculosis. The use of histopathology has been postulated to help differentiate between atypical and tuberculous infections.[124] In this retrospective study, the findings of ill-defined (nonpalisading) granulomas, irregular or serpiginous granulomas, a predominantly nonspecific granulomatous response, predominantly sarcoid-like granulomas, or lack of significant caseation were seen more commonly with nontuberculous lymphadenitis. Additionally, nontuberculous infections had neutrophils predominantly in the center of the necrosis, whereas in tuberculous infections, neutrophils were scattered throughout the specimen. A prospective study investigating these findings has not been published to date, and other authors have not noted similar patterns.[11]

In a Canadian study, the rate of atypical mycobacteria as a cause of lymphadenitis was 1.21 cases per 100,000 children, whereas the rate for tuberculosis was 0.3 case per 100,000 children.[147] Investigators from San Diego reported a marked increase in the number of infections in children.[125] Other authors around the world have reported a markedly increased incidence of infection with these organisms in immunocompetent children.[52] In one study, the incidence increased from one case between 1987 and 1990 to 85 cases between 1991 and 1993.[93] In a large study compiled by Lincoln and Gilbert[100] involving 243 children, more than 50 percent were younger than 3 years of age, and 80 percent were younger than 5 years. In contrast, one study showed that the mean age had increased to 5.2 years.[183]

Most patients have no systemic symptoms and normal chest radiographs; other laboratory studies generally are not helpful. The mean duration of swelling is approximately 6 weeks. Historically, the cervical nodes are affected most commonly in children, although a more recent study from Greece reported submandibular prominence.[107]

Infections are caused mainly by MAI and *M. scrofulaceum*. A large prospective study spanning 32 years from 1958 to 1990 showed that MAC has become the predominant etiologic agent and has surpassed *M. scrofulaceum* from earlier in the study.[189] A series of 190 patients from India showed, however, that 60 percent of the nontuberculous adenitis cases were caused by *M. scrofulaceum* followed by 40 percent by *M. avium* intracellulare.[77] Case reports involving *M. fortuitum* also have been published.[131] Lymphadenitis caused by *Mycobacterium haemophilum* is being diagnosed in immunocompetent children in increasing numbers.[7,138]

Samra and colleagues[138] showed that the BACTEC radiometric system or MB Redox broth (Heipha Diagnostika Biotest, Heidelberg, Germany) is superior to Löwenstein-Jensen (Heipha Diagnostika Biotest) media for isolation of *M. haemophilum*. This organism is thought to have been underdiagnosed previously because of the widespread use of Löwenstein-Jensen media. *Mycobacterium malmoense* also has been described as an etiologic agent of cervical lymphadenitis in children.[167] Haas and associates[62] have described *Mycobacterium heidelbergense*, a new agent of mycobacterial lymphadenitis in children.

The usefulness of mycobacterial antigens in skin testing for the diagnosis of atypical mycobacterial infection versus tuberculous lymphadenitis is controversial. The use of purified protein derivative type B (PPD-B) (*M. intracellulare*), PPD-Y (*M. kansasii*), PPD-G (*M. scrofulaceum*), and PPD-T (*M. tuberculosis*) was compared to discern whether children with active lymphadenitis caused by the atypical mycobacteria could be distinguished from children with tuberculosis.[74] Children with confirmed nontuberculous adenitis were six times more likely to have greater than 10-mm induration to PPD-B than were children with negative culture or biopsy results. In all groups except those with confirmed *M. tuberculosis*, responses to PPD-T were significantly smaller than responses to the nontuberculous mycobacterial antigens. The results of the study seem to indicate that the use of nontuberculous mycobacterial antigens could be helpful in diagnosing mycobacterial cervical adenopathy. The specificity for nontuberculous organisms is unknown, however.

Needle aspiration of an affected node can be a valuable diagnostic tool. Cultures for bacterial and mycobacterial etiologies should be performed, and recovery rates in children with cervical lymphadenitis range from 60 to 88 percent.[9,14,80,193] The aspirate should be inoculated onto aerobic and anaerobic media and Sabouraud agar and mycobacterial media (Löwenstein-Jensen slants or Middlebrook media). Use of the BACTEC system can be very helpful; mycobacteria can be isolated 12 to 17 days after inoculation.[152]

More recently, preoperative diagnosis of *M. avium* lymphadenitis was accomplished with the use of PCR of gastric aspirates in two children.[61] Further studies are needed to conclude whether PCR could be a noninvasive method of diagnosing this infection.

The best treatment of lymphadenitis caused by atypical myco-bacteria is complete excision of the involved lymph node.[108,172] Incision and drainage without excision result in a high rate of secondary drainage, and subsequent excision of the remaining tissue is required for cure.[4,137,144] Small uncontrolled trials have attempted to use antimicrobials alone for lymphadenitis caused by nontuberculous mycobacteria.[102] Preliminary results have been successful, but use of toxic agents for prolonged periods was required. Controlled trials have not been published.

ACQUIRED IMMUNODEFICIENCY SYNDROME AND ATYPICAL MYCOBACTERIA

Surveys have noted an increasing rate of nontuberculous infec-tion in children with AIDS.[73] Approximately 6 percent of adults and 4 percent of children with AIDS reported to the CDC had disseminated MAC infection as AIDS-defining disease.[20] Autopsy studies show that MAC infection is present in 20 to 50 percent of adult human immunodeficiency virus (HIV)–infected patients.[129,182,185] In a retrospective study from 1990 to 1996 in New York City, 26 percent of children had evidence of MAC infection at the time of their deaths.[78] MAC infection was thought to be the cause of death in 13 percent of the 54 children with HIV infection, and the mean age at death was 7.8 years. In two autopsy studies of opportunistic infection in HIV-infected chil-dren in Latin America and Argentina, only 2.7 percent and 3.4 percent had evidence of disseminated disease.[41,127] In these studies, 62 percent (Argentina) and 72 percent (Latin America) of the children studied were younger than 1 year of age. These data indicate that MAI infection is seen less commonly in younger children with HIV.

In the CDC study, MAC was the nontuberculous mycobac-terium most commonly isolated. *M. kansasii* and *M. scrofulaceum* were found in one case each. In adult studies, the incidence of infection with *M. kansasii* and *M. scrofulaceum* also is quite low.[38,72] More than 70 percent of children with MAC and AIDS had evidence of disseminated disease. Almost all had CD4+ counts less than 100 cells/mm³. Clinical findings included failure to maintain growth curves, anorexia, fever, abdominal pain, and anemia. The median age at diagnosis was 46 months, with a median of 9 months elapsing between the onset of symptoms and positive cultures. When nontuberculous mycobacterial infection was diagnosed in these patients, they survived less than 10 months. Blood cultures have 90 to 95 percent sensitivity in detecting disseminated MAC infection in adult patients with AIDS.[65]

MAI has been shown to infect the esophagus, stomach, and intestine of pediatric patients with AIDS.[79] Patients with exten-sive MAI infection of the small and large intestines have severe, persistent diarrhea.

Mycobacterium genavense has been shown to cause infection in children with HIV infection.[117] The children were febrile and had abdominal cramps and diarrhea. CD4+ lymphocyte counts were less than 400/mm³. The organism was found in numerous stool samples and lymph node specimens. Multiple-drug regimens that include amikacin, ethambutol, rifampin, and clarithromycin may be useful in treating this infection.

For treatment of MAC infection in HIV-infected children, combination therapy is recommended.[6] Clarithromycin (15 mg/kg/day divided into two oral doses, maximum of 500 mg) and ethambutol (15 to 20 mg/kg/day in a single dose, maximum of 1600 mg) should be included. Additionally, the use of rifabutin (5 to 10 mg/kg/day once daily, maximum of 300 mg), ciprofloxa-cin (20 to 30 mg/kg/day intravenously or orally once daily, maximum of 1.5 g), or azithromycin (10 mg/kg once daily) can

be considered. Because of their liquid form, clarithromycin and azithromycin have become available therapy for many infections in pediatric patients, including otitis media, pharyngitis, and skin infections.[85] The use of granulocyte colony-stimulating factor as an adjunct to antimicrobial therapy for disseminated MAC infec-tion has been reported,[121] but additional data are needed to deter-mine the usefulness of this agent.

For secondary prevention of recurrent disease, lifelong pro-phylaxis with clarithromycin is recommended (15 mg/kg/day in two divided doses, maximum of 500 mg), in combination with at least one of the following: ethambutol (15 to 20 mg/kg/day once daily), rifabutin (5 mg/kg/day once daily, maximum of 300 mg), or ciprofloxacin (20 to 30 mg/kg/day in two divided doses, maximum of 1.5 g).

The use of rifabutin or azithromycin (5 mg/kg/day once daily, maximum of 250 mg, or 20 mg/kg once weekly) for prophylaxis has been recommended based on adult studies in an attempt to delay and prevent MAC bacteremia in adults with CD4+ cell counts less than 100 cells/mm³. The U.S. Public Health Service and the Infectious Disease Society of America have published guidelines for the prevention of opportunistic infections, includ-ing disseminated MAC.[170] These guidelines incorporate age-specific CD4+ counts at which prophylaxis should be used: children 6 years or older, less than 50 cells/µL; children 2 to 6 years old, less than 75 cells/µL; children 1 to 2 years old, less than 500 cells/µL; and children younger than 12 months, less than 750 cells/µL. Azithromycin (20 mg/kg once weekly) seems to be effective. A phase I/II study of prophylactic rifabutin for prevention of disseminated MAC infection in children showed a side effect of bilateral, stellate, corneal deposits without associ-ated uveitis in 6 of 25 children.[149]

The emergence of resistance is a concern with the MAC prophylactic regimens in patients with AIDS. In some trials, 9 percent of adults receiving azithromycin prophylaxis and 5 percent of adults receiving clarithromycin prophylaxis had break-through MAC bacteremia. Of these cases, 11 percent and 58 percent of the azithromycin and clarithromycin, respectively, breakthrough isolates were macrolide-resistant.[5,64]

PULMONARY INFECTIONS

Reviews from the late 1970s showed that pulmonary disease caused by atypical mycobacteria usually was caused by *M. kansasii* and MAC.[26,54,132] MAC infection most commonly occurred during the sixth decade, whereas *M. kansasii* infection occurred in indi-viduals a decade younger. Men were affected most commonly, in ratios as high as 4:1. Chronic obstructive pulmonary disease as noted by radiographic findings was found in 50 to 60 percent of patients with atypical mycobacterial pulmonary infections. Bullous lung disease was seen in 24 to 39 percent. The lobar distribution and severity of disease were similar for atypical mycobacterial agents and *M. tuberculosis*, with one exception: *M. kansasii* was much more prone to produce unilateral disease, which occurred nearly 60 percent of the time compared with 35 percent of the time in MAC or *M. tuberculosis* infection. Typi-cally, disease begins in the posterior portions of the upper lobes. Progression to cavitary disease occurred in 87 percent of patients with *M. tuberculosis* and MAC infections and in 96 percent of patients with *M. kansasii* infection. Rare case reports of medias-tinal mass lesions in children caused by nontuberculous myco-bacteria have been published.[48]

Hilar and mediastinal adenopathy was an uncommon finding, particularly with MAC (4%) and *M. kansasii* (0.5%). Pleural effu-sions were rare, occurring in 6 percent of patients with MAC and 4 percent with *M. kansasii*. Treatment at that time generally involved three to four courses of drug therapy, including regimens of isonicotinic acid hydrazide, p-aminosalicylic acid, streptomycin, and rifampin. The American Thoracic Society recommends a four-drug regimen for MAC pulmonary infection in adults: isoniazid (300 mg), rifampin (600 mg), ethambutol (25 mg/kg for 2 months, then 15 mg/kg), and streptomycin (0.5 to 1 g five times each week for 8 to 12 weeks, then 0.5 to 1 g two or three times each week for 3 months, as tolerated).[177] Drugs are administered for 18 to 24 months, with a minimum of 12 months of culture negativity required while receiving therapy. A previous clinical investigation revealed success rates of 25 to 80 percent, and the best response rate was noted with a three-drug regimen of ethambutol, ethionamide, and cycloserine.[44] Resectional surgery seemed to have poor outcomes. For M. kansasii pulmonary infection, the American Thoracic Society recommendations include isoniazid (300 mg/day), ethambutol (15 mg/kg/day), and rifampin (600 mg/day) for 18 months in adults.

Patients with cystic fibrosis have been noted to have an increased incidence of infection with nontuberculous mycobacteria. Prevalence rates of 2 to 20 percent have been reported.[3,67,68,84] A study from France involving children aged 1 to 18 years old indicated that mycobacterial species were isolated from 6.6 percent of routine sputum samples, and that 1.9 percent had documented mycobacterial lung infection.[47] Mycobacterial infections are seen more commonly in older patients with cystic fibrosis. Frequent intravenous antibiotic use is a possible risk factor for colonization with nontuberculous mycobacteria.[166] Organisms most commonly found are MAC, M. kansasii, M. fortuitum, and M. chelonae. Mycobacterium abscessus has emerged as a clinically persistent pathogen in patients with cystic fibrosis, especially patients on steroid therapy for allergic bronchopulmonary aspergillosis.[46,116] Bacterial contamination, particularly with Pseudomonas aeruginosa, of the acid-fast bacilli cultures from patients with cystic fibrosis has been a major problem that has rendered isolation of mycobacteria more difficult.[150] Another confounding problem is the difficulty in differentiating infection from colonization in these patients.[84]

The American Thoracic Society recommends radiographic changes, isolation of multiple colonies of the same species, and the absence of other potential pathogens as criteria for the diagnosis of pathogenic infection with nontuberculous mycobacteria.[2] Discernment is even more difficult in the setting of the chronic lung disease seen in patients with cystic fibrosis. Kilby and associates[84] suggest that repeated isolation of nontuberculous mycobacteria associated with pulmonary cavities or infiltrates that do not improve with aggressive standard antibacterial treatment could indicate active mycobacterial disease in patients with cystic fibrosis.

M. xenopi has been described in adults as a cause of infection of the pulmonary tract.[148] The mean age at infection was 62 years, and it occurred in a mainly Canadian population. Eighty-six percent of the patients had underlying pulmonary pathology, including chronic obstructive pulmonary disease, previous pulmonary tuberculosis, carcinoma of the lung, sarcoidosis, and cystic fibrosis. Additionally, a case was reported of a 7-year-old boy with leukemia in whom pneumonia with M. xenopi developed and was treated successfully with 2 years of therapy that included ethambutol and clarithromycin.[95]

Mycobacterium simiae has been isolated in adults with underlying pulmonary abnormalities.[10,88] M. simiae is the most drug-resistant of all the nontuberculous mycobacteria. Some isolates are resistant even to all drugs tested.

Mycobacterium szulgai has been described in several case series as a cause of lung disease.[106,180] Disease occurred in elderly white men and resembled chronic tuberculosis. Therapeutic regimens effective against M. avium seemed to provide good clinical outcomes.

SKIN INFECTIONS

Mycobacterium marinum

M. marinum is photochromogenic and was identified as a pathogen in fish in 1926 by Aronson.[100] The skin lesions usually result from light trauma (abrasions) in swimming pools or other bodies of water when the surfaces of the pool are colonized by M. marinum.[34,113] Fish tanks also have been implicated and generally involve the upper limb or a finger.[8,162] Most cases occur in children aged 10 to 16 years old. The most common sites are the elbows, knees, and ankles. Cooler superficial portions of the body are affected most frequently. Other exposed body areas can be involved, depending on what part of the body has made contact with the surface containing the mycobacterium (e.g., the nose in divers).[114] Regional spread of lesions has been reported.[154]

The incubation period from exposure to formation of a small indurated area that ulcerates generally is 3 weeks. The lesion then crusts and forms a granuloma with a small crater. The lesions usually are painless and resolve in several months; occasionally, they can last longer. In contrast to other mycobacterial diseases, regional nodes are not involved.

Infection with this organism usually is benign. A main consequence is, however, that patients with M. marinum infection frequently have conversion of their PPD-T test to positive.[100] The natural reservoir for M. marinum, which requires a cool incubator (32° C), is in fish and other cold-blooded animals. Generally, only a few organisms may be isolated in some granulomas.

Treatment of M. marinum has been successful with rifampin and ethambutol,[171,190] and one report showed good results with rifampin alone.[40] An accompanying editorial cautioned against the use of rifampin alone, however, and recommended using rifampin with ethambutol.[17] The duration of therapy, according to the literature, varies from several weeks to 18 months. Generally, response to therapy is rapid, and treatment should be continued for 4 to 6 weeks after clinical resolution.[40]

Mycobacterium ulcerans

In 1948, MacCallum[105] reported the first cases of disease caused by Mycobacterium ulcerans. Most cases since then have occurred in remote, tropical, or subtropical areas of the world, including parts of Africa and Australia.[104,130] In a 1-year period, 23 cases of Buruli ulcer caused by M. ulcerans occurred in Lambarene (Gabon).[19] Cases also have been reported in Mexico.[100] The natural reservoir for M. ulcerans is unknown, although one report suggests the spines of a tall prickly grass known as Echinocloa pyrimidalis.[155] The lesions caused by M. ulcerans occur mainly on the cooler superficial portions of the body. Patients harboring this organism are in otherwise good health without underlying immunodeficiency.[27] Scraping of the skin by thorns or pieces of wood has been implicated as the route of inoculation in many of the cases. The organism is very fastidious, with growth seen only between 30° C and 35° C.

The incubation period for this painless infection also is approximately 3 weeks. Regional lymphadenitis rarely occurs with this organism. The infection has three distinct stages, and knowledge of them can be helpful in making the diagnosis and providing treatment. The disease begins as a hard, mobile nodule. It frequently is associated with pruritus, and in Zaire is termed mputa matadi (the itching stone). This stage is known as the pre-ulcerative stage.

In some patients, the infection resolves on its own, but in others, it progresses to the ulcerative stage. In contrast to M. marinum, in which the lesions are short-lived and do not progress past the ulcerative stage, the lesions of M. ulcerans usually last 6 to 9 months and frequently progress and lead to deformities of limbs that may require amputation.[100] The organisms can be isolated in large numbers from the periphery of ulcers adjacent to normal tissue, which again contrasts with infection by *M. marinum*, in which very few organisms are found in the lesions.

The infection generally involves subcutaneous adipose tissue and leads to areas of fat necrosis, which then proceeds to overlying necrosis of the adjacent skin. The lesions can become enormous, sometimes involving a complete limb. Although numerous organisms are seen in the progressing edge of the infection, little evidence of a cellular immune response is apparent. Additionally, anergy to skin reagents prepared from *M. ulcerans* (burulin) frequently is noted at this stage.[156] Finally, the next stage, called the *reactive phase*, is reached. Cellular infiltrates with granuloma formation occur in the lesion. The number of organisms in the lesion decreases dramatically, and a positive skin test reaction develops to the burulin. Infection with *M. ulcerans* also can cause conversion of a patient's PPD response to positive; however, conversion is seen in only approximately 50 percent of cases.[27] Finally, healing may occur, but with fibrosis left in its wake.

Treatment of *M. ulcerans* infection is anecdotal at best. Treatment choices are based on the stage of infection. Lesions in the pre-ulcerative stage are best treated with excision and primary closure.[57] Successful therapy in the anergic progressive stage is considered the most difficult and involves appropriate antimycobacterial therapy for the infection. Success has been reported with isonicotinic acid hydrazide and streptomycin or diaminodiphenylsulfone and oxytetracycline combinations[27] and sulfamethoxazole, rifampin, minocycline,[153] and clofazimine.[104] In the final stage, healing should be promoted with as little deformity or loss of function as possible, the use of skin grafting and splinting, and excision of fibrous tissue.[57,130] Disseminated infection in an immunocompetent child along with the development of multifocal osteomyelitis has been described.[69] (See also Chapter 109.)

Other Mycobacteria in Skin Disease

M. haemophilum has produced painful subcutaneous nodules in immunocompromised patients, particularly patients with renal transplants.[36,188] In addition, *M. haemophilum* has produced disseminated disease, including bacteremia, osteomyelitis, and pulmonary disease, in immunocompromised patients.[160] *M. chelonae* has been found to be a cause of disseminated cutaneous infection.[175] Steroid use is the predisposing factor for infection with this organism. *M. fortuitum* has been implicated in cutaneous lesions in a child involved in a motor scooter accident, with the subsequent development of lesions at the site of knee lacerations; regional adenopathy of the inguinal nodes also developed.[146] *M. fortuitum-chelonae* complex has been responsible for superficial skin abscesses in children.[13] *M. fortuitum* in adult studies also has been implicated in severe infections in immunocompromised hosts; these infections usually are rapidly disseminating, with high mortality.[188] *M. avium* has been isolated from an eyelid abscess with drainage.[143] Treatment of cutaneous disease caused by these organisms is difficult at best. Four- or five-drug therapy has been tried, but with poor results.

ORGANISMS SEEN IN CHILDREN

Specific organisms and treatment guidelines are discussed in the following sections. Table 108–3 provides a quick guide to some of the more commonly used antimycobacterial agents.

MYCOBACTERIUM AVIUM–INTRACELLULARE COMPLEX

MAC consists of *M. avium* and *M. intracellulare*. These organisms are slow-growing, obligate aerobes that require 2 to 6 weeks for colony formation on solid media. Colonies usually are smooth but may be rough and can be transparent or opaque. These organisms grow on routine bacterial media, but growth is achieved best on selective mycobacterial media, such as Löwenstein-Jensen medium or Middlebrook 7K10 and 7K11 agar. Nucleic acid hybridization probes using target sequences of ribosomal RNA are available commercially for rapid identification of clinical isolates.[99,115] MAC infection is diagnosed most commonly by culture of blood or bone marrow.

TABLE 108–3 Antimycobacterial Agents*

Drug	Dosage	Form
Amikacin (A)	15-20 mg/kg/day divided q8h	IV or IM
Azithromycin (Z)	500 mg bid (adults/adolescents); 10-12 mg/kg/day (children)	PO
Cefoxitin (X)	80-160 mg/kg/day divided q4-6h	IV or IM
Ciprofloxacin (C)	20-30 mg/kg/day divided q12h (adults only in U.S.)	PO or IV
Clarithromycin (CL)	15-30 mg/kg/day divided q12h	PO
Clofazimine (CLO)	1-2 mg/kg/day	PO
Doxycycline (D)	2-4 mg/kg/day divided q12h (>8 yr old)	PO, IV
Ethambutol (ETB)	15-25 mg/kg/day	PO
Ethionamide (ETH)	10-20 mg/kg/day divided q12h	PO
Isoniazid (I)	10-14 mg/kg/day	PO
Pyrazinamide (PZA)	15-30 mg/kg/day	PO
Rifabutin (RIB)	5-10 mg/kg/day; maximum of 300 mg/day (adults)*	PO
Rifampin (RIF)	10-20 mg/kg/day divided q12-24h	PO or IV
Streptomycin (S)	20-30 mg/kg/day	IM

Infections

Disseminated MAC: HIV infected: CL (or Z) + ETB (± RIB)
Disseminated MAC: HIV-negative, immunocompromised: RIF + ETB + INH + S or A
Mycobacterium abscessus: CL alone or A alone
Mycobacterium chelonae: A ± CLO or CL alone
Mycobacterium fortuitum: A + X + probenicid or A + C + sulfonamide
Mycobacterium kansasii: RIF + ETB + I
Mycobacterium marinum: ETB + RIF, or D or TMP-SMX

Not approved for use in children.
HIV, human immunodeficiency virus; MAC, M. avium complex; TMP-SMX, trimethoprim-sulfamethoxazole.
Data based on references 60, 73, 97, 98, 136, 171, 177, 179, 188, and 190.

In a study of 56 isolates from pediatric patients involving sequence analysis of the ribosomal internal transcribed spacer, Hazra and colleagues[66] showed that the closely related Mav-B and Mav-A sequevars caused most disease. Patients from geographically diverse areas of the United States (Boston, Miami, and Los Angeles) had isolates with closely related patterns. The finding of related strains causing disease in epidemiologically unrelated patients is most consistent with two hypotheses: a similar subset of *M. avium* strains is more virulent and more likely to cause disease in humans, and pathogenic strains are more prevalent in the environment.

M. avium was recognized in 1890 as the causative agent of disease in chickens.[188] *M. intracellulare* was designated in 1967 and at the time was difficult to distinguish routinely from *M. avium*—thus the name *M. avium-intracellulare*. Today, with the use of DNA probes, most seroagglutination types have been discerned between the two groups. *M. avium* is the most common nontuberculous mycobacterium causing disease in humans, but isolates from environmental sources are more likely to be *M. intracellulare*. Both organisms can be found in birds, soil, dust, and fresh or salt water. Infections caused by MAC strains isolated from adult patients with AIDS could be identified as either serotype 4 or 8, in contrast to patients without AIDS, in whom no predominant serotype has been identified.[83,192] Nearly all isolates of MAC from patients with AIDS have been identified as *M. avium*; in patients without AIDS, the rate of *M. avium* is approximately 55 percent, and the rate of *M. intracellulare* to 32 to 40 percent.[60,192]

Lung disease has been the major manifestation of MAC infection in nonimmunocompromised adults. Most investigators thought that MAC infection occurred mainly in patients with deficient immunity or underlying lung disease. Later reports seemed to indicate, however, that normal adult hosts are at risk for development of infection with MAC, and that rates are increasing.[76,126] Case reports involving children are lacking in detail because they usually appear within discussions of adult patients.[128]

Pediatric case reports of disseminated disease caused by MAI/MAC have appeared in the literature. Children have had ulcerative lesions of the colon[33]; mesenteric disease with abscess formation[143]; hematogenous spread to the liver, spleen, kidneys, and adrenal cortex; lesions of the epididymis[151]; bone lesions[174]; and skin lesions. Disseminated osteomyelitis rarely is caused by nontuberculous mycobacteria, but if it occurs, *M. intracellulare* most commonly is isolated.[25,86] Septic arthritis also has been reported in association with osteomyelitis.[51] Immunocompromised patients with disseminated MAI infection historically require multiple-drug therapy, including a combination of isoniazid, ethambutol, clofazimine, and rifabutin.[97] Some reports indicate, however, that disseminated disease in HIV-infected patients may respond to only two agents, as mentioned earlier in the AIDS section. The addition of other agents may be necessary because of the high incidence of resistant organisms. A preliminary report showed that interferon-γ may be effective when combined with conventional therapy in some patients who are refractory to standard chemotherapy alone.[71]

Bacterial peritonitis is a common occurrence in patients regularly undergoing ambulatory peritoneal dialysis for chronic renal failure. Reports of nontuberculous mycobacteria causing peritonitis have been noted.[63,122,184] In cases involving nontuberculous mycobacteria with foreign bodies, such as Tenckhoff catheters, the development of infected sinus tracts is frequent. Additionally, antituberculous drug regimens in these cases generally are unsuccessful. Although the mycobacteria were sensitive to the agents used, the patients continued to have sinus tract drainage without improvement, even after removal of the foreign body.

MYCOBACTERIUM SCROFULACEUM

M. scrofulaceum has many characteristics similar to *M. avium* and *M. intracellulare* and can be found in soil, water, and dairy products. This organism is associated most commonly with lymphadenitis in children 1 to 5 years old and rarely causes other manifestations in humans. Skin and bone lesions have been reported in two children chronically infected with *M. scrofulaceum* for 10 years.[43,181] Few data are available on chemotherapeutic agents for treatment of infection with this organism. Based on susceptibility patterns, three or more drugs may be necessary for treatment of serious disease. Lymphadenitis can be cured with complete excision of the lymph node.

MYCOBACTERIUM KANSASII

Of the photochromogens, *M. kansasii* is the one most commonly isolated in humans. In contrast to MAI and *M. scrofulaceum*, *M. kansasii* rarely is isolated in soil, but has been cultured from water and milk.[22,23] Chronic pulmonary infection is the most common manifestation of this disease and is seen mainly in adults, particularly adults with AIDS. A survey from Israel of 56 adults with *M. kansasii* pulmonary infection showed that 64 percent occurred in men, 59 percent had underlying lung disease, and none were HIV-infected.[145] Pulmonary disease occurs infrequently in children. Some children have a course similar to that of adults, with underlying pulmonary disease caused by previous tuberculosis or chronic pulmonary disease.[12,112] In contrast, other children have acute symptoms of classic bacterial pneumonia with an abrupt onset of fever and sputum production and lung consolidation on physical examination and radiographs.[12,21] Pleural effusions also can occur.

In contrast to some other nontuberculous organisms, *M. kansasii* is sensitive to most of the antituberculous drugs, particularly rifampin. Most authorities recommend the use of three drugs, including rifampin, isoniazid, and ethambutol. The treatment course usually requires a minimum of 12 months, with therapy for 24 months needed in some patients. A study of 18 patients showed that thrice-weekly clarithromycin, ethambutol, and rifampin was effective, with a mean follow-up of 46 months.[58] Patients with AIDS and *M. kansasii* infection have responded to this three-drug regimen, but the total duration of therapy is unknown at this time. In children with AIDS, the diagnosis of *M. kansasii* infection is rare, and the clinical response to therapy has been poor.[73] Cases have been reported in other immunocompromised children, including a 7-month-old boy from Texas with disseminated *M. kansasii* infection and numerous organisms found in his spleen at autopsy.[111] *M. kansasii* also has been reported to cause meningitis; the patients died despite the use of antimycobacterial therapy.[75,140]

MYCOBACTERIUM MALMOENSE

Buchholz and coworkers[18] reviewed infections with *M. malmoense* in the United States from 1993 to 1995. Only one of 73 patients was younger than 10 years. This patient had cervical lymphadenitis and was cured with surgical excision alone. This organism, which frequently is overlooked on standard Löwenstein-Jensen egg medium, grows at 25° C to 37° C. The organism is slow growing, and it may require 8 to 12 weeks for colonies to become visible on solid media. The BACTEC system was shown to be superior in isolating *M. malmoense* in one study of children with lymphadenitis.[70] Bone marrow involvement also was described in a patient with chronic granulocytic leukemia.[45] The aforementioned study by Buchholz and colleagues[18] showed that prolonged combination therapy with isoniazid, rifampin, ethambutol, and pyrazinamide after surgical excision was effective in some cases.

MYCOBACTERIUM CHELONAE AND MYCOBACTERIUM FORTUITUM

M. chelonae is the most important rapidly growing pathogenic mycobacterium, but its taxonomy is quite confusing.[56] Since Grange[56] made a presentation in 1981, the organism's taxonomy has continued to be in flux. The *M. chelonae* group consists of *M. chelonae* (formerly *M. chelonae* subsp. *chelonae*), *M. abscessus* (formerly *M. chelonae* subsp. *abscessus*), and a third biovariant known as *M. chelonae*–like organisms.[92] The *M. fortuitum* group consists of *M. fortuitum*, *Mycobacterium peregrinum*, and a third unnamed biovariant.[92] *M. fortuitum* is associated closely with *M. chelonae*. The two groups can be differentiated on the biochemical basis of nitrate reduction and iron uptake. Wallace and associates[175] have provided the largest series of patients with skin, soft tissue, and bone involvement with *M. chelonae*. Steroid use seemed to be the factor associated most commonly with the development of disease.

M. fortuitum and *M. chelonae* have been implicated in sternal wound infections and endocarditis and have occurred in outbreak-type settings.[91,136,163] Patients responded to surgical débridement and amikacin with cefoxitin. A case series from Hong Kong reported successful treatment of *M. fortuitum* sternotomy infections with the use of single daily dose ofloxacin as monotherapy in three patients.[194] Adult renal transplant patients also have been described with skin and subcutaneous tissue involvement caused by *M. chelonae*.[31] *M. chelonae*, likewise, has been described as an etiologic agent for otitis media, probably from contamination of ear, nose, and throat instruments with colonized water sources.[103]

M. abscessus, as stated earlier, is related closely to *M. chelonae* and should be designated as a separate species.[92] Manifestations of infection with this organism usually are related to pulmonary, cutaneous, or disseminated infections.[178] Clarithromycin may be effective for *M. chelonae* infection.[179] Maxson and associates[110] reported a case of osteomyelitis caused by *M. abscessus* that was controlled with long-term clarithromycin monotherapy.

Mycobacterium smegmatis, which resembles *M. fortuitum* except for the absence of a positive 3-day arylsulfatase test result, is a rapid grower that is responsible for skin and soft tissue infections.[176] A case of disseminated infection has been reported in a child with inherited interferon-γ receptor deficiency.[123]

Mycobacterium septicum is a newly described, rapidly growing species associated with catheter-related bacteremia.[142] It resembles *M. fortuitum* and *Mycobacterium senegalense*.

OTHER SITES OF INFECTION

Carpal tunnel syndrome in adults has been reported as being caused by *M. szulgai*, an uncommon scotochromogenic mycobacterium.[159] Effective treatment included débridement, ethambutol, and rifampin. Other infections in humans include choroiditis,[29] panniculitis,[139] genitourinary tract infection,[15,164] and synovitis.[161] Ear infections with nontuberculous mycobacteria also have been reported, as has mastoiditis.[49,119,158] More recently, infection of Broviac catheters in pediatric patients with leukemia and hemodialysis catheters has been described.[24,95] In all cases, removal of the catheter was required for resolution of the infection.

With the continued proliferation of immunocompromised patients because of AIDS and new treatment modalities that induce an immunocompromised state (e.g., organ transplantation, new immunosuppressive drugs), the atypical mycobacteria probably will continue to remain important pathogens. With newer isolation techniques and new technology such as DNA probes, the ability to diagnose these infections and understanding of the pathogenesis of the infections that these organisms produce should improve, as should the ability to treat these infections.

REFERENCES

1. Agy, M. B., Wassis, C. K., Plorde, J. J., et al.: Evaluation of four mycobacterial blood culture media: BACTEC 13A, Isolator/BACTEC 12B, Isolator/Middlebrook Agar and a biphasic medium. Diagn. Microbiol. Infect. Dis. 12:303-308, 1989.
2. Ahn, C. H., McLarty, J. W., Ahn, S. S., et al.: Diagnostic criteria for pulmonary disease caused by *Mycobacterium kansasii* and *Mycobacterium intracellulare*. Am. Rev. Respir. Dis. 125:388-391, 1982.
3. Aitken, M. L., Burke, W., McDonald, G., et al.: Nontuberculous mycobacterial disease in adult cystic fibrosis patients. Chest 103:1096-1099, 1993.
4. Altman, R. P., and Margileth, A. M.: Cervical lymphadenopathy from atypical mycobacteria: Diagnosis and surgical treatment. J. Pediatr. Surg. 10:419-422, 1975.
5. Alvarez-Elcoro, S., and Enzler, M. J.: The macrolides: Erythromycin, clarithromycin, and azithromycin. Mayo Clin. Proc. 74:613-634, 1999.
6. Antiretroviral therapy and medical management of pediatric HIV infection and 1997 USPHS/IDSA report on the prevention of opportunistic infections in persons infected with human immunodeficiency virus. Pediatrics 102(4 Pt. 2):999-1085, 1998.
7. Armstrong, K. L., James, R. W., Dawson, D. J., et al.: *Mycobacterium haemophilum* causing perihilar or cervical lymphadenitis in healthy children. J. Pediatr. 121:202-205, 1992.
8. Aubry, A., Chosidow, O., Caumes, E., et al.: Sixty-three cases of *Mycobacterium marinum* infection: Clinical features, treatment, and antibiotic susceptibility of causative isolates. Arch. Intern. Med. 162:1746-1752, 2002.
9. Barton, L. L., and Feigin, R. D.: Childhood cervical lymphadenitis: A reappraisal. J. Pediatr. 84:846-852, 1974.
10. Bell, R. C., Higuchi, J. H., Donovan, W. N., et al.: *Mycobacterium simiae*: Clinical features and follow-up of twenty-four patients. Am. Rev. Respir. Dis. 127:35-38, 1983.
11. Benjamin, D. R.: Granulomatous lymphadenitis in children. Arch. Pathol. Lab. Med. 111:750-753, 1987.
12. Bialkin, G., Pollak, A., and Weil, A. J.: Pulmonary infection with *Mycobacterium kansasii*. Am. J. Dis. Child. 101:739, 1961.
13. Blacklock, Z. M., and Dawson, D. J.: Atypical mycobacteria causing nonpulmonary disease in Queensland. Pathology 11:283-287, 1979.
14. Brook, I.: Aerobic and anaerobic bacteriology of cervical adenitis in children. Clin. Pediatr. (Phila.) 19:693-696, 1980.
15. Brooker, W. J., and Aufderheide, A. C.: Genitourinary tract infections due to atypical mycobacteria. J. Urol. 124:242-244, 1980.
16. Brooks, R. W., Parker, B. C., Gruft, H., et al.: Epidemiology of infection by nontuberculous mycobacteria. Am. Rev. Respir. Dis. 130:630-633, 1984.
17. Brown, J. W., III, and Sanders, C. V.: *Mycobacterium marinum* infections: A problem of recognition, not therapy? Arch. Intern. Med. 147:817-818, 1987.
18. Buchholz, U. T., McNeil, M. M., Keyes, L. E., and Good, R. C.: *Mycobacterium malmoense* infections in the United States, January 1993 through June 1995. Clin. Infect. Dis. 27:551-558, 1998.
19. Burchard, G. D., and Bierther, M.: Buruli ulcer: Clinical pathological study of 23 patients in Lambarene, Gabon. Trop. Med. Parasitol. 37:1-8, 1986.
20. Centers for Disease Control and Prevention: HIV/AIDS surveillance report. Feb.:1-23, 1993.
21. Chapman, J. S.: Varieties of tuberculosis in children. Minn. Med. 42:1773, 1959.
22. Chapman, J. S., Bernard, J. S., and Speight, M.: Isolation of mycobacteria from raw milk. Am. Rev. Respir. Dis. 91:351, 1965.
23. Chapman, J. S., and Speight, M.: Isolation of atypical mycobacteria from pasteurized milk. Am. Rev. Respir. Dis. 98:1052, 1968.
24. Chawla, P. G., and Nevins, T. E.: Management of hemodialysis catheter related bacteremia: A 10 year experience. Pediatr. Nephrol. 14:198-202, 2000.
25. Chicoine, L., La Pointe, N., Simoneau, R., et al.: "Anonymous" mycobacterial infection causing disseminated osteomyelitis and skin lesions. Can. Med. Assoc. J. 98:1059, 1968.
26. Christensen, E. E., Dietz, G. W., Ahn, C. H., et al.: Initial roentgenographic manifestations of pulmonary *Mycobacterium tuberculosis*, *M. kansasii*, and *M. intracellulare* infections. Chest 80:132-136, 1981.
27. Clancy, J. K., Dodge, O. G., Lunn, H. F., et al.: Mycobacterial skin ulcers in Uganda. Lancet 2:951-954, 1961.
28. Clarridge, J., Shawar, R., Shinnick, T., et al.: Large-scale use of polymerase chain reaction for detection of *Mycobacterium tuberculosis* in a routine mycobacteriology laboratory. J. Clin. Microbiol. 31:2049-2056, 1993.
29. Clever, V. G.: Choroidal involvement with *Mycobacterium intracellulare*. Ann. Ophthalmol. 12:1409-1411, 1980.
30. Colville, A.: Retrospective review of culture-positive mycobacterial lymphadenitis cases in children in Nottingham, 1979-1990. Eur. J. Clin. Microbiol. Infect. Dis. 12:192-195, 1993.

31. Cooper, J. F., Lichtenstein, M. J., Graham, B. S., et al.: *Mycobacterium chelonae*: A cause of nodular skin lesions with a proclivity for renal transplant recipients. Am. J. Med. *86*:173-177, 1989.

32. Currarino, G., Votteler, T. H., and Weinberg, A.: Atypical mycobacterial infection of intraparotid lymph nodes: Clinical and sialographic observations. Pediatr. Radiol. *6*:10-12, 1977.

33. Cuttino, J. T., and McCabe, A. M.: Pure granulomatous nocardiosis: A new fungus disease distinguished by intracellular parasitism. Am. J. Pathol. *25*:1, 1949.

34. Dailloux, M., Morlot, M., and Sirbat, C.: Etude des facteurs intervenant sur la presence des mycobacteries atypiques dans l'eau d'une piscine. Rev. Epidemiol. Sante Publique *28*:299-306, 1980.

35. Davidson, P. T.: Introduction (international conference on atypical mycobacteria). Rev. Infect. Dis. *3*:816-818, 1981.

36. Davis, B. R., Brumbach, M. T., Sanders, W. J., et al.: Skin lesions caused by *Mycobacterium haemophilum*. Ann. Intern. Med. *97*:723-724, 1982.

37. Deepe, G. S., Jr., Capparell, R., and Coonrod, J. D.: Atypical mycobacterial lymphadenitis in an adult. Chest *78*:882-883, 1980.

38. Delabie, J., DeWolfe-Peeters, C., Bobbaers, H., et al.: Immunophenotypic analysis of histocytes involved in AIDS-associated *Mycobacterium scrofulaceum* infection: Similarities with lepromatous lepra. Clin. Exp. Immunol. *85*:214-218, 1991.

39. Dhooge, I., Dhooge, C., De-Baets, F., et al.: Diagnostic and therapeutic management of atypical mycobacterial infections in children. Eur. Arch. Otorhinolaryngol. *250*:387-391, 1993.

40. Donta, S. T., Smith, P. W., Levitz, R. E., et al.: Therapy of *Mycobacterium marinum* infections. Arch. Intern. Med. *146*:902-904, 1986.

41. Drut, R., Anderson, V., Greco, M. A., et al.: Opportunistic infections in pediatric HIV infection: A study of 74 autopsy cases from Latin America. Pediatr. Pathol. Lab. Med. *17*:569-576, 1997.

42. Dunn, B. L., and Hodgson, D. J.: Atypical mycobacteria in milk. J. Appl. Bacteriol. *52*:373-376, 1982.

43. Dustin, P., Demol, P., Derks-Jacobovitz, D., et al.: Generalized fatal chronic infection by *Mycobacterium scrofulaceum* with severe amyloidosis in a child. Pathol. Res. Pract. *168*:237-248, 1980.

44. Dutt, A. K., and Stead, W. W.: Long-term results of medical treatment in *Mycobacterium intracellulare* infection. Am. J. Med. *67*:449-453, 1979.

45. Engervall, P., Bjorkholm, M., Petrini, B., et al.: Disseminated *Mycobacterium malmoense* infection in a patient with chronic granulocytic leukaemia. J. Intern. Med. *234*:231-233, 1993.

46. Esther, Jr., C. R., Henry, M. M., Molina, P. L., and Leigh, M. W.: Nontuberculous mycobacterial infection in young children with cystic fibrosis. Pediatr. Pulmonol. *40*:39-44, 2005.

47. Fauroux, B., Delaisi, B., Clement, A., et al.: Mycobacterial lung disease in cystic fibrosis: A prospective study. Pediatr. Infect. Dis. J. *16*:354-358, 1997.

48. Fergie, J. E., Milligan, T. W., Henderson, B. M., and Stafford, W. W.: Intrathoracic *Mycobacterium avium* complex infection in immunocompetent children: Case report and review. Clin. Infect. Dis. *24*:250-253, 1997.

49. Flint, D., Mahadevan, M., Gunn, R., and Brown, S.: Nontuberculous mycobacterial otomastoiditis in children: Four cases and a literature review. Int. J. Pediatr. Otorhinolaryngol. *51*:121-127, 1999.

50. Forbes, B., and Hicks, K.: Direct detection of *Mycobacterium tuberculosis* in respiratory specimens in a clinical laboratory by polymerase chain reaction. J. Clin. Microbiol. *31*:1688-1694, 1993.

51. Frosch, M., Roth, J., Ullrich, K., and Harms, E.: Successful treatment of *Mycobacterium avium* osteomyelitis and arthritis in a non-immunocompromised child. Scand. J. Infect. Dis. *32*:3328-3329, 2000.

52. Gill, M. J., Fanning, E. A., and Chomyc, S.: Childhood lymphadenitis in a harsh northern climate due to atypical mycobacteria. Scand. J. Infect. Dis. *19*:77-83, 1987.

53. Good, R. C., and Snider, D. E., Jr.: Isolation of nontuberculous mycobacteria in the United States, 1980. J. Infect. Dis. *146*:829-833, 1982.

54. Gorse, G. J., Fairshter, R. D., Friedly, G., et al.: Nontuberculous mycobacterial disease: Experience in a southern California hospital. Arch. Intern. Med. *143*:225-228, 1983.

55. Goto, M., Oka, S., Okuzumi, K., et al.: Evaluation of acridinium ester-labeled DNA probes for identification of *Mycobacterium tuberculosis* and *Mycobacterium avium-Mycobacterium intracellulare* complex in culture. J. Clin. Microbiol. *29*:2473-2476, 1991.

56. Grange, J. M.: *Mycobacterium chelonae*. Tubercle *62*:273-276, 1981.

57. Grange, J. M.: Mycobacteria and the skin. Int. J. Dermatol. *21*:497-503, 1982.

58. Griffith, D. E., Brown-Elliott, B. A., and Wallace, R. J., Jr.: Thrice-weekly clarithromycin-containing regimen for treatment of *Mycobacterium kansasii* lung disease: Results of a preliminary study. Clin. Infect. Dis. *37*:1178-1182, 2003.

59. Gruft, H., Falkinham, J. O., III, and Parker, B. C.: Recent experience in the epidemiology of disease caused by atypical mycobacteria. Rev. Infect. Dis. *3*:990-996, 1981.

60. Guthertz, L. S., Damsker, B., Bottone, E. J., et al.: *Mycobacterium avium* and *Mycobacterium intracellulare* infections in patients with and without AIDS. J. Infect. Dis. *160*:1037-1041, 1989.

61. Haas, W. H., Amthor, B., Engelmann, G., et al.: Preoperative diagnosis of *Mycobacterium avium* lymphadenitis in two immunocompetent children by polymerase chain reaction of gastric aspirates. Pediatr. Infect. Dis. J. *17*:1016-1020, 1998.

62. Haas, W. H., Butler, W. R., Kirshner, P., et al.: A new agent of mycobacterial lymphadenitis in children: *Mycobacterium heidelbergense* sp. nov. J. Clin. Microbiol. *35*:3203-3209, 1997.

63. Hakim, A., Hisam, N., and Reuman, P. D.: Environmental mycobacterial peritonitis complicating peritoneal dialysis: Three cases and review. Clin. Infect. Dis. *16*:426-431, 1993.

64. Havlir, D. V., Dube, M. P., Sattler, F. R., et al.: Prophylaxis against disseminated *Mycobacterium avium* complex with weekly azithromycin, daily rifabutin, or both. N. Engl. J. Med. *335*:392-398, 1996.

65. Havlir, D., Kemper, C. A., and Deresinski, S. C.: Reproducibility of lysis-centrifugation cultures for quantification of *Mycobacterium avium* complex bacteremia. J. Clin. Microbiol. *31*:1794-1798, 1993.

66. Hazra, R., Lee, S. H., Maslow, J. N., and Husson R. N.: Related strains of *Mycobacterium avium* cause disease in children with AIDS and in children with lymphadenitis. J. Infect. Dis. *181*:1298-1303, 2000.

67. Hjelt, K., Hojlyng, N., Howitz, P., et al.: The role of mycobacteria other than tuberculosis (MOTT) in patients with cystic fibrosis. Scand. J. Infect. Dis. *26*:569-576, 1994.

68. Hjelte, L., Petrini, B., Kallenius, G., et al.: Prospective study of mycobacterial infections in patients with cystic fibrosis. Thorax *45*:397-400, 1990.

69. Hofer, M., Hirschel, B., Kirschner, P., et al.: Brief report: Disseminated osteomyelitis from *Mycobacterium ulcerans* after a snakebite. N. Engl. J. Med. *328*:1007-1009, 1993.

70. Hoffner, S. E., Henriques, B., Petrini, B., et al.: *Mycobacterium malmoense*: An easily missed pathogen. J. Clin. Microbiol. *29*:2673-2674, 1991.

71. Holland, S. M., Eisenstein, E. M., Kuhns, D. B., et al.: Treatment of refractory disseminated nontuberculous mycobacterial infection with interferon gamma. N. Engl. J. Med. *330*:1348-1355, 1994.

72. Horsburgh, C. R., and Selik, R. M.: The epidemiology of disseminated nontuberculous mycobacterial infection in the acquired immunodeficiency syndrome (AIDS). Am. Rev. Respir. Dis. *139*:4-7, 1989.

73. Hoyt, L., Oleske, J., Holland, B., et al.: Nontuberculous mycobacteria in children with acquired immunodeficiency syndrome. Pediatr. Infect. Dis. J. *11*:354-360, 1992.

74. Huebner, R. E., Schein, M. F., Cauthen, G. M., et al.: Usefulness of skin testing with mycobacterial antigens in children with cervical lymphadenopathy. Pediatr. Infect. Dis. J. *11*:450-456, 1992.

75. Huempfner, H. R., Kingsolver, W. R., and Deuschle, K. W.: Tuberculous meningitis caused by both *Mycobacterium tuberculosis* and atypical mycobacteria. Am. Rev. Respir. Dis. *94*:612, 1966.

76. Iseman, M. D.: *Mycobacterium avium* complex and the normal host: The other side of the coin. N. Engl. J. Med. *321*:896-897, 1989.

77. Jindal, N., Devi, B., Aggarwal, A.: Mycobacterial cervical lymphadenitis in childhood. Indian J. Med. Sci. *57*:12-5, 2003.

78. Johann-Liang, R., Cervia, J. S., and Noel, G. J.: Characteristics of human immunodeficiency virus-infected children at the time of death: An experience in the 1990s. Pediatr. Infect. Dis. J. *16*:1145-1150, 1997.

79. Kahn, E.: Gastrointestinal manifestations in pediatric AIDS. Pediatr. Pathol. Lab. Med. *17*:171-208, 1997.

80. Kent, D. C.: Tuberculous lymphadenitis: Not a localized disease process. Am. J. Med. Sci. *254*:866-873, 1967.

81. Kiehn, T. E., and Cammarata, R.: Laboratory diagnosis of mycobacterial infections in patients with acquired immunodeficiency syndrome. J. Clin. Microbiol. *24*:708-711, 1986.

82. Kiehn, T. E., and Cammarata, R.: Comparative recoveries of *Mycobacterium avium-M. intracellulare* from isolator lysis-centrifugation and BACTEC 13A blood culture systems. J. Clin. Microbiol. *26*:760-761, 1988.

83. Kiehn, T. E., Edwards, F. F., Brannon, P., et al.: Infections caused by *Mycobacterium avium* complex in immunocompromised patients: Diagnosis by blood culture and fecal examination, antimicrobial susceptibility tests, and morphological and seroagglutination characteristics. J. Clin. Microbiol. *21*:168-173, 1985.

84. Kilby, J., Gilligan, P., Yankaskas, J., et al.: Nontuberculous mycobacteria in adult patients with cystic fibrosis. Chest *102*:70-75, 1992.

85. Klein, J. O.: Clarithromycin: Where do we go from here? Pediatr. Infect. Dis. J. *12*(Suppl.):148-151, 1993.

86. Koenig, M. G., Collins, R. D., and Heyssel, R. M.: Disseminated mycobacteriosis caused by Battey-type mycobacteria. Ann. Intern. Med. *64*:145, 1966.

87. Kox, L. F. F., Jansen, H. M., Kuijper, S., and Kolk, A. H. J.: Multiplex PCR assay for immediate identification of the infecting species in patients with mycobacterial disease. J. Clin. Microbiol. *35*:1492-1498, 1997.

88. Krasnow, I., and Gross, W.: *Mycobacterium simiae* infection in the United States. Am. Rev. Respir. Dis. *111*:357-360, 1975.

89. Kubica, G. P.: Current nomenclature of the mycobacteria. Bull. Int. Union Tuberc. *53*:192, 1978.

90. Kubica, G. P., and Wayne, L. G.: The Mycobacteria: A Sourcebook, Part A. New York, Marcel Dekker, 1984, pp. 38-41.

91. Kuritsky, J. N., Bullen, M. G., Broome, C. V., et al.: Sternal wound infections and endocarditis due to organisms of the *Mycobacterium fortuitum* complex. Ann. Intern. Med. 98:938-939, 1983.

92. Kusunoki, S., and Ezaki, T.: Proposal of *Mycobacterium peregrinum* sp. nov., nom. rev., and elevation of *Mycobacterium chelonae* subsp. abscessus (Kubica et al.) to species status: *Mycobacterium abscessus* comb. nov. Int. J. Syst. Bacteriol. *42*:240-245, 1992.

93. Kuth, G., Lamprecht, J., and Haase, G.: Cervical lymphadenitis due to mycobacteria other than tuberculosis: An emerging problem in children? J. Otorhinolaryngol. 57:36-38, 1995.

94. Lai, K. K., Stottmeier, K. D., Sherman, I. H., et al.: Mycobacterial cervical lymphadenopathy: Relation of etiologic agents to age. J. A. M. A. 251:1286-1288, 1984.

95. Levendoglu-Tugal, O., Munoz, J., Brudnicki, A., et al.: Infections due to nontuberculous mycobacteria in children with leukemia. Clin. Infect. Dis. 27:1227-1230, 1998.

96. Levin, M., Newport, M. J., D'Souza, S., et al.: Familial disseminated atypical mycobacterial infection in childhood: A human mycobacterial susceptibility gene? Lancet 345:79-83, 1995.

97. Levin, R. H., and Bolinger, A. M.: Treatment of nontuberculous mycobacterial infections in pediatric patients. Clin. Pharm. 7:545-551, 1988.

98. Lewis, L. L.: Nontuberculous mycobacterial infections. In Pizzo P. A., and Wilfert, C. M. (eds.): Pediatric AIDS: The Challenge of HIV Infection in Infants, Children, and Adolescents. 2nd ed. Baltimore, Williams & Wilkins, 1994, pp. 308-320.

99. Lim, S. D., Lopez, J., Ford, E., et al.: Genotypic identification of pathogenic Mycobacteria species by using a nonradioactive oligonucleotide probe. J. Clin. Microbiol. 29:1276-1278, 1991.

100. Lincoln, E. M., and Gilbert, L. A.: Disease in children due to mycobacteria other than Mycobacterium tuberculosis. Am. Rev. Respir. Dis. 105:683-714, 1972.

101. Lindberg, M. C., and Thomas, G. G.: Lymphadenitis due to atypical mycobacteria. Ala. Med. 59:19-21, 1989.

102. Losurdo, G., Castagnola, E., Cristina, E., et al.: Cervical lymphadenitis caused by nontuberculous mycobacteria in immunocompetent children: Clinical and therapeutic experience. Head Neck 20:245-249, 1998.

103. Lowry, P. W., Jarvis, W. R., Oberle, A. D., et al.: Mycobacterium chelonae causing otitis media in an ear-nose-and-throat practice. N. Engl. J. Med. 319:978-982, 1988.

104. Lunn, H. F., and Rees, R. J. W.: Treatment of mycobacterial skin ulcers in Uganda with a riminophenazine derivative (B663). Lancet 1:246, 1964.

105. MacCallum, P.: A new mycobacterial infection in man, I: Clinical aspects. J. Pathol. Bacteriol. 60:93, 1948.

106. Maloney, J. M., Gregg, C. R., Stephens, D. S., et al.: Infections caused by Mycobacterium szulgai in humans. Rev. Infect. Dis. 9:1120-1126, 1987.

107. Maltezou, H. C., Spyridis, P., and Kafetzis, D. A.: Nontuberculous mycobacterial lymphadenitis in children. Pediatr. Infect. Dis. J. 18:968-970, 1999.

108. Mandell, D. L., Wald, E. R., Michaels, M. G., and Dohar, J. E.: Management of nontuberculous mycobacterial cervical lymphadenitis. Arch. Otolaryngol. Head Neck Surg. 129:341-344, 2003.

109. Mankiewicz, E., and Majdaniw, O.: Atypical mycobacteria in tapwater. Can. J. Public Health 73:358-360, 1982.

110. Maxson, S., Schutze, G. E., and Jacobs, R. F.: Mycobacterium abscessus osteomyelitis: Treatment with clarithromycin. Infect. Dis. Clin. Pract. 3:203-206, 1994.

111. McCracken, G. H., Jr., and Reynolds, R. C.: Primary lymphopenic immunologic deficiency: Disseminated Mycobacterium kansasii infection. Am. J. Dis. Child. 120:143, 1970.

112. Merckx, J. J., Soule, E. H., and Karlson, A. G.: The histopathology of lesions caused by infection with unclassified acid-fast bacteria in man. Am. J. Clin. Pathol. 41:244, 1964.

113. Mollohan, C. S., and Romer, M. S.: Public health significance of swimming pool granuloma. Am. J. Public Health 51:883, 1961.

114. Morgan, J. K., and Blowers, R.: Swimming pool granuloma in Britain. Lancet 1:1034, 1964.

115. Musial, C. E., Tice, L. S., Stockman, L., et al.: Identification of mycobacteria from culture by using the Gen-Probe rapid diagnostic system for Mycobacterium avium complex and Mycobacterium tuberculosis complex. J. Clin. Microbiol. 26:2120-2123, 1988.

116. Mussaffi, H., Rivlin, J., Shalit, I., et al. Nontuberculous mycobacteria in cystic fibrosis associated with allergic bronchopulmonary aspergillosis and steroid therapy. Eur. Respir. J. 25:324-8, 2005.

117. Nadal, D., Caduff, R., Kraft, R., et al.: Invasive infection with Mycobacterium genavense in three children with the acquired immunodeficiency syndrome. Eur. J. Clin. Microbiol. Infect. Dis. 12:37-43, 1993.

118. Noordhoek, G. T., Kolk, A. H. J., Bjune, G., et al.: Sensitivity and specificity of PCR for detection of Mycobacterium tuberculosis: A blind comparison study among seven laboratories. J. Clin. Microbiol. 32:277-284, 1994.

119. Nylen, O., Alestig, K., Fasth, A., et al.: Infections of the ear with nontuberculous mycobacteria in three children. Pediatr. Infect. Dis. J. 13:653-656, 1994.

120. O'Brien, R. J.: The epidemiology of nontuberculous mycobacterial disease. Clin. Chest Med. 10:407-418, 1989.

121. Peacock, K. H., Lewis, L., and Lavoie, S.: Erosive mediastinal lymphadenitis associated with Mycobacterium avium infection in a pediatric acquired immunodeficiency syndrome patient. Pediatr. Infect. Dis. J. 19:576-578, 2000.

122. Perlino, C. A.: Mycobacterium avium complex: An unusual cause of peritonitis in patients undergoing continuous ambulatory peritoneal dialysis. Clin. Infect. Dis. 17:1083-1084, 1993.

123. Pierre-Audigier, C., Jouanguy, E., Lamhamedi, S., et al.: Fatal disseminated Mycobacterium smegmatis infection in a child with inherited interferon γ receptor deficiency. Clin. Infect. Dis. 24:982-984, 1997.

124. Pinder, S. E., and Colville, A.: Mycobacterial cervical lymphadenitis in children: Can histological assessment help differentiate infections caused by nontuberculous mycobacteria from Mycobacterium tuberculosis? Histopathology 22:59-64, 1993.

125. Pransky, S. M., Reismann, B. K., Kearns, D. B., et al.: Cervicofacial mycobacterial adenitis in children: Endemic to San Diego? Laryngoscope 100:920-925, 1990.

126. Prince, D. S., Peterson, D. D., Steiner, R. M., et al.: Infection with Mycobacterium avium complex in patients without predisposing conditions. N. Engl. J. Med. 321:863-868, 1989.

127. Quijano, G., Siminovich, M., and Drut, R.: Histopathologic findings in the lymphoid and reticuloendothelial system in pediatric HIV infection: A postmortem study. Pediatr. Pathol. Lab. Med. 17:845-856, 1997.

128. Reich, J. M., and Johnson, R. E.: Mycobacterium avium complex pulmonary disease: Incidence, presentation, and response to therapy in a community setting. Am. Rev. Respir. Dis. 143:1381-1385, 1991.

129. Reichert, C. M., O'Leary, T. J., Levens, D. L., et al.: Autopsy pathology in the acquired immune deficiency syndrome. Am. J. Pathol. 112:357-382, 1983.

130. Reid, I. S.: Mycobacterium ulcerans infection: A report of 13 cases at the Port Moresby General Hospital, Papua. Med. J. Aust. 1:427, 1967.

131. Rivron, M. J., Hughes, E. A., Sibert, J. R., et al.: Cervical lymphadenitis in childhood due to mycobacteria of the fortuitum group. Arch. Dis. Child. 54:312-313, 1979.

132. Rosenzweig, D. Y.: Pulmonary mycobacterial infections due to Mycobacterium intracellulare-avium complex: Clinical features and course in 100 consecutive cases. Chest 75:115-119, 1979.

133. Runyon, E. H.: Anonymous mycobacteria in pulmonary disease. Med. Clin. North Am. 43:273-290, 1959.

134. Runyon, E. H.: Pathogenic mycobacteria. Adv. Tuberc. Res. 14:235-287, 1965.

135. Runyon, E. H.: Mycobacteria: An overview. Rev. Infect. Dis. 3:819-821, 1981.

136. Safranek, T. J., Jarvis, W. R., Carson, L. A., et al.: Mycobacterium chelonae wound infections after plastic surgery employing contaminated gentian violet skin-marking solution. N. Engl. J. Med. 317:197-201, 1987.

137. Salyer, K. E., Votteler, T. P., and Dorman, G. W.: Surgical management of cervical adenitis due to atypical mycobacteria in children. J. A. M. A. 204:1037-1040, 1968.

138. Samra, Z., Kaufmann, L., Zeharia, A., et al.: Optimal detection and identification of Mycobacterium haemophilum in specimens from pediatric patients with cervical lymphadenopathy. J. Clin. Microbiol. 37:832-834, 1999.

139. Sanderson, T. L., Moskowitz, L., Hensley, G. T., et al.: Disseminated Mycobacterium avium-intracellulare infection appearing as a panniculitis. Arch. Pathol. Lab. Med. 106:112-114, 1982.

140. Sanford, J. P., and Barnett, J. A.: Atypical mycobacterial organisms as encountered in a general hospital and its clinics. In Chapman, J. S. (ed.): The Anonymous Mycobacteria in Human Disease. Springfield, IL, Charles C Thomas, 1960, p. 98.

141. Schaefer, W. B.: Incidence of the serotypes of Mycobacterium avium and atypical mycobacteria in human and animal diseases. Am. Rev. Respir. Dis. 97:18-23, 1968.

142. Schinsky, M. F., McNeil, M. M., Whitney, A. M., et al.: Mycobacterium septicum sp. nov., a new rapidly growing species associated with catheter-related bacteraemia. Int. J. Syst. Evolution. Microbiol. 2:575-581, 2000.

143. Schonell, M. E., Crofton, J. W., Stuart, A. E., et al.: Disseminated infection with Mycobacterium avium, I: Clinical features, treatment and pathology. Tubercle 49:12, 1968.

144. Schuit, K. E., and Powell, D. A.: Mycobacterial lymphadenitis in childhood. Am. J. Dis. Child. 132:675-677, 1978.

145. Shitrit, D., Baum, G. L., Priess, R., et al.: Pulmonary Mycobacterium kansasii infection in Israel, 1999-2004: Clinical features, drug susceptibility, and outcome. Chest 129:771-776, 2006.

146. Shocket, E., Drosd, R. E., and Tate, C. F., Jr.: Granuloma of the skin due to Mycobacterium fortuitum. South. Med. J. 57:1352, 1964.

147. Sigalet, D., Lees, G., and Fanning, A.: Atypical tuberculosis in the pediatric patient: Implications for the pediatric surgeon. J. Pediatr. Surg. 27:1381-1384, 1992.

148. Simor, A. E., Salit, I. E., and Vellend, H.: The role of Mycobacterium xenopi in human disease. Am. Rev. Respir. Dis. 129:435-438, 1984.

149. Smith, J. A., Mueller, B. U., Nussenblatt, R. B., and Whitcup, S. M.: Corneal endothelial deposits in children positive for human immunodeficiency virus receiving rifabutin prophylaxis for Mycobacterium avium complex bacteremia. Am. J. Ophthalmol. 127:164-169, 1999.

150. Smith, M. J., Efthimiou, J., Hodson, M. E., et al.: Mycobacterial isolations in young adults with cystic fibrosis. Thorax 39:369-375, 1984.

151. Snijder, J.: Morphological aspect of atypical mycobacterioses. In Selected Papers. Vol. 10. The Hague, Royal Netherlands Tuberculosis Association, 1967, p. 99.

152. Sommers, H. M., and Good, R. C.: Mycobacterium. In Lennette, E. H., Balows, A., Hausler, W. J., Jr., (eds.): Manual of Clinical Microbiology. 4th ed. Washington, D.C., American Society for Microbiology, 1985, pp. 216-240.

153. Song, M., Vincke, G., Vanachter, H., et al.: Treatment of cutaneous infection due to Mycobacterium ulcerans. Dermatologica 171:197-199, 1985.

154. Speight, E. L., and Williams, H. C.: Fish tank granuloma in a 14-month-old girl. Pediatr. Dermatol. 14:209-212, 1997.

155. Stanford, J. L., and Paul, R. C.: A preliminary report on some studies of environmental mycobacteria. Ann. Soc. Belg. Med. Trop. *53*:321, 1973.

156. Stanford, J. L., Revill, W. D. L., Gunthorpe, W. J., et al.: The production and preliminary investigation of burulin, a new skin test reagent for *Mycobacterium ulcerans* infection. J. Hyg. (Camb.) *74*:7, 1975.

157. Steadham, J. E.: High catalase strains of *Mycobacterium kansasii* isolated from water in Texas. J. Clin. Microbiol. *11*:496-498, 1980.

158. Stewart, M. G., Troendle-Atkins, J., Starke, J. R., et al.: Nontuberculous mycobacterial mastoiditis. Arch. Otolaryngol. Head Neck Surg. *121*:225-228, 1995.

159. Stratton, C. W., Phelps, D. B., and Reller, L. B.: Tuberculoid tenosynovitis and carpal tunnel syndrome caused by *Mycobacterium szulgai*. Am. J. Med. *65*:349-351, 1978.

160. Straus, W. L., Ostroff, S. M., Jernigan, D. B., et al.: Clinical and epidemiologic characteristics of *Mycobacterium haemophilum*, an emerging pathogen in immunocompromised patients. Ann. Intern. Med. *120*:118-125, 1994.

161. Sutker, W. L., Lankford, L. L., and Tompsett, R.: Granulomatous synovitis: The role of atypical mycobacteria. Rev. Infect. Dis. *1*:729-735, 1979.

162. Swift, S., and Cohen, H.: Granulomas of the skin due to *Mycobacterium balnei* after abrasions from a fish tank. N. Engl. J. Med. *267*:1244, 1962.

163. Syed, A. U., Hussain, R., Bhat, A. N., et al.: Mediastinitis due to *Mycobacterium fortuitum* infection following Fontan operation in a child. Scand. Cardiovasc. J. *31*:311-313, 1997.

164. Thomas, E., Hillman, B. J., and Stanisic, T.: Urinary tract infection with atypical mycobacteria. J. Urol. *124*:748-750, 1980.

165. Timpe, A., and Runyon, E. H.: Relationship of "atypical" acid-fast bacilli to human disease: Preliminary report. J. Lab. Clin. Med. *44*:202-209, 1954.

166. Torrens, J. K., Dawkins, P., Conway, S. P., and Moya, E.: Non-tuberculous mycobacteria in cystic fibrosis. Thorax *53*:182-185, 1998.

167. Tortoli, E., Piersimoni, C., Bartoloni, A., et al.: *Mycobacterium malmoense* in Italy: The modern Norman invasion? Eur. J. Epidemiol. *13*:341-346, 1997.

168. Tsukamura, M.: A review of the methods of identification and differentiation of mycobacteria. Rev. Infect. Dis. *3*:841-861, 1981.

169. Turneer, M., Van-Nerom, E., Nyabenda, J., et al.: Determination of humoral immunoglobulins M and G directed against mycobacterial antigen 60 failed to diagnose primary tuberculosis and mycobacterial adenitis in children. Am. J. Respir. Crit. Care Med. *150*:1508-1512, 1994.

170. 2002 USPHS guidelines for the prevention of opportunistic infections in persons infected with human immunodeficiency virus. U.S. Public Health Service (USPHS) and Infectious Diseases Society of America (IDSA). M. M. W. R. Morb. Mortal. Wkly. Rep. *51*(RR08):1-46, 2002.

171. Van Dyke, J. J., and Lake, K. B.: Chemotherapy for aquarium granuloma. J. A. M. A. *233*:1380-1381, 1975.

172. Venkatesh, V., Everson, N. W., and Johnstone, J. M.: Atypical mycobacterial lymphadenopathy in children: Is it underdiagnosed? J. R. Coll. Surg. Edinb. *39*:301-303, 1994.

173. Vestal, A. L.: Procedures for the Isolation and Identification of Mycobacteria. CDC Publication No. 76-8230. Washington, D.C., Department of Health, Education and Welfare, 1975.

174. Vollini, F., Cotton, R., and Lester, W.: Disseminated infection caused by Battey type mycobacteria. Am. J. Clin. Pathol. *43*:39, 1965.

175. Wallace, R. J., Brown B. A., and Onyi, G. O.: Skin, soft tissue, and bone infections due to *Mycobacterium chelonae*: Importance of prior corticosteroid

176. Wallace, R. J., Nash, D. R., Tsukamura, M., et al.: Human disease due to *Mycobacterium smegmatis*. J. Infect. Dis. *158*:52, 1988.

177. Wallace, R. J., Jr., O'Brien, R., Glassroth, J., et al.: Diagnosis and treatment of disease caused by nontuberculous mycobacteria. Am. Rev. Respir. Dis. *142*:940-953, 1990.

178. Wallace, R. J., Swenson, J. M., Silcox, V. A., et al.: Spectrum of disease due to rapidly growing mycobacteria. Rev. Infect. Dis. *5*:657-679, 1983.

179. Wallace, R. J., Tanner, D., Brennan, P. J., et al.: Clinical trial of clarithromycin for cutaneous (disseminated) infection due to *Mycobacterium chelonae*. Ann. Intern. Med. *119*:482-486, 1993.

180. Wayne, L. G., and Sramek, H. A.: Agents of newly recognized or infrequently encountered mycobacterial diseases. Clin. Microbiol. Rev. *5*:1-25, 1992.

181. Weed, L. A., Karlson, A. G., Ivins, J. C., et al.: Recurring migratory chronic osteomyelitis associated with saprophytic acid-fast bacilli: Report of a case of 10 years' duration apparently cured by surgery. Proc. Staff Meeting Mayo Clin. *31*:238, 1956.

182. Welch, K., Finkbeiner, W., Apers, C. E., et al.: Autopsy findings in the acquired immune deficiency syndrome. J. A. M. A. *252*:1152-1159, 1984.

183. White, M. P., Bangash, H., Goel, K. M., et al.: Non-tuberculous mycobacterial lymphadenitis. Arch. Dis. Child. *61*:368-371, 1986.

184. White, R., Abreo, K., Flanagan, R., et al.: Nontuberculous mycobacterial infections in continuous ambulatory peritoneal dialysis patients. Am. J. Kidney Dis. *22*:581-587, 1993.

185. Wilkes, M. S., Fortin, A. H., Felix, J. C., et al.: Value of necropsy in acquired immunodeficiency syndrome. Lancet *2*:85-88, 1988.

186. Wolinsky, E.: Nontuberculous mycobacteria and associated diseases. Am. Rev. Respir. Dis. *119*:107-159, 1979.

187. Wolinsky, E.: Mycobacteria: Significance of speciation and sensitivity tests. *In* Lorian, V. (ed.): Significance of Medical Microbiology in the Care of Patients. Baltimore, Williams & Wilkins, 1982, pp. 103-110.

188. Wolinsky, E.: Mycobacterial diseases other than tuberculosis. Clin. Infect. Dis. *15*:1-10, 1992.

189. Wolinsky, E.: Mycobacterial lymphadenitis in children: A prospective study of 105 nontuberculous cases with long-term follow-up. Clin. Infect. Dis. *20*:954-963, 1995.

190. Wolinsky, E., Gomez, F., and Zimpfer, F.: Sporotrichoid *Mycobacterium marinum* infection treated with rifampin-ethambutol. Am. Rev. Respir. Dis. *105*:964-967, 1972.

191. Woods, G. L., and Washington, J. A., II: Mycobacteria other than *Mycobacterium tuberculosis*: Review of microbiologic and clinical aspects. Rev. Infect. Dis. *9*:275-294, 1987.

192. Yakrus, M. A., and Good, R. C.: Geographic distribution frequency and specimen source of *Mycobacterium avium* complex serotypes isolated from patients with acquired immunodeficiency syndrome. J. Clin. Microbiol. *28*:926-929, 1990.

193. Yamauchi, T., Ferrieri, P., and Anthony, B. F.: The aetiology of acute cervical adenitis in children: Serological and bacteriological studies. J. Med. Microbiol. *13*:37-43, 1980.

194. Yew, W. W., Kwan, S. Y. L., Ma, W. K., et al.: Single daily-dose ofloxacin monotherapy for *Mycobacterium fortuitum* sternotomy infection. Chest *96*:1150-1152, 1989.

LEPROSY AND BURULI ULCER: THE MAJOR CUTANEOUS MYCOBACTERIOSES

Wayne M. Meyers ⊙ **Douglas S. Walsh**

Mycobacterial infections in humans date to at least the 10th millennium BCE. Bartels[15] in 1907 detected convincing evidence of tuberculosis in a Neolithic skeleton found near Heidelberg, Germany, and Ruffer[263] in 1910 noted Pott disease in an Egyptian mummy from approximately 1000 BCE. The origins of mycobacterial infections in humans are unknown, but most authorities speculate that domestication of animals in the Neolithic era promoted the transmission of mutants of *Mycobacterium tuberculosis* from livestock to humans. The origins of leprosy and Buruli ulcer and their respective etiologic agents are understood less well but may involve interplay among environmental mycobacteria, animals, and humans.[273] After tuberculosis, leprosy and Buruli ulcer are the second and third most common mycobacterial infections in humans. Leprosy and Buruli ulcer are the two most common cutaneous mycobacterioses.

Tuberculosis and other cutaneous mycobacterial infections are discussed in Chapters 107 and 108. This chapter is devoted to the two cutaneous mycobacterioses that are of greatest medical importance: leprosy and Buruli ulcer.

LEPROSY

Leprosy is a chronic infectious disease that is caused by *Mycobacterium leprae* and that principally affects the cooler parts of the body, especially the skin, upper respiratory tract, testes, eyes, and superficial segments of peripheral nerves.[27] Although leprosy has affected nearly every part of the world at some time, its geographic origin is only now being unraveled.[210]

The World Health Organization (WHO) reported that in 1999, approximately 800,000 patients were being treated for active leprosy and that also in 1999, 738,000 new patients were reported.[349] By 2005, the numbers had decreased to 220,000 and 296,000.[352] Many authorities consider that the total global prevalence of patients with active leprosy is much higher (1.5 to 2 million), however, and that new case rates are not rapidly declining.[11] Several more million patients experience serious sequelae.[168]

In the Middle Ages, leprosy was common in Europe and may have been transported to the Western Hemisphere by Portuguese and Spanish explorations beginning in the 15th century and later by slaves from Africa. At least two foci in the United States were established in the 19th century by specific immigrations: Asians brought leprosy to the Hawaiian Islands and started an epidemic in the highly susceptible Hawaiians[213] and Scandinavians introduced leprosy into the northern Midwest region of the United States.[178]

Patients with leprosy frequently experience severe stigmas, and, in Western cultures, this is attributable at least partially to a misunderstanding of what is called leprosy in the Old Testament.[28] Other cultures not influenced by Judaic laws and traditions have similar or more severe attitudes toward patients with leprosy. The Chinese literature indicates that in the 8th century BCE, patients with symptoms now recognized as symptoms of leprosy were stigmatized.[288] Because of enduring irrational attitudes based on the premise that relevant Old Testament references are to the same single disease now called leprosy, a brief explanation of "Old Testament leprosy" follows.

The Hebrew word *tsara'ath* was rendered *lepra* when the Old Testament was translated into Greek in the 3rd and 2nd centuries BCE. In preparing the Latin Vulgate version in AD 405, Jerome used the word *lepra* directly from the Greek. In the first English translation from the Vulgate in 1384, Wycliffe translated *lepra* as *leprosy*, perhaps because leprosy, then common in Europe and Great Britain, seemed to portray an image of an unholy and loathsome human condition. In the original text, *tsara'ath* was not a specific disease but probably a group of diseases, the identities of which are obscure, and the word more generally referred to ceremonial uncleanness. Old Testament *tsara'ath*, as described, for example, in Leviticus 13 and 14, had none of the distinctive clinical features of leprosy.

No rationale exists for attitudes toward leprosy that are based on Old Testament *tsara'ath*. Continuing efforts must be made to minimize the stigma peculiarly associated with leprosy. To help achieve this goal, the Fifth International Leprosy Congress in 1948 adopted a resolution to abandon the word *leper* for leprosy patient.[166] Some physicians prefer Hansen disease as a synonym for leprosy. Because of the stigma of leprosy, physicians must consider carefully the social implications of a diagnosis of leprosy, especially in children.

ORGANISM

M. leprae is a species in the order Actinomycetales and the family Mycobacteriaceae. This bacillus was seen first by Hansen in 1873 in Bergen, Norway, in lepromas from Norwegian patients, and this organism was the first reported bacterium causing chronic disease in humans.

M. leprae is an acid-fast bacillus (AFB) 0.3 to 0.5 μm wide by 4 to 7 μm long. The acid-fastness of *M. leprae* is weaker than that of other mycobacteria, but as in other mycobacteria, the acid-fastness is related to mycolic acid in the cell wall.[14] Viable, undamaged *M. leprae* organisms stain solidly, but degenerating bacilli first stain irregularly, then become granular, and eventually lose acid-fastness completely. The persistence of bacillary carcasses can be verified by silver staining techniques.[323] Staining quality provides a rapid method for determining the effectiveness of therapy. In vitro cultivation of *M. leprae* frequently is claimed, but all claims have been refuted or are as yet unsubstantiated.[152,256] Because *M. leprae* still cannot be cultivated, identification depends on criteria other than those used routinely for cultivable mycobacteria. Current criteria for *M. leprae* are the following: (1) It does not grow on routine laboratory media, (2) it infects the footpads of mice in a characteristic manner,[167,280] (3) acid-fastness is extractable with pyridine,[47] (4) the organism invades nerves of the host, (5) suspensions of dead bacilli produce a characteristic pattern of reactions when injected into the skin of patients (lepromin reaction) with the various clinical forms of leprosy, (6) it produces the species-specific antigen phenolic glycolipid-1 (PGL-1),[94] and (7) it exhibits species-specific DNA sequences.[344]

Electron micrographs of *M. leprae* reveal a cell wall 15 to 20 nm thick around a cytoplasmic membrane that gives rise to mesosomes extending into the cytoplasm. *M. leprae* divides by transverse fission. Its cell walls contain arabinogalactan, mycolates, peptidoglycan, and protein.[185]

The genome of *M. leprae* is small (3,268,203 base pairs) compared with that of *M. tuberculosis* (approximately 4.4 million base pairs).[41] Gene deletion and decay have markedly limited the metabolic activities of *M. leprae* and may contribute significantly to failure to cultivate the organism and to its long generation time in the mouse footpad (14 days).[25,76] In suitable hosts, the generation time of *M. leprae* has been speculated to be considerably shorter than 14 days.[117] Very young infants may have highly bacilliferous leprosy.[30,103] Localization of infections to the cooler parts of the body,[23] selective growth in the footpads of immunologically intact mice and in the ears of hamsters, and the high susceptibility of the armadillo (central body temperature of 32° C to 35° C [89.6° F to 95° F]) to disseminated infections all suggest that the optimal temperature for growth of *M. leprae* is less than 37° C (98.6° F).[189]

TRANSMISSION

The modes of transmission of *M. leprae* in nature have not been fully established. The frequency in children of a single early lesion in skin that usually is covered by clothing argues against the development of such lesions at the site of contact with *M. leprae*.[16] For many years, skin-to-skin contact between the patient and healthy subjects was considered the most important means of transmission, and this concept cannot be abandoned readily.[165] Intact skin of heavily infected patients discharges a few *M. leprae*, but ulcers in the skin may be a source of numerous bacilli. Skin-to-skin contact and fomites containing *M. leprae* could be sources of infection, but this mode has been minimized in recent years in favor of the nasorespiratory route.

That the nasal mucosa of lepromatous patients harbors massive numbers of *M. leprae* has been known since Hansen's original discovery, and studies suggest that the respiratory passages could be an important source of infecting bacilli.[66] *M. leprae* may bind to nasal mucosal cells by first binding fibronectin and attaching to fibronectin receptors on mucosal cells.[35] *M. leprae* organisms ejected in nose blowing remain viable under ambient conditions for 1 week,[58] and disseminated leprosy develops in immunosuppressed mice after the inhalation of aerosol that contains *M. leprae*.[250] Breast tissue and milk from lepromatous patients contain *M. leprae*, and infants may acquire infection from this source.[230]

Placental transmission of leprosy has been a subject of conjecture for some time, but evidence is growing for a significant influence of leprosy on fetal development and for intrauterine infection of the fetus. In a study of 116 pregnant leprosy patients in Ethiopia, the placentas were small, birth weights were low, and growth rates of the infants were retarded.[72] Mean birth weights of infants of lepromatous and healthy control mothers were 2558 and 3280 g. Estrogen excretion levels at 32 to 40 weeks' gestation are reduced in patients with leprosy, which suggests fetoplacental dysfunction.[74] Immunoglobulin A (IgA) and IgM antibodies for *M. leprae* are present in the cord blood of 30 to 50 percent of infants delivered by mothers with lepromatous leprosy.[186] Evidence is strong for synthesis of fetal antibodies to *M. leprae* or antigens thereof. Occasionally, *M. leprae* has been shown in placentas and cord blood.[127,313] *M. leprae*–specific IgA and IgM levels increased in infants of lepromatous mothers during the 3- to 24-month period after birth,[187] and two such infants had clinical leprosy at 9 and 17 months of age.[73]

Leprosy in young infants may be a common occurrence in areas of high endemicity.[103] In a report combining cases on file in the Leprosy Registry at the Armed Forces Institute of Pathology, cases cited in the literature, and personal observations by experienced leprologists, a total of at least 49 patients with leprosy younger than 1 year of age were identified.[30] In only half of these infants did the mother have leprosy or a history of leprosy. The youngest infant was 2.5 months old at the time the diagnosis was established. The fact that many of the mothers never had clinical leprosy suggests that they had an evanescent *M. leprae* bacteremia during gestation. A substantial bacteremia is a common finding in multibacillary disease[70,159] and is detectable in 15 percent of paucibacillary patients.[153]

The discoveries of a naturally acquired leprosy-like disease in recently captured wild armadillos in Louisiana,[331,333,334] chimpanzees,[69,107] a mangabey monkey from West Africa,[200] and a cynomolgus macaque from the Philippines provide reason to consider that leprosy is a zoonosis.[191,314,332] Reports of naturally acquired leprosy in armadillos range from 3 to 53 percent in the southern region of the United States.[137,305-307] In all these species, the histopathologic features resemble those in leprosy in humans, and the bacilli that cause the infection cannot be distinguished from *M. leprae*.[22,192,199] Leprosy has been transmitted successfully from the mangabey monkey to other mangabey, rhesus, and African green monkeys.[139,346]

Some authorities suggest that insects may ingest *M. leprae* during a blood meal from lepromatous patients and harbor viable bacteria. The natural transmission of leprosy by insects remains unproved, however, and generally is disregarded.

EPIDEMIOLOGY

The highest prevalence rates of leprosy are found in tropical Africa, South America, and Southeast Asia. Approximately 73 percent of all patients live in Southeast Asia (65% in India), 12 percent live in Africa, and 8 percent live in the Americas.[27] Based on limited whole-population surveys in endemic areas, the total number of active patients may exceed the number reported by WHO by a significant margin. The stigma of the disease and inefficiency in health care delivery systems contribute to this disparity in statistics.[164] In 1995, approximately 6000 patients with a history of leprosy resided in the United States,[129] with 101 new patients (L. Pfeifer, National Hansen's Disease Programs, Baton Rouge, LA, personal communication) reported in 1998, down from an annual high in recent times of 361 in 1985.

Most patients in the United States are immigrants, but a few indigenous patients regularly come from Hawaii, Louisiana, Texas, and other southeastern states.[160] No instances of secondary transmission from imported cases within the United States have been reported; immigrants with leprosy present no known public health risk to the population of the United States. The same situation probably is true for other nonendemic countries that receive many immigrants from endemic areas.

Hansen's discovery of the leprosy bacillus developed from his conviction that leprosy was a specific contagious disease, based on clinical and anatomic findings and, more importantly, on epidemiologic observations. In 1871 and 1872, he studied 69 families in western Norway in which several members had leprosy. The prevailing concept of that era was that leprosy was hereditary, but from data gathered on these families, Hansen showed that patients always had contact with another leprosy patient. Members of the same families with no such contacts were free of leprosy.[114] Hansen reasoned, after his pioneering observation of the leprosy bacillus in 1873, that the spread of leprosy depended on dissemination of this etiologic agent in a susceptible population.

The leprosy epidemic in Nauru in the central Pacific area shows how rapidly leprosy can spread in a leprosy-naive population.[108] Leprosy was introduced into this small island in 1912, and by 1924, one third of the 2500 inhabitants had leprosy.

The prevailing concept has been that an individual becomes infected only after experiencing repeated exposure. This concept now is doubted, and a single exposure may be sufficient in optimal conditions. One report describes leprosy transmission occurring after a single exposure from a patient to a surgeon who practiced in a leprosy non-endemic area.[2] In any patient-contact situation, the number of viable *M. leprae* being shed by the patient and the degree of susceptibility of the contact both may vary. Long periods of association may be necessary before optimal conditions for infection exist.

Lymphocyte transformation studies show that occupational contacts of leprosy patients in Ethiopia have the highest rate of sensitization (58%) to *M. leprae*, followed closely by household contacts (47%). Noncontacts living in endemic areas have a lower rate of sensitization, but approximately 29 percent of the population still is sensitized.[104]

Geographic, ethnic, and socioeconomic factors may contribute to the spread of leprosy by affecting the number of untreated or ineffectively treated bacillary-positive patients and the opportunities for exposure. The percentage of patients who harbor large numbers of bacilli—generally, patients with lepromatous leprosy—is related to ethnic background. In some Asian populations, 50 percent or more of patients with leprosy have lepromatous leprosy; in Africans, this figure is 5 to 10 percent. Socioeconomic factors are difficult to assess, and their relationship to the prevalence or clinical severity of leprosy is unknown. Nutritional status may or may not be important. The Nauru leprosy epidemic, indolent from 1912 through 1920, became rampant after a devastating epidemic of influenza (30% mortality) left a debilitated population with marked dietary deficiencies. During the next 4 years, the incidence of leprosy increased from 4 to 346 patients, but the role played by malnutrition is obscure.[108] Ryrie[264] in Malaya noted that during the Japanese occupation, the severity of leprosy worsened, which he attributed to a combination of malnutrition and psychic trauma. Skinsnes and Higa[289] drew similar conclusions from a study of mortality in leprosaria in China during World War II. Nonetheless, convincing evidence that the prevalence of leprosy is unusually high in chronically malnourished populations is lacking.

Improvements in housing and other living conditions may play a role in the declining prevalence of leprosy. No other factor satisfactorily explains the virtual disappearance of leprosy from northern Europe after the Middle Ages and from Scandinavia in the 20th century, long before any effective chemotherapy was available. If the disease is predominantly airborne, the construction of dwellings that provide less confined sleeping quarters in this era could have contributed in a major way to the disappearance of leprosy in northern Europe and Scandinavia. Consistent with this concept is the inadequate housing that prevails in all geographic areas in which leprosy is common today.

The presumed increased susceptibility of children is difficult to establish and may depend more on exposure to contagious patients and genetic predisposition than on other factors. The proportion of children among all detected patients is 20 to 30 percent.[95,222] Of the 615 known patients who were diagnosed in Louisiana between 1855 and 1970, 5 percent had disease onset at 0 to 9 years of age, and 19 percent were in the 10- to 19-year-old age group.[84] Lara,[162] in a study of 2000 children who lived in a leprosarium in the Philippines in an era when effective chemotherapy was unavailable, noted that leprosy developed in 470 (23%). Of these 470 patients, 254 were monitored closely, and in approximately 75 percent, the lesions healed spontaneously. Active, persistent disease developed in approximately 6 percent of the children who were heavily exposed to leprosy. In most populations studied, only 5 to 10 percent of individuals are susceptible to leprosy.

In adults, leprosy occurs more commonly in men than in women (2:1 to 3:1). In children, the sex ratio is approximately 1:1.

Genetic factors likely influence the susceptibility of some individuals to leprosy and the form of disease that develops.[27,85,88,89,282] Earlier studies found that if one twin has leprosy, the chance of leprosy developing in a monozygotic twin is 60 to 85 percent versus a 15 to 25 percent risk for dizygotic twins.[115] More recently, genome screening in Indian patients found an association with leprosy susceptibility on chromosome 10p13, near the gene for mannose receptor C, a phagocytic receptor on macrophages, and on chromosome 6, within the major histocompatibility complex (MHC).[284] Within the MHC, associations exist between leprosy and MHC class II genes in Indian patients, and with the tumor necrosis factor (TNF) gene in Brazilian patients.[279] Polymorphisms in the "promoter regions" of the interleukin-10 (IL-10) and TNF genes are associated with leprosy,[268] and the TNF promoter especially for the development of lepromatous or multibacillary leprosy.[262]

Certain human leukocyte antigens (HLA-DR) seem to be associated with specific forms of leprosy. HLA-DR2 and HLA-DR3 alleles are associated with tuberculoid disease, and HLA-DQ1 is associated with lepromatous disease.[50] In Suriname, HLA-DR3 is found frequently in mixed populations with tuberculoid leprosy and rarely in lepromatous patients; however, in Indians with tuberculoid leprosy, HLA-DR2 predominates.[317] HLA-DR antigens may influence the presentation of antigens of M. leprae to T cells and may affect the immune response to leprosy.[225]

Growing genetic evidence supports inter-population heterogeneity in leprosy susceptibility. On chromosome 6, within the leprosy susceptibility locus region q25-q26,[202] further investigation revealed a significant association between leprosy and 17 markers near the Parkinson disease gene *PARK2* and the co-regulated gene *PACRG* in Vietnamese and Brazilian families.[201] Having two of the alleles was associated with increased susceptibility to leprosy. In Malawi, a large case-control candidate gene study of leprosy susceptibility found that homozygotes for a silent T-to-C change in codon 352 of the vitamin D receptor gene were at higher risk, whereas homozygotes for the McCoy b blood group defining variant K1590E of the complement receptor 1 gene seemed to be protective.[88]

Toll-like receptors, molecules present on the surface of innate or native immune cells, mediate cytokine production on encountering a foreign invader, including mycobacteria, and ultimately may influence the pattern of specific immunity, which is especially relevant in leprosy.[180,258] Studies in Korea found that lepromatous leprosy occurred more commonly in patients with a mutation in the Toll-like receptor-2, associated with altered production of IL-10 and IL-12, underscoring the role early cytokine responses against *M. leprae* may play.[142-144] In African patients, polymorphisms in the *NRAMP1* gene, a gene that also is associated with cellular immunity to *M. leprae*, are associated with lepromatous leprosy,[184] as shown in the Mitsuda reaction.[7,245]

In Texas and Louisiana, the ratios of autochthonous to imported leprosy patients are the highest in the continental United States. Indigenous leprosy is highly prevalent in armadillos in only those two states,[23,290,332,334] and contact with such wild infected armadillos probably transmits leprosy to humans.[160,170,341] No cases of transmission of leprosy to humans from naturally infected mangabey monkeys or chimpanzees have been reported, but this potential exists.[107,193]

PATHOGENESIS AND PATHOLOGY

M. leprae causes disease by its ability to survive and multiply in macrophages (Fig. 109–1).[273] If macrophages of the host digest the bacilli early, disease is undetectable, or the patient has only minimal lesions. If the macrophages are totally incapable of destroying the organisms, a widely disseminated lepromatous leprosy follows. Survival of *M. leprae* in macrophages depends on the immune response of the patient; knowledge of immunity to *M. leprae* is necessary for understanding the mechanism of pathologic changes in leprosy.

IMMUNITY

The immunopathogenesis of leprosy can be understood by examining the spectral or polar nature of the condition, whereby polar tuberculoid disease is characterized by one or several well-demarcated lesions, borderline disease manifests with a modest number of medium-sized lesions, and lepromatous disease manifests with widespread poorly demarcated lesions (Table 109–1). Each type is associated with a different immunologic profile, especially within the lesions.

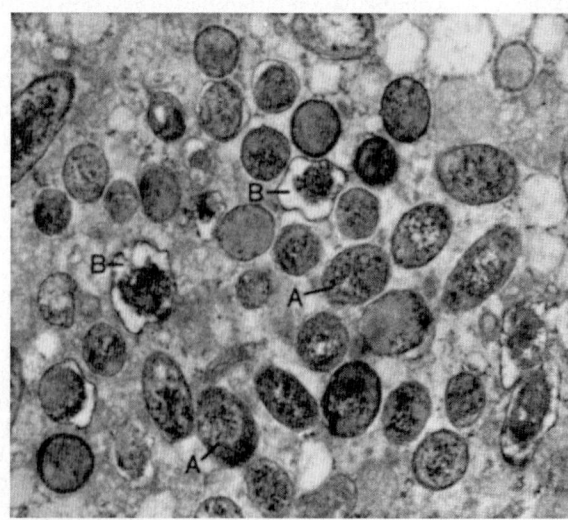

Figure 109–1 Electron micrograph of a portion of a globus of *M. leprae* within a histiocyte in a leproma in the skin. Cross sections of well-preserved (A) and degenerated (B) bacilli are presented (×45,000). *(Courtesy of Dr. S. C. Chang.)*

TABLE 109–1 Criteria for Classification of Leprosy

Group	Clinical Features	Histologic Features	Lepromin Reaction (Mitsuda)	Bacillary Density
Tuberculoid (TT)	A single or few anesthetic macules or plaques Borders well-defined Peripheral nerve involvement common	Epithelioid-lymphocyte granulomas, with or without giant cells, in skin and nerves No subepidermal clear zone Bacilli in nerves, but rare	Strongly positive	Rare
Borderline-tuberculoid (BT)	Lesions similar to those of TT, but more numerous Borders of lesions less distinct Satellite lesions sometimes present around larger lesions Peripheral nerve involvement common	Granulomas similar to those in TT Nerves are infiltrated Bacilli frequently found in nerves	Positive	Scanty
Borderline (BB)	More lesions than in BT Borders more vague Satellite lesions often seen Peripheral nerve involvement common	Epithelioid cells and histiocytic infiltrations focalized by lymphocytes Nerves show increased cellularity Bacilli readily found in nerves	Negative or weakly positive	Moderate
Borderline-lepromatous (BL)	Lesions are numerous and similar to those of BB Some nerve damage	Histiocytic infiltrations show a tendency to evolve toward epithelioid cells and foamy cells Lymphocytes present Nerves have less cellular infiltration Bacilli plentiful in nerves	Negative	Heavy
Lepromatous (LL)	Multiple, nonanesthetic, macular or papular, symmetrically distributed lesions No neural lesions until late Late complications of madarosis, leonine facies, testicular damage	Foamy histiocytes containing large numbers of bacilli Few or no lymphocytes Subepidermal clear zone Numerous bacilli in nerves and perineurium without significant intraneural cellular infiltration	Negative	Very heavy
Indeterminate (I)	Vaguely defined hypopigmented or erythematous macule	Often indistinguishable from "mild nonspecific dermatitis" Lymphocytes and histiocytes around skin appendages and nerves	Weakly positive or negative	Negative or scanty

The ability of an individual to resist *M. leprae* is assessed readily by the induration provoked by an intradermal injection of a suspension of killed *M. leprae* prepared from lepromatous tissue. Lepromatous nodules of patients were the traditional source, but now infected tissue from armadillos commonly is used.[194] The reagent is known as "lepromin," and the response is known as the "lepromin reaction." This reaction, first studied by Hayashi and later evaluated by Mitsuda,[204] has two components: an early response at 48 hours (Fernandez reaction) and a late response at 3 to 4 weeks (Mitsuda reaction). The Mitsuda reaction is the most consistent and is used by clinicians as an aid in classifying the clinical forms of leprosy.

Mitsuda reactions are strongly positive (>5 mm in diameter) in tuberculoid patients, weak or negative (0 to 2 mm) in lepromatous patients, and intermediate (3 to 5 mm) in borderline patients. The reactions are a direct measure of delayed hypersensitivity or cell-mediated immunity (CMI) to *M. leprae* antigens; lepromatous patients are anergic to *M. leprae*. The lepromin reaction has no value in establishing the diagnosis because a high percentage of any population is Mitsuda-positive. Even in children without leprosy, the Mitsuda reaction is positive in 20 percent of children younger than 5 years old and in two thirds

of children aged 7 to 9 years old.[112] Modifications of the lepromin reaction with the use of concentrated lepromin show that macrophages at the test site in lepromatous patients cannot clear *M. leprae* from the skin, whereas in tuberculoid patients, the bacilli are destroyed efficiently.[46]

Nonspecific factors participate in host defense against *M. leprae*. Complement promotes phagocytosis of leprosy bacilli.[271] After phagocytosis occurs, phagolysosomal fusion and intracellular killing ensue, perhaps by oxygen-independent mechanisms.

Although the precise mechanisms of specific immunity remain elusive, abundant experimental evidence indicates that in a lepromatous patient, CMI to *M. leprae* is markedly suppressed. Delayed hypersensitivity skin test reactions to many antigens often are depressed, but they are depressed most consistently and most severely to *M. leprae*.[32] The degree of suppression is gradually less pronounced in clinical forms of disease that are progressively nearer tuberculoid leprosy.[330]

A continuous decrease occurs in the sensitivity of peripheral blood lymphocytes to *M. leprae* that proceeds from tuberculoid to lepromatous patients.[217] Many investigators consider that the defect in CMI to *M. leprae* is in T-lymphocyte function or in the interaction of T lymphocytes with macrophages. Total numbers of circulating T lymphocytes are decreased in lepromatous patients,[75] but no consistent alteration occurs in the percent distribution of circulating T-cell subsets, particularly in the helper-suppressor (T_H1-T_H2) cell ratio.[246]

Within tuberculoid and lepromatous lesions, immunophenotypic and functional profiles of the infiltrating T cells differ markedly and are important factors in understanding the immunopathogenesis of leprosy.[208,209,244] In tuberculoid lesions, the CD4-to-CD8 T cell ratio is about 2:1, and the lesions are characterized by a T_H1 or T_H1-like profile, containing abundant mRNA transcripts for numerous proinflammatory cytokines that confer strong CMI, including IL-2, interferon-γ (IFN-γ), and IL-12.[356] Notably, CD4$^+$ T cells in tuberculoid lesions produce IFN-γ.[266] In lepromatous lesions, the CD4-to-CD8 ratio is approximately 1:2, and the lesions are characterized by a T_H2 or T_H2-like profile, containing mRNA transcripts for anti-inflammatory cytokines that include IL-4 and IL-10, factors associated with weak CMI, but strong humoral responses.[356] The CD8$^+$ T cells in lepromatous disease produce IL-4.[266] In contrast to Buruli ulcer (see later section on Buruli ulcer), induction of apoptosis in the lesions does not seem to play a major role in pathogenesis.[326] This immunologic dichotomy between tuberculoid and lepromatous lesions is consistent with the paradigm that robust CMI limits disease progression, and that humoral immunity has little or no effect.

The factors that determine whether a host generates a T_H1 or T_H2 response after having an infection with *M. leprae* are not completely understood. In addition to genetic predisposition (see section on epidemiology), an important immunologic factor may relate to host innate responses, when *M. leprae* is first encountered. Toll-like receptors on innate immune cells may recognize mycobacterial lipoproteins, generating cytokines that mediate specific or adoptive responses toward a T_H1 or T_H2 direction.[26,205]

In lepromatous lesions, T_H1 and T_H2 cells are admixed among the macrophages. Suppressor activity is generated by lepromin in vitro in peripheral leukocytes from lepromatous patients but not in cells from tuberculoid patients.[183] This suppressor activity also may be induced by the unique phenolic glycolipid (PGL-1) of *M. leprae*,[123,182] but it is unrelated to the type of leprosy.[241] PGL-1 abounds in the tissues of lepromatous patients. Secondary immunosuppression in advanced lepromatous leprosy may result from blockade of thymus-dependent areas of lymph nodes by *M. leprae*–laden macrophages.[309] Specific suppressor T-cell activity in immunosuppression in leprosy remains controversial.[147]

Macrophages of lepromatous patients are thought to have the capacity to kill, digest, and clear *M. leprae* if they are activated.[122] Patients with lepromatous leprosy fail to produce IL-2, but IL-2 restores the proliferation of lymphocytes in response to specific antigens.[116] Defective IFN-γ is produced by lymphocytes from lepromatous patients on stimulation by *M. leprae* antigens.[221] IL-2-bearing lymphocytes are reduced markedly in lepromatous infiltrations in tissues.[207] Suppressor T cells may influence IL-2 production in situ and reduce the proliferation of specifically sensitized T cells to release IFN-γ, with the result that macrophages are not activated. The injection of IFN-γ or recombinant IL-2 into the skin of lepromatous patients causes a local influx of CD4$^+$ T cells along with the formation of epithelioid and giant cells and a reduction in bacillary load.[146,320] IL-2 and IFN-γ, when available in quantity, may prove to be important immunotherapeutic agents for lepromatous leprosy. Therapy with IL-2 or IFN-γ induces the secretion of TNF-α; however, the activity of this toxic molecule may be inhibited by thalidomide or pentoxifylline.[145,302] Whether the increasing use of TNF-α antagonists such as infliximab, generally used for autoimmune disorders such as rheumatoid arthritis, would be associated with the develop-

ment of leprosy from latent infections and perhaps be useful in the management of leprosy reactions remains unclear.[80,274]

Immunoglobulin production (IgG, IgA, and IgM) usually is elevated only slightly in tuberculoid patients but is elevated markedly in lepromatous patients, consistent with the predominant T_H1 versus T_H2 responses.[33] The total number of B lymphocytes is increased in the blood of lepromatous patients, as is the circulating antibody to mycobacterial antigens.[92,219]

The role of immunologic processes in damage to nerves in leprosy is poorly understood. Some observations suggest that antineural antibodies in the sera of many patients, especially patients with lepromatous disease, are related to such damage.[228] TNF-α is associated with macrophage infiltration of peripheral nerves in reversal reactions.[155] Infected Schwann cells present antigens to T cells, rendering them targets for immune attack.[273]

HISTOPATHOLOGY

Biopsy specimens from well-defined lesions of leprosy should be taken from the active border and fixed in buffered 10 percent formalin or other suitable fixative. The Fite-Faraco staining method is used because the Ziehl-Neelsen stain does not show *M. leprae* optimally in tissue sections. A histopathologic diagnosis of leprosy must not be made unless the evidence is convincing. The pathologist must avoid making ambiguous evaluations, such as "consistent with leprosy." DNA probes specific for *M. leprae* are available and are useful in identifying leprosy bacilli in tissue or nasal secretions.[66,344] Specimens for DNA evaluation or polymerase chain reaction (PCR) amplification, techniques that have been steadily improved over the past decade, should be preserved in 70 percent ethyl alcohol.[37,86,109]

Indeterminate Leprosy

In indeterminate leprosy (Fig. 109–2), the immune potential of the patient is not portrayed clearly in the cellular reaction. Only a mild chronic inflammation is found, with small infiltrations of lymphocytes or histiocytes along neurovascular channels and sometimes around appendages (Fig. 109–3). If leprosy is suspected, all nerves in the dermis and subcutaneous tissue in numerous sections of the biopsy specimen must be searched for AFB, even if no inflammatory changes within the nerves are present. Sometimes AFB appear only in the arrector pili muscles or subepidermal zone.[252] A histopathologic diagnosis of leprosy cannot be made unreservedly in indeterminate leprosy without showing AFB. Molecular biologic studies are rarely helpful in diagnosing indeterminate leprosy.

Tuberculoid Leprosy

Patients with tuberculoid (TT) leprosy (Fig. 109–4) have a high level of CMI to *M. leprae*, which is reflected in the cellular reaction. Granulomata composed of epithelioid cells, Langhans giant cells, and lymphocytes are present in the dermis or subcutaneous tissue (Fig. 109–5A). Frequently, upper dermal granulomata invade the lower layers of the epidermis (see Fig. 109–5A). Damage to nerves is a distinctive feature—in old advanced lesions, all cutaneous nerves may be damaged beyond recognition (see Fig. 109–5B). Occasionally, S-100 immunostaining helps reveal a neural pattern of Schwann cells if a question exists of whether or not nerves are damaged. Schwann cells are increased in number in early lesions, and the nerves are invaded by mononuclear cells. Bacilli rarely are found, and often many sections must be searched to locate a single bacillus. The bacilli usually are within remnants of dermal nerves but sometimes are located just beneath the epidermis.

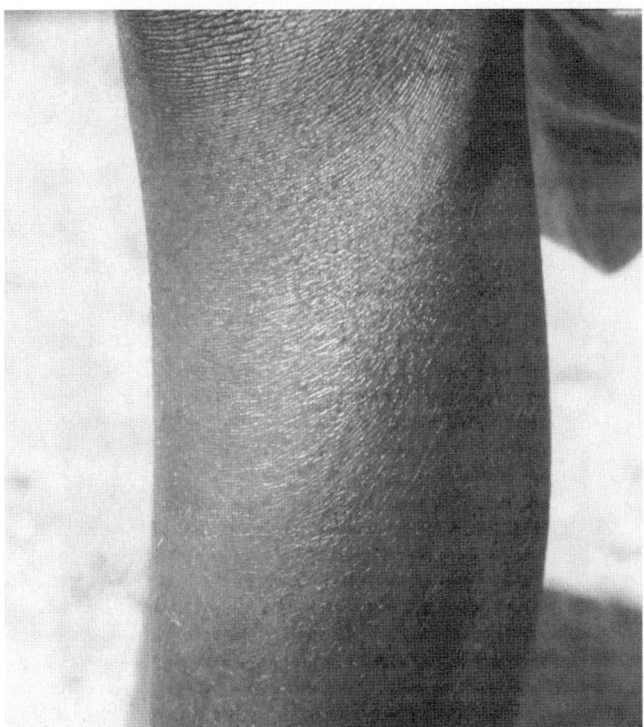

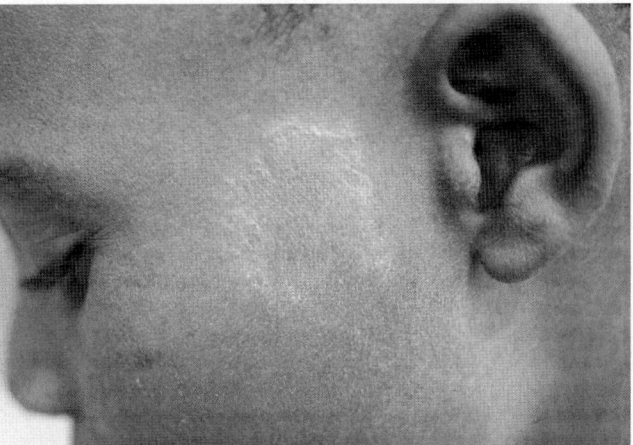

Figure 109–4 Tuberculoid leprosy in a 12-year-old Congolese boy. This was the only lesion, and it has a well-defined papulated border with central healing. (See companion Expert Consult web site for color version.)

Figure 109–2 Hypopigmented macule of indeterminate leprosy on the anterior surface of the leg of an Indian girl. (See companion Expert Consult web site for color version.)

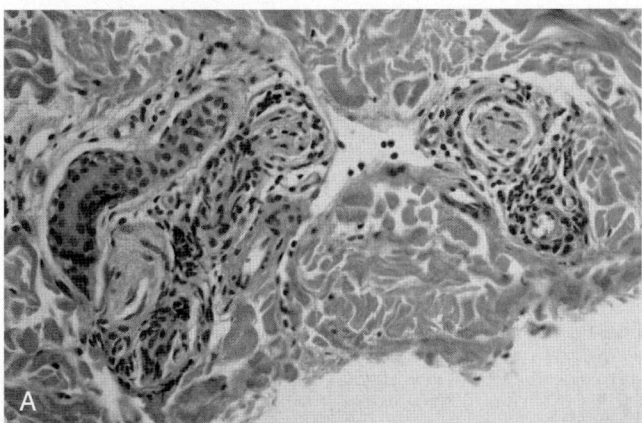

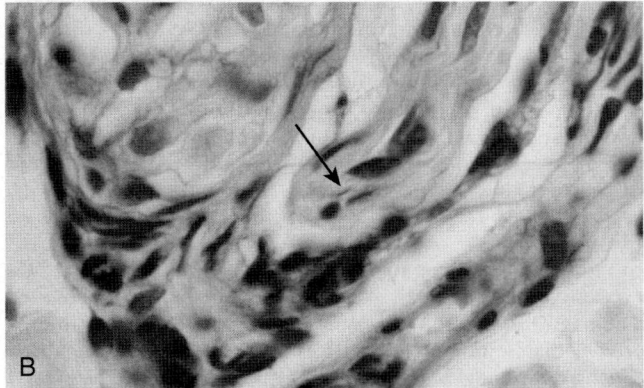

Figure 109–3 A, Indeterminate leprosy showing only mild infiltrations along neurovascular channels in the deep dermis (hematoxylin and eosin stain). **B,** Only a single acid-fast bacillus was found in one deep dermal nerve *(arrow)* after a search of multiple sections (Fite-Faraco stain). (See companion Expert Consult web site for color version.)

When major nerve trunks are involved, they contain typical tuberculoid infiltrates that eventually may replace the entire nerve. Occasionally, caseous "abscesses" are present in large nerves, but they are rare in children.

Borderline Leprosy

Borderline leprosy represents a broad spectrum of clinical (Fig. 109–6) and histopathologic variations (see Table 109–1). In the borderline-tuberculoid (BT) variety, strong CMI still is evident by the large numbers of epithelioid cells and lymphocytes. The nerves usually are damaged less and are identifiable more readily than in TT leprosy. *M. leprae* often remain rare but are seen more readily than in TT in nerves (Fig. 109–7) or in the subdermal zone. In the central portion of the borderline area of leprosy (BB), the epithelioid cells are not surrounded by large numbers of lymphocytes, and Langhans giant cells are uncommon. The subepidermal area is free of infiltrating cells, and nerves are not damaged severely, but the perineurium often is thickened by epithelioid cells. Some histopathologists do not recognize BB leprosy as an entity because there is usually a suggestion that the lesion is either on the BT or the borderline-lepromatous (BL) side of the spectrum of the disease.[136] BL lesions reveal a low level of CMI. The granulomata are composed mostly of macrophages, but contain many irregularly distributed lymphocytes. A few nests of epithelioid cells may be present. The perineurium of the nerves is infiltrated with cellular exudates. Nerves are easily identified and contain many bacilli.

Lepromatous Leprosy

Pre-lepromatous lesions show only a mild proliferation of macrophages around vessels, nerves, and appendages. AFB are few and often difficult to show.

Anergy to *M. leprae* becomes apparent early in the lepromatous lesion (Fig. 109–8), with the bacilli-laden macrophage (Virchow cell or lepra cell) being the predominant inflammatory cell. In early lesions, they tend to accumulate around vessels, nerves, and appendages, but they eventually may replace the entire dermis (Fig. 109–9A). The infected macrophages are supported by a delicate stroma and supplied by a rich network of capillaries. As the macrophages age, they become vacuolated (foamy), largely from their lipid content. In developing lesions, the intracellular bacilli are arranged in small bundles (see Fig.

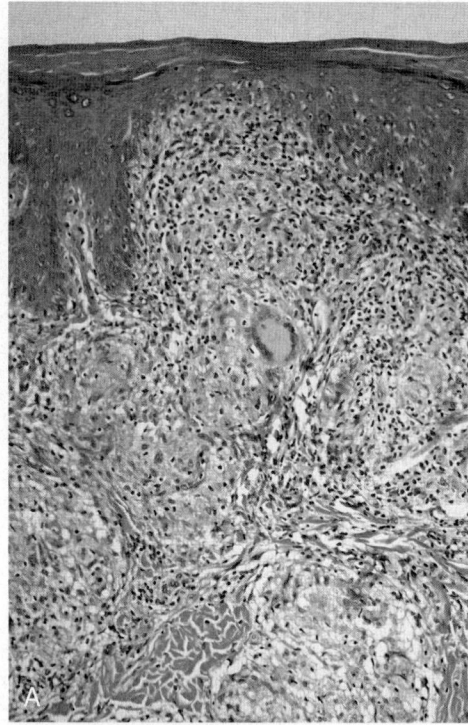

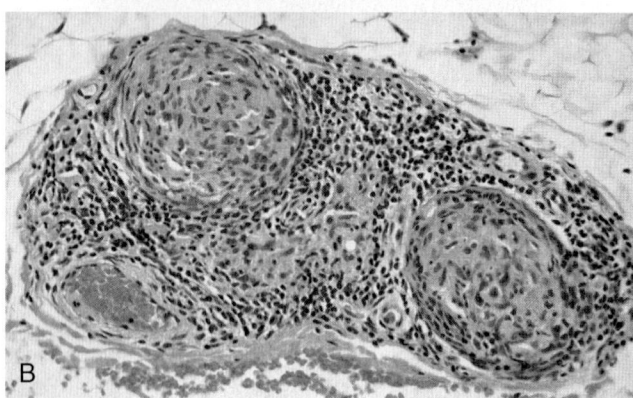

Figure 109–5 **A,** Tuberculoid leprosy with a dense granulomatous infiltration that invades the epidermis. Granulomata contain epithelioid cells, Langhans giant cells, and lymphocytes (hematoxylin and eosin stain). **B,** High magnification of a nerve bundle in the subcutaneous tissue of section in **A.** Granulomata have nearly completely destroyed the nerves. Remnants of nerves contained rare acid-fast bacilli (hematoxylin and eosin stain). (See companion Expert Consult web site for color version.)

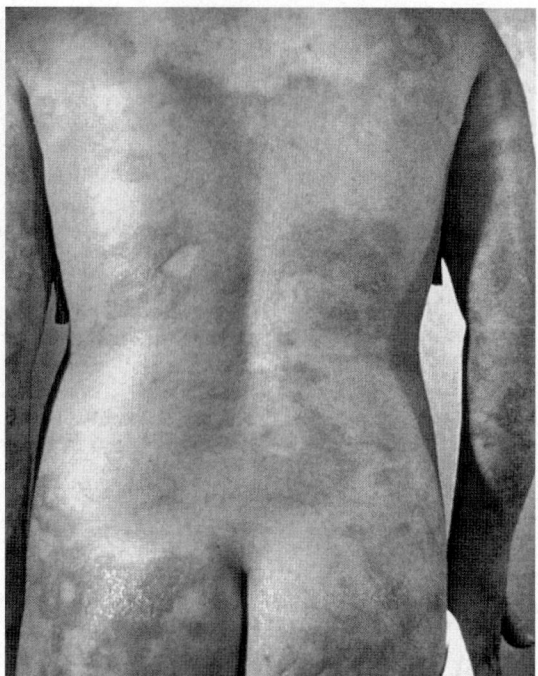

Figure 109–6 Borderline lepromatous leprosy in a Filipino. There are many plaques, some with well-defined borders and others vaguely defined. The erythematous plaques indicate that the patient is undergoing an upgrading reversal reaction (type 1). (See companion Expert Consult web site for color version.)

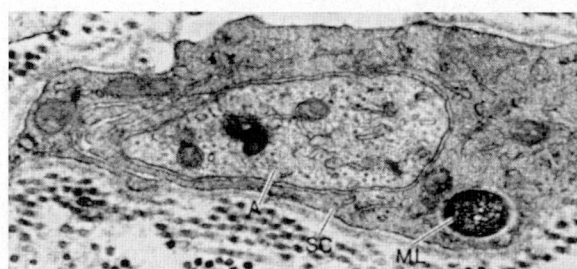

Figure 109–7 Electron micrograph of a portion of a damaged dermal nerve in borderline leprosy. A nonmyelinated axon (A) is surrounded by a Schwann cell (SC) that contains a single *M. leprae* bacillus (ML) (×60,000). *(Courtesy of Dr. S. C. Chang.)*

109–9B); in advanced lesions, dense masses of bacilli termed *globi* may replace nearly the entire cytoplasm of the macrophage. Infiltrating cells do not invade the epidermis but leave a narrow subepidermal clear zone. Many bacilli are found in the dermal nerves and frequently in endothelial cells, walls of blood vessels, arrector pili muscles, and epithelial cells of hair follicles.[215] Plasma cells vary in number and probably reflect B-lymphocyte hyperactivity.[92] Few lymphocytes are in a lepromatous lesion. Large nerve trunks may show typical lepromatous infiltrations.

Occasionally, in patients with lepromatous (LL) leprosy, elevated firm nodules form in the skin, especially in relapsing disease. Because of the characteristic histologic pattern of these lesions, in which the histiocytes resemble fibrocytes, this form is called *histoid leprosy*.[324] LL leprosy is disseminated widely, and lepromatous infiltrations frequently are found in the upper respiratory

tract as far down as the larynx and in the eyes and testes. In adults, the testes sometimes are densely infiltrated, with subsequent development of sterility and gynecomastia, but these complications are rare findings in children. Lymph nodes often are infiltrated by bacilli-laden macrophages, especially in the medulla and paracortical areas.

CLINICAL MANIFESTATIONS

The incubation period varies (usually 2 to 5 years), and no prodromal manifestations are well established. Some experienced clinicians working in areas of high prevalence recognize early signs of nerve involvement (localized paresthesia, itching, or numbness) before any visible lesions develop.

After the incubation period, various lesions appear. The nature of the lesions depends on the immune response of the patient to *M. leprae*. So far, no strain variations of the bacillus except in drug sensitivity have been detected.[342,343] Most clinicians

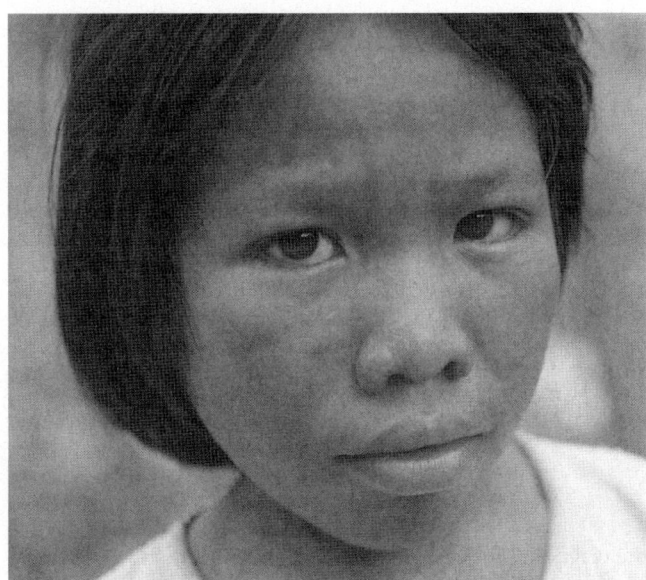

Figure 109–8 Advanced lepromatous leprosy in an adolescent Filipino. Skin of most of the face, especially the alae nasi, is diffusely thickened. Eyebrows are thinned. (See companion Expert Consult web site for color version.)

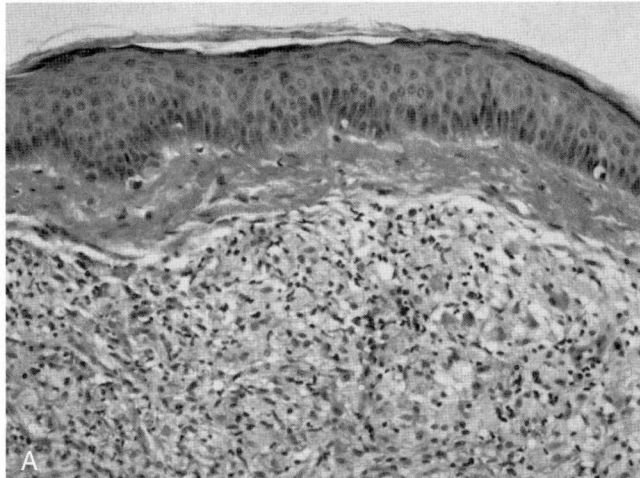

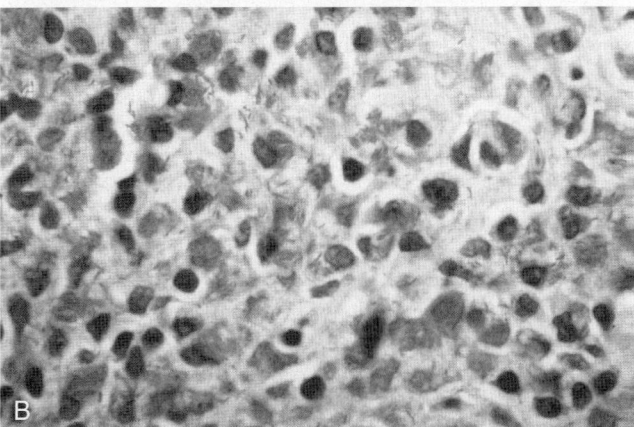

Figure 109–9 A, Advanced lepromatous leprosy showing replacement of dermis by foamy histiocytes and very few lymphocytes. Note thin subepidermal clear zone (hematoxylin and eosin stain). **B,** Higher magnification of same biopsy specimen showing clumps of *M. leprae* (globi) in histiocytes in a leproma in the skin (Fite-Faraco stain). (See companion Expert Consult web site for color version.)

today follow the classification scheme outlined by Ridley and Jopling (see Table 109–1).[253] Classification is important because it aids in establishing the prognosis and treatment program for the patient.

Virtually all patients with leprosy have peripheral neuropathy if cutaneous sensory changes are included, and approximately 25 percent have significant deformity. In experimental studies, the pathogenesis of peripheral neuritis in leprosy involves bacillation of the endothelial cells of epineural and perineural blood vessels and lymphatics.[272,273,275] Surface proteins of *M. leprae* may bind the bacillus to Schwann cells via lamimin.[243,283] Detailed discussions of peripheral neuropathy in leprosy can be found elsewhere.[265]

Ocular complications in leprosy are well known.[51,56,57,120] All patients with leprosy should be evaluated by an ophthalmologist at diagnosis and periodically thereafter, especially during any reactional episodes.

INDETERMINATE LEPROSY

An indeterminate lesion is the first manifestation of leprosy in most patients and may heal spontaneously, remain unchanged for months or years, or gradually progress toward TT or LL disease. Patients with indeterminate leprosy have a single or a few macules in the skin (see Fig. 109–2). The macule is defined poorly and is mildly hypopigmented in deeper pigmented skin and slightly erythematous in lighter skin. Skin texture, sensation, and sweating within early macules are normal or only slightly altered. Peripheral nerves are normal, and skin smears from lesions rarely contain bacilli. The definitive diagnosis can be made only by finding AFB in histopathologic sections.

TUBERCULOID LEPROSY

Patients with TT leprosy have a single or several asymmetrically distributed hypopigmented skin lesions (see Fig. 109–4). Tuberculoid lesions arise de novo or evolve from indeterminate macules. The lesion may be macular or infiltrated, but the borders always are sharply demarcated from the surrounding normal skin and frequently are finely papulated. Lesions range in size from less than 1 cm to large enough to cover entire regions such as the thigh or buttock. Many TT lesions heal spontaneously. In large, active lesions, the centers often are healed and repigmented, although somewhat atrophic.

In TT lesions, sensory loss with impaired sweating and eventual loss of hair occurs. On the face, because of its rich innervation, the detection of hypoesthesia in early lesions requires discriminating tests. Conversely, clinicians may mistakenly diagnose leprosy in areas of the body that normally are hypoesthetic (e.g., over the elbows or knees).

Involvement of peripheral nerves commonly occurs in TT leprosy (Fig. 109–10), and cutaneous nerves often can be palpated adjacent to or within lesions. The regional nerve trunks most commonly enlarged are the ulnar from the olecranon groove to midarm, lateral popliteal just distal to the head of the fibula, and posterior tibial in the medial aspect of the ankle. Enlarged or tender nerves anywhere should alert the clinician to the possibility of leprosy. Any readily palpable cutaneous nerve probably is enlarged, but evaluating the size of nerve trunks requires experience because of the wide range in normal size.

BORDERLINE LEPROSY

Borderline leprosy, sometimes called *dimorphous* or *intermediate leprosy*, has features of the LL and the TT forms and

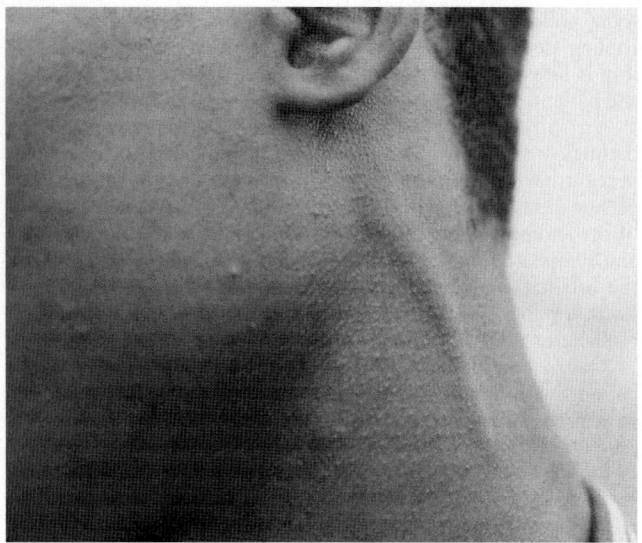

Figure 109–10 Enlargement of the great auricular nerve in an adolescent Congolese boy. A large macule of tuberculoid leprosy over the angle of the mandible is now nearly inactive and barely visible. (See companion Expert Consult web site for color version.)

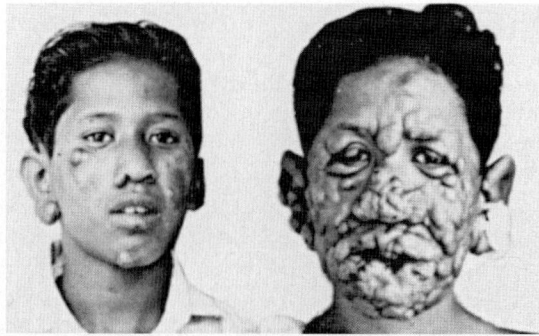

Figure 109–11 Progression of lepromatous leprosy in a Hawaiian boy. The photograph on the *left* was taken in 1931, when the patient was 13 years old, and the photograph on the *right* was taken 2 years later. No effective chemotherapy was available in that era.

represents a continuous spectrum of disease ranging from near-tuberculoid to near-lepromatous. It is an unstable form of leprosy and may evolve gradually toward TT leprosy by undergoing reversal reactions or be downgraded toward LL leprosy. Table 109–1 describes the three major subgroups of borderline leprosy: borderline-tuberculoid (BT), borderline (BB), and borderline-lepromatous (BL).

In BT leprosy, the number of lesions usually is greater than in TT leprosy, and the borders of each lesion, macule, or plaque are defined less sharply than in TT leprosy. Small satellite lesions may develop around larger macules or plaques. BL leprosy often manifests with widespread nodular infiltrations or plaques of varying size (see Fig. 109–6).

Damage to nerves and the resulting deformity develop early and often are widespread. Pain in nerves or neurotropic changes (e.g., sensory changes that lead to damaged hands or feet or a muscular weakness such as footdrop) frequently bring the patient to the physician. Severe damage to nerves occurs infrequently in young children, but can be disastrous. Prevention of this complication is an important goal of leprosy detection programs and of treatment of every patient with leprosy.

LEPROMATOUS LEPROSY

In LL leprosy, the bacilli multiply freely, and the disease disseminates widely, often before striking cutaneous manifestations develop, in contrast to the strict localization of lesions in TT leprosy. LL leprosy may evolve from indeterminate or BB leprosy or may be the first recognizable form. In its earliest form, LL leprosy manifests as "juvenile leprosy," a clinical entity delineated from observations of large numbers of children in homes for children of patients with leprosy in India.[214] This form, also called *pre-lepromatous leprosy*, is difficult to detect and frequently goes unrecognized until a more advanced stage develops. Skin texture may be altered slightly, but the vague macules with indistinct borders are detected only under appropriate lighting, preferably daylight. No changes in sensation or sweating occur in the macules, and frequently AFB are not detectable in smears from skin. Histopathologic sections may reveal a few bacilli to confirm

the diagnosis; however, if leprosy is suspected, the patient should be monitored until an explanation for the mild skin changes is found. If leprosy is present and not detected and treated, advanced forms of LL leprosy develop in many of these patients (Fig. 109–11).

The hypopigmented or slightly erythematous macules of early LL leprosy, similar to those of juvenile leprosy, are missed easily because they are vague and have slight, if any, sensory changes. These macules usually are small but gradually may coalesce and cover large areas of skin, even nearly the entire body. Clinical diagnosis often is missed, and over the course of a few years, advanced LL leprosy develops. If skin smears or biopsy specimens are taken in the macular stage, diagnosis is virtually ensured. If the disease is not diagnosed and treated in the macular stage, infiltration of the skin increases gradually, and nodules may develop. The skin is infiltrated most heavily in the cooler portions of the body, notably the ears (pinnae) and face. By this time, nerves usually are enlarged, with early signs of sensory loss in the hands and feet. Eyebrows are thinned and eventually lost, beginning at the lateral edges. These advanced changes of LL leprosy are not common findings in young children but are well known.

Patients of Latin American ancestry, especially patients from Mexico and Costa Rica, may contract the highly anergic diffuse form of LL leprosy called *Lucio leprosy*. The disease may be so diffuse that it is not recognized until sensory changes appear in the hands and feet, and the eyebrows and other body hair begin to disappear. In advanced forms of Lucio leprosy, a marked obstructive vasculitis in the skin is present, with the production of dermal infarcts and irregular ulcers (Lucio phenomenon).[163,247] Lucio leprosy has been reported in children 7 years old.[270]

NEURITIC LEPROSY

Rarely, leprosy involves one or more major nerve trunks unaccompanied by cutaneous lesions. These patients have anesthesia, paresis, or wasting of muscles in the affected area. Nerve trunks frequently are painful, enlarged, and tender. Leprosy must be suspected in patients with any peripheral neuritis that has these features. Chronic neuritis with pain and enlargement and tenderness of peripheral nerves often persists for years after the patient has completed chemotherapy for leprosy.[119] Large leprotic nerve abscesses are rare occurrences but are exquisitely painful and may require surgical intervention for drainage.[278] Most clinicians prefer to treat such lesions with corticosteroids.

REACTIONS

The course of leprosy, treated or nontreated, often is interrupted by acute episodes known as reactions, which fall into two general categories: reversal reactions (or type 1) and erythema nodosum leprosum (ENL) (or type 2).

REVERSAL REACTIONS

Reversal reactions complicate borderline leprosy and represent delayed hypersensitivity reactions, with an upgrading of CMI toward TT leprosy. Lesions become erythematous and edematous, and neuritis is a common manifestation (Fig. 109–12). Patients who are lepromin-positive and have IgM antibodies to PGL-1 are most at risk for having reversal reactions.[254] Proliferation of sensitized T lymphocytes initiates reversal reactions, releasing lymphokines that amplify the inflammatory response, calling in and activating macrophages.[259] Immunohistopathologic evidence has shown that effective chemotherapy for paucibacillary and multibacillary patients may activate CMI and provoke clinical or subclinical reversal reactions. Expression of HLA-DR is increased, which may enhance production of IFN-γ by lymphocytes in granulomata.[53] Histopathologically, edema is accompanied by an increase in the number of lymphocytes, often with epithelioid cells and giant cells. In severe reactions, necrosis may occur, almost always in nerves. Increased levels of TNF-α may partially explain this necrosis.[20] Cyclooxygenase-2 levels are elevated in nerves and blood vessels during reversal reactions, a finding that explains why nonsteroidal anti-inflammatory drugs, including selective cyclooxygenase-2 inhibitors, often improve the condition.[231]

Patients experiencing such reactions must be observed closely so that sensory loss and deformities are minimized. By repeated reversal reactions, borderline leprosy, even cases close to LL disease, may be upgraded gradually to TT leprosy, often with disastrous peripheral neuropathy.

Differentiating reversal reactions from relapsing lesions frequently is difficult and requires careful correlation of clinical and histopathologic findings. This correlation is becoming increasingly important in endemic areas, where shorter term chemotherapeutic regimens of fixed duration are used.[90,188] The following criteria for differentiating relapses and reversal reactions are suggested: A relapse involves an increased number of lesions, positive skin smears for AFB (for patients with BB and BL leprosy), tissue reaction inconsistent with a reversal reaction, and a favorable response to chemotherapy; a reversal reaction involves an exacerbation of existing lesions, skin smears negative for AFB, tissue reaction consistent with a reversal reaction, and a rapid response to anti-inflammatory drugs.

ERYTHEMA NODOSUM LEPROSUM

Formerly, ENL developed in approximately 50 percent of LL patients after they had undergone a few months of chemotherapy; however, with the addition of clofazimine to the standard therapeutic regimen, frequency of ENL is much reduced.[82] Tender erythematous subcutaneous nodules develop rapidly (Fig. 109–13); the nodules often are accompanied by fever and occasionally by synovitis and iridocyclitis.[234] ENL resembles the Arthus reaction and is thought to result from immune complex formation.[96] Immune complexes may form within lesions by the local release of antigens of *M. leprae* and could modulate the development of T-cell populations in situ. Numbers of helper T lymphocytes are increased in lesions of ENL.[206] Serum TNF-α is elevated in ENL.[20,269]

In the nodule, neutrophils and sometimes an intense vasculitis are present. Ulceration of the skin frequently accompanies severe ENL. Glomerulonephritis sometimes complicates ENL; secondary amyloidosis is a late sequela of repeated reactions and may be a consequence of the neutrophilic leukocytosis.[177] Although neutrophilic infiltration is considered by many physicians to be the hallmark of the tissue reaction, tissue from a rare patient with clinically typical ENL may not show neutrophils. In such patients,

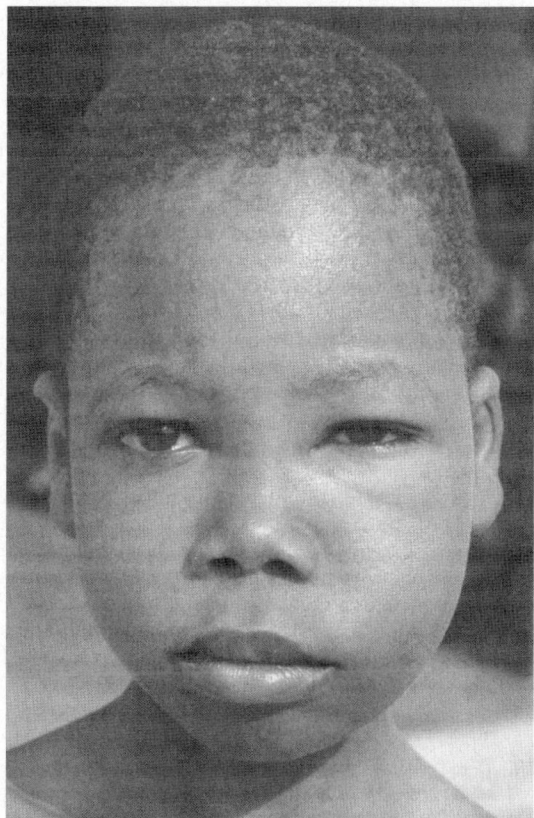

Figure 109–12 Reversal reaction (type 1) in an 8-year-old Congolese boy with borderline-tuberculoid leprosy. The left side of his face is swollen and displays mild palsy from facial nerve damage. The patient responded rapidly to oral steroid therapy. (See companion Expert Consult web site for color version.)

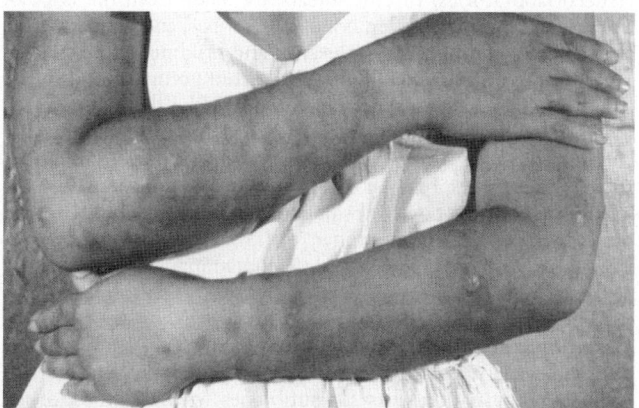

Figure 109–13 Erythema nodosum leprosum in a Filipino adolescent girl with lepromatous leprosy. (See companion Expert Consult web site for color version.)

demonstration of serum amyloid A and C-reactive protein may aid in establishing the diagnosis of ENL.[124] Occasional patients may have mixed reversal (upgrading) reactions and ENL. These patients usually have leprosy in the BL area of the spectrum.

DIAGNOSIS AND DIFFERENTIAL DIAGNOSIS

The cardinal signs of leprosy are hypoesthetic lesions of the skin, enlarged peripheral nerve or nerves, and AFB in skin smears. In the absence of another clear explanation, any one of these signs strongly suggests leprosy.

An experienced observer can establish a clinical diagnosis in most patients, except those with early leprosy, with a high degree of accuracy. Because leprosy is considered one of the "great imitators,"[329] however, histopathologic evaluation is strongly recommended to supplement and confirm the clinical diagnosis.

Patients with leprosy may be found in almost any geographic area, an awareness of which would minimize missed and delayed diagnoses, especially in areas of low prevalence. In the United States, the usual delay in establishing the diagnosis after the patient's first visit to a physician for symptoms related to leprosy is approximately 1.5 to 2 years. This delay often significantly worsens the prognosis.

History is important. Contact with patients with leprosy or residence in an endemic area raises suspicion of leprosy in a patient with a chronic lesion of the skin. Sensory loss or unexplained damage to hands or feet suggests damage to nerve trunks. Sometimes, a footdrop or clawhand brings the patient to a physician. Occasionally, patients with LL leprosy consult an otolaryngologist first because of a chronic stuffy nose.

Clinicians must evaluate sensory changes in a lesion by using the precautions already mentioned. The modalities usually tested are light touch with the use of a few fibers of cotton or calibrated nylon threads and heat-cold discrimination with the use of warm and cold water in test tubes. Much patience and repeated testing often are necessary in evaluating young children. Spontaneous sweating can be observed directly, or induced sweating can be evaluated. Hair may be completely preserved in early lesions but lost in advanced lesions.

The main nerve trunks must be palpated for tenderness and enlargement. Skin in the area of discrete lesions also must be palpated gently to detect enlargement of cutaneous nerves. In the world population, leprosy is the most common cause of peripheral neuropathy and must be considered in any patient with peripheral neuropathy.[265]

Obtaining and examining smears for AFB is an important diagnostic procedure and should be controlled carefully by experienced laboratories. Briefly, smears are made from the edge of discrete macules or plaques, nodules, ear lobes, and nasal mucosa. Skin smears are made by squeezing and holding a fold of skin between the thumb and forefinger to avoid getting blood in the smear and by making a short, shallow slit in the skin with a razor blade or scalpel. The instrument is turned at a right angle to the slit, and the edges of the incision are scraped. The cells and fluid thus obtained are spread on a slide, heat-fixed, and stained by the Ziehl-Neelsen method.[319] Evaluation of smears should not be done by researchers unfamiliar with their interpretation. An occasional AFB may be a harmless contaminant in the staining reagents.

The lepromin reaction is useless for the diagnosis of leprosy. Currently available skin tests with soluble *M. leprae* antigens are unreliable.[113] Enzyme-linked immunosorbent assays and gelatin particle agglutination tests for antibodies to the PGL-1 of *M. leprae* are available.[38,106,128] Although specificity for *M. leprae* is high, these tests detect antibodies to PGL-1 in only approximately 50 percent of paucibacillary patients. Other serologic tests for antibodies to *M. leprae*–specific epitopes on protein moieties

of the bacillus are being evaluated.[229] PGL-1 antigen is detectable in the serum and urine of most multibacillary patients.[223,357]

Reliance on DNA probes and PCR technology may prove useful in establishing the diagnosis of leprosy in tissue sections, skin smears, and nasal smears.[66,301,342,344] Because these methods can detect a single leprosy bacillus, interpreting results, particularly in highly endemic areas, is difficult. Careful clinicopathologic correlation is essential when basing a diagnosis on DNA findings.[315]

The differential diagnosis of leprosy in children is an extensive subject and can be discussed only briefly here. Superficial mycoses and postinflammatory changes commonly are confused with early leprosy. Changes in pigmentation may be caused by scars, birthmarks, and actinic dermatitis. In areas where dermal filariasis is endemic, vague macules in a black-skinned patient may appear identical to the early macules of leprosy.[29,179,190] Among the many infiltrated lesions of the skin that can resemble leprosy are leishmaniasis, lymphoma, granuloma annulare, granuloma multiforme (Mkar disease), lupus erythematosus, psoriasis, pityriasis rosea, sarcoidosis, and neurofibromatosis. Peripheral neuropathies that may simulate leprosy are those seen in Morvan syndrome, syringomyelia, lead intoxication, diabetes mellitus, primary amyloidosis of nerves, and familial hypertrophic neuropathy. Cardiolipin antibody assays of sera from patients with advanced LL leprosy frequently give false-positive reactions for syphilis.

PROGNOSIS

Without chemotherapy, the prognosis in all patients except those with limited and self-healing disease potentially is poor. Patients with borderline or advanced TT leprosy frequently become mutilated because of damage to nerves. Borderline patients can downgrade toward LL leprosy. In patients with LL leprosy, the disease is progressive and can cause death from laryngeal obstruction. Secondary amyloidosis is a frequent late sequela. Blindness may result from lagophthalmic keratitis or repeated episodes of iridocyclitis. General debility and deformity eventually prevent gainful employment in many patients.

With adequate specific chemotherapy and control of reactions, the prognosis is good in nearly all patients. If therapy is started early, the prognosis usually is excellent, and deformity and mutilation are prevented. Even after receiving successful chemotherapy, however, some patients continue to experience significant neuritis and loss of peripheral nerve function. Sometimes this "silent neuropathy" goes unnoticed by the patient and the physician.[59,338] Appropriate early attention to anesthetic hands and feet and restoration of function by reconstructive surgery can prevent most mutilation.

The lepromin test is a valuable prognostic tool because it measures the CMI potential of the host to acquisition of infection by *M. leprae*.[135] Patients with early macular lesions who are lepromin-negative have a poorer prognosis than patients who are lepromin-positive if treatment cannot be administered. Histopathologic evaluation made before instituting chemotherapy is important for determining the prognosis and, if available, should not be neglected.

TREATMENT

When a diagnosis of leprosy is established, chemotherapy must be initiated, and appropriate measures must be instituted for preventing or correcting deformity in patients with neurotropic changes.[40,91,161] The three chemotherapeutic agents most commonly used are dapsone, clofazimine, and rifampin.[212] Although WHO recommends only clinical findings for assessment of the therapeutic response in field programs, clinicians may wish to use additional evaluations. The effectiveness of chemotherapy is assessed readily in patients with LL or near-LL leprosy by the staining quality of *M. leprae* in skin smears. The response to chemotherapy in TT patients and most borderline patients is determined by the clinical response and by histopathologic evaluation. Viability of *M. leprae* in tissues is assessed in unusual cases in the mouse footpad.

Combined chemotherapy is being accepted increasingly for all forms of active leprosy. Although experimental data are limited,[281] the growing body of clinical data indicates that multidrug therapy has replaced monotherapy.[67,164] Monotherapy with any chemotherapeutic agent no longer is advised. The regimens recommended currently for multidrug therapy are given later, after a brief discussion of the most used individual drugs.

DAPSONE

In 1941, Faget and associates[81] at Carville, Louisiana, introduced the sulfones as the first chemotherapeutic agents regularly effective for leprosy and revolutionized the care of leprosy patients. The sulfone in common use is diaminodiphenylsulfone, or dapsone, available in the United States as Avlosulfon and Dapsone. Dapsone is an antimetabolite for *M. leprae* and is a bacteriostatic agent. The drug usually is given orally at 6 to 10 mg/kg body weight per week, divided into equal daily doses. The effect of dapsone on the bacilli is slow; 3 to 6 months of treatment is necessary to render bacilli from patients with LL leprosy noninfectious for the mouse footpad. Sulfone-resistant strains of *M. leprae* are being detected with increasing frequency,[337,338] and monotherapy with dapsone is not recommended. Dapsone usually is well tolerated but may provoke one or more of the following side reactions: dermatitis, anemia, hepatitis, or psychosis.[5]

CLOFAZIMINE

Clofazimine (Lamprene) is a bacteriostatic riminophenazine dye that has anti–*M. leprae* and anti-inflammatory activities, which render it a useful drug for the treatment of patients who are prone to having ENL reactions.[82] The mechanism of bacteriostasis may involve enhancement of oxygen-dependent killing of *M. leprae* and binding to bacterial DNA. The adult dose of clofazimine ranges from 50 to 300 mg daily, and some authorities recommend 1 mg/kg/day for children. The lower dosages are used for maintenance therapy when a good clinical response has been achieved, and the higher dosages may be needed to control ENL. The major side reactions to clofazimine are hyperpigmentation of skin and enteritis. Enteritis is experienced only at the higher dosages generally used for ENL. The hyperpigmentation subsides with the clinical improvement in leprosy, and hyperpigmentation and enteritis resolve after drug withdrawal. Although two instances of clofazimine-resistant *M. leprae* infection have been reported, the validity of these observations is uncertain.[148,336] For some time, clofazimine has been considered safe in pregnancy, but one report described three neonatal deaths in 15 observed pregnancies.[83] Whether the drug was associated with the deaths was not established. Monotherapy with clofazimine is not recommended.

RIFAMPIN

Rifampin is an antibiotic that inhibits bacterial DNA-dependent RNA polymerase and is rapidly bactericidal for *M. leprae*. A single large dose can render a highly positive LL patient noninfectious within 1 week. Dosages of 15 to 20 mg/kg/day have been given to children (maximal dose 600 mg/day). Optimal doses for chil-

dren with leprosy have not been reported. Adult doses range from 300 to 600 mg daily.[347] Many side reactions to rifampin have been described, and the relevant literature must be consulted.[32] Rifampin-resistant leprosy has been reported,[130,345] so monotherapy with rifampin is not recommended.

MULTIDRUG THERAPY

Because of the existence of drug-resistant *M. leprae*, combined drug regimens are mandatory for the treatment of all forms of leprosy.[77,281,337,338] The first large-scale multidrug therapy for leprosy was initiated in Malta in 1972. Rifampin, dapsone, prothionamide, and isoniazid were used. Evaluation of the patients approximately 20 years later revealed a single relapse; however, presumed "persisting" *M. leprae* organisms were detected.[93,141]

Combined drug therapy minimizes development of drug-resistant strains of *M. leprae* and may eliminate some "persisting" organisms. Persisting *M. leprae* are viable bacilli that can be isolated in small numbers from patients who are clinically responding well to therapy. These persisting *M. leprae* bacilli are sensitive to the drug in question when tested in the mouse footpad and may account for relapses when treatment is discontinued. Persisting *M. leprae* organisms have been detected after 5 years of therapy with rifampin, 6 years of clofazimine therapy, and 22 years of dapsone therapy.

In 1982, a WHO study group recommended the multidrug therapy regimens that are described hereafter.[348] Patients were divided into paucibacillary and multibacillary groups. Paucibacillary patients (usually indeterminate, TT, and BT) were defined originally as patients with negative skin smears at all sites or patients who have fewer than four lesions and no clinical peripheral neuritis. Subsequently, for field programs, paucibacillary patients are classified only as patients who have fewer than four lesions, without reference to skin smear evaluation. All other patients are multibacillary.

The multidrug therapy regimens were designed primarily for field programs, and they use pulsed supervised monthly rather than daily rifampin.[18] Multidrug therapy is well tolerated, and compliance in large-scale control programs has been satisfactory. The efficacy of multidrug therapy has been promising.[36,338] In two surveys involving approximately 112,000 multibacillary patients monitored for 9 years after receiving therapy, the cumulative risk of relapse was 0.77 percent. Anecdotal descriptions of certain groups of highly bacilliferous patients with relapse rates of 20 percent and recurrences developing 5 years or more after therapy have been reported.[132] These and other results suggest that therapeutic regimens for multibacillary patients should be given for longer than 2 years.

In most reports, relapse rates in paucibacillary patients exceed those in multibacillary patients. In our experience in evaluating histopathologic specimens, many patients classified clinically as paucibacillary were multibacillary. The potential for relapse after receiving multidrug therapy regimens must await long-term, large-scale follow-up results.[36,131] Peripheral neuropathy sometimes persists after completion of these therapeutic regimens.[4,119]

The trend since 2001 has been to reduce the duration of treatment and change the therapeutic regimens—even to the extreme of a single-dose regimen composed of rifampin, ofloxacin, and minocycline for single-lesion therapy. Many of these innovations are interwoven into WHO Elimination of Leprosy Program and have provoked critical concern by some authorities.[87,168,218,291]

Regimen for Paucibacillary Patients (Indeterminate, Tuberculoid, and Borderline-Tuberculoid)

In adults, rifampin, 600 mg once a month, plus dapsone, 100 mg daily, is given for 6 months, and treatment then is stopped. After the conclusion of multidrug therapy, the patient should be seen every 3 to 6 months. All apparent relapses require histopathologic examination for establishing whether the lesions represent relapses or reversal reactions. Relapsing patients must be treated again. The aforementioned multidrug therapy is not used alone in patients with concurrent tuberculosis.

Regimen for Multibacillary Patients (Lepromatous, Borderline-Lepromatous, and Borderline)

In adults, rifampin, 600 mg monthly; dapsone, 100 mg daily; and clofazimine, 50 mg daily, are given. If patient compliance is questionable, the rifampin and 300 mg of clofazimine should be given monthly under supervision, in addition to the 50 mg daily. These drugs must be given for 2 years. For patients in whom the hyperpigmentation caused by clofazimine is unacceptable, daily doses of 250 to 375 mg of prothionamide or ethionamide may be substituted for clofazimine. Another alternative therapy suggested by WHO for patients unwilling to accept the hyperpigmentation of clofazimine or who are noncompliant with other regimens consists of rifampin, 600 mg; ofloxacin, 400 mg; and minocycline, 100 mg, coined "ROM," all of which are administered on a single day, once monthly, for at least 2 years.[321]

Dosages of Multidrug Therapy for Children

Pediatric dosages of multidrug therapy are given in Table 109–2.[140]

Recommendations for the United States

The National Hansen's Disease Programs, Baton Rouge, Louisiana, recommends the following variations of WHO's recommended multidrug therapy regimens for adult patients in the United States:

- Paucibacillary disease: dapsone, 100 mg daily, plus rifampin, 600 mg daily, for 1 year.
- Multibacillary disease: dapsone, 100 mg daily, plus rifampin, 600 mg daily, and clofazimine, 50 mg daily, for 2 years. Minocycline, 100 mg daily, is substituted for clofazimine in patients who refuse to take clofazimine.
- Because the National Hansen's Disease Programs may change their recommendation for patient management, we advise clinicians in the United States to consult it before treating any patient with leprosy (telephone, 1-800-642-2477 or 1-225-756-3709, or e-mail, Mtemplet@hrsa.gov; it also has a website available at www.bphc.hrsa.gov/nhdp/).

OTHER DRUGS UNDER INVESTIGATION

Other potential antileprosy drugs that are undergoing advanced clinical evaluation and may gain general use include fluoroquinolones (pefloxacin and ofloxacin), the macrolide clarithromycin, and the tetracycline minocycline.[97,99,110,134]

TABLE 109–2 Dosage of Multidrug Therapy for Children with Leprosy

Weight (kg)	Percentage of Adult Dose
<15	25
15-30	50
30-45	75
>45	100

From Jopling, W. H.: Handbook of Leprosy. London, William Heinemann, 1984.

TREATMENT OF REACTIONS

Patients experiencing a reaction should be observed daily in the early stages and hospitalized if the symptoms are severe. Formerly, specific therapy was stopped or the dosage reduced during reactions, but these measures no longer are recommended.[348] Damage to eyes and neurotropic changes may ensue rapidly without immediate attention. Nerve tenderness and function must be assessed frequently during reactions. Acute inflammation of isolated lesions without damage to nerves is likely to be of little consequence except for cosmetic considerations, but the patient should be monitored closely.

Reversal (Type 1) Reaction

Patients with painful, tender nerves must receive immediate care, usually in the hospital. Analgesics are given, and the affected area is rested. Large daily doses of corticosteroids are started and tapered to a minimal effective dose until the reaction subsides. Conversion to alternate-day steroid regimens may be attempted when long-term treatment is necessary. Some clinicians use clofazimine for chronic reversal reactions, but it is not recommended for the initial treatment of reactions with acute neuritis. For reactions, clofazimine probably is consistently efficacious only for ENL.[126]

Erythema Nodosum Leprosum (Type 2) Reaction

Mild ENL is treated with analgesics; more severe ENL is treated with thalidomide or corticosteroids.[322] Pediatric doses of thalidomide in ENL have not been established, but the initial adult dose is 100 mg four times daily followed by a minimal effective dose, usually 100 mg daily. The teratogenic action of thalidomide demands that appropriate measures be taken in the treatment of fertile women. For the rare patient who does not respond to thalidomide or in fertile women, corticosteroids or clofazimine is used. Corticosteroids, if used, are administered in the usual dosage schedules, beginning with large doses and tapering to a minimal effective level. Some clinicians use an alternate-day regimen when long-term steroid therapy is necessary, minimizing the well-known side effects. A few studies suggest that pentoxifylline or pentoxifylline plus clofazimine is effective for ENL.[220,302,340]

Clofazimine is effective in most patients with ENL and does not have the disadvantages of thalidomide or corticosteroids. The anti-inflammatory action of clofazimine is not manifested until after 4 to 6 weeks of continuous use. The dosage must be adjusted to the minimal effective level.

Iridocyclitis requires emergency measures. Local corticosteroids must be added to systemic anti-inflammatory regimens. Ophthalmologic consultation should be obtained.

PREVENTION

Precise recommendations for the prevention of leprosy in individuals have not been formulated. Control programs today are based on the general principles that (1) the number of contagious patients is reduced by chemotherapy and (2) the surveillance of contacts detects early leprosy. To accomplish these goals, appropriate education of the public and medical personnel and population surveys in areas of higher prevalence must be implemented. In endemic areas, improved housing probably is a highly important preventive measure by reducing close contact of patients with healthy individuals.

The most important obstacles to improving control of leprosy include persistence of *M. leprae* in treated patients, the cost and toxicity of antileprotic medications, the long-term nature of therapeutic regimens, patient compliance, and the social stigma of leprosy.[249] For the total eradication of leprosy, zoonotic sources of *M. leprae* must be taken into account.[193]

CHEMOPROPHYLAXIS

Chemoprophylaxis with dapsone for close contacts has limited usefulness, but it is not recommended for large populations.[59] This recommendation is based on the probability that long-term use would be irregular, and dapsone-resistant *M. leprae* may develop.[347] Rifampin prophylaxis may have some value, at least in the short-term,[10] but the risk of increasing the rates of drug-resistant tuberculosis, or even leprosy, must be considered.

VACCINATION, IMMUNOPROPHYLAXIS, AND IMMUNOTHERAPY

WHO initiated an Immunology of Leprosy Program (IMMLEP) in 1974 with two primary goals: (1) development of a vaccine against leprosy and (2) development of reagents for detecting subclinical leprosy. Achievement of both goals could diminish profoundly the incidence of leprosy. *M. leprae*, or specific antigens thereof, for the IMMLEP studies were obtained from experimentally infected armadillos. Vaccines composed of heat-killed whole *M. leprae* alone or in combination with live bacille Calmette-Guérin (BCG) have been found to be safe and to induce delayed-type hypersensitivity to *M. leprae* in a high percentage of lepromin-negative individuals. Several other vaccines based on cultivable mycobacteria (*Mycobacterium vaccae*, *Mycobacterium* "w," and the Indian Cancer Research Centre bacillus) induce similar responses.[19,149,293]

Field trials of these vaccines for the immunoprophylaxis of leprosy have been conducted; however, because of the chronicity and low prevalence of the disease, meaningful evaluation of their efficacy would require extended follow-up observations.[21] Because infection-induced immunity is not observed regularly in leprosy, a reasonable doubt exists that vaccines containing only *M. leprae* would be protective. Combined vaccines of killed *M. leprae* and live BCG have been studied. Such vaccines convert lepromin-negative contacts of patients with leprosy to positive reactors and upgrade LL patients toward the tuberculoid region of the disease spectrum.[45,195] Vaccines based on cell wall fractions of *M. leprae* are being studied.[98] WHO does not recommend BCG vaccination for the prevention of leprosy.[17] This decision was based on the highly variable results of extensive studies in Burma, Papua New Guinea, and Uganda.[348] Another trial in India involving 270,000 individuals confirmed that during a 12.5-year follow-up, BCG vaccination was shown to be only approximately 25 percent effective against leprosy.[304]

Initial evaluations of a large-scale immunoprophylaxis trial of heat-killed *M. leprae* plus BCG vaccine in humans in Venezuela showed no better protection than did BCG alone 5 years after vaccination.[48] A randomized trial of a single BCG vaccination, repeated BCG, or BCG plus killed *M. leprae* involving 121,020 individuals in Malawi gave the following results over a 5- to 9-year follow-up: A single BCG vaccination afforded 50 percent protection against leprosy, a second BCG vaccination added appreciably to this protection, but the addition of killed *M. leprae* to BCG did not enhance protection against leprosy.[150]

LEPROSY AND ACQUIRED IMMUNODEFICIENCY SYNDROME

Because *M. tuberculosis*, *Mycobacterium avium–intracellulare*, and *Mycobacterium kansasii* are frequent opportunistic pathogens in patients with acquired immunodeficiency syndrome (AIDS), observations of AIDS in patients with leprosy are of interest.[312] In one study in Zambia, antibodies to human immunodeficiency virus (HIV) were found in 33 percent of new leprosy patients versus 7 percent of controls.[181] Perhaps the positivity of some of these patients with leprosy can be explained by cross-reactivity between antibodies to HIV-1 and the lipoarabinomannan of *M. leprae*.[151] In other populations in Africa, HIV infection constituted an overall risk factor of 2.2 for leprosy, with 4 to 23 percent of cases of multibacillary leprosy attributable to HIV co-infection.[24]

Other prospective studies show that HIV infection may not be a risk factor for acquisition of leprosy in some populations.[154,276] Only a few detailed clinicopathologic reports on individuals co-infected with *M. leprae* and HIV exist.[133,158,211] In these patients, no consistent deleterious effect of HIV infection on the clinical or pathologic findings of leprosy occurred. These observations are supported by a study of the parameters of CMI in co-infected patients in Brazil.[267] In these patients with borderline leprosy, the quality of the granulomata in the infiltrations of leprosy were not altered significantly despite low CD4+ T-cell counts. The incidence of reversal reactions (type 1) and neuritis is increased in multibacillary patients co-infected with HIV.[34] Perhaps, as previously and perceptively suggested,[169] observations in patients co-infected with HIV and *M. leprae* will lead to some revisions of the immunopathogenesis of leprosy.

BURULI ULCER

Mycobacterium ulcerans causes indolent, necrotizing cutaneous ulcers that are known classically as *Buruli ulcers*.[171,287,316] Other names for these lesions include Bairnsdale or Searles' ulcer in Australia and Kumusi ulcer in Papua New Guinea. Buruli ulcer seems most appropriate, however, because Clancey and colleagues[39] were the first to name the disease, after the site of the first large epidemic, which was located in Buruli County, Uganda.[68] Cook[49] in Uganda described lesions that fit Buruli ulcer in 1897. Today, researchers recognize that many infections with *M. ulcerans* are not manifested as ulcers, and *M. ulcerans* infection is a technically more appropriate name for the disease. A few infections have been acquired by North American or European travelers to endemic countries,[44,78,277] and patients with Buruli ulcers frequently come to European medical centers for treatment.[12,242]

WHO has recognized Buruli ulcer as a re-emerging infectious disease in western Africa with an important public health impact. WHO Global Buruli Ulcer Initiative has held annual meetings to evaluate all aspects of the disease since 1998, and in 2004, the World Health Assembly adopted a resolution for all member states to intensify research to develop tools for diagnosing, treating, and preventing Buruli ulcer.[351]

ORGANISM

MacCallum and associates[172] in 1948 in Australia were the first to isolate the etiologic agent in culture. *M. ulcerans* is strongly acid-fast, with an optimal growth temperature of 30° C to 32° C on routine mycobacteriologic media such as Löwenstein-Jensen medium. *M. ulcerans* is a slow-growing organism, and several months may be required to achieve isolation in primary culture. Microaerophilic conditions promote the growth of *M. ulcerans*, and the organism is strikingly sensitive to temperatures of 37° C or greater.[196,227] This temperature sensitivity often reduces rates of cultivation of the etiologic agent in laboratories remote from endemic areas.

M. ulcerans is the only mycobacterial pathogen of humans known to elaborate a necrotizing and immunosuppressive toxin.[55,233,248] This toxin is a polyketide and has been named *mycolactone*.[100,101] The genomic sequences of the plasmid-encoded synthases that produce mycolactone have been described more recently.[299] Animal studies and immunohistologic evaluations of human lesions indicate that at least one mechanism by which mycolactone mediates tissue destruction is by triggering massive levels of apoptosis.[102,328]

Although mycolactone is viewed as the dominant virulence factor of *M. ulcerans*, other factors may participate (e.g., phospholipases).[105] The phenolic mycosides of *M. ulcerans* and *Mycobacterium marinum* are identical, and sequences for the 16S rRNA gene differ by only one base pair.[54,255]

Specific insertion sequences for *M. ulcerans* have been characterized and are available for identification of the organism by PCR.[1,285,297] Variations in the 3′ end of the 16S rRNA gene sequence are related to geographic origin and are used to divide the organism into African, American, Asian, and Australian strains.[240]

TRANSMISSION AND EPIDEMIOLOGY

Endemic foci of *M. ulcerans* infections usually appear in rural settings near permanent wetlands in warm countries, especially in terrain subject to seasonal flooding. Reports of patients with Buruli ulcers have come from at least 27 countries, principally in the tropics.[335] A few patients live in nontropical climates, such as China,[79] Japan,[308] and southern Australia.[318] Today, the largest numbers of reported patients live in West Africa (Benin, Burkina Faso, Côte d'Ivoire, Ghana, Guinea, Liberia, and Nigeria).[238,316,335] In these countries, the disease is re-emerging rapidly, with an estimated total annual incidence exceeding 7000 patients. Other countries in which the disease is well known to be endemic include Malaysia, Indonesia, Papua New Guinea, Peru, Suriname, French Guiana, Cameroon, Equatorial Guinea, Gabon, Angola, Democratic Republic of Congo, and Uganda.[60,121,188,232]

Observers attribute this re-emergence to environmental factors such as deforestation, artificial topographic alterations (dams and irrigation systems), increasing populations engaged in basic manual agriculture in wetlands, and possibly climactic changes.[198] In North America, two cases of Buruli ulcer were reported in 2005 in central Mexico, the nearest location to the United States to date.[42]

Individuals of all ages are affected, but the highest frequencies are in children 15 years of age or younger—usually approximately 75 percent of all cases.[176] The sexes are affected equally, and a racial predilection is unknown.[61] Anecdotal observations of children in families of multiple parentage have suggested a possible genetic predisposition, now supported by molecular studies.[295] Seasonal variations in incidence occur in some foci.[118,251] Approximately 80 percent of the lesions are on the limbs, with the highest frequencies involving the lower extremities.

Although Buruli ulcer long has been associated with riverine environments, repeated long-term studies (1960 through 2005) on a large variety of flora, fauna, water, and mud samples from many endemic foci failed to reveal *M. ulcerans* in nature by culture.[13,71,235] After the development of molecular biologic techniques for the identification of *M. ulcerans*, the organism was detected in the environment in Australia by PCR.[260,261,296] With the increased understanding of this fastidious organism now available, researchers expected in 2001 that successful culture of *M. ulcerans* from nature would soon be achieved.[238] In 2006, two strains of *M. ulcerans* cultured from nature were reported.[287]

Although the ultimate source of *M. ulcerans* remains obscure, the organism has been discovered in aquatic insects, such as water bugs, firefly larvae, and beetles, obtained from stagnant water in

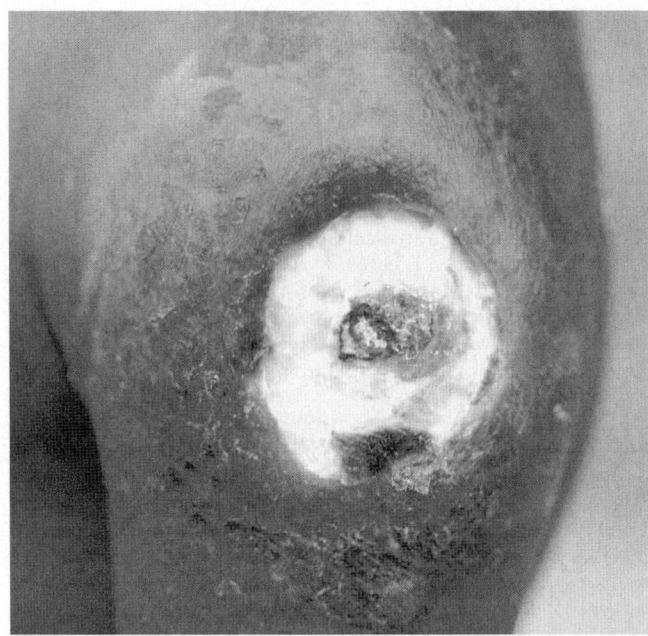

Figure 109–14 A major Buruli ulcer in the deltoid area of a 12-year-old Angolan boy. This pristine ulcer developed 3 months after a documented hypodermic anticholera vaccine injection at this site. Typical Buruli ulcer features are represented—undermining of borders, necrotic base, and induration of the adjacent skin. (See companion Expert Consult web site for color version.)

endemic areas of West Africa.[175,238,239] In some cases, the organisms were found only in the salivary glands of aquatic insects, supporting the notion that insect bites may play a role in transmitting *M. ulcerans*.[173,174]

Some authorities speculate that *M. ulcerans* is a saprophytic or commensal organism that thrives in the mud, flora, or fauna of the cool microaerophilic environment of the bottom of stagnant water, well protected from the lethal ultraviolet radiation that prevails in the tropics. Koalas and possums in Australia acquire infections in the wild that are typical of Buruli ulcer.[203,238]

Buruli ulcer rarely, if ever, is contagious. The distribution of patients, even in highly endemic foci, is random, suggesting that each patient is exposed to environmental sources, such as swamps where villagers work their gardens and obtain water for domestic use and especially where children play.

The mode or modes of transmission to humans have not yet been delineated completely; however, the most plausible route is by trauma at sites of skin recently contaminated by *M. ulcerans*.[71,197] Many patients give a history of specific antecedent penetrating trauma at the site of their initial lesion, which may include wounds from a gunshot or land mine, thrown stones, hypodermic injection, and even a human bite (Fig. 109–14).[64] The organism may be spread by aerosol from the surface of ponds or be carried by fomites or insects to skin surfaces. Insects may introduce *M. ulcerans* into the skin, but this means of transmission has not been proved. Although proposed by some authorities, transmission by nasorespiratory passage with a subsequent bacteremia seems to be unlikely.

PATHOGENESIS AND PATHOLOGY

The pathologic features of early *M. ulcerans* infection are determined primarily by two properties of the etiologic agent: optimal growth at 30° C to 33° C and elaboration of the toxin mycolactone. The temperature requirement tends to favor the development of lesions in the skin, and the toxin destroys tissues and suppresses immune responses. The spectrum of clinical and histopathologic forms of infection suggests that some patients have innate resistance, or resistance develops soon after infection is acquired, whereas others acquire resistance later or, occasionally, never.

A skin test with burulin, a purified sonicate of *M. ulcerans*, reveals that most patients do not have delayed-type hypersensitivity to *M. ulcerans* early in the course of the infection but mount a cellular response as healing begins.[292] Very few studies have investigated the immunology of Buruli ulcer. *M. ulcerans* profoundly suppresses B and T lymphocytes in vitro.[233] Mycolactone, a toxin of *M. ulcerans*, is thought to prevent sensitization of T lymphocytes to mycobacterial antigens and to inhibit production of TNF-γ by monocytes and IL-2 by T lymphocytes.[3,52,100,101,226] In a study of tissue sections of Buruli ulcer lesions, IL-10 was increased in ulcerative lesions without granulomata, whereas IFN-γ was abundant when granulomata were present.[156] These activities partly explain the immunologic unresponsiveness and reduced inflammatory reaction at the site of the lesion.

Based on the current understanding of the natural history of *M. ulcerans* infection, pathogenesis may proceed as follows: After inoculation of the etiologic agent deep into the skin or subcutaneous tissue, a latent phase occurs during which the mycobacterium proliferates slightly, probably initially intracellularly,[224] and begins to elaborate small amounts of toxin that causes necrosis, especially of fatty tissue. This necrosis provides a microaerophilic environment and perhaps nutrients favorable for the accelerated growth of *M. ulcerans* and elaboration of increased amounts of toxin. During this necrotic phase, no significant cellular response occurs.[43,44,68]

In some patients, at this stage, a subcutaneous nodule begins to develop, with clusters of *M. ulcerans* in the center surrounded by a zone of necrosis. In highly resistant patients, this lesion may self-heal, perhaps without ulceration, or form a small, sharply delineated ulcer. In others, the skin is undermined by the necrosis and eventually breaks down into larger ulcers with widely undermined skin. In the least resistant individuals, a nodule never develops, and the necrosis spreads rapidly and widely to cover large body surface areas, but ulceration, if it occurs at all, is a late event.

Eventually, the necrotic stage ceases in most patients, either because the toxin is neutralized or because production is interrupted. At this time, a granulomatous stage begins to develop, followed by healing and scarring. Some of the variability in clinical presentation and progression of the disease may be related to heterogeneity in the *M. ulcerans* genome and in the plasmid that encodes the production of mycolactone.[1,216,298,300]

Microscopically, the active ulcer shows extensive coagulation necrosis of the subcutaneous tissue down to and often including the fascia (Fig. 109–15).[111] The deep layers of necrosis reveal masses of AFB, often with mineralization and extensive vasculitis. Marked edema is present, and fat cells enlarge and die, with only their cellular ghost outlines remaining (Fig. 109–16). The dermis and surrounding tissue seldom contain AFB. Lesions sometimes provoke a reactive (contiguous) osteitis that leads to necrosis of cortical bone and osteomyelitis. Metastatic lesions may develop in the skin and bone from bacteremia and produce skin lesions distant from the original lesion and frequently focal or multifocal osteomyelitis. Regional lymph nodes may show massive necrosis and contain large numbers of AFB, especially in the capsule. Visceral organs are not known to be involved, but no necropsies of patients who died of disseminated disease have been reported.

An understanding of the pathogenesis and developing improved therapies for Buruli ulcer has been slowed by the lack of an experimental animal model that replicates the spectrum of features found in human disease. Laboratory rats and mice

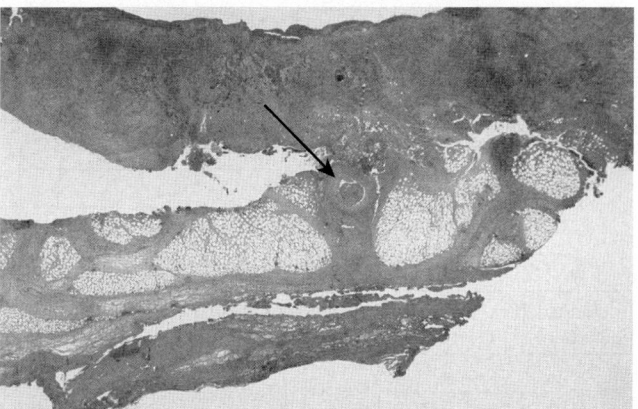

Figure 109–15 Histopathologic section of the undermined edge of a major Buruli ulcer. Note the coagulation necrosis of the entire panniculus and fascia, and vasculitis with thrombosis of a blood vessel (*arrow*) (hematoxylin and eosin stain). (See companion Expert Consult web site for color version.)

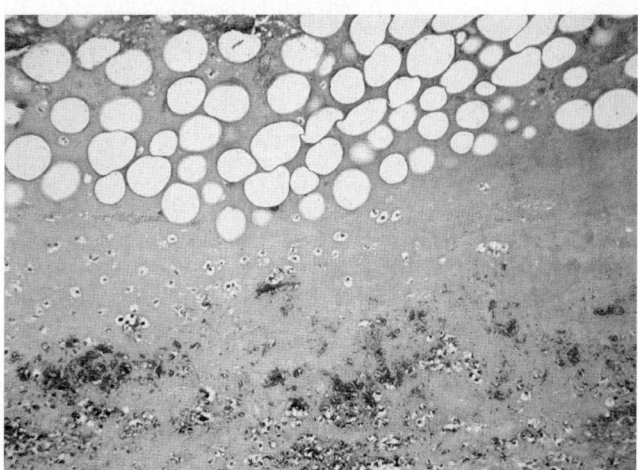

Figure 109–16 High magnification of the necrotic panniculus of a Buruli ulcer showing the dead fat cell "ghosts," coagulation necrosis, and masses of acid-fast bacilli (Ziehl-Neelsen stain). (See companion Expert Consult web site for color version.)

develop skin lesions after intradermal inoculation with *M. ulcerans*, but they lack the extensive ulceration found in human disease. Multimammate rats (*Mastomys natalensis*) rapidly develop systemic infections and die.[286] In the mouse footpad, *M. ulcerans* multiply, but necrosis without ulceration destroys the limb and causes death.[248] Guinea pigs develop inflammatory lesions at the inoculation sites that may resolve without formation of ulcers.[157,248] The nine-banded armadillo is susceptible to *M. ulcerans* and develops cutaneous lesions after experimental intradermal infection, approximating those of the human disease but is phylogenetically distant.[327] The cynomolgus monkey is moderately susceptible to experimental *M. ulcerans* infection and develops some of the clinical and histologic features of Buruli ulcer.[325]

CLINICAL MANIFESTATIONS

INCUBATION AND FORMS OF LESIONS

In one study of specific trauma related to lesions, the incubation period ranged from 2 weeks to 3 years, with a mean of 3 months.[197]

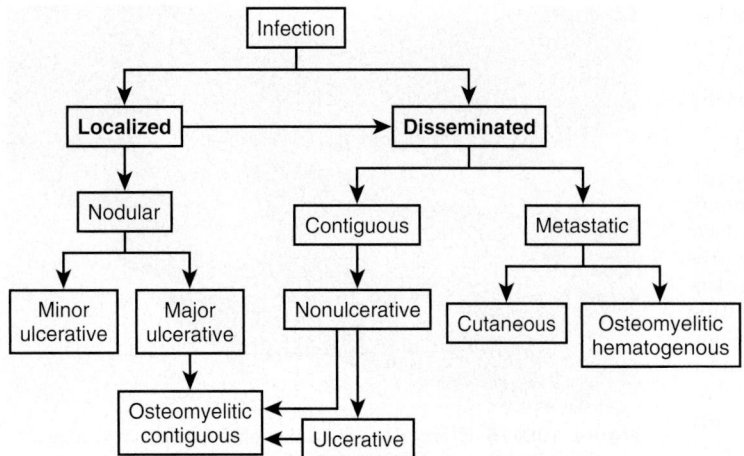

Figure 109–17 Proposed classification of clinical forms of *M. ulcerans* infections, indicating possible progression of lesions after the initial cutaneous infection. Without treatment, lesions may self-heal at any stage, or advance according to the schema shown at left.

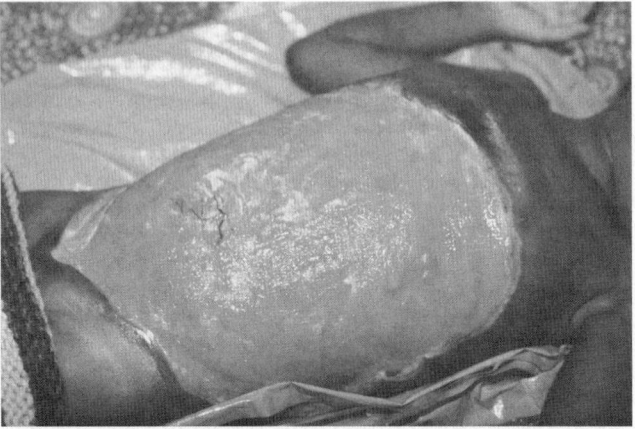

Figure 109–18 Edematous form of *M. ulcerans* infection in a 6-year-old Ghanaian girl after surgery to remove all necrotic tissue. There was never any ulceration. Note ablation of breast tissue. (See companion Expert Consult web site for color version.)

The following are the various forms of lesions of *M. ulcerans* infection according to WHO designations.[353,354] Figure 109–17 presents a proposed classification of the clinical forms of *M. ulcerans* disease and their possible inter-relationships.

Papule

The papular stage has been described only in patients from Australia. These papules are painless and elevated and measure up to 1 cm in diameter.

Nodule

Nodules are primarily subcutaneous and firm, measure approximately 2 cm in diameter, and are painless, although they are often pruritic. The overlying skin may be discolored. This stage is the initial one in most Africans, and in the Kikongo language, the disease is called *mputa matadi* because the nodule is a "rock-hard lesion."

Plaque

Plaques are firm, elevated, painless, well-defined lesions more than 2 cm in largest dimension. Their borders are irregular. This stage often is the one in which physicians initially see the patient, but the lesion may or may not arise from a nodule. The skin over

the lesion is reddened or discolored. These lesions may ulcerate in the late stages.

Edematous Form

Most edematous lesions do not begin in the nodular stage but spread directly from the initial nidus of infection. Spread often is rapid and wide and covers entire limbs or major portions of the trunk (Fig. 109–18). This type of lesion is characterized by diffuse nonpitting swelling and vague margins. Lesions are firm and frequently painful, with changes in color and scaling on the skin surface.

Ulcerative Forms

Classically, when fully developed, pristine ulcers have undermined edges surrounded by a zone of induration and often desquamation of the epidermis (see Fig. 109–14). In the base of the ulcerated area, a whitish necrotic slough and sometimes eschar develop. An oily exudate frequently oozes from the dependent area. Old ulcers tend to begin healing in the uppermost part while activity continues in the dependent portion. Collections of fluid in this area probably continue to support the growth of *M. ulcerans*, which sustains progression of the lesion.

The ulcerative forms are divided into major and minor ulcers. Both forms tend to self-heal. A major ulcer is large and chronic. Minor ulcers are small (1 to 2 cm in diameter), are sharply delineated, and heal early. Both ulcerative forms begin as subcutaneous nodules.

BONE INVOLVEMENT

Contiguous Osteomyelitis

Reactive osteitis occasionally develops beneath destroyed overlying skin and soft tissue. Bone becomes devitalized and necrotic, with the development of sequestra (Fig. 109–19).

Metastatic Osteomyelitis

M. ulcerans–specific osteomyelitis develops in approximately 10 percent of all patients, underscoring that Buruli ulcer should always be considered a potentially systemic disease.[242] Most likely, metastatic osteomyelitis is a result of lymphohematogenous spread of *M. ulcerans* from a distant, earlier cutaneous lesion (Fig. 109–20). The overlying skin ordinarily is intact, but swelling and inflammation occur over the site of bone involvement. If the

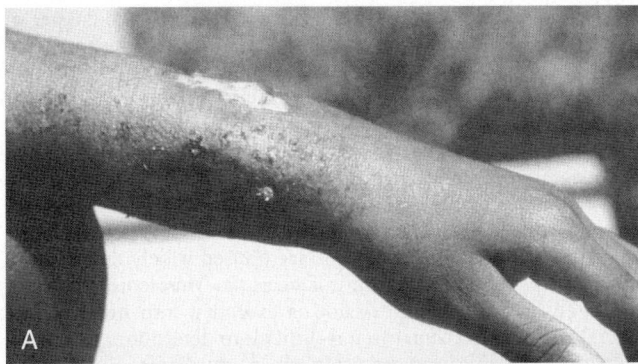

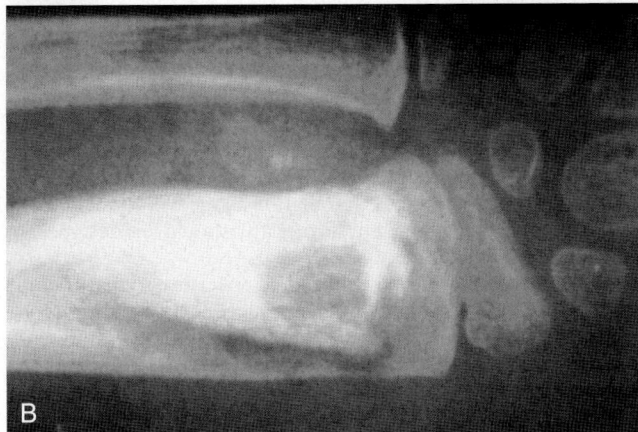

Figure 109–19 A, *M. ulcerans* infection in a young Congolese boy. Note swelling and ulcer on dorsum of forearm. (See companion Expert Consult web site for color version.) **B,** Radiograph of forearm shows reactive osteitis, necrosis of cortex of distal end of the radius, and early sequestration with osteomyelitis.

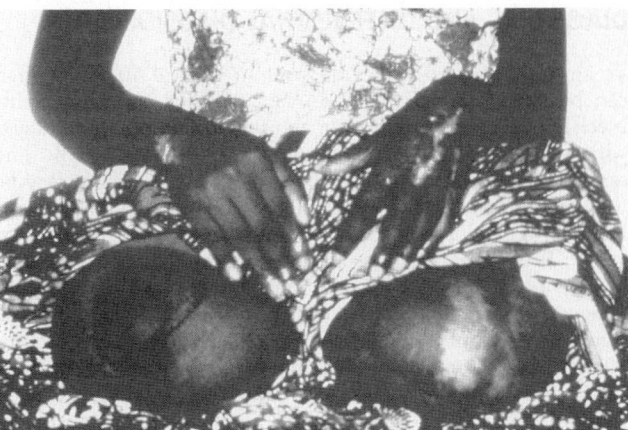

Figure 109–21 This 13-year-old girl in Benin initially had a cutaneous lesion of Buruli ulcer. Subsequently, metastatic spread to bones of the lower extremities occurred, resulting in bilateral high-thigh amputations. Note also the spread to bones of both wrists and left hand. (See companion Expert Consult web site for color version.)

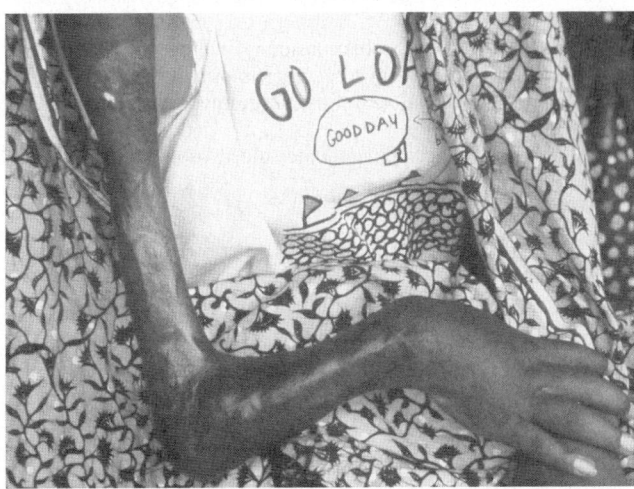

Figure 109–22 Ghanaian adolescent girl with healed *M. ulcerans* infection that extended from the wrist to the shoulder. The scarring resulted in contraction deformities of the wrist and elbow and disuse atrophy of the entire extremity. Appropriate physiotherapy would have minimized these sequelae. (See companion Expert Consult web site for color version.)

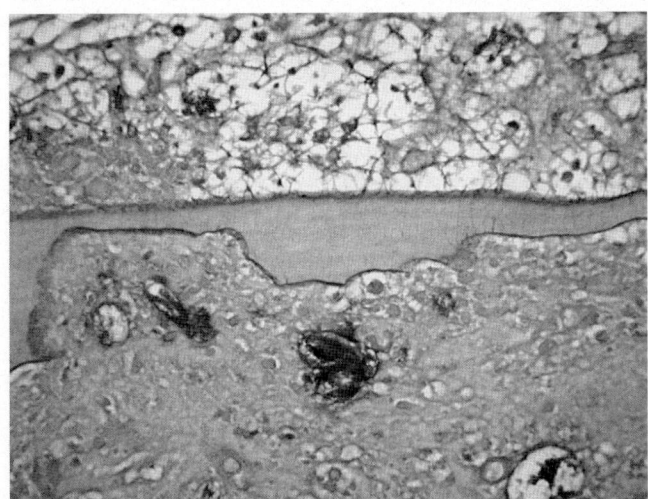

Figure 109–20 Ziehl-Neelsen–stained section shows metastatic osteomyelitis of the tibia in a 6-year-old boy in Benin. This lesion developed after *M. ulcerans* infection of the contralateral leg. Note necrosis of marrow, erosion of a trabecula, and many clusters of acid-fast bacilli (Ziehl-Neelsen stain). (See companion Expert Consult web site for color version.)

condition is suspected, and where available, bone scans may be helpful in diagnosis.[242] If the condition goes untreated, a draining fistula usually develops. Osteomyelitis often requires an amputation (Fig. 109–21).

Complications

Infection may traverse the deep fascia and damage tendons, nerves, joints, genitalia, and periorbital tissues, requiring subsequent enucleation of the eye. Healing leads to fibrosis and scarring and can severely limit movement, with attendant lifestyle alterations.[294] The scar may form keloids and often causes major contraction deformities, especially in lesions that cross joints (Fig. 109–22). Squamous cell carcinoma may develop in healed lesions, especially nonpigmented lesions. Skin grafting and physiotherapy prevent most of these complications. Most disease-related deaths result from septicemia, gas gangrene, or tetanus.

DIAGNOSIS AND DIFFERENTIAL DIAGNOSIS

To an experienced observer, an accurate clinical diagnosis often can be made with ease.[353,355] In the ulcerated forms, a Ziehl-Neelsen stain of exudate from the undermined edge obtained with a cotton swab reveals clusters of extracellular AFB. The same material, obtained by swab after decontamination, may be used for culture on Löwenstein-Jensen or other suitable mycobacterial media. The incubation temperature must be 30° C to 32° C. If culture cannot be performed locally, transport media may be inoculated with material from the cotton swab and maintained at 4° C while in transport to a specialized laboratory. The transport medium is composed of Middlebrook 7H9 broth supplemented with polymyxin B, amphotericin B, nalidixic acid, trimethoprim, azlocillin, and 0.5 percent agar. Molecular biologic analysis techniques consisting of PCR for the identification of *M. ulcerans* are available and increasing in popularity and convenience.[1,285,296] Tissue for histopathologic analysis should be obtained from the edge of the ulcer and must include all levels, including the fascia. Fixation in 4 percent buffered formalin is adequate.

Following are some differential diagnostic possibilities:

1. Papules—insect bites, verruca vulgaris, pityriasis, granuloma annulare
2. Nodules—lipoma, sebaceous cyst, onchocerciasis, furuncle
3. Plaques—leprosy, mycosis, necrobiosis, psoriasis
4. Edema—bacterial cellulitis, actinomycosis, elephantiasis, pyomyositis
5. Ulcers—tropical phagedenic ulcer, noma, stasis ulcer, leishmaniasis

PROGNOSIS

Without treatment, Buruli ulcer often leads to deforming depressed scars, contraction deformities, or amputation. The stigma of the deformities and the socioeconomic burden of the disease often are marked.[9] With early appropriate treatment, including excision and grafting, the prognosis usually is excellent. Metastatic lesions and local recurrences occur frequently enough, however, to warrant vigilant follow-up.[6]

TREATMENT

Treatment options for Buruli ulcer include antibiotics and surgical intervention. The choice is usually based on the morphology and extent of the lesions and the availability of antibiotics and surgical facilities. Current WHO guidelines are available.[350,354]

Briefly, antibiotic treatment as recommended by WHO, although still empiric, currently includes at least 8-week courses of daily oral rifampin (10 mg/kg) and streptomycin (15 mg/kg) given as an intramuscular injection. Rifampin is supplied in tablet and syrup forms, the latter being helpful for small children. Streptomycin and, to a lesser extent, rifampin, are associated with rare but important side effects, some of which require stopping treatment. For streptomycin, treatment should be stopped if hearing impairment or vertigo with nystagmus develops. For rifampin, treatment should be stopped if hepatitis, jaundice, or acute renal failure occurs, side effects that generally are associated with intermittent therapy of more than 10 mg/kg. Streptomycin also is contraindicated during pregnancy. In our opinion, antibiotic therapy for advanced lesions remains a subject for inquiry, and the above-described regimens do not constitute established recommendations at this time.

If surgical intervention is chosen, to minimize the danger of development of *M. ulcerans* bacteremia, many surgeons prescribe clarithromycin and rifampin 1 to 2 weeks before performing surgery and have the patients continue antibiotic therapy for several weeks after surgery. Although reasonable, this antibiotic complement to surgery is not of proven efficacy. Papules and pre-ulcerative nodules seldom are diagnosed, even in endemic areas; however, wide excision and primary closure usually are curative.[311]

Plaques and edematous forms are excised widely down to the fascia, or through the fascia if it is necrotic. Muscle usually is not damaged, but if so, the excision is extended into muscle. The lateral extent of excision often is difficult to determine. By careful palpation, the physician can establish an approximate limit of the disease. Exploratory incisions and blunt dissection may help determine the limit of induration and necrosis. Use of real-time PCR for determining the extent of disease is being evaluated.[257]

Very small ulcers can be excised and closed primarily, as for nodules. Large ulcers are excised widely. The required extent of surgery may be determined by exploratory lateral excision and blunt dissection. Split-skin autografting of surgical defects usually is performed after a bed of granulation tissue has formed. Postoperative care, including physiotherapy, should be designed to prevent contractures.

Bone lesions should be referred to specialists. Heat therapy without surgical excision has been successful for appropriate lesions, but must be applied assiduously with all necessary controls.[196] Recurrences after surgical treatment are frequent, but rates are not well established.[6]

PREVENTION

In an endemic tropical rural setting where children usually are scantily attired, prevention of contamination of the skin from environmental sources is virtually impossible. Wearing long trousers seems to prevent development of infection.[176] Protected water supplies in villages would reduce exposure; however, such protective measures usually are futile in rural areas of developing countries. Other risk factors have been analyzed extensively.[63]

Vaccination with BCG has a moderate protective effect against *M. ulcerans* infections for 6 to 12 months.[310] Studies are projected to determine whether repeated BCG vaccination may render the population more immune to *M. ulcerans* infection,[236,237] as was found for leprosy.[150] Other vaccines based on virulence factors of *M. ulcerans* (e.g., the toxin) also are being studied.[125]

HUMAN IMMUNODEFICIENCY VIRUS AND BURULI ULCER

Because Buruli ulcer primarily is a disease of children in rural areas, very few patients have been reported with Buruli ulcer and HIV infection.[8] Relevant reports available indicate, however, that HIV infection may render Buruli ulcer disease highly aggressive; rapidly spreading *M. ulcerans* osteomyelitis has developed in several patients with AIDS.[138,303]

REFERENCES

1. Ablordey, A., Kotlowski, R., Swings, J., et al.: PCR amplification with primers based on IS2404 and GC-rich repeated sequence reveals polymorphism in *Mycobacterium ulcerans*. J. Clin. Microbiol. *43*:448-451, 2005.
2. Achilles, E. G., Hagel, C., Vierbuchen, M., et al.: Leprosy accidentally transmitted from a patient to a surgeon in a nonendemic area. Ann. Intern. Med. *141*:W51, 2004.
3. Adusumilli, S., Mve-Obiang, A., Sparer, T., et al.: *Mycobacterium ulcerans* toxic macrolide, mycolactone modulates the host immune response and cellular location of *M. ulcerans* in vitro and in vivo. Cell. Microbiol. 7:1295-1304, 2005.

4. Agrawal, A., Pandit, L., Dalal, M., et al.: Neurological manifestations of Hansen's disease and their management. Clin. Neurol. Neurosurg. *107*:445-454, 2005.

5. Agrawal, S., and Agarwalla, A.: Dapsone hypersensitivity syndrome: A clinico-epidemiological review. J. Dermatol. *32*:883-889, 2005.

6. Aguiar, J., and Steunou, C.: Les ulcères de Buruli en zone rurale au Bénin pris en charge de 635 cas [Buruli ulcers in rural areas of Benin: management of 635 cases]. Med. Trop. (Mars.) *57*:83-90, 1997.

7. Alcais, A., Sanchez, F. O., Thuc, N. V., et al.: Granulomatous reaction to intradermal injection of lepromin (Mitsuda reaction) is linked to the human NRAMP1 gene in Vietnamese leprosy sibships. J. Infect. Dis. *181*:302-308, 2000.

8. Allen, S.: Buruli ulcer and HIV infection. Int. J. Dermatol. *31*:744-745, 1992.

9. Asiedu, K., and Etuaful, S.: Socioeconomic implications of Buruli ulcer in Ghana: A three-year review. Am. J. Trop. Med. Hyg. *59*:1015-1022, 1998.

10. Bakker, M. I., Hatta, M., Kwenang, A., et al.: Prevention of leprosy using rifampicin as chemoprophylaxis. Am. J. Trop. Med. Hyg. *72*:443-448, 2005.

11. Balagon, M. V., Cellona, R. V., Fajardo, T. T., Jr., et al.: Detection of new leprosy cases at a walk-in skin clinic in Cebu City, Philippines, highlights surveillance. Int. J. Dermatol. *38*:796-797, 1999.

12. Bär, W., Rusch-Gerdes, S., Richter, E., et al.: *Mycobacterium ulcerans* infection in a child from Angola: Diagnosis by direct detection and culture. Trop. Med. Int. Health *3*:189-196, 1998.

13. Barker, D. J. P., Clancey, J. K., and Rao, S. K.: Mycobacteria on vegetation in Uganda. East Afr. Med. J. *49*:667-671, 1972.

14. Barksdale, L., and Kim, K. S.: Mycobacterium. Bacteriol. Rev. *41*:217-372, 1977.

15. Bartels, P.: Tuberculose in der Jüngeren Steinzeit. Arch. Anthropol. *6*:243-255, 1907.

16. Bechelli, L. M., Garbajosa, P. G., Gyi, M. M., et al.: Site of early skin lesions in children with leprosy. Bull. World Health Organ. *48*:107-111, 1973.

17. Bechelli, L. M., Garbajosa, P. G., Gyi, M. M., et al.: BCG vaccination of children against leprosy: Seven-year findings of the controlled WHO trial in Burma. Bull. World Health Organ. *48*:323-334, 1973.

18. Becx-Bleuminck, M.: Operational aspects of multidrug therapy. Int. J. Lepr. Other Mycobact. Dis. *57*:540-551, 1989.

19. Bhatki, W. S., Chullawala, R. G., Chaturvedi, R. M., et al.: Lepromin conversion induced by a "sub-unit" vaccine from ICRC bacilli. Indian J. Med. Res. *87*:545-554, 1988.

20. Bhattacharya, S. N., Chattopadhaya, D., and Saha, K.: Tumor necrosis factor: Status in reactions in leprosy before and after treatment. Int. J. Dermatol. *32*:436-439, 1993.

21. Bhutani, L. K., Nath, I., and Mehra, N. K.: Grand round: Leprosy. Lancet *345*:697-703, 1995.

22. Binford, C. H., Meyers, W. M., and Walsh, G. P.: Leprosy: State of the art. J. A. M. A. *247*:2283-2292, 1982.

23. Binford, C. H., Meyers, W. M., Walsh, G. P., et al.: Naturally acquired leprosy-like disease in the nine-banded armadillo (*Dasypus novemcinctus*): Histopathologic and microbiologic studies of tissues. J. Reticuloendothel. Soc. *22*:377-388, 1977.

24. Borgdorff, M. W., van den Broek, J., Chum, H. J., et al.: HIV-1 infection as a risk factor for leprosy: A case-control study in Tanzania. Int. J. Lepr. Other Mycobact. Dis. *61*:556-562, 1993.

25. Brennan, P. J., and Vissa, V. D.: Genomic evidence for the retention of the essential mycobacterial cell wall in the otherwise defective *Mycobacterium leprae*. Lepr. Rev. *72*:415-428, 2001.

26. Brightbill, H. D., Libraty, D. H., Krutzik, S. R., et al.: Host defense mechanisms triggered by microbial lipoproteins through toll-like receptors. Science *285*:732-736, 1999.

27. Britton, W. J., and Lockwood, D. N.: Leprosy. Lancet *363*:1209-1219, 2004.

28. Brody, S. N.: The Disease of the Soul: Leprosy in Medieval Literature. Ithaca, NY, Cornell University Press, 1974.

29. Browne, S. G.: Onchocercal depigmentation. Trans. R. Soc. Trop. Med. Hyg. *54*:325-334, 1960.

30. Brubaker, M. L., Meyers, W. M., and Bourland, J.: Leprosy in children one year of age and under. Int. J. Lepr. Other Mycobact. Dis. *53*:517-523, 1985.

31. Bullock, W. E.: Studies of immune mechanisms in leprosy, I: Depression of delayed allergic response to skin test antigens. N. Engl. J. Med. *278*:298-304, 1968.

32. Bullock, W. E.: Rifampin in the treatment of leprosy. Rev. Infect. Dis. *5*(Suppl. 3):S606-S613, 1983.

33. Bullock, W. E., Ho, M. F., and Chen, M. J.: Studies of immune mechanisms in leprosy, II: Quantitative relationships of IgG, IgA, and IgM immunoglobulins. J. Lab. Clin. Med. *75*:863-870, 1970.

34. Bwire, R., and Kawuma, H. J. S.: Type 1 reactions in leprosy, neuritis and steroid therapy: The impact of the human immunodeficiency virus. Trans. R. Soc. Trop. Med. Hyg. *88*:315-316, 1994.

35. Byrd, S. R., Gelber, R., and Bermudez, L. E.: Roles of soluble fibronectin and β₁ integrin receptors in the binding of *Mycobacterium leprae* to nasal epithelial cells. Clin. Immunol. Immunopathol. *69*:266-271, 1993.

36. Cellona, R. V., Balagon, M. F., dela Cruz, E. C., et al.: Long-term efficacy of 2 year WHO multiple drug therapy (MDT) in multibacillary (MB) leprosy patients. Int. J. Lepr. Other Mycobact. Dis. *71*:308-319, 2003.

37. Chedore, P., Broukhanski, G., Shainhouse, Z., et al.: False-positive amplified *Mycobacterium tuberculosis* direct test results for samples containing *Mycobacterium leprae*. J. Clin. Microbiol. *44*:612-613, 2006.

38. Cho, S. N., Chatterjee, D., and Brennan, P. J.: A simplified serological test for leprosy based on a 3,6-di-O-methylglucose-containing synthetic antigen. Am. J. Trop. Med. Hyg. *35*:167-172, 1986.

39. Clancey, J. K., Dodge, O. G., Lunn, H. F., et al.: Mycobacterial skin ulcers in Uganda. Lancet *2*:951-954, 1961.

40. Cochrane, R. G., and Davey, T. F.: Leprosy in Theory and Practice. 2nd ed. Bristol, England, John Wright & Sons, 1964.

41. Cole, S. T., Eiglmeier, K., Parkhill, J., et al.: Massive gene decay in the leprosy bacillus. Nature *409*:1007-1011, 2001.

42. Coloma, J. N., Navarrete-Franco, G., Iribe, P., et al.: Ulcerative cutaneous mycobacteriosis due to *Mycobacterium ulcerans*: Report of two Mexican cases. Int. J. Lepr. Other Mycobact. Dis. *73*:5-12, 2005.

43. Connor, D. H., and Lunn, H. F.: Buruli ulceration: A clinicopathologic study of 38 Ugandans with *Mycobacterium ulcerans* infection. Arch. Pathol. *81*:183-189, 1966.

44. Connor, D. H., Meyers, W. M., and Krieg, R. E.: Infection by *Mycobacterium ulcerans*. *In* Connor, D. H., and Binford, C. H. (eds.): Pathology of Tropical and Extraordinary Diseases: An Atlas. Vol. 1. Washington, D.C., Armed Forces Institute of Pathology, 1976, p. 226.

45. Convit, J., Aranzazu, N., Ulrich, M., et al.: Immunotherapy with a mixture of *Mycobacterium leprae* and BCG in different forms of leprosy and in Mitsuda-negative contacts. Int. J. Lepr. Other Mycobact. Dis. *50*:415-424, 1982.

46. Convit, J., Avila, J. L., Goihman, M., et al.: A test for the determination of competency in clearing bacilli in leprosy patients. Bull. World Health Organ. *46*:821-826, 1972.

47. Convit, J., and Pinardi, M. E.: A simple method for the differentiation of *Mycobacterium leprae* from other mycobacteria through routine staining technics. Int. J. Lepr. Other Mycobact. Dis. *40*:130-132, 1972.

48. Convit, J., Sampson, C., Zuniga, M., et al.: Immunoprophylactic trial with combined *Mycobacterium leprae*/BCG vaccine against leprosy: Preliminary results. Lancet *339*:446-450, 1992.

49. Cook, A.: Mengo Hospital Notes. Kampala, Uganda, Makerere Medical School Library, 1897 (cited in B. M. J. *2*:37-39, 1970).

50. Cooke, G. S., and Hill, A. V.: Genetics of susceptibility to human infectious disease. Nat. Rev. Genet. *2*:967-977, 2001.

51. Courtright, P., Daniel, E., Sundarrao, et al.: Eye disease in multibacillary leprosy patients at the time of their leprosy diagnosis: Findings from the Longitudinal Study of Ocular Leprosy (LOSOL) in India, the Philippines and Ethiopia. Lepr. Rev. *73*:225-238, 2002.

52. Coutanceau, E., Marsollier, L., Brosch, R., et al.: Modulation of the host immune response by a transient intracellular stage of *Mycobacterium ulcerans*: The contribution of endogenous mycolactone toxin. Cell. Microbiol. *7*:1187-1196, 2005.

53. Cree, I. A., Coghill, G., Subedi, A. M., et al.: Effects of treatment on the histopathology of leprosy. J. Clin. Pathol. *48*:304-307, 1995.

54. Daffe, M., Varnerot, A., and Levy-Frebault, V. V.: The phenolic mycoside of *Mycobacterium ulcerans*: Structure and taxonomic implications. J. Gen. Microbiol. *138*:131-137, 1992.

55. Daniel, A. K., Lee, R. E., Portaels, F., et al.: Analysis of *Mycobacterium* species for the presence of a macrolide toxin, mycolactone. Infect. Immun. *72*:123-132, 2004.

56. Daniel, E., Ffytche, T. J., Kempen, J. H., et al.: Incidence of ocular complications in patients with multibacillary leprosy after completion of a 2 year course of multidrug therapy. Br. J. Ophthalmol. *90*:949-954, 2006.

57. Daniel, E., Ffytche, T. J., Sundar Rao, P. S., et al.: Incidence of ocular morbidity among multibacillary leprosy patients during a 2 year course of multidrug therapy. Br. J. Ophthalmol. *90*:568-573, 2006.

58. Davey, T. F., and Rees, R. J. W.: The nasal discharge in leprosy: Clinical and bacteriological aspects. Lepr. Rev. *45*:121-134, 1974.

59. Dayal, R., and Bharadwaj, V. P.: Prevention and early detection of leprosy in children. J. Trop. Pediatr. *41*:132-138, 1995.

60. Debacker, M., Aguiar, J., Steunou, C., et al.: *Mycobacterium ulcerans* disease (Buruli ulcer) in rural hospital, Southern Benin, 1997-2001. Emerg. Infect. Dis. *10*:1391-1398, 2004.

61. Debacker, M., Aguiar, J., Steunou, C., et al.: *Mycobacterium ulcerans* disease: Role of age and gender in incidence and morbidity. Trop. Med. Int. Health *9*:1297-1304, 2004.

62. Debacker, M., Aguiar, J., Steunou, C., et al.: Buruli ulcer recurrence, Benin. Emerg. Infect. Dis. *11*:584-589, 2005.

63. Debacker, M., Portaels, F., Aguiar, J., et al.: Risk factors for Buruli ulcer, Benin. Emerg. Infect. Dis. *12*:1325-1331, 2006.

64. Debacker, M., Zinsou, C., Aguiar, J., et al.: First case of *Mycobacterium ulcerans* disease (Buruli ulcer) following a human bite. Clin. Infect. Dis. *36*:e67-e68, 2003.

65. de Rijk, A. J., Gabre, S., Byass, P., et al.: Field evaluation of WHO-MDT of fixed duration at ALERT, Ethiopia: The AMFES project, II: Reaction and neuritis during and after MDT in PB and MB leprosy patients. Lepr. Rev. *65*:320-332, 1994.

66. de Wit, M. Y., Douglas, J. T., McFadden, J., et al.: Polymerase chain reaction for detection of *Mycobacterium leprae* in nasal swab specimens. J. Clin. Microbiol. *31*:502-506, 1993.

67. Dietrich, M., Gaus, W., Kern, P., et al.: An international randomized study with long-term follow-up of single versus combination chemotherapy of multibacillary leprosy. Antimicrob. Agents Chemother. 38:2249-2257, 1994.

68. Dodge, O. G.: Mycobacterial skin ulcers in Uganda: Histopathological and experimental aspects. J. Pathol. Bacteriol. 88:167-174, 1964.

69. Donham, K. J., and Leininger, J. R.: Spontaneous leprosy-like disease in a chimpanzee. J. Infect. Dis. 136:132-136, 1977.

70. Drutz, D. J., Chen, T. S., and Lu, W. H.: The continuous bacteremia of lepromatous leprosy. N. Engl. J. Med. 287:159-164, 1972.

71. Duker, A. A., Portaels, F., and Hale, M.: Pathways of Mycobacterium ulcerans infection: A review. Environ. Int. 32:567-573, 2006.

72. Duncan, M. E.: Babies of mothers with leprosy have small placentae, low birth weights and grow slowly. Br. J. Obstet. Gynaecol. 87:471-479, 1980.

73. Duncan, M. E., Melsom, R., Pearson, J. M., et al.: A clinical and immunological study of four babies of mothers with lepromatous leprosy, two of whom developed leprosy in infancy. Int. J. Lepr. Other Mycobact. Dis. 51:7-17, 1983.

74. Duncan, M. E., and Oakey, R. E.: Estrogen excretion in pregnant women with leprosy: Evidence of diminished fetoplacental function. Obstet. Gynecol. 60:82-86, 1982.

75. Dwyer, J. M., Bullock, W. E., and Fields, J. P.: Disturbances of the blood; T:B lymphocyte ratio in lepromatous leprosy. N. Engl. J. Med. 288:1036-1039, 1973.

76. Eiglmeier, K., Parkhill, J., Honore, N., et al.: The decaying genome of Mycobacterium leprae. Lepr. Rev. 72:387-398, 2001.

77. Ellard, G. A.: Rationale of the multidrug regimens recommended by a World Health Organization Study Group on Chemotherapy of Leprosy for Control Programs. Int. J. Lepr. Other Mycobact. Dis. 52:395-401, 1984.

78. Evans, M. R., Mawdsley, J., Bull, R., et al.: Buruli ulcer in a visitor to London. Br. J. Dermatol. 149:907-909, 2003.

79. Faber, W. R., Arias-Bouda, L. M., Zeegelaar, J. E., et al.: First reported case of Mycobacterium ulcerans infection in a patient from China. Trans. R. Soc. Trop. Med. Hyg. 94:277-279, 2000.

80. Faber, W. R., Jensema, A. J., and Goldschmidt, W. F.: Treatment of recurrent erythema nodosum leprosum with infliximab. N. Engl. J. Med. 355:739, 2006.

81. Faget, G. H., Pogge, R. C., Johansen, F. A., et al.: The Promin treatment of leprosy: A progress report. Public Health Rep. 58:1729-1741, 1943.

82. Fajardo, T. T., Abalos, R. M., dela Cruz, E. C., et al.: Clofazimine therapy for lepromatous leprosy: A historical perspective. Int. J. Dermatol. 38:70-74, 1999.

83. Farb, H., West, D. P., Pedvis-Leftick, A.: Clofazimine in pregnancy complicated by leprosy. Obstet. Gynecol. 59:122-123, 1982.

84. Feldman, R. A., and Sturdivant, M.: Leprosy in Louisiana 1855-1970: An epidemiologic study of long-term trends. Am. J. Epidemiol. 102:303-310, 1975.

85. Fernando, S. L., and Britton, W. J.: Genetic susceptibility to mycobacterial disease in humans. Immunol. Cell. Biol. 84:125-137, 2006.

86. Fiallo, P., Williams, D. L., Chan, G. P., et al.: Effects of fixation on polymerase chain reaction detection of Mycobacterium leprae. J. Clin. Microbiol. 30:3095-3098, 1992.

87. Fine, P. E., and Warndorff, D. K.: Leprosy by the year 2000—what is being eliminated? [editorial]. Lepr. Rev. 68:201-202, 1997.

88. Fitness, J., Floyd, S., Warndorff, D. K., et al.: Large-scale candidate gene study of leprosy susceptibility in the Karonga district of northern Malawi. Am. J. Trop. Med. Hyg. 71:330-340, 2004.

89. Fitness, J., Tosh, K., and Hill, A. V.: Genetics of susceptibility to leprosy. Genes Immun. 3:441-453, 2002.

90. Flageul, B., Wallach, D., Vignon-Pennamen, M. D., et al.: Late onset of a reversal reaction in borderline leprosy. J. Am. Acad. Dermatol. 20:857-860, 1989.

91. Fritschi, E. P.: Reconstructive Surgery in Leprosy. Bristol, England, John Wright & Sons, 1971.

92. Gajl-Peczalska, K. J., Lim, S. D., Jacobson, R. R., et al.: B lymphocytes in lepromatous leprosy. N. Engl. J. Med. 288:1033-1035, 1973.

93. Gatt, P.: The Malta experience, 1972-1992: 20 years after starting the eradication project in Malta. Int. J. Lepr. 61: suppl, 5A, 1993.

94. Gaylord, H., and Brennan, P. J.: Leprosy and the leprosy bacillus: Recent developments in characterization of antigens and immunology of the disease. Annu. Rev. Microbiol. 41:645-675, 1987.

95. Gehr, E.: Leprosy in childhood. Doc. Med. Geog. Trop. 9:101-124, 1957.

96. Gelber, R. H., Drutz, D. J., Epstein, W. V., et al.: Clinical correlates of C1Q-precipitating substances in the sera of patients with leprosy. Am. J. Trop. Med. Hyg. 23:471-475, 1974.

97. Gelber, R. H., Fukuda, K., Byrd, S., et al.: A clinical trial of minocycline in lepromatous leprosy. B. M. J. 304:91-92, 1992.

98. Gelber, R. H., Mehra, V., Bloom, B., et al.: Vaccination with pure Mycobacterium leprae proteins inhibits M. leprae multiplication in mouse footpads. Infect. Immun. 62:4250-4255, 1994.

99. Gelber, R. H., Murray, L. P., Siu, P., et al.: Efficacy of minocycline in single dose and at 100 mg twice daily for lepromatous leprosy. Int. J. Lepr. Other Mycobact. Dis. 62:568-573, 1994.

100. George, K. M., Barker, L. P., Welty, D. M., et al.: Partial purification and characterization of biological effects of a lipid toxin produced by Mycobacterium ulcerans. Infect. Immun. 66:587-593, 1998.

101. George, K. M., Chatterjee, D., Gunawardana, G., et al.: Mycolactone: A polyketide toxin from Mycobacterium ulcerans required for virulence. Science 283:854-857, 1999.

102. George, K. M., Pascopella, L., Welty, D. M., et al.: A Mycobacterium ulcerans toxin, mycolactone, causes apoptosis in guinea pig ulcers and tissue culture cells. Infect. Immun. 68:877-883, 2000.

103. Girdhar, B. K., Girdhar, A., Ramu, G., et al.: Borderline leprosy (BL) in an infant—report of a case and a brief review. Lepr. India 55:333-337, 1983.

104. Godal, T.: Growing points in leprosy research: (3) Immunological detection of sub-clinical infection in leprosy. Lepr. Rev. 45:22-30, 1974.

105. Gomez, A., Mve-Obiang, A., Vray, B., et al.: Detection of phospholipase C in nontuberculous mycobacteria and its possible role in hemolytic activity. J. Clin. Microbiol. 39:1396-1401, 2001.

106. Gonzalez-Abreu, E., Mora, N., Perez, M., et al.: Serodiagnosis of leprosy in patients' contacts by enzyme-linked immunosorbent assay. Lepr. Rev. 61:145-150, 1990.

107. Gormus, B. J., Xu, K. Y., Alford, P. L., et al.: A serologic study of naturally acquired leprosy in chimpanzees. Int. J. Lepr. Other Mycobact. Dis. 59:450-457, 1991.

108. Grant, A. M. B.: Leprosy at Nauru since 1928. Int. J. Lepr. 2:305-310, 1934.

109. Groathouse, N. A., Brown, S. E., Knudson, D. L., et al.: Isothermal amplification and molecular typing of the obligate intracellular pathogen Mycobacterium leprae isolated from tissues of unknown origins. J. Clin. Microbiol. 44:1502-1508, 2006.

110. Grosset, J. H.: Progress in the chemotherapy of leprosy. Int. J. Lepr. Other Mycobact. Dis. 62:268-277, 1994.

111. Guarner, J., Bartlett, J., Whitney, E. A., et al.: Histopathologic features of Mycobacterium ulcerans infection. Emerg. Infect. Dis. 9:651-656, 2003.

112. Guinto, R. S., Doull, J. A., and Mabalay, E. B.: The Mitsuda reaction in persons with and without household exposure to leprosy. Int. J. Lepr. 23:135-138, 1955.

113. Gupte, M. D., Anantharaman, D. S., Nagaraju, B., et al.: Experiences with Mycobacterium leprae soluble antigens in a leprosy endemic population. Lepr. Rev. 61:132-144, 1990.

114. Harboe, M.: The work and concepts of Armauer Hansen: How do they stand today? Ethiop. Med. J. 21:123-126, 1983.

115. Harboe, M.: The immunology of leprosy. In Hastings, R. C. (ed.): Leprosy (Medicine in the Tropics Series). Edinburgh, Churchill Livingstone, 1985, p. 53.

116. Haregewoin, A., Godal, T., Mustafa, A. S., et al.: T-cell conditioned media reverse T-cell unresponsiveness in lepromatous leprosy. Nature 303:342-344, 1983.

117. Hastings, R. C., and Morales, M. J.: Observations, calculations, and speculations on the growth and death of M. leprae in vivo. Int. J. Lepr. 50:579-582, 1982.

118. Hayman, J.: Clinical features of Mycobacterium ulcerans infection. Australas. J. Dermatol. 26:67-73, 1985.

119. Hietaharju, A., Croft, R., Alam, R., et al.: Chronic neuropathic pain in treated leprosy. Lancet 356:1080-1081, 2000.

120. Hogeweg, M., and Keunen, J. E.: Prevention of blindness in leprosy and the role of the Vision 2020 Programme. Eye 19:1099-1105, 2005.

121. Horsburgh, C. R., Jr., and Meyers, W. M.: Buruli ulcer. In Horsburgh, C. R., Jr., and Nelson, A. M. (eds.): Pathology of Emerging Infections. Washington, D.C., American Society for Microbiology, 1997, p. 119.

122. Horwitz, M. A., Levis, W. R., and Cohn, Z. A.: Defective production of monocyte-activating cytokines in lepromatous leprosy. J. Exp. Med. 159:666-678, 1984.

123. Hunter, S. W., Fujiwara, T., and Brennan, P. J.: Structure and antigenicity of the major specific glycolipid antigen of Mycobacterium leprae. J. Biol. Chem. 257:15072-15078, 1982.

124. Hussain, R., Lucas, S. B., Kifayet, A., et al.: Clinical and histological discrepancies in diagnosis of ENL reactions classified by assessment of acute phase proteins SAA and CRP. Int. J. Lepr. Other Mycobact. Dis. 63:222-230, 1995.

125. Huygen, K.: Prospects for vaccine development against Buruli disease. Expert Rev. Vaccines 2:561-569, 2003.

126. Imkamp, F. M. J. H.: Clofazimine (Lamprene or B663) in lepra reactions. Lepr. Rev. 52:135-140 1981.

127. Inaba, T.: Ueber die Histopathologischen und Bakteriologischen Untersuchungen der Plazenta bei Leprosen. La Lepro 9(Suppl. III), 1938.

128. Izumi, S., Fujiwara, T., Ikeda, M., et al.: Novel gelatin particle agglutination test for serodiagnosis of leprosy in the field. J. Clin. Microbiol. 28:525-529, 1990.

129. Jacobson, R. R.: Carville and Hansen's disease control: Past, present and future. Int. J. Lepr. Other Mycobact. Dis. 63:272-273, 1995.

130. Jacobson, R. R., and Hastings, R. C.: Rifampin-resistant leprosy. Lancet 2:1304-1305, 1976.

131. Jakeman, P.: Risk of relapse in multibacillary leprosy. Lancet 345:4-5, 1995.

132. Jamet, P., Ji, B.; and the Marchoux Chemotherapy Study Group: Relapse after long-term follow up of multibacillary patients treated by WHO multidrug regimen. Int. J. Lepr. Other Mycobact. Dis. 63:195-201, 1995.

133. Janssen, F., Wallach, D., Khuong, M. A., et al.: Association de maladie de Hansen et d'infection par le virus de l'immunodéficience humaine: Deux observations [Association of Hansen's disease and human deficiency virus infection: 2 cases]. Presse Med. 17:1652-1653, 1988.

134. Ji, B., Jamet, P., Perani, E. G., et al.: Powerful bactericidal activities of clarithromycin and minocycline against *Mycobacterium leprae* in lepromatous leprosy. J. Infect. Dis. *168*:188-190, 1993.

135. Job, C. K.: The Kellersberger Memorial Lecture 1983. The lepromin test and its role in the management of leprosy. Ethiop. Med. J. *21*:233-242, 1983.

136. Job, C. K., and Chacko, C. J. G.: A simplified 6 group classification of leprosy. Lepr. India *54*:26-32, 1982.

137. Job, C. K., Harris, E. B., Allen, J. L., et al.: A random survey of leprosy in wild nine-banded armadillos in Louisiana. Int. J. Lepr. Other Mycobact. Dis. *54*:453-457, 1986.

138. Johnson, R. C., Ifebe, D., Hans-Moevi, A., et al.: Disseminated *Mycobacterium ulcerans* disease in an HIV-positive patient: A case study. AIDS *16*:1704-1705, 2002.

139. Johnstone, P. A. S., Meyers, W. M., and Binford, C. H.: Recent advances in the development of nonhuman primates as animal models for leprosy. Scand. J. Lab. Anim. Sci. *16*(Suppl. 1):102-105, 1989.

140. Jopling, W. H.: Handbook of Leprosy. London, William Heinemann, 1984.

141. Jopling, W. H., Ridley, M. J., Bonnici, E., et al.: A follow-up investigation of the Malta Project. Lepr. Rev. *55*:247-253, 1984.

142. Kang, T. J., and Chae, G. T.: Detection of Toll-like receptor 2 (TLR2) mutation in the lepromatous leprosy patients. F. E. M. S. Immunol. Med. Microbiol. *31*:53-58, 2001.

143. Kang, T. J., Lee, S. B., and Chae, G. T.: A polymorphism in the Toll-like receptor 2 is associated with IL-12 production from monocyte in lepromatous leprosy. Cytokine *20*:56-62, 2002.

144. Kang, T. J., Yeum, C. E., Kim, B. C., et al.: Differential production of interleukin-10 and interleukin-12 in mononuclear cells from leprosy patients with a Toll-like receptor 2 mutation. Immunology *112*:674-680, 2004.

145. Kaplan, G.: Recent advances in cytokine therapy in leprosy. J. Infect. Dis. *167*(Suppl. 1):S18-S22, 1993.

146. Kaplan, G., Mathur, N. K., Job, C. K., et al.: Effect of multiple interferon gamma injections on the disposal of *Mycobacterium leprae*. Proc. Natl. Acad. Sci. U. S. A. *86*:8073-8077, 1989.

147. Kaplan, G., Sampaio, E. P., Walsh, G. P., et al.: Influence of *Mycobacterium leprae* and its soluble products on the cutaneous responsiveness of leprosy patients to antigen and recombinant interleukin 2. Proc. Natl. Acad. Sci. U. S. A. *86*:6269-6273, 1989.

148. Kar, H. K., Bhatia, V. N., and Harikrishnan, S.: Combined clofazimine- and dapsone-resistant leprosy: A case report. Int. J. Lepr. *54*:389-391, 1986.

149. Kar, H. K., Sharma, A. K., Misra, R. S., et al.: Reversal reaction in multibacillary leprosy patients following MDT with and without immunotherapy with a candidate for an antileprosy vaccine, *Mycobacterium w*. Lepr. Rev. *64*:219-226, 1993.

150. Karonga Prevention Trial Group: Randomised controlled trial of single BCG, repeated BCG, or combined BCG and killed *Mycobacterium leprae* vaccine for prevention of leprosy and tuberculosis in Malawi. Lancet *348*:17-24, 1996.

151. Kashala, O., Marlink, R., Ilunga, M., et al.: Infection with human immunodeficiency virus type 1 (HIV-1) and human T cell lymphotropic viruses among leprosy patients and contacts: Correlation between HIV-1 cross-reactivity and antibodies to lipoarabinomannan. J. Infect. Dis. *169*:296-304, 1994.

152. Kato, L.: Leprosy associated mycobacteria: Implications. Acta Leprol. 7:1-6, 1989.

153. Kaur, I., Kaur, S., Sharma, V. K., et al.: Bacillaemia and *Mycobacterium leprae* cell wall antigen in paucibacillary leprosy. Indian J. Lepr. *65*:283-288, 1993.

154. Kawuma, H. J. S., Bwire, R., and Adatu-Engwau, F.: Leprosy and infection with the human immunodeficiency virus in Uganda: A case-control study. Int. J. Lepr. *62*:521-526, 1994.

155. Khanolkar-Young, S., Rayment, N., Brickell, P. M., et al.: Tumour necrosis factor-alpha (TNF-alpha) synthesis is associated with the skin and peripheral nerve pathology of leprosy reversal reactions. Clin. Exp. Immunol. *99*:196-202, 1995.

156. Kiszewski, A. E., Becerril, E., Aguilar, L. D., et al.: The local immune response in ulcerative lesions of Buruli disease. Clin. Exp. Immunol. *143*:445-451, 2006.

157. Krieg, R. E., Hockmeyer, W. T., and Connor, D. H.: Toxin of *Mycobacterium ulcerans*: Production and effects in guinea pig skin. Arch. Dermatol. *110*:783-788, 1974.

158. Lamfers, E. J., Bastiaans, A. H., Mravunac, M., et al.: Leprosy in the acquired immunodeficiency syndrome. Ann. Intern. Med. *107*:111-112, 1987.

159. Lane, J. E., Balagon, M. V., Dela Cruz, E. C., et al.: *Mycobacterium leprae* in untreated lepromatous leprosy: More than skin deep. Clin. Exp. Dermatol. *31*:469-470, 2006.

160. Lane, J. E., Walsh, D. S., Meyers, W. M., et al.: Borderline tuberculoid leprosy in a woman from the state of Georgia with armadillo exposure. J. Am. Acad. Dermatol. *55*:714-716, 2006.

161. Languillon, J., and Carayon, A.: Précis de Léprologie. Paris, Masson, 1969.

162. Lara, C. B.: Leprosy in children: General considerations: Initial and early changes. Philipp. J. Lepr. *1*:22-57, 1966.

163. Latapi, F., and Zamora, A. C.: The "spotted" leprosy of Lucio: An introduction to its clinical and histological study. Int. J. Lepr. Other Mycobac. Dis. *16*:421-429, 1948.

164. Lechat, M. F.: Global evaluation of the introduction of multidrug therapy. Leprosy Epidemiology Bulletin No. 4. Brussels, Belgium, World Health Organization Collaborating Center for the Epidemiology of Leprosy, 1990.

165. Leiker, D. L.: On the mode of transmission of *Mycobacterium leprae*. Lepr. Rev. *48*:9-16, 1977.

166. Leprosy News and Notes: The words "leper" and "leprosy." Fifth International Leprosy Congress—1948. Int. J. Lepr. Other Mycobac. Dis. *16*:243, 1948.

167. Levy, L., and Ji, B.: The mouse foot-pad technique for cultivation of *Mycobacterium leprae*. Lepr. Rev. *77*:5-24, 2006.

168. Lockwood, D. N., and Suneetha, S.: Leprosy: Too complex a disease for a simple elimination paradigm. Bull. World Health Organ. *83*:230-235, 2005.

169. Lucas, S. B.: Human immunodeficiency virus and leprosy. Lepr. Rev. *64*:97-103, 1993.

170. Lumpkin, L. R., 3rd, Cox, G. F., and Wolf, J. E., Jr.: Leprosy in five armadillo handlers. J. Am. Acad. Dermatol. *9*:899-903, 1983.

171. Lupi, O., Madkan, V., and Tyring, S. K.: Tropical dermatology: Bacterial tropical diseases. J. Am. Acad. Dermatol. *54*:559-578; quiz 578-580, 2006.

172. MacCallum, P., Tolhurst, J. C., Buckle, G., et al.: A new mycobacterial infection in man. J. Pathol. Bacteriol. *60*:93-122, 1948.

173. Marsollier, L., Aubry, J., Coutanceau, E., et al.: Colonization of the salivary glands of *Naucoris cimicoides* by *Mycobacterium ulcerans* requires host plasmatocytes and a macrolide toxin, mycolactone. Cell. Microbiol. 7:935-943, 2005.

174. Marsollier, L., Aubry, J., Saint-André, J. P., et al.: Ecologie et transmission de *Mycobacterium ulcerans* [Ecology and transmission of *Mycobacterium ulcerans*]. Pathol. Biol. (Paris) *51*:490-495, 2003.

175. Marsollier, L., Robert, R., Aubry, J., et al.: Aquatic insects as a vector for *Mycobacterium ulcerans*. Appl. Environ. Microbiol. *68*:4623-4628, 2002.

176. Marston, B. J., Diallo, M. O., Horsburgh, C. R., Jr., et al.: Emergence of Buruli ulcer disease in the Daloa region of Côte d'Ivoire. Am. J. Trop. Med. Hyg. *52*:219-224, 1995.

177. McAdam, K. P., Anders, R. F., Smith, S. R., et al.: Association of amyloidosis with erythema nodosum leprosum reactions and recurrent neutrophil leucocytosis in leprosy. Lancet *2*:572-573, 1975.

178. McCoy, W.: History of leprosy in the United States. Am. J. Trop. Med. *18*:19-34, 1938.

179. McDougall, A. C., and Waudby, H.: Dermal microfilariasis and leprosy. Lepr. Rev. *48*:161-168, 1977.

180. McInturff, J. E., Modlin, R. L., and Kim, J.: The role of toll-like receptors in the pathogenesis and treatment of dermatological disease. J. Invest. Dermatol. *125*:1-8, 2005.

181. Meeran, K.: Prevalence of HIV infection among patients with leprosy and tuberculosis in rural Zambia. B. M. J. *298*:364-365, 1989.

182. Mehra, V., Brennan, P. J., Rada, E., et al.: Lymphocyte suppression in leprosy induced by unique *M. leprae* glycolipid. Nature *308*:194-196, 1984.

183. Mehra, V., Mason, L. H., Rothman, W., et al.: Delineation of a human T cell subset responsible for lepromin-induced suppression in leprosy patients. J. Immunol. *125*:1183-1188, 1980.

184. Meisner, S. J., Mucklow, S., Warner, G., et al.: Association of NRAMP1 polymorphism with leprosy type but not susceptibility to leprosy per se in west Africans. Am. J. Trop. Med. Hyg. *65*:733-735, 2001.

185. Melancon-Kaplan, J., Hunter, S. W., McNeil, M., et al.: Immunological significance of *Mycobacterium leprae* cell walls. Proc. Natl. Acad. Sci. U. S. A. *85*:1917-1921, 1988.

186. Melsom, R., Harboe, M., and Duncan, M. E.: IgA, IgM and IgG anti-*M. leprae* antibodies in babies of leprosy mothers during the first two years of life. Clin. Exp. Immunol. *49*:532-542, 1982.

187. Melsom, R., Harboe, M., Duncan, M. E., et al.: IgA and IgM antibodies against *Mycobacterium leprae* in cord sera and in patients with leprosy: An indicator of intrauterine infection in leprosy. Scand J. Immunol. *14*:343-352, 1981.

188. Meyers, W. M.: Mycobacterial infections of the skin (including leprosy, tuberculosis of the skin, Buruli ulcer, and less common mycobacterial infections). *In* Doerr, W., and Seifert, G. (eds.): Tropical Pathology. 2nd ed., Vol. 8. Berlin, Springer-Verlag, 1995, p. 291.

189. Meyers, W. M., Binford, C. H., Walsh, G. P., et al.: Animal models of leprosy. *In* Leive, L., and Schlessinger, D. (eds.): Microbiology—1984. Washington, D.C., American Society for Microbiology, 1984, p. 307.

190. Meyers, W. M., Connor, D. H., Harman, L. E., et al.: Human streptocerciasis: A clinico-pathologic study of 40 Africans (Zairians) including identification of the adult filaria. Am. J. Trop. Med. Hyg. *21*:528-545, 1972.

191. Meyers, W. M., Gormus, B. J., Walsh, G. P.: Nonhuman sources of leprosy. Int. J. Lepr. Other Mycobact. Dis. *60*:477-480, 1992.

192. Meyers, W. M., Gormus, B. J., Walsh, G. P.: Experimental leprosy. *In* Hastings, R. C. (ed.): Leprosy (Medicine in the Tropics Series). 2nd ed. Edinburgh, Churchill Livingstone, 1994, p. 385.

193. Meyers, W. M., Gormus, B. J., Walsh, G. P., et al.: Naturally acquired and experimental leprosy in nonhuman primates. Am. J. Trop. Med. Hyg. *44*:24-27, 1991.

194. Meyers, W. M., Kvernes, S., and Binford, C. H.: Comparison of reactions to human and armadillo lepromins in leprosy. Int. J. Lepr. Other Mycobact. Dis. *43*:218-225, 1975.

195. Meyers, W. M., McDougall, A. C., Fleury, R. N., et al.: Histologic responses in sixty multibacillary leprosy patients inoculated with autoclaved *Mycobacterium leprae* and live BCG. Int. J. Lepr. Other Mycobact. Dis. *56*:302-309, 1988.

196. Meyers, W. M., Shelly, W. M., and Connor, D. H.: Heat treatment of *Mycobacterium ulcerans* infections without surgical excision. Am. J. Trop. Med. Hyg. *23*:924-929, 1974.

197. Meyers, W. M., Shelly, W. M., Connor, D. H., et al.: Human *Mycobacterium ulcerans* infections developing at sites of trauma to skin. Am. J. Trop. Med. Hyg. *23*:919-923, 1974.

198. Meyers, W. M., Tignokpa, N., Priuli, G. B., et al.: *Mycobacterium ulcerans* infection (Buruli ulcer): First reported patients in Togo. Br. J. Dermatol. *134*:1116-1121, 1996.

199. Meyers, W. M., Walsh, G. P., Brown, H. L., et al.: Naturally acquired leprosy-like disease in the nine-banded armadillo (*Dasypus novemcinctus*): Reactions in leprosy patients to lepromins prepared from naturally infected armadillos. J. Reticuloendothel. Soc. *22*:369-375, 1977.

200. Meyers, W. M., Walsh, G. P., Brown, H. L., et al.: Leprosy in a mangabey monkey—naturally acquired infection. Int. J. Lepr. Other Mycobact. Dis. *53*:1-14, 1985.

201. Mira, M. T., Alcais, A., Nguyen, V. T., et al.: Susceptibility to leprosy is associated with PARK2 and PACRG. Nature *427*:636-640, 2004.

202. Mira, M. T., Alcais, A., Van Thuc, N., et al.: Chromosome 6q25 is linked to susceptibility to leprosy in a Vietnamese population. Nat. Genet. *33*:412-415, 2003.

203. Mitchell, P. J., Jerrett, I. V., and Slee, K. J.: Skin ulcers caused by *Mycobacterium ulcerans* in koalas near Bairnsdale, Australia. Pathology *16*:256-260, 1984.

204. Mitsuda, K.: On the value of a skin reaction to a suspension of leprous nodules. Reprinted in English in Int. J. Lepr. Other Mycobact. Dis. *21*:347-358, 1953. (First published in Japanese: Hifuka Hinyoka Zasshi [Jpn. J. Dermatol. Urol.] *19*:697-708, 1919.)

205. Modlin, R. L., Brightbill, H. D., and Godowski, P. J.: The toll of innate immunity on microbial pathogens. N. Engl. J. Med. *340*:1834-1835, 1999.

206. Modlin, R. L., Gebhard, J. F., Taylor, C. R., et al.: *In situ* characterization of T lymphocyte subsets in the reactional states of leprosy. Clin. Exp. Immunol. *53*:17-24, 1983.

207. Modlin, R. L., Hofman, F. M., Horwitz, D. A., et al.: *In situ* identification of cells in human leprosy granulomas with monoclonal antibodies to interleukin 2 and its receptor. J. Immunol. *132*:3085-3090, 1984.

208. Modlin, R. L., Hofman, F. M., Taylor, C. R., et al.: T lymphocyte subsets in the skin lesions of patients with leprosy. J. Am. Acad. Dermatol. *8*:182-189, 1983.

209. Modlin, R. L., Melancon-Kaplan, J., Young, S. M., et al.: Learning from lesions: Patterns of tissue inflammation in leprosy. Proc. Natl. Acad. Sci. U. S. A. *85*:1213-1217, 1988.

210. Monot, M., Honore, N., Garnier, T., et al.: On the origin of leprosy. Science *308*:1040-1042, 2005.

211. Moran, C. A., Nelson, A. M., Tuur, S. M., et al.: Leprosy in five human immunodeficiency virus-infected patients. Mod. Pathol. *8*:662-664, 1995.

212. Moschella, S. L.: An update on the diagnosis and treatment of leprosy. J. Am. Acad. Dermatol. *51*:417-426, 2004.

213. Mourit, A. A. M.: The Path of the Destroyer, A History of Leprosy in the Hawaiian Islands. Honolulu, Honolulu Star-Bulletin, 1916.

214. Muir, E.: Juvenile leprosy. Int. J. Lepr. Other Mycobact. Dis. *4*:45-48, 1936.

215. Mukherjee, A., and Meyers, W. M.: Endothelial cell bacillation in lepromatous leprosy: A case report. Lepr. Rev. *58*:419-424, 1987.

216. Mve-Obiang, A., Lee, R. E., Portaels, F., et al.: Heterogeneity of mycolactones produced by clinical isolates of *Mycobacterium ulcerans*: Implications for virulence. Infect. Immun. *71*:774-783, 2003.

217. Myrvang, B., Godal, T., Ridley, D. S., et al.: Immune responsiveness to *Mycobacterium leprae* and other mycobacterial antigens throughout the clinical and histopathological spectrum of leprosy. Clin. Exp. Immunol. *14*:541-553, 1973.

218. Naafs, B.: Treatment of leprosy: Science or politics? Trop. Med. Int. Health *11*:268-278, 2006.

219. Navalkar, R. G., Norlin, M., and Ouchterlony, O.: Characterization of leprosy sera with various mycobacterial antigens using double diffusion-in-gel analysis. Int. Arch. Allergy *28*:250-260, 1965.

220. Nery, J. A., Perisse, A. R., Sales, A. M., et al.: The use of pentoxifylline in the treatment of type 2 reactional episodes in leprosy. Indian J. Lepr. *72*:457-467, 2000.

221. Nogueira, N., Kaplan, G., Levy, E., et al.: Defective gamma interferon production in leprosy: Reversal with antigen and interleukin 2. J. Exp. Med. *158*:2165-2170, 1983.

222. Noussitou, F. M.: Leprosy in Children. Geneva, World Health Organization, 1976.

223. Olcen, P., Harboe, M., Warndorff, T., et al.: Antigens of *Mycobacterium Leprae* and anti-*M. leprae* antibodies in the urine of leprosy patients. Lepr. Rev. *54*:203-216, 1983.

224. Oliveira, M. S., Fraga, A. G., Torrado, E., et al.: Infection with *Mycobacterium ulcerans* induces persistent inflammatory responses in mice. Infect. Immun. *73*:6299-6310, 2005.

225. Ottenhoff, T. H. M.: State of the Art Lectures. Immunology of leprosy: Lessons from and for leprosy. Int. J. Lepr. Other Mycobact. Dis. *62*:108-121, 1994.

226. Pahlevan, A. A., Wright, D. J., Andrews, C., et al.: The inhibitory action of *Mycobacterium ulcerans* soluble factor on monocyte/T cell cytokine production and NF-kappa B function. J. Immunol. *163*:3928-3935, 1999.

227. Palomino, J. C., Obiang, A. M., Realini, L., et al.: Effect of oxygen on growth of *Mycobacterium ulcerans* growth in the BACTEC system. J. Clin. Microbiol. *36*:3420-3422, 1998.

228. Park, J. Y., Cho, S. N., Youn, J. K., et al.: Detection of antibodies to human nerve antigens in sera from leprosy patients by ELISA. Clin. Exp. Immunol. *87*:368-372, 1992.

229. Parkash, O., Chaturvedi, V., Girdhar, B. K., et al.: A study on performance of two serological assays for diagnosis of leprosy patients. Lepr. Rev. *66*:26-30, 1995.

230. Pedley, J. C.: The presence of *M. leprae* in human milk. Lepr. Rev. *38*:239-242, 1967.

231. Pesce, C., Grattarola, M., Menini, S., et al.: Cyclooxygenase 2 expression in vessels and nerves in reversal reaction leprosy. Am. J. Trop. Med. Hyg. *74*:1076-1077, 2006.

232. Phanzu, D. M., Bafende, E. A., Dunda, B. K., et al.: *Mycobacterium ulcerans* disease (Buruli ulcer) in a rural hospital in Bas-Congo, Democratic Republic of Congo, 2002-2004. Am. J. Trop. Med. Hyg. *75*:311-314, 2006.

233. Pimsler, M., Sponsler, T. A., and Meyers, W. M.: Immunosuppressive properties of the soluble toxin from *Mycobacterium ulcerans*. J. Infect. Dis. *157*:577-580, 1988.

234. Pocaterra, L., Jain, S., Reddy, R., et al.: Clinical course of erythema nodosum leprosum: An 11-year cohort study in Hyderabad, India. Am. J. Trop. Med. Hyg. *74*:868-879, 2006.

235. Portaels, F.: Contribution a l'étude des mycobactéries de l'environnement au Bas-Zaire. Ann. Soc. Belge. Med. Trop. *53*:373-387, 1973.

236. Portaels, F., Aguiar, J., Debacker, M., et al.: Prophylactic effect of *Mycobacterium bovis* BCG vaccination against osteomyelitis in children with *Mycobacterium ulcerans* disease (Buruli ulcer). Clin. Diagn. Lab. Immunol. *9*:1389-1391, 2002.

237. Portaels, F., Aguiar, J., Debacker, M., et al.: *Mycobacterium bovis* BCG vaccination as prophylaxis against *Mycobacterium ulcerans* osteomyelitis in Buruli ulcer disease. Infect. Immun. *72*:62-65, 2004.

238. Portaels, F., Chemlal, K., Elsen, P., et al.: *Mycobacterium ulcerans* in wild animals. Rev. Sci. Tech. Off. Int. Epiz. *20*:252-264, 2001.

239. Portaels, F., Elsen, P., Guimares-Peres, A., et al.: Insects in the transmission of *Mycobacterium ulcerans*. Lancet *353*:986, 1999.

240. Portaels, F., Fonteyene, P. A., de Beenhouwer, H., et al.: Variability in 3′ end of 16S rRNA sequence of *Mycobacterium ulcerans* is related to geographic origin of isolates. J. Clin. Microbiol. *34*:962-965, 1996.

241. Prasad, H. K., Mishra, R. S., and Nath, I.: Phenolic glycolipid-I of *Mycobacterium leprae* induces general suppression of in vitro concanavalin A responses unrelated to leprosy type. J. Exp. Med. *165*:239-244, 1987.

242. Pszolla, N., Sarkar, M. R., Strecker, W., et al.: Buruli ulcer: A systemic disease. Clin. Infect. Dis. *37*:e78-e82, 2003.

243. Rambukkana, A., Yamada, H., Zanazzi, G., et al.: Role of alpha-dystroglycan as a Schwann cell receptor for *Mycobacterium leprae*. Science *282*:2076-2079, 1998.

244. Rangdaeng, S., Scollard, D. M., Suriyanon, V., et al.: Studies of human leprosy lesions in situ using suction-induced blisters, 1: Cellular components of new, uncomplicated lesions. Int. J. Lepr. Other Mycobact. Dis. *57*:492-498, 1989.

245. Ranque, B., Alcais, A., Thuc, N. V., et al.: A recessive major gene controls the Mitsuda reaction in a region endemic for leprosy. J. Infect. Dis. *192*:1475-1482, 2005.

246. Rea, T. H., Bakke, A. C., Parker, J. W., et al.: Peripheral blood T lymphocyte subsets in leprosy. Int. J. Lepr. Other Mycobact. Dis. *52*:311-317, 1984.

247. Rea, T. H., and Jerskey, R. S.: Clinical and histologic variations among thirty patients with Lucio's phenomenon and pure and primitive diffuse lepromatosis (Latapi's lepromatosis). Int. J. Lepr. Other Mycobact. Dis. *73*:169-188, 2005.

248. Read, J. K., Heggie, C. M., Meyers, W. M., et al.: Cytotoxic activity of *Mycobacterium ulcerans*. Infect. Immun. *9*:1114-1122, 1974.

249. Recommendations of the International Task Force for Disease Eradication. M. M. W. R. Recomm. Rep. *42*(RR-16):1-38, 1993.

250. Rees, R. J. W., and McDougall, A. C.: Airborne infection with *Mycobacterium leprae* in mice. J. Med. Microbiol. *10*:63-68, 1977.

251. Revill, W. D. L., and Barker, D. J. P.: Seasonal distribution of mycobacterial skin ulcers. Br. J. Prev. Soc. Med. *26*:23-27, 1972.

252. Ridley, D. S.: Skin Biopsy in Leprosy. 2nd ed. Basel, Geigy, 1985.

253. Ridley, D. S., and Jopling, W. H.: Classification of leprosy according to immunity: A five-group system. Int. J. Lepr. Other Mycobact. Dis. *34*:255-273, 1966.

254. Roche, P. W., Theuvenet, W. L., and Britton, W. J.: Risk factors for type-1 reactions in borderline leprosy patients. Lancet *338*:654-657, 1991.

255. Rogall, T., Wolters, J., Flohr, T., et al.: Towards a phylogeny and definition of species at the molecular level within the genus *Mycobacterium*. Int. J. Syst. Bacteriol. *40*:323-330, 1990.

256. Rojas-Espinosa, O., and Løvik, M.: *Mycobacterium leprae* and *Mycobacterium lepraemurium* in domestic and wild animals. Rev. Sci. Tech. Off. Int. Epiz. *20*:219-251, 2001.

257. Rondini, S., Mensah-Quainoo, E., Troll, H., et al.: Development and application of real-time PCR assay for quantification of *Mycobacterium ulcerans* DNA. J. Clin. Microbiol. *41*:4231-4237, 2003.

258. Rook, G. A., Martinelli, R., and Brunet, L. R.: Innate immune responses to mycobacteria and the downregulation of atopic responses. Curr. Opin. Allergy Clin. Immunol. *3*:337-342, 2003.

259. Rook, G. A. W.: The immunology of leprosy. Tubercle *64*:297-312, 1983.

260. Ross, B. C., Johnson, P. D., Oppedisano, F., et al.: Detection of *Mycobacterium ulcerans* in environmental samples during an outbreak of ulcerative disease. Appl. Environ. Microbiol. *63*:4135-4138, 1997.

261. Ross, B. C., Marino, L., Oppedisano, F., et al.: Development of a PCR assay for rapid diagnosis of *Mycobacterium ulcerans* infection. J. Clin. Microbiol. *35*:1696-1700, 1997.

262. Roy, S., McGuire, W., Mascie-Taylor, C. G., et al.: Tumor necrosis factor promoter polymorphism and susceptibility to lepromatous leprosy. J. Infect. Dis. *176*:530-532, 1997.

263. Ruffer, M. A.: Pott'sche Krankeit an Einer Ägyptischen Mumie aus der Zeit der 21 Dynastie (um 1000 v. Chr.). Zur Historischen Biol d Krankheitserreger. Vol. 3. Giessen, Topelmann, 1910.

264. Ryrie, G. A.: Some impressions of Sungei Buloh Leper Hospital under Japanese occupation. Lepr. Rev. *18*:10-17, 1947.

265. Sabin, T. D., Swift, T. R., and Jacobson, R. R.: Peripheral Neuropathy. Philadelphia, W. B. Saunders, 1993.

266. Salgame, P., Abrams, J. S., Clayberger, C., et al.: Differing lymphokine profiles of functional subsets of human CD4 and CD8 T cell clones. Science *254*:279-282, 1991.

267. Sampaio, E. P., Caneshi, J. R., Nery, J. A., et al.: Cellular immune response to *Mycobacterium leprae* infection in human immunodeficiency virus-infected individuals. Infect. Immun. *63*:1848-1854, 1995.

268. Santos, A. R., Suffys, P. N., Vanderborght, P. R., et al.: Role of tumor necrosis factor-alpha and interleukin-10 promoter gene polymorphisms in leprosy. J. Infect. Dis. *186*:1687-1691, 2002.

269. Sarno, E. N., Grau, G. E., Vieira, L. M., et al.: Serum levels of tumour necrosis factor-alpha and interleukin-1 beta during leprosy reactional states. Clin. Exp. Immunol. *84*:103-108, 1991.

270. Saul, A., and Novales, J.: La lèpre de Lucio-Latapi et le phénomène de Lucio. Acta Leprol. *92*:115-132, 1983.

271. Schlesinger, L. S., and Horwitz, M. A.: Complement receptors and complement component C3 mediate phagocytosis of *Mycobacterium tuberculosis* and *Mycobacterium leprae*. Int. J. Lepr. Other Mycobact. Dis. *58*:200-201, 1990.

272. Scollard, D. M.: Endothelial cells and the pathogenesis of lepromatous neuritis: Insights from the armadillo model. Microbes Infect. *2*:1835-1843, 2000.

273. Scollard, D. M., Adams, L. B., Gillis, T. P., et al.: The continuing challenges of leprosy. Clin. Microbiol. Rev. *19*:338-381, 2006.

274. Scollard, D. M., Joyce, M. P., and Gillis, T. P.: Development of leprosy and type 1 leprosy reactions after treatment with infliximab: A report of 2 cases. Clin. Infect. Dis. *43*:e19-e22, 2006.

275. Scollard, D. M., McCormick, G., and Allen, J. L.: Localization of *Mycobacterium leprae* to endothelial cells of epineurial and perineurial blood vessels and lymphatics. Am. J. Pathol. *154*:1611-1620, 1999.

276. Sekar, B., Jayasheela, M., Chattopadhya, D., et al.: Prevalence of HIV infection and high-risk characteristics among leprosy patients of south India: A case-control study. Int. J. Lepr. Other Mycobact. Dis. *62*:527-531, 1994.

277. Semret, M., Koromihis, G., MacLean, J. D., et al.: *Mycobacterium ulcerans* infection (Buruli ulcer): First reported case in a traveler. Am. J. Trop. Med. Hyg. *61*:689-693, 1999.

278. Sethi, S. K., Solanki, R. S., and Mendiratta, V.: Leprotic nerve abcess. Appl. Radiol. *35*:44-47, 2006.

279. Shaw, M. A., Donaldson, I. J., Collins, A., et al.: Association and linkage of leprosy phenotypes with HLA class II and tumour necrosis factor genes. Genes Immun. *2*:196-204, 2001.

280. Shepard, C. C.: The experimental disease that follows the injection of human leprosy into footpads of mice. J. Exp. Med. *112*:445-454, 1960.

281. Shepard, C. C.: Combinations involving dapsone, rifampicin, clofazimine and ethionamide in the treatment of *M. leprae* infections in mice. Int. J. Lepr. Other Mycobact. Dis. *44*:135-139, 1976.

282. Shields, E. D., Russell, D. A., and Pericak-Vance, M. A.: Genetic epidemiology of the susceptibility to leprosy. J. Clin. Invest. *79*:1139-1143, 1987.

283. Shimoji, Y., Ng, V., Matsumura, K., et al.: A 21-kDa surface protein of *Mycobacterium leprae* binds peripheral nerve laminin-2 and mediates Schwann cell invasion. Proc. Natl. Acad. Sci. U. S. A. *96*:9857-9862, 1999.

284. Siddiqui, M. R., Meisner, S., Tosh, K., et al.: A major susceptibility locus for leprosy in India maps to chromosome 10p13. Nat. Genet. *27*:439-441, 2001.

285. Siegmund, V., Adjei, O., Racz, P., et al.: Dry-reagent-based PCR as a novel tool for laboratory confirmation of clinically diagnosed *Mycobacterium ulcerans*-associated disease in areas in the tropics where *M. ulcerans* is endemic. J. Clin. Microbiol. *43*:271-276, 2005.

286. Singh, N. B., Srivastava, A., Verma, V. K., et al.: *Mastomys natalensis*: A new animal model for *Mycobacterium ulcerans* research. Indian J. Exp. Biol. *22*:393-394, 1984.

287. Sizaire, V., Nackers, F., Comte, E., et al.: *Mycobacterium ulcerans* infection: Control, diagnosis, and treatment. Lancet Infect. Dis. *6*:288-296, 2006.

288. Skinsnes, O. K.: Leprosy in society, II: The pattern of concept and reaction to leprosy in Oriental antiquity. Lepr. Rev. *35*:106-122, 1964.

289. Skinsnes, O. K., and Higa, L. H.: The role of protein malnutrition in the pathogenesis of ulcerative "lazarine" leprosy. Int. J. Lepr. Other Mycobact. Dis. *44*:346-358, 1976.

290. Smith, J. H., Folse, D. S., Long, E. G., et al.: Leprosy in wild armadillos (*Dasypus novemcinctus*) of the Texas Gulf Coast: Epidemiology and mycobacteriology. J. Reticuloendothel. Soc. *34*:75-88, 1983.

291. Smith, W. C. S.: We need to know what is happening to the incidence of leprosy [editorial]. Lepr. Rev. *68*:195-200, 1997.

292. Stanford, J. L.: Biology of the Mycobacteria. New York, Academic Press, 1983.

293. Stanford, J. L., Rook, G. A., Bahr, G. M., et al.: *Mycobacterium vaccae* in immunoprophylaxis and immunotherapy of leprosy and tuberculosis. Vaccine *8*:525-530, 1990.

294. Stienstra, Y., Dijkstra, P. U., Van Wezel, M. J., et al.: Reliability and validity of the Buruli ulcer functional limitation score questionnaire. Am. J. Trop. Med. Hyg. *72*:449-452, 2005.

295. Stienstra, Y., van der Werf, T. S., Oosterom, E., et al.: Susceptibility to Buruli ulcer is associated with the SLC11A1 (NRAMP1) D543N polymorphism. Genes Immun. *7*:185-189, 2006.

296. Stinear, T., Davies, J. K., Jenkin, G. A., et al.: Identification of *Mycobacterium ulcerans* in the environment from regions in Southeast Australia in which it is endemic with sequence capture-PCR. Appl. Environ. Microbiol. *66*:3206-3213, 2000.

297. Stinear, T., Ross, B. C., Davies, J. K., et al.: Identification and characterization of IS2404 and IS2606: Two distinct repeated sequences for detection of *Mycobacterium ulcerans* by PCR. J. Clin. Microbiol. *37*:1018-1023, 1999.

298. Stinear, T. P., Hong, H., Frigui, W., et al.: Common evolutionary origin for the unstable virulence plasmid pMUM found in geographically diverse strains of *Mycobacterium ulcerans*. J. Bacteriol. *187*:1668-1676, 2005.

299. Stinear, T. P., Mve-Obiang, A., Small, P. L., et al.: Giant plasmid-encoded polyketide synthases produce the macrolide toxin of *Mycobacterium ulcerans*. Proc. Natl. Acad. Sci. U. S. A. *101*:1345-1349, 2004.

300. Stragier, P., Ablordey, A., Bayonne, L. M., et al.: Heterogeneity among *Mycobacterium ulcerans* isolates from Africa. Emerg. Infect. Dis. *12*:844-847, 2006.

301. Sung, K. J., Kim, S. B., Choi, J. H., et al.: Detection of *Mycobacterium leprae* DNA in formalin-fixed, paraffin-embedded samples from multibacillary and paucibacillary leprosy patients by polymerase chain reaction. Int. J. Dermatol. *32*:710-713, 1993.

302. Talhari, S., Orsi, A. T., Talhari, A. C., et al.: Pentoxifylline may be useful in the treatment of type 2 leprosy reaction. Lepr. Rev. *66*:261-263, 1995.

303. Toll, A., Gallardo, F., Ferran, M., et al.: Aggressive multifocal Buruli ulcer with associated osteomyelitis in an HIV-positive patient. Clin. Exp. Dermatol. *30*:649-651, 2005.

304. Tripathy, S. R.: BCG trial in leprosy. Indian J. Lepr. *56*:686-687, 1984.

305. Truman, R.: Leprosy in wild armadillos. Lepr. Rev. *76*:198-208, 2005.

306. Truman, R. W., Job, C. K., and Hastings, R. C.: Antibodies to the phenolic glycolipid-1 antigen for epidemiologic investigations of enzootic leprosy in armadillos (*Dasypus novemcinctus*). Lepr. Rev. *61*:19-24, 1990.

307. Truman, R. W., Kumaresan, J. A., McDonough, C. M., et al.: Seasonal and spatial trends in the detectability of leprosy in wild armadillos. Epidemiol. Infect. *106*:549-560, 1991.

308. Tsukamura, M., Kaneda, K., Imaeda, T., et al.: [A taxonomic study on a mycobacterium which caused a skin ulcer in a Japanese girl and resembled *Mycobacterium ulcerans*]. Kekkaku *64*:691-697, 1989.

309. Turk, J. L.: Cell-mediated immunological processes in leprosy. Lepr. Rev. *41*:207-222 1970.

310. Uganda Buruli Group: BCG vaccination against *Mycobacterium ulcerans* infection (Buruli ulcer). Lancet *1*:111-115, 1969.

311. Uganda Buruli Group: Clinical features and treatment of pre-ulcerative Buruli lesions (*Mycobacterium ulcerans* infection) B. M. J. *2*:390-393, 1970.

312. Ustianowski, A. P., Lawn, S. D., and Lockwood, D. N.: Interactions between HIV infection and leprosy: A paradox. Lancet Infect. Dis. *6*:350-360, 2006.

313. Valla, M. C.: Lèpre et grossesse. Lyon, France, Thèse de Médicine, 1976.

314. Valverde, C. R., Canfield, D., Tarara, R., et al.: Spontaneous leprosy in a wild-caught cynomolgus macaque. Int. J. Lepr. Other Mycobact. Dis. *66*:140-148, 1998.

315. van Beers, S. M., Izumi, S., Madjid, B., et al.: An epidemiological study of leprosy infection by serology and polymerase chain reaction. Int. J. Lepr. Other Mycobact. Dis. *62*:1-9, 1994.

316. van der Werf, T. S., Stienstra, Y., Johnson, R. C., et al.: *Mycobacterium ulcerans* disease. Bull. World Health Organ. *83*:785-791, 2005.

317. vanEden, W., deVries, R. R., D'Amaro, J., et al.: HLA-DR-associated genetic control of the type of leprosy in a population from Surinam. Hum. Immunol. *4*:343-350, 1982.

318. Veitch, M. G., Johnson, P. D., Flood, P. E., et al.: A large localized outbreak of *Mycobacterium ulcerans* infection on a temperate southern Australian island. Epidemiol. Infect. *119*:313-318, 1997.

319. Vettom, L., and Pritze, S.: Reliability of skin smear results: Experiences with quality control of skin smears in different routine services in leprosy control programmes. Lepr. Rev. *60*:187-196, 1989.

320. Villahermosa, L. G., Abalos, R. M., Walsh, D. S., et al.: Recombinant interleukin-2 in lepromatous leprosy lesions: Immunological and microbiological consequences. Clin. Exp. Dermatol. *22*:134-140, 1997.

321. Villahermosa, L. G., Fajardo, T. T., Jr., Abalos, R. M., et al.: Parallel assessment of 24 monthly doses of rifampin, ofloxacin, and minocycline versus two years of World Health Organization multi-drug therapy for multi-bacillary leprosy. Am. J. Trop. Med. Hyg. *70*:197-200, 2004.

322. Villahermosa, L. G., Fajardo, T. T., Jr., Abalos, R. M., et al.: A randomized, double-blind, double-dummy, controlled dose comparison of thalidomide for treatment of erythema nodosum leprosum. Am. J. Trop. Med. Hyg. *72*:518-526, 2005.

323. Wabitsch, K. R., and Meyers, W. M.: Histopathologic observations on the persistence of *Mycobacterium leprae* in the skin of multibacillary leprosy patients under chemotherapy. Lepr. Rev. *59*:341-346, 1988.

324. Wade, H. W.: The histoid variety of lepromatous leprosy. Int. J. Lepr. Other Mycobact. Dis. *31*:129-142, 1963.

325. Walsh, D. S., dela Cruz, E. C., Abalos, R. M., et al.: Clinical and histological features of skin lesions in a cynomolgus monkey experimentally infected with *Mycobacterium ulcerans* (Buruli ulcer) by intradermal inoculation. Am. J. Trop. Med. Hyg. 76:132-134, 2007.

326. Walsh, D. S., Lane, J. E., Abalos, R. M., et al.: TUNEL and limited immunophenotypic analyses of apoptosis in paucibacillary and multibacillary leprosy lesions. F. E. M. S. Immunol. Med. Microbiol. *41*:265-269, 2004.

327. Walsh, D. S., Meyers, W. M., Krieg, R. E., et al.: Transmission of *Mycobacterium ulcerans* to the nine-banded armadillo. Am. J. Trop. Med. Hyg. 61:694-697, 1999.

328. Walsh, D. S., Meyers, W. M., Portaels, F., et al.: High rates of apoptosis in human *Mycobacterium ulcerans* culture-positive Buruli ulcer skin lesions. Am. J. Trop. Med. Hyg. *73*:410-415, 2005.

329. Walsh, D. S., Prieto-Go, D., Abalos, R. M., et al.: Malignant T-cell lymphoma mimicking lepromatous leprosy. Clin. Exp. Dermatol. *26*:173-175, 2001.

330. Walsh, D. S., Villahermosa, L. G., Balagon, M. V., et al.: Cutaneous delayed-type hypersensitivity responsiveness in lepromatous and borderline lepromatous leprosy patients as determined by MULTITEST CMI. Southeast Asian J. Trop. Med. Public Health *30*:518-526, 1999.

331. Walsh, G. P., Meyers, W. M., and Binford, C. H.: Naturally acquired leprosy in the nine-banded armadillo: A decade of experience 1975-1985. J. Leukoc. Biol. *40*:645-656, 1986.

332. Walsh, G. P., Meyers, W. M., and Binford, C. H., et al.: Leprosy as a zoonosis: An update. Acta Leprol. 6:51-60, 1988.

333. Walsh, G. P., Storrs, E. E., Burchfield, H. P., et al.: Leprosy-like disease occurring naturally in armadillos. J. Reticuloendothel. Soc. *18*:347-351, 1975.

334. Walsh, G. P., Storrs, E. E., Meyers, W. M., et al.: Naturally acquired leprosy-like disease in the nine-banded armadillo (*Dasypus novemcinctus*): Recent epizootiologic findings. J. Reticuloendothel. Soc. 22:363-367, 1977.

335. Wansbrough-Jones, M., and Phillips, R.: Buruli ulcer: Emerging from obscurity. Lancet *367*:1849-1858, 2006.

336. Warndorff Van Diepen, T.: Clofazimine-resistant leprosy, a case report. Int. J. Lepr. Other Mycobact. Dis. *50*:139-142, 1982.

337. Waters, M. F. R.: The diagnosis and management of dapsone-resistant leprosy. Lepr. Rev. *48*:95-105, 1977.

338. Waters, M. F. R.: The treatment of leprosy. Tubercle *64*:221-232, 1983.

339. Waters, M. F. R.: Relapse following various types of multidrug therapy in multibacillary leprosy [editorial]. Lepr. Rev. 66:1-9, 1995.

340. Welsh, O., Gomez, M., Mancias, C., et al.: A new therapeutic approach to type II leprosy reaction. Int J. Dermatol. *38*:931-933, 1999.

341. West, B. C., Todd, J. R., Lary, C. H., et al.: Leprosy in six isolated residents of northern Louisiana: Time-clustered cases in an essentially nonendemic area. Arch. Intern. Med. *148*:1987-1992, 1988.

342. Williams, D. L., and Gillis, T. P.: A study of the relatedness of *Mycobacterium leprae* isolates using restriction fragment length polymorphism analysis. Acta Leprol 7(Suppl. 1):226-230, 1989.

343. Williams, D. L., and Gillis, T. P.: Molecular detection of drug resistance in *Mycobacterium leprae*. Lepr. Rev. *75*:118-130, 2004.

344. Williams, D. L., Gillis, T. P., Booth, R. J., et al.: The use of a specific DNA probe and polymerase chain reaction for the detection of *Mycobacterium leprae*. J. Infect. Dis. *162*:193-200, 1990.

345. Williams, D. L., Waguespack, C., Eisenach, K., et al.: Characterization of rifampin-resistance in pathogenic mycobacteria. Antimicrob. Agents Chemother. *38*:2380-2386, 1994.

346. Wolf, R. H., Gormus, B. J., Martin, L. N., et al.: Experimental leprosy in three species of monkeys. Science *227*:529-531, 1985.

347. World Health Organization: Expert Committee on Leprosy. World Health Organ. Tech. Rep. Ser. No. 607. Geneva, W. H. O., 1977.

348. World Health Organization: Chemotherapy of leprosy for control programmes. World Health Organ. Tech. Rep. Ser. No. 675. Geneva, W. H. O., 1982.

349. World Health Organization: Leprosy—global situation. Wkly. Epidemiol. Rec. No. 28 (July 14). Geneva, W. H. O., 2000.

350. World Health Organization: Provisional guidance on the role of specific antibiotics in the management of *Mycobacterium ulcerans* disease (Buruli ulcer) (WHO/CDS/CPE/GBUI/2004). Geneva, W. H. O., 2004.

351. World Health Organization: World Health Assembly, Seventh Plenary Meeting (A57/VR/7). Geneva, W. H. O., 2004.

352. World Health Organization: Global Leprosy Situation. Geneva, W. H. O., 2006.

353. World Health Organization; Asiedu, K., Scherpbier, R., and Raviglione, M. (eds.): Buruli Ulcer: *Mycobacterium ulcerans* Infection (WHO/CDS/CPE/GBUI/2000.1). Geneva, W. H. O., 2000.

354. World Health Organization; Buntine, J., and Croft, K. (eds.): The Management of *Mycobacterium ulcerans* Disease (Buruli Ulcer) (WHO/CDS/CPE/GBUI/2001.2). Geneva, W. H. O., 2001.

355. World Health Organization; Portaels, F., Johnson, P. D. R., and Meyers, W. M. (eds.): Diagnosis of *Mycobacterium ulcerans* Disease (Buruli Ulcer) (WHO/CDS/CPE/GBUI/2001.3). Geneva, W. H. O., 2001.

356. Yamamura, M., Uyemura, K., Deans, R. J., et al.: Defining protective responses to pathogens: Cytokine profiles in leprosy lesions. Science *254*:277-279, 1991.

357. Young, D. B., Harnisch, J. P., Knight, J., et al.: Detection of phenolic glycolipid I in sera from patients with lepromatous leprosy. J. Infect. Dis. *152*:1078-1081, 1985.

CHAPTER

110

NOCARDIA

Nada Harik ✪ Richard F. Jacobs

Nocardia spp. are obligate aerobic bacilli that exist throughout the world as soil and dust saprotrophs. These organisms are non–spore-forming, thin, branching, gram-positive, partially acid-fast, filamentous bacteria. Humans become infected with *Nocardia* by two primary routes: inhalation of contaminated airborne dust particles or traumatic implantation of the bacterium into subcutaneous tissue. Pulmonary disease is the form of nocardiosis recognized most commonly in the United States.[2] The pulmonary event may be subclinical or transient, or it may provoke an acute or chronic process mimicking staphylococcal or fungal pneumonia, tuberculosis, or carcinoma. Hematogenous dissemination may occur, especially in immunocompromised hosts. The central nervous system (CNS) is the most common site of dissemination, with involvement manifested most often as a brain abscess. Cutaneous nocardiosis may be acute, subacute, or chronic. This form of disease is seen predominantly in immunocompetent hosts, with *Nocardia brasiliensis* being the agent identified most frequently.

In 1888, Nocard, a veterinarian, noted an aerobic actinomycete in bovine farcy, a chronic wasting disease in cattle characterized by pulmonary abscesses and draining cutaneous sinus tracts. Eppinger first described human disease in 1890. The earliest pediatric case was documented in 1895 in a boy with pulmonary and subcutaneous infection.[5]

ORGANISM

Nocardia spp. are included among the aerobic actinomycetes. They are gram-positive bacteria that are filamentous and branched and grow more slowly than other aerobic and facultatively anaerobic bacteria. They commonly produce a fungus-like mycelium that fragments or breaks up into rod-shaped and short coccoid forms. *Nocardia* spp. grow well aerobically on a variety of simple media (e.g., blood agar, brain-heart infusion agar); adding carbon dioxide (10%) promotes more rapid growth. The organisms are inhibited by antibiotics and antifungal agents, so media containing such agents do not support the growth of *Nocardia*. Because of their growth on commonly used fungal media (e.g., Sabouraud dextrose agar) and on some mycobacterial media (e.g.,

Löwenstein-Jensen medium), many *Nocardia* samples may be misdirected to the mycology or mycobacteriology section of clinical laboratories for identification.

In the past, microscopic and colonial morphology, biochemical tests, chemotaxonomic methods, or antimicrobial susceptibility patterns were used to speciate *Nocardia.* 16S rRNA gene sequencing and polymerase chain reaction (PCR) restriction fragment length polymorphism (RFLP) analysis are the current methods most frequently used for speciation; use of these molecular techniques has resulted in changes in the nomenclature of *Nocardia* spp.[10,44]

More than 30 species of *Nocardia* of human clinical significance have been identified.[10] The term *Nocardia asteroides* complex formerly was used to account for the heterogeneity in antimicrobial resistance patterns seen among *N. asteroides.* Detailed molecular analyses and susceptibility testing have established clearly that *N. asteroides* complex represented many different *Nocardia* spp.[10] The most medically important species of *Nocardia* include *N. asteroides, Nocardia abscessus, Nocardia brevicatena/paucivorans* complex, *Nocardia farcinica, Nocardia nova* complex, *Nocardia brasiliensis, Nocardia otitidiscaviarum* complex, *Nocardia pseudobrasiliensis,* and *Nocardia transvalensis* complex.

Nocardia spp. grow best at temperatures of 25° C to 45° C; growth at higher temperatures may be used for differentiation. In pure culture, small, chalky white, heaped, wrinkled, or verrucous colonies appear in 3 to 5 days. Mature colonies usually are light orange and have a velvety appearance caused by the production of rudimentary aerial mycelia. They have the odor of a musty basement or freshly turned soil. Detection of colonies from clinical specimens, such as respiratory secretions, may require 2 to 4 weeks. In mixed culture, rapidly growing bacteria may obscure small *Nocardia* colonies. Use of modified Thayer-Martin medium may enhance recovery.[39]

Gram stain of a portion of a colony shows delicate, branching filaments no more than 1 μm in diameter. The delicate filaments may fragment and produce bacillary or coccoid forms. Many *Nocardia* spp. are partially acid-fast (i.e., compared with *Mycobacterium* spp., they retain fuchsin less tenaciously). A modified Ziehl-Neelsen or Kinyoun stain that decolorizes with 1 percent sulfuric acid instead of the more active acid alcohol is best for showing acid-fast *Nocardia* in clinical specimens. Acid-fastness is characteristic of *Nocardia* in tissue or primary colonial isolates but is lost quickly on subculture; not all pathogenic strains of *Nocardia* are acid-fast.[6] *N. asteroides* often survives the N-acetylcysteine digestion procedure (without sodium hydroxide) that is performed on sputum or bronchial washings; however, some positive sputum specimens may be rendered falsely negative.[38] Cultures of sputum and bronchial washings for isolation of *Nocardia* should be performed before and after the digestion procedure.

EPIDEMIOLOGY, TRANSMISSION, AND PATHOGENESIS

Nocardia spp. occasionally can be skin contaminants or upper respiratory tract saprotrophs.[21,44,53] Bronchial obstruction or decreased bronchociliary clearance predisposes to colonization.[44] The presence of signs and symptoms that correlate with nocardiosis can help ascertain the clinical significance of a positive *Nocardia* culture.

Most infections occur in the lungs, presumably via inhalation, with dissemination to the CNS occurring in one third of affected patients. Although nocardiosis occurs in immunocompetent individuals, 70 percent of patients are immunosuppressed by medications or underlying disease.[23] The typical patient has compromised cellular immunity (secondary to steroids, organ transplantation, cytotoxic chemotherapy, chronic granulomatous disease, chronic

alcoholism, diabetes mellitus, or human immunodeficiency virus [HIV] infection). Nocardiosis also is seen more commonly in patients with chronic pulmonary disease or a history of surgery or trauma.[35] Person-to-person communicability has not been a problem. The incidence of nocardiosis in the United States has been estimated to be approximately 500 to 1000 new cases per year.[3] This number most likely is an underrepresentation, however, given the marked increase in the number of immunocompromised individuals. In addition, nocardial infections can be difficult to recognize, resulting in underestimation of the true incidence of nocardiosis. Presumed nosocomial nocardiosis has been reported.

Cutaneous nocardiosis usually is an infection of immunocompetent hosts. *N. brasiliensis* is isolated from approximately 80 percent of cases of primary cutaneous or subcutaneous nocardiosis.[46] Traumatic implantation of aerobic actinomycetes into deep subcutaneous tissue may result in an indolent condition termed *actinomycotic mycetoma* (to distinguish it from the eumycotic mycetomas caused by true fungi). Mycetoma is a chronic, progressive infection that can extend to underlying bone. Actinomycotic mycetomas usually involve the lower extremities or hands and typically are caused by *Actinomadura* spp., non–acid-fast aerobic actinomycetes, or *Streptomyces* spp. Actinomycotic mycetomas caused by *Nocardia* frequently involve the chest and back. Mycetomas, the cause of which may be *N. brasiliensis,* have been described in Mexican and South American field workers. This *Nocardia* spp. also has been documented as an opportunistic pathogen prevalent in Florida, with a predilection for diabetics.[49]

In addition to the classic mycetoma, traumatic introduction of *Nocardia* spp. from soil may result in wound infections that occur after a more acute or subacute course. Over a 5-year period, 31 cases of localized cutaneous nocardiosis with *N. brasiliensis* were identified in immunocompetent children in South Texas.[19] The organism can be introduced into the skin by tick[31] and other insect bites[19,41] or by a cat scratch,[19,45] and result in cellulitis, pustules, or pyoderma; these conditions occasionally disseminate in immunocompromised individuals.[26,27] Post-traumatic endophthalmitis[20] and post-sternotomy mediastinitis[54,61] have been described.

Nocardiosis previously was considered a rare disease in humans; however, it is being recognized more frequently.[37] It has been diagnosed in individuals ranging from 4 weeks to 82 years of age, and, except in cases of cutaneous nocardiosis, almost all patients have one or more severe underlying diseases (e.g., lupus erythematosus, asthma, glomerulonephritis, ulcerative colitis, bronchiectasis, tuberculosis, rheumatoid arthritis, sarcoidosis). Patients with lymphoreticular neoplasms and transplant recipients seem to be particularly at risk. In addition, the risk of acquiring infection is increased in patients with chronic pulmonary disease and in any patient who is receiving long-term corticosteroid treatment. Infliximab treatment has been associated with the development of nocardial infection.[60] Severe infection with this catalase-positive organism may develop in children with chronic granulomatous disease.[24] Although *Nocardia* is not a surveillance organism for acquired immunodeficiency syndrome (AIDS), patients with AIDS may contract nocardiosis.[25] In a review of all cases (*n* = 25) of nocardiosis at an urban adult teaching hospital from 1999 to 2004, 76 percent of patients with nocardiosis also were infected with HIV; all had CD4+ counts less than 100 cells/mm[3].[12]

In a retrospective review of cases of pediatric nocardiosis admitted to Arkansas Children's Hospital, 5 children with nocardiosis were identified from more than 100,000 admissions in a 10-year period. Four of the five patients had received a transplant within the previous year. Three of these patients had pulmonary disease caused by *N. asteroides,* and one transplant recipient had skin involvement with *N. brasiliensis* at a central venous line site.

One immunocompetent 5-year-old boy contracted CNS infection caused by *N. asteroides* 2 months after incurring a penetrating brain injury.[22]

N. farcinica is a medically important pathogen.[48,59] In a series of 200 cases of *Nocardia* infection reported by Wallace and associates,[59] the isolates designated *N. farcinica* were from patients with severe illness, 56 percent of whom had disseminated infections. *N. farcinica* isolates were characterized by increased resistance to antimicrobials, specifically third-generation cephalosporins. Evidence from mouse models also indicates that *N. farcinica* seems to be more virulent than are other *Nocardia* spp.[16] Because the various species of *Nocardia* seem to have different pathogenicities, determination of the infecting species of *Nocardia* is important.

The immune response to *Nocardia* is multifaceted.[2] Neutrophils are mobilized to the site of infection and are the predominant cell type found in lesions. Neutrophils only inhibit the organisms, however, and limit the spread of infection until an adequate cell-mediated immune response develops, or until effective antimicrobial agents are administered. Immune T cells are vital in clearing *Nocardia* from the lung and preventing dissemination; many predisposing conditions for nocardiosis involve inadequate cell-mediated immunity. Activated macrophages induce cytotoxic T cells effective against *N. asteroides*. *Nocardia* may survive inside neutrophils and macrophages by inhibiting phagosome-lysosome fusion and by the production of catalase and superoxide dismutase, which inactivate the myeloperoxidase system. *Nocardia* organisms exhibit a differential ability to evade phagosome-lysosome fusion that depends on their state of growth, possibly related to specific cell wall mycolic acids detected only in log-phase cells.[4] Differential cell wall characteristics also may influence the ability of *Nocardia* organisms to exhibit specific organ tropism (e.g., the brain).[7] Antibody may play a role in host defense through enhancement of macrophage activities. Although antecedent conditions of nocardiosis frequently involve dysfunctional cellular immunity, other preconditions include neutrophil and immunoglobulin disorders.

PATHOLOGY

The lesions of nocardiosis are suppurative, whether in the lung or in subcutaneous tissue, and they involve primarily proliferation of neutrophils rather than formation of granulomas. Pulmonary nocardiosis in immunocompetent patients often resembles pulmonary actinomycosis in that it results in a chronic localized pneumonia that often abuts the pleura.[23] Indolent progressive fibrosis resembling fibronodular tuberculosis may occur. Nocardiosis is more aggressive in immunocompromised patients and is manifested as multifocal necrotizing pneumonia with confluent abscess formation. *Nocardia* spp. tend to invade the pleura and chest wall, with tissue planes disregarded in the process. Little evidence of encapsulation is characteristic of all organs invaded and probably accounts for the ready dissemination of organisms from the initial pulmonary focus.

N. asteroides organisms appear as delicate, beaded, branching filaments in tissue stained with Gram stain or modified acid-fast stain (Fig. 110–1). *Nocardia* spp. are invisible in hematoxylin and eosin preparations or in sections stained with periodic acid–Schiff for fungi. Methenamine silver preparations sometimes detect tissue organisms; overstaining with silver enhances visualization.

CLINICAL MANIFESTATIONS AND DIAGNOSIS

The most common manifestation of nocardiosis (>40% of all cases) in the United States is pulmonary disease in a patient with underlying immunosuppression.[14,42,44] Infection may remain

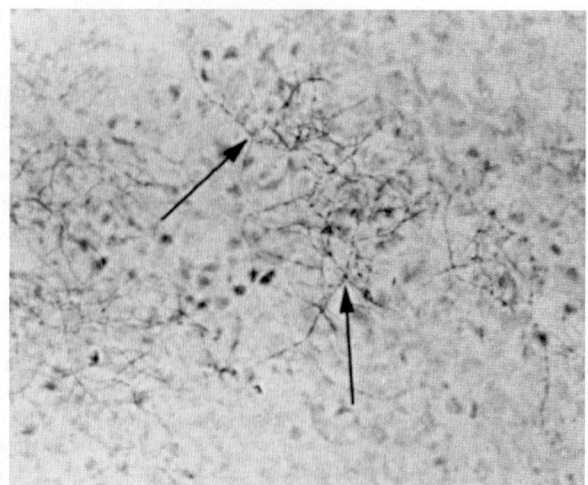

Figure 110–1 Appearance of *Nocardia asteroides* and *Nocardia brasiliensis (arrows)* in a properly decolorized acid-fast smear. Organisms appear as fragmented bacilli with stain concentrated in a beaded fashion along portions of the filaments (×160).

localized to the lung or may disseminate hematogenously to the CNS and skin and, more rarely, to almost any organ in the body. In high-risk patients, the diagnosis should be suspected when CNS manifestations, particularly signs of a brain tumor, abscess, or soft tissue swelling, develop in conjunction with a current or recent subacute or chronic pulmonary infection. Although sulfonamides are the most effective drugs for treatment of nocardiosis, invasive infections have been described in immunocompromised individuals receiving oral trimethoprim-sulfamethoxazole (TMP-SMX) as prophylaxis for *Pneumocystis* pneumonia[58] and in patients with chronic granulomatous disease who are receiving TMP-SMX prophylaxis.[50]

Clinical manifestations of pulmonary nocardiosis are not specific and include anorexia, weight loss, productive cough, pleural pain, dyspnea, and, occasionally, hemoptysis.[14] Untreated pulmonary nocardiosis usually runs a chronic course, similar to tuberculosis, but it also may clear spontaneously and obscure the source of subsequent metastatic infection. The diverse clinical and radiographic manifestations, including acute bronchopneumonia, lobar pneumonia or necrotizing pneumonia with single or multiple abscesses, and pleural empyema, may mimic more common pulmonary infections, such as mycobacterial, staphylococcal, and fungal pneumonia. Normal hosts or patients with only slightly impaired host defenses may have only mild respiratory tract symptoms of several months' duration.[17]

The CNS is the most common secondary site of infection, and such infection occurs in one third of patients.[2] Most experts recommend performing routine cranial computed tomography for patients with pulmonary nocardiosis even when they are asymptomatic because of the frequency of involvement of the CNS. Brain abscesses are the most common manifestation; meningitis is reported less frequently.[9]

Other reported clinical manifestations include tracheitis, peritonitis, iliopsoas abscess, hematogenous endophthalmitis, endocarditis, mediastinitis, septic arthritis, and osteomyelitis.[14] Traumatic inoculation may result in localized disease manifested as cellulitis, subcutaneous abscess, or a lymphocutaneous syndrome in which one or more cutaneous nodules are associated with regional adenopathy or suppurative lymphadenitis.[30] *Nocardia* spp. may cause cervicofacial disease and cervical adenitis in children.[29]

Bacteremic nocardiosis is reported rarely and usually is associated with endovascular foreign bodies in patients receiving long-term steroid therapy.[28] In a report of six cases of central venous catheter–related *Nocardia* bacteremia, four cases were in children 18 years or younger.[18] All six patients received antibiotic therapy; the catheter was retained in three of the six. Relapse occurred in one of the three patients in whom the catheter was not removed.[18]

The diagnosis of nocardiosis is established in one third of cases by sputum analysis and culture. Humoral methods used to diagnose nocardiosis generally lack specificity because of the high degree of serologic cross-reactivity that occurs among *Nocardia* spp. and between *Mycobacterium* and *Streptomyces* spp.[8] The probable decreased sensitivity for detection of an antibody response in immunocompromised individuals also likely is a limitation of serologic testing. It is important to notify the laboratory when nocardial infection is suspected so that steps can be taken to optimize its recognition and recovery. Although *Nocardia* colonies usually are evident by 3 to 5 days after culture, prolonged incubation may be necessary.

Although *Nocardia* spp. sometimes can be respiratory saprotrophs, withholding therapy from immunocompromised patients when cultures repeatedly are positive is difficult. Bronchoalveolar lavage or lung biopsy may be required to establish the diagnosis. Although these procedures are invasive, given the overlap in symptoms with other infectious and neoplastic processes and potential for rapid progression of disease, bronchoalveolar lavage or lung biopsy should be considered early in immunodeficient patients to establish a definitive diagnosis. The demonstration of tissue invasion confirms active infection. Tentative species identification of most *Nocardia* can be made by biochemical methods, by chemotaxonomic methods, or via antimicrobial susceptibility patterns. Only *N. brasiliensis*, *N. farcinica*, and *N. pseudobrasiliensis* can be identified reliably by these methods, however.[10] Molecular confirmation (e.g., DNA probes, PCR and PCR-RFLP molecular analyses, DNA sequencing, pyrosequencing, ribotyping) of species identification is the method of choice. Molecular testing by *hsp65* PCR and 16S restriction enzyme analysis identifies greater than 90 percent of currently recognized clinical species.[10]

TREATMENT AND PROGNOSIS

Sulfonamides have been the best-studied drugs for the treatment of nocardiosis.[47,50,57] In the United States, TMP-SMX, the only intravenous sulfonamide formulation available, has been the agent of choice for treatment of nocardiosis. TMP-SMX has been used successfully at doses of 15 mg/kg/day of TMP and 75 mg/kg/day of SMX, either parenterally or orally.[50,55,57] No prospective randomized trials have established the optimal antimicrobial therapy for nocardiosis, however. Recommended antimicrobial therapy regimens are based on efficacy in animal models of nocardiosis and in vitro susceptibility and synergy testing.[10] TMP-SMX as a single agent usually is sufficient for patients with cutaneous nocardiosis.

Many infectious disease specialists administer empiric combination drug therapy, consisting of TMP-SMX, amikacin, and a third-generation cephalosporin, or a carbapenem, for patients with severe disease, CNS nocardiosis, or disseminated disease, and for immunosuppressed patients because of documented treatment failure and mortality associated with sulfonamide monotherapy in those settings.[33,37,51] Currently, no *Nocardia* spp. are resistant to amikacin and a β-lactam in vitro; the use of both (plus TMP-SMX) ensures that all clinical isolates would be susceptible to at least one other drug.[10] Antimicrobial therapy can be narrowed to two agents when results of in vitro susceptibility testing become available. Because antimicrobial resistance patterns vary by species, clinical isolates identified initially as *Nocardia* should be speciated further using molecular techniques.

The 2003 Clinical and Laboratory Standards Institute document on susceptibility testing of mycobacteria and other aerobic actinomycetes recommends that all clinically significant isolates of *Nocardia* spp. be tested for susceptibility to multiple antimicrobial agents.[40] No published prospective clinical trials have correlated in vitro susceptibilities with clinical outcome for nocardiosis. Susceptibility testing is the best available guide for selecting appropriate combination therapy and alternative therapies if sulfonamides fail or cannot be given because of patient intolerance or allergy.

Clinical experience with minocycline, the tetracycline with best in vitro activity against *Nocardia*, has been encouraging. Amoxicillin-clavulanic acid has been effective in treating infections with *N. brasiliensis*, commonly a β-lactamase producer.[56] A case of acquired resistance to β-lactamase inhibitor antibiotics has been reported, however.[52] Other species with susceptibility to amoxicillin-clavulanic acid include *N. abscessus* and *N. farcinica*, whereas isolates of the *N. nova* complex are ampicillin susceptible/intermediate but resistant to amoxicillin-clavulanic acid.[10] Susceptibility of some *Nocardia* spp. to fluoroquinolones has been reported. In an in vitro study, the newer fluoroquinolones, gatifloxacin and moxifloxacin, generally were more active than was ciprofloxacin against isolates of *Nocardia*, especially against isolates of *N. farcinica* and *N. brasiliensis*.[10] A patient with disseminated *N. farcinica* nocardiosis initially treated with aspiration, TMP/SMX, and imipenem had recurrence of brain lesions after a change to monotherapy with moxifloxacin despite in vitro susceptibility to moxifloxacin.[15]

The oxazolidinone linezolid is the first antimicrobial shown to be active in vitro against all clinically important *Nocardia* spp.[11] Linezolid, which is available for oral administration, was used successfully to treat six patients with nocardiosis.[36] Linezolid-associated hematologic toxicity was seen in three of the six patients.[36] Myelosuppression may occur more commonly in individuals receiving linezolid for longer than 2 weeks. The use of linezolid for nocardial infection is limited by the prolonged treatment required for nocardiosis.

Clinical improvement typically is seen within 7 to 10 days after initiation of appropriate therapy.[35] Patients with unchanged or worsening symptoms after receiving 2 weeks of therapy should be reassessed thoroughly. Intravenous antibiotic therapy may be changed to an oral regimen after at least 3 to 6 weeks if clinical improvement is noted. The variable and chronic course of nocardiosis precludes determining precise therapeutic end-points. Metastatic lesions can appear during or after an otherwise effective course of sulfonamide therapy with maintenance of the recommended 100- to 150-μg/mL level in serum or plasma. Because the tendency for relapse or the late appearance of metastatic disease is a concern, therapy often is continued for many months. Patients with mycetomas may require 6 to 12 months of therapy; localized cutaneous nocardiosis usually is treated for 3 to 6 months. Therapy for 6 to 12 months is suggested for patients with serious infection. Therapy for 12 months is indicated for patients with CNS nocardiosis and for immunocompromised patients.[32] Patients with CNS disease should be monitored with serial neuroimaging studies. Patients with AIDS probably should be treated with suppressive therapy indefinitely.

Surgical drainage of abscesses is important because metastatic abscesses can appear in the face of adequate therapy until surgical drainage is achieved.[21] Select brain abscesses may respond to antimicrobial treatment without surgery.[34]

Despite specific therapy, the overall mortality rate is 25 to 40 percent.[43,44] Most reported cases involving dissemination to the CNS have been fatal.[43] Disseminated nocardiosis has a poor prognosis, with a mortality rate of greater than 85 percent in immunocompromised hosts.[3] Factors associated with increased mortality rates in one reported patient series were treatment with corticosteroids or antineoplastic agents, underlying Cushing disease, disseminated disease involving two or more noncontiguous organs or the CNS, and the presence of symptoms for less than 3 weeks before initial evaluation.

REFERENCES

1. Angeles, A. M., and Sugar, A. M.: Rapid diagnosis of nocardiosis with an enzyme immunoassay. J. Infect. Dis. 155:292-296, 1987.
2. Beaman, B. L., and Beaman, L.: Nocardia species: Host-parasite relationships. Clin. Microbiol. Rev. 7:213-264, 1994.
3. Beaman, B. L., Burnside, J., Edwards, B., and Causey, W.: Nocardial infections in the United States, 1972-1974. J. Infect. Dis.134:286-289, 1976.
4. Beaman, B. L., and Moring, S. E.: Relationship among cell wall composition, state of growth, and virulence of Nocardia asteroides GUH-2. Infect. Immun. 56:557-563, 1988.
5. Beckmeyer, W. J.: Nocardiosis: Report of a successfully treated case of cutaneous granuloma. Pediatrics 23:33-39, 1959.
6. Berd, D.: Laboratory identification of clinically important aerobic actinomycetes. Appl. Microbiol. 25:665-681, 1973.
7. Black, C. M., Paliescheskey, M., Beaman, B. L., et al.: Acidification of phagosome in murine macrophages: Blockage by Nocardia asteroides. J. Infect. Dis. 154:952-958, 1986.
8. Boiron, P., and Stynen, D.: Immunodiagnosis of nocardiosis. Gene 115:219-222, 1992.
9. Bross, J. E., and Gordon, G.: Nocardial meningitis case reports and review. Rev. Infect. Dis. 3:160-165, 1991.
10. Brown-Elliott, B. A., Brown, J. M., Conville, P. S., and Wallace, R. J., Jr.: Clinical and laboratory features of the Nocardia spp. based on current molecular taxonomy. Clin. Microbiol. Rev. 19:259-282, 2006.
11. Brown-Elliott, B. A., Ward, S. C., Crist, C. J., et al.: In vitro activities of linezolid against multiple Nocardia species. Antimicrob. Agents Chemother. 45:1295-1297, 2001.
12. Castro, J. G., and Espinoza, L.: Nocardia species infections in a large county hospital in Miami: 6 years experience. J. Infect. 54:358-361, 2006.
13. Causey, W. A.: Nocardia caviae: A report of 13 new isolations with clinical correlation. Appl. Microbiol. 28:193-198, 1974.
14. Curry, W. A.: Human nocardiosis: A clinical review with selected case reports. Arch. Intern. Med. 140:818-826, 1980.
15. Dahan, K., El Kabbaj, D., Venditto, M., et al.: Intracranial Nocardia recurrence during fluorinated quinolones therapy. Transpl. Infect. Dis. 8:161-165, 2006.
16. Desmond, E. P., and Flores, M.: Mouse pathogenicity studies of Nocardia asteroides complex species and clinical correlation with human isolates. F. E. M. S. Microbiol. Lett. 110:281-284, 1993.
17. Feigin, D. S.: Nocardiosis of the lung: Chest radiographic findings in 21 cases. Radiology 159:9-14, 1986.
18. Feng, Y.-H., Huang, W.-T., and Tsao, C.-J.: Venous access port-related Nocardia bacteremia with successful short-term antibiotics treatment. J. Chin. Med. Assoc. 67:416-418, 2004.
19. Fergie, J. E., and Purcell, K.: Nocardiosis in South Texas children. Pediatr. Infect. Dis. J. 20:711-714, 2001.
20. Ferry, A. P., Font, R. L., Weinberg, R. S., et al.: Nocardial endophthalmitis: Report of two cases studied histopathologically. Br. J. Ophthalmol. 72:55-61, 1988.
21. Frazier, A. R., Rosenow, E. C., III, and Roberts, G. D.: Nocardiosis: A review of 25 cases occurring during 24 months. Mayo Clin. Proc. 50:657-663, 1975.
22. Harik, N. K., Jacobs, R. F., and Darville, T.: Nocardiosis in children: Five cases. J. Invest. Med. 49:108, 2001.
23. Heffner, J. E.: Pleuropulmonary manifestations of actinomycosis and nocardiosis. Semin. Respir. Infect. 3:352-361, 1988.
24. Idriss, Z. H., Cunningham, R. J., and Wilfert, C. M.: Nocardiosis in children. Pediatrics 55:479-484, 1975.
25. Javalry, K., Horowitz, H. W., and Wormser, G. P.: Nocardiosis in patients with human immunodeficiency virus infection: Report of 2 cases and review of the literature. Medicine (Baltimore) 71:128-138, 1980.
26. Kahn, F. W., Gornick, C. C., and Tofte, R. W.: Primary cutaneous Nocardia asteroides infection with dissemination. Am. J. Med. 70:859-863, 1981.
27. Kalb, R. E., Kaplan, M. H., and Grosman, M. E.: Cutaneous nocardiosis. J. Am. Acad. Dermatol. 13:125-133, 1985.
28. Kontoyiannis, D. P., Ruoff, K., and Hooper, D. C.: Nocardia bacteremia: Report of 4 cases and review of the literature. Medicine (Baltimore) 77:255-267, 1998.
29. Lampe, R. M., Baker, C. J., Septimus, E. J., et al.: Cervicofacial nocardiosis in children. J. Pediatr. 99:593-595, 1981.
30. Law, B. L., and Marks, M. I.: Pediatric nocardiosis. Pediatrics 70:560-564, 1982.
31. Leggiadro, R. J., and Miller, R. B.: Cutaneous nocardiosis presenting as a tickborne infection. Pediatr. Infect. Dis. J. 6:421-422, 1987.
32. Lerner, P. I.: Nocardiosis. Clin. Infect. Dis. 22:891-903, 1996.
33. Long, P. F.: A retrospective study of Nocardia infections associated with the acquired immune deficiency syndrome (AIDS). Infection 22:362-364, 1994.
34. Mamelak, A. N., Obana, W. G., Flaherty, J. F., et al.: Nocardial brain abscess: Treatment strategies and factors influencing outcome. Neurosurgery 35:622-631, 1994.
35. McNeil, M. M., and Brown, J. M.: The medically important aerobic actinomycetes: Epidemiology and microbiology. Clin. Microbiol. Rev. 7:357-417, 1994.
36. Moylett, E. H., Pacheco, S. E., Brown-Elliott, B. A., et al.: Clinical experience with linezolid for the treatment of Nocardia infection. Clin. Infect. Dis. 36:313-318, 2003.
37. Murray, J. F., Finegold, S. M., Froman, S., et al.: The changing spectrum of nocardiosis. Am. Rev. Respir. Dis. 83:315-330, 1961.
38. Murray, P. R., Neeren, R. L., and Niles, A. C.: Effect of decontamination procedures on recovery of Nocardia spp. J. Clin. Microbiol. 25:2010-2011, 1987.
39. Murray, P. R., Niles, A. C., and Heeren, R. L.: Modified Thayer-Martin medium for recovery of Nocardia species from contaminated specimens. J. Clin. Microbiol. 26:1219-1220, 1988.
40. NCCLS: Susceptibility Testing of Mycobacteria, Nocardiae, and Other Aerobic Actinomycetes; Approved Standard. NCCLS document M24-A. Wayne, PA, NCCLS, 2003.
41. O'Conner, P. T., and Dire, D. J.: Cutaneous nocardiosis associated with insect bites. Cutis 50:301-302, 1992.
42. Palmer, D. L., Harvey, R. L., and Wheeler, J. K.: Diagnostic and therapeutic considerations in Nocardia asteroides infection. Medicine (Baltimore) 53:391-401, 1974.
43. Present, C. A., Wiernik, P. H., and Serpick, A. A.: Factors affecting survival in nocardiosis. Am. Rev. Respir. Dis. 108:1444-1451, 1973.
44. Rosett, W., and Hodges, G. R.: Recent experiences with nocardial infections. Am. J. Med. Sci. 276:279-285, 1978.
45. Sachs, M. K.: Lymphocutaneous Nocardia brasiliensis infection acquired from a cat scratch: Case report and review. Clin. Infect. Dis. 15:710-711, 1992.
46. Satterwhite, T. K., and Wallace, R. J., Jr.: Primary cutaneous nocardiosis. J. A. M. A. 242:333-336, 1979.
47. Schiff, T. A., McNeil, M. M., and Brown, J. M.: Cutaneous Nocardia farcinica infection in a nonimmunocompromised patient: Case report and review. Clin. Infect. Dis. 16:756-760, 1993.
48. Shetty, A. K., Arvin, A. M., and Gutierrez, K. M.: Nocardia farcinica pneumonia in chronic granulomatous disease. Pediatrics 104:961-964, 1999.
49. Smego, R. A., Jr., and Gallis, H. A.: The clinical spectrum of Nocardia brasiliensis infection in the United States. Rev. Infect. Dis. 6:164-180, 1984.
50. Smego, R. A., Jr., Moeller, M. G., and Gallis, H. A.: Trimethoprim-sulfamethoxazole therapy for Nocardia infections. Arch. Intern. Med. 143:711-718, 1983.
51. Stamm, A. M., McFall, D. W., and Dismukes, W. E.: Failure of sulfonamides and trimethoprim in the treatment of nocardiosis. Arch. Intern. Med. 143:383-385, 1983.
52. Steingrube, V. A., Wallace, R. J., Jr., Brown, B. A., et al.: Acquired resistance of Nocardia brasiliensis to clavulanic acid related to a change in β-lactamase following therapy with amoxicillin-clavulanic acid. Antimicrob. Agents Chemother. 35:524-528, 1991.
53. Stropnik, Z.: Isolation of Nocardia asteroides from human skin. Sabouraudia 4:41-44, 1965.
54. Thaler, F., Gotainer, B., Teodori, G., et al.: Mediastinitis due to Nocardia asteroides after cardiac transplantation. Intensive Care Med. 18:127-128, 1992.
55. van Burik, J.-A., Hackman, R. C., Nadeem, S. Q., et al.: Nocardiosis after bone marrow transplantation: A retrospective study. Clin. Infect. Dis. 22:1154-1160, 1997.
56. Wallace, R. J., Jr., Nash, D. R., Johnson, W. K., et al.: β-Lactam resistance in Nocardia brasiliensis is mediated by β-lactamase and reversed in the presence of clavulanic acid. J. Infect. Dis. 156:959-966, 1987.
57. Wallace, R. J., Jr., Septimus, E. J., Williams, T. W., et al.: Use of trimethoprim-sulfamethoxazole for treatment of infections due to Nocardia. Rev. Infect. Dis. 4:315-325, 1982.
58. Wallace, R. J., Jr., and Steele, L. C.: Susceptibility testing on Nocardia asteroides for the clinical laboratory. Diagn. Microbiol. Infect. Dis. 9:155-166, 1988.
59. Wallace, R. J., Jr., Tsukamura, M., Brown, B. A., et al.: Cefotaxime-resistant Nocardia asteroides strains are isolates of the controversial species Nocardia farcinica. J. Clin. Microbiol. 28:2726-2732, 1990.
60. Wallis, R. S., Broder, M. S., Wong, J. Y., et al.: Granulomatous infectious diseases associated with tumor necrosis factor antagonists. Clin. Infect. Dis. 38:1261-1265, 2004.
61. Yew, W. W., Wong, P. C., Kwan, S. Y. L., et al.: Two cases of Nocardia asteroides sternotomy infection treated with ofloxacin and a review of other active antimicrobial agents. J. Infect. Dis. 23:297-302, 1991.

MISCELLANEOUS GRAM-POSITIVE BACILLI

CHAPTER
111

Randall G. Fisher

The gram-positive rods encompass a vast number of species. They are widespread in the environment and are part of the normal flora of animals and humans. This chapter focuses on gram-positive bacilli seldom encountered as pathogens in healthy individuals. Many of these organisms show increasing prominence as causes of disease in immunocompromised patients.[12] Bacteria from the following genera are discussed: *Corynebacterium* (other than *Corynebacterium diphtheriae*) and *Rhodococcus*.

CORYNEBACTERIUM

The genus *Corynebacterium* comprises a wide number of organisms possessing little pathogenic potential, with some notable exceptions. The most infamous member of this genus, *C. diphtheriae* (see Chapter 101), is a cause of a potentially lethal pharyngeal infection with systemic manifestations. *Corynebacterium jeikeium* (formerly *Corynebacterium* group JK) can be a major nosocomial agent of bacteremia and endocarditis; other species commonly are associated with infections in animals and rarely cause invasive infection in humans.[70,98] For an exhaustive consideration of coryneform bacteria, the reader is referred to the review by Funke and colleagues.[41]

BACTERIOLOGY

Corynebacterium spp. derive their name from their club-like shape. Because of their resemblance to *C. diphtheriae*, they are included in the heterogeneous group of diphtheroids. Snapping division produces the angular and palisade arrangement of cells responsible for their characteristic gram-positive, "Chinese letters" microscopic appearance.[21] Organisms are facultatively anaerobic or aerobic and do not produce spores. They are nonmotile and catalase-positive and contain mycolic acid in their cell walls. Clinically relevant species include *C. diphtheriae*, *C. jeikeium*, *C. pseudotuberculosis*, *C. xerosis*, *Corynebacterium amycolatum*, *Corynebacterium pseudodiphtheriticum*, *Corynebacterium minutissimum*, *Corynebacterium striatum*, *Corynebacterium ulcerans*, and *Corynebacterium urealyticum*. Species can be differentiated according to biochemical tests and fermentation of sugars.[21,41,95]

EPIDEMIOLOGY

Corynebacterium spp. can be part of the normal skin and upper respiratory tract flora and commonly colonize hospitalized patients. Nosocomial acquisition of *C. jeikeium* has been characterized most completely. Thirty-five percent of hospitalized patients may be colonized with *C. jeikeium*, and the organism may be isolated at the time of admission.[42] The skin, groin, and rectum are common sites of recovery. Wounds and suppurative sites quickly become colonized.[42] Longer duration of hospitalization, receipt of broad-spectrum antimicrobial agents, and impaired skin integrity are risk factors for invasive infection. Hospital personnel caring for oncology patients have higher rates of hand colonization with pathogenic *Corynebacterium* spp. than do nurses caring for dermatology patients.[35] Transmission from patient to

patient in the hospital environment can occur, and selective antibiotic pressure has been shown to augment colonization with *Corynebacterium* spp.[68,78,128] Outbreaks of bacteremic infection have been reported in hematology wards,[92,110] and DNA restriction fragment analysis and hybridization techniques have been used to document spread.[68,89]

PATHOPHYSIOLOGY

C. jeikeium and *C. urealyticum* are lipophilic, which may account for their ability to proliferate on skin that has a higher lipid content; organisms have been isolated from sebum-filled eccrine gland biopsy specimens in an adolescent with malignancy.[59] Breach of the integrity of the skin is an important risk factor for acquisition of local infection and bacteremia with *Corynebacterium*. Plastic intravascular catheters increase the risk of infection.[93] Certain isolates of *C. pseudotuberculosis* and *C. ulcerans* can express diphtheria-like toxins,[126] which may confer virulence.

Some *Corynebacterium* spp., notably *C. jeikeium* and *C. urealyticum*, commonly show resistance to penicillins, cephalosporins, aminoglycosides, erythromycin, and tetracycline.[30,42,70,78,84,95,108] Strains with a significant DNA relationship to the *C. jeikeium*-type strain show penicillin resistance.[94] Resistant organisms have been noted to have significantly thickened cell walls compared with susceptible strains, but the functional importance of this feature is unknown.[14]

CLINICAL MANIFESTATIONS

Systemic infections with *Corynebacterium* spp. generally are not clinically distinguishable from serious infections caused by other pathogens. Immunocompromised patients are at the highest risk of developing disease caused by *Corynebacterium*,[51,97] but infections also have been described in neonates and immunocompromised older children.[13,30,62] Risk factors include male gender, neutropenia, broad-spectrum antibiotic exposure, and prolonged hospital stay.[92,110] Catalase production may be responsible for the rare infection with non-JK *Corynebacterium* spp. in children with chronic granulomatous disease.[62] *Corynebacterium* spp. are responsible for approximately 9 percent of early-onset and 4 percent of late-onset prosthetic valve endocarditis.[125]

C. jeikeium is a pathogen of particular concern. In 1976, this agent first was described as a cause of serious infection in four patients, including an 11-year-old boy with a ventriculoatrial shunt.[51] The other three patients had hematologic malignancies and were neutropenic at the time of infection. Immunocompromised patients, particularly patients with leukemia, are vulnerable to bacteremia. These high-risk subjects may show a local inflammatory lesion at the site of infection or a disseminated, hemorrhagic, or necrotic papular exanthem. Subcutaneous nodules also may be seen. *C. jeikeium* has been recovered from disseminated lesions in a 14-year-old boy with leukemia.[59] A literature review of 83 neutropenic patients (nearly all adults) with *C. jeikeium* sepsis found the following risk factors for development of infection: presence of a central venous catheter, being male, profound and prolonged neutropenia, and exposure to multiple antibiotics. Skin lesions were reported in 48 percent and pulmonary infiltrates in 36 percent of patients. The overall case-fatality rate was 34 percent, but it was reduced to 5 percent in patients with recovery of neutropenia.[119]

Infections with *C. jeikeium* also have been reported after trauma, ventriculoperitoneal shunting procedures,[2,64] orthopedic procedures,[20] bone marrow aspiration,[30] and central venous catheter placement.[30] *C. jeikeium* now is recognized to be one of the most common causes of prosthetic valve endocarditis in adults.[84] Cutaneous findings of bacteremia so commonly observed in patients with cancer generally are absent in patients with endocarditis.[26] In a series of 38 patients with *C. jeikeium* endocarditis, 74 percent of patients had prosthetic valves. The mortality rate was 33 percent and was not altered by valve replacement surgery.[82] Exit-site infections in patients on continuous ambulatory peritoneal dialysis also may be caused by *Corynebacterium* spp.; in the largest series published to date, *C. striatum* caused almost twice as many of these infections as did *C. jeikeium*. Most infections are manageable without removal of the dialysis catheter.[102]

Although primarily a pathogen in farm animals, *C. pseudotuberculosis* can cause localized suppurative granulomatous lymphadenitis in humans[70]; almost all cases are associated with animal contact, particularly sheep and goats.[43] Presentation and histology may mimic the much more common cat-scratch disease, and Gram stain and culture are required to differentiate the two entities.[70] Most cases have been reported from Australia.[88]

C. xerosis has been reported as a rare cause of endocarditis, arthritis, and ventriculoperitoneal shunt infection.[7,15] Most individuals with endocarditis have a prosthetic heart valve.[34,72] *C. xerosis* also can be a cause of eye infections in patients with superficial corneal foreign bodies; in one study of 101 patients, *C. xerosis* caused 3 of 15 culture-positive cases.[73] It also is an extremely rare cause of post-LASIK (laser-assisted in-situ keratomileusis) infectious keratitis.[29] Using chemical testing and molecular genetic investigation, Funke and colleagues[40] showed that many isolates tentatively identified as *C. xerosis* are actually *C. amycolatum*. *C. amycolatum* is much more likely to be multidrug-resistant than *C. xerosis*.[41] A case of fatal sepsis in a premature newborn caused by *C. amycolatum* has been reported.[13]

C. pseudodiphtheriticum, a commensal of the oropharynx, can cause pneumonia, bronchitis, or tracheitis.[1,22,25] Lung disease usually occurs in the context of underlying cardiopulmonary pathology or immunocompromise.[49] Onset typically is acute, but fever may be noticeably absent.[74] At least 18 cases of *C. pseudodiphtheriticum* endocarditis, including three infections in children with congenital heart disease, have been reported.[83] Infection of allograft material is a common finding; native heart valves may be involved but usually in the context of preexisting lesions or intravenous drug abuse. Three cases of exudative pharyngitis with a pseudomembrane mimicking diphtheria, including one in a 4-year-old girl from Arkansas, have been reported to be caused by *C. pseudodiphtheriticum*.[58] In one case, a surface swab from a draining wound after arthroscopy was reported to harbor "normal skin flora," but joint fluid grew the same organism, and it was finally identified as *C. pseudodiphtheriticum*. Treatment resulted in resolution of symptoms of septic arthritis.[63] Patients who are immunocompromised and have corneal epithelial defects can get severe eye infections with this organism.[69]

C. minutissimum traditionally has been regarded as the cause of the mild cutaneous disease erythrasma, which is characterized by scaly, pruritic red-brown patches, usually occurring in the axilla or groin. Although *C. minutissimum* may play a role, erythrasma probably is a polymicrobial process.[41] *C. minutissimum* is recognized as a rare nosocomial infectious complication of malignancy and dialysis and has been implicated in a case of pyelonephritis in an 8-month-old infant with posterior urethral valves.[24] An adult who developed native-valve endocarditis caused by *C. minutissimum* has been reported.[6]

C. striatum has been recovered from purulent sputum of hospitalized patients and from infected central venous catheter sites.[103] It also is a cause of exit-site infections in patients on long-term ambulatory peritoneal dialysis.[102] It has been reported as a cause of fatal pulmonary infection and endocarditis.[68,77,98] *C. striatum* was responsible for a nosocomial outbreak among 14 patients over a 12-month period in a surgical intensive care unit. Endotracheal intubation for longer than 24 hours was the only risk factor found to predispose to acquisition of infection.[17] *C. striatum* also has been reported as a cause of meningitis and ventriculoperitoneal shunt infections.[56,123]

C. ulcerans derives its name from its association with ulcerative pharyngitis. Although it is more commonly a pathogen of nonhuman primates,[87] infection can occur in humans after contact with an animal or consumption of contaminated raw milk.[11,27] Toxigenic strains of *C. ulcerans* can produce a syndrome indistinguishable from that caused by toxigenic *C. diphtheriae*.[4,5] Skin lesions that exactly mimic cutaneous diphtheria, caused by diphtheria toxin–secreting strains of *C. ulcerans*, also have been reported.[121]

C. urealyticum (formerly *Corynebacterium* group D2) is a cause of alkaline-encrusted cystitis and pyelitis, primarily in the elderly.[36,108] A case series of four children with encrusted cystitis and pyelitis has been published. The mean age was 9 years (range, 4 to 13 years). Treatment was with prolonged antibiotics and endoscopic debulking. Cure was effected in three of the four patients; the other patient was a renal transplant recipient who lost the graft.[80] Routine urine culture may miss the organism; it may grow with prolonged incubation of sheep's blood agar.[105] It is associated less commonly with infection at other sites and with bacteremia.[107] An 8-year-old boy with chemotherapy-induced neutropenia and a necrotic soft tissue infection of the scrotum caused by *C. urealyticum* has been reported.[99]

DIAGNOSIS

Diagnosis of *Corynebacterium* infection is based on isolation of the organism from clinical material. This organism commonly is accompanied by other pathogens. Similar to *Mycobacterium* and *Nocardia* spp., *Corynebacterium* organisms have mycolic acids in their cell wall. The chains are shorter, however, and the organisms are not acid-fast. *Corynebacterium* spp. may be difficult to distinguish from some *Rhodococcus* spp.[21] Colonies of *C. jeikeium* may show a metallic sheen when grown on agar.[51] Growth of *C. jeikeium* is enhanced by the addition of lipids to the medium. Most *Corynebacterium* spp. can be differentiated quickly from each other by sugar fermentation, hydrolysis of urea, and reduction of nitrate.[116] Selective media containing kanamycin or trimethoprim-sulfamethoxazole have been useful in the recovery of multidrug-resistant strains of *Corynebacterium*.[50] Erythrasma usually is diagnosed by the typical coral red fluorescence under Wood lamp examination.

TREATMENT

Empiric therapy for infection must account for the frequency of infection with *C. jeikeium*, which often are multiresistant to antibiotics but are susceptible to vancomycin.[41] In some series of immunocompromised patients, this organism is the most common *Corynebacterium* spp. encountered.[109,124] Vancomycin is recommended for empiric therapy of suspected *Corynebacterium* infection until susceptibilities are known. Treatment can be changed to a penicillin or cephalosporin, if appropriate. In vitro, *C. jeikeium* is sensitive to linezolid,[45] and most strains also are sensitive to quinupristin-dalfopristin[100] and daptomycin.[44] Linezolid is bacteriostatic against all species of *Corynebacterium*, and in vitro its activity is slower against *C. jeikeium* than it is against

C. striatum and *C. amycolatum*.[45] Clinical experience using these newer antimicrobial agents is lacking.

Two-drug therapy generally is recommended for treatment of *Corynebacterium* endocarditis; for gentamicin-susceptible strains, penicillin-gentamicin combinations have been shown to be synergistic, regardless of whether the strains are susceptible to penicillin.[84] Rarely, resistance to vancomycin is encountered. A woman with prosthetic valve endocarditis caused by a vancomycin-resistant *Corynebacterium* spp. was treated successfully with imipenem and ciprofloxacin.[10] Removal of infectious sources, such as central nervous system shunts and central venous catheters, may be required for cure. Scrupulous attention given to skin hygiene may reduce colonization of hospital personnel and the incidence of patient-to-patient transmission of pathogenic strains.[32,92] Management of toxigenic *C. ulcerans* infection is identical to that for infection caused by toxigenic *C. diphtheriae*, including the use of antitoxin.[5] Erythrasma usually responds to treatment with a macrolide.

RHODOCOCCUS

The genus *Rhodococcus* contains at least 15 species, of which *Rhodococcus equi* is the most clinically relevant to humans. Infections with other species are rare. Suppurative keratitis caused by *Rhodococcus ruber* after penetrating trauma has been described.[65] This organism derives its name from its role as a cause of pyogranulomatous pneumonia in young horses to occur.[90] It has assumed a prominent role as a cause of human pulmonary disease in immunocompromised patients, particularly in patients with acquired immunodeficiency syndrome (AIDS).[35,52,103] For a comprehensive discussion of this organism, the reader is referred to the review by Cornish and Washington.[23]

BACTERIOLOGY

R. equi is a catalase-positive, urease-positive, oxidase-negative, gram-positive rod. The organism assumes a more coccoid morphology in solid media and a more bacillary form in liquid media. Its cell wall contains mycolic acid, rendering it acid-fast when grown on Lowenstein-Jensen media and stained with Kinyoun stain.[46]

EPIDEMIOLOGY

R. equi is a soil organism, and its growth is enriched by the manure of herbivores. Despite the common occurrence of this pathogen as a cause of veterinary infections, exposure to animals apparently is not necessary for human infection to occur[90]; most reported human patients have not had farm or animal exposure.[52] Hospital outbreaks of infection associated with patient-to-patient transmission have not been reported. In a retrospective analysis of 24 cases of *R. equi* infection, however, six patients had shared a hospital room with a patient with *R. equi* pneumonia, raising the possibility of nosocomial transmission.[8] Most patients diagnosed with *Rhodococcus* infection are immunocompromised; AIDS is the most common underlying diagnosis, but infection also has been reported in transplant patients[9] and rarely in patients thought to be immunocompetent.[118]

PATHOPHYSIOLOGY

The prominence of pulmonary infection suggests that the respiratory tract is a common portal of entry. After gaining access to the lower respiratory tract, organisms are taken up by alveolar macrophages; Mac-1 macrophage receptors and complement are required for binding.[53] The appearance of pyogranulomatous lesions is consistent with the role of *R. equi* as an intracellular parasite containing mycolic acid, a possible virulence factor in the cell wall.[47,91] Surface 15- and 17-kd antigens expressed by an 85-kb plasmid seem to confer virulence in mice and foals,[111] and virulent strains seem to have an increased capacity for intracellular survival in macrophages.[54]

Most *R. equi* isolates from patients with AIDS express either the 15- to 17-kd antigens or a 20-kd antigen that seems to confer intermediate virulence. Most isolates from patients without AIDS express none of these antigens, however.[112] Other factors may play a role in promoting *Rhodococcus* disease in humans.[113] Death of parasitized macrophages may release enzymes, which contribute further to tissue damage. CD4+ lymphocytes are essential for pulmonary clearance of *R. equi* in a mouse model,[61] which may help to explain the high risk of infection associated with cellular immunodeficiency.

CLINICAL MANIFESTATIONS

Infection typically manifests as a subacute pneumonia developing over several weeks. Symptoms such as cough and fever are common, but progression of disease may be silent. Although most infections currently occur in patients with AIDS, malignancy and transplantation also pose risks. Pulmonary infection in children with leukemia has been described.[3,79] Infection may be accompanied by other pathogens, particularly in patients with AIDS.

Pulmonary infection often is pleura-based and associated with cavitation.[52] Empyema may occur as a complication. Computed tomography scan most frequently reveals pneumonia with cavitation, but other patterns, including "ground-glass" opacities, peribronchial nodules, and centrilobular nodules, may be seen.[75] Lung tissue showing malakoplakia, an unusual-appearing granulomatous inflammation with aggregates of histiocytes that contain concentrically layered basophilic inclusions, should raise suspicion of the presence of *R. equi* infection.[19,48,101]

Extrapulmonary disease is seen at diagnosis in 7 percent of patients with pneumonia.[120] Manifestations of infection include otitis/mastoiditis,[3,57,71] abscesses,[37] osteomyelitis,[16,38,86] meningitis,[28,104] pericarditis,[67] lymphadenitis,[67] and endophthalmitis.[33] The organism has been grown from a biopsy of a granulomatous skin lesion in an immunocompetent 7-year-old girl.[76] *R. equi* also has been reported as a cause of peritonitis in patients receiving long-term peritoneal dialysis.[18,114]

DIAGNOSIS

Diagnosis relies on isolation of *Rhodococcus* from clinical material. Although sputum specimens may be positive, bronchoalveolar lavage or lung biopsy may be required. Blood cultures may be positive in half or more of patients with AIDS and with focal pneumonic disease.[117] The physician should be alert to the possible coexistence of *R. equi* with other pathogens. In the laboratory, confusing this organism with *Corynebacterium*, acid-fast organisms, and other gram-positive coccobacilli has been shown to delay establishment of the diagnosis.[31] Positive findings on Gram stain and Kinyoun stain should be interpreted in the context of clinical information.[103] Organisms appear salmon-pink when grown on blood agar and orange on Lowenstein-Jensen medium.[12] Differentiating from acid-fast bacteria on smear sometimes can be difficult. Combined use of a siderophore detection medium, ethylene glycol degradation, and β-galactosidase activity may help differentiate *Rhodococcus* from *Nocardia* and rapid-growing mycobacteria.[39] DNA restriction fragment analysis and ribotyping show promise in aiding the identification and tracking of *Rhodococcus* spp.[66] A *Rhodococcus equi*-specific polymerase chain reaction has been used to confirm infection in some cases in which identification was difficult.[127]

TREATMENT

Clinical isolates commonly are resistant to penicillins and cephalosporins. Even if susceptible in vitro, β-lactam antibiotics should be avoided because of rapid development of resistance.[60] Erythromycin, clindamycin, rifampin, aminoglycosides, vancomycin, fluoroquinolones, and imipenem are active against *R. equi*.[85] Moxifloxacin is more active in vitro than is either ciprofloxacin or levofloxacin.[96] Synergy has been shown with various combinations of these agents. Including rifampin or erythromycin in a two-drug combination has been recommended because of penetrance of macrophages.[12,106] Combinations of antibiotics that included vancomycin were found to be most effective in clearing infection in a mouse model.[85] Cure rates in adults with lung infection are approximately 60 percent when antibiotic therapy alone is employed but may reach 75 percent when combined with surgical resection of infected pulmonary tissue.[52] Surgery has not been shown to increase survival rates, however.[8]

Pediatric patients generally have fared better than adults, but most reported cases in children have been in non-AIDS patients.[12] Relapse is a common occurrence, but the optimal duration of therapy to prevent relapse is unknown. For patients with AIDS, some authors recommend a minimum of 2 months of therapy followed by long-term suppressive therapy.[60] Relapse has been reported to occur at extrapulmonary sites in 13 percent of immunocom-promised patients,[120] often without reappearance of pulmonary disease. Treatment of *R. equi* peritonitis in patients receiving peritoneal dialysis has been reported to be successful with intraperitoneal imipenem or vancomycin for 14 days.[18,115] Removal of the peritoneal dialysis catheter may be required for cure.

Acknowledgments

The author thanks Dr. William Gruber and Dr. Thomas Boyce for their invaluable assistance with earlier versions of this chapter.

REFERENCES

1. Ahmed, K., Kawakami, K., Watanabe, K., et al.: *Corynebacterium pseudodiphtheriticum*: A respiratory tract pathogen. Clin. Infect. Dis. 20:41-46, 1995.
2. Allen, K. D., and Green, H. T.: Infections due to a "Group JK" *Corynebacterium*. J. Infect. 13:41-44, 1986.
3. Allen, V. D., Niec, A., Kerem, E., et al.: *Rhodococcus equi* pneumonia in a child with leukemia. Pediatr. Infect. Dis. J. 8:656-658, 1989.
4. Anonymous: Respiratory diphtheria caused by *Corynebacterium ulcerans*—Terre Haute, Indiana, 1996. M. M. W. R. Morb. Mortal. Wkly. Rep. 46:330-332, 1997.
5. Anonymous: Three cases of toxigenic *Corynebacterium ulcerans* infection. Commun. Dis. Rep. C. D. R. Wkly. 10:49, 52, 2000.
6. Aperis, G., and Moyssakis, I. *Corynebacterium minutissimum* endocarditis: A case report and review. J. Infect. 54:e79-e81, 2007.
7. Arisoy, E. S., Demmler, G. J., and Dunne, W. M., Jr.: *Corynebacterium xerosis* ventriculoperitoneal shunt infection in an infant: Report of a case and review of the literature. Pediatr. Infect. Dis. J. 12:536-538, 1993.
8. Arlotti, M., Zoboli, G., Moscatelli, G. L., et al.: *Rhodococcus equi* infection in HIV-positive subjects: A retrospective analysis of 24 cases. Scand. J. Infect. Dis. 28:463-467, 1996.
9. Ayra, B., Hussian, S., and Hariharan, S.: *Rhodococcus equi* pneumonia in a renal transplant patient: A case report and review of literature. Clin. Transplant. 18:748-752, 2004.
10. Barnass, S., Holland, K., and Tabaqchali, S.: Vancomycin-resistant *Corynebacterium* species causing prosthetic valve endocarditis successfully treated with imipenem and ciprofloxacin. J. Infect. 22:161-169., 1991.
11. Barrett, N. J.: Communicable disease associated with milk and dairy products in England and Wales: 1983-1984. J. Infect. 12:265-272, 1986.
12. Berkowitz, F. E.: The gram-positive bacilli: A review of the microbiology, clinical aspects, and antimicrobial susceptibilities of a heterogeneous group of bacteria. Pediatr. Infect. Dis. J. 13:1126-1138, 1994.
13. Berner, R., Pelz, K., Wilhelm, C., et al.: Fatal sepsis caused by *Corynebacterium amycolatum* in a premature infant. J. Clin. Microbiol. 35:1011-1012, 1997.
14. Blom, J., and Heltberg, O.: The ultrastructure of antibiotic-susceptible and multi-resistant strains of group JK diphtheroid rods isolated from clinical specimens. Acta Pathol. Microbiol. Immunol. Scand. B. 94:301-308, 1986.
15. Booth, L. V., Richards, R. H., and Chandran, D. R.: Septic arthritis caused by *Corynebacterium xerosis* following vascular surgery. Rev. Infect. Dis. 13:548-549, 1991.
16. Bouchou, K., Cathebras, P., Dumollard, J. M., et al.: Chronic osteitis due to *Rhodococcus equi* in an immunocompetent patient [letter]. Clin. Infect. Dis. 20:718-720, 1995.
17. Brandenburg, A. H., van Belkum, A., van Pelt, C., et al.: Patient-to-patient spread of a single strain of *Corynebacterium striatum* causing infections in a surgical intensive care unit. J. Clin. Microbiol. 34:2089-2094, 1996.
18. Brown, E., and Hendler, E.: *Rhodococcus* peritonitis in a patient treated with peritoneal dialysis. Am. J. Kidney Dis. 14:417-418, 1989.
19. Byard, R. W., Thorner, P. S., Edwards, V., et al.: Pulmonary malacoplakia in a child. Pediatr. Pathol. 10:417-424, 1990.
20. Claeys, G., Vershchraegen, G., DeSmet, L., et al.: *Corynebacterium* JK (Johnson-Kay strain) infection of a Kuntscher-nailed tibial fracture. Clin. Orthop. 202:227-229, 1986.
21. Collins, M. D., and Cummins, C. S.: *Corynebacterium. In* Garrity, G. M. (ed): Bergey's Manual of Systematic Bacteriology. New York, Springer, 1986, pp. 1266-1276.
22. Colt, H. G., Morris, J. F., Marston, B. J., et al.: Necrotizing tracheitis caused by *Corynebacterium pseudodiphtheriticum*: Unique case and review. Rev. Infect. Dis. 13:73-76, 1991.
23. Cornish, N., and Washington, J. A.: *Rhodococcus equi* infections: Clinical features and laboratory diagnosis. Curr. Clin. Top. Infect. Dis. 19:198-215, 1999.
24. Craig, J., Grigor, W., Doyle, B., et al.: Pyelonephritis caused by *Corynebacterium minutissimum*. Pediatr. Infect. Dis. J. 13:1151-1152, 1994.
25. Craig, T. J., Maguire, F. E., and Wallace, M. R.: Tracheobronchitis due to *Corynebacterium pseudodiphtheriticum*. South. Med. J. 84:504-506, 1991.
26. Dan, M., Somer, I., Knobel, B., et al.: Cutaneous manifestations of infection with *Corynebacterium* group JK. Rev. Infect. Dis. 10:1204-1207, 1988.
27. de Carpentier, J. P., Flanagan, P. M., Singh, I. P., et al.: Nasopharyngeal *Corynebacterium ulcerans*: A different diphtheria. J. Laryngol. Otol. 106:824-826, 1992.
28. DeMarais, P. L., and Kocka, F. E.: *Rhodococcus* meningitis in an immunocompetent host. Clin. Infect. Dis. 20:167-169, 1995.
29. deOliveira, G. C., Solari, H. P., Ciola, F. B., et al.: Corneal infiltrates after excimer laser photorefractive keratectomy and LASIK. J. Refract. Surg. 22:159-165, 2006.
30. Dietrich, M. C., Watson, D. C., and Kumar, M. L.: *Corynebacterium* group JK infections in children. Pediatr. Infect. Dis. J. 8:233-236, 1989.
31. Doig, C., Gill, M. J., and Church, D. L.: *Rhodococcus equi*—an easily missed opportunistic pathogen. Scand. J. Infect. Dis. 23:1-6, 1991.
32. Eagan, J. A., Blevins, A., and Armstrong, D.: Prevention of skin colonization and subsequent bacteremia with CDC-JK organisms in patients with cancer. Cancer Pract. 1:325-328, 1993.
33. Ebersole, L. L., and Paturzo, J. L.: Endophthalmitis caused by *Rhodococcus equi* Prescott serotype 4. J. Clin. Microbiol. 26:1221-1222, 1988.
34. Eliakim, R., Silkoff, P., Lugassy, G., et al.: *Corynebacterium xerosis* endocarditis. Arch. Intern. Med. 143:1995, 1983.
35. Emmons, W., Reichwein, B., and Winslow, D. L.: *Rhodococcus equi* infection in the patient with AIDS: Literature review and report of an unusual case. Rev. Infect. Dis. 13:91-96, 1991.
36. Estorc, J. J., de La Coussaye, J. E., Viel, E. J., et al.: Teicoplanin treatment of alkaline encrusted cystitis due to *Corynebacterium* group D2. Eur. J. Med. 1:183-184, 1992.
37. Fierer, J., Wolf, P., Seed, L., et al.: Non-pulmonary *Rhodococcus equi* infections in patients with acquired immune deficiency syndrome (AIDS). J. Clin. Pathol. 40:556-558, 1987.
38. Fischer, L., Sterneck, M., Albrecht, H., et al.: Vertebral osteomyelitis due to *Rhodococcus equi* in a liver transplant recipient. Clin. Infect. Dis. 26:749-752, 1998.
39. Fiss, E., and Brooks, G. F.: Use of a siderophore detection medium, ethylene glycol degradation, and beta-galactosidase activity in the early presumptive differentiation of *Nocardia, Rhodococcus, Streptomyces,* and rapidly growing *Mycobacterium* species. J. Clin. Microbiol. 29:1533-1535, 1991.
40. Funke, G., Lawson, P. A., Bernard, K. A., et al.: Most *Corynebacterium xerosis* strains identified in the routine clinical laboratory correspond to *Corynebacterium amycolatum*. J. Clin. Microbiol. 34:1124-1128, 1996.
41. Funke, G., von Graevenitz, A., Clarridge, J. E., 3rd, et al.: Clinical microbiology of coryneform bacteria. Clin. Microbiol. Rev. 10:125-159, 1997.
42. Gill, V. J., Manning, C., Lamson, M., et al.: Antibiotic-resistant group JK bacteria in hospitals. J. Clin. Microbiol. 13:472-477, 1981.
43. Goldberger, A. C., Lipsky, B. A., and Plorde, J. J.: Suppurative granulomatous lymphadenitis caused by *Corynebacterium ovis* (pseudotuberculosis). Am. J. Clin. Pathol. 76:486-490, 1981.

44. Goldstein, E. J., Citron, D. M., Merriam, C. V., et al.: In vitro activities of daptomycin, vancomycin, quinupristin-dalfopristin, linezolid, and five other antimicrobials against 307 gram-positive anaerobic and 31 *Corynebacterium* clinical isolates. Antimicrob. Agents Chemother. 47:1486, 2003.

45. Gomez-Garces, J. L., Alos, J. I., and Tamayo, J.: In vitro activity of linezolid and 12 other antimicrobials against coryneform bacteria. Int. J. Antimicrob. Agents. 29:688-692, 2007.

46. Goodfellow, M.: Rhodococcus. *In* Garrity, G. M. (ed): Bergey's Manual of Systematic Bacteriology. New York, Springer, 1986, pp. 1266-1276.

47. Gotoh, K., Mitsuyama, M., Imaizumi, S., et al.: Mycolic acid-containing gly-colipid as a possible virulence factor of *Rhodococcus equi* for mice. Microbiol. Immunol. 35:175-185, 1991.

48. Guerrero, M. F., Ramos, J. M., Renedo, G., et al.: Pulmonary malacoplakia associated with *Rhodococcus equi* infection in patients with AIDS: Case report and review. Clin. Infect. Dis. 28:1334-1336, 1999.

49. Gutierrez-Rodero, F., Ortiz de la Tabla, V., Martinez, C., et al.: *Corynebacterium pseudodiphtheriticum*: An easily missed respiratory pathogen in HIV-infected patients. Diagn. Microbiol. Infect. Dis. 33:209-216, 1999.

50. Hamilton, D. J., Ulness, B. K., Baugher, L. K., et al.: Comparison of a novel trimethoprim-sulfamethoxazole-containing medium (XT80) with kanamycin agar for isolation of antibiotic-resistant organisms from stool and rectal cultures of marrow transplant patients. J. Clin. Microbiol. 25:1886-1890, 1987.

51. Hande, K. R., Witebsky, F. G., Brown, M. S., et al.: Sepsis with a new species of *Corynebacterium*. Ann. Intern. Med. 85:423-426, 1976.

52. Harvey, R. L., and Sunstrum, J. C.: *Rhodococcus equi* infection in patients with and without human immunodeficiency virus infection. Rev. Infect. Dis. 13:139-145, 1991.

53. Hondalus, M. K., Diamond, M. S., Rosenthal, L. A., et al.: The intracellular bacterium *Rhodococcus equi* requires Mac-1 to bind to mammalian cells. Infect. Immun. 61:2919-2929, 1993.

54. Hondalus, M. K., and Mosser, D. M.: Survival and replication of *Rhodococcus equi* in macrophages. Infect. Immun. 62:4167-4175, 1994.

55. Horn, W. A., Larson, E. L., McGinley, K. J., et al.: Microbial flora on the hands of health care personnel: Differences in composition and antibacterial resistance. Infect. Control Hosp. Epidemiol. 9:189-193, 1988.

56. Hoy, C. M., Kerr, K., and Livingston, J. H.: Cerebrospinal fluid-shunt infection due to *Corynebacterium* striatum [letter; comment]. Clin. Infect. Dis. 25:1486-1487, 1997.

57. Ibarra, R., and Jinkins, J. R.: Severe otitis and mastoiditis due to *Rhodococcus equi* in a patient with AIDS: Case report. Neuroradiology. 41:699-701, 1999.

58. Izurieta, H. S., Strebel, P. M., Youngblood, T., et al.: Exudative pharyngitis possibly due to *Corynebacterium pseudodiphtheriticum*, a new challenge in the differential diagnosis of diphtheria [see comments]. Emerg. Infect. Dis. 3:65-68, 1997.

59. Jerdan, M. S., Shapiro, R. S., Smith, N. B., et al.: Cutaneous manifestations of *Corynebacterium* group JK sepsis. J. Am. Acad. Dermatol. 16:444-447, 1987.

60. Johnson, D. H., and Cunha, B. A.: *Rhodococcus equi* pneumonia. Semin. Respir. Infect. 12:57-60, 1997.

61. Kanaly, S. T., Hines, S. A., and Palmer, G. H.: Failure of pulmonary clearance of *Rhodococcus equi* infection in CD4+ T-lymphocyte-deficient transgenic mice. Infect. Immun. 61:4929-4932, 1993.

62. Kaplan, A., and Israel, F.: *Corynebacterium aquaticum* infection in a patient with chronic granulomatous disease. Am. J. Med. Sci. 296:57-58, 1988.

63. Kemp, M., Holtz, K., Andersen, K., and Christensen, J. J.: Demonstration by PCR and DNA sequencing of *Corynebacterium* pseudokiphtheriticum as a cause of joint infection and isolation of the same organism from a surface swab from the patient. J. Med. Microbiol. 54:689-691, 2005.

64. Keren, G., Geva, T., Bogokovsky, B., et al.: *Corynebacterium* Group JK pathogen in cerebrospinal fluid shunt infection: Report of two cases. J. Neurosurg. 68:648-650, 1988.

65. Lalitha, P., Srinivasan, M., and Prajna, V.: *Rhodococcus ruber* as a cause of keratitis. Cornea 25:238-239, 2006.

66. Lasker, B. A., Brown, J. M., and McNeil, M. M.: Identification and epidemiological typing of clinical and environmental isolates of the genus *Rhodococcus* with use of a digoxigenin-labeled rDNA gene probe. Clin. Infect. Dis. 15:223-233, 1992.

67. Lee-Chiong, T., Sadigh, M., Simms, M., et al.: Case reports: pericarditis and lymphadenitis due to *Rhodococcus equi*. Am. J. Med. Sci. 310:31-33, 1995.

68. Leonard, R. B., Nowowiejski, D. J., Warren, J. J., et al.: Molecular evidence of person-to-person transmission of a pigmented strain of *Corynebacterium* striatum in intensive care units. J. Clin. Microbiol. 32:164-169, 1994.

69. Li, A., and Lal, S.: *Corynebacterium pseudodiphtheriticum* keratitis and conjunctivitis: A case report. Clin. Exp. Ophthalmol. 28:60-61, 2000.

70. Lipsky, B. A., Goldberger, A. C., Tompkins, L. S., et al.: Infections caused by nondiphtheria corynebacteria. Rev. Infect. Dis. 4:1220-1235, 1982.

71. Lopes Cardoso, F. L., Machado, E. S., Souza, M. J., et al.: *Rhodococcus equi* mastoiditis in a patient with AIDS. Clin. Infect. Dis. 22:713, 1996.

72. Lortholary, O., Buu-Hoi, A., Fagon, J. Y., et al.: Mediastinitis due to multiple resistant *Corynebacterium xerosis*. Clin. Infect. Dis. 16:172, 1993.

73. Macedo Filho, E. T., Lago, A., Duarte, K., et al.: Superficial corneal foreign body: Laboratory and epidemiologic aspects. Arq. Bras. Oftalmol. 68:821-832, 2005.

74. Manzella, J. P., Kellogg, J. A., and Parsey, K. S.: *Corynebacterium pseudodiphtheriticum*: A respiratory tract pathogen in adults. Clin. Infect. Dis. 20:37-40, 1995.

75. Marchiori, E., de Mendonca, R. G., Capone, D., et al.: *Rhodococcus equi* infection in acquired immunodeficiency syndrome: Computed tomography aspects. J. Bras. Pneumool. 32:405-409, 2006.

76. Martin, T., Hogan, D. J., Murphy, F., et al.: *Rhodococcus* infection of the skin with lymphadenitis in a nonimmunocompromised girl. J. Am. Acad. Dermatol. 24:328-332, 1991.

77. Martinez-Martinez, L., Suarez, A. I., Ortega, M. C., et al.: Fatal pulmonary infection caused by *Corynebacterium* striatum. Clin. Infect. Dis. 19:806-807, 1994.

78. McGowan, J. E., Jr.: JK coryneforms: A continuing problem for hospital infection control. J. Hosp. Infect. 11(Suppl. A):358-366, 1988.

79. McGowan, K. L., and Mangano, M. F.: Infections with *Rhodococcus equi* in children. Diagn. Microbiol. Infect. Dis. 14:347-352, 1991.

80. Meria, P., Margaryan, M., Haddad, E., et al.: Encrusted cystitis and pyelitis in children: An unusual condition with potentially severe consequences. Urology 64:569-573, 2004.

81. Mills, A. E., Mitchell, R. D., and Lim, E. K.: *Corynebacterium pseudotuberculosis* is a cause of human necrotising granulomatous lymphadenitis. Pathology 29:231-233, 1997.

82. Mookadam, F., Cikes, M., Baddour, L. M., et al.: *Corynebacterium jeikeium* endocarditis: A systematic overview spanning four decades. Eur. J. Clin. Microbiol. Infect. Dis. 25:349-353, 2006.

83. Morris, A., and Guild, I.: Endocarditis due to *Corynebacterium pseudodiphtheriticum*: Five case reports, review, and antibiotic susceptibilities of nine strains. Rev. Infect. Dis. 13:887-892, 1991.

84. Murray, B. E., Karchmer, A. W., and Moellering, R. C., Jr.: Diphtheroid prosthetic valve endocarditis: A study of clinical features and infecting organisms. Am. J. Med. 69:838-848, 1980.

85. Nordmann, P., Kerestedjian, J. J. and Ronco, E.: Therapy of *Rhodococcus equi* disseminated infections in nude mice. Antimicrob. Agents Chemother. 36:1244-1248, 1992.

86. Novak, R. M., Polisky, E. L., Janda, W. M., et al.: Osteomyelitis caused by *Rhodococcus equi* in a renal transplant recipient. Infection 16:186-188, 1988.

87. Panaitescu, M., Maximescu, P., Michel, J., et al.: Respiratory pathogens in non-human primates with special reference to *Corynebacterium ulcerans*. Lab. Anim. 11:155-157, 1977.

88. Peel, M. M., Palmer, G. G., Stacpoole, A. M., et al.: Human lymphadenitis due to *Corynebacterium pseudotuberculosis*: Report of ten cases from Australia and review. Clin. Infect. Dis. 24:185-191, 1997.

89. Pitcher, D., Johnson, A., Allerberger, F., et al.: An investigation of nosocomial infection with *Corynebacterium jeikeium* in surgical patients using a ribosomal RNA gene probe. Eur. J. Clin. Microbiol. Infect. Dis. 9:643-648, 1990.

90. Prescott, J. F.: *Rhodococcus equi*: An animal and human pathogen. Clin. Microbiol. Rev. 4:20-34, 1991.

91. Prescott, J. F., Johnson, J. A., and Markham, R. J.: Experimental studies on the pathogenesis of *Corynebacterium equi* infection in foals. Can. J. Comp. Med. 44:280-288, 1980.

92. Quinn, J. P., Arnow, P. M., Weil, D., et al.: Outbreak of JK diphtheroid infections associated with environmental contamination. J. Clin. Microbiol. 19:668-671, 1984.

93. Riebel, W., Frantz, N., Adelstein, D., et al.: *Corynebacterium* JK: A cause of nosocomial device-related infection. Rev. Infect. Dis. 8:42-49, 1986.

94. Riegel, P., de Briel, D., Prevost, G., et al.: Genomic diversity among *Corynebacterium jeikeium* strains and comparison with biochemical characteristics and antimicrobial susceptibilities. J. Clin. Microbiol. 32:1860-1865, 1994.

95. Riley, P. S., Hollis, D. G., Utter, G. B., et al.: Characterization and identification of 95 diphtheroid (group JK) cultures isolated from clinical specimens. J. Clin. Microbiol. 9:418-424, 1979.

96. Rolston, K. V., Frisbee-Hume, S., Le Blanc, B., et al.: In vitro antimicrobial activity of moxifloxacin compared to other quinolones, against recent clinical bacterial isolates from hospitalized and community-based cancer patients. Diagn. Microbiol. Infect. Dis. 47:441-449, 2003.

97. Rozdzinski, E., Kern, W., Schmeiser, T., et al.: *Corynebacterium jeikeium* bacteremia at a tertiary care center. Infection 19:201-204, 1991.

98. Rufael, D. W., and Cohn, S. E.: Native valve endocarditis due to *Corynebacterium* striatum: Case report and review. Clin. Infect. Dis. 19:1054-1061, 1994.

99. Saavedra, J., Rodriguez, J. N., Fernandez-Jurado, A., et al.: A necrotic soft-tissue lesion due to *Corynebacterium urealyticum* in a neutropenic child. Clin. Infect. Dis. 22:851-852, 1996.

100. Sanchez Hernandez, J., Mora Peris, B., Yague Guirae, G., et al.: In vitro activity of new antibiotics against *Corynebacterium jeikeium*, *Corynebacterium amycolatum* and *Corynebacterium urealyticum*. Int. J. Antimicrob. Agents 22:492-496, 2003.

101. Scannell, K. A., Portoni, E. J., Finkle, H. I., et al.: Pulmonary malacoplakia and *Rhodococcus equi* infection in a patient with AIDS. Chest 97:1000-1001, 1990.

102. Schiffl, H., Mucke, C., and Lang, S. M.: Exit-site infections by non-diphtheria corynebacteria in CAPD. Perit. Dial. Int. 24:454-459, 2004.

103. Scott, M. A., Graham, B. S., Verrall, R., et al.: *Rhodococcus equi*—an increasingly recognized opportunistic pathogen: Report of 12 cases and review of 65 cases in the literature. Am. J. Clin. Pathol. 103:649-655, 1995.

104. Scotton, P. G., Tonon, E., Giobbia, M., et al.: *Rhodococcus equi* nosocomial meningitis cured by levofloxacin and shunt removal. Clin. Infect. Dis. 30:223-224, 2000.

105. Simoons-Smit, A. M., Savelkoul, P. H., Newling, D. W., and Vandenbroucke-Grauls, C. M.: Chronic cystitis caused by *Corynebacterium urealyticum* detected by polymerase chain reaction. Eur. J. Clin. Microbiol. Infect. Dis. *19*:949-952, 2000.

106. Sirera, G., Romeu, J., Clotet, B., et al.: Relapsing systemic infection due to *Rhodococcus equi* in a drug abuser seropositive for human immunodeficiency virus. Rev. Infect. Dis. *13*:509-510, 1991.

107. Soriano, F., Ponte, C., Ruiz, P., et al.: Non-urinary tract infections caused by multiply antibiotic-resistant *Corynebacterium* urealyticum. Clin. Infect. Dis. *17*:890-891, 1993.

108. Soriano, F., Ponte, C., Santamaria, M., et al.: *Corynebacterium* group D2 as a cause of alkaline-encrusted cystitis: Report of four cases and characterization of the organisms. J. Clin. Microbiol. *21*:788-792, 1985.

109. Soriano, F., Zapardiel, J., and Nieto, E.: Antimicrobial susceptibilities of *Corynebacterium* species and other non-spore-forming gram-positive bacilli to 18 antimicrobial agents. Antimicrob. Agents Chemother. *39*:208-214, 1995.

110. Stamm, W. E., Tompkins, L. S., Wagner, K. F., et al.: Infection due to *Corynebacterium* species in marrow transplant patients. Ann. Intern. Med. *91*:167-173, 1979.

111. Takai, S., Iie, M., Watanabe, Y., et al.: Virulence-associated 15- to 17-kilodalton antigens in *Rhodococcus equi*: Temperature-dependent expression and location of the antigens. Infect. Immun. *60*:2995-2997, 1992.

112. Takai, S., Imai, Y., Fukunaga, N., et al.: Identification of virulence-associated antigens and plasmids in *Rhodococcus equi* from patients with AIDS. J. Infect. Dis. *172*:1306-1311, 1995.

113. Tan, C., Prescott, J. F., Patterson, M. C., et al.: Molecular characterization of a lipid-modified virulence-associated protein of *Rhodococcus equi* and its potential in protective immunity. Can. J. Vet. Res. *59*:51-59, 1995.

114. Tang, S., Lo, C. Y., Lo, W. K., et al.: *Rhodococcus peritonitis* in continuous ambulatory peritoneal dialysis. Nephrol. Dial. Transplant. *11*:201-202, 1996.

115. Tang, S., Lo, C. Y., Lo, W. K., et al.: Optimal treatment regimen for CAPD peritonitis caused by *Rhodococcus* species [letter; comment]. Nephrol. Dial. Transplant. *12*:1080-1081, 1997.

116. Thompson, J. S., Gates-Davis, D. R., and Yong, D. C.: Rapid microbiochemical identification of *Corynebacterium* diphtheriae and other medically important corynebacteria. J. Clin. Microbiol. *18*:926-929, 1983.

117. Torres-Tortosa, M., Arrizabalaga, J., Villanueva, J. L., et al.: Prognosis and clinical evaluation of infection caused by *Rhodococcus equi* in HIV-infected patients: A multicenter study of 67 cases. Chest *123*:1970-1976, 2003.

118. Ulivieri, S., and Oliveri, G.: Cerebellar abscess due to *Rhodococcus equi* in an immunocompetent patient: Case report and literature review. J. Neurosurg. Sci. *50*:127-129, 2006.

119. van der Lelie, H., Leverstein-Van Hall, M., Mertens, M., et al.: *Corynebacterium* CDC group JK (*Corynebacterium jeikeium*) sepsis in haematological patients: A report of three cases and a systematic literature review. Scand. J. Infect. Dis. *27*:581-584, 1995.

120. Verville, T. D., Huycke, M. M., Greenfield, R. A., et al.: *Rhodococcus equi* infections of humans: 12 cases and a review of the literature. Medicine (Baltimore) *73*:119-132, 1994.

121. Wagner, J., Ignatius, R., Voss, S., et al.: Infection of the skin caused by *Corynebacterium ulcerans* and mimicking classical cutaneous diphtheria. Clin. Infect. Dis. *33*:1598-1600, 2001.

122. Watkins, D. A., Chahine, A., Creger, R. J., et al.: *Corynebacterium striatum*: A diphtheroid with pathogenic potential. Clin. Infect. Dis. *17*:21-25, 1993.

123. Weiss, K., Labbe, A. C., and Laverdiere, M.: *Corynebacterium striatum* meningitis: Case report and review of an increasingly important *Corynebacterium* species [see comments]. Clin. Infect. Dis. *23*:1246-1248, 1996.

124. Williams, D. Y., Selepak, S. T., and Gill, V. J.: Identification of clinical isolates of nondiphtherial *Corynebacterium* species and their antibiotic susceptibility patterns. Diagn. Microbiol. Infect. Dis. *17*:23-28, 1993.

125. Wilson, W. R., Danielson, G. K., Giuliani, E. R., et al.: Prosthetic valve endocarditis. Mayo Clin. Proc. *57*:155-161, 1982.

126. Wong, T. P., and Groman, N.: Production of diphtheria toxin by selected isolates of *Corynebacterium ulcerans* and *Corynebacterium pseudotuberculosis*. Infect. Immun. *43*:1114-1116, 1984.

127. Yoo, S. J., Sung, H., Chae, J. D., et al.: *Rhodococcus equi* pneumonia in a heart transplant recipient in Korea, with emphasis on microbial diagnosis. Clin. Microbiol. Infect. *9*:230-233, 2003.

128. Young, V. M., Meyers, W. F., Moody, M. R., et al.: The emergence of coryneform bacteria as a cause of nosocomial infections in compromised hosts. Am. J. Med. *70*:646-650, 1981.

CITROBACTER

Randall G. Fisher

Citrobacter, a genus of enteric gram-negative rods closely related to *Salmonella*, has been associated increasingly with human disease. Although *Citrobacter* strains usually are not considered normal inhabitants of the intestinal tract of humans and animals,[44,76] a study using 16S rDNA polymerase chain reaction showed that normal newborns are colonized with these organisms by day 6 of life.[52] They have been associated with urinary tract infections,[6,19,34,40,43,44] osteomyelitis,[43] diarrhea,[15,25,79] and invasive disease in the immunocompromised host.[32,34,43,44] As detailed in a review by Doran,[13] *Citrobacter* commonly is associated with sepsis, meningitis, and brain abscess in neonates.

BACTERIOLOGY

In 1931, Werkman and Gillen[76] proposed the generic term *Citrobacter* for citrate-positive coliaerogenes intermediates isolated from stool. This genus now includes 11 species, of which the most commonly identified are *Citrobacter freundii*, *Citrobacter koseri* (formerly *Citrobacter diversus*), and *Citrobacter farmeri* (formerly *Citrobacter amalonaticus*).[7] *Citrobacter* are straight, facultatively anaerobic bacilli possessing peritrichous flagellae that confer motility. In addition to using citrate, these organisms hydrolyze urea and ferment glucose, with production of gas.[65] They grow on ordinary media as gray, opaque, round colonies that produce a strong, fetid odor. In contrast to *Salmonella*, *Citrobacter* grows in the presence of potassium cyanide. Indole-negative strains that produce hydrogen sulfide are classified as *C. freundii*. Indole-positive, hydrogen sulfide–negative strains are differentiated by their ability to ferment malonate; *C. koseri* ferments malonate, whereas *C. farmeri* does not.[2] Antigenic schemata have been developed to classify the O somatic antigens of *Citrobacter*[20,24,79]; these antigens show cross-reactivity with O antigens of other Enterobacteriaceae.

EPIDEMIOLOGY

Meningitis caused by *Citrobacter* was reported first in 1960, with two cases of *C. freundii*.[29] In the decade from 1970 to 1979, 69 cases of *Citrobacter* meningitis were reported,[21] and 4 percent of neonatal meningitis cases reported in the First Neonatal Meningitis Cooperative Study Group were caused by *Citrobacter*.[48] *C. koseri* is the species usually isolated with meningitis; central nervous system (CNS) infection caused by *C. freundii* occurs less commonly.[13,21] Most of the cases in the United States are reported from southern states; biotype d or serotypes O2 and O1[21] are the most common isolates of *C. koseri* encountered.

Most cases of neonatal meningitis caused by this organism have been sporadic. The source of sporadic cases usually is unknown, but nine cases clearly have been documented to be vertically transmitted from mother to infant.[13] In addition, several well-documented nosocomial outbreaks of infection have been reported.[16,19,20,42,53,60,79] The source usually is the gastrointestinal tract or hands of nursery staff. One cluster was associated with contaminated formula.[71] When *Citrobacter* is introduced into the neonatal nursery, colonization may exceed 79 percent.[20] Parry and associates[53] described a nursery outbreak in which 11 of 128 infants were colonized with *C. koseri* over an observation period of 3 months; two of the colonized infants developed meningitis. Additional colonization of neonates seemed to be eliminated by removal of a nurse with persistent hand carriage of the organism.

In another outbreak,[79] introduction of *C. koseri* into the nursery was linked to an infant admitted with meningitis. Thirty-one percent of infants in the nursery subsequent to the index case were found to be colonized with *C. koseri* of the same serotype and biotype. A second infant from this study developed meningitis with the organism during the observation period. Umbilical colonization of infants in this cluster was more common than was rectal colonization, but rectal colonization was more persistent, lasting 4 months. Two nurses were found to have hand colonization with the organism, and the reintroduction of these bacteria into the nursery was linked to a pregnant nurse who had perineal cultures at delivery yielding the epidemic strain. She was implicated in the colonization of her own infant and three other neonates. Corresponding culture data from a reference hospital revealed an overall neonatal colonization rate with *Citrobacter* of 1 to 10 percent over a 5-year period, with no invasive disease.

Although *Citrobacter* has been isolated increasingly from debilitated adult patients,[77] particularly as a urinary tract,[34,43,44] soft tissue,[22,43,44] and bone[44] pathogen, *Citrobacter* infection in children is unusual after the first 2 months of life. One case of meningitis was reported in a teenager who lacked apparent risk factors or immunodeficiency.[59] In older children, *Citrobacter* spp. are more likely to cause opportunistic infection in an immunocompromised host or, occasionally, urinary tract infection. One study showed *Citrobacter* spp. to be responsible for 37 (1.4%) urinary tract infections in children over a 3-year period.[17] One quarter of infections were nosocomially acquired, and one third occurred in children with urinary tract abnormalities.

PATHOPHYSIOLOGY

Citrobacter infrequently colonizes the intestinal tract and perineum of humans.[34] Vertical transmission of strains shown to be identical by DNA typing shows that the newborn can acquire colonization at the time of passage through the birth canal of a colonized mother.[30,51] Onset of disease beyond the first week of life is related commonly to colonization of the infant in the nursery. As with other types of gram-negative neonatal meningitis, CNS infection results from bacteremia in a colonized infant, leading to seeding of the meninges.

The basis for the particular invasiveness of *Citrobacter* in the neonate and its propensity to cause multiple brain abscesses are largely unexplained. *Citrobacter* spp. possess the ability to invade, transcytose, and multiply within human brain microvascular endothelial cells in vitro.[3] Additionally, in the neonatal rat model, after being taken up into macrophages, *C. koseri* is able to survive phagolysosomal fusion and replicate therein.[72] Many strains of *C. koseri* seem to be able to produce brain pathology in the mouse, but the degree of damage seems to be related to virulence of the strain and the age of the mouse.[39,66] Differences in strains, related to the presence of an outer-membrane protein with a molecular weight of 32,000, have been associated with differences in brain histopathology in one infant rat model of *C. koseri* meningitis.[38] Strains isolated from cerebrospinal fluid (CSF) of infants with meningitis more commonly possess this outer-membrane protein than do strains isolated from other body sites.[39]

In an immunocompromised patient, broad use of antimicrobial agents may produce selective pressure, leading to increased colonization with *Citrobacter*. Increased bacterial density combined with a blunted immune response may result in invasive disease. Some strains of *C. freundii* have been shown to produce Shiga toxins (verotoxins) nearly identical to those produced by enterohemorrhagic strains of *Escherichia coli*.[63] At least one outbreak of gastroenteritis and the hemolytic-uremic syndrome caused by Shiga-toxin–producing *C. freundii* has been reported.[73]

CLINICAL MANIFESTATIONS

Citrobacter, similar to other neonatal pathogens, can cause early-onset and late-onset infection. In a review of 74 cases of neonatal meningitis caused by these bacteria,[21] the mean age of onset reported for early disease was 7 days; 85 percent of patients were included in this group. Fifteen percent of cases occurred after 3 weeks of age. Twenty-three (31%) of 74 patients were younger than 36 weeks' gestational age at birth, suggesting that preterm infants are at increased risk for acquisition of *Citrobacter* infection. Prematurity is even more common (71%) in cases that are proven to be vertically acquired.[13]

Clinical signs and symptoms are typical of neonatal sepsis. Fever, lethargy, poor feeding, vomiting, irritability, bulging fontanelle, seizures, and jaundice are common presenting features. Umbilical infection and surgical manipulation of colonized umbilical stumps occasionally have preceded development of bacteremia and meningitis.[53] The white blood cell count may show leukocytosis or leukopenia. CSF fluid findings are consistent with most types of neonatal bacterial meningitis and usually show polymorphonuclear cell elevation, elevated protein, and depressed glucose; gram-negative rods may be seen on smear. Although growing the organism in culture normally is not difficult, in one reported case standard cultures were negative, but the organism was recovered by direct inoculation of CSF into a BacTec blood culture bottle.[11] Of *Citrobacter* meningitis cases in which the results of blood cultures are reported, 80 percent document concurrent bacteremia.[13]

Citrobacter is a particularly devastating cause of neonatal meningitis. The most common *Citrobacter* spp. causing neonatal meningitis is *C. koseri*, which accounts for more than 80 percent of the cases.[13] CNS infection with this organism produces multiple brain abscesses with unusually high frequency.[21,27,35,39,41] In the extensive reviews by Graham and Band[21] and by Doran,[13] three quarters of *Citrobacter* meningitis cases resulted in intracerebral abscesses. By comparison, the incidence of abscess formation in non-*Citrobacter* gram-negative meningitis is reported to be as low as 10 percent.[21] The case-fatality rate for *Citrobacter* meningitis is approximately 30 percent, and at least three quarters of surviv-

ing infants have neurologic sequelae, such as mental retardation, hemiparesis, seizures, and developmental delay.[13]

The presence of brain abscess seems to contribute significantly to morbidity and mortality.[12,20,21] For unknown reasons, neonates with vertically acquired *Citrobacter* meningitis seem to be less likely to develop intracerebral abscesses.[13] At least three cases in which diffuse pneumocephalus developed in association with *Citrobacter* meningitis have been reported; in one, gas was noted to accumulate within the brain and in the anterior chamber of the eye, a condition known as *pneumatosis oculi*.[1,58] Rarely, *Citrobacter* infection in the neonatal period may lead to focal infection not involving the CNS. A case of septic arthritis and osteomyelitis of the shoulder in a 3-week-old infant has been reported.[31]

In adults, *Citrobacter* is isolated most commonly from the urinary tract.[34,43,44] In earlier studies, 5 to 12 percent of bacterial isolates from urinary tract infections in adult patients were *Citrobacter*.[15,78] More recently, in a health maintenance organization, *Citrobacter* spp. accounted for only 0.8 percent of 4342 isolates from women with acute uncomplicated cystitis.[26] *Citrobacter* spp. are a similarly uncommon cause of urinary tract infection in children.[17] Sputum is the second most common clinical specimen to yield *Citrobacter* in adults[34]; lung abscess,[18] pneumonia,[43,44] bronchitis,[32] and septic arthritis[43] have been reported. *Citrobacter* is an occasional cause of bacteremia in hospitalized patients, accounting for approximately 0.5 percent of blood culture isolates.[56,64] In one series, all 45 patients had at least one underlying disease, with malignancies (particularly intra-abdominal tumors) and hepatobiliary stones being the most frequent coexisting conditions.[64] Polymicrobial bacteremia occurred in one third of patients. The case-fatality rate was 18 percent.

Gastrointestinal disease occasionally has been attributed to *Citrobacter*, but frequent isolation of this agent from normal stools often renders this diagnosis equivocal. This genus was implicated first in an outbreak of mild gastroenteritis by Barnes and Cherry[5] in 1946, and an outbreak of watery diarrhea in a Virginia infant care unit included two infants in whom isolates of enterotoxin-liberating *Citrobacter* were obtained from the stool.[25] Some studies have found higher incidences of *Citrobacter* isolation from the stool of patients with enterocolitis syndrome than from stools of control patients.[79] Shiga-toxin (verotoxin)–producing *C. freundii* isolated from organically grown parsley was associated with an outbreak of diarrhea and hemolytic-uremic syndrome in a daycare setting.[73] *C. freundii* has been found as a cause of appendicitis in a healthy adult,[43] peritonitis in adults with liver disease or pancreatitis,[43] neutropenic colitis following chemotherapy for breast cancer,[10] and meningitis in adults as a complication of neurosurgery.[70] A case of Meleney gangrene occurring after cesarean section delivery has been reported.[69] A patient with diabetes developed necrotizing fasciitis caused by *C. freundii* associated with injury from a fish fin.[9] Bone and soft tissue infections occur[8,67]; 3 percent of *Citrobacter* pathogens were isolated from joint or bone in one adult series.[43]

DIAGNOSIS

Biochemical characteristics of *C. koseri* include lack of hydrogen sulfide production on triple-sugar iron agar, negative Voges-Proskauer reaction, use of citrate, motility, production of indole, decarboxylation of ornithine but not lysine, and production of acid from adonitol.[2] Identification of this organism as a pathogen in a nursery setting should heighten suspicion of its possible role in subsequent neonatal infections. *C. freundii* is indole-negative and hydrogen sulfide–positive, which differentiates it from *C. koseri*. *C. farmeri* differs from *C. koseri* because of the former's inability to ferment malonate. *C. freundii* and *C. farmeri* account for a significant portion of disease caused by *Citrobacter* in immunocompromised individuals and should be suspected particularly in this group of patients.[32]

Infants with invasive *Citrobacter* disease present in a similar fashion to infants with sepsis and meningitis of other causes. Such infants should undergo a thorough evaluation, including blood and urine culture and CSF studies. Brain imaging studies should be done when the diagnosis is established. Computed tomography is the most common test used, although ultrasound often is more feasible for an unstable neonate and may be nearly as sensitive in detecting abscesses.[41,49,80] Serial imaging studies should be done because abscesses may develop during the first few weeks of illness. In cases in which the CSF cultures are negative because of prior antimicrobial therapy, surgical aspiration of abscesses sometimes enables identification of the organism.

TREATMENT

Most *C. koseri* organisms are resistant to ampicillin (97% in one series)[43] and sensitive to aminoglycosides and third-generation cephalosporins.[13] A 4-year experience with neonatal septicemia caused by *C. koseri* has been described, however, in which all of 13 isolates were resistant to gentamicin, but susceptible to third-generation cephalosporins.[16] The resistance patterns of *C. freundii* were reported in a national surveillance study of nosocomial bloodstream infections.[56] Of the 23 *C. freundii* isolates tested, resistance to piperacillin, piperacillin/tazobactam, ceftriaxone, and ceftazidime was a common (39-48%) finding. Isolates generally were susceptible to the aminoglycosides and ciprofloxacin (91-96%), and all *C. freundii* tested were susceptible to cefepime and imipenem.

Some *Citrobacter* isolates contain chromosomally mediated group I β-lactamases. These bacteria possess a gene that, when triggered by exposure to cephalosporins or by spontaneous mutation, produces a cephalosporinase capable of inactivating cephalosporins.[33] Clinically, it manifests as treatment failure and emergence of drug resistance to various cephalosporins despite initial susceptibility.[45] In one study, the presence of group I β-lactamases was much more common with *C. freundii* (9 of 22 isolates) than with *C. koseri* (0 of 7 isolates).[33] Resistance was associated with previous receipt of an extended-spectrum, β-lactam antibiotic. Reliable estimates of the percentage of *Citrobacter* strains that contain the chromosomal resistance gene are difficult to obtain because most studies lump *Citrobacter*, *Enterobacter*, and *Serratia* isolates together. In one Korean study, of 152

Enterobacter/Citrobacter/Serratia isolates, 45 (30%) were derepressed AmpC mutants.[52] In an in vitro study, AmpC production was inducible in eight of nine clinical isolates of *C. freundii* and in one of three isolates of *C. koseri*. AmpC synthesis was stably derepressed in one of the nine *C. freundii* isolates.[14] Cefepime seems to be less likely to induce production of these β-lactamases and more resistant to hydrolysis by them,[62] although a highly cefepime-resistant strain has been described.[4] Ninety-nine percent of 3030 ceftazidime-resistant Enterobacteriaceae in a U.S. study retained susceptibility to imipenem, and 96.7 percent of ceftazidime-resistant *Citrobacter* isolates were susceptible to cefepime.[57] Many different types of β-lactamases, including a novel TEM-type (TEM-134),[54] the class A β-lactamase CKO,[55] and a VIM-1 metallo-β-lactamase, have been described in various isolates of *Citrobacter*.[75]

Treatment of *Citrobacter* meningitis often requires a multidisciplinary effort involving the neurosurgeon and the pediatrician. Although cerebral abscesses usually are aspirated or drained surgically, some patients are treated with antibiotics alone, and neither approach is clearly shown to be superior. When abscesses are inaccessible or small and not progressive, conservative management may be considered.[13] Ventriculostomy and craniectomy with open drainage of abscesses have been required in some children to effect bacteriologic cure, and placement of a shunt for hydrocephalus often is required.

Generally, antibiotic therapy for gram-negative neonatal meningitis has proved disappointing (see Chapter 78).[46,47] No evidence supports one combination of antibiotics over another in the treatment of *Citrobacter* meningitis. Usually a third-generation or fourth-generation cephalosporin or a carbapenem (usually meropenem) is used in combination with an aminoglycoside initially.[13] Chloramphenicol,[12,20,28] imipenem/cilastatin,[15,28] and trimethoprim-sulfamethoxazole[23] also have been used successfully.

Poor meningeal penetration of aminoglycosides in addition to the presence of intracranial abscesses renders antibiotic therapy for *Citrobacter* meningitis especially difficult. The ability of this organism to persist in the brain is shown by its recovery 4 years after neonatal infection.[15] Cranial computed tomography usually is used for evaluation of complications such as hydrocephalus and multicystic encephalomalacia (Fig. 112-1). Administration of antibiotics intrathecally or directly into abscess cavities has been tried but has not been shown convincingly to be beneficial.[23,24,27,37,42,50,61,68,74] In a randomized controlled trial, intraventricular administration of gentamicin in the treatment of neonates

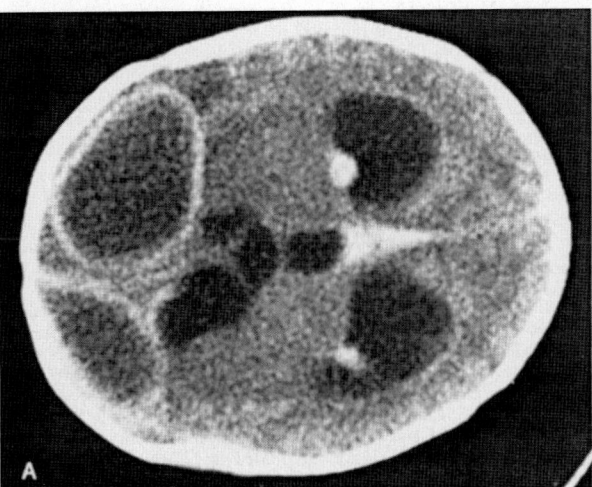
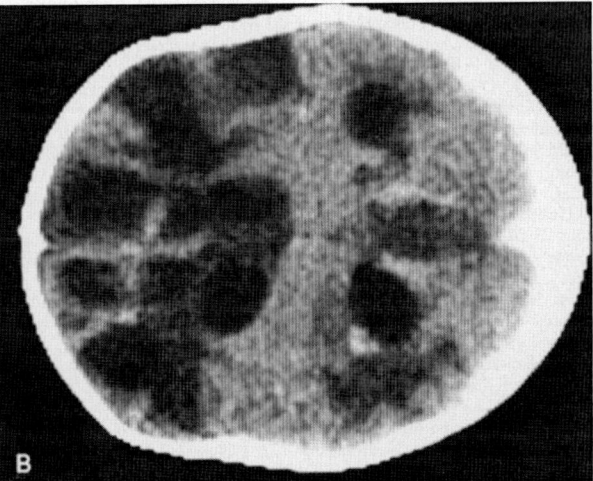

Figure 112–1 **A** and **B**, Computed tomography scans showing progressive abscess formation and encephalomalacia in an infant at 3 weeks of age (**A**) and 6 weeks of age (**B**), despite bacteriologic "cure" of *Citrobacter* meningitis.

with gram-negative meningitis was associated with a poorer outcome.[48]

Neonates with gram-negative meningitis should undergo repeat lumbar puncture approximately 72 hours after beginning therapy to document sterilization of CSF. Duration of therapy with intravenous antibiotics generally is a minimum of 21 days for gram-negative neonatal meningitis. For cases complicated by intracranial abscesses, prolonged therapy (usually 4 to 6 weeks after sterilization of CSF) is indicated.[13,56]

Scrupulous attention given to preventive infection control practices has been recommended to stem nursery outbreaks.[20,53,79] These prophylactic measures include care of skin and the umbilical cord, elimination of crowding with isolation of infected infants and carriers, and good handwashing practices. Exclusion of colonized personnel and temporary closing of the nursery have been followed by a reduction in neonatal *C. koseri* colonization. Although cohorting of colonized infants is a reasonable practice, multiple sources of introduction of *Citrobacter* may limit the efficacy of this approach in some outbreaks.[19]

Treatment of *Citrobacter* infection beyond the neonatal period requires choice of an appropriate antibiotic, with drainage of abscesses and appropriate débridement of wounds. Therapy should be guided by antimicrobial susceptibility testing. Outcome depends largely on the preceding debility of the host and location of the infection. Significant mortality is associated with immunocompromised patients with septicemia or pulmonary disease.[32,34,43,44,64]

Acknowledgments

The author thanks Dr. William Gruber and Dr. Thomas Boyce for their invaluable assistance with earlier versions of this chapter.

REFERENCES

1. Altmann, G., Sechter, I., Cahan, D., et al.: *Citrobacter diversus* isolated from clinical material. J. Clin. Microbiol. 3:390-392, 1976.
2. Alviedo, J. N., Sood, B. G., Aranda, J. V., and Becker, C.: Diffuse pneumocephalus in neonatal *Citrobacter* meningitis. Pediatrics 118:e1576-e1579, 2006.
3. Badger, J. L., Stins, M. F., and Kim, K. S.: *Citrobacter freundii* invades and replicates in human brain microvascular endothelial cells. Infect. Immun. 67:4208-4215, 1999.
4. Barnaud, G., Labia, R., Raskine, L., et al.: Extension of resistance to cefepime and cefpirome associated to a six amino acid deletion in the H-10 helix of the cephalosporinase of an *Enterobacter cloacae* clinical isolate. F. E. M. S. Microbiol. Lett. 195:185-190, 2001.
5. Barnes, L. A., and Cherry, C. B.: A group of paracolon organisms having apparent pathogenicity. Am. J. Public Health 36:481-483, 1946.
6. Barton, L. L., and Walentik, C.: *Citrobacter diversus* urinary tract infection. Am. J. Dis. Child. 136:467-468, 1982.
7. Brenner, D. J., O'Hara, C. M., Grimont, P. A., et al.: Biochemical identification of *Citrobacter* species defined by DNA hybridization and description of *Citrobacter gillenii* sp. nov. (formerly *Citrobacter* genomospecies 10) and *Citrobacter murliniae* sp. nov. (formerly *Citrobacter* genomospecies 11). J. Clin. Microbiol. 37:2619-2624, 1999.
8. Bruehl, C. L., and Listernick, R.: *Citrobacter freundii* septic arthritis. J. Paediatr. Child Health. 28:402-403, 1992.
9. Chuang, Y. M., Tseng, S. P., Teng, L. J., et al.: Emergence of cefotaxime resistance in *Citrobacter freundii* causing necrotizing fasciitis and osteomyelitis. J. Infect. 53:e161-e163, 2006.
10. Clemons, M. J., Valle, J. W., Harris, M., et al.: *Citrobacter freundii* and fatal neutropenic enterocolitis following adjuvant chemotherapy for breast cancer. Clin. Oncol. (R. Coll. Radiol.) 9:172-175, 1997.
11. Cohen-Wolkowicz, M., and Laufer, M.: Enhanced culture detection of *Citrobacter koseri* from cerebrospinal fluid in BacTec. Pediatr. Infect. Dis. J. 24:750, 2005.
12. Curless, R. G.: Neonatal intracranial abscess: Two cases caused by *Citrobacter* and a literature review. Ann. Neurol. 8:269-272, 1980.
13. Doran, T. I.: The role of *Citrobacter* in clinical disease of children: Review. Clin. Infect. Dis. 28:384-394, 1999.
14. Dunne, W. M., and Hardin, D. J.: Use of several inducer and substrate antibiotic combinations in a disk approximation assay format to screen for AmpC induction in patient isolates of *Pseudomonas aeruginosa*, *Enterobacter* spp., *Citrobacter* spp., and *Serratia* spp. J. Clin. Microbiol. 43:5945-5949, 2005.
15. Eppes, S. C., Woods, C. R., Mayer, A. S., et al.: Recurring *ventriculitis* due to *Citrobacter diversus*: Clinical and bacteriologic analysis. Clin. Infect. Dis. 17:437-440, 1993.
16. Giacoia, G. P., and West, K.: Sepsis with *Citrobacter diversus* in sick newborns. Am. J. Perinatol. 6:49-54, 1989.
17. Gill, M. A., and Schutze, G. E.: *Citrobacter* urinary tract infections in children. Pediatr. Infect. Dis. J. 18:889-892, 1999.
18. Gilman, R. M., Irwin, R. S., and Garrity, F. L.: Community-acquired *Citrobacter diversus* infections. Respir. Care 25:66-71, 1980.
19. Goering, R. V., Ehrenkranz, N. J., Sanders, C. C., et al.: Long term epidemiological analysis of *Citrobacter diversus* in a neonatal intensive care unit. Pediatr. Infect. Dis. J. 11:99-104, 1992.
20. Graham, D. R., Anderson, R. L., Ariel, F. E., et al.: Epidemic nosocomial meningitis due to *Citrobacter diversus* in neonates. J. Infect. Dis. 144:203-209, 1981.
21. Graham, D. R., and Band, J. D.: *Citrobacter diversus* brain abscess and meningitis in neonates. J. A. M. A. 245:1923-1925, 1981.
22. Grant, M. D., Horowitz, H. I., and Lorian, V.: Gangrenous ulcer and septicemia due to *Citrobacter*. N. Engl. J. Med. 280:1286-1287, 1969.
23. Greene, G. R., Heitlinger, L., and Madden, J. D.: *Citrobacter ventriculitis* in a neonate responsive to trimethoprim-sulfamethoxazole. Clin. Pediatr. (Phila.) 22:515-517, 1983.
24. Gross, R. J., Rowe, B., and Easton, J. A.: Neonatal meningitis caused by *Citrobacter koseri*. J. Clin. Pathol. 26:138-139, 1973.
25. Guerrant, R. L., Dickens, M. D., Wenzel, R. P., et al.: Toxigenic bacterial diarrhea: Nursery outbreak involving multiple bacterial strains. J. Pediatr. 89:885-891, 1976.
26. Gupta, K., Scholes, D., and Stamm, W. E.: Increasing prevalence of antimicrobial resistance among uropathogens causing acute uncomplicated cystitis in women [see comments]. J. A. M. A. 281:736-738, 1999.
27. Gwynn, C. M., and George, R. H.: Neonatal *Citrobacter* meningitis. Arch. Dis. Child. 48:455-458, 1973.
28. Haimi-Cohen, Y., Amir, J., Weinstock, A., et al.: The use of imipenem-cilastatin in neonatal meningitis caused by *Citrobacter diversus*. Acta Paediatr. 82:530-532, 1993.
29. Harris, D., and Cone, T. E., Jr.: *Escherichia freundii* meningitis: Report of two cases. J. Pediatr. 56:774-777, 1960.
30. Harvey, B. S., Koeuth, T., Versalovic, J., et al.: Vertical transmission of *Citrobacter diversus* documented by DNA fingerprinting. Infect. Control Hosp. Epidemiol. 16:564-569, 1995.
31. Hayani, K. C.: *Citrobacter koseri* osteomyelitis in an infant. Acta Paediatr. Jpn. 39:390-391, 1997.
32. Hodges, G. R., Degener, C. E., and Barnes, W. G.: Clinical significance of *Citrobacter* isolates. Am. J. Clin. Pathol. 70:37-40, 1978.
33. Jacobson, K. L., Cohen, S. H., Inciardi, J. F., et al.: The relationship between antecedent antibiotic use and resistance to extended-spectrum cephalosporins in group I beta-lactamase-producing organisms. Clin. Infect. Dis. 21:1107-1113, 1995.
34. Jones, S. R., Ragsdale, A. R., Kutscher, E., et al.: Clinical and bacteriologic observations on a recently recognized species of enterobacteriaceae, *Citrobacter diversus*. J. Infect. Dis. 128:563-565, 1973.
35. Kaplan, A. M., Itabashi, H. H., Yoshimori, R., et al.: Cerebral abscesses complicating neonatal *Citrobacter freundii* meningitis. West. J. Med. 127:418-422, 1977.
36. Kline, M. W.: *Citrobacter* meningitis and brain abscess in infancy: Epidemiology, pathogenesis, and treatment. J. Pediatr. 113:430-434, 1988.
37. Kline, M. W., and Kaplan, S. L.: *Citrobacter diversus* and neonatal brain abscess. Pediatr. Neurol. 3:178-180, 1987.
38. Kline, M. W., Kaplan, S. L., Hawkins, E. P., et al.: Pathogenesis of brain abscess formation in an infant rat model of *Citrobacter diversus* bacteremia and meningitis. J. Infect. Dis. 157:106-112, 1988.
39. Kline, M. W., Mason, E. O., Jr., and Kaplan, S. L.: Characterization of *Citrobacter diversus* strains causing neonatal meningitis. J. Infect. Dis. 157:101-105, 1988.
40. Lesseva, M. I., and Hadjiski, O. G.: Analysis of bacteriuria in patients with burns. Burns 21:3-6, 1995.
41. Levine, R. S., Rosenberg, H. K., Zimmerman, R. A., et al.: Complications of *Citrobacter* neonatal meningitis: Assessment by real-time cranial sonography correlated with CT. A. J. N. R. Am. J. Neuroradiol. 4:668-671, 1983.
42. Lin, F. C., Devoe, W. F., Morrison, C., et al.: Outbreak of neonatal *Citrobacter diversus* meningitis in a suburban hospital. Pediatr. Infect. Dis. J. 6:50-55, 1987.
43. Lipsky, B. A., Hook, E. W., 3rd, Smith, A. A., et al.: *Citrobacter* infections in humans: Experience at the Seattle Veterans Administration Medical Center and a review of the literature. Rev. Infect. Dis. 2:746-760, 1980.
44. Madrazo, A., Geiger, J., and Lauter, C. B.: *Citrobacter diversus* at Grace Hospital, Detroit, Michigan. Am. J. Med. Sci. 270:497-501, 1975.
45. Marshall, W. F., and Blair, J. E.: The cephalosporins. Mayo Clin. Proc. 74:187-195, 1999.
46. McCracken, G. H., Jr.: New developments in the management of children with bacterial meningitis. Pediatr. Infect. Dis. 3:S32-S34, 1984.

47. McCracken, G. H., Jr., and Mize, S. G.: A controlled study of intrathecal antibiotic therapy in gram-negative enteric meningitis of infancy: Report of the neonatal meningitis cooperative study group. J. Pediatr. *89*:66-72, 1976.
48. McCracken, G. H., Jr., Mize, S. G., and Threlkeld, N.: Intraventricular gentamicin therapy in gram-negative bacillary meningitis of infancy: Report of the Second Neonatal Meningitis Cooperative Study Group. Lancet *1*:787-791, 1980.
49. Meier, A., Chusid, M. J., and Sty, J. R.: Neonatal *Citrobacter* meningitis: Neurosonographic observations. J. Ultrasound Med. *17*:399-401, 1998.
50. Morgan, M. G., Stuart, C., Leanord, A. T., et al.: *Citrobacter diversus* brain abscess: Case reports and molecular epidemiology. J. Med. Microbiol. *36*:273-278, 1992.
51. Papasian, C. J., Kinney, J., Coffman, S., et al.: Transmission of *Citrobacter koseri* from mother to infant documented by ribotyping and pulsed-field gel electrophoresis. Diagn. Microbiol. Infect. Dis. *26*:63-67, 1996.
52. Park, H. K., Shim, S. S., Kim, S. Y., et al.: Molecular analysis of colonized bacteria in a human newborn infant gut. J. Microbiol. *43*:345-353, 2005.
53. Parry, M. F., Hutchinson, J. H., Brown, N. A., et al.: Gram-negative sepsis in neonates: A nursery outbreak due to hand carriage of *Citrobacter diversus*. Pediatrics *65*:1105-1109, 1980.
54. Perilli, M., Mugnaioli, C., Luzzaro, F., et al.: Novel TEM-type extended-spectrum beta-lactamase, TEM-134, in a *Citrobacter koseri* clinical isolate. Antimicrob. Agents Chemother. *49*:1564-1566, 2005.
55. Petrella, S., Renard, M., Ziental-Gelus, N., et al.: Characterization of the chromosomal class A beta-lactamase CKO from *Citrobacter koseri*. F. E. M. S. Micribiol. Lett. *254*:285-292, 2006.
56. Pfaller, M. A., Jones, R. N., Marshall, S. A., et al.: Inducible amp C beta-lactamase producing gram-negative bacilli from blood stream infections: Frequency, antimicrobial susceptibility, and molecular epidemiology in a national surveillance program (SCOPE). Diagn. Microbiol. Infect. Dis. *28*:211-219, 1997.
57. Pfaller, M. A., Sader, H. S., Fritsche, T. R., and Jones, R. N.: Antimicrobial activity of cefepime tested against ceftazidime-resistant Gram-negative clinical strains from North American Hospitals: Report from the SENTRY Antimicrobial Surveillance Program (1998-2004). Diagn. Microbiol. Infect. Dis. *56*:63-68, 2006.
58. Pooboni, S. K., Mathur, S. K., Dux, A., et al.: Pneumocephalus in neonatal meningitis: Diffuse, necrotizing meningoencephalitis in *Citrobacter* meningitis presenting with pneumatosis oculi and pneumocephalus. Pediatr. Crit. Care Med. *5*:393-395, 2004.
59. Prais, D., Nussinovitch, M., Harel, L., and Amir, I.: *Citrobacter koseri (diversus)* meningitis in an otherwise healthy adolescent. Scand. J. Infect. Dis. *35*:202-204, 2003.
60. Ribeiro, C. D., Davis, P., and Jones, D. M.: *Citrobacter koseri* meningitis in a special care baby unit. J. Clin. Pathol. *29*:1094-1096, 1976.
61. Rose, S. J.: Neonatal meningitis due to *Citrobacter koseri*. J. Perinat. Med. *7*:273-275, 1979.
62. Sanders, W. E., Jr., Tenney, J. H., and Kessler, R. E.: Efficacy of cefepime in the treatment of infections due to multiply resistant *Enterobacter* species. Clin. Infect. Dis. *23*:454-461, 1996.
63. Schmidt, H., Montag, M., Bockemuhl, J., et al.: Shiga-like toxin II-related cytotoxins in *Citrobacter freundii* strains from humans and beef samples. Infect. Immun. *61*:534-543, 1993.
64. Shih, C. C., Chen, Y. C., Chang, S. C., et al.: Bacteremia due to *Citrobacter* species: Significance of primary intraabdominal infection. Clin. Infect. Dis. *23*:543-549, 1996.
65. Smith, R. F., Dayton, S. L., and Chipps, D. D.: Recognition of *Citrobacter diversus* in the clinical laboratory. Appl. Microbiol. *25*:157-158, 1973.
66. Soriano, A. L., Russell, R. G., Johnson, D., et al.: Pathophysiology of *Citrobacter diversus* neonatal meningitis: Comparative studies in an infant mouse model. Infect. Immun. *59*:1352-1358, 1991.
67. Stricker, T., Frohlich, S., and Nadal, D.: Osteomyelitis and septic arthritis due to *Citrobacter reundii* and *Haemophilus influenzae* type b. J. Paediatr. Child Health *34*:90-91, 1998.
68. Tamborlane, W. V. F., and Soto, E. V.: Experience and reason—briefly recorded: *Citrobacter diversus* meningitis: A case report. Pediatrics *55*:739-741, 1975.
69. Tandon, A., Sharma, D., Dawar, P., et al.: Conservative debridement of postoperative Meleney's gangrene following a caesarean section. J. Wound Care. *15*:445-446, 2006.
70. Tang, L. M., Chen, S. T., and Lui, T. N.: *Citrobacter* meningitis in adults. Clin. Neurol. Neurosurg. *96*:52-57, 1994.
71. Thurm, V., and Gericke, B.: Identification of infant food as a vehicle in a nosocomial outbreak of *Citrobacter freundii*: Epidemiological subtyping by allozyme, whole-cell protein and antibiotic resistance. J. Appl. Bacteriol. *76*:553-558, 1994.
72. Townsend, S. M., Gonzalez-Gomez, I., Badger, J. L.: fliP influences *Citrobacter koseri* macrophage uptake, cytokine expression and brain abscess formation in the neonatal rat. J. Med. Microbiol. *55*:1631-1640, 2006.
73. Tschape, H., Prager, R., Streckel, W., et al.: Verotoxinogenic *Citrobacter freundii* associated with severe gastroenteritis and cases of haemolytic uraemic syndrome in a nursery school: Green butter as the infection source. Epidemiol. Infect. *114*:441-450, 1995.
74. Vogel, L. C., Ferguson, L., and Gotoff, S. P.: *Citrobacter* infections of the central nervous system in early infancy. J. Pediatr. *93*:86-88, 1978.
75. Weile, J., Gfroer, S., Schroeppel, K., et al.: First detection of a VIM-1 metallo-beta-lactamase in a carbapenem-resistant *Citrobacter freundii* clinical isolate in an acute hospital in Germany. Scand. J. Infect. Dis. *39*:264-266, 2007.
76. Werkman, C. H., and Gillen, G. F.: Bacteria producing trimethylene glycol. J. Bacteriol. *23*:167-182, 1932.
77. Werthamer, S., and Weiner, M.: Subacute bacterial endocarditis due to *Flavobacterium meningosepticum*. Am. J. Clin. Pathol. *57*:410-412, 1972.
78. Wientzen, R. L., McCracken, G. H., Jr., Petruska, M. L., et al.: Localization and therapy of urinary tract infections of childhood. Pediatrics. *63*:467-474, 1979.
79. Williams, W. W., Mariano, J., Spurrier, M., et al.: Nosocomial meningitis due to *Citrobacter diversus* in neonates: New aspects of the epidemiology. J. Infect. Dis. *150*:229-235, 1984.
80. Wilson, D. A., Nguyen, D. L., and Marshall, K.: Sonography of brain abscesses complicating *Citrobacter* neonatal meningitis. Am. J. Perinatol. *5*:37-39, 1988.

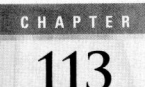

CHAPTER 113

ENTEROBACTER

Laura A. Sass ⊙ Randall G. Fisher

Enterobacter is a genus of Enterobacteriaceae that is an increasingly frequent cause of nosocomial pediatric infection. *Enterobacter* can cause infection of postsurgical wounds; meningitis; and infection of the gastrointestinal, urinary, and respiratory tracts. Development of resistance to antibiotics commonly used for treatment of infection is an increasingly common challenge. For a more detailed overview of *Enterobacter* spp., the reader is referred to the review by Sanders and Sanders.[132]

BACTERIOLOGY

Enterobacter spp. are named for their enteric recovery as gram-negative bacteria.[128] They commonly are found in soil, water, and sewage. They also are causes of botanical disease. These organisms are facultatively anaerobic and motile by peritrichous flagella, with the exception of *Enterobacter asburiae*. Most species yield positive results on malonate, citrate, sucrose fermentation, and Voges-Proskauer tests. *Enterobacter sakazakii* is distinguishable from the other species by its yellow-pigmented colonies. Taxonomic studies have led to several classifications of species contained in this genus. With the reclassification of *Enterobacter agglomerans* as *Pantoea agglomerans* (see Chapter 124), *Enterobacter cloacae*, *Enterobacter aerogenes*, and *E. sakazakii* are the most common species recovered from clinical material.[5,17,29,41,50,69,156,158]

Additional species in the *Enterobacter* genus rarely recovered from human infections include *Enterobacter amnigenus*, *E. asburiae*, *Enterobacter gergoviae*, *Enterobacter cancerogenus* (formerly *Enterobacter taylorae*), *Enterobacter kobei* (formerly NIH group 21), *E. cloacae* subsp. *dissolvens* (formerly *Enterobacter dissolvens*), *Enterobacter nimipressuralis*, and *Enterobacter hormaechei*.[1,53,99,100,109,128] NIH group 42 strains now have been proposed to become *Enterobacter cowanii*.[67] *Enterobacter intermedius* now has been reclassified to *Kluyvera intermedia* (formerly *Kluyvera cochleae*).[116] *Enterobacter ludwigii* is another new species isolated from clinical specimens that is closely related to *E. cloacae* complex.[65]

EPIDEMIOLOGY

Enterobacter is encountered most commonly as a hospital-acquired pathogen in patients with chronic illness.[5,17,29,41,69,156,158,165] A surveillance study at 50 American medical centers showed *Enterobacter* as the eighth most common cause of nosocomial bloodstream infections, accounting for 230 (5%) of 4725 isolates.[121] Of these, 71 percent were *E. cloacae*, 23 percent were *E. aerogenes*, and 6 percent were other species of *Enterobacter*. *Enterobacter* infections are particularly common in intensive care units (ICUs).[102] A report from the Centers for Disease Control and Prevention describing the epidemiology of health care–associated infections in 61 pediatric ICUs in the United States revealed that *Enterobacter* spp. were isolated with increasing frequency from patients with pneumonia and were the most common gram-negative isolates from bloodstream infections.[69] The frequency of *Enterobacter* spp. increased from 7 to 12 percent of reported pathogens over a 6-year period. *Enterobacter* spp. also were found to be second only to *Pseudomonas aeruginosa* in prevalence in health care–associated sinusitis.[129]

In another Centers for Disease Control and Prevention survey focusing on data from the National Nosocomial Infections Surveillance system, *Enterobacter* was one of the five pathogens most commonly encountered in ICUs, and accounted for 8.6 percent of reported infections.[69] During a 10-year period in six Brazilian neonatal ICUs, gram-negative pathogens accounted for more than half of all bloodstream infections, with *Enterobacter* spp. representing 2 percent.[32] In one pediatric hospital, *Enterobacter* spp. (primarily *E. cloacae*) were the most common cause of enteric bacteremia, and accounted for 14 percent of all bacteremic episodes occurring during a 3-year period.[5] Multiple outbreaks caused by *Enterobacter* have been described in neonatal ICUs.* *E. cloacae* has been found in some neonatal ICUs as the predominant pathogen, representing almost 40 percent of the bloodstream isolates.[93] In some series, one third of *Enterobacter* bacteremias are polymicrobial, which represents a greater prevalence than that of bacteremia caused by other gram-negative organisms.[20,50]

The most frequently cited risk factor for *Enterobacter* infection is the recent receipt of antibiotics, particularly third-generation cephalosporins.[3-5,16,23,50,70,154] Other risk factors include prolonged hospital stay, especially in an ICU, presence of serious underlying illness (e.g., burns, malignancy, and diabetes), prematurity in a neonate, immunosuppression, and the presence of a foreign device.[34,132,151]

Vertical spread of *Enterobacter* from mother to infant may occur at the time of birth.[48] Environmental sources implicated in outbreaks of infection have included intravenous fluids,[6,25,94,96,142,152,155,157] chronic hand dermatitis of a care provider,[11] contaminated infant formula,[7,14,30,33,108] blood gas machines,[2,82] contaminated transesophageal echocardiography probes,[72] cardioplegia ice,[22] therapeutic bed mattresses and mattress covers,[147] and rectal thermometers.[146]

Ribotyping, pulsed-field electrophoresis, and restriction-fragment polymorphism analysis of DNA from clinical isolates have been useful in discriminating possible sources of contamination and patient-to-patient transfer of individual strains.[15,22,29,30,33,57,60,84,132] Plasmid profiles often are of little value because many strains of *Enterobacter* possess few, if any,

plasmids.[132] Integrons, discrete mobile units of DNA that can confer antibiotic resistance, have been reported in *Enterobacter* spp. and are more common findings in infections acquired in a health care setting.[34]

Most cases are not outbreak-associated, and endogenous origin of infection is a more common means of acquisition than is the patient's environment.[121] This factor explains why recent antimicrobial use by the patient is such a strong predictor of infection.

PATHOPHYSIOLOGY

Newborns often are colonized by *Enterobacter* spp. in the gastrointestinal tract soon after birth,[13,113] and acquisition of hospital strains in immunocompromised newborns is common.[13,44,49,149] *Enterobacter* may contaminate the compromised respiratory tract. The oropharynx commonly is colonized by *Enterobacter* by the time the infant is 1 month of age; colonization rates generally are lower in breast-fed infants.[10] Newborns with gastrointestinal abnormalities requiring prolonged parenteral nutrition have higher rates of colonization with *Enterobacter* and a higher incidence of sepsis.[122] Other risk factors for increased *Enterobacter* colonization in neonates include prematurity and prior antibiotic use.[117] Enteric organisms are recovered less frequently from the oropharynx of healthy older children and adults, but increased colonization, including increased risk for third-generation cephalosporin–resistant strains, especially with prior cephalosporin treatment of at least 3 days, is noted during illness (see also Chapter 115).[160]

The ability of *Enterobacter* spp. to develop inducible resistance to penicillins and cephalosporins increases their pathogenic potential. All *Enterobacter* spp. possess an inducible chromosomally encoded class C (Bush group I) β-lactamase (*ampC*), which usually is produced in small amounts.[132] An inducible plasmid-encoded *ampC* (gene *bla*$_{ACT-1}$) also has been described and can be present in *Enterobacter* spp. and other Enterobacteriaceae.[130] Both enzymes have a high affinity for third-generation cephalosporins but a low maximum hydrolysis rate.[99] Consequently, β-lactamase mediates resistance to these antibiotics only when it is produced in large quantities or large numbers of plasmids are present.[88,127]

Resistance emerges after a mutation occurs in the *ampD* gene, which normally prevents high-level expression of β-lactamase.[68,71] Such mutants are considered "stably derepressed" and may be induced by exposure to β-lactam antibiotics, especially ampicillin and cephalosporins. Mutations in the *ampR* gene produce similar effects.[81] The addition of a β-lactamase inhibitor (e.g., clavulanic acid) does not increase the activity of β-lactam antibiotics against *Enterobacter* spp; rather, it may decrease the activity against the organism by inducing the class C β-lactamase, as can the presence of *ampR* mutants.[71,81,150]

Emergence of resistance can occur during therapy for an isolate that initially is shown to be susceptible.[62,132] Resistance can be detected 24 hours after initiation of therapy or may be delayed 2 to 3 weeks.[28] In addition, more reports of resistant strains of *Enterobacter* that produce plasmid-mediated, extended-spectrum β-lactamases (ESBL) have been published.[66,95,123] Various ESBL genes, including genes from the TEM, SHV, and CTX-M families, have been found.[26,114,138,171] This variation can complicate choosing antimicrobial agents because discerning the source of the β-lactam resistance in the clinical microbiology laboratory often is difficult without performing specific testing, such as the double disk diffusion method. A survey of 11 clinical laboratories in Germany to determine ESBL prevalence found that 40 percent of *E. cloacae* complex organisms were resistant to extended-spectrum cephalosporins, and only 6 percent carried ESBL

---

*See references 8, 46, 61, 82, 91, 120, 133, 147, 148, 161.

genes.[66] This finding is in contrast to other reports with prevalences of 36 percent in some Asia-Pacific regions.[12]

In one study, gram-negative fecal aerobic flora was eradicated completely after 24 hours of ceftriaxone therapy, only to be replaced within 10 days (mean 6.7 days) of therapy by *Pseudomonas aeruginosa*, *Enterobacter*, and *Citrobacter* resistant to all β-lactam antibiotics.[58] Although uncommon, the combination of reduced outer-membrane permeability and high-level β-lactamase production renders some clinical isolates of *Enterobacter* resistant to carbapenems (imipenem, meropenem, and ertapenem) and fourth-generation cephalosporins (cefepime).[18,37,85,87,99,119,139,144]

Other than the presence of endotoxin, factors responsible for the virulence of *Enterobacter* spp. are not well defined.[76,112] In vitro, it is possible to transfer and express an *Escherichia coli* enterotoxigenic plasmid in *Enterobacter*, implying the potential for transfer of virulence factors to *Enterobacter* spp. from other species.[170] Shiga-toxin–producing *E. cloacae* has been isolated from the stool of a 5-month-old girl with hemolytic-uremic syndrome.[115] *E. coli* OR:H9, which also produced Shiga toxin, also was isolated from the child's stool, rendering the cause of the child's symptoms unclear. Similar to other organisms associated with central venous catheter infections, *Enterobacter* spp. may adhere irreversibly to catheter material, promoting colonization and infection.[77,118] Certain ribotypes have been encountered more commonly as community or bloodstream isolates, indicating the presence of as yet undefined factors affecting virulence.[159] The propensity of *E. sakazakii* to produce neonatal meningitis complicated by abscesses and cerebral infarction is unexplained.[14,30,112,164] Proposed mechanisms have included brain capillary and intestinal endothelial cell invasion, persistence in human macrophages, and biofilm formation.[77,107,141]

CLINICAL MANIFESTATIONS

Infection caused by *Enterobacter* commonly is indistinguishable from illness caused by other enteric pathogens. Sources of infection include central venous catheters and the urinary and biliary tracts.[5,9,50,63,69,90] *Enterobacter* commonly colonizes the respiratory tract secretions of intubated patients, and it is implicated increasingly as a cause of nosocomial pneumonia.[69,129] It also is one of the most common causes of pneumonia after lung transplantation[92] and can be found as part of the oral flora in patients with strokes.[56] Neonatal infection warrants special mention because of the prominence of *E. sakazakii* as a cause of devastating meningitis.

Similar to *Citrobacter diversus* (see Chapter 112), *E. sakazakii* causes neonatal meningitis complicated by cerebral abscesses or infarctions.[14,30,39,74,164,166] Poor feeding, irritability, jaundice, a full anterior fontanelle, and fever or hypothermia are presenting features that are shared with other gram-negative causes of bacterial meningitis. The mortality rate has been reported to range from 33 to 80 percent, and almost all survivors experience severe neurologic complications, including quadriplegia, developmental impedance, and impaired sight and hearing.[39,164] This severe morbidity is consistent with the development of multiple cystic lesions of the brain in 50 percent of surviving neonates. Serial computed tomography scans commonly reveal evolution of lesions most consistent with initial cerebral infarction, rather than primary abscess formation.[51,83,164] Subsequent cystic lesions may be purulent abscesses, from which the organism can be cultured; alternatively, they sometimes represent sterile fluid collections.[24] Meningitis tended to develop in infants of greater gestational age and birth weight than in infants with only bacteremia, but they tended to be younger in chronologic age.[21]

Enterobacter also may be associated with necrotizing enterocolitis in the newborn, which became more apparent during the outbreaks of *E. sakazakii* associated with contaminated powdered infant formula.[83,145] *Enterobacter* spp. were the third most common isolate recovered from peritoneal fluid in a series of patients with necrotizing enterocolitis.[83,105]

In older immunocompromised children, bacteremia complicated by sepsis is a significant risk. Central venous catheterization and gastrointestinal tract pathology seem to pose greater risks for development of bacteremia than infection of the urinary tract.[5,29,50,90] Bacteremia is accompanied by shock in almost one third of patients, but disseminated intravascular coagulation occurs in less than 5 percent.[16,20,50] Seeding of metastatic foci is uncommon. Overall case-fatality rates with bacteremia vary but usually are approximately 30 percent.[132] Factors associated with a poor prognosis include age younger than 18 months, inadequacy of antimicrobial chemotherapy, septic shock, type of underlying disease, presence of pulmonary infection, thrombocytopenia, unknown primary site of infection, and requirement for intensive care.[16,20,36,50,73] Absence of fever during the course of infection may be a particularly ominous sign; four of five afebrile subjects died in one series.[16] One study found that the use of an aminoglycoside as part of the empiric antibiotic management was a factor contributing to survival of *Enterobacter* or *Citrobacter* bacteremia.[36]

Some *Enterobacter* spp. recovered from children with diarrhea have been reported to produce enterotoxin,[27] although a causative role in enteritis has not been established. Other presentations of *Enterobacter* infection include endophthalmitis,[78,101,103] endometritis,[54] wound infections,[50] diskitis,[124,136] endocarditis,[143] and osteomyelitis.[31,40,75,137] *Enterobacter* also has caused syndromes classically associated with other agents, such as gas gangrene,[45] childhood purpura fulminans,[59] ecthyma gangrenosum,[125] and necrotizing fasciitis.[80]

DIAGNOSIS

Diagnosis of infection caused by *Enterobacter* relies primarily on isolation of the organism in culture from clinical material. Motility, production of ornithine decarboxylase, and the absence of deoxyribonuclease help to distinguish the genus from *Klebsiella* and *Serratia*. The presence of yellow pigmented colonies can help identify *E. sakazakii*. Patterns of sugar fermentation and production of decarboxylase also distinguish the species. The ability to detect pathogens directly in tissue using biotinylated probes offers promise for rapidly establishing the diagnosis but remains primarily in the clinical research arena.[97] Other molecular techniques becoming available for rapid identification of bacteria include polymerase chain reaction (PCR)–single strand conformation polymorphism analysis using 16S ribosomal DNA. This technique allows the potential identification of pathogens to be made from a wide range of clinical specimens with low numbers of bacteria and shows promise for clinical applications.[162,168] In light of the increase of *E. sakazakii* invasive disease after ingestion of contaminated powdered infant formula, several techniques have been introduced for the rapid identification of this pathogen clinically and in foodstuffs. The use of a specific PCR amplification of the outer membrane protein A gene (*ompA*) is being investigated,[104] as is reverse-transcriptase PCR[89] and the use of selective media.[38] Ribotyping is a highly discriminatory and reproducible method for the typing of *E. cloacae*, the most common cause of infection.[52] Other useful molecular techniques include restriction endonuclease analysis of chromosomal DNA, pulsed-field gel electrophoresis, random amplification of polymorphic DNA, and amplification of short interspersed repetitive sequences.[132] Most often, molecular typing methods are used in concert with biotyping, serotyping, or bacteriocin typing.

TREATMENT

Treatment of *Enterobacter* infection is made problematic by inducible resistance to cephalosporins and intrinsic resistance to aminopenicillins, cefazolin, and cefoxitin.[19] The increasing recognition that *Enterobacter* spp. can carry ESBL plasmids in addition to expressing chromosomal *ampC* β-lactamases can be problematic using automated ESBL detection systems. The use of the double-disk synergy method for ESBL detection can indicate the presence of plasmid-mediated resistance but is challenging because high production of *ampC* can mask the inhibition of ESBL by clavulanic acid.[163]

Antibiotic resistance may be present at the time of initial isolation or may develop during therapy.[29,62] This problem is compounded by the common observation of resistance to extended-spectrum penicillins and, to a lesser extent, aminoglycosides. The risks for development of resistance to cephalosporins, piperacillin, and aminoglycosides have been reported to be higher at a tertiary care center than at a primary care hospital.[43] Previous administration of third-generation cephalosporins increases the risk of having multiresistant *Enterobacter* isolates in an initial positive blood culture.[5,28,106] Hospitalized newborns quickly may acquire multiresistant strains, even though they themselves have not been treated with cephalosporins.[13] Isolation of multiresistant *Enterobacter* spp. in blood culture is associated with a higher case-fatality rate compared with mortality after isolation of a more sensitive *Enterobacter*.[28,134] Although less common, resistance to imipenem has been reported.[42,85,140] Cefepime, a fourth-generation cephalosporin, generally maintains activity against *Enterobacter* spp. that possess the class C β-lactamase,[131] although minimum inhibitory concentrations may be higher.[99]

Emergence of cefepime resistance during therapy has been described in a liver transplant recipient with a hepatic abscess caused by *E. aerogenes*.[87] The accompanying editorial warns about the risk of failure using cefepime in patients who have high-density infections (e.g., poorly drained liver abscess) caused by ceftazidime-resistant strains of *Enterobacter*.[99] The presence of an SHV-type ESBL has been associated with cefepime resistance, highlighting the need to identify those strains.[138]

In a nationwide survey of nosocomial bloodstream infections, rates of *Enterobacter* resistance to third-generation cephalosporins (ceftazidime, ceftriaxone) and broad-spectrum semisynthetic penicillins (piperacillin) with or without a β-lactamase inhibitor (tazobactam) was high, ranging from 35 to 50 percent.[121] Cefepime and imipenem inhibited 97 to 100 percent of isolates. Susceptibility to aminoglycosides and fluoroquinolones ranged from 92 to 98 percent, and 85 to 96 percent of isolates were susceptible to trimethoprim-sulfamethoxazole. Fluoroquinolone resistance is now being reported and likely is plasmid-mediated.[111,169] Because resistance patterns may vary based on geographic location, local susceptibility data should be used to guide initial therapy.

Some investigators recommend initial combination therapy that includes an aminoglycoside plus either cefepime or a carbapenem (imipenem or meropenem), until results of susceptibility testing are available. Third-generation cephalosporins should be used with caution, even when initial susceptibility results seem favorable. When strains are resistant to gentamicin and tobramycin, amikacin may be a suitable alternative. Good responses to therapy and return of gentamicin susceptibility of hospital *Enterobacter* strains have occurred after routine substitution of amikacin for gentamicin.[126,135] Trimethoprim-sulfamethoxazole alone (or combined with an aminoglycoside) and quinolones seem to be good alternatives for the treatment of *Enterobacter* infections, including meningitis.[5,35,55,100,166] Fluoroquinolones may be another option, depending on local resistance rates. They have been reported to be effective in bone and joint infections, in combination with cefepime.[86] As newer antimicrobial agents become available, more testing will be required to determine their effectiveness. Tigecycline may have promise, but further studies are needed to determine its usefulness in clinical treatment.[153,167]

Enterobacter meningitis creates special concerns. As is common with other forms of neonatal enteric meningitis, even susceptible organisms often persist in cerebrospinal fluid for 5 days or longer.[74] Monotherapy with a cell wall–active agent seems to be less effective than combination therapy with an aminoglycoside. Trimethoprim-sulfamethoxazole also has been used successfully.[47,166] Intrathecal administration of antibiotics does not seem to be beneficial in infants,[98] but it has been used with some success in adults.[110] The physician should anticipate the potential development of cerebral abscesses, infarctions, and cysts in newborns with *E. sakazakii* infection. Serial computed tomography scans should be considered, and a neurosurgeon should be sought for drainage of abscesses and management of fluid accumulation.

REFERENCES

1. Abbott, S. L., and Janda, J. M.: *Enterobacter cancerogenus* ("*Enterobacter taylorae*") infections associated with severe trauma or crush injuries. Am. J. Clin. Pathol. *107*:359-361, 1997.
2. Acolet, D., Ahmet, Z., Houang, E., et al.: *Enterobacter cloacae* in a neonatal intensive care unit: Account of an outbreak and its relationship to use of third generation cephalosporins. J. Hosp. Infect. *28*:273-286, 1994.
3. al Ansari, N., McNamara, E. B., Cunney, R. J., et al.: Experience with *Enterobacter* bacteraemia in a Dublin teaching hospital. J. Hosp. Infect. *27*:69-72, 1994.
4. Anderson, E. L., and Hieber, J. P.: An outbreak of gentamicin-resistant *Enterobacter cloacae* infections in a pediatric intensive care unit. Infect. Control *4*:148-152, 1983.
5. Andresen, J., Asmar, B. I., and Dajani, A. S.: Increasing *Enterobacter* bacteremia in pediatric patients. Pediatr. Infect. Dis. J. *13*:787-792, 1994.
6. Anonymous: *Enterobacter cloacae* bloodstream infections associated with contaminated prefilled saline syringes—California, November 1998. M. M. W. R. Morb. Mortal. Wkly. Rep. *47*:959-960, 1998.
7. Anonymous: *Enterobacter sakazakii* infections associated with the use of powdered infant formula—Tennessee, 2001. M. M. W. R. Morb. Mortal. Wkly. Rep. *51*:297-300, 2002.
8. Archibald, L. K., Ramos, M., Arduino, M. J., et al.: *Enterobacter cloacae* and *Pseudomonas aeruginosa* polymicrobial bloodstream infections traced to extrinsic contamination of a dextrose multidose vial. J. Pediatr. *133*:640-644, 1998.
9. Ashkenazi, S., Even-Tov, S., Samra, Z., et al.: Uropathogens of various childhood populations and their antibiotic susceptibility. Pediatr. Infect. Dis. J. *10*:742-746, 1991.
10. Baltimore, R. S., Duncan, R. L., Shapiro, E. D., et al.: Epidemiology of pharyngeal colonization of infants with aerobic gram- negative rod bacteria. J. Clin. Microbiol. *27*:91-95, 1989.
11. Beck-Sague, C. M., Chong, W. H., Roy, C., et al.: Outbreak of surgical wound infections associated with total hip arthroplasty. Infect. Control Hosp. Epidemiol. *13*:526-534, 1992.
12. Bell, J. M., Turnidge, J. D., Jones, R. N., et al.: Prevalence of extended-spectrum beta-lactamase-producing *Enterobacter cloacae* in the Asia-Pacific region: Results from the SENTRY antimicrobial surveillance program, 1998 to 2001. Antimicrob. Agents Chemother. *47*:3989-3993, 2003.
13. Berkowitz, F. E., and Metchock, B.: Third generation cephalosporin-resistant gram-negative bacilli in the feces of hospitalized children. Pediatr. Infect. Dis. J. *14*:97-100, 1995.
14. Biering, G., Karlsson, S., Clark, N. C., et al.: Three cases of neonatal meningitis caused by *Enterobacter sakazakii* in powdered milk. J. Clin. Microbiol. *27*:2054-2056, 1989.
15. Bingen, E., Denamur, E., Lambert-Zechovsky, N., et al.: Rapid genotyping shows the absence of cross-contamination in *Enterobacter cloacae* nosocomial infections. J. Hosp. Infect. *21*:95-101, 1992.
16. Bodey, G. P., Elting, L. S., and Rodriguez, S.: Bacteremia caused by *Enterobacter*: 15 years of experience in a cancer hospital. Rev. Infect. Dis. *13*:550-558, 1991.
17. Bonadio, W. A., Margolis, D., and Tovar, M.: *Enterobacter cloacae* bacteremia in children: A review of 30 cases in 12 years. Clin. Pediatr. (Phila.) *30*:310-313, 1991.
18. Bornet, C., Davin-Regli, A., Bosi, C., et al.: Imipenem resistance of *Enterobacter aerogenes* mediated by outer membrane permeability. J. Clin. Microbiol. *38*:1048-1052, 2000.
19. Bouza, E., and Cercenado, E.: *Klebsiella* and *Enterobacter*: Antibiotic resistance and treatment implications. Semin. Respir. Infect. *17*:215-230, 2002.
20. Bouza, E., Garcia de la Torre, M., Erice, A., et al.: *Enterobacter* bacteremia: An analysis of 50 episodes. Arch. Intern. Med. *145*:1024-1027, 1985.
21. Bowen, A. B., and Braden, C. R.: Invasive *Enterobacter sakazakii* disease in infants. Emerg. Infect. Dis. *12*:1185-1189, 2006.

22. Breathnach, A. S., Riley, P. A., Shad, S., et al.: An outbreak of wound infection in cardiac surgery patients caused by *Enterobacter cloacae* arising from cardioplegia ice. J. Hosp. Infect. *64*:124-128, 2006.

23. Burchard, K. W., Barrall, D. T., Reed, M., et al.: *Enterobacter* bacteremia in surgical patients. Surgery *100*:857-862, 1986.

24. Burdette, J. H., and Santos, C.: *Enterobacter sakazakii* brain abscess in the neonate: The importance of neuroradiologic imaging. Pediatr. Radiol. *30*:33-34, 2000.

25. Campos, L. C., Lobianco, L. F., Seki, L. M., et al.: Outbreak of *Enterobacter hormaechei* septicemia in newborns caused by contaminated parenteral nutrition in Brazil. J. Hosp. Infect. *66*:95-97, 2007.

26. Cantón, R., Oliver, A., Coque, T. M., et al.: Epidemiology of extended-spectrum beta-lactamase-producing *Enterobacter* isolates in a Spanish hospital during a 12 year period. J. Clin. Microbiol. *40*:1237-1247, 2002.

27. Chatterjee, B. D., Thawani, G., and Sanyal, S. N.: Etiology of acute childhood diarrhoea in Calcutta. Trop. Gastroenterol. *10*:158-166, 1989.

28. Chow, J. W., Fine, M. J., Shlaes, D. M., et al.: *Enterobacter* bacteremia: Clinical features and emergence of antibiotic resistance during therapy. Ann. Intern. Med. *115*:585-590, 1991.

29. Chow, J. W., Yu, V. L., and Shlaes, D. M.: Epidemiologic perspectives on *Enterobacter* for the infection control professional. Am. J. Infect. Control *22*:195-201, 1994.

30. Clark, N. C., Hill, B. C., O'Hara, C. M., et al.: Epidemiologic typing of *Enterobacter sakazakii* in two neonatal nosocomial outbreaks. Diagn. Microbiol. Infect. Dis. *13*:467-472, 1990.

31. Corti, G., Panunzi, I., Losco, M., et al.: Postsurgical osteomyelitis caused by *Enterobacter sakazkii* in a healthy young man. J. Chemother. *19*:94-96, 2007.

32. Couto, R. C., Carvalho, E. A. A., Pedrosa, T. M. G., et al.: A 10 year prospective surveillance of nosocomial infections in neonatal intensive care units. Am. J. Infect. Control *35*:183-189, 2007.

33. Caubilla-Barron, J., Hurrell, E., Townsend, S., et al.: Genotypic and phenotypic analysis of *Enterobacter sakazakii* strains from a fatal outbreak in a neonatal intensive care unit in France. J. Clin. Microbiol. *45*:3979-3985, 2007.

34. Daikos, G. L., Kosmidis, C., Tassios, P. T., et al.: Enterobacteriaceae bloodstream infections: Presence of integrons, risk factors and outcome. Antimicrob. Agents Chemother. *51*:2366-2372, 2007.

35. D'Antuono, V. S., and Brown, I.: Successful treatment of enterobacter meningitis with ciprofloxacin. Clin. Infect. Dis. *26*:206-207, 1998.

36. Deal, E. N., Micek, S. T., Ritchie, D. J., et al.: Predictors of in-hospital mortality for bloodstream infections caused by *Enterobacter* species or *Citrobacter freundii*. Pharmacotherapy *27*:191-199, 2007.

37. De Gheldre, Y., Maes, N., Rost, F., et al.: Molecular epidemiology of an outbreak of multidrug-resistant *Enterobacter aerogenes* infections and in vivo emergence of imipenem resistance. J. Clin. Microbiol. *35*:152-160, 1997.

38. Derzelle, S., Dilasser, F., Maladen, V., et al.: Comparsion of three chromogenic media and evaluation of two molecular based identification systems for the detection of *Enterobacter sakazakii* from environmental samples from infant formulae factories. J. Food Prot. *70*:1678-1684, 2007.

39. Drudy, D., Mullane, N. R., Quinn, T., et al.: *Enterobacter sakazakii*: an emerging pathogen in powdered infant formula. Clin. Infect. Dis. *42*:996-1002, 2006.

40. Dubey, L., Krasinski, K., and Hernanz-Schulman, M.: Osteomyelitis secondary to trauma or infected contiguous soft tissue. Pediatr. Infect. Dis. J. *7*:26-34, 1988.

41. Ehni, W. F., Reller, L. B., and Ellison, R. T., 3rd: Bacteremia in granulocytopenic patients in a tertiary-care general hospital. Rev. Infect. Dis. *13*:613-619, 1991.

42. Ehrhardt, A. F., Sanders, C. C., Thomson, K. S., et al.: Emergence of resistance to imipenem in *Enterobacter* isolates masquerading as *Klebsiella pneumoniae* during therapy with imipenem/cilastatin. Clin. Infect. Dis. *17*:120-122, 1993.

43. Ellner, P. D., Fink, D. J., Neu, H. C., et al.: Epidemiologic factors affecting antimicrobial resistance of common bacterial isolates. J. Clin. Microbiol. *25*:1668-1674, 1987.

44. Fanaro, S., Chierici, R., Guerrini, P., et al.: Intestinal micorflora in early infancy: Composition and development. Acta Paediatr. Suppl. *91*:48-55, 2003.

45. Fata, F., Chittivelu, S., Tessler, S., et al.: Gas gangrene of the arm due to *Enterobacter cloacae* in a neutropenic patient. South. Med. J. *89*:1095-1096, 1996.

46. Fok, T. F., Lee, C. H., Wong, E. M., et al.: Risk factors for *Enterobacter* septicemia in a neonatal unit: Case-control study. Clin. Infect. Dis. *27*:1204-1209, 1998.

47. Foster, D., and Rhoney, D.: *Enterobacter* meningitis: Organism susceptibilities, antimicrobial therapy and related outcomes. Surg. Neurol. *63*:533-537, 2005.

48. Fryklund, B., Tullus, K., Berglund, B., et al.: Importance of the environment and the faecal flora of infants, nursing staff and parents as sources of gram-negative bacteria colonizing newborns in three neonatal wards. Infection *20*:253-257, 1992.

49. Fryklund, B., Tullus, K., and Burman, L. G.: Epidemiology of enteric bacteria in neonatal units—influence of procedures and patient variables. J. Hosp. Infect. *18*:15-21, 1991.

50. Gallagher, P. G.: *Enterobacter* bacteremia in pediatric patients. Rev. Infect. Dis. *12*:808-812, 1990.

51. Gallagher, P. G., and Ball, W. S.: Cerebral infarctions due to CNS infection with *Enterobacter sakazakii*. Pediatr. Radiol. *21*:135-136, 1991.

52. Garaizar, J., Kaufmann, M. E., and Pitt, T. L.: Comparison of ribotyping with conventional methods for the type identification of *Enterobacter cloacae*. J. Clin. Microbiol. *29*:1303-1307, 1991.

53. Gaston, M. A.: Enterobacter: An emerging nosocomial pathogen. J. Hosp. Infect. *11*:197-208, 1988.

54. Gibbs, R. S., Blanco, J. D., and Bernstein, S.: Role of aerobic gram-negative bacilli in endometritis after cesarean section. Rev. Infect. Dis. 7(Suppl. 4): S690-S695, 1985.

55. Goepp, J. G., Lee, C. K., Anderson, T., et al.: Use of ciprofloxacin in an infant with ventriculitis. J. Pediatr. *121*:303-305, 1992.

56. Gosney, M. A., Martin, M. V., Wright, A. E., et al.: *Enterobacter sakazakii* in the mouths of stroke patients and its association with aspiration pneumonia. Eur. J. Intern. Med. *17*:185-188, 2006.

57. Grattard, F., Pozzetto, B., Berthelot, P., et al.: Arbitrarily primed PCR, ribotyping, and plasmid pattern analysis applied to investigation of a nosocomial outbreak due to *Enterobacter cloacae* in a neonatal intensive care unit. J. Clin. Microbiol. *32*:596-602, 1994.

58. Guggenbichler, J. P., Kofler, J., and Allerberger, F.: The influence of third-generation cephalosporins on the aerobic intestinal flora. Infection *13*:S137-S139, 1985.

59. Gurses, N., and Ozkan, A.: Neonatal and childhood purpura fulminans: Review of seven cases. Cutis *41*:361-363, 1988.

60. Haertl, R., and Bandlow, G.: Molecular typing of *Enterobacter cloacae* by pulsed-field gel electrophoresis of genomic restriction fragments. J. Hosp. Infect. *25*:109-116, 1993.

61. Harbarth, S., Sudre, P., Dharan, S., et al.: Outbreak of *Enterobacter cloacae* related to understaffing, overcrowding, and poor hygiene practices. Infect. Control Hosp. Epidemiol. *20*:598-603, 1999.

62. Heusser, M. F., Patterson, J. E., Kuritza, A. P., et al.: Emergence of resistance to multiple beta-lactams in *Enterobacter cloacae* during treatment for neonatal meningitis with cefotaxime. Pediatr. Infect. Dis. J. *9*:509-512, 1990.

63. Hoffmann, H., Schmoldt, S., Trülzsch, K., et al.: Nosocomial urosepsis caused by *Enterobacter kobei* with aberrant phenotype. Diagn. Microbiol. Infect. Dis. *53*:143-147, 2005.

64. Hoffmann, H., Stindl, S., Ludwig, W., et al.: Reassignment of *Enterobacter dissolvens* to *Enterobacter cloacae* as *E. cloacae* subspecies dissolvens comb. nov. and emended description of *Enterobacter asburiae* and *Enterobacter kobei*. Syst. Appl. Microbiol. *28*:196-205, 2005.

65. Hoffmann, H., Stindl, S., Stumpf, A., et al.: Description of *Enterobacter ludwigii* sp. *nov.*, a novel *Enterobacter* species of clinical relevance. Syst. Appl. Microbiol. *28*:206-212, 2005.

66. Hoffmann, H., Stürenburg, E., Heesemann, J., et al.: Prevalence of extended-spectrum beta-lactamases in isolates of the *Enterobacter cloacae* complex from German hospitals. Clin. Microbiol. Infect. *12*:322-330, 2006.

67. Inouse, K., Sugiyama, K., Kosako, Y., et al.: *Enterobacter cowanii* sp. nov., a new species of the family Enterobacteriaceae. Curr. Microbiol. *41*:417-420, 2000.

68. Jacobs, C., Joris, B., Jamin, M., et al.: AmpD, essential for both β-lactamase regulation and cell wall recycling, is a novel cytosolic n-acetylmuramyl-L-alanine amidase. Mol. Microbiol. *15*:553-559, 1995.

69. Jarvis, W. R., and Martone, W. J.: Predominant pathogens in hospital infections. J. Antimicrob. Chemother. *29*(Suppl. A):19-24, 1992.

70. Johnson, M. P., and Ramphal, R.: Beta-lactam-resistant *Enterobacter* bacteremia in febrile neutropenic patients receiving monotherapy. J. Infect. Dis. *162*:981-983, 1990.

71. Kaneko, K., Okamoto, R., Nakano, R., et al.: Gene mutations responsible for overexpression of AmpC beta-lactamase in some clinical isolates of *Enterobacter cloacae*. J. Clin. Microbiol. *43*:2955-2958, 2005.

72. Kanemitsu, K., Endo, S., Oda, K., et al.: An increased incidence of *Enterobacter cloacae* in a cardiovascular ward. J. Hosp. Infect. *66*:130-134, 2007.

73. Kang, C. I., Kim, S. H., Park, W. B., et al.: Bloodstream infections caused by *Enterobacter* species: Predictors of 30 day mortality rate and impact of broad-spectrum cephalosporin resistance on outcome. Clin. Infect. Dis. *39*:812-818, 2004.

74. Kaplan, S. L., and Patrick, C. C.: Cefotaxime and aminoglycoside treatment of meningitis caused by gram-negative enteric organisms. Pediatr. Infect. Dis. J. *9*:810-814, 1990.

75. Klein, J. D., and Leach, K. A.: Pediatric pelvic osteomyelitis. Clin. Pediatr. (Phila.) *46*:787-790, 2007.

76. Keller, R., Pedroso, M. Z., Ritchmann, R., et al.: Occurrence of virulence-associated properties in *Enterobacter cloacae*. Infect. Immun. *66*:645-649, 1998.

77. Kim, H., Ryu, J. H., and Beuchat, L. R.: Attachment of and biofilm formation by *Enterobacter sakazakii* on stainless steel and enteral feeding tubes. Appl. Environ. Microbiol. *72*:5846-5856, 2006.

78. Korah, S., Braganza, A., Jacob, P., et al.: An "epidemic" of post cataract surgery endophthalmitis by a new organism. Indian J. Ophthalmol. *55*:464-466, 2007.

79. Kosako, Y., Tamura, K., Sakazaki, R., et al.: *Enterobacter kobei* sp. *nov.*, a new species of Enterobacteriaceae resembling *Enterobacter cloacae*. Curr. Microbiol. *33*:261-265, 1996.

80. Kronish, J. W., and McLeish, W. M.: Eyelid necrosis and periorbital necrotizing fasciitis: Report of a case and review of the literature. Ophthalmology *98*:92-98, 1991.

81. Kuga, A., Okamoto, R., and Inoue, M.: ampR gene mutations that greatly increase class C beta-lactamase activity in *Enterobacter cloacae*. Antimicrob. Agents Chemother. *44*:561-567, 2000.

82. Lacey, S. L., and Want, S. V.: An outbreak of *Enterobacter cloacae* associated with contamination of a blood gas machine. J. Infect. *30*:223-226, 1995.

83. Lai, K. K.: *Enterobacter sakazakii* infections among neonates, infants, children and adults. Medicine *80*:113-122, 2001.

84. Lambert-Zechovsky, N., Bingen, E., Denamur, E., et al.: Molecular analysis provides evidence for the endogenous origin of bacteremia and meningitis due to *Enterobacter cloacae* in an infant. Clin. Infect. Dis. *15*:30-32, 1992.

85. Lee, E. H., Nicolas, M. H., Kitzis, M. D., et al.: Association of two resistance mechanisms in a clinical isolate of *Enterobacter cloacae* with high-level resistance to imipenem. Antimicrob. Agents Chemother. *35*:1093-1098, 1991.

86. Legout, L., Senneville, E., Stern, R., et al.: Treatment of bone and joint infections caused by gram-negative bacilli with a cefepime-fluoroquinolone combination. Clin. Microbiol. Infect. *12*:1030-1033, 2006.

87. Limaye, A. P., Gautom, R. K., Black, D., et al.: Rapid emergence of resistance to cefepime during treatment. Clin. Infect. Dis. *25*:339-341, 1997.

88. Lindberg, F., and Normark, S.: Contribution of chromosomal beta-lactamases to beta-lactam resistance in enterobacteria. Rev. Infect. Dis. *8*(Suppl. 3):S292-S304, 1986.

89. Liu, Y., Cai, X., Zhang, X., et al.: Real time PCR using TaqMan and SYBR Green for detection of *Enterobacter sakazakii* in infant formula. J. Microbiol. Methods *65*:21-31, 2006.

90. Lohr, J. A., Donowitz, L. G., and Sadler, J. E., 3rd: Hospital-acquired urinary tract infection. Pediatrics *83*:193-199, 1989.

91. Loiwal, V., Kumar, A., Gupta, P., et al.: *Enterobacter aerogenes* outbreak in a neonatal intensive care unit. Pediatr. Int. *41*:157-161, 1999.

92. Low, D. E., Kaiser, L. R., Haydock, D. A., et al.: The donor lung: Infectious and pathologic factors affecting outcome in lung transplantation. J. Thorac. Cardiovasc. Surg. *106*:614-621, 1993.

93. Mahapatra, M. A., Ghosh, S. K., Mishra, S., et al.: *Enterobacter cloacae*: A predominant pathogen in neonatal septicemia. Indian J. Med. Microbiol. *20*:110-112, 2002.

94. Maki, D. G., Rhame, F. S., Mackel, D. C., et al.: Nationwide epidemic of septicemia caused by contaminated intravenous products, I: Epidemiologic and clinical features. Am. J. Med. *60*:471-485, 1976.

95. Manzur, A., Tubau, F., Pujol, M., et al.: Nosocomial outbreak due to extended-spectrum beta-lactamase-producing *Enterobacter cloacae* in a cardiothoracic intensive care unit. J. Clin. Microbiol. *45*:2365-2369, 2007.

96. Matsaniotis, N. S., Syriopoulou, V. P., Theodoridou, M. C., et al.: *Enterobacter* sepsis in infants and children due to contaminated intravenous fluids. Infect. Control *5*:471-477, 1984.

97. Matsuhisa, A., Saito, Y., Sakamoto, Y., et al.: Detection of bacteria in phagocyte-smears from septicemia-suspected blood by in situ hybridization using biotinylated probes. Microbiol. Immunol. *38*:511-517, 1994.

98. McCracken, G. H., Jr., and Mize, S. G.: A controlled study of intrathecal antibiotic therapy in gram-negative enteric meningitis of infancy: Report of the neonatal meningitis cooperative study group. J. Pediatr. *89*:66-72, 1976.

99. Medeiros, A. A.: Relapsing infection due to *Enterobacter* species: Lessons of heterogeneity. Clin. Infect. Dis. *25*:341-342, 1997.

100. Meis, J. F., Groot-Loonen, J., and Hoogkamp-Korstanje, J. A.: A brain abscess due to multiply-resistant *Enterobacter cloacae* successfully treated with meropenem. Clin. Infect. Dis. *20*:1567, 1995.

101. Milewski, S. A., and Klevjer-Anderson, P.: Endophthalmitis caused by *Enterobacter cloacae*. Ann. Ophthalmol. *25*:309-311, 1993.

102. Mireya, U. A., Marti, P. O., Xavier, K. V., et al.: Nosocomial infections in paediatric and neonatal intensive care units. J. Infect. *54*:212-220, 2007.

103. Mirza, G. E., Karakucuk, S., Doganay, M., et al.: Postoperative endophthalmitis caused by an *Enterobacter* species. J. Hosp. Infect. *26*:167-172, 1994.

104. Mohan Nair, M. K., and Venkitanarayanan, K. S.: Cloning and sequencing of the ompA gene of *Enterobacter sakazakii* and development of an ompA-targeted PCR for rapid detection of *Enterobacter sakazakii* in infant formula. Appl. Environ. Microbiol. *72*:2539-2546, 2006.

105. Mollitt, D. L., Tepas, J. J., 3rd, and Talbert, J. L.: The microbiology of neonatal peritonitis. Arch. Surg. *123*:176-179, 1988.

106. Muller, A., Lopez-Lozano, J. M., Bertrand, X., et al.: Relationship between ceftriaxone use and resistance to third-generation cephalosporins among clinical strains of *Enterobacter cloacae*. J. Antimicrob. Chemother. *54*:173-177, 2004.

107. Mohan Nair, M. K., and Venkitanarayanan, K.: Role of bacterial OmpA and host cytoskeleton in the invasion of human intestinal epithelial cells by *Enterobacter sakazakii*. Pediatr. Res. *62*:664-669, 2007.

108. Noriega, F. R., Kotloff, K. L., Martin, M. A., et al.: Nosocomial bacteremia caused by *Enterobacter sakazakiki* and *Leuconostoc mesenteroides* resulting from extrinsic contamination of infant formula. Pediatr. Infect. Dis. J. *9*:447-449, 1990.

109. O'Hara, C. M., Steigerwalt, A. G., Hill, B. C., et al.: *Enterobacter hormaechei*, a new species of the family Enterobacteriaceae formerly known as enteric group 75. J. Clin. Microbiol. *27*:2046-2049, 1989.

110. O'Neill, E., Humphreys, H., Phillips, J., et al.: Third-generation cephalosporin resistance among gram-negative bacilli causing meningitis in neurosurgical patients: Significant challenges in ensuring effective antibiotic therapy. J. Antimicrob. Chemother. *57*:356-359, 2006.

111. Paauw, A., Fluit, A. C., Verhoef, J., et al.: *Enterobacter cloacae* outbreak and emergence of quinolone resistance gene in a Dutch hospital. Emerg. Infect. Dis. *12*:807-812, 2006.

112. Pagotto, F. J., Nazarowec-White, M., Bidawid, S., et al.: *Enterobacter sakazakii*: Infectivity and enterotoxin production in vitro and in vivo. J. Food Prot. *66*:370-375, 2003.

113. Park, H. K., Shim, S. S., Kim, S. Y., et al.: Molecular analysis of colonized bacteria in a human newborn infant gut. J. Microbiol. *43*:345-353, 2005.

114. Park, Y. J., Park, S. Y., Oh, E. J., et al.: Occurrence of extended-spectrum beta-lactamases among choromosomal AmpC-producing *Enterobacter cloacae*, *Citrobacter freundii* and *Serratia marcescens* in Korea and investigation of screening criteria. Diagn. Microbiol. Infect. Dis. *51*:265-269, 2005.

115. Paton, A. W., and Paton, J. C.: *Enterobacter cloacae* producing a *Shiga*-like toxin II-related cytotoxin associated with a case of hemolytic-uremic syndrome. J. Clin. Microbiol. *34*:463-465, 1996.

116. Pavan, M. E., Franco, R. J., Rodriguez, J. M., et al.: Phylogenetic relationships of the genus *Kluyvera*: Transfer of *Enterobacter intermedius* Izard et al. 1980 to the genus *Kluyvera* as *Kluyvera intermedia* comb. nov. and reclassification of *Kluyvera cochleae* as a later synonym of *K. intermedia*. Int. J. Syst. Evol. Microbiol. *55*:437-442, 2005.

117. Penders, J., Thijs, C., and Vink, C.: Factors influencing the composition of the intestinal microbiota in early infancy. Pediatrics *118*:511-521, 2006.

118. Penner, J., Allerberger, F., Dierich, M. P., et al.: In vitro experiments on catheter-related infections due to gram-negative rods. Chemotherapy *39*:336-354, 1993.

119. Pérez, A., Canle, D., Latasa, C., et al.: Cloning, nucleotide sequencing, and analysis of the AcrAB-TolC efflux pump of *Enterobacter cloacae* and determination of its involvement in antibiotic resistance in a clinical isolate. Antimicrob. Agents Chemother. *51*:3247-3253, 2007.

120. Peters, S. M., Bryan, J., and Cole, M. F.: Enterobacterial repetitive intergenic consensus polymerase chain reaction typing of isolates of *Enterobacter cloacae* from an outbreak of infection in a neonatal intensive care unit. Am. J. Infect. Control *28*:123-129, 2000.

121. Pfaller, M. A., Jones, R. N., Marshall, S. A., et al.: Inducible amp C beta-lactamase producing gram-negative bacilli from blood stream infections: Frequency, antimicrobial susceptibility, and molecular epidemiology in a national surveillance program (SCOPE). Diagn. Microbiol. Infect. Dis. *28*:211-219, 1997.

122. Pierro, A., van Saene, H. K., Jones, M. O., et al.: Clinical impact of abnormal gut flora in infants receiving parenteral nutrition. Ann. Surg. *227*:547-552, 1998.

123. Pitout, J. D., Thomson, K. S., Hanson, N. D., et al.: Plasmid-mediated resistance to expanded-spectrum cephalosporins among *Enterobacter aerogenes* strains. Antimicrob. Agents Chemother. *42*:596-600, 1998.

124. Porter, P., and Wray, C. C.: *Enterobacter agglomerans* spondylodiscitis: A possible, unrecognized complication of tetracycline therapy. Spine *25*:1287-1289, 2000.

125. Rajan, R. K.: Spontaneous bacterial peritonitis with ecthyma gangrenosum due to *Escherichia coli*. J. Clin. Gastroenterol. *4*:145-148, 1982.

126. Raz, R., Sharir, R., Shmilowitz, L., et al.: The elimination of gentamicin-resistant gram-negative bacteria in a newborn intensive care unit. Infection *15*:32-34, 1987.

127. Reisbig, M. D., Hossain, A., and Hanson, N. D.: Factors influencing gene expression and resistance for Gram-negative organisms expressing plasmid-encoded *ampC* genes of *Enterobacter* origin. J. Antimicrob. Chemother. *51*:1141-1151, 2003.

128. Richard, C.: *Enterobacter*. *In* Garrity, G. M. (ed.): Bergey's Manual of Systematic Bacteriology. New York, Springer, 1984, pp. 465-467.

129. Richards, M. J., Edwards, J. R., Culver, D. H., et al.: Nosocomial infections in pediatric intensive care units in the United States. Pediatrics *103*:e39-e45, 1999.

130. Rottman, M., Benzerara, Y., Hanau-Berçot, B., et al.: Chromosomal ampC genes in *Enterobacter* species other than *Enterobacter cloacae*, and ancestral association of the ACT-1 plasmid-encoded cephalosporinase to *Enterobacter asburiae*. F. E. M. S. Microbiol. Lett. *210*:87-92, 2002.

131. Sanders, W. E., Jr., Tenney, J. H., and Kessler, R. E.: Efficacy of cefepime in the treatment of infections due to multiply resistant *Enterobacter* species. Clin. Infect. Dis. *23*:454-461, 1996.

132. Sanders, W. E., Jr., and Sanders, C. C.: *Enterobacter* spp.: Pathogens poised to flourish at the turn of the century. Clin. Microbiol. Rev. *10*:220-241, 1997.

133. Shi, Z. Y., Liu, P. Y., Lau, Y. J., et al.: Epidemiological typing of isolates from an outbreak of infection with multidrug-resistant *Enterobacter cloacae* by repetitive extragenic palindromic unit b1-primed PCR and pulsed-field gel electrophoresis. J. Clin. Microbiol. *34*:2784-2790, 1996.

134. Shlaes, D. M.: The clinical relevance of *Enterobacter* infections. Clin. Ther. *15*:21-28, 1993.

135. Shulman, S. T., and Yogev, R.: Treatment of pediatric infections with amikacin as first-line aminoglycoside. Am. J. Med. *79*:43-50, 1985.

136. Solans, R., Simeon, P., Cuenca, A., et al.: Infectious discitis caused by *Enterobacter cloacae*. Ann. Rheum. Dis. *51*:906-907, 1992.

137. Syrogiannopoulos, G. A., McCracken, G. H., Jr., and Nelson, J. D.: Osteoarticular infections in children with sickle cell disease. Pediatrics *78*:1090-1096, 1986.

138. Szabó, D., Bonomo, R. A., Silveira, F., et al.: SHV-type extended-spectrum beta-lactamase production is associated with reduced cefepime susceptibility in *Enterobacter cloacae*. J. Clin. Microbiol. *43*:5058-5064, 2005.

139. Szabó, D., Silveira, F., Hujer, A. M., et al.: Outer membrane changes and efflux pump expression together may confer resistance to ertapenem in *Enterobacter cloacae*. Antimicrob. Agents Chemother. *50*:2833-2835, 2006.

140. Thomson, K. S., Sanders, C. C. and Chmel, H.: Imipenem resistance in Enterobacter. Eur. J. Clin. Microbiol. Infect. Dis. 12:610-613, 1993.

141. Townsend, S. M., Hurrell, E., Gonzalez-Gomez, I., et al.: *Enterobacter saka-zakii* invades brain capillary endothelial cells, persists in human macrophages influencing cytokine secretion and induces severe brain pathology in the neonatal rat. Microbiology 153:3538-3547, 2007.

142. Tresoldi, A. T., Padoveze, M. C., Trabasso, P., et al.: *Enterobacter cloacae* sepsis outbreak in a newborn unit caused by contaminated total parenteral nutrition solution. Am. J. Infect. Control 28:258-261, 2000.

143. Tunkel, A. R., Fisch, M. J., Schlein, A., et al.: *Enterobacter* endocarditis. Scand. J. Infect. Dis. 24:233-240, 1992.

144. Tzouvelekis, L. S., Tzelepi, E., Kaufmann, M. E., et al.: Consecutive mutations leading to the emergence in vivo of imipenem resistance in a clinical strain of *Enterobacter aerogenes*. J. Med. Microbiol. 40:403-407, 1994.

145. vanAcker, J., deSmet, F., Muyldermans, G., et al.: Outbreak of necrotizing enterocolitis associated with *Enterobacter sakazakii* in powdered milk formula. J. Clin. Microbiol. 39:293-297, 2001.

146. van den Berg, R. W., Claahsen, H. L., Niessen, M., et al.: *Enterobacter cloacae* outbreak in the NICU related to disinfected thermometers. J. Hosp. Infect. 45:29-34, 2000.

147. van der Mee-Marquet, N., Girard, S., Lagarrigue, F., et al.: Multiresistant *Enterobacter cloacae* outbreak in an intensive care unit associated with therapeutic beds. Crit. Care. 10:405, 2006.

148. van Nierop, W. H., Duse, A. G., Stewart, R. G., et al.: Molecular epidemiology of an outbreak of *Enterobacter cloacae* in the neonatal intensive care unit of a provincial hospital in Gauteng, South Africa. J. Clin. Microbiol. 36:3085-3087, 1998.

149. van Rossem, M. C., de Waal, W. J., van Hannen, E. J., et al.: *Enterobacter* colonization in newborn infants: Predictors, follow-up and implications for infection control. J. Hosp. Infect. 67:142-148, 2007.

150. Varaldo, P. E., Biavasco, F., Mannelli, S., et al.: Distribution and antibiotic susceptibility of extraintestinal clinical isolates of *Klebsiella, Enterobacter* and *Serratia* species. Eur. J. Clin. Microbiol. Infect. Dis. 7:495-500, 1988.

151. Verhamme, K. M., DeCoster, W., DeRoo, L., et al.: Pathogens in early-onset and late-onset intensive care unit-acquired pneumonia. Infect. Control Hosp. Epidemiol. 28:389-397, 2007.

152. Vonberg, R. P., and Gastmeier, P.: Hospital-acquired infections related to contaminated substances. J. Hosp. Infect. 65:15-23, 2007.

153. Waites, K. B., Duffy, L. B., and Dowzicky, M. J.: Antimicrobial susceptibility among pathogens collected from hospitalized patients in the United States and in vitro activity of tigecycline, a new glycylcycline antimicrobial. Antimicrob. Agents Chemother. 50:3479-3484, 2006.

154. Walder, M., Haeggman, S., Tullus, K., et al.: A hospital outbreak of high-level beta-lactam-resistant *Enterobacter* spp.: Association more with ampicillin and cephalosporin therapy than with nosocomial transmission. Scand. J. Infect. Dis. 28:293-296, 1996.

155. Wang, S. A., Tokars, J. I., Bianchine, P. J., et al.: *Enterobacter cloacae* bloodstream infections traced to contaminated human albumin. Clin. Infect. Dis. 30:35-40, 2000.

156. Watanakunakorn, C., and Weber, J.: *Enterobacter* bacteremia: A review of 58 episodes. Scand. J. Infect. Dis. 21:1-8, 1989.

157. Watson, J. J., Jones, R. C., Siston, A. M., et al.: Outbreak of catheter-associated *Klebsiella oxytoca* and *Enterobacter cloacae* bloodstream infections in an oncology chemotherapy center. Arch. Intern. Med. 165:2639-2643, 2005.

158. Weischer, M., and Kolmos, H. J.: Retrospective 6-year study of enterobacter bacteraemia in a Danish university hospital. J. Hosp. Infect. 20:15-24, 1992.

159. Weischer, M., and Kolmos, H. J.: Ribotyping of selected isolates of *Enterobacter cloacae* and clinical data related to biotype, phage type, O-serotype, and ribotype. A. P. M. I. S. 101:879-886, 1993.

160. Wendt, C., Lin, D., and von Baum, H.: Risk factors for colonization with third-generation cephalosporin-resistant enterobacteriaceae. Infection 33:327-332, 2005.

161. Wenger, P. N., Tokars, J. I., Brennan, P., et al.: An outbreak of *Enterobacter hormaechei* infection and colonization in an intensive care nursery. Clin. Infect. Dis. 24:1243-1244, 1997.

162. Widjojoatmodjo, M. N., Fluit, A. C., and Verhoef, J.: Molecular identification of bacteria by fluorescence-based PCR-single-strand conformation polymorphism analysis of the 16S rRNA gene. J. Clin. Microbiol. 33:2601-2606, 1995.

163. Wiegand, I., Geiss, H. K., Mack, D., et al.: Detection of extended-spectrum beta-lactamases among Enterobacteriaceae by use of semiautomated microbiology systems and manual detection procedures. J. Clin. Microbiol. 45:1167-1174, 2007.

164. Willis, J., and Robinson, J. E.: Enterobacter sakazakii meningitis in neonates. Pediatr. Infect. Dis. J. 7:196-199, 1988.

165. Wisplinghoff, H., Bischoff, T., Tallent, S. M., et al.: Nosocomial bloodstream infections in US hospitals: Analysis of 24,179 cases from a prospective nationwide surveillance study. Clin. Infect. Dis. 39:309-317, 2004.

166. Wolff, M. A., Young, C. L., and Ramphal, R.: Antibiotic therapy for enterobacter meningitis: A retrospective review of 13 episodes and review of the literature. Clin. Infect. Dis. 16:772-777, 1993.

167. Woodford, N., Hill, R. L. R., and Livermore, D. M.: In vitro activity of tigecycline against carbapenem-susceptible and -resistant isolates of *Klebsiella* spp. and *Enterobacter* spp. J. Antimicrobiol. Chemother. 59:582-583, 2007.

168. Xu, J., Moore, J. E., Millar, B. C., et al.: Improved laboratory diagnosis of bacterial and fungal infections in patients with hematological malignancies using PCR and ribosomal RNA sequence analysis. Leuk. Lymphoma 45:1637-1641, 2004.

169. Xu, X., Wu, S., Ye, X., et al.: Prevalence and expression of the plasmid-mediated quinolone resistance determinant qnrA1. Antimicrob. Agents Chemother. 51:4105-4110, 2007.

170. Yamamoto, T., Honda, T., Miwatani, T., et al.: A virulence plasmid in *Escherichia coli* enterotoxigenic for humans: Intergenetic transfer and expression. J. Infect. Dis. 150:688-698, 1984.

171. Yu, W. L., Cheng, K. C., Chi, J. C., et al.: Characteristics and molecular epidemiology of extended-spectrum beta-lactamase-producing *Enterobacter cloacae* isolated from a district teaching hospital in Taiwan. Clin. Microbiol. Infect. 12:579-582, 2006.

DIARRHEA-CAUSING AND DYSENTERY-CAUSING *ESCHERICHIA COLI*

Andrea A. Berry ✪ **Jorge J. Velarde** ✪ **James P. Nataro**

Escherichia coli has long been recognized as the most common facultative anaerobe in the human gastrointestinal (GI) tract. Virtually all *Homo sapiens* (and most other mammals) harbor this bacterium. Yet within the *E. coli* biomass lurk highly evolved pathogenic subtypes that have adapted themselves to a new niche—human pathogenicity. These pathotypes may prefer the GI tract, the genitourinary tract, or disseminated sites (including the meninges)—the last almost exclusively in neonates. This chapter focuses on *E. coli* associated with enteric infections.

The first implication of *E. coli* with diarrhea occurred more than 75 years ago, when Adam[3] postulated the existence of a group of "dyspepsia" *E. coli* responsible for neonatal and infantile diarrhea. In the 1940s, Bray reported that many, but not all, *E. coli* from severe infant diarrhea cases in summer agglutinated with antiserum prepared from a diarrheal isolate, whereas *E. coli* organisms from other sources did not.[7] The isolate used by Bray to develop the antiserum was later serotyped by the Kauffman

scheme as O111:B4, one of the now classic serogroups of enteropathogenic *E. coli* (EPEC) (Table 114–1). Although this initial description was made possible by serologic fingerprinting, the advent of molecular biology rapidly produced a plethora of reports describing the several discrete *E. coli* pathotypes.

CAUSATIVE ORGANISMS

Six distinct diarrheogenic pathotypes are recognized currently on the basis of clinical, biochemical, and molecular/genetic criteria (Table 114–2), as follows:

1. Enterotoxigenic *E. coli* (ETEC), a major cause of traveler's diarrhea and infant diarrhea in developing countries, elaborates the heat-stable (ST) enterotoxin or the heat-labile (LT) enterotoxin, or both, and causes infection of the small intestine.

TABLE 114–1 Serotypes Characteristic of the Diarrheogenic Pathotypes of *Escherichia coli*

Enteropathogenic	Enterotoxigenic	Enteroinvasive	Enterohemorrhagic	Enteroaggregative
O44:H34	O6:H -, 12, 16, 40	O28:H -	O26:H11	Nontypeable
O55:H6, 7, 32	O8:H -, 42	O29:H -	O77:H18	Rough
O86:H2, 34	O25:H -, 42	O32:H -	O103:H2	O3:H2
O111:H2, 7, 12	O27:H7	O42:H -	O104:H21	O6:H1
O114:H2	O29:H21	O89:H -	O111:H8	O11:H16
O119:H6	O63:H -, 12	O112:H -	O113:H21	O15:H21
O124:H?	O78:H11, 12	O121:H -	O128:H2	O44:H18
O125:H21	O117:H4	O124:H -	O145:H -	O92:H23
O127:H4, 6, 21	O125:H30	O136:H -	O157:H -, 7	O111:H21
O128:H2, H21	O126:H10, 27	O144:H -	O178:H19	O126:H2, 27, H -
O142:H6, 34	O127:H2	O152:H -		
O158:H23	O128:H8, 35			
	O143:H -			
	O146:H39			
	O148:H28			
	O153:H45			
	O159:H4, 21			

TABLE 114–2 Relationship of *Escherichia coli* Virulence Genes to Clinical Patterns of Diarrhea

Pathogen Group*	Virulence Genes†									Clinical Disease
	EAF	A/E	LA	AA	LT/ST	CFA	Invasion Factors	Stx	ShET-2	
ETEC	–	–	–	–	+	+	–	–	–	Watery
EPEC	+	+	+	–	–	–	–	–	–	Watery
EHEC	–	+	–	–	–	–	–	+	–	Bloody (hemorrhagic colitis)
EIEC	–	–	–	–	–	–	+	–	+	Bloody (dysentery)
EAEC	–	–	–	+	+‡	–	–	–	–	Watery (persistent)

*ETEC, enterotoxigenic E. coli; EPEC, enteropathogenic E. coli; EHEC, enterohemorrhagic E. coli; EIEC, enteroinvasive E. coli; EAEC, enteroaggregative E. coli.
†EAF, EPEC adherence factor; A/E, attaching and effacing changes; LA, localized adherence pattern; AA, autoaggregative attaching pattern; LT/ST, heat-labile and heat-stable toxins; CFA, colonization factor antigens; invasion factors, chromosomal and plasmid factors mediating cell invasion; Stx, Shiga family cytotoxins; ShET-2, plasmid-encoded Shigella enterotoxin-2, highly homologous to the plasmid-encoded EIEC toxin.
‡Enteroaggregative stable toxin (EAST) is a member of the ST family.

2. EPEC, the original pathotype defined by Bray,[7] causes infant diarrhea in less-developed countries. The bacteria induce a characteristic attaching and effacing lesion in the small intestine. Classic EPEC requires the chromosomally encoded locus of enterocyte effacement (LEE) and a high-molecular-weight virulence plasmid termed EPEC adherence factor (EAF) plasmid.

3. Enterohemorrhagic *E. coli* (EHEC) causes outbreaks of hemorrhagic colitis and hemolytic-uremic syndrome (HUS) in temperate climates. The essential virulence factor is the Shiga toxin (Stx), which circulates through the bloodstream and acts by inhibition of protein synthesis in the target cell.

4. Enteroinvasive *E. coli* (EIEC) is an unusual cause of diarrhea and dysentery. It is similar to *Shigella* epidemiologically and pathogenetically and shares similar virulence genes.

5. Enteroaggregative *E. coli* (EAEC) causes diarrhea in individuals of all ages in industrialized countries and in less-developed areas and in travelers. The organism adheres to the intestinal mucosa and secretes several enterotoxins and cytotoxins.[95]

6. Diffusely adherent *E. coli* (DAEC) is the sixth category. The epidemiologic scenario for this organism has not been elucidated.

TRANSMISSION AND EPIDEMIOLOGY

Diarrheogenic *E. coli* strains are worldwide in distribution. The route of infection is fecal-oral, predominantly via contaminated food and water, although person-to-person transmission may

TABLE 114–3 Age-Related Patterns of *Escherichia coli* Diarrhea

Pathogen Classification	Age at Highest Risk	Characteristics of Diarrhea		
		Bloody	Watery	Inflammatory
EAEC	<6 mo	–	+++	–
EPEC	<1 yr	–	+++	–
ETEC	<1 yr	–	+++	–
EIEC	>2 yr	++	+	+++
EHEC	2-10 yr	+++	+	–

EAEC, enteroaggregative E. coli; EHEC, enterohemorrhagic E. coli; EIEC, enteroinvasive E. coli; EPEC, enteropathogenic E. coli; ETEC, enterotoxigenic E. coli.

occur with EHEC and possibly EPEC in infants.[111] As discussed subsequently, environmental contamination by EHEC is an emerging problem in industrialized countries, whereas ETEC continues to be ubiquitous worldwide. Table 114–3 lists the age-specific predilections of the various *E. coli* pathogens.

ENTEROTOXIGENIC *ESCHERICHIA COLI*

The infectious dose for ETEC is approximately 10^8 bacteria.[47] The incubation period is 14 to 50 hours.[107] Transmission typically occurs via contamination of food and water,[145] and person-to-person transmission is thought to be uncommon. In developing countries, contamination of food and water sources occurs commonly.[132] ETEC has been detected in the United States in numerous food samples, including cheese, hamburger, sausage, and seafood.[103,145] A domestic U.S. outbreak of diarrhea at Crater Lake National Park in Oregon was traced to ETEC organisms in the water supply.[143] Because large numbers of organisms are required for experimental infection, transmission probably would require multiplication of the inoculum within the vehicle, which probably contributes to the well-documented propensity of ETEC infection to occur in warm months.[132]

ETEC is a major cause of diarrhea in infants and children in the developing world.[64,132] The incidence typically increases during the first 6 months of life and decreases after 12 months. ETEC has been estimated to cause approximately 20 percent of diarrheal episodes in the developing world,[132] although this percentage varies substantially by location. A study in rural Egypt[134] found that ETEC accounted for 66 percent of all first episodes of diarrhea, with an incidence of 1.7 episodes per child-year during the first 6 months of life and 2.3 during the second 6 months. In Tehran,[148] researchers found that ETEC could be isolated from 15.5 percent of patients younger than 5 years old with diarrhea. The prevalence was 18 percent in Bangladesh[131] and 33 percent in Mexico.[36] A study in Hanoi[117] found, however, that only 2.2 percent of diarrheal episodes could be attributed to ETEC, and the frequency in Mongolia[150] was similarly low.

ETEC disease is primarily a childhood problem, with the incidence decreasing after the child reaches 5 years of age.[131,132] After infection with a particular ETEC strain, the host is resistant to disease but still may excrete the organism asymptomatically, a characteristic that contributes to the environmental burden.[111,162] Adults still may be susceptible to ETEC diarrhea.[64,132] In a study of elderly individuals in Dhaka, Bangladesh,[54] researchers found that 13 percent of adults older than 60 years with diarrhea were noted to have ETEC. Although the incidence of ETEC diarrhea decreases after age 5 years, the incidence seems to increase again in patients older than 15 years, and 25 percent of ETEC infections are seen in adults.[131,132]

ETEC is the most common cause of traveler's diarrhea, typically accounting for approximately 30 to 40 percent of cases.[2,84,152] Illness is acquired by ingestion of contaminated food or water. The diarrhea is acute and watery and typically resolves spontaneously without severe limitation of activities.[2] ETEC also has been implicated as the cause of diarrhea among cruise ship travelers, introduced when the ship docks in a foreign port.[40]

ETEC organisms are extremely diverse, and children in endemic areas experience multiple infections. The basis of immunity, which increases with repeated exposure, is unknown.[162] Strains producing ST cause more severe disease than strains producing only LT, and the former is not immunogenic. Colonization of the small intestinal mucosa is mediated by surface fimbriae called *colonization factor antigens* (CFAs), which are immunogenic and which may elicit some element of protective immunity.[135] Despite the existence of more than 20 CFAs, a few are overrepresented among clinical isolates; in a study from Bangladesh, 7 CFAs constituted greater than 75 percent of the CFAs isolated.[131] In an analysis of multiple studies, Wolf[180] suggested that most ETEC express CFA I, II, or IV. In some epidemiologic studies, most strains do not express known CFAs, however.[156]

ETEC is predominantly an infection of warm weather months in endemic areas, coincident with conditions promoting bacterial replication in the environment. Some sites report that a second peak occurs after the rainy season.[131,132]

ENTEROPATHOGENIC *ESCHERICHIA COLI*

Neter and associates[116] first coined the term EPEC to denote a group of *E. coli* serotypes associated with dramatic and highly lethal nursery outbreaks of diarrhea in the United States and the United Kingdom (see Table 114–1). We now recognize that these serotype antigens serve as surrogate markers for a package of chromosomal and plasmid-borne virulence genes, which together orchestrate enteric pathogenesis. The epidemiology of EPEC has changed since its original description was provided. Gone are the lethal outbreaks formerly reported in industrialized countries, to be replaced by sporadic endemic disease in resource-poor countries. The infection retains its dramatic predilection for infants and children younger than 24 months, is rarely seen in older children and adults, and is not a cause of traveler's diarrhea.[35,36,65,170] The basis of this age-dependent incidence is unknown.

Globally, EPEC is among the most common causes of infant diarrhea.[35,36,65,140] EPEC has a propensity to cause persistent infection and wasting, suggesting that its burden may comprise more than simple dehydration. Breast-feeding offers some protection against EPEC because of the presence of immune factors and oligosaccharides that inhibit adherence of EPEC to epithelial cells.[38] In industrialized countries such as the United States, EPEC generally is no longer considered to be a cause of endemic diarrhea, although EPEC may be present in infants immigrating from or visiting resource-poor settings. Rare indigenous cases may occur.[67] In an outpatient setting in the United States, 2 of 147 cases of non-dysenteric acute diarrhea were caused by EPEC.[27] In 166 Swiss children admitted to hospitals with diarrhea, 13 (7.8%) had EPEC isolated from stool cultures.[53]

As noted previously, EPEC strains of the classic serotypes (also known as typical EPEC) require the LEE chromosomal locus and the EAF plasmid to cause diarrhea. Controversy exists over whether or not so-called atypical EPEC (which are LEE-positive and EAF-negative) are a cause of diarrhea.[109] The description of an outbreak of diarrhea in Japan caused by an atypical EPEC strain suggests that at least some of these strains are pathogenic.[182]

ENTEROHEMORRHAGIC *ESCHERICHIA COLI*

Since its discovery in 1977, EHEC has emerged as an important and increasingly common human pathogen. The organisms may be excreted asymptomatically by cattle herds, and large outbreaks of human infection have been associated with the ingestion of undercooked hamburger and other foods contaminated indirectly by cattle manure. Careful prospective epidemiologic surveillance in Minnesota has revealed an increase in the incidence of EHEC from 0.5 to 2 per 100,000 children younger than 18 years old during the period 1979 to 1988,[101] similar to the incidence of EHEC determined in the state of Washington in the late 1980s: 2.1 per 100,000. In a multicenter study of mild acute diarrhea in outpatients in the United States, 5 (3.4%) of 147 cases were caused by EHEC,[27] a frequency similar to that in Swiss children hospitalized for community-acquired diarrhea.[53] Very young children are not commonly infected; rather, infection occurs most commonly and severely in children 2 to 10 years old or in the elderly.

Ground beef is identified as the most common source of EHEC infection. Several outbreaks have been associated with fast-food consumption.[133] In meat-processing plants where bulk ground beef is prepared for the fast-food industry, meat from one contaminated carcass can contaminate and distribute the organisms to a huge number of beef patties. Several other food sources of transmission that have been documented include other beef; produce, including spinach and lettuce; milk; water; and processed foods, including unpasteurized apple cider, mayonnaise, and dry fermented sausage. Person-to-person, cattle-to-person, and waterborne outbreaks have been described. Person-to-person spread as sequelae of point-source epidemics is common.[155] Many unusual modes of transmission linked with cattle have occurred and include poorly washed apples dropped in cow pastures and used to make cider, surface water supplies in proximity to areas where cattle graze, spread of aerosolized particles at agricultural fairs, and transmission by contact at petting zoos. Contaminated swimming holes have been implicated in several outbreaks.

A multistate outbreak of O157:H7 EHEC infections associated with the consumption of fresh bagged spinach occurred in the United States in 2006, affecting 26 states and resulting in 205 confirmed illnesses, 103 hospitalizations, 31 cases of HUS, and three deaths.[11,28] This outbreak exemplifies the widespread effect of a foodborne outbreak caused by the mass production and distribution of produce.

Strong epidemiologic evidence associates EHEC with HUS. In one series of patients from Canada, 60 percent of patients with HUS had either neutralizable free Shiga toxin (Stx) or Stx-producing *E. coli* in their stool, and 75 percent had serum antibody against Stx.[124] A review of O157:H7 outbreaks (defined as two or more cases) reported to the Centers for Disease Control and Prevention in the United States from 1982 to 2002 found 350 outbreaks representing 8598 cases, 1493 (17%) hospitalizations, 354 (4%) cases of HUS, and 40 (0.5%) deaths.[133] During a large outbreak of *E. coli* O157:H7 infection associated with fast-food restaurant hamburgers on the West Coast of the United States in 1993, of the 732 affected individuals identified, 195 were admitted to the hospital, HUS developed in 55 (7.5%), and 4 died.[67] Investigation of this outbreak showed that small numbers of bacteria (in the range of a few hundred) constituted an infectious dose. Among 93 cases of O157:H7 infection reported in Washington State in 1987, HUS or thrombotic thrombocytopenic purpura (TTP) developed in 11 (12%), for an approximate incidence of 0.23 per 100,000.[122]

The highest incidence of HUS occurs in children younger than 5 years, in whom the age-specific incidence ranged from 2.6 to 5.8 per 100,000 in Minnesota,[101] Washington,[122] and Oregon.[142] In the 2000 FoodNet Annual Report, *E. coli* O157:H7 accounted for 2 cases of HUS per 100,000, and more than 40 percent of cases with confirmed infection were hospitalized. The incidence of HUS in Argentina, 21.7 per 100,000, is four to eight times higher and is the highest reported incidence of HUS in the world.[99]

In the United Kingdom and the United States, HUS and TTP are associated predominantly with Stx2-producing *E. coli* O157:H7[101,123]; however, this finding may represent more facile detection of this serotype. In addition, the incidence of non-O157:H7 infections in the United States is increasing (serotypes associated with EHEC infection are presented in Table 114–1).[25,85,179] In Argentina, non-O157:H7, Stx2-producing strains are isolated most commonly.[99] Similarly, in Australia, other serotypes, especially O111, have been associated with major outbreaks and a significant number of HUS cases.[9] Many of these serotypes have been implicated in sporadic and outbreak disease in the United States[24] (e.g., an outbreak caused by O104:H21 acquired from contaminated milk[10]).

Non-O157:H7 EHEC infections have increased in prevalence in the United States and are now known to account for 20 to 50 percent of all EHEC infections.[85] Although some non-O157 strains are not pathogenic, others have been shown to cause disease as severe as that caused by O157:H7 strains, suggesting that a clinical suspicion for EHEC should be maintained even when testing for O157:H7 is negative.[85] Non-O157, Stx-producing *E. coli* infection was made a reportable disease in the United States in 2000.[25]

HUS occurs seasonally in the United States and Canada (most common during the summer months), although no specific seasonal risk factor or factors for infection with Stx-producing *E. coli* are known. Other epidemiologic data suggest that poor children are at lower risk for the development of HUS, perhaps because they already have immunity to EHEC or Stx toxins through early contact with the organisms in their environment.[32]

ENTEROINVASIVE *ESCHERICHIA COLI*

EIEC is closely related to *Shigella* microbiologically and pathogenetically. The pathotype typically is found in areas with a high burden of *Shigella*. The infectious dose may be higher than that of *Shigella*, and person-to-person transmission seldom is reported. Food-borne outbreaks occur sporadically.[66,100] The first description of EIEC as a pathotype occurred in 1971, when bloody diarrhea was traced to the consumption of French Camembert cheese contaminated with *E. coli* O124.[100] Small outbreaks or sporadic cases involving a limited number of serotypes have been reported from numerous countries, including the United States, France, Japan, and Brazil.[100,120,160,171,174] Prospective studies in Thailand using DNA probes for EIEC pathogenicity genes indicated that 6 percent of cases of dysentery may be caused by EIEC strains.[48] The epidemiology of the cases is complicated by the fact that in contrast to the initial descriptions of EIEC-associated disease, most EIEC infections probably are neither dysenteric nor characterized by bloody diarrhea but instead manifest as watery diarrhea with low-grade fever, similar to that caused by viral agents and ETEC.

Infection with 10^8 bacteria has been shown to be necessary for experimental dysentery in human volunteers,[47] a dose substantially higher than that for *Shigella* spp. ($\leq 10^4$ organisms). In a food-borne outbreak caused by a nontypeable EIEC, secondary person-to-person transmission was not reported.[160]

ENTEROAGGREGATIVE *ESCHERICHIA COLI*

EAEC was implicated first as a cause of diarrheal disease in studies of children in Chile, Mexico, and India.[18,19,37,112] The pathogenicity of at least some EAEC strains has been established by several observations. First, volunteer studies by Nataro and associates[108] revealed that some EAEC could elicit diarrhea in healthy subjects, whereas other strains may not be pathogenic. Second, EAEC strains have been implicated in outbreaks of diarrhea, the largest of which involved nearly 2700 schoolchildren in Japan.[72,82,183] Lastly, but most emphatically, a meta-analysis performed by Huang and colleagues[79] of more than 20 years of studies revealed convincingly that EAEC is a cause of diarrhea in infants; adults, especially those with human immunodeficiency virus and acquired immunodeficiency syndrome (AIDS) in developing countries; children in industrialized countries; and adult travelers to less-developed areas. In addition, a study from the United States by Nataro and colleagues[113] suggested that EAEC was the most frequent bacterial cause of diarrhea among all ages in Baltimore, Maryland, and New Haven, Connecticut.

Nonetheless, a persisting controversy surrounding EAEC epidemiology and pathogenesis is the definition of the pathotype. The meta-analysis described earlier implicated EAEC, as defined by the characteristic stacked-brick adherence pattern to epithelial cells in culture.[79] A study of infant diarrhea in Cincinnati suggested, however, that only strains hybridizing with an EAEC gene probe (see later) were truly associated with clinical diarrhea.[33] A full understanding of what constitutes a truly pathogenic EAEC strain is unavailable.

CLINICAL MANIFESTATIONS

Diarrhea-causing *E. coli* may be responsible for a variety of clinical syndromes because virtually all known mechanisms of diarrhea, including secretory toxins, cytotoxic toxins, invasion, and pathogenic adherence, are manifested by the various *E. coli* pathotypes. The clinical manifestations are largely a function of the complement of virulence genes (see Table 114–2), and identification of the essential pathogenicity genes provides the definitive diagnostic maneuver. As with other pathogens, invasive *E. coli* strains (i.e., EIEC) produce inflammatory diarrhea with fever, abdominal pain, nausea, vomiting, and leukocytes and blood in the stool. Noninvasive, cytotoxin-producing EHEC strains cause a frankly bloody diarrhea associated with leukocytosis but without fecal leukocytes or fever. Producers of LT or ST enterotoxins (i.e., ETEC) elicit brisk, watery diarrhea with the potential for significant dehydration.

ENTEROTOXIGENIC *ESCHERICHIA COLI*

ETEC causes watery, nonmucoid, nonbloody diarrhea in infants, older children, and adults, and it is a common cause of traveler's diarrhea.[132] The onset of diarrhea is abrupt, with an incubation period of 14 to 50 hours.[107] The frequency of stools varies from a few to more than 10 per day, and a striking absence of leukocytes is noted when the diarrheal stool is examined by light microscopy. Young affected children may vomit and commonly are febrile (38° C to 40° C), although adults typically are afebrile. ETEC disease cannot be distinguished clinically from most other causes of acute nonspecific watery diarrhea. The illness usually is self-limited to 3 to 5 days but occasionally lasts more than 1 week. Severely dehydrating illness that resembles clinical cholera can occur but is uncommon.

Variability in the clinical picture may be due to age differences and preexisting immunity, but it also may be attributed to differences in the infecting inoculum. DuPont and colleagues[47] produced mild diarrhea (three watery stools per day for 2 to 3 days) when 10^8 bacteria were fed to adult volunteers, whereas 10^{10} organisms caused more pronounced diarrhea (more than five stools per day for 4 to 5 days), with mucus but no blood observed in some subjects. Many subjects also had abdominal cramping, but no tenesmus was present, and all remained afebrile. This clinical picture is typical of traveler's diarrhea in adults.[104] ETEC diarrhea can result in severe dehydration necessitating aggressive fluid therapy.

ENTEROPATHOGENIC *ESCHERICHIA COLI*

EPEC diarrhea typically is copious and watery, without blood or fecal leukocytes.[97] Patients may have low-grade fever. In a Swiss study conducted with modern diagnostic methods, the mean age of 13 hospitalized children with EPEC diarrhea was 1.4 years (range 0.5-3 years).[53] Fever was low-grade, and vomiting occurred in 69 percent. Volume depletion was considered moderate in five and severe in two children. Although nursery outbreaks no longer occur commonly, severe illness still can develop in infants infected with EPEC,[83] with high mortality rates ranging from 25 to 70 percent.[43] The cause of death of patients in nursery outbreaks is not well documented. Investigations using an experimental EPEC infection model in adult volunteers (who are not naturally susceptible) revealed that watery diarrhea occurred 3 to 16 hours after inoculation and generally lasted less than 2 days. Diarrhea occasionally was copious and in some cases was associated with abdominal cramps, nausea, vomiting, malaise, and fever.[45] This clinical picture is consistent with disease caused by outbreaks of EPEC in adults and traveler's diarrhea caused by EPEC.

EPEC also has been implicated in chronic diarrhea in the United States and elsewhere, with serious nutritional consequences that may require total parenteral nutrition and hospital stays of 120 days.[144] In prospective studies of EPEC diarrhea in

young infants in Brazil[65] and Ethiopia,[169] fever, vomiting, and dehydration all were observed commonly. The clinical significance of chronic diarrhea may be increased by the underlying malnutrition of infants in resource-poor countries. In many settings, especially where effective oral rehydration programs are in place, chronic diarrhea and associated malnutrition are now more important causes of diarrheal deaths than are acute diarrhea and dehydration.[22]

In the course of the classic, severe nursery outbreaks caused by typical EPEC strains, the first signs and symptoms were mild and nonspecific, but they commonly were followed by vomiting and diarrhea of increasing severity. Stools contained neither mucus nor blood, and the volume fluctuated over a period of weeks. Plain abdominal radiographs revealed only nonspecific dilation of small bowel loops, although severe ileus not attributable to hypokalemia developed in many patients. Infected infants lost as much as 15 percent of body weight, leading to profound electrolyte disturbances and severe dehydration along with central nervous system manifestations, such as irritability, hypertonicity, convulsions, and coma. Circulatory collapse occurred despite adequate replacement of fluids and achievement of electrolyte balance. In an epidemic in Virginia, Belnap and O'Donnell[16] described fatal infections caused by *E. coli* O111:B4 occurring after 3 weeks of illness and associated with renal failure, coma, and signs of disseminated intravascular coagulation, but blood cultures typically remained negative. The fatality rate was age-dependent; although the overall mortality was 16 percent, the rate in neonates was 40 percent.

ENTEROHEMORRHAGIC *ESCHERICHIA COLI*

In 1971, a distinctive clinical diarrheal syndrome was recognized that was characterized by afebrile bloody diarrhea in addition to cramping and colonic inflammatory changes, usually right-sided.[138] In 1983, this illness was associated with an otherwise rare *E. coli* serotype, O157:H7, and a characteristic syndrome, hemorrhagic colitis, was defined.[139] O157:H7 subsequently was recognized as the most virulent prototype of a Stx-producing pathotype designated EHEC. EHEC now has been shown to cause a wide spectrum of diseases that may be confined to the GI tract or, in a sizable proportion (typically 5-10%), can become systemic.[15,165] After an incubation period of 3 to 4 days (range 1 to 8 days), the local GI illness usually begins with nonbloody diarrhea that can progress to bloody diarrhea after 1 or 2 days. Hemorrhagic colitis occurs in 50 to 90 percent of O157:H7 infections.[122,165]

Further progression may occur over the course of the next day or two and result in the passage of frank blood, the pathognomonic clinical feature of hemorrhagic colitis. Associated manifestations include vomiting in approximately 50 percent of patients and abdominal pain. Fever may occur but typically is low-grade. This clinical picture may be confused with other conditions, such as appendicitis, intussusception, inflammatory bowel disease, ischemic colitis, and diverticulitis. The difficulty in establishing the diagnosis can lead to inappropriate drug therapy or even surgery.[68,80]

A serious complication of hemorrhagic colitis is the development of HUS or TTP.[68] HUS is characterized by the triad of acute renal failure, thrombocytopenia, and hemolytic anemia and develops in approximately 10 to 20 percent of infected children younger than 10 years.[111] HUS is the most common cause of acquired renal failure in the United States.[172,173] The acute mortality rate is approximately 5 percent, and renal failure is expected to develop eventually in many more patients during the next several decades. After renal failure, cerebrovascular accident and colonic perforation are the most common serious sequelae. TTP and HUS have overlapping clinical features, but TTP generally occurs in older adults and is associated with prominent neurologic findings, including behavioral changes, altered consciousness or coma, and seizures, and fever.[77]

A prospective study in Canada identified E. coli O157:H7 in 15 percent of 125 patients with grossly bloody diarrhea over a 6-month period.[124] The age range was 15 months to 73 years; however, almost half of the patients were younger than 10 years old. The illness was similar to that described earlier, with a mean duration of 7.8 days, but it was significantly longer in children (9.1 ± 2 days) than in adults (6.6 ± 1.1 days). Sigmoidoscopy findings were abnormal in seven of eight adults examined, with hyperemic mucosa in six and superficial ulcerations in one. Biopsy samples showed mild mucosal inflammation in four of five patients. In another study, the findings on colonoscopy in 10 patients with hemorrhagic colitis caused by E. coli O157:H7 included severe inflammation (predominantly right-sided), marked edema, easy hemorrhage, and the frequent appearance of longitudinal ulcer-like lesions.[158]

Because local and systemic manifestations in EHEC infection are caused, at least partially, by Stx, the presence of these same toxins in the intestinal lumen in patients with non-O157:H7 infection puts them at risk for development of hemorrhagic colitis and HUS. No comparative data are available to assess the relative risk in O157:H7 and non-O157:H7 EHEC infection. Non-O157:H7 EHEC may cause similar clinical manifestations, with less aggressive transmission potential.

ENTEROINVASIVE ESCHERICHIA COLI

Naturally acquired EIEC infection causes a mild to moderately severe dysentery syndrome consisting of fever, malaise, diarrhea, tenesmus, and abdominal cramping.[47,174] Watery diarrhea usually occurs at the onset of the illness and progresses to mucoid diarrhea with streaks of blood or microscopic hematochezia but rarely to the classic small-volume, grossly bloody, dysenteric stool seen with Shigella infection. Of 204 cases reported in one study, grossly bloody stool occurred in only 4.[65] In two of these patients, sigmoidoscopy revealed superficial ulcerations in one and hyperemia alone in the second patient. As in Shigella infection, the stool reveals abundant polymorphonuclear cells, compatible with the inflammatory, invasive nature of the organism. Vomiting and dehydration can occur; the latter generally is mild in nature. Fever of 38° C to 39.5° C is a typical symptom that occurs early in association with malaise, myalgia, and headache and lasts for 2 to 3 days. In most instances, the diarrhea ceases in 1 week or less, but in some patients, it may continue for 2 weeks or more.

In adult volunteers with experimentally induced EIEC disease, febrile illness developed approximately 11 hours (range 8 to 24 hours) after the inoculum was ingested.[47] Chills, myalgia, headache, and profuse diarrhea or abdominal cramps and tenesmus rapidly followed. In 2 of 13 subjects, this picture was associated with systemic toxicity and transient hypotension consistent with bacteremia, even though blood cultures were negative for all patients. Clinical dysentery with bloody stools occurred in several subjects, and reddened, friable mucosa with multiple bleeding points was seen by sigmoidoscopy. Clinical illness was controlled quickly with parenteral ampicillin therapy.

ENTEROAGGREGATIVE ESCHERICHIA COLI

Descriptions of EAEC clinical features are derived from outbreak investigations, volunteer studies, and studies of traveler's diarrhea.[79] Most EAEC infections are accompanied by watery diarrhea, which may progress to persistent diarrhea that lasts 14 days or longer.[19,112] Bloody diarrhea is observed in a subset of patients.[37]

An EAEC strain was implicated in a school lunch outbreak in Tajimi City, Japan, in 1993.[82] Of 6636 children who ate the school lunch at 16 schools, 2697 (rate of attack 40.6%) reported GI symptoms. Major symptoms were abdominal pain (73.6%), nausea (51.1%), and diarrhea (39.9%). The incubation period for the onset of GI illness was 40 to 50 hours on average. Duration of symptoms was not reported. A nursery outbreak in Serbia involved 19 normal infants. All experienced watery diarrhea, which persisted beyond 2 weeks in three patients. A report of 17 pediatric patients with illness caused by EAEC of serotype O126:H27 in Israel suggested that patients typically manifested diarrhea (in all), vomiting (in 8), and fever (in 12, ≤40° C).[157] In this report, one 6-week-old infant developed diarrhea persisting for 40 days. Studies in travelers suggest that EAEC disease may be mildly inflammatory, although fever and fecal leukocytes are present in a few patients.[79]

PATHOGENESIS

ENTEROTOXIGENIC ESCHERICHIA COLI

ETEC was identified first as a porcine pathogen,[71,159] which elicited fluid secretion when injected into ligated ileal loops.[71] Two secretogenic activities were characterized: one could be inactivated by heating, and the other could not; the activities could be found both in the same strain or independently. These activities now have been assigned to two well-characterized enterotoxins, LT and ST. LT is genetically, structurally, and mechanistically similar to cholera toxin produced by Vibrio cholerae O1 strains.[63,111] ST is actually two distinct toxins: STa is associated with human disease, whereas STb causes disease only in animals.[90,130]

The essential pathogenic strategy for ETEC involves colonization of the proximal small intestine, followed by release of one or both of the enterotoxins. Colonization of the intestinal epithelium (Fig. 114–1) is mediated by proteinaceous, hair-like bacterial surface appendages called fimbriae (or pili), of which greater than 25 antigenic types are known to exist.[180] The adherence factors are termed colonization factor antigens (CFA) or coli surface antigens (Fig. 114–2).[60]

Human STa is a small, non-immunogenic molecule that is translated as a 72-amino acid polypeptide.[161] The first 19 amino acids serve as a signal sequence for secretion into the periplasmic space; a further cleavage event occurs after secretion, which results in the final 18- to 19-amino acid active peptide.[111,136] The sequence of the mature ST has six cysteine residues that form stabilizing disulfide bonds, contributing to the high stability of the toxin to heat and proteases.[184] The ST receptor on the apical surface of the intestinal epithelial cells is guanylate cyclase C. This receptor is a large transmembrane protein with an extracellular ligand-binding domain and intracellular catalytic domain; binding to guanylate cyclase C results in its activation, which is responsible for an increase in cellular cyclic guanosine monophosphate (cGMP).[153] cGMP is an intracellular signaling molecule that induces activation of apical chloride channels and inhibition of absorptive mechanisms.[57,69,105] ST exploits an endogenous signaling pathway, the natural agonist of which is the peptide guanylin, a natural controller of electrolyte homeostasis.[39]

The LT family of toxins includes LT-I, which has significant homology in structure and function with cholera toxin, and LT-II, which does not seem to cause human or animal disease.[111] LT-I shares 80 percent identity with cholera toxin and similarly has an A_1-B_5 stoichiometry.[62,111,163] The 28-kd A subunit is the catalytically active moiety, whereas the 11-kd B subunit pentamer mediates cell binding and entry. LT interacts mainly with G_{M1} gangliosides on the surface of the epithelial cells (although additional potential receptors have been identified).[111,168] The A

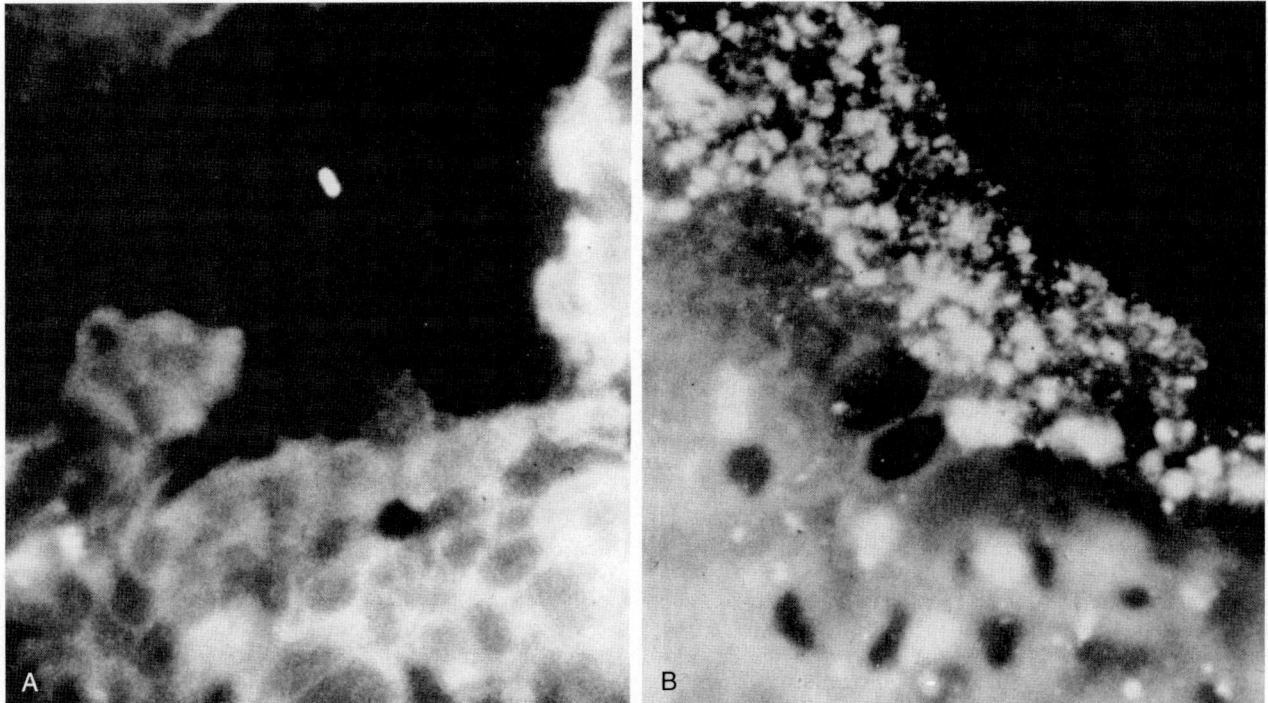

Figure 114–1 **A,** Laboratory-passaged avirulent *Escherichia coli* H10407 in infant rabbit intestine. No adherent, colonizing bacteria are seen. **B,** Fresh, virulent H10407 organisms at the same time interval in infant rabbit intestine are closely adherent to the brush border (indirect immunofluorescent stained section, ×1000). *(Courtesy of Drs. Dolores and Doyle Evans, Department of Microbiology, Baylor College of Medicine.)*

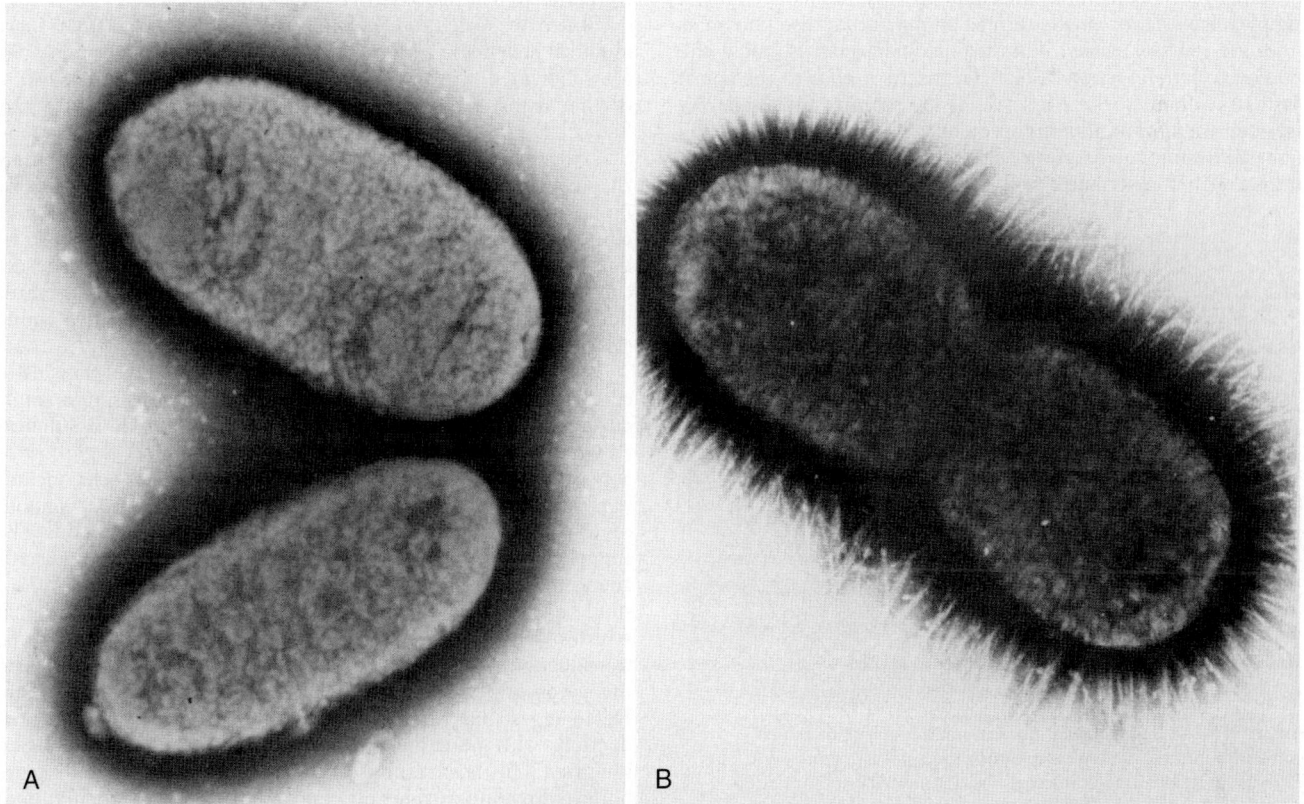

Figure 114–2 **A,** Electron micrograph of negatively stained cells of avirulent plasmid-cured *Escherichia coli* H10407. Note the bald appearance of the outer surface of the organism. **B,** Similar view of virulent, fresh *E. coli* H10407. Note the hairy surface of the organism as a result of CFA/I (×20,000). *(Courtesy of Drs. Dolores and Doyle Evans, Department of Microbiology, Baylor College of Medicine.)*

subunit is composed of two domains, termed A1 and A2, which are bound via a disulfide bond. A1 has an adenosine diphosphate–ribosyl transferase, which targets the cellular guanosine triphosphate binding protein G_s, a regulator of cellular cyclic adenosine monophosphate (cAMP) levels. Ribosylation of G_s leads to constitutive activation of adenylate cyclase, which greatly increases cAMP levels. Increased cAMP leads to increased phosphorylation of chloride channels, especially CFTR, by protein kinase A.[90,154]

ENTEROPATHOGENIC *ESCHERICHIA COLI*

EPEC pathogenesis is complex and only partly understood. In contrast to ETEC, it possesses no potent secretogenic toxin but rather induces changes to the enterocyte signal transduction environment, which transforms the enterocyte from an absorptive cell to a secretory cell. EPEC pathogenesis has been described as a multistep process. The first step comprises attachment to the small bowel mucosa, an event mediated by the EAF plasmid-encoded, bundle-forming pilus (BFP). BFP is a complex surface fimbrial structure that may undergo contraction, not only tethering the bacteria to the cell but also pulling itself close to the cell's apical membrane.[92] Approach of the bacteria is followed by induction of a characteristic lesion, called *attaching and effacing*. Under electron microscopy, the normal microvillus architecture is dissolved, and the bacterium adheres tightly (<20 nm distance) to the now undulating membrane. The bacteria may be observed sitting atop a cup or pedestal of protruding cell membrane (Fig. 114–3). This deceivingly simple phenotype is mediated and accompanied by a dizzying array of invisible changes to the cell's internal environment.[43]

Cellular changes are induced largely by a platoon of protein toxins that the bacterium injects directly into the cytoplasm of the target host cell. This injection process is mediated by a complex bacterial organelle termed an *injectisome*, also known as a *type III secretion system*. The first toxin injected is called the *translocated intimin receptor* (Tir). Tir inserts itself into the apical plasma membrane, where it serves as the receptor for the bacterial outer membrane adhesion protein called *intimin*. As its name suggests, intimin mediates very close attachment of the bacterium to the cell and contributes to the resulting cytoskeletal damage.

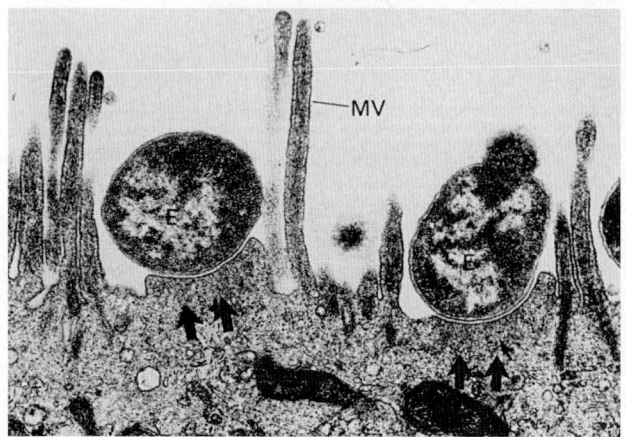

Figure 114–3 High-power electron micrograph of intestinal epithelium infected by typical enteropathogenic *Escherichia coli* strains *(E)*, with occasional intact microvilli *(MV)* and pedestal formation indicated by *double arrows*. This figure shows not only the structural alterations and loss of the brush border, but also the close apposition of the organisms to the epithelial cells. *(Courtesy of Ralph A. Gianella, Department of Medicine, University of Cincinnati School of Medicine.)*

The net effect of Tir, intimin, and other injected toxins is dissolution of the microfilament and microtubule networks, phosphorylation of membrane ion transporters, and disruption of tight junctions at the cell's periphery. Diarrhea apparently is caused by a combination of ion transport and paracellular leakage. Release of proinflammatory cytokines may complete the pathogenic cascade. The relative contributions of each of these events to EPEC disease are unknown.

EPEC adhere to HEp-2 epithelial cells in a characteristic localized pattern, which has been suggested as a diagnostic assay (Fig. 114–4).[43] Also, EPEC causes actin polymerization of target cells at sites of attachment, a virulence property readily detected in tissue culture (e.g., HEp-2 cells) by a fluorescent actin-staining test (Fig. 114–5).[91] As discussed subsequently, these phenotypic assays, although useful for pathogenesis studies, have largely been replaced by molecular diagnostic tests.

ENTEROHEMORRHAGIC *ESCHERICHIA COLI*

The cardinal pathogenic feature of the EHEC pathotype is the production of Stx, leading to the alternate name of Shiga-toxin–producing *E. coli*, accompanied by a cohort of accessory virulence factors. As with EPEC, these factors are encoded by the bacterial chromosome and a high-molecular-weight virulence plasmid. Stx is encoded on a lysogenic phage, which apparently is capable of infecting some nonpathogenic *E. coli* strains. The full package of virulence genes has been well characterized in serotype O157:H7; some evidence suggests that non-O157 pathogens share some, but not all, of the virulence traits, accounting for their reduced virulence and frequency. Stx toxins were discovered by Konowalchuk and associates,[93] who reported finding Vero cell toxic activity in culture filtrates of certain strains of *E. coli* isolated from patients with diarrhea (Stx occasionally has been referred to by the archaic synonym *Vero toxin*).

Stx toxins constitute a family of protein toxins that share identical enzymatic action and target cell binding specificity. Stx are subdivided into two families, Stx1 and Stx2, each consisting of the major Stx type and variants (i.e., Stx1c, Stx1d, Stx2c, Stx2c2, Stx2d$_{EH250}$, Stx2d$_{activatable}$, Stx2e, and Stx2f).[20] Stx2 and Stx2c have been associated with severe disease, including hemorrhagic colitis and HUS.[59,123] Stx2d$_{activatable}$ can be activated by mouse and human intestinal mucus and is associated with a severe clinical phenotype.[20] The greater pathogenicity of Stx2 may be due to greater accessibility of the active site on the Stx2 structure.[58] The *stx1* gene differs from the *Shigella stx* gene by three nucleotide changes, which result in a single conservative amino acid substitution in the A subunit: threonine to serine.[77]

Stx toxins have the same structure and mechanism of action. They have an A_1-B_5 stoichiometry, comprising a single enzymatically active A subunit and a pentamer of B subunits responsible for toxin binding. The B subunits bind to globotrioacyl ceramide (Gb$_3$) and related glycolipids on host cells, including epithelial enterocytes, vascular endothelial cells, smooth muscle cells, renal endothelial cells, and erythrocytes.[46,94] The catalytic A subunit cleaves the *N*-glycosidic bond in a specific adenosine of the 28S rRNA in the 60S ribosomal subunit.[49] This single cleavage event results in irreversible cessation of protein synthesis and ultimately leads to cell death via multiple signal transduction pathways.[34] Intestinal villus cells are susceptible to the action of Stx, which includes reduced absorption of sodium. Data suggest that Stx induces local inflammatory cytokine production, with potential effects on epithelial cell and mucosal integrity. This host response may induce a vicious cycle because both hydrogen peroxide and neutrophils augment production of Stx.[178]

Epidemiologic evidence strongly links Stx-producing strains to hemorrhagic colitis and to the associated systemic complica-

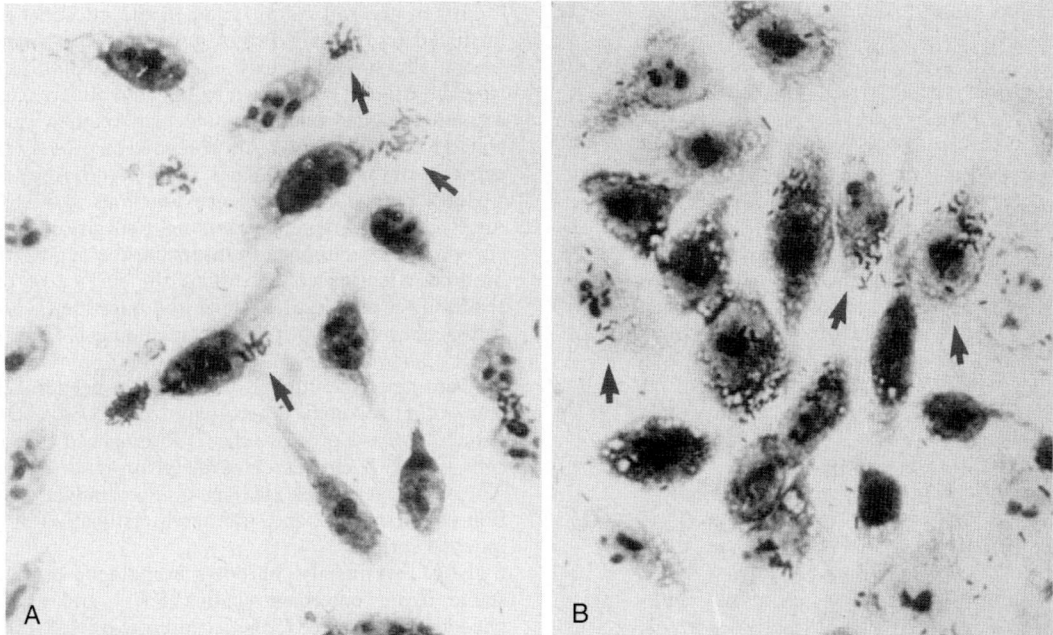

Figure 114–4 **A** and **B**, Patterns of adherence of *Escherichia coli* to HEp-2 cells in tissue culture. Typical enteropathogenic *E. coli* associates with HEp-2 cells in the pattern shown in **A**, termed localized adherence (LA). *Arrows* point to cells where growing microcolonies of bacteria are attached to focal areas of the cell membrane. Other *E. coli* organisms isolated from patients with diarrhea adhere over the entire HEp-2 cell membrane, as shown in the cells identified with *arrows* in **B**. This pattern of interaction is termed diffuse adherence (DA). Although the LA phenotype has been associated definitively with the capacity to induce diarrhea in experimental models, no convincing evidence of virulence in DA strains has been obtained to date.

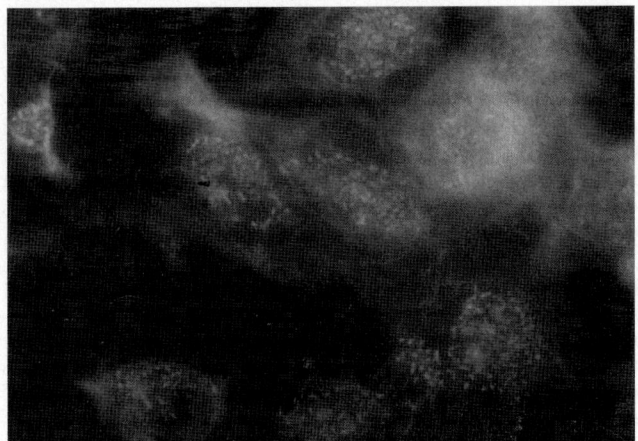

Figure 114–5 Some *Escherichia coli* strains have the capacity to attach to the eukaryotic cell membrane and induce polymerization of actin beneath the membrane. This property may be shown by the fluorescent actin staining test, in which polymerized F-actin is detected by a fluorescein-tagged mushroom toxin specific for this form of actin. In this figure, the bacteria are attached to HEp-2 cells, and the induced actin polymerization revealed by the fluorescent reagent highlights the organisms, which are seen as bright rods on the infected cells.

tions of HUS and TTP.[67,87,139] The mechanisms underlying HUS and TTP are uncertain but seem to be due to the effects of toxin on vascular endothelial cells, possibly in concert with lipopolysaccharide and a variety of cytokines, which initiate events resulting in endothelial cell injury and platelet thrombi and, subsequently, the characteristic thrombotic microangiopathy.[32,88,119] Other possible initiation factors include abnormal levels of von Willebrand factor, but whether this abnormality is a cause or a consequence

of disease is unknown.[106] Stx1 has been shown to decrease production of prostacyclins; however, the role of this event in the pathogenesis of HUS is uncertain.[88]

Similar to EPEC, EHEC express the intimin outer membrane protein and a type III secretion apparatus.[111] EHEC are capable of inducing complex cytoskeletal alterations similar to those caused by EPEC infection, although certain subtle differences are observed. EHEC infects the human colon, whereas EPEC is an infection of the small bowel. The genes encoding intimin, Tir, the type III secretion system, and secreted proteins reside on a 35-kb pathogenicity island called the LEE, which may be more crucial for EPEC than for EHEC for virulence.[46] A 60-Md plasmid, pO157, which contains genes encoding an enterohemolysin, is commonly found in O157:H7 strains, but its role in production of disease is unclear.[111] Subtilase cytotoxin (SubAB), a novel cytotoxin with an A_1-B_5 stoichiometry, was described more recently and associated with HUS in diverse EHEC strains in Australia and the United States.[90,127] SubAB is heat-stable, more toxic to vero cells than Stx, and lethal when injected in mice.[90,127] Cytotoxicity is the result of direct cleavage of an endoplasmic reticulum chaperone protein, BiP.[126]

ENTEROINVASIVE *ESCHERICHIA COLI*

In 1967, Trabulsi and coworkers[171] in Brazil and Sakazaki and associates[147] in Japan described the isolation of certain *E. coli* serotypes from patients with a disease resembling bacillary dysentery, but with cultures negative for *Shigella*. These isolates possessed a critical virulence hallmark associated with *Shigella*—the ability to invade intestinal and other epithelial cells (Fig. 114–6).[119] They have been called EIEC, and a limited number of serotypes, distinct from the EPEC O groups, but often crossreactive with *Shigella* O antigens, have been found to possess this property (see Table 114–1). The genetic and molecular basis of

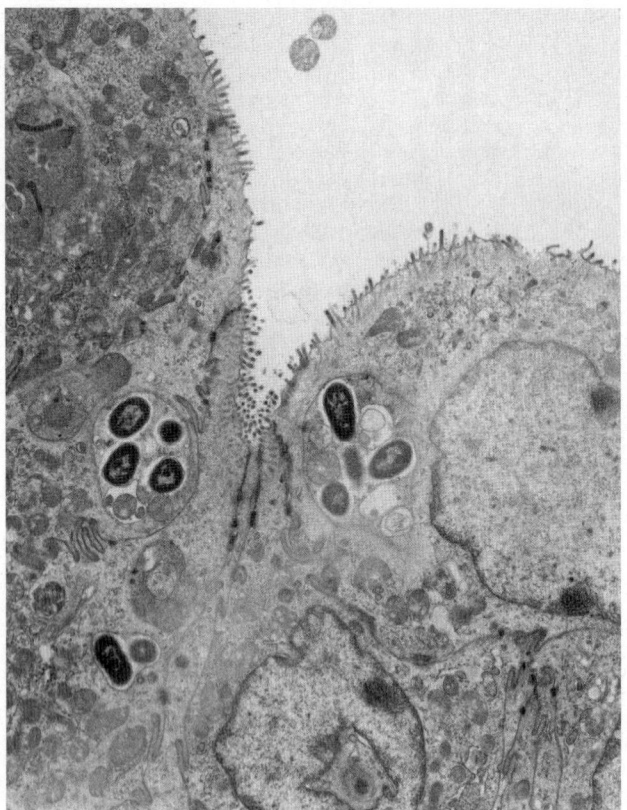

Figure 114–6 Electron micrograph of enteroinvasive *Escherichia coli* infection of intestinal mucosa. The intracellular location of the bacteria clearly is seen within membrane-bound vesicles in two adjacent infected cells. The pathogenesis of enteroinvasive *E. coli* infection involves the invasion of intestinal cells and local cell-to-cell spread, as shown here, by a mechanism identical to that of *Shigella* spp. *(Courtesy of Saul Tzipori, D.V.M., Department of Comparative Medicine, Tufts University School of Veterinary Medicine.)*

invasion by *Shigella* was well defined in the 1990s, and the same plasmid and chromosomal genes encoding invasion properties and mechanisms seem to be present in EIEC as well.[78,98,125,149]

The invasive process for EIEC is thought to be the same as that for *Shigella* spp. It has been well characterized and involves four main steps: (1) initial entry into cells, (2) intracellular multiplication, (3) intracellular and intercellular spread, and (4) host-cell killing. The process is complex and involves multiple genes on the invasion plasmid and the chromosome.[1] EIEC produces toxins reported to be structurally distinct from the Stx of *Shigella dysenteriae* type 1 and the Stx1 and Stx2 of EHEC.[55] Nonetheless, studies suggest that EIEC toxins possess many properties in common with the Stx family of toxins, including the ability to cause fluid secretion in animal models.[55] EIEC may contain a plasmid-borne gene that encodes a 63-kd protein called *ShET2* (Shigella enterotoxin 2); a mutation in this gene substantially decreases the enterotoxic activity of the parent strain.[114]

ENTEROAGGREGATIVE *ESCHERICHIA COLI*

The pathogenesis of EAEC includes adherence to the intestinal epithelium as a thick biofilm, accompanied by mucus hypersecretion, intestinal damage, and induction of an inflammatory response. Most of these phenotypes seem to be mediated by a set of bacterial cytotoxins and enterotoxins.[73]

Adherence and colonization of the intestinal epithelium are mediated by pili called *aggregative adherence fimbriae*, of which several allelic variants exist. EAEC may colonize the large and small intestines.[76] All known aggregative adherence fimbriae variants are encoded on high-molecular-weight virulence plasmids collectively termed *pAA*. Also encoded on pAA is a transcriptional activator of the fimbrial genes, called *AggR*. AggR is emerging as a global regulator of virulence functions in EAEC; also under AggR control is a gene encoding a surface protein nicknamed *dispersin*. In the absence of dispersin, the aggregative adherence fimbriae adhesins collapse onto the surface of the bacterium, rendering it unable to colonize the intestine (J. Nataro, unpublished). Several cryptic genes, including a large chromosomal locus, also are under AggR control.

Damage to the intestinal mucosa has been linked to the presence of a secreted enterotoxin called *Pet* (plasmid-encoded toxin).[52] Pet is a protease that is internalized by target epithelial cells, where it cleaves cytoskeletal proteins including spectrin. The net effect of these cleavage events is induction of fluid, secretion of electrolytes, and, ultimately, exfoliation of cells from the mucosal surface.[75]

EAEC strains also harbor a homologue of the ETEC heat-stable toxin, enteroaggregative ST,[151] and a chromosomally encoded toxin called *Shigella* enterotoxin 1.[56] Inflammation by EAEC has been linked to the expression of the bacterial flagellum, although studies in polarized epithelial monolayers suggest that additional factors under control of AggR also are required.[73]

DIAGNOSIS AND DIFFERENTIAL DIAGNOSIS

Diarrheogenic *E. coli* can be identified best by detecting their defining virulence genes. Although many molecular tests are described for this purpose, few laboratories in the United States use them. For most pathotypes, consultation with an expert, such as the senior author or the *E. coli* reference laboratories at the U.S. Centers for Disease Control and Prevention, is recommended. Detection of *E. coli* generally is indicated for severe and persistent diarrhea lacking any other diagnosis (particularly in returning travelers), or in the setting of diarrheal outbreaks of unknown cause. With the exception of EHEC, most infections caused by diarrheogenic pathotypes are self-limiting.

Because of the potential of EHEC to cause serious sequelae, establishing a specific diagnosis is of clinical and epidemiologic importance. The earlier in the course of illness that a stool specimen is obtained, the more likely that *E. coli* O157:H7 will be recovered[166]; recovery more than 7 days after onset of diarrhea is unusual. The laboratory can use sorbitol-MacConkey (SMAC) agar to screen colonies for lack of sorbitol fermentation or substrates such as 4-methylumbelliferyl-β-D-glucuronide (MUG) for the production of β-glucuronidase; *E. coli* O157:H7 is almost uniquely sorbitol-negative and glucuronidase-negative. These techniques have limited sensitivity, with the sensitivity of SMAC agar reported as 50 to 60 percent.[89] Some sorbitol-fermenting O157:H7 isolates and many other sorbitol-fermenting, non-O157 EHEC are capable of causing severe illness and HUS that are missed by sorbitol-MacConkey agar.

Detecting *Shiga* toxin in stool specimens, either directly or after overnight broth enrichment, currently is the most sensitive nonmolecular method for identifying EHEC.[89] These tests are more sensitive than are culture techniques and are not dependent on serotype. Commercial enzyme immunoassays for Stx have been approved by the U.S. Food and Drug Administration for either confirmation of isolates as toxin producers or rapid direct diagnosis based on the detection of Stx1 or Stx2 in stool.[17,110] Despite the detection of *Shiga* toxin by these rapid assays, isolation of the organism, usually performed at reference laboratories, remains crucial for serotyping and other epidemiologic purposes.

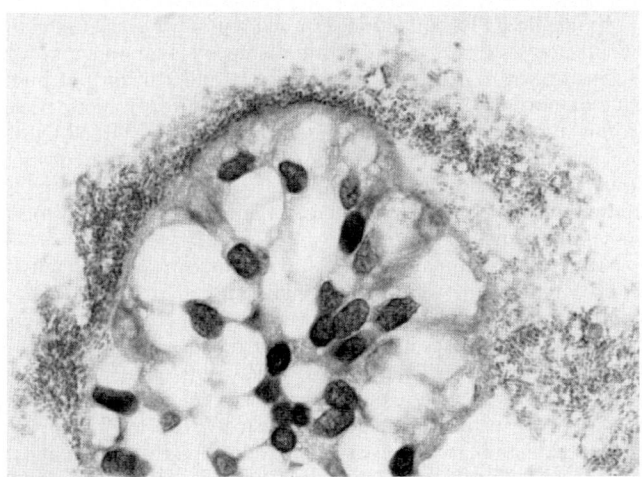

Figure 114–7 Enteroaggregative *Escherichia coli* (EAEC) infection of the gnotobiotic pig intestine. This photomicrograph shows the characteristic "stacked-brick" appearance of the aggregative organisms over the surface of the intestinal epithelium in vivo in the same manner described for EAEC adherence to HEp-2 cells in tissue culture. *(Courtesy of Saul Tzipori, D.V.M., Department of Comparative Medicine, Tufts University School of Veterinary Medicine.)*

Serotype-specific commercial antigen immunoassays also are available.[110]

Diagnosis of ETEC would require identifying the LT or ST genes in an isolate or, after isolation and growth in vitro, detecting their products by enzyme-linked immunosorbent assay. Polymerase chain reaction techniques are available that allow LT or ST genes to be detected directly from stool without the need for performing culture.[26] A retrospective diagnosis can be made by detecting an increase in antitoxin antibody, especially for LT. Enzyme-linked immunosorbent assay for CFA antigens of ETEC also could be useful.

EPEC can be detected reliably by DNA probes for the 60-Md EAF adherence plasmid or by adherence to cells in culture. The ability of *E. coli* to adhere to HEp-2 cells in culture in distinct morphologies led to the description of EPEC, EAEC, and DAEC as different pathotypes (see Fig. 114–3). After a 3-hour incubation of bacteria with cells, EPEC adheres to the cell in tight microcolonies, called the *localized adherence* pattern. Although it remains sensitive and specific for EPEC, this method has been replaced by molecular detection methods to detect the LEE island (via the intimin-encoding gene *eae*) and the EAF plasmid (often via detection of the BFP-encoding genes).[44]

EAEC can be detected by the presence of the aggregative adherence pattern in the Hep-2 adherence assay (Fig. 114–7). DNA probes and polymerase chain reaction are available to detect the AggR regulon, and these tests are likely to provide more specific detection of EAEC pathogens.[33]

EIEC is detected best using molecular techniques that are specific for detection of pathogenesis-related genes. Several multiplex polymerase chain reaction assays that allow the user to screen for multiple *E. coli* pathotypes simultaneously have been described.[13,128] They can be introduced readily into any molecular biology laboratory and produce excellent results.

PROGNOSIS

EPEC, EAEC, and ETEC do not cause systemic infections or complications except complications resulting from dehydration or the consequences of nutritional depletion. The prognosis is related directly to the availability and adequacy of fluid therapy. When this need is dealt with correctly in an otherwise healthy and well-nourished patient, the principal complication is the rare instance of monosaccharide intolerance. In infants or young children in developing countries with protein-energy malnutrition, however, chronic diarrhea and progressive worsening of nutritional status frequently are observed, sometimes resulting in mortality. When food is withheld from either well-nourished or poorly nourished children, hypoglycemia may occur and produce seizures, coma, or death. Rarely, loss of water in excess of salt causes hypertonic dehydration, with serum sodium concentrations greater than 160 mEq/L, a situation that may cause seizures, coma, and death.

As noted earlier, EAEC has been associated with persistent diarrhea lasting longer than 14 days in young infants and children. Persistent diarrhea leads to nutritional deterioration, may be difficult to control, and may culminate in death from sepsis or other infections. Inflammatory diarrhea caused by EIEC also results in nutritional deterioration, with significant protein losses occurring via the gut.

EHEC often is followed by HUS, neurologic and intestinal complications, and, especially in adults, TTP. Ten percent of patients may die early in the course of the systemic phase of either HUS or TTP. Although the renal failure of HUS generally is reversible with good management of fluid and electrolytes and the use of dialysis as needed, permanent damage to the kidneys is, contrary to earlier more optimistic assessments, likely to occur in 25 percent or more of patients over the course of 1 or 2 decades, and many of them require permanent dialysis or transplantation in the future.[61] The prognosis in TTP is related directly to initiation of plasmapheresis, which has been documented to reduce mortality rates significantly.[177] No such benefit has been noted in HUS.[177]

TREATMENT

In all age groups, the principal treatment of the intestinal manifestations of *E. coli* enteric infection is replacement of fluids and electrolytes; with maintenance of fluid balance, the disease is self-limited to 1 week or less in most patients and lasts no more than 2 weeks in nearly all patients. The earlier that fluid replacement therapy is begun, the better the prognosis, particularly when one considers that clinical signs of dehydration do not develop until a 5 percent loss of body weight occurs, and that sustained loss of more than 10 percent of body weight is incompatible with survival.

When shock is present (usually with altered consciousness and an absent or thready pulse) or oral rehydration is unsuccessful because of persistent vomiting, patients must be rehydrated by intravenous infusion of an isotonic electrolyte solution, such as lactated Ringer solution or normal saline. Three 20 mL/kg fluid boluses can be given back-to-back, with close monitoring of the patient's clinical status. When dehydration is less severe, initial replacement of losses usually can be accomplished by oral rehydration. Patients not in shock, who may have normal findings on physical examination or may manifest poor skin turgor, tachycardia, postural hypotension, and oliguria (along with irritability and a sunken fontanelle in the very young), should receive 50 to 120 mL/kg of fluid, depending on the severity of dehydration, as rapidly as they can be encouraged to drink, over 4 hours. Pulse, blood pressure, urine volume, skin turgor, general appearance, and thirst are monitored as indicators of response. Adults may need 1 L/hr to establish rehydration; adults as well as children may tire of drinking and fail to keep up with requirements.

Several prerequisites must be ensured for oral therapy: (1) the patient must not be in shock; (2) the patient must be fully conscious; (3) the patient must be able to drink (vomiting, particularly common in children, is not an absolute contraindication because frequent small oral feedings usually are largely retained; when the metabolic abnormality begins to reverse toward normal, vomiting ceases); (4) bowel sounds must be present; and (5) renal function must be normal. Current recommendations in the United States and Europe suggest the use of hypotonic fluid containing 30 to 60 mEq of sodium per liter, although specific attention given to sodium and potassium deficits may be required. In the developing world, where cholera is a common occurrence, the World Health Organization recommends that a solution containing 90 mEq of sodium be used for all cases of diarrhea because of the large sodium losses that occur in cholera, and the desire to avoid the need to choose among formulations because of difficulty in making an etiologic diagnosis. Rice-based solutions for oral rehydration currently are favored in many diarrheal centers because of their reduced osmotic load.[5]

A prospective cohort study comparing *E. coli* O157:H7 HUS patients who developed oligoanuric renal failure requiring dialysis with patients with non-oligoanuric renal failure found that the patients who required dialysis had received less intravascular volume expansion and sodium than had the patients who did not require dialysis, suggesting that intravascular volume expansion with isotonic fluid was protective for oligoanuric renal failure when given early in the course of O157 infection.[4] The authors advocate hospitalizing all children with suspected EHEC infection for volume expansion with isotonic fluids and close monitoring.

Although rehydration therapy is the cornerstone of management, antibiotic therapy should be considered in some cases. In most *E. coli*–associated diarrheal illnesses, the disease is mild and of short duration, and no specific antimicrobial therapy is required. Studies to address this issue have found antibiotics to be beneficial in some circumstances. In traveler's diarrhea secondary to ETEC, antibiotic therapy can shorten the duration of illness and decrease its severity.[8,51] Prophylactic antibiotic therapy probably carries more risk than benefit, however, and generally is not recommended. When antibiotics are used, trimethoprim-sulfamethoxazole (TMP-SMX) therapy presently is recommended for children with traveler's diarrhea caused by susceptible isolates; fluoroquinolones are the drugs of choice for adults when chemoprophylaxis is indicated.[137] A more recently approved antibiotic for adults, rifaximin, is not absorbed from the GI tract and shows promise as an effective treatment of ETEC.[50] The data in children are very limited, however, and use of rifaximin is not yet recommended in this population.

Children in developing countries with ETEC diarrhea also may benefit from receiving antibiotic therapy.[118] Resistance of ETEC to TMP-SMX was noted in U.S. troops in Saudi Arabia, where 44 percent of isolates were resistant.[121] EIEC infection theoretically would benefit even more from antibiotic therapy, given its pathogenic similarity to shigellosis and the known benefits of the early use of antibiotics. No controlled studies have validated this benefit for EIEC, however. In experimentally induced disease, DuPont and colleagues[47] reported that parenteral ampicillin produced a bacteriologic cure and rapid clinical response with defervescence and improvement of diarrhea in adults. TMP-SMX and ampicillin are the current drugs of choice, unless resistance is a problem.

Immunocompromised hosts, especially children with AIDS, may require prolonged antibiotic therapy for protracted or recrudescent diarrhea, even when it is caused by bacteria that normally produce only self-limited disease. Malnourished children and children with other serious underlying illness also fit this category. In these patients, systemic invasion may develop along with associated complications, including shock and renal failure. In addition, prolonged carrier states are common findings, with frequent relapses requiring long-term antibiotic therapy for suppression of relapse.

Epidemic EPEC infection, especially in newborns, seems to be affected favorably by antibiotic therapy.[115] The potential for this pathogen to cause prolonged disease and a history of high rates of mortality in neonates suggest the need for antibiotic trials in this age group. Based on limited data, either TMP-SMX or oral nonabsorbable antibiotics, such as gentamicin or colistin, usually are recommended, although antibiotic resistance is common and may alter the choice of antibiotics based on local susceptibility patterns.[14,176]

Antibiotic treatment of EHEC remains controversial but is not recommended. Antibiotics in clinical use do not improve the course or prevent sequelae, and they may exacerbate the illness by promoting release of Stx.[6,21,30] In vitro data suggest that subinhibitory concentrations of TMP-SMX and other antibiotics may increase expression of Stx,[86] perhaps related to enhanced release of toxin from damaged organisms.[14] The most rigorous prospective study to address this question found that the cohort who received antibiotics had a higher incidence of HUS (of 9 patients who received antibiotics, 5 developed HUS) than the cohort who did not (of 62 patients who did not receive antibiotics, 5 developed HUS; $p < 0.001$).[181] Other studies have found no association.[122]

Notably, no studies have used a randomized placebo-controlled design, so the association may reflect selection bias because both the use of antibiotics and systemic complications are associated with more severe disease. A meta-analysis[146] did not show a higher risk of HUS associated with antibiotics; however, this meta-analysis has been criticized because it included a study in which all of the patients received antibiotics[81] and because comparisons were made among different antibiotics, which may not induce similar sequelae.

Antimotility agents such as loperamide generally are not needed and should be used cautiously if prescribed, with great attention paid to dosage, especially in very young patients.[167] Dysentery is a contraindication to the use of antimotility agents, which may be a risk factor for the development of ileus and abdominal distention.[3] The prolonged use of antimotility agents is reported to be associated with more serious systemic complications of EHEC infection and is not recommended.[30,31]

In most instances of *E. coli* diarrhea, the clinician is left to make therapeutic decisions without knowing the etiologic agent responsible. For reasons already outlined, routine diagnostic microbiology laboratories cannot distinguish pathogenic from nonpathogenic *E. coli*, with the exception of classic EPEC serotypes and O157:H7 EHEC. Clinical decisions regarding the administration of antibiotic therapy are made on purely clinical grounds with criteria such as the history, duration, and severity of the illness; the age and immunologic competence of the patient; and the nature of the diarrheal stool (e.g., watery, inflammatory, bloody, or dysenteric). Empiric antimicrobial therapy is more justifiable for immunocompromised hosts, for patients with prolonged or severe illness or a history of relevant risk factors (e.g., specific food ingestion, travel, exposure to known contacts), and for cases of inflammatory or dysenteric illness.

A novel treatment approach was reported by DiCesare and associates,[42] who evaluated SP-303, a plant-derived product with antisecretory properties, in a randomized placebo-controlled study of acute diarrhea in 184 U.S. travelers to Mexico and Jamaica. SP-303 shortened the duration of traveler's diarrhea by 21 percent; ETEC was the etiologic agent of traveler's diarrhea in 19 percent of the subjects. Human breast milk contains oligosaccharides that can partially bind to ETEC and presumably block attachment to intestinal epithelial cells.[102] Bovine hyperimmune milk from cows immunized against ETEC and EPEC is not effective treatment or prophylaxis for ETEC or EPEC diarrhea.[29,164]

Research on alternative treatments of EHEC and prevention of HUS is ongoing. A synthetic verotoxin receptor, SYNSORB

Pk, was not shown to prevent death, dialysis, or serious extrarenal events in a trial of 145 children with EHEC-induced HUS.[175] Although antibodies against *E. coli* O157 intimin were protective for colonization and disease in a pig model,[41] plasmapheresis and intravenous immunoglobulin have not been shown to ameliorate HUS in humans.[141] Investigation of monoclonal antibodies directed against Stx are under way.[175] The complete genome sequence of *E. coli* O157:H7 is now known and may lead to greater understanding of the pathogenesis of hemorrhagic colitis and HUS and perhaps innovative approaches to treatment and prevention.[74]

PREVENTION

Epidemic nursery outbreaks of diarrhea in newborns can be controlled by the application of antiquated but still valid principles of preventive medicine. Prompt diagnosis and treatment and scrupulous attention given to details of handwashing and environmental sanitation to eliminate person-to-person transmission are still effective, whereas prophylactic antimicrobials have no role. Outbreaks in neonatal nurseries can be contained by epidemiologic control measures such as cohorting; by screening staff for carriage; and, if necessary, by closing the unit until it is decontaminated. In contrast, preventing sporadic cases of *E. coli* diarrhea is difficult. In communities with obvious deficits in water supply and feces disposal, correction of these problems would lead to a diminished incidence of diarrheal diseases in general.

For traveler's diarrhea, several studies indicate that prophylactic antibiotics can protect adult travelers, at least for a limited time.[70] The risk of selection of resistant organisms and drug side effects limits the use of antibiotic prophylaxis to short-term travelers with business or diplomatic missions that would be hindered significantly by an episode of diarrhea. Fluoroquinolones, tetracyclines, azithromycin, and rifaximin have been evaluated for prophylaxis and presumptive treatment, and all are efficacious. The use of tetracyclines is not recommended for children younger than 8 years, and toxicity concerns for fluoroquinolones are still present.[6] Some evidence has been presented for the efficacy of bismuth compounds, such as bismuth subsalicylate, for the prevention of ETEC diarrhea in adults. The concern for bismuth toxicity with prolonged use in young children would render it a problematic solution for pediatric *E. coli* diarrhea and its prevention.

ETEC vaccine development has been propelled by the observation that ETEC infection confers some protection from reinfection with the same strain,[162] also evident in the decreasing rates of infection in children older than 5 years.[132] The challenge is that greater than 25 CFAs have been identified, and strain serotypes vary tremendously across the world.[64] As noted previously, however, it also is known that certain serotypes and CFAs are most common (CFA I, II, and IV) and tend to co-segregate.[60,64,180] This factor would limit the antigenic variability needed in an effective vaccine. Most isolates of ETEC expressing only LT do not express fimbria colonization factors and would be unaffected by a CFA-based vaccine. Although no vaccine currently is licensed and available, several approaches have been attempted. Among the most successful to date is a vaccine composed of recombinant cholera toxin B (as a surrogate for the LTB toxin subunit) with four strains of formalin-killed ETEC expressing the most prevalent CFAs in developing countries. This vaccine was found to prevent 80 percent of ST ETEC diarrhea in travelers to developing countries.[132] It is available commercially in Europe and may provide limited, short-term protection in travelers.[96] In a study of Egyptian children, however, it was not efficacious in preventing disease.[23,132]

Other avenues of vaccine development that have been pursued include subunit vaccines. ST does not create a significant immune response; however, LT is a known adjuvant similar to cholera toxin and has been conjugated to ST.[23,64] Concerns for human use of this vaccine come, however, from the homology of ST to guanylin, which is produced endogenously.[23,39] Live, attenuated *Shigella* vaccine vectors also are being studied in an attempt to elicit a mucosal immune response. Researchers are studying new methods of delivering antigens to the mucosa, including encapsulation in microspheres and delivery in recombinant foods. A transcutaneous vaccine, composed of fimbrial antigens mixed with LT, has been shown to elicit serum antibodies in adult volunteers.[64] Work continues in this field in an attempt to decrease the incidence and severity of morbidity from dysentery in the developing world and from traveler's diarrhea.

Vaccine development for other diarrheogenic *E. coli* strains lags behind that for ETEC. Because EHEC-induced HUS is a rare disease, widespread human vaccination may not be cost-effective. Vaccine development for cattle, the major reservoir, is ongoing. A vaccine composed of type III secreted proteins resulted in decreased shedding of *E. coli* O157:H7 compared with controls, although prevalence of shedding increased over the study period. Repeat vaccination of cattle may serve as a mode to decrease human exposure to EHEC.[129]

REFERENCES

1. Acheson, D., and Keusch, G.: *Shigella* and enteroinvasive *Escherichia coli*. In Blaser, M. J., Smith, P. D., Ravdin, J. I., et al. (eds.): Infections of the Gastrointestinal Tract. New York, Raven Press, 1995, pp. 763-784.
2. Adachi, J. A., Ericsson, C. D., Jiang, Z. D., et al.: Natural history of enteroaggregative and enterotoxigenic *Escherichia coli* infection among US travelers to Guadalajara, Mexico. J. Infect. Dis. *185*:1681-1683, 2002.
3. Adam, A.: Biology of colon bacillus in dyspepsia, and its relation to pathogenesis and to intoxication. J. Kinderheilk *101*:295-314, 1923.
4. Ake, J. A., Jelacic, S., Ciol, M. A., et al.: Relative nephroprotection during *Escherichia coli* O157:H7 infections: Association with intravenous volume expansion. Pediatrics *115*:e673-e680, 2005.
5. Alam, N. H., Yunus, M., Faruque, A. S., et al.: Symptomatic hyponatremia during treatment of dehydrating diarrheal disease with reduced osmolarity oral rehydration solution. J. A. M. A. *296*:567-573, 2006.
6. Al-Qarawi, S., Fontaine, R. E., and Al-Qahtani, M. S.: An outbreak of hemolytic uremic syndrome associated with antibiotic treatment of hospital inpatients for dysentery. Emerg. Infect. Dis. *1*:138-140, 1995.
7. Anonymous: Bray's discovery of pathogenic *Esch. coli* as a cause of infantile gastroenteritis. Arch. Dis. Child. *48*:923-926, 1973.
8. Anonymous: Travelers' diarrhea. National Institutes of Health Consensus Development Conference, Bethesda, Maryland, January 28-30, 1985. Rev. Infect. Dis. *8*(Suppl. 2):S109-S233, 1986.
9. Anonymous: Community outbreak of hemolytic uremic syndrome attributable to *Escherichia coli* O111:NM—South Australia 1995. M. M. W. R. Morb. Mortal. Wkly. Rep. *44*:550-551, 557-558, 1995.
10. Anonymous: Outbreak of acute gastroenteritis attributable to *Escherichia coli* serotype O104:H21—Helena, Montana, 1994. M. M. W. R. Morb. Mortal. Wkly. Rep. *44*:501-503, 1995.
11. Anonymous: Ongoing multistate outbreak of *Escherichia coli* serotype O157:H7 infections associated with consumption of fresh spinach—United States, September 2006. M. M. W. R. Morb. Mortal. Wkly. Rep. *55*:1045-1046, 2006.
12. Anonymous: The use of systemic fluoroquinolones. Pediatrics *118*:1287-1292, 2006.
13. Aranda, K. R., Fabbricotti, S. H., Fagundes-Neto, U., et al.: Single multiplex assay to identify simultaneously enteropathogenic, enteroaggregative, enterotoxigenic, enteroinvasive and Shiga toxin-producing *Escherichia coli* strains in Brazilian children. F. E. M. S. Microbiol. Lett. *267*:145-150, 2007.
14. Ashkenazi, S., and Cleary, T. G.: Antibiotic treatment of bacterial gastroenteritis. Pediatr. Infect. Dis. J. *10*:140-148, 1991.
15. Bell, B. P., Griffin, P. M., Lozano, P., et al.: Predictors of hemolytic uremic syndrome in children during a large outbreak of *Escherichia coli* O157:H7 infections. Pediatrics *100*:E12, 1997.
16. Belnap, W. D., and O'Donnell, J. J.: Epidemic gastroenteritis due to *Escherichia coli* 0-111: A review of the literature, with the epidemiology, bacteriology, and clinical findings of a large outbreak. J. Pediatr. *47*:178-193, 1955.
17. Bettelheim, K. A., and Beutin, L.: Rapid laboratory identification and characterization of verocytotoxic (Shiga toxin producing) *Escherichia coli* (VTEC/STEC). J. Appl. Microbiol. *95*:205-217, 2003.
18. Bhan, M. K., Khoshoo, V., Sommerfelt, H., et al.: Enteroaggregative *Escherichia coli* and *Salmonella* associated with nondysenteric persistent diarrhea. Pediatr. Infect. Dis. J. *8*:499-502, 1989.

19. Bhan, M. K., Raj, P., Levine, M. M., et al.: Enteroaggregative *Escherichia coli* associated with persistent diarrhea in a cohort of rural children in India. J. Infect. Dis. *159*:1061-1064, 1989.

20. Bielaszewska, M., Friedrich, A. W., Aldick, T., et al.: Shiga toxin activatable by intestinal mucus in *Escherichia coli* isolated from humans: Predictor for a severe clinical outcome. Clin. Infect. Dis. *43*:1160-1167, 2006.

21. Bin Saeed, A. A., El Bushra, H. E., and Al-Hamdan, N. A.: Does treatment of bloody diarrhea due to *Shigella dysenteriae* type 1 with ampicillin precipitate hemolytic uremic syndrome? Emerg. Infect. Dis. *1*:134-137, 1995.

22. Black, R. E.: Persistent diarrhea in children of developing countries. Pediatr. Infect. Dis. J. *12*:751-761; discussion 762-764, 1993.

23. Boedeker, E. C.: Vaccines for enterotoxigenic *Escherichia coli*: Current status. Curr. Opin. Gastroenterol. *21*:15-19, 2005.

24. Bokete, T. N., O'Callahan, C. M., Clausen, C. R., et al.: Shiga-like toxin-producing *Escherichia coli* in Seattle children: A prospective study. Gastroenterology *105*:1724-1731, 1993.

25. Brooks, J. T., Sowers, E. G., Wells, J. G., et al.: Non-O157 Shiga toxin-producing *Escherichia coli* infections in the United States, 1983-2002. J. Infect. Dis. *192*:1422-1429, 2005.

26. Caeiro, J. P., Estrada-Garcia, M. T., Jiang, Z. D., et al.: Improved detection of enterotoxigenic *Escherichia coli* among patients with travelers' diarrhea, by use of the polymerase chain reaction technique. J. Infect. Dis. *180*:2053-2055, 1999.

27. Caeiro, J. P., Mathewson, J. J., Smith, M. A., et al.: Etiology of outpatient pediatric nondysenteric diarrhea: A multicenter study in the United States. Pediatr. Infect. Dis. J. *18*:94-97, 1999.

28. California Food Emergency Response Team: Investigation of an *Escherichia coli* O157:H7 Outbreak Associated with Dole Pre-Packaged Spinach. Sacramento, California, Department of Health Services, 2007.

29. Casswall, T. H., Sarker, S. A., Faruque, S. M., et al.: Treatment of enterotoxigenic and enteropathogenic *Escherichia coli*-induced diarrhoea in children with bovine immunoglobulin milk concentrate from hyperimmunized cows: A double-blind, placebo-controlled, clinical trial. Scand. J. Gastroenterol. *35*:711-718, 2000.

30. Cimolai, N., Carter, J. E., Morrison, B. J., et al.: Risk factors for the progression of *Escherichia coli* O157:H7 enteritis to hemolytic-uremic syndrome. J. Pediatr. *116*:589-592, 1990.

31. Cimolai, N., Morrison, B. J., and Carter, J. E.: Risk factors for the central nervous system manifestations of gastroenteritis-associated hemolytic-uremic syndrome. Pediatrics *90*:616-621, 1992.

32. Cleary, T. G., and Lopez, E. L.: The shiga-like toxin-producing *Escherichia coli* and hemolytic uremic syndrome. Pediatr. Infect. Dis. J. *8*:720-724, 1989.

33. Cohen, M. B., Nataro, J. P., Bernstein, D. I., et al.: Prevalence of diarrheagenic *Escherichia coli* in acute childhood enteritis: A prospective controlled study. J. Pediatr. *146*:54-61, 2005.

34. Colpoys, W. E., Cochran, B. H., Carducci, T. M., et al.: Shiga toxins activate translational regulation pathways in intestinal epithelial cells. Cell. Signal. *17*:891-899, 2005.

35. Cravioto, A., Reyes, R. E., Ortega, R., et al.: Prospective study of diarrhoeal disease in a cohort of rural Mexican children: Incidence and isolated pathogens during the first two years of life. Epidemiol. Infect. *101*:123-134, 1988.

36. Cravioto, A., Reyes, R. E., Trujillo, F., et al.: Risk of diarrhea during the first year of life associated with initial and subsequent colonization by specific enteropathogens. Am. J. Epidemiol. *131*:886-904, 1990.

37. Cravioto, A., Tello, A., Navarro, A., et al.: Association of *Escherichia coli* HEp-2 adherence patterns with type and duration of diarrhoea. Lancet *337*:262-264, 1991.

38. Cravioto, A., Tello, A., Villaf n, H., et al.: Inhibition of localized adhesion of enteropathogenic *Escherichia coli* to HEp-2 cells by immunoglobulin and oligosaccharide fractions of human colostrum and breast milk. J. Infect. Dis. *163*:1247-1255, 1991.

39. Currie, M. G., Fok, K. F., Kato, J., et al.: Guanylin: An endogenous activator of intestinal guanylate cyclase. Proc. Natl. Acad. Sci. U. S. A. *89*:947-951, 1992.

40. Daniels, N. A., Neimann, J., Karpati, A., et al.: Traveler's diarrhea at sea: Three outbreaks of waterborne enterotoxigenic *Escherichia coli* on cruise ships. J. Infect. Dis. *181*:1491-1495, 2000.

41. Dean-Nystrom, E. A., Gansheroff, L. J., Mills, M., et al.: Vaccination of pregnant dams with intimin(O157) protects suckling piglets from *Escherichia coli* O157:H7 infection. Infect. Immun. *70*:2414-2418, 2002.

42. DiCesare, D., DuPont, H. L., Mathewson, J. J., et al.: A double blind, randomized, placebo-controlled study of SP-303 (Provir) in the symptomatic treatment of acute diarrhea among travelers to Jamaica and Mexico. Am. J. Gastroenterol. *97*:2585-2588, 2002.

43. Donnenberg, M. S.: Enteropathogenic *Escherichia coli*. In Blaser, M. J., Smith, P. D., Ravdin, J. I., et al. (eds.): Infections of the Gastrointestinal Tract. New York, Raven Press, 1995, pp. 709-726.

44. Donnenberg, M. S., Giron, J. A., Nataro, J. P., et al.: A plasmid-encoded type IV fimbrial gene of enteropathogenic *Escherichia coli* associated with localized adherence. Mol. Microbiol. *6*:3427-3437, 1992.

45. Donnenberg, M. S., Tacket, C. O., James, S. P., et al.: Role of the *eaeA* gene in experimental enteropathogenic *Escherichia coli* infection. J. Clin. Invest. *92*:1412-1417, 1993.

46. Donnenberg, M. S., and Whittam, T. S.: Pathogenesis and evolution of virulence in enteropathogenic and enterohemorrhagic *Escherichia coli*. J. Clin. Invest. *107*:539-548, 2001.

47. DuPont, H. L., Formal, S. B., Hornick, R. B., et al.: Pathogenesis of *Escherichia coli* diarrhea. N. Engl. J. Med. *285*:1-9, 1971.

48. Echeverria, P., Sethabutr, O., Serichantalergs, O., et al.: *Shigella* and enteroinvasive *Escherichia coli* infections in households of children with dysentery in Bangkok. J. Infect. Dis. *165*:144-147, 1992.

49. Endo, Y., Tsurugi, K., Yutsudo, T., et al.: Site of action of a Vero toxin (VT2) from *Escherichia coli* O157:H7 and of Shiga toxin on eukaryotic ribosomes: RNA N-glycosidase activity of the toxins. Eur. J. Biochem. *171*(1-2):45-50, 1988.

50. Ericsson, C. D.: Travellers' diarrhoea. Int. J. Antimicrob. Agents *21*:116-124, 2003.

51. Ericsson, C. D., DuPont, H. L., Mathewson, J. J., et al.: Treatment of traveler's diarrhea with sulfamethoxazole and trimethoprim and loperamide. J. A. M. A. *263*:257-261, 1990.

52. Eslava, C., Navarro-Garcia, F., Czeczulin, J. R., et al.: Pet, an autotransporter enterotoxin from enteroaggregative *Escherichia coli*. Infect. Immun. *66*:3155-3163, 1998.

53. Essers, B., Burnens, A. P., Lanfranchini, F. M., et al.: Acute community-acquired diarrhea requiring hospital admission in Swiss children. Clin. Infect. Dis. *31*:192-196, 2000.

54. Faruque, A. S., Malek, M. A., Khan, A. I., et al.: Diarrhoea in elderly people: Aetiology, and clinical characteristics. Scand. J. Infect. Dis. *36*:204-208, 2004.

55. Fasano, A., Kay, B. A., Russell, R. G., et al.: Enterotoxin and cytotoxin production by enteroinvasive *Escherichia coli*. Infect. Immun. *58*:3717-3723, 1990.

56. Fasano, A., Noriega, F. R., Liao, F. M., et al.: Effect of shigella enterotoxin 1 (ShET1) on rabbit intestine in vitro and in vivo. Gut *40*:505-511, 1997.

57. Field, M., Graf, L. H., Jr., Laird, W. J., et al.: Heat-stable enterotoxin of *Escherichia coli*: In vitro effects on guanylate cyclase activity, cyclic GMP concentration, and ion transport in small intestine. Proc. Natl. Acad. Sci. U. S. A. *75*:2800-2804, 1978.

58. Fraser, M. E., Fujinaga, M., Cherney, M. M., et al.: Structure of shiga toxin type 2 (Stx2) from *Escherichia coli* O157:H7. J. Biol. Chem. *279*:27511-27517, 2004.

59. Friedrich, A. W., Bielaszewska, M., Zhang, W. L., et al.: *Escherichia coli* harboring Shiga toxin 2 gene variants: Frequency and association with clinical symptoms. J. Infect. Dis. *185*:74-84, 2002.

60. Gaastra, W., and Svennerholm, A.-M.: Colonization factors of human enterotoxigenic *Escherichia coli* (ETEC). Trends Microbiol. *4*:444-452, 1996.

61. Garg, A. X., Suri, R. S., Barrowman, N., et al.: Long-term renal prognosis of diarrhea-associated hemolytic uremic syndrome: A systematic review, meta-analysis, and meta-regression. J. A. M. A. *290*:1360-1370, 2003.

62. Gill, D. M., Clements, J. D., Robertson, D. C., et al.: Subunit number and arrangement in *Escherichia coli* heat-labile enterotoxin. Infect. Immun. *33*:677-682, 1981.

63. Gill, D. M., and Richardson, S. H.: Adenosine diphosphate-ribosylation of adenylate cyclase catalyzed by heat-labile enterotoxin of *Escherichia coli*: Comparison with cholera toxin. J. Infect. Dis. *141*:64-70, 1980.

64. Girard, M. P., Steele, D., Chaignat, C. L., et al.: A review of vaccine research and development: Human enteric infections. Vaccine *24*:2732-2750, 2006.

65. Gomes, T. A., Rassi, V., MacDonald, K. L., et al.: Enteropathogens associated with acute diarrheal disease in urban infants in Sao Paulo, Brazil. J. Infect. Dis. *164*:331-337, 1991.

66. Gordillo, M. E., Reeve, G. R., Pappas, J., et al.: Molecular characterization of strains of enteroinvasive *Escherichia coli* O143, including isolates from a large outbreak in Houston, Texas. J. Clin. Microbiol. *30*:889-893, 1992.

67. Griffin, P. M.: *Escherichia coli* O157:H7 and other enterohemorrhagic *Escherichia coli*. In Blaser, M. J., Smith, P. D., Ravdin, J. I., et al. (eds.): Infections of the Gastrointestinal Tract. New York, Raven Press, 1995, pp. 739-761.

68. Griffin, P. M., and Tauxe, R. V.: The epidemiology of infections caused by *Escherichia coli* O157:H7, other enterohemorrhagic *E. coli*, and the associated hemolytic uremic syndrome. Epidemiol. Rev. *13*:60-98, 1991.

69. Guandalini, S., Rao, M. C., Smith, P. L., et al.: cGMP modulation of ileal ion transport: In vitro effects of *Escherichia coli* heat-stable enterotoxin. Am. J. Physiol. *243*:G36-G41, 1982.

70. Guerrant, R. L., Van Gilder, T., Steiner, T. S., et al.: Practice guidelines for the management of infectious diarrhea. Clin. Infect. Dis. *32*:331-351, 2001.

71. Gyles, C. L., and Barnum, D. A.: A heat-labile enterotoxin from strains of *Escherichia coli* enteropathogenic for pigs. J. Infect. Dis. *120*:419-426, 1969.

72. Harada, T., Hiroi, M., Kawamori, F., et al.: A food poisoning diarrhea outbreak caused by enteroaggregative *Escherichia coli* serogroup O126:H27 in Shizuoka, Japan. Jpn. J. Infect. Dis. *60*(2-3):154-155, 2007.

73. Harrington, S. M., Dudley, E. G., and Nataro, J. P.: Pathogenesis of enteroaggregative *Escherichia coli* infection. F. E. M. S. Microbiol. Lett. *254*:12-18, 2006.

74. Hayashi, T., Makino, K., Ohnishi, M., et al.: Complete genome sequence of enterohemorrhagic *Escherichia coli* O157:H7 and genomic comparison with a laboratory strain K-12. DNA Res. *8*:11-22, 2001.

75. Henderson, I. R., Hicks, S., Navarro-Garcia, F., et al.: Involvement of the enteroaggregative *Escherichia coli* plasmid-encoded toxin in causing human intestinal damage. Infect. Immun. *67*:5338-5344, 1999.

76. Hicks, S., Candy, D. C., and Phillips, A. D.: Adhesion of enteroaggregative *Escherichia coli* to pediatric intestinal mucosa in vitro. Infect. Immun. *64*:4751-4760, 1996.

77. Hofmann, S. L.: Southwestern Internal Medicine Conference: Shiga-like toxins in hemolytic-uremic syndrome and thrombotic thrombocytopenic purpura. Am. J. Med. Sci. *306*:398-406, 1993.

78. Hromockyj, A. E., and Maurelli, A. T.: Identification of an *Escherichia coli* gene homologous to virR, a regulator of *Shigella* virulence. J. Bacteriol. *171*:2879-2881, 1989.

79. Huang, D. B., Nataro, J. P., DuPont, H. L., et al.: Enteroaggregative *Escherichia coli* is a cause of acute diarrheal illness: A meta-analysis. Clin. Infect. Dis. *43*:556-563, 2006.

80. Hunt, C. M., Harvey, J. A., Youngs, E. R., et al.: Clinical and pathological variability of infection by enterohaemorrhagic (Vero cytotoxin producing) *Escherichia coli*. J. Clin. Pathol. *42*:847-852, 1989.

81. Ikeda, K., Ida, O., Kimoto, K., et al.: Effect of early fosfomycin treatment on prevention of hemolytic uremic syndrome accompanying *Escherichia coli* O157:H7 infection. Clin. Nephrol. *52*:357-362, 1999.

82. Itoh, Y., Nagano, I., Kunishima, M., et al.: Laboratory investigation of enteroaggregative *Escherichia coli* O untypeable:H10 associated with a massive outbreak of gastrointestinal illness. J. Clin. Microbiol. *35*:2546-2550, 1997.

83. Jerse, A. E., Martin, W. C., Galen, J. E., et al.: Oligonucleotide probe for detection of the enteropathogenic *Escherichia coli* (EPEC) adherence factor of localized adherent EPEC. J. Clin. Microbiol. *28*:2842-2844, 1990.

84. Jiang, Z. D., Lowe, B., Verenkar, M. P., et al.: Prevalence of enteric pathogens among international travelers with diarrhea acquired in Kenya (Mombasa), India (Goa), or Jamaica (Montego Bay). J. Infect. Dis. *185*:497-502, 2002.

85. Johnson, K. E., Thorpe, C. M., and Sears, C. L.: The emerging clinical importance of non-O157 Shiga toxin-producing *Escherichia coli*. Clin. Infect. Dis. *43*:1587-1595, 2006.

86. Karch, H., Strockbine, N., and O'Brien, A. D.: Growth of *Escherichia coli* in the presence of trimethoprim-sulfamethoxazole facilitates detection of Shiga-like toxin producing strains by colony blot assay. F. E. M. S. Microbiol. Lett. *35*(2-3):141-145, 1986.

87. Karmali, M. A., Petric, M., Lim, C., et al.: The association between idiopathic hemolytic uremic syndrome and infection by verotoxin-producing *Escherichia coli*. J. Infect. Dis. *151*:775-782, 1985.

88. Kavi, J., and Wise, R.: Causes of the haemolytic uraemic syndrome. B. M. J. *298*:65-96, 1989.

89. Kehl, S. C.: Role of the laboratory in the diagnosis of enterohemorrhagic *Escherichia coli* infections. J. Clin. Microbiol. *40*:2711-2715, 2002.

90. Khaitan, A., Jandhyala, D. M., Thorpe, C. M., et al.: The operon encoding SubAB, a novel cytotoxin, is present in shiga toxin-producing *Escherichia coli* isolates from the United States. J. Clin. Microbiol. *45*:1374-1375, 2007.

91. Knutton, S., Baldwin, T., Williams, P. H., et al.: Actin accumulation at sites of bacterial adhesion to tissue culture cells: Basis of a new diagnostic test for enteropathogenic and enterohemorrhagic *Escherichia coli*. Infect. Immun. *57*:1290-1298, 1989.

92. Knutton, S., Shaw, R. K., Anantha, R. P., et al.: The type IV bundle-forming pilus of enteropathogenic *Escherichia coli* undergoes dramatic alterations in structure associated with bacterial adherence, aggregation and dispersal. Mol. Microbiol. *33*:499-509, 1999.

93. Konowalchuk, J., Speirs, J. I., and Stavric, S.: Vero response to a cytotoxin of *Escherichia coli*. Infect. Immun. *18*:775-779, 1977.

94. LeBlanc, J. J.: Implication of virulence factors in *Escherichia coli* O157:H7 pathogenesis. Crit. Rev. Microbiol. *29*:277-296, 2003.

95. Levine, M. M.: *Escherichia coli* infections. N. Engl. J. Med. *313*:445-447, 1985.

96. Levine, M. M.: Enteric infections and the vaccines to counter them: Future directions. Vaccine *24*:3865-3873, 2006.

97. Levine, M. M., and Edelman, R.: Enteropathogenic *Escherichia coli* of classic serotypes associated with infant diarrhea: Epidemiology and pathogenesis. Epidemiol. Rev. *6*:31-51, 1984.

98. Levine, M. M., Xu, J, G., Kaper, J. B., et al.: A DNA probe to identify enterohemorrhagic *Escherichia coli* of O157:H7 and other serotypes that cause hemorrhagic colitis and hemolytic uremic syndrome. J. Infect. Dis. *156*:175-182, 1987.

99. Lopez, E. L., Diaz, M., Grinstein, S., et al.: Hemolytic uremic syndrome and diarrhea in Argentine children: The role of Shiga-like toxins. J. Infect. Dis. *160*:469-475, 1989.

100. Marier, R., Wells, J. G., Swanson, R. C., et al.: An outbreak of enteropathogenic *Escherichia coli* foodborne disease traced to imported French cheese. Lancet *2*:1376-1378, 1973.

101. Martin, D. L., MacDonald, K. L., White, K. E., et al.: The epidemiology and clinical aspects of the hemolytic uremic syndrome in Minnesota. N. Engl. J. Med. *323*:1161-1167, 1990.

102. Martin-Sosa, S., Martin, M. J., and Hueso, P.: The sialylated fraction of milk oligosaccharides is partially responsible for binding to enterotoxigenic and uropathogenic *Escherichia coli* human strains. J. Nutr. *132*:3067-3072, 2002.

103. Mehlman, I. J., Fishbein, M., Gorbach, S. L., et al.: Pathogenicity of *Escherichia coli* recovered from food. J. Assoc. Off. Anal. Chem. *59*:67-80, 1976.

104. Merson, M. H., Morris, G. K., Sack, D. A., et al.: Travelers' diarrhea in Mexico: A prospective study of physicians and family members attending a congress. N. Engl. J. Med. *294*:1299-1305, 1976.

105. Mezoff, A. G., Giannella, R. A., Eade, M. N., et al.: *Escherichia coli* enterotoxin (STa) binds to receptors, stimulates guanyl cyclase, and impairs absorption in rat colon. Gastroenterology *102*:816-822, 1992.

106. Moake, J. L.: Haemolytic-uraemic syndrome: Basic science. Lancet *343*:393-397, 1994.

107. Nalin, D. R., McLaughlin, J. C., Rahaman, M., et al.: Enteropathogenic *Escherichia coli* and idiopathic diarrhoea in Bangladesh. Lancet *2*:1116-1119, 1975.

108. Nataro, J., Yikang, D., Cookson, S., et al.: Heterogeneity of enteroaggregative *Escherichia coli* virulence demonstrated in volunteers. J. Infect. Dis. *171*:465-468, 1995.

109. Nataro, J. P.: Atypical enteropathogenic *Escherichia coli*: Typical pathogens? Emerg. Infect. Dis. *12*:696, 2006.

110. Nataro, J. P., Bopp, C. A., Fields, P. I., et al.: *Escherichia, Shigella*, and *Salmonella*. In Murray, P. R., Baron, E. J., Jorgenson, J. H., et al. (eds.): *Manual of Clinical Microbiology*. Washington, D.C., American Society for Microbiology, 2007, pp. 670-687.

111. Nataro, J. P., and Kaper, J. B.: Diarrheagenic *Escherichia coli*. Clin. Microbiol. Rev. *11*:142-201, 1998.

112. Nataro, J. P., Kaper, J. B., Robins Browne, R., et al.: Patterns of adherence of diarrheagenic *Escherichia coli* to HEp-2 cells. Pediatr. Infect. Dis. J. *6*:829-831, 1987.

113. Nataro, J. P., Mai, V., Johnson, J., et al.: Diarrheagenic *Escherichia coli* infection in Baltimore, Maryland, and New Haven, Connecticut. Clin. Infect. Dis. *43*:402-407, 2006.

114. Nataro, J. P., Seriwatana, J., Fasano, A., et al.: Identification and cloning of a novel plasmid-encoded enterotoxin of enteroinvasive *Escherichia coli* and *Shigella* strains. Infect. Immun. *63*:4721-4728, 1995.

115. Nelson, J. D.: Duration of neomycin for enteropathogenic *Escherichia coli* diarrheal disease: A comparative study of 113 cases. Pediatrics *48*:248-258, 1971.

116. Neter, E., Korns, R. F., and Trussel, R. E.: Association of *Escherichia coli* serogroup O111 with two hospital outbreaks of epidemic diarrhea of the newborn infant in New York State during 1947. Pediatrics *12*:377-383, 1953.

117. Nguyen, T. V., Le Van, P., Le Huy, C., et al.: Detection and characterization of diarrheagenic *Escherichia coli* from young children in Hanoi, Vietnam. J. Clin. Microbiol. *43*:755-760, 2005.

118. Oberhelman, R. A., Laborde, D., Mera, R., et al.: Colonization with enteroadherent, enterotoxigenic and enterohemorrhagic *Escherichia coli* among day-care center attendees in New Orleans, Louisiana. Pediatr. Infect. Dis. J. *17*:1159-1162, 1998.

119. Obrig, T. G., Del Vecchio, P. J., Brown, J. E., et al.: Direct cytotoxic action of Shiga toxin on human vascular endothelial cells. Infect. Immun. *56*:2373-2378, 1988.

120. Ogawa, H., Nakamura, A., and Sakazaki, R.: Pathogenic properties of "enteropathogenic" *Escherichia coli* from diarrheal children and adults. Jpn. J. Med. Sci. Biol. *21*:333-349, 1968.

121. Oldfield, E. C., 3rd, Wallace, M. R., Hyams, K. C., et al.: Endemic infectious diseases of the Middle East. Rev. Infect. Dis. *13*(Suppl. 3):S199-S217, 1991.

122. Ostroff, S. M., Kobayashi, J. M., and Lewis, J. H.: Infections with *Escherichia coli* O157:H7 in Washington State: The first year of statewide disease surveillance. J. A. M. A. *262*:355-359, 1989.

123. Ostroff, S. M., Tarr, P. I., Neill, M. A., et al.: Toxin genotypes and plasmid profiles as determinants of systemic sequelae in *Escherichia coli* O157:H7 infections. J. Infect. Dis. *160*:994-998, 1989.

124. Pai, C. H., Gordon, R., Sims, H. V., et al.: Sporadic cases of hemorrhagic colitis associated with *Escherichia coli* O157:H7: Clinical, epidemiologic, and bacteriologic features. Ann. Intern. Med. *101*:738-742, 1984.

125. Pal, T., Formal, S. B., and Hale, T. L.: Characterization of virulence marker antigen of *Shigella* spp. and enteroinvasive *Escherichia coli*. J. Clin. Microbiol. *27*:561-563, 1989.

126. Paton, A. W., Beddoe, T., Thorpe, C. M., et al.: AB5 subtilase cytotoxin inactivates the endoplasmic reticulum chaperone BiP. Nature *443*:548-552, 2006.

127. Paton, A. W., Srimanote, P., Talbot, U. M., et al.: A new family of potent AB(5) cytotoxins produced by Shiga toxigenic *Escherichia coli*. J. Exp. Med. *200*:35-46, 2004.

128. Persson, S., Olsen, K. E., Scheutz, F., et al.: A method for fast and simple detection of major diarrhoeagenic *Escherichia coli* in the routine diagnostic laboratory. Clin. Microbiol. Infect. *13*:516-524, 2007.

129. Potter, A. A., Klashinsky, S., Li, Y., et al.: Decreased shedding of *Escherichia coli* O157:H7 by cattle following vaccination with type III secreted proteins. Vaccine *22*(3-4):362-369, 2004.

130. Qadri, F., Ahmed, T., Ahmed, F., et al.: Reduced doses of oral killed enterotoxigenic *Escherichia coli* plus cholera toxin B subunit vaccine is safe and immunogenic in Bangladeshi infants 6-17 months of age: Dosing studies in different age groups. Vaccine *24*:1726-1733, 2006.

131. Qadri, F., Das, S. K., Faruque, A. S., et al.: Prevalence of toxin types and colonization factors in enterotoxigenic *Escherichia coli* isolated during a 2-year period from diarrheal patients in Bangladesh. J. Clin. Microbiol. *38*:27-31, 2000.

132. Qadri, F., Svennerholm, A. M., Faruque, A. S., et al.: Enterotoxigenic *Escherichia coli* in developing countries: Epidemiology, microbiology, clinical features, treatment, and prevention. Clin. Microbiol. Rev. *18*:465-483, 2005.

133. Rangel, J. M., Sparling, P. H., Crowe, C., et al.: Epidemiology of *Escherichia coli* O157:H7 outbreaks, United States, 1982-2002. Emerg. Infect. Dis. *11*:603-609, 2005.

134. Rao, M. R., Abu-Elyazeed, R., Savarino, S. J., et al.: High disease burden of diarrhea due to enterotoxigenic *Escherichia coli* among rural Egyptian infants and young children. J. Clin. Microbiol. *41*:4862-4864, 2003.

135. Rao, M. R., Wierzba, T. F., Savarino, S. J., et al.: Serologic correlates of protection against enterotoxigenic *Escherichia coli* diarrhea. J. Infect. Dis. *191*:562-570, 2005.

136. Rasheed, J. K., Guzman-Verduzco, L. M., and Kupersztoch, Y. M.: Two precursors of the heat-stable enterotoxin of *Escherichia coli*: Evidence of extracellular processing. Mol. Microbiol. *4*:265-273, 1990.

137. Rendi-Wagner, P., and Kollaritsch, H.: Drug prophylaxis for travelers' diarrhea. Clin. Infect. Dis. *34*:628-633, 2002.

138. Riley, L. W.: The epidemiologic, clinical, and microbiologic features of hemorrhagic colitis. Annu. Rev. Microbiol. *41*:383-407, 1987.

139. Riley, L. W., Remis, R. S., Helgerson, S. D., et al.: Hemorrhagic colitis associated with a rare *Escherichia coli* serotype. N. Engl. J. Med. *308*:681-685, 1983.

140. Robins-Browne, R. M., Still, C. S., Miliotis, M. D., et al.: Summer diarrhoea in African infants and children. Arch. Dis. Child. *55*:923-928, 1980.

141. Robson, W. L., Fick, G. H., Jadavji, T., et al.: The use of intravenous gammaglobulin in the treatment of typical hemolytic uremic syndrome. Pediatr. Nephrol. *5*:289-292, 1991.

142. Rogers, M. F., Rutherford, G. W., Alexander, S. R., et al.: A population-based study of hemolytic-uremic syndrome in Oregon, 1979-1982. Am. J. Epidemiol. *123*:137-142, 1986.

143. Rosenberg, M. L., Koplan, J. P., Wachsmuth, I. K., et al.: Epidemic diarrhea at Crater Lake from enterotoxigenic *Escherichia coli*: A large waterborne outbreak. Ann. Intern. Med. *86*:714-718, 1977.

144. Rothbaum, R., McAdams, A. J., Giannella, R., et al.: A clinicopathological study of enterocyte-adherent *Escherichia coli*: A cause of protracted diarrhea in infants. Gastroenterology *83*:441-454, 1982.

145. Sack, R. B., Sack, D. A., Mehlman, I. J., et al.: Enterotoxigenic *Escherichia coli* isolated from food. J. Infect. Dis. *135*:313-317, 1977.

146. Safdar, N., Said, A., Gangnon, R. E., et al.: Risk of hemolytic uremic syndrome after antibiotic treatment of *Escherichia coli* O157:H7 enteritis: A meta-analysis. J. A. M. A. *288*:996-1001, 2002.

147. Sakazaki, R., Tamura, K., and Saito, M.: Enteropathogenic *Escherichia coli* associated with diarrhea in children and adults. Jpn. J. Med. Sci. Biol. *20*:387-399, 1967.

148. Salmanzadeh-Ahrabi, S., Habibi, E., Jaafari, F., et al.: Molecular epidemiology of *Escherichia coli* diarrhoea in children in Tehran. Ann. Trop. Paediatr. *25*:35-39, 2005.

149. Sansonetti, P. J.: Genetic and molecular basis of epithelial cell invasion by *Shigella* species. Rev. Infect. Dis. *13*(Suppl. 4):S285-S292, 1991.

150. Sarantuya, J., Nishi, J., Wakimoto, N., et al.: Typical enteroaggregative *Escherichia coli* is the most prevalent pathotype among *E. coli* strains causing diarrhea in Mongolian children. J. Clin. Microbiol. *42*:133-139, 2004.

151. Savarino, S. J., Fasano, A., Robertson, D. C., et al.: Enteroaggregative *Escherichia coli* elaborate a heat-stable enterotoxin demonstrable in an in vitro rabbit intestinal model. J. Clin. Invest. *87*:1450-1455, 1991.

152. Schultsz, C., Ende, J. V. D., Cobelens, F., et al.: Diarrheagenic *Escherichia coli* and acute and persistent diarrhea in returned travelers. J. Clin. Microbiol. *38*:3550-3554, 2000.

153. Schulz, S., Green, C. K., Yuen, P. S., et al.: Guanylyl cyclase is a heat-stable enterotoxin receptor. Cell *63*:941-948, 1990.

154. Sears, C. L., and Kaper, J. B.: Enteric bacterial toxins: Mechanisms of action and linkage to intestinal secretion. Microbiol. Rev. *60*:167-215, 1996.

155. Seto, E. Y., Soller, J. A., and Colford, J. M., Jr.: Strategies to reduce person-to-person transmission during widespread *Escherichia coli* O157:H7 outbreak. Emerg. Infect. Dis. *13*:860-866, 2007.

156. Shaheen, H. I., Khalil, S. B., Rao, M. R., et al.: Phenotypic profiles of enterotoxigenic *Escherichia coli* associated with early childhood diarrhea in rural Egypt. J. Clin. Microbiol. *42*:5588-5595, 2004.

157. Shazberg, G., Wolk, M., Schmidt, H., et al.: Enteroaggregative *Escherichia coli* serotype O126:H27, Israel. Emerg. Infect. Dis. *9*:1170-1173, 2003.

158. Shigeno, T., Akamatsu, T., Fujimori, K., et al.: The clinical significance of colonoscopy in hemorrhagic colitis due to enterohemorrhagic *Escherichia coli* O157:H7 infection. Endoscopy *34*:311-314, 2002.

159. Smith, H. W., and Linggood, M. A.: Observations on the pathogenic properties of the K88, Hly and Ent plasmids of *Escherichia coli* with particular reference to porcine diarrhoea. J. Med. Microbiol. *4*:467-485, 1971.

160. Snyder, J. D., Wells, J. G., Yashuk, J., et al.: Outbreak of invasive *Escherichia coli* gastroenteritis on a cruise ship. Am. J. Trop. Med. Hyg. *33*:281-284, 1984.

161. So, M., and McCarthy, B. J.: Nucleotide sequence of the bacterial transposon Tn1681 encoding a heat-stable (ST) toxin and its identification in enterotoxigenic *Escherichia coli* strains. Proc. Natl. Acad. Sci. U. S. A. *77*:4011-4015, 1980.

162. Steinsland, H., Valentiner-Branth, P., Gjessing, H. K., et al.: Protection from natural infections with enterotoxigenic *Escherichia coli*: Longitudinal study. Lancet *362*:286-291, 2003.

163. Streatfield, S. J., Sandkvist, M., Sixma, T. K., et al.: Intermolecular interactions between the A and B subunits of heat-labile enterotoxin from *Escherichia coli* promote holotoxin assembly and stability in vivo. Proc. Natl. Acad. Sci. U. S. A. *89*:12140-12144, 1992.

164. Tacket, C. O., Losonsky, G., Livio, S., et al.: Lack of prophylactic efficacy of an enteric-coated bovine hyperimmune milk product against enterotoxigenic *Escherichia coli* challenge administered during a standard meal. J. Infect. Dis. *180*:2056-2059, 1999.

165. Tarr, P. I., Gordon, C. A., and Chandler, W. L.: Shiga-toxin-producing *Escherichia coli* and haemolytic uraemic syndrome. Lancet *365*:1073-1086, 2005.

166. Tarr, P. I., Neill, M. A., Clausen, C. R., et al.: *Escherichia coli* O157:H7 and the hemolytic uremic syndrome: Importance of early cultures in establishing the etiology. J. Infect. Dis. *162*:553-556, 1990.

167. Taylor, D. N., Sanchez, J., Candler, W., et al.: Treatment of travelers' diarrhea: Ciprofloxacin plus loperamide compared with ciprofloxacin alone: A placebo-controlled, randomized trial. Ann. Intern. Med. *114*:731-734, 1991.

168. Teneberg, S., Hirst, T. R., Angstrom, J., et al.: Comparison of the glycolipid-binding specificities of cholera toxin and porcine *Escherichia coli* heat-labile enterotoxin: Identification of a receptor-active non-ganglioside glycolipid for the heat-labile toxin in infant rabbit small intestine. Glycoconj. J. *11*:533-540, 1994.

169. Thoren, A., Stintzing, G., Tufvesson, B., et al.: Aetiology and clinical features of severe infantile diarrhoea in Addis Ababa, Ethiopia. J. Trop. Pediatr. *28*:127-131, 1982.

170. Toledo, M. R., Alvariza Mdo, C., Murahovschi, J., et al.: Enteropathogenic *Escherichia coli* serotypes and endemic diarrhea in infants. Infect. Immun. *39*:586-589, 1983.

171. Trabulsi, L. R., Fernandes, M. R., and Zuliani, M. E.: Novas bacterias patogenicas para o intestino do homen. Rev. Inst. Med. Trop. Sao Paulo *9*:31-39, 1967.

172. Trachtman, H., and Christen, E.: Pathogenesis, treatment, and therapeutic trials in hemolytic uremic syndrome. Curr. Opin. Pediatr. *11*:162-168, 1999.

173. Trachtman, H., Cnaan, A., Christen, E., et al.: Effect of an oral Shiga toxin-binding agent on diarrhea-associated hemolytic uremic syndrome in children: A randomized controlled trial. J. A. M. A. *290*:1337-1344, 2003.

174. Tulloch, E. F., Jr., Ryan, K. J., Formal, S. B., et al.: Invasive enteropathic *Escherichia coli* dysentery: An outbreak in 28 adults. Ann. Intern. Med. *79*:13-17, 1973.

175. Tzipori, S., Sheoran, A., Akiyoshi, D., et al.: Antibody therapy in the management of shiga toxin-induced hemolytic uremic syndrome. Clin. Microbiol. Rev. *17*:926-941, 2004.

176. Vila, J., Vargas, M., Casals, C., et al.: Antimicrobial resistance of diarrheagenic *Escherichia coli* isolated from children under the age of 5 years from Ifakara, Tanzania. Antimicrob. Agents Chemother. *43*:3022-3024, 1999.

177. von Baeyer, H.: Plasmapheresis in thrombotic microangiopathy-associated syndromes: Review of outcome data derived from clinical trials and open studies. Ther. Apher. *6*:320-328, 2002.

178. Wagner, P. L., Acheson, D. W., and Waldor, M. K.: Human neutrophils and their products induce Shiga toxin production by enterohemorrhagic *Escherichia coli*. Infect. Immun. *69*:1934-1937, 2001.

179. Wickham, M. E., Lupp, C., Mascarenhas, M., et al.: Bacterial genetic determinants of non-O157 STEC outbreaks and hemolytic-uremic syndrome after infection. J. Infect. Dis. *194*:819-827, 2006.

180. Wolf, M. K.: Occurrence, distribution, and associations of O and H serogroups, colonization factor antigens, and toxins of enterotoxigenic *Escherichia coli*. Clin. Microbiol. Rev. *10*:569-584, 1997.

181. Wong, C. S., Jelacic, S., Habeeb, R. L., et al.: The risk of the hemolytic-uremic syndrome after antibiotic treatment of *Escherichia coli* O157:H7 infections. N. Engl. J. Med. *342*:1930-1936, 2000.

182. Yatsuyanagi, J., Saito, S., Miyajima, Y., et al.: Characterization of atypical enteropathogenic *Escherichia coli* strains harboring the astA gene that were associated with a waterborne outbreak of diarrhea in Japan. J. Clin. Microbiol. *41*:2033-2039, 2003.

183. Yatsuyanagi, J., Saito, S., Sato, H., et al.: Characterization of enteropathogenic and enteroaggregative *Escherichia coli* isolated from diarrheal outbreaks. J. Clin. Microbiol. *40*:294-297, 2002.

184. Yoshimura, S., Ikemura, H., Watanabe, H., et al.: Essential structure for full enterotoxigenic activity of heat-stable enterotoxin produced by enterotoxigenic *Escherichia coli*. F. E. B. S. Lett. *181*:138-142, 1985.

KLEBSIELLA

Randall G. Fisher

Klebsiella is a genus of Enterobacteriaceae, a frequent cause of nosocomial pediatric infection. Classically described by Friedländer[38] as a cause of pneumonia, *Klebsiella* can cause infections of the urinary tract, lung, and central venous catheters in high-risk newborns and immunocompromised older children.[18]

BACTERIOLOGY

Klebsiella organisms were named for Edwin Klebs, the noted German bacteriologist.[86] Distinguishing features of *Klebsiella* spp. include the absence of motility and the presence of a polysaccharide capsule that gives rise to large mucoid colonies on solid media. The organisms are oxidase-negative and citrate-positive; they ferment inositol and hydrolyze urea but do not produce ornithine decarboxylase or hydrogen sulfide. Acetoin and 2,3-butanediol predominate over acidic end-products during sugar fermentation (positive result on the Voges-Proskauer test). Four species of *Klebsiella* commonly are agreed on by microbiologists: *Klebsiella pneumoniae* (the most common human pathogen), *Klebsiella oxytoca* (a less common human pathogen), *Klebsiella terrigena*, and *Klebsiella planticola*. Previously, *K. planticola* was recovered almost exclusively from soil and aquatic environments; reports now suggest that this organism may be a relatively common neonatal pathogen in some parts of the world.[92,113] *K. planticola* may express virulence factors similar to those of *K. pneumoniae*.[93] Organisms are defined serologically by their capsular polysaccharide (K antigens) and lipopolysaccharide (O antigens). Significant cross-reactivity exists between the capsule of some pneumococci (e.g., 19F) and *Klebsiella*.[68] The reader is referred to a review by Podschun and Ullman[95] for a detailed description of *Klebsiella* spp.

EPIDEMIOLOGY

Friedländer[38] proposed that *K. pneumoniae* was the most common cause of community-acquired pneumonia, an observation that was refuted by Fraenkel's[36] observations on pneumococcal pneumonia. *K. pneumoniae* accounts for less than 10 percent of hospitalized cases of pneumonia in adults.[20] *Klebsiella* spp. now are in greatest evidence as opportunistic nosocomial pathogens of the urinary tract, respiratory tract, biliary tract, and bloodstream. In one survey of the Centers for Disease Control and Prevention, the infection rate of nosocomial *K. pneumoniae* was 16.7 infections per 10,000 patients discharged.[54] Hand-carriage generally is regarded as the common mode of transmission.[42] Environmental sources of *Klebsiella* spp. include contaminated blood-pressure monitoring equipment,[98] ventilator traps,[42] dialysate,[64] ultrasound coupling gel,[40] dextrose solution,[66] and hand disinfectant.[101] The emergence of plasmid-mediated, β-lactamase resistance can be responsible for the rapid spread of resistant organisms to susceptible patients in intensive care units (ICUs).[10,12] Outbreaks may be complex; patient-to-patient transmission of epidemic strains containing different plasmids may be interspersed with sporadic, nonepidemic *Klebsiella* infections.[12] *Klebsiella* spp. are second only to *Escherichia coli* as causes of sepsis,[41] with the highest rates of infection being reported from larger hospitals affiliated with medical schools.

Klebsiella spp. commonly are highlighted as pathogens of debilitated adults and alcoholics,[60] but by 1985, nearly 50 percent of reported outbreaks of *Klebsiella* were in neonatal ICUs.[54] Outbreaks in newborns continue to occur frequently worldwide.[2,7,24,30,49,90,100] Most outbreaks in newborns have been associated with *K. pneumoniae* infection, but scattered outbreaks of *K. oxytoca* infection in nurseries also have been reported.[6,112] A high percentage of infants in ICUs may become colonized with hospital strains of *Klebsiella*.[46] In one longitudinal study in which weekly rectal swabs were cultured, 80 (22%) of 368 neonates in an ICU harbored extended-spectrum β-lactamase (ESBL)–producing *Klebsiella* spp.[15] Infecting organisms have been isolated from care providers and from mothers of colonized infants.[24] One report described an outbreak among newborns associated with infestation of a neonatal unit by cockroaches colonized with infecting *Klebsiella* strains.[25] *Klebsiella* may spread from newborn units to adult units; interhospital and international spread of resistant strains has been described.[23,30,106]

Ribotyping, pulsed field gel electrophoresis, and DNA amplification techniques have proven valuable in characterizing *Klebsiella* strains associated with outbreaks.[70,108] Different ribotypes that share plasmids conferring antibiotic resistance can be responsible for pediatric infections in a particular institution.[12] Strains expressing ESBL may become endemic and may present a complex and diverse pattern of production of enzymes with resistance to β-lactamase inhibitors.[31,35] Although broad-spectrum resistance to β-lactams and carbapenems[72] has been described, some longitudinal studies have shown that the frequency of ESBLs in *K. pneumoniae* isolates is decreasing.[103]

PATHOPHYSIOLOGY

Pneumonias caused by *Klebsiella* most commonly arise from colonization of the upper respiratory tract, followed by aspiration of organisms to the lower respiratory tract. Some degree of gram-negative oropharyngeal colonization is a normal finding in newborns. The oropharynx of nearly one third of healthy newborns is colonized by gram-negative rods, including *Klebsiella*, by the time infants reach 1 month of age; colonization rates generally are lower in breast-fed infants.[9] Antibiotic pressure in high-risk newborns and older children has been observed to promote overgrowth of *Klebsiella*.[11,105] Enteric organisms are recovered less frequently from the oropharynx of healthy older children and adults; oral colonization with gram-negative rods is increased during illness,[57] after postoperative viral infections,[56,97] and in debilitated adults.[73] Increased adherence of gram-negative rods to oropharyngeal cells contributes to increased colonization.[56] Elastase made by polymorphonuclear cells contributes to such colonization by reducing the fibronectin coating of sugar receptors.[27] The capsule plays an initial role in interactions of epithelial cells but is not required for an adhesin interaction with the cell surface.[34] Adherence properties may be affected by plasmid content[29] and may be transferred between *E. coli* and *K. pneumoniae*.[53]

In animal models of sepsis, capsular polysaccharide (K antigens) is a virulence factor; monoclonal antibodies to the K antigens reduce the severity of illness in mice.[67] In a mouse model of urinary tract infection, the K antigens seemed to be more important in infection than was the lipopolysaccharide (O antigens), and clinical strains deficient in lipopolysaccharide retained virulence by resistance of capsule to complement.[3,19] In one series of adult patients, capsular type K2 frequently was associated with asymptomatic bacteriuria and cystitis, but not pyelonephritis; the presence of type 1 fimbriae bore a closer relationship to upper urinary tract infection.[94] In a retrospective study, patients bacteremic with hyperviscous strains were more likely to develop invasive localized disease, such as liver abscess, meningitis, pleural empyema, or endophthalmitis.[69] Neutrophils play an important role in clearance of *Klebsiella*, and phagocytosis is augmented by leukotrienes.[74]

CLINICAL MANIFESTATIONS

Klebsiella infection shows little clinical distinction from diseases produced by other enteric pathogens. The organism generally is less common than is group B streptococcus or *E. coli* as a cause of "early-onset" or "late-onset" infection in newborns.[43,77] Investigators from Spain,[49] however, reported one 7-year interval in which *K. pneumoniae* was the most common cause of bacteremia in newborns. Risk factors for neonatal *Klebsiella* infection include prematurity, presence of indwelling catheters, previous antibiotic treatment, and parenteral nutrition.[100] Infection in newborns is characterized by typical features of pneumonia, sepsis, and meningitis.[77] In one unusual case, *K. pneumoniae* bacteremia manifested on day 4 of life as a morbilliform maculopapular exanthem, more severe on the face. The infant was afebrile, but the mother had had fever in the peripartum period, and the amniotic fluid had been meconium stained.[21]

Although hepatic abscesses have been associated principally with adults with poorly controlled diabetes mellitus, one case report described a 32-week-gestation neonate with *K. pneumoniae* sepsis who developed a liver abscess large enough to be noted on physical examination as an abdominal "lump."[110] In adults, hepatic abscess occasionally is complicated by endophthalmitis or central nervous system infection, with devastating outcomes. A study from Taiwan found that infection with genotype K1 was the only significant risk factor for these complications.[33] This series also revealed that 8 (42%) of the 19 complicated K1 strain infections occurred in patients without identifiable underlying medical disease.[33] Other investigators have emphasized that serotype K2 also can be virulent in patients with liver abscess.[39] Careful study of the pathophysiology and epidemiology of complicated *K. pneumoniae* liver abscesses is ongoing, and the picture is likely to continue to be clarified.

Klebsiella spp. have been isolated commonly from blood and peritoneal fluid in outbreaks of necrotizing enterocolitis.[44,80] Less common manifestations in infants include toxic epidermal necrolysis,[47,89] conjunctivitis,[65] parotitis,[22] retropharyngeal abscess,[26] subdural hematoma,[84] psoas abscess,[4] and renal abscess.[111]

Klebsiella is an unusual cause of infection in an otherwise healthy older child. The classic Friedländer pneumonia that occurs in debilitated adults[38] is rare in children. The identification of pulmonary infection should suggest the possibility of underlying immunodeficiency or significant malnutrition, if not suspected previously.[52,58] If pneumonia caused by *Klebsiella* does occur, progression to lung abscesses should be anticipated.

Lung abscesses may develop within days to weeks after *Klebsiella* infection. Formation of abscesses occurs more frequently during *Klebsiella* pulmonary infection than during any other community-acquired infection.[20] A rare but devastating outcome is massive pulmonary gangrene, the rapid total destruction of part of the lung presumed to be due to vascular compromise. This complication is heralded by radiographs that show small cavities that later coalesce into a large cavity with an intracavitary mass of necrotic lung.[82,85] Some researchers have speculated that *Klebsiella* lung infection is accompanied by coincident anaerobic infection that contributes to or is primarily responsible for the pathology.[20]

Catheterization of the urinary tract can be associated with urinary tract *Klebsiella* infection, but bacteremia is an uncommon complication in an immunocompetent child.[28,71] Approximately 10 percent of nosocomial urinary tract infections observed in infants after surgery are caused by *Klebsiella*.[28] Focal renal infection progressing to renal abscess has been described.[63] *K. pneumoniae* bacteremia has been associated with lesions of the gastrointestinal tract, presence of an indwelling central venous catheter, and neutropenia. Patients with short-bowel syndrome seem to be at greater risk than are patients with inflammatory bowel disease or malignancy for development of catheter-associated *Klebsiella* or *Enterobacter* bacteremia. *K. pneumoniae* was a constituent of polymicrobial bacteremia in 15 such patients (26%).[14] Mortality rates have ranged from 5 to 20 percent, with higher death rates occurring in children infected with an aminoglycoside-resistant strain.[13,54] Pneumonia, shock, and disseminated intravascular coagulation are poor prognostic factors in children with underlying malignancy. Rare clinical presentations include multifocal osteomyelitis[62] and endophthalmitis.[75] Pediatric recipients of solid organ transplants may have high rates of acquisition of drug-resistant *Klebsiella*.[99] *Klebsiella* spp. have been described as a frequent pathogen in children and adults with sickle cell disease in West Africa.[1]

Of six patients with clinical and colonoscopic findings suggestive of antibiotic-associated hemorrhagic colitis (pseudomembranous enterocolitis) but negative evaluation for *Clostridium difficile*, five had stool cultures positive for *K. oxytoca*.[51] All five patients had been receiving penicillin therapy. *K. oxytoca* was cultured from only 1.6 percent of 385 healthy controls. Additionally, the disease could be reproduced in a rat model when rats were inoculated with *K. oxytoca* and administered amoxicillin-clavulanate, but disease was not seen if rats were not given the injection and the antibiotic treatment.[51]

DIAGNOSIS

Klebsiella spp. characteristically grow as large mucoid colonies on MacConkey agar. Citrate-containing media can be used to facilitate isolation of *Klebsiella* strains because these organisms can use citrate as a sole carbon source.[86] Serotyping with specific antisera usually is determined by countercurrent immunoelectrophoresis or a Quellung test.[8] In situ hybridization techniques have been used to identify *Klebsiella* in phagocytes from blood specimens,[76] and restriction-enzyme analysis and ribotyping of clinical isolates have been used to characterize nosocomial spread of antibiotic-resistant strains.[12,45] Conventional, commonly used microbiologic methods may misidentify some *Klebsiella* spp., particularly *K. planticola* and *K. terrigena*.[81] Rarely, blood cultures have required longer than 72 hours of incubation for radiometric detection of *Klebsiella*.[78]

TREATMENT

Empiric antimicrobial therapy should be guided by an understanding of antimicrobial susceptibilities of *Klebsiella* in the hospital. Therapy with a cephalosporin plus an aminoglycoside (rather than a cephalosporin alone) has been associated with a more favorable outcome in patients with cancer who are infected with susceptible strains.[13] Antimicrobial therapy of *Klebsiella* spp. is made problematic, however, by the resistance to penicillins and cephalosporins conferred by ESBL.[10,12,16,48] *Klebsiella* with ESBL are widely distributed, and regional differences in susceptibility occur.[59] Outer membrane protein changes and porin deficiencies of some strains can augment resistance to third-generation cephalosporins.[5,102] Some investigators have reported significant correlation between production of ESBL and resistance to ciprofloxacin.[88,107] Plasmid-mediated resistance to aminoglycosides also is common.[6,24,41,83] Endocarditis isolates that developed resistance to piperacillin-tazobactam and to ciprofloxacin during therapy have been reported.[114]

Effective treatment of multidrug-resistant isolates sometimes requires creativity or use of antibiotics no longer commonly employed. In one case report, a 15-year-old girl developed bacteremia with a meropenem-intermediate strain; bacteremia persisted despite thrice-daily administration of meropenem combined with gentamicin, to which the isolate was sensitive. Clearance was achieved eventually with meropenem administered as a continuous infusion.[32] In another case, bacteremia and peritonitis developed in a patient on continuous ambulatory peritoneal dialysis; infection persisted despite removal of the catheter and treatment with meropenem and amikacin (to which the isolate was intermediately resistant). Cure required a switch to intravenous polymyxin B.[87]

Antibiotic pressure is important in increasing the risk for development of resistant isolates.[96] In some nursery outbreaks, switching from gentamicin to amikacin has been associated with return of the susceptibility of *Klebsiella* isolates to gentamicin.[6,50] Imipenem or the combination of piperacillin and tazobactam may show good antimicrobial activity against multiply-resistant organisms.[55,91,96] The combination of β-lactamase and porin deficiency has been associated with resistance to imipenem,[17] and hyperproduction of some β-lactamases can limit the effectiveness of β-lactam–β-lactamase inhibitor combinations.[37] Experience with use of ciprofloxacin in young children is limited because of observations of irreversible cartilage injury in laboratory animals after administration of this quinolone. Successful treatment of a multidrug-resistant *K. pneumoniae* has been reported in a preterm infant, however, without observable short-term adverse effects.[61] Strict adherence to infection control policies that promote restricted antibiotic use, cohorting, and handwashing may help to prevent the spread of resistant *Klebsiella* strains.[6,24,46,79,104]

Acknowledgments

The author thanks Dr. William Gruber and Dr. Thomas Boyce for their invaluable assistance with earlier versions of this chapter.

REFERENCES

1. Aken'Ova, Y. A., Bakare, R. A., Okunade, M. A., and Olaniyi, J.: Bacterial causes of acute osteomyelitis in sickle cell anaemia: Changing infection profile. W. Afr. J. Med. *14*:255-258, 1995.
2. Akindele, J. A., and Gbadegesin, R. A.: Outbreak of neonatal *Klebsiella* septicaemia at the University College Hospital, Ibadan, Nigeria: Appraisal of predisposing factors and preventive measures. Trop. Geogr. Med. *46*:151-153, 1994.
3. Alvarez, D., Merino, S., Tomas, J. M., et al.: Capsular polysaccharide is a major complement resistance factor in lipopolysaccharide O side chain-deficient *Klebsiella pneumoniae* clinical isolates. Infect. Immun. *68*:953-955, 2000.
4. Andreou, A., Karasavvidou, A., Papadopoulou, F., and Koukoulidis, A.: Iliopsoas abscess in a neonate. Am. J. Perinatol. *14*:519-521, 1997.
5. Ardanuy, C., Linares, J., Dominguez, M. A., et al.: Outer membrane profiles of clonally related *Klebsiella pneumoniae* isolates from clinical samples and activities of cephalosporins and carbapenems. Antimicrob. Agents Chemother. *42*:1636-1640, 1998.
6. Aronsson, B., Eriksson, M., Herin, P., et al.: Gentamicin-resistant *Klebsiella* spp. and *Escherichia coli* in a neonatal intensive care unit. Scand. J. Infect. Dis. *23*:195-199, 1991.
7. Arredondo-Garcia, J. L., Diaz-Ramos, R., Solorzano-Santos, F., et al.: Neonatal septicaemia due to *K. pneumoniae*: Septicaemia due to *Klebsiella pneumoniae* in newborn infants: Nosocomial outbreak in an intensive care unit. Rev. Latinoam. Microbiol. *34*:11-16, 1992.
8. Ayling-Smith, B., and Pitt, T. L.: State of the art in typing: *Klebsiella* spp. J. Hosp. Infect. *16*:287-295, 1990.
9. Baltimore, R. S., Duncan, R. L., Shapiro, E. D., et al.: Epidemiology of pharyngeal colonization of infants with aerobic gram-negative rod bacteria. J. Clin. Microbiol. *27*:91-95, 1989.
10. Bauernfeind, A., Rosenthal, E., Eberlein, E., et al.: Spread of *Klebsiella pneumoniae* producing SHV-5 beta-lactamase among hospitalized patients. Infection *21*:18-22, 1993.
11. Bennet, R., Eriksson, M., Nord, C. E., et al.: Fecal bacterial microflora of newborn infants during intensive care management and treatment with five antibiotic regimens. Pediatr. Infect. Dis. *5*:533-539, 1986.
12. Bingen, E. H., Desjardins, P., Arlet, G., et al.: Molecular epidemiology of plasmid spread among extended broad-spectrum beta-lactamase-producing *Klebsiella pneumoniae* isolates in a pediatric hospital. J. Clin. Microbiol. *31*:179-184, 1993.
13. Bodey, G. P., Elting, L. S., Rodriquez, S., et al.: *Klebsiella* bacteremia: A 10-year review in a cancer institution. Cancer *64*:2368-2376, 1989.
14. Bonadio, W. A.: *Klebsiella pneumoniae* bacteremia in children: Fifty-seven cases in 10 years. Am. J. Dis. Child. *143*:1061-1063, 1989.
15. Boo, N. Y., Ng, S. F., and Lim, V. K.: A case-control study of risk factors associated with rectal colonization of extended-spectrum beta-lactamase producing *Klebsiella* sp. in newborn infants. J. Hosp. Infect. *61*:68-74, 2005.
16. Bradford, P. A., Cherubin C. E., Idemyor, V., et al.: Multiply resistant *Klebsiella pneumoniae* strains from two Chicago hospitals: Identification of the extended-spectrum TEM-12 and TEM-10 ceftazidime-hydrolyzing beta-lactamases in a single isolate. Antimicrob. Agents Chemother. *38*:761-766, 1994.
17. Bradford, P. A., Urban, C., Mariano, N., et al.: Imipenem resistance in *Klebsiella pneumoniae* is associated with the combination of ACT-1, a plasmid-mediated AmpC beta-lactamase, and the foss of an outer membrane protein. Antimicrob. Agents Chemother. *41*:563-569, 1997.
18. Brown, R. B., Cipriani, D., Schulte, M., et al.: Community-acquired bacteremias from tunneled central intravenous lines: Results from studies of a single vendor. Am. J. Infect. Control *22*:149-151, 1994.
19. Camprubi, S., Merino, S., Benedi, V. J., et al.: The role of the O-antigen lipopolysaccharide and capsule on an experimental *Klebsiella pneumoniae* infection of the rat urinary tract. FEMS Microbiol. Lett. *111*:9-13, 1993.
20. Carpenter, J. L.: *Klebsiella* pulmonary infections: Occurrence at one medical center and review. Rev. Infect. Dis. *12*:672-682, 1990.
21. Casacci, M., Carpentier, O., Truffert, P., et al.: Neonatal maculopapular exanthema revealing septicemia due to *Klebsiella pneumoniae* via maternofetal infection. Ann. Dermatol. Venereol. *133*:31-33, 2006.
22. Coban, A., Ince, Z., Ucsel, R., et al.: Neonatal suppurative parotitis: A vanishing disease? Eur. J. Pediatr. *152*:1004-1005, 1993.
23. Cookson, B., Johnson, A. P., Azadian, B., et al.: International inter- and intrahospital patient spread of a multiple antibiotic-resistant strain of *Klebsiella pneumoniae*. J. Infect. Dis. *171*:511-513, 1995.
24. Coovadia, Y. M., Johnson, A. P., Bhana, R. H., et al.: Multiresistant *Klebsiella pneumoniae* in a neonatal nursery: The importance of maintenance of infection control policies and procedures in the prevention of outbreaks. J. Hosp. Infect. *22*:197-205, 1992.
25. Cotton, M. F., Wasserman, E., Pieper, C. H., et al.: Invasive disease due to extended spectrum beta-lactamase-producing *Klebsiella pneumoniae* in a neonatal unit: The possible role of cockroaches. J. Hosp. Infect. *44*:13-17, 2000.
26. Coulthard, M., and Isaacs, D.: Retropharyngeal abscess. Arch. Dis. Child. *66*:1227-1230, 1991.
27. Dal Nogare, A. R., Toews, G. B., and Pierce, A. K.: Increased salivary elastase precedes gram-negative bacillary colonization in postoperative patients. Am. Rev. Respir. Dis. *135*:671-675, 1987.
28. Davies, H. D., Jones, E. L., Sheng, R. Y., et al.: Nosocomial urinary tract infections at a pediatric hospital. Pediatr. Infect. Dis. J. *11*:349-354, 1992.
29. Denoya, C. D., Trevisan, A. R., and Zorzopulos, J.: Adherence of multiresistant strains of *Klebsiella pneumoniae* to cerebrospinal fluid shunts: Correlation with plasmid content. J. Med. Microbiol. *21*:225-231, 1986.
30. Eisen, D., Russell, E. G., Tymms, M., et al.: Random amplified polymorphic DNA and plasmid analyses used in investigation of an outbreak of multiresistant *Klebsiella pneumoniae*. J. Clin. Microbiol. *33*:713-717, 1995.
31. Essack, S. Y., Hall, L. M., Pillay, D. G., et al.: Complexity and diversity of *Klebsiella pneumoniae* strains with extended-spectrum beta-lactamases isolated in 1994 and 1996 at a teaching hospital in Durban, South Africa. Antimicrob. Agents Chemother. *45*:88-95, 2001.
32. Falagas, M. E., Siempos, I. I., and Tsakoumis, I.: Cure of persistent, post-appendectomy *Klebsiella pneumoniae* septicemia with continuous intravenous administration of meropenem. Scand. J. Infect. Dis. *38*:807-810, 2006.
33. Fang, C. T., Lai, S. Y., Yi, W. C., et al.: *Klebsiella pneumoniae* genotype K1: An emerging pathogen that causes septic ocular or central nervous system complications from pyogenic liver abscess. Clin. Infect. Dis. *45*:284-293, 2007.
34. Favre-Bonte, S., Joly, B., and Forestier, C.: Consequences of reduction of *Klebsiella pneumoniae* capsule expression on interactions of this bacterium with epithelial cells. Infect. Immun. *67*:554-561, 1999.
35. Fiett, J., Palucha, A., Miaczynska, B., et al.: A novel complex mutant beta-lactamase, TEM-68, identified in a *Klebsiella pneumoniae* isolate from an outbreak of extended-spectrum beta-lactamase-producing klebsiellae. Antimicrob. Agents Chemother. *44*:1499-1505, 2000.
36. Fraenkel, A.: Bakteriologische mitteilungen. Leitsch. F. Klin. Med. *10*:401-411, 1886.
37. French, G. L., Shannon, K. P., and Simmons, N.: Hospital outbreak of *Klebsiella pneumoniae* resistant to broad-spectrum cephalosporins and beta-lactam-beta-lactamase inhibitor combinations by hyperproduction of SHV-5 beta-lactamase. J. Clin. Microbiol. *34*:358-363, 1996.

38. Friedländer, C.: Über die schizomyceten bei der acuten fibrosen pneumonie. Arch. Pathol. Anat. Physiol. Klin. Med. *87*:319-324, 1882.

39. Fung, C. P., and Siu, L. K.: Virulence of *Klebsiella pneumoniae* serotype K2 should not be underestimated in *K. pneumoniae* liver abscess. Clin. Infect. Dis. *45*:1530-1531, 2007.

40. Gaillot, O., Maruejouls, C., Abachin, E., et al.: Nosocomial outbreak of *Klebsiella pneumoniae* producing SHV-5 extended-spectrum beta-lactamase, originating from a contaminated ultrasonography coupling gel. J. Clin. Microbiol. *36*:1357-1360, 1998.

41. Garcia de la Torre, M., Romero-Vivas, J., Martinez-Beltran, J., et al.: *Klebsiella* bacteremia: An analysis of 100 episodes. Rev. Infect. Dis. 7:143-150, 1985.

42. Gorman, L. J., Sanai, L., Notman, A. W., et al.: Cross infection in an intensive care unit by *Klebsiella pneumoniae* from ventilator condensate. J. Hosp. Infect. *23*:27-34, 1993.

43. Grauel, E. L., Halle, E., Bollmann, R., et al.: Neonatal septicaemia: Incidence, etiology and outcome: A 6-year analysis. Acta Paediatr. Scand. *360*(Suppl.):113-119, 1989.

44. Gregersen, N., Van Nierop, W., Von Gottberg, A., et al.: *Klebsiella pneumoniae* with extended spectrum beta-lactamase activity associated with a necrotizing enterocolitis outbreak. Pediatr. Infect. Dis. J. *18*:963-967, 1999.

45. Haertl, R., and Bandlow, G.: Use of small fragment restriction endonuclease analysis (SF-REA) for epidemiological fingerprinting of *Klebsiella oxytoca*. Int. J. Med. Microbiol. Virol. Parasitol. Infect. Dis. *280*:312-318, 1994.

46. Hambraeus, A., Lagerqvist-Widh, A., Zettersten, U., et al.: Spread of *Klebsiella* in a neonatal ward. Scand. J. Infect. Dis. *23*:189-194, 1991.

47. Hawk, R. J., Storer, J. S., and Daum, R. S.: Toxic epidermal necrolysis in a 6-week-old infant. Pediatr. Dermatol. 2:197-200, 1985.

48. Heritage, J., Hawkey, P. M., Todd, N., et al.: Transposition of the gene encoding a TEM-12 extended-spectrum beta-lactamase. Antimicrob. Agents Chemother. *36*:1981-1986, 1992.

49. Hervas, J. A., Alomar, A., Salva, F., et al.: Neonatal sepsis and meningitis in Mallorca, Spain, 1977-1991. Clin. Infect. Dis. *16*:719-724, 1993.

50. Hesseling, P. B., Mouton, W. L., Henning, P. A., et al.: A prospective study of long-term use of amikacin in a paediatrics department: Indications, administration, side-effects, bacterial isolates and resistance. S. Afr. Med. J. *78*:192-195, 1990.

51. Hogenauer, C., Langner, C., Beubler, E., et al.: *Klebsiella oxytoca* as a causative organism of antibiotic-associated hemorrhagic colitis. N. Engl. J. Med. *355*:2418-2426, 2006.

52. Hughes, W. T.: Pneumonia in the immunocompromised child. Semin. Resp. Infect. 2:177-183, 1987.

53. Jallat, C., Darfeuille-Michaud, A., Girardeau, J. P., et al.: Self-transmissible R plasmids encoding CS31A among human *Escherichia coli* strains isolated from diarrheal stools. Infect. Immun. *62*:2865-2873, 1994.

54. Jarvis, W. R., Munn, V. P., Highsmith, A. K., et al.: The epidemiology of nosocomial infections caused by *Klebsiella pneumoniae*. Infect. Control 6:68-74, 1985.

55. Jett, B. D., Ritchie, D. J., Reichley, R., et al.: In vitro activities of various beta-lactam antimicrobial agents against clinical isolates of *Escherichia coli* and *Klebsiella* spp. resistant to oxyimino cephalosporins. Antimicrob. Agents Chemother. *39*:1187-1190, 1995.

56. Johanson, W. G., Higuchi, J. H., Chaudhuri, T. R., et al.: Bacterial adherence to epithelial cells in bacillary colonization of the respiratory tract. Am. Rev. Respir. Dis. *121*:55-63, 1980.

57. Johanson, W. G., Pierce, A. K., and Sanford, J. P.: Changing bacterial flora of hospitalized patients. N. Engl. J. Med. *281*:1137-1140, 1969.

58. Johnson, A. W., Osinusi, K., Aderele, W. I., et al.: Bacterial aetiology of acute lower respiratory infections in pre-school Nigerian children and comparative predictive features of bacteraemic and non-bacteraemic illnesses. J. Trop. Pediatr. *39*:97-106, 1993.

59. Jones, R. N., Jenkins, S. G., Hoban, D. J., et al.: In vitro efficacy of six cephalosporins tested against Enterobacteriaceae isolated at 38 North American medical centers participating in the SENTRY Antimicrobial Surveillance Program, 1997-1998. Int. J. Antimicrob. Agents *15*:111-118, 2000.

60. Jong, G. M., Hsiue, T. R., Chen, C. R., et al.: Rapidly fatal outcome of bacteremic *Klebsiella pneumoniae* pneumonia in alcoholics. Chest *107*:214-217, 1995.

61. Khaneja, M., Naprawa, J., Kumar, A., and Piecuch, S.: Successful treatment of late-onset infection due to resistant *Klebsiella pneumoniae* in an extremely low birth weight infant using ciprofloxacin. J. Perinatol. *19*:311-314, 1999.

62. Kishan, J., Mir, N. A., Elzouki, A. Y., et al.: Radiological case of the month: *Klebsiella* multifocal osteomyelitis. Am. J. Dis. Child. *142*:687-688, 1988.

63. Klar, A., Hurvitz, H., Berkun, Y., et al.: Focal bacterial nephritis (lobar nephronia) in children. J. Pediatr. *128*:850-853,1996.

64. Kolmos, H. J.: *Klebsiella pneumoniae* in a nephrological department. J. Hosp. Infect. 5:253-259, 1984.

65. Krohn, M. A., Hillier, S. L., Bell, T. A., et al.: The bacterial etiology of conjunctivitis in early infancy: Eye Prophylaxis Study Group. Am. J. Epidemiol. *138*:326-332, 1993.

66. Lalitha, M. K., Kenneth, J., Jana, A. K., et al.: Identification of an IV-dextrose solution as the source of an outbreak of *Klebsiella pneumoniae* sepsis in a newborn nursery. J. Hosp. Infect. *43*:70-73, 1999.

67. Lang, A. B., Bruderer, U., Senyk, G., et al.: Human monoclonal antibodies specific for capsular polysaccharides of *Klebsiella* recognize clusters of multiple serotypes. J. Immunol. *146*:3160-3164, 1991.

68. Lee, C. J.: Bacterial capsular polysaccharides: Biochemistry, immunity and vaccine. Mol. Immunol. *24*:1005-1019, 1987.

69. Lee, H. C., Chuang, Y. C., Yu, W. L., et al.: Clinical implications of hypermucoviscosity phenotype in *Klebsiella pneumoniae* isolates: Association with invasive syndrome in patients with community-acquired bacteremia. J. Intern. Med. *259*:606-614, 2006.

70. Lhopital, S., Bonacorsi, S., Meis, D., et al.: Molecular markers for differentiation of multiresistant *Klebsiella pneumoniae* isolates in a pediatric hospital. Infect. Control Hosp. Epidemiol. *18*:743-748, 1997.

71. Lohr, J. A., Donowitz, L. G., and Sadler, J. E.: Hospital-acquired urinary tract infection. Pediatrics *83*:193-199, 1989.

72. Lomaestro, B. M., Tobin, E. H., Shang, W., and Gootz, T.: The spread of *Klebsiella pneumoniae* carbapenemase-producing *K. pneumoniae* to upstate New York. Clin. Infect. Dis. *43*:e26-e28, 2006.

73. Mackowiak, P. A., Martin, R. M., Jones, S. R., et al.: Pharyngeal colonization by gram-negative bacilli in aspiration-prone persons. Arch. Intern. Med. *138*:1224-1227, 1978.

74. Mancuso, P., Nana-Sinkam, P., and Peters-Golden, M.: Leukotriene B4 augments neutrophil phagocytosis of *Klebsiella pneumoniae*. Infect. Immun. *69*:2011-2016, 2001.

75. Margo, C. E., Mames, R. N., and Guy, J. R.: Endogenous *Klebsiella* endophthalmitis: Report of two cases and review of the literature. Ophthalmology *101*:1298-1301, 1994.

76. Matsuhisa, A., Saito, Y., Sakamoto, Y., et al.: Detection of bacteria in phagocyte-smears from septicemia-suspected blood by in situ hybridization using biotinylated probes. Microbiol. Immunol. *38*:511-517, 1994.

77. McCracken, G. H. J., Mize, S. G., and Threlkeld, N.: Intraventricular gentamicin therapy in gram-negative bacillary meningitis of infancy: Report of the Second National Meningitis Cooperative Study Group. Lancet 1:787-791, 1980.

78. Meadow, W. L., and Schwartz, I. K.: Time course of radiometric detection of positive blood cultures in childhood. Pediatr. Infect. Dis. 5:333-336, 1986.

79. Meyer, K. S., Urban, C., Eagan, J. A., et al.: Nosocomial outbreak of *Klebsiella* infection resistant to late-generation cephalosporins. Ann. Intern. Med. *119*:353-358, 1993.

80. Mollitt, D. L., Tepas, J. J., and Talbert, J. L.: The microbiology of neonatal peritonitis. Arch. Surg. *123*:176-179, 1988.

81. Monnet, D., Freney, J., Brun, Y., et al.: Difficulties in identifying *Klebsiella* strains of clinical origin. Int. J. Med. Microbiol. *274*:456-464, 1991.

82. Moon, W. K., Im, J. G., Yeon, K. M., et al.: Complications of *Klebsiella* pneumonia: CT evaluation. J. Comput. Assist. Tomogr. *19*:176-181, 1995.

83. Nathoo, K. J., Mason, P. R., Gwanzura, L., et al.: Severe *Klebsiella* infection as a cause of mortality in neonates in Harare, Zimbabwe: Evidence from postmortem blood cultures. Pediatr. Infect. Dis. J. *12*:840-844, 1993.

84. Ng, P. C., Fok, T. F., Lee, C. H., et al.: Massive subdural haematoma: An unusual complication of septicaemia in preterm very low birthweight infants. J. Pediatr. Child Health *34*:296-298, 1998.

85. O'Reilly, G. V., Dee, P. M., and Otteni, G. V.: Gangrene of the lung: Successful medical management of three patients. Diagn. Radiol. *126*:575-579, 1978.

86. Orskov, I.: *Klebsiella*. In Krieg, N. R., and Holt, J. G. (eds.): Bergey's Manual of Systematic Bacteriology. Vol. 1. Baltimore, Williams & Wilkins, 1984, pp. 461-465.

87. Parchuri, S., Mohan, S., and Cunha, B. A.: Extended spectrum beta-lactamase-producing *Klebsiella pneumoniae* chronic ambulatory peritoneal dialysis peritonitis treated successfully with polymixin B. Heart Lung. *34*:360-363, 2005.

88. Paterson, D. L., Mulazimoglu, L., Casellas, J. M., et al.: Epidemiology of ciprofloxacin resistance and its relationship to extended-spectrum beta-lactamase production in *Klebsiella pneumoniae* isolates causing bacteremia. Clin. Infect. Dis. *30*:473-478, 2000.

89. Picard, E., Gillis, D., Klapholz, L., et al.: Toxic epidermal necrolysis associated with *Klebsiella pneumoniae* sepsis. Pediatr. Dermatol. *11*:331-334, 1994.

90. Pierce, J. R., Merenstein, G. B., and Stocker, J. T.: Immediate postmortem cultures in an intensive care nursery. Pediatr. Infect. Dis. J. 3:510-513, 1984.

91. Pillay, T., Pillay, D. G., Adhikari, M., and Sturm, A. W.: Piperacillin/tazobactam in the treatment of *Klebsiella pneumoniae* infections in neonates. Am. J. Perinatol. *15*:47-51, 1998.

92. Podschun, R., Acktun, H., Okpara, J., et al.: Isolation of *Klebsiella planticola* from newborns in a neonatal ward. J. Clin. Microbiol. *36*:2331-2332, 1998.

93. Podschun, R., Fischer, A., and Ullman, U.: Expression of putative virulence factors by clinical isolates of *Klebsiella planticola*. J. Med. Microbiol. *49*:115-119, 2000.

94. Podschun, R., Sievers, D., Fischer, A., et al.: Serotypes, hemagglutinins, siderophore synthesis, and serum resistance of *Klebsiella* isolates causing human urinary tract infections. J. Infect. Dis. *168*:1415-1421, 1993.

95. Podschun, R., and Ullmann, U.: *Klebsiella* spp. as nosocomial pathogens: Epidemiology, taxonomy, typing methods, and pathogenicity factors. Clin. Microbiol. Rev. *11*:589-603, 1998.

96. Quinn, J. P.: Clinical significance of extended-spectrum beta-lactamases. Eur. J. Clin. Microbiol. Infect. Dis. *13*(Suppl. 1):S39-S42, 1994.

97. Ramirez-Ronda, C. H., Fuxench-Lopez, Z., and Nevarez, M.: Increased pharyngeal bacterial colonization during viral illness. Arch. Intern. Med. *141*:1599-1603, 1981.

98. Ransjo, U., Good, Z., Jalakas. K., et al.: An outbreak of *Klebsiella oxytoca* septicemias associated with the use of invasive blood pressure monitoring equipment. Acta Anaesthesiol. Scand. *36*:289-291, 1992.

99. Rebuck, J. A., Olsen, K. M., Fey, P. D., et al.: Characterization of an outbreak due to extended-spectrum beta-lactamase-producing *Klebsiella pneumoniae* in a pediatric intensive care unit transplant population. Clin. Infect. Dis. *31*:1368-1372, 2000.

100. Reish, O., Ashkenazi, S., Naor, N., et al.: An outbreak of multiresistant *Klebsiella* in a neonatal intensive care unit. J. Hosp. Infect. *25*:287-291, 1993.

101. Reiss, I., Borkhardt, A., Fussle, R., et al.: Disinfectant contaminated with *Klebsiella oxytoca* as a source of sepsis in babies. Lancet *356*:310, 2000.

102. Rice, L. B., Carias, L. L., Hujer, A. M., et al.: High-level expression of chromosomally encoded SHV-1 beta-lactamase and an outer membrane protein change confer resistance to ceftazidime and piperacillin-tazobactam in a clinical isolate of *Klebsiella pneumoniae*. Antimicrob. Agents Chemother. *44*:362-367, 2000.

103. Romero, L., Lopez, L., Rodriguez-Bano, J., et al.: Long-term study of the frequency of *Escherichia coli* and *Klebsiella pneumoniae* isolates producing extended-spectrum beta-lactamases. Clin. Microbiol. Infect. *11*:625-631, 2005.

104. Royle, J., Halasz, S., Eagles, G., et al.: Outbreak of extended spectrum beta lactamase producing *Klebsiella pneumoniae* in a neonatal unit. Arch. Dis. Childh. Fetal Neonatal Ed. *80*:F64-F68, 1999.

105. Sakata, H., Fujita, K., and Yoshioka, H.: The effect of antimicrobial agents on fecal flora of children. Antimicrob. Agents Chemother. *29*:225-229, 1986.

106. Saurina, G., Quale, J. M., Manikal, V. M., et al.: Antimicrobial resistance in Enterobacteriaceae in Brooklyn, NY: Epidemiology and relation to antibiotic usage patterns. J. Antimicrob. Chemother. *45*:895-898, 2000.

107. Schumacher, H., Scheibel, J., and Moller, J. K.: Cross-resistance patterns among clinical isolates of *Klebsiella pneumoniae* with decreased susceptibility to cefuroxime. J. Antimicrob. Chemother. *46*:215-221, 2000.

108. Sechi, L. A., Spanu, T., Sanguinetti, M., et al.: Molecular analysis of *Klebsiella pneumoniae* strains isolated in pediatric wards by ribotyping, pulsed field gel electrophoresis and antimicrobial susceptibilities. New Microbiol. *24*:35-45, 2001.

109. Shannon, K., Fung, K., Stapleton, P., et al.: A hospital outbreak of extended-spectrum beta-lactamase-producing *Klebsiella pneumoniae* investigated by RAPD typing and analysis of the genetics and mechanisms of resistance. J. Hosp. Infect. *39*:291-300, 1998.

110. Sharma, S., Mohta, A., and Sharma, P.: Hepatic abscess in a preterm neonate. Indian Pediatr. *44*:226-228, 2007.

111. Sood, S. K., Mulvihill, D., and Daum, R. S.: Intrarenal abscess caused by *Klebsiella pneumoniae* in a neonate: Modern management and diagnosis. Am. J. Perinatol. *6*:367-370, 1989.

112. Tullus, K., Ayling-Smith, B., Kuhn, I., et al.: Nationwide spread of *Klebsiella oxytoca* K55 in Swedish neonatal special care wards. A. P. M. I. S. *100*:1008-1014, 1992.

113. Westbrook, G. L., O'Hara, C. M., Roman, S. B., and Miller, J. M.: Incidence and identification of *Klebsiella planticola* in clinical isolates with emphasis on newborns. J. Clin. Microbiol. *38*:1495-1497, 2000.

114. Zimhony, O., Chmelnitsky, I., Bardenstein, R., et al.: Endocarditis caused by extended-spectrum beta-lactamase-producing *Klebsiella pneumoniae*: Emergence of resistance to ciprofloxacin and piperacillin-tazobactam during treatment despite initial susceptibility. Antimicrob. Agents Chemother. *50*:3179-3182, 2006.

MORGANELLA MORGANII

Randall G. Fisher

Similar to *Proteus* and *Providencia* spp., *Morganella morganii* has emerged as an important nosocomial pathogen, most often associated with urinary tract or wound infections. Although most descriptions of infection are in adults, infections in children do occur.

BACTERIOLOGY

M. morganii (formerly *Proteus morganii*) is a motile gram-negative bacillus commonly found in the feces of humans, other mammals, and reptiles.[27] The organism was elevated to genus rank because of genetic differences from *Proteus*, with which it is otherwise biologically similar.[7] Most strains do not ferment lactose. *M. morganii*, *Proteus* spp., and *Providencia* spp. are distinguished from other Enterobacteriaceae by their ability to deaminate phenylalanine and lysine. Similar to *Proteus* and *Providencia* spp., *M. morganii* produces urease, but this enzyme is unrelated genetically and serologically to urease produced by the other two genera.[19,27] In contrast to *Proteus* spp., neither *Providencia* spp. nor *M. morganii* shows swarming activity on 1.5 percent agar[27]; *M. morganii* is ornithine-positive, whereas *Providencia* spp. are ornithine-negative. *M. morganii* organisms do not hydrolyze gelatin and do not produce hydrogen sulfide. For a detailed discussion of taxonomy and characterization of *M. morganii*, the reader is referred to the review by O'Hara and colleagues.[26]

EPIDEMIOLOGY

Similar to *Proteus* and *Providencia* spp., *M. morganii* organisms commonly are found in soil, sewage, and manure. Similar to *Proteus mirabilis*, *M. morganii* commonly invades the instrument-fitted urinary tract and surgical wounds; adults in inpatient surgical units have the greatest risk for colonization and infection.[1] Institutionalized elderly patients also are infected frequently with these organisms. Urinary tract colonization with *M. morganii* accompanying groin skin colonization in elderly individuals may account for the greater frequency of urinary tract infections in this population.[15] *M. morganii* accounted for nearly 10 percent of 145 consecutive complicated, multidrug-resistant urinary tract infections.[11] *Escherichia coli* and *P. mirabilis* account for most urinary tract infections in children, but *M. morganii* has been implicated in some cases of cystitis and pyelonephritis. In contrast to well-described nursery epidemics of *P. mirabilis* infection,[3,9] no *M. morganii* neonatal outbreaks have been described, and infections of the central nervous system are rare in newborns.[13,37] Ribotyping is a sensitive method for molecular characterization of isolates that may aid in analyzing outbreaks.[29]

PATHOPHYSIOLOGY

Factors that predispose the urinary tract to invasion by *P. mirabilis* and *Providencia* spp. also may favor *M. morganii* colonization and infection. These organisms all split urea, forming ammonium hydroxide and increasing local pH, which results in toxicity to renal cells and potentiation of urolithiasis.[6,25] The ability of *P. mirabilis* to regenerate more rapidly in urine with faster generation of alkaline pH compared with *M. morganii* may provide a selective advantage for the former organism in establishing itself as a urinary tract pathogen.[34]

CLINICAL MANIFESTATIONS

Urinary tract infection with *M. morganii* often is associated with an elevated urinary pH. Urolithiasis can occur, although perhaps less frequently than during *P. mirabilis* infection.[4] *M. morganii* has been recovered from less than 10 percent of adult bacteremic episodes, but mortality rates have exceeded 20 percent.[1] Approximately three fourths of all cases of adult *M. morganii* bacteremia are hospital-associated.[22] In a series of 132 patients with bacteremia from tribe Proteeae, preexisting biliary or hepatic disease (especially the presence of biliary drainage catheters) was associated with *Morganella* bacteremia.[22] Other reported complications identified in immunocompromised or instrument-fitted patients include meningitis,[17,23] arthritis,[21,33] empyema,[18] peritonitis,[18] and skin infection.[2] Many cases of postoperative *M. morganii* endophthalmitis and panophthalmitis have been reported, as have rare cases of endogenous endophthalmitis, all in adults.[10,36,38,39] *M. morganii* has been recovered alone or in combination with other organisms from surgical wounds[11] and soft tissue abscesses in children.[8] Perinatal bacterial sepsis and brain abscess have been described.[30-32,37] In three more recently reported cases of early-onset neonatal sepsis, premature rupture of membranes and maternal receipt of antepartum amoxicillin were documented.[5,14]

DIAGNOSIS

M. morganii produces a reddish brown pigment when cultured on nutrient media supplemented with 5 percent tryptophan.[27] Production of urease and deamination of tryptophan help to distinguish this bacterium from other organisms. In contrast to the closely related *Proteus* and *Providencia* spp., *M. morganii* generally ferments only glucose and mannose and does not produce a red color on lysine iron agar.[27] *M. morganii* may be missed or mistaken for other organisms in the common circumstance of polymicrobial infection in a catheterized patient. In one series, *M. morganii* was among the most common bacteriuric species in patients on long-term catheterization but commonly was missed by reference laboratories.[12] The clinical laboratory should be directed to look for this organism, particularly in circumstances of nosocomial urinary tract infection and sepsis.

TREATMENT

Effective treatment of local infections or septicemia relies on appropriate choice of an antibiotic, often including an aminoglycoside, combined with surgical débridement and drainage of abscesses, as necessary. Antimicrobial susceptibility can vary widely among *M. morganii* and the related *Proteus* and *Providencia* strains, emphasizing the importance of species identification and susceptibility testing.[28] Complex combinations of aminoglycoside resistance that differ by hospital and geographic region can occur.[24] Most isolates are intrinsically resistant to ampicillin and first-generation and second-generation cephalosporins. Some carry a chromosomal broad-spectrum AmpC β-lactamase that can be stably derepressed on treatment with third-generation cephalosporins, similar to *Enterobacter* spp. Most urinary tract infections respond to third-generation cephalosporins. Failure to clear bacteriuria should alert the physician to the possibility of urolithiasis or structural abnormality[4]; stone removal or surgical correction of anatomic defects often is required for cure. The approach to the treatment of sepsis or serious infection of non–urinary tract sites should be considered carefully in light of local susceptibility patterns, keeping in mind that isolates with AmpC β-lactamases may seem to be sensitive to cephalosporins on initial testing, only to develop resistance during therapy. Treatment failure, with prolonged culture-positive ventriculitis, has been described in an infant with *M. morganii* meningitis after initial therapy that included cefotaxime led to stable derepression of an AmpC β-lactamase, showing the potentially devastating clinical relevance of this phenomenon.[35] Aztreonam has shown effectiveness in therapy for 98 percent of multidrug-resistant strains.[11]

Acknowledgments

The author thanks Dr. William Gruber and Dr. Thomas Boyce for their invaluable assistance with earlier versions of this chapter.

REFERENCES

1. Adler, J. L., Burke, J. P., Martin, D. F., et al.: *Proteus* infection in a general hospital, II: Some clinical and epidemiological characteristics. Ann. Intern. Med. 75:531-536, 1971.
2. Bagel, J., and Grossman, M. E.: Hemorrhagic bullae associated with *Morganella morganii* septicemia. J. Am. Acad. Dermatol. 12:575-576, 1985.
3. Becker, A. H.: Infection due to *Proteus mirabilis* in a newborn nursery. Am. J. Dis. Child. 104:355-359, 1962.
4. Bensman, A., Roubach, L., Allouch, G., et al.: Urolithiasis in children: Presenting signs, etiology, bacteriology and localisation. Acta Paediatr. Scand. 72:879-883, 1983.
5. Boussemart, T., Piet-Duroux, S., Manouana, M., et al.: *Morganella morganii* and early-onset neonatal infection. Arch. Pediatr. 11:37-39, 2004.
6. Braude, A. I., and Siemienski, J.: Role of bacterial urease in experimental pyelonephritis. J. Bacteriol. 80:171-179, 1960.
7. Brenner, D. J., Farmer, J. J., III, Fanning, G. R., et al.: Deoxyribonucleic acid relatedness of *Proteus* and *Providencia* species. Int. J. Syst. Bacteriol. 28:269-282, 1978.
8. Brook, I., and Martin, W. J.: Aerobic and anaerobic bacteriology of perirectal abscess in children. Pediatrics 66:282-284, 1980.
9. Burke, J. P., Ingall, D., Klein, J. O., et al.: *Proteus mirabilis* infections in a hospital nursery traced to a human carrier. N. Engl. J. Med. 284:115-121, 1971.
10. Christensen, S. R., Hansen, A. B., LaCour, M., and Fledelius, H. C.: Bilateral endogenous bacterial endophthalmitis: A report of four cases. Acta Ophthalmol. Scand. 82:306-310, 2004.
11. Cox, C. E.: Aztreonam therapy for complicated urinary tract infections caused by multidrug-resistant bacteria. Rev. Infect. Dis. 7(Suppl. 4):S767-S771, 1985.
12. Damron, D. J., Warren, J. W., Chippendale, G. R., et al.: Do clinical microbiology laboratories report complete bacteriology in urine from patients with long-term urinary catheters? J. Clin. Microbiol. 24:400-404, 1986.
13. Darby, C. P., and Hill, O.: *Proteus morganii* meningitis treated with trimethoprim-sulfamethoxazole (co-trimoxazole) Clin. Pediatr. 14:669-672, 1975.
14. Dutta, S., and Narang, A.: Early onset neonatal sepsis due to *Morganella morganii*. Indian Pediatr. 41:1155-1157, 2004.
15. Ehrenkranz, N. J., Alfonso, B. C., Eckert, D. G., et al. *Proteeae* species bacteriuria accompanying *Proteeae* species groin skin carriage in geriatric outpatients. J. Clin. Microbiol. 27:1988-1991, 1989.
16. Haddad, J. J., Inglesby, T. V. J., and Addonizio, L.: Head and neck infections in pediatric cardiac transplant patients. Ear Nose Throat J. 74:422-425, 1995.
17. Isaacs, R. D., and Ellis-Pegler, R. B.: Successful treatment of *Morganella morganii* meningitis with pefloxacin mesylate. J. Antimicrob. Chemother. 20:769-770, 1987.
18. Isobe, H., Motomura, K., Kotou, K., et al.: Spontaneous bacterial empyema and peritonitis caused by *Morganella morganii*. J. Clin. Gastroenterol. 18:87-88, 1994.
19. Jones, B. D., and Mobley, H. L.: Genetic and biochemical diversity of ureases of *Proteus, Providencia,* and *Morganella* species isolated from urinary tract infection. Infect. Immun. 55:2198-2203, 1987.
20. Kaslow, R. A., Lindsey, J. O., Bison, A. L., et al.: Nosocomial infection with highly resistant *Proteus rettgeri*: Report of an epidemic. Am. J. Epidemiol. 104:278-286, 1976.
21. Katz, L. M., Lewis, R. J., and Borenstein, D. G.: Successful joint arthroplasty following *Proteus morganii* (*Morganella morganii*) septic arthritis: A four-year study. Arthritis Rheum. 30:583-585, 1987.
22. Kim, B. N., Kim, N. J., Kim, M. N., et al.: Bacteraemia due to tribe *Proteeae*: A review of 132 cases during a decade (1991-2000). Scand. J. Infect. Dis. 35:98-103, 2003.
23. Mastroianni, A., Coronado, O., and Chiodo, F.: *Morganella morganii* meningitis in a patient with AIDS. J. Infect. 29:356-357, 1994.
24. Miller, G. H., Sabatelli, F. J., Hare, R. S., et al.: The most frequent aminoglycoside resistance mechanisms—changes with time and geographic area: A reflection of aminoglycoside usage patterns? Aminoglycoside Resistance Study Groups. Clin. Infect. Dis. 24:S46-S62, 1997.
25. Musher, D. M., Griffith, D. P., Yawn, D., et al.: Role of urease in pyelonephritis resulting from urinary tract infection with *Proteus*. J. Infect. Dis. 131:177-181, 1975.
26. O'Hara, C. M., Brenner, F. W., and Miller, J. M.: Classification, identification, and clinical significance of *Proteus, Providencia,* and *Morganella*. Clin. Microbiol. Rev. 13:534-546, 2000.
27. Penner, J. L.: *Morganella. In* Krieg, N. R., and Holt, J. G. (eds.): Bergey's Manual of Systematic Bacteriology. Vol. 1. Baltimore, Williams & Wilkins, 1984, pp. 497-498.
28. Piccolomini, R., Cellini, L., Allocati, N., et al.: Comparative in vitro activities of 13 antimicrobial agents against *Morganella-Proteus-Providencia* group bacteria from urinary tract infections. Antimicrob. Agents Chemother. 31:1644-1647, 1987.

29. Pignato, S., Giammanco, G. M., Grimont, F., et al.: Molecular characterization of the genera *Proteus, Morganella,* and *Providencia* by ribotyping. J. Clin. Microbiol. *37*:2840-2847, 1999.
30. Ranu, S. S., Valencia, G. B., and Piecuch, S.: Fatal early onset infection in an extremely low birth weight infant due to *Morganella morganii.* J. Perinatol. *19*:533-535, 1999.
31. Rowen, J. L., and Lopez, S. M.: *Morganella morganii* early onset sepsis. Pediatr. Infect. Dis. J. *17*:1176-1177, 1998.
32. Salen, P. N., and Eppes, S.: *Morganella morganii:* A newly reported rare cause of neonatal sepsis. Acad. Emerg. Med. *4*:711-714, 1997.
33. Schonwetter, R. S., and Orson, F. M.: Chronic *Morganella morganii* arthritis in an elderly patient. J Clin. Microbiol. *26*:1414-1415, 1988.
34. Senior, B. W.: *Proteus morganii* is less frequently associated with urinary tract infections than *Proteus mirabilis:* An explanation. J. Med. Microbiol. *16*:317-322, 1983.
35. Sinha, A. K., Kempley, S. T., Price, E., et al.: Early onset *Morganella morganii* sepsis in a newborn infant with emergence of cephalosporin resistance caused by derepression of AmpC beta-lactamase production. Pediatr. Infect. Dis. J. *25*:376-377, 2006.
36. Tsanaktsidis, G., Agarwal, S. A., Maloof, A. J., et al.: Postoperative *Morganella morganii* endophthalmitis association with subclinical urinary tract infection. J. Cataract Refract. Surg. *29*:1011-1013, 2003.
37. Verboon-Maciolek, M., Vandertop, W. P., Peters, A. C., et al.: Neonatal brain abscess caused by *Morganella morganii.* Clin. Infect. Dis. *20*:471, 1995.
38. Wang, T. J., Huang, J. S., and Hsueh, P. R.: Acute postoperative *Morganella morganii* panopthalmitis. Eye *19*:713-715, 2005.
39. Zaninetti, M., Baglivo, E., and Safran, A. B.: *Morganella morganii* endophthalmitis after vitrectomy: Case report and review of the literature. Klin. Monatsbl. Augenheilkd. *220*:207-209, 2003.

PROTEUS

Randall G. Fisher

Proteus spp. are pathogens that are associated increasingly with pediatric illness. Neonatal meningitis and pediatric urinary tract infections are the most common childhood conditions in which these organisms are isolated, but infections of other organ systems have been described.

BACTERIOLOGY

Proteus spp. are motile, gram-negative bacilli that do not ferment lactose and are distinguished from other Enterobacteriaceae by their ability to deaminate phenylalanine and lysine. Rapid and abundant production of urease further differentiates *Proteus* spp. from *Providencia* spp.[33] *Proteus vulgaris* and *Proteus mirabilis* tend to form a thin, spreading growth (swarm) on the surface of moist agar media, often overgrowing other bacterial isolates. They also produce hydrogen sulfide and liquefy gelatin. *P. mirabilis* is distinguished from other *Proteus* spp. (e.g., *P. vulgaris*) by its inability to produce indole from tryptophan. Disparate DNA content and anomalous biochemical and serologic reactions have caused *Proteus morganii* to be renamed *Morganella morganii* (see Chapter 116),[33] and both terms for this organism appear in the clinical literature. For detailed discussion of taxonomy and characterization of *Proteus* spp., the reader is referred to the review by O'Hara and colleagues.[44]

EPIDEMIOLOGY

Proteus spp. commonly are found in soil, sewage, and manure. Although they are normal inhabitants of the colon and perineum, their numbers can be increased in individuals receiving antibiotic therapy.[30]

First reported by Buisine and Henninot in 1949,[12] neonatal meningitis caused by *P. mirabilis* accounts for approximately 4 percent of all neonatal meningitis cases.[41] Outbreaks in nurseries have been attributed to contaminated equipment and human carriers. Vertical transmission from mother to infant has been confirmed by DNA fingerprinting and ribotyping methods.[9] In Becker's series[6] of *P. mirabilis* neonatal meningitis, all affected infants came from the same nursery, and all were exposed to mist from an apparatus that yielded *P. mirabilis.* The importance of hand carriage was well documented by Burke and associates[13]; newborn umbilical colonization and invasive disease were linked to a single nurse from whom *P. mirabilis* was cultured from her

hands, rectum, and vagina. Ribotyping is a sensitive method for molecular characterization of isolates and may aid in analyzing outbreaks.[48]

Proteus infection after the first few months of life most commonly involves the urinary tract. Although *Escherichia coli* accounts for most urinary tract infections in children, *Proteus* spp. commonly are implicated in reported series of cystitis and pyelonephritis[8,22,31,65]; in a large pediatric series, they were the third most common cause of urinary tract infection, after *E. coli* and *Klebsiella pneumoniae.*[10] *P. mirabilis* is the most common species of *Proteus* isolated. *P. mirabilis* has been cultured more frequently from the urethra of uncircumcised than of circumcised male infants and has replaced *E. coli* as the most prevalent pathogen in one consecutive series of male patients presenting with initial urinary tract infection.[31,66]

Urinary tract infection with *Proteus* spp. is one of the most common presenting signs of urolithiasis in children,[18] and *P. mirabilis* supplants *E. coli* as the major urinary tract pathogen in children prone to renal stone formation.[8] Diagnosis of greater than 50 percent of pediatric urolithiasis cases is based on preceding urinary tract infection, and *Proteus* is responsible for 65 percent of these infections.[8] Isolation of this organism as a pathogen on urine culture should alert the physician to the possible presence of a urinary tract stone.

PATHOPHYSIOLOGY

Most cases of central nervous system infection caused by *Proteus* spp. occur in neonates and are thought to arise by bacteremic spread of the organism to the brain or meninges. Contiguous spread to the brain from localized infections is reported occasionally.[40] As is the case with *Citrobacter* meningitis, a propensity for formation of abscesses of the central nervous system remains unexplained. Rabbit models of *P. mirabilis* meningitis have shown that in vivo concentrations of gentamicin necessary to produce bacterial killing are 10 to 30 times higher than the concentrations predicted from in vitro susceptibility testing.[63] Reduced aminoglycoside effect may be secondary to depressed cerebrospinal fluid pH associated with *P. mirabilis* infection.[63] Whatever the mechanism, lack of effective antimicrobial activity in the ventricles accounts partly for the persistence of organisms at these sites.

Crystallization of urinary catheters and stents leads to obstruction of outflow of urine. Urease produced by *Proteus* infection causes calcium phosphate and magnesium phosphate to precipitate and accumulate in the catheter lumen.[62] This process is less likely to occur when the urine is dilute and acidic.[62] Mannose-resistant/*Proteus*-like fimbriae (often shortened to MR/P fimbriae) are important in the formation of biofilms on catheter material.[52] Methods of preventing this crystallization, including the use of low-energy acoustic waves generated by electrically activated piezo elements, which interferes with docking and attachment, are being studied.[26] More conventional approaches include coating the catheters with agarose[61] and impregnating catheters with chlorhexidine and triclosan.[21]

Numerous factors may predispose the urinary tract to invasion by *Proteus* spp. *Proteus* spp. split urea, forming ammonium hydroxide and increasing local pH, which results in toxicity to renal cells and potentiation of urolithiasis.[11,43] The ability of *P. mirabilis* to regenerate more rapidly in urine with faster generation of alkaline pH when compared with *M. morganii* (*P. morganii*) may provide a selective advantage for the former organism in establishing itself as a urinary tract pathogen.[55] Biochemically complex struvite ($MgNH_4PO_4$) stones provide a refuge for *Proteus* organisms and form a barrier to effective antimicrobial therapy.[8] Formation of struvite stones is a major cause of urinary bacterial persistence in women without azotemia,[60] and a similar case probably can be made for pediatric patients with urolithiasis. *P. mirabilis* ureases showed lower affinities for substrate, but hydrolyzed urea 6 to 25 times faster than enzymes from other species, which may explain the frequent association of this species with formation of stones.[27]

Organisms have been shown to be taken up by human renal epithelium, by an actin-independent mechanism.[14] Pili may enhance the virulence of *Proteus* in pyelonephritis by increasing adherence of organisms to the renal pelvis.[57] Flagella have been implicated in the spread of this organism in the urinary tract[36]; the ability to invade host uroepithelial cells is coupled closely with the ability of *P. mirabilis* to differentiate into hyperflagellated, filamentous swarm cells capable of rapid spread on the surface of moist agar media.[3] The role of fimbriae as a factor predisposing to ascending infection is less clear.[5,39] Swarming behavior might inherently assist ascending colonization of the urinary tract, as shown in a mouse model of infection.[4] A putative gene regulator for swarming behavior (RsbA) may act to identify environmental conditions that favor swarming.[7] The reader is referred to the review by Rozalski and colleagues[53] for a more in-depth review of *Proteus* virulence factors.

A growing body of literature suggests that adult rheumatoid arthritis may be triggered by infection of the urinary tract with *Proteus* spp. In one study, increased levels of total and class-specific IgG antibodies directed at three *Proteus* peptides were found in patients with rheumatoid arthritis, but not in controls.[51] Patients with active disease had measurable IgM, and a positive correlation was found between antibody indices and inflammatory markers.[51] These same investigators proposed measuring antibodies to *Proteus* hemolysin and urease as diagnostic tests for rheumatoid arthritis.[50] This association is still speculative and is being investigated; at this time, no suggestion has been made that juvenile rheumatoid arthritis is related in any way to *Proteus* infection.

CLINICAL MANIFESTATIONS

P. mirabilis can produce a broad spectrum of symptoms associated with neonatal infection. Most patients present with typical symptoms of early-onset neonatal sepsis, including nonspecific lethargy, fever, and poor feeding; manifestations of sepsis may include septic arthritis and osteomyelitis. A few patients present after the first week of life. Meningitis may occur with either early-onset or late-onset disease. Brain abscesses associated with subtle clini-

cal abnormalities rarely develop for weeks to months before presentation.[13] *Proteus* brain abscesses are associated with a high degree of mortality, frequent complications, and increased risks of neurologic deficits in survivors.[28,35,58] Hydrocephalus is a particularly frequent complication and should be anticipated. Destruction of the brain may progress to porencephaly or compartmentalization of ventricles and often requires surgical intervention.[28] Computed tomography is useful, especially in diagnosing and following progression of cerebral complications.[58]

Urinary tract infection with these bacteria involves predominantly younger patients and often is associated with an elevated urinary pH; clinical findings and urine abnormalities often are less striking than in patients with *E. coli* urinary tract infections.[31] Thirty percent of patients may show recurrent infection during the 12 months after receiving initial treatment.[31] Indwelling urinary catheters increase the risk of *Proteus* colonization and infection. Long-term indwelling urinary catheters or stents may become blocked by encrustations of aggregated struvite crystals; prolonged colonization with urease-producing *P. mirabilis* is associated with this complication.[34] *P. mirabilis* is the most common pathogen associated with xanthogranulomatous pyelonephritis,[2] which can mimic Wilms tumor and usually is not seen in childhood except in malnourished patients.

Proteus spp. often are implicated as agents of septicemia in adult patients and account for approximately 8 percent of gram-negative bacteremias in this group.[19,32] In 60 percent of *Proteus* bacteremic episodes in adults, the urinary tract has been determined to be the source[19]; no anatomic source is identified in 20 percent of cases of *Proteus* bacteremia. *P. mirabilis* and *P. vulgaris* are the species responsible for most cases of *Proteus* bacteremia. The overall incidence of gram-negative enteric bacteremia in pediatric patients is lower than that of adults; 5 percent of such cases are caused by *Proteus* spp.[19] As in adults, the genitourinary tract is the source identified most frequently.[19] Mortality rates average less than 40 percent and strongly depend on the severity of underlying disease in the host.[19,32]

Osteomyelitis,[29,47,63] pneumonia,[19,32,49] mastoiditis,[40] and wound infections[32] also occur. Rarely, native-valve endocarditis has been caused by *P. mirabilis*.[15] Severe multifocal osteomyelitis requiring bilateral above-knee amputation for cure has been reported in a patient with human immunodeficiency virus infection despite a reasonably good CD4+ cell count.[46] *Proteus* spp. have been isolated commonly from chronic suppurative otitis media on several different continents.[23,64] Reports that *Proteus* spp. are major pathogens of otogenic brain abscess in pediatric and adult patients support this association.[24,50] Pediatric osteomyelitis secondary to contiguous infection of traumatized soft tissue often is polymicrobial, and *Proteus* spp. have been implicated as co-pathogens in at least 10 percent of such cases.[47] Sickle cell anemia is a risk factor.[1,29]

DIAGNOSIS

Proteus is suspected readily because of its ability to swarm on the surface of moist agar. A selective medium developed for the isolation of protei relies on the ability of all members to produce a dark brown pigment in medium containing DL-tryptophan.[25] Production of urease, lack of indole production from tryptophan, and a positive result with ornithine decarboxylase testing distinguish *P. mirabilis* from *Providencia* spp. and other *Proteus* spp.[33]

TREATMENT

Treatment of meningitis caused by *Proteus* spp. should conform to standard regimens recommended for gram-negative meningitis. *P. mirabilis* usually is sensitive to ampicillin, however, and this drug alone or combined with an aminoglycoside often is suitable therapy when the identity and susceptibilities of the infecting organism are known.[54] A third-generation cephalosporin often is an alternative, but resistant extended-spectrum β-lactamase–producing strains and β-lactamase inhibitor–resistant strains have been described in pediatric patients.[17,36] Consecutive lumbar punctures should be performed for *Proteus* meningitis until cerebrospinal fluid cultures are sterile. A minimum of 2 weeks of antibiotic therapy is recommended after bacteriologic cure has been achieved. Ventricular aspiration or drainage of abscesses may be required to direct therapy, based on persistence of organisms at these sites. Open drainage of abscesses often is necessary, but resolution of abscess formation with the use of antibiotic therapy alone has been reported.[59] Intraventricular antibiotics are not of proven benefit in terms of mortality or morbidity but have been used to clear ventricular colonization. A 15-year-old boy with *Proteus* mastoiditis and meningitis has been treated successfully with intravenous trimethoprim-sulfamethoxazole.[40]

Effective treatment of local infections or septicemia relies on appropriate choice of antibiotics, often including an aminoglycoside, combined with surgical débridement and drainage of abscesses as necessary. Many experts recommended "double coverage"—a cell wall–active agent plus an aminoglycoside—especially when the infection is severe or is caused by an indole-positive strain. In a large, three-continent longitudinal survey, approximately 5 percent of *P. mirabilis* strains exhibited phenotypic extended-spectrum, β-lactamase resistance patterns.[20] In France, 59 percent of 1008 urinary *P. mirabilis* isolates were resistant to amoxicillin, 48 percent were resistant to piperacillin, 34 percent were resistant to amoxicillin-clavulanate, and 2.8 percent were resistant to piperacillin-tazobactam.[37] One third of isolates were resistant to trimethoprim-sulfamethoxazole.[37] Complex combinations of aminoglycoside resistance that differ by hospital and geographic region can occur.[42] In one study, amikacin retained better activity than did other aminoglycosides.[37] Most *P. mirabilis* urinary tract infections respond to ampicillin, but some organisms have been shown to acquire a plasmid-mediated β-lactamase.[38] Failure to clear bacteria should alert the physician to the possibility of urolithiasis or structural abnormality; removal of stones or surgical correction of anatomic defects often is required for cure.

Acknowledgments

The author thanks Dr. William Gruber and Dr. Thomas Boyce for their invaluable assistance with earlier versions of this chapter.

REFERENCES

1. Aken'Ova, Y. A., Bakare, R. A., Okunade, M. A., and Olaniyi, J.: Bacterial causes of acute osteomyelitis in sickle cell anaemia: Changing infection profile. W. Afr. J. Med. 14:255-258, 1995.
2. Al-Ghazo, M. A., Ghalayini, I. F., Matalka, I. I., et al.: Xanthogranulomatous pyelonephritis: analysis of 18 cases. Asian J. Surg. 29:257-261, 2006.
3. Allison, C., Coleman, N., Jones, P. L., et al.: Ability of *Proteus mirabilis* to invade human urothelial cells is coupled to motility and swarming differentiation. Infect. Immun. 60:4740-4746, 1992.
4. Allison, C., Emody, L., Coleman, N., et al.: The role of swarm cell differentiation and multicellular migration in the uropathogenicity of *Proteus mirabilis*. J. Infect. Dis. 169:1155-1158, 1994.
5. Bahrani, F. K., Massad, G., Lockatell, C. V., et al.: Construction of an MR/P fimbrial mutant of *Proteus mirabilis*: Role in virulence in a mouse model of ascending urinary tract infection. Infect. Immun. 62:3363-3371, 1994.
6. Becker, A. H.: Infection due to *Proteus mirabilis* in a newborn nursery. Am. J. Dis. Child. 104:355-359, 1962.
7. Belas, R., Schneider, R., and Melch, M.: Characterization of *Proteus mirabilis* precocious swarming mutants: Identification of rsbA, encoding a regulator of swarming behavior. J. Bacteriol. 180:6126-6139, 1998.
8. Bensman, A., Roubach, L., Allouch, G., et al.: Urolithiasis in children: Presenting signs, etiology, bacteriology and localisation. Acta Paediatr. Scand. 72:879-883, 1983.
9. Bingen, E., Boissinot, C., Desjardins, P., et al.: Arbitrarily primed polymerase chain reaction provides rapid differentiation of *Proteus mirabilis* isolates from a pediatric hospital. J. Clin. Microbiol. 31:1055-1059, 1993.
10. Bonsu, B. K., Shuler, L., Sawicki, L., et al.: Susceptibility of recent bacterial isolates to cefdinir and selected antibiotics among children with urinary tract infections. Acad. Emerg. Med. 13:76-81, 2006.
11. Braude, A. I., and Siemienski, J.: Role of bacterial urease in experimental pyelonephritis. J. Bacteriol. 80:171-179, 1960.
12. Buisine, A., and Henninot, E.: Les meningites a *Proteus* chez l'enfant. Ann. Biol. Clin. 7:448, 1949.
13. Burke, J. P., Ingall, D., Klein, J. O., et al.: *Proteus mirabilis* infections in a hospital nursery traced to a human carrier. N. Engl. J. Med. 284:115-121, 1971.
14. Chippendale, G. R., Warren, J. W., Trifillis, A. L., and Mobley, H. L.: Internalization of *Proteus mirabilis* by human renal epithelial cells. Infect. Immun. 62:3115-3121, 1994.
15. Claassen, D. O., Batsis, J. A., and Orenstein, R.: Proteus mirabilis: A rare cause of infective endocarditis. Scand. J. Infect. Dis. 39:373-375, 2007.
16. Darby, C. P., Conner, E., and Kyong, C. U.: *Proteus mirabilis* brain abscess in a neonate. Dev. Med. Child Neurol. 20:366-375, 1978.
17. de Champs, C., Bonnet, R., Sirot, D., et al.: Clinical relevance of *Proteus mirabilis* in hospital patients: A two year survey. J. Antimicrob. Chemother. 45:537-539, 2000.
18. Diamond, D. A.: Clinical patterns of paediatric urolithiasis. Br. J. Urol. 68:195-198, 1991.
19. duPont, H. L., and Spink, W. H.: Infections due to gram-negative organisms: An analysis of 860 patients with bacteremia at the University of Minnesota Medical Center, 1958-1966. Medicine 48:307-329, 1969.
20. Fedler, K. A., Biedenbach, D. J., and Jones, R. N.: Assessment of pathogen frequency and resistance patterns among pediatric patient isolates: Report from the 2004 SENTRY antimicrobial surveillance program on three continents. Diagn. Microbiol. Infect. Dis. 56:427-436, 2006.
21. Gaonkar, T. A., Caraos, L., and Modak, S.: Efficacy of a silicone urinary catheter impregnated with chlorhexidine and triclosan against colonization with *Proteus mirabilis* and other uropathogens. Infect. Control Hosp. Epidemiol. 28:596-598, 2007.
22. Ginsburg, C. M., and McCracken, G. H., Jr.: Urinary tract infections in young infants. Pediatrics 69:409-412, 1982.
23. Gul, H. C., Kurnaz, A., Turhan, V., et al.: Microorganisms isolated from middle ear cultures and their antibacterial susceptibility in patients with chronic suppurative otitis media. [Polish] Kulak Burun. Bogaz. Ihtis Derg. 16:164-168, 2006.
24. Hafidh, M. A., Keogh, I., Walsh, R. M., et al.: Otogenic intracranial complications: A 7-year retrospective review. Am. J. Otolaryngol. 27:390-395, 2006.
25. Hawkey, P. M., McCormick, A., and Simpson, R. A.: Selective and differential medium for the primary isolation of members of the Proteeae. J. Cin. Microbiol. 23:600-603, 1986.
26. Hazan, Z., Zumeris, J., Jacob, H., et al.: Effective prevention microbial biofilm formation on medical devices by low-energy surface acoustic waves. Antimicrob. Agents Chemother. 50:4144-4152, 2006.
27. Jones, B. D., and Mobley, H. L.: Genetic and biochemical diversity of ureases of *Proteus, Providencia*, and *Morganella* species isolated from urinary tract infection. Infect. Immun. 55:2198-2203, 1987.
28. Kalsbeck, J. E., DeSousa, A. L., Kleiman, M. B., et al.: Compartmentalization of the cerebral ventricles as a sequela of neonatal meningitis. J. Neurosurg. 52:547-552, 1980.
29. Kanfaoui, A., Graide, D., Petein, M., et al.: *Proteus mirabilis* osteomyelitis of the ribs in a girl with sickle cell anaemia. Eur. J. Pediatr. 158:767, 1999.
30. Kaslow, R. A., Lindsey, J. O., Bison, A. L., et al.: Nosocomial infection with highly resistant *Proteus rettgeri*: Report of an epidemic. Am. J. Epidemiol. 104:278-286, 1976.
31. Khan, A. J., Ubriani, R. S., Bombach, E., et al.: Initial urinary tract infection caused by *Proteus mirabilis* in infancy and childhood. J. Pediatr. 93:791-793, 1978.
32. Kreger, B. E., Craven, D. E., Carling, P. C., et al.: Gram-negative bacteremia, III: Reassessment of etiology, epidemiology and ecology in 612 patients. Am. J. Med. 68:332-343, 1980.
33. Krieg, N. R., and Holt, J. G. (eds.): Bergey's Manual of Systematic Bacteriology. Baltimore, Williams & Wilkins, 1984, pp. 491-494.
34. Kunin, C. M.: Blockage of urinary catheters: Role of microorganisms and constituents of the urine on formation of encrustations. J. Clin. Epidemiol. 42:835-842, 1989.
35. Levy, H. L., and Ingall, D.: Meningitis in neonates due to *Proteus mirabilis*. Am. J. Dis. Child. 114:320-324, 1967.
36. Luzzaro, F., Perilli, M., Amicosante, G., et al.: Properties of multidrug-resistant, ESBL-producing *Proteus mirabilis* isolates and possible role of beta-lactam/beta-lactamase inhibitor combinations. Int. J. Antimicrob. Agents 17:131-135, 2001.
37. Mahamat, A., Lavigne, J. P., Bouziges, N., et al.: Antimicrobial susceptibility of *Proteus mirabilis* urinary tract isolates from 1999 to 2005 at Nimes University Hospital. [French] Pathol. Biol. (Paris) 54:456-461, 2006.
38. Mariotte, S., Nordmann, P., and Nicolas, M. H.: Extended-spectrum beta-lactamase in *Proteus mirabilis*. J. Antimicrob. Chemother. 33:925-935, 1994.

39. Massad, G., Lockatell, C. V., Johnson, D. E., et al.: *Proteus mirabilis* fimbriae: Construction of an isogenic pmfA mutant and analysis of virulence in a CBA mouse model of ascending urinary tract infection. Infect. Immun. *62*:536-542, 1994.
40. McConville, J. H., and Manzella, J. P.: Parenteral trimethoprim/sulfamethoxazole for gram-negative bacillary meningitis. Am. J. Med. Sci. *287*:43-45, 1984.
41. McCracken, G. H., Jr.: New developments in the management of children with bacterial meningitis. Pediatr. Infect. Dis. *3*:S32-S34, 1984.
42. Miller, G. H., Sabatelli, F. J., Hare, R. S., et al.: The most frequent aminoglycoside resistance mechanisms—changes with time and geographic area: a reflection of aminoglycoside usage patterns? Aminoglycoside Resistance Study Groups. Clin. Infect. Dis. *24*:S46-S62, 1997.
43. Musher, D. M., Griffith, D. P., Yawn, D., et al.: Role of urease in pyelonephritis resulting from urinary tract infection with *Proteus*. J. Infect. Dis. *131*:177-181, 1975.
44. O'Hara, C. M., Brenner, F. W., and Miller, J. M.: Classification, identification, and clinical significance of *Proteus, Providencia*, and *Morganella*. Clin. Microbiol. Rev. *13*:534-546, 2000.
45. Pazin, G. J., and Braude, A. I.: Immobilizing antibodies in urine, 2: Prevention of ascending spread of *Proteus mirabilis*. Invest. Virol. *122*:129-133, 1974.
46. Petsatodis, G., Symeonidis, P. D., Karatagalis, D., and Pournaras, J.: Multifocal *Proteus mirabilis* osteomyelitis requiring bilateral amputation in an HIV-positive patient. J. Bone Joint Surg. Br. *89*:249-251, 2007.
47. Pichichero, M. E., and Friesen, H. A.: Polymicrobial osteomyelitis: Report of three cases and review of the literature. Rev. Infect. Dis. *4*:86-96, 1982.
48. Pignato, S., Giammanco, G. M., Grimont, F., et al.: Molecular characterization of the genera *Proteus, Morganella*, and *Providencia* by ribotyping. J. Clin. Microbiol. *37*:2840-2847, 1999.
49. Pine, J. R., and Hollman, J. L.: Elevated pleural fluid pH in *Proteus mirabilis* empyema. Chest *84*:109-111, 1983.
50. Rashid, T., Ebringer, A., Wilson, C., et al.: The potential use of antibacterial peptide antibody indices in the diagnosis of rheumatoid arthritis and ankylosing spondylitis. J. Clin. Rheumatol. *12*:1-2, 2006.
51. Rashid, T., Jayakumar, K. S., Binder, A., et al.: Rheumatoid arthritis patients have elevated antibodies to cross-reactive and non-cross reactive antigens from *Proteus* microbes. Clin. Exp. Rheumatol. *25*:259-267, 2007.
52. Rocha, S. P., Pelayo, J. S., and Elias, W. P.: Fimbriae of uropathogenic *Proteus mirabilis*. F. E. M. S. Immunol. Med. Microbiol. *51*:1-7, 2007.
53. Rozalski, A., Sidorczyk, Z., and Kotelko, K.: Potential virulence factors of *Proteus* bacilli. Microbiol. Mol. Biol. Rev. *61*:65-89, 1997.
54. Scherzer, A. L., Kaye, D., and Shinefield, H. R.: *Proteus mirabilis* meningitis: Report of two cases treated with ampicillin. J. Pediatr. *68*:731-740, 1966.
55. Senior, B. W.: *Proteus morganii* is less frequently associated with urinary tract infections than *Proteus mirabilis*: An explanation. J. Med. Microbiol. *16*:317-322, 1983.
56. Sennaroglu, L., and Sozeri, B.: Otogenic brain abscess: Review of 41 cases. Otolaryngol. Head Neck Surg. *123*:751-755, 2000.
57. Silverblatt, F. J.: Host-parasite interaction in the rat renal pelvis: A possible role for pili in the pathogenesis of pyelonephritis. J. Exp. Med. *140*:1696-1711, 1974.
58. Smith, M. L., and Mellor, D.: *Proteus mirabilis* meningitis and cerebral abscess in the newborn period. Arch. Dis. Child. *55*:308-310, 1980.
59. Spirer, Z., Jurgenson, U., Lazewnick, R., et al.: Complete recovery from an apparent brain abscess treated without neurosurgery: The importance of early CT scanning. Clin. Pediatr. *21*:106-109, 1982.
60. Stamey, T. A.: Pathogenesis and Treatment of Urinary Tract Infections. Baltimore, Williams & Wilkins, 1980.
61. Stickler, D. J., Lear, J. C., Morris, N. S., et. al.: Observations on the adherence of *Proteus mirabilis* onto polymer surfaces. J. Appl. Microbiol. *100*:1028-1033, 2006.
62. Stickler, D. J., and Morgan, S. D.: Modulation of crystalline *Proteus mirabilis* biofilm development on urinary catheters. J. Med. Microbiol. *55*:489-494, 2006.
63. Strausbaugh, L. J., and Sande, M. A.: Factors influencing the therapy of experimental *Proteus mirabilis* meningitis in rabbits. J. Infect. Dis. *137*:251-260, 1978.
64. Wariso, B. A., and Ibe, S. N.: Bacteriology of chronic discharging ears in Port Harcourt, Nigeria. West Afr. J. Med. *25*:219-222, 2006.
65. Wientzen, R. L., McCracken, G. H., Jr., Petruska, M. L., et al.: Localization and therapy of urinary tract infections of childhood. Pediatrics *63*:467-473, 1979.
66. Wiswell, T. E., Miller, G. M., Gelston, H. M., et al.: Effect of circumcision status on periurethral bacterial flora during the first year of life. J. Pediatr. *113*:442-446, 1988.

CHAPTER 118

PROVIDENCIA

Randall G. Fisher

The genus *Providencia* comprises pathogens most commonly associated with urinary tract infection. *Providencia* spp. are encountered most often as pathogens in hospitals or long-term care facilities and can be responsible for outbreaks of multidrug-resistant infection.[34]

BACTERIOLOGY

Providencia spp. (named after the city of Providence, RI) are motile gram-negative bacilli that do not ferment lactose and are distinguished from other Enterobacteriaceae by their ability to deaminate phenylalanine and lysine.[8,27] The genus distinguishes "urease-negative" organisms, *Providencia rettgeri, Providencia stuartii, Providencia alcalifaciens, Providencia rustigianii*, and *Providencia heimbachae*, from the otherwise biochemically similar "urease-positive" *Proteus* spp.[15,27] Urease is produced by most strains of *P. rettgeri* and by 15 percent or less of *P. stuartii* strains.[27] *Providencia* spp. also differ from other Proteeae in their ability to produce acid from inositol. Strains are differentiated further by reactivity with straight-chain hydroxy alcohols.[27] For a detailed discussion of taxonomy and characterization of *Providencia* spp., the reader is referred to the review by O'Hara and colleagues.[24]

EPIDEMIOLOGY

Providencia organisms are recovered uncommonly from stool in healthy humans, but they frequently colonize indwelling or condom urinary catheters, particularly in patients receiving antibiotic therapy.[5,10,16,34,35] In a Japanese study of patients with traveler's diarrhea, *Providencia* spp. were recovered, using a new selective medium, from 23 of 130 specimens tested.[36] *Providencia* spp. have been recognized as pathogens for more than 50 years[7]; *P. rettgeri* and *P. stuartii* are the most common species implicated in urinary tract infection.[10,12,13,21,35] Multiple biotypes of *P. stuartii* have been identified in hospital outbreaks, indicating the probability of multiple sources of colonization.[2] Ribotyping is a sensitive method for molecular characterization of isolates that may aid in analysis of outbreaks.[29]

PATHOPHYSIOLOGY

P. stuartii does not seem to have greater access to the urinary tract compared with other bacteria; in patients with long-term catheters, the incidence of bacteriuria caused by this organism is equivalent to that caused by other uropathogens.[34] Rather, *P. stuartii* manifests an extraordinary ability to persist within the catheterized urinary tract.[35] Bacteriuria may take weeks to months to clear. A mannose-resistant, *Klebsiella*-like hemagglutinin may play an important role in the persistence and adherence of *P. stuartii* to urinary tract catheters.[23]

Despite the similarities between *Proteus mirabilis* (the major pathogen responsible for urolithiasis in children)[4] and urease-producing *Providencia* spp., the latter organisms rarely are associated with formation of stones. *P. stuartii* occasionally produces urease with a higher affinity for substrate, but *P. mirabilis* ureases hydrolyze urea 6 to 25 times faster.[14] Restriction-enzyme analysis of genes coding for the respective enzymes shows significant divergence.[14] These differences may explain the more frequent association of *P. mirabilis* with formation of stones.

Some strains of *P. alcalifaciens* have been isolated more commonly in children with diarrhea, and enteropathogenicity has been shown in Hep 2 cells and a rabbit model.[2,3] Ex vivo *P. alcalifaciens* strains show the ability to translocate and to resist complement-mediated lysis.[33] In children with diarrhea, *P. alcalifaciens* often is associated with other enteric pathogens, so its role in pathogenesis remains unclear.[1]

CLINICAL MANIFESTATIONS

Although *Escherichia coli* and *Proteus* spp. account for most urinary tract infections in children, *Providencia* spp. have been reported as a cause of infection in children with spinal injury and long-term urinary tract catheterization.[17,21] Most infections have been described, however, in elderly patients or adults with spinal injury who require long-term urinary tract catheterization.[34] Clinical findings are typical of those associated with urinary tract infection. Bacteremia is uncommon but devastating.[18] In a study of 132 cases of bacteremia caused by members of the tribe Proteeae, only 8 were caused by *Providencia* spp., but four of those patients died of the infection.[18] A single case of endocarditis caused by *P. stuartii* has been reported.[19]

Eye infections caused by *P. rettgeri*, including conjunctivitis, dacryocystitis, keratitis, and endophthalmitis, have been reported. These infections generally occurred in patients with compromise in ocular surface or in immunity.[25]

Providencia spp. have been implicated in the so-called purple urine bag syndrome, in which an enzyme from the organism causes 3-indoxyl sulfate to be formed, which discolors the urine blue or blue-violet. This syndrome usually occurs in patients with indwelling cystotomy or nephrostomy tubes.[20,32]

DIAGNOSIS

Infection with *Providencia* spp. should be suspected when indole-positive, urease-negative, gram-negative rods, which oxidatively deaminate tryptophan, are isolated in culture. Because patients with long-term catheterization may be colonized with multiple organisms, *Providencia* spp. frequently are overlooked or misidentified.[7] Clinical laboratories should be encouraged to identify all bacterial colonies in patients with long-term catheterization in whom infection is suspected. Identification is particularly important because of the marked differences in susceptibility of uropathogens.[28]

TREATMENT

Empiric therapy should be guided by antimicrobial susceptibility testing of the patient's isolate and knowledge of susceptibilities of previously identified *Providencia* within the care facility. Removal of urinary tract catheters speeds eradication of these pathogens. Strains of *P. stuartii* and *P. rettgeri* commonly are resistant to many antibiotics. In a longitudinal Italian study of 223 *P. stuartii* isolates, 116 (52%) were extended-spectrum β-lactamase positive. The rate of extended-spectrum β-lactamase–positive isolates increased from 31 percent in 1999 to 62 percent in 2002.[31] Since the 1970s, multidrug resistance has emerged[26]; many strains are resistant to sulfonamides, trimethoprim, nitrofurantoin, nalidixic acid, penicillins, cephalosporins, and aminoglycosides; some singular strains are resistant to most antibiotics in common use.[28] Imipenem-resistant strains have now been described.[30] Much of the observed resistance seems to be plasmid-based[11]; quinolones and aztreonam have shown some promise in the treatment of such cases.[6,9] Complex combinations of aminoglycoside resistance that differ by hospital and geographic region can occur.[22] Organisms that are resistant to gentamicin and tobramycin may remain susceptible to amikacin.

Acknowledgments

The author thanks Dr. William Gruber and Dr. Thomas Boyce for their invaluable assistance with earlier versions of this chapter.

REFERENCES

1. Albert, M. J., Faruque, A. S., and Mahalanabis, D.: Association of *Providencia alcalifaciens* with diarrhea in children. J. Clin. Microbiol. 36:1433-1435, 1998.
2. Albert, M. J., Alam, K., Ansaruzzaman, M., et al.: Pathogenesis of *Providencia alcalifaciens*–induced diarrhea. Infect. Immun. 60:5017-5024, 1992.
3. Albert, M. J., Ansaruzzaman, M., Bhuiyan, N. A., et al.: Characteristics of invasion of HEp-2 cells by *Providencia alcalifaciens*. J. Med. Microbiol. 42:186-190, 1995.
4. Bensman, A., Roubach, L., Allouch, G., et al.: Urolithiasis in children: Presenting signs, etiology, bacteriology and localisation. Acta Paediatr. Scand. 72:879-883, 1983.
5. Breitenbucher, R. B.: Bacterial changes in the urine samples of patients with long-term indwelling catheters. Arch. Intern. Med. 144:1585-1588, 1984.
6. Cox, C. E.: Aztreonam therapy for complicated urinary tract infections caused by multidrug-resistant bacteria. Rev. Infect. Dis. 7(Suppl. 4):S767-S771, 1985.
7. Damron, D. J., Warren, J. W., Chippendale, G. R., et al.: Do clinical microbiology laboratories report complete bacteriology in urine from patients with long-term urinary catheters? J. Clin. Microbiol. 24:400-404, 1986.
8. Ewing, W. H., Tanner, K. E., and Dennard, D. A.: The Providence Group: An intermediate group of enteric bacteria. J. Infect. Dis. 94:134-140, 1954.
9. Fang, G. D., Brennen, C., Wagener, M., et al.: Use of ciprofloxacin versus use of aminoglycosides for therapy of complicated urinary tract infection: Prospective, randomized clinical and pharmacokinetic study. Antimicrob. Agents Chemother. 35:1849-1855, 1991.
10. Fierer, J., and Ekstrom, M.: An outbreak of *Providencia stuartii* urinary tract infections: Patients with condom catheters are a reservoir of the bacteria. J. A. M. A. 245:1553-1555, 1981.
11. Hawkey, P. M.: *Providencia stuartii*: A review of a multiply antibiotic-resistant bacterium. J. Antimicrob. Chemother. 13:209-226, 1984.
12. Hawkey, P. M., Penner, J. L., Potten, M. R., et al.: Prospective survey of fecal, urinary tract, and environmental colonization by *Providencia stuartii* in two geriatric wards. J. Clin. Microbiol. 16:422-426, 1982.
13. Hollick, G. E., Nolte, F. S., Calnan, B. J., et al.: Characterization of endemic *Providencia stuartii* isolates from patients with urinary devices. Eur. J. Clin. Microbiol. 3:521-525, 1984.
14. Jones, B. D., and Mobley, H. L.: Genetic and biochemical diversity of ureases of *Proteus*, *Providencia*, and *Morganella* species isolated from urinary tract infection. Infect. Immun. 55:2198-2203, 1987.
15. Jones, B. D., and Mobley, H. L.: *Proteus mirabilis* urease: Genetic organization, regulation, and expression of structural genes. J. Bacteriol. 170:3342-3349, 1988.
16. Kaslow, R. A., Lindsey, J. O., Bison, A. L., et al.: Nosocomial infection with highly resistant *Proteus rettgeri*: Report of an epidemic. Am. J. Epidemiol. 104:278-286, 1976.
17. Keren, G., and Tyrrel, D. L.: Gram-negative septicemia caused by *Providencia stuartii*. Int. J. Pediatr. Nephrol. 8:91-94, 1987.
18. Kim, B. M, Kim, N. J., Kim, M. N., et al.: Bacteremia due to tribe Proteeae: A review of 132 cases during a decade (1991-2000). Scand. J. Infect. Dis. 35:98-103, 2003.
19. Krake, P. R., and Tandon, N.: Infective endocarditis due to *Providencia stuartii*. South. Med. J. 97:1022-1023, 2004.
20. Lazimy, Y., Delotte, J., Machiavella, J. C., et al.: Purple urine bag syndrome: A case report. Prog. Urol. 17:864-865, 2007.
21. McHale, P. J., Walker, F., Scully, B., et al.: *Providencia stuartii* infections: A review of 117 cases over an eight-year period. J. Hosp. Infect. 2:155-165, 1981.

22. Miller, G. H., Sabatelli, F. J., Hare, R. S., et al.: The most frequent aminoglycoside resistance mechanisms—changes with time and geographic area: A reflection of aminoglycoside usage patterns? Aminoglycoside Resistance Study Groups. Clin. Infect. Dis. 24:S46-S62, 1997.
23. Mobley, H. L., Chippendale, G. R., Tenney, J. H., et al.: MR/K hemagglutination of Providencia stuartii correlates with adherence to catheters and with persistence in catheter-associated bacteriuria. J. Infect. Dis. 157:264-271, 1988.
24. O'Hara, C. M., Brenner, F. W., and Miller, J. M. Classification, identification, and clinical significance of Proteus, Providencia, and Morganella. Clin. Microbiol. Rev. 13:534-546, 2000.
25. Oreishi, A. F., Schechter, B. A., and Karp, C. L.: Ocular infections caused by Providencia rettgeri. Ophthalmology 113:1463-1466, 2006.
26. Overturf, G. D., Wilkins, J., and Ressler, R.: Emergence of resistant P. stuartii to multiple antibiotics: Specification and biochemical characterization of Providencia. J. Infect. Dis. 129:353-357, 1974.
27. Penner, J. L.: Providencia. In Krieg, N. R., and Holt, J. G. (eds.): Bergey's Manual of Systematic Bacteriology. Vol. 1. Baltimore, Williams & Wilkins, 1984, pp. 494-496.
28. Piccolomini, R., Cellini, L., Allocati, N., et al.: Comparative in vitro activities of 13 antimicrobial agents against Morganella-Proteus-Providencia group bacteria from urinary tract infections. Antimicrob. Agents Chemother. 31:1644-1647, 1987.
29. Pignato, S., Giammanco, G. M., Grimont, F., et al.: Molecular characterization of the genera Proteus, Morganella, and Providencia by ribotyping. J. Clin. Microbiol. 37:2840-2847, 1999.
30. Shiroto, K., Ishii, Y., Kimura, S., et al.: Metallo-beta-lactamase IMP-1 in Providencia rettgeri from two different hospitals in Japan. J. Med. Microbiol. 54:1065-1070, 2005.
31. Tumbarello, M., Citton, R., Spanu, T., et al.: ESBL-producing multidrug-resistant Providencia stuartii infections in a university hospital. J. Antimicrob. Chemother. 53:277-282, 2004.
32. Vaidyanathan, S., and Soni, B. M.: Bluish discolouration of urine drainage tube and bag in a female patient with spina bifida, paraplegia, and suprapubic cystostomy. Sci. World J. 3:1070-1072, 2007.
33. Vieira, A. B., Koh, I. H., and Guth, B. E.: Providencia alcalifaciens strains translocate from the gastrointestinal tract and are resistant to the lytic activity of serum complement. J. Med. Microbiol. 52:633-636, 2003.
34. Warren, J. W.: Providencia stuartii: A common cause of antibiotic-resistant bacteriuria in patients with long-term indwelling catheters. Rev. Infect. Dis. 8:61-67, 1986.
35. Warren, J. W., Tenney, J. H., Hoopes, J. M., et al.: A prospective microbiologic study of bacteriuria in patients with chronic indwelling urethral catheters. J. Infect. Dis. 146:719-723, 1982.
36. Yoh, M., Matsuyama, J., Ohnishi, M., et al.: Importance of Providencia species as a major cause of travellers' diarrhea. J. Med. Microbiol. 54:1077-1082, 2005.

CHAPTER 119

SHIGELLA

Theresa J. Ochoa ⊙ Thomas G. Cleary

HISTORICAL BACKGROUND

The term *dysentery* classically has been used to describe the frequent, painful passage of stools containing blood and mucus. The syndrome has been recognized since the time of Hippocrates. The differentiation of dysentery into bacillary and amebic forms followed the recognition by Shiga in 1898 that one form of dysentery was associated with a bacterium in the stools of affected individuals; their sera also were found to agglutinate the bacillus. In recognition of his achievement, the genus was eventually named after Shiga.

The most important subsequent advance has been the recognition of the molecular basis of *Shigella* virulence. In the 1960s, researchers showed that shigellae invade the corneal epithelium of guinea pigs and cause keratoconjunctivitis (Sereny test). Subsequently, Formal and colleagues[70] showed that *Shigella flexneri* invades the intestinal epithelium. Since 1980, Sansonetti and other investigators[201,203,204] have identified multiple plasmid and chromosomal virulence genes. *Shigella*-like enteroinvasive *Escherichia coli* have the same or closely related genes and produce a similar clinical syndrome.

ORGANISM

Shigellae are small, nonencapsulated gram-negative rods that are members of the family Enterobacteriaceae. Technically, they are *E. coli*, but for reasons of tradition and clinical usefulness, the designation as a separate genus has been preserved. Shigellae do not ferment lactose or do so slowly and are nonmotile (lack the H [flagellar] antigen). They lack urease and do not produce hydrogen sulfide on triple sugar iron media or gas during metabolism of carbohydrate.[62] The somatic antigen (or O antigen) side chains that determine serotype and serogroup are attached as multiple repeating units to the lipid A core and core oligosaccharides shared with other members of Enterobacteriaceae. Envelope or K antigens that are heat-labile also have been described, although their clinical relevance is uncertain.

SEROGROUP CLASSIFICATION

Four serogroups, or species, of *Shigella* are defined on the basis of serologic similarities and biochemical reactions. Group A (*Shigella dysenteriae*), mannitol nonfermenters, includes 13 serotypes having O antigens that do not cross-react immunologically. Two additional provisional serovars, types 14 and 15, also are pathogenic.[9] Serogroup D (*Shigella sonnei*), ornithine decarboxylase–positive, slow lactose fermenters, share the same lipopolysaccharide. *Shigella* strains that ferment mannitol (in contrast to *S. dysenteriae*) but do not decarboxylate ornithine or ferment lactose (in contrast to *S. sonnei*) are classified as serogroups B and C. Of these, the strains that express lipopolysaccharides that are related to each other immunologically are group B (*Shigella flexneri*), whereas the strains whose O antigens are unrelated to each other or to other shigellae are group C (*Shigella boydii*). Multiple serotypes of *S. flexneri* (15 serotypes and subtypes) and of *S. boydii* (18 serotypes) exist.

EPIDEMIOLOGY

An estimated 164.7 million cases of shigellosis occur annually, of which 99 percent occur in developing countries, with 1.1 million deaths, 61 percent of which involve children younger than 5 years old.[116] Generally, *Shigella* spp. are associated with 5 to 10 percent of all diarrhea cases and 30 percent of dysentery cases.[162] Although epidemic *Shigella* dysentery is the most dramatic manifestation of *Shigella* infections in developing countries, most infections are caused by endemic shigellosis. Endemic shigellosis is responsible for approximately 10 percent of all diarrheal episodes among children younger than 5 years of age in developing countries.[65] Despite the fact that severe dehydration usually is not seen in shigellosis, 75 percent of diarrheal deaths may be due to these infections.[162] According to surveillance reports of the Centers for Disease Control and Prevention, 10,000 to 15,000 cases of shigellosis have been documented each year during the last 30 years in the United States, for annual incidence rates of 5 to 10 per 100,000.[45]

Because shigellae are spread through a fecal-oral route, they are especially prevalent where hygiene is poor. The organisms can be cultured from around toilets in homes where shigellae have caused disease. Toilet paper does not prevent contamination of fingers. Shigellae are transmitted easily from person to person because the inoculum size required to cause disease is only 10 organisms in the case of *S. dysenteriae* serotype 1[60] and a few hundred organisms in the cases of *S. sonnei* and *S. flexneri*.[59] Handwashing and wearing gloves are mandatory procedures for individuals caring for patients with bacillary dysentery. Patients who lack the acid barrier provided by a normally functioning stomach because of prior gastrectomy or use of antacid are at increased risk of acquiring infection.

Shigellae survive for 30 days in foods such as milk, whole eggs, oysters, shrimp, and flour.[147] Epidemics usually are associated with exposure to contaminated water or food, although as might be predicted from the inoculum size, outbreaks related to swimming also occur.[137] Houseflies can be colonized with shigellae in their guts without illness and pass the organisms in their feces. Feces adherent to their legs can lead to contamination of food. Flies have been implicated in epidemics of shigellosis, particularly where the fly population is large. *Shigella* infection shows seasonal variation. In North America, few cases occur in the winter, whereas in tropical regions, the peak is during the rainy season. Shigellae are worldwide and thrive where susceptible individuals are grouped together (including institutions for retarded or mentally ill individuals, prisoner-of-war camps, Indian reservations, the military, daycare centers, and the developing world).[110,178,212] Spread within families is a common occurrence.

The species of *Shigella* causing most infections vary according to regions. In developed countries, *S. sonnei* is the most common species, followed by *S. flexneri* (approximately 70% *S. sonnei* and 25% *S. flexneri*); however, in the developing world, this pattern is reversed, with *S. flexneri* being more common than *S. sonnei*. *S. dysenteriae* serotype 1 occurs primarily in Africa, India, and Bangladesh. *S. boydii* is found primarily on the Indian subcontinent.[162]

Humans and other primates can be infected with shigellae, and an age-related risk of acquiring symptomatic shigellosis exists. In contrast to *Salmonella* spp., which cause disease most frequently in the first few months of life, shigellae infrequently cause illness in the first 6 months of life. The peak incidence occurs in children between 1 and 4 years of age, with fewer cases occurring in children aged 5 to 9 years old. Adults are at lower risk.

PATHOGENESIS

INVASIVENESS AND TOXIN PRODUCTION

The ability to invade mammalian cells is the most important virulence trait of *Shigella* spp.[74,122,129,159,169] Uptake by M cells overlying Peyer patches with ingestion by macrophages under the M cells induces production of cytokines and recruitment of polymorphonuclear leukocytes. Apoptosis is induced in macrophages after ingestion of shigellae; these events are accompanied by release of interleukin-1 (IL-1), IL-1β, and IL-18, which triggers other inflammatory events.[203,227,229] Polymorphonuclear leukocytes enter the gut lumen by moving between epithelial cells. The gaps between epithelial cells may be the portal of entry of bacteria into the epithelium. After penetration of intestinal epithelial cells, shigellae are located in vacuoles derived from the cytoplasmic membrane of the mucosal cells. The bacteria lyse these vacuoles, move intracellularly, multiply, kill the epithelial cells, and infect adjacent cells. Cell death is followed by formation of ulcerations and microabscesses in the colon. In contrast to *Salmonella* infection, *Shigella* infection rarely spreads beyond the

lamina propria, so bacteremia and metastatic infections are uncommon.

The genetic basis of virulence has been studied extensively.[170,174] Invasiveness is the result primarily of genes on a large 120- to 140-MDa (200- to 220-kb) virulence plasmid.[81,82,88,200-202,204] These genes encode a molecular apparatus called a type III secretion system that is capable of injecting bacterial proteins through bacterial and host membranes into host cells (translocation) or the extracellular milieu (secretion) to influence host biochemistry and cell physiology directly.[174] The invasive plasmid antigen (ipa) region includes genes for four polypeptides needed for invasion: *ipaA*, *ipaB*, *ipaC*, and *ipaD*. The proteins produced by these loci are recognized by the humoral immune system. The product of the *ipaB* locus is essential for induction of apoptosis in macrophages.[228] The mxi-spa region of the virulence plasmid is necessary for orientation of the ipa-encoded proteins into the outer membrane of the bacteria. The *virG* gene encodes a protein that causes intracellular and intercellular spread of shigellae after invasion of epithelial cells. The *virF* gene regulates a locus (*virB*) that is responsible for positive regulation of the ipa genes.[192]

Chromosomal loci also regulate virulence.[173] Chromosomal loci regulate expression of the virulence plasmid. The keratoconjunctivitis provocation (*kcpA*) gene is a positive regulator of the *virG* virulence plasmid gene that determines ability to spread within and between cells. The chromosomal *virR* gene is a temperature regulator that represses expression of ipa genes at 30° C, but not at 37° C.

Lipopolysaccharides (LPSs) play a role in resistance to nonspecific host defense mechanisms that are encountered during invasion of tissue. The *Shigella* LPS induces the trafficking of Toll-like receptor 4, the dominant mediator of the innate immune response.[42] Smooth colonies express the complete complex of LPS O side chains required for full virulence—ability to invade epithelial cells, to multiply within them, and to resist phagocytosis.[77,171] Rough colonial variants that lack complete LPS do not penetrate epithelial cells efficiently and are avirulent.

Some strains of *Shigella* spp. produce toxins that injure mammalian cells. A chromosomal locus in *S. dysenteriae* serotype 1 encodes a protein synthesis–inhibiting exotoxin (Shiga toxin) that is a major virulence factor in this serotype (and in the enterohemorrhagic *E. coli* serotypes that have the same or closely related genes).[25,207] This toxin is composed of a single copy of an A subunit (32,000 daltons) that is linked to five copies of B subunits (7790 daltons).[167] The B subunits bind to a glycolipid cell receptor, globotriaosylceramide, followed by internalization. The A subunit cleaves an adenine residue from the eukaryotic 28S ribosomal subunit. The resulting block in elongation factor 1–dependent binding of aminoacyl tRNA to the ribosome causes cell death through inhibition of protein synthesis.[167] Shiga toxin previously was considered to be a neurotoxin because its administration to mice or rabbits caused paralysis and death[37,44,92]; it now is thought to target primarily the vascular endothelium. It causes fluid accumulation in rabbit ileal loops[64,111] that probably is related to reduced fluid uptake by damaged villus cells.

The severity of *S. dysenteriae* serotype 1 infection relative to other *Shigella* serotypes is thought to be caused by production of Shiga toxin. Enterohemorrhagic *E. coli* serotypes, such as *E. coli* O157:H7, produce an identical (Shiga toxin 1) or similar (Shiga toxin 2) toxin and, similar to *S. dysenteriae* serotype 1, cause bloody diarrhea and hemolytic-uremic syndrome. Enteroinvasive *E. coli* serotypes do not produce these toxins.[50]

Shigella spp. also produce two enterotoxins, ShET-1 and ShET-2.[218] All *S. flexneri* 2a strains produce ShET-1, whereas only 3.3 percent of other *Shigella* serotypes and no enteroinvasive *E. coli* serotypes possess the gene for this toxin.[163] ShET-2 is produced by all *Shigella* spp.[218] Genes of an additional toxin, designated *Shigella* enterotoxin, or Sen, have been found in 75 percent of enteroinvasive *E. coli* serotypes and 83 percent of *Shigella* strains.[156] These enterotoxins may contribute to the high-volume, watery diarrhea often seen in the initial stages of the disease.[19] Vaccine studies using a mutant with deletions of these toxin genes have shown that one or both enterotoxins play a role in human disease.[117]

IMMUNE RESPONSE

Serum IgG, IgM, and IgA responses occur to the LPS and invasion plasmid antigens of shigellae.[166] Secretory IgA specific to both of these sets of antigens occurs in human milk and feces.[51] Protection is thought to be serotype-specific. The level of IgG antibodies to LPS present in an individual before infection occurs determines whether symptomatic shigellosis develops.[55] No clear proof currently exists about the role of antibodies to the invasion plasmid virulence proteins or to the toxins. Cell-mediated immunity against shigellae also may play a role in resolution of infection. Production of $\alpha\beta$ T cells and natural killer cells mediates interferon-γ production that may be essential to defense from *Shigella*.[124,222] Antibody-dependent cellular cytotoxicity against shigellae has been shown.

During infection, shigellae use effectors secreted via the type III secretion system to direct various cellular signaling pathways and to modify the innate immune activation of the host. More recent evidence indicates that a large part of the mucosal inflammation is initiated by intracellular sensing of bacterial peptidoglycan by cytosolic leucin-rich receptors of the NOD family in epithelial cells.[170,175] This causes activation of the nuclear factor κB and other terminal kinase pathways, with IL-8 appearing as a major chemokine mediating the inflammatory burst that is dominated by massive infiltration of the mucosa by polymorphonuclear leukocytes.[175] The levels of cytokines tumor necrosis factor-α, IL-1β, IL-1RA, IL-6, IL-8, and granulocyte-macrophage colony-stimulating factor in stool correlate with the severity of shigellosis. In contrast to other cytokines, interferon-γ and its receptor[186] are depressed early and increase during recovery. Fecal concentrations of tumor necrosis factor-α, IL-1β, IL-1RA, IL-6, IL-8, and granulocyte-macrophage colony-stimulating factor are significantly higher in patients with *S. dysenteriae* serotype 1 than in patients with *S. flexneri* infection.[189] Elevated tumor necrosis factor-α and IL-6 levels in stool and serum have been associated with complications during infection with *S. dysenteriae* serotype 1.[85] Infiltration of polymorphonuclear leukocytes and lymphocytes into the intestine is controlled by these cytokines. Epithelial cell production of IL-8[199] and a low IL-1RA-to-IL-1 ratio[11] are responsible for the severe inflammation. T lymphocytes with suppressor-cytotoxic and helper-inducer phenotypes are recruited into the epithelium and lamina propria during infection with *Shigella*, related partly to the induction of HLA-DR expression in the rectal mucosa.[187] Peripheral blood lymphocytes of infected individuals respond to *Shigella* antigens in vitro with production of interferon-γ and IL-10.[198]

Shigella spp. elicit an inflammatory response during multiplication within macrophages and epithelial cells. *Shigella* multiplication in macrophage cytoplasm induces cell death, which is achieved by two distinctive pathways: activation of caspase-1 by IpaB secreted by the type III secretion system, and translocation of lipid A from the cytosol, which occurs independent of caspase-1 and Toll-like receptor 4 activities.[170]

PATHOLOGY

The main morphologic changes of shigellosis (superficial ulcerations, focal hemorrhages, mucosal edema, erythema, and friability) occur in the colon where the organisms invade.[97,208] The rectosigmoid and distal segments of the colon typically are involved more severely than is the proximal colon. The epithelial cell damage may cause development of a pseudomembrane composed of thick, fibropurulent exudate tightly adherent to the necrotic ulcerated colonic mucosa. Pseudopolyposis also has been reported.[39] On microscopic examination, damage to epithelial cells, ulcerations, goblet cell depletion, and intense polymorphonuclear and mononuclear infiltration with crypt abscesses are seen. Rectal mucosa shows increased numbers of CD8$^+$ and $\gamma\delta^+$ T cells.[95] Vessels in the lamina propria are congested or thrombosed. Perforation of the colon usually does not occur as part of the colitis.[23] Evidence of inflammation and proinflammatory cytokines persists for at least 1 month after clinical resolution.[185] Histologic changes generally are more severe and persistent[96] with *S. dysenteriae* than with *S. flexneri*.[8]

CLINICAL MANIFESTATIONS

The incubation period ranges from 12 hours to a few days (if a low number of organisms is ingested). Onset of high fever, toxicity, and crampy abdominal pain is sudden. During the first 48 hours, high-volume watery diarrhea may occur (small bowel phase of disease); subsequently, low-volume, bloody, and mucous diarrhea develops in association with urgency and tenesmus (large bowel or "dysenteric" disease). In some cases, the watery diarrhea persists for several days, without subsequent development of dysentery. Other children present with bloody or mucous diarrhea.

Physical examination shows fever, signs of toxicity, tenderness over the lower abdominal quadrants, and hyperactive bowel sounds. Signs of dehydration may be present. Rectal examination reveals severe tenderness. Rectal prolapse may be present, particularly when diarrhea is associated with malnutrition.

The course without therapy typically lasts 7 to 10 days. Protein-losing enteropathy occurs during shigellosis; this enteropathy is severe with *S. dysenteriae* serotype 1.[32] In addition, anorexia related to fever and abdominal pain contributes further to malnutrition, particularly in *S. dysenteriae* type 1 infection.[184] These facts may explain partly the hypoproteinemia and adverse effect on growth of severe shigellosis. Malnutrition is associated with a more severe course of shigellosis. Fever may not develop, even when severe dysentery is present. Chronic infection may last for months, despite administration of appropriate antibiotic therapy. It may cause further deterioration of the nutritional status, which together with other complications (e.g., ileus, bacteremia, and pneumonia) is associated with overall increased mortality rates from shigellosis. Surgical complications of shigellosis are rare but are associated with significant morbidity and mortality because of delay in establishing the diagnosis. In a series of 57 children with surgical complications of shigellosis,[148] intestinal obstruction (53%), appendicitis (28%), and colonic perforation (17%) were the most common (Table 119–1).

Although the organism usually is excreted for only a few days or weeks (range 1 to 30 days), carriage for many months sometimes occurs.[52,130] The illness usually is acute; a chronic carrier state can occur in malnourished individuals. Asymptomatic infection of toddlers living in an endemic area occurs commonly. Most *Shigella* infections in Mexican children who were cultured each week from birth were not associated with symptoms.[80]

EXTRAINTESTINAL MANIFESTATIONS AND COMPLICATIONS

Multiple extraintestinal complications have been described with *Shigella* infection (see Table 119–1). Seizures have been reported in 10 to 45 percent of hospitalized children with culture-proven shigellosis.[17,21,24,57,68] In outpatient settings, the frequency of seizures is very low. Children who develop neurologic complaints

TABLE 119-1 Complications of Shigellosis

Abdominal
Persistent diarrhea
Post-dysenteric irritable bowel syndrome
Ileus, toxic megacolon, intestinal perforation
Protein-losing enteropathy, malnutrition
Surgical complications: intestinal perforation and obstruction, appendicitis, intra-abdominal abscesses

Neurologic
Seizures
Headache, lethargy, disorientation, hallucinations
Coma
Severe toxin encephalopathy or ekiri syndrome

Bacteremia
In malnourished children, young infants, and AIDS patients

Hemolytic-uremic syndrome
Only with *Shigella dysenteriae* serotype 1

Urogenital
Vulvovaginitis, urinary tract infections

Other
Conjunctivitis, keratitis, corneal ulcers
Reactive arthritis
Reiter syndrome
Hepatitis
Myocarditis

may have lethargy, severe headache, disorientation, hallucinations, or self-limited convulsions lasting less than 15 minutes.[15,18,21,152] Seizures are most likely to occur in very young patients, patients with a high peak body temperature, and patients with a family history of convulsive disorders.[17,118] Seizures can be focal, although usually they are generalized.

When symptoms related to the nervous system occur, they are likely to appear early in the illness, even preceding development of diarrhea. Death rarely has been described[90]; most children recover completely with no residual neurologic deficits.[18] In contrast, in Bangladesh, where seizures in shigellosis typically are associated with factors known to alter consciousness (e.g., hypoglycemia, hyponatremia, fever), mortality rates are high.[114] The pathogenesis of neurologic signs and symptoms during episodes of shigellosis is unclear. Hypoglycemia and electrolyte abnormalities are found in a few patients.[18] Direct invasion of the central nervous system during *Shigella* bacteremia is very rare.[223] Simple febrile seizures might explain convulsions in a few children with dysentery, but some children who have seizures during episodes of shigellosis do not experience seizures during other febrile infections and are outside the age range usually associated with febrile seizures.[18] Shiga toxin formerly was thought to cause the neurologic symptoms because it was considered to be a neurotoxin; however, data now clearly show that Shiga toxin is not responsible.[16]

Severe toxic encephalopathy has been described. This syndrome (ekiri), as originally described in Japan, was characterized by dysentery with hyperpyrexia, convulsions, sensory disturbances, and rapid progression to death.[193] The children died with cerebral edema early in the course of disease (6 to 48 hours after onset). Mild hyponatremia has been a common finding.[76] Children with ekiri did not have sepsis, disseminated intravascular coagulation, hemolytic-uremic syndrome, or severe dehydration. This toxic encephalopathy is rare. Whether this syndrome is part of a continuum of central nervous system dysfunctions with seizures and other encephalopathic symptoms or has a completely different pathogenesis is unclear.

Hemolytic-uremic syndrome (microangiopathic hemolytic anemia, thrombocytopenia, and acute renal failure) or isolated hemolysis has been reported, mainly after infections with *S. dysenteriae* serotype 1 and rarely after infection with *S. flexneri*.[182] Vascular endothelial cell damage by Shiga toxin is considered to be the initial event, although endotoxin absorbed from the gut also may play a role.[115]

Ileus that progresses to toxic megacolon with distended loops and eventual intestinal perforation occurs.[22] It is seen mainly with *S. dysenteriae* serotype 1 infection.

Septicemia in shigellosis is a rare occurrence except in malnourished children, young infants, and children with *S. dysenteriae* serotype 1 infections.[84,143,205] The mortality rate is at least twice as high in dysentery-associated sepsis as in shigellosis uncomplicated by bacteremia. The serogroup-related mortality risk in shigellemia has been reported to be 85 percent for infection with *S. dysenteriae*, 43 percent for infection with *S. flexneri*, and 25 percent for infection with *S. sonnei*; bacteremia rarely is reported with *S. boydii* infection.[141] In Bangladesh, *Shigella* bacteremia was found in 4 percent of patients.[213] When bacteremia occurs with dysentery, it is as likely to be caused by other enteric bacteria as by the *Shigella* itself. The occurrence of *Klebsiella*, *E. coli*, and other enteric pathogens in blood cultures of children with shigellosis presumably reflects loss of the barrier function during severe colitis.[158] *Shigella* bacteremia may be complicated by disseminated intravascular coagulation and multiorgan failure. Bronchopneumonia may develop in septicemic children,[4] but its pathogenesis is unclear. Children who die with shigellosis often have pneumonia at autopsy.[39]

Other extraintestinal infections rarely are caused by *Shigella* spp. Vaginitis with a bloody discharge (sometimes lasting for months in the absence of specific therapy) may occur, usually without concurrent or recent diarrhea.[56,154] *Shigella* cystitis, not always associated with diarrhea, has been described, usually in girls.[24] Conjunctivitis, keratitis, corneal ulcers, and iritis are other uncommon manifestations of shigellosis that usually are assumed to occur after autoinoculation.[24,216] Reactive arthritis or Reiter syndrome (arthritis, urethritis, conjunctivitis) may develop after episodes of shigellosis,[41] especially in adults who are HLA-B27-positive; reactive arthritis is uncommon in children. Hepatitis with mildly abnormal liver function test results has been described.[211] Myocarditis manifested clinically by hypotension despite fluid replacement, arrhythmia, heart block, or low voltage on electrocardiography and pathologically by interstitial lymphocytic infiltrates and focal necrosis has been described.[191] Post-dysenteric irritable bowel syndrome occurs in some patients after recovery.[221]

SHIGELLOSIS IN THE NEONATAL PERIOD

Bacillary dysentery is rare in newborns.[25,61,66,83,123] More than half of the reported neonatal cases occurred during the infants' first 3 days of life, consistent with fecal-oral transmission during delivery,[78,160] usually from a symptomatic mother. Although a neonate with shigellosis usually has only low-grade fever with diarrhea of variable severity,[5,120,150] septicemia[127,181] and chronic diarrhea are more common than in older children. Intestinal perforation has been reported in neonatal shigellosis.[210] Diarrhea more often is nonbloody in infants; fever also occurs less commonly than in older children.[94] Data on age-related mortality caused by shigellosis in developing countries suggest that the mortality rate of the neonate is more than twice that of older children.

SHIGELLOSIS IN ACQUIRED IMMUNODEFICIENCY SYNDROME

In patients with acquired immunodeficiency syndrome (AIDS), shigellosis not only is more common and more severe, but also is associated more often with bacteremia.[26,93] In contrast to the usual short, self-limited course of shigellosis, *Shigella* infection in patients with AIDS may be chronic and relapsing, despite appropriate antibiotic treatment.[121,206]

LABORATORY FINDINGS

The fecal leukocyte examination is helpful in evaluating a patient with fever and watery diarrhea. Direct microscopic examination of fecal mucus stained with methylene blue shows many polymorphonuclear leukocytes in patients with colitis, including most patients with shigellosis.[87] The blood leukocyte count in patients with shigellosis often is normal, although leukopenia or leukocytosis may occur.[13] The differential of the blood leukocyte count typically shows an increased percentage of band forms. Approximately one third of children with shigellosis have more bands than segmented neutrophils in their peripheral blood smear. A leukemoid reaction, with a peripheral leukocyte count greater than 50,000/mm³, has been reported, mainly with infections caused by *S. dysenteriae* serotype 1.[40] A leukemoid reaction has been reported in 10 percent of patients infected with the Shiga bacillus. When examination of cerebrospinal fluid is performed in children with neurologic symptoms, normal results usually are obtained, although some patients have a mild lymphocytic pleocytosis. Likewise, when electroencephalography is performed, the results usually are normal.[18]

DIAGNOSIS

Bacillary dysentery usually is suspected in children who present with bloody diarrhea, high fever, and generalized toxicity. Approximately half of children do not develop bloody diarrhea during the course of their disease. This fact is especially relevant in developed countries, where most infections are caused by *S. sonnei*. The presence of only watery diarrhea does not exclude the possibility of shigellosis in an ill patient with high fever.

ISOLATION TECHNIQUES

Proof of the diagnosis of suspected bacillary dysentery often is problematic. Definite diagnosis of *Shigella* infection depends on isolation of the organism from stool specimens or rectal swabs. The bacteria may not survive in fecal specimens during transit, however, and special selective media are necessary for isolation. Recovery of shigellae is easier early in the course of the disease than later because the number of viable organisms in stools decreases significantly during late stages of the disease. Even in adult volunteer studies, when appropriate stool cultures were obtained daily, cultures failed to isolate shigellae in approximately 20 percent of volunteers who had ingested the organism and developed diarrhea.

Several measures increase the likelihood of isolating *Shigella*. Specimens should be processed without delay. If a specimen cannot be processed immediately, a transport medium, such as buffered glycerol saline, should be used. More than one stool culture or rectal swab should be obtained and inoculated promptly onto at least two different culture media. Specimens should be plated lightly onto MacConkey, xylose-lysine-deoxycholate, or eosin–methylene blue agar, whereas a heavier plating is necessary for the more inhibitory *Shigella*-*Salmonella* medium.[151,215] After overnight incubation at 37° C, lactose-negative colonies are transferred to triple sugar iron and lysine iron agar slants and incubated again overnight. Slants showing characteristic reactions of alkaline red slants, acid butt, and production of gas are tested biochemically for presumptive identification and then serologically for definitive identification.

OTHER DIAGNOSTIC METHODS

Because presumptive identification of *Shigella* takes at least 48 hours and definite identification takes approximately 72 hours, attempts to develop rapid diagnostic methods are being made, especially because institution of early treatment is important in shigellosis. Identification of shigellae by specific DNA probes with use of either restriction fragments or synthetic oligonucleotides[161] based on detecting virulence genes located on the 120- to 140-MDa plasmid has been described. Because the invasion plasmids of shigellae, similar to other plasmids, may be lost spontaneously, a DNA probe derived from *S. flexneri ipaH* gene, a multicopy element that is found on the chromosome and on the invasion plasmid of shigellae, has been developed and found to be more sensitive than are probes used previously.[219] Use of polymerase chain reaction (PCR) in vitro amplification of nucleic acids, to detect shigellae directly from stool specimens, has been reported.[71] PCR can detect as few as 10 colony-forming units of *S. flexneri* in stool specimens, whereas the sensitivities of DNA probe hybridization (with no amplification) and standard biochemical methods are 10³ and 10⁶ colony-forming units. PCR for *ipaH* genes seems to be more sensitive than culture; 28 percent of patients with dysentery with a positive PCR assay result are culture negative.[73,99] Another new method for the identification of *Shigella* is microarray analysis using the *gyrB* genes.[106] This novel approach also renders it possible to identify simultaneously other enteric pathogens, such as *Salmonella* spp. and diarrheogenic *E. coli*.[106]

Serologic studies are not helpful in establishing the diagnosis of shigellosis in individual patients; humoral antibodies develop after clinical recovery. Serologic studies may be helpful, however, in epidemiologic studies to define spread of the disease in a population.[24]

Sigmoidoscopy and barium enema study are unnecessary, unless they are indicated to rule out other conditions. When these procedures are performed in patients with a possibility of having shigellosis, caution is necessary because of the diffuse acute colitis.

DIFFERENTIAL DIAGNOSIS

Colitis of any etiology manifesting with acute-onset bloody diarrhea with fever and abdominal cramps can mimic shigellosis. Etiologic agents to be considered include *Campylobacter* spp., *Salmonella* spp., *Clostridium difficile*, *Yersinia enterocolitica*, *Shigella* spp., *Vibrio parahaemolyticus*, enteroinvasive *E. coli*, enterohemorrhagic *E. coli* (e.g., serotype O157:H7), *Balantidium coli*, and *Entamoeba histolytica*. The initial presentation of inflammatory bowel disease can mimic shigellosis.

An etiologic diagnosis of acute colitis syndrome on the basis of clinical presentation is difficult to make, although some data suggest a specific causative agent. In developed countries, *Campylobacter* is the most common cause of acute infectious colitis. Shigellosis should be suspected when evidence exists of person-to-person spread, and when convulsions or other neurologic symptoms develop. In the first few months of life, *Salmonella* is the most common infectious cause of bloody diarrhea, and *Shigella* is very rare.

A history of previous antibiotic treatment suggests diarrhea related to *C. difficile*, and previous consumption of seafood suggests *V. parahaemolyticus*. *Yersinia* infections are found mainly in the cooler regions of Europe and North America; the disease may mimic acute appendicitis because of the right lower quadrant pain associated with mesenteric lymphadenitis.

Enterohemorrhagic *E. coli* infection often causes bloody diarrhea with little or no fever, in contrast to shigellosis, in which high fever is typical. Negative stool cultures for the mentioned bacterial pathogens may suggest infection by enteroinvasive *E. coli.* Amebiasis causes a colitis similar to the colitis caused by *Shigella*,[209] although it is of slower onset, with a lower degree of fever; the findings on fecal leukocyte examination are negative. The involvement of the colon with amebiasis is less diffuse than in shigellosis; areas of normal mucosa are found between ulcerations.

A prolonged course with negative cultures should raise concern about the possible presence of either ulcerative colitis or Crohn disease. When watery diarrhea is present, the list of possible etiologic agents is even longer, although many agents that cause watery diarrhea are associated with little or no fever and are not confused with shigellosis. The diagnosis usually cannot be made by clinical presentation alone and depends on culture results or other specific laboratory assays.

TREATMENT

FLUID ADMINISTRATION

Dehydration is less a problem with shigellosis than with rotavirus or toxigenic *E. coli* infection. Some children with shigellosis, particularly young infants, have dehydration during the course of the disease. The high-volume watery diarrhea seen early in the course of the disease may cause excess losses of fluids and electrolytes; likewise, in patients with severe colitis, systemic toxicity and vomiting may cause anorexia that interferes with fluid intake.

Assessment of the hydration status of the patient on admission is mandatory, with early institution of appropriate fluid and electrolyte therapy needed. The World Health Organization's oral rehydration therapy with glucose-electrolyte solutions usually is effective.[155] This solution contains 90 mEq/L of sodium, 20 mEq/L of potassium, 80 mEq/L of chloride, 30 mEq/L of bicarbonate or citrate, and 20 g/L of glucose. Oral rehydration therapy should be given with additional water containing no electrolytes to prevent hypernatremia; this therapy is particularly important in children too young to express their need for additional free water. In infants, 2 parts of oral rehydration solution should be followed by 1 part of water without electrolytes. Oral rehydration with commercially available solutions (e.g., Pedialyte) also is acceptable. Administration of intravenous fluid therapy is necessary in children who are comatose, have an ileus, or are in shock. Early (12 to 24 hours after oral fluids are begun) reinstitution of breast milk or other food is mandatory.

ANTIBIOTIC THERAPY

Children who have dysentery always should be treated empirically with antimicrobials. Antibiotic therapy for milder illness is controversial. World Health Organization guidelines suggest that presumptive shigellosis should be treated with antibiotics, the choice being decided by the antimicrobial susceptibility pattern of locally circulating *Shigella* strains (WHO/CDR/95.3). If after 2 days of therapy, the patient's condition improves, a full course of 5 days should be given. If the patient does not improve, the antibiotic should be changed. If with the second antibiotic, the patient does not show signs of improvement, the diagnosis must be reviewed, and stool microscopy, culture, and susceptibility testing should be performed.[162]

Appropriate antimicrobial therapy of shigellosis shortens the duration of fever and diarrhea, and it apparently also reduces the risk of developing complications.[12] Shedding of the organisms in stools stops within 1 to 2 days, so that intrafamilial spread may be decreased. Although use of antibiotics may favor emergence of resistant organisms, most authorities recommend that antibi-

otics be started when shigellosis first is suspected clinically, before culture confirmation of the infection is obtained. Therapy should be stopped or changed on the basis of culture results (e.g., another pathogen or a resistant *Shigella* strain is isolated) and clinical response.

The choice of antimicrobial agent is complicated by the increasing frequency of plasmid-mediated antibiotic resistance.[63,67,197] Organisms resistant to ampicillin, trimethoprim-sulfamethoxazole, tetracycline, and chloramphenicol have been reported from the Middle East,[1,6,10,19,64,86,105,224] Africa,[1,35,43,108,142,157] South America,[132,156,164,180] Europe,[25,46,101,107,119,139,220] Eurasia,[23,172,225] Asia,[2,7,34,112,131,133,135,138] and the South Pacific. Currently, ampicillin and trimethoprim-sulfamethoxazole are inappropriate for empiric therapy; they should be used only if the organism has been shown to be susceptible.[12]

Multiresistant strains also are found commonly in some parts of the United States. Among 344 *Shigella* isolates, from 1999 to 2001, 95 percent were resistant to one or more antimicrobial agents, and 70 percent were resistant to two or more agents. Ampicillin resistance occurred in 80 percent of isolates, and trimethoprim-sulfamethoxazole resistance occurred in approximately 50 percent of isolates. None of the isolates was resistant to ceftriaxone or gentamicin, and only one isolate (0.3%) was resistant to ciprofloxacin. Susceptibility testing against azithromycin was not performed.[176]

Multiresistant *Shigella* spp. are particularly likely to emerge in individuals who are exposed to multiple antibiotics[214] (e.g., patients with AIDS) and individuals who recently have traveled to areas with known resistance. Likewise, children in daycare centers are at risk of acquiring resistant organisms because the frequent use of antibiotics for otitis media may favor selection and emergence of resistant enteric organisms, and because crowding and poor hygiene facilitate transmission.[36]

Generally, shigellae are susceptible in vitro to azithromycin, ceftriaxone, cefotaxime, cefixime, nalidixic acid, and quinolones in the United States and elsewhere. In vitro susceptibility does not always predict clinical efficacy or superiority of one drug over another, however. The first-generation and second-generation cephalosporins are active in vitro but have been ineffective in clinical trials. Clinical studies have shown some drugs to be clearly superior to others when susceptibility data have suggested that either might work well.

Prevalent serotypes and resistance patterns vary from year to year in a given locale. Typically, rates of resistance are related to the severity of disease caused by a given serotype. The more likely an organism is to cause severe disease, the more likely that resistant strains will emerge. *S. dysenteriae* serotype 1 is more likely to be multiply resistant than *S. flexneri*; *S. flexneri* is more likely to be resistant than *S. sonnei*. In Africa[35,108] and Asia,[28,30,49,138,153] Shiga bacilli resistant to nalidixic acid and ciprofloxacin have been reported. Nalidixic acid–resistant *S. flexneri* also have been recognized occasionally.[48] Local resistance patterns, history of travel to an area of frequent resistance,[214] and severity of illness should determine treatment.

Given the frequent occurrence of resistant organisms, optimal empiric therapy in children with dysentery should be azithromycin, a third-generation cephalosporin, nalidixic acid, or ciprofloxacin (Table 119–2).[12,27,100,126,162,176] Although less well studied, ampicillin-sulbactam and pivmecillinam also have been shown to be effective in children. In children, oral cefixime seems to be superior to ampicillin-sulbactam.[89] Adults do not respond well to usual doses of cefixime.[196] Ampicillin, tetracycline, and chloramphenicol are used infrequently now for shigellosis.

Use of quinolones has been controversial in children. An oral fluoroquinolone (ciprofloxacin, norfloxacin) seems to be optimal for adults.[14,33,89,125,140,179,195] Limited data suggest that not all of these agents are equally effective, even when in vitro data suggest

TABLE 119–2 Antibiotic Treatment of Shigellosis in Children

Antibiotic	Dosage*	Comments
Ampicillin	100 mg/kg/day divided q6h PO, IV, or IM (maximum 4 g/day)	Currently of limited value because of the high frequency of resistance; it can be used when the organism is known to be susceptible
Trimethoprim-sulfamethoxazole	10 mg/kg/day of trimethoprim divided q12h PO (maximum 320/1600 mg/day)	Currently of limited value because of the high frequency of resistance; it can be used when the organism is known to be susceptible
Azithromycin	12 mg/kg/day once daily PO on day 1, followed by 6 mg/kg/day once daily on days 2-5 (maximum 500 mg/day)	Although limited published data in children, its use is recommended by many experts
Nalidixic acid	55 mg/kg/day divided q6h PO (maximum 2 g/day)	Not available in the United States; contraindicated in infants <3 mo old
Ciprofloxacin	15-30 mg/kg/day divided q12h PO (maximum 1.5 g/day)	Alternative when other options unavailable
Cefixime	8 mg/kg/day divided q12-24h PO (maximum 400 mg/day)	
Ceftriaxone	50 mg/kg/day IM or IV q24h (maximum 2 g/day)	Current drug of choice for empiric therapy of severe dysentery in children

*Treatment should be given for 5 days.

susceptibility. Norfloxacin is clinically superior to nalidixic acid in children and adults with shigellosis.[33,190] Nalidixic acid therapy is effective treatment,[194] although plasmid-mediated resistance to nalidixic acid of *S. dysenteriae* serotype 1 strains in Bangladesh[28,30,153] has emerged and spread rapidly. Various other quinolones have been effective in adult patients with shigellosis, but they are not approved for use in children younger than 17 years old because of potential damage to the cartilage of epiphyseal plates.[190] A considerable body of evidence from the long-term use of these drugs in children with cystic fibrosis has been accumulated, however, as has evidence from short-term use to treat typhoid fever and dysentery in children; no evidence of bone or joint toxicity or growth impairment has been found. Nalidixic acid does not cause arthropathy or limit growth when it is used for a short time.[165]

As resistance continues to increase, situations are likely to occur in which a quinolone is the only option for treatment of a child with severe shigellosis. Data for children suggest that norfloxacin at a dose of 10 to 15 mg/kg/day or ciprofloxacin at a dose of 10 mg/kg every 12 hours (maximum 500 mg/dose) for 5 days is effective therapy.[79,125,136,195] In adults, short-course therapy (1 or 2 days) with ciprofloxacin has been effective for treatment of infections caused by *Shigella* spp. other than *S. dysenteriae*, for which a 10-dose, 5-day regimen is superior.[31] Pediatric data suggest that even for *S. dysenteriae* serotype 1, a short course of ciprofloxacin (15 mg/kg/dose every 12 hours for 3 days) is as effective as a 5-day course.[226]

Because the patterns of antibiotic resistance of shigellae change, susceptibility testing should be performed on all clinical isolates, and the treatment should be changed accordingly. The recommended duration of antibiotic therapy for shigellosis usually is 5 days. Studies in adults and children have shown, however, that short-course treatment is nearly as effective as are multiple doses in terms of symptomatic improvement,[75,140] although eradication of the organism from stools is less likely to occur with a single-dose regimen.[102] Because a major goal of antibiotic therapy is to reduce person-to-person transmission, multiple doses are preferred.

After initiation of therapy, a resistant organism can be suspected in the event of persistence of fever, grossly bloody stools, or unchanged frequency of stools by day 3 of therapy.[98] Persistent presence of numerous fecal leukocytes (>50 per high-power field) and erythrocytes (>5 per high-power field) at day 5 also suggests resistance. These findings are important because morbidity and mortality rates are higher when the organism is not susceptible to the initial drug of choice.[105] Protein-losing enteropathy is a

more likely occurrence with resistant *Shigella* spp. if an inadequate agent has been used.[32]

ADJUNCTIVE THERAPY

As with other forms of infectious colitis, antimotility agents should be avoided. Antimotility drugs, such as diphenoxylate (Lomotil), prolong the duration of fever, diarrhea, and excretion of the organism.[58] It has been speculated that intestinal motility and the constant fluid flow are important host defense factors for clearing of the organism and recovery from the infection.

A high-protein diet during convalescence may be important, particularly in settings in which malnutrition, growth retardation, and hypoproteinemia is a major complication of shigellosis.[103,104,145] Vitamin A (200,000 IU) has been found to speed resolution of illness in a population in which vitamin A deficiency is a common finding.[91] Zinc supplementation in a population that is commonly deficient in this mineral improves development of shigella-specific antibody responses.[183,188]

PROGNOSIS

Most patients recover eventually with or without specific antimicrobial therapy, although illness may be prolonged and severe if it is not treated.[38] The mortality rate in developed countries is less than 1 percent, and life-threatening complications are rare events. With appropriate antibiotic therapy, defervescence usually occurs within 24 hours, and the diarrhea decreases dramatically in 2 or 3 days. If left untreated, the disease usually lasts 1 week or more. In developing countries, childhood shigellosis is associated with significant morbidity and mortality (10 to 30%),[29] particularly if it is caused by *S. dysenteriae* serotype 1. Children with malnutrition are particularly likely to have a complicated course.[47] Shigellosis in malnourished children often causes a vicious cycle of further impaired nutrition, and repeated infections may be associated with impaired growth. Young infants and children whose course is complicated by bacteremia also are at increased risk of dying.[168]

PREVENTION

In developed countries where person-to-person transmission of shigellae is the major mode of infection, personal hygiene measures are most important.[113] Special attention to hygiene should be given in daycare centers, which sometimes play a central role in community-wide outbreaks of shigellosis.[149] The close contact among children too young to control their excretions renders this setting ideal for fecal-oral spread of the organism. Children attending daycare centers frequently transmit infection to their families. Washing hands after defecating and before eating or preparing meals is important and helpful in preventing spread.[113] Daycare personnel who prepare food should avoid performing diaper-changing duties. Sick children should be excluded from the daycare center or cohorted, and mothers should be educated regarding the possibility of being infected by their children and the use of the necessary precautions. Proper cooking of potentially infected food, appropriate refrigeration, and exclusion of individuals with diarrhea from handling food are important precautions. Education of staff members in proper hygiene is essential to infection control.[177]

Patients with diarrhea in institutional and hospital settings should be isolated for prevention of outbreaks. Aggressive investigation and early initiation of appropriate antibiotic therapy in cases of bacillary dysentery are important measures in reducing excretion of virulent shigellae and stopping spread of the disease. Use of antibiotics for prophylaxis is not recommended.

In developing countries, a safe water supply and appropriate sanitation systems are important measures for reducing the risk of shigellosis. Chlorination of drinking water is important. Water stored in vessels that permit hand dipping has been defined as a risk factor.[217] Food prepared by street vendors also has been recognized as a risk factor. Prolonged breast-feeding is the best practical strategy for prevention of shigellosis (and most other enteric infections) in infants in most of the developing world.[3,53,144] Educational efforts to promote breast-feeding in these areas are key to children's survival. Human milk contains specific secretory IgA antibodies against *Shigella* LPS and virulence plasmid–coded antigens.[51] Lactoferrin and other nonspecific (non-antibody) factors in human milk, the effect of human milk on the type of intestinal flora, and the supply of an uncontaminated food source all may contribute to the protective effect of breast-feeding against diarrheal disease.

Epidemiologic data suggest that prior infection with shigellae confers resistance to subsequent illness caused by organisms of the same serotype. Serotype-specific (LPS-based) vaccines have been produced.[69,70] Although early studies showed that immunization by the parenteral route with killed vaccines was ineffective, interest in this approach continues. Polysaccharide conjugate vaccines[20,54] are now in phase 3 clinical trials.[128] Several oral, live organism–based *Shigella* vaccines have been studied. Avirulent mutants of *S. flexneri* that lack the ability to invade the intestinal mucosa are safe and effective in monkeys. Multiple doses of large numbers of organisms were required to protect humans, however. Attenuated vaccines prepared from streptomycin-dependent mutant strains were effective, but unstable.[146] Genetically attenuated *S. flexneri* strains conferred protection but caused diarrhea when fed to some volunteers. Prototype-attenuated *S. flexneri* strains CVD 1208[117] and WRSS[109] have provided encouraging results in early clinical trials. Two nonliving vaccine approaches include the oral administration of proteosomes[72] or of inactivated *Shigella* bacteria. No effective, licensed vaccine against shigellosis is available.[128,134]

Whatever prototype *Shigella* vaccines prove to be well tolerated, immunogenic, and protective, the final formulation will have to confer protection against multiple epidemiologically important serotypes, including *S. dysenteriae* 1 (the cause of epidemic Shiga), all *S. flexneri* serotypes and subtypes (the most important agents of endemic disease in developing countries), and *S. sonnei* (responsible for 5 to 15% of shigellosis in developing countries, an important cause of traveler's shigellosis, and of shigellosis in diarrhea in daycare centers in industrialized countries).[128]

REFERENCES

1. Adeleye, I. A.: Conjugal transferability of multiple antibiotic resistance in three genera of Enterobacteriaceae in Nigeria. J. Diarrhoeal Dis. Res. *10*:93-96, 1992.
2. Agarwal, S. K., Tewari, M., and Banerjee, G.: A study on transferable R-plasmids among *Shigella* species at Lucknow. J. Commun. Dis. *29*:351-354, 1997.
3. Ahmed, F., Clemens, J. D., Rao, M. R., et al.: Community-based evaluation of the effect of breast feeding on the risk of microbiologically confirmed or clinically presumptive shigellosis in Bangladeshi children. Pediatrics *90*:406-411, 1992.
4. Alam, A. N., Chowdhurg, A. A. K. M., Kabir, I. A. K. M., et al.: Association of pneumonia with under-nutrition and shigellosis. Indian Pediatr. *21*:609-613, 1984.
5. Aldrich, J. A., Flowers, R. P., and Hall, F. K.: *S. sonnei* septicemia in a neonate: A case report. J. Am. Osteopath. Assoc. *79*:93-98, 1979.
6. al-Eissa, Y., al-Zamil, F., al-Kharashi, M., et al.: The relative importance of *Shigella* in the aetiology of childhood gastroenteritis in Saudi Arabia. Scand. J. Infect. Dis. *24*:347-351, 1992.
7. Aleksic, S., Katz, A., Aleksic, V., et al.: Antibiotic resistance of *Shigella* strains isolated in the Federal Republic of Germany 1989-1990. Int. J. Med. Microbiol. Virol. Parasitol. Infect. Dis. *279*:484-493, 1993.
8. Anand, B. S., Malhotra, V., Bhattacharya, S. K., et al.: Rectal histology in acute bacillary dysentery. Gastroenterology *90*:654-660, 1986.
9. Ansaruzzaman, M., Kibriya, A. K. M. G., Rahman, A., et al.: Detection of provisional serovars of *S. dysenteriae* and designation as *S. dysenteriae* serotypes 14 and 15. J. Clin. Microbiol. *33*:1423-1425, 1995.
10. Araj, G. F., Uwaydah, M. M., and Alami, S. Y.: Antimicrobial susceptibility patterns of bacterial isolates at the American University Medical Center in Lebanon. Diagn. Microbiol. Infect. Dis. *20*:151-158, 1994.
11. Arondel, J., Singer, M., Matsukawa, A., et al.: Increased interleukin-1 (IL-1) and imbalance between IL-1 and IL-1 receptor antagonist during acute inflammation in experimental shigellosis. Infect. Immun. *67*:6056-6066, 1999.
12. Ashkenazi, S.: *Shigella* infections in children: New insights. Semin. Pediatr. Infect. Dis. *15*:246-52, 2004.
13. Ashkenazi, S., Amir, J., Dinari, T., et al.: The differential leukocyte count in acute gastroenteritis: An aid to early diagnosis. Clin. Pediatr. *22*:356-358, 1983.
14. Ashkenazi, S., Amir, J., Waisman, Y., et al.: A randomized double-blind study comparing cefixime and TMP/SMX in the treatment of childhood shigellosis. J. Pediatr. *123*:817-821, 1993.
15. Ashkenazi, S., Bellah, G., and Cleary, T. G.: Hallucinations as an initial manifestation of childhood shigellosis. J. Pediatr. *114*:95-97, 1989.
16. Ashkenazi, S., Cleary, K. R., Pickering, L. K., et al.: The association of Shiga toxin and other cytotoxins with the neurologic manifestations of shigellosis. J. Infect. Dis. *161*:961-965, 1990.
17. Ashkenazi, S., Dinari, G., Weitz, R., et al.: Convulsions in shigellosis: Evaluation of possible risk factors. Am. J. Dis. Child. *137*:985-987, 1983.
18. Ashkenazi, S., Dinari, G., Zevulunov, A., et al.: Convulsions in childhood shigellosis: Clinical and laboratory features in 153 children. Am. J. Dis. Child. *141*:208-210, 1987.
19. Ashkenazi, S., May-Zahav, M., Sulkes, J., et al.: Increasing antimicrobial resistance of *Shigella* isolates in Israel during the period 1984 to 1992. Antimicrob. Agents Chemother. *39*:819-823, 1995.
20. Ashkenazi, S., Passwell, J. H., Harlev, E., et al.: Safety and immunogenicity of *Shigella sonnei* and *Shigella flexneri* 2a O-specific polysaccharide conjugates in children. J. Infect. Dis. *179*:1565-1568, 1999.
21. Avital, A., Maayan, C., and Goitein, K. J.: Incidence of convulsions and encephalopathy in childhood *Shigella* infections. Clin. Pediatr. *21*:645-648, 1982.
22. Aysev, A. D., and Guriz, H.: Drug resistance of *Shigella* strains isolated in Ankara, Turkey, 1993-1996. Scand. J. Infect. Dis. *30*:351-353, 1998.
23. Azad, M. A., Islam, M., and Butler, T.: Colonic perforation of *S. dysenteriae* 1 infection. Pediatr. Infect. Dis. *5*:103-104, 1986.
24. Barrett-Connor, E., and Connor, J. D.: Extraintestinal manifestations of shigellosis. Am. J. Gastroenterol. *53*:234-245, 1970.
25. Barton, L. L., and Pickering, L. K.: Shigellosis in the first week of life. Pediatrics *52*:437-438, 1973.
26. Baskin, D. H., Lax, J. D., and Barenberg, D.: *Shigella* bacteremia in patients with the acquired immunodeficiency syndrome. Am. J. Gastroenterol. *82*:338-341, 1986.
27. Basualdo, W., and Arbo, A.: Randomized comparison of azithromycin versus cefixime for treatment of shigellosis in children. Pediatr. Infect. Dis. J. *22*:374-377, 2003.
28. Bennish, M., Eusof, A., and Kay, B.: Multiresistant *Shigella* infections in Bangladesh. Lancet *2*:441, 1985.
29. Bennish, M. L., Harris, J. R., Wojtyniak, B. J., et al.: Death in shigellosis: Incidence and risk factors in hospitalized patients. J. Infect. Dis. *161*:500-506, 1990.
30. Bennish, M. L., Salam, M. A., Hossain, M. A., et al.: Antimicrobial resistance of *Shigella* isolates in Bangladesh, 1983-1990: Increasing frequency of strains multiply resistant to ampicillin, trimethoprim-sulfamethoxazole, and nalidixic acid. Clin. Infect. Dis. *14*:1055-1060, 1992.

31. Bennish, M. L., Salam, M. A., Khan, W. A., et al.: Treatment of shigellosis, III: comparison of one- or two-dose ciprofloxacin with standard 5-day therapy. Ann. Intern. Med. *117*:727-734, 1992.

32. Bennish, M. L., Salam, M. A., and Wahed, M. A.: Enteric protein loss during shigellosis. Am. J. Gastroenterol. *88*:53-57, 1993.

33. Bhattacharya, K., Bhattacharya, M. K., Dutta, D., et al.: Double-blind, randomized clinical trial for safety and efficacy of norfloxacin for shigellosis in children. Acta Paediatr. *86*:319-320, 1997.

34. Bhattacharya, M. K., Bhattacharya, S. K., Paul, M., et al.: Shigellosis in Calcutta during 1990-1992: Antibiotic susceptibility pattern and clinical features. J. Diarrhoeal Dis. Res. *12*:121-124, 1994.

35. Bogaerts, J., Verhaegen, J., Munyabikali, J. P., et al.: Antimicrobial resistance and serotypes of *Shigella* isolates in Kigali, Rwanda (1983 to 1993): Increasing frequency of multiple resistance. Diagn. Microbiol. Infect. Dis. *28*:165-171, 1997.

36. Brian, M. J., Van, R., Townsend, I., et al.: Evaluation of the molecular epidemiology of an outbreak of multiply resistant *Shigella sonnei* in a day-care center by using pulsed-field gel electrophoresis and plasmid DNA analysis. J. Clin. Microbiol. *31*:2152-1256, 1993.

37. Bridgwater, F. A. J., Morgan, R. S., Rowson, K. E. K., et al.: The neurotoxin of *Shigella shigae*: Morphological and functional lesions produced in the central nervous system of rabbits. Br. J. Exp. Pathol. *36*:447, 1955.

38. Burry, V. F., Thurn, A. N., and Co, T. G.: Shigellosis: An analysis of 239 cases in a pediatric population. Mo. Med. *65*:671-674, 1968.

39. Butler, T., Dunn, D., Dahms, B., et al.: Causes of death and the histopathologic findings in fatal shigellosis. Pediatr. Infect. Dis. J. *8*:767-772, 1989.

40. Butler, T. C., Islam, M. R., and Bardhan, P. K.: The leukemoid reaction in shigellosis. *In* Rahaman, M. M., Greenough, W. B., Novak, N. R., et al. (eds.): Shigellosis: A Continuing Global Problem. Bangladesh, International Centre for Diarrhoeal Disease Research, 1983, p. 154.

41. Calin, A., and Fries, J. F.: An "experimental" epidemic of Reiter's syndrome revisited: Follow-up evidence on genetic and environmental factors. Ann. Intern. Med. *84*:564-566, 1976.

42. Cario, E.: Toll-like receptors and gastrointestinal diseases: From bench to bedside? Curr. Opin. Gastroenterol. *18*:696-704, 2002.

43. Casalino, M., Nicoletti, M., Salvia, A., et al.: Characterization of endemic *Shigella flexneri* strains in Somalia: Antimicrobial resistance, plasmid profiles, and serotype correlation. J. Clin. Microbiol. *32*:1179-1183, 1994.

44. Cavanagh, J. B., Howard, J. G., and Whitby, J. L.: The neurotoxin of *Shigella shigae*: A comparative study of the effects produced in various laboratory animals. Br. J. Exp. Pathol. *37*:272-276, 1956.

45. Centers for Disease Control and Prevention (CDC): Summary of notifiable diseases—United States, 2001. M. M. W. R. Morb. Mortal. Wkly. Rep. *50*: i-xxiv, 1-108, 2003.

46. Cheasty, T., Skinner, J. A., Rowe, B., and Threlfall, E. J.: Increasing incidence of antibiotic resistance in *Shigella*s from humans in England and Wales: Recommendations for therapy. Microb. Drug. Resist. *4*:57-60, 1998.

47. Chopra, M., Wilkinson, D., and Stirling, S.: Epidemic *Shigella* dysentery in children in northern KwaZulu-Natal. S. Afr. Med. J. *87*:48-51, 1997.

48. Chu, Y. W., Houang, E. T., Lyon, D. J., et al.: Antimicrobial resistance in *Shigella flexneri* and *Shigella sonnei* in Hong Kong, 1986 to 1995. Antimicrob. Agents Chemother. *42*:440-443, 1998.

49. Chunder, N., Bhattacharya, S. K., Biswas, D., et al.: Isolation of a fluoroquinolone resistant *Shigella* dysenteriae 1 strain from Calcutta. Indian J. Med. Res. *106*:494-496, 1997.

50. Cleary, T. G., and Murray, B. E.: Lack of Shiga-like cytotoxin production by enteroinvasive *E. coli*. J. Clin. Microbiol. *26*:2177-2179, 1988.

51. Cleary, T. G., Winsor, D. K., Reich, D., et al.: Human milk immunoglobulin A antibodies to *Shigella* virulence determinants. Infect. Immun. *57*:1675-1679, 1989.

52. Clemens, D., Ellis, C. J., and Allan, R. N.: Persistent shigellosis. Gut *29*:1277-1278, 1988.

53. Clemens, J. S., Stanton, B., Stohl, B., et al.: Breast-feeding as a determinant of severity of shigellosis. Am. J. Epidemiol. *123*:710-720, 1986.

54. Cohen, D., Ashkenazi, S., Green, M. S., et al.: Double-blind vaccine-controlled randomized efficacy trial of an investigational *Shigella sonnei* conjugate vaccine in young adults. Lancet *349*:155-159, 1997.

55. Cohen, D., Green, M. S., Block, C., et al.: Serum antibodies to lipopolysaccharide and natural immunity to shigellosis in an Israeli military population. J. Infect. Dis. *157*:1068-1071, 1988.

56. Davis, T. C.: Chronic vulvovaginitis in children due to *S. flexneri*. Pediatrics *56*:41-44, 1975.

57. Donald, W. D., Winkler, C. H., Jr., and Bargeron, L. M., Jr.: The occurrence of convulsions in children with *Shigella* gastroenteritis. J. Pediatr. *48*:323-327, 1956.

58. DuPont, H. L., and Hornick, R. B.: Adverse effect of Lomotil therapy in shigellosis. J. A. M. A. *226*:1525-1528, 1973.

59. DuPont, H. L., Hornick, R. B., Dawkins, A. T., et al.: The response of man to virulent *Shigella flexneri* 2a. J. Infect. Dis. *119*:296-299, 1969.

60. DuPont, H. L., Levine, M. M., Hornick, R. B., et al.: Inoculum size in shigellosis and implications for expected mode of transmission. J. Infect. Dis. *159*:1126-1128, 1989.

61. Emanuel, B., and Sherman, J. O.: Shigellosis in a neonate. Clin. Pediatr. *14*:725-726, 1975.

62. Ewing, W. H.: Edwards and Ewing's Identification of Enterobacteriaceae. 4th ed. New York, Elsevier Science, 1986.

63. Farrar, W. E., Eidson, M., Guerry, P., et al.: Interbacterial transfer of R-factor in the human intestine: In vitro acquisition of R-factor mediated kanamycin resistance by a multi-resistant strain of *S. sonnei*. J. Infect. Dis. *126*:27-33, 1972.

64. Fernandez, A., Sninsky, C. A., O'Brien, A. D., et al.: Purified *Shigella* enterotoxin does not alter intestinal motility. Infect. Immun. *43*:477-481, 1984.

65. Ferreccio, C., Prado, V., Ojeda, A., et al.: Epidemiologic patterns of acute diarrhea and endemic *Shigella* infections in children in a poor periurban setting in Santiago, Chile. Am. J. Epidemiol. *134*:614-627, 1991.

66. Floyd, T., Higgins, A. R., and Kader, M. A.: Studies in shigellosis, V: The relationship of age to the incidence of *Shigella* infections in Egyptian children, with special reference to shigellosis in the newborn and infant in the first six months of life. Am. J. Trop. Med. Hyg. *5*:119-130, 1956.

67. Fontaine, O.: Antibiotics in the management of shigellosis in children: What role for the quinolones? Rev. Infect. Dis. *11*:S1145-S1150, 1989.

68. Forbes, G.: Neurologic complications of systemic disease. Postgrad. Med. *15*:157, 1954.

69. Formal, S. B., Hale, T. L., and Kapfer, C.: *Shigella* vaccines. Rev. Infect. Dis. *11*:S547-S551, 1989.

70. Formal, S. B., Kent, T. H., Austin, S., et al.: Fluorescent-antibody and histological studies of vaccinated control monkeys challenged with *Shigella flexneri*. J. Bacteriol. *91*:2368-2376, 1966.

71. Frankel, G., Riley, L., Giron, J. A., et al.: Detection of *Shigella* in feces using DNA amplification. J. Infect. Dis. *161*:1252-1256, 1990.

72. Fries, L. F., Montemarano, A. D., Mallett, C. P., et al.: Safety and immunogenicity of a proteosome-*Shigella flexneri* 2a lipopolysaccharide vaccine administered intranasally to healthy adults. Infect. Immun. *69*:4545-4553, 2001.

73. Gaudio, P. A., Sethabutr, O., Echeverria, P., and Hoge, C. W.: Utility of a polymerase chain reaction diagnostic system in a study of the epidemiology of shigellosis among dysentery patients, family contacts, and well controls living in a shigellosis-endemic area. J. Infect. Dis. *176*:1013-1018, 1997.

74. Gemski, P., Jr., Takeuchi, A., Washington, O., et al.: Shigellosis due to *Shigella* dysenteriae, 1: Relative importance of mucosal invasion versus toxin production in pathogenesis. J. Infect. Dis. *126*:523-530, 1972.

75. Gilman, R. H., Spira, W., Rabbani, H., et al.: Single dose ampicillin therapy for severe shigellosis in Bangladesh. J. Infect. Dis. *143*:164-169, 1981.

76. Goren, A., Freier, S., and Passwell, J. H.: Lethal toxic encephalopathy due to childhood shigellosis in a developed country. Pediatrics *89*:1189-1193, 1992.

77. Gots, R. E., Formal, S. B., and Gianella, R. A.: Indomethacin inhibition of *Salmonella typhimurium*, *Shigella flexneri*, and cholera-mediated rabbit ileal secretion. J. Infect. Dis. *130*:280-284, 1974.

78. Greenberg, M., Frant, S., and Shapiro, R.: Bacillary dysentery acquired at birth. J. Pediatr. *17*:363-366, 1940.

79. Guerin, P. J., Brasher, C., Baron, E., et al.: Case management of a multidrug-resistant *Shigella* dysenteriae serotype 1 outbreak in a crisis context in Sierra Leone, 1999-2000. Trans. R. Soc. Trop. Med. Hyg. *98*:635-643, 2004.

80. Guerrero, L., Calva, J. J., Morrow, A. L., et al.: Asymptomatic *Shigella* infections in a cohort of Mexican children younger than two years of age. Pediatr. Infect. Dis. J. *13*:597-602, 1994.

81. Hale, T. L., Oaks, E. V., and Formal, S. B.: Identification and characterization of virulence-associated, plasmid-coded proteins of *Shigella* spp. and enteroinvasive *E. coli*. Infect. Immun. *50*:620-623, 1985.

82. Hale, T. L., Sansonetti, P., Schad, P. A., et al.: Characterization of virulence plasmids and plasmid-mediated outer membrane proteins in *Shigella flexneri*, *Shigella sonnei* and *Escherichia coli*. Infect. Immun. *40*:340-350, 1983.

83. Haltalin, K. C.: Neonatal shigellosis. Am. J. Dis. Child. *114*:603-611, 1967.

84. Haltalin, K. C., and Nelson, J. D.: Coliform septicemia complicating shigellosis in children. J. A. M. A. *192*:441-443, 1965.

85. Harenda de Silva, D. G., Mendis, L. N., Sheron, N., et al.: Concentrations of IL-6 and TNF in serum and stools of children with *S. dysenteriae* 1 infection. Gut *34*:194-198, 1993.

86. Harnett, N.: High-level resistance to trimethoprim, cotrimoxazole and other antimicrobial agents among clinical isolates of *Shigella* species in Ontario, Canada: An update. Epidemiol. Infect. *109*:463-472, 1992.

87. Harris, J. C., DuPont, H. L., and Hornick, R. B.: Fecal leukocytes in diarrheal illness. Ann. Intern. Med. *76*:697-703, 1972.

88. Harris, J. R., Wachsmuth, I. K., Davis, B. R., et al.: High molecular weight plasmid correlates with *Escherichia coli* enteroinvasiveness. Infect. Immun. *37*:1295-1298, 1982.

89. Helvaci, M., Bektaslar, D., Ozkaya, B., et al.: Comparative efficacy of cefixime and ampicillin-sulbactam in shigellosis in children. Acta Paediatr. Jpn. *40*:131-134, 1998.

90. Hoefnagel, D.: Fulminating, rapidly fatal shigellosis in children. N. Engl. J. Med. *258*:1256-1257, 1958.

91. Hossain, S., Biswas, R., Kabir, I., et al.: Single dose vitamin A treatment in acute shigellosis in Bangladesh children: Randomized double blind controlled trial. B. M. J. *316*:422-426, 1998.

92. Howard, J. G.: Observations on the intoxication produced in mice and rabbits by the neurotoxin of *Shigella shigae*. Br. J. Exp. Pathol. *36*:439-443, 1955.

93. Huebner, J., Czerwenka, W., Gruner, E., and von Graevenitz, A.: Shigellemia in AIDS patients: Case report and review of the literature. Infection *21*:122-124, 1993.

94. Huskins, W. C., Griffiths, J. K., Faruque, A. S. G., et al.: Shigellosis in neonates and young infants. J. Pediatr. *125*:14-22, 1994.

95. Islam, D., and Christensson, B.: Disease-dependent changes in T-cell populations in patients with shigellosis. A. P. M. I. S. *108*:251-260, 2000.

96. Islam, D., Veress, B., Bardhan, P. K., et al.: Quantitative assessment of IgG and IgA subclass producing cells in rectal mucosa during shigellosis. J. Clin. Pathol. *50*:513-520, 1997.

97. Islam, M. M., Azad, A. K., Bardhan, P. K., et al.: Pathology of shigellosis and its complications. Histopathology *24*:65-71, 1994.

98. Islam, M. R., Alam, A. N., Hussain, M. S., et al.: Effect of antimicrobial (nalidixic acid) therapy in shigellosis and predictive values of outcome variables in patients susceptible or resistant to it. J. Trop. Med. Hyg. *98*:121-125, 1995.

99. Islam, M. S., Hossain, M. S., Hasan, M. K., et al.: Detection of *Shigella* from stools of dysentery patients by culture and polymerase chain reaction techniques. J. Diarrhoeal Dis. Res. *16*:248-251, 1998.

100. Jain, S. K., Gupta, A., Glanz, B., et al.: Antimicrobial-resistant *Shigella sonnei*: Limited antimicrobial treatment options for children and challenges of interpreting in vitro azithromycin susceptibility. Pediatr. Infect. Dis. J. *24*:494-497, 2005.

101. Jensen, G., Wandall, D. A., Gaarslev, K., et al.: Antibiotic resistance in *Shigella* and *Salmonella* in a region of Lithuania. Eur. J. Clin. Microbiol. Infect. Dis. *15*:872-876, 1996.

102. Kabir, I., Butler, T., and Khanam, A.: Comparative efficacies of single intravenous doses of ceftriaxone and ampicillin for shigellosis in a placebo-controlled trial. Antimicrob. Agents Chemother. *29*:645-648, 1986.

103. Kabir, I., Butler, T., Underwood, L. E., et al.: Effects of a protein rich diet during convalescence from shigellosis on catch up growth, serum proteins, and insulin like growth factor I. Pediatr. Res. *32*:689-692, 1992.

104. Kabir, I., Rahman, M. M., Haider, R., et al.: Increased height gain of children fed a high-protein diet during convalescence from shigellosis: A six-month follow-up study. J. Nutr. *128*:1688-1691, 1998.

105. Kagalwalla, A. F., Khan, S. N., Kagalwalla, Y. A., et al.: Childhood shigellosis in Saudi Arabia. Pediatr. Infect. Dis. J. *11*:215-219, 1992.

106. Kakinuma, K., Fukushima, M., and Kawaguchi, R.: Detection and identification of *Escherichia coli*, *Shigella*, and *Salmonella* by microarrays using the gyrB gene. Biotechnol. Bioeng. *83*:721-728, 2003.

107. Kaminski, N., Bogomolski, V., and Stalnikowicz, R.: Acute bacterial diarrhoea in the emergency room: Therapeutic implications of stool culture results. J. Accid. Emerg. Med. *11*:168-171, 1994.

108. Kariuki, S., Muthotho, N., Kimari, J., et al.: Molecular typing of multi-drug resistant *Shigella* dysenteriae type 1 by plasmid analysis and pulsed-field gel electrophoresis. Trans. R. Soc. Trop. Med. Hyg. *90*:712-714, 1996.

109. Katz, D. E., Coster, T. S., Wolf, M. K., et al.: Two studies evaluating the safety and immunogenicity of a live, attenuated *Shigella flexneri* 2a vaccine (SC602) and excretion of vaccine organisms in North American volunteers. Infect. Immun. *72*:923-930, 2004.

110. Keusch, G. T., and Bennish, M. L.: Shigellosis: Recent progress, persisting problems and research issues. Pediatr. Infect. Dis. J. *8*:713-719, 1989.

111. Keusch, G. T., and Jacewicz, M.: The pathogenesis of *Shigella* diarrhea, V: relationship of Shiga enterotoxin, neurotoxin, and cytotoxin. J. Infect. Dis. *131*:S33, 1975.

112. Khalil, K., Khan, S. R., Mazhar, K., et al.: Occurrence and susceptibility to antibiotics of *Shigella* species in stools of hospitalized children with bloody diarrhea in Pakistan. Am. J. Trop. Med. Hyg. *58*:800-803, 1998.

113. Khan, M. U.: Interruption of shigellosis by handwashing. Trans. R. Soc. Trop. Med. Hyg. *76*:164-165, 1982.

114. Khan, W. A., Dhar, U., Salam, M. A., et al.: Central nervous system manifestations of childhood shigellosis: Prevalence, risk factors, and outcome. Pediatrics *103*:E18, 1999.

115. Koster, F., Levin, J., Walker, L., et al.: Hemolytic-uremic syndrome after shigellosis: Relation to endotoxemia and circulating immune complexes. N. Engl. J. Med. *298*:927-933, 1978.

116. Kotloff, K. L., Winickoff, J. P., Ivanoff, B., et al.: Global burden of *Shigella* infection: Implications for vaccine development and implementation of control strategies. Bull. World Health Organ. *77*:651-666, 1999.

117. Kotloff, K. L., Pasetti, M. F., Barry, E. M., et al.: Deletion in the *Shigella* enterotoxin genes further attenuates *Shigella flexneri* 2a bearing guanine auxotrophy in a phase 1 trial of CVD 1204 and CVD 1208. J. Infect. Dis. *190*:1745-1754, 2004.

118. Kowlessar, M., and Forbes, G. B.: The febrile convulsion in shigellosis. N. Engl. J. Med. *258*:520-523, 1958.

119. Kozlova, N. S.: Plasmids of antibiotic-resistant strains of *Shigella* isolated in Leningrad and Leningrad region. Antibiot. Khimioter. *38*:9-14, 1993.

120. Kraybill, E. N., and Controni, G.: Septicemia and enterocolitis due to *S. sonnei* in a newborn infant. Pediatrics *42*:529-531, 1968.

121. Kristjansson, M., Viner, B., and Maslow, J. N.: Polymicrobial and recurrent bacteremia with *Shigella* in a patient with AIDS. Scand. J. Infect. Dis. *26*:411-416, 1994.

122. LaBrec, E. H., Schneider, H., Magnani, T. J., et al.: Epithelial cell penetration as an essential step in the pathogenesis of bacillary dysentery. J. Bacteriol. *88*:1503-1518, 1964.

123. Landsberger, M.: Bacillary dysentery in a newborn infant. Arch. Pediatr. *59*:330-332, 1942.

124. Le-Barillec, K., Magalhaes, J. G., Corcuff, E., et al.: Roles for T and NK cells in the innate immune response to *Shigella flexneri*. J. Immunol. *175*:1735-1740, 2005.

125. Leibovitz, E., Janco, J., Piglansky, L., et al.: Oral ciprofloxacin vs. intramuscular ceftriaxone as empiric treatment of acute invasive diarrhea in children. Pediatr. Infect. Dis. J. *19*:1060-1067, 2000.

126. Leibovitz, E.: The use of fluoroquinolones in children. Curr. Opin. Pediatr. *18*:64-70, 2006.

127. Levin, S. E.: *Shigella* septicemia in the newborn infant. J. Pediatr. *71*:917-918, 1967.

128. Levine, M. M.: Enteric infections and the vaccines to counter them: Future directions. Vaccine *24*:3865-3873, 2006.

129. Levine, M. M., DuPont, H. L., Formal, S. B., et al.: Pathogenesis of *Shigella* dysenteriae 1 (Shiga) dysentery. J. Infect. Dis. *127*:261-270, 1973.

130. Levine, M. M., DuPont, H. L., Khodabandebou, M., et al.: Long-term *Shigella*-carrier state. N. Engl. J. Med. *288*:1169-1171, 1973.

131. Lim, Y. S., and Tay, L.: Serotype distribution and antimicrobial resistance of *Shigella* isolates in Singapore. J. Diarrhoeal Dis. Res. *9*:328-331, 1991.

132. Lima, A. A., Lima, N. L., Pinho, M. C., et al.: High frequency of strains multiply resistant to ampicillin, trimethoprim-sulfamethoxazole, streptomycin, chloramphenicol, and tetracycline isolated from patients with shigellosis in northeastern Brazil during the period 1988 to 1993. Antimicrob. Agents Chemother. *39*:256-259, 1995.

133. Lin, S. R., and Chang, S. F.: Drug resistance and plasmid profile of *Shigella* in Taiwan. Epidemiol. Infect. *108*:87-97, 1992.

134. Lindberg, A. A., and Pal, T.: Strategies for development of potential candidate *Shigella* vaccines. Vaccine *11*:168-179, 1993.

135. Ling, J. M., Shaw, P. C., Kam, K. M., et al.: Molecular studies of plasmids of multiply-resistant *Shigella* spp. in Hong Kong. Epidemiol. Infect. *110*:437-446, 1993.

136. Lolekha, S., Vibulbandhitkit, S., and Poonyarit, P.: Response to antimicrobial therapy for shigellosis in Thailand. Rev. Infect. Dis. *13*:S342-S346, 1991.

137. Makintubee, S., Mallonee, J., and Istre, G. R.: Shigellosis outbreak associated with swimming. Am. J. Public Health *77*:166-168, 1987.

138. Mamun, K. Z., Tabassum, S., Hussain, M. A., and Shears, P.: Antimicrobial susceptibility of *Shigella* from a rural community in Bangladesh. Ann. Trop. Med. Parasitol. *91*:643-647, 1997.

139. Maraki, S., Georgiladakis, A., Christidou, A., et al.: Antimicrobial susceptibilities and beta-lactamase production of *Shigella* isolates in Crete, Greece, during the period 1991-1995. A. P. M. I. S. *106*:879-883, 1998.

140. Martin, J. M., Pitetti, R., Maffei, F., et al.: Treatment of shigellosis with cefixime: Two days vs. five days. Pediatr. Infect. Dis. J. *19*:522-526, 2000.

141. Martin, T., Habbick, B. F., and Nyssen, J.: Shigellosis with bacteremia: A report of two cases and a review of the literature. Pediatr. Infect. Dis. *2*:21-26, 1983.

142. Mason, P. R., Nathoo, K. J., Wellington, M., et al.: Antimicrobial susceptibilities of *Shigella* dysenteriae type 1 isolated in Zimbabwe: Implications for the management of dysentery. Cent. Afr. J. Med. *41*:132-137, 1995.

143. Mata, L. G.: The Children of Santa Maria Cauque: A Prospective Field Study of Health and Growth. Cambridge, MIT Press, 1978.

144. Mata, L. J., Urrutia, J. J., Garcia, B., et al.: *Shigella* infections in breast fed Guatemalan Indian neonates. Am. J. Dis. Child. *117*:142-146, 1969.

145. Mazumder, R. N., Hoque, S. S., Ashraf, H., et al.: Early feeding of an energy dense diet during acute shigellosis enhances growth in malnourished children. J. Nutr. *127*:51-54, 1997.

146. Mel, D. M., Terzin, A. L., and Vuksic, L.: Studies on vaccination against bacillary dysentery, 3: Effective oral immunization against *Shigella flexneri* 2a in a field trial. Bull. World Health Organ. *32*:647-655, 1965.

147. Merson, M. H., Goldmann, D. A., Boyer, K. M., et al.: An outbreak of *Shigella sonnei* gastroenteritis on Colorado River raft trips. Am. J. Epidemiol. *100*:186-196, 1974.

148. Miron, D., Sochotnick, I., Yardeni, D., et al.: Surgical complications of shigellosis in children. Pediatr. Infect. Dis. J. *19*:898-900, 2000.

149. Mohle-Boetani, J. C., Stapleton, M., Finger, R., et al.: Community-wide shigellosis: Control of an outbreak and risk factors in child day care centers. Am. J. Public Health *85*:812-816, 1995.

150. Moore, E. E.: *Shigella sonnei* septicemia in a neonate. B. M. J. *1*:22-23, 1974.

151. Morris, G. K., Koehler, J. A., Gangarosa, E. J., et al.: Comparison of media for direct isolation and transport of *Shigella* from fecal specimens. Appl. Microbiol. *19*:434-437, 1970.

152. Mulligan, K., Nelson, S., Friedman, H. S., et al.: Shigellosis-associated encephalopathy. Pediatr. Infect. Dis. J. *11*:889-890, 1992.

153. Munshi, M. H., Sack, D. A., Haider, K., et al.: Plasmid-mediated resistance to nalidixic acid in *Shigella* dysenteriae type 1. Lancet *2*:419-421, 1987.

154. Murphy, T. V., and Nelson, J. D.: *Shigella* vaginitis: Report on 38 patients and review of the literature. Pediatrics *63*:511-516, 1979.

155. Nalin, D. R., and Cash, R. A.: Oral or nasogastric maintenance of cholera and other severe diarrhea in children. J. Pediatr. *78*:355-358, 1971.

156. Nataro, J. P., Seriwatana, J., Fasano, A., et al.: Identification and cloning of a novel plasmid encoded enterotoxin of enteroinvasive E. coli and *Shigella* strains. Infect. Immun. *63*:4721-4728, 1995.

157. Navia, M. M., Capitano, L., Ruiz, J., et al.: Typing and characterization of mechanisms of resistance of *Shigella* spp. isolated from feces of children under

5 years of age from Ifakara, Tanzania. J. Clin. Microbiol. *37*:3113-3117, 1999.
158. Neglia, T. G., Marr, T. J., and Davis, A. T.: *Shigella* dysentery with secondary *Klebsiella* sepsis. J. Pediatr. *63*:253-254, 1976.
159. Neill, R. J., Gemski, P., Formal, S. B., et al.: Deletion of Shiga toxin gene in a chlorate-resistant derivative of *Shigella* dysenteriae type 1 that retains virulence. J. Infect. Dis. *158*:737-741, 1988.
160. Neter, E.: *S. sonnei* infection at term and its transfer to the newborn. Obstet. Gynecol. *17*:517-519, 1961.
161. Newland, J. W., and Neill, R. J.: DNA probes for Shiga-like toxins I and II and for toxin-converting bacteriophages. J. Clin. Microbiol. *26*:1292-1297, 1988.
162. Niyogi, S. K.: Shigellosis. J. Microbiol. *43*:133-143, 2005.
163. Noriega, F. R., Liao, F. M., Formal, S. B., et al.: Prevalence of *Shigella* enterotoxin 1 among *Shigella* clinical isolates of diverse serotypes. J. Infect. Dis. *172*:1408-1410, 1995.
164. Notario, R., Morales, E., Carmelengo, E., et al.: Enteropathogenic microorganisms in children with acute diarrhea in 2 hospitals of Rosario, Argentina. Medicina (B. Aires) *53*:289-299, 1993.
165. Nuutinen, M., Turtinen, J., and Uhari, M.: Growth and joint symptoms in children treated with nalidixic acid. Pediatr. Infect. Dis. J. *13*:798-800, 1994.
166. Oaks, E. V., Hale, T. L., and Formal, S. B.: Serum immune response to *Shigella* protein antigens in rhesus monkeys and humans infected with *Shigella* spp. Infect. Immun. *53*:57-63, 1986.
167. O'Brien, A. D., and Holmes, R. K.: Shiga and Shiga-like toxins. Microbiol. Rev. *51*:206-220, 1987.
168. O'Connor, H. J., and O'Callaghan, U.: Fatal *S. sonnei* septicemia in an adult complemented by marrow aplasia and intestinal perforation. J. Infect. *3*:277-279, 1981.
169. Ogawa, H.: Experimental approach in studies on pathogenesis of bacillary dysentery: With special reference to the invasion of bacilli into intestinal mucosa. Acta Pathol. Jpn. *20*:261-277, 1970.
170. Ogawa, M., and Sasakawa, C.: Intracellular survival of *Shigella*. Cell Microbiol. *8*:177-184, 2006.
171. Okamura, N., Nagai, T., and Nakaya, R., et al.: HeLa cell invasiveness and O antigen of *Shigella flexneri* as separate and prerequisite attributes of virulence to evoke keratoconjunctivitis in guinea pigs. Infect. Immun. *39*:505-513, 1983.
172. Ozturk, M. K., Caksen, H., and Sumerkan, B.: Convulsions in childhood shigellosis and antimicrobial resistance patterns of *Shigella* isolates. Turk. J. Pediatr. *38*:183-188, 1996.
173. Pal, T., Newland, J. W., Tall, B. D., et al.: Intracellular spread of *Shigella flexneri* associated with the kcpA locus and a 140-kilodalton protein. Infect. Immun. *57*:477-486, 1989.
174. Parsot, C.: *Shigella* spp. and enteroinvasive *Escherichia coli* pathogenicity factors. F. E. M. S. Microbiol. Lett. *252*:11-18, 2005.
175. Phalipon, A., and Sansonetti, P. J.: *Shigella*'s ways of manipulating the host intestinal innate and adaptive immune system: A tool box for survival? Immunol. Cell Biol. *85*:119-129, 2007.
176. Pickering, L. K.: Antimicrobial resistance among enteric pathogens. Semin. Pediatr. Infect. Dis. *15*:71-77, 2004.
177. Pickering, L. K., Bartlett, A. V., and Woodward, W. E.: Acute infectious diarrhea among children in day care: Epidemiology and control. Rev. Infect. Dis. *8*:539-547, 1986.
178. Pickering, L. K., and Woodward, W. E.: Diarrhea in day care centers. Pediatr. Infect. Dis. *1*:47-52, 1982.
179. Prado, D., Lopez, E., Liu, H., et al.: Ceftibuten and TMP/SMX for treatment of *Shigella* and enteroinvasive *E. coli* disease. Pediatr. Infect. Dis. J. *11*:644-647, 1992.
180. Prado, V., Pidal, P., Arellano, C., et al: Antimicrobial multiresistance of *Shigella* sp strains in a semirural community of northern Santiago. Rev. Med. Chile *126*:1464-1471, 1998.
181. Ruderman, J. W., Stoller, K. P., and Pomerance, J. J.: Bloodstream invasion with *S. sonnei* in an asymptomatic newborn infant. Pediatr. Infect. Dis. *5*:379-380, 1986.
182. Rahaman, M. M., Jamiul Alam, A. K. M., Islam, M. R., et al.: Shiga bacillus dysentery associated with marked leukocytosis and erythrocyte fragmentation. Johns Hopkins Med. J. *136*:65-70, 1975.
183. Rahman, M. J., Sarker, P., Roy, S. K., et al.: Effects of zinc supplementation as adjunct therapy on the systemic immune responses in shigellosis. Am. J. Clin. Nutr. *81*:495-502, 2005.
184. Rahman, M. M., Kabir, I., Mahalanabis, D., et al.: Decreased food intake in children with severe dysentery due to *S. dysenteriae* 1 infection. Eur. J. Clin. Nutr. *46*:833-838, 1992.
185. Raqib, R., Lindberg, A. A., Wretlind, B., et al.: Persistence of local cytokine production in shigellosis in acute and convalescent stages. Infect. Immun. *63*:289-296, 1995.
186. Raqib, R., Ljungdahl, A., Lindberg, A. A., et al.: Local entrapment of interferon gamma in the recovery from *Shigella* dysenteriae type 1 infection. Gut *38*:328-336, 1996.
187. Raqib, R., Reinholt, F. P., Bardhan, P. K., et al.: Immunopathological patterns in the rectal mucosa of patients with shigellosis: Expression of HLA-DR antigens and T lymphocyte subsets. A. P. M. I. S. *102*:371-380, 1994.
188. Raqib, R., Roy, S. K., Rahman, M. J., et al.: Effect of zinc supplementation on immune and inflammatory responses in pediatric patients with shigellosis. Am. J. Clin. Nutr. *79*:444-450, 2004.

189. Raqib, R., Wretlind, B., Andersson, J., et al.: Cytokine secretion in acute shigellosis is correlated to disease activity and directed more to stool than to plasma. J. Infect. Dis. *171*:376-384, 1995.
190. Rogerie, F., Ott, D., Vandepitte, J., et al.: Comparisons of norfloxacin and nalidixic acid for treatment of dysentery caused by *S. dysenteriae* type 1 in adults. Antimicrob. Agents Chemother. *29*:883-886, 1986.
191. Rubenstein, J. S., Noah, Z. L., Zales, V. R., et al.: Acute myocarditis associated with *S. sonnei* gastroenteritis. J. Pediatr. *122*:82-84, 1993.
192. Sakai, T., Sasakawa, C., Makino, S., et al.: DNA sequence and product analysis of the virF locus responsible for Congo red binding and cell invasion in *Shigella flexneri* 2a. Infect. Immun. *54*:395-402, 1986.
193. Sakamoto, A., and Kamo, S.: Clinical, statistical observations on Ekiri and bacillary dysentery: A study of 785 cases. Ann. Paediatr. *186*:1-18, 1956.
194. Salam, M. A., and Bennish, M. L.: Therapy of shigellosis, 1: Randomized, double-blind trial of nalidixic acid in childhood shigellosis. Pediatrics *113*:901-907, 1988.
195. Salam, M. A., Dhar, U., Khan, W. A., and Bennish, M. L.: Randomised comparison of ciprofloxacin suspension and pivmecillinam for childhood shigellosis. Lancet *352*:522-527, 1998.
196. Salam, M. A., Seas, C., Khan, W. A., et al.: Treatment of shigellosis, IV: Cefixime is ineffective in shigellosis in adults. Ann. Intern. Med. *123*:505-508, 1995.
197. Salzman, T. C., Scher, C. D., and Moss, R.: *Shigella* with transferable drug resistance: Outbreak in a nursery for premature infants. J. Pediatr. *71*:21-26, 1967.
198. Samandari, T., Kotloff, K. L., Losonsky, G. A., et al.: Production of IFN-gamma and IL-10 to *Shigella* invasins by mononuclear cells from volunteers orally inoculated with a Shiga toxin-deleted *Shigella* dysenteriae type 1 strain. J. Immunol. *164*:2221-2232, 2000.
199. Sansonetti, P. J., Arondel, J., Huerre, M., et al.: Interleukin-8 controls bacterial transepithelial translocation at the cost of epithelial destruction in experimental shigellosis. Infect. Immun. *67*:1471-1480, 1999.
200. Sansonetti, P. J., Hale, T. L., Dammin, G. I., et al.: Alterations in the pathogenicity of *Escherichia coli* K-12 after transfer of plasmids and chromosomal genes from *Shigella flexneri*. Infect. Immun. *39*:1392-1402, 1983.
201. Sansonetti, P. J., Kopecko, D. J., and Formal, S. B.: *Shigella sonnei* plasmids: Evidence that a large plasmid is necessary for virulence. Infect. Immun. *34*:75-83, 1981.
202. Sansonetti, P. J., Kopecko, D. J., and Formal, S. B.: Involvement of a plasmid in the invasive ability of *Shigella flexneri*. Infect. Immun. *35*:852-860, 1982.
203. Sansonetti, P. J., Phalipon, A., Arondel, J., et al.: Caspase-1 activation of IL-1beta and IL-18 are essential for *Shigella flexneri*-induced inflammation. Immunity *12*:581-590, 2000.
204. Sasakawa, C., Kamata, K., Sakai, T., et al.: Molecular alteration of the 140-megadalton plasmid associated with the loss of virulence and Congo red binding activity in *Shigella flexneri*. Infect. Immun. *51*:470-475, 1986.
205. Scragg, J. N., Rubidge, C. J., and Appelbaum, P. C.: *Shigella* infection in African and Indian children with special reference to *Shigella* septicemia. J. Pediatr. *93*:796-797, 1978.
206. Simor, A. E., Poon, R., and Borczyk, A.: Chronic *Shigella flexneri* infection preceding development of acquired immunodeficiency syndrome. J. Clin. Microbiol. *27*:353-355, 1989.
207. Smith, H. R., Scotland, S. M., Chart, H., et al.: Vero cytotoxin production and presence of VT genes in strains of *Escherichia coli* and *Shigella*. F. E. M. S. Microbiol. Lett. *42*:173, 1987.
208. Speelman, P., Kabir, I., and Islam, M.: Distribution and spread of colonic lesions in shigellosis: A colonoscopic study. J. Infect. Dis. *150*:899-903, 1984.
209. Speelman, P., McGlaughlin, R., Kabir, I., et al.: Differential clinical features and stool findings in shigellosis and amoebic dysentery. Trans. R. Soc. Trop. Med. Hyg. *81*:549-551, 1987.
210. Starke, J. R., and Baker, C. J.: Neonatal shigellosis with bowel perforation. Pediatr. Infect. Dis. *4*:405-407, 1985.
211. Stern, M. S., and Gitnick, G. L.: *Shigella* hepatitis. J. A. M. A. *235*:2628, 1976.
212. Stoll, B. J., Glass, R. I., Huq, M. I., et al.: Surveillance of patients attending a diarrhoeal disease hospital in Bangladesh. B. M. J. *285*:1185-1188, 1982.
213. Struelens, M. J., Patte, D., Kabir, I., et al.: *Shigella* septicemia: Prevalence, presentation, risk factors, and outcome. J. Infect. Dis. *152*:784-790, 1985.
214. Tauxe, R. V., Puhr, N. D., Wells, J. G., et al.: Antimicrobial resistance of *Shigella* isolates in the USA: The importance of international travelers. J. Infect. Dis. *162*:1107-1111, 1990.
215. Taylor, W. I., and Harris, B.: Isolation of *Shigella*, II: Comparison of plating media and enrichment broths. Am. J. Clin. Pathol. *44*:471-475, 1965.
216. Tobias, J. D., Starke, J. R., and Tosi, M. F.: *Shigella* keratitis: A report of two cases and a review of the literature. Pediatr. Infect. Dis. *6*:79-81, 1987.
217. Tuttle, J., Ries, A. A., Chimba, R. M., et al.: Antimicrobial resistant epidemic *S. dysenteriae* type 1 in Zambia: Modes of transmission. J. Infect. Dis. *171*:371-375, 1995.
218. Vargas, M., Gascon, J., Jimenez De Anta, M. T., et al.: Prevalence of *Shigella* enterotoxins 1 and 2 among *Shigella* strains isolated from patients with traveler's diarrhea. J. Clin. Microbiol. *37*:3608-3611, 1999.
219. Venkatesan, M. M., Buyssee, J. M., and Kopecko, D. J.: Use of *Shigella flexneri* ipaC and ipaH gene sequences for the general identification of *Shigella* spp. and enteroinvasive *Escherichia coli*. J. Clin. Microbiol. *27*:2687-2691, 1989.

220. Vila, J., Gascon, J., Abdalla, S., et al.: Antimicrobial resistance of *Shigella* isolates causing traveler's diarrhea. Antimicrob. Agents Chemother. *38*:2668-2670, 1994.
221. Wang, L. H., Fang, X. C., and Pan, G. Z.: Bacillary dysentery as a causative factor of irritable bowel syndrome and its pathogenesis. Gut *53*:1096-101, 2004.
222. Way, S. S., Borczuk, A. C., Dominitz, R., and Goldberg, M. B.: An essential role for gamma interferon in innate resistance to *Shigella flexneri* infection. Infect. Immun. *66*:1342-1348, 1998.
223. Whitfield, C., and Humphries, J. M.: Meningitis and septicemia due to *Shigella* in a newborn infant. J. Pediatr. *70*:805-806, 1967.
224. Yolken, R. H., Ojeh, C., Khatri, I. A., et al.: Intestinal mucins inhibit rotavirus replication in an oligosaccharide-dependent manner. J. Infect. Dis. *169*:1002-1006, 1994.

225. Yurdakok, K., Sahin, N., Ozmert, E., and Berkman, E.: *Shigella* gastroenteritis: Clinical and epidemiological aspects, and antibiotic susceptibility. Acta Paediatr. Jpn. *39*:681-684, 1997.
226. Zimbabwe, Bangladesh, South Africa (Zimbasa) Dysentery Study Group: Multicenter, randomized, double blind clinical trial of short course versus standard course oral ciprofloxacin for *Shigella* dysenteriae type 1 dysentery in children. Pediatr. Infect. Dis. J. *21*:1136-1141, 2002.
227. Zychlinsky, A., Fitting, C., Cavaillon, J. M., et al.: IL-1 is released by murine macrophages during apoptosis induced by *S. flexneri*. J. Clin. Invest. *94*:1328-1332, 1994.
228. Zychlinsky, A., Kenny, B., Menard, R., et al.: IpaB mediates macrophage apoptosis induced by *S. flexneri*. Mol. Microbiol. *11*:619-627, 1994.
229. Zychlinsky, A., Perdomo, J. J., and Sansonetti, P. J.: Molecular and cellular mechanisms of tissue invasion by *S. flexneri*. Ann. N. Y. Acad. Sci. *730*:197-208, 1994.

SERRATIA

Randall G. Fisher

Similar to other members of Enterobacteriaceae, the genus *Serratia* contains species increasingly associated with opportunistic infection in the compromised host. One of the oldest bacterial organisms to be named,[105] *Serratia marcescens* is the chief species associated with disease in humans and has been associated with infection of the urinary tract, the respiratory tract, local wounds, and central venous catheters. Illness may be complicated by bacteremia and meningitis. Treatment of infection may be made exceptionally difficult because these organisms frequently are resistant to penicillins, cephalosporins, and aminoglycosides.

BACTERIOLOGY

S. marcescens can produce a red pigment resembling blood on contaminated foodstuffs. In the 6th century, the "miraculous" appearance of blood on food provoked superstition and scientific investigation. Troops were goaded into battle, and religious beliefs gained support because of the fortuitous growth of the saprophyte in bread.[105] In vitro, the red pigment produced by these strains is toxic to cancer cells but not to nonmalignant cell lines.[31]

In 1819, *S. marcescens* was named by Bizio, who correctly interpreted the discoloration of cornmeal to be due to a living organism.[69] The genus name honors the Italian physicist Serrafino Serrati, who Bizio thought had been slighted in favor of Robert Fulton as inventor of the steamboat; the species name *marcescens* was drawn from the Latin word meaning "to decay."

We now recognize the genus *Serratia* as straight, motile, catalase-positive, gram-negative rods. On solid agar, colonies are opaque; iridescent; and white, pink, or red. Organisms are Voges-Proskauer test-positive.[48] The genus may be distinguished from other enterobacteria (genera) by its use of caprylate or L-fucose as a sole carbon source, and its hydrolysis of gelatin.[48,100] Clinically relevant strains include *S. marcescens*, *Serratia liquefaciens*, *Serratia odorifera*, *Serratia ficara*, and *Serratia plymuthica*.[18,37] For a detailed review of the properties of *S. marcescens*, the reader is referred to the review by Hejazi and Falkiner.[49]

EPIDEMIOLOGY

S. marcescens was thought to be nonpathogenic in earlier times and was used as a biologic marker of transmission in 1906. In that year, N. H. Gordon, commissioned to study the atmospheric hygiene of the British House of Commons, gargled a liquid culture of *S. marcescens* and then quoted Shakespeare to an audience of agar plates in the otherwise empty House.[43,105] The organism subsequently was recovered from the plates, documenting the possibility of aerosol transmission of bacteria (Gordon reported no ill effects). The importance of *S. marcescens* as a biologic marker for hand-to-hand bacterial transmission, ascension of bacteria in the urinary tract in catheterized patients, and bacteremia after dental extraction is reviewed in detail by Yu.[105] Most remarkably, in investigations in 1950 and 1952 to judge the threat of biologic warfare to the United States, the Navy released *S. marcescens* into the Pacific, where it became aerosolized and drifted 80 m inland.[6] Although an epidemic of *S. marcescens* infection in a San Francisco hospital coincided with this event, subsequent serotype and biotype analyses cast doubt on any relationship to the Navy experiments.[36] Rather, the early San Francisco hospital experience heralded the increased frequency of nosocomial infections that would be observed in subsequent years.[105]

In some studies, *S. marcescens* is the organism most frequently isolated from contact lens solutions and contact lens cases.[82,107] Ex vivo mouse cornea studies show that the organism adheres to injured but not to intact corneas.[82] Commercial multipurpose disinfectant solutions all are active against the type strain but vary in their activity against actual clinical isolates. Polyquaternium-1–based solutions fared the worst in their activity against circulating strains.[52]

Sporadic nosocomial outbreaks of infection were reported first in the 1950s and 1960s.[66,83,103] Early outbreaks in a pediatric ward and neonatal nursery were attributed to contaminated intravenous solution and caps of bottles containing saline used to moisten umbilical cords.[66] As reviewed by Yu,[105] environmental sources before 1979 included disinfectants, water from ultrasonic nebulizers, respirators, arterial pressure monitors, and fiberoptic bronchoscopes. Environmental sources since have included suction traps,[74] intra-aortic pressure transducers,[11,101] contaminated handwashing brushes,[5] illicit intravenous drug paraphernalia,[27] contaminated urologic instruments,[34] colonized disinfectants or soaps,[35,64,67] contaminated infant parenteral nutrition fluid,[38] contaminated whole blood or blood products,[42,84] and inadequately sterilized breast milk pumps.[45]

Hand-to-hand transmission seems to be the primary mechanism of nosocomial spread. In one dramatic outbreak, spread of an organism with the same serotype, phage type, and antimicrobial sensitivity pattern was documented among four geographically separated teaching hospitals in the same region[89]; spread likely was due to passive carriage of *S. marcescens* on the hands of rotating personnel. By 1979, it was apparent that nosocomial increase in *S. marcescens* infection was becoming a worldwide concern.[18]

Outbreaks in neonatal units and pediatric wards have been widespread, persistent, and associated with high morbidity and mortality rates.[5,15,74,97] At the peak of one epidemic of invasive *S. marcescens* disease in a neonatal nursery, more than 90 percent of infants were colonized with the epidemic strain.[33] Increased rates of colonization have been associated with nearly 10-fold increases in rates of *S. marcescens* bacteremia and meningitis.[108] In a case-control study, neonates with *S. marcescens* bloodstream infection were at least three times more likely to have associated meningitis than were neonates whose blood cultures grew *Escherichia coli*.[13] Outbreaks of multidrug-resistant strains have been especially troublesome in surgical subspecialty wards, and an outbreak has been reported in a bone marrow transplant unit.[19,57]

Biotyping may be successful in characterizing isolates, which can be traced in the hospital environment.[47,96] Ribotyping or identification of a unique biochemical characteristic has proved useful for showing cross-contamination across hematology, gastroenterology, and neonatology units in a pediatric hospital.[12,39] Use of typing methods may be particularly important because drug-resistant and drug-susceptible isolates of *Serratia* organisms may co-circulate.[25] Banding differences from pulse field gel electrophoresis of DNA digests are restricted in number from outbreak strains; increases in banding pattern may reflect genetic drift over time.[8] Such DNA techniques have aided decisions regarding cohorting and closure of neonatal units and have been used to show cross-contamination of wards.[51,72] DNA amplification techniques offer promise for characterizing isolates in future outbreaks and defining antimicrobial susceptibility.[50,64,92]

PATHOPHYSIOLOGY

Pathologic findings of sepsis are similar to the findings of other gram-negative enteric bacilli. Postmortem examination of the lungs of patients with radiologic findings of *S. marcescens* pneumonia reveals a focal necrotizing pneumonia in most cases and hemorrhagic manifestations in some.[10]

Several properties may enhance virulence of *Serratia* organisms in human infection. The 56-kd protease of *S. marcescens* seems to possess properties of a virulence factor. It enhances vascular permeability through activation of the Hageman factor–kallikrein–kinin pathway in vivo.[65] The protease also has the capacity to degrade host proteins important in humoral immune response, such as immunoglobulins and fibronectin,[73] and inactivates the chemotactic effect of C5a.[78] *Serratia* hemolysin indirectly may increase vascular permeability, local edema, and granulocyte accumulation. Clinical strains seem to possess increased adherence properties compared with environmental isolates.[9] Compared with some enteric organisms, *Serratia* organisms adhere better to epithelial cells of the bladder, which may facilitate development of urinary tract infection.[29]

Cell-mediated immunity and humoral immunity may be important in protection from *Serratia* infection and illness. In a murine model of immunization against *S. marcescens*, only the transfer of antiserum and spleen cells from vaccinated mice increased bacterial clearance from the liver and survival after infection developed.[61]

Resistance of *S. marcescens* to aminoglycosides generally is plasmid-mediated. Resistance to aminoglycosides may be conferred by one of several genes producing acetylating, phosphorylating, or adenylating enzymes.[1,2,19,53,70] Risk of acquiring infection with aminoglycoside resistance increases with exposure to these agents.[44,106] In some patients, repeated hospitalizations have

shown greater importance, however, than aminoglycoside use as a risk factor for developing infection with resistant strains.[7] High levels of resistance to penicillins and cephalosporins are mediated by one or more plasmids. Cephalosporin resistance also may be derived chromosomally (see also Chapter 113).[25,40,68,81] Chromosomally mediated β-lactam resistance may be inducible in the presence of high levels of penicillin or cephalosporins, particularly when plasmid-derived β-lactamase is blocked by clavulanic acid.[20]

A group of researchers found and cloned a multidrug efflux pump of the major facilitator superfamily from *S. marcescens*.[94] Transposable plasmid elements may seem partly responsible for the rapid spread of multidrug resistance.[85,86,91] In one survey, 2.6 percent of *S. marcescens* isolates were deemed "multidrug resistant," defined as resistant to three or more classes of antimicrobials.[32] Plasmids conferring multidrug resistance are transferable from *S. marcescens* to *Klebsiella* spp. and may be responsible for sequential nosocomial outbreaks of different genera sharing common drug resistance patterns.[99]

CLINICAL MANIFESTATIONS

First described in a patient with bronchiectasis as a cause of "blood-tinged" sputum colored by the organism,[104] *S. marcescens* commonly is associated with urinary tract, respiratory tract, central venous catheter, and bacteremic infections.[2] Other species, including *S. liquefaciens*, *S. ficara*, *S. odorifera*, and *S. plymuthica*, are less common causes of disease.[13,23,30,37,93]

Chromogenic *S. marcescens* was responsible for the historically interesting and reportedly benign "red diaper syndrome," which persisted for 7 months in the infant of a genetics professor.[102] In at least one series, the organism has been identified as one of the top five causes of neonatal sepsis[46] and now is recognized as a major pathogen of compromised newborns. Disease in newborn intensive care units is associated commonly with high rates of underlying respiratory illness.[75] Other preexisting risk factors include necrotizing enterocolitis, surgical procedures, intravenous catheters, prolonged intubation, and cardiac disease.[13] Clinical illness shares features in common with other neonatal enteric pathogens; apnea, hypotension, and respiratory distress are seen frequently. Pneumonia with empyema has been reported.[56] Meningitis occurs as a complication in 24 percent of cases of neonatal bacteremia,[13] and antibiotic resistance may emerge during therapy for bacteremia or localized infection.[21] Significant brain injury caused by ventriculitis, brain abscesses, or porencephalic cysts is observed in most infants with meningitis.[21,62]

In older children and adults, *Serratia* spp. are isolated most frequently from the urinary tract.[2,89] Instrumentation, catheterization, and clustering of susceptibles are important risk factors.[7,22,53,87,90] By the 1970s, increased frequencies of serious infection, such as endocarditis, were noted in intravenous drug abusers.[27] In some series of respiratory and urinary tract infections, *S. marcescens* was observed to be associated more commonly with the complication of bacteremia than was any other enteric pathogen.[55,60] As is true of other causes of gram-negative sepsis, *Serratia* sepsis characterized by shock, pneumonia, or hemorrhage confers a substantially poorer prognosis.[16,88] The risk of these complications in cancer patients was observed by Saito and associates[88] to be lower, however, than their previous experience with other pathogens, such as *E. coli* and *Pseudomonas aeruginosa*. When predictive factors of mortality were sought in 385 subjects with nosocomial bacteremia, *S. marcescens* was not an independent predictor of death.[71] Other infections caused by *Serratia* include soft tissue infections, abscesses, endophthalmitis (including a case occurring after septicemia in an infant),[3,4] osteomyelitis and arthritis,[98] spinal epidural abscess, and peritonitis in dialysis patients.[26]

DIAGNOSIS

The diagnosis of *Serratia* infection relies primarily on isolation of organisms from clinical material. Nonspecific laboratory tests occasionally may be misleading. *Serratia* meningitis in a neonate may be accompanied by a normal cerebrospinal fluid white blood cell count or only a modest cerebrospinal fluid pleocytosis.[21] Although *S. marcescens* is famous historically because of its chromogenic potential, most strains are nonpigmented. Hydrolysis of gelatin distinguishes *S. marcescens* from *Klebsiella* and *Enterobacter* in the clinical microbiology laboratory. The presence of ornithine decarboxylase and fermentation of sorbitol but not arabinose helps to differentiate further *S. marcescens* from other *Serratia* spp.[48] Biotyping,[47] DNA and RNA detection techniques,[64] and antimicrobial susceptibilities[96] can be used to characterize strains.

TREATMENT

Empiric decisions about antibiotic treatment of *Serratia* infection should rely on knowledge of hospital flora. Therapy should be tailored when susceptibilities are known. In newborns, meningitis and its complications should be suspected, and interventions should be guided by imaging of the central nervous system. Imaging techniques may be useful in guiding needle aspiration of abscesses.[77] Recommended antibiotic therapy for neonatal meningitis is a cephalosporin and an aminoglycoside for susceptible strains. Mortality rates remain high (>45%) even with appropriate antibiotic management.[21]

In older children and adults, reported response rates for bacteremic infection have been 75 percent for patients who received appropriate antibiotics, 22 percent for patients who received inappropriate antibiotics, and 29 percent for patients who received no antibiotics.[88] Patients who continue to have positive blood culture results while receiving appropriate antibiotic therapy have a poor prognosis. Inclusion of a penicillin or cephalosporin for susceptible strains should be considered. In the review by Saito and associates[88] of 118 patients with *Serratia* bacteremia, patients who received only an aminoglycoside had the poorest response rate among those who received appropriate therapy; patients who received a cephalosporin, alone or in combination, fared better. *Serratia* organisms generally have proven susceptible to third-generation cephalosporins in more recent surveys of hospitals from North America.[54] The physician needs to be wary, however, of potential resistance to cephalosporins and penicillins owing to the production of extended-spectrum β-lactamases. An extended-spectrum, metallo-β-lactamase–mediating resistance to imipenem has been described,[80] but it is uncommon. Physicians should consider strongly empiric use of a carbapenem in combination with an aminoglycoside in critically ill patients.

Amikacin historically has been effective in the treatment of gentamicin-resistant strains.[28,63] In 1985, amikacin was recommended as a first-line antibiotic for treatment of pediatric nosocomial infection when *Serratia* spp. or other enterics with resistance potential were suspected.[95] Since the 1980s, however, outbreaks of *S. marcescens* infections caused by amikacin-resistant strains have been reported.[79] Quinolones have been used successfully for treatment of organisms resistant to other agents,[41] but resistance to these drugs also has been identified.[59]

Cohorting and attempts to remove environmental sources of infection have been successful in ending epidemics but typically require several months.[24] Rarely, neonatal intensive care units have been closed to admissions to halt epidemics.[17,74]

Acknowledgments

The author thanks Dr. William Gruber and Dr. Thomas Boyce for their invaluable assistance with earlier versions of this chapter.

REFERENCES

1. Acar, J. F.: Serratia marcescens infections. Infect. Control 7:273-278, 1986.
2. Acar, J. F., Witchitz, J. L., Goldstein, F., et al.: Susceptibility of aminoglycoside-resistant gram-negative bacilli to amikacin: Delineation of individual resistance patterns. J. Infect. Dis. 134(Suppl.):S280-S285, 1976.
3. al Hazzaa, S. A., Tabbara, K. F., and Gammon, J. A.: Pink hypopyon: A sign of Serratia marcescens endophthalmitis. Br. J. Ophthalmol. 76:764-765, 1992.
4. Alvarez, R., Adan, A., Martinez, J. A., et al.: Haematogenous Serratia marcescens endophthalmitis in an HIV-infected intravenous drug addict. Infection 18:29-30, 1990.
5. Anagnostakis, D., Fitsialos, J., Koutsia, C., et al.: A nursery outbreak of Serratia marcescens infection: Evidence of a single source of contamination. Am. J. Dis. Child. 135:413-414, 1981.
6. Anonymous: Biologic testing involving human subjects by the Department of Defense, 1977: Hearings before the Subcommittee on Health and Science Research of the United States Senate. Washington, D.C., Government Printing Office, 1977.
7. Arroyo, J. C., Milligan, W. L., Postic, B., et al.: Clinical, epidemiologic and microbiologic features of a persistent outbreak of amikacin-resistant Serratia marcescens. Infect. Control 2:367-372, 1981.
8. Aucken, H. M., Boquete, T., Kaufmann, M. E., and Pitt, T. L.: Interpretation of band differences to distinguish strains of Serratia marcescens by pulsed-field gel electrophoresis of XbaI DNA digests. Epidemiol. Infect. 125:63-70, 2000.
9. Aucken, H. M., and Pitt, T. L.: Antibiotic resistance and putative virulence factors of Serratia marcescens with respect to O and K serotypes. J. Med. Microbiol. 47:1105-1113, 1998.
10. Balikian, J. P., Herman, P. G., and Godleski, J. J.: Serratia pneumonia. Radiology 137:309-311, 1980.
11. Beck-Sague, C. M., and Jarvis, W. R.: Epidemic bloodstream infections associated with pressure transducers: A persistent problem. Infect. Control Hosp. Epidemiol. 10:54-59, 1989.
12. Bingen, E. H., Mariani-Kurkdjian, P., Lambert-Zechovsky, N. Y., et al.: Ribotyping provides efficient differentiation of nosocomial Serratia marcescens isolates in a pediatric hospital. J. Clin. Microbiol. 30:2088-2091, 1992.
13. Bizzarro, M. J., Dembry, L. M., Baltimore, R. S., and Gallagher, P. G.: Case-control analysis of endemic Serratia marcescens bacteremia in a neonatal intensive care unit. Arch. Dis. Child. Fetal Neonatal Ed. 92:F120-F126, 2007.
14. Bollet, C., Grimont, P., Gainnier, M., et al.: Fatal pneumonia due to Serratia proteamaculans subsp. quinovora. J. Clin. Microbiol. 31:444-445, 1993.
15. Bollmann, R., Halle, E., Sokolowska-Kohler, W., et al.: Nosocomial infections due to Serratia marcescens: Clinical findings, antibiotic susceptibility patterns and fine typing. Infection 17:294-300, 1989.
16. Bouza, E., Garcia de la Torre, M., Erice, A., et al.: Serratia bacteremia. Diagn. Microbiol. Infect. Dis. 7:237-247, 1987.
17. Braver, D. J., Hauser, G. J., Berns, L., et al.: Control of a Serratia marcescens outbreak in a maternity hospital. J. Hosp. Infection 10:129-137, 1987.
18. Brooks, H. J. Chambers, T. J., and Tabaqchali, S.: The increasing isolation of Serratia species from clinical specimens. J. Hyg. 82:31-40, 1979.
19. Bullock, D. W., Bidwell, J. L., Reeves, D. S., et al.: Outbreaks of hospital infection in southwest England caused by gentamicin-resistant Serratia marcescens. J. Hosp. Infect. 3:263-273, 1982.
20. Bush, K., Flamm, R. K., Ohringer, S., et al.: Effect of clavulanic acid on activity of beta-lactam antibiotics in Serratia marcescens isolates producing both a TEM beta-lactamase and a chromosomal cephalosporinase. Antimicrob. Agents Chemother. 35:2203-2208, 1991.
21. Campbell, J. R., Diacovo, T., and Baker, C. J.: Serratia marcescens meningitis in neonates. Pediatr. Infect. Dis. J. 11:881-886, 1992.
22. Cann, K. J., Johnstone, D., and Skene, A. I.: An outbreak of Serratia marcescens infection following urodynamic studies. J. Hosp. Infect. 9:291-293, 1987.
23. Chmel, H.: Serratia odorifera biogroup 1 causing an invasive human infection. J. Clin. Microbiol. 26:1244-1245, 1988.
24. Christensen, G. D., Korones, S. B., Reed, L., et al.: Epidemic Serratia marcescens in a neonatal intensive care unit: Importance of the gastrointestinal tract as a reservoir. Infect. Control 3:127-133, 1982.
25. Coleman, D., Falkiner, F. R., Carr, M. E., et al.: Simultaneous outbreaks of infection due to Serratia marcescens in a general hospital. J. Hosp. Infect. 5:270-282, 1984.
26. Connacher, A. A., Old, D. C., Phillips, G., et al.: Recurrent peritonitis caused by Serratia marcescens in a diabetic patient receiving continuous ambulatory peritoneal dialysis. J. Hosp. Infect. 11:155-160, 1988.

27. Cooper, R., and Mills, J.: *Serratia* endocarditis: A follow-up report. Arch. Intern. Med. *140*:199-202, 1980.
28. Craven, P. C., Jorgensen, J. H., Kaspar, R. L., et al.: Amikacin therapy of patients with multiply antibiotic-resistant *Serratia marcescens* infections: Development of increasing resistance during therapy. Am. J. Med. *62*:902-910, 1977.
29. Daifuku, R., and Stamm, W. E.: Bacterial adherence to bladder uroepithelial cells in catheter-associated urinary tract infection. N. Engl. J. Med. *314*:1208-1213, 1986.
30. Darbas, H., Jean-Pierre, H., and Paillisson, J.: Case report and review of septicemia due to *Serratia ficaria*. J. Clin. Microbiol. *32*:2285-2288, 1994.
31. Deorukhkar, A. A., Chander, R., Ghosh, S. B., and Sainis, K. B.: Identification of a red-pigmented bacterium producing a potent anti-tumor N-alkylated prodigiosin as *Serratia marcescens*. Res. Microbiol. *158*:399-404, 2007.
32. DiPersio, J. R., and Dowzicky, M. J.: Regional variations in multidrug resistance among Enterobacteriaceae in the USA and comparative activity of tigecycline, a new glycylcycline antimicrobial. Int. J. Antimicrob. Agents *29*:518-527, 2007.
33. Duggan, T. G., Leng, R. A., Hancock, B. M., et al.: *Serratia marcescens* in a newborn unit: Microbiological features. Pathology *16*:189-191, 1984.
34. Echols, R. M., Palmer, D. L., King, R. M., et al.: Multidrug-resistant *Serratia marcescens* bacteriuria related to urologic instrumentation. South. Med. J. *77*:173-177, 1984.
35. Ehrenkranz, N. J., Bolyard, E. A., Wiener, M., et al.: Antibiotic-sensitive *Serratia marcescens* infections complicating cardiopulmonary operations: Contaminated disinfectant as a reservoir. Lancet *2*:1289-1292, 1980.
36. Farmer, J. I., Davis, B. R., and Grimont, P. A. D.: Source of American *Serratia*. Lancet *2*:459-460, 1977.
37. Fitzgerald, P., Drew, J. H., and Kruszelnicki, I.: *Serratia*: A problem in a neonatal nursery. Aust. Paediatr. J. *20*:205-207, 1984.
38. Frean, J. A., Arntzen, L., Rosekilly, I., et al.: Investigation of contaminated parenteral nutrition fluids associated with an outbreak of *Serratia odorifera* septicaemia. J. Hosp. Infect. *27*:263-273, 1994.
39. Geiseler, P. J., Harris,.B., and Andersen, B. R.: Nosocomial outbreak of nitrate-negative *Serratia marcescens* infections. J. Clin. Microbiol. *15*:728-730, 1982.
40. Gianneli, D., Tzelepi, E., Tzouvelekis, L. S., et al.: Dissemination of cephalosporin-resistant *Serratia marcescens* strains producing a plasmidic SHV type beta-lactamase in Greek hospitals. Eur. J. Clin. Microbiol. Infect. Dis. *13*:764-767, 1994.
41. Goldstein, E. J., Alpert, M. L., Najem, A., et al.: Norfloxacin in the treatment of complicated and uncomplicated urinary tract infections: A comparative multicenter trial. Am. J. Med. *82*:65-69, 1987.
42. Gong, J., Hogman, C. F., Hambraeus, A., et al.: Transfusion-associated *Serratia marcescens* infection: Studies of the mechanism of action. Transfusion *33*:802-808, 1993.
43. Gordon, W. H.: Report on an investigation of the ventilation of the debating chamber of the House of Commons. Parliamentary Command Paper, p. 3035, 1906.
44. Graham, D. R., Clegg, H. W. D., Anderson, R. L., et al.: Gentamicin treatment associated with later nosocomial gentamicin-resistant *Serratia marcescens* infections. Infect. Control *2*:31-37, 1981.
45. Gransden, W. R., Webster, M., French, G. L., et. al.: An outbreak of *Serratia marcescens* transmitted by contaminated breast pumps in a special care baby unit. J. Hosp. Infect. *7*:149-154, 1986.
46. Grauel, E. L., Halle, E., Bollmann, R., et al.: Neonatal septicaemia: Incidence, etiology and outcome: A 6-year analysis. Acta Paediatr. Scand. *360*(Suppl.):113-119, 1989.
47. Grimont, P. A., and Grimont, F.: Biotyping of *Serratia marcescens* and its use in epidemiological studies. J. Clin. Microbiol *8*:73-83, 1978.
48. Grimont, P. A. D., and Grimont, F.: *Serratia. In* Krieg, N. R., and Holt, J. G. (eds.): Bergey's Manual of Systematic Bacteriology. Vol. 1. Baltimore, Williams & Wilkins, 1984, pp. 476-484.
49. Hejazi, A., and Falkiner, F. R.: *Serratia marcescens*. J. Med. Microbiol. *46*:903-912, 1997.
50. Hejazi, A., Keane, C. T., and Falkiner, F. R.: The use of RAPD-PCR as a typing method for *Serratia marcescens*. J. Med. Microbiol. *46*:913-919, 1997.
51. Hoyen, C., Rice, L., Conte, S., et al.: Use of real time pulsed field gel electrophoresis to guide interventions during a nursery outbreak of *Serratia marcescens* infection. Pediatr. Infect. Dis. J. *18*:357-360, 1999.
52. Hume, E. B., Zhu, H., Cole, N., et al.: Efficacy of contact lens multipurpose solutions against *Serratia marcescens*. Optom. Vis. Sci. *84*:316-320, 2007.
53. John, J. F. J., and McNeill, W. F.: Characteristics of *Serratia marcescens* containing a plasmid coding for gentamicin resistance in nosocomial infections. J. Infect. Dis. *143*:810-817, 1981.
54. Jones, R. N., Jenkins, S. G., Hoban, D. J., et al.: In vitro efficacy of six cephalosporins tested against Enterobacteriaceae isolated at 38 North American medical centres participating in the SENTRY Antimicrobial Surveillance Program, 1997-1998. Int. J. Antimicrob. Agents *15*:111-118, 2000.
55. Karnad, A., Alvarez, S., and Berk, S. L.: Pneumonia caused by gram-negative bacilli. Am. J. Med. *79*:61-67, 1985.
56. Khan, E. A., Wafelman, L. S., Garcia-Prats, J. A., and Taber, L. H.: *Serratia marcescens* pneumonia, empyema and pneumatocele in a preterm neonate. Pediatr. Infect. Dis. J. *16*:1003-1005, 1997.
57. Knowles, S., Herra, C., Devitt, E., et al.: An outbreak of multiply resistant *Serratia marcescens*: The importance of persistent carriage. Bone Marrow Transplant. *25*:873-877, 2000.
58. Konig, W., Faltin, Y., Scheffer, J., et al.: Role of cell-bound hemolysin as a pathogenicity factor for *Serratia* infections. Infect. Immun. *55*:2554-2561, 1987.
59. Korner, R. J., Nicol, A., Reeves, D. S., et al.: Ciprofloxacin-resistant *Serratia marcescens* endocarditis as a complication of non-Hodgkin's lymphoma. J. Infect. *29*:73-76, 1994.
60. Krieger, J. N., Kaiser, D. L., and Wenzel, R. P.: Urinary tract etiology of bloodstream infections in hospitalized patients. J. Infect. Dis. *148*:57-62, 1983.
61. Kumagai, Y., Okada, K., and Sawae, Y.: The effect of humoral and cell-mediated immunity in resistance to systemic *Serratia* infection. J. Med. Microbiol. *36*:245-249, 1992.
62. Lam, A. H., Berry, A., deSilva, M., et al.: Intracranial *Serratia* infection in preterm newborn infants. A. J. N. R. Am. J. Neuroradiol. *5*:447-451, 1984.
63. Leonard, J. M., McGee, Z. A., and Alford, R. H.: Gentamicin-resistant bacillary infection: Clinical features and amikacin therapy. Arch. Intern. Med. *138*:201-205, 1978.
64. Liu, P. Y., Lau, Y. J., Hu, B. S., et al.: Use of PCR to study epidemiology of *Serratia marcescens* isolates in nosocomial infection. J. Clin. Microbiol. *32*:1935-1938, 1994.
65. Matsumoto, K., Yamamoto, T., Kamata, R., et al.: Pathogenesis of serratial infection: Activation of the Hageman factor-prekallikrein cascade by serratial protease. J. Biochem. *96*:739-749, 1984.
66. McCormack, R. C., and Kunin, C. M.: Control of a single source nursery epidemic due to *Serratia marcescens*. Pediatrics *37*:750-755, 1966.
67. McNaughton, M., Mazinke, N., and Thomas, E.: Newborn conjunctivitis associated with triclosan 0.5 percent antiseptic intrinsically contaminated with *Serratia marcescens*. Can. J. Infect. Control *10*:7-8, 1995.
68. Medeiros, A. A., and O'Brien, T. F.: Contributions of R factors to the antibiotic resistance of hospital isolates of *Serratia*. Antimicrob. Agents Chemother. *8*:30-35, 1968.
69. Merlino, C. P.: Bartolomeo Bizio's letter to the most eminent priest, Angelo Bellani, concerning the phenomenon of the red-colored polenta. J. Bacteriol. *9*:527-543, 1924.
70. Meyer, R. D.: Patterns and mechanisms of emergence of resistance to amikacin. J. Infect. Dis. *136*:449-452, 1977.
71. Miller, P. J., and Wenzel, R. P.: Etiologic organisms as independent predictors of death and morbidity associated with bloodstream infections. J. Infect. Dis. *156*:471-477, 1987.
72. Miranda, G., Kelly, C., Solorzano, F., et al.: Use of pulsed-field gel electrophoresis typing to study an outbreak of infection due to *Serratia marcescens* in a neonatal intensive care unit. J. Clin. Microbiol. *34*:3138-3141, 1996.
73. Molla, A., Matsumoto, K., Oyamada, I., et al.: Degradation of protease inhibitors, immunoglobulins, and other serum proteins by *Serratia* protease and its toxicity to fibroblast in culture. Infect. Immun. *53*:522-529, 1986.
74. Montanaro, D., Grasso, G. M., Annino, I., et al.: Epidemiological and bacteriological investigation of *Serratia marcescens* epidemic in a nursery and in a neonatal intensive care unit. J. Hyg. *93*:67-78, 1984.
75. Newport, M. T., John, J. F., Michel, Y. M., et al.: Endemic *Serratia marcescens* infection in a neonatal intensive care nursery associated with gastrointestinal colonization. Pediatr. Infect. Dis. *4*:160-167, 1985.
76. Nicasio, A. M., Quintiliani, R., Jr., Deryke, C. A., et al.: Treatment of *Serratia marcescens* meningitis with prolonged infusion of meropenem. Ann. Pharmacother. *41*:1077-1081, 2007.
77. Obana, W. G., Cogen, P. H., Callen, P. W., et al.: Ultrasound-guided aspiration of a neonatal brain abscess. Child. Nerv. Syst. *7*:272-273; discussion 274, 1991.
78. Oda, T., Kojima, Y., Akaike, T., et al.: Inactivation of chemotactic activity of C5a by the serratial 56-kilodalton protease. Infect. Immun. *58*:1269-1272, 1990.
79. Okuda, T., Endo, N., Osada, Y., et al.: Outbreak of nosocomial urinary tract infections caused by *Serratia marcescens*. J. Clin. Microbiol. *20*:691-695, 1984.
80. Osano, E., Arakawa, Y., Wacharotayankun, R., et al.: Molecular characterization of an enterobacterial metallo beta-lactamase found in a clinical isolate of *Serratia marcescens* that shows imipenem resistance. Antimicrob. Agents Chemother. *38*:71-78, 1994.
81. Pagani, L., Luzzaro, F., Ronza, P., et al.: Outbreak of extended-spectrum beta-lactamase-producing *Serratia marcescens* in an intensive care unit. F. E. M. S. Immunol. Med. Microbiol. *10*:39-46, 1994.
82. Prabha, V., Singh, N., and Chopra, P.: Bacteriological evaluation of conjunctiva, contact lens storage cases and solutions during contact lens wear. Indian J. Pathol. Microbiol. *50*:101-103, 2007.
83. Rabinowitz, K., and Schiffrin, R.: A ward contamination by *Serratia marcescens*. Acta Med. Orient. *11*:181-184, 1952.
84. Roth, V. R., Arduino, M. J., Nobiletti, J., et al.: Transfusion-related sepsis due to *Serratia liquefaciens* in the United States. Transfusion *40*:931-935, 2000.
85. Rubens, C. E., Farrar, W. E. J., McGee, Z. A., et al.: Evolution of a plasmid mediating resistance to multiple antimicrobial agents during a prolonged epidemic of nosocomial infections. J. Infect. Dis. *143*:170-181, 1981.
86. Rubens, C. E., McNeill, W. F., and Farrar, W. E. J.: Evolution of multiple-antibiotic-resistance plasmids mediated by transposable plasmid deoxyribonucleic acid sequences. J. Bacteriol. *140*:713-719, 1979.

87. Rutala, W. A., Kennedy, V. A., Loflin, H. B., et al.: *Serratia marcescens* nosocomial infections of the urinary tract associated with urine measuring containers and urinometers. Am. J. Med. 70:659-663, 1981.

88. Saito, H., Elting, L., Bodey, G. P., et al.: *Serratia* bacteremia: Review of 118 cases. Rev. Infect. Dis. 11:912-920, 1989.

89. Schaberg, D. R., Alford, R. H., Anderson, R., et al.: An outbreak of nosocomial infection due to multiply resistant *Serratia marcescens*: Evidence of interhospital spread. J. Infect. Dis. 134:181-188, 1976.

90. Schaberg, D. R., Haley, R. W., Highsmith, A. K., et al.: Nosocomial bacteriuria: A prospective study of case clustering and antimicrobial resistance. Ann. Intern. Med. 93:420-424, 1980.

91. Schaberg, D. R., Rubens, C. E., Alford, R. H., et al.: Evolution of antimicrobial resistance and nosocomial infection: Lessons from the Vanderbilt experience. Am. J. Med. 70:445-448, 1981.

92. Senda, K., Arakawa, Y., Ichiyama, S., et al.: PCR detection of metallo-beta-lactamase gene (blaIMP) in gram-negative rods resistant to broad-spectrum beta-lactams. J. Clin. Microbiol. 34:2909-2913, 1996.

93. Serruys-Schoutens, E., Rost, F., and Depre, G.: A nosocomial epidemic of *Serratia liquefaciens* urinary tract infection after cystometry. Eur. J. Clin. Microbiol. 3:316-317, 1984.

94. Shahcheraghi, F., Minato, Y., Chen, J., et al.: Molecular cloning and characterization of a multidrug efflux pump, SmfY, from *Serratia marcescens*. Biol. Pharm. Bull. 30:798-800, 2007.

95. Shulman, S. T., and Yogev, R.: Treatment of pediatric infections with amikacin as first-line aminoglycoside. Am. J. Med. 79:43-50, 1985.

96. Sifuentes-Osornio, J., Ruiz-Palacios, G. M., and Groschel, D. H.: Analysis of epidemiologic markers of nosocomial *Serratia marcescens* isolates with special reference to the Grimont biotyping system. J. Clin. Microbiol. 23:230-234, 1986.

97. Stamm, W. E., Kolff, C. A., Dones, E. M., et al.: A nursery outbreak caused by *Serratia marcescens*: Scalp-vein needles as a portal of entry. J. Pediatr 89:96-99, 1976.

98. Svensson, O., Parment, P. A., and Blomgren, G.: Orthopaedic infections by *Serratia marcescens*: A report of seven cases. Scand. J. Infect. Dis. 19:69-75, 1987.

99. Thomas, F. E., Jackson, R. T., Melly, A., et al.: Sequential hospitalwide outbreaks of resistant *Serratia* and *Klebsiella* infections. Arch. Intern. Med. 137:581-584, 1977.

100. Verrall, R.: *Serratia marcescens*. Infect. Control 4:469-471, 1983.

101. Villarino, M. E., Jarvis, W. R., O'Hara, C., et al.: Epidemic of *Serratia marcescens* bacteremia in a cardiac intensive care unit. J. Clin. Microbiol. 27:2433-2436, 1989.

102. Waisman, H. A., and Stone, W. H.: The presence of *Serratia marcescens* as the predominating organism in the intestinal tract of the newborn: The occurrence of the "red diaper syndrome." Pediatrics 21:8-12, 1958.

103. Wheat, R. P., Zuckerman, A., and Rantz, L. A.: Infection due to chromobacteria: Report of eleven cases. Arch. Intern. Med. 88:461-466, 1951.

104. Woodward, H. M. M., and Clarke, K. B.: A case of infection in man by the *Bacterium prodigiosum*. Lancet 1:314-315, 1913.

105. Yu, V. L.: *Serratia marcescens*: Historical perspective and clinical review. N. Engl. J. Med. 300:887-893, 1979.

106. Yu, V. L., Oakes, C. A., Axnick, K. J., et al.: Patient factors contributing to the emergence of gentamicin-resistant *Serratia marcescens*. Am. J. Med. 66:468-472, 1979.

107. Yung, M. S., Boost, M., Cho, P, and Yap, M.: Microbial contamination of contact lenses and lens care accessories of soft contact lens wearers (university students) in Hong Kong. Ophthalmic Physiol. Opt. 27:11-21, 2007.

108. Zaidi, M., Sifuentes, J., Bobadilla, M., et al.: Epidemic of *Serratia marcescens* bacteremia and meningitis in a neonatal unit in Mexico City. Infect. Control Hosp. Epidemiol. 10:14-20, 1989.

SALMONELLA

121

Theresa J. Ochoa ⊕ Thomas G. Cleary

MICROBIOLOGY

The classification of *Salmonella* is confusing because multiple nomenclature systems are used (Table 121–1). In this chapter, we use the current designation of the Centers for Disease Control and Prevention, rather than either the complete name or the traditional clinical shorthand that referred to each of the 2463 serovars of *Salmonella* as though they were separate species. In hospital laboratories, *S.* ser. *Choleraesuis* and *S.* ser. *Typhi* are distinguished biochemically from other *Salmonella* spp. Serogroup, based on O (somatic) antigen, also usually is determined on initial isolation, and organisms that are not *S.* ser. *Typhi* or *S.* ser. *Choleraesuis* are reported as *Salmonella* serogroup A, B, C1, D1, and so on. Common *Salmonella* spp. and their serogroups are shown in Table 121–2.

Salmonella serotype is defined by the serogroup antigens, the flagellar (H) antigens, and the virulence (Vi) antigen. H antigens can be either phase 1 (nonspecific) or phase 2 (specific). The Vi antigen, a heat-labile polysaccharide found on *S.* ser. *Typhi*, *S.* ser. *Dublin*, and *S.* ser. *Paratyphi C*, may block agglutina-

TABLE 121–1 Examples of Current *Salmonella* Nomenclature

CDC Designation	Complete Name	Previous Designation
S. ser. Typhi	*S. enterica** subsp. *enterica* ser. Typhi	*S. typhi*
S. ser. Enteritidis	*S. enterica* subsp. *enterica* ser. Enteritidis	*S. enteritidis*
S. IIIa 18:z₄,z₂₃: -	*S. enterica* subsp. *arizonae* ser. 18:z₄,z₂₃: -	*Arizona hinshawii* ser. 7a, 7b:1,2,5: -
S. ser. Marina	*S. enterica* subsp. *houtenae* ser. Marina	*S. marina*

*S. choleraesuis and S. enteritidis also are designations commonly used for the species.
CDC, Centers for Disease Control and Prevention.

TABLE 121–2 *Salmonella* Species Included in Major Serogroups

Serogroup*	Representative Serotypes
A	*S.* ser. Paratyphi A
B	*S.* ser. Paratyphi B
	S. ser. Saint-Paul
	S. ser. Agona
	S. ser. Derby
	S. ser. Typhimurium
	S. ser. Heidelberg
C1	*S.* ser. Paratyphi C
	S. ser. Choleraesuis
	S. ser. Montevideo
	S. ser. Infantis
C2	*S.* ser. Newport
C3	*S.* ser. Santiago
D1	*S.* ser. Typhi
	S. ser. Enteritidis
	S. ser. Dublin
D2	*S.* ser. Strasbourg
E1	*S.* ser. Anatum
E2	*S.* ser. Newington
E3	*S.* ser. Illinois

*Human infections with organisms in serogroups E4, F, G1, G2, H, and I and the O antigens not given serogroup designation (O17 through O67) are uncommon.

tion caused by antibodies to O antigen. Serotyping generally is done in public health department laboratories. Although serotyping is an important epidemiologic tool for defining outbreaks, it is most useful when an unusual type is associated with disease. When a common serotype is associated with an outbreak (e.g., *S.* ser. *Typhimurium*), biochemical phenotype, antibiogram, plasmid characterization,[199] bacteriophage typing,[26,87] outer-membrane protein analysis, pulsed field gel electrophoresis, and randomly amplified polymorphic DNA may help deterimine whether a single-strain, common-source outbreak is in progress.

Six subgroups of *Salmonella* have been proposed on the basis of DNA relatedness. Most serotypes, including almost all of the serotypes important in human and animal disease, belong to subgroup I. The genus *Arizona* now is classified as a *Salmonella*.

Salmonellae are motile (owing to peritrichous flagella), non-encapsulated, gram-negative bacilli of the Enterobacteriaceae family. Most ferment glucose, maltose, and mannitol but do not use lactose or sucrose. All pathogenic *Salmonella* spp. other than *S.* ser. *Typhi* produce gas. *Salmonella* spp. are facultative anaerobes. Blood agar or chocolate agar supports their growth when they are present as the sole organisms in blood, cerebrospinal fluid, or joint fluid. For specimens containing mixed flora (e.g., stool), selective media such as Salmonella-Shigella (SS) agar or bismuth sulfate agar must be used.

EPIDEMIOLOGY

NONTYPHOIDAL *SALMONELLA*

Public Health Issues

In most of the world, the prevalence of *Salmonella* varies according to the water supply, waste disposal, food preparation practices, and climate. The incidence of nontyphoidal salmonellosis in the United States has been increasing steadily, however, despite implementation of good public health measures. During the last 40 years, a greater than sixfold increase in reported nontyphoidal *Salmonella* infection in the United States has occurred, with an estimate of 168,000 physician office visits, 15,000 hospitalizations, and 400 deaths annually during 1996 to 1999.[252] This increase reflects industrial-scale food production and distribution,[38] misuse of antimicrobial agents (in humans and animals) that alter the gastrointestinal flora and increase host susceptibility to *Salmonella*, and probably an increasing number of immunocompromised individuals in the population. More recently, an important decrease has occurred in the incidence of *S.* ser *Enteritidis* infections in the United States, as a result of targeted interventions, including on-farm control measures, refrigeration, and education,[153] highlighting the importance of these efforts to reduce the rate of *Salmonella* infection further.

Significance of Animal Reservoirs

In contrast to *Shigella* spp., which infect only primates, nontyphoidal *Salmonella* spp. infect a variety of animals (including poultry, livestock, and pet reptiles and rodents).[232] Animals and animal products (including meat and dairy products), water, and infected humans can be the source of infection. *Salmonella* is the number one cause of foodborne illness in the United States, and the second most common cause of death from foodborne pathogens.[146] Spread of resistant organisms from food animals to humans has been shown.[166] *Salmonella* spp. have been isolated from 50 percent of poultry,[28] 16 percent of pork, 5 percent of beef, and 40 percent of frozen egg products in retail stores. Undercooked eggs (e.g., in Caesar salad, egg-dipped bread,

homemade eggnog) may be contaminated by organisms on the shell surface or transovarially directly through the egg yolk. Grade A shell eggs have been implicated in more than 40 percent of more recent outbreaks.[146] Even in the absence of recognized outbreaks, eggs probably are important vehicles of infection; foods containing eggs that have been undercooked are more likely to have been consumed during the 3 days before illness in sporadic cases than in control cases.[112]

The risk of outbreaks occurring was shown when milk contaminated with *S.* ser. *Typhimurium* was distributed in Chicago, Illinois. Reports estimated that more than 150,000 people became ill, with more than 16,000 culture-confirmed cases, 2777 individuals hospitalized, and 14 fatalities.[21] Ice cream, cream cakes, and mayonnaise commonly have been incriminated as the source of infections. Fruits and vegetables rarely are vehicles.[36]

Some serotypes are associated with particular reservoirs. *S.* ser. *Dublin* is associated with dairy cattle and frequently is found in individuals who drink raw milk.[237] *S.* ser. *Choleraesuis* is associated with pigs. *S.* ser. *Typhimurium* is associated with contact with pet rodents.[232] Infection with *S.* ser. *Marina* is associated with contact with pet iguanas. *Salmonella* group F, *S.* ser. *Typhimurium*, *S.* ser. *Muenchen*, and *S.* ser. *Java* infections have been traced to pet turtles. Reptiles, including rattlesnakes, are important *S.* IIIa 18:z₄,z₂₃: (*Arizona hinshawii*) reservoirs.

Humans as a Reservoir

After infection occurs, nontyphoidal *Salmonella* spp. are excreted in feces for a median of 5 weeks. Children younger than 5 years old may excrete the organisms for 20 weeks after having an illness, but older children and adults usually excrete *Salmonella* for less than 8 weeks. *S.* ser. *Typhi* may be excreted chronically, particularly in the presence of gallbladder disease. Food handlers who are excreting *Salmonella* spp. represent an important risk group.

Bacterial Characteristics Favoring Survival

Salmonella spp. are hardy. They survive refrigeration and sometimes heating; they may remain viable at ambient or reduced temperatures for weeks. When contaminated foods are cooked for less than 12 minutes at temperatures less than 150° F (<65.5° C), salmonellae may remain viable. *Salmonella* spp. are killed by heating to 130° F (54.4° C) for 1 hour or 140° F (60° C) for 15 minutes. Salmonellae survive for hours on the hands of slaughterhouse workers.[183] The organisms have been found to survive in flour for nearly 1 year. *S.* ser. *Tennessee* has been reported to remain viable for 2 to 8 days on glass, stainless steel, enameled surfaces, rubber mattress, linen, and a rubber tabletop.[257] Nosocomial infections have been related to contaminated medical equipment (e.g., endoscopes) and diagnostic or pharmacologic preparations, particularly those of animal origin (e.g., pituitary extracts, bile salts, pancreatic extracts, pepsin, vitamins).

Relationship of Age to Risk of Disease

The highest incidence rates occur in children younger than 5 years of age, especially infants younger than 1 year, and in individuals older than 70 years. Nursery outbreaks often can be traced to an infected mother,[1,2,16,137] with subsequent spread occurring through health care personnel.[217,258] The mother of the index case can be symptomatic[82,155,207] or asymptomatic,[258] recovering from recent infection,[2,173,221] or a chronic carrier.[214] Low-birth-weight infants seem to be at higher risk than are full-term infants for acquiring *Salmonella* infection.[19,217,258] The source of infection occasionally is contaminated food, but more often it is fomites (delivery room resuscitators,[208] rectal thermometers,[123,158] suction devices,[133] water baths for heating formula,[199] soap dispensers,[165] scales,[6,20,258] tables,[258] air-conditioning filters,[258] and plumbing[162]). Outbreaks in nurseries often are extraordinarily difficult to stop. They have been reported to last months[158,177,258] to years.[82,162,234] Contamination sometimes can become so widespread that other areas of the hospital also experience cases.[156,219] These outbreaks occur far more commonly with *Salmonella* than with other bacterial enteropathogens. Such outbreaks sometimes are caused by multiresistant *Salmonella*.[137]

Seasonality

Salmonella infection occurs in warm months.

Inoculum Size Required to Cause Disease

The estimated inoculum size required to cause symptomatic disease in healthy adult volunteers is 10^5 to 10^{10} organisms,[25] but the number of organisms required to cause symptoms in infants and children probably is much lower. In contrast, large inocula are not required for *Shigella* infection, which occurs in adult volunteers exposed to only 10 organisms. In some outbreaks, very small inocula of *Salmonella* seem to have caused disease. Large inocula (e.g., 10^9 organisms) may cause severe symptoms, even in healthy children.[238] The incubation period usually is 6 to 72 hours, but it depends on inoculum size, bacterial virulence, and host immunocompetence. Communicability parallels the duration of fecal excretion. The probability of salmonellosis occuring is increased when a member of the household is infected. Infants especially may be susceptible to acquiring *Salmonella* infection directly or indirectly from ill family members. Infants also may acquire infection via exposure to raw meat while riding in a grocery cart or while having contact with infected pets.[127] In a retrospective review of 187 infants younger than 1 year old with *Salmonella* gastroenteritis, 39 percent had at least one family contact with diarrhea, and 71 percent of the contacts had stool cultures positive for *Salmonella*.[259] *Salmonella* spp. rarely have been isolated during studies of gastroenteritis in daycare centers, suggesting that larger inocula are required to cause illness in toddlers and older children.[44,142,186]

Antibiotic Selection Pressure

Since the mid-1960s, *Salmonella* spp. have become increasingly resistant to ampicillin, chloramphenicol, and trimethoprim-sulfamethoxazole (TMP-SMX). Multiresistant strains have included *S.* ser. *Typhimurium*, which is the most common serotype in Europe and the United States, and *S.* ser. *Heidelberg, S.* ser. *Agona, S.* ser. *Muenchen, S.* ser. *Enteritidis,* and *S.* ser. *Hadar.* Antibiotic resistance usually is transferable between organisms through plasmids that carry genes encoding resistance factors. More recent studies have revealed that some serotype-specific virulence plasmids form hybrid plasmids through recombination with resistance plasmids or acquire gene cassettes consisting of multiple resistance genes. Such evolutionary events provide a virulent strain with the advantage of survival in an unfavorable drug environment.[231] Patients who are infected with antibiotic-resistant strains are more likely to be hospitalized, to be very young, to be black, and to have been exposed recently to antibiotic agents.[138] Previous use of antimicrobial agents for treatment of other illnesses is a significant risk factor for acquiring multiresistant *Salmonella* infection.[148,200]

Perhaps the most important factor is the overuse and misuse of antibiotics in animals raised for food.[49,117,118,141,229] Subtherapeutic concentrations of antibiotics used to enhance growth and to prevent infection promote intestinal colonization by antibiotic-resistant bacteria, including *Salmonella*; these organisms may be found in feces and may contaminate meat at the time of slaughter. Plasmid analysis and antibiotic susceptibility patterns have linked *Salmonella* outbreaks to specific farms and slaughterhouses.[117,118,166]

SALMONELLA SER. TYPHI

The Centers for Disease Control and Prevention estimates that 21 million typhoid cases occur annually in the world, with an annual incidence varying from 100 to 1000 cases per 100,000 population.[55] The global mortality estimates from typhoid also have been revised downward from 600,000 to 200,000, on the basis of regional extrapolations.[55] *S.* ser. *Typhi* is the most common *Salmonella* isolate in many developing countries. Although the overall ratio of disease caused by *S.* ser. *Typhi* to disease caused by *S.* ser. *Paratyphi* is about 10:1, the proportion of *S. paratyphi* infections is increasing in some parts of the world.[23] The human immunodeficiency virus (HIV) and acquired immunodeficiency syndrome (AIDS) epidemic in Africa has been associated with a concomitant increase in community-acquired bacteremia caused by nontyphoidal *Salmonella*.[22,102] In the United States, approximately 1700 total cases were reported (1 case per 100,000) in 1955. In 1988, approximately 400 total cases were reported (0.018 case per 100,000). Approximately 28 percent of infections occurred in individuals 19 years old or younger. Frequently, the highest incidence is stated as occurring in individuals 5 to 12 years old. More recent population-based studies from South Asia and India suggest, however, that the incidence is highest in children younger than 5 years, with higher rates of complications and hospitalization.[23,224]

In the United States, individuals traveling to developing countries are a high-risk group; 62 to 81 percent of infections are related to foreign travel, especially to Mexico, India, the Philippines, Pakistan, El Salvador, and Haiti. Of these areas, the Indian subcontinent has the highest incidence of typhoid among travelers.[5,37,163,212]

Reservoir

Humans are the reservoir for *S.* ser. *Typhi;* infection implies direct or indirect contact with an infected person. Animal products transmit *S.* ser. *Typhi* if they are contaminated by infected humans during processing. The most common mode of transmission is food or water contaminated by human feces. Water-borne typhoid fever epidemics are especially important. Congenital transmission can occur from a bacteremic mother to her fetus transplacentally or at the time of delivery.

Relevance of Inoculum Size to Disease

As with nontyphoidal *Salmonella*, more than 10^5 organisms are required to cause clinical illness in adults.[120]

Antibiotic Resistance

The worldwide frequency of antibiotic-resistant *S.* ser. *Typhi* has been increasing since the 1960s[226] but remains much lower than that of nontyphoidal *Salmonella*. Extensive protracted outbreaks have been reported throughout Asia, the Middle East, and Central and South America. These outbreaks may have been related to widespread availability and inappropriate use of antimicrobial agents (especially chloramphenicol) as over-the-counter drugs in these areas. After sporadic outbreaks of chloramphenicol-resistant typhoid between 1970 and 1985, many strains of *S.* ser. *Typhi* developed plasmid-mediated, multidrug resistance to the three primary antimicrobials used (ampicillin, chloramphenicol, and co-trimoxazole).[205] This resistance was countered by the advent of oral quinolones, but chromosomally acquired quinolone resistance in *S.* ser. *Typhi* and *S.* ser. *Paratyphi* has been described more recently in various parts of Asia, possibly related to the widespread and indiscriminate use of quinolones.[197,223]

PATHOPHYSIOLOGY

Host susceptibility is understood most easily in terms of specific events in pathogenesis. Tables 121–3 and 121–4 show the rele-

TABLE 121–3 Susceptibility to *Salmonella* Species Infection

Patient Group at Risk	Mechanism
Newborn	Achlorhydria, rapid gastric emptying
	Poorly developed cell-mediated immunity
	Complement deficiency
	Immunoglobulin deficiency in premature infants
Sickle-cell anemia	Reticuloendothelial system overload owing to hemolysis
	Functional asplenia
	Tissue infarcts
	Defective opsonization
Neutropenia (congenital or acquired)	Polymorphonuclear neutrophils needed for killing
Chronic granulomatous disease	Defective killing by polymorphonuclear neutrophils
AIDS	Low CD4
	Effects of malnutrition on cell-mediated immunity
	Survival of organisms in macrophages (owing to *Salmonella* genes PhoP/PhoQ, spvA-D, R)
Organ transplantation, immunosuppression	Defective cell-mediated immunity
Gastrectomy	Loss of stomach acid barrier
Malaria	Reticuloendothelial overload during hemolysis
	Abnormal complement levels
	Abnormal macrophage function
Bartonellosis	Reticuloendothelial overload during hemolysis
Schistosomiasis	*Salmonella* sequestered in schistosomes protected from host defenses and antibiotics

TABLE 121–4 Putative Pathophysiologic Basis of Selected Clinical Features of Salmonellosis

Disease Manifestation	Mechanisms and Bacterial Genes
Bloody diarrhea	*sip* A-D mediated invasion and interleukin-8 mediated inflammation
Watery diarrhea	*stn* enterotoxin (cholera-like toxin)
	SopB-mediated intestinal inflammation and fluid secretion
	Serotypes that induce transepithelial polymorphonuclear leukocyte migration (e.g., *S.* ser. *Typhimurium*) are more likely to cause diarrhea than are serotypes that do not (e.g., *S.* ser. *Typhi*)
Bacteremia	*viaB* (Vi synthesis) capsular antigen interferes with C3 binding (*S.* ser. *Typhi*, *S.* ser. *Dublin*, *S.* ser. *Paratyphi C*)
	rck resistance to serum complement (virulence plasmid encoded)
	rfb encodes lipopolysaccharide synthesis; lipopolysaccharide contributes to persistence of bacteremia
Relapses, prolonged fever, failure of certain antibiotics	Survival in macrophages (*sseABC*, *spiC*, *mgtCB*, cytotoxin and virulence plasmid genes *spvRABCD*)

vance of specific host and bacterial virulence factors in salmonellosis. The outcome of ingestion of *Salmonella* depends on the bacteria and the host.

Various *Salmonella* strains can (1) adhere to, invade, and multiply in intestinal epithelium; (2) produce cholera toxin–like enterotoxin that increases cyclic adenosine monophosphate levels within intestinal crypt cells, causing a net efflux of electrolytes and water into the intestinal lumen; (3) be taken up by M cells overlying Peyer patches of the distal ileum and proximal colon; (4) survive in macrophages of Peyer patches, mesenteric lymph nodes, and the extraintestinal reticuloendothelial system; and (5) survive in the bloodstream.[80,81,90] Specific genes encode virulence factors necessary for each step in these processes.

Pathologic findings include hypertrophy and hyperplasia of the intestinal and mesenteric lymphoid tissues, liver, and spleen in *S.* ser. *Typhi* infection. In contrast, *S.* ser. *Typhimurium* and other nontyphoidal serotypes cause diffuse colitis, mucosal edema, and crypt abscesses as the major pathologic abnormalities.[28,58] Some virulence genes are shared by all *Salmonella* strains, whereas others are serotype-specific. Differences in invasiveness of various serotypes exist. *S.* ser. *Typhi*, *S.* ser. *Choleraesuis*, *S.* ser. *Heidelberg*,[122,160] and *S.* ser. *Dublin*[237] are more likely to enter the blood and to seed distant sites. Virulence plasmids have been identified in *S.* ser. *Typhi*, *S.* ser. *Typhimurium*, and *S.* ser. *Dublin*.[17] The presence of virulence plasmids seems to be more common in blood isolates of *S.* ser. *Typhimurium* than in fecal isolates (76% versus 42%).[79]

Nursery outbreaks of *Salmonella* have shown dramatically the variability in severity of illness related to strain or serotype. In nursery outbreaks of *S.* ser. *Oranienburg*[234] and *S.* ser. *Newport*,[137] grossly bloody stools were found in 76 to 90 percent of infected infants, with 10 to 11 percent febrile and only 9 to 11 percent asymptomatic. Watery, green, nonbloody diarrhea has been common with *S.* ser. *Typhimurium*,[2] *S.* ser. *Virchow*,[204] and *S.* ser. *Nienstedten*.[219] A high frequency of asymptomatic infections has been seen during nursery outbreaks with *S.* ser. *Heidelberg* (38% asymptomatic),[19] *S.* ser. *Virchow* (42% asymptomatic),[204] and *S.* ser. *Tennessee* (100% asymptomatic).[258]

Which genes are required for disease in humans versus animals remains unclear. *S.* ser. *Typhimurium* has genes that allow it to cause a nondiarrheal typhoidal illness in mice; in humans, it typically causes symptoms related primarily to intestinal involvement. An estimated more than 200 genes determine *S.* ser. *Typhimurium* virulence in mice. The clinical variability in host range and disease manifestations is due to the fact that *Salmonella* strains vary in their possession and expression of virulence genes.[154]

Of critical importance for in vivo virulence are the *Salmonella* pathogenicity islands (SPI), in particular SPI-1 and SPI-2. Both SPIs encode a molecular apparatus called *type III secretion system*, capable of injecting bacterial proteins through bacterial and host membranes into host cells (translocation) or the extracellular milieu (secretion) to influence host biochemistry and cell physiology directly.[47]

Genes relevant to the intestinal phase of illness are encoded primarily in SPI-1. The *invA-H* chromosomal genes are necessary for adherence to and invasion of intestinal mucosal cells[80]; most of the genes described so far seem to be involved in secretion or transport of virulence proteins.[104,248] Genes related to the *Shigella* invasion plasmid antigens (*ipaA-D*) have been described in *Salmonella* spp.[129,130]; these *Salmonella* genes (*sipA-D*) encode the proteins that interact with host cells to cause bacterial uptake and intracellular movement. Although initially characterized as an invasiveness island, SPI-1 has additional functions related to the activation of innate immune pathway, including (1) induction of polymorphonuclear recruitment across intestinal epithelium by the SPI-1 secreted effect SipA, (2) activation of nuclear factor-κB signaling by the concerted activity of SPI-1 translocated effectors, and (3) activation of caspase-1–mediated interleukin-1β (IL-1β)/IL-18 activation and proinflammatory cell death by the SPI-1 translocator effector SipB.[47]

The role of host cells in the invasion process is complex. After *S.* ser. *Typhimurium* comes in contact with epithelial cells, activation of epidermal growth factor receptor occurs, which activates a kinase that turns on phospholipase A$_2$ so that arachidonic acid is generated. Arachidonic acid is converted to leukotriene D$_4$, which opens calcium channels and causes membrane ruffling, cytoskeletal changes, and uptake of bacteria.[80] Nonphagocytic cells, including epithelial cells, are adapted poorly for killing of internalized bacteria. Not only do *Salmonella* spp. survive in vacuoles within epithelial cells, but they also can replicate actively.[81] *S.* ser. *Typhi* survives better in human than in mouse macrophages, whereas *S.* ser. *Typhimurium* survives better in mouse macrophages.[31,218] *Salmonella* is capable of infecting a wide variety of cells, including dendritic cells, macrophages, hepatocytes, neutrophils, colonocytes, and other epithelial cells. In vitro, within minutes of contact with cells, *Salmonella* organisms are internalized and take up residence in a unique membrane-bound compartment distinct from a phagosome or lysosome, the *Salmonella*-containing vacuole.[101]

SPI-2 is essential for intracellular parasitism and systemic virulence in murine typhoid and for evasion of phagocyte oxidase machinery of the host.[250] SPI-2 has additional roles in inflammatory disease, such as induction of cyclooxygenase and modulation of host cytokine expression and signaling.[244,245] SPI-2 is crucial for early and complete induction of enterocolitis and systemic disease.[47]

Several pathogen-associated molecular patterns of pathophysiologic importance are presented by *Salmonella* during infection, principally lipopolysaccharides and flagellin. The activation of toll-like receptor 4 in response to *Salmonella* lipopolysaccharides is essential for inducing host responses.[249] *Salmonella* flagellin is a potent inducer of host inflammation in polarized epithelial monolayers when delivered to the basolateral surface of the epithelium. When delivered there, *Salmonella* flagellin induces IL-8 secretion by stimulating basolateral toll-like receptor 5.[266] Flagellin stimulation of innate immune responses is crucial for intestinal inflammation but not for murine typhoid.[47]

The development of diarrhea depends on host and pathogen factors. An influx of polymorphonuclear leukocytes into the mucosa must occur for diarrhea to develop.[256] Neutropenic animals fail to develop fluid secretion when they are infected with *Salmonella*[255]; infiltration of leukocytes is thought to trigger production of prostaglandin because fluid secretion can be blocked by indomethacin.[91] A cholera toxin–like enterotoxin is made by approximately two thirds of *Salmonella* strains, including *S.* ser. *Typhimurium* and *S.* ser. *Typhi*.[125]

For most nontyphoidal *Salmonella* strains, infection does not extend beyond the lamina propria and the local lymphatics. In contrast, *S.* ser. *Typhi*, *S.* ser. *Dublin*, and *S.* ser. *Choleraesuis* rapidly invade the bloodstream with little intestinal involvement. Some virulence genes confer a survival advantage to the organisms if they get into the extraintestinal milieu. Vi capsular antigen present in *S.* ser. *Typhi*, *S.* ser. *Dublin*, and *S.* ser. *Paratyphi C* interferes with C3 binding. Mutations in lipopolysaccharide genes decrease invasiveness of *S.* ser. *Typhi* and *S.* ser. *Choleraesuis*, but not of *S.* ser. *Typhimurium*.[81,168] *S.* ser. *Dublin*, *S.* ser. *Typhimurium*, and *S.* ser. *Enteritidis* have virulence genes that confer resistance to complement by preventing the formation and insertion of the C5b-9 membrane attack complex. Patients with sickle-cell anemia have complement defects and defects in opsonization of *S.* ser. *Typhimurium*.[110] Newborns also have complement deficiencies that may explain the high frequency of *Salmonella* infection in newborns and the susceptibility of newborns to bacteremic complications seldom seen in normal hosts.

Multiple host defense strategies have evolved to deal with these virulence factors; host susceptibility often can be related directly to defects in these defense mechanisms. The host tries to kill ingested organisms in the stomach, to inhibit their growth in the gut, to limit their spread beyond the intestine, and to clear them by immune mechanisms.

At a pH of 2.0, most *Salmonella* spp. are killed rapidly.[89] When gastric pH is increased by oral administration of antacid, susceptibility increases.[88,120,200] A *Salmonella* inoculum ingested in water passes through the stomach more rapidly than when the same inoculum is ingested in food. Rapid transit through the small bowel decreases the contact time of organisms with the mucosa. Patients with decreased intestinal motility caused by medication or anatomic factors have increased severity and complications and may have a prolonged carrier state. Prior antimicrobial exposure increases the risk of incurring infection with antimicrobial-susceptible and antimicrobial-resistant strains of *Salmonella*.[182] The normal flora may compete for substrates, lower the local pH by production of short-chain fatty acids, and produce antibacterial substances such as colicins. Some patients with gastroenteritis have progression or exacerbation of symptoms when antibiotics are given.[203]

Salmonella organisms are able to survive in macrophages but not in polymorphonuclear leukocytes. Patients with neutropenia (e.g., congenital, related to chemotherapy) or neutrophil dysfunction (e.g., chronic granulomatous disease) are at high risk for development of disseminated infection. Patients who have been bacteremic with a nontyphoidal *Salmonella* strain are at increased risk for having a relapse if leukopenia is present.[85]

Cell-mediated immunity generally is thought to be more important than is humoral immunity in clearance of *Salmonella* organisms. T-cell activation of macrophages is necessary to kill intracellular *Salmonella* organisms.[150] Oral immunization with an attenuated typhoid vaccine primes lymphocytes to produce cytokines typical of a T$_H$1 response (high interferon-γ/low IL-4) to the flagellar antigen.[236] Healthy individuals vaccinated with either oral or parenteral typhoid vaccines develop antibody-dependent cellular cytotoxicity mediated by IgA, IgG, or both.[56] Studies of serum and secretory antibodies to O and H antigens have not shown protection, however; relapses of typhoid fever have occurred despite high antibody titers. Immunity may be short-lived. In a study of 14 individuals (17 to 28 years old) with acute typhoid fever, cell-mediated immunity persisted for 16 weeks; intestinal secretory IgA persisted for 48 weeks; and IgG, IgM, and anti-O and anti-H agglutinins persisted for 2 years, 16 weeks, 16 weeks, and 36 weeks, respectively.[216]

Cytokines play a crucial role in initiating and regulating the innate and adaptive immune response against *Salmonella*. These bacteria can trigger synthesis of cytokines and chemokines in epithelial cells, macrophages, and dendritic cells. The consequences of cytokine activation vary. Although interferon-γ, IL-12, tumor necrosis factor-α, IL-18, transforming growth factor-β, and CCL2 have protective functions during *Salmonella* infection, IL-4 and IL-10 interfere with host defenses.[70]

Impaired cell-mediated immunity probably explains the high frequency of bacteremia with nontyphoidal *Salmonella* strains in children with HIV infection[209] and with malnutrition.[225] Defective cell-mediated immunity can be congenital or acquired (tumors,[107] collagen vascular disease, organ transplantation,[72] chemotherapy, glucocorticosteroids).[195] Inherited deficiency in the IL-12/IL-23/interferon-γ pathway results in susceptibility to recurrent *Salmonella* and *Mycobacterium* infections.[64] Defects have been described in which patients have mutations in IL-12, IL-12 receptor, IL-23, IL-23 receptor, interferon-γ receptor, and STAT (signal transducer and activator of transcription). Complete and partial deficiency syndromes have been described.[10,11,128]

An increased risk of acquiring disease exists in settings in which reticuloendothelial function or cell-mediated immunity is impaired[171,228] or immature.[172] Hemolytic anemias are thought to cause reticuloendothelial overload. Children with sickle-cell anemia are at risk for developing bacteremia and osteomyelitis.[152,233,262,265] Children with sickle-cell and S-Thal also sometimes develop osteomyelitis.[48] Malaria predisposes to salmonellosis by multiple mechanisms.[147] Schistosomiasis predisposes to development of *Salmonella* infections and prolonged bacteremia[201]; reticuloendothelial cell killing of *Salmonella* is impaired, and *Salmonella* colonizes the schistosomes. Pili on *Salmonella* adhere to the surface of *Schistosoma mansoni* and *Schistosoma haematobium*.[144] In Gabonese children with bacteremic nontyphoidal *Salmonella* infection, rectal biopsy specimens showed the eggs of *Schistosoma intercalatum* in 90 percent of cases.[86]

Humoral immunity is less important. Preterm neonates who are infected with *S. ser. Typhimurium* may have a lower risk of developing complications (e.g., intestinal perforation, meningitis, endophthalmitis, sepsis, pyelitis), however, if they are given intravenous immunoglobulin plus cefoperazone than if given cefoperazone alone (16% versus 82%); the mortality rate also is decreased (12% versus 41%).[98]

CLINICAL MANIFESTATIONS

Salmonella spp. may cause acute or chronic asymptomatic infection. Symptomatic infections include acute gastroenteritis, bacteremia with or without local suppuration, and enteric fever.

ACUTE ASYMPTOMATIC INFECTION

Asymptomatic infections usually are identified by stool cultures obtained during prospective research studies or epidemiologic investigations. A study of Mexican infants showed that 74 percent of nontyphoidal *Salmonella* infections were asymptomatic.[54]

ACUTE GASTROENTERITIS

The most common clinical illness caused by *Salmonella* infection is gastroenteritis. Nausea, vomiting, and crampy abdominal pain begin 6 to 72 hours (median 24 hours) after ingestion of contaminated food or water. The abdominal pain may be severe enough to suggest appendicitis. Diarrhea usually is moderate in volume and, depending on the serotype, may contain blood. Headaches, malaise, myalgias, and fevers are common. These symptoms usually resolve in approximately 1 week without antibiotic therapy; symptoms may persist in very young patients and patients with underlying diseases. In neonates, loose, green, mucous stools or, less often, bloody diarrhea is seen; fever is common with *Salmonella* gastroenteritis during the first months of life.[122] Reactive arthritis develops in some adults after having otherwise uncomplicated *Salmonella* gastroenteritis; this complication rarely occurs in children.

BACTEREMIA WITH OR WITHOUT METASTATIC FOCAL INFECTION

Some *Salmonella* serotypes (e.g., *S. ser. Typhi*; *S. ser. Choleraesuis*; *S. ser. Paratyphi* A, B, and C; *S. ser. Heidelberg*; *S. ser. Typhimurium*; *S. ser. Enteritidis*; *S. ser. Saint-Paul*; *S. ser. Newport*; *S. ser. Panama*; *S. ser. Dublin*) have a propensity to invade the bloodstream; others (e.g., *S. ser. Tennessee*, *S. ser. Weltevreden*[261]) rarely seem to cause bacteremia. Fever, chills, diaphoresis, myalgias, anorexia, and weight loss may last for days or weeks. Stool cultures may be negative. A child sometimes can have afebrile diar-

rhea and yet be bacteremic for several days.[131] The true frequency of bacteremia is uncertain. Depending on the patient's age, geographic location, and nature of the study (prospective versus retrospective), 2 to 45 percent of infections are bacteremic.[57,122,160,172,225,241,261,263] Bacteremia probably occurs more commonly in newborns (in some studies 30 to 50%) than in older children,[122] although not all studies have reached this conclusion.[160] The true risk of bacteremia developing in the first year of life is likely to be 2 to 6 percent.[57,241]

Hemolytic anemia, especially sickle-cell anemia, is associated with a high risk of development of *Salmonella* bacteremia. Persistent or recurrent bacteremia occurs in patients with AIDS, schistosomiasis, and intravascular focal infection. Immunocompromised adults who become bacteremic with *Salmonella* are more likely to do so without having had a preceding gastroenteritis and to have a high mortality rate.[109] Children more typically are relatively immunocompetent; most often, they develop bacteremia associated with diarrhea and have a much better prognosis.[139,160] In a large study in African children, nontyphoidal *Salmonella* spp. were the second most common cause of community-acquired bacteremia in all children and in HIV-positive patients.[22] Even children with neoplastic disease may have a benign course when they are bacteremic with *Salmonella* spp.,[175] although the risk for development of focal infections during bacteremia is higher (36%) in children with underlying conditions than in previously healthy children (2.5%).[264]

Focal suppurative infections may occur almost anywhere; the most common sites are bones (particularly in sickle-cell anemia)[26,233,262] and the central nervous system.[29,66,134,145,202,264] Meningitis has a high morbidity, with acute hydrocephalus, seizures, ventriculitis, abscesses, subdural empyema, and cerebral infarction. Long-term neurologic sequelae include mental retardation, hemiparesis, chronic hydrocephalus, epilepsy, visual impairment, and athetosis.[48] Neurologic sequelae are particularly common in patients who have prolonged fever (>10 days) while receiving antibiotic therapy.[121] Mortality rates from meningitis have been 40 to 60 percent in the past, even with appropriate treatment; more recent data suggest that the mortality rate is now much lower. Relapses even after prolonged therapy occur commonly (reflecting the intracellular localization of *Salmonella* and the difficulty of achieving adequate intracellular levels of antibiotics). Of nontyphoidal *Salmonella* meningitis, 50 to 75 percent occurs in the first 4 months of life.[48]

The serotypes causing meningitis, including *S. ser. Typhimurium*, *S. ser. Heidelberg*, *S. ser. Enteritidis*, *S. ser. Saint-Paul*, *S. ser. Havana*, *S. ser. Oranienburg*, *S. ser. Newport*, and *S. ser. Panama*,[48,259] are serotypes commonly associated with bacteremia. In infants, complications include pneumonia,[19] osteomyelitis,[62,136,262] septic arthritis,[19,217] pericarditis,[108,159] pyelitis,[235] peritonitis,[2] otitis media,[2] mastitis,[169] cholecystitis,[106] endophthalmitis,[53] cutaneous abscesses,[192] and infected cephalohematoma.[62] In adults and occasionally in older children, femoral and distal aorta (mycotic aneurysms),[48] heart valves,[48] scrotum,[246] testicles,[48] prostate,[215] ovaries,[48] and fallopian tubes[215] also may be infected.

Hemolytic-uremic syndrome associated with *S. ser. Typhimurium*[67,157] and *S. ser. Typhi*[18] has been reported. Because the cytotoxins produced by various *Salmonella* strains are distinct immunologically from Shiga toxin produced by *Shigella dysenteriae* 1 and the Shiga toxins produced by enterohemorrhagic *Escherichia coli*,[12] the association of hemolytic-uremic syndrome with salmonellosis may represent undiagnosed dual infection with toxin-producing organisms.

ENTERIC FEVER

Enteric fever usually is caused by *S. ser. Typhi* and, less often, other invasive *Salmonella*, including *S. ser. Paratyphi* and *S. ser.*

Choleraesuis. In contrast to sepsis caused by other gram-negative bacilli, the onset of symptoms in enteric fever is insidious.[120] After an incubation period of 10 to 14 days (range 6 to 21 days), which generally is related to the inoculum size, fever, malaise, anorexia, and abdominal pain develop over 2 to 3 days. The incubation period tends to be shorter with paratyphoid fever. The temperature rises in small increments, usually reaching 40° C to 40.5° C by the end of the first week of illness. The temperature does not return to normal but rather rises to higher peaks each afternoon, with higher nadirs occurring each subsequent morning during the first week. Eventually, the fever is unremitting; spikes in temperature occur without return to normal.

Constipation occurs in approximately 50 percent of cases, whereas diarrhea occurs in approximately 30 percent of patients. When diarrhea develops, it usually does so after the patient has been febrile for several days. It is small in volume, resembles pea soup, and contains erythrocytes but usually is not grossly bloody. Fecal leukocytes are present in nearly all patients with diarrhea. Diarrhea occurs more commonly with paratyphoid than with typhoid fever.[242] Vomiting is mild and not sustained.

A dull, continuous frontal headache begins during the first 2 days of fever; headache is present in approximately 75 percent of patients. In adults, confusion or delirium occurs more commonly than does a normal mental status. Children commonly complain of headache; they often are drowsy, irritable, or delirious.[61] Mild arthralgia involving multiple joints and vague, poorly localized back pain occur in nearly 60 percent of patients.

Physical examination during the first week may show a relative bradycardia for the degree of fever. The patient has a dull, expressionless, toxic facies; coated tongue; a musty, "damp hay–like" odor; and a tender, doughy abdomen with slight guarding. Occasionally, a child may have a cough; it tends to be minimal and unimpressive. The skin is dry with little sweating. Meningismus may occur early in the illness.

During the second week, rose spots may appear on the abdomen or chest, and less often on the back, upper arms, and thighs. The spots typically begin between days 7 and 10 as crops of 10 to 15 lesions, each measuring 2 to 4 mm. More lesions may occur in paratyphoid. They are blanching, erythematous, slightly raised lesions that last approximately 3 days. Rose spots occur in a few patients and are difficult to recognize in dark-skinned individuals. New crops of rose spots may continue for 1 to 2 weeks.

The spleen becomes palpable, soft, and tender by early in the second week of illness. Respiratory symptoms may progress, and epistaxis occasionally may occur. If left untreated, enteric fever has a prolonged course, with continuous high temperature of 39.5° C to 40.5° C for up to 4 weeks, followed by a gradual return to normal, beginning during the third or fourth week. A rapid decrease in temperature late in illness suggests intestinal hemorrhage or perforation[24]; such a decline in temperature typically is followed by an increase a few hours later as peritonitis develops. Intestinal hemorrhage and intestinal perforation[24,33,92] may occur in the second to fourth week in 3 percent of patients with typhoid fever.[33] Late in the course of untreated typhoid, the mental status changes to a "coma vigil," in which the patient lies with open eyes, mutters, and is oblivious to the surroundings.

Complications occur in 10 to 15 percent of patients; most of these develop during the second or third week of illness. Many complications, of which gastrointestinal bleeding, intestinal perforation, and typhoid encephalopathy are the most important, have been described (Table 121–5).[140,178,180,194,260] Gastrointestinal bleeding is the most common, occurring in 10 percent of patients.[180] It results from erosion of a necrotic Peyer patch through the wall of an enteric vessel. Suppurative lymphadenitis,[126] tonsillitis,[126,215] infected prosthetic heart valves,[10] and pancreatitis[211] rarely occur. Patients who have thalassemia or

TABLE 121–5 Complications of Typhoid Fever

Abdominal
Gastrointestinal hemorrhage
Intestinal perforation
Hepatitis
Cholecystitis
Pancreatitis

Neuropsychiatric
Encephalopathy
Delirium
Psychosis
Meningitis
Impairment of coordination

Cardiovascular
Asymptomatic electrocardiographic changes
Myocarditis
Infected prosthetic valve
Shock

Respiratory
Bronchitis
Pneumonia

Hematologic
Anemia
Disseminated intravascular coagulation

Other
Focal abscess
Suppurative lymphadenitis
Pharyngitis
Tonsillitis
Osteomyelitis
Arthritis
Parotiditis
Orchitis
Pyelonephritis
Miscarriage
Relapse
Chronic carriage

Modified from Parry, C. M., Hien, T. T., Dougan, G., et al.: Typhoid fever. N. Engl. J. Med. 347:1770-1782, 2002.

glucose-6-phosphate dehydrogenase deficiency may have hemolysis during typhoid fever.[242]

The relapse rate is 5 to 20 percent, even when appropriate therapy has been given. Relapses typically occur 2 to 3 weeks after the resolution of fever and are milder than the initial illness. The *Salmonella* isolate from a patient in relapse usually has the same antibiotic susceptibility pattern as the isolate obtained from the patient during the original episode. Re-infection also may occur and can be distinguished from relapse by molecular typing.[253]

In some geographic areas, such as Indonesia, where an exceptionally virulent S. ser. *Typhi* is endemic, toxemia, delirium, obtundation, coma, and shock sometimes occur.[120,140] Some serotypes in Indonesia (e.g., H1-j) seem to be less virulent than others are, suggesting that properties of the flagellar antigen may be important to virulence.[105]

Typhoid fever varies in its clinical course. Variations on the classic theme include a completely afebrile course occurring in debilitated patients, a high spiking fever from the first day (particularly in children), a focal presentation (e.g., pneumonia, nephritis), and a severe course during relapses. Infants are said to be at higher risk for development of massive hepatomegaly, thrombocytopenia, and other complications.[193] The mortality rate is high in the neonatal period.[196] Children younger than 5 years old may have a nonspecific illness that is not recognized clinically as typhoid[224]; infants and toddlers often have a febrile illness misinterpreted as a "viral syndrome." In children younger than 2 years old, the fever may last for only 1 to 5 days, despite the presence of *S.* ser. *Typhi* or *S.* ser. *Paratyphi* in the blood; low-grade fever (temperature of 38.3° C to 38.8° C) and cough may be the only findings in such children.[77] The case-fatality rates are highest among children younger than 1 year and among elderly patients. The most important contributor to a poor outcome is probably a delay in instituting effective antibiotic treatment.[180]

Typhoid and nontyphoidal *Salmonella* infections during pregnancy increase the risk of spontaneous abortion.[165,230] Spontaneous abortion or premature labor usually can be prevented by early treatment.[222] Transmission of *S.* ser. *Typhi* rarely occurs in utero.[40] Typically, premature delivery occurs during the second to fourth week of untreated maternal typhoid fever.[103] In the pre-antibiotic era, 40 percent of women with typhoid delivered prematurely; the remainder carried to term, although only 17 percent of infants survived.[60] If infection occurs late in gestation and is treated appropriately, the infant may survive.

ASYMPTOMATIC CHRONIC CARRIER STATE

Chronic carriers excrete *Salmonella* organisms in stools for longer than 1 year after having gastroenteritis-enterocolitis or enteric fever. Approximately 1 to 4 percent of patients who recover from enteric fever caused by *S.* ser. *Typhi* chronically excrete the organism[164]; less than 1 percent of patients with nontyphoidal *Salmonella* excrete for a prolonged period.[30,39] Twenty-five percent of prolonged carriers have no history of typhoid.[180] Nontyphoidal infection is associated with excretion for a mean of 5 weeks, although children younger than 5 years old,[30] female patients, elderly patients, and patients with biliary tract disease are more likely to become carriers. The biliary tract is infected in almost all chronic carriers of *S.* ser. *Typhi*. As many as 10^6 organisms per 1 g of feces may be excreted.[164]

The significance of chronic excretion is that such patients serve as a source of infection to their contacts. Chronic carriers represent an epidemiologically important reservoir of *S.* ser. *Typhi*; they often are the source of outbreaks of typhoid fever. In the United States, although typhoid fever generally is imported, 30 percent of infections result from exposure to previously diagnosed or newly diagnosed chronic carriers.[212]

Patients who have a history of *S. haematobium* or tuberculous infections of the urinary tract may develop chronic urinary carriage after a bout of typhoid fever.[73,201] Other predisposing conditions include hydronephrosis, strictures, and kidney stones.

DIAGNOSIS

The symptoms in *Salmonella* gastroenteritis overlap sufficiently with symptoms seen in other diarrheal illnesses that laboratory studies generally are required to prove the diagnosis. On the rare occasions when proctoscopy has been done, typical findings have included mucosal edema, hyperemia, friability, and hemorrhages.[58] The fecal leukocyte examination is positive for polymorphonuclear leukocytes in 36 to 82 percent of nontyphoidal cases,[111,187] but this finding is nonspecific. Stool culture is preferable to swab culture, particularly for evaluation of long-term carriers. Overnight enrichment in selenite broth increases the yield from stool cultures. The optimal agar for isolation of the organism (SS agar, Hektoen enteric agar, MacConkey agar, xylose-lysine-deoxycholate agar, xylose-lysine-Tergitol 4 agar, brilliant green agar, or modified semisolid Rappaport Vassiliadis medium) is debated. Modified semisolid Rappaport Vassiliadis medium has a high yield but cannot be used for isolating *S.* ser. *Typhi* or nonmotile strains and has a lower specificity than SS agar.[210]

Salmonella organisms usually can be isolated readily from blood by use of conventional media if the patient is bacteremic. In patients with extraintestinal focal nontyphoidal infection, specimens from the affected areas may have positive Gram stains and grow the organism.

Enteric fever should be suspected on the basis of the setting and clinical course. Laboratory abnormalities are common but nonspecific findings. A normocytic, normochromic anemia and leukopenia or neutropenia, perhaps caused by hemophagocytosis in the bone marrow, often are present.[151] Clotting abnormalities consistent with disseminated intravascular coagulation (e.g., thrombocytopenia, hypofibrinogenemia) may occur[32] but usually are transient and not associated with clinically significant bleeding. In enteric fever, electrolyte values usually are normal, but increases in alkaline phosphatase, serum lactate dehydrogenase, serum aspartate aminotransferase, and serum cholesterol occur frequently. A transient proteinuria sometimes occurs during the first week of enteric fever.

Cultures from multiple sites should be submitted for suspected enteric fever; culture of bone marrow has the highest yield,[114,116,247] particularly if the patient has had antibiotic pretreatment. During the first week of typhoid fever, approximately 90 percent of patients have positive blood and bone marrow cultures, but negative stool and urine cultures. During subsequent weeks, the yield of blood and bone marrow cultures decreases as the yield of stool and urine cultures increases. Culture of duodenal fluid obtained by string capsules can be as sensitive as culture of bone marrow aspirates.[15,116,247] The overall frequencies of positive cultures during the course of typhoid are found in blood (40 to 54%), urine (7 to 10%), stool (approximately 35%), bone marrow (80 to 90%), rose spots (approximately 65%), and duodenal string test culture (58 to 85%).[93,116]

The Widal test measures antibodies against the O and H antigens of *S.* ser. *Typhi*. Although many patients with enteric fever may have a fourfold increase in the titer of paired sera during the second week of illness, false-negative and false-positive test results occur. Patients with acute or chronic liver disease and patients infected with other gram-negative enteric bacilli may develop cross-reacting antibodies. Recipients of the typhoid vaccine show positive Widal test results, which can be misleading. These titers may be more useful in children with typhoid who are living in a nonendemic area, such as the United States. Although patients who have a negative titer early in infection tend to maintain a negative titer, most develop titers of 1:80 or more.[50] Interpretation of Widal test results is aided by information about seropositivity in the population to which the patient belongs.[45,243] Some centers have found Widal's test helpful when it is used with locally determined cutoff points.[46,181]

Various diagnostic kits, including serologic tests such as passive hemagglutination, passive bacterial agglutination, latex particle agglutination slide tests, counterimmunoelectrophoresis, radioimmunoassay, and enzyme-linked immunosorbent assay with use of monoclonal antibodies, have been developed.[124] These commercial assays (Typhidot, Typhidot-M, Tubex) have not proved to be sufficiently robust in large-scale evaluations in community settings.[23] Molecular techniques used primarily in epidemiologic studies include DNA hybridization studies, phage typing, chromosome analysis, and plasmid analysis.

DIFFERENTIAL DIAGNOSIS

Salmonella gastroenteritis cannot be distinguished clinically from other infectious causes of acute diarrhea reliably, although history and epidemiology sometimes may suggest an etiologic agent. Bloody diarrhea with mucus can be caused by *Salmonella*, *Shigella*, enteroinvasive *E. coli*, enterohemorrhagic *E. coli*, *Campylobacter* spp., *Yersinia enterocolitica*, *Clostridium difficile*, *Trichuris trichiura*, and *Entamoeba histolytica*. Watery diarrhea may be caused by rotavirus or other viral enteropathogens or enterotoxin-producing bacterial pathogens. When abdominal pain and tenderness are severe, the differential diagnosis includes appendicitis, perforated viscus, and mesenteric adenitis.

Enteric fever can mimic other infections of the reticuloendothelial system, including Epstein-Barr virus infection, disseminated histoplasmosis, tuberculosis, ehrlichiosis, brucellosis, leptospirosis, tularemia, plague, malaria, systemic *Bartonella henselae* infection, and typhus. Noninfectious illnesses with prolonged fever that sometimes can be confused with typhoid include juvenile rheumatoid arthritis and other collagen vascular diseases, Kawasaki syndrome, and lymphomas. An early diagnosis often is difficult to establish because the findings are nonspecific. Findings that are particularly helpful in discriminating typhoid fever from other prolonged febrile illnesses include severe cough and chest pain (more typical of lobar pneumonia), diarrhea with grossly obvious blood (more typical of dysentery), acute onset of chills (more typical of malaria), and marked lower abdominal pain early in the febrile illness (more typical of bacillary dysentery, *Y. enterocolitica* infection, and salpingitis). For patients in countries where typhoid is not endemic, a history of travel is crucial.

TREATMENT

For children with salmonellosis for whom antibiotic treatment is appropriate, the interpretation of antimicrobial susceptibility studies is important. Drugs such as aminoglycosides, polymyxins, tetracyclines, and first-generation and second-generation cephalosporins (e.g., cephalothin, cefazolin, cefuroxime, cefamandole) have a poor clinical track record, despite apparent in vitro susceptibility. Table 121-6 shows the drugs that typically are useful in treatment of children with *Salmonella* infections. The emergence of *S.* ser. *Typhimurium* DT104 in the United States has led to a dramatic increase in multidrug-resistant (ampicillin, chloramphenicol, streptomycin, sulfonamides, tetracycline) organisms.[97] Most nontyphoidal *Salmonella* strains in the United States still are sensitive to ampicillin, chloramphenicol, amoxicillin–clavulanic acid, and TMP-SMX; ceftriaxone resistance, although described, is rare.[113]

GASTROENTERITIS

As with all forms of gastroenteritis, fluid and electrolyte replacement and maintenance are the first order of business. For most patients, oral rehydration is all that is necessary to treat *Salmonella* gastroenteritis. Generally, *Salmonella* gastroenteritis should not be treated with antibiotics because these agents do not shorten the course of illness. Multiple agents,[11] including ampicillin, amoxicillin,[132,170,184] neomycin,[13,184] chloramphenicol,[149]

TABLE 121-6 Antibiotics Commonly Used in the Treatment of *Salmonella* Infections

Drug	Dose
Ampicillin	200 mg/kg/day in 4 doses PO, IM, or IV
Trimethoprim-sulfamethoxazole (TMP-SMX)	10 mg/kg/day TMP, 50 mg/kg/day SMX in 2 doses PO or IV
Cefotaxime	100-200 mg/kg/day in 3 doses IM or IV
Ceftriaxone	50-100 mg/kg/day in 1 or 2 doses IM or IV
Cefixime	10-20 mg/kg/day in 1 or 2 doses PO
Chloramphenicol	50-75 mg/kg/day in 4 doses PO
Azithromycin	8-12 mg/kg/day in 1 dose PO
Ciprofloxacin	10-20 mg/kg/day in 2 doses PO or IV

TMP-SMX,[132,213] azithromycin,[43] cefixime,[43] ceftriaxone,[42] and ciprofloxacin, have been shown to be ineffective.[213] Antibiotics prolong excretion of *Salmonella*.[11,13,63,132,170,184] *Salmonella* serotypes typically have been grouped together for these treatment studies, however, as though they were all the same organism. Given the variability in expression of virulence genes, whether treatment may be useful for some serotypes that possess particular virulence traits remains an open question.

Exceptions to the generalization that *Salmonella* gastroenteritis should not be treated include children at high risk for developing complications, including children with underlying diseases or receiving therapies that impair host defenses. Examples of children who probably ought to be given antibiotics are infants 3 months old or younger; children with AIDS or malignant diseases; and children with hemolytic anemias, particularly sickle-cell anemia. Treatment of these patients is debatable; the data from neonates suggest that antibiotics make little difference in the course.[2,71,132,198,234] Because the risk of development of bacteremia is high, however, antibiotics likely will continue to be used in such settings. Because bacteremia occurs in a small fraction of infections, determining whether treatment of gastroenteritis prevents bacteremia is impossible without conducting a massive study.

When treatment is given, probably 5 days or fewer of antibiotics is indicated, barring complications. Although antibiotic resistance is an increasingly important problem, patients who require antibiotic therapy for *Salmonella* gastroenteritis not thought to be life-threatening usually should be given ampicillin or amoxicillin, pending susceptibility testing.

EXTRAINTESTINAL INFECTIONS

Any child who appears to be sufficiently toxic that bacteremia is suspected also should be started on antibiotic treatment until blood cultures exclude the diagnosis. For children with bacteremic nontyphoidal *Salmonella* and focal extraintestinal complications, a third-generation cephalosporin (e.g., ceftriaxone, cefotaxime) or chloramphenicol is an appropriate choice. If the patient seems to have a life-threatening infection, ampicillin should be used only if evidence exists that the pathogen is not ampicillin resistant. Children at high risk of having recurrence of bacteremia (children with congenital or acquired immunodeficiencies, such as AIDS) may require a third-generation cephalosporin or a fluoroquinolone to achieve cure; frequent recurrences of life-threatening infection sometimes necessitate use of lifelong maintenance therapy.[51,119]

Meningitis should be treated with a third-generation cephalosporin because these agents have good penetration into CSF; ampicillin and chloramphenicol use has been associated with higher relapse rates and lower cure rates than are third-generation cephalosporins.[134] Meningitis must be treated for at least 4 weeks; approximately three fourths of patients who have relapses have been treated for 3 weeks or less.[48] A bactericidal agent, such as ampicillin or a third-generation cephalosporin, is preferred for treatment of endovascular infections (e.g., endocarditis, mycotic aneurysm).

For extraintestinal infections, the duration of antibiotic treatment usually is 10 to 14 days in children with bacteremia, 4 to 6 weeks in children with acute osteomyelitis, and 4 weeks in children with meningitis. Collections of pus should be drained. Schistosomiasis, when present, must be treated to achieve resolution of the coincident *Salmonella* infection.

TYPHOID FEVER

The response to treatment with antibiotics is slow. Fever may persist for many days, even after bacteremia has resolved. The emergence and spread of multidrug-resistant *S.* ser. *Typhi* (MDRST) since 1989 has caused a shift in empiric therapy from chloramphenicol, TMP-SMX, or ampicillin to a fluoroquinolone in adults and a third-generation cephalosporin, such as ceftriaxone, azithromycin, or a fluoroquinolone, in children (Table 121-7). MDRST is particularly common in the Indian subcontinent, Southeast Asia, and Africa; strains resistant to ciprofloxacin are being recognized increasingly.[205]

In the United States, MDRST is less problematic than it is elsewhere; most strains are sensitive to ampicillin and chloramphenicol.[212] More recent data suggest that *S.* ser. *Typhi* is still sensitive consistently to ceftriaxone and ciprofloxacin, although nalidixic acid–resistant isolates are becoming more common in individuals who have traveled to the Indian subcontinent.[5] Such strains respond poorly to fluoroquinolones and may require several courses of treatment.[254] When the patient has a history of recent travel to an area with MDRST or of contact with an individual returning from such an area, the choice of empiric treatment should take this information into account. Third-generation cephalosporins are effective against *S.* ser. *Typhi* strains resistant to ampicillin, chloramphenicol, and TMP-SMX,[74,124,134,161,167,179,227,240] and are appropriate for children with suspected or proven MDRST. Some studies suggest that cefoperazone may have advantages in typhoid fever over chloramphenicol treatment (more rapid sterilization and defervescence),[179] perhaps related to its biliary excretion.[59] Data suggest that TMP-SMX may not be as effective as is ampicillin or chloramphenicol in typhoid fever.[94] Aztreonam also is less effective than is chloramphenicol for strains susceptible to both agents.[99]

Although 2 weeks of antibiotic treatment usually is given, data suggest that shorter courses with some drugs may be adequate. A short course of ceftriaxone (once daily for 3 to 5 days) is as effective and safe as is a 2- to 3-week course of chloramphenicol in adults and, on the basis of relatively small numbers, probably in children as well.[3,167] A 5-day course of ceftriaxone (50 to 70 mg/kg/day as a single dose) was associated with a significantly more rapid defervescence (average 3.9 days until afebrile) than

was oral cefixime (7.5 mg/kg/dose twice daily for 14 days) or intramuscular aztreonam (50 to 70 mg/kg/dose every 8 hours for 7 days); relapse rates were similar (approximately 5%).[96]

Strong evidence supports fluoroquinolones as the most effective drugs for the treatment of typhoid fever. These drugs have proved safe in all age groups, are rapidly effective, and are associated with lower rates of stool carriage than traditional first-line drugs. There are three main issues regarding the use of fluoroquinolones: (1) the potential for toxic effects in children, (2) the cost, and (3) the potential emergence of resistance.[180] In preclinical testing, the fluoroquinolones damaged the articular cartilage of young beagles. A considerable body of evidence exists from the long-term use of these drugs in children with cystic fibrosis and from short-term use to treat typhoid fever and dysentery in children. No bone or joint toxicity or growth impairment has been found. The production of generic fluoroquinolones in many countries has reduced the price considerably. The emergence of quinolone resistance in areas where the drugs are inexpensive and readily available is likely to be the greatest limitation on their use.[180]

Concerns about toxicity of fluoroquinolones in children have limited their use to situations in which infection is caused by an organism proved to be resistant to all of the usual antibiotics but sensitive to a fluoroquinolone. If a fluoroquinolone is used, ciprofloxacin or ofloxacin is superior to norfloxacin because it has inadequate oral bioavailability. Ciprofloxacin (500 mg twice daily for 10 days in adults) causes defervescence in an average of 4.2 days with infrequent relapses, even with MDRST.[7] Children with MDRST who have been treated with ciprofloxacin (10 mg/kg/ day) became afebrile in 3.3 days, and 94 percent achieved clinical cure, with no relapses or carriers detected on follow-up.[68] Ofloxacin (20 mg/kg twice daily for 10 days) is associated with more rapid defervescence than TMP-SMX.[220] Ofloxacin is associated with more rapid defervescence and better cure rates than cefixime.[35] Three days of ofloxacin (15 mg/kg/day in two doses for 3 days) causes defervescence more quickly than chloramphenicol (50 mg/kg/day in four doses for 14 days).[185] Very short courses of ofloxacin (2 or 3 days) may be followed by relapse,[251] however, especially if the organism is resistant to nalidixic acid.[174]

Other agents have been described that occasionally may be useful. Furazolidone (7.5 mg/kg/day) is nearly as effective as is chloramphenicol in strains susceptible to both drugs (86% versus 90% cure).[69] Despite low serum levels, azithromycin seems to be equivalent to chloramphenicol or ciprofloxacin; the high intracellular concentration in macrophages (>100 times serum levels) of azithromycin presumably accounts for its efficacy.[34,95] When MDRST is resistant to nalidixic acid, azithromycin is more effective than is ofloxacin.[41]

A 5-day course of oral azithromycin (20 mg/kg/day, maximum 1000 mg/day) is as effective as intravenous ceftriaxone (75 mg/ kg/day, maximum 2.5 g/day for 5 days).[84] Various nonantimicrobial measures should be considered as part of the management of *S.* ser. *Typhi* infections. Dexamethasone, although potentially increasing the relapse rate,[52] is indicated for patients with severe typhoid fever presenting with delirium, stupor, shock, or coma; the dose is 3 mg/kg initially and then eight doses of 1 mg/kg every 6 hours for 48 hours. This therapy reduces mortality rates from 35 to 55 percent to 10 percent.[115,191] Parenteral fluoroquinolones are probably the antibiotic of choice for severe infections, but no randomized trials of such treatment have been performed.[68] Antipyretics were thought at one time to be dangerous in typhoid fever[65]; whether this concern is correct is doubtful on the basis of more recent experience.[176]

Intestinal hemorrhage or perforation during enteric fever generally is considered to be an indication for surgical intervention.[24,33,92,143] Resection of 10 cm of intestine proximal and distal to the perforation seems to improve outcome compared with other surgical approaches.[14] Antibiotic coverage should be broad-

TABLE 121-7 Recommended Antibiotic Treatment of Typhoid Fever

Susceptibility	Antibiotic	Daily Dose (mg/kg)	Days
Full susceptible	Chloramphenicol, *or*	50-75	14-21
	Amoxicillin, *or*	75-100	14
	Trimethoprim-sulfamethoxazole, *or*	8/40	14
	Third-generation cephalosporin (e.g., cefixime), *or*	15-20	7-14
	Fluoroquinolone (e.g., ofloxacin or ciprofloxacin)	15	5-7
Multidrug-resistant	Azithromycin	8-10	7
	Third-generation cephalosporin (e.g., cefixime), *or*	15-20	7-14
	Fluoroquinolone (e.g., ofloxacin or ciprofloxacin)	15	5-7
Quinolone-resistant	Azithromycin, *or*	8-10	7
	Third-generation cephalosporin (e.g., cefixime), *or*	20	7-14
	Parenteral third-generation cephalosporin (e.g., ceftriaxone), *or*	75	10-14
	Fluoroquinolone (e.g., ofloxacin or ciprofloxacin)	20	10-14

ened to include anaerobes and gram-negative enterics when perforation occurs.[24]

CHRONIC CARRIERS

Generally, patients who are not food handlers probably should not be cultured or given special treatment after having a bout of gastroenteritis caused by a nontyphoidal *Salmonella* strain. Carriers of *S.* ser. *Typhi* should be decolonized to decrease the risk to close contacts. Carriers who have a normal gallbladder can be treated with high-dose intravenous ampicillin, oral ampicillin, or amoxicillin combined with probenecid for 6 weeks or, when a multiresistant organism is present, with a fluoroquinolone, such as norfloxacin[100] or ciprofloxacin.[78] Chronic carriers who cannot be decolonized are treated with cholecystectomy if cholelithiasis or cholecystitis is present; such patients should receive ampicillin intravenously for 7 to 10 days before and 30 days after cholecystectomy.

PREVENTION

PUBLIC HEALTH MEASURES

Recognition of an increased frequency of human infections with an unusual serotype should be followed by an epidemiologic investigation aimed at detecting the source and vehicle. Intervention to stop such outbreaks then can be attempted. Judicious use of antibiotics in dairy and livestock animals,[117] careful food processing and storage, and proper preparation of foods are helpful in decreasing transmission of infection. Appropriate sewage disposal, assurance of a safe water supply, prevention of sale of pet turtles, inspection of cosmetics for contamination, and adequate cleaning of medical equipment are important public health strategies. Families with small children should be informed of the risks associated with pet reptiles and encouraged to avoid such unnecessary risks.

PERSONAL HYGIENIC MEASURES

Person-to-person spread can be decreased by handwashing after defecating or changing diapers, frequent handwashing during preparation of foods that might be contaminated (e.g., meat), and excluding of infected individuals from food-handling tasks.

INFECTION CONTROL

Hospitalized children with *Salmonella* gastroenteritis should be isolated (enteric precautions) until stool cultures are negative. Children with extraintestinal infections should be isolated until stool studies exclude intestinal infection or colonization.

NURSERY OUTBREAKS

Neonatal *Salmonella* infection outbreaks should be investigated to determine the source. Cultures of fomites sometimes reveal a removable focus. Neonates and staff members caring for them should be cohorted during outbreaks, with use of enteric precautions in dealing with infants who are excreting the organism. Surveillance cultures should be done on feces of not only sick infants but also well infants to cohort more appropriately. With current early postpartum discharge policies, reporting *Salmonella* infections in infants is important in detecting outbreaks. Isolation and cohorting can be effective in controlling such outbreaks.[198]

BREAST-FEEDING

In the developing world, breast-feeding is key in prevention because human milk contains secretory IgA and other factors that protect infants from *Salmonella* spp.[27,76,83,188,189] In a case-control study conducted in the United States, breast-feeding was found also to have a strong protective effect against sporadic *Salmonella* infections.[206] Pediatric health care providers and community education programs should encourage mothers to breast-feed.

VACCINATION

Several vaccines have been developed for typhoid fever. Vaccination of children is indicated when the risk for development of typhoid fever is high (e.g., living with a chronic carrier or in an endemic area) but probably is underused.[239] Two vaccines are available: (1) an oral live attenuated Ty21a vaccine (Vivotif Berna; Swiss Serum and Vaccine Institute) and (2) a parenteral purified Vi capsular polysaccharide vaccine (Typhim Vi; Aventis Pasteur).[135,190]

The Ty21a vaccine has been evaluated in liquid and capsule forms. Ty21a oral vaccine is well tolerated; abdominal pain, nausea, vomiting, and rashes occur rarely. The form licensed in the United States is an enteric-coated capsule preparation meant to be given in four separate doses on alternate days taken 1 hour before meals. It is not recommended for children younger than 6 years of age. The four doses should be completed 1 week before potential exposure. Revaccination with the entire four-dose series is recommended every 5 years in high-risk settings. Because the Ty21a oral vaccine is a live-attenuated *Salmonella*, it should not be used in immunocompromised hosts or in individuals taking antibiotics at the time of receiving vaccination.[37] The antimalarial mefloquine inhibits growth of the attenuated organism, and vaccination should be delayed for 24 hours after its use. Malaria prophylaxis with atovaquone and proguanil does not interfere with immune response to Ty21a.[75]

Several large field trials suggest that the Vi capsular vaccine as a single 25-μg dose (0.5 mL) has an efficacy of 55 percent and 75 percent in adults and children older than 5 years.[4,190] Although fever, malaise, local pain, and tenderness occur with this vaccine, it has two major advantages over the Ty21a oral vaccines: It does not require refrigeration, and only a single dose is required for protection. It may be used in children 2 years of age. Vaccination must occur at least 2 weeks before exposure.

PROGNOSIS

Salmonella gastroenteritis usually is a self-limited disease in the normal host, although chronic diarrhea sometimes develops after an acute episode. Extraintestinal focal infections with nontyphoidal *Salmonella* strains are difficult to cure, particularly if they involve the meninges or occur in compromised hosts. *Salmonella* spp. meningitis may relapse if the course of treatment is too short. Likewise, bacteremia and focal infection recur after treatment in severely compromised hosts, particularly patients with AIDS. Relapse after typhoid fever has long been recognized as a risk.

REFERENCES

1. Abramson, H.: Infections with *S. typhimurium* in the newborn. Am. J. Dis. Child. 74:576-586, 1947.
2. Abroms, I. F., Cochran, W. D., Holmes, L. B., et al.: A *Salmonella newport* outbreak in a premature nursery with a one-year follow-up. Pediatrics 37:616-623, 1966.
3. Acharya, G., Butler, T., Ho, M., et al.: Treatment of typhoid fever: Randomized trial of a three-day course of ceftriaxone versus a fourteen-day course of chloramphenicol. Am. J. Trop. Med. Hyg. 52:162-165, 1995.

4. Acharya, I. L., Lowe, C. U., Thapa, R., et al.: Prevention of typhoid fever in Nepal with the Vi capsular polysaccharide of *Salmonella typhi*. N. Engl. J. Med. *317*:1101-1104, 1987.

5. Acker, M. L., Puhr, N. D., Tauxe, R. V., and Mintz, E. D.: Laboratory-based surveillance of *Salmonella* serotype *Typhi* infections in the United States: Antimicrobial resistance on the rise. J. A. M. A. *283*:2668-2673, 2000.

6. Adler, J. L., Anderson, R. L., Boring, J. R., et al.: A protracted hospital-associated outbreak of salmonellosis due to a multiple antibiotic-resistant strain of *S. indiana*. J. Pediatr. *77*:970-975, 1970.

7. Alam, M. N., Haq, S. A., Das, K. K., et al.: Efficacy of ciprofloxacin in enteric fever: Comparison of treatment duration in sensitive and multidrug resistant *Salmonella*. Am. J. Trop. Med. Hyg. *53*:306-311, 1995.

8. Altare, F., Durandy, A., Lammas, D., et al.: Impairment of mycobacterial immunity in human interleukin-12 receptor deficiency. Science *280*:1432-1438, 1998.

9. Altare, F., Lammas, D., Revy, P., et al.: Inherited interleukin 12 deficiency in a child with Bacille Calmette-Guérin and *Salmonella enteritidis* disseminated infection. J. Clin. Invest. *102*:2035-2040, 1998.

10. Alvarez-Elcoro, S., Soto-Ramirez, L., and Mateos-Mora, M.: *Salmonella* bacteremia in patients with prosthetic heart valves. Am. J. Med. *77*:61-66, 1984.

11. Aserkoff, B., and Bennett, J. V.: Effect of antibiotic therapy in acute salmonellosis on the fecal excretion of *Salmonellae*. N. Engl. J. Med. *281*:636-640, 1969.

12. Ashkenazi, S., Cleary, T. G., Murray, B. E., et al.: Quantitative analysis and partial characterization of cytotoxin production by *Salmonella* strains. Infect. Immun. *56*:3089-3094, 1988.

13. Association for Study of Infectious Diseases: Effect of neomycin in noninvasive *Salmonella* infections of the gastrointestinal tract. Lancet *2*:1159-1161, 1970.

14. Athie, C. G., Guizar, C. B., Alcantara, A. V., et al.: Twenty-five years of experience in the surgical treatment of perforation of the ileum caused by *Salmonella typhi* at the General Hospital of Mexico City, Mexico. Surgery *123*:632-636, 1998.

15. Avendano, A., Herrera, P., Horwitz, I., et al.: Duodenal string cultures: Practicality and sensitivity for diagnosing enteric fever in children. J. Infect. Dis. *153*:359-362, 1986.

16. Baine, W. B., Gangarosa, E. J., Bennett, J. V., et al.: Institutional salmonellosis. J. Infect. Dis. *128*:357-360, 1973.

17. Baird, G. D., Manning, E. J., and Jones, P. W.: Evidence for related virulence sequences in plasmids of *Salmonella dublin* and *Salmonella typhimurium*. J. Gen. Microbiol. *131*:1815-1823, 1985.

18. Baker, N. M., Mills, A. E., Rachman, I., et al.: Hemolytic uraemic syndrome in typhoid fever. B. M. J. *2*:84-87, 1974.

19. Bannerman, C. H.: *S. heidelberg* enteritis: An outbreak in the neonatal unit of Harare Central Hospital. Cent. Afr. J. Med. *31*:1-4, 1985.

20. Bate, J. G., and James, U.: *Salmonella typhimurium* infection dust-borne in a children's ward. Lancet *2*:713, 1958.

21. Bean, N. H., Griffin, P. M., Goulding, J. S., et al.: Foodborne disease outbreaks, 5-year summary, 1983-1987. M. M. W. R. Morb. Mortal. Wkly. Rep. *39*:15-57, 1990.

22. Berkley, J. A., Lowe, B. S., Mwangi, I., et al.: Bacteremia among children admitted to a rural hospital in Kenya. N. Engl. J. Med. *352*:39-47, 2005.

23. Bhutta, Z. A.: Current concepts in the diagnosis and treatment of typhoid fever. B. M. J. *333*:78-82, 2006.

24. Bitar, R., and Tarpley, J.: Intestinal perforation in typhoid fever: A historical and state-of-the-art review. Rev. Infect. Dis. *7*:257-270, 1985.

25. Blaser, M. J., and Newman, L. S.: A review of human salmonellosis, I: Infective dose. Rev. Infect. Dis. *4*:1096-1106, 1982.

26. Borecka, J., Hocmannova, M., and van Leeuwen, W. J.: Nosocomial infection of nurslings caused by multiple drug-resistant strain of *S. typhimurium*: Utilization of a new typing method based on lysogeny of strains. Zentralbl. Bakteriol. 1 Abt. Orig. A. *2336*:262, 1976.

27. Borgnolo, G., Barbone, F., Scornavacca, G., et al.: A case-control study of *Salmonella* gastrointestinal infection in Italian children. Acta Paediatr. *85*:804-808, 1996.

28. Boyd, J. F.: Pathology of the alimentary tract of *S. typhimurium* food poisoning. Gut *26*:935-944, 1985.

29. Bryan, J. P., Rocha, H., and Scheld, W. M.: Problems in salmonellosis: Rationale for clinical trials with newer β-lactam agents and quinolones. Rev. Infect. Dis. *8*:189-207, 1986.

30. Buchawald, D. S., and Blaser, M. J.: A review of human salmonellosis, II: Duration of excretion following infection with non-*typhi Salmonella*. Rev. Infect. Dis. *6*:345-356, 1984.

31. Buckmeier, N. A., and Heffron, F.: Intracellular survival of wild type *Salmonella typhimurium* and macrophage sensitive mutants in diverse populations of macrophages. Infect. Immun. *57*:1-7, 1989.

32. Butler, T., Bell, W. R., Levin, J., et al.: Typhoid fever: Studies of blood coagulation, bacteremia, and endotoxemia. Arch. Intern. Med. *138*:407-410, 1978.

33. Butler, T., Knight, J., Nath, S. K., et al.: Typhoid fever complicated by intestinal perforation: A persisting fatal disease requiring surgical management. Rev. Infect. Dis. *7*:244-256, 1985.

34. Butler, T., Sridhar, C. B., Daga, M. K., et al.: Treatment of typhoid fever with azithromycin versus chloramphenicol in a randomized multicenter trial in India. J. Antimicrob. Chemother. *44*:243-250, 1999.

35. Cao, X. T., Kneen, R., Nguyen, T. A., et al.: A comparative study of ofloxacin and cefixime for treatment of typhoid fever in children. The Dong Nai Pediatric Center Typhoid Study Group. Pediatr. Infect. Dis. J. *18*:245-248, 1999.

36. Centers for Disease Control: Update: *Salmonella enteritidis* infections and grade A shell eggs: United States 1989. M. M. W. R. Morb. Mortal. Wkly. Rep. *37*:490, 1989.

37. Centers for Disease Control: Typhoid immunization: Recommendations of the Immunization Practices Advisory Committee (ACIP). M. M. W. R. Morb. Mortal. Wkly. Rep. *39*:1-5, 1990.

38. Centers for Disease Control: Multistate outbreak of *Salmonella poona* infections: United States and Canada. M. M. W. R. Morb. Mortal. Wkly. Rep. *40*:549, 1991.

39. Challapalli, M., Cherubin, C., and Cunningham, D. G.: Lack of chronic carriage of *Salmonella typhimurium*. Pediatr. Infect. Dis. J. *8*:531-540, 1989.

40. Chin, K. C., Simmons, E. J., and Tarlow, M. J.: Neonatal typhoid fever. Arch. Dis. Child. *61*:1228-1230, 1986.

41. Chinh, N. T., Parry, C. M., Ly, N. T., et al.: A randomized controlled comparison of azithromycin and ofloxacin for treatment of multidrug-resistant or nalidixic acid-resistant enteric fever. Antimicrob. Agents Chemother. *44*:1855-1859, 2000.

42. Chiu, C. H., Lin, T. Y., and Ou, J. T.: A pilot study of seven days of ceftriaxone therapy for children with *Salmonella* enterocolitis. Chang. Gung. Yi. Xue. Za. Zhi. *20*:115-121, 1997.

43. Chiu, C. H., Lin, T. Y., and Ou, J. T.: A clinical trial comparing oral azithromycin, cefixime and no antibiotics in the treatment of acute uncomplicated *Salmonella* enteritis in children. J. Paediatr. Child Health *35*:372-374, 1999.

44. Chorba, T. L., Meriwether, R. A., Jenkins, B. R., et al.: Control of a non-foodborne outbreak of salmonellosis: Day care in isolation. Am. J. Public Health *77*:979-981, 1987.

45. Chow, C. B., Wang, P. S., Cheung, M. W., et al.: Diagnostic value of the Widal test in childhood typhoid fever. Pediatr. Infect. Dis. J. *6*:914-917, 1987.

46. Clegg, A., Passey, M., Omena, M., et al.: Re-evaluation of the Widal agglutination test in response to the changing pattern of typhoid fever in the highlands of Papua New Guinea. Acta Trop. *57*:255-263, 1994.

47. Coburn, B., Grassl, G. A., and Finlay, B. B.: *Salmonella*, the host and disease: A brief review. Immunol. Cell. Biol. *85*:112-118, 2007.

48. Cohen, J. I., Bartlett, J. A., and Corey, G. R.: Extra-intestinal manifestations of *Salmonella* infections. Medicine (Baltimore) *66*:349-388, 1987.

49. Cohen, M. L., and Tauxe, R. V.: Drug-resistant *Salmonella* in the United States: An epidemiologic perspective. Science *234*:964-969, 1986.

50. Colon, A. R., Gross, D. R., and Tamer, M. A.: Typhoid fever in children. Pediatrics *56*:606-609, 1975.

51. Connolly, M. J., Snow, M. N., and Ingham, H. R.: Ciprofloxacin treatment of recurrent *Salmonella* septicemia in a patient with acquired immune deficiency syndrome. J. Antimicrob. Chemother. *18*:647-648, 1986.

52. Cooles, P.: Adjuvant steroids and relapse of typhoid fever. J. Trop. Med. Hyg. *89*:229-231, 1986.

53. Corman, L. I., Poirier, R. H., Littlefield, C. A., et al.: Endophthalmitis due to *S. enteritidis*. J. Pediatr. *95*:1001-1002, 1979.

54. Cravioto, A., Reyes, R. E., Trujillo, F., et al.: Risk of diarrhea during the first year of life associated with initial and subsequent colonization by specific enteropathogens. Am. J. Epidemiol. *131*:886-904, 1990.

55. Crump, J. A., Luby, S. P., and Mintz, E. D.: The global burden of typhoid fever. Bull. World Health Organ. *82*:346-353, 2004.

56. D'Amelio, R., Tagliabue, A., Nencioni, L., et al.: Comparative analysis of immunological responses to oral (Ty21a) and parenteral (TAB) typhoid vaccines. Infect. Immun. *56*:2731-2735, 1988.

57. Davis, R. C.: *Salmonella* sepsis in infancy. Am. J. Dis. Child. *135*:1096-1099, 1981.

58. Day, D. W., Mandal, B. K., and Morson, B. C.: The rectal biopsy appearances in *Salmonella* colitis. Histopathology *2*:117-131, 1978.

59. Demmerich, B., Lode, H., Borner, K., et al.: Biliary excretion and pharmacokinetics of cefoperazone in humans. J. Antimicrob. Chemother. *12*:27-37, 1983.

60. Diddle, A. W., and Stephens, R. L.: Typhoid fever in pregnancy. Am. J. Obstet. Gynecol. *38*:300-305, 1939.

61. Dietrich, H. F.: Typhoid fever in children. J. Pediatr. *10*:191-201, 1937.

62. Diwan, N., and Sharma, K. B.: Isolation of *S. typhimurium* from cephalohematoma and osteomyelitis. Indian J. Med. Res. *67*:27-29, 1978.

63. Dixon, J. M. S.: Effect of antibiotic treatment on duration of excretion of *S. typhimurium* by children. B. M. J. *2*:1343-1345, 1965.

64. Doffinger, R., Patel, S., and Kumararatne, D. S.: Human immunodeficiencies that predispose to intracellular bacterial infections. Curr. Opin. Rheumatol. *17*:440-446, 2005.

65. Dowdle, E.: The reaction of patients with typhoid fever to the administration of aspirin. S. Afr. Med. J. *19*:474-477, 1956.

66. Dunn, D. W., McAllister, J., and Craft, J. C.: Brain abscess and empyema caused by *Salmonella*. Pediatr. Infect. Dis. *3*:54-57, 1984.

67. Dutta, P., Bhattacharya, S. K., Dutta, D., et al.: Hemolytic uremic syndrome following *Salmonella typhimurium* enteritis. Indian J. Pediatr. *56*:409-410, 1989.

68. Dutta, P., Rasaily, R., Saha, M. R., et al.: Ciprofloxacin for treatment of severe typhoid fever in children. Antimicrob. Agents Chemother. *37*:1197-1199, 1993.

69. Dutta, P., Rasaily, R., Saha, M. R., et al.: Randomized clinical trial of furazolidone for typhoid fever in children. Scand. J. Gastroenterol. *28*:168-172, 1993.

70. Eckmann, L., and Kagnoff, M. F.: Cytokines in host defense against *Salmonella*. Microbes Infect. *3*:1191-1200, 2001.

71. Edgar, W. M., and Lacey, B. W.: Infection with *S. heidelberg*: An outbreak presumably not foodborne. Lancet *1*:161, 1963.

72. Ejlertsen, T., and Aunsholt, N. A.: *Salmonella* bacteremia in renal transplant recipients. Scand. J. Infect. Dis. *21*:241-244, 1989.

73. Farid, Z., Bassily, S., Kent, D. C., et al.: Chronic urinary *Salmonella* carriers with intermittent bacteremia. J. Trop. Med. Hyg. *73*:153-157, 1970.

74. Farid, Z., Girgis, N., and Abu El Ella, A.: Successful treatment of typhoid fever in children with parenteral ceftriaxone. Scand. J. Infect. Dis. *19*:467-468, 1987.

75. Faucher, J. F., Binder, R., Missinou, M. A., et al.: Efficacy of atovaquone/proguanil for malaria prophylaxis in children and its effect on the immunogenicity of live oral typhoid and cholera vaccines. Clin. Infect. Dis. *35*:1147-1154, 2002.

76. Feachem, R. G., and Koblinsky, M. A.: Interventions for the control of diarrhoeal diseases among young children: Promotion of breastfeeding. Bull. World Health Organ. *62*:271, 1984.

77. Ferreccio, C., Levine, M. M., Manterola, A., et al.: Benign bacteremia caused by *S. typhi* and *paratyphi* in children younger than 2 years. J. Pediatr. *104*:899-901, 1984.

78. Ferreccio, C., Morris, J. G., and Valdivieso, C., et al.: Efficacy of ciprofloxacin in the treatment of chronic typhoid carriers. J. Infect. Dis. *157*:1235-1239, 1988.

79. Fierer, J., Krause, M., Tauxe, R., et al.: *Salmonella typhimurium* bacteremia: Association with the virulence plasmid. J. Infect. Dis. *166*:639-642, 1992.

80. Finlay, B. B.: Molecular and cellular mechanisms of *Salmonella* pathogenesis. Curr. Top. Microbiol. Immunol. *192*:163-185, 1994.

81. Finlay, B. B., and Falkow, S.: Comparison of the invasion strategies used by *S. choleraesuis*, *S. flexneri*, and *Y. enterocolitica* to enter cultured animal cells. Biochimie *70*:1089-1099, 1988.

82. Foley, A. R.: An outbreak of paratyphoid B fever in a nursery of a small hospital. Can. J. Public Health *38*:73, 1947.

83. France, G. L., Marmer, D. J., and Steele, R. W.: Breast-feeding and *Salmonella* infection. Am. J. Dis. Child. *134*:147-152, 1980.

84. Frenck, R. W., Jr., Mansour, A., Nakhla, I., et al.: Short-course azithromycin for the treatment of uncomplicated typhoid fever in children and adolescents. Clin. Infect. Dis. *38*:951-957, 2004.

85. Galofre, J., Moreno, A., Mensa, J., et al.: Analysis of factors influencing the outcome and development of septic metastasis or relapse in *Salmonella* bacteremia. Clin. Infect. Dis. *18*:873-878, 1994.

86. Gendrel, D., Kombila, M., Beaudoin-Leblevec, G., et al.: Nontyphoidal *Salmonella* septicemia in Gabonese children infected with *Schistosoma intercalatum*. Clin. Infect. Dis. *18*:103-105, 1994.

87. Gershman, M.: Single phage typing set for differentiating *Salmonella*. J. Clin. Microbiol. *5*:302-314, 1977.

88. Giannella, R. A., Broitman, S. A., and Zamcheck, N.: *Salmonella* enteritis, I: Role of reduced gastric secretion in pathogenesis. Dig. Dis. *16*:1000-1006, 1971.

89. Giannella, R. A., Broitman, S. A., and Zamcheck, N.: Influence of gastric acidity on bacterial and parasitic enteric infections: A perspective. Ann. Intern. Med. *78*:271-276, 1973.

90. Giannella, R. A., Formal, S. B., Dammin, G. J., et al.: Pathogenesis of salmonellosis: Studies of fluid secretion, mucosal invasion, and morphologic reaction in the rabbit ileum. J. Clin. Invest. *52*:441-453, 1973.

91. Giannella, R. A., Gots, R. E., Charney, A. N., et al.: Pathogenesis of *Salmonella*-mediated intestinal fluid secretion: Activation of adenylate cyclase and inhibition by indomethacin. Gastroenterology *69*:1238-1245, 1975.

92. Gibney, E. J.: Typhoid perforation. Br. J. Surg. *76*:887-889, 1989.

93. Gilman, R. H., Terminel, M., and Levine, M. M.: Relative efficacy of blood, urine, rectal swab, bone marrow, and rose spot cultures for recovery of *S. typhi* in typhoid fever. Lancet *1*:1211-1213, 1975.

94. Gilman, R. H., Terminel, M., Levine, M. M., et al.: Comparison of trimethoprim/sulfamethoxazole and amoxicillin in therapy of chloramphenicol-resistant and chloramphenicol-sensitive typhoid fever. J. Infect. Dis. *132*:630-636, 1975.

95. Girgis, N. I., Butler, T., Frenck, R. W., et al.: Azithromycin versus ciprofloxacin for treatment of uncomplicated typhoid in a randomized trial in Egypt that included patients with multidrug resistance. Antimicrob. Agents Chemother. *43*:1441-1444, 1999.

96. Girgis, N. I., Sultan, Y., Hammad, O., et al.: Comparison of the efficacy, safety and cost of cefixime, ceftriaxone and aztreonam in the treatment of multidrug resistant *S. typhi* septicemia in children. Pediatr. Infect. Dis. J. *14*:603-605, 1995.

97. Glynn, M. K., Bopp, C., Dewitt, W., et al.: Emergence of multidrug-resistant *Salmonella enterica* serotype *typhimurium* DT104 infections in the United States. N. Engl. J. Med. *338*:1333-1338, 1998.

98. Gokalp, A. S., Toksoy, H. B., Turkay, S., et al.: Intravenous immunoglobulin in the treatment of *Salmonella typhimurium* infections in preterm neonates. Clin. Pediatr. *33*:349-352, 1994.

99. Gotuzzo, E., Echevarria, J., Carrillo, C., et al.: Randomized comparison of aztreonam and chloramphenicol in treatment of typhoid fever. Antimicrob. Agents Chemother. *38*:558-562, 1994.

100. Gotuzzo, E., Guerra, J. G., Benavente, L., et al.: Use of norfloxacin to treat chronic typhoid carriers. J. Infect. Dis. *157*:1221-1225, 1988.

101. Gorvel, J. P., and Meresse, S.: Maturation steps of the *Salmonella*-containing vacuole. Microbes Infect. *3*:1299-1303, 2001.

102. Graham, S. M.: Salmonellosis in children in developing and developed countries and populations. Curr. Opin. Infect. Dis. *15*:507-512, 2002.

103. Griffith, J. P. C., and Ostheimer, M.: Typhoid fever in children. Am. J. Med. Sci. *124*:868-888, 1902.

104. Groisman, E. A., and Ochman, G.: Cognate gene clusters govern invasion of host epithelial cells by *S. typhimurium* and *Shigella flexneri*. E. M. B. O. J. *12*:3779-3787, 1993.

105. Grossman, D. A., Witham, N., Burr, D. H., et al.: Flagellar serotypes of *S. typhi* in Indonesia: Relationships among motility, invasiveness, and clinical illness. J. Infect. Dis. *171*:212-216, 1995.

106. Guthrie, K. J., and Montgomery, G. I.: Infections with *Bacterium enteritidis* in infancy with the triad of enteritis, cholecystitis and meningitis. J. Pathol. Bacteriol. *49*:393, 1939.

107. Hadfield, T. L., Monson, M. H., and Wachsmoth, I. K.: An outbreak of antibiotic-resistant *Salmonella* enteritidis in Liberia, West Africa. J. Infect. Dis. *151*:790-795, 1985.

108. Haggman, D. L., Rehm, S. J., Moodie, D. S., et al.: Non-typhoidal *Salmonella* pericarditis: A case report and review of the literature. Pediatr. Infect. Dis. J. *5*:259-264, 1986.

109. Han, T., Sokal, J. E., and Neter, E.: Salmonellosis in disseminated malignant diseases: A seven-year review (1959-1963). N. Engl. J. Med. *276*:1045, 1967.

110. Hand, W. L., and King, N. L.: Serum opsonization of *Salmonella* in sickle cell anemia. Am. J. Med. *64*:388-395, 1978.

111. Harris, J. C., DuPont, H. L., and Hornick, R. B.: Fecal leukocytes in diarrheal illness. Ann. Intern. Med. *76*:697-700, 1972.

112. Hedberg, C. W., David, M. J., White, K. E., et al.: Role of egg consumption in sporadic *Salmonella enteritidis* and *Salmonella typhimurium* infections in Minnesota. J. Infect. Dis. *167*:107-111, 1993.

113. Herikstat, H., Hayes, P., Hogan, J., et al.: Ceftriaxone-resistant *Salmonella* in the United States. Pediatr. Infect. Dis. J. *16*:904-905, 1997.

114. Hoffman, S. L., Edman, D. C., Punjabi, N. H., et al.: Bone marrow aspirate culture superior to streptokinase clot culture and 8 ml 1 : 10 blood-to-broth ratio blood culture for diagnosis of typhoid fever. Am. J. Trop. Med. Hyg. *35*:836-839, 1986.

115. Hoffman, S. L., Punjabi, N. H., Kumala, S., et al.: Reduction of mortality in chloramphenicol-treated severe typhoid fever by high dose dexamethasone. N. Engl. J. Med. *310*:82-88, 1984.

116. Hoffman, S. L., Punjabi, N. H., Rockhill, R. C., et al.: Duodenal string-capsule culture compared with bone marrow, blood, and rectal swab cultures for diagnosing typhoid and paratyphoid fever. J. Infect. Dis. *149*:157-161, 1984.

117. Holmberg, S. D.: Drug-resistant *Salmonella* species from animals fed antimicrobics. Infect. Dis. Newsl. *5*:25, 1986.

118. Holmberg, S. D., Osterholm, M. T., Senger, K. A., et al.: Drug-resistant *Salmonella* from animals fed antimicrobials. N. Engl. J. Med. *311*:617-622, 1984.

119. Hoppe, J. E., Dopfer, R., Huber, S., et al.: Eradication of *Salmonella dublin* in an immunodeficient child by combined use of ceftriaxone and ciprofloxacin after failure of either agent alone. Infection *17*:399-400, 1989.

120. Hornick, R. B., Griesman, S. E., Woodward, T. E., et al.: Typhoid fever: Pathogenesis and immunologic control, parts I and II. N. Engl. J. Med. *283*:686-691, 739-746, 1970.

121. Huang, L. T., Ko, S. F., and Lui, C. C.: *Salmonella* meningitis: Clinical experience with third-generation cephalosporin. Acta Paediatr. *86*:1056-1058, 1997.

122. Hyams, J. S., Durbin, W. A., Grand, R. J., et al.: *Salmonella* bacteremia in the first year of life. J. Pediatr. *96*:57-59, 1980.

123. Im, S. W. K., Chow, K., and Chau, P. Y.: Rectal thermometer-mediated cross-infection with *S. wadsworth* in a pediatric ward. J. Hosp. Infect. *2*:171-174, 1981.

124. Isomaki, O., Vuento, R., and Granfors, K.: Serological diagnosis of *Salmonella* infections by enzyme immunoassay. Lancet *1*:1411-1414, 1989.

125. Jiwa, S. F.: Probing for enterotoxigenicity among the salmonellae: An evaluation of biological assays. J. Clin. Microbiol. *14*:463-472, 1981.

126. Johnson, P. C., and Sabbaj, J.: Typhoid tonsillitis. J. A. M. A. *244*:362, 1980.

127. Jones, T. F., Ingram, L. A., Fullerton, K. E., et al.: A case-control study of the epidemiology of sporadic *Salmonella* infection in infants. Pediatrics *118*:2380-2387, 2006.

128. Jouanguy, E., Doffinger, R., Dupuis, S., et al.: IL-12 and IFN-γ in host defense against mycobacteria and *Salmonella* in mice and men. Curr. Opin. Immunol. *11*:346-351, 1999.

129. Kaniga, K., Trollinger, D., and Galan, J. E.: Identification of two targets of the type III protein secretion system encoded by the inv and spa loci of *Salmonella typhimurium* that have homology to the Shigella IpaD and IpaA proteins. J. Bacteriol. *177*:7078-7085, 1995.

130. Kaniga, K., Tucker, S., Trollinger, D., et al.: Homologs of the *Shigella* IpaB and IpaC invasins are required for *Salmonella typhimurium* entry into cultured epithelial cells. J. Bacteriol. *177*:3965-3971, 1995.

131. Katz, B. Z., and Shapiro, E. D.: Predictors of persistently positive blood cultures in children with "occult" *Salmonella bacteremia*. Pediatr. Infect. Dis. *5*:713-714, 1986.

132. Kazemi, M., Bumpert, T. G., and Marks, M. I.: A controlled trial comparing trimethoprim/sulfamethoxazole, ampicillin, and no therapy in the treatment of *Salmonella* gastroenteritis in children. J. Pediatr. *83*:646-650, 1973.

133. Khan, M. A., Abdur-Rab, M., Israr, N., et al.: Transmission of *S. worthington* by oropharyngeal suction in hospital neonatal unit. Pediatr. Infect. Dis. J. *10*:668-672, 1991.

134. Kinsella, T. R., Yoger, R., Shulman, S. T., et al.: Treatment of *Salmonella* meningitis and brain abscess with the new cephalosporins: Two case reports and a review of the literature. Pediatr. Infect. Dis. J. *6*:476-480, 1987.

135. Klugman, K. P., Gilbertson, I. T., Koornhof, H. J., et al.: Protective activity of Vi capsular polysaccharide vaccine against typhoid fever. Lancet *2*:1165-1169, 1987.

136. Konzert, W.: *Salmonella* osteomyelitis in reference to *S. typhimurium* epidemics in a newborn infant ward. Wien. Klin. Wochenschr. *81*:713-716, 1969.

137. Lamb, V. A., Mayhall, C. G., Spadora, A. C., et al.: Outbreak of *Salmonella typhimurium* gastroenteritis due to an imported strain resistant to ampicillin, chloramphenicol and trimethoprim/sulfamethoxazole in a nursery. J. Clin. Microbiol. *20*:1076-1079, 1984.

138. Lee, L. A., Puhr, N. D., Maloney, E. K., et al.: Increase in antimicrobial-resistant *Salmonella* infections in the US, 1989-1990. J. Infect. Dis. *170*:128-134, 1994.

139. Lee, S. C., Yang, P. H., Shieh, W. B., et al.: Bacteremia due to non-typhi *Salmonella*: Analysis of 64 cases and review. Clin. Infect. Dis. *19*:693-696, 1994.

140. Levine, M. M.: Typhoid fever and enteric fever. *In* Kass, E., and Platt, R. (eds.): Current Therapy in Infectious Diseases. Toronto, B.C., Decker, 1986.

141. Levy, S. B.: Man, animals, and antibiotic resistance. Pediatr. Infect. Dis. *4*:3-5, 1985.

142. Lieb, S., Gunn, R. A., and Taylor, D. N.: Salmonellosis in a day care center. J. Pediatr. *100*:1004, 1982.

143. Lizarralde, E.: Typhoid perforation of the ileum in children. J. Pediatr. Surg. *16*:1012-1016, 1981.

144. LoVerde, P. T., Amento, C., and Higashi, G. I.: Parasite-parasite interaction of *Salmonella typhimurium* and *Schistosoma*. J. Infect. Dis. *141*:177-185, 1980.

145. Low, L. C., Lam, B. C., Wong, W. T., et al.: *Salmonella* meningitis in infancy. Aust. Paediatr. J. *20*:225-228, 1984.

146. Lynch, M., Painter, J., Woodruff, R., and Braden, C.; Centers for Disease Control and Prevention: Surveillance for foodborne-disease outbreaks—United States, 1998-2002. M. M. W. R. Surveill. Summ. *55*:1-42, 2006.

147. Mabey, D. C., Brown, A., and Greenwood, B. M.: *Plasmodium falciparum* malaria and *Salmonella* infections in Gambian children. J. Infect. Dis. *155*:1319, 1987.

148. MacDonald, K. L., Cohen, M. L., Hargrett-Bean, N. T., et al.: Changes in antimicrobial resistance of *Salmonella* isolated from humans in the United States. J. A. M. A. *258*:1496-1499, 1987.

149. MacDonald, W. B., Friday, F., and McEacharn, M.: The effect of chloramphenicol in *Salmonella* enteritis in infancy. Arch. Dis. Child. *29*:238, 1954.

150. Mackaness, G. B., Blander, R. V., and Collins, F. M.: Host-parasite relations in mouse typhoid. J. Exp. Med. *124*:573-583, 1966.

151. Mallouh, A. A., and Sadi, A. R.: White blood cells and bone marrow in typhoid fever. Pediatr. Infect. Dis. J. *6*:527-529, 1987.

152. Mallouh, A. A., and Salamah, M. M.: Pattern of bacterial infections in homozygous sickle cell disease. Am. J. Dis. Child. *139*:820-826, 1985.

153. Marcus, R., Rabatsky-Ehr, T., Mohle-Boetani, J. C., et al.: Dramatic decrease in the incidence of *Salmonella* serotype *Enteritidis* infections in 5 FoodNet sites: 1996-1999. Clin. Infect. Dis. *38*(Suppl. 3):S135-S141, 2004.

154. Marcus, S. L., Brumell, J. H., Pfeifer, C. G., and Brett Finlay, B.: *Salmonella* pathogenicity islands: Big virulence in small packages. Microbes Infect. *2*:145-156, 2000.

155. Martyn-Jones, D. M., and Pantin, G. C.: Neonatal diarrhea due to *S. paratyphi*. Br. J. Clin. Pathol. *9*:128, 1956.

156. Marzetti, G., Laurenti, F., deCaro, M., et al.: *Salmonella münchen* infections in newborns and small infants. Clin. Pediatr. (Philadelphia) *12*:93-97, 1973.

157. Maudgil, A., Bhan, M. K., and Khoshoo, V.: Hemolytic uremic syndrome associated with *Salmonella typhimurium*. Indian Pediatr. *24*:608-609, 1987.

158. McAllister, T. A., Roud, J. A., and Marshall, A., et al.: Outbreak of *Salmonella eimsbuettel* in newborn infants spread by rectal thermometers. Lancet *1*:1262-1264, 1986.

159. McKinlay, B.: Infectious diarrhea of the newborn caused by an unclassified species of *Salmonella*. Am. J. Dis. Child. *54*:1252, 1937.

160. Meadow, W. L., Schneider, H., and Beem, M.: *Salmonella enteritidis* bacteremia in childhood. J. Infect. Dis. *152*:185-189, 1985.

161. Meloni, T., Marinaro, A. M., Desole, M. G., et al.: Ceftriaxone treatment of *Salmonella* enteric fever. Pediatr. Infect. Dis. J. *7*:734-735, 1986.

162. Mendis, N. M. P., de la Motte, P. U., Gunatillaka, P. D. P., et al.: Protracted infection with *S. bareilly* in a maternity hospital. J. Trop. Med. Hyg. *79*:142-150, 1976.

163. Mermin, J. H., Townes, J. M., Gerber, M., et al.: Typhoid fever in the United States, 1985-1994: Changing risks of international travel and increasing antimicrobial resistance. Arch. Intern. Med. *158*:633-638, 1998.

164. Merselis, J. G., Kaye, D., Connolly, C. S., et al.: Quantitative bacteriology of the typhoid carrier state. Am. J. Trop. Med. Hyg. *13*:425, 1964.

165. Michel, J., Malpuach, G., Godeneche, P., et al.: Clinical and bacteriological study of a salmonellosis epidemic in a hospital (*Salmonella oranienburg*). Pediatrie *25*:13-19, 1970.

166. Molbak, K., Baggesen, D. L., Aarestrup, F. M., et al.: An outbreak of multidrug-resistant, quinolone-resistant *Salmonella* enterica serotype *Typhimurium* DT104. N. Engl. J. Med. *34*:1420-1425, 1999.

167. Moosa, A., and Rubidge, C. J.: Once daily ceftriaxone vs. chloramphenicol for treatment of typhoid fever in children. Pediatr. Infect. Dis. J. *8*:696-699, 1989.

168. Mroczenski-Wildey, M. J., Di, F. J., and Cabello, F. C.: Invasion and lyssi of HeLa cell monolayers by *S. typhi*: The role of lipopolysaccharide. Microb. Pathog. *6*:143-152, 1989.

169. Nelson, J. D.: Suppurative mastitis in infants. Am. J. Dis. Child. *125*:458-459, 1973.

170. Nelson, J. D., Kusmiesz, H., Jackson, L. H., et al.: Treatment of *Salmonella* gastroenteritis with ampicillin, amoxicillin, or placebo. Pediatrics *65*:1125-1130, 1980.

171. Nelson, J. D., and McCracken, G. H.: What next? J. Pediatr. Infect. Dis. *16*:10-16, 1990.

172. Nelson, S. J., and Granoff, D.: *Salmonella* gastroenteritis in the first three months of life. Clin. Pediatr. *21*:709-712, 1982.

173. Neter, E.: Observation on the transmission of salmonellosis in man. Am. J. Public Health *40*:929, 1950.

174. Nguyen, T. C., Solomon, T., Mai, X. T., et al.: Short courses of ofloxacin for the treatment of enteric fever. Trans. R. Soc. Trop. Med. Hyg. *91*:347-349, 1997.

175. Novak, R., and Feldman, S.: Salmonellosis in children with cancer. Am. J. Dis. Child. *133*:298-300, 1979.

176. Noyola, D. E., Fernandez, M., and Kaplan, S. L.: Reevaluation of antipyretics in children with enteric fever. Pediatr. Infect. Dis. J. *17*:691-695, 1998.

177. Omland, T., and Gardborg, O.: *Salmonella* enteritidis infections in infancy with special reference to a small nosocomial epidemic. Acta Paediatr. Belg. *49*:583-590, 1960.

178. Ortiz-Neu, C., Marr, J. S., Cherubin, C. E., et al.: Bone and joint infections due to *Salmonella*. J. Infect. Dis. *138*:820-828, 1978.

179. Pape, J. W., Gerdes, H., Oriol, L., et al.: Typhoid fever: Successful therapy with cefoperazone. J. Infect. Dis. *153*:272-276, 1986.

180. Parry, C. M., Hien, T. T., Dougan, G., et al.: Typhoid fever. N. Engl. J. Med. *347*:1770-1782, 2002.

181. Parry, C. M., Hoa, N. T., Diep, T. S., et al.: Value of a single-tube Widal test in diagnosis of typhoid fever in Vietnam. J. Clin. Microbiol. *37*:2882-2886, 1999.

182. Pavia, A. T., Shipman, L. D., Wells, J. G., et al.: Epidemiologic evidence that prior antimicrobial exposure decreases resistance to infection by antimicrobial-sensitive *Salmonella*. J. Infect. Dis. *161*:255-260, 1990.

183. Pether, J. V., and Gilbert, R. J.: The survival of *Salmonella* on finger-tips and transfer of the organisms to foods. J. Hyg. (London) *69*:673-681, 1971.

184. Pettersson, T., Klemola, E., and Wager, O.: Treatment of acute cases of *Salmonella* infection and *Salmonella* carriers with ampicillin and neomycin. Acta Med. Scand. *175*:185, 1964.

185. Phongmany, S., Phetsouvanh, R., Sisouphone, S., et al.: A randomized comparison of oral chloramphenicol versus ofloxacin in the treatment of uncomplicated typhoid fever in Laos. Trans. R. Soc. Trop. Med. Hyg. *99*:451-458, 2005.

186. Pickering, L. K.: Bacterial and parasitic enteropathogens in day care. Semin. Pediatr. Infect. Dis. *1*:263, 1990.

187. Pickering, L. K., DuPont, H. L., Olarte, J., et al.: Fecal leukocytes in enteric infections. Am. J. Clin. Pathol. *68*:562-565, 1977.

188. Pickering, L. K., Kohl, S., and Cleary, T. G.: Humoral factors in breast milk that protect against diarrhea. *In* Jensen, R. G., and Neville, M. C. (eds.): Human Lactation. New York, Plenum, 1985, p. 63.

189. Pickering, L. K., and Ruiz-Palacios, G.: Antibodies in milk directed against specific enteropathogens. *In* Hamosh, A., and Goldman, A. S. (eds.): Human Lactation 2. New York, Plenum, 1986, p. 499.

190. Plotkin, S. A., and Bouveret-Le Cam, N.: A new typhoid vaccine composed of the Vi capsular polysaccharide. Arch. Intern. Med. *155*:2293-2299, 1995.

191. Punjabi, N. H., Hoffman, S. L., Edman, D. C., et al.: Treatment of severe typhoid fever in children with high dose dexamethasone. Pediatr. Infect. Dis. J. *7*:598-600, 1988.

192. Puri, V., Thirupuram, S., Khalil, A., et al.: Nosocomial *S. typhimurium* epidemic in a neonatal special care unit. Indian Pediatr. *17*:233-239, 1980.

193. Rajajee, S., Anandi, T. B., Subha, S., et al.: Patterns of resistant *S. typhi* infection in infants. J. Trop. Pediatr. *41*:52-54, 1995.

194. Ramachandran, S., Godfrey, J. J., and Perera, M. V.: Typhoid hepatitis. J. A. M. A. *230*:236-240, 1974.

195. Ramos, J. M., Garcia-Corbeira, P., Aguado, J. M., et al.: Clinical significance of primary vs. secondary bacteremia due to nontyphoid *Salmonella* in patients without AIDS. Clin. Infect. Dis. *19*:777-780, 1994.

196. Reed, R. P., and Klugman, K. P.: Neonatal typhoid fever. Pediatr. Infect. Dis. J. *13*:774-777, 1994.

197. Renuka, K., Sood, S., Das, B. K., and Kapil, A.: High-level ciprofloxacin resistance in *Salmonella enterica* serotype *Typhi* in India. J. Med. Microbiol. 54:999-1000, 2000.

198. Rice, P. A., Craven, P. C., and Wells, J. G.: *Salmonella heidelberg* enteritis and bacteremia: An epidemic on two pediatric wards. Am. J. Med. 60:509-516, 1976.

199. Riley, L. W., and Cohen, M. L.: Plasmid profiles and *Salmonella* epidemiology. Lancet 1:573, 1982.

200. Riley, L. W., Cohen, M. L., Seals, J. E., et al.: Importance of host factors in human salmonellosis caused by multi-resistant strains of *Salmonella*. J. Infect. Dis. 149:878-883, 1984.

201. Rocha, H., Kirk, J. W., and Hearey, C. D.: Prolonged *Salmonella* bacteremia in patients with *Schistosoma mansoni* infection. Arch. Intern. Med. 128:254-257, 1971.

202. Rodriguez, R. E., Valero, V., and Watanakunakorn, C.: *Salmonella* focal intracranial infections: Review of the world literature (1884-1984) and report of an unusual case. Rev. Infect. Dis. 8:31-41, 1986.

203. Rosenthal, S. L.: Exacerbation of *Salmonella* enteritis due to ampicillin. N. Engl. J. Med. 280:147-148, 1969.

204. Rowe, B., Giles, C., and Brown, G. L.: Outbreak of gastroenteritis due to S. *virchow* in a maternity hospital. B. M. J. 3:561-564, 1969.

205. Rowe, B., Ward, L. R., and Threlfall, E. J.: Multidrug-resistant *Salmonella typhi*: A worldwide epidemic. Clin. Infect. Dis. 24(Suppl. 1):S106-S109, 1997.

206. Rowe, S. Y., Rocourt, J. R., Shiferaw, B., et al.: Breast-feeding decreases the risk of sporadic salmonellosis among infants in FoodNet sites. Clin. Infect. Dis. 38(Suppl. 3):S262-S270, 2004.

207. Rubinstein, A. D., Feemster, R. F., and Smith, H. M.: Salmonellosis as a public health problem in wartime. Am. J. Public Health 34:841, 1944.

208. Rubinstein, A. D., and Fowler, R. N.: Salmonellosis of the newborn with transmission by delivery room resuscitators. Am. J. Public Health 45:1109, 1955.

209. Ruiz-Contreras, J., Ramos, J. T., Hernandez-Sampelayo, T., et al.: Sepsis in children with HIV infection. The Madrid HIV Pediatric Infection Collaborative Study Group. Pediatr. Infect. Dis. J. 14:522-526, 1995.

210. Ruiz-Gomez, J., Lorente Salinas, I., Perez Salmeron, J., et al.: Evaluation of methods for isolation of *Salmonella* species using modified Rappaport-Vassiliadis medium and *Salmonella-Shigella* agar. Eur. J. Clin. Microbiol. Infect. Dis. 17:791-793, 1998.

211. Russell, I. J., Forgacs, P., and Geraci, J. E.: Pancreatitis complicating typhoid fever. J. A. M. A. 235:753-754, 1976.

212. Ryan, C. A., Hargrett-Bean, N. T., and Blake, P. A.: *Salmonella typhi* infections in the United States, 1975-1984: Increasing role of foreign travel. Rev. Infect. Dis. 11:1-8, 1989.

213. Sanchez, C., Garcia Restoy, E., Garau, J., et al.: Ciprofloxacin and TMP/SMX versus placebo in acute uncomplicated *Salmonella* enteritis: A double-blind trial. J. Infect. Dis. 168:1304-1307, 1993.

214. Sanders, D. Y., Sinal, S. H., and Morrison, L.: Chronic salmonellosis in infancy. Clin. Pediatr. (Philadelphia) 13:640-643, 1974.

215. Saphra, I., and Winter, J. W.: Clinical manifestations of salmonellosis in man: An evaluation of 7779 human infections identified at the New York *Salmonella* Center. N. Engl. J. Med. 256:1128, 1957.

216. Sarasombath, S., Banchuin, N., Sukosol, T., et al.: Systemic and intestinal immunities after natural typhoid infection. J. Clin. Microbiol. 25:1088-1093, 1987.

217. Sasidharan, C. K., Rajagopal, K. C., Jayaram, C. K., et al.: S. *typhimurium* epidemic in newborn nursery. Indian J. Pediatr. 50:599-605, 1983.

218. Schwan, W. R., Huang, X., Hu, L., and Kopecko, D. J.: Differential bacterial survival, replication and apoptosis-inducing ability of *Salmonella* serovars within human and murine macrophages. Infect. Immun. 68:1005-1013, 2000.

219. Seals, J. E., Parrott, P. L., McGowan, J. E., et al.: Nursery salmonellosis: Delayed recognition due to unusually long incubation period. Infect. Control 4:205-208, 1983.

220. Secmeer, G., Kanra, G., Figen, G., et al.: Ofloxacin versus co-trimoxazole in the treatment of typhoid fever in children. Acta Paediatr. Jpn. 39:218-221, 1997.

221. Seligman, E.: Mass invasion of *Salmonella* in a babies ward. Ann. Paediatr. 172:406, 1949.

222. Seoud, M., Saade, G., Uwaydah, M., et al.: Typhoid fever in pregnancy. Obstet. Gynecol. 71:711-714, 1988.

223. Shirakawa, T., Acharya, B., Kinoshita, S., et al.: Decreased susceptibility to fluoroquinolones and gyrA gene mutation in the *Salmonella enterica* serovar *Typhi* and *Paratyphi* A isolated in Katmandu, Nepal, in 2003. Diagn. Microbiol. Infect. Dis. 54:299-303, 2006.

224. Sinha, A., Sazawal, S., Kumar, R., et al.: Typhoid fever in children aged less than 5 years. Lancet 354:734-737, 1999.

225. Sirinavin, S., Jayanetra, P., Lolekha, S., et al.: Predictors for extraintestinal infection in *Salmonella* enteritis in Thailand. Pediatr. Infect. Dis. J. 7:44-48, 1988.

226. Smith, S. M., Palumbo, P. E., and Edelson, P. J.: *Salmonella* strains resistant to multiple antibiotics: Therapeutic implications. Pediatr. Infect. Dis. 3:455-460, 1984.

227. Soe, G. B., and Overturf, G. D.: Treatment of typhoid fever and other systemic salmonellosis with cefotaxime, ceftriaxone, cefoperazone, and other newer cephalosporins. Rev. Infect. Dis. 9:719-736, 1987.

228. Sperber, S. J., and Schleupner, C. J.: Salmonellosis during infection with human immunodeficiency virus. Rev. Infect. Dis. 9:925-934, 1987.

229. Spika, J. S., Waterman, S. H., Soo Hoo, G. W., et al.: Chloramphenicol-resistant *Salmonella newport* traced through hamburger to dairy farms. N. Engl. J. Med. 316:565-570, 1987.

230. Stuart, B. M., and Pullen, R. L.: Typhoid: Clinical analysis of 360 cases. Arch. Intern. Med. 78:629, 1946.

231. Su, L. H., Chiu, C. H., Chu, C., Ou, J. T.: Antimicrobial resistance in nontyphoid *Salmonella* serotypes: A global challenge. Clin. Infect. Dis. 39:546-551, 2004.

232. Swanson, S. J., Snider, C., Braden, C. R., et al.: Multidrug-resistant *Salmonella enterica* serotype *Typhimurium* associated with pet rodents. N. Engl. J. Med. 356:21-28, 2007.

233. Syrogiannopoulos, G. A., McCracken, G. H., and Nelson, J. D.: Osteoarticular infections in children with sickle cell disease. Pediatrics 78:1090-1096, 1986.

234. Szanton, V. L.: Epidemic salmonellosis: A 30-month study of 80 cases of S. *oranienburg* infection. Pediatrics 20:794-808, 1957.

235. Szmuness, W., Sikorska, J., Szymanek, E., et al.: The microbiological and epidemiological properties of infections caused by S. *enteritidis*. J. Hyg. (London) 64:9-21, 1966.

236. Sztein, M. B., Wasserman, S. S., Tacket, C. O., et al.: Cytokine production patterns and lymphoproliferative responses in volunteers orally immunized with attenuated vaccine strains of S. *typhi*. J. Infect. Dis. 170:1508-1517, 1994.

237. Taylor, D. N., Beid, J. M., Munro, J. S., et al.: *Salmonella dublin* infections in the United States, 1979-1980. J. Infect. Dis. 146:322-327, 1982.

238. Taylor, D. N., Bopp, C., Birkness, K., et al.: An outbreak of salmonellosis associated with a fatality in a healthy child: A large dose and severe illness. Am. J. Epidemiol. 119:907-912, 1984.

239. Taylor, D. N., Levine, M. M., Kuppens, L., and Ivanoff, B.: Why are typhoid vaccines not recommended for epidemic typhoid fever? J. Infect. Dis. 180:2089-2090, 1999.

240. Ti, T. Y., Monteiro, E. H., Lam, S., et al.: Ceftriaxone therapy in bacteremic typhoid fever. Antimicrob. Agents Chemother. 28:540-543, 1985.

241. Torrey, S., Fleisher, G., and Jaffe, D.: Incidence of *Salmonella* bacteremia in infants with *Salmonella* gastroenteritis. J. Pediatr. 108:718-721, 1986.

242. Thisyakorn, U., Mansuwan, P., and Taylor, D. N.: Typhoid and paratyphoid fever in 192 hospitalized children in Thailand. Am. J. Dis. Child. 141:862-865, 1987.

243. Tsang, R. S., Chau, P. Y., Lam, S. K., et al.: Antibody response to the lipopolysaccharide and protein antigens of *Salmonella typhi* during typhoid infection. Clin. Exp. Immunol. 46:508-514, 1981.

244. Uchiya, K., and Nikai, T.: *Salmonella enterica* serovar *Typhimurium* infection induces cyclooxygenase 2 expression in macrophages: Involvement of *Salmonella* pathogenicity island 2. Infect. Immun. 72:6860-6869, 2004.

245. Uchiya, K., and Nikai, T.: *Salmonella* pathogenicity island 2-dependent expression of suppressor of cytokine signaling 3 in macrophages. Infect. Immun. 73:5587-5594, 2005.

246. Uwyyed, K., and Uromen, A.: Scrotal abscess with bacteremia caused by *Salmonella* group D after ritual circumcision. Pediatr. Infect. Dis. J. 9:65-66, 1990.

247. Vallenas, C., Hernandez, H., Kay, B., et al.: Efficacy of bone marrow, blood, stool, and duodenal contents cultures for bacteriologic confirmation of typhoid fever in children. Pediatr. Infect. Dis. 4:496-498, 1985.

248. Van Gijsegem, F., Genin, S., and Boucher, C.: Conservation of secretion pathways for pathogenicity determinants of plant and animal bacteria. Trends Microbiol. 1:175-180, 1993.

249. Vazquez-Torres, A., Vallance, B. A., Bergman, M. A., et al.: Toll-like receptor 4 dependence of innate and adaptive immunity to *Salmonella*: Importance of the Kupffer cell network. J. Immunol. 172:6202-6208, 2004.

250. Vazquez-Torres, A., Xu, Y., Jones-Carson, J., et al.: *Salmonella* pathogenicity island 2-dependent evasion of the phagocyte NADPH oxidase. Science 287:1655-1658, 2000.

251. Vinh, H., Duong, N. M., Phuong, Le. T., et al.: Comparative trial of short-course ofloxacin for uncomplicated typhoid fever in Vietnamese children. Ann. Trop. Paediatr. 25:17-22, 2005.

252. Voetsch, A. C., Angulo, F. J., Rabatsky-Her, T., et al.: Laboratory practices for stool-specimen culture for bacterial pathogens, including *Escherichia coli* O157:H7, in the FoodNet sites, 1995-2000. Clin. Infect. Dis. 38(Suppl. 3):S190-S197, 2004.

253. Wain, J., Hien, T. T., Connerton P., et al.: Molecular typing of multiple-antibiotic-resistant *Salmonella enterica* serovar *Typhi* from Vietnam: Application to acute and relapse cases of typhoid fever. J. Clin. Microbiol. 37:2466-2472, 1999.

254. Wain, J., Hoa, N. T., Ching, N. T., et al.: Quinolone-resistant *Salmonella typhi* in Viet Nam: Molecular basis of resistance and clinical response to treatment. Clin. Infect. Dis. 25:1404-1410, 1997.

255. Wallis, T. S., Hawker, R. J., Candy, D. C., et al.: Quantification of the leucocyte influx into rabbit ileal loops induced by strains of S. *typhimurium* of different virulence. J. Med. Microbiol. 30:149-156, 1989.

256. Wallis, T. S., Starkey, W. G., Stephen, J., et al.: The nature and role of mucosal damage in relation to *Salmonella typhimurium* induced fluid secretion in the rabbit ileum. J. Med. Microbiol. 22:39-49, 1986.

257. Watt, J., and Carlton, E.: Studies of the acute diarrheal diseases, XVI: an outbreak of *S. typhimurium* infection among newborn premature infants. Public Health Rep. *60*(Pt. I):734-810, 1945.
258. Watt, J., Wegman, M. E., Brown, O. W., et al.: Salmonellosis in a premature nursery unaccompanied by diarrheal diseases. Pediatrics *22*:689-705, 1958.
259. Wilson, R., Feldman, R. A., Davis, J., et al.: Salmonellosis in infants: The importance of intrafamilial transmission. Pediatrics *69*:436-438, 1982.
260. Winkler, A. P., and Gleich, S.: Acute acalculous cholecystitis caused by *Salmonella typhi* in an 11-year-old. Pediatr. Infect. Dis. J. *7*:125-128, 1988.
261. Wittler, R. R., and Bass, J. W.: Non-typhoidal *Salmonella* enteric infections and bacteremia. Pediatr. Infect. Dis. J. *8*:364-367, 1989.
262. Wright, J., Thomas, P., and Serjeant, G. R.: Septicemia caused by *Salmonella* infection: An overlooked complication of sickle cell disease. J. Pediatr. *130*:394-399, 1997.
263. Yamamoto, L. G., and Ashton, M. J.: *Salmonella* infections in infants in Hawaii. Pediatr. Infect. Dis. J. *7*:48-52, 1988.
264. Zaidi, E., Bachur, R., and Harper, M.: Non-typhi *Salmonella* bacteremia in children. Pediatr. Infect. Dis. J. *18*:1073-1077, 1999.
265. Zarkovsky, H. S., Gallagher, D., and Gill, F. M.: Bacteremia in sickle hemoglobinopathies. J. Pediatr. *109*:579-585, 1986.
266. Zeng, H., Wu, H., Sloane, V., et al.: Flagellin/TLR5 responses in epithelia reveal intertwined activation of inflammatory and apoptotic pathways. Am. J. Physiol. Gastrointest. Liver Physiol. *290*:G96-G108, 2006.

CHAPTER 122

PLAGUE *(YERSINIA PESTIS)*

Gary D. Overturf

HISTORY

Yersinia pestis has been responsible for the most devastating epidemics in human history. Possibly the first mention of plague dates back to approximately 1320 B.C.E., in I Samuel (Old Testament), Chapters 5 and 6. The next recorded outbreak may have been in 542 during Justinian's reign, when an estimated 100 million people died.[48] In 1346, plague appeared during the siege of the city of Kaffa in the Crimea, thereafter spreading throughout most of Europe, where it became known as the *black death*. One third of the population of Europe died in its aftermath. Between the 14th and 20th centuries, plague remained endemic in most of Europe and Russia, with resultant frequent outbreaks.[43]

In 1894, Yersin and Kitasato, working independently, first described the plague bacillus,[47] and the role played by rats and fleas in the spread of the disease became known. In 1900, plague was introduced into San Francisco by rats aboard ships docking there. The disease spread to ground squirrels and then to other wild animals of the American Southwest.[46] In 1943, effective antibiotics against *Y. pestis* became available. In the United States today, plague is rare, but it continues to be endemic in many parts of the world, leading to more recent outbreaks in Madagascar, Peru, and India. Although antibiotics have been effective in the treatment and prophylaxis of plague, plasmid-borne antibiotic resistance is being noted increasingly.[19] The potential of aerosolized *Y. pestis* as a biologic weapon is being scrutinized, leading to renewed interest in the understanding and study of this organism.[29]

BACTERIOLOGY

Y. pestis belongs in the family Enterobacteriaceae and is one of 10 *Yersinia* spp. It is a small, pleomorphic, nonmotile, gram-negative bacillus. With Wayson, Giemsa, and Gram stains, the bacillus takes on bipolar or safety-pin morphologic features.[17] *Y. pestis* grows at temperatures ranging from 0° C to 40° C (32° F to 104° F); the optimal temperature is 28° C (82.4° F). On first isolation at 35° C (95° F) on 5 percent blood agar, the colonies are pinpoint in size, growing to 1 to 2 mm after 2 days. They are nonhemolytic on 5 percent sheep blood agar.

Depending on the clinical nature of the disease, blood cultures, sputum samples, or aspirates of enlarged nodes should be examined for typical bacilli. The isolated bacilli can be identified by the following criteria. *Y. pestis*, the sole *Yersinia* spp. that is nonmotile at 37° C and 22° C (98.6° F and 71.6° F), also is the sole *Yersinia* spp. that is urease-negative, but it may be positive

in freshly isolated strains. The organism is positive for esculin, β-galactosidase, catalase, and methyl red. Oxidase, indole, and Voges-Proskauer reactions are negative. It ferments glucose, maltose, salicin, xylose, arabinose, dextrin, trehalose, and mannitol. It does not produce acid from lactose, sucrose, rhamnose, melibiose, adonitol, cellobiose, sorbose, or dulcitol. It does not use citrate, and it does not grow in potassium cyanide. *Y. pestis* is negative for lysine, ornithine decarboxylase, and arginine dihydrolase.[44,53]

Positive cultures show pinpoint colonies within 24 to 48 hours after inoculation. Many laboratories use fully automated or semiautomated identification systems (e.g., Vitek) that may not detect *Y. pestis*, often confusing *Y. pestis* and *Yersinia pseudotuberculosis* or *Yersinia enterocolitica* with plague bacillus. Nonautomated laboratories may require 6 days to identify the organism. Because of lack of standarized susceptibility testing procedures, suspected isolates must be referred to public health or other reference laboratories to comply with the select agent requirements of the Title II Enhanced Controls for Dangerous Biological Agents and Toxins Act.[29]

Several chromosomal-mediated virulence factors are responsible for the virulence of *Y. pestis*, including (1) an antiphagocytic capsular material known as fraction 1, (2) the endogenous purine synthesis that allows the organism to grow within macrophages, and (3) the ability to absorb iron from the medium. Several plasmids have been implicated in the development of other virulence factors. A plasmid of 9-kb pairs contains the determinant of secretory protein that kills other bacterial strains. A plasmid of 72-kb pairs, which all pathogenic *Y. pestis* strains contain, confers the requirement for environmental calcium to be present for the organism to grow at 37° C (98.6° F). When grown under this condition, *Y. pestis* produces V and W antigens that are necessary for virulence.[21] An exotoxin and an endotoxin have been found to contribute to the lethal effects of plague.[53]

TRANSMISSION

HOST

More than 200 mammalian species have been reported to be naturally infected with *Y. pestis*. Epidemics of plague usually are transmitted by the fleas of infected domestic rats, however. This form of spread is more likely to occur in urban, rat-infested, and crowded dwellings and may result in epidemics. In the United States, plague is transmitted sporadically to humans after contact with an enzootic sylvatic focus.[31] Infected wild rodents perpetuate the plague bacillus in a given ecosystem by virtue of their ability to withstand an inoculum of *Y. pestis* many times greater than that necessary to cause disease in humans or domestic animals. After inoculation, wild rodents may become bacteremic and infect fleas that feed on them; these fleas transmit the plague bacillus to another rodent. Hibernating animals are especially resistant to clinical infection. Animals inoculated before going into hibernation may survive through the winter and not die until after they come out of their burrows, reintroducing the bacillus in the new season.[26] Carnivores are relatively resistant to infection but contribute to the spread of the organism by transporting infected fleas from one area to another.[31]

The role of domestic animals in bridging the gap between sylvatic plague and human infection has been studied extensively.[41,47,51] Cats and dogs are susceptible to natural and experimental plague. Epizootics in cats have been observed in conjunction with plague epidemics in humans.[47] Experimentally infected cats develop severe systemic illness, with bacteremia and abscess formation at the site of the inoculum. Between 1977 and 1998, 23 cases of feline-associated human plague infection were reported.[22] Five of these cases were fatal; two of the patients presented with primary pneumonic plague, and one presented with septicemic plague. Many of these cases were misdiagnosed at presentation, leading to delays in treatment and, in some cases, fatalities. This diagnosis should be considered especially in the western states of Arizona, California, Colorado, and New Mexico. No seasonal variation in the occurrence of cat-associated illness was noted.[22]

Ten other cases reported in the literature of feline transmission of plague to humans involved four veterinarians.[18] Dogs also are susceptible, but the disease is milder.[51] Swine are resistant to plague, the only evidence of subclinical infection being the presence of antibodies to the fraction 1 antigen of *Y. pestis*. Domestic animals, by virtue of their intimate contact with wildlife and humans, may be responsible for some cases of human plague. This danger is accentuated by a dearth of symptoms in some animals.[41]

VECTOR

Plague is transmitted to humans by the bite of an infected flea, the skinning and evisceration of infected animals,[32] or the inhalation of infected droplets from a case of pneumonic plague.[35] Infrequent portals of entry include the conjunctiva[41] and the pharynx.[40,49]

The efficiency of the flea as a vector for human disease depends on the likelihood that the infected flea will feed on a person and that the flea will regurgitate the bacillus into the victim's bloodstream in the process of feeding.[31] Flea species vary in both of these attributes. Wild rodent fleas are reluctant to feed on humans and do it only under duress (e.g., when the natural host dies). Fleas of domestic animals are more likely to bite humans. The Oriental rat flea, *Xenopsylla cheopis*, is the most efficient transmitter of plague because of its willingness to bite people and its propensity for regurgitating large numbers of bacilli in the process.[31] When the Oriental rat flea ingests infected blood, the actions of a coagulase produced by *Y. pestis* and a trypsin-like enzyme present in the flea's stomach result in the formation of an infected clot that blocks the flea's proventriculus. In obstructing the flea's intestinal tract, the clot allows further replication of bacteria. When the flea tries to feed again, it regurgitates large numbers of plague bacilli. The formation and dissolution of the fibrin clot are temperature-dependent. At temperatures greater than 27° C (>80.6° F), a fibrinolytic enzyme is activated that dissolves the clot and allows the flea to dispose of the bacillus. One postulation is that this temperature-dependent phenomenon is responsible for the observed cyclic nature of urban plague epidemics, which tend to subside with the advent of hot weather.[7]

In contrast, fleas in which the intestinal tracts do not become blocked contribute to the endemicity of plague by harboring the organism and transmitting it in sublethal doses.[9] Sylvatic plague depends on the rodent flea as the vector. This flea, although not as efficient as the rat flea in transmitting the bacillus, may itself become a reservoir of *Y. pestis* by surviving for 12 to 15 months after the original host dies. In the new season, it reintroduces the plague bacillus into the new rodent population.[47] The observation that *Y. pestis* can survive in the soil during interepizootics suggests another possible mechanism of transmission of plague.[25]

EPIDEMIOLOGY

More recent studies have suggested that plague is an ancient disease of mammals; the plague bacterium emerged 1500 to 20,000 years ago as a clone that evolved from *Yersinia pseudotuberculosis* that first caused outbreaks in Africa.[1] The plague bacillus exists in enzootic cycles involving wild animals or domestic rats. In urban plague, the course of events usually is initiated by the introduction of the plague bacillus from an enzootic focus into a susceptible rat population. With humans and rats living in proximity, an epizootic in rats may be followed by an epidemic in humans.[47] The epidemic may subside with the advent of hot, humid weather[7] or the obliteration of the rat population.[47] Such epidemics rarely occur today but have been described in the former South Vietnam[4,33] and more recently in India.[13] Between 1985 and 1999, 23 countries reported a total of 29,020 cases of plague to the World Health Organization, with an average mortality rate of 11 percent; major epidemics and outbreaks occurred in Tanzania (1991), Zaire (1992, 1993), Peru (1993, 1994), India (1994), and Madagascar (1995), with fatality rates ranging from 4.6 to 22.3 percent.[55]

In the United States today, humans become infected most frequently by direct contact with a sylvatic reservoir of infection. Sporadic human cases usually result from working or hunting in a plague-infested area[31] and increasingly from living near foci of infection as suburban spread encroaches on the natural habitats of rodents.[14] In recent years, domestic animals, especially cats, have been responsible for a significant proportion of human cases. During 1990 to 2005, 107 cases of plague were reported in the United States, a median of 7 cases a year. By September 2006, 13 plague cases, with 2 deaths (case-fatality 15%), had been reported from four states (New Mexico, Colorado, California, and Texas). Such resurgences often occur after ecologic changes resulting in population increases in ground rodents such as prairie dogs, ground squirrels, mice, and rats in the American Southwest.[15]

Sylvatic plague epizootics occur in the summer. Most cases of rural plague occur between April and September. The rare occurrence of human plague in the winter usually is associated with hunting and direct exposure to infected tissues.[12,32]

The continental United States has a large enzootic focus that includes 130 counties in 15 western states. Surveillance for plague in rodents during the 1990s has identified infected animals farther east than ever before reported. The plague bacillus now has been isolated in wild rodents in eastern Montana, western Nebraska, western North Dakota, and eastern Texas.[14] Between 1925 and 1965, the number of reported cases in the United States averaged between two and three per year.[8,10] During the 1970s, 105 cases were reported.[32] The number of cases reported in 1980 through 1982 showed a similar increasing trend.[10] Between 1970 and 1979, 53 percent of cases were in females, in contrast to the period 1926 to 1969, when only 27 percent were in females. Approximately 60 percent of cases occur in individuals younger than 20 years.[32] Of 10 confirmed cases reported in the United States in 1993, however, the age distribution was 22 to 96 years. Five of the patients were older than 65 years.[14] Native Americans living on reservations in Arizona, New Mexico, and Utah are at increased risk. In the period 1970 to 1979, 35 percent of cases in these three states occurred in Native Americans.[10,32] Many of the patients were infected within 1 mile of their residence and almost all within their state of residence.[27] Seven of the 10 patients described in 1993 were exposed in their home sites, and one, a veterinarian, was exposed at work.[14]

Occasionally, plague has been acquired by a traveler in an endemic area who then traveled during the incubation period to a plague-free region of the country. This set of circumstances shows why all physicians need to be aware of the presenting symptoms and signs of plague and to obtain an accurate travel history.[34]

PATHOGENESIS AND PATHOLOGY

The portal of entry of the plague bacillus determines, to some extent, the form of disease. The most common portal of entry is the skin when it is bitten by an infected flea. Broken skin may provide access for direct inoculation while infected animals are being handled. After overcoming the skin barrier, the organisms move through the lymphatics to the regional lymph nodes, where they elicit an inflammatory response. The infection may be localized at this site, with subsequent formation of antibody and recovery. This clinical form is known as *pestis minor*. The bacillus commonly is disseminated through the bloodstream. Distant organ involvement may include the liver, spleen, kidneys, lungs, and meninges. Disseminated intravascular coagulation is common in fatal cases. Coagulation defects, including thrombocytopenia and elevated fibrin split products[4] and fibrin deposits in the glomeruli,[21,47] may be present. Bacteremia is not synonymous with severe disease and occurs commonly in mild cases.[47]

The major determinant of severity seems to be the presence of high levels of endotoxin. The toxin of *Y. pestis* has the biologic properties of typical endotoxin. When injected into experimental animals, it can cause the clinical symptoms and signs and pathologic changes characteristic of endotoxic shock and death. The quantity of endotoxin necessary to kill is estimated to be comparable to that present in a lethal dose of live bacteria.[2,54] The murine toxin of *Y. pestis* has a direct inhibitory effect in vitro on the respiration of heart mitochondria of rats and mice, whereas it has little or no effect on the mitochondria of rabbits, chimpanzees, dogs, and monkeys. The differing sensitivities in vitro correlate with the susceptibilities in vivo of these species to *Y. pestis* infection.[50]

Achieving high levels of toxin depends on the ability of the bacillus to replicate in the infected host. Resistance to phagocytosis had been assumed to be related to virulence. More recent experimental evidence has shown that virulent *Y. pestis* organisms are phagocytosed, but, in contrast to avirulent ones, are not killed. They continue to replicate freely in macrophages, allowing the accumulation of endotoxin.[30,50]

When the lung is the portal of entry, the disease usually is more fulminant. After being inhaled, bacilli replicate freely in the alveolar spaces. Severe pneumonia, endotoxemia, and septicemia ensue and, if untreated, cause death. In fatal cases, the thoracic lymph nodes show infarction, necrosis, and liquefaction, with pus formation. Edema and inflammation of the surrounding tissue are common.[47] The mucosa of trachea and bronchi is covered by bloody, frothy exudate. Submucosal hemorrhages and areas of necrosis may surround the trachea. The pleural surfaces contain hemorrhagic lesions and fibrinous adhesions. The lung parenchyma may be consolidated or show signs of acute edema.[47] The predominant histologic feature is an alveolar exudate consisting of histiocytes and polymorphonuclear leukocytes.[21]

Other organs also are involved. The kidneys may appear grossly hemorrhagic and contain areas of necrosis. Microscopic

examination reveals leukocytic infiltrates of congested veins and capillaries. Glomeruli with fibrin thrombi frequently are found in patients with disseminated intravascular coagulation.[21] Biopsy of purpuric skin lesions reveals subepithelial hemorrhages and fibrin deposit in the capillaries. These changes are indistinguishable from the changes seen in a generalized Shwartzman reaction.[4]

CLINICAL MANIFESTATIONS

The incubation period of *Y. pestis* generally is 3 to 4 days, but ranges from a few hours to 10 days. The onset of illness usually is abrupt, beginning with fever, malaise, weakness, and headache.[47,48] Fever is high, frequently accompanied by shaking chills.[41] The appearance of a visible and palpable bubo may be preceded by pain and tenderness at that site.[48]

On physical examination, the patient is "toxic," apprehensive, and tachycardic. The inoculation site in the skin may not be evident, or it may be marked by a carbuncle. In bubonic plague, typical large, fixed, edematous, and exquisitely tender nodes are present at one anatomic site.[33] In decreasing order of frequency, the areas of nodal involvement are the groin (including femoral and inguinal nodes), axilla, and neck.[47] Any lymph node may suppurate, sometimes presenting an atypical picture (e.g., if intra-abdominal nodes are involved, an acute abdominal emergency may be suspected).[48] Septicemia as an initial presentation of *Y. pestis* infection is common.[27] Twenty-five percent of the patients presented without adenopathy in the 71 confirmed cases of plague in New Mexico from 1980 to 1984. All patients with septicemic presentation had fever and chills, and most had tachycardia, tachypnea, and relative hypotension. Seventy-two percent had gastrointestinal symptoms. Plague pneumonia was twice as likely to occur among septicemic as among patients with bubonic plague. Septicemic patients were significantly older and more likely to die than were patients with a bubonic presentation. Although septicemic plague occurred more often in older patients, patients younger than 30 years with septicemic presentation were more likely to die.[27]

As a result of its nonspecific presentation, septicemic plague is difficult to diagnose early. Of 27 patients with plague admitted to Indian Medical Center in Gallup, New Mexico, between 1965 and 1989, 5 presented with a nonspecific febrile syndrome with upper respiratory symptoms. They were prescribed penicillin. Three of the five patients died. Another five patients presented with a nonspecific febrile syndrome associated with chills, myalgias, and anorexia. These patients were not treated initially with antibiotics, and three of the five died.[18] The index of suspicion must be high because early diagnosis is imperative for avoiding a high risk of mortality. Individuals presenting with what seems to be community-acquired, gram-negative sepsis and who reside in or have a history of recent travel to endemic areas of plague must be evaluated for and treated with antibiotics effective against *Y. pestis*.[39]

Gastrointestinal symptoms occur in patients with plague, especially patients with septicemic plague.[26] Between 1980 and 1984, more than half of the 71 patients with plague in New Mexico presented with gastrointestinal symptoms that sometimes preceded the appearance of the buboes in the bubonic cases. Common symptoms are abdominal pain, nausea, vomiting, and diarrhea. These symptoms are thought to be a general response of the body to gram-negative septicemia. Occasionally, hepatosplenomegaly and mesenteric or retroperitoneal lymphadenopathy have masqueraded as an acute abdomen.[28,34]

Neurologic manifestations caused by the effects of toxin on the brain are common. A patient with plague may have insomnia, delirium, stupor, weakness, staggering gait, vertigo, disorders of speech, and loss of memory.[38] *Y. pestis* meningitis is a rare occurrence, but it does occur. Children younger than 15 years old seem to be more susceptible, and septicemic patients are four times more likely to develop meningitis than are patients with bubonic plague. It often manifests while the patient is well into a course of antibiotic therapy for bubonic or septicemic plague.[3] When intravascular coagulation supervenes, renal involvement may be manifested by acute cortical or tubular necrosis. Hepatic involvement may be evidenced by mildly elevated liver enzymes.[47] Hantavirus pulmonary syndrome may mimic septicemic or pneumonic plague; they share similar geographic distribution, and patients for whom this diagnosis is contemplated should be treated with antibiotics to cover the possibility of plague.[45]

Primary pneumonic plague has identical constitutional symptoms but follows a fulminant course with a more pronounced pulmonary component. Within 20 to 24 hours after the onset of the illness, tachypnea, dyspnea, and cough productive of bloody mucopurulent sputum supervene. If early and effective treatment is not instituted, the patient usually dies.[47]

DIFFERENTIAL DIAGNOSIS

Because of the rare incidence of plague today, the diagnosis often is delayed or missed. Bubonic plague may be confused with other diseases affecting the skin and lymph nodes. The diagnosis of staphylococcal or streptococcal adenitis can be established easily by culture. Lymphogranuloma venereum is more indolent, has milder systemic symptoms, and is associated with anogenital ulcer. Syphilitic adenitis usually is nontender. With cat-scratch disease and *Pasteurella multocida* infections, the constitutional symptoms are few, and the patient typically has a history of animal exposure. Tularemia has a more gradual onset.[47] In their later stages, the ulcerated skin lesions of plague may resemble anthrax.[33]

DIAGNOSIS

The most important factor in promptly establishing the diagnosis of plague is having a high index of suspicion. Suspicion should trigger immediate notification to the local or state health department. The state reference laboratory can arrange for rapid diagnostic tests.

Bacterial staining of lymph node material by Giemsa, Wayson, or Wright stain often shows the typical bipolar plague organisms. In the septicemic form of the disease, similar bacterial staining of venous blood frequently permits visualization of the plague bacillus.[36] Fluorescent antibody staining of direct smears and tissues may provide a rapid, presumptive diagnosis of plague.[29] More recent rapid tests, such as enzyme-linked immunosorbent assay for F1 antigen and polymerase chain reaction, have shown promise in the laboratory or in outbreaks, but they are not widely available,[12] (*pla* and *caf1* genes).

TREATMENT

Therapeutic decisions cannot await culture results. All patients suspected to have plague should receive prompt antimicrobial therapy after appropriate blood and tissue have been obtained for cultures, fluorescent antibody staining, and serologic testing.

The sulfonamides and streptomycin proved effective when they were introduced first in the 1940s. Resistant strains to one or the other of these antibiotics soon appeared.[6,49] Despite the paucity of published trials in humans on antibiotic effectiveness, other than streptomycin and tetracycline, the Working Group on Civilian Biodefense Consensus Statement[29] recommends gentamicin as an effective alternative to streptomycin for patients needing parenteral antibiotics. Gentamicin has been used fre-

quently in recent years and has shown comparable outcomes to streptomycin in one case series.[3] In vitro and in vivo studies in mice corroborate its effectiveness against *Y. pestis* infections.[53]

For acutely ill patients thought to have plague infection, streptomycin and gentamicin are the drugs of choice. If available, streptomycin is given intramuscularly, 20 to 30 mg/kg/day in two divided doses.[38] Gentamicin is administered intravenously or intramuscularly, 7.5 mg/kg/day to children and 3 to 5 mg/kg/day to adults in three divided doses. Antibiotic susceptibility testing should be done because *Y. pestis* plasmid-mediated, multiple-antibiotic resistance has been described.[23]

When plague meningitis develops, chloramphenicol, 50 to 100 mg/kg/day (after administration of an initial dose of 25 mg/kg) intravenously in four divided doses, is the treatment of choice. Duration of therapy is determined by the length and severity of the illness. Treatment is continued for at least 7 days in patients with uncomplicated disease.[13]

Patients older than 8 years who do not require hospitalization receive tetracycline at a dose of 25 to 50 mg/kg/day every 4 to 6 hours up to a total daily dose of 1 g in children and 2 g in adults. When outpatient treatment is given, the patient should be observed closely for the first 3 days to ensure resolution of the disease.[13] Sulfonamides may be used for prophylaxis in pediatric patients as an alternative to the tetracycline class of antibiotics.[29] Doxycycline at a dose of 4 mg/kg/day (up to a maximum of 200 mg) divided into two doses may be substituted for tetracycline).

PROGNOSIS

In outbreaks of untreated plague, the mortality rate has ranged from 40 to 70 percent. Pneumonic plague almost invariably is fatal without treatment. With prompt specific antimicrobial therapy, the overall mortality rate for plague has decreased to 5 percent.[35] Complications during convalescence include polyarthritis, small lung abscesses, delayed suppuration of buboes,[33] and meningitis. *Staphylococcus aureus* and *Pseudomonas* spp. may superinfect involved lymph nodes.[48] Immunity usually ensues after clinical or asymptomatic infection occurs, but natural re-infection rarely has been observed.[48]

PREVENTION AND CONTROL

Institution of hygienic measures and eradication of rats from areas of human habitations have all but eliminated epidemics of urban plague. When epizootics occur in wild rodents, control measures must be directed against rodents and fleas. Vector control can be achieved by the use of insecticides in fields and housing areas. In plague-endemic areas, the public must be instructed to avoid burrows, not to handle sick or dead rodents, to deflea household pets, and to eliminate trash near living areas.[10] The immune status of domestic animals can be used as a surveillance tool to ascertain the presence of *Y. pestis* in the community. Dogs, cats, and swine develop antibodies to the fraction 1 antigen of *Y. pestis*.[41,51]

Patients with plague should be isolated with respiratory precautions until they are bacteriologically sterile. Contacts of patients with pneumonic plague should receive chemoprophylaxis with tetracycline at 25 to 50 mg/kg/day up to 2 g in adults and up to 1 g in children 8 years and older. Younger children receive trimethoprim-sulfamethoxazole at 40 mg/kg/day (sulfamethoxazole) in two equal doses orally.[29] The 6-day quarantine period for international travel for contacts of patients with plague does not guarantee the clearance of the bacillus from asymptomatic pharyngeal carriers.[6] Public and professional education in endemic zones is paramount for ensuring prompt reporting of human and animal cases.

Plague vaccines had been used since the late 19th century for individuals at high risk for occupational exposure. They are no longer being manufactured in the United States. Research in this area is continuing.[29]

REFERENCES

1. Achtmann, M., Zurth, K., Morelli, G., et al.: *Yersinia pestis*, the cause of plague, is a recent emerged clone of *Yersinia pseudotuberculosis*. Proc. Natl. Acad. Sci. U. S. A. *96*:14043-14048, 1999.
2. Albizo, J. M., and Surgalla, M. J.: Isolation and characterization of *Pasteurella pestis* endotoxin. Infect. Immun. *2*:229-236, 1970.
3. Becker, T. M., Poland, J. D., Quan, T. J., et al.: Plague meningitis: A retrospective analysis of cases reported in the United States, 1970-1979. West. J. Med. *147*:554-557, 1987.
4. Bonacorsi, S. P., Scavizzi, A., Guiyoule, J. H., et al.: Assessment of a fluoroquinolone, three beta-lactams, two aminoglycosides, and cycline in the treatment of murine *Yersinia pestis* infection. Antimicrob. Agents Chemother. *38*:481-486, 1994.
5. Butler, T.: A clinical study of bubonic plague. Am. J. Med. *53*:268-276, 1972.
6. Cantey, J. R.: Plague in Vietnam. Arch. Intern. Med. *133*:280-283, 1974.
7. Cavanaugh, D. C.: Specific effect of temperature upon transmission of the plague bacillus by the Oriental rat flea, *Xenopsylla cheopis*. Am. J. Trop. Med. Hyg. *20*:264-273, 1971.
8. Centers for Disease Control and Prevention: Plague: United States, 1976. M. M. W. R. Morb. Mortal. Wkly. Rep. *28*:159, 1977.
9. Centers for Disease Control and Prevention: Plague vaccine. M. M. W. R. Morb. Mortal. Wkly. Rep. *31*:301-303, 1982.
10. Centers for Disease Control and Prevention: Plague in the United States, 1982. M. M. W. R. Morb. Mortal. Wkly. Rep. *32*:19SS-24SS, 1983.
11. Centers for Disease Control and Prevention: Plague: Human plague in the United States, 1983. M. M. W. R. Morb. Mortal. Wkly. Rep. *32*:329-330, 1983.
12. Centers for Disease Control and Prevention: Plague: Winter plague Colorado, Washington, Texas, 1983-1984. M. M. W. R. Morb. Mortal. Wkly. Rep. *33*:145-148, 1984.
13. Centers for Disease Control and Prevention: Plague Treatment Guidelines. Fort Collins, CO, Bacteriologic Zoonoses Branch, Division of Vector-Borne Infectious Diseases.
14. Centers for Disease Control and Prevention: Human plague: United States, 1993-1994. M. M. W. R. Morb. Mortal. Wkly. Rep. *43*:242-246, 1994.
15. Centers for Disease Control and Prevention: Human plague—four states 2006. M. M. W. R. Morb. Mortal. Wkly. Rep. *55*:940-943, 2006.
16. Chanteau, S., Rahalison, L., Ratsitorahina, M., et al.: Early diagnosis of bubonic plague using F1 antigen capture ELISA assay and rapid immunogold dipstick. Int. J. Med. Microbiol. *290*:279-283, 2000.
17. Chen, T. H., and Elberg, S. S.: *Yersinia, Pasteurella*, and *Francisella. In* Braude, A. I., Davis, C. E., and Fierer, J. (eds.): Medical Microbiology and Infectious Diseases. Philadelphia, W. B. Saunders, 1981, pp. 393-399.
18. Crook, D., and Tempest, B.: Plague: A review of 27 cases. Arch. Intern. Med. *152*:1253-1256, 1992.
19. Dennis, D. T., and Hughes, J. M.: Multidrug resistance in plague. N. Engl. J. Med. *337*:702-704, 1997.
20. Eidson, M., Tierney, L., Rollag, O. J., et al.: Feline plague in New Mexico: Risk factors and transmission to humans. Am. J. Public Health *78*:1333-1335, 1988.
21. Finegold, M. J.: Pathogenesis of plague. Am. J. Med. *45*:549-555, 1968.
22. Gage, K. L., Dennis, D. T., Orloski, K. A., et al.: Cases of cat-associated human plague in the western US, 1977-1998. Clin. Infect. Dis. *30*:893-900, 2000.
23. Galimand, M., Guiyoule, A., Berbaud, G., et al.: Multidrug resistance in *Yersinia pestis* mediated by transferable plasmid. N. Engl. J. Med. *337*:677-680, 1997.
24. Ganem, D. E.: Plasmids and pestilence: Biological and clinical aspects of bubonic plague. West. J. Med. *144*:447-451, 1986.
25. Goldenberg, M. I., and Kartman, L.: Role of soil in the ecology of *Pasteurella pestis*. Bacteriol. Proc. *66*:54-57, 1966.
26. Hull, H. F., Montes, J. M., and Mann, J. M.: Plague masquerading as gastrointestinal illness. West. J. Med. *145*:485-487, 1986.
27. Hull, H. F., Montes, J. M., and Mann, J. M.: Septicemic plague in New Mexico. J. Infect. Dis. *155*:113-118, 1987.
28. Humphrey, M., McGiuney, R., Perkins, C., et al.: *Yersinia pestis*: A case of mistaken identity. Pediatr. Infect. Dis. J. *7*:365-366, 1988.
29. Inglesby, T. V., Dennis, D. T., Henderson, D. A., et al.: Plague as a biological weapon. J. A. M. A. *283*:2281-2290, 2000.
30. Janssen, W. A., and Surgalla, M. J.: Plague bacillus: Survival within host phagocytes. Science *163*:950-952, 1969.
31. Kartman, L., Goldenberg, M. I., and Hubbert, W. T.: Recent observations on the epidemiology of plague in the United States. Am. J. Public Health *56*:1554-1569, 1966.
32. Kaufmann, A. F., Boyce, J. M., and Martone, W. J.: Trends in human plague in the United States. J. Infect. Dis. *141*:522-524, 1980.
33. Legters, L. J., Cottingham, A. J., and Hunter, D. H.: Clinical and epidemiologic notes on a defined outbreak of plague in Vietnam. Am. J. Trop. Med. Hyg. *19*:639-652, 1970.
34. Leopold, J. C.: Septicemic plague in a 14-month old. Pediatr. Infect. Dis. J. *5*:108-110, 1986.
35. Maegraith, B. G.: Plague. *In* Adams, A. R., and Maegraith, B. G. (eds.): Clinical Tropical Diseases. Oxford, Blackwell Scientific, 1970, pp. 325-336.
36. Mann, J. M., Hull, H. F., Schmid, G. P., et al.: Plague and the peripheral smear. J. A. M. A. *251*:953, 1984.
37. Mann, J. M., Martone, W. J., Boyce, J. M., et al.: Endemic human plague in New Mexico: Risk factors associated with infection. J. Infect. Dis. *140*:397-401, 1979.
38. Mann, J. M., Schaudler, L., and Cushing, A.: Pediatric plague. Pediatrics *69*:762-767, 1982.
39. Mann, J. M., Schmid, G. P., Stoesz, P. A., et al.: Peripatetic plague. J. A. M. A. *247*:47-48, 1982.
40. Marshall, J. D., Guy, D. V., and Gibson, F. L.: Asymptomatic pharyngeal plague infection in Vietnam. Am. J. Trop. Med. Hyg. *16*:175-177, 1967.
41. Marshall, J. D., Harrison, D. N., Murr, J. A., et al.: The role of domestic animals in the epidemiology of plague, III: Experimental infection in swine. J. Infect. Dis. *125*:556-559, 1972.
42. Martin, A. R., Hurtado, F. P., Plessak, R. A., et al.: Plague meningitis. Pediatrics *40*:610-616, 1967.
43. McNeill, W. H. (ed.): Plagues and People. Garden City, NY, Anchor Press of Doubleday, 1976.
44. Mollaret, H. H., and Thal, E.: Yersinia. *In* Buchanan, R. E., and Gibbons, N. E. (eds.): Bergey's Manual of Determinative Bacteriology. 8th ed. Baltimore, Williams & Wilkins, 1974, pp. 330-332.
45. Peters, C. J., Simpson, G. L., and Levy, H.: Spectrum of hantavirus infection. Annu. Rev. Med. *50*:531-545, 1999.
46. Plague: Historical notes. Can. Med. Assoc. J. *119*:10, 1978.
47. Pollitzer, R.: Plague. W.H.O. Monogr. No. 22. Geneva, World Health Organization, 1954.
48. Reed, W. P., Palmer, D. L., Williams, R. C., et al.: Bubonic plague in the southwestern United States. Medicine (Baltimore) *49*:465-486, 1970.
49. Reiley, C. G., and Kates, E. D.: The clinical spectrum of plague in Vietnam. Arch. Intern. Med. *126*:990-994, 1970.
50. Rust, J. H., Jr., Cavanaugh, D. C., Kadis, S., et al.: Plague toxin: Its effect in vitro and in vivo. Science *142*:408-409, 1963.
51. Rust, J. H., Cavanaugh, D. C., O'Shita, R., et al.: The role of domestic animals in the epidemiology of plague, I: Experimental infection of dogs and cats. J. Infect. Dis. *124*:522-526, 1971.
52. Smith, M. D., Vinh, D. X., Nguyen, T. T., et al.: In vitro antimicrobial susceptibilities of strains of *Yersinia pestis*. Antimicrob. Agents Chemother. *39*:2153-2154, 1995.
53. Sonnenwirth, A. C.: Yersinia. *In* Lennette, E. H., Spaulding, E. H., and Trauant, J. P. (eds.): Manual of Clinical Microbiology. 2nd ed. Washington, D. C., American Society for Microbiology, 1974, pp. 222-229.
54. Walker, R. V., Bomes, M. G., and Thiggins, E. D.: Composition of and physiopathology produced by plague endotoxins. Nature *209*:1246, 1966.
55. World Heath Organization. Human plague in 1998 and 1999. Wkly Epidemiol Rec *75*:338-344, 2000.

CHAPTER

123 OTHER *YERSINIA* SPECIES

Charles R. Woods, Jr.

Yersinia spp. are gram-negative, coccobacillary organisms that are primarily zoonotic. The genus is a member of the family Enterobacteriaceae and consists of 11 species, 3 of which clearly are human pathogens:[69] *Yersinia pestis, Yersinia pseudotuberculosis* (both formerly included in the genus *Pasteurella*), and *Yersinia enteroco-* *litica. Y. pestis*, the causative agent of plague, is found in rodents and insect vectors and is discussed in Chapter 122.

Y. enterocolitica and *Y. pseudotuberculosis* are responsible for a variety of syndromes, some of which originally were called *pseudotuberculosis*. Infections caused by these enteropathogenic *Yer-*

sinia spp. now are collectively called *yersiniosis*, which is the focus of this chapter. Molecular phylogenetic analysis suggests that *Y. pestis* evolved from *Y. pseudotuberculosis* 1500 to 20,000 years ago.[4] The genomes of representative strains of the three pathogenic *Yersinia* spp. have been sequenced.[194]

During the past 3 decades, *Y. enterocolitica* has been recognized as an important human pathogen worldwide and is a common cause of gastroenteritis in some pediatric populations of the industrialized world.[1,47,56,118] *Y. enterocolitica* also has drawn attention because of its immunologic or postinfectious manifestations, which include reactive arthritis and erythema nodosum.[47] *Y. pseudotuberculosis*, although widespread in nature, is a much less common cause of human disease.[69] In Japan, it has been associated with clinical illness that sometimes has resembled Kawasaki disease.

HISTORICAL ASPECTS

In 1883, Malassez and Vignal[130] described a bacterium that produced a disease they named *pseudotuberculosis*. When injected into guinea pigs, the organism produced tuberculosis-like lesions. It grew at 4° C and multiplied better at 22° C than at 37° C. This observation was confirmed in 1910 by Albrecht,[11] who labeled the disease *enteritis follicularis suppurativa*. The first case of mesenteric adenitis, the most common syndrome produced by *Y. pseudotuberculosis*, was reported in 1913 by Saisawa.[173] A second instance of disease that indicated its capacity to produce death (bacteremia and multiple hepatic abscesses) was recorded in 1949 by Hassig and colleagues.[79] Masshoff[132] was the first to recover the organism from a culture of mesenteric lymph nodes of a patient with the clinical picture of acute appendicitis. Masshoff and Dolle[133] subsequently described the histologic picture produced by *Y. pseudotuberculosis*. In 1954, Knapp and Masshoff[106] first reported the clinical features of infection produced by this organism. Only 14 cases of this infection had been described up to that time.[55]

The existence of a species of *Yersinia* other than that causing pseudotuberculosis was suggested in 1933 by Gilbert,[62] who reported an unusual infection in animals. Schleifstein and Coleman[174,175] examined numerous organisms that were isolated between 1933 and 1957 from stool cultures of human cases of diarrhea from which *Salmonella* and *Shigella* organisms could not be recovered and that resembled the infections in animals reported by Gilbert. These investigators identified an organism that had not been described previously and named it *Bacterium enterocoliticum*. In 1964, it was named *Y. enterocolitica* by Frederiksen.[59]

The genus is named for A. J. Yersin, the French bacteriologist who first isolated the plague bacillus.[186] During the past 40 years, an extensive literature detailing the microbiology, pathology, epidemiology, molecular pathogenesis, and clinical features of disease caused by *Y. pseudotuberculosis* and *Y. enterocolitica* has accumulated.*

MICROBIOLOGY

Yersinia organisms are large (0.5 to 1 µm × 1 to 2 µm or larger), gram-negative, and ovoid or rod-shaped. *Y. enterocolitica* and *Y. pseudotuberculosis* are motile at 22° C to 25° C but not at 37° C. Similar to other members of Enterobacteriaceae, *Yersinia* organisms are facultative anaerobes and grow well on ordinary media. On Gram staining, *Y. pseudotuberculosis* appears as a large coccobacillus. Staining with methylene blue and carbol fuchsin discloses a bipolar (safety pin) morphology of most, but not all, strains. *Y. enterocolitica* is smaller and shows little, if any, bipolarity.[183,186]

Yersinia organisms may be confused with coliforms, such as *Escherichia coli, Morganella, Proteus, Shigella, Salmonella,* and *Providencia,* or with *Y. pestis, Brucella,* and *Achromobacter,* unless careful biochemical and physiologic studies are conducted. *Yersinia* organisms reduce nitrates and are oxidase-negative, catalase-positive, urease-positive, and citrate-negative. They ferment glucose, maltose, mannitol, glycerol, xylose, and fructose, producing acid but no gas with each sugar. *Yersinia* organisms usually do not ferment lactose but produce α-galactosidase. They do not ferment dulcitol, inositol, raffinose, or rhamnose. On lysine-iron agar slants, *Yersinia* organisms produce an alkaline slant with an acid butt. They do not produce hydrogen sulfide. The Voges-Proskauer reaction is negative at 37° C but may be positive at 25° C for some strains of *Y. enterocolitica*. All strains of *Y. pseudotuberculosis* and most strains of *Y. enterocolitica* isolated in Europe are indole-negative. Most strains of *Y. enterocolitica* found in the United States have been indole-positive.[50,66,88,146,151,183,186]

Although these two species of *Yersinia* share many properties, they are distinguishable on the basis of several biochemical activities, antigenic structure, and sensitivity to various *Yersinia* phages.[171] *Y. enterocolitica* produces an acid slant and acid butt on triple sugar iron agar caused by fermentation of sucrose, whereas *Y. pseudotuberculosis* produces an alkaline slant and an acid butt. *Y. enterocolitica* elaborates ornithine decarboxylase and ferments sucrose and amygdalin. *Y. pseudotuberculosis* does none of these, but it ferments adonitol, which *Y. enterocolitica* does not.[88,186]

Commercially available tests used to identify Enterobacteriaceae in clinical laboratories may not contain the biochemical reactions needed to identify specific *Yersinia* spp. Traditional macroscale biochemical testing may be required to distinguish *Y. enterocolitica* and *Y. pseudotuberculosis* from nonpathogenic *Yersinia* spp.[73,122] On solid culture media, colonies of the pathogenic species typically are small, smooth, opaque colonies. The colonies of nonpathogenic species are larger and more translucent.[100]

TYPING OF *YERSINIA* STRAINS

Biotyping and serotyping have been the predominant methods used to characterize strains of *Y. enterocolitica*. At least 54 to 60 serotypes of *Y. enterocolitica* exist on the basis of variability of somatic O antigens, but only 11 typically are associated with human disease.[21,23,56,69,197] Six biotypes of *Y. enterocolitica*, designated 1A, 1B, and 2 to 5, have been defined on the basis of differences in the following: lipase activity; salicin acid production; esculin hydrolysis; indole production; ornithine decarboxylase; Voges-Proskauer test; pyrazinamide activity; nitrate reduction; and fermentations of xylose, trehalose, sorbose, and inositol.[23,33,196]

Only a few serotype : biotype combinations are regarded as human pathogens: O:8, O:4, O:13a,13b, O:18, O:20, and O:21 (biotype 1B); O:9 and O:5,27 (biotype 2); O:1,2,3 and O:5,27 (biotype 3); O:3 (biotype 4); and O:2,3 (biotype 5).[202] These pathogenic strains, which carry *Yersinia* virulence plasmids (pYV), generally have negative test results for pyrazinamidase activity, esculin hydrolysis, and salicin fermentation. Nonpathogenic strains, generally of biotype 1A, have positive test results for each of them.[41,54,98] Data suggest that some biotype 1A strains that lack pYV and other *Yersinia* virulence factors also may cause gastroenteritis.[68,179]

Strains of *Y. enterocolitica* can be typed genetically by repetitive element-based (inter-repeat) polymerase chain reaction (PCR), arbitrarily primed PCR,[148] pulsed-field gel electrophoresis,[141] and

---

*See references 14, 21, 23, 24, 45, 47, 53, 55, 81, 82, 87, 92, 104-107, 118, 125, 137, 169, 183, 185, 186, 189, 200, 212.

ribotyping.[123] These methods allow distinction among strains within biotypes and serotypes and may be useful for outbreak and other epidemiologic investigations.

At least 11 antigenic groups of *Y. pseudotuberculosis* exist on the basis of variation of somatic O antigens. They have been labeled 1a, 1b, 2a, 2b, 2c, 3, 4a, 4b, 5a, 5b, and 6.[84,91,129] Type 2 is related antigenically to *Salmonella* group B, and type 4 is related to *Salmonella* groups D and H.[66] *Y. pseudotuberculosis* strains also can be typed by arbitrarily primed PCR.[129]

EPIDEMIOLOGY

Although most of the early reports of yersiniosis caused by *Y. pseudotuberculosis* and *Y. enterocolitica* came from northern Europe, these microbes have been identified with increasing frequency in all parts of the world,[13] with the possible exception of South America. During 1996 to 1998, the rate of foodborne disease caused by yersiniosis microbes in five areas of the United States was 1 per 100,000 population.[35]

YERSINIA ENTEROCOLITICA

Y. enterocolitica is distributed worldwide but is isolated most frequently in cooler climates.[138] Whether such geographic differences reflect differences in reservoirs or culinary practices that may enhance the risk of acquisition of this organism, or rather represent differences in surveillance for the disease and use of more sensitive culturing techniques in these areas, is unclear.[47] Increased frequency of infections during fall and winter has been reported from Europe[192] and the United States,[1] but no seasonality is evident among outbreaks of disease where more than three cases of *Y. enterocolitica* disease have been identified.[47]

Geographic differences in serotype distribution and frequency also exist. Sporadic infections caused by serotypes O:3 and O:9 are common in Europe,[9,85] but outbreaks rarely have occurred.[47] In North America, multiple serotypes have been responsible for sporadic disease,[18,22,33,65,177,181] but more recently serotype O:3 has become predominant.[33,51,118] Five outbreaks in the United States have been caused by serotype O:8, and two outbreaks in Canada have been caused by serotypes O:5 and O:5,27.[47] Disease caused by serotype O:8 has been reported in Europe.[85]

The true incidence and prevalence of *Y. enterocolitica* infection are unknown.[47] The reported proportional frequency of isolation of *Y. enterocolitica* from stool cultures from patients with diarrhea has ranged from 0 to 3.2 percent in series from Europe, the United States, and New Zealand (Table 123–1).[49,56,85,118,131,136,177] Symptomatic infection occurs more commonly in children. Most

series show a slight male predominance of approximately 1.3:1.[51,56,131,196] Surveillance at five FoodNet sites in the United States during 1996 to 1999 found that African-American infants had far higher rates than white infants, with a peak occurrence from November to February (Fig. 123–1).[162]

Animals and water sources are the primary environmental reservoirs for *Y. enterocolitica*, but the biotypes and serotypes of the strains found in them usually differ from those causing human disease.[33,47,177] Blood transfusions also may be a source of *Y. enterocolitica* infection.[34]

Animal Reservoirs

Y. enterocolitica strains have been isolated from a wide variety of mammals (dogs, pigs, sheep, rabbits, guinea pigs, cows, horses, chinchillas, monkeys), frogs, fish, flies, fleas, snails, crabs, and oysters. Birds do not seem to be a major reservoir for *Y. enterocolitica*, although avian isolates have been reported.[47,88,125]

Pigs seem to be an important reservoir for the human pathogenic serotypes O:3 and O:9 in Europe and Japan and serotype O:3 in North America and South Africa.[47,118,158] The biochemical and phage typing profiles of isolates from pigs are similar to those of strains commonly responsible for human infections.[200] *Y. enterocolitica* has been isolated from the tongue, tonsils, and cecal contents of swine and from pork, ham, and butcher shop cutting boards.[47,66] Pig farmers in Finland were 3 times and 2.4 times as likely to have seropositivity to serotypes O:3 and O:9 than were berry farmers.[176]

Wild rodents captured in areas of Japan where human infections caused by *Y. enterocolitica* serotype O:8 had occurred were shown to harbor isolates of the same serotype.[43] Two distinct serotype O:8 strains, defined by restriction enzyme analysis of the virulence plasmids, were isolated from humans and rodents. This finding suggests that rodents are a potential source of sporadic human infection in Japan.

Apparent transmission to humans from dogs and cats also has been reported. A fecal-oral or oral-oral route has been postulated but not confirmed. Little evidence supports airborne or insect vector–borne transmission.[47]

Foods and Water

In countries with high numbers of cases of yersiniosis, ingestion of raw pork has been common. Infection with serotypes O:3 and O:9 was highly associated with ingestion of raw pork during the 2 weeks preceding the illness in a case-control study.[192] In Belgium, laboratory surveillance that began in 1967 showed yearly increases in cases through 1986. After a media campaign was launched to dissuade people from eating raw or undercooked

TABLE 123–1   Percentage of Stool Cultures Yielding *Yersinia enterocolitica*

Country	Years	Population	Total Cultures	Percentage *Y. enterocolitica*
Canada[131]	1977-1978	Symptomatic children	6364	2.8
The Netherlands[85]	1982-1984	Enteritis patients <40 years old	827	2.9
Italy[136]	1981-1985	Children with diarrhea	2500	1.4*
New Zealand[56]	1988-1993	Patients with gastroenteritis	231,128	0.6
U.S. (Detroit, MI)[49]	May-November 1977	Children with diarrhea	1262	0
U.S. (New York State)[177]	1976-1980	Survey of cultures from a state laboratory, 6 hospitals, and several daycare centers	2487	0.9†
U.S.‡ (7 cities)[118]	November 1989-January 1990	All stool cultures submitted to 7 hospitals	4841	0.8
U.S. (St. Louis, MO)[103]	1998-2001	Children presenting to an emergency department with diarrhea	1626	0.1

Yearly percentages during the 5 years ranged from 0 to 4.4 percent.
†*This increased to 4 percent of 3035 isolates when cultures from an outbreak and other screenings were included.*
‡*Includes Detroit, MI.*

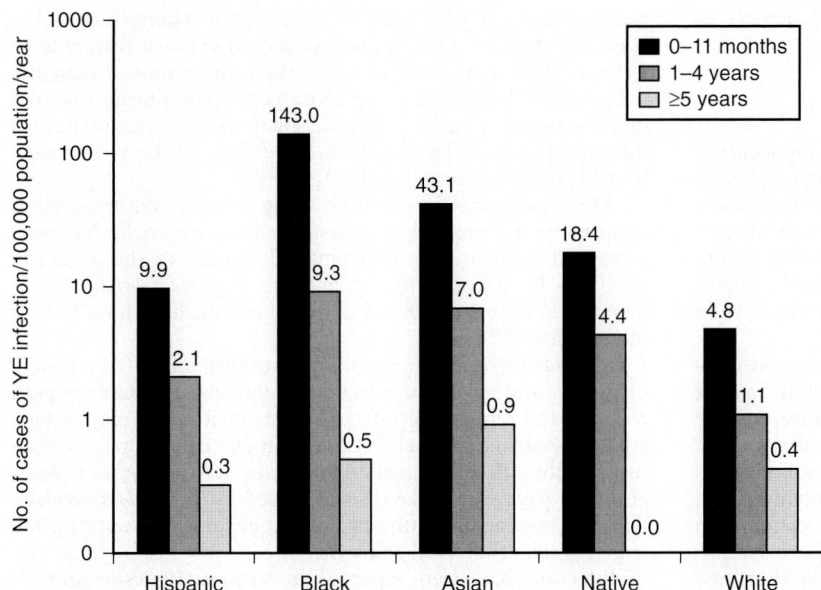

Figure 123-1 Adjusted incidence of *Yersinia enterocolitica* (YE) infection, by race and age. Average incidences are given over the 4-year surveillance period (1996 to 1999) by age group and adjusted race/ethnicity. *(From Ray, S. M., Ahuja, S. D., Blake, P. A., et al.: Population-based surveillance for* Yersinia enterocolitica *infections in FoodNet sites, 1996-1999: Higher risk for disease in infants and minority populations. Clin. Infect. Dis. 38:S181-S189, 2004.)*

pork or pork products and to educate consumers regarding good hygiene practices during food preparation, the number of isolations of *Y. enterocolitica* decreased from a high of 1469 in 1986 to 707 in 1996.[202] Changes in techniques for slaughtering also may have contributed to this decline. Preparation of chitterlings in the household was a risk factor for *Y. enterocolitica* infection among children in Michigan[1] and Illinois.[36]

Ingestion of water contaminated with serotype O:8 has led to sporadic cases and outbreaks.[47] Bean sprouts that had been immersed in contaminated water were the source of an outbreak in Pennsylvania in 1982. Ingestion of tofu (bean curd) packed in untreated spring water that subsequently was found to be contaminated with *Y. enterocolitica* caused 44 cases of symptomatic infection in Washington state in 1981 and 1982.[191] Serotypes commonly found in water samples rarely are isolated from humans with symptomatic disease, however.[33]

Contaminated milk has been implicated as the source of several large outbreaks of *Y. enterocolitica* infection.[19,47,197] Whipped cream and ice cream may harbor the organism. Contamination of milk products after pasteurization has been documented. *Y. enterocolitica* has been found in raw milk samples from cows and goats. Samples of beef, lamb, poultry, oysters, and a variety of vegetables also have been found to be contaminated with *Y. enterocolitica*.[30,47,66]

Serotypes O:3, O:4,33, O:5,27, O:7,8, O:8, O:10, O:13, and O:16 cause most human disease in North America but rarely are isolated in surveillance of water or food samples. Serotype O:8 strains have been cultured from cattle, milk, and water samples[146]; serotype O:4,33 strains have been isolated from pigs and cattle; and serotype O:4,32 strains have been found in cheese, ham, sausage, raw beef, and one pancake specimen.[33,177,197]

Incubation, Carriage, and Transmission in Humans

The incubation period of *Y. enterocolitica* enterocolitis ranges from 1 to 14 days, with a median of approximately 4 days.[33,47,118] The minimal infective dose of *Y. enterocolitica* is unknown. Ingestion of 3.5×10^9 organisms by a volunteer resulted in diarrhea in less than 1 day, but such large inocula are unlikely to be encountered clinically. The duration of excretion of the organism after development of infection in children ranges from 14 to 97 days (mean 42 days).[131] The impact, if any, of antibiotic treatment on the duration of carriage is unknown.

Transmission to household members occurs uncommonly, even among young children, who are at higher risk for development of symptomatic disease.[19,131,191] Six percent of household contacts developed disease in one outbreak,[191] but several large outbreaks with no secondary household cases have been reported.[47]

Yersinia enterocolitica and Blood Transfusion–Related Sepsis

Sporadic cases of *Y. enterocolitica* sepsis related to contamination of transfusions of red blood cells have been recognized since 1987 and have occurred in the United States, Europe, and Australia.[34] *Y. enterocolitica* is the most common cause of transfusion-related sepsis.[97] Among 20 cases from the United States, chills occurred in 16, fever occurred in 14, hypotension occurred in 13, and disseminated intravascular coagulation occurred in 7.[42] Death attributable to *Y. enterocolitica* infection occurred in 12, half of which occurred within 25 hours of receipt of the contaminated transfusion. Among the 20 donors, 13 had had gastrointestinal symptoms within the month before receiving a blood donation, and 16 had titers equal to or greater than 1:128 (considered positive).

In many cases of transfusion-related sepsis, the contaminated red blood cell units had been stored for 25 days or more.[80] After experimental inoculation of small numbers of *Y. enterocolitica* into packed cells kept at 4° C, the organisms continue to replicate, reaching concentrations of 100 colony-forming units (CFU)/mL in 7 days and 10^6 CFU/mL in 21 days. High levels of endotoxin can result from such replication and have been documented in samples from red blood cell units that led to transfusion-related sepsis.[42]

Human Outbreaks

Outbreaks of *Y. enterocolitica* disease have involved communities, families (with interfamily spread), hospitals, and schools. The sources of the organism have been various foods and animals, especially dogs. A review of these outbreaks suggests that infection may occur more commonly than has been recognized. Yersiniosis also resembles disease caused by *Salmonella* and *Shigella* organisms in many respects, including the environmental sources of the organisms, the clinical syndromes, and the occurrence of asymptomatic infection.

OUTBREAKS IN SCHOOLS AND COMMUNITIES

A community outbreak caused by a serotype O:8 strain occurred in New York state in 1976.[19] At least 222 children and employees had a yersiniosis-like illness during a 10-week period. Illness was associated with drinking chocolate milk that was contaminated after pasteurization during hand mixing with chocolate syrup. Transmission of infection from ill children to household contacts was not observed. School-related outbreaks also have occurred in Japan.[15,215]

In the summer of 1982, an estimated several thousand individuals in several southern states who consumed milk from a single dairy developed yersiniosis. A total of 172 culture-positive infections were confirmed, many as a result of hospitalization for illness. Seventeen patients underwent appendectomy; 24 others had extraintestinal spread of infection. The strain involved was designated serotype O:13a,13b.[197] An outbreak associated with consumption of pasteurized milk in Vermont and New Hampshire in 1995 probably resulted from contamination after pasteurization with a serotype O:8 strain, possibly from rinsing bottles with untreated well water.[5]

During November to December 2002, nine infants in the Chicago area developed gastroenteritis caused by *Y. enterocolitica*. Eight were African-American and were exposed to caretakers who had prepared chitterlings for holiday meals. All recovered, although six were hospitalized for a median of 5 days.[36]

FAMILY EPIDEMICS

In North Carolina, 21 individuals from four families were involved in an outbreak of yersiniosis that had an unusually high attack rate.[70] Of the 21 affected individuals, 18 were children aged 3 to 13 years; 16 of the 21 had diarrhea and fever, and 5 were asymptomatic. *Y. enterocolitica* was recovered from the spleen of the youngest child at autopsy. The diagnosis was established serologically in the others. A dog that had given birth to puppies that had died of a diarrheal illness a week before the families became ill seemed to be the source of the infection.

NOSOCOMIAL OUTBREAKS

A young child who was hospitalized in Finland with acute gastroenteritis was the source case of infection in a housekeeping worker and four nurses who cared for her.[195] The infecting strain was serotype O:9. Another hospital outbreak involved nine patients in Canada.[161] It was caused by a serotype O:5 strain. Person-to-person contact was considered the likely mode of transmission.

Prevention of Disease

During outbreaks, efforts should be made to identify environmental sources and vehicles of transmission.[47] A single environmental source can harbor multiple serotypes of *Y. enterocolitica*, such that resulting outbreaks may be polyclonal in nature.[191] Enteric precautions should be used for hospitalized patients with diarrhea caused by *Y. enterocolitica* (as with other causes of gastroenteritis).[47] At the population level, decreased consumption of raw or undercooked pork products potentially can reduce the incidence of infection.[192,202]

YERSINIA PSEUDOTUBERCULOSIS

Y. pseudotuberculosis may infect individuals of all ages, but at least 75 percent of patients with clinically apparent disease are children younger than 15 years old.[91,171] Infection in young infants has been reported.[91,208] Of 130 cases diagnosed in Great Britain from 1959 to 1970, boys were involved three times more frequently than girls.[125] Infections occur more commonly during the cold months of the year.[91,171] The seasonal winter peak of human infection produced by *Y. pseudotuberculosis* is similar to that seen in wild and domesticated animals.[104,105,171]

The attack rates for children living in rural and urban areas seem to be the same. *Y. pseudotuberculosis* occasionally has been recovered from healthy individuals. Exposure to the organism seems to be uncommon; antibody to *Y. pseudotuberculosis* was detected in only 1 of 2000 sera from individuals with no history of yersiniosis.[59,171]

Y. pseudotuberculosis is distributed worldwide in a large variety of animals and birds, but infection seldom occurs.[63] Guinea pigs, rodents, and rabbits are infected most often[125] and may experience a plaguelike illness.[63,88] Lesions in guinea pigs may be confused easily with lesions caused by *Y. pestis*. Rats and other rodents also may have plaguelike disease caused by *Y. pseudotuberculosis*. The microbe can be cultured from tongue, tonsils, intestines, and large organs of infected animals.[145]

Infection has been reported in various domestic animals (cattle, sheep, goats, cats, dogs, hamsters), commercially raised fur bearers (chinchillas, mink, coypu), and other wild or captive animals (rabbits, raccoons, foxes, deer, beavers, monkeys, puma, kangaroos). *Y. pseudotuberculosis* has been found in more than 50 species of birds,[75,99,125] and epizootics have occurred among turkeys, ducks, pigeons, and doves and in aviaries of canaries and finches. Strains obtained from animals and birds in the United States are predominantly of serotypes 1a, 1b, and 3.[125,171]

The incubation period for human disease ranges from 41 hours to 20 days.[91] In a food-associated outbreak in Finland, the median incubation period was 8 days (Fig. 123–2).[94] The organism can survive in fresh tap water for 46 days at room temperature and for 8 months at 4° C. It can survive at 4° C in meat for 145 days and in milk and bread for 2 to 3 weeks.[125]

A family outbreak of mesenteric adenitis caused by *Y. pseudotuberculosis* that involved four siblings aged 7 to 14 years has been reported.[160] A pet dog was shown to have increasing antibody titers at the time the children were ill.

Periodic outbreaks have been reported in Japan, northern Europe, and areas of the former Soviet Union. Sandwiches prepared by a single bakery were the primary risk factor for 67 cases that occurred in a 3-week period in Japan.[91] Drinking unchlorinated well water or mountain stream water has been the source of other outbreaks. Children were much more likely to have clinical disease than adults. More recent outbreaks in Finland have been associated with contaminated lettuce and grated carrots.[94]

PATHOLOGY

The diseases produced by *Y. enterocolitica* and *Y. pseudotuberculosis* are similar and share the histopathologic theme of involvement of the lymphoid tissues of the intestinal mucosa and mesentery.

YERSINIA ENTEROCOLITICA

Y. enterocolitica infection predominantly affects the gastrointestinal tract. The most severe clinical symptoms correlate with an acute terminal ileitis. The mucosal surface of the ileum and other involved sites may be inflamed diffusely. Ulcerations may occur throughout the gastrointestinal tract and may be small and superficial or extend to the muscularis propria. Mucosal and submucosal hyperplasia of Peyer patches occurs with scattered microabscess formation.

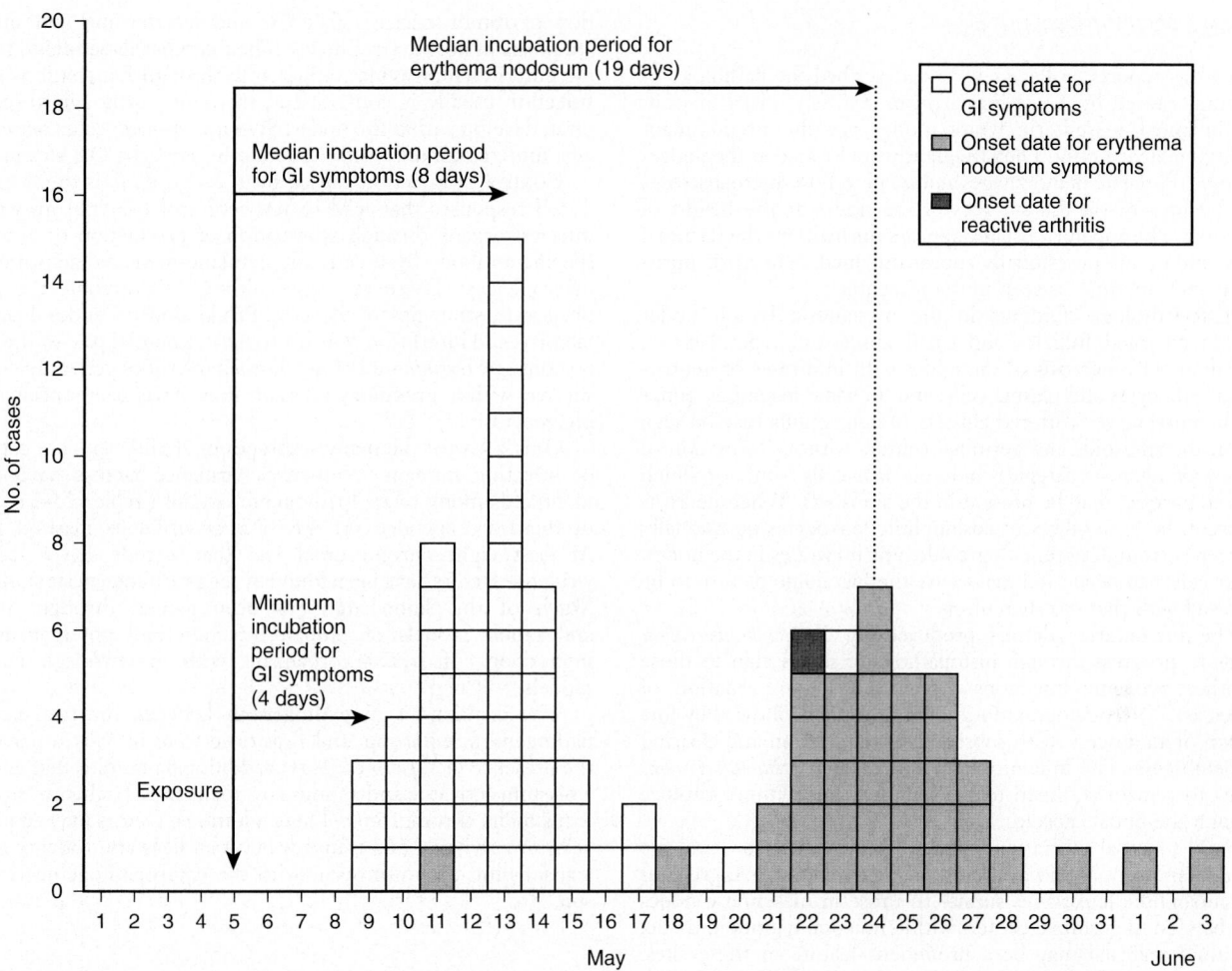

Figure 123–2 Distribution of incubation periods for *Yersinia pseudotuberculosis* infection to onset of gastrointestinal (GI) symptoms and erythema nodosum after point source exposure to contaminated carrots. Of 72 case patients with a known date of onset, 51 had GI symptoms and 38 had erythema nodosum only; 28 had GI symptoms and erythema nodosum and appear twice in the graph. *(From Jalava, K., Hakkinen, M., Valkonen, M., et al.: An outbreak of gastrointestinal illness and erythema nodosum from grated carrots contaminated with Yersinia pseudotuberculosis. J. Infect. Dis. 194:1209-1216, 2006.)*

Ulcers occur primarily over the sites of lymphoid tissue within the mucosa, which accounts for their more longitudinal appearance in the small intestine and an oval or punctate appearance in the stomach and colon. Ulcerations are characterized by necrosis of the epithelial layer. In the colon, the necrosis also may extend through the superficial third of the crypts. Large colonic ulcerations covered by pseudomembranes or mucoid debris are seen occasionally. Ulcerations may progress to perforation, with subsequent development of peritonitis or gastrointestinal hemorrhage in severe cases.[27,64,200,201]

The inflammatory response in the mucosa consists mainly of neutrophils and mononuclear cells. Lymphocytes and plasma cells also may be seen. Giant cells are not seen, although a granulomatous appearance can be imparted by the presence of plump epithelioid histiocytes. Numerous colonies of gram-negative bacteria often can be seen beneath the mucosal ulcerations and within the microabscesses that occur in the lymphoid tissues.[64,200,201]

The appendix usually appears normal on gross inspection, but small focal ulcerations frequently are present.[7] Large areas of necrosis are found occasionally, and acute, suppurative appendicitis has been reported.[27,96,131] Periappendicular inflammation

may result from a true appendicitis or an adjacent terminal ileitis.[200]

Mesenteric adenitis, the hallmark of infection caused by *Y. pseudotuberculosis*, also is a common feature of enterocolitis caused by *Y. enterocolitica*. The lymph nodes usually show numerous large pyroninophilic cells and mitotic figures in the cortical area and marginal sinuses. Small collections of leukocytes in the germinal centers are seen in some cases and suggest formation of microabscesses. In severe cases, extensive areas of necrosis circumscribed by a neutrophilic infiltrate may be seen. The sinusoids can become filled with neutrophils and mononuclear cells. The germinal centers often appear reactive.

The histopathologic appearance of the mesenteric adenitis of infection caused by *Y. enterocolitica* can resemble the adenitides caused by cat-scratch disease (*Bartonella henselae*), toxoplasmosis, infectious mononucleosis, and *Y. pseudotuberculosis*.[7,200,211] The necrotizing epithelioid granulomata that may be present in mesenteric adenitis caused by *Y. pseudotuberculosis* have not been described in infection caused by *Y. enterocolitica*. A more recent study of six cases suggests that biotype 1B strains may be more likely to cause suppurative inflammation, whereas biotype 2 through 5 strains may be more likely to cause granulomatous infection.[115]

YERSINIA PSEUDOTUBERCULOSIS

Numerous reports* collectively have described the pathology of infection caused by *Y. pseudotuberculosis*. Grossly enlarged, soft, and inflamed mesenteric lymph nodes are the predominant finding on laparotomy. They frequently are located at the ileocecal angle. Punctate hemorrhages and small, yellow microabscesses may be present on the surfaces of the nodes at the height of infection. The appendix usually appears normal, but the terminal ileum and cecum occasionally appear inflamed. A necrotic purulent mass sometimes is seen in the mesentery.

Histopathologic findings in the mesenteric lymph nodes include enlarged follicles and small abscesses; hyperplasia of reticulum cells; necrosis of the nodes with infiltrates of neutrophilic leukocytes and plasma cells; and, in some instances, punctate hemorrhages. Scattered clusters of neutrophils may be seen within the sinusoids and germinal centers without formation of abscess or necrosis. Atypical mononuclear cells, some of which may be mitotic, may be present in the sinusoids. When necrosis is absent, large numbers of eosinophilic leukocytes occasionally are seen surrounding reticulogranulocytic infiltrates in the nodes. Giant cells can occur and may cause the histologic picture to be confused with that of tuberculosis.

The mesenteric adenitis produced by *Y. pseudotuberculosis* seems to progress through histopathologic stages akin to those of other pyogenic infections that can lead to formation of abscesses.[50,71] Reticulogranulocytic infiltration is followed by formation of an abscess, with subsequent organization and clearing of the abscess. The inflammatory process of *Y. pseudotuberculosis* seems to remain confined to the lymph nodes without rupture through the nodal capsule.

Focal mucosal ulcerations may be seen in the ileum and are more likely to be found at the site of Peyer patches. Aggregates of neutrophilic leukocytes similar to those in mesenteric nodes may be seen in germinal centers within mucosal lymphoid tissue. Fibrinoid material may be a prominent feature at these sites. Small areas of necrosis surrounded by reticulum cells and leukocytes also may be present in the submucosal follicles.[57,105,107,207] Ulcerated lymphoid follicles in the intestinal wall are connected to the regional lymph nodes by a lymphangitis. This anatomic situation is analogous to the primary complex of tuberculosis.

Despite a clinical picture of acute appendicitis as the presenting feature of infection by *Y. pseudotuberculosis*, the appendix typically is grossly and microscopically normal. Inflammatory changes, when present, usually are in the form of a periappendicitis. Phlegmonous appendicitis can result from infection caused by *Y. pseudotuberculosis*, but is rare.[50,84]

PATHOGENESIS

The pathogenesis of infection by the two enteropathogenic *Yersinia* spp. has been studied extensively. After ingestion and successful transit to the small intestine have occurred, these *Yersinia* spp. are able to penetrate into the lamina propria primarily by passing through the cytoplasm of M cells that reside on the mucosal surface of Peyer patches. The bacteria are internalized in membrane-bound vacuoles in which they survive, but do not replicate. After reaching the lamina propria, the microbes multiply as extracellular microcolonies in lymph follicles and Peyer patches, where they may reach densities of 10^9 CFU/g of tissue.[52]

Neutrophils and macrophages infiltrate these sites in response to the infection, ultimately creating microabscesses, but *Y. enterocolitica* is able to resist phagocytosis and intracellular killing by neutrophils and macrophages. *Yersinia* spp. also inhibit produc-

tion of tumor necrosis factor-α and interferon-γ and induce apoptosis in host macrophages. The microbes disseminate to the mesenteric lymph nodes, apparently through lymphatic vessels. Infection usually is contained at this point, although abscesses often develop within the nodes. Systemic spread occurs occasionally, more commonly with infection by serotype O:8 strains.

Control of infection caused by *Y. enterocolitica* is the result of T-cell responses that lead to restriction of bacterial growth in infected organs through stimulation of production of *Yersinia*-specific antibody by B cells and cytokine-mediated activation of macrophages. These responses ultimately overcome the antiphagocyte strategies of *Yersinia*. Production of tumor necrosis factor-α and interferon-γ seems to be an essential part of the host response to *Yersinia* infections. *Yersinia* microbes generally do not survive within granulocytes after they have been successfully phagocytosed.[43,45,46,149]

Only a few of the many serotypes of *Yersinia* spp. are capable of infecting humans. Numerous virulence factors have been identified among these "pathogenic" strains (Table 123–2). Most of them are encoded on the *Yersinia* virulence plasmid pYV. At least eight chromosomal loci that encode novel *Yersinia* virulence factors have been found by tagged mutagenesis studies.[67] Much of this knowledge has been gained through mouse and rabbit models of human infection and observations of interactions of *Yersinia* organisms with in vitro cell culture models.[26,43,83,127,156]

The distinctions in pathogenesis between the two enteropathogenic *Yersinia* spp. and *Y. pestis* seem to be caused partly by the presence in *Y. pestis* of (1) two additional plasmids that encode a plasmin activator and a mouse exotoxin and (2) a hemin storage locus on its chromosome. These additional factors may enable *Y. pestis* to survive in and transmit between fleas and rodents. Such transmission does not occur with the enteropathogenic *Yersinia* spp.[167]

BACTERIAL DETERMINANTS OF MUCOSAL INVASION

Two outer-membrane proteins encoded by chromosomal genes permit entry into various mammalian cell types in vitro and are likely to be responsible for the ability of *Yersinia* to invade into and through the intestinal mucosal epithelium. They have been named *invasin* and the *attachment invasin locus protein* (Ail). All isolates of *Y. enterocolitica* that are virulent in humans contain DNA sequences that encode for invasin and Ail. Nonpathogenic strains do not contain the genetic code for Ail but most contain invasin genes that cannot be expressed because of chromosomal rearrangements. These proteins apparently are unique to the genus *Yersinia*.[92,135,153]

Invasin attaches to receptors in the β_1 integrin family and induces an actin-mediated endocytosis of the microbe. It binds to β_1-chain integrin receptors with approximately 100-fold higher affinity than do natural ligands, such as fibronectin. Such high-affinity binding triggers endocytosis-like internalization that involves clathrin.[46] Invasin is expressed maximally at ambient temperatures when the organism is in stationary phase. *Y. enterocolitica* microbes living in the environment probably exist in a stationary phase–like state and may be primed maximally for invasion of the host after ingestion. Invasin expression also can remain elevated at 37° C when the pH is 5.5, and such conditions are encountered during passage through the intestinal tract. Ail is expressed maximally at 37° C, functions as an adhesin and an invasion factor, and plays a role in the resistance of *Y. enterocolitica* to the bactericidal activity of human serum.[92,93,153]

High levels of β_1-chain integrin receptors are found on the luminal surface of M cells, which are antigen-sampling epithelial cells found in highest numbers overlying Peyer patches in the intestinal tract.[76] Flagellum-dependent motility seems

---

*See references 50, 55, 57, 87, 105, 126, 132, 133, 137, 160, 207.

TABLE 123-2   Known and Putative *Yersinia* Virulence Factors*

Stage of Pathogenesis	Determinant	Genomic Origin†	Function	Conditions of Expression
Gastric transit	Urease	Chromosome	Aids survival of gastric acidity	
Mucosal invasion	Invasin (inv)	Chromosome	Attachment, invasion via β₁ integrins; broad host/cell range	28° C
	Attachment invasion locus (AiL)	Chromosome	Attachment, lesser invasion factor; more host-specific than invasin; serum resistance	37° C
	Yersinia adhesin A (YadA)	Plasmid	Attachment, invasion; reduces opsonization by C3b by binding complement factor H; ? role in resistance to antibacterial polypeptides (e.g., bactericidal permeability-increasing protein)	37° C and *any* calcium concentration
Disruption of phagocyte function	Effector proteins (act on host cells)	Plasmid	Tyrosine phosphorylase that prevents phagocytosis by macrophages by preventing assembly of focal adhesion structures of phagocytes	37° C and low calcium concentration
	YopHᵈ		Phagocytosis resistance via induction of host cell actin filament rearrangements	
	YopE		Cysteine protease that inhibits mitogen-activated protein kinase and nuclear factor κB signaling via interruption of post-translational covalent additions of ubiquitin-like molecules to these enzymes. This prevents production of cytokines (tumor necrosis factor-α), inhibits the host immune response, and triggers apoptosis of macrophages. Inhibits kinase phosphorylation via an acetyltransferase function	
	YopJ/P		Serine kinase, causes rounding up of cells, specific target unknown	
	YpkA/YopO		Disruption of actin filaments	
	YopT		Role unclear. Inhibits thrombin-induced platelet activation in vitro but is delivered intracellularly during infection. Leads to depletion of natural killer cells and alters expression of interleukin-15 and interleukin-15 receptors	
	YopM			
	Host cell membrane attachment, pore insertion proteins	Plasmid	Pore formation in host cell membrane to allow translocation of effector proteins into the host cell. ? Suppression of interleukin-8 secretion by epithelial cells	37° C and low calcium concentration
	YopB and YopD		Controls translocation via modulating the size of the putative YopB, YopD pore in the host cell membrane	
	YopQ (YopK)		Involved in control of translocation, perhaps stabilizing contact between the bacterium and host cell membranes	
	YopN		Assists extrusion of Yops B and D to the host cell membrane. Homologue of the *Y. pestis* V antigen. Antibodies against V antigen seem to be protective at the serotype level	
	LcrVᵉ			
	Yop secretion apparatus (Ysc) (28 proteins in total)	Plasmid	Form a complex that spans the inner bacterial membrane (? gated pore/channel)	37° C and low calcium concentration
	YscD, YscR, YscU, and LcrD/YscV		Forms a pore in the outer bacterial membrane that may connect with the inner membrane pore	
	YscC secretin		ATPase that energizes Yop transfer across the membranes	
	YscN		Negative *yop* gene regulators that, when secreted, decrease in concentration in the bacterium, allowing *yop* expression	
	LcrQ (in *Y. pseudotuberculosis*), YscM1 and YscM2 (in *Y. enterocolitica*)			
	Cytosolic chaperones (Syc) (6 proteins in total)	Plasmid	Secretion/translocation pilots or antidegradation roles for effector proteins	37° C and low calcium concentration
Colonization of Peyer patches and lymph nodes	*Yersinia* phospholipase A	Plasmid	? Serum resistance, ? inhibition of phagocytosis	37° C and low calcium concentration
Iron metabolism	Yersiniabactin	Chromosome (high pathogenicity island)	Siderophore	37° C, iron starvation

TABLE 123–2   Known and Putative Yersinia Virulence Factors*—cont'd

Stage of Pathogenesis	Determinant	Genomic Origin†	Function	Conditions of Expression
Diarrhea	*Yersinia* heat-stable enterotoxin (Yst)	Chromosome	Fluid secretion in intestine. Precise role in pathogenesis of disease in humans is unclear, but found in clinical isolates from children with diarrhea	28° C (in vitro)
? Systemic invasion	O antigen	Chromosome	Component of lipopolysaccharide. ? Complement/serum resistance	

The pathogenesis/virulence roles of several gene products encoded on the Yersinia virulence plasmid pVY have yet to be determined, and additional functions may be identified for other gene products. Additional chromosomally encoded virulence factors are suspected, with investigations ongoing.
†*Plasmid refers to the Yersinia virulence plasmid pYV.*
Lcr, low calcium response; Yop, Yersinia outer membrane protein (although not all such designated proteins reside in the outer membrane).
Data from references 23, 44, 45, 67, 83, 102, 111, 119, 140, 149, 167, 179, 180, 214.

to be required for invasin-mediated invasion of cells by *Y. enterocolitica*.[213]

YERSINIA ADHESIN A

Yersinia adhesin A (YadA) is a multifunctional virulence factor of *Y. enterocolitica*. YadA is approximately 50 kd and probably forms tetrameric fibrillae on the microbial surface. Its gene resides on the pYV plasmid and is transcribed at 37° C independently of the calcium concentration. YadA binds to extracellular matrix proteins, such as collagen, and mediates adhesion to cells. It may play a role in translocation of Yop effector proteins into eukaryotic phagocytic cells. YadA also inhibits the terminal complement attack complex, reduces opsonization by C3b through binding of complement factor H, and contributes to the ability of *Y. enterocolitica* to resist killing by antimicrobial polypeptides of human granulocytes. YadA knockout mutants are far less virulent in mice than is the parent wild-type strain.[45,82,205]

VIRULENCE PLASMID AND TYPE III SECRETION SYSTEM

Pathogenic strains of *Y. enterocolitica* harbor a plasmid that consists of approximately 70 kb (denoted pYV) and encodes the low calcium response system of *Yersinia* spp., which involves a complex response to environmental conditions of 37° C and calcium concentrations of less than 2.5 mM, both of which describe the intracellular compartment of mammalian cells.[45,180] Plasmid-encoded factors are required for survival and extracellular multiplication after reaching Peyer patches. Plasmid-cured derivatives are ingested rapidly and killed by neutrophils in Peyer patches, whereas wild-type strains are able to proliferate and spread through the lamina propria to adjacent villi. Plasmid-encoded factors are not required for *Y. enterocolitica* to penetrate the intestinal mucosa.[82]

In DNA cross-hybridization studies, the pYVs of *Y. enterocolitica* serogroups O:9, O:3, and O:5 show 90 percent nucleotide identity with one another, 75 percent identity with the pYV of serogroup O:8, and 55 percent identity with the pYV of *Y. pestis* and *Y. pseudotuberculosis*. Despite the nucleotide divergence among the pYVs of the three *Yersinia* spp., the overall structures and most of the genes are highly similar among them. The *Yersinia* low calcium response plasmids are nonconjugative.[45,180]

The *Y. enterocolitica* pYV contains approximately 70 genes, of which approximately 53 have protein products with known or putative functions (many of these are listed among the virulence factors in Table 123–2). pYV encodes *Yersinia* adhesin A and a system of six effector proteins that are delivered into host cells (primarily phagocytic granulocytes) through a complex mechanism of regulatory proteins, secretion chaperones, and proteins that act as secretion channels or pores in the bacterial and host cell membranes. This system, called a type III secretion system, denotes secretion of the bacterial proteins only in response to contact with a mammalian cell. The effector proteins and several others involving pore formation are designated Yops (*Yersinia* outer-membrane proteins), although we now know that most of them do not reside in the outer membrane. Similar type III secretion systems are found in *Salmonella* and *Shigella* spp.[45,180]

The secretion system is composed partially of syringe-like organelles—called *Ysc injectisomes*—that develop when *Yersinia* organisms are incubated at mammalian body temperatures. These injectisomes are protein pumps that span the peptidoglycan layer and the two bacterial cell membranes, topped by a needle-like structure protruding outside the bacterium. Twenty-seven proteins are involved in the structure; 10 of them are located internally and appear to be similar to the basal body of a flagellum. The structure also includes an ATPase that functions as a proton pump. A homomultimeric ring-shaped structure extends through the outer membrane, with a central pore diameter of about 50 Å.[31]

As the injectisomes assemble, stocks of intracellular Yops are synthesized. Active transcription of Yop genes is limited to bacteria in close contact with eukaryotic cells. The secretion channel of the injectisome remains closed, with negative feedback mechanisms to prevent overproduction of Yops. On close contact with a phagocyte, the injectisome channels open, and secretion of effector Yops into the target cell begins.[31]

After secretion into a phagocytic cell occurs, Yop H, Yop E, Yop T, and YopO/YpkA disrupt its cytoskeletal dynamics, blocking phagocytosis (see Table 123–2). Other Yops inhibit production of tumor necrosis factor-α, interleukin-8, and other inflammatory chemokines and induce apoptosis of macrophages.[31]

SUMMARY OF YERSINIA PATHOGENESIS

Pathogenic strains of *Y. enterocolitica* require calcium concentrations equivalent to those of serum and extracellular fluids in humans for growth at body temperature. Plasmid proteins are synthesized maximally, however, at 37° C under conditions of low calcium concentrations, such as those found intracellularly. These regulatory effects of environmental calcium concentrations permit free growth of *Yersinia* organisms during extracellular life and production of factors that inhibit phagocytosis by macrophages and neutrophils when *Yersinia* organisms pass through the intracellular compartment during mucosal invasion or come into contact with these granulocytes.[43,45,82]

A model of how pathogenic *Yersinia* organisms living in cold (≤28° C) environmental reservoirs are able to establish infection in the mammalian host can be described at the molecular level (see Table 123–2). *Yersinia* microbes living in the environment express invasin, which renders them ready to attach and invade the intestinal mucosal M cells after ingestion. Expression of invasin continues at body temperature during gastric passage to the intestines. Survival of gastric acidity is assisted by a urease-producing system.

During intracellular passage through M cells in the small intestine, pYV genes are likely to be activated (conditions of low calcium, 37° C). YadA can be produced at body temperature and may assist in mucosal invasion. Transcytosis from the intestinal lumen to the lamina propria seems to occur by a clathrin-mediated process that probably is a normal function of the host cell, after internalization is triggered. Ail also is synthesized after ingestion occurs and probably promotes attachment to migrating cells in the lamina propria that may facilitate extracellular spread of the microbes to regional lymph nodes and perhaps the liver and spleen.

To survive this journey, *Yersinia* organisms must evade phagocytosis by macrophages and neutrophils. YadA can inhibit complement opsonization, reducing the likelihood that phagocytosis will occur. When contact between the microbe and a host granulocyte occurs, the previously activated type III secretion system (described earlier) encoded by the pYV plasmid comes into play. A contiguous pore is inserted into the granulocyte cell membrane (involving Yops B, D, Q, and N and LcrV). Effector proteins (Yops E, H, J/P, O/A, M, and T) then are translocated into the granulocyte cytoplasm, disrupting its abilities to ingest the bacterium and produce cytokines and triggering apoptotic cell death (see Table 123–2). Although this system of virulence factors is robust enough to facilitate short-lived infection that often causes mild to moderate clinical symptoms, the microbes that do not succumb to the innate immune response ultimately are contained and then eliminated by the adaptive host response.

IRON METABOLISM AND VIRULENCE

Iron is an essential growth factor for most bacteria, many of which release siderophores (high-affinity chelators) that bind ferric iron and then are taken up again through receptors by the microbe. *Y. enterocolitica* serotype O:8 and other biotype 1B strains synthesize a chromosomally encoded siderophore, designated *yersiniabactin*, which sits on the outer membrane of the bacterium. The presence of this siderophore decreases the concentration of environmental iron required for optimal growth and probably accounts for the increased virulence observed for serotype O:8 strains.[47,82] The gene encoding yersiniabactin and the genes required for its biosynthesis, transport, and regulation compose the core of what is termed a *high-pathogenicity island* because of the high lethality for mice that its presence confers.[159]

Serotypes O:8, O:4, O:13, O:18, O:20, and O:21 (all biotype 1B and historically considered "American" strains) are highly lethal to mice after intraperitoneal injection and are able to evoke a keratoconjunctivitis after inoculation into the conjunctival sac of guinea pigs (the positive Sereny test result). Oral infection in mice predominantly produces the features of mesenteric adenitis and systemic infection, rather than simple gastroenteritis, which is characteristic of human infection by American strains. The "European" serotypes, O:3, O:9, and O:5,27, yield a negative Sereny test result and cause mild diarrhea but not death in mice. The European serotypes of *Y. enterocolitica* do not produce yersiniabactin, but are able to use siderophores synthesized by other organisms.[43,82,135]

Deferoxamine, a *Streptomyces*-derived siderophore used clinically to treat iron overload states, can be used by *Y. enterocolitica* strains as a source of iron. The increased availability of ferric iron that exists in iron overload states, such as hemochromatosis and diseases such as thalassemia, that require frequent red blood cell transfusions also facilitates survival and growth of *Y. enterocolitica*. Iron overloading and deferoxamine are independent risk factors for development of systemic disease after intestinal infection with *Y. enterocolitica*.[47]

ENTEROTOXIN PRODUCTION

All enteropathogenic strains of *Y. enterocolitica* produce a heat-stable enterotoxin that closely resembles the heat-stable toxin of *E. coli*. Both enterotoxins induce increases in levels of cyclic guanosine monophosphate levels in intestinal epithelial cells. The *Y. enterocolitica* enterotoxin is not plasmid-encoded, and its presence does not correlate with the expression of other virulence phenotypes.[63] Because the enterotoxin is not produced in vitro at temperatures exceeding 30° C, production in the gastrointestinal tract and a causative role in diarrhea were thought to be unlikely.[47] Observations in the young rabbit oral infection model have shown, however, that enterotoxin-negative mutants did not induce diarrhea, and that the wild-type strain did. Clinical biotype 1A isolates from children with diarrhea in India produce *Y. enterocolitica* stable toxin-b. These findings suggest that *Yersinia* enterotoxins may play a role in causing the diarrhea frequently associated with *Y. enterocolitica* infection in children.[82,152,179]

GASTRIC ACIDITY AS A PROTECTIVE HOST FACTOR

Although *Y. enterocolitica* is able to grow under conditions at pH 5.0 to 9.0, optimal growth occurs at pH 7.0 to 8.0. Gastric acidity may play a protective role against some *Yersinia* inocula, although pathogenic *Yersinia* organisms produce a urease enzyme that facilitates survival. Therapeutic agents or clinical conditions that result in reduced gastric acidity may predispose patients to development of infection. *Y. enterocolitica* bacteremia has been reported after gastrectomy.[47,111]

CLINICAL MANIFESTATIONS

Clinical disease caused by *Y. enterocolitica* occurs far more frequently than that caused by *Y. pseudotuberculosis*.[56,120,121] Historically, diarrheal illness has been considered the hallmark of *Y. enterocolitica* and the pseudoappendicular syndrome of mesenteric adenitis indicative of *Y. pseudotuberculosis*. Each species can cause enterocolitis and mesenteric adenitis, however. Various other clinical infections and postinfection syndromes also are caused by these microbes. In a series of patients presenting with acute abdominal pain suggestive of appendicitis, the incidence of serologic evidence of *Yersinia* infection has ranged from 7 to 31 percent.[16]

YERSINIA ENTEROCOLITICA

The clinical features of the disease caused by *Y. enterocolitica*, primarily an acute enteritis, have been described by many investigators.* The clinical manifestations depend partly on the age and physiologic condition of the host.[47,131,160] Enterocolitis is the most common presentation and occurs most often in young children. The pseudoappendicular syndrome, which results primarily from mesenteric adenitis and mimics acute appendicitis, occurs more commonly in older children and young adults.[19,47,86,96,147,166]

---

*See references 17, 38, 47, 51, 74, 110, 117, 118, 127, 128, 131, 161, 166, 196, 212.

TABLE 123–3   Clinical Features of *Yersinia enterocolitica* Infection in Children

	Sweden,[17] 1967-1973	Finland,[128] 1974-1978	Canada,[51] 1972	Canada,[131] 1977-1978	U.S.,[118] 1989-1990	U.S.,[142] 1988-1991	Combined Totals
No.	31	35	40	57	37*	48	248
Age ≤5 yr	28	26	19	NS†	≥28	NS	≥101/142 (≥71%)
Fever (>38° C)	15	6	36	39	35	44	175/248 (71%)
Diarrhea	31	26	32	56	37	45	227/248 (92%)
Grossly bloody diarrhea	2	NS	7	NS	14	22	45/156 (29%)
Abdominal pain	4	6	20	31/48	NS	NS	61/154 (40%)
Vomiting	NS	12	12	22	18	23	87/217 (40%)
Rash‡	NS	2	2	NS	NS	NS	4/75 (5%)
Appendectomy	0	0	4	1	0	0	5/200 (2%)
Serotype O:3	31	NS	34	57	34	NS	156/165 (94%)

*All were black children; 7 different cities, 3-month period.
†More than half of these children were <2 years old.
‡Maculopapular rash or urticaria.
NS, not specified.

Enterocolitis

Y. enterocolitica enterocolitis is characterized by diarrhea and abdominal pain. The diarrhea usually persists for 7 to 14 days.[118,131,200] A range of 1 to 46 days of diarrhea has been reported.[109] Ten percent of cases may persist for 30 days or more,[131] and chronic diarrhea persisting for several months has been described.[51]

During the first week of symptoms, patients commonly have 3 to 10 stools per day, with a gradual decrease in frequency thereafter. Stools typically are greenish, exhibit variable consistency (usually watery or mucoid), and are not remarkably malodorous. Gross blood is noted in approximately 25 to 50 percent of patients. Vomiting occurs in 40 percent of cases. Nausea is a common symptom. The abdominal pain can be colicky, diffuse, or localized to the right lower quadrant or epigastrium. Fever occurs commonly and usually is low-grade, but may exceed 40° C; it usually resolves within 1 week.[1,128]

Most cases are self-limited, but some children require hospitalization. Among 60 children hospitalized in Michigan between 1990 and 1997, the mean number of hospital days required was 4 (range 1 to 17 days).[1]

Fecal leukocytes are present commonly but not universally. The peripheral white blood cell count may range from 5600/mm³ to more than 30,000/mm³. Most counts are greater than 15,000/mm³. Band forms often exceed 15 percent of the total. Infants frequently exhibit an immature-to-total neutrophil ratio greater than 0.5.[1,118,128] An absolute monocytosis may be seen in two thirds of patients.[113] Culture-negative cerebrospinal fluid pleocytosis can occur.[1]

Radiologic examination by upper gastrointestinal barium studies in 24 adult patients with severe diarrhea caused by *Y. enterocolitica* showed abnormalities of the terminal ileum in 21 cases.[201] Diffuse thickening of the mucosal folds was seen in 16 cases, and nodular filling defects were seen in 11. The radiographic appearance suggested the presence of one or more ulcerations of the terminal ileum in 11 patients. Dilation of the terminal ileum was noted in 12 patients, and extrinsic compression, presumably from enlarged lymph nodes, was present in 4. In some instances, the findings suggested the terminal ileitis of Crohn disease. Follow-up studies performed 2 months after acute illness showed decreased but persistent thickening of mucosal folds in eight patients. Barium enema studies were done in 15

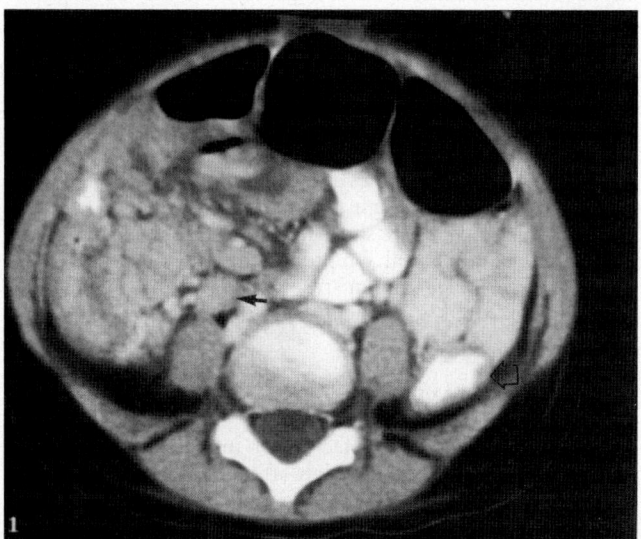

Figure 123–3 Mesenteric lymphadenopathy (*solid arrow*) and thickened bowel wall (*open arrow*) seen on computed tomography scan of a toddler with a 1-week history of severe abdominal pain, fever, vomiting, and nonbloody diarrhea. Stool culture on cefsulodin-irgasan-novobiocin agar yielded growth of *Yersinia enterocolitica*, serotype O:8. (*From Tuohy, A. M., O'Gorman, M., Byington, C., et al.: Yersinia enterocolitis mimicking Crohn's disease in a toddler. Pediatrics 104[issue 3]: e36, 1999.*)

patients and showed no striking abnormalities other than mucosal ulcerations, which were seen best on air-contrast studies.[200]

Mesenteric lymphadenopathy can be seen on computed tomography scans (Fig. 123–3).[199] Among 13 adults who had colonoscopy or sigmoidoscopy for severe diarrhea caused by *Y. enterocolitica*, abnormalities were seen in 8; the mucosa appeared diffusely swollen, erythematous, and friable in 6 individuals, and 2 had only small, 1- to 2-mm aphthoid ulcerations. Serial procedures showed macroscopic and microscopic healing of ulcers within 4 to 5 weeks.[201] Aphthoid ulcerations may be seen throughout the colon (Fig. 123–4).[199]

Pseudoappendicitis-Mesenteric Adenitis

The syndrome of pseudoappendicitis, characterized in most cases by a normal appendix and an intense suppurative mesenteric adenitis, has attracted considerable attention since it was reported first in 1953.[132,133] The first recognized cases were caused by *Y.*

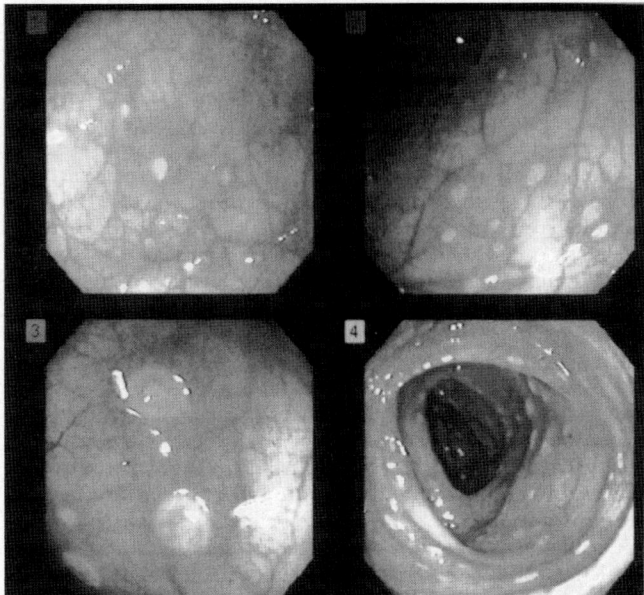

Figure 123–4 Multiple mucosal aphthoid ulcerations, 2 to 3 mm in size, as seen during colonoscopy in the child described in Figure 123–3. *(From Tuohy, A. M., O'Gorman, M., Byington, C., et al.: Yersinia enterocolitis mimicking Crohn's disease in a toddler. Pediatrics 104[issue 3]: e36, 1999.)*

pseudotuberculosis, but most cases reported in recent years have been caused by *Y. enterocolitica*.[28,95,117]

Fever, abdominal pain, right lower quadrant tenderness, and leukocytosis are the primary features of *Y. enterocolitica*–induced pseudoappendicular syndrome.[47,96] Some patients also have features of enterocolitis (nausea, vomiting, and diarrhea). The clinical presentation often is highly suggestive of acute appendicitis, such that laparotomy is required. Among a series of 581 patients in Scandinavia who underwent laparotomy for suspected appendicitis, 3.8 percent of cultures of stool or operative specimens yielded *Y. enterocolitica*.[147] Another 284 patients with similar symptoms were observed, and 5.6 percent of stool cultures from these cases yielded *Y. enterocolitica*. In a similar Scandinavian series of 205 patients who underwent appendectomy, 22 subsequently were diagnosed by serology as having *Y. enterocolitica* infection.[96] The findings on laparotomy usually are mesenteric lymphadenitis, terminal ileitis, and a normal or slightly inflamed appendix.[19,47,96,147]

A study of 40 cases of granulomatous appendicitis found evidence suggesting infection caused by *Y. enterocolitica* in 4 specimens, *Y. pseudotuberculosis* in 4 specimens, and both in 2 specimens by PCR analysis.[116] Two patients in the series subsequently were diagnosed as having Crohn disease, but causation cannot be inferred.

Asymptomatic Infection

In an unknown number of cases, infection by *Y. enterocolitica* is entirely asymptomatic. In a study of the distribution of antibodies to *Y. enterocolitica* in sera collected for various purposes in Ontario, Canada, from 4209 individuals who had no evidence of infection by this organism, specific antibody was present in 199 (serotype O:3 in 158 and serotype O:9 in 41).[196]

Other Presentations of Acute Infection

Bacteremia can occur[32,39,47,139] and may result in spread of infection to virtually any body site. Such events occur uncommonly and are seen more often in adults than in children. In children,

bacteremia occurs more commonly in infants than in older children.[1] The risk for development of bacteremia during gastroenteritis in infants younger than 3 months may be 30 percent.[142] Bacteremias may be transient and asymptomatic or lead to septic shock and death. Septic cases tend to occur among patients with underlying illnesses and are associated with mortality rates of 34 to 50 percent.[47]

Y. enterocolitica may cause focal infections in many extraintestinal sites, even in the absence of detectable bacteremia. Pharyngitis has been reported and occurs primarily in adults. Cervical adenopathy may be associated with *Y. enterocolitica* pharyngitis, and gastrointestinal symptoms may be absent.[47] One adult with pharyngitis died of associated septic shock.[168] Conjunctivitis and panophthalmitis caused by *Y. enterocolitica* have been described. Parinaud oculoglandular syndrome,[40] inguinal adenopathy,[208] and suppurative lymphadenitis[198] have been reported.

Cellulitis, soft tissue abscesses, and wound infections also have been reported. Cellulitis may have associated vesiculobullous lesions. An erysipelas-like rash, maculopapular rash, and urticaria also have been described in association with infection caused by *Y. enterocolitica*.[17,28,47,72,177,191,209]

Pancreatitis, cholecystitis, diverticulitis, and intestinal perforation have been described.[120,157] Peritonitis also can occur but is extremely rare,[163] especially considering the frequency of mesenteric adenitis. Pneumatosis intestinalis has been reported in an infant.[1] Pneumonia, pleural empyema, lung abscess, hepatic and splenic abscesses, urinary tract infection, and renal abscess also have been reported.[47] Glomerulonephritis that usually is transient has been reported.[48,60] Cases of meningitis, osteomyelitis, septic arthritis, pyomyositis (including psoas muscle abscess), endocarditis, mycotic aneurysm, and intravenous catheter–related infection caused by *Y. enterocolitica* have been described.[12,29,47,83,184,186] Thrombocytopenia[65] and hemolytic anemia[108] have occurred in association with infection caused by *Y. enterocolitica*.

Underlying Conditions That Predispose to Bacteremia

Y. enterocolitica bacteremias that occur in patients beyond early infancy most often occur in patients with chronic illnesses or iron overload states. Thalassemias are such conditions that occur most commonly in children.[38,58,101] Among 144 Italian children with thalassemia who were receiving deferoxamine therapy and frequent blood transfusions, 14 developed infection caused by *Y. enterocolitica* during a 12-month period.[38] Septicemia occurred in 5 of the 14 and was preceded by enterocolitis or mesenteric adenitis in each case. All 14 recovered after receiving 2 weeks of therapy with intravenous trimethoprim-sulfamethoxazole. A similar proportion of children with thalassemias observed in two centers in Canada between 1979 and 1994 also developed invasive disease caused by *Y. enterocolitica*.[6] Bacteremia can be associated temporally with blood transfusions in such patients, suggesting that transfusions may be the source of infection or predispose to development of infection in some cases.[120]

Hemochromatosis, cirrhosis, and other liver diseases may facilitate development of *Y. enterocolitica* bacteremia, also on the basis of excess availability of serum iron. Deferoxamine therapy itself is a risk factor for development of sepsis caused by *Y. enterocolitica* because of the ability of the microbe to extract iron from this compound. Immunosuppressive therapies, diabetes mellitus, and malnutrition also may predispose to development of *Y. enterocolitica* bacteremia.[47]

Postinfectious Syndromes

A reactive arthritis may occur 1 to 14 (usually 4 to 10) days after the cessation of acute illness.* Most such events occur in adults,

---

*See references 7, 8, 10, 13, 83, 86, 166, 193, 201, 210.

with a slight female predominance, but 8 of 74 cases in one series from Sweden were in children aged 11 to 20 years old (5 boys, 3 girls).[210] In a series from the Netherlands, 10 percent of children with yersiniosis, most of whom were aged 7 years old or older, developed arthritis.[86] The knees, ankles, and wrists are affected most commonly, and in approximately 50 percent of cases, only one or two joints are involved. Hands, fingers, toes, shoulders, hips, and elbows also may be involved. Pain usually is severe, and the arthritis is additive and usually not migratory. The inflammatory process is self-limited and may persist for 2 months or longer in two thirds of cases, with one third persisting for 4 months or longer.

The erythrocyte sedimentation rate exceeds 60 mm/hr in approximately 50 percent of cases. Joint effusions usually are inflammatory, but cell counts and differentials vary and occasionally mimic septic arthritis. Immune complexes have been found in joint fluid. Nonsteroidal anti-inflammatory drugs and corticosteroids, intra-articular and systemically administered, have been used for symptomatic relief for this process.[165]

Erythema nodosum also occurs as a postinfectious manifestation, more often in adults than in children. It can occur alone or in association with arthritis.[86] Tendinitis, myositis, myocarditis, urethritis, uveitis, and conjunctivitis also can occur in association with arthritis. Many but not all patients who develop these postinfectious reactions are HLA-B27 positive.[1] Some patients manifest full Reiter syndrome.[86,109,170,182] Acute glomerulonephritis has been linked to infection with serotype O:3 strains in one series of adults.[60]

Yersinia antigens, but not intact bacteria, have been found in synovial tissue obtained several weeks to months after onset of reactive arthritis. *Y. enterocolitica* is able to survive within in vitro cultures of human synovial cells for 6 weeks, with resultant deposition of residual antigen aggregates within the cells.[90] Synovial fluid–derived T cells from patients with *Y. enterocolitica*–induced reactive arthritis have been shown to respond to several *Y. enterocolitica* antigens: heat shock protein 60, urease beta subunit, ribosomal L2 protein, and a region of the plasmid-encoded tyrosine phosphatase YopH that is highly homologous to the catalytic domain of eukaryotic protein tyrosine phosphatases.[114,134,155]

Epitopes on *Yersinia*-produced proteins likely trigger cross-reactive immunologic recognition of host proteins that leads to chronic inflammation in susceptible individuals.[95] High levels of antibodies that react with 60 kd recombinant *Yersinia* heat shock protein have been found in HLA-B27–positive individuals with acute anterior uveitis or pars planitis.[31]

Antibodies against *Y. enterocolitica* have been detected in patients with disorders of the thyroid, including Graves disease, thyroid adenoma, and Hashimoto thyroiditis.[178] A Danish twin study found no increased risk of thyroid antibodies after *Y. enterocolitica* infection, however.[77] These observations may reflect autoantibodies that cross-react with *Yersinia* epitopes, rather than a causal link between yersiniosis and thyroid disease.[47,164]

Brachial plexus neuropathy and transverse myelitis, each occurring after the resolution of gastrointestinal symptoms caused by *Y. enterocolitica*, have been described in one patient.[187] Various chronic ailments have been described among a group of 160 Scandinavian patients observed for 4 to 14 years after having acute yersiniosis.[172] Ailments included persistent joint complaints, ankylosing spondylitis (in HLA-B27–positive patients), iridocyclitis, chronic hepatitis, chronic abdominal pain, rheumatoid arthritis, chronic nephritis, thyroid disease, and neurologic ailments. Observed deaths among these patients exceeded the expected number. These findings require confirmation before causal links can be considered.

YERSINIA PSEUDOTUBERCULOSIS

The pseudoappendicular syndrome that results from mesenteric adenitis is the primary disease produced by *Y. pseudotuberculosis*.* The chief complaint is abdominal pain, either diffuse or localized to the right lower quadrant. Fever (38° C to 40° C) almost always is present. Tenderness over the McBurney point usually is present. All of these symptoms are highly suggestive of acute appendicitis. Diarrhea may occur but often is absent. Mild leukocytosis occurs, but white blood cell counts usually are less than 20,000/mm[3]. The clinical course almost always is benign, with recovery usually beginning approximately the fifth day of illness. On laparotomy, the appendix is normal in most cases but occasionally appears inflamed or suppurative. The mesenteric lymph nodes are enlarged and may appear necrotic.

Efforts have been made to distinguish the pseudoappendicular syndrome caused by *Y. pseudotuberculosis* from that caused by *Y. enterocolitica*.[24,66] *Y. pseudotuberculosis* adenitis is less likely to have associated enterocolitis and may have a shorter febrile course, but no clear distinction can be made on clinical grounds alone.

A fulminant typhoidal or septicemic form of infection caused by *Y. pseudotuberculosis* can occur but seems to affect primarily older adults with debilitating conditions, such as diabetes or liver disease. This syndrome often is fatal.[105,171] Isolated cervical adenitis, liver abscess, and terminal ileitis have been described.[79,207] Subacute and recurrent disease can occur.[126]

Erythema nodosum[171] and nonsuppurative arthritis[37] also have been reported in association with infection caused by *Y. pseudotuberculosis*. In an outbreak related to eating contaminated grated carrots in Finland in 2003, erythema nodosum was seen in numerous patients with gastrointestinal illness.[94] Median time from exposure to development of gastrointestinal symptoms was 8 days. Median time from exposure to development of erythema nodosum was 19 days (see Fig. 123–2). One patient developed reactive arthritis in a similar time frame.

Yersinia pseudotuberculosis and Kawasaki Disease–like Illness

In Korea and Japan, *Y. pseudotuberculosis* strains have been responsible for a clinical syndrome that can mimic Kawasaki disease.[37] This manifestation of disease occurs primarily in outbreaks and has been described as scarlet fever–like.[150] A transient (2 to 3 days) erythematous maculopapular rash, strawberry tongue, conjunctivitis, and desquamation can occur, generally in association with gastrointestinal symptoms and fever. Erythema nodosum, lymphadenopathy, uveitis, and coronary aneurysms have occurred in some of these cases, as has acute interstitial nephritis, which can lead to transient renal failure.[3,112,150] Among a series of 33 patients (median age, 5 years) with such presentations, 20 had elevated antibody titers against *Y. pseudotuberculosis*–derived mitogen, which can function as a superantigen.[3] As in Kawasaki disease, Vβ3 T lymphocytes were increased in many of these patients compared with healthy control subjects.

DIFFERENTIAL DIAGNOSIS

The differential diagnosis of *Yersinia* enterocolitis includes viral and other bacterial causes of acute gastroenteritis. When the symptoms of mesenteric adenitis are predominant and severe, appendicitis and other causes of an acute abdomen must be considered. The acute terminal ileitis caused by *Yersinia* infections

---

*See references 20, 50, 55, 57, 66, 84, 89, 104, 105, 126, 150, 169, 171, 203, 207.

also can be similar to the gastrointestinal manifestations of Crohn disease, ulcerative colitis, cat-scratch disease, anisakiasis, amebiasis, actinomycosis, typhoid fever, and lymphoma.[64,86,150,200,207] Cases of infection caused by *Y. enterocolitica* with concomitant recovery of *Salmonella, Campylobacter,* and rotavirus antigen in stool specimens have been observed.[1]

DIAGNOSIS

The most effective approach to the diagnosis of yersiniosis is isolation of the organism from the stool of patients with enteritis caused by *Y. enterocolitica* or from the infected mesenteric lymph nodes of patients infected by *Y. pseudotuberculosis. Y. enterocolitica* occasionally can be recovered from involved mesenteric lymph nodes or the distal ileum.[47] Cultures of feces from individuals with acute suppurative mesenteric adenitis usually fail to grow either organism.

Isolating *Yersinia* organisms from extraintestinal specimens such as lymph nodes and blood is not difficult because they grow on ordinary media (e.g., blood agar) and on several selective and differential media employed for enteric bacteria. Isolating from fecal specimens is more difficult, however, because *Yersinia* multiply more slowly than other enteric bacteria at 37° C and have no characteristic colony morphology. Selective media have been developed, but many clinical laboratories culture stool specimens for *Yersinia* spp. only on request because of the costs of these media and the relatively low frequency of occurrences of these pathogens in the community.

Yersinia organisms grow well on MacConkey agar but are much smaller than are other enteric bacteria after standard incubation at 37° C. Cefsulodin-irgasan-novobiocin agar plates have been designed specifically for the isolation of *Yersinia* spp. from stool specimens. After being incubated for 48 hours, *Yersinia* colonies appear dark pink with translucent borders and occasionally are surrounded by a zone of precipitated bile. Cefsulodin-irgasan-novobiocin agar inhibits the growth of most other bacteria except for *Citrobacter* spp. (positive citrate reactions of which allow their distinction). If a dedicated medium for *Yersinia* isolation is not used, MacConkey agar can be examined after 24 hours at 35° C to 37° C for small colorless colonies that become much larger after an additional 24 hours of incubation at room temperature. Most *Y. enterocolitica* strains are lactose-negative.[69] *Yersinia* spp. can be differentiated readily from *Salmonella* spp. because the latter are motile at 37° C, urease-negative, citrate-positive, and lysine-positive. Most *Salmonella* strains also produce gas during fermentation and produce hydrogen sulfide. *Shigella* are urease-negative and lack motility at room temperature.[186]

Yersinia spp. grow faster at 37° C than at room temperature. Growth occurs readily at 22° C to 28° C, however, and these lower temperatures are recommended for primary isolation.[69] Because of the ability of *Yersinia* spp. to grow at even colder temperatures, specimens can be inoculated into phosphate-buffered saline, refrigerated at 4° C to 6° C, and subcultured periodically (up to 4 weeks) if the routine plates that were inoculated with the specimen remain negative. Such "cold enrichment" greatly enhances the isolation rate of *Yersinia* spp. and may be the most reliable method for isolating these organisms from fecal specimens. Many of the *Yersinia* isolates recovered by cold enrichment, however, represent either *Y. enterocolitica* serotypes, which usually are not associated with human disease, or other *Yersinia* spp., which have roles that remain unclear.

Pathologic or virulent *Yersinia* strains can be distinguished in most instances from nonpathogenic strains by three biochemical tests that are associated with absence of the virulence plasmid. The virulent strains lack pyrazinamidase activity, do not ferment salicin, and do not hydrolyze esculin. On Congo red–magnesium

oxalate agar during incubation at 36° C, fresh pathologic isolates (but not those that have been subcultured serially) grow as small red colonies, showing the virulence plasmid-determined properties of Congo red dye uptake and calcium-dependent growth.[54]

SEROLOGY

Serology can be performed with microtiter techniques and is most reliable for serotypes O:3 and O:9 of *Y. enterocolitica*. Antibody to the infecting serotype usually is absent at the onset of disease. Peak titers usually are reached 3 to 4 weeks after onset of clinical illness and decrease during the next 3 to 5 months. Low postconvalescent titers may persist for months. Microhemagglutination, complement fixation, and enzyme immunoassays are available in a few commercial laboratories.[25,69,200]

Agglutinin titers of 1:128 or higher for *Y. enterocolitica* in previously normal healthy individuals suggest infection. Titers of 1:200 or greater were present within 3 weeks of onset of illness in 62 of 65 Canadian children who had infection with serotype O:3. Fourfold increases in titer rarely were seen. Negative or minimal titers (≤1:32) do not rule out yersiniosis in infants or immunosuppressed patients. Serologic responses occur more commonly and are of higher titer among patients with extraintestinal systemic infection. Prozone reactions may occur at dilutions of 1:32 or lower. Marked cross-agglutination occurs between *Y. enterocolitica* serotype O:9 and *Brucella abortus, Morganella morganii,* and *Salmonella*.[25,131] Antibodies to *Y. pseudotuberculosis* often are detectable at the onset of clinical signs of infection and may be highest during the acute phase of illness.[84]

MOLECULAR TECHNIQUES

PCR assays have been developed for *Y. enterocolitica* and *Y. pseudotuberculosis* with use of primers that allow assessment of 16S rRNA sequences and of specific plasmid-encoded and chromosome-encoded genes.[37,116,143,144,204,206] PCR techniques have been used to identify *Yersinia* organisms in blood, tissue, stool, water, and food samples.[78,115]

TREATMENT

Most patients with yersiniosis do not require treatment because the disease usually is self-limited. Seriously ill patients generally have responded to treatment with chloramphenicol, gentamicin, or tetracyclines, but clinical success has not been uniform. Of these agents, tetracyclines have been the traditional agent of choice.[66,200] *Y. enterocolitica* isolates resistant to the tetracyclines have been reported in recent years, however. Two percent of a sample of *Y. enterocolitica* isolates from Canada in 1992 were resistant to tetracycline,[154] and 10 percent of a sample of *Y. enterocolitica* isolates from the Netherlands from 1982 to 1991 were resistant to doxycycline.[188]

More than 99 percent of 1060 isolates of *Y. enterocolitica* collected in Canada in the years 1972 to 1976, 1980, 1985, and 1990 were susceptible in vitro to piperacillin, cefotaxime, aztreonam, gentamicin, tobramycin, amikacin, trimethoprim-sulfamethoxazole, chloramphenicol, and ciprofloxacin. No evidence of decreasing susceptibility to any of these agents was found across the periods that were sampled. These results were mirrored by a study of 335 isolates obtained in the Netherlands from 1982 to 1991. All of these isolates were susceptible to ceftazidime, cefepime, imipenem, trimethoprim-sulfamethoxazole, ciprofloxacin, and ofloxacin. Aminoglycosides were effective against more than 99 percent, chloramphenicol was effective against 94 percent, and cefuroxime was effective against 90 percent. Seven multidrug-resistant isolates were present among the isolates from Canada, but none was found among the isolates from the Netherlands.[154,188]

Most *Y. enterocolitica* isolates, regardless of serotype, are resistant to ampicillin, ticarcillin, and first-generation cephalosporins. Most of them also are resistant to amoxicillin–clavulanic acid. Azithromycin was active in vitro against 50 percent of the 335 isolates in the Netherlands, but almost all isolates were resistant to erythromycin and clarithromycin.[154,188]

The decreasing effectiveness of tetracyclines in vitro raises the question of whether these agents should be the first choice for treatment of infection caused by *Y. enterocolitica*. A retrospective review of 43 cases (with patient ages ranging from 3 to 89 years) treated for *Y. enterocolitica* septicemia in France between 1985 and 1991 showed that third-generation cephalosporins were effective in 85 percent of cases in which they were used, although aminoglycosides or fluoroquinolones usually were administered concurrently.[61] Fluoroquinolones alone or in combination with other agents cured all 15 patients. Seven children with bacteremia and diarrhea in Michigan responded well to cefotaxime.[1]

In a double-blind, placebo-controlled trial of trimethoprim-sulfamethoxazole for treatment of children with gastroenteritis caused by *Y. enterocolitica*, the clinical course of illness was not shortened.[151] The children had been ill for a mean of 12 days before treatment was begun, however.

Systemic infections, extraintestinal focal infections, and enterocolitis in compromised hosts should be treated with antibiotics.[47] The in vitro susceptibilities and limited clinical data suggest that children with such infections should be treated with a third-generation cephalosporin, an aminoglycoside, or both. Trimethoprim-sulfamethoxazole also may be used.[38,86] Fluoroquinolones also probably would be effective. Cefotaxime and ceftriaxone were effective in treating bacteremia in a series of 12 children.[2]

Even fewer clinical and in vitro susceptibility data are available for *Y. pseudotuberculosis*. These infections probably can be managed identically to *Y. enterocolitica* infections. All isolates of *Y. enterocolitica* and *Y. pseudotuberculosis* should be examined for susceptibility to a variety of antibacterial drugs.

OTHER *YERSINIA* SPECIES

Eight other "non-*pestis*" *Yersinia* spp. (*Yersinia frederiksenii, Yersinia intermedia, Yersinia kristensenii, Yersinia aldovae, Yersinia bercovieri, Yersinia mollaretii, Yersinia rohdei,* and *Yersinia ruckeri*) occasionally have been isolated from clinical specimens, but their roles as human pathogens remain unclear.[69,177,189] Each except *Y. aldovae* has been isolated from humans worldwide, including individuals with gastrointestinal disorders.[189] These microbes also can be found in fresh-water sources, sewage, dogs, pigs, cattle, wild mammals, birds, reptiles, fish, and some foods, especially milk and meat products.

These organisms are similar biochemically to one another and have been termed atypical *Y. enterocolitica*.[47] None contains the *Yersinia* virulence plasmid pYV.[135] Some contain other large plasmids distinct from pYV, carriage of which may be associated with the ability to cause diarrhea in humans.[152,189] A heat-stable enterotoxin has been found in isolates of *Y. bercovieri*.[190] These *Yersinia* spp. can grow at 4° C and on cefsulodin-irgasan-novobiocin agar and can multiply in refrigerated foods.

These species occasionally may cause diarrhea and other gastrointestinal symptoms, especially in immunocompromised hosts or individuals with gastric acid suppression.[124] Use of cold enrichment techniques may enhance recovery of these organisms. Their isolation from clinical specimens neither should be disregarded nor should be deemed causative of clinical disease without careful epidemiologic considerations.[69] *Y. bercovieri, Y. mollaretii,* and *Y. rohdei* can be misidentified as *Y. enterocolitica* by commercial identification systems used in many clinical laboratories. Differences in colony morphology, pyrazinamide reactions (negative for *Y. enterocolitica*), and other biochemical tests can be used to distinguish them from *Y. enterocolitica*.[73,100]

REFERENCES

1. Abdel-Haq, N. M., Asmar, B. I., Abuhammour, W. M., and Brown, W. J.: *Yersinia enterocolitica* infection in children. Pediatr. Infect. Dis. J. *19*:954-958, 2000.
2. Abdel-Haq, N. M., Papadopol, R., Asmar, B. I., and Brown, W. J.: Antibiotic susceptibilities of *Yersinia enterocolitica* recovered from children over a 12-year period. Int. J. Antimicrob. Agents *27*:449-452, 2006.
3. Abe, J., Onimaru, M., Matsumoto, S., et al.: Clinical role for a superantigen in *Yersinia pseudotuberculosis* infection. J. Clin. Invest. *99*:1823-1830, 1997.
4. Achtman, M., Zurth, K., Morelli, G., et al.: *Yersinia pestis,* the cause of plague, is a recently emerged clone of *Yersinia pseudotuberculosis*. Proc. Natl. Acad. Sci. U. S. A. *96*:14043-14048, 1999.
5. Ackers, M. L., Schoenfeld, S., Markman, J., et al.: An outbreak of *Yersinia enterocolitica* O:8 infections associated with pasteurized milk. J. Infect. Dis. *181*:1834-1837, 2000.
6. Adamkiewicz, T. V., Berkovitch, M., Krishman, C., et al.: Infection due to *Yersinia enterocolitica* in a series of patients with β-thalassemia: Incidence and predisposing factors. Clin. Infect. Dis. *27*:1362-1366, 1998.
7. Ahlqvist, J., Ahvonen, P., Räsänen, J. A., et al.: Enteric infection with *Yersinia enterocolitica*: Large pyroninophilic cell reaction in mesenteric lymph nodes associated with early production of specific antibodies. Acta Pathol. Microbiol. Scand. *79A*:109-122, 1971.
8. Aho, K., Ahvonen, P., Lassus, A., et al.: HL-A 27 in reactive arthritis: A study of *Yersinia* arthritis and Reiter's disease. Arthritis Rheum. *17*:521-526, 1974.
9. Ahvonen, P.: Human yersiniosis in Finland, 1: Bacteriology and serology. Ann. Clin. Res. *4*:30-38, 1972.
10. Ahvonen, P., Sievers, K., and Aho, K.: Arthritis associated with *Yersinia enterocolitica* infection. Acta Rheumatol. Scand. *15*:232-253, 1969.
11. Albrecht, H.: Zur Aetiologie der Enteritis follicularis suppurativa. Wien. Klin. Wochenschr. *23*:991, 1910.
12. alMohsen, I., Luedtke, G., and English, B. K.: Invasive infections caused by *Yersinia enterocolitica* in infants. Pediatr. Infect. Dis. J. *16*:253-255, 1997.
13. Anonymous: Worldwide spread of infection with *Yersinia enterocolitica*. W. H. O. Chron. *30*:494-496, 1976.
14. Arvastson, B., Damgaard, K., and Winblad, S.: Clinical symptoms of infection with *Yersinia enterocolitica*. Scand. J. Infect. Dis. *3*:37-40, 1971.
15. Asakawa, Y., Akahane, S., Kheata, N., et al.: Two community outbreaks of human infection with *Yersinia enterocolitica*. J. Hyg. (Camb.) *71*:715-723, 1973.
16. Attwood, S. E., Healy, K., Caffarkey, M. T., et al.: *Yersinia* infection and abdominal pain. Lancet *1*:529-533, 1987.
17. Bergstrand, C. G., and Winblad, S.: Clinical manifestations of infection with *Yersinia enterocolitica* in children. Acta Paediatr. Scand. *63*:875-877, 1974.
18. Bissett, M. L.: *Yersinia enterocolitica* isolates from humans in California, 1968-1975. J. Clin. Microbiol. *4*:137-144, 1976.
19. Black, R. E., Jackson, R. J., Tsai, T., et al.: Epidemic *Yersinia enterocolitica* infection due to contaminated chocolate milk. N. Engl. J. Med. *298*:76-79, 1978.
20. Blattner, R. J.: Acute mesenteric lymphadenitis. J. Pediatr. *74*:479-481, 1969.
21. Bottone, E. J.: *Yersinia enterocolitica*: A panoramic view of a charismatic microorganism. Crit. Rev. Microbiol. *5*:211-241, 1977.
22. Bottone, E. J.: Current trends of *Yersinia enterocolitica* isolates in the New York City area. J. Clin. Microbiol. *17*:63-67, 1983.
23. Bottone, E. J.: *Yersinia enterocolitica*: Overview and epidemiologic correlates. Microbes Infect. *1*:323-333, 1999.
24. Bottone, E. J., Chester, B., Malowany, M. S., et al.: Unusual *Yersinia enterocolitica* isolates not associated with mesenteric lymphadenitis. Appl. Microbiol. *27*:858-861, 1974.
25. Bottone, E. J., and Sheehan, D. J.: *Yersinia enterocolitica*: Guidelines for serologic diagnosis of human infections. Rev. Infect. Dis. *5*:898-906, 1983.
26. Bovallius, A., and Nilsson, G.: Ingestion and survival of *Y. pseudotuberculosis* in HeLa cells. Can. J. Microbiol. *21*:1997-2007, 1975.
27. Bradford, W., Noce, P., and Gutman, L.: Pathologic features of enteric infection with *Yersinia enterocolitica*. Arch. Pathol. *98*:17-22, 1974.
28. Braunstein, H., Tucker, E. B., and Gibson, B. C.: Mesenteric lymphadenitis due to *Yersinia enterocolitica*: Report of a case. Am. J. Clin. Pathol. *55*:506-510, 1971.
29. Brennessel, D. J., Robbins, H., and Hindman, S.: Pyomyositis caused by *Yersinia enterocolitica*. J. Clin. Microbiol. *20*:293-294, 1984.
30. Brocklehurst, T. E., Zaman-Wong, C. H., and Lund, B. M.: A note on the microbiology of retail packs of prepared salad vegetables. J. Appl. Bacteriol. *63*:409-415, 1987.

31. Cancino-Diaz, J. C., Vargas-Rodriguez, L., Grinberg-Zylberbaum, N., et al.: High levels of IgG class antibodies to recombinant HSP60 kDA of *Yersinia enterocolitica* in sera of patients with uveitis. Br. J. Ophthalmol. *88*:247-250, 2004.

32. Caplan, L. M.: *Yersinia enterocolitica* septicemia. Am. J. Clin. Pathol. *69*:189, 1978.

33. Caprioli, T., Drapeau, A. J., and Kasatiya, S.: *Yersinia enterocolitica*: Serotypes and biotypes isolated from humans and the environment in Quebec, Canada. J. Clin. Microbiol. *8*:7-11, 1978.

34. Centers for Disease Control: *Yersinia enterocolitica* bacteremia and endotoxin shock associated with red blood cell transfusions-United States, 1991. M. M. W. R. Morb. Mortal. Wkly. Rep. *40*:176-178, 1991.

35. Centers for Disease Control and Prevention: Incidence of food-borne illnesses: Preliminary data from the Food-borne Diseases Active Surveillance Network (FoodNet)—United States, 1998. M. M. W. R. Morb. Mortal. Wkly. Rep. *48*:189-194, 1999.

36. Centers for Disease Control and Prevention: *Yersinia enterocolitica* gastroenteritis among infants exposed to chitterlings—Chicago, Illinois, 2002. M. M. W. R. Morb. Mortal. Wkly. Rep. *52*:956-958, 2003.

37. Cheong, H. I., Park, H. W., Koo, J. W., et al.: Diagnosis of *Yersinia pseudotuberculosis* infection by polymerase chain reaction. Pediatr. Infect. Dis. J. *15*:596-599, 1996.

38. Cherchi, B., Pacifico, L., Cossellu, S., et al.: Prospective study of *Yersinia enterocolitica* infection in thalassemic patients. Pediatr. Infect. Dis. J. *14*:579-584, 1995.

39. Chessum, B., Frengley, J. D., Fleck, D. G., et al.: Case of septicemia due to *Yersinia enterocolitica*. B. M. J. *3*:466, 1971.

40. Chin, G. N., and Noble, R. C.: Ocular involvement in *Yersinia enterocolitica* infections presenting as Parinaud's oculoglandular syndrome. Am. J. Ophthalmol. *83*:19-23, 1977.

41. Cimolai, N., Trombley, C., and Blair, G.: Implications of *Yersinia enterocolitica* biotyping. Arch. Dis. Child. *70*:19-21, 1994.

42. Cookson, S. T., Arduino, M. J., Aguero, S. M., et al.: *Yersinia enterocolitica*–contaminated red blood cells (RBCs): An emerging threat to blood safety. Abstract J99. Abstracts of the 36th Interscience Conference on Antimicrobial Agents and Chemotherapy, New Orleans, LA, American Society for Microbiology, 1996, p. 237.

43. Cornelis, G., Laroche, Y., Balligand, G., et al.: *Yersinia enterocolitica*, a primary model for bacterial invasiveness. Rev. Infect. Dis. *9*:64-86, 1987.

44. Cornelis, G. R.: *Yersinia* type III secretion: Send in the effectors. J. Cell Biol. *158*:401-408, 2002.

45. Cornelis, G. R., Boland, A., Boyd, A. P., et al.: The virulence plasmid of *Yersinia*, an antihost genome. Microbiol. Mol. Biol. Rev. *62*:1315-1352, 1998.

46. Cossart, P.: Subversion of the mammalian cell cytoskeleton by invasive bacteria. J. Clin. Invest. *100*(Suppl.):S33-S37, 1997.

47. Cover, T. L., and Aber, R. C.: *Yersinia enterocolitica*. N. Engl. J. Med. *321*:16-24, 1989.

48. Cusack, D., Martin, P., Schinittger, T., et al.: I.g.A. Nephropathy in association with *Yersinia enterocolitica*. Ir. J. Med. Sci. *152*:311-312, 1983.

49. Dajani, A., and Maurer, M.: Is *Yersinia enterocolitica* gastroenteritis a Canadian disease? J. Pediatr. *97*:165-166, 1980.

50. Daniels, J. J. H.: Enteric infections with *Pasteurella pseudotuberculosis*: An acute abdominal syndrome. J. Int. Coll. Surg. *38*:397-411, 1962.

51. Delorme, J., Laverdiere, M., Martineau, B., et al.: Yersiniosis in children. Can. Med. Assoc. J. *110*:281-284, 1974.

52. Dube, P. H., Handley, S. A., Lewis, J., and Miller, V. L.: Protective role of interleukin 6 during *Yersinia enterocolitica* infection is mediated through the modulation of inflammatory cytokines. Infect. Immun. *72*:3561-3570, 2004.

53. Fällman, M., Persson, C., and Wolf-Watz, H.: *Yersinia* proteins that target host cell signaling pathways. J. Clin. Invest. *100*(Suppl.):S15-S18, 1997.

54. Farmer, J. J., III, Carter, G. P., Miller, V. L., et al.: Pyrazinamidase, CR-MOX agar, salicin fermentation-esculin hydrolysis, and d-xylose fermentation for identifying pathogenic serotypes of *Yersinia enterocolitica*. J. Clin. Microbiol. *30*:2589-2594, 1992.

55. Feldman, W. H., and Karlson, A. G.: Pseudotuberculosis. *In* Hull, T. (ed.): Diseases Transmitted from Animals to Man. 5th ed. Springfield, IL, Charles C Thomas, 1963.

56. Fenwick, S. G., and McCarthy, M. D.: *Yersinia enterocolitica* is a common cause of gastroenteritis in Auckland. N. Z. Med. J. *108*:269-271, 1995.

57. Finlayson, N. B., and Fagundes, B.: *Pasteurella pseudotuberculosis* infection: Three cases in the United States. Am. J. Clin. Pathol. *55*:24-29, 1971.

58. Fontani, C., Valeri, M., and Pifferesi, M.: *Yersinia enterocolitica* septicemia in a girl with thalassemia major. Pediatr. Med. Clin. *10*:657-658, 1988.

59. Frederiksen, W.: Human pseudotuberculosis in Denmark. Symp. Series Immunobiol. Stand. *9*:137, 1968.

60. Friedberg, M., Denneberg, T., Brun, C., et al.: Glomerulonephritis in infections with *Yersinia enterocolitica* O-serotype 3. Acta Med. Scand. *209*:103-110, 1981.

61. Gayraud, M., Scavizzi, M. R., Mollaret, H. H., et al.: Antibiotic treatment of *Yersinia enterocolitica* septicemia: A retrospective review of 43 cases. Clin. Infect. Dis. *17*:405-410, 1993.

62. Gilbert, R.: Interesting cases and unusual specimens. Annual Report of the Division of Laboratory Research. Albany, NY, New York State Department of Health, 1933, p. 57.

63. Gillespie, J. H., and Timoney, J. F.: Hagan and Bruner's Infectious Diseases of Domestic Animals. 7th ed. Ithaca, NY, Comstock, 1981, pp. 96-97.

64. Gleason, T. H., and Patterson, S. D.: The pathology of *Yersinia enterocolitica* ileocolitis. Am. J. Surg. Pathol. *6*:347-355, 1982.

65. Glud, T. K., and Laursen, B.: *Yersinia enterocolitica* infection complicated by severe thrombocytopenia resistant to high-dose intravenous immunoglobulin. Acta Med. Scand. *217*:233-234, 1985.

66. Goodwin, C. S.: *Yersinia* infections including mesenteric adenitis, and gastrointestinal tuberculosis. *In* Goodwin, C. S. (ed.): Microbes and Infection of the Gut. Melbourne, Blackwell Scientific, 1984, pp. 241-251.

67. Gort, A. S., and Miller, V. L.: Identification and characterization of *Yersinia enterocolitica* genes induced during systemic infection. Infect. Immun. *68*:6635-6642, 2000.

68. Grant, T., Bennett-Wood, V., and Robins-Browne, R. M.: Characterization of the interaction between *Yersinia enterocolitica* biotype 1A and phagocytes and epithelial cells in vitro. Infect. Immun. *67*:4307-4375, 1999.

69. Gray, L. D.: *Escherichia, Salmonella, Shigella*, and *Yersinia*. *In* Murray, P. R. (ed.): Manual of Clinical Microbiology. 6th ed. Washington, D.C., ASM Press, 1995, pp. 450-456.

70. Gutman, L. T., Ottesen, E. A., Quan, T. J., et al.: An inter-familial outbreak of *Yersinia enterocolitica* enteritis. N. Engl. J. Med. *288*:1372-1377, 1973.

71. Haenselt, V.: Zur Kenntnis der abscedierenden reticulocytaren Lymphadenitis (Masshoff). Arzt. Wochenschr. *12*:509, 1957.

72. Hagan, A. G., Lassen, J., and Berge, L. N.: Erysipelas-like disease caused by *Yersinia enterocolitica*. Scand. J. Infect. Dis. *6*:101-102, 1974.

73. Hallanvuo, S., Peltola., J., Heiskanen, T., and Siitonen, A.: Simplified phenotypic scheme evaluated by 16S rRNA sequencing for differentiation between *Yersinia enterocolitica* and *Y. enterocolitica*-like species. J. Clin. Microbiol. *44*:1077-1080, 2006.

74. Hallstrom, K., Sairanen, E., and Ohela, K.: A pilot clinical study of yersinioses in South-Eastern Finland. Acta Med. Scand. *191*:485-491, 1972.

75. Hamasaki, S., Hayashidani, H., Keneko, K., et al.: A survey for *Yersinia pseudotuberculosis* in migratory birds in coastal Japan. J. Wildl. Dis. *25*:401-403, 1989.

76. Handley, S. A., Newberry, R. D., Miller, V. L.: *Yersinia enterocolitica* invasion-dependent and invasion-independent mechanisms of systemic dissemination. Infect. Immun. *73*:8453-8455, 2005.

77. Hansen, P. S., Wenzel, B. E., Brix, T. H., and Hegedus, L.: *Yersinia enterocolitica* infection does not confer an increased risk of thyroid antibodies: Evidence from a Danish twin study. Clin. Exp. Immunol. *146*:32-38, 2006.

78. HaoXuan, Z., JiDe, W., MingJun, Z., et al.: *Yersinia enterocolitica* identification in stool samples using real time PCR. Diagn. Microbiol. Infect. Dis. doi:10.1016/j.diagmicrobio. 2006.07.016.

79. Hassig, A., Karrer, J., and Pusterla, F.: Über Pseudotuberculoses beim Menschen. Schweiz. Med. Wochenschr. *79*:791, 1949.

80. Hastings, J. G. M., Batta, K., Gourevitch, D., et al.: Fatal transfusion reaction due to *Yersinia enterocolitica*. J. Hosp. Infect. *27*:75-79, 1993.

81. Hayashidani, H., Ohtomo, Y., Toyokawa, Y., et al.: Potential sources of sporadic human infection with *Yersinia enterocolitica* serovar O:8 in Aomori Prefecture, Japan. J. Clin. Microbiol. *33*:1253-1257, 1995.

82. Heesemann, J., Gaede, K., and Autenrieth, I. B.: Experimental *Yersinia enterocolitica* infection in rodents: A model for human yersiniosis. A. P. M. I. S. *101*:417-429, 1993.

83. Hewstone, A. S., and Davidson, G. P.: *Yersinia enterocolitica* septicaemia with arthritis in a thalassaemic child. Med. J. Aust. *1*:1035-1038, 1972.

84. Hnatko, S. I., and Rodin, A. E.: *Pasteurella pseudotuberculosis* infection in man. Can. Med. Assoc. J. *88*:1108-1112, 1963.

85. Hoogkamp-Korstanje, J. A. A., De Koning, J., and Samsom, J. P.: Incidence of human infection with *Yersinia enterocolitica* serotypes O3, O8, and O9 and the use of indirect immunofluorescence in diagnosis. J. Infect. Dis. *153*:138-141, 1986.

86. Hoogkamp-Korstanje, J. A. A., and Stolk-Engelaar, V. M. M.: *Yersinia enterocolitica* infection in children. Pediatr. Infect. Dis. J. *14*:771-775, 1995.

87. Horstebrock, R.: Zur Frage der "abscedierenden, retikulocytaren Lymphadenitis (Masshoff)." Zentralbl. Allg. Pathol. *91*:221, 1954.

88. Hubbert, W. T.: Yersiniosis in mammals and birds in the United States: Case reports and review. Am. J. Trop. Med. Hyg. *21*:458-463, 1972.

89. Hubbert, W. T., Petenyi, C. W., Glasgow, L. A., et al.: *Yersinia tuberculosis* infection in the United States: Septicemia, appendicitis, and mesenteric lymphadenitis. Am. J. Trop. Med. Hyg. *20*:679-684, 1971.

90. Huppertz, H., and Heesemann, J.: Experimental *Yersinia* infection of human synovial cells: Persistence of live bacteria and generation of bacterial antigen deposits including "ghosts," nucleic acid-free bacterial rods. Infect. Immun. *64*:1484-1487, 1996.

91. Inoue, H., Nakashima, H., Ishida, T., et al.: Three outbreaks of *Yersinia pseudotuberculosis* infections. Zentralbl. Bakteriol. Mikrobiol. Hyg. *186*:504-511, 1988.

92. Isberg, R. R.: Mammalian cell adhesion functions and cellular penetration of enteropathogenic *Yersinia* species. Mol. Microbiol. *3*:1449-1453, 1989.

93. Isberg, R. R., Voorhis, D. L., and Falkow, S.: Identification of invasin: A protein that allows enteric bacteria to penetrate cultured mammalian cells. Cell *50*:769-778, 1987.

94. Jalava, K., Hakkinen, M., Valkonen, M., et al.: An outbreak of gastrointestinal illness and erythema nodosum from grated carrots contaminated with *Yersinia pseudotuberculosis*. J. Infect. Dis. *194*:1209-1216, 2006.

95. Jansson, E., Wallgren, G. R., and Ahvonen, P.: *Yersinia enterocolitica* as a cause of acute mesenteric lymphadenitis. Acta Paediatr. Scand. *57*:448-450, 1968.

96. Jepsen, O. B., Korner, B., Lauritsen, K. B., et al.: *Yersinia enterocolitica* infection in patients with acute surgical abdominal disease: A prospective study. Scand. J. Infect. Dis. *8*:189-194, 1976.

97. Jones, B. L., and Hanson, M. F.: Prevention of transfusion of *Yersinia enterocolitica*. J. Hosp. Infect. *28*:236-238, 1994.

98. Kandolo, K., and Wauters, G.: Pyrazinamidase activity in *Yersinia enterocolitica* and related organisms. J. Clin. Microbiol. *21*:980-982, 1985.

99. Kato, Y., Ito, K., Kubo, Y., et al.: Occurrence of *Yersinia enterocolitica* in wild-living birds. Appl. Environ. Microbiol. *49*:198-200, 1985.

100. Kay, B. A., Wachsmuth, K., Gemski, P., et al.: Virulence and phenotypic characterization of *Yersinia enterocolitica* isolated from humans in the United States. J. Clin. Microbiol. *17*:128-138, 1983.

101. Kelly, D. A., Price, E., Jani, B., et al.: *Yersinia* enterocolitis vs. iron overload. J. Pediatr. Gastroenterol. Nutr. *6*:643-645, 1987.

102. Kerschen, E. J., Cohen, D. A., Kaplan, A. M., and Straley, S. C.: The plague virulence protein YopM targets the innate immune response by causing a global depletion of NK cells. Infect. Immun. *72*:4589-4602, 2004.

103. Klein, E. J., Boster, D. R., Stapp, J. R., et al.: Diarrhea etiology in a children's hospital emergency department: a prospective cohort study. Clin. Infect. Dis. *43*:807-813, 2006.

104. Knapp, W.: *Pasteurella pseudotuberculosis* als erreger einer mesenterialen Lymphadenitis beim Menschen. Zentralbl. Bakteriol. *161*:422-424, 1954.

105. Knapp, W.: Mesenteric adenitis due to *Pasteurella pseudotuberculosis* in young people. N. Engl. J. Med. *259*:776-778, 1958.

106. Knapp, W., and Masshoff, W.: Zur Ätiologie der abszedierenden retikulozytaren Lymphadenitis: Einer praktisch wichtigen, vielfach unter dem Bilde einer akuten Appendizitis verlaufenden Erkrankung. Dtsch. Med. Wochenschr. *79*:1266-1271, 1954.

107. Knapp, W., and Steuter, W.: Untersuchungen über den Nachweis komplementbindender und agglutinierender Antikorper gegen *Pasteurella pseudotuberculosis* in Sera infizierter und immunisierter Menschen and Tiere. Z. Immunitatsforsch. Exp. Ther. *113*:370-374, 1956.

108. Knorring, von, J., and Petterson, T.: Haemolytic anaemia complicating *Yersinia enterocolitica* infection: Report of a case. Scand. J. Haematol. *9*:149, 1972.

109. Kobayashi, S., Ogasawara, M., Maeda, K., et al.: Antibodies against *Yersinia enterocolitica* in patients with Reiter's syndrome. J. Lab. Clin. Med. *105*:380-389, 1985.

110. Kohl, S., Jacobson, J. A., and Nahmias, A.: *Yersinia enterocolitica* infections in children. J. Pediatr. *89*:77-79, 1976.

111. Koning-Ward, T. F., and Robins-Browne, R. M.: Analysis of the urease gene complex of members of the genus *Yersinia*. Gene *182*:225-228, 1996.

112. Koo, J. W., Park, S. N., Choi, S. M., et al.: Acute renal failure associated with *Yersinia pseudotuberculosis* infection in children. Pediatr. Nephrol. *10*:582-586, 1996.

113. Krogstad, P., Mendelman, P. M., Miller, V. L., et al.: Clinical and microbiologic characteristics of cutaneous infection with *Yersinia enterocolitica*. J. Infect. Dis. *165*:740-743, 1992.

114. Lahesmaa, R., Soderberg, C., Bliska, J., et al.: Pathogen antigen- and superantigen-reactive synovial fluid T cells in reactive arthritis. J. Infect. Dis. *172*:1290-1297, 1995.

115. Lamps, L. W., Havens, J. M., Gilbrech, L. J., and Scott, M. A.: Molecular biogrouping of pathogenic *Yersinia enterocolitica*: development of a diagnostic PCR assay with histologic correlation. Am. J. Clin. Pathol. *125*:658-664, 2006.

116. Lamps, L. W., Madhusudhan, K. T., Greenson, J. K., et al.: The role of *Yersinia enterocolitica* and *Yersinia pseudotuberculosis* in granulomatous appendicitis: A histologic and molecular study. Am. J. Surg. Pathol. *25*:508-515, 2001.

117. Larsen, J. H.: Human yersiniose. Ugeskr. Laeger *134*:431, 1972.

118. Lee, L. A., Taylor, J., Carter, G. P., et al.: *Yersinia enterocolitica* O:3: An emerging cause of pediatric gastroenteritis in the United States. J. Infect. Dis. *163*:660-663, 1991.

119. Lee, V. T., and Schneewind, O.: Type III secretion machines and the pathogenesis of enteric infections caused by *Yersinia* and *Salmonella* spp. Immunol. Rev. *168*:241-255, 1999.

121. Leino, R., Granfars, K., Havia, T., et al.: Yersiniosis as a gastrointestinal disease. Scand. J. Infect. Dis. *19*:63-68, 1987.

120. Leino, R., and Kalliomaki, J. L.: Yersiniosis as an internal disease. Ann. Intern. Med. *81*:458-461, 1974.

122. Linde, H.-J., Neubauer, H., Meyer, H., et al.: Identification of *Yersinia* species by the Vitek GNI Card. J. Clin. Microbiol. *37*:211-214, 1999.

123. Lobato, M. J., Landeras, E., González-Hevia, M. A., and Mendoza, M. C.: Genetic heterogeneity of clinical strains of *Yersinia enterocolitica* traced by ribotyping and relationships between ribotypes, serotypes, and biotypes. J. Clin. Microbiol. *36*:3297-3302, 1998.

124. Loftus, C. G., Harewood, G. C., Cockerill, F. R., III, and Murray, J. A.: Clinical features of patients with novel *Yersinia* species. Dig. Dis. Sci. *47*:2805-2810, 2002.

125. Mair, N. S.: Yersiniosis (infections due to *Yersinia pseudotuberculosis* and *Yersinia enterocolitica*). *In* Hubbert, W. T., McCollough, W. F., and Schnurrenberger, P. R. (eds.): Diseases Transmitted from Animals to Man. 6th ed. Springfield, IL, Charles C Thomas, 1975, pp. 174-185.

126. Mair, N. S., Mair, H. J., Stirk, E. M., et al.: Three cases of acute mesenteric lymphadenitis due to *Pasteurella pseudotuberculosis*. J. Clin. Pathol. *13*:432-439, 1960.

127. Maki, M., Gronroos, P., and Vesikari, T.: In vitro invasiveness of *Yersinia enterocolitica* isolated from children with diarrhea. J. Infect. Dis. *138*:677-680, 1978.

128. Maki, M., Vesikari, T., Rantala, I., et al.: Yersiniosis in children. Arch. Dis. Child. *55*:861-865, 1980.

129. Makino, S., Okada, Y., Maruyama, T., et al.: PCR-based random amplified polymorphic DNA fingerprinting of *Yersinia pseudotuberculosis* and its practical applications. J. Clin. Microbiol. *32*:65-69, 1994.

130. Malassez, L., and Vignal, W.: Tuberculos zoologique (forme ou aspect ou tuberculose sans bacillus). Arch. Physiol. Norm. Pathol. *53*:2, 1883.

131. Marks, M. I., Pai, C. H., Lafleur, L., et al.: *Yersinia enterocolitica* gastroenteritis: A prospective study of clinical, bacteriologic, and epidemiologic features. J. Pediatr. *96*:26-31, 1980.

132. Masshoff, W.: Eine neuartige Form der mesenterialen Lymphadenitis. Dtsch. Med. Wochenschr. *78*:532-535, 1953.

133. Masshoff, W., and Dolle, W.: Über eine besondere Form der sog. mesenterialen Lymphadenopathie: "Die abscedierende reticulocytare Lymphadenitis." Virchows Arch. Pathol. Anat. *323*:664-684, 1953.

134. Mertz, A. K. H., Ugrinovic, S., Lauster, R., et al.: Characterization of the synovial T cell response to various recombinant *Yersinia* antigens in *Yersinia enterocolitica*–triggered reactive arthritis. Arthritis Rheum. *41*:315-326, 1998.

135. Miller, V. L., Farmer, J. J., III, Hill, W. E., et al.: The ail locus is found uniquely in *Yersinia enterocolitica* serotypes commonly associated with disease. Infect. Immun. *57*:121-131, 1989.

136. Mingrone, M. G., Fantasia, M., Figura, N., et al.: Characteristics of *Yersinia enterocolitica* isolated from children with diarrhea in Italy. J. Clin. Microbiol. *25*:1301-1304, 1987.

137. Mollaret, H.-H.: Un domaine pathologique nouveau. Ann. Biol. Clin. *30*:1-5, 1972.

138. Mollaret, H. H., Bercovier, H., and Alonso, J. M.: Summary of the data received at the WHO Reference Center for *Yersinia enterocolitica*. Contrib. Microbiol. Immunol. *5*:174-184, 1979.

139. Mollaret, H.-H., Omland, T., Henriksen, S. D., et al.: Les septicemies humaines—"*Yersinia enterocolitica*": Propos de dix-sept cas recents. Presse Med. *19*:345, 1971.

140. Mukherjee, S., Keitany, G., Li, Y., et al.: *Yersinia* YopJ acetylates and inhibits kinase activation by blocking phosphorylation. Science *312*:1211-1214, 2006.

141. Najdenski, H., Iteman, I., and Carniel, E.: Efficient subtyping of pathogenic *Yersinia enterocolitica* strains by pulsed-field gel electrophoresis. J. Clin. Microbiol. *32*:2913-2920, 1994.

142. Naqvi, S. H., Swierkosz, E. M., Gerard, J., and Mills, J. R.: Presentation of *Yersinia enterocolitica* enteritis in children. Pediatr. Infect. Dis. J. *12*:386-389, 1993.

143. Neubauer, H., Hensel, A., Aleksic, S., and Meyer, H.: Evaluation of a *Yersinia* adhesion gene (yadA) specific PCR for the identification of enteropathogenic *Yersinia enterocolitica*. Int. J. Food Microbiol. *57*:225-227, 2000.

144. Neubauer, H., Hensel, A., Aleksic, S., and Meyer, H.: Identification of *Yersinia enterocolitica* within the genus *Yersinia*. Syst. Appl. Microbiol. *23*:58-62, 2000.

145. Nikolova, S., Tzvetkov, Y., Najdenski, H., and Vesselinova, A.: Isolation of pathogenic *Yersinia* from animals in Bulgaria. J. Vet. Med. B. Infect. Dis. Vet. Public Health *48*:203-209, 2001.

146. Nilehn, B.: Studies on *Yersinia enterocolitica*: With special reference to bacterial diagnosis and occurrence in human enteric disease. Acta Pathol. Microbiol. Scand. *206*(Suppl.):1-48, 1969.

147. Nilehn, B., and Sjostrom, B.: Studies on *Yersinia enterocolitica*: Occurrence in various groups of acute abdominal disease. Acta Pathol. Microbiol. Scand. *71*:612-628, 1967.

148. Odinot, P. T., Meis, J. F. G. M., Van Den Hurk, P. J. J. C., et al.: PCR-based characterization of *Yersinia enterocolitica*: Comparison with biotyping and serotyping. Epidemiol. Infect. *115*:269-277, 1995.

149. Orth, K., Xu, Z., Mudgett, M. B., et al.: Disruption of signaling by *Yersinia* effector YopJ, a ubiquitin-like protein protease. Science *290*:1594-1597, 2000.

150. Paff, J. R., Triplett, D. A., and Saari, T. N.: Clinical and laboratory aspects of *Yersinia pseudotuberculosis* infection with a report of two cases. Am. J. Clin. Pathol. *66*:101-110, 1976.

151. Pai, C. H., Gillis, F., Tuomanen, E., et al.: Placebo-controlled double-blind evaluation of trimethoprim-sulfamethoxazole treatment of *Yersinia enterocolitica* gastroenteritis. J. Pediatr. *104*:308-311, 1984.

152. Pai, C. H., and Mors, V.: Production of enterotoxin by *Yersinia enterocolitica*. Infect. Immun. *19*:908-911, 1978.

153. Pepe, J. C., Badger, J. L., and Miller, V. L.: Growth phase and low pH affect the thermal regulation of the *Yersinia enterocolitica* inv gene. Mol. Microbiol. *11*:123-125, 1994.

154. Preston, M. A., Brown, S., Borczyk, A. A., et al.: Antimicrobial susceptibility of pathogenic *Yersinia enterocolitica* isolated in Canada from 1972-1990. Antimicrob. Agents Chemother. *38*:2121-2124, 1994.

155. Probst, P., Hermann, E., Hermann-Meyer zum Buschenfelde, K., et al.: Identification of the *Yersinia enterocolitica* urease B subunit as a target anti-

gen for human synovial T lymphocytes in reactive arthritis. Infect. Immun. *61*:4507-4509, 1993.

156. Quan, T. J., Meek, J. L., Tsuchiya, K. R., et al.: Experimental pathogenicity of recent North American isolates of *Yersinia enterocolitica*. J. Infect. Dis. *129*:341-344, 1974.

157. Rabinovitz, M., Stremple, T. H., Granforo, K., et al.: *Yersinia enterocolitica* infections complicated by intestinal perforation. Arch. Intern. Med. *147*:1062-1063, 1987.

158. Rabson, A. R., and Koornhof, H. J.: *Yersinia enterocolitica* infections in South Africa. S. Afr. Med. J. *46*:798-803, 1972.

159. Rakin, A., Noelting, S., Schubert, S., and Heesemann, J.: Common and specific characteristics of the high-pathogenicity island of *Yersinia enterocolitica*. Infect. Immun. *67*:5265-5274, 1999.

160. Randall, K. J., and Mair, N. S.: Family outbreak of *Pasteurella pseudotuberculosis* infection. Lancet *1*:1042-1043, 1962.

161. Ratman, S., Mercer, E., Picco, B., et al.: A nosocomial outbreak due to *Yersinia enterocolitica* serotype O:5, biotype 1. J. Infect. Dis. *145*:242-247, 1982.

162. Ray, S. M., Ahuja, S. D., Blake, P. A., et al.: Population-based surveillance for *Yersinia enterocolitica* infections in FoodNet sites, 1996-1999: Higher risk for disease in infants and minority populations. Clin. Infect. Dis. *38*:S181-S189, 2004.

163. Reed, R. P., Robins-Browne, R. M., and Williams, M. L.: *Yersinia enterocolitica* peritonitis. Clin. Infect. Dis. *25*:1468-1469, 1997.

164. Resetkova, E., Notenboom, R., Arreaza, G., et al.: Seroreactivity to bacterial antigens is not a unique phenomenon in patients with autoimmune thyroid diseases in Canada. Thyroid *4*:269-274, 1994.

165. Rodnan, G. P., Schumacher, H. R., and Zvaifler, N. J.: Primer on the Rheumatic Diseases. 8th ed. Atlanta, GA, Arthritis Foundation, 1983, pp. 93-94.

166. Rodriguez, W. J., Controni, G., Cohen, G. J., et al.: *Yersinia enterocolitica* in children. J. A. M. A. *242*:1978-1980, 1979.

167. Roggenkamp, A., Geiger, A. M., Leitritz, L., et al.: Passive immunity to infection with *Yersinia* spp. mediated by anti-recombinant V antigen is dependent on polymorphism of V antigen. Infect. Immun. *65*:446-451, 1997.

168. Rose, E. B., Camp, C. J., and Antes, E. J.: Family outbreak of fatal *Yersinia enterocolitica* pharyngitis. Am. J. Med. *82*:636-637, 1987.

169. Ryser, R. J., and Hornick, R. B.: A review of "new" bacterial strains causing diarrhea. *In* Remington, J. S., and Swartz, M. N. (eds.): Clinical Topics in Infectious Diseases. New York, McGraw-Hill, 1981, pp. 184-210.

170. Saari, M., Make, M., Paivonsal, T., et al.: Acute anterior uveitis and conjunctivitis following *Yersinia* infection in children. Int. Ophthalmol. Med. *9*:237-241, 1986.

171. Saari, T. N., and Tripplet, D. A.: *Yersinia pseudotuberculosis* mesenteric adenitis. J. Pediatr. *85*:656-659, 1974.

172. Saebo, A., and Lassen, J.: *Yersinia enterocolitica*: An inducer of chronic inflammation. Int. J. Tissue React. *16*:51-57, 1994.

173. Saisasa, K.: Über die Pseudotuberkulose beim Menschen. Zeitschr. Hyg. *73*:353, 1913.

174. Schleifstein, J., and Coleman, M. B.: An identified microorganism resembling *B. ligneri* and *Past. pseudotuberculosis* and pathogenic for man. N. Y. State J. Med. *39*:1749, 1939.

175. Schleifstein, J., and Coleman, M. B.: *Bacterium enterocoliticum*. Annual Report, Division of Laboratories and Research. Albany, NY, New York State Department of Health, 1943, p. 56.

176. Seuri, M., and Granfors, K.: Antibodies against *Yersinia* among farmers and slaughterhouse workers. Scand. J. Work Environ. Health *18*:128-132, 1992.

177. Shayegani, M., DeForge, L., McGlynn, D. M., et al.: Characteristics of *Yersinia enterocolitica* and related species isolated from human and environmental sources. J. Clin. Microbiol. *14*:304-312, 1981.

178. Shenkman, L., and Bottone, E. J.: Antibodies to *Yersinia enterocolitica* in thyroid disease. Ann. Intern. Med. *85*:735-739, 1976.

179. Singh, I., and Virdi, J. S.: Production of *Yersinia* stable toxin (YST) and distribution of *yst* genes in biotype 1A strains of *Yersinia enterocolitica*. J. Med. Microbiol. *53*:1065-1068, 2004.

180. Snellings, N. J., Popek, M., and Lindler, L. E.: Complete DNA sequence of *Yersinia enterocolitica* serotype O:8 low-calcium-response plasmid reveals a new virulence plasmid-associated replicon. Infect. Immun. *69*:4627-4638, 2001.

181. Snyder, J. D., Christenson, E., and Feldman, R. A.: Human *Yersinia enterocolitica* infections in Wisconsin: Clinical, laboratory and epidemiologic features. Am. J. Med. *72*:768-774, 1982.

182. Solem, J., and Lassen, J.: Reiter's disease following *Yersinia enterocolitica* infection. Scand. J. Infect. Dis. *3*:83, 1971.

183. Sonnenwirth, A. C.: *Yersinia*. *In* Lennett, E. H., Spaulding, E. H., and Truant, J. P. (eds.): Manual of Clinical Microbiology. 2nd ed. Washington, D.C., American Society of Microbiology, 1954, pp. 222-229.

184. Sonnenwirth, A. C.: *Yersinia enterocolitica* as an etiologic agent in meningitis. Bact. Proc. Abstr. M. *128*:87, 1969.

185. Sonnenwirth, A. C.: *Yersinia enterocolitica*. N. Engl. J. Med. *283*:1468, 1970.

186. Sonnenwirth, A. C.: Isolation and characterization of *Yersinia enterocolitica*. Mt. Sinai. J. Med. *43*:736-745, 1976.

187. Sotaniemi, K. A.: Neurologic complications associated with yersiniosis. Neurology *33*:95-97, 1983.

188. Stolk-Engelaar, V. M. M., Meis, J. F. G. M., Mulder, J. A., et al.: In-vitro antimicrobial susceptibility of *Yersinia enterocolitica* isolates from stools of patients in The Netherlands from 1982-1991. J. Antimicrob. Chemother. *36*:839-843, 1995.

189. Sulakvelidze, A.: *Yersinia* other than *Y. enterocolitica*, *Y. pseudotuberculosis*, and *Y. pestis*: The ignored species. Microbes Infect. *2*:497-513, 2000.

190. Sulakvelidze, A., Kreger, A., Joseph, A., et al.: Production of enterotoxin by *Yersinia* bercovieri, a recently identified *Yersinia enterocolitica*-like species. Infect. Immun. *67*:968-971, 1999.

191. Tackett, C. O., Ballard, J., Harris, N., et al.: An outbreak of *Yersinia enterocolitica* infections caused by contaminated tofu (soybean curd). Am. J. Epidemiol. *121*:705-711, 1985.

192. Tauxe, R. V., Vandepitta, J., Mautero, G., et al.: *Yersinia enterocolitica* infections and pork: The missing link. Lancet *1*:1129-1133, 1987.

193. Thomas, A. F., Solomon, L., and Rabson, A.: Polyarthritis associated with *Yersinia enterocolitica* infection. S. Afr. Med. J. *49*:18-20, 1975.

194. Thomson, N. R., Howard, S., Wren, B. W., et al.: The complete genome sequence and comparative genome analysis of the high pathogenicity *Yersinia enterocolitica* strain 8081. PLoS Genet. *2*:2039-2051, 2006.

195. Toivanen, P., Toivanen, A., Olkkonen, L., et al.: Hospital outbreak of *Yersinia enterocolitica* infection. Lancet *1*:801-803, 1973.

196. Toma, S.: Survey on the incidence of *Yersinia enterocolitica* in the province of Ontario. Can. J. Public Health *64*:477-487, 1973.

197. Toma, S., Wauters, G., McClure, H. M., et al.: O:13a, 13b, a new pathogenic serotype of *Yersinia enterocolitica*. J. Clin. Microbiol. *20*:843-845, 1984.

198. Toshniwal, R., Kocka, F. E., and Kallick, C. A.: Suppurative lymphadenitis with *Yersinia enterocolitica*. Eur. J. Clin. Microbiol. *4*:587-588, 1985.

199. Tuohy, A. M., O'Gorman, M., Byington, C., et al.: *Yersinia* enterocolitis mimicking Crohn's disease in a toddler. Pediatrics *104*:e36, 1999.

200. Vantrappen, G., Geboes, K., and Ponette, E.: *Yersinia* enteritis. Med. Clin. North Am. *66*:639-653, 1982.

201. Vantrappen, G., Ponette, E., Geboes, K., et al.: *Yersinia* enteritis and enterocolitis: Gastroenterological aspects. Gastroenterology *72*:220-227, 1977.

202. Verhaegen, J., Charlier, J., Lemmens, P., et al.: Surveillance of human *Yersinia enterocolitica* infections in Belgium: 1967-1996. Clin. Infect. Dis. *27*:59-64, 1998.

203. Vilinskas, J., Tilton, R. C., and Kriz, J. J.: A new clinical entity: Human infection with *Yersinia* presenting as an acute abdomen. Am. J. Surg. *7*:568, 1971.

204. Vishnubhatla, A., Fung, D. Y., Oberst, R. D., et al.: Rapid 5′ nuclease (TaqMan) assay for detection of virulent strains of *Yersinia enterocolitica*. Appl. Environ. Microbiol. *66*:4131-4135, 2000.

205. Visser, L. G., Hiemstra, P. S., Van Den Barselaar, M. T., et al.: Role of YadA in resistance to killing of *Yersinia enterocolitica* by antimicrobial polypeptides of human granulocytes. Infect. Immun. *64*:1653-1658, 1996.

206. Waage, A. S., Vardund, T., Lund, V., and Kapperud, G.: Detection of low numbers of pathogenic *Yersinia enterocolitica* in environmental water and sewage samples by nested polymerase chain reaction. J. Appl. Microbiol. *87*:814-821, 1999.

207. Weber, J., Finlayson, N. B., and Mark, J. B. D.: Mesenteric lymphadenitis and terminal ileitis due to *Yersinia pseudotuberculosis*. N. Engl. J. Med. *283*:172-174, 1970.

208. Wilson, H. D., McCormick, J. S., and Feely, J. C.: *Yersinia enterocolitica* infection in a 4-month-old infant associated with infection in household dogs. J. Pediatr. *89*:767-769, 1976.

209. Winblad, S.: Erythema nodosum associated with infection with *Yersinia enterocolitica*. Scand. J. Infect. Dis. *1*:11-16, 1969.

210. Winblad, S.: Arthritis associated with *Yersinia enterocolitica* infections. Scand. J. Infect. Dis. *7*:191-195, 1975.

211. Winblad, S., Nilehn, B., and Jonsson, M.: Two further cases, bacteriologically verified, of human infection with "Pasteurella X" (syn. *Yersinia enterocolitica*). Acta Pathol. Microbiol. Scand. *67*:537-541, 1966.

212. Winblad, S., Nilehn, B., and Sternby, N. H.: *Yersinia enterocolitica* (Pasteurella X) in human enteric infections. B. M. J. *2*:1363-1366, 1966.

213. Young, G. M., Badger, J. L., and Miller, V. L.: Motility is required to initiate host cell invasion by *Yersinia enterocolitica*. Infect. Immun. *68*:4323-4326, 2000.

214. Zhang, L., Radziejewska-Lebrecht, J., Krajewska-Pietrasik, D., et al.: Molecular and chemical characterization of the lipopolysaccharide O-antigen and its role in the virulence of *Yersinia enterocolitica* serotype O:8. Mol. Microbiol. *23*:63-76, 1997.

215. Zen-Yoji, H., Maruyama, T., Sakai, S., et al.: An outbreak of enteritis due to *Yersinia enterocolitica* occurring at a junior high school. Jpn. J. Microbiol. *17*:220-222, 1973.

MISCELLANEOUS ENTEROBACTERIA

Randall G. Fisher

This chapter focuses on three less commonly isolated organisms of the family Enterobacteriaceae: *Edwardsiella tarda, Hafnia alvei,* and *Pantoea agglomerans.* Each of these organisms, although uncommon, can cause significant disease in certain clinical circumstances.[51]

EDWARDSIELLA TARDA

BACTERIOLOGY

E. tarda is a non–lactose-fermenting, gram-negative bacillus that is indole-positive and produces hydrogen sulfide. It ferments only glucose and maltose. The species name *tarda* reflects its biochemical inactivity. It usually is lysine-positive and ornithine decarboxylase–positive.[21] The organism resembles *Salmonella* biochemically and clinically.[33] *Salmonella* usually ferments mannitol, sorbitol, and rhamnose, however. The innate resistance of *Edwardsiella* to colistin also distinguishes it from *Salmonella.*[54] *E. tarda* grows well on usual differential media in the laboratory and produces smooth, glistening, semitranslucent colonies.

EPIDEMIOLOGY

E. tarda is an organism associated with fresh-water and marine life and has been isolated from turtles, fish, pelicans, alligators, seals, and toads.[33] It also is found in snakes and lizards. Case reports of human disease have implicated ornamental fish,[76] pet turtles,[55] snakes,[64] and catfish,[6,13,29] and injuries in fresh and brackish water.[70]

Patients with chronic liver disease, chronic ethanol abuse, steroid therapy, and hemoglobinopathy particularly are prone to developing infection with *E. tarda.*[33] Any condition associated with iron overload also is a potential risk factor. Serious infection with *E. tarda* in otherwise well individuals also can occur.[70]

Infection with *E. tarda* is global but occurs more commonly in tropical and subtropical climates, particularly Southeast Asia, Africa, and Latin America.[34] The elderly and the very young seem to be at increased risk for developing severe illness.[9] Asymptomatic carrier states have been documented well,[60] but no true epidemic has been reported, and person-to-person transmission has not been established directly.[19]

PATHOPHYSIOLOGY

Invasiveness of the organism in HeLa and HEp-2 cells,[61] siderophore production, the elaboration of a cell-associated hemolysin,[30] and resistance to complement-mediated lysis may contribute to virulence, although no clear associations have been made.[37] Hemolytic activity requires the presence of two genes, *ethA* and *ethB.* The *ethA* gene codes for the hemolysin, whereas the *ethB* gene codes for an activation/secretion protein, which is necessary for activation of the hemolysin. Transcription of the *ethB* gene is regulated by iron, which may explain the association between iron overload states and severe *E. tarda* infection.[30] Hemolysin activity seems to be necessary for cell entry and cytotoxicity.[73]

CLINICAL MANIFESTATIONS

Infections with *E. tarda* can be divided broadly into two types: intestinal and extraintestinal. Approximately 80 percent of infections are intestinal.[70] Gastrointestinal infection usually causes self-limited enteritis, with intermittent watery diarrhea and low-grade fever.[39] Nausea and vomiting usually are not seen. Occasionally, enterocolitis or a dysentery-like illness is noted.[47] Because most laboratories do not culture stool specimens specifically for *Edwardsiella,* most cases are unrecognized.

Wound infection is the most common extraintestinal infection. Most of the wounds are caused by fish fins or snakes; wounds sustained in automobile accidents also have been implicated.[33] Cellulitis or abscesses may be produced. Coinfection with other organisms, particularly *Aeromonas hydrophila,* is common.[29,70] One case of necrotizing fasciitis and myonecrosis in an immunocompetent man has been reported. Cultures obtained at surgical débridement yielded a pure growth of *E. tarda.*[70]

Septicemia with *E. tarda* is a rare but serious infection that carries a mortality rate of approximately 45 percent. Most patients with septicemia have underlying conditions, such as liver disease, iron overload, and immunosuppression. Septicemia occasionally follows a mild diarrheal illness.[13] Infants without other risk factors have been reported.[78] Septicemia manifests with high fever, shock, and, often, disseminated intravascular coagulation. Meningitis also has been reported.[59,68] Death sometimes occurs despite administration of appropriate antimicrobial therapy.

Other syndromes associated with *E. tarda* infection include an enteric fever–like illness,[13] multiple or solitary liver abscesses,[45,86] osteomyelitis,[64] septic arthritis,[6] cellulitis,[24] myonecrosis,[70] necrotizing fasciitis,[50] endocarditis,[56] uterine pyomyoma,[84] tubo-ovarian abscess,[62] and peritonitis.[13] A case of puerperal intrauterine infection in a woman without obvious risk factors has been reported; her infant was not affected.[52] Patients with sickle-cell disorders may be predisposed to bony infection with *E. tarda,* as they are with *Salmonella.*[68,83] Reported cases all are in patients with sickle-cell hemoglobinopathy, rather than homozygous sickle-cell disease.

DIAGNOSIS AND TREATMENT

Diagnosis rests on identification of *E. tarda* in culture. The major pitfall is mistaking it for *Salmonella.*

E. tarda is sensitive in vitro to most antibiotics used routinely in the treatment of gram-negative infections, including β-lactams, cephalosporins, aminoglycosides, and fluoroquinolones.[12] It also is sensitive to chloramphenicol, trimethoprim-sulfamethoxazole, and tetracycline.[72] Resistance to polymyxin B, colistin, and, occasionally, penicillin has been shown.[12,13] The organism almost universally elaborates a β-lactamase, but no resistance to β-lactams other than penicillin[12] and oxacillin[72] has been reported.

Gastrointestinal disease usually does not require treatment. Severe disease, such as septicemia or meningitis, probably should be treated with the combination of a β-lactam and an aminoglycoside,[33] even though synergy has not been shown.

HAFNIA ALVEI

BACTERIOLOGY

H. alvei is a facultatively anaerobic, gram-negative bacillus, formerly referred to as *Enterobacter hafnia*.[69] This indole-negative, catalase-positive, and oxidase-negative organism is positive for lysine and ornithine decarboxylases. It is motile at lower temperatures, but may be immotile at temperatures of 35° C and greater. *H. alvei* ferments mannitol, maltose, and sucrose. It grows well on blood or MacConkey agar as a nonlactose fermenter, producing gray-white, slightly elevated, glistening colonies.[20]

EPIDEMIOLOGY

H. alvei has been found in soil, dairy products, sewage, and the feces of humans and animals. Some question exists as to whether it is part of the endogenous microflora of the gut[65] or whether an asymptomatic "carrier" state exists. One study from Japan cultured *H. alvei* from 13 percent of healthy subjects[49]; other epidemiologic surveys have shown the incidence to be less than 2 percent.[66] Long regarded as a nonpathogen, *H. alvei* now has been associated clearly with enteritis and rarely has been isolated in pure culture from other sites, including blood, cerebrospinal fluid, peritoneal fluid, and urine. Infection seems to be opportunistic.

PATHOPHYSIOLOGY

The pathophysiology of *H. alvei* has been investigated most thoroughly with regard to its production of gastrointestinal symptoms,[2] although whether *H. alvei* is actually a diarrheagenic pathogen remains controversial. Albert and associates[3] showed that although *H. alvei* elaborated neither enterotoxins nor a Shiga-like toxin and was not invasive in HeLa cell assays or by Sereny test, it did produce diarrhea in experimental animals whether given parenterally or by mouth. Sections of intestines from infected animals showed lesions indistinguishable from those caused by enteropathogenic *Escherichia coli*. "Diarrheagenic strains" of *H. alvei* also were thought to differ from other strains in that they possessed the *eaeA* gene.[32] Janda and colleagues[36] first presented data suggesting that diarrheagenic *H. alvei* isolates were actually either unusual biotypes of *E. coli* or a new species in the genus *Escherichia*. Subsequently, the same group showed that organisms originally called *H. alvei* reported to produce attaching-effacing lesions and to possess the *eaeA* gene are actually a novel species, *Escherichia albertii*.[31] Information about the pathophysiology of extraintestinal infection is sparse.[35]

CLINICAL MANIFESTATIONS

Cases of diarrhea caused by *H. alvei* (possibly *E. albertii*) have been reported primarily in children.[2,3] Most patients with gastroenteritis secondary to *H. alvei/E. albertii* report 6 to 12 episodes of watery diarrhea per day, low-grade or no fever, and nausea with or without vomiting. Mucus sometimes is found in stools, but blood is not.[65,82] In most patients, symptoms last for a few days, but in some patients, symptoms persist for more than a week.[65] One patient with a reactive arthritis from *H. alvei/ E. albertii* enteritis has been reported.[57] A unique case has been reported of an 11-year-old girl who had a 3-day history of red lesions on the forehead, neck, and trunk associated with abdominal pain, emesis, and decreased urinary output, with one bloody diarrheal stool the day before admission, who then developed

hemolytic-uremic syndrome. Stool cultures repeatedly were negative for *E. coli* O157:H7, but positive for a toxigenic strain of *H. alvei* from two consecutive cultures.[15]

Traditionally, extraintestinal *H. alvei* infections were thought to occur mostly in hospitalized patients and to be hospital-acquired. In one large series, the organism was isolated from 80 samples collected from 61 patients; 57 (93%) patients had underlying illnesses, most commonly malignancies.[28] Nearly half of isolates were from the respiratory tract. Other sites included blood, skin, wounds, urine, and intra-abdominal abscesses. In 60 (75%) samples, other organisms were cultured concomitantly. In a more recent, larger study from Canada, two thirds of 138 isolates were of community onset, 112 (81%) were from the urinary tract, and 94 (68%) were from monomicrobial infections.[40] Older age and female gender were risk factors for development of infection.

One 20-day-old premature infant with necrotizing enterocolitis grew *H. alvei* from blood and stool.[25] Yeager and associates[85] reported four cases of pneumatosis intestinalis in patients after they had undergone bone marrow transplantation, and one of the four grew *H. alvei* in pure culture from blood. An 8-year-old boy with acquired immunodeficiency syndrome (AIDS) developed recurrent episodes of *H. alvei* bacteremia.[14] Both episodes were associated with fever and diarrhea; the second episode also was associated with pneumonia and pleural effusion, the cause of which is unclear. A well-documented case of pneumonia in a 54-year-old woman with AIDS has been reported in which the pleural fluid grew a pure culture of *H. alvei*.[22]

Wound abscess caused by *H. alvei* has been reported.[1] A 2-year-old liver transplant recipient developed hepatic abscess and bacteremia with *H. alvei* and *Enterococcus faecalis*.[7] One case of meningitis in a 1-year-old infant without known predisposing risk factors has been reported.[53] A case of a woman with rheumatoid arthritis who contracted endophthalmitis with *H. alvei* in mixed culture has been described; the woman used snake powder as a food seasoning.[11] Two case reports are described in the older literature of persistent bacteremia with this organism, alone and in mixed cultures. One of these patients was a previously well 13-year-old girl.[27]

DIAGNOSIS AND TREATMENT

Diagnosis is established by isolation of the organism from stools or from normally sterile body fluids. Gunthard and Pennekamp[28] reported the susceptibility results of 80 *H. alvei* isolates recovered from 61 patients over a 2.5-year period. All isolates tested were susceptible to ciprofloxacin. Isolates also were generally susceptible to tobramycin (99%), imipenem (99%), piperacillin (92%), trimethoprim-sulfamethoxazole (90%), ceftriaxone (88%), and ceftazidime (88%). Nearly all isolates were resistant to ampicillin and to amoxicillin-clavulanate.

H. alvei is constitutively cephalothin-resistant.[82] One report describes an inducible β-lactamase that rendered the isolate ceftazidime-resistant.[74] In one study, the antimicrobial susceptibility of *H. alvei* was compared with that of *E. albertii*, the organism with which *H. alvei* is confused most frequently. *E. albertii* isolates were naturally susceptible to all β-lactams except for penicillin and oxacillin; they also were susceptible to azithromycin. In contrast, *H. alvei* strains were naturally resistant to tetracycline, amoxicillin, amoxicillin-clavulanate, ampicillin-sulbactam, azithromycin, and the narrow-spectrum cephalosporins.[72]

Treatment probably is unnecessary for most cases of gastroenteritis. Treatment for invasive infection should be based on susceptibility testing. Empiric therapy with a third-generation cephalosporin and an aminoglycoside is reasonable pending susceptibility results.

PANTOEA AGGLOMERANS

First identified as a plant pathogen and named after Erwin Smith in 1917, the genus *Erwinia* has an extended domain as an infectious microbe, including production of disease in humans.[10,63,71] A member of this group of organisms, *Pantoea agglomerans* (*Enterobacter agglomerans*, *Erwinia herbicola*) has been established as a cause of conjunctivitis,[10] central nervous system infections,[10,69] urinary tract infections,[62,68] pneumonia,[4] and nosocomial infections secondary to contaminated intravenous fluids.[24,38]

BACTERIOLOGY

Species definition within *Erwinia* has been controversial and confusing. It has been suggested to rename the anaerogenic clinically relevant *Erwinia* of the *herbicola-lathryi* group *E. agglomerans* or *P. agglomerans*.[21,33,71] In clinical microbiology, both of the latter terms tend to be used interchangeably. This species consists of facultatively anaerobic, fermentative, hydrogen sulfide–negative, gram-negative rods; they do not possess oxidase, phenylalanine deaminase, proteinase, or arginine dehydrolase.[21] None decarboxylates ornithine.[33] They are motile, have peritrichous flagella, and produce a yellow pigment. Strains grow well at 37° C (98.6° F) on standard agar. When colonies are viewed microscopically after growth for 18 to 20 hours, characteristic biconvex spindle-shaped bodies and bacterial aggregates often can be seen.[10,69] Almost all strains isolated from clinical specimens and grown on agar slants show characteristic elongated, spheroidal aggregates,[69] called *symplasmata* by Cruickshank,[16] who first described them.

EPIDEMIOLOGY

Microorganisms of the genus *Erwinia* long have been recognized as phytopathogens producing dry necrosis, wilts, and soft rots in plants, and more recently they have been associated with disease in trout and leafhoppers.[63,71] *P. agglomerans* (*E. herbicola*) first was isolated in humans from stool specimens of patients with typhoid fever in the 1920s and given the name *Bacterium typhi flavum* because of the organism's alleged capacity to be transformed into *Salmonella typhi* in subculture. Identification of saprophytic human strains followed, and the biochemical and cultural identity of *B. typhi flavum* with the *E. herbicola-lathryi* group finally was established.[21]

The first reports of *P. agglomerans* as a human pathogen appeared in the 1960s. Subsequently, a nationwide outbreak of infection caused by this organism was traced to contaminated liners from caps of parenteral solution bottles.[43,44] The importance of this organism as a nosocomial cause of bacteremia is emphasized by the 17 percent mortality rate in patients receiving an infusion with the contaminated intravenous fluid.[43] A trend was noted for an increased mortality rate in infected individuals younger than 20 years old. In neonatal intensive care units, the situation seems to be even more dire; in one study, the mortality rate for infants with blood cultures positive for *P. agglomerans* was 88 percent (seven of eight).[77] Lipid-based medications support rapid bacterial growth at room temperature and, in the absence of strict aseptic handling have been implicated in more recent nosocomial *P. agglomerans* bloodstream infections.[8] *Pantoea* outbreaks also have been traced to contaminated blood products; prolonged storage of packed red blood cells at 4° C provides conditions that allow these organisms to grow and subsequently produce high concentrations of endotoxin.[5] Cotton used to filter heroin has been implicated as a source of infection ("cotton fever") in intravenous drug users.[23]

Outbreaks in pediatric hospitals caused by contaminated intravenous solutions also have been described.[48] At least one retrospective review of *Erwinia* organisms isolated from clinical specimens suggested a predisposition to infection in the pediatric age group[10]; however, other studies have noted no preference based on season, sex, age, or residence in hospitals.[71] A large pseudo-outbreak traced to contamination of cotton pledgets also has been reported.[38]

PATHOPHYSIOLOGY

The true incidence of clinical infection caused by *P. agglomerans* is difficult to ascertain because of the common association of this microbe with other organisms when obtained from clinical specimens. Nonetheless, the accumulation of case reports in which this organism is isolated in pure culture from infected material leaves little doubt that *P. agglomerans* can be a human pathogen, apart from its role as a nosocomial contaminant. This organism has little inherent invasiveness. Evidence for animal pathogenicity of *Erwinia* strains isolated from plants and humans is limited; 10^{13} washed organisms injected intraperitoneally into mice or guinea pigs do not cause symptoms, whereas inoculation of 10^{27} organisms leads to death within 36 hours.[16]

Most strains seem to act as saprophytes in humans,[79] but the organism has been isolated from purulent wounds of the extremities acquired through lacerations or thorn pricks, which suggests agricultural injury as a possible mode of infection.[79] Thorn injuries also have led to septic arthritis and osteomyelitis.[17] A delay of 4 to 6 weeks often occurs between the injury and the bone or joint infection. Most serious infections have occurred in individuals with a breach of host defenses (e.g., immunocompromised individuals or patients who received contaminated intravenous fluid).[16]

CLINICAL MANIFESTATIONS

P. agglomerans bacteremia often is associated with fever, shaking chills, and systemic toxicity characteristic of gram-negative sepsis. These symptoms frequently have been misinterpreted, however, in hospitalized patients who unknowingly were administered contaminated intravenous fluids.[44] Premature neonates with sepsis owing to *P. agglomerans* tend to have a rapidly progressive sepsis with prominent pulmonary involvement, including hemorrhage and acute respiratory distress syndrome. In the largest pediatric series reported to date, 21 of 53 (about 40%) *P. agglomerans* isolates from normally sterile sites were grown from central venous lines; of these, two thirds were polymicrobial.[17]

Eye and skin infections caused by *P. agglomerans* are particularly prominent. Bottone and Schneierson[10] included six cases of conjunctivitis, five of which occurred in infants, from whom this organism was isolated. Only two of the isolates were in pure culture, however, and a description of the clinical course of these children was not included in the report. *Erwinia* endophthalmitis has been associated with foreign body penetration of the eye in a 14-year-old boy.[58]

Skin infection in association with a casted fracture has been described in an elderly patient,[79] and wound infections from which this organism was isolated have been described subsequently, most often in association with agricultural injury.[79] Four isolates were obtained in mixed cultures from skin lesions of children younger than 5 years old, but their possible role in those infections was not confirmed.[10] In a recent series, 14 cases of abscesses required drainage; all 14 were polymicrobial.[17] *P. agglomerans* was the only organism isolated from six consecutive blood cultures in a 9-year-old boy with osteomyelitis.[46] A 13-year-old boy developed septic arthritis caused by *P. agglomerans* 1 month after sustaining a plant thorn injury to his knee.[18] A case of *P. agglomerans* spondylodiskitis has been reported.[63] In many cases of *P. agglomerans* osteomyelitis or septic arthritis, the patient is afebrile and blood cultures are negative. In addition, measures of inflammation and joint fluid findings may be largely unremarkable.[17] A high index of suspicion of *P. agglomerans* must be maintained when bone or joint infection follows plant thorn injury.

Primary lung disease caused by these bacteria is a rare occurrence; it has been reported in an adult with chronic bronchitis.[4] This organism is a very rare cause of meningitis. A contaminated incubator has been implicated in two cases of neonatal central nervous system infection,[75] and a cisternal tap revealed the presence of *P. agglomerans* in an unrelated newborn case whose clinical course was not described.[10] A 57-year-old man with tetralogy of Fallot and cyanosis had a brain abscess in which *P. agglomerans* organisms grew in pure culture.[80] Presenting manifestations included headaches, seizures, and left-sided weakness, which occurred over a 2-week period before admission. The patient recovered after undergoing drainage of the abscess and gentamicin therapy. One case of peritonitis in a patient on continuous ambulatory peritoneal dialysis has been reported; it was thought to be secondary to a rose thorn injury.[41]

DIAGNOSIS

Difficulty in identifying this organism is common; in March 1972, as part of a quality control program, *P. agglomerans* was sent as an unknown organism to 250 U.S. hospitals and was identified incorrectly 45 percent of the time.[44] Even when fully identified in isolates from human sources, *P. agglomerans* often is considered a contaminant or saprophyte. The organisms have been identified mistakenly as *Citrobacter, Escherichia coli, Flavobacterium,* and *Klebsiella.* In addition to routine microbiologic studies, identification of yellow-pigmented colonies and observation of the characteristic spindle-shaped bodies and symplasmata can aid in this differentiation. Symplasmata (elongated, spheroid aggregates) are seen best in the condensation water of slant cultures.[79] Spindle-shaped bodies termed *Wetzsteinformen* by German authors are observed best on standard agar with a low-power microscope lens.[71]

TREATMENT

Most localized infections respond to treatment that includes an aminoglycoside. The presence of persistent localized infection with this organism should prompt a search for an organic foreign body, given the organism's tendency to live as a saprophyte or as a pathogen in vegetable material. In addition to appropriate antimicrobial therapy, treatment of bacteremia should include removal of any potentially contaminated intravenous access. The physician should be alert to the possibility of a common source of infection in nosocomial outbreaks.[44] In view of the rarity of bacteremia caused by *P. agglomerans*, single sporadic cases should be investigated, and clusters of two or more cases should lead to immediate inquiry into possible sources of contamination. Formal surveillance programs have been the key to early recognition and abortion of epidemics.[44]

Acknowledgments

The author thanks Dr. William Gruber and Dr. Thomas Boyce for their invaluable assistance with earlier versions of this chapter.

REFERENCES

1. Agustin, E. T., and Cunha, B. A.: Buttock abscess due to *Hafnia alvei.* Clin. Infect. Dis. 20:1426, 1995. Letter.
2. Albert, M. J, Alam, K., Islam, M., et al.: *Hafnia alvei,* a probable cause of diarrhea in humans. Infect. Immun. 59:1507-1513, 1991.
3. Albert, M. J., Faruque, S. M., Ansaruzzaman, M., et al.: Sharing of virulence-associated properties at the phenotypic and genetic levels between enteropathogenic *Escherichia coli* and *Hafnia alvei.* J. Med. Microbiol. 37:310-314, 1992.
4. Al-Damluji, S., Dickinson, C. M., and Beck, A.: *Enterobacter agglomerans*: A new cause of primary pneumonia. Thorax 37:865-866, 1982.
5. Arduino, M. J., Bland, L. A., Tipple, M. A., et al.: Growth and endotoxin production of *Yersinia enterocolitica* and *Enterobacter agglomerans* in packed erythrocytes. J. Clin. Microbiol. 27:1483-1485, 1989.
6. Ashford, R. U., Sargeant, P. D., and Lum, G. D.: Septic arthritis of the knee caused by *Edwardsiella tarda* after a catfish puncture wound. Med. J. Aust. 168:443-444, 1998.
7. Barry, J. W., Dominguez, E. A., Boken, D. J., et al.: *Hafnia alvei* infection after liver transplantation. Clin. Infect. Dis. 24:1263-1264, 1997.
8. Bennett, S. N., McNeil, M. M., Bland, L. A., et al.: Postoperative infections traced to contamination of an intravenous anesthetic, propofol. N. Engl. J. Med. 333:147-154, 1995.
9. Bockemuhl, J., Pan-Urai, R., and Burkhardt, F.: *Edwardsiella tarda* associated with human disease. Pathol. Microbiol. 37:393-401, 1971.
10. Bottone, E., and Schneierson, S. S.: *Erwinia* species: An emerging human pathogen. Am. J. Clin. Pathol. 57:400-405, 1972.
11. Caravalho, J., Jr., McMillan, V. M., Ellis, R. B., et al.: Endogenous endophthalmitis due to *Salmonella arizonae* and *Hafnia alvei.* South. Med. J. 83:325-327, 1990.
12. Clark, R. B., Lister, P. D., and Janda, J. M.: In vitro susceptibilities of *Edwardsiella tarda* to 22 antibiotics and antibiotic-beta-lactamase-inhibitor agents. Diagn. Microbiol. Infect. Dis. 14:173-175, 1991.
13. Clarridge, J. E., Musher, D. M., Fainstein, V., et al.: Extraintestinal human infection caused by *Edwardsiella tarda.* J. Clin. Microbiol. 11:511-514, 1980.
14. Conte, M., Castagnola, E., Venzano, P., et al.: Bacteremia caused by *Hafnia alvei* in a human immunodeficiency virus-infected child. Pediatr. Infect. Dis. J. 15:182-183, 1996. Letter.
15. Crandall, C., Abbott, S. L., Zhao, Y. Q., et al.: Isolation of toxigenic *Hafnia alvei* from a probable case of hemolytic uremic syndrome. Infection 34:227-229, 2006.
16. Cruickshank, J. C.: A study of the so-called bacterium *Typhi flavum.* J. Hyg. 35:354-371, 1935.
17. Cruz, A. T., Cazacu, A. C., and Allen, C. H.: *Pantoea agglomerans,* a plant pathogen causing human disease. J. Clin. Microbiol. 45:1989-1992, 2007.
18. De Champs, C., Le Seaux, S., Dubost, J. J., et al.: Isolation of *Pantoea agglomerans* in two cases of septic monoarthritis after plant thorn and wood sliver injuries. J. Clin. Microbiol. 38:460-461, 2000.
19. Desenclos, J. C., Conti, L., Junejo, S., et al.: A cluster of *Edwardsiella tarda* infection in a day-care center in Florida. J. Infect. Dis. 162:782, 1990.
20. Englund, G. W.: Persistent septicemia due to *Hafnia alvei*: Report of a case. Am. J. Clin. Pathol. 51:717-719, 1969.
21. Ewing, W. H., and Fife, M. A.: *Enterobacter agglomerans* (Beijerinck) comb. nov. (the *herbicola-lathyri* bacteria). Int. J. Syst. Bacteriol. 22:4-11, 1972.
22. Fazal, B. A., Justman, J. E., Turett, G. S., et al.: Community-acquired *Hafnia alvei* infection. Clin. Infect. Dis. 24:527-528, 1997.
23. Ferguson, R., Feeney, C., and Chirurgi, V. A.: *Enterobacter agglomerans*-associated cotton fever. Arch. Intern. Med. 153:2381-2382, 1993.
24. Fournier, S., Pialoux, G., Feuillie, V., et al.: *Edwardsiella tarda* septicemia with cellulitis in a patient with AIDS. Eur. J. Clin. Microbiol. Infect. Dis. 16:551-553, 1997. Letter.
25. Ginsberg, H. G., and Goldsmith, J. P.: *Hafnia alvei* septicemia in an infant with necrotizing enterocolitis. J. Perinatol. 8:122-123, 1988.
26. Goncalves, C. R., Vaz, T. M., Leite, D., et al.: Molecular epidemiology of a nosocomial outbreak due to *Enterobacter cloacae* and *Enterobacter agglomerans* in Campinas, Sao Paulo, Brazil. Rev. Inst. Med. Trop. Sao Paulo 42:1-7, 2000.
27. Grajupa, L. A., Mukhopadhyay, D., and Grossman, B. J.: Chronic polymicrobial bacteremia. Clin. Pediatr. 14:280-283, 1975.
28. Gunthard, H., and Pennekamp, A.: Clinical significance of extraintestinal *Hafnia alvei* isolates from 61 patients and review of the literature. Clin. Infect. Dis. 22:1040-1045, 1996.
29. Hargreaves, J. E., and Lucey, D. R.: Life-threatening *Edwardsiella tarda* soft-tissue infection associated with catfish puncture wound. J. Infect. Dis. 162:1416-1417, 1990.
30. Hirono, I., Tange, N., and Aoki, T.: Iron-regulated haemolysin gene from *Edwardsiella tarda.* Mol. Microbiol. 24:851-856, 1997.
31. Huys, G., Crockaert, M., Janda, J. M., et al.: *Escherichia albertii* sp. Nov.: A diarrhoeogenic species isolated from stool specimens of Bangladeshi children. Int. J. Syst. Evol. Microbiol. 53:807-810, 2003.
32. Ismaili, A., Bourke, B., de Azavedo, J. C., et al.: Heterogeneity in phenotypic and genotypic characteristics among strains of *Hafnia alvei.* J. Clin. Microbiol. 34:2973-2979, 1996.
33. Janda, J. M., and Abbott, S. L.: Infections associated with the genus *Edwardsiella*: The role of *Edwardsiella tarda* in human disease. Clin. Infect. Dis. 17:742-748, 1993.

34. Janda, J. M., and Abbott, S. L.: Unusual food-borne pathogens: *Listeria monocytogenes*, *Aeromonas*, *Plesiomonas*, and *Edwardsiella* species. Clin. Lab. Med. 19:553-582, 1999.

35. Janda, J. M., and Abbott, S. L.: The genus *Hafnia*: From soup to nuts. Clin. Microbiol. Rev. 19:12-18, 2006.

36. Janda, J. M., Abbott, S. L., and Albert, M. J.: Prototypal diarrheagenic strains of *Hafnia alvei* are actually members of the genus *Escherichia*. J. Clin. Microbiol. 37:2399-2401, 1999.

37. Janda, J. M., Abbott, S. L., Kroske-Bystrom, S., et al.: Pathogenic properties of *Edwardsiella* species. J. Clin. Microbiol. 29:1997-2001, 1991.

38. Koo, H. S., Kim, J. S., Eom, J. S., et al.: Pseudooutbreak of *Pantoea* species bacteremia associated with contaminated cotton pledgets. Am. J. Infect. Control. 34:443-446, 2006.

39. Kourany, M., Vasquez, M. A., and Saenz, R.: Edwardsiellosis in man and animals in Panama: Clinical and epidemiological characteristics. Am. J. Trop. Med. Hyg. 26:1183-1190, 1977.

40. Laupland, K. B., Church, D. L., Ross, T., and Pitout, J. D.: Population-based laboratory surveillance of *Hafnia alvei* isolates in a large Canadian health region. Ann. Clin. Microbiol. Antimicrob. 5:12, 2006.

41. Lim, P. S., Chen, S. L., Tsai, C. Y., and Pai, M. A.: *Pantoea* peritonitis in a patient receiving chronic ambulatory peritoneal dialysis. Nephrology (Carlton). 11:97-99, 2006.

42. Lindh, E., Kjaeldgaard, P., Frederiksen, W., et al.: Phenotypical properties of *Enterobacter agglomerans* (*Pantoea agglomerans*) from human, animal and plant sources. A. P. M. I. S. 99:347-352, 1991.

43. Maki, D. G., and Martin, W. T.: Nationwide epidemic of septicemia caused by contaminated infusion products, IV: Growth of microbial pathogens in fluids for intravenous infusions. J. Infect. Dis. 131:267-272, 1975.

44. Maki, D. G., Rhame, F. S., Mackel, D. C., et al.: Nationwide epidemic of septicemia caused by contaminated intravenous products, I: epidemiologic and clinical features. Am. J. Med. 60:471-485, 1976.

45. Manchanda, V., Singh, N. P., Eideh, H. K., et al.: Liver abscess caused by *Edwardsiella tarda* biogroup 1 and identification of its epidemiological triad by ribotyping. Indian J. Med. Microbiol. 24:135-137, 2006.

46. Marklein, G., Waschkowski, G., and Reichertz, C.: [Septicaemia caused by *Erwinia herbicola* in an 8-year-old boy (author's transl)]. Klin. Padiatr. 193:394-397, 1981.

47. Marsh, P. K., and Gorbach, S. L.: Invasive enterocolitis caused by *Edwardsiella tarda*. Gastroenterology 82:336-338, 1982.

48. Matsaniotis, N. S., Syriopoulou, V. P., Theodoridou, M. C., et al.: *Enterobacter* sepsis in infants and children due to contaminated intravenous fluids. Infect. Control 5:471-477, 1984.

49. Matsumoto, H.: Studies on the *Hafnia* isolated from normal human. Jpn. J. Microbiol. 7:105-114, 1963.

50. Matsushima, S., Yajima, S., Taguchi, T., et al.: [A fulminating case of *Edwardsiella tarda* septicemia with necrotizing fasciitis]. Kansenshogaku Zasshi. 70:631-636, 1996.

51. Mayer, K. H., and Zinner, S. H.: Bacterial pathogens of increasing significance in hospital-acquired infections. Rev. Infect. Dis. 7(Suppl. 3):S371-S379, 1985.

52. Mikamo, H., Ninomiya, M., Sawamura, H., and Tamaya, T.: Puerperal intra-uterine infection caused by *Edwardsiella tarda*. J. Infect. Chemother. 9:341-343, 2003.

53. Mojtabaee, A., and Siadati, A.: Enterobacter *Hafnia* meningitis. J. Pediatr. 93:1062-1063, 1978.

54. Muyembe, T., Vandepitte, J., and Desmyter, J.: Natural colistin resistance in *Edwardsiella tarda*. Antimicrob. Agents Chemother. 4:521-524, 1973.

55. Nagel, P., Serritella, A., and Layden, T. J.: *Edwardsiella tarda* gastroenteritis associated with a pet turtle. Gastroenterology 82:1436-1437, 1982.

56. Nettles, R. E., and Sexton, D. J.: Successful treatment of *Edwardsiella tarda* prosthetic valve endocarditis in a patient with AIDS. Clin. Infect. Dis. 25:918-919, 1997.

57. Newmark, J. J., Hobbs, W. N., and Wilson, B. E.: Reactive arthritis associated with *Hafnia alvei* enteritis. Arthritis Rheum. 37:960, 1994.

58. Oesterle, C. S., Kronenberg, H. A., and Peyman, G. A.: Endophthalmitis caused by an *Erwinia* species. Arch. Ophthalmol. 95:824-825, 1977.

59. Okubadejo, O. A., and Alausa, K. O.: Neonatal meningitis caused by *Edwardsiella tarda*. B. M. J. 3:357-358, 1968.

60. Onogawa, T., Terayama, T., Zen-yoji, H., et al.: [Distribution of *Edwardsiella tarda* and hydrogen sulfide-producing *Escherichia coli* in healthy persons]. Kansenshogaku Zasshi. 50:10-17, 1976.

61. Phillips, A. D., Trabulsi, L. R., Dougan, G., et al.: *Edwardsiella tarda* induces plasma membrane ruffles on infection of HEp-2 cells. F. E. M. S. Microbiol. Lett. 161:317-323, 1998.

62. Pien, F. D., and Jackson, M. T.: Tuboovarian abscess caused by *Edwardsiella tarda*. Am. J. Obstet. Gynecol. 173:964-965, 1995.

63. Porter, P., and Wray, C. C.: *Enterobacter agglomerans* spondylodiscitis: A possible, unrecognized complication of tetracycline therapy. Spine 25:1287-1289, 2000.

64. Rao, K. R., Shah, J., Rajashekaraiah, K. R., et al.: *Edwardsiella tarda* osteomyelitis in a patient with SC hemoglobinopathy. South. Med. J. 74:288-292, 1981.

65. Reina, J., Hervas, J., and Borrell, N.: Acute gastroenteritis caused by *Hafnia alvei* in children. Clin. Infect. Dis. 16:443, 1993.

66. Ridell, J., Siitonen, A., Paulin, L., et al.: *Hafnia alvei* in stool specimens from patients with diarrhea and healthy controls. J. Clin. Microbiol. 32:2335-2337, 1994.

67. Ridell, J., Siitonen, A., Paulin, L., et al.: Characterization of *Hafnia alvei* by biochemical tests, random amplified polymorphic DNA PCR, and partial sequencing of 16S rRNA gene. J. Clin. Microbiol. 33:2372-2376, 1995.

68. Sachs, J. M., Pacin, M., and Counts, G. W.: Sickle hemoglobinopathy and *Edwardsiella tarda* meningitis. Am. J. Dis. Child. 128:387-388, 1974.

69. Sakazaki, R.: Genus IX: *Hafnia*. *In*: Garrity, G. M. (ed.): Bergey's Manual of Systematic Bacteriology. New York: Springer, 1984, pp. 484-486.

70. Slaven, E. M., Lopez, F. A., Hart, S. M., et al.: Myonecrosis caused by *Edwardsiella tarda*: A case report and case series of extraintestinal E. *tarda* infections. Clin. Infect. Dis. 32:1430-1433, 2001.

71. Starr, M. P., and Chatterjee, A. K.: The genus *Erwinia*: Enterobacteria pathogenic to plants and animals. Annu. Rev. Microbiol. 26:389-426, 1972.

72. Stock, I., and Wiedemann, B.: Natural antibiotic susceptibilities of *Edwardsiella tarda*, E. *ictaluri*, and E. *hoshinae*. Antimicrob. Agents Chemother. 45:2245-2255, 2001.

73. Strauss, E. J., Ghori, N., and Falkow, S.: An *Edwardsiella tarda* strain containing a mutation in a gene with homology to shlB and hpmB is defective for entry into epithelial cells in culture. Infect. Immun. 65:3924-3932, 1997.

74. Thomson, K. S., Sanders, C. C., and Washington, J. A., 2nd: Ceftazidime resistance in *Hafnia alvei*. Antimicrob. Agents Chemother. 37:1375-1376, 1993.

75. Urmenyi, A. M. C., and Franklin, A. W.: Neonatal death from pigmented coliform infection. Lancet 1:313-315, 1961.

76. Vandepitte, J., Lemmens, P., and de Swert, L.: Human edwardsiellosis traced to ornamental fish. J. Clin. Microbiol. 17:165-167, 1983.

77. Van Rostenberghe, H., Noraida, R., Wan Pauzi, W. I., et al.: The clinical picture of neonatal infection with *Pantoea* species. Jpn. J. Infect. Dis. 59:120-121, 2006.

78. Vohra, K., Torrijos, E., Jhaveri, R., et al.: Neonatal sepsis and meningitis caused by *Edwardsiella tarda*. Pediatr. Infect. Dis. J. 7:814-815, 1988.

79. von Graevenitz, A.: *Erwinia* species isolates. Ann. N. Y. Acad. Sci. 174:436-443, 1970.

80. Wechsler, A. M., Bottone, E., Lasser, R., et al.: Brain abscess caused by an *Erwinia* species: Report of a case and review of the literature. Am. J. Med. 51:680-684, 1971.

81. Werkman, C. H., and Gillen, G. F.: Bacterial producing trimethylene glycol. J. Bacteriol. 23:167-182, 1932.

82. Westblom, T. U., and Milligan, T. W.: Acute bacterial gastroenteritis caused by *Hafnia alvei*. Clin. Infect. Dis. 14:1271-1272, 1992.

83. Wilson, J. P., Waterer, R. R., Wofford, J. D., Jr., et al.: Serious infections with *Edwardsiella tarda*: A case report and review of the literature. Arch. Intern. Med. 149:208-210, 1989.

84. Yang, C. H., and Wang, C. K.: *Edwardsiella tarda* bacteraemia—complicated by acute pancreatitis and pyomyoma. J. Infect. 38:124-126, 1999.

85. Yeager, A. M., Kanof, M. E., Kramer, S. S., et al.: Pneumatosis intestinalis in children after allogeneic bone marrow transplantation. Pediatr. Radiol. 17:18-22, 1987.

86. Zighelboim, J., Williams, T. W., Jr., Bradshaw, M. W., et al.: Successful medical management of a patient with multiple hepatic abscesses due to *Edwardsiella tarda*. Clin. Infect. Dis. 14:117-120, 1992.

CHAPTER 125

AEROMONAS

Ralph D. Feigin ⊕ Roger K. Nicome

Aeromonas spp. were recognized for their role in disease first by Sanarelli in 1891. His findings associated aeromonads with bacteremic "red leg" disease in frogs.[131] Studies by Hill and associates in 1954 further linked the first human disease, acute fulminating metastatic myositis, with *Aeromonas* infection.[23] Generally, *Aeromonas* spp. have been considered opportunistic pathogens for humans; however, these organisms have been identified with increasing frequency as primary pathogens in normal individuals and in compromised hosts.

Aeromonas bacteria are ubiquitous. They are found as normal flora in nonfecal sewage and are isolated from tap water, canals, streams, and rivers. They also have been isolated from clinical and food samples. Aeromonads are pathogens for cold-blooded animals (fish, amphibians, and reptiles).

EPIDEMIOLOGY

Ewing and associates[46] and other investigators have isolated *Aeromonas* from tap water and from the water or sediments of rivers, especially during periods when the water temperature was relatively warm.[75,97,139] Hazen and colleagues[61] recovered *Aeromonas hydrophila* from 135 of 147 natural water sources in 30 states of the United States and reported that its density was higher in flowing (lotic) than in calm (lentic) water systems and lower in fresh-water than in saline systems; however, *Aeromonas* could not be recovered from waters in which the saline content approached that of sea water or from extremely polluted waters. Leclerc and Buttiaux[83] found *Aeromonas* in 30 percent of more than 9000 samples of drinking water in France. *Aeromonas* also have been recovered from hospital water supplies.[97,113,114] More recently, Pin and colleagues[116] isolated these organisms from clinical and food samples, including poultry, shellfish, pork, and beef, where they thrived even at low temperatures.

Aeromonas organisms survive readily on surfaces such as bench tops and moistened paper towels. Slotnick[144] recovered *Aeromonas* organisms from a moistened paper towel that had been allowed to dry 24 hours after the application of the organisms. When the towel was placed in a humidified closed environment, the period was extended to 2 weeks.

A. hydrophila may be found in the mouths of fish, alligators, turtles, tadpoles, and frogs.[65] It also has been found in the feces of guinea pigs and laboratory mice.[40] Ticks are another source of *Aeromonas*. Unusual sources of *Aeromonas* infection include contamination of home or hospital hemodialysis equipment,[71,121] tsunami-associated wound contamination,[64] and contamination of blood or blood products.[118,122] San Joaquin and colleagues[133] noted that *Aeromonas* organisms also have been found in ornamental aquaria belonging to patients with *Aeromonas*-associated gastroenteritis; however, they found that isolates from the aquaria differed in susceptibility testing from the gastrointestinal isolates, so the aquaria probably were not the sources of infection.

Aeromonas also have been isolated from a large proportion of ready-to-eat salads.[93] Of *Aeromonas* salad isolates, 35 percent were *A. hydrophila* or *Aeromonas sobria*. All isolates tested in this study had at least one marker of enteropathogenicity, including hemolysin and cytotoxin production. Nonetheless, few if any, cases of diarrhea have been associated with ingestion of these salads in immunocompetent hosts.

In 1988, California made infection by *Aeromonas* a reportable condition, permitting the first population-based study of the epidemiology of infection caused by this organism. The overall incidence rate for *Aeromonas* isolation was 10.6 cases per 1 million population. The gastrointestinal tract was the most common site of infection (81% of cases), followed by wounds (9%). Five (2%) of 219 patients with *Aeromonas* infection died; all had serious underlying medical conditions.[78] *A. hydrophila* has been placed on the U.S. Environmental Protection Agency Contaminant Candidate List of emerging pathogens in drinking water because it has the potential to grow in water distribution systems and to be resistant to chlorination.[14]

ETIOLOGIC AGENT

Aeromonas organisms are motile, asporogenic, gram-negative rods that contain a single polar flagellum. The organisms are oxidase-positive and catalase-positive and produce acid or gas during carbohydrate fermentation. They can grow at temperatures between 0° C and 41° C. Growth may occur within a pH range of 5.5 to 9. Lipase, gelatinase, DNase, and other exoenzymes are formed by these organisms.[45,138,156]

Aeromonads grow well on blood agar; most strains produce a large zone of beta-hemolysis on this medium, although nonhemolytic strains exist. *Aeromonas* colonies on blood agar have a ground-glass appearance and a fruity odor.[158] Aeromonads also grow on MacConkey, eosin-methylene blue, *Salmonella-Shigella*, and triple sugar iron media.

The sensitivity and specificity of various media for detection of *Aeromonas* spp. in fecal specimens have been evaluated.[103,126,155] Isolation is achieved readily on any of the following: pril-xylose-ampicillin agar, xylose-sodium, deoxycholate citrate agar, alkaline peptonic water, inositol–brilliant green bile salts agar, trypticase soy broth with ampicillin, and dextrin-fuchsin-sulfite agar.[155] The colonies appear almost colorless on these media, with the exception of growth on dextrin-fuchsin-sulfite agar, on which they appear dark red.

Mishva and associates[99] evaluated five selective agars. Of these, sheep blood agar with 30 mg of ampicillin/L (ASBA 30) permitted the greatest number of *Aeromonas* colonies to grow, while also inhibiting the competing fecal flora. They recommend that ASBA 30 be used with DNase–toluidine blue agar (DNTA) to detect the ampicillin-susceptible strains and the nonhemolytic strains. The combination of ASBA 30-DNTA allowed 98 percent of all isolates to be detected.

Strains of motile *Aeromonas* isolates can be identified to species level by use of the following tests: production of nitrate reductase; fermentation of D-glucose and trehalose; failure to use mucate; and the inability to produce acid from D-arabitol, dulcitol, erythritol, and xylose.[1] Detection of *Aeromonas* organisms by use of strain-specific fluorescent antibody has been described.[155] The technique is not satisfactory; only a small percentage of isolates react with prepared antisera, which suggests the presence of numerous serogroups. The use of a monoclonal antibody against *A. hydrophila* has been shown to overcome this problem, however.[38] This monoclonal antibody could prove beneficial in the future as a screening tool. Additionally, the study of selected housekeeping genes has been helpful in establishing phylogenetic relationships among members of the aeromonads.[147]

Aeromonas previously was considered a member of the Vibrionaceae family, which included the genera of *Vibrio* and *Plesiomonas*.[119] Molecular genetic techniques have identified that these three genera are not related evolutionarily, however, and aeromonads represent a family of their own.[34] *Aeromonas* have long been viewed as belonging to one of two major groups on the basis of their ability to grow at different temperatures. Mesophiles were strains that grew at 35° C to 37° C, and psychrophilic strains were more prevalent at lower temperatures (22° C to 28° C). These two groups could be distinguished not only by optimal growth conditions but also by elaboration of pigmentation on tyrosine agar and production of indole. The mesophilic strains are motile, and the psychrophilic strains are nonmotile.

Fourteen *Aeromonas* spp. have been recognized, and this number is expected to increase as new strains are isolated and identified.[1] Although the number of strains of psychrophilic *Aeromonas* spp. has remained stable, the number of various strains of mesophilic species isolated has increased. Several classification schemes within the genus are in use. The strains are classified based on biochemical assays or the use of genotyping techniques such as DNA-DNA hybridization and restriction fragment length polymorphism of the 16S rRNA, or both. Genetic techniques have been used to differentiate the genus into genomospecies or hybridization groups (HG), allowing more precise identification.[15]

Abbott and associates[1] classified *Aeromonas* based on the results of the Møeller decarboxylase and dihydrolase reactions. They also were able to place the strains they studied into complexes based on certain biochemical reactions. The *Aeromonas* strains that produced elastase, pectinase, and staphylosin were grouped into the *A. hydrophila* complex (*A. hydrophila*, *Aeromonas bestiarum*, *Aeromonas salmonicida*). Similarly, the *Aeromonas carviae* complex includes *A. caviae*, *Aeromonas media*, and *Aeromonas eucrenophil*, and the *Aeromonas sobria* complex comprises *Aeromonas veronii* HG8, *Aeromonas jandaei*, *Aeromonas schubertii*, and *Aeromonas trota*.

In addition, other species, including *Aeromonas media* (similar to *A. salmonicida*),[5] *A. veronii*,[63] *A. schubertii*,[22,62] *A. jandaei*,[20] *A. trota*,[21] *Aeromonas allosaccharophila*,[91] *Aeromonas encheleia*,[44] *A. bestiarum*,[6] *Aeromonas popoffii*,[68] and *A. eucrenophila*,[138] have been described. A new species, *Aeromonas culicicola*, was isolated more recently.[115] Other isolates include *Aeromonas enteropelogenes* and *Aeromonas ichthiosmia*, which seem to be similar to previously identified species.[33] Of the species isolated currently, *A. hydrophila*, *A. caviae*, and *A. veronii* have been associated most often with human infections.[69]

Aeromonas is confused most frequently with Enterobacteriaceae. The oxidase test always should be performed to aid in differentiation; *Aeromonas* organisms generally are oxidase-positive, whereas Enterobacteriaceae organisms are oxidase-negative. McGrath and associates[95] described oxidase-variable strains of *A. hydrophila*. These strains are oxidase-positive when grown on nonselective media but oxidase-negative when grown on differential or gram-negative media. Organic acid end-products of lactose fermentation can inhibit the oxidase reaction. Paik[110] also has shown that a platinum wire loop should be used for oxidase testing; use of an iron-containing loop can cause false-positive oxidase results.

Aeromonas is susceptible to ceftriaxone (8 µg/mL), chloramphenicol (2 to 4 µg/mL), gentamicin (0.5 to 2 µg/mL), streptomycin (16 µg/mL), and trimethoprim-sulfamethoxazole (<0.5/9.5 µg/mL).[46,47,108,109,123,155] Reinhardt and George[124] determined that the most active on a weight basis were ciprofloxacin, enoxacin, and norfloxacin; nalidixic acid and trimethoprim-sulfamethoxazole also possessed good activity. Neither sulfamethoxazole nor trimethoprim alone was active. In addition, they did not note appreciable differences in susceptibility among species or in susceptibility between fecal versus nonenteric isolates. In contrast, Motyl and colleagues[102] noted higher levels of resistance to various antibiotics among *A. hydrophila* strains compared with *A. sobria* or *A. caviae*, as judged by minimal inhibitory concentration. Susceptibility to cephalothin may serve as a useful criterion in the identification of *A. sobria*.[102,133]

Aeromonas organisms consistently are resistant to penicillin, ampicillin, carbenicillin, cephalothin, erythromycin, clindamycin, and vancomycin. Sawai and associates[137] showed that resistance to β-lactam antibiotics is caused by the production of a species-specific, chromosome-mediated β-lactamase. It is not R plasmid–mediated. In 1980, McNicol and coworkers[96] reported the recovery of *Aeromonas* isolates from the Chesapeake Bay that were resistant to tetracycline and polymyxin B. They also noted that 57 percent of isolates from Bangladesh had a multiple streptomycin-chloramphenicol-tetracycline resistance phenotype that correlated with the presence of a larger plasmid.

PATHOGENESIS

In addition to its pili, *A. hydrophila* produces numerous virulence factors, including extracellular toxins and enzymes that are involved in the pathogenesis of *A. hydrophila* infection. Some of the toxins elaborated by *A. hydrophila* include hemolysins, aerolysin, and enterotoxins.

Alpha-hemolysin is released from cells during a stationary growth phase. Alpha-hemolysin has a molecular weight of 50,000[87,88] to 65,000[88] and is stable at room temperature between pH 3.5 and 9.5. It is heat-labile. Alpha-hemolysin is cytotoxic to HeLa cells and human embryonic lung fibroblasts.[154] When injected into rabbit skin, it causes dermonecrosis. Intraperitoneal injection of alpha-hemolysin is lethal for rabbits and mice.

Beta-hemolysin has a molecular weight of 49,000 to 53,000 and is released near the end of the logarithmic phase of growth of the *Aeromonas* organism. It is heat-labile and resists destruction by trypsin and pronase.[88] It causes dermonecrosis of rabbit skin and is lethal for rabbits, rats, and mice. It is cytotoxic to HeLa cells and to human diploid lung fibroblasts.[152] It also has been shown to induce impairment in the intestinal epithelial barrier and to stimulate active chloride secretion in human colon cell monolayers, contributing to enteritis.[43]

Alpha-hemolysin and beta-hemolysin may be significant virulence factors. Most clinical isolates are beta-hemolytic, and hemolysis is a common feature of infection caused by *Aeromonas* spp. Alpha-hemolysin and beta-hemolysin in high concentrations produce hemorrhagic enteritis in a rabbit ileal loop; however, neither alpha-hemolysin nor beta-hemolysin is clearly established as a virulence factor in diarrheal disease.[89] Antibodies to either hemolysin neutralize both toxins.

Aerolysin is a pore-forming toxin that shares some homology with beta-hemolysin.[43] After inserting into its target cells, it disrupts ion gradients and membrane potentials, leading to cell lysis.[82] Caco-2 cells derived from human intestine have been shown to be very sensitive to the effects of aerolysin.[2]

In 1975, Sanyal and associates[135] showed that the enterotoxins from *A. hydrophila* were enterotoxigenic. Subsequently, enterotoxigenic *A. hydrophila* has been isolated from humans,[19,55-58,75,157] water sources, fish, and pigs.[16,108] Sha and colleagues[140] have characterized three enterotoxins from *A. hydrophila*. The cytotoxic enterotoxin has hemolytic, cytotoxic, and enterotoxic activities and has a molecular weight of 52,000. It is a pore-forming toxin that has been shown to cause fluid secretion and tissue damage in mouse ileal loops.[82] The other two are cytotonic enterotoxins. One has a molecular weight of 44,000 and is heat-labile. The second has a predicted molecular weight of 71,000 and is heat-stable. These cytotonic enterotoxins cause elevation of cyclic adenosine monophosphate and prostaglandin levels in Chinese hamster ovary cells and fluid secretion in rabbit ileal loops.[140] All three enterotoxins have been implicated in *A. hydrophila*–induced gastroenteritis. *Aeromonas* spp. also produce proteinase A and B, endopeptidase, staphylolytic enzyme, fibrinolysin, and leukocidin.[87] The precise relationship of these toxins and enzymes to the pathogenesis of human infection is unclear.

Strains of *Aeromonas* produce proteases, DNase, lecithinase, and elastase.[3] These extracellular enzymes may have pathologic significance. *Aeromonas* strains that possess hemolytic and cytotoxic capabilities and that are characterized as HG1/BD-2 type strains have been related strongly to patients with diarrheal disease.[81]

Antihemolysin and agglutinating and precipitating antibodies to *A. hydrophila* have been detected in patients with systemic *Aeromonas* infections but not in patients with superficial infections. Increases in the antihemolysin titer to 1:1280 and in the agglutinin titer to 1:640 have been noted.[24]

Burke and colleagues[18] found that many strains associated with diarrhea were able to hemagglutinate cells from human, horse, rat, and guinea pig. Of these strains, 68 percent displayed fucose-resistant hemagglutination. The investigators suggested that these properties may contribute to virulence.

Ketover and associates[76] showed that normal serum promotes phagocytosis and intracellular killing of *Aeromonas* organisms by normal white blood cells. In contrast, sera from two patients with fatal *Aeromonas* infections failed to do so. One patient had an increase in the serum opsonic antibody titer from less than 1:5 in the acute stage of disease to 1:5120 in the convalescent stage. These studies suggest that a specific opsonizing antibody that is present in normal serum and normal bactericidal activity of neutrophils are required to prevent invasive *A. hydrophila* infections.

The flexible type IV pili of *Aeromonas* are the predominant pili expressed on fecal isolates of diarrhea-associated species of *Aeromonas*. They represent a family of type IV pili that has been designated Bfp (bundle-forming pili). Kirov and associates[79] have presented compelling evidence to support the concept that Bfp are important intestinal colonization factors. More recently, this group also showed that *Aeromonas* flagella are adhesins for human intestinal cells, playing a role in its enteropathogenicity.

Serogroup analysis may be helpful in establishing which *Aeromonas* isolates can cause human disease. Serogroups O:11, O:34, and O:16 predominate as causes of clinical infection.[70]

Clear correlation between known virulence properties and enteropathogenicity in humans is lacking. This lack of a clear correlation has been attributed to the heterogeneity of *Aeromonas* spp., the great variety of *Aeromonas* virulence factors, and the loose association between virulence factors and the phenotype and genotype.[69] Consequently, many researchers have proposed a multifactorial pathogenesis with the involvement of numerous cellular and extracellular virulence factors.[29]

CLINICAL MANIFESTATIONS

Aeromonas spp. have been implicated as a cause of septicemia, gastroenteritis, peritonitis, skin and wound infections, osteomyelitis, septic arthritis, ocular infections, myositis, urinary tract infections, pneumonia, meningitis, and hemolytic-uremic syndrome in children. Most of these infections have been noted in normal and compromised hosts.[13,48,111,112]

Sepsis caused by *Aeromonas* spp. has been reported in children.* Because *Aeromonas* infection is not a reportable disease, the total number of affected children is unknown. Although septicemia caused by *Aeromonas* spp. has occurred in normal children, most children affected have had a disorder known to impair the normal host response to infection or a disorder in which the intact skin as a barrier to infection has been destroyed. *Aeromonas* infection has been noted in children with leukemia (particularly those with neutropenia), aplastic anemia, cirrhosis, hemoglobinopathies, malnutrition, burns, and renal failure.

The clinical manifestations of septicemia are similar to the manifestations noted in other gram-negative enteric bloodstream infections with high fever and shock. During the course of septicemia in some of these patients, ecthyma gangrenosum also has been noted. The reported case-fatality rate of 50 percent despite administration of antibiotic therapy presumably is related to the severity of the underlying disorders and not to an unusual virulence of the organism. The propensity for infection in the compromised host suggests that *Aeromonas* organisms are of low virulence for the human host. Bacteremia with *A. sobria* and *A. punctata* also has been described.[71,122,143]

Meningitis caused by *Aeromonas* spp. also has been reported in children.[49,50,159] In one reported review of 21 years' experience with gram-negative bacillary meningitis, *Aeromonas* spp. accounted for 2 percent of the cases.[154] The course was fulminant, and the patients died despite having received antibiotic therapy. All of these children could be considered immunocompromised as a result of sickle-cell anemia (a 23-month-old child) or age (neonates).

Gastrointestinal infections caused by *Aeromonas* spp. have been reported with greater frequency in pediatric patients. *A.*

hydrophila, *A. sobria*, *A. caviae*, and *A. punctata* have been recovered from stool specimens of patients with gastroenteritis.[19,28,51,71,101] In 1961, Martinez-Silva and colleagues[92] described an epidemic of enteritis in a newborn nursery affecting nine infants (eight as newborns and one at 7 days old). *Aeromonas* spp. were found in the stools of six of these infants. One newborn, the only patient with a pure growth of *Aeromonas* in a stool specimen, died. In 1964, Rosner[129] reported severe gastroenteritis in a child with growth of *A. hydrophila* from four stool cultures. In 1991, one study reported 224 cases of *Aeromonas* gastroenteritis in Iowa from January to June.[120] Taneja and associates[150] described an outbreak of diarrhea caused by *Aeromonas* spp. on a hematology-oncology ward in a pediatric hospital during March-April 2001 where 6 of 18 children were infected. *Aeromonas* spp. were found to be the sole enteropathogen in five of the six children. Aeromonads have been detected worldwide as the sole pathogen causing diarrhea in 2 to 20 percent of affected children and in only 0 to 2 percent of children without diarrhea.[29,39,56,151]

In an attempt to assess the role of *Aeromonas* spp. in diarrheal disease, numerous investigators have evaluated the fecal carriage rate of the organism.[60] Freij[50] described a study performed by other investigators who recovered *Aeromonas* from 0 of 300 adults and from 31 of 4426 (0.7%) children younger than 2 years. Pitarangsi and coworkers[117] reported carrier rates of 16 to 27 percent in various districts in Thailand and noted the same frequency of *A. hydrophila* in stools of Thais with and without diarrhea. In contrast, *A. hydrophila* was recovered from the stools of American Peace Corps volunteers more frequently when they had diarrhea than when their stool frequency was normal. Only three *Aeromonas* isolates were reported from 1685 rectal swab cultures obtained from 1217 children hospitalized for gastroenteritis in Manitoba, Canada. Bhat and colleagues[10] recovered *Aeromonas* organisms from 7 of 133 patients with acute diarrhea in a valley in India and found *Aeromonas* and *Plesiomonas shigelloides* in the well water commonly used by these individuals. Soltan Dallal and Moezardalan[148] isolated *Aeromonas* spp. from 14 of 310 Iranian children in a case-control study.

Gracey and associates[57,58] described a prospective study in Australia of 1156 children with diarrhea and an equal number of age-matched and sex-matched control subjects. Enterotoxigenic *Aeromonas* organisms were isolated from 10.2 percent of children with diarrhea compared with 0.6 percent of healthy children. *Aeromonas* was the only potential pathogen recovered in 6.5 percent of children with diarrhea. Cases of *Aeromonas* infection peaked during the summer months. The mean duration of diarrhea was 15.3 days, and 33 percent of the children required hospitalization. These investigators described three clinical syndromes of *Aeromonas* gastroenteritis: (1) watery diarrhea, vomiting, and low-grade fever in 41 percent; (2) diarrhea with blood and mucus in 22 percent; and (3) prolonged diarrhea of more than 2 weeks' duration in 37 percent.

Many investigators[4,27,104,106,132] have attempted to describe gastrointestinal infections caused by *Aeromonas* spp. Gluskin and associates[53] performed a 15-year study of the rate of *Aeromonas* spp. in gastroenteritis in hospitalized children. A total of 146 strains of *Aeromonas* spp. were isolated from 32,810 fecal specimens from 13,820 hospitalized patients. These isolates constituted 4 percent of all pathogenic bacterial strains cultured. Most of the cases of diarrhea (94%) occurred in children younger than 3 years old. The peak incidence occurred in infants aged 2 to 6 months. Bloody diarrhea occurred in 7 percent of children. Several investigators[4,132] have detected a larger number of cases of *Aeromonas*-associated diarrhea in the summer months than in other months, whereas Challapali and colleagues[27] found no seasonal patterns of *Aeromonas* isolation. The greatest number of cases occurred in children younger than 12 months to 3 years of age.

Symptoms included diarrhea, bloody stools, vomiting, abdominal cramps, mild dehydration, and fever. *Aeromonas*-associated

---

*See references 17, 32, 36, 59, 67, 76, 105, 111, 128, 136, 158-160.

diarrhea resembled other types of bacterial diarrhea, except that fecal leukocytes were absent in children with *Aeromonas*-associated diarrhea; in contrast, fecal leukocytes were found in 60 percent of children with other types of bacterial enteritis.[27] A cholera-like illness caused by enterotoxigenic *A. sobria* has been described.[28] Gastroenteritis caused by *A. sobria* and *A. hydrophila* tended to be acute, whereas diarrhea associated with *A. caviae* frequently was chronic, lasting 4 to 6 weeks in untreated patients.

San Joaquin and Pickett[132] described three patients with *A. caviae* diarrhea who originally presented with failure to thrive presumed to be secondary to formula intolerance. Diarrhea in these patients improved after administration of trimethoprim-sulfamethoxazole. Moyer[104] noted that although *A. caviae* is considered nonpathogenic, five pediatric patients with otitis media who were treated with penicillin or ampicillin subsequently developed diarrhea in which *A. caviae* was the only potential enteric pathogen. The prior therapy with antibiotics to which *Aeromonas* spp. are known to be resistant probably contributed to colonization of the gastrointestinal tract with *A. caviae* and subsequent development of diarrhea. These four patients also were treated successfully with trimethoprim-sulfamethoxazole.

Outbreaks of diarrhea associated with *Aeromonas* in daycare centers have been described.[39] *A. caviae*, *A. hydrophila*, and *A. sobria* were the strains recovered most commonly.

Complications of *Aeromonas* intestinal infection included gram-negative bacteremia, intussusception, internal hernia strangulation, hemolytic-uremic syndrome,[13,125] and failure to thrive. Peritonitis has been reported in a 5-year-old patient with a ruptured appendix.[67] No additional clinical information about this patient was provided.

A. hydrophila has been recovered from the skin or from wound infections of children.* Most of these patients have been normal hosts; three had leukemia. In 40 percent of these cases, *Aeromonas* organisms were not recovered from the lesion in pure culture. The lower extremity was involved in 75 percent of these cases. Exposure to water was noted in 40 percent of these cases; alligator bites, snakebites, stepping on glass, and burns were other presumed predisposing factors. Clinical manifestations included cellulitis, hemorrhagic blebs, and purulent diarrhea with fever and leukocytosis. Secondary bacteremia and osteomyelitis have been reported.[12]

We (R.D.F.) have recovered *Aeromonas* organisms from skin lesions that have been the result of tick bites. In each of these cases, a circumscribed area of purple discoloration has surrounded the bite, and nonpurulent drainage from the center of the lesion yielded the organism. These patients sought medical attention because the local lesion had persisted or had increased in size over the course of 1 to 2 weeks. *A. schubertii* also has been isolated from traumatic wound infections.[22]

Ecthyma gangrenosum caused by *A. hydrophila* has been described in several children with leukemia.[76,105,141] We (R.D.F.) have seen ecthyma gangrenosum in several children with *Aeromonas* septicemia who have had malignant or hepatobiliary disease. Clark and Chenoweth[31] isolated *A. hydrophila* from an 18-month-old boy and a 2-year-old boy, both of whom had liver transplants for biliary atresia and subsequently developed cholangitis. In both instances, these were polymicrobial infections.

Lopez and associates[90] described an 8-year-old child with acute myelogenous leukemia with bacteremia and osteomyelitis; *Aeromonas* organisms grew from a bone aspirate of this patient. Blatz[12] reported finding osteomyelitis and *Aeromonas* bacteremia in a previously healthy 16-year-old patient; a bone aspirate was not attempted. Septic arthritis caused by *A. hydrophila* also has been described in a child with leukemia; the organism was recov-

ered from the second metacarpophalangeal joint at autopsy.[36] Elwitigala and colleagues[42] also recovered *A. hydrophila* in a previously healthy 13-year-old girl who developed severe septic arthritis of the knee after injury sustained in a private fresh-water lake. This infection frequently is rapidly progressive.

Aeromonas has been recovered from the conjunctiva of a previously healthy 7-year-old boy whose eye had been penetrated by a safety pin[145] and from the anterior chamber of an 8-year-old boy who developed endophthalmitis after receiving a corneal laceration from a fishhook.[32] *A. sobria* endophthalmitis has been described in a 14-year-old patient after a penetrating eye injury occurred in which a cormorant pecked the patient's eye.[84]

Although numerous cases of *Aeromonas* urinary tract infections have been reported in adults, only a few cases have been reported in children. McCracken and Barkley[94] reported the recovery of *A. hydrophila* in pure culture from the urine of a 5-month-old boy with diarrhea. Bartolomé and colleagues[9] described a case of urinary tract infection associated with diarrhea in a newborn boy with bilateral ureterohydronephrosis and bladder involvement from posterior urethral valves. Ojeda-Vargas and associates[107] reported the case of an 18-year-old girl with severe pyelonephritis requiring admission to the intensive care unit. *A. hydrophila* and *Pseudomonas* were isolated from her urine cultures.

Myositis caused by *Aeromonas* also has been described in children. A 9-year-old girl and a 16-year-old boy required amputation of their legs as a result of *Aeromonas* myositis.[37,146] Necrosis of muscle was noted in both cases, and gas was seen on the radiographs before amputation in the 9-year-old girl. Fatal myofascial necrosis also has been reported in a patient with a history of aplastic anemia.[54] *A. hydrophila* also has been isolated from abscesses caused by snakebites.[72]

Pneumonia caused by *A. hydrophila* is a rare event in children. Kao and associates[74] reported that there have been a total of seven case reports in the literature so far, and four patients died of fulminant disease. Of the seven patients, four had accompanying medical conditions, including acute leukemia (two patients), cavernous hemangioma with thrombocytopenia (one patient), and nephrotic syndrome (one patient). One patient was the victim of a near-drowning, and two patients were previously healthy.[74,123,142] One of the previously healthy patients was described by Kao and associates[74] in their case report and literature review. The patient was a 5-year-old girl who presented with fulminant sepsis and pneumonia and quickly died. *A. hydrophila* was recovered from her blood, endotracheal aspirate, and postmortem pleural fluid. Neither a bone marrow aspirate nor an immunologic work-up was performed, so whether she had an underlying malignancy or immunodeficiency that might have contributed to her rapid demise is unknown. *A. hydrophila* has been isolated from lung abscess at autopsy of a 16-year-old girl with *A. hydrophila* septicemia and leukemia.[36]

DIAGNOSIS AND DIFFERENTIAL DIAGNOSIS

Aeromonas should be considered a possible cause of infection in children with any of the disorders previously noted. It always should be included as a possible cause of gastroenteritis, bacteremia, and skin infection in a compromised host. Generally, *Aeromonas* organisms are recognized only when they grow from body fluids or tissues that normally are sterile. The best methods for isolation of *Aeromonas* organisms have been described (see the section on etiologic agent).

A. hydrophila in food can be detected by an enzyme-linked immunosorbent assay and polymerase chain reaction.[11,98,153] These organisms also have been identified in environmental

---

*See references 9, 12, 37, 48, 67, 76, 94, 105, 112, 128, 141, 149, 155.

samples by use of 16S rDNA–targeted oligonucleotide primers.[41] Many sophisticated techniques, including rRNA sequencing, DNA-DNA reassociation techniques, and polymerase chain reaction, have been used to continue to identify and differentiate *Aeromonas* spp.[15,35,69,77]

TREATMENT AND PROGNOSIS

Aeromonas infection occurs infrequently; controlled studies to permit recommendation of one antibiotic over all others are unavailable. Penicillin-hydrolyzing β-lactamases have been detected in most strains of *Aeromonas*, rendering those strains resistant to ampicillin.[100] Piperacillin shows variable activity against *Aeromonas* spp., whereas ticarcillin-clavulanate generally is active. In vitro, *Aeromonas* organisms generally are susceptible to chloramphenicol, aminoglycosides, trimethoprim-sulfamethoxazole, aztreonam, quinolones, and the third-generation cephalosporins.[73,80,130]

In our (R.D.F.) experience, chloramphenicol or third-generation cephalosporins have proved efficacious. A drug to which the organism is sensitive should be provided (usually intravenously). The duration of administration depends on the site of infection and the clinical response to therapy. The occurrence of *Aeromonas* infections predominantly in compromised hosts accounts for the high case-fatality rate despite administration of an antibiotic agent to which the organism is susceptible.

REFERENCES

1. Abbott, S. L., Cheung, W. K., and Janda, J. M.: The genus *Aeromonas*: Biochemical characteristics, atypical reactions, and phenotypic identification schemes. J. Clin. Microbiol. *41*:2348-2357, 2003.
2. Abrami, L., Fivaz, M., Glauser, P. E., et al.: Sensitivity of polarized epithelial cells to the pore-forming toxin aerolysin. Infect. Immun. *71*:739-746, 2003.
3. Agarwal, R. K., Kapoor, K. N., and Kumar, A.: Virulence factors of Aeromonads—an emerging food borne pathogen problem. J. Commun. Dis. *30*:71-78, 1998.
4. Agger, W. A., McCormick, J. D., and Gurwith, M. J.: Clinical and microbial features of *Aeromonas hydrophila*–associated diarrhea. J. Clin. Microbiol. *21*:909-913, 1985.
5. Albert, M. J., Ansaruzzaman, M., Talukder, K. A., et al.: Prevalence of enterotoxin genes in *Aeromonas* spp. isolated from children with diarrhea, healthy controls, and the environment. J. Clin. Microbiol. *38*:3785-3790, 2000.
6. Ali, A., Carnahan, A. M., Altwegg, M., et al.: *Aeromonas bestiarum* sp. nov. (formerly genomospecies DNA group 2 *A. hydrophilia*), a new species isolated from non-human sources. Med. Microbiol. Lett. *5*:156-165, 1996.
7. Allen, D. A., Austin, B., and Colwell, R. R.: *Aeromonas media*, a new species isolated from river water. Int. J. Syst. Bacteriol. *33*:599, 1983.
8. Asao, T., Kozaki, S., Kato, K., et al.: Purification and characterization of an *Aeromonas hydrophila* hemolysin. J. Clin. Microbiol. *24*:228-232, 1986.
9. Bartolomé, R. M., Andreu, A., Xercavins, M., et al.: Urinary tract infection by *Aeromonas hydrophila* in a neonate. Infection *17*:172-173, 1989.
10. Bhat, P., Shanthakumari, S., and Rajan, D.: The characterization and significance of *Plesiomonas shigelloides* and *Aeromonas hydrophila* isolated from an epidemic of diarrhoea. Indian J. Med. Res. *62*:1051-1060, 1974.
11. Bin Kingombe, C. I., Huys, G., Howald, D., et al.: The usefulness of molecular techniques to assess the presence of *Aeromonas* spp. harboring virulence markers in foods. Int. J. Food Microbiol. *94*:113-121, 2004.
12. Blatz, D. J.: Open fracture of the tibia and fibula complicated by infection with *Aeromonas hydrophila*: A case report. J. Bone Joint Surg. Am. *61*:790-791, 1979.
13. Bogdanovic, R., Cobeljic, M., Markovic, M., et al.: Haemolytic-uraemic syndrome associated with *Aeromonas hydrophila* enterocolitis. Pediatr. Nephrol. *5*:293-295, 1991.
14. Borchardt, M. A., Stemper, M. E., Standridge, J. H.: Isolates from human diarrheic stool and groundwater compared by pulsed-field gel electrophoresis. Emerg. Infect. Dis. *9*:224-228, 2003.
15. Borrell, N., Acinas, S. G., Figueras, M. J., and Martinez-Murcia, A. J.: Identification of *Aeromonas* clinical isolates by restriction fragment length polymorphism of PCR-amplified 16S rRNA genes. J. Clin. Microbiol. *35*:1671-1674, 1997.
16. Boulanger, Y., Lallier, R., and Cousineau, G.: Isolation of enterotoxigenic *Aeromonas* from fish. Can. J. Microbiol. *23*:1161-1164, 1977.
17. Bulger, R. J., and Sherris, J. C.: The clinical significance of *Aeromonas hydrophila*: Report of two cases. Arch. Intern. Med. *118*:562-564, 1966.
18. Burke, V., Cooper, M., and Robinson, J.: Haemagglutination patterns of *Aeromonas* spp. related to species and source of strains. Aust. J. Exp. Biol. Med. Sci. *64*:563-570, 1986.
19. Burke, V., Gracey, M., Robinson, J., et al.: The microbiology of childhood gastroenteritis: *Aeromonas* species and other infective agents. J. Infect. Dis. *148*:68-74, 1983.
20. Carnahan, A., Fanning, G. R., and Joseph, S. W.: *Aeromonas jandaei* (formerly genospecies DNA group 9 *A. sobria*), new sucrose-negative species isolated from clinical specimens. J. Clin. Microbiol. *29*:560-564, 1991.
21. Carnahan, A. M., Chakraborty, T., Fanning, G. R., et al.: *Aeromonas trota* sp. nov., an ampicillin-susceptible species isolated from clinical specimens. J. Clin. Microbiol. *29*:1206-1210, 1991.
22. Carnahan, A. M., Marii, M. A., Fanning, G. R., et al.: Characterization of *Aeromonas schubertii* strains recently isolated from traumatic wound infections. J. Clin. Microbiol. *27*:1826-1830, 1989.
23. Caselitz, F. H.: How the *Aeromonas* story started in medical microbiology. Med. Microbiol. Lett. *5*:46-54, 1996.
24. Caselitz, F. H., Freitag, V., and Jannasch, G.: Demonstration of specific antibodies in sera of patients with infections caused by *Aeromonas hydrophila*. Zentralbl. Bakteriol. Mikrobiol. Hyg. A. *233*:347-354, 1975.
25. Chakraborty, T., Huhle, B., Bergbauer, H., and Goebel, W.: Cloning, expression, and mapping of the *Aeromonas hydrophila* aerolysin gene determinant in *Escherichia coli* K-12. J. Bacteriol. *167*:368-374, 1986.
26. Chakraborty, T., Montenegro, M. A., Sanyal, S. C., et al.: Cloning of enterotoxin gene from *Aeromonas hydrophila* provides conclusive evidence of production of a cytotonic enterotoxin. Infect. Immun. *46*:435-441, 1984.
27. Challapali, M., Tess, B. R., Cunningham, D. G., et al.: *Aeromonas*-associated diarrhea in children. Pediatr. Infect. Dis. *7*:693-698, 1988.
28. Champsaur, H., Andremont, A., Mathieu, D., et al.: Cholera-like illness due to *Aeromonas sobria*. J. Infect. Dis. *145*:248-254, 1982.
29. Chopra, A. K., and Houston, C. W.: Enterotoxins in *Aeromonas*-associated gastroenteritis. Microbes Infect. *1*:1129-1137, 1999.
30. Chopra, A. K., Houston, C. W., Peterson J. W., and Jin, G. F.: Cloning, expression, and sequence analysis of a cytolytic enterotoxin gene from *Aeromonas hydrophila*. Can. J. Microbiol. *39*:513-523, 1993.
31. Clark, N. M., and Chenoweth, C. E.: *Aeromonas* infection of the hepatobiliary system: Report of 15 cases and review of the literature. Clin. Infect. Dis. *37*:506-513, 2003.
32. Cohen, K. L., Holyk, P. R., McCarthy, L. R., et al.: *Aeromonas hydrophila* and *Plesiomonas shigelloides* endophthalmitis. Am. J. Ophthalmol. *96*:403-404, 1983.
33. Collins, M. D., Martinez-Murcia, A. J., and Cai, J.: *Aeromonas enteropelogenes* and *Aeromonas ichthiosmia* are identical to *Aeromonas trota* and *Aeromonas veronii*, respectively, as revealed by small-subunit rRNA sequence analysis. Int. J. Syst. Bacteriol. *43*:855-856, 1993.
34. Colwell, R. R., MacDonell, M. T., and DeLey, J.: Proposal to recognize the family Aeromonadaceae fam. nov. Int. J. Syst. Bacteriol. *36*:473-477, 1986.
35. Davin-Regli, A., Bollet, C., Chamorey, E., et al.: A cluster of cases of infections due to *Aeromonas hydrophila* revealed by combined RAPD and ERIC-PCR. J. Med. Microbiol. *47*:499-504, 1998.
36. Dean, H. M., and Post, R. M.: Fatal infection with *Aeromonas hydrophila* in a patient with acute myelogenous leukemia. Ann. Intern. Med. *66*:1177-1179, 1967.
37. Deepe, G. S., and Coonrod, J. D.: Fulminant wound infection with *Aeromonas hydrophila*. South. Med. J. *73*:1546-1547, 1980.
38. Delamare, A. P., Echeverrigaray S., Duarte, K. R., et al.: Production of a monoclonal antibody against *Aeromonas hydrophila* and its application to bacterial identification. J. Appl. Microbiol. *92*:936-940, 2002.
39. de la Morena, M. L., Van, R., Singh, K., et al.: Diarrhea associated with *Aeromonas* species in children in day care centers. J. Infect. Dis. *168*:215-218, 1993.
40. Dobrescu, L.: Enterotoxigenic *Aeromonas hydrophila* from a case of piglet diarrhea. Zentralbl. Veterinarmed. B. *25*:713-718, 1978.
41. Dorsch, M., Ashbolt, N. J., Cox, P. T., et al.: Rapid identification of *Aeromonas* species using 16S rDNA targeted oligonucleotide primers: A molecular approach based on screening of environmental isolates. J. Appl. Bacteriol. *77*:722-726, 1994.
42. Elwitigala, J. P., Higgs, D. S., Namnyak, S., et al.: Septic arthritis due to *Aeromonas hydrophila*: Case report and review of the literature. Int. J. Clin. Pract. *147*(Suppl.):121-124, 2005.
43. Epple, H. J., Mankertz, J., Ignatius, R., et al.: *Aeromonas hydrophila* beta-hemolysin induces active chloride secretion in colon epithelial cells (HT-29/B6). Infect. Immun. *72*:4848-4858, 2004.
44. Esteve, C., Gutierrez, M. C., and Ventosa, A.: *Aeromonas encheleia* sp. nov., isolated from European eels. Int. J. Syst. Bacteriol. *45*:462-466, 1995.
45. Ewing, W. H., and Hugh, R.: *Aeromonas*. *In* Lennette, E. H., Spaulding, E. H., and Truant, J. P. (eds.): Manual of Clinical Microbiology. 2nd ed. Washington, D.C., American Society for Microbiology, 1974, pp. 230-237.
46. Ewing, W. H., Hugh, R., and Johnson, J. G.: Studies on the *Aeromonas* Group. Public Health Service, Communicable Disease Center, 1961, pp. 1-8.
47. Fainstein, V., Weaver, S., and Bodey, G. P.: In vitro susceptibilities of *Aeromonas hydrophila* against new antibiotics. Antimicrob. Agents Chemother. *22*:513-514, 1982.

48. Fraire, A. E.: *Aeromonas hydrophila* infection. J. A. M. A. *239*:192, 1978.

49. Freij, B. J.: *Aeromonas*: Biology of the organism and diseases in children. Pediatr. Infect. Dis. *3*:164-175, 1984.

50. Freij, B. J.: Human disease other than gastroenteritis caused by *Aeromonas* and *Plesiomonas*. *Aeromonas* Symposium, Manchester, England, September 5-6, 1986, pp. 19-20.

51. Fritsche, D., Dahn, R., and Hoffmann, G.: *Aeromonas punctata subsp. caviae* as the causative agent of acute gastroenteritis. Zentralbl. Bakteriol. Mikrobiol. Hyg. A. *233*:232-235, 1975.

52. Gilbert, D. N., Sanford, J. P., Kutscher, E., et al.: Microbiologic study of wound infections in tornado casualties. Arch. Environ. Health *26*:125-130, 1973.

53. Gluskin, I., Batash, D., Shoseyov, D., et al.: A 15-year study of the role of *Aeromonas* spp. in gastroenteritis in hospitalised children. J. Med. Microbiol. *37*:315-318, 1992.

54. Gonzalez-Barca, E., Ardanuy, C., Carratala, J., et al.: Fatal myofascial necrosis due to imipenem-resistant *Aeromonas hydrophila*. Scand. J. Infect. Dis. *29*:91-92, 1997.

55. Goodwin, C. S., Harper, W. E. S., Steward, J. K., et al.: Enterotoxigenic *Aeromonas hydrophila* and diarrhoea in adults. Med. J. Aust. *1*:25-26, 1983.

56. Gracey, M.: Gastroenteritis in Australian children—studies on the aetiology of acute diarrhea. Ann. Trop. Pediatr. *8*:68-75, 1988.

57. Gracey, M., Burke, V., and Robinson, J.: *Aeromonas*-associated gastroenteritis. Lancet *2*:1304-1306, 1982.

58. Gracey, M., Burke, V., Rockhill, R. C., et al.: *Aeromonas* species as enteric pathogens. Lancet *1*:223-224, 1982.

59. Gupta, P., Ramachandran, V. G., and Seth, A.: Early onset neonatal septicemia caused by *Aeromonas hydrophilia*. Indian Pediatr. *33*:703-704, 1996.

60. Gurwith, M. J., and Williams, T. W.: Gastroenteritis in children: A two-year review in Manitoba, I: Etiology. J. Infect. Dis. *136*:239-247, 1977.

61. Hazen, T. E., Fliermans, C. B., and Hirsch, R. P.: Prevalence and distribution of *Aeromonas hydrophila* in the United States. Appl. Environ. Microbiol. *36*:731-738, 1978.

62. Hickman-Brenner, F. W., Fanning, G. R., Arduino, M. J., et al.: *Aeromonas schubertii*, a new mannitol-negative species found in human clinical specimens. J. Clin. Microbiol. *26*:1561-1564, 1988.

63. Hickman-Brenner, F. W., MacDonald, K. L., Steigerwalt, A. G., et al.: *Aeromonas veronii*, a new ornithine decarboxylase-positive species that may cause diarrhea. J. Clin. Microbiol. *25*:900-906, 1987.

64. Hiransuthikul, N., Tantisiriwat, W., Lertusahakul, K., et al.: Skin and soft tissue infections among tsunami survivors in southern Thailand. Clin. Infect. Dis. *41*:e93-e96, 2005.

65. Hird, D. W., Diesch, S. L., McKinnel, R. G., et al.: *Aeromonas hydrophila* in wild-caught frogs and tadpoles (*Rana pipiens*) in Minnesota. Lab. Anim. Sci. *31*:166-169, 1981.

66. Howard, S. P., and Buckley, J. T.: Molecular cloning and expression in *Escherichia coli* of the structural gene for the hemolytic toxin aerolysin from *Aeromonas hydrophila*. Mol. Gen. Genet. *204*:289-295, 1986.

67. Hunter, W. F., and Atkinson, H. M.: Infection due to *Aeromonas hydrophila*. Med. J. Aust. *1*:565, 1968.

68. Huys, G., Kampfer P., Altwegg, M., et al.: *Aeromonas popoffii* sp. nov., a mesophilic bacterium isolated from drinking water, production plants, and reservoirs. Int. J. Syst. Bacteriol. *47*:1165-1171, 1997.

69. Janda, J. M., and Abbott, S. L.: Evolving concepts regarding the genus *Aeromonas*: An expanding panorama of species, disease presentations, and unanswered questions. Clin. Infect. Dis. *27*:332-344, 1998.

70. Janda, J. M., Abbott, S. L., Khashe, S., et al.: Further studies on biochemical characteristics and serologic properties of the genus *Aeromonas*. J. Clin. Microbiol. *34*:1930-1933, 1996.

71. Janda, J. M., Bottone, E. J., and Reitano, M.: *Aeromonas* species in clinical microbiology: Significance, epidemiology and speciation. Diagn. Microbiol. Infect. Dis. *1*:221-228, 1983.

72. Jorge, M. T., Nishioka, S. de A., de Oliveira, R. B., et al.: *Aeromonas hydrophila* soft-tissue infection as a complication of snake bite: Report of three cases. Ann. Trop. Med. Parasitol. *92*:213-217, 1998.

73. Kampfer, P., Christmann, C., Swings, J., et al.: In vitro susceptibilities of *Aeromonas* genomic species to 69 antimicrobial agents. Syst. Appl. Microbiol. *22*:662-669, 1999.

74. Kao, H. T., Huang, Y. C., and Lin, T. Y.: Fatal bacteremic pneumonia caused by *Aeromonas hydrophila* in a previously healthy child. J. Microbiol. Immunol. Infect. *36*:209-211, 2003.

75. Kaper, J. B., Lockman, H., and Colwell, R. R.: *Aeromonas hydrophila*: Ecology and toxigenicity of isolates from an estuary. J. Appl. Bacteriol. *50*:359-377, 1981.

76. Ketover, B. P., Young, L. S., and Armstrong, D.: Septicemia due to *Aeromonas hydrophila*: Clinical and immunologic aspects. J. Infect. Dis. *127*:284-290, 1973.

77. Khan, A. A., and Cerniglia, C. E.: Rapid and sensitive method for the detection of *Aeromonas caviae* and *Aeromonas trota* by polymerase chain reaction. Lett. Appl. Microbiol. *24*:233-239, 1997.

78. King, G. E., Werner, S. B., and Kizer, K. W.: Epidemiology of *Aeromonas* infections in California. Clin. Infect. Dis. *15*:449-452, 1992.

79. Kirov, S. M., Barnett, T. C., Pepe, C. M., et al.: Investigation of the role of type IV *Aeromonas pilus* (Tap) in the pathogenesis of *Aeromonas* gastrointestinal infection. Infect. Immun. *68*:4040-4048, 2000.

80. Ko, W. C., Chiang, S. R., Lee, H. C., et al.: In vitro and in vivo activities of fluoroquinolones against *Aeromonas hydrophila*. Antimicrob. Agents Chemother. *47*:2217-2222, 2003.

81. Kuhn, I., Albert, M. J., Ansaruzzaman, M., et al.: Characterization of *Aeromonas* spp. isolated from humans with diarrhea, from healthy controls, and from surface water in Bangladesh. J. Clin. Microbiol. *35*:369-373, 1997.

82. Laohachai, K. N., Bahadi, R., Hardo, M. B., et al.: The role of bacterial and non-bacterial toxins in the induction of changes in membrane transport: Implications for diarrhea. Toxicon *42*:687-707, 2003.

83. Leclerc, H., and Buttiaux, R.: Fréquence des *Aeromonas* dans les eaux d'alimentation. Ann. Inst. Pasteur *103*:97-100, 1962.

84. Lee, L. R., O'Hagan, S., and Dal Pra, M.: *Aeromonas sobria* endophthalmitis. Aust. N. Z. J. Ophthalmol. *25*:299-300, 1997.

85. Ljungh, A., Eneroth, P., and Wadstrom, T.: Cytotonic enterotoxin from *Aeromonas hydrophila*. Toxicon *20*:787-794, 1982.

86. Ljungh, A., and Kronevi, T.: *Aeromonas hydrophila* toxins: Intestinal fluid accumulation and mucosal injury in animal models. Toxicon *20*:397-407, 1982.

87. Ljungh, A., and Wadstrom, T.: *Aeromonas* toxins. Pharmacol. Ther. *15*:339-354, 1982.

88. Ljungh, A., and Wadstrom, T.: Toxins of *Vibrio parahaemolyticus* and *Aeromonas hydrophila*. J. Toxicol. Toxin Rev. *1*:257-307, 1982-1983.

89. Ljungh, A., and Wadstrom, T.: *Aeromonas* and *Plesiomonas* as possible causes of diarrhea. Infection *13*:169-173, 1985.

90. Lopez, J. F., Quesada, J., and Saied, A.: Bacteremia and osteomyelitis due to *Aeromonas hydrophila*: A complication during treatment of acute leukemia. Am. J. Clin. Pathol. *50*:587-591, 1968.

91. Martinez-Murcia, A. J., Esteve, C., Garay, E., and Collins, M. D.: *Aeromonas allosaccharophila* sp. nov., a new mesophilic member of the genus *Aeromonas*. F. E. M. S. Microbiol. Lett. *91*:199-206, 1992.

92. Martinez-Silva, V. R., Guzmann-Urrego, M., and Caselitz, F. H.: Zur Frage der Bedeutung *Aeromonas* stammen bei Sauglingsenteritis. Z. Tropenmed. Parasitol. *12*:445-451, 1961.

93. Mattick, K. L., and Donovan, T. J.: The risk to public health of *Aeromonas* in ready-to-eat salad products. Commun. Dis. Public Health *1*:267-270, 1998.

94. McCracken, A. W., and Barkley, R.: Isolation of *Aeromonas* species from clinical sources. J. Clin. Pathol. *25*:970-975, 1972.

95. McGrath, V. A., Overman, S. B., and Overman, T. L.: Media-dependent oxidase reaction in a strain of *Aeromonas hydrophila*. J. Clin. Microbiol. *5*:112-113, 1977.

96. McNicol, L. A., Aziz, K. M. S., Huq, I., et al.: Isolation of drug-resistant *Aeromonas hydrophila* from aquatic environments. Antimicrob. Agents Chemother. *17*:477-483, 1980.

97. Meeks, M. V.: The genus *Aeromonas*: Methods for identification. Am. J. Med. Technol. *29*:361-378, 1963.

98. Merino, S., Camprubi, S., and Tomas, J. M.: Detection of *Aeromonas hydrophila* in food with an enzyme-linked immunosorbent assay. J. Appl. Bacteriol. *74*:149-154, 1993.

99. Mishva, S., Nair, G. B., and Bhadra, R. K.: Comparison of selective media for primary isolation of *Aeromonas* species from human and animal feces. J. Clin. Microbiol. *25*:2040-2043, 1987.

100. Morita, K., Watanabe, N., Kurata, S., et al.: β-Lactam resistance of motile *Aeromonas* isolates from clinical and environmental sources. Antimicrob. Agents Chemother. *38*:353-355, 1994.

101. Motyl, M. R., and Janda, J. M.: *Aeromonas* gastroenteritis: A two-year survey. Presented at the 23rd Interscience Conference on Antimicrobial Agents and Chemotherapy, Las Vegas, October 24-26, 1983.

102. Motyl, M. R., McKinley, G., and Janda, J. M.: In vitro susceptibilities of *Aeromonas hydrophila*, *Aeromonas sobria*, and *Aeromonas caviae* to 22 antimicrobial agents. Antimicrob. Agents Chemother. *28*:151-153, 1985.

103. Moulsdale, M. T.: Isolation of *Aeromonas* from faeces. Lancet *1*:351, 1983.

104. Moyer, N. P.: Clinical significance of *Aeromonas* species isolated from patients with diarrhea. J. Clin. Microbiol. *25*:2044-2048, 1987.

105. Moyes, C. D., Sykes, P. A., and Rayner, J. M.: *Aeromonas hydrophila* septicaemia producing ecthyma gangrenosum in a child with leukaemia. Scand. J. Infect. Dis. *9*:151-153, 1977.

106. Nygaard, G. S., Biosett, M. L., and Wood, R. M.: Laboratory identification of aeromonads from man to other animals. Appl. Microbiol. *19*:618-620, 1970.

107. Ojeda-Vargas, M., Gonzalez-Fernandez, M. A., Alfonso-Rodriguez, O., and Monzon-Moreno, C.: Infecciones del tracto urinario causadas por bacterias del género *Aeromonas*. Enferm. Infecc. Microbiol. Clin. *23*:181-182, 2005.

108. Olivier, G., Lallier, R., and Lariviere, S.: A toxigenic profile of *Aeromonas hydrophila* and *Aeromonas sobria* isolated from fish. Can. J. Microbiol. *27*:330-333, 1981.

109. Overman, T. L., and Janda, J. M.: Antimicrobial susceptibility patterns of *Aeromonas jandaei*, *A. schubertii*, *A. trota*, and *A. veronii* biotype *veronii*. J. Clin. Microbiol. *37*:706-708, 1999.

110. Paik, G.: Reagents, stains, and miscellaneous test procedures. *In* Lennette, E. H., Balows, A., Hausler, W. J., Jr., et al. (eds.): Manual of Clinical Microbiology. 3rd ed. Washington, D.C., American Society for Microbiology, 1980, pp. 1006-1007.

111. Pearson, T. A., Mitchell, C. A., and Hughes, W. T.: *Aeromonas hydrophila* septicemia. Am. J. Dis. Child. *123*:579-582, 1972.

112. Phillips, J. A., Bernhardt, H. E., and Rosenthal, S. G.: *Aeromonas hydrophila* infections. Pediatrics *53*:110-112, 1974.

113. Picard, B., Arlet, G., and Goullet, P.: Origin hydrique d'infections hôpitalières à *Aeromonas hydrophila.* Presse Med. *12*:700, 1983.

114. Picard, B., and Goullet, P.: Seasonal prevalence of nosocomial *Aeromonas hydrophila* infection related to *Aeromonas* in hospital water. J. Hosp. Infect. *10*:152-155, 1987.

115. Pidiyar, V., Kaznowski, A., Narayan, N. B., et al.: *Aeromonas culicicola* sp. nov. (MTC 3249), from the midgut of *Culex quinquifasiatus.* Int. J. Syst. Evol. Microbiol. *52*:1723-1728, 2002.

116. Pin, C., Benito, Y., Carcia, M. L., et al.: Influence of temperature, pH, sodium chloride, and sodium nitrate on the growth of clinical and food motile *Aeromonas* sp. strains. Arch. Lebensmittelhyg. *47*:35-56, 1996.

117. Pitarangsi, C., Escheverria, P., Whitmire, R., et al.: Enteropathogenicity of *Aeromonas hydrophila* and *Plesiomonas shigelloides*: Prevalence among individuals with and without diarrhea in Thailand. Infect. Immun. *35*:666-673, 1982.

118. Pittman, M.: A study of bacteria implicated in transfusion reactions and of bacteria isolated from blood products. J. Lab. Clin. Med. *42*:273-288, 1953.

119. Popoff, M.: Genus III: *Aeromonas* Kluyver and van Niel 1936. *In* Krieg, N. R., and Holt, J. G. (eds.): Bergey's Manual of Systematic Bacteriology. Baltimore, Williams & Wilkins, 1984, p. 545.

120. Quinn, J. P.: UHL enteric bacterial disease surveillance. Lab. Hotline *28*:2, 1991.

121. Ramsey, A. M., Rosenbaum, B. J., Yarbrough, C. L., et al.: *Aeromonas hydrophila* sepsis in patient undergoing hemodialysis therapy. J. A. M. A. *239*:128-129, 1978.

122. Raszeja, S., Krynski, S., Krueger, A., et al.: Blood contamination with *Aeromonas hydrophilus* as a cause of lethal post-transfusion complications. Pol. Tyg. Lek. *28*:1159-1162, 1973.

123. Reines, H. D., and Cook, F. V.: Pneumonia and bacteremia due to *Aeromonas hydrophila.* Chest *80*:264-267, 1981.

124. Reinhardt, J. F., and George, W. L.: Comparative in vitro activities of selected antimicrobial agents against *Aeromonas* species and *Plesiomonas shigelloides.* Antimicrob. Agents Chemother. *27*:643-645, 1985.

125. Robson, W. L. M., Leung, A. K. C., and Trevenen, C. L.: Haemolytic-uraemic syndrome associated with *Aeromonas hydrophila* enterocolitis. Pediatr. Nephrol. *6*:221-222, 1992.

126. Rogol, M., Sechter, I., Grinberg, L., et al.: Pril-xylose-ampicillin agar, a new selective medium for the isolation of *Aeromonas hydrophila.* J. Med. Microbiol. *12*:229-231, 1979.

127. Rose, J. M., Houston, C. W., Coppenhaver, D. H., et al.: Purification and chemical characterization of a cholera toxin-cross-reactive cytolytic enterotoxin produced by a human isolate of *Aeromonas hydrophila.* Infect. Immun. *57*:1165-1169, 1989.

128. Rosenthal, S. G., Bernhardt, H. E., and Phillips, J. A.: *Aeromonas hydrophila* wound infection. Plast. Reconstr. Surg. *53*:77-79, 1974.

129. Rosner, R.: *Aeromonas hydrophila* as the etiologic agent in a case of gastroenteritis. Am. J. Clin. Pathol. *42*:402-404, 1964.

130. Sader, H. S., and Jones, R. N.: Antimicrobial susceptibility of uncommonly isolated non-enteric Gram-negative bacilli. Int. J. Antimicrob. Agents *25*:95-109, 2005.

131. Sanarelli, G.: Über einem neuen Mikroorganismus des Wassers, welcher für Tieren mit veranderlichen und konstanter Temperatur Pathogen ist. Zentralbl. Bakteriol. Parasitenk. *9*:193-199, 222-228, 1891.

132. San Joaquin, V. H., and Pickett, D. A.: *Aeromonas*-associated gastroenteritis in children. Pediatr. Infect. Dis. *7*:53-57, 1988.

133. San Joaquin, V. H., Pickett, D. A., Welch, D. F., et al.: *Aeromonas* species in aquaria: A reservoir of gastrointestinal infections? J. Hosp. Infect. *13*:173-177, 1989.

134. San Joaquin, V. H., Scribner, R. K., Pickett, D. A., et al.: Antimicrobial susceptibility of *Aeromonas* species isolated from patients with diarrhea. Antimicrob. Agents Chemother. *30*:794-795, 1986.

135. Sanyal, S. C., Singh, S. J., and Sen, P. C.: Enteropathogenicity of *Aeromonas hydrophila* and *Plesiomonas shigelloides.* J. Med. Microbiol. *8*:195-198, 1975.

136. Sasu, D., and Apostica, E.: On a strain of *Aeromonas liquefaciens* isolated from blood. Microbiologia (Bucur) *12*:437-441, 1967.

137. Sawai, T., Takahashi, I., Nakagawa, H., et al.: Immunochemical comparison between an oxacillin-hydrolyzing penicillinase of *Aeromonas hydrophila* and those mediated by R plasmids. J. Bacteriol. *135*:281-282, 1978.

138. Schubert, R. H. W., and Hegazi, M.: *Aeromonas eucrenophila* species nova *Aeromonas caviae*: A later and illegitimate synonym of *Aeromonas punctata.* Zentralbl. Bakteriol. Mikrobiol. Hyg. A. *268*:34-39, 1988.

139. Seidler, R. J., Allen, D. A., Bockman, H., et al.: Isolation, enumeration and characterization of *Aeromonas* from polluted waters encountered in diving operations. Appl. Environ. Microbiol. *39*:1010-1018, 1980.

140. Sha, J., Kozlova, E. V., and Chopra, A. K.: Role of various enterotoxins in *Aeromonas hydrophila*–induced gastroenteritis: Generation of enterotoxin gene-deficient mutants and evaluation of their enterotoxic activity. Infect. Immun. *70*:1924-1935, 2002.

141. Shackelford, P. G., Ratzan, S. A., and Shearer, W. T.: Ecthyma gangrenosum produced by *Aeromonas hydrophila.* J. Pediatr. *83*:100-101, 1973.

142. Sirinavin, S., Likitnukul, S., and Lolekha, S.: *Aeromonas* septicemia in infants and children. Pediatr. Infect. Dis. *3*:122-125, 1984.

143. Skoll, P. J., Hudson, D. A., and Simpson, J. A.: *Aeromonas hydrophila* in burn patients. Burns *24*:350-353, 1998.

144. Slotnick, I. J.: *Aeromonas* species isolates. Ann. N. Y. Acad. Sci. *174*:503-510, 1970.

145. Smith, J. A.: Ocular *Aeromonas hydrophila.* Am. J. Ophthalmol. *89*:449-451, 1980.

146. Smith, J. A.: *Aeromonas hydrophila*: Analysis of 11 cases. Can. Med. Assoc. J. *122*:1270-1272, 1980.

147. Soler, L., Yanez, M. A., Chacon, M. R., et al.: Phylogenetic analysis of the genus *Aeromonas* based on two housekeeping genes. Int. J. Syst. Evol. Microbiol. *54*:1511-1519, 2004.

148. Soltan Dallal, M. M., and Moezardalan, K.: *Aeromonas* spp. associated with children's diarrhoea in Tehran: A case-control study. Ann. Trop. Paediatr. *24*:45-51, 2004.

149. Stephens, S., Rao, K. N. A., Kumar, M. S., et al.: Human infection with *Aeromonas* species: Varied clinical manifestations. Ann. Intern. Med. *83*:368-369, 1975.

150. Taneja, N., Khurana, S., Trehan, A., et al.: An outbreak of hospital acquired diarrhea due to *Aeromonas sobria.* Indian Pediatr. *41*:912-916, 2004.

151. Teka, T., Faruque, A. S., Hossain, M. I., and Fuchs, G. J.: *Aeromonas*-associated diarrhoea in Bangladeshi children: Clinical and epidemiological characteristics. Ann. Trop. Paediatr. *19*:15-20, 1999.

152. Thelestam, M., and Ljungh, A.: Membrane-damaging and cytotoxic effects on human fibroblasts of alpha- and beta-hemolysins from *Aeromonas hydrophila.* Infect. Immun. *34*:949-956, 1981.

153. Ullmann, D., Krause, G., Knabner, D., et al.: Isolation and characterization of potentially human pathogenic, cytotoxin-producing *Aeromonas* strains from retailed seafood in Berlin, Germany. J. Vet. Med. B. Infect. Dis. Vet. Public Health *52*:82-87, 2005.

154. Unhanand, M., Mustafa, M. M., McCracken, G. H., Jr., et al.: Gram-negative enteric bacillary meningitis: A twenty-one-year experience. J. Pediatr. *122*:15-21, 1993.

155. von Graevenitz, A.: *Aeromonas* and *Plesiomonas.* *In* Lennette, E. H., Balows, A., Hausler, W. H., et al. (eds.): Manual of Clinical Microbiology. 3rd ed. Washington, D.C., American Society for Microbiology, 1980, pp. 220-225.

156. von Graevenitz, A., and Bucher, C.: Evaluation of differential and selective media for isolation of *Aeromonas* and *Plesiomonas* spp. from human feces. J. Clin. Microbiol. *77*:16-21, 1983.

157. Wadstrom, T., Aust-Kettis, A., Habte, D., et al.: Enterotoxin-producing bacteria and parasites in stools of Ethiopian children with diarrhoeal disease. Arch. Dis. Child. *51*:865-870, 1976.

158. Washington, J. A., II: The role of *Aeromonas hydrophila* in clinical infection. *In* Holloway, W. J. (ed.): Infectious Disease Reviews. Vol. 2. Mount Kisco, N.Y., Futura Publishing, 1973, pp. 75-86.

159. Yadava, R., Seeler, R. A., Kalelkar, M., et al.: Fatal *Aeromonas hydrophila* sepsis and meningitis in a child with sickle cell anemia. Am. J. Dis. Child. *133*:753-754, 1979.

160. Zajc-Satler, J.: Morphological and biochemical studies of 27 strains belonging to the genus *Aeromonas* isolated from clinical sources. J. Med. Microbiol. *5*:263-265, 1972.

CHAPTER
126

PASTEURELLA MULTOCIDA
Barbara W. Stechenberg

In 1878, Kitt first isolated a bacterium of the *Pasteurella* group from wild hogs during an epidemic; 2 years later, Pasteur described the organism that causes fowl cholera. Since that time, the same organism has been implicated in rabbit septicemia, swine plague, hemorrhagic septicemia, and wildseuche (a fatal disease in deer). Hueppe applied the term *hemorrhagic septicemia* to this group of infectious diseases in lower animals because of the characteristic hemorrhagic areas scattered throughout most of the viscera. Original names for the causative organisms included *Pasteurella aviseptica*, *Pasteurella boviseptica*, *Pasteurella suiseptica*, and *Pasteurella lepiseptica*, but these organisms now are classified under the name *Pasteurella multocida*, a small, nonmotile, gram-negative rod.[38]

Although *P. multocida* primarily is a pathogen in animals, recognition of its potential for infection in humans has been increasing. Brugnatelli reported the first bacteriologically proven case in a human in 1913. Schipper[39] did an extensive review of the literature from 1930 through 1947 and reported only 40 cases of infection with *P. multocida*. Since then, an increasing number of human infections with *P. multocida* have been reported.

ORGANISM

P. multocida generally appears as a short, ovoid, gram-negative rod; however, it also may appear as coccobacilli with convex sides and rounded ends. The length ranges from 0.3 to 1.25 μm, and the diameter ranges from 0.15 to 0.25 μm. *P. multocida* may appear singly or in pairs, chains, or clusters. Healthy organisms stain easily with aniline dyes and are gram-negative. They may show bipolar staining, especially when smears are made directly from animal tissue or fluids. They become increasingly pleomorphic on subculture and may resemble enterics in broth. They do not grow on eosin–methylene blue, MacConkey, deoxycholate, or any other bile-containing agar. They are facultatively anaerobic and nonmotile. They do not require X or V factor for growth, an important differential point in distinguishing them from *Haemophilus influenzae*.

Colonies are nonhemolytic and translucent, usually 1 to 2 mm in diameter, and generally low, convex, and butyrous. Occasionally, they may be larger and mucoid. In a study of 30 strains isolated from humans, Heddleston and Wessman[17] reported that 9 of the cultures produced watery mucoid colonies, 4 produced iridescent colonies, 10 produced blue colonies, and 3 produced a mixture of iridescent and blue colonies. Colonies on blood agar are smaller, opaque, and grayish white. In broth cultures, turbidity, often with a flocculent sediment, is present.

Cultures tend to autoagglutinate in saline and have a peculiar odor described as musty, similar to semen or burning hair. They are catalase-positive, usually oxidase-positive, and indole-positive. They usually ferment galactose, glucose, fructose, mannitol, mannose, and sucrose without production of gas. Some variability occurs in the fermentation of other sugars. They reduce nitrates but have negative urease, methyl red, and Voges-Proskauer reactions. Using fermentation reactions, Oberhofer[31] developed a biotyping system in which correlation of biotype, 61 percent A and B, was found with cat-bite isolates but not with dog-bite isolates.

The pathogenicity of the organism varies; most mucoid and smooth colony-forming strains produce a capsule and usually are highly pathogenic for mice and rabbits. The capsule is antiphagocytic, resisting intracellular killing by neutrophils.

Nielsen and Rosdahl[29] have developed a bacteriophage typing system for typing toxigenic and nontoxigenic strains. DNA hybridization studies have led to a reclassification of the genus *Pasteurella*. *P. multocida* now includes three subspecies—*P. multocida* subsp. *multocida*, *P. multocida* subsp. *septica*, and *P. multocida* subsp. *gallicida*. Of 159 strains recovered from 46 infected humans, 95 were identified as *P. multocida* subsp. *multocida*, and 21 were identified as *P. multocida* subsp. *septica*; the remainder were divided among multiple other species.[16] The use of serology in conjunction with DNA fingerprinting can classify isolates for epidemiologic studies.[51]

Immunity to *P. multocida* can be shown in many animals, and vaccines have been developed with known efficacy, especially in birds and cattle. The precise mechanisms involved in this immunity and, more important, in natural immunity are being elucidated. Antibodies to somatic and capsular antigenic determinants develop within 2 weeks of development of clinical infection, with the capsular antibodies being longer lasting.[5] The precise role of these antibodies in human host defenses is unclear. Woolcock and Collins[52] developed models in pathogen-free mice that may help uncover these mechanisms. The efficacy of heat-killed vaccine has been shown to be considerable when multiple doses are used. With the use of an aerogenic mouse model for the stimulation of respiratory spread, however, the protection is reduced. Local instillation of the vaccine can be used with this model to develop local antibodies, but preliminary results show protection only with modest challenge doses.[3] A footpad inoculation model may help elucidate the mechanisms in local human infections.

TRANSMISSION

The organism is found in the oral flora of many different animals; 67 percent of cats may harbor this organism in their mouths or throats. Smith[40] found that *P. multocida* could be recovered from the tonsils of 54 percent of dogs and from the nose of 10 percent of dogs. Schipper[39] grew *P. multocida* from 14 percent of wild rats trapped in the Baltimore area. Hansmann and Tully[15] showed that *P. multocida* may remain as a commensal for prolonged periods in the mouth of a cat. They described a patient who had been bitten on two occasions 3 years apart by the same healthy pet cat; each time, an abscess caused by *P. multocida* developed. *P. multocida* also has been isolated from lion, tiger, panther, buffalo, mink, and opossum.[4,20]

Although verifying the mode of transmission has been easiest when an infection has been related specifically to a pet or farm animal, many cases of infection caused by *P. multocida* have been documented despite a negative history of such exposure. Respiratory infection with this organism has been described in veterinarians, farmers, milkmen, and individuals employed where animal tissues are processed. Meningitis caused by *P. multocida* has been described in a patient after undergoing brain surgery in which rabbit muscle was used for hemostasis.

The possibility of a reservoir of infection in humans with resultant interhuman transmission rarely has been considered. In a study of veterinary students, Smith[40] described 2 of 71 with positive throat isolations. The organisms were present in one student for a few days and in the other for the full 4 months of the study; both patients were asymptomatic. Several other cases of isolation of the organism from the human respiratory tract, many without associated symptoms or known animal contact, have been made.

In addition, interhuman spread by nasopharyngeal excretions, feces, and urine also may occur because the organism has been recovered from these sites. The female genital tract is another potential source, especially for cases of septicemia and meningitis that occur during pregnancy and in the newborn period.

Investigators of an outbreak in a chronic disease hospital showed that *P. multocida* may be viable on a hand towel for 24 hours. Although the source in this outbreak was not established, this finding may have implications for spread in other situations, particularly for pet owners.[23]

EPIDEMIOLOGY

P. multocida has been isolated from humans in all areas of North America and Europe, with some reports coming from other areas. In the United States, it is not a reportable organism, so incidence and prevalence data are unavailable. Lee and Buhr[26] have cited a seasonal variation in the number of reported cases related to dog bites, with the highest incidence being in the fall and winter months, possibly related to increased nasal carriage in dogs during that period. Other investigators have found no seasonal differences.[9,21]

No difference in attack rate has been found between the sexes. The attack rate is higher in individuals of both sexes in very young (0-4 years old) and in older (>55 years old) individuals.

PATHOGENESIS AND PATHOLOGY

In animals that are stressed, a benignly parasitic strain may invade the mucous membrane on which it is carried. With highly virulent strains, a picture of hemorrhagic septicemia may develop. It may be characterized by high fever, cardiac weakness, toxemia, and early death. Organisms can be cultured from the blood; autopsy findings may be minimal or include petechial hemorrhages on mucosal and serosal surfaces and in various organs. Less acute forms, such as a pneumonia with serofibrinous exudate in the interlobular septa of the lungs, a hemorrhagic gastroenteritis, and subacute and chronic infections such as otitis in the rabbit, may occur. The mechanisms by which these bacteria invade the mucosa and cause systemic disease continue to unfold. Key virulence factors are the capsule and lipopolysaccharide, with others still being identified.[16]

In humans, three major types of infections occur.[50] In the first and most common type, local infection occurs after a cat bite or scratch, a dog bite, or, rarely, the bite of another animal. Approximately 15 to 20 percent of dog-bite wounds and more than 50 percent of cat-bite wounds become infected. Many cases have been associated with non-bite exposure, such as licking.[11] These cases usually are characterized by a rapidly progressive, acute cellulitis with lymphangitis, local lymphadenitis, or both. Cat-bite wounds may progress to osteomyelitis of the underlying bone. This development is not because of any known predilection of *P. multocida* for the bone but because the sharp fangs of a cat deposit the organism on or under the periosteum.

The second type includes cases of chronic pulmonary infection in which the organism may be the only isolate or one of several organisms. Cases of bronchiectasis and empyema have been reported, usually in patients with underlying pulmonary disease. In a series of 28 cases of bronchiectasis in which the organism was recovered, it usually appeared as a secondary invader. It seems to have low pathogenicity in the respiratory tract until some other infection or physiologic disturbance decreases the natural resistance of the host, which enables active infection, most commonly liver disease such as cirrhosis, to occur. *Pasteurella* infection also may be septicemic or occur with meningitis. The pathology and pathogenesis are similar to those of other organisms.

CLINICAL MANIFESTATIONS

In cases of local infection from a scratch or bite, the usual clinical pattern shows swelling, erythema, and tenderness within a few hours of the bite; most symptoms occur within the first 24 hours. A gray serous or sanguinopurulent discharge from the puncture sites may be present. Signs of systemic toxic effects, such as chills and fever, may or may not be present; regional lymphadenopathy often is evident. Less commonly, the infection may be lower

grade and smoldering.[35] As noted, osteomyelitis and tenosynovitis most often occur after cat bites because of the sharpness of cats' teeth.

Lee and Buhr[26] found *P. multocida* to be the most common infecting organism in a report of 69 dog bites that had been cultured; 20 of the bites became grossly infected, and *P. multocida* was isolated from 10. Of 30 wounds that were sutured, 14 (47%) were infected with *P. multocida*. Other unusual localized infections include chronic skin ulcers, secondary infection of a gouty joint, and infection of a compound fracture site and an amputation site.[46] Preexisting joint disease seems to be a risk.

Clinical manifestations of patients having respiratory complaints are not unusual. Most of the isolates have been associated with chronic bronchitis, bronchiectasis, chronic sinusitis or otitis media, and pneumonia. Several cases of massive pulmonary abscesses, pleural effusion, and empyema also have been reported. Larsen and Holden[25] described a 14-year-old girl with chronic otitis media for 2 years who developed a *P. multocida* cerebellar abscess. A case of epiglottitis caused by this organism has been reported in an adult.[24] A child developed Ludwig angina after having a non-bite exposure.

In a report of 136 cases of *P. multocida* infection that were not related to animal bites, the most common site of infection after the respiratory tract was the abdomen; the organism was recovered from 10 patients with appendicitis. Eight isolates were from the female reproductive tract, four from the urine, and one from a chronic sacral abscess.[21] Whether these cases are secondary to ingestion of the organism or to hematogenous spread has not been determined. Raffi and colleagues[34] described three children with appendiceal peritonitis associated with *P. multocida*. The organism also has been seen in cases of peritoneal dialysis-associated peritonitis secondary to puncture of dialysis tubing.[27,28]

The disseminated infections are the other major clinical group of *Pasteurella* infections. Isolated bacteremia may be present[33]; however, most of these cases have been meningitis, many of which were mistaken for *Haemophilus influenzae* or *Neisseria meningitidis* infection because of the morphologic similarities among these organisms. In a review of the subject in 1967, Controni and Jones[7] noted 14 confirmed cases of *Pasteurella* meningitis; 11 occurred in adults, and 3 occurred in children. Eight of the 14 patients had a history of accidental or surgical trauma. The mortality rate was 50 percent, but only five patients were treated with antibiotics. Evaluation of the cerebrospinal fluid showed white blood cell counts ranging from 580/mm[3] to 5200/mm[3], all with a predominance of polymorphonuclear leukocytes. More recently, Green and coworkers[14] reviewed 29 cases of *P. multocida* meningitis in adults.

The first reported newborn with *Pasteurella* meningitis died at 88 hours of age.[1] The mother had a fever in the postpartum period, but her pretreatment cultures were lost, so verification of the source was impossible.[7] Since then, a case of *Pasteurella* chorioamnionitis associated with premature delivery and neonatal sepsis and death within 1.5 hours of delivery has been reported.[42] Gingival cultures of a pet cat that had scratched a mother numerous times during pregnancy also yielded *P. multocida*. Subsequently, several young infants with septicemia and meningitis caused by this organism survived without apparent sequelae after treatment with penicillin or ampicillin and gentamicin.[2,10,36,45] Pizey[32] reported another case of neonatal infection in a 3-week-old infant with septic arthritis. *P. multocida* infection may take a rapidly fatal course even in an older infant.[39] Clapp and associates[6] described two infants whose disease was associated with nontraumatic facial licking by pets, an avoidable exposure. In another report, a case of in utero infection at 12 weeks' gestation was described.[48] A newborn with meningitis and cervical spine osteomyelitis with full recovery has been reported.[18]

DIAGNOSIS AND TREATMENT

Although *P. multocida* is one of the more likely pathogens to cause infection of cat or dog bites, its clinical manifestations are not unusual. Diagnosis of *P. multocida* infection can be made definitively only by culture. It may resemble several other organisms morphologically, but identification should not be difficult to make. The fact that it does not require X and V factors for growth should distinguish it from *H. influenzae*. Its production of indole should differentiate it from the *Neisseria* group, and its inability to grow on MacConkey agar or a bile salt medium should distinguish it from *Acinetobacter* spp. and the enteric organisms.

The drug of choice for *P. multocida* infection is penicillin, to which the organism is exquisitely sensitive. This feature may be used as a rapid means of distinguishing it from *H. influenzae* or the enterics. Rare strains producing β-lactamase and resistance to penicillins have been recovered.[37] The organism usually is sensitive to a wide variety of other antibiotics, including ampicillin, other broad-spectrum penicillins (e.g., ticarcillin, piperacillin, mezlocillin), amoxicillin–clavulanic acid,[12] tetracyclines, parenteral cephalosporins (particularly second-generation and third-generation),[30] cefuroxime, cefpodoxime, and chloramphenicol. Semisynthetic penicillins (e.g., nafcillin, dicloxacillin), erythromycin, some orally administered cephalosporins (cephalexin, cefaclor), clindamycin, and aminoglycosides have relatively low activity against *P. multocida*.[8,13,41] Azithromycin seems to have acceptable activity,[6] as does ciprofloxacin.[22] Trimethoprim-sulfamethoxazole may be an alternative, particularly for patients unable to take a β-lactam antibiotic.[38] Surgical drainage or débridement also may be necessary. The duration of treatment depends on the primary disease process. Seven to 10 days generally is adequate for local infections.

PROGNOSIS AND PREVENTION

Proper cleansing and débridement of wounds caused by animal bites or scratches are important in prevention of *P. multocida* infection. Lee and Buhr[26] found that suturing wounds caused by dog bite was associated with a higher incidence of infection. Whether a wound is sutured often depends on the site and the potential cosmetic result. The use of prophylactic antibiotics to prevent infection after animal bites is controversial. Some experts recommend their use if a delay occurs in seeking medical assistance and for cat bites or for patients with immunocompromising conditions.

Limiting contact with wild and domestic animals that may harbor the organism probably is the only definitive way to prevent infection. Teaching proper handling of pets and keeping pets from licking infants and young children, particularly on the face, may help. No vaccine for human use is available.

Prognosis depends on the particular site of infection. With appropriate treatment, resolution usually occurs, but the healing process may be very slow, particularly in local infections with extension to the bone or tendons.[9,47]

REFERENCES

1. Bates, H. A., Controni, G., Elliott, N., et al.: Septicemia and meningitis in a newborn due to *Pasteurella multocida*. Clin. Pediatr. 4:668-670, 1965.
2. Bhave, S. A., Guy, L. M., and Rycroft, J. A.: *Pasteurella multocida* meningitis in an infant with recovery. B. M. J. 2:741-742, 1977.
3. Branson, D., and Bunkfeldt, F.: *Pasteurella multocida* in animal bites of humans. Am. J. Clin. Pathol. 48:552-555, 1967.
4. Burdge, D. R., Scheifele, D., and Speart, D. P.: Serious *Pasteurella multocida* infections from lion and tiger bites. J. A. M. A. 253:3296-3297, 1985.
5. Choudat, D., Paul, G., Legoff, C., et al.: Specific antibody responses to *Pasteurella multocida*. Scand. J. Infect. Dis. 19:453-457, 1987.
6. Clapp, W. C., Kleiman, M. B., Reynolds, J. K., et al.: *Pasteurella multocida* meningitis in infancy. Am. J. Dis. Child. 140:444-446, 1986.
7. Controni, G., and Jones, R. S.: *Pasteurella* meningitis: A review of the literature. Am. J. Med. Technol. 33:379-386, 1967.
8. Fass, R. J.: Erythromycin, clarithromycin and azithromycin: Use of frequency distribution curves, scattergrams and regression analyses to compare in vitro activities and describe cross-resistance. Antimicrob. Agents Chemother. 37:2080-2086, 1993.
9. Francis, D. P., Holmes, M. A., and Brandon, G.: *Pasteurella multocida*: Infection after domestic animal bites and scratches. J. A. M. A. 233:42-45, 1975.
10. Frutos, A. A., Levitsky, D., Scott, E. G., et al.: A case of septicemia and meningitis in an infant due to *Pasteurella multocida*. J. Pediatr. 92:853, 1978.
11. Goldstein, E. J. C.: Bite wounds and infection. Clin. Infect. Dis. 14:633-640, 1991.
12. Goldstein, E. J. C., and Citron, D. M.: Comparative activities of cefuroxime, amoxicillin-clavulanic acid, ciprofloxacin, enoxacin, and ofloxacin against aerobic and anaerobic bacteria isolated from bite wounds. Antimicrob. Agents Chemother. 32:1144-1148, 1988.
13. Goldstein, E. J. C., Citron, D. M., and Rechwald, G. A.: Lack of in vitro efficacy of oral forms of certain cephalosporins, erythromycin and oxacillin against *Pasteurella multocida*. Antimicrob. Agents Chemother. 32:213-215, 1988.
14. Green, B. T., Ramsey, K. M., and Nolan, P. E.: *Pasteurella multocida* meningitis: Case report and review of the last 11 y. Scand. J. Infect. Dis. 34:213-217, 2002.
15. Hansmann, G. H., and Tully, M.: Cat bite and scratch wounds with consequent *Pasteurella* infection of man. Am. J. Clin. Pathol. 15:312-318, 1945.
16. Harper, M., Boyce, J. D., and Adler, B.: *Pasteurella multocida* pathogenesis: 125 years after Pasteur. F. E. M. S. Microbiol. Lett. 265:1-10, 2006.
17. Heddleston, K. L., and Wessman, G.: Characteristics of *Pasteurella multocida* of human origin. J. Clin. Microbiol. 1:377-383, 1975.
18. Hirsh, D., Farrel, K., Reilly, C., and Dobson, S.: *Pasteurella multocida* meningitis and cervical spine osteomyelitis in a neonate. Pediatr. Infect. Dis. J. 23:1063-1065, 2004.
19. Holst, E., Rollof, J., Larsson, L., et al.: Characterization and distribution of *Pasteurella* species recovered from humans. J. Clin. Microbiol. 30:2984-2987, 1992.
20. Hubbert, W. T., and Rosen, M. N.: *Pasteurella multocida* infection due to animal bite. Am. J. Public Health 60:1103-1108, 1970.
21. Hubbert, W. T., and Rosen, M. N.: *Pasteurella multocida* infection in man unrelated to animal bite. Am. J. Public Health 60:1109-1117, 1970.
22. In vitro activity of oral antimicrobial agents against clinical isolates of *Pasturella multocida*. Diagn. Microbiol. Infect. Dis. 30:99-102, 1998.
23. Itoh, M., Tierno, P. M., Milstoc, M., et al.: A unique outbreak of *Pasteurella multocida* in a chronic disease hospital. Am. J. Public Health 70:1170-1173, 1980.
24. Johnson, R. H., and Rumans, L. W.: Unusual infections caused by *Pasteurella multocida*. J. A. M. A. 237:146-147, 1977.
25. Larsen, T. E., and Holden, F. A.: Isolation of *Pasteurella multocida* from an otogenic cerebellar abscess. Can. Med. Assoc. J. 101:629-630, 1969.
26. Lee, M. L. H., and Buhr, A. J.: Dog bites and local infection with *Pasteurella septica*. B. M. J. 1:169-171, 1960.
27. Loghman-Adham, M.: *Pasturella multocida* peritonitis in patients undergoing peritoneal dialysis. Pediatr. Nephrol. 11:353-354, 1997.
28. Malik, A., Aly, A., Mailey, K. S., and Bastani, B.: *Pasteurella multocida* peritoneal dialysis–associated peritonitis: A report of two cases and review of the literature. J. Nephrol. 18:791-793, 2005.
29. Nielsen, J. P., and Rosdahl, V. T.: Development and epidemiological applications of a bacteriophage typing system for typing *Pasteurella multocida*. J. Clin. Microbiol. 28:103-107, 1990.
30. Noel, G. T., and Teele, D. W.: In vitro activities of selected new and long-acting cephalosporins against *Pasteurella multocida*. Antimicrob. Agents Chemother. 29:344-345, 1986.
31. Oberhofer, T. R.: Characteristics and biotypes of *Pasteurella multocida* isolated from humans. J. Clin. Microbiol. 13:566-577, 1981.
32. Pizey, N. C. D.: Infection with *Pasteurella septica* in a child aged three weeks. Lancet 2:324-326, 1953.
33. Raffi, F., Barrier, J., Baron, D., et al.: *Pasteurella multocida* bacteremia: Report of thirteen cases over twelve years and review of the literature. Scand. J. Infect. Dis. 19:385-393, 1987.
34. Raffi, F., David, A., Mouzard, A., et al.: *Pasteurella multocida* appendiceal peritonitis: Report of three cases and review of the literature. Pediatr. Infect. Dis. 5:695-698, 1986.
35. Reinert, P., Canet, J., Pesnel, G., et al.: Une cause souvent ignorée d'arthrite subaiguë chez l'enfant; la pasteurellose à *P. multocida*. Arch. Fr. Pediatr. 29:99-104, 1972.
36. Repice, J. P., and Neter, E.: *Pasteurella multocida* meningitis in an infant with recovery. J. Pediatr. 86:91-93, 1975.
37. Rosenau, A., Labigne, A., Escande, F., et al.: Plasmid-mediated ROB-1 β-lactamase in *Pasteurella multocida* from a human specimen. Antimicrob. Agents Chemother. 35:2419-2422, 1991.
38. Sands, M., Ashley, R., and Brown, R.: Trimethoprim-sulfamethoxazole therapy of *Pasteurella multocida* infection. J. Infect. Dis. 160:353-354, 1989.
39. Schipper, G. J.: Unusual pathogenicity of *Pasteurella multocida* isolated from the throats of common wild rats. Bull. Johns Hopkins Hosp. 81:333-356, 1947.

40. Smith, J. E.: Studies on *Pasteurella septica*, I: Occurrence in nose and tonsils of dogs. J. Comp. Pathol. *65*:239-245, 1955.

41. Stevens, D. L., Higbee, J. W., Oberhofer, T. R., et al.: Antibiotic susceptibilities of human isolates of *Pasteurella multocida*. Antimicrob. Agents Chemother. *16*:322-324, 1979.

42. Strand, C. L., and Helfman, L.: *Pasteurella multocida* chorioamnionitis associated with premature delivery and neonatal sepsis and death. Am. J. Clin. Pathol. *55*:713-716, 1971.

43. Swartz, M. N., and Kunz, L. J.: *Pasteurella multocida* infection in man. N. Engl. J. Med. *261*:889-893, 1959.

44. Tessin, I., Brorson, J. E., and Trollfors, B.: Rapidly fatal *Pasteurella multocida* septicemia in infant following cat scratch. Pediatr. Infect. Dis. *6*:425-426, 1987.

45. Thompson, C. M., Pappu, L., Levkoff, A. H., et al.: Neonatal septicemia and meningitis due to *Pasteurella multocida*. Pediatr. Infect. Dis. *3*:559-561, 1984.

46. Tindall, J. P., and Harrison, C. M.: *Pasteurella multocida* infections following animal injuries, especially cat bites. Arch. Dermatol. *105*:412-416, 1972.

47. Torphy, D. E., and Ray, C. G.: *Pasteurella multocida* in dog and cat bite infections. Pediatrics *43*:295-297, 1969.

48. Waldor, M., Roberts, D., and Kazanjian, P.: In utero infections due to *Pasteurella multocida* in the first trimester of pregnancy: Case report and news. Clin. Infect. Dis. *14*:497-500, 1992.

49. Weber, D. J., and Hausen, A. R.: Infections resulting from animal bites. Infect. Dis. Clin. N. Am. *5*:663-680, 1991.

50. Weber, D. J., Wolfson, J. S., Swartz, M. N., et al.: *Pasteurella multocida* infections: Report of 34 cases and review of the literature. Medicine (Baltimore) *63*:133-154, 1984.

51. Wilson, M. A., Rimbler, R. B., and Hoffman, L. J.: Comparison of DNA fingerprints and somatic serotypes of serogroup B and E *Pasteurella multocida* isolates. J. Clin. Microbiol. *30*:1518-1524, 1992.

52. Woolcock, J. B., and Collins, F. M.: Immune mechanism in *Pasteurella multocida*–infected mice. Infect. Immun. *13*:949-958, 1976.

CHAPTER 127

CHOLERA

Matthew B. Laurens ✸ James P. Nataro

Cholera is a toxin-mediated diarrheal illness caused by the gram-negative organism *Vibrio cholerae*. Cholera is invariably a watery diarrhea syndrome that can range from mild and self-limiting to the severe life-threatening manifestation known as *cholera gravis*. Severe cholera can cause rapid intravascular volume depletion, shock, and death. The remarkable efficacy of rehydration therapy in preventing cholera deaths is one of the great triumphs of 20th century medicine.

Cholera may have existed since before the time of Hippocrates, and the infection continues to cause significant morbidity and mortality in areas where sanitation is poor. The infection is particularly prevalent in the Indian subcontinent and in parts of Africa. In 2005, a 30 percent increase in the global incidence of cholera was noted, mostly resulting from outbreaks in West Africa that accounted for 58 percent of all confirmed cases. The case-fatality rate decreased from 2.3 percent in 2004 to 1.7 percent in 2005.[6] This improvement likely is attributable to improved diagnostic tools and treatment, including availability of oral rehydration therapy and access to intravenous fluids for severe cases. On the forefront of prevention are the oral cholera vaccines, which have emerged as useful public health tools to combat the disease, especially in highly vulnerable transient populations.

HISTORY

Cholera has long been indigenous to the Ganges river valley in northern India. Although it exhibits a seasonal regularity, the annual epidemics are inconsistent, at times ravaging the population and at other times tolerable. In the absence of a known vertebrate reservoir or carrier state, the cause of this erratic pattern has remained mysterious until more recently.

With increased European incursion into the Indian subcontinent, the cyclical nature of cholera epidemics took on global proportions, occurring in a series of discrete pandemics through the 19th and 20th centuries. These disastrous events are largely responsible for the evolution of public health as an effective discipline. The first recorded cholera pandemic began in 1817, extending from India to southern Russia. During the second cholera pandemic, beginning in 1826, many jurisdictions were induced to establish local sanitation and health boards, eventually evolving into the first organized public health apparatus. During the London cholera epidemic of 1854, Dr. John Snow first showed the association of the disease with contaminated drinking water derived from the city's infamous Broad Street pump; this episode is widely considered the first scientific public health investigation. In 1866, an epidemic in New York City led to the creation of the first Board of Health in the United States, and cholera became the first reportable disease.

During the fifth pandemic in 1884, the causative bacterium, *V. cholerae*, finally was identified. The seventh pandemic began in Indonesia in the 1960s and marked the introduction of biotype *El Tor* strains. The seventh pandemic was the most widespread on record, involving Asia, Africa, southern Europe, and the Americas.[54] A new cholera serogroup O139 Bengal emerged in India and Bangladesh in the 1990s; it represents the first non-O1 serogroup isolated in association with an epidemic.[54]

MICROBIOLOGY

V. cholerae is a curved gram-negative rod that is classified by biochemical tests and subdivided into serogroups based on the somatic O antigen. It belongs to the family Vibrionaceae, which differs from the related family Enterobacteriaceae in being oxidase-positive and motile with a single flagellum. Vibrios are fermentative and oxidative in metabolism. They have few nutritional requirements and can grow in glucose as the sole source of carbon and energy. Most vibrios are marine organisms, and most grow best in 2 to 3 percent sodium chloride under aerobic conditions. Although neither the typical comma shape of *V. cholerae* nor its motility can be observed on Gram stain, both are apparent in wet mount even on fresh fecal samples, a characteristic that can be useful for rapidly establishing the diagnosis. A presumptive diagnosis of cholera can be made immediately by adding anti-*Vibrio* antiserum, which results in cessation of motility of only the homologous organism.

Numerous *Vibrio* spp. exist, most of which are nonpathogenic in humans. Within the species *V. cholerae* are more than 200 serogroups according to the antigenic characteristics of the lipopolysaccharide O antigen.[11] To date, only *V. cholerae* organisms carrying the somatic O antigens O1 and O139 are associated with epidemic disease. Some non-O1 *V. cholerae* serogroups are associated with sporadic diarrheal illness, which can be severe and sometimes invasive and inflammatory.

The O1 serogroup is divided further into two biotypes, Classical and El Tor, based on biochemical properties and phage susceptibilities. The Classical biotype traditionally is associated with a more severe disease, but the El Tor biotype may be better adapted to persistence in the environment and cause more persistent epidemics. The expression of genes conferring human virulence seems to be higher in the Classical biotype, whereas in the El Tor biotype, enhanced expression of genes for biofilm formation, chemotaxis, and transport of amino acids, peptides, and iron is higher.[11] Classical and El Tor biotypes are divided into three serotypes (Ogawa, Inaba, and Hikojima) based on their dominant heat-stable lipopolysaccharide somatic antigens. Media used to isolate cholera organisms in stool include thiosulfate citrate bile salts sucrose (TCBS) agar and tellurite taurocholate gelatin agar. The appearance of yellow ("popcorn") colonies on TCBS agar is considered to be highly suggestive of *V. cholerae*. The bacterium is confirmed further by its ability to grow in the presence (or absence) of salt and by serology.

PATHOGENESIS

The pathogenic paradigm of *V. cholerae* comprises colonization of the small bowel mucosa followed by release of one or more enterotoxins, the most potent of which is the oligomeric cholera toxin (CT) itself. The bacteria first must pass through the acidic gastric environment to reach the upper small intestine, and compromised gastric acidity is a classic risk factor for infection.[34] *V. cholerae* attaches to the intestinal mucosa by virtue of proteinaceous hairlike fimbriae, the most important of which apparently is the toxin-coregulated pilus.[54] Colonization is facilitated by chemotaxis and motility of the organism, accelerating its approach to the intestinal mucosa.

The infectious dose varies with gastric pH because the organism does not typically tolerate acidic conditions. When water is the source, 10^3 to 10^6 bacteria are needed to cause disease. Only 10^2 to 10^4 bacteria are required when ingested with food.[16,17]

V. cholerae organisms shed in the stool of an infected individual apparently are more virulent than are strains acquired from an environmental source, and serial passage through multiple patients may augment virulence further, partly accounting for the violent epidemics occurring throughout history.[42] On intestinal passage, genes required for acquiring nutrients and motility are up-regulated, whereas genes required for chemotaxis are down-regulated. This increased virulence is confirmed in an animal model in which *V. cholerae* shed by mice have a 10-fold lower infectious dose than organisms grown in vitro.[42] Reduced chemotaxis prevents dispersion in environmental waters and increases the clumping of the bacteria[14]; the resulting increased concentration of organisms also could contribute to the vigor of cholera outbreaks.

The principal secretogenic factor, the oligomeric protein toxin CT, is composed of five identical binding (B) subunits and one active (A) subunit. Similar in structure and function to the heat-labile toxin produced by enterotoxigenic *Escherichia coli*,[46] CT binds to the GM_1 ganglioside receptor on the surface of intestinal epithelial cells. The A subunit is transported into the cell, where it activates adenylate cyclase. As a result, cyclic adenosine monophosphate is up-regulated, causing an increase in chloride secretion from the intestinal crypt cells and a decrease in sodium chloride absorption by the villous cells. In addition to this mechanism, cholera toxin may have effects on prostaglandins and the enteric nervous system that may contribute to the voluminous diarrhea characteristic of the disease.[34] The loss of electrolytes is followed by water along the osmotic gradient into the intestinal lumen. The dramatic loss of fluid and electrolytes rapidly leads to decreased intravascular volume and the complications of hypovolemic shock and metabolic acidosis. Although CT is responsible for much of the pathogenicity associated with the organism, strains mutated in CT still elicit mild diarrhea.[34]

The genetics of *V. cholerae* provide insight into the organism's pathogenicity and spread. The genome comprises two circular chromosomes, the larger of which contains genes for growth and pathogenicity, whereas the smaller one contains elements of metabolism and regulation. The genes required for virulence can propagate laterally and among different strains. Required for pathogenicity are the CT genetic element and the vibrio pathogenicity island, which encodes the toxin-coregulated pilus. The CT-encoding genetic element can exist as a plasmid or as a prophage integrated into the chromosome. Transfer of genetic material can lead to the emergence of virulence in a previously avirulent organism, or it can lead to the emergence of a new epidemic strain. The O139 Bengal strain derived DNA from a more pathogenic O1 strain, resulting in the emergence of a new pathogen.[54]

EPIDEMIOLOGY

V. cholerae O1 is distinguished by its ability to cause explosive outbreaks and pandemics. Now truly pandemic, *V. cholerae* O1 occurs (although rarely) in the U.S. Gulf Coast region, where it is associated with consumption of shellfish. Cases were described in the wake of the severe hurricanes occurring in 2005.[5]

V. cholerae is isolated commonly from surface water of moderate salinity, where the bacterium associates itself with zooplankton and phytoplankton. Pathogenic *V. cholerae* exist in thick layers (biofilms) of partially dormant cells on plankton, which may be the infectious form first encountered by humans at the start of an epidemic. When human cases begin to occur in a community, direct contamination of food and water may occur, circumventing the need for the aquatic reservoir.[21] Although *V. cholerae* have been isolated from animals, their role in transmission is probably minimal.[56] Person-to-person transmission also seems to be uncommon.[47]

During acute cholera disease, infected individuals excrete 10^7 to 10^8 organisms per 1 g of stool.[38] If the infected individual survives the episode, shedding of organisms may continue for 1 to 2 weeks after recovery in the absence of antibiotic treatment, and in some cases may continue for even longer. Transient asymptomatic carriers often are found in the households of individuals affected with acute illness.[34] Although environmental reservoirs seem to be important in the initiation of epidemics, highly virulent strains seem to be more readily isolated from areas contaminated by human feces.[34] Clinical studies suggest that increased pathogenicity of organisms occurs after passage through the human intestine.[14]

A great deal of attention has been devoted to understanding the epidemiology of cholera during interepidemic periods, and findings suggest a complex interaction between humans and their environment. Seasonal patterns have long been recognized for cholera outbreaks, with a predilection for warmer months. *V. cholerae* can remain dormant in aquatic environments in a nonculturable but viable state.[32,61] When aquatic conditions are conducive to growth, *V. cholerae* proliferates.[19] Environmental conditions play an important role in the seasonal variations. In a 33-year observational study in Bangladesh, outbreaks were predicted by an increase in temperature and concentrations of cyanobacteria in local waters.[39] More recent climate changes in Bangladesh (El Nino/Southern Oscillation) are associated with 70 percent of the variance in cholera incidence seen during specific time intervals of heightened activity of climate change.[53]

More recent studies suggest that an increase in ocean water temperatures as a result of global warming has had an effect on cholera epidemics.[19,27,51] The ecology of vibrio-infecting phages also may affect the abundance of *V. cholerae* in the environment.[22]

Cholera classically is described as a water-borne illness, but it also can be transmitted via contaminated food. The incubation period depends on the inoculum, with lower inocula corresponding to a longer incubation period and decreased stool volumes.[34] Incubation generally is 1 to 3 days, with a range of several hours to 5 days. Symptoms usually last 2 to 3 days, and patients treated with antibiotics may be infectious for several days. Patients who are untreated remain infectious for 1 to 2 weeks. Although water-borne transmission is typical in developing countries of Asia and Africa, *V. cholerae* that is found in marine environments can be transmitted via undercooked shellfish.[20] Person-to-person transmission is rare, owing to the high infectious dose.

Factors that predispose the human host to cholera include age, immunity, blood type, reduced gastric acid production, and other factors that have not been determined. Age groups commonly affected by cholera typically include young children because susceptibility depends on the level of preexisting immunity. In endemic areas such as Bangladesh, cases of cholera are concentrated in the 2- to 9-year-old age category, followed by women of childbearing age.[34] The increased susceptibility of children is supported further by a more recent prospective study in Kolkata, India, which found that the burden of cholera was greatest in children younger than 2 years old and that cholera cases were more likely to have a household member with diarrhea.[58] Individuals with blood type O also are at increased risk of experiencing severe cholera for reasons not completely understood.[23,57,59] Host factors in addition to reduced gastric acidity also are thought to play a role because volunteers who received the same inoculum had large variations in the amount of stool they produced.[34]

Because of the potential for epidemic disease, cholera outbreaks should be reported to local and national health authorities. In 2004, five laboratory-confirmed cases of cholera were reported to the Centers for Disease Control and Prevention. Four were acquired outside the United States, and one occurred in Hawaii, thought to have been acquired through imported seafood.[33]

CLINICAL MANIFESTATIONS

Most individuals infected with *V. cholerae* have only mild symptoms, indistinguishable from symptoms caused by other enteric infections. Individuals who develop severe disease urgently need fluid resuscitation and replacement of ongoing losses. In areas where cholera is indigenous, the populations have developed a (generally healthy) respect for the potential life-threatening nature of diarrheal illness and seek early medical treatment. Of all causes of infectious diarrhea, stool volumes passed and the rapidity by which dehydration develops are greatest with cholera.[55] In severe disease, stool volume can exceed 250 mL/kg body weight in a 24-hour period.[44,52]

The most distinctive clinical feature of cholera is the painless passage of voluminous, watery stools. Termed "rice water stools"

because of the watery, colorless diarrhea dotted with mucus, cholera stools may have a fishy smell or may be nearly odorless. Other common symptoms include abdominal cramping and vomiting. Abdominal cramping is probably due to increased abdominal secretions and resulting small bowel distention. Vomiting commonly occurs a few hours after the onset of diarrhea, but it also occurs later in the course of the illness.[17,28,48]

Complications of cholera relate mostly to the massive loss of intravascular volume and electrolytes. If cholera is not treated promptly, diarrhea and vomiting eventually lead to dehydration, which is most often isotonic. Patients with severe cholera may experience vascular collapse, shock, and death rates of 50 percent,[54] starting within hours after the onset of diarrhea. Related to the massive loss of intravascular volume and hypoperfusion, bicarbonate losses in stool, and hyperphosphatemia, acidosis also may develop.[64,66] Compensatory tachypnea may be observed in patients with acidosis. In addition to bicarbonate losses in stool, potassium also is lost and may not be reflected in serum potassium levels; acidosis induces the shift of intracellular potassium into the intravascular space in exchange for hydrogen ions, resulting in decreased total body potassium and potentially normal serum potassium values. As the acidosis is corrected, serum hypokalemia may result. In cases complicated by severe malnutrition, in which body potassium stores already are depleted, hypokalemia may be quite severe and manifest as paralytic ileus. This hypokalemia rarely is associated with severe cardiac arrhythmias, but it may manifest as changes on electrocardiogram.

After dehydration, hypoglycemia is the second most common cause of death in pediatric patients with cholera.[10] At the International Center for Diarrheal Disease Research, Bangladesh, the mortality rate in pediatric patients with hypoglycemia caused by cholera was reported to be 15 percent compared with 1 percent mortality in patients with normoglycemia.[10] Although the precise mechanism of hypoglycemia is unknown, children who are malnourished and acutely ill have lower glycogen stores and impaired gluconeogenesis. Special attention should be given to monitor patients with concomitant malnutrition and cholera for hypoglycemia.

Severe cholera is diagnosed in individuals who present with clinical signs and symptoms of severe dehydration (loss of ≥15% of total body water, or loss of approximately 10% of body weight). Common signs of severe volume depletion include a combination of decreased skin turgor, depressed anterior fontanelle in infants, lack of tears and sunken eyes, dry mouth, anuria, tachycardia, decreased peripheral perfusion, and hypotension (Fig. 127–1). In

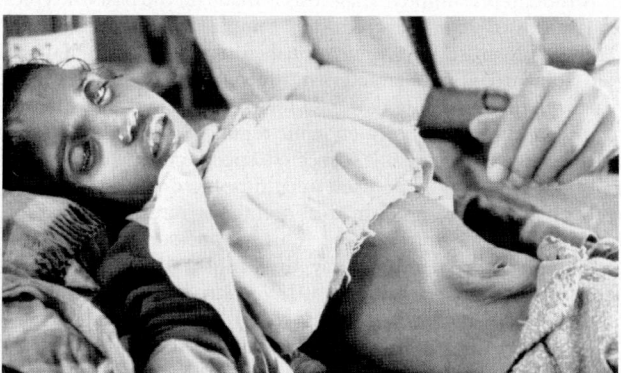

Figure 127–1 An adolescent girl with severe dehydration from cholera. Characteristic features include obtundation, sunken eyes, and "tenting" of the abdominal skin and subcutaneous tissues after firmly pinching the abdomen.

TABLE 127-1 Electrolyte Concentration in Cholera Stool and in Fluids Used for Rehydration and Replacement of Stool Losses

	Electrolyte Concentration (mmol/L)				
	Na⁺	Cl⁻	K⁺	HCO₃⁻	Osmolality
Cholera Stool					
Adults	130	100	20	44	300*
Infants and children	100	90	33	30	300*
Hydration Solutions					
WHO oral rehydration	90	80	20	30†	220‡
Intravenous					
Dhaka	133	98	13	48	273
Lactated Ringer	130	109	4	28§	251
5:4:1	129	97	11	44	281

*Osmolality includes unmeasured osmotically active molecules (primarily organic acids) in addition to electrolytes.
†As citrate.
‡From electrolytes only; also contains 111 mmol/L of glucose.
§As lactate.
WHO, World Health Organization.

some cases, mental status changes may be a sign of volume depletion, but more common are somnolence, restlessness, and lethargy. Table 127-1 summarizes the clinical findings associated with various degrees of clinical dehydration.

LABORATORY FINDINGS AND DIAGNOSIS

Laboratory abnormalities in patients with cholera relate to the massive loss of volume and electrolytes. The hypovolemic state can lead to hemoconcentration, causing increased hematocrit, serum specific gravity, serum protein, serum creatinine, and blood urea nitrogen.[64,66] Because of the loss of sodium that accompanies water loss, serum sodium is either slightly low[52] or normal.[34] As noted earlier, although potassium loss occurs in the stool, serum potassium may be normal, whereas total body potassium may be decreased. Acidosis caused by loss of bicarbonate in stool and lactic acidosis may result in a serum bicarbonate concentration of less than 15 mmol/L.[64,66] Serum creatinine and blood urea nitrogen also are elevated as a result of a decreased glomerular filtration rate. The common abnormalities of sodium, potassium, bicarbonate, and glucose mandate early determination of serum glucose and electrolytes as a guide to therapy.

Although presumptive diagnosis is made on the basis of typical oxidase-positive colonies from stool samples that agglutinate with O1 or O139 antiserum, conventional culture methods remain the gold standard. The characteristically motile organisms can be visualized directly using darkfield microscopy,[9] but few laboratories except those in cholera-endemic regions are experienced with this technique. If cholera is suspected, special culture media, such as TCBS agar, should be used to culture the organism.

In epidemic settings or in areas of intense transmission, a rapid vibrio dipstick test may be used. This is a one-step immunochromatographic test developed by the Institut Pasteur for rapid detection of cholera O1 and O139 from stool samples. The method has been tested in Madagascar, Bangladesh, and Mozambique, where the specificity ranged from 84 to 100 percent and sensitivity ranged from 94 to 100 percent.[49,65] It is especially advantageous because it requires minimal technical skill and can be read in 10 minutes.[49] This test also has been shown to be useful in detecting cholera from rectal swabs.[12,65] Confirmation of *V. cholerae* in stool also can be done through polymerase chain reaction amplification and use of oligoprobes.[31,43,63]

TREATMENT

The cornerstone of cholera management is fluid resuscitation. When fluid resuscitation is initiated, previous losses must be estimated and replaced, and ongoing losses must be quantified and replaced. Replacement fluids in children with cholera should be similar to fluids that are lost, such as Ringer lactate solution (Table 127-1).[4,30] The ideal solution contains amounts of bicarbonate and potassium sufficient to replace what is lost in stool.[8]

At the International Centre for Diarrhoeal Disease Research, Bangladesh, where thousands of cholera patients are treated annually, patients of all ages present with severe dehydration of rapid onset. Many present in hypovolemic shock. The extent of dehydration is determined as shown in Table 127-1. One or two intravenous catheters are inserted, and isotonic resuscitation solution is administered rapidly. The composition of the preferred solution at the Center (Dhaka solution) is listed in Table 127-1. The solution contains Na⁺, Cl⁻, K⁺, and HCO₃⁻, but no glucose. The complete estimated deficit is administered over 4 hours, whereupon ongoing losses and maintenance fluids are provided. Serum glucose and electrolytes are determined rapidly, with administration of glucose as needed based on these results.

Because severely dehydrated patients characteristically are anuric, concern may exist over early administration of potassium. The rapid onset of dehydration in cholera patients reduces this risk, however, and acute tubular necrosis rarely is seen.[52,66] A greater concern may be the rapid shift of potassium from the circulation on correction of acidosis. Patients treated in this manner respond dramatically. After the 4-hour resuscitation phase, most patients can begin to accept oral rehydration solution (ORS). Close attention to fluids and electrolytes is required for the duration of the diarrhea.

Although oral and intravenous rehydration methods are acceptable in theory for the management of cholera, the severity of losses renders intravenous rehydration the mainstay for treating cases of severe cholera. Not only do intravenous fluids allow predictable and rapid expansion of intravascular fluid volume to occur, they also ensure timely replacement of ongoing losses that may be difficult because of excessive purging.[50] Mild cases can be managed with ORS (see subsequently).

Because of the massive volumes of fluid that are lost during cholera gravis, the volume deficit frequently is underestimated, and rehydration therapy often is inadequate. Dehydration is not clinically apparent until a child has lost at least 5 percent of his or her body weight and can be diagnosed from the parent's history.

The use of a "cholera cot" is extremely helpful in quantifying ongoing fluid losses and for patient comfort (Fig. 127-2). It is constructed of a simple cot with a hole in the center through which a plastic sheet drains via a funnel into a graduated bucket below. This allows for accurate quantification of ongoing losses and permits the patient to remain horizontal, an important advantage if the patient is initially hypotensive. Attention given to tachycardia and signs of hypoperfusion in prostrate patients is essential.

The World Health Organization–approved oral rehydration salts (see Table 127-1) are recommended for patients with no detectable dehydration or mild dehydration, provided that the patient can drink sufficient quantities to replace the deficit and keep pace with ongoing losses. ORS also can be used for patients with severe dehydration to replace ongoing losses after initial intravenous replacement therapy. For cholera, ORS that is made with rice rather than with glucose, as carbohydrate seems to be more effective because it reduces the purging rate.[45,67] Food should be offered to patients as soon as they are able to eat and should not be restricted.

Effective use of ORS requires extra effort in treating pediatric patients with cholera. Parents need to be instructed to encourage and supervise ORS intake by the child, including taking small amounts frequently. Parents also need to be reassured that oral rehydration is still effective despite occasional vomiting.

A short course of antibiotics should be given to children with clinically significant cholera. This approach has been shown to shorten the duration of the illness and to decrease the amount of diarrhea.[25,54] Because of high resistance rates in some areas, the organism should be isolated and tested for susceptibility using standard methods for gram-negative enteric bacteria. Patients not treated with antibiotics may continue to shed organisms for 1 to 2 weeks after symptoms have abated.[34]

Treatment options for cholera in pediatric patients are derived from adult studies (Table 127–2). The treatment of choice for *V. cholerae* O1 and O139 is tetracycline for 3 days or a single dose of doxycycline for children older than 8 years.[3] This therapy generally is not recommended for children younger than 8 years old because of the risk of dental staining. This risk is cumulative, however, and the life-threatening nature of cholera may justify this risk. Trimethoprim-sulfamethoxazole is an alternative treat-ment for children younger than 8 years of age, although resis-tance may be present among O139 strains.[1] If tetracycline-resistant strains are encountered, other options include ampicillin, trimethoprim-sulfamethoxazole, erythromycin, and single-dose ciprofloxacin.[13,24,35,36] Single-dose azithromycin proved to be as effective as is a 3-day course of erythromycin in children 1 to 15 years old in Bangladesh.[37] Although transmission rates in endemic areas may decrease with prophylactic treatment of household members, this approach may promote resistance.[41] In the United States, where secondary transmission rates are low, prophylactic treatment of contacts is not recommended.

Antibiotic resistance to cholera seems to fluctuate with local usage patterns, showing alternating resistance and sensitivity. Conjugative plasmid–mediated, multiply-resistant *V. cholerae* O1 has been reported from several cholera endemic countries.[54] Appropriate antibiotics, usually prescribed before obtaining sen-sitivity testing results, should be administered according to local resistance patterns, and should be monitored for increased or decreased sensitivity patterns. *V. cholerae* O139 strains first appeared carrying a novel conjugative, self-transmissible, chro-mosomally integrating "SXT" element that conferred resistance to sulfamethoxazole, trimethoprim, chloramphenicol, and strep-tomycin. Multiple mechanisms of drug resistance are reported in *V. cholerae* and include proton-motive, force-dependent efflux and modifying enzymes.[7,26,62]

PREVENTION

Because contaminated food and water are the main routes of transmission of pathogenic *V. cholerae*, strategies to improve access to safe water sources and a clean food supply are the best methods of prevention. Proper sanitation methods also play a key role. During outbreaks, measures to increase awareness of cholera transmission and means to decrease spread should be communi-cated to the public; these measures include proper handwashing (especially after defecating), proper cooking of food, and identify-ing ill individuals so that they can be treated.

Vaccination is another method of preventing cholera. Paren-teral and oral vaccines have been developed. The whole-cell, killed parenteral vaccines stimulate short-term immunity to cholera, but they are not effective in young children. Because of limited efficacy and frequent local adverse reactions, this vaccine no longer is available.[29]

Two oral cholera vaccines, one composed of killed cholera bacteria and the other composed of a living attenuated organism, currently are licensed for use in children at least 2 years old.[29]

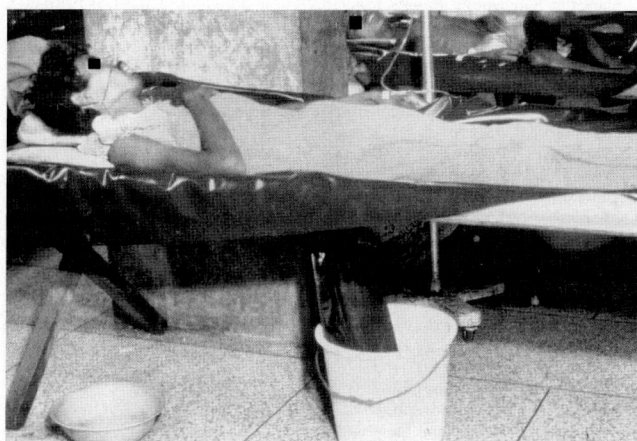

Figure 127–2 A cholera cot: a simple folding cot covered with plastic that has a hole and bucket for collecting the stool output, as used for the care of cholera patients at the International Centre for Diarrhoeal Disease Research, Bangladesh. The bucket is calibrated, and the volume of stool (and replacement fluids required) can be calculated easily. The plastic sheet is cleaned daily and between patients.

TABLE 127–2   Antimicrobial Therapy of Cholera*

Agent	Single Dose	Multiple Dose
Erythromycin	Not evaluated	40 mg/kg/day erythromycin base divided into 3 doses for 3 days; maximal dose 1 g/day
Azithromycin	20 mg/kg	
Furazolidone	7 mg/kg; maximal dose 300 mg†	5 mg/kg/day divided into 4 doses for 3 days; maximal dose 400 mg/day
Ciprofloxacin‡	30 mg/kg; maximal dose 1 g	30 mg/kg/day divided into 2 doses for 3 days; maximal dose 1 g/day
Trimethoprim-sulfamethoxazole	Not evaluated	8 mg trimethoprim/40 mg sulfamethoxazole/kg/day divided into 2 doses for 3 days; maximal doses 320 mg trimethoprim and 1.6 g sulfamethoxazole daily
Ampicillin	Not evaluated	50 mg/kg/day divided into 4 doses for 3 days; maximal dose 2 g/day

*Antimicrobial therapy is an adjunct to fluid therapy for cholera and is not an essential component. It reduces diarrhea volume and duration, however, by approximately 50 percent. The choice of antimicrobial agent is determined by the susceptibility pattern of local strains of Vibrio cholerae O1 or O139. Resistance to all agents except fluoroquinolones, such as ciprofloxacin, has been reported and is common in some areas.

†Single-dose therapy with these drugs has not been evaluated systematically in children, and recommendations are extrapolated from experience in adults.

‡The fluoroquinolones, such as ciprofloxacin, are not approved for use in children <18 years old in the United States because when given in high doses to juvenile animals, they cause arthropathy. Clinical experience indicates that this risk is very small in children when used for short courses of therapy.

The killed cholera vaccine (rBS-WC; marketed by SBL Vaccines [Sdna, Sweden] under the trade name Dukoral) consists of 1 mg of recombinant cholera toxin B subunit and approximately 1×10^{11} inactivated whole cells of the Classical and El Tor biotypes of *V. cholerae* O1, serotypes Inaba and Ogawa. The vaccine is approved for children older than 24 months of age and generally is well tolerated. The rBS-WC vaccine is supplied as 3-mL single-dose vials, each provided with a sachet of sodium bicarbonate buffer. The buffer solution is prepared by dissolving the sachet in 150 mL of water immediately before consumption. In one study, each dose of vaccine was mixed with 40 mL, 75 mL, or 150 mL of buffer solution for individuals 2 to 4 years, 5 to 11 years, or older than 11 years.[40] The vaccine must be refrigerated during shipping. Two doses administered at least 15 days apart are recommended. In a cohort of children and adults in Beira, Mozambique, studied during a cholera outbreak, receipt of one or more doses of rBS-WC vaccine was associated with 78 percent protection (95% confidence interval 39 to 92%; $P = 0.004$) against culture-confirmed cholera. Most vaccinees had received two doses. All of the cases were caused by infection with *V. cholerae* O1 El Tor Ogawa, and all occurred within 6 months of immunization. The vaccine was equally effective in children younger than 5 years old and older individuals. Protection induced by the killed vaccine persists for at least 3 years in adults, but it declines significantly after 6 months in children 2 to 5 years old.[18] The rBS-WC vaccine also may provide herd immunity in endemic settings.[2]

The live-attenuated cholera vaccine, CVD 103HgR, provided 100 percent protection against the homologous strain in challenge models for at least 6 months.[60] This vaccine also was proven to be effective in an outbreak of naturally occurring cholera in Micronesia[15]; a single dose of CVD 103HgR provided 79 percent protection (95% confidence interval 72.9 to 84.6%) against clinically defined cases of cholera during the 3-month post-vaccination period.

Both vaccines are available for travelers to developing countries with active transmission of cholera. The use of cholera vaccine in addition to initiation of proper sanitation methods should be considered in outbreaks in refugee camps, in relief and disaster workers, and in individuals who are traveling to endemic areas where access to medical care is limited.

Acknowledgments

The authors thank Dr. David Sack, Director of the International Centre for Diarrhoeal Disease Research, Bangladesh, for helpful discussions during the preparation of this chapter.

REFERENCES

1. Albert, M. J.: *Vibrio cholerae* O139 Bengal. J. Clin. Microbiol. 32:2345-2349, 1994.
2. Ali, M., Emch, M., Von, S. L., et al.: Herd immunity conferred by killed oral cholera vaccines in Bangladesh: A reanalysis 5. Lancet 366:44-49, 2005.
3. American Academy of Pediatrics. Cholera. *In*: Pickering, L. K., Baker, C. J., Long, S. S., McMillan, J. A. (eds.): Red Book: 2006 Report of the Committee on Infectious Diseases. 27th ed. Elk Grove Village, IL: American Academy of Pediatrics, 2006, pp. 725-727.
4. Anonymous. World Health Organization: Programme for Control of Diarrhoeal Disease: Guidelines for Cholera Control. Geneva, World Health Organization, 1991.
5. Anonymous. Two cases of toxigenic *Vibrio cholerae* O1 infection after Hurricanes Katrina and Rita—Louisiana, October 2005. M. M. W. R. Morb. Mortal. Wkly. Rep. 55:31-32, 2006.
6. Anonymous. Cholera 2005. Weekly epidemiological record 31[81], 297-308. Geneva, World Health Organization, 2006.
7. Baranwal, S., Dey, K., Ramamurthy, T., et al.: Role of active efflux in association with target gene mutations in fluoroquinolone resistance in clinical isolates of *Vibrio cholerae*. Antimicrob. Agents Chemother. 46:2676-2678, 2002.
8. Beisel, W. R., Atten, R. H., Lackwell, R. Q., and Enyajati, C.: The role of bicarbonate pathophysiology and therapy in asiatic cholera. Am. J. Med. 35:58-66, 1963.
9. Benenson, A. S., Islam, M. R., and Greenough, W. B., III: Rapid identification of *Vibrio cholerae* by darkfield microscopy. Bull. World Health Organ. 30:827-831, 1964.
10. Bennish, M. L.: Cholera: Pathophysiology, clinical features, and treatment. *In* Wachsmuth, I. K. B. P. A. a. O. O. (ed): *Vibrio cholerae* and Cholera: Molecular to Global Perspectives Washington, D.C., American Society of Microbiology, 1994, pp. 229-255.
11. Beyhan, S., Tischler, A. D., Camilli, A., and Yildiz, F. H.: Differences in gene expression between the classical and El Tor biotypes of *Vibrio cholerae* O1. Infect. Immun. 74:3633-3642, 2006.
12. Bhuiyan, N. A., Qadri, F., Faruque, A. S., et al.: Use of dipsticks for rapid diagnosis of cholera caused by *Vibrio cholerae* O1 and O139 from rectal swabs. J. Clin. Microbiol. 41:3939-3941, 2003.
13. Burans, J. P., Podgore, J., Mansour, M. M., et al.: Comparative trial of erythromycin and sulphatrimethoprim in the treatment of tetracycline-resistant *Vibrio cholerae* O1. Trans. R. Soc. Trop. Med. Hyg. 83:836-838, 1989.
14. Butler, S. M., Nelson, E. J., Chowdhury, N., et al.: Cholera stool bacteria repress chemotaxis to increase infectivity. Mol. Microbiol. 60:417-426, 2006.
15. Calain, P., Chaine, J. P., Johnson, E., et al.: Can oral cholera vaccination play a role in controlling a cholera outbreak? Vaccine 22:2444-2451, 2004.
16. Cash, R. A., Music, S. I., Libonati, J. P., et al.: Response of man to infection with *Vibrio cholerae*, II: Protection from illness afforded by previous disease and vaccine. J. Infect. Dis. 130:325-333, 1974.
17. Cash, R. A., Music, S. I., Libonati, J. P., et al.: Response of man to infection with *Vibrio cholerae*, I: Clinical, serologic, and bacteriologic responses to a known inoculum. J. Infect. Dis. 129:45-52, 1974.
18. Clemens, J. D., Sack, D. A., Harris, J. R., et al.: Field trial of oral cholera vaccines in Bangladesh: Results from three-year follow-up. Lancet 335:270-273, 1990.
19. Colwell, R. R., and Huq, A.: Environmental reservoir of *Vibrio cholerae*: The causative agent of cholera. Ann. N. Y. Acad. Sci. 740:44-54, 1994.
20. Colwell, R. R., Seidler, R. J., Kaper, J., et al.: Occurrence of *Vibrio cholerae* serotype O1 in Maryland and Louisiana estuaries. Appl. Environ. Microbiol. 41:555-558, 1981.
21. Faruque, S. M., Biswas, K., Udden, S. M., et al.: Transmissibility of cholera: In vivo-formed biofilms and their relationship to infectivity and persistence in the environment. Proc. Natl. Acad. Sci. U. S. A. 103:6350-6355, 2006.
22. Faruque, S. M., Naser, I. B., Islam, M. J., et al.: Seasonal epidemics of cholera inversely correlate with the prevalence of environmental cholera phages 6. Proc. Natl. Acad. Sci. U. S. A. 102:1702-1707, 2005.
23. Glass, R. I., Holmgren, J., Haley, C. E., et al.: Predisposition for cholera of individuals with O blood group: Possible evolutionary significance. Am. J. Epidemiol. 121:791-796, 1985.
24. Gotuzzo, E., Seas, C., Echevarria, J., et al.: Ciprofloxacin for the treatment of cholera: A randomized, double-blind, controlled clinical trial of a single daily dose in Peruvian adults. Clin. Infect. Dis. 20:1485-1490, 1995.
25. Greenough, W. B., Gordon, R. S., Jr., Rosenberg, I. S., et al.: Tetracycline in the treatment of cholera. Lancet 41:355-357, 1964.
26. Hall, R. M., and Collis, C. M.: Mobile gene cassettes and integrons: Capture and spread of genes by site-specific recombination. Mol. Microbiol. 15:593-600, 1995.
27. Harvell, C. D., Mitchell, C. E., Ward, J. R., et al.: Climate warming and disease risks for terrestrial and marine biota. Science 296:2158-2162, 2002.
28. Harvey, R. M., Enson, Y., Lewis, M. L., et al.: Hemodynamic studies on cholera: Effects of hypovolemia and acidosis. Circulation 37:709-728, 1968.
29. Hill, D. R., Ford, L., and Lalloo, D. G.: Oral cholera vaccines: Use in clinical practice. Lancet Infect. Dis. 6:361-373, 2006.
30. Hirschhorn, N.: The treatment of acute diarrhea in children: An historical and physiological perspective. Am. J. Clin. Nutr. 33:637-663, 1980.
31. Hoshino, K., Yamasaki, S., Mukhopadhyay, A. K., et al.: Development and evaluation of a multiplex PCR assay for rapid detection of toxigenic *Vibrio cholerae* O1 and O139. F. E. M. S. Immunol. Med. Microbiol. 20:201-207, 1998.
32. Huq, A., Colwell, R. R., Rahman, R., et al.: Detection of *Vibrio cholerae* O1 in the aquatic environment by fluorescent-monoclonal antibody and culture methods. Appl. Environ. Microbiol. 56:2370-2373, 1990.
33. Jajosky, R. A., Hall, P. A., Adams, D. A., et al.: Summary of notifiable diseases—United States, 2004. M. M. W. R. Morb. Mortal. Wkly. Rep. 53:1-79, 2006.
34. Kaper, J. B., Morris, J. G., Jr., and Levine, M. M.: Cholera. Clin. Microbiol. Rev. 8:48-86, 1995.
35. Khan, W. A., Begum, M., Salam, M. A., et al.: Comparative trial of five antimicrobial compounds in the treatment of cholera in adults. Trans. R. Soc. Trop. Med. Hyg. 89:103-106, 1995.
36. Khan, W. A., Bennish, M. L., Seas, C., et al.: Randomised controlled comparison of single-dose ciprofloxacin and doxycycline for cholera caused by *Vibrio cholerae* O1 or O139. Lancet 348:296-300, 1996.
37. Khan, W. A., Saha, D., Rahman, A., et al.: Comparison of single-dose azithromycin and 12-dose, 3-day erythromycin for childhood cholera: A randomised, double-blind trial. Lancet 360:1722-1727, 2002.
38. Levine, M. M., Kaper, J. B., Herrington, D., et al.: Volunteer studies of deletion mutants of *Vibrio cholerae* O1 prepared by recombinant techniques. Infect. Immun. 56:161-167, 1988.

39. Longini, I. M., Jr., Yunus, M., Zaman, K., et al.: Epidemic and endemic cholera trends over a 33-year period in Bangladesh. J. Infect. Dis. *186*:246-251, 2002.
40. Lucas, M. E., Deen, J. L., Von, S. L., et al.: Effectiveness of mass oral cholera vaccination in Beira, Mozambique. N. Engl. J. Med. *352*:757-767, 2005.
41. McCormack, W. M., Chowdhury, A. M., Jahangir, N., et al.: Tetracycline prophylaxis in families of cholera patients. Bull. World Health Organ. *38*:787-792, 1968.
42. Merrell, D. S., Butler, S. M., Qadri, F., et al.: Host-induced epidemic spread of the cholera bacterium. Nature *417*:642-645, 2002.
43. Miyagi, K., Matsumoto, Y., Hayashi, K., et al.: Successful application of enzyme-labeled oligonucleotide probe for rapid and accurate cholera diagnosis in a clinical laboratory. Microbiol. Immunol. *38*:301-304, 1994.
44. Molla, A. M., Rahman, M., Sarker, S. A., et al.: Stool electrolyte content and purging rates in diarrhea caused by rotavirus, enterotoxigenic *E. coli*, and *V. cholerae* in children. J. Pediatr. *98*:835-838, 1981.
45. Molla, A. M., Sarker, S. A., Hossain, M., et al.: Rice-powder electrolyte solution as oral-therapy in diarrhoea due to *Vibrio cholerae* and *Escherichia coli*. Lancet *1*:1317-1319, 1982.
46. Moseley, S. L., and Falkow, S.: Nucleotide sequence homology between the heat-labile enterotoxin gene of *Escherichia coli* and *Vibrio cholerae* deoxyribonucleic acid. J. Bacteriol. *144*:444-446, 1980.
47. Mosley, W. H., Alvero, M. G., Joseph, P. R., et al.: Studies of cholera El Tor in the Philippines, 4: Transmission of infection among neighbourhood and community contacts of cholera patients. Bull. World Health Organ. *33*:651-660, 1965.
48. Nalin, D. R., Levine, M. M., Hornick, R. B., et al.: The problem of emesis during oral glucose-electrolytes therapy given from the onset of severe cholera. Trans. R. Soc. Trop. Med. Hyg. *73*:10-14, 1979.
49. Nato, F., Boutonnier, A., Rajerison, M., et al.: One-step immunochromatographic dipstick tests for rapid detection of *Vibrio cholerae* O1 and O139 in stool samples. Clin. Diagn. Lab. Immunol. *10*:476-478, 2003.
50. Palmer, D. L., Koster, F. T., Islam, A. F., et al.: Comparison of sucrose and glucose in the oral electrolyte therapy of cholera and other severe diarrheas. N. Engl. J. Med. *297*:1107-1110, 1977.
51. Pascual, M., Rodo, X., Ellner, S. P., et al.: Cholera dynamics and El Nino-Southern Oscillation. Science *289*:1766-1769, 2000.
52. Rahman, O., Bennish, M. L., Alam, A. N., and Salam, M. A.: Rapid intravenous rehydration by means of a single polyelectrolyte solution with or without dextrose. J. Pediatr. *113*:654-660, 1988.
53. Rodo, X., Pascual, M., Fuchs, G., and Faruque, A. S.: ENSO and cholera: A nonstationary link related to climate change? Proc. Natl. Acad. Sci. U. S. A. *99*:12901-12906, 2002.
54. Sack, D. A., Sack, R. B., Nair, G. B., and Siddique, A. K.: Cholera. Lancet *363*:223-233, 2004.
55. Sanchez, J. L., Vasquez, B., Begue, R. E., et al.: Protective efficacy of oral whole-cell/recombinant-B-subunit cholera vaccine in Peruvian military recruits. Lancet *344*:1273-1276, 1994.
56. Sanyal, S. C., Singh, S. J., Tiwari, I. C., et al.: Role of household animals in maintenance of cholera infection in a community. J. Infect. Dis. *130*:575-579, 1974.
57. Shahinian, M. L., Passaro, D. J., Swerdlow, D. L., et al.: *Helicobacter pylori* and epidemic *Vibrio cholerae* O1 infection in Peru. Lancet *355*:377-378, 2000.
58. Sur, D., Deen, J. L., Manna, B., et al.: The burden of cholera in the slums of Kolkata, India: Data from a prospective, community based study. Arch. Dis. Child. *90*:1175-1181, 2005.
59. Swerdlow, D. L., Mintz, E. D., Rodriguez, M., et al.: Severe life-threatening cholera associated with blood group O in Peru: Implications for the Latin American epidemic. J. Infect. Dis. *170*:468-472, 1994.
60. Tacket, C. O., Losonsky, G., Nataro, J. P., et al.: Onset and duration of protective immunity in challenged volunteers after vaccination with live oral cholera vaccine CVD 103-HgR. J. Infect. Dis. *166*:837-841, 1992.
61. Tamplin, M. L., Gauzens, A. L., Huq, A., et al.: Attachment of *Vibrio cholerae* serogroup O1 to zooplankton and phytoplankton of Bangladesh waters. Appl. Environ. Microbiol. *56*:1977-1980, 1990.
62. Thungapathra, M., Amita, Sinha, K. K., et al.: Occurrence of antibiotic resistance gene cassettes aac(6′)-Ib, dfrA5, dfrA12, and ereA2 in class I integrons in non-O1, non-O139 *Vibrio cholerae* strains in India. Antimicrob. Agents Chemother. *46*:2948-2955, 2002.
63. Varela, P., Pollevick, G. D., Rivas, M., et al.: Direct detection of *Vibrio cholerae* in stool samples. J. Clin. Microbiol. *32*:1246-1248, 1994.
64. Wang, F., Butler, T., Rabbani, G. H., and Jones, P. K.: The acidosis of cholera: Contributions of hyperproteinemia, lactic acidemia, and hyperphosphatemia to an increased serum anion gap. N. Engl. J. Med. *315*:1591-1595, 1986.
65. Wang, X. Y., Ansaruzzaman, M., Vaz, R., et al.: Field evaluation of a rapid immunochromatographic dipstick test for the diagnosis of cholera in a high-risk population. B. M. C. Infect. Dis. *6*:17, 2006.
66. Watten, R. H., Morgan, F. M., Yachai, N., et al.: Water and electrolyte studies in cholera. J. Clin. Invest. *38*:1879-1889, 1959.
67. Zaman, K., Yunus, M., Rahman, A., et al.: Efficacy of a packaged rice oral rehydration solution among children with cholera and cholera-like illness. Acta Paediatr. *90*:505-510, 2001.

VIBRIO PARAHAEMOLYTICUS

David Y. Hyun

Vibrio parahaemolyticus is recognized worldwide as a cause of foodborne disease associated with consumption of seafood, in particular crustaceans and mollusks, and occasionally as a cause of wound infections and sepsis in immunocompromised hosts. *V. parahaemolyticus* was isolated first in Japan during a foodborne outbreak in 1951. Almost 10 years after it was first described, the organism was classified correctly in the genus *Vibrio*,[8] and its distribution in coastal waters and estuaries of temperate climates around the world was recognized. The regional differences in the incidence of this disease are related to patterns of consumption of marine products and practices of food preparation. In Japan and Taiwan, where fish and shellfish are a major source of dietary protein and frequently consumed raw, *V. parahaemolyticus* accounts for 10 to 40 percent of foodborne outbreaks.[57,73] In the United States, the first confirmed foodborne outbreak occurred in Maryland in 1971, secondary to consumption of contaminated crabmeat.[17] Since then, sporadic outbreaks have been reported,[5,6,17,18,55] showing the potential risk for development of infectious and toxic syndromes from marine products in the United States.[24]

BACTERIOLOGY

V. parahaemolyticus is a gram-negative, non–spore-forming, curved rod with rounded ends that possess a polar flagellum.[45] On surfaces or in viscous environments, *V. parahaemolyticus* can differentiate into swarmer cells equipped with additional shorter lateral peritrichous flagella.[44] *V. parahaemolyticus* is a facultative anaerobe with respiratory and fermentative metabolisms. Similar to most vibrios, it is an oxidase-positive nonfermenter of lactose.[7] It is arginine dihydrolase–negative and ornithine decarboxylase–positive. The requirement of sodium and enhancement of growth in a specific range of concentration differentiate it from *Vibrio cholerae* and *Vibrio mimicus*. The optimal sodium concentration range is 2 to 4 percent; a concentration greater than 8 percent inhibits its growth.[72]

V. parahaemolyticus produces round, blue-green colonies on the widely used *Vibrio*-selective thiosulfate citrate bile salt sucrose (TCBS) agar. This medium inhibits most fecal flora by the presence of bile salts and a highly alkaline pH. Direct plating on TCBS agar may be used for feces and other clinical specimens, but food samples that are not heavily contaminated require enrichment either in alkaline peptone water supplemented with 3 percent sodium chloride or in a strongly selective medium, such as glucose salt teepol broth.[72] The optimal pH for growth is in the neutral range, but *V. parahaemolyticus* can survive in alkaline media. Optimal growth temperatures are between 35° C and 39° C.[76] Growth is remarkable in conventional media and food-stuff, with generation times of only 8 minutes[36]; a significant number of organisms can be found after a short period of inappropriate storage. Growth is inhibited at temperatures of 44° C or greater. Degree of inactivation is greater with increased temperatures; a million-fold decline occurs in viable bacteria in shrimp homogenate kept at 100° C for only 1 minute.[70] In laboratory conditions with low temperature and nutrient supply, *V. parahaemolyticus* has been shown to enter a viable but nonculturable state, during which the organism no longer can be cultured on routine growth media, but its viability can be confirmed using direct microscopic assays.[25,74]

The genome of *V. parahaemolyticus* consists of two circular chromosomes. Genes for a type III secretion system (TTSS) were identified in a pathogenicity island on chromosome 2.[42] TTSS, which is considered a central virulence factor in salmonellae and shigellae, possesses needle-like structures, which facilitates direct injections of bacterial proteins into target host cell, and is related strongly to the pathogenicity of inflammatory diarrhea seen with *V. parahaemolyticus* infections. This finding suggests that the presence of TTSS in *V. parahaemolyticus* differentiates its pathogenicity from that of *V. cholerae*, which does not carry the genes.[42]

EPIDEMIOLOGY

In the United States, *V. parahaemolyticus* is found along the East, West, and Gulf coasts.[20,36] Water, sediments, suspended particulates, plankton, fish, and shellfish have been shown to harbor the organism.[4,47] The organisms are present in highest numbers in water at temperatures between 17° C and 35° C and containing 0.5 to 2.5 percent salinity.[34] Marked seasonal and geographic variations occur, with maximal mean concentrations occurring during late summer and spring along the Gulf Coast.[20] The seasonal distribution correlates with outbreaks, predominantly between June and October.[3]

Finfish and all types of shellfish products, including oysters, clams, crabs, and shrimp, may be involved in the transmission of the infection (Table 128–1).[34] The risk of acquiring infection is higher with molluscan shellfish because of their ability to concentrate contaminants and bacteria by filter feeding.[4,25,76] In oysters, the density of *V. parahaemolyticus* may be 100 times greater than in the surrounding water.[20] The levels of contamination of seafood generally are low in freshly collected oysters, with the highest mean density of only 160 bacteria/g found in the United States.[20] In Japan, higher counts (up to 10^3 to 10^4/g) have been reported in market shellfish.[13] The minimum infective dose is thought to be in the range of 10^5 to 10^7 organisms, based on volunteer feeding studies.[23] More recent outbreaks of illness caused by oysters that met bacteriologic safety standards have raised questions about current recommendations, however.[18]

During the period 1973 to 1987, only 23 of 1869 foodborne disease outbreaks with known bacterial etiology reported to the Centers for Disease Control and Prevention were caused by *V. parahaemolyticus*.[5] In 18 of these outbreaks, a shellfish was recognized as the food vehicle. No fatal cases were reported. Contributing factors included inadequate cooking (92%), improper holding temperature (75%), and food acquired from an unsafe source (75%).[5,6] Most of the affected individuals were adults, and no patterns of unusual susceptibility by age group or gender were noted. No evidence of secondary spread was found among family members. Between 1988 and 1997, 345 sporadic cases were reported to the Centers for Disease Control and Prevention. Most infections were related to eating raw oysters. Most of these infections (59%) were gastroenteritis.[19]

Until more recently, *V. parahaemolyticus* infections were casually associated with multiple serotypes and occurred as sporadic cases or localized outbreaks.[49] In 1996, a sudden increase in incidence was seen in India, and 50 to 80 percent of the cases were attributed to a single serotype, O3:K6.[54] Shortly thereafter, O3:K6 strains were isolated from clinical samples from other countries in Asia. In 1998, two outbreaks of gastroenteritis in the

TABLE 128–1 Selected Outbreaks of *Vibrio parahaemolyticus* Infection

Setting	Persons Ill/Exposed	Symptoms	Incubation	Resolution	Medical Attention/ Hospitalization	Vehicle	Risk Factor
Picnic[14]	351/631 (56%)	D (95%), C (82%), N (68%), V (61%), HA (41%), F (27%)	16 hr (4-42 hr)	4 days (<1-10 days)	60%/2%	Steamed crab	Cross-contamination, unrefrigerated food
Chronic hospital[14]	24/100 (24%)	D (100%), C (89%), N (72%), V (44%), HA (56%), F (33%)	18 hr (4-60 hr)	3 days (<1-7 days)	No data available	Crab salad	No data available
Shrimp boil[49]	~600/1200 (50%)	D, C, V, HA, F	23 hr (5-92 hr)	(few hr-1 wk)	1%/0%	Boiled shrimp	Storage temperature
International flight[43]	12/134 (9%)	D, C, V	(8-20 hr)	No data available	40%/25%	Cooked crab	Cross-contamination
Parish dinner[11]	~1000/1700 (59%)	D (95%), C (92%), N (72%), HA (47%), F (47%), V (12%)	16 hr (3-76 hr)	4.6 days (<1-8 days)	26%/7.4%	Shrimp	Cross-contamination, storage temperature
Pacific Northwest[47]	209 ill	D (99%), C (88%), N (52%), V (39%), F (33%)	15 hr (4-96 hr)	3 days mean	2 hospitalized, 1 death	Raw oysters	Uncooked oysters

C, cramps; D, diarrhea; F, fever; HA, headache; N, nausea; V, vomiting.

United States were associated with O3:K6.[19,56] By 2005, this pandemic clone was found in patients from Europe, South America, and Africa,[2,28,43] and other clones that genetically diverged from O3:K6, such as O4:K68 and O1:KUT, were isolated from clinical cases.[16]

PATHOGENESIS

The ability of certain strains of *V. parahaemolyticus* to produce beta-hemolysis on Wagatsuma agar, known as the Kanagawa phenomenon (KP), was first epidemiologically associated with human pathogenicity.[46] KP is observed in 88 to 96 percent of strains from clinical specimens and in 1 to 2 percent of strains from environmental sources.[23,36,68] Thermostable direct hemolysin (TDH) produces KP.[67] TDH has a molecular weight of 42,000, consisting of two subunits of 21,000,[47] and, in contrast to other hemolysins produced by *V. parahaemolyticus*, is not inactivated by heating at 100° C for 10 minutes. It is a pore-forming toxin that causes hemolysis by binding to and disrupting erythrocyte membranes.[30] TDH also has been shown to have enterotoxic activities, such as causing accumulation of fluid in rabbit ileal loop assays, invading intestinal mucosa,[15,71] and increasing intracellular calcium concentrations that trigger secretion of chloride by intestinal cells.[61,65,66] TDH is cytotoxic, lethal to small experimental animals, and cardiotoxic.[78]

Certain KP-negative isolates from outbreaks have been shown to produce TDH-related hemolysin (TRH).[32] Although TRH is heat-labile, it shares similarities with TDH, such as hemolysis, production of fluid accumulation in the rabbit ileal loop model, and induction of chloride secretion in human colonic epithelial cells.[31,65] Likewise, some variants closely related to the original TDH by molecular analysis (Vp TDH/I and Vp TDH/II) have been isolated from KP-negative strains.[48]

When the *tdh* and *trh* genes had been cloned and sequenced, researchers realized that certain strains possess the genetic material but are phenotypically incomplete. Strains with a typical hemolysin-positive phenotype carried two chromosome gene copies, whereas *tdh* gene–positive strains with weakly positive or negative hemolysin phenotype possessed only a single chromosome gene copy.[52] Less than 50 percent of *trh* gene–positive strains produce TRH when examined by enzyme-linked immunosorbent assay.[63] Low-level expression of the *tdh* genes may be the reason for the KP-negative phenotype.[53] The expression of the *tdh* genes is controlled by the Vp-toxRS operon. The basal production of mRNA and the degree of transcriptional activation seem to be related to differences in the nucleotide sequences and strength of the promoter region.[53]

Some studies suggest that virulence mechanisms in addition to TDH and TRH exist and that the mere presence of the *tdh* or *trh* genes does not reliably correlate with virulence of a given strain.[71,76] *V. parahaemolyticus* requires intestinal colonization factors to cause disease. A variety of pili and other potential colonization factors are present, but the evidence is too poor to implicate any of the candidate adhesins in virulence.[13] Adherence of *V. parahaemolyticus* to intestinal epithelial cells of rabbits[14] and human small intestine[27,75] seems to require binding to complex carbohydrates or hemagglutinins of the host. Also, *V. parahaemolyticus* appears to disrupt epithelial barrier function, regardless of TDH and TRH production.[41]

The occurrence of cases with grossly bloody stools[33,55] is indirect evidence of either invasiveness or production of cytotoxin. Invasion of Caco-2 cells in culture has been shown in approximately 20 percent of strains.[1] KP-positive and KP-negative strains from clinical specimens can invade and colonize the mucosal cells of the rabbit ileum, producing acute inflammation, degeneration, and erosion of the villi.[7] Vibrios can be cultured from tissue specimens of spleen, liver, and heart in experimental animals, indicating spread through the lymphatic or circulatory systems.[10]

CLINICAL MANIFESTATIONS

The spectrum of intestinal disease varies from a mild gastroenteritis to a dysenteric syndrome. The incubation period typically is 15 to 24 hours (range 4 to 96 hours)[3,64]; the variability presumably is related to the number of organisms ingested. Resolution is expected to occur in approximately 3 days,[47] but it varies from several hours to more than 10 days.[3,11] Fatigue may persist for a few days. Diarrhea (96%) and abdominal pain (95%) are the most frequent and earliest symptoms, accompanied by nausea, vomiting, and headache in 40 to 70 percent of cases. Chills and moderate fever are less frequent (20%) manifestations.[3,17] Diarrhea is watery and explosive,[12] with patients having up to 15 stools during the first day. Shock caused by loss of fluid is an exceptional event.[20] Mucus is observed frequently, but grossly bloody stool is seen less commonly.[8,33,40] Small superficial ulcerations on sigmoidoscopy may be present.[8] No difference in symptoms exists in cases associated with KP-negative strains.[30]

Extraintestinal infections occur. During the Vibrio Surveillance Program that started in 1989 in four Gulf Coast states, 18 to 34 percent of *V. parahaemolyticus* isolates were found to come from wound infections, and 3 to 5 percent were found to be associated with septicemia.[18,40] Wound infection occurs after contamination of skin lacerations with seawater or after direct trauma with pieces of shellfish, fishhooks, or utensils contaminated with seawater.[9] Superficial infection can extend to deeper soft tissue and may require radical surgical débridement. Septicemia is a concern in immunocompromised patients, particularly patients with leukemia[22] and patients with liver disease.[21,29] Bacteremia may develop after either wound infections[9,22] or ingestion of seafood.[29,60] Skin bullae,[29] intravascular hemolysis,[22] and disseminated intravascular coagulation[29] may complicate wound and bacteremic infections.

COMPLICATIONS

An acute diarrhea episode requires medical attention in 25 to 50 percent of cases during an outbreak, but less frequently requires hospitalization.[11,17,40,64] Children younger than 5 years old are more likely to require hospitalization compared with individuals older than 5 years.[69] Usually, no long-term sequelae occur. Severe dehydration, shock,[33,58] and death (0.04% of cases in Japan) can occur.[7,72] Primary septicemia,[38,40,60] septicemia secondary to wound infection,[9,22,38] and septicemia secondary to gastroenteritis[29,38] have higher mortality rates, especially in immunosuppressed patients or in patients with liver diseases.[9]

DIAGNOSIS

Epidemiologic data are the basis for the presumptive diagnosis. In a patient with compatible symptoms, a history of recent consumption of seafood should suggest this diagnosis. Leukocytosis and fecal leukocytes may be found.[8,33] A positive stool culture on selective media, such as TCBS agar, can confirm the clinical impression. Routine use of TCBS agar is not cost-effective, even in coastal areas, unless an appropriate clinical setting is available.[9,40,45] The use of a transport medium, such as Cary-Blair, is necessary if a delay in processing the sample is expected. Isolation of more than 10^5 *V. parahaemolyticus* from epidemiologically implicated food supports the diagnosis and identifies the vehicle.[45] A correlation between the serotype of the food and isolates from patients is not always present because multiple strains can contaminate a single food.[3] Adding an enrichment broth to the processing increases the yield of isolation.

For testing blood specimens, use of routine culture media followed by selective media is appropriate.[29,60] Immunoassays (enzyme-linked immunosorbent assay, immunoprecipitation in agar medium, reversed passive latex agglutination) are available in research laboratories and commercially in Japan (KAP-RPLA, Denka Seiken, Tokyo; BT test, Nissui Pharmaceutical, Tokyo) to detect the TDH. Strains producing TRH may be detected by cross-reactions.[77] Serologic methods (slide agglutination) can detect H antigens in lateral flagella.[62] Gene probe hybridization[51] and polymerase chain reaction with a sequence of a highly conserved DNA fragment[39] or targeting the *tdh* gene can be used to detect low numbers of the organism in environmental and clinical specimens. Histologic findings from duodenal and rectal biopsy samples from patients infected with *V. parahaemolyticus* were consistent with acute inflammatory response, showing epithelial degradation, polymorphonuclear neutrophil infiltration of villi and crypt cells, and hemorrhage.[59]

TREATMENT

Only supportive therapy and careful control of the fluid and electrolyte balances are required for the management of gastroenteritis. Oral rehydration usually is appropriate, although intravenous fluids may be required if massive losses of fluid occur.[8,33,58] Antibiotic therapy is unnecessary for this short-lived disease. In the unusual protracted episode, tetracycline or a fluoroquinolone may be beneficial for adults and older children.[7,8,36]

For wound infections and septicemia, antibiotics always are indicated. *V. parahaemolyticus* usually is susceptible to tetracycline. In addition, only a few strains are resistant to chloramphenicol, trimethoprim-sulfamethoxazole, third-generation cephalosporins, aztreonam, imipenem, fluoroquinolones, and aminoglycosides.[9,22,26,29] Penicillins are ineffective because of the presence of β-lactamases in 50 percent of isolates.[26,37] The older cephalosporins also have poor activity.[37]

PREVENTION AND CONTROL

Although ensuring the lack of contamination of seafood is impossible, avoiding food-handling errors should diminish the risk of infection. A recommendation for an acceptable upper limit of 100 colony-forming units per gram of *V. parahaemolyticus* in raw shrimp has been made by the International Commission on Microbiological Specification for Foods.[34] Thorough cooking eliminates the organism.[70] Heating seafood to 60° C for 15 minutes[23] or boiling for 7 minutes[11] seems to be adequate to reduce the risk of infection. When undercooked or raw seafood is consumed, adequate prior refrigeration to preclude multiplication of organisms is important. During the preparation of seafood, special attention should be paid to possible cross-contamination. Use of the same utensils, board surfaces, or containers for fresh and recently cooked seafood should be avoided.[58,70] Raw seafood consumption should be discouraged, particularly for individuals at high risk for development of septicemia.[21,38,40]

REFERENCES

1. Akeda, Y., Nagayama, K., Yamamoto, K., and Honda, T.: Invasive phenotype of *Vibrio parahaemolyticus*. J. Infect. Dis. *176*:822-824, 1997.
2. Ansaruzzaman, M., Lucas, M., Deen, J. L., et al.: Pandemic serovars (O3:K6 and O4:K68) of *Vibrio parahaemolyticus* associated with diarrhea in Mozambique: Spread of the pandemic into the African continent. J. Clin. Microbiol. *43*:2559-2562, 2005.
3. Barker, W. H., Jr.: *Vibrio parahaemolyticus* outbreaks in the United States. Lancet *1*:551-554, 1974.
4. Baross, J., and Liston, J.: Occurrence of *Vibrio parahaemolyticus* and related hemolytic vibrios in marine environments of Washington State. Appl. Microbiol. *20*:179-186, 1970.
5. Bean, N. H., and Griffin, P. M.: Foodborne disease outbreaks in the United States, 1973-1987: Pathogens, vehicles and trends. J. Food Protect. *53*:804-817, 1990.
6. Bean, N. H., Griffin, P. M., Goulding, J. S., et al.: Foodborne disease outbreaks, 5-year summary, 1983-1987. M. M. W. R. C. D. C. Surveill. Summ. *39*:15-57, 1990.
7. Blake, P. A.: Disease of humans (other than cholera) caused by vibrios. Annu. Rev. Microbiol. *34*:341-367, 1980.
8. Bolen, J. L., Zamiska, S. A., and Greenough, W. B.: Clinical features in enteritis due to *Vibrio parahaemolyticus*. Am. J. Med. *57*:638-641, 1974.
9. Bonner, J. R., Coker, A. S., Berryman, C. R., et al.: Spectrum of *Vibrio* infections in a Gulf Coast community. Ann. Intern. Med. *99*:464-469, 1983.
10. Boutin, B. K., Townsend, S. F., Scarpino, P. V., et al.: Demonstration of invasiveness of *Vibrio parahaemolyticus* in adult rabbits by immunofluorescence. Appl. Environ. Microbiol. *37*:647-653, 1979.
11. Caraway, C. T., Gregg, J., and McFarland, L.: *Vibrio parahaemolyticus* foodborne outbreak, Louisiana. M. M. W. R. Morb. Mortal. Wkly. Rep. *27*:345-346, 1978.
12. Carpenter, C. J.: More pathogenic vibrios. N. Engl. J. Med. *300*:39-41, 1979.
13. Chai, T. J., and Pace, J.: *Vibrio parahaemolyticus*. *In* Hui, Y., Gorham, J. R., and Murrel, K. D. (eds.): Foodborne Disease Handbook. New York, Marcel Dekker, 1994, pp. 395-425.
14. Chakrabarti, M. K., Sinha, A. K., and Biswas, T.: Adherence of *Vibrio parahaemolyticus* to rabbit intestinal epithelial cells in vitro. F. E. M. S. Microbiol. Lett. *84*:113-118, 1991.
15. Chatterjee, B. D., Mukherjee, A., and Sanyal, S. N.: Enteroinvasive model of *Vibrio parahaemolyticus*. Indian J. Med. Res. *79*:151-158, 1984.
16. Chowdhury, N. R., Chakraborty, S., Ramamurthy, T., et al.: Molecular evidence of clonal *Vibrio parahaemolyticus* pandemic strains. Emerg. Infect. Dis. *6*:631-636, 2000.
17. Dadisman, T. A., Nelson, R., Molenda, J. R., et al.: *Vibrio parahaemolyticus* gastroenteritis in Maryland, I: Clinical and epidemiological aspects. Am. J. Epidemiol. *96*:414-426, 1972.
18. Daniels, N. A., MacKinnon, L., Bishop, R., et al.: *Vibrio parahaemolyticus* infections in the United States, 1973-1998. J. Infect. Dis. *181*:1661-1666, 2000.
19. Daniels, N. A., Ray, B., Easton, A., et al.: Emergence of a new *Vibrio parahaemolyticus* serotype in raw oysters: A prevention quandary. J. A. M. A. *284*:1541-1545, 2000.
20. DePaola, A., Hopkins, L. H., Peeler, J. T., et al.: Incidence of *Vibrio parahaemolyticus* in U.S. coastal waters and oysters. Appl. Environ. Microbiol. *56*:2299-2302, 1990.
21. Desenclos, J. A., Klontz, K. C., Wolfe, L. E., et al.: The risk of *Vibrio* illness in the Florida raw oyster eating population, 1981-1988. Am. J. Epidemiol. *134*:290-297, 1991.
22. Dobroszycki, J., Sklarin, N. T., Szilagy, G., et al.: *Vibrio parahaemolyticus* septicemia in a patient with neutropenic leukemia. Clin. Infect. Dis. *15*:738-739, 1992.
23. Doyle, M. P.: Pathogenic *Escherichia coli*, *Yersinia enterocolitica*, and *Vibrio parahaemolyticus*. Lancet *336*:1111-1115, 1990.
24. Eastaugh, J., and Shepherd, S.: Infectious and toxic syndromes from fish and shellfish consumption. Arch. Intern. Med. *149*:1735-1740, 1989.
25. Franca, S. M., Gibbs, D. L., Samuels, P., et al.: *Vibrio parahaemolyticus* in Brazilian coastal waters. J. A. M. A. *244*:587-588, 1980.
26. French, G. L., Woo, M. L., Hui, Y. W., et al.: Antimicrobial susceptibilities of halophilic vibrios. J. Antimicrob. Chemother. *24*:183-194, 1989.
27. Gingras, S. P., and Howard, L. V.: Adherence of *Vibrio parahaemolyticus* to human epithelial cell lines. Appl. Environ. Microbiol. *39*:369-371, 1980.
28. Gonzalez-Escalona, N., Cachicas, V., Acevedo, C., et al.: *Vibrio parahaemolyticus* diarrhea, Chile, 1998 and 2004. Emerg. Infect. Dis. *11*:129-131, 2005.
29. Hally, R. J., Rubin, R. A., Fraimow, H. S., et al.: Fatal *Vibrio parahaemolyticus* septicemia in a patient with cirrhosis. Dig. Dis. Sci. *40*:1257-1260, 1995.
30. Honda, S. I., Goto, I., Minematsu, I., et al.: Gastroenteritis due to Kanagawa negative *Vibrio parahaemolyticus*. Lancet *1*:331-332, 1987.
31. Honda, T., Ni, Y., and Miwatani, T.: Purification and characterization of a hemolysin produced by a clinical isolate of Kanagawa phenomenon-negative *Vibrio parahaemolyticus* and related to the thermostable direct hemolysin. Infect. Immun. *56*:961-965, 1988.
32. Honda, T., Ni, Y., Miwatani, T., et al.: The thermostable direct hemolysin of *Vibrio parahaemolyticus* is a pore-forming toxin. Can. J. Microbiol. *38*:1175-1180, 1992.
33. Hughes, J. M., Boyce, J. M., Aleem, A. R., et al.: *Vibrio parahaemolyticus* enterocolitis in Bangladesh: Report of an outbreak. Am. J. Trop. Med. Hyg. *27*:106-112, 1978.
34. Janda, J. M., Powers, C., Bryant, R. G., et al.: Current perspective on the epidemiology and pathogenesis of clinically significant *Vibrio* spp. Clin. Microbiol. Rev. *1*:245-267, 1988.
35. Jiang, X., and Chai, T. J.: Survival of *Vibrio parahaemolyticus* at low temperatures under starvation conditions and subsequent resuscitation of viable, nonculturable cells. Appl. Environ. Microbiol. *62*:1300-1305, 1996.

36. Joseph, S. W., Colwell, R. R., and Kaper, J. B.: *Vibrio parahaemolyticus* and related halophilic vibrios. Crit. Rev. Microbiol. *10*:77-124, 1983.

37. Joseph, S. W., DeBell, R. M., and Brown, W. P.: In vitro response to chloramphenicol, tetracycline, ampicillin, gentamicin and beta-lactamase production by halophilic vibrios from human and environmental sources. Antimicrob. Agents Chemother. *13*:244-248, 1978.

38. Klontz, K. C.: Fatalities associated with *Vibrio parahaemolyticus* and *Vibrio cholerae* non-O1 infections in Florida (1981 to 1988). South. Med. J. *83*:500-502, 1990.

39. Lee, C. Y., Pan, S. F., and Chen, C. H.: Sequence of a cloned pR72H fragment and its use for detection of *Vibrio parahaemolyticus* in shellfish with the PCR. Appl. Environ. Microbiol. *61*:1311-1317, 1995.

40. Levine, W. C., and Griffin, P. M.: *Vibrio* infections on the Gulf Coast: Results of first year of regional surveillance. J. Infect. Dis. *167*:479-483, 1993.

41. Lynch, T., Livingstone, S., Buenaventura, E., et al.: *Vibrio parahaemolyticus* disruption of epithelial cell tight junctions occurs independently of toxin production. Infect. Immun. *73*:1275-1283, 2005.

42. Makino, K., Oshima, K., Kurokawa, K., et al.: Genome sequence of *Vibrio parahaemolyticus*: A pathogenic mechanism distinct from that of *V. cholerae*. Lancet *361*:743-749, 2003.

43. Martinez-Urtaza, J., Simental, L., Velasco, D., et al.: Pandemic *Vibrio parahaemolyticus* O3:K6, Europe. Emerg. Infect. Dis. *11*:1319-1320, 2005.

44. McCarter, L. L.: Dual flagellar systems enable motility under different circumstances. J. Mol. Microbiol. Biotechnol. 7:18-29, 2004.

45. McLaughlin, J. C.: *Vibrio. In* Murray, P. R., Baron, E. J., and Pfaller, M. A. (eds.): Manual of Clinical Microbiology. 6th ed. Washington, D.C., American Society for Microbiology, 1995, pp. 465-476.

46. Miyamoto, Y., Kato, T., Obara, Y., et al.: In vitro hemolytic characteristic of *Vibrio parahaemolyticus*: Its close correlation with human pathogenicity. J. Bacteriol. *100*:1147-1149, 1969.

47. Morris, J. G., Jr., and Black, R. E.: Cholera and other vibrios in the United States. N. Engl. J. Med. *312*:343-350, 1985.

48. Nagayama, K., Yamamoto, K., Mitawani, T., et al.: Characterization of a haemolysin related to Vp-TDH produced by a Kanagawa phenomenon-negative clinical isolate of *Vibrio parahaemolyticus*. J. Med. Microbiol. *42*:83-90, 1995.

49. Nair, G. B., and Hormazabal, J. C.: The *Vibrio parahaemolyticus* pandemic. Rev. Chilena Infectol. *22*:125-130, 2005.

50. Nasu, H., Iida, T., Sugahara, T., et al.: A filamentous phage associated with recent pandemic *Vibrio parahaemolyticus* O3:K6 strains. J. Clin. Microbiol. *38*:2156-2161, 2000.

51. Nishibuchi, M., Ishibashi, M., Takeda, Y., et al.: Detection of the thermostable direct hemolysin gene and related DNA sequences in *Vibrio parahaemolyticus* and other *Vibrio* species by the DNA colony hybridization test. Infect. Immun. *49*:481-486, 1985.

52. Nishibuchi, M., and Kaper, J. B.: Duplication and variation of the thermostable direct haemolysin (tdh) gene in *Vibrio parahaemolyticus*. Mol. Microbiol. *4*:87-99, 1990.

53. Nishibuchi, M., and Kaper, J. B.: Thermostable direct hemolysin gene of *Vibrio parahaemolyticus*: A virulence gene acquired by a marine bacterium. Infect. Immun. *63*:2093-2099, 1995.

54. Okuda, J., Ishibashi, M., Hayakawa, E., et al.: Emergence of a unique O3:K6 clone of *Vibrio parahaemolyticus* in Calcutta, India, and isolation of strains from the same clonal group from Southeast Asian travelers arriving in Japan. J. Clin. Microbiol. *35*:3150-3155, 1997.

55. Outbreak of *Vibrio parahaemolyticus* infections associated with eating raw oysters—Pacific Northwest, 1997. M. M. W. R. Morb. Mortal. Wkly. Rep. *47*:457-462, 1998.

56. Outbreak of *Vibrio parahaemolyticus* infection associated with eating raw oysters and clams harvested from Long Island Sound—Connecticut, New Jersey, and New York, 1998. M. M. W. R. Morb. Mortal. Wkly. Rep. *48*:48-51, 1999.

57. Pan, T., Wang, T., Lee, C., et al.: Foodborne disease outbreaks due to bacteria in Taiwan. J. Clin. Microbiol. *35*:1260-1262, 1997.

58. Peffers, A. S., Bailey, J., Barrow, G. I., et al.: *Vibrio parahaemolyticus* gastroenteritis and international air travel. Lancet *1*:143-145, 1973.

59. Qadri, F., Alam, M. S., Nishibuchi, M., et al.: Adaptive and inflammatory immune responses in patients infected with strains of *Vibrio parahaemolyticus*. J. Infect. Dis. *187*:1085-1096, 2003.

60. Rabinowitch, B. L., Nam, M. H., Levy, C. S., et al.: *Vibrio parahaemolyticus* septicemia associated with water skiing. Clin. Infect. Dis. *16*:339-340, 1993.

61. Raimondi, F., Kao, J. P., Fiorentini, C., et al.: Enterotoxicity and cytotoxicity of *Vibrio parahaemolyticus* thermostable direct hemolysin in in vitro systems. Infect. Immun. *68*:3180-3185, 2000.

62. Shinoda, S., Nakahara, N., Ninomiya, Y., et al.: Serological method for identification of *Vibrio parahaemolyticus* from marine samples. Appl. Environ. Microbiol. *45*:148-152, 1983.

63. Shirai, H., Ito, H., Hirayama, T., et al.: Molecular epidemiologic evidence for association of thermostable direct hemolysin (TDH) and TDH-related hemolysin of *Vibrio parahaemolyticus* with gastroenteritis. Infect. Immun. *58*:3568-3573, 1990.

64. Spearman, J. G., Tronca, E. L., Nichlos, E. M., et al.: Epidemiologic notes and reports, *Vibrio parahaemolyticus*, Louisiana. M. M. W. R. Morb. Mortal. Wkly. Rep. *21*:341-343, 1972.

65. Takahashi, A., Kenjyo, N., Imura, K., et al.: Cl⁻ secretion in colonic epithelial cells induced by the *Vibrio parahaemolyticus* hemolytic toxin related to thermostable direct hemolysin. Infect. Immun. *68*:5435-5438, 2000.

66. Takahashi, A., Sato, Y., Shiomi, Y., et al.: Mechanisms of chloride secretion induced by thermostable direct haemolysin of *Vibrio parahaemolyticus* in human colonic tissue and a human intestinal epithelial cell line. J. Med. Microbiol. *49*:801-810, 2000.

67. Takea, Y.: Thermostable direct hemolysin of *Vibrio parahaemolyticus*. Pharmacol. Ther. *19*:123-146, 1983.

68. Thompson, C. A., and Vanderzant, C.: Serological and hemolytic characteristics of *Vibrio parahaemolyticus* from marine sources. J. Food Sci. *41*:204-205, 1976.

69. Tuyet, D. T., Thiem, V. D., Von Seidlein, L., et al.: Clinical, epidemiological, and socioeconomic analysis of an outbreak of *Vibrio parahaemolyticus* in Khanh Hoa Province, Vietnam. J. Infect. Dis. *186*:1615-1620, 2002.

70. Twedt, R. M.: *Vibrio parahaemolyticus. In* Doyle, M. P. (ed.): Foodborne Bacterial Pathogens. New York, Marcel Dekker, 1989, pp. 543-568.

71. Twedt, R. M., Peerler, J. T., and Spaulding, P. L.: Effective ileal loop dose of Kanagawa-positive *Vibrio parahaemolyticus*. Appl. Environ. Microbiol. *40*:1012-1016, 1980.

72. Varmam, A. H.: *Vibrio. In* Varmam, A. H., and Evans, M. G. (eds.): Foodborne Pathogens. London, Wolfe Publishing, 1991, pp. 157-183.

73. *Vibrio parahaemolyticus*, Japan, 1996-1998. Wkly. Epidemiol. Rec. *74*:361-363, 1999.

74. Wong, H. C., and Wang, P.: Induction of viable but nonculturable state in *Vibrio parahaemolyticus* and its susceptibility to environmental stresses. J. Appl. Microbiol. *96*:359-366, 2004.

75. Yamamoto, T., and Yokota, T.: Adherence targets of *Vibrio parahaemolyticus* in human small intestines. Infect. Immun. *57*:2410-2419, 1989.

76. Yeung, P. S. M., and Boor, K. J.: Epidemiology, pathogenesis, and prevention of foodborne *Vibrio parahaemolyticus* infections. Foodborne Pathog. Dis. *1*:74-88, 2004.

77. Yoh, M., Kawakami, N., Funakoshi, Y., et al.: Evaluation of two assay kits for thermostable direct hemolysin (TDH) as an indicator of TDH-related hemolysin (TRH) produced by *Vibrio parahaemolyticus*. Microbiol. Immunol. *39*:157-159, 1995.

78. Zhang, X. H., and Austin, B.: Haemolysins in *Vibrio* species. J. Appl. Microbiol. *98*:1011-1019, 2005.

VIBRIO VULNIFICUS

Randall G. Fisher

BACTERIOLOGY

Vibrio vulnificus is a small, curvilinear, gram-negative rod of the family Vibrionaceae.[6] This facultative anaerobe is oxidase-positive and lysine-positive similar to other species of the genus *Vibrio*. Its major difference is that it ferments lactose, a feature that accounts for its original name, Lac + *Vibrio*. *V. vulnificus* is arginine-negative and ornithine-variable. This halophilic (salt-loving) organism grows in concentrations of sodium chloride of from 1 to 8 percent and seems to grow best at approximately 3 percent.[35]

EPIDEMIOLOGY

V. vulnificus, similar to *Vibrio parahaemolyticus*, is a marine organism that is a common inhabitant of off-shore waters, especially estuarial waters.[50] It has been isolated from sediment, plankton, water, finfish, crabs, and oysters. Peak recovery occurs in the summer and early fall,[17] possibly because at higher water temperatures *V. vulnificus* is released and rises to surface waters. There it attaches to plankton and shore fish and then is taken up and concentrated by filter-feeding mollusks and crustaceans.

V. vulnificus has been isolated from wild and commercial oysters throughout the world. It especially is prevalent in warm coastal waters. Reports about the survival of the organism in oysters stored at low temperatures are conflicting. Nilsson and associates[48] revealed, however, that even if *V. vulnificus* is rendered nonculturable by storage at low temperatures, it can be "resuscitated" by allowing the oysters to warm up to room temperature; this cycle could be carried out twice without any reduction in bacterial count. Because of the ubiquity of the organism in the marine environment and its ability to thrive under even the most careful conditions of sanitation, storage, and transport,[16,33] ensuring that commercial shellfish do not contain viable *V. vulnificus* is very difficult.

So-called heat shock shucking, during which the internal meat temperature exceeds 50° C for 1 to 4 minutes, reduces the *V. vulnificus* and total bacterial levels in oysters 10-fold to 10,000-fold compared with conventional processing.[22] A separate study confirms that low-temperature pasteurization, which brings oyster temperatures to 50° C for 10 to 15 minutes, reduces colony counts from greater than 100,000/g of oyster meat to undetectable levels.[2] Three-hour ice immersion is ineffective at reducing *V. vulnificus* and actually increases coliform counts in oysters.[53] High-pressure processing is a promising new approach to eliminating *V. vulnificus* from oysters; in preliminary studies, *V. vulnificus* could be reduced to undetectable levels by processing at 586 MPa with a 7-minute "come up" time.[36]

Disease in humans is initiated by contact with the organism. Contact occurs either through marine contamination of a wound or in the gastrointestinal tract after ingestion of the organism in raw shellfish, most commonly oysters.[6]

PATHOPHYSIOLOGY

V. vulnificus causes three distinct diseases in humans: wound infection and gastrointestinal infection, which may be self-limited or progress to septicemia. Local infection occurs after a wound is exposed to contaminated sea water. Wound infections with *V. vulnificus* are marked by rapid spread, the formation of bullae, and necrosis of involved tissues.[6] Marked edema and vascular thromboses occur in experimental and natural infection. *V. vulnificus* elaborates a cytolysin,[20,21,35] a collagenase,[56] and a protease,[46] which enhance its rapid spread in tissues. The protease activates the plasma kallikrein-kinin system to produce bradykinin[45]; histamine also is released locally. These factors account for the intense inflammatory reaction seen in these lesions. One group of researchers constructed an isolate that lacked a flagellum and found that its ability to adhere to cells was decreased, as was its lethality in mice.[39] Hemorrhagic complications may be due to the presence of a metalloprotease that interferes with blood homeostasis through prothrombin activation and fibrinolysis.[11]

In otherwise healthy individuals, a mild, self-limited gastrointestinal illness similar to that caused by *V. parahaemolyticus* has been described.[34] The most serious infection produced by *V. vulnificus* is primary septicemia, which occurs most commonly in patients with liver disease, after they have ingested the organism in raw shellfish.[6,51,52]

For patients with hepatic disease, the risk of acquiring septicemia is 40 to 80 times greater, and the case-fatality rate is 2.5 times higher than for otherwise healthy individuals.[24] *V. vulnificus*, similar to many other gram-negative organisms, requires iron for growth and grows better in an excess of iron.[64] It is able to extract iron from hemoglobin, even if it is complexed completely

to haptoglobin.[64,67] Liver damage, excess iron, and deferoxamine therapy all have been shown to decrease the median lethal dose (LD_{50}) of *V. vulnificus* in experimental animals. Deferoxamine alone decreased the LD_{50} by four orders of magnitude.[9] Iron overload almost certainly underlies *V. vulnificus* septicemia in patients who require repeated transfusions and deferoxamine therapy for anemia.[29,66] Some evidence indicates that alcoholism, even in the absence of demonstrable liver disease, is a risk factor for developing sepsis.[51] Fatal septicemia also has been reported in patients with other chronic diseases, such as diabetes mellitus and lymphomas.[52]

Virulence factors of the organism also have been described.[65] Virulent strains are resistant to the bactericidal activity of human serum,[37] probably because of the presence of a polysaccharide capsule.[1] Poor uptake of virulent strains into phagocytes[59] and opaqueness of the colony on agar have been correlated with the presence of the capsule.[55,65] No difference has been shown in the lipopolysaccharides of virulent versus avirulent strains.[5] The production of recalcitrant shock in patients with septicemia is secondary to toxins, loss of vascular tone, capillary leak, and possibly negative inotropy, as in other forms of gram-negative sepsis.

CLINICAL MANIFESTATIONS

Patients commonly present with wound infection or primary septicemia. Wound infection occurs after injury in sea water or after the contamination of a recently acquired wound with sea water. Often, the wound is caused by the shell of a crustacean or mollusk. Many patients with wound infections work in shellfish-related industries. Apparently, wound infection with *V. vulnificus* can develop from superficial wounds acquired within 24 hours of "uneventful" fish handling; the physiologic characteristics of human sweat may be conducive to the survival of the organism on the skin, allowing for later inoculation.[10] Cellulitis may develop and spread rapidly. Overlying skin often is covered with tense bullae. At débridement, the extent of necrosis may exceed presurgical expectations.[63] Primary wound infection may progress to systemic infection; for this reason, wound infection with *V. vulnificus* carries a mortality rate of 7 to 24 percent.[6,34]

Patients with primary septicemia generally give a history of recent (6 to 72 hours) consumption of raw seafood. Illness is marked by the rapid onset of fever, hypotension, and septic shock. Prodromal symptoms, such as malaise, chills, and fever, are common manifestations. Vomiting and diarrhea are seen in approximately 20 percent of patients.[7] Shock progresses quickly and is difficult to reverse. Secondary skin lesions develop in approximately half of patients[6] and may be bullous, petechial, or maculopapular. *V. vulnificus* frequently is isolated from cultures of secondary lesions, providing evidence of septicemic spread to those sites.[6] The mortality rate from primary septicemia has been reported to be 46 to 79 percent.[6,51]

In addition to causing the two above-mentioned syndromes, *V. vulnificus* has been reported as a cause of corneal ulcer,[60] myositis,[31] adult epiglottitis,[42] osteomyelitis,[61] endocarditis,[60] peritonitis,[26] tubo-ovarian abscess,[43] and meningitis.[29,51] In one case, a patient presented with endogenous endophthalmitis without systemic symptoms that developed after ingestion of raw seafood.[28] A case of fatal septicemia in which the presenting symptom was a compartment syndrome of the forearm has been described.[27]

Ninety percent of reported patients are 40 years old or older.[6,51] Childhood cases of septicemia have been associated with thalassemia major,[28] for which frequent transfusions and deferoxamine therapy are required. Wound infections in previously healthy children and adolescents have been reported. *V. vulnificus* also has been isolated from a premature infant's stool sample obtained on the infant's first day of life; the infant's mother worked as an oyster shucker.[4]

DIAGNOSIS

The diagnosis of *V. vulnificus* infection is made by isolating the organism from blood or tissue culture. It also may be recovered from stool specimens.[4,52] Agars designed specifically to aid in the growth and identification of *V. vulnificus* have been developed; cellobiose-colistin agar outperforms thiosulfate citrate bile salts sucrose agar (TCBS) for recovery of *V. vulnificus* from environmental samples.[25] From a practical standpoint, however, most hospital microbiology laboratories do not stock cellobiose-colistin agar. Of the commercially available media, *V. vulnificus* tends to grow best in thiosulfate citrate bile salts sucrose agar (TCBS),[6] but it also may be recovered from ordinary blood agar plates[3,54] or MacConkey plates.[6]

A very sensitive nested polymerase chain reaction technique that is capable of detecting 1 pg of bacterial DNA and one colony-forming unit of *V. vulnificus* has been described; it was positive in 94 percent of clinical samples that grew the bacteria in culture and was positive in 42 percent of culture-negative samples from patients with suspected *V. vulnificus* infection.[40] An enzyme immunoassay also has been developed.[59] Both of these methods are experimental and not yet available for routine clinical use.

The diagnosis of *V. vulnificus* wound infection or septicemia can be suspected on clinical grounds and appropriate therapy initiated while awaiting culture results. A history of ingestion of raw shellfish or contamination of a wound with either sea water or brackish inland waters[57] should be sought. *V. vulnificus* infection should be given high consideration in patients with hemosiderosis, anemia with transfusion therapy, liver disease, or other chronic diseases.

TREATMENT

For severe wound infections, performing surgical therapy as rapidly as possible is paramount. For primary septicemia, support of the patient's airway, along with aggressive pressor support and other adjunctive therapies for severe septic shock, is of primary concern. Secondarily, appropriate antibiotic treatment for *V. vulnificus* should be started as early as possible.

In vitro, the organism is susceptible to many antibiotics, including ampicillin, third-generation cephalosporins, tetracycline, chloramphenicol, and gentamicin.[6] Bowdre and associates[8] reported that, in mice, the minimum inhibitory concentrations obtained in the laboratory did not seem to correspond with response to therapy. In particular, the organism seemed to be exquisitely sensitive to cefotaxime in vitro (minimum inhibitory concentration 0.06 μg/mL); however, 9 of 10 mice treated with cefotaxime died of overwhelming infection. Anecdotal evidence indicates that this puzzling phenomenon may occur in humans as well; four of five patients reported by Chuang and associates[14] died, despite receiving therapy with third-generation cephalosporins at appropriate dosages. Similarly, although the organism is almost universally sensitive to gentamicin in the laboratory, case reports show a lack of response to this antibiotic. Of all the antibiotics to which the organism was sensitive in vitro, only tetracycline led to survival of mice in Bowdre's study; all 12 of the mice treated with tetracycline survived the infection.[8]

Case reports also show favorable outcomes with tetracycline or doxycycline[14] and chloramphenicol[14] and ciprofloxacin.[41] More recently, the combination of minocycline and cefotaxime has been shown to be synergistic in vitro, with the combination reducing the growth of *V. vulnificus* by six orders of magnitude compared with either drug alone.[13] Enhanced survival of mice infected with *V. vulnificus* and treated with minocycline plus cefotaxime provides an in vivo correlate of the in vitro results.[15] No data are available comparing the activity of minocycline versus that of tet-

racycline; nonetheless, the aforementioned evidence is sufficiently strong to suggest that either tetracycline or minocycline together with cefotaxime should be the treatment of choice for known or suspected *V. vulnificus* infection. Fluoroquinolones also may have a role in treatment. In vitro synergy studies show that the combination of ciprofloxacin and cefotaxime is synergistic for *V. vulnificus*,[32] and in a murine model, the newer fluoroquinolones (e.g., moxifloxacin) worked as well as combination therapy at preventing lethality in mice.[12] As yet, no human clinical data are available regarding the efficacy of third-generation fluoroquinolones.

The addition of modified Dakin solution (0.025% sodium hypochlorite) may have some utility in the treatment of skin and wound infections. An in vitro study of eight different topical antibiotic preparations showed that *V. vulnificus* was most sensitive to modified Dakin solution.[44] Although no controlled trial has been performed, a series of 10 patients with culture-proven *V. vulnificus* wound infections treated with doxycycline and topical modified Dakin solution, none of whom experienced progression of infection or required surgical débridement, has been reported.[62]

PREVENTION

Patients with severe anemia, liver disease, hemosiderosis, or other debilitating chronic diseases and patients on deferoxamine therapy should be advised against eating raw seafood of any kind. Patients with open wounds probably should avoid contact with sea water or brackish inland waters.

Acknowledgments

The author thanks Dr. William Gruber and Dr. Thomas Boyce for their invaluable assistance with earlier versions of this chapter.

REFERENCES

1. Amako, K., Okada, K., and Miake, S.: Evidence for the presence of a capsule in *Vibrio vulnificus*. J. Gen. Microbiol. *130*:2741-2743, 1984.
2. Andrews, L. S., Park, D. L., and Chen, Y. P.: Low temperature pasteurization to reduce the risk of vibrio infections from raw shell-stock oysters. Food Addit. Contam. *17*:787-791, 2000.
3. Armstrong, C. W., Lake, J. L., and Miller, G. B., Jr.: Extraintestinal infections due to halophilic *Vibrios*. South. Med. J. *76*:571-574, 1983.
4. Bachman, B., Boyd, W. P., Jr., Lieb, S., et al.: Marine noncholera *Vibrio* infections in Florida. South. Med. J. *76*:296-299, 1983.
5. Bahrani, K., and Oliver, J. D.: Studies on the lipopolysaccharide of a virulent and an avirulent strain of *Vibrio vulnificus*. Biochem. Cell. Biol. *68*:547-551, 1990.
6. Blake, P. A., Merson, M. H., Weaver, R. E., et al.: Disease caused by a marine *Vibrio*: Clinical characteristics and epidemiology. N. Engl. J. Med. *300*:1-5, 1979.
7. Blake, P. A., Weaver, R. E., and Hollis, D. G.: Disease of humans (other than cholera) caused by *Vibrios*. Ann. Rev. Microbiol. *34*:341-367, 1980.
8. Bowdre, J. H., Hull, J. H., and Cocchetto, D. M.: Antibiotic efficacy against *Vibrio vulnificus* in the mouse: Superiority of tetracycline. J. Pharmacol. Exp. Ther. *225*:595-598, 1983.
9. Brennaman, B., Soucy, D., and Howard, R. J.: Effect of iron and liver injury on the pathogenesis of *Vibrio vulnificus*. J. Surg. Res. *43*:527-531, 1987.
10. Calif, E., and Shalom, S.: Hand infections caused by delayed inoculation of *Vibrio vulnificus*: Does human skin serve as a potential reservoir of vibrios? Hand Surg. *9*:39-44, 2004.
11. Chang, A. K., Kim, H. Y, Park, J. E., et al.: Vibrio vulnificus secretes a broad-specificity metalloprotease capable of interfering with blood homeostasis through prothrombin activation and fibrinolysis. J. Bacteriol. *187*:6909-6916, 2005.
12. Chiang, S. R., and Chuang, Y. C.: *Vibrio vulnificus* infection: Clinical manifestations, pathogenesis, and antimicrobial therapy. J. Microbiol. Immunol. Infect. *36*:81-88, 2003.
13. Chuang, Y. C., Liu, J. W., Ko, W. C., et al.: In vitro synergism between cefotaxime and minocycline against *Vibrio vulnificus*. Antimicrob. Agents Chemother. *41*:2214-2217, 1997.
14. Chuang, Y. C., Yuan, C. Y., Lin, C. Y., et al.: *Vibrio vulnificus* infection in Taiwan: Report of 28 cases and review of clinical manifestations and treatment. Clin. Infect. Dis. *115*:271-276, 1992.

15. Chuang, Y. W., Ko, W. C., Wang, S. T., et al.: Minocycline and cefotaxime in the treatment of experimental murine *Vibrio vulnificus* infection. Antimicrob. Agents Chemother. *42*:1319-1322, 1998.

16. Cook, D. W.: Effect of time and temperature on multiplication of *Vibrio vulnificus* in postharvest Gulf Coast shellstock oysters. Appl. Environ. Microbiol. *60*:3483-3484, 1994.

17. DePaola, A., Capers, G. M., and Alexander, D.: Densities of *Vibrio vulnificus* in the intestines of fish from the U.S. Gulf Coast. Appl. Environ. Microbiol. *60*:984-988, 1994.

18. DiGaetano, M., Ball, S. F., and Straus, J. G.: *Vibrio vulnificus* corneal ulcer: Case reports. Arch. Ophthalmol. *107*:323-324, 1989.

19. Fang, F. C.: Use of tetracycline for treatment of *Vibrio vulnificus* infections. Clin. Infect. Dis. *15*:1071-1072, 1992.

20. Gray, L. D., and Kreger, A. S.: Purification and characterization of an extracellular cytolysin produced by *Vibrio vulnificus*. Infect. Immun. *48*:62-72, 1985.

21. Gray, L. D., and Kreger, A. S.: Mouse skin damage caused by cytolysin from *Vibrio vulnificus* and by *Vibrio vulnificus* infection. J. Infect. Dis. *155*:236-241, 1987.

22. Hesselman, D. M., Motes, M. L., and Lewis, J. P.: Effects of a commercial heat-shock process on *Vibrio vulnificus* in the American oyster, *Crassostrea virginica*, harvested from the Gulf Coast. J. Food Prot. *62*:1266-1269, 1999.

23. Hill, W. E., Keasler, S. P., Trucksess, M. W., et al.: Polymerase chain reaction identification of *Vibrio vulnificus* in artificially contaminated oysters. Appl. Environ. Microbiol. *57*:707-711, 1991.

24. Hlady, W. G., Mullen, R. C., and Hopkin, R. S.: *Vibrio vulnificus* from raw oysters: Leading cause of reported deaths from foodborne illness in Florida. J. Fla. Med. Assoc. *80*:536-538, 1993.

25. Hoi, L., Dalsgaard, I., and Dalsgaard, A.: Improved isolation of *Vibrio vulnificus* from seawater and sediment with cellobiose-colistin agar. Appl. Environ. Microbiol. *64*:1721-1724, 1998.

26. Holcombe, D. J.: *Vibrio vulnificus* peritonitis: A unique case. J. La. State Med. Soc. *143*:27-28, 1991.

27. Hui, K. C., Zhang, F., Komorowska-Timek, E., et al.: Compartment syndrome of the forearm as the initial symptom of systemic *Vibrio vulnificus* infection. J. Hand Surg. Am. *24*:715-717, 1999.

28. Jung, S. I., Shin, D. H., Park, K. H., et al.: *Vibrio vulnificus* endophthalmitis occurring after ingestion of raw seafood. J. Infect. *51*:e281-e283, 2005.

29. Katz, B. Z.: *Vibrio vulnificus* meningitis in a boy with thalassemia after eating raw oysters. Pediatrics *82*:784-786, 1988.

30. Kaysner, C. A., Tamplin, M. L., Wekell, M. M., et al.: Survival of *Vibrio vulnificus* in shellstock and shucked oysters (*Crassostrea gigas* and *Crassostrea virginica*) and effects of isolation medium on recovery. Appl. Environ. Microbiol. *55*:3072-3079, 1989.

31. Kelly, M. T., and McCormick, W. F.: Acute bacterial myositis caused by *Vibrio vulnificus*. J. A. M. A. *246*:72-73, 1981.

32. Kim, D. M., Lym, Y., Jang, S. J., et al.: In vitro efficacy of the combination of ciprofloxacin and cefotaxime against *Vibrio vulnificus*. Antimicrob. Agents Chemother. *49*:3489-3491, 2005.

33. Kizer, K. W.: *Vibrio vulnificus* hazard in patients with liver disease. West. J. Med. *161*:64-65, 1994.

34. Klontz, K. C., Lieb, S., Schreiber, M., et al.: Syndromes of *Vibrio vulnificus* infections: Clinical and epidemiologic features in Florida cases, 1981-1987. Ann. Intern. Med. *109*:318-323, 1988.

35. Koga, T., and Kawata, T.: Composition of the major outer membrane proteins of *Vibrio vulnificus* isolates: Effect of different growth media and iron deficiency. Microbiol. Immunol. *30*:193-201, 1986.

36. Koo, J., Jahncke, M. L., Reno, P. W., et al.: Inactivation of *Vibrio parahaemolyticus* and *Vibrio vulnificus* in phosphate-buffered saline and in inoculated whole oysters by high-pressure processing. J. Food Prot. *69*:596-601, 2006.

37. Kreger, A., DeChatelet, L., and Shirley, P.: Interaction of *Vibrio vulnificus* with human polymorphonuclear leukocytes: Association of virulence with resistance to phagocytosis. J. Infect. Dis. *144*:244-248, 1981.

38. Kreger, A. S., Kothary, M. H., and Gray, L. D.: Cytolytic toxins of *Vibrio vulnificus* and *Vibrio damsela*. Methods Enzymol. *165*:176-189, 1988.

39. Lee, J. H., Rho, J. B., Park, K. J, et al.: Role of flagellum and motility in pathogenesis of *Vibrio vulnificans*. Infect. Immun. *72*:4905-4910, 2004.

40. Lee, S. E., Kim, S. Y., Kim, S. J., et al.: Direct identification of *Vibrio vulnificus* in clinical specimens by nested PCR. J. Clin. Microbiol. *36*:2887-2892, 1998.

41. Meadors, M. C., and Pankey, G. A.: *Vibrio vulnificus* wound infection treated successfully with oral ciprofloxacin. J. Infect. *20*:88-89, 1990.

42. Mehtar, S., Bangham, L., Kalmanovitch, D., et al.: Adult epiglottitis due to *Vibrio vulnificus*. Br. Med. J. Clin. Res. *296*:827-828, 1988.

43. Midturi, J., Baker, D., Winn, R., and Fader, R.: Tubo-ovarian abscess caused by *Vibrio vulnificus*. Diagn. Microbiol. Infect. Dis. *51*:131-133, 2005.

44. Milner, S. M., and Heggers, J. P.: The use of a modified Dakin's solution (sodium hypochlorite) in the treatment of *Vibrio vulnificus* infection. Wild. Environ. Med. *10*:10-12, 1999.

45. Miyoshi, N., Miyoshi, S., Sugiyama, K., et al.: Activation of the plasma kallikrein-kinin system by *Vibrio vulnificus* protease. Infect. Immun. *55*:1936-1939, 1987.

46. Miyoshi, S., and Shinoda, S.: Role of the protease in the permeability enhancement by *Vibrio vulnificus*. Microbiol. Immunol. *32*:1025-1032, 1988.

47. Morris, J. G., Jr., and Tenney, J.: Antibiotic therapy for *Vibrio vulnificus* infection. J. A. M. A. *253*:1121-1122, 1985.

48. Nilsson, L., Oliver, J. D., and Kjelleberg, S.: Resuscitation of *Vibrio vulnificus* from the viable but nonculturable state. J. Bacteriol. *173*:5054-5059, 1991.

49. Oliver, J. D.: Lethal cold stress of *Vibrio vulnificus* in oysters. Appl. Environ. Microbiol. *41*:710-717, 1981.

50. Oliver, J. D., Warner, R. A., and Cleland, D. R.: Distribution of *Vibrio vulnificus* and other lactose-fermenting vibrios in the marine environment. Appl. Environ. Microbiol. *45*:985-998, 1983.

51. Park, S. D., Shon, H. S., and Joh, N. J.: *Vibrio vulnificus* septicemia in Korea: Clinical and epidemiologic findings in seventy patients. J. Am. Acad. Dermatol. *24*:397-403, 1991.

52. Pollak, S. J., Parrish, E. F., III, Barrett, T. J., et al.: *Vibrio vulnificus* septicemia: Isolation of organism from stool and demonstration of antibodies by indirect immunofluorescence. Arch. Intern. Med. *143*:837-838, 1983.

53. Quevedo, A. C., Smith, J. G., Rodrick, G. E., and Wright, A. C.: Ice immersion as a postharvest treatment of oysters for the reduction of *Vibrio vulnificus*. J. Food Prot. *68*:1192-1197, 2005.

54. Saraswathi, K., Barve, S. M., and Deodhar, L. P.: Septicaemia due to *Vibrio vulnificus*. Trans. R. Soc. Trop. Med. Hyg. *83*:714, 1989.

55. Simpson, L. M., White, V. K., Zane, S. F., et al.: Correlation between virulence and colony morphology in *Vibrio vulnificus*. Infect. Immun. *55*:269-272, 1987.

56. Smith, G. C., and Merkel, J. R.: Collagenolytic activity of *Vibrio vulnificus*: Potential contribution to its invasiveness. Infect. Immun. *35*:1155-1156, 1982.

57. Tacket, C. O., Barrett, T. J., Mann, J. M., et al.: Wound infections caused by *Vibrio vulnificus*, a marine *Vibrio*, in inland areas of the United States. J. Clin. Microbiol. *19*:197-199, 1984.

58. Tamplin, M. L., Martin, A. L., Ruple, A. D., et al.: Enzyme immunoassay for identification of *Vibrio vulnificus* in seawater, sediment, and oysters. Appl. Environ. Microbiol. *57*:1235-1240, 1991.

59. Tamplin, M. L., Specter, S., Rodrick, G. E., et al.: *Vibrio vulnificus* resists phagocytosis in the absence of serum opsonins. Infect. Immun. *49*:715-718, 1985.

60. Truwit, J. D., Badesch, D. B., Savage, A. M., et al.: *Vibrio vulnificus* bacteremia with endocarditis. South. Med. J. *80*:1457-1459, 1987.

61. Vartian, C. V., and Septimus, E. J.: Osteomyelitis caused by *Vibrio vulnificus*. J. Infect. Dis. *161*:363, 1990.

62. Wilhelmi, B. J., Calianos, T. A., 2nd, Appelt, E. A., et al.: Modified Dakin's solution for cutaneous vibrio infections. Ann. Plast. Surg. *43*:386-389, 1999.

63. Woo, M. L., Patrick, W. G., Simon, M. T., et al.: Necrotising fasciitis caused by *Vibrio vulnificus*. J. Clin. Pathol. *37*:1301-1304, 1984.

64. Wright, A. C., Simpson, L. M., and Oliver, J. D.: Role of iron in the pathogenesis of *Vibrio vulnificus* infections. Infect. Immun. *34*:503-507, 1981.

65. Yoshida, S., Ogawa, M., and Mizuguchi, Y.: Relation of capsular materials and colony opacity to virulence of *Vibrio vulnificus*. Infect. Immun. *47*:446-451, 1985.

66. Yoshida, S., Tanabe, T., Chiba, S., et al.: Fatal *Vibrio vulnificus* infection in a patient with aplastic anemia. Sangyo Ika Daigaku Zasshi *5*:95-100, 1983.

67. Zakaria-Meehan, Z., Massad, G., Simpson, L. M., et al.: Ability of *Vibrio vulnificus* to obtain iron from hemoglobin-haptoglobin complexes. Infect. Immun. *56*:275-277, 1988.

CHAPTER 130

MISCELLANEOUS NON-ENTEROBACTERIACEAE FERMENTATIVE BACILLI

Randall G. Fisher

This chapter discusses fermentative bacilli that are not of the family Enterobacteriaceae. Specifically, it examines *Chromobacterium violaceum*, *Plesiomonas shigelloides*, and *Pasteurella* organisms other than *Pasteurella multocida*.

CHROMOBACTERIUM VIOLACEUM

C. violaceum is a facultatively anaerobic, gram-negative rod that is a saprophyte of soil and water, especially in tropical and subtropical climates. It causes occasional illness in animals and, rarely, in humans. Infection with *C. violaceum*, when it does occur, is a serious disease with a high mortality rate.

BACTERIOLOGY

C. violaceum is a long, motile, gram-negative bacillus that appears singly or in pairs on Gram stain. It has a polar flagellum and one to four subpolar or lateral flagella, which antigenically are distinct from the polar flagellum.[73] Most isolates produce an insoluble pigment, violacein. This pigment is intense and makes colonies appear dark purple to black, especially on blood agar. Violacein induces apoptotic death in certain cell types in vitro, including leukemia and lymphoma cells.[57] The therapeutic potential of violacein and structural analogues is being explored. Violacein also has antibacterial, anti-trypanosomic, and weak antiviral effects.[7] *C. violaceum* grows readily on standard agar (any medium that contains tryptophan supports growth). The colonies are low convex, violet, smooth, and not gelatinous. Colonies produce hydrogen cyanide, so a faint almond odor may be present.[73]

C. violaceum is catalase-positive and oxidase-positive, although the latter may be difficult to interpret because of the production of pigment. Growing the organism anaerobically inhibits pigment formation.[45] Pigment also may be lost on subculture[65] or as effective treatment is initiated. *C. violaceum* has a fermentative, not oxidative, attack on carbohydrates. *C. violaceum* produces antimicrobial agents that have been shown to have activity against bacteria and trypanosomes.

EPIDEMIOLOGY

C. violaceum commonly is found in soil and water of areas with tropical or subtropical weather patterns. It also has been recovered from soil as far north as New Jersey.[17] Ten of the first 12 cases reported in the United States occurred in Florida; the other two were in Louisiana. Subsequently, one case from New Jersey[61] and one from Ohio[75] have been reported, along with more from southeastern states. All but one case occurred during summer.[65] Patients tend to be young, with a median age of 14 years.[65]

PATHOPHYSIOLOGY

Although *C. violaceum* is a common inhabitant of soil and water, human infection is rare. Disorders of neutrophil function are important risk factors. A disproportionately high number of *C. violaceum* infections have occurred in patients with chronic granulomatous disease.[52] *C. violaceum* infection in a child with another disorder of neutrophil function, polymorphonuclear leukocyte glucose-6-phosphate dehydrogenase deficiency, has been reported.[53] Organisms may show variable virulence, and differences in endotoxin activity, resistance to phagocytosis, and production of catalase and hydrogen peroxide have been observed between clinical and soil isolates.[58] An elastase activity, expressed through the entire life cycle and produced by a zinc metalloproteinase, may account for the propensity of *C. violaceum* to cause abscesses.[87] Because *C. violaceum* is a free-living organism that is exposed to diverse environmental conditions, it exploits a wide range of energy resources and is able to thrive in aerobic and anaerobic conditions.[16] It is equipped to be tolerant of harsh conditions, including acid and ultraviolet stress, temperature stress, heavy metal exposure, and antibiotic exposure.[37] The complete sequencing of its genome has allowed researchers to identify putative virulence genes that are likely involved in host cell adhesion, cell invasion, and cytolysis.[11]

The organism usually gains entrance to the body through cuts or abrasions that come in contact with contaminated soil or water. After entrance, a localized infection usually develops at or around the site of entry, which is commonly followed by dissemination of infection via the bloodstream to distant sites. Rapid débridement and appropriate antibiotic therapy may arrest the infection at the wound stage.[48] Two cases of systemic infection occurred in near-drowning victims. One case report describes fulminant infection and death in an immunocompetent host from *C. violaceum* sepsis that began as conjunctivitis after a fall that splattered mud into the patient's eye.[22] Numerous microabscesses are found in multiple organs, especially liver, lung, and kidneys. Spread to bone, joints, and the central nervous system also has been described.

CLINICAL MANIFESTATIONS

The pattern of illness in all reported patients is similar, with a contaminated inoculation site, localized disease, regional lymphadenopathy, and hematogenous spread to visceral organs. Progression of symptoms tends to be rapid after a variable incubation period.

Most patients have cutaneous lesions,[52] which are described as being nodular or pustular and sometimes with surrounding cellulitis.[80] They may progress to suppuration and drainage, or ulceration. Occasionally, classic ecthyma gangrenosum lesions have been described.[12] Regional lymphadenopathy is common; some of the nodes suppurate and require surgical drainage or removal.

Severe disease is heralded by high fever (39° C to 41° C), confusion or lethargy, abdominal pain, headaches, nausea and vomiting, and sometimes myalgias. Patients with systemic illness appear toxic. Hepatosplenomegaly develops frequently, and jaundice may be present. Progression from high fever and moderate toxicity to septic shock with disseminated intravascular coagulation and multisystem organ failure is precipitous. After the liver, the lung is the most common site of dissemination of infection, and evidence of pneumonia often is found. Adult respiratory distress syndrome is rare.[49] Brain and liver abscesses have been noted.[59] The overall mortality rate is 65 percent.[52] Rarely, there may be recurrence, which can prove fatal.[45,65] A review of all 25 pediatric cases reported between 1971 and 2005 revealed, counterintuitively, that the case-fatality rate was 12 of 16 (75%) in patients without chronic granulomatous disease and 0 of 9 in patients with a known diagnosis of chronic granulomatous disease.[71] Disseminated infection, bacteremia, and initiation of ineffective antibiotic therapy were associated with mortality.[71]

DIAGNOSIS

Diagnosis is made by recovery of the organism from blood, lymph nodes, skin lesions, or abscesses. Gram-negative bacilli sometimes can be seen in smears of material from skin lesions. Laboratory values reveal either very low or very high white blood cell counts with marked left shifts. Mild to moderate anemia is common. There may be elevated liver enzymes; evidence of early renal failure sometimes is present. The organism grows readily and is easy to identify if it produces the characteristic violet pigment. Nonpigmented forms exist in soil and have similar virulence in mice[72] but are recovered only rarely from clinical specimens.[75] Other cases may have been missed, however, because the nonpigmented forms often are misidentified as *Aeromonas hydrophila* or as pseudomonads.[72] Reports that *C. violaceum* infection causes a melioidosis-like illness were probably due to misidentification of *Burkholderia pseudomallei* by the API 20NE system.[38]

A clinical history of contamination of a wound with water or soil, especially in the southeastern United States or in Southeast Asia, with subsequent local infection, lymph node suppuration, and lack of response to conventional antibiotic therapy, should arouse suspicion of *C. violaceum* infection. The clinician particularly should be aware of the possibility of *C. violaceum* infection in patients with chronic granulomatous disease.

TREATMENT

C. violaceum is sensitive in vitro to chloramphenicol, gentamicin, fluorinated quinolones, tetracyclines, imipenem, trimethoprim-sulfamethoxazole, and semisynthetic penicillins. *C. violaceum* often is resistant to cephalosporins, penicillin, ampicillin, and the antistaphylococcal penicillins. All isolates are resistant to vancomycin and rifampin.[4] Some strains have been shown to elaborate a β-lactamase, which is chromosomal and inducible in vitro.[21] At least one case report gives in vivo evidence of inducible resistance to ceftazidime.[80] Laboratory evidence of susceptibility to erythromycin cannot be relied on. In vitro, the fluorinated quinolones have the highest activity.[4] Clinical experience with the fluoroquinolones in *C. violaceum* infection is scarce; an impressive case of a 4-month-old infant with severe disseminated *C. violaceum* infection who survived after therapy with trimethoprim-sulfamethoxazole and ciprofloxacin has been reported.[59] The review of 25 cases mentioned earlier found that all survivors had been given one or a combination of the following agents: ciprofloxacin, trimethoprim-sulfamethoxazole, chloramphenicol, or imipenem.[71]

Because infection with *C. violaceum* is rare and often rapidly fatal, optimal antimicrobial therapy is unknown. Duration of therapy also is unknown, but because of late recurrences, some authors recommend 3 to 4 weeks of intravenous therapy followed by 1 month or more of oral trimethoprim-sulfamethoxazole.[65]

PLESIOMONAS SHIGELLOIDES

Plesiomonas shigelloides is the only species for the genus *Plesiomonas*. These organisms are facultatively anaerobic, motile, gram-negative rods that are common inhabitants of surface water and fish. They have been implicated in gastrointestinal infections and, rarely, have been recovered from extraintestinal sites.

BACTERIOLOGY

These facultatively anaerobic, gram-negative rods are members of the family Vibrionaceae, although some authorities suggest they are related more closely to Enterobacteriaceae.[51] They are motile by means of a polar flagellum. They are lysine-positive, ornithine-positive, and arginine decarboxylase–positive. They can be distinguished from Enterobacteriaceae by oxidase positivity. They also are catalase-positive and indole-positive. They grow well on MacConkey agar but not on thiosulfate citrate bile salts sucrose. Growth may be enhanced by the use of selective media, such as trypticase soy broth with ampicillin[66] and inositol brilliant green–bile salts agar. Growth is maximal at 40° C to 44° C and completely inhibited at 8° C. Usually within 24 hours, 1- to 1.5-mm grayish, shiny, opaque colonies with a slightly raised center and a smooth surface are visible. A few isolates of *P. shigelloides* share a common O antigen with *Shigella sonnei*.

EPIDEMIOLOGY

The organism is a ubiquitous fresh-water inhabitant at temperatures greater than 8° C. It sometimes also is found in estuarial waters in temperate or tropical climates and can exist in sea water during the summer. It has been cultured from finfish, shellfish, pigs, birds, and dogs.[84] Although infection with *P. shigelloides* has been associated with ingestion of raw or improperly cooked fish (especially oysters), it is unknown what role, if any, other animals play in the ecology of the organism. Asymptomatic carriage of *P. shigelloides* is rare in developed countries,[68] but may be 15 percent in some parts of China.[84]

PATHOPHYSIOLOGY

Despite the ubiquity of the organism in nature, human infection is uncommon and has been recognized only more recently. Most often, infection is associated with gastroenteritis. Evidence for the role of *P. shigelloides* in the production of gastrointestinal symptoms is that it has been isolated much more frequently from patients with diarrhea than from healthy controls[35]; there have been some outbreaks, especially in Japan; it often is the only organism detected in the stools of patients with gastroenteritis[56]; and patients who have *P. shigelloides* growing from a stool culture recover more quickly with than without antibiotic therapy.[42] Acquisition of disease has been linked specifically to consumption of raw seafood or untreated water and to foreign travel, especially to Mexico.[33,55]

The mechanism by which the organism produces disease has been elusive. It is not enteroinvasive by laboratory tests, most investigators fail to find either a Shiga toxin or an enterotoxin,[1,33] no animal model of gastrointestinal disease has been found,[10] patients in the recovery phase do not show serologic evidence of infection, and inoculation of volunteers fails to produce illness.[33] In a suckling gnotobiotic piglet model in which the animals became septic, histology of the gastrointestinal tract showed neither destruction of cells nor invasion of tissues.[33] Neonatal BALB/c mice became chronically infected with *P. shigelloides*, however, and histopathologic findings included some cases of necrosis of the mucosal surface of the ileum and colon.[83]

Some potential virulence factors (i.e., a cholera-like toxin, a weak cytolysin, serum resistance, and a large [>150-kd] plasmid) have been described, but their exact roles in pathogenesis are uncertain; attempts to correlate these features with virulence have been fruitless.[1] Investigators have characterized a cytotoxin derived from *P. shigelloides* using strains from patients with a diarrheal illness. The cytotoxin is a complex of three lipopolysaccharide-binding proteins and lipopolysaccharide in a 6:5 ratio.[63] Cytotoxic activity was inhibited 80 percent in vitro by proteinase K or when incubated with anti-cholera toxin antibody. This cytotoxin produced a positive reaction in the suckling mouse assay, whereas the purified lipopolysaccharide exhibited almost no cytotoxicity.[63]

Transmission electron microscopy has provided investigators with the first definitive proof that *P. shigelloides* can adhere to and invade eukaryotic intestinal cells. Organisms attached to microvilli and plasma membranes of the cells; they also were seen within vacuoles in the cell cytoplasm, suggesting a phagocytotic entry mechanism.[78] In one in vitro system using Caco-2 cells, adherence occurred within 10 minutes, and internalization occurred within 60 minutes. Cytotoxicity was due to the induction of apoptosis.[81] In vitro, cell-free and cell-associated hemolysis is demonstrable,[29] and low levels of elastase, proteinase, histidine decarboxylase, and moderate levels of triacylglycerol lipase activity have been found.[15] Culture filtrates are capable of inducing vacuolation of a variety of mammalian cells in vitro.[20]

P. shigelloides rarely, but more clearly, is a pathogen in extraintestinal sites. Osteomyelitis, endophthalmitis, cholecystitis, pseudoappendicitis, spontaneous peritonitis,[3] meningitis,[77] and septicemia have been reported sporadically.[10] Most patients with septicemia have been immunocompromised hosts, but the organism has been isolated from blood cultures in otherwise healthy individuals.[39,64] The mode of infection in extraintestinal sites is unclear, but most cases are thought to arise from the gastrointestinal tract. The case of a newborn with *P. shigelloides* meningitis, septicemia, and endophthalmitis who was born to a mother who reported severe diarrhea after eating raw oysters 2 weeks before delivery raises the possibility of transplacental transmission.[54]

CLINICAL MANIFESTATIONS

Patients with *P. shigelloides* gastroenteritis complain of diarrhea, crampy abdominal pain, nausea and vomiting, headache, and fever. Symptoms usually begin 24 hours to 4 days after contact with the organism.[35] Diarrhea tends to be secretory, although some patients have symptoms more consistent with colitis.[42] Passage of blood, mucus, or both in the stools is a common manifestation, as is the presence of white blood cells by Wright stain.[35] Patients with *P. shigelloides* gastroenteritis tend to have disease that is more acute, associated with more severe abdominal pain, and of longer duration than patients with diseases caused by other enteropathogens.[42]

In one case-control study, 76 percent of patients were sick for more than 2 weeks, and 32 percent were sick for more than a month.[42] In contrast, a large Japanese study of returning travelers suggested that for most patients, the symptoms abated within approximately 3 days.[70] In a series of 38 pediatric cases in Bangladesh, 84 percent had secretory diarrhea and 71 percent had associated emesis. Only three patients (8%) had fever, and only five (13%) had diarrhea for 14 days or longer.[47] In a separate report, one child developed migratory polyarthritis during an otherwise typical case of culture-proven gastrointestinal infection. All symptoms and signs of arthritis disappeared when the gastrointestinal infection was treated with antibiotics.[30]

Localized extraintestinal infections have been reported but are rare. Two cases of severe polymicrobial endophthalmitis resulting from fishhook trauma progressed to enucleation.[13] Two cases of peritonitis associated with continuous ambulatory peritoneal dialysis were reported from Hong Kong. Both patients recovered with 10 days of receiving intraperitoneal cefazolin and tobramycin.[85] In one odd case, a woman presented with pyosalpinx from *P. shigelloides*, thought to have been acquired by swimming in contaminated water.[69]

Septicemia, meningitis, or both usually occur in immunocompromised hosts. Severe, rapidly progressive sepsis complicated by disseminated intravascular coagulation, adult respiratory distress syndrome, renal insufficiency, hepatic dysfunction, adrenal hemorrhage, and splenic abscess has occurred in patients with hemoglobinopathies and absence of splenic function, including thalassemia intermedia and sickle-cell disease.[6,82] Unusual sites of infection sometimes are noted in immunocompromised individuals, such as epididymo-orchitis in a patient with human immunodeficiency virus infection.[86] Newborns constitute most of the reported cases of *P. shigelloides* meningitis, in whom the mortality rate is 80 percent.[1] Septicemia also has a high mortality rate in adults, although otherwise well patients may recover with appropriate antimicrobial therapy.

DIAGNOSIS

A clinical history of foreign travel or of ingestion of raw seafood or untreated water should raise suspicion of possible *P. shigelloides*

infection, especially when the clinical illness matches the description just mentioned. Oxidase tests should be done on any predominant or solitary organisms to distinguish them from Enterobacteriaceae.[35] The organisms can be shown not to be aeromonads or pseudomonads by production of ornithine decarboxylase and fermentation of inositol. Selective medium can be used if the index of suspicion is high.

TREATMENT

Most strains of *P. shigelloides* produce a β-lactamase,[67] which seems to be specific for the penicillins. In one study, all isolates were resistant to ampicillin, ticarcillin, carbenicillin, and piperacillin.[26] *P. shigelloides* is universally susceptible to trimethoprim-sulfamethoxazole, the fluoroquinolones, most cephalosporins, carbapenems,[76] tetracycline,[76] and chloramphenicol. It is variably susceptible to the aminoglycosides and mostly resistant to erythromycin.

P. shigelloides gastroenteritis resolves without therapy, but the illness may be prolonged. Treatment seems to shorten the course.[42] Extraintestinal infections carry a poor prognosis and should be treated aggressively. For meningitis, the cephalosporins have good cerebrospinal fluid penetration and are effective therapy against most isolates.

OTHER *PASTEURELLA* ORGANISMS

The genus *Pasteurella* consists of a group of pleomorphic, gram-negative coccobacilli that are part of the normal flora of many animals. These organisms are frequent animal pathogens. *P. multocida* is a common human pathogen; it is discussed elsewhere (see Chapter 126). The other species of the genus *Pasteurella* are rare but occasionally serious causes of infection in humans.

BACTERIOLOGY

These organisms, similar to *P. multocida*, grow readily on most common laboratory media, including blood agar. Most of the species do not grow on MacConkey agar. They are non–spore-forming, nonmotile, aerobic, and facultatively anaerobic. These glucose-fermenting organisms all are oxidase-positive. Most are nitrate-positive and catalase-positive, and all except *Avibacterium gallinarum* (formerly *Pasteurella gallinarum*, see later) produce indole. They are small, coccoid or rod-shaped bacilli that may show prominent bipolar staining on Gram stain. Colonies are small, translucent, and gray. They may be smooth or rough. A browning discoloration may develop around them. Colonies are nonhemolytic. They have a distinctive musty or "mushroom" odor.[14]

The taxonomy of these organisms is confusing and continues to be revised. *Pasteurella ureae* and *Pasteurella pneumotropica* have been moved into the genus *Actinobacillus*. *Pasteurella haemolytica* has been reclassified into a new genus, *Mannheimia*.[8] *Pasteurella dagmatis* is the name now given to what formerly was called *P. new species*, or *P. gas*.[60] *Pasteurella gallinarum*, *Pasteurella avium*, and *Pasteurella volantium* have 96.8 percent sequence similarity and are phenotypically separate from other *Pasteurella* spp.; this feature has led to a proposal that they be moved into a new genus, *Avibacterium*.[9] Most experts agree that the genus *Pasteurella sensu stricto* should include *P. multocida*, *Pasteurella canis*, *Pasteurella stomatis*, *P. dagmatis*, and *Pasteurella* spp. B.[43] Clinically recovered species other than *P. multocida* include *Actinobacillus ureae*, *Mannheimia haemolytica*, *Actinobacillus pneumotropica*, *P. dagmatis*, *P. canis*, *Pasteurella aerogenes*, *Pasteurella bettyae*, *P.* "SP" group, and *P. stomatis. Pasteurella caballi* has caused wound infections after horse bites.[18] *A. gallinarum* is an extremely rare pathogen in humans.

PATHOPHYSIOLOGY

Infection with *Pasteurella* spp. has been divided clinically into three types: infection (1) from animal bites, (2) from animal contact,[25] and (3) without known animal contact.[16] Infections from animal bites include cellulitis, abscesses, tenosynovitis, and bone and joint infection, but infection can become generalized, especially in patients who are immunocompromised. Infections caused by animal contact can be similar to infections described earlier and are caused by animals licking broken skin or wounds. Sometimes pulmonary infections occur, possibly related to aerosolization of organisms. In some cases, these organisms have been reported as respiratory flora in patients with pets, but at present no proof exists that such colonization is an antecedent of infection.[23] Cases without known animal contact history constitute 3 to 30 percent[36,40] of all cases.

Infection usually occurs when the organisms are inoculated into deeper tissues either on animal teeth that break the skin or in animal saliva that comes in contact with nonintact skin. Bite wound infections often are polymicrobial. Infection in cases without known animal contact is harder to explain but definitely happens.[44] Most cases of serious infection occur in patients with underlying diseases, such as diabetes mellitus, chronic alcoholism, and other types of liver disease.[62] Central nervous system infection with these organisms has occurred after head trauma or neurosurgery in 10 of 11 reported cases.[44] One intrauterine death of the fetus of a 20-year-old woman who worked at a pig farm has been attributed to *P. aerogenes*.[79] Case reports of unusual infections with rare species of *Pasteurella*, such as fatal sepsis and meningitis in a 4-day-old infant caused by *A. (Pasteurella) gallinarum*,[2] should be considered doubtful unless molecular identification methods have been used.[32]

CLINICAL MANIFESTATIONS

Pasteurella infections produce pain, swelling, pus, and sometimes abscess formation at the site of inoculation, beginning within 24 to 36 hours. Clinically, these infections are indistinguishable from wound infections with *Staphylococcus aureus* or other gram-positive organisms. Gram stain may show the characteristic pleomorphic bacilli with bipolar staining. Growth on standard agar is rapid.

Patients with peritonitis,[62] meningitis,[44] osteomyelitis,[26] or infectious endocarditis[3] have symptoms typical of these diagnoses. Risk factors, such as household pet exposure, animal contact, animal bites, and comorbid conditions, should heighten suspicion of possible *Pasteurella* infection.

DIAGNOSIS

Establishing the diagnosis of *Pasteurella* infection can be difficult, not because the organism is fastidious or slow-growing, but because it often is misidentified. Other organisms of the same family (i.e., *Actinobacillus* spp. and *Haemophilus* spp.) have similar biochemical profiles and can be misidentified by commonly used systems, such as API. Lester and associates[50] reported that of 30 species firmly identified as *Pasteurella* by biochemical means, only three were identified correctly by the API 20E system. *Haemophilus aphrophilus* and *Actinobacillus actinomycetemcomitans* are sometimes misidentified as *P. gallinarum* by commercial systems.[24] Additionally, Hamilton-Miller[31] reported that four

strains of *Haemophilus influenzae* and three strains of *Haemophilus parainfluenzae* were identified falsely as *Pasteurella* spp. by API, and suggested that if the clinical history renders *Pasteurella* infection unlikely, tests for X and V factor requirements should be performed (see Chapter 145). Clinical case reports corroborate these laboratory observations.[19,62,74] Notifying the bacteriology laboratory of suspicion of *Pasteurella* infection is helpful.

TREATMENT

Penicillin has been considered the drug of choice for *Pasteurella* infection in the past and, despite some reports of penicillin resistance, still is effective against most strains. *Pasteurella* spp. also are susceptible to ampicillin, β-lactamase inhibitor combination drugs, tetracycline, and chloramphenicol. Truncated but fully functional tetracycline resistance genes have been identified in isolates from animal sources.[46] The aminoglycosides, erythromycin, clindamycin, cefadroxil, and cefaclor are not recommended. Dicloxacillin and cephalexin have poor activity against *Pasteurella* spp. and should not be used as monotherapy for animal bite wounds.[27] In one study of bite wound infections, ertapenem was found to be active against all *Pasteurella* spp.[28] Of fluoroquinolones tested in vitro against 75 clinical isolates of *Pasteurella* spp., levofloxacin was the most active.[34]

Acknowledgments

The author thanks Dr. William Gruber and Dr. Thomas Boyce for their invaluable assistance with earlier versions of this chapter.

REFERENCES

1. Abbott, S. L., Kokka, R. P., and Janda, J. M.: Laboratory investigations on the low pathogenic potential of *Plesiomonas shigelloides*. J. Clin. Microbiol. 29:148-153, 1991.
2. Ahmed, K., Sein, P. P., Shahnawaz, M., and Hoosen, A. A.: *Pasteurella gallinarum* neonatal meningitis. Clin. Microbiol. Infect. 8:55-57, 2002.
3. Alcaniz, J. P., de Cuenca Moron, B., Gomez Rubio, M., et al.: Spontaneous bacterial peritonitis due to *Plesiomonas shigelloides*. Am. J. Gastroenterol. 90:1529-1530, 1995.
4. Aldridge, K. E., Valainis, G. T., and Sanders, C. V.: Comparison of the in vitro activity of ciprofloxacin and twenty-four other antimicrobial agents against clinical strains of *Chromobacterium violaceum*. Diagn. Microbiol. Infect. Dis. 10:31-38, 1988.
5. al-Fadel Saleh, M., al-Madan, M. S., Erwa, H. H., et al.: First case of human infection caused by *Pasteurella gallinarum* causing infective endocarditis in an adolescent ten years after surgical correction for truncus arteriosus. Pediatrics 95:944-948, 1995.
6. Ampofo, K., Graham, P., Ratner, A., et al.: *Plesiomonas shigelloides* sepsis and splenic abscess in an adolescent with sickle-cell disease. Pediatr. Infect. Dis. J. 20:1178-1179, 2001.
7. Andrighetti-Frohner, C. R., Antonio, R. V., Creczynski-Pasa, T. B., et al.: Cytotoxicity and potential antiviral evaluation of violacein produced by *Chromobacterium violaceum*. Mem. Inst. Oswaldo. Cruz. 98:843-848, 2003.
8. Angen, O., Mutters, R., Caugant, D. A., et al.: Taxonomic relationships of the [*Pasteurella*] *haemolytica* complex as evaluted by DNA-DNA hybridizations and 16S rRNA sequencing with proposal of *Mannheimia haemolytica* gen. nov., comb. nov., *Mannheimia granulomatis* comb. nov., *Mannheimia glucosida* sp. nov., *Mannheimia ruminalis* sp. nov. and *Mannheimia varigena* sp. nov. Int. J. Syst. Bacteriol. 49:67-86, 1999.
9. Blackall, P. J., Christensen, H., Beckenham, T., et al.: Reclassification of *Pasteurella gallinarum*, [*Haemophilus*] *paragallinarum*, *Pasteurella avium* and *Pasteurella volantium* as *Avibacterium gallinarum* gen. nov., comb. nov., *Avibacterium paragallinarum* comb. nov., *Avibacterium avium* comb. nov. and *Avibacterium volantium* comb. nov. Int. J. Syst. Evol. Microbiol. 55:353-362, 2005.
10. Brendan, R. A., Miller, M. A., and Janda, J. M.: Clinical disease spectrum and pathogenic factors asssociated with *Plesiomonas shigelloides* infections in humans. Rev. Infect. Dis. 10:303-316, 1988.
11. Brito, C. F., Carvalho, C. B., Santos, F., et al.: *Chromobacterium violaceum* genome: Molecular mechanisms associated with pathogenicity. Genet. Mol. Res. 31:148-161, 2004.

12. Brown, K. L., Stein, A., and Morrell, D. S.: Ecthyma gangrenosum and septic shock syndrome secondary to *Chromobacterium violaceum*. J. Am. Acad. Dermatol. *54*(5 Suppl.):S224-S228, 2006.

13. Butt, A. A., Figueroa, J., and Martin, D. H.: Ocular infection caused by three unusual marine organisms. Clin. Infect. Dis. *24*:740-741, 1997.

14. Citron, D. M., Edelstein, M. A., Garcia, L. S., et al.: *Pasturella* and similar organisms. *In* Baron E. J., Peterson L. R., and Finegold, S. M. (eds.): Bailey and Scott's Diagnostic Microbiology. 9th ed. St. Louis, Mosby, 1994, pp. 420-423.

15. Ciznar, I., Hostacka, A., Gonzalez-Rey, C., and Krovacek, K.: Potential virulence-associated properties of *Plesiomonas shigelloides* strains. Folia Microbiol. *49*:543-548, 2004.

16. Creczynski-Pasa, T. B., and Antonio, R. V.: Energetic metabolism of *Chromobacterium violaceum*. Genet. Mol. Res. *31*:162-166, 2004.

17. Duma, R. J.: Aztreonam, the first monobactam. Ann. Intern. Med. *106*:766, 1987.

18. Escande, F., Vallee, E., and Aubart, F.: *Pasteurella caballi* infection following a horse bite. Zentralbl. Bakteriol. *285*:440-444, 1997.

19. Fajfar-Whetsone, C. J. T., Coleman, L., Biggs, D. R., et al.: *Pasteurella multocida* septicemia and subsequent *Pasteurella dagmatis* septicemia in a diabetic patient. J. Clin. Microbiol. *33*:202-204, 1995.

20. Falcon, R., Carbonell, G. V., Figueredo, P. M., et al.: Intracellular vacuolation induced by culture filtrates of *Plesiomonas shigelloides* isolated from environmental sources. J. Appl. Microbiol. *95*:273-278, 2003.

21. Farrar, W. E., Jr., and O'Dell, N. M.: Beta-lactamase activity in *Chromobacterium violaceum*. J. Infect. Dis. *134*:290-293, 1976.

22. Feldman, R. B., Stern, G. A., and Hood, I.: *Chromobacterium violaceum* infection of the eye. Arch. Ophthalmol. *102*:711-713, 1984.

23. Frebourg, N. B., Berthelot, G., Hocq, R., et al.: Septicemia due to *Pasteurella pneumotropica*: 16srRNA sequencing for diagnosis confirmation. J. Clin. Microbiol. *40*:687-689, 2002.

24. Fredericksen, W., and Tonning, B.: Possible misidentification of *Haemophilus aphrophilus* as *Pasteurella gallinarum*. Clin. Infect. Dis. *32*:987-988, 2001.

25. Furie, R. A., Cohen, R. P., Hartman, B. J., et al.: *Pasteurella multocida* infection: Report in urban setting and review of spectrum of human disease. N. Y. State Med. J. *80*:1597-1602, 1980.

26. Gadberry, J. L., Zipper, R., Taylor, J. A., et al.: *Pasteurella pneumotropica* isolated from bone and joint infections. J. Clin. Microbiol. *19*:926-927, 1984.

27. Goldstein, E. J. C., and Citron, D. M.: Comparative activities of cefuroxime, amoxicillin-clavulanic acid, ciprofloxacin, enoxacin, and ofloxacin against aerobic and anaerobic bacteria isolated from bite wounds. Antimicrob. Agents Chemother. *32*:1143-1148, 1988.

28. Goldstein, E. J., Citron, D. M., Merriam, C. V., et al.: Comparative in vitro activity of ertapenem and 11 other antimicrobial agents against aerobic and anaerobic pathogens isolated from skin and soft tissue animal and human bite wound infections. J. Antimicrob. Chemother. *48*:641-651, 2001.

29. Gonzalez-Rodriguez, N., Santos, J. A., Otero, A., and Garcia-Lopez, M. L.: Cell-associated hemolytic activity in environmental strains of *Plesiomonas shigelloides* expressing cell-free, iron-influenced extracellular hemolysin. J. Food Prot. *70*:885-890, 2007.

30. Gupta, S.: Migratory polyarthritis associated with *Plesiomonas shigelloides* infection. Scand. J. Rheumatol. *24*:323-325, 1995.

31. Hamilton-Miller, J. M.: A possible pitfall in the identification of *Pasteurella* spp. with the API system. J. Med. Microbiol. *39*:78-79, 1993.

32. Hamilton-Miller, J. M. T.: Distinguishing *Pasteurella* spp. from *Haemophilus* spp.: The problem revisited. Clin. Microbiol. Infect. *9*:243, 2003.

33. Herrington, D. A., Tzipori, S., Robins-Browne, R. M., et al.: In vitro and in vivo pathogenicity of *Plesiomonas shigelloides*. Infect. Immun. *55*:979-985, 1987.

34. Heurtin, C., Desbordes, L., Travert, M. F., et al.: Comparative study of the bacteriostatic and bactericidal activity of levofloxacin against *Pasteurella* strains isolated from man. Pathol. Biol. (Paris) *49*:606-611, 2001.

35. Holmberg, S. D., Wachsmuth, K., Hickman-Brenner, F. W., et al.: *Plesiomonas* enteric infections in the United States. Ann. Intern. Med. *105*:690-694, 1986.

36. Holst, E., Rollof, J., Larsson, L., et al.: Characterization and distribution of *Pasteurella* species recovered from infected humans. J. Clin. Microbiol. *30*:2984-2987, 1992.

37. Hungria, M., Nicolas, M. F., Guimaraes, C. T., et al.: Tolerance to stress and environmental adaptability of *Chromobacterium violaceum*. Genet. Mol. Res. *31*:102-116, 2004.

38. Inglis, T. J., Chiang, D., Lee, G. S., and Chor-Kiang, L.: Potential misidentification of *Burkholderia pseudomallei* by API 20NE. Pathology *30*:62-64, 1998.

39. Ingram, C. W., Morrison, A. J., Jr., and Levitz, R. E.: Gastroenteritis, sepsis, and osteomyelitis caused by *Plesiomonas shigelloides* in an immunocompetent host: Case report and review of the literature. J. Clin. Microbiol. *25*:1791-1793, 1987.

40. Jones, Jr., F. L., and Smull, C. E.: Infections in man due to *Pasteurella multocida*: Importance of human carrier. Pa. Med. J. *76*:41-44, 1985.

41. Kain, K. C., and Kelly, M. T.: Antimicrobial susceptibilities of *Plesiomonas shigelloides* from patients with diarrhea. Antimicrob. Agents Chemother. *33*:1609-1610, 1989.

42. Kain, K. C., and Kelly, M. T.: Clinical features, epidemiology, and treatment of *Plesiomonas shigelloides* diarrhea. J. Clin. Microbiol. *27*:998-1001, 1989.

43. Kainz, A., Lubitz, W., and Busse, H. J.: Genomic fingerprints, ARDRA profiles and quinone systems for classification of *Pasteurella sensu stricto*. Syst. Appl. Microbiol. *23*:494-503, 2000.

44. Kaka, S., Lunz, R., and Klugman, K. P.: *Actinobacillus (Pasteurella) ureae* meningitis in an HIV-positive patient. Diagn. Microbiol. Infect. Dis. *20*:105-107, 1994.

45. Kaufman, S. C., Ceraso, D., and Schugurensky, A.: First case report from Argentina of fatal septicemia caused by *Chromobacterium violaceum*. J. Clin. Microbiol. *23*:956-958, 1986.

46. Kehrenberg, C., and Schwartz, S.: Identification of a truncated, but functionally active tet(H) tetracycline resistance gene in *Pasteurella aerogenes* and *Pasteurella multocida*. F. E. M. S. Microbiol. Lett. *188*:191-195, 2000.

47. Khan, A. M., Faruque, A. S., Hossain, M. S., et al.: *Plesiomonas shigelloides*–associated diarrhea in Bangladeshi children: A hospital-based surveillance study. J. Trop. Pediatr. *50*:354-356, 2004.

48. Lee, J., Kim, J. S., Nahm, C. H., et al.: Two cases of *Chromobacterium violaceum* infection after injury in a subtropical region. J. Clin. Microbiol. *37*:2068-2070, 1999.

49. Leet, S., and Wright, B. D.: Fulminating chromobacterial septicemia presenting as respiratory distress syndrome. Thorax *36*:557-559, 1981.

50. Lester, A., Jarlov, J. O., Westh, H., et al.: *Pasteurella haemolytica* diagnosis questioned. J. Infect. *25*:334-335, 1992.

51. MacDonell, M. T., and Colwell, R. R.: Phylogeny of the Vibrionaceae, and recommendation for two new genera, *Listonella* and *Shewanella*. Syst. Appl. Microbiol. *6*:171-182, 1985.

52. Macher, A. M., Casale, T. B., and Fauci, A. S.: Chronic granulomatous disease of childhood and *Chromobacterium violaceum* infections in the southeastern United States. Ann. Intern. Med. *97*:51-55, 1982.

53. Mamlok, R. J., Mamlok, V., Mills, G. C., et al.: Glucose-6-phosphate dehydrogenase deficiency, neutrophil dysfunction, and *Chromobacterium violaceum* sepsis. J. Pediatr. *111*:852-854, 1987.

54. Marshman, W. E., and Lyons, C. J.: Congenital endophthalmitis following maternal shellfish ingestion. Aust. N. Z. J. Ophthalmol. *26*:161-163, 1998.

55. Martin, D. L., and Gustafson, T. L.: *Plesiomonas* gastroenteritis in Texas. J. A. M. A. *15*:2063, 1985.

56. McNeely, D., Ivy, P., Craft, J. C., et al.: *Plesiomonas*: Biology of the organism and disease in children. Pediatr. Infect. Dis. *3*:176-181, 1984.

57. Melo, P. S., Maria, S. S., Vidal, B. C., et al.: Violacein cytotoxicity and induction of apoptosis in V79 cells. In Vitro Cell Dev. Biol. Anim. *36*:539-543, 2000.

58. Miller, D. P., Blevins, W. T., Steele, D. B., et al.: A comparative study of virulent and avirulent strains of *Chromobacterium violaceum*. Can. J. Microbiol. *32*:249-255, 1988.

59. Moore, C. C., Lane, J. E., and Stephens, J. L.: Successful treatment of an infant with *Chromobacterium violaceum* sepsis. Clin. Infect. Dis. *32*:e107-e110, 2001.

60. Mutters, R., Ihm, P., Pohl, S., et al.: Reclassification of the genus *Pasteurella* Trivisan 1887 on the basis of deoxyribonucleic acid homology, with proposals for the new species *Pasteurella dagmatis*, *Pasteurella canis*, *Pasteurella stomatis*, *Pasteurella anatis*, and *Pasteurella langaa*. Int. J. Syst. Bacteriol. *35*:309, 1985.

61. Myers, J., Ragasa, D. A., and Eisole, C.: *Chromobacterium violaceum* septicemia in New Jersey. J. Med. Soc. N. J. *79*:213-214, 1982.

62. Noble, R. C., Marek, B. J., and Overman, S. B.: Spontaneous bacterial peritonitis caused by *Pasteurella ureae*. J. Clin. Microbiol. *25*:442-444, 1987.

63. Okawa, Y., Ohtomo, Y., Tsugawa, H., et al.: Isolation and characterization of a cytotoxin produced by *Plesiomonas shigelloides* P-1 strain. F. E. M. S. Microbiol. Lett. *239*:125-130, 2004.

64. Paul, R., Siitonen, A., and Karkkainen, P.: *Plesiomonas shigelloides* bacteremia in a healthy girl with mild gastroenteritis. J. Clin. Microbiol. *28*:1445-1446, 1990.

65. Ponte, R., and Jenkins, S. G.: Fatal *Chromobacterium violaceum* infections associated with exposure to stagnant waters. Pediatr. Infect. Dis. J. *11*:583-586, 1992.

66. Rahim, Z., and Kay, B. A.: Enrichment for *Plesiomonas shigelloides* from stools. J. Clin. Microbiol. *26*:789-790, 1988.

67. Reinhardt, J. F., and George, W. L.: Comparative in vitro activities of selected antimicrobial agents against *Aeromonas* species and *Plesiomonas shigelloides*. Antimicrob. Agents Chemother. *27*:643-645, 1985.

68. Rolston, K. V. I., and Hopfer, R. L.: Diarrhea due to *Plesiomonas shigelloides* in cancer patients. J. Clin. Microbiol. *20*:597-598, 1984.

69. Roth, T., Hentsch, C., Erard, P., and Tschantz, P.: Pyosalpinx: Not always a sexual transmitted disease? Pyosalpinx caused by *Plesiomonas shigelloides* in an immunocompetent host. Clin. Microbiol. Infect. *8*:803-805, 2002.

70. Shigematsu, M., Kaufmann, M. E., Charlett, A., et al.: An epidemiologic study of *Plesiomonas shigelloides* diarrhea among Japanese travellers. Epidemiol. Infect. *125*:523-530, 2000.

71. Sirinavin, S., Techasaensiri, C., Benjaponpitak, S., et al.: Invasive *Chromobacterium violaceum* infection in children: Case report and review. Pediatr. Infect. Dis. J. *24*:559-561, 2005.

72. Sivendra, R., and Tan, S. H.: Pathogenicity of unpigmented cultures of *Chromobacterium violaceum*. J. Clin. Microbiol. *5*:514-516, 1977.

73. Sneath, P. H. A. Genus *Chromobacterium*. *In* Krieg, N. R., and Holt, J. G. (eds.): Bergey's Manual of Systematic Bacteriology. Baltimore, Williams & Wilkins, 1984, pp. 580-582.

74. Sorbello, A. F., O'Donnell, J., Kaiser-Smith, J., et al.: Infective endocarditis due to *Pasteurella dagmatis*: Case report and review. Clin. Infect. Dis. *18*:336-338, 1994.

75. Sorenson, R. U., Jacobs, M. R., and Shurin, S. B.: *Chromobacterium violaceum* adenitis acquired in the northern United States as a complication of chronic granulomatous disease. Pediatr. Infect. Dis. J. *4*:701-702, 1985.

76. Stock, I., and Wiedemann, B.: Natural antimicrobial susceptibilities of *Plesiomonas shigelloides* strains. J. Antimicrob. Chemother. *48*:803-811, 2001.

77. Terpeluk, C., Goldman, A., Bartmann, P., et al.: *Plesiomonas shigelloides* sepsis and meningoencephalitis in a neonate. Eur. J. Pediatr. *151*:499-501, 1992.

78. Theodoropoulos, C., Wong, T. H., O'Brien, M., and Stenzel, D.: *Plesiomonas shigelloides* enters polarized human intestinal Caco-2 cells in an in vitro model system. Infect Immun. *69*:2260-2269, 2001.

79. Thorsen, P., Moller, B. R., Arpi, M., et al.: *Pasteurella aerogenes* isolated from stillbirth and mother. Lancet *343*:485-486, 1994.

80. Ti, T. Y., Tan, W. C., Chong, A. P. Y., et al.: Nonfatal and fatal infections caused by *Chromobacterium violaceum*. Clin. Infect. Dis. *17*:505-507, 1993.

81. Tsugawa, H., Ono, T., Murakami, H., and Okawa, Y.: Invasive phenotype and apoptosis induction of *Plesiomonas shigelloides* P-1 strain to Caco-2 cells. J. Appl. Microbiol. *99*:1235-1443, 2005.

82. Tzanetea, R., Konstantopoulos, K., Xanthaki, A., et al.: *Plesiomonas shigelloides* sepsis in a thalassemia intermedia patient. Scand. J. Infect. Dis. *34*:687-689, 2002.

83. Vitovec, J., Aldova, E., Vladik, P., and Krovacek, K.: Enteropathogenicity of *Plesiomonas shigelloides* and *Aeromonas* spp. in experimental mono- and coinfection with *Cryptosporidium parvum* in the intestine of neonatal BALB/c mice. Comp. Immunol. Microbiol. Infect. Dis. *24*:39-55, 2001.

84. Wang, S.: A study of the ecology of *Plesiomonas shigelloides* (Chinese). Chung-Hua Liu Hsing Ping Hsueh Tsa Chih Chin. J. Epidemiol. *12*:295-298, 1991.

85. Woo, P. C., Lau, S. K., Wong, S. S., and Yuen, K. Y.: Two cases of continuous ambulatory peritoneal dialysis–associated peritonitis due to *Plesiomonas shigelloides*. J. Clin. Microbiol. *42*:933-935, 2004.

86. Young, A. Z., Neujahr, D., and Estok, L.: Case report: Epididymo-orchitis and bacteremia caused by *Plesiomonas shigelloides* in an HIV-infected patient. AIDS Read. *11*:617-619, 2001.

87. Zims, M. M., Zimprich, C. A., Petermann, S. R., and Rust, L.: Expression and partial characterization of an elastase from *Chromobacterium violaceum*. Vet. Microbiol. *80*:63-74, 2001.

CHAPTER 131

ACINETOBACTER

Armando G. Correa

First recognized as a human pathogen in 1908,[66] the ubiquitous organism *Acinetobacter* has emerged as a rather common cause of nosocomial infections in immunocompromised hosts.[6] Some of the confusion regarding this organism may be attributed to the many changes in nomenclature that the members of this genus have undergone over the years. Names used in the past to identify this genus include *Herellea*, *Bacterium*, *Mima*, *Achromobacter*, *Alcaligenes*, *Neisseria*, *Micrococcus*, *Diplococcus*, *Moraxella*, and *Cytophaga*. Treatment of infection caused by *Acinetobacter* is complicated by its widespread multidrug resistance and the difficulty encountered in eradicating the organism.

THE ORGANISM

The genus *Acinetobacter* belongs to the family Neisseriaceae, which also includes the *Neisseria*, *Moraxella*, and *Kingella* genera. *Acinetobacter* is a gram-negative bacterium that typically appears as a rod 0.9 to 1.6 μm in diameter and 1.5 to 2.5 μm in length, but it may become spherical in the stationary phase of growth. It frequently occurs in pairs or short chains. Many strains are encapsulated. The organism has a strictly aerobic respiratory metabolism and does not grow under anaerobic conditions. It does not form spores or exhibit swimming mobility. *Acinetobacter* grows well in all common complex media between 20° C and 30° C, with optimal growth occurring between 33° C and 35° C, and it has no growth factor requirements.

Convex, grayish-white colonies 1 to 2.5 mm in diameter are typical findings. The colonies may appear mucoid if the strain is encapsulated. *Acinetobacter* is catalase-positive and may be differentiated readily from other closely related genera by virtue of its negative reaction to oxidase.

Formerly, the genus *Acinetobacter* contained the single species *Acinetobacter calcoaceticus* subdivided into two subspecies or biovars: *anitratus* and *lwoffii*.[31] However, in 1986, the taxonomy of the genus *Acinetobacter* was changed extensively on the basis of DNA hybridization studies,[10] and at least 32 genomic species have been proposed, of which 17 have been assigned species names.[17] Ten of these nomenspecies have been isolated from human specimens: *Acinetobacter baumannii*, *A. calcoaceticus*, *Acinetobacter haemolyticus*, *Acinetobacter johnsonii*, *Acinetobacter junii*, *Acinetobacter lwoffii*, *Acinetobacter radioresistens*, *Acinetobacter parvus*, *Acinetobacter schindleri*, and *Acinetobacter ursingi*.[17] Several unnamed genospecies also have

been isolated from human clinical samples and include genomic species 3, 13TU, 10, and 11.[17] These species may be difficult to differentiate in the clinical laboratory on the basis of their growth characteristics and biochemical activity. Because of their clinical relevance and antimicrobial resistance, four of these species, *A. baumannii*, *A. calcoaceticus*, and genomic species 3 and 13TU, are grouped under the term *A. baumannii-calcoaceticus* complex. Under the new classification, most *A. baumannii* strains represent organisms that were classified formerly as biovar *anitratus*, whereas *A. junii* and *A. lwoffii* previously were listed under the biovar *lwoffii*.

EPIDEMIOLOGY

Acinetobacter strains are distributed widely in nature and can be found in soil, fresh water, and sewage.[8,28] *Acinetobacter* also can be isolated from many animals, fresh meats, poultry, contaminated milk, and frozen foods.[8,28] The organism can be part of the bacterial flora of the skin in healthy individuals,[8,12] and the skin frequently becomes a reservoir for *Acinetobacter* in hospitalized patients and the health care staff.[6,8] It occasionally forms part of the normal flora of the oral cavity and the upper respiratory, genital, and lower gastrointestinal tracts.[8,12] Colonization by *Acinetobacter* is particularly common in patients who have undergone a tracheostomy.[52] The organism frequently can be found in the hospital environment, particularly in moist areas, such as in humidifiers, water sinks, and ventilators.[8] Nosocomial outbreaks have been linked to colonized medical equipment such as ventilator tubing and other respiratory equipment,[1,26] intravenous catheters,[8] gloves,[46] and mattresses.[59]

The frequency of occurrence of nosocomial infections by *Acinetobacter* is not easy to assess because the pathogenic role of this organism often has been underestimated. However, a national surveillance study conducted from 1974 to 1977 identified *Acinetobacter* as a pathogen in 0.76 percent of nosocomial infections.[49] The estimated rate of nosocomial infections caused by this organism was 3.11 per 10,000 patients discharged, and approximately 15 percent of 1372 reported episodes occurred in the pediatric age group.[49] By 1978, this rate increased by 14 percent and accounted for 1 percent of the bacterial isolates associated with nosocomial infections.[12] An unusual seasonal pattern was observed, with most infections occurring in late summer.[12,49] The cause of this increase is unknown. Pneumonia, tracheobronchitis, and infections of the urinary tract and surgical wounds were the entities observed most frequently.[49] In a national prospective survey of U.S. hospitals from 1995 through 2002, *Acinetobacter* spp. accounted for 1.3 percent of all nosocomial bloodstream infections and was associated with a crude mortality rate of 34 percent.[70] Data from SENTRY, an international surveillance program that monitors the frequency of occurrence and antimicrobial susceptibility of bacterial pathogens, revealed a significantly greater frequency of *Acinetobacter* infections in Latin America than in all other regions.[22] A higher prevalence rate of *Acinetobacter* infections was noted in patients ranging in age from birth to 10 years.[22] In the pediatric age group, neonates appear to be particularly susceptible to nosocomial infection with this organism (Table 131–1).[42]

More recently, *Acinetobacter* emerged as a particularly important pathogen in unusual situations such as earthquakes and war zones.[30] This prevalence was illustrated by reports of outbreaks of multidrug-resistant *Acinetobacter* infections associated with the U.S.-Iraq conflict.[56]

PATHOGENESIS

Limited information is available regarding the pathogenesis of *Acinetobacter* infections. The lipopolysaccharide of *Acinetobacter*, a normal constituent of the outer membrane of gram-negative bacteria, is capable of eliciting multiple pathogenic host responses. Strains producing exopolysaccharide have been shown to be more pathogenic than are nonproducers.[30] Nonspecific adherence factors, such as fimbriae, also have been described in *Acinetobacter*.[30] The role of quorum sensing as a regulatory mechanism for autoinduction of multiple virulence factors in *Acinetobacter* is currently under investigation.[30]

In animal models, *Acinetobacter* can enhance the virulence of other bacteria in mixed infections, perhaps by slime-induced inhibition of neutrophils.[44] Researchers have speculated that the ability of this organism to grow in an acidic pH at lower temperatures may enhance its ability to invade devitalized tissue.[2] The organism also may survive in a dry environment for as long as a week.[14]

CLINICAL MANIFESTATIONS

Acinetobacter can cause suppurative infection of virtually any organ, and the clinical manifestations typically are similar to those seen with other bacterial infections because no unique features are suggestive of *Acinetobacter* infection. The clinical mani-

festations also may depend on the underlying immune status of compromised hosts. Infections caused by *Acinetobacter* are rare occurrences in normal children.[18]

INTRACRANIAL INFECTION

Most cases of *Acinetobacter* meningitis are the result of a penetrating injury or occur after a neurosurgical procedure, although sporadic cases of meningitis have been reported in the absence of these factors. A cluster of eight children in whom *Acinetobacter* meningitis developed after the administration of intrathecal methotrexate was reported.[32] All patients had fever, headache, nausea, and vomiting, and lumbar puncture revealed cerebrospinal fluid (CSF) pleocytosis.

The earlier literature contains several reports of *Acinetobacter* meningitis developing in apparently normal children.[15,16,29,63,67] CSF pleocytosis with a predominance of segmented forms occurred commonly.[16] Because as many as 30 percent of these patients had a petechial rash and gram-negative diplococci on CSF smears, the diagnosis of meningococcal meningitis was made erroneously in most of these cases, thereby leading to a delay in the institution of appropriate therapy and possibly contributing to a mortality rate as high as 27 percent.[16]

Siegman-Igra and associates,[60] in a review of 25 cases of *Acinetobacter* meningitis secondary to invasive procedures that included some children, found that fever, leukocytosis, and neck stiffness, along with other clinical signs of central nervous system (CNS) infection, were common features. The CSF in these patients showed pleocytosis with a predominance of polymorphonuclear leukocytes, elevated protein concentration, and a low glucose level. Most of the infections were associated with indwelling ventriculostomy tubes or a fistula into the CSF space. Filka and colleagues[20] reported 10 cases of *Acinetobacter* meningitis that occurred over the course of a 7-year period in children who had undergone ventriculoperitoneal shunt insertion.

Researchers have suggested that an inherited or acquired complement deficiency may be associated with meningitis caused by *Acinetobacter*[19] because it is seen with *Neisseria meningitidis* and other related species. Treatment of CNS infections caused by *Acinetobacter* requires a minimum of 3 weeks of parenteral antibiotics.

BACTEREMIA

Acinetobacter bacteremia may occur as an isolated event or may be secondary to a primary infected site, such as the respiratory or urinary tract or a wound. Primary bacteremia appears to occur

TABLE 131–1 Illustrative Nosocomial Clusters of *Acinetobacter* Infection in Pediatric Patients

Country	Year	Type of Unit	Infected Children	Colonized Children	Presentation	Mortality (%)	Suspected Source
United Kingdom[42]	1981	NICU	4	0	Meningitis	0	None identified
United Kingdom[61]	1983	NICU	9	1	Pulmonary infection	22	Ambu bag
Japan[64]	1983-1986	NICU	19	52	Sepsis	11	Multiple sources
India[32]	1988	Oncology	8	N/A	Meningitis	38	Intrathecal needle
Germany[55]	1988	NICU	3	41	Sepsis	100	Humidifier
Israel[48]	1988-1990	NICU	9	N/A	Sepsis	44	None identified
United Kingdom[43]	1989	NICU	7	N/A	Sepsis	0	Intravenous fluids
Bahamas[40]	1996	NICU	8	1	Sepsis	37	Air conditioner
South Africa[47]	1997	NICU	9	N/A	Sepsis	22	Suction catheters
India[41]	1995	NICU	79	N/A	Sepsis	14	None identified
India[13]	1986-1990	NICU	26	N/A	Sepsis	42	None identified

N/A, data not available; NICU, neonatal intensive care unit.

more commonly in immunocompromised neonates, and clinical manifestations can vary from an absence of clinical signs of infection to fulminant septic shock and disseminated intravascular coagulation.[33,55] Thrombocytopenia has been reported to be a prominent feature in these neonates.[43,48] Pneumonia has been seen more commonly in early-onset sepsis.[41] Predisposing factors include low birth weight,[53,55] previous antibiotic therapy,[48,53,55] and the presence of indwelling catheters.[40,53]

Acinetobacter bacteremia in children with malignant diseases also has been noted to occur rarely. Fuchs and colleagues[21] reported 29 episodes of sepsis caused by this organism over the course of a 12-year period in an oncology center. All these children were febrile and appeared ill at the time of diagnosis, and a high association of *Acinetobacter* sepsis with the presence of intravascular catheters was noted. Surprisingly, no connection was found with the level of neutropenia.[21]

RESPIRATORY TRACT

Because *Acinetobacter* may be a transient colonizer of the pharynx in 7 percent of healthy children[5] and adults[23] and this rate is increased in hospitalized patients, the relative importance of *Acinetobacter* in comparison with other potential pathogens isolated from sputum is difficult to ascertain. The tracheobronchitis and pneumonia attributed to *Acinetobacter* are mostly nosocomial infections associated with the presence of an endotracheal tube or tracheostomy.[23] Pneumonias frequently are multilobar and occasionally may lead to cavitary destruction or pleural empyema.[23]

Community-acquired pneumonia caused by *A. baumannii* has been reported to occur in adults in the Northern Territory of Australia and other tropical regions.[4] This entity generally is seen in patients with diminished host defenses caused by alcoholism, cigarette smoking, or underlying pulmonary disease and is characterized by the rapid onset of fever, dyspnea, pleuritic chest pain, and purulent sputum. The mortality rate has been as high as 53 to 64 percent.[4]

MISCELLANEOUS

Urinary tract infections occur almost exclusively in patients with indwelling bladder catheters, usually are limited to the bladder, and generally are mild.[23] Burns, as well as traumatic and surgical wounds, frequently become colonized by *Acinetobacter* as a result of the ability of this organism to thrive on compromised tissue and foreign material.[23] Bacteremia may occur as a consequence of this colonization, which is often polymicrobial. *Acinetobacter* is a prominent cause of peritonitis in children undergoing peritoneal dialysis when gram-negative organisms are involved.[68]

Other rare infections caused by *Acinetobacter* that have been reported include suppurative otitis media,[50,63] cellulitis (frequently in association with trauma, a foreign body, or an animal bite),[23,50] synergistic necrotizing fasciitis,[3] native-valve and prosthetic-value endocarditis,[25] septic arthritis,[50] osteomyelitis,[63] and liver abscesses.[23] Ocular infections also have been documented.[38] A case of osteomyelitis occurring after a hamster bite in a child has been described.[39]

DIAGNOSIS

The diagnosis of *Acinetobacter* infection is made by culture of appropriate body fluids or tissue specimens. No serologic or antigen-detection tests are available. A selective medium containing MacConkey agar with cephaloridine has been used to culture skin specimens during investigation of outbreaks[61] because of its ability to inhibit most of the skin flora but not *Acinetobacter*.

Biotyping, phage typing, electrophoretic analysis of isoenzyme and cell wall proteins, plasmid analysis, polymerase chain reaction–based DNA fingerprinting, and restriction endonuclease digestion of DNA have been used for investigation of nosocomial outbreaks.[7] Antibiogram typing no longer is considered an effective method in the investigation of *Acinetobacter* epidemics because the susceptibility pattern may change rapidly within the same outbreak.[7,11]

TREATMENT

As with many other opportunistic gram-negative organisms, treatment of infections caused by *Acinetobacter* spp., particularly those of the *A. baumannii-calcoaceticus* complex,[57,65] have become more complicated by the rapid increase in resistance to the antibiotics used commonly in hospitals. Selection of an antibiotic regimen should be based on in vitro susceptibility testing and ideally should include both a β-lactam and an aminoglycoside, which may have synergistic activity[23] and prevent the emergence of resistance.[6]

Species of the *A. baumannii-calcoaceticus* complex have shown decreased susceptibility to ampicillin, broad-spectrum penicillins, cephalosporins, aminoglycosides, and ciprofloxacin.[22,57] Resistance to extended-spectrum cephalosporins may be the result of the presence of cephalosporinases (particularly the chromosomally encoded cephalosporinase AmpC),[9] other broad-spectrum β-lactamases, or changes in the outer-membrane porins and penicillin-binding proteins.[9,45] Resistance to aminoglycosides is mediated by aminoglycoside-modifying enzymes.[65] The carbapenems imipenem and meropenem appear to be the most active agents against *A. baumannii*,[60,65] but reports have found more than 10 percent of such strains to be resistant to these antibiotics in some areas,[22,37] and increasing numbers of nosocomial outbreaks of carbapenem-resistant *Acinetobacter* infections have been reported.[24,64,72] The incidence of carbapenem-resistant *Acinetobacter* strains has been particularly high in Latin America (11.4% of all isolates versus 4.8% in the United States).[22] Resistance to the carbapenems has been associated with the presence of serine and metallo-β-lactamases (carbapenemases). Of particular concern are the numerous carbapenem-hydrolyzing OXA enzymes that have emerged in *A. baumannii*.[9] Caution should be exercised when using imipenem at high dosage in children for the treatment of meningitis (i.e., 100 mg/kg/day) because of an unusually high rate of seizures.[71] Thus, meropenem is recommended for this indication. Ertapenem, a newer carbapenem antibiotic, has poor in vitro activity against *Acinetobacter*[35] and should not be used for the treatment of these infections. Combinations of a β-lactam antibiotic with a β-lactamase inhibitor, such as ampicillin-sulbactam, piperacillin-tazobactam, or ticarcillin-clavulanate, have been used for infections caused by carbapenem-resistant strains.[64,72]

The fluoroquinolones, in particular ciprofloxacin, have been used successfully to treat infections caused by multidrug-resistant *Acinetobacter* in children[41,47] and adults. Although ciprofloxacin has been approved for the treatment of complicated urinary tract infections in children, the other systemic fluoroquinolones are not approved for use in children younger than 16 years of age because of the theoretic concern for damage to growth cartilage. Of the quinolones currently available, gatifloxacin exhibits the best in vitro activity against *A. baumannii*, followed by levofloxacin and trovafloxacin.[27] Although 76 to 86 percent of sporadic isolates of *A. baumannii* are susceptible to the fluoroquinolones, only 32 to 55 percent of outbreak-related strains remain susceptible to this antibiotic class.[27] Topoisomerase mutations in both *gyrA* and *parC* have been identified in quinolone-resistant *A. baumannii*.[9] In some cases, the polymyxin drugs polymyxin B and colistin are the only therapeutic options for the treatment of multidrug-resistant *Acinetobacter* infection.[24,34] Efflux pumps capable of conferring resistance to multiple antibiotic classes have been identified in *Acinetobacter* spp.[9,51]

Tigecycline is the first member of the glycylcycline antimicrobial class to gain approval in the United States. Because this agent demonstrates in vitro activity against multidrug-resistant strains of *A. baumannii*, its potential use as an alternative therapy for severe infections caused by this organism is being investigated.[51] Data regarding the use of this agent in pediatric patients are lacking.

Imipenem, meropenem, amikacin, ciprofloxacin, ceftazidime, and ceftriaxone have exhibited good in vitro activity against isolates identified as species other than the *A. baumannii-calcoaceticus* complex.[57] In addition to antimicrobial therapy, prompt drainage of focal suppurative sites and removal of infected indwelling catheters are essential. Intraventricular administration of amikacin has been used in the treatment of CNS infections caused by this organism.[69]

PROGNOSIS

Because *Acinetobacter* strains often are resistant to the antibiotics used commonly, prompt recognition of the specific cause and institution of effective antibiotic therapy are critical to achieving a successful outcome. The reported mortality rate in a series of pediatric patients ranged from 0 percent to more than 50 percent (see Table 131–1), and the outcome appeared to correlate more closely with the underlying condition than with other factors such as polymicrobial bacteremia.[62] In a series of 58 infections caused by this organism that occurred over the course of a 2-year period from 1973 through 1974 at the Massachusetts General Hospital in Boston, the mortality rate was 23 percent.[23] A 1999 prospective study in the Slovak Republic revealed that the case-fatality rate for 157 episodes of *A. baumannii* bacteremia was significantly higher in adults than in children (34% vs. 12%).[33]

The nosocomial acquisition of multiresistant *A. baumannii-calcoaceticus* complex has been associated with high mortality rates and prolonged hospitalization in adult patients in intensive care units,[36,54] in contrast to the more benign clinical outcome usually seen with other species of *Acinetobacter*.[58]

PREVENTION

Nosocomial acquisition of *Acinetobacter* by high-risk compromised hosts can be prevented by placing emphasis on the control measures routinely used for endemic infections, such as careful handwashing by personnel, limitation of the frequency and duration of use of devices, proper isolation of colonized and infected patients, application of strict techniques for invasive procedures, and restricted use of antibiotics.[14,36,60]

REFERENCES

1. Ahmed, J., Brutus, A., D'Amato, R. F., et al.: *Acinetobacter calcoaceticus anitratus* outbreak in the intensive care unit traced to a peak flow meter. Am. J. Infect. Control 22:319-321, 1994.
2. Allen, D. M., and Hartman, B. J.: *Acinetobacter* species. *In* Mandell, G. L., Bennett, J. E., and Dolin, R. (eds.): Mandell, Douglas and Bennett's Principles and Practice of Infectious Diseases. 4th ed. New York, Churchill Livingstone, 1995, pp. 2009-2013.
3. Amsel, M. B., and Horrilleno, E.: Synergistic necrotizing fasciitis: A case of polymicrobial infection with *Acinetobacter calcoaceticus*. Curr. Surg. 42:370-372, 1985.
4. Anstey, N. M., Currie, B. J., and Withnall, K. M.: Community-acquired *Acinetobacter* pneumonia in the Northern Territory of Australia. Clin. Infect. Dis. 14:83-91, 1992.
5. Baltimore, R. S., Duncan, R. L., Shapiro, E. D., et al.: Epidemiology of pharyngeal colonization of infants with aerobic gram-negative rod bacteria. J. Clin. Microbiol. 27:91-95, 1989.
6. Bergogne-Berezin, E.: *Acinetobacter* spp., saprophytic organisms of increasing pathogenic importance. Zentrabl. Bakteriol. 81:389-405, 1994.
7. Bergogne-Berezin, E., and Joly-Guillou, M. L.: Hospital infection with *Acinetobacter* spp.: An increasing problem. J. Hosp. Infect. 18(Suppl. A):250-255, 1991.
8. Bergogne-Berezin, E., Joly-Guillou, M. L., and Vieu, J. F.: Epidemiology of nosocomial infections due to *Acinetobacter calcoaceticus*. J. Hosp. Infect. 10:105-113, 1987.
9. Bonomo, R. A., and Szabo, D.: Mechanisms of multidrug resistance in *Acinetobacter* species and *Pseudomonas aeruginosa*. Clin. Infect. Dis. 43(Suppl. 2):S49-S56, 2006.
10. Bouvet, P. J. M., and Grimont, P. A. D.: Taxonomy of the genus *Acinetobacter* with the recognition of *Acinetobacter baumannii* sp. nov., *Acinetobacter haemolyticus* sp. nov., *Acinetobacter johnsonii* sp. nov., and *Acinetobacter junii* sp. nov. and the emended descriptions of *Acinetobacter calcoaceticus* and *Acinetobacter lwoffii*. Int. J. Syst. Bacteriol. 36:228-240, 1986.
11. Carlquist, J. F., Conti, M., and Burke, J. P.: Progressive resistance in a single strain of *Acinetobacter calcoaceticus* recovered during a nosocomial outbreak. Am. J. Infect. Control 10:43-48, 1982.
12. Centers for Disease Control and Prevention: Nosocomial infections caused by *Acinetobacter calcoaceticus*: United States, 1978. M. M. W. R. Morb. Mortal Wkly. Rep. 28:177-179, 1979.
13. Christo, G. G., Shenoy, V., Matthai, J., et al.: *Acinetobacter* sepsis in neonates. Indian Pediatr. 30:1413-1416, 1993.
14. Crombach, W. H. J., Dijkshoorn, L., van Noort-Klaassen, M., et al.: Control of an epidemic spread of a multi-resistant strain of *Acinetobacter calcoaceticus* in a hospital. Intensive Care Med. 15:166-170, 1989.
15. DeBord, G. G.: *Mima polymorpha* in meningitis. J. Bacteriol. 55:764-765, 1948.
16. Donald, W. D., and Doak, W. M.: Mimeae meningitis and sepsis. J. A. M. A. 200:111-113, 1967.
17. Dortet, L., Legrand, P., Soussy, C. J., and Cattoir, V.: Bacterial identification, clinical significance, and antimicrobial susceptibilities of *Acinetobacter ursingii* and *Acinetobacter schindleri*, two frequently misidentified opportunistic pathogens. J. Clin. Microbiol. 44:4471-4478, 2006.
18. Feigin, R. D., and Shearer, W. T.: Opportunistic infection in children. III. In the normal host. J. Pediatr. 87:852-866, 1975.
19. Fijen, C. A. P., Kuijper, E. J., Tjia, H. G., et al.: Complement deficiency predisposes for meningitis due to nongroupable meningococci and *Neisseria*-related bacteria. Clin. Infect. Dis. 18:780-784, 1994.
20. Filka, J., Huttova, M., Schwartzova, D., et al.: Nosocomial meningitis due to *Acinetobacter calcoaceticus* in 10 children after ventriculoperitoneal shunt insertion. J. Hosp. Infect. 44:76-77, 2000.
21. Fuchs, G. J., Jaffe, N., and Pickering, L. K.: *Acinetobacter calcoaceticus* sepsis in children with malignancies. Pediatr. Infect. Dis. 5:545-549, 1986.
22. Gales, A. C., Jones, R. N., Forward, K. R., et al.: Emerging importance of multidrug-resistant *Acinetobacter* species and *Stenotrophomonas maltophilia* as pathogens in seriously ill patients: Geographic patterns, epidemiological features, and trends in the SENTRY antimicrobial surveillance program (1997-1999). Clin. Infect. Dis. 32(Suppl. 2):104-113, 2001.
23. Glew, R. H., Moellering R. C., and Kunz L. J.: Infections with *Acinetobacter calcoaceticus (Herellea vaginicola)*: Clinical and laboratory studies. Medicine (Baltimore) 56:79-97, 1977.
24. Go, E. S., Urban, C., Burns, J., et al.: Clinical and molecular epidemiology of *Acinetobacter* infections sensitive only to polymyxin B and sulbactam. Lancet 344:1329-1332, 1994.
25. Gradon, J. D., Chapnick, E. K., and Lutwick, L. I.: Infective endocarditis of a native valve due to *Acinetobacter*: Case report and review. Clin. Infect. Dis. 14:1145-1148, 1992.
26. Hartstein, A. I., Rashad, A. L., Liebler, J. M., et al.: Multiple intensive care unit outbreak of *Acinetobacter calcoaceticus* subspecies *anitratus* respiratory infection and colonization associated with contaminated, reusable ventilator circuits and resuscitation bags. Am. J. Med. 85:624-631, 1988.
27. Heinemann, B., Wisplinghoff, H., Edmond, M., and Seifert, H.: Comparative activities of ciprofloxacin, clinafloxacin, gatifloxacin, gemifloxacin, levofloxacin, moxifloxacin, and trovafloxacin against epidemiologically defined *Acinetobacter baumannii* strains. Antimicrob. Agents Chemother. 44:2211-2213, 2000.
28. Henriksen, S. D.: *Moraxella, Acinetobacter,* and the Mimeae. Bacteriol. Rev. 37:522-561, 1973.
29. Hermann, G., and Melnick, T.: *Mima polymorpha* meningitis in the young. Am. J. Dis. Child. 110:315-318, 1965.
30. Joly-Guillou, M. L.: Clinical impact and pathogenicity of *Acinetobacter*. Clin. Microbiol. Infect. 11:868-873, 2005.
31. Juni, E.: *Acinetobacter*. *In* Krieg, N. R. (ed.): Bergey's Manual of Systematic Bacteriology. Baltimore, Williams & Wilkins, 1984, pp. 303-306.
32. Kelkar, R., Gordon, S. M., Giri, N., et al.: Epidemic iatrogenic *Acinetobacter* spp. meningitis following administration of intrathecal methotrexate. J. Hosp. Infect. 14:233-243, 1989.
33. Koprnova, J., Svetlansky, I., Bilikova, E., et al.: *Acinetobacter baumannii* bacteremia in children. Pediatr. Infect. Dis. J. 20:1183, 2001.

34. Levin, A. S., Barone, A. A., Penco, J., et al.: Intravenous colistin as therapy for nosocomial infections caused by multidrug-resistant *Pseudomonas aeruginosa* and *Acinetobacter baumannii*. Clin. Infect. Dis. *28*:1008-1011, 1999.

35. Livermore, D. M., Carter, M. W., Bagel, S., et al.: In vitro activity of ertapenem (MK-0826) against recent clinical bacteria collected in Europe and Australia. Antimicrob. Agents Chemother. *45*:1860-1867, 2001.

36. Lortholary, O., Fagon, J. Y., Hoi, A. B., et al.: Nosocomial acquisition of multiresistant *Acinetobacter baumannii*: Risk factors and prognosis. Clin. Infect. Dis. *20*:790-796, 1995.

37. Manikal, V. M., Landman, D., Saurina, G., et al.: Endemic carbapenem-resistant *Acinetobacter* species in Brooklyn, New York: Citywide prevalence, interinstitutional spread, and relation to antibiotic usage. Clin. Infect. Dis. *31*:101-106, 2000.

38. Marcovich, A., and Levartovsky, S.: *Acinetobacter* exposure keratitis. Br. J. Ophthalmol. *78*:489-490, 1994.

39. Martin, R. W., Martin, D. L., and Levy, C. S.: *Acinetobacter* osteomyelitis from a hamster bite. Pediatr. Infect. Dis. J. *5*:364-365, 1988.

40. McDonald, L. C., Walker, M., Carson, L., et al.: Outbreak of *Acinetobacter* spp. bloodstream infections in a nursery associated with contaminated aerosols and air conditioners. Pediatr. Infect. Dis. J. *17*:716-722, 1998.

41. Mishra, A., Mishra, S., Jaganath, G., et al.: *Acinetobacter* sepsis in newborns. Indian Pediatr. *35*:2732, 1998.

42. Morgan, M. E. I., and Hart, C. A.: *Acinetobacter* meningitis: Acquired infection in a neonatal intensive care unit. Arch. Dis. Child. *657*:557-559, 1982.

43. Ng, P. C., Herrington, R. A., Beane, C. A., et al.: An outbreak of *Acinetobacter* septicaemia in a neonatal intensive care unit. J. Hosp. Infect. *14*:363-368, 1989.

44. Obana, Y.: Pathogenic significance of *Acinetobacter calcoaceticus*: Analysis of experimental infection in mice. Microbiol. Immunol. *30*:645-657, 1986.

45. Obara, M., and Nakae, T.: Mechanisms of resistance to β-lactam antibiotics in *Acinetobacter calcoaceticus*. J. Antimicrob. Chemother. *28*:791-800, 1991.

46. Patterson, J. E., Vecchio, J., Pantelick, E. L., et al.: Association of contaminated gloves with transmission of *Acinetobacter calcoaceticus* var. *anitratus* in an intensive care unit. Am. J. Med. *91*:479-483, 1991.

47. Pillay, T., Pillay, D. G., Adhikari, M., and Sturm, A. W.: An outbreak of neonatal infection with *Acinetobacter* linked to contaminated suction catheters. J. Hosp. Infect. *43*:299-304, 1999.

48. Regev, R., Dolfin, T., Zelig, I., et al.: *Acinetobacter* septicemia: A threat to neonates? Special aspects in a neonatal intensive care unit. Infection *21*:394-396, 1993.

49. Retailliau, H. F., Hightower, A. W., Dixon, R. E., et al.: *Acinetobacter calcoaceticus*: A nosocomial pathogen with an unusual seasonal pattern. J. Infect. Dis. *139*:371-375, 1979.

50. Reynolds, R. C., and Cluff, L. E.: Infection of men with Mimeae. Ann. Intern. Med. *58*:759-767, 1963.

51. Rice, L. B.: Challenges in identifying new antimicrobial agents effective for treating infections with *Acinetobacter baumannii* and *Pseudomonas aeruginosa*. Clin. Infect. Dis. *43*(Suppl. 2):S100-S105, 2006.

52. Rosenthal, S. L.: Sources of *Pseudomonas* and *Acinetobacter* species found in human culture materials. Am. J. Clin. Pathol. *62*:807-811, 1974.

53. Sakata, H., Fujita, K., Maruyama, S., et al.: *Acinetobacter calcoaceticus* biovar *anitratus* septicaemia in a neonatal intensive care unit: Epidemiology and control. J. Hosp. Infect. *14*:15-22, 1989.

54. Scerpella, E. G., Wanger, A. R., Armitige, L., et al.: Nosocomial outbreak caused by a multiresistant clone of *Acinetobacter baumannii*: Results of the case-control and molecular epidemiologic investigations. Infect. Control Hosp. Epidemiol. *16*:92-97, 1995.

55. Schloesser, R. L., Laufkoetter, E. A., Lehners, T., et al.: An outbreak of *Acinetobacter calcoaceticus* infection in a neonatal care unit. Infection *18*:230-233, 1990.

56. Scott, P., Deye, G., Srinivasan, A., et al.: An outbreak of multidrug-resistant *Acinetobacter baumannii-calcoaceticus* complex infection in the US Military Health Care System associated with military operations in Iraq. Clin. Infect. Dis. *44*:1577-1584, 2007.

57. Seifert, H., Baginski, R., Schulze, A., et al.: Antimicrobial susceptibility of *Acinetobacter* species. Antimicrob. Agents Chemother. *37*:750-753, 1993.

58. Seifert, H., Strate, A., Schulze, A., et al.: Bacteremia due to *Acinetobacter* species other than *Acinetobacter baumannii*. Infection *22*:379-385, 1994.

59. Sherertz, R. J., and Sullivan, M. L.: An outbreak of infections with *Acinetobacter calcoaceticus* in burn patients: Contamination of patients' mattresses. J. Infect. Dis. *151*:252-258, 1985.

60. Siegman-Igra, Y., Bar-Yosef, S., Gorea, A., et al.: Nosocomial *Acinetobacter* meningitis secondary to invasive procedures: Report of 25 cases and review. Clin. Infect. Dis. *17*:843-849, 1993.

61. Stone, J. W., and Das, B. C.: Investigation of an outbreak of infection with *Acinetobacter calcoaceticus* in a special care baby unit. J. Hosp. Infect. *6*:42-48, 1985.

62. Tilley, P. A. G., and Roberts, F. J.: Bacteremia with *Acinetobacter* species: Risk factors and prognosis in different clinical settings. Clin. Infect. Dis. *18*:896-900, 1994.

63. Torregrosa, M. V., and Ortiz, A.: Severe infections in children due to rare gram-negative bacilli (*Mima polymorpha* and *Bacillus anitratum*). J. Pediatr. *59*:35-41, 1961.

64. Urban, C., Go, E., Mariano, N., et al.: Effect of sulbactam on infections caused by imipenem-resistant *Acinetobacter calcoaceticus* biotype *anitratus*. *167*:448-451, 1993.

65. Vila, J., Marcos, A., Marco, F., et al.: In vitro antimicrobial production of β-lactamases, aminoglycoside-modifying enzymes, and chloramphenicol acetyltransferase by and susceptibility of clinical isolates of *Acinetobacter baumannii*. Antimicrob. Agents Chemother. *37*:138-141, 1993.

66. Von Lingelsheim, W.: Beitrage zur Aetiologie der epidemischen Genickstarre nach den Ergebnissen der letzten Jahre. Z. Hyg. Infektionskr. *59*:457-460, 1908.

67. Waite, C. L., and Kline, A. H.: *Mima polymorpha* meningitis. Am. J. Dis. Child. *98*:121-126, 1959.

68. Warady, B. A., Campoy, S. F., Gross, S. P., et al.: Peritonitis with continuous ambulatory peritoneal dialysis and continuous cycling peritoneal dialysis. J. Pediatr. *105*:726-729, 1984.

69. Wirt, T. C., McGee, Z. A., Oldfield, E. H., et al.: Intraventricular administration of amikacin for complicated gram-negative meningitis and ventriculitis. J. Neurosurg. *50*:95-99, 1979.

70. Wisplinghoff, H., Bischoff, T., Tallent, S. M., et al.: Nosocomial bloodstream infections in US hospitals: Analysis of 24,179 cases from a prospective nationwide surveillance study. Clin. Infect. Dis. *39*:309-317, 2004.

71. Wong, V. K., Wright, H. T., Ross, L. A., et al.: Imipenem/cilastatin treatment of bacterial meningitis in children. Pediatr. Infect. Dis. J. *10*:122-125, 1991.

72. Wood, C. A., and Reboli, A. C.: Infections caused by imipenem-resistant *Acinetobacter calcoaceticus* biotype *anitratus*. J. Infect. Dis. *168*:1602-1603, 1993.

CHAPTER

132

ACHROMOBACTER (ALCALIGENES)

Randall G. Fisher

Organisms of the genus *Achromobacter* are gram-negative bacilli that live in aqueous environments. Originally considered commensals, they increasingly are recognized as important, although rare, hospital pathogens. *Achromobacter* can be especially problematic in immunocompromised patients and in neonates, in whom infection can be life-threatening. These organisms have been isolated from such diverse clinical specimens as sputum, urine, feces, blood, cerebrospinal fluid, cornea, and peritoneal and pleural fluids.

BACTERIOLOGY

Achromobacter spp. are gram-negative, motile, indole-negative, obligate aerobes that are oxidase- and catalase-positive. They are considered to be nonfermenters because of their extremely limited action on carbohydrates. Most ferment xylose, and some ferment glucose. All reduce nitrate to nitrite. They are urease-, lysine-, and ornithine-negative. They grow well on both blood and MacConkey agar and produce colonies that are smooth and glistening and have a distinct edge. They alkalinize organic salts and amides, a property that led to the name *Alcaligenes*, which means *alkali producing*. *Alcaligenes faecalis* has a distinct, sweet odor that has been described as resembling that of green apples.[27]

Bacteriologically, these bacilli may be confused with other nonfermenting gram-negative organisms, especially *Pseudomonas* spp. Morphologically, however, they can be distinguished easily from pseudomonads by the presence of peritrichous flagella: *Pseudomonas* spp. have polar flagella.[23]

The taxonomy of these organisms is confusing and undergoes frequent changes. They were classified as *Achromobacter* spp., then reclassified as *Alcaligenes*; they have been reassigned the name *Achromobacter*. The genera *Achromobacter* and *Alcaligenes* are closely related and comprise many species, but clinically important ones are as follows: (1) *Achromobacter xylosoxidans*, which has two subspecies: *xylosoxidans* and *dentrificans*, the former of which is the most common cause of clinically recognizable infection; (2) *Alcaligenes faecalis*, which is a less common pathogen but has a distinct antimicrobial susceptibility pattern[5]; (3) and *Achromobacter piechaudii*, which has been isolated from clinical specimens[35] but is of doubtful significance. In the discussion that follows, the abbreviation *A. xylosoxidans* refers to *Achromobacter xylosoxidans* subspecies *xylosoxidans*.

EPIDEMIOLOGY

Like *Pseudomonas* spp., *Achromobacter* are water organisms and prefer aqueous environments and moist soil. They do not survive long on porous surfaces or fomites or if they become desiccated.[39] They also may be part of the normal flora of the ear and of the gastrointestinal and respiratory tracts of some people. These organisms establish a niche within the hospital environment and have been recovered from ventilators, humidifiers, "sterile" saline, intravenous fluids, and irrigation and dialysis solutions. *Achromobacter* spp. also have been recovered from infant formula,[16] children's soap bubbles,[32] well water,[45] and swimming pools.[25] Organisms also survive many disinfectants and have been cultured from chlorhexidine,[42] 1 percent eosin,[6] and alcohol- or quaternary amine–containing compounds.[39,42] Shigeta and associates[42] reported an outbreak of *A. xylosoxidans* ventriculitis secondary to contaminated chlorhexidine used on a surgical ward. Foley and colleagues[19] reported an outbreak accompanied by deaths in a neonatal intensive care unit secondary to contamination of saline used as an eyewash. Boukadida and coworkers[6] reported a neonatal death caused by meningitis contracted by dissemination after treatment of a diaper rash with 1 percent eosin. An outbreak of 37 cases (with 2 fatalities) that was caused by bacterial contamination of deionized water in a hemodialysis system was described by Reverdy and associates[36]. Surgical wound infection also has occurred wherein infection was suspected to be secondary to contaminated irrigation fluids used in surgery.[50] One outbreak of four cases in a hemodialysis unit was linked to an atomizer of 2.5 percent chlorhexidine used to disinfect the skin.[47] Three different kinds of pseudo-outbreaks have been described: in one, seven patients in a pediatric hospital were infected with *A. xylosoxidans*, but restriction fragment-length polymorphism analysis proved they all were genetically unrelated[4]; in another, *A. xylosoxidans* was isolated from three different clinical specimens but was later proven to be a contaminant of the saline used in their processing[22]; in a third, blood cultures were positive when drawn on the night shift because the nurses were cleaning the top of the blood culture bottles with a contaminated disinfectant.[44]

Studies have documented that *A. xylosoxidans* colonization of patients with cystic fibrosis is on the rise. In one large study, *A. xylosoxidans* was isolated from the sputum culture of 52 of 595 patients (8.7%).[7] In other studies, isolates of *A. xylosoxidans* at a single cystic fibrosis center were not genetically related, a finding implying no common source of infection and little or no patient-to-patient spread within the center.[14,49] However, colonization of multiple patients with identical strains also is well documented.[37] Environmental cultures at one cystic fibrosis center were positive for *A. xylosoxidans* only 0.8 percent of the time, whereas 22.8 percent of such cultures were positive for *Pseudomonas aeruginosa*.[18]

PATHOPHYSIOLOGY

Achromobacter spp. are weakly virulent bacteria. Medical care commonly provides the conduit through which organisms are introduced into their host, by way of indwelling catheters, endotracheal tubes, and so forth. The bacteria may take advantage of a weakened immune system and disseminate, causing sepsis, meningitis, and death. Preterm or small-for-gestational-age term infants are at particular risk for acquiring such severe *Achromobacter* infections.[19] Although most neonatal infections are considered to be nosocomial, vertical transmission from mother to baby may occur.[23] An increased incidence of infection has been reported for patients with neoplasms[28] and those receiving long-term steroid therapy.[26] Sporadic cases of *Achromobacter* infection in patients with idiopathic immunoglobulin M (IgM) deficiency,[15] Waldenström macroglobulinemia,[46] and systemic lupus erythematosus have been reported.[38] My colleagues and I have seen one boy with hyper-IgM syndrome in whom 14 separate episodes of *Achromobacter* bacteremia occurred; an exhaustive environmental search for a source was fruitless. The source was eventually proven to be deep infection of a cervical lymph node, and the episodes ceased when the node was removed.[51] *Achromobacter* infections occur in patients with acquired immunodeficiency syndrome (AIDS),[8,21] but whether this syndrome is an independent risk factor for infection is unclear.

In one study, patients with cystic fibrosis and colonized with *A. xylosoxidans* tended to be older (mean age, 20 years) and at baseline had worse lung function than did noncolonized controls; however, over the course of the study, the rate of decline of lung function did not differ between cases and controls.[10] In a second similar case-control study, lung function decline and growth parameters generally were not affected by colonization; however, a subset of patients had rapidly increasing antibody titers against *A. xylosoxidans*, and this group did experience more accelerated decline.[37]

In unusual circumstances, patients with neither overt underlying disease nor obvious immune deficiency will develop infection with *Achromobacter* spp. Most of these cases involve penetrating trauma. One case of corneal infection complicating epidemic keratoconjunctivitis in a normal host has been described.[33]

CLINICAL MANIFESTATIONS

Signs of sepsis or meningitis caused by *A. xylosoxidans* in the newborn are difficult to differentiate from other causes of bacterial sepsis. However, some babies may develop a distinctive rash in association with this infection, in which 1- to 2-cm, sharply demarcated red patches appear, especially in the head and neck region. This rash was noted in 29 of 33 newborns with *A. xylosoxidans* infection reported by Doxiadis and associates in 1960[12] and was seen again in a case reported in 1993.[6] *A. xylosoxidans* sepsis/meningitis tends to manifest later in life than do infections with the usual vertically acquired pathogens and may have a more insidious onset.[30] In some cases, cerebrospinal fluid profiles may resemble those usually associated with viral meningitis, with white blood cell counts in the hundreds and with monocytic predominance.[40] Neonatal *Achromobacter* sepsis or meningitis has an extremely poor prognosis; one series noted a mortality rate that approached 75 percent, and 36 percent of survivors had severe neurologic deficits.[19] The incidence of intracranial hemorrhage also was high.

Three large series of bloodstream infections with *A. xylosoxidans* all revealed a similar story: most cases are nosocomial, most patients have an underlying malignant disease, many are neutropenic or receiving high-dose steroids, and many patients have indwelling vascular catheters.[2,20,41] Polymicrobial bacteremia was not rare in these series. Mortality rates ranged from 15 percent[20] to 48 percent.[41] Risk factors for mortality were age greater than 65 years at diagnosis, neutropenia, nosocomial acquisition, and polymicrobial bacteremia. An earlier review of reported cases revealed that the case-fatality rate was lowest in patients with catheter-associated bacteremia and highest (65%) in those with pneumonia, meningitis, or endocarditis.[13]

One child developed osteomyelitis caused by *A. xylosoxidans* after stepping on a nail through old sneakers (a clinical situation classically associated with *Pseudomonas* infection)[24,25]; another developed *Achromobacter* infection as a consequence of a gunshot wound.[9] In the setting of a patient with an artificial heart valve, *A. xylosoxidans* endocarditis has been described.[34] In another case, endocarditis was associated with an abandoned pacemaker lead.[1] A case series of liver abscesses included three patients from whom *A. xylosoxidans* was isolated, all of whom shared a clinical pattern: history of cholecystectomy, "coral-like" multilobulated appearance on computed tomographic scanning, and epithelioid granulomas at the periphery of the abscesses.[3] *A. xylosoxidans* infection in older patients usually is not suspected on clinical grounds but rather in the context of a common-source outbreak or because of microbiologic clues. *A. faecalis* infection is less common and usually is part of a polymicrobial process.

DIAGNOSIS AND TREATMENT

Generally, the diagnosis of *Achromobacter* infections rests on recovery of the organism from clinical samples, although newer methods sometimes have been employed. In one case of culture-negative endophthalmitis, fluid obtained from the anterior chamber was subjected to polymerase chain reaction using a 16S rDNA primer set, finding a 214 base pair sequence from *A. xylosoxidans*.[48] These organisms often are mistaken for pseudomonads, and the clinician should suspect *A. xylosoxidans* when the laboratory reports an organism as a *Pseudomonas* spp. that is resistant to all aminoglycosides.[39] Key differentiation features include the antibiogram and the morphology of the organism, with its distinctive peritrichous flagella.

Achromobacter spp. typically are resistant to a large number of antibiotics, including ampicillin, aztreonam, aminoglycosides, first- and second-generation cephalosporins, tetracyclines, and rifampin. They variably are resistant to chloramphenicol, fluoroquinolones, macrolides, ureidopenicillins, and β-lactamase combination drugs.[5] *Achromobacter* spp. have been shown to produce β-lactamases, some of which are chromosomal, constitutive, and inducible[11] and some of which are on plasmids.[29] Some isolates overproduce β-lactamase,[11] which stoichiometrically can render β-lactamase inhibitors useless. In addition, their porins are small, thus rendering antibiotic entry difficult. Although there is no antibiotic to which all isolates have been shown to be sensitive,[34] most are sensitive in vitro to trimethoprim-sulfamethoxazole, imipenem, ceftazidime, and cefoperazone. Imipenem-resistant strains also have been discovered. These strains produced VIM-2, OXA-30, and a chromosomal AmpC β-lactamase.[43] Two case reports describe treatment failures of ceftazidime[31] and piperacillin[11] in clinical isolates that were sensitive at the time of isolation but developed resistance during the course of therapy.

Because resistance patterns vary from isolate to isolate, the combination of a third-generation cephalosporin, piperacillin, or imipenem with trimethoprim-sulfamethoxazole is reasonable empiric therapy for suspected *Achromobacter* infection, pending susceptibility results. In general, in vitro susceptibilities seem to correlate well with in vivo results,[28] but the risk of inducible resistance to β-lactam antibiotics should be acknowledged. One report described synergy in microbial killing with an aminoglycoside, even though the isolate was resistant to the same aminoglycoside when it was tested alone.[8] This phenomenon was confirmed by two-disk Kirby-Bauer approximation methods

using 11 clinical blood culture isolates; all were resistant to gentamicin, but 10 of 11 were inhibited synergistically when gentamicin was added to ticarcillin/clavulanate, and 9 of 11 displayed synergy when gentamicin was added to piperacillin or ceftazidime.[13]

Removal of infected catheters may speed recovery, although some patients have been treated successfully through indwelling lines.[8] Because of a high recurrence rate, experts in the care of patients with renal failure treated with continuous ambulatory peritoneal dialysis recommend removal of peritoneal catheters in patients who develop peritonitis with *A. xylosoxidans*.[17]

Acknowledgments

I would like to thank Dr. William Gruber and Dr. Thomas Boyce for their invaluable assistance with earlier versions of this chapter.

REFERENCES

1. Ahn, Y., Kim, N. H., Shin, D. H., et al.: Pacemaker lead endocarditis caused by *Achromobacter xylosoxidans*. J. Korean Med. Sci. 19:291-293, 2004.
2. Aisenberg, G., Rolston, K. V., and Safdar, A.: Bacteremia caused by *Achromobacter* and *Alcaligenes* species in 46 patients with cancer (1989-2003). Cancer 101:2134-2140, 2004.
3. Asano, K., Tada, S., Matsumoto, T., et al.: A novel bacterium *Achromobacter xylosoxidans* as a cause of liver abscess: Three case reports. J. Hepatol. 43:362-365, 2005.
4. Benaoudia, F., and Bengen, E.: Evidence for the genetic unrelatedness of nosocomial *Alcaligenes xylosoxidans* strains in a pediatric hospital. Infect. Control Hosp. Epidemiol. 18:132-134, 1997.
5. Bizet, C., Tekaia, F., and Phillipon, A.: In vitro susceptibility of *Alcaligenes faecalis* compared with those of other *Alcaligenes* species to antimicrobial agents including seven beta-lactams. J. Antimicrob. Chemother. 32:907-910, 1993.
6. Boukadida, J., Monastiri, K., Snoussi, N., et al.: Nosocomial neonatal meningitis by *Alcaligenes xylosoxidans* transmitted by aqueous eosin. Pediatr. Infect. Dis. J. 12:696-697, 1993.
7. Burns, J. L., Emerson, J., Stapp, J. R., et al: Microbiology of sputum from patients at cystic fibrosis centers in the United States. Clin. Infect. Dis. 27:158-163, 1998.
8. Cieslak, T. J., and Raszka, W. V.: Catheter-associated sepsis due to *Alcaligenes xylosoxidans* in a child with AIDS. Clin. Infect. Dis. 16:592-593, 1993.
9. D'Amato, R. F., Salemi, M., Mathews, A., et al.: *Achromobacter xylosoxidans* (*Alcaligenes xylosoxidans* subsp. *xylosoxidans*) meningitis associated with a gunshot wound. J. Clin. Microbiol. 26:2425-2426, 1988.
10. De Baets, F., Schelstraete, P., Van Daele, S., et al.: *Achromobacter xylosoxidans* in cystic fibrosis: Prevalence and clinical relevance. J. Cyst. Fibros. 6:75-78, 2007.
11. Decre, D., Arlet, G., Danglot, C., et al.: A beta-lactamase overproducing strain of *Alcaligenes dentrificans* subsp. *xylosoxidans* isolated from a case of meningitis. J. Antimicrob. Chemother. 30:769-779, 1992.
12. Doxiadis, S. A., Pavlatou, M., and Chryssostomidou, O.: *Bacillus foecalis alcaligenes* septicemia in the newborn. J. Pediatr. 56:648-654, 1960.
13. Duggan, J. M., Goldstein, S. J., Chenoweth, C. E., et al.: *Achromobacter xylosoxidans* bacteremia: Report of four cases and review of the literature. Clin. Infect. Dis. 23:569-576, 1996.
14. Dunne, W. M., Jr., and Maisch, S.: Epidemiological investigation of infections due to *Alcaligenes* species in children and patients with cystic fibrosis: Use of repetitive-element-sequence polymerase chain reaction. Clin. Infect. Dis. 20:836-841, 1995.
15. Dworzack, D. L., Murray, C. M., Hodges, G. R., et al.: Community acquired bacteremic *Achromobacter xylosoxidans* type IIIa: Pneumonia in a patient with idiopathic IgM deficiency. Am. J. Clin. Pathol. 70:712-717, 1978.
16. Edwards, L. D., Tan-Gatue, L. G., Levin, S., et al.: The problem of bacteriologically contaminated infant formulas in a newborn nursery. Clin. Pediatr. 13:63-65, 1974.
17. El-Shahawy, M. A., Kim, D., and Gadallah, M. F.: Peritoneal dialysis–associated peritonitis caused by *Alcaligenes xylosoxidans*. Am. J. Nephrol. 18:452-455, 1998.
18. Festini, F., Taccetti, G., Mannini, C., et al.: Patient risk of contact with respiratory pathogens from inanimate surfaces in a cystic fibrosis outpatient clinic: A prospective study over a four-year period. Pediatr. Pulmonol. 42:779-784, 2007.
19. Foley, J. F., Gravelle, C. R., Englehard, W. E., et al.: *Achromobacter* septicemia fatalities in prematures. Am. J. Dis. Child. 101:279-288, 1961.
20. Gomez-Cerezo, J., Suarez, I., Rios, J. J., et al.: *Achromobacter xylosoxidans* bacteremia: A 10-year analysis of 54 cases. Eur. J. Clin. Microbiol. Infect. Dis. 22:360-363, 2003.

21. Gradon, J. D., Mayrev, A. R., and Hayes, J.: Pulmonary abscess associated with *Alcaligenes xylosoxidans* in a patient with AIDS. Clin. Infect. Dis. *17*:1071-1072, 1993.

22. Granowitz, E. V., and Keenholtz, S. L.: A pseudoepidemic of *Alcaligenes xylosoxidans* attributable to contaminated saline. Am. J. Infect. Control. *83*:284-285, 1998.

23. Hearn, Y. R., and Gander, R. M.: *Achromobacter xylosoxidans*: An unusual neonatal pathogen. Am. J. Clin. Pathol. *96*:211-214, 1991.

24. Hoddy, D. M., and Barton, L. L.: Puncture wound–induced *Achromobacter xylosoxidans* osteomyelitis of the foot. Am. J. Dis. Child. *145*:599-600, 1991.

25. Holmes, B., Snell, J. J. S., and Lapage, S. P.: Strains of *Achromobacter xylosoxidans* from clinical material. J. Clin. Pathol. *30*:595-601, 1977.

26. Igra-Siegman, Y., Chmel, H., and Cobbs, C.: Clinical and laboratory characteristics of *Achromobacter xylosoxidans* infection. J. Clin. Microbiol. *11*:141-145, 1980.

27. Kersters, K., and DeLey, J.: Genus *Alcaligenes*. *In* Krieg, N. R., and Holt, J. G. (eds.): Bergey's Manual of Systematic Bacteriology. Baltimore, Williams & Wilkins, 1984, pp. 361-373.

28. Legrand, C., and Anqissie, E.: Bacteremia due to *Achromobacter xylosoxidans* in patients with cancer. Clin. Infect. Dis. *14*:479-484, 1992.

29. Levesque, R., Royu, P. H., Letarte, R., et al.: A plasmid-mediated cephalosporinase from *Achromobacter* species. J. Infect. Dis. *145*:753-761, 1982.

30. Mandell, W. F., Garvey, G. J., and Neu, H. C.: *Achromobacter xylosoxidans* bacteremia. Rev. Infect. Dis. *9*:1001-1005, 1987.

31. Manjra, A. I., Moosa, A., and Bhamjee, A.: Fatal neonatal meningitis and ventriculitis caused by multi-resistant *Achromobacter xylosoxidans*: A case report. S. Afr. Med. J. *76*:571-573, 1989.

32. McGarrity, G. J., and Coriell, L. L.: Bacterial contamination of children's soap bubbles. Am. J. Dis. Child. *125*:224-226, 1973.

33. Oh, J. Y., Shin, Y. J., and Wee, W. R.: A case of epidemic keratoconjunctivitis complicated by *Alcaligenes xylosoxidans* infection. Korean J. Ophthalmol. *19*:233-234, 2005.

34. Olson, D. A., and Hoeprich, P. D.: Postoperative infection of an aortic prosthesis with *Achromobacter xylosoxidans*. West. J. Med. *136*:153-157, 1982.

35. Peel, M. M., Hibberd, A. J., King, B. M., et al.: *Alcaligenes piechaudii* from chronic ear discharge. J. Clin. Microbiol. *26*:1580-1581, 1988.

36. Reverdy, M. E., Freney, J., Fleurette, J., et al.: Nosocomial colonization and infection by *Achromobacter xylosoxidans*. J. Clin. Microbiol. *19*:140-143, 1984.

37. Ronne Hansen, C., Pressler, T., Hoiby, N., and Gormsen, M.: Chronic infection with *Achromobacter xylosoxidans* in cystic fibrosis patients: A retrospective case control study. J. Cyst. Fibros. *5*:245-251, 2006.

38. San-Miguel, V. V., Lavery, J. P., York, J. C., et al.: *Achromobacter xylosoxidans* septic arthritis in a patient with systemic lupus erythematosus. Arthritis Rheum. *34*:1484-1485, 1991.

39. Schoch, P. E., and Cunha, B. A.: Nosocomial *Achromobacter xylosoxidans* infections. Infect. Control Hosp. Epidemiol. *9*:84-87, 1988.

40. Sepkowitz, D. V., Bostic, D. E., and Maslow, M. J.: *Achromobacter xylosoxidans* meningitis: Case report and review of the literature. Clin. Pediatr. *26*:483-485, 1987.

41. Shie, S. S., Huang, C. T., and Leu, H. S.: Characteristics of *Achromobacter xylosoxidans* bacteremia in northern Taiwan. J. Microbiol. Immunol. Infect. *38*:277-282, 2005.

42. Shigeta, S., Yasunaga, Y., Honsumi, K., et al.: Cerebral ventriculitis associated with *Achromobacter xylosoxidans*. J. Clin. Pathol. *70*:712-717, 1978.

43. Shin, K. S., Han, K., Lee, J., et al.: Imipenem-resistant *Achromobacter xylosoxidans* carrying blaVIM-2–containing class 1 integrin. Diagn. Microbiol. Infect. Dis. *53*:215-220, 2005.

44. Siebor, E., Llanes, C., Lafon, I., et al.: Presumed pseudobacteremia outbreak resulting from contamination of proportional disinfectant dispenser. Eur. J. Clin. Microbiol. Infect. Dis. *26*:195-198, 2007.

45. Spear, J. B., Fuhrer, J., and Kirby, B. D.: *Achromobacter xylosoxidans* (*Alcaligenes xylosoxidans* subsp. *xylosoxidans*) bacteremia associated with well-water source: Case report and review of the literature. J. Clin. Microbiol. *26*:598-599, 1988.

46. Taylor, P., and Fischbein, L.: Prosthetic knee infection due to *Achromobacter xylosoxidans*. J. Rheumatol. *19*:992-993, 1992.

47. Tena, D., Carranza, R., Barbera, J. R., et al.: Outbreak of long-term intravascular catheter-related bacteremia due to *Achromobacter xylosoxidans* subspecies *xylosoxidans* in a hemodialysis unit. Eur. J. Clin. Microbiol. Infect. Dis. *24*:727-732, 2005.

48. Uy, H. S., Matias, R., de la Cruz, F., and Natividad, F.: *Achromobacter xylosoxidans* endophthalmitis diagnosed by polymerase chain reaction and gene sequencing. Ocul. Immunol. Inflamm. *13*:463-467, 2005.

49. Vu-Thien, H., Moissenet, D., Valcin, M., et al.: Molecular epidemiology of *Burkholderia cepacia*, *Stenotrophomonas maltophilia*, and *Alcaligenes xylosoxidans* in a cystic fibrosis center. Eur. J. Clin. Microbiol. Infect. Dis. *15*:876-879, 1996.

50. Walsh, R. D., Klein, N. C., and Cunha, B. A.: *Achromobacter xylosoxidans* osteomyelitis. Clin. Infect. Dis. *16*:176-178, 1993.

51. Weitkamp, J. H., Tang, Y. W., Haas, D. W., et al.: Recurrent *Achromobacter xylosoxidans* bacteremia associated with persistent lymph node infection in a patient with hyper-immunoglobulin M syndrome. Clin. Infect. Dis. *31*:1183-1187, 2000.

CHAPTER 133

EIKENELLA CORRODENS

Randall G. Fisher

Eikenella corrodens is a facultatively anaerobic, fastidious gram-negative rod that is part of the normal flora of the mouth and the gastrointestinal and genitourinary tracts. Long regarded as a commensal, its pathogenicity no longer is in doubt. It frequently is a pathogen of periodontitis in both adults and children and is a common isolate from wounds that have been contaminated by oral secretions. It also has been recovered from pleuropulmonary infections, central nervous system infections, orbital cellulitis, peritonsillar abscesses, abdominal infections, osteomyelitis, and bloodstream infections, including endocarditis.

BACTERIOLOGY

In 1948, Hendriksen[17] described the organism and called it the *corroding bacillus* because it pitted the agar. It was characterized more fully in 1958 by Eiken,[10] who named it *Bacteroides corrodens*. In 1972, Jackson and Goodman[19] separated two species of corroding bacteria; the strict anaerobe kept the name *B. corrodens* (now called *Bacteroides ureolyticus*), and the facultative anaerobe was classified as *Eikenella*. It is a small, straight, nonmotile gram-negative rod that occasionally is coccobacillary. It is oxidase-positive and catalase-negative. Most strains are lysine- and ornithine decarboxylase-positive. The organism is nonfermentative, reduces nitrate to nitrite, and is urease- and indole-negative.

E. corrodens cell surface components vary from isolate to isolate; these differences probably relate to virulence.[6]

E. corrodens will grow either aerobically or anaerobically, but its growth is not rapid. Growth can be enhanced by 3 to 10 percent carbon dioxide. It grows on blood or chocolate agar but poorly or not at all on MacConkey agar. Selective medium, which contains clindamycin, may increase the yield. Colonies are small and grayish. They look slightly yellow when they are old. Although *E. corrodens* is nonhemolytic, a faint green appearance may be seen on blood agar. Approximately 50 percent will produce the characteristic pitting. They elaborate an odor that resembles that of bleach or hypochlorite.[18]

E. corrodens is a member of the so-called HACEK family of organisms, which have the following in common: (1) slow growth, (2) a requirement for carbon dioxide, and (3) a predilection for infecting heart valves. The other members of the family are *Haemophilus aphrophilus*, *Actinobacillus actinomycetemcomitans*, *Cardiobacterium hominis*, and *Kingella kingae*.

EPIDEMIOLOGY

Infection with *E. corrodens* occurs when mucosal or skin barriers are disrupted and the organism gains access to deeper tissues. Puncture of the skin with forks[32] or toothpicks[38] may result in deep-seated infections. One case of vertebral osteomyelitis that occurred after a woman accidentally inoculated the organism into the paravertebral space by penetration of a fish bone through the posterior pharynx has been reported.[28] In a similar case, a fish bone stuck in the throat for 2 months eventually led to a spinal epidural abscess.[21] Infection commonly occurs after clenched-fist injury as a result of fistfighting.[13] Hand infections in children are more likely to be secondary to digital biting or sucking.[15] Intravenous drug abusers are at risk for injection site and soft tissue abscesses,[14] bacteremia, and endocarditis.[9,31] Elderly persons and patients with advanced carcinomas are the other high-risk groups. However, children are at particularly high risk for serious *E. corrodens* infections.[37] Reports of thyroid abscesses[7,46] and purulent thyroiditis[36] all have been in children. In one review,[23] more than 20 percent of *E. corrodens* pleuropulmonary infections occurred in children younger than 14 years of age, and more than 50 percent of abdominal infections were reported in patients younger than 25 years of age.[8] *E. corrodens* orbital cellulitis,[16] empyema,[41] peritonsillar abscess,[25] paronychia,[1] and osteomyelitis[34,40] have been observed in children. A review of 54 cases of *E. corrodens* infection in children and adolescents revealed that 41 percent of pediatric infections occurred in the head and neck. The most common single site was the thyroid gland.[32]

PATHOPHYSIOLOGY

E. corrodens infections often are polymicrobial[44] and may include other anaerobes or gram-negative rods. However, *E. corrodens* is accompanied most frequently by recovery of alpha-hemolytic streptococci. In most reports, the streptococci were not speciated further, but Jacobs and associates[20] made a case for the *Streptococcus anginosus* group because of similarities between the two organisms (i.e., both are found in the mouth and gastrointestinal tract, both produce local suppurative infection, and both thrive in carbon dioxide-rich, oxygen-poor environments). Brooks and colleagues[4] also reported synergy of the two organisms in a rabbit model of skin infection. In vitro studies of *E. corrodens* co-cultivated with members of the *S. anginosus* group showed that a significant degree of co-aggregation occurs. Additionally, exponential growth of *Streptococcus constellatus* and *Streptococcus intermedius* occurs 6 hours into incubation when these species are grown in the presence of *E. corrodens*; in its absence, exponential growth does not occur until 25 hours after inoculation.[48]

The possible role of *E. corrodens* in periodontitis has not been delineated precisely. However, soluble products of *E. corrodens* induce gene expression and protein production of vascular endothelial growth factor and cause phosphorylation of mitogen-activated protein kinase in vitro, a process that leads to increased production of interleukin-8 and adhesion molecules.[49] This cascade of inflammatory responses could promote chronic periodontitis.

E. corrodens has a propensity toward formation of an abscess in any location, whether alone or in concert with other organisms. Such formation is a hallmark of central nervous system infection.[3] Of intra-abdominal infections reported by Danziger and associates,[8] 15 of 19 patients had abscesses. In two cases of orbital cellulitis reported by Hemady and coworkers,[16] both patients had subperiosteal abscesses. Deep or superficial skin abscesses reported in drug addicts[14] or in clenched-fist injury from fistfighting[13] often recur, even after presumed adequate drainage.[35]

CLINICAL MANIFESTATIONS

Infections with *E. corrodens* are indolent. The time from inoculation to onset of symptoms generally is 1 week or longer.[4] Many cases show initial improvement with treatment but relapse days later, even with appropriate therapy.[15,25,33,37] The head and neck are the most common sites of infection at all ages.[32]

Infection of periodontal sites may be associated with rapid progression and bone resorption thought to be secondary to surface-associated materials of *E. corrodens* and other organisms of periodontitis.[29] Craniofacial and neck infections tend to have prolonged morbidity; many require repeated drainage procedures and long courses of antimicrobial agents.[37] Central nervous system infections often are preceded by sinus infections but also have been seen in children with congenital heart disease.[2,45]

Pleuropulmonary infections are marked by fever, cough, and chest pain. Necrotizing pneumonia with multiple abscesses sometimes is seen. Effusions or empyema are noted in 30 percent, and cavitation is seen in 8 percent. Children with a predisposition toward aspiration may be at higher risk.[23] In one case, a bedridden 16-year-old girl developed a bronchopleural-cutaneous fistula complicating necrotizing pneumonia with empyema.[47]

Endocarditis is associated with large, friable vegetations and frequent emboli and often requires valve replacement.[11] Intravenous drug use has been implicated in approximately half of reported cases.

Abdominal *E. corrodens* infections are seen most commonly as complications of ruptured appendicitis but also have been associated with abdominal trauma and surgery. The clinical course is protracted.[8]

Chorioamnionitis leading to premature delivery has been documented infrequently. In one case, the infection precipitated the birth of twins at 23 weeks' gestation and led to the demise of one twin.[22,24,43]

Soft tissue infections tend to be severe. Many require wide débridement and skin grafting. Infection of underlying joints, tendons, or bones is not infrequent and can be necrotizing and even lead to amputation.[35]

DIAGNOSIS

Definitive diagnosis rests on recovery of *E. corrodens* in culture, which can be a difficult task because of the organism's slow growth. *Eikenella* tends to be overgrown by hardier species when it is part of a polymicrobial process and may be missed, especially if the isolate does not pit the agar. All the HACEK organisms can pit agar,[5] although not with the regularity of *E. corrodens*.

Many bacteriology laboratories have difficulty identifying and separating catalase-negative, oxidase-positive, gram-negative rods. Not surprisingly, one report noted that of 100 isolates of *E. corrodens* identified by the National Collection of Type Cultures, only 21 were sent in as probable *E. corrodens*.[5] Organisms that *E. corrodens* may be mistaken for include the other HACEK organisms, *H. paraphrophilus*, *Moraxella atlantae*, and *Actinobacillus ureae*.

TREATMENT

E. corrodens has a very unusual antimicrobial susceptibility pattern, in that although most isolates are sensitive to penicillin and ampicillin, they are resistant to semisynthetic penicillins, such as methicillin and nafcillin.[42] Additionally, these organisms uniformly are resistant to clindamycin and metronidazole,[18] drugs commonly used to treat anaerobic infections. They also variably are resistant to aminoglycosides.

Most isolates are sensitive to piperacillin, second- and third-generation cephalosporins, and tetracycline. In one report, all of 31 *Eikenella* isolates derived from normal oral flora were sensitive to azithromycin in vitro.[30] Although penicillin often is cited as the drug of choice, some strains produce β-lactamases. One report associated the β-lactamase with a transposon[26] and another with a plasmid[39]; one report found a chromosomal enzyme that was not inducible.[27] In addition, there are reports of intermediate resistance to penicillin, even in isolates that do not produce a β-lactamase.[12]

Incision and drainage of abscesses and débridement of necrotic tissue are essential to recovery from these infections. Therapy should be prolonged after patients apparently have recovered because early cessation of antibiotic therapy tends to be associated with relapse. If patients continue to have fever or other signs of infection days after appropriate therapy has been started, re-imaging of the infected area may be prudent to detect early reaccumulation of purulence.

Acknowledgments

I would like to thank Dr. William Gruber and Dr. Thomas Boyce for their invaluable assistance with earlier versions of this chapter.

REFERENCES

1. Barton, L. L., and Anderson, L. E.: Paronychia caused by HB-1 organisms. Pediatrics 54:372-373, 1974.
2. Brill, C. B., Pearlstein, L. S., Kaplan, M., et al.: Central nervous system infections caused by *Eikenella corrodens*. Arch. Neurol. 39:431-432, 1982.
3. Bronitsky, R., Heim, C. R., and McGee, Z. A.: Multifocal brain abscesses: Combined medical and neurosurgical therapy. South. Med. J. 75:1261-1263, 1982.
4. Brooks, G. F., O'Donoghue, J. M., and Rissing, J. P.: *Eikenella corrodens*: A recently recognized pathogen. Infections in medical-surgical patients and in association with methylphenidate abuse. Medicine (Baltimore) 53:325-342, 1974.
5. Chadwick, P. R., Malnick, H., and Ebizie, A. O.: *Haemophilus paraphrophilus* infection: A pitfall in laboratory diagnosis. J. Infect. 30:67-69, 1995.
6. Chen, C. K. C., and Wilson, M. E.: Outer membrane protein and lipopolysaccharide heterogeneity among *Eikenella corrodens* isolates. J. Infect. Dis. 162:664-671, 1990.
7. Cheng, A. F., Man, D. W. K., and French, G. L.: Thyroid abscess caused by *Eikenella corrodens*. J. Infect. 16:181-185, 1988.
8. Danziger, L. H., Schoonover, L. L., Kale, P., et al.: *Eikenella corrodens* as an intra-abdominal pathogen. Am. Surg. 60:296-299, 1994.
9. Decker, M. D., Graham, B. S., Hunter, E. B., et al.: Endocarditis and infections of intravascular devices due to *Eikenella corrodens*. Am. J. Med. Sci. 292:209-212, 1986.
10. Eiken, M.: Studies on an anaerobic, rod-shaped, gram-negative micro-organism: *Bacteroides corrodens*. Acta Pathol. Microbiol. Scand. 43:391-406, 1958.
11. Ellner, J. J., Rosenthal, M. S., Lerner, P. I., et al.: Infectious endocarditis caused by slow-growing, fastidious, gram negative bacteria. Medicine (Baltimore) 58:145-158, 1979.
12. Goldstein, E. J. C., and Citron, D. M.: Sensitivity of *Eikenella corrodens* to penicillin, apalcillin, and twelve new cephalosporins. Antimicrob. Agents Chemother. 26:947-948, 1984.
13. Goldstein, E. J. C., Miller, T. A., Citron, D. M., et al.: Infections following clenched-fist injury: A new perspective. J. Hand Surg. 3:455-457, 1978.
14. Gonzalez, M. H., Garst, J., Nourbush, P., et al.: Abscesses of the upper extremities from drug abuse by injection. J. Hand Surg. [Am.] 18:868-870, 1993.
15. Harness, N., and Blazar, P. E.: Causative microorganisms in surgically treated pediatric hand infections. J. Hand Surg. [Am.] 30:1294-1297, 2005.
16. Hemady, R., Zimmerman, A., Katzen, B. W., et al.: Orbital cellulitis caused by *Eikenella corrodens*. Am. J. Ophthalmol. 114:584-588, 1992.
17. Hendriksen, S. D.: Studies in gram-negative anaerobes. II. Gram-negative anaerobic rods with spreading colonies. Acta Pathol. Microbiol. Scand. 25:368-375, 1948.
18. Jackson, F. L., and Goodman, Y.: Genus *Eikenella*. *In* Krieg, N. R., and Holt, J. G. (eds.): Bergey's Manual of Systematic Bacteriology. Baltimore, Williams & Wilkins, 1984, pp. 591-597.
19. Jackson, F. L., and Goodman, Y. E.: Transfer of the facultatively anaerobic organism *Bacteroides corrodens* Eiken to a new genus, *Eikenella*. Int. J. Syst. Bacteriol. 22:73-77, 1972.
20. Jacobs, J. A., Algie, G. D., Cie, G. H., et al.: Association between *Eikenella corrodens* and streptococci. Clin. Infect. Dis. 16:173, 1993.
21. Jeon, S. H., Han, D. C., Lee, S. G., et al.: *Eikenella corrodens* cervical spine epidural abscess induced by a fish bone. J. Korean Med. Sci. 22:380-382, 2007.
22. Jeppson, K. G., and Reimer, L. G.: *Eikenella corrodens* amnionitis. Obstet. Gynecol. 78:503-505, 1991.
23. Joshi, N., O'Bryan, T., and Appelbaum, P. C.: Pleuropulmonary infections caused by *Eikenella corrodens*. Rev. Infect. Dis. 13:1207-1212, 1991.
24. Kostadinov, S., and Pinar, H.: Amniotic fluid infection syndrome and neonatal mortality caused by *Eikenella corrodens*. Pediatr. Dev. Pathol. 8:489-492, 2005.
25. Knudsen, T. D., and Simke, E. J.: *Eikenella corrodens*: An unexpected pathogen causing a persistent peritonsillar abscess. Ear Nose Throat J. 74:114-117, 1995.
26. Lacroix, J. M., and Walker, C. B.: Identification of a streptomycin resistance gene and a partial Tn3 transposon coding for a beta-lactamase in a periodontal strain of *Eikenella corrodens*. Antimicrob. Agents Chemother. 36:740-743, 1992.
27. Lacroix, J. M., and Wallar, C.: Characteristics of a beta-lactamase found in *Eikenella corrodens*. Antimicrob. Agents Chemother. 35:886-891, 1991.
28. Lehman, C. R., Deckey, J. E., Hu, S. S.: *Eikenella corrodens* vertebral osteomyelitis secondary to direct inoculation: A case report. Spine 25:1185-1187, 2000.
29. Meghji, S., Wilson, M., Barber, P., et al.: Bone resorbing activity of surface-associated material from *Actinobacillus actinomycetemcomitans* and *Eikenella corrodens*. J. Med. Microbiol. 41:197-203, 1994.
30. Merriam, C. V., Citron, D. M., Tyrrell, K. L., et al.: In vitro activity of azithromycin and nine comparator agents against 296 strains of oral anaerobes and 31 strains of *Eikenella corrodens*. Int. J. Antimicrob. Agents. 28:244-248, 2006.
31. Patrick, W. D., Brown, W. D., Bowmer, M. I., et al.: Infectious endocarditis due to *Eikenella corrodens*: Case report and review of the literature. Can. J. Infect. Dis. 1:139-142, 1990.
32. Paul, K., and Patel, S. S.: *Eikenella corrodens* infections in children and adolescents: Case reports and review of the literature. Clin. Infect. Dis. 33:54-61, 2001.
33. Perez-Pomata, M. T., Dominguez, J., Hercajo, P., et al.: Spleen abscess caused by *Eikenella corrodens*. Eur. J. Clin. Microbiol. Infect. Dis. 11:162-163, 1992.
34. Polin, K., and Shulman, S. T.: *Eikenella corrodens* osteomyelitis. Pediatrics 70:462-463, 1982.
35. Pollner, J. H., Khan, A., and Tuazon, C. U.: Severe soft tissue infection caused by *Eikenella corrodens*. Clin. Infect. Dis. 15:740-741, 1992.
36. Queen, J. S., Clegg, H. W., Council, J. C., et al.: Acute suppurative thyroiditis caused by *Eikenella corrodens*. J. Pediatr. Surg. 23:359-361, 1988.
37. Raffensperger, J. G.: *Eikenella corrodens* infections in children. J. Pediatr. Surg. 21:644-646, 1986.
38. Robinson, L. G., and Kourtis, A. P.: Tale of a toothpick: *Eikenella corrodens* osteomyelitis. Infection 28:332-333, 2000.
39. Rotger, R. E., Garcia-Valdes, E., and Trallero, E. P.: Characterization of a beta-lactamase–specifying plasmid isolated from *Eikenella corrodens* and its relationship to a commensal *Neisseria* plasmid. Antimicrob. Agents Chemother. 30:508-509, 1986.
40. Sagerman, S. D., and Lourie, G. M.: *Eikenella* osteomyelitis in a chronic nail biter: A case report. J. Hand Surg. [Am.] 20:71-72, 1995.
41. St. John, A., Belda, A. A., Matlow, A., et al.: *Eikenella corrodens* empyema in children. Am. J. Dis. Child. 135:415-417, 1981.
42. Sofianou, D., and Kolokotronis, A.: Susceptibility of *Eikenella corrodens* to antimicrobial agents. J. Chemother. 2:156-158, 1990.
43. Sporken, J. M. J., Muyfjens, H. L., and Vemer, H. M.: Intrauterine infection due to *Eikenella corrodens*. Acta Obstet. Gynecol. Scand. 64:683-684, 1985.
44. Suwanagool, S., Rothkopf, M. M., Smith, S. M., et al.: Pathogenicity of *Eikenella corrodens* in humans. Arch. Intern. Med. 143:2265-2268, 1983.
45. Swanston, W. H., Cameron, E. S., and Ramchaunder, V.: *Eikenella corrodens* brain abscess in a child with congenital heart disease. West Indian Med. J. 37:243-245, 1988.
46. Vichyanond, P., Howard, C. P., and Olson, L. C.: *Eikenella corrodens* as a cause of thyroid abscess. Am. J. Dis. Child. 137:971-973, 1983.
47. Wong, K. S., and Huang, Y. C.: Bronchopleural cutaneous fistula due to *Eikenella corrodens*. J. Pediatr. (Rio J.) 81:265-267, 2005.
48. Young, K. A., Allaker, R. P., Hardie, J. M., and Whiley, R. A.: Interactions between *Eikenella corrodens* and "*Streptococcus milleri*–group" organisms: Possible mechanisms of pathogenicity in mixed infections. Antonie Van Leeuwenhoek 69:371-373, 1996.
49. Yumoto, H., Yamada, M., Shinohara, C., et al.: Soluble products from *Eikenella corrodens* induce cell proliferation and expression of interleukin-8 and adhesion molecules in endothelial cells via mitogen-activated protein kinase pathways. Oral Microbiol. Immunol. 22:36-45, 2007.

CHAPTER 134
ELIZABETHKINGIA AND *CHRYSEOBACTERIUM* SPECIES

Randall G. Fisher

Members of the genus *Chryseobacterium* (formerly *Flavobacterium*) seldom are associated with human infection. Most disease occurs after exposure to a contaminated environmental source. In 1944, Shulmann and Johnson[50] reported a case of meningitis caused by a previously unidentified, gram-negative bacillus isolated from a 9-day-old premature infant. The term *Flavobacterium meningosepticum* was proposed for this organism by King[30] in 1959, based on her studies of bacterial isolates associated primarily with neonatal meningitis and septicemia. Although neonatal meningitis is the most common manifestation of human disease caused by this genus,[15,55] sepsis,[14,23,42,52] endocarditis, pneumonia,[44] septic arthritis with penetrating trauma or prosthesis,[22,31] and skin infection[19] (including one case of necrotizing fasciitis)[32] occur in individuals beyond the newborn period.[3]

BACTERIOLOGY

The taxonomy of these organisms is confusing because of frequent changes. All but one of the clinically relevant species of the original genus *Flavobacterium* were reclassified to the new genus *Chryseobacterium* in 1994.[59] Phylogenetic analysis based on 16S rRNA sequencing demonstrated that the organisms formerly classified as *Chryseobacterium meningosepticum* and *Chryseobacterium miricola* represent a separate lineage. Researchers proposed that these two organisms be moved to a new genus, named *Elizabethkingia* after the microbiologist who first described them.[29] The former *Flavobacterium odoratum*, rarely responsible for human disease, has been divided into two species (*odoratus* and *odoratimimus*) reclassified as members of the genus *Myroides*.[58] *Chryseobacterium indologenes* is the species isolated most frequently from human specimens, but it usually is not associated with significant disease. Therefore, this chapter focuses mainly on *Elizabethkingia meningosepticum*, which can cause severe infections, especially in newborns. These organisms are long, thin, catalase-positive, gram-negative rods with slightly swollen ends; they are nonmotile, oxidase-positive, weakly fermentative, and proteolytic and grow on solid agar as 1- to 2-mm, convex, glistening colonies of buttery consistency.[30] Yellow pigmentation is seen occasionally. Colonies do not demonstrate hemolysis on blood agar but may produce a lavender-green color in the surrounding media as a result of extensive proteolytic enzyme activity. *Elizabethkingia* is unable to grow on Salmonella-Shigella agar or Simmons citrate and lacks motility. These characteristics distinguish *Elizabethkingia* from *Pseudomonas*, with which it often is confused.[15] Similarly, utilization of glucose in an open tube of oxidation-fermentation media distinguishes *Elizabethkingia* from *Achromobacter faecalis*.[15] The clinically relevant species *E. meningosepticum* (also referred to interchangeably in the current literature by its old name *Chryseobacterium meningosepticum* and in the older literature as *Flavobacterium meningosepticum*) and *Flavobacterium IIB* (renamed *Flavobacterium balustinum*) are differentiated by the former's consistent liquefaction of gelatin and early utilization of mannitol and maltose and the latter's lack of these abilities.[30] *Myroides odoratus* and *Myroides odoratimimus* (*F. odoratum*), which have been identified most commonly as saprophytes in skin wounds,[26] characteristically are nonsaccharolytic and produce a fruity odor when they are grown on standard media.

EPIDEMIOLOGY

Elizabethkingia spp. and *Chryseobacteria* are distributed widely as saprophytes in fresh and salt water, as well as in the soil. *E. meningosepticum* has been identified as a pathogen in birds.[57] In hospitals, these organisms have been found to be ubiquitous colonizers of the patient's environment and have been isolated from flower vases,[54] ice machines,[52] vials of intravenous drugs,[42] and nebulizers.[16] In addition, tap water,[16] eyewashes,[45] tube feedings,[16] sink traps,[8] and hand cultures of hospital personnel[16] have yielded this organism. In some instances, these reservoirs have been implicated in nosocomial outbreaks of patient colonization and invasive disease.

Neonatal infection caused by *E. meningosepticum* has been reported frequently in the literature, often in association with nursery epidemics.[2,7,47] As with other neonatal pathogens, infants who are premature and small for gestational age seem to be at particular risk of infection. More than 50 percent of infected infants weigh less than 2500 g. Almost all cases occur within 3 weeks of birth, and more than 50 percent of these infants manifest illness before they are 7 days old.[15]

Nosocomial epidemics have occurred sporadically since the nursery outbreak reported by Brody and colleagues in 1958.[2,5,7,8] Cabrera and Davis[8] reported such an outbreak in detail in 1960. During a 3-month period, the bacteria were isolated from a total of 44 infants, of whom 14 had overt infection. Most colonized infants had organisms isolated from the nasopharynx. The only reservoir of infectious bacteria discovered was a faulty sink trap, beneath which cleaning materials for the nursery were stored. Repair of the defective trap and thorough cleansing and repainting of the nursery coincided with termination of the epidemic. More recently, clusters of neonatal and adult systemic infections caused by atypical strains of *E. meningosepticum* were reported from Taiwan. These strains initially were identified erroneously as *Aeromonas salmonicida*.[12]

Nursery outbreaks of *E. meningosepticum* have been traced to saline used to flush infants' eyes after administration of silver nitrate,[45] and organisms have been recovered from washbasins sinks, disinfectants, and suction devices in other epidemics.[8] Colonization of patients in a surgical intensive care unit was associated with tap water, sinks, ice machines, and washbasins yielding the bacteria.[16] Ribotyping and random amplified polymorphic DNA fingerprinting (RAPD) offer promise for more precise characterization of epidemics.[12,13]

PATHOPHYSIOLOGY

Elizabethkingia spp. and *Chryseobacterium* spp. generally are of low virulence. Rabbits administered 1-mL intravenous infections of 24-hour-old broth cultures demonstrated no mortality or morbidity; death rates were less than 30 percent in mice inoculated intracerebrally with "barely turbid" preparations.[30]

Most cases of invasive human disease are thought to be caused by environmental contamination with high numbers of *E. meningosepticum*, with spread to the compromised newborn or debilitated older patient. Some neonatal infections may be caused by colonization of the infant during passage through the birth canal of a colonized mother.[13] Intrapartum infection is supported by occurrence of symptoms as early as 10 hours after birth.[15] However, only 0.3 percent of genital swabs submitted from patients with suspected venereal disease yielded the organism.[41] Continuing reports of *E. meningosepticum* as a cause of neonatal infection in developing countries have been speculated to be related to use of contaminated groundwater for bathing of newborn infants and feminine genital hygiene.[15] The propensity for this organism to produce meningitis in the newborn is not understood, but infection may occur in association with heavy nasopharyngeal colonization, leading to subsequent bacteremia and seeding of the meninges.

Cases in older children have been related to insulin-dependent diabetes mellitus,[9] thalassemia major with splenectomy,[43] and oncologic disease with indwelling catheters.[40] Peritonitis in patients undergoing continuous ambulatory peritoneal dialysis, including a case series of 30 patients, also has been reported.[44]

In older individuals, *E. meningosepticum* and chryseobacteria primarily play the role of opportunists.[38,91] Heavy nosocomial colonization combined with a blunted immune response probably accounts for the immunocompromised patient's poor capacity to handle this otherwise noninvasive bacterium.

CLINICAL MANIFESTATIONS

Neonatal sepsis and meningitis caused by *E. meningosepticum* share signs and symptoms in common with other forms of neonatal bacterial infection. However, the development of meningitis may be insidious, and several days of illness often pass before its presentation[15,47]; this factor is consistent with the low virulence of *E. meningosepticum* in comparison with other agents of neonatal sepsis. Prognosis is extremely poor, and mortality rates may exceed 60 percent.[33] Fifty percent of survivors develop significant neurologic complications, often in association with hydrocephalus.[34]

These organisms are uncommon pathogens in adults, and childhood disease occurring beyond the newborn period is extremely rare. Among the 24 initial isolates of *E. meningosepticum* identified by King,[30] organisms were identified in a throat culture from an adult patient and in cerebrospinal fluid (CSF) from an 8-month-old infant. Bacteria formerly classified as *Flavobacterium IIB* (now known as *F. balustinum*) were isolated from the blood and CSF of several adult patients without clinical information.[27] Since their initial identification in 1959, these agents have been implicated as causes of meningitis,[38,47] postoperative bacteremia,[3,41] bacterial endocarditis,[61] pneumonia,[53,54] catheter-associated infection, septic arthritis, and skin infection.[19] *E. meningosepticum* is the clinically relevant species most commonly isolated, but *C. balustinum*, *M. odoratus* and *M. odoratimus* (*F. odoratum*), and other *Chryseobacterium* spp. have been implicated in human disease. *Elizabethkingia* and *Chryseobacterium* spp. accounted for 0.25 percent of infections in a large consecutive series of patients with human immunodeficiency virus infection. Risk factors included low CD4 counts and leukopenia.[37]

E. meningosepticum meningitis beyond the neonatal period typically occurs in immunocompromised patients. Adults with preexisting leukemia,[47] glomerulonephritis,[38] and squamous cell carcinoma[23] have been described as having meningitis caused by this organism. In a 56-year-old woman, meningitis with *E. meningosepticum* developed after she underwent transsphenoidal hypophysectomy[10]; in an 8-month-old male child with preceding severe neurologic damage, meningitis developed with bacteria designated by the Centers for Disease Control and Prevention as *Flavobacterium*-like organisms (IIE). In a 6-week-old infant, *E. meningosepticum* bacteremia and meningitis developed in association with a strangulated hernia.[15]

Elizabethkingia and *Chryseobacterium* spp. were isolated frequently from tracheal aspirates of patients in intensive care during a 70-month observation period; yet during that time, none of more than 2000 critically ill patients developed pneumonia attributable to these microbes.[16] However, true respiratory tract infection was identified in an intubated pediatric patient and in adults receiving aerosolized medications.[6,54]

Sporadic cases of bacteremia have been reported in adult patients.[23,35] Infection in immunocompromised patients can occur as a complication of relatively benign invasive procedures or as a localized infection.[35,51] Endocarditis was documented in intravenous drug abusers and in patients undergoing dialysis.[18,61] Postoperative bacteremia in eight adult patients was linked to contaminated intravenous medications infused during anesthesia.[42] Contaminated arterial catheters were implicated in an epidemic of *Chryseobacterium* bacteremia.[52] Four patients, including a 7-year-old boy, became bacteremic in an outbreak associated with contamination at the time of intracardiac surgery.[3] This organism also has been associated with bacteremia in pediatric burn patients.[49]

Chryseobacterium spp. also have been isolated from infected skin lesions manifesting as papules, sheet-like lesions, plaques, and deep panniculitis.[19] One fatal case of necrotizing fasciitis in a patient with diabetes mellitus and chronic heart failure was reported.[32] Infection may have been related to wound contamination during repair of an orthopedic injury. Chryseobacteria have been isolated from amputation stumps, but the bacteria may play a largely saprophytic role at these sites.[26]

DIAGNOSIS

Rapid identification of infection with these organisms is urgent, not only to ensure providing proper therapy for the patient, but also to hasten initiating appropriate infection control measures to forestall epidemic outbreaks. Identification of *E. meningosepticum* is hindered by characteristically long periods required for oxidation of carbohydrates and weak or delayed indole production. Cultures may be misidentified as species of *Achromobacter* or *Pseudomonas*.[15] Clinical isolation of an unidentified gram-negative rod that is catalase- and oxidase-positive and that shows multiple antibiotic resistance should raise suspicion of *E. meningosepticum* infection. Cultures should be kept for several days for observation for typical carbohydrate reactions, which confirm the diagnosis.[15,46] Pulse-field gel electrophoresis of DNA was used successfully to identify recurrence of intravenous catheter-associated infection in a 6-year-old boy with non-Hodgkin lymphoma.[4,48]

TREATMENT

Unfortunately, treatment of *E. meningosepticum* meningitis represents an especially difficult challenge for the physician. The organism is paradoxically likely to be sensitive to drugs commonly employed against gram-positive organisms (rifampin, vancomycin, clindamycin, trimethoprim-sulfamethoxazole) and resistant to those used to treat gram-negative infections (aminoglycosides, cephalosporins, tetracyclines, carbapenems). Most *Elizabethkingia* and *Chryseobacterium* spp. produce broad-spectrum metallo–β-lactamases. In *E. meningosepticum*, the enzyme is highly efficient at hydrolyzing carbapenems. Inactivation of cephalosporins displays a remarkable variability that is based on the affinity of the enzyme for the different compounds.[60] Delay in establishing a specific identification of the organism occurs commonly, so the physician knows only that the organism is gram-negative, often resulting in prolonged periods of suboptimal therapy because recommended empiric antimicrobial treatment of gram-negative neonatal meningitis usually consists of a third-generation cephalosporin or ampicillin and an aminoglycoside, drugs to which *E. meningosepticum* almost uniformly is resistant. Moreover, antimicrobial susceptibilities determined by disk diffusion must be interpreted with caution. Aber and associates[1] found clinical isolates in which specific strains were sensitive to gentamicin and rifampin by disk diffusion but were resistant by agar gel dilution susceptibility testing. Therefore, more direct methods of measuring the minimal inhibitory concentration than disk diffusion sensitivity should be used to determine the optimal microbial agents for therapy.

Probably as a consequence of difficulties encountered in providing rapid and effective antibacterial therapy, these organisms frequently persist for prolonged periods in CSF. Average persistence of *E. meningosepticum* in CSF is 19 days,[15] as compared with the 3.9 days described by McCracken[39] for most cases of gram-negative neonatal bacterial meningitis.

Studies of in vitro susceptibility data forced a reappraisal of the idea that vancomycin is a good first-line choice for the treatment of chryseobacterial infection. In one report, a literature review showed that only 65 percent of historic isolates were susceptible to vancomycin[4]; in another, a thorough search for a susceptible organism among 58 clinical isolates met with utter failure.[20] Ninety-seven percent of *E. meningosepticum* isolates were susceptible to rifampin. Clinically, drugs that have been used alone or in combination with some success have included erythromycin, vancomycin, trimethoprim-sulfamethoxazole, fluoroquinolones (especially sparfloxacin and levofloxacin), and rifampin.[56] Some of these agents have the potential disadvantage of poor penetration of CSF. Combined use of many of these drugs renders interpreting therapeutic response difficult. The 3 survivors among the 12 patients reported by George and associates[21] all received vancomycin intravenously, intrathecally, or both, as a part of their regimen. Hawley and Gump[24] reported a case of *E. meningosepticum* meningitis in a neonate who responded to systemic vancomycin after unsuccessful treatment with multiple antibiotics, including erythromycin.

Intraventricular erythromycin[17,47] or rifampin[11,33,34,47] has been used in conjunction with systemic administration of these drugs. In particular, Lee and associates[34] reported no deaths in seven infants with *E. meningosepticum* meningitis who were treated with intraventricular rifampin through an Ommaya reservoir at a dose of 2 to 5 mg every 24 hours combined with 40 mg/kg/day administered intravenously. Intraventricular administration continued until the CSF was sterile. However, colonization of the Ommaya reservoir was a common finding, and formation of a porencephalic cyst occurred in one patient. Chandrika and Adler[11] reported sterilization of ventricles in one afflicted neonate within 48 hours after institution of therapy with intraventricular and intravenous rifampin. Erythromycin has been used intraventricularly with limited success at 5 to 10 mg/day.[17,47] Rios and Associates[47] reported the successful addition of intraventricular rifampin to a failing regimen of intravenous and intraventricular erythromycin. Development of resistance during therapy has been demonstrated with erythromycin and rifampin[17,47]; persistence of organisms in the CSF despite administration of presumably adequate therapy should alert the physician to test for this possibility. Addition of trimethoprim-sulfamethoxazole may be of benefit with such an occurrence; this agent effected a bacteriologic cure in eight of nine infants with meningitis.[36] This agent usually is not recommended in the neonatal period because of possible displacement of bilirubin from albumin-binding sites. Bacterial eradication was achieved in 48 hours in two patients with meningitis who were treated with clindamycin, rifampin, and cefotaxime systemically and rifampin intraventricularly.[7]

As with other types of gram-negative meningitis, antimicrobial therapy should be continued for at least 2 weeks after sterilization of ventricular fluid has been achieved. Complications of hydrocephalus and the potential use of intraventricular therapy render the neurosurgeon an essential part of the management team. Historically, mortality has been in excess of 70 percent, no doubt in part because of delays in identifying the organism and the limited antibiotic spectrum available for effective therapy. More recent series of patients, although small, suggest some improvement in this statistic, but the rate of morbidity of hydrocephalus and neurologic deficits remains high.

Recovery has been the rule in immunocompetent older individuals infected with contaminated materials, often despite treatment with antibiotics to which the organism was insensitive, a finding highlighting the very low virulence of these organisms in immunocompetent adults.[38] However, significant mortality and morbidity often occur in immunocompromised individuals with bacteremia or meningitis. Use of chloramphenicol, vancomycin, levofloxacin, erythromycin, or rifampin has achieved some success in these patients, but the choice of antibiotic must be based on a detailed examination of the organism's susceptibility.[25,49]

Acknowledgments

I would like to thank Dr. William Gruber and Dr. Thomas Boyce for their invaluable assistance with earlier versions of this chapter.

REFERENCES

1. Aber, R. C., Wennersten, C., and Moellering, R. C., Jr.: Antimicrobial susceptibility of flavobacteria. Antimicrob. Agents Chemother. *14*:483-487, 1978.
2. Abrahamsen, T. G., Finne, P. H., and Lingaas, E: *Flavobacterium meningosepticum* infections in a neonatal intensive care unit. Acta Paediatr. Scand. *78*:51-55, 1989.
3. Berry, W. B., Morrow, A. G., Harrison, D. C., et al.: *Flavobacterium* septicemia following intracardiac operations. J. Thorac. Cardiovasc. Surg. *45*:476-481, 1963.
4. Bloch, K. C., Nadarajah, R., and Jacobs, R.: *Chryseobacterium meningosepticum*: An emerging pathogen among immunocompromised adults. Medicine (Baltimore) *76*:30-41, 1997.
5. Brody, J. A., Moore, H., and King, E. O.: Meningitis caused by an unclassified gram-negative bacterium in newborn infants. Am. J. Dis. Child. *96*:1-5, 1958.
6. Brown, R. B., Phillips, D., Barker, M. J., et al.: Outbreak of nosocomial *Flavobacterium meningosepticum* respiratory infections associated with use of aerosolized polymyxin B. Am. J. Infect. Control *17*:121-125, 1989.
7. Bruun, B., Jensen, E. T., Lundstrom, K., et al.: *Flavobacterium meningosepticum* infection in a neonatal ward. Eur. J. Clin. Microbiol. Infect. Dis. *8*:509-514, 1989.
8. Cabrera, H. A., and Davis, G. H.: Epidemic meningitis of the newborn caused by flavobacteria. I. Epidemiology and bacteriology. Am. J. Dis. Child. *101*:289-295, 1961.
9. Cascio, A., Stassi, G., Costa, G. B., et al.: Chryseobacterium indologenes bacteraemia in a diabetic child. J. Med. Microbiol. *54*:677-680, 2005.
10. Chan, K. H., Chau, P. Y., Wang, R. Y. C., et al.: Meningitis caused by *Flavobacterium meningosepticum* after transsphenoidal hypophysectomy with recovery. Surg. Neurol. *20*:294-296, 1983.
11. Chandrika, T., and Adler, S. P.: A case of neonatal meningitis due to *Flavobacterium meningosepticum* successfully treated with rifampin. Pediatr. Infect. Dis. *1*:40-41, 1982.
12. Chiu, C. H., Waddingdon, M., Greenberg, D., et al.: Atypical *Chryseobacterium meningosepticum* and meningitis and sepsis in newborns and the immunocompromised, Taiwan. Emerg. Infect. Dis. *6*:481-486, 2000.
13. Colding, H., Bangsborg, J., Fiehn, N. E., et al.: Ribotyping for differentiating *Flavobacterium meningosepticum* isolates from clinical and environmental sources. J. Clin. Microbiol. *32*:501-505, 1994.
14. Coyle-Gilchrist, M. M., Crew, P., and Roberts, G.: *Flavobacterium meningosepticum* in the hospital environment. J. Clin. Pathol. *29*:824-826, 1976.
15. Dooley, J. R., Nims, L. J., Lipp, V. H., et al.: Meningitis of infants caused by *Flavobacterium meningosepticum*. J. Trop. Pediatr. *26*:24-30, 1980.
16. du Moulin, G. C.: Airway colonization by *Flavobacterium* in an intensive care unit. J. Clin. Microbiol. *10*:155-160, 1979.
17. Ferlauto, J. J., and Wells, D. H.: *Flavobacterium meningosepticum* in the neonatal period. South. Med. J. *74*:757-759, 1981.
18. Ferrer, C., Jakob, E., Pastorino, G., et al.: Right-sided bacterial endocarditis due to *Flavobacterium odoratum* in a patient on chronic hemodialysis. Am. J. Nephrol. *15*:82-84, 1995.
19. Findlay, G. H., Hull, P. R., Smith, H. E., et al.: Cutaneous flavobacteriosis: Polymorphous skin granulomas from *Flavobacterium capsulatum*. S. Afr. Med. J. *64*:247-250, 1983.
20. Fraser, S. L., and Jorgensen, J. H.: Reappraisal of the antimicrobial susceptibilities of *Chryseobacterium* and *Flavobacterium* species and methods for reliable susceptibility testing. Antimicrob. Agents Chemother. *41*:2738-2741, 1997.

21. George, R. M., Cochran, C. P., and Wheeler, W. E: Epidemic meningitis of the newborn caused by flavobacteria. II. Clinical manifestations and treatment. Am. J. Dis. Child. *101*:296-304, 1961.

22. Gunnarsson, G., Baldursson, H., and Hilmarsdottir, I.: Septic arthritis caused by *Chryseobacterium meningosepticum* in an immunocompetent male. Scand. J. Infect. Dis. *34*:299-300, 2002.

23. Harrington, S. P., and Perlino, C. A.: *Flavobacterium meningosepticum* sepsis: Disease due to bacteria with unusual antibiotic susceptibility. South. Med. J. *74*:764-766, 1981.

24. Hawley, H. B., and Gump, D. W.: Vancomycin therapy of bacterial meningitis. Am. J. Dis. Child. *126*:261-264, 1973.

25. Hirsh, B. E., Wong, B., Kiehn, T. E., et al.: *Flavobacterium meningosepticum* bacteremia in an adult with acute leukemia: Use of rifampin to clear persistent infection. Diagn. Microbiol. Infect. Dis. *4*:65-69, 1986.

26. Holmes, B., Owen, R. J., and McMeekin, T. A.: Genus *Flavobacterium. In* Krieg, N. R., and Holt, J. G. (eds.): Bergey's Manual of Systematic Bacteriology. Vol. 1. Baltimore, Williams & Wilkins, 1984, pp. 353-360.

27. Holmes, B., Snell, J. J. S., and Lapage, S. P.: *Flavobacterium odoratum*: A species resistant to a wide range of antimicrobial agents. J. Clin. Pathol. *32*:73-77, 1979.

28. Hsueh P. R., Hsiue T. R., Wu J. J., et al.: *Flavobacterium indologenes* bacteremia: Clinical and microbiological characteristics. Clin. Infect. Dis. *23*:550-555, 1996.

29. Kim, K. K., Kim, M. D., Lim, J. H., et al.: Transfer of *Chryseobacterium meningosepticum* and *Chryseobacterium miricola* to *Elizabethkingia* gen. nov. as *Elizabethkingia meningoseptica* comb. nov. and *Elizabethkingia miricola* comb. nov. Int. J. Syst. Evol. Microbiol. *55*:1287-1293, 2005.

30. King, E. O.: Studies on a group of previously unclassified bacteria associated with meningitis in infants. Am. J. Clin. Pathol. *31*:241-247, 1959.

31. Kumar, R., and Stephens, J. L.: Septic arthritis caused by *Chryseobacterium meningosepticum* in an elbow joint prosthesis. South. Med. J. *97*:74-76, 2004.

32. Lee, C. C., Chen, P. L., Wang, L. R., et al.: Fatal case of community-acquired bacteremia and necrotizing fasciitis caused by *Chryseobacterium meningosepticum*: Case report and review of the literature. J. Clin. Microbiol. *44*:1181-1183, 2006.

33. Lee, E. L., Robinson, M. J., Thong, M. L., et al.: Rifamycin in neonatal flavobacteria meningitis. Arch. Dis. Child. *51*:209-213, 1976.

34. Lee, E. L., Robinson, M. J., Thong, M. L., et al.: Intraventricular chemotherapy in neonatal meningitis. J. Pediatr. *91*:991-995, 1977.

35. Lee, M., and Munoz, J.: Septicemia occurring after colonoscopic polypectomy in a splenectomized patient taking corticosteroids. Am. J. Gastroenterol. *89*:2245-2246, 1994.

36. Linder, N., Korman, S. H., Eyal, F., et al.: Trimethoprim-sulphamethoxazole in neonatal *Flavobacterium meningosepticum* infection. Arch. Dis. Child. *59*:582-584, 1984.

37. Manfredi, R., Nanetti, A., Ferri, M., et al.: *Flavobacterium* spp. organisms as opportunistic bacterial pathogens during advanced HIV disease. J. Infect. *39*:146-152, 1999.

38. Mani, R. M., Kuruvila, K. C., Batliwala, P. M., et al.: *Flavobacterium meningosepticum* as an opportunist. J. Clin. Pathol. *31*:220-222, 1978.

39. McCracken, G. H., Jr.: New developments in the management of children with bacterial meningitis. Pediatr. Infect. Dis. *3*(Suppl.):S32-S34, 1984.

40. Nulens, E., Bussels, B., Bols, A., et al.: Recurrent bacteremia by *Chryseobacterium indologenes* in an oncology patient with a totally implanted intravascular device. Clin. Microbiol. Infect. 7:391-393, 2001.

41. Olsen, H., and Raun, T.: *Flavobacterium meningosepticum* isolated from the genitals. Acta Pathol. Microbiol. Immunol. Scand. *79*:102-106, 1971.

42. Olsen, H., Frederiksen, W. C., and Siboni, K. E.: *Flavobacterium meningosepticum* in 8 non-fatal cases of postoperative bacteraemia. Lancet *1*:1294-1296, 1965.

43. Ozkalay, N., Anil, M., Agus, N., et al.: Community-acquired meningitis and sepsis caused by *Chryseobacterium meningosepticum* in a patient diagnosed with thalassemia major. J. Clin. Microbiol. *44*:3037-3039, 2006.

44. Perera, S., and Palasuntheram, C.: *Chryseobacterium meningosepticum* infections in a dialysis unit. Ceylon Med. J. *49*:57-60, 2004.

45. Plotkin, S. A., and McKitrick, J. C.: Nosocomial meningitis of the newborn caused by *Flavobacterium*. JAMA *198*:662-664, 1966.

46. Ratner, H.: *Flavobacterium meningosepticum*. Infect. Control *5*:237-239, 1984.

47. Rios, I., Klimek, J. J., Maderazo, E., et al.: *Flavobacterium meningosepticum* meningitis: Report of selected aspects. Antimicrob. Agents Chemother. *14*:444-447, 1978.

48. Sader, H. S., Jones, R. N., and Pfaller, M. A.: Relapse of catheter-related *Flavobacterium meningosepticum* bacteremia demonstrated by DNA macro-restriction analysis. Clin. Infect. Dis. *21*:997-1000, 1995.

49. Sheridan, R. L., Ryan, C. M., Pasternack, M. S., et al.: Flavobacterial sepsis in massively burned pediatric patients. Clin. Infect. Dis. *17*:185-187, 1993.

50. Shulman, B. H., and Johnson, M. S.: A case of meningitis in a premature infant due to a proteolytic gram-negative bacillus. J. Lab. Clin. Med. *29*:500-507, 1944.

51. Skapek, S. X., Jones, W. S., Hoffman, K. M., et al.: Sinusitis and bacteremia caused by *Flavobacterium meningosepticum* in a sixteen-year-old with Shwachman Diamond syndrome. Pediatr. Infect. Dis. *11*:411-413, 1992.

52. Stamm, W. F., Colella, J. J., Anderson, R. L., et al.: Indwelling arterial catheters as a source of nosocomial bacteremia. N. Engl. J. Med. *292*:1099-1102, 1975.

53. Sundin, D., Gold, B. D., Berkowitz, F. E., et al.: Community-acquired *Flavobacterium meningosepticum* meningitis, pneumonia and septicemia in a normal infant. Pediatr. Infect. Dis. *10*:73-76, 1991.

54. Teres, D.: ICU-acquired pneumonia due to *Flavobacterium meningosepticum*. JAMA *228*:732, 1974.

55. Thong, W. L., Puthucheary, S. D., and Lee, E. L.: *Flavobacterium meningosepticum* infection: An epidemiological study in a newborn nursery. J. Clin. Pathol. *34*:429-433, 1981.

56. Tizer, K. B., Cervia, J. S., Dunn, A. M., et al.: Successful combination vancomycin and rifampin therapy in a newborn with community-acquired *Flavobacterium meningosepticum* neonatal meningitis. Pediatr. Infect. Dis J. *14*:916-917, 1995.

57. Vancanneyt, M., Segers, P., Hauben, L., et al.: *Flavobacterium meningosepticum*, a pathogen in birds. J. Clin. Microbiol. *32*:2398-2403, 1994.

58. Vancanneyt, M., Segers, P., Torck, U., et al.: Reclassification of *Flavobacterium odoratum* (Stutzer 1929) strains to a new genus, *Myroides*, as *Myroides odoratus* comb. nov. and *Myroides odoratimimus* sp. nov. Int. J. Syst. Bacteriol. *46*:926-932, 1996.

59. Vandamme, P., Bernardet, J. F., Segers, P., et al.: New perspectives in the classification of the flavobacteria: Description of *Chryseobacterium* gen. Nov., *Bergeyella* gen. nov., and *Empedobacter* nom. rev. Int. J. Syst. Bacteriol. *44*:474-481, 1994.

60. Vessillier, S., Docquier, J. D., Rival, S., et al.: Overproduction and biochemical characterization of the *Chryseobacterium meningosepticum* BlaB metallo-beta-lactamase. Antimicrob. Agents Chemother. *46*:1921-1927, 2002.

61. Werthamer, S., and Weiner, M.: Subacute bacterial endocarditis due to *Flavobacterium meningosepticum*. Am. J. Clin. Pathol. *57*:410-412, 1972.

CHAPTER

135

PSEUDOMONAS AND RELATED GENERA

Michael T. Brady

The original classification of the genus *Pseudomonas* described a wide variety of aerobic gram-negative rods divided into five rRNA homology groups (homology groups I to V). The genus since has undergone extensive revision, with four of the five homology groups being reclassified into separate genera (Table 135–1).[83] This reclassification was accomplished by using DNA-rRNA hybridization, DNA-DNA hybridization, and 16S rRNA sequencing techniques.

Pseudomonas and related genera are aerobic, motile, non–spore-forming, nonfermentative, gram-negative bacilli that live in soil, in water, and on plants and animals. Most organisms of these genera are ubiquitous and rarely pathogenic in humans. Although the pseudomonads may produce disease in any individual, they usually are opportunists that more commonly cause disease in patients with burns, cystic fibrosis, malignant diseases, and immunodeficiency conditions; in recipients of immunosuppressive therapy; or in malnourished persons. The most important of the opportunistic pseudomonads is *Pseudomonas aeruginosa*. However, numerous other pseudomonads cause specific clinical syndromes in children.

TABLE 135-1 Recent Toxignomic Changes and Reclassification of *Pseudomonas* Homology Groups I to V That Cause Disease in Humans

Homology Group	Previous Designation	Current Designation
I		*Pseudomonas aeruginosa*
		Pseudomonas fluorescens
		Pseudomonas putida
		Pseudomonas stutzeri
		Pseudomonas mendocina
		Pseudomonas pseudoalcaligenes
		Pseudomonas alcaligenes
		Pseudomonas (CDC group 1)
	Chryseomonas luteola	*Pseudomonas luteola*
	Flavimonas oryzihabitans	*Pseudomonas oryzihabitans*
II	*Pseudomonas cepacia*	*Burkholderia cepacia*
	Pseudomonas gladioli	*Burkholderia gladioli*
	Pseudomonas mallei	*Burkholderia mallei*
	Pseudomonas pickettii	*Ralstonia pickettii*
	Pseudomonas pseudomallei	*Burkholderia pseudomallei*
III	*Pseudomonas acidovorans*	*Delftia acidovorans*
	Pseudomonas testosteroni	*Comamonas testosteroni*
	Pseudomonas delafieldii	*Acidovorax delafieldii*
	Hydrogenomonas facilis	*Acidovorax facilis*
IV	*Pseudomonas diminuta*	*Brevundimonas diminuta*
	Pseudomonas vesicularis	*Brevundimonas vesicularis*
V	*Xanthomonas maltophilia*	*Stenotrophomonas maltophilia*
		Stenotrophomonas africana

CDC, Centers for Disease Control and Prevention.
Data from Gilligan, P. H., and Whitier, S.: Burkholderia, Stenotrophomonas, Ralstonia, Brevundimonas, Comamonas, and Acidovorax. In Murray, P. R., Baron, J., Pfaller, M. A., et al. (eds.): Manual of Clinical Microbiology. 7th ed. Washington, D.C., ASM Press, 1999, pp. 526-538.

ETIOLOGY

Pseudomonas spp. usually are gram-negative obligate aerobes (oxygen as the terminal electron acceptor), but they can grow anaerobically in the presence of nitrates or arginine (terminal electron acceptors). They lack the phosphoenolpyruvate-hexose-phosphotransferase system and catabolize carbohydrates by the Entner-Doudoroff pathway. Because pseudomonads can use a wide variety of carbon sources (simple and complex carbohydrates, alcohols, and amino acids), they can survive and multiply in almost any moist environment containing minimal amounts of organic compounds.

P. aeruginosa is the most clinically important species of the genus *Pseudomonas*. It is an oxidase-positive, gram-negative rod varying in size from 0.5 to 0.8 μm by 1.5 to 3.0 μm. Most strains are motile by one or more polar, monotrichous flagella and display fine projections (pili or fimbriae). *P. aeruginosa* grows readily on standard laboratory media. It grows optimally at 37° C but not at 4° C. Clinical *Pseudomonas* isolates are oxidase-positive (except for *Pseudomonas luteola* and *Pseudomonas oryzihabitans*) and catalase-positive. On MacConkey agar, *Pseudomonas* spp. are identified as nonlactase fermenters. They do not ferment carbohydrates but do oxidize monosaccharides such as glucose and xylose, but not maltose. Strains from clinical specimens may produce beta-hemolysis on blood agar. More than 90 percent of *P. aeruginosa* organisms produce a bluish-green phenazine pigment (pyocyanin-blue pus), as well as fluorescein, a yellow-green fluorescent pigment. Occasional *Pseudomonas* strains also produce dark red (pyorubin) or black (pyomelanin) pigment. These pigments diffuse into and color the medium surrounding the colonies. Strains of *P. aeruginosa* can be differentiated from one another for epidemiologic purposes by serologic typing, phage typing, ribotyping, and pyocin (bacteriocin) typing.

EPIDEMIOLOGY

P. aeruginosa is a ubiquitous environmental organism found in soil, in water, and on vegetation, including the surface of many raw fruits and vegetables. It was recognized first as a pathogen when Gessard recovered it from green pus in 1882. Its minimal nutritional requirements and ability to grow in a wide variety of physical environments enhance the organism's ability to survive in numerous ecologic niches. *P. aeruginosa* is found infrequently as normal microflora of healthy humans. The gastrointestinal (GI) tract is the most frequent site of human colonization. As many as 5 to 30 percent of normal persons have *P. aeruginosa* in their GI tract, although it rarely is the predominant organism. The large intestine is the most frequent site of transient colonization after ingestion. Other moist body sites that may become colonized include the throat, nasal mucosa, axillae, perineum, and the respiratory tract of patients who have been hospitalized for extended periods, have foreign bodies in place (endotracheal tubes or tracheostomies), have poor mucociliary clearance, and have received broad-spectrum antibiotics or chemotherapy. In general, *P. aeruginosa* is an opportunistic and not a frank pathogen. Despite the ability to colonize skin and mucosal surfaces, it rarely results in persistent colonization, it does not produce specific toxic factors that damage host tissues, and it is not capable of invading normal skin or mucosa. *P. aeruginosa* proves most effective as a pathogen in situations in which the host's immune defenses are diminished or lacking (e.g., poor mucociliary clearance in children with cystic fibrosis, neutropenia in children receiving chemotherapy for cancer, damaged skin barriers in burned patients).

P. aeruginosa frequently enters the hospital environment on the clothes, skin, respiratory tract, or shoes of patients or hospital personnel; colonization of any moist environment ensues. Thus, these organisms may be found growing in distilled water, hospital kitchens and laundries, mops, shower heads, whirlpools, antiseptic solutions, eyedrops, irrigation fluid, dialysis fluid, and equipment used for dialysis and respiratory care or inhalation therapy. Transmission of *P. aeruginosa* from patient to patient or from hospital personnel to patient often is assumed but rarely is documented.[54,242] In hospitalized patients, the likelihood of *Pseudomonas* colonization increases with the duration of hospitalization.

Sources of *Pseudomonas* outside the hospital that may result in colonization with subsequent infection include swimming pools, water slides, hot tubs, contact lens solutions, cosmetics, illicit injectable drugs, and the inner soles of sneakers. *P. aeruginosa* commonly is found on the surface of many types of raw fruits and vegetables. Consumption of these foods by profoundly immunosuppressed children can result in GI colonization and potentially can lead to invasive disease.

The environmental distribution of most of the other *Pseudomonas* spp. and related genera is similar to that of *P. aeruginosa*. *Pseudomonas pseudoalcaligenes* has one of the more unusual habitats. This organism has been identified in metalworking fluid (a mixture of water and petroleum products) at concentrations as high as 10^8 organisms per milliliter or higher. Metalworkers are exposed to aerosols containing high concentrations (10^5 organisms per milliliter) of *P. pseudoalcaligenes*.[138] Despite the development of high antibody levels to *P. pseudoalcaligenes*, these metalworkers with long-term exposure do not have clinical evidence of any acute or chronic respiratory or systemic disease.

Burkholderia, formerly *Pseudomonas cepacia*, is a plant pathogen that is ubiquitous in nature and can be found in water, soil, and decaying organic matter.[124] *Burkholderia cepacia* is an obligate aerobic, gram-negative rod that is intrinsically resistant to a wide range of antimicrobial agents, including aminoglycosides and carboxypenicillins (e.g., ticarcillin, azlocillin, and piperacillin). Historically, it was regarded as an organism with low pathogenicity. However, *B. cepacia* has been identified increasingly as a cause of sporadic nosocomial outbreaks of infection in medical intensive care units. Outbreaks are far less common than with *P. aeruginosa*. When they occur, they have been traced to contaminated automated peritoneal dialysis machines, blood gas analyzers, povidone-iodine, and chlorhexidine.[20,21,88,215] *B. cepacia* can survive for extended periods in moist environments and even in the presence of disinfectants, including povidone-iodine.[6] Colonization of the respiratory tract, sometimes associated with endobronchial infection in patients with cystic fibrosis, is becoming a more common occurrence and is associated with increased morbidity and mortality. This organism also has become more important as a cause of infection and complications in patients with chronic granulomatous disease[219] and sickle-cell hemoglobinopathies.[22]

Stenotrophomonas maltophilia (formerly *Xanthomonas maltophilia*) is an aerobic gram-negative rod that grows readily on most bacteriologic media. *S. maltophilia* is being isolated with increasing frequency in hospitalized patients. Colonization of nonsterile sites such as the respiratory tract and wounds in the absence of clinical disease occurs commonly in hospitalized patients receiving long-term or broad-spectrum antibiotics. However, clinical illnesses such as pneumonia, urinary tract infections, endocarditis, bacteremia, meningitis, and peritonitis have been reported.[16,61,73,149,231] Isolation of *S. maltophilia* from the respiratory tract of patients with cystic fibrosis is increasing; in some centers, it is the second most frequent gram-negative bacterium isolated from sputum.[13,117]

Burkholderia pseudomallei is most prevalent in the tropical and subtropical areas of Southeast Asia and northern Australia. *B. pseudomallei* has been recovered frequently from rice paddy surface water in rice-growing areas of northern Thailand.[47,216]

PATHOGENESIS

The pathogenesis of *Pseudomonas* infections is multifactorial.[17,133] Although *P. aeruginosa* is not uncommonly a human saprophyte, it usually causes disease as an opportunistic pathogen. *P. aeruginosa* is a significant cause of infection in compromised hosts. Its ability to adapt to a variety of environments, its minimal nutritional requirements, and its propensity for the development of antibiotic resistance allow *P. aeruginosa* to survive in compromised patients. The requirement of oxygen for growth may account for the lack of invasiveness of these organisms after they have colonized and even infected the skin. *P. aeruginosa* possesses a variety of virulence factors, including an endotoxin, an enterotoxin, numerous extracellular enzymes, and cell-bound organelles such as flagella and pili. *P. aeruginosa* endotoxin is not as potent as are the endotoxins produced by other gram-negative organisms (2 to 3 mg needed to kill a 20-g mouse). However, *P. aeruginosa* endotoxin does protect the organism from the effects of complement and triggers cytokine pathways that lead to the sepsis syndrome and shock. This endotoxin may produce a diarrheal syndrome. A *Pseudomonas* enterotoxin also has been described, but its role in causing diarrhea in humans remains unclear.

The extracellular enzymes of *P. aeruginosa* include lecithinase, collagenase, lipase, elastase (LasA and LasB), caseinase, gelatinase, fibrinolysin, hemolysin, alkaline protease, phenazines, phospholipase C, exoenzyme S, exoenzyme U, and exotoxin A. The proteolytic enzymes may be responsible for localized necrosis of the skin or lung and for corneal ulceration. Exotoxin A is an adenosine-5′-diphosphate ribosyltransferase enzyme that inhibits the synthesis of eukaryotic cell protein (same mechanism as diphtheria toxin). Specific exotoxin A–deficient mutants of *P. aeruginosa* have reduced virulence in producing infection of the cornea or lung in mice and rats.[161,245] Exotoxin A also diminishes the activity of host phagocytes. Passive or active immunization against

exotoxin A significantly protects against experimental infection with exotoxin-producing strains of *P. aeruginosa*. Phospholipase C degrades phospholipids, which are plentiful in eukaryotic but not prokaryotic cell membranes. The hemolysis produced by *P. aeruginosa* may be caused by heat-labile phospholipase C and by a heat-stable moiety. Exoenzyme S is another virulence factor.

In patients with burn injuries, *P. aeruginosa* growing in the burned area produces exoenzyme S; *P. aeruginosa* on intact skin does not.[158] In burned patients in whom *Pseudomonas* sepsis develops, exoenzyme S can be found in the blood before the bacteria can be detected. *P. aeruginosa* strains that lack exoenzyme S production are less able to cause invasive disease.[198]

The various proteases also can degrade numerous plasma proteins such as complement and coagulation factors.[246] Solubilization and destruction of lecithin (surfactant) may play a role in the atelectasis seen in pulmonary infections caused by *P. aeruginosa*. A leukocidin also has been described that may in part be capsular material. The purified slime from *Pseudomonas* is nontoxic. Pigments produced by *P. aeruginosa* also are nontoxic.

Surface structures such as pili and fimbriae are involved in attachment of *P. aeruginosa* to the epithelial cells of mucosal surfaces. *P. aeruginosa* that lack flagella are less capable of dissemination from wounds and of causing bacteremia and pneumonia in animal models.[8,55,65] *P. aeruginosa* preferentially binds to normal respiratory mucin, in contrast to some members of the family Enterobacteriaceae.[234] Fibronectin may protect epithelial cells from bacterial attachment, but the ability to do so is reduced in patients with cystic fibrosis (high levels of protease in respiratory secretions) and after cellular injury (trauma after intubation and viral infection of the lower respiratory tract, especially influenza virus). The glycocalyx (extracellular slime layer) is important in allowing *P. aeruginosa* organisms to adhere to each other and form microcolonies, which impair phagocytosis and antibody and antibiotic activity.

The pathogenicity of *P. aeruginosa* also depends on its ability to resist phagocytosis. Fick and Reynolds[69] noted that in patients with cystic fibrosis, the opsonic function of immunoglobulin G (IgG) was reduced as a result of a molecular change in the Fc portion of the IgG molecule. This deficit was magnified in the lungs of patients with cystic fibrosis infected with *P. aeruginosa* because bacterial proteases can fragment IgG and further impair its opsonic activity, which already may be marginal. The persistent presence of *P. aeruginosa* in the lungs of patients with cystic fibrosis also may be related to the presence of one or more factors in their sputum that interfere with the bactericidal activity of fresh normal human serum against *P. aeruginosa*. These blocking factors have been shown to be IgG antibody that blocks the normal bactericidal IgM activity of human sera.[170,203]

Concentrations of IgG subclass immunoglobulins have been studied in patients with cystic fibrosis and compared with values obtained in age-matched healthy children and adults. Pressler and associates[176] noted that in 52 percent of patients with cystic fibrosis, at least one of the four IgG subclasses had an elevated serum concentration in comparison to controls. A significant correlation of elevated serum concentrations of IgG2 (and, to a lesser extent, IgG3) with decreased forced expiratory volume at 1 second was noted. Moss[147] found that patients with cystic fibrosis who were infected with *P. aeruginosa* had markedly elevated serum concentrations of IgG antibodies to the opsonic immunodeterminant, type-specific lipopolysaccharide. This elevation was distributed among all four IgG subclasses, with a significant shift toward IgG3. Sera from patients with cystic fibrosis who were colonized with *P. aeruginosa* had diminished opsonic capacity, but complement-dependent human neutrophil phagocytosis was not impaired. Serum concentrations of IgG4 but not IgG1, IgG2, or IgG3 were correlated inversely with opsonic capacity. On the basis of these data, Moss[147] suggested that high levels of IgG4 antibody to opsonic immunodeterminants may inhibit normal pulmonary clearance of *P. aeruginosa* by pulmonary macrophages in vivo.

P. aeruginosa produces two elastolytic enzymes: LasA and LasB. These enzymes are virulence factors produced during infection. They probably cause direct damage to lung tissue (elastin accounts for 30% of the protein of lung tissue) and interfere with immune clearance of *P. aeruginosa* from the lungs. Berger and associates[18] noted that elastase treatment of isolated polymorphonuclear leukocytes severely impaired the ability of the cells to kill opsonized *P. aeruginosa*. These investigators demonstrated proteolytic degradation of C3b receptors and suggested that it may contribute to the inability of patients with cystic fibrosis to eradicate *P. aeruginosa* from their lungs. Because several cell types, including macrophages, monocytes, B lymphocytes, and some T lymphocytes, all carry the same C3b receptor, the proteolytic activity may cleave this molecule from all these cells, thereby decreasing the phagocytic activity of monocytes and macrophages in these patients. Berger and colleagues[18] demonstrated that optimal interaction between the complement-derived opsonic ligands C3b and iC3b and their respective receptors does not occur in the milieu of the lungs of patients with cystic fibrosis who are infected with *Pseudomonas*. These workers suggested that both *Pseudomonas* and host proteases may contribute to the initiation of a cycle of events in which neutrophils entering the infected lung actually impair phagocytosis rather than eradicate the source of these infections. Breakdown of elastin in the walls of blood vessels possibly may be responsible for the intrapulmonary hemorrhage noted in individuals with cystic fibrosis.

The mucoid strains of *P. aeruginosa* isolated from the respiratory secretions of patients with cystic fibrosis produce large quantities of alginate (composed of acetylated D-mannuronic acid and L-glucuronic acid).[39,220] This polysaccharide polymer not only gives *P. aeruginosa* a mucoid appearance on agar but also has antiphagocytic activity. Alginate also can elicit a significant inflammatory immune response in the lungs of patients with cystic fibrosis that may contribute to the lung damage present after chronic *P. aeruginosa* lung infection.[140] Because of its viscous nature, alginate contributes to the thick bronchial secretions in the lungs of children with cystic fibrosis; these secretions obstruct small airways and impair mucociliary clearance and movement of phagocytic cells. Production of alginate by *P. aeruginosa* is regulated and inducible. Mucoid *P. aeruginosa* loses the mucoid trait when it is serially cultured on laboratory media. Nonmucoid isolates convert to the mucoid (alginate-producing) phenotype when they are inoculated into the lung in a rat model.[198]

The role of lipopolysaccharide in the virulence of *P. aeruginosa* also has been studied. The virulence of several strains of *P. aeruginosa* in burned mice was found to be related directly to lipopolysaccharide integrity.[44] Deficiency of the O side chain of lipopolysaccharide reduced virulence markedly.

S. maltophilia and *B. cepacia* are opportunistic organisms with virulence factors that include intrinsic resistance to many antimicrobials effective in treating infection with *Pseudomonas* spp., an ability to adhere to plastic materials,[111] and elaboration of exoenzymes such as elastase and gelatinase.[152] *B. cepacia* also resists nonoxidative neutrophil killing.[219] For both *S. maltophilia* and *B. cepacia*, the following factors increase the risk of colonization occurring with these organisms, as well as progression from colonization to infection: (1) prolonged hospitalization, especially in intensive care settings[138]; (2) administration of broad-spectrum antibiotics[221]; (3) malignant disease, particularly if associated with immunosuppressive therapy and neutropenia[112,221]; and (4) breaks in mucocutaneous defense barriers, chiefly by instrumentation or the use of invasive devices.[112]

CLINICAL MANIFESTATIONS

P. aeruginosa can produce disease in healthy, immunocompetent children.[64] Generally, when disease occurs in previously healthy children, the organism has been introduced into a minor wound contaminated with water, soil, or vegetative material. This contamination is followed by the development of localized cellulitis that typically progresses to an abscess that exudes green or blue pus. The skin lesions (whether caused by direct inoculation or secondary to septicemia) begin as pink macules that progress to small cutaneous hemorrhagic nodules and eventually to areas of necrosis with eschar formation surrounded by an intense red areola (ecthyma gangrenosum; Fig. 135–1). In addition to skin infections, previously healthy children may experience a number of localized and systemic infections, including septicemia, endocarditis, corneal infection, otitis externa, dacryocystitis, mastitis, mastoiditis, meningitis, pneumonia, diarrhea, necrotizing fasciitis, peritonitis, and urinary tract infection. *Pseudomonas* osteochondritis/osteomyelitis may develop after puncture wounds, particularly of the foot.[72] Systemic *P. aeruginosa* infections in healthy children can be life-threatening, with mortality rates reported as high as 55 percent.[232]

Outbreaks of dermatitis (folliculitis), plantar nodules (*Pseudomonas* hot-foot syndrome), otitis externa, mastitis, and urinary tract infections caused by *P. aeruginosa* have been reported in normal, healthy children after the use of community swimming pools, water slides, recreational whirlpools, or family-owned hot tubs.[63,64,71,85,197,214,236] Pruritic or painful skin lesions (5 to 30 mm) develop several hours to 5 days or longer (mean, 48 hours) after contact with these water sources. Skin lesions may be erythematous, macular, or pustular. In some cases, very tender nodules have been observed.[71] Illness may vary from a few scattered lesions in some patients to extensive truncal involvement in others. The rash is most severe in areas occluded by snug-fitting bathing suits. In some children, malaise, fever, otitis externa, vomiting, sore throat, conjunctivitis, rhinitis, pyuria, abdominal cramps, and swollen breasts may be associated with the dermal lesions.

Multiple serotypes of *P. aeruginosa* have been associated with these outbreaks. The use of whirlpool baths usually involves soaking in water for variable periods. Superhydration of skin and exposure to *P. aeruginosa* result in primary cutaneous infection.[92] Whirlpool water is heated to temperatures higher than 37.8° C (100° F) and frequently is not filtered, thereby allowing for the persistence of desquamated skin. Both these factors are conducive to growth of *P. aeruginosa*.

Otitis externa caused by *P. aeruginosa* has been reported in healthy competitive swimmers who swim repetitively in a pool contaminated with *P. aeruginosa*.[182] The organism also has been associated with a more malignant form of otitis externa manifested by high fever, necrosis of portions of the external ear, facial nerve paralysis, mastoiditis, and osteomyelitis of the temporal bone and basilar skull.[95,154] Rarely, *P. aeruginosa* meningitis results from progression of this infection.[173] Malignant otitis externa usually is associated with predisposing factors such as malnutrition, leukopenia (a disorder of leukocyte function), malignant disease, or diabetes mellitus. Successful management of this condition requires aggressive surgical débridement in addition to appropriate systemic antibiotic therapy.

P. aeruginosa is a common agent of chronic suppurative otitis media (with or without cholesteatoma) and acute and chronic mastoiditis.[33,109,159] Chronic suppurative otitis media is a complication of inadequately treated acute otitis media and is manifested by a perforated tympanic membrane with persistent otorrhea. Chronic suppurative otitis media also occurs in children with surgically induced perforations of the tympanic membrane by

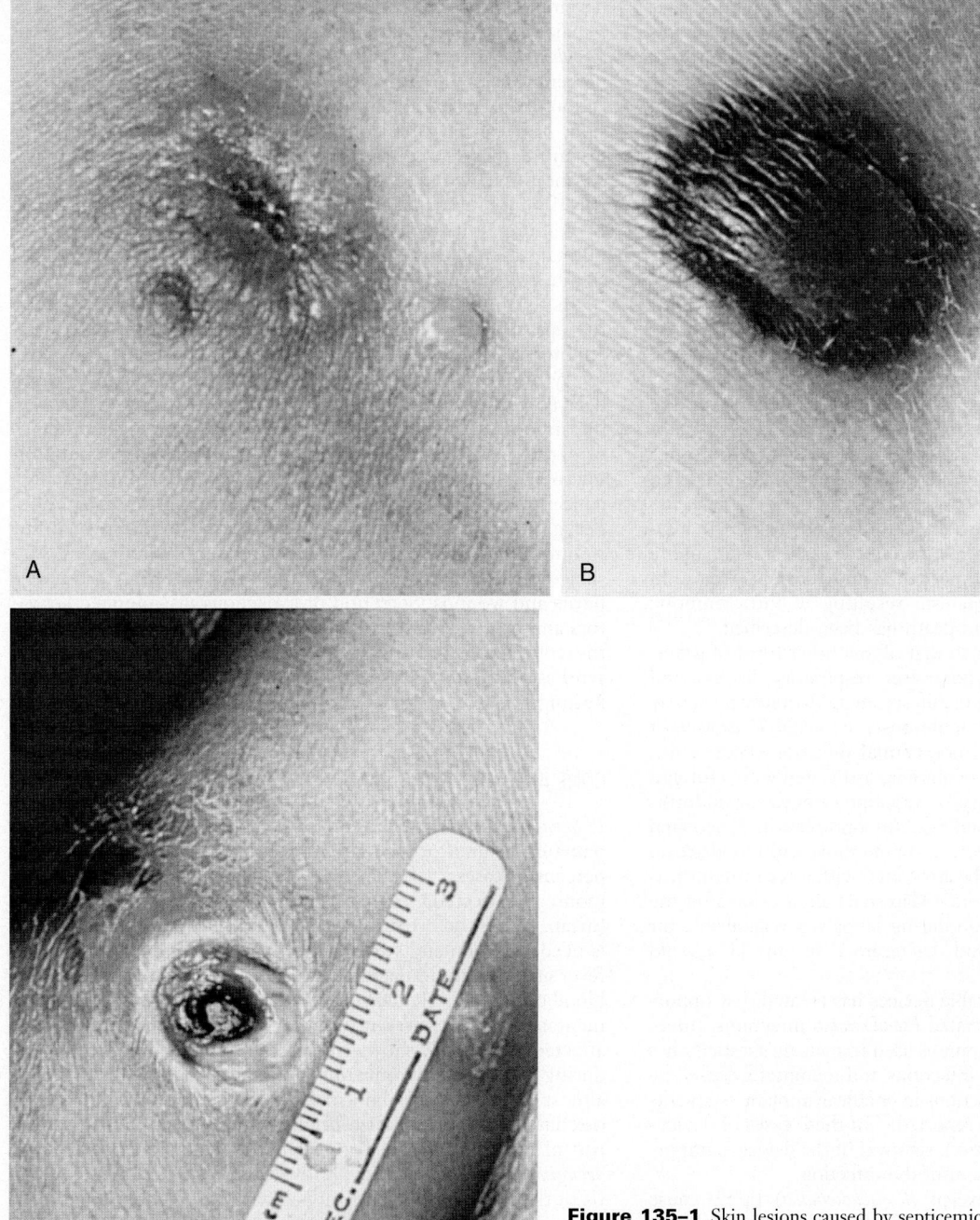

Figure 135–1 Skin lesions caused by septicemic *Pseudomonas aeruginosa* infection. **A,** A large macule has begun to undergo central necrosis and is surrounded by two smaller macules. **B,** A small cutaneous nodule representing the skin lesion of septicemic *P. aeruginosa*. **C,** A final stage of ecthyma gangrenosum in which a cutaneous hemorrhagic nodule has undergone central necrosis and eschar formation.

tympanostomy tubes and incompletely or inadequately treated otitis media. The etiologic microbial agents of acute otitis media in children with tympanostomy tubes differ from those in children with intact tympanic membranes. *P. aeruginosa* has been recovered from 12 percent of children with acute otitis media and

tympanostomy tubes.[190] When tympanostomy tubes become colonized with *P. aeruginosa*, eradication of the infection may be complicated by the production of a biofilm.[26] The presence of a biofilm reduces the effectiveness of conventional systemic and topical antimicrobial therapy. Outpatient therapy with oral antibiotics frequently is unsuccessful because of the lack of oral antimicrobial agents with antipseudomonal activity. Topical ciprofloxacin with or without dexamethasone has been shown to be effective and superior to oral amoxicillin/clavulanic acid in the treatment of acute otitis media in children with otorrhea through tympanostomy tubes.[53] Intravenous antibiotics targeting the bacterial agents isolated from middle ear aspirates may be needed to cure chronic suppurative otitis media. This therapy may preclude the necessity of performing tympanomastoid surgery, which becomes essential in patients with extensive granulation tissue and osteitis in the mastoid.

P. aeruginosa ear infections were reported after commercial ear piercing.[107] In these patients, upper ear cartilage was involved more commonly than was lobe piercing. Re-use of a "single-use" disinfectant bottle contaminated at a sink harboring *P. aeruginosa* was implicated.[107]

P. aeruginosa infection of the eye usually occurs after trauma or surgery, after deposition of a large inoculum topically, or by hematogenous spread. Using contaminated contact lens solution, using tap water during contact lens care, and endotracheal suctioning without covering the eyes of sedated or comatose patients have been implicated.[91,94] Infection of the cornea can result in ulceration, which may progress to more invasive disease, including endophthalmitis. Loss of vision may result, even if appropriate antimicrobial therapy is administered promptly.

P. aeruginosa may produce serious infections during the neonatal period. Septicemia may be noted in the earliest hours of life and is associated with high morbidity and mortality rates. In utero acquisition of the organism resulting in intra-amniotic infection, neonatal sepsis, and death has been described.[160,194,252] The clinical course is similar to that of any other form of gram-negative septicemia, with hypotension, respiratory distress, and skin lesions the predominant manifestations. Mortality rates may be as high as 80 percent.[102] Late-onset neonatal *P. aeruginosa* infection usually occurs as a nosocomial infection (bacteremia, urinary tract infection, and pneumonia) associated with a foreign body (e.g., indwelling urinary or vascular catheter or endotracheal tube) in hospitalized infants. An outbreak in a neonatal intensive care unit of *P. aeruginosa* pneumonia and bloodstream infection was determined to be associated with intermittent otitis externa in a health care worker.[253] Maternal colonization after the use of a hot tub for relaxation during labor was responsible for *P. aeruginosa* meningitis and bacteremia in an 11-day-old infant.[233]

Increasing use of implantable devices has created new opportunities for health care–associated *Pseudomonas* infections. Infections of intrathecal baclofen pumps used to manage spasticity has been associated with wound infections and meningitis caused by *P. aeruginosa*.[248] Delayed infections in cochlear implant recipients with *P. aeruginosa* have been reported.[79] In these cases of device-associated *Pseudomonas* infection, removal of the device is important for successful management of the infection.

Other pseudomonads (except *B. pseudomallei*) rarely cause disease in healthy persons. Reports in normal, healthy children, particularly when these children had been hospitalized in an intensive care unit,[24,204] include the following: pneumonia, keratitis,[129] and abscesses caused by *B. cepacia*; otitis media caused by *Shewanella putrefaciens*; abscesses caused by *Pseudomonas fluorescens*; otitis media, pneumonia, and osteomyelitis[34,192] caused by *Pseudomonas stutzeri*; post-traumatic leg ulcers[169] and brain abscess[227] caused by *Sphingomonas paucimobilis*; and cellulitis, pneumonia, septicemia, endocarditis, peritonitis, and meningitis caused by *S. maltophilia*. *S. maltophilia* septicemia and endocarditis have been associated with intravenous abuse of illicit drugs.[256] Peritonitis and septicemia caused by *B. cepacia*, *S. putrefaciens*, and *S. paucimobilis* have been associated with contamination of equipment used for peritoneal dialysis.[11,20,46,84]

BURNS AND WOUND INFECTION

The surface of wounds or burns frequently is populated by pseudomonads and other gram-negative organisms.[64] Colonization does not imply infection necessarily, but it is a prerequisite to development of invasive disease. Septicemia with *P. aeruginosa* is a major problem in burned patients; the mortality attributed to *Pseudomonas*-associated burn wound sepsis approaches 78 percent.[141] Systemic involvement may be related to the multiplication of organisms in devitalized surface areas, followed by invasion, or it can be associated with the prolonged intravenous or urinary catheterization required for the care of these persons. Antibiotics may diminish the susceptible microbiologic flora but permit more resistant selected strains of *P. aeruginosa* to flourish. In addition, the hydrotherapy that commonly is provided to burned patients promotes colonization of the burned area, as well as other sites.[228]

In burn patients, abnormalities in neutrophil function that precede the onset of septicemia have been described.[3] Killing of *Pseudomonas* by neutrophils is impaired. Burn injury also is associated with abnormal responses to antigens, delayed rejection of homografts, abnormal vascular responses, impaired delayed hypersensitivity responses, diminished uptake of particles by the reticuloendothelial system, and altered antimicrobial pharmacokinetics. Contamination of wounds with high concentrations of bacteria ($>10^5$ colony-forming units [CFUs] per gram of tissue) impedes contraction and healing of the wound.[167] In addition, *P. aeruginosa* produces numerous substances that can further inhibit the natural healing process of burns and wounds. Secretion of exogenous plasminogen activators and proteases breaks down proteins such as fibrin and halts the contraction process.[172] *P. aeruginosa* exotoxin A, a protein synthesis inhibitor, is also a potent cause of retardation of wound healing.[87]

BONE AND JOINT INFECTIONS

P. aeruginosa is the most common cause of osteomyelitis after puncture wounds of the foot and is responsible for more than 90 percent of cases.[27,62,144] The calcaneus or metatarsal bones commonly are affected.[43] Symptoms may be present for 2 to 40 days (mean, 9 days) before diagnosis is established and hospitalization is needed.[43] Pain and swelling are the most common symptoms; fever and wound drainage rarely are noted. Leukocytosis (white blood cell count $>10,000/mm^3$) and an elevated erythrocyte sedimentation rate are present in most patients. Radiographs of the affected foot usually show evidence of osteomyelitis at some time during the period of evaluation and treatment. Bone scan results almost universally are abnormal and frequently yield evidence of osteomyelitis before positive findings on radiographs. The inner pad of sneakers has been implicated as a possible source of *P. aeruginosa* in these patients.[72] However, *P. aeruginosa* osteomyelitis of the foot bones has developed when the puncture occurred through other types of footwear or while the child was barefoot.

Other *P. aeruginosa* infections of bones and joints are uncommon findings in children. When they do occur, they are the result of hematogenous spread of *P. aeruginosa* in patients who are intravenous drug abusers or who have urinary tract or pelvic infections. Although any bone or joint may be affected as a result of *P. aeruginosa* bacteremia, *P. aeruginosa* has a unique predilection for the vertebrae, sternoarticular joints, pelvis, and symphysis pubis. The clinical course of *P. aeruginosa* osteomyelitis or septic arthritis is more indolent than that occurring after infection with *Staphylococcus aureus*. Contiguous spread can occur after penetrating trauma, surgery, or overlying soft tissue infections, especially decubitus ulcers.

CYSTIC FIBROSIS

Cystic fibrosis is one of the most common lethal inherited diseases of children.[64] It is a generalized disorder of salt and water transport that affects the exocrine glands and is caused by mutations in the cystic fibrosis transmembrane conductance regulator (CFTR) gene.[118,191] The course and prognosis are determined largely by chronic infections of the airways with opportunistic bacteria. Death usually results from chronic obstructive pulmonary disease. *P. aeruginosa* can be recovered from cultures in most children with cystic fibrosis. Colonization with *P. aeruginosa* occurs more frequently in children with cystic fibrosis who require pancreatic enzyme supplementation. Recovery of *P. aeruginosa* from the sputum of a child with cystic fibrosis does not imply necessarily infection and the destructive pneumonitis related to this organism. Mucociliary clearance is impeded in patients with cystic fibrosis; as a consequence, they fail to cleanse the bronchopulmonary epithelium of inhaled particles, including bacteria.[118,146] Adherence of *P. aeruginosa* to the airways of children with cystic fibrosis may be enhanced by acidic environment that results from the hyperacidification of the trans-Golgi network caused by the dysfunctional CFTR in cystic fibrosis lung epithelial cells.[175] Colonization of the sputum of patients with cystic fibrosis may reflect the use of mist tents, inhalation therapy, exposure to colonized individuals in health care facilities, cystic fibrosis camps, or at home, and continuous use of broad-spectrum antibiotic therapy.[254] Colonization of the respiratory tract of patients with cystic fibrosis by mucoid strains of *P. aeruginosa* can be correlated with the patient's age, clinical score, extent of pulmonary function abnormalities, severity of changes on chest radiographs, and serum immunoglobulin levels.[68,70] Once *P. aeruginosa* is in the respiratory tract, it rarely is eradicated by antibiotic therapy.

Some observations, however, suggest that the relationship between *Pseudomonas* and patients with cystic fibrosis is more specific. Patients with cystic fibrosis almost always harbor an unusual mucoid *P. aeruginosa* phenotype that produces an excessive amount of capsular slime.[184] The tracheobronchial tree of 70 to 80 percent of these patients is colonized chronically, and the organism infrequently is eradicated either spontaneously or by antibiotic therapy.[80,210] The peculiar lung environment of a patient with cystic fibrosis is thought to trigger a switch to a cluster of genes that code for abundant production of the mucoid polysaccharide (alginate), thereby giving rise to the mucoid phenotype.[39,220] In contrast, mucoid strains of *P. aeruginosa* are recovered from only 0.5 to 1.7 percent of patients without cystic fibrosis. Chronic infection of the lungs in patients with cystic fibrosis causes additional genetic adaptations by *P. aeruginosa*. Chronic, persistent infection results in the loss of genes responsible for virulence factors required for initiation of acute infections.[213] The loss of these virulence factors is presumed to be beneficial for immune evasion. The immune system can recognize these virulence factors, thus leading to effective immune response. Loss of the virulence factors inhibits the immune response from eradicating *P. aeruginosa* from the airways.

Persistence of *P. aeruginosa* within the respiratory tract is aided by growth of the organism in microcolonies embedded in a biofilm of alginate.[93,168] This biofilm allows nutrients to pass while protecting the organism from host defense mechanisms, antibodies, and probably antibiotics.[118] In addition, investigators have noted that rabbit alveolar macrophages fail to phagocytize and kill the organism in the presence of serum from patients with cystic fibrosis. This phenomenon suggests that these patients have a specific, local defect in pulmonary resistance to *P. aeruginosa*.

A clustering of *P. aeruginosa* serotypes also occurs in isolates obtained from patients with cystic fibrosis. Homma type 8 strains may be recovered from 50 to 93 percent of patients with cystic fibrosis.

Bacterial infection in patients with cystic fibrosis is limited almost entirely to the respiratory tract, and pulmonary exacerbations with endobronchial disease are common findings. Infection of the pulmonary parenchyma rarely occurs. Rather, the epithelium of the airways and the submucosa are edematous and contain infiltrates of chronic inflammatory cells. Documentation of a pulmonary exacerbation in cystic fibrosis relies heavily on clinical impression (e.g., increase in the frequency of productive cough, increase in volume or a change in characteristics of the sputum, increase in the respiratory rate or dyspnea, and decrease in appetite, activity, or exercise tolerance). Fever and leukocytosis are present in a minority of patients and are associated with poorer pulmonary function test results and a worse prognostic score.[212] Concentrations of *P. aeruginosa*, DNA (derived from polymorphonuclear leukocytes and, to a lesser extent, from respiratory epithelial cells), and total protein in sputum are increased during pulmonary exacerbations and decrease significantly after administration of antimicrobial therapy.[212] Pulmonary infection in patients with cystic fibrosis generally is chronic. Bronchitis, bronchiolitis, and bronchiectasis can occur. Eventually, local necrotizing pneumonitis may be noted, in contrast to the overwhelming generalized necrotizing pneumonitis seen in immunosuppressed patients. Septicemia is a rare occurrence. However, bacteremia may develop in patients with indwelling venous catheters.

B. cepacia complex has emerged as an increasingly frequent agent of asymptomatic colonization, pneumonia, and septicemia in patients with cystic fibrosis. At least 10 distinct *Burkholderia* spp. are in the *B. cepacia* complex.[131] *Burkholderia cenocepacia* (genomovar III) is the most prevalent species, responsible for nearly half of all clinical isolates in the United States. This species is responsible for most of the cases of the "cepacia syndrome."[130] *Burkholderia multivorans* (genomovar II) accounts for approximately one third of clinical isolates in the United States and generally is thought to be less virulent than is *B. cenocepacia*.[105] A less common species, *Burkholderia dolosa* (genomovar IV), is associated with a rapid deterioration in lung function and decreased rates of survival.[105] Rates of colonization have been as high as 40 percent in some centers.[196] The increased frequency of colonization of the respiratory tract with *B. cepacia* in patients with cystic fibrosis has been associated with increased morbidity and mortality rates in some cystic fibrosis centers since the 1980s. The risk of colonization with *B. cepacia* complex increases with the severity of underlying disease and increasing age.[225] The source or mode of transmission of the organism has not been defined adequately.[131,226] However, more recent information supports person-to-person transmission.[103] Nosocomial transmission (patient-to-patient and contaminated inhalation therapy equipment) within cystic fibrosis centers and social contact, particularly at summer camps, appear to be important in the acquisition of new infection with *B. cepacia*. Once colonization with *B. cepacia* has been identified in patients with cystic fibrosis, three distinct clinical patterns have been noted: (1) chronic asymptomatic carriage (usually in association with *P. aeruginosa*); (2) progressive deterioration over the course of many months, with recurrent acute pulmonary exacerbations accompanied by fever, progressive weight loss, leukocytosis, and an elevated erythrocyte sedimentation rate; and (3) rapid, usually fatal, deterioration in pulmonary function associated with necrotizing pneumonia and, at times, bacteremia (cepacia syndrome).[98,130] The last complication can occur even in patients who were affected only mildly before acquiring *B. cepacia* infection.

B. cepacia has numerous important virulence factors, some of which may play a specific role in the clinical syndromes seen in patients with cystic fibrosis. *P. aeruginosa* enhances subsequent adhesion to epithelial surfaces by *B. cepacia*,[195] a property that may suggest a synergistic relationship between the two bacterial pathogens, particularly in patients with cystic fibrosis.[218] Additionally, *B. cepacia* strains from patients with the most severe progression of cystic fibrosis bind most avidly to mucin.[196]

S. maltophilia was reported first in respiratory cultures of patients with cystic fibrosis in 1975.[76] Since that time, the prevalence of isolation of *S. maltophilia* from patients with cystic fibrosis has been increasing; rates in the United States range from 1.8 to 8.7 percent,[51,148] and many European centers report higher rates. One center in Spain reported a prevalence rate of 30 percent.[12] The prognostic significance of *S. maltophilia* colonization in patients with cystic fibrosis is not certain. In general, new acquisition of *S. maltophilia* does not seem to be associated with an adverse clinical outcome.[51] However, prolonged colonization with *S. maltophilia*, particularly with high bacterial counts in excess of 10^5 to 10^6 CFUs/mL of sputum, may be associated with progressive deterioration in pulmonary function.[12,106]

MALIGNANCY

Children with leukemia, particularly those receiving immunosuppressive therapy and those who are neutropenic, are extremely susceptible to septicemia caused by *P. aeruginosa* and other pseudomonads.[64] Most pseudomonads, including *Pseudomonas putida*, have been reported as causes of septicemia in children with malignant disease.[4] Generally, infection results from invasion of the bloodstream by a colonizing *Pseudomonas* organism (e.g., from the GI tract). Anorexia, malaise, nausea, vomiting, diarrhea, and fever may be noted. Generalized vasculitis develops, and hemorrhagic necrotic lesions can be found in all organs, including the skin, where the lesions appear as purple nodules or ecchymotic areas that become gangrenous.[181] Other invasive *P. aeruginosa* infections noted in children receiving immunosuppressive chemotherapy include hemorrhagic gangrenous perirectal cellulitis or abscess, typhlitis, pre-septal cellulitis, and necrotizing fasciitis.[134,142,233]

Children undergoing treatment of malignant diseases are particularly vulnerable to bacterial infection. Chemotherapy and radiation therapy can disrupt mucocutaneous barriers and result in moderate to severe immunosuppression. Fergie and associates[66] described 98 children and adolescents with cancer in whom *P. aeruginosa* bacteremia developed; the rate of bacteremia was highest in patients with leukemia. Most cases occurred when patients had absolute neutrophil counts of less than 100/mm³. Mortality associated with *P. aeruginosa* bacteremia was higher in patients with solid tumors, an absolute neutrophil count of less than 100/mm³, perineal skin lesions, and bacteremia during remission or induction therapy rather than during a relapse.

The single most important factor that predisposes children with cancer to development of infection is granulocytopenia. The bactericidal capacity of children with leukemia and other neoplasms also may be impaired. Heat-stable opsonins specific for *P. aeruginosa* similarly may fall precipitously in children with acute leukemia who are receiving intensive combination chemotherapy. Fatal infections with *P. aeruginosa* may be related in part to a deficiency of this specific opsonin.

IMMUNOSUPPRESSION

Immunosuppressive agents may be used in the management of malignant diseases, transplantation, or collagen vascular disease. The location of the infectious process and the type of causative organisms depend somewhat on the underlying disease. Infection by *P. aeruginosa*, particularly pneumonia and septicemia, occurs more commonly in children receiving immunosuppressive therapy than in the normal, healthy population.

OTHER CONDITIONS THAT PREDISPOSE TO *PSEUDOMONAS* INFECTION

P. aeruginosa is a major cause of hospital-acquired infections in children. It is the leading cause of nosocomial respiratory tract infection in children undergoing mechanical ventilation or receiving inhalation therapy. Asymptomatic colonization of the upper and lower airways occurs commonly and should be distinguished from respiratory tract disease, tracheitis, and pneumonia. A predominance of gram-negative bacilli with an abundance of polymorphonuclear leukocytes on Gram stain of lower respiratory tract secretions, in conjunction with a positive culture for *P. aeruginosa*, strongly supports the role of *P. aeruginosa* as the causative agent for the lower respiratory tract infection. Absence of *P. aeruginosa* from lower respiratory tract secretions markedly reduces the likelihood that *P. aeruginosa* is in the lower respiratory tract.

P. aeruginosa septicemia occurs with increased frequency in children with indwelling vascular or urinary catheters.[223] In addition, septicemia may occur in children with congenital or acquired neutropenia or in persons with a functional deficit in polymorphonuclear leukocyte function. Urinary tract infections also have been associated with cystoscopic examination. *Pseudomonas* is a common cause of abscesses and meningitis in children with dermoid sinus tracts or dermoids extending down to or communicating with the meninges or neural tissue and in children with meningomyeloceles. *P. aeruginosa* may produce acute or subacute endocarditis in children with congenital cardiac lesions before or after they undergo cardiac surgery and in adolescents who inject illicit drugs intravenously. *P. aeruginosa* supraglottitis was reported in a 6-month-old child with severe combined immunodeficiency syndrome.[122]

Severe *P. aeruginosa* infections have been reported in children infected with human immunodeficiency virus (HIV), primarily after severe immunodeficiency has developed.[74,189] Risks for acquiring *P. aeruginosa* infection in HIV-infected individuals include hospital exposure, declining CD4+ cell count, and the use of dapsone or trimethoprim-sulfamethoxazole; azithromycin use was reported to be protective.[217] Bacteremia may occur with or without the presence of an indwelling vascular catheter. Fever, hypotension, skin lesions (papules or ecthyma gangrenosum), and pneumonia are common manifestations.[74] Mortality rates can be high, particularly when empiric antimicrobial therapy is inadequate for the treatment of severe, invasive *Pseudomonas* infection.

P. aeruginosa causes endocarditis on both native and prosthetic heart valves. Fortunately, it is an uncommon occurrence in children because its usual setting is in intravenous drug users. Obviously, *P. aeruginosa* needs to be considered in adolescents, particularly those with a history of intravenous drug use or at risk for acquiring HIV infection, and in infants, children, and adolescents with prosthetic valves or other intracardiac synthetic material. Tricuspid valve involvement occurs most commonly, but involvement of multiple valves is possible with *P. aeruginosa*; the manifestations are typical of subacute endocarditis. When the left side of the heart is involved (aortic or mitral valves), the patient has acute and more fulminant disease. Fever and heart murmur are almost universal findings.

DISEASE CAUSED BY OTHER PSEUDOMONADS

In addition to causing respiratory tract infection in patients with cystic fibrosis, *B. cepacia* can result in other infections, primarily in hospitalized or immunocompromised patients. Nosocomial pneumonia in ventilated patients, bacteremia, wound infections, urinary tract infections, meningitis, endocarditis, and skin lesions may be caused by *B. cepacia*. Fortunately, all these infections are uncommon occurrences in children.

S. maltophilia has been reported with an ever-expanding spectrum of clinical manifestations, most notably bacteremia, endocarditis, lower respiratory tract infection, urinary tract infection, wound infection, meningitis, conjunctivitis, keratitis, dacryocystitis, otitis media, and bone and joint infections. Lower respiratory tract colonization, at times associated with symptomatic disease, is the most common manifestation in children. In addition to its occurrence in children with cystic fibrosis, *S. maltophilia* may be isolated from the respiratory tract of hospitalized children, especially those with endotracheal tubes or tracheostomies. Although colonization usually is asymptomatic, occasionally, lower respiratory tract infection with *S. maltophilia* can result in respiratory deterioration, pneumonitis, and an increased risk of mortality.[119,145]

Bacteremia with *S. maltophilia* usually results from the presence of an intravascular device or an infection of the respiratory, GI, or urinary tracts. Pseudobacteremia with *S. maltophilia* arising from contamination of blood cultures that were performed with blood used to fill nonsterile tubes designed for coagulation studies has been reported.[99] Other infections with *S. maltophilia* in children occur primarily after trauma or instrumentation.

Melioidosis is a rare disease of Southeast Asia and northern Australia that increased in frequency in the United States when Americans returned from Vietnam,[37] Honduras,[37] or El Salvador,[36] and, rarely, after immigration by Southeast Asians.[47,163] The causative agent is *Burkholderia pseudomallei*, an environmental saprophyte of soil and water in the tropics, particularly in rice paddies. *B. pseudomallei* is a small, motile, pleomorphic gram-negative rod without a capsule that exhibits bipolar staining. It is an obligate aerobe that grows best at pH 7 and 37.0° C (98.6° F). Infection occurs after contact of abrasions or wounds with contaminated soil or water, inhalation of contaminated dust, or ingestion of contaminated water. Patients with poorly controlled diabetes, renal disease, or immunocompromised conditions caused by collagen vascular disease, hematologic malignant diseases, or immunosuppressive therapy appear to have an increased risk for development of disease after infection with *B. pseudomallei*.

Transmission most commonly occurs following percutaneous inoculation. Inhalation and ingestion are less common modes of transmission. Hematogenous spread occurs following local infection. Transmission from animals to humans has not been reported. The rat flea and the *Aedes aegypti* mosquito have been reported to infect animals with *B. pseudomallei*, but this route of infection has not been documented in human cases.[164] Human-to-human transmission has occurred during sexual or prolonged close contact.[121] Two cases of mother-to-child transmission of *B. pseudomallei* occurred through breast milk.[179] One mother had obvious mastitis.[179] An outbreak of melioidosis in Australia was traced to a potable water source from a water treatment plant that had irregularities in purification.[96]

Most infections with *B. pseudomallei* remain subclinical. Melioidosis can have a broad spectrum of clinical signs, and symptoms may be latent for months or years before the disease becomes clinically apparent. The initial clinical finding may be a single primary skin lesion (vesicle, pustule, bulla, urticaria) in a patient with no underlying disease. Septicemia occasionally occurs, and multiple abscesses may be noted in every organ of the body. The mortality rate associated with fulminant sepsis approaches 90 percent.[120] Meningitis, encephalitis, arthritis, nodular pulmonary densities, abscesses of liver,[7] lung, spleen, kidney, and bones, and endophthalmitis have been observed in both normal and compromised hosts after or concomitant with an episode of septicemia. The acute septicemic illness is indistinguishable from other types of septicemia caused by gram-negative organisms.

B. pseudomallei can cause myocarditis, pericarditis, endocarditis, intestinal abscess, cholecystitis, acute gastroenteritis, urinary

tract infection, septic arthritis, paraspinal abscess, osteomyelitis, hilar lymphadenopathy, and cervical lymphadenopathy. Parotitis was documented in 38 percent of 126 children with melioidosis in Thailand.[48] None of the 126 children with melioidosis had any apparent predisposition to infection.

Subacute melioidosis generally is characterized by an illness lasting weeks to months. Pulmonary infection in this form of disease is a common occurrence and may mimic tuberculosis. The disease can vary from mild bronchitis to severe, fulminant pneumonitis.[120] Consolidation and cavitation occur frequently.

Neonatal melioidosis has been reported in Thailand.[135] Infants with neonatal septicemia, meningitis, or both, caused by *B. pseudomallei*, have been described. The mode of transmission of this organism to these newborn infants is not always clear. A clear case of mother-to-child transmission of *B. pseudomallei* was reported.[1] The mother had acute melioidosis treated with ofloxacin at 32 weeks' gestation. Consolidation of the right lung of the infant occurred, and an abscess eventually developed. Postpartum cultures of the mother's cervix yielded *B. pseudomallei*.

Chronic melioidosis occurs more frequently in whites than in Asians.[139] Chronic melioidosis may involve every organ in the body, including the brain.[120] Melioidosis may become dormant, with exacerbations occurring years after primary infection when host defenses are impaired as a result of steroid use, burns, diabetes mellitus, or other processes. The longest latent period (24 years) was reported by Kingston.[113]

Melioidosis should be considered in any person who has been to Southeast Asia or northern Australia at any time and has fever of unknown origin, overwhelming sepsis, single or multiple abscesses, or any tuberculosis-like illness. The diagnosis is established by culture of blood, skin lesions, or purulent material from an abscess cavity or from other sites of infection.[125] The organism grows in media commonly used for isolation of gram-negative bacteria. On solid media, the colonies develop slowly (over a week) and have a characteristic daisy-head appearance. Alphahemolysis is noted on sheep blood agar. A selective medium (Ashdown medium) can increase the recovery rate of *B. pseudomallei* from clinical specimens containing mixed bacterial flora, such as throat, rectal, and sputum specimens.[9] *B. pseudomallei* produces a dry, wrinkled, and violet-purple colony with a pungent, earthy odor on Ashdown medium.[81]

Serologic tests are more useful in establishing the diagnosis of melioidosis in latent or asymptomatic forms of this disease.[2,136,156] Hemagglutination (HA), indirect HA, complement-fixation (CF) tests, and an enzyme-linked immunosorbent assay (ELISA) are available. Diagnostic titers are 1:40 or greater for the HA test and 1:10 or greater for the CF test. Because the sensitivity of these serologic tests varies, both should be performed. HA antibodies generally are present within 7 to 14 days after onset of the illness; the CF test yields positive results in 4 to 6 weeks. Maximal titers for both tests are reached in 4 to 6 months. Both HA and CF antibodies persist for 9 months to 2 years after the onset of disease. In the United States, the indirect HA test is used by the Centers for Disease Control and Prevention for the diagnosis of melioidosis. An ELISA that detects specific IgG and IgM antibody to *B. pseudomallei* was developed.[10] This assay proved more suitable than was an IgG indirect fluorescent antibody test in screening for melioidosis and also was more sensitive than was the indirect HA test for melioidosis. Gold blot detection of IgM- and IgG-specific antibodies has been developed[122] and allows serodiagnosis of melioidosis to be made more rapidly. *B. pseudomallei* can be detected in serum by an ELISA method.[244]

DIAGNOSIS AND DIFFERENTIAL DIAGNOSIS

The diagnosis of *Pseudomonas* infection depends on recovery of the organism from blood, cerebrospinal fluid (CSF), and urine obtained in a manner that avoids contamination by cutaneous flora (suprapubic aspiration or urethral catheterization is usually required for young children) and from joint fluid, peritoneal dialysis fluid, or purulent material obtained by aspiration of subcutaneous abscesses or areas of cellulitis. A diagnosis of *Pseudomonas* pneumonia can be made by needle aspiration of the lung and, less convincingly, by recovery of the organism from sputum obtained by postural drainage of a child with cystic fibrosis. Recovery of the organism from the surface of the skin or the throat, a tracheal aspirate, or bronchial secretions may reflect colonization and is not necessarily diagnostic of infection. The validity of a positive culture is enhanced when it is associated with a typical clinical syndrome (e.g., *P. aeruginosa* recovered from a skin lesion typical of whirlpool folliculitis). Isolation of *P. aeruginosa* from the respiratory tract, particularly when the specimen is obtained from an endotracheal tube in an intubated patient, is not an unusual occurrence. Differentiating colonization from infection is clinically important. Gram stain of respiratory secretions obtained by endotracheal suction typically reveals abundant gram-negative rods and polymorphonuclear leukocytes in the setting of a true lower respiratory tract infection caused by *P. aeruginosa* (tracheitis or pneumonitis). An absence of gram-negative rods or the presence of squamous epithelial cells, rather than polymorphonuclear leukocytes, indicates that either the patient does not have a lower respiratory tract infection or, if an infection is present, the etiologic agent is not likely to be *P. aeruginosa*.

Isolation of *Pseudomonas* spp. other than *P. aeruginosa* from clinical specimens occurs far less frequently. Recovery of these *Pseudomonas* spp. from sites that normally are sterile, such as blood or blood product containers, always should be considered clinically significant unless proved otherwise.

Pseudomonas and *Burkholderia* spp. are nutritionally versatile and grow well on most standard laboratory media (such as 5% sheep blood or chocolate agar). They grow optimally at 37° C and also at 42° C, but not at 4° C. All members of both genera grow in broth blood culture systems.[81] Isolation of *Pseudomonas* and *Burkholderia* from specimens with mixed bacterial flora is enhanced by using selective media such as MacConkey agar. Cetrimide, acetamide, nitrofurantoin, and 9-chloro-9[4-(diethylamino)phenyl]-9,10-dihydro-10-phenylacridine hydrochloride (C390) can be used for the isolation of *P. aeruginosa* from clinical as well as environmental specimens. Two media, PC (for *P. cepacia*)[81] and OFPBL (for oxidative-fermentative base-polymyxin B-bacitracin-lactose)[239] agar, inhibit *P. aeruginosa* and are useful for recovery of *B. cepacia* from the sputum of patients with cystic fibrosis.

P. aeruginosa usually is recognized easily on laboratory media by its characteristic colony morphology, diffusible pigment (when present), and odor (resembling sweet grapes or corn tacos). Colonies generally are spreading (sometimes overrunning other organisms in mixed infections) and flat. They usually have a metallic sheen. However, patients with cystic fibrosis typically have *P. aeruginosa* isolates with mucoid colony formation. *P. aeruginosa* can be identified reasonably by the presence of the following: (1) positive oxidase test, (2) triple sugar iron agar reaction of alkaline over no charge, (3) growth at 42° C, and (4) production of a bright blue to blue-green (and, to a lesser extent, red or brown) diffusible pigment on non–dye-containing agar such as Mueller-Hinton. Many laboratories rely on commercial systems for identifying *P. aeruginosa*. For pigmented *P. aeruginosa*, these systems are accurate 70 to 100 percent of the time (average, >90%).[77,186,188] The accuracy with nonpigmented *P. aeruginosa* is significantly less.[115]

The bluish, nodular skin lesions and the ulcers with ecchymotic and gangrenous centers and bright areolae (ecthyma gangrenosum) have been considered to be virtually pathognomonic of *P. aeruginosa* infection. Rarely, skin lesions that are clinically indistinguishable from those caused by *P. aeruginosa* develop after

septicemia secondary to *Aeromonas hydrophila*.[208] Cutaneous or disseminated infections with *Aspergillus* and *Fusarium* in immunocompromised patients also can cause the necrotic skin lesions of ecthyma gangrenosum.

Immunoglobulin antibodies to *P. aeruginosa* surface antigens in serum have been detected reliably by ELISA.[28] Detection of specific IgG and IgA antibodies is not clinically useful for establishing the diagnosis of acute *P. aeruginosa* infection. However, antibody titer increases were associated with active disease caused by *P. aeruginosa* in patients with cystic fibrosis. Antibody titers returned to baseline when *Pseudomonas* infection was controlled by effective antimicrobial therapy. Thus, this assay appears to help in differentiating between early infection and colonization. Antibodies to *P. aeruginosa* also may be detected by immunoblotting (Western blotting).[209] These methods may be sensitive and useful for determining the onset of *P. aeruginosa* infection in patients with cystic fibrosis.

TREATMENT

Systemic infections with *Pseudomonas* should be treated promptly with antibiotics to which the organism is susceptible in vitro.[23,185] Community-acquired *P. aeruginosa* infections typically are sensitive to antipseudomonal penicillins, aminoglycosides, ciprofloxacin, ceftazidime, meropenem, and imipenem. Susceptibility is less predictable for aztreonam, a monobactam. Nosocomially acquired *P. aeruginosa* is more likely to be antibiotic-resistant than are community-acquired strains. Response to treatment may be impaired, and prolonged treatment may be required when systemic infection occurs in an immunocompromised host. Unfortunately, *P. aeruginosa* has been developing resistance to many of the classes of drugs that previously were used to treat this organism. Multidrug-resistant and panresistant *P. aeruginosa* are occurring with increasing frequency, especially in critical care settings. *Multidrug resistance* may be defined when *P. aeruginosa* has diminished susceptibility to more than one of the following five drug classes: aminoglycosides, antipseudomonal cephalosporins, antipseudomonal carbapenems, antipseudomonal β-lactam–β-lactamase inhibitor combinations, and antipseudomonal fluoroquinolones.[165] *Panresistance* may be defined when *P. aeruginosa* has diminished susceptibility to antipseudomonal cephalosporins, antipseudomonal carbapenems, antipseudomonal fluoroquinolones, and antipseudomonal β-lactam–β-lactamase inhibitor combinations.[165] If *P. aeruginosa* organisms retain susceptibility to aminoglycosides while being resistant to the other drug classes, they still should be considered panresistant because aminoglycoside monotherapy in serious infections, especially in critically ill or immunocompromised patients, has a high failure rate.

Prior use of a specific antibiotic may predict the development of resistance to that antibiotic.[60,165] However, use of fluoroquinolones and, to a lesser extent, antipseudomonal β-lactam antibiotics predisposes to multidrug-resistant *P. aeruginosa*.[50,165] Combination therapy has been suggested as a means of reducing the development of resistance while the patient is receiving treatment. Some studies supported the benefit of combination therapy to reduce the development of resistance.[56,237] However, other studies found that antipseudomonal β-lactam antibiotics alone are as effective as is an antipseudomonal β-lactam antibiotic-aminoglycoside combination for preventing the emergence of antibiotic resistance.[166]

Pseudomonas spp. not only exhibit intrinsic resistance to numerous antibiotics but also have the ability to acquire genes encoding resistance determinants. Mechanisms of resistance include production of β-lactamases [AmpC cephalosporinases, PSE β-lactamases, OXA β-lactamases, TEM β-lactamases, SHV-type β-lactamases, PER-1 β-lactamases, and metallo-carbapenemases] and aminoglycoside modifying enzymes [AAC (6′)-I and APH (3′)-II], mutations in topoisomerases II and IV, up-regulation of efflux pumps, and diminished expression of outer-membrane proteins (porin).[165]

Table 135–2 provides dosages of some of the more commonly prescribed antipseudomonal antibiotics.[151] These dosages are only guidelines because the doses of some of these antibiotics may vary with different clinical situations and patient populations. Once-daily administration of aminoglycoside is being evaluated as a way to decrease nephrotoxicity and improve clinical efficacy. Aminoglycoside doses must be decreased, preferably by increasing the dosing interval, in patients with diminished creatinine clearance (e.g., renal impairment, neonates). Significantly higher doses (e.g., 7 to 12 mg/kg/day for gentamicin or tobramycin) may be required for patients with increased total plasma clearance, such as those with cystic fibrosis and burns. Therefore, aminoglycoside therapy must be individualized and doses guided by pharmacokinetic information. Extended-infusion (4-hour infusion every 8 hours) of β-lactam antibiotics (piperacillin-tazobactam) has been considered to enhance the duration of drug concentration that remains in excess of the minimal inhibitory concentration (MIC) of *P. aeruginosa*.[134]

Invasive infections, including septicemia caused by proven or suspected *P. aeruginosa* infection, should be treated with a β-lactam antibiotic (antipseudomonal penicillin, third- or fourth-generation cephalosporin, or carbapenem) combined with an aminoglycoside (gentamicin, tobramycin, netilmicin, or amikacin). The combination of an aminoglycoside and a β-lactam antibiotic may be synergistic against the organism. Rifampin (synergistic in vitro with anti-*Pseudomonas* penicillins and aminoglycosides) may be added to the combination therapy if the clinical response is not adequate. Monotherapy with the cell wall–active β-lactam antibiotics, as well as the fluoroquinolones, frequently leads to the development of antibiotic resistance during therapy as a result of a mutation.[15,205]

P. aeruginosa may be responsible for lower respiratory tract infections in neonates, infants, and children. Involvement of the airways in patients with cystic fibrosis and nosocomial tracheitis or pneumonitis in intubated patients are the most common manifestations. In patients with cystic fibrosis and in critically ill intubated patients, previous use of antimicrobial therapy results in a high frequency of antibiotic-resistant *P. aeruginosa*. Combination therapy with a β-lactam antibiotic and an aminoglycoside is synergistic in vitro and has superior clinical efficacy when compared with monotherapy, particularly with aminoglycosides alone.[89] Quinolones do not appear to be synergistic with either β-lactam antibiotics or aminoglycosides. However, in postpubertal children, quinolones can be used in combination therapy when antibiotic resistance reduces the potential benefit of either the β-lactam antibiotic or the aminoglycoside.

For empiric treatment of *P. aeruginosa* lower respiratory tract disease before antibiotic susceptibility test results are available, the choice of which β-lactam antibiotic and which aminoglycoside will be used should be based on the patient's previous antibiotic experience and knowledge of the usual pattern of antibiotic susceptibility and resistance in the patient's clinical environment. Once susceptibility testing has been completed, at least two effective antibiotics should be included in the patient's regimen. The dose and pharmacotherapeutics of the chosen antibiotics should be optimized. If the patient fails to respond to therapy or if clinical deterioration is noted, acquisition of antibiotic resistance should be anticipated. If antibiotic failure is likely, more than one new antibiotic should be substituted. Selection of the new antibiotic should be guided by previous susceptibility testing and the probable changes that resulted in antibiotic resistance.

The route of administration also may be important with aminoglycoside antibiotics. Penetration of aminoglycosides from blood into respiratory secretions is poor.[19] Topical application of aminoglycosides by aerosolization, particularly through an endotracheal tube, provides much higher concentrations in respiratory

TABLE 135–2   Dosages of Commonly Prescribed Antipseudomonal Antibiotics

Generic Name	Dosage (mg/kg/day)	Route	Interval	Pediatric Precaution
Antipseudomonal Penicillins				
Carbenicillin indanyl sodium	30-50	PO	q6h	SNE
Ticarcillin disodium	200-300	IV	q4-6h	
Ticarcillin/clavulanate	200-300 (ticarcillin)	IV	q4-6h	
Piperacillin	200-300	IV	q4-6h	PDNE
Piperacillin/tazobactam	240 (piperacillin)	IV	q4-6h	PDNE
Cephalosporins				
Ceftazidime	200-300	IV, IM	q6-8h	
Cefepime	100-150	IV, IM	q8-12h	
Aminoglycosides				
Gentamicin sulfate	3-7.5	IV, IM	q8h or q24h	
Tobramycin sulfate	3-7.5	IV, IM	q8h or q24h	
Netilmicin sulfate	3-7.5	IV, IM	q8h or q24h	
Amikacin sulfate	15-22.5	IV, IM	q8h or q24h	
Quinolones				
Ciprofloxacin	20-30	PO, IV	q12h	>18 yr*
Monobactams				
Aztreonam	90-120	IV, IM	q6-8h	SNE
Carbapenems				
Imipenem/cilastatin sodium	60-100	IV, IM	q6h	SNE
Meropenem	60 (meningitis: 120)	IV	q8h	

Safety in children younger than 18 years is not completely established, and use is recommended for specific infections (complicated urinary tract infections, pyelonephritis, and postexposure treatment of inhalation anthrax) and in circumstances in which the benefit outweighs the risk.

IM, intramuscular; IV, intravenous; PDNE, pediatric dose not yet established; PO, oral; SNE, safety in children not yet established.

Data from Bradley J. S., and Nelson J. D.: Nelson's Pocket Book of Pediatric Antimicrobial Therapy. 16th ed. Buenos Aires, Alliance for World Wide Editing, 2006-2007, pp. 94-112.

secretions. This approach results in faster bacteriologic eradication, but clinical efficacy varied in different studies.[30] Administration of aerosolized aminoglycosides to patients with cystic fibrosis resulted in improvement in pulmonary function tests, decreased concentrations of *P. aeruginosa* in sputum, and no significant apparent toxicity. This aerosol treatment did not increase the isolation of *B. cepacia*, *S. maltophilia*, or *Alcaligenes xylosoxidans*; however, isolation of the fungi *Candida albicans* and *Aspergillus* did increase.[31]

Aztreonam, a monobactam antibiotic, has excellent antipseudomonal activity but is not approved for use in pediatric patients. Fluoroquinolones are approved for use in patients younger than 18 years of age to treat complicated urinary tract infections and pyelonephritis and for post-exposure treatment for inhalation anthrax. Polymyxin B and colistin (polymyxin E), used previously, have been superseded largely by less toxic agents, but they may be useful in selected patients who are infected with strains resistant to the other agents. However, all *Burkholderia* spp. are resistant to polymyxin B.

Ciprofloxacin and the other quinolones have been evaluated for the treatment of acute and chronic *P. aeruginosa* infections in teenagers and adults with cystic fibrosis.[100,193,222,224] These antibiotics, which may be given orally or intravenously, proved to be effective, as judged by clinical scores and results of pulmonary function tests. In the United States, quinolone (ciprofloxacin, ofloxacin, norfloxacin, enoxacin, levofloxacin, lomefloxacin, sparfloxacin, and trovafloxacin) use is limited to specific infections until after puberty because these antibiotics may bind cartilage and arrest growth. The information available from clinical trials in Europe suggests that ciprofloxacin and the other quinolones may not be as harmful in children as they are in other juvenile animal species.[41,200,201] However, pefloxacin, a fluoroquinolone that had been used extensively in France, does cause arthropathy in children and adults. In addition, two other quinolones, alatrofloxacin and trovafloxacin, cause acute liver failure, and some cases resulted in patients' deaths. Ciprofloxacin may be considered in selected children when the risks associated with the use of this antibiotic are outweighed by the potential benefits associated with its clinical efficacy (e.g., multiresistant strains of *Pseudomonas*, substitution of an oral quinolone to avoid long-term intravenous therapy requiring an indwelling catheter). If ciprofloxacin is used in a patient younger than 18 years of age for infections other than those for which it is approved, the balance of the risks and benefits of administering ciprofloxacin and alternatives should be explained to the patient and parents or guardians. Ciprofloxacin may be administered in a dosage of 15 mg/kg every 12 hours orally or 10 to 15 mg/kg twice a day intravenously. The oral dosage should not exceed 1000 mg/day in patients who weigh less than 40 kg or 1500 mg/day in patients who weigh more than 40 kg.

Determining the optimal antibiotic therapy for patients with cystic fibrosis may be very problematic. Respiratory cultures may yield *P. aeruginosa* with many different colony morphotypes. These different morphotypes may have significantly different antibiograms. The accuracy of susceptibility testing is improved when different morphotypes are tested individually. However, it is labor-intensive and expensive.

After years of antibiotic exposure, patients with cystic fibrosis commonly are infected with *P. aeruginosa* that is resistant in vitro to all available antimicrobial agents. For these patients, aerosolized tobramycin may be used to yield tobramycin concentrations in the range of 100 to 200 µg/mL of respiratory secretion. Some of these panresistant *P. aeruginosa* strains may be susceptible in vivo when concentrations of tobramycin reach these high levels in respiratory secretions. Susceptibility testing of these panresistant organisms should be performed by either determining MICs or performing an E-test to ascertain whether the organism is susceptible at these higher levels, 100 to 200 µg/mL.[82] In addition

to management of resistant *P. aeruginosa*, aerosolized tobramycin given over a prolonged period (>1 year) may have the potential to eradicate *P. aeruginosa* temporarily from patients with cystic fibrosis who have newly acquired this organism.[180] Confirmation of the efficacy of prolonged antibiotic aerosol therapy may prove valuable because data indicate a poor outcome in children with cystic fibrosis who acquire *P. aeruginosa* by the age of 7 years.[157]

P. aeruginosa endocarditis requires aggressive medical and surgical therapy. Despite combination therapy with maximal β-lactam and aminoglycoside antibiotics, valve replacement (native and prosthetic) frequently is required for cure. When gentamicin or tobramycin is administered in three divided doses per day, peak concentrations should be maintained at 12 to 15 µg/mL. Quinolones should be reserved for patients intolerant of aminoglycosides or whose bacteria are resistant to aminoglycosides or for long-term suppression of *P. aeruginosa* prosthetic valve endocarditis.

Although fortunately uncommon, *P. aeruginosa* infection of the eye can be serious and sight-threatening. *P. aeruginosa* corneal ulcerations or keratitis may be seen in contact lens wearers or in intubated, sedated patients in intensive care units. Topical therapy with ticarcillin, piperacillin, tobramycin, gentamicin, amikacin, ciprofloxacin, or ofloxacin may be used and is effective. Clinical efficacy is improved by frequently clearing inflammatory debris and applying topical antibiotics. Initially, antibiotic solutions should be administered every 15 to 30 minutes. The frequency can be decreased gradually to four to six times a day when clinical improvement is apparent.

P. aeruginosa endophthalmitis frequently occurs after invasive eye surgery or penetrating injuries. Systemic, topical, and intraocular (anterior chamber and vitreous cavity) routes all are required. Even with aggressive medical intervention, return of retinal function seldom is achieved. The prognosis is worse when initiation of therapy is delayed. Ceftazidime, imipenem, and ciprofloxacin have greater intraocular penetration than do the aminoglycosides.[251]

P. aeruginosa meningitis or brain abscess should be treated with ceftazidime (200 mg/kg/day in four divided doses every 6 hours), and an aminoglycoside should be given intravenously. The initial empiric choice of the aminoglycoside should be guided by local susceptibility patterns. Concomitant intraventricular or intrathecal treatment with gentamicin may be required if initial intravenous therapy fails to sterilize the CSF. Gentamicin can be placed into the ventricular or lumbar CSF in a total dose of 1 to 5 mg once each day (the dose is independent of body weight). Meropenem has good penetration into CSF and can be used when the *P. aeruginosa* is ceftazidime-resistant. Meropenem is the preferred carbapenem because the high doses of imipenem required to treat central nervous system (CNS) infections may be associated with CNS toxicity. Fluoroquinolones such as parenteral ciprofloxacin or pefloxacin and aztreonam are possible alternatives in the treatment of *P. aeruginosa* CNS infections if more conventional therapy has failed. However, experience with these agents for CNS infections is limited.[112,127,158,207]

Skin abscesses or abscesses in other locations caused by *P. aeruginosa* should be incised and drained.[181] Failure to do so may result in a poor response despite prolonged systemic antibiotic treatment. Osteomyelitis of foot bones requires surgical débridement in every case. A course of 10 to 14 days of appropriate antibiotics appears to be adequate if surgery has removed the infected tissue effectively.[98] The adequacy of surgical débridement and clinical improvement can be monitored by serial sedimentation rates.[43] *P. aeruginosa* infection of foreign bodies (vascular, peritoneal, and CNS catheters) may require removal of the foreign material to cure the infection, particularly if a tunnel or exit-site infection exists.

Pseudomonas folliculitis and plantar nodules generally are self-limited and do not usually require specific antimicrobial therapy.

More severe cases can be treated by the topical application of any of the following: 2.5 percent acetic acid compresses (vinegar is 5% acetic acid), gentamicin ointment, topical 0.1 percent polymyxin B, or silver sulfadiazine (Silvadene).

The β-lactam antibiotics (antipseudomonal penicillins, cephalosporins, carbapenems), monobactams, and ciprofloxacin are rapidly bactericidal to *P. aeruginosa*.[75] The combination of an aminoglycoside with any of these antibiotics is unlikely to have a significant effect on the initial clinical response rate. However, a reduction in the emergence of drug-resistant *P. aeruginosa* clones is the major potential benefit of combination therapy that includes an aminoglycoside. Combination therapy with two β-lactam antibiotics is inappropriate for serious *Pseudomonas* infections because the induction of β-lactamase may result in resistance to both antibiotics.

Antibiotic resistance is an important factor in patients with serious *Pseudomonas* infections that do not respond to antibiotic therapy. As the quintessential opportunist, *Pseudomonas* has acquired various means to resist the activity of antibiotics. *P. aeruginosa* produces numerous different β-lactamase enzymes. Plasmid-mediated β-lactamases are responsible for resistance to antipseudomonal penicillins but not to the cephalosporins or carbapenems.[42] The most clinically relevant β-lactamases produced by *P. aeruginosa* are encoded primarily chromosomally rather than located on plasmids. Cephalosporinases, classified as class I β-lactamases,[187] produced by *P. aeruginosa* increase on exposure to any of the β-lactam antibiotics (de-repression of the β-lactamase gene).[199] However, the propensity to induce β-lactamase varies among the β-lactam antibiotics.[45] Imipenem and cefoxitin are strong inducers of β-lactamase.[57] All antipseudomonal penicillins, cephalosporins, and aztreonam are susceptible to the class I β-lactamase produced by *P. aeruginosa*.[155]

Clavulanate and tazobactam are β-lactamase inhibitors effective against plasmid-encoded class III and class V β-lactamases and the chromosomally encoded class II β-lactamases found in *P. aeruginosa* and some other gram-negative bacteria. However, these β-lactamase inhibitors not only are ineffective against the common class I β-lactamase of *Pseudomonas* but also are potent inducers of the β-lactamase gene. Use of these β-lactamase inhibitors will not enhance the activity of ticarcillin (Timentin) or piperacillin (Zosyn) against *Pseudomonas* and may actually increase the likelihood of emergence of resistant strains.

Pseudomonas strains with chromosomally encoded class I β-lactamase may not produce detectable β-lactamase until they are exposed to β-lactam antibiotics. These β-lactamase–encoded strains may appear sensitive to β-lactam antibiotics on in vitro sensitivity testing before antibiotic use. However, administration of β-lactam antibiotics to patients colonized or infected with these strains results in the induction of β-lactamase production and emergence of resistance. For this reason, repeat in vitro sensitivity testing of clinical isolates of *Pseudomonas* a few days after the administration of β-lactam antibiotics may reveal reduced sensitivity to β-lactams.

Whereas imipenem and meropenem resist the β-lactamases commonly produced by *Pseudomonas*, resistance to carbapenems can result through the loss of an outer-membrane porin that allows carbapenems to enter *Pseudomonas*.[32] The permeability of other β-lactam antibiotics also may be reduced when this outer-membrane porin is lost. Although chemically distinct from imipenem or meropenem, fluoroquinolones such as ciprofloxacin may induce decreased permeability to both antibiotics.[178] Plasmid-mediated metallo-β-lactamases that confer resistance to imipenem have been described.[143,206,238] Fortunately, these metallo-β-lactamases are identified only rarely in *P. aeruginosa*. Continued use of carbapenems may pressure an increase in these β-lactamases in the future. *S. maltophilia* is resistant innately to imipenem.

Tobramycin is the most active aminoglycoside against *P. aeruginosa*, whereas amikacin induces the lowest frequency of resistant strains. Resistance to aminoglycosides usually results from enzyme-mediated antibiotic modification.[52] The various aminoglycoside-modifying enzymes have different substrate affinities. Therefore, resistance to one aminoglycoside through aminoglycoside-modifying enzymes does not predict resistance to others necessarily. Resistance is less common to amikacin than to other aminoglycosides.[78,250] Aminoglycoside-modifying enzymes usually are coded by plasmid-mediated genes, but they occasionally can be coded by genes on the bacterial chromosome.[52] Plasmid-encoded resistance supports rapid transference among strains within an institution. *P. aeruginosa* also can become resistant to aminoglycosides by decreasing the intracellular uptake of aminoglycosides or by modification of intracellular ribosomal attachment.[49,57] These mechanisms of resistance generally cause cross-resistance for all aminoglycosides.

Ciprofloxacin, a bacterial DNA gyrase inhibitor, is the most effective of the quinolones used against *P. aeruginosa*. Alteration of the binding site of DNA gyrase and decreased penetration of ciprofloxacin through the *Pseudomonas* cell membrane can result in resistant strains.[57,127]

Multidrug resistance is not an unusual occurrence in *P. aeruginosa*, and it may arise after treatment with a single antibiotic. The induction and production of β-lactamase may act synergistically with diminished outer-membrane permeability.[251] In addition, facilitation of energy-dependent efflux of antibiotics by *P. aeruginosa* can result in simultaneous resistance to quinolones, β-lactams, tetracycline, and chloramphenicol.[174,251]

In addition to antibiotic resistance, other clinical factors can adversely affect aminoglycoside activity against *Pseudomonas*. The acidic environment in tissue infected with *P. aeruginosa* can inactivate aminoglycosides.[25] Aminoglycosides may fail to reach therapeutic tissue levels because of poor penetration into bronchial secretions and lung tissue.[19] For patients with tracheitis (e.g., intubated patients) or endobronchial disease (e.g., cystic fibrosis), aminoglycosides and, less frequently, colistin have been administered by aerosol.[202] This route of delivery allows for greater availability of the antibiotic at the site of the infection, with enhanced safety because of negligible absorption into the systemic circulation. Doses of gentamicin and tobramycin of 2.5 to 8 mg/kg can be given safely by aerosol three times a day, with a maximum of 300 mg/dose. Resistance may emerge after prolonged courses.

Antibiotic therapy for *B. cepacia* infection is very challenging and should be guided by results of in vitro susceptibility testing. Unfortunately, *B. cepacia* frequently is resistant to many commonly used antipseudomonal antibiotic agents, particularly the aminoglycosides. Antibiotics that may have activity against *B. cepacia* include ceftazidime, cefoperazone, ureidopenicillins, quinolones, trimethoprim-sulfamethoxazole, and chloramphenicol. Susceptibility to carbapenems and minocycline varies; meropenem has greater in vitro activity against *B. cepacia* than does imipenem.[58] Typically, *B. cepacia* isolates from patients with cystic fibrosis are more antibiotic-resistant than are isolates from other patient populations. Combination therapy with two or three antibiotics may be required to achieve a clinical response. Combinations of β-lactam agents with aminoglycosides may provide synergy clinically, even when the *B. cepacia* strain isolated is aminoglycoside-resistant. *B. cepacia* may be sensitive to minocycline.[119] Minocycline may be considered to have an adjunctive role in the management of *B. cepacia* infection in patients with cystic fibrosis. However, resistance to minocycline commonly develops with prolonged therapy (3 to 13 months).[119]

S. maltophilia also exhibits significant antibiotic resistance to the common antipseudomonal agents. Trimethoprim-sulfamethoxazole, chloramphenicol, ceftazidime, cefoperazone, ticarcillin plus clavulanic acid, and ciprofloxacin may be active against this organism whether these drugs are used alone or in combinations. *S. maltophilia* is resistant to antipseudomonal penicillins, imipenem, and aminoglycosides. A combination of trimethoprim-sulfamethoxazole and ticarcillin-clavulanate has been recommended as the most appropriate initial therapy for serious infections that are suspected or known to be caused by *S. maltophilia*.[230] For patients with catheter-related infections, removal of the catheter offers the greatest opportunity for cure.[61]

The most active antibiotics against *B. pseudomallei* are imipenem, piperacillin-tazobactam, piperacillin, ceftazidime, ticarcillin-clavulanate, ampicillin-sulbactam, tetracycline, and chloramphenicol.[216] Piperacillin, ceftazidime, and imipenem are not bactericidal in vitro.[216] Ciprofloxacin seems to be of limited value because of a high rate of resistance.

Chronic melioidosis can be treated with chloramphenicol over a period of many months or with tetracycline. Trimethoprim-sulfamethoxazole was recommended previously, but most strains currently are resistant.

For acute systemic melioidosis, ceftazidime (120 mg/kg/day) or chloramphenicol (50 to 75 mg/kg/day) plus an aminoglycoside (amikacin, 15 to 20 mg/kg/day) and sulfisoxazole (120 to 150 mg/kg/day) should be administered for a period of 4 weeks. When third-generation cephalosporins have been used, cefoperazone and ceftazidime have shown greater activity against *B. pseudomallei* than have other third-generation cephalosporin agents. Ceftazidime was compared with chloramphenicol, doxycycline, and trimethoprim-sulfamethoxazole for the treatment of severe melioidosis.[241] Ceftazidime, in a dosage of 120 mg/kg/day intravenously in three divided doses every 8 hours, was associated with a 50 percent lower overall mortality rate when compared with other forms of therapy. These results suggest that ceftazidime combined with an aminoglycoside and sulfisoxazole now should be considered the treatment of choice for severe melioidosis.

Soft tissue infections should be treated for 4 to 6 months with tetracycline (in children older than 8 years) provided in a dosage of 50 mg/kg/day in four divided doses. In younger children, trimethoprim-sulfamethoxazole (8 mg/kg/day of trimethoprim and 40 mg/kg/day of sulfamethoxazole) in two divided doses may be used. Most penicillins are ineffective.[59,216] The duration of therapy must be guided by clinical and laboratory findings; therapy for 4 weeks to many months may be required in patients with osteomyelitis. Relapses are common occurrences and should be treated as one would treat the first episode.[38]

PREVENTION

Prevention of infection with pseudomonads depends, in part, on a continuous surveillance program of the hospital environment that is designed to identify and subsequently eradicate sources of pseudomonads as quickly as possible. Transmission of health care–associated *P. aeruginosa* frequently can be traced back to colonization of the water distribution system of the health care institution. Biofilm colonization of faucets can be particularly problematic. However, eradication of *P. aeruginosa* from the water distribution system has not been successful, even after using high water temperatures, copper and silver ionization, or microfilters at faucets or after removing colonized faucets. Because *P. aeruginosa* cannot be eradicated from the environment, other infection control measures, especially good hand hygiene and the use of sterile water to wash patients and patient supplies, should be emphasized. Pseudomonads can grow to a concentration of 10^6 organisms per milliliter in distilled water that appears to be perfectly clear. Growth of pseudomonads in distilled water, disinfectants, and medications is the factor most commonly incriminated in single-source outbreaks of *Pseudomonas* infection in hospitals. Prevention of the follicular dermatitis caused by *P.*

aeruginosa contamination of whirlpools or hot tubs should be possible by maintaining the pool water at a pH of 7.2 to 7.8 and free allowable chlorine concentrations at 0.4 to 1.5 ppm.[35]

Outbreaks of *Pseudomonas* infection in newborn nurseries have been reported.[24] Generally, infection has been transmitted by the hands of personnel from washbasin surfaces and by suction catheter rinse solution to the newborn infants. Strict attention given to handwashing, particularly with a liquid iodophor handwashing agent before and between contact with newborn infants, may prevent or interdict epidemic disease. Growth of *Pseudomonas* on suction catheters can be prevented by rinsing the catheter in an acetic acid solution.

Daily replacement of all apparatus used for intravenous administration greatly reduces the hazard of extrinsic contamination by *Pseudomonas* and other gram-negative organisms. When intravenous administration is indicated, a small metal needle is preferable to a plastic catheter because these needles have been associated with a lower rate of septicemia and phlebitis. Meticulous care is required in the preparation of solutions for total parenteral alimentation and in the insertion and care of catheters.

The risk of developing *Pseudomonas* infection in a burned patient also can be minimized by careful protective isolation and by the topical application of silver nitrate (0.5%) solution or 10 percent mafenide acetate cream. Débridement for removal of devitalized tissue also is imperative.

Pseudomonas infection of dermal abnormalities that communicate with the cerebrospinal axis can be prevented by careful evaluation and early surgical repair. Providing antibiotic prophylaxis of *Pseudomonas* urinary tract infection is difficult without a suitable oral antipseudomonal antibiotic for children. Identification and surgical correction of obstructive lesions of the urinary tract minimize or prevent the development of *Pseudomonas* infection of the urinary tract.

Cohorting plus isolation of patients with cystic fibrosis who are colonized with multiresistant strains of *P. aeruginosa* or *B. cepacia* has been suggested as a means of reducing nosocomial transmission of these organisms.[67] However, the proper manner of handling patients with these organisms has not been established. Any attempt to reduce transmission should be based on measures with proven efficacy and must also consider the potential consequences of strict isolation or segregation on this population, which spends so much time at health care facilities.

In patients with cystic fibrosis and in certain immunocompromised patients, high rates of *P. aeruginosa* colonization and infection and ever-increasing antibiotic resistance render active or passive immunization (or both) against *P. aeruginosa* desirable. Since the 1980s, an understanding of the human immune response to *P. aeruginosa* and the immune responses that may provide protection against infection or disease has increased considerably. Naturally occurring immunity generally is ineffective. Certain naturally generated antibodies may even be detrimental.[240] These antibodies may form antigen-antibody complexes that increase pulmonary inflammation and direct lung damage. Even if neutralizing antibodies could be administered passively or developed after vaccine administration, the large quantities of mucoid exopolysaccharide produced by *P. aeruginosa* could possibly mask many of the antigens targeted for antibody neutralization or opsonization.

Despite the aforementioned difficulties, numerous investigations of candidates for *P. aeruginosa* vaccines are ongoing. Purified bacterial proteins, including flagellar antigen, outer membrane proteins, lipopolysaccharide-O, several inactivated bacterial toxins, high-molecular-weight polysaccharide antigen and glycoconjugate, and killed whole-cell vaccine preparations, have been tested. Many of the candidate vaccines have been shown to be safe, immunogenic, and capable of generating protective immunity in various animal systems.[177] To date, evidence of protective efficacy in humans has not been established definitively for any of these vaccines. Some studies have demonstrated the efficacy of active immunization of burned patients with specific strains of *Pseudomonas* or the administration of hyperimmune globulin in the prevention of *Pseudomonas* septicemia.[3,103] *P. aeruginosa* vaccine also has been suggested as a possible method for preventing or delaying this disease in patients with acute leukemia or cystic fibrosis.[124,171]

The route of vaccine delivery may be important in creating the optimal immune response. Data from experimental animals suggest that vaccine antigens administered parenterally stimulate IgG and IgM antibodies; antigens administered orally induce IgA and IgG at mucosal surfaces. For patients whose disease occurs after mucosal colonization (e.g., cystic fibrosis), oral administration of a *P. aeruginosa* vaccine could be the preferred route of administration to develop the optimal immune response at the site of *P. aeruginosa* infection.

Purified bacterial proteins and lipopolysaccharide from *B. cepacia* are in the initial vaccine research and development stages. Whether these *B. cepacia* vaccine candidates will enter preclinical or phase I clinical trials is yet to be determined.

PROGNOSIS

The prognosis depends largely on the nature of the underlying disease process. Septicemia is the leading cause of death in children with leukemia; *Pseudomonas* is responsible for half of these deaths. Four variables independently influence the outcome of *Pseudomonas* septicemia: (1) the development of septic shock, (2) inappropriate antibiotic therapy, (3) granulocyte counts less than 500/mm^3, and (4) the development of septic metastases.[17] Most deaths in children with cystic fibrosis are caused by pulmonary insufficiency. *Pseudomonas* can be recovered from the lungs of almost every one of these patients, and, in many, it has been responsible for their deaths.

REFERENCES

1. Abbink, F. C., Orendi, J. M., and DeBeaufort, A. J.: Mother-to-child transmission of *Burkholderia pseudomallei*. N. Engl. J. Med. *344*:1171, 2001.
2. Alexander, A. D., Huxsoll, D. L., Warner, A. R., et al.: Serological diagnosis of human melioidosis with indirect hemagglutination and complement fixation titers. Appl. Microbiol. *20*:825-833, 1970.
3. Alexander, J. W., and Fisher, M. W.: Immunization against *Pseudomonas* in infection after thermal injury. J. Infect. Dis. *130*(Suppl.):152-158, 1974.
4. Anaissie, E., Fainstein, V., Miller, P., et al.: *Pseudomonas putida*: Newly recognized pathogen in patients with cancer. Am. J. Med. *82*:1191-1194, 1987.
5. Ancel, A. M., Borque, C., and del Castello, F.: Pseudomonas sepsis in children without previous medical problems. Pediatr. Infect. Dis. J. *12*:258-260, 1993.
6. Anderson, R. L., Vess, R. W., Carr, J. H., et al.: Investigations of intrinsic *Pseudomonas cepacia* contamination in commercially manufactured povidone-iodine. Infect. Control Hosp. Epidemiol. *12*:297-302, 1991.
7. Apisarnthanarak, A., Apisarnthanarak, P., and Mundy, L. M.: Computed tomography characteristic of *Burkholderia pseudomallei* liver abscess. Clin. Infect. Dis. *42*:989-993, 2006.
8. Arora, S. K., Neely, A. N., Blair, B., et al.: Role of motility and flagellin glycosylation in the pathogenesis of *Pseudomonas aeruginosa* burn wound infections. Infect. Immun. *73*:4395, 2005.
9. Ashdown, L. R.: An improved screening technique for isolation of *Pseudomonas pseudomallei* from clinical specimens. Pathology *1*:293-297, 1979.
10. Ashdown, L. R., Johnson, R. W., Koehler, J. M., et al.: Enzyme-linked immunosorbent assay for the diagnosis of clinical and subclinical melioidosis. J. Infect. Dis. *160*:253-260, 1989.
11. Baddour, L. M., Kraus, A. P., Jr., and Smalley, D. L.: Peritonitis due to *Pseudomonas paucimobilis* during ambulatory peritoneal dialysis. South. Med. J. *78*:336, 1985.
12. Ballestero, S., Virseda, I., Escobar, H., et al.: *Stenotrophomonas maltophilia* in cystic fibrosis patients. Eur. J. Clin. Microbiol. Infect. *14*:728-729, 1995.
13. Bauernfeind, A., Bertele, R. M., Harms, K., et al.: Qualitative and quantitative microbiological analysis of sputa of 102 patients with cystic fibrosis. Infection *15*:270-277, 1987.
14. Baussano, I., Tardivo, I., Bellezza-Fontana, R., et al.: Neonatal screening for cystic fibrosis does not affect time to first infection with *Pseudomonas aeruginosa*. Pediatrics *118*:888-895, 2006.
15. Bell, S. M., Pham, J. M., and Lanzarone, J. Y. M.: Mutation of *Pseudomonas aeruginosa* to piperacillin resistance mediated by β-lactamase production. J. Antimicrob. Chemother. *15*:665-670, 1985.
16. Berbari, N., Johnson, D. H., and Cunha, B. A.: *Xanthomonas maltophilia* peritonitis in a patient undergoing peritoneal dialysis. Heart Lung *22*:282-283, 1993.
17. Bergan, T.: Pathogenetic factors of *Pseudomonas aeruginosa*. Scand. J. Infect. Dis. *29*(Suppl.):7-12, 1981.
18. Berger, M., Sorensen, R. U., Tosi, M. F., et al.: Complement receptor expression on neutrophils at an inflammatory site, the *Pseudomonas*-infected lung in cystic fibrosis. J. Clin. Invest. *84*:1302-1313, 1989.
19. Bergogne-Berezin, E.: Pharmacokinetics of antibiotics in respiratory secretions. *In* Pennington, J. E. (ed.): Respiratory Infection: Diagnosis and Management. 2nd ed. New York, Raven Press, 1988, p. 608.
20. Berkelman, R. L., Godley, J., Weber, J. A., et al.: *Pseudomonas cepacia* peritonitis associated with contamination of automatic peritoneal dialysis machines. Ann. Intern. Med. *96*:456-458, 1982.
21. Berkelman, R. L., Lewis, S., Allen, J. R., et al.: Pseudobacteremia attributed to contamination of povidone-iodine with *Pseudomonas cepacia*. Ann. Intern. Med. *95*:32-36, 1981.
22. Berry, M. D., and Asmar, B. I.: *Pseudomonas cepacia* bacteremia in children with sickle cell hemoglobinopathies. Pediatr. Infect. Dis. J. *10*:696-699, 1991.
23. Bisbe, J., Gatell, J. M., Puig, J., et al.: *Pseudomonas aeruginosa* bacteremia: Univariate and multivariate analyses in 133 episodes. Rev. Infect. Dis. *10*:629-635, 1988.
24. Bobo, R. A., Newton, E. J., Jones, L. F., et al.: Nursery outbreak of *Pseudomonas aeruginosa*: Epidemiologic conclusions from five different typing methods. Appl. Microbiol. *25*:414-420, 1973.
25. Bodem, C. R., Lampton, L. M., Miller, D. P., et al.: Relevance to aminoglycoside activity in gram-negative bacillary pneumonia. Am. Rev. Respir. Dis. *127*:39-41, 1983.
26. Bothwell, M. R., Smith, A. L., and Phillips, T.: Recalcitrant otorrhea due to *Pseudomonas* biofilm. Otolaryngol. Head Neck Surg. *149*:599-601, 2003.
27. Brand, R. A., and Black, H.: *Pseudomonas* osteomyelitis following puncture wounds in children. J. Bone Joint Surg. Am. *56*:1637-1642, 1974.
28. Brett, M. M., Ghoneim, A. T. M., and Littlewood, J. M.: Prediction and diagnosis of early *Pseudomonas aeruginosa* infection in cystic fibrosis: A follow-up study. J. Clin. Microbiol. *26*:1565-1570, 1988.
29. Briscoe, D., Rubowitz, A., and Assia E.: Changing bacterial isolates and antibiotic sensitivities of purulent dacryocystitis. Orbit *24*:29-32, 2005.
30. Brown, R. B., Kruse, J. A., Counts, G. W. A., et al.: Double-blind study of endotracheal tobramycin in treatment of gram-negative bacterial pneumonia. Antimicrob. Agents Chemother. *34*:269-272, 1990.
31. Burns, J. L., Van Dalfsen, J. M., Shawar, R. M., et al.: Effect of chronic intermittent administration of inhaled tobramycin on respiratory microbiologic flora in patients with cystic fibrosis. J. Infect. Dis. *179*:1190-1196, 1999.
32. Buscher, K. H., Cullman, W., Dick, W., et al.: Imipenem resistance in *Pseudomonas aeruginosa* resulting from diminished expression of an outer membrane protein. Antimicrob. Agents Chemother. *31*:703-708, 1987.
33. Butbul-Aviel, Y., Miron, D., Halevy, R., et al.: Acute mastoiditis in children: *Pseudomonas aeruginosa* as a leading pathogen. Int. J. Pediatr. Otorhinolaryngol. *67*:277-281, 2003.
34. Carratala, J., Salazar, A., Mascaro, J., et al.: Community-acquired pneumonia due to *Pseudomonas stutzeri*. Clin. Infect. Dis. *14*:792, 1992.
35. Centers for Disease Control: Swimming Pools: Safety and Disease Control through Proper Design and Operation. D. H. H. S. publication number (C. D. C.) 98-411. Washington, D.C., U.S. Government Printing Office, 1979.
36. Centers for Disease Control and Prevention: Laboratory exposure to *Burkholderia pseudomallei*: Los Angeles, California, 2003. M. M. W. R. Morb. Mortal. Wkly. Rep. *53*:988-990, 2004.
37. Centers for Disease Control and Prevention: Imported melioidosis reported in Florida. M. M. W. R. Morb. Mortal. Wkly. Rep. *55*:873-876, 2006.
38. Chaowagul, W., Suputtamongkol, Y., Dance, D. A. B., et al.: Relapse in melioidosis: Incidence and risk factors. J. Infect. Dis. *168*:1181-1185, 1993.
39. Chitnis, C. E., and Ohman, D. E.: Genetic analysis of the alginate biosynthetic gene cluster of *Pseudomonas aeruginosa* shows evidence of an operonic structure. Mol. Microbiol. *8*:583-590, 1993.
40. Chusid, M. J., and Hillman, S. M.: Community acquired *Pseudomonas* sepsis in previously healthy infants. Pediatr. Infect. Dis. J. *6*:681-684, 1987.
41. Chysky, V., Kapila, K., Hullmann, R., et al.: Safety of ciprofloxacin in children: Worldwide clinical experiences based on compassionate use. Emphasis on joint evaluation. Infection *19*:289-296, 1991.
42. Craig, W. A., and Ebert, S. C.: Antimicrobial therapy in *Pseudomonas aeruginosa* infections. *In* Baltch, A. L., and Smith, R. P. (eds): *Pseudomonas aeruginosa* Infections and Treatment. New York, Marcel Dekker, 1994, pp. 441-518.
43. Crosby, L. A., and Powell, D. A.: The potential value of the sedimentation rate in monitoring treatment outcome in puncture-wound–related *Pseudomonas* osteomyelitis. Clin. Orthop. Relat. Res. *188*:172-176, 1984.
44. Cryz, S. J., Jr., Pitt, T. L., Furer, E., et al.: Role of lipopolysaccharides in virulence of *Pseudomonas aeruginosa*. Infect. Immun. *44*:508-513, 1984.

45. Cullman, W., Buscher, K. H., and Dick, W.: Selection and properties of *Pseudomonas aeruginosa* variants resistant to beta-lactam antibiotics. Eur. J. Clin. Microbiol. 6:467-473, 1987.
46. Dan, M., Gutman, R., and Biro, A.: Peritonitis caused by *Pseudomonas putrefaciens* in patients undergoing continuous ambulatory peritoneal dialysis. Clin. Infect. Dis. 14:359-360, 1992.
47. Dance, D. A.: Melioidosis: The tip of the iceberg? Clin. Microbiol. Rev. 4:52-60, 1991.
48. Dance, D. A., Davis, T. M. E., Wattanagoon, Y., et al.: Acute suppurative parotitis caused by *Pseudomonas pseudomallei* in children. J. Infect. Dis. 159:654-660, 1989.
49. Davis, B. D.: Mechanism of bactericidal action of aminoglycosides. Microbiol. Rev. 51:341-350, 1987.
50. Defez, C., Fabbro-Peray, P., Bouziges, N., et al.: Risk factors for multidrug-resistant *Pseudomonas aeruginosa* nosocomial infection. J. Hosp. Infect. 57:209-216, 2004.
51. Demko, C., Doershuk, C., and Stern, R.: Thirteen year experience with *Xanthomonas maltophilia* in patients with cystic fibrosis. Pediatr. Pulmonol. 25:304-308, 1998.
52. Dever, L. A., and Dermody, T. S.: Mechanisms of bacterial resistance to antibiotics. Arch. Intern. Med. 151:886-895, 1991.
53. Dohar, J., Giles, W., Roland, P., et al.: Topical ciprofloxacin/dexamethasone superior to oral amoxicillin/clavulanic acid in acute otitis media with otorrhea through tympanostomy tubes. Pediatrics 118:e561-e569, 2006.
54. Doring, G., Herz, M., Ortelt, J., et al.: Molecular epidemiology of *Pseudomonas aeruginosa* in an intensive care unit. Epidemiol. Infect. 110:427-436, 1993.
55. Drake, D., and Montie, T.: Flagella, motility and invasive virulence of *Pseudomonas aeruginosa*. J. Gen. Microbiol. 134:43, 1988.
56. Drusano, G. L., Sorgel, F., Quinn, J., et al.: Impact of pharmacodynamic dosing of meropenem on emergence of resistance during treatment of ventilator-associated pneumonia: A prospective clinical trial. Abstract K-127. *In* Program and Abstracts of the 45th Interscience Conference on Antimicrobial Agents and Chemotherapy, Washington, D.C. Washington, D.C., American Society of Microbiology, 2005, p. 298.
57. Dunn, M., and Wunderink, R. G.: Ventilator-associated pneumonia caused by *Pseudomonas* infection. Clin. Chest Med. 16:95-109, 1995.
58. Edwards, J. R., and Turner, P. J.: Laboratory data which differentiates meropenem and imipenem. Scand. J. Infect. Dis. 96(Suppl.):5-10, 1995.
59. Eickhoff, T. C., Bennett, J. V., and Hayes, P. J.: *Pseudomonas pseudomallei*: Susceptibility to chemotherapeutic agents. J. Infect. Dis. 121:95-102, 1970.
60. El Amari, E. B., Charnot, E., Auckenthaler, R., et al.: Influence of previous exposure to antibiotic therapy on the susceptibility pattern of *Pseudomonas aeruginosa* bacteremia isolates. Clin. Infect. Dis. 33:1859-1864, 2001.
61. Elting, L. S., and Bodey, G. P.: Septicemia due to *Xanthomonas* species and non-*aeruginosa Pseudomonas* species: Incidence of catheter-related infections. Medicine (Baltimore) 69:296-306, 1990.
62. Faden, H., and Grossi, M.: Acute osteomyelitis in children: Reassessment of etiologic agents and their clinical characteristics. Am. J. Dis. Child. 145:65-69, 1991.
63. Feder, H. M., Jr., Grant-Kels, J. M., and Tilton, R. C.: *Pseudomonas* whirlpool dermatitis. Clin. Pediatr. (Phila.) 22:638-642, 1983.
64. Feigin, R. D., and Shearer, W. T.: Opportunistic infection in children. Parts I, II, and III. J. Pediatr. 87:507-514, 677-694, 852-866, 1975.
65. Feldman, J., Bryan, R., Rajan, S., et al.: Role of flagella in pathogenesis of *Pseudomonas aeruginosa* pulmonary infection. Infect. Immun. 66:43, 1998.
66. Fergie, J. E., Sherma, S. J., Lott, L., et al.: *Pseudomonas aeruginosa* bacteremia in immunocompromised children: Analysis of factors associated with a poor outcome. Clin. Infect. Dis. 18:390-394, 1994.
67. Festini, F., Buzzetti, R., Bassi, C., et al.: Isolation measures for prevention of infection with respiratory pathogens in cystic fibrosis: A systemic review. J. Hosp. Infect. 64:1-6, 2006.
68. Fick, R. B., Jr.: Pathogenetic mechanisms in cystic fibrosis lung disease: A paradigm for inflammatory airways disease. J. Lab. Clin. Med. 121:632-634, 1993.
69. Fick, R. B., and Reynolds, H. Y.: *Pseudomonas* respiratory infection in cystic fibrosis: A possible defect in opsonic IgG antibody? Bull. Eur. Physiopathol. Respir. 19:151-161, 1983.
70. Fick, R. B., Jr., Sonoda, F., and Hornick, D. B.: Emergence and persistence of *Pseudomonas aeruginosa* in the cystic fibrosis airway. Semin. Respir. Infect. 7:168-178, 1992.
71. Fiorillo, L., Zucker, M., Sawyer, D., and Lin, A. N.: The *Pseudomonas* hot-foot syndrome. N. Engl. J. Med. 345:335-338, 2001.
72. Fisher, M. C., Goldsmith, J. F., and Gilligan, P. H.: Sneakers as a source of *Pseudomonas aeruginosa* in children with osteomyelitis following puncture wounds. J. Pediatr. 106:607-609, 1985.
73. Fisher, M. C., Long, S. S., Roberts, E. M., et al.: *Pseudomonas maltophilia* bacteremia in children undergoing open heart surgery. JAMA 246:1571-1574, 1981.
74. Flores, G., Stavola, J. J., and Noel, G. J.: Bacteremia due to *Pseudomonas aeruginosa* in children with AIDS. Clin. Infect. Dis. 16:706-708, 1993.
75. Fox, R. C., Williams, G. J., Wunderink, R. G., et al.: Followup bronchoscopy predicts therapeutic outcome in ventilated patients with nosocomial pneumonia. Abstract. Am. Rev. Respir. Dis. 143:109, 1991.
76. Fredrekson, B.: *Stenotrophomonas (Xanthomonas) maltophilia* at the Danish Cystic Fibrosis Centre 1974-1993. Abstract. Pediatr. Pulmonol. 20(Suppl. 12):287, 1995.
77. Geiss, H. R., and Geiss, M.: Evaluation of a new commercial system for the identification of Enterobacteriaceae and non-fermentative bacteria. Eur. J. Clin. Microbiol. Infect. Dis. 11:610-616, 1992.
78. Gerding, D. N., and Larson, T. A.: Aminoglycoside resistance in gram-negative bacilli during increased amikacin use. Am. J. Med. 79:1-7, 1985.
79. Germiller, J. A., El-Kashlan, K., and Shah, U. K.: Chronic *Pseudomonas* infections of cochlear implants. Otol. Neurotol. 26:196-201, 2005.
80. Gilligan, P. H.: Microbiology of airway disease in patients with cystic fibrosis. Clin. Microbiol. Rev. 4:35-51, 1991.
81. Gilligan, P. H.: *Pseudomonas* and *Burkholderia*. *In* Murray, P. R., Baron, E. J., Pfaller, M. A., et al. (eds.): Manual of Clinical Microbiology. 6th ed. Washington, D.C., ASM Press, 1995, pp. 509-519.
82. Gilligan, P. H.: Report on the consensus document for microbiology and infectious diseases in cystic fibrosis. Clin. Microbiol. Newsl. 18:83-87, 1996.
83. Gilligan, P. H., and Whittier, S.: *Burkholderia, Stenotrophomonas, Ralstonia, Brevundimonas, Comamonas*, and *Acidovorax*. *In* Murray, P. R., Baron, E. J., Pfaller, M. A., et al. (eds.): Manual of Clinical Microbiology. 7th ed. Washington, D.C., ASM Press, 1999, pp. 526-538.
84. Glupczynski, Y., Hansen, W., Dratwa, M., et al.: *Pseudomonas paucimobilis* peritonitis in patients treated by peritoneal dialysis. J. Clin. Microbiol. 20:1225-1226, 1984.
85. Gustafson, T. L., Band, J. D., Hutcheson, R. H., Jr., et al.: *Pseudomonas* folliculitis: An outbreak and review. Rev. Infect. Dis. 5:1-8, 1983.
86. Hatchette, T. F., Gupta, R., and Marrie, T. J.: *Pseudomonas aeruginosa* community-acquired pneumonia in previously healthy adults: Case report and review of the literature. Clin. Infect. Dis. 31:1349-1356, 2000.
87. Heggers, J. P., Haydon, S., Ko, F., et al.: *Pseudomonas aeruginosa* exotoxin A: Its role in retardation of wound healing. The 1992 Lindberg Award. J. Burn Care Rehabil. 13:512-518, 1992.
88. Henderson, D. K., Baptiste, R., Parillo, J., et al.: Indolent epidemic of *Pseudomonas cepacia* bacteremia and pseudobacteremia in an intensive care unit traced to a contaminated blood gas analyzer. Am. J. Med. 84:75-81, 1988.
89. Hilf, M., Yu, V. L., Sharp, J., et al.: Antibiotic therapy for *Pseudomonas aeruginosa* bacteremia: Outcome correlation in a prospective study of 200 patients. Am. J. Med. 87:540-556, 1989.
90. Hilton, E., Adams, A. A., Uliss, A., et al.: Nosocomial bacterial eye infections in intensive-care units. Lancet 1:1318-1320, 1983.
91. Hioyo-Tomoka, M. T., Marples, R. R., and Klingman, A. M.: *Pseudomonas* infection in superhydrated skin. Arch. Dermatol. 107:723-727, 1973.
92. Hoiby, N., and Koch, C.: *Pseudomonas aeruginosa* infection in cystic fibrosis and its management. Thorax 45:881-884, 1990.
93. Holland, S. P., Pulido, J. S., Shires, T. K., et al.: *Pseudomonas aeruginosa* ocular infections. *In* Fick, R. B., Jr. (ed.): *Pseudomonas aeruginosa*: The Opportunist. Boca Raton, FL, CRC Press, 1993, pp. 159-176.
94. Horn, K. L., and Gherini, S.: Malignant external otitis of childhood. Ann. J. Otol. 2:402-404, 1981.
95. Huang, Y. C., Lin, T. Y., and Wang, C. H.: Community acquired *Pseudomonas aeruginosa* sepsis in previously healthy infants and children: Analysis of forty-three episodes. Pediatr. Infect. Dis. J. 21:1049-1052, 2002.
96. Inglis, T. J. J., Garrow, S., Henderson, M., et al.: *Burkholderia pseudomallei* traced to water treatment plant in Australia. Emerg. Infect. Dis. 6:56-59, 2000.
97. Isles, A., Maclusky, I., Corey, M., et al.: *Pseudomonas cepacia* infection in cystic fibrosis: An emerging problem. J. Pediatr. 104:206-210, 1984.
98. Jacobs, R. F., McCarthy, R. E., and Elser, J. M.: *Pseudomonas* osteochondritis complicating puncture wounds of the foot in children: A 10-year evaluation. J. Infect. Dis. 160:657-661, 1989.
99. Jang, T. N., Wang, F. D., Wang, L. H., et al.: *Xanthomonas maltophilia* bacteremia: An analysis of 32 cases. J. Formos. Med. Assoc. 91:1170-1176, 1992.
100. Jensen, T., Pedersen, S. S., Nielsen, C. H., et al.: The efficacy and safety of ciprofloxacin and ofloxacin in chronic *Pseudomonas aeruginosa* infection in cystic fibrosis. J. Antimicrob. Chemother. 20:585-594, 1987.
101. Jiang, J. H., Chiu, N. C., Huang, F. Y., et al.: Neonatal sepsis in the neonatal intensive care unit: Characteristics of early versus late onset. J. Microbiol. Immunol. Infect. 37:301-306, 2004.
102. John, M., Ecclestone, E., Hunter, E., et al.: Epidemiology of *Pseudomonas cepacia* colonization among patients with cystic fibrosis. Pediatr. Pulmonol. 18:108-113, 1994.
103. Jones, C. E., Alexander, J. W., and Fisher, M. W.: Clinical evaluation of *Pseudomonas* hyperimmune globulin. J. Surg. Res. 14:87-96, 1973.
104. Kalish, L. A., Waltz, D. A., Dovey, M., et al.: Impact of *Burkholderia dolosa* on lung function and survival in cystic fibrosis. Am. J. Respir. Crit. Care Med. 173:421-425, 2006.
105. Kavpati, F., Malmborg, A. S., Alfredsson, H., et al.: Bacterial colonization with *Xanthomonas maltophilia*: A retrospective study in a cystic fibrosis patient population. Infection 22:258-263, 1994.
106. Keene, W. E., Markum, A. C., and Samadpour, M.: Outbreak of *Pseudomonas aeruginosa* infections caused by commercial piercing of upper ear cartilage. JAMA 291:981-985, 2004.
107. Kemmerich, B., Small, G., and Pennington, J. E.: Comparative evaluation of ciprofloxacin, enoxacin, and ofloxacin in experimental *Pseudomonas aeruginosa* infections. Antimicrob. Chemother. 29:395-399, 1986.

108. Kenna, M. A., Bluestone, C. D., Reilly, J. S., et al.: Medical management of chronic suppurative otitis media without cholesteatoma in children. Laryngoscope 96:146-151, 1986.

109. Kercsmar, C. M., Stern, R. C., Reed, M. D., et al.: Ceftazidime in cystic fibrosis: Pharmacokinetics and therapeutic response. J. Antimicrob. Chemother. 12(Suppl. A):289-295, 1983.

110. Kerr, K. G., Anson, J. J., Patmore, R., Snith, G.: Intravenous line infections. J. Hosp. Infect. 26:73-75, 1994.

111. Khardori, N., Elting, L., Wong, E., et al.: Nosocomial infections due to *Xanthomonas maltophilia* (*Pseudomonas maltophilia*) in patients with cancer. Rev. Infect. Dis. 12:997-1003, 1990.

112. Kilpatrick, M., Girgis, N., Farid, Z., et al.: Aztreonam for treating meningitis caused by gram-negative rods. Scand. J. Infect. Dis. 23:125-126, 1991.

113. Kingston, C. W.: Chronic or latent melioidosis. Med. J. Aust. 2:618-621, 1971.

114. Kiska, D. L., and Gilligan, P. H.: *Pseudomonas. In* Murray, P. R., Baron, E. J., Pfaller, M. A., et al. (eds.): Manual of Clinical Microbiology. 7th ed. Washington, D.C., ASM Press, 1999, pp. 517-525.

115. Kiska, D. L., Kerr, A., Jones, M. C., et al.: Accuracy of four commercial systems for identification of *Burkholderia cepacia* and other gram-negative non-fermenting bacilli recovered from patients with cystic fibrosis. J. Clin. Microbiol. 34:886-891, 1996.

116. Klinger, J. D., and Thomassen, M. J.: Occurrence and antimicrobial susceptibility of gram-negative nonfermentative bacilli in cystic fibrosis patients. Diagn. Microbiol. Infect. Dis. 3:149-158, 1985.

117. Kock, C., and Koiby, N.: Pathogenesis of cystic fibrosis. Lancet 341:1065-1069, 1993.

118. Kollef, M., Silver, H. P., Murphy, M., and Trouillon, E.: The effect of late-onset ventilator pneumonia in determining patient mortality. Chest 108:1655-1662, 1995.

119. Kurlandsky, L. E., and Fader, R. C.: In vitro activity of minocycline against respiratory pathogens from patients with cystic fibrosis. Pediatr. Pulmonol. 29:210-212, 2000.

120. Kurukularathe, C., and Barzaga, R.: Melioidosis. Infect. Dis. Pract. Clinicians 24:37-40, 2000.

121. Kynakorn, M., Petchlai, B., Khupulsup, K., et al.: Gold blot for detection of immunoglobulin M (IgM)–specific antibodies for rapid serodiagnosis of melioidosis. J. Clin. Microbiol. 29:2065-2067, 1991.

122. Lacroix, J., Gauthier, M., Lapointe, N., et al.: *Pseudomonas aeruginosa* supraglottitis in a six-month-old child with severe combined immunodeficiency syndrome. Pediatr. Infect. Dis. J. 7:739-741, 1988.

123. Laing, F. P., Ramotar, K., Read, R. R., et al.: Molecular epidemiology of *Xanthomonas maltophilia* colonization and infection in the hospital environment. J. Clin. Microbiol. 33:513-518, 1995.

124. Lang, A. B., Ruedberg, A., Schoeni, M. H., et al.: Vaccination of cystic fibrosis patients against *Pseudomonas aeruginosa* reduces the proportion of patients infected and delays time to infection. Pediatr. Infect. Dis. J. 23:504-510, 2004.

125. Leelarasamee, A., and Bovornkitti, S.: Melioidosis: Review and update. Rev. Infect. Dis. 11:413-425, 1989.

126. Legakis, N. J., Tzouvelekis, L. S., Makris, A., et al.: Outer membrane alterations in multiresistant mutants of *Pseudomonas aeruginosa*. Antimicrob. Agents Chemother. 33:124-127, 1989.

127. Lentnek, A. L., and Williams, R. R.: Aztreonam in the treatment of gram-negative bacterial meningitis. Rev. Infect. Dis. 13(Suppl. 7):586-590, 1991.

128. Levy, J. H., and Katz, H. R.: *Pseudomonas cepacia* keratitis. Cornea 8:67-71, 1989.

129. Lipuma, J. J.: *Burkholderia* and emerging pathogens in cystic fibrosis. Semin. Respir. Crit. Care Med. 24:681-692, 2003.

130. Lipuma, J. J., Mortensen, J. E., Dasen, S. E., et al.: Ribotype analysis of *Pseudomonas cepacia* from cystic fibrosis treatment centers. J. Pediatr. 113:859-862, 1988.

131. Lipuma, J. J., Spilker, T., Gill, L. H., et al.: Disproportionate distributions of *Burkholderia cepacia* complex species and transmissibility markers in cystic fibrosis. Am. J. Respir. Crit. Care Med. 164:92-96, 2001.

132. Liu, P. V.: Biology of *Pseudomonas aeruginosa*. Hosp. Pract. 82:139-147, 1976.

133. Lo, W. T., Cheng, S. N., Wang, C. C., and Chu, M. L.: Extensive necrotizing fasciitis caused by *Pseudomonas aeruginosa* in a child with acute myeloid leukaemia: Case report and literature review. Eur. J. Pediatr. 164:113-114, 2005.

134. Lodise, T., Lomaestro, B., and Drusano, L.: Piperacillin-tazobactam for *Pseudomonas aeruginosa* infection: Clinical implications of an extended dosing strategy. Clin. Infect. Dis. 44:357-363, 2007.

135. Lumbiganon, P., Pengsaa, K., Puapermpoonsiri, S., et al.: Neonatal melioidosis: A report of 5 cases. Pediatr. Infect. Dis. J. 7:634-636, 1988.

136. Malizia, W. F., West, G. A., Brundage, W. G., et al.: Melioidosis: Laboratory studies. Health Lab. Sci. 6:27-39, 1969.

137. Marshall, W. F., Keating, M. R., Anhalt, J. P., and Steckelberg, J. M.: *Xanthomonas maltophilia*: An emerging nosocomial pathogen. Mayo Clin. Proc. 64:1097-1104, 1989.

138. Mattsby-Baltzer, I., Edebo, L., Jarvholm, B., and Lavenius, B.: Serum antibodies to *Pseudomonas pseudoalcaligenes* in metal workers exposed to infected metal-working fluids. Int. Arch. Allergy Appl. Immunol. 88:304-311, 1989.

139. Mayer, J. H., and Finnlayson, M. H.: Chronic melioidosis: A case with bone and pulmonary lesions. S. Afr. Med. J. 18:109, 1944.

140. McCubbin, M., and Fick, R. B., Jr.: Pathogenesis of *Pseudomonas* lung disease in cystic fibrosis. *In* Fick, R. B., Jr. (ed.): *Pseudomonas aeruginosa*: The Opportunist. Boca Raton, FL, CRC Press, 1993, pp. 189-211.

141. McManus, A. J., Mason, A. D., Jr., McManus, W. F., and Pruitt, B. A., Jr.: Twenty-five year review of *Pseudomonas aeruginosa* bacteremia in a burn center. Eur. J. Clin. Microbiol. 4:219-223, 1985.

142. Milstone, A. M., Ruff, A. J., Yeamans, C. H., et al.: *Pseudomonas aeruginosa* preseptal cellulitis and bacteremia in a pediatric oncology patient. Pediatr. Blood Cancer 45:353, 2005.

143. Minami, S., Akama, M., Araki, H., et al.: Imipenem and cephem resistant *Pseudomonas aeruginosa* carrying plasmid coding for class B beta-lactamase. J. Antimicrob. Chemother. 37:433-444, 1996.

144. Minnefor, A. B., Olson, M. I., and Cawer, D. H.: *Pseudomonas* osteomyelitis following puncture wounds of the foot. Pediatrics 47:598-601, 1971.

145. Morrison, A. J., Jr., Hoffmann, K. K., and Wenzel, R. P.: Associated mortality and clinical characteristics of nosocomial *Pseudomonas maltophilia* in a university hospital. J. Clin. Microbiol. 24:52-55, 1986.

146. Mortensen, J., Hansen, A., Falk, M., et al.: Reduced effect of inhaled beta-2-adrenergic agonists on lung mucociliary clearance in patients with cystic fibrosis. Chest 103:805-811, 1993.

147. Moss, R. B.: The role of IgG subclass antibodies in chronic infection: The case of cystic fibrosis. N. Engl. Reg. Allergy Proc. 9:57-61, 1988.

148. Moss, R. B.: Cystic fibrosis: Pathogenesis, pulmonary function and treatment. Clin. Infect. Dis. 21:839-851, 1995.

149. Muder, R. R., Yu, V. L., Dummer, J. S., et al.: Infections caused by *Pseudomonas maltophilia*: Expanding clinical spectrum. Arch. Intern. Med. 147:1672-1674, 1987.

150. Mull, C. C., Scarfone, R. J., and Conway, D.: Ecthyma gangrenosum as a manifestation of *Pseudomonas* sepsis in a previously healthy child. Ann. Emerg. Med., 36:383-387, 2000.

151. Nelson, J. D., and Bradley, J. S.: Pocketbook of Pediatric Antimicrobial Therapy. 16th ed. Baltimore, Williams & Wilkins, 2006-2007, pp. 94-112.

152. Nelson, J. W., Butler, S. L., Kreig, D., and Govan, J. R.: Virulence factors of *Burkholderia cepacia*. FEMS Immunol. Med. Microbiol. 8:89-97, 1994.

153. Neo, E. N., Haritharan, T., Thambidorai, C. R., and Suresh, V.: *Pseudomonas* necrotizing fasciitis in an immunocompetent infant. Pediatr. Infect. Dis. J. 24:942-943, 2005.

154. Neu, H. C.: The role of *Pseudomonas aeruginosa* in infections. J. Antimicrob. Chemother. 11(Suppl. B):1-13, 1983.

155. Neu, H. C.: Carbapenems: Special properties contributing to their activity. Am. J. Med. 78:33-40, 1985.

156. Niggs, C., and Johnston, M. M.: Complement fixation test in experimental clinical and subclinical melioidosis. J. Bacteriol. 82:159-168, 1961.

157. Nixon, G. M., Armstrong, D. S., Carzino, R., et al.: Clinical outcome after early *Pseudomonas aeruginosa* infection in cystic fibrosis. J. Pediatr. 138:699-704, 2001.

158. Norby, S. R.: 4-Quinolones in the treatment of infections of the central nervous system. Rev. Infect. Dis. 10(Suppl. 1):253-255, 1988.

159. Nussinovitch, M., Yoeli, R., Elishkevitz, K., and Varsano, I.: Acute mastoiditis in children: Epidemiologic, clinical, microbiologic, and therapeutic aspects over past years. Clin. Pediatr. 43:261-267, 2004.

160. O'Boyle, J. D., Heslinger, K. A., and Hier-Duffin, S. L.: *Pseudomonas aeruginosa* as an unusual cause of intraamniotic infection, fulminant neonatal sepsis and neonatal death: A case report. J. Reprod. Med. 41:534-536, 1996.

161. Ohman, D. E., Burns, R. P., and Iglewski, B. H.: Corneal infections in mice with toxin A and elastase mutants of *Pseudomonas aeruginosa*. J. Infect. Dis. 142:547-555, 1980.

162. Ortì, A., Escrig, R., Perez-Tamarit, D., et al.: *Pseudomonas aeruginosa* infection in a previously healthy infant. Clin. Pediatr. 41:525-528, 2002.

163. Patamasucon, P., Pitchyangkura, C., and Fischer, G. W.: Melioidosis in childhood. J. Pediatr. 87:133-136, 1975.

164. Patamasucon, P., Schaad, U. B., and Nelson, J. D.: Melioidosis. J. Pediatr. 100:175-182, 1982.

165. Paterson, D. L.: The epidemiological profile of infections with multidrug-resistant *Pseudomonas aeruginosa* and *Acinetobacter* species. Clin. Infect. Dis. 43:543-548, 2006.

166. Paul, M., Silbiger, I., Grozinsky, S., et al.: Beta lactam antibiotic monotherapy versus beta lactam-aminoglycoside antibiotic combination therapy for sepsis. Cochrane Database Syst. Rev. 1:CD003344, 2006.

167. Peacock, E. E.: Wound Repair. 3rd ed. Philadelphia, W. B. Saunders, 1984, pp. 38-55.

168. Pedersen, S. S.: Lung infection with alginate-producing, mucoid *Pseudomonas aeruginosa* in cystic fibrosis. APMIS Suppl. 28:1-79, 1992.

169. Peel, M. M., Davis, J. M., Armstrong, W. L. H., et al.: *Pseudomonas paucimobilis* from a leg ulcer on a Japanese seaman. J. Clin. Microbiol. 9:561-564, 1979.

170. Penketh, A. R., Pitt, T. L., Hodson, M. E., et al.: Bactericidal activity of serum from cystic fibrosis patients for *Pseudomonas aeruginosa*. J. Med. Microbiol. 16:91-408, 1983.

171. Pennington, J. E., Reynolds, H. Y., Wood, R. E., et al.: Use of *Pseudomonas aeruginosa* vaccine in patients with acute leukemia and cystic fibrosis. Am. J. Med. 58:629-636, 1975.

172. Perry, A. W., Sutkin, H. S., Gottlieb, L. D., et al.: Skin graft survival: The bacterial answer. Ann. Plast. Surg. 22:479-483, 1989.

173. Pollack, M.: *Pseudomonas aeruginosa. In* Mandell, G. L., Douglas, R. G., Jr., and Bennett, J. E. (eds.): Principles and Practice of Infectious Diseases. 3rd ed. New York, Churchill Livingstone, 1990, pp. 1673-1691.

174. Poore, K.: Bacterial multidrug resistance-emphasis on efflux mechanisms and *Pseudomonas aeruginosa.* J. Antimicrob. Chemother. *34*:453-456, 1994.

175. Poschet, J. F., Boucher, J. C., Tatterson, L., et al.: Molecular basis for defective glycosylation and *Pseudomonas* pathogenesis in cystic fibrosis lung. Proc. Natl. Acad. Sci. U. S. A. *98*:13972-13977, 2001.

176. Pressler, T., Mansa, B., Jensen, T., et al.: Increased IgG2 and IgG3 concentration is associated with advanced *Pseudomonas aeruginosa* infection and poor pulmonary function in cystic fibrosis. Acta Pediatr. Scand. 77:576-582, 1988.

177. *Pseudomonas aeruginosa. In* Gerber, M. A. (ed.): The Jordan Report 2000: Accelerated Development of Vaccines. Bethesda, MD, Division of Microbiology and Infectious Diseases, National Institute of Allergy and Infectious Diseases, National Institutes of Health, 2000, pp. 60-62.

178. Radberg, G., Nilsson, L. E., and Svensson, S.: Development of quinolone-imipenem cross resistance in *Pseudomonas aeruginosa* during exposure to ciprofloxacin. Antimicrob. Agents Chemother. *34*:2142-2147, 1990.

179. Ralph, A., McBride, J., and Currie, B.: Transmission of *Burkholderia Pseudomallei* via breast milk in northern Australia. Pediatr. Infect. Dis. J. *23*:1169-1171, 2004.

180. Ratjen, F., Doring, G., and Nikolaizik, W. H.: Effect of inhaled tobramycin in early *Pseudomonas aeruginosa* colonization in patients with cystic fibrosis. Lancet *358*:983-984, 2001.

181. Reed, R. K., Larter, W. E., Sieber, O. F., Jr., et al.: Peripheral nodular lesions in *Pseudomonas* sepsis: The importance of incision and drainage. J. Pediatr. *88*:977-979, 1976.

182. Reid, T. M. S., and Porter, I. A.: An outbreak of otitis externa in competitive swimmers due to *Pseudomonas aeruginosa.* J. Hyg. (Camb.) *86*:357-362, 1981.

183. Reymond, J., Frey, B., and Birrer, P.: Infection invasive à *Pseudomonas aeruginosa* et ecthyma gangrenosum chez un enfant sans facteurs de risques. Arch. Pediatr. *3*:569-572, 1996.

184. Reynolds, H. Y., DiSant'Agnese, P. A., and Zierdt, C. H.: Mucoid *Pseudomonas aeruginosa.* JAMA *236*:2190-2192, 1976.

185. Reynolds, H. Y., Levine, A. S., Wood, R. E., et al.: *Pseudomonas aeruginosa* infections: Persisting problems and current research to find new therapies. Ann. Intern. Med. *82*:819-831, 1975.

186. Rhoads, S., Marinelli, L., Imperative, C. A., and Machamkin, I.: Comparison of the MicroScan Walkaway System and Vitek System for identification of gram-negative bacteria. J. Clin. Microbiol. *33*:3044-3046, 1995.

187. Richmond, H. M., and Sykes, R. B.: The β-lactamases of gram-negative bacilli and their possible physiologic role. Adv. Microb. Physiol. *9*:31-88, 1973.

188. Robinson, A., McCarter, Y. S., and Tetreault, J.: Comparison of crystal enteric/non-fermenter system, API 20E system and Vitek Autonomicrobic System for identification of gram-negative bacilli. J. Clin. Microbiol. *33*:364-370, 1995.

189. Roiliders, E., Butler, K. M., Husson, R. N., et al.: *Pseudomonas* infections in children with human immunodeficiency virus infection. Pediatr. Infect. Dis. J. *11*:547-553, 1992.

190. Roland, P. S., Parry, D. A., and Stroman, D. W.: Microbiology of acute otitis media with tympanostomy tubes. Otolaryngol. Head Neck Surg. *133*:585-595, 2005.

191. Romling, V., Fiedler, B., Bosshammer, J., et al.: Epidemiology of chronic *Pseudomonas aeruginosa* in cystic fibrosis. J. Infect. Dis. *170*:616-621, 1994.

192. Rowley, A. H., Dias, L. D., Chadwick, E. G., et al.: *Pseudomonas stutzeri:* An unusual cause of calcaneal *Pseudomonas* osteomyelitis. Pediatr. Infect. Dis. J. *6*:296-297, 1987.

193. Rubio, T. T.: Ciprofloxacin: Comparative data in cystic fibrosis. Am. J. Med. *82*(Suppl. 4A):185-188, 1987.

194. Ruvalo, C., and Bauer, C. R.: Intrauterinely acquired *Pseudomonas* infection in the neonate. Clin. Pediatr. (Phila.) *21*:664-667, 1982.

195. Saiman, L., Cacalano, G., and Prince, A.: *Pseudomonas cepacia* adherence to respiratory epithelial cells is enhanced by *Pseudomonas aeruginosa.* Infect. Immun. *58*:2578-2584, 1990.

196. Sajjan, U. S., Karmali, M. A., and Forstner, J. F.: Binding of *Pseudomonas cepacia* to normal human intestinal mucin and respiratory mucin for patients with cystic fibrosis. J. Clin. Invest. *89*:648-656, 1992.

197. Salmen, P., Dwyer, D. M., Vorse, H., et al.: Whirlpool-associated *Pseudomonas aeruginosa* urinary tract infections. JAMA *15*:2025-2026, 1983.

198. Salyers, A. A., and Whitt, D. D.: *Pseudomonas aeruginosa. In* Salyers, A. A., and Whitt, D. D. (eds.): Bacterial Pathogenesis: A Molecular Approach. Washington, D.C., American Society for Microbiology Press, 1994, pp. 260-272.

199. Sanders, C. C., and Sanders, W. E.: Type I β-lactamases of gram-negative bacteria: Interactions with β-lactam antibiotics. J. Infect. Dis. *154*:792-800, 1986.

200. Schaad, U. B., Sander, E., Wedgwood, J., et al.: Morphologic studies for skeletal toxicity after prolonged ciprofloxacin therapy in two juvenile cystic fibrosis patients. Pediatr. Infect. Dis. J. *11*:1047-1049, 1992.

201. Schaad, U. B., Stoupis, C., Wedgwood, J., et al.: Clinical, radiologic and magnetic resonance monitoring for skeletal toxicity in pediatric patients with cystic fibrosis receiving a three-month course of ciprofloxacin. Pediatr. Infect. Dis. J. *10*:723-729, 1991.

202. Schaad, U. B., Wedgwood-Krucko, J., Suter, S., et al.: Efficacy of inhaled amikacin as adjunct to intravenous combination therapy (ceftazidime and amikacin) in cystic fibrosis. J. Pediatr. *111*:599-605, 1987.

203. Schiller, N. L., and Millard, R. L.: *Pseudomonas*-infected cystic fibrosis patient sputum inhibits the bactericidal activity of normal human sputum. Pediatr. Res. *17*:747-752, 1983.

204. Schoch, P. E., and Cunha, B. A.: *Pseudomonas maltophilia.* Infect. Control *8*:169-172, 1987.

205. Scully, B. E., Parry, M. F., Nev, H. C., et al.: Oral ciprofloxacin therapy of infections due to *Pseudomonas aeruginosa.* Lancet *1*:819-822, 1986.

206. Senda, C. C., Arakawa, Y., Nakashina, K., et al.: Multifocal outbreaks of metallo-beta-lactamase producing *Pseudomonas aeruginosa* resistant to broad spectrum beta-lactams, including carbapenem. Antimicrob. Agents Chemother. *40*:349-353, 1996.

207. Sesev, S., Rosen, N., Joseph, G., et al.: Pefloxacin efficacy in gram-negative bacillary meningitis. J. Antimicrob. Chemother. *26*(Suppl. B):187-192, 1990.

208. Shackelford, P. G., Ratzan, S. A., and Shearer, W. T.: Ecthyma gangrenosum produced by *Aeromonas hydrophila.* J. Pediatr. *83*:100-101, 1973.

209. Shand, G. H., Pedersen, S. S., Tilling, R., et al.: Use of immunoblot detection of serum antibodies in the diagnosis of chronic *Pseudomonas aeruginosa* lung infection in cystic fibrosis. J. Med. Microbiol. *27*:169-177, 1988.

210. Sharma, G. D., Tosi, M. F., Stern, R. C., et al.: Progression of pulmonary disease after disappearance of *Pseudomonas* in cystic fibrosis. Am. J. Respir. Crit. Care Med. *152*:169-173, 1995.

211. Simon, P. R.: *Pseudomonas* bacteraemia in a previously healthy 2-year-old boy. Clin. Pediatr. *28*:336, 1989.

212. Smith, A. L., Redding, G., Doershuk, C., et al.: Sputum changes associated with therapy for endobronchial exacerbation in cystic fibrosis. J. Pediatr. *112*:547-554, 1988.

213. Smith, E. E., Buckley, D. G., Wu, Z., et al.: Genetic adaptation by *Pseudomonas aeruginosa* to the airways of cystic fibrosis patients. Proc. Natl. Acad. Sci. U. S. A. *103*:8305-8306, 2006.

214. Smith, G. L.: Methods for preventing *Pseudomonas* folliculitis. Cutis *29*:378-381, 1982.

215. Sobel, J. D., Hashman, N., Reinherz, G., et al.: Nosocomial *Pseudomonas cepacia* infection associated with chlorhexidine contamination. Am. J. Med. *73*:183-186, 1982.

216. Sookpranee, T., Sookpranee, M., Mellencamp, M. A., et al.: *Pseudomonas pseudomallei*, a common pathogen in Thailand that is resistant to bactericidal effects of many antibiotics. Antimicrob. Agents Chemother. *35*:484-489, 1991.

217. Sorvillo, F., Beall, G., Turner, P. A., et al.: Incidence and determinants of *Pseudomonas aeruginosa* infection among persons with HIV: Association with hospital exposure. Am. J. Infect. Control *29*:79-84, 2001.

218. Speert, D. P.: Understanding *Burkholderia cepacia*: Epidemiology, genomovars and virulence. Infect. Med. *18*:49-56, 2001.

219. Speert, D. P., Bond, M., Woodman, R. C., and Curnutte, J. J.: Infection with *Pseudomonas cepacia* in chronic granulomatous disease: Role of nonoxidative killing by neutrophils in host defense. J. Infect. Dis. *170*:1524-1531, 1994.

220. Speert, D. P., Farmer, S. W., Campbell, M. E., et al.: Conversion of *Pseudomonas aeruginosa* to the phenotype characteristic of strains from patients with cystic fibrosis. J. Clin. Microbiol. *28*:188-194, 1990.

221. Spencer, R. C.: The emergence of epidemic, multiple-antibiotic-resistant *Stenotrophomonas (Xanthomonas) maltophilia* and *Burkholderia (Pseudomonas) cepacia.* J. Hosp. Infect. *30*(Suppl.):453-465, 1995.

222. Steen, H. J., Scott, E. M., Stevenson, M. I., et al.: Clinical and pharmacokinetic aspects of ciprofloxacin in the treatment of acute exacerbations of *Pseudomonas* infection in cystic fibrosis patients. J. Antimicrob. Chemother. *24*:787-795, 1989.

223. Strand, C. L., Bryant, J. K., Morgan, J. W., et al.: Nosocomial *Pseudomonas aeruginosa* urinary tract infections. JAMA *248*:1615-1618, 1982.

224. Strandvik, B., Hjelte, L., Lindblad, A., et al.: Comparison of efficacy and tolerance of intravenously and orally administered ciprofloxacin in cystic fibrosis patients with acute exacerbations of lung infection. Scand. J. Infect. Dis. *60*(Suppl.):84-88, 1989.

225. Tablan, O. C., Martone, W. J., Doershuk, C. F., et al.: Colonization of the respiratory tract with *Pseudomonas cepacia* in cystic fibrosis: Risk factors and outcomes. Chest *9*:527-532, 1987.

226. Tablan, O. C., Martone, W. J., and Jarvis, W. R.: The epidemiology of *Pseudomonas cepacia* in patients with cystic fibrosis. Eur. J. Epidemiol. *3*:336-342, 1987.

227. Tiffany, K. K., and Kline, M. W.: Mixed flora brain abscess with *Pseudomonas paucimobilis* after a penetrating lawn dart injury. Pediatr. Infect. Dis. J. *7*:667-669, 1988.

228. Tredget, E. E., Shankowsky, H. A., Joffe, A. M., et al.: Epidemiology of infections with *Pseudomonas aeruginosa* in burn patients: The role of hydrotherapy. Clin. Infect. Dis. *15*:941-949, 1992.

229. Ugwumadu, A. H., Manyonda, I. T., and Hay, P. E.: Chorioamnionitis due to *Pseudomonas aeruginosa*: A complication of prolonged antibiotic therapy for premature rupture of membranes. Br. J. Obstet. Gynaecol. *103*:1049-1056, 1996.

230. Vartivarian, S., and Anaissie, E.: *Stenotrophomonas maltophilia* and *Burkholderia cepacia. In* Mandell, G. L., Bennett, J. E., and Dolin, R. (eds.): Principles and Practice of Infectious Diseases. 5th ed. Philadelphia, Churchill Livingstone, 2000, pp. 2235-2237.

231. Victo, M. A., Arpi, M., Bruun, B., et al.: *Xanthomonas maltophilia* bacteremia in immunocompromised hematologic patients. Scand. J. Infect. Dis. *26*:163-170, 1994.

232. Viola, L., Langer, A., Pulitanò, S., et al.: Serious *Pseudomonas aeruginosa* infection in healthy children: Case report and review of the literature. Pediatr. Int. *48*:330-333, 2006.

233. Virgili, A., Colombo, E., Serino, R., et al.: Necrotizing fasciitis from *Pseudomonas aeruginosa* in infantile actue lymphoblastic leukaemia. Acta Derm. Venereol. *85*:538-539, 2005.

234. Vishwanath, S., and Ramphal, R.: Adherence of *Pseudomonas aeruginosa* to human tracheobronchial mucin. Infect. Immun. *45*:197-202, 1984.

235. Vochem, M., Vogt, M., and Doring, G.: Sepsis in a newborn due to *Pseudomonas aeruginosa* from a contaminated tub bath. N. Engl. J. Med. *345*:378, 2001.

236. Vogt, R., LaRue, D., Parry, M. F., et al.: *Pseudomonas aeruginosa* skin infections in persons using a whirlpool in Vermont. J. Clin. Microbiol. *15*:571-574, 1982.

237. Wade, J. C.: Antibiotic therapy for the febrile granulocytopenic cancer patient: Combination therapy vs. monotherapy. Rev. Infect. Dis. *11*(Suppl.): S1572-S1581, 1989.

238. Watanabe, M., Iyobe, S., Inoue, M., and Mitsuhashi, S.: Transferable imipenem resistance in *Pseudomonas aeruginosa*. Antimicrob. Chemother. *35*:147-151, 1991.

239. Welch, D. F., Muszynski, M. J., Pai, C. H., et al.: Selective and differential medium for recovery of *Pseudomonas cepacia* from the respiratory tracts of patients with cystic fibrosis. J. Clin. Microbiol. *25*:1730-1734, 1987.

240. Wheeler, W. B., Williams, R. N., Matthew, W. J., and Colten, H. R.: Progression of cystic fibrosis lung disease as a function of serum immunoglobulin G levels: A 5-year longitudinal study. J. Pediatr. *104*:695-699, 1984.

241. White, N. J., Dance, D. A., Chaowagul, W., et al.: Halving of mortality of severe melioidosis by ceftazidime. Lancet *2*:697-701, 1989.

242. Widmer, A. F., Wenzel, R. P., Trilla, A., et al.: Outbreak of *Pseudomonas aeruginosa* infections in a surgical intensive care unit: Probable transmission via hands of a health care worker. Clin. Infect. Dis. *16*:372-376, 1993.

243. Wong, S. N., Tam, A. Y. C., Yung, R. W. Y., et al.: *Pseudomonas* septicaemia in apparently healthy children. Acta Paediatr. Scand. *80*:515-520, 1991.

244. Wongratanacheewin, S., Tattawasart, U., and Lulitanond, V.: An avidin-biotin enzyme-linked immunosorbent assay for the detection of *Pseudomonas pseudomallei* antigens. Trans. R. Trop. Med. Hyg. *84*:429-430, 1990.

245. Woods, D. E., Cryz, S. J., Friedman, R. L., et al.: Contribution of toxin A and elastase to virulence of *Pseudomonas aeruginosa* in chronic lung infections of rats. Infect. Immun. *36*:1223-1228, 1982.

246. Wretlind, B., and Pavlovskis, O. R.: The role of proteases and exotoxin A in the pathogenicity of *Pseudomonas aeruginosa* infections. Scand. J. Infect. Dis. Suppl. *29*:13-19, 1981.

247. Wu, B. Y., Peng, C. T., Tsai, C. H., and Chiu, H. H.: Community-acquired *Pseudomonas aeruginosa* bacteraemia and sepsis in previously healthy infants. Acta Paediatr. Taiwan *40*:233-236, 1999.

248. Wunderlich, C. A., and Krach, L. E.: Gram-negative meningitis and infections in individuals treated with intrathecal baclofen for spasticity: A retrospective study. Dev. Med. Child Neurol. *48*:450-455, 2006.

249. Yeung, C. K., and Lee, K. H.: Community acquired fulminant *Pseudomonas* infection of the gastrointestinal tract in previously healthy infants. J. Paediatr. Child Health *34*:584-587, 1998.

250. Young, E. J., Sewell, M. C., Koza, M. A., et al.: Antibiotic resistance patterns during aminoglycoside restriction. Am. J. Med. *290*:223-227, 1985.

251. Yu, V. L., Paterson, D. L.: *Pseudomonas aeruginosa*. *In* Yu, V. L., Merigan, T. C., and Barriere, S. L. (eds.): Antimicrobial Therapy and Vaccines. Baltimore, Williams & Wilkins, 1999, pp. 348-358.

252. Zachariah, M., Vyjayanthi, S., and Bell-Thomas, S.: Umbilical vein varix thrombosis: A rare pathology. J. Obstet. Gynaecol. *24*:581, 2004.

253. Zawacki, A., O'Rourke, E., Potter-Bynoe, G., et al.: An outbreak of *Pseudomonas aeruginosa* pneumonia and bloodstream infection associated with intermittent otitis externa in a healthcare worker. Infect. Control Hosp. Epidemiol. *25*:1083-1089, 2004.

254. Zimakoff, J., Hoiby, N., Rosendal, K., et al.: Epidemiology of *Pseudomonas aeruginosa* infection and the role of contamination of the environment in a cystic fibrosis clinic. J. Hosp. Infect. *4*:31-40, 1983.

255. Zomorrodi, A., and Walk, E.R.: Ecthyma gangrenosum: Considerations in a previously healthy child. Pediatr. Infect. Dis. J. *21*:1161-1164, 2002.

256. Zuravleff, J. J., and Yu, V. L.: Infections caused by *Pseudomonas maltophilia* with emphasis on bacteremia: Case reports and review of the literature. Rev. Infect. Dis. *4*:1236-1246, 1982.

STENOTROPHOMONAS (XANTHOMONAS) MALTOPHILIA

CHAPTER 136

Carlos A. Sattler

Stenotrophomonas maltophilia is a gram-negative bacillus that previously belonged to the *Pseudomonas* and subsequently the *Xanthomonas* genus. In 1993, the new genus *Stenotrophomonas* was proposed, resulting in the most recent reclassification of this bacterium.[75] *S. maltophilia* is an opportunistic pathogen that has emerged as a significant cause of nosocomially acquired infection. It rarely is a cause of infection in healthy, immunocompetent children.

BACTERIOLOGY

S. maltophilia is an aerobic, nonfermentative, gram-negative bacillus that is oxidase-negative and lysine decarboxylase-positive. In addition, key features that allow identification of *S. maltophilia* include oxidation of glucose and maltose, as well as a positive DNase reaction.[40] Optimal growth occurs at 35° C; on sheep blood agar, colonies appear rough and lavender green and have a distinct ammonia-like odor. Morphologically, the organism is a straight bacillus, 0.7 to 1.8 μm long, that is motile by means of multiple polar flagella. It grows well on standard culture media, including blood agar and chocolate agar, as well as in broth blood culture systems, within the standard 5-day incubation period. Because of the hardy nature of this organism, standard collection, transport, and storage procedures are sufficient. The use of selective media such as MacConkey agar allows for *S. maltophilia* to be isolated from polymicrobial specimens, although

for highly contaminated samples such as feces, the addition of antibiotics such as imipenem, vancomycin, and amphotericin B to the media should be considered.[54]

EPIDEMIOLOGY

S. maltophilia is a free-living, ubiquitous organism, the natural habitats for which include water, soil, and plants. The ability to survive in an aqueous milieu has allowed *S. maltophilia* to occupy a niche in the hospital environment. It has been cultured from dialysis fluids,[9] ventilators and other respiratory equipment,[24,55,81] and preoperative surgical brushes.[74] Several reports have linked nosocomial outbreaks of *S. maltophilia* to contamination of hospital water sources such as faucet aerators,[96] taps, and sinks,[55] as well as disinfectant solutions.[99] Intestinal colonization with *S. maltophilia* has been described in hospitalized oncology patients with diarrhea and could represent a potential source of nosocomial infection.[4] Other reports have described cases of nosocomial cross-infection occurring in neonatal and pediatric intensive care units.[36,44,59] In addition, cases of "pseudoinfection" caused by contamination of blood collection tubes have been described.[84]

Infection with *S. maltophilia* generally is hospital acquired.[37,83] Predisposing factors associated with colonization and infection by *S. maltophilia* include the presence of a severe, debilitating underlying illness, particularly malignancy; immune suppression (including human immunodeficiency virus infection); exposure to broad-spectrum antibiotics (particularly to carbapenems, quino-lones, or broad-spectrum cephalosporins); prolonged exposure to antibiotics; the presence of a central venous catheter; neutro-penia; severe mucositis; prolonged hospital stay; stay in an intensive care unit; tracheostomy; mechanical ventilation; chronic obstructive pulmonary disease; or a combination of these factors.[5,12,13,21,30,65,72,73,89,94] Among children, predisposing factors are similar to those found in adults.[83] S. maltophilia is being iso-lated from clinical samples with increasing frequency.[5,29,56,64,68,83] This increase probably is related to advances in medical care that allow for a rise in the survival rate of severely ill patients, who are at highest risk for acquiring infection with this organism and who require more frequent use of invasive medical equipment, including indwelling lines, as well as broad-spectrum antimicro-bials to which the organism is not susceptible.

PATHOPHYSIOLOGY

Like many pseudomonads, S. maltophilia is an organism with low virulence and limited invasiveness. An intact host immune system is an important deterrent to acquisition of a severe and even life-threatening infection; septicemia and death occur in patients with underlying debilitating illnesses. S. maltophilia elaborates a wide range of extracellular enzymes, including DNase, RNase, fibri-nolysin, lipase, hyaluronidase, protease, and elastase, which may play a role in the pathogenesis of disease processes associated with S. maltophilia.[23] The pathogenesis of S. maltophilia infection also may be related to the development of cytotoxic activity.[33] In addition, S. maltophilia has been found to adhere to plastic mate-rials, including intravenous catheters, and to produce biofilm, properties that may account for the relatively high incidence of catheter-related bloodstream infections caused by this organ-ism.[20,23,31] S. maltophilia is inherently resistant to several classes of antibiotics. Colonization with S. maltophilia, especially in the respiratory tract, is not an uncommon finding. In debilitated patients, exposure to broad-spectrum antimicrobials, many of which are ineffective against this bacterium, may allow over-growth of colonizing organisms that subsequently gain access to sterile body sites and cause infection. Portals of infection include indwelling devices such as central venous catheters, peritoneal dialysis or urinary tract catheters, the respiratory tract, and the gastrointestinal tract.

CLINICAL MANIFESTATIONS

S. maltophilia once was regarded as a microorganism with very limited pathogenicity that was unlikely to cause infection except in the most debilitated patients.[37] However, not only the incidence but also the severity of infection and the spectrum of clinical manifestations caused by this bacterium have increased. The most common site of isolation of S. maltophilia is the respira-tory tract, particularly in hospitalized, mechanically ventilated patients. Attributing a causative role to S. maltophilia occasionally is difficult when the organism is isolated only from respiratory secretions, particularly as part of a mixed culture. Most critically ill, mechanically ventilated patients have abnormal chest radiographs, and differentiating infectious from noninfectious infiltrates may be very difficult. Nonetheless, S. maltophilia has unequivocally been associated with pneumonia, which may be severe and which may occur in patients who are not receiving mechanical ventilation.[1,34,39] Occasionally, the pathogen may be associated with massive, fatal pulmonary hemorrhage in adult patients with malignant disease,[28] and it is a cause of ventilator-associated pneumonia.[62] In adults with pneumonia, the development of secondary bacteremia signals a grave prognosis.[29]

S. maltophilia bloodstream infections usually are catheter-associated.[10,55,57,58,69,93] In a series of 32 episodes of bacteremia in children, all were related to the presence of a central venous catheter, although in 10 episodes, the primary source was not the catheter.[83] In a series of 217 episodes of S. maltophilia blood-stream infections occurring in patients with cancer who had central venous catheters, secondary bacteremia generally occurred in patients who were neutropenic, had concurrent pneumonia, or were critically ill, and it was associated with a worse outcome compared with patients who had central venous catheter–related bacteremia.[10] Frequently, S. maltophilia is isolated as part of a polymicrobial bloodstream infection, particularly when the central venous catheter is the origin of the infection. In children, the severity of illness appears to be similar regardless of whether S. maltophilia is isolated in a monomicrobial or mixed blood culture.[83] Malignant disease is the most common underlying illness in patients with bacteremia, and many patients have con-comitant neutropenia. Bloodstream infections caused by S. malto-philia can be severe. In a pediatric series, 31 percent of the patients initially were seen in septic shock, and the attributable mortality rate was 6.3 percent.[83] In another pediatric series of 32 episodes of bacteremia occurring in 31 children, the crude mortality rate was 40.6 percent.[100] However, the death rate associated with S. maltophilia bloodstream infection is, in general, higher in adults.[55,56,66,69]

S. maltophilia endocarditis is a rare occurrence. It has been associated with intravenous drug abuse and frequently occurs after replacement of a prosthetic valve.[6,46,70,101] Surgical therapy often is required, although cure with medical treatment alone has been reported. No cases of endocarditis caused by this organism in children have been reported.

Urinary tract infections caused by S. maltophilia almost invari-ably occur in patients with structural abnormalities of the urinary tract, indwelling urinary catheters, or underlying illnesses. Infec-tion may be severe and associated with sepsis and septic shock.[91]

Skin and soft tissue infections caused by S. maltophilia have occurred in patients who have had work-related injuries and wounds contaminated with soil and plant material, such as occur in injuries associated with use of lawn mowers.[18,27,41] In the hos-pital setting, S. maltophilia frequently is cultured from wounds and surgical sites, although determining the clinical significance of this organism in children, particularly when it is isolated in mixed culture, often is difficult.[83] In adult patients with cancer, tender, erythematous nodular skin lesions have been described in association with S. maltophilia bacteremia and probably represent metastatic infectious foci.[92] In 2006, the first reported cases of metastatic soft tissue involvement, including nodular skin lesions and pyomyositis, in pediatric patients with bacteremia were described.[87,100] All these patients had severe underlying dis-eases, particularly hematologic malignancies, associated with neutropenia.

S. maltophilia has been implicated as a cause of conjunctivitis and keratitis in the setting of ocular surface compromise resulting from trauma, the use of soft contact lenses, or previous infection with human herpes simplex virus.[79] Endophthalmitis occurring after ophthalmologic surgical interventions also has been described.[15,48,51]

Meningitis caused by S. maltophilia is an extremely rare occur-rence and usually is nosocomial and associated with neurosurgical procedures and infection of intraventricular devices.[78] However, spontaneous meningitis in four infants was reported.[61,71,82]

S. maltophilia is the fourth most common organism isolated from the bronchial secretions of patients with cystic fibrosis, after Pseudomonas aeruginosa, Staphylococcus aureus, and Haemophilus influenzae.[88] The incidence and prevalence of S. maltophilia iso-lated from the respiratory secretions of patients with cystic fibro-sis are increasing,[53,86] although they are not uniform across all cystic fibrosis centers.[21] *S. maltophilia* is recovered from the sputum of an estimated 10 percent of patients with cystic fibrosis in the Untied States and from as many as 25 percent of such patients in Europe.[95] The origin of the bacterium is uncertain; evidence suggests that it may be acquired both in the hospital and in the community.[21] Colonization may be transient or persistent, with chronic colonization occurring more frequently in older patients.[88] Case-control studies identified greater exposure to antipseudomonal antibiotics, oral ciprofloxacin, inhaled aminoglycosides, and oral corticosteroids, as well as more hospitalization days, and isolation of *Aspergillus fumigatus* from the sputum as risk factors for colonization with *S. maltophilia*.[26,63,86] Unlike with *Burkholderia cepacia* infection, no evidence of patient-to-patient transmission of *S. maltophilia* has been found, nor does the organism appear to be associated with rapid deterioration of pulmonary function in patients with cystic fibrosis.[25,42] Cases of *S. maltophilia* bacteremia have not been reported in patients with cystic fibrosis, with the exception of one patient who died of sepsis caused by this bacterium on the first day after undergoing lung transplantation.[52] The clinical significance of isolation of *S. maltophilia* from the sputum of patients with cystic fibrosis and its role in the deterioration in lung function is uncertain. Its presence may represent more a marker of severe, advanced disease than causally related respiratory deterioration.[22,43]

Other infections caused by *S. maltophilia* include peritoneal catheter exit-site infections and peritonitis in patients undergoing peritoneal dialysis,[19,85] as well as cholangitis,[76] osteochondritis,[7] mastoiditis,[47] bursitis,[77] sinusitis,[45] liver abscess,[80] osteomyelitis,[58] and necrotizing ulcerative gingivitis.[67]

DIAGNOSIS

The diagnosis of infection is established by isolating the organism from normally sterile sites in the presence of a compatible clinical picture. However, growth of *S. maltophilia* from normally sterile samples actually may represent an episode of pseudoinfection caused by the ability of this organism to contaminate and survive in hospital equipment such as blood collection tubes and antiseptic solutions. Because *S. maltophilia* is a common colonizer of hospitalized patients, isolation from nonsterile sites such as sputum or wounds is more difficult to interpret, particularly when the organism is isolated in mixed culture. Because nosocomial outbreaks have been reported, isolation of *S. maltophilia* from other patients in a hospital setting should alert the physician to the possibility of *Stenotrophomonas* infection. Infection control offices should be notified after the organism has been isolated.

Occasionally, *B. cepacia* is misidentified as *S. maltophilia*, especially in patients with cystic fibrosis.[11] *S. maltophilia* is oxidase-negative and DNase-positive. These tests should be repeated when identification of the organism is in doubt. Because of the serious clinical implications of misidentification in this group of patients, molecular analysis of the isolates should be considered if results remain uncertain.[98]

TREATMENT

Providing antibiotic therapy for *S. maltophilia* is difficult for several reasons. This organism displays multiple resistance mechanisms that confer broad antibiotic resistance, including resistance to β-lactam antibiotic agents. Mechanisms of resistance include the production of two chromosomally encoded, inducible β-lactamases designated L1 and L2. The former is a β-lactamase inhibitor–resistant metalloenzyme that hydrolyzes a broad range of β-lactam antibiotics, including carbapenems such as imipenem and meropenem. L2 is a cephalosporinase and, unlike L1, is susceptible to β-lactamase inhibitors.[23] Other mechanisms of resis-

tance include reduced antibiotic uptake, the main mechanism providing aminoglycoside resistance, and an antibiotic efflux system that confers multidrug resistance.[3,103] In addition, in vitro antibiotic susceptibility testing is plagued by numerous methodologic problems. Several factors, including the time of incubation and the composition of the medium, affect the interpretation of test results. Furthermore, poor reproducibility among different testing methods has been described.[14] The Clinical and Laboratory Standards Institute (CLSI, formerly the National Committee for Clinical Laboratory Standards) has established standards for antibiotic susceptibility testing, including testing by both disk diffusion and broth or agar dilution (minimum inhibitory concentration [MIC] evaluation).[17] For the disk diffusion method, the CLSI recommends testing only trimethoprim-sulfamethoxazole, levofloxacin, and minocycline. In the case of broth or agar dilution, the CLSI recommends testing trimethoprim-sulfamethoxazole (susceptible: 2/38 μg/mL; resistant: 4/76 μg/mL), ceftazidime (susceptible: 8 μg/mL; intermediate: 16 μg/mL; resistant: 32 μg/mL), chloramphenicol (susceptible: 8 μg/mL; intermediate: 16 μg/mL; resistant: 32 μg/mL), levofloxacin (susceptible: 2 μg/mL; intermediate: 4 μg/mL; resistant: 8 μg/mL), minocycline (susceptible: 4 μg/mL; intermediate: 8 μg/mL; resistant: 16 μg/mL), and ticarcillin-clavulanate (susceptible: 16/2 μg/mL; intermediate: 32/2-64/2 μg/mL; resistant: 128/2 μg/mL). However, no controlled clinical studies have determined the most effective antibiotic regimen or duration of treatment.

Antibiotic susceptibility studies and clinical observation suggest that the most active antibiotic against *S. maltophilia* is trimethoprim-sulfamethoxazole, and most authorities agree that it is the drug of choice. It is bacteriostatic, however, a property that may have clinical implications in immunosuppressed patients. In addition, resistant strains are being identified with increasing frequency.[2,66,90] Other antibiotics that have shown good in vitro activity include ticarcillin-clavulanate, doxycycline, minocycline, and tigecycline, although clinical experience with the latter three drugs is limited.[23,49] The activity of early fluoroquinolones such as ciprofloxacin and ofloxacin varies widely, and emergence of resistance during treatment has been reported.[16] Newer quinolones, including levofloxacin and gatifloxacin, appear to have better activity in vitro against *S. maltophilia*,[32,50,60,97] but their activity decreases against multiresistant strains, and the development of resistance during the course of treatment has been described.[8,58] In addition, geographic variations in antibiotic resistance rates have been reported.[35]

Bloodstream infections can be severe, particularly in immunosuppressed patients. Combination antibiotic therapy with trimethoprim-sulfamethoxazole and ticarcillin-clavulanate for bloodstream infections by isolates that are susceptible has been advocated by some authorities and is supported by in vitro pharmacodynamic model data.[69,90,102] Other combinations have shown varying efficacy and correlation between in vitro and in vivo findings, which have not always been consistent.[23] In cases of catheter-related bloodstream infection, removal of the catheter has been associated with improved outcome, irrespective of the appropriateness of antibiotic therapy.[29,83] Nonetheless, successful treatment without removal of the catheter,[69] as well as an association of inappropriate antibiotic therapy and death,[66] has been described. In cases of serious infection such as bacteremia or severe pneumonia, combination antibiotic therapy should be considered when in vitro and in vivo evidence suggest that rapid emergence of resistance may occur during treatment.[38]

Appropriate management of patients from whom *S. maltophilia* is isolated from nonsterile sites, particularly in mixed culture, is not always clear because some isolates may represent colonization or contamination of the sample. In a pediatric study describing nonrespiratory infections in children, 6 of 16 patients with *S. maltophilia* that was cultured from sites other than the bloodstream were treated with antibiotics not active in vitro, and 5 of these children were "cured."[83] Nonetheless, in adults, *S. maltophilia* has been associated unquestionably with severe infection at sites other than the bloodstream, and death caused by *S. maltophilia* infection has been associated with inappropriate initial antibiotic therapy.[72]

REFERENCES

1. Aisenberg, G., Rolston, K. V., Dickey, B. F., et al.: *Stenotrophomonas maltophilia* pneumonia in cancer patients without traditional risk factors for infection, 1997-2004. Eur. J. Clin. Microbiol. Infect. Dis. 26:13-20, 2007.
2. Al-Jasser, A. M.: *Stenotrophomonas maltophilia* resistant to trimethoprim-sulfamethoxazole: An increasing problem. Ann. Clin. Microbiol. Antimicrob. 5:23, 2006.
3. Alonso, A., and Martinez, J. L.: Expression of multidrug efflux pump SmeDEF by clinical isolates of *Stenotrophomonas maltophilia*. Antimicrob. Agents Chemother. 45:1879-1881, 2001.
4. Apisarnthanarak, A., Fraser, V. J., Dunne, W. M., et al.: *Stenotrophomonas maltophilia* intestinal colonization in hospitalized oncology patients with diarrhea. Clin. Infect. Dis. 37:1131-1135, 2003.
5. Apisarnthanarak, A., Mayfield, J. L., Garison, T., et al.: Risk factors for *Stenotrophomonas maltophilia* bacteremia in oncology patients: A case-control study. Infect. Control Hosp. Epidemiol. 24:269-274, 2003.
6. Aydin, K., Koksal, I., Kaygusuz, S., et al.: Endocarditis caused by *Stenotrophomonas maltophilia*. Scand. J. Infect. Dis. 32:427-430, 2000.
7. Baltimore, R. S., and Jenson, H. B.: Puncture wound osteochondritis of the foot caused by *Pseudomonas maltophilia*. Pediatr. Infect. Dis. J. 9:143-144, 1990.
8. Bellido, J. L., Hernandez, F. J., Zufiaurre, M. N., and Garcia-Rodriguez, J. A.: In vitro activity of newer fluoroquinolones against *Stenotrophomonas maltophilia*. J. Antimicrob. Chemother. 46:334-335, 2000.
9. Berbari, N., Johnson, D. H., and Cunha, B. A.: *Xanthomonas maltophilia* peritonitis in a patient undergoing peritoneal dialysis. Heart Lung 22:282-283, 1993.
10. Boktour, M., Hanna, H., Ansari, S., et al.: Central venous catheter and *Stenotrophomonas maltophilia* bacteremia in cancer patients. Cancer 106:1967-1973, 2006.
11. Burdge, D. R., Noble, M. A., Campbell, M. E., et al.: *Xanthomonas maltophilia* misidentified as *Pseudomonas cepacia* in cultures of sputum from patients with cystic fibrosis: A diagnostic pitfall with major clinical implications. Clin. Infect. Dis. 20:445-448, 1995.
12. Calza, L., Manfredi, R., and Chiodo, F.: *Stenotrophomonas (Xanthomonas) maltophilia* as an emerging opportunistic pathogen in association with HIV infection: A 10-year surveillance study. Infection 31:155-161, 2003.
13. Carmeli, Y., and Samore, M. H.: Comparison of treatment with imipenem vs. ceftazidime as a predisposing factor for nosocomial acquisition of *Stenotrophomonas maltophilia*: A historical cohort study. Clin. Infect. Dis. 24:1131-1134, 1997.
14. Carroll, K. C., Cohen, S., Nelson, R., et al.: Comparison of various in vitro susceptibility methods for testing *Stenotrophomonas maltophilia*. Diagn. Microbiol. Infect. Dis. 32:229-235, 1998.
15. Chen, S., Stroh, E. M., Wald, K., and Jalkh, A.: *Xanthomonas maltophilia* endophthalmitis after implantation of sustained-release ganciclovir. Am. J. Ophthalmol. 114:772-773, 1992.
16. Cheng, A. F., Li, M. K., Ling, T. K., and French, G. L.: Emergence of ofloxacin-resistant *Citrobacter freundii* and *Pseudomonas maltophilia* after ofloxacin therapy. J. Antimicrob. Chemother. 20:283-285, 1987.
17. Clinical and Laboratory Standards Institute (CLSI): Performance Standards for Antimicrobial Susceptibility Testing: Seventeenth Informational Supplement. CLSI document M100-S17. Wayne, PA, CLSI, 2007.
18. Daley, A. J., and McIntyre, P. B.: *Stenotrophomonas maltophilia* and lawn mower injuries in children. J. Trauma 48:536-537, 2000.
19. Dapena, F., Selgas, R., Garcia-Perea, A., et al.: Clinical significance of exit-site infections due to *Xanthomonas* in CAPD patients: A comparison with *Pseudomonas* infection. Nephrol. Dial. Transplant. 9:1774-1777, 1994.
20. de Oliveira-Garcia, D., Dall'Agnol, M., Rosales, M., et al.: Fimbriae and adherence of *Stenotrophomonas maltophilia* to epithelial cells and to abiotic surfaces. Cell. Microbiol. 5:625-636, 2003.
21. del Toro, M. D., Rodríguez-Bano, J., Herrero, M., et al.: Clinical epidemiology of *Stenotrophomonas maltophilia* colonization and infection: A multicenter study. Medicine (Baltimore) 81:228-239, 2002.
22. Demko, C. A., Stern, R. C., and Doershuk, C. F.: *Stenotrophomonas maltophilia* in cystic fibrosis: Incidence and prevalence. Pediatr. Pulmonol. 25:304-308, 1998.
23. Denton, M., and Kerr, K. G.: Microbiological and clinical aspects of infection associated with *Stenotrophomonas maltophilia*. Clin. Microbiol. Rev. 11:57-80, 1998.
24. Denton, M., Rajgopal, A., Mooney, L., et al.: *Stenotrophomonas maltophilia* contamination of nebulizers used to deliver aerosolized therapy to inpatients with cystic fibrosis. J. Hosp. Infect. 55:180-183, 2003.
25. Denton, M., Todd, N. J., Kerr, K. G., et al.: Molecular epidemiology of *Stenotrophomonas maltophilia* isolated from clinical specimens from patients with cystic fibrosis and associated environmental samples. J. Clin. Microbiol. 36:1953-1958, 1998.
26. Denton, M., Todd, N. J., and Littlewood, J. M.: Role of anti-pseudomonal antibiotics in the emergence of *Stenotrophomonas maltophilia* in cystic fibrosis patients. Eur. J. Clin. Microbiol. Infect. Dis. 15:402-405, 1996.
27. Dyte, P. H., and Gillians, J. A.: *Pseudomonas maltophilia* infection in an abattoir worker. Med. J. Aust. 1:444-445, 1977.
28. Elsner, H. A., Duhrsen, U., Hollwitz, B., et al.: Fatal pulmonary hemorrhage in patients with acute leukemia and fulminant pneumonia caused by *Stenotrophomonas maltophilia*. Ann. Hematol. 74:155-161, 1997.
29. Elting, L. S., and Bodey, G. P.: Septicemia due to *Xanthomonas* species and non-*aeruginosa Pseudomonas* species: Increasing incidence of catheter-related infections. Medicine (Baltimore) 69:296-306, 1990.
30. Elting, L. S., Khardori, N., Bodey, G. P., and Fainstein, V.: Nosocomial infection caused by *Xanthomonas maltophilia*: A case-control study of predisposing factors. Infect. Control Hosp. Epidemiol. 11:134-138, 1990.
31. Elvers, K. T., Leeming, K., Moore, C. P., and Lappin-Scott, H. M.: Bacterial-fungal biofilms in flowing water photo-processing tanks. J. Appl. Microbiol. 84:607-618, 1998.
32. Fedler, K. A., Biedenbach, D. J., and Jones, R. N.: Assessment of pathogen frequency and resistance patterns among pediatric patient isolates: Report from the 2004 SENTRY Antimicrobial Surveillance Program on 3 continents. Diagn. Microbiol. Infect. Dis. 56:427-436, 2006.
33. Figueiredo, P. M., Furumura, M. T., Santos, A. M., et al.: Cytotoxic activity of clinical *Stenotrophomonas maltophilia*. Lett. Appl. Microbiol. 43:443-449, 2006.
34. Fujita, J., Yamadori, I., Xu, G., et al.: Clinical features of *Stenotrophomonas maltophilia* pneumonia in immunocompromised patients. Respir. Med. 90:35-38, 1996.
35. Gales, A. C., Jones, R. N., Forward, K. R., et al.: Emerging importance of multidrug-resistant *Acinetobacter* species and *Stenotrophomonas maltophilia* as pathogens in seriously ill patients: Geographic patterns, epidemiological features, and trends in the SENTRY Antimicrobial Surveillance Program (1997-1999). Clin. Infect. Dis. 32(Suppl 2):104-113, 2001.
36. Garcia de Viedma, D., Marin, M., Cercenado, E., et al.: Evidence of nosocomial *Stenotrophomonas maltophilia* cross-infection in a neonatology unit analyzed by three molecular typing methods. Infect. Control Hosp. Epidemiol. 20:816-820, 1999.
37. Gardner, P., Griffin, W. B., Swartz, M. N., et al.: Nonfermentative gram negative bacilli of nosocomial interest. Am. J. Med. 48:735-749, 1970.
38. Garrison, M. W., Anderson, D. E., Campbell, D. M., et al.: *Stenotrophomonas maltophilia*: Emergence of multidrug-resistant strains during therapy and in an in vitro pharmacodynamic chamber model. Antimicrob. Agents Chemother. 40:2859-2864, 1996.
39. Gasparetto, E. L., Bertholdo, D. B., Davaus, T., et al.: *Stenotrophomonas maltophilia* pneumonia after bone marrow transplantation: Case report with emphasis on the high-resolution CT findings. Br. J. Radiol. 80:e19-e20, 2007.
40. Gilligan, P. H., and Whittier, S.: *Burkholderia, Stenotrophomonas, Ralstonia, Brevundimonas, Comamonas, Acidovorax.* In Murray, P. R., Baron, E. J., Pfaller, M. A., et al. (eds.): Manual of Clinical Microbiology. 7th ed. Washington, D.C., American Society for Microbiology, 1999, pp. 526-538.
41. Gordon, G., Indeck, M., Bross, J., et al.: Injury from silage wagon accident complicated by mucormycosis. J. Trauma 28:866-867, 1988.
42. Goss, C. H., Mayer-Hamblett, N., Aitken, M. L., et al.: Association between *Stenotrophomonas maltophilia* and lung function in cystic fibrosis. Thorax 59:955-959, 2004.
43. Goss, C. H., Otto, K., Aitken, M. L., et al.: Detecting *Stenotrophomonas maltophilia* does not reduce survival of patients with cystic fibrosis. Am. J. Respir. Crit. Care Med. 166:356-361, 2002.
44. Gulcan, H., Kuzucu, C., and Durmaz, R.: Nosocomial *Stenotrophomonas maltophilia* cross-infection: Three cases in newborns. Am. J. Infect. Control 32:365-368, 2004.
45. Gunnarsson, G., and Steinsson, K.: Sinusitis due to *Stenotrophomonas maltophilia*. Scand. J. Infect. Dis. 34:136-137, 2001.
46. Gutierrez Rodero, F., Masia, M. M., Cortes, J., et al.: Endocarditis caused by *Stenotrophomonas maltophilia*: Case report and review. Clin. Infect. Dis. 23:1261-1265, 1996.
47. Harlowe, H. D.: Acute mastoiditis following *Pseudomonas maltophilia* infection: Case report. Laryngoscope 82:882-883, 1972.
48. Horio, N., Horiguchi, M., Murakami, K., et al.: *Stenotrophomonas maltophilia* endophthalmitis after intraocular lens implantation. Graefes Arch. Clin. Exp. Ophthalmol. 238:299-301, 2000.
49. Insa, R., Cercenado, E., Goyanes, M. J., et al.: In vitro activity of tigecycline against clinical isolates of *Acinetobacter baumannii* and *Stenotrophomonas maltophilia*. J. Antimicrob. Chemother. 59:583-585, 2007.
50. Jones, R. N., Sader, H. S., and Beach, M. L.: Contemporary in vitro spectrum of activity summary for antimicrobial agents tested against 18569 strains non-fermentative gram-negative bacilli isolated in the SENTRY Antimicrobial Surveillance Program (1997-2001). Int. J. Antimicrob. Agents 22:551-556, 2003.

51. Kaiser, G. M., Tso, P. C., Morris, R., and McCurdy, D.: *Xanthomonas maltophilia* endophthalmitis after cataract extraction. Am. J. Ophthalmol. *123*:410-411, 1997.
52. Kanj, S. S., Tapson, V., Davis, R. D., et al.: Infections in patients with cystic fibrosis following lung transplantation. Chest *112*:924-930, 1997.
53. Karpati, F., Malmborg, A. S., Alfredsson, H., et al.: Bacterial colonisation with *Xanthomonas maltophilia*: A retrospective study in a cystic fibrosis patient population. Infection *22*:258-263, 1994.
54. Kerr, K. G., Denton, M., Todd, N., et al.: A new selective differential medium for isolation of *Stenotrophomonas maltophilia*. Eur. J. Clin. Microbiol. Infect. Dis. *15*:607-610, 1996.
55. Khardori, N., Elting, L., Wong, E., et al.: Nosocomial infections due to *Xanthomonas maltophilia (Pseudomonas maltophilia)* in patients with cancer. Rev. Infect. Dis. *12*:997-1003, 1990.
56. Krcmery, V., Jr., Pichna, P., Oravcova, E., et al.: *Stenotrophomonas maltophilia* bacteraemia in cancer patients: Report on 31 cases. J. Hosp. Infect. *34*:75-77, 1996.
57. Lai, C. H., Wong, W. W., Chin, C., et al.: Central venous catheter-related *Stenotrophomonas maltophilia* bacteraemia and associated relapsing bacteraemia in haematology and oncology patients. Clin. Microbiol. Infect. *12*:986-991, 2006.
58. Landrum, M. L., Conger, N. G., and Forgione, M. A.: Trimethoprim-sulfamethoxazole in the treatment of *Stenotrophomonas maltophilia* osteomyelitis. Clin. Infect. Dis. *40*:1551-1552, 2005.
59. Lanotte, P., Cantagrel, S., Mereghetti, L., et al.: Spread of *Stenotrophomonas maltophilia* colonization in a pediatric intensive care unit detected by monitoring tracheal bacterial carriage and molecular typing. Clin. Microbiol. Infect. *9*:1142-1147, 2003.
60. Lanzafame, A., Bonfiglio, G., Santini, L., et al.: In vitro activity of levofloxacin against recent gram-negative nosocomial pathogens. Chemotherapy *51*:44-50, 2005.
61. Lo, W. T., Wang, C. C., Lee, C. M., et al.: Successful treatment of multiresistant *Stenotrophomonas maltophilia* meningitis with ciprofloxacin in a preterm infant. Eur. J. Pediatr. *161*:680-682, 2002.
62. Maningo, E., and Watanakunakorn, C.: *Xanthomonas maltophilia* and *Pseudomonas cepacia* in lower respiratory tracts of patients in critical care units. J. Infect. *31*:89-92, 1995.
63. Marchac, V., Equi, A., Le Bihan-Benjamin, C., et al.: Case-control study of *Stenotrophomonas maltophilia* acquisition in cystic fibrosis patients. Eur. Respir. J. *23*:98-102, 2004.
64. Marshall, W. F., Keating, M. R., Anhalt, J. P., and Steckelberg, J. M.: *Xanthomonas maltophilia*: An emerging nosocomial pathogen. Mayo Clin. Proc. *64*:1097-1104, 1989.
65. Metan, G., Hayran, M., Hascelik, G., et al.: Which patient is a candidate for empirical therapy against *Stenotrophomonas maltophilia* bacteraemia? An analysis of associated risk factors in a tertiary care hospital. Scand. J. Infect. Dis. *38*:527-531, 2006.
66. Micozzi, A., Venditti, M., Monaco, M., et al.: Bacteremia due to *Stenotrophomonas maltophilia* in patients with hematologic malignancies. Clin. Infect. Dis. *31*:705-711, 2000.
67. Miyairi, I., Franklin, J. A., Andreansky, M., et al.: Acute necrotizing ulcerative gingivitis and bacteremia caused by *Stenotrophomonas maltophilia* in an immunocompromised host. Pediatr. Infect. Dis. *24*:181-183, 2005.
68. Morrison, A. J., Jr., Hoffmann, K. K., and Wenzel, R. P.: Associated mortality and clinical characteristics of nosocomial *Pseudomonas maltophilia* in a university hospital. J. Clin. Microbiol. *24*:52-55, 1986.
69. Muder, R. R., Harris, A. P., Muller, S., et al.: Bacteremia due to *Stenotrophomonas (Xanthomonas) maltophilia*: A prospective, multicenter study of 91 episodes. Clin. Infect. Dis. *22*:508-512, 1996.
70. Munter, R. G., Yinnon, A. M., Schlesinger, Y., and Hershko, C.: Infective endocarditis due to *Stenotrophomonas (Xanthomonas) maltophilia*. Eur. J. Clin. Microbiol. Infect. Dis. *17*:353-356, 1998.
71. Nguyen, M. H., and Muder, R. R.: Meningitis due to *Xanthomonas maltophilia*: Case report and review. Clin. Infect. Dis. *19*:325-326, 1994.
72. Nseir, S., Di Pompeo, C., Brisson, H., et al.: Intensive care unit-acquired *Stenotrophomonas maltophilia*: incidence, risk factors, and outcome. Crit. Care *10*:1-9, 2006.
73. Nseir, S., Di Pompeo, C., Cavestri, B., et al.: Multiple-drug-resistant bacteria in patients with severe acute exacerbation of chronic obstructive pulmonary disease: Prevalence, risk factors, and outcome. Crit. Care Med. *34*:2959-2966, 2006.
74. Oie, S., and Kamiya, A.: Microbial contamination of brushes used for preoperative shaving. J. Hosp. Infect. *21*:103-110, 1992.
75. Palleroni, N. J., and Bradbury, J. F.: *Stenotrophomonas*, a new bacterial genus for *Xanthomonas maltophilia* (Hugh 1980) Swings et al. 1983. Int. J. Syst. Bacteriol. *43*:606-609, 1993.
76. Papadakis, K. A., Vartivarian, S. E., Vassilaki, M. E., and Anaissie, E. J.: *Stenotrophomonas maltophilia*: An unusual cause of biliary sepsis. Clin. Infect. Dis. *21*:1032-1034, 1995.
77. Papadakis, K. A., Vartivarian, S. E., Vassilaki, M. E., and Anaissie, E. J.: Septic prepatellar bursitis caused by *Stenotrophomonas (Xanthomonas) maltophilia*. Clin. Infect. Dis. *22*:388-389, 1996.
78. Papadakis, K. A., Vartivarian, S. E., Vassilaki, M. E., and Anaissie, E. J.: *Stenotrophomonas maltophilia* meningitis: Report of two cases and review of the literature. J. Neurosurg. *87*:106-108, 1997.
79. Penland, R. L., and Wilhelmus, K. R.: *Stenotrophomonas maltophilia* ocular infections. Arch. Ophthalmol. *114*:433-436, 1996.
80. Petri, A., Tiszlavicz, L., Nagy, E., et al.: Liver abscess caused by *Stenotrophomonas maltophilia*: Report of a case. Surg. Today *33*:224-228, 2003.
81. Rogues, A. M., Maugein, J., Allery, A., et al.: Electronic ventilator temperature sensors as a potential source of respiratory tract colonization with *Stenotrophomonas maltophilia*. J. Hosp. Infect. *49*:289-292, 2001.
82. Sarvamangala Devi, J. N., Venkatesh, A., and Shivananda, P. G.: Neonatal infections due to *Pseudomonas maltophilia*. Indian Pediatr. *21*:72-74, 1984.
83. Sattler, C. A., Mason, E. O., Jr., and Kaplan, S. L.: Nonrespiratory *Stenotrophomonas maltophilia* infection at a children's hospital. Clin. Infect. Dis. *31*:1321-1330, 2000.
84. Semel, J. D., Trenholme, G. M., Harris, A. A., et al.: *Pseudomonas maltophilia* pseudosepticemia. Am. J. Med. *64*:403-406, 1978.
85. Szeto, C. C., Li, P. K., Leung, C. B., et al.: *Xanthomonas maltophilia* peritonitis in uremic patients receiving continuous ambulatory peritoneal dialysis. Am. J. Kidney Dis. *29*:91-95, 1997.
86. Talmaciu, I., Varlotta, L., Mortensen, J., and Schidlow, D. V.: Risk factors for emergence of *Stenotrophomonas maltophilia* in cystic fibrosis. Pediatr. Pulmonol. *30*:10-15, 2000.
87. Teo, W. Y., Chan, M. Y., Lam, C. M., et al.: Skin manifestation of *Stenotrophomonas maltophilia* infection: A case report and review article. Ann. Acad. Med. Singapore *35*:897-900, 2006.
88. Valdezate, S., Vindel, A., Maiz, L., et al.: Persistence and variability of *Stenotrophomonas maltophilia* in cystic fibrosis patients, Madrid, 1991-1998. Emerg. Infect. Dis. *7*:113-122, 2001.
89. Van Couwenberghe, C. J., Farver, T. B., and Cohen, S. H.: Risk factors associated with isolation of *Stenotrophomonas (Xanthomonas) maltophilia* in clinical specimens. Infect. Control Hosp. Epidemiol. *18*:316-321, 1997.
90. Vartivarian, S., Anaissie, E., Bodey, G., et al.: A changing pattern of susceptibility of *Xanthomonas maltophilia* to antimicrobial agents: Implications for therapy. Antimicrob. Agents Chemother. *38*:624-627, 1994.
91. Vartivarian, S. E., Papadakis, K. A., and Anaissie, E. J.: *Stenotrophomonas (Xanthomonas) maltophilia* urinary tract infection: A disease that is usually severe and complicated. Arch. Intern. Med. *156*:433-435, 1996.
92. Vartivarian, S. E., Papadakis, K. A., Palacios, J. A., et al.: Mucocutaneous and soft tissue infections caused by *Xanthomonas maltophilia*: A new spectrum. Ann. Intern. Med. *121*:969-973, 1994.
93. Victor, M. A., Arpi, M., Bruun, B., et al.: *Xanthomonas maltophilia* bacteremia in immunocompromised hematological patients. Scand. J. Infect. Dis. *26*:163-170, 1994.
94. Villarino, M. E., Stevens, L. E., Schable, B., et al.: Risk factors for epidemic *Xanthomonas maltophilia* infection/colonization in intensive care unit patients. Infect. Control Hosp. Epidemiol. *13*:201-206, 1992.
95. Waters, V. and Ratjen, F.: Multidrug-resistant organisms in cystic fibrosis: Management and infection-control issues. Expert Rev. Anti Infect. Ther. *4*:807-819, 2006.
96. Weber, D. J., Rutala, W. A., Blanchet, C. N., et al.: Faucet aerators: A source of patient colonization with *Stenotrophomonas maltophilia*. Am. J. Infect. Control *27*:59-63, 1999.
97. Weiss, K., Restieri, C., De Carolis, E., et al.: Comparative activity of new quinolones against 326 clinical isolates of *Stenotrophomonas maltophilia*. J. Antimicrob. Chemother. *45*:363-365, 2000.
98. Whitby, P. W., Carter, K. B., Burns, J. L., et al.: Identification and detection of *Stenotrophomonas maltophilia* by rRNA-directed PCR. J. Clin. Microbiol. *38*:4305-4309, 2000.
99. Wishart, M. M., and Riley, T. V.: Infection with *Pseudomonas maltophilia* hospital outbreak due to contaminated disinfectant. Med. J. Aust. *2*:710-712, 1976.
100. Wu, P. S., Lu, C. Y., Chang, L. Y., et al.: *Stenotrophomonas maltophilia* bacteremia in pediatric patients: A 10-year analysis. J. Microbiol. Immunol. Infect. *39*:144-149, 2006.
101. Yu, V. L., Rumans, L. W., Wing, E. J., et al.: *Pseudomonas maltophilia* causing heroin-associated infective endocarditis. Arch. Intern. Med. *138*:1667-1671, 1978.
102. Zelenitsky S. A., Iacovides, H., Ariano, R. E., et al.: Antibiotic combinations significantly more active than monotherapy in an in vitro infection model of *Stenotrophomonas maltophilia*. Diagn. Microbiol. Infect. Dis. *51*:39-43, 2005.
103. Zhang, L., Li, X. Z., and Poole, K. Multiple antibiotic resistance in *Stenotrophomonas maltophilia*: Involvement of a multidrug efflux system. Antimicrob. Agents Chemother. *44*:287-293, 2000.

SUBSECTION 5

Gram-Negative Coccobacilli

CHAPTER

137

ACTINOBACILLUS ACTINOMYCETEMCOMITANS

Suzanne Whitworth ✪ Richard F. Jacobs

Actinobacillus actinomycetemcomitans is a fastidious, non–spore-forming, nonmotile, facultatively anaerobic gram-negative rod that frequently complicates actinomycosis caused by *Actinomyces israelii*. In addition to being associated with actinomycosis, it has been implicated as a pathogen in periodontal disease and is part of the oral flora. Infection by this bacterium often is not resolved by the normal host, possibly because of inefficient phagocytosis and a weak oxidative burst response of neutrophils.[7] In addition, the bacterium has several virulence factors, including induction of apoptosis and tissue destruction.[3] This organism is characterized by slow growth in culture and a requirement for incubation in an atmosphere enhanced with carbon dioxide.[4] Other bacterial species concomitantly isolated in human actinomycosis are *Eikenella corrodens, Fusobacterium, Bacteroides, Capnocytophaga, Staphylococcus, Streptococcus,* and members of Enterobacteriaceae.

A. actinomycetemcomitans is a pathogen in at least 30 percent of actinomycotic infections[4] (see Chapter 161). Failure to recognize this organism and to treat it adequately has resulted in clinical relapse and deterioration in patients infected with actinomycosis.[5,13] Severe forms of periodontitis, particularly localized aggressive periodontitis, also are associated with this pathogen, and studies have shown that this organism is related strongly to children in the 10- to 19-year age group.[9] This type of periodontitis is characterized by rapid loss of attachment and bone around the permanent incisors and permanent molars. Treatment consists of local débridement and antibiotic therapy, usually metronidazole alone or in combination with amoxicillin. *A. actinomycetemcomitans* also is an important pathogen in Papillon-Lefèvre syndrome, an autosomal recessive disorder characterized by prepubertal periodontitis and palmar-plantar hyperkeratosis.[8] Additionally, it is one of the HACEK (HACEK also includes *Haemophilus aphrophilus, Cardiobacterium hominis, E. corrodens,* and *Kingella kingae*) organisms that have a propensity for infecting heart valves. The endocarditis caused by this organism usually is insidious, with fever occurring in fewer than 50 percent of cases.[4] This organism also has been reported to cause pericarditis, meningitis, brain abscess, parotitis, synovitis, osteomyelitis, urinary tract infection, pneumonia, and empyema.[4] Cases of endophthalmitis[1,11] and cavernous sinus infection also have been reported.[12]

A. actinomycetemcomitans can be cultured on blood and chocolate agar, but it grows poorly on MacConkey agar. Cultures require incubation in an enhanced carbon dioxide atmosphere. Growth of the organism in a blood culture may take as long as 9 days in patients with endocarditis, and thus cultures should be held longer. On Gram stain, the organism appears coccoid to coccobacillary. Molecular techniques based on non-amplification nucleic acid probes or on polymerase chain reaction can provide rapid and accurate identification of *A. actinomycetemcomitans.*[10] Because of the frequency of co-infection with this organism in cases of actinomycosis, attempts always should be made to isolate this organism in these patients.

A. actinomycetemcomitans is susceptible to the newer cephalosporins, rifampin, trimethoprim-sulfamethoxazole, aminoglycosides, quinolones, tetracycline, azithromycin, and chloramphenicol. It is susceptible also to penicillin and ampicillin in vitro, but test results do not necessarily correlate with clinical outcome. Vancomycin, erythromycin, and clindamycin have very little activity against this organism. Treatment of aggressive periodontal disease consists of local débridement and antibiotic therapy with metronidazole and amoxicillin, which appear to be effective at suppressing *A. actinomycetemcomitans* to less than the level of detection.[2] Endocarditis caused by this organism has been treated successfully with a combination of ampicillin and gentamicin.[6] Cefotaxime or ceftriaxone is also acceptable.

REFERENCES

1. Binder, M. I., Chua, J., Kaiser, P. K., et al.: *Actinobacillus actinomycetemcomitans* endogenous endophthalmitis: Report of two cases and review of the literature. Scand. J. Infect. Dis. 35:133-136, 2003.
2. Dorfer, C. E.: Antimicrobials for the treatment of aggressive periodontitis. Oral Dis. 9(Suppl. 1):51-53, 2003.
3. Henderson, B., Wilson, M., Sharp, L., Ward, J. M.: *Actinobacillus actinomycetemcomitans.* J. Med. Microbiol. 51:1013-1020, 2002.
4. McGowan, J. E., and Steinberg, J. P.: Other gram-negative bacilli. *In* Mandell, G. L., Bennett, J. E., and Dolin, R. (eds.): Principles and Practices of Infectious Disease. New York, Churchill Livingstone, 1995, pp. 2106-2107.
5. Morris, J. F., and Sewell, D. L.: Necrotizing pneumonia caused by mixed infection with *Actinobacillus actinomycetemcomitans* and *Actinomyces israelii:* Case report and review. Clin. Infect. Dis. 18:450-452, 1994.
6. Paturel, L., Casalta, J. P., Habib, G., et al.: *Actinobacillus actinomycetemcomitans* endocarditis. Clin. Microbiol. Infect. 10:98-118, 2004.
7. Permpanich, P., Kowolik, M. J., and Galli, D. M.: Resistance of fluorescent-labelled *Actinobacillus actinomycetemcomitans* strains to phagocytosis and killing by human neutrophils. Cell. Microbiol. 8:72-84, 2006.
8. Rudiger, S., Petersilka, G., and Flemmig, T. F.: Combined systemic and local antimicrobial therapy of periodontal disease in Papillon-Lefevre syndrome. J. Clin. Periodontol. 26:847-854, 1999.
9. Savitt, E. D., and Kent, R. L.: Distribution of *Actinobacillus actinomycetemcomitans* and *Porphyromonas gingivalis.* J. Periodontol. 62:490-494, 1991.
10. Slots, J.: *Actinobacillus actinomycetemcomitans* and *Porphyromonas gingivalis* in periodontal disease: Introduction. Periodontol. 2000 20:7-13, 1999.
11. Sullivan, P., Clark, W. L., and Kaiser, P. K.: Bilateral endogenous endophthalmitis caused by HACEK microorganism. Am. J. Ophthalmol. 133:144-145, 2002.
12. Tobias, S., Lee, J. H., and Tomford, J. W.: Rare *Actinobacillus* infection of the cavernous sinus causing painful ophthalmoplegia: Case report. Neurosurgery 51:807-809, 2002.
13. Tyrrell, J., Noone, P., and Prichard, J. S.: Thoracic actinomycosis complicated by *Actinobacillus actinomycetemcomitans:* Case report and review of literature. Respir. Med. 86:341-343, 1992.

BARTONELLOSIS

CHAPTER 138

Barbara W. Stechenberg

Bartonellosis is a term that has been used to describe a geographically distinct disease caused by *Bartonella bacilliformis*. Recent advances in molecular biology have led to the reclassification of several bacterial pathogens, and the family Bartonellaceae, genus *Bartonella*, has expanded from a single species, *B. bacilliformis*, to include 16 validated species, 8 of which have been known to be pathogenic in humans. Of the members of the genus *Rochalimaea* that have been reclassified as *Bartonella* spp., *Bartonella henselae* is the cause of cat-scratch disease (see Chapter 151). Manifestations of *Bartonella* infection other than classic bartonellosis seldom occur in children and are discussed briefly.

BARTONELLOSIS (CARRIÓN DISEASE)

Bartonellosis is a disease unusual in its manifestations and rich in its history. The organism, *B. bacilliformis*, causes two illnesses that are both clinically and temporally distinctive. Besides producing subclinical asymptomatic infection, this organism can cause Oroya fever, a disease characterized by severe febrile hemolytic anemia, or verruga peruana, an eruption of hemangioma-like lesions. The eponym *Carrión disease* is used to designate the two forms collectively. The disease is restricted in its distribution to an area in South America that includes parts of Peru, Ecuador, and Colombia.

The origin of this disease in the history of the region probably considerably precedes the first written documentation of the disorder. The first written account of bartonellosis is attributed to Gago de Vadillo, who published a treatise on the subject in 1630, a century after the arrival of the first Spaniards. In 1764, Cosme Bueno first described the vector of this disease and of cutaneous leishmaniasis as the uta or sandfly.[13] The era of the mid-1800s was a period of increasing wealth in Peru because of a new industry, the mining of guano, or bird manure. With this increase came the building of a railroad from Callao to Oroya and nearly 10,000 workers from Chile, Bolivia, and China, none of whom had previous contact with or immunity to Carrión disease.[17] An epidemic that took the lives of hundreds of workers ensued. A cavalry unit of black soldiers sent to round up deserters quickly fell ill with the disease. A physician caring for them was so impressed with the rapidity and the profound anemia of the disease that he said, "It turned the blacks to whites," a remark henceforth frequently associated with the disease.[30]

In 1885, a Peruvian medical student (Carrión) was collecting data on the geographic distribution and clinical features of verruga peruana. Because of concern about the difficulty in diagnosing the pre-eruption period of verruga, he inoculated himself with material taken from a patient with verruga. He experienced his first symptoms 21 days after inoculation and then went on to exhibit the classic signs and symptoms of Oroya fever. Carrión realized the significance of his experiment 3 days before he died; he had proved the unitary origin of the two illnesses. In 1905, Alberto Barton, a Peruvian physician, described the etiologic agent *(B. bacilliformis)*, but several years passed before this organism was accepted as the cause of Oroya fever and was named in his honor.

THE ORGANISM

B. bacilliformis is small, 0.2 to 1.0 μm wide by 0.3 to 2.0 μm long. It stains easily with Giemsa (purple) and is a gram-negative and motile organism, with a brush of 10 or more unipolar flagella. In tissues, the organism stains black with silver-impregnated stains, such as Warthin-Starry stain. On electron microscopy, the contrast between *B. bacilliformis* and other members of the genus *Bartonella* is striking. Cultured *B. bacilliformis* organisms show the retracted cytoplasm and cell walls typical of bacteria.[22] They are rod shaped in young culture and become mostly coccoid in older culture. These organisms are obligate aerobes that grow best at 28° C in semisolid nutrient agar with 10 percent rabbit serum and 0.5 percent rabbit hemoglobin. Growth is subsurface, usually occurring in 7 to 10 days. The organism is pathogenic only for human beings and other primates, and only one antigenic type exists. Analysis of 16S rRNA sequences shows that *B. bacilliformis* is in the alpha$_2$ subgroup of proteobacteria and that its closest relatives are *Bartonella quintana* and *Brucella abortus*.[5]

EPIDEMIOLOGY

The distribution of the disease historically has been restricted to the mountain valleys of the Andes Mountains in Peru, Ecuador, and Colombia. Within these regions, the disease usually is seen only between the altitudes of 500 and 3200 m above sea level and primarily in valleys that are at right angles to the prevailing wind. This interesting geographic distribution reflects the habits of *Lutzomyia verrucarum*, the sandfly vector, which is seen only at these altitudes. One usually acquires the disease at twilight or soon thereafter because of the feeding habits of the insects. Within the region, the disease is endemic, with sporadic epidemic outbreaks that continue to occur.[12] Recent outbreaks have occurred in nonendemic populations in the surrounding area.[16] Several isolated reports of anemia with *Bartonella*-like organisms have been reported: three cases from Thailand in 1966 and one case from the Sudan in 1969.

PATHOPHYSIOLOGY

After inoculation by the sandfly, *Bartonella* organisms enter the endothelial cells of the blood vessels, where they proliferate during the incubation period. Microscopically, masses of organisms may be noted within the cytoplasm of the cells lining the blood vessels and lymph channels, and their numbers cause them to bulge into the lumen of the vessel. The organisms may be found within reticuloendothelial cells, particularly in the lymph nodes, but also in the liver, spleen, bone marrow, kidneys, adrenals, pancreas, and, more rarely, the skin, heart, and lungs.[11]

The organisms then re-enter the bloodstream and parasitize erythrocytes (red blood cells [RBCs]). Binding of *B. bacilliformis* to RBCs causes indentations and deformation of the membrane; membrane fusion is induced, and the organisms then enter the intracellular vacuoles, where they replicate.[4] The resulting anemia is caused primarily by destruction of these parasitized cells. Because as many as 90 percent of cells may be infected, profound, rapid anemia is a common symptom; the life span of infected RBCs is markedly shortened, particularly in the first few days. All parasitized cells are not destroyed, and no hemolysins or agglutinins have been recovered.[27] *B. bacilliformis* can be demonstrated easily with Giemsa stain. In earlier studies, considerable controversy ensued regarding whether the parasites were within or on the surface of RBCs; Cuadra and Takano[9] showed that they are located predominantly within the cells. In the recovery phase of the anemia, the rod-shaped organisms change to a more coccoid form and rapidly disappear from the blood.

A patient who survives the acute phase of Oroya fever may or may not experience cutaneous manifestations of the disease, which appear as nodular, hemangiomatous lesions ranging in size from a few millimeters to several centimeters. Light microscopy reveals angioblastic and histiocytic hyperplasia of the dermis. Numerous newly formed small vessels with endothelial cell proliferation are found. Mast cells, lymphocytes, and macrophages are present.[1] Electron microscopy demonstrates that the bacterial organisms are located in the verruga, extracellularly in the fine fibrous interstitium. Two types of histiocytic cells are found in the verruga: a more numerous one, which is clear and has many lysosomes, ribosomes, mitochondria, and cytoplasm, and a darker one, with numerous lamellar membranous structures in the cytoplasm.[26] Studies have substantiated the presence of activity in *B. bacilliformis* that stimulates endothelial cells in vitro and is angiogenic in vivo. This finding may explain the similar pathogenesis of verruca and bacillary angiomatosis produced by other *Bartonella* spp.[1]

CLINICAL MANIFESTATIONS

The incubation period varies from 2 to 14 weeks, with a mean of 3 weeks. The difficulty in determining the duration of the incubation period results from the variable symptoms of the disease. Some patients are totally asymptomatic, and disease is detected only by blood culture or on serologic survey.[16] In a population-based cohort study, 0.5 percent of participants had asymptomatic bacteremia.[7] Other patients are not anemic, but symptoms such as headache, malaise, and occasional fever develop, and *B. bacilliformis* is recovered from blood cultures. Still others have severe anemia (Oroya fever). Patients with hemolytic anemia are febrile, and organisms may parasitize the RBCs. The anemia develops rapidly. Patients are deeply apathetic and have a peculiar discoloration of their skin and sclerae secondary to the combination of slight icterus and severe anemia.[28] Tachycardia and soft hemic murmurs are noted; occasionally, peripheral vascular collapse occurs. Headache, vertigo, restlessness, tinnitus, and occasionally angina pectoris may be present. Clouding of the sensorium and delirium are rather common findings; these effects usually are mild but may progress to overt psychosis. The temperature usually fluctuates between 37.5° C and 38.5° C (99.5° F and 101.3° F); higher elevations in temperature may be caused by intercurrent infection. Physical examination discloses generalized lymphadenopathy and nonpainful hepatomegaly.[18]

The anemia is macrocytic and usually hypochromic, with anisocytosis and poikilocytosis. The RBC count may drop to as low as 500,000/mm³ in the first 2 to 4 weeks of illness. Reticulocytes may increase to 50 percent. The pathognomonic sign of the disease is the presence of *B. bacilliformis* within Giemsa-stained RBCs as red-violet rods. The leukocyte count may be normal, low, or elevated.

The "critical stage" of the anemia is the period of transition when the organism suddenly disappears from the RBCs.[28] During this time, *Bartonella* organisms change from the rod shape to more coccoid forms, the number of parasitized RBCs decreases, and the degree of anemia decreases; accordingly, the RBC count increases, and less hyperbilirubinemia is present. Clinically, fever decreases, and the patient stabilizes.[28] In some cases, the illness may become more severe, a finding that suggests the development of intercurrent infection (usually with *Salmonella*). Although this complication may occur at any time, it does so most commonly during the transitional period and may be noted in as many as 40 percent of patients.[8]

In the pre-eruptive stage, patients may complain of pain in their joints, bones, and muscles, as well as cramps and paresthe-sias. Inflammatory reactions such as phlebitis, parotitis, pleuritis, erythema nodosum, and encephalitis may occur. The anemia and lymphadenopathy of the invasive stage disappear.

The appearance of red cutaneous nodules, or verruga, is pathognomonic of the disease in the eruptive stage. Usually, these lesions are present in the skin, but they may be found in mesenchymatous tissue. They vary greatly in number and size, from small nodules to disfiguring zonular (hemangioma-like) lesions. They rarely cause symptoms; however, larger lesions may require surgical excision. This stage may last from several months to a year and may be the sole manifestation of the disease, particularly in school-aged children in endemic areas.

DIAGNOSIS

The diagnosis is based on clinical manifestations, in conjunction with a Giemsa-stained blood smear showing typical organisms, or on blood cultures. In the pre-anemic stage or in patients without the typical anemia who reside in an endemic area, the diagnosis can be based on blood culture alone. The presence of typical verruga in patients from an endemic area is pathognomonic of the disease. Immunoglobulin M antibody may be present in both stages of the disease, as well as in some healthy persons.[12,14] Persons with typical Oroya fever who are treated with antibiotics may not have an antibody response.[12,14] More recently, an indirect fluorescent antibody assay has shown promise for evaluating patients in both the acute and convalescent phases of the disease.[6] The differential diagnosis in the initial phase includes typhoid fever, malaria, tuberculosis, leptospirosis, brucellosis, and meningitis, as well as hematologic malignant disease and aplastic or hemolytic anemia. The eruptive phase may resemble hemangiomata, bacillary angiomatosis, Kaposi sarcoma, and other nodular diseases.

TREATMENT

B. bacilliformis is sensitive to many antibiotics, including penicillin, tetracycline, streptomycin, and chloramphenicol. With treatment, the fever usually abates by 24 hours; the rod-shaped organisms change to more coccoid forms and soon disappear from the blood.

The choice of antibiotic may be guided by considerations other than simple eradication of *B. bacilliformis*, including the risk of developing intercurrent infection. Chloramphenicol is considered the drug of choice because it also is useful in the treatment of salmonellosis.[33] Occasional patients need the addition of another antibiotic, usually a β-lactam.[29] Blood transfusions may be helpful during the period of severe anemia, especially if blood is obtained from patients who have recently recovered from the disease.[27]

Treatment of verruga peruana usually is not necessary unless particularly large zonular lesions interfere with function; in these persons, surgery may be necessary. Treatment is considered when patients have more than 10 cutaneous lesions, if the lesions are particularly erythematous or violaceous, or if the onset of lesions was less than 1 month before presentation.[18] Oral rifampin, ciprofloxacin (not approved for children), or tetracycline may be used to aid in healing of the cutaneous lesions.[17,29]

PROGNOSIS

The mortality rate in untreated bartonellosis was estimated in the past at approximately 40 percent. However, the more recent fatality rate has been approximately 9 percent in patients admitted to the hospital.[17] Intercurrent *Salmonella* infection increases the mortality rate. In one population-based study, the fatality rate was 0.7 percent.[14,16] With the use of chloramphenicol, the prognosis is much improved. Permanent immunity develops in most patients.

PREVENTION

Dichlorodiphenyltrichloroethane (DDT) has been effective in controlling the disease by eliminating the vector *Lutzomyia verrucarum*. Persons can protect themselves by leaving endemic areas at night and using insect repellents. No vaccine of demonstrable efficacy has been developed.

TRENCH FEVER (*BARTONELLA QUINTANA*)

Trench fever was described first in Russia and was recognized as causing a severe epidemic during World War I, with more than a million troops infected.[3] The human body louse, *Pediculus humanus* variety *corporis*, is the vector, and humans are the only known reservoir.

The incubation period is extremely variable (from 4 to 35 days, with an average of 22 days). Symptoms also are highly variable. Four major fever patterns have been described: (1) a single febrile episode; (2) a single febrile period lasting 4 to 5 days; (3) three to eight recurrent febrile episodes, each lasting 4 to 5 days (sometimes for a year or more); and (4) persistent fever lasting 2 to 6 weeks.[10,31] Associated signs and symptoms may include conjunctival injection, retro-orbital pain, myalgias, arthralgias, headache, bone pain (especially in the shins), and splenomegaly. Chronic bacteremia following clinical improvement is common.[10]

In a non-epidemic situation, establishing the diagnosis of trench fever is impossible because the manifestations are not distinctive. The relapsing form can mimic malaria or *Borrelia recurrentis* relapsing fever. A history of body louse infestation or association with an epidemic should heighten suspicion. *B. quintana* can be cultured from blood by using a modification that includes culturing on epithelial cells. Serologic testing is available; however, cross-reactions with *B. henselae* occur. No controlled trials of treatment have been performed, but dramatic defervescence has been noted with the use of tetracycline and chloramphenicol.[15,31]

BACILLARY ANGIOMATOSIS AND BACILLARY PELIOSIS HEPATIS

Both *B. henselae* and *B. quintana* can cause disease in immunocompromised persons, primarily adults with acquired immunodeficiency syndrome (AIDS) or cancer or recipients of organ transplants. Lesions of bacillary angiomatosis are the most easily recognized form of *Bartonella* infection in immunocompromised patients. They are seen predominantly in patients with AIDS and with very low CD4 counts.[13,15] The vasoproliferative lesions may be cutaneous or subcutaneous and pathologically resemble the verruga of *B. bacilliformis*. Most characteristically, these lesions are red with a collarette of scale, but the clinical findings can be diverse. The differential diagnosis includes Kaposi sarcoma, pyogenic granuloma, and verruga peruana, and deep soft tissue masses may develop. Trauma may result in ulceration or bleeding. Osseous lesions occur in the long bones and can be very painful. A 12-year-old child with lymphocytic leukemia and bacillary angiomatosis has been reported.[19]

Bacillary peliosis hepatis was described first in 1990.[21] It is seen primarily in patients infected with human immunodeficiency virus (HIV) who have fever and abdominal pain. Vascular prolif-

erative lesions develop, primarily in the liver and spleen. The differential diagnosis includes hepatic Kaposi sarcoma, lymphoma, extrapulmonary pneumocystosis, and infection with *Mycobacterium avium-intracellulare*. Both bacillary angiomatosis and bacillary peliosis hepatis have been treated successfully with antimicrobial therapy, including erythromycin, newer macrolides such as azithromycin or clarithromycin, or, as an alternative, doxycycline.[15,21,31]

ENDOCARDITIS

B. henselae, *B. quintana*, and *Bartonella elizabethae* all have been reported to cause bacteremia or endocarditis. The symptoms and signs are similar to those of other causes of endocarditis, although prolonged fever, night sweats, and profound weight loss may occur.[32] Many of the immunocompetent patients reported have been homeless. Cases also have been described in immunocompromised persons, particularly HIV-infected patients. *Bartonella* organisms may be a significant cause of culture-negative endocarditis.[2,23,24,32] Two children have been reported with central nervous system infection associated with *B. quintana*.[20]

Special culturing techniques, including the use of Isolator tubes, and prolonged incubation, as well as serology, histopathology of valvular tissue, and polymerase chain reaction, may be helpful.[34] Initial treatment of culture-negative endocarditis with ceftriaxone and gentamicin is effective for *Bartonella* organisms. A retrospective analysis of 101 patients with endocarditis[25] showed a benefit with the use of an aminoglycoside as part of a treatment regimen for a minimum of 14 days. If *Bartonella* is proven, doxycycline with gentamicin are recommended.

REFERENCES

1. Arias-Stella, J., Lieberman, P. H., Erlandson, R. A., et al.: Histology, immunohistochemistry and ultrastructure of the verruga in Carrión's disease. Am. J. Surg. Pathol. *10*:595-610, 1986.
2. Baorto, E., Payne, R. M., Slater, L. N., et al.: Culture-negative endocarditis caused by *Bartonella henselae*. J. Pediatr. *132*:1051-1054, 1998.
3. Bass, J. W., Vincent, J. M., and Person, D. A.: The expanding spectrum of *Bartonella* infections. I. Bartonellosis and trench fever. Pediatr. Infect. Dis. J. *16*:2-10, 1997.
4. Benson, N. A., Kar, S., McLaughlin, G., et al.: Entry of *Bartonella* into erythrocytes. Infect. Immun. *54*:347-353, 1986.
5. Brenner, D. J., O'Connor, S. P., Hollis, D. G., et al: Molecular characterization and proposal of a neotype strain for *Bartonella bacilliformis*. J. Clin. Microbiol. *29*:1299-1302, 1991.
6. Chamberlain, J., Laughlin, L., Gordon, S., et al.: Serodiagnosis of *Bartonella bacilliformis* infection by indirect fluorescence antibody assay. J. Clin. Microbiol. *38*:4269-4271, 2000.
7. Chamberlain, J., Laughlin, L., Romero, S., et al.: Epidemiology of endemic *Bartonella bacilliformis*: A prospective cohort study in a Peruvian mountain valley community. J. Infect. Dis. *186*:983-990, 2002.
8. Cuadra, M.: Salmonellosis complication in human bartonellosis. Tex. Rep. Biol. Med. *14*:97-113, 1956.
9. Cuadra, M., and Takano, J.: The relationship of *Bartonella* to the red blood cell as revealed by electron microscopy. Blood *33*:708-716, 1969.
10. Foucault, C., Brouqui, P., and Raoult, D.: *Bartonella quintana* characteristics and clinical management. Emerg. Infect. Dis. *12*:217-223, 2006.
11. Garcia, F. U., Wojta, J., and Hoover, R. L.: Interactions between live *Bartonella bacilliformis* and endothelial cells. J. Infect. Dis. *165*:1138-1141, 1992.
12. Gray, G. C., Johnson, A. A., Thornton, S. A., et al.: An epidemic of Oroya fever in the Peruvian Andes. Am. J. Trop. Hyg. *42*:215-221, 1990.
13. Herrer, A., and Christensen, H.: Implication of *Phlebotomus* sand flies as vectors of bartonellosis and leishmaniasis as early as 1764. Science *190*:154-155, 1975.
14. Knobloch, J., Solano, L., Alvarez, O., et al.: Antibodies to *Bartonella* as determined by fluorescence antibody test, indirect hemagglutination and ELISA. Trop. Med. Parasitol. *36*:183-185, 1985.
15. Koehler, J. E.: *Bartonella* infections. Adv. Pediatr. Infect. Dis. *11*:1-27, 1996.
16. Kosek, M., Lavarello, R., Gilman, R. H., et al.: Natural history of infection with *Bartonella bacilliformis* in a nonendemic population. J. Infect. Dis. *182*:865-872, 2000.
17. Maguiña, C., and Gotuzzo, E.: Bartonellosis new and old. Infect. Dis. Clin. North Am. *14*:1-22, 2000.

18. Maguiña, C., Garcia, P., Gotuzzo, E., et al.: Bartonellosis (Carrion's disease) in the modern era. Clin. Infect. Dis. 33:772-779, 2001.
19. Myers, S. A., Prose, N. S., Barcia, J. A., et al.: Bacillary angiomatosis in a child undergoing chemotherapy. J. Pediatr. 121:574-578, 1992.
20. Parrott, J. H., Dure, L., Sullender, W., et al.: Central nervous system infection associated with *Bartonella quintana*: A report of two cases. Pediatrics 100:403-408, 1997.
21. Perkocha, L. A., Geaghan, S. M., Yen, T. S. B., et al.: Clinical and pathological features of bacillary peliosis hepatis in association with human immunodeficiency virus infection. N. Engl. J. Med. 323:1581-1586, 1990.
22. Peters, D., and Wigand, R.: Bartonellaceae. Bacteriol. Rev. 19:150-155, 1955.
23. Posfay Barbe, K., Jaeggi, E., Ninet, B., et al.: *Bartonella quintana* endocarditis in a child. N. Engl. J. Med. 342:1841-1842, 2000.
24. Raoult, D., Fournier, P. E., Drancourt, M., et al.: Diagnosis of 22 new cases of *Bartonella* endocarditis. Ann. Intern. Med. 127:249, 1997.
25. Raoult, D., Fournier, P. E., Vandenesch, F., et al.: Outcome and treatment of *Bartonella* endocarditis. Arch. Intern. Med. 163:226-230, 2003.
26. Recavarren, S., and Lumbreras, H.: Pathogenesis of the verruga of Carrión's disease. Am. J. Pathol. 66:461-464, 1972.
27. Reynafarje, C., and Ramos, J.: The hemolytic anemia of human bartonellosis. Blood 17:562-578, 1961.
28. Ricketts, W. E.: Clinical manifestations of Carrión's disease. Arch. Intern. Med. 84:751-781, 1949.
29. Rolain, J. M., Brouqui, P., Koehler, J. E., et al.: Recommendations for treatment of human infections caused by *Bartonella* species. Antimicrob. Agents Chemother. 48:1921-1933, 2004.
30. Schultz, M. G.: A history of bartonellosis (Carrión's disease). Am. J. Trop. Med. Hyg. 17:503-515, 1968.
31. Spach, D. H., and Koehler, J. E.: *Bartonella*-associated infections. Infect. Dis. Clin. North Am. 12:137-155, 1998.
32. Spach, D. H., Kanter, A. S., Dougherty, M. J., et al.: *Bartonella (Rochalimaea)* species as a cause of apparent "culture negative" endocarditis. Clin. Infect. Dis. 20:1044-1047, 1995.
33. Urteaga, O., and Payne, E.: Treatment of the acute febrile phase of Carrión's disease with chloramphenicol. Am. J. Trop. Med. 4:507-511, 1955.
34. Zeaiter, Z., Fournier, P. E., Greub, G., et al.: Diagnosis of *Bartonella* endocarditis by a real-time nested PCR assay using serum. J. Clin. Microbiol. 41:919-925, 2003.

CHAPTER
139   BRUCELLOSIS
Edward J. Young

Brucellosis is a disease of animals (zoonosis) that is transmittable to humans.[76] Humans are accidental hosts, and human-to-human transmission rarely occurs. Brucellosis is distributed worldwide, and an estimated 500,000 human cases occur annually.[78] Programs to eradicate the disease in animals have reduced the incidence of human infection in many countries; however, brucellosis remains enzootic in large parts of the world.[117] Although brucellosis was once considered a rare occurrence in children, it now is recognized that persons of all ages are susceptible, especially in areas where *Brucella melitensis* is endemic.[38]

HISTORY

Brucellosis was one of many indistinguishable fevers until 1859, when J. A. Marston, a Royal Army Medical Corps physician, provided the first accurate description of the disease among troops stationed on Malta during the Crimean War.[62] During the 19th century, brucellosis was known by various names, including Malta fever, Mediterranean fever, and undulant fever.[72] Although the disease caused considerable morbidity and mortality in British military personnel stationed throughout the Mediterranean, the cause was not immediately apparent. In 1886, David Bruce,[16] another Royal Army Medical Corps surgeon, isolated a microorganism from spleen tissue of victims of Malta fever. Termed *Micrococcus* (later renamed *Brucella*) *melitensis*, the organism could be found in the blood, urine, and feces of patients with Malta fever. Between 1904 and 1907, Bruce headed the Mediterranean Fever Commission, which studied aspects of the disease in Malta. Themistocles Zammit, a Maltese physician working with the Commission, first identified native goats as the reservoir of brucellosis and their unpasteurized milk as the vehicle of transmission to humans.[108] When fresh goat's milk was replaced with tinned condensed milk in the military mess, the incidence of brucellosis among military personnel declined precipitously.[97] In 1897, Almroth Wright applied the newly devised agglutination assay to the serologic diagnosis of Malta fever.[112]

Unlike *B. melitensis* that was initially isolated from human tissue, other *Brucella* spp. were recognized for the disease they caused in animals. In 1897, Bernhard Bang,[13] a Danish veterinarian, isolated the "abortion bacillus" (later, *Brucella abortus*) from placental tissue of cattle suffering contagious abortions. *Brucella*

suis was isolated around 1914 by F. M. Hayes and J. Traum[45] at the Bureau of Animal Industry. The bacteriologist Alice Evans[36] finally recognized the relatedness of these disparate bacteria in 1918. After Evans' work was confirmed, K. F. Meyer and E. B. Shaw proposed the name *Brucella* for the genus to honor Bruce.[43]

Additional *Brucella* spp. were isolated from sheep (*Brucella ovis*) and from desert wood rats (*Brucella neotomae*), but to date they have not been shown to cause illness in humans. *Brucella canis* was isolated from kennel-bred dogs in 1968 by Carmichael and Brunner,[19] although it appears to be a rare cause of human brucellosis.[102,109] Since the late 1990s, at least two previously unrecognized species of *Brucella* have been isolated from marine mammals.[15,47] Tentatively named *Brucella cetaceae* (from cetaceans) and *Brucella pinnepediae* (from pinnepeds),[23] their role as human pathogens remains to be clarified.[63,91]

ETIOLOGY

The brucellae are small, fastidious, nonmotile, non–spore forming, gram-negative coccobacilli that lack native plasmids. The outer cell membrane resembles other gram-negative bacilli with a dominant lipopolysaccharide (LPS) component. Their metabolism is oxidative, and all strains are aerobic. Some strains require carbon dioxide for growth, especially for primary isolation. Brucellae are always catalase-positive, but oxidase activity varies among biovars. Most strains reduce nitrate to nitrite, but some do not. Production of hydrogen sulfide also varies, as does urease activity.[28] Various media, including chocolate, trypticase soy, and serum dextrose agars, support the growth of brucellae. Growth in vitro characteristically is slow, and when brucellosis is suspected, cultures should not be discarded before 28 days.

Brucellae belong to the alpha-2 subdivision of the Proteobacteria phylogenetically related to plant pathogens and symbionts, such as *Agrobacterium* and *Rhizobium*, and to intracellular animal parasites, such as *Bartonella* and *Rickettsia*.[22] On the basis of DNA-DNA hybridization and genome sequencing, the genus *Brucella* comprises a single species.[31,44,79] Despite genetic homology greater than 90 percent, the *Brucella* nomen species show a remarkable preference for certain natural hosts. Consequently, the traditional nomen species classification is retained for epidemiologic purposes (Table 139-1).

TABLE 139–1 Nomen-Species Classification of *Brucella* Species

Species	Biovars	Natural Hosts	Pathogenicity for Humans
B. abortus	1-6, 9	Cattle, other Bovidae	Yes
B. melitensis	1-3	Goats, sheep	Yes
B. suis	1-3	Swine	Yes
	4	Reindeer, caribou	Yes
	5	Rodents	Yes
B. canis	—	Dogs, other canines	Yes
B. neotomae	—	Desert wood rats	No
B. ovis	—	Sheep	No
*B. maris**			
*B. pinnipediae**		Pinnipeds	?
*B. cetaceae**		Cetaceans	?

*Tentative designations.
?Still unresolved.

EPIDEMIOLOGY

Historically in the United States, brucellosis was linked to the livestock industry, and *B. abortus* was the predominant species causing human illness. Farmers, ranchers, meat inspectors, and veterinarians were at highest risk of acquiring infection, usually through direct contact with infected animals. With the virtual elimination of bovine brucellosis by way of test-and-slaughter practices and immunization of susceptible cattle, the epidemiology of brucellosis changed, especially in states that border Mexico. *Brucella melitensis* replaced *B. abortus* as the major cause of human disease, and foodborne transmission replaced direct contact with animals as the primary mode of infection.[20,105] On the Mexican border, human brucellosis occurs at a rate eight times higher than the national average in the United States,[33] and unpasteurized goat's milk cheese is a common vehicle of transmission.[104,121] Human infection caused by *B. suis* traditionally has been an abattoir-associated infection,[18] but in recent years, the hunting of feral swine has become a risk when hunters are contaminated with the blood of infected animals.[99] Personnel working in clinical or research laboratories also are at risk, and brucellosis continues to be the most commonly reported laboratory-associated bacterial infection.[85,113]

Brucellosis once was thought to be an uncommon or mild disease in children, but susceptibility now is recognized in persons of all ages.[90] Conditions for the transmission of brucellosis from animals to humans vary among countries and cultures. Where farm animals traditionally are raised in the home, contact with children occurs frequently. Moreover, foodborne infection is not limited to any age or sex and can occur without direct contact with animals. Childhood brucellosis occurs more commonly in locations where *B. melitensis* is enzootic.[38,60]

The clinical manifestations of brucellosis in children do not differ from those in adults,[101] although unfamiliarity with the disease can delay diagnosis.[3,21] Human-to-human transmission of brucellosis is a rare occurrence, but evidence of venereal transfer has been documented.[88,98] Rare cases associated with bone marrow transplantation have been reported.[35] Few cases of brucellosis have been reported in patients infected with the human immunodeficiency virus.[68]

Spontaneous abortion is a common manifestation of brucellosis in animals in which brucellae localize within the reproductive organs of both sexes. Brucellosis in pregnant women can lead to abortion if the infection is unrecognized and untreated.[75] In a retrospective study from Saudi Arabia, intrauterine death and spontaneous abortion occurred in 46 percent of 92 women with brucellosis.[52] This rate was significantly higher than the rate of spontaneous abortion in women without brucellosis. When the infection is diagnosed early, pregnant women can

be treated successfully without compromising their ability to carry the pregnancy to term or to conceive again. On rare occasions, transplacental transmission can lead to neonatal brucellosis.[69]

PATHOGENESIS

The incubation period for brucellosis varies; however, symptoms generally appear within 2 to 3 weeks after acquisition of infection. Disease caused by *B. melitensis* and *B. suis* tends to be more severe than is illness caused by *B. abortus* or *B. canis*.[105] Morbidity can be considerable, but death occurs in only approximately 1 percent of cases, usually from complications such as neurobrucellosis or endocarditis.[117] Although no racial or genetic differences in susceptibility are known in humans, innate immunity has been demonstrated in various animals.[103] Normal human serum has limited bactericidal activity against brucellae, but complement opsonizes the organism for phagocytosis by neutrophils.[122] Brucellae are facultative intracellular pathogens that are able to survive and multiply within phagocytic cells of the host. The mechanisms by which brucellae evade killing by neutrophils is not completely understood; however, virulent strains contain a potent superoxide dismutase enzyme and nucleotides (adenine and guanosine monophosphate) that inhibit phagolysosome fusion, degranulation, and activation of the myeloperoxidase-halide system.[29] Brucellae that survive neutrophils killing enter the lymphatics, where they are ingested by monocytes and fixed macrophages of the reticuloendothelial system (RES). Survival within mononuclear phagocytes appears to depend on specific proteins, including stress proteins that block tumor necrosis factor-α (TNF-α), increase cyclic adenosine monophosphate, and prolong the life of the host cell by inhibiting apoptosis.[49,56] Intracellular killing of brucellae occurs when macrophages become "activated" by specifically committed T lymphocytes. This T-helper (T_H1) response involves cytokines, including interleukin-2, interferon-?, and TNF.[114]

CLINICAL MANIFESTATIONS

The spectrum of human brucellosis ranges from subclinical (diagnosed by serology) to chronic (characterized by recurrent symptoms over many years).[120] The disease is characterized by a plethora of nonspecific somatic complaints, such as fatigue, anorexia, nausea, weight loss, sweats, and depression. In contrast, there is a paucity of physical findings, notably fever, and occasionally hepatosplenomegaly. The infection can involve any organ or organ system of the body. Sometimes, symptoms related to a single organ predominate, in which case the disease is termed *localized*.[26] Not unexpectedly, localization often involves organs rich in elements of the RES.

Osteoarticular complications are the most frequent localized manifestations of brucellosis, and in children monoarticular arthritis involving the hips, knees, and sacroiliac predominates.[12,41,59,71] Spondylitis, osteomyelitis, and inflammatory arthropathy also have been described, but they occur less often in children than in adults.[53,93] Brucella is a rare cause of prosthetic joint infection.[110]

Neurobrucellosis comprises a variety of nervous system complications including meningitis/encephalitis, myelitis, radiculitis, peripheral and cranial neuropathies, and demyelinating syndromes.[64] Although most patients complain of headache and weakness, direct invasion of the central nervous system occurs in less than 5 percent of cases.[14,70] Analysis of cerebrospinal fluid (CSF) in cases of *Brucella* meningitis reveals lymphocytic pleocytosis, elevated protein, and normal or low glucose. Organisms are rarely seen on Gram stain or culture from CSF; however, antibodies to *Brucella* are present, and their finding in CSF is diagnostic.[7]

Gastrointestinal complaints frequently reported include anorexia, nausea, vomiting, abdominal discomfort, and weight loss.[67,90] Rare cases of ileitis,[81] colitis,[48,100] and peritonitis[2] have been reported.

The liver is the largest organ of the RES, and it probably always is involved in brucellosis, even when transaminase levels are normal or only slightly elevated.[25] Rarely, acute hepatitis occurs with hepatic enzyme levels resembling viral hepatitis.[57] The liver histology in patients infected with *B. abortus* is characterized by epithelioid granulomas indistinguishable from sarcoidosis.[96] In contrast, infection with *B. melitensis* can result in a spectrum of lesions ranging from diffuse hepatitis to granulomas.[115,118] Infection with *B. suis* (and *B. melitensis*) also can result in suppurative abscess that may become chronic.[11,27,107]

Genitourinary tract involvement usually manifests as orchitis or epididymo-orchitis and can be mistaken for testicular cancer.[74] Rare cases of interstitial nephritis, membranous nephropathy, and glomerulonephritis also have been reported.[106]

Respiratory tract localization of brucellosis is reported in approximately 7 percent of cases.[77] Lung lesions attributed to brucellosis include hilar adenopathy, lobar pneumonia, lung nodules, pleural effusion, and thoracic empyema.[58]

Cardiovascular lesions of brucellosis include endocarditis, myocarditis, pericarditis, and aneurysms of the aorta and cerebral blood vessels.[84] Both native valve endocarditis and prosthetic valve endocarditis have been described, and the aortic valve is involved most often. Delays in establishing a diagnosis can result in life-threatening complications such as valve rupture, myocardial abscess, and sinus of Valsalva fistula. Treatment of *Brucella* endocarditis generally requires the combination of antibiotics in addition to valve surgery.[46,51]

Ocular lesions, most notably uveitis, have been described in patients with brucellosis. Other eye lesions that have been reported include endophthalmitis, optic neuritis, episcleritis, nummular keratitis, and chorioretinitis. The pathogenesis of some of the lesions is a matter of conjecture because brucellae rarely are isolated from the eye.[5,34,50]

Cutaneous lesions attributed to brucellosis include contact dermatitis, rashes, abscess, and vasculitis.[66] On occasion, brucellae have been cultured from subcutaneous papules.[60]

Hematologic abnormalities such as anemia, leukopenia, and thrombocytopenia are common occurrences in the course of brucellosis.[30] These changes generally are mild and resolve promptly with antimicrobial therapy. On occasion, thrombocytopenia can be severe, resulting in hemorrhage into the skin and from mucosal sites.[123] The origin of this complication likely is multifactorial, including hypersplenism, disseminated intravascular coagulation, bone marrow suppression and hemophagocytosis, and immune mechanisms.

DIAGNOSIS

The symptoms of brucellosis are nonspecific. Therefore, the importance of obtaining a detailed history including occupation, avocations, travel, animal exposure, and food habits cannot be overemphasized. Routine laboratory tests generally are not helpful; however, characteristic hematologic findings (normal or low white blood cell count) can suggest the possibility of brucellosis.[4]

A definitive diagnosis of brucellosis is made by isolating a *Brucella* sp. from blood, bone marrow, or other tissue. The rate of positive blood cultures varies from 15 to 70 percent depending on the methods used and the period of in vitro incubation.[42] Bone marrow culture was reported to be more sensitive than blood culture before the introduction of newer isolation techniques.[32,65]

Nucleic acid amplification tests using a variety of gene sequences are being applied with some success to the rapid diagnosis of brucellosis.[73,83,111]

In the absence of bacteriologic confirmation, a presumptive diagnosis can be made by measuring the titer of specific antibodies in serum.[116] Human brucellosis is characterized by an initial production of immunoglobulin M (IgM) antibodies followed by a switch to IgG synthesis within the second week of infection. Treatment results in a gradual decline in both antibody isotypes; however, the persistence of IgG antibodies is associated with relapse or chronic infection.[80] Consequently, the pattern of immunoglobulin isotypes is important in differentiating active from treated disease.[39,116] This distinction is made by performing the serum agglutination test with and without 2-mercaptoethanol or dithiothreitol, agents used to destroy the agglutinability of IgM while preserving agglutination by IgG.[17] Alternatively, a more direct way to measure IgM and IgG antibodies is the indirect enzyme-linked immunosorbent assay (ELISA) employing anti-IgM and anti-IgG conjugates.[61]

Most serologic tests for brucellosis employ smooth LPS (S-LPS), the immunodominant cell wall antigen capable of detecting antibodies to all smooth species (*B. abortus*, *B. melitensis*, *B. suis*). Because *B. canis* is naturally rough and lacks S-LPS, antibodies against this organism are detected with antigen prepared from rough species (*B. canis* or *B. ovis*).[82] Various cell wall and cytoplasmic proteins have been studied as potential serodiagnostic antigens.[40] However, none has proved superior to LPS-based assays. More recently, a latex agglutination assay using S-LPS has been shown to be simple to run and rapid and to have good sensitivity and specificity.[1]

TREATMENT

Antimicrobial therapy lessens morbidity, shortens the course of illness, and reduces the incidence of complications of brucellosis.[119] Numerous drugs are active against *Brucella* spp., but the results of in vitro sensitivity tests do not always correlate with clinical effectiveness. Because the rate of relapse with single-drug therapy is high, successful treatment of brucellosis requires combination therapy for prolonged periods of time.[93,94] The tetracyclines remain the most effective antibiotics against brucellae with minimal inhibitory concentrations (MICs) lower than 1 µg/mL. Aminoglycosides (streptomycin and gentamicin) have been shown to enhance the killing of brucellae in vitro by numerous antibiotics.[89] Traditionally, the combination of tetracycline HCl administered for 6 weeks and streptomycin given for 2 to 3 weeks provided the highest cure rates in patients with brucellosis.[10] Currently, the preferred regimen is doxycycline (for adults 200 mg/day orally for 45 days) in combination with gentamicin (5 mg/kg/day as a single daily dose intramuscularly for the first 7 days).[86,92]

Rifampin also shows good in vitro activity against *Brucella* spp., and in 1986 the World Health Organization recommended the combination of doxycycline (200 mg/day orally for 45 days) and rifampin (600 to 900 mg/day orally for 45 days) as the treatment of choice. Although this regimen has been used successfully, subsequent studies have shown the superiority of the combination of doxycycline and an aminoglycoside.[95]

Children who are older than 8 years can be treated as adults. Because tetracycline is contraindicated for children younger than 8 years old and for pregnant women, alternative treatments have been sought. A regimen of trimethoprim-sulfamethoxazole (TMP-SMZ; co-trimoxazole) in a fixed combination (80 mg TMP, 400 mg SMZ twice daily for 45 days) in addition to gentamicin (5 mg/kg/day as a single daily dose for 7 days) has yielded satisfactory results.[90] Alternatively, the combination of TMP-SMZ and rifampin (15 mg/kg once daily) administered for either 6 or 8 weeks gave comparable results.[87] Similarly, pregnant women can be treated successfully with TMP-SMZ in combination with rifampin without causing adverse drug effects in the newborn.[52]

The quinolones are active against *Brucella* spp. in vitro, but the MIC values vary for each compound and to some extent for *Brucella* isolates.[37] In clinical practice, however, results have been disappointing.[54,119] Consequently, quinolones are not recommended alone for treating brucellosis, and their role in combination therapy awaits well-designed clinical trials.

The optimal treatment for complications of brucellosis such as meningitis and endocarditis has not been defined with certainty. Doxycycline crosses the blood-brain barrier more effectively than does generic tetracycline, and it has been used in combination with other drugs (e.g., rifampin, TMP-SMZ) for neurobrucellosis.[64,70] Third-generation cephalosporins achieve high concentrations in CSF, but the sensitivity of brucellae varies, and in general, β-lactam drugs are not effective when they are used alone.[55] On occasion, patients with *Brucella* endocarditis have been treated successfully with antimicrobial therapy alone; however, most patients have required valve replacement surgery.[6]

RELAPSE AND CHRONIC BRUCELLOSIS

Most patients with brucellosis recover completely within a few weeks to months after receiving adequate therapy. Despite receiving appropriate treatment, some patients suffer a relapse characterized by recurrence of symptoms and re-isolation of brucellae from their blood.[9] Obviously, relapse occurs more frequently if the full course of treatment is not completed, and taking oral antibiotics for 6 weeks can tax a patient's compliance. With few exceptions, relapse is *not* caused by antibiotic-resistant strains of *Brucella*.[8]

Even with appropriate treatment, some patients experience delayed recovery and continue to have nonspecific complaints, notably fatigue. Such patients have no objective evidence of infection, such as fever, and their antibody titers decline as expected. Whether this condition represents a variant of the chronic fatigue syndrome is not clear, but additional antibiotic therapy does not improve their recovery.[24] Rarely, chronic brucellosis results from a persisting focus of infection such as osteomyelitis or a deep tissue abscess. Such patients have fever or other objective signs of infection, and levels of IgG antibodies in the serum remain elevated. Scanning techniques (e.g., technetium 99m bone scan, gallium 67 scan, computed tomography, or magnetic resonance imaging) can be useful in localizing an occult focus of infection.

REFERENCES

1. Abdoel, T. H., and Smits, H. L.: Rapid latex agglutination test for the serodiagnosis of human brucellosis. Diagn. Microbiol. Infect. Dis. *57*:123-128, 2007.
2. Akritidis, N., and Pappas, G.: Ascites caused by brucellosis: a report of two cases. Scand. J. Infect. Dis. *36*:110-112, 2001.
3. Al-Eissa, Y.: Unusual suppurative complications of brucellosis in children. Acta Pediatr. *82*:987-992, 1993.
4. Al-Eissa, Y., and Al-Nasser, M.: Haematological manifestations of childhood brucellosis. Infection *21*:23-26, 1993.
5. Al-Kaff, A. S.: Ocular brucellosis. Int. Ophthalmol. Clin. *35*:139-145, 1995.
6. Al-Kasab, S., Al-Fagih, M. R., Al-Yousef, S., et al.: *Brucella* infective endocarditis: Successful combined medical and surgical therapy. J. Thorac. Surg. *95*:862-870, 1988.
7. Araj, G. F., Lulu, A. R., Saadah, M. A., et al.: Rapid diagnosis of central nervous system brucellosis by ELISA. J. Neuroimmunol. *12*:173-182, 1986.
8. Ariza, J., Bosch, J., Gudiol, F., et al.: Relevance of in vitro antimicrobial susceptibility of *Brucella melitensis* to relapse rate in human brucellosis. Antimicrob. Agents Chemother. *30*:958-960, 1986.
9. Ariza, J., Corredoira, J., Pallares, R., et al.: Characteristics of and risk factors for relapse of brucellosis in humans. Clin. Infect. Dis. *20*:1241-1249, 1995.
10. Ariza, J., Gudiol, F., Pallares, R., et al.: Treatment of human brucellosis with doxycycline plus rifampin or doxycycline plus streptomycin: A randomized, double-blind study. Ann. Intern. Med. *117*:23-30, 1992.
11. Ariza, J., Pigrau, C., Cañas, C., et al.: Current understanding and management of chronic hepatosplenic suppurative brucellosis. Clin. Infect. Dis. *32*:1024-1033, 2001.
12. Ariza, J., Pujol, M., Valverde, J., et al.: Brucellar sacroiliitis: Findings in 63 episodes and current relevance. Clin. Infect. Dis. *16*:761-765, 1993.
13. Bang, B.: Die Aetiologie des seuchenhaften ("infectiosen") Verwerfens. Z. Thiermed. *1*:241-278, 1897.
14. Bouza, E., Garcia-de-la-Torre, M., Parras, F., et al.: Brucellar meningitis. Rev. Infect. Dis. *9*:810-822, 1987.
15. Bricker, B. J., Ewalt, D. R., MacMillan, A. P., et al.: Molecular characterization of *Brucella* strains isolated from marine mammals. J. Clin. Microbiol. *38*:1258-1262, 2000.
16. Bruce, D.: Note on the discovery of a micro-organism in Malta fever. Practitioner *39*:161, 1887.
17. Buchanan, T. M., and Faber, L. C.: 2-Mercaptoethanol *Brucella* agglutination test: Usefulness for predicting recovery from brucellosis. J. Clin. Microbiol. *11*:691-693, 1980.
18. Buchanan, T. M., Faber, L. C., and Feldman, R. A.: Brucellosis in the United States, 1960-1972: An abattoir-associated disease. Part I. Clinical features and therapy. Medicine (Baltimore) *53*:403-413, 1974.
19. Carmichael, L. E., and Brunner, D. W.: Characteristics of a newly recognized species of *Brucella* responsible for infectious canine abortion. Cornell Vet. *58*:579-592, 1968.
20. Chomel, B. B., De Bess, E. E., Mangiamele, D. M., et al.: Changing trends in the epidemiology of human brucellosis in California from 1973 to 1992: A shift toward foodborne transmission. J. Infect. Dis. *170*:1216-1223, 1994.
21. Chusid, M. J., Perzigian, R. W., Dunne, M., et al.: Brucellosis: An unusual cause of a child's fever of unknown origin. Wisc. Med. J. *88*:11-13, 1989.
22. Cloeckaert, A., and Vizcaino, N.: DNA polymorphism and taxonomy of *Brucella* species. *In* López-Goñi, I., and Moriyón, I. (eds.): Brucella: Molecular and Cellular Biology. Norfolk, UK, Horizon Books, 2004, pp. 1-24.
23. Cloeckaert, A., Grayon, M., Grépinet, O., et al.: Classification of *Brucella* strains isolated from marine mammals by infrequent restriction site-PCR and development of specific PCR identification tests. Microbes Infect. *5*:593-602, 2003.
24. Cluff, L. E.: Medical aspects of delayed convalescence. Rev. Infect. Dis. *13*(Suppl. 1):138-140, 1991.
25. Cohen, F. B., Robins, B., and Lipstein, W.: Isolation of *Brucella abortus* by percutaneous liver biopsy. N. Engl. J. Med. *257*:228-230, 1957.
26. Colmenero, J. D., Regnera, J. M., Martos, F., et al.: Complications associated with *Brucella melitensis* infection: A study of 530 cases. Medicine (Baltimore) *75*:195-211, 1996.
27. Colmenero, J. D., Suarez-Muñoz, M. A., Queipo-Ortuño, M. I., et al.: Late reactivation of calcified granuloma in a patient with chronic suppurative brucellosis. Eur. J. Microbiol. Infect. Dis. *21*:897-899, 2002.
28. Corbel, M. J.: Brucellosis: An overview. Emerg. Infect. Dis. *3*:213-221, 1997.
29. Corbel, M. J.: Recent advances in brucellosis. J. Med. Microbiol. *46*:101-103, 1997.
30. Crosby, E., Liosa, L., Miro Quesada, M., et al.: Hematologic changes in brucellosis. J. Infect. Dis. *150*:419-424, 1984.
31. Del Vecchio, V. G., Kapatral, V., Redkar, R. J., et al.: The genome sequence of the facultative intracellular pathogen *Brucella melitensis*. Proc. Natl. Acad. Sci. U. S. A. *99*:443-448, 2002.
32. Doern, G. V.: Detection of selected fastidious bacteria. Clin. Infect. Dis. *30*:166-173, 2000.
33. Doyle, T. J., and Bryan, R. T.: Infectious disease morbidity in the U.S. region bordering Mexico, 1990-1998. J. Infect. Dis. *182*:1503-1510, 2000.
34. Elrazak, M. A.: *Brucella* optic neuritis. Arch. Intern. Med. *151*:776-778, 1991.
35. Ertem, M., Kurekci, A. E., Aysev, D., et al.: Brucellosis transmitted by bone marrow transplantation. Bone Marrow Transplant. *26*:225-226, 2000.
36. Evans, A. C.: Further studies on *Bacterium abortus* and related bacteria. II. A comparison of *Bacterium abortus* and *Bacterium bronchisepticus* and with the agent which causes Malta fever. J. Infect. Dis. *22*:580-587, 1918.
37. Falagas, M. E., and Bliziotis, I. A.: Quinolones for treatment of human brucellosis: Critical review of the evidence from microbiological and clinical studies. Antimicrob. Agents Chemother. *50*:22-33, 2006.
38. Feiz, J., Sabbaghian, H., and Mirali, M.: Brucellosis due to *B. melitensis* in children. Clin. Pediatr. (Phila.) *12*:904-907, 1978.
39. Gazazo, E., Lahoz, J. G., Subiza, J. L., et al.: Changes in IgM and IgG antibody concentrations in brucellosis over time: Importance for diagnosis and follow-up. J. Infect. Dis. *159*:219-225, 1989.
40. Goldbaum, F. A., Velikovsky, C. A., Baldi, P. C., et al.: The 18-kDa cytoplasmic protein of *Brucella* species—an antigen useful for diagnosis—is a lumazine synthetase. J. Med. Microbiol. *48*:833-839, 1999.
41. Gotuzzo, E., Alarcon, G. S., and Bocanegra, T. S.: Articular involvement in human brucellosis: A retrospective analysis of 304 cases. Semin. Arthritis Rheum. *12*:245-255, 1982.
42. Gotuzzo, E., Carrillo, C., Guerra, J., et al.: An evaluation of diagnostic methods for brucellosis: The value of bone marrow culture. J. Infect. Dis. *153*:122-125, 1986.

43. Hall, W. H.: History of *Brucella* as a human pathogen. *In* Young, E. J., and Corbel, M. J. (eds.): Brucellosis: Clinical and Laboratory Aspects. Boca Raton, FL, CRC Press, 1989, pp. 1-9.

44. Halling, S. M., Paterson-Burch, B. D., Bricker, B. J., et al.: Completion of the genome sequence of *Brucella abortus* and comparison to the highly similar genomes of *Brucella melitensis* and *Brucella suis*. J. Bacteriol. *187*:2715-2726, 2005.

45. Hayes, F. M., and Traum, J.: Preliminary report of abortion in swine caused by *Br. abortus* (Bang). Mod. Vet. Pract. *1*:58-65, 1929.

46. Jacobs, F., Abramowicz, D., Vereerstraeten, P., et al.: *Brucella* endocarditis: The role of combined medical and surgical treatment. Rev. Infect. Dis. *12*:740-744, 1990.

47. Jahans, K. L., Foster, G., and Broughton, E. S.: The characterisation of *Brucella* strains isolated from marine mammals. Vet. Microbiol. *57*:373-382, 1997.

48. Jorens, P. G., Michielsen, P. P., Van den Enden, E. J., et al.: A rare cause of colitis: *Brucella melitensis*. Dis. Colon Rectum *34*:194-196, 1991.

49. Jubier-Maurin, V., Loisel, S., Liautard, J.-P., et al.: The intramacrophagic environment of *Brucella* spp. and their replicative niche. *In* López-Goñi, I., and Moriyón, I. (eds.): Brucella: Molecular and Cellular Biology. Norfolk, UK, Horizon Bioscience, 2004, pp. 313-340.

50. Karapinar, B., Yilmaz, D., Vardar, F., et al.: Unusual presentation of brucellosis in a child: Acute blindness. Acta Paediatr. *94*:378-380, 2005.

51. Kazaz, H., Celkan, M. A., Ustunsoy, H., et al.: Mitral annuloplasty with biodegradable ring for infective endocarditis: A new tool for the surgeon for valve repair in childhood. Interact. Cardiovasc. Thorac. Surg. *4*:378-380, 2005.

52. Khan, M. Y., Mah, M. M., and Memish, Z. A.: Brucellosis in pregnant women. Clin. Infect. Dis. *32*:1172-1177, 2001.

53. Khateeb, M. I., Araj, G. F., Majeed, S. A., et al.: *Brucella* arthritis: A study of 96 cases in Kuwait. Ann. Rheum. Dis. *49*:994-998, 1990.

54. Lang, R, and Rubinstein, E.: Quinolones for the treatment of brucellosis. J. Antimicrob. Chemother. *29*:357-363, 1992.

55. Lang, R. Dugan, R., Potasman, I., et al.: Failure of ceftriaxone in the treatment of acute brucellosis. Clin. Infect. Dis. *14*:506-509, 1992.

56. Lin, J., and Ficht, T. A.: Protein synthesis in *Brucella abortus* induced during macrophage infection. Infect. Immun. *63*:1409-1414, 1995.

57. Losurdo, G., Timitilli, A., Tasso, L., et al.: Acute hepatitis due to *Brucella* in a 2-year-old child. Arch. Dis. Child. *71*:387, 1994.

58. Lubani, M. M., Lulu, A. R., Araj, G. F., et al.: Pulmonary brucellosis. Q. J. Med. *71*:319-324, 1989.

59. Lubani, M. M., Sharda, D., and Helin, I.: *Brucella* arthritis in children. Infection *14*:233-236, 1986.

60. Mantur, B. G., Akki, A. S., Mangalgi, S. S., et al.: Childhood brucellosis: A microbiological, epidemiological and clinical study. J. Trop. Pediatr. *50*:153-157, 2004.

61. Marrodan, T., Nenova-Poliakova, R., Rubio, M., et al.: Evaluation of three methods to measure anti-*Brucella* IgM antibodies and interference of IgA in the interpretation of mercaptan-based tests. Diagn. Microbiol. *50*:663-666, 2001.

62. Marston, J. A.: Report of fever (Malta). R. Army Med. Dept. Rep. *3*:520-521, 1863.

63. McDonald, W. L., Jamaludin, R., Mackereth, G., et al.: Characterization of a *Brucella* sp. strain as a marine-mammal type despite isolation from a patient with spinal osteomyelitis in New Zealand. J. Clin. Microbiol. *44*:4363-4370, 2006.

64. McLean, D. R., Russell, N., and Khan, M. Y.: Neurobrucellosis: Clinical and therapeutic features. Clin. Infect. Dis. *15*:582-590, 1992.

65. Memish, Z., Mah, M. W., Al Mahmoud, S., et al.: *Brucella* bacteremia: Clinical and laboratory observations in 160 patients. J. Infect. *40*:59-63, 2000.

66. Milionis, H., Christou, L., and Elisaf, M.: Cutaneous manifestations in brucellosis: Case report and review of the literature. Infection *28*:124-126, 2000.

67. Mohamed, A. E. S., Ven, D., Madkour, M. M., et al.: Alimentary tract presentations of brucellosis. Ann. Saudi Med. *6*:27-31, 1986.

68. Moreno, S., Ariza, J., Espinosa, F. J., et al.: Brucellosis in patients infected with the human immunodeficiency virus. Eur. J. Clin. Microbiol. Infect. Dis. *17*:319-326, 1998.

69. Mosayebi, Z., Movahedian, A. H., Ghayomi, A., et al.: Congenital brucellosis in a preterm neonate. Indian Pediatr. *42*;599-601, 2005.

70. Mousa, A. R. M., Koshy, T. S., Araj, G. F., et al.: *Brucella* meningitis: Presentation, diagnosis, and treatment. A prospective study of ten cases. Q. J. Med. *60*:873-885, 1986.

71. Mousa, A. R. M., Muhtaseb, S. A., Almudallal, D. S., et al.: Osteoarticular complications of brucellosis: A study of 169 cases. Rev. Infect. Dis. *9*:531-543, 1987.

72. Naudi, J. R.: Brucellosis: The Malta Experience. A Celebration 1905-2005. Malta, Enterprise Group, 2005.

73. Navarro, E., Segura, J. C., Castaño, M. J., et al.: Use of real-time quantitative polymerase chain reaction to monitor the evolution of *Brucella melitensis* DNA load during therapy and post-therapy follow-up in patients with brucellosis. Clin. Infect. Dis. *42*:1266-1273, 2006.

74. Navarro-Martínez, A., Solera, J., Corredoira, J., et al.: Epididymoorchitis due to *Brucella melitensis*: A retrospective study of 59 patients. Clin. Infect. Dis. *33*:2017-2022, 2001.

75. Oscherwitz, S. L.: Brucellar bacteremia in pregnancy. Clin. Infect. Dis. *21*:714-715, 1995.

76. Pappas, G., Akritidis, N., Bosilkovski, M., and Tsianos, E.: Brucellosis. N. Engl. J. Med. *352*:2325-2336, 2005.

77. Pappas, G., Bosilkovski, M., Akritidis, N., et al.: Brucellosis and the respiratory system. Clin. Infect. Dis. *37*:95e-99e, 2003.

78. Pappas, G., Papadimitriou, P., Akritidis, N., et al.: The new global map of human brucellosis. Lancet Infect. Dis. *6*:91-99, 2006.

79. Paulsen, I. T., Seshadri, R., Nelson, K. E., et al.: The *Brucella suis* genome reveals fundamental similarities between animal and plant pathogens and symbionts. Proc. Natl. Acad. Sci. U. S. A. *99*:13148-13153, 2002.

80. Pellicer, T., Ariza, J., Foz, A., et al.: Specific antibodies detected during relapse of human brucellosis. J. Infect. Dis. *157*:918-924, 1988.

81. Petrella, R., and Young, E. J.: Acute *Brucella* ileitis. Am. J. Gastroenterol. *83*:80-82, 1988.

82. Polt, S. S., and Schaefer, J. A.: A microagglutination test for human *Brucella canis* antibodies. Am. J. Clin. Pathol. *77*:740-744, 1982.

83. Probert, W. S., Schrader, K. N., Khuong, N. Y., et al.: Real-time multiplex PCR assay for detection of *Brucella* spp., *B. abortus* and *B. melitensis*. J. Clin. Microbiol. *42*:1290-1293, 2004.

84. Reguera, J. M., Alarcon, A., Miralles, F., et al.: *Brucella* endocarditis: Clinical, diagnostic, and therapeutic approach. Eur. J. Clin. Microbiol. Infect. Dis. *22*:647-650, 2003.

85. Robichaud, S., Libman, M., Behr, M., et al.: Prevention of laboratory-acquired brucellosis. Clin. Infect. Dis. *38*:e119-e122, 2004.

86. Roushan, M. R. H., Mohraz, M., Hajiahmadi, M., et al.: Efficacy of gentamicin plus doxycycline versus streptomycin plus doxycycline in the treatment of brucellosis in humans. Clin. Infect. Dis. *42*:1075-1080, 2006.

87. Roushan, M. R. H., Mohaz, M., Janmohammadi, N., et al.: Efficacy of cotrimoxazole and rifampin for 6 or 8 weeks of therapy in childhood brucellosis. Pediatr. Infect. Dis. J. *25*:544-545, 2006.

88. Rubin, B., Band, J. D., Wong, P., et al.: Person-to-person transmission of *Brucella melitensis*. Lancet *337*:14-15, 1991.

89. Rubinstein, E., Lang, R., Shasha, B., et al.: In vitro susceptibility of *Brucella melitensis* to antibiotics. Antimicrob. Agents Chemother. *35*:1925-1927, 1991.

90. Sharda, D. C., and Lubani, M.: A study of brucellosis in childhood. Clin. Pediatr. *25*:492-495, 1986.

91. Sohn, A. H., Probert, W. S., Glaser, C. A., et al.: Human neurobrucellosis with intracerebral granuloma caused by a marine mammal *Brucella* spp. Emerg. Infect. Dis. *9*:485-488, 2003.

92. Solera, J., Geijo, P., Largo, J., et al.: A randomized, double-blind study to assess the optimal duration of doxycycline treatment for human brucellosis. Clin. Infect. Dis. *39*:1776-1782, 2004.

93. Solera, J., Lozano, E., Martinez-Alfaro, E., et al.: Brucellar spondylitis: Review of 35 cases and literature survey. Clin. Infect. Dis. *29*:1440-1449, 1999.

94. Solera, J., Martinez-Alfaro, E., and Espinosa, A.: Recognition and optimum treatment of brucellosis. Drugs *53*:245-256, 1997.

95. Solera, J., Rodríguez-Zapata, M., Geijo, P., et al.: Doxycycline-rifampin versus doxycycline-streptomycin in treatment of human brucellosis due to *Brucella melitensis*. Antimicrob. Agents Chemother. *39*:2061-2067, 1995.

96. Spink, W. W.: The Nature of Brucellosis. Minneapolis, University of Minnesota Press, 1956.

97. Spink, W. W., Hoffbauer, F. W., Walker, W. W., et al.: Histopathology of the liver in human brucellosis. J. Lab. Clin. Med. *34*:40-58, 1949.

98. Stantic-Pavlinic, M., Cec, V., and Mehk, J: Brucellosis in spouses and the possibility of interhuman infection. Infection *11*:313-314, 1983.

99. Starnes, C. T., Talwani, R., Horvath, J. A., et al.: Brucellosis in two hunt club members in South Carolina. J. S. C. Med. Assoc. *100*:113-115, 2004.

100. Stermer, E., Levy, N., Potasman, I., et al.: Brucellosis as a cause of severe colitis. Am. J. Gastroenterol. *86*:917-919, 1991.

101. Street, L., Grant, W. W., and Alva, J. D.: Brucellosis in childhood. Pediatrics *55*:416-421, 1975.

102. Swenson, R. M., Carmichael, L. E., and Cundy, K. R.: Human infection with *Brucella canis*. Ann. Intern. Med. *76*:435-438, 1972.

103. Templeton, J. W., and Adams, L. G.: Natural resistance to bovine brucellosis. *In* Adams, L. G. (ed.): Advances in Brucellosis Research. College Station, TX, Texas A&M University Press, 1990, pp. 144-150.

104. Thapar, M. K., and Young, E. J.: Urban outbreak of goat cheese brucellosis. Pediatr. Infect. Dis. J. *5*:640-643, 1986.

105. Troy, S. B., Rickman, L. S., and Davis, C. E.: Brucellosis in San Diego: Epidemiology and species-related differences in acute clinical presentation. Medicine (Baltimore) *84*:174-187, 2005.

106. Ustun, I., Ozcakar, L., Arda, N., et al.: *Brucella* glomerulonephritis: Case report and review of the literature. South. Med. J. *98*:1216-1217, 2005.

107. Vallejo, J. G., Stevens, A. M., Dutton, R. V., et al.: Hepatosplenic abscesses due to *Brucella melitensis*: Report of a case involving a child and review of the literature. Clin. Infect. Dis. *22*:485-489, 1996.

108. Vassallo, D. J.: The saga of brucellosis: Controversy over credit for linking Malta fever with goat's milk. Lancet *348*:804-808, 1996.

109. Wanke, M. M.: Canine brucellosis. Anim. Reprod. Sci. *82-83*:195-207, 2004.

110. Weil, Y., Mattan, Y., Liebergall, M., et al.: *Brucella* prosthetic joint infection: A report of 3 cases and a review of the literature. Clin. Infect. Dis. *36*:e81-e86, 2003.

111. Whatmore, A. M., Murphy, T. J., Shankster, S., et al.: Use of amplified fragment length polymorphism to identify and type *Brucella* isolates of medical and veterinary interest. J. Clin. Microbiol. *43*:761-769, 2005.

112. Wright, A. E., and Semple, D.: On the employment of dead bacteria in the serum diagnosis of typhoid and Malta fever. Br. Med. J. *1*:1214-1215, 1897.
113. Yagupsky, P., and Baron, E. J.: Laboratory exposure to brucellae and implications for bioterrorism. Emerg. Infect. Dis. *11*:1180-1185, 2005.
114. Yingst, S., and Hoover, D. L.: T cell immunity to brucellosis. Crit. Rev. Microbiol. *29*:313-331, 2003.
115. Young, E. J.: *Brucella melitensis* hepatitis: The absence of granulomas. Ann. Intern. Med. *91*:414-415, 1979.
116. Young, E. J.: Serologic diagnosis of human brucellosis: Analysis of 214 cases by agglutination tests and review of the literature. Clin. Infect. Dis. *13*:359-372, 1991.
117. Young, E. J.: An overview of human brucellosis. Clin. Infect. Dis. *21*:283-290, 1995.
118. Young, E. J. Brucellosis. *In* Connor, D. H., Chandler, F. W., Manz, H. J., et al. (eds.): Pathology of Infectious Diseases. Stamford, CT, Appleton & Lange, 1997, pp.447-452.
119. Young, E. J.: *Brucella* species. *In* Yu, V., Weber, R., and Raoult, D. (eds.): Antimicrobial Therapy and Vaccines. 2nd ed., Vol. I: Microbes. New York, Apple Trees Productions, 2002, pp.121-140.
120. Young, E. J.: *Brucella* species. *In* Mandell, G. L., Bennett, J. E., and Dolin, R. (eds.): Principles and Practice of Infectious Diseases. 6th ed. Philadelphia, Elsevier Churchill Livingstone 2005, pp. 2669-2674.
121. Young, E. J., and Suvannoparrat, U.: Brucellosis outbreak attributed to ingestion of unpasteurized goat cheese. Arch. Intern. Med. *135*:240-243, 1975.
122. Young, E. J., Borchert, M., Kretzer, F. L., et al.: Phagocytosis and killing of *Brucella* by human polymorphonuclear leukocytes. J. Infect. Dis. *151*:682-690, 1985.
123. Young, E. J., Tarry, A., Genta, R. M., et al.: Thrombocytopenic purpura associated with brucellosis: Report of 2 cases and literature review. Clin. Infect. Dis. *31*:904-909, 2000.

PERTUSSIS AND OTHER *BORDETELLA* INFECTIONS

140

James D. Cherry ✪ Ulrich Heininger

Pertussis (whooping cough) is an acute infectious illness of the respiratory tract caused by *Bordetella pertussis* and, less frequently, by *Bordetella parapertussis*.[49,55,68,174,257] The illness occurs worldwide and affects all age groups, but it is recognized primarily in children; it is most serious in young, unprotected infants.[85,168,257]

HISTORY

Unlike other severe epidemic infectious diseases of children (e.g., smallpox, poliomyelitis, and measles), pertussis lacks an ancient history.[184] The first observation of pertussis occurred in France in 1414, and the first epidemic was noted in Paris in 1578.[68,77,221] This epidemic and the clinical characteristics of the cases were described in 1640 by Guillaume de Baillou.

Pertussis was noted as *the kink* (a Scottish term synonymous with *fit* or *paroxysm*) and *kindhoest* (a Teutonic word meaning *child's cough*) in the Middle Ages.[58,184] In 1669, Sydenham named the illness *pertussis* (meaning *violent cough*).[221] Isolation of *B. pertussis*, the main causative agent of pertussis, was reported by Bordet and Gengou in 1906.[30,31]

Vaccines consisting of killed whole *B. pertussis* organisms were developed shortly after the bacterium was isolated, and the first results of protection were reported by Madsen in 1925.[246] The mouse protection test, developed and reported by Kendrick and collaborators[209] in 1947, allowed vaccine production to be standardized. Comprehensive studies conducted by the British Medical Research Council[264] in the 1940s and 1950s demonstrated a correlation between the potency of pertussis vaccines as determined by the mouse protection test and their clinical efficacy in children. As a consequence, immunization against pertussis, most commonly in combination with diphtheria and tetanus toxoids (DTP), became part of routine vaccination programs in many countries throughout the world.

Concern about a relationship between pertussis vaccination and temporally associated serious adverse events (e.g., sudden infant death syndrome and a variety of neurologic illnesses) led to a sharp decline in vaccination rates in Japan and several European countries during the 1970s.[49,55,68,213] This concern, along with well-documented high rates of unpleasant local and systemic reactions, led to the development of new acellular vaccines. These vaccines cause reactions less frequently and have been used in Japan since 1981 and in many developed countries since the mid 1990s.[162,213,391,408]

B. bronchiseptica, which causes cough illnesses in a number of animals as well as humans, was first isolated some time around 1910 by Ferry[115], McGowan, and perhaps others who were studying dogs with distemper.[257,260] *B. parapertussis* was isolated first from children with pertussis in the 1930s, and *Bordetella holmesii* was noted in nasopharyngeal specimens from patients with pertussis-like illnesses in Massachusetts during the period from 1995 through 1998.[32,104,105,258,427]

MICROBIOLOGY

The genus *Bordetella* contains nine species: *B. pertussis*, *B. parapertussis*$_{bu}$ (adapted to humans), *B. parapertussis*$_{ov}$ (ovine-adapted *B. parapertussis*), *B. bronchiseptica*, *Bordetella avium*, *Bordetella hinzii*, *B. holmesii*, *Bordetella trematum*, and *Bordetella petrii*.[81,174,257] *B. pertussis* infects exclusively humans. *B. parapertussis* also is a human pathogen, but it has been recovered from sheep ("ovine") as well.[322] Both *B. pertussis* and *B. parapertussis* are respiratory pathogens. *B. bronchiseptica* primarily is an animal pathogen that causes atrophic rhinitis and pneumonia in pigs, kennel cough in dogs, pneumonia in cats, and respiratory illnesses in other animals.[81,132,377] This organism also is the occasional cause of respiratory illness in humans.[72,89,143,299,344,361,377,378,423] *B. avium* is an important cause of respiratory illness in turkeys and other birds.[211]

Three additional species of *Bordetella* have been recognized to infect humans: *B. holmesii* and *B. hinzii* have been isolated from blood cultures, primarily in patients with underlying chronic illness.[80,234,380,414] *B. holmesii* also has been isolated from the human respiratory tract, and *B. trematum* has been found in wounds and ear infections.[258,395,427] *B. petrii* has been isolated from the environment and is capable of anaerobic growth.[403]

The genus *Bordetella* consists of gram-negative, pleomorphic, aerobic bacilli that are grouped together on the basis of genotypic characteristics, and species are differentiated by phenotypic characteristics. Selected differential characteristics of the four *Bordetella* spp. that cause respiratory illnesses in humans are presented in Table 140–1. All species have relatively simple requirements, but *B. pertussis* is quite fastidious and is inhibited by constituents in common laboratory media such as fatty acids, metal ions, sulfides, and peroxides.[239,394] For laboratory growth, *B. pertussis* requires the addition of "protective substances" such as charcoal, blood, or starch, whereas the other species are less fastidious and may grow in blood or MacConkey agars.

TABLE 140–1 Selected Differential Characteristics of *Bordetella* Species That Cause Respiratory Illnesses in Humans

Organism	Catalase	Oxidase	Nitrate reduction	Urease production	Motility
B. pertussis	+	+	–	–	–
B. parapertussis	+	–	–	+†	–
B. bronchiseptica	+	+	+	+‡	+
B. holmesii	+	–	–	–	–

*+, activity; –, not present
†At 24 hours.
‡At 4 hours.
From Loeffelholz, M. J.: Bordetella. In Murray, P. R., Baron, E. J., Jorgensen, J. H. (eds.): Manual of Clinical Microbiology. 8th ed. Washington, D.C., American Society for Microbiology, 2003, pp.780-788.

The genomes of representative strains of *B. pertussis*, *B. parapertussis*, and *B. bronchiseptica* have been sequenced.[312,324] The genome sizes are as follows: *B. pertussis*, 4,086,186 bp; *B. parapertussis*, 4,773,551 bp; and *B. bronchiseptica*, 5,338,400 bp. *B. pertussis* has 3816 predicted genes, whereas *B. parapertussis* and *B. bronchiseptica* have 4404 and 5007 predicted genes, respectively. Pseudogenes occur most commonly in *B. pertussis* (358) and *B. parapertussis* (220) and are uncommon in *B. bronchiseptica* (18). *B. pertussis* has three insertion sequence elements (IS): IS 481 (238 copies), IS 1002 (6 copies), and IS 1663 (17 copies). *B. parapertussis* has IS 1001 (22 copies) and IS 1002 (90 copies). The sequenced RB50 *B. bronchiseptica* strain contained no IS elements, but studies of other *B. bronchiseptica* strains found strains with IS 481, IS 1001, and IS 1663.[95,122,328]

ETIOLOGY OF PERTUSSIS (WHOOPING COUGH)

B. pertussis and *B. parapertussis* are the etiologic agents of pertussis, but approximately 95 percent of illnesses are caused by *B. pertussis*.[133,174,325] In rare instances, *B. bronchiseptica*, which normally is enzootic in pigs, dogs, cats, rodents, and other animals, has been isolated from humans with pertussis-like cough illnesses.[72,89,143,299,344,361,377,378,423] From 1995 to 1998, *B. holmesii* was isolated from the nasopharynx of 33 individuals in Massachusetts suspected of having pertussis, most of them adolescents and young adults.[258] In contrast to all other *Bordetella* spp., this organism is susceptible to cephalexin, an antibiotic that frequently is added to *Bordetella* culture media.[302] This addition may explain why the organism has not been noted in patients with pertussis in other laboratory studies.

Adenoviruses have been isolated from children with pertussis, and some researchers have suggested that several adenoviral types on occasion may cause a pertussis-like illness.[14,76,78,295] However, the data of Nelson and associates[295] and Baraff and coworkers,[14] as well as our own observations, lead us to suggest that mixed infections are occurring and that the classic symptoms are caused by *B. pertussis* and not infection with an adenovirus. At variance with our view are data presented by Wirsing von König and associates.[421] These investigators noted pertussis-like illnesses caused by viral or *Mycoplasma pneumoniae* infections in 83 patients in whom pertussis laboratory studies were performed and were negative. These authors serologically identified 33 adenoviral illnesses, 18 illnesses caused by parainfluenza viruses, 15 illnesses caused by *M. pneumoniae*, and 14 caused by respiratory syncytial virus (RSV). In young infants, co-infection with an adenovirus and perhaps RSV may lead to more severe disease.[20,227] Infection with human bocavirus also may cause an illness with a paroxysmal cough.[9] Of 54 children with laboratory confirmed bocavirus infections, 85 percent had cough, and 19 percent had paroxysmal coughing episodes.

Physicians often suggest that *Chlamydia trachomatis* can cause a pertussis-like illness. However, in our opinion, the repetitive cough of *C. trachomatis* is distinctly different from the paroxysmal cough of *B. pertussis* infection, and thus illnesses caused by the two agents usually should not be confused clinically. Infections with *Chlamydia pneumoniae* and *M. pneumoniae* also cause long-lasting illness with cough.[87,149,421] Although infection with these agents in older children and adults can be confused with *B. pertussis* infection, true paroxysms typical of pertussis rarely occur.

ANTIGENIC AND BIOLOGICALLY ACTIVE COMPONENTS OF *BORDETELLA PERTUSSIS*

B. pertussis contains a variety of components that are antigenic or biologically active (Table 140–2).* With the exception of tracheal cytotoxin (TCT), all known virulence factors produced by *B. pertussis* are regulated by the single genetic locus *bvgAS*.[81] Under certain conditions, such as an environmental temperature of 37° C, *bvgAS* is active, toxins and adhesins are produced, and the organism is virulent in a mouse model (*bvg*+ phase). In the *bvg*- phase, a different set of genes (*vrg*, *vir* repressed genes) are expressed, and *B. pertussis* is avirulent in mice in this phase.[411] The switch from *bvg*+ to *bvg*- is a phenomenon common to all *Bordetella* spp. and is associated with a change in phenotype. An intermediate phase with reduced virulence and expression of specific proteins also has been characterized. Although still speculative, the intermediate phase may have some function in transmission of the organism.[81,367]

Fimbriae

Fimbriae (FIM) are protein projections on the surface of *B. pertussis*.[257,279,281,325,334,335] They are highly immunogenic, and antibody to them, as well as to other antigens, causes agglutination of the organism. Two fimbrial antigens (FIM 2 and 3) are the main agglutinogens; endotoxin and pertactin (PRN) also are agglutinogens.[52,334]

In the past, typing of *B. pertussis* strains was based on the agglutination patterns noted with specific antisera.[57,106,325,334] Six specific agglutinogens were recognized, and typing was based on the presence or absence of agglutination by each specific antiserum. More recently, researchers recognized that two of the agglutinogens (agglutinogens 2 and 3) are fimbrial in location (FIM 2 and 3) and that agglutinogens 4, 5, and 6 are minor antigens.[325,334] All *B. pertussis* strains contain agglutinogen 1. The nature of this agglutinogen is not known.[334] It could be lipopolysaccharide (LPS) or PRN, but because the original serotyping scheme was based on heat-labile antigens, it probably was not LPS.[33,229,382]

FIM function as adhesins, but some studies suggest that in infection they are not the primary adhesins but serve to sustain the attachment established by other attachment factors.[68,335,387,412] An in vitro study by Rodriguez and associates[336] suggested that the effect of FIM on attachment was the result of bacterial agglutination. In the mouse model system, immunization with purified FIM resulted in protection against infection when challenged with *B. pertussis*.[206] Data from two trials in which serologic correlates of immunity were studied indicated that antibody to FIM was important in protection.[69,372]

---

*See references 7, 52, 68, 81, 82, 130, 157, 162, 175, 179-181, 210, 238, 243, 248, 255, 257, 274, 281, 296, 345, 355, 387, 390, 405, 412, 432.

TABLE 140–2 Biologically Active and Antigenic Components of *Bordetella pertussis*

Component	Characteristic
Adhesions	
Fimbriae (FIM)	Two serologic types (types 2 and 3); antibody to specific types causes agglutination of the organism; organisms may contain fimbriae 2, fimbriae 3, fimbriae 2 and 3, or neither fimbriae 2 nor fimbriae 3
Filamentous hemagglutinin (FHA)	220-kd surface-associated and secreted protein; highly immunogenic
Pertactin (PRN)	A 69-kd outer-membrane protein that is the most important adhesin; antibody to pertactin causes agglutination of the organism
Vag8	95-kd outer-membrane protein
BrkA	73-kd surface-associated N-terminal passenger domain with 30-kd outer-membrane C-terminal protein; confers serum resistance and protection against antimicrobial peptides in *B. pertussis*
SphB1	Subtilisin-like Ser protease/lipoprotein required for FHA maturation
Tracheal colonization factor (TcfA)	60-kd secreted protein
Toxins	
Pertussis toxin (PT; also called lymphocytosis-promoting factor)	A classic bacterial toxin with an enzymatically active A subunit and a B oligomer-binding protein; effects in an animal model system include histamine sensitization, promotion of lymphocytosis, stimulation of insulin secretion, and adjuvant and mitogenic activity; it is an envelope protein that is also an important adhesin; it adversely affects host immune cell function
Adenylate cyclase toxin (ACT)	Calmodulin-activated RTX family toxin with dual adenylate cyclase/hemolysin activity; acts as an antiphagocytic factor during infection
Dermonecrotic toxin (DNT)	160-kd heat-labile secreted toxin; induces necrosis in vitro
Tracheal cytotoxin	Disaccharide-tetrapeptide monomeric byproduct of peptidoglycan synthesis; causes mitochondrial bloating, disruption of tight junctions, damage to cilia, and interleukin-1α and nitric oxide production
Lipopolysaccharide (LPS) (endotoxin)	An envelope toxin with activities similar to endotoxins of other gram-negative bacteria; a significant cause of reactions to whole-cell pertussis vaccines; antibody to LPS causes agglutination of the organism

Filamentous Hemagglutinin

Filamentous hemagglutinin (FHA) is a component of the cell wall of all *Bordetella* spp.[25,68,81,214,248,257,387] It is highly immunogenic and is the dominant attachment factor for *Bordetella* in animal model systems.[257,345,354] However, because FHA is released in large amounts from the cell surface, its role as an adhesin must be questioned. Adhesins typically remain associated with the bacterial surface to promote maximum attachment. FHA is a component of most acellular component (DTaP) vaccines.[102] However, the importance of antibody to FHA and protection from disease is not clear. Some data indicate that a vaccine containing both pertussis toxin (PT) and FHA had an efficacy greater than that

of a vaccine containing only toxoided PT.[370] However, in two studies in which serologic correlates of immunity were evaluated, researchers found that FHA made no contribution to protection.[69,372] Finally, one whole-cell component DTP vaccine in which vaccinees did not mount an antibody response to FHA was, nonetheless, highly efficacious.[166,362]

Pertactin

PRN is a 69-kd outer-membrane protein that is, in our opinion, the most important adhesin of *B. pertussis*.[25,225,302,303] Antibody to PRN has a strong protective effect in aerosol-challenge studies in mice.[48,355] In the two vaccine efficacy trials in which serologic correlates of immunity were evaluated, researchers found that antibody to PRN was most important in protection.[69,372] In addition, the vaccine efficacy trials conducted in the 1990s, in which mild disease and typical disease were evaluated, revealed that DTaP vaccines that contained PRN in addition to PT and FHA clearly were significantly more effective.[56,65,145,257] Another study revealed that anti-PRN antibodies were required for efficient phagocytosis of *B. pertussis* by host immune cells.[176]

Other Autotransporters

In addition to PRN are several other surface-associated proteins (Vag8, BrkA, SphB1, and TcfA) that are considered to belong to the autotransformer family.[257] All likely contribute to attachment to host cells, but their potential adhesive functions have not been investigated directly.

Pertussis Toxin

PT is an adenosine diphosphate–ribosylating toxin synthesized and secreted exclusively by *B. pertussis*. It is an A-B toxin with an enzymatically active A subunit (S_1) and a B oligomer (S_{2-5}) binding portion.* PT inactivates G proteins, a process resulting in disruption of signaling pathways and leading to histamine sensitization, enhancement of insulin secretion in response to regulatory signals, and both suppressive and stimulatory immunologic effects in animal model systems.[257] The various effects of PT in animal model systems and in humans were reviewed in depth previously by one of us (J. D. C.).[68,257] In contrast to animal studies, histamine sensitization does not appear to happen in children, but PT does cause an increase in plasma insulin levels.[68,257] PT also is responsible for leukocytosis with lymphocytosis in *B. pertussis* infections. PT is a strong adjuvant in several immunologic systems in animals, but in DTP-vaccinated persons (DTP vaccines contain small amounts of active toxin), only the enhancement of serum antibody responses to antigens of other vaccines has been demonstrated. In mouse and rat models, PT inhibits chemotaxis and migration of neutrophils, monocytes/macrophages, and lymphocytes to infection sites, and PT also functions as an adhesin in the adherence of *B. pertussis* to human macrophages and ciliated respiratory epithelial cells.

In 1979, researchers suggested that pertussis was a single-toxin disease, a suggestion that led to the idea that pertussis could be prevented by a PT vaccine in a manner similar to the success achieved with diphtheria toxoid in diphtheria.[52,319,320] Although convincing arguments to the contrary have been presented, this idea persists.[332] The most compelling evidence that pertussis from *B. pertussis* infection is not a PT disease is as follows: identical illness results from *B. parapertussis* infection, and this organism does not express PT.[52,174]

PT does contribute to morbidity in *B. pertussis* infections, as indicated by the severity of illness, which tends to be greater than

---

*See references 7, 8, 68, 81, 125, 196, 225, 257, 319, 320, 389.

that caused by *B. parapertussis* infection. In particular, the frequent finding of extreme leukocytosis caused by PT in neonates and young infants with fatal pertussis is noteworthy.

Adenylate Cyclase Toxin

Adenylate cyclase toxin (ACT) is an extracytoplasmic enzyme that impairs host immune cell function and may contribute to local tissue damage in the respiratory tract.[68,81,181,212,257,413] ACT enters phagocytic cells (particularly polymorphonuclear neutrophils) and, once inside, is activated by calmodulin and catalyzes the production of supraphysiologic amounts of cyclic adenosine monophosphate from adenosine triphosphate, which intoxicates these cells.[257]

Dermonecrotic Toxin

Dermonecrotic toxin (DNT) is a heat-labile toxin described by Bordet and Gengou[31] in 1909. This cytoplasmic protein causes skin necrosis in laboratory animals,[293] and it may contribute to local tissue damage in the respiratory tract.

Tracheal Cytotoxin

TCT is a disaccharide-tetrapeptide monomer of peptidoglycan.[81,130] It causes local damage to respiratory epithelium and may affect host neutrophil function adversely.[86,130] The cytopathology caused by TCT probably is the result of increases in nitric oxide.[81]

Lipopolysaccharide (Endotoxin)

The LPS of *B. pertussis* is similar to the endotoxins of other gram-negative bacteria.[46,68,81] Its function in disease is unknown, but it may act as an adhesin.[89] LPS is a major cause of reactions to whole-cell pertussis vaccines.[13] LPS is a significant agglutinogen. Antibody to LPS reduces colonization of *B. pertussis* in the lungs and trachea of mice after aerosol challenge.[289]

EPIDEMIOLOGY

Today, considerable misinformation is circulating with regard to the epidemiology of pertussis. The main reason for misinformation is the failure to recognize the significant differences in the dynamics of reported pertussis compared with the dynamics of

B. pertussis infections.[60,61] The two different epidemiologies are the (1) epidemiology of reported clinical pertussis and (2) the epidemiology of *B. pertussis* infection.

OBSERVED (REPORTED PERTUSSIS)

Pertussis is one of the most highly communicable diseases; when it has been introduced into a susceptible population, attack rates of 100 percent in susceptible individuals have been recorded.[220] Infants and young children have the highest risk of acquiring the disease.

Incidence

The incidence of reported pertussis and its mortality are affected markedly by the use of pertussis vaccine. In the prevaccine era in the United States, the average attack rate of reported pertussis was 157 per 100,000 population, versus 230 per 100,000 population in England and Wales.[49] Previous studies, however, suggested that reported cases represent only between 15 and 25 percent of cases that actually occur.[159,203,205,368]

With the introduction and widespread use of pertussis vaccines, the attack rate in the United State fell approximately 150-fold from 1943 to 1976. For the 7-year period from 1976 to 1982, the attack rate in the United States remained between 0.5 and 1.0 per 100,000 population (Fig. 140–1). From 1982 to 2005, the attack rate curve shifted modestly upward and reached a rate of 8.9 per 100,000 in 2004.[61] Possible reasons for the resurgence of reported pertussis that have been suggested are (1) increased vaccine failures resulting from genetic changes in *B. pertussis*, (2) increased vaccine failures related to vaccines of lessened potency, (3) greater awareness of pertussis, and (4) the availability of better laboratory tests.[60,61,65,74,138,145] Of these possibilities, it is our opinion that greater awareness is the most important. Also of probable importance is that, in general, DTaP vaccines are less efficacious than are DTP vaccines, which, in particular, may be a contributing factor relating to the increase in reported pertussis in older children and adolescents.

Pertussis epidemics in the prevaccine era occurred at 2- to 5-year intervals (average, 3.2 years), and these cycles have continued in the vaccine era. As noted by Fine and Clarkson,[116,118] this continuation of the same cycles today as occurred in the prevaccine era indicates that, although immunization has controlled disease, it has not reduced transmission of the organism in the population.[49,54,57]

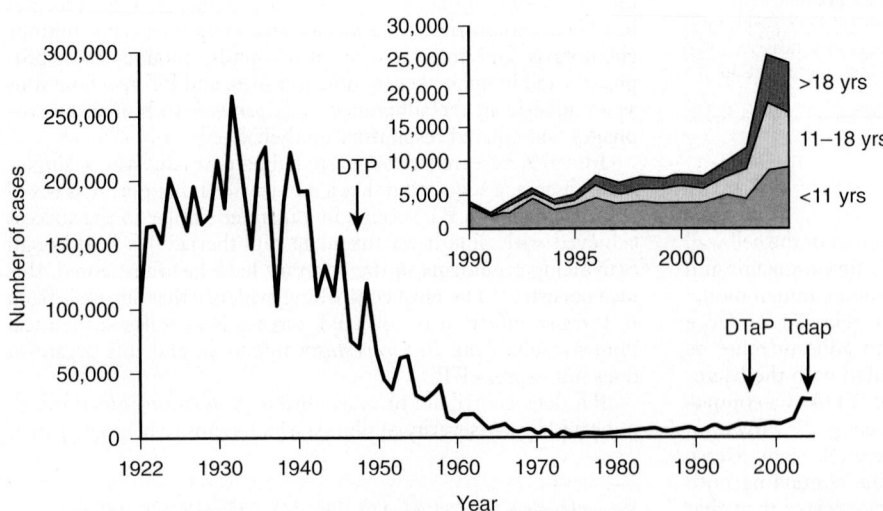

Figure 140–1 Number of reported cases of pertussis by year, United States, 1922 to 2005. DTaP, diphtheria-tetanus-acellular pertussis; Tdap, tetanus-diphtheria-acellular pertussis component vaccine. (*Data from Centers for Disease Control and Prevention, Atlanta.*)

In the prevaccine era, the following percentages of cases by age were noted in Massachusetts: younger than 1 year, 7.5 percent; 1 to 4 years, 41.1 percent; 5 to 9 years, 46.0 percent; 10 to 14 years, 4.1 percent; and 15 years and older, 0.9 percent.[30] Associated with the marked reduction in reported cases of pertussis in the United States resulting from widespread pediatric immunization, a major shift occurred in the percentages by age category.[30] During the period from 1978 to 1981, the age distributions were as follows: younger than 1 year, 53.5 percent; 1 to 4 years, 26.5 percent; 5 to 9 years, 8.2 percent; 10 to 14 years, 5.4 percent; and 15 years or older, 6.5 percent. In contrast, U.S. data for 2005 revealed the following: younger than 1 year, 16 percent; 1 to 4 years, 9 percent; 5 to 9 years, 10 percent; 10 to 19 years, 31 percent; and 20 years or older, 28 percent (unknown age, 6%). Today, pertussis in adolescents and adults is an important source of *B. pertussis* infection in unimmunized or partially immunized children.* Disease in adolescents and adults usually is not recognized as pertussis, even though the cough frequently is paroxysmal and the illness persists for weeks.[57,251,323,352]

In a study in university students, members of our group found that 26 percent of students with a cough illness of 6 days' duration or longer had *Bordetella* infections, none of which had been diagnosed correctly clinically.[278] The findings in this study led to the suggestion that *B. pertussis* infections are endemic in adults and are responsible for cyclic outbreaks in susceptible children. More recent studies in the United States, Germany, and elsewhere support this hypothesis.†

Morbidity and Mortality

During the first 30 years of the 20th century, pertussis was an important cause of death in the United States.[221] The number of deaths from pertussis in the United States between 1926 and 1930 was 36,013,[133] and most of these deaths occurred in children younger than 1 year of age. The pertussis death rate curve in the United States declined throughout the 20th century. In infants, the mortality rate decreased approximately fivefold from 1900 to 1944. During the next 35 years, it declined more than 85-fold.[286,287] Today, most of the deaths caused by pertussis occur in unimmunized infants younger than 6 months of age.[144,257] During 1990 to 1996, 57 deaths attributed to pertussis were reported in the United States.[144] Of these 57 patients, 49 were younger than 6 months old. Young maternal age and preterm delivery were risk factors for fatal disease. Currently in the United States, approximately 10 to 20 deaths are reported each year.[39,42,144,402,425]

Of importance is that deaths caused by pertussis frequently are misdiagnosed as deaths from other respiratory infectious illnesses.[49,171,300] For example, in England and Wales during the epidemic from 1977 to 1979 and at the beginning of the epidemic in 1982, 32 deaths were reported to be caused by pertussis.[49] However, when the excess deaths from other respiratory infectious illnesses were examined, approximately 362 additional deaths appeared to be caused by pertussis.

The morbidity caused by pertussis in recent years can be gleaned from numerous reports. The numbers of pertussis-related hospitalizations, complications, and deaths in the United States during 1990 to 1996 were reviewed in 1999 by Güris and colleagues.[144] Of the 31,837 cases analyzed, 31.7 percent of these patients were hospitalized, 9.5 percent had pneumonia, 1.4 percent had seizures, 0.2 percent had encephalopathy, and 0.2 percent died. The most severe morbidity occurred in infants younger than 6 months of age. Of this group, 72.2 percent were hospitalized, 17.3 percent had pneumonia, 2.1 percent had seizures, 0.5 percent had encephalopathy, and 0.5 percent died.

During the period from 2000 to 2004, 12,174 cases in infants were reported.[44] Of this group, 62.8 percent were hospitalized, 55.8 percent had apnea, 12.7 percent had pneumonia, 1.5 percent had seizures, and 0.8 percent died.

In adolescents with reported pertussis, 0 to 2 percent are hospitalized, and 2 percent have pneumonia.[45] In a review of data from seven studies of reported adult pertussis, the following findings were noted: hospitalization, 3 to 12 percent; seizures, 0 to 0.6 percent; rib fracture, 0 to 4 percent; and pneumonia, 0.6 to 8 percent.[44]

A pertussis surveillance system was introduced in conjunction with a large pertussis vaccine efficacy trial in several regions of Germany in 1990. The initial results of this ongoing surveillance study were published in 1993.[164] Of 601 culture-proven cases, 12.3 percent occurred in infants, and 86.2 percent occurred in children younger than 6 years of age. Serious complications were reported in 22 of 275 patients with follow-up. These complications included pneumonia in 5.5 percent, apnea in 2.2 percent, and cardiorespiratory failure in 0.4 percent.

In a follow-up report of the same study, 1 of 185 culture-confirmed cases in infants was fatal.[168] In another German study from 1993 to 1996, Herzig and associates[178] noted 116 hospitalized pertussis patients with the following complications: pneumonia in 81 percent, apnea requiring assisted ventilation in 15 percent, seizures in 14 percent, encephalopathy in 5 percent, and death in 2 percent. In Canada from 1991 to 1997, Halperin and colleagues[156] analyzed the complications of pertussis in 1082 hospitalized children younger than 2 years of age and noted that 9.4 percent had pneumonia, 3 percent had atelectasis, 2.3 percent had seizures, 0.59 percent had encephalopathy, 0.8 percent had inguinal or umbilical hernias, 1.3 percent had more than a 5 percent weight loss, and 0.9 percent died.

Season, Geography, and Sex

Pertussis occurs throughout the world.[68] Historically, epidemic pertussis had no seasonal pattern.[49] However, in the present vaccine era in North America, pertussis usually occurs in the summer and fall.[110,134,144,257,294] In the past, the incidence of pertussis was greater in female than in male patients.[49,133,409] Between 1980 and 1996, this female preponderance was observed again, but only in older age groups.[110,144] In 2004, 25,827 cases were reported in the United States, and of these patients, 11,199 (45%) were male and 13,879 (55%) were female (sex not identified in 749 cases).[41] In the large study in Germany, 1263 (50.7%) of the 2493 subjects were female.[168]

Transmission

Transmission is thought to occur by droplets from a coughing patient that reach the upper respiratory tract of a susceptible person. Indirect spread also possibly occurs. A symptomatic patient could contaminate the environment with respiratory secretions. The hands of the new host-to-be make contact with the secretions and then may inoculate the respiratory tract.[68] Attack rates in susceptible household contacts range from 70 to 100 percent.[49,68] Antibody studies indicate that asymptomatic infections also occur in contacts.[91,240,241] These asymptomatic infections are likely to be short-lived and probably are not important with regard to contagion. Transmissibility is greatest early in the illness, that is, during the catarrhal and early paroxysmal phases.

BORDETELLA PERTUSSIS INFECTION

The cyclic pattern of reported pertussis is similar today to what it was in the pre-vaccine era.[257] This pattern is different from that

---

*See references 27, 44, 57, 60, 61, 66, 219, 236, 237, 285, 294, 392.
†See references 26, 57, 60, 61, 91, 94, 280, 352, 420, 426.

seen with other diseases that have been brought under control by universal immunization.[57,60,61,278] An example is measles. As this disease was brought under control, the interepidemic cycle lengthened because circulation of the measles virus in the population had been reduced. In contrast, with pertussis, immunization controlled disease but did not decrease the circulation of *B. pertussis*.[118,119] In the 1970s, Nelson[294] noted that the source of *B. pertussis* infection in hospitalized infants most often was an adult. This observation led many investigators to suspect that *B. pertussis* infections were endemic in adolescents and adults.[57,278] Sporadic infection in the adolescent and adult reservoir is the major source of *B. pertussis* infections in nonimmune children. The cyclic pattern occurs because it takes a few years for a significant number of susceptible members of the population to develop so that an outbreak will result from the sustained transmission.

Our present understanding of the importance of adolescent and adult *B. pertussis* infections has been the result of the ability to diagnose infection serologically by measuring immunoglobulin G (IgG) and IgA antibodies to PT by enzyme-linked immunosorbent assay (ELISA).[60,61,257,278] During the last 20 years, numerous studies in adolescent and adult populations have contributed to our understanding of *B. pertussis* epidemiology.

Studies of prolonged cough illnesses in adolescents and adults suggest that between 13 and 20 percent of the illnesses are caused by *B. pertussis* infection.* Many studies have looked at overall infection rates by determining significant IgG or IgA titer rises to PT in persons who have two or more serum samples collected over extended periods.[60,61,83,94,182,257,407] These studies suggest that between 1 and 6.7 percent of adolescents and adults have a *B. pertussis* infection each year. In another large study in the Netherlands, which used a combination of serologic surveys, an incidence of infection of 6.6 percent per year for persons between the ages of 3 and 79 years was estimated.[92] The incidence in children 3 to 4 years of age was 3.3 percent. It then increased gradually to a peak of 10.8 percent in those 20 to 24 years of age. Other age-specific incidences were 6.5 percent in persons 25 to 55 years old and 4.0 percent in those older than 55 years of age.

The specific rates of cough illnesses caused by *B. pertussis* were determined in two prospective specific population-based studies.[373,406] In the first study, the rate was 500 per 100,000 (0.5%), and in the second, it was 370 per 100,000 (0.37%). In addition, the retrospective serologic analysis of a respiratory disease study in adults older than 65 years suggested a rate as high as 1.5 percent.[182] This high value assumes that all respiratory illnesses with cough during the 4-month periods of seroconversion were the result of *B. pertussis* infection.

PATHOLOGY

Data on pathology of *B. pertussis* infections have been determined mainly by postmortem study in fatal cases.[49,68,73,221,235,249,311,358] However, information relating to uncomplicated pertussis can be gleaned from experiments using rhesus and ringtail monkeys.[221,347] In these studies, pure cultures of *B. pertussis* have been obtained from between the cilia of the smaller bronchi and bronchioli. Endobronchitis and peribronchitis are noted, and the bronchi contain leukocytes, mucus, and debris.

In a recent study of autopsy material from is infants (≤4 months old), the consistent histopathologic features were necrotizing bronchiolitis and pneumonia, intra-alveolar hemorrhage and fibrinous edema, and abundant intra-alveolar macrophages.[311] Angiolymphatic aggregates of mixed leukocytes in the intralobular septa and pleurae were seen in 86 percent of the specimens. Intact *Bordetella* were noted in cilia of the trachea, bronchi, and bronchioles and within airways and alveoli. They also were noted intracellularly in alveolar macrophages and respiratory epithelium. Six of the respiratory specimens had evidence of co-infections with one or more other agents (cytomegalovirus, 1 child; RSV, 2 children; *Streptococcus pneumoniae*, 2 children; *Streptococcus pyogenes*, 2 patients; *Moraxella catarrhalis*, 1 child; and viridans streptococci, 1 child).

Pathologic changes in the brain and liver also have been described. Microscopic or gross cerebral hemorrhage may be noted, and cortical atrophy has been observed. These changes most likely are the result of anoxic brain damage. In some studies of pertussis encephalopathy, findings suggested meningoencephalitis, with perivascular cuffs of lymphocytes within cerebral gray matter and pleocytosis.[422] However, the studies in which inflammation was demonstrated were performed before modern virologic techniques became available. Probably, the neurologic findings in these instances were caused by interactions with neurotropic viruses or other infectious agents and were not the result of *B. pertussis* infection.[68] Fatty infiltration of the liver has been noted in patients with pertussis encephalopathy.

PATHOGENESIS AND IMMUNITY

After the patient is exposed to *B. pertussis*, the pathogenesis of infection depends on four important steps: attachment, evasion of host defenses, local damage, and systemic disease.* The biologically active antigenic components of *B. pertussis* listed in Table 140–2 have various roles in pathogenesis.

Infection is initiated in the respiratory tract by the attachment of *B. pertussis* organisms to the cilia of ciliated epithelial cells.[412] Adhesins (FHA, PT, FIM, LPS, TcfA, Vag8, BrkA, and PRN) facilitate this attachment.[81,210,291,325,387,412] Because of the redundancy of protein adhesins, determining the importance of the individual proteins and ascertaining a primary adhesin or adhesins have been difficult.[257] In animal model systems, FHA is an important adhesin; however, data from two vaccine efficacy trials in which serologic correlates of immunity were studied suggested that FHA may not be necessary if other adhesins are present.[69,372] Data from one of these efficacy trials noted that a DTP vaccine that contained a minimal amount of FHA and generated a minimal anti-FHA response had greater efficacy than did a DTaP vaccine that contained a large amount of FHA and generated a vigorous antibody response to FHA.[166,362] However, in a study in which a PT toxoid vaccine was compared with a two-component PT/FHA vaccine, researchers found that the two-component vaccine was more efficacious.[1,369-371] This finding suggests that in the absence of antibody to other adhesins, antibody to FHA contributes to protection.

Of the other attachment proteins, data relating to human infection are available for PRN and FIM only. In the two trials that looked at serologic correlates of immunity, researchers found in both that antibody to PRN was most important and that antibody to FIM was also important.[66,372] Studies suggest that FHA and PRN may act synergistically.[25,214,225] Because the FIM of some gram-negative bacteria are important for attachment, researchers have assumed that *B. pertussis* FIM are important in attachment. However, in one tissue culture study, FIM did not mediate the attachment of organisms to cells.[390] In a more recent study, investigators found that FIM played a role in attachment in persistent infection.[281] Furthermore, antibodies against FIM were shown to provide protection against colonization with *B. pertussis* in the murine respiratory tract.[417]

---

*See references 26, 60, 61, 127, 202, 257, 278, 297, 338, 352, 373, 401, 420, 426.

*See references 68, 81, 130, 179, 257, 289, 291, 293, 325, 412.

Both ACT and PT adversely affect immune cell function and, therefore, allow infection, once initiated, to continue.[68,181,291] PT prevents migration of lymphocytes and macrophages to areas of infection and adversely affects phagocytosis and intracellular killing. ACT enters phagocytic cells and catalyzes excessive production of cyclic adenosine monophosphate, which intoxicates neutrophils and results in a decrease in phagocytosis.

TCT, DNT, and ACT all have been implicated as contributors to local tissue damage in the respiratory tract.[68,130,293] Of these toxins, TCT is likely to be the most important.[130] In hamster tracheal organ cultures, TCT selectively destroys ciliated cells in a manner similar to that seen in *B. pertussis* infection, and the pathologic process is similar to that noted in human pertussis autopsy studies. As noted in Table 140–2, several other *Bordetella* virulence factors have been described and have been characterized to some extent in mouse models.[81,114,120,210,257,428] Determination of their precise roles, however, requires further investigation.

Pertussis is a unique illness in that it has only one manifestation of systemic disease in uncomplicated infection: leukocytosis with lymphocytosis caused by PT.[68,174,194] T and B lymphocytes increase to a similar extent in the circulation.[24] In contrast to the situation in *B. pertussis* infection, lymphocytosis is not a characteristic of *B. parapertussis* infection because this organism does not liberate PT. The most important systemic complication of pertussis is encephalopathy, the mechanism for which is not known. The most likely explanation is anoxia associated with coughing paroxysms.

Some investigators have suggested that pertussis is a toxin-mediated disease caused by PT.[319,320] Although some researchers continue to entertain this idea,[332] little evidence supports it. Undoubtedly, PT is a fascinating protein with multiple activities in experimental animals, such as histamine sensitization, promotion of lymphocytosis, effects on glucose metabolism, and induction of adjuvant and mitogenic activity.[68,125,257,291] However, in infections in humans, the main effects that appear to be caused by PT are lymphocytosis and mild, compensated hyperinsulinemia. PT has been suggested to be the cause of the prolonged cough in pertussis. However, because persistent cough is a major manifestation of *B. bronchiseptica* infection in dogs and of *B. parapertussis* infection in children, and because neither organism liberates PT, this hypothesis should be refuted.[174,257,302]

Cell-mediated immune function is altered by *B. pertussis* infection. In some studies, cell-mediated immunity was depressed, whereas in others it was augmented.[307]

Various antibodies develop after exposure of the human host to infection with *B. pertussis*. The development of agglutinins, hemagglutination-inhibiting antibodies, and bactericidal antibodies has been described.[49] ELISA techniques have demonstrated class-specific antibodies (IgA, IgE, IgG, and IgM) to many of the specific proteins of *B. pertussis*.[161,250,308] These antibodies develop after infection and, with the exception of IgA antibodies, also after immunization. Neutralizing antibody to PT likewise develops after both infection and immunization.[152,308] Specific IgA antibodies to PT and FHA also can be demonstrated in nasopharyngeal secretions and saliva.[136,429]

At present, both *B. pertussis* infection and immunization with whole-cell or acellular pertussis vaccines clearly elicit protection of varying degree and duration against pertussis. The prevailing opinion throughout the last century was that immunity acquired from having *B. pertussis* infection is lifelong, whereas vaccine-induced immunity is relatively short-lived. Although the latter clearly is true,[118] studies performed by members of our research group suggest that the former opinion regarding infection-induced immunity is wrong.[55,58,67,257,352,399] Proceeding from the knowledge that IgA antibodies to pertussis antigens (PT, FHA, and PRN) result from infection and not from primary vaccination, our group studied the prevalence of these antibodies in the

sera of young German and American men of similar ages.[67] In Germany, routine childhood immunization was not carried out during the 1970s and 1980s, and pertussis was epidemic. To our surprise, the rate and mean values of IgA antibodies in the two populations were similar, thus suggesting that adult infection rates were similar. In another study in Germany, we found that *Bordetella* infections were common occurrences in adults, often in persons with a known history of childhood pertussis.[352]

The nature of immunity in pertussis is not known. The consensus has been that serum antibodies greater than some unknown concentration to one or more of the pertussis antigens are responsible for protection.[91] Antibodies to PT, FHA, and PRN have been shown to be protective in animal model systems.[25,82,225,345,355] However, no serologic correlates of immunity had been established until recently, although several large vaccine trials have been performed since the late 1980s.[1,138,145,231,357,362,385] In a nested household contact study, our group was able to evaluate the roles of IgG antibodies to PT, FHA, PRN, and FIM 2 by determining pre-exposure imputed values in children at the time of household exposure to *B. pertussis* infection by using both classification tree and logistic regression methods.[69] The imputed geometric mean antibody values to PT, PRN, and FIM 2 were higher in non-cases than in cases. In the classification tree analysis, however, only antibodies against PRN contributed significantly to protection. Specifically, subjects with an imputed PRN value of less than 7 EU/mL had a 67 percent likelihood of infection. Logistic regression analysis also found that PRN values of 8 EU/mL or more were associated with prevention of illness after household exposure. In accordance with our findings, data from a Swedish study indicate that antibody values of 5 EU/mL or more to PRN and FIM 2/3 correlated with protection.[372]

In addition to humoral responses to several *B. pertussis* antigens, evidence exists that cell-mediated immune responses to PT, FHA, and PRN also occur.[10,247,275-277,340,341,384,415,431] Studies in a murine respiratory infection model suggest that cellular immunity plays an important role in bacterial clearance and augments the effects of antibody by predominantly T-helper 1 (T_H1) cell stimulation.[275,276] Studies in humans demonstrate a cellular immune response shortly after natural infection with *B. pertussis*, with PT, FHA, and PRN preferentially inducing the synthesis of T_H1 cells.[415] Immunization with a whole-cell pertussis vaccine results in a T_H1 response, whereas the response to acellular vaccines is more heterogeneous and involves both T_H1 and T_H2 cells.[315] Persistent memory T and B cells and anamnestic antibody responses are important in long-term immunity.[247]

Immunity developed after having *B. pertussis* infection or receiving vaccination with a whole-cell pertussis vaccine does not protect against illness caused by *B. parapertussis*, and, similarly, infection with *B. parapertussis* does not induce protection against disease caused by *B. pertussis*.[222,381] However, in our vaccine efficacy trial in Germany, the results showed some evidence that the acellular pertussis multicomponent vaccine, which contained a large amount of FHA, offered some protection against *B. parapertussis* infections, whereas the whole-cell vaccine, which contained minimal amounts of FHA, did not.[172] Although *B. pertussis* infection is a localized infection involving ciliated cells of the respiratory track, bacteremia has been noted in immunocompromised adults.[40,201,386]

CLINICAL MANIFESTATIONS

The *clinical* manifestations of *B. pertussis* infection have considerable variation that depends on age, previous immunization or infection, the presence of passively acquired antibody, and perhaps other factors such as the degree of exposure, host genetic and acquired factors, and the genotype of the organism. The incubation period for pertussis generally varies between 6 and 20 days; most cases have an onset 7 to 10 days after exposure. However, after household exposure, 22 percent of secondary cases were noted to have an onset more than 4 weeks after the onset of illness in the primary case.[166]

CLASSIC ILLNESS

Classic illness occurs as a primary infection in unimmunized children between the ages of 1 and 10 years.[58,68,133,307] The illness usually lasts 6 to 12 weeks and has three stages: catarrhal, paroxysmal, and convalescent. The initial illness is characterized by rhinorrhea, lacrimation, and mild cough suggesting a common cold. Body temperature usually is normal. The severity of the cough gradually increases over a period of 1 to 2 weeks, but pertussis usually is not suspected until the cough becomes paroxysmal.

After the catarrhal period, the coughs increase in severity and number. Repetitive series of 5 to 10 or more forceful coughs during a single expiration can be noted. These paroxysms are followed by a sudden massive inspiratory effort, and a characteristic whoop may occur as air is forcefully inhaled through a narrowed glottis. Cyanosis, bulging eyes, protrusion of the tongue, salivation, lacrimation, and distention of neck veins occur during paroxysms. Several paroxysmal coughing episodes with their associated massive inspiratory effort may occur sequentially until the child succeeds in dislodging the obstructing mucus. The production of purulent sputum does not occur. Post-tussive vomiting is a common occurrence. Paroxysms may strike several times per hour, and they occur during both day and night.

The paroxysmal episodes are exhausting, and patients frequently appear dazed and apathetic. Weight loss may occur as a result of vomiting and also because eating and drinking may be resisted, given that they trigger attacks. Attacks also may be triggered by yawning, sneezing, or physical exertion. Between attacks, the patient may appear normal and usually is in no distress.

Common and important complications of classic pertussis include pneumonia, otitis media, seizures, and encephalopathy. Pneumonia may be caused by *B. pertussis* or secondary bacterial invaders. Atelectasis may develop as a result of the mucus plugs. The forcefulness of the paroxysms can cause rupture of the alveoli and can produce interstitial or subcutaneous emphysema.

Otitis media is a common occurrence and frequently is caused by *S. pneumoniae*. Pertussis also has been associated with activation of latent tuberculosis. Convulsions and coma may be observed. These findings may be a reflection of cerebral hypoxia related to asphyxia. Rarely, subarachnoid and intraventricular hemorrhage may occur. Tetanic seizures may be associated with the severe alkalosis that results from the loss of gastric contents caused by persistent vomiting.

Other complications that have been noted include ulcer of the frenulum of the tongue, epistaxis, melena, subconjunctival hemorrhage, subdural hematoma, spinal epidural hematoma, rupture of the diaphragm, umbilical hernia, inguinal hernia, rectal prolapse, dehydration, meningoencephalitis, the syndrome of inappropriate antidiuretic hormone secretion, apnea, rib fracture, and nutritional disturbances.[37,58,198,256,323,359,410]

The convalescent stage, which usually lasts 1 to 2 weeks, is characterized by a decreasing frequency and severity of coughing episodes, whooping, and vomiting. All patients with classic pertussis caused by primary infection have leukocytosis secondary to lymphocytosis. Fever and pharyngitis are not usual manifestations in pertussis, and, therefore, a search for a secondary cause should be undertaken when these findings occur. Except for the observation of typical paroxysms, physical examination in pertussis usually is unrewarding. Diffuse rhonchi may be noted on auscultation.

Infection with *B. parapertussis* causes an illness that is similar to that caused by *B. pertussis*, but generally it is less severe and of shortened duration.[174]

MILD ILLNESS AND ASYMPTOMATIC INFECTION

Mild, nonclassic illness is common in *B. pertussis* infection.[91,164,168,348] It occurs in previously vaccinated children and also as a primary infection in nonvaccinated children. In a study in which physicians sent nasopharyngeal specimens from children with cough illness, regardless of whether the illness was typical of pertussis, to our laboratory,[164] 247 culture-positive cases were noted. Of these patients, 47 percent had a total duration of cough illness of 28 days or less. In 26 percent, the duration of cough was less than 3 weeks. Most of these cases occurred in unvaccinated children. In a 6-year, similar study involving 2592 culture-positive, previously unvaccinated children, 38 percent had a duration of cough illness of 28 days or less, and in 17 percent, the duration was 21 days or less.[168] In a study in which both culture and polymerase chain reaction (PCR) were used for establishing the diagnosis of *B. pertussis* infection, many mild cases were found to be PCR-positive and culture-negative.[348] Of these cases, only 68 percent had a cough illness lasting 4 weeks or longer, and only 57 percent and 32 percent had paroxysmal cough and whoop, respectively.

In studies of household contacts, asymptomatic infections in family members are common occurrences.[91,240,241] Deen and associates[91] found that 52 (46%) of 114 household contacts who remained well had laboratory evidence of *B. pertussis* infection. In another study, 21 of 399 healthy infants who were controls had PCR-positive nasopharyngeal samples.[167]

INFANTS

Pertussis in infancy is a unique experience.[257] Its spectrum of clinical manifestations varies by age, immunization, and the presence or absence of transplacentally acquired antibody.* Most deaths resulting from *B. pertussis* infection occur in neonates and early infancy, and morbidity is most severe in infants.† From 1997 through 2000, 8276 cases of pertussis were reported in infants in the United States.[39] Of this group, 59 percent were hospitalized, 11 percent had pneumonia, 1 percent had seizures, 0.2 percent had encephalopathy, and 0.7 percent died. Eighty-seven percent of these infant cases occurred in children younger than 6 months of age.

The source of infection in infants usually is a family member.[16,27,85,91,107,217] In a study of 616 infant cases, the source was identified in 43 percent.[27] A family member was the source 75 percent of the time, and the mother was the most common source (32%). Of the source persons, 56 percent were adults, and 20 percent were 10 to 19 years of age.

B. pertussis infection in neonates is particularly severe, with a death rate of between 1 and 3 percent.[20,73,144,171,173,189,233,261] A common initial finding is apnea, and typical coughing is not observed. Seizures in association with apnea caused by hypoxia occur frequently. Severe pulmonary hypertension is a relatively common problem in pertussis in the first 4 months of life.[88,97,135,142,148,311,317,360,416] The severity of disease and the risk of death correlate directly with the white blood cell count and, in particular, the number of lymphocytes.[20,73,88,142,171,261,269,311,317] White blood cell counts in the range of 30,000 to more than 100,000 cells/mL are common findings. Co-infection with

---

*See references 20, 49, 68, 73, 107, 110, 171, 217, 261, 294, 300.
†See references 16, 20, 73, 84, 85, 88, 129, 135, 142, 144, 147, 148, 167, 171, 173, 189, 227, 257, 259, 261, 269, 294, 300, 311, 317, 321, 337, 358, 360, 379, 402, 416.

respiratory viruses (RSV, adenovirus, influenza viruses) and respiratory bacterial pathogens (*S. pneumoniae, Haemophilus influenzae*) are relatively frequent.[20,85,227,311,358]

Whoop is a rare manifestation of illness in infants, and other respiratory manifestations frequently are confused with those caused by respiratory viruses.[49] *B. pertussis* infection has been noted in association with sudden infant death syndrome (SIDS), but whether a cause-and-effect relationship exists is not clear.[167,173,233,300] Nichol and Gardner,[300] in a study in England, found that many deaths attributed to SIDS were, in fact, related to *B. pertussis* infection. Using PCR, we found *B. pertussis* DNA in nasopharyngeal specimens from 9 (18%) of 51 infants who had sudden, unexpected deaths.[173] In a subsequent study, we collected specimens for PCR from 254 infants who experienced sudden, unexplained deaths and from 441 healthy matched controls.[167] The rate of PCR-positive results in the sudden death cases was 5.1 percent; it was 5.3 percent in the controls. In a careful follow-up histopathologic study with unique immunohistochemical staining of specimens from a subset of these fatal cases, we could find no evidence of specific *B. pertussis* pulmonary infection or pathologic features.[310]

ADULTS

Increased awareness of adult pertussis has occurred since the 1970s.* Unrecognized pertussis cases in adults often are the source from which infants and children become infected.[20,27,57,73,171,261,294,352] All adults previously have been exposed to *B. pertussis* antigens by immunization, infection, or both,[67,91,94,257] and this exposure tends to modify their illness. In a U.S. study, the following cough characteristics were noted in 31 university students with laboratory evidence of *Bordetella* infection: the median duration was 21 days before initial evaluation, 94 percent had one or more coughing episodes per hour, and 90 percent of the coughs had a staccato or paroxysmal quality.[278] Despite these findings, pertussis was not suspected in any of the students, and clinical diagnoses by the primary care providers included upper respiratory tract infection (39%), bronchitis (48%), and other diagnoses (16%). Although specific records were not available, most of these students probably were vaccinated as children and almost certainly had previous, unrecognized infections.[67,91]

In contrast to these findings in the United States, in a study in Germany, adults were found to be more likely to have typical pertussis, even though the epidemiologic data suggested that all had a previous infection, and 26 percent of 64 patients with laboratory evidence of infection recalled having had pertussis during childhood.[67,352] Rates of clinical manifestations in the 64 laboratory-confirmed cases were as follows: paroxysms, 70 percent; whoop, 38 percent; post-tussive phlegm, 66 percent; and post-tussive vomiting, 17 percent. The clinical diagnosis in 39 percent was definite or probable pertussis; only 14 percent were thought not to have pertussis. Of note is that the clinical diagnosis was not made by primary care physicians but by a small team of specially trained central investigators with high awareness for pertussis.

In a German household contact study, similar findings were noted: 80 percent of 79 adults with laboratory-confirmed *B. pertussis* infection coughed for 3 or more weeks, and 63 percent had spasmodic cough for 3 or more weeks.[323] In addition, in 53 percent of patients, coughing was followed by choking or vomiting. However, only 8 percent of the adults in this study had whoops. Complications that were observed included pneumonia,

rib fracture, inguinal hernia, and severe weight loss. Unique sweating episodes are reported in approximately 5 percent of adults, and fainting can occur in association with coughing.[93,323]

DIAGNOSIS

DIFFERENTIAL DIAGNOSIS

In typical pertussis, the clinical diagnosis should be apparent based on the paroxysmal cough with post-tussive vomiting and whooping and lack of significant fever. However, the cause of the illness can be *B. pertussis* or *B. parapertussis*. A history of contact with a known case (laboratory confirmed) will help to establish the diagnosis in a patient with mild or atypical illness. The presence of leukocytosis with lymphocytosis in a child with a cough illness or the presence of apnea in an infant is a strong indication that the illness is caused by *B. pertussis* and not *B. parapertussis*. In a matched-control comparison, none of 11 children with culture-proven *B. parapertussis* infection versus 7 of 22 (32%) with *B. pertussis* infection had lymphocytosis of 10,000 or more cells/mL.[174] Lymphocytosis of 10,000 or more cells/mL is observed in few other diseases.

Many other infectious agents cause illnesses with prolonged and repetitive cough that can be confused with *B. pertussis* or *B. parapertussis* infections.[257] In particular, *M. pneumoniae, C. pneumoniae*, adenoviruses, bocavirus, and other respiratory viruses all can cause prolonged cough illnesses.* In addition, coughing episodes may be seen in children with asthma, bronchiolitis, bacterial pneumonia, cystic fibrosis, *Coccidioides immitis* infection, and other fungal pulmonary infections and tuberculosis. Another problem is the cough associated with sinusitis, which can be confused with *B. pertussis* infection. The cough associated with gastroesophageal reflux also can be confused with pertussis, as can cough associated with an airway foreign body.

SPECIFIC DIAGNOSIS

A laboratory diagnosis of pertussis caused by either *B. pertussis* or *B. parapertussis* can be made by culturing the organisms on appropriate media, by identifying their presence by direct fluorescent antibody testing (DFA) or PCR, and by demonstrating the presence of specific antibodies. *Bordetella* spp. can be recovered from nasopharyngeal specimens, with the highest rate of isolation occurring within the first 3 weeks of cough.[164,374] Specimens for culture can be collected by swabbing the nasopharynx, by nasopharyngeal washing, or by nasopharyngeal aspiration.[68,150] In general, nasopharyngeal aspiration gives the highest yield of positive cultures.

B. pertussis and *B. parapertussis* are recovered most easily by direct plating of the specimen from the patient onto selective media.[68,70,186,239] Specific swabs (calcium alginate or Dacron) and media (Regan-Lowe or Bordet-Gengou agar and modified Stainer-Scholte broth) are required, and laboratory personnel should be experienced in isolating the organisms. If cultures cannot be inoculated directly, the use of Regan-Lowe transport medium is recommended. In classic disease, the culture or a DFA study will be positive in approximately 80 percent of cases if the specimen is obtained within 2 weeks of the onset of cough and antibiotics have not been administered previously.[165,308] DFA has been used for the diagnosis of pertussis caused by *B. pertussis* or *B. parapertussis* during the last 40 years.[257,290,363] It is rapid and inexpensive, but it lacks sensitivity and specificity; it does not employ amplification for sensitivity, and it lacks specificity because

---

*See references 26, 27, 41, 42, 44, 45, 57, 60, 61, 91-94, 110, 127, 144, 182, 200, 202, 219, 257, 278, 280, 294, 297, 323, 333, 338, 352, 373, 383, 407, 420, 426.

*See references 9, 14, 49, 68, 76, 78, 87, 149, 295, 421.

of cross-reactions with other organisms of the nasopharyngeal flora.[109]

Since the late 1980s, numerous PCR assays with primers derived from four different chromosomal regions have been developed for the diagnosis of *B. pertussis* and *B. parapertussis* infections, and they have been evaluated in multiple studies by comparison with culture and clinically typical pertussis.*

PCR has the advantage of having much higher sensitivity than that of conventional culture. In a prospective study in which swabs for PCR and culture were obtained simultaneously from 555 subjects with cough illnesses, the use of PCR increased the identification of *B. pertussis* infection almost fourfold, from 28 to 111.[348] Only a few studies have been reported in which the sensitivity and the specificity of PCR for the diagnosis of *B. pertussis* infection were determined by comparison with serologically identified cases.[169,230,232,329,397] In a study that our group performed, we compared PCR results with serologic diagnosis and found that PCR had a sensitivity of 61 percent and a specificity of 88 percent.[118] Similar findings have been noted in other studies.[230,232,330,397] At present, the most commonly used primers for the diagnosis of pertussis include IS 481 and IS 1001.[257] IS 481 occurs in the genomes of *B. pertussis* and *B. holmesii* but not in *B. parapertussis*. IS 1001 occurs in the genomes of *B. parapertussis* and *B. holmesii* but not in *B. pertussis*. The genome of *B. bronchiseptica* generally contains neither IS 481 nor IS 1001. However, in two recent studies, *B. bronchiseptica* strains were found to contain IS 1001 in their genomes.[122,328] False-positive results are a potential problem with the use of PCR for establishing the diagnosis of pertussis and other respiratory illnesses.[3,262,290] False-positive results can occur if specimens are opened in the pertussis laboratory before transport to the PCR laboratory.[257] False-positive results also can result from contamination of the air in a room in which the previous patient had pertussis. Moreover, as noted earlier, *B. bronchiseptica* can be mistaken for *B. parapertussis* when the IS 1001 primer is used.[122,328] Therefore, rigorous internal and external laboratory controls are necessary.

Obtaining a routine laboratory diagnosis of *B. pertussis* infection in adults or in other atypical cases is hampered by the problem that medical care usually is not sought until the third or fourth week of the illness, and antibiotics frequently have been administered before the possibility of pertussis was considered.[278,352] During the last 2 decades, the most significant advance in the diagnosis of pertussis has been the development of ELISA.[257]

Natural infection with *B. pertussis* is followed by a rise in serum concentrations of IgA, IgG, and IgM antibodies to specific antigens of the organism, as well as to preparations of the whole organism.[79,123,154,250,268,278,308,362,400] In contrast to natural infection, primary immunization of children induces mainly IgM and IgG antibodies.

Serologic testing for *B. pertussis* infection in the clinical setting is neither standardized nor widely available.[68,308] In the research setting, the use of ELISA has contributed significantly to establishing the diagnosis of *B. pertussis* infection in many patients with negative cultures.[94,151,240,241,278,280,352,426] Most useful has been the determination of IgG and IgA antibodies to PT and FHA. The most reliable proof of acute infection is the demonstration of a significant increase in antibody values between acute-phase and convalescent-phase serum specimens. Frequently, because collection of acute-phase specimens is delayed and, therefore, the acute-phase values already are elevated, significant increases between first and second serum specimens cannot be demonstrated. However, a diagnosis frequently can be established on the basis of a high value or values on a single serum speci-

men.[91,278,352,419,426] Because *B. parapertussis* infection induces cross-reacting antibodies to *B. pertussis* FHA, the use of this antigen alone cannot differentiate *B. pertussis* from *B. parapertussis* infection.[137,362]

Measurement of agglutinating antibodies also is useful for establishing the diagnosis of *B. pertussis* infection, and, because the test is simple, inexpensive, and accurate, it can be used in the clinical setting.[91,170,278,308,352] Unfortunately, its sensitivity is low.

Today in clinical practice, the laboratory diagnosis of pertussis should be approached as follows: In all cases in which the cough illness is of less than 2 weeks' duration in adolescents and adults or 3 weeks' duration in children, a nasopharyngeal specimen should be obtained for culture or PCR. In adults who have had cough for greater than 2 weeks' duration, single serum ELISA is the preferred method. This method also can be used in children if they have not been immunized within 2 years. At present, many commercial laboratories offer single serum diagnostic tests for *B. pertussis*, and almost all the offered tests lack specificity. Any test that employs the whole organism in the test is fraught with false-positive results. Tests that report specific IgM antibodies also are unreliable. The greatest sensitivity and specificity for the serologic diagnosis of *B. pertussis* infection are achieved by ELISA or an ELISA-like test with the measurement of IgG and IgA antibodies to PT. Single high values of IgG or IgA antibodies to PT are indicative of infection.[257] In our opinion, a sensitive and specific test is available from Focus Diagnostics, Cypress, California.[326]

Not all infected persons develop antibody responses to PT. In children, approximately 25 percent lack an adequate response, as do approximately 10 percent of adolescents and adults.[63,362]

An ELISA also has been developed for the detection of IgA antibody to *B. pertussis* in nasopharyngeal secretions and as an indicator of recent infection.[131,136,429] *B. pertussis* IgA appears in nasopharyngeal secretions during the second or third week of illness and persists for at least 3 months.[131] However, the appearance of secretory IgA may be delayed in children younger than 1 year of age.[292] This antibody is not induced by primary parenteral *B. pertussis* vaccination. Detection with the use of ELISA of *B. pertussis* IgA in secretions may be a diagnostic aid in culture-negative patients whose symptoms have persisted for longer than 3 weeks. To our knowledge, this test is not clinically available.

TREATMENT

Several antibiotics have in vitro efficacy against *B. pertussis*.[14,17-19,23,43,187,190-192] The first choice for treatment since the 1970s has been oral erythromycin; this ameliorates the symptoms if it is given early during the course of the illness and eliminates the organism from the nasopharynx within a few days, thereby shortening the period of contagiousness.[23] The dose for children is 40 to 50 mg/kg/day given every 6 hours for 14 days; the dose for adults is 2 g/day given every 6 hours for 14 days. A 7-day course of erythromycin estolate was shown in a large study in Canada to be as efficacious as 14 days of treatment.[153] The newer macrolides, azithromycin (10 mg/kg on day 1 and 5 mg/kg on days 2 to 5 as a single dose for 5 days for children and 500 mg on day 1 and 250 mg on days 2 to 5 for adults) or clarithromycin (15 to 20 mg/kg/day in two divided doses for 7 days for children and 1 g/day in two doses for 7 days for adults), also can be expected to be effective.[6,43] Although rare, the use of erythromycin in young infants is associated with hypertrophic pyloric stenosis, so parents need to be educated about the symptoms of this potential risk.[38,185,284] Because of this risk, the Centers for Disease Control and Prevention (CDC) recommends treating neonates with azithromycin rather than erythromycin.[43] Trimethoprim-sulfamethoxazole can be used as an alternative agent in those who

---

*See references 98, 108, 111, 128, 141, 160, 169, 193, 215, 228, 230, 232, 253, 262, 304, 329, 330, 348, 349, 396-398, 430.

cannot tolerate erythromycin.[192] The first erythromycin-resistant strain of *B. pertussis* was isolated from a 2-month-old male infant in Yuma County, Arizona, in June 1994.[227] The isolate was highly resistant, with a minimal inhibitory concentration (MIC) greater than 64 µg/mL (the usual MIC of erythromycin is 0.02 to 0.1 µg/mL). More recently, two more resistant *B. pertussis* strains were recovered from cases in California and Utah.[216,224] At present, no evidence of a pattern of emerging macrolide resistance has been seen, but because PCR rather than culture is becoming the diagnostic method of choice in many laboratories, the chance of missing resistant strains is a possible problem.

Patients infected with *B. parapertussis* and *B. holmesii* also can be treated with macrolides, but *B. bronchiseptica* usually is resistant to erythromycin so that alternative therapy is necessary.[257] *B. bronchiseptica* strains usually are sensitive to aminoglycosides, extended-spectrum, third-generation penicillins, tetracyclines, quinolones, and trimethoprim-sulfamethoxazole.

Historically, no infectious disease has a greater list of remedies lauded as beneficial but without objective evidence of effectiveness.[62] Supportive care includes avoidance of factors that provoke attacks of coughing and maintenance of hydration and nutrition. In the hospital, gentle suction to remove secretions and well-humidified oxygen may be required, particularly in infants with pneumonia and significant respiratory distress. In severe infections in neonates and young infants, assisted ventilation may be necessary.

However, infants who develop pulmonary hypertension with respiratory and cardiovascular failure respond poorly to aggressive therapy (pulmonary artery vasodilators and extracorporeal membrane oxygenation [ECMO]) and have high mortality rates. Because data suggest that the pulmonary hypertension results from the extreme leukocytosis with lymphocytosis, which is always present in fatal cases, our opinion is that leukocyte-reducing measures such as exchange transfusion should be implemented.[96,142,317,337]

The use of corticosteroids has received attention in the treatment of pertussis. Cortisone treatment in the murine model of pertussis increased the mortality rate.[195] In contrast, Zoumboulakis and associates[433] suggested that a 7-day course of steroids and erythromycin reduced the number of coughing paroxysms and episodes of vomiting significantly, in addition to shortening the duration of symptoms. Unfortunately, this study was not controlled rigorously.

The use of salbutamol has also been suggested as having some value, but definitive studies are needed to confirm the efficacy of this mode of treatment.[34] Pillay and Swingler[318] reviewed the symptomatic treatment of pertussis and found no statistically significant benefit for the use of diphenhydramine, dexamethasone, or salbutamol.

PROGNOSIS

The prognosis in pertussis is related to the patient's age. In older children and adults, the prognosis is good, but infants have a significant risk of death and development of encephalopathy.* In addition, long-term follow-up suggests that apnea or seizures at the time of disease may be associated with subsequent intellectual impairment.[376] The present availability of pediatric intensive care units and assisted ventilation has reduced the rate of mortality in infants who receive medical care.[171] Unfortunately, many deaths occur outside the hospital. No evidence has shown that pertussis impairs ventilatory function later in life.[204]

---

*See references 16, 20, 73, 84, 85, 110, 129, 142, 144, 189, 259, 261, 269, 321, 337, 358, 379, 402.

PREVENTION

VACCINE EFFICACY

Whole-Cell Vaccines

The first pertussis vaccines were developed in the 1920s, and effective vaccines have enjoyed worldwide use since the 1940s.[49,63,68,257] After World War II, extensive vaccine trials were organized by the British Medical Research Council.[263-265] Based on these studies, as well as smaller studies in England, the United States, and other countries, DTP vaccine use became routine in many countries.[119]

The pertussis attack rate was relatively constant in the United States in the pre-vaccine era between 1922 and 1942 (see Fig. 140–1). From 1943 to 1976, a 150-fold reduction in the attack rate was noted in association with widespread childhood pertussis immunization.

The existence of a relationship between vaccine use and disease control also was supported by data from England and Wales. The pertussis attack rate declined between 1958 and 1973 and increased dramatically between 1977 and 1983 after a marked decrease occurred in the number of vaccinations administered, beginning in 1974.[49] The attack rate decreased with the widespread use of vaccine and increased when vaccine use decreased. Moreover, the attack rate after the decrease in vaccine use was increased most markedly in the newly susceptible cohort of children younger than 4 years of age. Until recently, English children received their pertussis immunization only in the first year of life, and protection is not long-lasting.

In the 1980s, numerous household contact studies were performed.[91,309,313-315] In a study from 1982 to 1983 involving 440 household contacts aged 6 months to 9 years, the secondary attack rate in unvaccinated contacts was compared with the rate in children who had received three or more DTP doses. Vaccine efficacy was found to be 91.4 percent. A similar study conducted during the period 1979 to 1981 revealed an efficacy of 82.4 percent.

In another study, Onorato and associates[309] noted that the calculated efficacy varied markedly according to the clinical case definition. Efficacy against any cough illness was 63 percent, whereas it was 83 percent if a cough duration of 21 or more days was required.

In the 1990s, the most definite studies of DTP vaccine efficacy were carried out in four countries.[138,145,166,231,351,357,362] In these trials, the efficacy of the candidate DTaP vaccines was compared with the efficacy of DTP vaccines; the controls were subjects who received DT. With the exception of one lot of one DTP vaccine (Connaught, USA), which had poor immunogenicity, the DTP vaccines were more efficacious than were the DTaP vaccines. The poor efficacy of the Connaught DTP vaccine probably was the result of an unusual low potency lot of this vaccine rather than a generic problem with this vaccine.[257] In a case-control study in the United States, the efficacy of the Connaught vaccine was similar to that of the Wyeth-Lederle DTP vaccine, which, in the controlled trial in Germany, had a high level of efficacy.[28] Finally, in a large comparative trial, the DTP vaccine from England (Evans vaccine) had efficacy greater than those of the three DTaP vaccines with which it was compared.[146,306]

Acellular Vaccines

Research in the 1970s showed that three *B. pertussis* antigens (PT, FHA, LPS) were liberated into the medium during culture and that these antigens could be concentrated and separated by density gradient centrifugation.[68,179] This finding allowed for the development and production of vaccines by six manufacturers in Japan.[64,213,301,346] All six vaccines had minimal or no endotoxin but different amounts of PT and FHA. In addition, some of the vaccines were found to contain FIM 2 and PRN.

Despite limited proof of efficacy, the six vaccines were put into routine use in Japan in 1981, and they have controlled, to some degree, epidemic pertussis during the ensuing decades. However, because adequate data were not available on any single vaccine or on vaccine use in young infants, many extensive trials were performed subsequently in Europe, Africa, and Japan.[1,288]

After extensive analysis of the data was conducted on the original efficacy trial in Sweden in the mid-1980s, calculated efficacy was found to vary significantly, depending on the clinical case definition and the laboratory methods.[1,29,151,369-371] Therefore, researchers decided that a universal primary case definition should be developed for use in all subsequent efficacy trials so that different vaccines in different trials could be compared.

A World Health Organization (WHO) committee met in Geneva in January 1991, and a primary case definition was developed.[424] This definition and minor variations of it were used in the efficacy trials in the 1990s. The WHO case definition is as follows: (1) an illness with 21 days or more of spasmodic cough and either culture-confirmed infection with *B. pertussis* or serologic evidence of infection with *B. pertussis* as indicated by a significant rise in IgA or IgG antibody by ELISA against PT or FHA in paired sera or (2) contact with a case of culture-confirmed pertussis in the household with onset within 28 days before or after the onset of cough in the study vaccinee. Not all members of the WHO committee, including one of us (J. D. C.), agreed with this primary case definition because its use results in the elimination of many laboratory-confirmed cases from efficacy calculations.[56,164,168,369-371] With this definition, vaccines that lessen the severity of disease but are poor at preventing mild disease will be overrated.

In 1994 and 1995, seven efficacy trials with candidate DTaP vaccines in four countries were completed,[138,145,231,351,357,362,385] and an additional trial in Sweden was completed in 1997.[306] As noted in Table 140–3, the nine vaccines are different in the number of antigens that they contain, as well as in the concentrations of the specific antigens. In all efficacy studies, confounding factors may affect the results. In general, double-blind studies with placebo and whole-cell vaccine controls are ideal. However, placebo control was not ethical in countries in which DTP vaccine was recommended. Therefore, studies in Germany and Senegal used various methods to obtain efficacy data in spite of the lack of a

blinded diphtheria-tetanus (DT) toxoid group. Observer bias can affect the results of all studies, including those with double-blind control. For example, a less efficacious vaccine that prevents typical disease but not mild disease can be determined to be more efficacious than it actually is if the study observers believe they "know pertussis" and dismiss atypical cases as being other respiratory illnesses and do not obtain cultures or conduct prospective follow-up.[71]

In general, household contact studies, unless they are nested analyses in prospective cohort studies, also are subject to observer bias, and case-control studies result in significantly inflated efficacy percentages.[56,65,71,117,119,288] In cohort studies, observer bias by parents can be reduced by frequent prospective telephone contact with study families. Finally, serologic diagnosis, as well as diagnosis by culture, increases the identification of mild cases, which are more likely to occur in vaccinees than in control subjects.

A summary of the efficacy data for 10 acellular pertussis vaccines evaluated in the 8 trials performed in the 1990s and the earlier 1980s Swedish trial is presented in Table 140–4. The data

TABLE 140–3 Pertussis Antigens in Nine Diphtheria-Tetanus-Acellular Pertussis Vaccines Evaluated in Eight Efficacy Trials (1990 to 1997)

Vaccine*	Pertussis Toxin (µg/Dose)	Filamentous Hemagglutinin (µg/Dose)	Pertactin (µg/Dose)	Fimbriae (µg/Dose)
Certiva[†]	40			
Tripedia[†]	23.4	23.4		
Triavax	25	25		
SKB-2[‡]	25	25		
Acelluvax	5	2.5	2.5	
INFANRIX[†]	25	25	8	
Acel-Immune[†]	3.5	35	2	0.8[§]
Daptacel[†]	10	5	3	5[‖]
CCL DTaP5[¶]	20	20	3	5[‖]

*Product name.
[†]Licensed in the United States.
[‡]No product name.
[§]Fimbriae 2.
[‖]Fimbriae 2 and 3.
[¶]No product name. However, is available in Canada with IPV as Quadracel and in Canada and the United States with IPV and Hib as Pentacel.

TABLE 140–4 Vaccine Efficacy Data for 10 Acellular Pertussis Vaccines Evaluated in Eight Trials Carried Out in the 1990s and the Earlier 1980s Swedish Trials

Location/References	Design	Vaccine	Schedule	Typical Pertussis (%)	Mild and Typical Pertussis (%)
Sweden, Stockholm[1,29,369]	Double-blind prospective cohort	JNIH-6	2 doses (2-3 mo apart starting at 5-11 mo of age)	84*	42
		JNIH-7		90	–7
Sweden, Göteborg[†385]	Double-blind prospective cohort	Certiva	3 doses (3, 5, 12 mo)	71	54
Sweden, Stockholm[145]	Double-blind prospective cohort	SKB-2	3 doses (2, 4, 6 mo)	59	42
		Daptacel		85	78
Italy, Rome[138]	Double-blind prospective cohort	Acelluvax	3 doses (2, 4, 6 mo)	84	71
		INFANRIX		84	71
Germany, Erlangen[362]	Prospective cohort	Acel-Immune	4 doses (3, 4½, 6, 15-18 mo)	83	72
Germany, Mainz[351]	Household contact	INFANRIX	3 doses (3, 4, 5 mo)	89	81
Germany, Munich[‡231]	Case control	Tripedia	4 doses (2, 4, 6, 15-25 mo)	80, 93	—
Senegal[§357]	Household contact	Triavax	3 doses	31, 74	—

*Efficacy against typical pertussis based on positive culture without serologic analysis.
[†]Significant observer bias occurred in this trial.[56]
[‡]Laboratory diagnosis based on culture only; 80 percent efficacy was against cough illness of 21 or more days, and 93 percent efficacy was against the World Health Organization (WHO) case definition.
[§]Thirty-one percent efficacy based on 21 days or more of cough illness; 74 percent efficacy was against the WHO case definition.

in this table indicate that three- and four-component vaccines (vaccines containing PRN and FIM as well as PT and FHA) have greater efficacy against *B. pertussis* illness (mild and typical) than do the PT or PT/FHA vaccines. The apparent high efficacy of the two-component vaccine (Tripedia) in the Munich study[231] can be explained by the type of study (case-control study), significant observer bias, and the lack of serologic diagnosis. However, in the post-licensure effectiveness case-control study done in the United States from 1998 to 2001, investigators found that the two-component vaccine (Tripedia) was slightly more effective than the four-component vaccine (Acel-Immune).[28] This finding suggests that a vaccine without PRN was more effective than was a vaccine that contained PRN. However, it is our understanding that this "two-component" vaccine also contained some PRN and perhaps some fimbrial protein as well. The final study, done in Stockholm, was a comparative study without a DT control group.[305] In this trial, in which vaccines were administered to children at 3, 5, and 12 months of age, the efficacy of CCL DTaP5 (five-component) was significantly better than that of Acelluvax (three-component vaccine) and was not significantly different from that of the comparative DTP vaccine (Evans vaccine). Acelluvax had greater efficacy than did the two-component vaccine SKB-2.

Follow-up studies of the various efficacy trials have been done in Sweden, Italy, and Germany, and all suggest sustained protection.[146,242,305,342,343] Of particular importance in this regard is the most recent report by Gustafsson and associates,[146] in which the large cohort vaccinated at 3, 5, and 12 months in the 1993 to 1996 trial were followed from October 1997 to September 2004. Overall, good protection lasted for approximately 5 years. The tabular data in this report suggest that Acelluvax (three-component vaccine) had efficacy similar to that of CCL DTaP5 (five-component vaccine). However, when all the data from the original trial and the present follow up data are combined, the overall attack rate in those children who had received the five-component vaccine was lower (47.5/100,000) than that in children who had received the three-component vaccine (59.7/100,000). This difference was not significantly different, however. Most notable is that the Evans DTP vaccine had greater sustained efficacy than did either Acelluvax or CCL DTaP5. In summary, it appears that DTaP vaccines that contain PRN have relatively good efficacy for approximately 5 years, but that (with the exception of one lot of one DTP vaccine), in general, DTP vaccines are more efficacious.[138,145,146,231,306,342,351,357,362]

In recent years, two acellular pertussis component, diphtheria, and tetanus toxoid vaccines (Tdap vaccines) have been developed for use in adolescents and adults.[44,45,59,112,113,163] These two vaccines are Adacel and BOOSTRIX, and their components are presented in Table 140–5. Both these vaccines elicit vigorous antibody responses to the antigens that they contain after a single dose. These responses are significantly greater than those observed in infants at 7 months of age after they have received three doses of the DTaP vaccines (Daptacel and INFANRIX) of the two manufacturers.

TABLE 140–5   Antigenic Composition of Adacel and BOOSTRIX per 0.5 mL

Antigen	Adacel	BOOSTRIX
Diphtheria toxoid	2 Lf	2.5 Lf
Tetanus toxoid	5 Lf	5 Lf
Pertussis toxin toxoid (PT)	2.5 µg	8 µg
Filamentous hemagglutinin (FHA)	5 µg	8 µg
Pertactin (PRN)	3 µg	2.5 µg
Fimbriae 2/3 (FIM 2, 3)	5 µg	—

Lf, flocculation units.

In a double-blind efficacy trial in adolescents and adults, an acellular pertussis vaccine (without diphtheria and tetanus toxoids) with the same concentrations of PT, FHA, and PRN as BOOSTRIX had an efficacy of 92 percent.[406] No similar efficacy trial was done with Adacel or its acellular pertussis components. However, extensive epidemiologic data from Canada, where Adacel has been used since 2003, show a marked reduction of pertussis in adolescents.[207]

ADVERSE EVENTS

Whole-Cell Vaccines

Local reactions and relatively mild systemic complaints are frequent occurrences after pertussis immunization. Less commonly, severe neurologic illness and death have been noted in temporal association with DTP immunization.

The largest study in the United States designed to assess the risk of relatively common and uncommon reactions to pertussis vaccine was performed by Baraff and associates.[11-13,75] This study was conducted between January 1978 and December 1979. Reactions in children who received either DTP or DT immunization were compared. A total of 15,752 DTP immunizations and 784 DT immunizations were given to children aged birth to 6 years of age. These children were evaluated for reactions that occurred within 48 hours of vaccine administration. All common local and systemic reactions occurred more frequently in the DTP recipients than in the DT group. Differences between the common reactions in the two groups were all highly significant ($p < .005$).

Redness at the injection site occurred in 37.4 percent of DTP recipients and in 7.6 percent of DT vaccinees. Fever (≥38° C [100.4° F]) was noted in 46.5 percent of DTP recipients. A temperature of 39° C (102.2° F) or higher occurred in 6.1 percent of DTP recipients, but in only 0.7 percent of DT recipients. Drowsiness, fretfulness, vomiting, anorexia, and persistent crying were other reactions recorded in 3.1 percent (persistent crying) to 53.4 percent (fretfulness) of DTP recipients versus 0.7 percent (persistent crying) to 22.6 percent (fretfulness) of DT vaccinees. In general, rates of local reactions, but not those of systemic reactions (except fever), increase from dose to dose in an immunization series.

In addition to these reactions, 0.1 percent of DTP recipients in this study were reported by the parents to have a high-pitched, unusual cry; 0.06 percent had convulsions, and 0.06 percent had hypotonic-hyporesponsive episodes (shock, collapse). No children in the control group (DT recipients) had similar reactions; however, the control group was of modest size (784 DT recipients), so statistical significance could not be assigned to any of these relatively uncommon events.

Because convulsions in young children are the result of many different etiologic factors, the cause-and-effect relationship with pertussis vaccine is less clear. However, inasmuch as fever develops in almost half of all DTP vaccinees and febrile convulsions are not uncommon events, a reasonable assumption is that many convulsions that occur in temporal association with DTP vaccination are induced by the immunization. Three studies have noted a significant association between pertussis immunization and febrile convulsions.[15,356,404] Approximately 1 per 1000 vaccinees older than 6 months of age will have a first febrile seizure after receiving pertussis immunization. The concomitant use of acetaminophen (15 mg/kg per dose at the time of immunization and every 4 hours for 24 hours) and DTP vaccine has been suggested as a means of reducing the incidence of febrile convulsions in vaccinees.[226]

Neurologic disease and death occurring in temporal association with pertussis immunization have been of major concern throughout the vaccine era. During the last 60 years, several case series and individual cases of neurologic illness occurring after receipt of pertussis immunization were reported; by 1979, more than 1000 cases of alleged neurologic damage induced by pertussis vaccine were reported.[22,36,47,49,218,252,418] Few of these reports had evidence of an adequate search for other possible causes of the neurologic disease, and in none were data available for rate calculations.

From 1967 to 1980, several attempts were made to determine the frequency of neurologic disease after receipt of pertussis immunization.[2,49,100,101,121,158,366,375] However, because controls were not included in any of the population evaluations, all rate estimates included children with temporally related events that had other causes.

A carefully designed prospective case-control study (National Childhood Encephalopathy Study [NCES]) of all hospital admissions of children aged 2 to 35 months with acute serious neurologic disorders in England, Wales, and Scotland was undertaken between 1976 and 1979.[4,21,245,270-273] The results of this study for the first time revealed an apparent statistical association between pertussis immunization and neurologic illness. Researchers found that a child who had received DTP vaccine within the previous 3 to 7 days was two to five times more likely to have neurologic disease than was a child who was not immunized during the same interval. The causal relationship between DTP immunization and neurologic illness noted in this study must be questioned, however, because both cases and controls had an equal frequency of immunization during the month preceding the index date. A more appropriate interpretation of the results is that they do not indicate cause and effect; rather, the DTP immunization calls attention to or brings out something that will occur anyway, but just moves it forward in time ("trigger effect").[50,51]

Infantile spasms, an identifiable seizure disorder of infancy, usually has its onset in the 6-month period from 2 to 7 months of age; therefore, that some cases occur after DTP immunization is not surprising. Simple calculations indicate that approximately 12 percent of all patients destined to have infantile spasms between 2 and 7 months of age will have an onset of illness within 7 days after receiving DTP immunization. The temporal association between DTP immunization and infantile spasms has led many people to assume a cause-and-effect relationship. However, controlled data from the NCES in Great Britain provide strong evidence against a causative role for pertussis vaccine in infantile spasms.[21] In another study, Melchior[266] in Denmark noted that the time of onset of infantile spasms was not altered when the time of pertussis immunization was changed from 5, 6, 7, and 15 months of age to 5 weeks, 9 weeks, and 10 months of age. In both periods, 42 percent of patients had their onset during the first 4 months of life.

Data from the NCES were reanalyzed with the exclusion of cases of infantile spasm.[271,273] From these analyses, the risk of permanent brain damage occurring from pertussis immunization has been suggested to be 1 per 330,000 vaccine doses, and the risk of any encephalopathy has been estimated to be 1 per 140,000 vaccinations. However, a review of the NCES data by other investigators indicates that both rate estimates are incorrect. Specifically, Stephenson[365] showed that the 1 per 140,000 rate for all encephalopathy is an artifact resulting from the inclusion of 9 children with febrile convulsions. Similarly, MacRae[244] noted that the increased relative risk that was observed within 7 days of receiving immunization (which was used to calculate the risk of brain damage of 1 per 330,000 immunizations) was offset by a decreased relative risk over the subsequent 3-week period. This finding, similar to the original study data and the infantile spasm data, indicates not a cause-and-effect relationship but rather a redistribution of events over time.

In the United States, the major neurologic illness that was noted in temporal association with DTP immunization was the first seizure of what turned out to be severe epilepsy. By chance alone, this association may occur 400 times a year in the United States. Four carefully performed studies that included approximately 330,000 children and 1 million immunizations have examined the possibility that pertussis immunization is a causative factor in epilepsy; no evidence of a causative role has been found.[51,126,140,356,404] More recently, two large studies in the United States and Canada found no evidence of a causal association with DTP immunization and encephalopathy.[282,327]

Similar to infantile spasms, SIDS also occurs in early life; therefore, that cases are noted to occur after administration of DTP immunization again is not surprising. Hoffman and associates[183] performed an extensive prospective case-control study of risk factors in SIDS from October 1978 through December 1979. In this study of 800 cases, investigators found that DTP immunization was not a risk factor for development of the syndrome. Other good, controlled studies have yielded similar results.[68,139] No evidence has demonstrated that DTP vaccinees have an increased risk of developing asthma later in life.[177]

Acellular Vaccines

An extensive amount of reactogenicity information has been generated in phase II and phase III studies with all licensed DTaP vaccines.[90,138,145,231,331,350,388] Because endotoxin has been removed from all DTaP vaccines, one is not surprised that all are less reactogenic than are DTP vaccines. In a double-blind study, the reactogenicity of 13 DTaP vaccines was presented and was compared with the reactogenicity of a DTP vaccine.[90] This study involved 2200 infants; 113 to 217 received an acellular product, and 370 received the whole-cell vaccine. Study participants received three doses of vaccine at 2, 4, and 6 months of age. Overall, all monitored reactions except vomiting occurred less frequently and were less severe in DTaP recipients than in DTP recipients. Specific results from this study are presented in Table 140-6. As can be seen, local redness and swelling and fever increased in frequency from the first to the third dose, whereas the complaint of drowsiness decreased.

In our efficacy trial in Germany with Acel-Immune, we monitored reactions in more than 8000 children after receipt of four doses of vaccine at 3, 4½, 6, and 15 to 18 months.[353,388] For the first three vaccine doses, the findings were similar to those noted in Table 140-6. After the fourth dose, the frequency of occurrence of local erythema and induration and fever increased considerably in comparison with their frequencies after the third dose. Ten percent of DTaP recipients had local erythema of 2.4 cm or greater, and 28 percent had temperatures of 38° C or higher. Other investigators also noted an increased frequency and severity of local reactions occurring after administration of the fourth and fifth doses of DTaP vaccines.[165,199,316,331,350] Of particular concern is the observation of extensive swelling of the thigh with booster doses of some DTaP vaccines.[331,350] Rennels and associates[331] found that this swelling occurred more commonly after immunization with DTaP vaccines containing high amounts of diphtheria toxoid. With Acel-Immune, a vaccine with a low diphtheria toxoid content, we noted that 15.4 percent of subjects had induration of more than 5 cm but less than 10 cm after receiving a fifth dose; swelling of the entire limb was not noted.[165]

In five of the 1990s efficacy trials, the occurrence of less common, more severe events (persistent crying, seizures, and hypotonic-hyporesponsive episodes) was monitored. A summary of these data is presented in Table 140-7. As can be seen, temporally related persistent crying, hypotonic-hyporesponsive episodes, and seizures were rare events after receipt of immunization with DTaP vaccines. In a large active surveillance program (IMPACT), researchers found that risks of having febrile seizures and hypotonic-hyporesponsive episodes after receiving pertussis-

TABLE 140–6   Summary of Reactogenicity Data from the Nationwide Multicenter Acellular Pertussis Trial

Event	DTaP 1st Dose (%)	DTaP 2nd Dose (%)	DTaP 3rd Dose (%)	DTP 1st Dose (%)	DTP 2nd Dose (%)	DTP 3rd Dose (%)
Local						
Redness	13.5	17.1	21.5	49.4	47.7	47.6
Swelling	8.7	12.1	13.3	39.7	34.1	35.7
Pain	3.8	2.0	2.1	27.3	18.7	15.8
Systemic						
Fever (Temp. ≥100.1° F)	4.2	11.3	15.8	27.3	34.1	37.7
Fussiness	6.6	7.7	6.7	20.1	23.5	17.3
Drowsiness	29.9	17.6	12.9	43.5	31.0	24.6
Anorexia	9.3	8.9	8.9	19.5	16.5	14.3
Vomiting	6.3	4.5	4.2	7.0	4.5	5.3
Use of antipyretic	39.3	36.7	36.3	60.5	59.8	61.4

DTaP, diphtheria-tetanus-acellular pertussis; DTP, diphtheria-tetanus-pertussis.
Data from Decker, M. D., Edwards, K. M., Steinhoff, M. C., et al.: Comparison of 13 acellular pertussis vaccines: Adverse reactions. Pediatrics 96:557-566, 1995.

TABLE 140–7   Rates* of Severe Events after Diphtheria-Tetanus-Acellular Pertussis Vaccines in the 1990s Efficacy Trials

Vaccine	Persistent Crying (≥3 hr)	Hypotonic-Hyporesponsive Episodes	Seizures
Certiva	0	0	0.4
Tripedia	0.1	0.05	0.02
SKB-2	0.8	0	0.3
Acelluvax	1.9	0.07	0
INFANRIX	1.3	0	0.07
Acel-Immune	2.0	0	0.1
Daptacel	1.5	0.1	0

Rates per 1000 doses.
Data from references 138, 145, 231, 385, and 388.

containing vaccines decreased significantly after the introduction of DTaP vaccines in Canada.[223]

SCHEDULES AND CONTRAINDICATIONS

Immunization schedules with whole-cell vaccines have varied throughout the world and to great measure were determined by concern relating to true and perceived reactions.[49,68] An immunization schedule involving only three doses given to infants at 2, 3, and 4 months of age has been quite effective in controlling pertussis-related morbidity and mortality in the United Kingdom.[393] However, the five-dose schedule used in the United States resulted in lower attack rates in preschool- and school-aged children.[49,68]

The recommendation for the DTaP vaccine in the United States is that it be given in the same five-dose schedule as recommended for DTP vaccines.[391] However, follow-up data from the 1990s efficacy trials, as well as reactogenicity data, suggest that administration of this "one size fits all" approach could be modified.[138,145,146,305,342,343,350,382,385] Our findings with Acel-Immune suggest that the present five-dose schedule is appropriate.[242,362] Conversely, data from other trials suggest that administration of the fourth dose of some vaccines can be postponed until the child is 4 to 6 years of age, or the third dose can be moved back to the child's second year of life.[146,305,306,342,343,382,385] These changes would not be expected to decrease efficacy but would decrease troubling local reactions with booster doses.

Acellular pertussis component quadrivalent (DTaP, IPV), pentavalent (DTaP, IPV, HBV; DTaP, IPV, Hib), and hexava-

lent (DTaP, IPV, HBV, Hib) vaccines have been developed and are available in many countries. In the United States, the following multicomponent vaccines are available: DTaP/Hib (TriHIBit for the fourth dose of DTaP and Hib series), DTaP/IPV/HBV (PEDIARIX), and DTaP, IPV, Hib (Pentacel). In general, multicomponent vaccine use should be encouraged to reduce the number of injections that a child receives.

In addition to providing childhood immunization, the availability of adolescent and adult Tdap vaccines allows the vaccination of adolescents and adults to be conducted.* At present, the schedule for the use of Tdap vaccines varies in different countries.[112,113,163] The most common recommendation is for universal immunization of preadolescents and adolescents and the selective immunization of adults. However, our opinion is that a universal program involving all preadolescents or adolescents and adults every 10 years will be necessary to prevent the transmission of *B. pertussis* effectively to unimmunized infants and to prevent the continued circulation of *B. pertussis* in a population.

Over the years, pertussis vaccine recommendations have undergone many changes. In particular, contraindications to vaccine are evolving continually. An important note, however, is that few scientific data support any of the present contraindications. The primary goal of national immunization programs is to vaccinate all infants and children. If excessive contraindications and their overinterpretation lead to a large number of unimmunized children, the programs will fail, and the children in greatest need of protection will contract pertussis. In the United States, the most recent recommendations of the Committee on Infectious Diseases of the American Academy of Pediatrics generally should be followed. However, individual case-by-case decisions often need to be made.

ISOLATION AND PROPHYLACTIC MEASURES

Erythromycin, azithromycin, or clarithromycin treatment in the index case shortens the duration of communicability of the organisms and thus limits spread of the disease. During the first few days of treatment, contact with susceptible persons should be avoided. In general, close contacts (household members, those in daycare centers, playmates) of the index case should be protected from infection. Such protection can be implemented by the prophylactic use of erythromycin for 14 days, azithromycin for 5

*See references 44, 45, 53, 54, 57, 59-61, 112, 113, 155, 163, 208, 257, 339.

days, or clarithromycin for 7 days.[6,43,257,364] Active immunization of all exposed persons (children, adolescents, and adults) who are not adequately vaccinated also should be conducted.

The use of prophylactic antibiotics in adolescents and adults in exposure situations such as classrooms and hospital settings frequently is recommended. This approach often involves many people and considerable expense.

In our experience, the side effects of erythromycin and other macrolides are such that adult compliance is poor. Therefore, our opinion is that erythromycin and other macrolides should not be used prophylactically but only for treatment at the first sign of respiratory illness in those exposed.

OTHER *BORDETELLA* INFECTIONS

BORDETELLA PARAPERTUSSIS

B. parapertussis infection in children can cause unrecognized infection, mild pertussis, or typical pertussis.[257] We studied 38 children with *B. parapertussis* illnesses and compared their illnesses with those occurring in 76 children with *B. pertussis* illnesses.[174] The results were as follows (*B. pertussis/B. parapertussis*), in percentages: cough for longer than 4 weeks, 57 percent/37 percent (p = .06); whooping, 80 percent/59 percent (p = .07); whooping for longer than 2 weeks, 26 percent/18 percent (p = .05); paroxysms, 90 percent/83 percent; post-tussive vomiting, 47 percent/42 percent; and mean leukocyte and lymphocyte counts, 12,500 per mm[3] and 7600 per mm[3]/7800 per mm[3] and 3500 per mm[3] (p < .0001), respectively. In another study in Italy, children with *B. parapertussis* infection had the following rates of findings: cough, 100 percent; paroxysms, 76 percent; whooping, 33 percent; post-tussive vomiting, 42 percent; apnea, 29 percent; and cyanosis, 12 percent.[254] All of these rates except cough and paroxysms were lower in children with *B. parapertussis* infections than in children with *B. pertussis* infections. Concomitant infections with *B. pertussis* and *B. parapertussis* are not rare.[188,197,267]

Before and during the early pertussis vaccine era, pertussis caused by *B. parapertussis* was considerably less common than that caused by *B. pertussis*.[257] For example, during a 16-year period in the Grand Rapids area of Michigan, 4483 cases of pertussis were caused by *B. pertussis*, and 106 cases were caused by *B. parapertussis*.[103] More recently, during the DTaP vaccine efficacy trials in Europe, the comparative rates of illness caused by *B. pertussis* or *B. parapertussis* were examined. In our trial in Germany, the rate of pertussis caused by *B. parapertussis* infection in control children was 0.9 cases per 100 person years.[362] Of 130 culture-confirmed cases, 21 percent were caused by *B. parapertussis*. The percentage of cases caused by *B. parapertussis* in five other trials varied from 2.1 to 20 percent.[254]

During the last 30 years in the United States, pertussis caused by *B. parapertussis* has been an uncommon occurrence. However, during 2004 and 2005, 493 culture-positive cases of pertussis were noted by the Wisconsin State Laboratory of Hygiene.[298] Of these cases, 14 percent were caused by *B. parapertussis*.

BORDETELLA BRONCHISEPTICA

In 1911, McGowan[260] observed that laboratory workers exposed to various animals with *B. bronchiseptica* infections on occasion had respiratory illness. In 1926, a 5-year-old girl with a pertussis-like illness was found to be infected with *B. bronchiseptica*.[35] Her illness commenced about 10 to 12 days after she had been given a rabbit with mild "snuffles." Otherwise healthy children who became infected with *B. bronchiseptica* after being exposed to farm animals or pets usually have pertussis-like illnesses.[257]

B. bronchiseptica causes respiratory infections in at least 18 different mammals.[81] Most notable are atrophic rhinitis in pigs, kennel cough (rhinotracheitis) in dogs, and bronchopneumonia in rabbits and other laboratory animals. Occasional infections in humans have been noted during the last 35 years, with the majority occurring in immunocompromised adults.[5,99,423] Most recent reports have noted *B. bronchiseptica* infections in patients with acquired immunodeficiency syndrome (AIDS). Respiratory infections have ranged from mild upper respiratory illnesses to pneumonia. In patients with AIDS, the pneumonia frequently is cavitary. Sinusitis and bronchitis also occur.

BORDETELLA HINZII

B. hinzii has been recovered from an adult patient with cystic fibrosis during pulmonary exacerbations throughout a 3-year period.[124] Bacteremia has been noted in a patient with AIDS.[80]

BORDETELLA HOLMESII

B. holmesii has been isolated from the nasopharyngeal specimens of 33 patients suspected of having pertussis.[427] Twenty-three of the cases were investigated further, and 19 (82%) of these patients were adolescents, 2 (9%) were adults, and 2 (9%) were children. All had cough: 61 percent had paroxysms, 26 percent had post-tussive vomiting, and 9 percent had whoop. *B. holmesii* also has been isolated from a 10-month-old boy with bacteremia and from patients with septicemia, endocarditis, and respiratory failure.[283,380]

BORDETELLA TREMATUM

B. trematum has been isolated from wounds and ear infections.[395]

REFERENCES

1. Ad Hoc Group for the Study of Pertussis Vaccines: Placebo-controlled trial of two acellular pertussis vaccines in Sweden: Protective efficacy and adverse events. Lancet *1*:955-960, 1988.
2. Advisory Panel of the Committee on Safety of Medicines: The collection of data relating to adverse reactions in pertussis vaccine. *In* Whooping Cough: Reports from the Committee on Safety of Medicines and the Joint Committee on Vaccination and Immunisation. London, Department of Health and Social Security, Her Majesty's Stationery Office, 1981, p. 27.
3. Aintablian, N., Walpita, P., and Sawyer, M.: Detection of *Bordetella pertussis* and respiratory syncytial virus in air samples from hospital rooms. Infect. Control Hosp. Epidemiol. *19*:918-923, 1998.
4. Alderslade, R., Bellman, M. H., Rawson, N. S. B., et al.: The National Childhood Encephalopathy Study. *In* Whooping Cough: Reports From the Committee on Safety of Medicines and the Joint Committee on Vaccination and Immunisation. London, Department of Health and Social Security, Her Majesty's Stationery Office, 1981, p. 79.
5. Amador, C., Chiner, E., Calpe, J. L., et al.: Pneumonia due to *Bordetella bronchiseptica* in a patient with AIDS. Rev. Infect. Dis. *13*:771-772, 1991.
6. American Academy of Pediatrics: Active immunization: Pertussis. *In* Pickering L. K. (ed.): 2006 Red Book: Report of the Committee on Infectious Diseases. 25th ed. Elk Grove Village, IL, American Academy of Pediatrics, 2006, pp. 1-51, 498-520.
7. Arciniega, J. L., Shahin, R. D., Burnette, W. N., et al.: Contribution of the B oligomer to the protective activity of genetically attenuated pertussis toxin. Infect. Immun. *59*:3407-3410, 1991.
8. Arico, B., and Rappuoli, R.: *Bordetella parapertussis* and *Bordetella bronchiseptica* contain transcriptionally silent pertussis toxin genes. J. Bacteriol. *169*:2847-2853, 1987.
9. Arnold, J. C., Singh, K. K., Spector, S. A., et al.: Human bocavirus: Prevalence and clinical spectrum at a children's hospital. Clin. Infect. Dis. *43*:283-288, 2006.
10. Ausiello, C. M., Lande, R., Urbani, F., et al.: Cell-mediated immunity and antibody responses to *Bordetella pertussis* antigens in children with a history of

pertussis infection and in recipients of an acellular pertussis vaccine. J. Infect. Dis. *181*:1989-1995, 2000.

11. Baraff, L. J., and Cherry, J. D.: Nature and rates of adverse reactions associated with pertussis immunization. *In* Manclark, C. R., and Hill, J. C. (eds.): International Symposium on Pertussis. Publication No. (N. I. H.) 79-1830. Washington, D.C., U.S. Dept. of Health, Education, and Welfare, U.S. Government Printing Office, 1979, p. 291.

12. Baraff, L. J., Manclark, C. R., Cherry, J. D., et al.: Analyses of adverse reactions to diphtheria and tetanus toxoids and pertussis vaccine by vaccine lot, endotoxin content, pertussis vaccine potency and percentage of mouse weight gain. Pediatr. Infect. Dis. J. *8*:502-507, 1989.

13. Baraff, L. J., Cody, C. L., and Cherry, J. D.: DTP-associated reactions: An analysis by injection site, manufacturer, prior reactions, and dose. Pediatrics *73*:31-36, 1984.

14. Baraff, L. J., Wilkins, J., and Wehrle, P. F.: The role of antibiotics, immunizations and adenoviruses in pertussis. Pediatrics *61*:224-230, 1978.

15. Barlow, W. E., Davis, R. L., Glasser, J. W., et al.: The risk of seizures after receipt of whole-cell pertussis or measles, mumps, and rubella vaccine. N. Engl. J. Med. *345*:656-662, 2001.

16. Baron, S., Njamkepo, E., Grimprel, E., et al.: Epidemiology of pertussis in French hospitals in 1993 and 1994: Thirty years after a routine use of vaccination. Pediatr. Infect. Dis. J. *17*:412-418, 1998.

17. Bass, J. W.: Pertussis: Current status of prevention and treatment. Pediatr. Infect. Dis. J. *4*:614-619, 1985.

18. Bass, J. W.: Erythromycin for treatment and prevention of pertussis. Pediatr. Infect. Dis. J. *5*:154-157, 1986.

19. Bass, J. W., Klenk, E. L., Kotheimer, J. B., et al.: Antimicrobial treatment of pertussis. J. Pediatr. *75*:768-781, 1969.

20. Beiter, A., Lewis, K., Pineda, E. F., et al.: Unrecognized maternal peripartum pertussis with subsequent fatal neonatal pertussis. Obstet. Gynecol. *82*:691-693, 1993.

21. Bellman, M. H., Ross, E. M., and Miller, D. L.: Infantile spasms and pertussis immunisation. Lancet *1*:1031-1034, 1983.

22. Berg, J. M.: Neurological complications of pertussis immunization. Br. Med. J. *2*:24, 1958.

23. Bergquist, S., Bernander, S., Dahnsjo, H., et al.: Erythromycin in the treatment of pertussis: A study of bacteriologic and clinical effects. Pediatr. Infect. Dis. J. *6*:458-461, 1987.

24. Bernales, R., Eastman, J., and Kaplan, J.: Quantitation of circulating T and B lymphocytes in children with whooping cough. Pediatr. Res. *10*:965-967, 1976.

25. Bhargava, A., Leininger, E., Roberts, M., et al.: Filamentous hemagglutinin and the 69-kDa protein, pertactin, promote adherence of *Bordetella pertussis* to epithelial cells and macrophages. Paper presented at the Sixth International Symposium on Pertussis, Bethesda, MD, September 26-28, 1990, pp. 137-138.

26. Birkebaek, N. H., Kristiansen, M., Seefeldt, T., et al.: *Bordetella pertussis* and chronic cough in adults. Clin. Infect. Dis. *29*:1239-1242, 1999.

27. Bisgard, K. M., Pascual, F. B., Ehresmann, K. R., et al.: Infant pertussis: Who was the source? Pediatr. Infect. Dis. J. *23*:985-989, 2004.

28. Bisgard, K. M., Rhodes, P., Connelly, B. L., et al.: Pertussis vaccine effectiveness among children 6 to 59 months of age in the United States, 1998-2001. Pediatrics *116*:e285-e294, 2005.

29. Blackwelder, W. C., Storsaeter, J., Olin, P., et al.: Acellular pertussis vaccines. Am. J. Dis. Child. *145*:1285-1289, 1991.

30. Bordet, J., and Gengou, O.: Le microbe de la coqueluche. Ann. Inst. Pasteur (Paris) *20*:48-68, 1906.

31. Bordet, J., and Gengou, O.: L'endotoxin coquelucheuse. Ann. Inst. Pasteur (Paris) *23*:415-419, 1909.

32. Bradford, W. L., and Slavin, B.: An organism resembling *Haemophilus* pertussis with special reference to color changes produced by its growth upon certain media. Am. J. Public Health. *27*:1277-1282, 1937.

33. Brennan, M. J., Li, Z. M., Cowell, J. L, et al.: Identification of a 69-kilodalton nonfimbrial protein as an agglutinogen of *Bordetella pertussis*. Infect. Immun. *56*:3189-3195, 1988.

34. Broomhall, J., and Herxheimer, A.: Treatment of whooping cough: The facts. Arch. Dis. Child. *59*:185-187, 1984.

35. Brown, J. H.: *Bacillus bronchisepticus* infection in a child with symptoms of pertussis. Bull. Johns Hopkins Hosp. *38*:147-153, 1926.

36. Byers, R. K., and Moll, F. C.: Encephalopathies following prophylactic pertussis vaccine. Pediatrics *1*:437-457, 1948.

37. Celermajor, J. M., and Brown, J.: The neurological complications of pertussis. Med. J. Aust. *1*:1066-1069, 1966.

38. Centers for Disease Control and Prevention: Hypertrophic pyloric stenosis in infants following pertussis prophylaxis with erythromycin: Knoxville, Tennessee, 1999. M. M. W. R. Morb. Mortal. Wkly. Rep. *48*:1117-1140, 1999.

39. Centers for Disease Control and Prevention: Pertussis: United States, 1997-2000. M. M. W. R. Morb. Mortal. Wkly. Rep. *51*:73-76, 2002.

40. Centers for Disease Control and Prevention: Fatal case of unsuspected pertussis diagnosed from a blood culture: Minnesota, 2003. M. M. W. R. Morb. Mortal. Wkly. Rep. *53*:131-132, 2004.

41. Centers for Disease Control and Prevention: Summary of notifiable diseases: United States, 2004. M. M. W. R. Morb. Mortal. Wkly. Rep. *53*:1-80, 2004.

42. Centers for Disease Control and Prevention: Pertussis: United States, 2001-2003. M. M. W. R. Morb. Mortal. Wkly. Rep. *54*:1283-1286, 2005.

43. Centers for Disease Control and Prevention: Recommended antimicrobial agents for the treatment and postexposure prophylaxes of pertussis: 2005 CDC guidelines. M. M. W. R. Morb. Mortal. Wkly. Rep. *54*:1-16, 2005.

44. Centers for Disease Control and Prevention: Preventing tetanus, diphtheria, and pertussis among adults: Use of tetanus toxoid, reduced diphtheria toxoid and acellular pertussis vaccine. M. M. W. R. Morb. Mortal. Wkly. Rep. *55*:1-33, 2006.

45. Centers for Disease Control and Prevention: Preventing tetanus, diphtheria, and pertussis among adolescents: Use of tetanus toxoid, reduced diphetheria toxoid and acellular pertussis vaccines. M. M. W. R. Morb. Mortal. Wkly. Rep. *55*:1-34, 2006.

46. Chaby, R., and Caroff, M.: Lipopolysaccharides of *Bordetella pertussis* endotoxin. *In* Wardlaw, A. C., and Parton, R. (eds.): Pathogenesis and Immunity in Pertussis. New York, John Wiley & Sons, 1988, pp. 247-272.

47. Chakravorty, A. P.: Blindness after use of triple antigen. Br. Med. J. *1*:105, 1963.

48. Charles, I. G., Li, J. L., Roberts, M., et al.: Identification and characterization of a protective immunodominant B cell epitope of pertactin (P.69) from *Bordetella pertussis*. Eur. J. Immunol. *21*:1147-1153, 1991.

49. Cherry, J. D.: The epidemiology of pertussis and pertussis immunization in the United Kingdom and the United States: A comparative study. Curr. Probl. Pediatr. *14*:1-78, 1984.

50. Cherry, J. D.: Pertussis and the vaccine controversy. *In* Root, R. K., Griffiss, J. M., Warren, K. S., et al. (eds.): Immunization. New York, Churchill Livingstone, 1989, pp. 47-63.

51. Cherry, J. D.: Pertussis vaccine encephalopathy: It is time to recognize it as the myth that it is. JAMA *263*:1679-1680, 1990.

52. Cherry, J. D.: Pertussis: The trials and tribulations of old and new pertussis vaccines. Vaccine *10*:1033-1038, 1992.

53. Cherry, J. D.: Acellular pertussis vaccines: A solution to the pertussis problem. J. Infect. Dis. *168*:21-24, 1993.

54. Cherry, J. D.: Strategies for Diphtheria, Tetanus, and Pertussis (DTP) Immunization: Report of the 104th Ross Conference on Pediatric Research. Columbus, OH, Ross Products Division, Abbott Laboratories, 1994, pp. 218-225.

55. Cherry, J. D.: Historical review of pertussis and the classical vaccine. J. Infect. Dis. *174*(Suppl.):259-263, 1996.

56. Cherry, J. D.: Comparative efficacy of acellular pertussis vaccines: An analysis of recent trials. Pediatr. Infect. Dis. J. *16*(Suppl.):90-96, 1997.

57. Cherry, J. D.: Epidemiological, clinical, and laboratory aspects of pertussis in adults. Clin. Infect. Dis. *28*(Suppl 2):112-117, 1999.

58. Cherry, J. D.: Pertussis in the preantibiotic and prevaccine era, with emphasis on adult pertussis. Clin. Infect. Dis. *28*(Suppl. 2):107-111, 1999.

59. Cherry, J. D.: Pertussis vaccines for adolescents and adults. Pediatrics. *116*:755-756, 2005.

60. Cherry, J. D.: The epidemiology of pertussis: A comparison of the epidemiology of the disease pertussis with the epidemiology of *Bordetella pertussis* infection. Pediatr. Infect. Dis. J. *115*:1422-1427, 2005.

61. Cherry, J. D.: Epidemiology of pertussis. Pediatr. Infect. Dis. J. *25*:361-362, 2006.

62. Cherry, J. D.: Historical perspective on pertussis and use of vaccines to prevent it. Microbe *2*:139-144, 2007.

63. Cherry, J. D.: Unpublished observation.

64. Cherry, J. D., and Mortimer, E. A.: Acellular and whole-cell pertussis vaccines in Japan: Report of a visit by US scientists. JAMA *257*:1375-1376, 1987.

65. Cherry, J. D., and Olin, P.: Commentaries: The science and fiction of pertussis vaccines. Pediatrics *104*:1381-1384, 1999.

66. Cherry, J. D., Baraff, L. J., and Hewlett, E.: The past, present, and future of pertussis: The role of adults in epidemiology and future control. West. J. Med. *150*:319-328, 1989.

67. Cherry, J. D., Beer, T., Chartrand, S. A., et al.: Comparison of antibody values to *Bordetella pertussis* antigens in young German and American men. Clin. Infect. Dis. *20*:1271-1274, 1995.

68. Cherry, J. D., Brunell, P. A., Golden, G. S., et al.: Report of the Task Force on Pertussis and Pertussis Immunization: 1988. Pediatrics *81*(Suppl.):939-984, 1988.

69. Cherry, J. D., Gornbein J., Heininger, U., et al.: A search for serologic correlates of immunity to *Bordetella pertussis* cough illnesses. Vaccine *16*:1901-1906, 1998.

70. Cherry, J. D., Grimprel, E., Guiso, N., et al.: Defining pertussis epidemiology: Clinical, microbiologic and serologic perspectives. Pediatr. Infect. Dis. J. *24*(Suppl.):S25-S34.

71. Cherry, J. D., Heininger, U., Stehr, K., et al.: The effect of investigator compliance (observer bias) on calculated efficacy in a pertussis vaccine trial. Pediatrics *102*:909-912, 1998.

72. Choy, K. W., Wulffraat, N. M., Wolfs, T. F. W., et al.: *Bordetella bronchiseptica* respiratory infection in a child after a bone marrow transplantation. Pediatr. Infect. Dis. J. *18*:481-482, 1999.

73. Christie, C. D. C., and Baltimore, R. S.: Pertussis in neonates. Am. J. Dis. Child. *143*:1199-1202, 1989.

74. Christie, C. D. C., Marx, M. L., Marchant, C. D., et al.: The 1993 epidemic of pertussis in Cincinnati: Resurgence of disease in a highly immunized population of children. N. Engl. J. Med. *331*:16-21, 1994.

75. Cody, C. L., Baraff, L. J., Cherry, J. D., et al.: Nature and rates of adverse reactions associated with DTP and DT immunizations in infants and children. Pediatrics 68:650-660, 1981.

76. Collier, A. M., Connor, J. T., and Irving, W. R., Jr.: Generalized type 5 adenovirus infection associated with the pertussis syndrome. J. Pediatr. 69:1073-1978, 1966.

77. Cone, T. E., Jr.: Whooping cough is first described as a disease *sui generis* by Baillou in 1640. Pediatrics 46:522, 1970.

78. Connor, J. D.: Evidence for an etiological role of adenoviral infection in pertussis syndrome. N. Engl. J. Med. 283:390-394, 1970.

79. Conway, S. P., Balfour, A. H., and Ross, H.: Serologic diagnosis of whooping cough by enzyme-linked immunosorbent assay. Pediatr. Infect. Dis. J. 7:570-574, 1988.

80. Cookson, B. T., Vandamme, P., Carlson, L. C., et al.: Bacteremia caused by a novel *Bordetella* species, "*B. hinzii.*" J. Clin. Microbiol. 32:2569-2571, 1994.

81. Cotter, P. A., and Miller, J. F.: *Bordetella. In* Groisman, E. A. (ed.): Principles of Bacterial Pathogenesis. San Diego, Academic Press, 2001, pp. 619-674.

82. Cowell, J. L., Sato, Y., Sato, H., et al.: Separation, purification and properties of the filamentous hemagglutinin and the leukocytosis promoting factor-hemagglutinin from *Bordetella pertussis. In* Robbins, J. B., Hill, J. C., and Sadoff, G. (eds.): Seminars in Infectious Disease. Vol. IV. Bacterial Vaccines: International Symposium on Bacterial Vaccines. New York, Thieme-Stratton, 1982, pp. 371-379.

83. Cromer, B. A., Goydos, J., Hackell, J., et al.: Unrecognized pertussis infection in adolescents. Am. J. Dis. Child. 147:575-577. 1993.

84. Crowcroft, N. S., Andrews, N., Rooney, C., et al.: Deaths from pertussis are underestimated in England. Arch. Dis. Child. 86:336-8, 2002.

85. Crowcroft, N. S., Booy, R., Harrison, T., et al.: Severe and unrecognised: Pertussis in UK infants. Arch. Dis. Child. 88:802-6, 2003.

86. Cundell, D. R., Kanthakumar, K., Taylor, G. W., et al.: Effect of tracheal cytotoxin from *Bordetella pertussis* on human neutrophil function in vitro. Infect. Immun. 62:639-643, 1994.

87. Davis, S. F., Sutter, R. W., Strebel, P. M., et al.: Concurrent outbreaks of pertussis and *Mycoplasma pneumoniae* infection: Clinical and epidemiological characteristics of illnesses manifested by cough. Clin. Infect. Dis. 20:621-628, 1995.

88. De Berry, B. B., Lynch, J. E., Chung, D. H., et al.: Pertussis with severe pulmonary hypertension and leukocytosis treated with extracorporeal memebrane oxygenation. Pediatr. Surg. Int. 21:692-694, 2005.

89. Decker, G. R., Lavelle, J. P., Kuman, P. N., et al.: Pneumonia due to *Bordetella bronchiseptica* in a patient with AIDS. Rev. Infect. Dis. 13:1250-1251, 1991.

90. Decker, M. D., Edwards, K. M., Steinhoff, M. C., et al.: Comparison of 13 acellular pertussis vaccines: Adverse reactions. Pediatrics 96:557-566, 1995.

91. Deen, J. L., Mink, C. M., Cherry, J. D., et al.: A household contact study of *Bordetella pertussis* infections in adults. Clin. Infect. Dis. 21:1211-1219, 1995.

92. De Melker, H. E., Versteegh, F. G. A., Schellekens, J. F. P., et al.: The incidence of *Bordetella pertussis* infections estimated in the population from a combination of serological surveys. J. Infect. 53:106-13, 2006.

93. De Serres, G., Shadmani, R., Duval, B., et al.: Morbidity of pertussis in adolescents and adults. J. Infect. Dis. 182:174-179, 2000.

94. Deville, J. G., Cherry, J. D., Christenson, P. D., et al.: Frequency of unrecognized *Bordetella pertussis* infections in adults. Clin. Infect. Dis. 21:639-642, 1995.

95. Diavatopoulos, D. A., Cummings, C. A., Schouls, L. M., et al.: *Bordetella pertussis*, the causative agent of whooping cough, evolved from a distinct, human-associated lineage of *B. bronchiseptica*. PLoS. Pathog. 1:0373-0383, 2005.

96. Donoso, A. F., Cruces, P. I., Camacho, J. F., et al.: Exchange transfusion to reverse severe pertussis-induced cardiogenic shock. Pediatr. Infect. Dis. J. 25:846-848, 2006.

97. Donoso, A., León, J., Ramírez, M., et al.: Pertussis and fatal pulmonary hypertension: A discouraged entity. Scand. J. Infect. Dis. 37:145-8, 2005.

98. Douglas, E., Coote, J. G., Parton, R., et al.: Identification of *Bordetella pertussis* in nasopharyngeal swabs by PCR amplification of a region of the adenylate cyclase gene. J. Med. Microbiol. 38:140-144, 1993.

99. Dworkin, M. S., Sullivan, P. S., Buskin, S. E., et al.: *Bordetella bronchiseptica* infection in human immunodeficiency virus-infected patients. Clin. Infect. Dis. 28:1095-1099, 1999.

100. Edsall, G.: Present status of pertussis vaccination. Practitioner 215:310-314, 1975.

101. Edsall, G.: Comment. *In* International Symposium on Pertussis, Bilthoven, 1969: Immunobiologic Standards. Vol. 13. New York, S. Karger, 1979, p. 170.

102. Edwards, K. M., and Decker, M. D.: Pertussis vaccine. Vaccines 4:484-485, 2004.

103. Eldering, G., and Kendrick, P.: Incidence of parapertussis in the Grand Rapids area as indicated by 16 years' experience with diagnostic cultures. Am. J. Public Health 42:27-31, 1952.

104. Eldering, G., and Kendrick, P.: A group of cultures resembling both *Bacillus pertussis* and *Bacillus bronchisepticus* but identical with neither. J. Bacteriol. 33:71, 1937.

105. Eldering, G., and Kendrick, P.: *Bacillus parapertussis*: A species resembling both *Bacillus pertussis* and *Bacillus bronchiseptica* but identical with neither. J. Bacteriol. 35:561-572, 1938.

106. Eldering, G., Hornbeck, C., and Baker, J.: Serological study of *Bordetella pertussis* and related species. J. Bacteriol. 74:133-136, 1957.

107. Elliot, E., McIntyre, P., Ridley, G., et al.: National study of infants hospitalized with pertussis in the acellular vaccine era. Pediatr. Infect. Dis. J. 23:246-52, 2004.

108. Erlandsson, A., Backman, A., Nygren, M., et al. Quantification of *Bordetella pertussis* in clinical samples by colorimetric detection of competitive PCR products. A. P. M. I. S. 106:1041-1048, 1998.

109. Ewanowich, C. A., Chui, L. W., Paranchych, M. G., et al.: Major outbreaks of pertussis in northern Alberta, Canada: Analysis of discrepant direct fluorescent-antibody and culture results by using polymerase chain reaction methodology. J. Clin. Microbiol. 31:1715-1725, 1993.

110. Farizo, K. M., Cochi, S. L., Zell, E. R., et al.: Epidemiological features of pertussis in the United States, 1980-1989. Clin. Infect. Dis. 14:708-719, 1992.

111. Farrell, D. J., McKeon, M., Daggard, G., et al.: Rapid-cycle PCR method to detect *Bordetella pertussis* that fulfills all consensus recommendations for use of PCR in diagnosis of pertussis. J. Clin. Microbiol. 38:4499-4502, 2000.

112. Food and Drug Administration: Product approval information-licensing action, package insert: BOOSTRIX. Tetanus toxoid, reduced diphtheria toxoid and acellular pertussis vaccine, adsorbed. GlaxoSmithKline Biologicals. Rockville, MD: U.S. Department of Health and Human Services, Food and Drug Administration, Center for Biologics Evaluation and Research, 2005. Available at http://www.fda.gov/cber/label/tdapgla122905LB.pdf.

113. Food and Drug Administration: Product approval information-licensing action, package insert: Tetanus toxoid, reduced diphtheria toxoid and acellular pertussis vaccine adsorbed ADACEL. Sanofi Pasteur. Rockville, MD: U.S. Department of Health and Human Services, Food and Drug Administration, Center for Biologics Evaluation and Research, 2006. Available at http://www.fda.gov/cber/label/tdapave012306LB.pdf.

114. Fernandez, R. C., and Weiss, A. A.: Cloning and sequencing of a *Bordetella pertussis* serum resistance locus. Infect. Immun. 62:4727-4738, 1994.

115. Ferry, N. S.: *Bacillus bronchisepticus (bronchicanis)*: The cause of distemper in dogs and a similar disease in other animals. Vet. J. 68:376-391, 1912.

116. Fine, P. E. M.: Epidemiological considerations for whooping cough eradication. *In* Wardlaw, A. C., and Parton, R. (eds.): Pathogenesis and Immunity in Pertussis. New York, John Wiley & Sons, 1988, pp. 451-467.

117. Fine, P. E. M.: Implications of different study designs for the evaluation of acellular pertussis vaccines. Dev. Biol. Stand. 89:123-133, 1997.

118. Fine, P. E. M., and Clarkson, J. A.: The recurrence of whooping cough: Possible implications for assessment of vaccine efficacy. Lancet 1:666-669, 1982.

119. Fine, P. E. M., and Clarkson, J. A.: Reflections on the efficacy of pertussis vaccines. Rev. Infect. Dis. 9:866-883, 1987.

120. Finn, T. M., and Stevens, L. A.: Tracheal colonization factor: A *Bordetella pertussis* secreted virulence determinant. Mol. Microbiol. 16:625-634, 1995.

121. Foege, W. H.: Statement read before the Subcommittee on Investigations and General Oversight Committee on Labor and Human Resources, United States Senate, Washington, D.C., May 7, 1982.

122. Friedman, L. E., Messina, M. T., Santoferrara, L., et al.: Characterization of *Bordetella bronchiseptica* strains using phenotypic and genotypic markers. Vet. Microbiol. 117:313-320, 2006.

123. Friedman, R. L.: Pertussis: The disease and new diagnostic methods. Clin. Microbiol. Rev. 1:365-376, 1988.

124. Funke, G., Hess, T., von Graevenitz, A., et al.: Characteristics of *Bordetella hinzii* strains isolated from a cystic fibrosis patient over a 3-year period. J. Clin. Microbiol. 34:966-969, 1996.

125. Furman, B. L., Sidey, F. M., and Smith, M.: Metabolic disturbances produced by pertussis toxin. *In* Wardlaw, A. C., and Parton, R. (eds.): Pathogenesis and Immunity in Pertussis. New York, John Wiley & Sons, 1988, pp. 147-172.

126. Gale, J. L., Thapa, P. B., Wassilak, S. G. F., et al.: Risk of serious acute neurological illness after immunization with diphtheria-tetanus-pertussis vaccine: A population-based case-control study. JAMA 271:37-41, 1994.

127. Gilberg, S., Njamkepo, E., Du Chatelet, I. P., et al.: Evidence of *Bordetella pertussis* infection in adults presenting with persistent cough in a French area with very high whole-cell vaccine coverage. J. Infect. Dis. 186:415-418, 2002.

128. Glare, E. M., Paton, J. C., Premier, R. R., et al.: Analysis of a repetitive DNA sequence from *Bordetella pertussis* and its application to the diagnosis of pertussis using the polymerase chain reaction. J. Clin. Microbiol. 28:1982-1987, 1990.

129. Gil, A., Oyaguez, I., Carrasco, P., et al.: Hospital admissions for pertussis in Spain, 1995-1998. Vaccine 19:4791-4794, 2001.

130. Goldman, W. E.: Tracheal cytotoxin of *Bordetella pertussis. In* Wardlaw, A. C., and Parton, R. (eds.): Pathogenesis and Immunity in Pertussis. New York, John Wiley & Sons, 1988, pp. 237-246.

131. Goodman, Y. E., Wort, A. J., and Jackson, F. L.: Enzyme-linked immunosorbent assay for detection of pertussis immunoglobulin A in nasopharyngeal secretions as an indicator of recent infection. J. Clin. Microbiol. 13:286-292, 1981.

132. Goodnow, R. A.: Biology of *Bordetella bronchiseptica*. Microbiol. Rev. 44:722-738, 1980.

133. Gordon, J. E., and Hood, R. I.: Whooping cough and its epidemiological anomalies. Am. J. Med. Sci. 222:333-361, 1951.

134. Gordon, M., Davies, H. D., and Gold, R.: Clinical and microbiologic features of children presenting with pertussis to a Canadian pediatric hospital during an eleven-year period. Pediatr. Infect. Dis. J. 13:617-622, 1994.

135. Goulin, G. D., Kaya, K. M., and Bradley, J. S.: Severe pulmonary hypertension associated with shock and death in infants infected with *Bordetella pertussis*. Crit. Care Med. *21*:1791-1794, 1993.
136. Granström, G., Askelof, P., and Granström, M.: Specific immunoglobulin A to *Bordetella pertussis* antigens in mucosal secretion for rapid diagnosis of whooping cough. J. Clin. Microbiol. *26*:869-874, 1988.
137. Granström, M., Lindberg, A. A., Askelof, P., Hederstedt, B.: Detection of antibodies in human serum against fimbrial haemagglutinin of *Bordetella pertussis* by enzyme-linked immunosorbent assay. J. Med. Microbiol. *15*:85-96, 1982.
138. Greco, D., Salmaso, S., Mastrantonio, P., et al.: A controlled trial of two acellular vaccines and one whole-cell vaccine against pertussis. N. Engl. J. Med. *334*:341-348, 1996.
139. Griffin, M. R., Ray, W. A., Livengood, J. R., et al.: Risk of sudden infant death syndrome after immunization with the diphtheria-tetanus-pertussis vaccine. N. Engl. J. Med. *319*:618-623, 1988.
140. Griffin, M. R., Ray, W. A., Mortimer, E. A., et al.: Risk of seizures and encephalopathy after immunization with the diphtheria-tetanus-pertussis vaccine. JAMA *263*:1641-1645, 1990.
141. Grimpel, E., Begue, P., Anjak, I., et al.: Comparison of polymerase chain reaction, culture and Western immunoblot serology for diagnosis of *Bordetella pertussis* infection. J. Clin. Microbiol. *31*:2745-2750, 1993.
142. Grzeszczak, M. J., Churchwell, K. B., Edwards, K. M., et al.: Leukapheresis therapy for severe infantile pertussis with myocardial and pulmonary failure. Pediatr. Crit. Care Med. 7:580-582, 2006.
143. Gueirard, P., Weber, C., Coustumier, A. L., et al.: Human *Bordetella bronchiseptica* infection related to contact with infected animals: Persistence of bacteria in host. J. Clin. Microbiol. *33*:2002-2006, 1995.
144. Güris, D., Strebel, P. M., Bardenheier, B., et al.: Changing epidemiology of pertussis in the United States: Increasing reported incidence among adolescents and adults, 1990-1996. Clin. Infect. Dis. *28*:1230-1237, 1999.
145. Gustafsson, L., Hallander, H. O., Olin, P., et al.: A controlled trial of a two-component acellular, a five-component acellular, and a whole-cell pertussis vaccine. N. Engl. J. Med. *334*:349-355, 1996.
146. Gustafsson, L., Hessel, L., Storsaeter, J., et al.: Long-term follow-up of Swedish children vaccinated with acellular pertussis vaccines at 3, 5, and 12 months of age indicates the need for a booster dose at 5 to 7 years of age. Pediatrics *118*:978-984, 2006.
147. Hackman, R., Perrin, D. G., Karmali, M., et al.: Fatal *Bordetella pertussis* infection: Report of two cases with novel pathologic findings. Pediatr. Pathol. *16*:643-653, 1996.
148. Halasa, N. B., Barr, F. E., Johnson, J. E., et al.: Fatal pulmonary hypertension associated with pertussis in infants: Does extracorporeal membrane oxygenation have a role? Pediatrics *112*:1274-1278, 2003.
149. Hallander, H. O., Gnarpe, J., Gnarpe, H., et al.: *Bordetella pertussis, Bordetella parapertussis, Mycoplasma pneumoniae, Chlamydia pneumoniae* and persistent cough in children. Scand. J. Infect. Dis. *31*:281-286, 1999.
150. Hallander, H. O., Reizenstein, I., Renemar, B., et al.: Comparison of nasopharyngeal aspirates with swabs for culture of *Bordetella pertussis*. J. Clin. Microbiol. *31*:50-52, 1993.
151. Hallander, H. O., Storsaeter, J., and Mollby, R.: Evaluation of serologic and nasopharyngeal cultures for diagnosis of pertussis in a vaccine efficacy trial. J. Infect. Dis. *163*:1046-1054, 1991.
152. Halperin, S. A., Bortolussi, R., Kasina, A., et al.: Use of a Chinese hamster ovary cell cytotoxicity assay for the rapid diagnosis of pertussis. J. Clin. Microbiol. *28*:32-38, 1990.
153. Halperin, S. A., Bortolussi, R., Langley, J. M., et al.: Seven days of erythromycin estolate is as effective as fourteen days for the treatment of *Bordetella pertussis* infections. Pediatrics *100*:65-71, 1997.
154. Halperin, S. A., Bortolussi, R., MacLean, D., et al.: Persistence of pertussis in an immunized population: Results of the Nova Scotia Enhanced Pertussis Surveillance Program. J. Pediatr. *115*:686-693, 1989.
155. Halperin, S. A., Smith, B., Russell, M., et al.: Adult formulation of a five component acellular pertussis vaccine combined with diphtheria and tetanus toxoids and inactivated poliovirus vaccine is safe and immunogenic in adolescents and adults. Pediatr. Infect. Dis. J. *19*:276-283, 2000.
156. Halperin, S. A., Wang, E. E. L., Law, B., et al.: Epidemiological features of pertussis in hospitalized patients in Canada, 1991-1997: Report of the Immunization Monitoring Program-Active (IMPACT). Clin. Infect. Dis. *28*:1238-1243, 1999.
157. Hannah, J. H., Menozzi, F. D., Renauld, G., et al.: Sulfated glycoconjugate receptors for the *Bordetella pertussis* adhesin filamentous hemagglutinin (FHA) and mapping of the heparin-binding domain on FHA. Infect. Immun. *62*:5010-5019, 1994.
158. Hannik, C. A., and Cohen, H.: Pertussis vaccine experience in the Netherlands. *In* Manclark, C. R., and Hill, J. C. (eds.): International Symposium on Pertussis. Publication No. (N. I. H.) 79-1830. Washington, D.C., U.S. Dept. of Health, Education, and Welfare, U.S. Government Printing Office, 1979, p. 279.
159. Haward, R. A.: Scale of undernotification of infectious diseases by general practitioners. Lancet *1*:873-874, 1973.
160. He, Q., Mertsola, J., Soini, H., et al.: Sensitive and specific polymerase chain reaction assays for detection of *Bordetella pertussis* in nasopharyngeal specimens. J. Pediatr. *124*:421-426, 1994.
161. Hedenskog, S., Bjorksten, B., Blennow, M., et al.: Immunoglobulin E response to pertussis toxin in whooping cough and after immunization with a whole-cell and an acellular pertussis vaccine. Int. Arch. Allergy Appl. Immunol. *89*:156-161, 1989.
162. Heininger, U.: Recent progress in clinical and basic pertussis research. Eur. J. Pediatr. *160*:203-213, 2001.
163. Heininger, U., and Cherry, J. D.: Pertussis immunization in adolescents and adults: *Bordetella pertussis* epidemiology should guide vaccination recommendations. Expert Opin. Biol. Ther. *6*:1-13, 2006.
164. Heininger, U., Cherry, J. D., Eckhardt, T., et al.: Clinical and laboratory diagnosis of pertussis in the regions of a large vaccine efficacy trial in Germany. Pediatr. Infect. Dis. J. *12*:504-509, 1993.
165. Heininger, U., Cherry, J. D., Lugauer, S., et al.: Reactogenicity data following fourth and fifth doses of the Wyeth-Lederle Takeda acellular pertussis component vaccine: The Erlangen trial. Paper presented at the Acellular Pertussis Vaccine Conference, Bethesda, MD, November 12-14, 2000.
166. Heininger, U., Cherry, J. D., Stehr, K., et al.: Comparative efficacy of the Lederle/Takeda acellular pertussis component DTP (DTaP) vaccine and Lederle whole-cell component DTP vaccine in German infants following household exposure. Pediatrics *102*:546-553, 1998.
167. Heininger, U., Kleemann, W. J., Cherry, J. D., et al.: A controlled study of the relationship between *Bordetella pertussis* infection and sudden unexpected deaths in German infants. Pediatrics *114*:e9-e15, 2004.
168. Heininger, U., Klich, K., Stehr, K., et al.: Clinical findings in *Bordetella pertussis* infections: Results of a prospective multicenter surveillance study. Pediatrics *100*:e10, 1997.
169. Heininger, U., Schläpfer, G., Cherry, J. D., et al.: Clinical validation of a polymerase chain reaction assay for the diagnosis of pertussis by comparison with serology, culture, and symptoms during a large pertussis vaccine efficacy trial. Pediatrics *105*:e31, 2000.
170. Heininger, U., Schmitt-Grohè, S., Cherry, J. D., et al.: Der Mikroagglutinationstest: Ein einfaches und sensitives Verfahren zur Serodiagnostik von Pertussis. Klin. Paediatr. *207*:277-280, 1995.
171. Heininger, U., Stehr, K., and Cherry, J. D.: Serious pertussis overlooked in infants. Eur. J. Pediatr. *151*:342-343, 1992.
172. Heininger, U., Stehr, K., Christenson, P., et al.: Evidence of efficacy of the Lederle/Takeda acellular pertussis component diphtheria and tetanus toxoids and pertussis vaccine but not the Lederle whole-cell component diphtheria and tetanus toxoids and pertussis vaccine against *Bordetella parapertussis* infection. Clin. Infect. Dis. *28*:602-604, 1999.
173. Heininger, U., Stehr, K., Schläpfer, G., et al.: *Bordetella pertussis* infections and sudden unexpected deaths in children. Eur. J. Pediatr. *155*:551-553, 1996.
174. Heininger, U., Stehr, K., Schmitt-Grohè, S., et al.: Clinical characteristics of illness caused by *Bordetella parapertussis* compared with illness caused by *Bordetella pertussis*. Pediatr. Infect. Dis. J. *13*:306-309, 1994.
175. Heiss, L. N., Lancaster, J. R., Corbett, J. A., et al.: Epithelial autotoxicity of nitric oxide: Role in the respiratory cytopathology of pertussis. Proc. Natl. Acad. Sci. U. S. A. *91*:267-270, 1994.
176. Hellwig, S. M., Rodriguez, M. E., Berbers, G. A., et al.: Crucial role of antibodies to pertactin in *Bordetella pertussis* immunity. J. Infect. Dis. *188*:738-742, 2003.
177. Henderson, J., North, K., Griffiths, M., et al.: Pertussis vaccination and wheezing illnesses in young children: Prospective cohort study. BMJ *318*:1173-1176, 1999.
178. Herzig, P., Hartmann, C., Fischer, D., et al.: Pertussis complications in Germany: 3 years of hospital-based surveillance during the introduction of acellular vaccines. Infection *26*:227-231, 1998.
179. Hewlett, E. L., and Cherry, J. D.: New and improved vaccines against pertussis. *In* Woodrow, G. C., and Levine, M. M. (eds.): New Generation Vaccines. New York, Marcel Dekker, 1990, pp. 231-250.
180. Hewlett, E. L., and Cherry, J. D.: New and improved vaccines against pertussis. In Levine, M. M., Woodrow, G. C., Kaper, J. B., and Cobon, G. S. (eds.): New Generation Vaccines. 2nd ed. New York, Marcel Dekker, 1997, pp. 387-416.
181. Hewlett, E. L., and Gordon, V. M.: Adenylate cyclase toxin of *Bordetella pertussis*. *In* Wardlaw, A. C., and Parton, R. (eds.): Pathogenesis and Immunity in Pertussis. New York, John Wiley & Sons, 1988, pp. 193-209.
182. Hodder, S. L., Cherry, J. D., Mortimer, E. A., et al.: Antibody responses to *Bordetella pertussis* antigens and clinical correlations in elderly community residents. Clin. Infect. Dis. *31*:7-14, 2000.
183. Hoffman, H. J., Hunter, J. C., Damus, K., et al.: Diphtheria-tetanus-pertussis immunization and sudden infant death: Results of the National Institute of Child Health and Human Development Cooperative Epidemiological Study of Sudden Infant Death Syndrome Risk Factors. Pediatrics 79:598-611, 1987.
184. Holmes, W. H.: Bacillary and Rickettsial Infections Acute and Chronic, a Textbook: Black Death to White Plague. New York, Macmillan, 1940, pp. 395-414.
185. Honein, M. A., Paulozzi, L. J., Himelright, I. M., et al.: Infantile hypertrophic pyloric stenosis after pertussis prophylaxis with erythromycin: A case review and cohort study. Lancet *354*:2101-2105, 1999.
186. Hoppe, J. E.: Methods for isolation of *Bordetella pertussis* from patients with whooping cough. Eur. J. Clin. Microbiol. Infect. Dis. 7:616-620, 1988.
187. Hoppe, J.: State of art in antibacterial susceptibility of *Bordetella pertussis* and antibiotic treatment of pertussis. Infection *26*:242-246, 1998.

188. Hoppe, J. E.: Update on respiratory infection caused by *Bordetella parapertussis*. Pediatr. Infect. Dis. J. *18*:375-381, 1999.

189. Hoppe, J.: Neonatal pertussis. Pediatr. Infect. Dis. J. *19*:244-247, 2000.

190. Hoppe, J., and Eichhorn, A.: Activity of new macrolides against *Bordetella pertussis* and *Bordetella parapertussis*. Eur. J. Clin. Microbiol. Infect. Dis. 8:653-654, 1989.

191. Hoppe, J., and Haug, A.: Antimicrobial susceptibility of *Bordetella pertussis*. Part I. Infection *16*:126-130, 1988.

192. Hoppe, J., Halm, U., Hagedorn, H., et al.: Comparison of erythromycin ethyl-succinate and co-trimoxazole for treatment of pertussis. Infection *17*:227-231, 1989.

193. Houard, S., Hackel, C., Herzog, A., et al.: Specific identification of *Bordetella pertussis* by the polymerase chain reaction. Res. Microbiol. *140*:477-484, 1989.

194. Hudnall, S. D., Molina, C. P.: Marked increase in L-selectin–negative T cells in neonatal pertussis: The lymphocytosis explained? Am. J. Clin. Pathol. *114*:35-40, 2000.

195. Iida, T., Kunitani, A., Komase, Y., et al.: Studies on experimental infection with *Bordetella pertussis*: Effect of cortisone on the infection and immunity in mice. Jpn. J. Exp. Med. *33*:283-295, 1983.

196. Irons, L. I., and Gorringe, A. R.: Pertussis toxin: Production, purification, molecular structure, and assay. *In* Wardlaw, A. C., and Parton, R. (eds.): Pathogenesis and Immunity in Pertussis. New York, John Wiley & Sons, 1988, pp. 95-120.

197. Iwata, S., Aoyama, T., Iwai, H., et al.: Mixed outbreak of *Bordetella pertussis* and *Bordetella parapertussis* in an apartment house. Dev. Biol. Stand. *73*:333-341, 1991.

198. Jackson, F. E.: Spontaneous spinal epidural hematoma coincident with whooping cough. J. Neurosurg. *20*:715-717, 1963.

199. Jackson, L. A., Carste, B. A., Malais, D., et al.: Retrospective population-based assessment of medically attended injection site reactions, seizures, allergic responses and febrile episodes after acellular pertussis vaccine combined with diphtheria and tetanus toxoids. Pediatr. Inf. Dis. J. *21*:781-785, 2002.

200. Jackson, L. A., Cherry, J. D., Wang, S. P., et al.: Frequency of serological evidence of *Bordetella* infections and mixed infections with other respiratory pathogens in university students with cough illnesses. Clin. Infect. Dis. *31*:3-6, 2000.

201. Janda, W. M., Santos, E., Stevens, J., et al.: Unexpected isolation of *Bordetella pertussis* from a blood culture. J. Clin. Microbiol. *32*:2851-2853, 1994.

202. Jensen, D. L., Gray, G. C., Putnam, S. D., et al.: Evaluation of pertussis in U.S. Marine Corps trainees. Clin. Infect. Dis. *25*:1099-1107, 1997.

203. Jenkinson, D.: Whooping cough: What proportion of cases is notified in an epidemic? BMJ *287*:183-185, 1983.

204. Johnston, I. D., Strachan, D. P., Anderson, H. R., et al.: Effect of pneumonia and whooping cough in childhood on adult lung function. N. Engl. J. Med. *338*:581-587, 1998.

205. Joint Committee on Vaccination and Immunisation: The whooping cough epidemic, 1977-79. *In* Whooping Cough: Reports from the Committee on Safety in Medicine and the Joint Committee on Vaccination and Immunisation. London, Department of Health and Social Security, Her Majesty's Stationery Office, 1981, p. 170.

206. Jones, D. H., McBride, B. W., Jeffery, H., et al.: Protection of mice from *Bordetella pertussis* respiratory infection using microencapsulated pertussis fimbriae. Vaccine *13*:675-681, 1995.

207. Kandola, K., Lea, A., and Santos, M.: Pertussis rates in Northwest Territories after introducing adult formulation acellular vaccine. Can. J. Infect. Dis. Med. Microbiol. *15*:351, 2004. Abstract.

208. Keitel, W. A., Muenz, L. R., Decker, M. D., et al.: A randomized clinical trial of acellular pertussis vaccines in healthy adults: Dose-response comparisons of 5 vaccines and implications for booster immunization. J. Infect. Dis. *180*:397-403, 1999.

209. Kendrick, P. L., Eldering, G., Dixon, M. K., et al.: Mouse protection tests in the study of pertussis vaccines. Am. J. Public Health *37*:803-810, 1947.

210. Kerr, J. R., and Matthews, R. C.: *Bordetella pertussis* infection: Pathogenesis, diagnosis, management, and the role of protective immunity. Eur. J. Clin. Microbiol. Infect. Dis. *19*:77-88, 2000.

211. Kersters, K., Hinz, K. H., Hertle, A., et al.: *Bordetella avium* sp. nov., isolated from the respiratory tracts of turkeys and other birds. Int. J. Syst. Bacteriol. *34*:56-70, 1984.

212. Khelef, N., Sakamoto, H., and Guiso, N.: Both adenylate cyclase and hemolytic activities are required by *Bordetella pertussis* to initiate infection. Microbiol. Pathog. *12*:227-235, 1992.

213. Kimura, M., and Kuno-Sakai, H.: Pertussis vaccines in Japan. Acta Paediatr. Jpn. *30*:143-153, 1988.

214. Kimura, A., Mountzouros, K. T., Relman, D. A., et al.: *Bordetella pertussis* filamentous hemagglutinin: Evaluation as a protective antigen and colonization factor in a mouse respiratory infection model. Infect. Immun. *58*:7-16, 1990.

215. Knorr, L., Fox, J. D., Tilley, P. A. G., et al.: Evaluation of real-time PCR for diagnosis of *Bordetella pertussis* infection. BMC Infect. Dis. *6*:1-12, 2006.

216. Korgenski, E. K., Daly, J. A.: Surveillance and detection of erythromycin resistance in *Bordetella pertussis* isolates recovered from a pediatric population in the Intermountain West region of the United States. J. Clin. Microbiol. *35*:2989-2991, 1997.

217. Kowalzik, F., Barbosa, A., Fernandes, V. R., et al.: Prospective multinational study of pertussis infection in hospitalized infants and their household contacts. Pediatr. Infect. Dis. *26*:238-242, 2007.

218. Kulenkampff, M., Schwartzman, J. S., and Wilson, J.: Neurological complications of pertussis inoculation. Arch. Dis. Child. *49*:46, 1974.

219. Kurt, T. L., Yeager, A. S., Guenette, S., et al.: Spread of pertussis by hospital staff. JAMA *221*:264-267, 1972.

220. Lambert, H. J.: Epidemiology of a small pertussis outbreak in Kent County, Michigan. Public Health Rep. *80*:365-369, 1965.

221. Lapin, J. H.: Whooping Cough. Springfield, IL, Charles C Thomas, 1943.

222. Lautrop, H.: Observations on parapertussis in Denmark 1950-1957. Acta Pathol. Microbiol. Scand. *43*:255-266, 1958.

223. Le Saux, N., Barrowman, N. J., Moore, D. L., et al.: Decrease in hospital admissions for febrile seizures and reports of hypotonic-hyporesponsive episodes presenting to hospital emergency departments since switching to acellular pertussis vaccine in Canada: A report from IMPACT. Pediatrics *112*:348-353, 2003.

224. Lee, B.: Progressive respiratory distress in an infant treated for presumed pertussis. Pediatr. Infect. Dis. J. *19*:475, 492-493, 2000.

225. Leininger, E., Kenimer, J. G., and Brennan, M. J.: Surface proteins of *Bordetella pertussis*: Role in adherence. Paper presented at the Sixth International Symposium on Pertussis, Bethesda, MD, September 26-28, 1990, pp. 25-26.

226. Lewis, K., Cherry, J. D., Sachs, M. H., et al.: The effect of prophylactic acetaminophen administration on reactions to DTP vaccination. Am. J. Dis. Child. *142*:62-65, 1988.

227. Lewis, K., Saubolle, M. A., Tenover, F. C., et al.: Pertussis caused by an erythromycin-resistant strain of *Bordetella pertussis*. Pediatr. Infect. Dis. J. *14*:388-391, 1995.

228. Li, A. M, Jansen, D. L., Finn, T. M., et al.: Identification of *Bordetella pertussis* infection by shared-primer PCR. J. Clin. Microbiol. *32*:783-789, 1994.

229. Li, Z. M., Cowell, J. L., and Brennan, M. J.: Agglutinating monoclonal antibodies that specifically recognize lipooligosaccharide A of *Bordetella pertussis*. Infect. Immun. *56*:699-702, 1988.

230. Lichtinghagen, R., Diedrich-Glaubitz, R., and von Hörsten, B.: Identification of *B. pertussis* in nasopharyngeal swabs using the polymerase chain reaction: Evaluation of detection methods. Eur. J. Clin. Chem. Clin. Biochem. *32*:161-167, 1994.

231. Liese, J. G., Meschievitz, C. K., Harzer, E., et al.: Efficacy of a two-component acellular pertussis vaccine in infants. Pediatr. Infect. Dis. J. *16*:1038-1044, 1997.

232. Lind-Brandberg, L., Welinder-Olsson, C., Lagergard, T., et al.: Evaluation of PCR for diagnosis of *Bordetella pertussis* and *Bordetella parapertussis* infections. J. Clin. Microbiol. *36*:679-683, 1998.

233. Lindgren, C., Milerad, J., and Lagercrantz, H.: Sudden infant death and prevalence of whooping cough in the Swedish and Norwegian communities. Eur. J. Pediatr. *156*:405-409, 1997.

234. Lindquist, S. W., Weber, D. J., Mangum, M. E., et al.: *Bordetella holmesii sepsis* in an asplenic adolescent. Pediatr. Infect. Dis. J. *14*:813-815, 1995.

235. Linnemann, C. C., Jr.: Host-parasite interactions in pertussis. *In* Manclark, C. R., and Hill, J. C. (eds.): International Symposium on Pertussis. Publication No. (N. I. H.) 79-1830. Washington, D.C., U.S. Dept. of Health, Education, and Welfare, U.S. Government Printing Office, 1979, pp. 3-18.

236. Linnemann, C. C., Jr., and Nasenbeny, J.: Pertussis in the adult. Annu. Rev. Med. *28*:179-185, 1977.

237. Linnemann, C. C., Jr., Ramundo, N., Perlstein, P. H., et al.: Use of pertussis vaccine in an epidemic involving hospital staff. Lancet *2*:540-543, 1975.

238. Locht, C., Bertin, P., Menozzi, F. D., et al.: The filamentous haemagglutinin, a multifaceted adhesin produced by virulent *Bordetella* spp. Mol. Microbiol. *9*:653-660, 1993.

239. Loeffelholz, M. J.: Bordetella. *In* Murray, P. R., Baron, E. J., Jorgensen, J. H. (eds.): Manual of Clinical Microbiology. 8th ed. Washington, D.C., American Society for Microbiology, 2003, pp.780-788.

240. Long, S., Lischner, H., Deforest, A., et al.: Serologic evidence of subclinical pertussis in immunized children. Pediatr. Infect. Dis. J. *9*:700-705, 1990.

241. Long, S., Welkon, C., and Clark, J.: Widespread silent transmission of pertussis in families: Antibody correlates of infection and symptomatology. J. Infect. Dis. *161*:480-486, 1990.

242. Lugauer, S., Heininger, U., Cherry, J. D., et al.: Long-term clinical effectiveness of an acellular pertussis component vaccine and a whole cell pertussis component vaccine. Eur. J. Pediatr. *161*:142-146, 2002.

243. Luker, K. E., Collier, J. L., Kolodziej, E. W., et al.: *Bordetella pertussis* tracheal cytotoxin and other muramyl peptides: Distinct structure-activity relationships for respiratory epithelial cytopathology. Proc. Natl. Acad. Sci. U. S. A. *90*:2365-2369, 1993.

244. MacRae, K. D.: Epidemiology, encephalopathy, and pertussis vaccine. *In* FEMS-Symposium Pertussis: Proceedings of a Conference Organized by the Society of Microbiology and Epidemiology of the GDR. Berlin, April 20-22, 1988.

245. Madge, N., Diamond, J., Miller, D., et al.: The national childhood encephalopathy study: A 10-year follow-up. Dev. Med. Child Neurol. *68*(Suppl.):1-119, 1993.

246. Madsen, T.: Whooping cough: Its bacteriology, diagnosis, prevention and treatment. Boston Med. Surg. J. *192*:50-60, 1925.

247. Mahon, B. P., Brady, M. T., and Mills, K. H. G.: Protection against *Bordetella pertussis* in mice in the absence of detectable circulating antibody: Implications for long-term immunity in children. J. Infect. Dis. *181*:2087-2091, 2000.

248. Makhov, A. M., Hannah, J. H., Brennan, M. J., et al.: Filamentous hemagglutinin of *Bordetella pertussis*: A bacterial adhesin formed as a 50-nm monomeric rigid rod based on a 19-residue repeat motif rich in beta strains and turns. J. Mol. Biol. *241*:110-124, 1994.

249. Mallory, F. B., and Hornor, A. A.: Pertussis: The histological lesion in the respiratory tract. J. Med. Res. *27*:115-123, 1912.

250. Manclark, C. R., Meade, B. D., and Burstyn, D. G.: Serological response to *Bordetella pertussis*. *In* Rose, N. R., Friedman, H., and Fahey, J. L. (eds.): Manual of Clinical Laboratory Immunology. 3rd ed. Washington, D.C., American Society for Microbiology, 1986, pp. 388-394.

251. Mannerstedt, G.: Pertussis in adults. J. Pediatr. *5*:596-600, 1934.

252. Martin, G. I., and Weintraub, M. I.: Brachial neuritis and seventh nerve palsy: A rare hazard of DPT vaccination. Clin. Pediatr. (Phila.) *12*:506-507, 1973.

253. Mastrantonio, P., Stefanelli, P., and Giuliano, M.: Polymerase chain reaction for the detection of *Bordetella pertussis* in clinical nasopharyngeal aspirates. J. Med. Microbiol. *44*:261-266, 1996.

254. Mastrantonio, P., Stefanelli, P. and Giuliano, M.: *Bordetella parapertussis* infection in children: Epidemiology, clinical symptoms, and molecular characteristics of isolates. J. Clin. Microbiol. *36*:999-1002, 1998.

255. Masure, H. R.: The adenylate cyclase toxin contributes to the survival of *Bordetella pertussis* within human macrophages. Microb. Pathog. *14*:253-260, 1993.

256. Matherne, P., Matson, J., and Marks, M. I.: Pertussis complicated by the syndrome of inappropriate antidiuretic hormone secretion. Clin. Pediatr. (Phila.) *25*:46-48, 1986.

257. Mattoo, S., and Cherry, J. D.: Molecular pathogenesis, epidemiology, and clinical manifestations of respiratory infections due to *Bordetella pertussis* and other *Bordetella* subspecies. Clin. Microbiol. Rev. *18*:326-382, 2005.

258. Mazengia, E., Silva, E. A., Peppe, J. A., et al.: Recovery of *Bordetella holmesii* from patients with pertussis-like symptoms: Use of pulsed-field gel electrophoresis to characterize circulating strains. J. Clin. Microbiol. *38*:2330-2333, 2000.

259. McEniery, J. A., Delbridge, R. G., and Reith, D. M.: Infant pertussis deaths and the management of cardiovascular compromise. J. Paediatr. Child Health *40*:230-232, 2004.

260. McGowan, J. P.: Some observations on a laboratory epidemic, principally among dogs and cats, in which the animals affected presented the symptoms of the disease called "distemper." J. Pathol. Bacteriol. *15*:372-430, 1911.

261. McGregor, J., Ogle, J., and Curry-Kane, G.: Perinatal pertussis. Obstet. Gynecol. *68*:582-586, 1986.

262. Meade, B. D., and Bollen, A.: Recommendations for use of the polymerase chain reaction in the diagnosis of *Bordetella pertussis* infections. J. Med. Microbiol. *41*:51-55, 1994.

263. Medical Research Council: The prevention of whooping cough by vaccination. Br. Med. J. *1*:1463-1471, 1951.

264. Medical Research Council: Vaccination against whooping cough: Relation between protection in children and results of laboratory tests. Br. Med. J. *2*:454-462, 1956.

265. Medical Research Council: Vaccination against whooping cough. Br. Med. J. *1*:994-1000, 1959.

266. Melchior, J. C.: Infantile spasms and early immunization against whooping cough: Danish survey from 1970 to 1975. Arch. Dis. Child. *52*:134, 1977.

267. Mertsola, J.: Mixed outbreak of *Bordetella pertussis* and *Bordetella parapertussis* infection in Finland. Eur. J. Clin. Microbiol. *4*:123-128,1985.

268. Mertsola, J., Ruuskanen, O., Kuronen, T., et al.: Serologic diagnosis of pertussis: Evaluation of pertussis toxin and other antigens in enzyme-linked immunosorbent assay. J. Infect. Dis. *161*:966-971, 1990.

269. Mikelova, L. K., Halperin, S. A., Scheifele D., et al.: Predictors of death in infants hospitalized with pertussis: A case-control study of 16 pertussis deaths in Canada. J. Pediatr. *143*:576-81, 2003.

270. Miller, D., Madge, N., Diamond, J., et al.: Pertussis immunisation and serious acute neurological illnesses in children. BMJ *307*:1171-1176, 1993.

271. Miller, D., Ross, E. M., Alderslade, R., et al.: Pertussis immunisation and serious acute neurological illness in children. BMJ *282*:1595-1597, 1981.

272. Miller, D., Wadsworth, J., Diamond, J., et al.: Pertussis vaccine and whooping cough as risk factors in acute neurological illness and death in young children. Dev. Biol. Stand. *61*:389-394, 1985.

273. Miller, D., Wadsworth, J., and Ross, E.: Severe neurological illness: Further analyses of the British National Childhood Encephalopathy Study. Tokai J. Exp. Clin. Med. *13*(Suppl.):145-155, 1988.

274. Miller, J. J., Jr., Silverberg, R. J., Saito, T. M., et al.: An agglutinative reaction for *Hemophilus pertussis*. II. Its relation to clinical immunity. J. Pediatr. *22*:644-651, 1943.

275. Mills, K. H. G., and Redhead, K.: Cellular immunity in pertussis. J. Med. Microbiol. *39*:163-164, 1993.

276. Mills, K. H. G., Barnard, A., Watkins, J., et al.: Cell-mediated immunity to *Bordetella pertussis*: Role of Th1 cells in bacterial clearance in a murine respiratory infection model. Infect. Immun. *61*:399-410, 1993.

277. Minh, N. N. T., He, Q., Edelman, K., et al.: Cell-mediated immune responses to antigens of *Bordetella pertussis* and protection against pertussis in school children. Pediatr. Infect. Dis. J. *18*:366-370, 1999.

278. Mink, C., Cherry, J. D., Christenson, P., et al.: A search for *Bordetella pertussis* infection in university students. Clin. Infect. Dis. *14*:464-471, 1992.

279. Mink, C., O'Brien, C. H., Wassilak, S., et al.: Isotype and antigen specificity of pertussis agglutinins following whole-cell pertussis vaccination and infection with *Bordetella pertussis*. Infect. Immun. *62*:1118-1120, 1994.

280. Mink, C., Sirota, N. M., and Nugent, S.: Outbreak of pertussis in a fully immunized adolescent and adult population. Arch. Pediatr. Adolesc. Med. *148*:153-157, 1994.

281. Mooi, F. A., van der Heide, H. G. J., Wellems, R., et al.: *Bordetella pertussis* fimbriae: Role in pathogenesis and mechanism of phase variation. Paper presented at the Sixth International Symposium on Pertussis, Bethesda, MD, September 26-28, 1990, p. 63.

282. Moore, D. L., Le Saux, N., Scheifele, D., et al.: Lack of evidence of encephalopathy related to pertussis vaccine: Active surveillance by IMPACT, Canada, 1993-2002. Pediatr. Infect. Dis. J. *23*:568-571, 2004.

283. Morris, J. T., and Myers, M.: Bacteremia due to *Bordetella holmesii*. Clin. Infect. Dis. *27*:912-913, 1998.

284. Morrison, W.: Infantile hypertrophic pyloric stenosis in infants treated with azithromycin. Pediatr. Infect. Dis. J. *26*:186-188, 2007.

285. Mortimer, E. A., Jr.: Pertussis and its prevention: A family affair. J. Infect. Dis. *161*:473-479, 1990.

286. Mortimer, E. A., Jr., and Jones, P. K.: An evaluation of pertussis vaccine. Rev. Infect. Dis. *1*:927-932, 1979.

287. Mortimer, E. A., Jr., and Jones, P. K.: Pertussis vaccine in the United States: The benefit-risk ratio. *In* Manclark, C. R., and Hill, J. C. (eds.): International Symposium on Pertussis. Publication No. (N. I. H.) 79-1830. Washington, D.C., U.S. Dept. of Health, Education, and Welfare, U.S. Government Printing Office, 1979, p. 250.

288. Mortimer, E. A., Jr., Kimura, M., Cherry, J. D., et al.: Protective efficacy of the Takeda acellular pertussis vaccine combined with diphtheria and tetanus toxoids following household exposure of Japanese children. Am. J. Dis. Child. *144*:899-904, 1990.

289. Mountzouros, K. T., Kimura, A., and Cowell, J. L.: A bactericidal monoclonal antibody specific for the lipooligosaccharide of *Bordetella pertussis* reduces colonization of the respiratory tract of mice after aerosol infection with *B. pertussis*. Infect. Immun. *60*:5316-5318, 1992.

290. Müller, F., Hoppe, J. E., and Wirsing von König, C. H.: Laboratory diagnosis of pertussis: State of the art in 1997. J. Clin. Microbiol. *135*:2435-2443, 1997.

291. Munoz, J. J.: Action of pertussigen (pertussis toxin) on the host immune system. *In* Wardlaw, A. C., and Parton, R. (eds.): Pathogenesis and Immunity in Pertussis. New York, John Wiley & Sons, 1988, pp. 173-192.

292. Nagel, J., and Poot-Scholtens, E. J.: Serum IgA antibody to *Bordetella pertussis* as an indicator of infection. J. Med. Microbiol. *16*:417-426, 1983.

293. Nakase, Y., and Endoh, M.: Heat-labile toxin of *Bordetella pertussis*. *In* Wardlaw, A. C., and Parton, R. (eds.): Pathogenesis and Immunity in Pertussis. New York, John Wiley & Sons, 1988, pp. 217-229.

294. Nelson, J. D.: The changing epidemiology of pertussis in young infants: The role of adults as reservoirs of infection. Am. J. Dis. Child. *132*:371-375, 1978.

295. Nelson, K. E., Gavitt, F., Batt, M. D., et al.: The role of adenoviruses in the pertussis syndrome. J. Pediatr. *86*:335-341, 1975.

296. Nencioni, L., Pizza, M., Volpini, G., et al.: Properties of the B oligomer of pertussis toxin. Infect. Immun. *59*:4732-4734, 1991.

297. Nennig, M. E., Shinefield, H. R., Edwards, K. M., et al.: Prevalence and incidence of adult pertussis in an urban population. JAMA *275*:1672-1674, 1996.

298. Newman, A., Davis, J. P., and Warshaner, D.: Personal communication. 2006.

299. Ng, V. L., Boggs, J. M., York, M. K., et al.: Recovery of *Bordetella bronchiseptica* from patients with AIDS. Clin. Infect. Dis. *15*:376-377, 1992.

300. Nicoll, A., and Gardner, A.: Whooping cough and unrecognised postperinatal mortality. Arch. Dis. Child. *63*:41-47, 1988.

301. Noble, G. R., Bernier, R. H., Esber, E. C., et al.: Acellular and whole cell pertussis vaccines in Japan: Report of a visit by U.S. scientists. JAMA *257*:1351-1356, 1987.

302. Novotny, P.: Pathogenesis in *Bordetella* species. J. Infect. Dis. *161*:581-582, 1990.

303. Novotny, P., Chubb, A. P., Cownley, K., et al.: Biologic and protective properties of the 69-kDa outer membrane protein of *Bordetella pertussis*: A novel formulation for an acellular pertussis vaccine. J. Infect. Dis. *164*:114-122, 1991.

304. Olcen, P., Backman, A., Johansson, B., et al.: Amplification of DNA by the polymerase chain reaction for the efficient diagnosis of pertussis. Scand. J. Infect. Dis. *24*:339-345, 1992.

305. Olin, P., Gustafsson, L., Barreto, L., et al.: Declining pertussis incidence in Sweden following the introduction of acellular pertussis vaccine. Vaccine *21*:2015-2021, 2003.

306. Olin, P., Rasmussen, F., Gustafsson, L., et al.: Randomised controlled trial of two-component, three-component, and five-component acellular pertussis vaccines compared with whole-cell pertussis vaccine. Lancet *350*:1569-1577, 1997.

307. Olsen, L. C.: Pertussis. Medicine (Baltimore) *54*:427-469, 1975.

308. Onorato, I. M., and Wassilak, S. G. F.: Laboratory diagnosis of pertussis: The state of the art. Pediatr. Infect. Dis. J. *6*:145-151, 1987.

309. Onorato, I. M., Wassilak, S. G., and Meade, B.: Efficacy of whole-cell pertussis vaccine in preschool children in the United States. JAMA 20:2745-2749, 1992.

310. Paddock, C. D., Cherry, J. D., Heininger, U. Unpublished data.

311. Paddock, C. D., Sanden, G. N., Cherry, J. D., et al.: The pathology and pathogenesis of fatal *Bordetella pertussis* infection in infants. Clin. Infect. Dis. J. 47:328-338, 2008.

312. Parkhill, J., Sebaihia, M., Preston, A., et al.: Comparative analysis of the genome sequence of *Bordetella pertussis*, *Bordetella parapertussis* and *Bordetella bronchiseptica*. Nat. Genet. 35:32-40, 2003.

313. Pertussis: Maryland, 1982. M. M. W. R. Morb. Mortal. Wkly. Rep. 32:297-300, 305, 1983.

314. Pertussis surveillance, 1979-1981. M. M. W. R. Morb. Mortal. Wkly. Rep. 31:333-336, 1982.

315. Pertussis: United States, 1982 and 1983. M. M. W. R. Morb. Mortal. Wkly. Rep. 33:573-575, 1984.

316. Pichichero, M. E., Edwards, K. M., Anderson, E. L., et al.: Safety and immunogenicity of six acellular pertussis vaccines and one whole-cell pertussis vaccine given as a fifth dose in four- to six-year-old children. Pediatrics 105:e11, 2000.

317. Pierce, C., Klein, N., and Peters, M.: Is leukocytosis a predictor of mortality in severe pertussis infection? Intensive Care Med. 26:1512-1514, 2000.

318. Pillay, V., and Swingler, G.: Symptomatic treatment of the cough in whooping cough. Cochrane Database Syst. Rev. 4:CD003257, 2003.

319. Pittman, M.: Pertussis toxin: The cause of the harmful effects and prolonged immunity of whooping cough: A hypothesis. Rev. Infect. Dis. 1:401-412, 1979.

320. Pittman, M.: The concept of pertussis as a toxin-mediated disease. Pediatr. Infect. Dis. 3:467-486, 1984.

321. Pooboni, S., Roberts, N., Westrope, C., et al.: Extracorporeal life support in pertussis. Pediatr. Pulmonol. 36:310-315, 2003.

322. Porter, J. F., Connor, K., and Donachie, W.: Isolation and characterization of *Bordetella parapertussis*–like bacteria from ovine lungs. Microbiolology 140:255-261, 1994.

323. Postels-Multani, S., Schmitt, H. J., Wirsing von König, C. H., et al.: Symptoms and complications of pertussis in adults. Infection 23:139-142, 1995.

324. Preston, A., Parkhill, J., and Maskell, D. J.: The Bordetellae: Lessons from genomics. Nat. Rev. Microbiol. 2:379-390, 2004.

325. Preston, N. W.: Pertussis today. *In* Wardlaw, A. C., and Parton, R. (eds.): Pathogenesis and Immunity in Pertussis. New York, John Wiley & Sons, 1988, pp. 1-18.

326. Prince, H. E., Lapé-Nixon, M., and Matud, J.: Evaluation of a Tetraplex Microsphere Assay for *Bordetella pertussis* antibodies. Clin. Vaccine Immunol. 13:266-270, 2006.

327. Ray, P., Hayward, J., Michelson, D., et al.: Encephalopathy after whole-cell pertussis or measles vaccination. Pediatr. Infect. Dis. J. 25:768-773, 2006.

328. Register, K. B., and Sanden, G. N.: Prevalence and sequence variants of IS*481* in *Bordetella bronchiseptica*: Implications for IS*481*-based detection of *Bordetella pertussis*. J. Clin. Microbiol. 44:4577-4583, 2006.

329. Reizenstein, E., Johanson, B., Mardin, L., et al.: Diagnostic evaluation of polymerase chain reaction discriminative for *Bordetella pertussis*, *B. parapertussis*, and *B. bronchiseptica*. Diagn. Microbiol. Infect. Dis. 17:185-191, 1993.

330. Reizenstein, E., Lindberg, L., Möllby, R., et al.: Validation of nested *Bordetella* PCR in a pertussis vaccine trial. J. Clin. Microbiol. 34:810-815, 1996.

331. Rennels, M. B., Deloria, M. A., Pichichero, M. E., et al.: Extensive swelling after booster doses of acellular pertussis-tetanus-diphtheria vaccines. Pediatrics 105:e12, 2000.

332. Robbins, J. B., Pittman, M., Trollfors, B., et al.: Primum non nocere: A pharmacologically inert pertussis toxoid alone should be the next pertussis vaccine. Pediatr. Infect. Dis. J. 12:795-807, 1993.

333. Robertson, P. W., Goldberg, H., Jarvie, B. H., et al.: *Bordetella pertussis* infection: A cause of persistent cough in adults. Med. J. Aust. 146:522-525, 1987.

334. Robinson, A., Ashworth, L. A. E., and Irons, L. I.: Serotyping *Bordetella pertussis* strains. Vaccine 7:491-494, 1989.

335. Robinson, A., Irons, L. I., Seabrook, R. N., et al.: Structure-function studies of *Bordetella pertussis* fimbriae. *In* Manclark, C. R. (ed.): Proceedings of the Sixth International Symposium on Pertussis. D. H. H. S. Publication No. (F. D. A.) 90. Bethesda, MD, Department of Health and Human Services, U.S. Public Health Service, 1990, pp. 126-135.

336. Rodriguez, M. E., Hellwig, S. M. M., Vidakovics, M. L. A. P., et al.: *Bordetella pertussis* attachment to respiratory epithelial cells can be impaired by fimbriae-specific antibodies. Immunol. Med. Microbiol. 46:39-47, 2006.

337. Romano, M. J., Weber, M. D., Weisse, M. E., et al.: Pertussis pneumonia, hypoxemia, hyperleukocytosis, and pulmonary hypertension: improvement in oxygenation after a double volume exchange transfusion. Pediatrics 114:e264-e266, 2004.

338. Rosenthal, S., Strebel, P., Cassiday, P., et al.: Pertussis infection among adults during the 1993 outbreak in Chicago. J. Infect. Dis. 171:1650-1652, 1995.

339. Rothstein, E. P., Anderson, E. L., Decker, M. D., et al.: An acellular pertussis vaccine in healthy adults: Safety and immunogenicity. Pennridge Pediatric Associates. Vaccine 17:2999-3006, 1999.

340. Ryan, M., Murphy, G., Gothefors, L., et al.: *Bordetella pertussis* respiratory infection in children is associated with preferential activation of type 1 T helper cells. J. Infect. Dis. 175:1246-1250, 1997.

341. Ryan, M., Murphy, G., Ryan, E., et al.: Distinct T-cell subtypes induced with whole cell and acellular pertussis vaccines in children. Immunology 93:1-10, 1998.

342. Salmaso, S., Mastrantonio, P., Tozzi, A., E., et al.: Sustained efficacy during the first 6 years of life of 3-component acellular pertussis vaccines administered in infancy: The Italian experience. Pediatrics 108:1-7, 2001.

343. Salmaso, S., Mastrantonio, P., Wassilak, S. G. F., et al.: Persistence of protection through 33 months of age provided by immunization in infancy with two three-component acellular pertussis vaccines. Vaccine 13:1270-1275, 1998.

344. Sans, M. B., Bonal, J., Bonet, J., et al.: *Bordetella bronchiseptica* septicemia in a hemodialysis patient. Nephron 59:676, 1991.

345. Sato, H., and Sato, Y.: *Bordetella pertussis* infection in mice: Correlation of specific antibodies against two antigens, pertussis toxin, and filamentous hemagglutinin with mouse protectivity in an intracerebral or aerosol challenge system. Infect. Immun. 46:415-421, 1984.

346. Sato, Y., Kimura, M., and Fukumi, H.: Development of a pertussis component vaccine in Japan. Lancet 1:122-6, 1984.

347. Sauer, L. W., and Hambrecht, L.: Experimental whooping cough. Am. J. Dis. Child. 37:732-744, 1929.

348. Schläpfer, G., Cherry, J. D., Heininger, U., et al.: Polymerase chain reaction identification of *Bordetella pertussis* infections in vaccinees and family members in a pertussis vaccine efficacy trial in Germany. Pediatr. Infect. Dis. J. 14:209-214, 1995.

349. Schläpfer, G., Senn, H. P., Berger, R., et al.: Use of the polymerase chain reaction to detect *Bordetella pertussis* in patients with mild or typical symptoms of infection. Eur. J. Clin. Microbiol. Infect. Dis. 12:459-463, 1993.

350. Schmitt, H. J., Beutel K., Schuind A, et al.: Reactogenicity and immunogenicity of a booster dose of a combined diphtheria, tetanus, and tricomponent acellular pertussis vaccine at fourteen to twenty-eight months of age. J. Pediatr. 130:616-623, 1997.

351. Schmitt, H. J., Wirsing von König, C. H., Neiss, A., et al.: Efficacy of acellular pertussis vaccine in early childhood after household exposure. JAMA 275:37-41, 1996.

352. Schmitt-Grohè, S., Cherry, J. D., Heininger, U., et al.: Pertussis in German adults. Clin. Infect. Dis. 27:860-866, 1995.

353. Schmitt-Grohè, S., Stehr, K., Cherry, J. D., et al.: Minor adverse events in a comparative efficacy trial in Germany in infants receiving either the Lederle/Takeda acellular pertussis component DTP (DTaP) vaccine, the Lederle whole-cell component DTP (DTP) or DT vaccine. Dev. Biol. Stand. 89:113-118, 1997.

354. Shahin, R. D., Amsbaugh, D. F., and Leef, M. F.: Mucosal immunization with filamentous hemagglutinin protects against *Bordetella pertussis* respiratory infection. Infect. Immun. 60:1482-1488, 1992.

355. Shahin, R. D., Brennan, M. J., Meade, B. D., et al.: Characterization of the protective capacity and immunogenicity of the 69-kD outer membrane protein of *Bordetella pertussis*. J. Exp. Med. 171:63-73, 1990.

356. Shields, W. D., Nielsen, C., Buch, D., et al.: Relationship of pertussis immunization to the onset of neurologic disorders: A retrospective epidemiologic study. J. Pediatr. 113:801-805, 1988.

357. Simonond, F., Preziosi, M. P., Yam, A., et al.: A randomized double-blind trial comparing a two-component acellular to a whole-cell pertussis vaccine in Senegal. Vaccine 15:1606-1612, 1997.

358. Smith, C., and Vyas, H.: Early infantile pertussis: Increasingly prevalent and potentially fatal. Eur. J. Pediatr. 159:898-900, 2000.

359. Southall, D. P., Thomas, M. G., and Lambert, H. P.: Severe hypoxaemia in pertussis. Arch. Dis. Child. 63:598-605, 1988.

360. Sreenan, C. D., and Osiovich, H.: Neonatal pertussis requiring extracorporeal membrane oxygenation. Pediatr. Surg. Int. 17:201-203, 2001.

361. Stefanelli, P., Mastrantonio, P., Hausman, S. Z., et al.: Molecular characterization of two *Bordetella bronchiseptica* strains isolated from children with coughs. J. Clin. Microbiol. 35:1550-1555, 1997.

362. Stehr, K., Cherry, J. D., Heininger, U., et al.: A comparative efficacy trial in Germany in infants who received either the Lederle/Takeda acellular pertussis component DTP (DTaP) vaccine, the Lederle whole-cell component DTP vaccine or DT vaccine. Pediatrics 101:1-11, 1998.

363. Steketee, R. W., Burstyn, D. G., Wassilak, S. G. F., et al.: A comparison of laboratory and clinical methods for diagnosing pertussis in an outbreak in a facility for the developmentally disabled. J. Infect. Dis. 157:441-449, 1988.

364. Steketee, R. W., Wassilak, S. G. F., Adkins, W. N., Jr., et al.: Evidence for a high attack rate and efficacy of erythromycin prophylaxis in a pertussis outbreak in a facility for the developmentally disabled. J. Infect. Dis. 157:434-440, 1988.

365. Stephenson, J. B. P.: A neurologist looks at neurological disease temporally related to DTP immunization. Tokai J. Exp. Clin. Med. 13(Suppl.):157-164, 1988.

366. Stewart, G. T.: Vaccination against whooping-cough: Efficacy versus risks. Lancet 1:234, 1977.

367. Stockbauer, K. E., Fuchslocher B., Miller, J. F., et al.: Identification and characterization of BipA, a *Bordetella* Bvg-intermediate phase protein. Mol. Microbiol. 39:65-78, 2001.

368. Stocks, P.: Studies in the Population of England and Wales 1944-47. Studies on Medical and Population Subjects. No. 2. London, His Majesty's Stationery Office, 1949.

369. Storsaeter, J., and Olin, P.: Relative efficacy of two acellular pertussis vaccines during three years of passive surveillance. Vaccine 10:142-144, 1992.

370. Storsaeter, J., Blackwelder, W. C., and Hallander, H. O.: Pertussis antibodies, protection, and vaccine efficacy after household exposure. Am. J. Dis. Child. 146:167-172, 1992.

371. Storsaeter, J., Hallander, H., Farrington, C. P., et al.: Secondary analyses of the efficacy of two acellular pertussis vaccines evaluated in a Swedish phase III trial. Vaccine 8:457-461, 1990.

372. Storsaeter, J., Hallander, H. O., Gustafsson, L., et al.: Levels of anti-pertussis antibodies related to protection after household exposure to *Bordetella pertussis*. Vaccine 16:1907-1916, 1998.

373. Strebel, P., Nordin, J., Edwards, K., et al.: Population-based incidence of pertussis among adolescents and adults, Minnesota, 1995-1996. J. Infect. Dis. 183:1353-1359, 2001.

374. Strebel, P. M., Cochi, S. L., Farizo, K. M., et al.: Pertussis in Missouri: Evaluation of nasopharyngeal culture, direct fluorescent antibody testing, and clinical case definitions in the diagnosis of pertussis. Clin. Infect. Dis. 16:276-285, 1993.

375. Ström, J.: Further experience of reactions, especially of a cerebral nature, in conjunction with triple vaccination: A study based on vaccinations in Sweden 1959-65. Br. Med. J. 4:320, 1967.

376. Swansea Research Unit of the Royal College of General Practitioners: Study of intellectual performance of children in ordinary schools after certain serious complications of whooping cough. BMJ 295:1044-1047, 1987.

377. Switzer, W. P., Mare, C. J., and Hubbard, E. D.: Incidence of *Bordetella bronchisepticum* in wildlife and man in Iowa. Am. J. Vet. Res. 27:1134-1136, 1966.

378. Tamion, F., Girault, C., Chevron, V., et al.: *Bordetella bronchoseptica* pneumonia with shock in an immunocompetent patient. Scand. J. Infect. Dis. 28:137-138, 1996.

379. Tanaka, M., Vitek, C. R., Pascual, F. B., et al.: Trends in pertussis among infants in the United States, 1980-1999. JAMA 290:2968-2975, 2003.

380. Tang, Y. W., Hopkins, M. K., Kolbert, C. P., et al.: *Bordetella holmesii*–like organisms associated with septicemia, endocarditis and respiratory failure. Clin. Infect. Dis. 26:389-392, 1998.

381. Taranger, J., Trollfors, B., Lagergard, T., et al.: Parapertussis infection followed by pertussis infection. Lancet 2:1703, 1994.

382. Taranger, J., Trollfors, B., Lagergard, T., et al.: Unchanged efficacy of a pertussis toxoid vaccine throughout the two years after the third vaccination of infants. Pediatr. Infect. Dis. J. 16:180-184, 1997.

383. Thomas, P. F., McIntyre, P. B., and Jalaludin, B. B.: Survey of pertussis morbidity in adults in western Sydney. Med. J. Aust. 173:74-76, 2000.

384. Tomoda, T. Ogura, H., and Kurashige, T.: Immune responses to *Bordetella pertussis* infection and vaccination. J. Infect. Dis. 163:559-563, 1991.

385. Trollfors, B., Taranger, J., Lagergard, T., et al.: A placebo-controlled trial of a pertussis-toxoid vaccine. N. Engl. J. Med. 333:1045-1050, 1995.

386. Troseid, M., Jonassen, T. O., and Steinbakk, M.: Isolation of *Bordetella pertussi* in blood culture from a patient with multiple myeloma. J. Infect. 52:e11-e13, 2006.

387. Tuomanen, E.: *Bordetella pertussis* adhesins. *In* Wardlaw, A. C., and Parton, R. (eds.): Pathogenesis and Immunity in Pertussis. New York, John Wiley & Sons, 1988, pp. 75-94.

388. Überall, M. A., Stehr, K., Cherry, J. D., et al.: Severe adverse events in a comparative efficacy trial in Germany in infants receiving either the Lederle/Takeda acellular pertussis component DTP (DTaP) vaccine, the Lederle whole-cell component DTP (DTP) or DT vaccine. Dev. Biol. Stand. 89:83-89, 1997.

389. Ui, M.: The multiple biological activities of pertussis toxin. *In* Wardlaw, A. C., and Parton, R. (eds.): Pathogenesis and Immunity in Pertussis. New York, John Wiley & Sons, 1988, pp. 121-146.

390. Urisu, A., Cowell, J. L., and Manclark, C. R.: Filamentous hemagglutinin has a major role in mediating adherence of *Bordetella pertussis* to human WiDr cells. Infect. Immun. 52:695-701, 1986.

391. Use of diphtheria toxoid-tetanus toxoid-acellular pertussis vaccine as a five-dose series: Supplemental recommendations of the Advisory Committee on Immunization Practices (ACIP). M. M. W. R. Recomm. Rep. 49:1-8, 2000.

392. Valenti, W. M., Pincus, P. H., and Messner, M. K.: Nosocomial pertussis: Possible spread by a hospital visitor. Am. J. Dis. Child. 134:520-521, 1980.

393. Van Buynder, P. G., Owen, D., Vurdien, J. E., et al.: *Bordetella pertussis* surveillance in England and Wales: 1995-7. Epidemiol. Infect. 123:403-411, 1999.

394. Vancanneyt, M., Vandamme, P., and Kersters, K.: Differentiation of *Bordetella pertussis*, *B. parapertussis*, and *B. bronchiseptica* by whole-cell protein electrophoresis and fatty acid analysis. Int. J. Syst. Bacteriol. 45:843-847, 1995.

395. Vandamme, P., Heyndrickx, M., Vancanneyt, M., et al.: *Bordetella trematum* sp. nov., isolated from wounds and ear infections in humans, and reassessment of *Alcaligenes denitrificans* Rüger and Tan 1983. Int. J. Syst. Bacteriol. 46:849-858, 1996.

396. van der Zee, A., Agterberg, C., Peeters, M., et al.: Polymerase chain reaction assay for pertussis: Simultaneous detection and discrimination of *Bordetella pertussis* and *Bordetella parapertussis*. J. Clin. Microbiol. 31:2134-2140, 1993.

397. van der Zee, A., Agterberg, C., Peeters, M., et al.: A clinical validation of *Bordetella pertussis* and *Bordetella parapertussis* polymerase chain reaction: Comparison with culture and serology using samples from patients with suspected whooping cough from a highly immunized population. J. Infect. Dis. 174:89-96, 1996.

398. Van Kruijssen, A. M., Templeton K. E., van der Plas, R. N., et al.: Detection of respiratory pathogens by real-time PCR in children with clinical suspicion of pertussis. Eur. J. Pediatr. 166:1189-1191, 2007.

399. Versteegh, F. G. A., Schellekens, J. F. P., Nagelkerke, A. F., et al.: Laboratory-confirmed reinfections with *Bordetella pertussis*. Acta Paediatr. 91:95-99, 2002.

400. Viljanen, M. K., Ruuskanen, O., Granberg, C., et al.: Serological diagnosis of pertussis: IgM, IgA, and IgG antibodies against *Bordetella pertussis* measured by enzyme-linked immunosorbent assay (ELISA). Scand. J. Infect. Dis. 14:117-122, 1982.

401. Vincent, J. M., Cherry, J. D., Nauschuetz, W. F., et al.: Prolonged afebrile nonproductive cough illnesses in American soldiers in Korea: A serological search for causation. Clin. Infect. Dis. 30:534-539, 2000.

402. Vitek, C. R., Pascual, F. B., Baughman, A. L., et al.: Increase in deaths from pertussis among young infants in the United States in the 1990s. Pediatr. Infect. Dis. J. 22:628-634, 2003.

403. Von Wintzingerode, F., Schattke, A., Siddiqui, R. A., et al.: *Bordetella petrii* sp. nov., isolated from an anaerobic bioreactor, and emended description of the genus *Bordetella*. Int. J. Syst. Evol. Microbiol. 51:1257-1265, 2001.

404. Walker, A. M., Jick, H., Perera, D. R., et al.: Neurologic events following diphtheria-tetanus-pertussis immunization. Pediatrics 81:345-349, 1988.

405. Walker, K. E., and Weiss, A. A.: Characterization of the dermonecrotic toxin in members of the genus *Bordetella*. Infect. Immun. 62:3817-3828, 1994.

406. Ward, J. I., Cherry, J. D., Chang, S., et al.: Efficacy of an acellular pertussis vaccine among adolescents and adults. N. Engl. J. Med. 353:1555-1563, 2005.

407. Ward, J. I., Cherry, J. D., Chang, S., et al.: *Bordetella pertussis* infections in vaccinated and unvaccinated adolescents and adults, as assessed in a national prospective randomized acellular pertussis vaccine trial (APERT). Clin. Infect. Dis. 43:151-157, 2006.

408. Wärngård, O., Nilsson, L., Fåhraeus, C., et al.: Catch-up primary vaccination with acellular pertussis vaccines in 3-4-year-old children-reactogenicity and serological response. Vaccine 16:480-484, 1998.

409. Washburn, T. C., Medearis, D. N., and Childs, B.: Sex differences in susceptibility to infection. Pediatrics 35:57-67, 1965.

410. Watts, E. C., and Acosta, C.: Pertussis and bilateral subdural hematomas. Am. J. Dis. Child. 118:518-519, 1969.

411. Weiss, A. A., and Falkow, S.: Genetic analysis of phase variation in *Bordetella pertussis*. Infect. Immun. 43:263-269, 1984.

412. Weiss, A. A., and Hewlett, E. L.: Virulence factors of *Bordetella pertussis*. Annu. Rev. Microbiol. 40:661-686, 1986.

413. Weiss, A. A., Hewlett, E. L., Myers, G. A., et al.: Pertussis toxin and extracytoplasmic adenylate cyclase as virulence factors of *Bordetella pertussis*. J. Infect. Dis. 2:219-222, 1984.

414. Weyant, R. S., Hollis, D. G., Weaver, R. E., et al.: *Bordetella holmesii* sp. nov., a new gram-negative species associated with septicemia. J. Clin. Microbiol. 33:1-7, 1995.

415. Wiertz, E. J. H., Loggen, H. G., Walvoort, H. D., et al.: In vitro induction of antigen specific antibody synthesis and proliferation of T lymphocytes with acellular pertussis vaccines, pertussis toxin and filamentous hemagglutinin in humans. J. Biol. Stand. 17:181-190, 1989.

416. Williams, G. D., Numa, A., Sokol, J., et al.: ECLS in pertussis: Does it have a role? Intensive Care Med. 24:1089-1092, 1998.

417. Willems, R. J. L., Kamerbeek, J., Geuijen, C. A. W., et al.: The efficacy of a whole cell pertussis vaccine and fimbriae against *Bordetella pertussis* and *Bordetella parapertussis* infections in a respiratory mouse model. Vaccine 16:410-416, 1998.

418. Wilson, G. S.: The Hazards of Immunization. London, Althone Press, 1967.

419. Wirsing von König, C. H., Gounis, D., Laukamp, S., et al.: Evaluation of a single-sample serological technique for diagnosing pertussis in unvaccinated children. Eur. J. Clin. Microbiol. Infect. Dis. 18:341-345, 1999.

420. Wirsing von König, C. H., Postels-Multani, S., Bock, H. L., et al.: Pertussis in adults: Frequency of transmission after household exposure. Lancet 346:1326-1329, 1995.

421. Wirsing von König, C. H., Rott, H., Bogaerts, H., et al.: A serologic study of organisms possibly associated with pertussis-like coughing. Pediatr. Infect. Dis. J. 17:645-649, 1998.

422. Woolf, A. L., and Caplin, H.: Whooping cough encephalitis. Arch. Dis. Child. 3:87-91, 1956.

423. Woolfrey, B. F., and Moody, J. A.: Human infections associated with *Bordetella bronchiseptica*. Clin. Microbiol. Rev. 4:243-255, 1991.

424. World Health Organization: World Health Organization Meeting on Case Definition of Pertussis, Geneva, January 10-11, 1991, MIM/EPI/PERT/9.1. Geneva, World Health Organization, 1991.

425. Wortis, N., Strebel, P. M., Wharton, M., et al.: Pertussis deaths: Report of 23 cases in the United States, 1992 and 1993. Pediatrics 97:607-612, 1996.

426. Wright, S. W., Edwards, K. M., Decker, M. D., et al.: Pertussis infections in adults with persistent cough. JAMA 273:1044-1046, 1995.

427. Yih, W. K., Silva, E. A., Ida, J., et al.: *Bordetella holmesii*–like organisms isolated from Massachusetts patients with pertussis-like symptoms. Emerg. Infect. Dis. 5:441-443, 1999.

428. Yuk, M. H., Harvill, E. T., Miller, J. F., et al.: The BvgAS virulence control system regulates type III secretion in *Bordetella bronchiseptica*. Mol. Microbiol. 28:945-959, 1998.

429. Zackrisson, G., Lagergard, T., Trollfors, B., et al.: Immunoglobulin A antibodies to pertussis toxin and filamentous hemagglutinin in saliva from patients with pertussis. J. Clin. Microbiol. 28:1502-1505, 1990.

430. Zee, A., Agterberg, C., Peeters, M., et al.: Polymerase chain reaction assay for pertussis: Simultaneous detection and discrimination of *Bordetella pertussis* and *Bordetella parapertussis*. J. Clin. Microbiol. *31*:2134-2140, 1993.
431. Zepp, F., Knuf, M., Habermehl, P., et al.: Pertussis-specific cell-mediated immunity in infants after vaccination with a tricomponent acellular pertussis vaccine. Infect. Immun. *64*:4078-4084, 1996.
432. Zhang, Y. L., and Sekura, R. D.: Purification and characterization of the heat-labile toxin of *Bordetella pertussis*. Infect. Immun. *59*:3754-3759, 1991.
433. Zoumboulakis, D., Anagnostakis, D., Albams, V., et al.: Steroids in treatment of pertussis: A controlled clinical trial. Arch. Dis. Child. *48*:51-54, 1973.

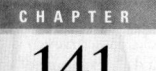

CHAPTER 141
CALYMMATOBACTERIUM GRANULOMATIS
Mariam R. Chacko

Granuloma inguinale is caused by *Calymmatobacterium granulomatis*. It was described first by McLeod in 1882, and *C. granulomatis* was isolated by Donovan in 1905. This disease has been known through the years by many different names, the most common being granuloma inguinale, donovanosis, and granuloma venereum.[30]

THE ORGANISM

C. granulomatis is an encapsulated gram-negative rod measuring 1.5×0.7 mm. Although some of its characteristics resemble those of *Klebsiella* and *Enterobacter*, *C. granulomatis* is considered a unique species distinct from other related organisms belonging to the subclass Proteobacteria.[21,30,31] However, the biochemical and bacteriologic characteristics of the organism have not been identified.[30,31]

Study of the organism reveals a complex cell envelope. In addition to having regular bacterial structures such as a mesosome, ribosomes, and nuclear material, the cytoplasm contains electron-dense granules; transmission electron microscopy shows an outer membrane, middle electron-opaque layer, and an inner plasma membrane. The organisms are enclosed mainly in large histiocytic cells and occasionally in polymorphonuclear cells and plasma cells. They multiply intracellularly to approximately 30 in number and eventually cause cell rupture.[7,30]

EPIDEMIOLOGY

Granuloma inguinale occurs predominantly in young and older adults and is a cause of genital ulcerative disease in tropical and subtropical regions of the world. As with all genital ulcerative diseases, granuloma inguinale has been given greater attention as a risk factor for development of human immunodeficiency virus (HIV) infection.[37] In South Africa, the prevalence of granuloma inguinale in patients with genital ulcer disease is reported to be approximately 10 percent.[34]

Granuloma inguinale is a rare occurrence in children. In the early 1950s, 4 percent of 1- to 4-year-old children in a Papua New Guinea population were found to have granuloma inguinale. Although the mode of transmission in adolescents and adults is considered to be sexual, the mode of transmission of the disease in these children was thought to be by skin-to-skin contact from sitting on the laps of infected adults.[30] More recent case reports show that otitis media, mastoiditis, neck mass, and cervical lymphadenopathy have been described as the initial manifestations of donovanosis in infants and children.[3,14,15] The modes of transmission in these cases are thought to be perinatal and by skin-to-skin contact.[3,14,15]

Granuloma inguinale has been reported since the early 1990s as endemic in South Africa, Papua New Guinea, India, and the Aboriginal community of Australia.[29] A resurgence of the disease was reported in the late 1980s in Durban, South Africa. After a rapid test for donovanosis was introduced in the early 1990s, the number of cases reported by the Durban Health Department in South Africa increased substantially.[27] As a result of the availability of the rapid test and implementation of an HIV/STI (sexually transmitted infections) initiative, the number of new cases of donovanosis in Australia decreased dramatically; five cases were reported in 2005.[2] In 1994, after 4 decades, a case of granuloma inguinale was reported in China.[13]

Granuloma inguinale is not a common occurrence in Europe or the United States today. However, the prevalence increased in developed countries in the 1990s, especially among migrant and poor people living in metropolitan areas. For example, three cases of granuloma inguinale were reported in Rome between 1993 and 2001, with most of them diagnosed in 2000 and 2001.[26] Until 1952, more than a thousand cases a year were reported to the Center for Disease Control (now the Centers for Disease Control and Prevention [CDC]). Since 1952, the prevalence of this disease declined rapidly; between 1971 and 1981, 50 to 90 cases a year were reported. Except for an isolated surge of 97 cases in 1990, fewer than 50 cases a year have been reported since 1982, and in 1993, 19 cases (15 male and 4 female) were reported. In 2000, no cases were reported in the United States.[5] Granuloma inguinale was detected in a white adolescent girl in California in 1985.[16] In 1991, nongenital granuloma inguinale was diagnosed in a man with testicular carcinoma in Texas.[25] In 1992, three unrelated cases of granuloma inguinale, seen within a period of a few weeks, were reported in Toronto; two occurred in immigrants, and one occurred in a native-born Canadian. The first patient was a recent immigrant from El Salvador, and the second patient had immigrated several years previously and had a history of sexual activity with a Jamaican who had immigrated recently. The sexual partner of the third case had come from Turkey.[18] Although the prevalence of the disease is low, this disease needs to be suspected in North America and Europe because of international travel and immigration. Granuloma inguinale usually occurs more commonly in male than in female patients. However, in adolescents, the disease can develop more commonly in girls than in boys. This ratio probably is a reflection of sexual activity between adolescent girls and adult men.[28]

The risk factors and mode of transmission of granuloma inguinale are not clear. The disease generally is considered sexually transmitted. However, in many cases, granuloma inguinale cannot be detected in the sexual partners of infected persons. Nonetheless, numerous studies have reported the disease in 12 to 50 percent of marital or steady sexual partners.[30] Anal intercourse also has been associated with rectal and penile lesions of granuloma inguinale.[22] O'Farrell and associates[35] studied the patterns of sexual behavior in men and women with genital ulcer disease and found that patients with granuloma inguinale and secondary syphilis were more likely than were patients with other genital ulcer diseases to have had sexual intercourse despite the presence of ulcers. Studies reported from India and South Africa have noted a preponderance of granuloma inguinale cases in uncircumcised male patients with poor genital hygiene.[28]

Coexistence of granuloma inguinale with other sexually transmitted diseases occurs commonly. Syphilis has been described in as many as 23 percent of patients with granuloma inguinale. In one report, HIV-1 antibodies were found in as many as 8 percent of male patients with granuloma inguinale.[25,37]

PATHOGENESIS AND PATHOLOGY

The primary lesion in granuloma inguinale is an indurated nodule that erodes through the skin and becomes a granulomatous heaped ulcer. Adjacent lesions form and eventually coalesce, especially in the perineal area. Secondary infection of lesions may occur and may aggravate the tissue destruction and cause scarring. *C. granulomatis* organisms invade mononuclear endothelial cells. Extensive acanthosis and dense dermal infiltrates of mainly plasma cells and histiocytes have been observed in the indurated nodules. Polymorphonuclear cell infiltration also occurs, but lymphocytes are rare findings when secondary infection develops. The pathognomonic feature of granuloma inguinale is a large, infected mononuclear cell, 25 to 90 μm in diameter, that contains many intracytoplasmic cysts filled with deep-staining Donovan bodies. Metastatic spread to the bones, joints, liver, and lymphatics occasionally occurs.[30]

A possible link between human leukocyte antigen (HLA)-B57 and granuloma inguinale infection may exist; class I, class II, and DQ antigens have been detected in the genital ulcers of individuals with granuloma inguinale.[32] Circulating lymphocytes and tissue-level lymphocyte subpopulations in granuloma inguinale have been studied.[40,41] T-lymphocyte and B-lymphocyte infiltration in tissues is almost identical, without any significant difference in ulcerogranulomatous and hypertrophic variants. Both total leukocyte and absolute lymphocyte counts are increased in the ulcerogranulomatous variant of granuloma inguinale. Total T lymphocytes, CD4, CD8, and CD22 levels, and the CD4/CD8 ratio all are increased significantly in the ulcerogranulomatous variant. In contrast, the hypertrophic variant causes a significant elevation only in the CD4/CD8 ratio. This finding suggests a greater cell-mediated immune response in the ulcerogranulomatous variant of granuloma inguinale and is consistent with the paucity of Donovan bodies in smears obtained from patients with this variant.[40,41]

CLINICAL MANIFESTATIONS

The incubation period of granuloma inguinale usually is less than 2 weeks but may be as long as 3 months. The disease begins as one or more subcutaneous nodules that erode through the skin to produce clean, large, beefy-red, granulomatous ulcers that bleed easily. The lesions are sharply defined and painless, and the ulcers feel hard when palpated. The disease usually is limited to local tissue; therefore, constitutional symptoms are unlikely to be present. Autoinoculation is a common manifestation that produces "kissing" lesions. When left untreated at this early stage, the disease progresses and causes extensive mutilating lesions (see Chapter 48).[30]

The morphology of the cutaneous lesions of granuloma inguinale can vary, depending on the stage of the disease. The exuberant or hypertrophic stage appears before secondary infection develops. It consists of large, vegetating masses with overgrowth of granulation tissue, usually in the perianal region. The ulcerative stage is accompanied by secondary infection. In this stage, large, spreading, shallow necrotic ulcers with a foul odor may be

noted. The cicatricial stage results after prolonged healing and is characterized by fibrosis, scarring, depigmentation, keloid formation, elephantiasis, and stenosis of the vagina, urethra, and anus. In patients in Durban, ulcerogranulomatous lesions occurred far more commonly than did hypertrophic and necrotic lesions. Although lymphadenopathy is an unusual occurrence in granuloma inguinale, pseudobuboes and pseudoelephantiasis of the genitals (massive edema) may be seen. Pseudobuboes are the result of deep, inguinal granulomata; pseudoelephantiasis is caused by cutaneous extension of lesions and inflammation.[10,25,30]

The genitalia are involved in 90 percent of cases, the inguinal region in 10 percent, the anal region in 5 to 10 percent, and extragenital sites in 1 to 5 percent. In male patients, lesions usually occur on the prepuce and also can occur on the coronal sulcus and frenulum of the penis.[30,31]

As ulcers enlarge, they can be mutilating and can lead to urethral stenosis. The most common clinical manifestation in pregnant and nonpregnant women is vulvar ulceration. Genital tract bleeding is the next most common finding in nonpregnant women. Multiple sites of genital ulceration (vulva, vagina, and cervix) have been noted only in nonpregnant women.[10,28,30] Extragenital sites, through hematogenous spread, have been reported in the mouth, chin, axillae, abdomen including the pelvic cavity, and foot.[9,11,23,30,38,39,42] These distant sites usually are associated with a primary lesion in the genital area.[30] Lesions in the oral cavity have been described after apparently successful treatment of genital lesions.[9] Donovanosis ulcers may take longer to heal in HIV-positive individuals, and greater destruction of tissue may be noted as well.[30,31]

In endemic areas, unusual manifestations of granuloma inguinale may cause confusion with a wide variety of diseases and can result in misdiagnosis. The differential diagnosis includes carcinoma, secondary syphilis, necrotic ulcerations of amebiasis, tuberculosis, and filariasis. In addition, secondary infection can confuse the diagnosis.[17,30]

DIAGNOSIS

Generally, granuloma inguinale is diagnosed on clinical grounds. The accuracy of a clinical diagnosis of granuloma inguinale can be as high as 63 percent in male patients and 83 percent in female patients. When compared with other genital ulcers, the ulcers are larger in granuloma inguinale, are painless, bleed easily to touch, and usually are not associated with inguinal lymphadenopathy.[36]

The diagnosis of granuloma inguinale can be confirmed by identification of Donovan bodies on a stained crush specimen from the lesion (see Fig. 48–22). Examination of appropriately stained specimens from active lesions remains the most reliable diagnostic test. Light-microscopic examination of biopsy specimens that have been fixed in formalin and embedded in wax is less reliable. Donovan bodies rarely are seen by this method.[30,36]

The common stain used to identify Donovan bodies is Wright-Giemsa blue-black stain. Sections that are formalin-fixed or stained with hematoxylin and eosin are less useful for detecting Donovan bodies. If donovanosis is suspected, a swab for this condition should be taken first, before swabs for other organisms, so that an adequate amount of cellular material can be obtained.[20,30,33] When *C. granulomatis* organisms are likely to be scarce or when smear or crush specimens are likely to be nondiagnostic, one should consider obtaining a biopsy of the lesion. Accordingly, a biopsy specimen preferably stained with Giemsa or silver is recommended in very early, very sclerotic, or heavily superinfected specimens.[20,30,33]

Successful isolation of *C. granulomatis* by culture on human epithelial cell lines with a modified *Chlamydia* culture technique has been reported from South Africa and Australia.[4] Polymerase chain reaction (PCR) techniques for *C. granulomatis* also have been developed and further refined into a colorimetric detection system for use in diagnostic laboratories.

Donovan bodies have been identified on Papanicolaou smears from the cervix.[8] Serologic and skin tests for granuloma inguinale are highly sensitive but not specific. A serologic test using the indirect immunofluorescence technique has been evaluated and found to have a sensitivity of 100 percent, a specificity of 98 percent, a positive predictive value of 89 percent, and a negative predictive value of 100 percent in diagnosing granuloma inguinale. In the absence of culture methods for *C. granulomatis*, this test may prove helpful in the diagnosis of established lesions and not early ulcers.[12]

TREATMENT

Antibiotics with strong activity against *C. granulomatis* are those effective in the treatment of gram-negative bacilli or those whose lipid solubility ensures good intracellular penetration. The CDC recommends treatment of adolescents and adults with doxycycline, 100 mg orally twice a day for a minimum of 3 weeks, until lesions are healed.[5] Alternative regimens include the following: azithromycin, 1 g orally weekly for at least 3 weeks; or ciprofloxacin, 750 mg orally twice a day for at least 3 weeks; or erythromycin, 500 mg orally four times a day for at least 3 weeks; or trimethoprim-sulfamethoxazole, one double-strength tablet (160 mg/800 U) orally, twice a day for at least 3 weeks.[5] Children younger than 9 years of age can be treated with oral azithromycin suspension (10 mg/kg daily) trimethoprim-sulfamethoxazole (10 mg/kg/day trimethoprim), or erythromycin (30 to 50 mg/kg/day).[6]

Clinical response to antibiotics should be noted within a week of treatment; the lesions should become paler and less friable. After a week of treatment, the lesions become smaller, and total healing of the area takes 3 to 5 weeks. Relapse occurs in approximately 10 percent of cases, especially if use of the antibiotic is discontinued before the primary lesion has healed completely. Donovan bodies may reappear within 7 to 10 days.[30] Treatment can fail in patients with coexisting HIV infection, and more intensive and prolonged antibiotic therapy may be needed. As compared with HIV-negative patients, the mean duration to complete ulcer healing in these patients is significantly longer: 25.7 days versus 16.8 days.[19]

Merianos and associates[24] reported the possible effectiveness of ceftriaxone for chronic, recurrent granuloma inguinale. Patients in this study had been suffering from the disease for 1 to 5 years and had received 4 to 19 courses of antibiotics. A single daily intramuscular injection of 1 g of ceftriaxone diluted in 2 mL of 1 percent lidocaine was administered for 7 to 26 days. Clinical improvement was dramatic in most lesions; one third of patients recovered completely without a recurrence after receiving daily doses of ceftriaxone for 7 to 10 days. Patients with mild recurrences responded to additional ceftriaxone or short courses of oral antibiotics.[24] Vulvectomy is reserved for infections that have not responded to antibiotic treatment or for patients with severe vulvar elephantiasis.[10]

PROGNOSIS

Healing is complete in patients who seek treatment early in the course of the disease and who comply with their medication and follow-up regimens. O'Farrell[28] noted complete healing of lesions in 24 percent of patients who complied with follow-up. Complications of granuloma inguinale include pseudoelephantiasis, urethral stricture, and pelvic abscess, which may require surgery.

Another complication is the acquisition of HIV infection and granuloma inguinale, especially when patients with ulcerations that are left untreated for a prolonged period have sexual contact with an HIV-positive partner.[28,30]

The severe, mutilating complications of granuloma inguinale are primarily a result of delayed treatment or poor compliance with medication. In Durban, South Africa, almost half of the male patients had ulcerations for 1 to 6 months before they sought medical care, and 16 percent had ulcerations for 1 to 3 weeks. In contrast, approximately 25 percent of female patients had ulcerations for 1 to 6 months, and 50 percent had ulcerations for 1 to 3 weeks.[28] Delayed medical attention may be related to limited education, ignorance of sexually transmitted diseases, absence of suitable medical facilities, or embarrassment in seeking treatment because of extensive genital lesions.

PREVENTION

Sexual partners of persons with the disease should be traced, examined, and treated. Treatment of granuloma inguinale when the nodule first appears is associated with a benign course. Thus, community-based eradication that targets men with granuloma inguinale in endemic areas should be implemented. Programs should be aimed at identification of lesions, provision of early treatment, and prevention of severe complications. Teaching the importance of personal genital hygiene, such as instruction on simple retraction of the foreskin in men and cleansing the penis with soap and water, also is effective.[28,30]

REFERENCES

1. Bassa, A. G., Hoosen, A. A., Moodley, J., et al.: Granuloma inguinale (donovanosis) in women: An analysis of 61 cases from Durban, South Africa. Sex. Transm. Dis. *20*:164-167, 1993.
2. Bowden, F. J., on behalf of the National Donovanosis Eradication Advisory Committee: Donovanosis in Australia: Going, going. . . . Sex. Transm. Infect. *81*:365-366, 2005.
3. Bowden, F. J., Bright, A., Rode, J. W., and Brewster, D.: Donovanosis causing cervical lymphadenopathy in a five-month-old boy. Pediatr. Infect. Dis. *19*:167-169, 2000.
4. Carter, J., Hutton, S., Sriprakash, K. S., et al.: Culture of the causative organism of donovanosis (*Calymmatobacterium granulomatis*) in MEP-2 cells. J. Clin. Microbiol. *35*:2915-2917, 1997.
5. Centers for Disease Control and Prevention: Sexually Transmitted Disease Surveillance: 2004. Atlanta, Centers for Disease Control and Prevention, Public Health Service, U.S. Department of Health and Human Services, 2005.
6. Centers for Disease Control and Prevention: Sexually transmitted disease treatment guidelines: 2006. M. M. W. R. Recomm. Rep. *55(No.RR-11)*:1-94, 2006.
7. Chandra, M., and Jain, A. K.: Fine structure of *Calymmatobacterium granulomatis* with particular reference to the surface structure. Indian J. Med. Res. *93*:225-231, 1991.
8. DeBoer, A., DeBoer, F., and Van Der Merwe, J.: Cytologic identification of Donovan bodies in granuloma inguinale. Acta Cytol. *28*:126-128, 1984.
9. Doddridge, M., and Muirhead, R.: Donovanosis of the oral cavity: Case report. Aust. Dent. J. *39*:203-205, 1994.
10. Faro, S.: Lymphogranuloma venereum, chancroid, and granuloma inguinale. Obstet. Gynecol. Clin. North Am. *16*:517-530, 1989.
11. Fletcher, H. M., Rattray, C. A., Hanchard, B., et al.: Disseminated donovanosis (granuloma inguinale) with osteomyelitis of both wrists. West Indian Med. J. *51*:194-196, 2002.
12. Freinkel, A. L., Dangor, Y., Koornhof, H. J., et al.: A serological test for granuloma inguinale. Genitourin. Med. *68*:269-272, 1992.
13. Gao, Y., Ni, K., Hu, B., and Zheng, K.: Granuloma inguinale: First case reported in the last four decades in China. Int. J. Dermatol. *35*:758-759, 1996.
14. Govender, D., Hadley, G. P., and Donnellan, R.: Granuloma inguinale (donovanosis) as a neck mass in an infant. Pediatr. Surg. Int. *15*:129-131, 1999.
15. Govender, D., Naidoo, K., and Chetty, R.: Granuloma inguinale (donovanosis): An usual cause of otitis media and mastoiditis in children. Am. J. Clin. Pathol. *108*:510-514, 1997.
16. Growden, W. A., Lebherz, T. B., Moore, J. G., et al.: Granuloma inguinale in a white teenager: A diagnosis easily forgotten, poorly pursued. West. J. Med. *143*:105-108, 1985.
17. Gupta, S., Ajith, C., Kanwar, A. J., et al.: Genital elephantiasis and sexually transmitted infections revisited. Int. J. STD AIDS *17*:157-166, 2006.

18. Hacker, P., Fisher, B. K., Dekoven, J., et al.: Granuloma inguinale: Three cases diagnosed in Toronto, Canada. Int. J. Dermatol. *31*:696-699, 1992.
19. Jamkhedkar, P. P., Hira, S. K., Shroff, H. J., et al.: Clinico-epidemiologic features of granuloma inguinale in the era of acquired immune deficiency syndrome. Sex. Transm. Infect. *25*:196-200, 1998.
20. Joseph, A. K., and Rosen, T.: Laboratory techniques used in the diagnosis of chancroid, granuloma inguinale and lymphogranuloma venereum. Dermatol. Clin. *12*:1-8, 1994.
21. Kharsany, A. B., Hoosen, A. A., Kiepala, P., et al.: Phylogenetics analysis of *Calymmatobacterium granulomatis* based on 16S sequence. J. Med. Microbiol. *48*:841-847, 1999.
22. Marmell, M.: Donovanosis of the anus in the male: An epidemiologic consideration. Br. J. Vener. Dis. *34*:213-218, 1958.
23. Mein, J., Russell, C., Know, J., et al.: Intrapelvic donovanosis presenting as a psoas abscess in two patients. Sex. Transm. Infect. *75*:75-76, 1999.
24. Merianos, A., Gilles, M., and Chuah, J.: Ceftriaxone in the treatment of chronic donovanosis in central Australia. Genitourin. Med. *70*:84-89, 1994.
25. Morris, L. F., Cohen, P. R., and Dodd, L. G.: Nongenital granuloma inguinale in an oncology patient. Am. J. Clin. Oncol. *17*:456-460, 1994.
26. Morrone, A., Toma, L., Franco, G., et al.: Donovanosis in developed countries: Neglected or misdiagnosed disease? Int. J. STD AIDS *14*:288-89, 2003.
27. O'Farrell, N.: Trends in reported cases of donovanosis in Durban, South Africa. Genitourin. Med. *68*:366-369, 1992.
28. O'Farrell, N.: Clinico-epidemiological study of donovanosis in Durban, South Africa. Genitourin. Med. *69*:108-111, 1993.
29. O'Farrell, N.: Global eradication of donovanosis: An opportunity for limiting the spread of HIV-1 infection. Genitourin. Med. *71*:27-31, 1995.
30. O'Farrell, N.: Donovanosis. *In* Holmes, K. K., Sparling, P. E., Mardh, P. A., et al. (eds.): Sexually Transmitted Disease. New York, McGraw-Hill, 1999, pp. 525-531.
31. O'Farrell, N.: Donovanosis: An update. Int. J. STD AIDS *12*:423-427, 2001.
32. O'Farrell, N., and Hammond, M.: HLA antigens in donovanosis (granuloma inguinale). Genitourin. Med. *67*:400-402, 1991.
33. O'Farrell, N., Hoosen, A. A., Coetzee, K. D., et al.: A rapid stain for the diagnosis of granuloma inguinale. Genitourin. Med. *66*:200-201, 1990.
34. O'Farrell, N., Hoosen, A. A., Coetzee, K. D., et al.: Genital ulcer disease in men in Durban, South Africa. Genitourin. Med. *67*:327-330, 1991.
35. O'Farrell, N., Hoosen, A. A., Coetzee, K. D., et al.: Sexual behavior in Zulu men and women with genital ulcer disease. Genitourin. Med. *68*:245-248, 1992.
36. O'Farrell, N., Hoosen, A. A., Coetzee, K. D., et al.: Genital ulcer disease: Accuracy of clinical diagnosis and strategies to improve control in Durban, South Africa. Genitourin. Med. *70*:7-11, 1994.
37. O'Farrell, N., Windsor, I., and Becker, P.: HIV-1 infection among heterosexual attenders at a sexually transmitted diseases clinic in Durban. S. Afr. Med. J. *80*:17-20, 1991.
38. Rao, M. V., Thappa, D. M., Jaisaukar, T. J., and Ratnakar, C.: Extragenital donovanosis of the foot. Sex. Transm. Infect. *74*:298-299, 1998.
39. Sanders, C. T.: Extragenital donovanosis in a patient with AIDS. Sex. Transm. Infect. *74*:142-143, 1998.
40. Sehgal, V. N., Gupta, M. M., and Jain, V. K.: Tissue level lymphocyte subpopulations in donovanosis. Int. J. Dermatol. *30*:857-859, 1991.
41. Sehgal, V. N., Sharma, H. K., and Sharma, V. K.: Characterization of circulating lymphocytes by monoclonal antibodies in donovanosis. J. Dermatol. *18*:181-183, 1991.
42. Veeranna, S., and Raghu, T.Y.: Oral donovanosis. Int. J. STD AIDS *13*:855-856, 2002.

CHAPTER 142

CAMPYLOBACTER JEJUNI

Norma Pérez ⊙ Gloria P. Heresi ⊙ James R. Murphy

Campylobacter jejuni is a frequent cause of enteritis and less often of extraintestinal infection in humans. Since it first was recognized as a common human pathogen in the 1970s, appreciation of this agent's importance as a cause of disease has been increasing steadily. *C. jejuni* is one of the most frequent bacterial causes of human enteritis in the United States and is a leading cause of bacterial foodborne diarrheal disease throughout the world.[4,10,200] Immunoreactive complications may develop after infection.[157,169]

HISTORY

The pathologic consequences of infection with members of the group of bacteria that includes *C. jejuni* were recognized first in 1909 from studies of abortions in sheep.[130] In 1947, the sheep abortion–associated organism *Vibrio fetus* was isolated from a blood culture from a pregnant woman who had an influenza-like illness and delivered a stillborn infant with a necrotic, infarcted placenta.[219] In 1957, King[112,113] hypothesized that *V. fetus*–related organisms could be associated with human enteric disease. Butzler and colleagues[31] showed that bacteria similar to *V. fetus* were present in the stools of children with diarrhea. This observation was confirmed rapidly and repeatedly.[21,33,67,189,202] Major differences in biochemical activities, growth characteristics, and DNA base nucleotide content between true vibrios and *V. fetus* led to the establishment of the new genus *Campylobacter*.[217] The genome of a representative *C. jejuni* was published in 2000.[154] Information gleaned from this and comparative analyses of additional isolates have markedly advanced knowledge of these agents.[63,85]

THE ORGANISM

C. jejuni is a gram-negative rod that may vary in width from 0.2 to 0.9 μm and in length from 0.5 to 5.0 μm.[214] The rods may be short and S-shaped or longer spirals (Fig. 142–1). The organism grows best in cultures maintained at 42° C under microaerophilic conditions (5%-10% oxygen). *C. jejuni* belongs to rRNA superfamily VI, a specialized subgroup of gram-negative bacteria that

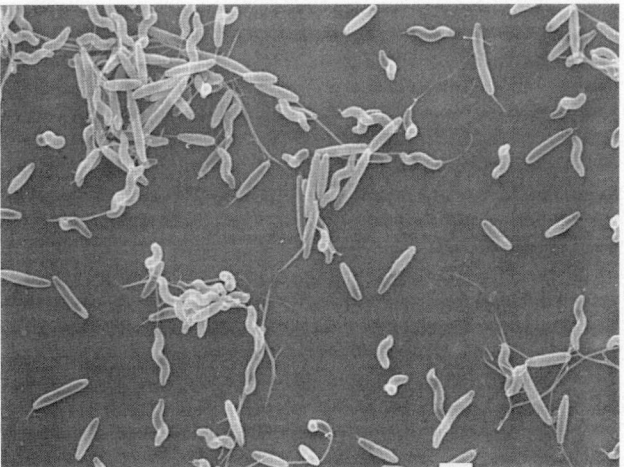

Figure 142–1 Scanning electron microscopy of *Campylobacter jejuni* strain 20-01. *(From Baqar, S., and Rice, B.: Campylobacter jejuni enteritis. Clin. Infect. Dis. 33:901-905, 2001.)*

also includes *Arcobacter* and *Helicobacter*. *C. jejuni* usually is motile, with either a single polar flagellum or two flagella, one at each end of the rod; nonmotile variants exist, and spores are not formed. Organisms obtained from stressed cultures may be coccoid or spherical. The species *C. jejuni* has two subspecies: *C. jejuni jejuni* and *C. jejuni doylei*. *C. jejuni doylei* can be differentiated from *C. jejuni jejuni* by the failure of *C. jejuni doylei* to grow at 42° C, lack of nitrate reduction, and sensitivity to cephalothin. For brevity, we refer to *C. jejuni jejuni* as *C. jejuni*. The spectrum of disease recognized as caused by *C. jejuni* is expanding.[5]

C. jejuni has a circular chromosome of 1.64 million base pairs (30.6% guanosine and cytosine).[154] Marked differences in pathogenic surrogates (motility, colonization of chicks, invasion, and translocation of cultured cells) are associated with variable chromosomal sequences within different passage sequences for a single isolate, and unique chromosomal sequences are associated with known pathogenic isolates of *C. jejuni*. Genomic analyses demonstrate that substantial differences exist among organisms classified by conventional means as *C. jejuni* and that some of these differences are associated with the capacity to cause disease in humans.[63,85,153] Genomic sequence analyses have yielded a catalogue of phase-variable surface structures (including lipo-oligosaccharide and capsule) that appear to relate to pathogenesis and immunity,[58,154] a lack of classical operon structure, repetitive DNA, and an unexpected capacity to produce polysaccharide.[154] Populations of *C. jejuni* are nonclonal, and interstrain exchange of genetic material occurs.[41]

EPIDEMIOLOGY

Human infection with *C. jejuni* occurs worldwide.[19] *C. jejuni* persists in zoonotic niches (Table 142-1), and most human infections are thought to arise from these reservoirs. Chickens and contaminated water are the main sources of campylobacteriosis in developed countries. The organism is a common commensal of the gastrointestinal tract of cattle, pigs, dogs, cats, and most birds used as human food,[25,185] and transmission from these sources occurs. In the United States, *C. jejuni* infection peaks in late summer and early fall (Fig. 142-2). Fresh-water bathing sites may yield *Campylobacter* organisms that are epidemiologically linked to human infections.[145,181,182] Dairy cows in the United Kingdom have higher concentrations of *Campylobacter* organisms in spring and autumn, but the concentration of *Campylobacter* organisms in beef cattle at slaughter does not change with season; as many as 90 percent of beef cattle may be stool-positive for *Campylobacter*.[196] In subtropical areas, the peak incidence of isolation of *C. jejuni* often is associated with the rainy season. In most tropical climates, rates of isolation are similar year-round. Studies in volunteers show an incubation period of 2 to 4 days after challenges ranging from 800 to 100 million colony-forming units.[18] Fecal shedding of *C. jejuni* by humans may last a median of 2 to 3 weeks, with a range of 3 days to several months.[33,109,149]

The distribution of *C. jejuni* infections within populations is linked to the level of industrialization. In industrialized countries, *C. jejuni* infection is found often in children and adults with enteritis and seldom in healthy individuals.[200] In less industrial-

TABLE 142-1 Illustrative Studies of Isolation of *Campylobacter jejuni* from Animal Sources

Animal	Sample	Location and Reference	Sample Size	Positive*
Chicken	Processing plants, shops	Japan[211]	156	67.9
	Flocks on farms	England[94]	49	76.0
	Flocks on farms	Russia[197]	370	31.5
	Giblets	Egypt[111]	50	23.5
	Eggs from 23 farms	United States[15]	276	0.0
	Live birds	United States[15]	10	90.0
	Processing plants, carcasses	United States[193]	325	78.5
Duck	Giblets	Egypt[111]	50	19.0
	At reservoir	United States[148]	113	73.0
Goose	At reservoir	United States[148]	94	5.0
Turkey	Giblets	Egypt[111]	50	14.5
	Feces	United Kingdom[183]	5000	100.0
Squab	Giblets	Egypt[111]	50	4.0
Crane	At reservoir	United States[148]	91	81.0
Pig	Pork at processing plants, shops	Japan[211]	94	2.1
Cow	Beef at processing plants, shops	Japan	52	0.0
	Rectal swabs	United Kingdom[93]	668	72.0
	Farms	Canada[220]	78	13.0
	Milk cows	United States[48]	78	68.0
	Milk, bulk tanks	United States[48]	108	0.9
	Housed indoors, feces	Switzerland[29]	395	38.5
	Outdoors, feces	Switzerland[29]	395	13.3
Goat	Rectal swabs	Ghana[1]	72	33.3
Sheep	Rectal swabs	Ghana[1]	13	23.0
Sheep	Liver	New Zealand[38]	272	66.2
Cat	Domestic, rectal swabs	United States[66]	430	1.0
	Zoo, rectal swab (species-positive)	United States[66]	15	6.7
	Feces	United States[83]	206	1.0
Monkey	Stool	United States[137]	50	77.0
	Stool	Indonesia[76]	50	36.0
Dog	Rectal swabs of puppies	Denmark[76]	72	22.2
	Fecal culture of puppies	United States[224]	4	100.0
Birds	Feces of migrating passerines	Sweden[151]	101	3.0
Pigeons, feral	Rectal swabs, feces	Norway[121]	200	3.0
Penguin	Feces	South Georgia Island[27]	100	3.0

Percent positive. In instances in which studies reported ranges of percent positive, the highest rate is recorded.

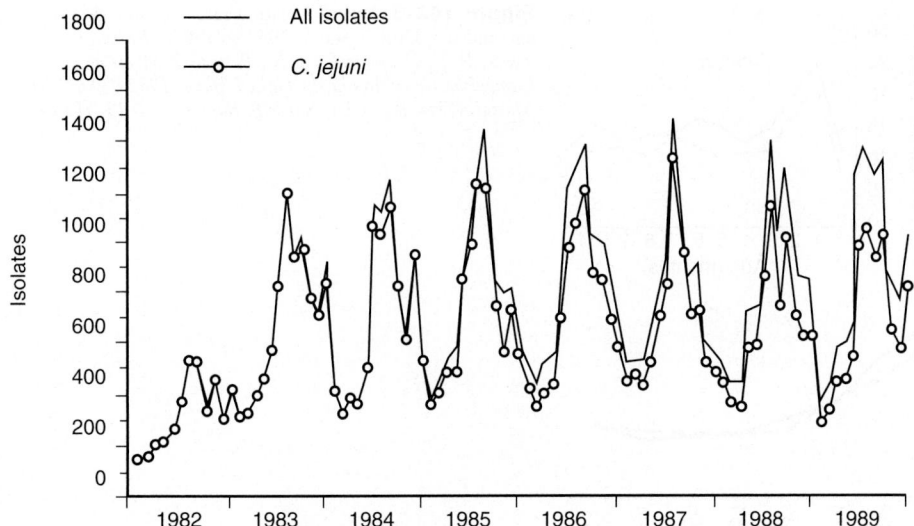

Figure 142–2 Reported human *Campylobacter* isolates by month in the United States, 1982 to 1989. *(From Tauxe, R. V.: Epidemiology of Campylobacter jejuni infections in the United States and other industrialized countries. In Nachamkin, I., Blaser, M. J., and Tompkins, L. S. [eds.]: Campylobacter jejuni: Current Strategy and Future Trends. Washington, D.C., American Society for Microbiology, 1992, pp. 9-19.)*

TABLE 142–2   Selected Longitudinal Studies of Frequency of *Campylobacter jejuni* Infection in Children

Location	No. of Children	Isolation of *C. jejuni* from Children*	
		With Diarrhea	**Without Diarrhea**
Guatemala[167]	321	12.1	8.1
Czechoslovakia[86]	5831	10.1	NR
Mexico[33]	179	0.4	1.7
Thailand[203]	411	0.4	1.1

*Results are reported as percent of stools positive.
NR, not reported.

TABLE 142–3   Selected Cross-Sectional Studies of Frequency of *Campylobacter jejuni* Infection in Children

Location	Frequency of Isolation of *C. jejuni* from Children: Percentage of Stools with *C. jejuni* (Number of Children Studied)	
	With Diarrhea	**Without Diarrhea**
South Africa[26]	35.0 (78)	16.0 (63)
Zaire[43]	14.4 (416)	3.0 (200)
Rwanda[42]	9.3 (150)	0.0 (58)
Zaire[31]	8.6 (70)	0.0 (30)
Cameroon[116]	7.7 (272)	3.2 (157)
Bangladesh[78]	25.5 (102)	8.6 (93)
China[226]	18.7 (48)	8.6 (104)
China[46]	11.9 (303)	4.6 (953)
Kuwait[184]	7.0 (621)	0.0 (152)
India[141]	4.0 (607)	0.9 (529)
Saudi Arabia[37]	1.0 (7369)	0.1 (1130)
Belgium[31]	5.1 (800)	1.3 (1000)
Canada[149]	4.3 (1004)	0.0 (176)
Chile[56]	10.0 (299)	6.0 (304)

tion rate of 5.5 per 100,000 person-years (with *C. jejuni* accounting for 99% of the *Campylobacter* isolates; Fig. 142–3).[202] Population-based isolation rates of *Campylobacter* in the United States range from 28 to 1560 per 100,000 per year.[201,202] The rate of death attributable to *Campylobacter* is estimated between 100 and 124 per year in the United States.[8,9] The case mortality rate is between 0.10[131] and 0.23 percent.[81] It is possible that the mortality rate is higher. A registry-based study demonstrated about fivefold and twofold increases in mortality rates for the first 30 days or first year, respectively, after developing *Campylobacter* infection.[81] Population-based studies in England, the United States, and Sweden showed a bimodal age distribution, with a peak of illness occurring in children younger than 5 years of age and a second peak at 15 to 29 years of age.[172,202] The highest isolation rate occurs in the first year of life (see Fig. 142–3).

In less industrialized regions, *Campylobacter* is found in association with childhood diarrhea in 8 to 45 percent of cases, but it is isolated at similar rates from healthy children.[33,39,64] The highest rates of *Campylobacter* isolation are in children younger than 5 years of age.[33] As many as 75 percent of *Campylobacter* infections occurring during the first year of life are asymptomatic.[39]

In industrialized regions, most sporadic cases occur because of handling, preparation, and consumption of contaminated raw or undercooked poultry.[21,32,44,87,184,192,202] Raw milk and contaminated water less frequently are sources (see Table 142–1).[90,96,133,204,222] Poor kitchen hygiene plays a role in transmission; the risk of acquiring infection is inversely related to the frequency of using soap to clean cutting boards.[202] Barbecues represent a special hazard because they permit easy transfer of bacteria from raw meat to hands and other food and from there to the mouth.[33] Sporadic cases of *C. jejuni* infection occur much more frequently than do outbreaks.

Campylobacter is transmitted usually by a contaminated food or water vehicle. However, direct transmission of the agent may occur, usually to individuals with direct exposure to reservoir animals or to those who process contaminated animal products.[30] Person-to-person spread may occur in areas of high contamination, such as where diapered children are present.[155] In addition, intrapartum transmission is documented.[30,218] Asymptomatic mothers may transmit the infection to their newborns.[30]

In developing countries, transmission is multifactorial. Free-roaming poultry, toddlers, unsafe water supply, and lack of adequate disposal of excreta are documented sources.[69] However, proving that *Campylobacter* cause disease in regions where the

ized areas, *C. jejuni* is isolated frequently from children, even in the absence of enteritis (Tables 142–2 and 142–3).

In industrialized countries, *C. jejuni* has been isolated from between 1 and 13 percent of children with diarrhea, and the prevalence of infection in healthy individuals has been reported to be between 0 and 1.5 percent.[21,31,170,189,200] A 5-year, laboratory-based national surveillance of *Campylobacter* spp. showed an isola-

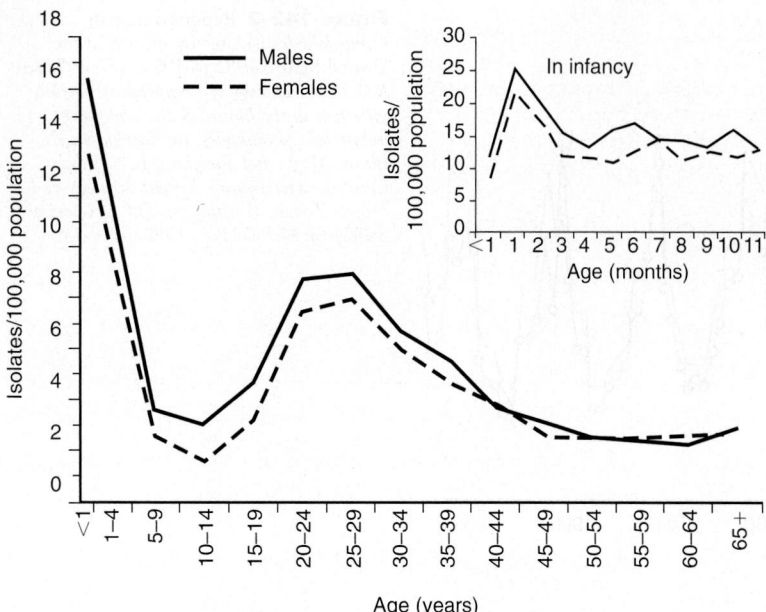

Figure 142–3 Annual isolation rates of *Campylobacter* by age and sex, United States, 1982 to 1986. *(From Tauxe, R. V., Hargrett-Bean, N., Patton, C. M., et al.: Campylobacter isolates in the United States, 1982-1986. Morb. Mortal. Wkly. Rep. CDC Surveill. Summ. 37:1-13, 1988.)*

agent is environmentally pervasive is difficult. Confounders include statistically indistinguishable rates of isolation from diarrhea cases and matched controls (see Table 142–2) and direct evidence that the presence in a household of a *Campylobacter* shared between humans and chickens is associated with protection from diarrhea.[144] Improved knowledge of the immune responses that protect from *Campylobacter* infection and disease and knowledge of the components of *Campylobacter* required to cause disease are needed to understand the agent's epidemiology better.

Because of the biochemical inactivity of *Campylobacter* organisms, discriminating species and subspecies by conventional chemotaxonomic methods is problematic. The consequences of this difficulty include ambiguities in epidemiologic investigations and low resolution in studies of mechanisms of virulence and immunity. Effort is being invested in devising genotyping schemes.[47,146,223]

PATHOLOGY

Most *C. jejuni* infections are not associated with illness or notable pathologic features. When illness does occur, watery diarrhea, invasive enteritis, or systemic infection may result. The spectrum of pathology reflects this range of manifestations. Acute watery diarrhea may occur in the absence of grossly visible pathologic features. Acute inflammation of the colon and rectum is the hallmark of *C. jejuni* invasive enteritis,[125] although hemorrhagic jejunitis and ileitis may also occur.[54,109,113,189] In patients who have undergone proctoscopy, normal mucosa is found in approximately 50 percent; in the remainder, mucosal edema, congestion, friability, and granularity are seen. The spectrum of histologic changes ranges from minimal edema with acute and chronic inflammatory cells and no vascular congestion to moderate inflammation and cryptitis to crypt abscess formation.[12] Acute appendicitis, mesenteric lymphadenitis, and ileocolitis have been reported in patients who have undergone appendectomies while they were infected with *C. jejuni*.[23] *C. jejuni* infection is at low frequency a precursor to immunoreactive complications wherein disease results from immunologic effectors generated in response to infection that damage neurons. The demonstration that, after adjustments for co-morbidities, *Campylobacter* infection is associated with increased mortality over the course of a 1-year period

after infection suggests that as yet unidentified severe late disease occurs.[81] *C. jejuni* is one of a few microbes that have been hypothesized as triggering a common mechanism leading to lymphomas.[75]

PATHOGENESIS

The mechanisms by which *C. jejuni* causes diarrhea, dysentery, and, less frequently, systemic disease are not understood well. Evidence consistent with the production of a heat-labile enterotoxin has been presented.[73,100,123,174] However, this toxic activity is not universally associated with isolates from individuals who have *C. jejuni* illness. Some strains produce a cytotoxin,[101,124] but its relevance to disease has not been established. Some *C. jejuni* can invade various cultured cell lines.[32,55] Motility, surface structures, and molecular adaptations have been associated with capacity to cause disease,[13,14,60,61,74,82,107,136] but the pattern of their expression in disease-associated isolates is not uniform. Dogs,[166] rhesus,[57] rabbits,[195] mice,[57] and hamsters[92] have been evaluated as models of *Campylobacter* enteritis, but none faithfully reproduces the disease seen in humans. A mouse intranasal challenge model[16] has been developed for use in studies of *C. jejuni* invasiveness, and a ferret model[17] has been developed for studies of *C. jejuni*-induced diarrhea.

In vitro studies demonstrate a capacity to disrupt tight junctions of intestinal epithelial cell monolayers and preferentially induce proinflammatory cytokine responses. These capacities and the demonstrated microtubule-dependent eucaryotic cell evasion mechanism[114] may contribute to establishment and maintenance of *C. jejuni* in the gut.[36]

IMMUNITY

The preponderance of evidence of protective acquired immune responses to *C. jejuni* comes from studies of children in developing countries. Such children have more frequent symptomatic infections at younger ages; with increasing age, the rate of symptomatic infection decreases.* The number of *C. jejuni* organisms

---

*See references 20, 22, 24, 102, 103, 105, 127, 198, 203, 205.

excreted per gram of stool of infected individuals also declines with increasing age,[205] as does the duration of excretion of the organism.[203] These phenomena parallel increasing titers of *Campylobacter*-specific antibodies.[22,24,102,127,198,205,210] Additional inferential evidence includes that breast-feeding is associated with reduced frequency of *C. jejuni* diarrhea.[173,213] Adult volunteers who became ill after a first challenge were protected from illness after repeat challenge with a homologous strain,[18] and resistance related to the presence of anti *Campylobacter* antibodies. Prolonged, severe, and sometimes recurrent infections occur in immunodeficient patients.[128,132,161] Hypogammaglobulinemic patients have difficulty clearing *Campylobacter* organisms. Patients with late-stage acquired immunodeficiency syndrome (AIDS) are at increased risk of acquiring severe relapsing *Campylobacter* infection; patients with early stages of human immunodeficiency virus (HIV) infection and high CD4 counts are not at risk. Immunity to disease may not protect against asymptomatic colonization. The bacterial components against which the protective immune responses are directed are not known. The sum of this evidence forms the basis for attempts to develop *C. jejuni* vaccines.

Very little information is available on cellular immune responses to *C. jejuni*. Cellular responses may play an important role in facilitating the formation of antibody and in clearing intracellular *C. jejuni* from eukaryotic cells.

Despite the mass of evidence indicating protective roles for immune responses, the *Campylobacter* components against which protective immune responses are targeted are not known. Similarly, attempts to relate classic serotyping schemes, flagellar types, or presence or absence of virulence factors with disease-causing capacity have yielded associations of poor strength. The completion of the genome sequence of *C. jejuni*, NCTC 11168, in 2000[154] enabled studies to be pursued that are beginning to explain the relationships between bacterial components and immune responses. The *Campylobacter* glycome is remarkably plastic,[108] and *Campylobacter* spp. produce a surprising variety of carbohydrates ($\approx$8% of the genome is dedicated to the biosynthesis of surface carbohydrates). Furthermore, multiple mechanisms exist for sequence variation for genes encoding the glycome. In a clinical trial, researchers demonstrated that passage of *C. jejuni* in volunteers can be associated with phase variation in lipo-oligosaccharide.[165]

CLINICAL MANIFESTATIONS

C. jejuni produces a spectrum of manifestations, the most common of which is enteritis. Bacteremia, other systemic manifestations, and perinatal infections occur infrequently.

ENTERITIS

Children with *Campylobacter* enteritis may have unformed stools, watery diarrhea, inflammatory diarrhea, or a combination of these symptoms.[5,21,23,33,109,149,189] Inflammatory diarrhea can be so severe that it is misdiagnosed as inflammatory bowel disease.[189] Inflammatory diarrhea is a more common occurrence in industrialized countries, and secretory watery diarrhea more typically occurs in developing areas. Patients with ciprofloxacin-resistant strains have longer duration of diarrhea than do patients infected with sensitive strains.[143]

Most cases of enteric illness subside within 7 days, although 20 to 30 percent last for 2 weeks and a few (5-10%) may persist longer, with a relapsing course lasting for weeks.[109,149] In one third to one half of patients, the initial symptoms are periumbilical cramping, intense abdominal pain, malaise, myalgia, and headache. An acute abdomen or appendicitis may be sus-

pected at first[34] because acute abdominal pain occasionally may be the only initial symptom; pseudoappendicitis or mesenteric adenitis and terminal ileitis can be found.[158] The pain may be mild and intermittent for several weeks, and vomiting is a common occurrence. Secretory diarrhea with 10 or more profuse, watery stools per day may be present. Because this course occurs commonly in younger children, dehydration frequently (10%) is an outcome. Relapse of symptoms may occur.

The symptoms of inflammatory diarrhea are similar to those caused by *Shigella*, invasive *Escherichia coli*, and *Salmonella* and consist of generalized malaise, fever, abdominal cramps, tenesmus, bloody stools, and the presence of fecal leukocytes on light microscopy.[125] Fever without other symptoms may develop and can be associated with febrile seizures.[225] Toxic megacolon with massive bleeding may occur.[71,106,179] In neonates, blood-streaked formed stools or hematochezia may be associated with the isolation of *C. jejuni*.[71,106] The abdomen is tender, especially in the right lower quadrant. Splenomegaly occurs rarely.

EXTRAINTESTINAL INFECTIONS

Bacteremia with *C. jejuni* occurs much less commonly than does enteritis. Bacteremia was recognized first in malnourished children, patients with chronic illness or immunodeficiency, and patients at the extremes of age.[2,72,132,168] Cirrhosis, cancer, immunosuppressive therapy, and HIV infection commonly are underlying conditions in patients with bacteremia.[162] These findings led to the view that *C. jejuni* bacteremia was a disease of the relatively immunoincompetent patient. However, most *C. jejuni* blood isolates are from healthy individuals who often have histories of recent gastrointestinal disease.[190] The average incidence of *Campylobacter* bacteremia in England and Wales is 1.5 per 1000 intestinal *Campylobacter* infections. The Centers for Disease Control and Prevention (CDC) reports that only 0.4 percent of *C. jejuni* isolates in the United States are from blood cultures.[202] Most *C. jejuni* strains are susceptible to killing by serum, a finding that perhaps explains the transient nature of the bacteremia and its tendency to resolve without specific therapy. In HIV-infected patients, *Campylobacter* bacteremia occurs more frequently and with increased morbidity and higher mortality rates.[126,162,206] Fatal cases have been reported in the absence of enteric disease.[126]

The main reason for the increased recognition of extraintestinal *Campylobacter* infections appears to be the growing application of appropriate microbiologic culture methods. The incidence of *C. jejuni* bacteremia probably remains underestimated. Typically, blood cultures are not performed in individuals with the primary complaint of diarrhea. Rarely,[164] cholecystitis, urinary tract infection,[40] pancreatitis,[62] hepatitis,[115] and meningitis[49,210] can result from *Campylobacter* infection.

PERINATAL INFECTIONS

Occasionally, abortion or stillbirth, premature labor, neonatal sepsis, and meningitis caused by *C. jejuni* have been described.[156] *Campylobacter*-associated second trimester abortion generally is preceded by mild gastroenteritis.[138,187] The placenta may have areas of necrosis, infarction, microabscesses, and inflammation. The most likely route of placental/fetal infection is through the bloodstream, although a case with possible ascending spread has been reported.[45] Infected infants often are premature. Illness in neonates generally is mild or asymptomatic, but symptomatic gastroenteritis and asymptomatic bloody diarrhea caused by *C. jejuni* have been reported in newborn infants.[28,149] Bacteremia and meningitis also may occur.[68,210] The source of the organism in these cases usually has been the mother, who may be symptomatic or asymptomatic at the time of delivery.[28,186]

IMMUNOREACTIVE COMPLICATIONS

An episode of *C. jejuni* infection may be followed by immunoreactive complications such as Guillain-Barré syndrome (GBS),[79,80,104,134,171] Reiter syndrome,[99,160,163] reactive arthritis,[51,164,177] and erythema nodosum.[11,59,194] A preceding *C. jejuni* infection has been documented by serologic methods or stool culture in 12 to 60 percent of patients with GBS.[3,79,80,91,110,134] *C. jejuni* infection is the most common identified causal factor for GBS.[140,169] However, the risk of development of this syndrome after having a *C. jejuni* infection is less than 1 percent.[4] *Campylobacter*-associated GBS is associated with axonal degeneration and poorer outcome than in GBS associated with other causes.[169] During the 2 months after a symptomatic episode of *C. jejuni* infection, the likelihood of GBS is approximately 100 times (30.4 per 100,000) higher than the risk in the general population (0.3 per 100,000).[129] In a nested case-control study from 1991 to 2001 using data from the United Kingdom General Practice Research Database, 20 percent of GBS cases were attributable to *Campylobacter*.[199] GBS syndrome appears to be an age-related risk; one study found no cases in patients less than 20 years of age, 14 per 100,000 in patients aged 20 to 59 years, and 248 per 100,000 infections in those older than 60 years of age.[129] Certain serotypes of *C. jejuni* are associated more frequently with the subsequent development of GBS.[6,117]

Molecular mimicry between G_{M1} ganglioside and *C. jejuni* lipo-oligosaccharide is established as one of the causes of GBS.[227] A positive correlation of serologic evidence of *C. jejuni* and the presence of antibody to G_{M1} has been described.[70,98] Lipopolysaccharide extracted from *C. jejuni* was found to have core oligosaccharide resembling human ganglioside G_{M1}. Pure motor neuropathy with a tendency for more distal weakness and sparing of the cranial nerves has been associated with *C. jejuni* infection in patients with anti-G_{M1} antibody.[4,209] *Campylobacter* carrying the cst-II sialy transferase gene is associated with the development of GBS and Fisher syndrome and gene polymorphisms may determine which syndrome develops after having a case of *C. jejuni* enteritis.[227] Cases of Miller-Fisher syndrome, a polyneuritis variant characterized by ophthalmoplegia, areflexia, and cerebellar ataxia, also have been reported in association with *C. jejuni* infection.[97,228] Patients with Miller-Fisher syndrome often have antibodies to ganglioside G_{Q1b}. Reactive arthritis may be associated with *Campylobacter* enteritis, especially in adults with human leukocyte antigen (HLA)-B27.[51,177]

Campylobacter reactive arthritis may occur in 1 to 5 percent of patients infected.[164] The arthritis starts a few days to several weeks after the episode of diarrhea. Involvement of joints can be monarticular or multiple, as well as migratory, and both large and small joints can be affected. Synovial fluid is sterile, and fever and leukocytosis are absent; the duration ranges from 1 week to several months. The course is self-limited, and the prognosis is good.[77]

Severe, persistent, and relapsing *C. jejuni* infections have been reported in patients with immune deficiencies, including congenital and acquired hypogammaglobulinemia and malnutrition.[2,89,132] In patients with AIDS, increased frequency and severity of *C. jejuni* infection have been reported; the severity correlates inversely with the CD4 count.[120,159,161]

DIAGNOSIS

The initial characteristics of *C. jejuni* enteritis are not sufficiently unique to permit the diagnosis to be established on clinical grounds. The differential diagnosis should include *Shigella*, *Salmonella*, invasive *E. coli*, *E. coli* O157:H7, *Yersinia enterocolitica*, *Aeromonas*, and *Vibrio parahaemolyticus* infections, and amebiasis. Consideration should be given to pseudomembranous colitis

caused by *Clostridium difficile* if the patient has been receiving antibiotic therapy. Fecal leukocytes are found in as many as 75 percent of cases of *Campylobacter* enteritis; gross or occult fecal blood is present in 50 percent.[18,21,125] White blood cell counts usually are normal, although a shift to the left may occur. Mild elevations in alanine aminotransferase, alkaline phosphatase, and the sedimentation rate are observed in as many as 25 percent of patients.

Methods for demonstrating *C. jejuni* include direct microscopy,[150,152] bacteriologic culture, antigen detection by electroimmunoassay (EIA) or enzyme-linked immunosorbent assay (ELISA),[84,178,212] DNA probes,[207] polymerase chain reaction (PCR),[98,118,147,216] and serology.[5] Detection of antigen by EIA is nearly as sensitive and specific as is culture. ELISA using recombinant P18 and P39 as antigens has demonstrated 91.9 percent sensitivity and 99 percent specificity.[178] PCR enables some culture-negative *Campylobacter* infections to be diagnosed.[118,119] Serologic tests appear useful for epidemiologic investigations but are not recommended for routine diagnosis.

C. jejuni can be detected by darkfield and phase-contrast examination of fresh suspensions of stool. The distinguishing characteristic of *Campylobacter* is darting motility. Gram stain of stool showing *Vibrio* forms is said to be useful in making a presumptive diagnosis.[176] Using the direct carbol-fuchsin Gram-stain method, Wang and Murdoch[221] reported 89 percent sensitivity and 99.7 percent specificity when examining stool samples of *Campylobacter*-infected patients. The indirect fluorescent antibody test can be used for identification of *Campylobacter* on smears; however, standardized reagents for this procedure are not available from commercial sources.

Establishing a definitive diagnosis of *C. jejuni* infection requires the demonstration of *C. jejuni* in stool or in a tissue sample. Unfortunately, not all laboratories culture for *C. jejuni*, despite its frequency. Culture of *C. jejuni* from stool requires special methods and special media. It can be accomplished with media that contain antibiotics[52] to which *Campylobacter* organisms are resistant. If culturing is to be done on medium free of antibiotics, diluted stool samples should be passed through a cellulose acetate membrane filter to reduce the number of other enteric microorganisms.[68] Inoculated plates should be incubated in 5 percent oxygen and 10 percent carbon dioxide at 42° C. Colony formation may not be grossly visible until 72 hours after plating. Identification of colonies as *C. jejuni/coli* is based on a Gram stain showing characteristic morphology and positive catalase and oxidase reactions. Hydrolysis of hippurate establishes an isolate as meeting the conventional inclusion criteria for *C. jejuni*. Routine media usually are adequate for isolation of *Campylobacter* from normally sterile body fluids and tissues. PCR analysis performed on fixed, routinely processed colon biopsies is an excellent diagnostic method for detecting *C. jejuni* from focal active colitis cases. An advantage of the PCR on tissue is that it can be done retrospectively from the paraffin block.[180]

TREATMENT

Most *C. jejuni* organisms are susceptible to macrolides, aminoglycosides, chloramphenicol, imipenem, and clindamycin and are resistant to cephalosporins, tetracyclines, rifampin, penicillins, trimethoprim, and vancomycin.[188,215] However, the development of resistance to macrolides is starting to emerge, with case reports worldwide.[65] Patterns of antibiotic resistance in *C. jejuni* show regional differences. In the past, quinolones were used as empiric therapy for adult traveler's diarrhea because of their good microbiologic activity against *Campylobacter*, *Shigella*, and *Salmonella* strains.[4,50,175]

However, since the late 1980s, *Campylobacter* strains have become increasingly resistant to fluoroquinolones worldwide,

TABLE 142-4 Antibiotic Resistance Pattern of *Campylobacter jejuni* Isolates

| Location | Study Years | No. Tested | Percentage of Isolates Resistant to | | | |
			Erythromycin	Fluoroquinolones	Tetracycline	Gentamicin
Netherlands[177]	1994-1997	1315	2	11-29	7-15	ND
Minnesota[172]	1994-1998	4953	ND	1.3-10.2	ND	ND
Spain, Barcelona[149]	1995-1998	909	5	81	72	1
Canada[53]	1995-1997	158	0	12.7	56	ND
Spain[158]	1997-1998	537	3.2	75	ND	0.4
Taiwan[106]	1994-1996	93	10	52	95	1
Thailand[73]	1995	57	ND	84	ND	ND

ND, no data.

except in Australia (Table 142–4). The emergence of resistance has been associated with the use of quinolones such as sarafloxacin, difloxacin, and enrofloxacin in veterinary medicine in Europe and the United States.[52,53,95,191] The association of human infection with fluoroquinolone-resistant *Campylobacter* spp. and consumption of poultry prompted the U.S. Food and Drug Administration (FDA) to withdraw enrofloxacin for use in poultry, effective September 2005.[142] Despite this measure, it will take time for fluoroquinolone-sensitive *Campylobacter* spp. to be reestablished in the environment.

In general, patients with quinolone-resistant isolates have a longer duration of diarrhea than do patients with fluoroquinolone-sensitive isolates.[191] Fluoroquinolone resistance in *C. jejuni* appears to be related to mutations in the genes encoding subunits of DNA gyrase.[88] The frequency of erythromycin-resistant *Campylobacter* isolates is low[175] (see Table 142–4); therefore, it remains the drug of choice in adults, as in children. Most patients with *C. jejuni* enteritis have mild symptoms and do not require antibiotic therapy. For these patients, oral rehydration and replacement of electrolytes are sufficient. Patients who may benefit from antibiotic therapy are those with fever, bloody stool, and symptoms lasting longer than a week.[5] Patients with HIV infection or other immunodeficiency syndromes should be treated.

Data on antibiotic treatment are controversial. A recent meta-analysis on the effects of antibiotic treatment on duration of symptoms caused by *Campylobacter* spp. looked at 11 randomized control trials. It concluded that antibiotic therapy (with erythromycin, ciprofloxacin, or norfloxacin) shortened the duration of intestinal symptoms by less than 2 days, especially if these drugs were given early in the course of disease.[208] In addition, antibiotic therapy shortened the excretion of *Campylobacter* spp. from feces.[208] All immunocompromised and bacteremic patients with *C. jejuni* infections should be treated with an appropriate antibiotic such as gentamicin, imipenem, or both drugs.[5]

PREVENTION

Tactics for prevention of *Campylobacter*iosis include breastfeeding and avoidance of raw food and food that has been cooked under conditions that permit the survival of bacteria or that has been handled in such a way that bacterial contamination may occur. Risks of foodborne illnesses including campylobacteriosis transmitted by restaurant-prepared meals may be reduced by mandating that food-service employees obtain training in food safety (e.g., thorough handwashing with soap and water after handling raw poultry or meat, cooking poultry to 180° F or until meat is no longer pink and juices run clear, separating raw poultry from other foods during preparation).[7]

A 24-month (2002 to 2004), population-based surveillance case-control study by FoodNet in the United States evaluated infants with laboratory confirmed *Campylobacter* infection and

identified risk factors associated with their infection. Identified risk factors include drinking well water, eating fruits and vegetables prepared at home, having a pet with diarrhea in the home, visiting or living on a farm, riding in a shopping cart next to meat or poultry, and traveling outside the United States.[61] Prevention measures should then be targeted at the potential source. An interesting finding is that attendance at a daycare center did not pose an increased risk in this study.

Selected microorganisms may displace *Campylobacter* from its ecologic niches. This finding may prove useful in reducing *Campylobacter* contamination of food animals.[35,122,135,139] Attempts to develop vaccines against *Campylobacter*iosis continue, but no product is in advanced development.

REFERENCES

1. Abrahams, C. A., Agbodaze, D., Nakano, T., et al.: Prevalence and antibiogram of *Campylobacter jejuni* in domestic animals in rural Ghana. Arch. Environ. Health *45*:59-62, 1990.
2. Ahnen, D. J., and Brown, W. R.: *Campylobacter* enteritis in immune-deficient patients. Ann. Intern. Med. *96*:187-188, 1982.
3. Allos, B. M.: Association between *Campylobacter* infection and Guillain-Barré syndrome. J. Infect. Dis. *176*(Suppl. 2):S125-128, 1997.
4. Allos, B. M.: *Campylobacter jejuni* Infections: Update on emerging issues and trends. Clin. Infect. Dis. *32*:1201-1206, 2001.
5. Allos, B. M., and Blaser, M. J.: *Campylobacter jejuni* and the expanding spectrum of related infections. Clin. Infect. Dis. *20*:1092-1099, quiz 1100-1091, 1995.
6. Allos, B. M., Lippy, F. T., Carlsen, A,. et al.: *Campylobacter jejuni* strains from patients with Guillain-Barré syndrome. Emerg. Infect. Dis. *4*:263-268, 1998.
7. Anonymous: From the Centers for Disease Control and Prevention: Outbreak of *Campylobacter* enteritis associated with cross-contamination of food: Oklahoma, 1996. JAMA *279*:1341, 1998.
8. Anonymous: *Campylobacter* Infections. U.S. Department of Health and Human Services, 2005.
9. Anonymous: Fact Sheets: Foodborne Illness and Diseases. U.S. Department of Agriculture, 2007.
10. Anonymous: Preliminary FoodNet data on the incidence of infection with pathogens transmitted commonly through food: 10 states, 2006. M. M. W. R. Morb. Mortal. Wkly. Rep. *56*:336-339, 2007.
11. Anton, E.: [Reactive arthritis and erythema nodosum caused by *Campylobacter jejuni*]. Enferm. Infecc. Microbiol. Clin. *16*:387-388, 1998.
12. Babakhani, F. K., Bradley, G. A., and Joens, L. A.: Newborn piglet model for *Campylobacter*iosis. Infect. Immun. *61*:3466-3475, 1993.
13. Bacon, D. J., Alm, R. A., Burr, D. H., et al.: Involvement of a plasmid in virulence of *Campylobacter jejuni* 81-176. Infect. Immun. *68*:4384-4390, 2000.
14. Bacon DJ, Alm RA, Hu L, et al.: DNA sequence and mutational analyses of the pVir plasmid of *Campylobacter jejuni* 81-176. Infect. Immun. *70*:6242-6250, 2002.
15. Baker, R. C., Paredes, M. D., and Qureshi, R. A.: Prevalence of *Campylobacter jejuni* in eggs and poultry meat in New York State. Poult. Sci. *66*:1766-1770, 1987.
16. Baqar, S., Bourgeois, A. L., Schultheiss, P. J., et al.: Safety and immunogenicity of a prototype oral whole-cell killed *Campylobacter* vaccine administered with a mucosal adjuvant in non-human primates. Vaccine *13*:22-28, 1995.
17. Bell, J. A., and Manning, D. D.: A domestic ferret model of immunity to *Campylobacter jejuni*-induced enteric disease. Infect. Immun. *58*:1848-1852, 1990.

18. Black, R. E., Levine, M. M., Clements, M. L., et al.: Experimental *Campylobacter jejuni* infection in humans. J. Infect. Dis. *157*:472-479, 1988.

19. Blaser, M. J.: Epidemiologic and clinical features of *Campylobacter jejuni* infections. J. Infect. Dis. *176*(Suppl. 2):S103-S105, 1997.

20. Blaser, M. J., and Duncan, D. J.: Human serum antibody response to *Campylobacter jejuni* infection as measured in an enzyme-linked immunosorbent assay. Infect. Immun. *44*:292-298, 1984.

21. Blaser, M. J., Berkowitz, I. D., LaForce, F. M., et al.: *Campylobacter* enteritis: Clinical and epidemiologic features. Ann. Intern. Med. *91*:179-185, 1979.

22. Blaser, M. J., Duncan, D. J., Osterholm, M. T., et al.: Serologic study of two clusters of infection due to *Campylobacter jejuni*. J. Infect. Dis. *147*:820-823, 1983.

23. Blaser, M. J., Parsons, R. B., Wang, W. L.: Acute colitis caused by *Campylobacter fetus* ss. *jejuni*. Gastroenterology *78*:448-453, 1980.

24. Blaser, M. J., Taylor, D. N., and Echeverria, P.: Immune response to *Campylobacter jejuni* in a rural community in Thailand. J. Infect. Dis. *153*:249-254, 1986.

25. Blaser, M. J., Taylor, D. N., and Feldman, R. A.: Epidemiology of *Campylobacter jejuni* infections. Epidemiol. Rev. *5*:157-176, 1983.

26. Bokkenheuser, V. D., Richardson, N. J., Bryner, J. H., et al.: Detection of enteric campylobacteriosis in children. J. Clin. Microbiol. *9*:227-232, 1979.

27. Broman, T., Bergstrom, S., On, S. L., et al.: Isolation and characterization of *Campylobacter jejuni* subsp. *jejuni* from macaroni penguins (*Eudyptes chrysolophus*) in the subantarctic region. Appl. Environ. Microbiol. *66*:449-452, 2000.

28. Buck, G. E., Kelly, M. T., Pichanick, A. M., et al.: *Campylobacter jejuni* in newborns: A cause of asymptomatic bloody diarrhea. Am. J. Dis. Child. *136*:744, 1982.

29. Busato, A., Hofer, D., Lentze, T., et al.: Prevalence and infection risks of zoonotic enteropathogenic bacteria in Swiss cow-calf farms. Vet. Microbiol. *69*:251-263, 1999.

30. Butzler, J. P.: *Campylobacter*, from obscurity to celebrity. Clin. Microbiol. Infect. *10*:868-876, 2004.

31. Butzler, J. P., Dekeyser, P., Detrain, M., et al.: Related vibrio in stools. J. Pediatr. *82*:493-495, 1973.

32. Butzler, J. P., and Skirrow, M. B.: *Campylobacter* enteritis. Clin. Gastroenterol. *8*:737-765, 1979.

33. Calva, J. J., Ruiz-Palacios, G. M., Lopez-Vidal, A. B., et al.: Cohort study of intestinal infection with *Campylobacter* in Mexican children. Lancet *1*:503-506, 1988.

34. Chan, F. T., Stringel, G., and Mackenzie, A. M.: Isolation of *Campylobacter jejuni* from an appendix. J. Clin. Microbiol. *18*:422-424, 1983.

35. Chang, M. H., and Chen, T. C.: Reduction of *Campylobacter jejuni* in a simulated chicken digestive tract by Lactobacilli cultures. J. Food Prot. *63*:1594-1597, 2000.

36. Chen, M. L., Ge, Z., Fox, J. G., et al.: Disruption of tight junctions and induction of proinflammatory cytokine responses in colonic epithelial cells by *Campylobacter jejuni*. Infect. Immun. *74*:6581-6589, 2006.

37. Chowdhury, M. N., and al-Eissa, Y. A.: *Campylobacter* gastroenteritis in children in Riyadh, Saudi Arabia. J. Trop. Pediatr. *38*:158-161, 1992.

38. Cornelius, A. J., Nicol, C., and Hudson, J. A.: *Campylobacter* spp. in New Zealand raw sheep liver and human Campylobacteriosis cases. Int. J. Food Microbiol. *99*:99-105, 2005.

39. Cravioto, A., Reyes, R. E., Trujillo, F., et al.: Risk of diarrhea during the first year of life associated with initial and subsequent colonization by specific enteropathogens. Am. J. Epidemiol. *131*:886-904, 1990.

40. Davies, J. S., and Penfold, J. B.: *Campylobacter* urinary infection. Lancet *1*:1091-1092, 1979.

41. de Boer, P., Wagenaar, J. A., Achterberg, R. P., et al.: Generation of *Campylobacter jejuni* genetic diversity in vivo. Mol. Microbiol. *44*:351-359, 2002.

42. De Mol, P., and Bosmans, E.: *Campylobacter* enteritis in Central Africa. Lancet *1*:604, 1978.

43. De Mol, P., Brasseur, D., and Lauwers, S.: An important enteropathogen in a tropical area. *In* The 20th Interscience Conference on Antimicrobial Agents and Chemotherapy. New Orleans: American Society for Microbiology, 1980.

44. Deming, M. S., Tauxe, R. V., Blake, P. A., et al.: *Campylobacter* enteritis at a university: Transmission from eating chicken and from cats. Am. J. Epidemiol. *126*:526-534, 1987.

45. Denton, K. J., and Clarke, T.: Role of *Campylobacter jejuni* as a placental pathogen. J. Clin. Pathol. *45*:171-172, 1992.

46. Desheng, L., Zhixin, C., and Bolun, W.: Age distribution of diarrhoeal and healthy children infected with *Campylobacter jejuni*. J. Trop. Med. Hyg. *95*:218-220, 1992.

47. Dingle, K. E., Colles, F. M., Wareing, D. R., et al.: Multilocus sequence typing system for *Campylobacter jejuni*. J. Clin. Microbiol. *39*:14-23, 2001.

48. Doyle, M. P., and Roman, D. J.: Prevalence and survival of *Campylobacter jejuni* in unpasteurized milk. Appl. Environ. Microbiol. *44*:1154-1158, 1982.

49. Dronda, F., Garcia-Arata, I., Navas, E., et al.: Meningitis in adults due to *Campylobacter fetus* subspecies fetus. Clin. Infect. Dis. *27*:906-907, 1998.

50. DuPont, H. L.: Use of quinolones in the treatment of gastrointestinal infections. Eur. J. Clin. Microbiol. Infect. *10*:325-329, 1991.

51. Ebright, J. R., and Ryan, L. M.: Acute erosive reactive arthritis associated with *Campylobacter jejuni*-induced colitis. Am. J. Med. *76*:321-323, 1984.

52. Endtz, H. P., Ruijs, G. J., Zwinderman, A. H., et al.: Comparison of six media, including a semisolid agar, for the isolation of various *Campylobacter* species from stool specimens. J. Clin. Microbiol. *29*:1007-1010, 1991.

53. Engberg, J., Aarestrup, F. M., Taylor, D. E., et al.: Quinolone and macrolide resistance in *Campylobacter jejuni* and *C. coli*: Resistance mechanisms and trends in human isolates. Emerg. Infect. Dis. *7*:24-34, 2001.

54. Evans, R. G., and Dadswell, J. V.: Human vibriosis. Br. Med. J. *3*:240, 1967.

55. Falkow, S.: Bacterial entry into eukaryotic cells. Cell *65*:1099-1102, 1991.

56. Figueroa, G., Galeno, H., Troncoso, M., et al.: Prospective study of *Campylobacter jejuni* infection in Chilean infants evaluated by culture and serology. J. Clin. Microbiol. *27*:1040-1044, 1989.

57. Fitzgeorge, R. B., Baskerville, A., and Lander, K. P.: Experimental infection of rhesus monkeys with a human strain of *Campylobacter jejuni*. J. Hyg. (Lond.) *86*:343-351, 1981.

58. Fouts, D. E., Mongodin, E. F., Mandrell, R. E., et al.: Major structural differences and novel potential virulence mechanisms from the genomes of multiple *Campylobacter* species. PLoS. Biol. *3*:e15, 2005.

59. Frohli, P., Hanselmann, R., and Koelz, H. R.: [Erythema nodosum in *Campylobacter jejuni* colitis.] Schweiz. Med. Wochenschr. *120*:946-947, 1990.

60. Fry, B. N., Feng, S., Chen, Y. Y., et al.: The galE gene of *Campylobacter jejuni* is involved in lipopolysaccharide synthesis and virulence. Infect. Immun. *68*:2594-2601, 2000.

61. Fullerton, K. E., Ingram, L. A., Jones, T. F., et al.: Sporadic *Campylobacter* infection in infants: A population-based surveillance case-control study. Pediatr. Infect. Dis. J. *26*:19-24, 2007.

62. Gallagher, P., Chadwick, P., Jones, D. M., et al.: Acute pancreatitis associated with *Campylobacter* infection. Br. J. Surg. *68*:383, 1981.

63. Gaynor, E. C., Cawthraw, S., Manning, G., et al.: The genome-sequenced variant of *Campylobacter jejuni* NCTC 11168 and the original clonal clinical isolate differ markedly in colonization, gene expression, and virulence-associated phenotypes. J. Bacteriol. *186*:503-517, 2004.

64. Georges-Courbot, M. C., Beraud-Cassel, A. M., Gouandjika, I., et al.: Prospective study of enteric *Campylobacter* infections in children from birth to 6 months in the Central African Republic. J. Clin. Microbiol. *25*:836-839, 1987.

65. Gibreel, A., and Taylor, D. E.: Macrolide resistance in *Campylobacter jejuni* and *Campylobacter coli*. J. Antimicrob. Chemother. *58*:243-255, 2006.

66. Gifford, D. H., Shane, S. M., and Smith, R. E.: Prevalence of *Campylobacter jejuni* in Felidae in Baton Rouge, Louisiana. Int. J. Zoonoses *12*:67-73, 1985.

67. Glass, R. I., Stoll, B. J., Huq, M. I., et al.: Epidemiologic and clinical features of endemic *Campylobacter jejuni* infection in Bangladesh. J. Infect. Dis. *148*:292-296, 1983.

68. Goossens, H., Henocque, G., Kremp, L., et al.: Nosocomial outbreak of *Campylobacter jejuni* meningitis in newborn infants. Lancet *2*:146-149, 1986.

69. Grados, O., Bravo, N., Black, R. E., et al.: Paediatric *Campylobacter* diarrhoea from household exposure to live chickens in Lima, Peru. Bull. World Health Organ. *66*:369-374, 1988.

70. Gregson, N. A., Koblar, S., and Hughes, R. A.: Antibodies to gangliosides in Guillain-Barré syndrome: Specificity and relationship to clinical features. Q. J. Med. *86*:111-117, 1993.

71. Guandalini, S., Cucchiara, S., de Ritis, G., et al.: *Campylobacter* colitis in infants. J. Pediatr. *102*:72-74, 1983.

72. Guerrant, R. L., Lahita, R. G., Winn, W. C., Jr., et al.: *Campylobacter*iosis in man: Pathogenic mechanisms and review of 91 bloodstream infections. Am. J. Med. *65*:584-592, 1978.

73. Guerrant, R. L., Wanke, C. A., Pennie, R. A., et al.: Production of a unique cytotoxin by *Campylobacter jejuni*. Infect. Immun. *55*:2526-2530, 1987.

74. Guerry, P., Ewing, C. P., Hickey, T. E., et al.: Sialylation of lipooligosaccharide cores affects immunogenicity and serum resistance of *Campylobacter jejuni*. Infect. Immun. *68*:6656-6662, 2000.

75. Guidoboni, M., Ferreri, A. J., Ponzoni, M., et al.: Infectious agents in mucosa-associated lymphoid tissue–type lymphomas: Pathogenic role and therapeutic perspectives. Clin. Lymphoma Myeloma *6*:289-300, 2006.

76. Hald, B., and Madsen, M.: Healthy puppies and kittens as carriers of *Campylobacter* spp., with special reference to *Campylobacter upsaliensis*. J. Clin. Microbiol. *35*:3351-3352, 1997.

77. Hannu, T., Kauppi, M., Tuomala, M., et al.: Reactive arthritis following an outbreak of *Campylobacter jejuni* infection. J. Rheumatol. *31*:528-530, 2004.

78. Haq, J. A., and Rahman, K. M.: *Campylobacter jejuni* as a cause of acute diarrhoea in children: a study at an urban hospital in Bangladesh. J. Trop. Med. Hyg. *94*:50-54, 1991.

79. Hartung, H. P., Pollard, J. D., Harvey, G. K., et al.: Immunopathogenesis and treatment of the Guillain-Barré syndrome: Part I. Muscle Nerve *18*:137-153, 1995.

80. Hartung, H. P., Pollard, J. D., Harvey, G. K., et al.: Immunopathogenesis and treatment of the Guillain-Barré syndrome. Part II. Muscle Nerve *18*:154-164, 1995.

81. Helms, M., Vastrup, P., Gerner-Smidt, P., et al.: Short and long term mortality associated with foodborne bacterial gastrointestinal infections: Registry based study. BMJ *326*:357, 2003.

82. Hendrixson, D. R., and DiRita, V. J.: Identification of *Campylobacter jejuni* genes involved in commensal colonization of the chick gastrointestinal tract. Mol. Microbiol. *52*:471-484, 2004.

83. Hill, S. L., Cheney, J. M., Taton-Allen, G. F., et al.: Prevalence of enteric zoonotic organisms in cats. J. Am. Vet. Med. Assoc. *216*:687-692, 2000.

84. Hindiyeh, M., Jense, S., Hohmann, S., et al.: Rapid detection of *Campylobacter jejuni* in stool specimens by an enzyme immunoassay and surveillance for *Campylobacter* upsaliensis in the greater Salt Lake City area. J. Clin. Microbiol. *38*:3076-3079, 2000.

85. Hofreuter, D., Tsai, J., Watson, R. O., et al.: Unique features of a highly pathogenic *Campylobacter jejuni* strain. Infect. Immun. *74*:4694-4707, 2006.

86. Hofstetr, A., Dvorakova, A., Nikodymova, I., et al.: [A 3-year follow-up study of the incidence of *Campylobacter*iosis in a pediatric population]. Cesk. Pediatr. *45*:651-654, 1990.

87. Hood, A. M., Pearson, A. D., and Shahamat, M.: The extent of surface contamination of retailed chickens with *Campylobacter jejuni* serogroups. Epidemiol. Infect. *100*:17-25, 1988.

88. Hooper, D. C.: Emerging mechanisms of fluoroquinolone resistance. Emerg. Infect. Dis. *7*:337-341, 2001.

89. Hossain, M. A., Kabir, I., Albert, M. J., et al.: *Campylobacter jejuni* bacteraemia in children with diarrhoea in Bangladesh: Report of six cases. J. Diarrhoeal Dis. Res. *10*:101-104, 1992.

90. Hudson, P. J., Vogt, R. L., Brondum, J., et al.: Isolation of *Campylobacter jejuni* from milk during an outbreak of *Campylobacter*iosis. J. Infect. Dis. *150*:789, 1984.

91. Hughes, R. A., and Rees, J. H.: Guillain-Barré syndrome. Curr. Opin. Neurol. *7*:386-392, 1994.

92. Humphrey, C. D., Montag, D. M., and Pittman, F. E.: Experimental infection of hamsters with *Campylobacter jejuni*. J. Infect. Dis. *151*:485-493, 1985.

93. Humphrey, T. J., and Beckett, P.: *Campylobacter jejuni* in dairy cows and raw milk. Epidemiol. Infect. *98*:263-269, 1987.

94. Humphrey, T. J., Henley, A., and Lanning, D. G.: The colonization of broiler chickens with *Campylobacter jejuni*: Some epidemiological investigations. Epidemiol. Infect. *110*:601-607, 1993.

95. Humphrey, T. J., Jorgensen, F., Frost, J. A., et al.: Prevalence and subtypes of ciprofloxacin-resistant *Campylobacter* spp. in commercial poultry flocks before, during, and after treatment with fluoroquinolones. Antimicrob. Agents Chemother. *49*:690-698, 2005.

96. Hutchinson, D. N., Bolton, F. J., Hinchliffe, P. M., et al.: Evidence of udder excretion of *Campylobacter jejuni* as the cause of milk-borne *Campylobacter* outbreak. J. Hyg. (Lond.) *94*:205-215, 1985.

97. Ichikawa, H., Sugita, K., Fukui, T., et al.: [Fisher's syndrome following *Campylobacter jejuni* enteritis: A case report and review of the literature.] Rinsho Shinkeigaku *35*:391-395, 1995.

98. Jacobs, B. C., van Doorn, P., Schmitz, P. I., et al.: *Campylobacter jejuni* infections and anti-GM1 antibodies in Guillain-Barré syndrome. Ann, Neurol, *40*:181-187, 1996.

99. Johnsen, K., Ostensen, M., Melbye, A. C., et al.: HLA-B27-negative arthritis related to *Campylobacter jejuni* enteritis in three children and two adults. Acta Med. Scand. *214*:165-168, 1983.

100. Johnson, W, M., and Lior, H.: Toxins produced by *Campylobacter jejuni* and *Campylobacter coli*. Lancet *1*:229-230, 1984.

101. Johnson, W, M., and Lior, H.: Cytotoxic and cytotonic factors produced by *Campylobacter jejuni*, *Campylobacter coli*, and *Campylobacter laridis*. J. Clin. Microbiol. *24*:275-281, 1986.

102. Jones, D. M., Eldridge, J., and Dale, B.: Serological response to *Campylobacter jejuni/coli* infection. J. Clin. Pathol. *33*:767-769, 1980.

103. Jones, D. M., Robinson, D. A., and Eldridge, J.: Serological studies in two outbreaks of *Campylobacter jejuni* infection. J. Hyg. (Lond.) *87*:163-170, 1981.

104. Kaldor, J., and Speed, B. R.: Guillain-Barré syndrome and *Campylobacter jejuni*: A serological study. Br. Med. J. (Clin. Res. Ed.) *288*:1867-1870, 1984.

105. Kaldor, J., Pritchard, H., Serpell, A., et al.: Serum antibodies in *Campylobacter* enteritis. J. Clin. Microbiol. *18*:1-4, 1983.

106. Kalkay, M. N., Ayanian, Z. S., Lehaf, E. A., et al.: *Campylobacter*-induced toxic megacolon. Am. J. Gastroenterol. *78*:557-559, 1983.

107. Kanipes, M. I., Holder, L. C., and Corcoran, A. T., et al.: A deep-rough mutant of *Campylobacter jejuni* 81-176 is noninvasive for intestinal epithelial cells. Infect. Immun. *72*:2452-2455, 2004.

108. Karlyshev, A. V., Ketley, J. M., and Wren, B. W.: The *Campylobacter jejuni* glycome. FEMS Microbiol. Rev. *29*:377-390, 2005.

109. Karmali, M. A., and Fleming, P. C.: *Campylobacter* enteritis. Can. Med. Assoc. J. *120*:1525-1532, 1979.

110. Kendall, E. J., and Tanner, E. I.: *Campylobacter* enteritis in general practice. J. Hyg. (Lond.) *88*:155-163, 1982.

111. Khalafalla, F. A.: *Campylobacter jejuni* in poultry giblets. Zentralbl. Veterinarmed. B *37*:31-34, 1990.

112. King, E.: Human infections with *Vibrio fetus* and a closely related *Vibrio*. J. Infect. Dis. *101*:119-128, 1957.

113. King, E.: The laboratory recognition of *Vibrio fetus* and a closely related *Vibrio* isolated from cases of human vibriosis. Ann. N. Y. Acad. Sci. *98*:700-711, 1962.

114. Kopecko, D. J., Hu, L., and Zaal, K. J.: *Campylobacter jejuni*: Microtubule-dependent invasion. Trends Microbiol. *9*:389-396, 2001.

115. Korman, T. M., Varley, C. C., and Spelman, D. W.: Acute hepatitis associated with *Campylobacter jejuni* bacteraemia. Eur. J. Clin. Microbiol. Infect. Dis. *16*:678-681, 1997.

116. Koulla-Shiro, S., Loe, C., and Ekoe, T.: Prevalence of *Campylobacter* enteritis in children from Yaounde (Cameroon). Cent. Afr. J. Med. *41*:91-94, 1995.

117. Kuroki, S., Saida, T., Nukina, M., et al.: *Campylobacter jejuni* strains from patients with Guillain-Barré syndrome belong mostly to Penner serogroup

118. Lawson, A. J., Logan, J. M., O'Neill, G. L., et al.: Large-scale survey of *Campylobacter* species in human gastroenteritis by PCR and PCR–enzyme-linked immunosorbent assay. J. Clin. Microbiol. *37*:3860-3864, 1999.

119. Lawson, A. J., Shafi, M. S., Pathak, K., et al.: Detection of *Campylobacter* in gastroenteritis: Comparison of direct PCR assay of faecal samples with selective culture. Epidemiol. Infect. *121*:547-553, 1998.

120. Leyes, M., Vara, F., Reina, J., et al.: [*Campylobacter* gastroenteritis in patients with human immunodeficiency virus infection.] Enferm. Infecc. Microbiol. Clin. *12*:332-336, 1994.

121. Lillehaug, A., Monceyron Jonassen, C., Bergsjo, B., et al.: Screening of feral pigeon (*Colomba livia*), mallard (*Anas platyrhynchos*) and graylag goose (*Anser anser*) populations for *Campylobacter* spp., *Salmonella* spp., avian influenza virus and avian paramyxovirus. Acta Vet. Scand. *46*:193-202, 2005.

122. Ljungh, A., and Wadstrom, T.: Lactic acid bacteria as probiotics. Curr. Issues Intest. Microbiol. *7*:73-89, 2006.

123. Madden, J. M., McCardell, B. A., and Shah, D. B.: Cytotoxin production by members of genus *Vibrio*. Lancet *2*:1217-1218, 1984.

124. Mahajan, S., and Rodgers, F. G.: Isolation, characterization, and host-cell-binding properties of a cytotoxin from *Campylobacter jejuni*. J. Clin. Microbiol. *28*:1314-1320, 1990.

125. Maki, M., Maki, R., and Vesikari, T.: Faecal leucocytes in *Campylobacter*-associated diarrhoea in infants. Acta Paediatr. Scand. *68*:271-272, 1979.

126. Manfredi, R., Nanetti, A., Ferri, M., et al.: Fatal *Campylobacter jejuni* bacteraemia in patients with AIDS. J. Med. Microbiol. *48*:601-603, 1999.

127. Martin, P. M., Mathiot, J., Ipero, J., et al.: Immune response to *Campylobacter jejuni* and *Campylobacter coli* in a cohort of children from birth to 2 years of age. Infect. Immun. *57*:2542-2546, 1989.

128. Martinez, R. M., Figueras, M. P., Ramos, C., et al.: [*Campylobacter jejuni* and HIV infection.] Enferm. Infecc. Microbiol. Clin. *12*:90-94, 1994.

129. McCarthy, N., and Giesecke, J.: Incidence of Guillain-Barré syndrome following infection with *Campylobacter jejuni*. Am. J. Epidemiol. *153*:610-614, 2001.

130. McFadyean, F., and Stockman, S.: Report to the Departmental Committee Appointed by the Board of Agriculture and Fisheries to Inquire into Epizootic Abortion. III Abortion in Sheep. London: His Majesty's Stationary Office, 1913.

131. Mead, P. S., Slutsker, L., Dietz, V., et al.: Food-related illness and death in the United States. Emerg. Infect. Dis. *5*:607-625, 1999.

132. Melamed, I., Bujanover, Y., Igra, Y. S., et al.: *Campylobacter* enteritis in normal and immunodeficient children. Am. J. Dis. Child. *137*:752-753, 1983.

133. Mentzing, L. O.: Waterborne outbreaks of *Campylobacter* enteritis in central Sweden. Lancet *2*:352-354, 1981.

134. Mishu, B., and Blaser, M. J.: Role of infection due to *Campylobacter jejuni* in the initiation of Guillain-Barre syndrome. Clin. Infect. Dis. *17*:104-108, 1993.

135. Morishita, T. Y., Aye, P. P., Harr, B. S., et al.: Evaluation of an avian-specific probiotic to reduce the colonization and shedding of *Campylobacter jejuni* in broilers. Avian Dis. *41*:850-855, 1997.

136. Morooka, T., Umeda, A., and Amako, K.: Motility as an intestinal colonization factor for *Campylobacter jejuni*. J. Gen. Microbiol. *131*:1973-1980, 1985.

137. Morton, W. R., Bronsdon, M., Mickelsen, G., et al.: Identification of *Campylobacter jejuni* in *Macaca fascicularis* imported from Indonesia. Lab. Anim. Sci. *33*:187-188, 1983.

138. Moscuna, M., Gross, Z., Korenblum, R., et al.: Septic abortion due to *Campylobacter jejuni*. Eur. J. Clin. Microbiol. Infect. Dis. *8*:800-801, 1989.

139. Moyen, E. N., Bonneville, F., and Fauchere, J. L.: [Modification of intestinal colonization and translocation of *Campylobacter jejuni* by erythromycin and an extract of *Lactobacillus acidophilus* in axenic mice.] Ann. Inst. Pasteur Microbiol. *137A*:199-207, 1986.

140. Nachamkin, I., Allos, B. M., and Ho, T.: *Campylobacter* species and Guillain-Barré syndrome. Clin. Microbiol. Rev. *11*:555-567, 1998.

141. Nath, G., Shukla, B. N., Reddy, D. C., et al.: A community study on the aetiology of childhood diarrhoea with special reference to *Campylobacter jejuni* in a semiurban slum of Varanasi, India. J. Diarrhoeal Dis. Res. *11*:165-168, 1993.

142. Nelson, J. M., Chiller, T. M., Powers, J. H., et al.: Fluoroquinolone-resistant *Campylobacter* species and the withdrawal of fluoroquinolones from use in poultry: a public health success story. Clin. Infect. Dis. *44*:977-980, 2007.

143. Nelson, J. M., Smith, K. E., Vugia, D. J., et al.: Prolonged diarrhea due to ciprofloxacin-resistant *Campylobacter* infection. J. Infect. Dis. *190*:1150-1157, 2004.

144. Oberhelman, R. A., Gilman, R. H., Sheen, P., et al.: *Campylobacter* transmission in a Peruvian shantytown: A longitudinal study using strain typing of *Campylobacter* isolates from chickens and humans in household clusters. J. Infect. Dis. *187*:260-269, 2003.

145. Obiri-Danso, K., and Jones, K.: Distribution and seasonality of microbial indicators and thermophilic campylobacters in two freshwater bathing sites on the River Lune in northwest England. J. Appl. Microbiol. *87*:822-832, 1999.

146. On, S. L.: Identification methods for campylobacters, helicobacters, and related organisms. Clin. Microbiol. Rev. *9*:405-422, 1996.

147. Oyofo, B. A., Soderquist, R., Lesmana, M., et al.: Norwalk-like virus and bacterial pathogens associated with cases of gastroenteritis onboard a US Navy ship. Am. J. Trop. Med. Hyg. *61*:904-908, 1999.

148. Pacha, R. E., Clark, G. W., Williams, E. A., et al.: Migratory birds of central Washington as reservoirs of *Campylobacter jejuni*. Can. J. Microbiol. *34*:80-82, 1988.

149. Pai, C. H., Sorger, S., Lackman, L., et al.: *Campylobacter* gastroenteritis in children. J. Pediatr. *94*:589-591, 1979.

150. Paisley, J. W., Mirrett, S., Lauer, B. A., et al.: Dark-field microscopy of human feces for presumptive diagnosis of *Campylobacter fetus* subsp. *jejuni enteritis*. J. Clin. Microbiol. *15*:61-63, 1982.

151. Palmgren, H., Sellin, M., Bergstrom, S., et al.: Enteropathogenic bacteria in migrating birds arriving in Sweden. Scand. J. Infect. Dis. *29*:565-568, 1997.

152. Park, C. H., Hixon, D. L., Polhemus, A. S., et al.: A rapid diagnosis of *Campylobacter* enteritis by direct smear examination. Am. J. Clin. Pathol. *80*:388-390, 1983.

153. Parker, C. T., Quinones, B., Miller, W. G., et al.: Comparative genomic analysis of *Campylobacter jejuni* strains reveals diversity due to genomic elements similar to those present in *C. jejuni* strain RM1221. J. Clin. Microbiol. *44*:4125-4135, 2006.

154. Parkhill, J., Wren, B. W., Mungall, K., et al.: The genome sequence of the food-borne pathogen *Campylobacter jejuni* reveals hypervariable sequences. Nature *403*:665-668, 2000.

155. Pearson, A. D., and Healing, T. D.: The surveillance and control of *Campylobacter* infection. Commun Dis Rep CDR Rev *2*:R133-139, 1992.

156. Pepersack, F., Prigogyne, T., Butzler, J. P., et al.: *Campylobacter jejuni* post-transfusional septicaemia. Lancet *2*:911, 1979.

157. Perera, V. N., Nachamkin, I., Ung, H., et al.: Molecular mimicry in *Campylobacter jejuni*: Role of the lipo-oligosaccharide core oligosaccharide in inducing anti-ganglioside antibodies. FEMS Immunol. Med. Microbiol. *50*:27-36, 2007.

158. Perkins, D. J., and Newstead, G. L.: *Campylobacter jejuni* enterocolitis causing peritonitis, ileitis and intestinal obstruction. Aust. N. Z. J. Surg. *64*:55-58, 1994.

159. Perlman, D. M., Ampel, N. M., Schifman, R. B., et al.: Persistent *Campylobacter jejuni* infections in patients infected with the human immunodeficiency virus (HIV). Ann. Intern. Med. *108*:540-546, 1988.

160. Peterson, M. C.: Rheumatic manifestations of *Campylobacter jejuni* and *C. fetus* infections in adults. Scand. J. Rheumatol. *23*:167-170, 1994.

161. Peterson, M. C., Farr, R. W., and Castiglia, M.: Prosthetic hip infection and bacteremia due to *Campylobacter jejuni* in a patient with AIDS. Clin. Infect. Dis. *16*:439-440, 1993.

162. Pigrau, C., Bartolome, R., Almirante, B., et al.: Bacteremia due to *Campylobacter* species: clinical findings and antimicrobial susceptibility patterns. Clin. Infect. Dis. *25*:1414-1420, 1997.

163. Ponka, A., Martio, J., and Kosunen, T. U.: Reiter's syndrome in association with enteritis due to *Campylobacter fetus* ssp. *jejuni*. Ann. Rheum. Dis. *40*:414-415, 1981.

164. Pope, J. E., Krizova, A., Garg, A. X., et al.: *Campylobacter* reactive arthritis: A systematic review. Semin. Arthritis Rheum. *37*:48-55, 2007.

165. Prendergast, M. M., Tribble, D. R., Baqar, S., et al.: In vivo phase variation and serologic response to lipooligosaccharide of *Campylobacter jejuni* in experimental human infection. Infect. Immun. *72*:916-922, 2004.

166. Prescott, J. F., Barker, I. K., Manninen, K. I., et al.: *Campylobacter jejuni* colitis in gnotobiotic dogs. Can. J. Comp. Med. *45*:377-383, 1981.

167. Ramiro Cruz, J., Cano, F., Bartlett, A. V., et al.: Infection, diarrhea, and dysentery caused by *Shigella* species and *Campylobacter jejuni* among Guatemalan rural children. Pediatr. Infect. Dis. J. *13*:216-223, 1994.

168. Reed, R. P., Friedland, I. R., Wegerhoff, F. O., et al.: *Campylobacter* bacteremia in children. Pediatr. Infect. Dis. J. *15*:345-348, 1996.

169. Rees, J. H., Soudain, S. E., Gregson, N. A., et al.: *Campylobacter jejuni* infection and Guillain-Barré syndrome. N. Engl. J. Med. *333*:1374-1379, 1995.

170. Rettig, P. J.: *Campylobacter* infections in human beings. J. Pediatr. *94*:855-864, 1979.

171. Rhodes, K. M., and Tattersfield, A. E.: Guillain-Barré syndrome associated with *Campylobacter* infection. Br. Med. J. (Clin. Res. Ed.) *285*:173-174, 1982.

172. Riley, L. W., and Finch, M. J.: Results of the first year of national surveillance of *Campylobacter* infections in the United States. J. Infect. Dis. *151*:956-959, 1985.

173. Ruiz-Palacios, G. M., Calva, J. J., Pickering, L. K., et al.: Protection of breast-fed infants against *Campylobacter* diarrhea by antibodies in human milk. J. Pediatr. *116*:707-713, 1990.

174. Ruiz-Palacios, G. M., Torres, J., Torres, N. I., et al.: Cholera-like enterotoxin produced by *Campylobacter jejuni*: Characterisation and clinical significance. Lancet *2*:250-253, 1983.

175. Sanchez, R., Fernandez-Baca, V., Diaz, M. D., et al.: Evolution of susceptibilities of *Campylobacter* spp. to quinolones and macrolides. Antimicrob. Agents Chemother. *38*:1879-1882, 1994.

176. Sazie, E. S., and Titus, A. E.: Rapid diagnosis of *Campylobacter* enteritis. Ann. Intern. Med. *96*:62-63, 1982.

177. Schaad, U. B.: Reactive arthritis associated with *Campylobacter* enteritis. Pediatr. Infect. Dis. *1*:328-332, 1982.

178. Schmidt-Ott, R., Brass, F., Scholz, C., et al.: Improved serodiagnosis of *Campylobacter jejuni* infections using recombinant antigens. J. Med. Microbiol. *54*:761-767, 2005.

179. Schneider, A., Runzi, M., Peitgen, K., et al.: *Campylobacter jejuni*-induced severe colitis: A rare cause of toxic megacolon. Z. Gastroenterol. *38*:307-309, 2000.

180. Schneider, E. N., Havens, J. M., Scott, M. A., et al.: Molecular diagnosis of *Campylobacter jejuni* infection in cases of focal active colitis. Am. J. Surg. Pathol. *30*:782-785, 2006.

181. Schonberg-Norio, D., Sarna, S., Hanninen, M. L., et al.: Strain and host characteristics of *Campylobacter jejuni* infections in Finland. Clin. Microbiol. Infect. *12*:754-760, 2006.

182. Schonberg-Norio, D., Takkinen, J., Hanninen, M. L., et al.: Swimming and *Campylobacter* infections. Emerg. Infect. Dis. *10*:1474-1477, 2004.

183. Schumer, W., Wong, T. P., Wallace, S., et al.: Standard linear plans in single channel high dose rate brachytherapy: A dosimetric analysis. Med. Dosim. *23*:307-310, 1998.

184. Shanker, S., Rosenfield, J. A., Davey, G. R., et al.: *Campylobacter jejuni*: Incidence in processed broilers and biotype distribution in human and broiler isolates. Appl. Environ. Microbiol. *43*:1219-1220, 1982.

185. Simbert, R.: Genus *Campylobacter*. *In* Krieg, N. R., and Holt, H. (eds.): Manual of Systematic Bacteriology. Vol. 1. Baltimore, Williams & Wilkins, 1984, p. 111.

186. Simor, A. E., and Ferro, S.: *Campylobacter jejuni* infection occurring during pregnancy. Eur. J. Clin. Microbiol. Infect. Dis. *9*:142-144, 1990.

187. Simor, A. E., Karmali, M. A., Jadavji, T., et al.: Abortion and perinatal sepsis associated with *Campylobacter* infection. Rev. Infect. Dis. *8*:397-402, 1986.

188. Sjogren, E., Kaijser, B., and Werner, M.: Antimicrobial susceptibilities of *Campylobacter jejuni* and *Campylobacter coli* isolated in Sweden: A 10-year follow-up report. Antimicrob. Agents Chemother. *36*:2847-2849, 1992.

189. Skirrow, M. B.: *Campylobacter* enteritis: A "new" disease. Br. Med. J. *2*:9-11, 1977.

190. Skirrow, M. B., Jones, D. M., Sutcliffe, E., et al.: *Campylobacter* bacteraemia in England and Wales, 1981-91. Epidemiol. Infect. *110*:567-573, 1993.

191. Smith, K. E., Besser, J. M., Hedberg, C. W., et al.: Quinolone-resistant *Campylobacter jejuni* infections in Minnesota, 1992-1998: Investigation team. N. Engl. J. Med. *340*:1525-1532, 1999.

192. Smith, M. V., 2nd, and Muldoon, P. J.: *Campylobacter fetus* subspecies *jejuni* (*Vibrio fetus*) from commercially processed poultry. Appl. Microbiol. *27*:995-996, 1974.

193. Son, I., Englen, M. D., Berrang, M. E., et al.: Prevalence of *Arcobacter* and *Campylobacter* on broiler carcasses during processing. Int. J. Food Microbiol. *113*:16-22, 2007.

194. Sota Busselo, I., Onate Vergara, E., Perez-Yarza, E. G., et al.: [Erythema nodosum: etiological changes in the last two decades.] An. Pediatr. (Barc.) *61*:403-407, 2004.

195. Spira, W. M., Sack, R. B., and Froehlich, J. L.: Simple adult rabbit model for *Vibrio cholerae* and enterotoxigenic *Escherichia coli* diarrhea. Infect. Immun. *32*:739-747, 1981.

196. Stanley, K. N., Wallace, J. S., Currie, J. E., et al.: The seasonal variation of thermophilic *Campylobacters* in beef cattle, dairy cattle and calves. J. Appl. Microbiol. *85*:472-480, 1998.

197. Stern, N. J., Bannov, V. A., Svetoch, E. A., et al.: Distribution and characterization of *Campylobacter* spp. from Russian poultry. J. Food Prot. *67*:239-245, 2004.

198. Svedhem, A., Gunnarsson, H., and Kaijser, B.: Diffusion-in-gel enzyme-linked immunosorbent assay for routine detection of IgG and IgM antibodies to *Campylobacter jejuni*. J. Infect. Dis. *148*:82-92, 1983.

199. Tam, C. C., O'Brien, S. J., Petersen, I., et al.: Guillain-Barré syndrome and preceding infection with *Campylobacter*, influenza and Epstein-Barr virus in the General Practice Research Database. PLoS. ONE *2*:e344, 2007.

200. Tauxe, R. V.: Epidemiology of *Campylobacter jejuni* infections in the United States and other industrialized countries. *In* Nachamkin, I., Blaser, M. J., and Tompkins, L. S. (eds.): *Campylobacter jejuni*: Current Strategy and Future Trends. Washington, D.C.: American Society for Microbiology, 1992, pp. 9-19.

201. Tauxe, R. V., Deming, M. S., and Blake, P. A.: *Campylobacter jejuni* infections on college campuses: A national survey. Am. J. Public Health *75*:659-660, 1985.

202. Tauxe, R. V., Hargrett-Bean, N., Patton, C. M., et al.: *Campylobacter* isolates in the United States, 1982-1986. M. M. W. R. CDC Surveill. Summ. *37*:1-13, 1988.

203. Taylor, D. N., Echeverria, P., Pitarangsi, C., et al.: Influence of strain characteristics and immunity on the epidemiology of *Campylobacter* infections in Thailand. J. Clin. Microbiol. *26*:863-868, 1988.

204. Taylor, D. N., McDermott, K. T., Little, J. R., et al.: *Campylobacter* enteritis from untreated water in the Rocky Mountains. Ann. Intern. Med. *99*:38-40, 1983.

205. Taylor, D. N., Perlman, D. M., Echeverria, P. D., et al.: *Campylobacter* immunity and quantitative excretion rates in Thai children. J. Infect. Dis. *168*:754-758, 1993.

206. Tee, W., and Mijch, A.: *Campylobacter jejuni* bacteremia in human immunodeficiency virus (HIV)–infected and non-HIV-infected patients: Comparison of clinical features and review. Clin. Infect. Dis. *26*:91-96, 1998.

207. Tenover, F. C., Carlson, L., Barbagallo, S., et al.: DNA probe culture confirmation assay for identification of thermophilic *Campylobacter* species. J. Clin. Microbiol. *28*:1284-1287, 1990.

208. Ternhag, A., Asikainen, T., Giesecke, J., et al.: A meta-analysis on the effects of antibiotic treatment on duration of symptoms caused by infection with *Campylobacter* species. Clin. Infect. Dis. *44*:696-700, 2007.

209. Teunis, P. F., Nagelkerke, N. J., and Haas, C. N.: Dose response models for infectious gastroenteritis. Risk Anal. *19*:1251-1260, 1999.

210. Thomas, K., Chan, K. N., and Ribeiro, C. D.: *Campylobacter jejuni/coli* meningitis in a neonate. Br. Med. J. *280*:1301-1302, 1980.

211. Tokumaru, M., Konuma, H., Umesako, M., et al.: Rates of detection of *Salmonella* and *Campylobacter* in meats in response to the sample size and the infection level of each species. Int. J. Food Microbiol. *13*:41-46, 1991.
212. Tolcin, R., LaSalvia, M. M., Kirkley, B. A., et al.: Evaluation of the Alexon-trend ProSpecT *Campylobacter* microplate assay. J. Clin. Microbiol. *38*:3853-3855, 2000.
213. Torres, O., and Cruz, J. R.: Protection against *Campylobacter* diarrhea: Role of milk IgA antibodies against bacterial surface antigens. Acta Paediatr. *82*:835-838, 1993.
214. Vandamme, P., and De Ley, J.: Proposal for a new family, *Campylobacter*aceae. Int. J. Syst. Bacteriol. *41*:451-455, 1991.
215. Vanhoof, R., Gordts, B., Dierickx, R., et al.: Bacteriostatic and bactericidal activities of 24 antimicrobial agents against *Campylobacter fetus* subsp. *jejuni*. Antimicrob. Agents Chemother. *18*:118-121, 1980.
216. Vanniasinkam, T., Lanser, J. A., and Barton, M. D.: PCR for the detection of *Campylobacter* spp. in clinical specimens. Lett. Appl. Microbiol. *28*:52-56, 1999.
217. Vernon, M., and Chatelain, R.: Taxonomic study of the genus *Campylobacter* and designation of the neotype strain for the type species, *Campylobacter* fetus. Int. J. Syst. Bacteriol. *23*:122-134, 1973.
218. Vesikari, T., Huttunen, L., and Maki, R.: Perinatal *Campylobacter* fetus ss *jejuni* enteritis. Acta Paediatr. Scand. *70*:261-263, 1981.
219. Vinzent, R., Dumas, J., and Picard, N.: Septicemia grave au cours de la grossesse due à vibrion: Avortement consecutif. Bull. Acad. Natl. Med. *131*:122-134, 1947.
220. Waltner-Toews, D., Martin, S. W., and Meek, A. H.: An epidemiological study of selected calf pathogens on Holstein dairy farms in southwestern Ontario. Can. J. Vet. Res. *50*:307-313, 1986.
221. Wang, H., and Murdoch, D. R.: Detection of *Campylobacter* species in faecal samples by direct Gram stain microscopy. Pathology *36*:343-344, 2004.
222. Warner, D. P., Bryner, J. H., and Beran, G. W.: Epidemiologic study of campylobacteriosis in Iowa cattle and the possible role of unpasteurized milk as a vehicle of infection. Am. J. Vet. Res. *47*:254-258, 1986.
223. Wassenaar, T. M., and Newell, D. G.: Genotyping of *Campylobacter* spp. Appl. Environ. Microbiol. *66*:1-9, 2000.
224. Wolfs, T. F., Duim, B., Geelen, S. P., et al.: Neonatal sepsis by *Campylobacter jejuni*: Genetically proven transmission from a household puppy. Clin. Infect. Dis. *32*:E97-E99, 2001.
225. Wright, E. P., and Seager, J.: Convulsions associated with *Campylobacter* enteritis. Br. Med. J. *281*:454, 1980.
226. Young, D. M., Biao, J., Zheng, Z., et al.: Isolation of *Campylobacter jejuni* in Hunan, the People's Republic of China: Epidemiology and comparison of Chinese and American methodology. Diagn. Microbiol. Infect. Dis. *5*:143-149, 1986.
227. Yuki, N., and Koga, M.: Bacterial infections in Guillain-Barré and Fisher syndromes. Curr. Opin. Neurol. *19*:451-457, 2006.
228. Yuki, N., Ichikawa, H., and Doi, A.: Fisher syndrome after *Campylobacter jejuni* enteritis: Human leukocyte antigen and the bacterial serotype. J. Pediatr. *126*:55-57, 1995.

CHAPTER 143

OTHER *CAMPYLOBACTER* SPECIES

Robert J. Leggiadro

Although they are not isolated as frequently as are *Campylobacter jejuni* and *Campylobacter coli*, the "other" *Campylobacter* spp. are gaining recognition as human pathogens. *Campylobacter fetus*, a classic cause of perinatal infection, also is an infrequent cause of bacteremia in immunocompromised hosts. *Campylobacter upsaliensis*, *Campylobacter lari*, and *Campylobacter hyointestinalis* are associated primarily with diarrheal disease. Populations affected by these three species include normal as well as immunosuppressed hosts, especially persons infected with human immunodeficiency virus (HIV), with or without a history of animal exposure. The clinical spectrum of these organisms should expand as the special diagnostic tests needed to identify them become more widely available.

HISTORY

McFadyean and Stockman[59] first described the organisms now known as campylobacters in 1913. These *Vibrio*-like organisms were implicated as a cause of epizootic abortion in sheep, and a few years later, Smith[82] reported their association with bovine abortion as well and gave them the name *Vibrio fetus*. Although never confirmed microbiologically, these organisms are thought to have been *C. fetus* according to current nomenclature.[49] Vinzent and associates[94] first reported *Campylobacter* infection in humans in 1947. These investigators described a pregnant woman with *V. fetus* bacteremia who subsequently aborted at 6 months' gestation. In addition to pregnancy, gastrectomy, tooth extraction, heart disease, diabetes, and cirrhosis were predisposing conditions in King's 1957 review of 15 patients with *V. fetus* bacteremia.[51]

Many reports describing "new" *Campylobacter* spp. were published in the 1980s and early 1990s. *C. upsaliensis* was reported to be a pathogen in dogs and humans.[69,77] *C. lari*, a common isolate from healthy seagulls, was found to be a cause of gastrointestinal and extraintestinal disease in humans.[4,87] Originally identified in the intestines of swine with proliferative ileitis, *C. hyointestinalis* was reported first as a human pathogen in a homosexual man with proctitis.[26] The hydrogen-requiring campylobacters, *Campylo-*

bacter concisus,[93] *Campylobacter rectus*,[72] and *Campylobacter curvus*, have been associated with periodontal disease. *Campylobacter sputorum* has been identified in abscesses,[64] as well as in bacteremia,[41,88] and *Campylobacter mucosalis* was reported in two children with diarrhea.[27]

Once called *Campylobacter*-like organisms, *Helicobacter cinaedi* and *Helicobacter fennelliae* now are classified in the *Helicobacter* genus.[66] These pathogens cause enteritis and proctocolitis in homosexual men and, on occasion, bacteremia.[68,90] Two former *Campylobacter* spp., *Arcobacter butzleri* and *Arcobacter cryaerophilus*, are associated with abortion and enteritis in cattle and pigs, in addition to bacteremia and diarrhea in humans.[50]

MICROBIOLOGY

Campylobacter is a Greek word meaning "curved rod." Members of this genus are gram-negative, curved, S-shaped or spiral, non–spore-forming rods that are 0.2 to 0.9 μm wide and 0.5 to 5 μm long.[64] Organisms are motile by means of a single polar flagellum, but some have a flagellum at each pole.[37] They are microaerophilic and have a respiratory type of metabolism.[64] Campylobacters are oxidase-positive and reduce nitrates but do not ferment or oxidize carbohydrates.[70] Although most grow at 37° C, *C. jejuni*, the *Campylobacter* sp. most commonly identified in humans, grows optimally at 42° C.[2]

Most *Campylobacter* spp. require a microaerobic atmosphere containing approximately 5 percent oxygen, 10 percent carbon dioxide, and 85 percent nitrogen for optimal recovery.[64] Some species such as *C. sputorum*, *C. concisus*, *C. mucosalis*, *C. curvus*, *C. rectus*, and *C. hyointestinalis* may require hydrogen for primary isolation and growth. Many different selective media for isolation of *Campylobacter* spp. have been developed, but because of species differences in antibiotic resistance patterns, no single formulation isolates all species of clinical importance.[37] For example, *C. jejuni* and *C. coli* are resistant to cephalothin, whereas *C. fetus* is susceptible. A filtration method with nonselective media may be used to complement direct culture on selective media for the detection of antibiotic-susceptible *Campylobacter* spp. Because of their small

TABLE 143-1   Growth and Biochemical Characteristics of Species of the Genus *Campylobacter*

Species	25° C	37° C	42° C	Anaerobically	In CO_2 Inhibitor	Glycine 1%	Bile 1%	Growth Charcoal Casein Deoxycholate
C. lari	−	+	+	+	+	+	+	+
C. upsaliensis	−	+	+	+	+	−	+	+
C. fetus	+	+	(−)	−	+	+	−	−
C. hyointestinalis	(+)	+*	+	+	+	+	NA	NA
C. concisus	−	+	+	+	+	+	NA	NA
C. mucosalis	+	+	+	+	+	+	NA	NA
C. sputorum†	-	+	+	+	+	+	+	+

*Best at 35° C.
†*C. sputorum has three biovars with different biochemical characteristics.*
+, positive; −, negative; (+), most strains positive; (−), most strains negative; NA, data not available or found; R, resistant; S, susceptible; TSI, triple sugar iron.
Adapted from Ruiz-Palacios, G., and Pickering, L. K.: Campylobacter and Helicobacter infections. In Feigin, R. D., and Cherry, J. D. (eds.): Textbook of Pediatric Infectious Diseases. 3rd ed. Philadelphia, W. B. Saunders, 1992, pp. 1072-2084.

size and motility, campylobacters may pass through filters with pores of 0.45 to 0.65 μm, whereas other enteric flora are retained.[2,64]

Although colonies may appear on plates within 24 to 48 hours, growth of campylobacters from stool may take as long as 72 to 96 hours. Primary isolation from blood may require 2 weeks.[2] Gram stain of young cultures reveals vibrioid forms, and longer incubation may yield spherical or coccoid bodies. *Campylobacter* spp. usually can be distinguished from one another on the basis of biochemical tests and growth characteristics (Table 143–1). Although the significant pathogens *C. jejuni*, *C. coli*, and *C. lari* cannot be discriminated reliably by the use of 16s rDNA data, these sequences provide a substantially improved basis for the identification and differentiation of *Campylobacter* spp.[36] Many investigators have applied molecular techniques to identify enteric campylobacters directly from stool.[9]

EPIDEMIOLOGY

Much needs to be learned about the epidemiology of *Campylobacter* spp. other than *C. jejuni* and *C. coli*, a group of organisms that made up only about 1 percent of *Campylobacter* spp. reported to the Centers for Disease Control and Prevention (CDC) from 1982 to 1986.[12] However, this study found that age-specific isolation rates of *C. fetus* parallel those of *C. jejuni* and *C. coli*; rates peak in infancy and increase in young adulthood, and *C. fetus* increases substantially in elderly persons. Seasonal distribution patterns of *C. jejuni*, *C. coli*, and *C. fetus* also were similar, with peaks occurring in warm months. In this surveillance study, *C. jejuni* and *C. coli* isolates were predominantly from stool, whereas 54 percent of *C. fetus* isolates with a known source were from blood.[12] The epidemiology and antimicrobial susceptibilities of 111 *C. fetus* strains isolated from 103 patients from 1983 to 2000 in Quebec, Canada, were determined.[91] The isolation site was blood in 69 percent of the patients, stools in 20 percent, and other body fluids, including aorta, bile, synovial fluid, cerebrospinal fluid, tubo-ovarian abscess, ascites, and pleural fluid, in 11 percent of these patients.[91]

C. fetus, an important cause of sporadic abortion in cattle and sheep, may be isolated from the intestines and genital tracts of these animals.[70] Contaminated food and water are the suspected sources of infection for sheep, cattle, and other animals, including goats, pigs, cats, dogs, hamsters, guinea pigs, antelopes, chickens, and turkeys.[30] A *C. fetus* strain with markers of reptile origin was isolated from the blood of a febrile patient with precursor T-cell acute lymphoblastic leukemia.[92] Although the source of *C. fetus* infection in humans generally is not apparent,[38] a 1970 review of *Vibrio fetus* infection in humans found that one third of patients

had recent contact with animals or animal products and one third denied such contact; no information was available on the remaining third.[8]

C. fetus bacteremia generally occurs in immunosuppressed hosts (especially elderly men), pregnant women, and neonates.[73,89] Predisposing conditions include alcoholism or cirrhosis, diabetes mellitus, heart disease, malignancy, splenectomy, and corticosteroid or other immunosuppressive therapy.[21,45,73] *C. fetus* is not considered a major cause of gastroenteritis, perhaps because of the failure of this organism to grow in stool specimens evaluated by routine laboratory methods for *C. jejuni* and *C. coli*.[12,70]

The epidemiology of human *C. fetus* infection as a foodborne, perinatal infection was reflected in the original report by Vinzent and colleagues[94] that described a 39-year-old pregnant woman who had a history of drinking raw milk from a cow that recently had aborted a pregnancy; this woman contracted a flulike syndrome in the sixth month of pregnancy. Two blood cultures grew *C. fetus*, and after 5 weeks of illness, a stillborn infant was delivered. In addition to raw milk,[96] raw beef liver[84] and "nutritional therapy" (raw fruit, vegetable juice, and calves' liver, along with coffee enemas) have been associated with *C. fetus* infection.[13] The last report described nine patients with malignant disease and one with systemic lupus erythematosus in whom *C. fetus* sepsis was associated with such therapy. Nine patients received their "nutritional therapy" in Mexico, and one died.[13]

First associated with human disease in a homosexual man with proctitis, *C. hyointestinalis* (*hyos*, "hog"; *intestinalis*, "pertaining to the intestines") originally was isolated from the intestines of swine with proliferative ileitis.[26,70] *C. hyointestinalis* also has been isolated from the stool of persons with nonbloody, watery diarrhea.[23] Two of these patients were homosexual men, the third was an elderly woman who had been traveling in Egypt, and the fourth was an infant from a large farm family that drank raw milk. These organisms are closer to *C. fetus* by DNA hybridization than are any other catalase-positive *Campylobacter* spp. and are resistant to nalidixic acid but susceptible to cephalothin.[76]

C. lari, frequently isolated from apparently healthy seagulls, is nalidixic acid resistant and thermophilic.[81] The name is derived from *laridis*, "of a sea bird," although seagulls do not play a direct role in its epidemiology.[87] Epidemiologically and microbiologically similar to *C. jejuni*, *C. lari* has been reported to cause enteritis in patients with and without a history of animal exposure and bacteremia in two elderly patients with multiple myeloma and permanent pacemakers.[62,65,79,87] A waterborne outbreak of *C. lari*–associated gastroenteritis also has been reported.[10]

Catalase-negative or weak *Campylobacter* spp. that are hippurate-negative and thermotolerant were isolated first from dogs in 1983.[77] This *C. upsaliensis* group is associated with gastroenteritis, breast abscess, spontaneous abortion, and bacteremia in normal

						Susceptibility	
Oxidase	Catalase	Urease	Hippurate	Nitrate	H₂S (TSI)	Nalidixic Acid	Cephalothin
+	+	–	–	+	–	R	R
+	(–)	–	–	+	–	S	S
+	+	–	–	+	–	R	S
+	+	–	–	+	+	R	S
+	–	–	–	+	+	R	R
+	–	–	–	+	+	R	S
+	–	–	–	+	+	R	S

TABLE 143–2   Clinical Features Associated with Infection by "Atypical" *Campylobacter* and Related Species Implicated as Causes of Human Illness

Species	Common Clinical Features	Less Common Clinical Features	Additional Information
C. fetus	Bacteremia, sepsis, meningitis, vascular infections	Diarrhea, relapsing fevers	Not usually isolated from media containing cephalothin
C. upsaliensis	Watery diarrhea, low-grade fever, abdominal pain	Bacteremia, abscesses, abortion, hemolytic-uremic syndrome	Difficult to isolate because of cephalothin susceptibility
C. lari	Abdominal pain, diarrhea	Colitis, appendicitis, bacteremia	Seagulls frequently colonized; organism often transmitted to humans by contaminated water
C. hyointestinalis	Watery or bloody diarrhea, vomiting, abdominal pain	Bacteremia	Causes proliferative enteritis in swine
C. sputorum	Pulmonary, perianal, groin, knee, and axillary abscesses	Bacteremia	Three clinically relevant biovars: *C. sputorum* subspecies *sputorum*, *C. sputorum* subspecies *bubulus*, and *C. mucosalis*
H₂-requiring *Campylobacter**	Periodontitis	Diarrhea, osteomyelitis, bacteremia	Uncertain role as human pathogen

**Includes C. rectus, C. curvus, and C. concisus.*
Adapted from Allos, B. M., Blaser, M. J.: Campylobacter jejuni and the expanding spectrum of related infections. Clin. Infect. Dis. 20:1092-1099, 1995.

hosts, as well as opportunistic infections in immunocompromised persons.[39,42,69] Conditions predisposing to *C. upsaliensis* bacteremia include gallbladder surgery, ectopic pregnancy, kwashiorkor, and acquired immunodeficiency syndrome (AIDS).[69] Young puppies and kittens are potential transmitters of *C. upsaliensis*,[40] and an outbreak in a childcare center suggesting direct transmission between humans also has been described.[35,48] In a sample of *Campylobacter* recovered from patients with campylobacteriosis in Los Angeles County, California, in 1998, the second most frequently isolated species was *C. upsaliensis* (6 [4%] of 155 isolates).[55] Of the six patients with *C. upsaliensis* isolates, five had pets, including three dogs, a cat, and a turtle, at home.[55] Routine selective media for *Campylobacter* spp. may fail to detect this organism, which is slow growing and susceptible to cephalothin.[34,56,95] Filtration methods may improve the yield from stool cultures.[9,34,35,47,48,58,83]

PATHOGENESIS AND IMMUNITY

Information on the pathogenic and immune mechanisms involved in *Campylobacter* infections other than those caused by *C. jejuni* and *C. coli* is scarce. Much of what is known has been learned from animal, clinical, and epidemiologic data. The association of *Campylobacter* bacteremia with hypogammaglobulinemia, HIV infection, kwashiorkor, pregnancy, and malignancy indicates the importance of both humoral and cell-mediated immunity in host defense against this genus.[2,17,56,65,80,98] The predilection of *C. fetus*

for endovascular surfaces in adults and the central nervous system in neonates also is well documented.[22,78]

In pregnant animals, *C. fetus* bacteremia occurs after ingestion of the organism, with subsequent development of infection of the placenta and fetus.[60,67] Examination of infected animal placentas has revealed necrosis, infarction, and microabscesses, along with disruption of the placental circulation.[18] Placental changes similar to these have been described in humans after preterm maternal bacteremia, consistent with infection as a result of hematogenous rather than ascending spread.[80] Ascending infection with premature rupture of membranes and amnionitis in the absence of maternal bacteremia has resulted in stillbirth or early-onset disease.[28,44] Contamination of the baby at the time of vaginal delivery is important in the pathogenesis of neonatal sepsis and meningitis with *C. fetus* in live-born infants.[57,97]

Bacteremia may occur more commonly with *C. fetus* than with *C. jejuni* because the former is resistant to the bactericidal effects of human serum, whereas the latter is susceptible.[6] A surface-layer protein that covers *C. fetus* functions as a capsule and appears to be an important virulence property of the organism.[5] It inhibits C3b binding, and this action explains both the serum resistance and the phagocytic resistance of *C. fetus*.[7]

CLINICAL MANIFESTATIONS

The clinical spectrum of non-*jejuni* or non-*coli Campylobacter* infections varies with the age of the patient and the individual species (Table 143–2). *C. fetus* is responsible for most reported disease patterns, including prenatal, neonatal, bacteremic, and focal infections, caused by this "other *Campylobacter*" group of organisms.[89] Pregnancies complicated by maternal infection with *C. fetus* may result in abortion, stillbirth, and prematurity.[22,71,80] Live-born infants may suffer from sepsis and meningitis with a high case-fatality rate.

Mothers may have fever and chills with bacteremia alone or with diarrhea. Maternal blood, placenta, cervix, vaginal, and stool cultures have yielded *C. fetus* in reported perinatal cases.[22,57,80,97] Maternal outcome is excellent.

Torphy and Bond[89] reviewed eight infants 12 hours to 22 days old with reported *C. fetus* disease. The initial symptoms, including fever, cough, respiratory distress, vomiting, diarrhea, cyanosis, convulsions, and jaundice, were consistent with neonatal sepsis. Meningitis developed in all eight infants, and six died. Four were premature, and three of them had an onset of illness at 2 days of age or younger and died during the first week of life. However, a subsequent review reported three additional neonatal patients who survived *C. fetus* meningitis after contracting the disease at 1 to 3 days of age.[97] Hemorrhagic infarction and necrosis, as well as cystic degeneration of the cerebral cortex, are the cerebral lesions most commonly reported in *Campylobacter* meningitis.[97]

Descriptions of *C. fetus* infection in children outside the neonatal age group are rare.[52,96,98] One was a 2½-year-old child with *V. fetus* bacteremia who had low-grade fever for 3 weeks and a cervical mass on the day of admission and was treated successfully with penicillin.[96] Her past history included drinking raw cow's milk and untested well water. A 16-month-old girl from India whose father operated a dairy business was admitted for evaluation of fever lasting 10 days and seizures for 5 days before admission.[52] Her provisional diagnosis was encephalitis, and a blood culture grew *V. fetus*. No antibiotics were administered, and the patient recovered uneventfully. The authors of the report emphasized the undulant nature of *C. fetus* infection, similar to that of brucellosis. *C. fetus* bacteremia also was detected in a nearly 5-year-old boy with agammaglobulinemia who had a 3-week history of anorexia, lethargy, fever, and, more recently, hepatitis.[98] Blood culture grew *C. fetus*, and liver biopsy demonstrated hepatitis with multiple areas of severe focal necrosis, bridging necrosis, and Kupffer cell hyperplasia. He responded rapidly to ampicillin therapy.

Most reported patients with *C. fetus* infection are men older than 45 years of age who have bacteremia with or without focal infection.[21,73,89] Most of them have underlying conditions such as diabetes, malignant disease, and hepatorenal or cardiovascular disease.[38,45] Typically, illness begins with fever, malaise, and headache. Chills and night sweats are prominent, as is weight loss in prolonged illness. Diarrhea, nausea, vomiting, and abdominal pain occur in as many as 38 percent of cases, and hepatosplenomegaly or jaundice develops in two thirds.[38,98] Pulmonary involvement is a rare finding.[8,38]

Three patterns of invasive *C. fetus* disease have been described.[74] Clinical manifestations of the first localized infection accompanied by septicemia include meningitis,[11,57] endocarditis,[25] pericarditis,[63] thrombophlebitis,[14] mycotic aneurysm,[74] cellulitis,[29,45] gluteal abscess,[20] septic arthritis,[54] salpingitis,[11] and peritonitis.[86] The second form is transient asymptomatic bacteremia, which may be self-limited.[38,73,75] Prolonged and recurrent bacteremia, with waxing and waning symptoms as spontaneous relapses and remissions occur, is the third pattern of invasive *C. fetus* infection.[8,19,46,75,98]

The vascular tropism of *C. fetus*, especially in the presence of preexisting vessel damage, is well recognized.[14,63,98] Possible explanations for this predilection include a surface receptor on the organism with an affinity for vascular endothelium that results in endothelial damage and subsequent thrombus formation. In addition, the organism's microaerophilic growth requirements may be favored by venous oxygen tensions.[63] Previous valvular heart disease is a common finding in endocarditis.[25] *Campylobacter* infection of prosthetic devices is rare, with only four cases of *C. fetus* and one infection each of *C. lari* and *C. upsaliensis* described in the literature.[16]

A report from the CDC reviewed clinical and epidemiologic information on 12 patients with *C. upsaliensis* isolates from 1980 to 1986.[69] Eight isolates were from blood, and three were from stool. Ages of the 12 patients ranged from 6 months to 83 years. Two infants with *C. upsaliensis* bacteremia that responded to amoxicillin therapy were included. One was a 10-month-old child who had fever, leukocytosis, and a history of culture-negative diarrhea, bronchiolitis, and *Klebsiella* bacteremia 3 months previously. The second was a 6½-month-old infant with fever, respiratory distress, and erythematous tympanic membranes. A 14-month-old child who lived on a farm with a private well and several household dogs and cats had a history of pica, including dirt from ground where chickens roamed. Stool culture obtained for evaluation of febrile, watery diarrhea yielded *C. upsaliensis*, and he recovered after receiving erythromycin therapy.[69]

Underlying medical problems in adults with *C. upsaliensis* bacteremia included peptic ulcer disease and partial large-bowel resection for a benign tumor, perforated gallbladder with peritonitis, AIDS, corticosteroid therapy, ruptured ectopic pregnancy, and cirrhosis with pancreatic insufficiency and partial gastrectomy.[69] One adult with a *C. upsaliensis* stool isolate was a 35-year-old woman with relapsing acute myelogenous leukemia. She was ill with fever and blood-tinged, watery diarrhea while thrombocytopenic and neutropenic. A healthy, 20-year-old student with a history of drinking raw milk and swimming in fresh-water lakes and rivers was the second adult reported with a *C. upsaliensis* stool isolate. He had fever, severe cramping abdominal pain, and nonbloody, watery diarrhea of 3 weeks' duration that responded to oral erythromycin.[69]

Kwashiorkor and gastroenteritis were the predominant clinical features in a retrospective series of 16 pediatric patients with *C. upsaliensis* bacteremia from South Africa.[56] The age range was 2 to 36 months, with a mean age of 15.5 months. The authors suggested that *C. upsaliensis* bacteremia was secondary to intestinal infection with the same organism, but no confirmatory stool culture data were available.[56] A gastrointestinal source also was postulated for the *C. upsaliensis* isolated from a breast abscess in a previously healthy, 46-year-old woman.[31] Hemolytic-uremic syndrome was reported in a 14-year-old girl with *C. upsaliensis* gastroenteritis.[15]

C. upsaliensis was the only organism isolated from 83 patients in a large stool culture survey using a filtration system for *Campylobacter* in Belgium.[35] Ninety-two percent of patients had diarrhea, which was of acute onset in most cases. Vomiting (14%) and fever (7%) were uncommon occurrences, and symptoms generally abated in less than a week. Gross or occult blood was identified in 25 percent of cases, and neutrophils were seen on fecal smear in approximately 20 percent. Erythromycin (11 patients) or amoxicillin (2 patients) eradicated the organism, with resolution of symptoms in all 13 patients treated with antibiotics.[35] Australian workers identified *C. upsaliensis* in 19 (0.1%) of 18,516 stool specimens from August 1992 to March 1999 at the Royal Children's Hospital in Melbourne.[48] Infection with *C. upsaliensis* was associated with milder disease than was infection with *C. jejuni*; patients with *C. upsaliensis* infection had significantly less fever, diarrhea, and rectal bleeding.

Six clinical *C. lari* isolates were referred to the national *Campylobacter* reference laboratory at the CDC in 1982 and 1983.[87] Clinical illness associated with these isolates included enteritis in four patients, severe crampy abdominal pain in a 7-year-old girl, and terminal bacteremia in a 71-year-old man with multiple myeloma and chronic renal failure. The ages of the four patients with enteritis were 8 months, 3 years, 22 years, and 39 years. Diarrhea was watery or mucoid, and fever was an unusual occurrence. Potential exposure included consuming chicken, having contact with house pets, drinking untreated surface water, and eating raw oysters. *C. lari* colitis also developed in an HIV-infected woman.[24]

C. hyointestinalis has been isolated from the stool specimens of adult and pediatric patients experiencing nonbloody, watery diarrhea[23] and from a rectal culture of a homosexual man with proctitis.[26] Over a 4-year period, 20 strains of *C. curvus* were isolated from two separate and distinct clinical settings: a hospital survey of infectious causes of bloody diarrhea and an outbreak of Brainerd (chronic) diarrhea in northern California.[1] *C. curvus* also was reported to cause polymicrobial liver and lung abscesses in two patients with cancer, respectively. *C. rectus* was reported in a polymicrobial breast abscess in a patient with lymphoma.[1] The clinical features of other *Campylobacter* spp. are presented in Table 143–2.

DIAGNOSIS

Confirmation of infection with *C. fetus* and *Campylobacter* spp. other than *C. jejuni* and *C. coli* is based on positive culture results from clinical specimens.[2] *C. fetus* has been isolated from blood, cerebrospinal fluid, joint effusions, bile, urine, and pleural and pericardial fluid in standard culture media.[38] Blood cultures generally are positive within 4 to 14 days. Isolation of *C. fetus* and "other" *Campylobacter* spp. from stool requires incubation at 37° C and media without cephalosporins. Filtration techniques also may be warranted to detect these strains in stool cultures.

TREATMENT

Gentamicin, erythromycin, and imipenem are bactericidal for *C. fetus*, as is ampicillin to a lesser extent.[25,32,43,61,91] Cefotaxime, ticarcillin, amikacin, chloramphenicol, clindamycin, tetracycline, and ciprofloxacin have variable activity against different *C. fetus* strains.[25,91] Reported synergistic antimicrobial combinations in vitro include ampicillin and gentamicin or cefazolin and imipenem with gentamicin.[25,85]

Erythromycin continues to be the drug of choice for most patients with *Campylobacter* diarrhea.[2] The newer macrolide azithromycin, which has a broader spectrum of activity than does erythromycin, is effective therapy for *Campylobacter* enteritis, as well as for diarrhea caused by *Salmonella*, *Shigella*, *Vibrio cholerae*, and *Escherichia coli*, thus rendering it a useful drug in the treatment of traveler's diarrhea.[53] Increasing *Campylobacter* resistance to quinolones related to expanded use in humans and in animals used for food, especially chickens, diminished the usefulness of quinolones such as ciprofloxacin in the treatment of *Campylobacter* gastroenteritis in adults.[2,24,53]

Gentamicin, imipenem, ampicillin, and cefotaxime are therapeutic options in treating *Campylobacter* bacteremia and other extraintestinal infections.[2,3,25,43,91,97] Synergistic combination therapy is indicated for patients with meningitis and endocarditis, in which bactericidal activity is critical.[2,61] Patients with *Campylobacter* in their stool who are being treated for an extraintestinal *Campylobacter* infection with gentamicin should be prescribed supplemental oral therapy because gentamicin is ineffective against *Campylobacter* in the gut.[2]

Prolonged antimicrobial therapy and follow-up blood cultures are warranted for patients with *C. fetus* bacteremia because of the relapsing nature of the illness.[63,75] Chloramphenicol should be used with caution in treating *C. fetus* meningitis because clinical outcome and in vitro susceptibility results for this drug have been disappointing.[57,61]

REFERENCES

1. Abbott, S. L., Waddington, M., Lindquist, D., et al.: Description of *Campylobacter curvus* and *C. curvus*–like strains associated with sporadic episodes of bloody gastroenteritis and Brainerd's diarrhea. J. Clin. Microbiol. *43*:585-588, 2005.
2. Allos, B. M., and Blaser, M. J.: *Campylobacter jejuni* and the expanding spectrum of related infections. Clin. Infect. Dis. *20*:1092-1099, 1995.
3. American Academy of Pediatrics: *Campylobacter* infections. *In* Pickering, L. K. (ed.): 2000 Redbook: Report of the Committee on Infectious Diseases. 25th ed. Elk Grove Village, IL, American Academy of Pediatrics, 2000, pp. 196-198.
4. Benjamin, J., Leaper, S., Owen, R. J., et al.: Description of *Campylobacter laridis*, a new species comprising the nalidixic acid resistant thermophilic *Campylobacter* (NARTC) group. Curr. Microbiol. *8*:231, 1983.
5. Blaser, M. J., Smith, P. F., Hopkins, J. A., et al.: Pathogenesis of *Campylobacter fetus* infections: Serum resistance associated with high molecular weight surface proteins. J. Infect. Dis. *135*:696-706, 1987.
6. Blaser, M. J., Smith, P. F., and Kohler, P. A.: Susceptibility of *Campylobacter* isolates to the bactericidal activity in human serum. J. Infect. Dis. *151*:227-235, 1985.
7. Blaser, M. J., Smith, P. F., Repine, J. E., et al.: Pathogenesis of *Campylobacter fetus* infections: Failure of C3b to bind explains serum and phagocytosis resistance. J. Clin. Invest. *81*:1434-1444, 1988.
8. Bokkenheuser, V.: *Vibrio fetus* infection in man. I. Ten new cases and some epidemiologic observations. Am. J. Epidemiol. *91*:400-409, 1970.
9. Bourke, B., Chan, V. L., and Sherman, P.: *Campylobacter upsaliensis*: Waiting in the wings. Clin. Microbiol. Rev. *11*:440-449, 1998.
10. Broczyk, A., Thompson, S., Smith, D., and Lior, H.: Water-borne outbreak of *Campylobacter laridis*–associated gastroenteritis. Letter. Lancet *1*:164-165, 1987.
11. Brown, W. J., and Sautter, R.: *Campylobacter fetus* septicemia with concurrent salpingitis. J. Clin. Microbiol. *6*:72-75, 1977.
12. *Campylobacter* isolates in the United States, 1982-1986. Morb. Mortal. Wkly. Rep. CDC Surveill. Summ. *37*:1-13, 1988.
13. *Campylobacter* sepsis associated with "nutrition therapy." M. M. W. R. Morb. Mortal. Wkly. Rep. *30*:294-295, 1981.
14. Carbone, K. M., Heinrich, M. C., and Quinn, T. C.: Thrombophlebitis and cellulitis due to *Campylobacter fetus* ssp. fetus: Report of four cases and a review of the literature. Medicine (Baltimore) *64*:244-250, 1985.
15. Carter, J. E., and Cimolai, N.: Hemolytic-uremic syndrome associated with acute *Campylobacter upsaliensis* gastroenteritis. Nephron *74*:489, 1996.
16. Chambers, S. T., Morpeth, S. C., and Laird, H. M.: *Campylobacter fetus* prosthetic hip joint infection: Successful management with device retention and review. J. Infect. *50*:258-261, 2005.
17. Chusid, M. J., Wortman, D. W., and Dunne, W. M.: "*Campylobacter upsaliensis*" sepsis in a boy with acquired hypogammaglobulinemia. Diagn. Microbiol. Infect. Dis. *13*:367-369, 1990.
18. Coid, C. R., and Fox, H.: Short review: Campylobacters as placental pathogens. Placenta *4*:295-305, 1983.
19. Collins, H. S., Blevins, A., and Benter, E.: Protracted bacteremia and meningitis due to *Vibrio fetus*. Arch. Intern. Med. *113*:361, 1964.
20. de Otero, J., Pigrau, C., Buti, M., et al.: Isolation of *Campylobacter fetus* subspecies fetus from a gluteal abscess. Clin. Infect. Dis. *19*:557-558, 1994.
21. Dronda, F., Garcia-Arata, I., Navas, E., and de Rafael, L.: Meningitis in adults due to *Campylobacter fetus* subspecies fetus. Clin. Infect. Dis. *27*:906-907, 1998.
22. Eden, A. N.: Perinatal mortality caused by *Vibrio fetus*. J. Pediatr. *68*:297, 1966.
23. Edmonds, P., Patton, C. M., Griffin, P. M., et al.: *Campylobacter hyointestinalis* associated with human gastrointestinal disease in the United States. J. Clin. Microbiol. *25*:685-691, 1987.
24. Evans, T. G., and Riley, D.: *Campylobacter laridis* colitis in a human immunodeficiency virus–positive patient treated with a quinolone. Clin. Infect. Dis. *15*:172-173, 1992.
25. Farrugia, D. C., Eykyn, S. J., and Smyth, E. G.: *Campylobacter fetus* endocarditis: Two case reports and review. Clin. Infect. Dis. *18*:443-446, 1994.
26. Fennell, C. L., Rompalo, A. M., Totten, P. A., et al.: Isolation of *Campylobacter hyointestinalis* from a human. J. Clin. Microbiol. *24*:146-148, 1986.
27. Figura, N., Guglielmetti, P., Zanchi, A., et al.: Two cases of *Campylobacter mucosalis* enteritis in children. J. Clin. Microbiol. *31*:727-728, 1993.
28. Forbes, J. D., and Scheifele, D. W.: Early onset *Campylobacter* sepsis in a neonate. Pediatr. Infect. Dis. J. *6*:494, 1987.
29. Francioli, P., Hertzstein, J., Grob, J., et al.: *Campylobacter fetus* subspecies fetus bacteremia. Arch. Intern. Med. *145*:289-292, 1985.
30. Franklin, B., and Ulmer, D. D.: Human infection with *Vibrio fetus*. West. J. Med. *120*:200-204, 1974.
31. Gaudreau, C., and Lamothe, F.: *Campylobacter upsaliensis* isolated from a breast abscess. J. Clin. Microbiol. *30*:1354-1356, 1992.
32. Goossens, H., Coignau, H., Vlaes, L., et al.: In vitro evaluation of antibiotic combinations against *Campylobacter fetus*. J. Antimicrob. Chemother. *24*:195-201, 1989.
33. Goossens, H., Giesendorf, A. S., Vandamme, P., et al.: Investigation of an outbreak of *Campylobacter upsaliensis* in day care centers in Brussels: Analysis of relationships among isolates by phenotypic and genotypic typing methods. J. Infect. Dis. *172*:1298-1305, 1995.

34. Goossens, H., Pot, B., Vlaes, L., et al.: Characterization and description of *Campylobacter upsaliensis* isolated from human feces. J. Clin. Microbiol. *28*:1039-1046, 1990.

35. Goossens, H., Vlaes, L., DeBoeck, M., et al.: Is "*Campylobacter upsaliensis*" an unrecognised cause of human diarrhoea? Lancet *335*:584-586, 1990.

36. Gorkiewicz, G., Feierl, G., Schober, C., et al. Species-specific identification of campylobacters by partial 16s rRNA gene sequencing. J. Clin. Microbiol. *41*:2537-2546, 2003.

37. Griffiths, P. L., and Park, R. W. A.: Campylobacters associated with human diarrhoeal disease. J. Appl. Bacteriol. *69*:281-301, 1990.

38. Guerrant, R. L., Lahita, R. G., Winn, W. C., et al.: Campylobacteriosis in man: Pathogenic mechanisms and review of 91 bloodstream infections. Am. J. Med. *65*:584-592, 1978.

39. Gurgani, T., and Diker, K. S.: Abortion associated with *Campylobacter upsaliensis*. J. Clin. Microbiol. *32*:3093-3094, 1994.

40. Hald, B., and Madsen, M.: Healthy puppies and kittens as carriers of *Campylobacter* spp., with special reference to *Campylobacter upsaliensis*. J. Clin. Microbiol. *35*:3351-3352, 1997.

41. Han, X. Y., Tarrand, J. J., and Rice, D. C.: Oral *Campylobacter* species involved in extraoral abscess: A report of three cases. J. Clin. Microbiol. *43*:2513-2515, 2005.

42. Hanna, J. N., Enbom, R. M., and Murphy, D. M.: *Campylobacter upsaliensis* bacteraemia in an Aboriginal child. Med. J. Aust. *160*:655-656, 1994.

43. Herve, J., Aissa, N., Legrand, P., et al. *Campylobacter fetus* meningitis in a diabetic adult cured by imipenem. Eur. J. Clin. Microbiol. Infect. Dis. *23*:722-724, 2004.

44. Hood, M., and Todd, J. M.: *Vibrio fetus*: A cause of human abortion. Am. J. Obstet. Gynecol. *80*:506, 1960.

45. Ichiyama, S., Hirai, S., Minami, T., et al.: *Campylobacter fetus* subspecies *fetus* cellulitis associated with bacteremia in debilitated hosts. Clin. Infect. Dis. *27*:252-255, 1998.

46. Jackson, J. F., Hinton, P., and Allison, F., Jr.: Human vibriosis: Report of a patient with relapsing febrile illness due to *Vibrio fetus*. Am. J. Med. *28*:986, 1960.

47. Jenkin, G. A., and Tee, W.: *Campylobacter upsaliensis*–associated diarrhea in human immunodeficiency virus–infected patients. Clin. Infect. Dis. *27*:816-821, 1998.

48. Jimenez, S. G., Heine, R. G., Ward, P. B., et al.: *Campylobacter upsaliensis* gastroenteritis in childhood. Pediatr. Infect. Dis. J. *18*:988-992, 1999.

49. Karmali, M A., Allen, A. K., and Fleming, P. C.: Differentiation of catalase-positive campylobacters with special reference to morphology. Int. J. Syst. Bacteriol. *31*:64, 1981.

50. Kiehlbauch, J. A., Brenner, D. J., Nicholson, M. A., et al.: *Campylobacter butzleri* sp. nov. isolated from humans and animals with diarrheal illness. J. Clin. Microbiol. *29*:376-385, 1991.

51. King, E. O.: Human infections with *Vibrio fetus* and a closely related vibrio. J. Infect. Dis. *101*:119, 1957.

52. Koshi, G., Samuel, B. T., Malati, J., et al.: *Vibrio fetus* encephalitis with bacteremia in a child. Indian J. Med. Res. 57:1232-1239, 1969.

53. Kuschner, R. A., Trofa, A. F., Thomas, R. J., et al.: Use of azithromycin for the treatment of *Campylobacter* enteritis in travelers to Thailand, an area where ciprofloxacin resistance is prevalent. Clin. Infect. Dis. *21*:536, 1995.

54. Kutner, L. J., and Arnold, W. D.: Septic arthritis due to *Vibrio fetus*. J. Bone. Joint Surg. Am. *52*:161-164, 1970.

55. Labarca, J. A., Sturgeon, J., Borenstein, L., et at. *Campylobacter upsaliensis*: Another pathogen for consideration in the United States. Clin. Infect. Dis. *34*: e59-e60, 2002.

56. Lastovica, A. J., LeRoux, E., and Penner, J. L.: *Campylobacter upsaliensis* isolated from blood cultures of pediatric patients. J. Clin. Microbiol. 27:657-659, 1989.

57. Lee, M. M., Welliver, R. C., and La Scolea, L. J.: *Campylobacter* meningitis in childhood. Pediatr. Infect. Dis. *4*:544-547, 1985.

58. Lindblom, G.-B., Sjogren, E., Hansson-Westberg, J., et al.: *Campylobacter upsaliensis*, *C. sputorum sputorum* and *C. concisus* as common causes of diarrhea in Swedish children. Scand. J. Infect. Dis. *27*:187-188, 1995.

59. McFadyean, F., and Stockman, S.: Report of the Departmental Committee Appointed by the Board of Agriculture and Fisheries to Inquire into Epizootic Abortion, London, 1909-1913. Vol. 3. London, His Majesty's Stationary Office, 1913, p. 1.

60. Miller, V. A., Jensen, R., and Gilroy, J. J.: Bacteremia in pregnant sheep following oral administration of *Vibrio fetus*. Am. J. Vet. Res. *20*:677, 1959.

61. Morooka, T., Oda, T., and Shigeoka, H.: In vitro evaluation of antibiotics for treatment of meningitis caused by *Campylobacter fetus* subspecies *fetus*. Pediatr. Infect. Dis. J. *8*:653-654, 1989.

62. Morris, C. N., Scully, B., and Garvey, G. J.: *Campylobacter lari* associated with permanent pacemaker infection and bacteremia. Clin. Infect. Dis. 27:220-221, 1998.

63. Morrison, V. A., Lloyd, B. D., Chia, J. K. S., et al.: Cardiovascular and bacteremic manifestations of *Campylobacter fetus* infection: Case report and review. Rev. Infect. Dis. *12*:387-392, 1990.

64. Nachamkin, I.: *Campylobacter* and *Arcobacter*. *In* Murray, P. R., Baron, E. J., Pfaller, M. A., et al. (eds.): Manual of Clinical Microbiology. 6th ed. Washington, D.C., ASM Press, 1995, pp. 483-491.

65. Nachamkin, I., Stowell, C., Skalina, D., et al.: *Campylobacter laridis* causing bacteremia in an immunosuppressed patient. Ann. Intern. Med. *101*:55-57, 1984.

66. Orlicek, S. L., Welch, D. F., and Kuhls, T. L.: Septicemia and meningitis caused by a *Helicobacter cinaedi* in a neonate. J. Clin. Microbiol. *31*:569-571, 1993.

67. Osburn, B. I., and Hoskins, R. K.: Experimentally induced *Vibrio fetus* var. *intestinalis* infection in pregnant cows. Am. J. Vet. Res. *31*:1733-1741, 1970.

68. Pasternak, J., Bolivar, R., Hopfer, R. L., et al.: Bacteremia caused by *Campylobacter*-like organisms in two male homosexuals. Ann. Intern. Med. *101*:339-341, 1984.

69. Patton, C. M., Shaffer, N., Edmonds, P., et al.: Human disease associated with *Campylobacter upsaliensis* (catalase-negative or weakly positive *Campylobacter* species) in the United States. J. Clin. Microbiol. 27:66-73, 1989.

70. Penner, J. L.: The genus *Campylobacter*: A decade of progress. Clin. Microbiol. Rev. *1*:157-172, 1988.

71. Premature labor and neonatal sepsis caused by *Campylobacter fetus*, subsp. fetus: Ontario. M. M. W. R. Morb. Mortal. Wkly. Rep. *33*:483-484, 1984.

72. Rams, T. E., Feik, D., and Slots, J.: *Campylobacter rectus* in human periodontitis. Oral Microbiol. Immunol. *8*:230-235, 1993.

73. Rettig, P. J.: *Campylobacter* infections in human beings. J. Pediatr. *94*:855-864, 1979.

74. Righter, J., and Woods, J. M.: *Campylobacter* and endovascular lesions. Can. J. Surg. *28*:451-452, 1985.

75. Righter, J., Wells, W. A., Hart, G. D., et al.: Relapsing septicemia caused by *Campylobacter fetus* subsp *fetus*. Can. Med. Assoc. J. *128*:686-689, 1983.

76. Roop, R. M., II, Smibert, R. M., Johnson, J. L., et al.: Differential characteristics of catalase positive campylobacters correlated with DNA homology groups. Can. J. Microbiol. *30*:938-951, 1984.

77. Sanstedt, K., Ursing, J., and Walder, M.: Thermotolerant *Campylobacter* with no or weak catalase activity isolated from dogs. Curr. Microbiol. *8*:209, 1983.

78. Schmidt, U., Chmel, H., Kaminski, Z., et al.: The clinical spectrum of *Campylobacter fetus* infections: Report of five cases and review of the literature. Q. J. Med. *49*:431-432, 1980.

79. Simor, A. E., and Wilcox, L.: Enteritis associated with *Campylobacter laridis*. J. Clin. Microbiol. *25*:10-12, 1987.

80. Simor, A. E., Karmali, M. A., Jadavji, T., et al.: Abortion and perinatal sepsis associated with *Campylobacter* infection. Rev. Infect. Dis. *8*:397-402, 1986.

81. Skirrow, M. B., and Benjamin, J.: Differentiation of enteropathogenic *Campylobacter*. J Clin Pathol *33*:1122, 1980.

82. Smith, T.: Spirilla associated with disease of the fetal membranes in cattle. J. Exp. Med. *28*:701, 1918.

83. Snijders, F., Kuijper, E. J., deWever, B., et al.: Prevalence of *Campylobacter*-associated diarrhea among patients infected with human immunodeficiency virus. Clin. Infect. Dis. *24*:1107-1113, 1997.

84. Soonattrakul, W., Andersen, B. R., and Brynor, J. H.: Raw liver as a possible source of *Vibrio fetus* septicemia in man. Am. J. Med. Sci. *261*:245, 1981.

85. Spelhaug, D. R., Gilchrist, M. J. R., and Washington, J. A., II: Bactericidal activity of antibiotics against *Campylobacter fetus* subspecies intestinalis. J. Infect. Dis. *143*:500, 1981.

86. Targan, S. R., Chow, A. W., and Guze, L. B.: Spontaneous peritonitis of cirrhosis due to *Campylobacter fetus*. Gastroenterology 71:311-313, 1976.

87. Tauxe, R. V., Patton, C. M., Edmonds, P., et al.: Illness associated with *Campylobacter laridis*, a newly recognized *Campylobacter* species. J. Clin. Microbiol. *21*:222-225, 1985.

88. Tee, W., Luppino, M., and Rambaldo, S.: Bacteremia due to *Campylobacter sputorum* biovar sputorum. Clin. Infect. Dis. *27*:1544-1545, 1998.

89. Torphy, D. E., and Bond, W. W.: *Campylobacter fetus* infections in children. Pediatrics *64*:898-903, 1979.

90. Totten, P. A., Fennell, C. L., Tenover, F. C., et al.: *Campylobacter cinaedi* (sp. nov.) and *Campylobacter fennelliae* (sp. nov.): Two new *Campylobacter* species associated with enteric disease in homosexual men. J. Infect. Dis. *151*:131-139, 1985.

91. Tremblay, C., Gandreu, C., and Lorange, M.: Epidemiology and antimicrobial susceptibilities of 111 *Campylobacter fetus* subsp. *fetus* strains isolated in Quebec, Canada, from 1983 to 2000. J. Clin. Microbiol. *41*:463-466, 2003.

92. Tu, Z.-C., Zeitlin, G., Gaguer, J.-P., et al.: *Campylobacter fetus* of reptile origin as a human pathogen. J. Clin. Microbiol. *42*:4405-4405, 2004.

93. Vandamme, P., Falsen, E., Pot, B., et al.: Identification of EF group 22 campylobacters from gastroenteritis cases as *Campylobacter concisus*. J. Clin. Microbiol. 27:1775-1781, 1989.

94. Vinzent, R., Dumas, J., and Picard, N.: Septicemie grave au cours de la grossesse, due à un vibrion: Avortement consecutif. Bull. Acad. Natl. Med. (Paris) *131*:90, 1947.

95. Walmsley, S. L., and Karmali, M. A.: Direct isolation of atypical thermophilic *Campylobacter* species from human feces on selective agar medium. J. Clin. Microbiol. 27:668-670, 1989.

96. Willis, M. D., and Austin, W. J.: Human *Vibrio fetus* infection: Report of two dissimilar cases. Am. J. Dis. Child. *112*:459-462, 1966.

97. Wong, S., Tam, A. Y., and Yeun, K.: *Campylobacter* infection in the neonate: Case report and review of the literature. Pediatr. Infect. Dis. J. *9*:665, 1990.

98. Wyatt, R. A., Younoszai, K., Anuras, S., et al.: *Campylobacter fetus* septicemia and hepatitis in a child with agammaglobulinemia. J. Pediatr. *91*:441-442, 1977.

INDEX

Note: Page numbers followed by *f* and *t* indicate figures and tables, respectively. Numbers in **boldface** indicate main discussions. Numbers followed by *n* indicate footnotes.

Fever (*Continued*)
severity, and risk of occult
bacteremia or serious bacterial
infection, 852
in Sindbis fever, 2324
sustained, 855
in toxic shock syndrome, 867, 868*f*,
871
treatment, 108–109
indications for, 108–109
in Venezuelan equine encephalitis,
2312
in Western equine encephalitis, 2306
Yale Observation Score for, 853
Fever of unknown origin (FUO), 851,
854–860
causes
in children, 856, 857*t*
common disorders as, 854
infectious, 856–859
localized, 858–859
systemic, 856–858
noninfectious, 856, 859–860
rare, 854
clinical evaluation of child with,
855–856
definition, 851, 854
diagnostic approach to, 855–856
and fever without source, distinction
between, 851
history-taking in, 855
laboratory evaluation in, 856
prognosis for, 854
Fever without source (FWS), **851–854**
causes, noninfectious, 852
clinical management, 853–854
definition, 851
empiric antibiotic therapy for,
853–854
and fever of unknown origin,
distinction between, 851
incidence, 852
and occult bacteremia, 852
in onset of chronic disease, 852
in prodromal stage of acute
infection, 852
FFI. *See* Fatal familial insomnia
FHA. *See* Filamentous hemagglutinin
(FHA)
Fibrinogen, microbial adherence to, 5
Fibrinolytics, intrapleural instillation,
in empyema, 311
Fibromyalgia
enteroviruses and, 2140
human parvovirus B19 infection and,
1908
Fibrosing cholestatic hepatitis, 1982
Fièvre boutonneuse, animal sources,
3453*t*
Fifth disease, 755, 796. *See also*
Erythema infectiosum; Human
parvovirus B19
historical perspective on, 1902
Fiibronectin, microbial adherence to, 5
Filamentous hemagglutinin (FHA), 4–
5, 5*f*
binding domains, 4–5, 5*f*
synthesis, 4
Filarial worms, 2840, **2991–2994**
animal sources, 3454*t*
Filariasis. *See also* Brugia malayi;
Brugia timori; Loa loa; Wuchereria
bancrofti
animal sources, 3454*t*
cutaneous manifestations, 768*t*
drug therapy for, 3311*t*–3312*t*
lymphatic, 2991–2992
vectors for, 2838*t*
Filobasidiella spp., classification, 2716
Filopodia, 14
Filoviridae, 1895, 1896*f*, 1897*t*, 2524,
3513
genera, 2524
taxonomy, 1901*f*
Filovirus(es), virology, 2524

FimA adhesin, 4
Fimbriae. *See* Pilus (pl., pili)
FimH adhesin, 10
Finegoldia spp., 1886
Finegoldia magna, 1886
Finlaya spp., as dengue vector, 2348
Fire ant bite, cutaneous manifestations,
769*t*
First-pass effect, definition, 3159
Fish, raw, infectious diseases associated
with, 624–625
Fish tapeworm, 624, 2840, **3005–3006**
animal sources, 3455*t*
drug therapy for, 3319*t*
Fishnet dermatitis
clinical manifestations, 766*t*
cutaneous manifestations, 766*t*
Fitz-Hugh–Curtis syndrome, 611, 1377
Flagella-mediated attachment, in
biofilm formation, 8, 9*f*
Flagellates, 2837
of blood and tissues, 2839–2840
intestinal, 2838–2839
non-intestinal, 2839
Flagellin
Salmonella, 1571
Toll-like receptors and, 24
Flagyl. *See* Metronidazole
Flamazine. *See* Silver sulfadiazine
Flammacerium. *See* Cerium nitrate–
silver sulfadiazine
Flare, of anterior uveitis, 823
Flatworms, 2837
Flaviviridae, 1896*f*, 1898*t*, 2325, 2332,
2344, 2347, 3513
taxonomy, 1901*f*
Flavivirus, 1898*t*, 2332, 2344, 2347,
2356
infection, cutaneous manifestations,
762
Flavobacterium spp. *See also*
Chryseobacterium spp.
in animal bites, 790*t*
taxonomy, 1192*t*
Flavobacterium balustinum, 1648
Flavobacterium IIB, 1648–1649
Flavobacterium meningosepticum, 1648
Flavobacterium odoratum, 1648
Flea(s), and plague, 1582–1583, 1585
Flea bite, cutaneous manifestations,
769*t*
Fleas
dog, as helminthic vector, 2838*t*
human, as helminthic vector, 2838*t*
rat, as helminthic vector, 2838*t*
Flexal virus, 2515, 2515*f*–2516*f*
infection, 2518
Flora
indigenous, **110–117**
adverse effects, 114
by anatomic site, 112–114, 112*t*
beneficial effects, 114, 1863
neonatal acquisition, 111, 1863
normal, 110
exogenous influences on, 111–112,
1863
of skin, 784
resident, 110, 784
by anatomic site, 112–114, 112*t*
transient, 784
by anatomic site, 112–114, 112*t*
Florida horse leeches, 2831
Flow cytometry, for malaria diagnosis,
2911
Fluconazole, 800–801, **3282–3284**
adverse effects and side effects,
2780*t*, 3283
antifungal activity, 3281
for *Blastoschizomyces capitatus*
infection, 2827
for candidiasis, 2746
for cryptococcosis, 2780–2781, 2780*t*
drug interactions with, 3283–3284
for fungal meningitis, 487
for fungal peritonitis, 2822–2823

Fluconazole (*Continued*)
for histoplasmosis, 2797–2798, 2797*t*
indications for, 3274*t*, 3276*t*, 3284,
3296*t*
for neonatal candidiasis, **960**
for paracoccidioidomycosis, 2771
pharmacodynamics, 3282–3283
pharmacokinetics, 3283, 3283*t*
for *Pichia* infection, 2826
prophylaxis, for neonatal candidiasis,
961
for sporotrichosis, 2812
structure, 3280, 3281*f*
for trichosporonosis, 2825
Flucytosine, **3278–3280**
adverse effects and side effects,
2780*t*, 3280
antifungal activity, 3278, 3279*f*
for *Blastoschizomyces capitatus*
infection, 2827
for cryptococcosis, 2780–2781, 2780*t*
drug interactions with, 3280
indications for, 3280
for neonatal candidiasis, **960**
pharmacodynamics, 3278–3279
pharmacokinetics, 3279–3280, 3279*f*
for *Pichia* infection, 2826
for *Rhodotorula* infection, 2826
for *Saccharomyces cerevisiae* infection,
2827
for sporotrichal meningitis, 2812
structure, 3278, 3278*f*
Fluid and electrolyte therapy, in
diarrheal disease, 640, 640*t*
Fluid management
in cholera, 1622–1623, 1622*t*
in shock, 842–843
in toxic shock syndrome, 869–870
Flukes, 2841, 3015. *See also* Clonorchis
sinensis; Fasciola hepatica;
Opisthorchis viverrini; Paragonimus
westermani
hermaphroditic, drug therapy for,
3312*t*
intestinal, **3016–3017**
drug therapy for, 3312*t*
liver, **3017–3020**
lung, 3020–3022
Fluorescent treponemal antibody
absorption test (FTA-ABS), 1836–
1837, 1836*t*
Fluoroquinolones, **3205–3206**
activity in vitro, 3205
adverse effects and side effects, 3206
as antileprosy drugs, 1492
clinical pharmacology, 3205–3206
dosage schedules for infants and
children, 3216*t*
indications for, 3205–3206
mechanism of action, 3205
pharmacokinetics, 3205
resistance to, 1281
mechanisms of, 3205
Fluorouracil, structure, 3278, 3278*f*
Fly bite, cutaneous manifestations, 769*t*
Foamy viruses, 2588
Focal adhesions, 10
Focal epithelial hyperplasia, 1932*t*,
1937–1938, 1938*f*
Folate, 73–74
Folliculitis, 785*t*, **787–788**
in immunocompromised host, 788
Fomites, 123
Fonsecaea spp., classification, 2716
Fonsecaea pedrosoi, 803, 2828, 2828*f*
Food, and absorption of oral
antibiotics, 3218
Food poisoning, **621–653**
chemical causes, 623–625, 624*t*
clostridial, 1858–1859
prevention, 1861
prognosis for, 1860
treatment, 1860
staphylococcal, 628*t*, 630
Food sanitation, 3472

Foodborne disease, **621–653**
Internet resources on, 625
Vibrio parahaemolyticus in, 628*t*, 631,
1625–1629
Food-borne illness(es)
epidemiology, 3472, 3473*t*
prevention, 3472
public health considerations with,
3465
Foot and mouth disease
animal sources, 3457*t*
clinical manifestations, 758*t*
cutaneous manifestations, 758*t*
Foreign body(ies)
infections associated with,
791–792
and risk of toxic shock syndrome,
866
vaginal, 582, 582*f*
Foreign body infection
biofilms and, 8
staphylococcal, 7
Foreign body reactions, 1109
Forest yaws, 2921*t*
Formula feeding
disadvantages, 84, 1863–1864
and infant botulism, 1863–1865
Forssman (F) antigen, pneumococcal,
1290
Fort Detrick (Maryland), 3508–3509
Fort Morgan virus, 2304
Fosamprenavir, 2635
Foscarnet, **3260–3261**
adverse effects and side effects,
3261
for CMV infection, 2034–2035,
2034*f*
dosage and administration, 3253*t*,
3260–3261
indications for, 3253*t*, 3260
mechanism of action, 3260
pharmacokinetics, 3260
resistance to, 3260
spectrum of activity, 3260
structure, 3260, 3260*f*
Fournier gangrene, 790
Fractalkine, 25
France, Toscana virus in, 2583
Francisella tularensis, **1725–1734**
animal sources, 3451*t*
bacteriology, 1725–1726
as bioweapon, 3512
historical perspective on, 3509
disease production by, 1728
ecogenetics, 1727
genome, 1726
geographic distribution, 1725–1726
historical perspective on, 1725
infection. *See* Tularemia
interactions with host, 1727–1728
invasion, 1728
pleural effusions caused by, 328
pneumonia, 303
reservoirs, 1726–1727
subspecies *holarctica* (Jellison type B),
1725
subspecies *novicida*, 1725
subspecies *tularensis* (Jellison type A),
1725
taxonomy, 1194*t*, 1725
type IV pili, 1726
F-ratio, 3562
Frequency distribution, 3558–3559,
3559*f*
Frequency matching, 3563
Friedländer pneumonia, 1542
Frontofacial monoblock advancement,
1135
Fruit bat(s), Ebola virus in, 2528
FTC. *See* Emtricitabine
F-test, 3562
Fumagillin, 2889
Functional antibody deficiencies,
sinopulmonary infections in,
274

Immune globulin(s) (Continued)
adverse effects and side effects, 3404
in antibody immunodeficiency, 3404
inhibition of vaccine antibody response, 3406
pharmacology, 3403–3404
for prevention of infectious disease, 3402t, 3404
intrathecal administration, 3408
intratracheal, 3407–3408
intravenous, 3401, 3402t, 3403, **3404–3407**
administration, 3405
adverse effects and side effects, 3405–3406
in antibody deficiencies, 3407
aseptic meningitis caused by, 3405
immediate reactions to
in IgA-deficient patients, 3405
severe, 3405
inhibition of vaccine antibody response, 3406
pathogen transmission by, 3406
pharmacology, 3404–3405
in primary immunodeficiencies, 3406, 3406t
renal complications, 3405
thrombotic complications, 3406
local application, 3408
oral administration, 3407
for pediatric traveler, 3050t
in secondary immunodeficiencies, 3406t, 3408–3410
special, 3401, 3402t
standard, 3401, 3402t
subcutaneous, 3401, 3402t, 3403, **3407**
Immune reconstitution inflammatory syndrome (IRIS), 1446–1447, 2781, 2790
management, 1447
progressive multifocal leukoencephalopathy in, 2629
and tuberculosis, 1446–1447
Immune response, 21–65. See also Adaptive immunity; Cell-mediated immunity (CMI); Innate immunity
complement and, 29
genetic variations in, 65
and infectious disease, 124–125
normal, 23–27
to respiratory syncytial virus, 2467–2468, 2467f
in Ross River virus infection, 2321–2322
Immune system, developing, HIV and, 2621–2622, 2622f
Immunity
and infectious disease, 124–125
microbial evasion of, 14–16
passive. See also Passive immunization
principles, 3401–3402
Immunization(s). See also Vaccine(s)
active, agents for, **3340–3400**
in cystic fibrosis, 356–357
DPT series, for international adoptees, 3071
and Guillain-Barré syndrome, 539–540
for heart transplant recipient, 1055
for hematopoietic stem cell transplant recipient, 1043–1044, 1043t
for HIV-infected (AIDS) patients, 2636, 2636t
informed consent for, 3342–3344
for international adoptees, 3071, 3071t
for international travel, 3043–3050, 3046t–3051t, 3348, 3349t
in immunocompromised children, 3062

Immunization(s) (Continued)
lapsed, 3342
malnutrition and, 99
passive. See Passive immunization
patient information about, 3342–3344
record keeping for, 3342–3344
reportable events after, 3342–3344, 3343t
routine, for pediatric travelers, 3043–3045, 3046t–3049t
schedules for, 3340–3341
recommended, 3344, 3345f–3347f
Immunoadsorption, in Guillain-Barré syndrome, 544
Immunoassay(s), for Chagas disease, 2936
Immunocompromised host. See Immunocompromised patient(s)
Immunocompromised patient(s)
acalculous cholecystitis in, 685
Acremonium infection in, 2831
appendicitis in, 699
aspergillosis in, 2718–2719
atypical mycobacterial infections in, 1469
bacillary angiomatosis in, 1677
bacillary peliosis hepatis in, 1677
bacteremia in
etiology, 837
treatment, 844–845
blastomycosis in, 2735
cholangitis in, 682
coccidioidomycosis in, 2756
Corynebacterium infection in, 1509
cryptococcosis in, 806
ocular findings in, 826
cytomegalovirus (CMV) infection in, 2025–2026, 2029–2030
enterococcal infections in, 1260
fusariosis in, 806
Fusarium infection in, 2830, 2830f
herpes zoster ophthalmicus in, 819
human metapneumovirus infection in, clinical manifestations, 2491
infections in, cutaneous manifestations, 776
listeriosis in, 1420–1421
measles in, 776, 2441–2442
microsporidial keratoconjunctivitis in, 823
molluscum contagiosum in, 795–796
molluscum contagiosum of eyelid in, 812
Moraxella catarrhalis infection in, 1348
mumps vaccine and, 2459
Mycoplasma infections in, 2702–2703
ocular aspergillosis in, 826
ocular candidiasis in, 826
orbital cellulitis in, 816–817
Paecilomyces infection in, 2831
pharyngitis in, 164–165, 164t
pneumococcal infections in, **1315**
treatment, 1320–1321
progressive disseminated histoplasmosis in, 2789
respiratory syncytial virus infection in, 2471–2472
Rhodococcus in, 1511–1512
salmonellosis in, 1570t
sepsis/septic shock in
empiric antibiotic therapy for, 844, 844t
viridans streptococci in, 1279–1280, 1282
streptococcal infection in, prognosis for, 1232
as travelers, special considerations for, 3061–3063
Ureaplasma infections in, 2702–2703
West Nile virus infection in, 2336
Immunodeficiency(ies)
autoimmune endocrinopathies with, 1031
and bacterial pneumonia, 306

Immunodeficiency(ies) (Continued)
bacterial pneumonia in, chemoprophylaxis for, 312
and Epstein-Barr virus infection, 2054–2055
evaluation for, 52–54
history-taking in, 52–53, 52t
indications for, 1021, 1022t
laboratory studies in, 53–54
physical examination in, 53
fever of unknown origin in, 858
fungal infections in, 22
and fungal pneumonia, 306
heritable, **40–51**
in HIV-infected (AIDS) patients, origin of, 2623–2624
indications of, 1021, 1022t
infection in
evaluation for, 54
prevention, 54
treatment, 54
infections in, characteristics, 1021–1022
and infectious esophagitis, 617
initial evaluation for, 1021–1025
invasive fungal sinusitis in, 2824
and lung abscess, 337
management, 54
medical history-taking in, 1021–1022
and mucormycosis, 2815
mumps vaccine and, 2459
parasitic infestations in, 23
pathophysiology, 2621–2622, 2622f
patient/family education about, 54
phaeohyphomycosis in, 2828
pharyngitis in, 164t
primary, **40–51, 1021–1037**
common pathogens in, 1022, 1022t
epidemiology, 1021
genetics, 1021–1022
laboratory tests for, 1023–1025, 1023t
management, 1025, 1025t
advances in (future directions for), 54
physical examination in, 1022–1023
screening tests for, 1023, 1023t
severity, 1021
sex ratio, 1022
X-linked, 1022, 1022t
rabies prophylaxis in, 2504
rubella immunization and, 2291
Scedosporium infection in, 2829
secondary, 51–52, 1021
causes, 1021
sinopulmonary infections in, 274
sporotrichosis in, 2811
and viral pneumonia, 306
Immunofluorescence assay (IFA)
for Toscana virus, 2584–2585
for Toxoplasma, 828
for virologic diagnosis, 3534–3535
Immunogenicity, 121
Immunoglobulin(s), 36–37. See also Agammaglobulinemia; Intravenous immunoglobulin(s) (IVIG); Transient hypogammaglobulinemia of infancy
abnormalities, in congenital toxoplasmosis, 974
anti-Cryptosporidium, therapy with, 2875
antigen-binding site, 36, 36f
antiviral, in neonatal infection, 903t, 904–905
in breast milk, 83
constant regions, 36, 36f
deficiency
fever of unknown origin in, 858
with increased IgM. See Hyper-IgM syndrome
diversity, 37

Immunoglobulin(s) (Continued)
fetal, kinetics of, 904, 904f
IgA. See also IgA deficiency; Selective IgA deficiency
of fetus and newborn, 38f, 39, 39t
properties, 37
secretory, in breast milk, 83
IgD
of fetus and newborn, 38f, 39, 39t
properties, 37
IgE. See also Hyper-IgE syndrome
of fetus and newborn, 38f, 39, 39t
properties, 37
IgG. See also IgG subclass deficiency
antiviral, in neonatal infection, 903t, 904
and complement activation, 27
in congenital toxoplasmosis, 974–975, 974t
of fetus and newborn, 38–39, 38f, 39t
passive transfer of, to fetus, 39
properties, 37
IgM
antiviral, in neonatal infection, 903t, 904–905
and complement activation, 27
in congenital toxoplasmosis, 974–975, 974t
of fetus and newborn, 38f, 39, 39t
properties, 37
in rubella, 2287–2288
isotype switching, 37
isotypes, 36–37
in leprosy, 1484
neonatal, kinetics of, 904, 904f
in newborn, 38–39, 39t
in parasitic infestations, 23
in serum, age-related levels of, 38–39, 38f, 39t
structure, 36–37, 36f
therapy with, mumps vaccine and, 2459
variable regions, 36, 36f
Immunohistochemistry, for retroviral detection, 2594
Immunologic synapse, 32
Immunology of Leprosy Program (IMMLEP), 1493
Immunomodulators, **3323–3337**
for C. neoformans, 961
for HPV infection, 1942
for neonatal candidiasis, **961**
Immunoprophylaxis, active, **3340–3400**
Immunoregulatory disorder(s), intravenous immunoglobulin for, 3410–3411, 3411t
Immunoscintigraphy, in endocarditis, 372
Immunosuppressed patient. See Immunocompromised patient(s)
Immunosuppressive therapy
interactions with antibiotics, 1054, 1055t
in myocarditis, 413–414
pancreatitis caused by, 707
Impetigo
bullous, **785–786**, 785t, 786f
clinical manifestations, 765t
cutaneous manifestations, 765t, 767f
clinical manifestations, 765t
cutaneous manifestations, 765t
of eyelids, 811
microbiology, 1226
nonbullous, **784–785**, 785t
pathogenesis, 7–8
simple superficial, **784–785**, 785t
streptococcal
clinical manifestations, 1229
diagnosis, 1231
epidemiology, 1227
geographic distribution, 1227
pathogenesis, 1227

Mycobacterium genavense, 1188*t*
infection, in HIV-infected (AIDS) patients, 1472
Mycobacterium gordonae, 1188*t,* 1469
growth characteristics, 1470*t*
laboratory identification, 1471
Mycobacterium haemophilum, 1188*t*
disseminated disease, in immunocompromised patients, 1474
infection, cervical lymphadenitis in, 187
lymphadenitis, 1471
skin infection, 1474
Mycobacterium heidelbergense, 1188*t*
lymphadenitis, 1471
Mycobacterium interjectum
infection, cervical lymphadenitis in, 187
taxonomy, 1188*t*
Mycobacterium intracellulare, 1188*t*
Mycobacterium kansasii, 1188*t,* 1469–1470
growth characteristics, 1470*t*
infection
antimycobacterial therapy for, 1474*t*
cervical lymphadenitis in, 187
in children, **1475**
in HIV-infected (AIDS) patients, 1472
laboratory identification, 1471
pulmonary infections, 1472–1473
in cystic fibrosis, 1473
Mycobacterium lentiflavum
infection, cervical lymphadenitis in, 187
taxonomy, 1188*t*
Mycobacterium leprae, 1188*t,* 1480.
See also Leprosy
animal sources, 3452*t*
antibiotic resistance, 1491
corneal infection, 826
host defense against, 1482–1484
immune response to, 1481–1484
infection
clinical manifestations, 767*t*
cutaneous manifestations, 767*t*
drug therapy for, 1452
microbiology, 1480
pathogenicity, 1481–1484, 1482*f*
transmission, 1480–1481
vaccine, 1493
Mycobacterium malmoense, 1188*t*
infection
cervical lymphadenitis in, 187
in children, **1475–1476**
lymphadenitis, 1471
Mycobacterium marinum, 1188*t,* 1469–1470, 3504
animal sources, 3452*t*
growth characteristics, 1470*t*
infection, antimycobacterial therapy for, 1474*t*
skin infection, **1473**
in water-contaminated wounds, 791*t*
Mycobacterium microti, 1188*t,* 1469
Mycobacterium mucogenicum
infection, hepatitis in, 673
taxonomy, 1188*t*
Mycobacterium peregrinum, 1188*t,* 1476
Mycobacterium scrofulaceum, 1188*t,* 1469–1470
growth characteristics, 1470*t*
infection
cervical lymphadenitis in, 187
in children, **1475**
in HIV-infected (AIDS) patients, 1472
lymphadenitis, 1471
Mycobacterium senegalense, 1188*t,* 1476
Mycobacterium septicum, infection, in children, 1476
Mycobacterium simiae, 1188*t*
pulmonary infections, 1473

Mycobacterium smegmatis, 1188*t*
infection, in children, 1476
Mycobacterium szulgai, 1188*t,* 1476
growth characteristics, 1470*t*
pulmonary infections, 1473
Mycobacterium terrae, 1188*t,* 1469
Mycobacterium tuberculosis, 1188*t,* 1426–1427
animal sources, 3452*t*
anti-apoptotic mechanisms, 12
arthritis, 743
in breast milk, 84
cervical adenitis, 186, 186*t*
cholangitis, 678
esophagitis, 617
growth characteristics, 1470*t*
host defense against, 1431
immune response to, 1431
infection
cutaneous manifestations, 767*t*
gastrointestinal involvement in, in HIV-infected (AIDS) patients, 699
in HIV-infected (AIDS) patients, **2626**
in lung transplant recipient, 1062–1063
retroperitoneal involvement in, 723
infections, in daycare settings, 3485–3486
interactions with macrophages, 11–12
intracellular survival, molecular mechanisms, 11–12
laboratory identification, 1471
lymphadenitis, 1471
mastoiditis, 238, 240
mgtC gene, 11
microbiology, 1470*t*
mother-to-child transmission, 1445
pericarditis, 391
peritonitis, 715
pleural effusions caused by, 328
portal of entry, 1431, 1431*t*
pulmonary infections, 1472–1473
Mycobacterium ulcerans, 1188*t*
growth characteristics, 1470*t*
in human bites, 791
infection
animal models, 1495
bone involvement in, 1496–1498
clinical forms of, classification, 1495–1496, 1496*f*
complications, 1496–1497, 1497*f*
contiguous osteomyelitis in, 1496, 1497*f,* 1498
diagnosis, 1498
edematous, 1496, 1496*f,* 1498
metastatic osteomyelitis in, 1496–1497, 1497*f,* 1498
nodules of, 1496, 1498
papules of, 1496, 1498
plaque of, 1496, 1498
prevention, 1498
treatment, 1498
ulcerative, 1496, 1498. *See also* Buruli ulcer
microbiology, 1493–1494
skin infection, **1473–1474**
transmission, 1494
vaccine, 1494
virulence factors, 1494
Mycobacterium xenopi, 1188*t,* 1469–1470
growth characteristics, 1470*t*
pulmonary infections, 1473
Mycograb, for neonatal candidiasis, 961
Mycolactone, 1494
Mycolic acid, 35
Mycoplasma spp. (mycoplasmas), 1195*t,* **2685–2714**
culture, 552
endocarditis, 375

Mycoplasma spp. (mycoplasmas) *(Continued)*
historical perspective on, 2685
infection
cutaneous manifestations, 763, 764*t*
in HIV-infected (AIDS) patients, 2702
in immunocompromised patients, 2702–2703
neonatal, **945–951**
in renal transplant recipient, 1102
myocarditis, 400*t*
pancreatitis, 708*t,* 710
pharyngitis, 161–165, 163*t*
and pleural effusion/empyema, 327
pneumonia, **288–301,** 290*t*
pneumonial encephalopathy, differential diagnosis, 2564
sinusitis, 203–205, 204*t*
taxonomy, 1195*t,* 2685
in vaginal flora, 979
Mycoplasma amphoriforme, 1195*t,* 2685, 2686*t*
Mycoplasma arginini, 2702–2703
Mycoplasma buccale, 1195*t,* 2685, 2686*t*
Mycoplasma faucium, 1195*t,* 2685, 2686*t*
Mycoplasma fermentans, 1195*t,* 2685, 2686*t,* **2702**
Mycoplasma genitalium, 1195*t,* 2685, 2686*t,* 2689, **2702**
urethritis, 550
Mycoplasma hominis, 1195*t,* 2685, 2686*t,* 2689, **2701–2702**
antibiotic resistance, 947
antibiotic susceptibility, 947
and bronchopulmonary dysplasia, 1011
epidemiology, 945
infection
clinical manifestations, 2701–2702
diagnosis, 2702
epidemiology, 2701
neonatal, **945–951**
clinical manifestations, 945–947
diagnosis, 947
prevention, 948
systemic, 947
treatment, 947–948
in renal transplant recipient, 1102
treatment, 2702
mediastinitis, 437
morphologic forms, 2701
neonatal meningitis, 497, 507
pneumonia, 288–301, 290*t*
transmission, 945
vertical, 945
and *Trichomonas vaginalis* co-infection, 2862
urethritis, 550
Mycoplasma hyorhinis, 2689
Mycoplasma lipophilum, 1195*t,* 2685, 2686*t*
Mycoplasma mycoides, 2689
Mycoplasma orale, 1195*t,* 2686*t,* 2689
Mycoplasma penetrans, 1195*t,* 2685, 2686*t,* **2702**
Mycoplasma pirum, 1195*t,* 2685, 2686*t,* **2702**
Mycoplasma pneumoniae, 1195*t,* 2685, **2685–2700,** 2686*t*
and acalculous gallbladder disease, 685
acute transverse myelitis, 532
animal susceptibility to, 2687
antigenic composition, 2686–2687
arthritis, 2696
bronchiolitis, 278, 278*t,* **2693**
bronchitis, 269–272, 270*t,* **2693**
bullous hemorrhagic myringitis, 2693
and chronic obstructive pulmonary disease, 2693–2694
co-infection with other pathogens, 2697

Mycoplasma pneumoniae (Continued)
common cold, 2692–2693
composition, 2686
croup, 2693
culture, 2698–2699
enanthem, 2694–2695, 2694*t*
encephalitis, 507, 2696–2697
exanthem, 2694–2695, 2694*t*
geographic distribution, 2688
growth characteristics, 2686
infection
cardiac involvement in, 2695
clinical manifestations, 764*t,* 2690–2697
cutaneous manifestations, 763, 764*t,* 774, 775*t,* 2694–2695, 2694*t*
diagnosis, 2698–2699
differential diagnosis, 2698
disease associations, 2697
epidemic pattern, 2687
epidemiology, 2687–2688
gastrointestinal findings in, 2696
hematologic findings in, 2695–2696
hepatic involvement in, 2696
immunology, 2689–2690
incidence, 2687–2688
incubation period for, 2688
mucocutaneous manifestations, 2694–2695, 2695*t*
neurologic complications, 497–498, 2696–2697
pathogenesis, 2688–2689
pathology, 2689
prevention, 2699–2700
recurrence, 2697
in renal transplant recipient, 1102
serology, 2698
sex distribution, 2688
splenic infarct in, 2696
treatment, 2699
infectious asthma, 2693
meningitis, 2697
morphology, 2685–2686
motility, 2686
multiplication, 2686
nasopharyngitis, 2693
otitis media, 2693
pancreatitis, 710, 2696
pericarditis, 391
pertussis-like syndrome, 1684
pharyngitis, 2693
physical properties, 2686
pneumonia, 288–301, 290*t,* **2690–2692,** 2691*t*
treatment, 310
respiratory diseases other than pneumonia, 2692–2694
rhabdomyolysis, 2696
sinusitis, 2693
Mycoplasma primatum, 1195*t,* 2685, 2686*t*
Mycoplasma pulmonis, 2689
Mycoplasma salivarium, 1195*t,* 2686*t,* 2689
Mycoplasma spermatophilum, 1195*t,* 2686*t*
Mycoses. *See also* Fungal infection(s)
caused by non-fungal organisms, 2831–2832
endemic
in lung transplant recipient, 1069
pulmonary, 2716
miscellaneous, 2821–2836
etiologies, 2824–2832
organisms implicated in, 2821, 2822*t*
Mycosis fungoides, HTLV-I and, 2599
Mycostatin. *See* Nystatin
Mycotic aneurysm
candidal, 2744
in yersiniosis, 1597

Nocardia otitidiscaviarum complex, 1505
Nocardia paucivorans, 1188*t*
Nocardia pseudobrasiliensis, 1188*t*, 1505
  laboratory identification, 1507
Nocardia transvalensis, 1188*t*
  infection, in renal transplant
    recipient, 1103
Nocardia transvalensis complex, 1505
Nocardiosis
  clinical manifestations, 1506–1507
  CNS involvement in, 1506
  cutaneous, 785*t*, 1504, 1506
  diagnosis, 1506–1507
  disseminated, 1504, 1506
  epidemiology, 1505–1506
  in heart transplant recipient, after
    sixth postoperative month,
    1053
  hepatitis in, 673
  historical perspective on, 1504
  in HIV-infected (AIDS) patients,
    1505
  mediastinitis in, 437
  mortality rate for, 1507–1508
  pathogenesis, 1504–1505
  pathology, 1506, 1506*f*
  prognosis for, 1507–1508
  pulmonary, 1504, 1506
  transmission, 1505
  treatment, 1507
Nodaviridae, 1896*f*
Noma, 990
Non-Hodgkin's lymphoma (NHL)
  B-cell, in HIV-infected (AIDS)
    patients, 2629
  in HIV-infected (AIDS) patients,
    2055
  prognosis for, 2062
  T-cell, HTLV-I and, 2599
Non-nucleoside reverse transcriptase
    inhibitors
  HIV-2 resistance to, 2611
  for HIV-infected (AIDS) patients,
    2635
  mechanism of action, 2610–2611,
    2635
Nonparametric test, 3561
Nonrandom error, 3557
Nonsteroidal anti-inflammatory drugs
    (NSAIDs), pancreatitis caused by,
    707
Nontuberculous mycobacteria,
    1469–1479
  colonization, in cystic fibrosis, 1063
  infection
    clinical manifestations, 1471–1474
    in cystic fibrosis, 348, **352**
      pulmonary exacerbation,
        treatment, 354–355
    in lung transplant recipient,
      1063–1064
    in renal transplant recipient,
      1102–1103
    in soil-contaminated wounds, 791,
      791*t*
Norepinephrine, secretion, in response
    to infectious illness, 77
Norfloxacin, clinical pharmacology,
    3205–3206
Normal (statistical), 3564
Normal distribution, 3564
Normal flora. *See* Flora
Norovirus, 1898*t*, 2213, **2217–2220**.
    See also Calicivirus(es)
  gastroenteritis, 623*t*, 631*t*, 632
  genome, 2216
  and health care–associated infections,
    3089–3090
  hosts, 2214–2215, 2215*t*
  infection
    in daycare settings, 3487
    diagnosis, 639
    laboratory diagnosis, 3533*t*
    prototype strains, 2214–2215,
      2215*t*

Norovirus (Continued)
  taxonomy, 2214, 2215*f*
  traveler's diarrhea, 626–627
North American blastomycosis, 805
North American liver fluke, 2841
  drug therapy for, 3312*t*
North Asian tick typhus, animal
    sources, 3453*t*
North Asian tick-borne rickettsiosis,
    764*t*
Norwalk agent, 2213
Norwalk virus, 1898*t*, 2215, 2215*t*
Norwegian scabies, 3035–3036
  in HTLV-I–associated immune
    dysfunction, 2604
Nose
  flora, 112*t*, 113
  specimen collection from, for
    virologic diagnosis, 2528*t*, 3529
Nosema spp., 635, 2886
Nosema conorii, 2888
Nosema corneum, 2886, 2888–2889
  drug therapy for, 3317*t*
Nosema ocularum, 2839, 2886, 2888
Nosocomial infection(s). *See* Health
    care–associated infection(s)
Novirhabdovirus, 1896*f*
Noxafil. *See* Posaconazole
NRTIs. *See* Nucleoside reverse
    transcriptase inhibitors (NRTIs)
NTED. *See* Neonatal toxic shock
    syndrome-like exanthematous
    disease
NTM. *See* Nontuberculous
    mycobacteria
Nuchal rigidity
  in St. Louis encephalitis, 2327
  in Venezuelan equine encephalitis,
    2312
Nuclear factor κB
  inhibitors, 24
  in Toll-like receptor signaling, 24
Nuclear factor κB–enhancing
    modulator (NEMO), deficiency in,
    1032, 1032*f*
Nuclear imaging
  in cholangitis, 679
  in myocarditis, 410
  of pyomyositis, 750, 750*f*
Nucleic acid(s)
  detection, for virologic diagnosis,
    3536–3540, 3537*t*
  viral, 1899*f*–1901*f*
Nucleic acid amplification
  in bacterial respiratory infection,
    3518
  in diagnosis of gonorrhea, 1380–
    1381, 1380*t*
  in diagnosis of urethritis, 551–552
Nucleocapsid, viral, 1899*f*–1901*f*
Nucleoside analogues. *See* Nucleoside
    reverse transcriptase inhibitors
    (NRTIs)
Nucleoside reverse transcriptase
    inhibitors (NRTIs), 2633–2635
  activity against HIV-2, 2610
  HIV-1 resistance to, 2610
  mechanism of action, 2610
  pancreatitis caused by, 707
Nucleotide reverse transcriptase
    inhibitors (NtRTIs)
  adverse effects and side effects, 2635
  for HIV-infected (AIDS) patients,
    2635
  mechanism of action, 2635
Null hypothesis, 3560
Nursing bottle caries, treatment, 151
Nutrition
  for burn patient, 1148–1149
  for critically ill patients
    composition, 92–93
    route for, 92–93
  effect of, on resistance to infection,
    96–99

Nutrition *(Continued)*
  for HIV-infected (AIDS) patients,
    91–92, 2629
  and infection
    interaction, **81–104**
    WHO report on, 81
  in preterm infants, 93–94
Nutritional deficiency(ies), 87–91
  and childhood mortality, 81
  in HIV-infected (AIDS) patients,
    2629
  and infection, 81
NV. *See* Norwalk virus
NVP. *See* Nevirapine
Nystatin, topical, for burn wound,
    1147–1148
Nystatin A1, structure, 3272*f*, 3273

O

O antigen, 838
Obesity
  adenoviral infection and, 1953, 1961
  and infections, 95–96
  prevention, 99
Obsessive-compulsive disorder (OCD),
    426
Obstetric complications, and neonatal
    sepsis, 985
Obstructive airway disease, 275
Obturator sign, 744, 744*f*
Occupational exposure(s), and
    pulmonary disease, 275
Occupational health, for health care
    workers, 3126–3127
Occupational Safety and Health
    Administration (OSHA), and
    prevention/control of health care–
    associated infections, 3121–3122
*Ochlerotatus triseriatus. See also Aedes
    triseriatus*
  and La Crosse encephalitis virus,
    2559, 2565
Ochroconus gallopavum, 2828
3OC12-HSL, in acyl-homoserine
    lactone quorum-sensing system, 8
Ockelbo fever, 2324
Ockelbo strain, of Sindbis virus, 2324
Octreotide, nonspecific antidiarrheal
    therapy with, 641–642, 641*t*
Ocular infections, 811–825
  Acinetobacter in, 1640
  Aeromonas and, 1611–1612
  neonatal, candidal, 956, 958
Ocular larva migrans, 2840
Ocular prostheses, infectious
    complications, 1110–1111
Oculocerebrorenal syndrome, 903
Odds ratio, 3557
Odontogenic infection(s)
  anatomical considerations in, 147–
    150, 148*f*–150*f*
  complications, 154–156, 154*f*–156*f*
  intracranial complications, 156
  orbital complications, 156
  periapical, treatment, 151, 152*t*
  treatment, 150–155
Odynophagia
  in esophagitis, 617–618
  in HIV-infected (AIDS) patients,
    617
Oesophagostomum spp., 2840, 2990
Oesophagostomum bifurcum, 2840, 2990
  drug therapy for, 3318*t*
Oestrus ovis, uveitis caused by, 827
Ofloxacin
  as antileprosy drug, 1492
  clinical pharmacology, 3205–3206
  resistance to, 1281
Oil of lemon eucalyptus, 2309
OKT3. *See* Muromonab
Old Testament leprosy *(tsara'ath)*,
    1480
Old World hookworm, 2840
Oliguria, in toxic shock syndrome, 867,
    868*f*

Oliveros virus, 2515, 2515*f*–2516*f*
  receptors for, 2519
Omalizumab, 3402*t*
Omenn syndrome, physical findings in,
    1022
Omniserum test, 1281
Omphalitis, **1008**, 1022
  bacterial
    complications, 983
    pathogenesis, 983
  neonatal, treatment, 993–995, 993*t*
  sequelae, 1008
  streptococcal, 1229
Omsk hemorrhagic fever
  animal sources, 3459*t*
  and health care–associated infections,
    3094
Onchocerca volvulus, 768*t*, 827, 2840,
    2992–2993. *See also* Filariasis
  drug therapy for, 3312*t*
  keratitis, 823
  laboratory diagnosis, 3547–3551,
    3547*t*
  vector for, 2838*t*
Onchocerciasis, 823, **2992–2993**
  cutaneous manifestations, 768*t*
  ocular involvement in, 827
  vector for, 2838*t*
Oncovirinae, 2588
Oncovirus(es), 2587, **2594–2606**. *See
    also* Human T-cell lymphotropic
    virus (HTLV); Retrovirus(es)
  accessory genes, 2589–2590
  genetic stability, 2591
  regulatory genes, 2589–2590
  replication, 2591
    expression phase, 2591–2593,
      2592*f*
    infection phase, 2591–2592, 2592*f*
  virology, 2588
One-compartment open model, in
    pharmacokinetics, definition, 3158
One-tailed analysis, 3560
Onychomycosis, 800, 800*f*, 801
  Candida, 801
  Fusarium, 2830
O'nyong-nyong, **2323**
  clinical manifestations, 758*t*
  cutaneous manifestations, 758*t*
Oophoritis, **612**
  cytomegalovirus, 612
  mumps, 612, 2456
Oospores, motile (fungal), 2715
OPAT. *See* Outpatient parenteral
    antimicrobial therapy
Open reading frames (ORFs),
    oncoviral, 2589–2590
Ophiostoma spp., classification, 2716
Ophthalmia neonatorum, **819–821**,
    941, 1006–1007, 1366
  antimicrobial prophylaxis for, **3228**
  chemoprophylaxis for, 3467, 3468*t*
  chlamydial, chemoprophylaxis for,
    3467–3469, 3468*t*
  and clinical characteristics, 820, 820*t*
  clinical manifestations, 820, 820*t*
  gonococcal, 820, 820*t*, 1006–1007,
    1373–1374
    chemoprophylaxis for, 3467–3469,
      3468*t*
    clinical manifestations, 1374,
      1375*f*
    epidemiology, 1373
    prevention, 1373–1374
  herpetic, 820–821, 820*t*
  prevention, 821
Ophthalmomyiasis, 827
Opisthorchiasis, **3018–3020**
Opisthorchis spp., laboratory diagnosis,
    3547–3551, 3547*t*
Opisthorchis felineus
  animal sources, 3455*t*
  cholangitis, 678
Opisthorchis sinensis, 2841
  cholangitis, 678

Population structure, and infectious disease, 126

Por1, and microbial resistance to complement, 14

Pork tapeworm, 2840, **2999–3000**
drug therapy for, 3319*t*

Porphyromonas spp., 1193*t*, 1885*t*, 1887–1890
antibiotic susceptibility, 1887*t*
necrotizing fasciitis, 790

Porphyromonas asaccharolytica, 1193*t*
Bartholin duct abscess, 593

Porphyromonas endodontalis, 1193*t*, 1887

Porphyromonas gingivalis, 1193*t*, 1887

Porrocaecum spp., 2840

Portal hypertension, in schistosomiasis, 3027

Portal vein, septic thrombophlebitis, in peritonitis, 718–719

Portugal, Toscana virus in, 2583

Posaconazole, 3280, **3287–3288**
adverse effects and side effects, 3287
approval status, 3288
for aspergillosis, 2727
for candidiasis, 2746
clinical efficacy, 3287–3288
dosage and administration, 3288
drug interactions with, 3287
for histoplasmosis, 2798
indications for, 3275*t*–3276*t*
for *Paecilomyces* infection, 2831
for phaeohyphomycosis, 2828
pharmacodynamics, 3287
pharmacokinetics, 3287, 3287*t*
for *Pseudallescheria boydii* infection, 2829
structure, 3282*f*
for trichosporonosis, 2825
for zygomycosis, 2818

Positive end-expiratory pressure, in ARDS, 884–885, 889

Post-antibiotic effect, 3171–3172

Post-antibiotic leukocyte enhancement, 3171–3172

Posterior synechiae, 823

Postinfectious encephalomyelitis, 519. *See also* Acute disseminated encephalomyelitis

Postinfectious neuralgic amyotrophy, human parvovirus B19 infection and, 1909

Post-β-lactamase inhibitor effect, 3171–3172

Postoperative infection(s), antimicrobial prophylaxis for, 3235–3236, 3235*t*

Post-polio syndrome, 2151

Post-transplant lymphoproliferative disorder (PTLD), 2046
clinical manifestations, 2054
Epstein-Barr virus and, 2054
histopathology, 2047
in liver/intestinal transplant recipient, 1089–1090, 1089*t*
in lung transplant recipient, 1070–1072
prevention, 2062
prognosis for, 2062
in renal transplant recipient, 1099–1100
treatment, 2060

Potassium iodide, for entomophthoromycosis, 2819

Pott abscess, 1442

Pott disease, 1442

Povidone-iodine
for burn wound, 1148
for prevention of ophthalmia neonatorum, 821

Powassan virus, 2329
animal sources, 3459*t*

Poxviridae, 1895, 1896*f*, 1897*t*, 2101
taxonomy, 1900*f*

Poxvirus(es), **2101–2108**. *See also* Monkeypox; Smallpox (variola) virus; Vaccinia
classification, 2101, 2101*t*
infection
diagnosis, 2106
differential diagnosis, 2106
laboratory diagnosis, 3533*t*
properties, 2101
structure, 2101

PPLO. *See* Pleuropneumonia-like organisms (PPLO)

Praomys spp., Ebola virus–like nucleocapsids in, 2527

Praziquantel, for schistosomiasis, 3029–3030

Precocious puberty, in congenital toxoplasmosis, 974

Pregnancy
blastomycosis in, 2736
eastern equine encephalitis in, 2302
human parvovirus B19 infection in, 928–929, 1902, 1905, **1909,** 1912
prevention, 1912
and infectious disease, 124
malaria in, **2904**
malnutrition in, 82
measles in, 914, 2438
teratogenicity, 895–896, 897*t*, 2438
mumps in, 2457
mumps vaccine contraindicated in, 2458–2459
outcomes, gonococcal infections and, 1370*t*
rabies vaccination in, 2503
rubella exposure in, management, 2288
rubella immunization in, inadvertent, 2291
rubella in, management, 2288–2289
rubella prevention in, 2288
severe acute respiratory syndrome in, 2537
tuberculosis and, 1446
Western equine encephalitis in, 2307

Pre-integration complex, retroviral, 2592, 2592*f*

Premature neonates
early passage of meconium, 990
fungal dermatitis in, 802
fungal infections in, 951
group B streptococcal infection in, 985
HBIG prophylaxis for, 3423
immune globulins for, 3409
listeriosis in, 990
phaeohyphomycosis in, 2828
response to vaccination, 39
sinopulmonary infections in, 274–275

Prematurity
and group B streptococcal infection, 984
poliomyelitis and, 2148
viral infections causing, 895, 897*t*, 2141–2142

Preseptal cellulitis, 814
intracranial infection associated with, 815
nontraumatic, 814–815
and orbital cellulitis, concurrent, 815
post-traumatic, 814
severity index for, 815

Presumed ocular histoplasmosis syndrome, 2790

Preterm infant(s), nutrition in, 93–94

Prevalence, definition, 118, 127

Prevalence rate, 128, 3559

Prevotella spp., 1193*t*, 1885*t*, 1886–1890
antibiotic susceptibility, 1887*t*
mediastinitis, 436
necrotizing fasciitis, 790

Prevotella bivia, 1193*t*, 1887, 1889

Prevotella buccae, 1193*t*, 1887

Prevotella corporis, 1193*t*, 1886

Prevotella denticola, 1194*t*, 1886

Prevotella disiens, 1194*t*, 1887, 1889

Prevotella heparinolytica, 1194*t*, 1887

Prevotella intermedia, 1194*t*, 1886–1887

Prevotella loescheii, 1194*t*, 1886

Prevotella melaninogenica, 1194*t*, 1886–1887
in human bites, 791

Prevotella nigrescens, 1194*t*, 1887

Prevotella oralis, 1194*t*, 1887
renal abscess, 569

Prevotella oris, 1194*t*, 1887

Priapsim, in rabies, 2499

Primaquine
chemoprophylaxis, 2916*t*, 2917
for malaria, **2914**

Primary sclerosing cholangitis (PSC), 680

Primate T-cell lymphotropic virus (PTLV)
PTLV-1, 1898*t*
PTLV-2, 1898*t*

Primates, as dengue hosts, 2348

Prion(s), 1898*t*
protease-resistant, 2646–2647, 2649

Prion disease(s), 508, **2642–2653**
animal sources, 3459*t*
clinical manifestations, 2648, 2648*t*
diagnosis, 2648–2649
epidemiology, 2643–2645
historical perspective on, 2642–2643
pathogenesis, 2645–2647, 2648*t*
pathology, 2645–2647
prevention, 2649
transmission, 2643–2645

PRNP gene, 2642–2644, 2646

PRNT. *See* Plaque reduction neutralization test (PRNT)

PRO 2000, 2633

Probiotics
for acute gastroenteritis, 626, 1003
for antibiotic-associated colitis, 658
antidiarrheal therapy with, 641–642, 641*t*
precautions with, 1003, 2826–2827

Procaine penicillin, for streptococcal infections, 1232

Procalcitonin
as marker for infection, 78
secretion, 78
serum levels
clinical significance, 843, 992
in sepsis neonatorum, 992
in septic shock, 841

Proctitis, 639, 639*t*
in boys, 575
gonococcal, 1378
in premenarcheal girls, 582–583

Product-limit method, 3557

Progressive disseminated histoplasmosis. *See* Histoplasmosis, progressive disseminated

Progressive multifocal leukoencephalopathy (PML), 508
clinical manifestations, 1925–1927
CNS manifestations, 1925, 1926*f*
epidemiology, 1924–1925
historical perspective on, 1923–1924
in HIV-infected (AIDS) patients, 1925, 1926*f*, 1928
in immune reconstitution syndrome, 2629
laboratory diagnosis, 1927
renal manifestations, 1925–1926

Progressive outer retinal necrosis, 824

Progressive rubella panencephalitis, 2283, 2286

Proguanil, 2917

Properdin, deficiency, and meningococcal disease, 1352

Propionibacterium spp., 1880–1886, 1885*t*, 1888
antibiotic susceptibility, 1891
dacryocystitis, 814

Propionibacterium acnes, 1189*t*, 1885–1886, 1888–1889
arthritis, 743
in normal flora, 784

Propionibacterium avidum, 1189*t*, 1885–1886

Propionibacterium granulosum, 1189*t*, 1885–1886

Propionibacterium propionicum, 1189*t*, 1885–1886. *See also* *Propionibacterium propionicus*

Propionibacterium propionicus, 1189*t*, 1881

Propioniferax innocua, 1885

Propofol, pancreatitis caused by, 707

Proportion, definition, 3559

Prospect Hill virus, 2548*t*
reservoir for, 2549

Prostaphlin. *See* Oxacillin

Prostate cancer, 1939

Prostatic secretions, specimen collection, for fungal diagnosis, 3524*t*

Prostatitis, **573–575**
acute, 573–574
chronic, 573–574
bacterial, 574
nonbacterial, 574
gonococcal, 553

Prostatodynia, 573–574

Prosthetic devices
coagulase-negative staphylococcal infection, 1218–1219
infectious complications, **1108–1134**
interaction of host with, 1109
interaction of microbes with, 1109–1110
permanent, 1109*t*
temporary, 1109*t*

Protease, retroviral, 2588*f*, 2589, 2593, 2611

Protease inhibitors (PIs), **2635–2636**
activity against HIV-2, 2611
adverse effects and side effects, 2629, 2635
mechanism of action, 2611, 2635
nutritional/metabolic effects, 91

Proteasome, 33, 34*f*

Protein(s)
dietary, intake, 82
somatic, catabolism, 69–70
synthesis, in infection, 69–70

Protein binding (drug)
definition, 3159
developmental changes (ontogeny) and, 3161, 3162*t*

Protein C
activated, 24
recombinant human, 846
therapy with
for ARDS, 890
in meningococcal infections, 1358–1359, 1359*t*
recombinant, therapy with, in meningococcal infections, 1359
in septic shock, 841

Protein-calorie malnutrition, **81–82**
control of, 82
defects of PMN chemotaxis in, 48
in HIV-infected (AIDS) patients, 92
and infection, 81
prevention, 82

Protein-losing enteropathy, immune globulins for, 3408

Proteinuria, in HIV-infected (AIDS) patients, 2630

Proteoglycans
and chemokines, 25
microbial adherence to, 5

Urinary tract infection(s) (UTI) *(Continued)*
dysfunctional voiding and, 555
enterococcal, 1261
clinical manifestations, 1262
treatment, 1268
epidemiology, 554–555, 1021
fever of unknown origin in, 854
imahing in, 560, 561*t*
infectious, differential diagnosis, 557–558
Klebsiella, 1542
Leuconostoc in, 1343
neonatal
bacterial, **1003–1004**
clinical manifestations, 1003
diagnosis, 1003–1004
etiology, 1003
treatment, 1004
treatment, 993–995, 993*t*
noninfectious, differential diagnosis, 558
nutritional status and, 97
pathogenesis, 555–556
pediococcal, 1344
physical examination in, 556, 557*t*
prevention, 566
prognosis for, 565–566
quinolone-resistant organisms in, 3145–3146
recurrence, 565–566
recurrent, antimicrobial prophylaxis for, **3232**
in renal transplant recipient, 1103
early, 1097
late, 1104
risk factors for, 554–555
sexual activity and, 555
site of, determination, 560–562
staphylococcal, 1219
Stenotrophomonas maltophilia, 1670
streptococcal, 1235
TMP-SMX–resistant, **3140**
treatment, 562–565
in uncircumcised boys, 554
virulence factors in, 555–556
work-up for, 557, 557*t*
in yersiniosis, 1597
Urine
microscopy, 559–560
specimen collection
for fungal diagnosis, 3524*t*
for virologic diagnosis, 3528*t*, 3529, 3529*t*
Urine culture
in bacterial infection, 1003–1004, 3520–3521
in fever of unknown origin, 856
Urine dipsticks, 560
Urine specimen
catheter collection, 559, 559*t*
clean catch, 559, 559*t*
collection, 558–559, 558*f*–559*f*, 559*t*
suprapubic aspiration, 558–559, 558*f*–559*f*, 559*t*
Urogenital specimens, for diagnosis of parasitic disease, 3551
Urolithiasis, pediatric, *Proteus* and, 1547, 1551
Uropathogenic *Escherichia coli* (UPEC)
intracellular bacterial communities, 9*f*
invasion by, 10
P pilus, 2, 7–9
tissue tropism, 7–9
Uropathogens, quinolone resistance, 3145–3146
Urticaria, 761*f*–762*f*, 773, 773*t*
papular, 773
Usutu virus, 2332
Uta, 2921*t*
animal sources, 3456*t*
Uterine infection, clostridial, 1859
prevention, 1860–1861
treatment, 1860

UTIs. *See* Urinary tract infection(s) (UTI)
Uukuniemi virus, 1897*t*
UUKV. *See Uukuniemi virus*
Uvea, infections involving, 823–827. *See also* Uveitis
Uveal tract, anatomy, 823
Uveitis
anterior, 823–824
EBV-related, 827
in leishmaniasis, 827
nongranulomatous, poststreptococcal, 827
in sporotrichosis, 827
bacterial, 825–826
definition, 823
epidemiology, 824
fungal, 826–827
helminthic, 827
herpes simplex, 824
herpes zoster, 824
in herpes zoster ophthalmicus, 819
in HIV-infected (AIDS) patients, 825
HTLV-I–associated, 2587, **2601–2602**
human parvovirus B19 infection and, 1908
infectious causes, 823–824
in insect-induced disease, 827
intermediate
definition, 823
in Lyme disease, 825
in leptospirosis, 826
neonatal, 820
posterior, 823–824
postinfectious, 827
poststreptococcal, 827
protozoal, 827
psoterior, definition, 823
signs and symptoms, 823
tuberculous, 826
viral, 824–825
in West Nile virus infection, 2337
Uvulitis, **176–177**
clinical manifestations, 176, 176*f*
diagnosis, 176
differential diagnosis, 177
epidemiology, 176
etiology, 176
pathogenesis, 176
treatment, 177

V

V (variable) segments, 35
Vaccine(s), **3340–3351**. *See also* Immunization(s); *specific vaccine*
and acute transverse myelitis, 529–531, 531*t*
administration routes for, 3341–3342, 3341*t*
advances in (future directions for), 16
antibody response to, inhibition by immune globulin, 3406
available in United States, 3340, 3341*t*
combination, **3383–3384**, 3383*t*
contraindications to, 3344
and diabetes, 3350
disease associated with, immunodeficiency and, 1022
dose, 3342
efficacy, 3340, 3340*t*
assessment of, methods for, 3566
for hematopoietic stem cell transplant recipient, 1043–1044, 1043*t*
ideal, characteristics, 3340
infant's response to, maternal antibodies and, 39
intramuscular administration, 3341–3342, 3342*t*
investigational, 3391–3392

Vaccine(s) *(Continued)*
live and inactivated, spacing, 3342, 3342*t*
misconceptions about, 3348, 3349*t*
multiple, simultaneous administration, 3342, 3342*t*
precautions with, 3344
protective efficacy, assessment of, methods for, 3566
recommendations for, 3344, 3345*f*–3347*f*
recommended for routine administration, 3351–3383
references on, 3350–3351
related to bioterrorism, 3391
safety, 3348–3350
with selective indications for children and adolescents, **3384–3390**
thimerosal-containing, and neurodevelopmental disorders, 3350
travel-related, 3050*t*–3051*t*
use in special circumstances, 3344–3348
Vaccine programs
implementation, 3344, 3348*t*
standards for, 3344, 3348*t*
Vaccine-preventable disease(s), reduction in, 3340, 3340*t*
Vaccinia, 762, 2101, 2101*t*. *See also* Smallpox vaccine
arthritis, 745
congenital, 896, 896*t*
pathogenesis, 895
contact transmission, prevention, 2098
disseminated, clinical manifestations, 757*t*
effects on fetus/neonate, 897*t*
historical perspective on, 119
infection
clinical manifestations, 757*t*
congenital, 898
cutaneous manifestations, 757*t*
progressive, 2097
teratogenicity, 896
Vaccinia immune globulin, 2097*t*, 2098–2099, 3402*t*, **3433–3434**
intramuscular, 2098, **3433–3434**
intravenous, 2098, **3433–3434**
Vaccinia necrosum, 2097, 3433
Vaccinia vaccination "take," clinical manifestations, 757*t*
Vaccinia virus, 1897*t*, **2104–2105**
recombinant, 2105
Vacuolar myelopathy, in HIV-infected (AIDS) patients, 531–532
VACV. *See* Vaccinia virus
Vaejovis carolinianus, 3038
Vaginal discharge
neonatal, 577, 577*f*
pubertal, 577, 578*f*
Vaginal flora, 112*t*, 114, 979
normal, 576–577, 576*t*
and risk of toxic shock syndrome, 866–867
Vaginal specimen collection, for fungal diagnosis, 3524*t*
Vaginal specimens, obtaining, in young girls, 578–579, 579*f*
Vaginitis
candidal, 2743
in premenarcheal girls, 579*t*, 585–586, 586*f*
chlamydial, in premenarcheal girls, 583–584
fungal, 2826
gonococcal, 1366
in prepubertal girls, 1375–1376
streptococcal, 1229
Trichomonas vaginalis, clinical manifestations, 2863–2864

Valacyclovir, **3256**
adverse effects and side effects, 3256
for CMV infection, 2034–2035
dosage and administration, 3253*t*, 3256
for HSV infection, 2012–2015, 2013*t*, 2016
indications for, 3253*t*, 3256
mechanism of action, 3256
pharmacokinetics, 3256
resistance to, 3256
spectrum of activity, 3256
for varicella, 2083
Valganciclovir, **3259–3260**
adverse effects and side effects, 3260
for CMV infection, 2034–2035
dosage and administration, 3253*t*, 3260
indications for, 3253*t*, 3260
mechanism of action, 3259
pharmacokinetics, 3260
resistance to, 3259
spectrum of activity, 3259
Validity, of epidemiologic study, 3554
Valproic acid, pancreatitis caused by, 707
Vancomycin
activity in vitro, 3195
adverse effects and side effects, 3196
anti-anaerobic activity, 1892
clinical pharmacology, **3194–3196**
for *Clostridium difficile* diarrhea and colitis, 657–658, 658*t*
contraindications to, 1270, 1270*t*
for *Corynebacterium* infection, 1510–1511
dosage schedules, for neonates, 980*t*
based on postconceptual age, 3217*t*
dosage schedules for infants and children, 3216*t*
for enterococcal infections, 1268
indications for, 1270, 1270*t*, 3195–3196
mechanism of action, 3194
for meningococcal infections, 1358
pharmacokinetics, 3195
developmental changes (ontogeny) and, 3162*t*
prophylaxis, for viridans streptococcal infection, 1282–1283
resistance to
enterococcal, 1343, **3142–3144**, 3144*t*. *See also* Vancomycin-resistant enterococci (VRE); Vancomycin-resistant *Enterococus faecium* (VREF)
prevention, 1270–1271, 1270*t*
in *Leuconostoc* spp., 1343
mechanisms of, 3194–3195
in pediococci, 1344
streptococcal, 1281
for staphylococcal infections, 1220
in infants and children, 1205*t*
in neonates, 1206*t*
for streptococcal infections, 1236
tolerance, 1300, 3194
for viridans streptococcal infection, 1281–1282
Vancomycin-resistant enterococci (VRE), 1266, 1266*t*–1267*t*, 1267, **3142–3144**, 3144*t*
infections
epidemiology, 1258, 1260–1261
in HIV-infected (AIDS) patients, 1261
nosocomial, 1258, 1260
controlling spread of, 1271
in neonates, 1264
prevention, 1271
prevention, 1258
risk factors for, 1260
treatment, 1268–1270
newer options for, 1269–1270

Vitamin D
  deficiency, **90**
  in HIV-infected (AIDS) patients, 74
Vitamin E, 73–74
  deficiency, **90**
Vitrectomy, for postoperative
    endophthalmitis, 831
Vitreous body, 823
Vitritis
  in loiasis, 827
  of toxoplasmosis, 828
  in West Nile virus infection, 2337
Vitronectin, microbial adherence to, 5
Vittaforma spp., 2886
Vittaforma corneae, 2839, 2888
  drug therapy for, 3317*t*
Voiding, dysfunctional
  management, 564
  and urinary tract infections, 555, 564
Voiding cystourethrography, 562, 562*f*
Volume of distribution, definition,
    3159
Volume replacement, in septic shock,
    842
Vomiting
  in coxsackievirus infection, 2121*t*,
    2130
  in echoviral infection, 2121*t*, 2130
  in neonatal enteroviral infection,
    2143*t*, 2144
  in pancreatitis, 706
  in Reye syndrome, 693–694
  in toxic shock syndrome, 867, 868*f*
Voriconazole, 3280, **3288–3290**
  antifungal activity of, 2818
  approval status, 3289
  for aspergillosis, 2727–2729
  for *Blastoschizomyces capitatus*
    infection, 2827
  for candidiasis, 2746
  clinical efficacy, 3289
  dosage and administration, 3289–
    3290, 3289*t*
  drug interactions with, 3289
  for fusariosis, 2831
  for histoplasmosis, 2798
  indications for, 3274*t*–3275*t*
  for mycotic keratitis, 2822
  for neonatal candidiasis, **960**
  for *Paecilomyces* infection, 2831
  pharmacodynamics, 3288
  pharmacokinetics, 3288–3289
  for *Pseudallescheria boydii* infection,
    2829
  and risk of zygomycosis, 2815
  for *Saccharomyces cerevisiae* infection,
    2827
  safety, 3289
  for *Scedosporium prolificans* infection,
    2829
  structure, 3282*f*
  susceptible organisms, 960
  for trichosporonosis, 2825
VP16, and immediate early gene
    activation, 15–16
VRE. *See* Vancomycin-resistant
    enterococci (VRE)
VREF. *See* Vancomycin-resistant
    Enterococcus faecium (VREF)
VRSA. *See* Vancomycin-resistant
    Staphylococcus aureus (VRSA)
VSIV. *See* Vesicular stomatitis Indiana
    virus
Vulvar cancer, 1932*t*
Vulvar vestibulitis, 606
Vulvovaginitis
  amebic, in premenarcheal girls, 579*t*,
    588
  candidal, in premenarcheal girls,
    579*t*, 585–586, 586*f*
  diphtheritic, in premenarcheal girls,
    579*t*, 588
  gonococcal, 579*t*, 582–583
    epidemiology, 1368
    in prepubertal girls, 1375–1376

Vulvovaginitis *(Continued)*
  group A streptococcal, in
    premenarcheal girls, 579*t*, 587
  mycotic (fungal)
    postmenarcheal, 594–595
      treatment, 595
    in premenarcheal girls, 579*t*, 585–
      586, 586*f*
  nasopharyngeal bacteria and, in
    premenarcheal girls, 579*t*, 587
  nongonococcal neisserial, in
    premenarcheal girls, 579*t*,
    586–587
  nonspecific, postmenarcheal, 596
    treatment, 596
  postmenarcheal, 594–596
  premenarcheal, 577–588
    etiologic factors, 578, 579*t*
    foreign bodies and, 582, 582*f*
    nonspecific, 579–582, 579*t*
    pinworm and, 581–582, 581*f*
    poor perineal hygiene and, 580–
      581, 581*f*
    in prepubertal girls, causes, 1376
  Shigella, in premenarcheal girls,
    579*t*, 587–588
  skin infections and, in premenarcheal
    girls, 579*t*, 587
  specific infections causing, 579*t*,
    582–588
  trichomonal, cutaneous
    manifestations, 768*t*
VUR. *See* Vesicoureteral reflux
VZIG. *See* Varicella-zoster immune
    globulin (VZIG)
VZV. *See* Varicella-zoster virus (VZV)

W

Wangiella dermatitidis, 2828
Wart(s), 755, **795**, 1931, 1933
  anogenital, 1932*t*, 1933, **1935–1936**
    in adolescent, 599, 599*f*
    in premenarcheal patient, 598–
      599, 599*f*
    in sexually abused children, 590*t*,
      592
  butcher's, 1932*t*
  clinical manifestations, 756*t*
  common, 1932*t*
  cutaneous (skin), 1932*t*, 1933,
    1934–1935
  filiform, 1932*t*
  flat, 1932*t*
  in immunocompromised patients,
    1932*t*
  mosaic, 1932*t*
  mucosal, 1932*t*
  plantar, 1932*t*
  treatment, 795
Warthin-Finkelday giant cells, 2431
Wasting syndrome, in HIV-infected
    (AIDS) patients, 2629
Water
  atypical mycobacteria in, 1469
  diseases and infections associated
    with, 625, 3471–3472
  drinking, diseases and infections
    associated with, 3471–3472
  recreational, diseases and infections
    associated with, 3471–3472
  safety
    chemical treatment for,
      3473–3474
    heat treatment for, 3473
    in international travel, 3473–3474
Water-borne illness(es), public health
    considerations with, 3465,
    3471–3472
Waterhouse-Friderichsen syndrome,
    1358
Weakness, in toxic shock syndrome,
    867, 868*f*
Webster, Noah, 119
WEE. *See* Western equine encephalitis
    (WEE)

Wegener granulomatosis
  diagnosis, 331
  human parvovirus B19 infection and,
    1908
Wegner sign, 1833
Weight loss
  in HIV-infected (AIDS) patients,
    91–92
  in infective endocarditis, 370, 370*t*
  in Whipple disease, 663
Weil syndrome, clinical manifestations,
    1817–1818
Weissella spp., 1343
Wesselsbron virus, animal sources,
    3459*t*
West African trypanosomiasis, 2840,
    2936
  drug therapy for, 3320*t*
  vector for, 2838*t*
West Nile virus, 1898*t*, **2331–2343**
  animal sources, 3459*t*
  antibodies to, detection, 2338–2339
  in breast milk, 897, 2334
  culture, 2338
  E glycoprotein, 2332–2333
  effects on fetus/neonate, 897*t*
  encephalitis, 496–499, 506, 2334–
    2335, 2335*t*, 2336
    clinical manifestations, 2337
    differential diagnosis, 2329
    pathogenesis, 2335–2336
  enzootic life cycle, 2333
  flaccid paralysis syndrome,
    2335–2336
    clinical manifestations, 2337
    neuroimaging in, 2338
  genome, 2332, 2332*f*
  genotype/lineages, 2333
  geographic distribution, 2332, 2334,
    2335*f*
  historical perspective on, 2331–2332
  hosts for, 2333
  immune response to, 2336
  infection
    asymptomatic, 2336
    CCR5 deficiency and, 8
    in children, epidemiology, 2334–
      2335, 2335*t*
    clinical manifestations, 758*t*,
      2336–2337
    congenital, 896*t*, 930, 2334
    cutaneous manifestations, 758*t*,
      762
    differential diagnosis, 2329
    electrodiagnostic studies in, 2338
    epidemiology, 2333–2335
    epizootic, 2333
    in immunocompromised host,
      2336
    laboratory findings in, 2338
    maternal, in pregnancy, 930
    neonatal, 930
    neuroimaging in, 2338
    neuroinvasive, 2334–2335,
      2335*t*
      neuroimaging in, 2338
      pathogenesis, 2335–2336
      risk factors for, 2336
    neuropathology, 2339
    non-neurologic manifestations,
      2336
    ocular manifestations, 2337
    outcomes with, 2337
    pathogenesis, 2335–2336
    postnatal, 896*t*
    prevention, 2339–2440
    in renal transplant recipient,
      1102
    seasonal patterns, 2308, 2333
    severe, risk factors for, 2336
    severity of, factors affecting, 2336
    subclinical, 2336
    treatment, 2339
    in United States, 1999-2005,
      2334, 2335*t*

West Nile virus *(Continued)*
  initial outbreak, as model of
    potential bioterrorist attack,
    3509
  in lung transplant recipient, 1074
  meningitis, 496–499, 2335, 2335*t*,
    2336
    clinical manifestations, 2336–2337
  meningoencephalitis, 2334–2335,
    2335*t*, 2336
    pathogenesis, 2335–2336
  mortality rates for, 2334, 2335*t*
  prM protein, 2332–2333
  reverse transcription–polymerase
    chain reaction (RT-PCR)
    detection, 2338
  seasonal patterns, 2308
  seroprevalence, in children,
    2333–2334
  transmission, 2324, 2326
    maternal-fetal, 2334
    maternal-infant, 2334
    non–vector-borne, 2334
    in organ transplantation, 2334
    transfusion-associated, 2334
    vector-borne, 2333–2334
    vertical, 2334
  virology, 2332–2333, 2332*f*
  virulence, genotype/lineage and,
    2333
West Nile virus vaccine, 2330, 2440
Western blot
  for HIV, 2631, 2631*t*
  for retroviruses, 2594
Western equine encephalitis (WEE),
    2304–2310
  animal sources, 3459*t*
  antigenic complex, viruses of, 2304
  attack rates
    age and, 2305–2306, 2306*f*
    population density and, 2306,
      2306*f*
    in rural areas, 2306, 2306*t*, 2307*f*
    sex-specific, 2306, 2306*f*
  case-fatality rate in, 2308
  clinical manifestations, 2306–2307
  congenital, 896, 896*t*
  diagnosis, 2308
  differential diagnosis, 2308
  epidemiology, 2305–2306,
    2305*f*–2306*f*
  etiologic agent, 2304
  pathogenesis, 2307–2308
  pathology, 2307
  predictive indicators, 2309
  in pregnancy, 2307
  prevention, 2309
  prognosis for, 2308
  risk factors for, 2305–2306, 2306*f*
  seasonal patterns, 2305, 2306*f*, 2327*f*
  sequelae, 2308
  serology in, 2308
  treatment, 2309
Western equine encephalitis (WEE)
    vaccine, 2309
Western equine encephalitis (WEE)
    virus, 1898*t*, 2324
  ecology o, 2304–2305
  effects on fetus/neonate, 897*t*
  geographic distribution, 2304
  hosts for, 2304
  overwintering mechanism, 2305
  sylvatic subtype, 2304
  vectors for, 2304–2305, 2326
Wetzsteinformen, 1607
Wheezing
  human coronavirus and, 2535
  recurrent, 284–285
    infectious causes, 278, 278*t*
Whipple disease, **660–666**
  clinical manifestations, 663–664,
    663*t*
  CNS findings in, 663, 663*t*
  cutaneous findings in, 664
  diagnosis, 664–665